ICD-10-CM
Expert for
Hospitals

The Complete Official Code Set

2016

Publisher's Notice

The *ICD-10-CM Expert for Hospitals: The Complete Official Code Set* is designed to be an accurate and authoritative source regarding coding and every reasonable effort has been made to ensure accuracy and completeness of the content. However, Optum360 makes no guarantee, warranty, or representation that this publication is accurate, complete, or without errors. It is understood that Optum360 is not rendering any legal or other professional services or advice in this publication and that Optum360 bears no liability for any results or consquences that may arise from the use of this book.

Our Commitment to Accuracy

Optum360 is committed to producing accurate and reliable materials.

To report corrections, please visit www.optumcoding.com/accuracy or email accuracy@optum.com. You can also reach customer service by calling 1.800.464.3649, option 1.

Acknowledgments

Lauri Gray, RHIT, CPC, AHIMA-Approved ICD-10-CM/PCS Trainer, *Product Manager*
Karen Schmidt, BSN, *Technical Director*
Stacy Perry, *Manager, Desktop Publishing*
Anita Schmidt, BS, RHIT, AHIMA-Approved ICD-10-CM/PCS Trainer, *Clinical Technical Editor*
Peggy Willard, CCS, AHIMA-Approved ICD-10-CM/PCS Trainer, *Clinical Technical Editor*
Karen Krawzik, RHIT, CCS, AHIMA-Approved ICD-10-CM/PCS Trainer, *Clinical Technical Editor*
Lisa Singley, *Project Manager*
Tracy Betzler, *Senior Desktop Publishing Specialist*
Hope M. Dunn, *Senior Desktop Publishing Specialist*
Katie Russell, *Desktop Publishing Specialist*
Kate Holden, *Editor*

Anita Schmidt, BS, RHIT, AHIMA-Approved ICD-10-CM/PCS Trainer

Ms. Schmidt has expertise in Level I adult and pediatric trauma hospital coding, specializing in ICD-9-CM, DRG, and CPT coding. Her experience includes analysis of medical record documentation and assignment of ICD-9-CM codes and DRGs, and CPT code assignments for same-day surgery cases. She has conducted coding training and auditing, including DRG validation, conducted electronic health record training, and worked with clinical documentation specialists to identify documentation needs and potential areas for physician education. Ms. Schmidt is an AHIMA-approved ICD-10-CM/PCS trainer, and is an active member of the American Health Information Management Association (AHIMA) and the Minnesota Health Information Management Association (MHIMA).

Peggy Willard, CCS, AHIMA-Approved ICD-10-CM/PCS Trainer

Ms. Willard has several years of experience in Level I Adult and Pediatric Trauma hospital coding, specializing in ICD-9-CM, DRG, and CPT coding. She has been extensively trained in ICD-10-CM and PCS. Her recent experience includes in-depth analysis of medical record documentation, ICD-10-CM code assignment, and DRG shifts based on ICD-10-CM code assignment. Ms. Willard's expertise includes conducting coding audits, conducting coding training for coding staff and clinical documentation specialists, and creating internal ICD-10-CM coding guidelines/tips. Ms. Willard is an active member of the American Health Information Management Association (AHIMA) and the Minnesota Health Information Management Association (MHIMA).

Karen Krawzik, RHIT, CCS, AHIMA-Approved ICD-10-CM/PCS Trainer

Ms. Krawzik has expertise in ICD-10-CM, ICD-9-CM, and CPT/HCPCS coding. Her coding experience includes inpatient, ambulatory surgery, and ancillary and emergency room records. She has served as a DRG analyst and auditor of commercial and government payer claims, and as a contract administrator. Most recently she was responsible for the conversion of the ICD-9-CM code set to ICD-10 and for analyzing audit results, identifying issues and trends, and developing remediation plans. Ms. Krawzik is credentialed by the American Health Information Management Association (AHIMA) as a Certified Coding Specialist (CCS) and is an AHIMA-approved ICD-10-CM/PCS trainer. She is an active member of AHIMA and the Missouri Health Information Management Association.

Contents

Preface

ICD-10-CM Official Preface

This 2016 update of the International Classification of Diseases, 10th revision, Clinical Modification (ICD-10-CM) is being published by the United States government in recognition of its responsibility to promulgate this classification throughout the United States for morbidity coding. The International Statistical Classification of Diseases and Related Health Problems, 10th Revision (ICD-10), published by the World Health Organization (WHO), is the foundation of ICD-10-CM. ICD-10 continues to be the classification used in cause-of-death coding in the United States. The ICD-10-CM is comparable with the ICD-10. The WHO Collaborating Center for the Family of International Classifications in North America, housed at the National Center for Health Statistics (NCHS), has responsibility for the implementation of ICD and other WHO-FIC classifications and serves as a liaison with the WHO, fulfilling international obligations for comparable classifications and the national health data needs of the United States. The historical background of ICD and ICD-10 can be found in the Introduction to the International Classification of Diseases and Related Health Problems (ICD-10), 2008, World Health Organization, Geneva, Switzerland.

ICD-10-CM is the United States' clinical modification of the World Health Organization's ICD-10. The term clinical is used to emphasize the modification's intent: to serve as a useful tool in the area of classification of morbidity data for indexing of medical records, medical care review, and ambulatory and other medical care programs, as well as for basic health statistics. To describe the clinical picture of the patient the codes must be more precise than those needed only for statistical groupings and trend analysis.

Characteristics of ICD-10-CM

ICD-10-CM far exceeds its predecessors in the number of concepts and codes provided. The disease classification has been expanded to include health-related conditions and to provide greater specificity at the 6th and 7th character level. The 6th and 7th characters are not optional and are intended for use in recording the information documented in the clinical record.

Introduction

History of ICD-10-CM

The ICD-10-CM classification system was developed by the National Center for Health Statistics (NCHS) as a clinical modification to the ICD-10 system developed by the World Health Organization (WHO), primarily as a unique system for use in the United States for morbidity and mortality reporting. Although ICD-10 replaced ICD-9 for use in coding and classifying of mortality data from death certificates beginning January 1, 1999, ICD-10-CM implementation was postponed many years until legislation to replace ICD-9-CM, volumes 1 and 2, with ICD-10-CM was approved.

ICD-10 is the copyrighted product of the World Health Organization (WHO), which has authorized the development of a clinical modification (CM) of ICD-10 for use in the United States. However, all modifications to the ICD-10 must conform to WHO conventions for ICD. The development of ICD-10-CM included comprehensive evaluation by a Technical Advisory Panel and extensive consultation with physician groups, clinical coders, and other industry experts.

The ICD-10-CM draft and crosswalk between ICD-9-CM and ICD-10-CM were made available on the Centers for Medicare and Medicaid Services (CMS) website for public comment. The initial public comment period extended from December 1997 through February 1998. A field test for ICD-10-CM was conducted in the summer of 2003 jointly by The American Hospital Association (AMA) and the American Health Information Management Association (AHIMA). Public comments and suggestions were reviewed and additional modifications to ICD-10-CM were made. Revisions were made to ICD-10-CM based on the established update process for ICD-10-CM (the ICD-10-CM Coordination and Maintenance Committee) and the World Health Organization's ICD-10 (the Update and Revision Committee).

These revisions to ICD-10-CM have included:

- information relevant to ambulatory and managed care encounters
- expanded injury codes
- creation of combination diagnosis/symptom codes to reduce the number of codes needed to fully describe a condition
- the addition of 6th and 7th character classifications
- incorporation of common 4th and 5th character classifications
- classifications specific to laterality
- classification refinement for increased data granularity

This new structure allows for further expansion than was possible with the ICD-9-CM classification system.

The Department of Health and Human Services (HHS) published the final rule regarding the adoption of both ICD-10-CM and ICD-10-PCS in the January 16, 2009, *Federal Register* (45 CFR part 162 [CMS—0013—F]). The initial compliance date for implementation of ICD-10-CM and ICD-10-PCS as a replacement for ICD-9-CM was set at October 1, 2013. On April 17, 2012, the Department of Health and Human Services (HHS) released a notice to postpone the date by which certain health care entities have to comply with International Classification of Diseases, 10th Revision diagnosis and procedure codes (ICD-10). The compliance date for implementation of ICD-10-CM and ICD-10-PCS as a replacement for ICD-9-CM was changed to October 1, 2014. On April 1, 2014, Congress enacted the Protecting Access to Medicare Act of 2014, which contained a provision to delay the implementation of ICD-10-CM/PCS by a least one year, prohibiting the Department of Health and Human Services (HHS) from adopting the ICD-10-CM/PCS code sets as the mandatory standard until at least October 1, 2015.

ICD-10-CM for Hospitals: The Complete Official Code Set

ICD-10-CM for Hospitals: The Complete Official Code Set 2016 includes many of the enhancements described below in direct response to requests from our subscribers. Many of these enhancements were introduced in the Optum360 *ICD-9-CM for Hospitals* and users will find many of the conventions, icons, color bars, and other enhancements familiar since many of these features are similar to the hallmark color coding and symbols of our ICD-9-CM code books.

As you review the content, you will find the following:

- Optum360 Exclusive feature—Check Placeholder Alert symbol, indicating the need for one or more "filler" x character assignments in the 5th and/or 6th character position to appropriately assign a required character in the 7th character position

- Optum360 Exclusive feature—Key word differentiation by the use of a green font that highlights the differentiating terms in similar code descriptions in a given category

- Optum360 Exclusive feature — Exclusive *following* references and Check Additional Character symbol in the indexes. The *following* references (designed and used exclusively by Optum360) help coders locate those alphanumeric codes that are out of sequence in the tabular section.

- Optum360 Exclusive feature — Exclusive shaded guides in the index help users easily follow the indent levels for the subterms under a main term.

- Illustrations at the back of the book feature anatomy and terminology included in the ICD-10-CM classification system

- Optum360 Exclusive feature – Detailed muscle/tendon tables that correspond with codes in chapters 13 and 19

- The complete ICD-10-CM official guidelines for coding and reporting, published by the U.S. Department of Health and Human Services and approved by the cooperating parties (American Health Information Management Association, National Center for Health Statistics, Centers for Medicare and Medicaid Services, American Hospital Association)

- Optum360 Exclusive feature – Official chapter-specific guidelines with coding examples at the beginning of each chapter

- Exclusive color coding, symbols, and footnotes that alert coders to coding and reimbursement issues, including the majority of the Medicare code edits and identification of conditions that significantly affect DRG assignment

- The complication and comorbidity (CC) exclusion list, integrated beneath the applicable codes, which makes it easier to determine complications and comorbidities excluded with a particular principal diagnosis

- All official ICD-10-CM codes, indexes, notes, footnotes, and symbols

- Icons and definitions to differentiate between the two types of Excludes notes

- Check 4th, 5th, 6th, and 7th character symbols identify codes that require the addition of a 4th, 5th, 6th, or 7th character for code specificity and validity

- Color coding and symbol legend at the bottom of each page

Please review "How to Use *ICD-10-CM for Hospitals*" in this manual to learn about the features that will help you assign and report correct codes, ensuring appropriate reimbursement.

How to Use ICD-10-CM for Hospitals 2016

This International Classification of Diseases, 10th Revision, Clinical Modification (ICD-10-CM) is being published by the United States Government in recognition of its responsibility to promulgate this classification throughout the United States for morbidity coding. This code book represents an adaptation of ICD-10 which was created specifically for use in the United States. Future revisions to ICD-10-CM will be made based on the established update process for ICD-10-CM (the ICD-10-CM Coordination and Maintenance Committee) and the World Health Organization's ICD-10 (the Update and Revision Committee). ICD-10-CM has been approved for implementation on October 1, 2015.

Steps to Correct Coding

1. Before beginning to use this code book, review section I.A., "Conventions for the ICD-10-CM" and section I.B., "General Coding Guidelines" of the ICD-10-CM Official Guidelines for Coding and Reporting 2016.

2. Look up the main term in the alphabetic index and scan the subterm entries as appropriate. Review continued lines and additional subterms that may appear in the next column or on the next page.

3. Note all parenthetical terms (nonessential modifiers) that help in code selection but do not affect code assignment. Shaded vertical guidelines in the Index are provided to help determine the indentation level for each subterm in relation to the main terms.

4. Pay close attention to the following instructions in the Index:

    –   "see", "see also", and "see category" cross-references

    –   "with"/"without" notes

    –   "omit code" notes

    –   "due to" subterms

    –   other instructions found in note boxes, such as "code by site"

    –   *Following* references and Check Additional Character symbol in the indexes. The *following* references (designed and used exclusively by Optum360) help coders locate those alphanumeric codes that are out of sequence in the tabular section.

5. Do not code from the alphabetic index without verifying the accuracy of the code in the Tabular List. Locate the code in the alphanumerically arranged Tabular List.

6. To determine the appropriateness of the code selection and proper coding, read all instructional material:

    –   "includes" and both types of "excludes" notes

    –   "use additional code" and "code first underlying disease"

    –   instructions

    –   "code also"

    –   4th, 5th, and 6th character requirements and 7th character extension requirements

    –   CC Exclusions

    –   age and sex symbols

7. Consult the official ICD-10-CM guidelines, which govern the use of specific codes. These guidelines provide both general and chapter-specific coding guidance.

8. Confirm and assign the correct code.

Organization

This book is organized in the following manner:

Introduction

The introductory material in this book includes the ICD-10-CM Official Preface, the history of ICD-10-CM as well as an overview of the classification system.

Official ICD-10-CM Conventions and Guidelines

This section provides an explanation of the conventions and guidelines regulating the appropriate assignment and reporting of ICD-10-CM codes. This coding guidance is presented by the National Center for Health Statistics (NCHS), a governmental agency of the Centers for Disease Control and Prevention (CDC), within the United States Department of Health and Human Services (DHHS).

Alphabetic Index to Diseases

The Alphabetic Index to Diseases is arranged in alphabetic order by disease — by specific illness, injury, eponym, abbreviation, or other descriptive diagnostic term. The Index also lists diagnostic terms for other reasons for encounters with health care professionals.

Neoplasm Table

The Neoplasm Table provides the proper code based upon histology of the neoplasm and site.

Table of Drugs and Chemicals

The Table of Drugs and Chemicals is also included within the Alphabetic Index.

The Table of Drugs and Chemicals lists the drug and the specific codes that identify the drug and the intent. No additional external cause of injury and poisoning code is assigned in ICD-10-CM.

Index to External Causes

The alphabetic index to External Causes of injuries is arranged in alphabetic order by main term indicating the event.

Tabular List of Diseases

ICD-10-CM codes and descriptors are arranged numerically within the Tabular List of diseases within 21 separate chapters according to body system or nature of injury and disease. Classifications which were previously considered supplemental to ICD-9-CM (e.g., V codes and E codes) are incorporated into the Tabular Listing of ICD-10-CM as individual chapters. Chapters 20 External Causes of Morbidity and 21 Factors Influencing Health Status and Contact with Health Services include chapter-specific guidelines.

Appendixes

The resources described below have been included as appendixes for the *ICD-10-CM Expert for Hospitals: The Complete Official Code Set*. These resources further instruct the inpatient coder on the appropriate application of the ICD-10-CM code set.

Appendix A: 10 Steps to Correct Coding

This step-by-step tutorial walks the coder through the process of locating the correct code in the Alphabetic Index and verifying it in the tabular section while following applicable conventions and guidelines. Detailed examples are provided and explained along with advice for proper sequencing.

Appendix B: Valid 3-character ICD-10-CM Codes

The user may consult this table to confirm that no further specificity, such as the use of 4th, 5th, 6th, or 7th characters or placeholders (x), is necessary. All ICD-10-CM codes that are valid at the three-character level are listed.

Appendix C: Pharmacology List 2016

This reference helps users select the most accurate code for drug classifications for adverse effects and poisonings, in addition to alerting the coder of potential chronic conditions in a patient record by identifying various medications used and their actions. This list is not all-inclusive but discusses many commonly used drugs.

Appendix D: Z Codes for Long-Term Drug Use with Associated Drugs

This resource correlates Z codes that are used to identify current long-term drug use with a list of drugs that are typically categorized to that class of drug.

Note: These tables are not all-inclusive but list some of the more commonly used drugs.

Appendix E: Major Complication and Comorbidity (MCC) Code List

This is a full listing of conditions considered to be major complications and/or comorbidities that when present as a secondary diagnosis may affect DRG assignment under the Medicare Severity DRG (MS-DRG) system, version 32.0.

Appendix F: Complication and Comorbidity (CC) Code List

This is a full listing of conditions considered to be complications and/or comorbidities that when present as a secondary diagnosis may affect DRG assignment under the MS-DRG system, version 32.0.

Appendix G: Lists of Principal Diagnoses That Are Their Own CC and Their Own MCC

This listing displays those ICD-10-CM combination codes that may function as their own CC or MCC when sequenced as a principal diagnosis based on the MS-DRG system, version 32.0.

Appendix H: Present on Admission (POA) Tutorial

This tutorial walks the coder through the process of assigning the appropriate present-on-admission (POA) indicator for inpatient codes based on the POA reporting guidelines. Detailed scenarios for a variety of situations are provided and discussed.

Appendix I: Hospital Acquired Conditions

This comprehensive table displays codes that identify conditions that are considered reasonably preventable when occurring during the hospital admission and may prevent the case from grouping to a higher-paying MS-DRG. Many of these HACs are conditional and are based on reporting the specific diagnosis code(s) in combination with certain procedure codes, which are also noted in this table.

Illustrations

This section includes illustrations of normal anatomy with ICD-10-CM specific terminology.

Use of Official Sources

The *ICD-10-CM for Hospitals* contains the official U.S. Department of Health and Human Services, Tenth Revision, Clinical Modification (ICD-10-CM) codes, effective for the current year.

The color coding, footnotes, and symbols, which identify coding and reimbursement issues, are derived from official federal government sources, including the Medicare Code Edits (MCE), version 32.

Overview of ICD-10-CM Official Conventions

This is an overview of the ICD-10-CM official conventions, which are general rules for the use of the classification system, independent of the guidelines. The official conventions and instructions of the classification, which take precedence over the guidelines, are incorporated within the Alphabetic Index and Tabular List as instructional notes and are applicable regardless of the health care setting. For the full version of the official conventions, see the ICD-10-CM Official Guidelines for Coding and Reporting 2016, section I.A., which is included in this book.

Format

ICD-10-CM is divided into two main parts: the Index, an alphabetical list of terms and their corresponding code, and the Tabular List, a sequential, alphanumeric list of codes divided into chapters based on body system or condition. The Index contains the Index to Diseases and Injuries (main index) and the Index to External Causes of Injury. Also included in the main Index is the Neoplasm Table and a Table of Drugs and Chemicals.

The Tabular List contains categories, subcategories, and valid codes.

ICD-10-CM is an alphanumeric classification system. The 1st character of a three-character category is a letter. The 2nd and 3rd characters may be numbers or alpha characters. A three-character category without further subclassification is equivalent to a valid three-character code. Subcategories are either four or five characters. Subcategory characters include either letters or numbers. Codes may be three, four, five, six, or seven characters in length, in which each level of subdivision after a category is a subcategory. The final level of subdivision is a valid code. The final character in a code may be either a letter or a number.

The ICD-10-CM uses the letter "X" as a placeholder. A placeholder "X" is used as a 5th character placeholder at certain six-character codes to allow for future expansion, without disturbing the 6th character structure. For instance, an initial encounter for accidental poisoning by penicillin is coded to T36.ØX1A. The "X" in the 5th character position is a placeholder, or filler character.

Similarly, certain categories have applicable 7th character extensions. In these cases, the 7th character extension is required for all codes within the category, or as otherwise instructed in the Tabular List notations. 7th character extensions must always be the last character in the data field. If a code is not a full six characters in length, a dummy placeholder "X" must be used to fill in the empty characters when a 7th character extension is required.

Punctuation

[ ]   In the Tabular List, brackets are used to enclose synonyms, alternative wording, or explanatory phrases. In the Index, brackets are used to identify manifestation codes.

( )   Parentheses are used in both the Index and Tabular List to enclose nonessential modifiers; supplementary words that may be present or absent in the statement of a disease or procedure without affecting the code number to which it is assigned.

:   Colons are used in the Tabular List after an incomplete term that needs one or more of the modifiers following the colon to make it assignable to a given category.

Abbreviations

NEC

The abbreviation NEC, "Not elsewhere classifiable" represents "other specified" in the ICD-10-CM. An Index entry that states NEC directs the coder to an "other specified" code in the Tabular List. Codes titled "Other" or "Other specified" in the Tabular List (usually a code with a 4th or 6th character 8 and 5th character 9) are for use when the information in the medical record provides detail for which a specific code does not exist.

NOS

The abbreviation NOS, "Not otherwise specified," in the Tabular List may be interpreted as "unspecified." Codes in the Tabular List with "Unspecified" in the title (usually a code with a 4th or 6th character 9 and 5th character Ø) are for use when the information in the medical record is insufficient to assign a more specific code.

Typeface

Boldface

Boldface type is used for main term entries in the Alphabetic Index, and all codes and descriptions in the Tabular List.

General Notes

The following conventions and notes appear only in the Tabular List of Diseases:

Includes Notes

The word `INCLUDES` appears immediately under certain categories to further define, clarify, or give examples of the content of a code category.

Inclusion Terms

Lists of inclusion terms are included under certain codes. These terms indicate some of the conditions for which that code number may be used. Inclusion terms may be synonyms with the code title, or, in the case of "other specified" codes, the terms may also provide a list of various conditions included within a classification code. The inclusion terms are not exhaustive. The Index may provide additional terms that may also be assigned to a given code.

Excludes Notes

ICD-10-CM has two types of excludes notes. Each note has a different definition for use. However, they are similar in that they both indicate that codes excluded from each other are independent of each other.

Excludes 1

An `EXCLUDES 1` note is a "pure" excludes. It means "NOT CODED HERE!" An Excludes 1 note indicates mutually exclusive codes; two conditions that cannot be reported together. For example, a congenital form of a disease may not be reported with the acquired form of the same condition. The code excluded should never be reported with the applicable codes listed above the excludes notation.

Excludes 2

An `EXCLUDES 2` note means "NOT INCLUDED HERE." An Excludes 2 note indicates that although the excluded condition is not part of the condition it is excluded from, a patient may have both conditions at the same time. Therefore, when an Excludes 2 note appears under a code, it may be acceptable to use both the code and the excluded code together if supported by the medical documentation.

Default Codes

In the Index, the default code is the code listed next to the main term. The default code represents the condition most commonly associated with the main term. This code may be assigned when documentation does not facilitate reporting a more specific code. Alternatively, it may provide an unspecified code for the condition.

Syndromes

Follow the Alphabetic Index guidance when coding syndromes. In the absence of index guidance, assign codes for the documented manifestations of the syndrome.

And

When the term "and" is used in a narrative statement or code title, it may be interpreted as "and/or."

With

The word "with" should be interpreted to mean "associated with or "due to" when it appears in a code title, the Alphabetic Index, or an instructional note in the Tabular List.

Instructional Notes Used in the Tabular List

In the tabular section, the following instructional notes appear in red type for emphasis:

Code First/Use additional code:

These instructional notes provide sequencing instruction. They may appear independently of each other or to designate certain etiology/manifestation paired codes. These instructions signal the coder that an additional code should be reported to provide a more complete picture of that diagnosis.

In etiology/manifestation coding, ICD-10-CM requires the underlying condition to be sequenced first, followed by the manifestation. In these situations, codes with "In diseases classified elsewhere" in the code description are never permitted as a first-listed or principal diagnosis code and must be sequenced following the underlying condition code.

Code Also:

A code also note alerts the coder that more than one code may be required to fully describe the condition. Code sequencing is discretionary. Factors that may determine sequencing include severity and reason for the encounter.

Additional Conventions

Color-coding and symbols are included to alert the coder to important reimbursement issues affected by the diagnosis code assignment. Some codes may carry more than one color and/or symbol. For a quick reference to the color codes and their meanings, refer to the color/symbol legend located at the bottom of each page in the Tabular Listing.

Additional Characters Required

√4ᵗʰ This symbol indicates that the code requires a 4th character.

√5ᵗʰ This symbol indicates that the code requires a 5th character.

√6ᵗʰ This symbol indicates that the code requires a 6th character.

√7ᵗʰ This symbol indicates that the code requires a 7th character.

√x7ᵗʰ This symbol indicates that the code requires a 7th character following the placeholder "X". Codes with fewer than six characters that require a 7th character must contain placeholder "X" to fill in the empty character(s).

Italics

Italicized type is used for all exclusion notes and to identify manifestation codes, those codes that should not be reported as first-listed (principal) diagnoses.

Color Coding

Note

NOTE The term "Note" appears as an icon and precedes the instructional information. These notes function as an alert, to highlight coding instruction within the text.

Key Word

Green font is used throughout the Tabular List of Diseases to differentiate the key words that appear in similar code descriptions in a given category or subcategory.

For example, refer to the list of codes below from category C7A:

C7A.Ø2Ø   Malignant carcinoid tumor of the **appendix**

C7A.Ø21   Malignant carcinoid tumor of the **cecum**

C7A.Ø22   Malignant carcinoid tumor of the **ascending colon**

C7A.Ø23   Malignant carcinoid tumor of the **transverse colon**

C7A.Ø24   Malignant carcinoid tumor of the **descending colon**

C7A.Ø25   Malignant carcinoid tumor of the **sigmoid colon**

C7A.Ø29   Malignant carcinoid tumor of the large intestine, **unspecified portion**

The portion of the code description that appears in bold font above appears in green font in the Tabular List, to assist the coder in quickly identifying the key terms and in identifying the correct code. This convention is especially useful when the codes describe laterality, such as the following codes from category H4Ø.22:

H4Ø.221   Chronic angle-closure glaucoma, **right** eye

H4Ø.222   Chronic angle-closure glaucoma, **left** eye

H4Ø.223   Chronic angle-closure glaucoma, **bilateral**

H4Ø.229   Chronic angle-closure glaucoma, **unspecified** eye

The key word convention is only used in those categories in which there are multiple codes with very similar descriptions with only a few words that differentiate them.

Medicare Code Edits

Medicare Administrative Contractors (MACs) and many payers use Medicare code edits to check the coding accuracy on claims. The coding edit information in this manual is effective from October 1, 2015, to September 30, 2016, and reflects those edits used for acute care hospital inpatient admission. This ICD-10 version of the Medicare Code Editor (MCE) is version 32.

The Medicare code edits are listed below:

- Invalid diagnosis or procedure code
- External causes of morbidity codes as principal diagnosis
- Duplicate of PDx
- *Age conflict
- *Sex conflict
- *Manifestation code as principal diagnosis
- Nonspecific principal diagnosis (Discontinued as of 10/1/07)
- *Questionable principal diagnosis
- *Unacceptable principal diagnosis
- Nonspecific O.R. procedure (Discontinued as of 10/1/07)
- Noncovered procedure
- Open biopsy check (Discontinued as of 10/1/10)
- Bilateral procedure (Discontinued as of ICD-10 implementation)
- Invalid age
- Invalid sex
- Invalid discharge status
- Limited coverage
- *Wrong procedure performed

Starred edits above that are related to diagnosis issues are identified in this manual by color bars, symbols, or footnotes as described below.

Age and Sex Edit Symbols

The age and sex edits below are used to detect inconsistencies between the patient's age and/or sex and the patient's diagnosis. The following edit symbols appear in the Tabular List of diseases to the right of the code description.

Newborn Age: 0   N

These diagnoses are intended for newborns and neonates and the patient's age must be 0 years.

Pediatric Age: 0-17   P

These diagnoses are intended for children and the patient's age must between 0 and 17 years.

Maternity Age: 12-55   M

These diagnoses are intended for childbearing patients between the age of 12 and 55 years.

Adult Age: 15-124   A

These diagnoses are intended for the patients between the age of 15 and 124 years.

Male diagnosis only   ♂

Female diagnosis only   ♀

Manifestation Code

These codes appear in italic type, with a ***blue color bar*** over the title. A manifestation code cannot be reported as a first-listed or principal diagnosis. By definition, a manifestation code represents a demonstration of some aspect of an underlying disease, which is separately classifiable. In the alphabetic index, these codes are listed as the secondary code in brackets. The underlying disease code is listed first.

Unacceptable PDx

These codes will appear with a **gray color bar** over the code title. These codes do not describe a current illness or injury, but a circumstance which influences a patient's health status. They are considered an unacceptable principal diagnosis for *inpatient* admission.

Questionable admission diagnoses will also appear with a gray color bar over the code title along with a reference to footnote 13. These codes, although not unacceptable as a PDx, may be considered a "questionable admission" when used as PDx in an acute care hospital.

Hospital Acquired Condition (HAC)

These codes will appear with a **yellow color bar** over the code title. These codes identify conditions that are high cost or high volume or both, are either a complication or comorbidity (CC) or major complication or comorbidity (MCC) that as a secondary diagnosis results in assignment of a case to a higher-paying MS-DRG. These conditions are reasonably preventable through the application of evidence-based guidelines. If the condition is not present on admission (meaning it developed during the hospital admission), the case will not group to the higher-paying MS-DRG based solely upon the reporting of the HAC code. Many of these HACs are conditional, and are based on reporting the specific diagnosis code(s) in combination with certain procedure codes, notated in footnotes.

Wrong Procedure Performed Edit

The Wrong Surgery Edit was created to identify cases in which wrong surgeries occurred. Any claim with a code from the Y65.51-Y65.53 will be denied and returned to the provider. A surgical or other invasive procedure is considered to be a wrong procedure if:

- The procedure was performed on the wrong site
- The procedure was performed on the wrong patient, or
- The incorrect procedure was performed on a patient.

Other Notations in the Tabular

CC Condition   `CC`

This symbol designates a complication or comorbidity diagnosis that may affect DRG assignment. A complication or comorbidity diagnosis, CC condition, is defined as a significant acute disease, a significant acute manifestation of a chronic disease, an advanced or end stage chronic disease, or a chronic disease associated with systemic physiological decompensation and debility that have consistently greater impact on hospital resources.

A CC icon most often appears to the right of the code description.

MCC Condition   `MCC`

This symbol designates a major complication or comorbidity diagnosis that may affect DRG assignment. An MCC condition meets the same criteria as a CC condition but is associated with a higher acuity level and hospital resource consumption is expected to be higher than that for a CC condition. There are fewer conditions that meet the criteria as an MCC than those for a CC condition.

Similar to a CC icon, an MCC icon appears to the right of the code description.

CC Excludes Notations

Many distinct CC Excludes notations appear directly below the code to which they relate. However, in some cases the CC Excludes information is identical for all codes within a category or subcategory. In those cases, the CC Excludes notation is listed once, at the beginning of the category or subcategory. For example:

G43.6   **Persistent migraine aura with cerebral infarction**

> **CC Excl: For CC codes in subcategory G43.6, unless otherwise noted:** G43.601-G43.619, I63.00-I66.9

There are four codes with a CC designation in subcategory G43.6; the CC Excludes notation above applies to all four codes.

Optum360 ICD-10-CM coding manuals include references to a previously designated CC Excludes notation, and those CC or MCC codes for which there are no excluded conditions. Refer to examples below:

K67   **Disorders of peritoneum in infectious diseases classified elsewhere**
> **CC Excl:** See code: K65

A17.83   **Tuberculosis neuritis**
> **CC Excl:** No Excl

By definition of being a condition which acts as its own CC or MCC, PDxCC or PDxMCC, the CC exclusion concept (the two conditions being too interrelated) does not apply. However, if a condition carries separate PDxCC/PDxMCC and MCC/CC designations, a CC excludes notation will appear for the CC or MCC designation.

PDxCC or PDxMCC Condition   `PDxCC` `PDxMCC`

When the MS-DRG system was translated from ICD-9-CM to ICD-10-CM, some significant differences existed. One involved the assignment of two codes in ICD-9-CM, one for an underlying condition, and one for a related acute manifestation. In ICD-10-CM, only one combination code was necessary to replicate the same clinical concept. However, in ICD-9-CM, one of the two codes acted as a CC or MCC for the other. To address this situation, CMS has introduced the concept of certain ICD-10-CM diagnosis codes acting as their own CC or MCC when sequenced as a principal diagnosis. For example, refer to the table below:

ICD-9 PDx	ICD-9 SDx	CC Level	ICD-10 Code with CC or MCC
415.19 Other pulm embolism	415.0 Acute cor pulmonale	MCC	I26.09 Other pulm embolism with acute cor pulmonale

In the ICD-9-CM MS-DRG system, diagnosis code 415.0 acts as an MCC for code 415.19, grouping the case to the highest weighted DRG in its subgroup. In the ICD-10-CM MS-DRG system, the same clinical concept, represented by code I26.09 is sequenced as the principal diagnosis and the code functions as its own MCC. Codes which function as their own CC or MCC when sequenced as a principal diagnosis are designated with the PDxCC or PDxMCC icon to the right of the code description.

HIV   `HIV`

This symbol indicates that the condition is considered a major HIV related diagnosis. When the condition is coded in combination with a diagnosis of human immunodeficiency virus (HIV), code B20, the case will move from MS-DRG 977 to MS-DRGs 974-976.

Bracketed Codes

Some of the ICD-10-CM or ICD-10-PCS referenced codes that appear in this manual use bracketing as a space-saving convention. The numbers or letters within the brackets correspond to all appropriate, valid characters for the character position where the bracket appears. For example:

S04.01[1,2,9] Injury of optic nerve, [right, left, unspecified] eye

The bracketed code above represents three distinct codes:

S04.011   Injury of optic nerve, right eye

S04.012   Injury of optic nerve, left eye

S04.019   Injury of optic nerve, unspecified eye

Similarly, ICD-10-PCS codes may be represented in the same way:

OSU[A,E,R,S] ØBZ Supplement [Right, Left Hip Joint; Acetabular, Femoral Surface] with Resurfacing Device, Open Approach

The bracketed code above represents four distinct codes:

ØSUAØBZ   Supplement Right Hip Joint, Acetabular Surface with Resurfacing Device, Open Approach

ØSUEØBZ   Supplement Left Hip Joint, Acetabular Surface with Resurfacing Device, Open Approach

ØSURØBZ   Supplement Right Hip Joint, Femoral Surface with Resurfacing Device, Open Approach

ØSUSØBZ   Supplement Left Hip Joint, Femoral Surface with Resurfacing Device, Open Approach

Bracketed codes are most often found in CC Excludes notations, as well as in footnotes related to hospital acquired conditions (HACs).

Footnotes

All footnotes are identified by a numerical superscript that appears to the upper left of the code. For example:

10 I49.01   Ventricular fibrillation

The footnote 10 indicates "MCC = Only if patient is discharged alive." This means that ventricular fibrillation is considered a major complication or comorbidity that may affect DRG assignment only if the patient is discharged alive. Otherwise ventricular fibrillation is assigned as a non-MCC condition.

The following list identifies the meaning of each footnote number in the Tabular List of diseases:

1   [HAC 06: Catheter-Associated Urinary Tract Infection (UTI)] This condition represents a hospital acquired condition (HAC) when reported as a secondary diagnosis along with a secondary diagnosis of T83.51XA (Infection and inflammatory reaction due to indwelling urinary catheter, initial encounter) and neither are present on admission.

2   [HAC 11: Surgical Site Infection Following Bariatric Surgery] This condition represents a hospital acquired condition (HAC) when reported as the principal diagnosis along with a secondary diagnosis of K68.11 or K95.01 or K95.81 (surgical site infection) or T81.4XXA (Infection following a procedure, initial encounter) and in combination with one of the following procedure codes, which represent bariatric procedures: ØD16[0,4,8][7,J,K,Z][9,A,B,L] or ØDV64CZ. The secondary diagnosis code is not present on admission.

3   [HAC 10: Deep Vein Thrombosis (DVT)/Pulmonary Embolism (PE) with Total Knee or Hip Replacement] This condition represents a hospital acquired condition (HAC) when reported as a secondary diagnosis in combination with one of the following procedural codes that represent total knee or hip replacement: ØSR[9,B]Ø[1,2,3,4,J][9,A,Z]; ØSR[9,B]Ø[7,K]Z; ØSR[A,E]Ø[0,1,3,J][9,A,Z]; ØSR[A,E]Ø[7,K]Z; ØSR[C,D,T,U,V,W]Ø[7,K]Z; ØSR[C,D,T,U,V,W]ØJ[9,A,Z]; ØSR[R,S]Ø[1,3,J][9,A,Z]; ØSR[R,S]Ø[7,K]Z; ØSU[9,B]ØBZ; ØSU[A,E,R,S]ØBZ. The secondary diagnosis code is not present on admission.

4   [HAC 11: Surgical Site Infection Following Bariatric Surgery] This condition represents a hospital acquired condition (HAC) when reported as a secondary diagnosis along with PDx E66.01 (Morbid

obesity) and in combination with one of the following procedure codes, which represent bariatric procedures: ØD16[0,4,8][7,J,K,Z][9,A,B,L] or ØDV64CZ. The secondary diagnosis code is not present on admission.

5   [HAC 08: Surgical Site Infection — Mediastinitis after Coronary Bypass Graft (CABG)] This condition represents a hospital acquired condition (HAC) when reported as a secondary diagnosis in combination with one of the following procedure codes, which represent Coronary Bypass Graft (CABG): 021[0,1,2,3][0,4][9,A,J,K][3,8,9,C,F,W]; 021[0,1,2,3][0,4]Z[3,8,9,C,F]. The secondary diagnosis code is not present on admission.

6   [HAC 12: Surgical Site Infection — Certain Orthopedic Procedures of Spine, Shoulder and Elbow] This condition represents a hospital acquired condition (HAC) when reported as a secondary diagnosis in combination with one of the following procedure codes, which represent spine, shoulder, and elbow procedures: ØRG[0,1,2,4,6,7,8,A][0,3,4][7,A,J,K,Z][0,1,J]; ØRG[E,F,G,H,J,K][0,3,4][4,7,J,K,Z]Z; ØRG[L,M][0,3,4][4,5,7,J,K,Z]Z; ØRQ[E,F,G,H,J,K,L,M][0,3,4,X]ZZ; ØRU[E,F,G,H,J,K,L,M][0,3,4][7,J,K]Z; ØSG[0,1,3][0,3,4][7,A,J,K,Z][0,1,J]; ØSG[7,8][0,3,4][4,7,J,K,Z]Z. The secondary diagnosis code is not present on admission.

7   This condition represents a hospital acquired condition (HAC) only when reported as the initial encounter (7th character A, B, or C) and the diagnosis is not present upon admission.

8   [HAC 13: Surgical Site Infection (SSI) Following Cardiac Implantable Electronic Device (CIED) Procedures] This condition represents a hospital acquired condition (HAC) when reported as a secondary diagnosis in combination with one of the following procedure codes: 02H43[J,K,M]Z; 02H[6,7]3[J,M]Z; 02H[K,L]3JZ; 02HN[0,3,4][J,M]Z; 02PA[0,3,4]MZ; 02PAXMZ; 02WA[0,3,4]MZ; ØJH[6,8][0,3][4,5,6,7,8,9,P]Z; ØJPT[0,3]PZ; ØJWT[0,3]PZ. The secondary diagnosis is not present upon admission.

9   [HAC 14: Iatrogenic Pneumothorax w/ Venous Catheterization] This condition represents a hospital acquired condition (HAC) when reported as a secondary diagnosis in combination with one of the following procedure codes: 05H[M,N,P,Q]33Z or ØJH63XZ. The secondary diagnosis is not present upon admission.

10   These codes are considered major complication/comorbidity (MCC) conditions and may affect MS-DRG assignment only if the patient is discharged alive.

11   These codes indicate that the wrong procedure was performed on the patient and reimbursement may be affected.

12   This condition represents an unacceptable PDx only when reported as the initial encounter (7th character A).

13   These codes, although not unacceptable as PDx, would be considered questionable as a PDx for acute care hospital admissions.

14   This code is considered an unacceptable PDx unless a relevant secondary diagnosis is also reported.

15   This condition represents a hospital acquired condition (HAC) only when reported as the initial encounter for an open fracture (7th character B or C specific to category) and the diagnosis is not present upon admission.

16   This condition is considered an MCC only when reported as an initial encounter for an open fracture (7th character B or C specific to category).

17   This condition is considered a CC only when reported as an initial encounter for a fracture (7th character A, B, or C specific to category) or a subsequent encounter for nonunion or malunion fracture (7th character K, M, N, P, Q, or R specific to category).

18   This condition is considered a CC only when reported as a subsequent encounter for a nonunion or malunion fracture (7th character K, M, N, P, Q, or R specific to category).

19   This condition is considered a CC only when reported as an initial encounter for a closed fracture (7th character A) **OR** a subsequent encounter for nonunion or malunion fracture (7th character K, M, N, P, Q, or R specific to category).

20   This condition is considered a CC only when reported as an initial encounter for an open fracture (7th character B or C specific to category) **OR** a subsequent encounter for nonunion or malunion fracture (7th character K, M, N, P, Q, or R specific to category).

Muscle and Tendon Table

ICD-10-CM categorizes certain muscles and tendons in the upper and lower extremities by their action (e.g., extension or flexion) as well as their anatomical location. The Muscle/Tendon Table is provided at the beginning of chapter 13 and chapter 19 as a resource to assist users when code selection is dependent depends on the action of the muscle and/or tendon. The categories and/or subcategories that relate to this table are identified by a purple diamond icon ✦, which refers the user to a footnote at the bottom of the page indicating the use of the table. Please note that this table is not all-inclusive and proper code assignment should be based on the provider's documentation.

Other Notations in the Index

▽   Subterms under main terms may continue to next column or page. This warning statement is a reminder to always check for additional subterms and information that may continue onto the next page or column before making a final selection.

Following References

The Index includes following references to assist in locating "out-of-sequence" codes in the Tabular List. "Out-of-sequence" codes contain an alphabetic character (letter) in the 3rd or 4th character position. These codes are placed according to the classification rules — the placement of the codes according to condition — not according to alphabetic or numeric sequencing rules.

Example:

Carcinoma (malignant) (*see also* Neoplasm, by site, malignant)
neuroendocrine (*see also* Tumor, neuroendocrine)
    high grade, any site C7A.1 (*following* C75)
    poorly differentiated, any site C7A.1 (*following* C75)

In the tabular rubric, C7A is included after rubric C75 and before C76.

Gout, chronic (*see also* Gout, gouty) M1A.9
    drug-induced M1A.20 (*following* M08)
      ankle M1A.27-(*following* M08)
      elbow M1A.22-(*following* M08)

In the tabular rubric, M1A is included after rubric M08 and before M10.

ICD-10-CM Official Guidelines for Coding and Reporting 2016

Narrative changes appear in **bold** text.

Items <u>underlined</u> have been moved within the guidelines since the 2014 version.

Italics are used to indicate revisions to heading changes.

The Centers for Medicare and Medicaid Services (CMS) and the National Center for Health Statistics (NCHS), two departments within the U.S. Federal Government's Department of Health and Human Services (DHHS) provide the following guidelines for coding and reporting using the International Classification of Diseases, 10th Revision, Clinical Modification (ICD-10-CM). These guidelines should be used as a companion document to the official version of the ICD-10-CM as published on the NCHS website. The ICD-10-CM is a morbidity classification published by the United States for classifying diagnoses and reason for visits in all health care settings. The ICD-10-CM is based on the ICD-10, the statistical classification of disease published by the World Health Organization (WHO).

These guidelines have been approved by the four organizations that make up the Cooperating Parties for the ICD-10-CM: the American Hospital Association (AHA), the American Health Information Management Association (AHIMA), CMS, and NCHS.

These guidelines are a set of rules that have been developed to accompany and complement the official conventions and instructions provided within the ICD-10-CM itself. The instructions and conventions of the classification take precedence over guidelines. These guidelines are based on the coding and sequencing instructions in the Tabular List and Alphabetic Index of ICD-10-CM, but provide additional instruction. Adherence to these guidelines when assigning ICD-10-CM diagnosis codes is required under the Health Insurance Portability and Accountability Act (HIPAA). The diagnosis codes (Tabular List and Alphabetic Index) have been adopted under HIPAA for all healthcare settings. A joint effort between the healthcare provider and the coder is essential to achieve complete and accurate documentation, code assignment, and reporting of diagnoses and procedures. These guidelines have been developed to assist both the healthcare provider and the coder in identifying those diagnoses and procedures that are to be reported. The importance of consistent, complete documentation in the medical record cannot be overemphasized. Without such documentation accurate coding cannot be achieved. The entire record should be reviewed to determine the specific reason for the encounter and the conditions treated.

The term encounter is used for all settings, including hospital admissions. In the context of these guidelines, the term provider is used throughout the guidelines to mean physician or any qualified health care practitioner who is legally accountable for establishing the patient's diagnosis. Only this set of guidelines, approved by the Cooperating Parties, is official.

The guidelines are organized into sections. Section I includes the structure and conventions of the classification and general guidelines that apply to the entire classification, and chapter-specific guidelines that correspond to the chapters as they are arranged in the classification. Section II includes guidelines for selection of principal diagnosis for non-outpatient settings. Section III includes guidelines for reporting additional diagnoses in non-outpatient settings. Section IV is for outpatient coding and reporting. It is necessary to review all sections of the guidelines to fully understand all of the rules and instructions needed to code properly.

Section I. Conventions, general coding guidelines and chapter specific guidelines

The conventions, general guidelines and chapter-specific guidelines are applicable to all health care settings unless otherwise indicated. The conventions and instructions of the classification take precedence over guidelines.

A. Conventions for the ICD-10-CM

The conventions for the ICD-10-CM are the general rules for use of the classification independent of the guidelines. These conventions are incorporated within the Alphabetic Index and Tabular List of the ICD-10-CM as instructional notes.

1. **The Alphabetic Index and Tabular List**
   The ICD-10-CM is divided into the Alphabetic Index, an alphabetical list of terms and their corresponding code, and the Tabular List, a structured chronological list of codes divided into chapters based on body system or condition. The Alphabetic Index consists of the following parts: the Index of Diseases and Injury, the Index of External Causes of Injury, the Table of Neoplasms and the Table of Drugs and Chemicals.

   See Section I.C2. General guidelines

   See Section I.C.19. Adverse effects, poisoning, underdosing and toxic effects

2. **Format and Structure**
   The ICD-10-CM Tabular List contains categories, subcategories and codes. Characters for categories, subcategories and codes may be either a letter or a number. All categories are 3 characters. A three-character category that has no further subdivision is equivalent to a code. Subcategories are either 4 or 5 characters. Codes may be 3, 4, 5, 6 or 7 characters. That is, each level of subdivision after a category is a subcategory. The final level of subdivision is a code. Codes that have applicable 7th characters are still referred to as codes, not subcategories. A code that has an applicable 7th character is considered invalid without the 7th character.

   The ICD-10-CM uses an indented format for ease in reference.

3. **Use of codes for reporting purposes**
   For reporting purposes only codes are permissible, not categories or subcategories, and any applicable 7th character is required.

4. **Placeholder character**
   The ICD-10-CM utilizes a placeholder character "X". The "X" is used as a placeholder at certain codes to allow for future expansion. An example of this is at the poisoning, adverse effect and underdosing codes, categories T36-T50.

   Where a placeholder exists, the X must be used in order for the code to be considered a valid code.

5. **7th Characters**
   Certain ICD-10-CM categories have applicable 7th characters. The applicable 7th character is required for all codes within the category, or as the notes in the Tabular List instruct. The 7th character must always be the 7th character in the data field. If a code that requires a 7th character is not 6 characters, a placeholder X must be used to fill in the empty characters.

6. **Abbreviations**
   a. **Alphabetic Index abbreviations**
      NEC   "Not elsewhere classifiable"

This abbreviation in the Alphabetic Index represents "other specified". When a specific code is not available for a condition, the Alphabetic Index directs the coder to the "other specified" code in the Tabular List.

   NOS   "Not otherwise specified"
          This abbreviation is the equivalent of unspecified.

   b. **Tabular List abbreviations**
      NEC   "Not elsewhere classifiable"
             This abbreviation in the Tabular List represents "other specified". When a specific code is not available for a condition the Tabular List includes an NEC entry under a code to identify the code as the "other specified" code.

      NOS   "Not otherwise specified"
             This abbreviation is the equivalent of unspecified.

7. **Punctuation**
   [ ] Brackets are used in the Tabular List to enclose synonyms, alternative wording or explanatory phrases. Brackets are used in the Alphabetic Index to identify manifestation codes.

   ( ) Parentheses are used in both the Alphabetic Index and Tabular List to enclose supplementary words that may be present or absent in the statement of a disease or procedure without affecting the code number to which it is assigned. The terms within the parentheses are referred to as nonessential modifiers. The nonessential modifiers in the Alphabetic Index to Diseases apply to subterms following a main term except when a nonessential modifier and a subentry are mutually exclusive, the subentry takes precedence. For example, in the ICD-10-CM Alphabetic Index under the main term Enteritis, "acute" is a nonessential modifier and "chronic" is a subentry. In this case, the nonessential modifier "acute" does not apply to the subentry "chronic".

   :   Colons are used in the Tabular List after an incomplete term which needs one or more of the modifiers following the colon to make it assignable to a given category.

8. **Use of "and"**
   See Section I.A.14. Use of the term "And"

9. **Other and Unspecified codes**
   a. **"Other" codes**
      Codes titled "other" or "other specified" are for use when the information in the medical record provides detail for which a specific code does not exist. Alphabetic Index entries with NEC in the line designate "other" codes in the Tabular List. These Alphabetic Index entries represent specific disease entities for which no specific code exists so the term is included within an "other" code.

   b. **"Unspecified" codes**
      Codes titled "unspecified" are for use when the information in the medical record is insufficient to assign a more specific code. For those categories for which an unspecified code is not provided, the "other specified" code may represent both other and unspecified.

      See Section I.B.18 Use of Signs/Symptom/Unspecified Codes

10. **Includes Notes**
    This note appears immediately under a three character code title to further define, or give examples of, the content of the category.

11. **Inclusion Terms**
    List of terms is included under some codes. These terms are the conditions for which that code is to be used. The terms may be synonyms of the code title, or, in the case of "other specified" codes, the terms are a list of the various conditions assigned to that code. The inclusion terms are not necessarily exhaustive. Additional terms found only in the Alphabetic Index may also be assigned to a code.

12. **Excludes Notes**
    The ICD-10-CM has two types of excludes notes. Each type of note has a different definition for use but they are all similar in that they indicate that codes excluded from each other are independent of each other.

    a. **Excludes1**
       A type 1 Excludes note is a pure excludes note. It means "NOT CODED HERE!" An Excludes1 note indicates that the code excluded should never be used at the same time as the code above the Excludes1 note. An Excludes1 is used when two conditions cannot occur together, such as a congenital form versus an acquired form of the same condition.

b. **Excludes2**

A type 2 Excludes note represents "Not included here". An excludes2 note indicates that the condition excluded is not part of the condition represented by the code, but a patient may have both conditions at the same time. When an Excludes2 note appears under a code, it is acceptable to use both the code and the excluded code together, when appropriate.

13. **Etiology/manifestation convention ("code first", "use additional code" and "in diseases classified elsewhere" notes)**

Certain conditions have both an underlying etiology and multiple body system manifestations due to the underlying etiology. For such conditions, the ICD-10-CM has a coding convention that requires the underlying condition be sequenced first followed by the manifestation. Wherever such a combination exists, there is a "use additional code" note at the etiology code, and a "code first" note at the manifestation code. These instructional notes indicate the proper sequencing order of the codes, etiology followed by manifestation.

In most cases the manifestation codes will have in the code title, "in diseases classified elsewhere." Codes with this title are a component of the etiology/ manifestation convention. The code title indicates that it is a manifestation code. "In diseases classified elsewhere" codes are never permitted to be used as first-listed or principal diagnosis codes. They must be used in conjunction with an underlying condition code and they must be listed following the underlying condition. See category F02, Dementia in other diseases classified elsewhere, for an example of this convention.

There are manifestation codes that do not have "in diseases classified elsewhere" in the title. For such codes, there is a "use additional code" note at the etiology code and a "code first" note at the manifestation code and the rules for sequencing apply.

In addition to the notes in the Tabular List, these conditions also have a specific Alphabetic Index entry structure. In the Alphabetic Index both conditions are listed together with the etiology code first followed by the manifestation codes in brackets. The code in brackets is always to be sequenced second.

An example of the etiology/manifestation convention is dementia in Parkinson's disease. In the Alphabetic Index, code G20 is listed first, followed by code F02.80 or F02.81 in brackets. Code G20 represents the underlying etiology, Parkinson's disease, and must be sequenced first, whereas codes F02.80 and F02.81 represent the manifestation of dementia in diseases classified elsewhere, with or without behavioral disturbance.

"Code first" and "Use additional code" notes are also used as sequencing rules in the classification for certain codes that are not part of an etiology/ manifestation combination.

See Section I.B.7. Multiple coding for a single condition.

14. **"And"**

The word "and" should be interpreted to mean either "and" or "or" when it appears in a title.

For example, cases of "tuberculosis of bones", "tuberculosis of joints" and "tuberculosis of bones and joints" are classified to subcategory A18.0, Tuberculosis of bones and joints.

15. **"With"**

The word "with" should be interpreted to mean "associated with" or "due to" when it appears in a code title, the Alphabetic Index, or an instructional note in the Tabular List.

The word "with" in the Alphabetic Index is sequenced immediately following the main term, not in alphabetical order.

16. **"See" and "See Also"**

The "see" instruction following a main term in the Alphabetic Index indicates that another term should be referenced. It is necessary to go to the main term referenced with the "see" note to locate the correct code.

A "see also" instruction following a main term in the Alphabetic Index instructs that there is another main term that may also be referenced that may provide additional Alphabetic Index entries that may be useful. It is not necessary to follow the "see also" note when the original main term provides the necessary code.

17. **"Code also note"**

A "code also" note instructs that two codes may be required to fully describe a condition, but this note does not provide sequencing direction.

18. **Default codes**

A code listed next to a main term in the ICD-10-CM Alphabetic Index is referred to as a default code. The default code represents that condition that is most commonly associated with the main term, or is the unspecified code for the condition. If a condition is documented in a medical record (for example, appendicitis) without any additional information, such as acute or chronic, the default code should be assigned.

B. General Coding Guidelines

1. **Locating a code in the ICD-10-CM**

To select a code in the classification that corresponds to a diagnosis or reason for visit documented in a medical record, first locate the term in the Alphabetic Index, and then verify the code in the Tabular List. Read and be guided by instructional notations that appear in both the Alphabetic Index and the Tabular List.

It is essential to use both the Alphabetic Index and Tabular List when locating and assigning a code. The Alphabetic Index does not always provide the full code. Selection of the full code, including laterality and any applicable 7th character can only be done in the Tabular List. A dash (-) at the end of an Alphabetic Index entry indicates that additional characters are required. Even if a dash is not included at the Alphabetic Index entry, it is necessary to refer to the Tabular List to verify that no 7th character is required.

2. **Level of Detail in Coding**

Diagnosis codes are to be used and reported at their highest number of characters available.

ICD-10-CM diagnosis codes are composed of codes with 3, 4, 5, 6 or 7 characters. Codes with three characters are included in ICD-10-CM as the heading of a category of codes that may be further subdivided by the use of fourth and/or fifth characters and/or sixth characters, which provide greater detail.

A three-character code is to be used only if it is not further subdivided. A code is invalid if it has not been coded to the full number of characters required for that code, including the 7th character, if applicable.

3. **Code or codes from A00.0 through T88.9, Z00-Z99.8**

The appropriate code or codes from A00.0 through T88.9, Z00-Z99.8 must be used to identify diagnoses, symptoms, conditions, problems, complaints or other reason(s) for the encounter/visit.

4. **Signs and symptoms**

Codes that describe symptoms and signs, as opposed to diagnoses, are acceptable for reporting purposes when a related definitive diagnosis has not been established (confirmed) by the provider. Chapter 18 of ICD-10-CM, Symptoms, Signs, and Abnormal Clinical and Laboratory Findings, Not Elsewhere Classified (codes R00.0 - R99) contains many, but not all codes for symptoms.

See Section I.B.18 Use of Signs/Symptom/Unspecified Codes

5. **Conditions that are an integral part of a disease process**

Signs and symptoms that are associated routinely with a disease process should not be assigned as additional codes, unless otherwise instructed by the classification.

6. **Conditions that are not an integral part of a disease process**

Additional signs and symptoms that may not be associated routinely with a disease process should be coded when present.

7. **Multiple coding for a single condition**

In addition to the etiology/manifestation convention that requires two codes to fully describe a single condition that affects multiple body systems, there are other single conditions that also require more than one code. "Use additional code" notes are found in the Tabular List at codes that are not part of an etiology/manifestation pair where a secondary code is useful to fully describe a condition. The sequencing rule is the same as the etiology/manifestation pair, "use additional code" indicates that a secondary code should be added.

For example, for bacterial infections that are not included in chapter 1, a secondary code from category B95, Streptococcus, Staphylococcus, and Enterococcus, as the cause of diseases classified elsewhere, or B96, Other bacterial agents as the cause of diseases classified elsewhere, may be required to identify the bacterial organism causing the infection. A "use additional code" note will normally be found at the infectious disease code, indicating a need for the organism code to be added as a secondary code.

"Code first" notes are also under certain codes that are not specifically manifestation codes but may be due to an underlying cause. When there is a "code first" note and an underlying condition is present, the underlying condition should be sequenced first.

"Code, if applicable, any causal condition first", notes indicate that this code may be assigned as a principal diagnosis when the causal condition is unknown or not applicable. If a causal condition is known, then the code for that condition should be sequenced as the principal or first-listed diagnosis.

Multiple codes may be needed for sequela, complication codes and obstetric codes to more fully describe a condition. See the specific guidelines for these conditions for further instruction.

8. Acute and Chronic Conditions
If the same condition is described as both acute (subacute) and chronic, and separate subentries exist in the Alphabetic Index at the same indentation level, code both and sequence the acute (subacute) code first.

9. Combination Code
A combination code is a single code used to classify:

Two diagnoses, or

A diagnosis with an associated secondary process (manifestation)

A diagnosis with an associated complication

Combination codes are identified by referring to subterm entries in the Alphabetic Index and by reading the inclusion and exclusion notes in the Tabular List.

Assign only the combination code when that code fully identifies the diagnostic conditions involved or when the Alphabetic Index so directs. Multiple coding should not be used when the classification provides a combination code that clearly identifies all of the elements documented in the diagnosis. When the combination code lacks necessary specificity in describing the manifestation or complication, an additional code should be used as a secondary code.

10. Sequela (Late Effects)
A sequela is the residual effect (condition produced) after the acute phase of an illness or injury has terminated. There is no time limit on when a sequela code can be used. The residual may be apparent early, such as in cerebral infarction, or it may occur months or years later, such as that due to a previous injury. Examples of sequela include: scar formation resulting from a burn, deviated septum due to a nasal fracture, and infertility due to tubal occlusion from old tuberculosis. Coding of sequela generally requires two codes sequenced in the following order: the condition or nature of the sequela is sequenced first. The sequela code is sequenced second.

An exception to the above guidelines are those instances where the code for the sequela is followed by a manifestation code identified in the Tabular List and title, or the sequela code has been expanded (at the fourth, fifth or sixth character levels) to include the manifestation(s). The code for the acute phase of an illness or injury that led to the sequela is never used with a code for the late effect.

See Section I.C.9. Sequelae of cerebrovascular disease

See Section I.C.15. Sequelae of complication of pregnancy, childbirth and the puerperium

See Section I.C.19. Application of 7th characters for Chapter 19

11. Impending or Threatened Condition
Code any condition described at the time of discharge as "impending" or "threatened" as follows:

If it did occur, code as confirmed diagnosis.

If it did not occur, reference the Alphabetic Index to determine if the condition has a subentry term for "impending" or "threatened" and also reference main term entries for "Impending" and for "Threatened."

If the subterms are listed, assign the given code.

If the subterms are not listed, code the existing underlying condition(s) and not the condition described as impending or threatened.

12. Reporting Same Diagnosis Code More than Once
Each unique ICD-10-CM diagnosis code may be reported only once for an encounter. This applies to bilateral conditions when there are no distinct codes identifying laterality or two different conditions classified to the same ICD-10-CM diagnosis code.

13. Laterality
Some ICD-10-CM codes indicate laterality, specifying whether the condition occurs on the left, right or is bilateral. If no bilateral code is provided and the condition is bilateral, assign separate codes for both the left and right side. If the side is not identified in the medical record, assign the code for the unspecified side.

14. Documentation for BMI, Non-pressure ulcers, and Pressure Ulcer Stages
For the Body Mass Index (BMI), depth of non-pressure chronic ulcers and pressure ulcer stage codes, code assignment may be based on medical record documentation from clinicians who are not the patient's provider (i.e., physician or other qualified healthcare practitioner legally accountable for establishing the patient's diagnosis), since this information is typically documented by other clinicians involved in the care of the patient (e.g., a dietitian often documents the BMI and nurses often documents the pressure ulcer stages). However, the associated diagnosis (such as overweight, obesity, or pressure ulcer) must be documented by the patient's provider. If there is conflicting medical record documentation, either from the same clinician or different clinicians, the patient's attending provider should be queried for clarification.

The BMI codes should only be reported as secondary diagnoses. As with all other secondary diagnosis codes, the BMI codes should only be assigned when they meet the definition of a reportable additional diagnosis (see Section III, Reporting Additional Diagnoses).

15. Syndromes
Follow the Alphabetic Index guidance when coding syndromes. In the absence of Alphabetic Index guidance, assign codes for the documented manifestations of the syndrome.

Additional codes for manifestations that are not an integral part of the disease process may also be assigned when the condition does not have a unique code.

16. Documentation of Complications of Care
Code assignment is based on the provider's documentation of the relationship between the condition and the care or procedure. The guideline extends to any complications of care, regardless of the chapter the code is located in. It is important to note that not all conditions that occur during or following medical care or surgery are classified as complications. There must be a cause-and-effect relationship between the care provided and the condition, and an indication in the documentation that it is a complication. Query the provider for clarification, if the complication is not clearly documented.

17. Borderline Diagnosis
If the provider documents a "borderline" diagnosis at the time of discharge, the diagnosis is coded as confirmed, unless the classification provides a specific entry (e.g., borderline diabetes). If a borderline condition has a specific index entry in ICD-10-CM, it should be coded as such. Since borderline conditions are not uncertain diagnoses, no distinction is made between the care setting (inpatient versus outpatient). Whenever the documentation is unclear regarding a borderline condition, coders are encouraged to query for clarification.

18. Use of Sign/Symptom/Unspecified Codes
Sign/symptom and "unspecified" codes have acceptable, even necessary, uses. While specific diagnosis codes should be reported when they are supported by the available medical record documentation and clinical knowledge of the patient's health condition, there are instances when signs/symptoms or unspecified codes are the best choices for accurately reflecting the healthcare encounter. Each healthcare encounter should be coded to the level of certainty known for that encounter.

If a definitive diagnosis has not been established by the end of the encounter, it is appropriate to report codes for sign(s) and/or symptom(s) in lieu of a definitive diagnosis. When sufficient clinical information isn't known or available about a particular health condition to assign a more specific code, it is acceptable to report the appropriate "unspecified" code (e.g., a diagnosis of pneumonia has been determined, but not the specific type). Unspecified codes should be reported when they are the codes that most accurately reflects what is known about the patient's condition at the time of that particular encounter. It would be inappropriate to select a specific code that is not supported by the medical record documentation or conduct medically unnecessary diagnostic testing in order to determine a more specific code.

C. Chapter-Specific Coding Guidelines

In addition to general coding guidelines, there are guidelines for specific diagnoses and/or conditions in the classification. Unless otherwise indicated, these guidelines apply to all health care settings. Please refer to Section II for guidelines on the selection of principal diagnosis.

1. **Chapter 1: Certain Infectious and Parasitic Diseases (A00-B99)**
   a. **Human immunodeficiency virus (HIV) infections**
      1) **Code only confirmed cases**
         Code only confirmed cases of HIV infection/illness. This is an exception to the hospital inpatient guideline Section II, H.

         In this context, "confirmation" does not require documentation of positive serology or culture for HIV; the provider's diagnostic statement that the patient is HIV positive, or has an HIV-related illness is sufficient.

      2) **Selection and sequencing of HIV codes**
         (a) **Patient admitted for HIV-related condition**
            If a patient is admitted for an HIV-related condition, the principal diagnosis should be B20, Human immunodeficiency virus [HIV] disease followed by additional diagnosis codes for all reported HIV-related conditions.

         (b) **Patient with HIV disease admitted for unrelated condition**
            If a patient with HIV disease is admitted for an unrelated condition (such as a traumatic injury), the code for the unrelated condition (e.g., the nature of injury code) should be the principal diagnosis. Other diagnoses would be B20 followed by additional diagnosis codes for all reported HIV-related conditions.

         (c) **Whether the patient is newly diagnosed**
            Whether the patient is newly diagnosed or has had previous admissions/encounters for HIV conditions is irrelevant to the sequencing decision.

         (d) **Asymptomatic human immunodeficiency virus**
            Z21, Asymptomatic human immunodeficiency virus [HIV] infection status, is to be applied when the patient without any documentation of symptoms is listed as being "HIV positive," "known HIV," "HIV test positive," or similar terminology. Do not use this code if the term "AIDS" is used or if the patient is treated for any HIV-related illness or is described as having any condition(s) resulting from his/her HIV positive status; use B20 in these cases.

         (e) **Patients with inconclusive HIV serology**
            Patients with inconclusive HIV serology, but no definitive diagnosis or manifestations of the illness, may be assigned code R75, Inconclusive laboratory evidence of human immunodeficiency virus [HIV].

         (f) **Previously diagnosed HIV-related illness**
            Patients with any known prior diagnosis of an HIV-related illness should be coded to B20. Once a patient has developed an HIV-related illness, the patient should always be assigned code B20 on every subsequent admission/encounter. Patients previously diagnosed with any HIV illness (B20) should never be assigned to R75 or Z21, Asymptomatic human immunodeficiency virus [HIV] infection status.

         (g) **HIV infection in pregnancy, childbirth and the puerperium**
            During pregnancy, childbirth or the puerperium, a patient admitted (or presenting for a health care encounter) because of an HIV-related illness should receive a principal

diagnosis code of O98.7-, Human immunodeficiency [HIV] disease complicating pregnancy, childbirth and the puerperium, followed by B20 and the code(s) for the HIV-related illness(es). Codes from Chapter 15 always take sequencing priority.

Patients with asymptomatic HIV infection status admitted (or presenting for a health care encounter) during pregnancy, childbirth, or the puerperium should receive codes of O98.7- and Z21.

(h) **Encounters for testing for HIV**
   If a patient is being seen to determine his/her HIV status, use code Z11.4, Encounter for screening for human immunodeficiency virus [HIV]. Use additional codes for any associated high risk behavior.

   If a patient with signs or symptoms is being seen for HIV testing, code the signs and symptoms. An additional counseling code Z71.7, Human immunodeficiency virus [HIV] counseling, may be used if counseling is provided during the encounter for the test.

   When a patient returns to be informed of his/her HIV test results and the test result is negative, use code Z71.7, Human immunodeficiency virus [HIV] counseling.

   If the results are positive, see previous guidelines and assign codes as appropriate.

b. **Infectious agents as the cause of diseases classified to other chapters**
   Certain infections are classified in chapters other than Chapter 1 and no organism is identified as part of the infection code. In these instances, it is necessary to use an additional code from Chapter 1 to identify the organism. A code from category B95, Streptococcus, Staphylococcus, and Enterococcus as the cause of diseases classified to other chapters, B96, Other bacterial agents as the cause of diseases classified to other chapters, or B97, Viral agents as the cause of diseases classified to other chapters, is to be used as an additional code to identify the organism. An instructional note will be found at the infection code advising that an additional organism code is required.

c. **Infections resistant to antibiotics**
   Many bacterial infections are resistant to current antibiotics. It is necessary to identify all infections documented as antibiotic resistant. Assign a code from category Z16, Resistance to antimicrobial drugs, following the infection code only if the infection code does not identify drug resistance.

d. **Sepsis, severe sepsis, and septic shock**
   1) **Coding of sepsis and severe sepsis**
      (a) **Sepsis**
         For a diagnosis of sepsis, assign the appropriate code for the underlying systemic infection. If the type of infection or causal organism is not further specified, assign code A41.9, Sepsis, unspecified organism.

         A code from subcategory R65.2, Severe sepsis, should not be assigned unless severe sepsis or an associated acute organ dysfunction is documented.

         (i) Negative or inconclusive blood cultures and sepsis
            Negative or inconclusive blood cultures do not preclude a diagnosis of sepsis in patients with clinical evidence of the condition, however, the provider should be queried.

         (ii) Urosepsis
            The term urosepsis is a nonspecific term. It is not to be considered synonymous with sepsis. It has no default code in the Alphabetic Index. Should a provider use this term, he/she must be queried for clarification.

         (iii) Sepsis with organ dysfunction
            If a patient has sepsis and associated acute organ dysfunction or multiple organ dysfunction (MOD), follow the instructions for coding severe sepsis.

         (iv) Acute organ dysfunction that is not clearly associated with the sepsis
            If a patient has sepsis and an acute organ dysfunction, but the medical record documentation indicates that

the acute organ dysfunction is related to a medical condition other than the sepsis, do not assign a code from subcategory R65.2, Severe sepsis. An acute organ dysfunction must be associated with the sepsis in order to assign the severe sepsis code. If the documentation is not clear as to whether an acute organ dysfunction is related to the sepsis or another medical condition, query the provider.

(b) Severe sepsis

The coding of severe sepsis requires a minimum of 2 codes: first a code for the underlying systemic infection, followed by a code from subcategory R65.2, Severe sepsis. If the causal organism is not documented, assign code A41.9, Sepsis, unspecified organism, for the infection. Additional code(s) for the associated acute organ dysfunction are also required.

Due to the complex nature of severe sepsis, some cases may require querying the provider prior to assignment of the codes.

2) Septic shock

(a) Septic shock generally refers to circulatory failure associated with severe sepsis, and therefore, it represents a type of acute organ dysfunction.

For cases of septic shock, the code for the systemic infection should be sequenced first, followed by code R65.21, Severe sepsis with septic shock or code T81.12, Postprocedural septic shock. Any additional codes for the other acute organ dysfunctions should also be assigned. As noted in the sequencing instructions in the Tabular List, the code for septic shock cannot be assigned as a principal diagnosis.

3) Sequencing of severe sepsis

If severe sepsis is present on admission, and meets the definition of principal diagnosis, the underlying systemic infection should be assigned as principal diagnosis followed by the appropriate code from subcategory R65.2 as required by the sequencing rules in the Tabular List. A code from subcategory R65.2 can never be assigned as a principal diagnosis.

When severe sepsis develops during an encounter (it was not present on admission) the underlying systemic infection and the appropriate code from subcategory R65.2 should be assigned as secondary diagnoses.

Severe sepsis may be present on admission but the diagnosis may not be confirmed until sometime after admission. If the documentation is not clear whether severe sepsis was present on admission, the provider should be queried.

4) Sepsis and severe sepsis with a localized infection

If the reason for admission is both sepsis or severe sepsis and a localized infection, such as pneumonia or cellulitis, a code(s) for the underlying systemic infection should be assigned first and the code for the localized infection should be assigned as a secondary diagnosis. If the patient has severe sepsis, a code from subcategory R65.2 should also be assigned as a secondary diagnosis. If the patient is admitted with a localized infection, such as pneumonia, and sepsis/severe sepsis doesn't develop until after admission, the localized infection should be assigned first, followed by the appropriate sepsis/severe sepsis codes.

5) Sepsis due to a postprocedural infection

(a) Documentation of causal relationship

As with all postprocedural complications, code assignment is based on the provider's documentation of the relationship between the infection and the procedure.

(b) Sepsis due to a postprocedural infection

For such cases, the postprocedural infection code, such as T80.2, Infections following infusion, transfusion, and therapeutic injection, T81.4, Infection following a procedure, T88.0, Infection following immunization, or O86.0, Infection of obstetric surgical wound, should be coded first, followed by the code for the specific infection. If the patient has severe sepsis, the appropriate code from subcategory R65.2 should also be

assigned with the additional code(s) for any acute organ dysfunction.

(c) Postprocedural infection and postprocedural septic shock

In cases where a postprocedural infection has occurred and has resulted in severe sepsis the code for the precipitating complication such as code T81.4, Infection following a procedure, or O86.0, Infection of obstetrical surgical wound should be coded first followed by code R65.20, Severe sepsis without septic shock. A code for the systemic infection should also be assigned.

If a postprocedural infection has resulted in postprocedural septic shock, the code for the precipitating complication such as code T81.4, Infection following a procedure, or O86.0, Infection of obstetrical surgical wound should be coded first followed by code T81.12-, Postprocedural septic shock. A code for the systemic infection should also be assigned.

6) Sepsis and severe sepsis associated with a noninfectious process (condition)

In some cases a noninfectious process (condition), such as trauma, may lead to an infection which can result in sepsis or severe sepsis. If sepsis or severe sepsis is documented as associated with a noninfectious condition, such as a burn or serious injury, and this condition meets the definition for principal diagnosis, the code for the noninfectious condition should be sequenced first, followed by the code for the resulting infection. If severe sepsis is present, a code from subcategory R65.2 should also be assigned with any associated organ dysfunction(s) codes. It is not necessary to assign a code from subcategory R65.1, Systemic inflammatory response syndrome (SIRS) of non-infectious origin, for these cases.

If the infection meets the definition of principal diagnosis, it should be sequenced before the non-infectious condition. When both the associated non-infectious condition and the infection meet the definition of principal diagnosis, either may be assigned as principal diagnosis.

Only one code from category R65, Symptoms and signs specifically associated with systemic inflammation and infection, should be assigned. Therefore, when a non-infectious condition leads to an infection resulting in severe sepsis, assign the appropriate code from subcategory R65.2, Severe sepsis.

Do not additionally assign a code from subcategory R65.1, Systemic inflammatory response syndrome (SIRS) of non-infectious origin.

See Section I.C.18. SIRS due to non-infectious process

7) Sepsis and septic shock complicating abortion, pregnancy, childbirth, and the puerperium

See Section I.C.15. Sepsis and septic shock complicating abortion, pregnancy, childbirth and the puerperium

8) Newborn sepsis

See Section I.C.16. f. Bacterial sepsis of Newborn

e. Methicillin resistant *Staphylococcus aureus* (MRSA) conditions

1) Selection and sequencing of MRSA codes

(a) Combination codes for MRSA infection

When a patient is diagnosed with an infection that is due to methicillin resistant *Staphylococcus aureus* (MRSA), and that infection has a combination code that includes the causal organism (e.g., sepsis, pneumonia) assign the appropriate combination code for the condition (e.g., code A41.02, Sepsis due to Methicillin resistant *Staphylococcus aureus* or code J15.212, Pneumonia due to Methicillin resistant *Staphylococcus aureus*). Do not assign code B95.62, Methicillin resistant *Staphylococcus aureus* infection as the cause of diseases classified elsewhere, as an additional code because the combination code includes the type of infection and the MRSA organism. Do not assign a code from subcategory Z16.11, Resistance to penicillins, as an additional diagnosis.

See Section C.1. for instructions on coding and sequencing of sepsis and severe sepsis.

(b) **Other codes for MRSA infection**

When there is documentation of a current infection (e.g., wound infection, stitch abscess, urinary tract infection) due to MRSA, and that infection does not have a combination code that includes the causal organism, assign the appropriate code to identify the condition along with code B95.62, Methicillin resistant *Staphylococcus aureus* infection as the cause of diseases classified elsewhere for the MRSA infection. Do not assign a code from subcategory Z16.11, Resistance to penicillins.

(c) **Methicillin susceptible *Staphylococcus aureus* (MSSA) and MRSA colonization**

The condition or state of being colonized or carrying MSSA or MRSA is called colonization or carriage, while an individual person is described as being colonized or being a carrier. Colonization means that MSSA or MSRA is present on or in the body without necessarily causing illness. A positive MRSA colonization test might be documented by the provider as "MRSA screen positive" or "MRSA nasal swab positive".

Assign code Z22.322, Carrier or suspected carrier of Methicillin resistant *Staphylococcus aureus*, for patients documented as having MRSA colonization. Assign code Z22.321, Carrier or suspected carrier of Methicillin susceptible *Staphylococcus aureus*, for patient documented as having MSSA colonization. Colonization is not necessarily indicative of a disease process or as the cause of a specific condition the patient may have unless documented as such by the provider.

(d) **MRSA colonization and infection**

If a patient is documented as having both MRSA colonization and infection during a hospital admission, code Z22.322, Carrier or suspected carrier of Methicillin resistant *Staphylococcus aureus*, and a code for the MRSA infection may both be assigned.

2. **Chapter 2: Neoplasms (C00-D49)**

General guidelines

Chapter 2 of the ICD-10-CM contains the codes for most benign and all malignant neoplasms. Certain benign neoplasms, such as prostatic adenomas, may be found in the specific body system chapters. To properly code a neoplasm it is necessary to determine from the record if the neoplasm is benign, in-situ, malignant, or of uncertain histologic behavior. If malignant, any secondary (metastatic) sites should also be determined.

Primary malignant neoplasms overlapping site boundaries

A primary malignant neoplasm that overlaps two or more contiguous (next to each other) sites should be classified to the subcategory/code .8 ('overlapping lesion'), unless the combination is specifically indexed elsewhere. For multiple neoplasms of the same site that are not contiguous such as tumors in different quadrants of the same breast, codes for each site should be assigned.

Malignant neoplasm of ectopic tissue

Malignant neoplasms of ectopic tissue are to be coded to the site of origin mentioned, e.g., ectopic pancreatic malignant neoplasms involving the stomach are coded to pancreas, unspecified (C25.9).

The neoplasm table in the Alphabetic Index should be referenced first. However, if the histological term is documented, that term should be referenced first, rather than going immediately to the Neoplasm Table, in order to determine which column in the Neoplasm Table is appropriate. For example, if the documentation indicates "adenoma," refer to the term in the Alphabetic Index to review the entries under this term and the instructional note to "see also neoplasm, by site, benign." The table provides the proper code based on the type of neoplasm and the site. It is important to select the proper column in the table that corresponds to the type of neoplasm. The Tabular List should then be referenced to verify that the correct code has been selected from the table and that a more specific site code does not exist.

See Section I.C.21. Factors influencing health status and contact with health services, Status, for information regarding Z15.0, codes for genetic susceptibility to cancer.

a. **Treatment directed at the malignancy**

If the treatment is directed at the malignancy, designate the malignancy as the principal diagnosis.

The only exception to this guideline is if a patient admission/encounter is solely for the administration of chemotherapy, immunotherapy or radiation therapy, assign the appropriate Z51.- code as the first-listed or principal diagnosis, and the diagnosis or problem for which the service is being performed as a secondary diagnosis.

b. **Treatment of secondary site**

When a patient is admitted because of a primary neoplasm with metastasis and treatment is directed toward the secondary site only, the secondary neoplasm is designated as the principal diagnosis even though the primary malignancy is still present.

c. **Coding and sequencing of complications**

Coding and sequencing of complications associated with the malignancies or with the therapy thereof are subject to the following guidelines:

1) **Anemia associated with malignancy**

When admission/encounter is for management of an anemia associated with the malignancy, and the treatment is only for anemia, the appropriate code for the malignancy is sequenced as the principal or first-listed diagnosis followed by the appropriate code for the anemia (such as code D63.0, Anemia in neoplastic disease).

2) **Anemia associated with chemotherapy, immunotherapy and radiation therapy**

When the admission/encounter is for management of an anemia associated with an adverse effect of the administration of chemotherapy or immunotherapy and the only treatment is for the anemia, the anemia code is sequenced first followed by the appropriate codes for the neoplasm and the adverse effect (T45.1X5, Adverse effect of antineoplastic and immunosuppressive drugs).

When the admission/encounter is for management of an anemia associated with an adverse effect of radiotherapy, the anemia code should be sequenced first, followed by the appropriate neoplasm code and code Y84.2, Radiological procedure and radiotherapy as the cause of abnormal reaction of the patient, or of later complication, without mention of misadventure at the time of the procedure.

3) **Management of dehydration due to the malignancy**

When the admission/encounter is for management of dehydration due to the malignancy and only the dehydration is being treated (intravenous rehydration), the dehydration is sequenced first, followed by the code(s) for the malignancy.

4) **Treatment of a complication resulting from a surgical procedure**

When the admission/encounter is for treatment of a complication resulting from a surgical procedure, designate the complication as the principal or first-listed diagnosis if treatment is directed at resolving the complication.

d. **Primary malignancy previously excised**

When a primary malignancy has been previously excised or eradicated from its site and there is no further treatment directed to that site and there is no evidence of any existing primary malignancy, a code from category Z85, Personal history of malignant neoplasm, should be used to indicate the former site of the malignancy. Any mention of extension, invasion, or metastasis to another site is coded as a secondary malignant neoplasm to that site. The secondary site may be the principal or first-listed with the Z85 code used as a secondary code.

e. **Admissions/Encounters involving chemotherapy, immunotherapy and radiation therapy**

1) **Episode of care involves surgical removal of neoplasm**

When an episode of care involves the surgical removal of a neoplasm, primary or secondary site, followed by adjunct chemotherapy or radiation treatment during the same episode of care, the code for the neoplasm should be assigned as principal or first-listed diagnosis.

2) **Patient admission/encounter solely for administration of chemotherapy, immunotherapy and radiation therapy**

If a patient admission/encounter is solely for the administration of chemotherapy, immunotherapy or radiation therapy assign code Z51.0, Encounter for antineoplastic radiation therapy, or Z51.11, Encounter for antineoplastic chemotherapy, or Z51.12, Encounter for antineoplastic immunotherapy as the first-listed or principal diagnosis. If a patient receives more than one of these therapies during the same admission more than one of these codes may be assigned, in any sequence.

The malignancy for which the therapy is being administered should be assigned as a secondary diagnosis.

3) **Patient admitted for radiation therapy, chemotherapy or immunotherapy and develops complications**

When a patient is admitted for the purpose of radiotherapy, immunotherapy or chemotherapy and develops complications such as uncontrolled nausea and vomiting or dehydration, the principal or first-listed diagnosis is Z51.0, Encounter for antineoplastic radiation therapy, or Z51.11, Encounter for antineoplastic chemotherapy, or Z51.12, Encounter for antineoplastic immunotherapy followed by any codes for the complications.

f. **Admission/encounter to determine extent of malignancy**

When the reason for admission/encounter is to determine the extent of the malignancy, or for a procedure such as paracentesis or thoracentesis, the primary malignancy or appropriate metastatic site is designated as the principal or first-listed diagnosis, even though chemotherapy or radiotherapy is administered.

g. **Symptoms, signs, and abnormal findings listed in Chapter 18 associated with neoplasms**

Symptoms, signs, and ill-defined conditions listed in Chapter 18 characteristic of, or associated with, an existing primary or secondary site malignancy cannot be used to replace the malignancy as principal or first-listed diagnosis, regardless of the number of admissions or encounters for treatment and care of the neoplasm.

See section I.C.21. Factors influencing health status and contact with health services, Encounter for prophylactic organ removal.

h. **Admission/encounter for pain control/management**

See Section I.C.6. for information on coding admission/encounter for pain control/management.

i. **Malignancy in two or more noncontiguous sites**

A patient may have more than one malignant tumor in the same organ. These tumors may represent different primaries or metastatic disease, depending on the site. Should the documentation be unclear, the provider should be queried as to the status of each tumor so that the correct codes can be assigned.

j. **Disseminated malignant neoplasm, unspecified**

Code C80.0, Disseminated malignant neoplasm, unspecified, is for use only in those cases where the patient has advanced metastatic disease and no known primary or secondary sites are specified. It should not be used in place of assigning codes for the primary site and all known secondary sites.

k. **Malignant neoplasm without specification of site**

Code C80.1, Malignant (primary) neoplasm, unspecified, equates to Cancer, unspecified. This code should only be used when no determination can be made as to the primary site of a malignancy. This code should rarely be used in the inpatient setting.

l. **Sequencing of neoplasm codes**

1) **Encounter for treatment of primary malignancy**

If the reason for the encounter is for treatment of a primary malignancy, assign the malignancy as the principal/first-listed diagnosis. The primary site is to be sequenced first, followed by any metastatic sites.

2) **Encounter for treatment of secondary malignancy**

When an encounter is for a primary malignancy with metastasis and treatment is directed toward the metastatic (secondary) site(s) only, the metastatic site(s) is designated as the principal/first-listed diagnosis. The primary malignancy is coded as an additional code.

3) **Malignant neoplasm in a pregnant patient**

When a pregnant woman has a malignant neoplasm, a code from subcategory O9A.1-, Malignant neoplasm complicating pregnancy, childbirth, and the puerperium, should be sequenced first, followed by the appropriate code from Chapter 2 to indicate the type of neoplasm.

4) **Encounter for complication associated with a neoplasm**

When an encounter is for management of a complication associated with a neoplasm, such as dehydration, and the treatment is only for the complication, the complication is coded first, followed by the appropriate code(s) for the neoplasm.

The exception to this guideline is anemia. When the admission/encounter is for management of an anemia associated with the malignancy, and the treatment is only for anemia, the appropriate code for the malignancy is sequenced as the principal or first-listed diagnosis followed by code D63.0, Anemia in neoplastic disease.

5) **Complication from surgical procedure for treatment of a neoplasm**

When an encounter is for treatment of a complication resulting from a surgical procedure performed for the treatment of the neoplasm, designate the complication as the principal/first-listed diagnosis. See guideline regarding the coding of a current malignancy versus personal history to determine if the code for the neoplasm should also be assigned.

6) **Pathologic fracture due to a neoplasm**

When an encounter is for a pathological fracture due to a neoplasm, and the focus of treatment is the fracture, a code from subcategory M84.5, Pathological fracture in neoplastic disease, should be sequenced first, followed by the code for the neoplasm.

If the focus of treatment is the neoplasm with an associated pathological fracture, the neoplasm code should be sequenced first, followed by a code from M84.5 for the pathological fracture.

m. **Current malignancy versus personal history of malignancy**

When a primary malignancy has been excised but further treatment, such as an additional surgery for the malignancy, radiation therapy or chemotherapy is directed to that site, the primary malignancy code should be used until treatment is completed.

When a primary malignancy has been previously excised or eradicated from its site, there is no further treatment (of the malignancy) directed to that site, and there is no evidence of any existing primary malignancy, a code from category Z85, Personal history of malignant neoplasm, should be used to indicate the former site of the malignancy.

See Section I.C.21. Factors influencing health status and contact with health services, History (of)

n. **Leukemia, multiple myeloma, and malignant plasma cell neoplasms in remission versus personal history**

The categories for leukemia, and category C90, Multiple myeloma and malignant plasma cell neoplasms, have codes indicating whether or not the leukemia has achieved remission. There are also codes Z85.6, Personal history of leukemia, and Z85.79, Personal history of other malignant neoplasms of lymphoid, hematopoietic and related tissues. If the documentation is unclear, as to whether the leukemia has achieved remission, the provider should be queried.

See Section I.C.21. Factors influencing health status and contact with health services, History (of)

o. **Aftercare following surgery for neoplasm**

See Section I.C.21. Factors influencing health status and contact with health services, Aftercare

p. **Follow-up care for completed treatment of a malignancy**

See Section I.C.21. Factors influencing health status and contact with health services, Follow-up

q. **Prophylactic organ removal for prevention of malignancy**

See Section I.C. 21, Factors influencing health status and contact with health services, Prophylactic organ removal

r. **Malignant neoplasm associated with transplanted organ**
A malignant neoplasm of a transplanted organ should be coded as a transplant complication. Assign first the appropriate code from category T86.-, Complications of transplanted organs and tissue, followed by code C80.2, Malignant neoplasm associated with transplanted organ. Use an additional code for the specific malignancy.

3. **Chapter 3: Disease of the blood and blood-forming organs and certain disorders involving the immune mechanism (D50-D89)**
Reserved for future guideline expansion

4. **Chapter 4: Endocrine, Nutritional, and Metabolic Diseases (E00-E89)**
a. **Diabetes mellitus**
The diabetes mellitus codes are combination codes that include the type of diabetes mellitus, the body system affected, and the complications affecting that body system. As many codes within a particular category as are necessary to describe all of the complications of the disease may be used. They should be sequenced based on the reason for a particular encounter. Assign as many codes from categories E08 – E13 as needed to identify all of the associated conditions that the patient has.

1) **Type of diabetes**
The age of a patient is not the sole determining factor, though most type 1 diabetics develop the condition before reaching puberty. For this reason type 1 diabetes mellitus is also referred to as juvenile diabetes.

2) **Type of diabetes mellitus not documented**
If the type of diabetes mellitus is not documented in the medical record the default is E11.-, Type 2 diabetes mellitus.

3) **Diabetes mellitus and the use of insulin**
If the documentation in a medical record does not indicate the type of diabetes but does indicate that the patient uses insulin, code E11, Type 2 diabetes mellitus, should be assigned. Code Z79.4, Long-term (current) use of insulin, should also be assigned to indicate that the patient uses insulin. Code Z79.4 should not be assigned if insulin is given temporarily to bring a type 2 patient's blood sugar under control during an encounter.

4) **Diabetes mellitus in pregnancy and gestational diabetes**
See Section I.C.15. Diabetes mellitus in pregnancy.

See Section I.C.15. Gestational (pregnancy induced) diabetes

5) **Complications due to insulin pump malfunction**
(a) **Underdose of insulin due to insulin pump failure**
An underdose of insulin due to an insulin pump failure should be assigned to a code from subcategory T85.6, Mechanical complication of other specified internal and external prosthetic devices, implants and grafts, that specifies the type of pump malfunction, as the principal or first-listed code, followed by code T38.3x6-, Underdosing of insulin and oral hypoglycemic [antidiabetic] drugs. Additional codes for the type of diabetes mellitus and any associated complications due to the underdosing should also be assigned.

(b) **Overdose of insulin due to insulin pump failure**
The principal or first-listed code for an encounter due to an insulin pump malfunction resulting in an overdose of insulin, should also be T85.6-, Mechanical complication of other specified internal and external prosthetic devices, implants and grafts, followed by code T38.3X1-, Poisoning by insulin and oral hypoglycemic [antidiabetic] drugs, accidental (unintentional).

6) **Secondary diabetes mellitus**
Codes under categories E08, Diabetes mellitus due to underlying condition, E09, Drug or chemical induced diabetes mellitus, and E13, Other specified diabetes mellitus, identify complications/manifestations associated with secondary diabetes mellitus. Secondary diabetes is always caused by another condition or event (e.g., cystic fibrosis, malignant neoplasm of pancreas, pancreatectomy, adverse effect of drug, or poisoning).

(a) **Secondary diabetes mellitus and the use of insulin**
For patients who routinely use insulin, code Z79.4, Long-term (current) use of insulin, should also be assigned. Code Z79.4 should not be assigned if insulin is given temporarily to bring a patient's blood sugar under control during an encounter.

(b) **Assigning and sequencing secondary diabetes codes and its causes**
The sequencing of the secondary diabetes codes in relationship to codes for the cause of the diabetes is based on the Tabular List instructions for categories E08, E09 and E13.

(i) **Secondary diabetes mellitus due to pancreatectomy**
For postpancreatectomy diabetes mellitus (lack of insulin due to the surgical removal of all or part of the pancreas), assign code E89.1, Postprocedural hypoinsulinemia. Assign a code from category E13 and a code from subcategory Z90.41-, Acquired absence of pancreas, as additional codes.

(ii) **Secondary diabetes due to drugs**
Secondary diabetes may be caused by an adverse effect of correctly administered medications, poisoning or sequela of poisoning.
See section I.C.19.e for coding of adverse effects and poisoning, and section I.C.20 for external cause code reporting.

5. **Chapter 5: Mental, Behavioral and Neurodevelopmental disorders (F01 – F99)**
a. **Pain disorders related to psychological factors**
Assign code F45.41, for pain that is exclusively related to psychological disorders. As indicated by the Excludes 1 note under category G89, a code from category G89 should not be assigned with code F45.41.

Code F45.42, Pain disorders with related psychological factors, should be used with a code from category G89, Pain, not elsewhere classified, if there is documentation of a psychological component for a patient with acute or chronic pain.
See Section I.C.6. Pain

b. **Mental and behavioral disorders due to psychoactive substance use**
1) **In remission**
Selection of codes for "in remission" for categories F10-F19, Mental and behavioral disorders due to psychoactive substance use (categories F10-F19 with -.21) requires the provider's clinical judgment. The appropriate codes for "in remission" are assigned only on the basis of provider documentation (as defined in the Official Guidelines for Coding and Reporting).

2) **Psychoactive substance use, abuse and dependence**
When the provider documentation refers to use, abuse and dependence of the same substance (e.g. alcohol, opioid, cannabis, etc.), only one code should be assigned to identify the pattern of use based on the following hierarchy:

- If both use and abuse are documented, assign only the code for abuse
- If both abuse and dependence are documented, assign only the code for dependence
- If use, abuse and dependence are all documented, assign only the code for dependence
- If both use and dependence are documented, assign only the code for dependence.

3) **Psychoactive substance use**
As with all other diagnoses, the codes for psychoactive substance use (F10.9-, F11.9-, F12.9-, F13.9-, F14.9-, F15.9-, F16.9-) should only be assigned based on provider documentation and when they meet the definition of a reportable diagnosis (see Section III, Reporting Additional Diagnoses). The codes are to be used only when the psychoactive substance use is associated with a mental or behavioral disorder, and such a relationship is documented by the provider.

6. **Chapter 6: Diseases of Nervous System (G00-G99)**
   a. **Dominant/nondominant side**

   Codes from category G81, Hemiplegia and hemiparesis, and subcategories, G83.1, Monoplegia of lower limb, G83.2, Monoplegia of upper limb, and G83.3, Monoplegia, unspecified, identify whether the dominant or nondominant side is affected. Should the affected side be documented, but not specified as dominant or nondominant, and the classification system does not indicate a default, code selection is as follows:

   - For ambidextrous patients, the default should be dominant.
   - If the left side is affected, the default is non-dominant.
   - If the right side is affected, the default is dominant.

   b. **Pain - Category G89**
   1) **General coding information**

   Codes in category G89, Pain, not elsewhere classified, may be used in conjunction with codes from other categories and chapters to provide more detail about acute or chronic pain and neoplasm-related pain, unless otherwise indicated below.

   If the pain is not specified as acute or chronic, post-thoracotomy, postprocedural, or neoplasm-related, do not assign codes from category G89.

   A code from category G89 should not be assigned if the underlying (definitive) diagnosis is known, unless the reason for the encounter is pain control/ management and not management of the underlying condition.

   When an admission or encounter is for a procedure aimed at treating the underlying condition (e.g., spinal fusion, kyphoplasty), a code for the underlying condition (e.g., vertebral fracture, spinal stenosis) should be assigned as the principal diagnosis. No code from category G89 should be assigned.

   (a) **Category G89 codes as principal or first-listed diagnosis**

   Category G89 codes are acceptable as principal diagnosis or the first-listed code:

   - When pain control or pain management is the reason for the admission/encounter (e.g., a patient with displaced intervertebral disc, nerve impingement and severe back pain presents for injection of steroid into the spinal canal). The underlying cause of the pain should be reported as an additional diagnosis, if known.

   - When a patient is admitted for the insertion of a neurostimulator for pain control, assign the appropriate pain code as the principal or first-listed diagnosis. When an admission or encounter is for a procedure aimed at treating the underlying condition and a neurostimulator is inserted for pain control during the same admission/encounter, a code for the underlying condition should be assigned as the principal diagnosis and the appropriate pain code should be assigned as a secondary diagnosis.

   (b) **Use of category G89 codes in conjunction with site specific pain codes**
   (i) **Assigning category G89 and site-specific pain codes**

   Codes from category G89 may be used in conjunction with codes that identify the site of pain (including codes from chapter 18) if the category G89 code provides additional information. For example, if the code describes the site of the pain, but does not fully describe whether the pain is acute or chronic, then both codes should be assigned.

   (ii) **Sequencing of category G89 codes with site-specific pain codes**

   The sequencing of category G89 codes with site-specific pain codes (including chapter 18 codes), is dependent on the circumstances of the encounter/admission as follows:

   - If the encounter is for pain control or pain management, assign the code from category G89 followed by the code identifying the specific site of

   pain (e.g., encounter for pain management for acute neck pain from trauma is assigned code G89.11, Acute pain due to trauma, followed by code M54.2, Cervicalgia, to identify the site of pain).

   - If the encounter is for any other reason except pain control or pain management, and a related definitive diagnosis has not been established (confirmed) by the provider, assign the code for the specific site of pain first, followed by the appropriate code from category G89.

   2) **Pain due to devices, implants and grafts**
   See Section I.C.19. Pain due to medical devices

   3) **Postoperative pain**

   The provider's documentation should be used to guide the coding of postoperative pain, as well as *Section III. Reporting Additional Diagnoses* and *Section IV. Diagnostic Coding and Reporting in the Outpatient Setting.*

   The default for post-thoracotomy and other postoperative pain not specified as acute or chronic is the code for the acute form.

   Routine or expected postoperative pain immediately after surgery should not be coded.

   (a) **Postoperative pain not associated with specific postoperative complication**

   Postoperative pain not associated with a specific postoperative complication is assigned to the appropriate postoperative pain code in category G89.

   (b) **Postoperative pain associated with specific postoperative complication**

   Postoperative pain associated with a specific postoperative complication (such as painful wire sutures) is assigned to the appropriate code(s) found in Chapter 19, Injury, poisoning, and certain other consequences of external causes. If appropriate, use additional code(s) from category G89 to identify acute or chronic pain (G89.18 or G89.28).

   4) **Chronic pain**

   Chronic pain is classified to subcategory G89.2. There is no time frame defining when pain becomes chronic pain. The provider's documentation should be used to guide use of these codes.

   5) **Neoplasm related pain**

   Code G89.3 is assigned to pain documented as being related, associated or due to cancer, primary or secondary malignancy, or tumor. This code is assigned regardless of whether the pain is acute or chronic.

   This code may be assigned as the principal or first-listed code when the stated reason for the admission/encounter is documented as pain control/pain management. The underlying neoplasm should be reported as an additional diagnosis.

   When the reason for the admission/encounter is management of the neoplasm and the pain associated with the neoplasm is also documented, code G89.3 may be assigned as an additional diagnosis. It is not necessary to assign an additional code for the site of the pain.

   See Section I.C.2 for instructions on the sequencing of neoplasms for all other stated reasons for the admission/encounter (except for pain control/pain management).

   6) **Chronic pain syndrome**

   Central pain syndrome (G89.0) and chronic pain syndrome (G89.4) are different than the term "chronic pain," and therefore codes should only be used when the provider has specifically documented this condition.

   See Section I.C.5. Pain disorders related to psychological factors

7. **Chapter 7: Diseases of Eye and Adnexa (H00-H59)**
   a. **Glaucoma**
   1) **Assigning glaucoma codes**

   Assign as many codes from category H40, Glaucoma, as needed to identify the type of glaucoma, the affected eye, and the glaucoma stage.

   2) **Bilateral glaucoma with same type and stage**

   When a patient has bilateral glaucoma and both eyes are documented as being the same type and stage, and there is a code for bilateral glaucoma, report only the code for the type of glaucoma, bilateral, with the seventh character for the stage.

When a patient has bilateral glaucoma and both eyes are documented as being the same type and stage, and the classification does not provide a code for bilateral glaucoma (i.e. subcategories H40.10, H40.11 and H40.20) report only one code for the type of glaucoma with the appropriate seventh character for the stage.

3) Bilateral glaucoma stage with different types or stages
When a patient has bilateral glaucoma and each eye is documented as having a different type or stage, and the classification distinguishes laterality, assign the appropriate code for each eye rather than the code for bilateral glaucoma.

When a patient has bilateral glaucoma and each eye is documented as having a different type, and the classification does not distinguish laterality (i.e. subcategories H40.10, H40.11 and H40.20), assign one code for each type of glaucoma with the appropriate seventh character for the stage.

When a patient has bilateral glaucoma and each eye is documented as having the same type, but different stage, and the classification does not distinguish laterality (i.e. subcategories H40.10, H40.11 and H40.20), assign a code for the type of glaucoma for each eye with the seventh character for the specific glaucoma stage documented for each eye.

4) Patient admitted with glaucoma and stage evolves during the admission
If a patient is admitted with glaucoma and the stage progresses during the admission, assign the code for highest stage documented.

5) Indeterminate stage glaucoma
Assignment of the seventh character "4" for "indeterminate stage" should be based on the clinical documentation. The seventh character "4" is used for glaucomas whose stage cannot be clinically determined. This seventh character should not be confused with the seventh character "0", unspecified, which should be assigned when there is no documentation regarding the stage of the glaucoma.

8. Chapter 8: Diseases of Ear and Mastoid Process (H60-H95)
Reserved for future guideline expansion

9. Chapter 9: Diseases of Circulatory System (I00-I99)
a. Hypertension
1) Hypertension with heart disease
Heart conditions classified to I50.- or I51.4-I51.9, are assigned to, a code from category I11, Hypertensive heart disease, when a causal relationship is stated (due to hypertension) or implied (hypertensive). Use an additional code from category I50, Heart failure, to identify the type of heart failure in those patients with heart failure.

The same heart conditions (I50.-, I51.4-I51.9) with hypertension, but without a stated causal relationship, are coded separately. Sequence according to the circumstances of the admission/encounter.

2) Hypertensive chronic kidney disease
Assign codes from category I12, Hypertensive chronic kidney disease, when both hypertension and a condition classifiable to category N18, Chronic kidney disease (CKD), are present. Unlike hypertension with heart disease, ICD-10-CM presumes a cause-and-effect relationship and classifies chronic kidney disease with hypertension as hypertensive chronic kidney disease.

The appropriate code from category N18 should be used as a secondary code with a code from category I12 to identify the stage of chronic kidney disease.

See Section I.C.14. Chronic kidney disease.

If a patient has hypertensive chronic kidney disease and acute renal failure, an additional code for the acute renal failure is required.

3) Hypertensive heart and chronic kidney disease
Assign codes from combination category I13, Hypertensive heart and chronic kidney disease, when both hypertensive

kidney disease and hypertensive heart disease are stated in the diagnosis. Assume a relationship between the hypertension and the chronic kidney disease, whether or not the condition is so designated. If heart failure is present, assign an additional code from category I50 to identify the type of heart failure.

The appropriate code from category N18, Chronic kidney disease, should be used as a secondary code with a code from category I13 to identify the stage of chronic kidney disease.

See Section I.C.14. Chronic kidney disease.

The codes in category I13, Hypertensive heart and chronic kidney disease, are combination codes that include hypertension, heart disease and chronic kidney disease. The Includes note at I13 specifies that the conditions included at I11 and I12 are included together in I13. If a patient has hypertension, heart disease and chronic kidney disease then a code from I13 should be used, not individual codes for hypertension, heart disease and chronic kidney disease, or codes from I11 or I12.

For patients with both acute renal failure and chronic kidney disease an additional code for acute renal failure is required.

4) Hypertensive cerebrovascular disease
For hypertensive cerebrovascular disease, first assign the appropriate code from categories I60-I69, followed by the appropriate hypertension code.

5) Hypertensive retinopathy
Subcategory H35.0, Background retinopathy and retinal vascular changes, should be used with a code from category I10 – I15, Hypertensive disease to include the systemic hypertension. The sequencing is based on the reason for the encounter.

6) Hypertension, secondary
Secondary hypertension is due to an underlying condition. Two codes are required: one to identify the underlying etiology and one from category I15 to identify the hypertension. Sequencing of codes is determined by the reason for admission/encounter.

7) Hypertension, transient
Assign code R03.0, Elevated blood pressure reading without diagnosis of hypertension, unless patient has an established diagnosis of hypertension. Assign code O13.-, Gestational [pregnancy-induced] hypertension without significant proteinuria, or O14.-, Pre-eclampsia, for transient hypertension of pregnancy.

8) Hypertension, controlled
This diagnostic statement usually refers to an existing state of hypertension under control by therapy. Assign the appropriate code from categories I10-I15, Hypertensive diseases.

9) Hypertension, uncontrolled
Uncontrolled hypertension may refer to untreated hypertension or hypertension not responding to current therapeutic regimen. In either case, assign the appropriate code from categories I10-I15, Hypertensive diseases.

b. Atherosclerotic coronary artery disease and angina
ICD-10-CM has combination codes for atherosclerotic heart disease with angina pectoris. The subcategories for these codes are I25.11, Atherosclerotic heart disease of native coronary artery with angina pectoris and I25.7, Atherosclerosis of coronary artery bypass graft(s) and coronary artery of transplanted heart with angina pectoris.

When using one of these combination codes it is not necessary to use an additional code for angina pectoris. A causal relationship can be assumed in a patient with both atherosclerosis and angina pectoris, unless the documentation indicates the angina is due to something other than the atherosclerosis.

If a patient with coronary artery disease is admitted due to an acute myocardial infarction (AMI), the AMI should be sequenced before the coronary artery disease.

See Section I.C.9. Acute myocardial infarction (AMI)

c. Intraoperative and postprocedural cerebrovascular accident
Medical record documentation should clearly specify the cause-and-effect relationship between the medical intervention and the

cerebrovascular accident in order to assign a code for intraoperative or postprocedural cerebrovascular accident.

Proper code assignment depends on whether it was an infarction or hemorrhage and whether it occurred intraoperatively or postoperatively. If it was a cerebral hemorrhage, code assignment depends on the type of procedure performed.

d. Sequelae of cerebrovascular disease

1) Category I69, sequelae of cerebrovascular disease

Category I69 is used to indicate conditions classifiable to categories I60-I67 as the causes of sequela (neurologic deficits), themselves classified elsewhere. These "late effects" include neurologic deficits that persist after initial onset of conditions classifiable to categories I60-I67. The neurologic deficits caused by cerebrovascular disease may be present from the onset or may arise at any time after the onset of the condition classifiable to categories I60-I67.

Codes from category I69, Sequelae of cerebrovascular disease, that specify hemiplegia, hemiparesis and monoplegia identify whether the dominant or nondominant side is affected. Should the affected side be documented, but not specified as dominant or nondominant, and the classification system does not indicate a default, code selection is as follows:

- For ambidextrous patients, the default should be dominant.
- If the left side is affected, the default is non-dominant.
- If the right side is affected, the default is dominant.

2) Codes from category I69 with codes from I60-I67

Codes from category I69 may be assigned on a health care record with codes from I60-I67, if the patient has a current cerebrovascular disease and deficits from an old cerebrovascular disease.

3) Codes from category I69 and Personal history of transient ischemic attack (TIA) and cerebral infarction (Z86.73)

Codes from category I69 should not be assigned if the patient does not have neurologic deficits.

See Section I.C.21. 4. History (of) for use of personal history codes

e. Acute myocardial infarction (AMI)

1) ST elevation myocardial infarction (STEMI) and non ST elevation myocardial infarction (NSTEMI)

The ICD-10-CM codes for acute myocardial infarction (AMI) identify the site, such as anterolateral wall or true posterior wall. Subcategories I21.0-I21.2 and code I21.3 are used for ST elevation myocardial infarction (STEMI). Code I21.4, Non-ST elevation (NSTEMI) myocardial infarction, is used for non ST elevation myocardial infarction (NSTEMI) and nontransmural MIs.

If NSTEMI evolves to STEMI, assign the STEMI code. If STEMI converts to NSTEMI due to thrombolytic therapy, it is still coded as STEMI.

For encounters occurring while the myocardial infarction is equal to, or less than, four weeks old, including transfers to another acute setting or a postacute setting, and the patient requires continued care for the myocardial infarction, codes from category I21 may continue to be reported. For encounters after the 4 week time frame and the patient is still receiving care related to the myocardial infarction, the appropriate aftercare code should be assigned, rather than a code from category I21. For old or healed myocardial infarctions not requiring further care, code I25.2, Old myocardial infarction, may be assigned.

2) Acute myocardial infarction, unspecified

Code I21.3, ST elevation (STEMI) myocardial infarction of unspecified site, is the default for the unspecified term acute myocardial infarction. If only STEMI or transmural MI without the site is documented, query the provider as to the site, or assign code I21.3.

3) AMI documented as nontransmural or subendocardial but site provided

If an AMI is documented as nontransmural or subendocardial, but the site is provided, it is still coded as a subendocardial AMI.

See Section I.C.21.3 for information on coding status post administration of tPA in a different facility within the last 24 hrs.

4) Subsequent acute myocardial infarction

A code from category I22, Subsequent ST elevation (STEMI) and non ST elevation (NSTEMI) myocardial infarction, is to be used when a patient who has suffered an AMI has a new AMI within the 4 week time frame of the initial AMI. A code from category I22 must be used in conjunction with a code from category I21. The sequencing of the I22 and I21 codes depends on the circumstances of the encounter.

10. Chapter 10: Diseases of the Respiratory System (J00-J99)

a. Chronic Obstructive Pulmonary Disease [COPD] and Asthma

1) Acute exacerbation of chronic obstructive bronchitis and asthma

The codes in categories J44 and J45 distinguish between uncomplicated cases and those in acute exacerbation. An acute exacerbation is a worsening or a decompensation of a chronic condition. An acute exacerbation is not equivalent to an infection superimposed on a chronic condition, though an exacerbation may be triggered by an infection.

b. Acute Respiratory Failure

1) Acute respiratory failure as principal diagnosis

A code from subcategory J96.0, Acute respiratory failure, or subcategory J96.2, Acute and chronic respiratory failure, may be assigned as a principal diagnosis when it is the condition established after study to be chiefly responsible for occasioning the admission to the hospital, and the selection is supported by the Alphabetic Index and Tabular List. However, chapter-specific coding guidelines (such as obstetrics, poisoning, HIV, newborn) that provide sequencing direction take precedence.

2) Acute respiratory failure as secondary diagnosis

Respiratory failure may be listed as a secondary diagnosis if it occurs after admission, or if it is present on admission, but does not meet the definition of principal diagnosis.

3) Sequencing of acute respiratory failure and another acute condition

When a patient is admitted with respiratory failure and another acute condition, (e.g., myocardial infarction, cerebrovascular accident, aspiration pneumonia), the principal diagnosis will not be the same in every situation. This applies whether the other acute condition is a respiratory or nonrespiratory condition. Selection of the principal diagnosis will be dependent on the circumstances of admission. If both the respiratory failure and the other acute condition are equally responsible for occasioning the admission to the hospital, and there are no chapter-specific sequencing rules, the guideline regarding two or more diagnoses that equally meet the definition for principal diagnosis (Section II, C.) may be applied in these situations.

If the documentation is not clear as to whether acute respiratory failure and another condition are equally responsible for occasioning the admission, query the provider for clarification.

c. Influenza due to certain identified influenza viruses

Code only confirmed cases of influenza due to certain identified influenza viruses (category J09), and due to other identified influenza virus (category J10). This is an exception to the hospital inpatient guideline Section II, H. (Uncertain Diagnosis).

In this context, "confirmation" does not require documentation of positive laboratory testing specific for avian or other novel influenza A or other identified influenza virus. However, coding should be based on the provider's diagnostic statement that the patient has avian influenza, or other novel influenza A, for category J09, or has another particular identified strain of influenza, such as H1N1 or H3N2, but not identified as novel or variant, for category J10.

If the provider records "suspected" or "possible" or "probable" avian influenza, or novel influenza, or other identified influenza, then the appropriate influenza code from category J11, Influenza due to unidentified influenza virus, should be assigned. A code from category J09, Influenza due to certain identified influenza viruses, should not be assigned nor should a code from category J10, Influenza due to other identified influenza virus.

d. **Ventilator associated pneumonia**

1) **Documentation of ventilator associated pneumonia**
As with all procedural or postprocedural complications, code assignment is based on the provider's documentation of the relationship between the condition and the procedure.

Code J95.851, Ventilator associated pneumonia, should be assigned only when the provider has documented ventilator associated pneumonia (VAP). An additional code to identify the organism (e.g., Pseudomonas aeruginosa, code B96.5) should also be assigned. Do not assign an additional code from categories J12-J18 to identify the type of pneumonia.

Code J95.851 should not be assigned for cases where the patient has pneumonia and is on a mechanical ventilator and the provider has not specifically stated that the pneumonia is ventilator-associated pneumonia. If the documentation is unclear as to whether the patient has a pneumonia that is a complication attributable to the mechanical ventilator, query the provider.

2) **Ventilator associated pneumonia develops after admission**
A patient may be admitted with one type of pneumonia (e.g., code J13, Pneumonia due to Streptococcus pneu- monia) and subsequently develop VAP. In this instance, the principal diagnosis would be the appro- priate code from categories J12-J18 for the pneumonia diagnosed at the time of admission. Code J95.851, Ventilator assoc- iated pneumonia, would be assigned as an additional diagnosis when the provider has also documented the presence of ventilator associated pneumonia.

11. **Chapter 11: Diseases of the Digestive System (K00-K95)**
Reserved for future guideline expansion

12. **Chapter 12: Diseases of the Skin and Subcutaneous Tissue (L00-L99)**
a. **Pressure ulcer stage codes**
1) **Pressure ulcer stages**
Codes from category L89, Pressure ulcer, are combination codes that identify the site of the pressure ulcer as well as the stage of the ulcer.

The ICD-10-CM classifies pressure ulcer stages based on severity, which is designated by stages 1-4, unspecified stage and unstageable.

Assign as many codes from category L89 as needed to identify all the pressure ulcers the patient has, if applicable.

2) **Unstageable pressure ulcers**
Assignment of the code for unstageable pressure ulcer (L89.--0) should be based on the clinical documentation. These codes are used for pressure ulcers whose stage cannot be clinically determined (e.g., the ulcer is covered by eschar or has been treated with a skin or muscle graft) and pressure ulcers that are documented as deep tissue injury but not documented as due to trauma. This code should not be confused with the codes for unspecified stage (L89.--9). When there is no documentation regarding the stage of the pressure ulcer, assign the appropriate code for unspecified stage (L89.--9).

3) **Documented pressure ulcer stage**
Assignment of the pressure ulcer stage code should be guided by clinical documentation of the stage or documentation of the terms found in the Alphabetic Index. For clinical terms describing the stage that are not found in the Alphabetic Index, and there is no documentation of the stage, the provider should be queried.

4) **Patients admitted with pressure ulcers documented as healed**
No code is assigned if the documentation states that the pressure ulcer is completely healed.

5) **Patients admitted with pressure ulcers documented as healing**
Pressure ulcers described as healing should be assigned the appropriate pressure ulcer stage code based on the documentation in the medical record. If the documentation does not provide information about the stage of the healing pressure ulcer, assign the appropriate code for unspecified stage.

If the documentation is unclear as to whether the patient has a current (new) pressure ulcer or if the patient is being treated for a healing pressure ulcer, query the provider.

6) **Patient admitted with pressure ulcer evolving into another stage during the admission**
If a patient is admitted with a pressure ulcer at one stage and it progresses to a higher stage, assign the code for the highest stage reported for that site.

13. **Chapter 13: Diseases of the Musculoskeletal System and Connective Tissue (M00-M99)**
a. **Site and laterality**
Most of the codes within Chapter 13 have site and laterality designations. The site represents the bone, joint or the muscle involved. For some conditions where more than one bone, joint or muscle is usually involved, such as osteoarthritis, there is a "multiple sites" code available. For categories where no multiple site code is provided and more than one bone, joint or muscle is involved, multiple codes should be used to indicate the different sites involved.

1) **Bone versus joint**
For certain conditions, the bone may be affected at the upper or lower end, (e.g., avascular necrosis of bone, M87, Osteoporosis, M80, M81). Though the portion of the bone affected may be at the joint, the site designation will be the bone, not the joint.

b. **Acute traumatic versus chronic or recurrent musculoskeletal conditions**
Many musculoskeletal conditions are a result of previous injury or trauma to a site, or are recurrent conditions. Bone, joint or muscle conditions that are the result of a healed injury are usually found in chapter 13. Recurrent bone, joint or muscle conditions are also usually found in chapter 13. Any current, acute injury should be coded to the appropriate injury code from chapter 19. Chronic or recurrent conditions should generally be coded with a code from chapter 13. If it is difficult to determine from the documentation in the record which code is best to describe a condition, query the provider.

c. **Coding of Pathologic Fractures**
7th character A is for use as long as the patient is receiving active treatment for the fracture. Examples of active treatment are: surgical treatment, emergency department encounter, evaluation and continuing treatment by the same or a different physician. While the patient may be seen by a new or different provider over the course of treatment for a pathological fracture, assignment of the 7th character is based on whether the patient is undergoing active treatment and not whether the provider is seeing the patient for the first time.

7th character, D is to be used for encounters after the patient has completed active treatment. The other 7th characters, listed under each subcategory in the Tabular List, are to be used for subsequent encounters for treatment of problems associated with the healing, such as malunions, nonunions, and sequelae.

Care for complications of surgical treatment for fracture repairs during the healing or recovery phase should be coded with the appropriate complication codes.

See Section I.C.19. Coding of traumatic fractures.

d. **Osteoporosis**
Osteoporosis is a systemic condition, meaning that all bones of the musculoskeletal system are affected. Therefore, site is not a component of the codes under category M81, Osteoporosis without current pathological fracture. The site codes under category M80, Osteoporosis with current pathological fracture, identify the site of the fracture, not the osteoporosis.

1) **Osteoporosis without pathological fracture**
Category M81, Osteoporosis without current pathological fracture, is for use for patients with osteoporosis who do not currently have a pathologic fracture due to the osteoporosis, even if they have had a fracture in the past. For patients with a history of osteoporosis fractures, status code Z87.310, Personal history of (healed) osteoporosis fracture, should follow the code from M81.

2) **Osteoporosis with current pathological fracture**
Category M80, Osteoporosis with current pathological fracture, is for patients who have a current pathologic fracture at the time of an encounter. The codes under M80 identify the site of the fracture. A code from category M80, not a traumatic fracture code, should be used for any patient with known osteoporosis who suffers a fracture, even if the patient had a minor fall or trauma, if that fall or trauma would not usually break a normal, healthy bone.

14. **Chapter 14: Diseases of Genitourinary System (N00-N99)**
a. **Chronic kidney disease**
1) **Stages of chronic kidney disease (CKD)**
The ICD-10-CM classifies CKD based on severity. The severity of CKD is designated by stages 1-5. Stage 2, code N18.2, equates to mild CKD; stage 3, code N18.3, equates to moderate CKD; and stage 4, code N18.4, equates to severe CKD. Code N18.6, End stage renal disease (ESRD), is assigned when the provider has documented end-stage-renal disease (ESRD).

If both a stage of CKD and ESRD are documented, assign code N18.6 only.

2) **Chronic kidney disease and kidney transplant status**
Patients who have undergone kidney transplant may still have some form of chronic kidney disease (CKD) because the kidney transplant may not fully restore kidney function. Therefore, the presence of CKD alone does not constitute a transplant complication. Assign the appropriate N18 code for the patient's stage of CKD and code Z94.0, Kidney transplant status. If a transplant complication such as failure or rejection or other transplant complication is documented, see section I.C.19.g for information on coding complications of a kidney transplant. If the documentation is unclear as to whether the patient has a complication of the transplant, query the provider.

3) **Chronic kidney disease with other conditions**
Patients with CKD may also suffer from other serious conditions, most commonly diabetes mellitus and hypertension. The sequencing of the CKD code in relationship to codes for other contributing conditions is based on the conventions in the Tabular List.

See I.C.9. Hypertensive chronic kidney disease.

See I.C.19. Chronic kidney disease and kidney transplant complications.

15. **Chapter 15: Pregnancy, Childbirth, and the Puerperium (O00-O9A)**
a. **General Rules for Obstetric Cases**
1) **Codes from chapter 15 and sequencing priority**
Obstetric cases require codes from chapter 15, codes in the range O00-O9A, Pregnancy, Childbirth, and the Puerperium. Chapter 15 codes have sequencing priority over codes from other chapters. Additional codes from other chapters may be used in conjunction with chapter 15 codes to further specify conditions. Should the provider document that the pregnancy is incidental to the encounter, then code Z33.1, Pregnant state, incidental, should be used in place of any chapter 15 codes. It is the provider's responsibility to state that the condition being treated is not affecting the pregnancy.

2) **Chapter 15 codes used only on the maternal record**
Chapter 15 codes are to be used only on the maternal record, never on the record of the newborn.

3) **Final character for trimester**
The majority of codes in Chapter 15 have a final character indicating the trimester of pregnancy. The timeframes for the trimesters are indicated at the beginning of the chapter. If trimester is not a component of a code it is because the condition always occurs in a specific trimester, or the concept of trimester of pregnancy is not applicable. Certain codes have characters for only certain trimesters because the condition does not occur in all trimesters, but it may occur in more than just one.

Assignment of the final character for trimester should be based on the provider's documentation of the trimester (or number of weeks) for the current admission/encounter. This applies to the assignment of trimester for pre-existing conditions as well as

those that develop during or are due to the pregnancy. The provider's documentation of the number of weeks may be used to assign the appropriate code identifying the trimester.

Whenever delivery occurs during the current admission, and there is an "in childbirth" option for the obstetric complication being coded, the "in childbirth" code should be assigned.

4) **Selection of trimester for inpatient admissions that encompass more than one trimesters**
In instances when a patient is admitted to a hospital for complications of pregnancy during one trimester and remains in the hospital into a subsequent trimester, the trimester character for the antepartum complication code should be assigned on the basis of the trimester when the complication developed, not the trimester of the discharge. If the condition developed prior to the current admission/encounter or represents a pre-existing condition, the trimester character for the trimester at the time of the admission/encounter should be assigned.

5) **Unspecified trimester**
Each category that includes codes for trimester has a code for "unspecified trimester." The "unspecified trimester" code should rarely be used, such as when the documentation in the record is insufficient to determine the trimester and it is not possible to obtain clarification.

6) **7th character for fetus identification**
Where applicable, a 7th character is to be assigned for certain categories (O31, O32, O33.3 - O33.6, O35, O36, O40, O41, O60.1, O60.2, O64, and O69) to identify the fetus for which the complication code applies.

Assign 7th character "0":
- For single gestations
- When the documentation in the record is insufficient to determine the fetus affected and it is not possible to obtain clarification.
- When it is not possible to clinically determine which fetus is affected.

b. **Selection of OB principal or first-listed diagnosis**
1) **Routine outpatient prenatal visits**
For routine outpatient prenatal visits when no complications are present, a code from category Z34, Encounter for supervision of normal pregnancy, should be used as the first-listed diagnosis. These codes should not be used in conjunction with chapter 15 codes.

2) **Prenatal outpatient visits for high-risk patients**
For routine prenatal outpatient visits for patients with high-risk pregnancies, a code from category O09, Supervision of high-risk pregnancy, should be used as the first-listed diagnosis. Secondary chapter 15 codes may be used in conjunction with these codes if appropriate.

3) **Episodes when no delivery occurs**
In episodes when no delivery occurs, the principal diagnosis should correspond to the principal complication of the pregnancy which necessitated the encounter. Should more than one complication exist, all of which are treated or monitored, any of the complications codes may be sequenced first.

4) **When a delivery occurs**
When a delivery occurs, the principal diagnosis should correspond to the main circumstances or complication of the delivery. In cases of cesarean delivery, the selection of the principal diagnosis should be the condition established after study that was responsible for the patient's admission. If the patient was admitted with a condition that resulted in the performance of a cesarean procedure, that condition should be selected as the principal diagnosis. If the reason for the admission/encounter was unrelated to the condition resulting in the cesarean delivery, the condition related to the reason for the admission/encounter should be selected as the principal diagnosis.

5) **Outcome of delivery**
A code from category Z37, Outcome of delivery, should be included on every maternal record when a delivery has occurred. These codes are not to be used on subsequent records or on the newborn record.

c. **Pre-existing conditions versus conditions due to the pregnancy**
Certain categories in Chapter 15 distinguish between conditions of the mother that existed prior to pregnancy (pre-existing) and those that are a direct result of pregnancy. When assigning codes from Chapter 15, it is important to assess if a condition was pre-existing prior to pregnancy or developed during or due to the pregnancy in order to assign the correct code.

Categories that do not distinguish between pre-existing and pregnancy-related conditions may be used for either. It is acceptable to use codes specifically for the puerperium with codes complicating pregnancy and childbirth if a condition arises postpartum during the delivery encounter.

d. **Pre-existing hypertension in pregnancy**
Category O10, Pre-existing hypertension complicating pregnancy, childbirth and the puerperium, includes codes for hypertensive heart and hypertensive chronic kidney disease. When assigning one of the O10 codes that includes hypertensive heart disease or hypertensive chronic kidney disease, it is necessary to add a secondary code from the appropriate hypertension category to specify the type of heart failure or chronic kidney disease.
See Section I.C.9. Hypertension.

e. **Fetal conditions affecting the management of the mother**
1) **Codes from categories O35 and O36**
Codes from categories O35, Maternal care for known or suspected fetal abnormality and damage, and O36, Maternal care for other fetal problems, are assigned only when the fetal condition is actually responsible for modifying the management of the mother, i.e., by requiring diagnostic studies, additional observation, special care, or termination of pregnancy. The fact that the fetal condition exists does not justify assigning a code from this series to the mother's record.

2) **In utero surgery**
In cases when surgery is performed on the fetus, a diagnosis code from category O35, Maternal care for known or suspected fetal abnormality and damage, should be assigned identifying the fetal condition. Assign the appropriate procedure code for the procedure performed.

No code from Chapter 16, the perinatal codes, should be used on the mother's record to identify fetal conditions. Surgery performed in utero on a fetus is still to be coded as an obstetric encounter.

f. **HIV Infection in pregnancy, childbirth and the puerperium**
During pregnancy, childbirth or the puerperium, a patient admitted because of an HIV-related illness should receive a principal diagnosis from subcategory O98.7-, Human immunodeficiency [HIV] disease complicating pregnancy, childbirth and the puerperium, followed by the code(s) for the HIV-related illness(es).

Patients with asymptomatic HIV infection status admitted during pregnancy, childbirth, or the puerperium should receive codes of O98.7- and Z21, Asymptomatic human immunodeficiency virus [HIV] infection status.

g. **Diabetes mellitus in pregnancy**
Diabetes mellitus is a significant complicating factor in pregnancy. Pregnant women who are diabetic should be assigned a code from category O24, Diabetes mellitus in pregnancy, childbirth, and the puerperium, first, followed by the appropriate diabetes code(s) (E08-E13) from Chapter 4.

h. **Long term use of insulin**
Code Z79.4, Long-term (current) use of insulin, should also be assigned if the diabetes mellitus is being treated with insulin.

i. **Gestational (pregnancy induced) diabetes**
Gestational (pregnancy induced) diabetes can occur during the second and third trimester of pregnancy in women who were not diabetic prior to pregnancy. Gestational diabetes can cause complications in the pregnancy similar to those of pre-existing diabetes mellitus. It also puts the woman at greater risk of developing diabetes after the pregnancy. Codes for gestational diabetes are in subcategory O24.4, Gestational diabetes mellitus. No other code from category O24, Diabetes mellitus in pregnancy, childbirth, and the puerperium, should be used with a code from O24.4.

The codes under subcategory O24.4 include diet controlled and insulin controlled. If a patient with gestational diabetes is treated with both diet and insulin, only the code for insulin-controlled is required.

Code Z79.4, Long-term (current) use of insulin, should not be assigned with codes from subcategory O24.4.

An abnormal glucose tolerance in pregnancy is assigned a code from subcategory O99.81, Abnormal glucose complicating pregnancy, childbirth, and the puerperium.

j. **Sepsis and septic shock complicating abortion, pregnancy, childbirth and the puerperium**
When assigning a chapter 15 code for sepsis complicating abortion, pregnancy, childbirth, and the puerperium, a code for the specific type of infection should be assigned as an additional diagnosis. If severe sepsis is present, a code from subcategory R65.2, Severe sepsis, and code(s) for associated organ dysfunction(s) should also be assigned as additional diagnoses.

k. **Puerperal sepsis**
Code O85, Puerperal sepsis, should be assigned with a secondary code to identify the causal organism (e.g., for a bacterial infection, assign a code from category B95-B96, Bacterial infections in conditions classified elsewhere). A code from category A40, Streptococcal sepsis, or A41, Other sepsis, should not be used for puerperal sepsis. If applicable, use additional codes to identify severe sepsis (R65.2-) and any associated acute organ dysfunction.

l. **Alcohol and tobacco use during pregnancy, childbirth and the puerperium**
1) **Alcohol use during pregnancy, childbirth and the puerperium**
Codes under subcategory O99.31, Alcohol use complicating pregnancy, childbirth, and the puerperium, should be assigned for any pregnancy case when a mother uses alcohol during the pregnancy or postpartum. A secondary code from category F10, Alcohol related disorders, should also be assigned to identify manifestations of the alcohol use.

2) **Tobacco use during pregnancy, childbirth and the puerperium**
Codes under subcategory O99.33, Smoking (tobacco) complicating pregnancy, childbirth, and the puerperium, should be assigned for any pregnancy case when a mother uses any type of tobacco product during the pregnancy or postpartum. A secondary code from category F17, Nicotine dependence, or code Z72.0, Tobacco use, should also be assigned to identify the type of nicotine dependence.

m. **Poisoning, toxic effects, adverse effects and underdosing in a pregnant patient**
A code from subcategory O9A.2, Injury, poisoning and certain other consequences of external causes complicating pregnancy, childbirth, and the puerperium, should be sequenced first, followed by the appropriate injury, poisoning, toxic effect, adverse effect or underdosing code, and then the additional code(s) that specifies the condition caused by the poisoning, toxic effect, adverse effect or underdosing.
See Section I.C.19. Adverse effects, poisoning, underdosing and toxic effects.

n. **Normal delivery, code O80**
1) **Encounter for full term uncomplicated delivery**
Code O80 should be assigned when a woman is admitted for a full-term normal delivery and delivers a single, healthy infant without any complications antepartum, during the delivery, or postpartum during the delivery episode. Code O80 is always a principal diagnosis. It is not to be used if any other code from chapter 15 is needed to describe a current complication of the antenatal, delivery, or perinatal period. Additional codes from other chapters may be used with code O80 if they are not related to or are in any way complicating the pregnancy.

2) Uncomplicated delivery with resolved antepartum complication

Code O80 may be used if the patient had a complication at some point during the pregnancy, but the complication is not present at the time of the admission for delivery.

3) Outcome of delivery for O80

Z37.0, Single live birth, is the only outcome of delivery code appropriate for use with O80.

o. The peripartum and postpartum periods

1) Peripartum and postpartum periods

The postpartum period begins immediately after delivery and continues for six weeks following delivery. The peripartum period is defined as the last month of pregnancy to five months postpartum.

2) Peripartum and postpartum complication

A postpartum complication is any complication occurring within the six-week period.

3) Pregnancy-related complications after 6 week period

Chapter 15 codes may also be used to describe pregnancy-related complications after the peripartum or postpartum period if the provider documents that a condition is pregnancy related.

4) Admission for routine postpartum care following delivery outside hospital

When the mother delivers outside the hospital prior to admission and is admitted for routine postpartum care and no complications are noted, code Z39.0, Encounter for care and examination of mother immediately after delivery, should be assigned as the principal diagnosis.

5) Pregnancy associated cardiomyopathy

Pregnancy associated cardiomyopathy, code O90.3, is unique in that it may be diagnosed in the third trimester of pregnancy but may continue to progress months after delivery. For this reason, it is referred to as peripartum cardiomyopathy. Code O90.3 is only for use when the cardiomyopathy develops as a result of pregnancy in a woman who did not have pre-existing heart disease.

p. Code O94, Sequelae of complication of pregnancy, childbirth, and the puerperium

1) Code O94

Code O94, Sequelae of complication of pregnancy, childbirth, and the puerperium, is for use in those cases when an initial complication of a pregnancy develops a sequelae requiring care or treatment at a future date.

2) After the initial postpartum period

This code may be used at any time after the initial postpartum period.

3) Sequencing of code O94

This code, like all late effect codes, is to be sequenced following the code describing the sequelae of the complication.

q. *Termination of Pregnancy and Spontaneous abortions*

1) Abortion with Liveborn Fetus

When an attempted termination of pregnancy results in a liveborn fetus, assign code Z33.2, Encounter for elective termination of pregnancy and a code from category Z37, Outcome of Delivery.

2) Retained Products of Conception following an abortion

Subsequent encounters for retained products of conception following a spontaneous abortion or elective termination of pregnancy are assigned the appropriate code from category O03, Spontaneous abortion, or codes O07.4, Failed attempted termination of pregnancy without complication and Z33.2, Encounter for elective termination of pregnancy. This advice is appropriate even when the patient was discharged previously with a discharge diagnosis of complete abortion.

3) Complications leading to abortion

Codes from Chapter 15 may be used as additional codes to identify any documented complications of the pregnancy in conjunction with codes in categories in O07 and O08.

r. Abuse in a pregnant patient

For suspected or confirmed cases of abuse of a pregnant patient, a code(s) from subcategories O9A.3, Physical abuse complicating pregnancy, childbirth, and the puerperium, O9A.4, Sexual abuse complicating pregnancy, childbirth, and the puerperium, and O9A.5, Psychological abuse complicating pregnancy, childbirth, and the puerperium, should be sequenced first, followed by the appropriate codes (if applicable) to identify any associated current injury due to physical abuse, sexual abuse, and the perpetrator of abuse.

See Section I.C.19. Adult and child abuse, neglect and other maltreatment.

16. Chapter 16: Certain Conditions Originating in the Perinatal Period (P00- P96)

For coding and reporting purposes the perinatal period is defined as before birth through the 28th day following birth. The following guidelines are provided for reporting purposes

a. General Perinatal Rules

1) Use of Chapter 16 codes

Codes in this chapter are <u>never</u> for use on the maternal record. Codes from Chapter 15, the obstetric chapter, are never permitted on the newborn record. Chapter 16 codes may be used throughout the life of the patient if the condition is still present.

2) Principal diagnosis for birth record

When coding the birth episode in a newborn record, assign a code from category Z38, Liveborn infants according to place of birth and type of delivery, as the principal diagnosis. A code from category Z38 is assigned only once, to a newborn at the time of birth. If a newborn is transferred to another institution, a code from category Z38 should not be used at the receiving hospital.

A code from category Z38 is used only on the newborn record, not on the mother's record.

3) Use of codes from other chapters with codes from Chapter 16

Codes from other chapters may be used with codes from chapter 16 if the codes from the other chapters provide more specific detail. Codes for signs and symptoms may be assigned when a definitive diagnosis has not been established. If the reason for the encounter is a perinatal condition, the code from chapter 16 should be sequenced first.

4) Use of Chapter 16 codes after the perinatal period

Should a condition originate in the perinatal period, and continue throughout the life of the patient, the perinatal code should continue to be used regardless of the patient's age.

5) Birth process or community acquired conditions

If a newborn has a condition that may be either due to the birth process or community acquired and the documentation does not indicate which it is, the default is due to the birth process and the code from Chapter 16 should be used. If the condition is community-acquired, a code from Chapter 16 should not be assigned.

6) Code all clinically significant conditions

All clinically significant conditions noted on routine newborn examination should be coded. A condition is clinically significant if it requires:

- clinical evaluation; or
- therapeutic treatment; or
- diagnostic procedures; or
- extended length of hospital stay; or
- increased nursing care and/or monitoring; or
- has implications for future health care needs

Note: The perinatal guidelines listed above are the same as the general coding guidelines for "additional diagnoses", except for the final point regarding implications for future health care needs. Codes should be assigned for conditions that have been specified by the provider as having implications for future health care needs.

b. **Observation and Evaluation of Newborns for Suspected Conditions not Found**
Reserved for future expansion

c. **Coding Additional Perinatal Diagnoses**

1) **Assigning codes for conditions that require treatment**
Assign codes for conditions that require treatment or further investigation, prolong the length of stay, or require resource utilization.

2) **Codes for conditions specified as having implications for future health care needs**
Assign codes for conditions that have been specified by the provider as having implications for future health care needs.

Note: This guideline should not be used for adult patients.

d. **Prematurity and Fetal Growth Retardation**
Providers utilize different criteria in determining prematurity. A code for prematurity should not be assigned unless it is documented. Assignment of codes in categories P05, Disorders of newborn related to slow fetal growth and fetal malnutrition, and P07, Disorders of newborn related to short gestation and low birth weight, not elsewhere classified, should be based on the recorded birth weight and estimated gestational age. Codes from category P05 should not be assigned with codes from category P07.

When both birth weight and gestational age are available, two codes from category P07 should be assigned, with the code for birth weight sequenced before the code for gestational age.

e. **Low birth weight and immaturity status**
Codes from category P07, Disorders of newborn related to short gestation and low birth weight, not elsewhere classified, are for use for a child or adult who was premature or had a low birth weight as a newborn and this is affecting the patient's current health status.
See Section I.C.21. Factors influencing health status and contact with health services, Status.

f. **Bacterial Sepsis of Newborn**
Category P36, Bacterial sepsis of newborn, includes congenital sepsis. If a perinate is documented as having sepsis without documentation of congenital or community acquired, the default is congenital and a code from category P36 should be assigned. If the P36 code includes the causal organism, an additional code from category B95, Streptococcus, Staphylococcus, and Enterococcus as the cause of diseases classified elsewhere, or B96, Other bacterial agents as the cause of diseases classified elsewhere, should not be assigned. If the P36 code does not include the causal organism, assign an additional code from category B96. If applicable, use additional codes to identify severe sepsis (R65.2-) and any associated acute organ dysfunction.

g. **Stillbirth**
Code P95, Stillbirth, is only for use in institutions that maintain separate records for stillbirths. No other code should be used with P95. Code P95 should not be used on the mother's record.

17. **Chapter 17: Congenital malformations, deformations, and chromosomal abnormalities (Q00-Q99)**
Assign an appropriate code(s) from categories Q00-Q99, Congenital malformations, deformations, and chromosomal abnormalities when a malformation/deformation or chromosomal abnormality is documented. A malformation/deformation/or chromosomal abnormality may be the principal/first-listed diagnosis on a record or a secondary diagnosis.

When a malformation/deformation/or chromosomal abnormality does not have a unique code assignment, assign additional code(s) for any manifestations that may be present.

When the code assignment specifically identifies the malformation/deformation or chromosomal abnormality, manifestations that are an inherent component of the anomaly should not be coded separately. Additional codes should be assigned for manifestations that are not an inherent component.

Codes from Chapter 17 may be used throughout the life of the patient. If a congenital malformation or deformity has been corrected, a personal history code should be used to identify the history of the malformation or deformity. Although present at birth, malformation/deformation/or chromosomal abnormality may not be identified until later in life. Whenever the condition is diagnosed by the physician, it is appropriate

to assign a code from codes Q00-Q99.For the birth admission, the appropriate code from category Z38, Liveborn infants, according to place of birth and type of delivery, should be sequenced as the principal diagnosis, followed by any congenital anomaly codes, Q00- Q99.

18. **Chapter 18: Symptoms, signs, and abnormal clinical and laboratory findings, not elsewhere classified (R00-R99)**
Chapter 18 includes symptoms, signs, abnormal results of clinical or other investigative procedures, and ill-defined conditions regarding which no diagnosis classifiable elsewhere is recorded. Signs and symptoms that point to a specific diagnosis have been assigned to a category in other chapters of the classification.

a. **Use of symptom codes**
Codes that describe symptoms and signs are acceptable for reporting purposes when a related definitive diagnosis has not been established (confirmed) by the provider.

b. **Use of a symptom code with a definitive diagnosis code**
Codes for signs and symptoms may be reported in addition to a related definitive diagnosis when the sign or symptom is not routinely associated with that diagnosis, such as the various signs and symptoms associated with complex syndromes. The definitive diagnosis code should be sequenced before the symptom code.

Signs or symptoms that are associated routinely with a disease process should not be assigned as additional codes, unless otherwise instructed by the classification.

c. **Combination codes that include symptoms**
ICD-10-CM contains a number of combination codes that identify both the definitive diagnosis and common symptoms of that diagnosis. When using one of these combination codes, an additional code should not be assigned for the symptom.

d. **Repeated falls**
Code R29.6, Repeated falls, is for use for encounters when a patient has recently fallen and the reason for the fall is being investigated.

Code Z91.81, History of falling, is for use when a patient has fallen in the past and is at risk for future falls. When appropriate, both codes R29.6 and Z91.81 may be assigned together.

e. **Coma scale**
The coma scale codes (R40.2-) can be used in conjunction with traumatic brain injury codes, acute cerebrovascular disease or sequelae of cerebrovascular disease codes. These codes are primarily for use by trauma registries, but they may be used in any setting where this information is collected. The coma scale codes should be sequenced after the diagnosis code(s).

These codes, one from each subcategory, are needed to complete the scale. The 7th character indicates when the scale was recorded. The 7th character should match for all three codes.

At a minimum, report the initial score documented on presentation at your facility. This may be a score from the emergency medicine technician (EMT) or in the emergency department. If desired, a facility may choose to capture multiple Glasgow coma scale scores.

Assign code R40.24, Glasgow coma scale, total score, when only the total score is documented in the medical record and not the individual score(s).

f. **Functional quadriplegia**
Functional quadriplegia (code R53.2) is the lack of ability to use one's limbs or to ambulate due to extreme debility. It is not associated with neurologic deficit or injury, and code R53.2 should not be used for cases of neurologic quadriplegia. It should only be assigned if functional quadriplegia is specifically documented in the medical record.

g. **SIRS due to non-infectious process**
The systemic inflammatory response syndrome (SIRS) can develop as a result of certain non-infectious disease processes, such as trauma, malignant neoplasm, or pancreatitis. When SIRS is documented with a noninfectious condition, and no subsequent infection is documented, the code for the underlying condition, such as an injury, should be assigned, followed by code R65.10, Systemic inflammatory response syndrome (SIRS) of non-infectious origin without acute organ dysfunction, or code R65.11, Systemic inflammatory response syndrome (SIRS) of non-infectious origin with acute organ dysfunction. If an associated acute organ dysfunction is documented, the appropriate code(s) for the specific

type of organ dysfunction(s) should be assigned in addition to code R65.11. If acute organ dysfunction is documented, but it cannot be determined if the acute organ dysfunction is associated with SIRS or due to another condition (e.g., directly due to the trauma), the provider should be queried.

h. Death NOS

Code R99, Ill-defined and unknown cause of mortality, is only for use in the very limited circumstance when a patient who has already died is brought into an emergency department or other healthcare facility and is pronounced dead upon arrival. It does not represent the discharge disposition of death.

19. Chapter 19: Injury, poisoning, and certain other consequences of external causes (S00-T88)

a. Application of 7th Characters in Chapter 19

Most categories in chapter 19 have a 7th character requirement for each applicable code. Most categories in this chapter have three 7th character values (with the exception of fractures): A, initial encounter, D, subsequent encounter and S, sequela. Categories for traumatic fractures have additional 7th character values. While the patient may be seen by a new or different provider over the course of treatment for an injury, assignment of the 7th character is based on whether the patient is undergoing active treatment and not whether the provider is seeing the patient for the first time.

For complication codes, active treatment refers to treatment for the condition described by the code, even though it may be related to an earlier precipitating problem. For example, code T84.50XA, Infection and inflammatory reaction due to unspecified internal joint prosthesis, initial encounter, is used when active treatment is provided for the infection, even though the condition relates to the prosthetic device, implant or graft that was placed at a previous encounter.

7th character "A", initial encounter is used while the patient is receiving active treatment for the condition. Examples of active treatment are: surgical treatment, emergency department encounter, and evaluation and continuing treatment by the same or a different physician.

7th character "D" subsequent encounter is used for encounters after the patient has received active treatment of the condition and is receiving routine care for the condition during the healing or recovery phase. Examples of subsequent care are: cast change or removal, an x-ray to check healing status of fracture, removal of external or internal fixation device, medication adjustment, other aftercare and follow up visits following treatment of the injury or condition.

The aftercare Z codes should not be used for aftercare for conditions such as injuries or poisonings, where 7th characters are provided to identify subsequent care. For example, for aftercare of an injury, assign the acute injury code with the 7th character "D" (subsequent encounter).

7th character "S", sequela, is for use for complications or conditions that arise as a direct result of a condition, such as scar formation after a burn. The scars are sequelae of the burn. When using 7th character "S", it is necessary to use both the injury code that precipitated the sequela and the code for the sequela itself. The "S" is added only to the injury code, not the sequela code. The 7th character "S" identifies the injury responsible for the sequela. The specific type of sequela (e.g. scar) is sequenced first, followed by the injury code.

See Section I.B.10 Sequelae, (Late Effects)

b. Coding of injuries

When coding injuries, assign separate codes for each injury unless a combination code is provided, in which case the combination code is assigned. Code T07, Unspecified multiple injuries should not be assigned in the inpatient setting unless information for a more specific code is not available. Traumatic injury codes (S00-T14.9) are not to be used for normal, healing surgical wounds or to identify complications of surgical wounds.

The code for the most serious injury, as determined by the provider and the focus of treatment, is sequenced first.

1) Superficial injuries

Superficial injuries such as abrasions or contusions are not coded when associated with more severe injuries of the same site.

2) Primary injury with damage to nerves/blood vessels

When a primary injury results in minor damage to peripheral nerves or blood vessels, the primary injury is sequenced first with additional code(s) for injuries to nerves and spinal cord (such as category S04), and/or injury to blood vessels (such as category S15). When the primary injury is to the blood vessels or nerves, that injury should be sequenced first.

c. Coding of Traumatic Fractures

The principles of multiple coding of injuries should be followed in coding fractures. Fractures of specified sites are coded individually by site in accordance with both the provisions within categories S02, S12, S22, S32, S42, S49, S52, S59, S62, S72, S79, S82, S89, S92 and the level of detail furnished by medical record content.

A fracture not indicated as open or closed should be coded to closed. A fracture not indicated whether displaced or not displaced should be coded to displaced.

More specific guidelines are as follows:

1) Initial vs. Subsequent Encounter for Fractures

Traumatic fractures are coded using the appropriate 7th character for initial encounter (A, B, C) while the patient is receiving active treatment for the fracture. Examples of active treatment are: surgical treatment, emergency department encounter, and evaluation and continuing (ongoing) treatment by the same or different physician. The appropriate 7th character for initial encounter should also be assigned for a patient who delayed seeking treatment for the fracture or nonunion.

Fractures are coded using the appropriate 7th character for subsequent care for encounters after the patient has completed active treatment of the fracture and is receiving routine care for the fracture during the healing or recovery phase. Examples of fracture aftercare are: cast change or removal, an x-ray to check healing status of fracture, removal of external or internal fixation device, medication adjustment, and follow-up visits following fracture treatment.

Care for complications of surgical treatment for fracture repairs during the healing or recovery phase should be coded with the appropriate complication codes.

Care of complications of fractures, such as malunion and nonunion, should be reported with the appropriate 7th character for subsequent care with nonunion (K, M, N,) or subsequent care with malunion (P, Q, R).

Malunion/nonunion: The appropriate 7th character for initial encounter should also be assigned for a patient who delayed seeking treatment for the fracture or nonunion.

A code from category M80, not a traumatic fracture code, should be used for any patient with known osteoporosis who suffers a fracture, even if the patient had a minor fall or trauma, if that fall or trauma would not usually break a normal, healthy bone.

See Section I.C.13. Osteoporosis.

The aftercare Z codes should not be used for aftercare for traumatic fractures. For aftercare of a traumatic fracture, assign the acute fracture code with the appropriate 7th character.

2) Multiple fractures sequencing

Multiple fractures are sequenced in accordance with the severity of the fracture.

d. Coding of burns and corrosions

The ICD-10-CM makes a distinction between burns and corrosions. The burn codes are for thermal burns, except sunburns, that come from a heat source, such as a fire or hot appliance. The burn codes are also for burns resulting from electricity and radiation. Corrosions are burns due to chemicals. The guidelines are the same for burns and corrosions.

Current burns (T20-T25) are classified by depth, extent and by agent (X code). Burns are classified by depth as first degree (erythema), second degree (blistering), and third degree (full-thickness involvement). Burns of the eye and internal organs (T26-T28) are classified by site, but not by degree.

1) Sequencing of burn and related condition codes
Sequence first the code that reflects the highest degree of burn when more than one burn is present.

a. When the reason for the admission or encounter is for treatment of external multiple burns, sequence first the code that reflects the burn of the highest degree.

b. When a patient has both internal and external burns, the circumstances of admission govern the selection of the principal diagnosis or first-listed diagnosis.

c. When a patient is admitted for burn injuries and other related conditions such as smoke inhalation and/or respiratory failure, the circumstances of admission govern the selection of the principal or first-listed diagnosis.

2) Burns of the same local site
Classify burns of the same local site (three-character category level, T20-T28) but of different degrees to the subcategory identifying the highest degree recorded in the diagnosis.

3) Non-healing burns
Non-healing burns are coded as acute burns.

Necrosis of burned skin should be coded as a non-healed burn.

4) Infected burn
For any documented infected burn site, use an additional code for the infection.

5) Assign separate codes for each burn site
When coding burns, assign separate codes for each burn site. Category T30, Burn and corrosion, body region unspecified is extremely vague and should rarely be used.

6) Burns and corrosions classified according to extent of body surface involved
Assign codes from category T31, Burns classified according to extent of body surface involved, or T32, Corrosions classified according to extent of body surface involved, when the site of the burn is not specified or when there is a need for additional data. It is advisable to use category T31 as additional coding when needed to provide data for evaluating burn mortality, such as that needed by burn units. It is also advisable to use category T31 as an additional code for reporting purposes when there is mention of a third-degree burn involving 20 percent or more of the body surface.

Categories T31 and T32 are based on the classic "rule of nines" in estimating body surface involved: head and neck are assigned nine percent, each arm nine percent, each leg 18 percent, the anterior trunk 18 percent, posterior trunk 18 percent, and genitalia one percent. Providers may change these percentage assignments where necessary to accommodate infants and children who have proportionately larger heads than adults, and patients who have large buttocks, thighs, or abdomen that involve burns.

7) Encounters for treatment of sequela of burns
Encounters for the treatment of the late effects of burns or corrosions (i.e., scars or joint contractures) should be coded with a burn or corrosion code with the 7th character "S" for sequela.

8) Sequelae with a late effect code and current burn
When appropriate, both a code for a current burn or corrosion with 7th character "A" or "D" and a burn or corrosion code with 7th character "S" may be assigned on the same record (when both a current burn and sequelae of an old burn exist). Burns and corrosions do not heal at the same rate and a current healing wound may still exist with sequela of a healed burn or corrosion.

See Section I.B.10 Sequela (Late Effects)

9) Use of an external cause code with burns and corrosions
An external cause code should be used with burns and corrosions to identify the source and intent of the burn, as well as the place where it occurred.

e. Adverse effects, poisoning, underdosing and toxic effects
Codes in categories T36-T65 are combination codes that include the substance that was taken as well as the intent. No additional external cause code is required for poisonings, toxic effects, adverse effects and underdosing codes.

1) Do not code directly from the Table of Drugs
Do not code directly from the Table of Drugs and Chemicals. Always refer back to the Tabular List.

2) Use as many codes as necessary to describe
Use as many codes as necessary to describe completely all drugs, medicinal or biological substances.

3) If the same code would describe the causative agent
If the same code would describe the causative agent for more than one adverse reaction, poisoning, toxic effect or underdosing, assign the code only once.

4) If two or more drugs, medicinal or biological substances
If two or more drugs, medicinal or biological substances are reported, code each individually unless a combination code is listed in the Table of Drugs and Chemicals.

5) The occurrence of drug toxicity is classified in ICD-10-CM as follows:

(a) Adverse effect
When coding an adverse effect of a drug that has been correctly prescribed and properly administered, assign the appropriate code for the nature of the adverse effect followed by the appropriate code for the adverse effect of the drug (T36-T50). The code for the drug should have a 5th or 6th character "5" (for example T36.0X5-) Examples of the nature of an adverse effect are tachycardia, delirium, gastrointestinal hemorrhaging, vomiting, hypokalemia, hepatitis, renal failure, or respiratory failure.

(b) Poisoning
When coding a poisoning or reaction to the improper use of a medication (e.g., overdose, wrong substance given or taken in error, wrong route of administration), first assign the appropriate code from categories T36-T50. The poisoning codes have an associated intent as their 5th or 6th character (accidental, intentional self-harm, assault and undetermined. Use additional code(s) for all manifestations of poisonings.

If there is also a diagnosis of abuse or dependence of the substance, the abuse or dependence is assigned as an additional code.

Examples of poisoning include:

(i) Error was made in drug prescription

Errors made in drug prescription or in the administration of the drug by provider, nurse, patient, or other person.

(ii) Overdose of a drug intentionally taken

If an overdose of a drug was intentionally taken or administered and resulted in drug toxicity, it would be coded as a poisoning.

(iii) Nonprescribed drug taken with correctly prescribed and properly administered drug

If a nonprescribed drug or medicinal agent was taken in combination with a correctly prescribed and properly administered drug, any drug toxicity or other reaction resulting from the interaction of the two drugs would be classified as a poisoning.

(iv) Interaction of drug(s) and alcohol

When a reaction results from the interaction of a drug(s) and alcohol, this would be classified as poisoning.

See Section I.C.4. if poisoning is the result of insulin pump malfunctions.

(c) Underdosing
Underdosing refers to taking less of a medication than is prescribed by a provider or a manufacturer's instruction. For underdosing, assign the code from categories T36-T50 (fifth or sixth character "6").

Codes for underdosing should never be assigned as principal or first-listed codes. If a patient has a relapse or exacerbation of the medical condition for which the drug is prescribed because of the reduction in dose, then the medical condition itself should be coded.

Noncompliance (Z91.12-, Z91.13-) or complication of care (Y63.61, Y63.8-Y63.9) codes are to be used with an underdosing code to indicate intent, if known.

(d) Toxic effects

When a harmful substance is ingested or comes in contact with a person, this is classified as a toxic effect. The toxic effect codes are in categories T51-T65.

Toxic effect codes have an associated intent: accidental, intentional self-harm, assault and undetermined.

f. Adult and child abuse, neglect and other maltreatment

Sequence first the appropriate code from categories T74.- (Adult and child abuse, neglect and other maltreatment, confirmed) or T76.- (Adult and child abuse, neglect and other maltreatment, suspected) for abuse, neglect and other maltreatment, followed by any accompanying mental health or injury code(s).

If the documentation in the medical record states abuse or neglect it is coded as confirmed (T74.-). It is coded as suspected if it is documented as suspected (T76.-).

For cases of confirmed abuse or neglect an external cause code from the assault section (X92-Y08) should be added to identify the cause of any physical injuries. A perpetrator code (Y07) should be added when the perpetrator of the abuse is known. For suspected cases of abuse or neglect, do not report external cause or perpetrator code.

If a suspected case of abuse, neglect or mistreatment is ruled out during an encounter code Z04.71, Encounter for examination and observation following alleged physical adult abuse, ruled out, or code Z04.72, Encounter for examination and observation following alleged child physical abuse, ruled out, should be used, not a code from T76.

If a suspected case of alleged rape or sexual abuse is ruled out during an encounter code Z04.41, Encounter for examination and observation following alleged physical adult abuse, ruled out, or code Z04.42, Encounter for examination and observation following alleged rape or sexual abuse, ruled out, should be used, not a code from T76.

See Section I.C.15. Abuse in a pregnant patient.

g. Complications of care

1) General guidelines for complications of care

(a) Documentation of complications of care

See Section I.B.16. for information on documentation of complications of care.

2) Pain due to medical devices

Pain associated with devices, implants or grafts left in a surgical site (for example painful hip prosthesis) is assigned to the appropriate code(s) found in Chapter 19, Injury, poisoning, and certain other consequences of external causes. Specific codes for pain due to medical devices are found in the T code section of the ICD-10-CM. Use additional code(s) from category G89 to identify acute or chronic pain due to presence of the device, implant or graft (G89.18 or G89.28).

3) Transplant complications

(a) Transplant complications other than kidney

Codes under category T86, Complications of transplanted organs and tissues, are for use for both complications and rejection of transplanted organs. A transplant complication code is only assigned if the complication affects the function of the transplanted organ. Two codes are required to fully describe a transplant complication: the appropriate code from category T86 and a secondary code that identifies the complication.

Pre-existing conditions or conditions that develop after the transplant are not coded as complications unless they affect the function of the transplanted organs.

See I.C.21. for transplant organ removal status

See I.C.2. for malignant neoplasm associated with transplanted organ.

(b) Kidney transplant complications

Patients who have undergone kidney transplant may still have some form of chronic kidney disease (CKD) because the kidney transplant may not fully restore kidney function. Code T86.1- should be assigned for documented complications of a kidney transplant, such as transplant failure or rejection or other transplant complication. Code T86.1- should not be assigned for post kidney transplant patients who have chronic kidney (CKD) unless a transplant complication such as transplant failure or rejection is documented. If the documentation is unclear as to whether the patient has a complication of the transplant, query the provider.

Conditions that affect the function of the transplanted kidney, other than CKD, should be assigned a code from subcategory T86.1, Complications of transplanted organ, Kidney, and a secondary code that identifies the complication.

For patients with CKD following a kidney transplant, but who do not have a complication such as failure or rejection, *see section I.C.14. Chronic kidney disease and kidney transplant status.*

4) Complication codes that include the external cause

As with certain other T codes, some of the complications of care codes have the external cause included in the code. The code includes the nature of the complication as well as the type of procedure that caused the complication. No external cause code indicating the type of procedure is necessary for these codes.

5) Complications of care codes within the body system chapters

Intraoperative and postprocedural complication codes are found within the body system chapters with codes specific to the organs and structures of that body system. These codes should be sequenced first, followed by a code(s) for the specific complication, if applicable.

20. Chapter 20: External Causes of Morbidity (V00-Y99)

The external causes of morbidity codes should never be sequenced as the first- listed or principal diagnosis.

External cause codes are intended to provide data for injury research and evaluation of injury prevention strategies. These codes capture how the injury or health condition happened (cause), the intent (unintentional or accidental; or intentional, such as suicide or assault), the place where the event occurred the activity of the patient at the time of the event, and the person's status (e.g., civilian, military).

There is no national requirement for mandatory ICD-10-CM external cause code reporting. Unless a provider is subject to a state-based external cause code reporting mandate or these codes are required by a particular payer, reporting of ICD-10-CM codes in Chapter 20, External Causes of Morbidity, is not required. In the absence of a mandatory reporting requirement, providers are encouraged to voluntarily report external cause codes, as they provide valuable data for injury research and evaluation of injury prevention strategies.

a. General External Cause Coding Guidelines

1) Used with any code in the range of A00.0-T88.9, Z00-Z99

An external cause code may be used with any code in the range of A00.0-T88.9, Z00-Z99, classification that is a health condition due to an external cause. Though they are most applicable to injuries, they are also valid for use with such things as infections or diseases due to an external source, and other health conditions, such as a heart attack that occurs during strenuous physical activity.

2) External cause code used for length of treatment

Assign the external cause code, with the appropriate 7th character (initial encounter, subsequent encounter or sequela) for each encounter for which the injury or condition is being treated.

Most categories in chapter 20 have a 7th character requirement for each applicable code. Most categories in this chapter have three 7th character values: A, initial encounter, D, subsequent encounter and S, sequela. While the patient may be seen by a new or different provider over the course of treatment for an injury or condition, assignment of the 7th character for external cause should match the 7th character of the code assigned for the associated injury or condition for the encounter.

3) **Use the full range of external cause codes**
Use the full range of external cause codes to completely describe the cause, the intent, the place of occurrence, and if applicable, the activity of the patient at the time of the event, and the patient's status, for all injuries, and other health conditions due to an external cause.

4) **Assign as many external cause codes as necessary**
Assign as many external cause codes as necessary to fully explain each cause. If only one external code can be recorded, assign the code most related to the principal diagnosis.

5) **The selection of the appropriate external cause code**
The selection of the appropriate external cause code is guided by the Alphabetic Index of External Causes and by Inclusion and Exclusion notes in the Tabular List.

6) **External cause code can never be a principal diagnosis**
An external cause code can never be a principal (first-listed) diagnosis.

7) **Combination external cause codes**
Certain of the external cause codes are combination codes that identify sequential events that result in an injury, such as a fall which results in striking against an object. The injury may be due to either event or both. The combination external cause code used should correspond to the sequence of events regardless of which caused the most serious injury.

8) **No external cause code needed in certain circumstances**
No external cause code from Chapter 20 is needed if the external cause and intent are included in a code from another chapter (e.g. T36.0X1- Poisoning by penicillins, accidental (unintentional)).

b. **Place of Occurrence Guideline**
Codes from category Y92, Place of occurrence of the external cause, are secondary codes for use after other external cause codes to identify the location of the patient at the time of injury or other condition.

Generally, a place of occurrence code is assigned only once, at the initial encounter for treatment. However, in the rare instance that a new injury occurs during hospitalization, an additional place of occurrence code may be assigned. No 7th characters are used for Y92.

Do not use place of occurrence code Y92.9 if the place is not stated or is not applicable.

c. **Activity code**
Assign a code from category Y93, Activity code, to describe the activity of the patient at the time the injury or other health condition occurred.

An activity code is used only once, at the initial encounter for treatment. Only one code from Y93 should be recorded on a medical record. An activity code should be used in conjunction with a place of occurrence code, Y92.

The activity codes are not applicable to poisonings, adverse effects, misadventures or sequela.

Do not assign Y93.9, Unspecified activity, if the activity is not stated.

A code from category Y93 is appropriate for use with external cause and intent codes if identifying the activity provides additional information about the event.

d. **Place of occurrence, activity, and status codes used with other external cause code**
When applicable, place of occurrence, activity, and external cause status codes are sequenced after the main external cause code(s). Regardless of the number of external cause codes assigned, there should be only one place of occurrence code, one activity code, and one external cause status code assigned to an encounter.

e. **If the reporting format limits the number of external cause codes**
If the reporting format limits the number of external cause codes that can be used in reporting clinical data, report the code for the cause/intent most related to the principal diagnosis. If the format permits capture of additional external cause codes, the cause/intent, including medical misadventures, of the additional events should be reported rather than the codes for place, activity, or external status.

f. **Multiple external cause coding guidelines**
More than one external cause code is required to fully describe the external cause of an illness or injury. The assignment of external cause codes should be sequenced in the following priority:

If two or more events cause separate injuries, an external cause code should be assigned for each cause. The first-listed external cause code will be selected in the following order:

External codes for child and adult abuse take priority over all other external cause codes.

See Section I.C.19., Child and Adult abuse guidelines.

External cause codes for terrorism events take priority over all other external cause codes except child and adult abuse.

External cause codes for cataclysmic events take priority over all other external cause codes except child and adult abuse and terrorism.

External cause codes for transport accidents take priority over all other external cause codes except cataclysmic events, child and adult abuse and terrorism.

Activity and external cause status codes are assigned following all causal (intent) external cause codes.

The first-listed external cause code should correspond to the cause of the most serious diagnosis due to an assault, accident, or self-harm, following the order of hierarchy listed above.

g. **Child and adult abuse guideline**
Adult and child abuse, neglect and maltreatment are classified as assault. Any of the assault codes may be used to indicate the external cause of any injury resulting from the confirmed abuse.

For confirmed cases of abuse, neglect and maltreatment, when the perpetrator is known, a code from Y07, Perpetrator of maltreatment and neglect, should accompany any other assault codes.

See Section I.C.19. Adult and child abuse, neglect and other maltreatment

h. **Unknown or undetermined intent guideline**
If the intent (accident, self-harm, assault) of the cause of an injury or other condition is unknown or unspecified, code the intent as accidental intent. All transport accident categories assume accidental intent.

1) **Use of undetermined intent**
External cause codes for events of undetermined intent are only for use if the documentation in the record specifies that the intent cannot be determined.

i. **Sequelae (Late Effects) of External Cause Guidelines**
1) **Sequelae external cause codes**
Sequela are reported using the external cause code with the 7th character "S" for sequela. These codes should be used with any report of a late effect or sequela resulting from a previous injury.

See Section I.B.10 Sequela (Late Effects)

2) **Sequela external cause code with a related current injury**
A sequela external cause code should never be used with a related current nature of injury code.

3) **Use of sequela external cause codes for subsequent visits**
Use a late effect external cause code for subsequent visits when a late effect of the initial injury is being treated. Do not use a late effect external cause code for subsequent visits for follow-up care (e.g., to assess healing, to receive rehabilitative therapy) of the injury when no late effect of the injury has been documented.

j. **Terrorism guidelines**
1) **Cause of injury identified by the Federal Government (FBI) as terrorism**
When the cause of an injury is identified by the Federal Government (FBI) as terrorism, the first-listed external cause code should be a code from category Y38, Terrorism. The definition of terrorism employed by the FBI is found at the

inclusion note at the beginning of category Y38. Use additional code for place of occurrence (Y92.-). More than one Y38 code may be assigned if the injury is the result of more than one mechanism of terrorism.

2) **Cause of an injury is suspected to be the result of terrorism**
When the cause of an injury is suspected to be the result of terrorism a code from category Y38 should not be assigned. Suspected cases should be classified as assault.

3) **Code Y38.9, terrorism, secondary effects**
Assign code Y38.9, Terrorism, secondary effects, for conditions occurring subsequent to the terrorist event. This code should not be assigned for conditions that are due to the initial terrorist act.

It is acceptable to assign code Y38.9 with another code from Y38 if there is an injury due to the initial terrorist event and an injury that is a subsequent result of the terrorist event.

k. **External cause status**
A code from category Y99, External cause status, should be assigned whenever any other external cause code is assigned for an encounter, including an Activity code, except for the events noted below. Assign a code from category Y99, External cause status, to indicate the work status of the person at the time the event occurred. The status code indicates whether the event occurred during military activity, whether a non-military person was at work, whether an individual including a student or volunteer was involved in a non-work activity at the time of the causal event.

A code from Y99, External cause status, should be assigned, when applicable, with other external cause codes, such as transport accidents and falls. The external cause status codes are not applicable to poisonings, adverse effects, misadventures or late effects.

Do not assign a code from category Y99 if no other external cause codes (cause, activity) are applicable for the encounter.

An external cause status code is used only once, at the initial encounter for treatment. Only one code from Y99 should be recorded on a medical record.

Do not assign code Y99.9, Unspecified external cause status, if the status is not stated.

21. **Chapter 21: Factors influencing health status and contact with health services (Z00-Z99)**
Note: The chapter specific guidelines provide additional information about the use of Z codes for specified encounters.

a. **Use of Z codes in any healthcare setting**
Z codes are for use in any healthcare setting. Z codes may be used as either a first-listed (principal diagnosis code in the inpatient setting) or secondary code, depending on the circumstances of the encounter. Certain Z codes may only be used as first-listed or principal diagnosis.

b. **Z Codes indicate a reason for an encounter**
Z codes are not procedure codes. A corresponding procedure code must accompany a Z code to describe any procedure performed.

c. **Categories of Z Codes**
1) **Contact/Exposure**
Category Z20 indicates contact with, and suspected exposure to, communicable diseases. These codes are for patients who do not show any sign or symptom of a disease but are suspected to have been exposed to it by close personal contact with an infected individual or are in an area where a disease is epidemic.

Category Z77, Other contact with and (suspected) exposures hazardous to health, indicates contact with and suspected exposures hazardous to health.

Contact/exposure codes may be used as a first-listed code to explain an encounter for testing, or, more commonly, as a secondary code to identify a potential risk.

2) **Inoculations and vaccinations**
Code Z23 is for encounters for inoculations and vaccinations. It indicates that a patient is being seen to receive a prophylactic inoculation against a disease. Procedure codes are required to identify the actual administration of the injection and the type(s) of immunizations given. Code Z23 may be used as a

secondary code if the inoculation is given as a routine part of preventive health care, such as a well-baby visit.

3) **Status**
Status codes indicate that a patient is either a carrier of a disease or has the sequelae or residual of a past disease or condition. This includes such things as the presence of prosthetic or mechanical devices resulting from past treatment. A status code is informative, because the status may affect the course of treatment and its outcome. A status code is distinct from a history code. The history code indicates that the patient no longer has the condition.

A status code should not be used with a diagnosis code from one of the body system chapters, if the diagnosis code includes the information provided by the status code. For example, code Z94.1, Heart transplant status, should not be used with a code from subcategory T86.2, Complications of heart transplant. The status code does not provide additional information. The complication code indicates that the patient is a heart transplant patient.

For encounters for weaning from a mechanical ventilator, assign a code from subcategory J96.1, Chronic respiratory failure, followed by code Z99.11, Dependence on respirator [ventilator] status.

The status Z codes/categories are:

Z14   Genetic carrier
Genetic carrier status indicates that a person carries a gene, associated with a particular disease, which may be passed to offspring who may develop that disease. The person does not have the disease and is not at risk of developing the disease.

Z15   Genetic susceptibility to disease
Genetic susceptibility indicates that a person has a gene that increases the risk of that person developing the disease.
Codes from category Z15 should not be used as principal or first-listed codes. If the patient has the condition to which he/she is susceptible, and that condition is the reason for the encounter, the code for the current condition should be sequenced first. If the patient is being seen for follow-up after completed treatment for this condition, and the condition no longer exists, a follow-up code should be sequenced first, followed by the appropriate personal history and genetic susceptibility codes. If the purpose of the encounter is genetic counseling associated with procreative management, code Z31.5, Encounter for genetic counseling, should be assigned as the first-listed code, followed by a code from category Z15. Additional codes should be assigned for any applicable family or personal history.

Z16   Resistance to antimicrobial drugs
This code indicates that a patient has a condition that is resistant to antimicrobial drug treatment. Sequence the infection code first.

Z17   Estrogen receptor status
Z18   Retained foreign body fragments
Z21   Asymptomatic HIV infection status
This code indicates that a patient has tested positive for HIV but has manifested no signs or symptoms of the disease.

Z22   Carrier of infectious disease
Carrier status indicates that a person harbors the specific organisms of a disease without manifest symptoms and is capable of transmitting the infection.

Z28.3 Underimmunization status
Z33.1 Pregnant state, incidental
This code is a secondary code only for use when the pregnancy is in no way complicating the reason for visit. Otherwise, a code from the obstetric chapter is required.

Z66   Do not resuscitate

This code may be used when it is documented by the provider that a patient is on do not resuscitate status at any time during the stay.

Z67   Blood type

Z68   Body mass index (BMI)

Z74.Ø1   Bed confinement status

Z76.82   Awaiting organ transplant status

Z78   Other specified health status

Code Z78.1, Physical restraint status, may be used when it is documented by the provider that a patient has been put in restraints during the current encounter. Please note that this code should not be reported when it is documented by the provider that a patient is temporarily restrained during a procedure.

Z79   Long-term (current) drug therapy

Codes from this category indicate a patient's continuous use of a prescribed drug (including such things as aspirin therapy) for the long-term treatment of a condition or for prophylactic use. It is not for use for patients who have addictions to drugs. This subcategory is not for use of medications for detoxification or maintenance programs to prevent withdrawal symptoms in patients with drug dependence (e.g., methadone maintenance for opiate dependence). Assign the appropriate code for the drug dependence instead.

Assign a code from Z79 if the patient is receiving a medication for an extended period as a prophylactic measure (such as for the prevention of deep vein thrombosis) or as treatment of a chronic condition (such as arthritis) or a disease requiring a lengthy course of treatment (such as cancer). Do not assign a code from category Z79 for medication being administered for a brief period of time to treat an acute illness or injury (such as a course of antibiotics to treat acute bronchitis).

Z88   Allergy status to drugs, medicaments and biological substances

Except: Z88.9, Allergy status to unspecified drugs, medicaments and biological substances status

Z89   Acquired absence of limb

Z90   Acquired absence of organs, not elsewhere classified

Z91.Ø-   Allergy status, other than to drugs and biological substances

Z92.82   Status post administration of tPA (rtPA) in a different facility within the last 24 hours prior to admission to a current facility

Assign code Z92.82, Status post administration of tPA (rtPA) in a different facility within the last 24 hours prior to admission to current facility, as a secondary diagnosis when a patient is received by transfer into a facility and documentation indicates they were administered tissue plasminogen activator (tPA) within the last 24 hours prior to admission to the current facility.

This guideline applies even if the patient is still receiving the tPA at the time they are received into the current facility.

The appropriate code for the condition for which the tPA was administered (such as cerebrovascular disease or myocardial infarction) should be assigned first.

Code Z92.82 is only applicable to the receiving facility record and not to the transferring facility record.

Z93   Artificial opening status

Z94   Transplanted organ and tissue status

Z95   Presence of cardiac and vascular implants and grafts

Z96   Presence of other functional implants

Z97   Presence of other devices

Z98   Other postprocedural states

Assign code Z98.85, Transplanted organ removal status, to indicate that a transplanted organ has been previously removed. This code should not be assigned for the encounter in which the transplanted organ is removed. The complication necessitating removal of the transplant organ should be assigned for that encounter.

See section I.C19. for information on the coding of organ transplant complications.

Z99   Dependence on enabling machines and devices, not elsewhere classified

Note: Categories Z89-Z90 and Z93-Z99 are for use only if there are no complications or malfunctions of the organ or tissue replaced, the amputation site or the equipment on which the patient is dependent.

4)   **History (of)**

There are two types of history Z codes, personal and family. Personal history codes explain a patient's past medical condition that no longer exists and is not receiving any treatment, but that has the potential for recurrence, and therefore may require continued monitoring.

Family history codes are for use when a patient has a family member(s) who has had a particular disease that causes the patient to be at higher risk of also contracting the disease.

Personal history codes may be used in conjunction with follow-up codes and family history codes may be used in conjunction with screening codes to explain the need for a test or procedure. History codes are also acceptable on any medical record regardless of the reason for visit. A history of an illness, even if no longer present, is important information that may alter the type of treatment ordered.

The history Z code categories are:

Z80   Family history of primary malignant neoplasm

Z81   Family history of mental and behavioral disorders

Z82   Family history of certain disabilities and chronic diseases (leading to disablement)

Z83   Family history of other specific disorders

Z84   Family history of other conditions

Z85   Personal history of malignant neoplasm

Z86   Personal history of certain other diseases

Z87   Personal history of other diseases and conditions

Z91.4-   Personal history of psychological trauma, not elsewhere classified

Z91.5   Personal history of self-harm

Z91.8-   Other specified personal risk factors, not elsewhere classified

Exception:

Z91.83, Wandering in diseases classified elsewhere

Z92   Personal history of medical treatment

Except: Z92.Ø, Personal history of contraception

Except: Z92.82, Status post administration of tPA (rtPA) in a different facility within the last 24 hours prior to admission to a current facility

5)   **Screening**

Screening is the testing for disease or disease precursors in seemingly well individuals so that early detection and treatment can be provided for those who test positive for the disease (e.g., screening mammogram).

The testing of a person to rule out or confirm a suspected diagnosis because the patient has some sign or symptom is a diagnostic examination, not a screening. In these cases, the sign or symptom is used to explain the reason for the test.

A screening code may be a first-listed code if the reason for the visit is specifically the screening exam. It may also be used as an additional code if the screening is done during an office visit for other health problems. A screening code is not necessary if the screening is inherent to a routine examination, such as a pap smear done during a routine pelvic examination.

Should a condition be discovered during the screening then the code for the condition may be assigned as an additional diagnosis.

The Z code indicates that a screening exam is planned. A procedure code is required to confirm that the screening was performed.

The screening Z codes/categories:

Z11   Encounter for screening for infectious and parasitic diseases

Z12   Encounter for screening for malignant neoplasms

Z13   Encounter for screening for other diseases and disorders

       Except: Z13.9, Encounter for screening, unspecified

Z36   Encounter for antenatal screening for mother

6) **Observation**

There are two observation Z code categories. They are for use in very limited circumstances when a person is being observed for a suspected condition that is ruled out. The observation codes are not for use if an injury or illness or any signs or symptoms related to the suspected condition are present. In such cases the diagnosis/symptom code is used with the corresponding external cause code.

The observation codes are to be used as principal diagnosis only. Additional codes may be used in addition to the observation code but only if they are unrelated to the suspected condition being observed.

Codes from subcategory Z03.7, Encounter for suspected maternal and fetal conditions ruled out, may either be used as a first-listed or as an additional code assignment depending on the case. They are for use in very limited circumstances on a maternal record when an encounter is for a suspected maternal or fetal condition that is ruled out during that encounter (for example, a maternal or fetal condition may be suspected due to an abnormal test result). These codes should not be used when the condition is confirmed. In those cases, the confirmed condition should be coded. In addition, these codes are not for use if an illness or any signs or symptoms related to the suspected condition or problem are present. In such cases the diagnosis/symptom code is used.

Additional codes may be used in addition to the code from subcategory Z03.7, but only if they are unrelated to the suspected condition being evaluated.

Codes from subcategory Z03.7 may not be used for encounters for antenatal screening of mother. *See Section I.C.21.c.5, Screening.*

For encounters for suspected fetal condition that are inconclusive following testing and evaluation, assign the appropriate code from category O35, O36, O40 or O41.

The observation Z code categories:

Z03   Encounter for medical observation for suspected diseases and conditions ruled out

Z04   Encounter for examination and observation for other reasons

       Except: Z04.9, Encounter for examination and observation for unspecified reason

7) **Aftercare**

Aftercare visit codes cover situations when the initial treatment of a disease has been performed and the patient requires continued care during the healing or recovery phase, or for the long-term consequences of the disease. The aftercare Z code should not be used if treatment is directed at a current, acute disease. The diagnosis code is to be used in these cases. Exceptions to this rule are codes Z51.0, Encounter for antineoplastic radiation therapy, and codes from subcategory Z51.1, Encounter for antineoplastic chemotherapy and immunotherapy. These codes are to be first-listed, followed by the diagnosis code when a patient's encounter is solely to receive radiation therapy, chemotherapy, or immunotherapy for the treatment of a neoplasm. If the reason for the encounter is more than one type of antineoplastic therapy, code Z51.0 and a code from subcategory Z51.1 may be assigned together, in

which case one of these codes would be reported as a secondary diagnosis.

The aftercare Z codes should also not be used for aftercare for injuries. For aftercare of an injury, assign the acute injury code with the appropriate 7th character (for subsequent encounter).

The aftercare codes are generally first-listed to explain the specific reason for the encounter. An aftercare code may be used as an additional code when some type of aftercare is provided in addition to the reason for admission and no diagnosis code is applicable. An example of this would be the closure of a colostomy during an encounter for treatment of another condition.

Aftercare codes should be used in conjunction with other aftercare codes or diagnosis codes to provide better detail on the specifics of an aftercare encounter visit, unless otherwise directed by the classification. Should a patient receive multiple types of antineoplastic therapy during the same encounter, code Z51.0, Encounter for antineoplastic radiation therapy, and codes from subcategory Z51.1, Encounter for antineoplastic chemotherapy and immunotherapy, may be used together on a record. The sequencing of multiple aftercare codes depends on the circumstances of the encounter.

Certain aftercare Z code categories need a secondary diagnosis code to describe the resolving condition or sequelae. For others, the condition is included in the code title.

Additional Z code aftercare category terms include fitting and adjustment, and attention to artificial openings.

Status Z codes may be used with aftercare Z codes to indicate the nature of the aftercare. For example code Z95.1, Presence of aortocoronary bypass graft, may be used with code Z48.812, Encounter for surgical aftercare following surgery on the circulatory system, to indicate the surgery for which the aftercare is being performed. A status code should not be used when the aftercare code indicates the type of status, such as using Z43.0, Encounter for attention to tracheostomy, with Z93.0, Tracheostomy status.

The aftercare Z category/codes:

Z42   Encounter for plastic and reconstructive surgery following medical procedure or healed injury

Z43   Encounter for attention to artificial openings

Z44   Encounter for fitting and adjustment of external prosthetic device

Z45   Encounter for adjustment and management of implanted device

Z46   Encounter for fitting and adjustment of other devices

Z47   Orthopedic aftercare

Z48   Encounter for other postprocedural aftercare

Z49   Encounter for care involving renal dialysis

Z51   Encounter for other aftercare

8) **Follow-up**

The follow-up codes are used to explain continuing surveillance following completed treatment of a disease, condition, or injury. They imply that the condition has been fully treated and no longer exists. They should not be confused with aftercare codes, or injury codes with a 7th character for subsequent encounter, that explain ongoing care of a healing condition or its sequelae. Follow-up codes may be used in conjunction with history codes to provide the full picture of the healed condition and its treatment. The follow-up code is sequenced first, followed by the history code.

A follow-up code may be used to explain multiple visits. Should a condition be found to have recurred on the follow-up visit, then the diagnosis code for the condition should be assigned in place of the follow-up code.

The follow-up Z code categories:

Z08   Encounter for follow-up examination after completed treatment for malignant neoplasm

Z09   Encounter for follow-up examination after completed treatment for conditions other than malignant neoplasm

Z39   Encounter for maternal postpartum care and examination

9) Donor

Codes in category Z52, Donors of organs and tissues, are used for living individuals who are donating blood or other body tissue. These codes are only for individuals donating for others, not for self-donations. They are not used to identify cadaveric donations.

10) Counseling

Counseling Z codes are used when a patient or family member receives assistance in the aftermath of an illness or injury, or when support is required in coping with family or social problems. They are not used in conjunction with a diagnosis code when the counseling component of care is considered integral to standard treatment.

The counseling Z codes/categories:

Z30.0-   Encounter for general counseling and advice on contraception

Z31.5   Encounter for genetic counseling

Z31.6-   Encounter for general counseling and advice on procreation

Z32.2   Encounter for childbirth instruction

Z32.3   Encounter for childcare instruction

Z69   Encounter for mental health services for victim and perpetrator of abuse

Z70   Counseling related to sexual attitude, behavior and orientation

Z71   Persons encountering health services for other counseling and medical advice, not elsewhere classified

Z76.81 Expectant mother prebirth pediatrician visit

11) Encounters for obstetrical and reproductive services

See Section I.C.15. Pregnancy, Childbirth, and the Puerperium, for further instruction on the use of these codes.

Z codes for pregnancy are for use in those circumstances when none of the problems or complications included in the codes from the Obstetrics chapter exist (a routine prenatal visit or postpartum care). Codes in category Z34, Encounter for supervision of normal pregnancy, are always first-listed and are not to be used with any other code from the OB chapter.

Codes in category Z3A, Weeks of gestation, may be assigned to provide additional information about the pregnancy. The date of the admission should be used to determine weeks of gestation for inpatient admissions that encompass more than one gestational week.

The outcome of delivery, category Z37, should be included on all maternal delivery records. It is always a secondary code.

Z codes for family planning (contraceptive) or procreative management and counseling should be included on an obstetric record either during the pregnancy or the postpartum stage, if applicable.

Z codes/categories for obstetrical and reproductive services:

Z30   Encounter for contraceptive management

Z31   Encounter for procreative management

Z32.2   Encounter for childbirth instruction

Z32.3   Encounter for childcare instruction

Z33   Pregnant state

Z34   Encounter for supervision of normal pregnancy

Z36   Encounter for antenatal screening of mother

Z3A   Weeks of gestation

Z37   Outcome of delivery

Z39   Encounter for maternal postpartum care and examination

Z76.81 Expectant mother prebirth pediatrician visit

12) Newborns and Infants

See Section I.C.16. Newborn (Perinatal) Guidelines, for further instruction on the use of these codes.

Newborn Z codes/categories:

Z76.1   Encounter for health supervision and care of foundling

Z00.1- Encounter for routine child health examination

Z38   Liveborn infants according to place of birth and type of delivery

13) Routine and administrative examinations

The Z codes allow for the description of encounters for routine examinations, such as, a general check-up, or, examinations for administrative purposes, such as, a pre-employment physical. The codes are not to be used if the examination is for diagnosis of a suspected condition or for treatment purposes. In such cases the diagnosis code is used. During a routine exam, should a diagnosis or condition be discovered, it should be coded as an additional code. Pre-existing and chronic conditions and history codes may also be included as additional codes as long as the examination is for administrative purposes and not focused on any particular condition.

Some of the codes for routine health examinations distinguish between "with" and "without" abnormal findings. Code assignment depends on the information that is known at the time the encounter is being coded. For example, if no abnormal findings were found during the examination, but the encounter is being coded before test results are back, it is acceptable to assign the code for "without abnormal findings." When assigning a code for "with abnormal findings," additional code(s) should be assigned to identify the specific abnormal finding(s).

Pre-operative examination and pre-procedural laboratory examination Z codes are for use only in those situations when a patient is being cleared for a procedure or surgery and no treatment is being given.

The Z codes/categories for routine and administrative examinations:

Z00   Encounter for general examination without complaint, suspected or reported diagnosis

Z01   Encounter for other special examination without complaint, suspected or reported diagnosis

Z02   Encounter for administrative examination

        Except: Z02.9, Encounter for administrative examinations, unspecified

Z32.0- Encounter for pregnancy test

14) Miscellaneous Z codes

The miscellaneous Z codes capture a number of other health care encounters that do not fall into one of the other categories. Certain of these codes identify the reason for the encounter; others are for use as additional codes that provide useful information on circumstances that may affect a patient's care and treatment.

Prophylactic Organ Removal

For encounters specifically for prophylactic removal of an organ (such as prophylactic removal of breasts due to a genetic susceptibility to cancer or a family history of cancer), the principal or first-listed code should be a code from category Z40, Encounter for prophylactic surgery, followed by the appropriate codes to identify the associated risk factor (such as genetic susceptibility or family history).

If the patient has a malignancy of one site and is having prophylactic removal at another site to prevent either a new primary malignancy or metastatic disease, a code for the malignancy should also be assigned in addition to a code from subcategory Z40.0, Encounter for prophylactic surgery for risk factors related to malignant neoplasms. A Z40.0 code should not be assigned if the patient is having organ removal for treatment of a malignancy, such as the removal of the testes for the treatment of prostate cancer.

Miscellaneous Z codes/categories:

Z28   Immunization not carried out

Except: Z28.3, Underimmunization status

Z40   Encounter for prophylactic surgery

Z41   Encounter for procedures for purposes other than remedying health state

Except: Z41.9, Encounter for procedure for purposes other than remedying health state, unspecified

Z53   Persons encountering health services for specific procedures and treatment, not carried out

Z55   Problems related to education and literacy

Z56   Problems related to employment and unemployment

Z57   Occupational exposure to risk factors

Z58   Problems related to physical environment

Z59   Problems related to housing and economic circumstances

Z60   Problems related to social environment

Z62   Problems related to upbringing

Z63   Other problems related to primary support group, including family circumstances

Z64   Problems related to certain psychosocial circumstances

Z65   Problems related to other psychosocial circumstances

Z72   Problems related to lifestyle

Z73   Problems related to life management difficulty

Z74   Problems related to care provider dependency

Except: Z74.01, Bed confinement status

Z75   Problems related to medical facilities and other health care

Z76.0   Encounter for issue of repeat prescription

Z76.3   Healthy person accompanying sick person

Z76.4   Other boarder to healthcare facility

Z76.5   Malingerer [conscious simulation]

Z91.1-   Patient's noncompliance with medical treatment and regimen

Z91.83   Wandering in diseases classified elsewhere

Z91.89   Other specified personal risk factors, not elsewhere classified

15) Nonspecific Z codes

Certain Z codes are so non-specific, or potentially redundant with other codes in the classification, that there can be little justification for their use in the inpatient setting. Their use in the outpatient setting should be limited to those instances when there is no further documentation to permit more precise coding. Otherwise, any sign or symptom or any other reason for visit that is captured in another code should be used.

Nonspecific Z codes/categories:

Z02.9   Encounter for administrative examinations, unspecified

Z04.9   Encounter for examination and observation for unspecified reason

Z13.9   Encounter for screening, unspecified

Z41.9   Encounter for procedure for purposes other than remedying health state, unspecified

Z52.9   Donor of unspecified organ or tissue

Z86.59   Personal history of other mental and behavioral disorders

Z88.9   Allergy status to unspecified drugs, medicaments and biological substances status

Z92.0   Personal history of contraception

16) Z codes that may only be principal/first-listed diagnosis

The following Z codes/categories may only be reported as the principal/first-listed diagnosis, except when there are multiple encounters on the same day and the medical records for the encounters are combined:

Z00   Encounter for general examination without complaint, suspected or reported diagnosis

Except: Z00.6

Z01   Encounter for other special examination without complaint, suspected or reported diagnosis

Z02   Encounter for administrative examination

Z03   Encounter for medical observation for suspected diseases and conditions ruled out

Z04   Encounter for examination and observation for other reasons

Z33.2   Encounter for elective termination of pregnancy

Z31.81   Encounter for male factor infertility in female patient

Z31.82   Encounter for Rh incompatibility status

Z31.83   Encounter for assisted reproductive fertility procedure cycle

Z31.84   Encounter for fertility preservation procedure

Z34   Encounter for supervision of normal pregnancy

Z39   Encounter for maternal postpartum care and examination

Z38   Liveborn infants according to place of birth and type of delivery

Z42   Encounter for plastic and reconstructive surgery following medical procedure or healed injury

Z51.0   Encounter for antineoplastic radiation therapy

Z51.1-   Encounter for antineoplastic chemotherapy and immunotherapy

Z52   Donors of organs and tissues

Except: Z52.9, Donor of unspecified organ or tissue

Z76.1   Encounter for health supervision and care of foundling

Z76.2   Encounter for health supervision and care of other healthy infant and child

Z99.12   Encounter for respirator [ventilator] dependence during power failure

Section II. Selection of Principal Diagnosis

The circumstances of inpatient admission always govern the selection of principal diagnosis.

The principal diagnosis is defined in the Uniform Hospital Discharge Data Set (UHDDS) as "that condition established after study to be chiefly responsible for occasioning the admission of the patient to the hospital for care."

The UHDDS definitions are used by hospitals to report inpatient data elements in a standardized manner. These data elements and their definitions can be found in the July 31, 1985, Federal Register (Vol. 50, No, 147), pp. 31038-40.

Since that time the application of the UHDDS definitions has been expanded to include all non- outpatient settings (acute care, short term, long term care and psychiatric hospitals; home health agencies; rehab facilities; nursing homes, etc).

In determining principal diagnosis, coding conventions in the ICD-10-CM, the Tabular List and Alphabetic Index take precedence over these official coding guidelines.

(See Section I.A., Conventions for the ICD-10-CM)

The importance of consistent, complete documentation in the medical record cannot be overemphasized. Without such documentation the application of all coding guidelines is a difficult, if not impossible, task.

A. Codes for symptoms, signs, and ill-defined conditions

Codes for symptoms, signs, and ill-defined conditions from Chapter 18 are not to be used as principal diagnosis when a related definitive diagnosis has been established.

B. Two or more interrelated conditions, each potentially meeting the definition for principal diagnosis

When there are two or more interrelated conditions (such as diseases in the same ICD-10-CM chapter or manifestations characteristically associated with a certain disease) potentially meeting the definition of principal diagnosis, either condition may be sequenced first, unless the circumstances of the admission, the therapy provided, the Tabular List, or the Alphabetic Index indicate otherwise.

C. Two or more diagnoses that equally meet the definition for principal diagnosis

In the unusual instance when two or more diagnoses equally meet the criteria for principal diagnosis as determined by the circumstances of admission, diagnostic workup and/or therapy provided, and the Alphabetic Index, Tabular List, or another coding guidelines does not provide sequencing direction, any one of the diagnoses may be sequenced first.

D. Two or more comparative or contrasting conditions

In those rare instances when two or more contrasting or comparative diagnoses are documented as "either/or" (or similar terminology), they are coded as if the diagnoses were confirmed and the diagnoses are sequenced according to the circumstances of the admission. If no further determination can be made as to which diagnosis should be principal, either diagnosis may be sequenced first.

E. A symptom(s) followed by contrasting/ comparative diagnoses

GUIDELINE HAS BEEN DELETED EFFECTIVE OCTOBER 1, 2014

F. Original treatment plan not carried out

Sequence as the principal diagnosis the condition, which after study occasioned the admission to the hospital, even though treatment may not have been carried out due to unforeseen circumstances.

G. Complications of surgery and other medical care

When the admission is for treatment of a complication resulting from surgery or other medical care, the complication code is sequenced as the principal diagnosis. If the complication is classified to the T80-T88 series and the code lacks the necessary specificity in describing the complication, an additional code for the specific complication should be assigned.

H. Uncertain diagnosis

If the diagnosis documented at the time of discharge is qualified as "probable", "suspected", "likely", "questionable", "possible", or "still to be ruled out", or other similar terms indicating uncertainty, code the condition as if it existed or was established. The bases for these guidelines are the diagnostic workup, arrangements for further workup or observation, and initial therapeutic approach that correspond most closely with the established diagnosis.

Note: This guideline is applicable only to inpatient admissions to short-term, acute, long-term care and psychiatric hospitals.

I. Admission from observation unit

1. **Admission Following Medical Observation**
    When a patient is admitted to an observation unit for a medical condition, which either worsens or does not improve, and is subsequently admitted as an inpatient of the same hospital for this same medical condition, the principal diagnosis would be the medical condition which led to the hospital admission.

2. **Admission Following Post-Operative Observation**
    When a patient is admitted to an observation unit to monitor a condition (or complication) that develops following outpatient surgery, and then is subsequently admitted as an inpatient of the same hospital, hospitals should apply the Uniform Hospital Discharge Data Set (UHDDS) definition of principal diagnosis as "that condition established after study to be chiefly responsible for occasioning the admission of the patient to the hospital for care."

J. Admission from outpatient surgery

When a patient receives surgery in the hospital's outpatient surgery department and is subsequently admitted for continuing inpatient care at the same hospital, the following guidelines should be followed in selecting the principal diagnosis for the inpatient admission:

*   If the reason for the inpatient admission is a complication, assign the complication as the principal diagnosis.
*   If no complication, or other condition, is documented as the reason for the inpatient admission, assign the reason for the outpatient surgery as the principal diagnosis.
*   If the reason for the inpatient admission is another condition unrelated to the surgery, assign the unrelated condition as the principal diagnosis.

K. Admissions/Encounters for Rehabilitation

When the purpose for the admission/encounter is rehabilitation, sequence first the code for the condition for which the service is being performed. For example, for an admission/encounter for rehabilitation for right-sided dominant hemiplegia following a cerebrovascular infarction, report code I69.351, Hemiplegia and hemiparesis following cerebral infarction affecting right dominant side, as the first-listed or principal diagnosis.

If the condition for which the rehabilitation service is no longer present, report the appropriate aftercare code as the first-listed or principal diagnosis. For example, if a patient with severe degenerative osteoarthritis of the hip, underwent hip replacement and the current encounter/admission is for rehabilitation, report code Z47.1, Aftercare following joint replacement surgery, as the first-listed or principal diagnosis.

See Section I.C.21.c.7, Factors influencing health states and contact with health services, Aftercare.

Section III. Reporting Additional Diagnoses

GENERAL RULES FOR OTHER (ADDITIONAL) DIAGNOSES

For reporting purposes the definition for "other diagnoses" is interpreted as additional conditions that affect patient care in terms of requiring:

> clinical evaluation; or
>
> therapeutic treatment; or
>
> diagnostic procedures; or
>
> extended length of hospital stay; or
>
> increased nursing care and/or monitoring.

The UHDDS item #11-b defines Other Diagnoses as "all conditions that coexist at the time of admission, that develop subsequently, or that affect the treatment received and/or the length of stay. Diagnoses that relate to an earlier episode which have no bearing on the current hospital stay are to be excluded." UHDDS definitions apply to inpatients in acute care, short-term, long term care and psychiatric hospital setting. The UHDDS definitions are used by acute care short-term hospitals to report inpatient data elements in a standardized manner. These data elements and their definitions can be found in the July 31, 1985, Federal Register (Vol. 50, No, 147), pp. 31038-40.

Since that time the application of the UHDDS definitions has been expanded to include all non-outpatient settings (acute care, short term, long term care and psychiatric hospitals; home health agencies; rehab facilities; nursing homes, etc.).

The following guidelines are to be applied in designating "other diagnoses" when neither the Alphabetic Index nor the Tabular List in ICD-10-CM provide direction. The listing of the diagnoses in the patient record is the responsibility of the attending provider.

A. **Previous conditions**
    If the provider has included a diagnosis in the final diagnostic statement, such as the discharge summary or the face sheet, it should ordinarily be coded. Some providers include in the diagnostic statement resolved conditions or diagnoses and status-post procedures from previous admission that have no bearing on the current stay. Such conditions are not to be reported and are coded only if required by hospital policy.

    However, history codes (categories Z80-Z87) may be used as secondary codes if the historical condition or family history has an impact on current care or influences treatment.

B. **Abnormal findings**
    Abnormal findings (laboratory, x-ray, pathologic, and other diagnostic results) are not coded and reported unless the provider indicates their clinical significance. If the findings are outside the normal range and the attending provider has ordered other tests to evaluate the condition or prescribed treatment, it is appropriate to ask the provider whether the abnormal finding should be added.

    Please note: This differs from the coding practices in the outpatient setting for coding encounters for diagnostic tests that have been interpreted by a provider.

C. **Uncertain Diagnosis**
    If the diagnosis documented at the time of discharge is qualified as "probable", "suspected", "likely", "questionable", "possible", or "still to be ruled out" or other similar terms indicating uncertainty, code the condition as if it existed or was established. The bases for these guidelines are the diagnostic workup, arrangements for further workup

or observation, and initial therapeutic approach that correspond most closely with the established diagnosis.

Note: This guideline is applicable only to inpatient admissions to short-term, acute, long-term care and psychiatric hospitals.

Section IV. Diagnostic Coding and Reporting Guidelines for Outpatient Services

These coding guidelines for outpatient diagnoses have been approved for use by hospitals/ providers in coding and reporting hospital-based outpatient services and provider-based office visits.

Information about the use of certain abbreviations, punctuation, symbols, and other conventions used in the ICD-10-CM Tabular List (code numbers and titles), can be found in Section IA of these guidelines, under "Conventions Used in the Tabular List." Section I.B. contains general guidelines that apply to the entire classification. Section I.C. contains chapter-specific guidelines that correspond to the chapters as they are arranged in the classification. Information about the correct sequence to use in finding a code is also described in Section I.

The terms encounter and visit are often used interchangeably in describing outpatient service contacts and, therefore, appear together in these guidelines without distinguishing one from the other.

Though the conventions and general guidelines apply to all settings, coding guidelines for outpatient and provider reporting of diagnoses will vary in a number of instances from those for inpatient diagnoses, recognizing that:

The Uniform Hospital Discharge Data Set (UHDDS) definition of principal diagnosis applies only to inpatients in acute, short-term, long-term care and psychiatric hospitals.

Coding guidelines for inconclusive diagnoses (probable, suspected, rule out, etc.) were developed for inpatient reporting and do not apply to outpatients.

A. Selection of first-listed condition

In the outpatient setting, the term first-listed diagnosis is used in lieu of principal diagnosis.

In determining the first-listed diagnosis the coding conventions of ICD-10-CM, as well as the general and disease specific guidelines take precedence over the outpatient guidelines.

Diagnoses often are not established at the time of the initial encounter/visit. It may take two or more visits before the diagnosis is confirmed.

The most critical rule involves beginning the search for the correct code assignment through the Alphabetic Index. Never begin searching initially in the Tabular List as this will lead to coding errors.

1. **Outpatient surgery**
When a patient presents for outpatient surgery (same day surgery), code the reason for the surgery as the first-listed diagnosis (reason for the encounter), even if the surgery is not performed due to a contraindication.

2. **Observation stay**
When a patient is admitted for observation for a medical condition, assign a code for the medical condition as the first-listed diagnosis.

When a patient presents for outpatient surgery and develops complications requiring admission to observation, code the reason for the surgery as the first reported diagnosis (reason for the encounter), followed by codes for the complications as secondary diagnoses.

B. Codes from A00.0 through T88.9, Z00-Z99
The appropriate code(s) from A00.0 through T88.9, Z00-Z99 must be used to identify diagnoses, symptoms, conditions, problems, complaints, or other reason(s) for the encounter/visit.

C. Accurate reporting of ICD-10-CM diagnosis codes
For accurate reporting of ICD-10-CM diagnosis codes, the documentation should describe the patient's condition, using terminology which includes specific diagnoses as well as symptoms, problems, or reasons for the encounter. There are ICD-10-CM codes to describe all of these.

D. Codes that describe symptoms and signs
Codes that describe symptoms and signs, as opposed to diagnoses, are acceptable for reporting purposes when a diagnosis has not been established (confirmed) by the provider. Chapter 18 of ICD-10-CM, Symptoms, Signs, and Abnormal Clinical and Laboratory Findings Not Elsewhere Classified (codes R00-R99) contain many, but not all codes for symptoms.

E. Encounters for circumstances other than a disease or injury
ICD-10-CM provides codes to deal with encounters for circumstances other than a disease or injury. The Factors Influencing Health Status and Contact with Health Services codes (Z00-Z99) are provided to deal with occasions when circumstances other than a disease or injury are recorded as diagnosis or problems.

See Section I.C.21. Factors influencing health status and contact with health services.

F. Level of Detail in Coding

1. **ICD-10-CM codes with 3, 4, 5, 6 or 7 characters**
ICD-10-CM is composed of codes with 3, 4, 5, 6 or 7 characters. Codes with three characters are included in ICD-10-CM as the heading of a category of codes that may be further subdivided by the use of fourth, fifth, sixth or seventh characters to provide greater specificity.

2. **Use of full number of *characters* required for a code**
A three-character code is to be used only if it is not further subdivided. A code is invalid if it has not been coded to the full number of characters required for that code, including the 7th character extension, if applicable.

G. ICD-10-CM code for the diagnosis, condition, problem, or other reason for encounter/visit
List first the ICD-10-CM code for the diagnosis, condition, problem, or other reason for encounter/visit shown in the medical record to be chiefly responsible for the services provided. List additional codes that describe any coexisting conditions. In some cases the first-listed diagnosis may be a symptom when a diagnosis has not been established (confirmed) by the physician.

H. Uncertain diagnosis
Do not code diagnoses documented as "probable", "suspected," "questionable," "rule out," or "working diagnosis" or other similar terms indicating uncertainty. Rather, code the condition(s) to the highest degree of certainty for that encounter/visit, such as symptoms, signs, abnormal test results, or other reason for the visit.

Please note: This differs from the coding practices used by short-term, acute care, long-term care and psychiatric hospitals.

I. Chronic diseases
Chronic diseases treated on an ongoing basis may be coded and reported as many times as the patient receives treatment and care for the condition(s)

J. Code all documented conditions that coexist
Code all documented conditions that coexist at the time of the encounter/visit, and require or affect patient care treatment or management. Do not code conditions that were previously treated and no longer exist. However, history codes (categories Z80-Z87) may be used as secondary codes if the historical condition or family history has an impact on current care or influences treatment.

K. Patients receiving diagnostic services only
For patients receiving diagnostic services only during an encounter/visit, sequence first the diagnosis, condition, problem, or other reason for encounter/visit shown in the medical record to be chiefly responsible for the outpatient services provided during the encounter/visit. Codes for other diagnoses (e.g., chronic conditions) may be sequenced as additional diagnoses.

For encounters for routine laboratory/radiology testing in the absence of any signs, symptoms, or associated diagnosis, assign Z01.89, Encounter for other specified special examinations. If routine testing is performed during the same encounter as a test to evaluate a sign, symptom, or diagnosis, it is appropriate to assign both the Z code and the code describing the reason for the non-routine test.

For outpatient encounters for diagnostic tests that have been interpreted by a physician, and the final report is available at the time of coding, code any confirmed or definitive diagnosis(es) documented in the interpretation. Do not code related signs and symptoms as additional diagnoses.

Please note: This differs from the coding practice in the hospital inpatient setting regarding abnormal findings on test results.

L. Patients receiving therapeutic services only

For patients receiving therapeutic services only during an encounter/visit, sequence first the diagnosis, condition, problem, or other reason for encounter/visit shown in the medical record to be chiefly responsible for the outpatient services provided during the encounter/visit. Codes for other diagnoses (e.g., chronic conditions) may be sequenced as additional diagnoses.

The only exception to this rule is that when the primary reason for the admission/encounter is chemotherapy or radiation therapy, the appropriate Z code for the service is listed first, and the diagnosis or problem for which the service is being performed listed second.

M. Patients receiving preoperative evaluations only

For patients receiving preoperative evaluations only, sequence first a code from subcategory Z01.81, Encounter for pre-procedural examinations, to describe the pre-op consultations. Assign a code for the condition to describe the reason for the surgery as an additional diagnosis. Code also any findings related to the pre-op evaluation.

N. Ambulatory surgery

For ambulatory surgery, code the diagnosis for which the surgery was performed. If the postoperative diagnosis is known to be different from the preoperative diagnosis at the time the diagnosis is confirmed, select the postoperative diagnosis for coding, since it is the most definitive.

O. Routine outpatient prenatal visits

See Section I.C.15. Routine outpatient prenatal visits.

P. Encounters for general medical examinations with abnormal findings

The subcategories for encounters for general medical examinations, Z00.0-, provide codes for with and without abnormal findings. Should a general medical examination result in an abnormal finding, the code for general medical examination with abnormal finding should be assigned as the first-listed diagnosis. A secondary code for the abnormal finding should also be coded.

Q. Encounters for routine health screenings

See Section I.C.21. Factors influencing health status and contact with health services, Screening

Appendix I. Present on Admission Reporting Guidelines

Introduction

These guidelines are to be used as a supplement to the *ICD-10-CM Official Guidelines for Coding and Reporting* to facilitate the assignment of the Present on Admission (POA) indicator for each diagnosis and external cause of injury code reported on claim forms (UB-04 and 837 Institutional).

These guidelines are not intended to replace any guidelines in the main body of the *ICD-10-CM Official Guidelines for Coding and Reporting*. The POA guidelines are not intended to provide guidance on when a condition should be coded, but rather, how to apply the POA indicator to the final set of diagnosis codes that have been assigned in accordance with Sections I, II, and III of the official coding guidelines. Subsequent to the assignment of the ICD-10-CM codes, the POA indicator should then be assigned to those conditions that have been coded.

As stated in the Introduction to the *ICD-10-CM Official Guidelines for Coding and Reporting*, a joint effort between the healthcare provider and the coder is essential to achieve complete and accurate documentation, code assignment, and reporting of diagnoses and procedures. The importance of consistent, complete documentation in the medical record cannot be overemphasized. Medical record documentation from any provider involved in the care and treatment of the patient may be used to support the determination of whether a condition was present on admission or not. In the context of the official coding guidelines, the term "provider" means a physician or any qualified healthcare practitioner who is legally accountable for establishing the patient's diagnosis.

These guidelines are not a substitute for the provider's clinical judgment as to the determination of whether a condition was/was not present on admission. The provider should be queried regarding issues related to the linking of signs/symptoms, timing of test results, and the timing of findings.

General Reporting Requirements

All claims involving inpatient admissions to general acute care hospitals or other facilities that are subject to a law or regulation mandating collection of present on admission information.

Present on admission is defined as present at the time the order for inpatient admission occurs -- conditions that develop during an outpatient encounter, including emergency department, observation, or outpatient surgery, are considered as present on admission.

POA indicator is assigned to principal and secondary diagnoses (as defined in Section II of the Official Guidelines for Coding and Reporting) and the external cause of injury codes.

Issues related to inconsistent, missing, conflicting or unclear documentation must still be resolved by the provider.

If a condition would not be coded and reported based on UHDDS definitions and current official coding guidelines, then the POA indicator would not be reported.

Reporting Options

Y –	Yes
N –	No
U –	Unknown
W –	Clinically undetermined
	Unreported/Not used (or "1" for Medicare usage) – (Exempt from POA reporting)

Reporting Definitions

Y –	present at the time of inpatient admission
N –	not present at the time of inpatient admission
U –	documentation is insufficient to determine if condition is present on admission
W –	provider is unable to clinically determine whether condition was present on admission or not

Timeframe for POA Identification and Documentation

There is no required timeframe as to when a provider (per the definition of "provider" used in these guidelines) must identify or document a condition to be present on admission. In some clinical situations, it may not be possible for a provider to make a definitive diagnosis (or a condition may not be recognized or reported by the patient) for a period of time after admission. In some cases it may be several days before the provider arrives at a definitive diagnosis. This does not mean that the condition was not present on admission. Determination of whether the condition was present on admission or not will be based on the applicable POA guideline as identified in this document, or on the provider's best clinical judgment.

If at the time of code assignment the documentation is unclear as to whether a condition was present on admission or not, it is appropriate to query the provider for clarification.

Assigning the POA Indicator

Condition is on the "Exempt from Reporting" list

Leave the "present on admission" field blank if the condition is on the list of ICD-10-CM codes for which this field is not applicable. This is the only circumstance in which the field may be left blank.

POA Explicitly Documented

Assign "Y" for any condition the provider explicitly documents as being present on admission.

Assign "N" for any condition the provider explicitly documents as not present at the time of admission.

Conditions diagnosed prior to inpatient admission

Assign "Y" for conditions that were diagnosed prior to admission (example: hypertension, diabetes mellitus, asthma).

Conditions diagnosed during the admission but clearly present before admission

Assign "Y" for conditions diagnosed during the admission that were clearly present but not diagnosed until after admission occurred.

Diagnoses subsequently confirmed after admission are considered present on admission if at the time of admission they are documented as suspected, possible, rule out, differential diagnosis, or constitute an underlying cause of a symptom that is present at the time of admission.

Condition develops during outpatient encounter prior to inpatient admission

Assign "Y" for any condition that develops during an outpatient encounter prior to a written order for inpatient admission.

Documentation does not indicate whether condition was present on admission

Assign "U" when the medical record documentation is unclear as to whether the condition was present on admission. "U" should not be routinely assigned and used only in very limited circumstances. Coders are encouraged to query the providers when the documentation is unclear.

Documentation states that it cannot be determined whether the condition was or was not present on admission

Assign "W" when the medical record documentation indicates that it cannot be clinically determined whether or not the condition was present on admission.

Chronic condition with acute exacerbation during the admission

If a single code identifies both the chronic condition and the acute exacerbation, see POA guidelines pertaining to combination codes.

If a single code only identifies the chronic condition and not the acute exacerbation (e.g., acute exacerbation of chronic leukemia), assign "Y."

Conditions documented as possible, probable, suspected, or rule out at the time of discharge

If the final diagnosis contains a possible, probable, suspected, or rule out diagnosis, and this diagnosis was based on signs, symptoms or clinical findings suspected at the time of inpatient admission, assign "Y."

If the final diagnosis contains a possible, probable, suspected, or rule out diagnosis, and this diagnosis was based on signs, symptoms or clinical findings that were not present on admission, assign "N".

Conditions documented as impending or threatened at the time of discharge

If the final diagnosis contains an impending or threatened diagnosis, and this diagnosis is based on symptoms or clinical findings that were present on admission, assign "Y".

If the final diagnosis contains an impending or threatened diagnosis, and this diagnosis is based on symptoms or clinical findings that were not present on admission, assign "N".

Acute and Chronic Conditions

Assign "Y" for acute conditions that are present at time of admission and N for acute conditions that are not present at time of admission.

Assign "Y" for chronic conditions, even though the condition may not be diagnosed until after admission.

If a single code identifies both an acute and chronic condition, see the POA guidelines for combination codes.

Combination Codes

Assign "N" if any part of the combination code was not present on admission (e.g., COPD with acute exacerbation and the exacerbation was not present on admission; gastric ulcer that does not start bleeding until after admission; asthma patient develops status asthmaticus after admission).

Assign "Y" if all parts of the combination code were present on admission (e.g., patient with acute prostatitis admitted with hematuria).

If the final diagnosis includes comparative or contrasting diagnoses, and both were present, or suspected, at the time of admission, assign "Y".

For infection codes that include the causal organism, assign "Y" if the infection (or signs of the infection) was present on admission, even though the culture results may not be known until after admission (e.g., patient is admitted with pneumonia and the provider documents pseudomonas as the causal organism a few days later).

Same Diagnosis Code for Two or More Conditions

When the same ICD-10-CM diagnosis code applies to two or more conditions during the same encounter (e.g. two separate conditions classified to the same ICD-10-CM diagnosis code):

Assign "Y" if all conditions represented by the single ICD-10-CM code were present on admission (e.g. bilateral unspecified age-related cataracts).

Assign "N" if any of the conditions represented by the single ICD-10-CM code was not present on admission (e.g. traumatic secondary and recurrent hemorrhage and seroma is assigned to a single code T79.2, but only one of the conditions was present on admission).

Obstetrical conditions

Whether or not the patient delivers during the current hospitalization does not affect assignment of the POA indicator. The determining factor for POA assignment is whether the pregnancy complication or obstetrical condition described by the code was present at the time of admission or not.

If the pregnancy complication or obstetrical condition was present on admission (e.g., patient admitted in preterm labor), assign "Y".

If the pregnancy complication or obstetrical condition was not present on admission (e.g., 2nd degree laceration during delivery, postpartum hemorrhage that occurred during current hospitalization, fetal distress develops after admission), assign "N".

If the obstetrical code includes more than one diagnosis and any of the diagnoses identified by the code were not present on admission assign "N". (e.g., Category O11, Pre-existing hypertension with pre-eclampsia).

Perinatal conditions

Newborns are not considered to be admitted until after birth. Therefore, any condition present at birth or that developed in utero is considered present at admission and should be assigned "Y". This includes conditions that occur during delivery (e.g., injury during delivery, meconium aspiration, exposure to streptococcus B in the vaginal canal).

Congenital conditions and anomalies

Assign "Y" for congenital conditions and anomalies except for categories Q00-Q99, Congenital anomalies, which are on the exempt list. Congenital conditions are always considered present on admission.

External cause of injury codes

Assign "Y" for any external cause code representing an external cause of morbidity that occurred prior to inpatient admission (e.g., patient fell out of bed at home, patient fell out of bed in emergency room prior to admission).

Assign "N" for any external cause code representing an external cause of morbidity that occurred during inpatient hospitalization (e.g., patient fell out of hospital bed during hospital stay, patient experienced an adverse reaction to a medication administered after inpatient admission).

Categories and Codes Exempt from Diagnosis Present on Admission Requirement

Note: "Diagnosis present on admission" for these code categories are exempt because they represent circumstances regarding the healthcare encounter or factors influencing health status that do not represent a current disease or injury or are always present on admission.

B90–B94	Sequelae of infectious and parasitic diseases
E64	Sequelae of malnutrition and other nutritional deficiences
I25.2	Old myocardial infarction
I69	Sequelae of cerebrovascular disease
O09	Supervision of high risk pregnancy
O66.5	Attempted application of vacuum extractor and forceps
O80	Encounter for full-term uncomplicated delivery
O94	Sequelae of complication of pregnancy, childbirth, and the puerperium
P00	Newborn (suspected to be) affected by maternal conditions that may be unrelated to present pregnancy
Q00-Q99	Congenital malformations, deformations and chromosomal abnormalities

S00-T88.9	Injury, poisoning and certain other consequences of external causes with 7th character representing subsequent encounter or sequela	Z00	Encounter for general examination without complaint, suspected or reported diagnosis
V00-V09	Pedestrian injured in transport accident	Z01	Encounter for other special examination without complaint, suspected or reported diagnosis
	Except:V00.81-, Accident with wheelchair (powered) V00.83-, Accident with motorized mobility scooter	Z02	Encounter for administrative examination
V10-V19	Pedal cycle rider injured in transport accident	Z03	Encounter for medical observation for suspected diseases and conditions ruled out
V20-V29	Motorcycle rider injured in transport accident	Z08	Encounter for follow-up examination following completed treatment for malignant neoplasm
V30-V39	Occupant of three-wheeled motor vehicle injured in transport accident	Z09	Encounter for follow-up examination after completed treatment for conditions other than malignant neoplasm
V40-V49	Car occupant injured in transport accident	Z11	Encounter for screening for infectious and parasitic diseases
V50-V59	Occupant of pick-up truck or van injured in transport accident	Z11.8	Encounter for screening for other infectious and parasitic diseases
V60-V69	Occupant of heavy transport vehicle injured in transport accident	Z12	Encounter for screening for malignant neoplasms
V70-V79	Bus occupant injured in transport accident	Z13	Encounter for screening for other diseases and disorders
V80-V89	Other land transport accidents	Z13.4	Encounter for screening for certain developmental disorders in childhood
V90-V94	Water transport accidents	Z13.5	Encounter for screening for eye and ear disorders
V95-V97	Air and space transport accidents		
V98-V99	Other and unspecified transport accidents	Z13.6	Encounter for screening for cardiovascular disorders
W09	Fall on and from playground equipment	Z13.83	Encounter for screening for respiratory disorder NEC
W14	Fall from tree	Z13.89	Encounter for screening for other disorder
W15	Fall from cliff	Z14	Genetic carrier
W17.0	Fall into well	Z15	Genetic susceptibility to disease
W17.1	Fall into storm drain or manhole	Z17	Estrogen receptor status
W18.01	Striking against sports equipment with subsequent fall	Z18	Retained foreign body fragments
W21	Striking against or struck by sports equipment	Z22	Carrier of infectious disease
W30	Contact with agricultural machinery	Z23	Encounter for immunization
W31	Contact with other and unspecified machinery	Z28	Immunization not carried out and underimmunization status
W32-W34	Accidental handgun discharge and malfunction	Z28.3	Underimmunization status
W35-W40	Exposure to inanimate mechanical forces	Z30	Encounter for contraceptive management
W52	Crushed, pushed or stepped on by crowd or human stampede	Z31	Encounter for procreative management
W56	Contact with nonvenomous marine animal	Z34	Encounter for supervision of normal pregnancy
W58	Contact with crocodile or alligator	Z36	Encounter for antenatal screening of mother
W61	Contact with birds (domestic) (wild)	Z37	Outcome of delivery
W62	Contact with nonvenomous amphibians	Z38	Liveborn infants according to place of birth and type of delivery
W89	Exposure to man-made visible and ultraviolet light	Z39	Encounter for maternal postpartum care and examination
X02	Exposure to controlled fire in building or structure	Z41	Encounter for procedures for purposes other than remedying health state
X03	Exposure to controlled fire, not in building or structure	Z42	Encounter for plastic and reconstructive surgery following medical procedure or healed injury
X04	Exposure to ignition of highly flammable material		
X52	Prolonged stay in weightless environment	Z43	Encounter for attention to artificial openings
X71	Intentional self-harm by drowning and submersion	Z44	Encounter for fitting and adjustment of external prosthetic device
	Except: X71.0-, Intentional self-harm by drowning and submersion while in bath tub	Z45	Encounter for adjustment and management of implanted device
X72	Intentional self-harm by handgun discharge	Z46	Encounter for fitting and adjustment of other devices
X73	Intentional self-harm by rifle, shotgun and larger firearm discharge	Z47.8	Encounter for other orthopedic aftercare
		Z49	Encounter for care involving renal dialysis
X74	Intentional self-harm by other and unspecified firearm and gun discharge	Z51	Encounter for other aftercare
		Z51.5	Encounter for palliative care
X75	Intentional self-harm by explosive material	Z51.8	Encounter for other specified aftercare
X76	Intentional self-harm by smoke, fire and flames	Z52	Donors of organs and tissues
X77	Intentional self-harm by steam, hot vapors and hot objects	Z59	Problems related to housing and economic circumstances
X81	Intentional self-harm by jumping or lying in front of moving object	Z63	Other problems related to primary support groupincluding family circumstances
X82	Intentional self-harm by crashing of motor vehicle		
X83	Intentional self-harm by other specified means	Z65	Problems related to other psychosocial circumstances
Y03	Assault by crashing of motor vehicle	Z65.8	Other specified problems related to psychosocial circumstances
Y07	Perpetrator of assault, maltreatment and neglect	Z67.1-Z67.9	Blood type
Y08.8	Assault by strike by sports equipment	Z68	Body mass index (BMI)
Y21	Drowning and submersion, undetermined intent	Z72	Problems related to lifestyle
Y22	Handgun discharge, undetermined intent	Z74.01	Bed confinement status
Y23	Rifle, shotgun and larger firearm discharge, undetermined intent	Z76	Persons encountering health services in other circumstances
Y24	Other and unspecified firearm discharge, undetermined intent	Z77.110-Z77.128	Environmental pollution and hazards in the physical environment
Y30	Falling, jumping or pushed from a high place, undetermined intent	Z78	Other specified health status
		Z79	Long term (current) drug therapy
Y32	Assault by crashing of motor vehicle, undetermined intent	Z80	Family history of primary malignant neoplasm
Y36	Operations of war	Z81	Family history of mental and behavioral disorders
Y37	Military operations	Z82	Family history of certain disabilities and chronic diseases (leading to disablement)
Y92	Place of occurrence of the external cause		
Y93	Activity code	Z83	Family history of other specific disorders
Y99	External cause status		

Z84	Family history of other conditions	Z92	Personal history of medical treatment
Z85	Personal history of primary malignant neoplasm	Z93	Artificial opening status
Z86	Personal history of certain other diseases	Z94	Transplanted organ and tissue status
Z87	Personal history of other diseases and conditions	Z95	Presence of cardiac and vascular implants and grafts
Z87.828	Personal history of other (healed) physical injury and trauma	Z97	Presence of other devices
Z87.891	Personal history of nicotine dependence	Z98	Other postprocedural states
Z88	Allergy status to drugs, medicaments and biological substances	Z99	Dependence on enabling machines and devices, not elsewhere classified
Z89	Acquired absence of limb		
Z90.710	Acquired absence of both cervix and uterus		
Z91.0	Allergy status, other than to drugs and biological substances		
Z91.4	Personal history of psychological trauma, not elsewhere classified		
Z91.5	Personal history of self-harm		
Z91.8	Other specified risk factors, not elsewhere classified		

A

Aarskog's syndrome Q87.1
Abandonment — *see* Maltreatment
Abasia (-astasia) (hysterical) F44.4
Abderhalden-Kaufmann-Lignac syndrome (cystinosis) E72.04
Abdomen, abdominal (*see also* condition)
  acute R10.0
  angina K55.1
  muscle deficiency syndrome Q79.4
Abdominalgia — *see* Pain, abdominal
Abduction contracture, hip or other joint — *see* Contraction, joint
Aberrant (congenital) (*see also* Malposition, congenital)
  adrenal gland Q89.1
  artery (peripheral) Q27.8
    basilar NEC Q28.1
    cerebral Q28.3
    coronary Q24.5
    digestive system Q27.8
    eye Q15.8
    lower limb Q27.8
    precerebral Q28.1
    pulmonary Q25.79
    renal Q27.2
    retina Q14.1
    specified site NEC Q27.8
    subclavian Q27.8
    upper limb Q27.8
    vertebral Q28.1
  breast Q83.8
  endocrine gland NEC Q89.2
  hepatic duct Q44.5
  pancreas Q45.3
  parathyroid gland Q89.2
  pituitary gland Q89.2
  sebaceous glands, mucous membrane, mouth, congenital Q38.6
  spleen Q89.09
  subclavian artery Q27.8
  thymus (gland) Q89.2
  thyroid gland Q89.2
  vein (peripheral) NEC Q27.8
    cerebral Q28.3
    digestive system Q27.8
    lower limb Q27.8
    precerebral Q28.1
    specified site NEC Q27.8
    upper limb Q27.8
Aberration
  distantial — *see* Disturbance, visual
  mental F99
Abetalipoproteinemia E78.6
Abiotrophy R68.89
Ablatio, ablation
  retinae — *see* Detachment, retina
Ablepharia, ablepharon Q10.3
Abnormal, abnormality, abnormalities (*see also* Anomaly)
  acid-base balance (mixed) E87.4
  albumin R77.0
  alphafetoprotein R77.2
  alveolar ridge K08.9
  anatomical relationship Q89.9
  apertures, congenital, diaphragm Q79.1
  auditory perception H93.29- ☑
    diplacusis — *see* Diplacusis
    hyperacusis — *see* Hyperacusis
    recruitment — *see* Recruitment, auditory
    threshold shift — *see* Shift, auditory threshold
  autosomes Q99.9
    fragile site Q95.5
  basal metabolic rate R94.8
  biosynthesis, testicular androgen E29.1
  bleeding time R79.1
  blood level (of)
    cobalt R79.0
    copper R79.0
    iron R79.0
    lithium R78.89

Abnormal, abnormality, abnormalities — *continued*
  blood level — *continued*
    magnesium R79.0
    mineral NEC R79.0
    zinc R79.0
  blood pressure
    elevated R03.0
    low reading (nonspecific) R03.1
  blood sugar R73.09
  blood-gas level R79.81
  bowel sounds R19.15
    absent R19.11
    hyperactive R19.12
  brain scan R94.02
  breathing R06.9
  caloric test R94.138
  cerebrospinal fluid R83.9
    cytology R83.6
    drug level R83.2
    enzyme level R83.0
    hormones R83.1
    immunology R83.4
    microbiology R83.5
    nonmedicinal level R83.3
    specified type NEC R83.8
  chemistry, blood R79.9
    C-reactive protein R79.82
    drugs — *see* Findings, abnormal, in blood
    gas level R79.81
    minerals R79.0
    pancytopenia D61.818
    PTT R79.1
    specified NEC R79.89
    toxins — *see* Findings, abnormal, in blood
  chest sounds (friction) (rales) R09.89
  chromosome, chromosomal Q99.9
    with more than three X chromosomes, female Q97.1
    analysis result R89.8
      bronchial washings R84.8
      cerebrospinal fluid R83.8
      cervix uteri NEC R87.89
      nasal secretions R84.8
      nipple discharge R89.8
      peritoneal fluid R85.89
      pleural fluid R84.8
      prostatic secretions R86.8
      saliva R85.89
      seminal fluid R86.8
      sputum R84.8
      synovial fluid R89.8
      throat scrapings R84.8
      vagina R87.89
      vulva R87.89
      wound secretions R89.8
    dicentric replacement Q93.2
    ring replacement Q93.2
    sex Q99.8
      female phenotype Q97.9
        specified NEC Q97.8
      male phenotype Q98.9
        specified NEC Q98.8
      structural male Q98.6
    specified NEC Q99.8
  clinical findings NEC R68.89
  coagulation D68.9
    newborn, transient P61.6
    profile R79.1
    time R79.1
  communication — *see* Fistula
  conjunctiva, vascular H11.41- ☑
  coronary artery Q24.5
  cortisol-binding globulin E27.8
  course, eustachian tube Q17.8
  creatinine clearance R94.4
  cytology
    anus R85.619
      atypical squamous cells cannot exclude high grade squamous intraepithelial lesion (ASC-H) R85.611
      atypical squamous cells of undetermined significance (ASC-US) R85.610

Abnormal, abnormality, abnormalities — *continued*
  cytology — *continued*
    anus — *continued*
      cytologic evidence of malignancy R85.614
      high grade squamous intraepithelial lesion (HGSIL) R85.613
      human papillomavirus (HPV) DNA test
        high risk positive R85.81
        low risk postive R85.82
      inadequate smear R85.615
      low grade squamous intraepithelial lesion (LGSIL) R85.612
      satisfactory anal smear but lacking transformation zone R85.616
      specified NEC R85.618
      unsatisfactory smear R85.615
    female genital organs — *see* Abnormal, Papanicolaou (smear)
  dark adaptation curve H53.61
  dentofacial NEC — *see* Anomaly, dentofacial
  development, developmental Q89.9
    central nervous system Q07.9
  diagnostic imaging
    abdomen, abdominal region NEC R93.5
    biliary tract R93.2
    breast R92.8
    central nervous system NEC R90.89
    cerebrovascular NEC R90.89
    coronary circulation R93.1
    digestive tract NEC R93.3
    gastrointestinal (tract) R93.3
    genitourinary organs R93.8
    head R93.0
    heart R93.1
    intrathoracic organ NEC R93.8
    limbs R93.6
    liver R93.2
    lung (field) R91.8
    musculoskeletal system NEC R93.7
    retroperitoneum R93.5
    site specified NEC R93.8
    skin and subcutaneous tissue R93.8
    skull R93.0
    urinary organs R93.4
  direction, teeth, fully erupted M26.30
  ear ossicles, acquired NEC H74.39- ☑
    ankylosis — *see* Ankylosis, ear ossicles
    discontinuity — *see* Discontinuity, ossicles, ear
    partial loss — *see* Loss, ossicles, ear (partial)
  Ebstein Q22.5
  echocardiogram R93.1
  echoencephalogram R90.81
  echogram — *see* Abnormal, diagnostic imaging
  electrocardiogram [ECG] [EKG] R94.31
  electroencephalogram [EEG] R94.01
  electrolyte — *see* Imbalance, electrolyte
  electromyogram [EMG] R94.131
  electro-oculogram [EOG] R94.110
  electrophysiological intracardiac studies R94.39
  electroretinogram [ERG] R94.111
  erythrocytes
    congenital, with perinatal jaundice D58.9
  feces (color) (contents) (mucus) R19.5
  finding — *see* Findings, abnormal, without diagnosis
  fluid
    amniotic — *see* Abnormal, specimen, specified
    cerebrospinal — *see* Abnormal, cerebrospinal fluid
    peritoneal — *see* Abnormal, specimen, digestive organs
    pleural — *see* Abnormal, specimen, respiratory organs
    synovial — *see* Abnormal, specimen, specified
    thorax (bronchial washings) (pleural fluid) — *see* Abnormal, specimen, respiratory organs
    vaginal — *see* Abnormal, specimen, female genital organs
  form
    teeth K00.2
    uterus — *see* Anomaly, uterus
  function studies
    auditory R94.120
    bladder R94.8

Abnormal, abnormality, abnormalities — *continued*
- function studies — *continued*
  - brain R94.09
  - cardiovascular R94.30
  - ear R94.128
  - endocrine NEC R94.7
  - eye NEC R94.118
  - kidney R94.4
  - liver R94.5
  - nervous system
    - central NEC R94.09
    - peripheral NEC R94.138
  - pancreas R94.8
  - placenta R94.8
  - pulmonary R94.2
  - special senses NEC R94.128
  - spleen R94.8
  - thyroid R94.6
  - vestibular R94.121
- gait — *see* Gait
  - hysterical F44.4
- gastrin secretion E16.4
- globulin R77.1
  - cortisol-binding E27.8
  - thyroid-binding E07.89
- glomerular, minor (*see also* N00-N07 with fourth character .0) N05.0
- glucagon secretion E16.3
- glucose tolerance (test) (non-fasting) R73.09
- gravitational (G) forces or states (effect of) T75.81 ☑
- hair (color) (shaft) L67.9
  - specified NEC L67.8
- hard tissue formation in pulp (dental) K04.3
- head movement R25.0
- heart
  - rate R00.9
    - specified NEC R00.8
  - shadow R93.1
  - sounds NEC R01.2
- hemoglobin (disease) (*see also* Disease, hemoglobin) D58.2
  - trait — *see* Trait, hemoglobin, abnormal
- histology NEC R89.7
- immunological findings R89.4
  - in serum R76.9
    - specified NEC R76.8
- increase in appetite R63.2
- involuntary movement — *see* Abnormal, movement, involuntary
- jaw closure M26.51
- karyotype R89.8
- kidney function test R94.4
- knee jerk R29.2
- leukocyte (cell) (differential) NEC D72.9
- liver
- loss of
  - height R29.890
  - weight R63.4
- mammogram NEC R92.8
  - calcification (calculus) R92.1
  - microcalcification R92.0
- Mantoux test R76.11
- movement (disorder) (*see also* Disorder, movement)
  - head R25.0
  - involuntary R25.9
    - fasciculation R25.3
    - of head R25.0
    - spasm R25.2
    - specified type NEC R25.8
    - tremor R25.1
- myoglobin (Aberdeen) (Annapolis) R89.7
- neonatal screening P09
- oculomotor study R94.113
- palmar creases Q82.8
- Papanicolaou (smear)
  - anus R85.619
    - atypical squamous cells cannot exclude high grade squamous intraepithelial lesion (ASC-H) R85.611
    - atypical squamous cells of undetermined significance (ASC-US) R85.610
    - cytologic evidence of malignancy R85.614
    - high grade squamous intraepithelial lesion (HGSIL) R85.613
    - human papillomavirus (HPV) DNA test
      - high risk positive R85.81
      - low risk positve R85.82

Abnormal, abnormality, abnormalities — *continued*
- Papanicolaou — *continued*
  - anus — *continued*
    - inadequate smear R85.615
    - low grade squamous intraepithelial lesion (LGSIL) R85.612
    - satisfactory anal smear but lacking transformation zone R85.616
    - specified NEC R85.618
    - unsatisfactory smear R85.615
  - bronchial washings R84.6
  - cerebrospinal fluid R83.6
  - cervix R87.619
    - atypical squamous cells cannot exclude high grade squamous intraepithelial lesion (ASC-H) R87.611
    - atypical squamous cells of undetermined significance (ASC-US) R87.610
    - cytologic evidence of malignancy R87.614
    - high grade squamous intraepithelial lesion (HGSIL) R87.613
    - inadequate smear R87.615
    - low grade squamous intraepithelial lesion (LGSIL) R87.612
    - non-atypical endometrial cells R87.618
    - satisfactory cervical smear but lacking transformation zone R87.616
    - specified NEC R87.618
    - thin preparaton R87.619
    - unsatisfactory smear R87.615
  - nasal secretions R84.6
  - nipple discharge R89.6
  - peritoneal fluid R85.69
  - pleural fluid R84.6
  - prostatic secretions R86.6
  - saliva R85.69
  - seminal fluid R86.6
  - sites NEC R89.6
  - sputum R84.6
  - synovial fluid R89.6
  - throat scrapings R84.6
  - vagina R87.629
    - atypical squamous cells cannot exclude high grade squamous intraepithelial lesion (ASC-H) R87.621
    - atypical squamous cells of undetermined significance (ASC-US) R87.620
    - cytologic evidence of malignancy R87.624
    - high grade squamous intraepithelial lesion (HGSIL) R87.623
    - inadequate smear R87.625
    - low grade squamous intraepithelial lesion (LGSIL) R87.622
    - specified NEC R87.628
    - thin preparation R87.629
    - unsatisfactory smear R87.625
  - vulva R87.69
  - wound secretions R89.6
- partial thromboplastin time (PTT) R79.1
- pelvis (bony) — *see* Deformity, pelvis
- percussion, chest (tympany) R09.89
- periods (grossly) — *see* Menstruation
- phonocardiogram R94.39
- plantar reflex R29.2
- plasma
  - protein R77.9
    - specified NEC R77.8
  - viscosity R70.1
- pleural (folds) Q34.0
- posture R29.3
- product of conception O02.9
  - specified type NEC O02.89
- prothrombin time (PT) R79.1
- pulmonary
  - artery, congenital Q25.79
  - function, newborn P28.89
  - test results R94.2
- pulsations in neck R00.2
- pupillary H21.56- ☑
  - function (reaction) (reflex) — *see* Anomaly, pupil, function
- radiological examination — *see* Abnormal, diagnostic imaging
- red blood cell(s) (morphology) (volume) R71.8
- reflex — *see* Reflex
- renal function test R94.4
- response to nerve stimulation R94.130

Abnormal, abnormality, abnormalities — *continued*
- retinal correspondence H53.31
- retinal function study R94.111
- rhythm, heart (*see also* Arrhythmia)
- saliva — *see* Abnormal, specimen, digestive organs
- scan
  - kidney R94.4
  - liver R93.2
  - thyroid R94.6
- secretion
  - gastrin E16.4
  - glucagon E16.3
- semen, seminal fluid — *see* Abnormal, specimen, male genital organs
- serum level (of)
  - acid phosphatase R74.8
  - alkaline phosphatase R74.8
  - amylase R74.8
  - enzymes R74.9
    - specified NEC R74.8
  - lipase R74.8
  - triacylglycerol lipase R74.8
- shape
  - gravid uterus — *see* Anomaly, uterus
- sinus venosus Q21.1
- size, tooth, teeth K00.2
- spacing, tooth, teeth, fully erupted M26.30
- specimen
  - digestive organs (peritoneal fluid) (saliva) R85.9
    - cytology R85.69
    - drug level R85.2
    - enzyme level R85.0
    - histology R85.7
    - hormones R85.1
    - immunology R85.4
    - microbiology R85.5
    - nonmedicinal level R85.3
    - specified type NEC R85.89
  - female genital organs (secretions) (smears) R87.9
    - cytology R87.69
      - cervix R87.619
        - human papillomavirus (HPV) DNA test
          - high risk positive R87.810
          - low risk positive R87.820
        - inadequate (unsatisfactory) smear R87.615
        - non-atypical endometrial cells R87.618
        - specified NEC R87.618
      - vagina R87.629
        - human papillomavirus (HPV) DNA test
          - high risk positive R87.811
          - low risk positive R87.821
        - inadequate (unsatisfactory) smear R87.625
      - vulva R87.69
    - drug level R87.2
    - enzyme level R87.0
    - histological R87.7
    - hormones R87.1
    - immunology R87.4
    - microbiology R87.5
    - nonmedicinal level R87.3
    - specified type NEC R87.89
  - male genital organs (prostatic secretions) (semen) R86.9
    - cytology R86.6
    - drug level R86.2
    - enzyme level R86.0
    - histological R86.7
    - hormones R86.1
    - immunology R86.4
    - microbiology R86.5
    - nonmedicinal level R86.3
    - specified type NEC R86.8
  - nipple discharge — *see* Abnormal, specimen, specified
  - respiratory organs (bronchial washings) (nasal secretions) (pleural fluid) (sputum) R84.9
    - cytology R84.6
    - drug level R84.2
    - enzyme level R84.0
    - histology R84.7
    - hormones R84.1
    - immunology R84.4
    - microbiology R84.5
    - nonmedicinal level R84.3
    - specified type NEC R84.8

Abnormal, abnormality, abnormalities — *continued*
 specimen — *continued*
 specified organ, system and tissue NOS R89.9
 cytology R89.6
 drug level R89.2
 enzyme level R89.0
 histology R89.7
 hormones R89.1
 immunology R89.4
 microbiology R89.5
 nonmedicinal level R89.3
 specified type NEC R89.8
 synovial fluid — *see* Abnormal, specimen, specified
 thorax (bronchial washings) (pleural fluids) — *see* Abnormal, specimen, respiratory organs
 vagina (secretion) (smear) R87.629
 vulva (secretion) (smear) R87.69
 wound secretion — *see* Abnormal, specimen, specified
 spermatozoa — *see* Abnormal, specimen, male genital organs
 sputum (amount) (color) (odor) R09.3
 stool (color) (contents) (mucus) R19.5
 bloody K92.1
 guaiac positive R19.5
 synchondrosis Q78.8
 thermography (*see also* Abnormal, diagnostic imaging) R93.8
 thyroid-binding globulin E07.89
 tooth, teeth (form) (size) K00.2
 toxicology (findings) R78.9
 transport protein E88.09
 tumor marker NEC R97.8
 ultrasound results — *see* Abnormal, diagnostic imaging
 umbilical cord complicating delivery O69.9 ☑
 urination NEC R39.19
 urine (constituents) R82.90
 bile R82.2
 cytological examination R82.8
 drugs R82.5
 fat R82.0
 glucose R81
 heavy metals R82.6
 hemoglobin R82.3
 histological examination R82.8
 ketones R82.4
 microbiological examination (culture) R82.7
 myoglobin R82.1
 positive culture R82.7
 protein — *see* Proteinuria
 specified substance NEC R82.99
 chromoabnormality NEC R82.91
 substances nonmedical R82.6
 uterine hemorrhage — *see* Hemorrhage, uterus
 vectorcardiogram R94.39
 visually evoked potential (VEP) R94.112
 white blood cells D72.9
 specified NEC D72.89
 X-ray examination — *see* Abnormal, diagnostic imaging
Abnormity (any organ or part) — *see* Anomaly
Abocclusion M26.29
 hemolytic disease (newborn) P55.1
 incompatibility reaction ABO — *see* Complication(s), transfusion, incompatibility reaction, ABO
Abolition, language R48.8
Aborter, habitual or recurrent — *see* Loss (of), pregnancy, recurrent
Abortion (complete) (spontaneous) O03.9
 with
 retained products of conception — *see* Abortion, incomplete
 attempted (elective) (failed) O07.4
 complicated by O07.30
 afibrinogenemia O07.1
 cardiac arrest O07.36
 chemical damage of pelvic organ(s) O07.34
 circulatory collapse O07.31
 cystitis O07.38
 defibrination syndrome O07.1
 electrolyte imbalance O07.33
 embolism (air) (amniotic fluid) (blood clot) (fat) (pulmonary) (septic) (soap) O07.2
 endometritis O07.0
 genital tract and pelvic infection O07.0
 hemolysis O07.1

Abortion — *continued*
 attempted — *continued*
 complicated by — *continued*
 hemorrhage (delayed) (excessive) O07.1
 infection
 genital tract or pelvic O07.0
 urinary tract tract O07.38
 intravascular coagulation O07.1
 laceration of pelvic organ(s) O07.34
 metabolic disorder O07.33
 oliguria O07.32
 oophoritis O07.0
 parametritis O07.0
 pelvic peritonitis O07.0
 perforation of pelvic organ(s) O07.34
 renal failure or shutdown O07.32
 salpingitis or salpingo-oophoritis O07.0
 sepsis O07.37
 shock O07.31
 specified condition NEC O07.39
 tubular necrosis (renal) O07.32
 uremia O07.32
 urinary tract infection O07.38
 venous complication NEC O07.35
 embolism (air) (amniotic fluid) (blood clot) (fat) (pulmonary) (septic) (soap) O07.2
 complicated (by) (following) O03.80
 afibrinogenemia O03.6
 cardiac arrest O03.86
 chemical damage of pelvic organ(s) O03.84
 circulatory collapse O03.81
 cystitis O03.88
 defibrination syndrome O03.6
 electrolyte imbalance O03.83
 embolism (air) (amniotic fluid) (blood clot) (fat) (pulmonary) (septic) (soap) O03.7
 endometritis O03.5
 genital tract and pelvic infection O03.5
 hemolysis O03.6
 hemorrhage (delayed) (excessive) O03.6
 infection
 genital tract or pelvic O03.5
 urinary tract O03.88
 intravascular coagulation O03.6
 laceration of pelvic organ(s) O03.84
 metabolic disorder O03.83
 oliguria O03.82
 oophoritis O03.5
 parametritis O03.5
 pelvic peritonitis O03.5
 perforation of pelvic organ(s) O03.84
 renal failure or shutdown O03.82
 salpingitis or salpingo-oophoritis O03.5
 sepsis O03.87
 shock O03.81
 specified condition NEC O03.89
 tubular necrosis (renal) O03.82
 uremia O03.82
 urinary tract infection O03.88
 venous complication NEC O03.85
 embolism (air) (amniotic fluid) (blood clot) (fat) (pulmonary) (septic) (soap) O03.7
 failed — *see* Abortion, attempted
 habitual or recurrent N96
 with current abortion — *see* categories O03-O06
 without current pregnancy N96
 care in current pregnancy O26.2- ☑
 incomplete (spontaneous) O03.4
 complicated (by) (following) O03.30
 afibrinogenemia O03.1
 cardiac arrest O03.36
 chemical damage of pelvic organ(s) O03.34
 circulatory collapse O03.31
 cystitis O03.38
 defibrination syndrome O03.1
 electrolyte imbalance O03.33
 embolism (air) (amniotic fluid) (blood clot) (fat) (pulmonary) (septic) (soap) O03.2
 endometritis O03.0
 genital tract and pelvic infection O03.0
 hemolysis O03.1
 hemorrhage (delayed) (excessive) O03.1
 infection
 genital tract or pelvic O03.0
 urinary tract O03.38
 intravascular coagulation O03.1
 laceration of pelvic organ(s) O03.34
 metabolic disorder O03.33

Abortion — *continued*
 incomplete — *continued*
 complicated — *continued*
 oliguria O03.32
 oophoritis O03.0
 parametritis O03.0
 pelvic peritonitis O03.0
 perforation of pelvic organ(s) O03.34
 renal failure or shutdown O03.32
 salpingitis or salpingo-oophoritis O03.0
 sepsis O03.37
 shock O03.31
 specified condition NEC O03.39
 tubular necrosis (renal) O03.32
 uremia O03.32
 urinary infection O03.38
 venous complication NEC O03.35
 embolism (air) (amniotic fluid) (blood clot) (fat) (pulmonary) (septic) (soap) O03.2
 induced (encounter for) Z33.2
 complicated by O04.80
 afibrinogenemia O04.6
 cardiac arrest O04.86
 chemical damage of pelvic organ(s) O04.84
 circulatory collapse O04.81
 cystitis O04.88
 defibrination syndrome O04.6
 electrolyte imbalance O04.83
 embolism (air) (amniotic fluid) (blood clot) (fat) (pulmonary) (septic) (soap) O04.7
 endometritis O04.5
 genital tract and pelvic infection O04.5
 hemolysis O04.6
 hemorrhage (delayed) (excessive) O04.6
 infection
 genital tract or pelvic O04.5
 urinary tract O04.88
 intravascular coagulation O04.6
 laceration of pelvic organ(s) O04.84
 metabolic disorder O04.83
 oliguria O04.82
 oophoritis O04.5
 parametritis O04.5
 pelvic peritonitis O04.5
 perforation of pelvic organ(s) O04.84
 renal failure or shutdown O04.82
 salpingitis or salpingo-oophoritis O04.5
 sepsis O04.87
 shock O04.81
 specified condition NEC O04.89
 tubular necrosis (renal) O04.82
 uremia O04.82
 urinary tract infection O04.88
 venous complication NEC O04.85
 embolism (air) (amniotic fluid) (blood clot) (fat) (pulmonary) (septic) (soap) O04.7
 missed O02.1
 spontaneous — *see* Abortion (complete) (spontaneous)
 threatened O20.0
 threatened (spontaneous) O20.0
 tubal O00.1
Abortus fever A23.1
Aboulomania F60.7
Abrami's disease D59.8
Abramov-Fiedler myocarditis (acute isolated myocarditis) I40.1
Abrasion T14.8
 abdomen, abdominal (wall) S30.811 ☑
 alveolar process S00.512 ☑
 ankle S90.51- ☑
 antecubital space — *see* Abrasion, elbow
 anus S30.817 ☑
 arm (upper) S40.81- ☑
 auditory canal — *see* Abrasion, ear
 auricle — *see* Abrasion, ear
 axilla — *see* Abrasion, arm
 back, lower S30.810 ☑
 breast S20.11- ☑
 brow S00.81 ☑
 buttock S30.810 ☑
 calf — *see* Abrasion, leg
 canthus — *see* Abrasion, eyelid
 cheek S00.81 ☑
 internal S00.512 ☑
 chest wall — *see* Abrasion, thorax
 chin S00.81 ☑
 clitoris S30.814 ☑

Abrasion — *continued*
cornea S05.0- ☑
costal region — *see* Abrasion, thorax
dental K03.1
digit(s)
  foot — *see* Abrasion, toe
  hand — *see* Abrasion, finger
ear S00.41- ☑
elbow S50.31- ☑
epididymis S30.813 ☑
epigastric region S30.811 ☑
epiglottis S10.11 ☑
esophagus (thoracic) S27.818 ☑
  cervical S10.11 ☑
eyebrow — *see* Abrasion, eyelid
eyelid S00.21- ☑
face S00.81 ☑
finger(s) S60.41- ☑
  index S60.41- ☑
  little S60.41- ☑
  middle S60.41- ☑
  ring S60.41- ☑
flank S30.811 ☑
foot (except toe(s) alone) S90.81- ☑
  toe — *see* Abrasion, toe
forearm S50.81- ☑
  elbow only — *see* Abrasion, elbow
forehead S00.81 ☑
genital organs, external
  female S30.816 ☑
  male S30.815 ☑
groin S30.811 ☑
gum S00.512 ☑
hand S60.51- ☑
head S00.91 ☑
  ear — *see* Abrasion, ear
  eyelid — *see* Abrasion, eyelid
  lip S00.511 ☑
  nose S00.31 ☑
  oral cavity S00.512 ☑
  scalp S00.01 ☑
  specified site NEC S00.81 ☑
heel — *see* Abrasion, foot
hip S70.21- ☑
inguinal region S30.811 ☑
interscapular region S20.419 ☑
jaw S00.81 ☑
knee S80.21- ☑
labium (majus) (minus) S30.814 ☑
larynx S10.11 ☑
leg (lower) S80.81- ☑
  knee — *see* Abrasion, knee
  upper — *see* Abrasion, thigh
lip S00.511 ☑
lower back S30.810 ☑
lumbar region S30.810 ☑
malar region S00.81 ☑
mammary — *see* Abrasion, breast
mastoid region S00.81 ☑
mouth S00.512 ☑
nail
  finger — *see* Abrasion, finger
  toe — *see* Abrasion, toe
nape S10.81 ☑
nasal S00.31 ☑
neck S10.91 ☑
  specified site NEC S10.81 ☑
  throat S10.11 ☑
nose S00.31 ☑
occipital region S00.01 ☑
oral cavity S00.512 ☑
orbital region — *see* Abrasion, eyelid
palate S00.512 ☑
palm — *see* Abrasion, hand
parietal region S00.01 ☑
pelvis S30.810 ☑
penis S30.812 ☑
perineum
  female S30.814 ☑
  male S30.810 ☑
periocular area — *see* Abrasion, eyelid
phalanges
  finger — *see* Abrasion, finger
  toe — *see* Abrasion, toe
pharynx S10.11 ☑
pinna — *see* Abrasion, ear

Abrasion — *continued*
popliteal space — *see* Abrasion, knee
prepuce S30.812 ☑
pubic region S30.810 ☑
pudendum
  female S30.816 ☑
  male S30.815 ☑
sacral region S30.810 ☑
scalp S00.01 ☑
scapular region — *see* Abrasion, shoulder
scrotum S30.813 ☑
shin — *see* Abrasion, leg
shoulder S40.21- ☑
skin NEC T14.8
sternal region S20.319 ☑
submaxillary region S00.81 ☑
submental region S00.81 ☑
subungual
  finger(s) — *see* Abrasion, finger
  toe(s) — *see* Abrasion, toe
supraclavicular fossa S10.81 ☑
supraorbital S00.81 ☑
temple S00.81 ☑
temporal region S00.81 ☑
testis S30.813 ☑
thigh S70.31- ☑
thorax, thoracic (wall) S20.91 ☑
  back S20.41- ☑
  front S20.31- ☑
throat S10.11 ☑
thumb S60.31- ☑
toe(s) (lesser) S90.416 ☑
  great S90.41- ☑
tongue S00.512 ☑
tooth, teeth (dentifrice) (habitual) (hard tissues) (occupational) (ritual) (traditional) K03.1
trachea S10.11 ☑
tunica vaginalis S30.813 ☑
tympanum, tympanic membrane — *see* Abrasion, ear
uvula S00.512 ☑
vagina S30.814 ☑
vocal cords S10.11 ☑
vulva S30.814 ☑
wrist S60.81- ☑

Abrism — *see* Poisoning, food, noxious, plant
Abruptio placentae O45.9- ☑
  with
    afibrinogenemia O45.01- ☑
    coagulation defect O45.00- ☑
      specified NEC O45.09- ☑
    disseminated intravascular coagulation O45.02- ☑
    hypofibrinogenemia O45.01- ☑
  specified NEC O45.8- ☑
Abruption, placenta — *see* Abruptio placentae
Abscess (connective tissue) (embolic) (fistulous) (infective) (metastatic) (multiple) (pernicious) (pyogenic) (septic) L02.91
  with
    diverticular disease (intestine) K57.80
      with bleeding K57.81
      large intestine K57.20
        with
          bleeding K57.21
          small intestine K57.40
            with bleeding K57.41
      small intestine K57.00
        with
          bleeding K57.01
          large intestine K57.40
            with bleeding K57.41
    lymphangitis — *code by* site under Abscess
  abdomen, abdominal
    cavity K65.1
    wall L02.211
  abdominopelvic K65.1
  accessory sinus — *see* Sinusitis
  adrenal (capsule) (gland) E27.8
  alveolar K04.7
    with sinus K04.6
  amebic A06.4
    brain (and liver or lung abscess) A06.6
    genitourinary tract A06.82
    liver (without mention of brain or lung abscess) A06.4
    lung (and liver) (without mention of brain abscess) A06.5
    specified site NEC A06.89

Abscess — *continued*
  amebic — *continued*
    spleen A06.89
  anerobic A48.0
  ankle — *see* Abscess, lower limb
  anorectal K61.2
  antecubital space — *see* Abscess, upper limb
  antrum (chronic) (Highmore) — *see* Sinusitis, maxillary
  anus K61.0
  apical (tooth) K04.7
    with sinus (alveolar) K04.6
  appendix K35.3
  areola (acute) (chronic) (nonpuerperal) N61
    puerperal, postpartum or gestational — *see* Infection, nipple
  arm (any part) — *see* Abscess, upper limb
  artery (wall) I77.89
  atheromatous I77.2
  auricle, ear — *see* Abscess, ear, external
  axilla (region) L02.41- ☑
    lymph gland or node L04.2
  back (any part, except buttock) L02.212
  Bartholin's gland N75.1
    with
      abortion — *see* Abortion, by type complicated by, sepsis
      ectopic or molar pregnancy O08.0
    following ectopic or molar pregnancy O08.0
  Bezold's — *see* Mastoiditis, acute
  bilharziasis B65.1
  bladder (wall) — *see* Cystitis, specified type NEC
  bone (subperiosteal) (*see also* Osteomyelitis, specified type NEC)
    accessory sinus (chronic) — *see* Sinusitis
    chronic or old — *see* Osteomyelitis, chronic
    jaw (lower) (upper) M27.2
    mastoid — *see* Mastoiditis, acute, subperiosteal
    petrous — *see* Petrositis
    spinal (tuberculous) A18.01
      nontuberculous — *see* Osteomyelitis, vertebra
  bowel K63.0
  brain (any part) (cystic) (otogenic) G06.0
    amebic (with abscess of any other site) A06.6
    gonococcal A54.82
    pheomycotic (chromomycotic) B43.1
    tuberculous A17.81
  breast (acute) (chronic) (nonpuerperal) N61
    newborn P39.0
    puerperal, postpartum, gestational — *see* Mastitis, obstetric, purulent
  broad ligament N73.2
    acute N73.0
    chronic N73.1
  Brodie's (localized) (chronic) M86.8X- ☑
  bronchi J98.09
  buccal cavity K12.2
  bulbourethral gland N34.0
  bursa M71.00
    ankle M71.07- ☑
    elbow M71.02- ☑
    foot M71.07- ☑
    hand M71.04- ☑
    hip M71.05- ☑
    knee M71.06- ☑
    multiple sites M71.09
    pharyngeal J39.1
    shoulder M71.01- ☑
    specified site NEC M71.08
    wrist M71.03- ☑
  buttock L02.31
  canthus — *see* Blepharoconjunctivitis
  cartilage — *see* Disorder, cartilage, specified type NEC
  cecum K35.3
  cerebellum, cerebellar G06.0
    sequelae G09
  cerebral (embolic) G06.0
    sequelae G09
  cervical (meaning neck) L02.11
    lymph gland or node L04.0
  cervix (stump) (uteri) — *see* Cervicitis
  cheek (external) L02.01
    inner K12.2
  chest J86.9
    with fistula J86.0
    wall L02.213
  chin L02.01
  choroid — *see* Inflammation, chorioretinal

Abscess — *continued*
circumtonsillar J36
cold (lung) (tuberculous) (*see also* Tuberculosis, abscess, lung)
  articular — *see* Tuberculosis, joint
colon (wall) K63.0
colostomy K94.02
conjunctiva — *see* Conjunctivitis, acute
cornea H16.31- ☑
corpus
  cavernosum N48.21
  luteum — *see* Oophoritis
Cowper's gland N34.0
cranium G06.0
cul-de-sac (Douglas') (posterior) — *see* Peritonitis, pelvic, female
cutaneous — *see* Abscess, by site
dental K04.7
  with sinus (alveolar) K04.6
dentoalveolar K04.7
  with sinus K04.6
diaphragm, diaphragmatic K65.1
Douglas' cul-de-sac or pouch — *see* Peritonitis, pelvic, female
Dubois A50.59
ear (middle) (*see also* Otitis, media, suppurative)
  acute — *see* Otitis, media, suppurative, acute
  external H60.0- ☑
entamebic — *see* Abscess, amebic
enterostomy K94.12
epididymis N45.4
epidural G06.2
  brain G06.0
  spinal cord G06.1
epiglottis J38.7
epiploon, epiploic K65.1
erysipelatous — *see* Erysipelas
esophagus K20.8
ethmoid (bone) (chronic) (sinus) J32.2
external auditory canal — *see* Abscess, ear, external
extradural G06.2
  brain G06.0
    sequelae G09
  spinal cord G06.1
extraperitoneal K68.19
eye — *see* Endophthalmitis, purulent
eyelid H00.03- ☑
face (any part, except ear, eye and nose) L02.01
fallopian tube — *see* Salpingitis
fascia M72.8
fauces J39.1
fecal K63.0
femoral (region) — *see* Abscess, lower limb
filaria, filarial — *see* Infestation, filarial
finger (any) (*see also* Abscess, hand)
  nail — *see* Cellulitis, finger
foot L02.61- ☑
forehead L02.01
frontal sinus (chronic) J32.1
gallbladder K81.0
genital organ or tract
  female (external) N76.4
  male N49.9
    multiple sites N49.8
    specified NEC N49.8
gestational mammary O91.11- ☑
gestational subareolar O91.11- ☑
gingival K05.21
gland, glandular (lymph) (acute) — *see* Lymphadenitis, acute
gluteal (region) L02.31
gonorrheal — *see* Gonococcus
groin L02.214
gum K05.21
hand L02.51- ☑
head NEC L02.811
  face (any part, except ear, eye and nose) L02.01
heart — *see* Carditis
heel — *see* Abscess, foot
helminthic — *see* Infestation, helminth
hepatic (cholangitic) (hematogenic) (lymphogenic) (pylephlebitic) K75.0
  amebic A06.4
hip (region) — *see* Abscess, lower limb
ileocecal K35.3
ileostomy (bud) K94.12

Abscess — *continued*
iliac (region) L02.214
  fossa K35.3
infraclavicular (fossa) — *see* Abscess, upper limb
inguinal (region) L02.214
  lymph gland or node L04.1
intestine, intestinal NEC K63.0
  rectal K61.1
intra-abdominal (*see also* Abscess, peritoneum) K65.1
  postoperative T81.4 ☑
    retroperitoneal K68.11
intracranial G06.0
intramammary — *see* Abscess, breast
intraorbital — *see* Abscess, orbit
intraperitoneal K65.1
intrasphincteric (anus) K61.4
intraspinal G06.1
intratonsillar J36
ischiorectal (fossa) K61.3
jaw (bone) (lower) (upper) M27.2
joint — *see* Arthritis, pyogenic or pyemic
  spine (tuberculous) A18.01
    nontuberculous — *see* Spondylopathy, infective
kidney N15.1
  with calculus N20.0
    with hydronephrosis N13.6
  puerperal (postpartum) O86.21
knee (*see also* Abscess, lower limb)
  joint M00.9
labium (majus) (minus) N76.4
lacrimal
  caruncle — *see* Inflammation, lacrimal, passages, acute
  gland — *see* Dacryoadenitis
  passages (duct) (sac) — *see* Inflammation, lacrimal, passages, acute
lacunar N34.0
larynx J38.7
lateral (alveolar) K04.7
  with sinus K04.6
leg (any part) — *see* Abscess, lower limb
lens H27.8
lingual K14.0
  tonsil J36
lip K13.0
Littre's gland N34.0
liver (cholangitic) (hematogenic) (lymphogenic) (pylephlebitic) (pyogenic) K75.0
  amebic (due to Entamoeba histolytica) (dysenteric) (tropical) A06.4
    with
      brain abscess (and liver or lung abscess) A06.6
      lung abscess A06.5
loin (region) L02.211
lower limb L02.41- ☑
lumbar (tuberculous) A18.01
  nontuberculous L02.212
lung (miliary) (putrid) J85.2
  with pneumonia J85.1
    due to specified organism (see Pneumonia, in (due to))
  amebic (with liver abscess) A06.5
    with
      brain abscess A06.6
      pneumonia A06.5
lymph, lymphatic, gland or node (acute) (*see also* Lymphadenitis, acute)
  mesentery I88.0
malar M27.2
mammary gland — *see* Abscess, breast
marginal, anus K61.0
mastoid — *see* Mastoiditis, acute
maxilla, maxillary M27.2
  molar (tooth) K04.7
    with sinus K04.6
  premolar K04.7
  sinus (chronic) J32.0
mediastinum J85.3
meibomian gland — *see* Hordeolum
meninges G06.2
mesentery, mesenteric K65.1
mesosalpinx — *see* Salpingitis
mons pubis L02.215
mouth (floor) K12.2
muscle — *see* Myositis, infective
myocardium I40.0

Abscess — *continued*
nabothian (follicle) — *see* Cervicitis
nasal J32.9
nasopharyngeal J39.1
navel L02.216
  newborn P38.9
    with mild hemorrhage P38.1
    without hemorrhage P38.9
neck (region) L02.11
  lymph gland or node L04.0
nephritic — *see* Abscess, kidney
nipple N61
  associated with
    lactation — *see* Pregnancy, complicated by, pregnancy — *see* Pregnancy, complicated by
nose (external) (fossa) (septum) J34.0
  sinus (chronic) — *see* Sinusitis
omentum K65.1
operative wound T81.4 ☑
orbit, orbital — *see* Cellulitis, orbit
otogenic G06.0
ovary, ovarian (corpus luteum) — *see* Oophoritis
oviduct — *see* Oophoritis
palate (soft) K12.2
  hard M27.2
palmar (space) — *see* Abscess, hand
pancreas (duct) — *see* Pancreatitis, acute
parafrenal N48.21
parametric, parametrium N73.2
  acute N73.0
  chronic N73.1
paranephric N15.1
parapancreatic — *see* Pancreatitis, acute
parapharyngeal J39.0
pararectal K61.1
parasinus — *see* Sinusitis
parauterine (*see also* Disease, pelvis, inflammatory) N73.2
paravaginal — *see* Vaginitis
parietal region (scalp) L02.811
parodontal K05.21
parotid (duct) (gland) K11.3
  region K12.2
pectoral (region) L02.213
pelvis, pelvic
  female — *see* Disease, pelvis, inflammatory
  male, peritoneal K65.1
penis N48.21
  gonococcal (accessory gland) (periurethral) A54.1
perianal K61.0
periapical K04.7
  with sinus (alveolar) K04.6
periappendicular K35.3
pericardial I30.1
pericecal K35.3
pericemental K05.21
pericholecystic — *see* Cholecystitis, acute
pericoronal K05.21
peridental K05.21
perimetric (*see also* Disease, pelvis, inflammatory) N73.2
perinephric, perinephritic — *see* Abscess, kidney
perineum, perineal (superficial) L02.215
  urethra N34.0
periodontal (parietal) K05.21
  apical K04.7
periosteum, periosteal (*see also* Osteomyelitis, specified type NEC)
  with osteomyelitis (*see also* Osteomyelitis, specified type NEC)
    acute — *see* Osteomyelitis, acute
    chronic — *see* Osteomyelitis, chronic
peripharyngeal J39.0
peripleuritic J86.9
  with fistula J86.0
periprostatic N41.2
perirectal K61.1
perirenal (tissue) — *see* Abscess, kidney
perisinuous (nose) — *see* Sinusitis
peritoneum, peritoneal (perforated) (ruptured) K65.1
  with appendicitis K35.3
  pelvic
    female — *see* Peritonitis, pelvic, female
    male K65.1
  postoperative T81.4 ☑
  puerperal, postpartum, childbirth O85
  tuberculous A18.31
peritonsillar J36

▽ **Subterms under main terms may continue to next column or page**   ☑ **Additional Character Required — Refer to the Tabular List for Character Selection**   5

Abscess — Abscess

Abscess — *continued*
 perityphlic K35.3
 periureteral N28.89
 periurethral N34.0
   gonococcal (accessory gland) (periurethral) A54.1
 periuterine (*see also* Disease, pelvis, inflammatory) N73.2
 perivesical — *see* Cystitis, specified type NEC
 petrous bone — *see* Petrositis
 phagedenic NOS L02.91
   chancroid A57
 pharynx, pharyngeal (lateral) J39.1
 pilonidal L05.01
 pituitary (gland) E23.6
 pleura J86.9
   with fistula J86.0
 popliteal — *see* Abscess, lower limb
 postcecal K35.3
 postlaryngeal J38.7
 postnasal J34.0
 postoperative (any site) T81.4 ☑
   retroperitoneal K68.11
 postpharyngeal J39.0
 posttonsillar J36
 post-typhoid A01.09
 pouch of Douglas — *see* Peritonitis, pelvic, female
 premammary — *see* Abscess, breast
 prepatellar — *see* Abscess, lower limb
 prostate N41.2
   gonococcal (acute) (chronic) A54.22
 psoas muscle K68.12
 puerperal — *code by* site under Puerperal, abscess
 pulmonary — *see* Abscess, lung
 pulp, pulpal (dental) K04.0
 rectovaginal septum K63.0
 rectovesical — *see* Cystitis, specified type NEC
 rectum K61.1
 renal — *see* Abscess, kidney
 retina — *see* Inflammation, chorioretinal
 retrobulbar — *see* Abscess, orbit
 retrocecal K65.1
 retrolaryngeal J38.7
 retromammary — *see* Abscess, breast
 retroperitoneal NEC K68.19
   postprocedural K68.11
 retropharyngeal J39.0
 retrouterine — *see* Peritonitis, pelvic, female
 retrovesical — *see* Cystitis, specified type NEC
 root, tooth K04.7
   with sinus (alveolar) K04.6
 round ligament (*see also* Disease, pelvis, inflammatory) N73.2
 rupture (spontaneous) NOS L02.91
 sacrum (tuberculous) A18.01
   nontuberculous M46.28
 salivary (duct) (gland) K11.3
 scalp (any part) L02.811
 scapular — *see* Osteomyelitis, specified type NEC
 sclera — *see* Scleritis
 scrofulous (tuberculous) A18.2
 scrotum N49.2
 seminal vesicle N49.0
 septal, dental K04.7
   with sinus (alveolar) K04.6
 serous — *see* Periostitis
 shoulder (region) — *see* Abscess, upper limb
 sigmoid K63.0
 sinus (accessory) (chronic) (nasal) (*see also* Sinusitis)
   intracranial venous (any) G06.0
 Skene's duct or gland N34.0
 skin — *see* Abscess, by site
 specified site NEC L02.818
 spermatic cord N49.1
 sphenoidal (sinus) (chronic) J32.3
 spinal cord (any part) (staphylococcal) G06.1
   tuberculous A17.81
 spine (column) (tuberculous) A18.01
   epidural G06.1
   nontuberculous — *see* Osteomyelitis, vertebra
 spleen D73.3
   amebic A06.89
 stitch T81.4 ☑
 subarachnoid G06.2
   brain G06.0
   spinal cord G06.1
 subareolar — *see* Abscess, breast
 subcecal K35.3

Abscess — *continued*
 subcutaneous (*see also* Abscess, by site)
   pheomycotic (chromomycotic) B43.2
 subdiaphragmatic K65.1
 subdural G06.2
   brain G06.0
     sequelae G09
   spinal cord G06.1
 subgaleal L02.811
 subhepatic K65.1
 sublingual K12.2
   gland K11.3
 submammary — *see* Abscess, breast
 submandibular (region) (space) (triangle) K12.2
   gland K11.3
 submaxillary (region) L02.01
   gland K11.3
 submental L02.01
   gland K11.3
 subperiosteal — *see* Osteomyelitis, specified type NEC
 subphrenic K65.1
   postoperative T81.4 ☑
 suburethral N34.0
 sudoriparous L75.8
 supraclavicular (fossa) — *see* Abscess, upper limb
 suprapelvic, acute N73.0
 suprarenal (capsule) (gland) E27.8
 sweat gland L74.8
 tear duct — *see* Inflammation, lacrimal, passages, acute
 temple L02.01
 temporal region L02.01
 temporosphenoidal G06.0
 tendon (sheath) M65.00
   ankle M65.07- ☑
   foot M65.07- ☑
   forearm M65.03- ☑
   hand M65.04- ☑
   lower leg M65.06- ☑
   pelvic region M65.05- ☑
   shoulder region M65.01- ☑
   specified site NEC M65.08
   thigh M65.05- ☑
   upper arm M65.02- ☑
 testis N45.4
 thigh — *see* Abscess, lower limb
 thorax J86.9
   with fistula J86.0
 throat J39.1
 thumb (*see also* Abscess, hand)
   nail — *see* Cellulitis, finger
 thymus (gland) E32.1
 thyroid (gland) E06.0
 toe (any) (*see also* Abscess, foot)
   nail — *see* Cellulitis, toe
 tongue (staphylococcal) K14.0
 tonsil(s) (lingual) J36
 tonsillopharyngeal J36
 tooth, teeth (root) K04.7
   with sinus (alveolar) K04.6
   supporting structures NEC K05.21
 trachea J39.8
 trunk L02.219
   abdominal wall L02.211
   back L02.212
   chest wall L02.213
   groin L02.214
   perineum L02.215
   umbilicus L02.216
 tubal — *see* Salpingitis
 tuberculous — *see* Tuberculosis, abscess
 tubo-ovarian — *see* Salpingo-oophoritis
 tunica vaginalis N49.1
 umbilicus L02.216
 upper
   limb L02.41- ☑
   respiratory J39.8
 urethral (gland) N34.0
 urinary N34.0
 uterus, uterine (wall) (*see also* Endometritis)
   ligament (*see also* Disease, pelvis, inflammatory) N73.2
   neck — *see* Cervicitis
 uvula K12.2
 vagina (wall) — *see* Vaginitis
 vaginorectal — *see* Vaginitis

Abscess — *continued*
 vas deferens N49.1
 vermiform appendix K35.3
 vertebra (column) (tuberculous) A18.01
   nontuberculous — *see* Osteomyelitis, vertebra
 vesical — *see* Cystitis, specified type NEC
 vesico-uterine pouch — *see* Peritonitis, pelvic, female
 vitreous (humor) — *see* Endophthalmitis, purulent
 vocal cord J38.3
 von Bezold's — *see* Mastoiditis, acute
 vulva N76.4
 vulvovaginal gland N75.1
 web space — *see* Abscess, hand
 wound T81.4 ☑
 wrist — *see* Abscess, upper limb
Absence (of) (organ or part) (complete or partial)
 adrenal (gland) (congenital) Q89.1
   acquired E89.6
 albumin in blood E88.09
 alimentary tract (congenital) Q45.8
   upper Q40.8
 alveolar process (acquired) — *see* Anomaly, alveolar
 ankle (acquired) Z89.44- ☑
 anus (congenital) Q42.3
   with fistula Q42.2
 aorta (congenital) Q25.4
 appendix, congenital Q42.8
 arm (acquired) Z89.20- ☑
   above elbow Z89.22- ☑
     congenital (with hand present) — *see* Agenesis, arm, with hand present
       and hand — *see* Agenesis, forearm, and hand
   below elbow Z89.21- ☑
     congenital (with hand present) — *see* Agenesis, arm, with hand present
       and hand — *see* Agenesis, forearm, and hand
   congenital — *see* Defect, reduction, upper limb
   shoulder (following explantation of shoulder joint prosthesis) (joint) (with or without presence of antibiotic-impregnated cement spacer) Z89.23- ☑
   congenital (with hand present) — *see* Agenesis, arm, with hand present
 artery (congenital) (peripheral) Q27.8
   brain Q28.3
   coronary Q24.5
   pulmonary Q25.79
   specified NEC Q27.8
   umbilical Q27.0
 atrial septum (congenital) Q21.1
 auditory canal (congenital) (external) Q16.1
 auricle (ear), congenital Q16.0
 bile, biliary duct, congenital Q44.5
 bladder (acquired) Z90.6
   congenital Q64.5
 bowel sounds R19.11
 brain Q00.0
   part of Q04.3
 breast(s) (and nipple(s)) (acquired) Z90.1- ☑
   congenital Q83.8
 broad ligament Q50.6
 bronchus (congenital) Q32.4
 canaliculus lacrimalis, congenital Q10.4
 cerebellum (vermis) Q04.3
 cervix (acquired) (with uterus) Z90.710
   with remaining uterus Z90.712
   congenital Q51.5
 chin, congenital Q18.8
 cilia (congenital) Q10.3
   acquired — *see* Madarosis
 clitoris (congenital) Q52.6
 coccyx, congenital Q76.49
 cold sense R20.8
 congenital
   lumen — *see* Atresia
   organ or site NEC — *see* Agenesis
   septum — *see* Imperfect, closure
 corpus callosum Q04.0
 cricoid cartilage, congenital Q31.8
 diaphragm (with hernia), congenital Q79.1
 digestive organ(s) or tract, congenital Q45.8
   acquired NEC Z90.49
   upper Q40.8
 ductus arteriosus Q28.8
 duodenum (acquired) Z90.49
   congenital Q41.0

Absence — *continued*
- ear, congenital Q16.9
  - acquired H93.8- ☑
  - auricle Q16.0
  - external Q16.0
  - inner Q16.5
  - lobe, lobule Q17.8
  - middle, except ossicles Q16.4
    - ossicles Q16.3
  - ossicles Q16.3
- ejaculatory duct (congenital) Q55.4
- endocrine gland (congenital) NEC Q89.2
  - acquired E89.89
- epididymis (congenital) Q55.4
  - acquired Z90.79
- epiglottis, congenital Q31.8
- esophagus (congenital) Q39.8
  - acquired (partial) Z90.49
- eustachian tube (congenital) Q16.2
- extremity (acquired) Z89.9
  - congenital Q73.0
  - knee (following explanation of knee joint prosthesis) (joint) (with or without presence of antibiotic-impregnated cement spacer) Z89.52- ☑
  - lower (above knee) Z89.619
    - below knee Z89.51- ☑
  - upper — *see* Absence, arm
- eye (acquired) Z90.01
  - congenital Q11.1
  - muscle (congenital) Q10.3
- eyeball (acquired) Z90.01
- eyelid (fold) (congenital) Q10.3
  - acquired Z90.01
- face, specified part NEC Q18.8
- fallopian tube(s) (acquired) Z90.79
  - congenital Q50.6
- family member (causing problem in home) NEC (*see also* Disruption, family) Z63.32
- femur, congenital — *see* Defect, reduction, lower limb, longitudinal, femur
- fibrinogen (congenital) D68.2
  - acquired D65
- finger(s) (acquired) Z89.02- ☑
  - congenital — *see* Agenesis, hand
- foot (acquired) Z89.43- ☑
  - congenital — *see* Agenesis, foot
- forearm (acquired) — *see* Absence, arm, below elbow
- gallbladder (acquired) Z90.49
  - congenital Q44.0
- gamma globulin in blood D80.1
  - hereditary D80.0
- genital organs
  - acquired (female) (male) Z90.79
  - female, congenital Q52.8
    - external Q52.71
    - internal NEC Q52.8
  - male, congenital Q55.8
- genitourinary organs, congenital NEC
  - female Q52.8
  - male Q55.8
- globe (acquired) Z90.01
  - congenital Q11.1
- glottis, congenital Q31.8
- hand and wrist (acquired) Z89.11- ☑
  - congenital — *see* Agenesis, hand
- head, part (acquired) NEC Z90.09
- heat sense R20.8
- hip (following explanation of hip joint prosthesis) (joint) (with or without presence of antibiotic-impregnated cement spacer) Z89.62- ☑
- hymen (congenital) Q52.4
- ileum (acquired) Z90.49
  - congenital Q41.2
- immunoglobulin, isolated NEC D80.3
  - IgA D80.2
  - IgG D80.3
  - IgM D80.4
- incus (acquired) — *see* Loss, ossicles, ear
  - congenital Q16.3
- inner ear, congenital Q16.5
- intestine (acquired) (small) Z90.49
  - congenital Q41.9
    - specified NEC Q41.8
  - large Z90.49
    - congenital Q42.9
      - specified NEC Q42.8
- iris, congenital Q13.1

Absence — *continued*
- jejunum (acquired) Z90.49
  - congenital Q41.1
- joint
  - acquired
    - hip (following explanation of hip joint prosthesis) (with or without presence of antibiotic-impregnated cement spacer) Z89.62- ☑
    - knee (following explanation of knee joint prosthesis) (with or without presence of antibiotic-impregnated cement spacer) Z89.52- ☑
    - shoulder (following explanation of shoulder joint prosthesis) (with or without presence of antibiotic-impregnated cement spacer) Z89.23- ☑
  - congenital NEC Q74.8
- kidney(s) (acquired) Z90.5
  - congenital Q60.2
    - bilateral Q60.1
    - unilateral Q60.0
- knee (following explanation of knee joint prosthesis) (joint) (with or without presence of antibiotic-impregnated cement spacer) Z89.52- ☑
- labyrinth, membranous Q16.5
- larynx (congenital) Q31.8
  - acquired Z90.02
- leg (acquired) (above knee) Z89.61- ☑
  - below knee (acquired) Z89.51- ☑
  - congenital — *see* Defect, reduction, lower limb
- lens (acquired) (*see also* Aphakia)
  - congenital Q12.3
  - post cataract extraction Z98.4- ☑
- limb (acquired) — *see* Absence, extremity
- lip Q38.6
- liver (congenital) Q44.7
- lung (fissure) (lobe) (bilateral) (unilateral) (congenital) Q33.3
  - acquired (any part) Z90.2
- menstruation — *see* Amenorrhea
- muscle (congenital) (pectoral) Q79.8
  - ocular Q10.3
- neck, part Q18.8
- neutrophil — *see* Agranulocytosis
- nipple(s) (with breast(s)) (acquired) Z90.1- ☑
  - congenital Q83.2
- nose (congenital) Q30.1
  - acquired Z90.09
- organ
  - of Corti, congenital Q16.5
  - or site, congenital NEC Q89.8
    - acquired NEC Z90.89
- osseous meatus (ear) Q16.4
- ovary (acquired)
  - bilateral Z90.722
  - congenital
    - bilateral Q50.02
    - unilateral Q50.01
  - unilateral Z90.721
- oviduct (acquired)
  - bilateral Z90.722
  - congenital Q50.6
  - unilateral Z90.721
- pancreas (congenital) Q45.0
  - acquired Z90.410
    - complete Z90.410
    - partial Z90.411
    - total Z90.410
- parathyroid gland (acquired) E89.2
  - congenital Q89.2
- patella, congenital Q74.1
- penis (congenital) Q55.5
  - acquired Z90.79
- pericardium (congenital) Q24.8
- pituitary gland (congenital) Q89.2
  - acquired E89.3
- prostate (acquired) Z90.79
  - congenital Q55.4
- pulmonary valve Q22.0
- punctum lacrimale (congenital) Q10.4
- radius, congenital — *see* Defect, reduction, upper limb, longitudinal, radius
- rectum (congenital) Q42.1
  - with fistula Q42.0
  - acquired Z90.49
- respiratory organ NOS Q34.9

Absence — *continued*
- rib (acquired) Z90.89
  - congenital Q76.6
- sacrum, congenital Q76.49
- salivary gland(s), congenital Q38.4
- scrotum, congenital Q55.29
- seminal vesicles (congenital) Q55.4
  - acquired Z90.79
- septum
  - atrial (congenital) Q21.1
  - between aorta and pulmonary artery Q21.4
  - ventricular (congenital) Q20.4
- sex chromosome
  - female phenotype Q97.8
  - male phenotype Q98.8
- skull bone (congenital) Q75.8
  - with
    - anencephaly Q00.0
    - encephalocele — *see* Encephalocele
    - hydrocephalus Q03.9
      - with spina bifida — *see* Spina bifida, by site, with hydrocephalus
    - microcephaly Q02
- spermatic cord, congenital Q55.4
- spine, congenital Q76.49
- spleen (congenital) Q89.01
  - acquired Z90.81
- sternum, congenital Q76.7
- stomach (acquired) (partial) Z90.3
  - congenital Q40.2
- superior vena cava, congenital Q26.8
- teeth, tooth (congenital) K00.0
  - acquired (complete) K08.109
    - class I K08.101
    - class II K08.102
    - class III K08.103
    - class IV K08.104
    - due to
      - caries K08.139
        - class I K08.131
        - class II K08.132
        - class III K08.133
        - class IV K08.134
      - periodontal disease K08.129
        - class I K08.121
        - class II K08.122
        - class III K08.123
        - class IV K08.124
      - specified NEC K08.199
        - class I K08.191
        - class II K08.192
        - class III K08.193
        - class IV K08.194
      - trauma K08.119
        - class I K08.111
        - class II K08.112
        - class III K08.113
        - class IV K08.114
    - partial K08.409
      - class I K08.401
      - class II K08.402
      - class III K08.403
      - class IV K08.404
      - due to
        - caries K08.439
          - class I K08.431
          - class II K08.432
          - class III K08.433
          - class IV K08.434
        - periodontal disease K08.429
          - class I K08.421
          - class II K08.422
          - class III K08.423
          - class IV K08.424
        - specified NEC K08.499
          - class I K08.491
          - class II K08.492
          - class III K08.493
          - class IV K08.494
        - trauma K08.419
          - class I K08.411
          - class II K08.412
          - class III K08.413
          - class IV K08.414
- tendon (congenital) Q79.8
- testis (congenital) Q55.0
  - acquired Z90.79

Absence — *continued*
- thumb (acquired) Z89.Ø1- ☑
  - congenital — *see* Agenesis, hand
- thymus gland Q89.2
- thyroid (gland) (acquired) E89.Ø
  - cartilage, congenital Q31.8
  - congenital EØ3.1
- toe(s) (acquired) Z89.42- ☑
  - with foot — *see* Absence, foot and ankle
  - congenital — *see* Agenesis, foot
  - great Z89.41- ☑
- tongue, congenital Q38.3
- trachea (cartilage), congenital Q32.1
- transverse aortic arch, congenital Q25.4
- tricuspid valve Q22.4
- umbilical artery, congenital Q27.Ø
- upper arm and forearm with hand present, congenital — *see* Agenesis, arm, with hand present
- ureter (congenital) Q62.4
  - acquired Z9Ø.6
- urethra, congenital Q64.5
- uterus (acquired) Z9Ø.71Ø
  - with cervix Z9Ø.71Ø
  - with remaining cervical stump Z9Ø.711
  - congenital Q51.Ø
- uvula, congenital Q38.5
- vagina, congenital Q52.Ø
- vas deferens (congenital) Q55.4
  - acquired Z9Ø.79
- vein (peripheral) congenital NEC Q27.8
  - cerebral Q28.3
  - digestive system Q27.8
  - great Q26.8
  - lower limb Q27.8
  - portal Q26.5
  - precerebral Q28.1
  - specified site NEC Q27.8
  - upper limb Q27.8
- vena cava (inferior) (superior), congenital Q26.8
- ventricular septum Q2Ø.4
- vertebra, congenital Q76.49
- vulva, congenital Q52.71
- wrist (acquired) Z89.12- ☑

Absorbent system disease I87.8
Absorption
- carbohydrate, disturbance K9Ø.4
- chemical — *see* Table of Drugs and Chemicals
  - through placenta (newborn) PØ4.9
    - environmental substance PØ4.6
    - nutritional substance PØ4.5
    - obstetric anesthetic or analgesic drug PØ4.Ø
- drug NEC — *see* Table of Drugs and Chemicals
  - addictive
    - through placenta (newborn) PØ4.49
      - cocaine PØ4.41
  - medicinal
    - through placenta (newborn) PØ4.1
  - through placenta (newborn) PØ4.1
    - obstetric anesthetic or analgesic drug PØ4.Ø
- fat, disturbance K9Ø.4
  - pancreatic K9Ø.3
- noxious substance — *see* Table of Drugs and Chemicals
- protein, disturbance K9Ø.4
- starch, disturbance K9Ø.4
- toxic substance — *see* Table of Drugs and Chemicals
- uremic — *see* Uremia

Abstinence symptoms, syndrome
- alcohol F1Ø.239
  - with delirium F1Ø.231
- cocaine F14.23
- neonatal P96.1
- nicotine — *see* Dependence, drug, nicotine, with, withdrawal
- opioid F11.93
  - with dependence F11.23
- psychoactive NEC F19.939
  - with
    - delirium F19.931
    - dependence F19.239
      - with
        - delirium F19.231
        - perceptual disturbance F19.232
      - uncomplicated F19.23Ø
    - perceptual disturbance F19.932
  - uncomplicated F19.93Ø

Abstinence symptoms, syndrome — *continued*
- sedative F13.939
  - with
    - delirium F13.931
    - dependence F13.239
      - with
        - delirium F13.231
        - perceptual disturbance F13.232
      - uncomplicated F13.23Ø
    - perceptual disturbance F13.932
  - uncomplicated F13.93Ø
- stimulant NEC F15.93
  - with dependence F15.23
Abulia R68.89
Abulomania F6Ø.7
Abuse
- adult — *see* Maltreatment, adult
  - as reason for
    - couple seeking advice (including offender) Z63.Ø
- alcohol (non-dependent) F1Ø.1Ø
  - with
    - anxiety disorder F1Ø.18Ø
    - intoxication F1Ø.129
      - with delirium F1Ø.121
      - uncomplicated F1Ø.12Ø
    - mood disorder F1Ø.14
    - other specified disorder F1Ø.188
    - psychosis F1Ø.159
      - delusions F1Ø.15Ø
      - hallucinations F1Ø.151
    - sexual dysfunction F1Ø.181
    - sleep disorder F1Ø.182
    - unspecified disorder F1Ø.19
  - counseling and surveillance Z71.41
- amphetamine (or related substance) — *see* Abuse, drug, stimulant NEC
- analgesics (non-prescribed) (over the counter) F55.8
- antacids F55.Ø
- antidepressants — *see* Abuse, drug, psychoactive NEC
- anxiolytic — *see* Abuse, drug, sedative
- barbiturates — *see* Abuse, drug, sedative
- caffeine — *see* Abuse, drug, stimulant NEC
- cannabis, cannabinoids — *see* Abuse, drug, cannabis
- child — *see* Maltreatment, child
- cocaine — *see* Abuse, drug, cocaine
- drug NEC (non-dependent) F19.1Ø
  - with sleep disorder F19.182
  - amphetamine type — *see* Abuse, drug, stimulant NEC
  - analgesics (non-prescribed) (over the counter) F55.8
  - antacids F55.Ø
  - antidepressants — *see* Abuse, drug, psychoactive NEC
  - anxiolytics — *see* Abuse, drug, sedative
  - barbiturates — *see* Abuse, drug, sedative
  - caffeine — *see* Abuse, drug, stimulant NEC
  - cannabis F12.1Ø
    - with
      - anxiety disorder F12.18Ø
      - intoxication F12.129
        - with
          - delirium F12.121
          - perceptual disturbance F12.122
        - uncomplicated F12.12Ø
      - other specified disorder F12.188
      - psychosis F12.159
        - delusions F12.15Ø
        - hallucinations F12.151
      - unspecified disorder F12.19
  - cocaine F14.1Ø
    - with
      - anxiety disorder F14.18Ø
      - intoxication F14.129
        - with
          - delirium F14.121
          - perceptual disturbance F14.122
        - uncomplicated F14.12Ø
      - mood disorder F14.14
      - other specified disorder F14.188
      - psychosis F14.159
        - delusions F14.15Ø
        - hallucinations F14.151
      - sexual dysfunction F14.181
      - sleep disorder F14.182
      - unspecified disorder F14.19
    - counseling and surveillance Z71.51

Abuse — *continued*
- drug — *continued*
  - hallucinogen F16.1Ø
    - with
      - anxiety disorder F16.18Ø
      - flashbacks F16.183
      - intoxication F16.129
        - with
          - delirium F16.121
          - perceptual disturbance F16.122
        - uncomplicated F16.12Ø
      - mood disorder F16.14
      - other specified disorder F16.188
      - perception disorder, persisting F16.183
      - psychosis F16.159
        - delusions F16.15Ø
        - hallucinations F16.151
      - unspecified disorder F16.19
  - hashish — *see* Abuse, drug, cannabis
  - herbal or folk remedies F55.1
  - hormones F55.3
  - hypnotics — *see* Abuse, drug, sedative
  - inhalant F18.1Ø
    - with
      - anxiety disorder F18.18Ø
      - dementia, persisting F18.17
      - intoxication F18.129
        - with delirium F18.121
        - uncomplicated F18.12Ø
      - mood disorder F18.14
      - other specified disorder F18.188
      - psychosis F18.159
        - delusions F18.15Ø
        - hallucinations F18.151
      - unspecified disorder F18.19
  - laxatives F55.2
  - LSD — *see* Abuse, drug, hallucinogen
  - marihuana — *see* Abuse, drug, cannabis
  - morphine type (opioids) — *see* Abuse, drug, opioid
  - opioid F11.1Ø
    - with
      - intoxication F11.129
        - with
          - delirium F11.121
          - perceptual disturbance F11.122
        - uncomplicated F11.12Ø
      - mood disorder F11.14
      - other specified disorder F11.188
      - psychosis F11.159
        - delusions F11.15Ø
        - hallucinations F11.151
      - sexual dysfunction F11.181
      - sleep disorder F11.182
      - unspecified disorder F11.19
  - PCP (phencyclidine) (or related substance) — *see* Abuse, drug, hallucinogen
  - psychoactive NEC F19.1Ø
    - with
      - amnestic disorder F19.16
      - anxiety disorder F19.18Ø
      - dementia F19.17
      - intoxication F19.129
        - with
          - delirium F19.121
          - perceptual disturbance F19.122
        - uncomplicated F19.12Ø
      - mood disorder F19.14
      - other specified disorder F19.188
      - psychosis F19.159
        - delusions F19.15Ø
        - hallucinations F19.151
      - sexual dysfunction F19.181
      - sleep disorder F19.182
      - unspecified disorder F19.19
  - sedative, hypnotic or anxiolytic F13.1Ø
    - with
      - anxiety disorder F13.18Ø
      - intoxication F13.129
        - with delirium F13.121
        - uncomplicated F13.12Ø
      - mood disorder F13.14
      - other specified disorder F13.188
      - psychosis F13.159
        - delusions F13.15Ø
        - hallucinations F13.151
      - sexual dysfunction F13.181
      - sleep disorder F13.182
      - unspecified disorder F13.19

☑ Additional Character Required — Refer to the Tabular List for Character Selection ▽ Subterms under main terms may continue to next column or page

Abuse — *continued*
  drug — *continued*
    solvent — *see* Abuse, drug, inhalant
    steroids F55.3
    stimulant NEC F15.10
      with
        anxiety disorder F15.180
        intoxication F15.129
          with
            delirium F15.121
            perceptual disturbance F15.122
          uncomplicated F15.120
        mood disorder F15.14
        other specified disorder F15.188
        psychosis F15.159
          delusions F15.150
          hallucinations F15.151
        sexual dysfunction F15.181
        sleep disorder F15.182
        unspecified disorder F15.19
    tranquilizers — *see* Abuse, drug, sedative
    vitamins F55.4
  hallucinogens — *see* Abuse, drug, hallucinogen
  hashish — *see* Abuse, drug, cannabis
  herbal or folk remedies F55.1
  hormones F55.3
  hypnotic — *see* Abuse, drug, sedative
  inhalant — *see* Abuse, drug, inhalant
  laxatives F55.2
  LSD — *see* Abuse, drug, hallucinogen
  marihuana — *see* Abuse, drug, cannabis
  morphine type (opioids) — *see* Abuse, drug, opioid
  non-psychoactive substance NEC F55.8
    antacids F55.0
    folk remedies F55.1
    herbal remedies F55.1
    hormones F55.3
    laxatives F55.2
    steroids F55.3
    vitamins F55.4
  opioids — *see* Abuse, drug, opioid
  PCP (phencyclidine) (or related substance) — *see* Abuse, drug, hallucinogen
  physical (adult) (child) — *see* Maltreatment
  psychoactive substance — *see* Abuse, drug, psychoactive NEC
  psychological (adult) (child) — *see* Maltreatment
  sedative — *see* Abuse, drug, sedative
  sexual — *see* Maltreatment
  solvent — *see* Abuse, drug, inhalant
  steroids F55.3
  vitamins F55.4
Acalculia R48.8
  developmental F81.2
Acanthamebiasis (with) B60.10
  conjunctiva B60.12
  keratoconjunctivitis B60.13
  meningoencephalitis B60.11
  other specified B60.19
Acanthocephaliasis B83.8
Acanthocheilonemiasis B74.4
Acanthocytosis E78.6
Acantholysis L11.9
Acanthosis (acquired) (nigricans) L83
  benign Q82.8
  congenital Q82.8
  seborrheic L82.1
    inflamed L82.0
  tongue K14.3
Acapnia E87.3
Acarbia E87.2
Acardia, acardius Q89.8
Acardiacus amorphus Q89.8
Acardiotrophia I51.4
Acariasis B88.0
  scabies B86
Acarodermatitis (urticarioides) B88.0
Acarophobia F40.218
Acatalasemia, acatalasia E80.3
Acathisia (drug induced) G25.71
Accelerated atrioventricular conduction I45.6
Accentuation of personality traits (type A) Z73.1
Accessory (congenital)
  adrenal gland Q89.1
  anus Q43.4
  appendix Q43.4
  atrioventricular conduction I45.6

Accessory — *continued*
  auditory ossicles Q16.3
  auricle (ear) Q17.0
  biliary duct or passage Q44.5
  bladder Q64.79
  blood vessels NEC Q27.9
    coronary Q24.5
  bone NEC Q79.8
  breast tissue, axilla Q83.1
  carpal bones Q74.0
  cecum Q43.4
  chromosome(s) NEC (nonsex) Q92.9
    with complex rearrangements NEC Q92.5
      seen only at prometaphase Q92.8
    13 — *see* Trisomy, 13
    18 — *see* Trisomy, 18
    21 — *see* Trisomy, 21
    partial Q92.9
    sex
      female phenotype Q97.8
  coronary artery Q24.5
  cusp(s), heart valve NEC Q24.8
    pulmonary Q22.3
  cystic duct Q44.5
  digit(s) Q69.9
  ear (auricle) (lobe) Q17.0
  endocrine gland NEC Q89.2
  eye muscle Q10.3
  eyelid Q10.3
  face bone(s) Q75.8
  fallopian tube (fimbria) (ostium) Q50.6
  finger(s) Q69.0
  foreskin N47.8
  frontonasal process Q75.8
  gallbladder Q44.1
  genital organ(s)
    female Q52.8
      external Q52.79
      internal NEC Q52.8
    male Q55.8
  genitourinary organs NEC Q89.8
    female Q52.8
    male Q55.8
  hallux Q69.2
  heart Q24.8
    valve NEC Q24.8
      pulmonary Q22.3
  hepatic ducts Q44.5
  hymen Q52.4
  intestine (large) (small) Q43.4
  kidney Q63.0
  lacrimal canal Q10.6
  leaflet, heart valve NEC Q24.8
  ligament, broad Q50.6
  liver Q44.7
    duct Q44.5
  lobule (ear) Q17.0
  lung (lobe) Q33.1
  muscle Q79.8
  navicular of carpus Q74.0
  nervous system, part NEC Q07.8
  nipple Q83.3
  nose Q30.8
  organ or site not listed — *see* Anomaly, by site
  ovary Q50.31
  oviduct Q50.6
  pancreas Q45.3
  parathyroid gland Q89.2
  parotid gland (and duct) Q38.4
  pituitary gland Q89.2
  preauricular appendage Q17.0
  prepuce N47.8
  renal arteries (multiple) Q27.2
  rib Q76.6
    cervical Q76.5
  roots (teeth) K00.2
  salivary gland Q38.4
  sesamoid bones Q74.8
    foot Q74.2
    hand Q74.0
  skin tags Q82.8
  spleen Q89.09
  sternum Q76.7
  submaxillary gland Q38.4
  tarsal bones Q74.2
  teeth, tooth K00.1
  tendon Q79.8
  thumb Q69.1

Accessory — *continued*
  thymus gland Q89.2
  thyroid gland Q89.2
  toes Q69.2
  tongue Q38.3
  tooth, teeth K00.1
  tragus Q17.0
  ureter Q62.5
  urethra Q64.79
  urinary organ or tract NEC Q64.8
  uterus Q51.2
  vagina Q52.10
  valve, heart NEC Q24.8
    pulmonary Q22.3
  vertebra Q76.49
  vocal cords Q31.8
  vulva Q52.79
Accident
  birth — *see* Birth, injury
  cardiac — *see* Infarct, myocardium
  cerebral I63.9
  cerebrovascular (embolic) (ischemic) (thrombotic) I63.9
    aborted I63.9
    hemorrhagic — *see* Hemorrhage, intracranial, intracerebral
    old (without sequelae) Z86.73
      with sequelae (of) — *see* Sequelae, infarction, cerebral
  coronary — *see* Infarct, myocardium
  craniovascular I63.9
  vascular, brain I63.9
Accidental — *see* condition
Accommodation (disorder) (*see also* condition)
  hysterical paralysis of F44.89
  insufficiency of H52.4
  paresis — *see* Paresis, of accommodation
  spasm — *see* Spasm, of accommodation
Accouchement — *see* Delivery
Accreta placenta O43.21- ☑
Accretio cordis (nonrheumatic) I31.0
Accretions, tooth, teeth K03.6
Acculturation difficulty Z60.3
Accumulation secretion, prostate N42.89
Acephalia, acephalism, acephalus, acephaly Q00.0
Acephalobrachia monster Q89.8
Acephalochirus monster Q89.8
Acephalogaster Q89.8
Acephalostomus monster Q89.8
Acephalothorax Q89.8
Acerophobia F40.298
Acetonemia R79.89
  in Type 1 diabetes E10.10
    with coma E10.11
Acetonuria R82.4
Achalasia (cardia) (esophagus) K22.0
  congenital Q39.5
  pylorus Q40.0
  sphincteral NEC K59.8
Ache(s) — *see* Pain
Acheilia Q38.6
Achillobursitis — *see* Tendinitis, Achilles
Achillodynia — *see* Tendinitis, Achilles
Achlorhydria, achlorhydric (neurogenic) K31.83
  anemia D50.8
  diarrhea K31.83
  psychogenic F45.8
  secondary to vagotomy K91.1
Achluophobia F40.228
Acholia K82.8
Acholuric jaundice (familial) (splenomegalic) (*see also* Spherocytosis)
  acquired D59.8
Achondrogenesis Q77.0
Achondroplasia (osteosclerosis congenita) Q77.4
Achroma, cutis L80
Achromat (ism), achromatopsia (acquired) (congenital) H53.51
Achromia, congenital — *see* Albinism
Achromia parasitica B36.0
Achylia gastrica K31.89
  psychogenic F45.8
Acid
  burn — *see* Corrosion
  deficiency
    amide nicotinic E52
    ascorbic E54
    folic E53.8

Acid — *continued*
  deficiency — *continued*
    nicotinic E52
    pantothenic E53.8
  intoxication E87.2
  peptic disease K3Ø
  phosphatase deficiency E83.39
  stomach K3Ø
    psychogenic F45.8
Acidemia E87.2
  argininosuccinic E72.22
  isovaleric E71.11Ø
  metabolic (newborn) P19.9
    first noted before onset of labor P19.Ø
    first noted during labor P19.1
    noted at birth P19.2
  methylmalonic E71.12Ø
  pipecolic E72.3
  propionic E71.121
Acidity, gastric (high) K3Ø
  psychogenic F45.8
Acidocytopenia — *see* Agranulocytosis
Acidocytosis D72.1
Acidopenia — *see* Agranulocytosis
Acidosis (lactic) (respiratory) E87.2
  in Type 1 diabetes E10.10
    with coma E10.11
  kidney, tubular N25.89
  lactic E87.2
  metabolic NEC E87.2
    with respiratory acidosis E87.4
    late, of newborn P74.Ø
  mixed metabolic and respiratory, newborn P84
  newborn P84
  renal (hyperchloremic) (tubular) N25.89
  respiratory E87.2
    complicated by
      metabolic
        acidosis E87.4
        alkalosis E87.4
Aciduria
  argininosuccinic E72.22
  glutaric (type I) E72.3
    type II E71.313
    type III E71.5- ☑
  orotic (congenital) (hereditary) (pyrimidine deficiency)
    E79.8
    anemia D53.Ø
Acladiosis (skin) B36.Ø
Aclasis, diaphyseal Q78.6
Acleistocardia Q21.1
Aclusion — *see* Anomaly, dentofacial, malocclusion
Acne L70.9
  artificialis L70.8
  atrophica L70.2
  cachecticorum (Hebra) L70.8
  conglobata L70.1
  cystic L70.Ø
  decalvans L66.2
  excoriée des jeunes filles L70.5
  frontalis L70.2
  indurata L70.Ø
  infantile L70.4
  keloid L73.Ø
  lupoid L70.2
  necrotic, necrotica (miliaris) L70.2
  neonatal L70.4
  nodular L70.Ø
  occupational L70.8
  picker's L70.5
  pustular L70.Ø
  rodens L70.2
  rosacea L71.9
  specified NEC L70.8
  tropica L70.3
  varioliformis L70.2
  vulgaris L70.Ø
Acnitis (primary) A18.4
Acosta's disease T70.29 ☑
Acoustic — *see* condition
Acousticophobia F40.298
Acquired (*see also* condition)
  immunodeficiency syndrome (AIDS) B2Ø
Acrania Q00.Ø
Acroangiodermatitis I78.9
Acroasphyxia, chronic I73.89
Acrobystitis N47.7
Acrocephalopolysyndactyly Q87.Ø

Acrocephalosyndactyly Q87.Ø
Acrocephaly Q75.Ø
Acrochondrohyperplasia — *see* Syndrome, Marfan's
Acrocyanosis I73.8 ☑
  newborn P28.2
    meaning transient blue hands and feet — *omit code*
Acrodermatitis L30.8
  atrophicans (chronica) L90.4
  continua (Hallopeau) L40.2
  enteropathica (hereditary) E83.2
  Hallopeau's L40.2
  infantile papular L44.4
  perstans L40.2
  pustulosa continua L40.2
  recalcitrant pustular L40.2
Acrodynia — *see* Poisoning, mercury
Acromegaly, acromegalia E22.Ø
Acromelalgia I73.81
Acromicria, acromikria Q79.8
Acronyx L60.Ø
Acropachy, thyroid — *see* Thyrotoxicosis
Acroparesthesia (simple) (vasomotor) I73.89
Acropathy, thyroid — *see* Thyrotoxicosis
Acrophobia F40.241
Acroposthitis N47.7
Acroscleriasis, acroscleroderma, acrosclerosis — *see* Sclerosis, systemic
Acrosphacelus I96
Acrospiroma, eccrine — *see* Neoplasm, skin, benign
Acrostealgia — *see* Osteochondropathy
Acrotrophodynia — *see* Immersion
ACTH ectopic syndrome E24.3
Actinic — *see* condition
Actinobacillosis, actinobacillus A28.8
  mallei A24.Ø
  muris A25.1
Actinomyces israelii (infection) — *see* Actinomycosis
Actinomycetoma (foot) B47.1
Actinomycosis, actinomycotic A42.9
  with pneumonia A42.Ø
  abdominal A42.1
  cervicofacial A42.2
  cutaneous A42.89
  gastrointestinal A42.1
  pulmonary A42.Ø
  sepsis A42.7
  specified site NEC A42.89
Actinoneuritis G62.82
Action, heart
  disorder I49.9
  irregular I49.9
    psychogenic F45.8
Activated protein C resistance D68.51
Active — *see* condition
Acute (*see also* condition)
  abdomen R10.Ø
  gallbladder — *see* Cholecystitis, acute
Acyanotic heart disease (congenital) Q24.9
Acystia Q64.5
Adair-Dighton syndrome (brittle bones and blue sclera, deafness) Q78.Ø
Adamantinoblastoma — *see* Ameloblastoma
Adamantinoma (*see also* Cyst, calcifying odontogenic)
  long bones C40.90
    lower limb C40.2- ☑
    upper limb C40.0- ☑
  malignant C41.1
    jaw (bone) (lower) C41.1
      upper C41.Ø
  tibial C40.2- ☑
Adamantoblastoma — *see* Ameloblastoma
Adams-Stokes (-Morgagni) disease or syndrome I45.9
Adaption reaction — *see* Disorder, adjustment
Addiction (*see also* Dependence) F19.2Ø
  alcohol, alcoholic (ethyl) (methyl) (wood) (without remission) F10.2Ø
    with remission F10.21
  drug — *see* Dependence, drug
  ethyl alcohol (without remission) F10.2Ø
    with remission F10.21
  heroin — *see* Dependence, drug, opioid
  methyl alcohol (without remission) F10.2Ø
    with remission F10.21
  methylated spirit (without remission) F10.2Ø
    with remission F10.21

Addiction — *continued*
  morphine (-like substances) — *see* Dependence, drug, opioid
  nicotine — *see* Dependence, drug, nicotine
  opium and opioids — *see* Dependence, drug, opioid
  tobacco — *see* Dependence, drug, nicotine
Addison-Biermer anemia (pernicious) D51.Ø
Addisonian crisis E27.2
Addison's
  anemia (pernicious) D51.Ø
  disease (bronze) or syndrome E27.1
    tuberculous A18.7
  keloid L94.Ø
Addison-Schilder complex E71.528
Additional (*see also* Accessory)
  chromosome(s) Q99.8
    21 — *see* Trisomy, 21
  sex — *see* Abnormal, chromosome, sex
Adduction contracture, hip or other joint — *see* Contraction, joint
Adenitis (*see also* Lymphadenitis)
  acute, unspecified site L04.9
  axillary I88.9
    acute L04.2
    chronic or subacute I88.1
  Bartholin's gland N75.8
  bulbourethral gland — *see* Urethritis
  cervical I88.9
    acute L04.Ø
    chronic or subacute I88.1
  chancroid (Hemophilus ducreyi) A57
  chronic, unspecified site I88.1
  Cowper's gland — *see* Urethritis
  due to Pasteurella multocida (p. septica) A28.Ø
  epidemic, acute B27.09
  gangrenous L04.9
  gonorrheal NEC A54.89
  groin I88.9
    acute L04.1
    chronic or subacute I88.1
  infectious (acute) (epidemic) B27.09
  inguinal I88.9
    acute L04.1
    chronic or subacute I88.1
  lymph gland or node, except mesenteric I88.9
    acute — *see* Lymphadenitis, acute
    chronic or subacute I88.1
  mesenteric (acute) (chronic) (nonspecific) (subacute) I88.Ø
  parotid gland (suppurative) — *see* Sialoadenitis
  salivary gland (any) (suppurative) — *see* Sialoadenitis
  scrofulous (tuberculous) A18.2
  Skene's duct or gland — *see* Urethritis
  strumous, tuberculous A18.2
  subacute, unspecified site I88.1
  sublingual gland (suppurative) — *see* Sialoadenitis
  submandibular gland (suppurative) — *see* Sialoadenitis
  submaxillary gland (suppurative) — *see* Sialoadenitis
  tuberculous — *see* Tuberculosis, lymph gland
  urethral gland — *see* Urethritis
  Wharton's duct (suppurative) — *see* Sialoadenitis
Adenoacanthoma — *see* Neoplasm, malignant, by site
Adenoameloblastoma — *see* Cyst, calcifying odontogenic
Adenocarcinoid (tumor) — *see* Neoplasm, malignant, by site
Adenocarcinoma (*see also* Neoplasm, malignant, by site)
  acidophil
    specified site — *see* Neoplasm, malignant, by site
    unspecified site C75.1
  adrenal cortical C74.0- ☑
  alveolar — *see* Neoplasm, lung, malignant
  apocrine
    breast — *see* Neoplasm, breast, malignant
    in situ
      breast D05.8- ☑
      specified site NEC — *see* Neoplasm, skin, in situ
      unspecified site D04.9
    specified site NEC — *see* Neoplasm, skin, malignant
    unspecified site C44.99
  basal cell
    specified site — *see* Neoplasm, skin, malignant
    unspecified site C08.9
  basophil
    specified site — *see* Neoplasm, malignant, by site

Adenocarcinoma — *continued*
  basophil — *continued*
    unspecified site C75.1
  bile duct type C22.1
    liver C22.1
    specified site NEC — *see* Neoplasm, malignant, by site
    unspecified site C22.1
  bronchiolar — *see* Neoplasm, lung, malignant
  bronchioloalveolar — *see* Neoplasm, lung, malignant
  ceruminous C44.29- ☑
  cervix, in situ (*see also* Carcinoma, cervix uteri, in situ) D06.9
  chromophobe
    specified site — *see* Neoplasm, malignant, by site
    unspecified site C75.1
  diffuse type
    specified site — *see* Neoplasm, malignant, by site
    unspecified site C16.9
  duct
    infiltrating
      with Paget's disease — *see* Neoplasm, breast, malignant
      specified site — *see* Neoplasm, malignant, by site
        unspecified site (female) C50.91- ☑
          male C50.92- ☑
    specified site — *see* Neoplasm, malignant, by site
    unspecified site
      female C56.9
      male C61
  eosinophil
    specified site — *see* Neoplasm, malignant, by site
    unspecified site C75.1
  follicular
    with papillary C73
    moderately differentiated C73
    specified site — *see* Neoplasm, malignant, by site
    trabecular C73
    unspecified site C73
    well differentiated C73
  Hurthle cell C73
  in
    adenomatous
      polyposis coli C18.9
  infiltrating duct
    with Paget's disease — *see* Neoplasm, breast, malignant
    specified site — *see* Neoplasm, by site, malignant
    unspecified site (female) C50.91- ☑
      male C50.92- ☑
  inflammatory
    specified site — *see* Neoplasm, by site, malignant
    unspecified site (female) C50.91- ☑
      male C50.92- ☑
  intestinal type
    specified site — *see* Neoplasm, by site, malignant
    unspecified site C16.9
  intracystic papillary
  intraductal
    breast D05.1- ☑
    noninfiltrating
      breast D05.1- ☑
      papillary
        with invasion
          specified site — *see* Neoplasm, by site, malignant
          unspecified site (female) C50.91- ☑
            male C50.92- ☑
        breast D05.1- ☑
        specified site NEC — *see* Neoplasm, in situ, by site
        unspecified site D05.1- ☑
      specified site NEC — *see* Neoplasm, in situ, by site
      unspecified site D05.1- ☑
    papillary
      with invasion
        specified site — *see* Neoplasm, malignant, by site
        unspecified site (female) C50.91- ☑
          male C50.92- ☑
      breast D05.1- ☑
      specified site — *see* Neoplasm, in situ, by site
      unspecified site D05.1- ☑
    specified site NEC — *see* Neoplasm, in situ, by site
    unspecified site D05.1- ☑

Adenocarcinoma — *continued*
  islet cell
    with exocrine, mixed
      specified site — *see* Neoplasm, malignant, by site
      unspecified site C25.9
    pancreas C25.4
    specified site NEC — *see* Neoplasm, malignant, by site
    unspecified site C25.4
  lobular
    in situ
      breast D05.0- ☑
      specified site NEC — *see* Neoplasm, in situ, by site
      unspecified site D05.0- ☑
    specified site — *see* Neoplasm, malignant, by site
    unspecified site (female) C50.91- ☑
      male C50.92- ☑
  mucoid (*see also* Neoplasm, malignant, by site)
    cell
      specified site — *see* Neoplasm, malignant, by site
      unspecified site C75.1
  nonencapsulated sclerosing C73
  papillary
    with follicular C73
    follicular variant C73
    intraductal (noninfiltrating)
      with invasion
        specified site — *see* Neoplasm, malignant, by site
        unspecified site (female) C50.91- ☑
          male C50.92- ☑
      breast D05.1- ☑
      specified site NEC — *see* Neoplasm, in situ, by site
      unspecified site D05.1- ☑
    serous
      specified site — *see* Neoplasm, malignant, by site
      unspecified site C56.9
  papillocystic
    specified site — *see* Neoplasm, malignant, by site
    unspecified site C56.9
  pseudomucinous
    specified site — *see* Neoplasm, malignant, by site
    unspecified site C56.9
  renal cell C64- ☑
  sebaceous — *see* Neoplasm, skin, malignant
  serous (*see also* Neoplasm, malignant, by site)
    papillary
      specified site — *see* Neoplasm, malignant, by site
      unspecified site C56.9
  sweat gland — *see* Neoplasm, skin, malignant
  water-clear cell C75.0
Adenocarcinoma-in-situ (*see also* Neoplasm, in situ, by site)
  breast D05.9- ☑
Adenofibroma
  clear cell — *see* Neoplasm, benign, by site
  endometrioid D27.9
    borderline malignancy D39.10
    malignant C56- ☑
  mucinous
    specified site — *see* Neoplasm, benign, by site
    unspecified site D27.9
  papillary
    specified site — *see* Neoplasm, benign, by site
    unspecified site D27.9
  prostate — *see* Enlargement, enlarged, prostate
  serous
    specified site — *see* Neoplasm, benign, by site
    unspecified site D27.9
  specified site — *see* Neoplasm, benign, by site
  unspecified site D27.9
Adenofibrosis
  breast — *see* Fibroadenosis, breast
  endometrioid N80.0
Adenoiditis (chronic) J35.02
  with tonsillitis J35.03
  acute J03.90
    recurrent J03.91
    specified organism NEC J03.80
      recurrent J03.81

Adenoiditis — *continued*
  acute — *continued*
    staphylococcal J03.80
      recurrent J03.81
    streptococcal J03.00
      recurrent J03.01
Adenoids — *see* condition
Adenolipoma — *see* Neoplasm, benign, by site
Adenolipomatosis, Launois-Bensaude E88.89
Adenolymphoma
  specified site — *see* Neoplasm, benign, by site
  unspecified site D11.9
Adenoma (*see also* Neoplasm, benign, by site)
  acidophil
    specified site — *see* Neoplasm, benign, by site
    unspecified site D35.2
  acidophil-basophil, mixed
    specified site — *see* Neoplasm, benign, by site
    unspecified site D35.2
  adrenal (cortical) D35.00
    clear cell D35.00
    compact cell D35.00
    glomerulosa cell D35.00
    heavily pigmented variant D35.00
    mixed cell D35.00
  alpha-cell
    pancreas D13.7
    specified site NEC — *see* Neoplasm, benign, by site
    unspecified site D13.7
  alveolar D14.30
  apocrine
    breast D24- ☑
    specified site NEC — *see* Neoplasm, skin, benign, by site
    unspecified site D23.9
  basal cell D11.9
  basophil
    specified site — *see* Neoplasm, benign, by site
    unspecified site D35.2
  basophil-acidophil, mixed
    specified site — *see* Neoplasm, benign, by site
    unspecified site D35.2
  beta-cell
    pancreas D13.7
    specified site NEC — *see* Neoplasm, benign, by site
    unspecified site D13.7
  bile duct D13.4
    common D13.5
    extrahepatic D13.5
    intrahepatic D13.4
    specified site NEC — *see* Neoplasm, benign, by site
    unspecified site D13.4
  black D35.00
  bronchial D38.1
    cylindroid type — *see* Neoplasm, lung, malignant
  ceruminous D23.2- ☑
  chief cell D35.1
  chromophobe
    specified site — *see* Neoplasm, benign, by site
    unspecified site D35.2
  colloid
    specified site — *see* Neoplasm, benign, by site
    unspecified site D34
  duct
  eccrine, papillary — *see* Neoplasm, skin, benign
  endocrine, multiple
    single specified site — *see* Neoplasm, uncertain behavior, by site
    two or more specified sites D44- ☑
    unspecified site D44.9
  endometrioid (*see also* Neoplasm, benign)
    borderline malignancy — *see* Neoplasm, uncertain behavior, by site
  eosinophil
    specified site — *see* Neoplasm, benign, by site
    unspecified site D35.2
  fetal
    specified site — *see* Neoplasm, benign, by site
    unspecified site D34
  follicular
    specified site — *see* Neoplasm, benign, by site
    unspecified site D34
  hepatocellular D13.4
  Hurthle cell D34
  islet cell
    pancreas D13.7
    specified site NEC — *see* Neoplasm, benign, by site
    unspecified site D13.7

Index

Adenocarcinoma — Adenoma

Adenoma — *continued*
  liver cell D13.4
  macrofollicular
    specified site — *see* Neoplasm, benign, by site
    unspecified site D34
  malignant, malignum — *see* Neoplasm, malignant, by site
  microcystic
    pancreas D13.7
    specified site NEC — *see* Neoplasm, benign, by site
    unspecified site D13.7
  microfollicular
    specified site — *see* Neoplasm, benign, by site
    unspecified site D34
  mucoid cell
    specified site — *see* Neoplasm, benign, by site
    unspecified site D35.2
  multiple endocrine
    single specified site — *see* Neoplasm, uncertain behavior, by site
    two or more specified sites D44- ☑
    unspecified site D44.9
  nipple D24- ☑
  papillary (*see also* Neoplasm, benign, by site)
    eccrine — *see* Neoplasm, skin, benign, by site
  Pick's tubular
    specified site — *see* Neoplasm, benign, by site
    unspecified site
      female D27.9
      male D29.20
  pleomorphic
    carcinoma in — *see* Neoplasm, salivary gland, malignant
      specified site — *see* Neoplasm, malignant, by site
      unspecified site C08.9
  polypoid (*see also* Neoplasm, benign)
    adenocarcinoma in — *see* Neoplasm, malignant, by site
    adenocarcinoma in situ — *see* Neoplasm, in situ, by site
  prostate — *see* Neoplasm, benign, prostate
  rete cell D29.20
  sebaceous — *see* Neoplasm, skin, benign
  Sertoli cell
    specified site — *see* Neoplasm, benign, by site
    unspecified site
      female D27.9
      male D29.20
  skin appendage — *see* Neoplasm, skin, benign
  sudoriferous gland — *see* Neoplasm, skin, benign
  sweat gland — *see* Neoplasm, skin, benign
  testicular
    specified site — *see* Neoplasm, benign, by site
    unspecified site
      female D27.9
      male D29.20
  tubular (*see also* Neoplasm, benign, by site)
    adenocarcinoma in — *see* Neoplasm, malignant, by site
    adenocarcinoma in situ — *see* Neoplasm, in situ, by site
    Pick's
      specified site — *see* Neoplasm, benign, by site
      unspecified site
        female D27.9
        male D29.20
  tubulovillous (*see also* Neoplasm, benign, by site)
    adenocarcinoma in — *see* Neoplasm, malignant, by site
    adenocarcinoma in situ — *see* Neoplasm, in situ, by site
  villous — *see* Neoplasm, uncertain behavior, by site
    adenocarcinoma in — *see* Neoplasm, malignant, by site
    adenocarcinoma in situ — *see* Neoplasm, in situ, by site
  water-clear cell D35.1
Adenomatosis
  endocrine (multiple) E31.20
    single specified site — *see* Neoplasm, uncertain behavior, by site
  erosive of nipple D24- ☑
  pluriendocrine — *see* Adenomatosis, endocrine
  pulmonary D38.1
    malignant — *see* Neoplasm, lung, malignant
    specified site — *see* Neoplasm, benign, by site

Adenomatosis — *continued*
  unspecified site D12.6
Adenomatous
  goiter (nontoxic) E04.9
    with hyperthyroidism — *see* Hyperthyroidism, with, goiter, nodular
    toxic — *see* Hyperthyroidism, with, goiter, nodular
Adenomyoma (*see also* Neoplasm, benign, by site)
  prostate — *see* Enlarged, prostate
Adenomyometritis N80.0
Adenomyosis N80.0
Adenopathy (lymph gland) R59.9
  generalized R59.1
  inguinal R59.0
  localized R59.0
  mediastinal R59.0
  mesentery R59.0
  syphilitic (secondary) A51.49
  tracheobronchial R59.0
    tuberculous A15.4
      primary (progressive) A15.7
  tuberculous (*see also* Tuberculosis, lymph gland)
    tracheobronchial A15.4
      primary (progressive) A15.7
Adenosalpingitis — *see* Salpingitis
Adenosarcoma — *see* Neoplasm, malignant, by site
Adenosclerosis I88.8
Adenosis (sclerosing) breast — *see* Fibroadenosis, breast
Adenovirus, as cause of disease classified elsewhere B97.0
Adentia (complete) (partial) — *see* Absence, teeth
Adherent (*see also* Adhesions)
  labia (minora) N90.89
  pericardium (nonrheumatic) I31.0
    rheumatic I09.2
  placenta (with hemorrhage) O72.0
    without hemorrhage O73.0
  prepuce, newborn N47.0
  scar (skin) L90.5
  tendon in scar L90.5
Adhesions, adhesive (postinfective) K66.0
  with intestinal obstruction K56.5
  abdominal (wall) — *see* Adhesions, peritoneum
  appendix K38.8
  bile duct (common) (hepatic) K83.8
  bladder (sphincter) N32.89
  bowel — *see* Adhesions, peritoneum
  cardiac I31.0
    rheumatic I09.2
  cecum — *see* Adhesions, peritoneum
  cervicovaginal N88.1
    congenital Q52.8
    postpartal O90.89
      old N88.1
  cervix N88.1
  ciliary body NEC — *see* Adhesions, iris
  clitoris N90.89
  colon — *see* Adhesions, peritoneum
  common duct K83.8
  congenital (*see also* Anomaly, by site)
    fingers — *see* Syndactylism, complex, fingers
    omental, anomalous Q43.3
    peritoneal Q43.3
    tongue (to gum or roof of mouth) Q38.3
  conjunctiva (acquired) H11.21- ☑
    congenital Q15.8
  cystic duct K82.8
  diaphragm — *see* Adhesions, peritoneum
  due to foreign body — *see* Foreign body
  duodenum — *see* Adhesions, peritoneum
  ear
    middle H74.1- ☑
  epididymis N50.8
  epidural — *see* Adhesions, meninges
  epiglottis J38.7
  eyelid H02.59
  female pelvis N73.6
  gallbladder K82.8
  globe H44.89
  heart I31.0
    rheumatic I09.2
  ileocecal (coil) — *see* Adhesions, peritoneum
  ileum — *see* Adhesions, peritoneum
  intestine (*see also* Adhesions, peritoneum)
    with obstruction K56.5
  intra-abdominal — *see* Adhesions, peritoneum

Adhesions, adhesive — *continued*
  iris H21.50- ☑
    anterior H21.51- ☑
    goniosynechiae H21.52- ☑
    posterior H21.54- ☑
    to corneal graft T85.89 ☑
  joint — *see* Ankylosis
    knee M23.8X ☑
    temporomandibular M26.61
  labium (majus) (minus), congenital Q52.5
  liver — *see* Adhesions, peritoneum
  lung J98.4
  mediastinum J98.5
  meninges (cerebral) (spinal) G96.12
    congenital Q07.8
    tuberculous (cerebral) (spinal) A17.0
  mesenteric — *see* Adhesions, peritoneum
  nasal (septum) (to turbinates) J34.89
  ocular muscle — *see* Strabismus, mechanical
  omentum — *see* Adhesions, peritoneum
  ovary N73.6
    congenital (to cecum, kidney or omentum) Q50.39
  paraovarian N73.6
  pelvic (peritoneal)
    female N73.6
      postprocedural N99.4
    male — *see* Adhesions, peritoneum
    postpartal (old) N73.6
    tuberculous A18.17
  penis to scrotum (congenital) Q55.8
  periappendiceal (*see also* Adhesions, peritoneum)
  pericardium (nonrheumatic) I31.0
    focal I31.8
    rheumatic I09.2
    tuberculous A18.84
  pericholecystic K82.8
  perigastric — *see* Adhesions, peritoneum
  periovarian N73.6
  periprostatic N42.89
  perirectal — *see* Adhesions, peritoneum
  perirenal N28.89
  peritoneum, peritoneal (postinfective) (postprocedural) K66.0
    with obstruction (intestinal) K56.5
    congenital Q43.3
    pelvic, female N73.6
      postprocedural N99.4
    postpartal, pelvic N73.6
    to uterus N73.6
  peritubal N73.6
  periureteral N28.89
  periuterine N73.6
  perivesical N32.89
  perivesicular (seminal vesicle) N50.8
  pleura, pleuritic J94.8
    tuberculous NEC A15.6
  pleuropericardial J94.8
  postoperative (gastrointestinal tract) K66.0
    with obstruction K91.3
    due to foreign body accidentally left in wound — *see* Foreign body, accidentally left during a procedure
    pelvic peritoneal N99.4
    urethra — *see* Stricture, urethra, postprocedural
    vagina N99.2
  postpartal, old (vulva or perineum) N90.89
  preputial, prepuce N47.5
  pulmonary J98.4
  pylorus — *see* Adhesions, peritoneum
  sciatic nerve — *see* Lesion, nerve, sciatic
  seminal vesicle N50.8
  shoulder (joint) — *see* Capsulitis, adhesive
  sigmoid flexure — *see* Adhesions, peritoneum
  spermatic cord (acquired) N50.8
    congenital Q55.4
  spinal canal G96.12
  stomach — *see* Adhesions, peritoneum
  subscapular — *see* Capsulitis, adhesive
  temporomandibular M26.61
  tendinitis (*see also* Tenosynovitis, specified type NEC)
    shoulder — *see* Capsulitis, adhesive
  testis N44.8
  tongue, congenital (to gum or roof of mouth) Q38.3
    acquired K14.8
  trachea J39.8
  tubo-ovarian N73.6
  tunica vaginalis N44.8

Adhesions, adhesive — *continued*
- uterus N73.6
  - internal N85.6
  - to abdominal wall N73.6
- vagina (chronic) N89.5
  - postoperative N99.2
- vitreomacular H43.82- ☑
- vitreous H43.89
- vulva N90.89

Adiaspiromycosis B48.8

Adie (-Holmes) **pupil or syndrome** — *see* Anomaly, pupil, function, tonic pupil

Adiponecrosis neonatorum P83.8

Adiposis (*see also* Obesity)
- cerebralis E23.6
- dolorosa E88.2

Adiposity (*see also* Obesity)
- heart — *see* Degeneration, myocardial
- localized E65

Adiposogenital dystrophy E23.6

Adjustment
- disorder — *see* Disorder, adjustment
- implanted device — *see* Encounter (for), adjustment (of)
- prosthesis, external — *see* Fitting
- reaction — *see* Disorder, adjustment

Administration of tPA (rtPA) in a different facility within the last 24 hours prior to admission to current facility Z92.82

Admission (for) (*see also* Encounter (for))
- adjustment (of)
  - artificial
    - arm Z44.00- ☑
      - complete Z44.01- ☑
      - partial Z44.02- ☑
    - eye Z44.2 ☑
    - leg Z44.10- ☑
      - complete Z44.11- ☑
      - partial Z44.12- ☑
  - brain neuropacemaker Z46.2
    - implanted Z45.42
  - breast
    - implant Z45.81 ☑
    - prosthesis (external) Z44.3 ☑
  - colostomy belt Z46.89
  - contact lenses Z46.0
  - cystostomy device Z46.6
  - dental prosthesis Z46.3
  - device NEC
    - abdominal Z46.89
    - implanted Z45.89
      - cardiac Z45.09
        - defibrillator (with synchronous cardiac pacemaker) Z45.02
        - pacemaker Z45.018
          - pulse generator Z45.010
      - hearing device Z45.328
        - bone conduction Z45.320
        - cochlear Z45.321
      - infusion pump Z45.1
      - nervous system Z45.49
        - CSF drainage Z45.41
        - hearing device — *see* Admission, adjustment, device, implanted, hearing device
        - neuropacemaker Z45.42
        - visual substitution Z45.31
      - specified NEC Z45.89
      - vascular access Z45.2
      - visual substitution Z45.31
    - nervous system Z46.2
      - implanted — *see* Admission, adjustment, device, implanted, nervous system
    - orthodontic Z46.4
    - prosthetic Z44.9
      - arm — *see* Admission, adjustment, artificial, arm
      - breast Z44.3 ☑
      - dental Z46.3
      - eye Z44.2 ☑
      - leg — *see* Admission, adjustment, artificial, leg
      - specified type NEC Z44.8

Admission — *continued*
- adjustment — *continued*
  - device — *continued*
    - substitution
      - auditory Z46.2
        - implanted — *see* Admission, adjustment, device, implanted, hearing device
      - nervous system Z46.2
        - implanted — *see* Admission, adjustment, device, implanted, nervous system
      - visual Z46.2
        - implanted Z45.31
    - urinary Z46.6
  - hearing aid Z46.1
    - implanted — *see* Admission, adjustment, device, implanted, hearing device
  - ileostomy device Z46.89
  - intestinal appliance or device NEC Z46.89
  - neuropacemaker (brain) (peripheral nerve) (spinal cord) Z46.2
    - implanted Z45.42
  - orthodontic device Z46.4
  - orthopedic (brace) (cast) (device) (shoes) Z46.89
  - pacemaker
    - cardiac Z45.018
      - pulse generator Z45.010
    - nervous system Z46.2
      - implanted Z45.42
  - portacath (port-a-cath) Z45.2
  - prosthesis Z44.9
    - arm — *see* Admission, adjustment, artificial, arm
    - breast Z44.3 ☑
    - dental Z46.3
    - eye Z44.2 ☑
    - leg — *see* Admission, adjustment, artificial, leg
    - specified NEC Z44.8
  - spectacles Z46.0
- aftercare (*see also* Aftercare) Z51.89
  - postpartum
    - immediately after delivery Z39.0
    - routine follow-up Z39.2
  - radiation therapy (antineoplastic) Z51.0
- attention to artificial opening (of) Z43.9
  - artificial vagina Z43.7
  - colostomy Z43.3
  - cystostomy Z43.5
  - enterostomy Z43.4
  - gastrostomy Z43.1
  - ileostomy Z43.2
  - jejunostomy Z43.4
  - nephrostomy Z43.6
  - specified site NEC Z43.8
    - intestinal tract Z43.4
    - urinary tract Z43.6
  - tracheostomy Z43.0
  - ureterostomy Z43.6
  - urethrostomy Z43.6
- breast augmentation or reduction Z41.1
- breast reconstruction following mastectomy Z42.1
- change of
  - dressing (nonsurgical) Z48.00
  - neuropacemaker device (brain) (peripheral nerve) (spinal cord) Z46.2
    - implanted Z45.42
  - surgical dressing Z48.01
- circumcision, ritual or routine (in absence of diagnosis) Z41.2
- clinical research investigation (control) (normal comparison) (participant) Z00.6
- contraceptive management Z30.9
- cosmetic surgery NEC Z41.1
- counseling (*see also* Counseling)
  - dietary Z71.3
  - HIV Z71.7
  - human immunodeficiency virus Z71.7
  - nonattending third party Z71.0
  - procreative management NEC Z31.69
- delivery, full-term, uncomplicated O80
  - cesarean, without indication O82
- dietary surveillance and counseling Z71.3
- ear piercing Z41.3
- examination at health care facility (adult) (*see also* Examination) Z00.00
  - with abnormal findings Z00.01

Admission — *continued*
- examination at health care facility (*see also* Examination) — *continued*
  - clinical research investigation (control) (normal comparison) (participant) Z00.6
  - dental Z01.20
    - with abnormal findings Z01.21
  - donor (potential) Z00.5
  - ear Z01.10
    - with abnormal findings NEC Z01.118
  - eye Z01.00
    - with abnormal findings Z01.01
  - general, specified reason NEC Z00.8
  - hearing Z01.10
    - with abnormal findings NEC Z01.118
  - postpartum checkup Z39.2
  - psychiatric (general) Z00.8
    - requested by authority Z04.6
  - vision Z01.00
    - with abnormal findings Z01.01
- fitting (of)
  - artificial
    - arm — *see* Admission, adjustment, artificial, arm
    - eye Z44.2 ☑
    - leg — *see* Admission, adjustment, artificial, leg
  - brain neuropacemaker Z46.2
    - implanted Z45.42
  - breast prosthesis (external) Z44.3 ☑
  - colostomy belt Z46.89
  - contact lenses Z46.0
  - cystostomy device Z46.6
  - dental prosthesis Z46.3
  - dentures Z46.3
  - device NEC
    - abdominal Z46.89
    - nervous system Z46.2
      - implanted — *see* Admission, adjustment, device, implanted, nervous system
    - orthodontic Z46.4
    - prosthetic Z44.9
      - breast Z44.3 ☑
      - dental Z46.3
      - eye Z44.2 ☑
    - substitution
      - auditory Z46.2
        - implanted — *see* Admission, adjustment, device, implanted, hearing device
      - nervous system Z46.2
        - implanted — *see* Admission, adjustment, device, implanted, nervous system
      - visual Z46.2
        - implanted Z45.31
  - hearing aid Z46.1
  - ileostomy device Z46.89
  - intestinal appliance or device NEC Z46.89
  - neuropacemaker (brain) (peripheral nerve) (spinal cord) Z46.2
    - implanted Z45.42
  - orthodontic device Z46.4
  - orthopedic device (brace) (cast) (shoes) Z46.89
  - prosthesis Z44.9
    - arm — *see* Admission, adjustment, artificial, arm
    - breast Z44.3 ☑
    - dental Z46.3
    - eye Z44.2 ☑
    - leg — *see* Admission, adjustment, artificial, leg
    - specified type NEC Z44.8
  - spectacles Z46.0
- follow-up examination Z09
- intrauterine device management Z30.431
  - initial prescription Z30.014
- mental health evaluation Z00.8
  - requested by authority Z04.6
- observation — *see* Observation
- Papanicolaou smear, cervix Z12.4
  - for suspected malignant neoplasm Z12.4
- plastic and reconstructive surgery following medical procedure or healed injury NEC Z42.8
- plastic surgery, cosmetic NEC Z41.1
- postpartum observation
  - immediately after delivery Z39.0
  - routine follow-up Z39.2
- poststerilization (for restoration) Z31.0
  - aftercare Z31.42

Admission — *continued*
  procreative management Z31.9
  prophylactic (measure)
    organ removal Z40.00
      breast Z40.01
      ovary Z40.02
      specified organ NEC Z40.09
      testes Z40.09
    vaccination Z23
  psychiatric examination (general) Z00.8
    requested by authority Z04.6
  radiation therapy (antineoplastic) Z51.0
  reconstructive surgery following medical procedure
      or healed injury NEC Z42.8
  removal of
    cystostomy catheter Z43.5
    drains Z48.03
    dressing (nonsurgical) Z48.00
    intrauterine contraceptive device Z30.432
    neuropacemaker (brain) (peripheral nerve) (spinal
        cord) Z46.2
      implanted Z45.42
    staples Z48.02
    surgical dressing Z48.01
    sutures Z48.02
    ureteral stent Z46.6
  respirator [ventilator] use during power failure Z99.12
  restoration of organ continuity (poststerilization) Z31.0
    aftercare Z31.42
  sensitivity test (*see also* Test, skin)
    allergy NEC Z01.82
    Mantoux Z11.1
  tuboplasty following previous sterilization Z31.0
    aftercare Z31.42
  vasoplasty following previous sterilization Z31.0
    aftercare Z31.42
  vision examination Z01.00
    with abnormal findings Z01.01
  waiting period for admission to other facility Z75.1
Adnexitis (suppurative) — *see* Salpingo-oophoritis
Adolescent X-linked adrenoleukodystrophy E71.521
Adrenal (gland) — *see* condition
Adrenalism, tuberculous A18.7
Adrenalitis, adrenitis E27.8
  autoimmune E27.1
  meningococcal, hemorrhagic A39.1
Adrenarche, premature E27.0
Adrenocortical syndrome — *see* Cushing's, syndrome
Adrenogenital syndrome E25.9
  acquired E25.8
  congenital E25.0
  salt loss E25.0
Adrenogenitalism, congenital E25.0
Adrenoleukodystrophy E71.529
  neonatal E71.511
  X-linked E71.529
    Addison only phenotype E71.528
    Addison-Schilder E71.528
    adolescent E71.521
    adrenomyeloneuropathy E71.522
    childhood cerebral E71.520
    other specified E71.528
Adrenomyeloneuropathy E71.522
Adventitious bursa — *see* Bursopathy, specified type
    NEC
Adverse effect — *see* Table of Drugs and Chemicals,
    categories T36-T50, with 6th character 5
Advice — *see* Counseling
Adynamia (episodica) (hereditary) (periodic) G72.3
Aeration lung imperfect, newborn — *see* Atelectasis
Aerobullosis T70.3 ☑
Aerocele — *see* Embolism, air
Aerodermectasia
  subcutaneous (traumatic) T79.7 ☑
Aerodontalgia T70.29 ☑
Aeroembolism T70.3 ☑
Aerogenes capsulatus infection A48.0
Aero-otitis media T70.0 ☑
Aerophagy, aerophagia (psychogenic) F45.8
Aerophobia F40.228
Aerosinusitis T70.1 ☑
Aerotitis T70.0 ☑
Affection — *see* Disease
Afibrinogenemia (*see also* Defect, coagulation) D68.8
  acquired D65
  congenital D68.2
  following ectopic or molar pregnancy O08.1

Afibrinogenemia — *continued*
  in abortion — *see* Abortion, by type, complicated by,
      afibrinogenemia
  puerperal O72.3
African
  sleeping sickness B56.9
  tick fever A68.1
  trypanosomiasis B56.9
    gambian B56.0
    rhodesian B56.1
Aftercare (*see also* Care) Z51.89
  following surgery (for) (on)
    amputation Z47.81
    attention to
      drains Z48.03
      dressings (nonsurgical) Z48.00
        surgical Z48.01
      sutures Z48.02
    circulatory system Z48.812
    delayed (planned) wound closure Z48.1
    digestive system Z48.815
    explantation of joint prosthesis (staged procedure)
      hip Z47.32
      knee Z47.33
      shoulder Z47.31
    genitourinary system Z48.816
    joint replacement Z47.1
    neoplasm Z48.3
    nervous system Z48.811
    oral cavity Z48.814
    organ transplant
      bone marrow Z48.290
      heart Z48.21
      heart-lung Z48.280
      kidney Z48.22
      liver Z48.23
      lung Z48.24
      multiple organs NEC Z48.288
      specified NEC Z48.298
    orthopedic NEC Z47.89
    planned wound closure Z48.1
    removal of internal fixation device Z47.2
    respiratory system Z48.813
    scoliosis Z47.82
    sense organs Z48.810
    skin and subcutaneous tissue Z48.817
    specified body system
      circulatory Z48.812
      digestive Z48.815
      genitourinary Z48.816
      nervous Z48.811
      oral cavity Z48.814
      respiratory Z48.813
      sense organs Z48.810
      skin and subcutaneous tissue Z48.817
      teeth Z48.814
    specified NEC Z48.89
    spinal Z48.89
    teeth Z48.814
  fracture — *code to* fracture with seventh character D
  involving
    removal of
      drains Z48.03
      dressings (nonsurgical) Z48.00
      staples Z48.02
      surgical dressings Z48.01
      sutures Z48.02
    neuropacemaker (brain) (peripheral nerve) (spinal
        cord) Z46.2
      implanted Z45.42
    orthopedic NEC Z47.89
  postprocedural — *see* Aftercare, following surgery
After-cataract — *see* Cataract, secondary
Agalactia (primary) O92.3
  elective, secondary or therapeutic O92.5
Agammaglobulinemia (acquired (secondary)) (nonfa-
    milial) D80.1
  with
    immunoglobulin-bearing B-lymphocytes D80.1
    lymphopenia D81.9
  autosomal recessive (Swiss type) D80.0
  Bruton's X-linked D80.0
  common variable (CVAgamma) D80.1
  congenital sex-linked D80.0
  hereditary D80.0
  lymphopenic D81.9
  Swiss type (autosomal recessive) D80.0

Agammaglobulinemia — *continued*
  X-linked (with growth hormone deficiency)(Bruton)
      D80.0
Aganglionosis (bowel) (colon) Q43.1
Age (old) — *see* Senility
Agenesis
  adrenal (gland) Q89.1
  alimentary tract (complete) (partial) NEC Q45.8
    upper Q40.8
  anus, anal (canal) Q42.3
    with fistula Q42.2
  aorta Q25.4
  appendix Q42.8
  arm (complete) Q71.0- ☑
    with hand present Q71.1- ☑
  artery (peripheral) Q27.9
    brain Q28.3
    coronary Q24.5
    pulmonary Q25.79
    specified NEC Q27.8
    umbilical Q27.0
  auditory (canal) (external) Q16.1
  auricle (ear) Q16.0
  bile duct or passage Q44.5
  bladder Q64.5
  bone Q79.9
  brain Q00.0
    part of Q04.3
  breast (with nipple present) Q83.8
    with absent nipple Q83.0
  bronchus Q32.4
  canaliculus lacrimalis Q10.4
  carpus — *see* Agenesis, hand
  cartilage Q79.9
  cecum Q42.8
  cerebellum Q04.3
  cervix Q51.5
  chin Q18.8
  cilia Q10.3
  circulatory system, part NOS Q28.9
  clavicle Q74.0
  clitoris Q52.6
  coccyx Q76.49
  colon Q42.9
    specified NEC Q42.8
  corpus callosum Q04.0
  cricoid cartilage Q31.8
  diaphragm (with hernia) Q79.1
  digestive organ(s) or tract (complete) (partial) NEC
      Q45.8
    upper Q40.8
  ductus arteriosus Q28.8
  duodenum Q41.0
  ear Q16.9
    auricle Q16.0
    lobe Q17.8
  ejaculatory duct Q55.4
  endocrine (gland) NEC Q89.2
  epiglottis Q31.8
  esophagus Q39.8
  eustachian tube Q16.2
  eye Q11.1
    adnexa Q15.8
  eyelid (fold) Q10.3
  face
    bones NEC Q75.8
    specified part NEC Q18.8
  fallopian tube Q50.6
  femur — *see* Defect, reduction, lower limb, longitudi-
      nal, femur
  fibula — *see* Defect, reduction, lower limb, longitudi-
      nal, fibula
  finger (complete) (partial) — *see* Agenesis, hand
  foot (and toes) (complete) (partial) Q72.3- ☑
  forearm (with hand present) — *see* Agenesis, arm,
      with hand present
    and hand Q71.2- ☑
  gallbladder Q44.0
  gastric Q40.2
  genitalia, genital (organ(s))
    female Q52.8
      external Q52.71
      internal NEC Q52.8
    male Q55.8
  glottis Q31.8
  hair Q84.0
  hand (and fingers) (complete) (partial) Q71.3- ☑

☑ **Additional Character Required — Refer to the Tabular List for Character Selection**   ▽ **Subterms under main terms may continue to next column or page**

Agenesis — continued
heart Q24.8
  valve NEC Q24.8
    pulmonary Q22.0
hepatic Q44.7
humerus — see Defect, reduction, upper limb
hymen Q52.4
ileum Q41.2
incus Q16.3
intestine (small) Q41.9
  large Q42.9
    specified NEC Q42.8
iris (dilator fibers) Q13.1
jaw M26.09
jejunum Q41.1
kidney(s) (partial) Q60.2
  bilateral Q60.1
  unilateral Q60.0
labium (majus) (minus) Q52.71
labyrinth, membranous Q16.5
lacrimal apparatus Q10.4
larynx Q31.8
leg (complete) Q72.0- ☑
  with foot present Q72.1- ☑
  lower leg (with foot present) — see Agenesis, leg,
    with foot present
    and foot Q72.2- ☑
lens Q12.3
limb (complete) Q73.0
  lower — see Agenesis, leg
  upper — see Agenesis, arm
lip Q38.0
liver Q44.7
lung (fissure) (lobe) (bilateral) (unilateral) Q33.3
mandible, maxilla M26.09
metacarpus — see Agenesis, hand
metatarsus — see Agenesis, foot
muscle Q79.8
  eyelid Q10.3
  ocular Q15.8
musculoskeletal system NEC Q79.8
nail(s) Q84.3
neck, part Q18.8
nerve Q07.8
nervous system, part NEC Q07.8
nipple Q83.2
nose Q30.1
nuclear Q07.8
organ
  of Corti Q16.5
  or site not listed — see Anomaly, by site
osseous meatus (ear) Q16.1
ovary
  bilateral Q50.02
  unilateral Q50.01
oviduct Q50.6
pancreas Q45.0
parathyroid (gland) Q89.2
parotid gland(s) Q38.4
patella Q74.1
pelvic girdle (complete) (partial) Q74.2
penis Q55.5
pericardium Q24.8
pituitary (gland) Q89.2
prostate Q55.4
punctum lacrimale Q10.4
radioulnar — see Defect, reduction, upper limb
radius — see Defect, reduction, upper limb, longitudinal, radius
rectum Q42.1
  with fistula Q42.0
renal Q60.2
  bilateral Q60.1
  unilateral Q60.0
respiratory organ NEC Q34.8
rib Q76.6
roof of orbit Q75.8
round ligament Q52.8
sacrum Q76.49
salivary gland Q38.4
scapula Q74.0
scrotum Q55.29
seminal vesicles Q55.4
septum
  atrial Q21.1
  between aorta and pulmonary artery Q21.4
  ventricular Q20.4
shoulder girdle (complete) (partial) Q74.0

Agenesis — continued
skull (bone) Q75.8
  with
    anencephaly Q00.0
    encephalocele — see Encephalocele
    hydrocephalus Q03.9
      with spina bifida — see Spina bifida, by site,
        with hydrocephalus
    microcephaly Q02
spermatic cord Q55.4
spinal cord Q06.0
spine Q76.49
spleen Q89.01
sternum Q76.7
stomach Q40.2
submaxillary gland(s) (congenital) Q38.4
tarsus — see Agenesis, foot
tendon Q79.8
testicle Q55.0
thymus (gland) Q89.2
thyroid (gland) E03.1
  cartilage Q31.8
tibia — see Defect, reduction, lower limb, longitudinal,
  tibia
tibiofibular — see Defect, reduction, lower limb,
  specified type NEC
toe (and foot) (complete) (partial) — see Agenesis,
  foot
tongue Q38.3
trachea (cartilage) Q32.1
ulna — see Defect, reduction, upper limb, longitudinal,
  ulna
upper limb — see Agenesis, arm
ureter Q62.4
urethra Q64.5
urinary tract NEC Q64.8
uterus Q51.0
uvula Q38.5
vagina Q52.0
vas deferens Q55.4
vein(s) (peripheral) Q27.9
  brain Q28.3
  great NEC Q26.8
  portal Q26.5
vena cava (inferior) (superior) Q26.8
vermis of cerebellum Q04.3
vertebra Q76.49
vulva Q52.71
Ageusia R43.2
Agitated — see condition
Agitation R45.1
Aglossia (congenital) Q38.3
Aglossia-adactylia syndrome Q87.0
Aglycogenosis E74.00
Agnosia (body image) (other senses) (tactile) R48.1
  developmental F88
  verbal R48.1
    auditory R48.1
      developmental F80.2
    developmental F80.2
  visual (object) R48.3
Agoraphobia F40.00
  with panic disorder F40.01
  without panic disorder F40.02
Agrammatism R48.8
Agranulocytopenia — see Agranulocytosis
Agranulocytosis (chronic) (cyclical) (genetic) (infantile)
  (periodic) (pernicious) (see also Neutropenia) D70.9
  congenital D70.0
  cytoreductive cancer chemotherapy sequela D70.1
  drug-induced D70.2
    due to cytoreductive cancer chemotherapy D70.1
  due to infection D70.3
  secondary D70.4
    drug-induced D70.2
      due to cytoreductive cancer chemotherapy
        D70.1
Agraphia (absolute) R48.8
  with alexia R48.0
  developmental F81.81
Ague (dumb) — see Malaria
Agyria Q04.3
Ahumada-del Castillo syndrome E23.0
Aichomophobia F40.298
AIDS (related complex) B20
Ailment heart — see Disease, heart
Ailurophobia F40.218
Ainhum (disease) L94.6

AIPHI (acute idiopathic pulmonary hemorrhage in infants
  (over 28 days old)) R04.81
Air
anterior mediastinum J98.2
compressed, disease T70.3 ☑
conditioner lung or pneumonitis J67.7
embolism (artery) (cerebral) (any site) T79.0 ☑
  with ectopic or molar pregnancy O08.2
  due to implanted device NEC — see Complications,
    by site and type, specified NEC
  following
    abortion — see Abortion by type, complicated
      by, embolism
    ectopic or molar pregnancy O08.2
    infusion, therapeutic injection or transfusion
      T80.0 ☑
  in pregnancy, childbirth or puerperium — see
    Embolism, obstetric
  traumatic T79.0 ☑
hunger, psychogenic F45.8
rarefied, effects of — see Effect, adverse, high altitude
sickness T75.3 ☑
Airplane sickness T75.3 ☑
Akathisia (drug-induced) (treatment-induced) G25.71
  neuroleptic induced (acute) G25.71
Akinesia R29.898
Akinetic mutism R41.89
Akureyri's disease G93.3
Alactasia, congenital E73.0
Alagille's syndrome Q44.7
Alastrim B03
Albers-Schönberg syndrome Q78.2
Albert's syndrome — see Tendinitis, Achilles
Albinism, albino E70.30
  with hematologic abnormality E70.339
    Chédiak-Higashi syndrome E70.330
    Hermansky-Pudlak syndrome E70.331
    other specified E70.338
  I E70.320
  II E70.321
  ocular E70.319
    autosomal recessive E70.311
    other specified E70.318
    X-linked E70.310
  oculocutaneous E70.329
    other specified E70.328
    tyrosinase (ty) negative E70.320
    tyrosinase (ty) positive E70.321
  other specified E70.39
Albinismus E70.30
Albright (-McCune)(-Sternberg) syndrome Q78.1
Albuminous — see condition
Albuminuria, albuminuric (acute) (chronic) (subacute)
  (see also Proteinuria) R80.9
  complicating pregnancy — see Proteinuria, gestational
    with
      gestational hypertension — see Pre-eclampsia
      pre-existing hypertension — see Hypertension,
        complicating pregnancy, pre-existing,
        with, pre-eclampsia
  gestational — see Proteinuria, gestational
    with
      gestational hypertension — see Pre-eclampsia
      pre-existing hypertension — see Hypertension,
        complicating pregnancy, pre-existing,
        with, pre-eclampsia
  orthostatic R80.2
  postural R80.2
  pre-eclamptic — see Pre-eclampsia
  scarlatinal A38.8
Albuminurophobia F40.298
Alcaptonuria E70.29
Alcohol, alcoholic, alcohol-induced
  addiction (without remission) F10.20
    with remission F10.21
  amnestic disorder, persisting F10.96
    with dependence F10.26
  brain syndrome, chronic F10.97
    with dependence F10.27
  cardiopathy I42.6
  counseling and surveillance Z71.41
    family member Z71.42
  delirium (acute) (tremens) (withdrawal) F10.231
    with intoxication F10.921
    in
      abuse F10.121
      dependence F10.221

Alcohol, alcoholic, alcohol-induced — continued
- dementia F10.97
  - with dependence F10.27
- deterioration F10.97
  - with dependence F10.27
- hallucinosis (acute) F10.951
  - in
    - abuse F10.151
    - dependence F10.251
- insanity F10.959
- intoxication (acute) (without dependence) F10.129
  - with
    - delirium F10.121
    - dependence F10.229
      - with delirium F10.221
      - uncomplicated F10.220
    - uncomplicated F10.120
- jealousy F10.988
- Korsakoff's, Korsakov's, Korsakow's F10.26
- liver K70.9
  - acute — see Disease, liver, alcoholic, hepatitis
- mania (acute) (chronic) F10.959
- paranoia, paranoid (type) psychosis F10.950
- pellagra E52
- poisoning, accidental (acute) NEC — see Table of Drugs and Chemicals, alcohol, poisoning
- psychosis — see Psychosis, alcoholic
- withdrawal (without convulsions) F10.239
  - with delirium F10.231

Alcoholism (chronic) (without remission) F10.20
- with
  - psychosis — see Psychosis, alcoholic
  - remission F10.21
- Korsakov's F10.96
  - with dependence F10.26

Alder (-Reilly) **anomaly or syndrome** (leukocyte granulation) D72.0

Aldosteronism E26.9
- familial (type I) E26.02
- glucocorticoid-remediable E26.02
- primary (due to (bilateral) adrenal hyperplasia) E26.09
- primary NEC E26.09
- secondary E26.1
- specified NEC E26.89

Aldosteronoma D44.10

Aldrich (-Wiskott) **syndrome** (eczema-thrombocytopenia) D82.0

Alektorophobia F40.218

Aleppo boil B55.1

Aleukemic — see condition

Aleukia
- congenital D70.0
- hemorrhagica D61.9
  - congenital D61.09
- splenica D73.1

Alexia R48.0
- developmental F81.0
- secondary to organic lesion R48.0

Algoneurodystrophy M89.00
- ankle M89.07- ☑
- foot M89.07- ☑
- forearm M89.03- ☑
- hand M89.04- ☑
- lower leg M89.06- ☑
- multiple sites M89.0- ☑
- shoulder M89.01- ☑
- specified site NEC M89.08
- thigh M89.05- ☑
- upper arm M89.02- ☑

Algophobia F40.298

Alienation, mental — see Psychosis

Alkalemia E87.3

Alkalosis E87.3
- metabolic E87.3
  - with respiratory acidosis E87.4
- respiratory E87.3

Alkaptonuria E70.29

Allen-Masters syndrome N83.8

Allergy, allergic (reaction) (to) T78.40 ☑
- air-borne substance NEC (rhinitis) J30.89
- alveolitis (extrinsic) J67.9
  - due to
    - Aspergillus clavatus J67.4
    - Cryptostroma corticale J67.6
    - organisms (fungal, thermophilic actinomycete) growing in ventilation (air conditioning) systems J67.7

Allergy, allergic — continued
- alveolitis — continued
  - specified type NEC J67.8
- anaphylactic reaction or shock T78.2 ☑
- angioneurotic edema T78.3 ☑
- animal (dander) (epidermal) (hair) (rhinitis) J30.81
- bee sting (anaphylactic shock) — see Toxicity, venom, arthropod, bee
- biological — see Allergy, drug
- colitis K52.2
- dander (animal) (rhinitis) J30.81
- dandruff (rhinitis) J30.81
- dental restorative material (existing) K08.55
- dermatitis — see Dermatitis, contact, allergic
- diathesis — see History, allergy
- drug, medicament & biological (any) (external) (internal) T78.40 ☑
  - correct substance properly administered — see Table of Drugs and Chemicals, by drug, adverse effect
  - wrong substance given or taken NEC (by accident) — see Table of Drugs and Chemicals, by drug, poisoning
- due to pollen J30.1
- dust (house) (stock) (rhinitis) J30.89
  - with asthma — see Asthma, allergic extrinsic
- eczema — see Dermatitis, contact, allergic
- epidermal (animal) (rhinitis) J30.81
- feathers (rhinitis) J30.89
- food (any) (ingested) NEC T78.1 ☑
  - anaphylactic shock — see Shock, anaphylactic, due to food
  - dermatitis — see Dermatitis, due to, food
  - dietary counseling and surveillance Z71.3
  - in contact with skin L23.6
  - rhinitis J30.5
  - status (without reaction) Z91.018
    - eggs Z91.012
    - milk products Z91.011
    - peanuts Z91.010
    - seafood Z91.013
    - specified NEC Z91.018
- gastrointestinal K52.2
- grain J30.1
- grass (hay fever) (pollen) J30.1
  - asthma — see Asthma, allergic extrinsic
- hair (animal) (rhinitis) J30.81
- history (of) — see History, allergy
- horse serum — see Allergy, serum
- inhalant (rhinitis) J30.89
  - pollen J30.1
- kapok (rhinitis) J30.89
- medicine — see Allergy, drug
- milk protein K52.2
- nasal, seasonal due to pollen J30.1
- pneumonia J82
- pollen (any) (hay fever) J30.1
  - asthma — see Asthma, allergic extrinsic
- primrose J30.1
- primula J30.1
- purpura D69.0
- ragweed (hay fever) (pollen) J30.1
  - asthma — see Asthma, allergic extrinsic
- rose (pollen) J30.1
- seasonal NEC J30.2
- Senecio jacobae (pollen) J30.1
- serum (see also Reaction, serum) T80.69 ☑
  - anaphylactic shock T80.59 ☑
- shock (anaphylactic) T78.2 ☑
  - due to
    - administration of blood and blood products T80.51 ☑
    - adverse effect of correct medicinal substance properly administered T88.6 ☑
    - immunization T80.52 ☑
    - serum NEC T80.59 ☑
    - vaccination T80.52 ☑
- specific NEC T78.49 ☑
- tree (any) (hay fever) (pollen) J30.1
  - asthma — see Asthma, allergic extrinsic
- upper respiratory J30.9
- urticaria L50.0
- vaccine — see Allergy, serum
- wheat — see Allergy, food

Allescheriasis B48.2

Alligator skin disease Q80.9

Allocheiria, allochiria R20.8

Almeida's disease — see Paracoccidioidomycosis

Alopecia (hereditaria) (seborrheica) L65.9
- androgenic L64.9
  - drug-induced L64.0
  - specified NEC L64.8
- areata L63.9
  - ophiasis L63.2
  - specified NEC L63.8
  - totalis L63.0
  - universalis L63.1
- cicatricial L66.9
  - specified NEC L66.8
- circumscripta L63.9
- congenital, congenitalis Q84.0
- due to cytotoxic drugs NEC L65.8
- mucinosa L65.2
- postinfective NEC L65.8
- postpartum L65.0
- premature L64.8
- specific (syphilitic) A51.32
- specified NEC L65.8
- syphilitic (secondary) A51.32
- totalis (capitis) L63.0
- universalis (entire body) L63.1
- X-ray L58.1

Alpers' disease G31.81

Alpine sickness T70.29 ☑

Alport syndrome Q87.81

ALTE (apparent life threatening event) **in newborn and infant** R68.13

Alteration (of), **Altered**
- awareness, transient R40.4
- mental status R41.82
- pattern of family relationships affecting child Z62.898
- sensation
  - following
    - cerebrovascular disease I69.998
      - cerebral infarction I69.398
      - intracerebral hemorrhage I69.198
      - nontraumatic intracranial hemorrhage NEC I69.298
      - specified disease NEC I69.898
      - subarachnoid hemorrhage I69.098

Alternating — see condition

Altitude, high (effects) — see Effect, adverse, high altitude

Aluminosis (of lung) J63.0

Alveolitis
- allergic (extrinsic) — see Pneumonitis, hypersensitivity
- due to
  - Aspergillus clavatus J67.4
  - Cryptostroma corticale J67.6
- fibrosing (cryptogenic) (idiopathic) J84.112
- jaw M27.3
- sicca dolorosa M27.3

Alveolus, alveolar — see condition

Alymphocytosis D72.810
- thymic (with immunodeficiency) D82.1

Alymphoplasia, thymic D82.1

Alzheimer's disease or sclerosis — see Disease, Alzheimer's

Amastia (with nipple present) Q83.8
- with absent nipple Q83.0

Amathophobia F40.228

Amaurosis (acquired) (congenital) (see also Blindness)
- fugax G45.3
- hysterical F44.6
- Leber's congenital H35.50
- uremic — see Uremia

Amaurotic idiocy (infantile) (juvenile) (late) E75.4

Amaxophobia F40.248

Ambiguous genitalia Q56.4

Amblyopia (congenital) (ex anopsia) (partial) (suppression) H53.00- ☑
- anisometropic — see Amblyopia, refractive
- deprivation H53.01- ☑
- hysterical F44.6
- nocturnal (see also Blindness, night)
  - vitamin A deficiency E50.5
- refractive H53.02- ☑
- strabismic H53.03- ☑
- tobacco H53.8
- toxic NEC H53.8
- uremic — see Uremia

Ameba, amebic (histolytica) (see also Amebiasis)
- abscess (liver) A06.4

16

☑ Additional Character Required — Refer to the Tabular List for Character Selection   ▽ Subterms under main terms may continue to next column or page

Amebiasis A06.9
  with abscess — *see* Abscess, amebic
  acute A06.0
  chronic (intestine) A06.1
    with abscess — *see* Abscess, amebic
  cutaneous A06.7
  cutis A06.7
  cystitis A06.81
  genitourinary tract NEC A06.82
  hepatic — *see* Abscess, liver, amebic
  intestine A06.0
  nondysenteric colitis A06.2
  skin A06.7
  specified site NEC A06.89
Ameboma (of intestine) A06.3
Amelia Q73.0
  lower limb — *see* Agenesis, leg
  upper limb — *see* Agenesis, arm
Ameloblastoma (*see also* Cyst, calcifying odontogenic)
  long bones C40.9- ☑
    lower limb C40.2- ☑
    upper limb C40.0- ☑
  malignant C41.1
    jaw (bone) (lower) C41.1
      upper C41.0
  tibial C40.2- ☑
Amelogenesis imperfecta K00.5
  nonhereditaria (segmentalis) K00.4
Amenorrhea N91.2
  hyperhormonal E28.8
  primary N91.0
  secondary N91.1
Amentia — *see* Disability, intellectual
  Meynert's (nonalcoholic) F04
American
  leishmaniasis B55.2
  mountain tick fever A93.2
Ametropia — *see* Disorder, refraction
Amianthosis J61
Amimia R48.8
Amino-acid disorder E72.9
  anemia D53.0
Aminoacidopathy E72.9
Aminoaciduria E72.9
Amnesia R41.3
  anterograde R41.1
  auditory R48.8
  dissociative F44.0
  hysterical F44.0
  postictal in epilepsy — *see* Epilepsy
  psychogenic F44.0
  retrograde R41.2
  transient global G45.4
Amnes(t)ic syndrome (post-traumatic) F04
  induced by
    alcohol F10.96
      with dependence F10.26
    psychoactive NEC F19.96
      with
        abuse F19.16
        dependence F19.26
    sedative F13.96
      with dependence F13.26
Amnion, amniotic — *see* condition
Amnionitis — *see* Pregnancy, complicated by
Amok F68.8
Amoral traits F60.89
Ampulla
  lower esophagus K22.8
  phrenic K22.8
Amputation (*see also* Absence, by site, acquired)
  neuroma (postoperative) (traumatic) — *see* Complications, amputation stump, neuroma
  stump (surgical)
    abnormal, painful, or with complication (late) — *see* Complications, amputation stump
    healed or old NOS Z89.9
  traumatic (complete) (partial)
    arm (upper) (complete) S48.91- ☑
      at
        elbow S58.01- ☑
          partial S58.02- ☑
        shoulder joint (complete) S48.01- ☑
          partial S48.02- ☑
      between
        elbow and wrist (complete) S58.11- ☑
          partial S58.12- ☑

Amputation — *continued*
  traumatic — *continued*
    arm — *continued*
      between — *continued*
        shoulder and elbow (complete) S48.11- ☑
          partial S48.12- ☑
      partial S48.92- ☑
    breast (complete) S28.21- ☑
      partial S28.22- ☑
    clitoris (complete) S38.211 ☑
      partial S38.212 ☑
    ear (complete) S08.11- ☑
      partial S08.12- ☑
    finger (complete) (metacarpophalangeal) S68.11- ☑
      index S68.11- ☑
      little S68.11- ☑
      middle S68.11- ☑
      partial S68.12- ☑
        index S68.12- ☑
        little S68.12- ☑
        middle S68.12- ☑
        ring S68.12- ☑
      ring S68.11- ☑
      thumb — *see* Amputation, traumatic, thumb
      transphalangeal (complete) S68.61- ☑
        index S68.61- ☑
        little S68.61- ☑
        middle S68.61- ☑
        partial S68.62- ☑
          index S68.62- ☑
          little S68.62- ☑
          middle S68.62- ☑
          ring S68.62- ☑
        ring S68.61- ☑
    foot (complete) S98.91- ☑
      at ankle level S98.01- ☑
        partial S98.02- ☑
      midfoot S98.31- ☑
        partial S98.32- ☑
      partial S98.92- ☑
    forearm (complete) S58.91- ☑
      at elbow level (complete) S58.01- ☑
        partial S58.02- ☑
      between elbow and wrist (complete) S58.11- ☑
        partial S58.12- ☑
      partial S58.92- ☑
    genital organ(s) (external)
      female (complete) S38.211 ☑
        partial S38.212 ☑
      male
        penis (complete) S38.221 ☑
          partial S38.222 ☑
        scrotum (complete) S38.231 ☑
          partial S38.232 ☑
        testes (complete) S38.231 ☑
          partial S38.232 ☑
    hand (complete) (wrist level) S68.41- ☑
      finger(s) alone — *see* Amputation, traumatic, finger
      partial S68.42- ☑
      thumb alone — *see* Amputation, traumatic, thumb
      transmetacarpal (complete) S68.71- ☑
        partial S68.72- ☑
    head
      ear — *see* Amputation, traumatic, ear
      nose (partial) S08.812 ☑
        complete S08.811 ☑
      part S08.89 ☑
        scalp S08.0 ☑
    hip (and thigh) (complete) S78.91- ☑
      at hip joint (complete) S78.01- ☑
        partial S78.02- ☑
      between hip and knee (complete) S78.11- ☑
        partial S78.12- ☑
      partial S78.92- ☑
    labium (majus) (minus) (complete) S38.21- ☑
      partial S38.21- ☑
    leg (lower) S88.91- ☑
      at knee level S88.01- ☑
        partial S88.02- ☑
      between knee and ankle S88.11- ☑
        partial S88.12- ☑
      partial S88.92- ☑

Amputation — *continued*
  traumatic — *continued*
    nose (partial) S08.812 ☑
      complete S08.811 ☑
    penis (complete) S38.221 ☑
      partial S38.222 ☑
    scrotum (complete) S38.231 ☑
      partial S38.232 ☑
    shoulder — *see* Amputation, traumatic, arm
      at shoulder joint — *see* Amputation, traumatic, arm, at shoulder joint
    testes (complete) S38.231 ☑
      partial S38.232 ☑
    thigh — *see* Amputation, traumatic, hip
    thorax, part of S28.1
      breast — *see* Amputation, traumatic, breast
    thumb (complete) (metacarpophalangeal) S68.01- ☑
      partial S68.02- ☑
      transphalangeal (complete) S68.51- ☑
        partial S68.52- ☑
    toe (lesser) S98.13- ☑
      great S98.11- ☑
        partial S98.12- ☑
      more than one S98.21- ☑
        partial S98.22- ☑
      partial S98.14- ☑
    vulva (complete) S38.211 ☑
      partial S38.212 ☑
Amputee (bilateral) (old) Z89.9
Amsterdam dwarfism Q87.1
Amusia R48.8
  developmental F80.89
Amyelencephalus, amyelencephaly Q00.0
Amyelia Q06.0
Amygdalitis — *see* Tonsillitis
Amygdalolith J35.8
Amyloid heart (disease) E85.4 [I43]
Amyloidosis (generalized) (primary) E85.9
  with lung involvement E85.4 [J99]
  familial E85.2
  genetic E85.2
  heart E85.4 [I43]
  hemodialysis-associated E85.3
  liver E85.4 [K77]
  localized E85.4
  neuropathic heredofamilial E85.1
  non-neuropathic heredofamilial E85.0
  organ limited E85.4
  Portuguese E85.1
  pulmonary E85.4 [J99]
  secondary systemic E85.3
  skin (lichen) (macular) E85.4 [L99]
  specified NEC E85.8
  subglottic E85.4 [J99]
Amylopectinosis (brancher enzyme deficiency) E74.03
Amylophagia — *see* Pica
Amyoplasia congenita Q79.8
Amyotonia M62.89
  congenita G70.2
Amyotrophia, amyotrophy, amyotrophic G71.8
  congenita Q79.8
  diabetic — *see* Diabetes, amyotrophy
  lateral sclerosis G12.21
  neuralgic G54.5
  spinal progressive G12.21
Anacidity, gastric K31.83
  psychogenic F45.8
Anaerosis of newborn P28.89
Analbuminemia E88.09
Analgesia — *see* Anesthesia
Analphalipoproteinemia E78.6
Anaphylactic
  purpura D69.0
  shock or reaction — *see* Shock, anaphylactic
Anaphylactoid shock or reaction — *see* Shock, anaphylactic
Anaphylactoid syndrome of pregnancy O88.01- ☑
Anaphylaxis — *see* Shock, anaphylactic
Anaplasia cervix (*see also* Dysplasia, cervix) N87.9
Anaplasmosis, human A77.49
Anarthria R47.1
Anasarca R60.1
  cardiac — *see* Failure, heart, congestive
  lung J18.2
  newborn P83.2
  nutritional E43

Anasarca — continued
pulmonary J18.2
renal N04.9
Anastomosis
aneurysmal — see Aneurysm
arteriovenous ruptured brain I60.8
intestinal K63.89
complicated NEC K91.89
involving urinary tract N99.89
retinal and choroidal vessels (congenital) Q14.8
Anatomical narrow angle H40.03- ☑
Ancylostoma, ancylostomiasis (braziliense) (caninum) (ceylanicum) (duodenale) B76.0
Necator americanus B76.1
Andersen's disease (glycogen storage) E74.09
Anderson-Fabry disease E75.21
Andes disease T70.29 ☑
Andrews' disease (bacterid) L08.89
Androblastoma
benign
specified site — see Neoplasm, benign, by site
unspecified site
female D27.9
male D29.20
malignant
specified site — see Neoplasm, malignant, by site
unspecified site
female C56.9
male C62.90
specified site — see Neoplasm, uncertain behavior, by site
tubular
with lipid storage
specified site — see Neoplasm, benign, by site
unspecified site
female D27.9
male D29.20
specified site — see Neoplasm, benign, by site
unspecified site
female D27.9
male D29.20
unspecified site
female D39.10
male D40.10
Androgen insensitivity syndrome (see also Syndrome, androgen insensitivity) E34.50
Androgen resistance syndrome (see also Syndrome, androgen insensitivity) E34.50
Android pelvis Q74.2
with disproportion (fetopelvic) O33.3 ☑
causing obstructed labor O65.3
Androphobia F40.290
Anectasis, pulmonary (newborn) — see Atelectasis
Anemia (essential) (general) (hemoglobin deficiency) (infantile) (primary) (profound) D64.9
with (due to) (in)
disorder of
anaerobic glycolysis D55.2
pentose phosphate pathway D55.1
koilonychia D50.9
achlorhydric D50.8
achrestic D53.1
Addison (-Biermer) (pernicious) D51.0
agranulocytic — see Agranulocytosis
amino-acid-deficiency D53.0
aplastic D61.9
congenital D61.09
drug-induced D61.1
due to
drugs D61.1
external agents NEC D61.2
infection D61.2
radiation D61.2
idiopathic D61.3
red cell (pure) D60.9
chronic D60.0
congenital D61.01
specified type NEC D60.8
transient D60.1
specified type NEC D61.89
toxic D61.2
aregenerative
congenital D61.09
asiderotic D50.9
atypical (primary) D64.9
Baghdad spring D55.0
Balantidium coli A07.0
Biermer's (pernicious) D51.0

Anemia — continued
blood loss (chronic) D50.0
acute D62
bothriocephalus B70.0 [D63.8]
brickmaker's B76.9 [D63.8]
cerebral I67.89
childhood D58.9
chlorotic D50.8
chronic
blood loss D50.0
hemolytic D58.9
idiopathic D59.9
simple D53.9
chronica congenita aregenerativa D61.09
combined system disease NEC D51.0 [G32.0]
due to dietary vitamin B12 deficiency D51.3 [G32.0]
complicating pregnancy, childbirth or puerperium — see Pregnancy, complicated by (management affected by), anemia
congenital P61.4
aplastic D61.09
due to isoimmunization NOS P55.9
dyserythropoietic, dyshematopoietic D64.4
following fetal blood loss P61.3
Heinz body D58.2
hereditary hemolytic NOS D58.9
pernicious D51.0
spherocytic D58.0
Cooley's (erythroblastic) D56.1
cytogenic D51.0
deficiency D53.9
6-PGD D55.1
2, 3 diphosphoglycurate mutase D55.2
2, 3 PG D55.2
6 phosphogluconate dehydrogenase D55.1
amino-acid D53.0
combined B12 and folate D53.1
enzyme D55.9
drug-induced (hemolytic) D59.2
glucose-6-phosphate dehydrogenase (G6PD) D55.0
glycolytic D55.2
nucleotide metabolism D55.3
related to hexose monophosphate (HMP) shunt pathway NEC D55.1
specified type NEC D55.8
erythrocytic glutathione D55.1
folate D52.9
dietary D52.0
drug-induced D52.1
folic acid D52.9
dietary D52.0
drug-induced D52.1
G SH D55.1
G6PD D55.0
GGS-R D55.1
glucose-6-phosphate dehydrogenase D55.0
glutathione reductase D55.1
glyceraldehyde phosphate dehydrogenase D55.2
hexokinase D55.2
iron D50.9
secondary to blood loss (chronic) D50.0
nutritional D53.9
with
poor iron absorption D50.8
specified deficiency NEC D53.8
phosphofructo-aldolase D55.2
phosphoglycerate kinase D55.2
PK D55.2
protein D53.0
pyruvate kinase D55.2
transcobalamin II D51.2
triose-phosphate isomerase D55.2
vitamin B12 NOS D51.9
dietary D51.3
due to
intrinsic factor deficiency D51.0
selective vitamin B12 malabsorption with proteinuria D51.1
pernicious D51.0
specified type NEC D51.8
Diamond-Blackfan (congenital hypoplastic) D61.01
dibothriocephalus B70.0 [D63.8]
dimorphic D53.1
diphasic D53.1
Diphyllobothrium (Dibothriocephalus) B70.0 [D63.8]
due to (in) (with)
antineoplastic chemotherapy D64.81

Anemia — continued
due to — continued
blood loss (chronic) D50.0
acute D62
chemotherapy, antineoplastic D64.81
chronic disease classified elsewhere NEC D63.8
chronic kidney disease D63.1
deficiency
amino-acid D53.0
copper D53.8
folate (folic acid) D52.9
dietary D52.0
drug-induced D52.1
molybdenum D53.8
protein D53.0
zinc D53.8
dietary vitamin B12 deficiency D51.3
disorder of
glutathione metabolism D55.1
nucleotide metabolism D55.3
drug — see Anemia, by type (see also Table of Drugs and Chemicals)
end stage renal disease D63.1
enzyme disorder D55.9
fetal blood loss P61.3
fish tapeworm (D.latum) infestation B70.0 [D63.8]
hemorrhage (chronic) D50.0
acute D62
impaired absorption D50.9
loss of blood (chronic) D50.0
acute D62
myxedema E03.9 [D63.8]
Necator americanus B76.1 [D63.8]
prematurity P61.2
selective vitamin B12 malabsorption with protein-uria D51.1
transcobalamin II deficiency D51.2
Dyke-Young type (secondary) (symptomatic) D59.1
dyserythropoietic (congenital) D64.4
dyshematopoietic (congenital) D64.4
Egyptian B76.9 [D63.8]
elliptocytosis — see Elliptocytosis
enzyme-deficiency, drug-induced D59.2
epidemic (see also Ancylostomiasis) B76.9 [D63.8]
erythroblastic
familial D56.1
newborn (see also Disease, hemolytic) P55.9
of childhood D56.1
erythrocytic glutathione deficiency D55.1
erythropoietin-resistant anemia (EPO resistant anemia) D63.1
Faber's (achlorhydric anemia) D50.9
factitious (self-induced blood letting) D50.0
familial erythroblastic D56.1
Fanconi's (congenital pancytopenia) D61.09
favism D55.0
fish tapeworm (D. latum) infestation B70.0 [D63.8]
folate (folic acid) deficiency D52.9
glucose-6-phosphate dehydrogenase (G6PD) deficiency D55.0
glutathione-reductase deficiency D55.1
goat's milk D52.0
granulocytic — see Agranulocytosis
Heinz body, congenital D58.2
hemolytic D58.9
acquired D59.9
with hemoglobinuria NEC D59.6
autoimmune NEC D59.1
infectious D59.4
specified type NEC D59.8
toxic D59.4
acute D59.9
due to enzyme deficiency specified type NEC D55.8
Lederer's D59.1
autoimmune D59.1
drug-induced D59.0
chronic D58.9
idiopathic D59.9
cold type (secondary) (symptomatic) D59.1
congenital (spherocytic) — see Spherocytosis
due to
cardiac conditions D59.4
drugs (nonautoimmune) D59.2
autoimmune D59.0
enzyme disorder D55.9
drug-induced D59.2

Anemia — Aneurysm

Aneurysm — *continued*
arteriosclerotic I72.9
　cerebral I67.1
　　ruptured — *see* Hemorrhage, intracranial,
　　　subarachnoid
arteriovenous (congenital) (*see also* Malformation, ar-
　teriovenous)
　acquired I77.0
　　brain I67.1
　　coronary I25.41
　　pulmonary I28.0
　brain Q28.2
　　ruptured I60.8
　peripheral — *see* Malformation, arteriovenous,
　　peripheral
　precerebral vessels Q28.0
　specified site NEC (*see also* Malformation, arteriove-
　　nous)
　　acquired I77.0
basal — *see* Aneurysm, brain
berry (congenital) (nonruptured) I67.1
　ruptured I60.7
brain I67.1
　arteriosclerotic I67.1
　　ruptured — *see* Hemorrhage, intracranial,
　　　subarachnoid
　arteriovenous (congenital) (nonruptured) Q28.2
　　acquired I67.1
　　　ruptured I60.8
　　ruptured I60.8
　berry (congenital) (nonruptured) I67.1
　　ruptured (*see also* Hemorrhage, intracranial,
　　　subarachnoid) I60.7
　congenital Q28.3
　　ruptured I60.7
　meninges I67.1
　　ruptured I60.8
　miliary (congenital) (nonruptured) I67.1
　　ruptured (*see also* Hemorrhage, intracranial,
　　　subarachnoid) I60.7
　mycotic I33.0
　ruptured — *see* Hemorrhage, intracranial, subarach-
　　noid
　syphilitic (hemorrhage) A52.05
cardiac (false) (*see also* Aneurysm, heart) I25.3
carotid artery (common) (external) I72.0
　internal (intracranial) I67.1
　　extracranial portion I72.0
　ruptured into brain I60.0- ☑
　syphilitic A52.09
　　intracranial A52.05
cavernous sinus I67.1
　arteriovenous (congenital) (nonruptured) Q28.3
　　ruptured I60.8
celiac I72.8
central nervous system, syphilitic A52.05
cerebral — *see* Aneurysm, brain
chest — *see* Aneurysm, thorax
circle of Willis I67.1
　congenital Q28.3
　　ruptured I60.6
　ruptured I60.6
common iliac artery I72.3
congenital (peripheral) Q27.8
　brain Q28.3
　　ruptured I60.7
　coronary Q24.5
　digestive system Q27.8
　lower limb Q27.8
　pulmonary Q25.79
　retina Q14.1
　specified site NEC Q27.8
　upper limb Q27.8
conjunctiva — *see* Abnormality, conjunctiva, vascular
conus arteriosus — *see* Aneurysm, heart
coronary (arteriosclerotic) (artery) I25.41
　arteriovenous, congenital Q24.5
　congenital Q24.5
　ruptured — *see* Infarct, myocardium
　syphilitic A52.06
　vein I25.89
cylindroid (aorta) I71.9
　ruptured I71.8
　syphilitic A52.01
ductus arteriosus Q25.0
endocardial, infective (any valve) I33.0
femoral (artery) (ruptured) I72.4
gastroduodenal I72.8

Aneurysm — *continued*
gastroepiploic I72.6
heart (wall) (chronic or with a stated duration of over
　4 weeks) I25.3
　valve — *see* Endocarditis
hepatic I72.8
iliac (common) (artery) (ruptured) I72.3
infective I72.9
　endocardial (any valve) I33.0
innominate (nonsyphilitic) I72.8
　syphilitic A52.09
interauricular septum — *see* Aneurysm, heart
interventricular septum — *see* Aneurysm, heart
intrathoracic (nonsyphilitic) I71.2
　ruptured I71.1
　syphilitic A52.01
lower limb I72.4
lung (pulmonary artery) I28.1
mediastinal (nonsyphilitic) I72.8
　syphilitic A52.09
miliary (congenital) I67.1
　ruptured — *see* Hemorrhage, intracerebral, sub-
　　arachnoid, intracranial
mitral (heart) (valve) I34.8
mural — *see* Aneurysm, heart
mycotic I72.9
　endocardial (any valve) I33.0
　ruptured, brain — *see* Hemorrhage, intracerebral,
　　subarachnoid
myocardium — *see* Aneurysm, heart
neck I72.0
pancreaticoduodenal I72.8
patent ductus arteriosus Q25.0
peripheral NEC I72.8
　congenital Q27.8
　　digestive system Q27.8
　　lower limb Q27.8
　　specified site NEC Q27.8
　　upper limb Q27.8
popliteal (artery) (ruptured) I72.4
precerebral, congenital (nonruptured) Q28.1
pulmonary I28.1
　arteriovenous Q25.72
　　acquired I28.0
　syphilitic A52.09
　valve (heart) — *see* Endocarditis, pulmonary
racemose (peripheral) I72.9
　congenital — *see* Aneurysm, congenital
radial I72.1
Rasmussen NEC A15.0
renal (artery) I72.2
retina (*see also* Disorder, retina, microaneurysms)
　congenital Q14.1
　diabetic — *see* Diabetes, microaneurysms, retinal
sinus of Valsalva Q25.4
specified NEC I72.8
spinal (cord) I72.8
　syphilitic (hemorrhage) A52.09
splenic I72.8
subclavian (artery) (ruptured) I72.8
　syphilitic A52.09
superior mesenteric I72.8
syphilitic (aorta) A52.01
　central nervous system A52.05
　congenital (late) A50.54 [I79.0]
　spine, spinal A52.09
thoracoabdominal (aorta) I71.6
　ruptured I71.5
　syphilitic A52.01
thorax, thoracic (aorta) (arch) (nonsyphilitic) I71.2
　ruptured I71.1
　syphilitic A52.01
traumatic (complication) (early), specified site — *see*
　Injury, blood vessel
tricuspid (heart) (valve) I07.8
ulnar I72.1
upper limb (ruptured) I72.1
valve, valvular — *see* Endocarditis
venous (*see also* Varix) I86.8
　congenital Q27.8
　　digestive system Q27.8
　　lower limb Q27.8
　　specified site NEC Q27.8
　　upper limb Q27.8
ventricle — *see* Aneurysm, heart
visceral NEC I72.8

Angelman syndrome Q93.5
Anger R45.4

Angiectasis, angiectopia I99.8
Angiitis I77.6
　allergic granulomatous M30.1
　hypersensitivity M31.0
　necrotizing M31.9
　　specified NEC M31.8
　nervous system, granulomatous I67.7
Angina (attack) (cardiac) (chest) (heart) (pectoris) (syn-
　drome) (vasomotor) I20.9
　with
　　atherosclerotic heart disease — *see* Arteriosclerosis,
　　　coronary (artery),
　　documented spasm I20.1
　abdominal K55.1
　accelerated — *see* Angina, unstable
　agranulocytic — *see* Agranulocytosis
　angiospastic — *see* Angina, with documented spasm
　aphthous B08.5
　crescendo — *see* Angina, unstable
　croupous J05.0
　cruris I73.9
　de novo effort — *see* Angina, unstable
　diphtheritic, membranous A36.0
　equivalent I20.8
　exudative, chronic J37.0
　following acute myocardial infarction I23.7
　gangrenous diphtheritic A36.0
　intestinal K55.1
　Ludovici K12.2
　Ludwig's K12.2
　malignant diphtheritic A36.0
　membranous J05.0
　　diphtheritic A36.0
　　Vincent's A69.1
　mesenteric K55.1
　monocytic — *see* Mononucleosis, infectious
　of effort — *see* Angina, specified NEC
　phlegmonous J36
　　diphtheritic A36.0
　post-infarctional I23.7
　pre-infarctional — *see* Angina, unstable
　Prinzmetal — *see* Angina, with documented spasm
　progressive — *see* Angina, unstable
　pseudomembranous A69.1
　pultaceous, diphtheritic A36.0
　spasm-induced — *see* Angina, with documented
　　spasm
　specified NEC I20.8
　stable I20.9
　stenocardia — *see* Angina, specified NEC
　stridulous, diphtheritic A36.2
　tonsil J36
　trachealis J05.0
　unstable I20.0
　variant — *see* Angina, with documented spasm
　Vincent's A69.1
　worsening effort — *see* Angina, unstable
Angioblastoma — *see* Neoplasm, connective tissue,
　uncertain behavior
Angiocholecystitis — *see* Cholecystitis, acute
Angiocholitis (*see also* Cholecystitis, acute) K83.0
Angiodysgenesis spinalis G95.19
Angiodysplasia (cecum) (colon) K55.20
　with bleeding K55.21
　duodenum (and stomach) K31.819
　　with bleeding K31.811
　stomach (and duodenum) K31.819
　　with bleeding K31.811
Angioedema (allergic) (any site) (with urticaria) T78.3 ☑
　hereditary D84.1
Angioendothelioma — *see* Neoplasm, uncertain behav-
　ior, by site
　benign D18.00
　　intra-abdominal D18.03
　　intracranial D18.02
　　skin D18.01
　　specified site NEC D18.09
　bone — *see* Neoplasm, bone, malignant
　Ewing's — *see* Neoplasm, bone, malignant
Angioendotheliomatosis C85.8- ☑
Angiofibroma (*see also* Neoplasm, benign, by site)
　juvenile
　　specified site — *see* Neoplasm, benign, by site
　　unspecified site D10.6
Angiohemophilia (A) (B) D68.0
Angioid streaks (choroid) (macula) (retina) H35.33

Angiokeratoma — *see* Neoplasm, skin, benign
  corporis diffusum E75.21
Angioleiomyoma — *see* Neoplasm, connective tissue,
  benign
Angiolipoma (*see also* Lipoma)
  infiltrating — *see* Lipoma
Angioma (*see also* Hemangioma, by site)
  capillary I78.1
  hemorrhagicum hereditaria I78.0
  intra-abdominal D18.03
  intracranial D18.02
  malignant — *see* Neoplasm, connective tissue, malig-
    nant
  plexiform D18.00
    intra-abdominal D18.03
    intracranial D18.02
    skin D18.01
    specified site NEC D18.09
  senile I78.1
  serpiginosum L81.7
  skin D18.01
  specified site NEC D18.09
  spider I78.1
  stellate I78.1
  venous Q28.3
Angiomatosis Q82.8
  bacillary A79.89
  encephalotrigeminal Q85.8
  hemorrhagic familial I78.0
  hereditary familial I78.0
  liver K76.4
Angiomyolipoma — *see* Lipoma
Angiomyoliposarcoma — *see* Neoplasm, connective
  tissue, malignant
Angiomyoma — *see* Neoplasm, connective tissue, benign
Angiomyosarcoma — *see* Neoplasm, connective tissue,
  malignant
Angiomyxoma — *see* Neoplasm, connective tissue, uncertain behavior
Angioneurosis F45.8
Angioneurotic edema (allergic) (any site) (with urticaria)
  T78.3 ☑
  hereditary D84.1
Angiopathia, angiopathy I99.9
  cerebral I67.9
    amyloid E85.4 [I68.0]
  diabetic (peripheral) — *see* Diabetes, angiopathy
  peripheral I73.9
    diabetic — *see* Diabetes, angiopathy
    specified type NEC I73.89
  retinae syphilitica A52.05
  retinalis (juvenilis)
    diabetic — *see* Diabetes, retinopathy
    proliferative — *see* Retinopathy, proliferative
Angiosarcoma (*see also* Neoplasm, connective tissue,
  malignant)
  liver C22.3
Angiosclerosis — *see* Arteriosclerosis
Angiospasm (peripheral) (traumatic) (vessel) I73.9
  brachial plexus G54.0
  cerebral G45.9
  cervical plexus G54.2
  nerve
    arm — *see* Mononeuropathy, upper limb
      axillary G54.0
      median — *see* Lesion, nerve, median
      ulnar — *see* Lesion, nerve, ulnar
    axillary G54.0
    leg — *see* Mononeuropathy, lower limb
    median — *see* Lesion, nerve, median
    plantar — *see* Lesion, nerve, plantar
    ulnar — *see* Lesion, nerve, ulnar
Angiospastic disease or edema I73.9
Angiostrongyliasis
  due to
    Parastrongylus
      cantonensis B83.2
      costaricensis B81.3
  intestinal B81.3
Anguillulosis — *see* Strongyloidiasis
Angulation
  cecum — *see* Obstruction, intestine
  coccyx (acquired) (*see also* subcategory) M43.8 ☑
    congenital NEC Q76.49

Angulation — *continued*
  femur (acquired) (*see also* Deformity, limb, specified
    type NEC, thigh)
    congenital Q74.2
  intestine (large) (small) — *see* Obstruction, intestine
  sacrum (acquired) (*see also* subcategory) M43.8 ☑
    congenital NEC Q76.49
  sigmoid (flexure) — *see* Obstruction, intestine
  spine — *see* Dorsopathy, deforming, specified NEC
  tibia (acquired) (*see also* Deformity, limb, specified
    type NEC, lower leg)
    congenital Q74.2
  ureter N13.5
    with infection N13.6
  wrist (acquired) (*see also* Deformity, limb, specified
    type NEC, forearm)
    congenital Q74.0
Angulus infectiosus (lips) K13.0
Anhedonia R45.84
Anhidrosis L74.4
Anhydration, anhydremia E86.0
  with
    hypernatremia E87.0
    hyponatremia E87.1
Anhydremia E86.0
  with
    hypernatremia E87.0
    hyponatremia E87.1
Anidrosis L74.4
Aniridia (congenital) Q13.1
Anisakiasis (infection) (infestation) B81.0
Anisakis larvae infestation B81.0
Aniseikonia H52.32
Anisocoria (pupil) H57.02
  congenital Q13.2
Anisocytosis R71.8
Anisometropia (congenital) H52.31
Ankle — *see* condition
Ankyloblepharon (eyelid) (acquired) (*see also* Blepharophimosis)
  filiforme (adnatum) (congenital) Q10.3
  total Q10.3
Ankyloglossia Q38.1
Ankylosis (fibrous) (osseous) (joint) M24.60
  ankle M24.67- ☑
  arthrodesis status Z98.1
  cricoarytenoid (cartilage) (joint) (larynx) J38.7
  dental K03.5
  ear ossicles H74.31- ☑
  elbow M24.62- ☑
  foot M24.67- ☑
  hand M24.64- ☑
  hip M24.65- ☑
  incostapedial joint (infectional) — *see* Ankylosis, ear
    ossicles
  jaw (temporomandibular) M26.61
  knee M24.66- ☑
  lumbosacral (joint) M43.27
  postoperative (status) Z98.1
  produced by surgical fusion, status Z98.1
  sacro-iliac (joint) M43.28
  shoulder M24.61- ☑
  spine (joint) (*see also* Fusion, spine)
    spondylitic — *see* Spondylitis, ankylosing
  surgical Z98.1
  temporomandibular M26.61
  tooth, teeth (hard tissues) K03.5
  wrist M24.63- ☑
Ankylostoma — *see* Ancylostoma
Ankylostomiasis — *see* Ancylostomiasis
Ankylurethria — *see* Stricture, urethra
Annular (*see also* condition)
  detachment, cervix N88.8
  organ or site, congenital NEC — *see* Distortion
  pancreas (congenital) Q45.1
Anodontia (complete) (partial) (vera) K00.0
  acquired K08.10 ☑
Anomaly, anomalous (congenital) (unspecified type)
  Q89.9
  abdominal wall NEC Q79.59
  acoustic nerve Q07.8
  adrenal Q89.1
  Alder (-Reilly) (leukocyte granulation) D72.0
  alimentary tract Q45.9
    upper Q40.9

Anomaly, anomalous — *continued*
  alveolar M26.70
    hyperplasia M26.79
      mandibular M26.72
      maxillary M26.71
    hypoplasia M26.79
      mandibular M26.74
      maxillary M26.73
    ridge (process) M26.79
    specified NEC M26.79
  ankle (joint) Q74.2
  anus Q43.9
  aorta (arch) NEC Q25.4
    coarctation (preductal) (postductal) Q25.1
  aortic cusp or valve Q23.9
  appendix Q43.8
  apple peel syndrome Q41.1
  aqueduct of Sylvius Q03.0
    with spina bifida — *see* Spina bifida, with hydro-
      cephalus
  arm Q74.0
  arteriovenous NEC
    coronary Q24.5
    gastrointestinal Q27.33
      acquired — *see* Angiodysplasia
  artery (peripheral) Q27.9
    basilar NEC Q28.1
    cerebral Q28.3
    coronary Q24.5
    digestive system Q27.8
    eye Q15.8
    great Q25.9
      specified NEC Q25.8
    lower limb Q27.8
    peripheral Q27.9
      specified NEC Q27.8
    pulmonary NEC Q25.79
    renal Q27.2
    retina Q14.1
    specified site NEC Q27.8
    subclavian Q27.8
    umbilical Q27.0
    upper limb Q27.8
    vertebral NEC Q28.1
  aryteno-epiglottic folds Q31.8
  atrial
    bands or folds Q20.8
    septa Q21.1
  atrioventricular
    excitation I45.6
    septum Q21.0
  auditory canal Q17.8
  auricle
    ear Q17.8
      causing impairment of hearing Q16.9
    heart Q20.8
  Axenfeld's Q15.0
  back Q89.9
  band
    atrial Q20.8
    heart Q24.8
    ventricular Q24.8
  Bartholin's duct Q38.4
  biliary duct or passage Q44.5
  bladder Q64.70
    absence Q64.5
    diverticulum Q64.6
    exstrophy Q64.10
      cloacal Q64.12
      extroversion Q64.19
      specified type NEC Q64.19
      supravesical fissure Q64.11
    neck obstruction Q64.31
    specified type NEC Q64.79
  bone Q79.9
    arm Q74.0
    face Q75.9
    leg Q74.2
    pelvic girdle Q74.2
    shoulder girdle Q74.0
    skull Q75.9
      with
        anencephaly Q00.0
        encephalocele — *see* Encephalocele
        hydrocephalus Q03.9
          with spina bifida — *see* Spina bifida, by
            site, with hydrocephalus
        microcephaly Q02

Anomaly, anomalous — *continued*
- brain (multiple) Q04.9
  - vessel Q28.3
- breast Q83.9
- broad ligament Q50.6
- bronchus Q32.4
- bulbus cordis Q21.9
- bursa Q79.9
- canal of Nuck Q52.4
- canthus Q10.3
- capillary Q27.9
- cardiac Q24.9
  - chambers Q20.9
    - specified NEC Q20.8
  - septal closure Q21.9
    - specified NEC Q21.8
  - valve NEC Q24.8
    - pulmonary Q22.3
- cardiovascular system Q28.8
- carpus Q74.0
- caruncle, lacrimal Q10.6
- cascade stomach Q40.2
- cauda equina Q06.3
- cecum Q43.9
- cerebral Q04.9
  - vessels Q28.3
- cervix Q51.9
- Chédiak-Higashi (-Steinbrinck) (congenital gigantism of peroxidase granules) E70.330
- cheek Q18.9
- chest wall Q67.8
  - bones Q76.9
- chin Q18.9
- chordae tendineae Q24.8
- choroid Q14.3
  - plexus Q07.8
- chromosomes, chromosomal Q99.9
  - D (1) — *see* condition, chromosome 13
  - E (3) — *see* condition, chromosome 18
  - G — *see* condition, chromosome 21
  - sex
    - female phenotype Q97.8
    - gonadal dysgenesis (pure) Q99.1
    - Klinefelter's Q98.4
    - male phenotype Q98.9
    - Turner's Q96.9
  - specified NEC Q99.8
- cilia Q10.3
- circulatory system Q28.9
- clavicle Q74.0
- clitoris Q52.6
- coccyx Q76.49
- colon Q43.9
- common duct Q44.5
- communication
  - coronary artery Q24.5
  - left ventricle with right atrium Q21.0
- concha (ear) Q17.3
- connection
  - portal vein Q26.5
  - pulmonary venous Q26.4
    - partial Q26.3
    - total Q26.2
  - renal artery with kidney Q27.2
- cornea (shape) Q13.4
- coronary artery or vein Q24.5
- cranium — *see* Anomaly, skull
- cricoid cartilage Q31.8
- cystic duct Q44.5
- dental
  - alveolar — *see* Anomaly, alveolar
  - arch relationship M26.20
    - specified NEC M26.29
- dentofacial M26.9
  - alveolar — *see* Anomaly, alveolar
  - dental arch relationship M26.20
    - specified NEC M26.29
  - functional M26.50
    - specified NEC M26.59
  - jaw size M26.00
    - macrogenia M26.05
    - mandibular
      - hyperplasia M26.03
      - hypoplasia M26.04
    - maxillary
      - hyperplasia M26.01
      - hypoplasia M26.02
    - microgenia M26.06

Anomaly, anomalous — *continued*
- dentofacial — *continued*
  - jaw size — *continued*
    - specified type NEC M26.09
  - jaw-cranial base relationship M26.10
    - asymmetry M26.12
      - maxillary M26.11
    - specified type NEC M26.19
  - malocclusion M26.4
    - dental arch relationship NEC M26.29
    - jaw size — *see* Anomaly, dentofacial, jaw size
    - jaw-cranial base relationship — *see* Anomaly, dentofacial, jaw-cranial base relationship
  - specified type NEC M26.89
  - temporomandibular joint M26.60
    - adhesions M26.61
    - ankylosis M26.61
    - arthralgia M26.62
    - articular disc M26.63
    - specified type NEC M26.69
  - tooth position, fully erupted M26.30
    - specified NEC M26.39
- dermatoglyphic Q82.8
- diaphragm (apertures) NEC Q79.1
- digestive organ(s) or tract Q45.9
  - lower Q43.9
  - upper Q40.9
- distance, interarch (excessive) (inadequate) M26.25
- distribution, coronary artery Q24.5
- ductus
  - arteriosus Q25.0
  - botalli Q25.0
- duodenum Q43.9
- dura (brain) Q04.9
  - spinal cord Q06.9
- ear (external) Q17.9
  - causing impairment of hearing Q16.9
  - inner Q16.5
  - middle (causing impairment of hearing) Q16.4
  - ossicles Q16.3
- Ebstein's (heart) (tricuspid valve) Q22.5
- ectodermal Q82.9
- Eisenmenger's (ventricular septal defect) Q21.8
- ejaculatory duct Q55.4
- elbow Q74.0
- endocrine gland NEC Q89.2
- epididymis Q55.4
- epiglottis Q31.8
- esophagus Q39.9
- eustachian tube Q17.8
- eye Q15.9
  - anterior segment Q13.9
    - specified NEC Q13.89
  - posterior segment Q14.9
    - specified NEC Q14.8
  - ptosis (eyelid) Q10.0
  - specified NEC Q15.8
- eyebrow Q18.8
- eyelid Q10.3
  - ptosis Q10.0
- face Q18.9
  - bone(s) Q75.9
- fallopian tube Q50.6
- fascia Q79.9
- femur NEC Q74.2
- fibula NEC Q74.2
- finger Q74.0
- fixation, intestine Q43.3
- flexion (joint) NOS Q74.9
  - hip or thigh Q65.89
- foot NEC Q74.2
  - varus (congenital) Q66.3
- foramen
  - Botalli Q21.1
  - ovale Q21.1
- forearm Q74.0
- forehead Q75.8
- form, teeth K00.2
- fovea centralis Q14.1
- frontal bone — *see* Anomaly, skull
- gallbladder (position) (shape) (size) Q44.1
- Gartner's duct Q52.4
- gastrointestinal tract Q45.9
- genitalia, genital organ(s) or system
  - female Q52.9
    - external Q52.70
    - internal NOS Q52.9

Anomaly, anomalous — *continued*
- genitalia, genital organ(s) or system — *continued*
  - male Q55.9
    - hydrocele P83.5
    - specified NEC Q55.8
- genitourinary NEC
  - female Q52.9
  - male Q55.9
- Gerbode Q21.0
- glottis Q31.8
- granulation or granulocyte, genetic (constitutional) (leukocyte) D72.0
- gum Q38.6
- gyri Q07.9
- hair Q84.2
- hand Q74.0
- hard tissue formation in pulp K04.3
- head — *see* Anomaly, skull
- heart Q24.9
  - auricle Q20.8
  - bands or folds Q24.8
  - fibroelastosis cordis I42.4
  - obstructive NEC Q22.6
  - patent ductus arteriosus (Botalli) Q25.0
  - septum Q21.9
    - auricular Q21.1
    - interatrial Q21.1
    - interventricular Q21.0
      - with pulmonary stenosis or atresia, dextra-position of aorta and hypertrophy of right ventricle Q21.3
    - specified NEC Q21.8
    - ventricular Q21.0
      - with pulmonary stenosis or atresia, dextra-position of aorta and hypertrophy of right ventricle Q21.3
  - tetralogy of Fallot Q21.3
  - valve NEC Q24.8
    - aortic
      - bicuspid valve Q23.1
      - insufficiency Q23.1
      - stenosis Q23.0
        - subaortic Q24.4
    - mitral
      - insufficiency Q23.3
      - stenosis Q23.2
    - pulmonary Q22.3
      - atresia Q22.0
      - insufficiency Q22.2
      - stenosis Q22.1
        - infundibular Q24.3
        - subvalvular Q24.3
    - tricuspid
      - atresia Q22.4
      - stenosis Q22.4
  - ventricle Q20.8
- heel NEC Q74.2
- Hegglin's D72.0
- hemianencephaly Q00.0
- hemicephaly Q00.0
- hemicrania Q00.0
- hepatic duct Q44.5
- hip NEC Q74.2
- hourglass stomach Q40.2
- humerus Q74.0
- hydatid of Morgagni
  - female Q50.5
  - male (epididymal) Q55.4
    - testicular Q55.29
- hymen Q52.4
- hypersegmentation of neutrophils, hereditary D72.0
- hypophyseal Q89.2
- ileocecal (coil) (valve) Q43.9
- ileum Q43.9
- ilium NEC Q74.2
- integument Q84.9
  - specified NEC Q84.8
- interarch distance (excessive) (inadequate) M26.25
- intervertebral cartilage or disc Q76.49
- intestine (large) (small) Q43.9
  - with anomalous adhesions, fixation or malrotation Q43.3
- iris Q13.2
- ischium NEC Q74.2
- jaw — *see* Anomaly, dentofacial
  - alveolar — *see* Anomaly, alveolar
- jaw-cranial base relationship — *see* Anomaly, dento-facial, jaw-cranial base relationship

Anomaly, anomalous — *continued*
- jejunum Q43.8
- joint Q74.9
  - specified NEC Q74.8
- Jordan's D72.0
- kidney(s) (calyx) (pelvis) Q63.9
  - artery Q27.2
  - specified NEC Q63.8
- Klippel-Feil (brevicollis) Q76.1
- knee Q74.1
- labium (majus) (minus) Q52.70
- labyrinth, membranous Q16.5
- lacrimal apparatus or duct Q10.6
- larynx, laryngeal (muscle) Q31.9
  - web (bed) Q31.0
- lens Q12.9
- leukocytes, genetic D72.0
  - granulation (constitutional) D72.0
- lid (fold) Q10.3
- ligament Q79.9
  - broad Q50.6
  - round Q52.8
- limb Q74.9
  - lower NEC Q74.2
    - reduction deformity — *see* Defect, reduction, lower limb
  - upper Q74.0
- lip Q38.0
- liver Q44.7
  - duct Q44.5
- lower limb NEC Q74.2
- lumbosacral (joint) (region) Q76.49
  - kyphosis — *see* Kyphosis, congenital
  - lordosis — *see* Lordosis, congenital
- lung (fissure) (lobe) Q33.9
- mandible — *see* Anomaly, dentofacial
- maxilla — *see* Anomaly, dentofacial
- May (-Hegglin) D72.0
- meatus urinarius NEC Q64.79
- meningeal bands or folds Q07.9
  - constriction of Q07.8
  - spinal Q06.9
- meninges Q07.9
  - cerebral Q04.8
  - spinal Q06.9
- meningocele Q05.9
- mesentery Q45.9
- metacarpus Q74.0
- metatarsus NEC Q74.2
- middle ear Q16.4
  - ossicles Q16.3
- mitral (leaflets) (valve) Q23.9
  - insufficiency Q23.3
  - specified NEC Q23.8
  - stenosis Q23.2
- mouth Q38.6
- Müllerian (*see also* Anomaly, by site)
  - uterus NEC Q51.818
- multiple NEC Q89.7
- muscle Q79.9
  - eyelid Q10.3
- musculoskeletal system, except limbs Q79.9
- myocardium Q24.8
- nail Q84.6
- narrowness, eyelid Q10.3
- nasal sinus (wall) Q30.8
- neck (any part) Q18.9
- nerve Q07.9
  - acoustic Q07.8
  - optic Q07.8
- nervous system (central) Q07.9
- nipple Q83.9
- nose, nasal (bones) (cartilage) (septum) (sinus) Q30.9
  - specified NEC Q30.8
- ocular muscle Q15.8
- omphalomesenteric duct Q43.0
- opening, pulmonary veins Q26.4
- optic
  - disc Q14.2
  - nerve Q07.8
- opticociliary vessels Q13.2
- orbit (eye) Q10.7
- organ Q89.9
  - of Corti Q16.5
- origin
  - artery
    - innominate Q25.8
    - pulmonary Q25.79

Anomaly, anomalous — *continued*
- origin — *continued*
  - artery — *continued*
    - renal Q27.2
    - subclavian Q25.8
- osseous meatus (ear) Q16.1
- ovary Q50.39
- oviduct Q50.6
- palate (hard) (soft) NEC Q38.5
- pancreas or pancreatic duct Q45.3
- papillary muscles Q24.8
- parathyroid gland Q89.2
- paraurethral ducts Q64.79
- parotid (gland) Q38.4
- patella Q74.1
- Pelger-Huët (hereditary hyposegmentation) D72.0
- pelvic girdle NEC Q74.2
- pelvis (bony) NEC Q74.2
  - rachitic E64.3
- penis (glans) Q55.69
- pericardium Q24.8
- peripheral vascular system Q27.9
- Peter's Q13.4
- pharynx Q38.8
- pigmentation L81.9
  - congenital Q82.8
- pituitary (gland) Q89.2
- pleural (folds) Q34.0
- portal vein Q26.5
  - connection Q26.5
- position, tooth, teeth, fully erupted M26.30
  - specified NEC M26.39
- precerebral vessel Q28.1
- prepuce Q55.69
- prostate Q55.4
- pulmonary Q33.9
  - artery NEC Q25.79
  - valve Q22.3
    - atresia Q22.0
    - insufficiency Q22.2
    - specified type NEC Q22.3
    - stenosis Q22.1
      - infundibular Q24.3
      - subvalvular Q24.3
  - venous connection Q26.4
    - partial Q26.3
    - total Q26.2
- pupil Q13.2
  - function H57.00
    - anisocoria H57.02
    - Argyll Robertson pupil H57.01
    - miosis H57.03
    - mydriasis H57.04
    - specified type NEC H57.09
    - tonic pupil H57.05- ☑
- pylorus Q40.3
- radius Q74.0
- rectum Q43.9
- reduction (extremity) (limb)
  - femur (longitudinal) — *see* Defect, reduction, lower limb, longitudinal, femur
  - fibula (longitudinal) — *see* Defect, reduction, lower limb, longitudinal, fibula
  - lower limb — *see* Defect, reduction, lower limb
  - radius (longitudinal) — *see* Defect, reduction, upper limb, longitudinal, radius
  - tibia (longitudinal) — *see* Defect, reduction, lower limb, longitudinal, tibia
  - ulna (longitudinal) — *see* Defect, reduction, upper limb, longitudinal, ulna
  - upper limb — *see* Defect, reduction, upper limb
- refraction — *see* Disorder, refraction
- renal Q63.9
  - artery Q27.2
  - pelvis Q63.9
    - specified NEC Q63.8
- respiratory system Q34.9
  - specified NEC Q34.8
- retina Q14.1
- rib Q76.6
  - cervical Q76.5
- Rieger's Q13.81
- rotation — *see* Malrotation
  - hip or thigh Q65.89
- round ligament Q52.8
- sacroiliac (joint) NEC Q74.2
- sacrum NEC Q76.49
  - kyphosis — *see* Kyphosis, congenital

Anomaly, anomalous — *continued*
- sacrum — *continued*
  - lordosis — *see* Lordosis, congenital
- saddle nose, syphilitic A50.57
- salivary duct or gland Q38.4
- scapula Q74.0
- scrotum — *see* Malformation, testis and scrotum
- sebaceous gland Q82.9
- seminal vesicles Q55.4
- sense organs NEC Q07.8
- sex chromosomes NEC (*see also* Anomaly, chromosomes)
  - female phenotype Q97.8
  - male phenotype Q98.9
- shoulder (girdle) (joint) Q74.0
- sigmoid (flexure) Q43.9
- simian crease Q82.8
- sinus of Valsalva Q25.4
- skeleton generalized Q78.9
- skin (appendage) Q82.9
- skull Q75.9
  - with
    - anencephaly Q00.0
    - encephalocele — *see* Encephalocele
    - hydrocephalus Q03.9
      - with spina bifida — *see* Spina bifida, by site, with hydrocephalus
    - microcephaly Q02
- specified organ or site NEC Q89.8
- spermatic cord Q55.4
- spine, spinal NEC Q76.49
  - column NEC Q76.49
    - kyphosis — *see* Kyphosis, congenital
    - lordosis — *see* Lordosis, congenital
  - cord Q06.9
  - nerve root Q07.8
- spleen Q89.09
  - agenesis Q89.01
- stenonian duct Q38.4
- sternum NEC Q76.7
- stomach Q40.3
- submaxillary gland Q38.4
- tarsus NEC Q74.2
- tendon Q79.9
- testis — *see* Malformation, testis and scrotum
- thigh NEC Q74.2
- thorax (wall) Q67.8
  - bony Q76.9
- throat Q38.8
- thumb Q74.0
- thymus gland Q89.2
- thyroid (gland) Q89.2
  - cartilage Q31.8
- tibia NEC Q74.2
  - saber A50.56
- toe Q74.2
- tongue Q38.3
- tooth, teeth K00.9
  - eruption K00.6
  - position, fully erupted M26.30
  - spacing, fully erupted M26.30
- trachea (cartilage) Q32.1
- tragus Q17.9
- tricuspid (leaflet) (valve) Q22.9
  - atresia or stenosis Q22.4
  - Ebstein's Q22.5
- Uhl's (hypoplasia of myocardium, right ventricle) Q24.8
- ulna Q74.0
- umbilical artery Q27.0
- union
  - cricoid cartilage and thyroid cartilage Q31.8
  - thyroid cartilage and hyoid bone Q31.8
  - trachea with larynx Q31.8
- upper limb Q74.0
- urachus Q64.4
- ureter Q62.8
  - obstructive NEC Q62.39
    - cecoureterocele Q62.32
    - orthotopic ureterocele Q62.31
- urethra Q64.70
  - absence Q64.5
  - double Q64.74
  - fistula to rectum Q64.73
  - obstructive Q64.39
    - stricture Q64.32
  - prolapse Q64.71
  - specified type NEC Q64.79
- urinary tract Q64.9

Anomaly, anomalous — *continued*
  uterus Q51.9
    with only one functioning horn Q51.4
  uvula Q38.5
  vagina Q52.4
  valleculae Q31.8
  valve (heart) NEC Q24.8
    coronary sinus Q24.5
    inferior vena cava Q24.8
    pulmonary Q22.3
    sinus coronario Q24.5
    venae cavae inferioris Q24.8
  vas deferens Q55.4
  vascular Q27.9
    brain Q28.3
    ring Q25.4
  vein(s) (peripheral) Q27.9
    brain Q28.3
    cerebral Q28.3
    coronary Q24.5
    developmental Q28.3
    great Q26.9
      specified NEC Q26.8
  vena cava (inferior) (superior) Q26.9
  venous — *see* Anomaly, vein(s)
  venous return Q26.8
  ventricular
    bands or folds Q24.8
    septa Q21.0
  vertebra Q76.49
    kyphosis — *see* Kyphosis, congenital
    lordosis — *see* Lordosis, congenital
  vesicourethral orifice Q64.79
  vessel(s) Q27.9
    optic papilla Q14.2
    precerebral Q28.1
  vitelline duct Q43.0
  vitreous body or humor Q14.0
  vulva Q52.70
  wrist (joint) Q74.0
Anomia R48.8
Anonychia (congenital) Q84.3
  acquired L60.8
Anophthalmos, anophthalmus (congenital) (globe) Q11.1
  acquired Z90.01
Anopia, anopsia H53.46- ☑
  quadrant H53.46- ☑
Anorchia, anorchism, anorchidism Q55.0
Anorexia R63.0
  hysterical F44.89
  nervosa F50.00
    atypical F50.9
    binge-eating type F50.2
      with purging F50.02
    restricting type F50.01
Anorgasmy, psychogenic (female) F52.31
  male F52.32
Anosmia R43.0
  hysterical F44.6
  postinfectional J39.8
Anosognosia R41.89
Anosteoplasia Q78.9
Anovulatory cycle N97.0
Anoxemia R09.02
  newborn P84
Anoxia (pathological) R09.02
  altitude T70.29 ☑
  cerebral G93.1
    complicating
      anesthesia (general) (local) or other sedation T88.59 ☑
        in labor and delivery O74.3
        in pregnancy O29.21- ☑
        postpartum, puerperal O89.2
      delivery (cesarean) (instrumental) O75.4
    during a procedure G97.81
    newborn P84
    resulting from a procedure G97.82
  due to
    drowning T75.1 ☑
    high altitude T70.29 ☑
  heart — *see* Insufficiency, coronary
  intrauterine P84
  myocardial — *see* Insufficiency, coronary
  newborn P84
  spinal cord G95.11

Anoxia — *continued*
  systemic (by suffocation) (low content in atmosphere) — *see* Asphyxia, traumatic
Anteflexion — *see* Anteversion
Antenatal
  care (normal pregnancy) Z34.90
  screening (encounter for) of mother Z36
Antepartum — *see* condition
Anterior — *see* condition
Antero-occlusion M26.220
Anteversion
  cervix — *see* Anteversion, uterus
  femur (neck), congenital Q65.89
  uterus, uterine (cervix) (postinfectional) (postpartal, old) N85.4
    congenital Q51.818
    in pregnancy or childbirth — *see* Pregnancy, complicated by
Anthophobia F40.228
Anthracosilicosis J60
Anthracosis (lung) (occupational) J60
  lingua K14.3
Anthrax A22.9
  with pneumonia A22.1
  cerebral A22.8
  colitis A22.2
  cutaneous A22.0
  gastrointestinal A22.2
  inhalation A22.1
  intestinal A22.2
  meningitis A22.8
  pulmonary A22.1
  respiratory A22.1
  sepsis A22.7
  specified manifestation NEC A22.8
Anthropoid pelvis Q74.2
  with disproportion (fetopelvic) O33.0
Anthropophobia F40.10
  generalized F40.11
Antibodies, maternal (blood group) — *see* Isoimmunization, affecting management of pregnancy
  anti-D — *see* Isoimmunization, affecting management of pregnancy, Rh
  newborn P55.0
Antibody
  anticardiolipin R76.0
    with
      hemorrhagic disorder D68.312
      hypercoagulable state D68.61
  antiphosphatidylglycerol R76.0
    with
      hemorrhagic disorder D68.312
      hypercoagulable state D68.61
  antiphosphatidylinositol R76.0
    with
      hemorrhagic disorder D68.312
      hypercoagulable state D68.61
  antiphosphatidylserine R76.0
    with
      hemorrhagic disorder D68.312
      hypercoagulable state D68.61
  antiphospholipid R76.0
    with
      hemorrhagic disorder D68.312
      hypercoagulable state D68.61
Anticardiolipin syndrome D68.61
Anticoagulant, circulating (intrinsic) (*see also* Disorder, hemorrhagic) D68.318
  drug-induced (extrinsic) (*see also* Disorder, hemorrhagic) D68.32
Antidiuretic hormone syndrome E22.2
Antimonial cholera — *see* Poisoning, antimony
Antiphospholipid
  antibody
    with hemorrhagic disorder D68.312
    syndrome D68.61
Antisocial personality F60.2
Antithrombinemia — *see* Circulating anticoagulants
Antithromboplastinemia D68.318
Antithromboplastinogenemia D68.318
Antitoxin complication or reaction — *see* Complications, vaccination
Antlophobia F40.228
Antritis J32.0
  maxilla J32.0
    acute J01.00
      recurrent J01.01

Antritis — *continued*
  stomach K29.60
    with bleeding K29.61
Antrum, antral — *see* condition
Anuria R34
  calculous (impacted) (recurrent) (*see also* Calculus, urinary) N20.9
  following
    abortion — *see* Abortion by type complicated by, renal failure
    ectopic or molar pregnancy O08.4
  newborn P96.0
  postprocedural N99.0
  postrenal N13.8
  traumatic (following crushing) T79.5 ☑
Anus, anal — *see* condition
Anusitis K62.89
Anxiety F41.9
  depression F41.8
  episodic paroxysmal F41.0
  generalized F41.1
  hysteria F41.8
  neurosis F41.1
  panic type F41.0
  reaction F41.1
  separation, abnormal (of childhood) F93.0
  specified NEC F41.8
  state F41.1
Aorta, aortic — *see* condition
Aortectasia — *see* Ectasia, aorta
  with aneurysm — *see* Aneurysm, aorta
Aortitis (nonsyphilitic) (calcific) I77.6
  arteriosclerotic I70.0
  Doehle-Heller A52.02
  luetic A52.02
  rheumatic — *see* Endocarditis, acute, rheumatic
  specific (syphilitic) A52.02
  syphilitic A52.02
    congenital A50.54 [I79.1]
Apathetic thyroid storm — *see* Thyrotoxicosis
Apathy R45.3
Apeirophobia F40.228
Apepsia K30
  psychogenic F45.8
Aperistalsis, esophagus K22.0
Apertognathia M26.29
Apert's syndrome Q87.0
Aphagia R13.0
  psychogenic F50.9
Aphakia (acquired) (postoperative) H27.0- ☑
  congenital Q12.3
Aphasia (amnestic) (global) (nominal) (semantic) (syntactic) R47.01
  acquired, with epilepsy (Landau-Kleffner syndrome) — *see* Epilepsy, specified NEC
  auditory (developmental) F80.2
  developmental (receptive type) F80.2
    expressive type F80.1
    Wernicke's F80.2
  following
    cerebrovascular disease I69.920
      cerebral infarction I69.320
      intracerebral hemorrhage I69.120
      nontraumatic intracranial hemorrhage NEC I69.220
      specified disease NEC I69.820
      subarachnoid hemorrhage I69.020
  primary progressive G31.01 [F02.80]
    with behavioral disturbance G31.01 [F02.81]
  progressive isolated G31.01 [F02.80]
    with behavioral disturbance G31.01 [F02.81]
  sensory F80.2
  syphilis, tertiary A52.19
  Wernicke's (developmental) F80.2
Aphonia (organic) R49.1
  hysterical F44.4
  psychogenic F44.4
Aphthae, aphthous (*see also* condition)
  Bednar's K12.0
  cachectic K14.0
  epizootic B08.8
  fever B08.8
  oral (recurrent) K12.0
  stomatitis (major) (minor) K12.0
  thrush B37.0
  ulcer (oral) (recurrent) K12.0
    genital organ(s) NEC
      female N76.6

Aphthae, aphthous — *continued*
  ulcer — *continued*
    genital organ(s) — *continued*
      male N50.8
    larynx J38.7
Apical — *see* condition
Apiphobia F40.218
Aplasia (*see also* Agenesis)
  abdominal muscle syndrome Q79.4
  alveolar process (acquired) — *see* Anomaly, alveolar
    congenital Q38.6
  aorta (congenital) Q25.4
  axialis extracorticalis (congenita) E75.29
  bone marrow (myeloid) D61.9
    congenital D61.01
  brain Q00.0
    part of Q04.3
  bronchus Q32.4
  cementum K00.4
  cerebellum Q04.3
  cervix (congenital) Q51.5
  congenital pure red cell D61.01
  corpus callosum Q04.0
  cutis congenita Q84.8
  erythrocyte congenital D61.01
  extracortical axial E75.29
  eye Q11.1
  fovea centralis (congenital) Q14.1
  gallbladder, congenital Q44.0
  iris Q13.1
  labyrinth, membranous Q16.5
  limb (congenital) Q73.8
    lower — *see* Defect, reduction, lower limb
    upper — *see* Agenesis, arm
  lung, congenital (bilateral) (unilateral) Q33.3
  pancreas Q45.0
  parathyroid-thymic D82.1
  Pelizaeus-Merzbacher E75.29
  penis Q55.5
  prostate Q55.4
  red cell (with thymoma) D60.9
    acquired D60.9
      due to drugs D60.9
    adult D60.9
    chronic D60.0
    congenital D61.01
    constitutional D61.01
    due to drugs D60.9
    hereditary D61.01
    of infants D61.01
    primary D61.01
    pure D61.01
      due to drugs D60.9
    specified type NEC D60.8
    transient D60.1
  round ligament Q52.8
  skin Q84.8
  spermatic cord Q55.4
  spleen Q89.01
  testicle Q55.0
  thymic, with immunodeficiency D82.1
  thyroid (congenital) (with myxedema) E03.1
  uterus Q51.0
  ventral horn cell Q06.1
Apnea, apneic (of) (spells) R06.81
  newborn NEC P28.4
    obstructive P28.4
    sleep (central) (obstructive) (primary) P28.3
    prematurity P28.4
  sleep G47.30
    central (primary) G47.31
      in conditions classified elsewhere G47.37
    obstructive (adult) (pediatric) G47.33
    primary central G47.31
    specified NEC G47.39
Apneumatosis, newborn P28.0
Apocrine metaplasia (breast) — *see* Dysplasia, mammary, specified type NEC
Apophysitis (bone) (*see also* Osteochondropathy)
  calcaneus M92.8
  juvenile M92.9
Apoplectiform convulsions (cerebral ischemia) I67.82
Apoplexia, apoplexy, apoplectic
  adrenal A39.1
  heart (auricle) (ventricle) — *see* Infarct, myocardium
  heat T67.0 ☑
  hemorrhagic (stroke) — *see* Hemorrhage, intracranial

Apoplexia, apoplexy, apoplectic — *continued*
  meninges, hemorrhagic — *see* Hemorrhage, intracranial, subarachnoid
  uremic N18.9 [I68.8]
Appearance
  bizarre R46.1
  specified NEC R46.89
  very low level of personal hygiene R46.0
Appendage
  epididymal (organ of Morgagni) Q55.4
  intestine (epiploic) Q43.8
  preauricular Q17.0
  testicular (organ of Morgagni) Q55.29
Appendicitis (pneumococcal) (retrocecal) K37
  with
    perforation or rupture K35.2
    peritoneal abscess K35.3
    peritonitis NEC K35.3
      generalized (with perforation or rupture) K35.2
      localized (with perforation or rupture) K35.3
  acute (catarrhal) (fulminating) (gangrenous) (obstructive) (retrocecal) (suppurative) K35.80
    with
      peritoneal abscess K35.3
      peritonitis NEC K35.3
        generalized (with perforation or rupture) K35.2
        localized (with perforation or rupture) K35.3
    specified NEC K35.89
  amebic A06.89
  chronic (recurrent) K36
  exacerbation — *see* Appendicitis, acute
  gangrenous — *see* Appendicitis, acute
  healed (obliterative) K36
  interval K36
  neurogenic K36
  obstructive K36
  recurrent K36
  relapsing K36
  subacute (adhesive) K36
  subsiding K36
  suppurative — *see* Appendicitis, acute
  tuberculous A18.32
Appendicopathia oxyurica B80
Appendix, appendicular (*see also* condition)
  epididymis Q55.4
  Morgagni
    female Q50.5
    male (epididymal) Q55.4
      testicular Q55.29
  testis Q55.29
Appetite
  depraved — *see* Pica
  excessive R63.2
  lack or loss (*see also* Anorexia) R63.0
    nonorganic origin F50.8
    psychogenic F50.8
  perverted (hysterical) — *see* Pica
Apple peel syndrome Q41.1
Apprehension state F41.1
Apprehensiveness, abnormal F41.9
Approximal wear K03.0
Apraxia (classic) (ideational) (ideokinetic) (ideomotor) (motor) (verbal) R48.2
  following
    cerebrovascular disease I69.990
      cerebral infarction I69.390
      intracerebral hemorrhage I69.190
      nontraumatic intracranial hemorrhage NEC I69.290
      specified disease NEC I69.890
      subarachnoid hemorrhage I69.090
  oculomotor, congenital H51.8
Aptyalism K11.7
Apudoma — *see* Neoplasm, uncertain behavior, by site
Aqueous misdirection H40.83- ☑
Arabicum elephantiasis — *see* Infestation, filarial
Arachnitis — *see* Meningitis
Arachnodactyly — *see* Syndrome, Marfan's
Arachnoiditis (acute) (adhesive) (basal) (brain) (cerebrospinal) — *see* Meningitis
Arachnophobia F40.210
Arboencephalitis, Australian A83.4
Arborization block (heart) I45.5
ARC (AIDS-related complex) B20
Arches — *see* condition
Arcuate uterus Q51.810

Arcuatus uterus Q51.810
Arcus (cornea) senilis — *see* Degeneration, cornea, senile
Arc-welder's lung J63.4
Areflexia R29.2
Areola — *see* condition
Argentaffinoma (*see also* Neoplasm, uncertain behavior, by site)
  malignant — *see* Neoplasm, malignant, by site
  syndrome E34.0
Argininemia E72.21
Arginosuccinic aciduria E72.22
Argyll Robertson phenomenon, pupil or syndrome (syphilitic) A52.19
  atypical H57.09
  nonsyphilitic H57.09
Argyria, argyriasis
  conjunctival H11.13- ☑
  from drug or medicament — *see* Table of Drugs and Chemicals, by substance
Argyrosis, conjunctival H11.13- ☑
Arhinencephaly Q04.1
Ariboflavinosis E53.0
Arm — *see* condition
Arnold-Chiari disease, obstruction or syndrome (type II) Q07.00
  with
    hydrocephalus Q07.02
      with spina bifida Q07.03
    spina bifida Q07.01
      with hydrocephalus Q07.03
  type III — *see* Encephalocele
  type IV Q04.8
Aromatic amino-acid metabolism disorder E70.9
  specified NEC E70.8
Arousals, confusional G47.51
Arrest, arrested
  cardiac I46.9
    complicating
      abortion — *see* Abortion, by type, complicated by, cardiac arrest
      anesthesia (general) (local) or other sedation — *see* Table of Drugs and Chemicals, by drug
        in labor and delivery O74.2
        in pregnancy O29.11- ☑
        postpartum, puerperal O89.1
      delivery (cesarean) (instrumental) O75.4
    due to
      cardiac condition I46.2
      specified condition NEC I46.8
    intraoperative I97.71- ☑
    newborn P29.81
    postprocedural I97.12- ☑
      obstetric procedure O75.4
  cardiorespiratory — *see* Arrest, cardiac
  circulatory — *see* Arrest, cardiac
  deep transverse O64.0 ☑
  development or growth
    bone — *see* Disorder, bone, development or growth
    child R62.50
    tracheal rings Q32.1
  epiphyseal
    complete
      femur M89.15- ☑
      humerus M89.12- ☑
      tibia M89.16- ☑
      ulna M89.13- ☑
      forearm M89.13- ☑
        specified NEC M89.13- ☑
        ulna — *see* Arrest, epiphyseal, by type, ulna
      lower leg M89.16- ☑
        specified NEC M89.168
        tibia — *see* Arrest, epiphyseal, by type, tibia
    partial
      femur M89.15- ☑
      humerus M89.12- ☑
      tibia M89.16- ☑
      ulna M89.13- ☑
      specified NEC M89.18
  granulopoiesis — *see* Agranulocytosis
  growth plate — *see* Arrest, epiphyseal
  heart — *see* Arrest, cardiac
  legal, anxiety concerning Z65.3
  physeal — *see* Arrest, epiphyseal
  respiratory R09.2
    newborn P28.81

Index

Arrest, arrested — Arteriosclerosis, arteriosclerotic

Arrest, arrested — *continued*
  sinus I45.5
  spermatogenesis (complete) — *see* Azoospermia
    incomplete — *see* Oligospermia
  transverse (deep) O64.0 ☑
Arrhenoblastoma
  benign
    specified site — *see* Neoplasm, benign, by site
    unspecified site
      female D27.9
      male D29.20
  malignant
    specified site — *see* Neoplasm, malignant, by site
    unspecified site
      female C56.9
      male C62.90
  specified site — *see* Neoplasm, uncertain behavior,
    by site
  unspecified site
    female D39.10
    male D40.10
Arrhythmia (auricle) (cardiac) (juvenile) (nodal) (reflex)
    (sinus) (supraventricular) (transitory) (ventricle) I49.9
  block I45.9
  extrasystolic I49.49
  newborn
    bradycardia P29.12
    occurring before birth P03.819
      before onset of labor P03.810
      during labor P03.811
    tachycardia P29.11
  psychogenic F45.8
  specified NEC I49.8
  vagal R55
  ventricular re-entry I47.0
Arrillaga-Ayerza syndrome (pulmonary sclerosis with
    pulmonary hypertension) I27.0
Arsenical pigmentation L81.8
  from drug or medicament — *see* Table of Drugs and
    Chemicals
Arsenism — *see* Poisoning, arsenic
Arterial — *see* condition
Arteriofibrosis — *see* Arteriosclerosis
Arteriolar sclerosis — *see* Arteriosclerosis
Arteriolith — *see* Arteriosclerosis
Arteriolitis I77.6
  necrotizing, kidney I77.5
  renal — *see* Hypertension, kidney
Arteriolosclerosis — *see* Arteriosclerosis
Arterionephrosclerosis — *see* Hypertension, kidney
Arteriopathy I77.9
Arteriosclerosis, arteriosclerotic (diffuse) (obliterans)
    (of) (senile) (with calcification) I70.90
  aorta I70.0
  arteries of extremities — *see* Arteriosclerosis, extrem-
    ities
  brain I67.2
  bypass graft
    coronary — *see* Arteriosclerosis, coronary, bypass
      graft
    extremities — *see* Arteriosclerosis, extremities,
      bypass graft
  cardiac — *see* Disease, heart, ischemic, atherosclerotic
  cardiopathy — *see* Disease, heart, ischemic,
    atherosclerotic
  cardiorenal — *see* Hypertension, cardiorenal
  cardiovascular — *see* Disease, heart, ischemic,
    atherosclerotic
  carotid (*see also* Occlusion, artery, carotid) I65.2- ☑
  central nervous system I67.2
  cerebral I67.2
  cerebrovascular I67.2
  coronary (artery) I25.10
    bypass graft I25.810
      with
        angina pectoris I25.709
          with documented spasm I25.701
          specified type NEC I25.708
          unstable I25.700
        ischemic chest pain I25.709
      autologous artery I25.810
        with
          angina pectoris I25.729
            with documented spasm I25.721
            specified type I25.728
            unstable I25.720
          ischemic chest pain I25.729

Arteriosclerosis, arteriosclerotic — *continued*
  coronary — *continued*
    bypass graft — *continued*
      autologous vein I25.810
        with
          angina pectoris I25.719
            with documented spasm I25.711
            specified type I25.718
            unstable I25.710
          ischemic chest pain I25.719
      nonautologous biological I25.810
        with
          angina pectoris I25.739
            with documented spasm I25.731
            specified type I25.738
            unstable I25.730
          ischemic chest pain I25.739
      specified type NEC I25.810
        with
          angina pectoris I25.799
            with documented spasm I25.791
            specified type I25.798
            unstable I25.790
          ischemic chest pain I25.799
    due to
      calcified coronary lesion (severely) I25.84
      lipid rich plaque I25.83
    native vessel
      with
        angina pectoris I25.119
          with documented spasm I25.111
          specified type NEC I25.118
          unstable I25.110
        ischemic chest pain I25.119
    transplanted heart I25.811
      bypass graft I25.812
        with
          angina pectoris I25.769
            with documented spasm I25.761
            specified type I25.768
            unstable I25.760
          ischemic chest pain I25.769
      native coronary artery I25.811
        with
          angina pectoris I25.759
            with documented spasm I25.751
            specified type I25.758
            unstable I25.750
          ischemic chest pain I25.759
  extremities (native arteries) I70.209
    bypass graft I70.309
      autologous vein graft I70.409
        leg I70.409
          with
            gangrene (and intermittent claudica-
              tion, rest pain and ulcer)
              I70.469
            intermittent claudication I70.419
            rest pain (and intermittent claudica-
              tion) I70.429
          bilateral I70.403
            with
              gangrene (and intermittent clau-
                dication, rest pain and ul-
                cer) I70.463
             intermittent claudication I70.463
             rest pain (and intermittent claudi-
              cation) I70.423
            specified type NEC I70.493
          left I70.402
            with
              gangrene (and intermittent clau-
                dication, rest pain and ul-
                cer) I70.462
             intermittent claudication I70.412
             rest pain (and intermittent claudi-
              cation) I70.422
             ulceration (and intermittent
              claudication and rest pain)
              I70.449
             ankle I70.443
             calf I70.442
             foot site NEC I70.445
             heel I70.444
             lower leg NEC I70.448
             midfoot I70.444
             thigh I70.441
            specified type NEC I70.492

Arteriosclerosis, arteriosclerotic — *continued*
  extremities — *continued*
    bypass graft — *continued*
      autologous vein graft — *continued*
        leg — *continued*
          right I70.401
            with
              gangrene (and intermittent clau-
                dication, rest pain and ul-
                cer) I70.461
             intermittent claudication I70.411
             rest pain (and intermittent claudi-
              cation) I70.421
             ulceration (and intermittent
              claudication and rest pain)
              I70.439
             ankle I70.433
             calf I70.432
             foot site NEC I70.435
             heel I70.434
             lower leg NEC I70.438
             midfoot I70.434
             thigh I70.431
            specified type NEC I70.491
        specified type NEC I70.499
      specified NEC I70.408
        with
          gangrene (and intermittent claudica-
            tion, rest pain and ulcer)
            I70.468
          intermittent claudication I70.418
          rest pain (and intermittent claudica-
            tion) I70.428
          ulceration (and intermittent claudica-
            tion and rest pain) I70.45
        specified type NEC I70.498
    leg I70.309
      with
        gangrene (and intermittent claudication,
          rest pain and ulcer) I70.369
        intermittent claudication I70.319
        rest pain (and intermittent claudication)
          I70.329
      bilateral I70.303
        with
          gangrene (and intermittent claudica-
            tion, rest pain and ulcer)
            I70.363
          intermittent claudication I70.313
          rest pain (and intermittent claudica-
            tion) I70.323
        specified type NEC I70.393
      left I70.302
        with
          gangrene (and intermittent claudica-
            tion, rest pain and ulcer)
            I70.362
          intermittent claudication I70.312
          rest pain (and intermittent claudica-
            tion) I70.322
          ulceration (and intermittent claudica-
            tion and rest pain) I70.349
          ankle I70.343
          calf I70.342
          foot site NEC I70.345
          heel I70.344
          lower leg NEC I70.348
          midfoot I70.344
          thigh I70.341
        specified type NEC I70.392
      right I70.301
        with
          gangrene (and intermittent claudica-
            tion, rest pain and ulcer)
            I70.361
          intermittent claudication I70.311
          rest pain (and intermittent claudica-
            tion) I70.321
          ulceration (and intermittent claudica-
            tion and rest pain I70.339
          ankle I70.333
          calf I70.332
          foot site NEC I70.335
          heel I70.334
          lower leg NEC I70.338
          midfoot I70.334
          thigh I70.331
        specified type NEC I70.391

Arteriosclerosis, arteriosclerotic — *continued*
  extremities — *continued*
    bypass graft — *continued*
      leg — *continued*
        specified type NEC I70.399
      nonautologous biological graft I70.509
        leg I70.509
          with
            gangrene (and intermittent claudication, rest pain and ulcer) I70.569
            intermittent claudication I70.519
            rest pain (and intermittent claudication) I70.529
          bilateral I70.503
            with
              gangrene (and intermittent claudication, rest pain and ulcer) I70.563
              intermittent claudication I70.513
              rest pain (and intermittent claudication) I70.523
            specified type NEC I70.593
          left I70.502
            with
              gangrene (and intermittent claudication, rest pain and ulcer) I70.562
              intermittent claudication I70.512
              rest pain (and intermittent claudication) I70.522
              ulceration (and intermittent claudication and rest pain) I70.549
                ankle I70.543
                calf I70.542
                foot site NEC I70.545
                heel I70.544
                lower leg NEC I70.548
                midfoot I70.544
                thigh I70.541
            specified type NEC I70.592
          right I70.501
            with
              gangrene (and intermittent claudication, rest pain and ulcer) I70.561
              intermittent claudication I70.511
              rest pain (and intermittent claudication) I70.521
              ulceration (and intermittent claudication and rest pain) I70.539
                ankle I70.533
                calf I70.532
                foot site NEC I70.535
                heel I70.534
                lower leg NEC I70.538
                midfoot I70.534
                thigh I70.531
            specified type NEC I70.591
        specified type NEC I70.599
      specified NEC I70.508
        with
          gangrene (and intermittent claudication, rest pain and ulcer) I70.568
          intermittent claudication I70.518
          rest pain (and intermittent claudication) I70.528
          ulceration (and intermittent claudication and rest pain) I70.55
        specified type NEC I70.598
      nonbiological graft I70.609
        leg I70.609
          with
            gangrene (and intermittent claudication, rest pain and ulcer) I70.669
            intermittent claudication I70.619
            rest pain (and intermittent claudication) I70.629
          bilateral I70.603
            with
              gangrene (and intermittent claudication, rest pain and ulcer) I70.663
              intermittent claudication I70.613

Arteriosclerosis, arteriosclerotic — *continued*
  extremities — *continued*
    bypass graft — *continued*
      nonbiological graft — *continued*
        leg — *continued*
          bilateral — *continued*
            with — *continued*
              rest pain (and intermittent claudication) I70.623
            specified type NEC I70.693
          left I70.602
            with
              gangrene (and intermittent claudication, rest pain and ulcer) I70.662
              intermittent claudication I70.612
              rest pain (and intermittent claudication) I70.622
              ulceration (and intermittent claudication and rest pain) I70.649
                ankle I70.643
                calf I70.642
                foot site NEC I70.645
                heel I70.644
                lower leg NEC I70.648
                midfoot I70.644
                thigh I70.641
            specified type NEC I70.692
          right I70.601
            with
              gangrene (and intermittent claudication, rest pain and ulcer) I70.661
              intermittent claudication I70.611
              rest pain (and intermittent claudication) I70.621
              ulceration (and intermittent claudication and rest pain) I70.639
                ankle I70.633
                calf I70.632
                foot site NEC I70.635
                heel I70.634
                lower leg NEC I70.638
                midfoot I70.634
                thigh I70.631
            specified type NEC I70.691
          specified type NEC I70.699
        specified NEC I70.608
          with
            gangrene (and intermittent claudication, rest pain and ulcer) I70.668
            intermittent claudication I70.618
            rest pain (and intermittent claudication) I70.628
            ulceration (and intermittent claudication and rest pain) I70.65
          specified type NEC I70.698
      specified graft NEC I70.709
        leg I70.709
          with
            gangrene (and intermittent claudication, rest pain and ulcer) I70.769
            intermittent claudication I70.719
            rest pain (and intermittent claudication) I70.729
          bilateral I70.703
            with
              gangrene (and intermittent claudication, rest pain and ulcer) I70.763
              intermittent claudication I70.713
              rest pain (and intermittent claudication) I70.723
            specified type NEC I70.793
          left I70.702
            with
              gangrene (and intermittent claudication, rest pain and ulcer) I70.762
              intermittent claudication I70.712
              rest pain (and intermittent claudication) I70.722

Arteriosclerosis, arteriosclerotic — *continued*
  extremities — *continued*
    bypass graft — *continued*
      specified graft — *continued*
        leg — *continued*
          left — *continued*
            with — *continued*
              ulceration (and intermittent claudication and rest pain) I70.749
                ankle I70.743
                calf I70.742
                foot site NEC I70.745
                heel I70.744
                lower leg NEC I70.748
                midfoot I70.744
                thigh I70.741
            specified type NEC I70.792
          right I70.701
            with
              gangrene (and intermittent claudication, rest pain and ulcer) I70.761
              intermittent claudication I70.711
              rest pain (and intermittent claudication) I70.721
              ulceration (and intermittent claudication and rest pain) I70.739
                ankle I70.733
                calf I70.732
                foot site NEC I70.735
                heel I70.734
                lower leg NEC I70.738
                midfoot I70.734
                thigh I70.731
            specified type NEC I70.791
         specified type NEC I70.799
        specified NEC I70.708
          with
            gangrene (and intermittent claudication, rest pain and ulcer) I70.768
            intermittent claudication I70.718
            rest pain (and intermittent claudication) I70.728
            ulceration (and intermittent claudication and rest pain) I70.75
          specified type NEC I70.798
      specified NEC I70.308
        with
          gangrene (and intermittent claudication, rest pain and ulcer) I70.368
          intermittent claudication I70.318
          rest pain (and intermittent claudication) I70.328
          ulceration (and intermittent claudication and rest pain) I70.35
        specifiec type NEC I70.398
    leg I70.209
      with
        gangrene (and intermittent claudication, rest pain and ulcer) I70.269
        intermittent claudication I70.219
        rest pain (and intermittent claudication) I70.229
      bilateral I70.203
        with
          gangrene (and intermittent claudication, rest pain and ulcer) I70.263
          intermittent claudication I70.213
          rest pain (and intermittent claudication) I70.223
          specified type NEC I70.293
      left I70.202
        with
          gangrene (and intermittent claudication, rest pain and ulcer) I70.262
          intermittent claudication I70.212
          rest pain (and intermittent claudication) I70.222
          ulceration (and intermittent claudication and rest pain) I70.249
            ankle I70.243
            calf I70.242
            foot site NEC I70.245
            heel I70.244
            lower leg NEC I70.248

Arteriosclerosis, arteriosclerotic — *continued*
extremities — *continued*
  leg — *continued*
    left — *continued*
      with — *continued*
        ulceration — *continued*
          midfoot I70.244
          thigh I70.241
        specified type NEC I70.292
    right I70.201
      with
        gangrene (and intermittent claudication, rest pain and ulcer) I70.261
        intermittent claudication I70.211
        rest pain (and intermittent claudication) I70.221
        ulceration (and intermittent claudication and rest pain) I70.239
          ankle I70.233
          calf I70.232
          foot site NEC I70.235
          heel I70.234
          lower leg NEC I70.238
          midfoot I70.234
          thigh I70.231
        specified type NEC I70.291
      specified type NEC I70.299
    specified site NEC I70.208
      with
        gangrene (and intermittent claudication, rest pain and ulcer) I70.268
        intermittent claudication I70.218
        rest pain (and intermittent claudication) I70.228
        ulceration (and intermittent claudication and rest pain) I70.25
      specified type NEC I70.298
generalized I70.91
heart (disease) — *see* Arteriosclerosis, coronary (artery),
kidney — *see* Hypertension, kidney
medial — *see* Arteriosclerosis, extremities
mesenteric (artery) K55.1
Mönckeberg's — *see* Arteriosclerosis, extremities
myocarditis I51.4
peripheral (of extremities) — *see* Arteriosclerosis, extremities
pulmonary (idiopathic) I27.0
renal (arterioles) (*see also* Hypertension, kidney)
  artery I70.1
retina (vascular) I70.8 [H35.0-] ☑
specified artery NEC I70.8
spinal (cord) G95.19
vertebral (artery) I67.2
Arteriospasm I73.9
Arteriovenous — *see* condition
Arteritis I77.6
allergic M31.0
aorta (nonsyphilitic) I77.6
  syphilitic A52.02
aortic arch M31.4
brachiocephalic M31.4
brain I67.7
  syphilitic A52.04
cerebral I67.7
  in systemic lupus erythematosus M32.19
  listerial A32.89
  syphilitic A52.04
  tuberculous A18.89
coronary (artery) I25.89
  rheumatic I01.8
    chronic I09.89
  syphilitic A52.06
cranial (left) (right), giant cell M31.6
deformans — *see* Arteriosclerosis
giant cell NEC M31.6
  with polymyalgia rheumatica M31.5
necrosing or necrotizing M31.9
  specified NEC M31.8
nodosa M30.0
obliterans — *see* Arteriosclerosis
pulmonary I28.8
rheumatic — *see* Fever, rheumatic
senile — *see* Arteriosclerosis
suppurative I77.2
syphilitic (general) A52.09
  brain A52.04
  coronary A52.06

Arteritis — *continued*
syphilitic — *continued*
  spinal A52.09
temporal, giant cell M31.6
young female aortic arch syndrome M31.4
Artery, arterial (*see also* condition)
abscess I77.89
single umbilical Q27.0
Arthralgia (allergic) (*see also* Pain, joint)
in caisson disease T70.3 ☑
temporomandibular M26.62
Arthritis, arthritic (acute) (chronic) (nonpyogenic) (subacute) M19.90
allergic — *see* Arthritis, specified form NEC
ankylosing (crippling) (spine) (*see also* Spondylitis, ankylosing)
  sites other than spine — *see* Arthritis, specified form NEC
atrophic — *see* Osteoarthritis
  spine — *see* Spondylitis, ankylosing
back — *see* Spondylopathy, inflammatory
blennorrhagic (gonococcal) A54.42
Charcot's — *see* Arthropathy, neuropathic
  diabetic — *see* Diabetes, arthropathy, neuropathic
  syringomyelic G95.0
chylous (filarial) (*see also* category M01) B74.9
climacteric (any site) NEC — *see* Arthritis, specified form NEC
crystal (-induced) — *see* Arthritis, in, crystals
deformans — *see* Osteoarthritis
degenerative — *see* Osteoarthritis
due to or associated with
  acromegaly E22.0
  brucellosis — *see* Brucellosis
  caisson disease T70.3 ☑
  diabetes — *see* Diabetes, arthropathy
  dracontiasis (*see also* category M01) B72
  enteritis NEC
    regional — *see* Enteritis, regional
  erysipelas (*see also* category M01) A46
  erythema
    epidemic A25.1
    nodosum L52
  filariasis NOS B74.9
  glanders A24.0
  helminthiasis (*see also* category M01) B83.9
  hemophilia D66 [M36.2]
  Henoch- (Schönlein) purpura D69.0 [M36.4]
  human parvovirus (*see also* category M01) B97.6
  infectious disease NEC M01 ☑
  leprosy (*see also* category M01) (*see also* Leprosy) A30.9
  Lyme disease A69.23
  mycobacteria (*see also* category M01) A31.8
  parasitic disease NEC (*see also* category M01) B89
  paratyphoid fever (see also category M01) (*see also* Fever, paratyphoid) A01.4
  rat bite fever (*see also* category M01) A25.1
  regional enteritis — *see* Enteritis, regional
  respiratory disorder NOS J98.9
  serum sickness (*see also* Reaction, serum) T80.69 ☑
  syringomyelia G95.0
  typhoid fever A01.04
epidemic erythema A25.1
febrile — *see* Fever, rheumatic
gonococcal A54.42
gouty (acute) — *see* Gout, idiopathic
in (due to)
  acromegaly (*see also* subcategory M14.8-) E22.0
  amyloidosis (*see also* subcategory M14.8-) E85.4
  bacterial disease (*see also* subcategory M01) A49.9
  Behçet's syndrome M35.2
  caisson disease (*see also* subcategory M14.8-) T70.3 ☑
  coliform bacilli (Escherichia coli) — *see* Arthritis, in, pyogenic organism NEC
  crystals M11.9
    dicalcium phosphate — *see* Arthritis, in, crystals, specified type NEC
    hydroxyapatite M11.0- ☑
    pyrophosphate — *see* Arthritis, in, crystals, specified type NEC
    specified type NEC M11.80
      ankle M11.87- ☑
      elbow M11.82- ☑
      foot joint M11.87- ☑
      hand joint M11.84- ☑

Arthritis, arthritic — *continued*
in — *continued*
  crystals — *continued*
    specified type — *continued*
      hip M11.85- ☑
      knee M11.86- ☑
      multiple sites M11.8- ☑
      shoulder M11.81- ☑
      vertebrae M11.88
      wrist M11.83- ☑
  dermatoarthritis, lipoid E78.81
  dracontiasis (dracunculiasis) (*see also* category M01) B72
  endocrine disorder NEC (*see also* subcategory M14.8-) E34.9
  enteritis, infectious NEC (*see also* category M01) A09
    specified organism NEC (*see also* category M01) A08.8
  erythema
    multiforme (*see also* subcategory M14.8-) L51.9
    nodosum (*see also* subcategory M14.8-) L52
  gout — *see* Gout, idiopathic
  helminthiasis NEC (*see also* category M01) B83.9
  hemochromatosis (*see also* subcategory M14.8-) E83.118
  hemoglobinopathy NEC D58.2 [M36.3]
  hemophilia NEC D66 [M36.2]
  Hemophilus influenzae M00.8- ☑ [B96.3]
  Henoch (-Schönlein) purpura D69.0 [M36.4]
  hyperparathyroidism NEC (*see also* subcategory M14.8-) E21.3
  hypersensitivity reaction NEC T78.49 ☑ [M36.4]
  hypogammaglobulinemia (*see also* subcategory M14.8-) D80.1
  hypothyroidism NEC (*see also* subcategory M14.8-) E03.9
  infection — *see* Arthritis, pyogenic or pyemic
    spine — *see* Spondylopathy, infective
  infectious disease NEC M01 ☑
  leprosy (*see also* category M01) A30.9
  leukemia NEC C95.9- ☑ [M36.1]
  lipoid dermatoarthritis E78.81
  Lyme disease A69.23
  Mediterranean fever, familial (*see also* subcategory M14.8-) E85.0
  Meningococcus A39.83
  metabolic disorder NEC (*see also* subcategory M14.8-) E88.9
  multiple myelomatosis C90.0- ☑ [M36.1]
  mumps B26.85
  mycosis NEC (*see also* category M01) B49
  myelomatosis (multiple) C90.0- ☑ [M36.1]
  neurological disorder NEC G98.0
  ochronosis (*see also* subcategory M14.8-) E70.29
  O'nyong-nyong (*see also* category M01) A92.1
  parasitic disease NEC (*see also* category M01) B89
  paratyphoid fever (*see also* category M01) A01.4
  Pseudomonas — *see* Arthritis, pyogenic, bacterial NEC
  psoriasis L40.50
  pyogenic organism NEC — *see* Arthritis, pyogenic, bacterial NEC
  Reiter's disease — *see* Reiter's disease
  respiratory disorder NEC (*see also* subcategory M14.8-) J98.9
  reticulosis, malignant (*see also* subcategory M14.8-) C86.0
  rubella B06.82
  Salmonella (arizonae) (cholerae-suis) (enteritidis) (typhimurium) A02.23
  sarcoidosis D86.86
  specified bacteria NEC — *see* Arthritis, pyogenic, bacterial NEC
  sporotrichosis B42.82
  syringomyelia G95.0
  thalassemia NEC D56.9 [M36.3]
  tuberculosis — *see* Tuberculosis, arthritis
  typhoid fever A01.04
  urethritis, Reiter's — *see* Reiter's disease
  viral disease NEC (*see also* category M01) B34.9
infectious or infective (*see also* Arthritis, pyogenic or pyemic)
  spine — *see* Spondylopathy, infective
juvenile M08.90
  with systemic onset — *see* Still's disease
  ankle M08.97- ☑

☑ **Additional Character Required** — Refer to the Tabular List for Character Selection   Ⓦ **Subterms under main terms may continue to next column or page**

Arthritis, arthritic — *continued*
  juvenile — *continued*
    elbow M08.92- ☑
    foot joint M08.97- ☑
    hand joint M08.94- ☑
    hip M08.95- ☑
    knee M08.96- ☑
    multiple site M08.99
    pauciarticular M08.40
      ankle M08.47- ☑
      elbow M08.42- ☑
      foot joint M08.47- ☑
      hand joint M08.44- ☑
      hip M08.45- ☑
      knee M08.46- ☑
      shoulder M08.41- ☑
      vertebrae M08.48
      wrist M08.43- ☑
    psoriatic L40.54
    rheumatoid — *see* Arthritis, rheumatoid, juvenile
    shoulder M08.91- ☑
    specified type NEC M08.80
      ankle M08.87- ☑
      elbow M08.82- ☑
      foot joint M08.87- ☑
      hand joint M08.84- ☑
      hip M08.85- ☑
      knee M08.86- ☑
      multiple site M08.89
      shoulder M08.81- ☑
      specified joint NEC M08.88
      vertebrae M08.88
      wrist M08.83- ☑
    wrist M08.93- ☑
  meaning osteoarthritis — *see* Osteoarthritis
  meningococcal A39.83
  menopausal (any site) NEC — *see* Arthritis, specified
    form NEC
  mutilans (psoriatic) L40.52
  mycotic NEC (*see also* category M01) B49
  neuropathic (Charcot) — *see* Arthropathy, neuropathic
    diabetic — *see* Diabetes, arthropathy, neuropathic
    nonsyphilitic NEC G98.0
    syringomyelic G95.0
  ochronotic (*see also* subcategory M14.8-) E70.29
  palindromic (any site) — *see* Rheumatism, palindromic
  pneumococcal M00.10
    ankle M00.17- ☑
    elbow M00.12- ☑
    foot joint — *see* Arthritis, pneumococcal, ankle
    hand joint M00.14- ☑
    hip M00.15- ☑
    knee M00.16- ☑
    multiple site M00.19
    shoulder M00.11- ☑
    vertebra M00.18
    wrist M00.13- ☑
  postdysenteric — *see* Arthropathy, postdysenteric
  postmeningococcal A39.84
  postrheumatic, chronic — *see* Arthropathy,
    postrheumatic, chronic
  primary progressive (*see also* Arthritis, specified form
    NEC)
    spine — *see* Spondylitis, ankylosing
  psoriatic L40.50
  purulent (any site except spine) — *see* Arthritis, pyo-
    genic or pyemic
    spine — *see* Spondylopathy, infective
  pyogenic or pyemic (any site except spine) M00.9
    bacterial NEC M00.80
      ankle M00.87- ☑
      elbow M00.82- ☑
      foot joint — *see* Arthritis, pyogenic, bacterial
        NEC, ankle
      hand joint M00.84- ☑
      hip M00.85- ☑
      knee M00.86- ☑
      multiple site M00.89
      shoulder M00.81- ☑
      vertebra M00.88
      wrist M00.83- ☑
    pneumococcal — *see* Arthritis, pneumococcal
    spine — *see* Spondylopathy, infective
    staphylococcal — *see* Arthritis, staphylococcal
    streptococcal — *see* Arthritis, streptococcal NEC
      pneumococcal — *see* Arthritis, pneumococcal

Arthritis, arthritic — *continued*
  reactive — *see* Reiter's disease
  rheumatic (*see also* Arthritis, rheumatoid)
    acute or subacute — *see* Fever, rheumatic
  rheumatoid M06.9
    with
      carditis — *see* Rheumatoid, carditis
      endocarditis — *see* Rheumatoid, carditis
      heart involvement NEC — *see* Rheumatoid,
        carditis
      lung involvement — *see* Rheumatoid, lung
      myocarditis — *see* Rheumatoid, carditis
      myopathy — *see* Rheumatoid, myopathy
      pericarditis — *see* Rheumatoid, carditis
      polyneuropathy — *see* Rheumatoid, polyneu-
        ropathy
      rheumatoid factor — *see* Arthritis, rheumatoid,
        seropositive
      splenoadenomegaly and leukopenia — *see*
        Felty's syndrome
      vasculitis — *see* Rheumatoid, vasculitis
      visceral involvement NEC — *see* Rheumatoid,
        arthritis, with involvement of organs NEC
    juvenile (with or without rheumatoid factor)
      M08.00
      ankle M08.07- ☑
      elbow M08.02- ☑
      foot joint M08.07- ☑
      hand joint M08.04- ☑
      hip M08.05- ☑
      knee M08.06- ☑
      multiple site M08.09
      shoulder M08.01- ☑
      vertebra M08.08
      wrist M08.03- ☑
    seronegative M06.00
      ankle M06.07- ☑
      elbow M06.02- ☑
      foot joint M06.07- ☑
      hand joint M06.04- ☑
      hip M06.05- ☑
      knee M06.06- ☑
      multiple site M06.09
      shoulder M06.01- ☑
      vertebra M06.08
      wrist M06.03- ☑
    seropositive M05.9
      without organ involvement M05.70
        ankle M05.77- ☑
        elbow M05.72- ☑
        foot joint M05.77- ☑
        hand joint M05.74- ☑
        hip M05.75- ☑
        knee M05.76- ☑
        multiple sites M05.79
        shoulder M05.71- ☑
        vertebra — *see* Spondylitis, ankylosing
        wrist M05.73- ☑
      specified NEC M05.80
        ankle M05.87- ☑
        elbow M05.82- ☑
        foot joint M05.87- ☑
        hand joint M05.84- ☑
        hip M05.85- ☑
        knee M05.86- ☑
        multiple sites M05.89
        shoulder M05.81- ☑
        vertebra — *see* Spondylitis, ankylosing
        wrist M05.83- ☑
    specified type NEC M06.80
      ankle M06.87- ☑
      elbow M06.82- ☑
      foot joint M06.87- ☑
      hand joint M06.84- ☑
      hip M06.85- ☑
      knee M06.86- ☑
      multiple site M06.89
      shoulder M06.81- ☑
      vertebra M06.88
      wrist M06.83- ☑
    spine — *see* Spondylitis, ankylosing
  rubella B06.82
  scorbutic (*see also* subcategory M14.8-) E54
  senile or senescent — *see* Osteoarthritis

Arthritis, arthritic — *continued*
  septic (any site except spine) — *see* Arthritis, pyogenic
    or pyemic
    spine — *see* Spondylopathy, infective
  serum (nontherapeutic) (therapeutic) — *see*
    Arthropathy, postimmunization
  specified form NEC M13.80
    ankle M13.87- ☑
    elbow M13.82- ☑
    foot joint M13.87- ☑
    hand joint M13.84- ☑
    hip M13.85- ☑
    knee M13.86- ☑
    multiple site M13.89
    shoulder M13.81- ☑
    specified joint NEC M13.88
    wrist M13.83- ☑
  spine (*see also* Spondylopathy, inflammatory)
    infectious or infective NEC — *see* Spondylopathy,
      infective
    Marie-Strümpell — *see* Spondylitis, ankylosing
    pyogenic — *see* Spondylopathy, infective
    rheumatoid — *see* Spondylitis, ankylosing
    traumatic (old) — *see* Spondylopathy, traumatic
    tuberculous A18.01
  staphylococcal M00.00
    ankle M00.07- ☑
    elbow M00.02- ☑
    foot joint — *see* Arthritis, staphylococcal, ankle
    hand joint M00.04- ☑
    hip M00.05- ☑
    knee M00.06- ☑
    multiple site M00.09
    shoulder M00.01- ☑
    vertebra M00.08
    wrist M00.03- ☑
  streptococcal NEC M00.20
    ankle M00.27- ☑
    elbow M00.22- ☑
    foot joint — *see* Arthritis, streptococcal, ankle
    hand joint M00.24- ☑
    hip M00.25- ☑
    knee M00.26- ☑
    multiple site M00.29
    shoulder M00.21- ☑
    vertebra M00.28
    wrist M00.23- ☑
  suppurative — *see* Arthritis, pyogenic or pyemic
  syphilitic (late) A52.16
    congenital A50.55 [M12.80]
  syphilitica deformans (Charcot) A52.16
  temporomandibular M26.69
  toxic of menopause (any site) — *see* Arthritis, specified
    form NEC
  transient — *see* Arthropathy, specified form NEC
  traumatic (chronic) — *see* Arthropathy, traumatic
  tuberculous A18.02
    spine A18.01
  uratic — *see* Gout, idiopathic
  urethritica (Reiter's) — *see* Reiter's disease
  vertebral — *see* Spondylopathy, inflammatory
  villous (any site) — *see* Arthropathy, specified form
    NEC
Arthrocele — *see* Effusion, joint
Arthrodesis status Z98.1
Arthrodynia (*see also* Pain, joint)
Arthrodysplasia Q74.9
Arthrofibrosis, joint — *see* Ankylosis
Arthrogryposis (congenital) Q68.8
  multiplex congenita Q74.3
Arthrokatadysis M24.7
Arthropathy (*see also* Arthritis) M12.9
  Charcot's — *see* Arthropathy, neuropathic
    diabetic — *see* Diabetes, arthropathy, neuropathic
    syringomyelic G95.0
  cricoarytenoid J38.7
  crystal (-induced) — *see* Arthritis, in, crystals
  diabetic NEC — *see* Diabetes, arthropathy
  distal interphalangeal, psoriatic L40.51
  enteropathic M07.60
    ankle M07.67- ☑
    elbow M07.62- ☑
    foot joint M07.67- ☑
    hand joint M07.64- ☑
    hip M07.65- ☑
    knee M07.66- ☑

▽ Subterms under main terms may continue to next column or page   ☑ Additional Character Required — Refer to the Tabular List for Character Selection   29

Arthritis, arthritic — Arthropathy

Arthropathy — *continued*
 enteropathic — *continued*
  multiple site M07.69
  shoulder M07.61- ☑
  vertebra M07.68
  wrist M07.63- ☑
 following intestinal bypass M02.00
  ankle M02.07- ☑
  elbow M02.02- ☑
  foot joint M02.07- ☑
  hand joint M02.04- ☑
  hip M02.05- ☑
  knee M02.06- ☑
  multiple site M02.09
  shoulder M02.01- ☑
  vertebra M02.08
  wrist M02.03- ☑
 gouty (*see also* Gout, idiopathic)
  in (due to)
   Lesch-Nyhan syndrome E79.1 [M14.8-] ☑
   sickle-cell disorders D57- [M14.8-] ☑
 hemophilic NEC D66 [M36.2]
  in (due to)
   hyperparathyroidism NEC E21.3 [M14.8-] ☑
   metabolic disease NOS E88.9 [M14.8-] ☑
 in (due to)
  acromegaly E22.0 [M14.8-] ☑
  amyloidosis E85.4 [M14.8-] ☑
  blood disorder NOS D75.9 [M36.3]
  diabetes — *see* Diabetes, arthropathy
  endocrine disease NOS E34.9 [M14.8-] ☑
  erythema
   multiforme L51.9 [M14.8-] ☑
   nodosum L52 [M14.8-] ☑
  hemochromatosis E83.118 [M14.8-] ☑
  hemoglobinopathy NEC D58.2 [M36.3]
  hemophilia NEC D66 [M36.2]
  Henoch-Schönlein purpura D69.0 [M36.4]
  hyperthyroidism E05.90 [M14.8-] ☑
  hypothyroidism E03.9 [M14.8-] ☑
  infective endocarditis I33.0 [M12.80]
  leukemia NEC C95.9- [M36.1] ☑
  malignant histiocytosis C96.A [M36.1]
  metabolic disease NOS E88.9 [M14.8-] ☑
  multiple myeloma C90.0- ☑ [M36.1]
  neoplastic disease NOS (*see also* Neoplasm)
   D49.9 [M36.1]
  nutritional deficiency (*see also* subcategory
   M14.8-) E63.9
  psoriasis NOS L40.50
  sarcoidosis D86.86
  syphilis (late) A52.77
   congenital A50.55 [M12.80]
  thyrotoxicosis (*see also* subcategory M14.8-) E05.90
  ulcerative colitis K51.90 [M07.60]
  viral hepatitis (postinfectious) NEC B19.9 [M12.80]
  Whipple's disease (*see also* subcategory M14.8-)
   K90.81
 Jaccoud — *see* Arthropathy, postrheumatic, chronic
 juvenile — *see* Arthritis, juvenile
  psoriatic L40.54
 mutilans (psoriatic) L40.52
 neuropathic (Charcot) M14.60
  ankle M14.67- ☑
  diabetic — *see* Diabetes, arthropathy, neuropathic
  elbow M14.62- ☑
  foot joint M14.67- ☑
  hand joint M14.64- ☑
  hip M14.65- ☑
  knee M14.66- ☑
  multiple site M14.69
  nonsyphilitic NEC G98.0
  shoulder M14.61- ☑
  syringomyelic G95.0
  vertebra M14.68
  wrist M14.63- ☑
 osteopulmonary — *see* Osteoarthropathy, hypertrophic, specified NEC
 postdysenteric M02.10
  ankle M02.17- ☑
  elbow M02.12- ☑
  foot joint M02.17- ☑
  hand joint M02.14- ☑
  hip M02.15- ☑
  knee M02.16- ☑
  multiple site M02.19
  shoulder M02.11- ☑

Arthropathy — *continued*
 postdysenteric — *continued*
  vertebra M02.18
  wrist M02.13- ☑
 postimmunization M02.20
  ankle M02.27- ☑
  elbow M02.22- ☑
  foot joint M02.27- ☑
  hand joint M02.24- ☑
  hip M02.25- ☑
  knee M02.26- ☑
  multiple site M02.29
  shoulder M02.21- ☑
  vertebra M02.28
  wrist M02.23- ☑
 postinfectious NEC B99 ☑ [M12.80]
  in (due to)
   enteritis due to Yersinia enterocolitica
    A04.6 [M12.80]
   syphilis A52.77
   viral hepatitis NEC B19.9 [M12.80]
 postrheumatic, chronic (Jaccoud) M12.00
  ankle M12.07- ☑
  elbow M12.02- ☑
  foot joint M12.07- ☑
  hand joint M12.04- ☑
  hip M12.05- ☑
  knee M12.06- ☑
  multiple site M12.09
  shoulder M12.01- ☑
  specified joint NEC M12.08
  vertebrae M12.08
  wrist M12.03- ☑
 psoriatic NEC L40.59
  interphalangeal, distal L40.51
 reactive M02.9
  in (due to)
   infective endocarditis I33.0 [M02.9]
  specified type NEC M02.80
   ankle M02.87- ☑
   elbow M02.82- ☑
   foot joint M02.87- ☑
   hand joint M02.84- ☑
   hip M02.85- ☑
   knee M02.86- ☑
   multiple site M02.89
   shoulder M02.81- ☑
   vertebra M02.88
   wrist M02.83- ☑
 specified form NEC M12.80
  ankle M12.87- ☑
  elbow M12.82- ☑
  foot joint M12.87- ☑
  hand joint M12.84- ☑
  hip M12.85- ☑
  knee M12.86- ☑
  multiple site M12.89
  shoulder M12.81- ☑
  specified joint NEC M12.88
  vertebrae M12.88
  wrist M12.83- ☑
 syringomyelic G95.0
 tabes dorsalis A52.16
 tabetic A52.16
 transient — *see* Arthropathy, specified form NEC
 traumatic M12.50
  ankle M12.57- ☑
  elbow M12.52- ☑
  foot joint M12.57- ☑
  hand joint M12.54- ☑
  hip M12.55- ☑
  knee M12.56- ☑
  multiple site M12.59
  shoulder M12.51- ☑
  specified joint NEC M12.58
  vertebrae M12.58
  wrist M12.53- ☑
Arthropyosis — *see* Arthritis, pyogenic or pyemic
Arthrosis (deformans) (degenerative) (localized) (*see also*
 Osteoarthritis) M19.90
 spine — *see* Spondylosis
Arthus' phenomenon or reaction T78.41 ☑
 due to
  drug — *see* Table of Drugs and Chemicals, by drug
Articular — *see* condition
Articulation, reverse (teeth) M26.24

Artificial
 insemination complication — *see* Complications, artificial, fertilization
 opening status (functioning) (without complication)
  Z93.9
  anus (colostomy) Z93.3
  colostomy Z93.3
  cystostomy Z93.50
   appendico-vesicostomy Z93.52
   cutaneous Z93.51
   specified NEC Z93.59
  enterostomy Z93.4
  gastrostomy Z93.1
  ileostomy Z93.2
  intestinal tract NEC Z93.4
  jejunostomy Z93.4
  nephrostomy Z93.6
  specified site NEC Z93.8
  tracheostomy Z93.0
  ureterostomy Z93.6
  urethrostomy Z93.6
  urinary tract NEC Z93.6
  vagina Z93.8
 vagina status Z93.8
Arytenoid — *see* condition
Asbestosis (occupational) J61
Ascariasis B77.9
 with
  complications NEC B77.89
  intestinal complications B77.0
  pneumonia, pneumonitis B77.81
Ascaridosis, ascaridiasis — *see* Ascariasis
Ascaris (infection) (infestation) (lumbricoides) — *see*
 Ascariasis
Ascending — *see* condition
ASC-H (atypical squamous cells cannot exclude high
 grade squamous intraepithelial lesion on cytologic
 smear)
 anus R85.611
 cervix R87.611
 vagina R87.621
Aschoff's bodies — *see* Myocarditis, rheumatic
Ascites (abdominal) R18.8
 cardiac I50.9
 chylous (nonfilarial) I89.8
  filarial — *see* Infestation, filarial
 due to
  cirrhosis, alcoholic K70.31
  hepatitis
   alcoholic K70.11
   chronic active K71.51
  S. japonicum B65.2
 heart I50.9
 malignant R18.0
 pseudochylous R18.8
 syphilitic A52.74
 tuberculous A18.31
ASC-US (atypical squamous cells of undetermined significance on cytologic smear)
 anus R85.610
 cervix R87.610
 vagina R87.620
Aseptic — *see* condition
Asherman's syndrome N85.6
Asialia K11.7
Asiatic cholera — *see* Cholera
Asimultagnosia (simultanagnosia) R48.3
Askin's tumor — *see* Neoplasm, connective tissue, malignant
Asocial personality F60.2
Asomatognosia R41.4
Aspartylglucosaminuria E77.1
Asperger's disease or syndrome F84.5
Aspergilloma — *see* Aspergillosis
Aspergillosis (with pneumonia) B44.9
 bronchopulmonary, allergic B44.81
 disseminated B44.7
 generalized B44.7
 pulmonary NEC B44.1
  allergic B44.81
  invasive B44.0
 specified NEC B44.89
 tonsillar B44.2
Aspergillus (flavus) (fumigatus) (infection) (terreus) —
 see Aspergillosis
Aspermatogenesis — *see* Azoospermia
Aspermia (testis) — *see* Azoospermia

Asphyxia, asphyxiation (by) R09.01
- antenatal P84
- birth P84
- bunny bag — *see* Asphyxia, due to, mechanical threat to breathing, trapped in bed clothes
- crushing S28.0 ☑
- drowning T75.1 ☑
- gas, fumes, or vapor — *see* Table of Drugs and Chemicals
- inhalation — *see* Inhalation
- intrauterine P84
- local I73.00
  - with gangrene I73.01
- mucus (*see also* Foreign body, respiratory tract, causing asphyxia)
- newborn P84
- pathological R09.01
- postnatal P84
  - mechanical — *see* Asphyxia, due to, mechanical threat to breathing
- prenatal P84
- reticularis R23.1
- strangulation — *see* Asphyxia, due to, mechanical threat to breathing
- submersion T75.1 ☑
- traumatic T71.9 ☑
  - due to
    - crushed chest S28.0 ☑
    - foreign body (in) — *see* Foreign body, respiratory tract, causing asphyxia
    - low oxygen content of ambient air T71.20 ☑
      - due to
        - being trapped in
          - low oxygen environment T71.29 ☑
            - in car trunk T71.221 ☑
              - circumstances undetermined T71.224 ☑
              - done with intent to harm by
                - another person T71.223 ☑
                - self T71.222 ☑
            - in refrigerator T71.231 ☑
              - circumstances undetermined T71.234 ☑
              - done with intent to harm by
                - another person T71.233 ☑
                - self T71.232 ☑
        - cave-in T71.21 ☑
    - mechanical threat to breathing (accidental) T71.191 ☑
      - circumstances undetermined T71.194 ☑
      - done with intent to harm by
        - another person T71.193 ☑
        - self T71.192 ☑
      - hanging T71.161 ☑
        - circumstances undetermined T71.164 ☑
        - done with intent to harm by
          - another person T71.163 ☑
          - self T71.162 ☑
      - plastic bag T71.121 ☑
        - circumstances undetermined T71.124 ☑
        - done with intent to harm by
          - another person T71.123 ☑
          - self T71.122 ☑
      - smothering
        - in furniture T71.151 ☑
          - circumstances undetermined T71.154 ☑
          - done with intent to harm by
            - another person T71.153 ☑
            - self T71.152 ☑
        - under
          - another person's body T71.141 ☑
            - circumstances undetermined T71.144 ☑
            - done with intent to harm T71.143 ☑
          - pillow T71.111 ☑
            - circumstances undetermined T71.114 ☑
            - done with intent to harm by
              - another person T71.113 ☑
              - self T71.112 ☑
        - trapped in bed clothes T71.131 ☑
          - circumstances undetermined T71.134 ☑
          - done with intent to harm by
            - another person T71.133 ☑
            - self T71.132 ☑

Asphyxia, asphyxiation — *continued*
- vomiting, vomitus — *see* Foreign body, respiratory tract, causing asphyxia

Aspiration
- amniotic (clear) fluid (newborn) P24.10
  - with
    - pneumonia (pneumonitis) P24.11
    - respiratory symptoms P24.11
- blood
  - newborn (without respiratory symptoms) P24.20
    - with
      - pneumonia (pneumonitis) P24.21
      - respiratory symptoms P24.21
    - specified age NEC — *see* Foreign body, respiratory tract
- bronchitis J69.0
- food or foreign body (with asphyxiation) — *see* Asphyxia, food
- liquor (amnii) (newborn) P24.10
  - with
    - pneumonia (pneumonitis) P24.11
    - respiratory symptoms P24.11
- meconium (newborn) (without respiratory symptoms) P24.00
  - with
    - pneumonitis (pneumonitis) P24.01
    - respiratory symptoms P24.01
- milk (newborn) (without respiratory symptoms) P24.30
  - with
    - pneumonia (pneumonitis) P24.31
    - respiratory symptoms P24.31
  - specified age NEC — *see* Foreign body, respiratory tract
- mucus (*see also* Foreign body, by site, causing asphyxia)
  - newborn P24.10
    - with
      - pneumonia (pneumonitis) P24.11
      - respiratory symptoms P24.11
- neonatal P24.9
  - specific NEC (without respiratory symptoms) P24.80
    - with
      - pneumonia (pneumonitis) P24.81
      - respiratory symptoms P24.81
- newborn P24.9
  - specific NEC (without respiratory symptoms) P24.80
    - with
      - pneumonia (pneumonitis) P24.81
      - respiratory symptoms P24.81
- pneumonia J69.0
- pneumonitis J69.0
- syndrome of newborn — *see* Aspiration, by substance, with pneumonia
- vernix caseosa (newborn) P24.80
  - with
    - pneumonia (pneumonitis) P24.81
    - respiratory symptoms P24.81
- vomitus (*see also* Foreign body, respiratory tract)
  - newborn (without respiratory symptoms) P24.30
    - with
      - pneumonia (pneumonitis) P24.31
      - respiratory symptoms P24.31

Asplenia (congenital) Q89.01
- postsurgical Z90.81

Assam fever B55.0

Assault, sexual — *see* Maltreatment

Assmann's focus NEC A15.0

Astasia (-abasia) (hysterical) F44.4

Asteatosis cutis L85.3

Astereognosia, astereognosis R48.1

Asterixis R27.8
- in liver disease K71.3

Asteroid hyalitis — *see* Deposit, crystalline

Asthenia, asthenic R53.1
- cardiac (*see also* Failure, heart) I50.9
  - psychogenic F45.8
- cardiovascular (*see also* Failure, heart) I50.9
  - psychogenic F45.8
- heart (*see also* Failure, heart) I50.9
  - psychogenic F45.8
- hysterical F44.4
- myocardial (*see also* Failure, heart) I50.9
  - psychogenic F45.8
- nervous F48.8
- neurocirculatory F45.8
- neurotic F48.8
- psychogenic F48.8
- psychoneurotic F48.8

Asthenia, asthenic — *continued*
- psychophysiologic F48.8
- reaction (psychophysiologic) F48.8
- senile R54

Asthenopia (*see also* Discomfort, visual)
- hysterical F44.6
- psychogenic F44.6

Asthenospermia — *see* Abnormal, specimen, male genital organs

Asthma, asthmatic (bronchial) (catarrh) (spasmodic) J45.909
- with
  - chronic obstructive bronchitis J44.9
    - with
      - acute lower respiratory infection J44.0
      - exacerbation (acute) J44.1
  - chronic obstructive pulmonary disease J44.9
    - with
      - acute lower respiratory infection J44.0
      - exacerbation (acute) J44.1
  - exacerbation (acute) J45.901
  - hay fever — *see* Asthma, allergic extrinsic
  - rhinitis, allergic — *see* Asthma, allergic extrinsic
  - status asthmaticus J45.902
- allergic extrinsic J45.909
  - with
    - exacerbation (acute) J45.901
    - status asthmaticus J45.902
- atopic — *see* Asthma, allergic extrinsic
- cardiac — *see* Failure, ventricular, left
- cardiobronchial I50.1
- childhood J45.909
  - with
    - exacerbation (acute) J45.901
    - status asthmaticus J45.902
- chronic obstructive J44.9
  - with
    - acute lower respiratory infection J44.0
    - exacerbation (acute) J44.1
- collier's J60
- cough variant J45.991
- detergent J69.8
- due to
  - detergent J69.8
  - inhalation of fumes J68.3
- eosinophilic J82
- extrinsic, allergic — *see* Asthma, allergic extrinsic
- grinder's J62.8
- hay — *see* Asthma, allergic extrinsic
- heart I50.1
- idiosyncratic — *see* Asthma, nonallergic
- intermittent (mild) J45.20
  - with
    - exacerbation (acute) J45.21
    - status asthmaticus J45.22
- intrinsic, nonallergic — *see* Asthma, nonallergic
- Kopp's E32.8
- late-onset J45.909
  - with
    - exacerbation (acute) J45.901
    - status asthmaticus J45.902
- mild intermittent J45.20
  - with
    - exacerbation (acute) J45.21
    - status asthmaticus J45.22
- mild persistent J45.30
  - with
    - exacerbation (acute) J45.31
    - status asthmaticus J45.32
- Millar's (laryngismus stridulus) J38.5
- miner's J60
- mixed J45.909
  - with
    - exacerbation (acute) J45.901
    - status asthmaticus J45.902
- moderate persistent J45.40
  - with
    - exacerbation (acute) J45.41
    - status asthmaticus J45.42
- nervous — *see* Asthma, nonallergic
- nonallergic (intrinsic) J45.909
  - with
    - exacerbation (acute) J45.901
    - status asthmaticus J45.902
- persistent
  - mild J45.30
    - with
      - exacerbation (acute) J45.31

Asthma, asthmatic — *continued*
  persistent — *continued*
    mild — *continued*
      with — *continued*
        status asthmaticus J45.32
    moderate J45.40
      with
        exacerbation (acute) J45.41
        status asthmaticus J45.42
    severe J45.50
      with
        exacerbation (acute) J45.51
        status asthmaticus J45.52
  platinum J45.998
  pneumoconiotic NEC J64
  potter's J62.8
  predominantly allergic J45.909
  psychogenic F54
  pulmonary eosinophilic J82
  red cedar J67.8
  Rostan's I50.1
  sandblaster's J62.8
  sequoiosis J67.8
  severe persistent J45.50
    with
      exacerbation (acute) J45.51
      status asthmaticus J45.52
  specified NEC J45.998
  stonemason's J62.8
  thymic E32.8
  tuberculous — *see* Tuberculosis, pulmonary
  Wichmann's (laryngismus stridulus) J38.5
  wood J67.8
Astigmatism (compound) (congenital) H52.20- ☑
  irregular H52.21- ☑
  regular H52.22- ☑
Astraphobia F40.220
Astroblastoma
  specified site — *see* Neoplasm, malignant, by site
  unspecified site C71.9
Astrocytoma (cystic)
  anaplastic
    specified site — *see* Neoplasm, malignant, by site
    unspecified site C71.9
  fibrillary
    specified site — *see* Neoplasm, malignant, by site
    unspecified site C71.9
  fibrous
    specified site — *see* Neoplasm, malignant, by site
    unspecified site C71.9
  gemistocytic
    specified site — *see* Neoplasm, malignant, by site
    unspecified site C71.9
  juvenile
    specified site — *see* Neoplasm, malignant, by site
    unspecified site C71.9
  pilocytic
    specified site — *see* Neoplasm, malignant, by site
    unspecified site C71.9
  piloid
    specified site — *see* Neoplasm, malignant, by site
    unspecified site C71.9
  protoplasmic
    specified site — *see* Neoplasm, malignant, by site
    unspecified site C71.9
  specified site NEC — *see* Neoplasm, malignant, by site
  subependymal D43.2
    giant cell
      specified site — *see* Neoplasm, uncertain behavior, by site
      unspecified site D43.2
    specified site — *see* Neoplasm, uncertain behavior, by site
    unspecified site D43.2
  unspecified site C71.9
Astroglioma
  specified site — *see* Neoplasm, malignant, by site
  unspecified site C71.9
Asymbolia R48.8
Asymmetry (*see also* Distortion)
  between native and reconstructed breast N65.1
  face Q67.0
  jaw (lower) — *see* Anomaly, dentofacial, jaw-cranial base relationship, asymmetry
Asynergia, asynergy R27.8
  ventricular I51.89
Asystole (heart) — *see* Arrest, cardiac

At risk
  for falling Z91.81
Ataxia, ataxy, ataxic R27.0
  acute R27.8
  brain (hereditary) G11.9
  cerebellar (hereditary) G11.9
    with defective DNA repair G11.3
    alcoholic G31.2
    early-onset G11.1
    in
      alcoholism G31.2
      myxedema E03.9 [G13.2]
      neoplastic disease (*see also* Neoplasm) D49.9 [G13.1]
      specified disease NEC G32.81
    late-onset (Marie's) G11.2
  cerebral (hereditary) G11.9
  congenital nonprogressive G11.0
  family, familial — *see* Ataxia, hereditary
  following
    cerebrovascular disease I69.993
      cerebral infarction I69.393
      intracerebral hemorrhage I69.193
      nontraumatic intracranial hemorrhage NEC I69.293
      specified disease NEC I69.893
      subarachnoid hemorrhage I69.093
  Friedreich's (heredofamilial) (cerebellar) (spinal) G11.1
  gait R26.0
    hysterical F44.4
  general R27.8
  gluten M35.9 [G32.81]
    with celiac disease K90.0 [G32.81]
  hereditary G11.9
    with neuropathy G60.2
    cerebellar — *see* Ataxia, cerebellar
    spastic G11.4
    specified NEC G11.8
    spinal (Friedreich's) G11.1
  heredofamilial — *see* Ataxia, hereditary
  Hunt's G11.1
  hysterical F44.4
  locomotor (progressive) (syphilitic) (partial) (spastic) A52.11
    diabetic — *see* Diabetes, ataxia
  Marie's (cerebellar) (heredofamilial) (late- onset) G11.2
  nonorganic origin F44.4
  nonprogressive, congenital G11.0
  psychogenic F44.4
  Roussy-Lévy G60.0
  Sanger-Brown's (hereditary) G11.2
  spastic hereditary G11.4
  spinal
    hereditary (Friedreich's) G11.1
    progressive (syphilitic) A52.11
  spinocerebellar, X-linked recessive G11.1
  telangiectasia (Louis-Bar) G11.3
Ataxia-telangiectasia (Louis-Bar) G11.3
Atelectasis (massive) (partial) (pressure) (pulmonary) J98.11
  newborn P28.10
    due to resorption P28.11
    partial P28.19
    primary P28.0
    secondary P28.19
  primary (newborn) P28.0
  tuberculous — *see* Tuberculosis, pulmonary
Atelocardia Q24.9
Atelomyelia Q06.1
Atheroembolism
  of
    extremities
      lower I75.02- ☑
      upper I75.01- ☑
    kidney I75.81
    specified NEC I75.89
Atheroma, atheromatous (*see also* Arteriosclerosis) I70.90
  aorta, aortic I70.0
    valve (*see also* Endocarditis, aortic) I35.8
  aorto-iliac I70.0
  artery — *see* Arteriosclerosis
  basilar (artery) I67.2
  carotid (artery) (common) (internal) I67.2
  cerebral (arteries) I67.2
  coronary (artery) I25.10
    with angina pectoris — *see* Arteriosclerosis, coronary (artery),

Atheroma, atheromatous — *continued*
  degeneration — *see* Arteriosclerosis
  heart, cardiac — *see* Disease, heart, ischemic, atherosclerotic
  mitral (valve) I34.8
  myocardium, myocardial — *see* Disease, heart, ischemic, atherosclerotic
  pulmonary valve (heart) (*see also* Endocarditis, pulmonary) I37.8
  tricuspid (heart) (valve) I36.8
  valve, valvular — *see* Endocarditis
  vertebral (artery) I67.2
Atheromatosis — *see* Arteriosclerosis
Atherosclerosis (*see also* Arteriosclerosis)
  coronary
    artery I25.10
      with angina pectoris — *see* Arteriosclerosis, coronary (artery),
      due to
        calcified coronary lesion (severely) I25.84
        lipid rich plaque I25.83
    transplanted heart I25.811
      bypass graft I25.812
        with angina pectoris — *see* Arteriosclerosis, coronary (artery),
      native coronary artery I25.811
        with angina pectoris — *see* Arteriosclerosis, coronary (artery),
Athetosis (acquired) R25.8
  bilateral (congenital) G80.3
  congenital (bilateral) (double) G80.3
  double (congenital) G80.3
  unilateral R25.8
Athlete's
  foot B35.3
  heart I51.7
Athrepsia E41
Athyrea (acquired) (*see also* Hypothyroidism)
  congenital E03.1
Atonia, atony, atonic
  bladder (sphincter) (neurogenic) N31.2
  capillary I78.8
  cecum K59.8
    psychogenic F45.8
  colon — *see* Atony, intestine
  congenital P94.2
  esophagus K22.8
  intestine K59.8
    psychogenic F45.8
  stomach K31.89
    neurotic or psychogenic F45.8
  uterus (during labor) O62.2
    with hemorrhage (postpartum) O72.1
    postpartum (with hemorrhage) O72.1
      without hemorrhage O75.89
Atopy — *see* History, allergy
Atransferrinemia, congenital E88.09
Atresia, atretic
  alimentary organ or tract NEC Q45.8
    upper Q40.8
  ani, anus, anal (canal) Q42.3
    with fistula Q42.2
  aorta (arch) (ring) Q25.2
  aortic (orifice) (valve) Q23.0
    arch Q25.2
    congenital with hypoplasia of ascending aorta and defective development of left ventricle (with mitral stenosis) Q23.4
    in hypoplastic left heart syndrome Q23.4
  aqueduct of Sylvius Q03.0
    with spina bifida — *see* Spina bifida, with hydrocephalus
  artery NEC Q27.8
    cerebral Q28.3
    coronary Q24.5
    digestive system Q27.8
    eye Q15.8
    lower limb Q27.8
    pulmonary Q25.5
    specified site NEC Q27.8
    umbilical Q27.0
    upper limb Q27.8
  auditory canal (external) Q16.1
  bile duct (common) (congenital) (hepatic) Q44.2
    acquired — *see* Obstruction, bile duct
  bladder (neck) Q64.39
    obstruction Q64.31
  bronchus Q32.4

☑ **Additional Character Required** — Refer to the Tabular List for Character Selection   ▽ Subterms under main terms may continue to next column or page

Atresia, atretic — *continued*
cecum Q42.8
cervix (acquired) N88.2
   congenital Q51.828
   in pregnancy or childbirth — *see* Anomaly, cervix, in pregnancy or childbirth
      causing obstructed labor O65.5
choana Q30.0
colon Q42.9
   specified NEC Q42.8
common duct Q44.2
cricoid cartilage Q31.8
cystic duct Q44.2
   acquired K82.8
      with obstruction K82.0
digestive organs NEC Q45.8
duodenum Q41.0
ear canal Q16.1
ejaculatory duct Q55.4
epiglottis Q31.8
esophagus Q39.0
   with tracheoesophageal fistula Q39.1
eustachian tube Q17.8
fallopian tube (congenital) Q50.6
   acquired N97.1
follicular cyst N83.0
foramen of
   Luschka Q03.1
      with spina bifida — *see* Spina bifida, with hy-
         drocephalus
   Magendie Q03.1
      with spina bifida — *see* Spina bifida, with hy-
         drocephalus
gallbladder Q44.1
genital organ
   external
      female Q52.79
      male Q55.8
   internal
      female Q52.8
      male Q55.8
glottis Q31.8
gullet Q39.0
   with tracheoesophageal fistula Q39.1
heart valve NEC Q24.8
   pulmonary Q22.0
   tricuspid Q22.4
hymen Q52.3
   acquired (postinfective) N89.6
ileum Q41.2
intestine (small) Q41.9
   large Q42.9
      specified NEC Q42.8
iris, filtration angle Q15.0
jejunum Q41.1
lacrimal apparatus Q10.4
larynx Q31.8
meatus urinarius Q64.33
mitral valve Q23.2
   in hypoplastic left heart syndrome Q23.4
nares (anterior) (posterior) Q30.0
nasopharynx Q34.8
nose, nostril Q30.0
   acquired J34.89
organ or site NEC Q89.8
osseous meatus (ear) Q16.1
oviduct (congenital) Q50.6
   acquired N97.1
parotid duct Q38.4
   acquired K11.8
pulmonary (artery) Q25.5
   valve Q22.0
pulmonic Q22.0
pupil Q13.2
rectum Q42.1
   with fistula Q42.0
salivary duct Q38.4
   acquired K11.8
sublingual duct Q38.4
   acquired K11.8
submandibular duct Q38.4
   acquired K11.8
submaxillary duct Q38.4
   acquired K11.8
thyroid cartilage Q31.8
trachea Q32.1
tricuspid valve Q22.4

Atresia, atretic — *continued*
ureter Q62.10
   pelvic junction Q62.11
   vesical orifice Q62.12
ureteropelvic junction Q62.11
ureterovesical orifice Q62.12
urethra (valvular) Q64.39
   stricture Q64.32
urinary tract NEC Q64.8
uterus Q51.818
   acquired N85.8
vagina (congenital) Q52.4
   acquired (postinfectional) (senile) N89.5
vas deferens Q55.3
vascular NEC Q27.8
   cerebral Q28.3
   digestive system Q27.8
   lower limb Q27.8
   specified site NEC Q27.8
   upper limb Q27.8
vein NEC Q27.8
   digestive system Q27.8
   great Q26.8
   lower limb Q27.8
   portal Q26.5
   pulmonary Q26.3
   specified site NEC Q27.8
   upper limb Q27.8
vena cava (inferior) (superior) Q26.8
vesicourethral orifice Q64.31
vulva Q52.79
   acquired N90.5
Atrichia, atrichosis — *see* Alopecia
Atrophia (*see also* Atrophy)
cutis senilis L90.8
   due to radiation L57.8
gyrata of choroid and retina H31.23
senilis R54
   dermatological L90.8
      due to radiation (nonionizing) (solar) L57.8
unguium L60.3
   congenita Q84.6
Atrophie blanche (en plaque) (de Milian) L95.0
Atrophoderma, atrophodermia (of) L90.9
diffusum (idiopathic) L90.4
maculatum L90.8
   et striatum L90.8
      due to syphilis A52.79
   syphilitic A51.39
neuriticum L90.8
Pasini and Pierini L90.3
pigmentosum Q82.1
reticulatum symmetricum faciei L66.4
senile L90.8
   due to radiation (nonionizing) (solar) L57.8
vermiculata (cheeks) L66.4
Atrophy, atrophic (of)
adrenal (capsule) (gland) E27.49
   primary (autoimmune) E27.1
alveolar process or ridge (edentulous) K08.20
anal sphincter (disuse) N81.84
appendix K38.8
arteriosclerotic — *see* Arteriosclerosis
bile duct (common) (hepatic) K83.8
bladder N32.89
   neurogenic N31.8
blanche (en plaque) (of Milian) L95.0
bone (senile) NEC (*see also* Disorder, bone, specified type NEC)
   due to
      tabes dorsalis (neurogenic) A52.11
brain (cortex) (progressive) G31.9
   frontotemporal circumscribed G31.01 [F02.80]
      with behavioral disturbance G31.01 [F02.81]
   senile NEC G31.1
breast N64.2
   obstetric — *see* Disorder, breast, specified type NEC
buccal cavity K13.79
cardiac — *see* Degeneration, myocardial
cartilage (infectional) (joint) — *see* Disorder, cartilage, specified NEC
cerebellar — *see* Atrophy, brain
cerebral — *see* Atrophy, brain
cervix (mucosa) (senile) (uteri) N88.8
   menopausal N95.8
Charcot-Marie-Tooth G60.0

Atrophy, atrophic — *continued*
choroid (central) (macular) (myopic) (retina) H31.10- ☑
   diffuse secondary H31.12- ☑
   gyrate H31.23
   senile H31.11- ☑
ciliary body — *see* Atrophy, iris
conjunctiva (senile) H11.89
corpus cavernosum N48.89
cortical — *see* Atrophy, brain
cystic duct K82.8
Déjérine-Thomas G23.8
disuse NEC — *see* Atrophy, muscle
Duchenne-Aran G12.21
ear H93.8- ☑
edentulous alveolar ridge K08.20
endometrium (senile) N85.8
   cervix N88.8
enteric K63.89
epididymis N50.8
eyeball — *see* Disorder, globe, degenerated condition, atrophy
eyelid (senile) — *see* Disorder, eyelid, degenerative
facial (skin) L90.9
fallopian tube (senile) N83.32
   with ovary N83.33
fascioscapulohumeral (Landouzy- Déjérine) G71.0
fatty, thymus (gland) E32.8
gallbladder K82.8
gastric K29.40
   with bleeding K29.41
gastrointestinal K63.89
glandular I89.8
globe H44.52- ☑
gum K06.0
hair L67.8
heart (brown) — *see* Degeneration, myocardial
hemifacial Q67.4
   Romberg G51.8
infantile E41
   paralysis, acute — *see* Poliomyelitis, paralytic
intestine K63.89
iris (essential) (progressive) H21.26- ☑
   specified NEC H21.29
kidney (senile) (terminal) (*see also* Sclerosis, renal) N26.1
   congenital or infantile Q60.5
      bilateral Q60.4
      unilateral Q60.3
   hydronephrotic — *see* Hydronephrosis
lacrimal gland (primary) H04.14- ☑
   secondary H04.15- ☑
Landouzy-Déjérine G71.0
laryngitis, infective J37.0
larynx J38.7
Leber's optic (hereditary) H47.22
lip K13.0
liver (yellow) K72.90
   with coma K72.91
   acute, subacute K72.00
      with coma K72.01
   chronic K72.10
      with coma K72.11
lung (senile) J98.4
macular (dermatological) L90.8
   syphilitic, skin A51.39
      striated A52.79
mandible (edentulous) K08.20
   minimal K08.21
   moderate K08.22
   severe K08.23
maxilla K08.20
   minimal K08.24
   moderate K08.25
   severe K08.26
muscle, muscular (diffuse) (general) (idiopathic) (primary) M62.50
   ankle M62.57- ☑
   Duchenne-Aran G12.21
   foot M62.57- ☑
   forearm M62.53- ☑
   hand M62.54- ☑
   infantile spinal G12.0
   lower leg M62.56- ☑
   multiple sites M62.59
   myelopathic — *see* Atrophy, muscle, spinal
   myotonic G71.11
   neuritic G58.9
   neuropathic (peroneal) (progressive) G60.0

Atrophy, atrophic — *continued*
  muscle, muscular — *continued*
    pelvic (disuse) N81.84
    peroneal G60.0
    progressive (bulbar) G12.21
      adult G12.1
      infantile (spinal) G12.0
      spinal G12.9
        adult G12.1
        infantile G12.0
    pseudohypertrophic G71.0
    shoulder region M62.51- ☑
    specified site NEC M62.58
    spinal G12.9
      adult form G12.1
      Aran-Duchenne G12.21
      childhood form, type II G12.1
      distal G12.1
      hereditary NEC G12.1
      infantile, type I (Werdnig-Hoffmann) G12.0
      juvenile form, type III (Kugelberg- Welander) G12.1
      progressive G12.21
      scapuloperoneal form G12.1
      specified NEC G12.8
    syphilitic A52.78
    thigh M62.55- ☑
    upper arm M62.52- ☑
  myocardium — *see* Degeneration, myocardial
  myometrium (senile) N85.8
    cervix N88.8
  myopathic NEC — *see* Atrophy, muscle
  myotonia G71.11
  nail L60.3
  nasopharynx J31.1
  nerve (*see also* Disorder, nerve)
    abducens — *see* Strabismus, paralytic, sixth nerve
    accessory G52.8
    acoustic or auditory H93.3 ☑
    cranial G52.9
      eighth (auditory) H93.3 ☑
      eleventh (accessory) G52.8
      fifth (trigeminal) G50.8
      first (olfactory) G52.0
      fourth (trochlear) — *see* Strabismus, paralytic, fourth nerve
      second (optic) H47.20
      sixth (abducens) — *see* Strabismus, paralytic, sixth nerve
      tenth (pneumogastric) (vagus) G52.2
      third (oculomotor) — *see* Strabismus, paralytic, third nerve
      twelfth (hypoglossal) G52.3
    hypoglossal G52.3
    oculomotor — *see* Strabismus, paralytic, third nerve
    olfactory G52.0
    optic (papillomacular bundle) G52.0
      syphilitic (late) A52.15
        congenital A50.44
    pneumogastric G52.2
    trigeminal G50.8
    trochlear — *see* Strabismus, paralytic, fourth nerve
    vagus (pneumogastric) G52.2
  neurogenic, bone, tabetic A52.11
  nutritional E41
  old age R54
  olivopontocerebellar G23.8
  optic (nerve) H47.20
    glaucomatous H47.23- ☑
    hereditary H47.22
    primary H47.21- ☑
    specified type NEC H47.29- ☑
    syphilitic (late) A52.15
      congenital A50.44
  orbit H05.31- ☑
  ovary (senile) N83.31
    with fallopian tube N83.33
  oviduct (senile) — *see* Atrophy, fallopian tube
  palsy, diffuse (progressive) G12.22
  pancreas (duct) (senile) K86.8
  parotid gland K11.0
  pelvic muscle N81.84
  penis N48.89
  pharynx J39.2
  pluriglandular E31.8
    autoimmune E31.0
  polyarthritis M15.9

Atrophy, atrophic — *continued*
  prostate N42.89
  pseudohypertrophic (muscle) G71.0
  renal (*see also* Sclerosis, renal) N26.1
  retina, retinal (postinfectional) H35.89
  rhinitis J31.0
  salivary gland K11.0
  scar L90.5
  sclerosis, lobar (of brain) G31.09 [F02.80]
    with behavioral disturbance G31.09 [F02.81]
  scrotum N50.8
  seminal vesicle N50.8
  senile R54
    due to radiation (nonionizing) (solar) L57.8
  skin (patches) (spots) L90.9
    degenerative (senile) L90.8
    due to radiation (nonionizing) (solar) L57.8
    senile L90.8
  spermatic cord N50.8
  spinal (acute) (cord) G95.89
    muscular — *see* Atrophy, muscle, spinal
    paralysis G12.20
      acute — *see* Poliomyelitis, paralytic
      meaning progressive muscular atrophy G12.21
  spine (column) — *see* Spondylopathy, specified NEC
  spleen (senile) D73.0
  stomach K29.40
    with bleeding K29.41
  striate (skin) L90.6
    syphilitic A52.79
  subcutaneous L90.9
  sublingual gland K11.0
  submandibular gland K11.0
  submaxillary gland K11.0
  Sudeck's — *see* Algoneurodystrophy
  suprarenal (capsule) (gland) E27.49
    primary E27.1
  systemic affecting central nervous system in
      myxedema E03.9 [G13.2]
      neoplastic disease (*see also* Neoplasm) D49.9 [G13.1]
      specified disease NEC G13.8
  tarso-orbital fascia, congenital Q10.3
  testis N50.0
  thenar, partial — *see* Syndrome, carpal tunnel
  thymus (fatty) E32.8
  thyroid (gland) (acquired) E03.4
    with cretinism E03.1
    congenital (with myxedema) E03.1
  tongue (senile) K14.8
    papillae K14.4
  trachea J39.8
  tunica vaginalis N50.8
  turbinate J34.89
  tympanic membrane (nonflaccid) H73.82- ☑
    flaccid H73.81- ☑
  upper respiratory tract J39.8
  uterus, uterine (senile) N85.8
    cervix N88.8
    due to radiation (intended effect) N85.8
      adverse effect or misadventure N99.89
  vagina (senile) N95.2
  vas deferens N50.8
  vascular I99.8
  vertebra (senile) — *see* Spondylopathy, specified NEC
  vulva (senile) N90.5
  Werdnig-Hoffmann G12.0
  yellow — *see* Failure, hepatic
Attack, attacks
  with alteration of consciousness (with automatisms) — *see* Epilepsy, localization-related, symptomatic, with complex partial seizures
  without alteration of consciousness — *see* Epilepsy, localization-related, symptomatic, with simple partial seizures
  Adams-Stokes I45.9
  akinetic — *see* Epilepsy, generalized, specified NEC
  angina — *see* Angina
  atonic — *see* Epilepsy, generalized, specified NEC
  benign shuddering G25.83
  cataleptic — *see* Catalepsy
  coronary — *see* Infarct, myocardium
  cyanotic, newborn P28.2
  drop NEC R55
  epileptic — *see* Epilepsy
  heart — *see* infarct, myocardium
  hysterical F44.9

Attack, attacks — *continued*
  jacksonian — *see* Epilepsy, localization-related, symptomatic, with simple partial seizures
  myocardium, myocardial — *see* Infarct, myocardium
  myoclonic — *see* Epilepsy, generalized, specified NEC
  panic F41.0
  psychomotor — *see* Epilepsy, localization-related, symptomatic, with complex partial seizures
  salaam — *see* Epilepsy, spasms
  schizophreniform, brief F23
  shuddering, benign G25.83
  Stokes-Adams I45.9
  syncope R55
  transient ischemic (TIA) G45.9
    specified NEC G45.8
  unconsciousness R55
    hysterical F44.89
  vasomotor R55
  vasovagal (paroxysmal) (idiopathic) R55
Attention (to)
  artificial
    opening (of) Z43.9
      digestive tract NEC Z43.4
        colon Z43.3
        ilium Z43.2
        stomach Z43.1
      specified NEC Z43.8
      trachea Z43.0
      urinary tract NEC Z43.6
        cystostomy Z43.5
        nephrostomy Z43.6
        ureterostomy Z43.6
        urethrostomy Z43.6
      vagina Z43.7
  colostomy Z43.3
  cystostomy Z43.5
  deficit disorder or syndrome F98.8
    with hyperactivity — *see* Disorder, attention-deficit hyperactivity
  gastrostomy Z43.1
  ileostomy Z43.2
  jejunostomy Z43.4
  nephrostomy Z43.6
  surgical dressings Z48.01
  sutures Z48.02
  tracheostomy Z43.0
  ureterostomy Z43.6
  urethrostomy Z43.6
Attrition
  gum K06.0
  tooth, teeth (excessive) (hard tissues) K03.0
Atypical, atypism (*see also* condition)
  cells (on cytolgocial smear) (endocervical) (endometrial) (glandular)
    cervix R87.619
    vagina R87.629
  cervical N87.9
  endometrium N85.9
    hyperplasia N85.00
  parenting situation Z62.9
Auditory — *see* condition
Aujeszky's disease B33.8
Aurantiasis, cutis E67.1
Auricle, auricular (*see also* condition)
  cervical Q18.2
Auriculotemporal syndrome G50.8
Austin Flint murmur (aortic insufficiency) I35.1
Australian
  Q fever A78
  X disease A83.4
Autism, autistic (childhood) (infantile) F84.0
  atypical F84.9
Autodigestion R68.89
Autoerythrocyte sensitization (syndrome) D69.2
Autographism L50.3
Autoimmune
  disease (systemic) M35.9
  inhibitors to clotting factors D68.311
  lymphoproliferative syndrome [ALPS] D89.82
  thyroiditis E06.3
Autointoxication R68.89
Automatism G93.89
  with temporal sclerosis G93.81
  epileptic — *see* Epilepsy, localization-related, symptomatic, with complex partial seizures
  paroxysmal, idiopathic — *see* Epilepsy, localization-related, symptomatic, with complex partial seizures

Autonomic, autonomous
   bladder (neurogenic) N31.2
   hysteria seizure F44.5
Autosensitivity, erythrocyte D69.2
Autosensitization, cutaneous L30.2
Autosome — *see* condition by chromosome involved
Autotopagnosia R48.1
Autotoxemia R68.89
Autumn — *see* condition
Avellis' syndrome G46.8
Aversion
   oral R63.3
     newborn P92.- ☑
     nonorganic origin F98.2 ☑
   sexual F52.1
Aviator's
   disease or sickness — *see* Effect, adverse, high altitude
   ear T70.0 ☑
Avitaminosis (multiple) (*see also* Deficiency, vitamin)
   E56.9
   B E53.9
     with
       beriberi E51.11
       pellagra E52
   B2 E53.0
   B6 E53.1
   B12 E53.8
   D E55.9
     with rickets E55.0
   G E53.0
   K E56.1
   nicotinic acid E52
AVNRT (atrioventricular nodal re-entrant tachycardia)
   I47.1
AVRT (atrioventricular nodal re-entrant tachycardia) I47.1
Avulsion (traumatic)
   blood vessel — *see* Injury, blood vessel
   bone — *see* Fracture, by site
   cartilage (*see also* Dislocation, by site)
     symphyseal (inner), complicating delivery O71.6
   external site other than limb — *see* Wound, open, by
     site
   eye S05.7- ☑
   head (intracranial)
     external site NEC S08.89 ☑
     scalp S08.0 ☑
   internal organ or site — *see* Injury, by site
   joint (*see also* Dislocation, by site)
     capsule — *see* Sprain, by site
   kidney S37.06- ☑
   ligament — *see* Sprain, by site
   limb (*see also* Amputation, traumatic, by site)
     skin and subcutaneous tissue — *see* Wound, open,
       by site
   muscle — *see* Injury, muscle
   nerve (root) — *see* Injury, nerve
   scalp S08.0 ☑
   skin and subcutaneous tissue — *see* Wound, open, by
     site
   spleen S36.032 ☑
   symphyseal cartilage (inner), complicating delivery
     O71.6
   tendon — *see* Injury, muscle
   tooth S03.2 ☑
Awareness of heart beat R00.2
Axenfeld's
   anomaly or syndrome Q15.0
   degeneration (calcareous) Q13.4
Axilla, axillary (*see also* condition)
   breast Q83.1
Axonotmesis — *see* Injury, nerve
Ayerza's disease or syndrome (pulmonary artery sclerosis with pulmonary hypertension) I27.0
Azoospermia (organic) N46.01
   due to
     drug therapy N46.021
     efferent duct obstruction N46.023
     infection N46.022
     radiation N46.024
     specified cause NEC N46.029
     systemic disease N46.025
Azotemia R79.89
   meaning uremia N19
Aztec ear Q17.3
Azygos
   continuation inferior vena cava Q26.8
   lobe (lung) Q33.1

B

Baastrup's disease — *see* Kissing spine
Babesiosis B60.0
Babington's disease (familial hemorrhagic telangiecta-
   sia) I78.0
Babinski's syndrome A52.79
Baby
   crying constantly R68.11
   floppy (syndrome) P94.2
Bacillary — *see* condition
Bacilluria N39.0
Bacillus (*see also* Infection, bacillus)
   abortus infection A23.1
   anthracis infection A22.9
   coli infection (*see also* Escherichia coli) B96.20
   Flexner's A03.1
   mallei infection A24.0
   Shiga's A03.0
   suipestifer infection — *see* Infection, salmonella
Back — *see* condition
Backache (postural) M54.9
   sacroiliac M53.3
   specified NEC M54.89
Backflow — *see* Reflux
Backward reading (dyslexia) F81.0
Bacteremia R78.81
   with sepsis — *see* Sepsis
Bactericholia — *see* Cholecystitis, acute
Bacterid, bacteride (pustular) L40.3
Bacterium, bacteria, bacterial
   agent NEC, as cause of disease classified elsewhere
     B96.89
   in blood — *see* Bacteremia
   in urine — *see* Bacteriuria
Bacteriuria, bacteruria N39.0
   asymptomatic N39.0
Bacteroides
   fragilis, as cause of disease classified elsewhere B96.6
Bad
   heart — *see* Disease, heart
   trip
     due to drug abuse — *see* Abuse, drug, hallucino-
       gen
     due to drug dependence — *see* Dependence, drug,
       hallucinogen
Baelz's disease (cheilitis glandularis apostematosa) K13.0
Baerensprung's disease (eczema marginatum) B35.6
Bagasse disease or pneumonitis J67.1
Bagassosis J67.1
Baker's cyst — *see* Cyst, Baker's
Bakwin-Krida syndrome (craniometaphyseal dysplasia)
   Q78.5
Balancing side interference M26.56
Balanitis (circinata) (erosiva) (gangrenosa) (phagedenic)
   (vulgaris) N48.1
   amebic A06.82
   candidal B37.42
   due to Haemophilus ducreyi A57
   gonococcal (acute) (chronic) A54.09
   xerotica obliterans N48.0
Balanoposthitis N47.6
   gonococcal (acute) (chronic) A54.09
   ulcerative (specific) A63.8
Balanorrhagia — *see* Balanitis
Balantidiasis, balantidiosis A07.0
Bald tongue K14.4
Baldness (*see also* Alopecia)
   male-pattern — *see* Alopecia, androgenic
Balkan grippe A78
Balloon disease — *see* Effect, adverse, high altitude
Balo's disease (concentric sclerosis) G37.5
Bamberger-Marie disease — *see* Osteoarthropathy,
   hypertrophic, specified type NEC
Bancroft's filariasis B74.0
Band(s)
   adhesive — *see* Adhesions, peritoneum
   anomalous or congenital (*see also* Anomaly, by site)
     heart (atrial) (ventricular) Q24.8
     intestine Q43.3
     omentum Q43.3
   cervix N88.1
   constricting, congenital Q79.8
   gallbladder (congenital) Q44.1
   intestinal (adhesive) — *see* Adhesions, peritoneum

Band(s) — *continued*
   obstructive
     intestine K56.5
     peritoneum K56.5
   periappendiceal, congenital Q43.3
   peritoneal (adhesive) — *see* Adhesions, peritoneum
   uterus N73.6
     internal N85.6
   vagina N89.5
Bandemia D72.825
Bandl's ring (contraction), complicating delivery O62.4
Bangkok hemorrhagic fever A91
Bang's disease (brucella abortus) A23.1
Bankruptcy, anxiety concerning Z59.8
Bannister's disease T78.3 ☑
   hereditary D84.1
Banti's disease or syndrome (with cirrhosis) (with portal
   hypertension) K76.6
Bar, median, prostate — *see* Enlargement, enlarged,
   prostate
Barcoo disease or rot — *see* Ulcer, skin
Barlow's disease E54
Barodontalgia T70.29 ☑
Baron Münchausen syndrome — *see* Disorder, facti-
   tious
Barosinusitis T70.1 ☑
Barotitis T70.0 ☑
Barotrauma T70.29 ☑
   odontalgia T70.29 ☑
   otitic T70.0 ☑
   sinus T70.1 ☑
Barraquer (-Simons) **disease or syndrome** (progressive
   lipodystrophy) E88.1
Barré-Guillain disease or syndrome G61.0
Barrel chest M95.4
Barré-Liéou syndrome (posterior cervical sympathetic)
   M53.0
Barrett's
   disease — *see* Barrett's, esophagus
   esophagus K22.70
     with dysplasia K22.719
       high grade K22.711
       low grade K22.710
     without dysplasia K22.70
   syndrome — *see* Barrett's, esophagus
   ulcer K22.10
     with bleeding K22.11
     without bleeding K22.10
Bársony (-Polgár) (-Teschendorf) **syndrome** (corkscrew
   esophagus) K22.4
Barth syndrome E78.71
Bartholinitis (suppurating) N75.8
   gonococcal (acute) (chronic) (with abscess) A54.1
Bartonellosis A44.9
   cutaneous A44.1
   mucocutaneous A44.1
   specified NEC A44.8
   systemic A44.0
Barton's fracture S52.56- ☑
Bartter's syndrome E26.81
Basal — *see* condition
Basan's (hidrotic) ectodermal dysplasia Q82.4
Baseball finger — *see* Dislocation, finger
Basedow's disease (exophthalmic goiter) — *see* Hyper-
   thyroidism, with, goiter
Basic — *see* condition
Basilar — *see* condition
Bason's (hidrotic) ectodermal dysplasia Q82.4
Basopenia — *see* Agranulocytosis
Basophilia D72.824
Basophilism (cortico-adrenal) (Cushing's) (pituitary)
   E24.0
Bassen-Kornzweig disease or syndrome E78.6
Bat ear Q17.5
Bateman's
   disease B08.1
   purpura (senile) D69.2
Bathing cramp T75.1 ☑
Bathophobia F40.248
Batten (-Mayou) **disease** E75.4
   retina E75.4 [H36]
Batten-Steinert syndrome G71.11
Battered — *see* Maltreatment
Battey Mycobacterium infection A31.0
Battle exhaustion F43.0
Battledore placenta O43.19- ☑

Baumgarten-Cruveilhier cirrhosis, disease or syndrome K74.69
Bauxite fibrosis (of lung) J63.1
Bayle's disease (general paresis) A52.17
Bazin's disease (primary) (tuberculous) A18.4
Beach ear — see Swimmer's, ear
Beaded hair (congenital) Q84.1
Béal conjunctivitis or syndrome B30.2
Beard's disease (neurasthenia) F48.8
Beat(s)
  atrial, premature I49.1
  ectopic I49.49
  elbow — see Bursitis, elbow
  escaped, heart I49.49
  hand — see Bursitis, hand
  knee — see Bursitis, knee
  premature I49.40
    atrial I49.1
    auricular I49.1
    supraventricular I49.1
Beau's
  disease or syndrome — see Degeneration, myocardial
  lines (transverse furrows on fingernails) L60.4
Bechterev's syndrome — see Spondylitis, ankylosing
Becker's
  cardiomyopathy I42.8
  disease
    idiopathic mural endomyocardial disease I42.3
    myotonia congenita, recessive form G71.12
  dystrophy G71.0
  pigmented hairy nevus D22.5
Beck's syndrome (anterior spinal artery occlusion) I65.8
Beckwith-Wiedemann syndrome Q87.3
Bed confinement status Z74.01
Bed sore — see Ulcer, pressure, by site
Bedbug bite(s) — see Bite(s), by site, superficial, insect
Bedclothes, asphyxiation or suffocation by — see Asphyxia, traumatic, due to, mechanical, trapped
Bednar's
  aphthae K12.0
  tumor — see Neoplasm, malignant, by site
Bedridden Z74.01
Bedsore — see Ulcer, pressure, by site
Bedwetting — see Enuresis
Bee sting (with allergic or anaphylactic shock) — see Toxicity, venom, arthropod, bee
Beer drinker's heart (disease) I42.6
Begbie's disease (exophthalmic goiter) — see Hyperthyroidism, with, goiter
Behavior
  antisocial
    adult Z72.811
    child or adolescent Z72.810
  disorder, disturbance — see Disorder, conduct
  disruptive — see Disorder, conduct
  drug seeking Z72.89
  inexplicable R46.2
  marked evasiveness R46.5
  obsessive-compulsive R46.81
  overactivity R46.3
  poor responsiveness R46.4
  self-damaging (life-style) Z72.89
  sleep-incompatible Z72.821
  slowness R46.4
  specified NEC R46.89
  strange (and inexplicable) R46.2
  suspiciousness R46.5
  type A pattern Z73.1
  undue concern or preoccupation with stressful events R46.6
  verbosity and circumstantial detail obscuring reason for contact R46.7
Behçet's disease or syndrome M35.2
Behr's disease — see Degeneration, macula
Beigel's disease or morbus (white piedra) B36.2
Bejel A65
Bekhterev's syndrome — see Spondylitis, ankylosing
Belching — see Eructation
Bell's
  mania F30.8
  palsy, paralysis G51.0
    infant or newborn P11.3
  spasm G51.3
Bence Jones albuminuria or proteinuria NEC R80.3
Bends T70.3 ☑
Benedikt's paralysis or syndrome G46.3

Benign (see also condition)
  prostatic hyperplasia — see Hyperplasia, prostate
Bennett's fracture (displaced) S62.21- ☑
Benson's disease — see Deposit, crystalline
Bent
  back (hysterical) F44.4
  nose M95.0
    congenital Q67.4
Bereavement (uncomplicated) Z63.4
Bergeron's disease (hysterical chorea) F44.4
Berger's disease — see Nephropathy, IgA
Beriberi (dry) E51.11
  heart (disease) E51.12
  polyneuropathy E51.11
  wet E51.12
    involving circulatory system E51.11
Berlin's disease or edema (traumatic) S05.8X- ☑
Berlock (berloque) **dermatitis** L56.2
Bernard-Horner syndrome G90.2
Bernard-Soulier disease or thrombopathia D69.1
Bernhardt (-Roth) **disease** — see Mononeuropathy, lower limb, meralgia paresthetica
Bernheim's syndrome — see Failure, heart, congestive
Bertielliasis B71.8
Berylliosis (lung) J63.2
Besnier-Boeck (-Schaumann) **disease** — see Sarcoidosis
Besnier's
  lupus pernio D86.3
  prurigo L20.0
Bestiality F65.89
Best's disease H35.50
Betalipoproteinemia, broad or floating E78.2
Beta-mercaptolactate-cysteine disulfiduria E72.09
Betting and gambling Z72.6
  pathological (compulsive) F63.0
Bezoar T18.9 ☑
  intestine T18.3 ☑
  stomach T18.2 ☑
Bezold's abscess — see Mastoiditis, acute
Bianchi's syndrome R48.8
Bicornate or bicornis uterus Q51.3
  in pregnancy or childbirth O34.59- ☑
    causing obstructed labor O65.5
Bicuspid aortic valve Q23.1
Biedl-Bardet syndrome Q87.89
Bielschowsky (-Jansky) disease E75.4
Biermer's (pernicious) anemia or disease D51.0
Biett's disease L93.0
Bifid (congenital)
  apex, heart Q24.8
  clitoris Q52.6
  kidney Q63.8
  nose Q30.2
  patella Q74.1
  scrotum Q55.29
  toe NEC Q74.2
  tongue Q38.3
  ureter Q62.8
  uterus Q51.3
  uvula Q35.7
Biforis uterus (suprasimplex) Q51.3
Bifurcation (congenital)
  gallbladder Q44.1
  kidney pelvis Q63.8
  renal pelvis Q63.8
  rib Q76.6
  tongue, congenital Q38.3
  trachea Q32.1
  ureter Q62.8
  urethra Q64.74
  vertebra Q76.49
Big spleen syndrome D73.1
Bigeminal pulse R00.8
Bilateral — see condition
Bile
  duct — see condition
  pigments in urine R82.2
Bilharziasis (see also Schistosomiasis)
  chyluria B65.9
  cutaneous B65.3
  galacturia B65.0
  hematochyluria B65.0
  intestinal B65.1
  lipemia B65.9
  lipuria B65.0
  oriental B65.2
  piarhemia B65.9

Bilharziasis — continued
  pulmonary NOS B65.9 [J99]
    pneumonia B65.9 [J17]
  tropical hematuria B65.0
  vesical B65.0
Biliary — see condition
Bilirubin metabolism disorder E80.7
  specified NEC E80.6
Bilirubinemia, familial nonhemolytic E80.4
Bilirubinuria R82.2
Biliuria R82.2
Bilocular stomach K31.2
Binswanger's disease I67.3
Biparta, bipartite
  carpal scaphoid Q74.0
  patella Q74.1
  vagina Q52.10
Bird
  face Q75.8
  fancier's disease or lung J67.2
Birth
  complications in mother — see Delivery, complicated
  compression during NOS P15.9
  defect — see Anomaly
  immature (less than 37 completed weeks) — see Preterm, newborn
    extremely (less than 28 completed weeks) — see Immaturity, extreme
  inattention, at or after — see Maltreatment, child, neglect
  injury NOS P15.9
    basal ganglia P11.1
    brachial plexus NEC P14.3
    brain (compression) (pressure) P11.2
    central nervous system NOS P11.9
    cerebellum P11.1
    cerebral hemorrhage P10.1
    external genitalia P15.5
    eye P15.3
    face P15.4
    fracture
      bone P13.9
        specified NEC P13.8
      clavicle P13.4
      femur P13.2
      humerus P13.3
      long bone, except femur P13.3
      radius and ulna P13.3
      skull P13.0
      spine P11.5
      tibia and fibula P13.3
    intracranial P11.2
      laceration or hemorrhage P10.9
        specified NEC P10.8
    intraventricular hemorrhage P10.2
    laceration
      brain P10.1
      by scalpel P15.8
      peripheral nerve P14.9
    liver P15.0
    meninges
      brain P11.1
      spinal cord P11.5
    nerve
      brachial plexus P14.3
      cranial NEC (except facial) P11.4
      facial P11.3
      peripheral P14.9
      phrenic (paralysis) P14.2
    paralysis
      facial nerve P11.3
      spinal P11.5
    penis P15.5
    rupture
      spinal cord P11.5
    scalp P12.9
    scalpel wound P15.8
    scrotum P15.5
    skull NEC P13.1
      fracture P13.0
    specified type NEC P15.8
    spinal cord P11.5
    spine P11.5
    spleen P15.1
    sternomastoid (hematoma) P15.2
    subarachnoid hemorrhage P10.3
    subcutaneous fat necrosis P15.6
    subdural hemorrhage P10.0

Birth — *continued*
  injury — *continued*
    tentorial tear P10.4
    testes P15.5
    vulva P15.5
  lack of care, at or after — *see* Maltreatment, child, neglect
  neglect, at or after — *see* Maltreatment, child, neglect
  palsy or paralysis, newborn, NOS (birth injury) P14.9
  premature (infant) — *see* Preterm, newborn
  shock, newborn P96.89
  trauma — *see* Birth, injury
  weight
    4000 grams to 4499 grams P08.1
    4500 grams or more P08.0
    low (2499 grams or less) — *see* Low, birthweight
      extremely (999 grams or less) — *see* Low, birthweight, extreme
Birthmark Q82.5
Birt-Hogg-Dube syndrome Q87.89
Bisalbuminemia E88.09
Biskra's button B55.1
Bite(s) (animal) (human)
  abdomen, abdominal
    wall S31.159 ☑
      with penetration into peritoneal cavity S31.659 ☑
      epigastric region S31.152 ☑
        with penetration into peritoneal cavity S31.652 ☑
      left
        lower quadrant S31.154 ☑
          with penetration into peritoneal cavity S31.654 ☑
        upper quadrant S31.151 ☑
          with penetration into peritoneal cavity S31.651 ☑
      periumbilic region S31.155 ☑
        with penetration into peritoneal cavity S31.655 ☑
      right
        lower quadrant S31.153 ☑
          with penetration into peritoneal cavity S31.653 ☑
        upper quadrant S31.150 ☑
          with penetration into peritoneal cavity S31.650 ☑
      superficial NEC S30.871 ☑
        insect S30.861 ☑
  alveolar (process) — *see* Bite, oral cavity
  amphibian (venomous) — *see* Venom, bite, amphibian
  animal (*see also* Bite, by site)
    venomous — *see* Venom
  ankle S91.05- ☑
    superficial NEC S90.57- ☑
      insect S90.56- ☑
  antecubital space — *see* Bite, elbow
  anus S31.835 ☑
    superficial NEC S30.877 ☑
      insect S30.867 ☑
  arm (upper) S41.15- ☑
    lower — *see* Bite, forearm
    superficial NEC S40.87- ☑
      insect S40.86- ☑
  arthropod NEC — *see* Venom, bite, arthropod
  auditory canal (external) (meatus) — *see* Bite, ear
  auricle, ear — *see* Bite, ear
  axilla — *see* Bite, arm
  back (*see also* Bite, thorax, back)
    lower S31.050 ☑
      with penetration into retroperitoneal space S31.051 ☑
    superficial NEC S30.870 ☑
      insect S30.860 ☑
  bedbug — *see* Bite(s), by site, superficial, insect
  breast S21.05- ☑
    superficial NEC S20.17- ☑
      insect S20.16- ☑
  brow — *see* Bite, head, specified site NEC
  buttock S31.805 ☑
    left S31.825 ☑
    right S31.815 ☑
    superficial NEC S30.870 ☑
      insect S30.860 ☑
  calf — *see* Bite, leg
  canaliculus lacrimalis — *see* Bite, eyelid

Bite(s) — *continued*
  canthus, eye — *see* Bite, eyelid
  centipede — *see* Toxicity, venom, arthropod, centipede
  cheek (external) S01.45- ☑
    internal — *see* Bite, oral cavity
    superficial NEC S00.87 ☑
      insect S00.86 ☑
  chest wall — *see* Bite, thorax
  chigger B88.0
  chin — *see* Bite, head, specified site NEC
  clitoris — *see* Bite, vulva
  costal region — *see* Bite, thorax
  digit(s)
    hand — *see* Bite, finger
    toe — *see* Bite, toe
  ear (canal) (external) S01.35- ☑
    superficial NEC S00.47- ☑
      insect S00.46- ☑
  elbow S51.05- ☑
    superficial NEC S50.37- ☑
      insect S50.36- ☑
  epididymis — *see* Bite, testis
  epigastric region — *see* Bite, abdomen
  epiglottis — *see* Bite, neck, specified site NEC
  esophagus, cervical S11.25 ☑
    superficial NEC S10.17 ☑
      insect S10.16 ☑
  eyebrow — *see* Bite, eyelid
  eyelid S01.15- ☑
    superficial NEC S00.27- ☑
      insect S00.26- ☑
  face NEC — *see* Bite, head, specified site NEC
  finger(s) S61.259 ☑
    with
      damage to nail S61.359 ☑
    index S61.258 ☑
      with
        damage to nail S61.358 ☑
      left S61.251 ☑
        with
          damage to nail S61.351 ☑
      right S61.250 ☑
        with
          damage to nail S61.350 ☑
      superficial NEC S60.478 ☑
        insect S60.46- ☑
    little S61.25- ☑
      with
        damage to nail S61.35- ☑
      superficial NEC S60.47- ☑
        insect S60.46- ☑
    middle S61.25- ☑
      with
        damage to nail S61.35- ☑
      superficial NEC S60.47- ☑
        insect S60.46- ☑
    ring S61.25- ☑
      with
        damage to nail S61.35- ☑
      superficial NEC S60.47- ☑
        insect S60.46- ☑
    superficial NEC S60.479 ☑
      insect S60.469 ☑
    thumb — *see* Bite, thumb
  flank — *see* Bite, abdomen, wall
  flea — *see* Bite, by site, superficial, insect
  foot (except toe(s) alone) S91.35- ☑
    superficial NEC S90.87- ☑
      insect S90.86- ☑
    toe — *see* Bite, toe
  forearm S51.85- ☑
    elbow only — *see* Bite, elbow
    superficial NEC S50.87- ☑
      insect S50.86- ☑
  forehead — *see* Bite, head, specified site NEC
  genital organs, external
    female S31.552 ☑
      superficial NEC S30.876 ☑
        insect S30.866 ☑
      vagina and vulva — *see* Bite, vulva
    male S31.551 ☑
      penis — *see* Bite, penis
      scrotum — *see* Bite, scrotum
      superficial NEC S30.875 ☑
        insect S30.865 ☑

Bite(s) — *continued*
  genital organs, external — *continued*
    male — *continued*
      testes — *see* Bite, testis
  groin — *see* Bite, abdomen, wall
  gum — *see* Bite, oral cavity
  hand S61.45- ☑
    finger — *see* Bite, finger
    superficial NEC S60.57- ☑
      insect S60.56- ☑
    thumb — *see* Bite, thumb
  head S01.95 ☑
    cheek — *see* Bite, cheek
    ear — *see* Bite, ear
    eyelid — *see* Bite, eyelid
    lip — *see* Bite, lip
    nose — *see* Bite, nose
    oral cavity — *see* Bite, oral cavity
    scalp — *see* Bite, scalp
    specified site NEC S01.85 ☑
      superficial NEC S00.87 ☑
        insect S00.86 ☑
    superficial NEC S00.97 ☑
      insect S00.96 ☑
    temporomandibular area — *see* Bite, cheek
  heel — *see* Bite, foot
  hip S71.05- ☑
    superficial NEC S70.27- ☑
      insect S70.26- ☑
  hymen S31.45 ☑
  hypochondrium — *see* Bite, abdomen, wall
  hypogastric region — *see* Bite, abdomen, wall
  inguinal region — *see* Bite, abdomen, wall
  insect — *see* Bite, by site, superficial, insect
  instep — *see* Bite, foot
  interscapular region — *see* Bite, thorax, back
  jaw — *see* Bite, head, specified site NEC
  knee S81.05- ☑
    superficial NEC S80.27- ☑
      insect S80.26- ☑
  labium (majus) (minus) — *see* Bite, vulva
  lacrimal duct — *see* Bite, eyelid
  larynx S11.015 ☑
    superficial NEC S10.17 ☑
      insect S10.16 ☑
  leg (lower) S81.85- ☑
    ankle — *see* Bite, ankle
    foot — *see* Bite, foot
    knee — *see* Bite, knee
    superficial NEC S80.87- ☑
      insect S80.86- ☑
    toe — *see* Bite, toe
    upper — *see* Bite, thigh
  lip S01.551 ☑
    superficial NEC S00.571 ☑
      insect S00.561 ☑
  lizard (venomous) — *see* Venom, bite, reptile
  loin — *see* Bite, abdomen, wall
  lower back — *see* Bite, back, lower
  lumbar region — *see* Bite, back, lower
  malar region — *see* Bite, head, specified site NEC
  mammary — *see* Bite, breast
  marine animals (venomous) — *see* Toxicity, venom, marine animal
  mastoid region — *see* Bite, head, specified site NEC
  mouth — *see* Bite, oral cavity
  nail
    finger — *see* Bite, finger
    toe — *see* Bite, toe
  nape — *see* Bite, neck, specified site NEC
  nasal (septum) (sinus) — *see* Bite, nose
  nasopharynx — *see* Bite, head, specified site NEC
  neck S11.95 ☑
    involving
      cervical esophagus — *see* Bite, esophagus, cervical
      larynx — *see* Bite, larynx
      pharynx — *see* Bite, pharynx
      thyroid gland S11.15 ☑
      trachea — *see* Bite, trachea
    specified site NEC S11.85 ☑
      superficial NEC S10.87 ☑
        insect S10.86 ☑
    superficial NEC S10.97 ☑
      insect S10.96 ☑

Bite(s) — *continued*
  neck — *continued*
    throat S11.85 ☑
      superficial NEC S10.17 ☑
        insect S10.16 ☑
  nose (septum) (sinus) S01.25 ☑
    superficial NEC S00.37 ☑
      insect S00.36 ☑
  occipital region — *see* Bite, scalp
  oral cavity S01.552 ☑
    superficial NEC S00.572 ☑
      insect S00.562 ☑
  orbital region — *see* Bite, eyelid
  palate — *see* Bite, oral cavity
  palm — *see* Bite, hand
  parietal region — *see* Bite, scalp
  pelvis S31.050 ☑
    with penetration into retroperitoneal space
        S31.051 ☑
    superficial NEC S30.870 ☑
      insect S30.860 ☑
  penis S31.25 ☑
    superficial NEC S30.872 ☑
      insect S30.862 ☑
  perineum
    female — *see* Bite, vulva
    male — *see* Bite, pelvis
  periocular area (with or without lacrimal passages) —
        see Bite, eyelid
  phalanges
    finger — *see* Bite, finger
    toe — *see* Bite, toe
  pharynx S11.25 ☑
    superficial NEC S10.17 ☑
      insect S10.16 ☑
  pinna — *see* Bite, ear
  poisonous — *see* Venom
  popliteal space — *see* Bite, knee
  prepuce — *see* Bite, penis
  pubic region — *see* Bite, abdomen, wall
  rectovaginal septum — *see* Bite, vulva
  red bug B88.0
  reptile NEC (*see also* Venom, bite, reptile)
    nonvenomous — *see* Bite, by site
    snake — *see* Venom, bite, snake
  sacral region — *see* Bite, back, lower
  sacroiliac region — *see* Bite, back, lower
  salivary gland — *see* Bite, oral cavity
  scalp S01.05 ☑
    superficial NEC S00.07 ☑
      insect S00.06 ☑
  scapular region — *see* Bite, shoulder
  scrotum S31.35 ☑
    superficial NEC S30.873 ☑
      insect S30.863 ☑
  sea-snake (venomous) — *see* Toxicity, venom, snake,
        sea snake
  shin — *see* Bite, leg
  shoulder S41.05- ☑
    superficial NEC S40.27- ☑
      insect S40.26- ☑
  snake (*see also* Venom, bite, snake)
    nonvenomous — *see* Bite, by site
  spermatic cord — *see* Bite, testis
  spider (venomous) — *see* Toxicity, venom, spider
    nonvenomous — *see* Bite, by site, superficial, insect
  sternal region — *see* Bite, thorax, front
  submaxillary region — *see* Bite, head, specified site
        NEC
  submental region — *see* Bite, head, specified site NEC
  subungual
    finger(s) — *see* Bite, finger
    toe — *see* Bite, toe
  superficial — *see* Bite, by site, superficial
  supraclavicular fossa S11.85 ☑
  supraorbital — *see* Bite, head, specified site NEC
  temple, temporal region — *see* Bite, head, specified
        site NEC
  temporomandibular area — *see* Bite, cheek
  testis S31.35 ☑
    superficial NEC S30.873 ☑
      insect S30.863 ☑
  thigh S71.15- ☑
    superficial NEC S70.37- ☑
      insect S70.36- ☑

Bite(s) — *continued*
  thorax, thoracic (wall) S21.95 ☑
    back S21.25- ☑
      with penetration into thoracic cavity S21.45- ☑
    breast — *see* Bite, breast
    front S21.15- ☑
      with penetration into thoracic cavity S21.35- ☑
    superficial NEC S20.97 ☑
      back S20.47- ☑
      front S20.37- ☑
      insect S20.96 ☑
        back S20.46- ☑
        front S20.36- ☑
  throat — *see* Bite, neck, throat
  thumb S61.05- ☑
    with
      damage to nail S61.15- ☑
    superficial NEC S60.37- ☑
      insect S60.36- ☑
  thyroid S11.15 ☑
    superficial NEC S10.87 ☑
      insect S10.86 ☑
  toe(s) S91.15- ☑
    with
      damage to nail S91.25- ☑
    great S91.15- ☑
      with
        damage to nail S91.25- ☑
    lesser S91.15- ☑
      with
        damage to nail S91.25- ☑
    superficial NEC S90.47- ☑
      great S90.47- ☑
      insect S90.46- ☑
        great S90.46- ☑
  tongue S01.552 ☑
  trachea S11.025 ☑
    superficial NEC S10.17 ☑
      insect S10.16 ☑
  tunica vaginalis — *see* Bite, testis
  tympanum, tympanic membrane — *see* Bite, ear
  umbilical region S31.155 ☑
  uvula — *see* Bite, oral cavity
  vagina — *see* Bite, vulva
  venomous — *see* Venom
  vocal cords S11.035 ☑
    superficial NEC S10.17 ☑
      insect S10.16 ☑
  vulva S31.45 ☑
    superficial NEC S30.874 ☑
      insect S30.864 ☑
  wrist S61.55- ☑
    superficial NEC S60.87- ☑
      insect S60.86- ☑
Biting, cheek or lip K13.1
Biventricular failure (heart) I50.9
Björck (-Thorson) **syndrome** (malignant carcinoid) E34.0
Black
  death A20.9
  eye S00.1- ☑
  hairy tongue K14.3
  heel (foot) S90.3- ☑
  lung (disease) J60
  palm (hand) S60.22- ☑
Blackfan-Diamond anemia or syndrome (congenital
      hypoplastic anemia) D61.01
Blackhead L70.0
Blackout R55
Bladder — *see* condition
Blast (air) (hydraulic) (immersion) (underwater)
  blindness S05.8X- ☑
  injury
    abdomen or thorax — *see* Injury, by site
    ear (acoustic nerve trauma) — *see* Injury, nerve,
          acoustic, specified type NEC
    syndrome NEC T70.8 ☑
Blastoma — *see* Neoplasm, malignant, by site
  pulmonary — *see* Neoplasm, lung, malignant
Blastomycosis, blastomycotic B40.9
  Brazilian — *see* Paracoccidioidomycosis
  cutaneous B40.3
  disseminated B40.7
  European — *see* Cryptococcosis
  generalized B40.7
  keloidal B48.0
  North American B40.9

Blastomycosis, blastomycotic — *continued*
  primary pulmonary B40.0
  pulmonary B40.2
    acute B40.0
    chronic B40.1
  skin B40.3
  South American — *see* Paracoccidioidomycosis
  specified NEC B40.89
Bleb(s) R23.8
  emphysematous (lung) (solitary) J43.9
  endophthalmitis H59.43
  filtering (vitreous), after glaucoma surgery Z98.83
  inflamed (infected), postprocedural H59.40
    stage 1 H59.41
    stage 2 H59.42
    stage 3 H59.43
  lung (ruptured) J43.9
    congenital — *see* Atelectasis
    newborn P25.8
  subpleural (emphysematous) J43.9
Blebitis, postprocedural H59.40
  stage 1 H59.41
  stage 2 H59.42
  stage 3 H59.43
Bleeder (familial) (hereditary) — *see* Hemophilia
Bleeding (*see also* Hemorrhage)
  anal K62.5
  anovulatory N97.0
  atonic, following delivery O72.1
  capillary I78.8
    puerperal O72.2
  contact (postcoital) N93.0
  due to uterine subinvolution N85.3
  ear — *see* Otorrhagia
  excessive, associated with menopausal onset N92.4
  familial — *see* Defect, coagulation
  following intercourse N93.0
  gastrointestinal K92.2
  hemorrhoids — *see* Hemorrhoids
  intermenstrual (regular) N92.3
    irregular N92.1
  intraoperative — *see* Complication, intraoperative,
        hemorrhage
  irregular N92.6
  menopausal N92.4
  newborn, intraventricular — *see* Newborn, affected
        by, hemorrhage, intraventricular
  nipple N64.59
  nose R04.0
  ovulation N92.3
  postclimacteric N95.0
  postcoital N93.0
  postmenopausal N95.0
  postoperative — *see* Complication, postprocedural,
        hemorrhage
  preclimacteric N92.4
  puberty (excessive, with onset of menstrual periods)
        N92.2
  rectum, rectal K62.5
    newborn P54.2
  tendencies — *see* Defect, coagulation
  throat R04.1
  tooth socket (post-extraction) K91.840
  umbilical stump P51.9
  uterus, uterine NEC N93.9
    climacteric N92.4
    dysfunctional of functional N93.8
    menopausal N92.4
    preclimacteric or premenopausal N92.4
    unrelated to menstrual cycle N93.9
  vagina, vaginal (abnormal) N93.9
    dysfunctional or functional N93.8
    newborn P54.6
  vicarious N94.89
Blennorrhagia, blennorrhagic — *see* Gonorrhea
Blennorrhea (acute) (chronic) (*see also* Gonorrhea)
  inclusion (neonatal) (newborn) P39.1
  lower genitourinary tract (gonococcal) A54.00
  neonatorum (gonococcal ophthalmia) A54.31
Blepharelosis — *see* Entropion
Blepharitis (angularis) (ciliaris) (eyelid) (marginal)
      (nonulcerative) H01.009
  herpes zoster B02.39
  left H01.006
    lower H01.005
    upper H01.004
  right H01.003
    lower H01.002

Blepharitis — *continued*
  right — *continued*
    upper H01.001
  squamous H01.029
    left H01.026
      lower H01.025
      upper H01.024
    right H01.023
      lower H01.022
      upper H01.021
  ulcerative H01.019
    left H01.016
      lower H01.015
      upper H01.014
    right H01.013
      lower H01.012
      upper H01.011
Blepharochalasis H02.30
  congenital Q10.0
  left H02.36
    lower H02.35
    upper H02.34
  right H02.33
    lower H02.32
    upper H02.31
Blepharoclonus H02.59
Blepharoconjunctivitis H10.50- ☑
  angular H10.52- ☑
  contact H10.53- ☑
  ligneous H10.51- ☑
Blepharophimosis (eyelid) H02.529
  congenital Q10.3
  left H02.526
    lower H02.525
    upper H02.524
  right H02.523
    lower H02.522
    upper H02.521
Blepharoptosis H02.40- ☑
  congenital Q10.0
  mechanical H02.41- ☑
  myogenic H02.42- ☑
  neurogenic H02.43- ☑
  paralytic H02.43- ☑
Blepharopyorrhea, gonococcal A54.39
Blepharospasm G24.5
  drug induced G24.01
Blighted ovum O02.0
Blind (*see also* Blindness)
  bronchus (congenital) Q32.4
  loop syndrome K90.2
    congenital Q43.8
  sac, fallopian tube (congenital) Q50.6
  spot, enlarged — *see* Defect, visual field, localized, scotoma, blind spot area
  tract or tube, congenital NEC — *see* Atresia, by site
Blindness (acquired) (congenital) (both eyes) H54.0
  blast S05.8X- ☑
  color — *see* Deficiency, color vision
  concussion S05.8X- ☑
  cortical H47.619
    left brain H47.612
    right brain H47.611
  day H53.11
  due to injury (current episode) S05.9- ☑
    sequelae — *code to* injury with seventh character S
  eclipse (total) — *see* Retinopathy, solar
  emotional (hysterical) F44.6
  face H53.16
  hysterical F44.6
  legal (both eyes) (USA definition) H54.8
  mind R48.8
  night H53.60
    abnormal dark adaptation curve H53.61
    acquired H53.62
    congenital H53.63
    specified type NEC H53.69
    vitamin A deficiency E50.5
  one eye (other eye normal) H54.40
    left (normal vision on right) H54.42
      low vision on right H54.12
    low vision, other eye H54.10
    right (normal vision on left) H54.41
      low vision on left H54.11
  psychic R48.8
  river B73.01
  snow — *see* Photokeratitis

Blindness — *continued*
  sun, solar — *see* Retinopathy, solar
  transient — *see* Disturbance, vision, subjective, loss, transient
  traumatic (current episode) S05.9- ☑
  word (developmental) F81.0
    acquired R48.0
    secondary to organic lesion R48.0
Blister (nonthermal)
  abdominal wall S30.821 ☑
  alveolar process S00.522 ☑
  ankle S90.52- ☑
  antecubital space — *see* Blister, elbow
  anus S30.827 ☑
  arm (upper) S40.82- ☑
  auditory canal — *see* Blister, ear
  auricle — *see* Blister, ear
  axilla — *see* Blister, arm
  back, lower S30.820 ☑
  beetle dermatitis L24.89
  breast S20.12- ☑
  brow S00.82 ☑
  calf — *see* Blister, leg
  canthus — *see* Blister, eyelid
  cheek S00.82 ☑
    internal S00.522 ☑
  chest wall — *see* Blister, thorax
  chin S00.82 ☑
  costal region — *see* Blister, thorax
  digit(s)
    foot — *see* Blister, toe
    hand — *see* Blister, finger
  due to burn — *see* Burn, by site, second degree
  ear S00.42- ☑
  elbow S50.32- ☑
  epiglottis S10.12 ☑
  esophagus, cervical S10.12 ☑
  eyebrow — *see* Blister, eyelid
  eyelid S00.22- ☑
  face S00.82 ☑
  fever B00.1
  finger(s) S60.429 ☑
    index S60.42- ☑
    little S60.42- ☑
    middle S60.42- ☑
    ring S60.42- ☑
  foot (except toe(s) alone) S90.82- ☑
    toe — *see* Blister, toe
  forearm S50.82- ☑
    elbow only — *see* Blister, elbow
  forehead S00.82 ☑
  fracture — *omit code*
  genital organ
    female S30.826 ☑
    male S30.825 ☑
  gum S00.522 ☑
  hand S60.52- ☑
  head S00.92 ☑
    ear — *see* Blister, ear
    eyelid — *see* Blister, eyelid
    lip S00.521 ☑
    nose S00.32 ☑
    oral cavity S00.522 ☑
    scalp S00.02 ☑
    specified site NEC S00.82 ☑
  heel — *see* Blister, foot
  hip S70.22- ☑
  interscapular region S20.429 ☑
  jaw S00.82 ☑
  knee S80.22- ☑
  larynx S10.12 ☑
  leg (lower) S80.82- ☑
    knee — *see* Blister, knee
    upper — *see* Blister, thigh
  lip S00.521 ☑
  malar region S00.82 ☑
  mammary — *see* Blister, breast
  mastoid region S00.82 ☑
  mouth S00.522 ☑
  multiple, skin, nontraumatic R23.8
  nail
    finger — *see* Blister, finger
    toe — *see* Blister, toe
  nasal S00.32 ☑
  neck S10.92 ☑
    specified site NEC S10.82 ☑

Blister — *continued*
  neck — *continued*
    throat S10.12 ☑
  nose S00.32 ☑
  occipital region S00.02 ☑
  oral cavity S00.522 ☑
  orbital region — *see* Blister, eyelid
  palate S00.522 ☑
  palm — *see* Blister, hand
  parietal region S00.02 ☑
  pelvis S30.820 ☑
  penis S30.822 ☑
  periocular area — *see* Blister, eyelid
  phalanges
    finger — *see* Blister, finger
    toe — *see* Blister, toe
  pharynx S10.12 ☑
  pinna — *see* Blister, ear
  popliteal space — *see* Blister, knee
  scalp S00.02 ☑
  scapular region — *see* Blister, shoulder
  scrotum S30.823 ☑
  shin — *see* Blister, leg
  shoulder S40.22- ☑
  sternal region S20.329 ☑
  submaxillary region S00.82 ☑
  submental region S00.82 ☑
  subungual
    finger(s) — *see* Blister, finger
    toe(s) — *see* Blister, toe
  supraclavicular fossa S10.82 ☑
  supraorbital S00.82 ☑
  temple S00.82 ☑
  temporal region S00.82 ☑
  testis S30.823 ☑
  thermal — *see* Burn, second degree, by site
  thigh S70.32- ☑
  thorax, thoracic (wall) S20.92 ☑
    back S20.42- ☑
    front S20.32- ☑
  throat S10.12 ☑
  thumb S60.32- ☑
  toe(s) S90.42- ☑
    great S90.42- ☑
  tongue S00.522 ☑
  trachea S10.12 ☑
  tympanum, tympanic membrane — *see* Blister, ear
  upper arm — *see* Blister, arm (upper)
  uvula S00.522 ☑
  vagina S30.824 ☑
  vocal cords S10.12 ☑
  vulva S30.824 ☑
  wrist S60.82- ☑
Bloating R14.0
Bloch-Sulzberger disease or syndrome Q82.3
Block, blocked
  alveolocapillary J84.10
  arborization (heart) I45.5
  arrhythmic I45.9
  atrioventricular (incomplete) (partial) I44.30
    with atrioventricular dissociation I44.2
    complete I44.2
      congenital Q24.6
    congenital Q24.6
    first degree I44.0
    second degree (types I and II) I44.1
    specified NEC I44.39
    third degree I44.2
    types I and II I44.1
  auriculoventricular — *see* Block, atrioventricular
  bifascicular (cardiac) I45.2
  bundle-branch (complete) (false) (incomplete) I45.4
    bilateral I45.2
    left I44.7
      with right bundle branch block I45.2
      hemiblock I44.60
        anterior I44.4
        posterior I44.5
      incomplete I44.7
        with right bundle branch block I45.2
    right I45.10
      with
        left bundle branch block I45.2
        left fascicular block I45.2
      specified NEC I45.19
    Wilson's type I45.19
  cardiac I45.9

Block, blocked — *continued*
  conduction I45.9
    complete I44.2
  fascicular (left) I44.60
    anterior I44.4
    posterior I44.5
    right I45.0
    specified NEC I44.69
  foramen Magendie (acquired) G91.1
    congenital Q03.1
      with spina bifida — *see* Spina bifida, by site,
        with hydrocephalus
  heart I45.9
    bundle branch I45.4
      bilateral I45.2
    complete (atrioventricular) I44.2
    congenital Q24.6
    first degree (atrioventricular) I44.0
    second degree (atrioventricular) I44.1
    specified type NEC I45.5
    third degree (atrioventricular) I44.2
  hepatic vein I82.0
  intraventricular (nonspecific) I45.4
    bundle branch
      bilateral I45.2
  kidney N28.9
    postcystoscopic or postprocedural N99.0
  Mobitz (types I and II) I44.1
  myocardial — *see* Block, heart
  nodal I45.5
  organ or site, congenital NEC — *see* Atresia, by site
  portal (vein) I81
  second degree (types I and II) I44.1
  sinoatrial I45.5
  sinoauricular I45.5
  third degree I44.2
  trifascicular I45.3
  tubal N97.1
  vein NOS I82.90
  Wenckebach (types I and II) I44.1
Blockage — *see* Obstruction
Blocq's disease F44.4
Blood
  constituents, abnormal R78.9
  disease D75.9
  donor — *see* Donor, blood
  dyscrasia D75.9
    with
      abortion — *see* Abortion, by type, complicated
        by, hemorrhage
      ectopic pregnancy O08.1
      molar pregnancy O08.1
    following ectopic or molar pregnancy O08.1
    newborn P61.9
    puerperal, postpartum O72.3
  flukes NEC — *see* Schistosomiasis
  in
    feces K92.1
      occult R19.5
    urine — *see* Hematuria
  mole O02.0
  occult in feces R19.5
  pressure
    decreased, due to shock following injury T79.4 ☑
    examination only Z01.30
    fluctuating I99.8
    high — *see* Hypertension
      borderline R03.0
      incidental reading, without diagnosis of hyper-
        tension R03.0
    low (*see also* Hypotension)
      incidental reading, without diagnosis of hy-
        potension R03.1
  spitting — *see* Hemoptysis
  staining cornea — *see* Pigmentation, cornea, stromal
  transfusion
    reaction or complication — *see* Complications,
      transfusion
  type
    A (Rh positive) Z67.10
      Rh negative Z67.11
    AB (Rh positive) Z67.30
      Rh negative Z67.31
    B (Rh positive) Z67.20
      Rh negative Z67.21
    O (Rh positive) Z67.40
      Rh negative Z67.41
    Rh (positive) Z67.90

Blood — *continued*
  type — *continued*
    Rh (positive) Z67.90
      negative Z67.91
  vessel rupture — *see* Hemorrhage
  vomiting — *see* Hematemesis
Blood-forming organs, disease D75.9
Bloodgood's disease — *see* Mastopathy, cystic
Bloom (-Machacek)(-Torre) **syndrome** Q82.8
Blount's disease or osteochondrosis — *see* Osteochondrosis, juvenile, tibia
Blue
  baby Q24.9
  diaper syndrome E72.09
  dome cyst (breast) — *see* Cyst, breast
  dot cataract Q12.0
  nevus D22.9
  sclera Q13.5
    with fragility of bone and deafness Q78.0
  toe syndrome I75.02- ☑
Blueness — *see* Cyanosis
Blues, postpartal O90.6
  baby O90.6
Blurring, visual H53.8
Blushing (abnormal) (excessive) R23.2
BMI — *see* Body, mass index
Boarder, hospital NEC Z76.4
  accompanying sick person Z76.3
  healthy infant or child Z76.2
    foundling Z76.1
Bockhart's impetigo L01.02
Bodechtel-Guttman disease (subacute sclerosing panencephalitis) A81.1
Boder-Sedgwick syndrome (ataxia-telangiectasia)
  G11.3
Body, bodies
  Aschoff's — *see* Myocarditis, rheumatic
  asteroid, vitreous — *see* Deposit, crystalline
  cytoid (retina) — *see* Occlusion, artery, retina
  drusen (degenerative) (macula) (retinal) (*see also* De-
    generation, macula, drusen)
    optic disc — *see* Drusen, optic disc
  foreign — *see* Foreign body
  loose
    joint, except knee — *see* Loose, body, joint
      knee M23.4- ☑
    sheath, tendon — *see* Disorder, tendon, specified
      type NEC
  mass index (BMI)
    adult
      19 or less Z68.1
      20.0-20.9 Z68.20
      21.0-21.9 Z68.21
      22.0-22.9 Z68.22
      23.0-23.9 Z68.23
      24.0-24.9 Z68.24
      25.0-25.9 Z68.25
      26.0-26.9 Z68.26
      27.0-27.9 Z68.27
      28.0-28.9 Z68.28
      29.0-29.9 Z68.29
      30.0-30.9 Z68.30
      31.0-31.9 Z68.31
      32.0-32.9 Z68.32
      33.0-33.9 Z68.33
      34.0-34.9 Z68.34
      35.0-35.9 Z68.35
      36.0-36.9 Z68.36
      37.0-37.9 Z68.37
      38.0-38.9 Z68.38
      39.0-39.9 Z68.39
      40.0-44.9 Z68.41
      45.0-49.9 Z68.42
      50.0-59.9 Z68.43
      60.0-69.9 Z68.44
      70 and over Z68.45
    pediatric
      5th percentile to less than 85th percentile for
        age Z68.52
      85th percentile to less than 95th percentile for
        age Z68.53
      less than fifth percentile for age Z68.51
      greater than or equal to ninety-fifth percentile
        for age Z68.54
  Mooser's A75.2
  rice (*see also* Loose, body, joint)
    knee M23.4- ☑
  rocking F98.4

Boeck's
  disease or sarcoid — *see* Sarcoidosis
  lupoid (miliary) D86.3
Boerhaave's syndrome (spontaneous esophageal rup-
  ture) K22.3
Boggy
  cervix N88.8
  uterus N85.8
Boil (*see also* Furuncle, by site)
  Aleppo B55.1
  Baghdad B55.1
  Delhi B55.1
  lacrimal
    gland — *see* Dacryoadenitis
    passages (duct) (sac) — *see* Inflammation, lacrimal,
      passages, acute
  Natal B55.1
  orbit, orbital — *see* Abscess, orbit
  tropical B55.1
Bold hives — *see* Urticaria
Bombé, iris — *see* Membrane, pupillary
Bone — *see* condition
Bonnevie-Ullrich syndrome Q87.1
Bonnier's syndrome H81.8 ☑
Bonvale dam fever T73.3 ☑
Bony block of joint — *see* Ankylosis
BOOP (bronchiolitis obliterans organized pneumonia)
  J84.89
Borderline
  diabetes mellitus R73.09
  hypertension R03.0
  osteopenia M85.8- ☑
  pelvis, with obstruction during labor O65.1
  personality F60.3
Borna disease A83.9
Bornholm disease B33.0
Boston exanthem A88.0
Botalli, ductus (patent) (persistent) Q25.0
Botulism (foodborne intoxication) A05.1
  infant A48.51
  non-foodborne A48.52
  wound A48.52
Bouba — *see* Yaws
Bouchard's nodes (with arthropathy) M15.2
Bouffée délirante F23
Bouillaud's disease or syndrome (rheumatic heart
  disease) I01.9
Bourneville's disease Q85.1
Boutonniere deformity (finger) — *see* Deformity, finger,
  boutonniere
Bouveret (-Hoffmann) **syndrome** (paroxysmal tachycar-
  dia) I47.9
Bovine heart — *see* Hypertrophy, cardiac
Bowel — *see* condition
Bowen's
  dermatosis (precancerous) — *see* Neoplasm, skin, in
    situ
  disease — *see* Neoplasm, skin, in situ
  epithelioma — *see* Neoplasm, skin, in situ
  type
    epidermoid carcinoma-in-situ — *see* Neoplasm,
      skin, in situ
    intraepidermal squamous cell carcinoma — *see*
      Neoplasm, skin, in situ
Bowing
  femur (*see also* Deformity, limb, specified type NEC,
    thigh)
    congenital Q68.3
  fibula (*see also* Deformity, limb, specified type NEC,
    lower leg)
    congenital Q68.4
  forearm — *see* Deformity, limb, specified type NEC,
    forearm
  leg(s), long bones, congenital Q68.5
  radius — *see* Deformity, limb, specified type NEC,
    forearm
  tibia (*see also* Deformity, limb, specified type NEC,
    lower leg)
    congenital Q68.4
Bowleg(s) (acquired) M21.16- ☑
  congenital Q68.5
  rachitic E64.3
Boyd's dysentery A03.2
Brachial — *see* condition
Brachycardia R00.1
Brachycephaly Q75.0

☑ **Additional Character Required — Refer to the Tabular List for Character Selection** ▽ **Subterms under main terms may continue to next column or page**

Bradley's disease A08.19
Bradyarrhythmia, cardiac I49.8
Bradycardia (sinoatrial) (sinus) (vagal) R00.1
  neonatal P29.12
  reflex G90.09
  tachycardia syndrome I49.5
Bradykinesia R25.8
Bradypnea R06.89
Bradytachycardia I49.5
Brailsford's disease or osteochondrosis — *see* Osteo-
    chondrosis, juvenile, radius
Brain (*see also* condition)
  death G93.82
  syndrome — *see* Syndrome, brain
Branched-chain amino-acid disorder E71.2
Branchial — *see* condition
  cartilage, congenital Q18.2
Branchiogenic remnant (in neck) Q18.0
Brandt's syndrome (acrodermatitis enteropathica) E83.2
Brash (water) R12
Bravais-jacksonian epilepsy — *see* Epilepsy, localiza-
    tion-related, symptomatic, with simple partial
    seizures
Braxton Hicks contractions — *see* False, labor
Brazilian leishmaniasis B55.2
BRBPR K62.5
Break, retina (without detachment) H33.30- ☑
  with retinal detachment — *see* Detachment, retina
  horseshoe tear H33.31- ☑
  multiple H33.33- ☑
  round hole H33.32- ☑
Breakdown
  device, graft or implant (*see also* Complications, by
    site and type, mechanical) T85.618 ☑
    arterial graft NEC — *see* Complication, cardiovas-
      cular device, mechanical, vascular
    breast (implant) T85.41 ☑
    catheter NEC T85.618 ☑
      cystostomy T83.010 ☑
      dialysis (renal) T82.41 ☑
        intraperitoneal T85.611 ☑
      infusion NEC T82.514 ☑
        spinal (epidural) (subdural) T85.610 ☑
      urinary (indwelling) T83.018 ☑
    electronic (electrode) (pulse generator) (stimulator)
      bone T84.310 ☑
      cardiac T82.119 ☑
        electrode T82.110 ☑
        pulse generator T82.111 ☑
        specified type NEC T82.118 ☑
      nervous system — *see* Complication, prosthetic
        device, mechanical, electronic nervous
        system stimulator
      urinary — *see* Complication, genitourinary,
        device, urinary, mechanical
    fixation, internal (orthopedic) NEC — *see* Compli-
      cation, fixation device, mechanical
    gastrointestinal — *see* Complications, prosthetic
      device, mechanical, gastrointestinal device
    genital NEC T83.418 ☑
      intrauterine contraceptive device T83.31 ☑
      penile prosthesis T83.410 ☑
    heart NEC — *see* Complication, cardiovascular de-
      vice, mechanical
    joint prosthesis — *see* Complications..., joint pros-
      thesis,internal, mechanical, by site
    ocular NEC — *see* Complications, prosthetic device,
      mechanical, ocular device
    orthopedic NEC — *see* Complication, orthopedic,
      device, mechanical
    specified NEC T85.618 ☑
    sutures, permanent T85.612 ☑
      used in bone repair — *see* Complications, fixa-
        tion device, internal (orthopedic), me-
        chanical
    urinary NEC (*see also* Complication, genitourinary,
      device, urinary, mechanical)
      graft T83.21 ☑
    vascular NEC — *see* Complication, cardiovascular
      device, mechanical
    ventricular intracranial shunt T85.01 ☑
  nervous F48.8
  perineum O90.1
  respirator J95.850
    specified NEC J95.859
  ventilator

Breakdown — *continued*
  ventilator J95.850
    specified NEC J95.859
Breast (*see also* condition)
  buds E30.1
    in newborn P96.89
  dense R92.2
  nodule N63
Breath
  foul R19.6
  holder, child R06.89
  holding spell R06.89
  shortness R06.02
Breathing
  labored — *see* Hyperventilation
  mouth R06.5
    causing malocclusion M26.5 ☑
  periodic R06.3
    high altitude G47.32
Breathlessness R06.81
Breda's disease — *see* Yaws
Breech presentation (mother) O32.1 ☑
  causing obstructed labor O64.1 ☑
  footling O32.8 ☑
    causing obstructed labor O64.8 ☑
  incomplete O32.8 ☑
    causing obstructed labor O64.8 ☑
Breisky's disease N90.4
Brennemann's syndrome I88.0
Brenner
  tumor (benign) D27.9
    borderline malignancy D39.1- ☑
    malignant C56 ☑
    proliferating D39.1- ☑
Bretonneau's disease or angina A36.0
Breus' mole O02.0
Brevicollis Q76.49
Brickmakers' anemia B76.9 [D63.8]
Bridge, myocardial Q24.5
Bright red blood per rectum (BRBPR) K62.5
Bright's disease (*see also* Nephritis)
  arteriosclerotic — *see* Hypertension, kidney
Brill (-Zinsser) **disease** (recrudescent typhus) A75.1
  flea-borne A75.2
  louse-borne A75.1
Brill-Symmers' disease C82.90
Brion-Kayser disease — *see* Fever, parathyroid
Briquet's disorder or syndrome F45.0
Brissaud's
  infantilism or dwarfism E23.0
  motor-verbal tic F95.2
Brittle
  bones disease Q78.0
  nails L60.3
    congenital Q84.6
Broad (*see also* condition)
  beta disease E78.2
  ligament laceration syndrome N83.8
Broad- or floating-betalipoproteinemia E78.2
Brock's syndrome (atelectasis due to enlarged lymph
    nodes) J98.19
Brocq-Duhring disease (dermatitis herpetiformis) L13.0
Brodie's abscess or disease M86.8X- ☑
Broken
  arches (*see also* Deformity, limb, flat foot)
  arm (meaning upper limb) — *see* Fracture, arm
  back — *see* Fracture, vertebra
  bone — *see* Fracture
  implant or internal device — *see* Complications, by
    site and type, mechanical
  leg (meaning lower limb) — *see* Fracture, leg
  nose S02.2 ☑
  tooth, teeth — *see* Fracture, tooth
Bromhidrosis, bromidrosis L75.0
Bromidism, bromism G92
  chronic (dependence) F13.20
  due to
    correct substance properly administered — *see*
      Table of Drugs and Chemicals, by drug, ad-
      verse effect
    overdose or wrong substance given or taken —
      see Table of Drugs and Chemicals, by drug,
      poisoning
Bromidrosiphobia F40.298
Bronchi, bronchial — *see* condition
Bronchiectasis (cylindrical) (diffuse) (fusiform) (localized)
  (saccular) J47.9

Bronchiectasis — *continued*
  with
    acute
      bronchitis J47.0
      lower respiratory infection J47.0
    exacerbation (acute) J47.1
  congenital Q33.4
  tuberculous NEC — *see* Tuberculosis, pulmonary
Bronchiolectasis — *see* Bronchiectasis
Bronchiolitis (acute) (infective) (subacute) J21.9
  with
    bronchospasm or obstruction J21.9
    influenza, flu or grippe — *see* Influenza, with, res-
      piratory manifestations NEC
  chemical (chronic) J68.4
    acute J68.0
  chronic (fibrosing) (obliterative) J44.9
  due to
    external agent — *see* Bronchitis, acute, due to
    human metapneumovirus J21.1
    respiratory syncytial virus J21.0
    specified organism NEC J21.8
  fibrosa obliterans J44.9
  influenzal — *see* Influenza, with, respiratory manifes-
    tations NEC
  obliterans J42
    with organizing pneumonia (BOOP) J84.89
  obliterative (chronic) (subacute) J44.9
    due to chemicals, gases, fumes or vapors (inhala-
      tion) J68.4
    due to fumes or vapors J68.4
  respiratory, interstitial lung disease J84.115
Bronchitis (diffuse) (fibrinous) (hypostatic) (infective)
  (membranous) J40
  with
    influenza, flu or grippe — *see* Influenza, with, res-
      piratory manifestations NEC
    obstruction (airway) (lung) J44.9
    tracheitis (15 years of age and above) J40
      acute or subacute J20.9
      chronic J42
      under 15 years of age J20.9
  acute or subacute (with bronchospasm or obstruction)
    J20.9
    with
      bronchiectasis J47.0
      chronic obstructive pulmonary disease J44.0
    chemical (due to gases, fumes or vapors) J68.0
    due to
      fumes or vapors J68.0
      Haemophilus influenzae J20.1
      Mycoplasma pneumoniae J20.0
      radiation J70.0
      specified organism NEC J20.8
      Streptococcus J20.2
      virus
        coxsackie J20.3
        echovirus J20.7
        parainfluenzae J20.4
        respiratory syncytial J20.5
        rhinovirus J20.6
    viral NEC J20.8
  allergic (acute) J45.909
    with
      exacerbation (acute) J45.901
      status asthmaticus J45.902
  arachidic T17.528 ☑
  aspiration (due to fumes or vapors) J68.0
  asthmatic J45.9 ☑
    chronic J44.9
      with
        acute lower respiratory infection J44.0
        exacerbation (acute) J44.1
  capillary — *see* Pneumonia, broncho
  caseous (tuberculous) A15.5
  Castellani's A69.8
  catarrhal (15 years of age and above) J40
    acute — *see* Bronchitis, acute
    chronic J41.0
    under 15 years of age J20.9
  chemical (acute) (subacute) J68.0
    chronic J68.4
    due to fumes or vapors J68.0
      chronic J68.4
  chronic J42
    with
      airways obstruction J44.9
      tracheitis (chronic) J42

Bronchitis — *continued*
chronic — *continued*
asthmatic (obstructive) J44.9
catarrhal J41.0
chemical (due to fumes or vapors) J68.4
due to
chemicals, gases, fumes or vapors (inhalation)
J68.4
radiation J70.1
tobacco smoking J41.0
emphysematous J44.9
mucopurulent J41.1
non-obstructive J41.0
obliterans J44.9
obstructive J44.9
purulent J41.1
simple J41.0
croupous — *see* Bronchitis, acute
due to gases, fumes or vapors (chemical) J68.0
emphysematous (obstructive) J44.9
exudative — *see* Bronchitis, acute
fetid J41.1
grippal — *see* Influenza, with, respiratory manifestations NEC
in those under 15 years age — *see* Bronchitis, acute
chronic — *see* Bronchitis, chronic
influenzal — *see* Influenza, with, respiratory manifestations NEC
mixed simple and mucopurulent J41.8
moulder's J62.8
mucopurulent (chronic) (recurrent) J41.1
acute or subacute J20.9
simple (mixed) J41.8
obliterans (chronic) J44.9
obstructive (chronic) (diffuse) J44.9
pituitous J41.1
pneumococcal, acute or subacute J20.2
pseudomembranous, acute or subacute — *see* Bronchitis, acute
purulent (chronic) (recurrent) J41.1
acute or subacute — *see* Bronchitis, acute
putrid J41.1
senile (chronic) J42
simple and mucopurulent (mixed) J41.8
smokers' J41.0
spirochetal NEC A69.8
subacute — *see* Bronchitis, acute
suppurative (chronic) J41.1
acute or subacute — *see* Bronchitis, acute
tuberculous A15.5
under 15 years of age — *see* Bronchitis, acute
chronic — *see* Bronchitis, chronic
viral NEC, acute or subacute (*see also* Bronchitis, acute)
J20.8
Bronchoalveolitis J18.0
Bronchoaspergillosis B44.1
Bronchocele meaning goiter E04.0
Broncholithiasis J98.09
tuberculous NEC A15.5
Bronchomalacia J98.09
congenital Q32.2
Bronchomycosis NOS B49 [J99]
candidal B37.1
Bronchopleuropneumonia — *see* Pneumonia, broncho
Bronchopneumonia — *see* Pneumonia, broncho
Bronchopneumonitis — *see* Pneumonia, broncho
Bronchopulmonary — *see* condition
Bronchopulmonitis — *see* Pneumonia, broncho
Bronchorrhagia (see Hemoptysis)
Bronchorrhea J98.09
acute J20.9
chronic (infective) (purulent) J42
Bronchospasm (acute) J98.01
with
bronchiolitis, acute J21.9
bronchitis, acute (conditions in J20) — *see* Bronchi-
tis, acute
due to external agent — *see* condition, respiratory,
acute, due to
exercise induced J45.990
Bronchospirochetosis A69.8
Castellani A69.8
Bronchostenosis J98.09
Bronchus — *see* condition
Brontophobia F40.220
Bronze baby syndrome P83.8
Brooke's tumor — *see* Neoplasm, skin, benign

Brown enamel of teeth (hereditary) K00.5
Brown's sheath syndrome H50.61- ☑
Brown-Séquard disease, paralysis or syndrome
G83.81
Bruce sepsis A23.0
Brucellosis (infection) A23.9
abortus A23.1
canis A23.3
dermatitis A23.9
melitensis A23.0
mixed A23.8
sepsis A23.9
melitensis A23.0
specified NEC A23.8
suis A23.2
Bruck-de Lange disease Q87.1
Bruck's disease — *see* Deformity, limb
Brugsch's syndrome Q82.8
Bruise (skin surface intact) (*see also* Contusion)
with
open wound — *see* Wound, open
internal organ — *see* Injury, by site
newborn P54.5
scalp, due to birth injury, newborn P12.3
umbilical cord O69.5 ☑
Bruit (arterial) R09.89
cardiac R01.1
Brush burn — *see* Abrasion, by site
Bruton's X-linked agammaglobulinemia D80.0
Bruxism
psychogenic F45.8
sleep related G47.63
Bubbly lung syndrome P27.0
Bubo I88.8
blennorrhagic (gonococcal) A54.89
chancroidal A57
climatic A55
due to Haemophilus ducreyi A57
gonococcal A54.89
indolent (nonspecific) I88.8
inguinal (nonspecific) I88.8
chancroidal A57
climatic A55
due to H. ducreyi A57
infective I88.8
scrofulous (tuberculous) A18.2
soft chancre A57
suppurating — *see* Lymphadenitis, acute
syphilitic (primary) A51.0
congenital A50.07
tropical A55
virulent (chancroidal) A57
Bubonic plague A20.0
Bubonocele — *see* Hernia, inguinal
Buccal — *see* condition
Buchanan's disease or osteochondrosis M91.0
Buchem's syndrome (hyperostosis corticalis) M85.2
Bucket-handle fracture or tear (semilunar cartilage)
— *see* Tear, meniscus
Budd-Chiari syndrome (hepatic vein thrombosis) I82.0
Budgerigar fancier's disease or lung J67.2
Buds
breast E30.1
in newborn P96.89
Buerger's disease (thromboangiitis obliterans) I73.1
Bulbar — *see* condition
Bulbus cordis (left ventricle) (persistent) Q21.8
Bulimia (nervosa) F50.2
atypical F50.9
normal weight F50.9
Bulky
stools R19.5
uterus N85.2
Bulla (e) R23.8
lung (emphysematous) (solitary) J43.9
newborn P25.8
Bullet wound (*see also* Wound, open)
fracture — *code as* Fracture, by site
internal organ — *see* Injury, by site
Bundle
branch block (complete) (false) (incomplete) — *see*
Block, bundle-branch
of His — *see* condition
Bunion — *see* Deformity, toe, hallux valgus
Buphthalmia, buphthalmos (congenital) Q15.0
Burdwan fever B55.0
Bürger-Grütz disease or syndrome E78.3

Buried
penis (congenital) Q55.64
acquired N48.83
roots K08.3
Burke's syndrome K86.8
Burkitt
cell leukemia C91.0- ☑
lymphoma (malignant) C83.7- ☑
small noncleaved, diffuse C83.7- ☑
spleen C83.77
undifferentiated C83.7- ☑
tumor C83.7- ☑
type
acute lymphoblastic leukemia C91.0- ☑
undifferentiated C83.7- ☑
Burn (electricity) (flame) (hot gas, liquid or hot object)
(radiation) (steam) (thermal) T30.0
abdomen, abdominal (muscle) (wall) T21.02 ☑
first degree T21.12 ☑
second degree T21.22 ☑
third degree T21.32 ☑
above elbow T22.039 ☑
first degree T22.139 ☑
left T22.032 ☑
first degree T22.132 ☑
second degree T22.232 ☑
third degree T22.332 ☑
right T22.031 ☑
first degree T22.131 ☑
second degree T22.231 ☑
third degree T22.331 ☑
second degree T22.239 ☑
third degree T22.339 ☑
acid (caustic) (external) (internal) — *see* Corrosion, by
site
alimentary tract NEC T28.2 ☑
esophagus T28.1 ☑
mouth T28.0 ☑
pharynx T28.0 ☑
alkaline (caustic) (external) (internal) — *see* Corrosion,
by site
ankle T25.019 ☑
first degree T25.119 ☑
left T25.012 ☑
first degree T25.112 ☑
second degree T25.212 ☑
third degree T25.312 ☑
multiple with foot — *see* Burn, lower, limb, multiple, ankle and foot
right T25.011 ☑
first degree T25.111 ☑
second degree T25.211 ☑
third degree T25.311 ☑
second degree T25.219 ☑
third degree T25.319 ☑
anus — *see* Burn, buttock
arm (lower) (upper) — *see* Burn, upper, limb
axilla T22.049 ☑
first degree T22.149 ☑
left T22.042 ☑
first degree T22.142 ☑
second degree T22.242 ☑
third degree T22.342 ☑
right T22.041 ☑
first degree T22.141 ☑
second degree T22.241 ☑
third degree T22.341 ☑
second degree T22.249 ☑
third degree T22.349 ☑
back (lower) T21.04 ☑
first degree T21.14 ☑
second degree T21.24 ☑
third degree T21.34 ☑
upper T21.03 ☑
first degree T21.13 ☑
second degree T21.23 ☑
third degree T21.33 ☑
blisters — *code as* Burn, second degree, by site
breast(s) — *see* Burn, chest wall
buttock(s) T21.05 ☑
first degree T21.15 ☑
second degree T21.25 ☑
third degree T21.35 ☑
calf T24.039 ☑
first degree T24.139 ☑

Burn — *continued*
  calf — *continued*
    left T24.032 ☑
      first degree T24.132 ☑
      second degree T24.232 ☑
      third degree T24.332 ☑
    right T24.031 ☑
      first degree T24.131 ☑
      second degree T24.231 ☑
      third degree T24.331 ☑
    second degree T24.239 ☑
    third degree T24.339 ☑
  canthus (eye) — *see* Burn, eyelid
  caustic acid or alkaline — *see* Corrosion, by site
  cervix T28.3 ☑
  cheek T20.06 ☑
    first degree T20.16 ☑
    second degree T20.26 ☑
    third degree T20.36 ☑
  chemical (acids) (alkalines) (caustics) (external) (internal) — *see* Corrosion, by site
  chest wall T21.01 ☑
    first degree T21.11 ☑
    second degree T21.21 ☑
    third degree T21.31 ☑
  chin T20.03 ☑
    first degree T20.13 ☑
    second degree T20.23 ☑
    third degree T20.33 ☑
  colon T28.2 ☑
  conjunctiva (and cornea) — *see* Burn, cornea
  cornea (and conjunctiva) T26.1- ☑
    chemical — *see* Corrosion, cornea
  corrosion (external) (internal) — *see* Corrosion, by site
  deep necrosis of underlying tissue — *code as* Burn, third degree, by site
  dorsum of hand T23.069 ☑
    first degree T23.169 ☑
    left T23.062 ☑
      first degree T23.162 ☑
      second degree T23.262 ☑
      third degree T23.362 ☑
    right T23.061 ☑
      first degree T23.161 ☑
      second degree T23.261 ☑
      third degree T23.361 ☑
    second degree T23.269 ☑
    third degree T23.369 ☑
  due to ingested chemical agent — *see* Corrosion, by site
  ear (auricle) (external) (canal) T20.01 ☑
    first degree T20.11 ☑
    second degree T20.21 ☑
    third degree T20.31 ☑
  elbow T22.029 ☑
    first degree T22.129 ☑
    left T22.022 ☑
      first degree T22.122 ☑
      second degree T22.222 ☑
      third degree T22.322 ☑
    right T22.021 ☑
      first degree T22.121 ☑
      second degree T22.221 ☑
      third degree T22.321 ☑
    second degree T22.229 ☑
    third degree T22.329 ☑
  epidermal loss — *code as* Burn, second degree, by site
  erythema, erythematous — *code as* Burn, first degree, by site
  esophagus T28.1 ☑
  extent (percentage of body surface)
    less than 10 percent T31.0
    10-19 percent T31.10
      with 0-9 percent third degree burns T31.10
      with 10-19 percent third degree burns T31.11
    20-29 percent T31.20
      with 0-9 percent third degree burns T31.20
      with 10-19 percent third degree burns T31.21
      with 20-29 percent third degree burns T31.22
    30-39 percent T31.30
      with 0-9 percent third degree burns T31.30
      with 10-19 percent third degree burns T31.31
      with 20-29 percent third degree burns T31.32
      with 30-39 percent third degree burns T31.33
    40-49 percent T31.40
      with 0-9 percent third degree burns T31.40

Burn — *continued*
  extent — *continued*
    40-49 percent — *continued*
      with 10-19 percent third degree burns T31.41
      with 20-29 percent third degree burns T31.42
      with 30-39 percent third degree burns T31.43
      with 40-49 percent third degree burns T31.44
    50-59 percent T31.50
      with 0-9 percent third degree burns T31.50
      with 10-19 percent third degree burns T31.51
      with 20-29 percent third degree burns T31.52
      with 30-39 percent third degree burns T31.53
      with 40-49 percent third degree burns T31.54
      with 50-59 percent third degree burns T31.55
    60-69 percent T31.60
      with 0-9 percent third degree burns T31.60
      with 10-19 percent third degree burns T31.61
      with 20-29 percent third degree burns T31.62
      with 30-39 percent third degree burns T31.63
      with 40-49 percent third degree burns T31.64
      with 50-59 percent third degree burns T31.65
      with 60-69 percent third degree burns T31.66
    70-79 percent T31.70
      with 0-9 percent third degree burns T31.70
      with 10-19 percent third degree burns T31.71
      with 20-29 percent third degree burns T31.72
      with 30-39 percent third degree burns T31.73
      with 40-49 percent third degree burns T31.74
      with 50-59 percent third degree burns T31.75
      with 60-69 percent third degree burns T31.76
      with 70-79 percent third degree burns T31.77
    80-89 percent T31.80
      with 0-9 percent third degree burns T31.80
      with 10-19 percent third degree burns T31.81
      with 20-29 percent third degree burns T31.82
      with 30-39 percent third degree burns T31.83
      with 40-49 percent third degree burns T31.84
      with 50-59 percent third degree burns T31.85
      with 60-69 percent third degree burns T31.86
      with 70-79 percent third degree burns T31.87
      with 80-89 percent third degree burns T31.88
    90 percent or more T31.90
      with 0-9 percent third degree burns T31.90
      with 10-19 percent third degree burns T31.91
      with 20-29 percent third degree burns T31.92
      with 30-39 percent third degree burns T31.93
      with 40-49 percent third degree burns T31.94
      with 50-59 percent third degree burns T31.95
      with 60-69 percent third degree burns T31.96
      with 70-79 percent third degree burns T31.97
      with 80-89 percent third degree burns T31.98
      with 90 percent or more third degree burns T31.99
  extremity — *see* Burn, limb
  eye(s) and adnexa T26.4- ☑
    with resulting rupture and destruction of eyeball T26.2- ☑
    conjunctival sac — *see* Burn, cornea
    cornea — *see* Burn, cornea
    lid — *see* Burn, eyelid
    periocular area — *see* Burn, eyelid
    specified site NEC T26.3- ☑
  eyeball — *see* Burn, eye
  eyelid(s) T26.0- ☑
    chemical — *see* Corrosion, eyelid
  face — *see* Burn, head
  finger T23.029 ☑
    first degree T23.129 ☑
    left T23.022 ☑
      first degree T23.122 ☑
      second degree T23.222 ☑
      third degree T23.322 ☑
    multiple sites (without thumb) T23.039 ☑
      with thumb T23.049 ☑
        first degree T23.149 ☑
        left T23.042 ☑
          first degree T23.142 ☑
          second degree T23.242 ☑
          third degree T23.342 ☑
        right T23.041 ☑
          first degree T23.141 ☑
          second degree T23.241 ☑
          third degree T23.341 ☑
      second degree T23.249 ☑
      third degree T23.349 ☑
    first degree T23.139 ☑

Burn — *continued*
  finger — *continued*
    multiple sites — *continued*
      left T23.032 ☑
        first degree T23.132 ☑
        second degree T23.232 ☑
        third degree T23.332 ☑
      right T23.031 ☑
        first degree T23.131 ☑
        second degree T23.231 ☑
        third degree T23.331 ☑
      second degree T23.239 ☑
      third degree T23.339 ☑
    right T23.021 ☑
      first degree T23.121 ☑
      second degree T23.221 ☑
      third degree T23.321 ☑
    second degree T23.229 ☑
    third degree T23.329 ☑
  flank — *see* Burn, abdominal wall
  foot T25.029 ☑
    first degree T25.129 ☑
    left T25.022 ☑
      first degree T25.122 ☑
      second degree T25.222 ☑
      third degree T25.322 ☑
    multiple with ankle — *see* Burn, lower, limb, multiple, ankle and foot
    right T25.021 ☑
      first degree T25.121 ☑
      second degree T25.221 ☑
      third degree T25.321 ☑
    second degree T25.229 ☑
    third degree T25.329 ☑
  forearm T22.019 ☑
    first degree T22.119 ☑
    left T22.012 ☑
      first degree T22.112 ☑
      second degree T22.212 ☑
      third degree T22.312 ☑
    right T22.011 ☑
      first degree T22.111 ☑
      second degree T22.211 ☑
      third degree T22.311 ☑
    second degree T22.219 ☑
    third degree T22.319 ☑
  forehead T20.06 ☑
    first degree T20.16 ☑
    second degree T20.26 ☑
    third degree T20.36 ☑
  fourth degree — *code as* Burn, third degree, by site
  friction — *see* Burn, by site
  from swallowing caustic or corrosive substance NEC — *see* Corrosion, by site
  full thickness skin loss — *code as* Burn, third degree, by site
  gastrointestinal tract NEC T28.2 ☑
    from swallowing caustic or corrosive substance T28.7 ☑
  genital organs
    external
      female T21.07 ☑
        first degree T21.17 ☑
        second degree T21.27 ☑
        third degree T21.37 ☑
      male T21.06 ☑
        first degree T21.16 ☑
        second degree T21.26 ☑
        third degree T21.36 ☑
    internal T28.3 ☑
      from caustic or corrosive substance T28.8 ☑
  groin — *see* Burn, abdominal wall
  hand(s) T23.009 ☑
    back — *see* Burn, dorsum of hand
    finger — *see* Burn, finger
    first degree T23.109 ☑
    left T23.002 ☑
      first degree T23.102 ☑
      second degree T23.202 ☑
      third degree T23.302 ☑
    multiple sites with wrist T23.099 ☑
      first degree T23.199 ☑
      left T23.092 ☑
        first degree T23.192 ☑
        second degree T23.292 ☑
        third degree T23.392 ☑

Burn — *continued*
  hand(s) — *continued*
    multiple sites with wrist — *continued*
      right T23.091 ☑
        first degree T23.191 ☑
        second degree T23.291 ☑
        third degree T23.391 ☑
      second degree T23.299 ☑
      third degree T23.399 ☑
    palm — *see* Burn, palm
    right T23.001 ☑
      first degree T23.101 ☑
      second degree T23.201 ☑
      third degree T23.301 ☑
    second degree T23.209 ☑
    third degree T23.309 ☑
    thumb — *see* Burn, thumb
  head (and face) (and neck) T20.00 ☑
    cheek — *see* Burn, cheek
    chin — *see* Burn, chin
    ear — *see* Burn, ear
    eye(s) only — *see* Burn, eye
    first degree T20.10 ☑
    forehead — *see* Burn, forehead
    lip — *see* Burn, lip
    multiple sites T20.09 ☑
      first degree T20.19 ☑
      second degree T20.29 ☑
      third degree T20.39 ☑
    neck — *see* Burn, neck
    nose — *see* Burn, nose
    scalp — *see* Burn, scalp
    second degree T20.20 ☑
    third degree T20.30 ☑
  hip(s) — *see* Burn, lower, limb
  inhalation — *see* Burn, respiratory tract
    caustic or corrosive substance (fumes) — *see* Corrosion, respiratory tract
  internal organ(s) T28.40 ☑
    alimentary tract T28.2 ☑
      esophagus T28.1 ☑
    eardrum T28.41 ☑
    esophagus T28.1 ☑
    from caustic or corrosive substance (swallowing) NEC — *see* Corrosion, by site
    genitourinary T28.3 ☑
    mouth T28.0 ☑
    pharynx T28.0 ☑
    respiratory tract — *see* Burn, respiratory tract
    specified organ NEC T28.49 ☑
  interscapular region — *see* Burn, back, upper
  intestine (large) (small) T28.2 ☑
  knee T24.029 ☑
    first degree T24.129 ☑
    left T24.022 ☑
      first degree T24.122 ☑
      second degree T24.222 ☑
      third degree T24.322 ☑
    right T24.021 ☑
      first degree T24.121 ☑
      second degree T24.221 ☑
      third degree T24.321 ☑
    second degree T24.229 ☑
    third degree T24.329 ☑
  labium (majus) (minus) — *see* Burn, genital organs, external, female
  lacrimal apparatus, duct, gland or sac — *see* Burn, eye, specified site NEC
  larynx T27.0 ☑
    with lung T27.1 ☑
  leg(s) (lower) (upper) — *see* Burn, lower, limb
  lightning — *see* Burn, by site
  limb(s)
    lower (except ankle or foot alone) — *see* Burn, lower, limb
    upper — *see* Burn, upper limb
  lip(s) T20.02 ☑
    first degree T20.12 ☑
    second degree T20.22 ☑
    third degree T20.32 ☑
  lower
    back — *see* Burn, back
    limb T24.009 ☑
      ankle — *see* Burn, ankle
      calf — *see* Burn, calf
      first degree T24.109 ☑

Burn — *continued*
  lower — *continued*
    limb — *continued*
      foot — *see* Burn, foot
      hip — *see* Burn, thigh
      knee — *see* Burn, knee
      left T24.002 ☑
        first degree T24.102 ☑
        second degree T24.202 ☑
        third degree T24.302 ☑
      multiple sites, except ankle and foot T24.099 ☑
        ankle and foot T25.099 ☑
          first degree T25.199 ☑
          left T25.092 ☑
            first degree T25.192 ☑
            second degree T25.292 ☑
            third degree T25.392 ☑
          right T25.091 ☑
            first degree T25.191 ☑
            second degree T25.291 ☑
            third degree T25.391 ☑
          second degree T25.299 ☑
          third degree T25.399 ☑
        first degree T24.199 ☑
        left T24.092 ☑
          first degree T24.192 ☑
          second degree T24.292 ☑
          third degree T24.392 ☑
        right T24.091 ☑
          first degree T24.191 ☑
          second degree T24.291 ☑
          third degree T24.391 ☑
        second degree T24.299 ☑
        third degree T24.399 ☑
      right T24.001 ☑
        first degree T24.101 ☑
        second degree T24.201 ☑
        third degree T24.301 ☑
      second degree T24.209 ☑
      thigh — *see* Burn, thigh
      third degree T24.309 ☑
      toe — *see* Burn, toe
  lung (with larynx and trachea) T27.1 ☑
  mouth T28.0 ☑
  neck T20.07 ☑
    first degree T20.17 ☑
    second degree T20.27 ☑
    third degree T20.37 ☑
  nose (septum) T20.04 ☑
    first degree T20.14 ☑
    second degree T20.24 ☑
    third degree T20.34 ☑
  ocular adnexa — *see* Burn, eye
  orbit region — *see* Burn, eyelid
  palm T23.059 ☑
    first degree T23.159 ☑
    left T23.052 ☑
      first degree T23.152 ☑
      second degree T23.252 ☑
      third degree T23.352 ☑
    right T23.051 ☑
      first degree T23.151 ☑
      second degree T23.251 ☑
      third degree T23.351 ☑
    second degree T23.259 ☑
    third degree T23.359 ☑
  partial thickness — *code as* Burn, unspecified degree, by site
  pelvis — *see* Burn, trunk
  penis — *see* Burn, genital organs, external, male
  perineum
    female — *see* Burn, genital organs, external, female
    male — *see* Burn, genital organs, external, male
  periocular area — *see* Burn, eyelid
  pharynx T28.0 ☑
  rectum T28.2 ☑
  respiratory tract T27.3 ☑
    larynx — *see* Burn, larynx
    specified part NEC T27.2 ☑
    trachea — *see* Burn, trachea
  sac, lacrimal — *see* Burn, eye, specified site NEC
  scalp T20.05 ☑
    first degree T20.15 ☑
    second degree T20.25 ☑
    third degree T20.35 ☑

Burn — *continued*
  scapular region T22.069 ☑
    first degree T22.169 ☑
    left T22.062 ☑
      first degree T22.162 ☑
      second degree T22.262 ☑
      third degree T22.362 ☑
    right T22.061 ☑
      first degree T22.161 ☑
      second degree T22.261 ☑
      third degree T22.361 ☑
    second degree T22.269 ☑
    third degree T22.369 ☑
  sclera — *see* Burn, eye, specified site NEC
  scrotum — *see* Burn, genital organs, external, male
  shoulder T22.059 ☑
    first degree T22.159 ☑
    left T22.052 ☑
      first degree T22.152 ☑
      second degree T22.252 ☑
      third degree T22.352 ☑
    right T22.051 ☑
      first degree T22.151 ☑
      second degree T22.251 ☑
      third degree T22.351 ☑
    second degree T22.259 ☑
    third degree T22.359 ☑
  stomach T28.2 ☑
  temple — *see* Burn, head
  testis — *see* Burn, genital organs, external, male
  thigh T24.019 ☑
    first degree T24.119 ☑
    left T24.012 ☑
      first degree T24.112 ☑
      second degree T24.212 ☑
      third degree T24.312 ☑
    right T24.011 ☑
      first degree T24.111 ☑
      second degree T24.211 ☑
      third degree T24.311 ☑
    second degree T24.219 ☑
    third degree T24.319 ☑
  thorax (external) — *see* Burn, trunk
  throat (meaning pharynx) T28.0 ☑
  thumb(s) T23.019 ☑
    first degree T23.119 ☑
    left T23.012 ☑
      first degree T23.112 ☑
      second degree T23.212 ☑
      third degree T23.312 ☑
    multiple sites with fingers T23.049 ☑
      first degree T23.149 ☑
      left T23.042 ☑
        first degree T23.142 ☑
        second degree T23.242 ☑
        third degree T23.342 ☑
      right T23.041 ☑
        first degree T23.141 ☑
        second degree T23.241 ☑
        third degree T23.341 ☑
      second degree T23.249 ☑
      third degree T23.349 ☑
    right T23.011 ☑
      first degree T23.111 ☑
      second degree T23.211 ☑
      third degree T23.311 ☑
    second degree T23.219 ☑
    third degree T23.319 ☑
  toe T25.039 ☑
    first degree T25.139 ☑
    left T25.032 ☑
      first degree T25.132 ☑
      second degree T25.232 ☑
      third degree T25.332 ☑
    right T25.031 ☑
      first degree T25.131 ☑
      second degree T25.231 ☑
      third degree T25.331 ☑
    second degree T25.239 ☑
    third degree T25.339 ☑
  tongue T28.0 ☑
  tonsil(s) T28.0 ☑
  trachea T27.0 ☑
    with lung T27.1 ☑

Index

Burn — *continued*
  trunk T21.00 ☑
    abdominal wall — *see* Burn, abdominal wall
    anus — *see* Burn, buttock
    axilla — *see* Burn, upper limb
    back — *see* Burn, back
    breast — *see* Burn, chest wall
    buttock — *see* Burn, buttock
    chest wall — *see* Burn, chest wall
    first degree T21.10 ☑
    flank — *see* Burn, abdominal wall
    genital
      female — *see* Burn, genital organs, external, female
      male — *see* Burn, genital organs, external, male
    groin — *see* Burn, abdominal wall
    interscapular region — *see* Burn, back, upper
    labia — *see* Burn, genital organs, external, female
    lower back — *see* Burn, back
    penis — *see* Burn, genital organs, external, male
    perineum
      female — *see* Burn, genital organs, external, female
      male — *see* Burn, genital organs, external, male
    scapula region — *see* Burn, scapular region
    scrotum — *see* Burn, genital organs, external, male
    second degree T21.20 ☑
    specified site NEC T21.09 ☑
      first degree T21.19 ☑
      second degree T21.29 ☑
      third degree T21.39 ☑
    testes — *see* Burn, genital organs, external, male
    third degree T21.30 ☑
    upper back — *see* Burn, back, upper
    vulva — *see* Burn, genital organs, external, female
  unspecified site with extent of body surface involved specified
    less than 10 per cent T31.0
    10-19 per cent (0-9 percent third degree) T31.10
      with 10-19 percent third degree T31.11
    20-29 per cent (0-9 percent third degree) T31.20
      with
        10-19 percent third degree T31.21
        20-29 percent third degree T31.22
    30-39 per cent (0-9 percent third degree) T31.30
      with
        10-19 percent third degree T31.31
        20-29 percent third degree T31.32
        30-39 percent third degree T31.33
    40-49 per cent (0-9 percent third degree) T31.40
      with
        10-19 percent third degree T31.41
        20-29 percent third degree T31.42
        30-39 percent third degree T31.43
        40-49 percent third degree T31.44
    50-59 per cent (0-9 percent third degree) T31.50
      with
        10-19 percent third degree T31.51
        20-29 percent third degree T31.52
        30-39 percent third degree T31.53
        40-49 percent third degree T31.54
        50-59 percent third degree T31.55
    60-69 per cent (0-9 percent third degree) T31.60
      with
        10-19 percent third degree T31.61
        20-29 percent third degree T31.62
        30-39 percent third degree T31.63
        40-49 percent third degree T31.64
        50-59 percent third degree T31.65
        60-69 percent third degree T31.66
    70-79 per cent (0-9 percent third degree) T31.70
      with
        10-19 percent third degree T31.71
        20-29 percent third degree T31.72
        30-39 percent third degree T31.73
        40-49 percent third degree T31.74
        50-59 percent third degree T31.75
        60-69 percent third degree T31.76
        70-79 percent third degree T31.77
    80-89 per cent (0-9 percent third degree) T31.80
      with
        10-19 percent third degree T31.81
        20-29 percent third degree T31.82
        30-39 percent third degree T31.83
        40-49 percent third degree T31.84
        50-59 percent third degree T31.85
        60-69 percent third degree T31.86
        70-79 percent third degree T31.87

Burn — *continued*
  unspecified site with extent of body surface involved specified — *continued*
    80-89 per cent — *continued*
      with — *continued*
        80-89 percent third degree T31.88
    90 per cent or more (0-9 percent third degree) T31.90
      with
        10-19 percent third degree T31.91
        20-29 percent third degree T31.92
        30-39 percent third degree T31.93
        40-49 percent third degree T31.94
        50-59 percent third degree T31.95
        60-69 percent third degree T31.96
        70-79 percent third degree T31.97
        80-89 percent third degree T31.98
        90-99 percent third degree T31.99
  upper limb T22.00 ☑
    above elbow — *see* Burn, above elbow
    axilla — *see* Burn, axilla
    elbow — *see* Burn, elbow
    first degree T22.10 ☑
    forearm — *see* Burn, forearm
    hand — *see* Burn, hand
    interscapular region — *see* Burn, back, upper
    multiple sites T22.099 ☑
      first degree T22.199 ☑
      left T22.092 ☑
        first degree T22.192 ☑
        second degree T22.292 ☑
        third degree T22.392 ☑
      right T22.091 ☑
        first degree T22.191 ☑
        second degree T22.291 ☑
        third degree T22.391 ☑
      second degree T22.299 ☑
      third degree T22.399 ☑
    scapular region — *see* Burn, scapular region
    second degree T22.20 ☑
    shoulder — *see* Burn, shoulder
    third degree T22.30 ☑
    wrist — *see* Burn, wrist
  uterus T28.3 ☑
  vagina T28.3 ☑
  vulva — *see* Burn, genital organs, external, female
  wrist T23.079 ☑
    first degree T23.179 ☑
    left T23.072 ☑
      first degree T23.172 ☑
      second degree T23.272 ☑
      third degree T23.372 ☑
    multiple sites with hand T23.099 ☑
      first degree T23.199 ☑
      left T23.092 ☑
        first degree T23.192 ☑
        second degree T23.292 ☑
        third degree T23.392 ☑
      right T23.091 ☑
        first degree T23.191 ☑
        second degree T23.291 ☑
        third degree T23.391 ☑
      second degree T23.299 ☑
      third degree T23.399 ☑
    right T23.071 ☑
      first degree T23.171 ☑
      second degree T23.271 ☑
      third degree T23.371 ☑
    second degree T23.279 ☑
    third degree T23.379 ☑
Burnett's syndrome E83.52
Burning
  feet syndrome E53.9
  sensation R20.8
  tongue K14.6
Burn-out (state) Z73.0
Burns' disease or osteochondrosis — *see* Osteochondrosis, juvenile, ulna
Bursa — *see* condition
Bursitis M71.9
  Achilles — *see* Tendinitis, Achilles
  adhesive — *see* Bursitis, specified NEC
  ankle — *see* Enthesopathy, lower limb, ankle, specified type NEC
  calcaneal — *see* Enthesopathy, foot, specified type NEC

Bursitis — *continued*
  collateral ligament, tibial — *see* Bursitis, tibial collateral
  due to use, overuse, pressure (*see also* Disorder, soft tissue, due to use, specified type NEC)
    specified NEC — *see* Disorder, soft tissue, due to use, specified NEC
  Duplay's M75.0 ☑
  elbow NEC M70.3- ☑
    olecranon M70.2- ☑
  finger — *see* Disorder, soft tissue, due to use, specified type NEC, hand
  foot — *see* Enthesopathy, foot, specified type NEC
  gonococcal A54.49
  gouty — *see* Gout, idiopathic
  hand M70.1- ☑
  hip NEC M70.7- ☑
    trochanteric M70.6- ☑
  infective NEC M71.10
    abscess — *see* Abscess, bursa
    ankle M71.17- ☑
    elbow M71.12- ☑
    foot M71.17- ☑
    hand M71.14- ☑
    hip M71.15- ☑
    knee M71.16- ☑
    multiple sites M71.19
    shoulder M71.11- ☑
    specified site NEC M71.18
    wrist M71.13- ☑
  ischial — *see* Bursitis, hip
  knee NEC M70.5- ☑
    prepatellar M70.4- ☑
  occupational NEC (*see also* Disorder, soft tissue, due to, use)
  olecranon — *see* Bursitis, elbow, olecranon
  pharyngeal J39.1
  popliteal — *see* Bursitis, knee
  prepatellar M70.4- ☑
  radiohumeral M77.8
  rheumatoid M06.20
    ankle M06.27- ☑
    elbow M06.22- ☑
    foot joint M06.27- ☑
    hand joint M06.24- ☑
    hip M06.25- ☑
    knee M06.26- ☑
    multiple site M06.29
    shoulder M06.21- ☑
    vertebra M06.28
    wrist M06.23- ☑
  scapulohumeral — *see* Bursitis, shoulder
  semimembranous muscle (knee) — *see* Bursitis, knee
  shoulder M75.5- ☑
    adhesive — *see* Capsulitis, adhesive
  specified NEC M71.50
    ankle M71.57- ☑
    due to use, overuse or pressure — *see* Disorder, soft tissue, due to, use
    elbow M71.52- ☑
    foot M71.57- ☑
    hand M71.54- ☑
    hip M71.55- ☑
    knee M71.56- ☑
    shoulder — *see* Bursitis, shoulder
    specified site NEC M71.58
    tibial collateral M76.4- ☑
    wrist M71.53- ☑
  subacromial — *see* Bursitis, shoulder
  subcoracoid — *see* Bursitis, shoulder
  subdeltoid — *see* Bursitis, shoulder
  syphilitic A52.78
  Thornwaldt, Tornwaldt J39.2
  tibial collateral — *see* Bursitis, tibial collateral
  toe — *see* Enthesopathy, foot, specified type NEC
  trochanteric (area) — *see* Bursitis, hip, trochanteric
  wrist — *see* Bursitis, hand
Bursopathy M71.9
  specified type NEC M71.80
    ankle M71.87- ☑
    elbow M71.82- ☑
    foot M71.87- ☑
    hand M71.84- ☑
    hip M71.85- ☑
    knee M71.86- ☑
    multiple sites M71.89
    shoulder M71.81- ☑

Burn — Bursopathy

Bursopathy — *continued*
 specified type — *continued*
  specified site NEC M71.88
  wrist M71.83- ☑
Burst stitches or sutures (complication of surgery)
 T81.31 ☑
 external operation wound T81.31 ☑
 internal operation wound T81.32 ☑
Buruli ulcer A31.1
Bury's disease L95.1
Buschke's
 disease B45.3
 scleredema — *see* Sclerosis, systemic
Busse-Buschke disease B45.3
Buttock — *see* condition
Button
 Biskra B55.1
 Delhi B55.1
 oriental B55.1
Buttonhole deformity (finger) — *see* Deformity, finger, boutonniere
Bwamba fever A92.8
Byssinosis J66.0
Bywaters' syndrome T79.5 ☑

C

Cachexia R64
 cancerous R64
 cardiac — *see* Disease, heart
 dehydration E86.0
  with
   hypernatremia E87.0
   hyponatremia E87.1
 due to malnutrition R64
 exophthalmic — *see* Hyperthyroidism
 heart — *see* Disease, heart
 hypophyseal E23.0
 hypopituitary E23.0
 lead — *see* Poisoning, lead
 malignant R64
 marsh — *see* Malaria
 nervous F48.8
 old age R54
 paludal — *see* Malaria
 pituitary E23.0
 renal N28.9
 saturnine — *see* Poisoning, lead
 senile R54
 Simmonds' E23.0
 splenica D73.0
 strumipriva E03.4
 tuberculous NEC — *see* Tuberculosis
Café, au lait spots L81.3
Caffey's syndrome Q78.8
Caisson disease T70.3 ☑
Cake kidney Q63.1
Caked breast (puerperal, postpartum) O92.79
Calabar swelling B74.3
Calcaneal spur — *see* Spur, bone, calcaneal
Calcaneo-apophysitis M92.8
Calcareous — *see* condition
Calcicosis J62.8
Calciferol (vitamin D) deficiency E55.9
 with rickets E55.0
Calcification
 adrenal (capsule) (gland) E27.49
  tuberculous E35 [B90.8]
 aorta I70.0
 artery (annular) — *see* Arteriosclerosis
 auricle (ear) — *see* Disorder, pinna, specified type NEC
 basal ganglia G23.8
 bladder N32.89
  due to Schistosoma hematobium B65.0
 brain (cortex) — *see* Calcification, cerebral
 bronchus J98.09
 bursa M71.40
  ankle M71.47- ☑
  elbow M71.42- ☑
  foot M71.47- ☑
  hand M71.44- ☑
  hip M71.45- ☑
  knee M71.46- ☑
  multiple sites M71.49
  shoulder M75.3- ☑
  specified site NEC M71.48
  wrist M71.43- ☑

Calcification — *continued*
 cardiac — *see* Degeneration, myocardial
 cerebral (cortex) G93.89
  artery I67.2
 cervix (uteri) N88.8
 choroid plexus G93.89
 conjunctiva — *see* Concretion, conjunctiva
 corpora cavernosa (penis) N48.89
 cortex (brain) — *see* Calcification, cerebral
 dental pulp (nodular) K04.2
 dentinal papilla K00.4
 fallopian tube N83.8
 falx cerebri G96.19
 gallbladder K82.8
 general E83.59
 heart (*see also* Degeneration, myocardial)
  valve — *see* Endocarditis
 idiopathic infantile arterial (IIAC) Q28.8
 intervertebral cartilage or disc (postinfective) — *see* Disorder, disc, specified NEC
 intracranial — *see* Calcification, cerebral
 joint — *see* Disorder, joint, specified type NEC
 kidney N28.89
  tuberculous N29 [B90.1]
 larynx (senile) J38.7
 lens — *see* Cataract, specified NEC
 lung (active) (postinfectional) J98.4
  tuberculous B90.9
 lymph gland or node (postinfectional) I89.8
  tuberculous (*see also* Tuberculosis, lymph gland) B90.8
 mammographic R92.1
 massive (paraplegic) — *see* Myositis, ossificans, in, quadriplegia
 medial — *see* Arteriosclerosis, extremities
 meninges (cerebral) (spinal) G96.19
 metastatic E83.59
 Mönckeberg's — *see* Arteriosclerosis, extremities
 muscle M61.9
  due to burns — *see* Myositis, ossificans, in, burns
  paralytic — *see* Myositis, ossificans, in, quadriplegia
  specified type NEC M61.40
   ankle M61.47- ☑
   foot M61.47- ☑
   forearm M61.43- ☑
   hand M61.44- ☑
   lower leg M61.46- ☑
   multiple sites M61.49
   pelvic region M61.45- ☑
   shoulder region M61.41- ☑
   specified site NEC M61.48
   thigh M61.45- ☑
   upper arm M61.42- ☑
 myocardium, myocardial — *see* Degeneration, myocardial
 ovary N83.8
 pancreas K86.8
 penis N48.89
 periarticular — *see* Disorder, joint, specified type NEC
 pericardium (*see also* Pericarditis) I31.1
 pineal gland E34.8
 pleura J94.8
  postinfectional J94.8
  tuberculous NEC B90.9
 pulpal (dental) (nodular) K04.2
 sclera H15.89
 spleen D73.89
 subcutaneous L94.2
 suprarenal (capsule) (gland) E27.49
 tendon (sheath) (*see also* Tenosynovitis, specified type NEC)
  with bursitis, synovitis or tenosynovitis — *see* Tendinitis, calcific
 trachea J39.8
 ureter N28.89
 uterus N85.8
 vitreous — *see* Deposit, crystalline
Calcified — *see* Calcification
Calcinosis (interstitial) (tumoral) (universalis) E83.59
 with Raynaud's phenomenon, esophageal dysfunction, sclerodactyly, telangiectasia (CREST syndrome) M34.1
 circumscripta (skin) L94.2
 cutis L94.2
Calciphylaxis (*see also* Calcification, by site) E83.59
Calcium
 deposits — *see* Calcification, by site

Calcium — *continued*
 metabolism disorder E83.50
 salts or soaps in vitreous — *see* Deposit, crystalline
Calciuria R82.99
Calculi — *see* Calculus
Calculosis, intrahepatic — *see* Calculus, bile duct
Calculus, calculi, calculous
 ampulla of Vater — *see* Calculus, bile duct
 anuria (impacted) (recurrent) (*see also* Calculus, urinary) N20.9
 appendix K38.1
 bile duct (common) (hepatic) K80.50
  with
   calculus of gallbladder — *see* Calculus, gallbladder and bile duct
   cholangitis K80.30
    with
     cholecystitis — *see* Calculus, bile duct, with cholecystitis
     obstruction K80.31
    acute K80.32
     with
      chronic cholangitis K80.36
       with obstruction K80.37
      obstruction K80.33
    chronic K80.34
     with
      acute cholangitis K80.36
       with obstruction K80.37
      obstruction K80.35
   cholecystitis (with cholangitis) K80.40
    with obstruction K80.41
    acute K80.42
     with
      chronic cholecystitis K80.46
       with obstruction K80.47
      obstruction K80.43
    chronic K80.44
     with
      acute cholecystitis K80.46
       with obstruction K80.47
      obstruction K80.45
   obstruction K80.51
 biliary (*see also* Calculus, gallbladder)
  specified NEC K80.80
   with obstruction K80.81
 bilirubin, multiple — *see* Calculus, gallbladder
 bladder (encysted) (impacted) (urinary) (diverticulum) N21.0
 bronchus J98.09
 calyx (kidney) (renal) — *see* Calculus, kidney
 cholesterol (pure) (solitary) — *see* Calculus, gallbladder
 common duct (bile) — *see* Calculus, bile duct
 conjunctiva — *see* Concretion, conjunctiva
 cystic N21.0
  duct — *see* Calculus, gallbladder
 dental (subgingival) (supragingival) K03.6
 diverticulum
  bladder N21.0
  kidney N20.0
 epididymis N50.8
 gallbladder K80.20
  with
   bile duct calculus — *see* Calculus, gallbladder and bile duct
   cholecystitis K80.10
    with obstruction K80.11
    acute K80.00
     with
      chronic cholecystitis K80.12
       with obstruction K80.13
      obstruction K80.01
    chronic K80.10
     with
      acute cholecystitis K80.12
       with obstruction K80.13
      obstruction K80.11
   specified NEC K80.18
    with obstruction K80.19
  obstruction K80.21
 gallbladder and bile duct K80.70
  with
   cholecystitis K80.60
    with obstruction K80.61
    acute K80.62
     with
      chronic cholecystitis K80.66
       with obstruction K80.67

Calculus, calculi, calculous — *continued*
  gallbladder and bile duct — *continued*
    with — *continued*
      cholecystitis — *continued*
        acute — *continued*
          with — *continued*
            obstruction K80.63
        chronic K80.64
          with
            acute cholecystitis K80.66
              with obstruction K80.67
            obstruction K80.65
        obstruction K80.71
  hepatic (duct) — *see* Calculus, bile duct
  ileal conduit N21.8
  intestinal (impaction) (obstruction) K56.49
  kidney (impacted) (multiple) (pelvis) (recurrent)
    (staghorn) N20.0
    with calculus, ureter N20.2
    congenital Q63.8
  lacrimal passages — *see* Dacryolith
  liver (impacted) — *see* Calculus, bile duct
  lung J98.4
  mammographic R92.1
  nephritic (impacted) (recurrent) — *see* Calculus, kidney
  nose J34.89
  pancreas (duct) K86.8
  parotid duct or gland K11.5
  pelvis, encysted — *see* Calculus, kidney
  prostate N42.0
  pulmonary J98.4
  pyelitis (impacted) (recurrent) N20.0
    with hydronephrosis N13.2
  pyelonephritis (impacted) (recurrent) N20 ☑
    with hydronephrosis N13.2
  renal (impacted) (recurrent) — *see* Calculus, kidney
  salivary (duct) (gland) K11.5
  seminal vesicle N50.8
  staghorn — *see* Calculus, kidney
  Stensen's duct K11.5
  stomach K31.89
  sublingual duct or gland K11.5
    congenital Q38.4
  submandibular duct, gland or region K11.5
  submaxillary duct, gland or region K11.5
  suburethral N21.8
  tonsil J35.8
  tooth, teeth (subgingival) (supragingival) K03.6
  tunica vaginalis N50.8
  ureter (impacted) (recurrent) N20.1
    with calculus, kidney N20.2
      with hydronephrosis N13.2
        with infection N13.6
  urethra (impacted) N21.1
  urinary (duct) (impacted) (passage) (tract) N20.9
    with hydronephrosis N13.2
      with infection N13.6
    in (due to)
    lower N21.9
      specified NEC N21.8
  vagina N89.8
  vesical (impacted) N21.0
  Wharton's duct K11.5
  xanthine E79.8 [N22]
Calicectasis N28.89
Caliectasis N28.89
California
  disease B38.9
  encephalitis A83.5
Caligo cornea — *see* Opacity, cornea, central
Callositas, callosity (infected) L84
Callus (infected) L84
  bone — *see* Osteophyte
  excessive, following fracture — *code as* Sequelae of fracture
Calorie deficiency or malnutrition (*see also* Malnutrition) E46
Calvé-Perthes disease — *see* Legg-Calvé-Perthes disease
Calvé's disease — *see* Osteochondrosis, juvenile, spine
Calvities — *see* Alopecia, androgenic
Cameroon fever — *see* Malaria
Camptocormia (hysterical) F44.4
Camurati-Engelmann syndrome Q78.3
Canal (*see also* condition)
  atrioventricular common Q21.2
Canaliculitis (lacrimal) (acute) (subacute) H04.33- ☑
  Actinomyces A42.89

Canaliculitis — *continued*
  chronic H04.42- ☑
Canavan's disease E75.29
Canceled procedure (surgical) Z53.9
  because of
    contraindication Z53.09
      smoking Z53.01
    left against medical advice (AMA) Z53.21
    patient's decision Z53.20
      for reasons of belief or group pressure Z53.1
      specified reason NEC Z53.29
    specified reason NEC Z53.8
Cancer (*see also* Neoplasm, by site, malignant)
  bile duct type liver C22.1
  blood — *see* Leukemia
  breast (*see also* Neoplasm, breast, malignant)
    C50.91- ☑
  hepatocellular C22.0
  lung (*see also* Neoplasm, lung, malignant) C34.90
  ovarian (*see also* Neoplasm ovary, malignant) C56.9
  unspecified site (primary) C80.1
Cancer (o)**phobia** F45.29
Cancerous — *see* Neoplasm, malignant, by site
Cancrum oris A69.0
Candidiasis, candidal B37.9
  balanitis B37.42
  bronchitis B37.1
  cheilitis B37.83
  congenital P37.5
  cystitis B37.41
  disseminated B37.7
  endocarditis B37.6
  enteritis B37.82
  esophagitis B37.81
  intertrigo B37.2
  lung B37.1
  meningitis B37.5
  mouth B37.0
  nails B37.2
  neonatal P37.5
  onychia B37.2
  oral B37.0
  osteomyelitis B37.89
  otitis externa B37.84
  paronychia B37.2
  perionyxis B37.2
  pneumonia B37.1
  proctitis B37.82
  pulmonary B37.1
  pyelonephritis B37.49
  sepsis B37.7
  skin B37.2
  specified site NEC B37.89
  stomatitis B37.0
  systemic B37.7
  urethritis B37.41
  urogenital site NEC B37.49
  vagina B37.3
  vulva B37.3
  vulvovaginitis B37.3
Candidid L30.2
Candidosis — *see* Candidiasis
Candiru infection or infestation B88.8
Canities (premature) L67.1
  congenital Q84.2
Canker (mouth) (sore) K12.0
  rash A38.9
Cannabinosis J66.2
Canton fever A75.9
Cantrell's syndrome Q87.89
Capillariasis (intestinal) B81.1
  hepatic B83.8
Capillary — *see* condition
Caplan's syndrome — *see* Rheumatoid, lung
Capsule — *see* condition
Capsulitis (joint) (*see also* Enthesopathy)
  adhesive (shoulder) M75.0- ☑
  hepatic K65.8
  labyrinthine — *see* Otosclerosis, specified NEC
  thyroid E06.9
Caput
  crepitus Q75.8
  medusae I86.8
  succedaneum P12.81
Car sickness T75.3 ☑
Carapata (disease) A68.0
Carate — *see* Pinta

Carbon lung J60
Carbuncle L02.93
  abdominal wall L02.231
  anus K61.0
  auditory canal, external — *see* Abscess, ear, external
  auricle ear — *see* Abscess, ear, external
  axilla L02.43- ☑
  back (any part) L02.232
  breast N61
  buttock L02.33
  cheek (external) L02.03
  chest wall L02.233
  chin L02.03
  corpus cavernosum N48.21
  ear (any part) (external) (middle) — *see* Abscess, ear, external
  external auditory canal — *see* Abscess, ear, external
  eyelid — *see* Abscess, eyelid
  face NEC L02.03
  femoral (region) — *see* Carbuncle, lower limb
  finger — *see* Carbuncle, hand
  flank L02.231
  foot L02.63- ☑
  forehead L02.03
  genital — *see* Abscess, genital
  gluteal (region) L02.33
  groin L02.234
  hand L02.53- ☑
  head NEC L02.831
  heel — *see* Carbuncle, foot
  hip — *see* Carbuncle, lower limb
  kidney — *see* Abscess, kidney
  knee — *see* Carbuncle, lower limb
  labium (majus) (minus) N76.4
  lacrimal
    gland — *see* Dacryoadenitis
    passages (duct) (sac) — *see* Inflammation, lacrimal, passages, acute
  leg — *see* Carbuncle, lower limb
  lower limb L02.43- ☑
  malignant A22.0
  navel L02.236
  neck L02.13
  nose (external) (septum) J34.0
  orbit, orbital — *see* Abscess, orbit
  palmar (space) — *see* Carbuncle, hand
  partes posteriores L02.33
  pectoral region L02.233
  penis N48.21
  perineum L02.235
  pinna — *see* Abscess, ear, external
  popliteal — *see* Carbuncle, lower limb
  scalp L02.831
  seminal vesicle N49.0
  shoulder — *see* Carbuncle, upper limb
  specified site NEC L02.838
  temple (region) L02.03
  thumb — *see* Carbuncle, hand
  toe — *see* Carbuncle, foot
  trunk L02.239
    abdominal wall L02.231
    back L02.232
    chest wall L02.233
    groin L02.234
    perineum L02.235
    umbilicus L02.236
  umbilicus L02.236
  upper limb L02.43- ☑
  urethra N34.0
  vulva N76.4
Carbunculus — *see* Carbuncle
Carcinoid (tumor) — *see* Tumor, carcinoid
Carcinoidosis E34.0
Carcinoma (malignant) (*see also* Neoplasm, by site, malignant)
  acidophil
    specified site — *see* Neoplasm, malignant, by site
    unspecified site C75.1
  acidophil-basophil, mixed
    specified site — *see* Neoplasm, malignant, by site
    unspecified site C75.1
  adnexal (skin) — *see* Neoplasm, skin, malignant
  adrenal cortical C74.0- ☑
  alveolar — *see* Neoplasm, lung, malignant
    cell — *see* Neoplasm, lung, malignant
  ameloblastic C41.1
    upper jaw (bone) C41.0

Carcinoma — *continued*
  apocrine
    breast — *see* Neoplasm, breast, malignant
    specified site NEC — *see* Neoplasm, skin, malignant
    unspecified site C44.99
  basal cell (pigmented) (*see also* Neoplasm, skin, malignant) C44.91
    fibro-epithelial — *see* Neoplasm, skin, malignant
    morphea — *see* Neoplasm, skin, malignant
    multicentric — *see* Neoplasm, skin, malignant
  basaloid
  basal-squamous cell, mixed — *see* Neoplasm, skin, malignant
  basophil
    specified site — *see* Neoplasm, malignant, by site
    unspecified site C75.1
  basophil-acidophil, mixed
    specified site — *see* Neoplasm, malignant, by site
    unspecified site C75.1
  basosquamous — *see* Neoplasm, skin, malignant
  bile duct
    with hepatocellular, mixed C22.0
    liver C22.1
    specified site NEC — *see* Neoplasm, malignant, by site
    unspecified site C22.1
  branchial or branchiogenic C10.4
  bronchial or bronchogenic — *see* Neoplasm, lung, malignant
  bronchiolar — *see* Neoplasm, lung, malignant
  bronchioloalveolar — *see* Neoplasm, lung, malignant
  C cell
    specified site — *see* Neoplasm, malignant, by site
    unspecified site C73
  ceruminous C44.29- ☑
  cervix uteri
    in situ D06.9
      endocervix D06.0
      exocervix D06.1
      specified site NEC D06.7
  chorionic
    specified site — *see* Neoplasm, malignant, by site
    unspecified site
      female C58
      male C62.90
  chromophobe
    specified site — *see* Neoplasm, malignant, by site
    unspecified site C75.1
  cloacogenic
    specified site — *see* Neoplasm, malignant, by site
    unspecified site C21.2
  diffuse type
    specified site — *see* Neoplasm, malignant, by site
    unspecified site C16.9
  duct (cell)
    with Paget's disease — *see* Neoplasm, breast, malignant
    infiltrating
      with lobular carcinoma (in situ)
        specified site — *see* Neoplasm, malignant, by site
        unspecified site (female) C50.91- ☑
          male C50.92- ☑
      specified site — *see* Neoplasm, malignant, by site
      unspecified site (female) C50.91- ☑
        male C50.92- ☑
  ductal
    with lobular
      specified site — *see* Neoplasm, malignant, by site
      unspecified site (female) C50.91- ☑
        male C50.92- ☑
  ductular, infiltrating
    specified site — *see* Neoplasm, malignant, by site
    unspecified site (female) C50.91- ☑
      male C50.92- ☑
  embryonal
    liver C22.7
  endometrioid
    specified site — *see* Neoplasm, malignant, by site
    unspecified site
      female C56.9
      male C61
  eosinophil
    specified site — *see* Neoplasm, malignant, by site
    unspecified site C75.1

Carcinoma — *continued*
  epidermoid (*see also* Neoplasm, skin, malignant)
    in situ, Bowen's type — *see* Neoplasm, skin, in situ
  fibroepithelial, basal cell — *see* Neoplasm, skin, malignant
  follicular
    with papillary (mixed) C73
    moderately differentiated C73
    pure follicle C73
    specified site — *see* Neoplasm, malignant, by site
    trabecular C73
    unspecified site C73
    well differentiated C73
  generalized, with unspecified primary site C80.0
  glycogen-rich — *see* Neoplasm, breast, malignant
  granulosa cell C56- ☑
  hepatic cell C22.0
  hepatocellular C22.0
    with bile duct, mixed C22.0
    fibrolamellar C22.0
  hepatocholangiolitic C22.0
  Hurthle cell C73
  in
    adenomatous
      polyposis coli C18.9
    pleomorphic adenoma — *see* Neoplasm, salivary glands, malignant
    situ — *see* Carcinoma-in-situ
  infiltrating
    duct
      with lobular
        specified site — *see* Neoplasm, malignant, by site
        unspecified site (female) C50.91- ☑
          male C50.92- ☑
      with Paget's disease — *see* Neoplasm, breast, malignant
      specified site — *see* Neoplasm, malignant
      unspecified site (female) C50- ☑
        male C50.92- ☑
    ductular
      specified site — *see* Neoplasm, malignant
      unspecified site (female) C50.91- ☑
        male C50.92- ☑
    lobular
      specified site — *see* Neoplasm, malignant
      unspecified site (female) C50.91- ☑
        male C50.92- ☑
  inflammatory
    specified site — *see* Neoplasm, malignant
    unspecified site (female) C50.91- ☑
      male C50.92- ☑
  intestinal type
    specified site — *see* Neoplasm, malignant, by site
    unspecified site C16.9
  intracystic
    noninfiltrating — *see* Neoplasm, in situ, by site
  intraductal (noninfiltrating)
    with Paget's disease — *see* Neoplasm, breast, malignant
    breast D05.1- ☑
    papillary
      with invasion
        specified site — *see* Neoplasm, malignant, by site
        unspecified site (female) C50.91- ☑
          male C50.92- ☑
      breast D05.1- ☑
      specified site NEC — *see* Neoplasm, in situ, by site
      unspecified site (female) D05.1- ☑
    specified site NEC — *see* Neoplasm, in situ, by site
    unspecified site (female) D05.1- ☑
  intraepidermal — *see* Neoplasm, in situ
    squamous cell, Bowen's type — *see* Neoplasm, skin, in situ
  intraepithelial — *see* Neoplasm, in situ, by site
    squamous cell — *see* Neoplasm, in situ, by site
  intraosseous C41.1
    upper jaw (bone) C41.0
  islet cell
    with exocrine, mixed
      specified site — *see* Neoplasm, malignant, by site
      unspecified site C25.9
    pancreas C25.4

Carcinoma — *continued*
  islet cell — *continued*
    specified site NEC — *see* Neoplasm, malignant, by site
    unspecified site C25.4
  juvenile, breast — *see* Neoplasm, breast, malignant
  large cell
    small cell
      specified site — *see* Neoplasm, malignant, by site
      unspecified site C34.90
  Leydig cell (testis)
    specified site — *see* Neoplasm, malignant, by site
    unspecified site
      female C56.9
      male C62.90
  lipid-rich (female) C50.91- ☑
    male C50.92- ☑
  liver cell C22.0
  liver NEC C22.7
  lobular (infiltrating)
    with intraductal
      specified site — *see* Neoplasm, malignant, by site
      unspecified site (female) C50.91- ☑
        male C50.92- ☑
    noninfiltrating
      breast D05.0- ☑
      specified site NEC — *see* Neoplasm, in situ, by site
      unspecified site D05.0- ☑
    specified site — *see* Neoplasm, malignant, by site
    unspecified site (female) C50.91- ☑
      male C50.92- ☑
  medullary
    with
      amyloid stroma
        specified site — *see* Neoplasm, malignant, by site
        unspecified site C73
      lymphoid stroma
        specified site — *see* Neoplasm, malignant, by site
        unspecified site (female) C50.91- ☑
          male C50.92- ☑
  Merkel cell C4A.9 (*following* C43)
    anal margin C4A.51 (*following* C43)
    anal skin C4A.51 (*following* C43)
    canthus C4A.1- ☑ (*following* C43)
    ear and external auricular canal C4A.2- ☑ (*following* C43)
    external auricular canal C4A.2- ☑ (*following* C43)
    eyelid, including canthus C4A.1- ☑ (*following* C43)
    face C4A.30 (*following* C43)
      specified NEC C4A.39 (*following* C43)
    hip C4A.7- ☑ (*following* C43)
    lip C4A.0 (*following* C43)
    lower limb, including hip C4A.7- ☑ (*following* C43)
    neck C4A.4 (*following* C43)
    nodal presentation C7B.1 (*following* C75)
    nose C4A.31 (*following* C43)
    overlapping sites C4A.8 (*following* C43)
    perianal skin C4A.51 (*following* C43)
    scalp C4A.4 (*following* C43)
    secondary C7B.1 (*following* C75)
    shoulder C4A.6- ☑ (*following* C43)
    skin of breast C4A.52 (*following* C43)
    trunk NEC C4A.59 (*following* C43)
    upper limb, including shoulder C4A.6- ☑ (*following* C43)
    visceral metastatic C7B.1 (*following* C75)
  metastatic — *see* Neoplasm, secondary, by site
  metatypical — *see* Neoplasm, skin, malignant
  morphea, basal cell — *see* Neoplasm, skin, malignant
  mucoid
    cell
      specified site — *see* Neoplasm, malignant, by site
      unspecified site C75.1
  neuroendocrine (*see also* Tumor, neuroendocrine)
    high grade, any site C7A.1 (*following* C75)
    poorly differentiated, any site C7A.1 (*following* C75)
  nonencapsulated sclerosing C73
  noninfiltrating
    intracystic — *see* Neoplasm, in situ, by site
    intraductal
      breast D05.1- ☑

☑ **Additional Character Required — Refer to the Tabular List for Character Selection**   ▼ Subterms under main terms may continue to next column or page

Carcinoma — *continued*
  noninfiltrating — *continued*
    intraductal — *continued*
      papillary
        breast D05.1- ☑
        specified site NEC — *see* Neoplasm, in situ, by site
        unspecified site D05.1- ☑
      specified site — *see* Neoplasm, in situ, by site
      unspecified site D05.1- ☑
    lobular
      breast D05.0- ☑
      specified site NEC — *see* Neoplasm, in situ, by site
      unspecified site (female) D05.0- ☑
  oat cell
    specified site — *see* Neoplasm, malignant, by site
    unspecified site C34.90
  odontogenic C41.1
    upper jaw (bone) C41.0
  papillary
    with follicular (mixed) C73
    follicular variant C73
    intraductal (noninfiltrating)
      with invasion
        specified site — *see* Neoplasm, malignant, by site
        unspecified site (female) C50.91- ☑
          male C50.92- ☑
      breast D05.1- ☑
      specified site NEC — *see* Neoplasm, in situ, by site
      unspecified site D05.1- ☑
    serous
      specified site — *see* Neoplasm, malignant, by site
      surface
        specified site — *see* Neoplasm, malignant, by site
        unspecified site C56.9
      unspecified site C56.9
  papillocystic
    specified site — *see* Neoplasm, malignant, by site
    unspecified site C56.9
  parafollicular cell
    specified site — *see* Neoplasm, malignant, by site
    unspecified site C73
  pilomatrix — *see* Neoplasm, skin, malignant
  pseudomucinous
    specified site — *see* Neoplasm, malignant, by site
    unspecified site C56.9
  renal cell C64- ☑
  Schmincke — *see* Neoplasm, nasopharynx, malignant
  Schneiderian
    specified site — *see* Neoplasm, malignant, by site
    unspecified site C30.0
  sebaceous — *see* Neoplasm, skin, malignant
  secondary (*see also* Neoplasm, secondary, by site)
    Merkel cell C7B.1 (*following* C75)
  secretory, breast — *see* Neoplasm, breast, malignant
  serous
    papillary
      specified site — *see* Neoplasm, malignant, by site
      unspecified site C56.9
    surface, papillary
      specified site — *see* Neoplasm, malignant, by site
      unspecified site C56.9
  Sertoli cell
    specified site — *see* Neoplasm, malignant, by site
    unspecified site C62.90
      female C56.9
      male C62.90
  skin appendage — *see* Neoplasm, skin, malignant
  small cell
    fusiform cell
      specified site — *see* Neoplasm, malignant, by site
      unspecified site C34.90
    intermediate cell
      specified site — *see* Neoplasm, malignant, by site
      unspecified site C34.90
    large cell
      specified site — *see* Neoplasm, malignant, by site

Carcinoma — *continued*
  small cell — *continued*
    large cell — *continued*
      unspecified site C34.90
    solid
      with amyloid stroma
        specified site — *see* Neoplasm, malignant, by site
        unspecified site C73
      microinvasive
        specified site — *see* Neoplasm, malignant, by site
        unspecified site C53.9
  sweat gland — *see* Neoplasm, skin, malignant
  theca cell C56.- ☑
  thymic C37
  unspecified site (primary) C80.1
  water-clear cell C75.0
Carcinoma-in-situ (*see also* Neoplasm, in situ, by site)
  breast NOS D05.9- ☑
    specified type NEC D05.8- ☑
  epidermoid (*see also* Neoplasm, in situ, by site)
    with questionable stromal invasion
      cervix D06.9
      specified site NEC — *see* Neoplasm, in situ, by site
      unspecified site D06.9
    Bowen's type — *see* Neoplasm, skin, in situ
  intraductal
    breast D05.1- ☑
    specified site NEC — *see* Neoplasm, in situ, by site
    unspecified site D05.1- ☑
  lobular
    with
      infiltrating duct
        breast (female) C50.91- ☑
          male C50.92- ☑
        specified site NEC — *see* Neoplasm, malignant
        unspecified site (female) C50.91- ☑
          male C50.92- ☑
      intraductal
        breast D05.8- ☑
        specified site NEC — *see* Neoplasm, in situ, by site
        unspecified site (female) D05.8- ☑
    breast D05.0- ☑
    specified site NEC — *see* Neoplasm, in situ, by site
    unspecified site D05.0- ☑
  squamous cell (*see also* Neoplasm, in situ, by site)
    with questionable stromal invasion
      cervix D06.9
      specified site NEC — *see* Neoplasm, in situ, by site
      unspecified site D06.9
Carcinomaphobia F45.29
Carcinomatosis C80.0
  peritonei C78.6
  unspecified site (primary) (secondary) C80.0
Carcinosarcoma — *see* Neoplasm, malignant, by site
  embryonal — *see* Neoplasm, malignant, by site
Cardia, cardial — *see* condition
Cardiac (*see also* condition)
  death, sudden — *see* Arrest, cardiac
  pacemaker
    in situ Z95.0
    management or adjustment Z45.018
  tamponade I31.4
Cardialgia — *see* Pain, precordial
Cardiectasis — *see* Hypertrophy, cardiac
Cardiochalasia K21.9
Cardiomalacia I51.5
Cardiomegalia glycogenica diffusa E74.02 [I43]
Cardiomegaly (*see also* Hypertrophy, cardiac)
  congenital Q24.8
  glycogen E74.02 [I43]
  idiopathic I51.7
Cardiomyoliposis I51.5
Cardiomyopathy (familial) (idiopathic) I42.9
  alcoholic I42.6
  amyloid E85.4 [I43]
  arteriosclerotic — *see* Disease, heart, ischemic, atherosclerotic
  beriberi E51.12
  cobalt-beer I42.6
  congenital I42.4
  congestive I42.0

Cardiomyopathy — *continued*
  constrictive NOS I42.5
  dilated I42.0
  due to
    alcohol I42.6
    beriberi E51.12
    cardiac glycogenosis E74.02 [I43]
    drugs I42.7
    external agents NEC I42.7
    Friedreich's ataxia G11.1
    myotonia atrophica G71.11 [I43]
    progressive muscular dystrophy G71.0
  glycogen storage E74.02 [I43]
  hypertensive — *see* Hypertension, heart
  hypertrophic (nonobstructive) I42.2
    obstructive I42.1
      congenital Q24.8
  in
    Chagas' disease (chronic) B57.2
      acute B57.0
    sarcoidosis D86.85
  ischemic I25.5
  metabolic E88.9 [I43]
    thyrotoxic E05.90 [I43]
      with thyroid storm E05.91 [I43]
  newborn I42.8
    congenital I42.4
  nutritional E63.9 [I43]
    beriberi E51.12
  obscure of Africa I42.8
  peripartum O90.3
  postpartum O90.3
  restrictive NEC I42.5
  rheumatic I09.0
  secondary I42.9
  stress induced I51.81
  takotsubo I51.81
  thyrotoxic E05.90 [I43]
    with thyroid storm E05.91 [I43]
  toxic NEC I42.7
  tuberculous A18.84
  viral B33.24
Cardionephritis — *see* Hypertension, cardiorenal
Cardionephropathy — *see* Hypertension, cardiorenal
Cardionephrosis — *see* Hypertension, cardiorenal
Cardiopathia nigra I27.0
Cardiopathy (*see also* Disease, heart) I51.9
  idiopathic I42.9
  mucopolysaccharidosis E76.3 [I52]
Cardiopericarditis — *see* Pericarditis
Cardiophobia F45.29
Cardiorenal — *see* condition
Cardiorrhexis — *see* Infarct, myocardium
Cardiosclerosis — *see* Disease, heart, ischemic, atherosclerotic
Cardiosis — *see* Disease, heart
Cardiospasm (esophagus) (reflex) (stomach) K22.0
  congenital Q39.5
    with megaesophagus Q39.5
Cardiostenosis — *see* Disease, heart
Cardiosymphysis I31.0
Cardiovascular — *see* condition
Carditis (acute) (bacterial) (chronic) (subacute) I51.89
  meningococcal A39.50
  rheumatic — *see* Disease, heart, rheumatic
  rheumatoid — *see* Rheumatoid, carditis
  viral B33.20
Care (of) (for) (following)
  child (routine) Z76.2
  family member (handicapped) (sick)
    creating problem for family Z63.6
    provided away from home for holiday relief Z75.5
    unavailable, due to
      absence (person rendering care) (sufferer) Z74.2
      inability (any reason) of person rendering care Z74.2
  foundling Z76.1
  holiday relief Z75.5
  improper — *see* Maltreatment
  lack of (at or after birth) (infant) — *see* Maltreatment, child, neglect
  lactating mother Z39.1
  palliative Z51.5
  postpartum
    immediately after delivery Z39.0
    routine follow-up Z39.2
  respite Z75.5

Care — *continued*
- unavailable, due to
  - absence of person rendering care Z74.2
  - inability (any reason) of person rendering care Z74.2
  - well-baby Z76.2
Caries
- bone NEC A18.03
- dental K02.9
  - arrested (coronal) (root) K02.3
  - chewing surface
    - limited to enamel K02.51
    - penetrating into dentin K02.52
    - penetrating into pulp K02.53
  - coronal surface
    - chewing surface
      - limited to enamel K02.51
      - penetrating into dentin K02.52
      - penetrating into pulp K02.53
    - pit and fissure surface
      - limited to enamel K02.51
      - penetrating into dentin K02.52
      - penetrating into pulp K02.53
    - smooth surface
      - limited to enamel K02.61
      - penetrating into dentin K02.62
      - penetrating into pulp K02.63
  - pit and fissure surface
    - limited to enamel K02.51
    - penetrating into dentin K02.52
    - penetrating into pulp K02.53
  - root K02.7
  - smooth surface
    - limited to enamel K02.61
    - penetrating into dentin K02.62
    - penetrating into pulp K02.63
- external meatus — *see* Disorder, ear, external, specified type NEC
- hip (tuberculous) A18.02
- initial (tooth)
  - chewing surface K02.51
  - pit and fissure surface K02.51
  - smooth surface K02.61
- knee (tuberculous) A18.02
- labyrinth H83.8 ☑
- limb NEC (tuberculous) A18.03
- mastoid process (chronic) — *see* Mastoiditis, chronic tuberculous A18.03
- middle ear H74.8 ☑
- nose (tuberculous) A18.03
- orbit (tuberculous) A18.03
- ossicles, ear — *see* Abnormal, ear ossicles
- petrous bone — *see* Petrositis
- root (dental) (tooth) K02.7
- sacrum (tuberculous) A18.01
- spine, spinal (column) (tuberculous) A18.01
- syphilitic A52.77
  - congenital (early) A50.02 [M90.80]
- tooth, teeth — *see* Caries, dental
- tuberculous A18.03
- vertebra (column) (tuberculous) A18.01
Carious teeth — *see* Caries, dental
Carneous mole O02.0
Carnitine insufficiency E71.40
Carotid body or sinus syndrome G90.01
Carotidynia G90.01
Carotinemia (dietary) E67.1
Carotinosis (cutis) (skin) E67.1
Carpal tunnel syndrome — *see* Syndrome, carpal tunnel
Carpenter's syndrome Q87.0
Carpopedal spasm — *see* Tetany
Carr-Barr-Plunkett syndrome Q97.1
Carrier (suspected) of
- amebiasis Z22.1
- bacterial disease NEC Z22.39
  - diphtheria Z22.2
  - intestinal infectious NEC Z22.1
    - typhoid Z22.0
  - meningococcal Z22.31
  - sexually transmitted Z22.4
  - specified NEC Z22.39
  - staphylococcal (Methicillin susceptible) Z22.321
    - Methicillin resistant Z22.322
  - streptococcal Z22.338
    - group B Z22.330
  - typhoid Z22.0
- cholera Z22.1
- diphtheria Z22.2

Carrier of — *continued*
- gastrointestinal pathogens NEC Z22.1
- genetic Z14.8
  - cystic fibrosis Z14.1
  - hemophilia A (asymptomatic) Z14.01
    - symptomatic Z14.02
- gonorrhea Z22.4
- HAA (hepatitis Australian-antigen) Z22.59
- HB (c)(s)-AG Z22.51
- hepatitis (viral) Z22.50
  - Australia-antigen (HAA) Z22.59
  - B surface antigen (HBsAg) Z22.51
    - with acute delta- (super)infection B17.0
  - C Z22.52
  - specified NEC Z22.59
- human T-cell lymphotropic virus type-1 (HTLV-1) infection Z22.6
- infectious organism Z22.9
  - specified NEC Z22.8
- meningococci Z22.31
- Salmonella typhosa Z22.0
- serum hepatitis — *see* Carrier, hepatitis
- staphylococci (Methicillin susceptible) Z22.321
  - Methicillin resistant Z22.322
- streptococci Z22.338
  - group B Z22.330
- syphilis Z22.4
- typhoid Z22.0
- venereal disease NEC Z22.4
Carrion's disease A44.0
Carter's relapsing fever (Asiatic) A68.1
Cartilage — *see* condition
Caruncle (inflamed)
- conjunctiva (acute) — *see* Conjunctivitis, acute
- labium (majus) (minus) N90.89
- lacrimal — *see* Inflammation, lacrimal, passages
- myrtiform N89.8
- urethral (benign) N36.2
Cascade stomach K31.2
Caseation lymphatic gland (tuberculous) A18.2
Cassidy (-Scholte) syndrome (malignant carcinoid) E34.0
Castellani's disease A69.8
Castration, traumatic, male S38.231 ☑
Casts in urine R82.99
Cat
- cry syndrome Q93.4
- ear Q17.3
- eye syndrome Q92.8
Catabolism, senile R54
Catalepsy (hysterical) F44.2
- schizophrenic F20.2
Cataplexy (idiopathic) — *see* Narcolepsy
Cataract (cortical) (immature) (incipient) H26.9
- with
  - neovascularization — *see* Cataract, complicated
- age-related — *see* Cataract, senile
- anterior
  - and posterior axial embryonal Q12.0
  - pyramidal Q12.0
- associated with
  - galactosemia E74.21 [H28]
  - myotonic disorders G71.19 [H28]
- blue Q12.0
- central Q12.0
- cerulean Q12.0
- complicated H26.20
  - with
    - neovascularization H26.21- ☑
    - ocular disorder H26.22- ☑
    - glaucomatous flecks H26.23- ☑
- congenital Q12.0
- coraliform Q12.0
- coronary Q12.0
- crystalline Q12.0
- diabetic — *see* Diabetes, cataract
- drug-induced H26.3- ☑
- due to
  - ocular disorder — *see* Cataract, complicated
  - radiation H26.8
- electric H26.8
- extraction status Z98.4- ☑
- glass-blower's H26.8
- heat ray H26.8
- heterochromic — *see* Cataract, complicated
- hypermature — *see* Cataract, senile, morgagnian type
- in (due to)
  - chronic iridocyclitis — *see* Cataract, complicated

Cataract — *continued*
- in — *continued*
  - diabetes — *see* Diabetes, cataract
  - endocrine disease E34.9 [H28]
  - eye disease — *see* Cataract, complicated
  - hypoparathyroidism E20.9 [H28]
  - malnutrition-dehydration E46 [H28]
  - metabolic disease E88.9 [H28]
  - myotonic disorders G71.19 [H28]
  - nutritional disease E63.9 [H28]
- infantile — *see* Cataract, presenile
- irradiational — *see* Cataract, specified NEC
- juvenile — *see* Cataract, presenile
- malnutrition-dehydration E46 [H28]
- morgagnian — *see* Cataract, senile, morgagnian type
- myotonic G71.19 [H28]
- myxedema E03.9 [H28]
- nuclear
  - embryonal Q12.0
  - sclerosis — *see* Cataract, senile, nuclear
- presenile H26.00- ☑
  - combined forms H26.06- ☑
  - cortical H26.01- ☑
  - lamellar — *see* Cataract, presenile, cortical
  - nuclear H26.03- ☑
  - specified NEC H26.09
  - subcapsular polar (anterior) H26.04- ☑
    - posterior H26.05- ☑
  - zonular — *see* Cataract, presenile, cortical
- secondary H26.40
  - Soemmering's ring H26.41- ☑
  - specified NEC H26.49- ☑
  - to eye disease — *see* Cataract, complicated
- senile H25.9
  - brunescens — *see* Cataract, senile, nuclear
  - combined forms H25.81- ☑
  - coronary — *see* Cataract, senile, incipient
  - cortical H25.01- ☑
  - hypermature — *see* Cataract, senile, morgagnian type
  - incipient (mature) (total) H25.09- ☑
    - cortical — *see* Cataract, senile, cortical
    - subcapsular — *see* Cataract, senile, subcapsular
  - morgagnian type (hypermature) H25.2- ☑
  - nuclear (sclerosis) H25.1- ☑
  - polar subcapsular (anterior) (posterior) — *see* Cataract, senile, incipient
  - punctate — *see* Cataract, senile, incipient
  - specified NEC H25.89
  - subcapsular polar (anterior) H25.03- ☑
    - posterior H25.04- ☑
- snowflake — *see* Diabetes, cataract
- specified NEC H26.8
- toxic — *see* Cataract, drug-induced
- traumatic H26.10- ☑
  - localized H26.11- ☑
  - partially resolved H26.12- ☑
  - total H26.13- ☑
- zonular (perinuclear) Q12.0
Cataracta (*see also* Cataract)
- brunescens — *see* Cataract, senile, nuclear
- centralis pulverulenta Q12.0
- cerulea Q12.0
- complicata — *see* Cataract, complicated
- congenita Q12.0
- coralliformis Q12.0
- coronaria Q12.0
- diabetic — *see* Diabetes, cataract
- membranacea
  - accreta — *see* Cataract, secondary
  - congenita Q12.0
- nigra — *see* Cataract, senile, nuclear
- sunflower — *see* Cataract, complicated
Catarrh, catarrhal (acute) (febrile) (infectious) (inflammation) (*see also* condition) J00
- bronchial — *see* Bronchitis
- chest — *see* Bronchitis
- chronic J31.0
- due to congenital syphilis A50.03
- enteric — *see* Enteritis
- eustachian H68.009
- fauces — *see* Pharyngitis
- gastrointestinal — *see* Enteritis
- gingivitis K05.00
  - nonplaque induced K05.01
  - plaque induced K05.00
- hay — *see* Fever, hay

☑ Additional Character Required — Refer to the Tabular List for Character Selection   ▽ Subterms under main terms may continue to next column or page

Catarrh, catarrhal — *continued*
  intestinal — *see* Enteritis
  larynx, chronic J37.0
  liver B15.9
    with hepatic coma B15.0
  lung — *see* Bronchitis
  middle ear, chronic — *see* Otitis, media, nonsuppurative, chronic, serous
  mouth K12.1
  nasal (chronic) — *see* Rhinitis
  nasobronchial J31.1
  nasopharyngeal (chronic) J31.1
    acute J00
  pulmonary — *see* Bronchitis
  spring (eye) (vernal) — *see* Conjunctivitis, acute, atopic
  summer (hay) — *see* Fever, hay
  throat J31.2
  tubotympanal (*see also* Otitis, media, nonsuppurative)
    chronic — *see* Otitis, media, nonsuppurative, chronic, serous
Catatonia (schizophrenic) F20.2
Catatonic
  disorder due to known physiologic condition F06.1
  schizophrenia F20.2
  stupor R40.1
Cat-scratch (*see also* Abrasion)
  disease or fever A28.1
Cauda equina — *see* condition
Cauliflower ear M95.1- ☑
Causalgia (upper limb) G56.4- ☑
  lower limb G57.7- ☑
Cause
  external, general effects T75.89 ☑
Caustic burn — *see* Corrosion, by site
Cavare's disease (familial periodic paralysis) G72.3
Cave-in, injury
  crushing (severe) — *see* Crush
  suffocation — *see* Asphyxia, traumatic, due to low oxygen, due to cave-in
Cavernitis (penis) N48.29
Cavernositis N48.29
Cavernous — *see* condition
Cavitation of lung (*see also* Tuberculosis, pulmonary)
  nontuberculous J98.4
Cavities, dental — *see* Caries, dental
Cavity
  lung — *see* Cavitation of lung
  optic papilla Q14.2
  pulmonary — *see* Cavitation of lung
Cavovarus foot, congenital Q66.1
Cavus foot (congenital) Q66.7
  acquired — *see* Deformity, limb, foot, specified NEC
Cazenave's disease L10.2
Cecitis K52.9
  with perforation, peritonitis, or rupture K65.8
Cecum — *see* condition
Celiac
  artery compression syndrome I77.4
  disease K90.0
  infantilism K90.0
Cell(s), **cellular** (*see also* condition)
  in urine R82.99
Cellulitis (diffuse) (phlegmonous) (septic) (suppurative) L03.90
  abdominal wall L03.311
  anaerobic A48.0
  ankle — *see* Cellulitis, lower limb
  anus K61.0
  arm — *see* Cellulitis, upper limb
  auricle (ear) — *see* Cellulitis, ear
  axilla L03.11- ☑
  back (any part) L03.312
  broad ligament
    acute N73.0
  buttock L03.317
  cervical (meaning neck) L03.221
  cervix (uteri) — *see* Cervicitis
  cheek (external) L03.211
    internal K12.2
  chest wall L03.313
  chronic L03.90
  clostridial A48.0
  corpus cavernosum N48.22
  digit
    finger — *see* Cellulitis, finger
    toe — *see* Cellulitis, toe

Cellulitis — *continued*
  Douglas' cul-de-sac or pouch
    acute N73.0
  drainage site (following operation) T81.4 ☑
  ear (external) H60.1- ☑
  eosinophilic (granulomatous) L98.3
  erysipelatous — *see* Erysipelas
  external auditory canal — *see* Cellulitis, ear
  eyelid — *see* Abscess, eyelid
  face NEC L03.211
  finger (intrathecal) (periosteal) (subcutaneous) (subcuticular) L03.01- ☑
  foot — *see* Cellulitis, lower limb
  gangrenous — *see* Gangrene
  genital organ NEC
    female (external) N76.4
    male N49.9
      multiple sites N49.8
      specified NEC N49.8
  gluteal (region) L03.317
  gonococcal A54.89
  groin L03.314
  hand — *see* Cellulitis, upper limb
  head NEC L03.811
    face (any part, except ear, eye and nose) L03.211
  heel — *see* Cellulitis, lower limb
  hip — *see* Cellulitis, lower limb
  jaw (region) L03.211
  knee — *see* Cellulitis, lower limb
  labium (majus) (minus) — *see* Vulvitis
  lacrimal passages — *see* Inflammation, lacrimal, passages
  larynx J38.7
  leg — *see* Cellulitis, lower limb
  lip K13.0
  lower limb L03.11- ☑
    toe — *see* Cellulitis, toe
  mouth (floor) K12.2
  multiple sites, so stated L03.90
  nasopharynx J39.1
  navel L03.316
    newborn P38.9
      with mild hemorrhage P38.1
      without hemorrhage P38.9
  neck (region) L03.221
  nose (septum) (external) J34.0
  orbit, orbital H05.01- ☑
  palate (soft) K12.2
  pectoral (region) L03.313
  pelvis, pelvic (chronic)
    female (*see also* Disease, pelvis, inflammatory) N73.2
      acute N73.0
    following ectopic or molar pregnancy O08.0
    male K65.0
  penis N48.22
  perineal, perineum L03.315
  perirectal K61.1
  peritonsillar J36
  periurethral N34.0
  periuterine (*see also* Disease, pelvis, inflammatory) N73.2
    acute N73.0
  pharynx J39.1
  rectum K61.1
  retroperitoneal K68.9
  round ligament
    acute N73.0
  scalp (any part) L03.811
  scrotum N49.2
  seminal vesicle N49.0
  shoulder — *see* Cellulitis, upper limb
  specified site NEC L03.818
  submandibular (region) (space) (triangle) K12.2
    gland K11.3
  submaxillary (region) K12.2
    gland K11.3
  thigh — *see* Cellulitis, lower limb
  thumb (intrathecal) (periosteal) (subcutaneous) (subcuticular) — *see* Cellulitis, finger
  toe (intrathecal) (periosteal) (subcutaneous) (subcuticular) L03.03- ☑
  tonsil J36
  trunk L03.319
    abdominal wall L03.311
    back (any part) L03.312
    buttock L03.317
    chest wall L03.313

Cellulitis — *continued*
  trunk — *continued*
    groin L03.314
    perineal, perineum L03.315
    umbilicus L03.316
  tuberculous (primary) A18.4
  umbilicus L03.316
  upper limb L03.11- ☑
    axilla — *see* Cellulitis, axilla
    finger — *see* Cellulitis, finger
    thumb — *see* Cellulitis, finger
  vaccinal T88.0 ☑
  vocal cord J38.3
  vulva — *see* Vulvitis
  wrist — *see* Cellulitis, upper limb
Cementoblastoma, benign — *see* Cyst, calcifying odontogenic
Cementoma — *see* Cyst, calcifying odontogenic
Cementoperiostitis — *see* Periodontitis
Cementosis K03.4
Central auditory processing disorder H93.25
Central pain syndrome G89.0
Cephalematocele, cephal (o)hematocele
  newborn P52.8
    birth injury P10.8
  traumatic — *see* Hematoma, brain
Cephalematoma, cephalhematoma (calcified)
  newborn (birth injury) P12.0
  traumatic — *see* Hematoma, brain
Cephalgia, cephalalgia (*see also* Headache)
  histamine G44.009
    intractable G44.001
    not intractable G44.009
  trigeminal autonomic (TAC) NEC G44.099
    intractable G44.091
    not intractable G44.099
Cephalic — *see* condition
Cephalitis — *see* Encephalitis
Cephalocele — *see* Encephalocele
Cephalomenia N94.89
Cephalopelvic — *see* condition
Cerclage (with cervical incompetence) in pregnancy — *see* Incompetence, cervix, in pregnancy
Cerebellitis — *see* Encephalitis
Cerebellum, cerebellar — *see* condition
Cerebral — *see* condition
Cerebritis — *see* Encephalitis
Cerebro-hepato-renal syndrome Q87.89
Cerebromalacia — *see* Softening, brain
  sequelae of cerebrovascular disease I69.398
Cerebroside lipidosis E75.22
Cerebrospasticity (congenital) G80.1
Cerebrospinal — *see* condition
Cerebrum — *see* condition
Ceroid-lipofuscinosis, neuronal E75.4
Cerumen (accumulation) (impacted) H61.2- ☑
Cervical (*see also* condition)
  auricle Q18.2
  dysplasia in pregnancy — *see* Abnormal, cervix, in pregnancy or childbirth
  erosion in pregnancy — *see* Abnormal, cervix, in pregnancy or childbirth
  fibrosis in pregnancy — *see* Abnormal, cervix, in pregnancy or childbirth
  fusion syndrome Q76.1
  rib Q76.5
  shortening (complicating pregnancy) O26.87- ☑
Cervicalgia M54.2
Cervicitis (acute) (chronic) (nonvenereal) (senile (atrophic)) (subacute) (with ulceration) N72
  with
    abortion — *see* Abortion, by type complicated by genital tract and pelvic infection
    ectopic pregnancy O08.0
    molar pregnancy O08.0
  chlamydial A56.09
  gonococcal A54.03
  herpesviral A60.03
  puerperal (postpartum) O86.11
  syphilitic A52.76
  trichomonal A59.09
  tuberculous A18.16
Cervicocolpitis (emphysematosa) (see also Cervicitis) N72
Cervix — *see* condition
Cesarean delivery, previous, affecting management of pregnancy O34.21

Céstan (-Chenais) paralysis or syndrome G46.3
Céstan-Raymond syndrome I65.8
Cestode infestation B71.9
  specified type NEC B71.8
Cestodiasis B71.9
Chabert's disease A22.9
Chacaleh E53.8
Chafing L30.4
Chagas' (-Mazza) disease (chronic) B57.2
  with
    cardiovascular involvement NEC B57.2
    digestive system involvement B57.30
      megacolon B57.32
      megaesophagus B57.31
      other specified B57.39
    megacolon B57.32
    megaesophagus B57.31
    myocarditis B57.2
    nervous system involvement B57.40
      meningitis B57.41
      meningoencephalitis B57.42
      other specified B57.49
    specified organ involvement NEC B57.5
  acute (with) B57.1
    cardiovascular NEC B57.0
    myocarditis B57.0
Chagres fever B50.9
Chairridden Z74.09
Chalasia (cardiac sphincter) K21.9
Chalazion H00.19
  left H00.16
    lower H00.15
    upper H00.14
  right H00.13
    lower H00.12
    upper H00.11
Chalcosis (see also Disorder, globe, degenerative, chalcosis)
  cornea — see Deposit, cornea
  crystalline lens — see Cataract, complicated
  retina H35.89
Chalicosis (pulmonum) J62.8
Chancre (any genital site) (hard) (hunterian) (mixed) (primary) (seronegative) (seropositive) (syphilitic) A51.0
  congenital A50.07
  conjunctiva NEC A51.2
  Ducrey's A57
  extragenital A51.2
  eyelid A51.2
  lip A51.2
  nipple A51.2
  Nisbet's A57
  of
    carate A67.0
    pinta A67.0
    yaws A66.0
  palate, soft A51.2
  phagedenic A57
  simple A57
  soft A57
    bubo A57
    palate A51.2
  urethra A51.0
  yaws A66.0
Chancroid (anus) (genital) (penis) (perineum) (rectum) (urethra) (vulva) A57
Chandler's disease (osteochondritis dissecans, hip) — see Osteochondritis, dissecans, hip
Change(s) (in) (of) (see also Removal)
  arteriosclerotic — see Arteriosclerosis
  bone (see also Disorder, bone)
    diabetic — see Diabetes, bone change
  bowel habit R19.4
  cardiorenal (vascular) — see Hypertension, cardiorenal
  cardiovascular — see Disease, cardiovascular
  circulatory I99.9
  cognitive (mild) (organic) R41.89
  color, tooth, teeth
    during formation K00.8
    posteruptive K03.7
  contraceptive device Z30.433
  corneal membrane H18.30
    Bowman's membrane fold or rupture H18.31- ☑
    Descemet's membrane
      fold H18.32- ☑
      rupture H18.33- ☑
  coronary — see Disease, heart, ischemic

Change(s) — continued
  degenerative, spine or vertebra — see Spondylosis
  dental pulp, regressive K04.2
  dressing (nonsurgical) Z48.00
    surgical Z48.01
  heart — see Disease, heart
  hip joint — see Derangement, joint, hip
  hyperplastic larynx J38.7
  hypertrophic
    nasal sinus J34.89
    turbinate, nasal J34.3
    upper respiratory tract J39.8
  indwelling catheter Z46.6
  inflammatory (see also Inflammation)
    sacroiliac M46.1
  job, anxiety concerning Z56.1
  joint — see Derangement, joint
  life — see Menopause
  mental status R41.82
  minimal (glomerular) (see also N00-N07 with fourth character .0) N05.0
  myocardium, myocardial — see Degeneration, myocardial
  of life — see Menopause
  pacemaker Z45.018
    pulse generator Z45.010
  personality (enduring) F68.8
    due to (secondary to)
      general medical condition F07.0
    secondary (nonspecific) F60.89
  regressive, dental pulp K04.2
  renal — see Disease, renal
  retina H35.9
    myopic H44.2- ☑
  sacroiliac joint M53.3
  senile (see also condition) R54
  sensory R20.8
  skin R23.9
    acute, due to ultraviolet radiation L56.9
      specified NEC L56.8
    chronic, due to nonionizing radiation L57.9
      specified NEC L57.8
    cyanosis R23.0
    flushing R23.2
    pallor R23.1
    petechiae R23.3
    specified change NEC R23.8
    swelling — see Mass, localized
    texture R23.4
  trophic
    arm — see Mononeuropathy, upper limb
    leg — see Mononeuropathy, lower limb
  vascular I99.9
  vasomotor I73.9
  voice R49.9
    psychogenic F44.4
    specified NEC R49.8
Changing sleep-work schedule, affecting sleep G47.26
Changuinola fever A93.1
Chapping skin T69.8 ☑
Charcot-Marie-Tooth disease, paralysis or syndrome G60.0
Charcot's
  arthropathy — see Arthropathy, neuropathic
  cirrhosis K74.3
  disease (tabetic arthropathy) A52.16
  joint (disease) (tabetic) A52.16
    diabetic — see Diabetes, with, arthropathy
    syringomyelic G95.0
  syndrome (intermittent claudication) I73.9
CHARGE association Q89.8
Charley-horse (quadriceps) M62.831
  traumatic (quadriceps) S76.11- ☑
Charlouis' disease — see Yaws
Cheadle's disease E54
Checking (of)
  cardiac pacemaker (battery) (electrode(s)) Z45.018
    pulse generator Z45.010
  intrauterine contraceptive device Z30.431
Check-up — see Examination
Chédiak-Higashi (-Steinbrinck) **syndrome** (congenital gigantism of peroxidase granules) E70.330
Cheek — see condition
Cheese itch B88.0
Cheese-washer's lung J67.8
Cheese-worker's lung J67.8

Cheilitis (acute) (angular) (catarrhal) (chronic) (exfoliative) (gangrenous) (glandular) (infectional) (suppurative) (ulcerative) (vesicular) K13.0
  actinic (due to sun) L56.8
    other than from sun L59.8
  candidal B37.83
Cheilodynia K13.0
Cheiloschisis — see Cleft, lip
Cheilosis (angular) K13.0
  with pellagra E52
  due to
    vitamin B2 (riboflavin) deficiency E53.0
Cheiromegaly M79.89
Cheiropompholyx L30.1
Cheloid — see Keloid
Chemical burn — see Corrosion, by site
Chemodectoma — see Paraganglioma, nonchromaffin
Chemosis, conjunctiva — see Edema, conjunctiva
Chemotherapy (session) (for)
  cancer Z51.11
  neoplasm Z51.11
Cherubism M27.8
Chest — see condition
Cheyne-Stokes breathing (respiration) R06.3
Chiari's
  disease or syndrome (hepatic vein thrombosis) I82.0
  malformation
    type I G93.5
    type II — see Spina bifida
  net Q24.8
Chicago disease B40.9
Chickenpox — see Varicella
Chiclero ulcer or sore B55.1
Chigger (infestation) B88.0
Chignon (disease) B36.8
  newborn (from vacuum extraction) (birth injury) P12.1
Chilaiditi's syndrome (subphrenic displacement, colon) Q43.3
Chilblain(s) (lupus) T69.1 ☑
Child
  custody dispute Z65.3
Childbirth — see Delivery
Childhood
  cerebral X-linked adrenoleukodystrophy E71.520
  period of rapid growth Z00.2
Chill(s) R68.83
  with fever R50.9
  without fever R68.83
  congestive in malarial regions B54
Chilomastigiasis A07.8
Chimera 46,XX/46,XY Q99.0
Chin — see condition
Chinese dysentery A03.9
Chionophobia F40.228
Chitral fever A93.1
Chlamydia, chlamydial A74.9
  cervicitis A56.09
  conjunctivitis A74.0
  cystitis A56.01
  endometritis A56.11
  epididymitis A56.19
  female
    pelvic inflammatory disease A56.11
    pelviperitonitis A56.11
  orchitis A56.19
  peritonitis A74.81
  pharyngitis A56.4
  proctitis A56.3
  psittaci (infection) A70
  salpingitis A56.11
  sexually-transmitted infection NEC A56.8
  specified NEC A74.89
  urethritis A56.01
  vulvovaginitis A56.02
Chlamydiosis — see Chlamydia
Chloasma (skin) (idiopathic) (symptomatic) L81.1
  eyelid H02.719
    hyperthyroid E05.90 [H02.719]
      with thyroid storm E05.91 [H02.719]
    left H02.716
      lower H02.715
      upper H02.714
    right H02.713
      lower H02.712
      upper H02.711
Chloroma C92.3- ☑

Chlorosis D50.9
Egyptian B76.9 [D63.8]
miner's B76.9 [D63.8]
Chlorotic anemia D50.8
Chocolate cyst (ovary) N80.1
Choked
disc or disk — *see* Papilledema
on food, phlegm, or vomitus NOS — *see* Foreign body, by site
while vomiting NOS — *see* Foreign body, by site
Chokes (resulting from bends) T70.3 ☑
Choking sensation R09.89
Cholangiectasis K83.8
Cholangiocarcinoma
with hepatocellular carcinoma, combined C22.0
liver C22.1
specified site NEC — *see* Neoplasm, malignant, by site
unspecified site C22.1
Cholangiohepatitis K83.8
due to fluke infestation B66.1
Cholangiohepatoma C22.0
Cholangiolitis (acute) (chronic) (extrahepatic) (gangrenous) (intrahepatic) K83.0
paratyphoidal — *see* Fever, paratyphoid
typhoidal A01.09
Cholangioma D13.4
malignant — *see* Cholangiocarcinoma
Cholangitis (ascending) (primary) (recurrent) (sclerosing) (secondary) (stenosing) (suppurative) K83.0
with calculus, bile duct — *see* Calculus, bile duct, with cholangitis
chronic nonsuppurative destructive K74.3
Cholecystectasia K82.8
Cholecystitis K81.9
with
calculus, stones in
bile duct (common) (hepatic) — *see* Calculus, bile duct, with cholecystitis
cystic duct — *see* Calculus, gallbladder, with cholecystitis
gallbladder — *see* Calculus, gallbladder, with cholecystitis
choledocholithiasis — *see* Calculus, bile duct, with cholecystitis
cholelithiasis — *see* Calculus, gallbladder, with cholecystitis
acute (emphysematous) (gangrenous) (suppurative) K81.0
with
calculus, stones in
cystic duct — *see* Calculus, gallbladder, with cholecystitis, acute
gallbladder — *see* Calculus, gallbladder, with cholecystitis, acute
choledocholithiasis — *see* Calculus, bile duct, with cholecystitis, acute
cholelithiasis — *see* Calculus, gallbladder, with cholecystitis, acute
chronic cholecystitis K81.2
with gallbladder calculus K80.12
with obstruction K80.13
chronic K81.1
with acute cholecystitis K81.2
with gallbladder calculus K80.12
with obstruction K80.13
emphysematous (acute) — *see* Cholecystitis, acute
gangrenous — *see* Cholecystitis, acute
paratyphoidal, current A01.4
suppurative — *see* Cholecystitis, acute
typhoidal A01.09
Cholecystolithiasis — *see* Calculus, gallbladder
Choledochitis (suppurative) K83.0
Choledocholith — *see* Calculus, bile duct
Choledocholithiasis (common duct) (hepatic duct) — *see* Calculus, bile duct
cystic — *see* Calculus, gallbladder
typhoidal A01.09
Cholelithiasis (cystic duct) (gallbladder) (impacted) (multiple) — *see* Calculus, gallbladder
bile duct (common) (hepatic) — *see* Calculus, bile duct
hepatic duct — *see* Calculus, bile duct
specified NEC K80.80
with obstruction K80.81
Cholemia (*see also* Jaundice)
familial (simple) (congenital) E80.4
Gilbert's E80.4
Choleperitoneum, choleperitonitis K65.3

Cholera (Asiatic) (epidemic) (malignant) A00.9
antimonial — *see* Poisoning, antimony
classical A00.0
due to Vibrio cholerae 01 A00.9
biovar cholerae A00.0
biovar eltor A00.1
el tor A00.1
el tor A00.1
Cholerine — *see* Cholera
Cholestasis NEC K83.1
with hepatocyte injury K71.0
due to total parenteral nutrition (TPN) K76.89
pure K71.0
Cholesteatoma (ear) (middle) (with reaction) H71.9- ☑
attic H71.0- ☑
external ear (canal) H60.4- ☑
mastoid H71.2- ☑
postmastoidectomy cavity (recurrent) — *see* Complications, postmastoidectomy, recurrent cholesteatoma
recurrent (postmastoidectomy) — *see* Complications, postmastoidectomy, recurrent cholesteatoma
tympanum H71.1- ☑
Cholesteatosis, diffuse H71.3- ☑
Cholesteremia E78.0
Cholesterin in vitreous — *see* Deposit, crystalline
Cholesterol
deposit
retina H35.89
vitreous — *see* Deposit, crystalline
elevated (high) E78.0
with elevated (high) triglycerides E78.2
screening for Z13.220
imbibition of gallbladder K82.4
Cholesterolemia (essential) (familial) (hereditary) (pure) E78.0
Cholesterolosis, cholesterosis (gallbladder) K82.4
cerebrotendinous E75.5
Cholocolic fistula K82.3
Choluria R82.2
Chondritis M94.8X9
aurical H61.03- ☑
costal (Tietze's) M94.0
external ear H61.03- ☑
patella, posttraumatic — *see* Chondromalacia, patella
pinna H61.03- ☑
purulent M94.8X- ☑
tuberculous NEC A18.02
intervertebral A18.01
Chondroblastoma (*see also* Neoplasm, bone, benign)
malignant — *see* Neoplasm, bone, malignant
Chondrocalcinosis M11.20
ankle M11.27- ☑
elbow M11.22- ☑
familial M11.10
ankle M11.17- ☑
elbow M11.12- ☑
foot joint M11.17- ☑
hand joint M11.14- ☑
hip M11.15- ☑
knee M11.16- ☑
multiple site M11.19
shoulder M11.11- ☑
vertebrae M11.18
wrist M11.13- ☑
foot joint M11.27- ☑
hand joint M11.24- ☑
hip M11.25- ☑
knee M11.26- ☑
multiple site M11.29
shoulder M11.21- ☑
specified type NEC M11.20
ankle M11.27- ☑
elbow M11.22- ☑
foot joint M11.27- ☑
hand joint M11.24- ☑
hip M11.25- ☑
knee M11.26- ☑
multiple site M11.29
shoulder M11.21- ☑
vertebrae M11.28
wrist M11.23- ☑
vertebrae M11.28
wrist M11.23- ☑
Chondrodermatitis nodularis helicis or anthelicis — *see* Perichondritis, ear

Chondrodysplasia Q78.9
with hemangioma Q78.4
calcificans congenita Q77.3
fetalis Q77.4
metaphyseal (Jansen's) (McKusick's) (Schmid's) Q78.5
punctata Q77.3
Chondrodystrophy, chondrodystrophia (familial) (fetalis) (hypoplastic) Q78.9
calcificans congenita Q77.3
myotonic (congenital) G71.13
punctata Q77.3
Chondroectodermal dysplasia Q77.6
Chondrogenesis imperfecta Q77.4
Chondrolysis M94.35- ☑
Chondroma (*see also* Neoplasm, cartilage, benign)
juxtacortical — *see* Neoplasm, bone, benign
periosteal — *see* Neoplasm, bone, benign
Chondromalacia (systemic) M94.20
acromioclavicular joint M94.21- ☑
ankle M94.27- ☑
elbow M94.22- ☑
foot joint M94.27- ☑
glenohumeral joint M94.21- ☑
hand joint M94.24- ☑
hip M94.25- ☑
knee M94.26- ☑
patella M22.4- ☑
multiple sites M94.29
patella M22.4- ☑
rib M94.28
sacroiliac joint M94.259
shoulder M94.21- ☑
sternoclavicular joint M94.21- ☑
vertebral joint M94.28
wrist M94.23- ☑
Chondromatosis (*see also* Neoplasm, cartilage, uncertain behavior)
internal Q78.4
Chondromyxosarcoma — *see* Neoplasm, cartilage, malignant
Chondro-osteodysplasia (Morquio-Brailsford type) E76.219
Chondro-osteodystrophy E76.29
Chondro-osteoma — *see* Neoplasm, bone, benign
Chondropathia tuberosa M94.0
Chondrosarcoma — *see* Neoplasm, cartilage, malignant
juxtacortical — *see* Neoplasm, bone, malignant
mesenchymal — *see* Neoplasm, connective tissue, malignant
myxoid — *see* Neoplasm, cartilage, malignant
Chordee (nonvenereal) N48.89
congenital Q54.4
gonococcal A54.09
Chorditis (fibrinous) (nodosa) (tuberosa) J38.2
Chordoma — *see* Neoplasm, vertebral (column), malignant
Chorea (chronic) (gravis) (posthemiplegic) (senile) (spasmodic) G25.5
with
heart involvement I02.0
active or acute (conditions in I01-) I02.0
rheumatic I02.9
with valvular disorder I02.0
rheumatic heart disease (chronic) (inactive)(quiescent) — *code to* rheumatic heart condition involved
drug-induced G25.4
habit F95.8
hereditary G10
Huntington's G10
hysterical F44.4
minor I02.9
with heart involvement I02.0
progressive G25.5
hereditary G10
rheumatic (chronic) I02.9
with heart involvement I02.0
Sydenham's I02.9
with heart involvement — *see* Chorea, with rheumatic heart disease
nonrheumatic G25.5
Choreoathetosis (paroxysmal) G25.5
Chorioadenoma (destruens) D39.2
Chorioamnionitis O41.12- ☑
Chorioangioma D26.7

Choriocarcinoma — see Neoplasm, malignant, by site
  combined with
    embryonal carcinoma — see Neoplasm, malignant,
      by site
    other germ cell elements — see Neoplasm, malig-
      nant, by site
    teratoma — see Neoplasm, malignant, by site
  specified site — see Neoplasm, malignant, by site
  unspecified site
    female C58
    male C62.90
Chorioencephalitis (acute) (lymphocytic) (serous) A87.2
Chorioepithelioma — see Choriocarcinoma
Choriomeningitis (acute) (lymphocytic) (serous) A87.2
Chorionepithelioma — see Choriocarcinoma
Chorioretinitis (see also Inflammation, chorioretinal)
  disseminated (see also Inflammation, chorioretinal,
    disseminated)
    in neurosyphilis A52.19
  Egyptian B76.9 [D63.8]
  focal (see also Inflammation, chorioretinal, focal)
  histoplasmic B39.9 [H32]
  in (due to)
    histoplasmosis B39.9 [H32]
    syphilis (secondary) A51.43
      late A52.71
    toxoplasmosis (acquired) B58.01
      congenital (active) P37.1 [H32]
    tuberculosis A18.53
  juxtapapillary, juxtapapillaris — see Inflammation,
    chorioretinal, focal, juxtapapillary
  leprous A30.9 [H32]
  miner's B76.9 [D63.8]
  progressive myopia (degeneration) H44.2- ☑
  syphilitic (secondary) A51.43
    congenital (early) A50.01 [H32]
    late A50.32
    late A52.71
  tuberculous A18.53
Chorioretinopathy, central serous H35.71- ☑
Choroid — see condition
Choroideremia H31.21
Choroiditis — see Chorioretinitis
Choroidopathy — see Disorder, choroid
Choroidoretinitis — see Chorioretinitis
Choroidoretinopathy, central serous — see Chori-
  oretinopathy, central serous
Christian-Weber disease M35.6
Christmas disease D67
Chromaffinoma (see also Neoplasm, benign, by site)
  malignant — see Neoplasm, malignant, by site
Chromatopsia — see Deficiency, color vision
Chromhidrosis, chromidrosis L75.1
Chromoblastomycosis — see Chromomycosis
Chromoconversion R82.91
Chromomycosis B43.9
  brain abscess B43.1
  cerebral B43.1
  cutaneous B43.0
  skin B43.0
  specified NEC B43.8
  subcutaneous abscess or cyst B43.2
Chromophytosis B36.0
Chromosome — see Anomaly, by chromosome involved
  D (1) — see Anomaly, chromosome 13
  E (3) — see Anomaly, chromosome 18
  G — see Anomaly, chromosome 21
Chromotrichomycosis B36.8
Chronic — see condition
  fracture — see Fracture, pathological
Churg-Strauss syndrome M30.1
Chyle cyst, mesentery I89.8
Chylocele (nonfilarial) I89.8
  filarial (see also Infestation, filarial) B74.9 [N51]
  tunica vaginalis N50.8
    filarial (see also Infestation, filarial) B74.9 [N51]
Chylomicronemia (fasting) (with hyperprebetalipopro-
  teinemia) E78.3
Chyloperikardium I31.3
  acute I30.9
Chylothorax (nonfilarial) I89.8
  filarial (see also Infestation, filarial) B74.9 [J91.8]
Chylous — see condition
Chyluria (nonfilarial) R82.0
  due to
    bilharziasis B65.0

Chyluria — continued
  due to — continued
    Brugia (malayi) B74.1
      timori B74.2
    schistosomiasis (bilharziasis) B65.0
    Wuchereria (bancrofti) B74.0
  filarial — see Infestation, filarial
Cicatricial (deformity) — see Cicatrix
Cicatrix (adherent) (contracted) (painful) (vicious) (see
  also Scar) L90.5
  adenoid (and tonsil) J35.8
  alveolar process M26.79
  anus K62.89
  auricle — see Disorder, pinna, specified type NEC
  bile duct (common) (hepatic) K83.8
  bladder N32.89
  bone — see Disorder, bone, specified type NEC
  brain G93.89
  cervix (postoperative) (postpartal) N88.1
  common duct K83.8
  cornea H17.9
    tuberculous A18.59
  duodenum (bulb), obstructive K31.5
  esophagus K22.2
  eyelid — see Disorder, eyelid function
  hypopharynx J39.2
  lacrimal passages — see Obstruction, lacrimal
  larynx J38.7
  lung J98.4
  middle ear H74.8 ☑
  mouth K13.79
  muscle M62.89
    with contracture — see Contraction, muscle NEC
  nasopharynx J39.2
  palate (soft) K13.79
  penis N48.89
  pharynx J39.2
  prostate N42.89
  rectum K62.89
  retina — see Scar, chorioretinal
  semilunar cartilage — see Derangement, meniscus
  seminal vesicle N50.8
  skin L90.5
    infected L08.89
    postinfective L90.5
    tuberculous B90.8
  specified site NEC L90.5
  throat J39.2
  tongue K14.8
  tonsil (and adenoid) J35.8
  trachea J39.8
  tuberculous NEC B90.9
  urethra N36.8
  uterus N85.8
  vagina N89.8
    postoperative N99.2
  vocal cord J38.3
  wrist, constricting (annular) L90.5
CIDP (chronic inflammatory demyelinating polyneuropathy) G61.81
CIN — see Neoplasia, intraepithelial, cervix
Cinchonism — see Deafness, ototoxic
  correct substance properly administered — see Table
    of Drugs and Chemicals, by drug, adverse effect
  overdose or wrong substance given or taken — see
    Table of Drugs and Chemicals, by drug, poison-
    ing
Circle of Willis — see condition
Circular — see condition
Circulating anticoagulants (see also Disorder, hemorrhagic) D68.318
  due to drugs (see also Disorder, hemorrhagic) D68.32
  following childbirth O72.3
Circulation
  collateral, any site I99.8
  defective (lower extremity) I99.8
    congenital Q28.9
  embryonic Q28.9
  failure (peripheral) R57.9
    newborn P29.89
  fetal, persistent P29.3
  heart, incomplete Q28.9
Circulatory system — see condition
Circulus senilis (cornea) — see Degeneration, cornea,
  senile
Circumcision (in absence of medical indication) (ritual)
  (routine) Z41.2
Circumscribed — see condition

Circumvallate placenta O43.11- ☑
Cirrhosis, cirrhotic (hepatic) (liver) K74.60
  alcoholic K70.30
    with ascites K70.31
  atrophic — see Cirrhosis, liver
  Baumgarten-Cruveilhier K74.69
  biliary (cholangiolitic) (cholangitic) (hypertrophic)
    (obstructive) (pericholangiolitic) K74.5
    due to
      Clonorchiasis B66.1
      flukes B66.3
    primary K74.3
    secondary K74.4
  cardiac (of liver) K76.1
  Charcot's K74.3
  cholangiolitic, cholangitic, cholostatic (primary) K74.3
  congestive K76.1
  Cruveilhier-Baumgarten K74.69
  cryptogenic (liver) K74.69
  due to
    hepatolenticular degeneration E83.01
    Wilson's disease E83.01
    xanthomatosis E78.2
  fatty K76.0
    alcoholic K70.0
  Hanot's (hypertrophic) K74.3
  hepatic — see Cirrhosis, liver
  hypertrophic K74.3
  Indian childhood K74.69
  kidney — see Sclerosis, renal
  Laennec's K70.30
    with ascites K70.31
    alcoholic K70.30
      with ascites K70.31
    nonalcoholic K74.69
  liver K74.60
    alcoholic K70.30
      with ascites K70.31
      fatty K70.0
    congenital P78.81
    syphilitic A52.74
  lung (chronic) J84.10
  macronodular K74.69
    alcoholic K70.30
      with ascites K70.31
  micronodular K74.69
    alcoholic K70.30
      with ascites K70.31
  mixed type K74.69
  monolobular K74.3
  nephritis — see Sclerosis, renal
  nutritional K74.69
    alcoholic K70.30
      with ascites K70.31
  obstructive — see Cirrhosis, biliary
  ovarian N83.8
  pancreas (duct) K86.8
  pigmentary E83.110
  portal K74.69
    alcoholic K70.30
      with ascites K70.31
  postnecrotic K74.69
    alcoholic K70.30
      with ascites K70.31
  pulmonary J84.10
  renal — see Sclerosis, renal
  spleen D73.2
  stasis K76.1
  Todd's K74.3
  unilobar K74.3
  xanthomatous (biliary) K74.5
    due to xanthomatosis (familial) (metabolic) (prima-
      ry) E78.2
Cistern, subarachnoid R93.0
Citrullinemia E72.23
Citrullinuria E72.23
Civatte's disease or poikiloderma L57.3
Clam digger's itch B65.3
Clammy skin R23.1
Clap — see Gonorrhea
Clarke-Hadfield syndrome (pancreatic infantilism)
  K86.8
Clark's paralysis G80.9
Clastothrix L67.8
Claude Bernard-Horner syndrome G90.2
  traumatic — see Injury, nerve, cervical sympathetic
Claude's disease or syndrome G46.3
Claudicatio venosa intermittens I87.8

54

☑ **Additional Character Required** — Refer to the Tabular List for Character Selection   ▽ Subterms under main terms may continue to next column or page

Claudication, intermittent I73.9
  cerebral (artery) G45.9
  spinal cord (arteriosclerotic) G95.19
    syphilitic A52.09
  venous (axillary) I87.8
Claustrophobia F40.240
Clavus (infected) L84
Clawfoot (congenital) Q66.89
  acquired — see Deformity, limb, clawfoot
Clawhand (acquired) (see also Deformity, limb, clawhand)
  congenital Q68.1
Clawtoe (congenital) Q66.89
  acquired — see Deformity, toe, specified NEC
Clay eating — see Pica
Cleansing of artificial opening — see Attention to, artificial, opening
Cleft (congenital) (see also Imperfect, closure)
  alveolar process M26.79
  branchial (cyst) (persistent) Q18.2
  cricoid cartilage, posterior Q31.8
  lip (unilateral) Q36.9
    with cleft palate Q37.9
      hard Q37.1
        with soft Q37.5
      soft Q37.3
        with hard Q37.5
    bilateral Q36.0
      with cleft palate Q37.8
        hard Q37.0
          with soft Q37.4
        soft Q37.2
          with hard Q37.4
    median Q36.1
  nose Q30.2
  palate Q35.9
    with cleft lip (unilateral) Q37.9
      bilateral Q37.8
    hard Q35.1
      with
        cleft lip (unilateral) Q37.1
          bilateral Q37.0
        soft Q35.5
          with cleft lip (unilateral) Q37.5
            bilateral Q37.4
    medial Q35.5
    soft Q35.3
      with
        cleft lip (unilateral) Q37.3
          bilateral Q37.2
        hard Q35.5
          with cleft lip (unilateral) Q37.5
            bilateral Q37.4
  penis Q55.69
  scrotum Q55.29
  thyroid cartilage Q31.8
  uvula Q35.7
Cleidocranial dysostosis Q74.0
Cleptomania F63.2
Clicking hip (newborn) R29.4
Climacteric (female) (see also Menopause)
  arthritis (any site) NEC — see Arthritis, specified form NEC
  depression (single episode) F32.8
  male (symptoms) (syndrome) NEC N50.8
  paranoid state F22
  polyarthritis NEC — see Arthritis, specified form NEC
  symptoms (female) N95.1
Clinical research investigation (clinical trial) (control subject) (normal comparison) (participant) Z00.6
Clitoris — see condition
Cloaca (persistent) Q43.7
Clonorchiasis, clonorchis infection (liver) B66.1
Clonus R25.8
Closed bite M26.29
Clostridium (C.) **perfringens, as cause of disease classified elsewhere** B96.7
Closure
  congenital, nose Q30.0
  cranial sutures, premature Q75.0
  defective or imperfect NEC — see Imperfect, closure
  fistula, delayed — see Fistula
  foramen ovale, imperfect Q21.1
  hymen N89.6
  interauricular septum, defective Q21.1
  interventricular septum, defective Q21.0
  lacrimal duct (see also Stenosis, lacrimal, duct)
    congenital Q10.5

Closure — continued
  nose (congenital) Q30.0
    acquired M95.0
  of artificial opening — see Attention to, artificial, opening
  vagina N89.5
  valve — see Endocarditis
  vulva N90.5
Clot (blood) (see also Embolism)
  artery (obstruction) (occlusion) — see Embolism
  bladder N32.89
  brain (intradural or extradural) — see Occlusion, artery, cerebral
  circulation I74.9
  heart (see also Infarct, myocardium)
    not resulting in infarction I24.0
  vein — see Thrombosis
Clouded state R40.1
  epileptic — see Epilepsy, specified NEC
  paroxysmal — see Epilepsy, specified NEC
Cloudy antrum, antra J32.0
Clouston's (hidrotic) **ectodermal dysplasia** Q82.4
Clubbed nail pachydermoperiostosis M89.40 [L62]
Clubbing of finger(s) (nails) R68.3
Clubfinger R68.3
  congenital Q68.1
Clubfoot (congenital) Q66.89
  acquired — see Deformity, limb, clubfoot
  equinovarus Q66.0
  paralytic — see Deformity, limb, clubfoot
Clubhand (congenital) (radial) Q71.4- ☑
  acquired — see Deformity, limb, clubhand
Clubnail R68.3
  congenital Q84.6
Clump, kidney Q63.1
Clumsiness, clumsy child syndrome F82
Cluttering F80.81
Clutton's joints A50.51 [M12.80]
Coagulation, intravascular (diffuse) (disseminated) (see also Defibrination syndrome)
  complicating abortion — see Abortion, by type, complicated by, intravascular coagulation
  following ectopic or molar pregnancy O08.1
Coagulopathy (see also Defect, coagulation)
  consumption D65
  intravascular D65
  newborn P60
Coalition
  calcaneo-scaphoid Q66.89
  tarsal Q66.89
Coalminer's
  elbow — see Bursitis, elbow, olecranon
  lung or pneumoconiosis J60
Coalworker's lung or pneumoconiosis J60
Coarctation
  aorta (preductal) (postductal) Q25.1
  pulmonary artery Q25.71
Coated tongue K14.3
Coats' disease (exudative retinopathy) — see Retinopathy, exudative
Cocainism — see Dependence, drug, cocaine
Coccidioidomycosis B38.9
  cutaneous B38.3
  disseminated B38.7
  generalized B38.7
  meninges B38.4
  prostate B38.81
  pulmonary B38.2
    acute B38.0
    chronic B38.1
  skin B38.3
  specified NEC B38.89
Coccidioidosis — see Coccidioidomycosis
Coccidiosis (intestinal) A07.3
Coccydynia, coccygodynia M53.3
Coccyx — see condition
Cochin-China diarrhea K90.1
Cockayne's syndrome Q87.1
Cocked up toe — see Deformity, toe, specified NEC
Cock's peculiar tumor L72.3
Codman's tumor — see Neoplasm, bone, benign
Coenurosis B71.8
Coffee-worker's lung J67.8
Cogan's syndrome H16.32- ☑
  oculomotor apraxia H51.8
Coitus, painful (female) N94.1
  male N53.12

Coitus, painful — continued
  psychogenic F52.6
Cold J00
  with influenza, flu, or grippe — see Influenza, with, respiratory manifestations NEC
  agglutinin disease or hemoglobinuria (chronic) D59.1
  bronchial — see Bronchitis
  chest — see Bronchitis
  common (head) J00
  effects of T69.9 ☑
    specified effect NEC T69.8 ☑
  excessive, effects of T69.9 ☑
    specified effect NEC T69.8 ☑
  exhaustion from T69.8 ☑
  exposure to T69.9 ☑
    specified effect NEC T69.8 ☑
  head J00
  injury syndrome (newborn) P80.0
  on lung — see Bronchitis
  rose J30.1
  sensitivity, auto-immune D59.1
  virus J00
Coldsore B00.1
Colibacillosis A49.8
  as the cause of other disease (see also Escherichia coli) B96.20
  generalized A41.50
Colic (bilious) (infantile) (intestinal) (recurrent) (spasmodic) R10.83
  abdomen R10.83
    psychogenic F45.8
  appendix, appendicular K38.8
  bile duct — see Calculus, bile duct
  biliary — see Calculus, bile duct
  common duct — see Calculus, bile duct
  cystic duct — see Calculus, gallbladder
  Devonshire NEC — see Poisoning, lead
  gallbladder — see Calculus, gallbladder
  gallstone — see Calculus, gallbladder
    gallbladder or cystic duct — see Calculus, gallbladder
  hepatic (duct) — see Calculus, bile duct
  hysterical F45.8
  kidney N23
  lead NEC — see Poisoning, lead
  mucous K58.9
    with diarrhea K58.0
    psychogenic F54
  nephritic N23
  painter's NEC — see Poisoning, lead
  pancreas K86.8
  psychogenic F45.8
  renal N23
  saturnine NEC — see Poisoning, lead
  ureter N23
  urethral N36.8
    due to calculus N21.1
  uterus NEC N94.89
    menstrual — see Dysmenorrhea
  worm NOS B83.9
Colicystitis — see Cystitis
Colitis (acute) (catarrhal) (chronic) (noninfective) (hemorrhagic) (see also Enteritis) K52.9
  allergic K52.2
  amebic (acute) (see also Amebiasis) A06.0
    nondysenteric A06.2
  anthrax A22.2
  bacillary — see Infection, Shigella
  balantidial A07.0
  Clostridium difficile A04.7
  coccidial A07.3
  collagenous K52.89
  cystica superficialis K52.89
  dietary counseling and surveillance (for) Z71.3
  dietetic K52.2
  drug-induced K52.1
  due to radiation K52.0
  eosinophilic K52.82
  food hypersensitivity K52.2
  giardial A07.1
  granulomatous — see Enteritis, regional, large intestine
  infectious — see Enteritis, infectious
  ischemic K55.9
    acute (fulminant) (subacute) K55.0
    chronic K55.1
    due to mesenteric artery insufficiency K55.1

Colitis — *continued*
  ischemic — *continued*
    fulminant (acute) K55.0
  left sided K51.50
    with
      abscess K51.514
      complication K51.519
        specified NEC K51.518
      fistula K51.513
      obstruction K51.512
      rectal bleeding K51.511
  lymphocytic K52.89
  membranous
    psychogenic F54
  microscopic (collagenous) (lymphocytic) K52.89
  mucous — *see* Syndrome, irritable, bowel
    psychogenic F54
  noninfective K52.9
    specified NEC K52.89
  polyposa — *see* Polyp, colon, inflammatory
  protozoal A07.9
  pseudomembranous A04.7
  pseudomucinous — *see* Syndrome, irritable, bowel
  regional — *see* Enteritis, regional, large intestine
  segmental — *see* Enteritis, regional, large intestine
  septic — *see* Enteritis, infectious
  spastic K58.9
    with diarrhea K58.0
    psychogenic F54
  staphylococcal A04.8
    foodborne A05.0
  subacute ischemic K55.0
  thromboulcerative K55.0
  toxic NEC K52.1
    due to Clostridium difficile A04.7
  transmural — *see* Enteritis, regional, large intestine
  trichomonal A07.8
  tuberculous (ulcerative) A18.32
  ulcerative (chronic) K51.90
    with
      complication K51.919
        abscess K51.914
        fistula K51.913
        obstruction K51.912
        rectal bleeding K51.911
        specified complication NEC K51.918
    enterocolitis — *see* Enterocolitis, ulcerative
    ileocolitis — *see* Ileocolitis, ulcerative
    mucosal proctocolitis — *see* Proctocolitis, mucosal
    proctitis — *see* Proctitis, ulcerative
    pseudopolyposis — *see* Polyp, colon, inflammatory
    psychogenic F54
    rectosigmoiditis — *see* Rectosigmoiditis, ulcerative
    specified type NEC K51.80
      with
        complication K51.819
          abscess K51.814
          fistula K51.813
          obstruction K51.812
          rectal bleeding K51.811
          specified complication NEC K51.818
Collagenosis, collagen disease (nonvascular) (vascular) M35.9
  cardiovascular I42.8
  reactive perforating L87.1
  specified NEC M35.8
Collapse R55
  adrenal E27.2
  cardiorespiratory R57.0
  cardiovascular R57.0
    newborn P29.89
  circulatory (peripheral) R57.9
    during or after labor and delivery O75.1
    following ectopic or molar pregnancy O08.3
    newborn P29.89
  during or
    after labor and delivery O75.1
    resulting from a procedure, not elsewhere classified T81.10 ☑
  external ear canal — *see* Stenosis, external ear canal
  general R55
  heart — *see* Disease, heart
  heat T67.1 ☑
  hysterical F44.89
  labyrinth, membranous (congenital) Q16.5

Collapse — *continued*
  lung (*see also* Atelectasis) J98.19
    pressure due to anesthesia (general) (local) or other sedation T88.2 ☑
    during labor and delivery O74.1
    in pregnancy O29.02-
    postpartum, puerperal O89.09
  myocardial — *see* Disease, heart
  nervous F48.8
  neurocirculatory F45.8
  nose M95.0
  postoperative T81.10 ☑
  pulmonary (*see also* Atelectasis) J98.19
    newborn — *see* Atelectasis
  trachea J39.8
  tracheobronchial J98.09
  valvular — *see* Endocarditis
  vascular (peripheral) R57.9
    during or after labor and delivery O75.1
    following ectopic or molar pregnancy O08.3
    newborn P29.89
  vertebra M48.50- ☑
    cervical region M48.52- ☑
    cervicothoracic region M48.53- ☑
    in (due to)
      metastasis — *see* Collapse, vertebra, in, specified disease NEC
      osteoporosis (*see also* Osteoporosis) M80.88 ☑
        cervical region M80.88 ☑
        cervicothoracic region M80.88 ☑
        lumbar region M80.88 ☑
        lumbosacral region M80.88 ☑
        multiple sites M80.88 ☑
        occipito-atlanto-axial region M80.88 ☑
        sacrococcygeal region M80.88 ☑
        thoracic region M80.88 ☑
        thoracolumbar region M80.88 ☑
      specified disease NEC M48.50- ☑
        cervical region M48.52- ☑
        cervicothoracic region M48.53- ☑
        lumbar region M48.56- ☑
        lumbosacral region M48.57- ☑
        occipito-atlanto-axial region M48.51- ☑
        sacrococcygeal region M48.58- ☑
        thoracic region M48.54- ☑
        thoracolumbar region M48.55- ☑
    lumbar region M48.56- ☑
    lumbosacral region M48.57- ☑
    occipito-atlanto-axial region M48.51- ☑
    sacrococcygeal region M48.58- ☑
    thoracic region M48.54- ☑
    thoracolumbar region M48.55- ☑
Collateral (*see also* condition)
  circulation (venous) I87.8
  dilation, veins I87.8
Colles' fracture S52.53- ☑
Collet (-Sicard) syndrome G52.7
Collier's asthma or lung J60
Collodion baby Q80.2
Colloid nodule (of thyroid) (cystic) E04.1
Coloboma (iris) Q13.0
  eyelid Q10.3
  fundus Q14.8
  lens Q12.2
  optic disc (congenital) Q14.2
    acquired H47.31- ☑
Coloenteritis — *see* Enteritis
Colon — *see* condition
Colonization
  MRSA (Methicillin resistant Staphylococcus aureus) Z22.322
  MSSA (Methicillin susceptible Staphylococcus aureus) Z22.321
  status — *see* Carrier (suspected) of
Coloptosis K63.4
Color blindness — *see* Deficiency, color vision
Colostomy
  attention to Z43.3
  fitting or adjustment Z46.89
  malfunctioning K94.03
  status Z93.3
Colpitis (acute) — *see* Vaginitis
Colpocele N81.5
Colpocystitis — *see* Vaginitis
Colpospasm N94.2
Column, spinal, vertebral — *see* condition

Coma R40.20
  with
    motor response (none) R40.231 ☑
      abnormal R40.233 ☑
      extension R40.232 ☑
      flexion withdrawal R40.234 ☑
      localizes pain R40.235 ☑
      obeys commands R40.236 ☑
    opening of eyes (never) R40.211 ☑
      in response to
        pain R40.212 ☑
        sound R40.213 ☑
      spontaneous R40.214 ☑
    verbal response (none) R40.221 ☑
      confused conversation R40.224 ☑
      inappropriate words R40.223 ☑
      incomprehensible words R40.222 ☑
      oriented R40.225 ☑
  eclamptic — *see* Eclampsia
  epileptic — *see* Epilepsy
  Glasgow, scale score — *see* Glasgow coma scale
  hepatic — *see* Failure, hepatic, by type, with coma
  hyperglycemic (diabetic) — *see* Diabetes, coma
  hyperosmolar (diabetic) — *see* Diabetes, coma
  hypoglycemic (diabetic) — *see* Diabetes, coma, hypoglycemic
    nondiabetic E15
  in diabetes — *see* Diabetes, coma
  insulin-induced — *see* Coma, hypoglycemic
  myxedematous E03.5
  newborn P91.5
  persistent vegetative state R40.3
  specified NEC, without documented Glasgow coma scale score, or with partial Glasgow coma scale score reported R40.244
Comatose — *see* Coma
Combat fatigue F43.0
Combined — *see* condition
Comedo, comedones (giant) L70.0
Comedocarcinoma (*see also* Neoplasm, breast, malignant)
  noninfiltrating
    breast D05.8- ☑
    specified site — *see* Neoplasm, in situ, by site
    unspecified site D05.8- ☑
Comedomastitis — *see* Ectasia, mammary duct
Comminuted fracture — *code as* Fracture, closed
Common
  arterial trunk Q20.0
  atrioventricular canal Q21.2
  atrium Q21.1
  cold (head) J00
  truncus (arteriosus) Q20.0
  variable immunodeficiency — *see* Immunodeficiency, common variable
  ventricle Q20.4
Commotio, commotion (current)
  brain — *see* Injury, intracranial, concussion
  cerebri — *see* Injury, intracranial, concussion
  retinae S05.8X- ☑
  spinal cord — *see* Injury, spinal cord, by region
  spinalis — *see* Injury, spinal cord, by region
Communication
  between
    base of aorta and pulmonary artery Q21.4
    left ventricle and right atrium Q20.5
    pericardial sac and pleural sac Q34.8
    pulmonary artery and pulmonary vein, congenital Q25.72
  congenital between uterus and digestive or urinary tract Q51.7
Compartment syndrome (deep) (posterior) (traumatic) T79.A0 ☑ (*following* T79.7)
  abdomen T79.A3 ☑ (*following* T79.7)
  lower extremity (hip, buttock, thigh, leg, foot, toes) T79.A2 ☑ (*following* T79.7)
  nontraumatic
    abdomen M79.A3 (*following* M79.7)
    lower extremity (hip, buttock, thigh, leg, foot, toes) M79.A2- ☑ (*following* M79.7)
    specified site NEC M79.A9 (*following* M79.7)
    upper extremity (shoulder, arm, forearm, wrist, hand, fingers) M79.A1- ☑ (*following* M79.7)
  specified site NEC T79.A9 ☑ (*following* T79.7)
  upper extremity (shoulder, arm, forearm, wrist, hand, fingers) T79.A1- ☑ (*following* T79.7)

Compensation
  failure — *see* Disease, heart
  neurosis, psychoneurosis — *see* Disorder, factitious
Complaint (*see also* Disease)
  bowel, functional K59.9
    psychogenic F45.8
  intestine, functional K59.9
    psychogenic F45.8
  kidney — *see* Disease, renal
  miners' J60
Complete — *see* condition
Complex
  Addison-Schilder E71.528
  cardiorenal — *see* Hypertension, cardiorenal
  Costen's M26.69
  disseminated mycobacterium avium- intracellulare
    (DMAC) A31.2
  Eisenmenger's (ventricular septal defect) I27.89
  hypersexual F52.8
  jumped process, spine — *see* Dislocation, vertebra
  primary, tuberculous A15.7
  Schilder-Addison E71.528
  subluxation (vertebral) M99.19
    abdomen M99.19
    acromioclavicular M99.17
    cervical region M99.11
    cervicothoracic M99.11
    costochondral M99.18
    costovertebral M99.18
    head region M99.10
    hip M99.15
    lower extremity M99.16
    lumbar region M99.13
    lumbosacral M99.13
    occipitocervical M99.10
    pelvic region M99.15
    pubic M99.15
    rib cage M99.18
    sacral region M99.14
    sacrococcygeal M99.14
    sacroiliac M99.14
    specified NEC M99.19
    sternochondral M99.18
    sternoclavicular M99.17
    thoracic region M99.12
    thoracolumbar M99.12
    upper extremity M99.17
  Taussig-Bing (transposition, aorta and overriding pul-
    monary artery) Q20.1
Complication(s) (from) (of)
  accidental puncture or laceration during a procedure
    (of) — *see* Complications, intraoperative (in-
    traprocedural), puncture or laceration
  amputation stump (surgical) (late) NEC T87.9
    dehiscence T87.81
    infection or inflammation T87.40
      lower limb T87.4- ☑
      upper limb T87.4- ☑
    necrosis T87.50
      lower limb T87.5- ☑
      upper limb T87.5- ☑
    neuroma T87.30
      lower limb T87.3- ☑
      upper limb T87.3- ☑
    specified type NEC T87.89
  anastomosis (and bypass) (*see also* Complications,
    prosthetic device or implant)
    intestinal (internal) NEC K91.89
      involving urinary tract N99.89
    urinary tract (involving intestinal tract) N99.89
    vascular — *see* Complications, cardiovascular de-
      vice or implant
  anesthesia, anesthetic (*see also* Anesthesia, complica-
    tion) T88.59 ☑
    brain, postpartum, puerperal O89.2
    cardiac
      in
        labor and delivery O74.2
        pregnancy O29.19- ☑
      postpartum, puerperal O89.1
    central nervous system
      in
        labor and delivery O74.3
        pregnancy O29.29- ☑
      postpartum, puerperal O89.2
    difficult or failed intubation T88.4 ☑
      in pregnancy O29.6- ☑

Complication(s) — *continued*
  anesthesia, anesthetic (*see also* Anesthesia, complica-
    tion) — *continued*
    failed sedation (conscious) (moderate) during
      procedure T88.52 ☑
    hyperthermia, malignant T88.3 ☑
    hypothermia T88.51 ☑
    intubation failure T88.4 ☑
    malignant hyperthermia T88.3 ☑
    pulmonary
      in
        labor and delivery O74.1
        pregnancy NEC O29.09- ☑
      postpartum, puerperal O89.09
    shock T88.2 ☑
    spinal and epidural
      in
        labor and delivery NEC O74.6
          headache O74.5
        pregnancy NEC O29.5X- ☑
      postpartum, puerperal NEC O89.5
        headache O89.4
  anti-reflux device — *see* Complications, esophageal
    anti-reflux device
  aortic (bifurcation) graft — *see* Complications, graft,
    vascular
  aortocoronary (bypass) graft — *see* Complications,
    coronary artery (bypass) graft
  aortofemoral (bypass) graft — *see* Complications, ex-
    tremity artery (bypass) graft
  arteriovenous
    fistula, surgically created T82.9 ☑
      embolism T82.818 ☑
      fibrosis T82.828 ☑
      hemorrhage T82.838 ☑
      infection or inflammation T82.7 ☑
      mechanical
        breakdown T82.510 ☑
        displacement T82.520 ☑
        leakage T82.530 ☑
        malposition T82.520 ☑
        obstruction T82.590 ☑
        perforation T82.590 ☑
        protrusion T82.590 ☑
      pain T82.848 ☑
      specified type NEC T82.898 ☑
      stenosis T82.858 ☑
      thrombosis T82.868 ☑
    shunt, surgically created T82.9 ☑
      embolism T82.818 ☑
      fibrosis T82.828 ☑
      hemorrhage T82.838 ☑
      infection or inflammation T82.7 ☑
      mechanical
        breakdown T82.511 ☑
        displacement T82.521 ☑
        leakage T82.531 ☑
        malposition T82.521 ☑
        obstruction T82.591 ☑
        perforation T82.591 ☑
        protrusion T82.591 ☑
      pain T82.848 ☑
      specified type NEC T82.898 ☑
      stenosis T82.858 ☑
      thrombosis T82.868 ☑
  arthroplasty — *see* Complications, joint prosthesis
  artificial
    fertilization or insemination N98.9
      attempted introduction (of)
        embryo in embryo transfer N98.3
        ovum following in vitro fertilization N98.2
      hyperstimulation of ovaries N98.1
      infection N98.0
      specified NEC N98.8
    heart T82.9 ☑
      embolism T82.817 ☑
      fibrosis T82.827 ☑
      hemorrhage T82.837 ☑
      infection or inflammation T82.7 ☑
      mechanical
        breakdown T82.512 ☑
        displacement T82.522 ☑
        leakage T82.532 ☑
        malposition T82.522 ☑
        obstruction T82.592 ☑
        perforation T82.592 ☑

Complication(s) — *continued*
  artificial — *continued*
    heart — *continued*
      mechanical — *continued*
        protrusion T82.592 ☑
      pain T82.847 ☑
      specified type NEC T82.897 ☑
      stenosis T82.857 ☑
      thrombosis T82.867 ☑
    opening
      cecostomy — *see* Complications, colostomy
      colostomy — *see* Complications, colostomy
      cystostomy — *see* Complications, cystostomy
      enterostomy — *see* Complications, enterosto-
        my
      gastrostomy — *see* Complications, gastrostomy
      ileostomy — *see* Complications, enterostomy
      jejunostomy — *see* Complications, enterostomy
      nephrostomy — *see* Complications, stoma,
        urinary tract
      tracheostomy — *see* Complications, tracheosto-
        my
      ureterostomy — *see* Complications, stoma,
        urinary tract
      urethrostomy — *see* Complications, stoma,
        urinary tract
  balloon implant or device
    gastrointestinal T85.9 ☑
      embolism T85.81 ☑
      fibrosis T85.82 ☑
      hemorrhage T85.83 ☑
      infection and inflammation T85.79 ☑
      pain T85.84 ☑
      specified type NEC T85.89 ☑
      stenosis T85.85 ☑
      thrombosis T85.86 ☑
    vascular (counterpulsation) T82.9 ☑
      embolism T82.818 ☑
      fibrosis T82.828 ☑
      hemorrhage T82.838 ☑
      infection or inflammation T82.7 ☑
      mechanical
        breakdown T82.513 ☑
        displacement T82.523 ☑
        leakage T82.533 ☑
        malposition T82.523 ☑
        obstruction T82.593 ☑
        perforation T82.593 ☑
        protrusion T82.593 ☑
      pain T82.848 ☑
      specified type NEC T82.898 ☑
      stenosis T82.858 ☑
      thrombosis T82.868 ☑
  bariatric procedure
    gastric band procedure K95.09
      infection K95.01
    specified procedure NEC K95.89
      infection K95.81
  bile duct implant (prosthetic) T85.9 ☑
    embolism T85.81 ☑
    fibrosis T85.82 ☑
    hemorrhage T85.83 ☑
    infection and inflammation T85.79 ☑
    mechanical
      breakdown T85.510 ☑
      displacement T85.520 ☑
      malfunction T85.510 ☑
      malposition T85.520 ☑
      obstruction T85.590 ☑
      perforation T85.590 ☑
      protrusion T85.590 ☑
      specified NEC T85.590 ☑
    pain T85.84 ☑
    specified type NEC T85.89 ☑
    stenosis T85.85 ☑
    thrombosis T85.86 ☑
  bladder device (auxiliary) — *see* Complications, geni-
    tourinary, device or implant, urinary system
  bleeding (postoperative) — *see* Complication, postop-
    erative, hemorrhage
    intraoperative — *see* Complication, intraoperative,
      hemorrhage
  blood vessel graft — *see* Complications, graft, vascular
  bone
    device NEC T84.9 ☑
      embolism T84.81 ☑

Complication(s) — *continued*
bone — *continued*
  device — *continued*
    fibrosis T84.82 ☑
    hemorrhage T84.83 ☑
    infection or inflammation T84.7 ☑
    mechanical
      breakdown T84.318 ☑
      displacement T84.328 ☑
      malposition T84.328 ☑
      obstruction T84.398 ☑
      perforation T84.398 ☑
      protrusion T84.398 ☑
    pain T84.84 ☑
    specified type NEC T84.89 ☑
    stenosis T84.85 ☑
    thrombosis T84.86 ☑
  graft — *see* Complications, graft, bone
  growth stimulator (electrode) — *see* Complications, electronic stimulator device, bone
  marrow transplant — *see* Complications, transplant, bone, marrow
brain neurostimulator (electrode) — *see* Complications, electronic stimulator device, brain
breast implant (prosthetic) T85.9 ☑
  capsular contracture T85.44 ☑
  embolism T85.81 ☑
  fibrosis T85.82 ☑
  hemorrhage T85.83 ☑
  infection and inflammation T85.79 ☑
  mechanical
    breakdown T85.41 ☑
    displacement T85.42 ☑
    leakage T85.43 ☑
    malposition T85.42 ☑
    obstruction T85.49 ☑
    perforation T85.49 ☑
    protrusion T85.49 ☑
    specified NEC T85.49 ☑
  pain T85.84 ☑
  specified type NEC T85.89 ☑
  stenosis T85.85 ☑
  thrombosis T85.86 ☑
bypass (*see also* Complications, prosthetic device or implant)
  aortocoronary — *see* Complications, coronary artery (bypass) graft
  arterial (*see also* Complications, graft, vascular)
    extremity — *see* Complications, extremity artery (bypass) graft
cardiac (*see also* Disease, heart)
  device, implant or graft T82.9 ☑
    embolism T82.817 ☑
    fibrosis T82.827 ☑
    hemorrhage T82.837 ☑
    infection or inflammation T82.7 ☑
      valve prosthesis T82.6 ☑
    mechanical
      breakdown T82.519 ☑
        specified device NEC T82.518 ☑
      displacement T82.529 ☑
        specified device NEC T82.528 ☑
      leakage T82.539 ☑
        specified device NEC T82.538 ☑
      malposition T82.529 ☑
        specified device NEC T82.528 ☑
      obstruction T82.599 ☑
        specified device NEC T82.598 ☑
      perforation T82.599 ☑
        specified device NEC T82.598 ☑
      protrusion T82.599 ☑
        specified device NEC T82.598 ☑
    pain T82.847 ☑
    specified type NEC T82.897 ☑
    stenosis T82.857 ☑
    thrombosis T82.867 ☑
cardiovascular device, graft or implant T82.9 ☑
  aortic graft — *see* Complications, graft, vascular
  arteriovenous
    fistula, artificial — *see* Complication, arteriovenous, fistula, surgically created
    shunt — *see* Complication, arteriovenous, shunt, surgically created
  artificial heart — *see* Complication, artificial, heart
  balloon (counterpulsation) device — *see* Complication, balloon implant, vascular

Complication(s) — *continued*
cardiovascular device, graft or implant — *continued*
  carotid artery graft — *see* Complications, graft, vascular
  coronary bypass graft — *see* Complication, coronary artery (bypass) graft
  dialysis catheter (vascular) — *see* Complication, catheter, dialysis
  electronic T82.9 ☑
    electrode T82.9 ☑
      embolism T82.817 ☑
      fibrosis T82.827 ☑
      hemorrhage T82.837 ☑
      infection T82.7 ☑
      mechanical
        breakdown T82.110 ☑
        displacement T82.120 ☑
        leakage T82.190 ☑
        obstruction T82.190 ☑
        perforation T82.190 ☑
        protrusion T82.190 ☑
        specified type NEC T82.190 ☑
      pain T82.847 ☑
      specified NEC T82.897 ☑
      stenosis T82.857 ☑
      thrombosis T82.867 ☑
    embolism T82.817 ☑
    fibrosis T82.827 ☑
    hemorrhage T82.837 ☑
    infection T82.7 ☑
    mechanical
      breakdown T82.119 ☑
      displacement T82.129 ☑
      leakage T82.199 ☑
      obstruction T82.199 ☑
      perforation T82.199 ☑
      protrusion T82.199 ☑
      specified type NEC T82.199 ☑
    pain T82.847 ☑
    pulse generator T82.9 ☑
      embolism T82.817 ☑
      fibrosis T82.827 ☑
      hemorrhage T82.837 ☑
      infection T82.7 ☑
      mechanical
        breakdown T82.111 ☑
        displacement T82.121 ☑
        leakage T82.191 ☑
        obstruction T82.191 ☑
        perforation T82.191 ☑
        protrusion T82.191 ☑
        specified type NEC T82.191 ☑
      pain T82.847 ☑
      specified NEC T82.897 ☑
      stenosis T82.857 ☑
      thrombosis T82.867 ☑
  specified condition NEC T82.897 ☑
  specified device NEC T82.9 ☑
    embolism T82.817 ☑
    fibrosis T82.827 ☑
    hemorrhage T82.837 ☑
    infection T82.7 ☑
    mechanical
      breakdown T82.118 ☑
      displacement T82.128 ☑
      leakage T82.198 ☑
      obstruction T82.198 ☑
      perforation T82.198 ☑
      protrusion T82.198 ☑
      specified type NEC T82.198 ☑
    pain T82.847 ☑
    specified NEC T82.897 ☑
    stenosis T82.857 ☑
    thrombosis T82.867 ☑
  stenosis T82.857 ☑
  thrombosis T82.867 ☑
  extremity artery graft — *see* Complication, extremity artery (bypass) graft
  femoral artery graft — *see* Complication, extremity artery (bypass) graft
  heart
    transplant — *see* Complication, transplant, heart
    valve — *see* Complication, prosthetic device, heart valve

Complication(s) — *continued*
cardiovascular device, graft or implant — *continued*
  heart — *continued*
    valve — *see* Complication, prosthetic device, heart valve — *continued*
      graft — *see* Complication, heart, valve, graft
  heart-lung transplant — *see* Complication, transplant, heart, with lung
  infection or inflammation T82.7 ☑
  umbrella device — *see* Complication, umbrella device, vascular
  vascular graft (or anastomosis) — *see* Complication, graft, vascular
carotid artery (bypass) graft — *see* Complications, graft, vascular
catheter (device) NEC (*see also* Complications, prosthetic device or implant)
  cystostomy T83.9 ☑
    embolism T83.81 ☑
    fibrosis T83.82 ☑
    hemorrhage T83.83 ☑
    infection and inflammation T83.59 ☑
    mechanical
      breakdown T83.010 ☑
      displacement T83.020 ☑
      leakage T83.030 ☑
      malposition T83.020 ☑
      obstruction T83.090 ☑
      perforation T83.090 ☑
      protrusion T83.090 ☑
      specified NEC T83.090 ☑
    pain T83.84 ☑
    specified type NEC T83.89 ☑
    stenosis T83.85 ☑
    thrombosis T83.86 ☑
  dialysis (vascular) T82.9 ☑
    embolism T82.818 ☑
    fibrosis T82.828 ☑
    hemorrhage T82.838 ☑
    infection and inflammation T82.7 ☑
    intraperitoneal — *see* Complications, catheter, intraperitoneal
    mechanical
      breakdown T82.41 ☑
      displacement T82.42 ☑
      leakage T82.43 ☑
      malposition T82.42 ☑
      obstruction T82.49 ☑
      perforation T82.49 ☑
      protrusion T82.49 ☑
    pain T82.848 ☑
    specified type NEC T82.898 ☑
    stenosis T82.858 ☑
    thrombosis T82.868 ☑
  epidural infusion T85.9 ☑
    embolism T85.81 ☑
    fibrosis T85.82 ☑
    hemorrhage T85.83 ☑
    infection and inflammation T85.79 ☑
    mechanical
      breakdown T85.610 ☑
      displacement T85.620 ☑
      leakage T85.630 ☑
      malfunction T85.610 ☑
      malposition T85.620 ☑
      obstruction T85.690 ☑
      perforation T85.690 ☑
      protrusion T85.690 ☑
      specified NEC T85.690 ☑
    pain T85.84 ☑
    specified type NEC T85.89 ☑
    stenosis T85.85 ☑
    thrombosis T85.86 ☑
  intraperitoneal dialysis T85.9 ☑
    embolism T85.81 ☑
    fibrosis T85.82 ☑
    hemorrhage T85.83 ☑
    infection and inflammation T85.71 ☑
    mechanical
      breakdown T85.611 ☑
      displacement T85.621 ☑
      leakage T85.631 ☑
      malfunction T85.611 ☑
      malposition T85.621 ☑
      obstruction T85.691 ☑

Complication(s) — *continued*
  catheter (*see also* Complications, prosthetic device or implant) — *continued*
    intraperitoneal dialysis — *continued*
      mechanical — *continued*
        perforation T85.691 ☑
        protrusion T85.691 ☑
        specified NEC T85.691 ☑
      pain T85.84 ☑
      specified type NEC T85.89 ☑
      stenosis T85.85 ☑
      thrombosis T85.86 ☑
    intravenous infusion T82.9 ☑
      embolism T82.818 ☑
      fibrosis T82.828 ☑
      hemorrhage T82.838 ☑
      infection or inflammation T82.7 ☑
      mechanical
        breakdown T82.514 ☑
        displacement T82.524 ☑
        leakage T82.534 ☑
        malposition T82.524 ☑
        obstruction T82.594 ☑
        perforation T82.594 ☑
        protrusion T82.594 ☑
      pain T82.848 ☑
      specified type NEC T82.898 ☑
      stenosis T82.858 ☑
      thrombosis T82.868 ☑
    subdural infusion T85.9 ☑
      embolism T85.81 ☑
      fibrosis T85.82 ☑
      hemorrhage T85.83 ☑
      infection and inflammation T85.79 ☑
      mechanical
        breakdown T85.610 ☑
        displacement T85.620 ☑
        leakage T85.630 ☑
        malfunction T85.610 ☑
        malposition T85.620 ☑
        obstruction T85.690 ☑
        perforation T85.690 ☑
        protrusion T85.690 ☑
        specified NEC T85.690 ☑
      pain T85.84 ☑
      specified type NEC T85.89 ☑
      stenosis T85.85 ☑
      thrombosis T85.86 ☑
    urethral, indwelling T83.9 ☑
      displacement T83.028 ☑
      embolism T83.81 ☑
      fibrosis T83.82 ☑
      hemorrhage T83.83 ☑
      infection and inflammation T83.51 ☑
      leakage T83.038 ☑
      malposition T83.028 ☑
      mechanical
        breakdown T83.018 ☑
      obstruction (mechanical) T83.098 ☑
      pain T83.84 ☑
      perforation T83.098 ☑
      protrusion T83.098 ☑
      specified type NEC T83.098 ☑
      stenosis T83.85 ☑
      thrombosis T83.86 ☑
    urinary (indwelling) — *see* Complications, catheter, urethral, indwelling
  cecostomy (stoma) — *see* Complications, colostomy
  cesarean delivery wound NEC O90.89
    disruption O90.0
    hematoma O90.2
    infection (following delivery) O86.0
  chemotherapy (antineoplastic) NEC T88.7 ☑
  chin implant (prosthetic) — *see* Complication, prosthetic device or implant, specified NEC
  circulatory system I99.8
    intraoperative I97.88
    postprocedural I97.89
      following cardiac surgery I97.19- ☑
        postcardiotomy syndrome I97.0
      hypertension I97.3
      lymphedema after mastectomy I97.2
      postcardiotomy syndrome I97.0
      specified NEC I97.89
  colostomy (stoma) K94.00
    hemorrhage K94.01

Complication(s) — *continued*
  colostomy — *continued*
    infection K94.02
    malfunction K94.03
    mechanical K94.03
    specified complication NEC K94.09
  contraceptive device, intrauterine — *see* Complications, intrauterine, contraceptive device
  cord (umbilical) — *see* Complications, umbilical cord
  corneal graft — *see* Complications, graft, cornea
  coronary artery (bypass) graft T82.9 ☑
    atherosclerosis — *see* Arteriosclerosis, coronary (artery),
    embolism T82.818 ☑
    fibrosis T82.828 ☑
    hemorrhage T82.838 ☑
    infection and inflammation T82.7 ☑
    mechanical
      breakdown T82.211 ☑
      displacement T82.212 ☑
      leakage T82.213 ☑
      malposition T82.212 ☑
      obstruction T82.218 ☑
      perforation T82.218 ☑
      protrusion T82.218 ☑
      specified NEC T82.218 ☑
    pain T82.848 ☑
    specified type NEC T82.897 ☑
    stenosis T82.858 ☑
    thrombosis T82.868 ☑
  counterpulsation device (balloon), intra-aortic — *see* Complications, balloon implant, vascular
  cystostomy (stoma) N99.518
    catheter — *see* Complications, catheter, cystostomy
    hemorrhage N99.510
    infection N99.511
    malfunction N99.512
    specified type NEC N99.518
  delivery (*see also* Complications, obstetric) O75.9
    procedure (instrumental) (manual) (surgical) O75.4
    specified NEC O75.89
  dialysis (peritoneal) (renal) (*see also* Complications, infusion)
    catheter (vascular) — *see* Complication, catheter, dialysis
      peritoneal, intraperitoneal — *see* Complications, catheter, intraperitoneal
  dorsal column (spinal) neurostimulator — *see* Complications, electronic stimulator device, spinal cord
  drug NEC T88.7 ☑
  ear procedure (*see also* Disorder, ear)
    intraoperative H95.88
      hematoma — *see* Complications, intraoperative, hemorrhage (hematoma) (of), ear
      hemorrhage — *see* Complications, intraoperative, hemorrhage (hematoma) (of), ear
      laceration — *see* Complications, intraoperative, puncture or laceration..., ear
      specified NEC H95.88
    postoperative H95.89
      external ear canal stenosis H95.81- ☑
      hematoma — *see* Complications, postprocedural, hemorrhage (hematoma) (of), ear
      hemorrhage — *see* Complications, postprocedural, hemorrhage (hematoma) (of), ear
      postmastoidectomy — *see* Complications, postmastoidectomy
      specified NEC H95.89
  ectopic pregnancy O08.9
    damage to pelvic organs O08.6
    embolism O08.2
    genital infection O08.0
    hemorrhage (delayed) (excessive) O08.1
    metabolic disorder O08.5
    renal failure O08.4
    shock O08.3
    specified type NEC O08.0
    venous complication NEC O08.7
  electronic stimulator device
    bladder (urinary) — *see* Complications, electronic stimulator device, urinary
    bone T84.9 ☑
      breakdown T84.310 ☑
      displacement T84.320 ☑
      embolism T84.81 ☑
      fibrosis T84.82 ☑

Complication(s) — *continued*
  electronic stimulator device — *continued*
    bone — *continued*
      hemorrhage T84.83 ☑
      infection or inflammation T84.7 ☑
      malfunction T84.310 ☑
      malposition T84.320 ☑
      mechanical NEC T84.390 ☑
      obstruction T84.390 ☑
      pain T84.84 ☑
      perforation T84.390 ☑
      protrusion T84.390 ☑
      specified type NEC T84.89 ☑
      stenosis T84.85 ☑
      thrombosis T84.86 ☑
    brain T85.9 ☑
      embolism T85.81 ☑
      fibrosis T85.82 ☑
      hemorrhage T85.83 ☑
      infection and inflammation T85.79 ☑
      mechanical
        breakdown T85.110 ☑
        displacement T85.120 ☑
        leakage T85.190 ☑
        malposition T85.120 ☑
        obstruction T85.190 ☑
        perforation T85.190 ☑
        protrusion T85.190 ☑
        specified NEC T85.190 ☑
      pain T85.84 ☑
      specified type NEC T85.89 ☑
      stenosis T85.85 ☑
      thrombosis T85.86 ☑
    cardiac (defibrillator) (pacemaker) — *see* Complications, cardiovascular device or implant, electronic
    muscle T84.9 ☑
      breakdown T84.418 ☑
      displacement T84.428 ☑
      embolism T84.81 ☑
      fibrosis T84.82 ☑
      hemorrhage T84.83 ☑
      infection or inflammation T84.7 ☑
      mechanical NEC T84.498 ☑
      pain T84.84 ☑
      specified type NEC T84.89 ☑
      stenosis T84.85 ☑
      thrombosis T84.86 ☑
    nervous system T85.9 ☑
      brain — *see* Complications, electronic stimulator device, brain
      embolism T85.81 ☑
      fibrosis T85.82 ☑
      hemorrhage T85.83 ☑
      infection and inflammation T85.79 ☑
      mechanical
        breakdown T85.118 ☑
        displacement T85.128 ☑
        leakage T85.199 ☑
        malposition T85.128 ☑
        obstruction T85.199 ☑
        perforation T85.199 ☑
        protrusion T85.199 ☑
        specified NEC T85.199 ☑
      pain T85.84 ☑
      peripheral nerve — *see* Complications, electronic stimulator device, peripheral nerve
      specified type NEC T85.89 ☑
      spinal cord — *see* Complications, electronic stimulator device, spinal cord
      stenosis T85.85 ☑
      thrombosis T85.86 ☑
    peripheral nerve T85.9 ☑
      embolism T85.81 ☑
      fibrosis T85.82 ☑
      hemorrhage T85.83 ☑
      infection and inflammation T85.79 ☑
      mechanical
        breakdown T85.111 ☑
        displacement T85.121 ☑
        leakage T85.191 ☑
        malposition T85.121 ☑
        obstruction T85.191 ☑
        perforation T85.191 ☑
        protrusion T85.191 ☑
        specified NEC T85.191 ☑

⬇ **Subterms under main terms may continue to next column or page**   ☑ **Additional Character Required — Refer to the Tabular List for Character Selection**   **59**

Complication — Complication

Index

Complication — Complication

Complication(s) — *continued*
electronic stimulator device — *continued*
  peripheral nerve — *continued*
    pain T85.84 ☑
    specified type NEC T85.89 ☑
    stenosis T85.85 ☑
    thrombosis T85.86 ☑
  spinal cord T85.9 ☑
    embolism T85.81 ☑
    fibrosis T85.82 ☑
    hemorrhage T85.83 ☑
    infection and inflammation T85.79 ☑
    mechanical
      breakdown T85.112 ☑
      displacement T85.122 ☑
      leakage T85.192 ☑
      malposition T85.122 ☑
      obstruction T85.192 ☑
      perforation T85.192 ☑
      protrusion T85.192 ☑
      specified NEC T85.192 ☑
    pain T85.84 ☑
    specified type NEC T85.89 ☑
    stenosis T85.85 ☑
    thrombosis T85.86 ☑
  urinary T83.9 ☑
    embolism T83.81 ☑
    fibrosis T83.82 ☑
    hemorrhage T83.83 ☑
    infection and inflammation T83.59 ☑
    mechanical
      breakdown T83.110 ☑
      displacement T83.120 ☑
      malposition T83.120 ☑
      perforation T83.190 ☑
      protrusion T83.190 ☑
      specified NEC T83.190 ☑
    pain T83.84 ☑
    specified type NEC T83.89 ☑
    stenosis T83.85 ☑
    thrombosis T83.86 ☑
electroshock therapy T88.9 ☑
  specified NEC T88.8 ☑
endocrine E34.9
  postprocedural
    adrenal hypofunction E89.6
    hypoinsulinemia E89.1
    hypoparathyroidism E89.2
    hypopituitarism E89.3
    hypothyroidism E89.0
    ovarian failure E89.40
      asymptomatic E89.40
      symptomatic E89.41
    specified NEC E89.89
    testicular hypofunction E89.5
endodontic treatment NEC M27.59
enterostomy (stoma) K94.10
  hemorrhage K94.11
  infection K94.12
  malfunction K94.13
  mechanical K94.13
  specified complication NEC K94.19
episiotomy, disruption O90.1
esophageal anti-reflux device T85.9 ☑
  embolism T85.81 ☑
  fibrosis T85.82 ☑
  hemorrhage T85.83 ☑
  infection and inflammation T85.79 ☑
  mechanical
    breakdown T85.511 ☑
    displacement T85.521 ☑
    malfunction T85.511 ☑
    malposition T85.521 ☑
    obstruction T85.591 ☑
    perforation T85.591 ☑
    protrusion T85.591 ☑
    specified NEC T85.591 ☑
  pain T85.84 ☑
  specified type NEC T85.89 ☑
  stenosis T85.85 ☑
  thrombosis T85.86 ☑
esophagostomy K94.30
  hemorrhage K94.31
  infection K94.32
  malfunction K94.33
  mechanical K94.33

Complication(s) — *continued*
esophagostomy — *continued*
  specified complication NEC K94.39
extracorporeal circulation T80.90 ☑
extremity artery (bypass) graft T82.9 ☑
  arteriosclerosis — *see* Arteriosclerosis, extremities,
    bypass graft
  embolism T82.818 ☑
  fibrosis T82.828 ☑
  hemorrhage T82.838 ☑
  infection and inflammation T82.7 ☑
  mechanical
    breakdown T82.318 ☑
      femoral artery T82.312 ☑
    displacement T82.328 ☑
      femoral artery T82.322 ☑
    leakage T82.338 ☑
      femoral artery T82.332 ☑
    malposition T82.328 ☑
      femoral artery T82.322 ☑
    obstruction T82.398 ☑
      femoral artery T82.392 ☑
    perforation T82.398 ☑
      femoral artery T82.392 ☑
    protrusion T82.398 ☑
      femoral artery T82.392 ☑
  pain T82.848 ☑
  specified type NEC T82.898 ☑
  stenosis T82.858 ☑
  thrombosis T82.868 ☑
eye H57.9
  corneal graft — *see* Complications, graft, cornea
  implant (prosthetic) T85.9 ☑
    embolism T85.81 ☑
    fibrosis T85.82 ☑
    hemorrhage T85.83 ☑
    infection and inflammation T85.79 ☑
    mechanical
      breakdown T85.318 ☑
      displacement T85.328 ☑
      leakage T85.398 ☑
      malposition T85.328 ☑
      obstruction T85.398 ☑
      perforation T85.398 ☑
      protrusion T85.398 ☑
      specified NEC T85.398 ☑
    pain T85.84 ☑
    specified type NEC T85.89 ☑
    stenosis T85.85 ☑
    thrombosis T85.86 ☑
  intraocular lens — *see* Complications, intraocular
    lens
  orbital prosthesis — *see* Complications, orbital
    prosthesis
female genital N94.9
  device, implant or graft NEC — *see* Complications,
    genitourinary, device or implant, genital tract
femoral artery (bypass) graft — *see* Complication, extremity artery (bypass) graft
fixation device, internal (orthopedic) T84.9 ☑
  infection and inflammation T84.60 ☑
    arm T84.61- ☑
      humerus T84.61- ☑
      radius T84.61- ☑
      ulna T84.61- ☑
    leg T84.629 ☑
      femur T84.62- ☑
      fibula T84.62- ☑
      tibia T84.62- ☑
    specified site NEC T84.89 ☑
    spine T84.63 ☑
  mechanical
    breakdown
      limb T84.119 ☑
        carpal T84.210 ☑
        femur T84.11- ☑
        fibula T84.11- ☑
        humerus T84.11- ☑
        metacarpal T84.210 ☑
        metatarsal T84.213 ☑
        phalanx
          foot T84.213 ☑
          hand T84.210 ☑
        radius T84.11- ☑
        tarsal T84.213 ☑
        tibia T84.11- ☑

Complication(s) — *continued*
fixation device, internal — *continued*
  mechanical — *continued*
    breakdown — *continued*
      limb — *continued*
        ulna T84.11- ☑
      specified bone NEC T84.218 ☑
      spine T84.216 ☑
    displacement
      limb T84.129 ☑
        carpal T84.220 ☑
        femur T84.12- ☑
        fibula T84.12- ☑
        humerus T84.12- ☑
        metacarpal T84.220 ☑
        metatarsal T84.223 ☑
        phalanx
          foot T84.223 ☑
          hand T84.220 ☑
        radius T84.12- ☑
        tarsal T84.223 ☑
        tibia T84.12- ☑
        ulna T84.12- ☑
      specified bone NEC T84.228 ☑
      spine T84.226 ☑
    malposition — *see* Complications, fixation de-
      vice, internal, mechanical, displacement
    obstruction — *see* Complications, fixation de-
      vice, internal, mechanical, specified type
      NEC
    perforation — *see* Complications, fixation de-
      vice, internal, mechanical, specified type
      NEC
    protrusion — *see* Complications, fixation de-
      vice, internal, mechanical, specified type
      NEC
    specified type NEC
      limb T84.199 ☑
        carpal T84.290 ☑
        femur T84.19- ☑
        fibula T84.19- ☑
        humerus T84.19- ☑
        metacarpal T84.290 ☑
        metatarsal T84.293 ☑
        phalanx
          foot T84.293 ☑
          hand T84.290 ☑
        radius T84.19- ☑
        tarsal T84.293 ☑
        tibia T84.19- ☑
        ulna T84.19- ☑
      specified bone NEC T84.298 ☑
      vertebra T84.296 ☑
  specified type NEC T84.89 ☑
    embolism T84.81 ☑
    fibrosis T84.82 ☑
    hemorrhage T84.83 ☑
    pain T84.84 ☑
    specified complication NEC T84.89 ☑
    stenosis T84.85 ☑
    thrombosis T84.86 ☑
following
  acute myocardial infarction NEC I23.8
    aneurysm (false) (of cardiac wall) (of heart wall)
      (ruptured) I23.3
    angina I23.7
    atrial
      septal defect I23.1
      thrombosis I23.6
    cardiac wall rupture I23.3
    chordae tendinae rupture I23.4
    defect
      septal
        atrial (heart) I23.1
        ventricular (heart) I23.2
    hemopericardium I23.0
    papillary muscle rupture I23.5
    rupture
      cardiac wall I23.3
        with hemopericardium I23.0
      chordae tendineae I23.4
      papillary muscle I23.5
    specified NEC I23.8
    thrombosis
      atrium I23.6
      auricular appendage I23.6
      ventricle (heart) I23.6

☑ **Additional Character Required — Refer to the Tabular List for Character Selection**   ▽ Subterms under main terms may continue to next column or page

Complication(s) — *continued*
  following — *continued*
    acute myocardial infarction — *continued*
      ventricular
        septal defect I23.2
        thrombosis I23.6
    ectopic or molar pregnancy O08.9
      cardiac arrest O08.81
      sepsis O08.82
      specified type NEC O08.89
      urinary tract infection O08.83
    termination of pregnancy — *see* Abortion
  gastrointestinal K92.9
    bile duct prosthesis — *see* Complications, bile duct implant
    esophageal anti-reflux device — *see* Complications, esophageal anti-reflux device
    postoperative
      colostomy — *see* Complications, colostomy
      dumping syndrome K91.1
      enterostomy — *see* Complications, enterostomy
      gastrostomy — *see* Complications, gastrostomy
      malabsorption NEC K91.2
      obstruction K91.3
      postcholecystectomy syndrome K91.5
      specified NEC K91.89
      vomiting after GI surgery K91.0
    prosthetic device or implant
      bile duct prosthesis — *see* Complications, bile duct implant
      esophageal anti-reflux device — *see* Complications, esophageal anti-reflux device
      specified type NEC
        embolism T85.81 ☑
        fibrosis T85.82 ☑
        hemorrhage T85.83 ☑
        mechanical
          breakdown T85.518 ☑
          displacement T85.528 ☑
          malfunction T85.518 ☑
          malposition T85.528 ☑
          obstruction T85.598 ☑
          perforation T85.598 ☑
          protrusion T85.598 ☑
          specified NEC T85.598 ☑
        pain T85.84 ☑
        specified complication NEC T85.89 ☑
        stenosis T85.85 ☑
        thrombosis T85.86 ☑
  gastrostomy (stoma) K94.20
    hemorrhage K94.21
    infection K94.22
    malfunction K94.23
    mechanical K94.23
    specified complication NEC K94.29
  genitourinary
    device or implant T83.9 ☑
      genital tract T83.9 ☑
        infection or inflammation T83.6 ☑
        intrauterine contraceptive device — *see* Complications, intrauterine, contraceptive device
        mechanical — *see* Complications, by device, mechanical
        mesh — *see* Complications, mesh
        penile prosthesis — *see* Complications, prosthetic device, penile
        specified type NEC T83.89 ☑
          embolism T83.81 ☑
          fibrosis T83.82 ☑
          hemorrhage T83.83 ☑
          pain T83.84 ☑
          specified complication NEC T83.89 ☑
          stenosis T83.85 ☑
          thrombosis T83.86 ☑
        vaginal mesh — *see* Complications, mesh
      urinary system T83.9 ☑
        cystostomy catheter — *see* Complication, catheter, cystostomy
        electronic stimulator — *see* Complications, electronic stimulator device, urinary
        indwelling urethral catheter — *see* Complications, catheter, urethral, indwelling
        infection or inflammation T83.59 ☑
          indwelling urinary catheter T83.51 ☑

Complication(s) — *continued*
  genitourinary — *continued*
    device or implant — *continued*
      urinary system — *continued*
        kidney transplant — *see* Complication, transplant, kidney
        organ graft — *see* Complication, graft, urinary organ
        specified type NEC T83.89 ☑
          embolism T83.81 ☑
          fibrosis T83.82 ☑
          hemorrhage T83.83 ☑
          mechanical T83.198 ☑
            breakdown T83.118 ☑
            displacement T83.128 ☑
            malfunction T83.118 ☑
            malposition T83.128 ☑
            obstruction T83.198 ☑
            perforation T83.198 ☑
            protrusion T83.198 ☑
            specified NEC T83.198 ☑
          pain T83.84 ☑
          specified complication NEC T83.89 ☑
          stenosis T83.85 ☑
          thrombosis T83.86 ☑
        sphincter implant — *see* Complications, implant, urinary sphincter
    postprocedural
      pelvic peritoneal adhesions N99.4
      renal failure N99.0
      specified NEC N99.89
      stoma — *see* Complications, stoma, urinary tract
      urethral stricture — *see* Stricture, urethra, postprocedural
      vaginal
        adhesions N99.2
        vault prolapse N99.3
  graft (bypass) (patch) (*see also* Complications, prosthetic device or implant)
    aorta — *see* Complications, graft, vascular
    arterial — *see* Complication, graft, vascular
    bone T86.839
      failure T86.831
      infection T86.832
      mechanical T84.318 ☑
        breakdown T84.318 ☑
        displacement T84.328 ☑
        protrusion T84.398 ☑
        specified type NEC T84.398 ☑
      rejection T86.830
      specified type NEC T86.838
    carotid artery — *see* Complications, graft, vascular
    cornea T86.849
      failure T86.841
      infection T86.842
      mechanical T85.398 ☑
        breakdown T85.318 ☑
        displacement T85.328 ☑
        protrusion T85.398 ☑
        specified type NEC T85.398 ☑
      rejection T86.840
      retroprosthetic membrane T85.398 ☑
      specified type NEC T86.848
    femoral artery (bypass) — *see* Complication, extremity artery (bypass) graft
    genital organ or tract — *see* Complications, genitourinary, device or implant, genital tract
    muscle T84.9 ☑
      breakdown T84.410 ☑
      displacement T84.420 ☑
      embolism T84.81 ☑
      fibrosis T84.82 ☑
      hemorrhage T84.83 ☑
      infection and inflammation T84.7 ☑
      mechanical NEC T84.490 ☑
      pain T84.84 ☑
      specified type NEC T84.89 ☑
      stenosis T84.85 ☑
      thrombosis T84.86 ☑
    nerve — *see* Complication, prosthetic device or implant, specified NEC
    skin — *see* Complications, prosthetic device or implant, skin graft
    tendon T84.9 ☑
      breakdown T84.410 ☑

Complication(s) — *continued*
  graft (*see also* Complications, prosthetic device or implant) — *continued*
    tendon — *continued*
      displacement T84.420 ☑
      embolism T84.81 ☑
      fibrosis T84.82 ☑
      hemorrhage T84.83 ☑
      infection and inflammation T84.7 ☑
      mechanical NEC T84.490 ☑
      pain T84.84 ☑
      specified type NEC T84.89 ☑
      stenosis T84.85 ☑
      thrombosis T84.86 ☑
    urinary organ T83.9 ☑
      embolism T83.81 ☑
      fibrosis T83.82 ☑
      hemorrhage T83.83 ☑
      infection and inflammation T83.59 ☑
        indwelling urinary catheter T83.51 ☑
      mechanical
        breakdown T83.21 ☑
        displacement T83.22 ☑
        leakage T83.23 ☑
        malposition T83.22 ☑
        obstruction T83.29 ☑
        perforation T83.29 ☑
        protrusion T83.29 ☑
        specified NEC T83.29 ☑
      pain T83.84 ☑
      specified type NEC T83.89 ☑
      stenosis T83.85 ☑
      thrombosis T83.86 ☑
    vascular T82.9 ☑
      embolism T82.818 ☑
      femoral artery — *see* Complication, extremity artery (bypass) graft
      fibrosis T82.828 ☑
      hemorrhage T82.838 ☑
      mechanical
        breakdown T82.319 ☑
          aorta (bifurcation) T82.310 ☑
          carotid artery T82.311 ☑
          specified vessel NEC T82.318 ☑
        displacement T82.329 ☑
          aorta (bifurcation) T82.320 ☑
          carotid artery T82.321 ☑
          specified vessel NEC T82.328 ☑
        leakage T82.339 ☑
          aorta (bifurcation) T82.330 ☑
          carotid artery T82.331 ☑
          specified vessel NEC T82.338 ☑
        malposition T82.329 ☑
          aorta (bifurcation) T82.320 ☑
          carotid artery T82.321 ☑
          specified vessel NEC T82.328 ☑
        obstruction T82.399 ☑
          aorta (bifurcation) T82.390 ☑
          carotid artery T82.391 ☑
          specified vessel NEC T82.398 ☑
        perforation T82.399 ☑
          aorta (bifurcation) T82.390 ☑
          carotid artery T82.391 ☑
          specified vessel NEC T82.398 ☑
        protrusion T82.399 ☑
          aorta (bifurcation) T82.390 ☑
          carotid artery T82.391 ☑
          specified vessel NEC T82.398 ☑
      pain T82.848 ☑
      specified complication NEC T82.898 ☑
      stenosis T82.858 ☑
      thrombosis T82.868 ☑
  heart I51.9
    assist device
      infection and inflammation T82.7 ☑
    following acute myocardial infarction — *see* Complications, following, acute myocardial infarction
    postoperative — *see* Complications, circulatory system
    transplant — *see* Complication, transplant, heart and lung(s) — *see* Complications, transplant, heart, with lung
    valve
      graft (biological) T82.9 ☑
        embolism T82.817 ☑

Complication(s) — *continued*
   heart — *continued*
     valve — *continued*
      graft — *continued*
       fibrosis T82.827 ☑
       hemorrhage T82.837 ☑
       infection and inflammation T82.7 ☑
       mechanical T82.228 ☑
        breakdown T82.221 ☑
        displacement T82.222 ☑
        leakage T82.223 ☑
        malposition T82.222 ☑
        obstruction T82.228 ☑
        perforation T82.228 ☑
        protrusion T82.228 ☑
       pain T82.847 ☑
       specified type NEC T82.897 ☑
       stenosis T82.857 ☑
       thrombosis T82.867 ☑
      prosthesis T82.9 ☑
       embolism T82.817 ☑
       fibrosis T82.827 ☑
       hemorrhage T82.837 ☑
       infection or inflammation T82.6 ☑
       mechanical T82.09 ☑
        breakdown T82.01 ☑
        displacement T82.02 ☑
        leakage T82.03 ☑
        malposition T82.02 ☑
        obstruction T82.09 ☑
        perforation T82.09 ☑
        protrusion T82.09 ☑
       pain T82.847 ☑
       specified type NEC T82.897 ☑
        mechanical T82.09 ☑
       stenosis T82.857 ☑
       thrombosis T82.867 ☑
   hematoma
     intraoperative — *see* Complication, intraoperative, hemorrhage
     postprocedural — *see* Complication, postprocedural, hemorrhage
   hemodialysis — *see* Complications, dialysis
   hemorrhage
     intraoperative — *see* Complication, intraoperative, hemorrhage
     postprocedural — *see* Complication, postprocedural, hemorrhage
   ileostomy (stoma) — *see* Complications, enterostomy
   immunization (procedure) — *see* Complications, vaccination
   implant (*see also* Complications, by site and type)
     urinary sphincter T83.9 ☑
      embolism T83.81 ☑
      fibrosis T83.82 ☑
      hemorrhage T83.83 ☑
      infection and inflammation T83.59 ☑
      mechanical
       breakdown T83.111 ☑
       displacement T83.121 ☑
       leakage T83.191 ☑
       malposition T83.121 ☑
       obstruction T83.191 ☑
       perforation T83.191 ☑
       protrusion T83.191 ☑
       specified NEC T83.191 ☑
      pain T83.84 ☑
      specified type NEC T83.89 ☑
      stenosis T83.85 ☑
      thrombosis T83.86 ☑
   infusion (procedure) T80.90 ☑
     air embolism T80.0 ☑
     blood — *see* Complications, transfusion
     catheter — *see* Complications, catheter
     infection T80.29 ☑
     pump — *see* Complications, cardiovascular, device or implant
     sepsis T80.29 ☑
     serum reaction (*see also* Reaction, serum) T80.69 ☑
      anaphylactic shock (*see also* Shock, anaphylactic) T80.59 ☑
     specified type NEC T80.89 ☑
   inhalation therapy NEC T81.81 ☑
   injection (procedure) T80.90 ☑
     drug reaction — *see* Reaction, drug
     infection T80.29 ☑

Complication(s) — *continued*
   injection — *continued*
     sepsis T80.29 ☑
     serum (prophylactic) (therapeutic) — *see* Complications, vaccination
     specified type NEC T80.89 ☑
     vaccine (any) — *see* Complications, vaccination
   inoculation (any) — *see* Complications, vaccination
   insulin pump
     infection and inflammation T85.72 ☑
     mechanical
      breakdown T85.614 ☑
      displacement T85.624 ☑
      leakage T85.633 ☑
      malposition T85.624 ☑
      obstruction T85.694 ☑
      perforation T85.694 ☑
      protrusion T85.694 ☑
      specified NEC T85.694 ☑
   intestinal pouch NEC K91.858
   intraocular lens (prosthetic) T85.9 ☑
     embolism T85.81 ☑
     fibrosis T85.82 ☑
     hemorrhage T85.83 ☑
     infection and inflammation T85.79 ☑
     mechanical
      breakdown T85.21 ☑
      displacement T85.22 ☑
      malposition T85.22 ☑
      obstruction T85.29 ☑
      perforation T85.29 ☑
      protrusion T85.29 ☑
      specified NEC T85.29 ☑
     pain T85.84 ☑
     specified type NEC T85.89 ☑
     stenosis T85.85 ☑
     thrombosis T85.86 ☑
   intraoperative (intraprocedural)
     cardiac arrest
      during cardiac surgery I97.710
      during other surgery I97.711
     cardiac functional disturbance NEC
      during cardiac surgery I97.790
      during other surgery I97.791
     hemorrhage (hematoma) (of)
      circulatory system organ or structure
       during cardiac bypass I97.411
       during cardiac catheterization I97.410
       during other circulatory system procedure I97.418
       during other procedure I97.42
      digestive system organ
       during procedure on digestive system K91.61
       during procedure on other organ K91.62
      ear
       during procedure on ear and mastoid process H95.21
       during procedure on other organ H95.22
      endocrine system organ or structure
       during procedure on endocrine system organ or structure E36.01
       during procedure on other organ E36.02
      eye and adnexa
       during ophthalmic procedure H59.11- ☑
       during other procedure H59.12- ☑
      genitourinary organ or structure
       during procedure on genitourinary organ or structure N99.61
       during procedure on other organ N99.62
      mastoid process
       during procedure on ear and mastoid process H95.21
       during procedure on other organ H95.22
      musculoskeletal structure
       during musculoskeletal surgery M96.810
       during non-orthopedic surgery M96.811
       during orthopedic surgery M96.810
      nervous system
       during a nervous system procedure G97.31
       during other procedure G97.32
      respiratory system
       during other procedure J95.62
       during procedure on respiratory system organ or structure J95.61
      skin and subcutaneous tissue
       during a dermatologic procedure L76.01

Complication(s) — *continued*
   intraoperative — *continued*
     hemorrhage — *continued*
      skin and subcutaneous tissue — *continued*
       during a procedure on other organ L76.02
      spleen
       during a procedure on other organ D78.02
       during a procedure on the spleen D78.01
     puncture or laceration (accidental) (unintentional) (of)
      brain
       during a nervous system procedure G97.48
       during other procedure G97.49
      circulatory system organ or structure
       during circulatory system procedure I97.51
       during other procedure I97.52
      digestive system
       during procedure on digestive system K91.71
       during procedure on other organ K91.72
      ear
       during procedure on ear and mastoid process H95.31
       during procedure on other organ H95.32
      endocrine system organ or structure
       during procedure on endocrine system organ or structure E36.11
       during procedure on other organ E36.12
      eye and adnexa
       during ophthalmic procedure H59.21- ☑
       during other procedure H59.22- ☑
      genitourinary organ or structure
       during procedure on genitourinary organ or structure N99.71
       during procedure on other organ N99.72
      mastoid process
       during procedure on ear and mastoid process H95.31
       during procedure on other organ H95.32
      musculoskeletal structure
       during musculoskeletal surgery M96.820
       during non-orthopedic surgery M96.821
       during orthopedic surgery M96.820
      nervous system
       during a nervous system procedure G97.48
       during other procedure G97.49
      respiratory system
       during other procedure J95.72
       during procedure on respiratory system organ or structure J95.71
      skin and subcutaneous tissue
       during a dermatologic procedure L76.11
       during a procedure on other organ L76.12
      spleen
       during a procedure on other organ D78.12
       during a procedure on the spleen D78.11
     specified NEC
      circulatory system I97.88
      digestive system K91.81
      ear H95.88
      endocrine system E36.8
      eye and adnexa H59.88
      genitourinary system N99.81
      mastoid process H95.88
      musculoskeletal structure M96.89
      nervous system G97.81
      respiratory system J95.88
      skin and subcutaneous tissue L76.81
      spleen D78.81
   intraperitoneal catheter (dialysis) (infusion) — *see* Complications, catheter, intraperitoneal
   intrauterine
     contraceptive device
      embolism T83.81 ☑
      fibrosis T83.82 ☑
      hemorrhage T83.83 ☑
      infection and inflammation T83.6 ☑
      mechanical
       breakdown T83.31 ☑
       displacement T83.32 ☑
       malposition T83.32 ☑
       obstruction T83.39 ☑
       perforation T83.39 ☑
       protrusion T83.39 ☑
       specified NEC T83.39 ☑
      pain T83.84 ☑
      specified type NEC T83.89 ☑
      stenosis T83.85 ☑

☑ **Additional Character Required — Refer to the Tabular List for Character Selection**   ▽ **Subterms under main terms may continue to next column or page**

Complication(s) — *continued*
  intrauterine — *continued*
    contraceptive device — *continued*
      thrombosis T83.86 ☑
    procedure (fetal), to newborn P96.5
  jejunostomy (stoma) — *see* Complications, enterostomy
  joint prosthesis, internal T84.9 ☑
    breakage (fracture) T84.01- ☑
    dislocation T84.02- ☑
    fracture T84.01- ☑
    infection or inflammation T84.50 ☑
      hip T84.5- ☑
      knee T84.5- ☑
      specified joint NEC T84.59 ☑
    instability T84.02- ☑
    malposition — *see* Complications, joint prosthesis, mechanical, displacement
    mechanical
      breakage, broken T84.01- ☑
      dislocation T84.02- ☑
      fracture T84.01- ☑
      instability T84.02- ☑
      leakage — *see* Complications, joint prosthesis, mechanical, specified NEC
      loosening T84.039 ☑
        hip T84.03- ☑
        knee T84.03- ☑
        specified joint NEC T84.038 ☑
      obstruction — *see* Complications, joint prosthesis, mechanical, specified NEC
      perforation — *see* Complications, joint prosthesis, mechanical, specified NEC
      periprosthetic
        fracture T84.049 ☑
          hip T84.04- ☑
          knee T84.04- ☑
          other specified joint T84.048 ☑
        osteolysis T84.059 ☑
          hip T84.05- ☑
          knee T84.05- ☑
          other specified joint T84.058 ☑
      protrusion — *see* Complications, joint prosthesis, mechanical, specified NEC
      specified complication NEC T84.099 ☑
        hip T84.09- ☑
        knee T84.09- ☑
        other specified joint T84.098 ☑
      subluxation T84.02- ☑
      wear of articular bearing surface T84.069 ☑
        hip T84.06- ☑
        knee T84.06- ☑
        other specified joint T84.068 ☑
    specified joint NEC T84.89 ☑
      embolism T84.81 ☑
      fibrosis T84.82 ☑
      hemorrhage T84.83 ☑
      pain T84.84 ☑
      specified complication NEC T84.89 ☑
      stenosis T84.85 ☑
      thrombosis T84.86 ☑
    subluxation T84.02- ☑
  kidney transplant — *see* Complications, transplant, kidney
  labor O75.9
    specified NEC O75.89
  liver transplant (immune or nonimmune) — *see* Complications, transplant, liver
  lumbar puncture G97.1
    cerebrospinal fluid leak G97.0
    headache or reaction G97.1
  lung transplant — *see* Complications, transplant, lung
    and heart — *see* Complications, transplant, lung, with heart
  male genital N50.9
    device, implant or graft — *see* Complications, genitourinary, device or implant, genital tract
    postprocedural or postoperative — *see* Complications, genitourinary, postprocedural
    specified NEC N99.89
  mastoid (process) procedure
    intraoperative H95.88
      hematoma — *see* Complications, intraoperative, hemorrhage (hematoma) (of), mastoid process

Complication(s) — *continued*
  mastoid procedure — *continued*
    intraoperative — *continued*
      hemorrhage — *see* Complications, intraoperative, hemorrhage (hematoma) (of), mastoid process
      laceration — *see* Complications, intraoperative, puncture or laceration, mastoid process
      specified NEC H95.88
    postmastoidectomy — *see* Complications, postmastoidectomy
    postoperative H95.89
      external ear canal stenosis H95.81
      hematoma — *see* Complications, postprocedural, hemorrhage (hematoma) (of), mastoid process
      hemorrhage — *see* Complications, postprocedural, hemorrhage (hematoma) (of), mastoid process
      postmastoidectomy — *see* Complications, postmastoidectomy
      specified NEC H95.89
  mastoidectomy cavity — *see* Complications, postmastoidectomy
  mechanical — *see* Complications, by site and type, mechanical
  medical procedures (*see also* Complication(s), intraoperative) T88.9 ☑
  metabolic E88.9
    postoperative E89.89
      specified NEC E89.89
  molar pregnancy NOS O08.9
    damage to pelvic organs O08.6
    embolism O08.2
    genital infection O08.0
    hemorrhage (delayed) (excessive) O08.1
    metabolic disorder O08.5
    renal failure O08.4
    shock O08.3
    specified type NEC O08.0
    venous complication NEC O08.7
  musculoskeletal system (*see also* Complication, intraoperative (intraprocedural), by site)
    device, implant or graft NEC — *see* Complications, orthopedic, device or implant
    internal fixation (nail) (plate) (rod) — *see* Complications, fixation device, internal
    joint prosthesis — *see* Complications, joint prosthesis
    post radiation M96.89
      kyphosis M96.3
      scoliosis M96.5
      specified complication NEC M96.89
    postoperative (postprocedural) M96.89
      with osteoporosis — *see* Osteoporosis
      fracture following insertion of device — *see* Fracture, following insertion of device, joint prosthesis or bone plate
      joint instability after prosthesis removal M96.89
      lordosis M96.4
      postlaminectomy syndrome NEC M96.1
        kyphosis M96.3
      pseudarthrosis M96.0
      specified complication NEC M96.89
  nephrostomy (stoma) — *see* Complications, stoma, urinary tract, external NEC
  nervous system G98.8
    central G96.9
    device, implant or graft (*see also* Complication, prosthetic device or implant, specified NEC)
    electronic stimulator (electrode(s)) — *see* Complications, electronic stimulator device
    ventricular shunt — *see* Complications, ventricular shunt
    electronic stimulator (electrode(s)) — *see* Complications, electronic stimulator device
    postprocedural G97.82
      intracranial hypotension G97.2
      specified NEC G97.82
      spinal fluid leak G97.0
  newborn, due to intrauterine (fetal) procedure P96.5
  nonabsorbable (permanent) sutures — *see* Complications, sutures, permanent
  obstetric O75.9
    procedure (instrumental) (manual) (surgical)
      specified NEC O75.4
    specified NEC O75.89

Complication(s) — *continued*
  obstetric — *continued*
    surgical wound NEC O90.89
      hematoma O90.2
      infection O86.0
    ocular lens implant — *see* Complications, intraocular lens
    ophthalmologic
      postprocedural bleb — *see* Blebitis
    orbital prosthesis T85.9 ☑
      embolism T85.81 ☑
      fibrosis T85.82 ☑
      hemorrhage T85.83 ☑
      infection and inflammation T85.79 ☑
      mechanical
        breakdown T85.31- ☑
        displacement T85.32- ☑
        malposition T85.32- ☑
        obstruction T85.39- ☑
        perforation T85.39- ☑
        protrusion T85.39- ☑
        specified NEC T85.39- ☑
      pain T85.84 ☑
      specified type NEC T85.89 ☑
      stenosis T85.85 ☑
      thrombosis T85.86 ☑
    organ or tissue transplant (partial) (total) — *see* Complications, transplant
    orthopedic (*see also* Disorder, soft tissue)
      device or implant T84.9 ☑
        bone
          device or implant — *see* Complication, bone, device NEC
          graft — *see* Complication, graft, bone
        breakdown T84.418 ☑
        displacement T84.428 ☑
        electronic bone stimulator — *see* Complications, electronic stimulator device, bone
        embolism T84.81 ☑
        fibrosis T84.82 ☑
        fixation device — *see* Complication, fixation device, internal
        hemorrhage T84.83 ☑
        infection or inflammation T84.7 ☑
        joint prosthesis — *see* Complication, joint prosthesis, internal
        malfunction T84.418 ☑
        malposition T84.428 ☑
        mechanical NEC T84.498 ☑
        muscle graft — *see* Complications, graft, muscle
        obstruction T84.498 ☑
        pain T84.84 ☑
        perforation T84.498 ☑
        protrusion T84.498 ☑
        specified complication NEC T84.89 ☑
        stenosis T84.85 ☑
        tendon graft — *see* Complications, graft, tendon
        thrombosis T84.86 ☑
      fracture (following insertion of device) — *see* Fracture, following insertion of orthopedic implant, joint prosthesis or bone plate
      postprocedural M96.89
        fracture — *see* Fracture, following insertion of orthopedic implant, joint prosthesis or bone plate
        postlaminectomy syndrome NEC M96.1
          kyphosis M96.3
          lordosis M96.4
        postradiation
          kyphosis M96.2
          scoliosis M96.5
        pseudarthrosis post-fusion M96.0
        specified type NEC M96.89
    pacemaker (cardiac) — *see* Complications, cardiovascular device or implant, electronic
    pancreas transplant — *see* Complications, transplant, pancreas
    penile prosthesis (implant) — *see* Complications, prosthetic device, penile
    perfusion NEC T80.90 ☑
    perineal repair (obstetrical) NEC O90.89
      disruption O90.1
      hematoma O90.2
      infection (following delivery) O86.0
    phototherapy T88.9 ☑
      specified NEC T88.8 ☑

Complication(s) — *continued*
- postmastoidectomy NEC H95.19- ☑
  - cyst, mucosal H95.13- ☑
  - granulation H95.12- ☑
  - inflammation, chronic H95.11- ☑
  - recurrent cholesteatoma H95.0- ☑
- postoperative — *see* Complications, postprocedural
  - circulatory — *see* Complications, circulatory system
  - ear — *see* Complications, ear
  - endocrine — *see* Complications, endocrine
  - eye — *see* Complications, eye
  - lumbar puncture G97.1
    - cerebrospinal fluid leak G97.0
  - nervous system (central) (peripheral) — *see* Complications, nervous system
  - respiratory system — *see* Complications, respiratory system
- postprocedural (*see also* Complications, surgical procedure)
  - cardiac arrest
    - following cardiac surgery I97.120
    - following other surgery I97.121
  - cardiac functional disturbance NEC
    - following cardiac surgery I97.190
    - following other surgery I97.191
  - cardiac insufficiency
    - following cardiac surgery I97.110
    - following other surgery I97.111
  - chorioretinal scars following retinal surgery H59.81- ☑
  - following cataract surgery
    - cataract (lens) fragments H59.02- ☑
    - cystoid macular edema H59.03- ☑
    - specified NEC H59.09- ☑
    - vitreous (touch) syndrome H59.01- ☑
  - heart failure
    - following cardiac surgery I97.130
    - following other surgery I97.131
  - hemorrhage (hematoma) (of)
    - circulatory system organ or structure
      - following a cardiac bypass I97.611
      - following a cardiac catheterization I97.610
      - following other circulatory system procedure I97.618
      - following other procedure I97.62
    - digestive system
      - following procedure on digestive system K91.840
      - following procedure on other organ K91.841
    - ear
      - following other procedure H95.42
      - following procedure on ear and mastoid process H95.41
    - endocrine system
      - following endocrine system procedure E89.810
      - following other procedure E89.811
    - eye and adnexa
      - following ophthalmic procedure H59.31- ☑
      - following other procedure H59.32- ☑
    - genitourinary organ or structure
      - following procedure on genitourinary organ or structure N99.820
      - following procedure on other organ N99.821
    - mastoid process
      - following other procedure H95.42
      - following procedure on ear and mastoid process H95.41
    - musculoskeletal structure
      - following musculoskeletal surgery M96.830
      - following non-orthopedic surgery M96.831
      - following orthopedic surgery M96.830
    - nervous system
      - following a nervous system procedure G97.51
      - following other procedure G97.52
    - respiratory system
      - following a respiratory system procedure J95.830
      - following other procedure J95.831
    - skin and subcutaneous tissue
      - following a dermatologic procedure L76.21
      - following a procedure on other organ L76.22
    - spleen
      - following procedure on other organ D78.22
      - following procedure on the spleen D78.21

Complication(s) — *continued*
- postprocedural (*see also* Complications, surgical procedure) — *continued*
  - specified NEC
    - circulatory system I97.89
    - digestive K91.89
    - ear H95.89
    - endocrine E89.89
    - eye and adnexa H59.89
    - genitourinary N99.89
    - mastoid process H95.89
    - metabolic E89.89
    - musculoskeletal structure M96.89
    - nervous system G97.82
    - respiratory system J95.89
    - skin and subcutaneous tissue L76.82
    - spleen D78.89
- pregnancy NEC — *see* Pregnancy, complicated by
- prosthetic device or implant T85.9
  - bile duct — *see* Complications, bile duct implant
  - breast — *see* Complications, breast implant
  - cardiac and vascular NEC — *see* Complications, cardiovascular device or implant
  - corneal transplant — *see* Complications, graft, cornea
  - electronic nervous system stimulator — *see* Complications, electronic stimulator device
  - epidural infusion catheter — *see* Complications, catheter, epidural
  - esophageal anti-reflux device — *see* Complications, esophageal anti-reflux device
  - genital organ or tract — *see* Complications, genitourinary, device or implant, genital tract
  - heart valve — *see* Complications, heart, valve, prosthesis
  - infection or inflammation T85.79 ☑
    - intestine transplant T86.892
    - liver transplant T86.43
    - lung transplant T86.812
    - pancreas transplant T86.892
    - skin graft T86.822
  - intraocular lens — *see* Complications, intraocular lens
  - intraperitoneal (dialysis) catheter — *see* Complications, catheter, intraperitoneal
  - joint — *see* Complications, joint prosthesis, internal
  - mechanical NEC T85.698 ☑
    - dialysis catheter (vascular) (*see also* Complication, catheter, dialysis, mechanical)
      - peritoneal — *see* Complication, catheter, intraperitoneal, mechanical
    - gastrointestinal device T85.598 ☑
    - ocular device T85.398 ☑
    - subdural (infusion) catheter T85.690 ☑
    - suture, permanent T85.692 ☑
      - that for bone repair — *see* Complications, fixation device, internal (orthopedic), mechanical
    - ventricular shunt
      - breakdown T85.01 ☑
      - displacement T85.02 ☑
      - leakage T85.03 ☑
      - malposition T85.02 ☑
      - obstruction T85.09 ☑
      - perforation T85.09 ☑
      - protrusion T85.09 ☑
      - specified NEC T85.09 ☑
  - mesh
    - erosion (to surrounding organ or tissue) T83.718 ☑
      - vaginal (into pelvic floor muscles) T83.711 ☑
    - exposure (into surrounding organ or tissue) T83.728 ☑
      - vaginal (into vagina) (through vaginal wall) T83.721 ☑
  - orbital — *see* Complications, orbital prosthesis
  - penile T83.9 ☑
    - embolism T83.81 ☑
    - fibrosis T83.82 ☑
    - hemorrhage T83.83 ☑
    - infection and inflammation T83.6 ☑
    - mechanical
      - breakdown T83.410 ☑
      - displacement T83.420 ☑
      - leakage T83.490 ☑
      - malposition T83.420 ☑

Complication(s) — *continued*
- prosthetic device or implant — *continued*
  - penile — *continued*
    - mechanical — *continued*
      - obstruction T83.490 ☑
      - perforation T83.490 ☑
      - protrusion T83.490 ☑
      - specified NEC T83.490 ☑
    - pain T83.84 ☑
    - specified type NEC T83.89 ☑
    - stenosis T83.85 ☑
    - thrombosis T83.86 ☑
  - prosthetic materials NEC
    - erosion (to surrounding organ or tissue) T83.718 ☑
      - vaginal (into pelvic floor muscles) T83.711 ☑
    - exposure (into surrounding organ or tissue) T83.728 ☑
      - vaginal (into vagina) (through vaginal wall) T83.721 ☑
  - skin graft T86.829
    - artificial skin or decellularized allodermis
      - embolism T85.81 ☑
      - fibrosis T85.82 ☑
      - hemorrhage T85.83 ☑
      - infection and inflammation T85.79 ☑
      - mechanical
        - breakdown T85.613 ☑
        - displacement T85.623 ☑
        - malfunction T85.613 ☑
        - malposition T85.623 ☑
        - obstruction T85.693 ☑
        - perforation T85.693 ☑
        - protrusion T85.693 ☑
        - specified NEC T85.693 ☑
      - pain T85.84 ☑
      - specified type NEC T85.89 ☑
      - stenosis T85.85 ☑
      - thrombosis T85.86 ☑
    - failure T86.821
    - infection T86.822
    - rejection T86.820
    - specified NEC T86.828
  - specified NEC T85.9 ☑
    - embolism T85.81 ☑
    - fibrosis T85.82 ☑
    - hemorrhage T85.83 ☑
    - infection and inflammation T85.79 ☑
    - mechanical
      - breakdown T85.618 ☑
      - displacement T85.628 ☑
      - leakage T85.638 ☑
      - malfunction T85.618 ☑
      - malposition T85.628 ☑
      - obstruction T85.698 ☑
      - perforation T85.698 ☑
      - protrusion T85.698 ☑
      - specified NEC T85.698 ☑
    - pain T85.84 ☑
    - specified type NEC T85.89 ☑
    - stenosis T85.85 ☑
    - thrombosis T85.86 ☑
  - subdural infusion catheter — *see* Complications, catheter, subdural
  - sutures — *see* Complications, sutures
  - urinary organ or tract NEC — *see* Complications, genitourinary, device or implant, urinary system
  - vascular — *see* Complications, cardiovascular device or implant
  - ventricular shunt — *see* Complications, ventricular shunt (device)
- puerperium — *see* Puerperal
- puncture, spinal G97.1
  - cerebrospinal fluid leak G97.0
  - headache or reaction G97.1
- pyelogram N99.89
- radiation
  - kyphosis M96.2
  - scoliosis M96.5
- reattached
  - extremity (infection) (rejection)
    - lower T87.1X- ☑
    - upper T87.0X- ☑
  - specified body part NEC T87.2

64

☑ **Additional Character Required** — Refer to the Tabular List for Character Selection   ▽ **Subterms under main terms may continue to next column or page**

Complication — Complication

Complication(s) — *continued*
  reconstructed breast
    asymmetry between native and reconstructed breast N65.1
    deformity N65.0
    disproportion between native and reconstructed breast N65.1
    excess tissue N65.0
    misshappen N65.0
  reimplant NEC (*see also* Complications, prosthetic device or implant)
    limb (infection) (rejection) — *see* Complications, reattached, extremity
    organ (partial) (total) — *see* Complications, transplant
    prosthetic device NEC — *see* Complications, prosthetic device
  renal N28.9
    allograft — *see* Complications, transplant, kidney
    dialysis — *see* Complications, dialysis
  respirator
    mechanical J95.850
      specified NEC J95.859
  respiratory system J98.9
    device, implant or graft — *see* Complication, prosthetic device or implant, specified NEC
    lung transplant — *see* Complications, prosthetic device or implant, lung transplant
    postoperative J95.89
      air leak J95.812
      Mendelson's syndrome (chemical pneumonitis) J95.4
      pneumothorax J95.811
      pulmonary insufficiency (acute) (after nonthoracic surgery) J95.2
        chronic J95.3
        following thoracic surgery J95.1
      respiratory failure (acute) J95.821
        acute and chronic J95.822
      specified NEC J95.89
      subglottic stenosis J95.5
      tracheostomy complication — *see* Complications, tracheostomy
    therapy T81.89 ☑
  sedation during labor and delivery O74.9
    cardiac O74.2
    central nervous system O74.3
    pulmonary NEC O74.1
  shunt (*see also* Complications, prosthetic device or implant)
    arteriovenous — *see* Complications, arteriovenous, shunt
    ventricular (communicating) — *see* Complications, ventricular shunt
  skin
    graft T86.829
      failure T86.821
      infection T86.822
      rejection T86.820
      specified type NEC T86.828
  spinal
    anesthesia — *see* Complications, anesthesia, spinal
    catheter (epidural) (subdural) — *see* Complications, catheter
    puncture or tap G97.1
      cerebrospinal fluid leak G97.0
      headache or reaction G97.1
  stent
    bile duct — *see* Complications, bile duct prosthesis
    urinary T83.9 ☑
      embolism T83.81 ☑
      fibrosis T83.82 ☑
      hemorrhage T83.83 ☑
      infection and inflammation T83.59 ☑
      mechanical
        breakdown T83.112 ☑
        displacement T83.122 ☑
        leakage T83.192 ☑
        malposition T83.122 ☑
        obstruction T83.192 ☑
        perforation T83.192 ☑
        protrusion T83.192 ☑
        specified NEC T83.192 ☑
      pain T83.84 ☑
      specified type NEC T83.89 ☑
      stenosis T83.85 ☑
      thrombosis T83.86 ☑

Complication(s) — *continued*
  stoma
    digestive tract
      colostomy — *see* Complications, colostomy
      enterostomy — *see* Complications, enterostomy
      esophagostomy — *see* Complications, esophagostomy
      gastrostomy — *see* Complications, gastrostomy
    urinary tract N99.538
      cystostomy — *see* Complications, cystostomy
      external NOS N99.528
        hemorrhage N99.520
        infection N99.521
        malfunction N99.522
        specified type NEC N99.528
      hemorrhage N99.530
      infection N99.531
      malfunction N99.532
      specified type NEC N99.538
  stomach banding — *see* Complication(s), bariatric procedure
  stomach stapling — *see* Complication(s), bariatric procedure
  surgical material, nonabsorbable — *see* Complication, suture, permanent
  surgical procedure (on) T81.9 ☑
    amputation stump (late) — *see* Complications, amputation stump
    cardiac — *see* Complications, circulatory system
    cholesteatoma, recurrent — *see* Complications, postmastoidectomy, recurrent cholesteatoma
    circulatory (early) — *see* Complications, circulatory system
    digestive system — *see* Complications, gastrointestinal
    dumping syndrome (postgastrectomy) K91.1
    ear — *see* Complications, ear
    elephantiasis or lymphedema I97.89
      postmastectomy I97.2
    emphysema (surgical) T81.82 ☑
    endocrine — *see* Complications, endocrine
    eye — *see* Complications, eye
    fistula (persistent postoperative) T81.83 ☑
    foreign body inadvertently left in wound (sponge) (suture) (swab) — *see* Foreign body, accidentally left during a procedure
    gastrointestinal — *see* Complications, gastrointestinal
    genitourinary NEC N99.89
    hematoma
      intraoperative — *see* Complication, intraoperative, hemorrhage
      postprocedural — *see* Complication, postprocedural, hemorrhage
    hemorrhage
      intraoperative — *see* Complication, intraoperative, hemorrhage
      postprocedural — *see* Complication, postprocedural, hemorrhage
    hepatic failure K91.82
    hyperglycemia (postpancreatectomy) E89.1
    hypoinsulinemia (postpancreatectomy) E89.1
    hypoparathyroidism (postparathyroidectomy) E89.2
    hypopituitarism (posthypophysectomy) E89.3
    hypothyroidism (post-thyroidectomy) E89.0
    intestinal obstruction K91.3
    intracranial hypotension following ventricular shunting (ventriculostomy) G97.2
    lymphedema I97.89
      postmastectomy I97.2
    malabsorption (postsurgical) NEC K91.2
      osteoporosis — *see* Osteoporosis, postsurgical malabsorption
    mastoidectomy cavity NEC — *see* Complications, postmastoidectomy
    metabolic E89.89
      specified NEC E89.89
    musculoskeletal — *see* Complications, musculoskeletal system
    nervous system (central) (peripheral) — *see* Complications, nervous system
    ovarian failure E89.40
      asymptomatic E89.40
      symptomatic E89.41

Complication(s) — *continued*
  surgical procedure — *continued*
    peripheral vascular — *see* Complications, surgical procedure, vascular
    postcardiotomy syndrome I97.0
    postcholecystectomy syndrome K91.5
    postcommissurotomy syndrome I97.0
    postgastrectomy dumping syndrome K91.1
    postlaminectomy syndrome NEC M96.1
      kyphosis M96.3
    postmastectomy lymphedema syndrome I97.2
    postmastoidectomy cholesteatoma — *see* Complications, postmastoidectomy, recurrent cholesteatoma
    postvagotomy syndrome K91.1
    postvalvulotomy syndrome I97.0
    pulmonary insufficiency (acute) J95.2
      chronic J95.3
      following thoracic surgery J95.1
    reattached body part — *see* Complications, reattached
    respiratory — *see* Complications, respiratory system
    shock (hypovolemic) T81.19 ☑
    spleen (postoperative) D78.89
      intraoperative D78.81
    stitch abscess T81.4 ☑
    subglottic stenosis (postsurgical) J95.5
    testicular hypofunction E89.5
    transplant — *see* Complications, organ or tissue transplant
    urinary NEC N99.89
    vaginal vault prolapse (posthysterectomy) N99.3
    vascular (peripheral)
      artery T81.719 ☑
        mesenteric T81.710 ☑
        renal T81.711 ☑
        specified NEC T81.718 ☑
      vein T81.72 ☑
    wound infection T81.4 ☑
  suture, permanent (wire) NEC T85.9 ☑
    with repair of bone — *see* Complications, fixation device, internal
    embolism T85.81 ☑
    fibrosis T85.82 ☑
    hemorrhage T85.83 ☑
    infection and inflammation T85.79 ☑
    mechanical
      breakdown T85.612 ☑
      displacement T85.622 ☑
      malfunction T85.612 ☑
      malposition T85.622 ☑
      obstruction T85.692 ☑
      perforation T85.692 ☑
      protrusion T85.692 ☑
      specified NEC T85.692 ☑
    pain T85.84 ☑
    specified type NEC T85.89 ☑
    stenosis T85.85 ☑
    thrombosis T85.86 ☑
  tracheostomy J95.00
    granuloma J95.09
    hemorrhage J95.01
    infection J95.02
    malfunction J95.03
    mechanical J95.03
    obstruction J95.03
    specified type NEC J95.09
    tracheo-esophageal fistula J95.04
  transfusion (blood) (lymphocytes) (plasma) T80.92 ☑
    air embolism T80.0 ☑
    circulatory overload E87.71
    febrile nonhemolytic transfusion reaction R50.84
    hemochromatosis E83.111
    hemolysis T80.89 ☑
    hemolytic reaction (antigen unspecified) T80.919 ☑
    incompatibility reaction (antigen unspecified) T80.919 ☑
      ABO T80.30 ☑
        delayed serologic (DSTR) T80.39 ☑
        hemolytic transfusion reaction (HTR) (unspecified time after transfusion) T80.319 ☑
          acute (AHTR) (less than 24 hours after transfusion) T80.310 ☑

🔺 Subterms under main terms may continue to next column or page   ☑ Additional Character Required — Refer to the Tabular List for Character Selection   65

Complication — Complication

Complication(s) — *continued*
  transfusion — *continued*
    incompatibility reaction — *continued*
      ABO — *continued*
        hemolytic transfusion reaction — *contin-ued*
          delayed (DHTR) (24 hours or more after transfusion) T80.311 ☑
          specified NEC T80.39 ☑
      acute (antigen unspecified) T80.910 ☑
      delayed (antigen unspecified) T80.911 ☑
      delayed serologic (DSTR) T80.89 ☑
      non-ABO (minor antigens (Duffy) (Kell) (Kidd) (Lewis) (M) (N) (P) (S)) T80.A0 ☑ *(following T80.4)*
        delayed serologic (DSTR) T80.A9 ☑ *(following T80.4)*
        hemolytic transfusion reaction (HTR) (unspecified time after transfusion) T80.A19 ☑ *(following T80.4)*
          acute (AHTR) (less than 24 hours after transfusion) T80.A10 ☑ *(following T80.4)*
          delayed (DHTR) (24 hours or more after transfusion) T80.A11 ☑ *(following T80.4)*
          specified NEC T80.A9 ☑ *(following T80.4)*
      Rh (antigens (C) (c) (D) (E) (e)) (factor) T80.40 ☑
        delayed serologic (DSTR) T80.49 ☑
        hemolytic transfusion reaction (HTR) (unspecified time after transfusion) T80.419 ☑
          acute (AHTR) (less than 24 hours after transfusion) T80.410 ☑
          delayed (DHTR) (24 hours or more after transfusion) T80.411 ☑
          specified NEC T80.49 ☑
    infection T80.29 ☑
    reaction NEC T80.89 ☑
    sepsis T80.29 ☑
    shock T80.89 ☑
  transplant T86.90
    bone T86.839
      failure T86.831
      infection T86.832
      rejection T86.830
      specified type NEC T86.838
    bone marrow T86.00
      failure T86.02
      infection T86.03
      rejection T86.01
      specified type NEC T86.09
    cornea T86.849
      failure T86.841
      infection T86.842
      rejection T86.840
      specified type NEC T86.848
    failure T86.92
    heart T86.20
      with lung T86.30
      cardiac allograft vasculopathy T86.290
        failure T86.32
        infection T86.33
        rejection T86.31
        specified type NEC T86.39
      failure T86.22
      infection T86.23
      rejection T86.21
      specified type NEC T86.298
    infection T86.93
    intestine T86.859
      failure T86.851
      infection T86.852
      rejection T86.850
      specified type NEC T86.858
    kidney T86.10
      failure T86.12
      infection T86.13
      rejection T86.11
      specified type NEC T86.19
    liver T86.40
      failure T86.42
      infection T86.43
      rejection T86.41
      specified type NEC T86.49
    lung T86.819
      with heart T86.30
        failure T86.32

Complication(s) — *continued*
  transplant — *continued*
    lung — *continued*
      with heart — *continued*
        infection T86.33
        rejection T86.31
        specified type NEC T86.39
      failure T86.811
      infection T86.812
      rejection T86.810
      specified type NEC T86.818
    malignant neoplasm C80.2
    pancreas T86.899
      failure T86.891
      infection T86.892
      rejection T86.890
      specified type NEC T86.898
    peripheral blood stem cells T86.5
    post-transplant lymphoproliferative disorder (PTLD) D47.Z1 *(following D47.4)*
    rejection T86.91
    skin T86.829
      failure T86.821
      infection T86.822
      rejection T86.820
      specified type NEC T86.828
    specified
      tissue T86.899
        failure T86.891
        infection T86.892
        rejection T86.890
        specified type NEC T86.898
      type NEC T86.99
    stem cell (from peripheral blood) (from umbilical cord) T86.5
    umbilical cord stem cells T86.5
  trauma (early) T79.9 ☑
    specified NEC T79.8 ☑
  ultrasound therapy NEC T88.9 ☑
  umbilical cord NEC
    complicating delivery O69.9 ☑
      specified NEC O69.89 ☑
  umbrella device, vascular T82.9 ☑
    embolism T82.818 ☑
    fibrosis T82.828 ☑
    hemorrhage T82.838 ☑
    infection or inflammation T82.7 ☑
    mechanical
      breakdown T82.515 ☑
      displacement T82.525 ☑
      leakage T82.535 ☑
      malposition T82.525 ☑
      obstruction T82.595 ☑
      perforation T82.595 ☑
      protrusion T82.595 ☑
    pain T82.848 ☑
    specified type NEC T82.898 ☑
    stenosis T82.858 ☑
    thrombosis T82.868 ☑
  urethral catheter — *see* Complications, catheter, urethral, indwelling
  vaccination T88.1 ☑
    anaphylaxis NEC T80.52 ☑
    arthropathy — *see* Arthropathy, postimmunization
    cellulitis T88.0 ☑
    encephalitis or encephalomyelitis G04.02
    infection (general) (local) NEC T88.0 ☑
    meningitis G03.8
    myelitis G04.89
    protein sickness T80.62 ☑
    rash T88.1 ☑
    reaction (allergic) T88.1 ☑
      serum T80.62 ☑
    sepsis T88.0 ☑
    serum intoxication, sickness, rash, or other serum reaction NEC T80.62 ☑
      anaphylactic shock T80.52 ☑
    shock (allergic) (anaphylactic) T80.52 ☑
    vaccinia (generalized) (localized) T88.1 ☑
  vas deferens device or implant — *see* Complications, genitourinary, device or implant, genital tract
  vascular I99.9
    device or implant T82.9 ☑
      embolism T82.818 ☑
      fibrosis T82.828 ☑
      hemorrhage T82.838 ☑
      infection or inflammation T82.7 ☑

Complication(s) — *continued*
  vascular — *continued*
    device or implant — *continued*
      mechanical
        breakdown T82.519 ☑
          specified device NEC T82.518 ☑
        displacement T82.529 ☑
          specified device NEC T82.528 ☑
        leakage T82.539 ☑
          specified device NEC T82.538 ☑
        malposition T82.529 ☑
          specified device NEC T82.528 ☑
        obstruction T82.599 ☑
          specified device NEC T82.598 ☑
        perforation T82.599 ☑
          specified device NEC T82.598 ☑
        protrusion T82.599 ☑
          specified device NEC T82.598 ☑
      pain T82.848 ☑
      specified type NEC T82.898 ☑
      stenosis T82.858 ☑
      thrombosis T82.868 ☑
    dialysis catheter — *see* Complication, catheter, dialysis
    following infusion, therapeutic injection or transfusion T80.1 ☑
    graft T82.9 ☑
      embolism T82.818 ☑
      fibrosis T82.828 ☑
      hemorrhage T82.838 ☑
      mechanical
        breakdown T82.319 ☑
          aorta (bifurcation) T82.310 ☑
          carotid artery T82.311 ☑
          specified vessel NEC T82.318 ☑
        displacement T82.329 ☑
          aorta (bifurcation) T82.320 ☑
          carotid artery T82.321 ☑
          specified vessel NEC T82.328 ☑
        leakage T82.339 ☑
          aorta (bifurcation) T82.330 ☑
          carotid artery T82.331 ☑
          specified vessel NEC T82.338 ☑
        malposition T82.329 ☑
          aorta (bifurcation) T82.320 ☑
          carotid artery T82.321 ☑
          specified vessel NEC T82.328 ☑
        obstruction T82.399 ☑
          aorta (bifurcation) T82.390 ☑
          carotid artery T82.391 ☑
          specified vessel NEC T82.398 ☑
        perforation T82.399 ☑
          aorta (bifurcation) T82.390 ☑
          carotid artery T82.391 ☑
          specified vessel NEC T82.398 ☑
        protrusion T82.399 ☑
          aorta (bifurcation) T82.390 ☑
          carotid artery T82.391 ☑
          specified vessel NEC T82.398 ☑
      pain T82.848 ☑
      specified complication NEC T82.898 ☑
      stenosis T82.858 ☑
      thrombosis T82.868 ☑
    postoperative — *see* Complications, postoperative, circulatory
  vena cava device (filter) (sieve) (umbrella) — *see* Complications, umbrella device, vascular
  ventilation therapy NEC T81.81 ☑
  ventilator
    mechanical J95.850
      specified NEC J95.859
  ventricular (communicating) shunt (device) T85.9 ☑
    embolism T85.81 ☑
    fibrosis T85.82 ☑
    hemorrhage T85.83 ☑
    infection and inflammation T85.79 ☑
    mechanical
      breakdown T85.01 ☑
      displacement T85.02 ☑
      leakage T85.03 ☑
      malposition T85.02 ☑
      obstruction T85.09 ☑
      perforation T85.09 ☑
      protrusion T85.09 ☑
      specified NEC T85.09 ☑
    pain T85.84 ☑

☑ **Additional Character Required** — Refer to the Tabular List for Character Selection   ▽ **Subterms under main terms may continue to next column or page**

Complication(s) — *continued*
  ventricular shunt — *continued*
    specified type NEC T85.89 ☑
    stenosis T85.85 ☑
    thrombosis T85.86 ☑
  wire suture, permanent (implanted) — *see* Complications, suture, permanent
Compressed air disease T70.3 ☑
Compression
  with injury — *code by Nature of injury*
  artery I77.1
    celiac, syndrome I77.4
  brachial plexus G54.0
  brain (stem) G93.5
    due to
      contusion (diffuse) — *see* Injury, intracranial, diffuse
        focal — *see* Injury, intracranial, focal
      injury NEC — *see* Injury, intracranial, diffuse
      traumatic — *see* Injury, intracranial, diffuse
  bronchus J98.09
  cauda equina G83.4
  celiac (artery) (axis) I77.4
  cerebral — *see* Compression, brain
  cervical plexus G54.2
  cord
    spinal — *see* Compression, spinal
    umbilical — *see* Compression, umbilical cord
  cranial nerve G52.9
    eighth H93.3 ☑
    eleventh G52.8
    fifth G50.8
    first G52.0
    fourth — *see* Strabismus, paralytic, fourth nerve
    ninth G52.1
    second — *see* Disorder, nerve, optic
    seventh G52.8
    sixth — *see* Strabismus, paralytic, sixth nerve
    tenth G52.2
    third — *see* Strabismus, paralytic, third nerve
    twelfth G52.3
  diver's squeeze T70.3 ☑
  during birth (newborn) P15.9
  esophagus K22.2
  eustachian tube — *see* Obstruction, eustachian tube, cartilaginous
  facies Q67.1
  fracture — *see* Fracture
  heart — *see* Disease, heart
  intestine — *see* Obstruction, intestine
  laryngeal nerve, recurrent G52.2
    with paralysis of vocal cords and larynx J38.00
      bilateral J38.02
      unilateral J38.01
  lumbosacral plexus G54.1
  lung J98.4
  lymphatic vessel I89.0
  medulla — *see* Compression, brain
  nerve (*see also* Disorder, nerve) G58.9
    arm NEC — *see* Mononeuropathy, upper limb
    axillary G54.0
    cranial — *see* Compression, cranial nerve
    leg NEC — *see* Mononeuropathy, lower limb
    median (in carpal tunnel) — *see* Syndrome, carpal tunnel
    optic — *see* Disorder, nerve, optic
    plantar — *see* Lesion, nerve, plantar
    posterior tibial (in tarsal tunnel) — *see* Syndrome, tarsal tunnel
    root or plexus NOS (in) G54.9
      intervertebral disc disorder NEC — *see* Disorder, disc, with, radiculopathy
      with myelopathy — *see* Disorder, disc, with, myelopathy
      neoplastic disease (*see also* Neoplasm) D49.9 [G55]
      spondylosis — *see* Spondylosis, with radiculopathy
    sciatic (acute) — *see* Lesion, nerve, sciatic
    sympathetic G90.8
    traumatic — *see* Injury, nerve
    ulnar — *see* Lesion, nerve, ulnar
    upper extremity NEC — *see* Mononeuropathy, upper limb
  spinal (cord) G95.20
    by displacement of intervertebral disc NEC (*see also* Disorder, disc, with, myelopathy)

Compression — *continued*
  spinal — *continued*
    nerve root NOS G54.9
      due to displacement of intervertebral disc NEC — *see* Disorder, disc, with, radiculopathy
      with myelopathy — *see* Disorder, disc, with, myelopathy
    specified NEC G95.29
    spondylogenic (cervical) (lumbar, lumbosacral) (thoracic) — *see* Spondylosis, with myelopathy NEC
    anterior — *see* Syndrome, anterior, spinal artery, compression
    traumatic — *see* Injury, spinal cord, by region
  subcostal nerve (syndrome) — *see* Mononeuropathy, upper limb, specified NEC
  sympathetic nerve NEC G90.8
  syndrome T79.5 ☑
  trachea J39.8
  ulnar nerve (by scar tissue) — *see* Lesion, nerve, ulnar
  umbilical cord
    complicating delivery O69.2 ☑
      cord around neck O69.1 ☑
      prolapse O69.0 ☑
      specified NEC O69.2 ☑
  ureter N13.5
  vein I87.1
  vena cava (inferior) (superior) I87.1
Compulsion, compulsive
  gambling F63.0
  neurosis F42
  personality F60.5
  states F42
  swearing F42
    in Gilles de la Tourette's syndrome F95.2
  tics and spasms F95.9
Concato's disease (pericardial polyserositis) A19.9
  nontubercular I31.1
  pleural — *see* Pleurisy, with effusion
Concavity chest wall M95.4
Concealed penis Q55.69
Concern (normal) **about sick person in family** Z63.6
Concrescence (teeth) K00.2
Concretio cordis I31.1
  rheumatic I09.2
Concretion (*see also* Calculus)
  appendicular K38.1
  canaliculus — *see* Dacryolith
  clitoris N90.89
  conjunctiva H11.12- ☑
  eyelid — *see* Disorder, eyelid, specified type NEC
  lacrimal passages — *see* Dacryolith
  prepuce (male) N47.8
  salivary gland (any) K11.5
  seminal vesicle N50.8
  tonsil J35.8
Concussion (brain) (cerebral) (current) S06.0X- ☑
  blast (air) (hydraulic) (immersion) (underwater)
    abdomen or thorax — *see* Injury, blast, by site
    ear with acoustic nerve injury — *see* Injury, nerve, acoustic, specified type NEC
  cauda equina S34.3 ☑
  conus medullaris S34.02 ☑
  ocular S05.8X- ☑
  spinal (cord)
    cervical S14.0 ☑
    lumbar S34.01 ☑
    sacral S34.02 ☑
    thoracic S24.0 ☑
  syndrome F07.81
Condition — *see* Disease
Conditions arising in the perinatal period — *see* Newborn, affected by
Conduct disorder — *see* Disorder, conduct
Condyloma A63.0
  acuminatum A63.0
  gonorrheal A54.09
  latum A51.31
  syphilitic A51.31
    congenital A50.07
  venereal, syphilitic A51.31
Conflagration (*see also* Burn)
  asphyxia (by inhalation of gases, fumes or vapors) (*see also* Table of Drugs and Chemicals) T59.9- ☑
Conflict (with) (*see also* Discord)
  family Z73.9

Conflict — *continued*
  marital Z63.0
    involving divorce or estrangement Z63.5
  parent-child Z62.820
    parent-adopted child Z62.821
    parent-biological child Z62.820
    parent-foster child Z62.822
  social role NEC Z73.5
Confluent — *see* condition
Confusion, confused R41.0
  epileptic F05
  mental state (psychogenic) F44.89
  psychogenic F44.89
  reactive (from emotional stress, psychological trauma) F44.89
Confusional arousals G47.51
Congelation T69.9 ☑
Congenital (*see also* condition)
  aortic septum Q25.4
  intrinsic factor deficiency D51.0
  malformation — *see* Anomaly
Congestion, congestive
  bladder N32.89
  bowel K63.89
  brain G93.89
  breast N64.59
  bronchial J98.09
  catarrhal J31.0
  chest R09.89
  chill, malarial — *see* Malaria
  circulatory NEC I99.8
  duodenum K31.89
  eye — *see* Hyperemia, conjunctiva
  facial, due to birth injury P15.4
  general R68.89
  glottis J37.0
  heart — *see* Failure, heart, congestive
  hepatic K76.1
  hypostatic (lung) — *see* Edema, lung
  intestine K63.89
  kidney N28.89
  labyrinth H83.8 ☑
  larynx J37.0
  liver K76.1
  lung R09.89
    active or acute — *see* Pneumonia
  malaria, malarial — *see* Malaria
  nasal R09.81
  nose R09.81
  orbit, orbital (*see also* Exophthalmos)
    inflammatory (chronic) — *see* Inflammation, orbit
  ovary N83.8
  pancreas K86.8
  pelvic, female N94.89
  pleural J94.8
  prostate (active) N42.1
  pulmonary — *see* Congestion, lung
  renal N28.89
  retina H35.81
  seminal vesicle N50.1
  spinal cord G95.19
  spleen (chronic) D73.2
  stomach K31.89
  trachea — *see* Tracheitis
  urethra N36.8
  uterus N85.8
    with subinvolution N85.3
  venous (passive) I87.8
  viscera R68.89
Congestive — *see* Congestion
Conical
  cervix (hypertrophic elongation) N88.4
  cornea — *see* Keratoconus
  teeth K00.2
Conjoined twins Q89.4
Conjugal maladjustment Z63.0
  involving divorce or estrangement Z63.5
Conjunctiva — *see* condition
Conjunctivitis (staphylococcal) (streptococcal) NOS H10.9
  Acanthamoeba B60.12
  acute H10.3- ☑
    atopic H10.1- ☑
    chemical (*see also* Corrosion, cornea) H10.21- ☑
    mucopurulent H10.02- ☑
      follicular H10.01- ☑
    pseudomembranous H10.22- ☑

Constriction — *continued*
  gallbladder — *see* Obstruction, gallbladder
  intestine — *see* Obstruction, intestine
  larynx J38.6
    congenital Q31.8
      specified NEC Q31.8
      subglottic Q31.1
  organ or site, congenital NEC — *see* Atresia, by site
  prepuce (acquired) (congenital) N47.1
  pylorus (adult hypertrophic) K31.1
    congenital or infantile Q40.0
    newborn Q40.0
  ring dystocia (uterus) O62.4
  spastic (*see also* Spasm)
    ureter N13.5
  ureter N13.5
    with infection N13.6
  urethra — *see* Stricture, urethra
  visual field (peripheral) (functional) — *see* Defect, visual field
Constrictive — *see* condition
Consultation
  without complaint or sickness Z71.9
    feared complaint unfounded Z71.1
    specified reason NEC Z71.89
  medical — *see* Counseling, medical
  religious Z71.81
  specified reason NEC Z71.89
  spiritual Z71.81
Consumption — *see* Tuberculosis
Contact (with) (*see also* Exposure (to))
  acariasis Z20.7
  AIDS virus Z20.6
  air pollution Z77.110
  algae and algae toxins Z77.121
  algae bloom Z77.121
  anthrax Z20.810
  aromatic amines Z77.020
  aromatic (hazardous) compounds NEC Z77.028
  aromatic dyes NOS Z77.028
  arsenic Z77.010
  asbestos Z77.090
  bacterial disease NEC Z20.818
  benzene Z77.021
  blue-green algae bloom Z77.121
  body fluids (potentially hazardous) Z77.21
  brown tide Z77.121
  chemicals (chiefly nonmedicinal) (hazardous) NEC Z77.098
  cholera Z20.09
  chromium compounds Z77.018
  communicable disease Z20.9
    bacterial NEC Z20.818
    specified NEC Z20.89
    viral NEC Z20.828
  cyanobacteria bloom Z77.121
  dyes Z77.098
  Escherichia coli (E. coli) Z20.01
  fiberglass — *see* Table of Drugs and Chemicals, fiberglass
  German measles Z20.4
  gonorrhea Z20.2
  hazardous metals NEC Z77.018
  hazardous substances NEC Z77.29
  hazards in the physical environment NEC Z77.128
  hazards to health NEC Z77.9
  HIV Z20.6
  HTLV-III/LAV Z20.6
  human immunodeficiency virus (HIV) Z20.6
  infection Z20.9
    specified NEC Z20.89
  infestation (parasitic) NEC Z20.7
  intestinal infectious disease NEC Z20.09
    Escherichia coli (E. coli) Z20.01
  lead Z77.011
  meningococcus Z20.811
  mold (toxic) Z77.120
  nickel dust Z77.018
  noise Z77.122
  parasitic disease Z20.7
  pediculosis Z20.7
  pfiesteria piscicida Z77.121
  poliomyelitis Z20.89
  pollution
    air Z77.110
    environmental NEC Z77.118
    soil Z77.112
    water Z77.111

Contact — *continued*
  polycyclic aromatic hydrocarbons Z77.028
  rabies Z20.3
  radiation, naturally occurring NEC Z77.123
  radon Z77.123
  red tide (Florida) Z77.121
  rubella Z20.4
  sexually-transmitted disease Z20.2
  smallpox (laboratory) Z20.89
  syphilis Z20.2
  tuberculosis Z20.1
  uranium Z77.012
  varicella Z20.820
  venereal disease Z20.2
  viral disease NEC Z20.828
  viral hepatitis Z20.5
  water pollution Z77.111
Contamination, food — *see* Intoxication, foodborne
Contraception, contraceptive
  advice Z30.09
  counseling Z30.09
  device (intrauterine) (in situ) Z97.5
    causing menorrhagia T83.83 ☑
    checking Z30.431
    complications — *see* Complications, intrauterine, contraceptive device
    in place Z97.5
    initial prescription Z30.014
    reinsertion Z30.433
    removal Z30.432
    replacement Z30.433
  emergency (postcoital) Z30.012
  initial prescription Z30.019
    injectable Z30.013
    intrauterine device Z30.014
    pills Z30.011
    postcoital (emergency) Z30.012
    specified type NEC Z30.018
    subdermal implantable Z30.019
  maintenance Z30.40
    examination Z30.8
    injectable Z30.42
    intrauterine device Z30.431
    pills Z30.41
    specified type NEC Z30.49
    subdermal implantable Z30.49
  management Z30.9
    specified NEC Z30.8
  postcoital (emergency) Z30.012
  prescription Z30.019
    repeat Z30.40
  sterilization Z30.2
  surveillance (drug) — *see* Contraception, maintenance
Contraction(s), contracture, contracted
  Achilles tendon (*see also* Short, tendon, Achilles)
    congenital Q66.89
  amputation stump (surgical) (flexion) (late) (next proximal joint) T87.89
  anus K59.8
  bile duct (common) (hepatic) K83.8
  bladder N32.89
    neck or sphincter N32.0
  bowel, cecum, colon or intestine, any part — *see* Obstruction, intestine
  Braxton Hicks — *see* False, labor
  breast implant, capsular T85.44 ☑
  bronchial J98.09
  burn (old) — *see* Cicatrix
  cervix — *see* Stricture, cervix
  cicatricial — *see* Cicatrix
  conjunctiva, trachomatous, active A71.1
    sequelae (late effect) B94.0
  Dupuytren's M72.0
  eyelid — *see* Disorder, eyelid function
  fascia (lata) (postural) M72.8
    Dupuytren's M72.0
    palmar M72.0
    plantar M72.2
  finger NEC (*see also* Deformity, finger)
    congenital Q68.1
    joint — *see* Contraction, joint, hand
  flaccid — *see* Contraction, paralytic
  gallbladder K82.0
  heart valve — *see* Endocarditis
  hip — *see* Contraction, joint, hip
  hourglass
    bladder N32.89
      congenital Q64.79

Contraction(s), contracture, contracted — *continued*
  hourglass — *continued*
    gallbladder K82.0
      congenital Q44.1
    stomach K31.89
      congenital Q40.2
      psychogenic F45.8
    uterus (complicating delivery) O62.4
  hysterical F44.4
  internal os — *see* Stricture, cervix
  joint (abduction) (acquired) (adduction) (flexion) (rotation) M24.50
    ankle M24.57- ☑
    congenital NEC Q68.8
      hip Q65.89
    elbow M24.52- ☑
    foot joint M24.57- ☑
    hand joint M24.54- ☑
    hip M24.55- ☑
      congenital Q65.89
    hysterical F44.4
    knee M24.56- ☑
    shoulder M24.51- ☑
    wrist M24.53- ☑
  kidney (granular) (secondary) N26.9
    congenital Q63.8
    hydronephritic — *see* Hydronephrosis Page N26.2
    pyelonephritic — *see* Pyelitis, chronic
    tuberculous A18.11
  ligament (*see also* Disorder, ligament)
    congenital Q79.8
  muscle (postinfective) (postural) NEC M62.40
    with contracture of joint — *see* Contraction, joint
    ankle M62.47- ☑
    congenital Q79.8
      sternocleidomastoid Q68.0
    extraocular — *see* Strabismus
    eye (extrinsic) — *see* Strabismus
    foot M62.47- ☑
    forearm M62.43- ☑
    hand M62.44- ☑
    hysterical F44.4
    ischemic (Volkmann's) T79.6 ☑
    lower leg M62.46- ☑
    multiple sites M62.49
    pelvic region M62.45- ☑
    posttraumatic — *see* Strabismus, paralytic
    psychogenic F45.8
      conversion reaction F44.4
    shoulder region M62.41- ☑
    specified site NEC M62.48
    thigh M62.45- ☑
    upper arm M62.42- ☑
  neck — *see* Torticollis
  ocular muscle — *see* Strabismus
  organ or site, congenital NEC — *see* Atresia, by site
  outlet (pelvis) — *see* Contraction, pelvis
  palmar fascia M72.0
  paralytic
    joint — *see* Contraction, joint
    muscle (*see also* Contraction, muscle NEC)
    ocular — *see* Strabismus, paralytic
  pelvis (acquired) (general) M95.5
    with disproportion (fetopelvic) O33.1
      causing obstructed labor O65.1
    inlet O33.2
    mid-cavity O33.3 ☑
    outlet O33.3 ☑
  plantar fascia M72.2
  premature
    atrium I49.1
    auriculoventricular I49.49
    heart I49.49
    junctional I49.2
    supraventricular I49.1
    ventricular I49.3
  prostate N42.89
  pylorus NEC (*see also* Pylorospasm)
    psychogenic F45.8
  rectum, rectal (sphincter) K59.8
  ring (Bandl's) (complicating delivery) O62.4
  scar — *see* Cicatrix
  spine — *see* Dorsopathy, deforming
  sternocleidomastoid (muscle), congenital Q68.0

Contraction(s), contracture, contracted —
continued
- stomach K31.89
  - hourglass K31.89
    - congenital Q40.2
    - psychogenic F45.8
  - psychogenic F45.8
- tendon (sheath) M62.40
  - with contracture of joint — *see* Contraction, joint
  - Achilles — *see* Short, tendon, Achilles
  - ankle M62.47- ☑
    - Achilles — *see* Short, tendon, Achilles
  - foot M62.47- ☑
  - forearm M62.43- ☑
  - hand M62.44- ☑
  - lower leg M62.46- ☑
  - multiple sites M62.49
  - neck M62.48
  - pelvic region M62.45- ☑
  - shoulder region M62.41- ☑
  - specified site NEC M62.48
  - thigh M62.45- ☑
  - thorax M62.48
  - trunk M62.48
  - upper arm M62.42- ☑
- toe — *see* Deformity, toe, specified NEC
- ureterovesical orifice (postinfectional) N13.5
  - with infection N13.6
- urethra (*see also* Stricture, urethra)
  - orifice N32.0
- uterus N85.8
  - abnormal NEC O62.9
  - clonic (complicating delivery) O62.4
  - dyscoordinate (complicating delivery) O62.4
  - hourglass (complicating delivery) O62.4
  - hypertonic O62.4
  - hypotonic NEC O62.2
  - inadequate
    - primary O62.0
    - secondary O62.1
  - incoordinate (complicating delivery) O62.4
  - poor O62.2
  - tetanic (complicating delivery) O62.4
- vagina (outlet) N89.5
- vesical N32.89
  - neck or urethral orifice N32.0
- visual field — *see* Defect, visual field, generalized
- Volkmann's (ischemic) T79.6 ☑

Contusion (skin surface intact) T14.8
- abdomen, abdominal (muscle) (wall) S30.1 ☑
- adnexa, eye NEC S05.8X- ☑
- adrenal gland S37.812 ☑
- alveolar process S00.532 ☑
- ankle S90.0- ☑
- antecubital space — *see* Contusion, forearm
- anus S30.3 ☑
- arm (upper) S40.02- ☑
  - lower (with elbow) — *see* Contusion, forearm
- auditory canal — *see* Contusion, ear
- auricle — *see* Contusion, ear
- axilla — *see* Contusion, arm, upper
- back (*see also* Contusion, thorax, back)
  - lower S30.0 ☑
- bile duct S36.13 ☑
- bladder S37.22 ☑
- bone NEC T14.8
- brain (diffuse) — *see* Injury, intracranial, diffuse
  - focal — *see* Injury, intracranial, focal
- brainstem S06.38- ☑
- breast S20.0- ☑
- broad ligament S37.892 ☑
- brow S00.83 ☑
- buttock S30.0 ☑
- canthus, eye S00.1- ☑
- cauda equina S34.3 ☑
- cerebellar, traumatic S06.37- ☑
- cerebral S06.33- ☑
  - left side S06.32- ☑
  - right side S06.31- ☑
- cheek S00.83 ☑
  - internal S00.532 ☑
- chest (wall) — *see* Contusion, thorax
- chin S00.83 ☑
- clitoris S30.23 ☑
- colon — *see* Injury, intestine, large, contusion
- common bile duct S36.13 ☑

Contusion — *continued*
- conjunctiva S05.1- ☑
  - with foreign body (in conjunctival sac) — *see* Foreign body, conjunctival sac
- conus medullaris (spine) S34.139 ☑
- cornea — *see* Contusion, eyeball
  - with foreign body — *see* Foreign body, cornea
- corpus cavernosum S30.21 ☑
- cortex (brain) (cerebral) — *see* Injury, intracranial, diffuse
  - focal — *see* Injury, intracranial, focal
- costal region — *see* Contusion, thorax
- cystic duct S36.13
- diaphragm S27.802 ☑
- duodenum S36.420 ☑
- ear S00.43- ☑
- elbow S50.0- ☑
  - with forearm — *see* Contusion, forearm
- epididymis S30.22 ☑
- epigastric region S30.1 ☑
- epiglottis S10.0 ☑
- esophagus (thoracic) S27.812 ☑
  - cervical S10.0 ☑
- eyeball S05.1- ☑
- eyebrow S00.1- ☑
- eyelid (and periocular area) S00.1- ☑
- face NEC S00.83 ☑
- fallopian tube S37.529 ☑
  - bilateral S37.522 ☑
  - unilateral S37.521 ☑
- femoral triangle S30.1 ☑
- finger(s) S60.00 ☑
  - with damage to nail (matrix) S60.10 ☑
  - index S60.02- ☑
    - with damage to nail S60.12- ☑
  - little S60.05- ☑
    - with damage to nail S60.15- ☑
  - middle S60.03- ☑
    - with damage to nail S60.13- ☑
  - ring S60.04- ☑
    - with damage to nail S60.14- ☑
  - thumb — *see* Contusion, thumb
- flank S30.1 ☑
- foot (except toe(s) alone) S90.3- ☑
  - toe — *see* Contusion, toe
- forearm S50.1- ☑
  - elbow only — *see* Contusion, elbow
- forehead S00.83 ☑
- gallbladder S36.122 ☑
- genital organs, external
  - female S30.202 ☑
  - male S30.201 ☑
- globe (eye) — *see* Contusion, eyeball
- groin S30.1 ☑
- gum S00.532 ☑
- hand S60.22- ☑
  - finger(s) — *see* Contusion, finger
  - wrist — *see* Contusion, wrist
- head S00.93 ☑
  - ear — *see* Contusion, ear
  - eyelid — *see* Contusion, eyelid
  - lip S00.531 ☑
  - nose S00.33 ☑
  - oral cavity S00.532 ☑
  - scalp S00.03 ☑
  - specified part NEC S00.83 ☑
- heel — *see* Contusion, foot
- hepatic duct S36.13 ☑
- hip S70.0- ☑
- ileum S36.428 ☑
- iliac region S30.1 ☑
- inguinal region S30.1 ☑
- interscapular region S20.229 ☑
- intra-abdominal organ S36.92 ☑
  - colon — *see* Injury, intestine, large, contusion
  - liver S36.112 ☑
  - pancreas — *see* Contusion, pancreas
  - rectum S36.62 ☑
  - small intestine — *see* Injury, intestine, small, contusion
  - specified organ NEC S36.892 ☑
  - spleen — *see* Contusion, spleen
  - stomach S36.32 ☑
- iris (eye) — *see* Contusion, eyeball
- jaw S00.83 ☑
- jejunum S36.428 ☑

Contusion — *continued*
- kidney S37.01- ☑
  - major (greater than 2 cm) S37.02- ☑
  - minor (less than 2 cm) S37.01- ☑
- knee S80.0- ☑
- labium (majus) (minus) S30.23 ☑
- lacrimal apparatus, gland or sac S05.8X- ☑
- larynx S10.0 ☑
- leg (lower) S80.1- ☑
  - knee — *see* Contusion, knee
- lens — *see* Contusion, eyeball
- lip S00.531 ☑
- liver S36.112 ☑
- lower back S30.0 ☑
- lumbar region S30.0 ☑
- lung S27.329 ☑
  - bilateral S27.322 ☑
  - unilateral S27.321 ☑
- malar region S00.83 ☑
- mastoid region S00.83 ☑
- membrane, brain — *see* Injury, intracranial, diffuse
  - focal — *see* Injury, intracranial, focal
- mesentery S36.892 ☑
- mesosalpinx S37.892 ☑
- mouth S00.532 ☑
- muscle — *see* Contusion, by site
- nail
  - finger — *see* Contusion, finger, with damage to nail
  - toe — *see* Contusion, toe, with damage to nail
- nasal S00.33 ☑
- neck S10.93 ☑
  - specified site NEC S10.83 ☑
  - throat S10.0 ☑
- nerve — *see* Injury, nerve
- newborn P54.5
- nose S00.33 ☑
- occipital
  - lobe (brain) — *see* Injury, intracranial, diffuse
    - focal — *see* Injury, intracranial, focal
  - region (scalp) S00.03 ☑
- orbit (region) (tissues) S05.1- ☑
- ovary S37.429 ☑
  - bilateral S37.422 ☑
  - unilateral S37.421 ☑
- palate S00.532 ☑
- pancreas S36.229 ☑
  - body S36.221 ☑
  - head S36.220 ☑
  - tail S36.222 ☑
- parietal
  - lobe (brain) — *see* Injury, intracranial, diffuse
    - focal — *see* Injury, intracranial, focal
  - region (scalp) S00.03 ☑
- pelvic organ S37.92 ☑
  - adrenal gland S37.812 ☑
  - bladder S37.22 ☑
  - fallopian tube — *see* Contusion, fallopian tube
  - kidney — *see* Contusion, kidney
  - ovary — *see* Contusion, ovary
  - prostate S37.822 ☑
  - specified organ NEC S37.892 ☑
  - ureter S37.12 ☑
  - urethra S37.32 ☑
  - uterus S37.62 ☑
- pelvis S30.0 ☑
- penis S30.21 ☑
- perineum
  - female S30.23 ☑
  - male S30.0 ☑
- periocular area S00.1- ☑
- peritoneum S36.81 ☑
- periurethral tissue — *see* Contusion, urethra
- pharynx S10.0 ☑
- pinna — *see* Contusion, ear
- popliteal space — *see* Contusion, knee
- prepuce S30.21 ☑
- prostate S37.822 ☑
- pubic region S30.1 ☑
- pudendum
  - female S30.202 ☑
  - male S30.201 ☑
- quadriceps femoris — *see* Contusion, thigh
- rectum S36.62 ☑
- retroperitoneum S36.892 ☑
- round ligament S37.892 ☑

☑ Additional Character Required — Refer to the Tabular List for Character Selection   ▽ **Subterms under main terms may continue to next column or page**

Contusion — *continued*
  sacral region S30.0 ☑
  scalp S00.03 ☑
    due to birth injury P12.3
  scapular region — *see* Contusion, shoulder
  sclera — *see* Contusion, eyeball
  scrotum S30.22 ☑
  seminal vesicle S37.892 ☑
  shoulder S40.01- ☑
  skin NEC T14.8
  small intestine — *see* Injury, intestine, small, contusion
  spermatic cord S30.22 ☑
  spinal cord — *see* Injury, spinal cord, by region
    cauda equina S34.3 ☑
    conus medullaris S34.139 ☑
  spleen S36.029 ☑
    major S36.021 ☑
    minor S36.020 ☑
  sternal region S20.219 ☑
  stomach S36.32 ☑
  subconjunctival S05.1- ☑
  subcutaneous NEC T14.8
  submaxillary region S00.83 ☑
  submental region S00.83 ☑
  subperiosteal NEC T14.8
  subungual
    finger — *see* Contusion, finger, with damage to nail
    toe — *see* Contusion, toe, with damage to nail
  supraclavicular fossa S10.83 ☑
  supraorbital S00.83 ☑
  suprarenal gland S37.812 ☑
  temple (region) S00.83 ☑
  temporal
    lobe (brain) — *see* Injury, intracranial, diffuse
      focal — *see* Injury, intracranial, focal
    region S00.83 ☑
  testis S30.22 ☑
  thigh S70.1- ☑
  thorax (wall) S20.20 ☑
    back S20.22- ☑
    front S20.21- ☑
  throat S10.0 ☑
  thumb S60.01- ☑
    with damage to nail S60.11- ☑
  toe(s) (lesser) S90.12- ☑
    with damage to nail S90.22- ☑
    great S90.11- ☑
      with damage to nail S90.21- ☑
      specified type NEC S90.221 ☑
  tongue S00.532 ☑
  trachea (cervical) S10.0 ☑
    thoracic S27.52 ☑
  tunica vaginalis S30.22 ☑
  tympanum, tympanic membrane — *see* Contusion, ear
  ureter S37.12 ☑
  urethra S37.32 ☑
  urinary organ NEC S37.892 ☑
  uterus S37.62 ☑
  uvula S00.532 ☑
  vagina S30.23 ☑
  vas deferens S37.892 ☑
  vesical S37.22 ☑
  vocal cord(s) S10.0 ☑
  vulva S30.23 ☑
  wrist S60.21- ☑
Conus (congenital) (any type) Q14.8
  cornea — *see* Keratoconus
  medullaris syndrome G95.81
Conversion hysteria, neurosis or reaction F44.9
Converter, tuberculosis (test reaction) R76.11
Conviction (legal), **anxiety concerning** Z65.0
  with imprisonment Z65.1
Convulsions (idiopathic) (*see also* Seizure(s)) R56.9
  apoplectiform (cerebral ischemia) I67.82
  benign neonatal (familial) — *see* Epilepsy, generalized, idiopathic
  dissociative F44.5
  epileptic — *see* Epilepsy
  epileptiform, epileptoid — *see* Seizure, epileptiform
  ether (anesthetic) — *see* Table of Drugs and Chemicals, by drug
  febrile R56.00
    with status epilepticus G40.901

Convulsions — *continued*
  febrile — *continued*
    complex R56.01
      with status epilepticus G40.901
    simple R56.00
  hysterical F44.5
  infantile P90
    epilepsy — *see* Epilepsy
  jacksonian — *see* Epilepsy, localization-related, symptomatic, with simple partial seizures
  myoclonic G25.3
  neonatal, benign (familial) — *see* Epilepsy, generalized, idiopathic
  newborn P90
  obstetrical (nephritic) (uremic) — *see* Eclampsia
  paretic A52.17
  post traumatic R56.1
  psychomotor — *see* Epilepsy, localization-related, symptomatic, with complex partial seizures
  recurrent R56.9
  reflex R25.8
  scarlatinal A38.8
  tetanus, tetanic — *see* Tetanus
  thymic E32.8
Convulsive (*see also* Convulsions)
Cooley's anemia D56.1
Coolie itch B76.9
Cooper's
  disease — *see* Mastopathy, cystic
  hernia — *see* Hernia, abdomen, specified site NEC
Copra itch B88.0
Coprophagy F50.8
Coprophobia F40.298
Coproporphyria, hereditary E80.29
Cor
  biloculare Q20.8
  bovis, bovinum — *see* Hypertrophy, cardiac
  pulmonale (chronic) I27.81
    acute I26.09
  triatriatum, triatrium Q24.2
  triloculare Q20.8
    biatrium Q20.4
    biventriculare Q21.1
Corbus' disease (gangrenous balanitis) N48.1
Cord (*see also* condition)
  around neck (tightly) (with compression)
    complicating delivery O69.1 ☑
  bladder G95.89
    tabetic A52.19
Cordis ectopia Q24.8
Corditis (spermatic) N49.1
Corectopia Q13.2
Cori's disease (glycogen storage) E74.03
Corkhandler's disease or lung J67.3
Corkscrew esophagus K22.4
Corkworker's disease or lung J67.3
Corn (infected) L84
Cornea (*see also* condition)
  donor Z52.5
  plana Q13.4
Cornelia de Lange syndrome Q87.1
Cornu cutaneum L85.8
Cornual gestation or pregnancy O00.8
Coronary (artery) — *see* condition
Coronavirus, as cause of disease classified elsewhere B97.29
  SARS-associated B97.21
Corpora (*see also* condition)
  amylacea, prostate N42.89
  cavernosa — *see* condition
Corpulence — *see* Obesity
Corpus — *see* condition
Corrected transposition Q20.5
Corrosion (injury) (acid) (caustic) (chemical) (lime) (external) (internal) T30.4
  abdomen, abdominal (muscle) (wall) T21.42 ☑
    first degree T21.52 ☑
    second degree T21.62 ☑
    third degree T21.72 ☑
  above elbow T22.439 ☑
    first degree T22.539 ☑
    left T22.432 ☑
      first degree T22.532 ☑
      second degree T22.632 ☑
      third degree T22.732 ☑
    right T22.431 ☑
      first degree T22.531 ☑

Corrosion — *continued*
  above elbow — *continued*
    right — *continued*
      second degree T22.631 ☑
      third degree T22.731 ☑
    second degree T22.639 ☑
    third degree T22.739 ☑
  alimentary tract NEC T28.7 ☑
  ankle T25.419 ☑
    first degree T25.519 ☑
    left T25.412 ☑
      first degree T25.512 ☑
      second degree T25.612 ☑
      third degree T25.712 ☑
    multiple with foot — *see* Corrosion, lower, limb, multiple, ankle and foot
    right T25.411 ☑
      first degree T25.511 ☑
      second degree T25.611 ☑
      third degree T25.711 ☑
    second degree T25.619 ☑
    third degree T25.719 ☑
  anus — *see* Corrosion, buttock
  arm(s) (meaning upper limb(s)) — *see* Corrosion, upper limb
  axilla T22.449 ☑
    first degree T22.549 ☑
    left T22.442 ☑
      first degree T22.542 ☑
      second degree T22.642 ☑
      third degree T22.742 ☑
    right T22.441 ☑
      first degree T22.541 ☑
      second degree T22.641 ☑
      third degree T22.741 ☑
    second degree T22.649 ☑
    third degree T22.749 ☑
  back (lower) T21.44 ☑
    first degree T21.54 ☑
    second degree T21.64 ☑
    third degree T21.74 ☑
    upper T21.43 ☑
      first degree T21.53 ☑
      second degree T21.63 ☑
      third degree T21.73 ☑
  blisters — *code as* Corrosion, second degree, by site
  breast(s) — *see* Corrosion, chest wall
  buttock(s) T21.45 ☑
    first degree T21.55 ☑
    second degree T21.65 ☑
    third degree T21.75 ☑
  calf T24.439 ☑
    first degree T24.539 ☑
    left T24.432 ☑
      first degree T24.532 ☑
      second degree T24.632 ☑
      third degree T24.732 ☑
    right T24.431 ☑
      first degree T24.531 ☑
      second degree T24.631 ☑
      third degree T24.731 ☑
    second degree T24.639 ☑
    third degree T24.739 ☑
  canthus (eye) — *see* Corrosion, eyelid
  cervix T28.8 ☑
  cheek T20.46 ☑
    first degree T20.56 ☑
    second degree T20.66 ☑
    third degree T20.76 ☑
  chest wall T21.41 ☑
    first degree T21.51 ☑
    second degree T21.61 ☑
    third degree T21.71 ☑
  chin T20.43 ☑
    first degree T20.53 ☑
    second degree T20.63 ☑
    third degree T20.73 ☑
  colon T28.7 ☑
  conjunctiva (and cornea) — *see* Corrosion, cornea
  cornea (and conjunctiva) T26.6- ☑
  deep necrosis of underlying tissue — *code as* Corrosion, third degree, by site
  dorsum of hand T23.469 ☑
    first degree T23.569 ☑

Corrosion — *continued*
  dorsum of hand — *continued*
    left T23.462 ☑
      first degree T23.562 ☑
      second degree T23.662 ☑
      third degree T23.762 ☑
    right T23.461 ☑
      first degree T23.561 ☑
      second degree T23.661 ☑
      third degree T23.761 ☑
    second degree T23.669 ☑
    third degree T23.769 ☑
  ear (auricle) (external) (canal) T20.41 ☑
    drum T28.91 ☑
    first degree T20.51 ☑
    second degree T20.61 ☑
    third degree T20.71 ☑
  elbow T22.429 ☑
    first degree T22.529 ☑
    left T22.422 ☑
      first degree T22.522 ☑
      second degree T22.622 ☑
      third degree T22.722 ☑
    right T22.421 ☑
      first degree T22.521 ☑
      second degree T22.621 ☑
      third degree T22.721 ☑
    second degree T22.629 ☑
    third degree T22.729 ☑
  entire body — *see* Corrosion, multiple body regions
  epidermal loss — *code as* Corrosion, second degree, by site
  epiglottis T27.4 ☑
  erythema, erythematous — *code as* Corrosion, first degree, by site
  esophagus T28.6 ☑
  extent (percentage of body surface)
    less than 10 per cent T32.0
    10-19 per cent (0-9 percent third degree) T32.10
      with 10-19 percent third degree T32.11
    20-29 per cent (0-9 percent third degree) T32.20
      with
        10-19 percent third degree T32.21
        20-29 percent third degree T32.22
    30-39 per cent (0-9 percent third degree) T32.30
      with
        10-19 percent third degree T32.31
        20-29 percent third degree T32.32
        30-39 percent third degree T32.33
    40-49 per cent (0-9 percent third degree) T32.40
      with
        10-19 percent third degree T32.41
        20-29 percent third degree T32.42
        30-39 percent third degree T32.43
        40-49 percent third degree T32.44
    50-59 per cent (0-9 percent third degree) T32.50
      with
        10-19 percent third degree T32.51
        20-29 percent third degree T32.52
        30-39 percent third degree T32.53
        40-49 percent third degree T32.54
        50-59 percent third degree T32.55
    60-69 per cent (0-9 percent third degree) T32.60
      with
        10-19 percent third degree T32.61
        20-29 percent third degree T32.62
        30-39 percent third degree T32.63
        40-49 percent third degree T32.64
        50-59 percent third degree T32.65
        60-69 percent third degree T32.66
    70-79 per cent (0-9 percent third degree) T32.70
      with
        10-19 percent third degree T32.71
        20-29 percent third degree T32.72
        30-39 percent third degree T32.73
        40-49 percent third degree T32.74
        50-59 percent third degree T32.75
        60-69 percent third degree T32.76
        70-79 percent third degree T32.77
    80-89 per cent (0-9 percent third degree) T32.80
      with
        10-19 percent third degree T32.81
        20-29 percent third degree T32.82
        30-39 percent third degree T32.83
        40-49 percent third degree T32.84
        50-59 percent third degree T32.85
        60-69 percent third degree T32.86

Corrosion — *continued*
  extent — *continued*
    80-89 per cent — *continued*
      with — *continued*
        70-79 percent third degree T32.87
        80-89 percent third degree T32.88
    90 per cent or more (0-9 percent third degree) T32.90
      with
        10-19 percent third degree T32.91
        20-29 percent third degree T32.92
        30-39 percent third degree T32.93
        40-49 percent third degree T32.94
        50-59 percent third degree T32.95
        60-69 percent third degree T32.96
        70-79 percent third degree T32.97
        80-89 percent third degree T32.98
        90-99 percent third degree T32.99
  extremity — *see* Corrosion, limb
  eye(s) and adnexa T26.9-
    with resulting rupture and destruction of eyeball T26.7- ☑
    conjunctival sac — *see* Corrosion, cornea
    cornea — *see* Corrosion, cornea
    lid — *see* Corrosion, eyelid
    periocular area — *see* Corrosion eyelid
    specified site NEC T26.8- ☑
  eyeball — *see* Corrosion, eye
  eyelid(s) T26.5- ☑
  face — *see* Corrosion, head
  finger T23.429 ☑
    first degree T23.529 ☑
    left T23.422 ☑
      first degree T23.522 ☑
      second degree T23.622 ☑
      third degree T23.722 ☑
    multiple sites (without thumb) T23.439 ☑
      with thumb T23.449 ☑
        first degree T23.549 ☑
        left T23.442 ☑
          first degree T23.542 ☑
          second degree T23.642 ☑
          third degree T23.742 ☑
        right T23.441 ☑
          first degree T23.541 ☑
          second degree T23.641 ☑
          third degree T23.741 ☑
        second degree T23.649 ☑
        third degree T23.749 ☑
    first degree T23.539 ☑
    left T23.432 ☑
      first degree T23.532 ☑
      second degree T23.632 ☑
      third degree T23.732 ☑
    right T23.431 ☑
      first degree T23.531 ☑
      second degree T23.631 ☑
      third degree T23.731 ☑
    second degree T23.639 ☑
    third degree T23.739 ☑
    right T23.421 ☑
      first degree T23.521 ☑
      second degree T23.621 ☑
      third degree T23.721 ☑
    second degree T23.629 ☑
    third degree T23.729 ☑
  flank — *see* Corrosion, abdomen
  foot T25.429 ☑
    first degree T25.529 ☑
    left T25.422 ☑
      first degree T25.522 ☑
      second degree T25.622 ☑
      third degree T25.722 ☑
    multiple with ankle — *see* Corrosion, lower, limb, multiple, ankle and foot
    right T25.421 ☑
      first degree T25.521 ☑
      second degree T25.621 ☑
      third degree T25.721 ☑
    second degree T25.629 ☑
    third degree T25.729 ☑
  forearm T22.419 ☑
    first degree T22.519 ☑
    left T22.412 ☑
      first degree T22.512 ☑
      second degree T22.612 ☑

Corrosion — *continued*
  forearm — *continued*
    left — *continued*
      third degree T22.712 ☑
    right T22.411 ☑
      first degree T22.511 ☑
      second degree T22.611 ☑
      third degree T22.711 ☑
    second degree T22.619 ☑
    third degree T22.719 ☑
  forehead T20.46 ☑
    first degree T20.56 ☑
    second degree T20.66 ☑
    third degree T20.76 ☑
  fourth degree — *code as* Corrosion, third degree, by site
  full thickness skin loss — *code as* Corrosion, third degree, by site
  gastrointestinal tract NEC T28.7 ☑
  genital organs
    external
      female T21.47 ☑
        first degree T21.57 ☑
        second degree T21.67 ☑
        third degree T21.77 ☑
      male T21.46 ☑
        first degree T21.56 ☑
        second degree T21.66 ☑
        third degree T21.76 ☑
    internal T28.8 ☑
  groin — *see* Corrosion, abdominal wall
  hand(s) T23.409 ☑
    back — *see* Corrosion, dorsum of hand
    finger — *see* Corrosion, finger
    first degree T23.509 ☑
    left T23.402 ☑
      first degree T23.502 ☑
      second degree T23.602 ☑
      third degree T23.702 ☑
    multiple sites with wrist T23.499 ☑
      first degree T23.599 ☑
      left T23.492 ☑
        first degree T23.592 ☑
        second degree T23.692 ☑
        third degree T23.792 ☑
      right T23.491 ☑
        first degree T23.591 ☑
        second degree T23.691 ☑
        third degree T23.791 ☑
      second degree T23.699 ☑
      third degree T23.799 ☑
    palm — *see* Corrosion, palm
    right T23.401 ☑
      first degree T23.501 ☑
      second degree T23.601 ☑
      third degree T23.701 ☑
    second degree T23.609 ☑
    third degree T23.709 ☑
    thumb — *see* Corrosion, thumb
  head (and face) (and neck) T20.40 ☑
    cheek — *see* Corrosion, cheek
    chin — *see* Corrosion, chin
    ear — *see* Corrosion, ear
    eye(s) only — *see* Corrosion, eye
    first degree T20.50 ☑
    forehead — *see* Corrosion, forehead
    lip — *see* Corrosion, lip
    multiple sites T20.49 ☑
      first degree T20.59 ☑
      second degree T20.69 ☑
      third degree T20.79 ☑
    neck — *see* Corrosion, neck
    nose — *see* Corrosion, nose
    scalp — *see* Corrosion, scalp
    second degree T20.60 ☑
    third degree T20.70 ☑
  hip(s) — *see* Corrosion, lower, limb
  inhalation — *see* Corrosion, respiratory tract
  internal organ(s) (*see also* Corrosion, by site) T28.90 ☑
    alimentary tract T28.7 ☑
      esophagus T28.6 ☑
    esophagus T28.6 ☑
    genitourinary tract T28.8 ☑
    mouth T28.5 ☑
    pharynx T28.5 ☑
    specified organ NEC T28.99 ☑

Corrosion — *continued*
  interscapular region — *see* Corrosion, back, upper
  intestine (large) (small) T28.7 ☑
  knee T24.429 ☑
    first degree T24.529 ☑
    left T24.422 ☑
      first degree T24.522 ☑
      second degree T24.622 ☑
      third degree T24.722 ☑
    right T24.421 ☑
      first degree T24.521 ☑
      second degree T24.621 ☑
      third degree T24.721 ☑
    second degree T24.629 ☑
    third degree T24.729 ☑
  labium (majus) (minus) — *see* Corrosion, genital organs, external, female
  lacrimal apparatus, duct, gland or sac — *see* Corrosion, eye, specified site NEC
  larynx T27.4 ☑
    with lung T27.5 ☑
  leg(s) (meaning lower limb(s)) — *see* Corrosion, lower limb
  limb(s)
    lower — *see* Corrosion, lower, limb
    upper — *see* Corrosion, upper limb
  lip(s) T20.42 ☑
    first degree T20.52 ☑
    second degree T20.62 ☑
    third degree T20.72 ☑
  lower
    back — *see* Corrosion, back
    limb T24.409 ☑
      ankle — *see* Corrosion, ankle
      calf — *see* Corrosion, calf
      first degree T24.509 ☑
      foot — *see* Corrosion, foot
      hip — *see* Corrosion, thigh
      knee — *see* Corrosion, knee
      left T24.402 ☑
        first degree T24.502 ☑
        second degree T24.602 ☑
        third degree T24.702 ☑
      multiple sites, except ankle and foot T24.499 ☑
        ankle and foot T25.499 ☑
          first degree T25.599 ☑
          left T25.492 ☑
            first degree T25.592 ☑
            second degree T25.692 ☑
            third degree T25.792 ☑
          right T25.491 ☑
            first degree T25.591 ☑
            second degree T25.691 ☑
            third degree T25.791 ☑
          second degree T25.699 ☑
          third degree T25.799 ☑
        first degree T24.599 ☑
        left T24.492 ☑
          first degree T24.592 ☑
          second degree T24.692 ☑
          third degree T24.792 ☑
        right T24.491 ☑
          first degree T24.591 ☑
          second degree T24.691 ☑
          third degree T24.791 ☑
        second degree T24.699 ☑
        third degree T24.799 ☑
      right T24.401 ☑
        first degree T24.501 ☑
        second degree T24.601 ☑
        third degree T24.701 ☑
      second degree T24.609 ☑
      thigh — *see* Corrosion, thigh
      third degree T24.709 ☑
  lung (with larynx and trachea) T27.5 ☑
  mouth T28.5 ☑
  neck T20.47 ☑
    first degree T20.57 ☑
    second degree T20.67 ☑
    third degree T20.77 ☑
  nose (septum) T20.44 ☑
    first degree T20.54 ☑
    second degree T20.64 ☑
    third degree T20.74 ☑
  ocular adnexa — *see* Corrosion, eye
  orbit region — *see* Corrosion, eyelid

Corrosion — *continued*
  palm T23.459 ☑
    first degree T23.559 ☑
    left T23.452 ☑
      first degree T23.552 ☑
      second degree T23.652 ☑
      third degree T23.752 ☑
    right T23.451 ☑
      first degree T23.551 ☑
      second degree T23.651 ☑
      third degree T23.751 ☑
    second degree T23.659 ☑
    third degree T23.759 ☑
  partial thickness — *code as* Corrosion, unspecified degree, by site
  pelvis — *see* Corrosion, trunk
  penis — *see* Corrosion, genital organs, external, male
  perineum
    female — *see* Corrosion, genital organs, external, female
    male — *see* Corrosion, genital organs, external, male
  periocular area — *see* Corrosion, eyelid
  pharynx T28.5 ☑
  rectum T28.7 ☑
  respiratory tract T27.7 ☑
    larynx — *see* Corrosion, larynx
    specified part NEC T27.6 ☑
    trachea — *see* Corrosion, larynx
  sac, lacrimal — *see* Corrosion, eye, specified site NEC
  scalp T20.45 ☑
    first degree T20.55 ☑
    second degree T20.65 ☑
    third degree T20.75 ☑
  scapular region T22.469 ☑
    first degree T22.569 ☑
    left T22.462 ☑
      first degree T22.562 ☑
      second degree T22.662 ☑
      third degree T22.762 ☑
    right T22.461 ☑
      first degree T22.561 ☑
      second degree T22.661 ☑
      third degree T22.761 ☑
    second degree T22.669 ☑
    third degree T22.769 ☑
  sclera — *see* Corrosion, eye, specified site NEC
  scrotum — *see* Corrosion, genital organs, external, male
  shoulder T22.459 ☑
    first degree T22.559 ☑
    left T22.452 ☑
      first degree T22.552 ☑
      second degree T22.652 ☑
      third degree T22.752 ☑
    right T22.451 ☑
      first degree T22.551 ☑
      second degree T22.651 ☑
      third degree T22.751 ☑
    second degree T22.659 ☑
    third degree T22.759 ☑
  stomach T28.7 ☑
  temple — *see* Corrosion, head
  testis — *see* Corrosion, genital organs, external, male
  thigh T24.419 ☑
    first degree T24.519 ☑
    left T24.412 ☑
      first degree T24.512 ☑
      second degree T24.612 ☑
      third degree T24.712 ☑
    right T24.411 ☑
      first degree T24.511 ☑
      second degree T24.611 ☑
      third degree T24.711 ☑
    second degree T24.619 ☑
    third degree T24.719 ☑
  thorax (external) — *see* Corrosion, trunk
  throat (meaning pharynx) T28.5 ☑
  thumb(s) T23.419 ☑
    first degree T23.519 ☑
    left T23.412 ☑
      first degree T23.512 ☑
      second degree T23.612 ☑
      third degree T23.712 ☑

Corrosion — *continued*
  thumb(s) — *continued*
    multiple sites with fingers T23.449 ☑
      first degree T23.549 ☑
      left T23.442 ☑
        first degree T23.542 ☑
        second degree T23.642 ☑
        third degree T23.742 ☑
      right T23.441 ☑
        first degree T23.541 ☑
        second degree T23.641 ☑
        third degree T23.741 ☑
      second degree T23.649 ☑
      third degree T23.749 ☑
    right T23.411 ☑
      first degree T23.511 ☑
      second degree T23.611 ☑
      third degree T23.711 ☑
    second degree T23.619 ☑
    third degree T23.719 ☑
  toe T25.439 ☑
    first degree T25.539 ☑
    left T25.432 ☑
      first degree T25.532 ☑
      second degree T25.632 ☑
      third degree T25.732 ☑
    right T25.431 ☑
      first degree T25.531 ☑
      second degree T25.631 ☑
      third degree T25.731 ☑
    second degree T25.639 ☑
    third degree T25.739 ☑
  tongue T28.5 ☑
  tonsil(s) T28.5 ☑
  total body — *see* Corrosion, multiple body regions
  trachea T27.4 ☑
    with lung T27.5 ☑
  trunk T21.40 ☑
    abdominal wall — *see* Corrosion, abdominal wall
    anus — *see* Corrosion, buttock
    axilla — *see* Corrosion, upper limb
    back — *see* Corrosion, back
    breast — *see* Corrosion, chest wall
    buttock — *see* Corrosion, buttock
    chest wall — *see* Corrosion, chest wall
    first degree T21.50 ☑
    flank — *see* Corrosion, abdominal wall
    genital
      female — *see* Corrosion, genital organs, external, female
      male — *see* Corrosion, genital organs, external, male
    groin — *see* Corrosion, abdominal wall
    interscapular region — *see* Corrosion, back, upper
    labia — *see* Corrosion, genital organs, external, female
    lower back — *see* Corrosion, back
    penis — *see* Corrosion, genital organs, external, male
    perineum
      female — *see* Corrosion, genital organs, external, female
      male — *see* Corrosion, genital organs, external, male
    scapular region — *see* Corrosion, upper limb
    scrotum — *see* Corrosion, genital organs, external, male
    second degree T21.60 ☑
    shoulder — *see* Corrosion, upper limb
    specified site NEC T21.49 ☑
      first degree T21.59 ☑
      second degree T21.69 ☑
      third degree T21.79 ☑
    testes — *see* Corrosion, genital organs, external, male
    third degree T21.70 ☑
    upper back — *see* Corrosion, back, upper
    vagina T28.8 ☑
    vulva — *see* Corrosion, genital organs, external, female
  unspecified site with extent of body surface involved specified
    less than 10 per cent T32.0
    10-19 per cent (0-9 percent third degree) T32.10
      with 10-19 percent third degree T32.11

Corrosion — *continued*
  unspecified site with extent of body surface involved
    specified — *continued*
    20-29 per cent (0-9 percent third degree) T32.20
      with
        10-19 percent third degree T32.21
        20-29 percent third degree T32.22
    30-39 per cent (0-9 percent third degree) T32.30
      with
        10-19 percent third degree T32.31
        20-29 percent third degree T32.32
        30-39 percent third degree T32.33
    40-49 per cent (0-9 percent third degree) T32.40
      with
        10-19 percent third degree T32.41
        20-29 percent third degree T32.42
        30-39 percent third degree T32.43
        40-49 percent third degree T32.44
    50-59 per cent (0-9 percent third degree) T32.50
      with
        10-19 percent third degree T32.51
        20-29 percent third degree T32.52
        30-39 percent third degree T32.53
        40-49 percent third degree T32.54
        50-59 percent third degree T32.55
    60-69 per cent (0-9 percent third degree) T32.60
      with
        10-19 percent third degree T32.61
        20-29 percent third degree T32.62
        30-39 percent third degree T32.63
        40-49 percent third degree T32.64
        50-59 percent third degree T32.65
        60-69 percent third degree T32.66
    70-79 per cent (0-9 percent third degree) T32.70
      with
        10-19 percent third degree T32.71
        20-29 percent third degree T32.72
        30-39 percent third degree T32.73
        40-49 percent third degree T32.74
        50-59 percent third degree T32.75
        60-69 percent third degree T32.76
        70-79 percent third degree T32.77
    80-89 per cent (0-9 percent third degree) T32.80
      with
        10-19 percent third degree T32.81
        20-29 percent third degree T32.82
        30-39 percent third degree T32.83
        40-49 percent third degree T32.84
        50-59 percent third degree T32.85
        60-69 percent third degree T32.86
        70-79 percent third degree T32.87
        80-89 percent third degree T32.88
    90 per cent or more (0-9 percent third degree)
      T32.90
      with
        10-19 percent third degree T32.91
        20-29 percent third degree T32.92
        30-39 percent third degree T32.93
        40-49 percent third degree T32.94
        50-59 percent third degree T32.95
        60-69 percent third degree T32.96
        70-79 percent third degree T32.97
        80-89 percent third degree T32.98
        90-99 percent third degree T32.99
  upper limb (axilla) (scapular region) T22.40 ☑
    above elbow — *see* Corrosion, above elbow
    axilla — *see* Corrosion, axilla
    elbow — *see* Corrosion, elbow
    first degree T22.50 ☑
    forearm — *see* Corrosion, forearm
    hand — *see* Corrosion, hand
    interscapular region — *see* Corrosion, back, upper
    multiple sites T22.499 ☑
      first degree T22.599 ☑
      left T22.492 ☑
        first degree T22.592 ☑
        second degree T22.692 ☑
        third degree T22.792 ☑
      right T22.491 ☑
        first degree T22.591 ☑
        second degree T22.691 ☑
        third degree T22.791 ☑
      second degree T22.699 ☑
      third degree T22.799 ☑
    scapular region — *see* Corrosion, scapular region
    second degree T22.60 ☑
    shoulder — *see* Corrosion, shoulder
    third degree T22.70 ☑

Corrosion — *continued*
  upper limb — *continued*
    wrist — *see* Corrosion, hand
  uterus T28.8 ☑
  vagina T28.8 ☑
  vulva — *see* Corrosion, genital organs, external, female
  wrist T23.479 ☑
    first degree T23.579 ☑
    left T23.472 ☑
      first degree T23.572 ☑
      second degree T23.672 ☑
      third degree T23.772 ☑
    multiple sites with hand T23.499 ☑
      first degree T23.599 ☑
      left T23.492 ☑
        first degree T23.592 ☑
        second degree T23.692 ☑
        third degree T23.792 ☑
      right T23.491 ☑
        first degree T23.591 ☑
        second degree T23.691 ☑
        third degree T23.791 ☑
      second degree T23.699 ☑
      third degree T23.799 ☑
    right T23.471 ☑
      first degree T23.571 ☑
      second degree T23.671 ☑
      third degree T23.771 ☑
    second degree T23.679 ☑
    third degree T23.779 ☑
Corrosive burn — *see* Corrosion
Corsican fever — *see* Malaria
Cortical — *see* condition
Cortico-adrenal — *see* condition
Coryza (acute) J00
  with grippe or influenza — *see* Influenza, with, respiratory manifestations NEC
  syphilitic
    congenital (chronic) A50.05
Costen's syndrome or complex M26.69
Costiveness — *see* Constipation
Costochondritis M94.0
Cot death R99
Cotard's syndrome F22
Cotia virus B08.8
Cotton wool spots (retinal) H35.81
Cotungo's disease — *see* Sciatica
Cough (affected) (chronic) (epidemic) (nervous) R05
  with hemorrhage — *see* Hemoptysis
  bronchial R05
    with grippe or influenza — *see* Influenza, with, respiratory manifestations NEC
  functional F45.8
  hysterical F45.8
  laryngeal, spasmodic R05
  psychogenic F45.8
  smokers' J41.0
  tea taster's B49
Counseling (for) Z71.9
  abuse NEC
    perpetrator Z69.82
    victim Z69.81
  alcohol abuser Z71.41
    family Z71.42
  child abuse
    nonparental
      perpetrator Z69.021
      victim Z69.020
    parental
      perpetrator Z69.011
      victim Z69.010
  consanguinity Z71.89
  contraceptive Z30.09
  dietary Z71.3
  drug abuser Z71.51
    family member Z71.52
  family Z71.89
  fertility preservation (prior to cancer therapy) (prior to removal of gonads) Z31.62
  for non-attending third party Z71.0
    related to sexual behavior or orientation Z70.2
  genetic NEC Z31.5
  health (advice) (education) (instruction) — *see* Counseling, medical
  human immunodeficiency virus (HIV) Z71.7
  impotence Z70.1
  insulin pump use Z46.81

Counseling — *continued*
  medical (for) Z71.9
    boarding school resident Z59.3
    consanguinity Z71.89
    feared complaint and no disease found Z71.1
    human immunodeficiency virus (HIV) Z71.7
    institutional resident Z59.3
    on behalf of another Z71.0
      related to sexual behavior or orientation Z70.2
    person living alone Z60.2
    specified reason NEC Z71.89
  natural family planning
    procreative Z31.61
    to avoid pregnancy Z30.02
  perpetrator (of)
    abuse NEC Z69.82
    child abuse
      non-parental Z69.021
      parental Z69.011
    rape NEC Z69.82
    spousal abuse Z69.12
  procreative NEC Z31.69
    fertility preservation (prior to cancer therapy) (prior to removal of gonads) Z31.62
    using natural family planning Z31.61
  promiscuity Z70.1
  rape victim Z69.81
  religious Z71.81
  sex, sexual (related to) Z70.9
    attitude(s) Z70.0
    behavior or orientation Z70.1
    combined concerns Z70.3
    non-responsiveness Z70.1
    on behalf of third party Z70.2
    specified reason NEC Z70.8
  specified reason NEC Z71.89
  spiritual Z71.81
  spousal abuse (perpetrator) Z69.12
    victim Z69.11
  substance abuse Z71.89
    alcohol Z71.41
    drug Z71.51
    tobacco Z71.6
  tobacco use Z71.6
  use (of)
    insulin pump Z46.81
  victim (of)
    abuse Z69.81
    child abuse
      by parent Z69.010
      non-parental Z69.020
    rape NEC Z69.81
Coupled rhythm R00.8
Couvelaire syndrome or uterus (complicating delivery) O45.8X- ☑
Cowperitis — *see* Urethritis
Cowper's gland — *see* condition
Cowpox B08.010
  due to vaccination T88.1 ☑
Coxa
  magna M91.4- ☑
  plana M91.2- ☑
  valga (acquired) (*see also* Deformity, limb, specified type NEC, thigh)
    congenital Q65.81
    sequelae (late effect) of rickets E64.3
  vara (acquired) (*see also* Deformity, limb, specified type NEC, thigh)
    congenital Q65.82
    sequelae (late effect) of rickets E64.3
Coxalgia, coxalgic (nontuberculous) (*see also* Pain, joint, hip)
  tuberculous A18.02
Coxitis — *see* Monoarthritis, hip
Coxsackie (virus) (infection) B34.1
  as cause of disease classified elsewhere B97.11
  carditis B33.20
  central nervous system NEC A88.8
  endocarditis B33.21
  enteritis A08.39
  meningitis (aseptic) A87.0
  myocarditis B33.22
  pericarditis B33.23
  pharyngitis B08.5
  pleurodynia B33.0
  specific disease NEC B33.8
Crabs, meaning pubic lice B85.3
Crack baby P04.41

☑ Additional Character Required — Refer to the Tabular List for Character Selection ▽ Subterms under main terms may continue to next column or page

Cracked nipple N64.Ø
  associated with
    lactation O92.13
    pregnancy O92.11- ☑
    puerperium O92.12
Cracked tooth KØ3.81
Cradle cap L21.Ø
Craft neurosis F48.8
Cramp(s) R25.2
  abdominal — *see* Pain, abdominal
  bathing T75.1 ☑
  colic R1Ø.83
    psychogenic F45.8
  due to immersion T75.1 ☑
  fireman T67.2 ☑
  heat T67.2 ☑
  immersion T75.1 ☑
  intestinal — *see* Pain, abdominal
    psychogenic F45.8
  leg, sleep related G47.62
  limb (lower) (upper) NEC R25.2
    sleep related G47.62
  linotypist's F48.8
    organic G25.89
  muscle (limb) (general) R25.2
    due to immersion T75.1 ☑
    psychogenic F45.8
  occupational (hand) F48.8
    organic G25.89
  salt-depletion E87.1
  sleep related, leg G47.62
  stoker's T67.2 ☑
  swimmer's T75.1 ☑
  telegrapher's F48.8
    organic G25.89
  typist's F48.8
    organic G25.89
  uterus N94.89
    menstrual — *see* Dysmenorrhea
  writer's F48.8
    organic G25.89
Cranial — *see* condition
Craniocleidodysostosis Q74.Ø
Craniofenestria (skull) Q75.8
Craniolacunia (skull) Q75.8
Craniopagus Q89.4
Craniopathy, metabolic M85.2
Craniopharyngeal — *see* condition
Craniopharyngioma D44.4
Craniorachischisis (totalis) QØØ.1
Cranioschisis Q75.8
Craniostenosis Q75.Ø
Craniosynostosis Q75.Ø
Craniotabes (cause unknown) M83.8
  neonatal P96.3
  rachitic E64.3
  syphilitic A5Ø.56
Cranium — *see* condition
Craw-craw — *see* Onchocerciasis
Creaking joint — *see* Derangement, joint, specified type NEC
Creeping
  eruption B76.9
  palsy or paralysis G12.22
Crenated tongue K14.8
Creotoxism AØ5.9
Crepitus
  caput Q75.8
  joint — *see* Derangement, joint, specified type NEC
Crescent or conus choroid, congenital Q14.3
CREST syndrome M34.1
Cretin, cretinism (congenital) (endemic) (nongoitrous) (sporadic) EØØ.9
  pelvis
    with disproportion (fetopelvic) O33.Ø
      causing obstructed labor O65.Ø
  type
    hypothyroid EØØ.1
    mixed EØØ.2
    myxedematous EØØ.1
    neurological EØØ.Ø
Creutzfeldt-Jakob disease or syndrome (with dementia) A81.ØØ
  familial A81.Ø9
  iatrogenic A81.Ø9
  specified NEC A81.Ø9
  sporadic A81.Ø9

Creutzfeldt-Jakob disease or syndrome — *continued*
  variant (vCJD) A81.Ø1
Crib death R99
Cribriform hymen Q52.3
Cri-du-chat syndrome Q93.4
Crigler-Najjar disease or syndrome E8Ø.5
Crime, victim of Z65.4
Crimean hemorrhagic fever A98.Ø
Criminalism F6Ø.2
Crisis
  abdomen R1Ø.Ø
  acute reaction F43.Ø
  addisonian E27.2
  adrenal (cortical) E27.2
  celiac K9Ø.4
  Dietl's N13.8
  emotional (*see also* Disorder, adjustment)
    acute reaction to stress F43.Ø
    specific to childhood and adolescence F93.8
  glaucomatocyclitic — *see* Glaucoma, secondary, inflammation
  heart — *see* Failure, heart
  nitritoid I95.2
    correct substance properly administered — *see* Table of Drugs and Chemicals, by drug, adverse effect
    overdose or wrong substance given or taken — *see* Table of Drugs and Chemicals, by drug, poisoning
  oculogyric H51.8
    psychogenic F45.8
  Pel's (tabetic) A52.11
  psychosexual identity F64.2
  renal N28.Ø
  sickle-cell D57.ØØ
    with
      acute chest syndrome D57.Ø1
      splenic sequestration D57.Ø2
  state (acute reaction) F43.Ø
  tabetic A52.11
  thyroid — *see* Thyrotoxicosis with thyroid storm
  thyrotoxic — *see* Thyrotoxicosis with thyroid storm
Crocq's disease (acrocyanosis) I73.89
Crohn's disease — *see* Enteritis, regional
Crooked septum, nasal J34.2
Cross syndrome E7Ø.328
Crossbite (anterior) (posterior) M26.24
Cross-eye — *see* Strabismus, convergent concomitant
Croup, croupous (catarrhal) (infectious) (inflammatory) (nondiphtheritic) JØ5.Ø
  bronchial J2Ø.9
  diphtheritic A36.2
  false J38.5
  spasmodic J38.5
    diphtheritic A36.2
  stridulous J38.5
    diphtheritic A36.2
Crouzon's disease Q75.1
Crowding, tooth, teeth, fully erupted M26.31
CRST syndrome M34.1
Cruchet's disease A85.8
Cruelty in children (*see also* Disorder, conduct)
Crural ulcer — *see* Ulcer, lower limb
Crush, crushed, crushing T14.8
  abdomen S38.1- ☑
  ankle S97.Ø- ☑
  arm (upper) (and shoulder) S47.- ☑
  axilla — *see* Crush, arm
  back, lower S38.1- ☑
  buttock S38.1- ☑
  cheek SØ7.Ø- ☑
  chest S28.Ø ☑
  cranium SØ7.1 ☑
  ear SØ7.Ø- ☑
  elbow S57.Ø- ☑
  extremity
    lower
      ankle — *see* Crush, ankle
      below knee — *see* Crush, leg
      foot — *see* Crush, foot
      hip — *see* Crush, hip
      knee — *see* Crush, knee
      thigh — *see* Crush, thigh
      toe — *see* Crush, toe
    upper
      below elbow S67.9- ☑

Crush, crushed, crushing — *continued*
  extremity — *continued*
    upper — *continued*
      elbow — *see* Crush, elbow
      finger — *see* Crush, finger
      forearm — *see* Crush, forearm
      hand — *see* Crush, hand
      thumb — *see* Crush, thumb
      upper arm — *see* Crush, arm
      wrist — *see* Crush, wrist
  face SØ7.Ø ☑
  finger(s) S67.1- ☑
    with hand (and wrist) — *see* Crush, hand, specified site NEC
    index S67.19- ☑
    little S67.19- ☑
    middle S67.19- ☑
    ring S67.19- ☑
    thumb — *see* Crush, thumb
  foot S97.8- ☑
    toe — *see* Crush, toe
  forearm S57.8- ☑
  genitalia, external
    female S38.ØØ2 ☑
      vagina S38.Ø3 ☑
      vulva S38.Ø3 ☑
    male S38.ØØ1 ☑
      penis S38.Ø1 ☑
      scrotum S38.Ø2 ☑
      testis S38.Ø2 ☑
  hand (except fingers alone) S67.2- ☑
    with wrist S67.4- ☑
  head SØ7.9 ☑
    specified NEC SØ7.8 ☑
  heel — *see* Crush, foot
  hip S77.Ø- ☑
    with thigh S77.2- ☑
  internal organ (abdomen, chest, or pelvis) NEC T14.8
  knee S87.Ø- ☑
  labium (majus) (minus) S38.Ø3 ☑
  larynx S17.Ø ☑
  leg (lower) S87.8- ☑
    knee — *see* Crush, knee
  lip SØ7.Ø ☑
  lower
    back S38.1 ☑
    leg — *see* Crush, leg
  neck S17.9 ☑
  nerve — *see* Injury, nerve
  nose SØ7.Ø ☑
  pelvis S38.1 ☑
  penis S38.Ø1 ☑
  scalp SØ7.8 ☑
  scapular region — *see* Crush, arm
  scrotum S38.Ø2 ☑
  severe, unspecified site T14.8
  shoulder (and upper arm) — *see* Crush, arm
  skull SØ7.1 ☑
  syndrome (complication of trauma) T79.5 ☑
  testis S38.Ø2 ☑
  thigh S77.1- ☑
    with hip S77.2- ☑
  throat S17.8 ☑
  thumb S67.Ø- ☑
    with hand (and wrist) — *see* Crush, hand, specified site NEC
  toe(s) S97.1Ø- ☑
    great S97.11- ☑
    lesser S97.12- ☑
  trachea S17.Ø ☑
  vagina S38.Ø3 ☑
  vulva S38.Ø3 ☑
  wrist S67.3- ☑
    with hand S67.4- ☑
Crusta lactea L21.Ø
Crusts R23.4
Crutch paralysis — *see* Injury, brachial plexus
Cruveilhier-Baumgarten cirrhosis, disease or syndrome K74.69
Cruveilhier's atrophy or disease G12.8
Crying (constant) (continuous) (excessive)
  child, adolescent, or adult R45.83
  infant (baby) (newborn) R68.11
Cryofibrinogenemia D89.2
Cryoglobulinemia (essential) (idiopathic) (mixed) (primary) (purpura) (secondary) (vasculitis) D89.1

Cryoglobulinemia — *continued*
  with lung involvement D89.1 [J99]
Cryptitis (anal) (rectal) K62.89
Cryptococcosis, cryptococcus (infection) (neoformans)
    B45.9
  bone B45.3
  cerebral B45.1
  cutaneous B45.2
  disseminated B45.7
  generalized B45.7
  meningitis B45.1
  meningocerebralis B45.1
  osseous B45.3
  pulmonary B45.0
  skin B45.2
  specified NEC B45.8
Cryptopapillitis (anus) K62.89
Cryptophthalmos Q11.2
  syndrome Q87.0
Cryptorchid, cryptorchism, cryptorchidism Q53.9
  bilateral Q53.20
    abdominal Q53.21
    perineal Q53.22
  unilateral Q53.10
    abdominal Q53.11
    perineal Q53.12
Cryptosporidiosis A07.2
  hepatobiliary B88.8
  respiratory B88.8
Cryptostromosis J67.6
Crystalluria R82.99
Cubitus
  congenital Q68.8
  valgus (acquired) M21.0- ☑
    congenital Q68.8
    sequelae (late effect) of rickets E64.3
  varus (acquired) M21.1- ☑
    congenital Q68.8
    sequelae (late effect) of rickets E64.3
Cultural deprivation or shock Z60.3
Curling esophagus K22.4
Curling's ulcer — *see* Ulcer, peptic, acute
Curschmann (-Batten) (-Steinert) **disease or syndrome**
    G71.11
Curse, Ondine's — *see* Apnea, sleep
Curvature
  organ or site, congenital NEC — *see* Distortion
  penis (lateral) Q55.61
  Pott's (spinal) A18.01
  radius, idiopathic, progressive (congenital) Q74.0
  spine (acquired) (angular) (idiopathic) (incorrect)
      (postural) — *see* Dorsopathy, deforming
    congenital Q67.5
    due to or associated with
        Charcot-Marie-Tooth disease (*see also* subcate-
            gory M49.8) G60.0
        osteitis
            deformans M88.88
            fibrosa cystica (*see also* subcategory M49.8)
                E21.0
        tuberculosis (Pott's curvature) A18.01
    sequelae (late effect) of rickets E64.3
    tuberculous A18.01
Cushingoid due to steroid therapy E24.2
  correct substance properly administered — *see* Table
      of Drugs and Chemicals, by drug, adverse effect
  overdose or wrong substance given or taken — *see*
      Table of Drugs and Chemicals, by drug, poison-
      ing
Cushing's
  syndrome or disease E24.9
    drug-induced E24.2
    iatrogenic E24.2
    pituitary-dependent E24.0
    specified NEC E24.8
  ulcer — *see* Ulcer, peptic, acute
Cusp, Carabelli — *omit code*
Cut (external) (*see also* Laceration)
  muscle — *see* Injury, muscle
Cutaneous (*see also* condition)
  hemorrhage R23.3
  larva migrans B76.9
Cutis (*see also* condition)
  hyperelastica Q82.8
    acquired L57.4
  laxa (hyperelastica) — *see* Dermatolysis
  marmorata R23.8

Cutis — *continued*
  osteosis L94.2
  pendula — *see* Dermatolysis
  rhomboidalis nuchae L57.2
  verticis gyrata Q82.8
    acquired L91.8
Cyanosis R23.0
  due to
    patent foramen botalli Q21.1
    persistent foramen ovale Q21.1
  enterogenous D74.8
  paroxysmal digital — *see* Raynaud's disease
    with gangrene I73.01
  retina, retinal H35.89
Cyanotic heart disease I24.9
  congenital Q24.9
Cycle
  anovulatory N97.0
  menstrual, irregular N92.6
Cyclencephaly Q04.9
Cyclical vomiting (*see also* Vomiting, cyclical) G43.A0
      (*following* G43.7)
  psychogenic F50.8
Cyclitis (*see also* Iridocyclitis) H20.9
  chronic — *see* Iridocyclitis, chronic
  Fuchs' heterochromic H20.81- ☑
  granulomatous — *see* Iridocyclitis, chronic
  lens-induced — *see* Iridocyclitis, lens-induced
  posterior H30.2- ☑
Cycloid personality F34.0
Cyclophoria H50.54
Cyclopia, cyclops Q87.0
Cyclopism Q87.0
Cyclosporiasis A07.4
Cyclothymia F34.0
Cyclothymic personality F34.0
Cyclotropia H50.41- ☑
Cylindroma (*see also* Neoplasm, malignant, by site)
  eccrine dermal — *see* Neoplasm, skin, benign
  skin — *see* Neoplasm, skin, benign
Cylindruria R82.99
Cynanche
  diphtheritic A36.2
  tonsillaris J36
Cynophobia F40.218
Cynorexia R63.2
Cyphosis — *see* Kyphosis
Cyprus fever — *see* Brucellosis
Cyst (colloid) (mucous) (simple) (retention)
  adenoid (infected) J35.8
  adrenal gland E27.8
    congenital Q89.1
  air, lung J98.4
  allantoic Q64.4
  alveolar process (jaw bone) M27.40
  amnion, amniotic O41.8X- ☑
  anterior
    chamber (eye) — *see* Cyst, iris
    nasopalatine K09.1
  antrum J34.1
  anus K62.89
  apical (tooth) (periodontal) K04.8
  appendix K38.8
  arachnoid, brain (acquired) G93.0
    congenital Q04.6
  arytenoid J38.7
  Baker's M71.2- ☑
    ruptured M66.0
    tuberculous A18.02
  Bartholin's gland N75.0
  bile duct (common) (hepatic) K83.5
  bladder (multiple) (trigone) N32.89
  blue dome (breast) — *see* Cyst, breast
  bone (local) NEC M85.60
    aneurysmal M85.50
      ankle M85.57- ☑
      foot M85.57- ☑
      forearm M85.53- ☑
      hand M85.54- ☑
      jaw M27.49
      lower leg M85.56- ☑
      multiple site M85.59
      neck M85.58
      rib M85.58
      shoulder M85.51- ☑
      skull M85.58
      specified site NEC M85.58

Cyst — *continued*
  bone — *continued*
    aneurysmal — *continued*
      thigh M85.55- ☑
      toe M85.57- ☑
      upper arm M85.52- ☑
      vertebra M85.58
    solitary M85.40
      ankle M85.47- ☑
      fibula M85.46- ☑
      foot M85.47- ☑
      hand M85.44- ☑
      humerus M85.42- ☑
      jaw M27.49
      neck M85.48
      pelvis M85.45- ☑
      radius M85.43- ☑
      rib M85.48
      shoulder M85.41- ☑
      skull M85.48
      specified site NEC M85.48
      tibia M85.46- ☑
      toe M85.47- ☑
      ulna M85.43- ☑
      vertebra M85.48
    specified type NEC M85.60
      ankle M85.67- ☑
      foot M85.67- ☑
      forearm M85.63- ☑
      hand M85.64- ☑
      jaw M27.40
        developmental (nonodontogenic) K09.1
        odontogenic K09.0
        latent M27.0
      lower leg M85.66- ☑
      multiple site M85.69
      neck M85.68
      rib M85.68
      shoulder M85.61- ☑
      skull M85.68
      specified site NEC M85.68
      thigh M85.65- ☑
      toe M85.67- ☑
      upper arm M85.62- ☑
      vertebra M85.68
  brain (acquired) G93.0
    congenital Q04.6
    hydatid B67.99 [G94]
    third ventricle (colloid), congenital Q04.6
  branchial (cleft) Q18.0
  branchiogenic Q18.0
  breast (benign) (blue dome) (pedunculated) (solitary)
      N60.0- ☑
    involution — *see* Dysplasia, mammary, specified
        type NEC
    sebaceous — *see* Dysplasia, mammary, specified
        type NEC
  broad ligament (benign) N83.8
  bronchogenic (mediastinal) (sequestration) J98.4
    congenital Q33.0
  buccal K09.8
  bulbourethral gland N36.8
  bursa, bursal NEC M71.30
    with rupture — *see* Rupture, synovium
    ankle M71.37- ☑
    elbow M71.32- ☑
    foot M71.37- ☑
    hand M71.34- ☑
    hip M71.35- ☑
    multiple sites M71.39
    pharyngeal J39.2
    popliteal space — *see* Cyst, Baker's
    shoulder M71.31- ☑
    specified site NEC M71.38
    wrist M71.33- ☑
  calcifying odontogenic D16.5
    upper jaw (bone) (maxilla) D16.4
  canal of Nuck (female) N94.89
    congenital Q52.4
  canthus — *see* Cyst, conjunctiva
  carcinomatous — *see* Neoplasm, malignant, by site
  cauda equina G95.89
  cavum septi pellucidi — *see* Cyst, brain
  celomic (pericardium) Q24.8
  cerebellopontine (angle) — *see* Cyst, brain
  cerebellum — *see* Cyst, brain
  cerebral — *see* Cyst, brain

☑ **Additional Character Required** — Refer to the Tabular List for Character Selection   ↪ Subterms under main terms may continue to next column or page

Cyst — continued
  cervical lateral Q18.1
  cervix NEC N88.8
    embryonic Q51.6
    nabothian N88.8
  chiasmal optic NEC — see Disorder, optic, chiasm
  chocolate (ovary) N80.1
  choledochus, congenital Q44.4
  chorion O41.8X- ☑
  choroid plexus G93.0
  ciliary body — see Cyst, iris
  clitoris N90.7
  colon K63.89
  common (bile) duct K83.5
  congenital NEC Q89.8
    adrenal gland Q89.1
    epiglottis Q31.8
    esophagus Q39.8
    fallopian tube Q50.4
    kidney Q61.00
      more than one (multiple) Q61.02
        specified as polycystic Q61.3
          adult type Q61.2
          infantile type NEC Q61.19
            collecting duct dilation Q61.11
      solitary Q61.01
    larynx Q31.8
    liver Q44.6
    lung Q33.0
    mediastinum Q34.1
    ovary Q50.1
    oviduct Q50.4
    periurethral (tissue) Q64.79
    prepuce Q55.69
    salivary gland (any) Q38.4
    sublingual Q38.6
    submaxillary gland Q38.6
    thymus (gland) Q89.2
    tongue Q38.3
    ureterovesical orifice Q62.8
    vulva Q52.79
  conjunctiva H11.44- ☑
  cornea H18.89- ☑
  corpora quadrigemina G93.0
  corpus
    albicans N83.29
    luteum (hemorrhagic) (ruptured) N83.1
  Cowper's gland (benign) (infected) N36.8
  cranial meninges G93.0
  craniobuccal pouch E23.6
  craniopharyngeal pouch E23.6
  cystic duct K82.8
  Cysticercus — see Cysticercosis
  Dandy-Walker Q03.1
    with spina bifida — see Spina bifida
  dental (root) K04.8
    developmental K09.0
    eruption K09.0
    primordial K09.0
  dentigerous (mandible) (maxilla) K09.0
  dermoid — see Neoplasm, benign, by site
    with malignant transformation C56.- ☑
    implantation
      external area or site (skin) NEC L72.0
      iris — see Cyst, iris, implantation
      vagina N89.8
      vulva N90.7
    mouth K09.8
    oral soft tissue K09.8
    sacrococcygeal — see Cyst, pilonidal
  developmental K09.1
    odontogenic K09.0
    oral region (nonodontogenic) K09.1
    ovary, ovarian Q50.1
  dura (cerebral) G93.0
    spinal G96.19
  ear (external) Q18.1
  echinococcal — see Echinococcus
  embryonic
    cervix uteri Q51.6
    fallopian tube Q50.4
    vagina Q51.6
  endometrium, endometrial (uterus) N85.8
    ectopic — see Endometriosis
  enterogenous Q43.8
  epidermal, epidermoid (inclusion) (see also Cyst, skin) L72.0
    mouth K09.8

Cyst — continued
  epidermal, epidermoid (see also Cyst, skin) — continued
    oral soft tissue K09.8
  epididymis N50.3
  epiglottis J38.7
  epiphysis cerebri E34.8
  epithelial (inclusion) L72.0
  epoophoron Q50.5
  eruption K09.0
  esophagus K22.8
  ethmoid sinus J34.1
  external female genital organs NEC N90.7
  eyelid (sebaceous) H02.829
    infected — see Hordeolum
    left H02.826
      lower H02.825
      upper H02.824
    right H02.823
      lower H02.822
      upper H02.821
  eye NEC H57.8
    congenital Q15.8
  fallopian tube N83.8
    congenital Q50.4
  fimbrial (twisted) Q50.4
  fissural (oral region) K09.1
  follicle (graafian) (hemorrhagic) N83.0
    nabothian N88.8
  follicular (atretic) (hemorrhagic) (ovarian) N83.0
    dentigerous K09.0
    odontogenic K09.0
    skin L72.9
      specified NEC L72.8
  frontal sinus J34.1
  gallbladder K82.8
  ganglion — see Ganglion
  Gartner's duct Q52.4
  gingiva K09.0
  gland of Moll — see Cyst, eyelid
  globulomaxillary K09.1
  graafian follicle (hemorrhagic) N83.0
  granulosal lutein (hemorrhagic) N83.1
  hemangiomatous D18.00
    intra-abdominal D18.03
    intracranial D18.02
    skin D18.01
    specified site NEC D18.09
  hydatid (see also Echinococcus) B67.90
    brain B67.99 [G94]
    liver (see also Cyst, liver, hydatid) B67.8
    lung NEC B67.99 [J99]
    Morgagni
      female Q50.5
      male (epididymal) Q55.4
        testicular Q55.29
    specified site NEC B67.99
  hymen N89.8
    embryonic Q52.4
  hypopharynx J39.2
  hypophysis, hypophyseal (duct) (recurrent) E23.6
    cerebri E23.6
  implantation (dermoid)
    external area or site (skin) NEC L72.0
    iris — see Cyst, iris, implantation
    vagina N89.8
    vulva N90.7
  incisive canal K09.1
  inclusion (epidermal) (epithelial) (epidermoid) (squamous) L72.0
    not of skin — code under Cyst, by site
  intestine (large) (small) K63.89
  intracranial — see Cyst, brain
  intraligamentous (see also Disorder, ligament)
    knee — see Derangement, knee
  intrasellar E23.6
  iris H21.309
    exudative H21.31- ☑
    idiopathic H21.30- ☑
    implantation H21.32- ☑
    parasitic H21.33- ☑
    pars plana (primary) H21.34- ☑
      exudative H21.35- ☑
  jaw (bone) M27.40
    aneurysmal M27.49
    developmental (odontogenic) K09.0
    fissural K09.1
    hemorrhagic M27.49

Cyst — continued
  jaw — continued
    traumatic M27.49
  joint NEC — see Disorder, joint, specified type NEC
  kidney (acquired) N28.1
    calyceal — see Hydronephrosis
    congenital Q61.00
    more than one (multiple) Q61.02
      specified as polycystic Q61.3
        adult type (autosomal dominant) Q61.2
        infantile type (autosomal recessive) NEC Q61.19
          collecting duct dilation Q61.11
    pyelogenic — see Hydronephrosis
    simple N28.1
    solitary (single) Q61.01
      acquired N28.1
  labium (majus) (minus) N90.7
    sebaceous N90.7
  lacrimal (see also Disorder, lacrimal system, specified NEC)
    gland H04.13- ☑
    passages or sac — see Disorder, lacrimal system, specified NEC
  larynx J38.7
  lateral periodontal K09.0
  lens H27.8
    congenital Q12.8
  lip (gland) K13.0
  liver (idiopathic) (simple) K76.89
    congenital Q44.6
    hydatid B67.8
      granulosus B67.0
      multilocularis B67.5
  lung J98.4
    congenital Q33.0
    giant bullous J43.9
  lutein N83.1
  lymphangiomatous D18.1
  lymphoepithelial, oral soft tissue K09.8
  macula — see Degeneration, macula, hole
  malignant — see Neoplasm, malignant, by site
  mammary gland — see Cyst, breast
  mandible M27.40
    dentigerous K09.0
    radicular K04.8
  maxilla M27.40
    dentigerous K09.0
    radicular K04.8
  medial, face and neck Q18.8
  median
    anterior maxillary K09.1
    palatal K09.1
  mediastinum, congenital Q34.1
  meibomian (gland) — see Chalazion
    infected — see Hordeolum
  membrane, brain G93.0
  meninges (cerebral) G93.0
    spinal G96.19
  meniscus, knee — see Derangement, knee, meniscus, cystic
  mesentery, mesenteric K66.8
    chyle I89.8
  mesonephric duct
    female Q50.5
    male Q55.4
  milk N64.89
  Morgagni (hydatid)
    female Q50.5
    male (epididymal) Q55.4
      testicular Q55.29
  mouth K09.8
  Müllerian duct Q50.4
    appendix testis Q55.29
    cervix Q51.6
    fallopian tube Q50.4
    female Q50.4
    male Q55.29
    prostatic utricle Q55.4
    vagina (embryonal) Q52.4
  multilocular (ovary) D39.10
    benign — see Neoplasm, benign, by site
  myometrium N85.8
  nabothian (follicle) (ruptured) N88.8
  nasoalveolar K09.1
  nasolabial K09.1
  nasopalatine (anterior) (duct) K09.1
  nasopharynx J39.2

☝ Subterms under main terms may continue to next column or page   ☑ Additional Character Required — Refer to the Tabular List for Character Selection   77

Cyst — Cyst

Cyst — *continued*
 neoplastic — *see* Neoplasm, uncertain behavior, by site
  benign — *see* Neoplasm, benign, by site
 nervous system NEC G96.8
 neuroenteric (congenital) Q06.8
 nipple — *see* Cyst, breast
 nose (turbinates) J34.1
  sinus J34.1
 odontogenic, developmental K09.0
 omentum (lesser) K66.8
  congenital Q45.8
 ora serrata — *see* Cyst, retina, ora serrata
 oral
  region K09.9
   developmental (nonodontogenic) K09.1
    specified NEC K09.8
  soft tissue K09.9
   specified NEC K09.8
 orbit H05.81- ☑
 ovary, ovarian (twisted) N83.20
  adherent N83.20
  chocolate N80.1
  corpus
   albicans N83.29
   luteum (hemorrhagic) N83.1
  dermoid D27.9
  developmental Q50.1
  due to failure of involution NEC N83.20
  endometrial N80.1
  follicular (graafian) (hemorrhagic) N83.0
  hemorrhagic N83.20
  in pregnancy or childbirth O34.8- ☑
   with obstructed labor O65.5
  multilocular D39.10
  pseudomucinous D27.9
  retention N83.29
  serous N83.20
  specified NEC N83.29
  theca lutein (hemorrhagic) N83.1
  tuberculous A18.18
 oviduct N83.8
 palate (median) (fissural) K09.1
 palatine papilla (jaw) K09.1
 pancreas, pancreatic (hemorrhagic) (true) K86.2
  congenital Q45.2
  false K86.3
 paralabral
  hip M24.85- ☑
  shoulder S43.43- ☑
 paramesonephric duct Q50.4
  female Q50.4
  male Q55.29
 paranephric N28.1
 paraphysis, cerebri, congenital Q04.6
 parasitic B89
 parathyroid (gland) E21.4
 paratubal N83.8
 paraurethral duct N36.8
 paroophoron Q50.5
 parotid gland K11.6
 parovarian Q50.5
 pelvis, female N94.89
  in pregnancy or childbirth O34.8- ☑
   causing obstructed labor O65.5
 penis (sebaceous) N48.89
 periapical K04.8
 pericardial (congenital) Q24.8
  acquired (secondary) I31.8
 pericoronal K09.0
 periodontal K04.8
  lateral K09.0
 peripelvic (lymphatic) N28.1
 peritoneum K66.8
  chylous I89.8
 periventricular, acquired, newborn P91.1
 pharynx (wall) J39.2
 pilar L72.11
 pilonidal (infected) (rectum) L05.91
  with abscess L05.01
  malignant C44.59- ☑
 pituitary (duct) (gland) E23.6
 placenta O43.19- ☑
 pleura J94.8
 popliteal — *see* Cyst, Baker's
 porencephalic Q04.6
  acquired G93.0
 postanal (infected) — *see* Cyst, pilonidal

Cyst — *continued*
 postmastoidectomy cavity (mucosal) — *see* Complications, postmastoidectomy, cyst
 preauricular Q18.1
 prepuce N47.4
  congenital Q55.69
 primordial (jaw) K09.0
 prostate N42.83
 pseudomucinous (ovary) D27.9
 pupillary, miotic H21.27- ☑
 radicular (residual) K04.8
 radiculodental K04.8
 ranular K11.8
 Rathke's pouch E23.6
 rectum (epithelium) (mucous) K62.89
 renal — *see* Cyst, kidney
 residual (radicular) K04.8
 retention (ovary) N83.29
  salivary gland K11.6
 retina H33.19- ☑
  ora serrata H33.11- ☑
  parasitic H33.12- ☑
 retroperitoneal K68.9
 sacrococcygeal (dermoid) — *see* Cyst, pilonidal
 salivary gland or duct (mucous extravasation or retention) K11.6
 Sampson's N80.1
 sclera H15.89
 scrotum L72.9
  sebaceous L72.3
 sebaceous (duct) (gland) L72.3
  breast — *see* Dysplasia, mammary, specified type NEC
  eyelid — *see* Cyst, eyelid
  genital organ NEC
   female N94.89
   male N50.8
  scrotum L72.3
 semilunar cartilage (knee) (multiple) — *see* Derangement, knee, meniscus, cystic
 seminal vesicle N50.8
 serous (ovary) N83.20
 sinus (accessory) (nasal) J34.1
 Skene's gland N36.8
 skin L72.9
  breast — *see* Dysplasia, mammary, specified type NEC
  epidermal, epidermoid L72.0
  epithelial L72.0
  eyelid — *see* Cyst, eyelid
  genital organ NEC
   female N90.7
   male N50.8
  inclusion L72.0
  scrotum L72.9
  sebaceous L72.3
  sweat gland or duct L74.8
 solitary
  bone — *see* Cyst, bone, solitary
  jaw M27.40
  kidney N28.1
 spermatic cord N50.8
 sphenoid sinus J34.1
 spinal meninges G96.19
 spleen NEC D73.4
  congenital Q89.09
  hydatid (*see also* Echinococcus) B67.99 [D77]
 Stafne's M27.0
 subarachnoid intrasellar R93.0
 subcutaneous, pheomycotic (chromomycotic) B43.2
 subdural (cerebral) G93.0
  spinal cord G96.19
 sublingual gland K11.6
 submandibular gland K11.6
 submaxillary gland K11.6
 suburethral N36.8
 suprarenal gland E27.8
 suprasellar — *see* Cyst, brain
 sweat gland or duct L74.8
 synovial (*see also* Cyst, bursa)
  ruptured — *see* Rupture, synovium
 tarsal — *see* Chalazion
 tendon (sheath) — *see* Disorder, tendon, specified type NEC
 testis N44.2
  tunica albuginea N44.1
 theca lutein (ovary) N83.1
 Thornwaldt's J39.2

Cyst — *continued*
 thymus (gland) E32.8
 thyroglossal duct (infected) (persistent) Q89.2
 thyroid (gland) E04.1
 thyrolingual duct (infected) (persistent) Q89.2
 tongue K14.8
 tonsil J35.8
 tooth — *see* Cyst, dental
 Tornwaldt's J39.2
 trichilemmal (proliferating) L72.12
 trichodermal L72.12
 tubal (fallopian) N83.8
  inflammatory — *see* Salpingitis, chronic
 tubo-ovarian N83.8
  inflammatory N70.13
 tunica
  albuginea testis N44.1
  vaginalis N50.8
 turbinate (nose) J34.1
 Tyson's gland N48.89
 urachus, congenital Q64.4
 ureter N28.89
 ureterovesical orifice N28.89
 urethra, urethral (gland) N36.8
 uterine ligament N83.8
 uterus (body) (corpus) (recurrent) N85.8
  embryonic Q51.818
   cervix Q51.6
 vagina, vaginal (implantation) (inclusion) (squamous cell) (wall) N89.8
  embryonic Q52.4
 vallecula, vallecular (epiglottis) J38.7
 vesical (orifice) N32.89
 vitreous body H43.89
 vulva (implantation) (inclusion) N90.7
  congenital Q52.79
  sebaceous gland N90.7
 vulvovaginal gland N90.7
 wolffian
  female Q50.5
  male Q55.4
Cystadenocarcinoma — *see* Neoplasm, malignant, by site
 bile duct C22.1
 endometrioid — *see* Neoplasm, malignant, by site
  specified site — *see* Neoplasm, malignant, by site
  unspecified site
   female C56.9
   male C61
 mucinous
  papillary
   specified site — *see* Neoplasm, malignant, by site
   unspecified site C56.9
  specified site — *see* Neoplasm, malignant, by site
  unspecified site C56.9
 papillary
  mucinous
   specified site — *see* Neoplasm, malignant, by site
   unspecified site C56.9
  pseudomucinous
   specified site — *see* Neoplasm, malignant, by site
   unspecified site C56.9
  serous
   specified site — *see* Neoplasm, malignant, by site
   unspecified site C56.9
  specified site — *see* Neoplasm, malignant, by site
  unspecified site C56.9
 pseudomucinous
  papillary
   specified site — *see* Neoplasm, malignant, by site
   unspecified site C56.9
  specified site — *see* Neoplasm, malignant, by site
  unspecified site C56.9
 serous
  papillary
   specified site — *see* Neoplasm, malignant, by site
   unspecified site C56.9
  specified site — *see* Neoplasm, malignant, by site
  unspecified site C56.9
Cystadenofibroma
 clear cell — *see* Neoplasm, benign, by site
 endometrioid D27.9

☑ **Additional Character Required — Refer to the Tabular List for Character Selection**   ▼ **Subterms under main terms may continue to next column or page**

Cystadenofibroma — *continued*
  endometrioid D27.9
    borderline malignancy D39.1- ☑
    malignant C56.- ☑
  mucinous
    specified site — *see* Neoplasm, benign, by site
    unspecified site D27.9
  serous
    specified site — *see* Neoplasm, benign, by site
    unspecified site D27.9
  specified site — *see* Neoplasm, benign, by site
  unspecified site D27.9
Cystadenoma (*see also* Neoplasm, benign, by site)
  bile duct D13.4
  endometrioid — *see* Neoplasm, benign, by site
    borderline malignancy — *see* Neoplasm, uncertain
      behavior, by site
  malignant — *see* Neoplasm, malignant, by site
  mucinous
    borderline malignancy
      ovary C56.- ☑
      specified site NEC — *see* Neoplasm, uncertain
        behavior, by site
      unspecified site C56.9
    papillary
      borderline malignancy
        ovary C56.- ☑
        specified site NEC — *see* Neoplasm, uncer-
          tain behavior, by site
        unspecified site C56.9
      specified site — *see* Neoplasm, benign, by site
      unspecified site D27.9
    specified site — *see* Neoplasm, benign, by site
    unspecified site D27.9
  papillary
    borderline malignancy
      ovary C56.- ☑
      specified site NEC — *see* Neoplasm, uncertain
        behavior, by site
      unspecified site C56.9
    lymphomatosum
      specified site — *see* Neoplasm, benign, by site
      unspecified site D11.9
    mucinous
      borderline malignancy
        ovary C56.- ☑
        specified site NEC — *see* Neoplasm, uncer-
          tain behavior, by site
        unspecified site C56.9
      specified site — *see* Neoplasm, benign, by site
      unspecified site D27.9
    pseudomucinous
      borderline malignancy
        ovary C56.- ☑
        specified site NEC — *see* Neoplasm, uncer-
          tain behavior, by site
        unspecified site C56.9
      specified site — *see* Neoplasm, benign, by site
      unspecified site D27.9
    serous
      borderline malignancy
        ovary C56.- ☑
        specified site NEC — *see* Neoplasm, uncer-
          tain behavior, by site
        unspecified site C56.9
      specified site — *see* Neoplasm, benign, by site
      unspecified site D27.9
    specified site — *see* Neoplasm, benign, by site
    unspecified site D27.9
  pseudomucinous
    borderline malignancy
      ovary C56.- ☑
      specified site NEC — *see* Neoplasm, uncertain
        behavior, by site
      unspecified site C56.9
    papillary
      borderline malignancy
        ovary C56.- ☑
        specified site NEC — *see* Neoplasm, uncer-
          tain behavior, by site
        unspecified site C56.9
      specified site — *see* Neoplasm, benign, by site
      unspecified site D27.9
    specified site — *see* Neoplasm, benign, by site

Cystadenoma — *continued*
  pseudomucinous — *continued*
    unspecified site D27.9
  serous
    borderline malignancy
      ovary C56.- ☑
      specified site NEC — *see* Neoplasm, uncertain
        behavior, by site
      unspecified site C56.9
    papillary
      borderline malignancy
        ovary C56.- ☑
        specified site NEC — *see* Neoplasm, uncer-
          tain behavior, by site
        unspecified site C56.9
      specified site — *see* Neoplasm, benign, by site
      unspecified site D27.9
    specified site — *see* Neoplasm, benign, by site
    unspecified site D27.9
Cystathionine synthase deficiency E72.11
Cystathioninemia E72.19
Cystathioninuria E72.19
Cystic (*see also* condition)
  breast (chronic) — *see* Mastopathy, cystic
  corpora lutea (hemorrhagic) N83.1
  duct — *see* condition
  eyeball (congenital) Q11.0
  fibrosis — *see* Fibrosis, cystic
  kidney (congenital) Q61.9
    adult type Q61.2
    infantile type NEC Q61.19
      collecting duct dilatation Q61.11
    medullary Q61.5
  liver, congenital Q44.6
  lung disease J98.4
    congenital Q33.0
  mastitis, chronic — *see* Mastopathy, cystic
  medullary, kidney Q61.5
  meniscus — *see* Derangement, knee, meniscus, cystic
  ovary N83.20
Cysticercosis, cysticerciasis B69.9
  with
    epileptiform fits B69.0
    myositis B69.81
  brain B69.0
  central nervous system B69.0
  cerebral B69.0
  ocular B69.1
  specified NEC B69.89
Cysticercus cellulose infestation — *see* Cysticercosis
Cystinosis (malignant) E72.04
Cystinuria E72.01
Cystitis (exudative) (hemorrhagic) (septic) (suppurative)
  N30.90
  with
    fibrosis — *see* Cystitis, chronic, interstitial
    hematuria N30.91
    leukoplakia — *see* Cystitis, chronic, interstitial
    malakoplakia — *see* Cystitis, chronic, interstitial
    metaplasia — *see* Cystitis, chronic, interstitial
    prostatitis N41.3
  acute N30.00
    with hematuria N30.01
    of trigone N30.30
      with hematuria N30.31
  allergic — *see* Cystitis, specified type NEC
  amebic A06.81
  bilharzial B65.9 [N33]
  blennorrhagic (gonococcal) A54.01
  bullous — *see* Cystitis, specified type NEC
  calculous N21.0
  chlamydial A56.01
  chronic N30.20
    with hematuria N30.21
    interstitial N30.10
      with hematuria N30.11
    of trigone N30.30
      with hematuria N30.31
    specified NEC N30.20
      with hematuria N30.21
  cystic (a) — *see* Cystitis, specified type NEC
  diphtheritic A36.85
  echinococcal
    granulosus B67.39

Cystitis — *continued*
  echinococcal — *continued*
    multilocularis B67.69
  emphysematous — *see* Cystitis, specified type NEC
  encysted — *see* Cystitis, specified type NEC
  eosinophilic — *see* Cystitis, specified type NEC
  follicular — *see* Cystitis, of trigone
  gangrenous — *see* Cystitis, specified type NEC
  glandularis — *see* Cystitis, specified type NEC
  gonococcal A54.01
  incrusted — *see* Cystitis, specified type NEC
  interstitial (chronic) — *see* Cystitis, chronic, interstitial
  irradiation N30.40
    with hematuria N30.41
  irritation — *see* Cystitis, specified type NEC
  malignant — *see* Cystitis, specified type NEC
  of trigone N30.30
    with hematuria N30.31
  panmural — *see* Cystitis, chronic, interstitial
  polyposa — *see* Cystitis, specified type NEC
  prostatic N41.3
  puerperal (postpartum) O86.22
  radiation — *see* Cystitis, irradiation
  specified type NEC N30.80
    with hematuria N30.81
  subacute — *see* Cystitis, chronic
  submucous — *see* Cystitis, chronic, interstitial
  syphilitic (late) A52.76
  trichomonal A59.03
  tuberculous A18.12
  ulcerative — *see* Cystitis, chronic, interstitial
Cystocele (-urethrocele)
  female N81.10
    with prolapse of uterus — *see* Prolapse, uterus
    lateral N81.12
    midline N81.11
    paravaginal N81.12
  in pregnancy or childbirth O34.8- ☑
    causing obstructed labor O65.5
  male N32.89
Cystolithiasis N21.0
Cystoma (*see also* Neoplasm, benign, by site)
  endometrial, ovary N80.1
  mucinous
    specified site — *see* Neoplasm, benign, by site
    unspecified site D27.9
  serous
    specified site — *see* Neoplasm, benign, by site
    unspecified site D27.9
  simple (ovary) N83.29
Cystoplegia N31.2
Cystoptosis N32.89
Cystopyelitis — *see* Pyelonephritis
Cystorrhagia N32.89
Cystosarcoma phyllodes D48.6- ☑
  benign D24- ☑
  malignant — *see* Neoplasm, breast, malignant
Cystostomy
  attention to Z43.5
  complication — *see* Complications, cystostomy
  status Z93.50
    appendico-vesicostomy Z93.52
    cutaneous Z93.51
    specified NEC Z93.59
Cystourethritis — *see* Urethritis
Cystourethrocele (*see also* Cystocele)
  female N81.10
    with uterine prolapse — *see* Prolapse, uterus
    lateral N81.12
    midline N81.11
    paravaginal N81.12
  male N32.89
Cytomegalic inclusion disease
  congenital P35.1
Cytomegalovirus infection B25.9
Cytomycosis (reticuloendothelial) B39.4
Cytopenia D75.9
  refractory
    with multilineage dysplasia D46.A (*following* D46.2)
      and ring sideroblasts (RCMD RS) D46.B (*follow-*
        ing D46.2)
Czerny's disease (periodic hydrarthrosis of the knee) —
    see Effusion, joint, knee

D

Da Costa's syndrome F45.8
Daae (-Finsen) **disease** (epidemic pleurodynia) B33.0
Dabney's grip B33.0
Dacryoadenitis, dacryadenitis H04.00- ☑
  acute H04.01- ☑
  chronic H04.02- ☑
Dacryocystitis H04.30- ☑
  acute H04.32- ☑
  chronic H04.41- ☑
  neonatal P39.1
  phlegmonous H04.31- ☑
  syphilitic A52.71
    congenital (early) A50.01
  trachomatous, active A71.1
    sequelae (late effect) B94.0
Dacryocystoblenorrhea — see Inflammation, lacrimal, passages, chronic
Dacryocystocele — see Disorder, lacrimal system, changes
Dacryolith, dacryolithiasis H04.51- ☑
Dacryoma — see Disorder, lacrimal system, changes
Dacryopericystitis — see Dacryocystitis
Dacryops H04.11- ☑
Dacryostenosis (see also Stenosis, lacrimal)
  congenital Q10.5
Dactylitis
  bone — see Osteomyelitis
  sickle-cell D57.00
    Hb C D57.219
    Hb SS D57.00
    specified NEC D57.819
  skin L08.9
  syphilitic A52.77
  tuberculous A18.03
Dactylolysis spontanea (ainhum) L94.6
Dactylosymphysis Q70.9
  fingers — see Syndactylism, complex, fingers
  toes — see Syndactylism, complex, toes
Damage
  arteriosclerotic — see Arteriosclerosis
  brain (nontraumatic) G93.9
    anoxic, hypoxic G93.1
      resulting from a procedure G97.82
    child NEC G80.9
    due to birth injury P11.2
  cardiorenal (vascular) — see Hypertension, cardiorenal
  cerebral NEC — see Damage, brain
  coccyx, complicating delivery O71.6
  coronary — see Disease, heart, ischemic
  eye, birth injury P15.3
  liver (nontraumatic) K76.9
    alcoholic K70.9
    due to drugs — see Disease, liver, toxic
    toxic — see Disease, liver, toxic
  medication T88.7 ☑
  pelvic
    joint or ligament, during delivery O71.6
    organ NEC
      during delivery O71.5
      following ectopic or molar pregnancy O08.6
  renal — see Disease, renal
  subendocardium, subendocardial — see Degeneration, myocardial
  vascular I99.9
Dana-Putnam syndrome (subacute combined sclerosis with pernicious anemia) — see Degeneration, combined
Danbolt (-Cross) **syndrome** (acrodermatitis enteropathica) E83.2
Dandruff L21.0
Dandy-Walker syndrome Q03.1
  with spina bifida — see Spina bifida
Danlos' syndrome Q79.6
Darier (-White) **disease** (congenital) Q82.8
  meaning erythema annulare centrifugum L53.1
Darier-Roussy sarcoid D86.3
Darling's disease or histoplasmosis B39.4
Darwin's tubercle Q17.8

Dawson's (inclusion body) **encephalitis** A81.1
De Beurmann (-Gougerot) **disease** B42.1
De la Tourette's syndrome F95.2
De Lange's syndrome Q87.1
De Morgan's spots (senile angiomas) I78.1
De Quervain's
  disease (tendon sheath) M65.4
  syndrome E34.51
  thyroiditis (subacute granulomatous thyroiditis) E06.1
De Toni-Fanconi (-Debré) **syndrome** E72.09
  with cystinosis E72.04
Dead
  fetus, retained (mother) O36.4 ☑
    early pregnancy O02.1
  labyrinth H83.2 ☑
  ovum, retained O02.0
Deaf nonspeaking NEC H91.3
Deafmutism (acquired) (congenital) NEC H91.3
  hysterical F44.6
  syphilitic, congenital (see also subcategory) H94.8
    A50.09
Deafness (acquired) (complete) (hereditary) (partial) H91.9- ☑
  with blue sclera and fragility of bone Q78.0
  auditory fatigue — see Deafness, specified type NEC
  aviation T70.0 ☑
    nerve injury — see Injury, nerve, acoustic, specified type NEC
  boilermaker's H83.3 ☑
  central — see Deafness, sensorineural
  conductive H90.2
    and sensorineural, mixed H90.8
      bilateral H90.6
    bilateral H90.0
    unilateral H90.1- ☑
  congenital H90.5
    with blue sclera and fragility of bone Q78.0
  due to toxic agents — see Deafness, ototoxic
  emotional (hysterical) F44.6
  functional (hysterical) F44.6
  high frequency H91.9- ☑
  hysterical F44.6
  low frequency H91.9- ☑
  mental R48.8
  mixed conductive and sensorineural H90.8
    bilateral H90.6
    unilateral H90.7- ☑
  nerve — see Deafness, sensorineural
  neural — see Deafness, sensorineural
  noise-induced (see also subcategory) H83.3 ☑
    nerve injury — see Injury, nerve, acoustic, specified type NEC
  nonspeaking H91.3
  ototoxic H91.0 ☑
  perceptive — see Deafness, sensorineural
  psychogenic (hysterical) F44.6
  sensorineural H90.5
    and conductive, mixed H90.8
      bilateral H90.6
    bilateral H90.3
    unilateral H90.4- ☑
  sensory — see Deafness, sensorineural
  specified type NEC H91.8 ☑
  sudden (idiopathic) H91.2- ☑
  syphilitic A52.15
  transient ischemic H93.01- ☑
  traumatic — see Injury, nerve, acoustic, specified type NEC
  word (developmental) H93.25
Death (cause unknown) (of) (unexplained) (unspecified cause) R99
  brain G93.82
  cardiac (sudden) (with successful resuscitation) — code to underlying disease
    family history of Z82.41
    personal history of Z86.74
  family member (assumed) Z63.4
Debility (chronic) (general) (nervous) R53.81
  congenital or neonatal NOS P96.9
  nervous R53.81
  old age R54
  senile R54

Débove's disease (splenomegaly) R16.1
Decalcification
  bone — see Osteoporosis
  teeth K03.89
Decapsulation, kidney N28.89
Decay
  dental — see Caries, dental
  senile R54
  tooth, teeth — see Caries, dental
Deciduitis (acute)
  following ectopic or molar pregnancy O08.0
Decline (general) — see Debility
  cognitive, age-associated R41.81
Decompensation
  cardiac (acute) (chronic) — see Disease, heart
  cardiovascular — see Disease, cardiovascular
  heart — see Disease, heart
  hepatic — see Failure, hepatic
  myocardial (acute) (chronic) — see Disease, heart
  respiratory J98.8
Decompression sickness T70.3 ☑
Decrease (d)
  absolute neutrophile count — see Neutropenia
  blood
    platelets — see Thrombocytopenia
    pressure R03.1
      due to shock following
        injury T79.4 ☑
        operation T81.19 ☑
  estrogen E28.39
    postablative E89.40
      asymptomatic E89.40
      symptomatic E89.41
  fragility of erythrocytes D58.8
  function
    lipase (pancreatic) K90.3
    ovary in hypopituitarism E23.0
    parenchyma of pancreas K86.8
    pituitary (gland) (anterior) (lobe) E23.0
      posterior (lobe) E23.0
  functional activity R68.89
  glucose R73.09
  hematocrit R71.0
  hemoglobin R71.0
  leukocytes D72.819
    specified NEC D72.818
  libido R68.82
  lymphocytes D72.810
  platelets D69.6
  respiration, due to shock following injury T79.4 ☑
  sexual desire R68.82
  tear secretion NEC — see Syndrome, dry eye
  tolerance
    fat K90.4
    glucose R73.09
    pancreatic K90.3
    salt and water E87.8
  vision NEC H54.7
  white blood cell count D72.819
    specified NEC D72.818
Decubitus (ulcer) — see Ulcer, pressure, by site
  cervix N86
Deepening acetabulum — see Derangement, joint, specified type NEC, hip
Defect, defective Q89.9
  3-beta-hydroxysteroid dehydrogenase E25.0
  11-hydroxylase E25.0
  21-hydroxylase E25.0
  abdominal wall, congenital Q79.59
  antibody immunodeficiency D80.9
  aorticopulmonary septum Q21.4
  atrial septal (ostium secundum type) Q21.1
    following acute myocardial infarction (current complication) I23.1
    ostium primum type Q21.2
  atrioventricular
    canal Q21.2
    septum Q21.2
  auricular septal Q21.1
  bilirubin excretion NEC E80.6
  biosynthesis, androgen (testicular) E29.1
  bulbar septum Q21.0

☑ **Additional Character Required — Refer to the Tabular List for Character Selection**　　▽ **Subterms under main terms may continue to next column or page**

Defect, defective — *continued*
- catalase E80.3
- cell membrane receptor complex (CR3) D71
- circulation I99.9
  - congenital Q28.9
  - newborn Q28.9
- coagulation (factor) (*see also* Deficiency, factor) D68.9
  - with
    - ectopic pregnancy O08.1
    - molar pregnancy O08.1
  - acquired D68.4
  - antepartum with hemorrhage — *see* Hemorrhage, antepartum, with coagulation defect
  - due to
    - liver disease D68.4
    - vitamin K deficiency D68.4
  - hereditary NEC D68.2
  - intrapartum O67.0
  - newborn, transient P61.6
  - postpartum O72.3
  - specified type NEC D68.8
- complement system D84.1
- conduction (heart) I45.9
  - bone — *see* Deafness, conductive
- congenital, organ or site not listed — *see* Anomaly, by site
- coronary sinus Q21.1
- cushion, endocardial Q21.2
- degradation, glycoprotein E77.1
- dental bridge, crown, fillings — *see* Defect, dental restoration
- dental restoration K08.50
  - specified NEC K08.59
- dentin (hereditary) K00.5
- Descemet's membrane, congenital Q13.89
- developmental (*see also* Anomaly)
  - cauda equina Q06.3
- diaphragm
  - with elevation, eventration or hernia — *see* Hernia, diaphragm
  - congenital Q79.1
    - with hernia Q79.0
    - gross (with hernia) Q79.0
- ectodermal, congenital Q82.9
- Eisenmenger's Q21.8
- enzyme
  - catalase E80.3
  - peroxidase E80.3
- esophagus, congenital Q39.9
- extensor retinaculum M62.89
- fibrin polymerization D68.2
- filling
  - bladder R93.4
  - kidney R93.4
  - stomach R93.3
  - ureter R93.4
- Gerbode Q21.0
- glycoprotein degradation E77.1
- Hageman (factor) D68.2
- hearing — *see* Deafness
- high grade F70
- interatrial septal Q21.1
- interauricular septal Q21.1
- interventricular septal Q21.0
  - with dextroposition of aorta, pulmonary stenosis and hypertrophy of right ventricle Q21.3
  - in tetralogy of Fallot Q21.3
- learning (specific) — *see* Disorder, learning
- lymphocyte function antigen-1 (LFA-1) D84.0
- lysosomal enzyme, post-translational modification E77.0
- major osseous M89.70
  - ankle M89.77- ☑
  - carpus M89.74- ☑
  - clavicle M89.71- ☑
  - femur M89.75- ☑
  - fibula M89.76- ☑
  - fingers M89.74- ☑
  - foot M89.77- ☑
  - forearm M89.73- ☑
  - hand M89.74- ☑
  - humerus M89.72- ☑
  - lower leg M89.76- ☑
  - metacarpus M89.74- ☑
  - metatarsus M89.77- ☑
  - multiple sites M89.79
  - pelvic region M89.75- ☑
  - pelvis M89.75- ☑

Defect, defective — *continued*
- major osseous — *continued*
  - radius M89.73- ☑
  - scapula M89.71- ☑
  - shoulder region M89.71- ☑
  - specified NEC M89.78
  - tarsus M89.77- ☑
  - thigh M89.75- ☑
  - tibia M89.76- ☑
  - toes M89.77- ☑
  - ulna M89.73- ☑
- mental — *see* Disability, intellectual
- modification, lysosomal enzymes, post-translational E77.0
- obstructive, congenital
  - renal pelvis Q62.39
  - ureter Q62.39
    - atresia — *see* Atresia, ureter
    - cecoureterocele Q62.32
    - megaureter Q62.2
    - orthotopic ureterocele Q62.31
- osseous, major M89.70
  - ankle M89.77- ☑
  - carpus M89.74- ☑
  - clavicle M89.71- ☑
  - femur M89.75- ☑
  - fibula M89.76- ☑
  - fingers M89.74- ☑
  - foot M89.77- ☑
  - forearm M89.73- ☑
  - hand M89.74- ☑
  - humerus M89.72- ☑
  - lower leg M89.76- ☑
  - metacarpus M89.74- ☑
  - metatarsus M89.77- ☑
  - multiple sites M89.9
  - pelvic region M89.75- ☑
  - pelvis M89.75- ☑
  - radius M89.73- ☑
  - scapula M89.71- ☑
  - shoulder region M89.71- ☑
  - specified NEC M89.78
  - tarsus M89.77- ☑
  - thigh M89.75- ☑
  - tibia M89.76- ☑
  - toes M89.77- ☑
  - ulna M89.73- ☑
- osteochondral NEC (*see also* Deformity) M95.8
- ostium
  - primum Q21.2
  - secundum Q21.1
- peroxidase E80.3
- placental blood supply — *see* Insufficiency, placental
- platelets, qualitative D69.1
  - constitutional D68.0
- postural NEC, spine — *see* Dorsopathy, deforming
- reduction
  - limb Q73.8
    - lower Q72.9- ☑
      - absence — *see* Agenesis, leg
        - foot — *see* Agenesis, foot
      - longitudinal
        - femur Q72.4- ☑
        - fibula Q72.6- ☑
        - tibia Q72.5- ☑
      - specified type NEC Q72.89- ☑
      - split foot Q72.7- ☑
    - specified type NEC Q73.8
    - upper Q71.9- ☑
      - absence — *see* Agenesis, arm
        - forearm — *see* Agenesis, forearm
        - hand — *see* Agenesis, hand
      - lobster-claw hand Q71.6- ☑
      - longitudinal
        - radius Q71.4- ☑
        - ulna Q71.5- ☑
      - specified type NEC Q71.89- ☑
- renal pelvis Q63.8
  - obstructive Q62.39
- respiratory system, congenital Q34.9
- restoration, dental K08.50
  - specified NEC K08.59
- retinal nerve bundle fibers H35.89
- septal (heart) NOS Q21.9
  - acquired (atrial) (auricular) (ventricular) (old) I51.0

Defect, defective — *continued*
- septal — *continued*
  - atrial Q21.1
    - concurrent with acute myocardial infarction — *see* Infarct, myocardium
    - following acute myocardial infarction (current complication) I23.1
    - ventricular (*see also* Defect, ventricular septal) Q21.0
  - sinus venosus Q21.1
- speech R47.9
  - developmental F80.9
  - specified NEC R47.89
- Taussig-Bing (aortic transposition and overriding pulmonary artery) Q20.1
- teeth, wedge K03.1
- vascular (local) I99.9
  - congenital Q27.9
- ventricular septal Q21.0
  - concurrent with acute myocardial infarction — *see* Infarct, myocardium
  - following acute myocardial infarction (current complication) I23.2
  - in tetralogy of Fallot Q21.3
- vision NEC H54.7
- visual field H53.40
  - bilateral
    - heteronymous H53.47
    - homonymous H53.46- ☑
  - generalized contraction H53.48- ☑
  - localized
    - arcuate H53.43- ☑
    - scotoma (central area) H53.41- ☑
      - blind spot area H53.42- ☑
    - sector H53.43- ☑
    - specified type NEC H53.45- ☑
- voice R49.9
  - specified NEC R49.8
- wedge, tooth, teeth (abrasion) K03.1

Deferentitis N49.1
- gonorrheal (acute) (chronic) A54.23

Defibrination (syndrome) D65
- antepartum — *see* Hemorrhage, antepartum, with coagulation defect, disseminated intravascular coagulation
- following ectopic or molar pregnancy O08.1
- intrapartum O67.0
- newborn P60
- postpartum O72.3

Deficiency, deficient
- 3-beta hydroxysteroid dehydrogenase E25.0
- 5-alpha reductase (with male pseudo-hermaphroditism) E29.1
- 11-hydroxylase E25.0
- 21-hydroxylase E25.0
- abdominal muscle syndrome Q79.4
- AC globulin (congenital) (hereditary) D68.2
  - acquired D68.4
- accelerator globulin (Ac G) (blood) D68.2
- acid phosphatase E83.39
- activating factor (blood) D68.2
- adenosine deaminase (ADA) D81.3
- aldolase (hereditary) E74.19
- alpha-1-antitrypsin E88.01
- amino-acids E72.9
- anemia — *see* Anemia
- aneurin E51.9
- antibody with
  - hyperimmunoglobulinemia D80.6
  - near-normal immunoglobins D80.6
- antidiuretic hormone E23.2
- anti-hemophilic
  - factor (A) D66
    - B D67
    - C D68.1
  - globulin (AHG) NEC D66
- antithrombin (antithrombin III) D68.59
- ascorbic acid E54
- attention (disorder) (syndrome) F98.8
  - with hyperactivity — *see* Disorder, attention-deficit hyperactivity
- autoprothrombin
  - C D68.2
  - I D68.2
  - II D67
- beta-glucuronidase E76.29
- biotin E53.8
- biotin-dependent carboxylase D81.819

Defect, defective — Deficiency, deficient

Deficiency, deficient — *continued*
biotinidase D81.810
brancher enzyme (amylopectinosis) E74.03
C1 esterase inhibitor (C1-INH) D84.1
calciferol E55.9
  with
    adult osteomalacia M83.8
    rickets — *see* Rickets
calcium (dietary) E58
calorie, severe E43
  with marasmus E41
    and kwashiorkor E42
cardiac — *see* Insufficiency, myocardial
carnitine E71.40
  due to
    hemodialysis E71.43
    inborn errors of metabolism E71.42
    Valproic acid therapy E71.43
  iatrogenic E71.43
  muscle palmityltransferase E71.314
  primary E71.41
  secondary E71.448
carotene E50.9
central nervous system G96.8
ceruloplasmin (Wilson) E83.01
choline E53.8
Christmas factor D67
chromium E61.4
clotting (blood) (*see also* Deficiency, coagulation factor) D68.9
clotting factor NEC (hereditary) (*see also* Deficiency, factor) D68.2
coagulation NOS D68.9
  with
    ectopic pregnancy O08.1
    molar pregnancy O08.1
  acquired (any) D68.4
  antepartum hemorrhage — *see* Hemorrhage, antepartum, with coagulation defect
  clotting factor NEC (*see also* Deficiency, factor) D68.2
  due to
    hyperprothrombinemia D68.4
    liver disease D68.4
    vitamin K deficiency D68.4
  newborn, transient P61.6
  postpartum O72.3
  specified NEC D68.8
cognitive F09
color vision H53.50
  achromatopsia H53.51
  acquired H53.52
  deuteranomaly H53.53
  protanomaly H53.54
  specified type NEC H53.59
  tritanomaly H53.55
combined glucocorticoid and mineralocorticoid E27.49
contact factor D68.2
copper (nutritional) E61.0
corticoadrenal E27.40
  primary E27.1
craniofacial axis Q75.0
cyanocobalamin E53.8
debrancher enzyme (limit dextrinosis) E74.03
dehydrogenase
  long chain/very long chain acyl CoA E71.310
  medium chain acyl CoA E71.311
  short chain acyl CoA E71.312
diet E63.9
dihydropyrimidine dehydrogenase (DPD) E88.89
disaccharidase E73.9
edema — *see* Malnutrition, severe
endocrine E34.9
energy-supply — *see* Malnutrition
enzymes, circulating NEC E88.09
ergosterol E55.9
  with
    adult osteomalacia M83.8
    rickets — *see* Rickets
essential fatty acid (EFA) E63.0
factor (*see also* Deficiency, coagulation)
  Hageman D68.2
  I (congenital) (hereditary) D68.2
  II (congenital) (hereditary) D68.2
  IX (congenital) (functional) (hereditary) (with functional defect) D67
  multiple (congenital) D68.8
    acquired D68.4

Deficiency, deficient — *continued*
factor (*see also* Deficiency, coagulation) — *continued*
  V (congenital) (hereditary) D68.2
  VII (congenital) (hereditary) D68.2
  VIII (congenital) (functional) (hereditary) (with functional defect) D66
    with vascular defect D68.0
  X (congenital) (hereditary) D68.2
  XI (congenital) (hereditary) D68.1
  XII (congenital) (hereditary) D68.2
  XIII (congenital) (hereditary) D68.2
femoral, proximal focal (congenital) — *see* Defect, reduction, lower limb, longitudinal, femur
fibrinase D68.2
fibrinogen (congenital) (hereditary) D68.2
  acquired D65
fibrin-stabilizing factor (congenital) (hereditary) D68.2
  acquired D68.4
folate E53.8
folic acid E53.8
foreskin N47.3
fructokinase E74.11
fructose 1,6-diphosphatase E74.19
fructose-1-phosphate aldolase E74.19
galactokinase E74.29
galactose-1-phosphate uridyl transferase E74.29
gammaglobulin in blood D80.1
  hereditary D80.0
glass factor D68.2
glucocorticoid E27.49
  mineralocorticoid E27.49
glucose-6-phosphatase E74.01
glucose-6-phosphate dehydrogenase anemia D55.0
glucuronyl transferase E80.5
glycogen synthetase E74.09
gonadotropin (isolated) E23.0
growth hormone (idiopathic) (isolated) E23.0
Hageman factor D68.2
hemoglobin D64.9
hepatophosphorylase E74.09
homogentisate 1,2-dioxygenase E70.29
hormone
  anterior pituitary (partial) NEC E23.0
    growth E23.0
  growth (isolated) E23.0
  pituitary E23.0
  testicular E29.1
hypoxanthine- (guanine)-phosphoribosyltransferase (HG- PRT) (total H-PRT) E79.1
immunity D84.9
  cell-mediated D84.8
    with thrombocytopenia and eczema D82.0
  combined D81.9
  humoral D80.9
  IgA (secretory) D80.2
  IgG D80.3
  IgM D80.4
immuno — *see* Immunodeficiency
immunoglobulin, selective
  A (IgA) D80.2
  G (IgG) (subclasses) D80.3
  M (IgM) D80.4
inositol (B complex) E53.8
intrinsic
  factor (congenital) D51.0
  sphincter N36.42
    with urethral hypermobility N36.43
iodine E61.8
  congenital syndrome — *see* Syndrome, iodine-deficiency, congenital
iron E61.1
  anemia D50.9
kalium E87.6
kappa-light chain D80.8
labile factor (congenital) (hereditary) D68.2
  acquired D68.4
lacrimal fluid (acquired) (*see also* Syndrome, dry eye)
  congenital Q10.6
lactase
  congenital E73.0
  secondary E73.1
Laki-Lorand factor D68.2
lecithin cholesterol acyltransferase E78.6
lipocaic K86.8
lipoprotein (familial) (high density) E78.6
liver phosphorylase E74.09
lysosomal alpha-1, 4 glucosidase E74.02

Deficiency, deficient — *continued*
magnesium E61.2
major histocompatibility complex
  class I D81.6
  class II D81.7
manganese E61.3
menadione (vitamin K) E56.1
  newborn P53
mental (familial) (hereditary) — *see* Disability, intellectual
methylenetetrahydrofolate reductase (MTHFR) E72.12
mineralocorticoid E27.49
  with glucocorticoid E27.49
mineral NEC E61.8
molybdenum (nutritional) E61.5
moral F60.2
multiple nutrient elements E61.7
muscle
  carnitine (palmityltransferase) E71.314
  phosphofructokinase E74.09
myoadenylate deaminase E79.2
myocardial — *see* Insufficiency, myocardial
myophosphorylase E74.04
NADH diaphorase or reductase (congenital) D74.0
NADH-methemoglobin reductase (congenital) D74.0
natrium E87.1
niacin (amide) (-tryptophan) E52
nicotinamide E52
nicotinic acid E52
number of teeth — *see* Anodontia
nutrient element E61.9
  multiple E61.7
  specified NEC E61.8
nutrition, nutritional E63.9
  sequelae — *see* Sequelae, nutritional deficiency
  specified NEC E63.8
ornithine transcarbamylase E72.4
ovarian E28.39
oxygen — *see* Anoxia
pantothenic acid E53.8
parathyroid (gland) E20.9
perineum (female) N81.89
phenylalanine hydroxylase E70.1
phosphoenolpyruvate carboxykinase E74.4
phosphofructokinase E74.19
phosphomannomutase E74.8
phosphomannose isomerase E74.8
phosphomannosyl mutase E74.8
phosphorylase kinase, liver E74.09
pituitary hormone (isolated) E23.0
plasma thromboplastin
  antecedent (PTA) D68.1
  component (PTC) D67
platelet NEC D69.1
  constitutional D68.0
polyglandular E31.8
  autoimmune E31.0
potassium (K) E87.6
prepuce N47.3
proaccelerin (congenital) (hereditary) D68.2
  acquired D68.4
proconvertin factor (congenital) (hereditary) D68.2
  acquired D68.4
protein (*see also* Malnutrition) E46
  anemia D53.0
  C D68.59
  S D68.59
prothrombin (congenital) (hereditary) D68.2
  acquired D68.4
Prower factor D68.2
pseudocholinesterase E88.09
PTA (plasma thromboplastin antecedent) D68.1
PTC (plasma thromboplastin component) D67
purine nucleoside phosphorylase (PNP) D81.5
pyracin (alpha) (beta) E53.1
pyridoxal E53.1
pyridoxamine E53.1
pyridoxine (derivatives) E53.1
pyruvate
  carboxylase E74.4
  dehydrogenase E74.4
riboflavin (vitamin B2) E53.0
salt E87.1
secretion
  ovary E28.39
  salivary gland (any) K11.7
  urine R34
selenium (dietary) E59

Deficiency, deficient — *continued*
serum antitrypsin, familial E88.01
short stature homeobox gene (SHOX)
  with
    dyschondrosteosis Q78.8
    short stature (idiopathic) E34.3
    Turner's syndrome Q96.9
sodium (Na) E87.1
SPCA (factor VII) D68.2
sphincter, intrinsic N36.42
  with urethral hypermobility N36.43
stable factor (congenital) (hereditary) D68.2
  acquired D68.4
Stuart-Prower (factor X) D68.2
sucrase E74.39
sulfatase E75.29
sulfite oxidase E72.19
thiamin, thiaminic (chloride) E51.9
  beriberi (dry) E51.11
    wet E51.12
thrombokinase D68.2
  newborn P53
thyroid (gland) — *see* Hypothyroidism
tocopherol E56.0
tooth bud K00.0
transcobalamine II (anemia) D51.2
vanadium E61.6
vascular I99.9
vasopressin E23.2
viosterol — *see* Deficiency, calciferol
vitamin (multiple) NOS E56.9
  A E50.9
    with
      Bitot's spot (corneal) E50.1
      follicular keratosis E50.8
      keratomalacia E50.4
      manifestations NEC E50.8
      night blindness E50.5
      scar of cornea, xerophthalmic E50.6
      xeroderma E50.8
      xerophthalmia E50.7
      xerosis
        conjunctival E50.0
          and Bitot's spot E50.1
        cornea E50.2
          and ulceration E50.3
    sequelae E64.1
  B (complex) NOS E53.9
    with
      beriberi (dry) E51.11
        wet E51.12
      pellagra E52
  B1 NOS E51.9
    beriberi (dry) E51.11
      with circulatory system manifestations E51.11
      wet E51.12
  B2 (riboflavin) E53.0
  B6 E53.1
  B12 E53.8
  C E54
    sequelae E64.2
  D E55.9
    with
      adult osteomalacia M83.8
      rickets — *see* Rickets
    25-hydroxylase E83.32
  E E56.0
  folic acid E53.8
  G E53.0
  group B E53.9
    specified NEC E53.8
  H (biotin) E53.8
  K E56.1
    of newborn P53
  nicotinic E52
  P E56.8
  PP (pellagra-preventing) E52
  specified NEC E56.8
  thiamin E51.9
    beriberi — *see* Beriberi
zinc, dietary E60

Deficit (*see also* Deficiency)
attention and concentration R41.840
  disorder — *see* Attention, deficit
cognitive communication R41.841

Deficit — *continued*
cognitive NEC R41.89
  following
    cerebral infarction I69.31
    cerebrovascular disease I69.91
      specified disease NEC I69.81
    intracerebral hemorrhage I69.11
    nontraumatic intracranial hemorrhage NEC I69.21
    subarachnoid hemorrhage I69.01
concentration R41.840
executive function R41.844
frontal lobe R41.844
neurologic NEC R29.818
  ischemic
    reversible (RIND) I63.9
      prolonged (PRIND) I63.9
oxygen R09.02
prolonged reversible ischemic neurologic (PRIND) I63.9
psychomotor R41.843
visuospatial R41.842

Deflection
radius — *see* Deformity, limb, specified type NEC, forearm
septum (acquired) (nasal) (nose) J34.2
spine — *see* Curvature, spine
turbinate (nose) J34.2

Defluvium
capillorum — *see* Alopecia
ciliorum — *see* Madarosis
unguium L60.8

Deformity Q89.9
abdomen, congenital Q89.9
abdominal wall
  acquired M95.8
  congenital Q79.59
acquired (unspecified site) M95.9
adrenal gland Q89.1
alimentary tract, congenital Q45.9
  upper Q40.9
ankle (joint) (acquired) (*see also* Deformity, limb, lower leg)
  abduction — *see* Contraction, joint, ankle
  congenital Q68.8
  contraction — *see* Contraction, joint, ankle
  specified type NEC — *see* Deformity, limb, foot, specified NEC
anus (acquired) K62.89
  congenital Q43.9
aorta (arch) (congenital) Q25.4
  acquired I77.89
aortic
  arch, acquired I77.89
  cusp or valve (congenital) Q23.8
    acquired (*see also* Endocarditis, aortic) I35.8
arm (acquired) (upper) (*see also* Deformity, limb, upper arm)
  congenital Q68.8
  forearm — *see* Deformity, limb, forearm
artery (congenital) (peripheral) NOS Q27.9
  acquired I77.89
  coronary (acquired) I25.9
    congenital Q24.5
  umbilical Q27.0
atrial septal Q21.1
auditory canal (external) (congenital) (*see also* Malformation, ear, external)
  acquired — *see* Disorder, ear, external, specified type NEC
auricle
  ear (congenital) (*see also* Malformation, ear, external)
    acquired — *see* Disorder, pinna, deformity
back — *see* Dorsopathy, deforming
bile duct (common) (congenital) (hepatic) Q44.5
  acquired K83.8
biliary duct or passage (congenital) Q44.5
  acquired K83.8
bladder (neck) (trigone) (sphincter) (acquired) N32.89
  congenital Q64.79
bone (acquired) NOS M95.9
  congenital Q79.9
  turbinate M95.0
brain (congenital) Q04.9
  acquired G93.89
  reduction Q04.3
breast (acquired) N64.89
  congenital Q83.9

Deformity — *continued*
breast — *continued*
  reconstructed N65.0
bronchus (congenital) Q32.4
  acquired NEC J98.09
bursa, congenital Q79.9
canaliculi (lacrimalis) (acquired) (*see also* Disorder, lacrimal system, changes)
  congenital Q10.6
canthus, acquired — *see* Disorder, eyelid, specified type NEC
capillary (acquired) I78.8
cardiovascular system, congenital Q28.9
caruncle, lacrimal (acquired) (*see also* Disorder, lacrimal system, changes)
  congenital Q10.6
cascade, stomach K31.2
cecum (congenital) Q43.9
  acquired K63.89
cerebral, acquired G93.89
  congenital Q04.9
cervix (uterus) (acquired) NEC N88.8
  congenital Q51.9
cheek (acquired) M95.2
  congenital Q18.9
chest (acquired) (wall) M95.4
  congenital Q67.8
  sequelae (late effect) of rickets E64.3
chin (acquired) M95.2
  congenital Q18.9
choroid (congenital) Q14.3
  acquired H31.8
  plexus Q07.8
    acquired G96.19
cicatricial — *see* Cicatrix
cilia, acquired — *see* Disorder, eyelid, specified type NEC
clavicle (acquired) M95.8
  congenital Q68.8
clitoris (congenital) Q52.6
  acquired N90.89
clubfoot — *see* Clubfoot
coccyx (acquired) — *see* subcategory M43.8 ☑
colon (congenital) Q43.9
  acquired K63.89
concha (ear), congenital (*see also* Malformation, ear, external)
  acquired — *see* Disorder, pinna, deformity
cornea (acquired) H18.70
  congenital Q13.4
  descemetocele — *see* Descemetocele
  ectasia — *see* Ectasia, cornea
  specified NEC H18.79- ☑
  staphyloma — *see* Staphyloma, cornea
coronary artery (acquired) I25.9
  congenital Q24.5
cranium (acquired) — *see* Deformity, skull
cricoid cartilage (congenital) Q31.8
  acquired J38.7
cystic duct (congenital) Q44.5
  acquired K82.8
Dandy-Walker Q03.1
  with spina bifida — *see* Spina bifida
diaphragm (congenital) Q79.1
  acquired J98.6
digestive organ NOS Q45.9
ductus arteriosus Q25.0
duodenal bulb K31.89
duodenum (congenital) Q43.9
  acquired K31.89
dura — *see* Deformity, meninges
ear (acquired) (*see also* Disorder, pinna, deformity)
  congenital (external) Q17.9
    internal Q16.5
    middle Q16.4
      ossicles Q16.3
    ossicles Q16.3
ectodermal (congenital) NEC Q84.9
ejaculatory duct (congenital) Q55.4
  acquired N50.8
elbow (joint) (acquired) (*see also* Deformity, limb, upper arm)
  congenital Q68.8
  contraction — *see* Contraction, joint, elbow
endocrine gland NEC Q89.2
epididymis (congenital) Q55.4
  acquired N50.8

Deformity — *continued*
pelvis, pelvic (acquired) (bony) M95.5
  with disproportion (fetopelvic) O33.0
    causing obstructed labor O65.0
  congenital Q74.2
  rachitic sequelae (late effect) E64.3
penis (glans) (congenital) Q55.69
  acquired N48.89
pericardium (congenital) Q24.8
  acquired — *see* Pericarditis
pharynx (congenital) Q38.8
  acquired J39.2
pinna, acquired (*see also* Disorder, pinna, deformity)
  congenital Q17.9
pituitary (congenital) Q89.2
posture — *see* Dorsopathy, deforming
prepuce (congenital) Q55.69
  acquired N47.8
prostate (congenital) Q55.4
  acquired N42.89
pupil (congenital) Q13.2
  acquired — *see* Abnormality, pupillary
pylorus (congenital) Q40.3
  acquired K31.89
rachitic (acquired), old or healed E64.3
radius (acquired) (*see also* Deformity, limb, forearm)
  congenital Q68.8
rectum (congenital) Q43.9
  acquired K62.89
reduction (extremity) (limb), congenital (*see also* condition and site) Q73.8
  brain Q04.3
  lower — *see* Defect, reduction, lower limb
  upper — *see* Defect, reduction, upper limb
renal — *see* Deformity, kidney
respiratory system (congenital) Q34.9
rib (acquired) M95.4
  congenital Q76.6
  cervical Q76.5
rotation (joint) (acquired) — *see* Deformity, limb, specified site NEC
  congenital Q74.9
  hip — *see* Deformity, limb, specified type NEC, thigh
    congenital Q65.89
sacroiliac joint (congenital) — *see* subcategory Q74.2
  acquired — *see* subcategory M43.8 ☑
sacrum (acquired) — *see* subcategory M43.8 ☑
saddle
  back — *see* Lordosis
  nose M95.0
    syphilitic A50.57
salivary gland or duct (congenital) Q38.4
  acquired K11.8
scapula (acquired) M95.8
  congenital Q68.8
scrotum (congenital) (*see also* Malformation, testis and scrotum)
  acquired N50.8
seminal vesicles (congenital) Q55.4
  acquired N50.8
septum, nasal (acquired) J34.2
shoulder (joint) (acquired) — *see* Deformity, limb, upper arm
  congenital Q74.0
  contraction — *see* Contraction, joint, shoulder
sigmoid (flexure) (congenital) Q43.9
  acquired K63.89
skin (congenital) Q82.9
skull (acquired) M95.2
  congenital Q75.8
    with
      anencephaly Q00.0
      encephalocele — *see* Encephalocele
      hydrocephalus Q03.9
        with spina bifida — *see* Spina bifida, by site, with hydrocephalus
      microcephaly Q02
soft parts, organs or tissues (of pelvis)
  in pregnancy or childbirth NEC O34.8- ☑
    causing obstructed labor O65.5
spermatic cord (congenital) Q55.4
  acquired N50.10
  torsion — *see* Torsion, spermatic cord
spinal — *see* Dorsopathy, deforming
  column (acquired) — *see* Dorsopathy, deforming
  congenital Q67.5

Deformity — *continued*
spinal — *see* Dorsopathy, deforming — *continued*
  cord (congenital) Q06.9
    acquired G95.89
  nerve root (congenital) Q07.9
spine (acquired) (*see also* Dorsopathy, deforming)
  congenital Q67.5
  rachitic E64.3
  specified NEC — *see* Dorsopathy, deforming, specified NEC
spleen
  acquired D73.89
  congenital Q89.09
Sprengel's (congenital) Q74.0
sternocleidomastoid (muscle), congenital Q68.0
sternum (acquired) M95.4
  congenital NEC Q76.7
stomach (acquired) Q40.3
  acquired K31.89
submandibular gland (congenital) Q38.4
submaxillary gland (congenital) Q38.4
  acquired K11.8
talipes — *see* Talipes
testis (congenital) (*see also* Malformation, testis and scrotum)
  acquired N44.8
  torsion — *see* Torsion, testis
thigh (acquired) (*see also* Deformity, limb, thigh)
  congenital NEC Q68.8
thorax (acquired) (wall) M95.4
  congenital Q67.8
  sequelae of rickets E64.3
thumb (acquired) (*see also* Deformity, finger)
  congenital NEC Q68.1
thymus (tissue) (congenital) Q89.2
thyroid (gland) (congenital) Q89.2
  cartilage Q31.8
    acquired J38.7
tibia (acquired) (*see also* Deformity, limb, specified type NEC, lower leg)
  congenital NEC Q68.8
  saber (syphilitic) A50.56
toe (acquired) M20.6- ☑
  congenital Q66.9
  hallux rigidus M20.2- ☑
  hallux valgus M20.1- ☑
  hallux varus M20.3- ☑
  hammer toe M20.4- ☑
  specified NEC M20.5X- ☑
tongue (congenital) Q38.3
  acquired K14.8
tooth, teeth K00.2
trachea (rings) (congenital) Q32.1
  acquired J39.8
transverse aortic arch (congenital) Q25.4
tricuspid (leaflets) (valve) I07.8
  atresia or stenosis Q22.4
  Ebstein's Q22.5
trunk (acquired) M95.8
  congenital Q89.9
ulna (acquired) (*see also* Deformity, limb, forearm)
  congenital NEC Q68.8
urachus, congenital Q64.4
ureter (opening) (congenital) Q62.8
  acquired N28.89
urethra (congenital) Q64.79
  acquired N36.8
urinary tract (congenital) Q64.9
  urachus Q64.4
uterus (congenital) Q51.9
  acquired N85.8
uvula (congenital) Q38.5
vagina (acquired) N89.8
  congenital Q52.4
valgus NEC M21.00
  ankle M21.07- ☑
  elbow M21.02- ☑
  hip M21.05- ☑
  knee M21.06- ☑
valve, valvular (congenital) (heart) Q24.8
  acquired — *see* Endocarditis
varus NEC M21.10
  ankle M21.17- ☑
  elbow M21.12- ☑
  hip M21.15 ☑
  knee M21.16- ☑
  tibia — *see* Osteochondrosis, juvenile, tibia

Deformity — *continued*
vas deferens (congenital) Q55.4
  acquired N50.8
vein (congenital) Q27.9
  great Q26.9
vertebra — *see* Dorsopathy, deforming
vertical talus (congenital) Q66.80
  left foot Q66.82
  right foot Q66.81
vesicourethral orifice (acquired) N32.89
  congenital NEC Q64.79
vessels of optic papilla (congenital) Q14.2
visual field (contraction) — *see* Defect, visual field
vitreous body, acquired H43.89
vulva (congenital) Q52.79
  acquired N90.89
wrist (joint) (acquired) (*see also* Deformity, limb, forearm)
  congenital Q68.8
  contraction — *see* Contraction, joint, wrist

Degeneration, degenerative
adrenal (capsule) (fatty) (gland) (hyaline) (infectional) E27.8
amyloid (*see also* Amyloidosis) E85.9
anterior cornua, spinal cord G12.29
anterior labral S43.49- ☑
aorta, aortic I70.0
  fatty I77.89
aortic valve (heart) — *see* Endocarditis, aortic
arteriovascular — *see* Arteriosclerosis
artery, arterial (atheromatous) (calcareous) (*see also* Arteriosclerosis)
  cerebral, amyloid E85.4 [I68.0]
  medial — *see* Arteriosclerosis, extremities
articular cartilage NEC — *see* Derangement, joint, articular cartilage, by site
atheromatous — *see* Arteriosclerosis
basal nuclei or ganglia G23.9
  specified NEC G23.8
bone NEC — *see* Disorder, bone, specified type NEC
brachial plexus G54.0
brain (cortical) (progressive) G31.9
  alcoholic G31.2
  arteriosclerotic I67.2
  childhood G31.9
    specified NEC G31.89
  cystic G31.89
    congenital Q04.6
  in
    alcoholism G31.2
    beriberi E51.2
    cerebrovascular disease I67.9
    congenital hydrocephalus Q03.9
      with spina bifida (*see also* Spina bifida)
    Fabry-Anderson disease E75.21
    Gaucher's disease E75.22
    Hunter's syndrome E76.1
    lipidosis
      cerebral E75.4
      generalized E75.6
    mucopolysaccharidosis — *see* Mucopolysaccharidosis
    myxedema E03.9 [G32.89]
    neoplastic disease (*see also* Neoplasm) D49.6 [G32.89]
    Niemann-Pick disease E75.249 [G32.89]
    sphingolipidosis E75.3 [G32.89]
    vitamin B12 deficiency E53.8 [G32.89]
  senile NEC G31.1
breast N64.89
Bruch's membrane — *see* Degeneration, choroid
capillaries (fatty) I78.8
  amyloid E85.8 [I79.8]
cardiac (*see also* Degeneration, myocardial)
  valve, valvular — *see* Endocarditis
cardiorenal — *see* Hypertension, cardiorenal
cardiovascular (*see also* Disease, cardiovascular)
  renal — *see* Hypertension, cardiorenal
cerebellar NOS G31.9
  alcoholic G31.2
  primary (hereditary) (sporadic) G11.9
cerebral — *see* Degeneration, brain
cerebrovascular I67.9
  due to hypertension I67.4
cervical plexus G54.2
cervix N88.8
  due to radiation (intended effect) N88.8
    adverse effect or misadventure N99.89

Index

Deformity — Degeneration, degenerative

Degeneration, degenerative — *continued*
- chamber angle H21.21- ☑
- changes, spine or vertebra — *see* Spondylosis
- chorioretinal (*see also* Degeneration, choroid)
  - hereditary H31.20
- choroid (colloid) (drusen) H31.10- ☑
  - atrophy — *see* Atrophy, choroidal
  - hereditary — *see* Dystrophy, choroidal, hereditary
- ciliary body H21.22- ☑
- cochlear — *see* subcategory H83.8 ☑
- combined (spinal cord) (subacute) E53.8 [G32.0]
  - with anemia (pernicious) D51.0 [G32.0]
    - due to dietary vitamin B12 deficiency D51.3 [G32.0]
  - in (due to)
    - vitamin B12 deficiency E53.8 [G32.0]
    - anemia D51.9 [G32.0]
- conjunctiva H11.10
  - concretions — *see* Concretion, conjunctiva
  - deposits — *see* Deposit, conjunctiva
  - pigmentations — *see* Pigmentation, conjunctiva
  - pinguecula — *see* Pinguecula
  - xerosis — *see* Xerosis, conjunctiva
- cornea H18.40
  - calcerous H18.43
    - band keratopathy H18.42- ☑
  - familial, hereditary — *see* Dystrophy, cornea
  - hyaline (of old scars) H18.49
  - keratomalacia — *see* Keratomalacia
  - nodular H18.45- ☑
  - peripheral H18.46- ☑
  - senile H18.41- ☑
  - specified type NEC H18.49
- cortical (cerebellar) (parenchymatous) G31.89
  - alcoholic G31.2
  - diffuse, due to arteriopathy I67.2
- corticobasal G31.85
- cutis L98.8
  - amyloid E85.4 [L99]
- dental pulp K04.2
- disc disease — *see* Degeneration, intervertebral disc NEC
- dorsolateral (spinal cord) — *see* Degeneration, combined
- extrapyramidal G25.9
- eye, macular (*see also* Degeneration, macula)
  - congenital or hereditary — *see* Dystrophy, retina
- facet joints — *see* Spondylosis
- fatty
  - liver NEC K76.0
    - alcoholic K70.0
- grey matter (brain) (Alpers') G31.81
- heart (*see also* Degeneration, myocardial)
  - amyloid E85.4 [I43]
  - atheromatous — *see* Disease, heart, ischemic, atherosclerotic
  - ischemic — *see* Disease, heart, ischemic
- hepatolenticular (Wilson's) E83.01
- hepatorenal K76.7
- hyaline (diffuse) (generalized)
  - localized — *see* Degeneration, by site
- infrapatellar fat pad M79.4
- intervertebral disc NOS
  - with
    - myelopathy — *see* Disorder, disc, with, myelopathy
    - radiculitis or radiculopathy — *see* Disorder, disc, with, radiculopathy
  - cervical, cervicothoracic — *see* Disorder, disc, cervical, degeneration
    - with
      - myelopathy — *see* Disorder, disc, cervical, with myelopathy
      - neuritis, radiculitis or radiculopathy — *see* Disorder, disc, cervical, with neuritis
  - lumbar region M51.36
    - with
      - myelopathy M51.06
      - neuritis, radiculitis, radiculopathy or sciatica M51.16
  - lumbosacral region M51.37
    - with
      - neuritis, radiculitis, radiculopathy or sciatica M51.17
  - sacrococcygeal region M53.3

Degeneration, degenerative — *continued*
- intervertebral disc — *continued*
  - thoracic region M51.34
    - with
      - myelopathy M51.04
      - neuritis, radiculitis, radiculopathy M51.14
  - thoracolumbar region M51.35
    - with
      - myelopathy M51.05
      - neuritis, radiculitis, radiculopathy M51.15
- intestine, amyloid E85.4
- iris (pigmentary) H21.23- ☑
- ischemic — *see* Ischemia
- joint disease — *see* Osteoarthritis
- kidney N28.89
  - amyloid E85.4 [N29]
  - cystic, congenital Q61.9
  - fatty N28.89
  - polycystic Q61.3
    - adult type (autosomal dominant) Q61.2
    - infantile type (autosomal recessive) NEC Q61.19
      - collecting duct dilatation Q61.11
- Kuhnt-Junius (*see also* Degeneration, macula) H35.32
- lens — *see* Cataract
- lenticular (familial) (progressive) (Wilson's) (with cirrhosis of liver) E83.01
- liver (diffuse) NEC K76.89
  - amyloid E85.4 [K77]
  - cystic K76.89
    - congenital Q44.6
  - fatty NEC K76.0
    - alcoholic K70.0
  - hypertrophic K76.89
  - parenchymatous, acute or subacute K72.00
    - with coma K72.01
  - pigmentary K76.89
  - toxic (acute) K71.9
- lung J98.4
- lymph gland I89.8
  - hyaline I89.8
- macula, macular (acquired) (age-related) (senile) H35.30
  - angioid streaks H35.33
  - atrophic age-related H35.31
  - congenital or hereditary — *see* Dystrophy, retina
  - cystoid H35.35- ☑
  - drusen H35.36- ☑
  - exudative H35.32
  - hole H35.34- ☑
  - nonexudative H35.31
  - puckering H35.37- ☑
  - toxic H35.38- ☑
- membranous labyrinth, congenital (causing impairment of hearing) Q16.5
- meniscus — *see* Derangement, meniscus
- mitral — *see* Insufficiency, mitral
- Mönckeberg's — *see* Arteriosclerosis, extremities
- motor centers, senile G31.1
- multi-system G90.3
- mural — *see* Degeneration, myocardial
- muscle (fatty) (fibrous) (hyaline) (progressive) M62.89
  - heart — *see* Degeneration, myocardial
- myelin, central nervous system G37.9
- myocardial, myocardium (fatty) (hyaline) (senile) I51.5
  - with rheumatic fever (conditions in I00) I09.0
    - active, acute or subacute I01.2
      - with chorea I02.0
    - inactive or quiescent (with chorea) I09.0
  - hypertensive — *see* Hypertension, heart
  - rheumatic — *see* Degeneration, myocardial, with rheumatic fever
  - syphilitic A52.06
- nasal sinus (mucosa) J32.9
  - frontal J32.1
  - maxillary J32.0
- nerve — *see* Disorder, nerve
- nervous system G31.9
  - alcoholic G31.2
  - amyloid E85.4 [G99.8]
  - autonomic G90.9
  - fatty G31.89
  - specified NEC G31.89
- nipple N64.89
- olivopontocerebellar (hereditary) (familial) G23.8
- osseous labyrinth — *see* subcategory H83.8 ☑
- ovary N83.8
  - cystic N83.20
  - microcystic N83.20

Degeneration, degenerative — *continued*
- pallidal pigmentary (progressive) G23.0
- pancreas K86.8
  - tuberculous A18.83
- penis N48.89
- pigmentary (diffuse) (general)
  - localized — *see* Degeneration, by site
  - pallidal (progressive) G23.0
- pineal gland E34.8
- pituitary (gland) E23.6
- popliteal fat pad M79.4
- posterolateral (spinal cord) — *see* Degeneration, combined
- pulmonary valve (heart) I37.8
- pulp (tooth) K04.2
- pupillary margin H21.24- ☑
- renal — *see* Degeneration, kidney
- retina H35.9
  - hereditary (cerebroretinal) (congenital) (juvenile) (macula) (peripheral) (pigmentary) — *see* Dystrophy, retina
  - Kuhnt-Junius (*see also* Degeneration, macula) H35.32
  - macula (cystic) (exudative) (hole) (nonexudative) (pseudohole) (senile) (toxic) — *see* Degeneration, macula
  - peripheral H35.40
    - lattice H35.41- ☑
    - microcystoid H35.42- ☑
    - paving stone H35.43- ☑
    - secondary
      - pigmentary H35.45- ☑
      - vitreoretinal H35.46- ☑
    - senile reticular H35.44- ☑
  - pigmentary (primary) (*see also* Dystrophy, retina)
    - secondary — *see* Degeneration, retina, peripheral, secondary
  - posterior pole — *see* Degeneration, macula
- saccule, congenital (causing impairment of hearing) Q16.5
- senile R54
  - brain G31.1
  - cardiac, heart or myocardium — *see* Degeneration, myocardial
  - motor centers G31.1
  - vascular — *see* Arteriosclerosis
- sinus (cystic) (*see also* Sinusitis)
  - polypoid J33.1
- skin L98.8
  - amyloid E85.4 [L99]
  - colloid L98.8
- spinal (cord) G31.89
  - amyloid E85.4 [G32.89]
  - combined (subacute) — *see* Degeneration, combined
  - dorsolateral — *see* Degeneration, combined
  - familial NEC G31.89
  - fatty G31.89
  - funicular — *see* Degeneration, combined
  - posterolateral — *see* Degeneration, combined
  - subacute combined — *see* Degeneration, combined
  - tuberculous A17.81
- spleen D73.0
  - amyloid E85.4 [D77]
- stomach K31.89
- striatonigral G23.2
- suprarenal (capsule) (gland) E27.8
- synovial membrane (pulpy) — *see* Disorder, synovium, specified type NEC
- tapetoretinal — *see* Dystrophy, retina
- thymus (gland) E32.8
  - fatty E32.8
- thyroid (gland) E07.89
- tricuspid (heart) (valve) I07.9
- tuberculous NEC — *see* Tuberculosis
- turbinate J34.89
- uterus (cystic) N85.8
- vascular (senile) — *see* Arteriosclerosis
  - hypertensive — *see* Hypertension
- vitreoretinal, secondary — *see* Degeneration, retina, peripheral, secondary, vitreoretinal
- vitreous (body) H43.81- ☑
- Wallerian — *see* Disorder, nerve
- Wilson's hepatolenticular E83.01

☑ **Additional Character Required** — Refer to the Tabular List for Character Selection   ⬇ Subterms under main terms may continue to next column or page

Deglutition
- paralysis R13.0
  - hysterical F44.4
- pneumonia J69.0

Degos' disease I77.89

Dehiscence (of)
- amputation stump T87.81
- cesarean wound O90.0
- closure of
  - cornea T81.31 ☑
  - craniotomy T81.32 ☑
  - fascia (muscular) (superficial) T81.32 ☑
  - internal organ or tissue T81.32 ☑
  - laceration (external) (internal) T81.33 ☑
  - ligament T81.32 ☑
  - mucosa T81.31 ☑
  - muscle or muscle flap T81.32 ☑
  - ribs or rib cage T81.32 ☑
  - skin and subcutaneous tissue (full-thickness) (superficial) T81.31 ☑
  - skull T81.32 ☑
  - sternum (sternotomy) T81.32 ☑
  - tendon T81.32 ☑
  - traumatic laceration (external) (internal) T81.33 ☑
- episiotomy O90.1
- operation wound NEC T81.31 ☑
  - external operation wound (superficial) T81.31 ☑
  - internal operation wound (deep) T81.32 ☑
- perineal wound (postpartum) O90.1
- traumatic injury wound repair T81.33 ☑
- wound T81.30 ☑
  - traumatic repair T81.33 ☑

Dehydration E86.0
- hypertonic E87.0
- hypotonic E87.1
- newborn P74.1

Déjérine-Roussy syndrome G89.0

Déjérine-Sottas disease or neuropathy (hypertrophic) G60.0

Déjérine-Thomas atrophy G23.8

Delay, delayed
- any plane in pelvis
  - complicating delivery O66.9
- birth or delivery NOS O63.9
- closure, ductus arteriosus (Botalli) P29.3
- coagulation — see Defect, coagulation
- conduction (cardiac) (ventricular) I45.9
- delivery, second twin, triplet, etc O63.2
- development R62.50
  - global F88
  - intellectual (specific) F81.9
  - language F80.9
    - due to hearing loss F80.4
  - learning F81.9
  - pervasive F84.9
  - physiological R62.50
    - specified stage NEC R62.0
  - reading F81.0
  - sexual E30.0
  - speech F80.9
    - due to hearing loss F80.4
  - spelling F81.81
- gastric emptying K30
- menarche E30.0
- menstruation (cause unknown) N91.0
- milestone R62.0
- passage of meconium (newborn) P76.0
- primary respiration P28.9
- puberty (constitutional) E30.0
- separation of umbilical cord P96.82
- sexual maturation, female E30.0
- sleep phase syndrome G47.21
- union, fracture — see Fracture, by site
- vaccination Z28.9

Deletion(s)
- autosome Q93.9
  - identified by fluorescence in situ hybridization (FISH) Q93.89
  - identified by in situ hybridization (ISH) Q93.89
- chromosome
  - with complex rearrangements NEC Q93.7
  - part of NEC Q93.5
  - seen only at prometaphase Q93.89
  - short arm
    - 22q11.2 Q93.81
    - 4 Q93.3
    - 5p Q93.4

Deletion(s) — continued
- chromosome — continued
  - specified NEC Q93.89
- long arm chromosome 18 or 21 Q93.89
  - with complex rearrangements NEC Q93.7
- microdeletions NEC Q93.88

Delhi boil or button B55.1

Delinquency (juvenile) (neurotic) F91.8
- group Z72.810

Delinquent immunization status Z28.3

Delirium, delirious (acute or subacute) (not alcohol- or drug-induced) (with dementia) R41.0
- alcoholic (acute) (tremens) (withdrawal) F10.921
  - with intoxication F10.921
    - in
      - abuse F10.121
      - dependence F10.221
- due to (secondary to)
  - alcohol
    - intoxication F10.921
      - in
        - abuse F10.121
        - dependence F10.221
    - withdrawal F10.231
  - amphetamine intoxication F15.921
    - in
      - abuse F15.121
      - dependence F15.221
  - anxiolytic
    - intoxication F13.921
      - in
        - abuse F13.121
        - dependence F13.221
    - withdrawal F13.231
  - cannabis intoxication (acute) F12.921
    - in
      - abuse F12.121
      - dependence F12.221
  - cocaine intoxication (acute) F14.921
    - in
      - abuse F14.121
      - dependence F14.221
  - general medical condition F05
  - hallucinogen intoxication F16.921
    - in
      - abuse F16.121
      - dependence F16.221
  - hypnotic
    - intoxication F13.921
      - in
        - abuse F13.121
        - dependence F13.221
    - withdrawal F13.231
  - inhalant intoxication (acute) F18.921
    - in
      - abuse F18.121
      - dependence F18.221
  - multiple etiologies F05
  - opioid intoxication (acute) F11.921
    - in
      - abuse F11.121
      - dependence F11.221
  - phencyclidine intoxication (acute) F16.921
    - in
      - abuse F16.121
      - dependence F16.221
  - psychoactive substance NEC intoxication (acute) F19.921
    - in
      - abuse F19.121
      - dependence F19.221
  - sedative
    - intoxication F13.921
      - in
        - abuse F13.121
        - dependence F13.221
    - withdrawal F13.231
  - unknown etiology F05
- exhaustion F43.0
- hysterical F44.89
- postprocedural (postoperative) F05
- puerperal F05
- thyroid — see Thyrotoxicosis with thyroid storm
- traumatic — see Injury, intracranial
- tremens (alcohol-induced) F10.231
  - sedative-induced F13.231

Delivery (childbirth) (labor)
- arrested active phase O62.1

Delivery — continued
- cesarean (for)
  - without indication O82
  - abnormal
    - pelvis (bony) (deformity) (major) NEC with disproportion (fetopelvic) O33.0
      - with obstructed labor O65.0
    - presentation or position O32.9 ☑
  - abruptio placentae (see also Abruptio placentae) O45.9-
  - acromion presentation O32.2 ☑
  - atony, uterus O62.2
  - breech presentation O32.1 ☑
    - incomplete O32.8 ☑
  - brow presentation O32.3 ☑
  - cephalopelvic disproportion O33.9
  - cerclage O34.3- ☑
  - chin presentation O32.3 ☑
  - cicatrix of cervix O34.4- ☑
  - contracted pelvis (general)
    - inlet O33.2
    - outlet O33.3 ☑
  - cord presentation or prolapse O69.0 ☑
  - cystocele O34.8- ☑
  - deformity (acquired) (congenital)
    - pelvic organs or tissues NEC O34.8- ☑
    - pelvis (bony) NEC O33.0
  - disproportion NOS O33.9
  - eclampsia — see Eclampsia
  - face presentation O32.3 ☑
  - failed
    - forceps O66.5
    - induction of labor O61.9
      - instrumental O61.1
      - mechanical O61.1
      - medical O61.0
      - specified NEC O61.8
      - surgical O61.1
    - trial of labor NOS O66.40
      - following previous cesarean delivery O66.41
    - vacuum extraction O66.5
    - ventouse O66.5
  - fetal-maternal hemorrhage O43.01- ☑
  - hemorrhage (intrapartum) O67.9
    - with coagulation defect O67.0
    - specified cause NEC O67.8
  - high head at term O32.4 ☑
  - hydrocephalic fetus O33.6 ☑
  - incarceration of uterus O34.51- ☑
  - incoordinate uterine action O62.4
  - increased size, fetus O33.5 ☑
  - inertia, uterus O62.2
    - primary O62.0
    - secondary O62.1
  - lateroversion, uterus O34.59- ☑
  - mal lie O32.9 ☑
  - malposition
    - fetus O32.9 ☑
    - pelvic organs or tissues NEC O34.8- ☑
    - uterus NEC O34.59- ☑
  - malpresentation NOS O32.9 ☑
  - oblique presentation O32.2 ☑
  - occurring after 37 completed weeks of gestation but before 39 completed weeks gestation due to (spontaneous) onset of labor O75.82
  - oversize fetus O33.5 ☑
  - pelvic tumor NEC O34.8- ☑
  - placenta previa O44.1- ☑
    - without hemorrhage O44.0- ☑
  - placental insufficiency O36.51- ☑
  - planned, occurring after 37 completed weeks of gestation but before 39 completed weeks gestation due to (spontaneous) onset of labor O75.82
  - polyp, cervix O34.4- ☑
    - causing obstructed labor O65.5
  - poor dilatation, cervix O62.0
  - pre-eclampsia O14.9- ☑
    - mild O14.0- ☑
    - moderate O14.0- ☑
    - severe
      - with hemolysis, elevated liver enzymes and low platelet count (HELLP) O14.2- ☑
  - previous
    - cesarean delivery O34.21
    - surgery (to)
      - cervix O34.4- ☑

Index

Delivery — Delivery

Delivery — *continued*
  cesarean — *continued*
    previous — *continued*
      surgery — *continued*
        gynecological NEC O34.8- ☑
        rectum O34.7- ☑
        uterus O34.29
        vagina O34.6- ☑
      prolapse
        arm or hand O32.2 ☑
        uterus O34.52- ☑
      prolonged labor NOS O63.9
      rectocele O34.8- ☑
      retroversion
        uterus O34.53- ☑
      rigid
        cervix O34.4- ☑
        pelvic floor O34.8- ☑
        perineum O34.7- ☑
        vagina O34.6- ☑
        vulva O34.7- ☑
      sacculation, pregnant uterus O34.59- ☑
      scar(s)
        cervix O34.4- ☑
        cesarean delivery O34.21
        uterus O34.29
      Shirodkar suture in situ O34.3- ☑
      shoulder presentation O32.2 ☑
      stenosis or stricture, cervix O34.4- ☑
      streptococcus B carrier state O99.824
      transverse presentation or lie O32.2 ☑
      tumor, pelvic organs or tissues NEC O34.8- ☑
        cervix O34.4- ☑
      umbilical cord presentation or prolapse O69.0 ☑
    completely normal case O80
    complicated O75.9
      by
        abnormal, abnormality (of)
          forces of labor O62.9
            specified type NEC O62.8
          glucose O99.814
          uterine contractions NOS O62.9
        abruptio placentae (*see also* Abruptio placentae) O45.9- ☑
        abuse
          physical O9A.32 (*following* O99)
          psychological O9A.52 (*following* O99)
          sexual O9A.42 (*following* O99)
        adherent placenta O72.0
          without hemorrhage O73.0
        alcohol use O99.314
        anemia (pre-existing) O99.02
        anesthetic death O74.8
        annular detachment of cervix O71.3
        atony, uterus O62.2
        attempted vacuum extraction and forceps O66.5
        Bandl's ring O62.4
        bariatric surgery status O99.844
        biliary tract disorder O26.62
        bleeding — *see* Delivery, complicated by, hemorrhage
        blood disorder NEC O99.12
        cervical dystocia (hypotonic) O62.2
          primary O62.0
          secondary O62.1
        circulatory system disorder O99.42
        compression of cord (umbilical) NEC O69.2 ☑
        condition NEC O99.89
        contraction, contracted ring O62.4
        cord (umbilical)
          around neck
            with compression O69.1 ☑
            without compression O69.81 ☑
          bruising O69.5 ☑
          complication O69.9 ☑
            specified NEC O69.89 ☑
          compression NEC O69.2 ☑
          entanglement O69.2 ☑
            without compression O69.82 ☑
          hematoma O69.5 ☑
          presentation O69.0 ☑
          prolapse O69.0 ☑
          short O69.3 ☑
          thrombosis (vessels) O69.5 ☑
          vascular lesion O69.5 ☑
        Couvelaire uterus O45.8X- ☑

Delivery — *continued*
  complicated — *continued*
    by — *continued*
      damage to (injury to) NEC
        perineum O71.82
        periurethral tissue O71.82
        vulva O71.82
      delay following rupture of membranes (spontaneous) — *see* Pregnancy, complicated by, premature rupture of membranes
      depressed fetal heart tones O76
      diabetes O24.92
        gestational O24.429
          diet controlled O24.420
          insulin controlled O24.424
        pre-existing O24.32
          specified NEC O24.82
          type 1 O24.02
          type 2 O24.12
      diastasis recti (abdominis) O71.89
      dilatation
        bladder O66.8
        cervix incomplete, poor or slow O62.0
      disease NEC O99.89
      disruptio uteri — *see* Delivery, complicated by, rupture, uterus
      drug use O99.324
      dysfunction, uterus NOS O62.9
        hypertonic O62.4
        hypotonic O62.2
          primary O62.0
          secondary O62.1
        incoordinate O62.4
      eclampsia O15.1
      embolism (pulmonary) — *see* Embolism, obstetric
      endocrine, nutritional or metabolic disease NEC O99.284
      failed
        attempted vaginal birth after previous cesarean delivery O66.41
        induction of labor O61.9
          instrumental O61.1
          mechanical O61.1
          medical O61.0
          specified NEC O61.8
          surgical O61.1
        trial of labor O66.40
      female genital mutilation O65.5
      fetal
        abnormal acid-base balance O68
        acidemia O68
        acidosis O68
        alkalosis O68
        death, early O02.1
        deformity O66.3
        heart rate or rhythm (abnormal) (non-reassuring) O76
        hypoxia O77.8
        stress O77.9
          due to drug administration O77.1
          electrocardiographic evidence of O77.8
          specified NEC O77.8
          ultrasound evidence of O77.8
      fever during labor O75.2
      gastric banding status O99.844
      gastric bypass status O99.844
      gastrointestinal disease NEC O99.62
      gestational diabetes O24.429
        diet controlled O24.420
        insulin (and diet) controlled O24.424
      gonorrhea O98.22
      hematoma O71.7
        ischial spine O71.7
        pelvic O71.7
        vagina O71.7
        vulva or perineum O71.7
      hemorrhage (uterine) O67.9
        associated with
          afibrinogenemia O67.0
          coagulation defect O67.0
          hyperfibrinolysis O67.0
          hypofibrinogenemia O67.0
        due to
          low-lying placenta O44.1- ☑
          placenta previa O44.1- ☑

Delivery — *continued*
  complicated — *continued*
    by — *continued*
      hemorrhage — *continued*
        due to — *continued*
          premature separation of placenta (normally implanted) (*see also* Abruptio placentae) O45.9- ☑
          retained placenta O72.0
          uterine leiomyoma O67.8
        placenta NEC O67.8
        postpartum NEC (atonic) (immediate) O72.1
          with retained or trapped placenta O72.0
          delayed O72.2
          secondary O72.2
          third stage O72.0
      hourglass contraction, uterus O62.4
      hypertension, hypertensive (pre-existing) — *see* Hypertension, complicated by, childbirth (labor)
      hypotension O26.5- ☑
      incomplete dilatation (cervix) O62.0
      incoordinate uterus contractions O62.4
      inertia, uterus O62.2
        during latent phase of labor O62.0
        primary O62.0
        secondary O62.1
      infection (maternal) O98.92
        carrier state NEC O99.834
        gonorrhea O98.22
        human immunodeficiency virus (HIV) O98.72
        sexually transmitted NEC O98.32
        specified NEC O98.82
        syphilis O98.12
        tuberculosis O98.02
        viral hepatitis O98.42
        viral NEC O98.52
      injury (to mother) (*see also* Delivery, complicated, by, damage to) O71.9
        nonobstetric O9A.22 (*following* O99)
          caused by abuse — *see* Delivery, complicated by, abuse
      intrauterine fetal death, early O02.1
      inversion, uterus O71.2
      laceration (perineal) O70.9
        anus (sphincter) O70.4
          with third degree laceration O70.2
            with mucosa O70.3
            without third degree laceration O70.4
        bladder (urinary) O71.5
        bowel O71.5
        cervix (uteri) O71.3
        fourchette O70.0
        hymen O70.0
        labia O70.0
        pelvic
          floor O70.1
          organ NEC O71.5
        perineum, perineal O70.9
          first degree O70.0
          fourth degree O70.3
          muscles O70.1
          second degree O70.1
          skin O70.0
          slight O70.0
          third degree O70.2
        peritoneum (pelvic) O71.5
        rectovaginal (septum) (without perineal laceration) O71.4
          with perineum O70.2
            with anal or rectal mucosa O70.3
        specified NEC O71.89
        sphincter ani — *see* Delivery, complicated, by, laceration, anus (sphincter)
        urethra O71.5
        uterus O71.81
          before labor O71.81
        vagina, vaginal (deep) (high) (without perineal laceration) O71.4
          with perineum O70.0
            muscles, with perineum O70.1
        vulva O70.0
      liver disorder O26.62
      malignancy O9A.12 (*following* O99)
      malnutrition O25.2

☑ **Additional Character Required** — Refer to the Tabular List for Character Selection   ▽ **Subterms under main terms may continue to next column or page**

Delivery — *continued*
  complicated — *continued*
    by — *continued*
      malposition, malpresentation
        without obstruction (*see also* Delivery,
          complicated by, obstruction) O32.9 ☑
          breech O32.1 ☑
          compound O32.6 ☑
          face (brow) (chin) O32.3 ☑
          footling O32.8 ☑
          high head O32.4 ☑
          oblique O32.2 ☑
          specified NEC O32.8 ☑
          transverse O32.2 ☑
          unstable lie O32.0 ☑
      placenta (with hemorrhage) O44.1- ☑
        without hemorrhage O44.0- ☑
      uterus or cervix O65.5
      meconium in amniotic fluid O77.0
      mental disorder NEC O99.344
      metrorrhexis — *see* Delivery, complicated by,
        rupture, uterus
      nervous system disorder O99.354
      obesity (pre-existing) O99.214
      obesity surgery status O99.844
      obstetric trauma O71.9
        specified NEC O71.89
      obstructed labor
        due to
          breech (complete) (frank) presentation
            O64.1 ☑
            incomplete O64.8 ☑
          brow presenation O64.3
          buttock presentation O64.1 ☑
          chin presentation O64.2 ☑
          compound presentation O64.5 ☑
          contracted pelvis O65.1
          deep transverse arrest O64.0 ☑
          deformed pelvis O65.0 ☑
          dystocia (fetal) O66.9
            due to
              conjoined twins O66.3
              fetal
                abnormality NEC O66.3
                ascites O66.3
                hydrops O66.3
                meningomyelocele O66.3
                sacral teratoma O66.3
                tumor O66.3
              hydrocephalic fetus O66.3
            shoulder O66.0
          face presentation O64.2 ☑
          fetopelvic disproportion O65.4
          footling presentation O64.8 ☑
          impacted shoulders O66.0
          incomplete rotation of fetal head
            O64.0 ☑
          large fetus O66.2
          locked twins O66.1
          malposition O64.9 ☑
            specified NEC O64.8 ☑
          malpresentation O64.9 ☑
            specified NEC O64.8 ☑
          multiple fetuses NEC O66.6
          pelvic
            abnormality (maternal) O65.9
              organ O65.5
              specified NEC O65.8
            contraction
              inlet O65.2
              mid-cavity O65.3
              outlet O65.3
          persistent (position)
            occipitoiliac O64.0 ☑
            occipitoposterior O64.0 ☑
            occipitosacral O64.0 ☑
            occipitotransverse O64.0 ☑
          prolapsed arm O64.4 ☑
          shoulder presentation O64.4 ☑
        specified NEC O66.8
      pathological retraction ring, uterus O62.4
      penetration, pregnant uterus by instrument
        O71.1
      perforation — *see* Delivery, complicated by,
        laceration

Delivery — *continued*
  complicated — *continued*
    by — *continued*
      placenta, placental
        ablatio (*see also* Abruptio placentae)
          O45.9- ☑
        abnormality O43.9- ☑
          specified NEC O43.89- ☑
        abruptio (*see also* Abruptio placentae)
          O45.9- ☑
        accreta O43.21- ☑
        adherent (with hemorrhage) O72.0
          without hemorrhage O73.0
        detachment (premature) (*see also* Abruptio
          placentae) O45.9- ☑
        disorder O43.9-
          specified NEC O43.89- ☑
        hemorrhage NEC O67.8
        increta O43.22- ☑
        low (implantation) O44.1- ☑
          without hemorrhage O44.0- ☑
        malformation O43.10- ☑
        malposition O44.1- ☑
          without hemorrhage O44.0- ☑
        percreta O43.23- ☑
        previa (central) (lateral) (low) (marginal)
          (partial) (total) O44.1- ☑
          without hemorrhage O44.0- ☑
        retained (with hemorrhage) O72.0
          without hemorrhage O73.0
        separation (premature) O45.9- ☑
          specified NEC O45.8X- ☑
        vicious insertion O44.1- ☑
      precipitate labor O62.3
      premature rupture, membranes (*see also* Preg-
        nancy, complicated by, premature rup-
        ture of membranes) O42.90
      prolapse
        arm or hand O32.2 ☑
        cord (umbilical) O69.0 ☑
        foot or leg O32.8 ☑
        uterus O34.52- ☑
      prolonged labor O63.9
        first stage O63.0
        second stage O63.1
      protozoal disease (maternal) O98.62
      respiratory disease NEC O99.52
      retained membranes or portions of placenta
        O72.2
        without hemorrhage O73.1
      retarded birth O63.9
      retention of secundines (with hemorrhage)
        O72.0
        without hemorrhage O73.0
        partial O72.2
          without hemorrhage O73.1
      rupture
        bladder (urinary) O71.5
        cervix O71.3
        pelvic organ NEC O71.5
        urethra O71.5
        uterus (during or after labor) O71.1
          before labor O71.0- ☑
      separation, pubic bone (symphysis pubis) O71.6
      shock O75.1
      shoulder presentation O64.4 ☑
      skin disorder NEC O99.72
      spasm, cervix O62.4
      stenosis or stricture, cervix O65.5
      streptococcus B carrier state O99.824
      subluxation of symphysis (pubis) O26.72
      syphilis (maternal) O98.12
      tear — *see* Delivery, complicated by, laceration
      tetanic uterus O62.4
      trauma (obstetrical) (*see also* Delivery, compli-
        cated, by, damage to) O71.9
        non-obstetric O9A.22 (*following* O99)
        periurethral O71.82
        specified NEC O71.89
      tuberculosis (maternal) O98.02
      tumor, pelvic organs or tissues NEC O65.5
      umbilical cord around neck
        with compression O69.1 ☑
        without compression O69.81 ☑
      uterine inertia O62.2
        during latent phase of labor O62.0
        primary O62.0

Delivery — *continued*
  complicated — *continued*
    by — *continued*
      uterine inertia — *continued*
        secondary O62.1
      vasa previa O69.4 ☑
      velamentous insertion of cord O43.12- ☑
      specified complication NEC O75.89
    delayed NOS O63.9
      following rupture of membranes
        artificial O75.5
      second twin, triplet, etc. O63.2
    forceps, low following failed vacuum extraction O66.5
    missed (at or near term) O36.4 ☑
    normal O80
    obstructed — *see* Delivery, complicated by, obstruc-
      tion
    precipitate O62.3
    preterm (*see also* Pregnancy, complicated by, preterm
      labor) O60.10 ☑
    spontaneous O80
    term pregnancy NOS O80
    uncomplicated O80
    vaginal, following previous cesarean delivery O34.21
Delusions (paranoid) — *see* Disorder, delusional
Dementia (degenerative (primary)) (old age) (persisting)
  F03.90
  with
    aggressive behavior F03.91
    behavioral disturbance F03.91
    combative behavior F03.91
    Lewy bodies G31.83 [F02.80]
      with behavioral disturbance G31.83 [F02.81]
    Parkinsonism G31.83 [F02.80]
      with behavioral disturbance G31.83 [F02.81]
    Parkinson's disease G20 [F02.80]
      with behavioral disturbance G20 [F02.81]
    violent behavior F03.91
  alcoholic F10.97
    with dependence F10.27
  Alzheimer's type — *see* Disease, Alzheimer's
  arteriosclerotic — *see* Dementia, vascular
  atypical, Alzheimer's type — *see* Disease, Alzheimer's,
    specified NEC
  congenital — *see* Disability, intellectual
  frontal (lobe) G31.09 [F02.80]
    with behavioral disturbance G31.09 [F02.81]
  frontotemporal G31.09 [F02.80]
    with behavioral disturbance G31.09 [F02.81]
    specified NEC G31.09 [F02.80]
      with behavioral disturbance G31.09 [F02.81]
  in (due to)
    with behavioral disturbance G31.83 [F02.81]
    alcohol F10.97
      with dependence F10.27
    Alzheimer's disease — *see* Disease, Alzheimer's
    arteriosclerotic brain disease — *see* Dementia,
      vascular
    cerebral lipidoses E75.- ☑ [F02.80]
      with behavioral disturbance E75.- ☑ [F02.81]
    Creutzfeldt-Jakob disease (*see also* Creutzfeldt-
      Jakob disease or syndrome (with dementia))
      A81.00
    epilepsy G40.- ☑ [F02.80]
      with behavioral disturbance G40.- ☑ [F02.81]
    hepatolenticular degeneration E83.01 [F02.80]
      with behavioral disturbance E83.01 [F02.81]
    human immunodeficiency virus (HIV) disease
      B20 [F02.80]
      with behavioral disturbance B20 [F02.81]
    Huntington's disease or chorea G10
    hypercalcemia E83.52 [F02.80]
      with behavioral disturbance E83.52 [F02.81]
    hypothyroidism, acquired E03.9 [F02.80]
      with behavioral disturbance E03.9 [F02.81]
      due to iodine deficiency E01.8 [F02.80]
        with behavioral disturbance E01.8 [F02.81]
    inhalants F18.97
      with dependence F18.27
    multiple
      etiologies F03 ☑
      sclerosis G35 [F02.80]
        with behavioral disturbance G35 [F02.81]
    neurosyphilis A52.17 [F02.80]
      with behavioral disturbance A52.17 [F02.81]
      juvenile A50.49 [F02.80]
        with behavioral disturbance A50.49 [F02.81]

Dementia — continued
in — continued
　niacin deficiency E52 [F02.80]
　　with behavioral disturbance E52 [F02.81]
　paralysis agitans G20 [F02.80]
　　with behavioral disturbance G20 [F02.81]
　Parkinson's disease G20 [F02.80]
　pellagra E52 [F02.80]
　　with behavioral disturbance E52 [F02.81]
　Pick's G31.01 [F02.80]
　　with behavioral disturbance G31.01 [F02.81]
　polyarteritis nodosa M30.0 [F02.80]
　　with behavioral disturbance M30.0 [F02.81]
　psychoactive drug F19.97
　　with dependence F19.27
　　inhalants F18.97
　　　with dependence F18.27
　　sedatives, hypnotics or anxiolytics F13.97
　　　with dependence F13.27
　　sedatives, hypnotics or anxiolytics F13.97
　　　with dependence F13.27
　systemic lupus erythematosus M32.- ☑ [F02.80]
　　with behavioral disturbance M32.- ☑ [F02.81]
　trypanosomiasis
　　African B56.9 [F02.80]
　　　with behavioral disturbance B56.9 [F02.81]
　unknown etiology F03 ☑
　vitamin B12 deficiency E53.8 [F02.80]
　　with behavioral disturbance E53.8 [F02.81]
　volatile solvents F18.97
　　with dependence F18.27
infantile, infantilis F84.3
Lewy body G31.83 [F02.80]
　with behavioral disturbance G31.83 [F02.81]
multi-infarct — see Dementia, vascular
paralytica, paralytic (syphilitic) A52.17 [F02.80]
　with behavioral disturbance A52.17 [F02.81]
　juvenilis A50.45
paretic A52.17
praecox — see Schizophrenia
presenile F03 ☑
　Alzheimer's type — see Disease, Alzheimer's, early
　　onset
primary degenerative F03 ☑
progressive, syphilitic A52.17
senile F03 ☑
　with acute confusional state F05
　Alzheimer's type — see Disease, Alzheimer's, late
　　onset
　depressed or paranoid type F03 ☑
vascular (acute onset) (mixed) (multi-infarct) (subcortical) F01.50
　with behavioral disturbance F01.51
Demineralization, bone — see Osteoporosis
Demodex folliculorum (infestation) B88.0
Demophobia F40.248
Demoralization R45.3
Demyelination, demyelinization
central nervous system G37.9
　specified NEC G37.8
corpus callosum (central) G37.1
disseminated, acute G36.9
　specified NEC G36.8
global G35
in optic neuritis G36.0
Dengue (classical) (fever) A90
hemorrhagic A91
sandfly A93.1
Dennie-Marfan syphilitic syndrome A50.45
Dens evaginatus, in dente or invaginatus K00.2
Dense breasts R92.2
Density
increased, bone (disseminated) (generalized) (spotted)
　— see Disorder, bone, density and structure,
　　specified type NEC
lung (nodular) J98.4
Dental (see also condition)
examination Z01.20
　with abnormal findings Z01.21
restoration
　aesthetically inadequate or displeasing K08.56
　defective K08.50
　　specified NEC K08.59
　failure of marginal integrity K08.51
　failure of periodontal anatomical integrity K08.54
Dentia praecox K00.6
Denticles (pulp) K04.2
Dentigerous cyst K09.0

Dentin
irregular (in pulp) K04.3
opalescent K00.5
secondary (in pulp) K04.3
sensitive K03.89
Dentinogenesis imperfecta K00.5
Dentinoma — see Cyst, calcifying odontogenic
Dentition (syndrome) K00.7
delayed K00.6
difficult K00.7
precocious K00.6
premature K00.6
retarded K00.6
Dependence (on) (syndrome) F19.20
with remission F19.21
alcohol (ethyl) (methyl) (without remission) F10.20
　with
　　amnestic disorder, persisting F10.26
　　anxiety disorder F10.280
　　dementia, persisting F10.27
　　intoxication F10.229
　　　with delirium F10.221
　　　uncomplicated F10.220
　　mood disorder F10.24
　　psychotic disorder F10.259
　　　with
　　　　delusions F10.250
　　　　hallucinations F10.251
　　remission F10.21
　　sexual dysfunction F10.281
　　sleep disorder F10.282
　　specified disorder NEC F10.288
　　withdrawal F10.239
　　　with
　　　　delirium F10.231
　　　　perceptual disturbance F10.232
　　　　uncomplicated F10.230
　counseling and surveillance Z71.41
amobarbital — see Dependence, drug, sedative
amphetamine(s) (type) — see Dependence, drug,
　stimulant NEC
amytal (sodium) — see Dependence, drug, sedative
analgesic NEC F55.8
anesthetic (agent) (gas) (general) (local) NEC — see
　Dependence, drug, psychoactive NEC
anxiolytic NEC — see Dependence, drug, sedative
barbital(s) — see Dependence, drug, sedative
barbiturate(s) (compounds) (drugs classifiable to T42)
　— see Dependence, drug, sedative
benzedrine — see Dependence, drug, stimulant NEC
bhang — see Dependence, drug, cannabis
bromide(s) NEC — see Dependence, drug, sedative
caffeine — see Dependence, drug, stimulant NEC
cannabis (sativa) (indica) (resin) (derivatives) (type) —
　see Dependence, drug, cannabis
chloral (betaine) (hydrate) — see Dependence, drug,
　sedative
chlordiazepoxide — see Dependence, drug, sedative
coca (leaf) (derivatives) — see Dependence, drug, cocaine
cocaine — see Dependence, drug, cocaine
codeine — see Dependence, drug, opioid
combinations of drugs F19.20
dagga — see Dependence, drug, cannabis
demerol — see Dependence, drug, opioid
dexamphetamine — see Dependence, drug, stimulant
　NEC
dexedrine — see Dependence, drug, stimulant NEC
dextromethorphan — see Dependence, drug, opioid
dextromoramide — see Dependence, drug, opioid
dextro-nor-pseudo-ephedrine — see Dependence,
　drug, stimulant NEC
dextrorphan — see Dependence, drug, opioid
diazepam — see Dependence, drug, sedative
dilaudid — see Dependence, drug, opioid
D-lysergic acid diethylamide — see Dependence, drug,
　hallucinogen
drug NEC F19.20
　with sleep disorder F19.282
　cannabis F12.20
　　with
　　　anxiety disorder F12.280
　　　intoxication F12.229
　　　　with
　　　　　delirium F12.221
　　　　　perceptual disturbance F12.222
　　　　uncomplicated F12.220

Dependence — continued
drug — continued
　cannabis — continued
　　with — continued
　　　other specified disorder F12.288
　　　psychosis F12.259
　　　　delusions F12.250
　　　　hallucinations F12.251
　　　unspecified disorder F12.29
　　in remission F12.21
　cocaine F14.20
　　with
　　　anxiety disorder F14.280
　　　intoxication F14.229
　　　　with
　　　　　delirium F14.221
　　　　　perceptual disturbance F14.222
　　　　uncomplicated F14.220
　　　mood disorder F14.24
　　　other specified disorder F14.288
　　　psychosis F14.259
　　　　delusions F14.250
　　　　hallucinations F14.251
　　　sexual dysfunction F14.281
　　　sleep disorder F14.282
　　　unspecified disorder F14.29
　　　withdrawal F14.23
　　in remission F14.21
　　withdrawal symptoms in newborn P96.1
　counseling and surveillance Z71.51
　hallucinogen F16.20
　　with
　　　anxiety disorder F16.280
　　　flashbacks F16.283
　　　intoxication F16.229
　　　　with delirium F16.221
　　　　uncomplicated F16.220
　　　mood disorder F16.24
　　　other specified disorder F16.288
　　　perception disorder, persisting F16.283
　　　psychosis F16.259
　　　　delusions F16.250
　　　　hallucinations F16.251
　　　unspecified disorder F16.29
　　in remission F16.21
　in remission F19.21
　inhalant F18.20
　　with
　　　anxiety disorder F18.280
　　　dementia, persisting F18.27
　　　intoxication F18.229
　　　　with delirium F18.221
　　　　uncomplicated F18.220
　　　mood disorder F18.24
　　　other specified disorder F18.288
　　　psychosis F18.259
　　　　delusions F18.250
　　　　hallucinations F18.251
　　　unspecified disorder F18.29
　　in remission F18.21
　nicotine F17.200
　　with disorder F17.209
　　　remission F17.201
　　　specified disorder NEC F17.208
　　　withdrawal F17.203
　　chewing tobacco F17.220
　　　with disorder F17.229
　　　　remission F17.221
　　　　specified disorder NEC F17.228
　　　　withdrawal F17.223
　　cigarettes F17.210
　　　with disorder F17.219
　　　　remission F17.211
　　　　specified disorder NEC F17.218
　　　　withdrawal F17.213
　　specified product NEC F17.290
　　　with disorder F17.299
　　　　remission F17.291
　　　　specified disorder NEC F17.298
　　　　withdrawal F17.293
　opioid F11.20
　　with
　　　intoxication F11.229
　　　　with
　　　　　delirium F11.221
　　　　　perceptual disturbance F11.222
　　　　uncomplicated F11.220
　　　mood disorder F11.24

☑ **Additional Character Required — Refer to the Tabular List for Character Selection**　　　🔺 **Subterms under main terms may continue to next column or page**

Dependence — continued
 drug — continued
  opioid — continued
   with — continued
    other specified disorder F11.288
    psychosis F11.259
     delusions F11.250
     hallucinations F11.251
    sexual dysfunction F11.281
    sleep disorder F11.282
    unspecified disorder F11.29
    withdrawal F11.23
   in remission F11.21
  psychoactive NEC F19.20
   with
    amnestic disorder F19.26
    anxiety disorder F19.280
    dementia F19.27
    intoxication F19.229
     with
      delirium F19.221
      perceptual disturbance F19.222
     uncomplicated F19.220
    mood disorder F19.24
    other specified disorder F19.288
    psychosis F19.259
     delusions F19.250
     hallucinations F19.251
    sexual dysfunction F19.281
    sleep disorder F19.282
    unspecified disorder F19.29
    withdrawal F19.239
     with
      delirium F19.231
      perceptual disturbance F19.232
     uncomplicated F19.230
  sedative, hypnotic or anxiolytic F13.20
   with
    amnestic disorder F13.26
    anxiety disorder F13.280
    dementia, persisting F13.27
    intoxication F13.229
     with delirium F13.221
     uncomplicated F13.220
    mood disorder F13.24
    other specified disorder F13.288
    psychosis F13.259
     delusions F13.250
     hallucinations F13.251
    sexual dysfunction F13.281
    sleep disorder F13.282
    unspecified disorder F13.29
    withdrawal F13.239
     with
      delirium F13.231
      perceptual disturbance F13.232
     uncomplicated F13.230
   in remission F13.21
  stimulant NEC F15.20
   with
    anxiety disorder F15.280
    intoxication F15.229
     with
      delirium F15.221
      perceptual disturbance F15.222
     uncomplicated F15.220
    mood disorder F15.24
    other specified disorder F15.288
    psychosis F15.259
     delusions F15.250
     hallucinations F15.251
    sexual dysfunction F15.281
    sleep disorder F15.282
    unspecified disorder F15.29
    withdrawal F15.23
   in remission F15.21
 ethyl
  alcohol (without remission) F10.20
   with remission F10.21
  bromide — see Dependence, drug, sedative
  carbamate F19.20
  chloride F19.20
  morphine — see Dependence, drug, opioid
 ganja — see Dependence, drug, cannabis
 glue (airplane) (sniffing) — see Dependence, drug, inhalant
 glutethimide — see Dependence, drug, sedative

Dependence — continued
 hallucinogenics — see Dependence, drug, hallucinogen
 hashish — see Dependence, drug, cannabis
 hemp — see Dependence, drug, cannabis
 heroin (salt) (any) — see Dependence, drug, opioid
 hypnotic NEC — see Dependence, drug, sedative
 Indian hemp — see Dependence, drug, cannabis
 inhalants — see Dependence, drug, inhalant
 khat — see Dependence, drug, stimulant NEC
 laudanum — see Dependence, drug, opioid
 LSD (-25) (derivatives) — see Dependence, drug, hallucinogen
 luminal — see Dependence, drug, sedative
 lysergic acid — see Dependence, drug, hallucinogen
 maconha — see Dependence, drug, cannabis
 marihuana — see Dependence, drug, cannabis
 meprobamate — see Dependence, drug, sedative
 mescaline — see Dependence, drug, hallucinogen
 methadone — see Dependence, drug, opioid
 methamphetamine(s) — see Dependence, drug, stimulant NEC
 methaqualone — see Dependence, drug, sedative
 methyl
  alcohol (without remission) F10.20
   with remission F10.21
  bromide — see Dependence, drug, sedative
  morphine — see Dependence, drug, opioid
  phenidate — see Dependence, drug, stimulant NEC
  sulfonal — see Dependence, drug, sedative
 morphine (sulfate) (sulfite) (type) — see Dependence, drug, opioid
 narcotic (drug) NEC — see Dependence, drug, opioid
 nembutal — see Dependence, drug, sedative
 neraval — see Dependence, drug, sedative
 neravan — see Dependence, drug, sedative
 neurobarb — see Dependence, drug, sedative
 nicotine — see Dependence, drug, nicotine
 nitrous oxide F19.20
 nonbarbiturate sedatives and tranquilizers with similar effect — see Dependence, drug, sedative
 on
  artificial heart (fully implantable) (mechanical) Z95.812
  aspirator Z99.0
  care provider (because of) Z74.9
   impaired mobility Z74.09
   need for
    assistance with personal care Z74.1
    continuous supervision Z74.3
   no other household member able to render care Z74.2
   specified reason NEC Z74.8
  machine Z99.89
   enabling NEC Z99.89
   specified type NEC Z99.89
  renal dialysis (hemodialysis) (peritoneal) Z99.2
  respirator Z99.11
  ventilator Z99.11
  wheelchair Z99.3
 opiate — see Dependence, drug, opioid
 opioids — see Dependence, drug, opioid
 opium (alkaloids) (derivatives) (tincture) — see Dependence, drug, opioid
 oxygen (long-term) (supplemental) Z99.81
 paraldehyde — see Dependence, drug, sedative
 paregoric — see Dependence, drug, opioid
 PCP (phencyclidine) (see also Abuse, drug, hallucinogen) F16.20
 pentobarbital — see Dependence, drug, sedative
 pentobarbitone (sodium) — see Dependence, drug, sedative
 pentothal — see Dependence, drug, sedative
 peyote — see Dependence, drug, hallucinogen
 phencyclidine (PCP) (and related substances) (see also Abuse, drug, hallucinogen) F16.20
 phenmetrazine — see Dependence, drug, stimulant NEC
 phenobarbital — see Dependence, drug, sedative
 polysubstance F19.20
 psilocibin, psilocin, psilocyn, psilocyline — see Dependence, drug, hallucinogen
 psychostimulant NEC — see Dependence, drug, stimulant NEC
 secobarbital — see Dependence, drug, sedative
 seconal — see Dependence, drug, sedative

Dependence — continued
 sedative NEC — see Dependence, drug, sedative
 specified drug NEC — see Dependence, drug
 stimulant NEC — see Dependence, drug, stimulant NEC
 substance NEC — see Dependence, drug
 supplemental oxygen Z99.81
 tobacco — see Dependence, drug, nicotine
  counseling and surveillance Z71.6
 tranquilizer NEC — see Dependence, drug, sedative
 vitamin B6 E53.1
 volatile solvents — see Dependence, drug, inhalant
Dependency
 care-provider Z74.9
 passive F60.7
 reactions (persistent) F60.7
Depersonalization (in neurotic state) (neurotic) (syndrome) F48.1
Depletion
 extracellular fluid E86.9
 plasma E86.1
 potassium E87.6
  nephropathy N25.89
 salt or sodium E87.1
  causing heat exhaustion or prostration T67.4 ☑
  nephropathy N28.9
 volume NOS E86.9
Deployment (current) (military) status Z56.82
 in theater or in support of military war, peacekeeping and humanitarian operations Z56.82
 personal history of Z91.82
  military war, peacekeeping and humanitarian deployment (current or past conflict) Z91.82
 returned from Z91.82
Depolarization, premature I49.40
 atrial I49.1
 junctional I49.2
 specified NEC I49.49
 ventricular I49.3
Deposit
 bone in Boeck's sarcoid D86.89
 calcareous, calcium — see Calcification
 cholesterol
  retina H35.89
  vitreous (body) (humor) — see Deposit, crystalline
 conjunctiva H11.11- ☑
 cornea H18.00- ☑
  argentous H18.02- ☑
  due to metabolic disorder H18.03- ☑
  Kayser-Fleischer ring H18.04- ☑
  pigmentation — see Pigmentation, cornea
 crystalline, vitreous (body) (humor) H43.2- ☑
 hemosiderin in old scars of cornea — see Pigmentation, cornea, stromal
 metallic in lens — see Cataract, specified NEC
 skin R23.8
 tooth, teeth (betel) (black) (green) (materia alba) (orange) (tobacco) K03.6
 urate, kidney — see Calculus, kidney
Depraved appetite — see Pica
Depressed
 HDL cholesterol E78.6
Depression (acute) (mental) F32.9
 agitated (single episode) F32.2
 anaclitic — see Disorder, adjustment
 anxiety F41.8
  persistent F34.1
 arches (see also Deformity, limb, flat foot)
 atypical (single episode) F32.8
 basal metabolic rate R94.8
 bone marrow D75.89
 central nervous system R09.2
 cerebral R29.818
  newborn P91.4
 cerebrovascular I67.9
 chest wall M95.4
 climacteric (single episode) F32.8
 endogenous (without psychotic symptoms) F33.2
  with psychotic symptoms F33.3
 functional activity R68.89
 hysterical F44.89
 involutional (single episode) F32.8
 major F32.9
  with psychotic symptoms F32.3
  recurrent — see Disorder, depressive, recurrent
 manic-depressive — see Disorder, depressive, recurrent

Depression — *continued*
  masked (single episode) F32.8
  medullary G93.89
  menopausal (single episode) F32.8
  metatarsus — *see* Depression, arches
  monopolar F33.9
  nervous F34.1
  neurotic F34.1
  nose M95.0
  postnatal F53
  postpartum F53
  post-psychotic of schizophrenia F32.8
  post-schizophrenic F32.8
  psychogenic (reactive) (single episode) F32.9
  psychoneurotic F34.1
  psychotic (single episode) F32.3
    recurrent F33.3
  reactive (psychogenic) (single episode) F32.9
    psychotic (single episode) F32.3
  recurrent — *see* Disorder, depressive, recurrent
  respiratory center G93.89
  seasonal — *see* Disorder, depressive, recurrent
  senile F03 ☑
  severe, single episode F32.2
  situational F43.21
  skull Q67.4
  specified NEC (single episode) F32.8
  sternum M95.4
  visual field — *see* Defect, visual field
  vital (recurrent) (without psychotic symptoms) F33.2
    with psychotic symptoms F33.3
    single episode F32.2
Deprivation
  cultural Z60.3
  effects NOS T73.9 ☑
    specified NEC T73.8 ☑
  emotional NEC Z65.8
    affecting infant or child — *see* Maltreatment, child, psychological
  food T73.0 ☑
  protein — *see* Malnutrition
  sleep Z72.820
  social Z60.4
    affecting infant or child — *see* Maltreatment, child, psychological
  specified NEC T73.8 ☑
  vitamins — *see* Deficiency, vitamin
  water T73.1 ☑
Derangement
  ankle (internal) — *see* Derangement, joint, ankle
  cartilage (articular) NEC — *see* Derangement, joint, articular cartilage, by site
    recurrent — *see* Dislocation, recurrent
  cruciate ligament, anterior, current injury — *see* Sprain, knee, cruciate, anterior
  elbow (internal) — *see* Derangement, joint, elbow
  hip (joint) (internal) (old) — *see* Derangement, joint, hip
  joint (internal) M24.9
    ankylosis — *see* Ankylosis
    articular cartilage M24.10
      ankle M24.17- ☑
      elbow M24.12- ☑
      foot M24.17- ☑
      hand M24.14- ☑
      hip M24.15- ☑
      knee NEC M23.9- ☑
      loose body — *see* Loose, body
      shoulder M24.11- ☑
      wrist M24.13- ☑
    contracture — *see* Contraction, joint
    current injury (*see also* Dislocation)
      knee, meniscus or cartilage — *see* Tear, meniscus
    dislocation
      pathological — *see* Dislocation, pathological
      recurrent — *see* Dislocation, recurrent
    knee — *see* Derangement, knee
    ligament — *see* Disorder, ligament
    loose body — *see* Loose, body
    recurrent — *see* Dislocation, recurrent
    specified type NEC M24.80
      ankle M24.87- ☑
      elbow M24.82- ☑
      foot joint M24.87- ☑
      hand joint M24.84- ☑
      hip M24.85- ☑

Derangement — *continued*
  joint — *continued*
    specified type — *continued*
      shoulder M24.81- ☑
      wrist M24.83- ☑
    temporomandibular M26.69
  knee (recurrent) M23.9- ☑
    ligament disruption, spontaneous M23.60- ☑
      anterior cruciate M23.61- ☑
      capsular M23.67- ☑
      instability, chronic M23.5- ☑
      lateral collateral M23.64- ☑
      medial collateral M23.63- ☑
      posterior cruciate M23.62- ☑
    loose body M23.4- ☑
    meniscus M23.30- ☑
      cystic M23.00- ☑
        lateral M23.002
          anterior horn M23.04- ☑
          posterior horn M23.05- ☑
          specified NEC M23.06- ☑
        medial M23.005
          anterior horn M23.01- ☑
          posterior horn M23.02- ☑
          specified NEC M23.03- ☑
      degenerate — *see* Derangement, knee, meniscus, specified NEC
      detached — *see* Derangement, knee, meniscus, specified NEC
      due to old tear or injury M23.20- ☑
        lateral M23.20- ☑
          anterior horn M23.24- ☑
          posterior horn M23.25- ☑
          specified NEC M23.26- ☑
        medial M23.20- ☑
          anterior horn M23.21- ☑
          posterior horn M23.22- ☑
          specified NEC M23.23- ☑
      retained — *see* Derangement, knee, meniscus, specified NEC
      specified NEC M23.30- ☑
        lateral M23.30- ☑
          anterior horn M23.34- ☑
          posterior horn M23.35- ☑
          specified NEC M23.36- ☑
        medial M23.30- ☑
          anterior horn M23.31- ☑
          posterior horn M23.32- ☑
          specified NEC M23.33- ☑
      old M23.8X- ☑
      specified NEC — *see* subcategory M23.8 ☑
  low back NEC — *see* Dorsopathy, specified NEC
  meniscus — *see* Derangement, knee, meniscus
  mental — *see* Psychosis
  patella, specified NEC — *see* Disorder, patella, derangement NEC
  semilunar cartilage (knee) — *see* Derangement, knee, meniscus, specified NEC
  shoulder (internal) — *see* Derangement, joint, shoulder
Dercum's disease E88.2
Derealization (neurotic) F48.1
Dermal — *see* condition
Dermaphytid — *see* Dermatophytosis
Dermatitis (eczematous) L30.9
  ab igne L59.0
  acarine B88.0
  actinic (due to sun) L57.8
    other than from sun L59.8
  allergic — *see* Dermatitis, contact, allergic
  ambustionis, due to burn or scald — *see* Burn
  amebic A06.7
  ammonia L22
  arsenical (ingested) L27.8
  artefacta L98.1
    psychogenic F54
  atopic L20.9
    psychogenic F54
    specified NEC L20.89
  autoimmune progesterone L30.8
  berlock, berloque L56.2
  blastomycotic B40.3
  blister beetle L24.89
  bullous, bullosa L13.9
    mucosynechial, atrophic L12.1
    seasonal L30.8

Dermatitis — *continued*
  bullous, bullosa — *continued*
    specified NEC L13.8
  calorica L59.0
    due to burn or scald — *see* Burn
  caterpillar L24.89
  cercarial B65.3
  combustionis L59.0
    due to burn or scald — *see* Burn
  congelationis T69.1 ☑
  contact (occupational) L25.9
    allergic L23.9
      due to
        adhesives L23.1
        cement L23.5
        chemical products NEC L23.5
        chromium L23.0
        cosmetics L23.2
        dander (cat) (dog) L23.81
        drugs in contact with skin L23.3
        dyes L23.4
        food in contact with skin L23.6
        hair (cat) (dog) L23.81
        insecticide L23.5
        metals L23.0
        nickel L23.0
        plants, non-food L23.7
        plastic L23.5
        rubber L23.5
        specified agent NEC L23.89
    due to
      cement L25.3
      chemical products NEC L25.3
      cosmetics L25.0
      dander (cat) (dog) L23.81
      drugs in contact with skin L25.1
      dyes L25.2
      food in contact with skin L25.4
      hair (cat) (dog) L23.81
      plants, non-food L25.5
      specified agent NEC L25.8
    irritant L24.9
      due to
        cement L25.3
        chemical products NEC L24.5
        cosmetics L24.3
        detergents L24.0
        drugs in contact with skin L24.4
        food in contact with skin L24.6
        oils and greases L24.1
        plants, non-food L24.7
        solvents L24.2
        specified agent NEC L24.89
  contusiformis L52
  diabetic — *see* E08-E13 with .620
  diaper L22
  diphtheritica A36.3
  dry skin L85.3
  due to
    acetone (contact) (irritant) L24.2
    acids (contact) (irritant) L24.5
    adhesive(s) (allergic) (contact) (plaster) L23.1
      irritant L24.5
    alcohol (irritant) (skin contact) (substances in category T51) L24.2
      taken internally L27.8
    alkalis (contact) (irritant) L24.5
    arsenic (ingested) L27.8
    carbon disulfide (contact) (irritant) L24.2
    caustics (contact) (irritant) L24.5
    cement (contact) L25.3
    cereal (ingested) L27.2
    chemical(s) NEC L25.3
      taken internally L27.8
    chlorocompounds L24.2
    chromium (contact) (irritant) L24.81
    coffee (ingested) L27.2
    cold weather L30.8
    cosmetics (contact) L25.0
      allergic L23.2
      irritant L24.3
    cyclohexanes L24.2
    dander (cat) (dog) L23.81
    Demodex species B88.0
    Dermanyssus gallinae B88.0
    detergents (contact) (irritant) L24.0
    dichromate L24.81

☑ **Additional Character Required — Refer to the Tabular List for Character Selection**   ꟷ **Subterms under main terms may continue to next column or page**

Dermatitis — continued
  due to — continued
    drugs and medicaments (generalized) (internal use) L27.0
      external — see Dermatitis, due to, drugs, in contact with skin
      in contact with skin L25.1
        allergic L23.3
        irritant L24.4
      localized skin eruption L27.1
      specified substance — see Table of Drugs and Chemicals
    dyes (contact) L25.2
      allergic L23.4
      irritant L24.89
    epidermophytosis — see Dermatophytosis
    esters L24.2
    external irritant NEC L24.9
    fish (ingested) L27.2
    flour (ingested) L27.2
    food (ingested) L27.2
      in contact with skin L25.4
    fruit (ingested) L27.2
    furs (allergic) (contact) L23.81
    glues — see Dermatitis, due to, adhesives
    glycols L24.2
    greases NEC (contact) (irritant) L24.1
    hair (cat) (dog) L23.81
    hot
      objects and materials — see Burn
      weather or places L59.0
    hydrocarbons L24.2
    infrared rays L59.8
    ingestion, ingested substance L27.9
      chemical NEC L27.8
      drugs and medicaments — see Dermatitis, due to, drugs
      food L27.2
      specified NEC L27.8
    insecticide in contact with skin L24.5
    internal agent L27.9
      drugs and medicaments (generalized) — see Dermatitis, due to, drugs
      food L27.2
    irradiation — see Dermatitis, due to, radioactive substance
    ketones L24.2
    lacquer tree (allergic) (contact) L23.7
    light (sun) NEC L57.8
      acute L56.8
      other L59.8
    Liponyssoides sanguineus B88.0
    low temperature L30.8
    meat (ingested) L27.2
    metals, metal salts (contact) (irritant) L24.81
    milk (ingested) L27.2
    nickel (contact) (irritant) L24.81
    nylon (contact) (irritant) L24.5
    oils NEC (contact) (irritant) L24.1
    paint solvent (contact) (irritant) L24.2
    petroleum products (contact) (irritant) (substances in T52.0) L24.2
    plants NEC (contact) L25.5
      allergic L23.7
      irritant L24.7
    plasters (adhesive) (any) (allergic) (contact) L23.1
      irritant L24.5
    plastic (contact) L25.3
    preservatives (contact) — see Dermatitis, due to, chemical, in contact with skin
    primrose (allergic) (contact) L23.7
    primula (allergic) (contact) L23.7
    radiation L59.8
      nonionizing (chronic exposure) L57.8
      sun NEC L57.8
        acute L56.8
    radioactive substance L58.9
      acute L58.0
      chronic L58.1
    radium L58.9
      acute L58.0
      chronic L58.1
    ragweed (allergic) (contact) L23.7
    Rhus (allergic) (contact) (diversiloba) (radicans) (toxicodendron) (venenata) (verniciflua) L23.7
    rubber (contact) L24.5
    Senecio jacobaea (allergic) (contact) L23.7

Dermatitis — continued
  due to — continued
    solvents (contact) (irritant) (substances in category T52) L24.2
    specified agent NEC (contact) L25.8
      allergic L23.89
      irritant L24.89
    sunshine NEC L57.8
      acute L56.8
    tetrachlorethylene (contact) (irritant) L24.2
    toluene (contact) (irritant) L24.2
    turpentine (contact) L24.2
    ultraviolet rays (sun NEC) (chronic exposure) L57.8
      acute L56.8
    vaccine or vaccination L27.0
      specified substance — see Table of Drugs and Chemicals
    varicose veins — see Varix, leg, with, inflammation
    X-rays L58.9
      acute L58.0
      chronic L58.1
  dyshydrotic L30.1
  dysmenorrheica N94.6
  escharotica — see Burn
  exfoliative, exfoliativa (generalized) L26
    neonatorum L00
  eyelid (see also Dermatosis, eyelid)
    allergic H01.119
      left H01.116
        lower H01.115
        upper H01.114
      right H01.113
        lower H01.112
        upper H01.111
    contact — see Dermatitis, eyelid, allergic
    due to
      Demodex species B88.0
      herpes (zoster) B02.39
        simplex B00.59
    eczematous H01.139
      left H01.136
        lower H01.135
        upper H01.134
      right H01.133
        lower H01.132
        upper H01.131
  facta, factitia, factitial L98.1
    psychogenic F54
  flexural NEC L20.82
  friction L30.4
  fungus B36.9
    specified type NEC B36.8
  gangrenosa, gangrenous infantum L08.0
  harvest mite B88.0
  heat L59.0
  herpesviral, vesicular (ear) (lip) B00.1
  herpetiformis (bullous) (erythematous) (pustular) (vesicular) L13.0
    juvenile L12.2
    senile L12.0
  hiemalis L30.8
  hypostatic, hypostatica — see Varix, leg, with, inflammation
  infectious eczematoid L30.3
  infective L30.3
  irritant — see Dermatitis, contact, irritant
  Jacquet's (diaper dermatitis) L22
  Leptus B88.0
  lichenified NEC L28.0
  medicamentosa (generalized) (internal use) — see Dermatitis, due to drugs
  mite B88.0
  multiformis L13.0
    juvenile L12.2
  napkin L22
  neurotica L13.0
  nummular L30.0
  papillaris capillitii L73.0
  pellagrous E52
  perioral L71.0
  photocontact L56.2
  polymorpha dolorosa L13.0
  pruriginosa L13.0
  pruritic NEC L30.8
  psychogenic F54
  purulent L08.0
  pustular
    contagious B08.02

Dermatitis — continued
  pustular — continued
    subcorneal L13.1
  pyococcal L08.0
  pyogenica L08.0
  repens L40.2
  Ritter's (exfoliativa) L00
  Schamberg's L81.7
  schistosome B65.3
  seasonal bullous L30.8
  seborrheic L21.9
    infantile L21.1
    specified NEC L21.8
  sensitization NOS L23.9
  septic L08.0
  solare L57.8
  specified NEC L30.8
  stasis I87.2
    with varicose ulcer — see Varix, leg, with ulcer, with inflammation
    due to postthrombotic syndrome — see Syndrome, postthrombotic
  suppurative L08.0
  traumatic NEC L30.4
  trophoneurotica L13.0
  ultraviolet (sun) (chronic exposure) L57.8
    acute L56.8
  varicose — see Varix, leg, with, inflammation
  vegetans L10.1
  verrucosa B43.0
  vesicular, herpesviral B00.1
Dermatoarthritis, lipoid E78.81
Dermatochalasis, eyelid H02.839
  left H02.836
    lower H02.835
    upper H02.834
  right H02.833
    lower H02.832
    upper H02.831
Dermatofibroma (lenticulare) — see Neoplasm, skin, benign
  protuberans — see Neoplasm, skin, uncertain behavior
Dermatofibrosarcoma (pigmented) (protuberans) — see Neoplasm, skin, malignant
Dermatographia L50.3
Dermatolysis (exfoliativa) (congenital) Q82.8
  acquired L57.4
  eyelids — see Blepharochalasis
  palpebrarum — see Blepharochalasis
  senile L57.4
Dermatomegaly NEC Q82.8
Dermatomucosomyositis M33.10
  with
    myopathy M33.12
    respiratory involvement M33.11
    specified organ involvement NEC M33.19
Dermatomycosis B36.9
  furfuracea B36.0
  specified type NEC B36.8
Dermatomyositis (acute) (chronic) (see also Dermatopolymyositis)
  in (due to) neoplastic disease (see also Neoplasm) D49.9 [M36.0]
Dermatoneuritis of children — see Poisoning, mercury
Dermatophilosis A48.8
Dermatophytid L30.2
Dermatophytide — see Dermatophytosis
Dermatophytosis (epidermophyton) (infection) (Microsporum) (tinea) (Trichophyton) B35.9
  beard B35.0
  body B35.4
  capitis B35.0
  corporis B35.4
  deep-seated B35.8
  disseminated B35.8
  foot B35.3
  granulomatous B35.8
  groin B35.6
  hand B35.2
  nail B35.1
  perianal (area) B35.6
  scalp B35.0
  specified NEC B35.8
Dermatopolymyositis M33.90
  with
    myopathy M33.92
    respiratory involvement M33.91
    specified organ involvement NEC M33.99

Dermatopolymyositis — *continued*
 in neoplastic disease (*see also* Neoplasm)
  D49.9 [M36.0]
 juvenile M33.00
  with
   myopathy M33.02
   respiratory involvement M33.01
   specified organ involvement NEC M33.09
 specified NEC M33.10
  myopathy M33.12
  respiratory involvement M33.11
  specified organ involvement NEC M33.19
Dermatopolyneuritis — *see* Poisoning, mercury
Dermatorrhexis Q79.6
 acquired L57.4
Dermatosclerosis (*see also* Scleroderma)
 localized L94.0
Dermatosis L98.9
 Andrews' L08.89
 Bowen's — *see* Neoplasm, skin, in situ
 bullous L13.9
  specified NEC L13.8
 exfoliativa L26
 eyelid (noninfectious)
  dermatitis — *see* Dermatitis, eyelid
  discoid lupus erythematosus — *see* Lupus, erythematosus, eyelid
  xeroderma — *see* Xeroderma, acquired, eyelid
 factitial L98.1
 febrile neutrophilic L98.2
 gonococcal A54.89
 herpetiformis L13.0
  juvenile L12.2
 linear IgA L13.8
 menstrual NEC L98.8
 neutrophilic, febrile L98.2
 occupational — *see* Dermatitis, contact
 papulosa nigra L82.1
 pigmentary L81.9
  progressive L81.7
  Schamberg's L81.7
 psychogenic F54
 purpuric, pigmented L81.7
 pustular, subcorneal L13.1
 transient acantholytic L11.1
Dermographia, dermographism L50.3
Dermoid (cyst) (*see also* Neoplasm, benign, by site)
 with malignant transformation C56- ☑
 due to radiation (nonionizing) L57.8
Dermopathy
 infiltrative with thyrotoxicosis — *see* Thyrotoxicosis
 nephrogenic fibrosing L90.8
Dermophytosis — *see* Dermatophytosis
Descemetocele H18.73- ☑
Descemet's membrane — *see* condition
Descending — *see* condition
Descensus uteri — *see* Prolapse, uterus
Desert
 rheumatism B38.0
 sore — *see* Ulcer, skin
Desertion (newborn) — *see* Maltreatment
Desmoid (extra-abdominal) (tumor) — *see* Neoplasm,
 connective tissue, uncertain behavior
 abdominal D48.1
Despondency F32.9
Desquamation, skin R23.4
Destruction, destructive (*see also* Damage)
 articular facet (*see also* Derangement, joint, specified
  type NEC)
  knee M23.8X- ☑
  vertebra — *see* Spondylosis
 bone (*see also* Disorder, bone, specified type NEC)
  syphilitic A52.77
 joint (*see also* Derangement, joint, specified type NEC)
  sacroiliac M53.3
 rectal sphincter K62.89
 septum (nasal) J34.89
 tuberculous NEC — *see* Tuberculosis
 tympanum, tympanic membrane (nontraumatic) —
  see Disorder, tympanic membrane, specified
  NEC
 vertebral disc — *see* Degeneration, intervertebral disc
Destructiveness (*see also* Disorder, conduct)
 adjustment reaction — *see* Disorder, adjustment
Desultory labor O62.2
Detachment
 cartilage — *see* Sprain

Detachment — *continued*
 cervix, annular N88.8
  complicating delivery O71.3
 choroid (old) (postinfectional) (simple) (spontaneous)
  H31.40- ☑
  hemorrhagic H31.41- ☑
  serous H31.42- ☑
 ligament — *see* Sprain
 meniscus (knee) (*see also* Derangement, knee, meniscus, specified NEC)
  current injury — *see* Tear, meniscus
  due to old tear or injury — *see* Derangement, knee,
   meniscus, due to old tear
 retina (without retinal break) (serous) H33.2- ☑
  with retinal:
   break H33.00- ☑
    giant H33.03- ☑
    multiple H33.02- ☑
    single H33.01- ☑
   dialysis H33.04- ☑
  pigment epithelium — *see* Degeneration, retina,
   separation of layers, pigment epithelium
   detachment
  rhegmatogenous — *see* Detachment, retina, with
   retinal, break
  specified NEC H33.8
  total H33.05- ☑
  traction H33.4- ☑
 vitreous (body) H43.81 ☑
Detergent asthma J69.8
Deterioration
 epileptic F06.8
 general physical R53.81
 heart, cardiac — *see* Degeneration, myocardial
 mental — *see* Psychosis
 myocardial, myocardium — *see* Degeneration, myocardial
 senile (simple) R54
Deuteranomaly (anomalous trichromat) H53.53
Deuteranopia (complete) (incomplete) H53.53
Development
 abnormal, bone Q79.9
 arrested R62.50
  bone — *see* Arrest, development or growth, bone
  child R62.50
  due to malnutrition E45
 defective, congenital (*see also* Anomaly, by site)
  cauda equina Q06.3
  left ventricle Q24.8
   in hypoplastic left heart syndrome Q23.4
  valve Q24.8
   pulmonary Q22.3
 delayed (*see also* Delay, development) R62.50
  arithmetical skills F81.2
  language (skills) (expressive) F80.1
  learning skill F81.9
  mixed skills F88
  motor coordination F82
  reading F81.0
  specified learning skill NEC F81.89
  speech F80.9
  spelling F81.81
  written expression F81.81
 imperfect, congenital (*see also* Anomaly, by site)
  heart Q24.9
  lungs Q33.6
 incomplete
  bronchial tree Q32.4
  organ or site not listed — *see* Hypoplasia, by site
  respiratory system Q34.9
 sexual, precocious NEC E30.1
 tardy, mental (*see also* Disability, intellectual) F79
Developmental — *see* condition
 testing, child — *see* Examination, child
Devergie's disease (pityriasis rubra pilaris) L44.0
Deviation (in)
 conjugate palsy (eye) (spastic) H51.0
 esophagus (acquired) K22.8
 eye, skew H51.8
 midline (jaw) (teeth) (dental arch) M26.29
  specified site NEC — *see* Malposition
 nasal septum J34.2
  congenital Q67.4
 opening and closing of the mandible M26.53
 organ or site, congenital NEC — *see* Malposition,
  congenital
 septum

Deviation — *continued*
 septum (nasal) (acquired) J34.2
  congenital Q67.4
 sexual F65.9
  bestiality F65.89
  erotomania F52.8
  exhibitionism F65.2
  fetishism, fetishistic F65.0
   transvestism F65.1
  frotteurism F65.81
  masochism F65.51
  multiple F65.89
  necrophilia F65.89
  nymphomania F52.8
  pederosis F65.4
  pedophilia F65.4
  sadism, sadomasochism F65.52
  satyriasis F52.8
  specified type NEC F65.89
  transvestism F64.1
  voyeurism F65.3
 teeth, midline M26.29
 trachea J39.8
 ureter, congenital Q62.61
Device
 cerebral ventricle (communicating) in situ Z98.2
 contraceptive — *see* Contraceptive, device
 drainage, cerebrospinal fluid, in situ Z98.2
Devic's disease G36.0
Devil's
 grip B33.0
 pinches (purpura simplex) D69.2
Devitalized tooth K04.99
Devonshire colic — *see* Poisoning, lead
Dextraposition, aorta Q20.3
 in tetralogy of Fallot Q21.3
Dextrinosis, limit (debrancher enzyme deficiency)
 E74.03
Dextrocardia (true) Q24.0
 with
  complete transposition of viscera Q89.3
  situs inversus Q89.3
Dextrotransposition, aorta Q20.3
d-glycericacidemia E72.59
Dhat syndrome F48.8
Dhobi itch B35.6
Di George's syndrome D82.1
Di Guglielmo's disease C94.0- ☑
Diabetes, diabetic (mellitus) (sugar) E11.9
 with
  amyotrophy E11.44
  arthropathy NEC E11.618
  autonomic (poly)neuropathy E11.43
  cataract E11.36
  Charcot's joints E11.610
  chronic kidney disease E11.22
  circulatory complication NEC E11.59
  complication E11.8
   specified NEC E11.69
  dermatitis E11.620
  foot ulcer E11.621
  gangrene E11.52
  gastroparesis E11.43
  glomerulonephrosis, intracapillary E11.21
  glomerulosclerosis, intercapillary E11.21
  hyperglycemia E11.65
  hyperosmolarity E11.00
   with coma E11.01
  hypoglycemia E11.649
   with coma E11.641
  kidney complications NEC E11.29
  Kimmelstiel-Wilson disease E11.21
  loss of protective sensation (LOPS) — *see* Diabetes,
   by type, with neuropathy
  mononeuropathy E11.41
  myasthenia E11.44
  necrobiosis lipoidica E11.620
  nephropathy E11.21
  neuralgia E11.42
  neurologic complication NEC E11.49
  neuropathic arthropathy E11.610
  neuropathy E11.40
  ophthalmic complication NEC E11.39
  oral complication NEC E11.638
  periodontal disease E11.630
  peripheral angiopathy E11.51
   with gangrene E11.52
  polyneuropathy E11.42

☑ **Additional Character Required — Refer to the Tabular List for Character Selection**
  Subterms under main terms may continue to next column or page

Diabetes, diabetic — *continued*
  with — *continued*
    renal complication NEC E11.29
    renal tubular degeneration E11.29
    retinopathy E11.319
      with macular edema E11.311
      nonproliferative E11.329
        with macular edema E11.321
        mild E11.329
          with macular edema E11.321
        moderate E11.339
          with macular edema E11.331
        severe E11.349
          with macular edema E11.341
      proliferative E11.359
        with macular edema E11.351
    skin complication NEC E11.628
    skin ulcer NEC E11.622
  bronzed E83.110
  complicating pregnancy — *see* Pregnancy, complicated by, diabetes
  dietary counseling and surveillance Z71.3
  due to drug or chemical E09.9
    with
      amyotrophy E09.44
      arthropathy NEC E09.618
      autonomic (poly)neuropathy E09.43
      cataract E09.36
      Charcot's joints E09.610
      chronic kidney disease E09.22
      circulatory complication NEC E09.59
      complication E09.8
        specified NEC E09.69
      dermatitis E09.620
      foot ulcer E09.621
      gangrene E09.52
      gastroparesis E09.43
      glomerulonephrosis, intracapillary E09.21
      glomerulosclerosis, intercapillary E09.21
      hyperglycemia E09.65
      hyperosmolarity E09.00
        with coma E09.01
      hypoglycemia E09.649
        with coma E09.641
      ketoacidosis E09.10
        with coma E09.11
      kidney complications NEC E09.29
      Kimmelstein-Wilson disease E09.21
      mononeuropathy E09.41
      myasthenia E09.44
      necrobiosis lipoidica E09.620
      nephropathy E09.21
      neuralgia E09.42
      neurologic complication NEC E09.49
      neuropathic arthropathy E09.610
      neuropathy E09.40
      ophthalmic complication NEC E09.39
      oral complication NEC E09.638
      periodontal disease E09.630
      peripheral angiopathy E09.51
        with gangrene E09.52
      polyneuropathy E09.42
      renal complication NEC E09.29
      renal tubular degeneration E09.29
      retinopathy E09.319
        with macular edema E09.311
        nonproliferative E09.329
          with macular edema E09.321
          mild E09.329
            with macular edema E09.321
          moderate E09.339
            with macular edema E09.331
          severe E09.349
            with macular edema E09.341
        proliferative E09.359
          with macular edema E09.351
      skin complication NEC E09.628
      skin ulcer NEC E09.622
  due to underlying condition E08.9
    with
      amyotrophy E08.44
      arthropathy NEC E08.618
      autonomic (poly)neuropathy E08.43
      cataract E08.36
      Charcot's joints E08.610
      chronic kidney disease E08.22
      circulatory complication NEC E08.59

Diabetes, diabetic — *continued*
  due to underlying condition — *continued*
    with — *continued*
      complication E08.8
        specified NEC E08.69
      dermatitis E08.620
      foot ulcer E08.621
      gangrene E08.52
      gastroparesis E08.43
      glomerulonephrosis, intracapillary E08.21
      glomerulosclerosis, intercapillary E08.21
      hyperglycemia E08.65
      hyperosmolarity E08.00
        with coma E08.01
      hypoglycemia E08.649
        with coma E08.641
      ketoacidosis E08.10
        with coma E08.11
      kidney complications NEC E08.29
      Kimmelstein-Wilson disease E08.21
      mononeuropathy E08.41
      myasthenia E08.44
      necrobiosis lipoidica E08.620
      nephropathy E08.21
      neuralgia E08.42
      neurologic complication NEC E08.49
      neuropathic arthropathy E08.610
      neuropathy E08.40
      ophthalmic complication NEC E08.39
      oral complication NEC E08.638
      periodontal disease E08.630
      peripheral angiopathy E08.51
        with gangrene E08.52
      polyneuropathy E08.42
      renal complication NEC E08.29
      renal tubular degeneration E08.29
      retinopathy E08.319
        with macular edema E08.311
        nonproliferative E08.329
          with macular edema E08.321
          mild E08.329
            with macular edema E08.321
          moderate E08.339
            with macular edema E08.331
          severe E08.349
            with macular edema E08.341
        proliferative E08.359
          with macular edema E08.351
      skin complication NEC E08.628
      skin ulcer NEC E08.622
  gestational (in pregnancy) O24.419
    affecting newborn P70.0
    diet controlled O24.410
    in childbirth O24.429
      diet controlled O24.420
      insulin (and diet) controlled O24.424
    insulin (and diet) controlled O24.414
    puerperal O24.439
      diet controlled O24.430
      insulin (and diet) controlled O24.434
  hepatogenous E13.9
  inadequately controlled — *code to* Diabetes, by type, with hyperglycemia
  insipidus E23.2
    nephrogenic N25.1
    pituitary E23.2
    vasopressin resistant N25.1
  insulin dependent — *code to* type of diabetes
  juvenile-onset — *see* Diabetes, type 1
  ketosis-prone — *see* Diabetes, type 1
  latent R73.09
  neonatal (transient) P70.2
  non-insulin dependent — *code to* type of diabetes
  out of control — *code to* Diabetes, by type, with hyperglycemia
  phosphate E83.39
  poorly controlled — *code to* Diabetes, by type, with hyperglycemia
  postpancreatectomy — *see* Diabetes, specified type NEC
  postprocedural — *see* Diabetes, specified type NEC
  secondary diabetes mellitus NEC — *see* Diabetes, specified type NEC
  specified type NEC E13.9
    with
      amyotrophy E13.44
      arthropathy NEC E13.618
      autonomic (poly)neuropathy E13.43

Diabetes, diabetic — *continued*
  specified type — *continued*
    with — *continued*
      cataract E13.36
      Charcot's joints E13.610
      chronic kidney disease E13.22
      circulatory complication NEC E13.59
      complication E13.8
        specified NEC E13.69
      dermatitis E13.620
      foot ulcer E13.621
      gangrene E13.52
      gastroparesis E13.43
      glomerulonephrosis, intracapillary E13.21
      glomerulosclerosis, intercapillary E13.21
      hyperglycemia E13.65
      hyperosmolarity E13.00
        with coma E13.01
      hypoglycemia E13.649
        with coma E13.641
      ketoacidosis E13.10
        with coma E13.11
      kidney complications NEC E13.29
      Kimmelstein-Wilson disease E13.21
      mononeuropathy E13.41
      myasthenia E13.44
      necrobiosis lipoidica E13.620
      nephropathy E13.21
      neuralgia E13.42
      neurologic complication NEC E13.49
      neuropathic arthropathy E13.610
      neuropathy E13.40
      ophthalmic complication NEC E13.39
      oral complication NEC E13.638
      periodontal disease E13.630
      peripheral angiopathy E13.51
        with gangrene E13.52
      polyneuropathy E13.42
      renal complication NEC E13.29
      renal tubular degeneration E13.29
      retinopathy E13.319
        with macular edema E13.311
        nonproliferative E13.329
          with macular edema E13.321
          mild E13.329
            with macular edema E13.321
          moderate E13.339
            with macular edema E13.331
          severe E13.349
            with macular edema E13.341
        proliferative E13.359
          with macular edema E13.351
      skin complication NEC E13.628
      skin ulcer NEC E13.622
  steroid-induced — *see* Diabetes, due to, drug or chemical
  type 1 E10.9
    with
      amyotrophy E10.44
      arthropathy NEC E10.618
      autonomic (poly)neuropathy E10.43
      cataract E10.36
      Charcot's joints E10.610
      chronic kidney disease E10.22
      circulatory complication NEC E10.59
      complication E10.8
        specified NEC E10.69
      dermatitis E10.620
      foot ulcer E10.621
      gangrene E10.52
      gastroparesis E10.43
      glomerulonephrosis, intracapillary E10.21
      glomerulosclerosis, intercapillary E10.21
      hyperglycemia E10.65
      hypoglycemia E10.649
        with coma E10.641
      ketoacidosis E10.10
        with coma E10.11
      kidney complications NEC E10.29
      Kimmelstein-Wilson disease E10.21
      mononeuropathy E10.41
      myasthenia E10.44
      necrobiosis lipoidica E10.620
      nephropathy E10.21
      neuralgia E10.42
      neurologic complication NEC E10.49
      neuropathic arthropathy E10.610
      neuropathy E10.40

Diabetes, diabetic — *continued*
  type 1 — *continued*
    with — *continued*
      ophthalmic complication NEC E10.39
      oral complication NEC E10.638
      periodontal disease E10.630
      peripheral angiopathy E10.51
        with gangrene E10.52
      polyneuropathy E10.42
      renal complication NEC E10.29
      renal tubular degeneration E10.29
      retinopathy E10.319
        with macular edema E10.311
        nonproliferative E10.329
          with macular edema E10.321
          mild E10.329
            with macular edema E10.321
          moderate E10.339
            with macular edema E10.331
          severe E10.349
            with macular edema E10.341
        proliferative E10.359
          with macular edema E10.351
      skin complication NEC E10.628
      skin ulcer NEC E10.622
  type 2 E11.9
    with
      amyotrophy E11.44
      arthropathy NEC E11.618
      autonomic (poly)neuropathy E11.43
      cataract E11.36
      Charcot's joints E11.610
      chronic kidney disease E11.22
      circulatory complication NEC E11.59
      complication E11.8
        specified NEC E11.69
      dermatitis E11.620
      foot ulcer E11.621
      gangrene E11.52
      gastroparesis E11.43
      glomerulonephrosis, intracapillary E11.21
      glomerulosclerosis, intercapillary E11.21
      hyperglycemia E11.65
      hyperosmolarity E11.00
        with coma E11.01
      hypoglycemia E11.649
        with coma E11.641
      kidney complications NEC E11.29
      Kimmelstiel-Wilson disease E11.21
      mononeuropathy E11.41
      myasthenia E11.44
      necrobiosis lipoidica E11.620
      nephropathy E11.21
      neuralgia E11.42
      neurologic complication NEC E11.49
      neuropathic arthropathy E11.610
      neuropathy E11.40
      ophthalmic complication NEC E11.39
      oral complication NEC E11.638
      periodontal disease E11.630
      peripheral angiopathy E11.51
        with gangrene E11.52
      polyneuropathy E11.42
      renal complication NEC E11.29
      renal tubular degeneration E11.29
      retinopathy E11.319
        with macular edema E11.311
        nonproliferative E11.329
          with macular edema E11.321
          mild E11.329
            with macular edema E11.321
          moderate E11.339
            with macular edema E11.331
          severe E11.349
            with macular edema E11.341
        proliferative E11.359
          with macular edema E11.351
      skin complication NEC E11.628
      skin ulcer NEC E11.622
Diacyclothrombopathia D69.1
Diagnosis deferred R69
Dialysis (intermittent) (treatment)
  noncompliance (with) Z91.15
  renal (hemodialysis) (peritoneal), status Z99.2
  retina, retinal — *see* Detachment, retina, with retinal, dialysis
Diamond-Blackfan anemia (congenital hypoplastic) D61.01

Diamond-Gardener syndrome (autoerythrocyte sensitization) D69.2
Diaper rash L22
Diaphoresis (excessive) R61
Diaphragm — *see* condition
Diaphragmalgia R07.1
Diaphragmatitis, diaphragmitis J98.6
Diaphysial aclasis Q78.6
Diaphysitis — *see* Osteomyelitis, specified type NEC
Diarrhea, diarrheal (disease) (infantile) (inflammatory) R19.7
  achlorhydric K31.83
  allergic K52.2
  amebic (*see also* Amebiasis) A06.0
    with abscess — *see* Abscess, amebic
    acute A06.0
    chronic A06.1
    nondysenteric A06.2
  bacillary — *see* Dysentery, bacillary
  balantidial A07.0
  cachectic NEC K52.89
  Chilomastix A07.8
  choleriformis A00.1
  chronic (noninfectious) K52.9
  coccidial A07.3
  Cochin-China K90.1
    strongyloidiasis B78.0
  Dientamoeba A07.8
  dietetic K52.2
  drug-induced K52.1
  due to
    bacteria A04.9
      specified NEC A04.8
    Campylobacter A04.5
    Capillaria philippinensis B81.1
    Clostridium difficile A04.7
    Clostridium perfringens (C) (F) A04.8
    Cryptosporidium A07.2
    drugs K52.1
    Escherichia coli A04.4
      enteroaggregative A04.4
      enterohemorrhagic A04.3
      enteroinvasive A04.2
      enteropathogenic A04.0
      enterotoxigenic A04.1
      specified NEC A04.4
    food hypersensitivity K52.2
    Necator americanus B76.1
    S. japonicum B65.2
    specified organism NEC A08.8
      bacterial A04.8
      viral A08.39
    Staphylococcus A04.8
    Trichuris trichiuria B79
    virus — *see* Enteritis, viral
    Yersinia enterocolitica A04.6
  dysenteric A09
  endemic A09
  epidemic A09
  flagellate A07.9
  Flexner's (ulcerative) A03.1
  functional K59.1
    following gastrointestinal surgery K91.89
    psychogenic F45.8
  Giardia lamblia A07.1
  giardial A07.1
  hill K90.1
  infectious A09
  malarial — *see* Malaria
  mite B88.0
  mycotic NEC B49
  neonatal (noninfectious) P78.3
  nervous F45.8
  neurogenic K59.1
  noninfectious K52.9
  postgastrectomy K91.1
  postvagotomy K91.1
  protozoal A07.9
    specified NEC A07.8
  psychogenic F45.8
  specified
    bacterium NEC A04.8
    virus NEC A08.39
  strongyloidiasis B78.0
  toxic K52.1
  trichomonal A07.8
  tropical K90.1
  tuberculous A18.32

Diarrhea, diarrheal — *continued*
  viral — *see* Enteritis, viral
Diastasis
  cranial bones M84.88
    congenital NEC Q75.8
  joint (traumatic) — *see* Dislocation
  muscle M62.00
    ankle M62.07- ☑
    congenital Q79.8
    foot M62.07- ☑
    forearm M62.03- ☑
    hand M62.04- ☑
    lower leg M62.06- ☑
    pelvic region M62.05- ☑
    shoulder region M62.01- ☑
    specified site NEC M62.08
    thigh M62.05- ☑
    upper arm M62.02- ☑
  recti (abdomen)
    complicating delivery O71.89
    congenital Q79.59
Diastema, tooth, teeth, fully erupted M26.32
Diastematomyelia Q06.2
Diataxia, cerebral G80.4
Diathesis
  allergic — *see* History, allergy
  bleeding (familial) D69.9
  cystine (familial) E72.00
  gouty — *see* Gout
  hemorrhagic (familial) D69.9
    newborn NEC P53
  spasmophilic R29.0
Diaz's disease or osteochondrosis (juvenile) (talus) — *see* Osteochondrosis, juvenile, tarsus
Dibothriocephalus, dibothriocephaliasis (latus) (infection) (infestation) B70.0
  larval B70.1
Dicephalus, dicephaly Q89.4
Dichotomy, teeth K00.2
Dichromat, dichromatopsia (congenital) — *see* Deficiency, color vision
Dichuchwa A65
Dicroceliasis B66.2
Didelphia, didelphys — *see* Double uterus
Didymytis N45.1
  with orchitis N45.3
Dietary
  inadequacy or deficiency E63.9
  surveillance and counseling Z71.3
Dietl's crisis N13.8
Dieulafoy lesion (hemorrhagic)
  duodenum K31.82
  esophagus K22.8
  intestine (colon) K63.81
  stomach K31.82
Difficult, difficulty (in)
  acculturation Z60.3
  feeding R63.3
    newborn P92.9
      breast P92.5
      specified NEC P92.8
    nonorganic (infant or child) F98.29
  intubation, in anesthesia T88.4 ☑
  mechanical, gastroduodenal stoma K91.89
    causing obstruction K91.3
  reading (developmental) F81.0
    secondary to emotional disorders F93.9
  spelling (specific) F81.81
    with reading disorder F81.89
    due to inadequate teaching Z55.8
  swallowing — *see* Dysphagia
  walking R26.2
  work
    conditions NEC Z56.5
    schedule Z56.3
Diffuse — *see* condition
Digestive — *see* condition
Dihydropyrimidine dehydrogenase disease (DPD) E88.89
Diktyoma — *see* Neoplasm, malignant, by site
Dilaceration, tooth K00.4
Dilatation
  anus K59.8
    venule — *see* Hemorrhoids
  aorta (focal) (general) — *see* Ectasia, aorta
    with aneurysm — *see* Aneurysm, aorta
  artery — *see* Aneurysm

Index

Diabetes, diabetic — Dilatation

Dilatation — continued
bladder (sphincter) N32.89
- congenital Q64.79
blood vessel I99.8
bronchial J47.9
- with
- - exacerbation (acute) J47.1
- - lower respiratory infection J47.0
calyx (due to obstruction) — see Hydronephrosis
capillaries I78.8
cardiac (acute) (chronic) (see also Hypertrophy, cardiac)
- congenital Q24.8
- - valve NEC Q24.8
- - - pulmonary Q22.3
- valve — see Endocarditis
cavum septi pellucidi Q06.8
cervix (uteri) (see also Incompetency, cervix)
- incomplete, poor, slow complicating delivery O62.0
colon K59.3
- congenital Q43.1
- psychogenic F45.8
common duct (acquired) K83.8
- congenital Q44.5
cystic duct (acquired) K82.8
- congenital Q44.5
duct, mammary — see Ectasia, mammary duct
duodenum K59.8
esophagus K22.8
- congenital Q39.5
- due to achalasia K22.0
eustachian tube, congenital Q17.8
gallbladder K82.8
gastric — see Dilatation, stomach
heart (acute) (chronic) (see also Hypertrophy, cardiac)
- congenital Q24.8
- valve — see Endocarditis
ileum K59.8
- psychogenic F45.8
jejunum K59.8
- psychogenic F45.8
kidney (calyx) (collecting structures) (cystic) (parenchyma) (pelvis) (idiopathic) N28.89
lacrimal passages or duct — see Disorder, lacrimal system, changes
lymphatic vessel I89.0
mammary duct — see Ectasia, mammary duct
Meckel's diverticulum (congenital) Q43.0
- malignant — see Table of Neoplasms, small intestine, malignant
myocardium (acute) (chronic) — see Hypertrophy, cardiac
organ or site, congenital NEC — see Distortion
pancreatic duct K86.8
pericardium — see Pericarditis
pharynx J39.2
prostate N42.89
pulmonary
- artery (idiopathic) I28.8
- valve, congenital Q22.3
pupil H57.04
rectum K59.3
saccule, congenital Q16.5
salivary gland (duct) K11.8
sphincter ani K62.89
stomach K31.89
- acute K31.0
- psychogenic F45.8
submaxillary duct K11.8
trachea, congenital Q32.1
ureter (idiopathic) N28.82
- congenital Q62.2
- due to obstruction N13.4
urethra (acquired) N36.8
vasomotor I73.9
vein I86.8
ventricular, ventricle (acute) (chronic) (see also Hypertrophy, cardiac)
- cerebral, congenital Q04.8
venule NEC I86.8
vesical orifice N32.89

Dilated, dilation — see Dilatation
Diminished, diminution
hearing (acuity) — see Deafness
sense or sensation (cold) (heat) (tactile) (vibratory) R20.8
vision NEC H54.7
vital capacity R94.2
Diminuta taenia B71.0

Dimitri-Sturge-Weber disease Q85.8
Dimple
parasacral, pilonidal or postanal — see Cyst, pilonidal
Dioctophyme renalis (infection) (infestation) B83.8
Dipetalonemiasis B74.4
Diphallus Q55.69
Diphtheria, diphtheritic (gangrenous) (hemorrhagic) A36.9
- carrier (suspected) Z22.2
- cutaneous A36.3
- faucial A36.0
- infection of wound A36.3
- laryngeal A36.2
- myocarditis A36.81
- nasal, anterior A36.89
- nasopharyngeal A36.1
- neurological complication A36.89
- pharyngeal A36.0
- specified site NEC A36.89
- tonsillar A36.0
Diphyllobothriasis (intestine) B70.0
- larval B70.1
Diplacusis H93.22- ☑
Diplegia (upper limbs) G83.0
- congenital (cerebral) G80.8
- facial G51.0
- lower limbs G82.20
- spastic G80.1
Diplococcus, diplococcal — see condition
Diplopia H53.2
Dipsomania F10.20
- with
- - psychosis — see Psychosis, alcoholic
- - remission F10.21
Dipylidiasis B71.1
Direction, teeth, abnormal, fully erupted M26.30
Dirofilariasis B74.8
Dirt-eating child F98.3
Disability, disabilities
heart — see Disease, heart
intellectual F79
- with
- - autistic features F84.9
- - mild (I.Q. 50-69) F70
- - moderate (I.Q. 35-49) F71
- - profound (I.Q. under 20) F73
- - severe (I.Q. 20-34) F72
- - specified level NEC F78
- knowledge acquisition F81.9
- learning F81.9
- limiting activities Z73.6
- spelling, specific F81.81
Disappearance of family member Z63.4
Disarticulation — see Amputation
- meaning traumatic amputation — see Amputation, traumatic
Discharge (from)
- abnormal finding in — see Abnormal, specimen
- breast (female) (male) N64.52
- diencephalic autonomic idiopathic — see Epilepsy, specified NEC
- ear (see also Otorrhea)
- - blood — see Otorrhagia
- excessive urine R35.8
- nipple N64.52
- penile R36.9
- postnasal R09.82
- prison, anxiety concerning Z65.2
- urethral R36.9
- - without blood R36.0
- - hematospermia R36.1
- vaginal N89.8
Discitis, diskitis M46.40
- cervical region M46.42
- cervicothoracic region M46.43
- lumbar region M46.46
- lumbosacral region M46.47
- multiple sites M46.49
- occipito-atlanto-axial region M46.41
- pyogenic — see Infection, intervertebral disc, pyogenic
- sacrococcygeal region M46.48
- thoracic region M46.44
- thoracolumbar region M46.45
Discoid
- meniscus (congenital) Q68.6
- semilunar cartilage (congenital) — see Derangement, knee, meniscus, specified NEC

Discoloration
nails L60.8
teeth (posteruptive) K03.7
- during formation K00.8
Discomfort
chest R07.89
visual H53.14- ☑
Discontinuity, ossicles, ear H74.2- ☑
Discord (with)
- boss Z56.4
- classmates Z55.4
- counselor Z64.4
- employer Z56.4
- family Z63.8
- fellow employees Z56.4
- in-laws Z63.1
- landlord Z59.2
- lodgers Z59.2
- neighbors Z59.2
- probation officer Z64.4
- social worker Z64.4
- teachers Z55.4
- workmates Z56.4
Discordant connection
- atrioventricular (congenital) Q20.5
- ventriculoarterial Q20.3
Discrepancy
- centric occlusion maximum intercuspation M26.55
- leg length (acquired) — see Deformity, limb, unequal length
- - congenital — see Defect, reduction, lower limb
- uterine size date O26.84- ☑
Discrimination
- ethnic Z60.5
- political Z60.5
- racial Z60.5
- religious Z60.5
- sex Z60.5
Disease, diseased (see also Syndrome)
- absorbent system I87.8
- acid-peptic K30
- Acosta's T70.29 ☑
- Adams-Stokes (-Morgagni) (syncope with heart block) I45.9
- Addison's anemia (pernicious) D51.0
- adenoids (and tonsils) J35.9
- adrenal (capsule) (cortex) (gland) (medullary) E27.9
- - hyperfunction E27.0
- - specified NEC E27.8
- ainhum L94.6
- airway
- - obstructive, chronic J44.9
- - - due to
- - - - cotton dust J66.0
- - - - specific organic dusts NEC J66.8
- - reactive — see Asthma
- akamushi (scrub typhus) A75.3
- Albers-Schönberg (marble bones) Q78.2
- Albert's — see Tendinitis, Achilles
- alimentary canal K63.9
- alligator-skin Q80.9
- - acquired L85.0
- alpha heavy chain C88.3
- alpine T70.29 ☑
- altitude T70.20 ☑
- alveolar ridge
- - edentulous K06.9
- - - specified NEC K06.8
- alveoli, teeth K08.9
- Alzheimer's G30.9 [F02.80]
- - with behavioral disturbance G30.9 [F02.81]
- - early onset G30.0 [F02.80]
- - - with behavioral disturbance G30.0 [F02.81]
- - late onset G30.1 [F02.80]
- - - with behavioral disturbance G30.1 [F02.81]
- - specified NEC G30.8 [F02.80]
- - - with behavioral disturbance G30.8 [F02.81]
- amyloid — see Amyloidosis
- Andersen's (glycogenosis IV) E74.09
- Andes T70.29 ☑
- Andrews' (bacterid) L08.89
- angiospastic I73.9
- - cerebral G45.9
- - vein I87.8
- anterior
- - chamber H21.9
- - horn cell G12.29

Index / **Disease, diseased — Disease, diseased**

Disease, diseased — *continued*
antiglomerular basement membrane (anti- GBM) anti-body M31.0
  tubulo-interstitial nephritis N12
antral — *see* Sinusitis, maxillary
anus K62.9
  specified NEC K62.89
aorta (nonsyphilitic) I77.9
  syphilitic NEC A52.02
aortic (heart) (valve) I35.9
  rheumatic I06.9
Apollo B30.3
aponeuroses — *see* Enthesopathy
appendix K38.9
  specified NEC K38.8
aqueous (chamber) H21.9
Arnold-Chiari — *see* Arnold-Chiari disease
arterial I77.9
  occlusive — *see* Occlusion, by site
    due to stricture or stenosis I77.1
arteriocardiorenal — *see* Hypertension, cardiorenal
arteriolar (generalized) (obliterative) I77.9
arteriorenal — *see* Hypertension, kidney
arteriosclerotic (*see also* Arteriosclerosis)
  cardiovascular — *see* Disease, heart, ischemic, atherosclerotic
  coronary (artery) — *see* Disease, heart, ischemic, atherosclerotic
  heart — *see* Disease, heart, ischemic, atherosclerotic
artery I77.9
  cerebral I67.9
  coronary I25.10
    with angina pectoris — *see* Arteriosclerosis, coronary (artery)
arthropod-borne NOS (viral) A94
  specified type NEC A93.8
atticoantral, chronic H66.20
  left H66.22
    with right H66.23
  right H66.21
    with left H66.23
auditory canal — *see* Disorder, ear, external
auricle, ear NEC — *see* Disorder, pinna
Australian X A83.4
autoimmune (systemic) NOS M35.9
  hemolytic (cold type) (warm type) D59.1
    drug-induced D59.0
  thyroid E06.3
aviator's — *see* Effect, adverse, high altitude
Ayala's Q78.5
Ayerza's (pulmonary artery sclerosis with pulmonary hypertension) I27.0
Babington's (familial hemorrhagic telangiectasia) I78.0
bacterial A49.9
  specified NEC A48.8
  zoonotic A28.9
    specified type NEC A28.8
Baelz's (cheilitis glandularis apostematosa) K13.0
bagasse J67.1
balloon — *see* Effect, adverse, high altitude
Bang's (brucella abortus) A23.1
Bannister's T78.3 ☑
barometer makers' — *see* Poisoning, mercury
Barraquer (-Simons') (progressive lipodystrophy) E88.1
Barrett's — *see* Barrett's, esophagus
Bartholin's gland N75.9
basal ganglia G25.9
  degenerative G23.9
    specified NEC G23.8
  specified NEC G25.89
Basedow's (exophthalmic goiter) — *see* Hyperthyroidism, with, goiter (diffuse)
Bateman's B08.1
Batten-Steinert G71.11
Battey A31.0
Beard's (neurasthenia) F48.8
Becker
  idiopathic mural endomyocardial I42.3
  myotonia congenita G71.12
Begbie's (exophthalmic goiter) — *see* Hyperthyroidism, with, goiter (diffuse)
behavioral, organic F07.9
Beigel's (white piedra) B36.2
Benson's — *see* Deposit, crystalline
Bernard-Soulier (thrombopathy) D69.1
Bernhardt (-Roth) — *see* Mononeuropathy, lower limb, meralgia paresthetica

Disease, diseased — *continued*
Biermer's (pernicious anemia) D51.0
bile duct (common) (hepatic) K83.9
  with calculus, stones — *see* Calculus, bile duct
  specified NEC K83.8
biliary (tract) K83.9
  specified NEC K83.8
Billroth's — *see* Spina bifida
bird fancier's J67.2
black lung J60
bladder N32.9
  in (due to)
    schistosomiasis (bilharziasis) B65.0 [N33]
  specified NEC N32.89
bleeder's D66
blood D75.9
  forming organs D75.9
  vessel I99.9
Bloodgood's — *see* Mastopathy, cystic
Bodechtel-Guttmann (subacute sclerosing panencephalitis) A81.1
bone (*see also* Disorder, bone)
  aluminum M83.4
  fibrocystic NEC
    jaw M27.49
bone-marrow D75.9
Borna A83.9
Bornholm (epidemic pleurodynia) B33.0
Bouchard's (myopathic dilatation of the stomach) K31.0
Bouillaud's (rheumatic heart disease) I01.9
Bourneville (-Brissaud) (tuberous sclerosis) Q85.1
Bouveret (-Hoffmann) (paroxysmal tachycardia) I47.9
bowel K63.9
  functional K59.9
    psychogenic F45.8
brain G93.9
  arterial, artery I67.9
  arteriosclerotic I67.2
  congenital Q04.9
  degenerative — *see* Degeneration, brain
  inflammatory — *see* Encephalitis
  organic G93.9
    arteriosclerotic I67.2
  parasitic NEC B71.9 [G94]
  senile NEC G31.1
  specified NEC G93.89
breast (*see also* Disorder, breast) N64.9
  cystic (chronic) — *see* Mastopathy, cystic
  fibrocystic — *see* Mastopathy, cystic
  Paget's
    female, unspecified side C50.91- ☑
    male, unspecified side C50.92- ☑
  specified NEC N64.89
Breda's — *see* Yaws
Bretonneau's (diphtheritic malignant angina) A36.0
Bright's — *see* Nephritis
  arteriosclerotic — *see* Hypertension, kidney
Brill's (recrudescent typhus) A75.1
Brill-Zinsser (recrudescent typhus) A75.1
Brion-Kayser — *see* Fever, paratyphoid
broad
  beta E78.2
  ligament (noninflammatory) N83.9
    inflammatory — *see* Disease, pelvis, inflammatory
    specified NEC N83.8
Brocq-Duhring (dermatitis herpetiformis) L13.0
Brocq's
  meaning
    dermatitis herpetiformis L13.0
    prurigo L28.2
bronchopulmonary J98.4
bronchus NEC J98.09
bronze Addison's E27.1
  tuberculous A18.7
budgerigar fancier's J67.2
Buerger's (thromboangiitis obliterans) I73.1
bullous L13.9
  chronic of childhood L12.2
  specified NEC L13.8
Bürger-Grütz (essential familial hyperlipemia) E78.3
bursa — *see* Bursopathy
caisson T70.3 ☑
California — *see* Coccidioidomycosis
capillaries I78.9
  specified NEC I78.8
Carapata A68.0

Disease, diseased — *continued*
cardiac — *see* Disease, heart
cardiopulmonary, chronic I27.9
cardiorenal (hepatic) (hypertensive) (vascular) — *see* Hypertension, cardiorenal
cardiovascular (atherosclerotic) I25.10
  with angina pectoris — *see* Arteriosclerosis, coronary (artery),
  congenital Q28.9
  hypertensive — *see* Hypertension, heart
  newborn P29.9
    specified NEC P29.89
  renal (hypertensive) — *see* Hypertension, cardiorenal
  syphilitic (asymptomatic) A52.00
cartilage — *see* Disorder, cartilage
Castellani's A69.8
cat-scratch A28.1
Cavare's (familial periodic paralysis) G72.3
cecum K63.9
celiac (adult) (infantile) K90.0
cellular tissue L98.9
central core G71.2
cerebellar, cerebellum — *see* Disease, brain
cerebral (*see also* Disease, brain)
  degenerative — *see* Degeneration, brain
cerebrospinal G96.9
cerebrovascular I67.9
  acute I67.89
    embolic I63.4- ☑
    thrombotic I63.3- ☑
  arteriosclerotic I67.2
  specified NEC I67.89
cervix (uteri) (noninflammatory) N88.9
  inflammatory — *see* Cervicitis
  specified NEC N88.8
Chabert's A22.9
Chandler's (osteochondritis dissecans, hip) — *see* Osteochondritis, dissecans, hip
Charlouis — *see* Yaws
Chédiak-Steinbrinck (-Higashi) (congenital gigantism of peroxidase granules) E70.330
chest J98.9
Chiari's (hepatic vein thrombosis) I82.0
Chicago B40.9
Chignon B36.8
chigo, chigoe B88.1
childhood granulomatous D71
Chinese liver fluke B66.1
chlamydial A74.9
  specified NEC A74.89
cholecystic K82.9
choroid H31.9
  specified NEC H31.8
Christmas D67
chronic bullous of childhood L12.2
chylomicron retention E78.3
ciliary body H21.9
  specified NEC H21.89
circulatory (system) NEC I99.8
  newborn P29.9
  syphilitic A52.00
    congenital A50.54
coagulation factor deficiency (congenital) — *see* Defect, coagulation
coccidioidal — *see* Coccidioidomycosis
cold
  agglutinin or hemoglobinuria D59.1
    paroxysmal D59.6
  hemagglutinin (chronic) D59.1
collagen NOS (nonvascular) (vascular) M35.9
  specified NEC M35.8
colon K63.9
  functional K59.9
    congenital Q43.2
  ischemic K55.0
combined system — *see* Degeneration, combined
compressed air T70.3 ☑
Concato's (pericardial polyserositis) A19.9
  nontubercular I31.1
  pleural — *see* Pleurisy, with effusion
conjunctiva H11.9
  chlamydial A74.0
  specified NEC H11.89
  viral B30.9
    specified NEC B30.8

☑ **Additional Character Required** — Refer to the Tabular List for Character Selection   Subterms under main terms may continue to next column or page

Disease, diseased — *continued*

connective tissue, systemic (diffuse) M35.9
   in (due to)
      hypogammaglobulinemia D80.1 [M36.8]
      ochronosis E70.29 [M36.8]
   specified NEC M35.8
Conor and Bruch's (boutonneuse fever) A77.1
Cooper's — *see* Mastopathy, cystic
Cori's (glycogenosis III) E74.03
corkhandler's or corkworker's J67.3
cornea H18.9
   specified NEC H18.89- ✅
coronary (artery) — *see* Disease, heart, ischemic, atherosclerotic
   congenital Q24.5
   ostial, syphilitic (aortic) (mitral) (pulmonary) A52.03
corpus cavernosum N48.9
   specified NEC N48.89
Cotugno's — *see* Sciatica
coxsackie (virus) NEC B34.1
cranial nerve NOS G52.9
Creutzfeldt-Jakob — *see* Creutzfeldt-Jakob disease or syndrome
Crocq's (acrocyanosis) I73.89
Crohn's — *see* Enteritis, regional
Curschmann G71.11
cystic
   breast (chronic) — *see* Mastopathy, cystic
   kidney, congenital Q61.9
   liver, congenital Q44.6
   lung J98.4
      congenital Q33.0
cytomegalic inclusion (generalized) B25.9
   with pneumonia B25.0
   congenital P35.1
cytomegaloviral B25.9
   specified NEC B25.8
Czerny's (periodic hydrarthrosis of the knee) — *see* Effusion, joint, knee
Daae (-Finsen) (epidemic pleurodynia) B33.0
Darling's — *see* Histoplasmosis capsulati
de Quervain's (tendon sheath) M65.4
   thyroid (subacute granulomatous thyroiditis) E06.1
Débove's (splenomegaly) R16.1
deer fly — *see* Tularemia
Degos' I77.89
demyelinating, demyelinizating (nervous system) G37.9
   multiple sclerosis G35
   specified NEC G37.8
dense deposit (*see also* N00-N07 with fourth character .6) N05.6
deposition, hydroxyapatite — *see* Disease, hydroxyapatite deposition
Devergie's (pityriasis rubra pilaris) L44.0
Devic's G36.0
diaphorase deficiency D74.0
diaphragm J98.6
diarrheal, infectious NEC A09
digestive system K92.9
   specified NEC K92.89
disc, degenerative — *see* Degeneration, intervertebral disc
discogenic (*see also* Displacement, intervertebral disc NEC)
   with myelopathy — *see* Disorder, disc, with, myelopathy
diverticular — *see* Diverticula
Dubois (thymus) A50.59 [E35]
Duchenne-Griesinger G71.0
Duchenne's
   muscular dystrophy G71.0
   pseudohypertrophy, muscles G71.0
ductless glands E34.9
Duhring's (dermatitis herpetiformis) L13.0
duodenum K31.9
   specified NEC K31.89
Dupré's (meningism) R29.1
Dupuytren's (muscle contracture) M72.0
Durand-Nicholas-Favre (climatic bubo) A55
Duroziez's (congenital mitral stenosis) Q23.2
ear — *see* Disorder, ear
Eberth's — *see* Fever, typhoid
Ebola (virus) A98.4
Ebstein's heart Q22.5
Echinococcus — *see* Echinococcus
echovirus NEC B34.1
Eddowes' (brittle bones and blue sclera) Q78.0

Disease, diseased — *continued*

edentulous (alveolar) ridge K06.9
   specified NEC K06.8
Edsall's T67.2 ✅
Eichstedt's (pityriasis versicolor) B36.0
Ellis-van Creveld (chondroectodermal dysplasia) Q77.6
end stage renal (ESRD) N18.6
   due to hypertension I12.0
endocrine glands or system NEC E34.9
endomyocardial (eosinophilic) I42.3
English (rickets) E55.0
enteroviral, enterovirus NEC B34.1
   central nervous system NEC A88.8
epidemic B99.9
   specified NEC B99.8
epididymis N50.9
Erb (-Landouzy) G71.0
Erdheim-Chester (ECD) E88.89
esophagus K22.9
   functional K22.4
   psychogenic F45.8
   specified NEC K22.8
Eulenburg's (congenital paramyotonia) G71.19
eustachian tube — *see* Disorder, eustachian tube
external
   auditory canal — *see* Disorder, ear, external
   ear — *see* Disorder, ear, external
extrapyramidal G25.9
   specified NEC G25.89
eye H57.9
   anterior chamber H21.9
   inflammatory NEC H57.8
   muscle (external) — *see* Strabismus
   specified NEC H57.8
   syphilitic — *see* Oculopathy, syphilitic
eyeball H44.9
   specified NEC H44.89
eyelid — *see* Disorder, eyelid
   specified NEC — *see* Disorder, eyelid, specified type NEC
eyeworm of Africa B74.3
facial nerve (seventh) G51.9
   newborn (birth injury) P11.3
Fahr (of brain) G23.8
Fahr Volhard (of kidney) I12.- ✅
fallopian tube (noninflammatory) N83.9
   inflammatory — *see* Salpingo-oophoritis
   specified NEC N83.8
familial periodic paralysis G72.3
Fanconi's (congenital pancytopenia) D61.09
fascia NEC (*see also* Disorder, muscle)
   inflammatory — *see* Myositis
   specified NEC M62.89
Fauchard's (periodontitis) — *see* Periodontitis
Favre-Durand-Nicolas (climatic bubo) A55
Fede's K14.0
Feer's — *see* Poisoning, mercury
female pelvic inflammatory (*see also* Disease, pelvis, inflammatory) N73.9
   syphilitic (secondary) A51.42
   tuberculous A18.17
Fernels' (aortic aneurysm) I71.9
fibrocaseous of lung — *see* Tuberculosis, pulmonary
fibrocystic — *see* Fibrocystic disease
Fiedler's (leptospiral jaundice) A27.0
fifth B08.3
file-cutter's — *see* Poisoning, lead
fish-skin Q80.9
   acquired L85.0
Flajani (-Basedow) (exophthalmic goiter) — *see* Hyperthyroidism, with, goiter (diffuse)
flax-dresser's J66.1
fluke — *see* Infestation, fluke
foot and mouth B08.8
foot process N04.9
Forbes' (glycogenosis III) E74.03
Fordyce-Fox (apocrine miliaria) L75.2
Fordyce's (ectopic sebaceous glands) (mouth) Q38.6
Forestier's (rhizomelic pseudopolyarthritis) M35.3
   meaning ankylosing hyperostosis — *see* Hyperostosis, ankylosing
Fothergill's
   neuralgia — *see* Neuralgia, trigeminal
   scarlatina anginosa A38.9
Fournier (gangrene) N49.3
   female N76.89
fourth B08.8
Fox (-Fordyce) (apocrine miliaria) L75.2

Disease, diseased — *continued*

Francis' — *see* Tularemia
Franklin C88.2
Frei's (climatic bubo) A55
Friedreich's
   combined systemic or ataxia G11.1
   myoclonia G25.3
frontal sinus — *see* Sinusitis, frontal
fungus NEC B49
Gaisböck's (polycythemia hypertonica) D75.1
gallbladder K82.9
   calculus — *see* Calculus, gallbladder
   cholecystitis — *see* Cholecystitis
   cholesterolosis K82.4
   fistula — *see* Fistula, gallbladder
   hydrops K82.1
   obstruction — *see* Obstruction, gallbladder
   perforation K82.2
   specified NEC K82.8
gamma heavy chain C88.2
Gamna's (siderotic splenomegaly) D73.2
Gamstorp's (adynamia episodica hereditaria) G72.3
Gandy-Nanta (siderotic splenomegaly) D73.2
ganister J62.8
gastric — *see* Disease, stomach
gastroesophageal reflux (GERD) K21.9
   with esophagitis K21.0
gastrointestinal (tract) K92.9
   amyloid E85.4
   functional K59.9
      psychogenic F45.8
   specified NEC K92.89
Gee (-Herter) (-Heubner) (-Thaysen) (nontropical sprue) K90.0
genital organs
   female N94.9
   male N50.9
Gerhardt's (erythromelalgia) I73.81
Gibert's (pityriasis rosea) L42
Gierke's (glycogenosis I) E74.01
Gilles de la Tourette's (motor-verbal tic) F95.2
gingiva K06.9
   specified NEC K06.8
gland (lymph) I89.9
Glanzmann's (hereditary hemorrhagic thrombasthenia) D69.1
glass-blower's (cataract) — *see* Cataract, specified NEC
   salivary gland hypertrophy K11.1
Glisson's — *see* Rickets
globe H44.9
   specified NEC H44.89
glomerular (*see also* Glomerulonephritis)
   with edema — *see* Nephrosis
   acute — *see* Nephritis, acute
   chronic — *see* Nephritis, chronic
   minimal change N05.0
   rapidly progressive N01.9
glycogen storage E74.00
   Andersen's E74.09
   Cori's E74.03
   Forbes' E74.03
   generalized E74.00
   glucose-6-phosphatase deficiency E74.01
   heart E74.02 [I43]
   hepatorenal E74.09
   Hers' E74.09
   liver and kidney E74.09
   McArdle's E74.04
   muscle phosphofructokinase E74.09
   myocardium E74.02 [I43]
   Pompe's E74.02
   Tauri's E74.09
   type 0 E74.09
   type I E74.01
   type II E74.02
   type III E74.03
   type IV E74.09
   type V E74.04
   type VI-XI E74.09
   Von Gierke's E74.01
Goldstein's (familial hemorrhagic telangiectasia) I78.0
gonococcal NOS A54.9
graft-versus-host (GVH) D89.813
   acute D89.810
   acute on chronic D89.812
   chronic D89.811
grainhandler's J67.8
granulomatous (childhood) (chronic) D71

Disease, diseased — *continued*
- Graves' (exophthalmic goiter) — *see* Hyperthyroidism, with, goiter (diffuse)
- Griesinger's — *see* Ancylostomiasis
- Grisel's M43.6
- Gruby's (tinea tonsurans) B35.0
- Guillain-Barré G61.0
- Guinon's (motor-verbal tic) F95.2
- gum K06.9
- gynecological N94.9
- H (Hartnup's) E72.02
- Haff — *see* Poisoning, mercury
- Hageman (congenital factor XII deficiency) D68.2
- hair (color) (shaft) L67.9
  - follicles L73.9
    - specified NEC L73.8
- Hamman's (spontaneous mediastinal emphysema) J98.2
- hand, foot and mouth B08.4
- Hansen's — *see* Leprosy
- Hantavirus, with pulmonary manifestations B33.4
  - with renal manifestations A98.5
- Harada's H30.81- ☑
- Hartnup (pellagra-cerebellar ataxia-renal aminoaciduria) E72.02
- Hart's (pellagra-cerebellar ataxia-renal aminoaciduria) E72.02
- Hashimoto's (struma lymphomatosa) E06.3
- Hb — *see* Disease, hemoglobin
- heart (organic) I51.9
  - with
    - pulmonary edema (acute) (*see also* Failure, ventricular, left) I50.1
    - rheumatic fever (conditions in I00)
      - active I01.9
        - with chorea I02.0
          - specified NEC I01.8
      - inactive or quiescent (with chorea) I09.9
        - specified NEC I09.89
  - amyloid E85.4 [I43]
  - aortic (valve) I35.9
  - arteriosclerotic or sclerotic (senile) — *see* Disease, heart, ischemic, atherosclerotic
  - artery, arterial — *see* Disease, heart, ischemic, atherosclerotic
  - beer drinkers' I42.6
  - beriberi (wet) E51.12
  - black I27.0
  - congenital Q24.9
    - cyanotic Q24.9
    - specified NEC Q24.8
  - coronary — *see* Disease, heart, ischemic
  - cryptogenic I51.9
  - fibroid — *see* Myocarditis
  - functional I51.89
    - psychogenic F45.8
  - glycogen storage E74.02 [I43]
  - gonococcal A54.83
  - hypertensive — *see* Hypertension, heart
  - hyperthyroid (*see also* Hyperthyroidism) E05.90 [I43]
    - with thyroid storm E05.91 [I43]
  - ischemic (chronic or with a stated duration of over 4 weeks) I25.9
    - atherosclerotic (of) I25.10
      - with angina pectoris — *see* Arteriosclerosis, coronary (artery)
      - coronary artery bypass graft — *see* Arteriosclerosis, coronary (artery), cardiomyopathy I25.5
    - diagnosed on ECG or other special investigation, but currently presenting no symptoms I25.6
    - silent I25.6
    - specified form NEC I25.89
  - kyphoscoliotic I27.1
  - meningococcal A39.50
    - endocarditis A39.51
    - myocarditis A39.52
    - pericarditis A39.53
  - mitral I05.9
    - specified NEC I05.8
  - muscular — *see* Degeneration, myocardial
  - psychogenic (functional) F45.8
  - pulmonary (chronic) I27.9
    - in schistosomiasis B65.9 [I52]
    - specified NEC I27.89

Disease, diseased — *continued*
- heart — *continued*
  - rheumatic (chronic) (inactive) (old) (quiescent) (with chorea) I09.9
    - active or acute I01.9
      - with chorea (acute) (rheumatic) (Sydenham's) I02.0
    - specified NEC I09.89
  - senile — *see* Myocarditis
  - syphilitic A52.06
    - aortic A52.03
      - aneurysm A52.01
    - congenital A50.54 [I52]
  - thyrotoxic (*see also* Thyrotoxicosis) E05.90 [I43]
    - with thyroid storm E05.91 [I43]
  - valve, valvular (obstructive) (regurgitant) (*see also* Endocarditis)
    - congenital NEC Q24.8
    - pulmonary Q22.3
  - vascular — *see* Disease, cardiovascular
- heavy chain NEC C88.2
  - alpha C88.3
  - gamma C88.2
  - mu C88.2
- Hebra's
  - pityriasis
    - maculata et circinata L42
    - rubra pilaris L44.0
  - prurigo L28.2
- hematopoietic organs D75.9
- hemoglobin or Hb
  - abnormal (mixed) NEC D58.2
    - with thalassemia D56.9
  - AS genotype D57.3
  - Bart's D56.0
  - C (Hb-C) D58.2
    - with other abnormal hemoglobin NEC D58.2
    - elliptocytosis D58.1
    - Hb-S D57.2- ☑
    - sickle-cell D57.2- ☑
    - thalassemia D56.8
  - Constant Spring D58.2
  - D (Hb-D) D58.2
  - E (Hb-E) D58.2
  - E-beta thalassemia D56.5
  - elliptocytosis D58.1
  - H (Hb-H) (thalassemia) D56.0
    - with other abnormal hemoglobin NEC D56.9
    - Constant Spring D56.0
  - I thalassemia D56.9
  - M D74.0
  - S or SS D57.1
  - SC D57.2- ☑
  - SD D57.8- ☑
  - SE D57.8- ☑
  - spherocytosis D58.0
  - unstable, hemolytic D58.2
- hemolytic (newborn) P55.9
  - autoimmune (cold type) (warm type) D59.1
  - drug-induced D59.0
  - due to or with
    - incompatibility
      - ABO (blood group) P55.1
      - blood (group) (Duffy) (K(ell)) (Kidd) (Lewis) (M) (S) NEC P55.8
      - Rh (blood group) (factor) P55.0
      - Rh negative mother P55.0
    - specified type NEC P55.8
  - unstable hemoglobin D58.2
- hemorrhagic D69.9
  - newborn P53
- Henoch (-Schönlein) (purpura nervosa) D69.0
- hepatic — *see* Disease, liver
- hepatolenticular E83.01
- heredodegenerative NEC
  - spinal cord G95.89
- herpesviral, disseminated B00.7
- Hers' (glycogenosis VI) E74.09
- Herter (-Gee) (-Heubner) (nontropical sprue) K90.0
- Heubner-Herter (nontropical sprue) K90.0
- high fetal gene or hemoglobin thalassemia D56.9
- Hildenbrand's — *see* Typhus
- hip (joint) M25.9
  - congenital Q65.89
  - suppurative M00.9
  - tuberculous A18.02
- His (-Werner) (trench fever) A79.0

Disease, diseased — *continued*
- Hodgson's I71.2
  - ruptured I71.1
- Holla — *see* Spherocytosis
- hookworm B76.9
  - specified NEC B76.8
- host-versus-graft D89.813
  - acute D89.810
  - acute on chronic D89.812
  - chronic D89.811
- human immunodeficiency virus (HIV) B20
- Huntington's G10
- Hutchinson's (cheiropompholyx) — *see* Hutchinson's disease
- hyaline (diffuse) (generalized)
  - membrane (lung) (newborn) P22.0
    - adult J80
- hydatid — *see* Echinococcus
- hydroxyapatite deposition M11.00
  - ankle M11.07- ☑
  - elbow M11.02- ☑
  - foot joint M11.07- ☑
  - hand joint M11.04- ☑
  - hip M11.05- ☑
  - knee M11.06- ☑
  - multiple site M11.09
  - shoulder M11.01- ☑
  - vertebra M11.08
  - wrist M11.03- ☑
- hyperkinetic — *see* Hyperkinesia
- hypertensive — *see* Hypertension
- hypophysis E23.7
- Iceland G93.3
- I-cell E77.0
- immune D89.9
- immunoproliferative (malignant) C88.9
  - small intestinal C88.3
  - specified NEC C88.8
- inclusion B25.9
  - salivary gland B25.9
- infectious, infective B99.9
  - congenital P37.9
    - specified NEC P37.8
    - viral P35.9
      - specified type NEC P35.8
  - specified NEC B99.8
- inflammatory
  - penis N48.29
    - abscess N48.21
    - cellulitis N48.22
  - prepuce N47.7
    - balanoposthitis N47.6
  - tubo-ovarian — *see* Salpingo-oophoritis
- intervertebral disc (*see also* Disorder, disc)
  - with myelopathy — *see* Disorder, disc, with, myelopathy
  - cervical, cervicothoracic — *see* Disorder, disc, cervical
  - with
    - myelopathy — *see* Disorder, disc, cervical, with myelopathy
    - neuritis, radiculitis or radiculopathy — *see* Disorder, disc, cervical, with neuritis
    - specified NEC — *see* Disorder, disc, cervical, specified type NEC
  - lumbar (with)
    - myelopathy M51.06
    - neuritis, radiculitis, radiculopathy or sciatica M51.16
    - specified NEC M51.86
  - lumbosacral (with)
    - neuritis, radiculitis, radiculopathy or sciatica M51.17
    - specified NEC M51.87
  - specified NEC — *see* Disorder, disc, specified NEC
  - thoracic (with)
    - myelopathy M51.04
    - neuritis, radiculitis or radiculopathy M51.14
    - specified NEC M51.84
  - thoracolumbar (with)
    - myelopathy M51.05
    - neuritis, radiculitis or radiculopathy M51.15
    - specified NEC M51.85
- intestine K63.9
  - functional K59.9
    - psychogenic F45.8
    - specified NEC K59.8
  - organic K63.9

☑ **Additional Character Required** — Refer to the Tabular List for Character Selection   🔻 Subterms under main terms may continue to next column or page

Disease, diseased — *continued*
  intestine — *continued*
    protozoal A07.9
    specified NEC K63.89
  iris H21.9
    specified NEC H21.89
  iron metabolism or storage E83.10
  island (scrub typhus) A75.3
  itai-itai — *see* Poisoning, cadmium
  Jakob-Creutzfeldt — *see* Creutzfeldt-Jakob disease or syndrome
  jaw M27.9
    fibrocystic M27.49
    specified NEC M27.8
  jigger B88.1
  joint (*see also* Disorder, joint)
    Charcot's — *see* Arthropathy, neuropathic (Charcot)
    degenerative — *see* Osteoarthritis
      multiple M15.9
      spine — *see* Spondylosis
    hypertrophic — *see* Osteoarthritis
    sacroiliac M53.3
    specified NEC — *see* Disorder, joint, specified type NEC
    spine NEC — *see* Dorsopathy
    suppurative — *see* Arthritis, pyogenic or pyemic
  Jourdain's (acute gingivitis) K05.00
    nonplaque induced K05.01
    plaque induced K05.00
  Kaschin-Beck (endemic polyarthritis) M12.10
    ankle M12.17- ☑
    elbow M12.12- ☑
    foot joint M12.17- ☑
    hand joint M12.14- ☑
    hip M12.15- ☑
    knee M12.16- ☑
    multiple site M12.19
    shoulder M12.11- ☑
    vertebra M12.18
    wrist M12.13- ☑
  Katayama B65.2
  Kedani (scrub typhus) A75.3
  Keshan E59
  kidney (functional) (pelvis) N28.9
    chronic N18.9
      hypertensive — *see* Hypertension, kidney
      stage 1 N18.1
      stage 2 (mild) N18.2
      stage 3 (moderate) N18.3
      stage 4 (severe) N18.4
      stage 5 N18.5
    complicating pregnancy — *see* Pregnancy, complicated by, renal disease
    cystic (congenital) Q61.9
    fibrocystic (congenital) Q61.8
    hypertensive — *see* Hypertension, kidney
    in (due to)
      schistosomiasis (bilharziasis) B65.9 [N29]
    multicystic Q61.4
    polycystic Q61.3
      adult type Q61.2
      childhood type NEC Q61.19
        collecting duct dilatation Q61.11
  Kimmelstiel (-Wilson) (intercapillary polycystic (congenital) glomerulosclerosis) — *see* E08-E13 with .21
  Kinnier Wilson's (hepatolenticular degeneration) E83.01
  kissing — *see* Mononucleosis, infectious
  Klebs' (*see also* Glomerulonephritis) N05- ☑
  Klippel-Feil (brevicollis) Q76.1
  Köhler-Pellegrini-Stieda (calcification, knee joint) — *see* Bursitis, tibial collateral
  Kok Q89.8
  König's (osteochondritis dissecans) — *see* Osteochondritis, dissecans
  Korsakoff's (nonalcoholic) F04
    alcoholic F10.96
      with dependence F10.26
  Kostmann's (infantile genetic agranulocytosis) D70.0
  kuru A81.81
  Kyasanur Forest A98.2
  labyrinth, ear — *see* Disorder, ear, inner
  lacrimal system — *see* Disorder, lacrimal system
  Lafora's — *see* Epilepsy, generalized, idiopathic
  Lancereaux-Mathieu (leptospiral jaundice) A27.0
  Landry's G61.0

Disease, diseased — *continued*
  Larrey-Weil (leptospiral jaundice) A27.0
  larynx J38.7
  legionnaires' A48.1
    nonpneumonic A48.2
  Lenegre's I44.2
  lens H27.9
    specified NEC H27.8
  Lev's (acquired complete heart block) I44.2
  Lewy body (dementia) G31.83 [F02.80]
    with behavioral disturbance G31.83 [F02.81]
  Lichtheim's (subacute combined sclerosis with pernicious anemia) D51.0
  Lightwood's (renal tubular acidosis) N25.89
  Lignac's (cystinosis) E72.04
  lip K13.0
  lipid-storage E75.6
    specified NEC E75.5
  Lipschütz's N76.6
  liver (chronic) (organic) K76.9
    alcoholic (chronic) K70.9
      acute — *see* Disease, liver, alcoholic, hepatitis
      cirrhosis K70.30
        with ascites K70.31
      failure K70.40
        with coma K70.41
      fatty liver K70.0
      fibrosis K70.2
      hepatitis K70.10
        with ascites K70.11
      sclerosis K70.2
    cystic, congenital Q44.6
    drug-induced (idiosyncratic) (toxic) (predictable) (unpredictable) — *see* Disease, liver, toxic
    end stage K72.90
      due to hepatitis — *see* Hepatitis
    fatty, nonalcoholic (NAFLD) K76.0
      alcoholic K70.0
    fibrocystic (congenital) Q44.6
    fluke
      Chinese B66.1
      oriental B66.1
      sheep B66.3
    glycogen storage E74.09 [K77]
    in (due to)
      schistosomiasis (bilharziasis) B65.9 [K77]
    inflammatory K75.9
      alcoholic K70.1 ☑
      specified NEC K75.89
    polycystic (congenital) Q44.6
    toxic K71.9
      with
        cholestasis K71.0
        cirrhosis (liver) K71.7
        fibrosis (liver) K71.7
        focal nodular hyperplasia K71.8
        hepatic granuloma K71.8
        hepatic necrosis K71.10
          with coma K71.11
        hepatitis NEC K71.6
          acute K71.2
          chronic
            active K71.50
              with ascites K71.51
            lobular K71.4
            persistent K71.3
        lupoid K71.50
          with ascites K71.51
        peliosis hepatis K71.8
        veno-occlusive disease (VOD) of liver K71.8
    veno-occlusive K76.5
  Lobo's (keloid blastomycosis) B48.0
  Lobstein's (brittle bones and blue sclera) Q78.0
  Ludwig's (submaxillary cellulitis) K12.2
  lumbosacral region M53.87
  lung J98.4
    black J60
    congenital Q33.9
    cystic J98.4
      congenital Q33.0
    fibroid (chronic) — *see* Fibrosis, lung
    fluke B66.4
      oriental B66.4
    in
      amyloidosis E85.4 [J99]
      sarcoidosis D86.0
      Sjögren's syndrome M35.02

Disease, diseased — *continued*
  lung — *continued*
    in — *continued*
      systemic
        lupus erythematosus M32.13
        sclerosis M34.81
    interstitial J84.9
      of childhood, specified NEC J84.848
      respiratory bronchiolitis J84.115
      specified NEC J84.89
    obstructive (chronic) J44.9
      with
        acute
          bronchitis J44.0
          exacerbation NEC J44.1
          lower respiratory infection J44.0
        alveolitis, allergic J67.9
        asthma J44.9
        bronchiectasis J47.9
          with
            exacerbation (acute) J47.1
            lower respiratory infection J47.0
        bronchitis J44.9
          with
            exacerbation (acute) J44.1
            lower respiratory infection J44.0
        emphysema J44.9
        hypersensitivity pneumonitis J67.9
      decompensated J44.1
        with
          exacerbation (acute) J44.1
    polycystic J98.4
      congenital Q33.0
    rheumatoid (diffuse) (interstitial) — *see* Rheumatoid, lung
  Lutembacher's (atrial septal defect with mitral stenosis) Q21.1
  Lyme A69.20
  lymphatic (gland) (system) (channel) (vessel) I89.9
  lymphoproliferative D47.9
    specified NEC D47.Z9 (*following* D47.4)
    T-gamma D47.Z9 (*following* D47.4)
    X-linked D82.3
  Magitot's M27.2
  malarial — *see* Malaria
  malignant (*see also* Neoplasm, malignant, by site)
  Manson's B65.1
  maple bark J67.6
  maple-syrup-urine E71.0
  Marburg (virus) A98.3
  Marion's (bladder neck obstruction) N32.0
  Marsh's (exophthalmic goiter) — *see* Hyperthyroidism, with, goiter (diffuse)
  mastoid (process) — *see* Disorder, ear, middle
  Mathieu's (leptospiral jaundice) A27.0
  Maxcy's A75.2
  McArdle (-Schmid-Pearson) (glycogenosis V) E74.04
  mediastinum J98.5
  medullary center (idiopathic) (respiratory) G93.89
  Meige's (chronic hereditary edema) Q82.0
  meningococcal — *see* Infection, meningococcal
  mental F99
    organic F09
  mesenchymal M35.9
  mesenteric embolic K55.0
  metabolic, metabolism E88.9
    bilirubin E80.7
  metal-polisher's J62.8
  metastatic (*see also* Neoplasm, secondary, by site) C79.9
  microvascular - code to condition
  microvillus
    atrophy Q43.8
    inclusion (MVD) Q43.8
  middle ear — *see* Disorder, ear, middle
  Mikulicz' (dryness of mouth, absent or decreased lacrimation) K11.8
  Milroy's (chronic hereditary edema) Q82.0
  Minamata — *see* Poisoning, mercury
  minicore G71.2
  Minor's G95.19
  Minot's (hemorrhagic disease, newborn) P53
  Minot-von Willebrand-Jürgens (angiohemophilia) D68.0
  Mitchell's (erythromelalgia) I73.81
  mitral (valve) I05.9
    nonrheumatic I34.9
  mixed connective tissue M35.1

Disease, diseased — *continued*
  moldy hay J67.0
  Monge's T70.29 ☑
  Morgagni-Adams-Stokes (syncope with heart block) I45.9
  Morgagni's (syndrome) (hyperostosis frontalis interna) M85.2
  Morton's (with metatarsalgia) — *see* Lesion, nerve, plantar
  Morvan's G60.8
  motor neuron (bulbar) (familial) (mixed type) (spinal) G12.20
    amyotrophic lateral sclerosis G12.21
    progressive bulbar palsy G12.22
    specified NEC G12.29
  moyamoya I67.5
  mu heavy chain disease C88.2
  multicore G71.2
  muscle (*see also* Disorder, muscle)
    inflammatory — *see* Myositis
    ocular (external) — *see* Strabismus
  musculoskeletal system, soft tissue — *see also* Disorder, soft tissue
    specified NEC — *see* Disorder, soft tissue, specified type NEC
  mushroom workers' J67.5
  mycotic B49
  myelodysplastic, not classified C94.6
  myeloproliferative, not classified C94.6
    chronic D47.1
  myocardium, myocardial (*see also* Degeneration, myocardial) I51.5
    primary (idiopathic) I42.9
  myoneural G70.9
  Naegeli's D69.1
  nails L60.9
    specified NEC L60.8
  Nairobi (sheep virus) A93.8
  nasal J34.9
  nemaline body G71.2
  nerve — *see* Disorder, nerve
  nervous system G98.8
    autonomic G90.9
    central G96.9
      specified NEC G96.8
    congenital Q07.9
    parasympathetic G90.9
    specified NEC G98.8
    sympathetic G90.9
    vegetative G90.9
  neuromuscular system G70.9
  Newcastle B30.8
  Nicolas (-Durand)-Favre (climatic bubo) A55
  nipple N64.9
    Paget's C50.01- ☑
      female C50.01- ☑
      male C50.02- ☑
  Nishimoto (-Takeuchi) I67.5
  nonarthropod-borne NOS (viral) B34.9
    enterovirus NEC B34.1
  nonautoimmune hemolytic D59.4
    drug-induced D59.2
  Nonne-Milroy-Meige (chronic hereditary edema) Q82.0
  nose J34.9
  nucleus pulposus — *see* Disorder, disc
  nutritional E63.9
  oast-house-urine E72.19
    ocular
      herpesviral B00.50
      zoster B02.30
  obliterative vascular I77.1
  Ohara's — *see* Tularemia
  Opitz's (congestive splenomegaly) D73.2
  Oppenheim-Urbach (necrobiosis lipoidica diabeticorum) — *see* E08-E13 with .620
  optic nerve NEC — *see* Disorder, nerve, optic
  orbit — *see* Disorder, orbit
  Oriental liver fluke B66.1
  Oriental lung fluke B66.4
  Ormond's N13.5
  Oropouche virus A93.0
  Osler-Rendu (familial hemorrhagic telangiectasia) I78.0
  osteofibrocystic E21.0
  Otto's M24.7
  outer ear — *see* Disorder, ear, external
  ovary (noninflammatory) N83.9
    cystic N83.20
    inflammatory — *see* Salpingo-oophoritis

Disease, diseased — *continued*
  ovary — *continued*
    polycystic E28.2
    specified NEC N83.8
  Owren's (congenital) — *see* Defect, coagulation
  pancreas K86.9
    cystic K86.2
    fibrocystic E84.9
    specified NEC K86.8
  panvalvular I08.9
    specified NEC I08.8
  parametrium (noninflammatory) N83.9
  parasitic B89
    cerebral NEC B71.9 [G94]
    intestinal NOS B82.9
    mouth B37.0
    skin NOS B88.9
    specified type — *see* Infestation
    tongue B37.0
  parathyroid (gland) E21.5
    specified NEC E21.4
  Parkinson's G20
  parodontal K05.6
  Parrot's (syphilitic osteochondritis) A50.02
  Parry's (exophthalmic goiter) — *see* Hyperthyroidism, with, goiter (diffuse)
  Parson's (exophthalmic goiter) — *see* Hyperthyroidism, with, goiter (diffuse)
  Paxton's (white piedra) B36.2
  pearl-worker's — *see* Osteomyelitis, specified type NEC
  Pellegrini-Stieda (calcification, knee joint) — *see* Bursitis, tibial collateral
  pelvis, pelvic
    female NOS N94.9
      specified NEC N94.89
    gonococcal (acute) (chronic) A54.24
    inflammatory (female) N73.9
      acute N73.0
      chronic N73.1
      specified NEC N73.8
      syphilitic (secondary) A51.42
        late A52.76
      tuberculous A18.17
    organ, female N94.9
    peritoneum, female NEC N94.89
  penis N48.9
    inflammatory N48.29
      abscess N48.21
      cellulitis N48.22
    specified NEC N48.89
  periapical tissues NOS K04.90
  periodontal K05.6
    specified NEC K05.5
  periosteum — *see* Disorder, bone, specified type NEC
  peripheral
    arterial I73.9
    autonomic nervous system G90.9
    nerves — *see* Polyneuropathy
    vascular NOS I73.9
  peritoneum K66.9
    pelvic, female NEC N94.89
    specified NEC K66.8
  persistent mucosal (middle ear) H66.20
    left H66.22
      with right H66.23
    right H66.21
      with left H66.23
  Petit's — *see* Hernia, abdomen, specified site NEC
  pharynx J39.2
    specified NEC J39.2
  Phocas' — *see* Mastopathy, cystic
  photochromogenic (acid-fast bacilli) (pulmonary) A31.0
    nonpulmonary A31.9
  Pick's G31.01 [F02.80]
    with behavioral disturbance G31.01 [F02.81]
  pigeon fancier's J67.2
  pineal gland E34.8
  pink — *see* Poisoning, mercury
  Pinkus' (lichen nitidus) L44.1
  pinworm B80
  Piry virus A93.8
  pituitary (gland) E23.7
  pituitary-snuff-taker's J67.8
  pleura (cavity) J94.9
    specified NEC J94.8
  pneumatic drill (hammer) T75.21 ☑

Disease, diseased — *continued*
  Pollitzer's (hidradenitis suppurativa) L73.2
  polycystic
    kidney or renal Q61.3
      adult type Q61.2
      childhood type NEC Q61.19
        collecting duct dilatation Q61.11
    liver or hepatic Q44.6
    lung or pulmonary J98.4
      congenital Q33.0
    ovary, ovaries E28.2
    spleen Q89.09
  polyethylene T84.05- ☑
  Pompe's (glycogenosis II) E74.02
  Posadas-Wernicke B38.9
  Potain's (pulmonary edema) — *see* Edema, lung
  prepuce N47.8
    inflammatory N47.7
      balanoposthitis N47.6
  Pringle's (tuberous sclerosis) Q85.1
  prion, central nervous system A81.9
    specified NEC A81.89
  prostate N42.9 (congenital) Q61.3
    specified NEC N42.89
  protozoal B64
    acanthamebiasis — *see* Acanthamebiasis
    African trypanosomiasis — *see* African trypanosomiasis
    babesiosis B60.0
    Chagas disease — *see* Chagas disease
    intestine, intestinal A07.9
    leishmaniasis — *see* Leishmaniasis
    malaria — *see* Malaria
    naegleriasis B60.2
    pneumocystosis B59
    specified organism NEC B60.8
    toxoplasmosis — *see* Toxoplasmosis
  pseudo-Hurler's E77.0
  psychiatric F99
  psychotic — *see* Psychosis
  Puente's (simple glandular cheilitis) K13.0
  puerperal (*see also* Puerperal) O90.89
  pulmonary (*see also* Disease, lung)
    artery I28.9
    chronic obstructive J44.9
      with
        acute bronchitis J44.0
        exacerbation (acute) J44.1
        lower respiratory infection (acute) J44.0
      decompensated J44.1
        with
          exacerbation (acute) J44.1
    heart I27.9
      specified NEC I27.89
    hypertensive (vascular) I27.0
    valve I37.9
      rheumatic I09.89
  pulp (dental) NOS K04.90
  pulseless M31.4
  Putnam's (subacute combined sclerosis with pernicious anemia) D51.0
  Pyle (-Cohn) (craniometaphyseal dysplasia) Q78.5
  ragpicker's or ragsorter's A22.1
  Raynaud's — *see* Raynaud's disease
  reactive airway — *see* Asthma
  Reclus' (cystic) — *see* Mastopathy, cystic
  rectum K62.9
    specified NEC K62.89
  Refsum's (heredopathia atactica polyneuritiformis) G60.1
  renal (functional) (pelvis) (*see also* Disease, kidney) N28.9
    with
      edema — *see* Nephrosis
      glomerular lesion — *see* Glomerulonephritis
        with edema — *see* Nephrosis
      interstitial nephritis N12
    acute N28.9
    chronic (*see also* Disease, kidney, chronic) N18.9
    cystic, congenital Q61.9
    diabetic — *see* E08-E13 with .22
    end-stage (failure) N18.6
      due to hypertension I12.0
    fibrocystic (congenital) Q61.8
    hypertensive — *see* Hypertension, kidney
    lupus M32.14
    phosphate-losing (tubular) N25.0

Disease, diseased — *continued*
  renal (*see also* Disease, kidney) — *continued*
    polycystic (congenital) Q61.3
      adult type Q61.2
      childhood type NEC Q61.19
        collecting duct dilatation Q61.11
    rapidly progressive N01.9
    subacute N01.9
  Rendu-Osler-Weber (familial hemorrhagic telangiectasia) I78.0
  renovascular (arteriosclerotic) — *see* Hypertension, kidney
  respiratory (tract) J98.9
    acute or subacute NOS J06.9
      due to
        chemicals, gases, fumes or vapors (inhalation) J68.3
          external agent J70.9
            specified NEC J70.8
          radiation J70.0
          smoke inhalation J70.5
      noninfectious J39.8
    chronic NOS J98.9
      due to
        chemicals, gases, fumes or vapors J68.4
          external agent J70.9
            specified NEC J70.8
          radiation J70.1
      newborn P27.9
        specified NEC P27.8
    due to
      chemicals, gases, fumes or vapors J68.9
        acute or subacute NEC J68.3
        chronic J68.4
      external agent J70.9
        specified NEC J70.8
    newborn P28.9
      specified type NEC P28.89
    upper J39.9
      acute or subacute J06.9
      noninfectious NEC J39.8
      specified NEC J39.8
      streptococcal J06.9
  retina, retinal H35.9
    Batten's or Batten-Mayou E75.4 [H36]
    specified NEC H35.89
  rheumatoid — *see* Arthritis, rheumatoid
  rickettsial NOS A79.9
    specified type NEC A79.89
  Riga (-Fede) (cachectic aphthae) K14.0
  Riggs' (compound periodontitis) — *see* Periodontitis
  Ritter's L00
  Rivalta's (cervicofacial actinomycosis) A42.2
  Robles' (onchocerciasis) B73.01
  Roger's (congenital interventricular septal defect) Q21.0
  Rosenthal's (factor XI deficiency) D68.1
  Ross River B33.1
  Rossbach's (hyperchlorhydria) K30
  Rotes Quérol — *see* Hyperostosis, ankylosing
  Roth (-Bernhardt) — *see* Mononeuropathy, lower limb, meralgia paresthetica
  Runeberg's (progressive pernicious anemia) D51.0
  sacroiliac NEC M53.3
  salivary gland or duct K11.9
    inclusion B25.9
    specified NEC K11.8
    virus B25.9
  sandworm B76.9
  Schimmelbusch's — *see* Mastopathy, cystic
  Schmorl's — *see* Schmorl's disease or nodes
  Schönlein (-Henoch) (purpura rheumatica) D69.0
  Schottmüller's — *see* Fever, paratyphoid
  Schultz's (agranulocytosis) — *see* Agranulocytosis
  Schwalbe-Ziehen-Oppenheim G24.1
  Schwartz-Jampel G71.13
  sclera H15.9
    specified NEC H15.89
  scrofulous (tuberculous) A18.2
  scrotum N50.9
  sebaceous glands L73.9
  semilunar cartilage, cystic (*see also* Derangement, knee, meniscus, cystic)
  seminal vesicle N50.9
  serum NEC (*see also* Reaction, serum) T80.69 ☑
  sexually transmitted A64
    anogenital
      herpesviral infection — *see* Herpes, anogenital

Disease, diseased — *continued*
  sexually transmitted — *continued*
    anogenital — *continued*
      warts A63.0
    chancroid A57
    chlamydial infection — *see* Chlamydia
    gonorrhea — *see* Gonorrhea
    granuloma inguinale A58
    specified organism NEC A63.8
    syphilis — *see* Syphilis
    trichomoniasis — *see* Trichomoniasis
  Sézary C84.1- ☑
  shimamushi (scrub typhus) A75.3
  shipyard B30.0
  sickle-cell D57.1
    with crisis (vasoocclusive pain) D57.00
      with
        acute chest syndrome D57.01
        splenic sequestration D57.02
    elliptocytosis D57.8- ☑
    Hb-C D57.20
      with crisis (vasoocclusive pain) D57.219
        with
          acute chest syndrome D57.211
          splenic sequestration D57.212
      without crisis D57.20
    Hb-SD D57.80
      with crisis D57.819
        with
          acute chest syndrome D57.811
          splenic sequestration D57.812
    Hb-SE D57.80
      with crisis D57.819
        with
          acute chest syndrome D57.811
          splenic sequestration D57.812
    specified NEC D57.80
      with crisis D57.819
        with
          acute chest syndrome D57.811
          splenic sequestration D57.812
    spherocytosis D57.80
      with crisis D57.819
        with
          acute chest syndrome D57.811
          splenic sequestration D57.812
    thalassemia D57.40
      with crisis (vasoocclusive pain) D57.419
        with
          acute chest syndrome D57.411
          splenic sequestration D57.412
      without crisis D57.40
  silo-filler's J68.8
    bronchitis J68.0
    pneumonitis J68.0
    pulmonary edema J68.1
  simian B B00.4
  Simons' (progressive lipodystrophy) E88.1
  sin nombre virus B33.4
  sinus — *see* Sinusitis
  Sirkari's B55.0
  sixth B08.20
    due to human herpesvirus 6 B08.21
    due to human herpesvirus 7 B08.22
  skin L98.9
    due to metabolic disorder NEC E88.9 [L99]
    specified NEC L98.8
  slim (HIV) B20
  small vessel I73.9
  Sneddon-Wilkinson (subcorneal pustular dermatosis) L13.1
  South African creeping B88.0
  spinal (cord) G95.9
    congenital Q06.9
    specified NEC G95.89
  spine (*see also* Spondylopathy)
    joint — *see* Dorsopathy
    tuberculous A18.01
  spinocerebellar (hereditary) G11.9
    specified NEC G11.8
  spleen D73.9
    amyloid E85.4 [D77]
    organic D73.9
    polycystic Q89.09
    postinfectional D73.89
  sponge-diver's — *see* Toxicity, venom, marine animal, sea anemone
  Startle Q89.8

Disease, diseased — *continued*
  Steinert's G71.11
  Sticker's (erythema infectiosum) B08.3
  Stieda's (calcification, knee joint) — *see* Bursitis, tibial collateral
  Stokes' (exophthalmic goiter) — *see* Hyperthyroidism, with, goiter (diffuse)
  Stokes-Adams (syncope with heart block) I45.9
  stomach K31.9
    functional, psychogenic F45.8
    specified NEC K31.89
  stonemason's J62.8
  storage
    glycogen — *see* Disease, glycogen storage
    mucopolysaccharide — *see* Mucopolysaccharidosis
  striatopallidal system NEC G25.89
  Stuart-Prower (congenital factor X deficiency) D68.2
  Stuart's (congenital factor X deficiency) D68.2
  subcutaneous tissue — *see* Disease, skin
  supporting structures of teeth K08.9
    specified NEC K08.8
  suprarenal (capsule) (gland) E27.9
    hyperfunction E27.0
    specified NEC E27.8
  sweat glands L74.9
    specified NEC L74.8
  Sweeley-Klionsky E75.21
  Swift (-Feer) — *see* Poisoning, mercury
  swimming-pool granuloma A31.1
  Sylvest's (epidemic pleurodynia) B33.0
  sympathetic nervous system G90.9
  synovium — *see* Disorder, synovium
  syphilitic — *see* Syphilis
  systemic tissue mast cell C96.2
  tanapox (virus) B08.71
  Tangier E78.6
  Tarral-Besnier (pityriasis rubra pilaris) L44.0
  Tauri's E74.09
  tear duct — *see* Disorder, lacrimal system
  tendon, tendinous (*see also* Disorder, tendon)
    nodular — *see* Trigger finger
  terminal vessel I73.9
  testis N50.9
  thalassemia Hb-S — *see* Disease, sickle-cell, thalassemia
  Thaysen-Gee (nontropical sprue) K90.0
  Thomsen G71.12
  throat J39.2
    septic J02.0
  thromboembolic — *see* Embolism
  thymus (gland) E32.9
    specified NEC E32.8
  thyroid (gland) E07.9
    heart (*see also* Hyperthyroidism) E05.90 [I43]
      with thyroid storm E05.91 [I43]
    specified NEC E07.89
  Tietze's M94.0
  tongue K14.9
    specified NEC K14.8
  tonsils, tonsillar (and adenoids) J35.9
  tooth, teeth K08.9
    hard tissues K03.9
      specified NEC K03.89
    pulp NEC K04.99
    specified NEC K08.8
  Tourette's F95.2
  trachea NEC J39.8
  tricuspid I07.9
    nonrheumatic I36.9
  triglyceride-storage — *see* Disease, glycogen storage
  trophoblastic — *see* Mole, hydatidiform
  tsutsugamushi A75.3
  tube (fallopian) (noninflammatory) N83.9
    inflammatory — *see* Salpingitis
    specified NEC N83.8
  tuberculous NEC — *see* Tuberculosis
  tubo-ovarian (noninflammatory) N83.9
    inflammatory — *see* Salpingo-oophoritis
    specified NEC N83.8
  tubotympanic, chronic — *see* Otitis, media, suppurative, chronic, tubotympanic
  tubulo-interstitial N15.9
    specified NEC N15.8
  tympanum — *see* Disorder, tympanic membrane
  Uhl's Q24.8
  Underwood's (sclerema neonatorum) P83.0
  Unverricht (-Lundborg) — *see* Epilepsy, generalized, idiopathic

Disease, diseased — continued
Urbach-Oppenheim (necrobiosis lipoidica diabeticorum) — see E08-E13 with .620
ureter N28.9
in (due to)
schistosomiasis (bilharziasis) B65.0 [N29]
urethra N36.9
specified NEC N36.8
urinary (tract) N39.9
bladder N32.9
specified NEC N32.89
specified NEC N39.8
uterus (noninflammatory) N85.9
infective — see Endometritis
inflammatory — see Endometritis
specified NEC N85.8
uveal tract (anterior) H21.9
posterior H31.9
vagabond's B85.1
vagina, vaginal (noninflammatory) N89.9
inflammatory NEC N76.89
specified NEC N89.8
valve, valvular I38
multiple I08.9
specified NEC I08.8
van Creveld-von Gierke (glycogenosis I) E74.01
vas deferens N50.9
vascular I99.9
arteriosclerotic — see Arteriosclerosis
ciliary body NEC — see Disorder, iris, vascular
hypertensive — see Hypertension
iris NEC — see Disorder, iris, vascular
obliterative I77.1
peripheral I73.9
occlusive I99.8
peripheral (occlusive) I73.9
in diabetes mellitus — see E08-E13 with .51
vasomotor I73.9
vasospastic I73.9
vein I87.9
venereal (see also Disease, sexually transmitted) A64
chlamydial NEC A56.8
anus A56.3
genitourinary NOS A56.2
pharynx A56.4
rectum A56.3
fifth A55
sixth A55
specified nature or type NEC A63.8
vertebra, vertebral (see also Spondylopathy)
disc — see Disorder, disc
vibration — see Vibration, adverse effects
viral, virus (see also Disease, by type of virus) B34.9
arbovirus NOS A94
arthropod-borne NOS A94
congenital P35.9
specified NEC P35.8
Hanta (with renal manifestations) (Dobrava) (Puumala) (Seoul) A98.5
with pulmonary manifestations (Andes) (Bayou)
(Bermejo) (Black Creek Canal) (Choclo)
(Juquitiba) (Laguna negra) (Lechiguanas)
(New York) (Oran) (Sin nombre) B33.4
Hantaan (Korean hemorrhagic fever) A98.5
human immunodeficiency (HIV) B20
Kunjin A83.4
nonarthropod-borne NOS B34.9
Powassan A84.8
Rocio (encephalitis) A83.6
Sin nombre (Hantavirus) (cardio)-pulmonary syndrome) B33.4
Tahyna B33.8
vesicular stomatitis A93.8
vitreous H43.9
specified NEC H43.89
vocal cord J38.3
Volkmann's, acquired T79.6 ☑
von Eulenburg's (congenital paramyotonia) G71.19
von Gierke's (glycogenosis I) E74.01
von Graefe's — see Strabismus, paralytic, ophthalmoplegia, progressive
von Willebrand (-Jürgens) (angiohemophilia) D68.0
Vrolik's (osteogenesis imperfecta) Q78.0
vulva (noninflammatory) N90.9
inflammatory NEC N76.89
specified NEC N90.89
Wallgren's (obstruction of splenic vein with collateral
circulation) I87.8

Disease, diseased — continued
Wassilieff's (leptospiral jaundice) A27.0
wasting NEC R64
due to malnutrition E41
Waterhouse-Friderichsen A39.1
Wegner's (syphilitic osteochondritis) A50.02
Weil's (leptospiral jaundice of lung) A27.0
Weir Mitchell's (erythromelalgia) I73.81
Werdnig-Hoffmann G12.0
Wermer's E31.21
Werner-His (trench fever) A79.0
Werner-Schultz (neutropenic splenomegaly) D73.81
Wernicke-Posadas B38.9
whipworm B79
white blood cells D72.9
specified NEC D72.89
white matter R90.82
white-spot, meaning lichen sclerosus et atrophicus
L90.0
penis N48.0
vulva N90.4
Wilkie's K55.1
Wilkinson-Sneddon (subcorneal pustular dermatosis)
L13.1
Willis' — see Diabetes
Wilson's (hepatolenticular degeneration) E83.01
woolsorter's A22.1
yaba monkey tumor B08.72
yaba pox (virus) B08.72
zoonotic, bacterial A28.9
specified type NEC A28.8
Disfigurement (due to scar) L90.5
Disgerminoma — see Dysgerminoma
DISH (diffuse idiopathic skeletal hyperostosis) — see
Hyperostosis, ankylosing
Disinsertion, retina — see Detachment, retina
Dislocatable hip, congenital Q65.6
Dislocation (articular)
with fracture — see Fracture
acromioclavicular (joint) S43.10- ☑
with displacement
100%-200% S43.12- ☑
more than 200% S43.13- ☑
inferior S43.14- ☑
posterior S43.15- ☑
ankle S93.0- ☑
astragalus — see Dislocation, ankle
atlantoaxial S13.121 ☑
atlantooccipital S13.111 ☑
atloidooccipital S13.111 ☑
breast bone S23.29 ☑
capsule, joint — code by site under Dislocation
carpal (bone) — see Dislocation, wrist
carpometacarpal (joint) NEC S63.05- ☑
thumb S63.04- ☑
cartilage (joint) — code by site under Dislocation
cervical spine (vertebra) — see Dislocation, vertebra,
cervical
chronic — see Dislocation, recurrent
clavicle — see Dislocation, acromioclavicular joint
coccyx S33.2 ☑
congenital NEC Q68.8
coracoid — see Dislocation, shoulder
costal cartilage S23.29 ☑
costochondral S23.29 ☑
cricoarytenoid articulation S13.29 ☑
cricothyroid articulation S13.29 ☑
dorsal vertebra — see Dislocation, vertebra, thoracic
ear ossicle — see Discontinuity, ossicles, ear
elbow S53.10- ☑
congenital Q68.8
pathological — see Dislocation, pathological NEC,
elbow
radial head alone — see Dislocation, radial head
recurrent — see Dislocation, recurrent, elbow
traumatic S53.10- ☑
anterior S53.11- ☑
lateral S53.14- ☑
medial S53.13- ☑
posterior S53.12- ☑
specified type NEC S53.19- ☑
eye, nontraumatic — see Luxation, globe
eyeball, nontraumatic — see Luxation, globe
femur
distal end — see Dislocation, knee
proximal end — see Dislocation, hip

Dislocation — continued
fibula
distal end — see Dislocation, ankle
proximal end — see Dislocation, knee
finger S63.25- ☑
index S63.25- ☑
interphalangeal S63.27- ☑
distal S63.29- ☑
index S63.29- ☑
little S63.29- ☑
middle S63.29- ☑
ring S63.29- ☑
index S63.27- ☑
little S63.27- ☑
middle S63.27- ☑
proximal S63.28- ☑
index S63.28- ☑
little S63.28- ☑
middle S63.28- ☑
ring S63.28- ☑
ring S63.27- ☑
little S63.25- ☑
metacarpophalangeal S63.26- ☑
index S63.26- ☑
little S63.26- ☑
middle S63.26- ☑
ring S63.26- ☑
middle S63.25- ☑
recurrent — see Dislocation, recurrent, finger
ring S63.25- ☑
thumb — see Dislocation, thumb
foot S93.30- ☑
recurrent — see Dislocation, recurrent, foot
specified site NEC S93.33- ☑
tarsal joint S93.31- ☑
tarsometatarsal joint S93.32- ☑
toe — see Dislocation, toe
fracture — see Fracture
glenohumeral (joint) — see Dislocation, shoulder
glenoid — see Dislocation, shoulder
habitual — see Dislocation, recurrent
hip S73.00- ☑
anterior S73.03- ☑
obturator S73.02- ☑
central S73.04- ☑
congenital (total) Q65.2
bilateral Q65.1
partial Q65.5
bilateral Q65.4
unilateral Q65.3- ☑
unilateral Q65.0- ☑
developmental M24.85- ☑
pathological — see Dislocation, pathological NEC,
hip
posterior S73.01- ☑
recurrent — see Dislocation, recurrent, hip
humerus, proximal end — see Dislocation, shoulder
incomplete — see Subluxation, by site
incus — see Discontinuity, ossicles, ear
infracoracoid — see Dislocation, shoulder
innominate (pubic junction) (sacral junction) S33.39 ☑
acetabulum — see Dislocation, hip
interphalangeal (joint(s))
finger S63.279 ☑
distal S63.29- ☑
index S63.29- ☑
little S63.29- ☑
middle S63.29- ☑
ring S63.29- ☑
index S63.27- ☑
little S63.27- ☑
middle S63.27- ☑
proximal S63.28- ☑
index S63.28- ☑
little S63.28- ☑
middle S63.28- ☑
ring S63.28- ☑
ring S63.27- ☑
foot or toe — see Dislocation, toe
thumb S63.12- ☑
distal joint S63.14- ☑
proximal joint S63.13- ☑
jaw (cartilage) (meniscus) S03.0 ☑
joint prosthesis — see Complications, joint prosthesis,
mechanical, displacement, by site
knee S83.106 ☑

☑ **Additional Character Required** — Refer to the Tabular List for Character Selection   ⬚ Subterms under main terms may continue to next column or page

Dislocation — *continued*
  knee S83.106 ☑
    cap — *see* Dislocation, patella
    congenital Q68.2
    old M23.8X- ☑
    patella — *see* Dislocation, patella
    pathological — *see* Dislocation, pathological NEC, knee
    proximal tibia
      anteriorly S83.11- ☑
      laterally S83.14- ☑
      medially S83.13- ☑
      posteriorly S83.12- ☑
    recurrent (*see also* Derangement, knee, specified NEC)
    specified type NEC S83.19- ☑
  lacrimal gland H04.16- ☑
  lens (complete) H27.10
    anterior H27.12- ☑
    congenital Q12.1
    ocular implant — *see* Complications, intraocular lens
    partial H27.11- ☑
    posterior H27.13- ☑
    traumatic S05.8X- ☑
  ligament — *code by* site under Dislocation
  lumbar (vertebra) — *see* Dislocation, vertebra, lumbar
  lumbosacral (vertebra) (*see also* Dislocation, vertebra, lumbar)
    congenital Q76.49
  mandible S03.0 ☑
  meniscus (knee) — *see* Tear, meniscus
    other sites - code by site under Dislocation
  metacarpal (bone)
    distal end — *see* Dislocation, finger
    proximal end S63.06- ☑
  metacarpophalangeal (joint)
    finger S63.26- ☑
      index S63.26- ☑
      little S63.26- ☑
      middle S63.26- ☑
      ring S63.26- ☑
      thumb S63.11- ☑
  metatarsal (bone) — *see* Dislocation, foot
  metatarsophalangeal (joint(s)) — *see* Dislocation, toe
  midcarpal (joint) S63.03- ☑
  midtarsal (joint) — *see* Dislocation, foot
  neck S13.20 ☑
    specified site NEC S13.29 ☑
    vertebra — *see* Dislocation, vertebra, cervical
  nose (septal cartilage) S03.1 ☑
  occipitoatloid S13.111 ☑
  old — *see* Derangement, joint, specified type NEC
  ossicles, ear — *see* Discontinuity, ossicles, ear
  partial — *see* Subluxation, by site
  patella S83.006 ☑
    congenital Q74.1
    lateral S83.01- ☑
    recurrent (nontraumatic) M22.0- ☑
      incomplete M22.1- ☑
    specified type NEC S83.09- ☑
  pathological NEC M24.30
    ankle M24.37- ☑
    elbow M24.32- ☑
    foot joint M24.37- ☑
    hand joint M24.34- ☑
    hip M24.35- ☑
    knee M24.36- ☑
    lumbosacral joint — *see* subcategory M53.2 ☑
    pelvic region — *see* Dislocation, pathological, hip
    sacroiliac — *see* subcategory M53.2 ☑
    shoulder M24.31- ☑
    wrist M24.33- ☑
  pelvis NEC S33.30 ☑
    specified NEC S33.39 ☑
  phalanx
    finger or hand — *see* Dislocation, finger
    foot or toe — *see* Dislocation, toe
  prosthesis, internal — *see* Complications, prosthetic device, by site, mechanical
  radial head S53.006 ☑
    anterior S53.01- ☑
    posterior S53.02- ☑
    specified type NEC S53.09- ☑
  radiocarpal (joint) S63.02- ☑
  radiohumeral (joint) — *see* Dislocation, radial head

Dislocation — *continued*
  radioulnar (joint)
    distal S63.01- ☑
    proximal — *see* Dislocation, elbow
  radius
    distal end — *see* Dislocation, wrist
    proximal end — *see* Dislocation, radial head
  recurrent M24.40
    ankle M24.47- ☑
    elbow M24.42- ☑
    finger M24.44- ☑
    foot joint M24.47- ☑
    hand joint M24.44- ☑
    hip M24.45- ☑
    knee M24.46- ☑
      patella — *see* Dislocation, patella, recurrent
    patella — *see* Dislocation, patella, recurrent
    sacroiliac — *see* subcategory M53.2 ☑
    shoulder M24.41- ☑
    toe M24.47- ☑
    vertebra (*see also* subcategory) M43.5 ☑
      atlantoaxial M43.4
        with myelopathy M43.3
    wrist M24.43- ☑
  rib (cartilage) S23.29 ☑
  sacrococcygeal S33.2 ☑
  sacroiliac (joint) (ligament) S33.2 ☑
    congenital Q74.2
    recurrent — *see* subcategory M53.2 ☑
  sacrum S33.2 ☑
  scaphoid (bone) (hand) (wrist) — *see* Dislocation, wrist
    foot — *see* Dislocation, foot
  scapula — *see* Dislocation, shoulder, girdle, scapula
  semilunar cartilage, knee — *see* Tear, meniscus
  septal cartilage (nose) S03.1 ☑
  septum (nasal) (old) J34.2
  sesamoid bone — *code by* site under Dislocation
  shoulder (blade) (ligament) (joint) (traumatic) S43.006 ☑
    acromioclavicular — *see* Dislocation, acromioclavicular
    chronic — *see* Dislocation, recurrent, shoulder
    congenital Q68.8
    girdle S43.30- ☑
      scapula S43.31- ☑
      specified site NEC S43.39- ☑
    humerus S43.00- ☑
      anterior S43.01- ☑
      inferior S43.03- ☑
      posterior S43.02- ☑
    pathological — *see* Dislocation, pathological NEC, shoulder
    recurrent — *see* Dislocation, recurrent, shoulder
    specified type NEC S43.08- ☑
  spine
    cervical — *see* Dislocation, vertebra, cervical
    congenital Q76.49
    due to birth trauma P11.5
    lumbar — *see* Dislocation, vertebra, lumbar
    thoracic — *see* Dislocation, vertebra, thoracic
  spontaneous — *see* Dislocation, pathological
  sternoclavicular (joint) S43.206 ☑
    anterior S43.21- ☑
    posterior S43.22- ☑
  sternum S23.29 ☑
  subglenoid — *see* Dislocation, shoulder
  symphysis pubis S33.4 ☑
  talus — *see* Dislocation, ankle
  tarsal (bone(s)) (joint(s)) — *see* Dislocation, foot
  tarsometatarsal (joint(s)) — *see* Dislocation, foot
  temporomandibular (joint) S03.0 ☑
  thigh, proximal end — *see* Dislocation, hip
  thorax S23.20 ☑
    specified site NEC S23.29 ☑
    vertebra — *see* Dislocation, vertebra
  thumb S63.10- ☑
    interphalangeal joint — *see* Dislocation, interphalangeal (joint), thumb
    metacarpophalangeal joint — *see* Dislocation, metacarpophalangeal (joint), thumb
  thyroid cartilage S13.29 ☑
  tibia
    distal end — *see* Dislocation, ankle
    proximal end — *see* Dislocation, knee
  tibiofibular (joint)
    distal — *see* Dislocation, ankle

Dislocation — *continued*
  tibiofibular — *continued*
    superior — *see* Dislocation, knee
  toe(s) S93.106 ☑
    great S93.10- ☑
      interphalangeal joint S93.11- ☑
      metatarsophalangeal joint S93.12- ☑
    interphalangeal joint S93.119 ☑
    lesser S93.106 ☑
      interphalangeal joint S93.11- ☑
      metatarsophalangeal joint S93.12- ☑
    metatarsophalangeal joint S93.12- ☑
  tooth S03.2 ☑
  trachea S23.29 ☑
  ulna
    distal end S63.07- ☑
    proximal end — *see* Dislocation, elbow
  ulnohumeral (joint) — *see* Dislocation, elbow
  vertebra (articular process) (body) (traumatic)
    cervical S13.101 ☑
      atlantoaxial joint S13.121 ☑
      atlantooccipital joint S13.111 ☑
      atloidooccipital joint S13.111 ☑
      joint between
        C0 and C1 S13.111 ☑
        C1 and C2 S13.121 ☑
        C2 and C3 S13.131 ☑
        C3 and C4 S13.141 ☑
        C4 and C5 S13.151 ☑
        C5 and C6 S13.161 ☑
        C6 and C7 S13.171 ☑
        C7 and T1 S13.181 ☑
      occipitoatloid joint S13.111 ☑
    congenital Q76.49
    lumbar S33.101 ☑
      joint between
        L1 and L2 S33.111 ☑
        L2 and L3 S33.121 ☑
        L3 and L4 S33.131 ☑
        L4 and L5 S33.141 ☑
    nontraumatic — *see* Displacement, intervertebral disc
    partial — *see* Subluxation, by site
    recurrent NEC — *see* subcategory M43.5 ☑
    thoracic S23.101 ☑
      joint between
        T1 and T2 S23.111 ☑
        T2 and T3 S23.121 ☑
        T3 and T4 S23.123 ☑
        T4 and T5 S23.131 ☑
        T5 and T6 S23.133 ☑
        T6 and T7 S23.141 ☑
        T7 and T8 S23.143 ☑
        T8 and T9 S23.151 ☑
        T9 and T10 S23.153 ☑
        T10 and T11 S23.161 ☑
        T11 and T12 S23.163 ☑
        T12 and L1 S23.171 ☑
  wrist (carpal bone) S63.006 ☑
    carpometacarpal joint — *see* Dislocation, carpometacarpal (joint)
    distal radioulnar joint — *see* Dislocation, radioulnar (joint), distal
    metacarpal bone, proximal — *see* Dislocation, metacarpal (bone), proximal end
    midcarpal — *see* Dislocation, midcarpal (joint)
    radiocarpal joint — *see* Dislocation, radiocarpal (joint)
    recurrent — *see* Dislocation, recurrent, wrist
    specified site NEC S63.09- ☑
    ulna — *see* Dislocation, ulna, distal end
  xiphoid cartilage S23.29 ☑
Disorder (of) (*see also* Disease)
  acantholytic L11.9
    specified NEC L11.8
  acute
    psychotic — *see* Psychosis, acute
    stress F43.0
  adjustment (grief) F43.20
    with
      anxiety F43.22
        with depressed mood F43.23
      conduct disturbance F43.24
        with emotional disturbance F43.25
      depressed mood F43.21
        with anxiety F43.23

Index

Disorder — Disorder

Disorder — *continued*
  adjustment — *continued*
    with — *continued*
      other specified symptom F43.29
    adrenal (capsule) (gland) (medullary) E27.9
      specified NEC E27.8
  adrenogenital E25.9
    drug-induced E25.8
    iatrogenic E25.8
    idiopathic E25.8
  adult personality (and behavior) F69
    specified NEC F68.8
  affective (mood) — *see* Disorder, mood
  aggressive, unsocialized F91.1
  alcohol-related F10.99
    with
      amnestic disorder, persisting F10.96
      anxiety disorder F10.980
      dementia, persisting F10.97
      intoxication F10.929
        with delirium F10.921
        uncomplicated F10.920
      mood disorder F10.94
      other specified F10.988
      psychotic disorder F10.959
        with
          delusions F10.950
          hallucinations F10.951
      sexual dysfunction F10.981
      sleep disorder F10.982
  allergic — *see* Allergy
  alveolar NEC J84.09
  amino-acid
    cystathioninuria E72.19
    cystinosis E72.04
    cystinuria E72.01
    glycinuria E72.09
    homocystinuria E72.11
    metabolism — *see* Disturbance, metabolism,
      amino-acid
      specified NEC E72.8
    neonatal, transitory P74.8
    renal transport NEC E72.09
    transport NEC E72.09
  amnesic, amnestic
    alcohol-induced F10.96
      with dependence F10.26
    due to (secondary to) general medical condition
      F04
    psychoactive NEC-induced F19.96
      with
        abuse F19.16
        dependence F19.26
    sedative, hypnotic or anxiolytic-induced F13.96
      with dependence F13.26
  anaerobic glycolysis with anemia D55.2
  anxiety F41.9
    due to (secondary to)
      alcohol F10.980
      amphetamine F15.980
        in
          abuse F15.180
          dependence F15.280
      anxiolytic F13.980
        in
          abuse F13.180
          dependence F13.280
      caffeine F15.980
        in
          abuse F15.180
          dependence F15.280
      cannabis F12.980
        in
          abuse F12.180
          dependence F12.280
      cocaine F14.980
        in
          abuse F14.180
          dependence F14.180
      general medical condition F06.4
      hallucinogen F16.980
        in
          abuse F16.180
          dependence F16.280
      hypnotic F13.980
        in
          abuse F13.180
          dependence F13.280

Disorder — *continued*
  anxiety — *continued*
    due to — *continued*
      inhalant F18.980
        in
          abuse F18.180
          dependence F18.280
      phencyclidine F16.980
        in
          abuse F16.180
          dependence F16.280
      psychoactive substance NEC F19.980
        in
          abuse F19.180
          dependence F19.280
      sedative F13.980
        in
          abuse F13.180
          dependence F13.280
      volatile solvents F18.980
        in
          abuse F18.180
          dependence F18.280
    generalized F41.1
    mixed
      with depression (mild) F41.8
      specified NEC F41.3
    organic F06.4
    phobic F40.9
      of childhood F40.8
    specified NEC F41.8
  aortic valve — *see* Endocarditis, aortic
  aromatic amino-acid metabolism E70.9
    specified NEC E70.8
  arteriole NEC I77.89
  artery NEC I77.89
  articulation — *see* Disorder, joint
  attachment (childhood)
    disinhibited F94.2
    reactive F94.1
  attention-deficit hyperactivity (adolescent) (adult)
    (child) F90.9
    combined type F90.2
    hyperactive type F90.1
    inattentive type F90.0
    specified type NEC F90.8
  attention-deficit without hyperactivity (adolescent)
    (adult) (child) F90.0
  auditory processing (central) H93.25
  autistic F84.0
  autonomic nervous system G90.9
    specified NEC G90.8
  avoidant, child or adolescent F40.10
  balance
    acid-base E87.8
      mixed E87.4
    electrolyte E87.8
    fluid NEC E87.8
  behavioral (disruptive) — *see* Disorder, conduct
  beta-amino-acid metabolism E72.8
  bile acid and cholesterol metabolism E78.70
    Barth syndrome E78.71
    other specified E78.79
    Smith-Lemli-Opitz syndrome E78.72
  bilirubin excretion E80.6
  binocular
    movement H51.9
      convergence
        excess H51.12
        insufficiency H51.11
      internuclear ophthalmoplegia — *see* Ophthal-
        moplegia, internuclear
      palsy of conjugate gaze H51.0
      specified type NEC H51.8
    vision NEC — *see* Disorder, vision, binocular
  bipolar (I) F31.9
    current episode
      depressed F31.9
        with psychotic features F31.5
        without psychotic features F31.30
          mild F31.31
          moderate F31.32
          severe (without psychotic features) F31.4
            with psychotic features F31.5
      hypomanic F31.0
      manic F31.9
        with psychotic features F31.2

Disorder — *continued*
  bipolar — *continued*
    current episode — *continued*
      manic — *continued*
        without psychotic features F31.10
          mild F31.11
          moderate F31.12
          severe (without psychotic features)
            F31.13
            with psychotic features F31.2
        mixed F31.60
          mild F31.61
          moderate F31.62
          severe (without psychotic features) F31.63
            with psychotic features F31.64
        severe depression (without psychotic features)
          F31.4
          with psychotic features F31.5
    in remission (currently) F31.70
      in full remission
        most recent episode
          depressed F31.76
          hypomanic F31.72
          manic F31.74
          mixed F31.78
      in partial remission
        most recent episode
          depressed F31.75
          hypomanic F31.71
          manic F31.73
          mixed F31.77
    organic F06.30
    single manic episode F30.9
      mild F30.11
      moderate F30.12
      severe (without psychotic symptoms) F30.13
        with psychotic symptoms F30.2
    specified NEC F31.89
  bipolar II F31.81
  bladder N32.9
    functional NEC N31.9
    in schistosomiasis B65.0 [N33]
    specified NEC N32.89
  bleeding D68.9
  blood D75.9
    in congenital early syphilis A50.09 [D77]
  body dysmorphic F45.22
  bone M89.9
    continuity M84.9
      specified type NEC M84.80
        ankle M84.87- ☑
        fibula M84.86- ☑
        foot M84.87- ☑
        hand M84.84- ☑
        humerus M84.82- ☑
        neck M84.88
        pelvis M84.859
        radius M84.83- ☑
        rib M84.88
        shoulder M84.81- ☑
        skull M84.88
        thigh M84.85- ☑
        tibia M84.86- ☑
        ulna M84.83- ☑
        vertebra M84.88
    density and structure M85.9
      cyst (see also Cyst, bone, specified type NEC)
        aneurysmal — *see* Cyst, bone, aneurysmal
        solitary — *see* Cyst, bone, solitary
      diffuse idiopathic skeletal hyperostosis — *see*
        Hyperostosis, ankylosing
      fibrous dysplasia (monostotic) — *see* Dysplasia,
        fibrous, bone
      fluorosis — *see* Fluorosis, skeletal
      hyperostosis of skull M85.2
      osteitis condensans — *see* Osteitis, condensans
      specified type NEC M85.8- ☑
        ankle M85.87- ☑
        foot M85.87- ☑
        forearm M85.83- ☑
        hand M85.84- ☑
        lower leg M85.86- ☑
        multiple sites M85.89
        neck M85.88
        rib M85.88
        shoulder M85.81- ☑
        skull M85.88
        thigh M85.85- ☑

☑ **Additional Character Required** — **Refer to the Tabular List for Character Selection**　　▽ **Subterms under main terms may continue to next column or page**

Disorder — *continued*
 bone — *continued*
  density and structure — *continued*
   specified type — *continued*
    upper arm M85.82- ☑
    vertebra M85.88
  development and growth NEC M89.20
   carpus M89.24- ☑
   clavicle M89.21- ☑
   femur M89.25- ☑
   fibula M89.26- ☑
   finger M89.24- ☑
   humerus M89.22- ☑
   ilium M89.259
   ischium M89.259
   metacarpus M89.24- ☑
   metatarsus M89.27- ☑
   multiple sites M89.29
   neck M89.28
   radius M89.23- ☑
   rib M89.28
   scapula M89.21- ☑
   skull M89.28
   tarsus M89.27- ☑
   tibia M89.26- ☑
   toe M89.27- ☑
   ulna M89.23- ☑
   vertebra M89.28
  specified type NEC M89.8X- ☑
 brachial plexus G54.0
 branched-chain amino-acid metabolism E71.2
  specified NEC E71.19
 breast N64.9
  agalactia — *see* Agalactia
  associated with
   lactation O92.70
    specified NEC O92.79
   pregnancy O92.20
    specified NEC O92.29
   puerperium O92.20
    specified NEC O92.29
  cracked nipple — *see* Cracked nipple
  galactorrhea — *see* Galactorrhea
  hypogalactia O92.4
  lactation disorder NEC O92.79
  mastitis — *see* Mastitis
  nipple infection — *see* Infection, nipple
  retracted nipple — *see* Retraction, nipple
  specified type NEC N64.89
 Briquet's F45.0
 bullous, in diseases classified elsewhere L14
 cannabis use
  due to drug abuse — *see* Abuse, drug, cannabis
  due to drug dependence — *see* Dependence, drug, cannabis
 carbohydrate
  absorption, intestinal NEC E74.39
  metabolism (congenital) E74.9
   specified NEC E74.8
 cardiac, functional I51.89
 carnitine metabolism E71.40
 cartilage M94.9
  articular NEC — *see* Derangement, joint, articular cartilage
  chondrocalcinosis — *see* Chondrocalcinosis
  specified type NEC M94.8X- ☑
   articular — *see* Derangement, joint, articular cartilage
   multiple sites M94.8X0
 catatonic
  due to (secondary to) known physiological condition F06.1
  organic F06.1
 central auditory processing H93.25
 cervical
  region NEC M53.82
  root (nerve) NEC G54.2
 character NOS F60.9
 childhood disintegrative NEC F84.3
 cholesterol and bile acid metabolism E78.70
  Barth syndrome E78.71
  other specified E78.79
  Smith-Lemli-Opitz syndrome E78.72
 choroid H31.9
  atrophy — *see* Atrophy, choroid
  degeneration — *see* Degeneration, choroid
  detachment — *see* Detachment, choroid

Disorder — *continued*
 choroid — *continued*
  dystrophy — *see* Dystrophy, choroid
  hemorrhage — *see* Hemorrhage, choroid
  rupture — *see* Rupture, choroid
  scar — *see* Scar, chorioretinal
  solar retinopathy — *see* Retinopathy, solar
  specified type NEC H31.8
 ciliary body — *see* Disorder, iris
  degeneration — *see* Degeneration, ciliary body
 coagulation (factor) (*see also* Defect, coagulation) D68.9
  newborn, transient P61.6
 coccyx NEC M53.3
 cognitive F09
  due to (secondary to) general medical condition F09
  persisting R41.89
   due to
    alcohol F10.97
     with dependence F10.27
    anxiolytics F13.97
     with dependence F13.27
    hypnotics F13.97
     with dependence F13.27
    sedatives F13.97
     with dependence F13.27
    specified substance NEC F19.97
     with
      abuse F19.17
      dependence F19.27
 communication F80.9
 conduct (childhood) F91.9
  adjustment reaction — *see* Disorder, adjustment
  adolescent onset type F91.2
  childhood onset type F91.1
  compulsive F63.9
  confined to family context F91.0
  depressive F91.8
  group type F91.2
  hyperkinetic — *see* Disorder, attention-deficit hyperactivity
  oppositional defiance F91.3
  socialized F91.2
  solitary aggressive type F91.1
  specified NEC F91.8
  unsocialized (aggressive) F91.1
 conduction, heart I45.9
 congenital glycosylation (CDG) E74.8
 conjunctiva H11.9
  infection — *see* Conjunctivitis
 connective tissue, localized L94.9
  specified NEC L94.8
 conversion — *see* Disorder, dissociative
 convulsive (secondary) — *see* Convulsions
 cornea H18.9
  deformity — *see* Deformity, cornea
  degeneration — *see* Degeneration, cornea
  deposits — *see* Deposit, cornea
  due to contact lens H18.82- ☑
   specified as edema — *see* Edema, cornea
  edema — *see* Edema, cornea
  keratitis — *see* Keratitis
  keratoconjunctivitis — *see* Keratoconjunctivitis
  membrane change — *see* Change, corneal membrane
  neovascularization — *see* Neovascularization, cornea
  scar — *see* Opacity, cornea
  specified type NEC H18.89- ☑
  ulcer — *see* Ulcer, cornea
 corpus cavernosum N48.9
 cranial nerve — *see* Disorder, nerve, cranial
 cyclothymic F34.0
 defiant oppositional F91.3
 delusional (persistent) (systematized) F22
  induced F24
 depersonalization F48.1
 depressive F32.9
  major F32.9
   with psychotic symptoms F32.3
   in remission (full) F32.5
    partial F32.4
   recurrent F33.9
   single episode F32.9
    mild F32.0
    moderate F32.1

Disorder — *continued*
 depressive — *continued*
  major — *continued*
   single episode — *continued*
    severe (without psychotic symptoms) F32.2
     with psychotic symptoms F32.3
   organic F06.31
   recurrent F33.9
    current episode
     mild F33.0
     moderate F33.1
     severe (without psychotic symptoms) F33.2
      with psychotic symptoms F33.3
    in remission F33.40
     full F33.42
     partial F33.41
    specified NEC F33.8
   single episode — *see* Episode, depressive
 developmental F89
  arithmetical skills F81.2
  coordination (motor) F82
  expressive writing F81.81
  language F80.9
   expressive F80.1
   mixed receptive and expressive F80.2
   receptive type F80.2
   specified NEC F80.89
  learning F81.9
   arithmetical F81.2
   reading F81.0
  mixed F88
  motor coordination or function F82
  pervasive F84.9
   specified NEC F84.8
  phonological F80.0
  reading F81.0
  scholastic skills (*see also* Disorder, learning)
   mixed F81.89
  specified NEC F88
  speech F80.9
   articulation F80.0
   specified NEC F80.89
  written expression F81.81
 diaphragm J98.6
 digestive (system) K92.9
  newborn P78.9
   specified NEC P78.89
  postprocedural — *see* Complication, gastrointestinal
  psychogenic F45.8
 disc (intervertebral) M51.9
  with
   myelopathy
    cervical region M50.00
    cervicothoracic region M50.03
    high cervical region M50.01
    lumbar region M51.06
    mid-cervical region M50.02
    sacrococcygeal region M53.3
    thoracic region M51.04
    thoracolumbar region M51.05
   radiculopathy
    cervical region M50.10
    cervicothoracic region M50.13
    high cervical region M50.11
    lumbar region M51.16
    lumbosacral region M51.17
    mid-cervical region M50.12
    sacrococcygeal region M53.3
    thoracic region M51.14
    thoracolumbar region M51.15
  cervical M50.90
   with
    myelopathy M50.00
     C2-C3 M50.01
     C3-C4 M50.01
     C4-C5 M50.02
     C5-C6 M50.02
     C6-C7 M50.02
     C7-T1 M50.03
     cervicothoracic region M50.03
     high cervical region M50.01
     mid-cervical region M50.02
    neuritis, radiculitis or radiculopathy M50.10
     C2-C3 M50.11
     C3-C4 M50.11
     C4-C5 M50.12
     C5-C6 M50.12

Disorder — *continued*
  disc — *continued*
    cervical — *continued*
      with — *continued*
        neuritis, radiculitis or radiculopathy — *continued*
          C6-C7 M50.12
          C7-T1 M50.13
          cervicothoracic region M50.13
          high cervical region M50.11
          mid-cervical region M50.12
        C2-C3 M50.91
        C3-C4 M50.91
        C4-C5 M50.92
        C5-C6 M50.92
        C6-C7 M50.92
        C7-T1 M50.93
        cervicothoracic region M50.93
        degeneration M50.30
          C2-C3 M50.31
          C3-C4 M50.31
          C4-C5 M50.32
          C5-C6 M50.32
          C6-C7 M50.32
          C7-T1 M50.33
          cervicothoracic region M50.33
          high cervical region M50.31
          mid-cervical region M50.32
        displacement M50.20
          C2-C3 M50.21
          C3-C4 M50.21
          C4-C5 M50.22
          C5-C6 M50.22
          C6-C7 M50.22
          C7-T1 M50.23
          cervicothoracic region M50.23
          high cervical region M50.21
          mid-cervical region M50.22
        high cervical region M50.91
        mid-cervical region M50.92
        specified type NEC M50.80
          C2-C3 M50.81
          C3-C4 M50.81
          C4-C5 M50.82
          C5-C6 M50.82
          C6-C7 M50.82
          C7-T1 M50.83
          cervicothoracic region M50.83
          high cervical region M50.81
          mid-cervical region M50.82
      specified NEC
        lumbar region M51.86
        lumbosacral region M51.87
        sacrococcygeal region M53.3
        thoracic region M51.84
        thoracolumbar region M51.85
  disinhibited attachment (childhood) F94.2
  disintegrative, childhood NEC F84.3
  disruptive behavior F98.9
  dissocial personality F60.2
  dissociative F44.9
    affecting
      motor function F44.4
        and sensation F44.7
      sensation F44.6
        and motor function F44.7
    brief reactive F43.0
    due to (secondary to) general medical condition F06.8
    mixed F44.7
    organic F06.8
    other specified NEC F44.89
  double heterozygous sickling — *see* Disease, sickle-cell
  dream anxiety F51.5
  drug induced hemorrhagic D68.32
  drug related F19.99
    abuse — *see* Abuse, drug
    dependence — *see* Dependence, drug
  dysmorphic body F45.1
  dysthymic F34.1
  ear H93.9- ☑
    bleeding — *see* Otorrhagia
    deafness — *see* Deafness
    degenerative H93.09- ☑
    discharge — *see* Otorrhea

Disorder — *continued*
  ear — *continued*
    external H61.9- ☑
      auditory canal stenosis — *see* Stenosis, external ear canal
      exostosis — *see* Exostosis, external ear canal
      impacted cerumen — *see* Impaction, cerumen
      otitis — *see* Otitis, externa
      perichondritis — *see* Perichondritis, ear
      pinna — *see* Disorder, pinna
      specified type NEC H61.89- ☑
    inner H83.9- ☑
      vestibular dysfunction — *see* Disorder, vestibular function
    middle H74.9- ☑
      adhesive H74.1- ☑
      ossicle — *see* Abnormal, ear ossicles
      polyp — *see* Polyp, ear (middle)
      specified NEC, in diseases classified elsewhere H75.8- ☑
    postprocedural — *see* Complications, ear, procedure
    specified NEC, in diseases classified elsewhere H94.8- ☑
  eating (adult) (psychogenic) F50.9
    anorexia — *see* Anorexia
    bulimia F50.2
    child F98.29
      pica F98.3
      rumination disorder F98.21
    pica F50.8
      childhood F98.3
  electrolyte (balance) NEC E87.8
    with
      abortion — *see* Abortion by type complicated by specified condition NEC
      ectopic pregnancy O08.5
      molar pregnancy O08.5
    acidosis (metabolic) (respiratory) E87.2
    alkalosis (metabolic) (respiratory) E87.3
  elimination, transepidermal L87.9
    specified NEC L87.8
  emotional (persistent) F34.9
    of childhood F93.9
      specified NEC F93.8
  endocrine E34.9
    postprocedural E89.89
      specified NEC E89.89
  erectile (male) (organic) (*see also* Dysfunction, sexual, male, erectile) N52.9
    nonorganic F52.21
  erythematous — *see* Erythema
  esophagus K22.9
    functional K22.4
    psychogenic F45.8
  eustachian tube H69.9- ☑
    infection — *see* Salpingitis, eustachian
    obstruction — *see* Obstruction, eustachian tube
    patulous — *see* Patulous, eustachian tube
    specified NEC H69.8- ☑
  extrapyramidal G25.9
    in deseases classified elsewhere — *see* category G26
    specified type NEC G25.89
  eye H57.9
    postprocedural — *see* Complication, postprocedural, eye
  eyelid H02.9
    cyst — *see* Cyst, eyelid
    degenerative H02.70
      chloasma — *see* Chloasma, eyelid
      madarosis — *see* Madarosis
      specified type NEC H02.79
      vitiligo — *see* Vitiligo, eyelid
      xanthelasma — *see* Xanthelasma
    dermatochalasis — *see* Dermatochalasis
    edema — *see* Edema, eyelid
    elephantiasis — *see* Elephantiasis, eyelid
    foreign body, retained — *see* Foreign body, retained, eyelid
    function H02.59
      abnormal innervation syndrome — *see* Syndrome, abnormal innervation
      blepharochalasis — *see* Blepharochalasis
      blepharoclonus — *see* Blepharoclonus
      blepharophimosis — *see* Blepharophimosis
      blepharoptosis — *see* Blepharoptosis

Disorder — *continued*
  eyelid — *continued*
    function — *continued*
      lagophthalmos — *see* Lagophthalmos
      lid retraction — *see* Retraction, lid
      hypertrichosis — *see* Hypertrichosis, eyelid
      specified type NEC H02.89
    vascular H02.879
      left H02.876
        lower H02.875
        upper H02.874
      right H02.873
        lower H02.872
        upper H02.871
  factitious F68.10
    with predominantly
      physical symptoms F68.12
        with psychological symptoms F68.13
      psychological symptoms F68.11
        with physical symptoms F68.13
  factor, coagulation — *see* Defect, coagulation
  fatty acid
    metabolism E71.30
      specified NEC E71.39
    oxidation
      LCAD E71.310
      MCAD E71.311
      SCAD E71.312
      specified deficiency NEC E71.318
  feeding (infant or child) (*see also* Disorder, eating) R63.3
  feigned (with obvious motivation) Z76.5
    without obvious motivation — *see* Disorder, factitious
  female
    hypoactive sexual desire F52.0
    orgasmic F52.31
    sexual arousal F52.22
  fibroblastic M72.9
    specified NEC M72.8
  fluency
    adult onset F98.5
    childhood onset F80.81
    following
      cerebral infarction I69.323
      cerebrovascular disease I69.923
        specified disease NEC I69.823
      intracerebral hemorrhage I69.123
      nontraumatic intracranial hemorrhage NEC I69.223
      subarachnoid hemorrhage I69.023
    in conditions classified elsewhere R47.82
  fluid balance E87.8
  follicular (skin) L73.9
    specified NEC L73.8
  fructose metabolism E74.10
    essential fructosuria E74.11
    fructokinase deficiency E74.11
    fructose-1, 6-diphosphatase deficiency E74.19
    hereditary fructose intolerance E74.12
    other specified E74.19
  functional polymorphonuclear neutrophils D71
  gallbladder, biliary tract and pancreas in diseases classified elsewhere K87
  gamma-glutamyl cycle E72.8
  gastric (functional) K31.9
    motility K30
    psychogenic F45.8
    secretion K30
  gastrointestinal (functional) NOS K92.9
    newborn P78.9
    psychogenic F45.8
  gender-identity or -role F64.9
    childhood F64.2
    effect on relationship F66
    of adolescence or adulthood (nontranssexual) F64.1
    specified NEC F64.8
    uncertainty F66
  genitourinary system
    female N94.9
    male N50.9
    psychogenic F45.8
  globe H44.9
    degenerated condition H44.50
      absolute glaucoma H44.51- ☑
      atrophy H44.52- ☑
      leucocoria H44.53- ☑
    degenerative H44.30

☑ **Additional Character Required** — Refer to the Tabular List for Character Selection   🔻 **Subterms under main terms may continue to next column or page**

Disorder — *continued*
  globe — *continued*
    degenerative H44.3Ø
      chalcosis H44.31- ☑
      myopia H44.2- ☑
      siderosis H44.32- ☑
      specified type NEC H44.39- ☑
    endophthalmitis — *see* Endophthalmitis
    foreign body, retained — *see* Foreign body, intraocular, old, retained
    hemophthalmos — *see* Hemophthalmos
    hypotony H44.4Ø
      due to
        ocular fistula H44.42- ☑
        specified disorder NEC H44.43- ☑
      flat anterior chamber H44.41- ☑
      primary H44.44- ☑
    luxation — *see* Luxation, globe
    specified type NEC H44.89
  glomerular (in) NØ5.9
    amyloidosis E85.4 [NØ8]
    cryoglobulinemia D89.1 [NØ8]
    disseminated intravascular coagulation D65 [NØ8]
    Fabry's disease E75.21 [NØ8]
    familial lecithin cholesterol acyltransferase deficiency E78.6 [NØ8]
    Goodpasture's syndrome M31.Ø
    hemolytic-uremic syndrome D59.3
    Henoch (-Schönlein) purpura D69.Ø [NØ8]
    malarial malaria B52.Ø
    microscopic polyangiitis M31.7 [NØ8]
    multiple myeloma C9Ø.Ø- ☑ [NØ8]
    mumps B26.83
    schistosomiasis B65.9 [NØ8]
    sepsis NEC A41.- ☑ [NØ8]
      streptococcal A4Ø.- ☑ [NØ8]
    sickle-cell disorders D57.- ☑ [NØ8]
    strongyloidiasis B78.9 [NØ8]
    subacute bacterial endocarditis I33.Ø [NØ8]
    syphilis A52.75
    systemic lupus erythematosus M32.14
    thrombotic thrombocytopenic purpura M31.1 [NØ8]
    Waldenström macroglobulinemia C88.Ø [NØ8]
    Wegener's granulomatosis M31.31
  gluconeogenesis E74.4
  glucosaminoglycan metabolism — *see* Disorder, metabolism, glucosaminoglycan
  glycine metabolism E72.5Ø
    d-glycericacidemia E72.59
    hyperhydroxyprolinemia E72.59
    hyperoxaluria E72.53
    hyperprolinemia E72.59
    non-ketotic hyperglycinemia E72.51
    oxalosis E72.53
    oxaluria E72.53
    sarcosinemia E72.59
    trimethylaminuria E72.52
  glycoprotein metabolism E77.9
    specified NEC E77.8
  habit (and impulse) F63.9
    involving sexual behavior NEC F65.9
    specified NEC F63.89
  heart action I49.9
  hematological D75.9
    newborn (transient) P61.9
      specified NEC P61.8
  hematopoietic organs D75.9
  hemorrhagic NEC D69.9
    drug-induced D68.32
    due to
      extrinsic circulating anticoagulants D68.32
      increase in
        anti-IIa D68.32
        anti-Xa D68.32
      intrinsic
        circulating anticoagulants D68.318
        increase in
          anti-IXa D68.318
          antithrombin D68.318
          anti-VIIIa D68.318
          anti-XIa D68.318
    following childbirth O72.3
  hemostasis — *see* Defect, coagulation
  histidine metabolism E7Ø.4Ø
    histidinemia E7Ø.41
    other specified E7Ø.49

Disorder — *continued*
  hyperkinetic — *see* Disorder, attention-deficit hyperactivity
  hyperleucine-isoleucinemia E71.19
  hypervalinemia E71.19
  hypoactive sexual desire F52.Ø
  hypochondriacal F45.2Ø
    body dysmorphic F45.22
    neurosis F45.21
    other specified F45.29
  identity
    dissociative F44.81
    of childhood F93.8
  immune mechanism (immunity) D89.9
    specified type NEC D89.89
  impaired renal tubular function N25.9
    specified NEC N25.89
  impulse (control) F63.9
  inflammatory
    pelvic, in diseases classified elsewhere — *see* category N74
    penis N48.29
      abscess N48.21
      cellulitis N48.22
  integument, newborn P83.9
    specified NEC P83.8
  intermittent explosive F63.81
  internal secretion pancreas — *see* Increased, secretion, pancreas, endocrine
  intestine, intestinal
    carbohydrate absorption NEC E74.39
      postoperative K91.2
    functional NEC K59.9
      postoperative K91.89
    psychogenic F45.8
    vascular K55.9
      chronic K55.1
      specified NEC K55.8
  intraoperative (intraprocedural) — *see* Complications, intraoperative
  involuntary emotional expression (IEED) FØ7.89
  iris H21.9
    adhesions — *see* Adhesions, iris
    atrophy — *see* Atrophy, iris
    chamber angle recession — *see* Recession, chamber angle
    cyst — *see* Cyst, iris
    degeneration — *see* Degeneration, iris
    in diseases classified elsewhere H22
    iridodialysis — *see* Iridodialysis
    iridoschisis — *see* Iridoschisis
    miotic pupillary cyst — *see* Cyst, pupillary
    pupillary
      abnormality — *see* Abnormality, pupillary
      membrane — *see* Membrane, pupillary
    specified type NEC H21.89
    vascular NEC H21.1X- ☑
  iron metabolism E83.1Ø
    specified NEC E83.19
  isovaleric acidemia E71.11Ø
  jaw, developmental M27.Ø
    temporomandibular — *see* Anomaly, dentofacial, temporomandibular joint
  joint M25.9
    derangement — *see* Derangement, joint
    effusion — *see* Effusion, joint
    fistula — *see* Fistula, joint
    hemarthrosis — *see* Hemarthrosis
    instability — *see* Instability, joint
    osteophyte — *see* Osteophyte
    pain — *see* Pain, joint
    psychogenic F45.8
    specified type NEC M25.8Ø
      ankle M25.87- ☑
      elbow M25.82- ☑
      foot joint M25.87- ☑
      hand joint M25.84- ☑
      hip M25.85- ☑
      knee M25.86- ☑
      shoulder M25.81- ☑
      wrist M25.83- ☑
    stiffness — *see* Stiffness, joint
  ketone metabolism E71.32
  kidney N28.9
    functional (tubular) N25.9
    in
      schistosomiasis B65.9 [N29]

Disorder — *continued*
  kidney — *continued*
    tubular function N25.9
      specified NEC N25.89
  lacrimal system HØ4.9
    changes HØ4.69
      fistula — *see* Fistula, lacrimal
    gland HØ4.19
      atrophy — *see* Atrophy, lacrimal gland
      cyst — *see* Cyst, lacrimal, gland
      dacryops — *see* Dacryops
      dislocation — *see* Dislocation, lacrimal gland
      dry eye syndrome — *see* Syndrome, dry eye
      infection — *see* Dacryoadenitis
      granuloma — *see* Granuloma, lacrimal
      inflammation — *see* Inflammation, lacrimal
      obstruction — *see* Obstruction, lacrimal
    specified NEC HØ4.89
  lactation NEC O92.79
  language (developmental) F8Ø.9
    expressive F8Ø.1
    mixed receptive and expressive F8Ø.2
    receptive F8Ø.2
  late luteal phase dysphoric N94.89
  learning (specific) F81.9
    acalculia R48.8
    alexia R48.Ø
    mathematics F81.2
    reading F81.Ø
    specified NEC F81.89
    spelling F81.81
    written expression F81.81
  lens H27.9
    aphakia — *see* Aphakia
    cataract — *see* Cataract
    dislocation — *see* Dislocation, lens
    specified type NEC H27.8
  ligament M24.2Ø
    ankle M24.27- ☑
    attachment, spine — *see* Enthesopathy, spinal
    elbow M24.22- ☑
    foot joint M24.27- ☑
    hand joint M24.24- ☑
    hip M24.25- ☑
    knee — *see* Derangement, knee, specified NEC
    shoulder M24.21- ☑
    vertebra M24.28
    wrist M24.23- ☑
  ligamentous attachments (*see also* Enthesopathy)
    spine — *see* Enthesopathy, spinal
  lipid
    metabolism, congenital E78.9
    storage E75.6
      specified NEC E75.5
  lipoprotein
    deficiency (familial) E78.6
    metabolism E78.9
      specified NEC E78.89
  liver K76.9
    malarial B54 [K77]
  low back (*see also* Dorsopathy, specified NEC)
  lumbosacral
    plexus G54.1
    root (nerve) NEC G54.4
  lung, interstitial, drug-induced J7Ø.4
    acute J7Ø.2
    chronic J7Ø.3
  lymphoproliferative, post-transplant (PTLD) D47.Z1 (*following* D47.4)
  lysine and hydroxylysine metabolism E72.3
  male
    erectile (organic) (*see also* Dysfunction, sexual, male, erectile) N52.9
      nonorganic F52.21
    hypoactive sexual desire F52.Ø
    orgasmic F52.32
  manic F3Ø.9
    organic FØ6.33
  mastoid (*see also* Disorder, ear, middle)
    postprocedural — *see* Complications, ear, procedure
  meniscus — *see* Derangement, knee, meniscus
  menopausal N95.9
    specified NEC N95.8
  menstrual N92.6
    psychogenic F45.8
    specified NEC N92.5

Disorder — *continued*
mental (or behavioral) (nonpsychotic) F99
  due to (secondary to)
    amphetamine
      due to drug abuse — *see* Abuse, drug,
        stimulant
      due to drug dependence — *see* Depen-
        dence, drug, stimulant
    brain disease, damage and dysfunction F09
    caffeine use
      due to drug abuse — *see* Abuse, drug,
        stimulant
      due to drug dependence — *see* Depen-
        dence, drug, stimulant
    cannabis use
      due to drug abuse — *see* Abuse, drug,
        cannabis
      due to drug dependence — *see* Depen-
        dence, drug, cannabis
    general medical condition F09
    sedative or hypnotic use
      due to drug abuse — *see* Abuse, drug,
        sedative
      due to drug dependence — *see* Depen-
        dence, drug, sedative
    tobacco (nicotine) use — *see* Dependence,
      drug, nicotine
  following organic brain damage F07.9
    frontal lobe syndrome F07.0
    personality change F07.0
    postconcussional syndrome F07.81
    specified NEC F07.89
  infancy, childhood or adolescence F98.9
  neurotic — *see* Neurosis
  organic or symptomatic F09
  presenile, psychotic F03 ☑
  problem NEC
  psychoneurotic — *see* Neurosis
  psychotic — *see* Psychosis
  puerperal F53
  senile, psychotic NEC F03 ☑
metabolic, amino acid, transitory, newborn P74.8
metabolism NOS E88.9
  amino-acid E72.9
    aromatic E70.9
      albinism — *see* Albinism
      histidine E70.40
        histidinemia E70.41
        other specified E70.49
      hyperphenylalaninemia E70.1
        classical phenylketonuria E70.0
      other specified E70.8
      tryptophan E70.5
      tyrosine E70.20
        hypertyrosinemia E70.21
        other specified E70.29
    branched chain E71.2
      3-methylglutaconic aciduria E71.111
      hyperleucine-isoleucinemia E71.19
      hypervalinemia E71.19
      isovaleric acidemia E71.110
      maple syrup urine disease E71.0
      methylmalonic acidemia E71.120
      organic aciduria NEC E71.118
      other specified E71.19
      proprionate NEC E71.128
      proprionic acidemia E71.121
    glycine E72.50
      d-glycericacidemia E72.59
      hyperhydroxyprolinemia E72.59
      hyperoxaluria E72.53
      hyperprolinemia E72.59
      non-ketotic hyperglycinemia E72.51
      other specified E72.59
      sarcosinemia E72.59
      trimethylaminuria E72.52
    hydroxylysine E72.3
    lysine E72.3
    ornithine E72.4
    other specified E72.8
      beta-amino acid E72.8
      gamma-glutamyl cycle E72.8
    straight-chain E72.8
    sulfur-bearing E72.10
      homocystinuria E72.11
      methylenetetrahydrofolate reductase defi-
        ciency E72.12
      other specified E72.19

Disorder — *continued*
metabolism — *continued*
  bile acid and cholesterol metabolism E78.70
  bilirubin E80.7
    specified NEC E80.6
  calcium E83.50
    hypercalcemia E83.52
    hypocalcemia E83.51
    other specified E83.59
  carbohydrate E74.9
    specified NEC E74.8
  cholesterol and bile acid metabolism E78.70
  congenital E88.9
  copper E83.00
    specified type NEC E83.09
    Wilson's disease E83.01
  cystinuria E72.01
  fructose E74.10
  galactose E74.20
  glucosaminoglycan E76.9
    mucopolysaccharidosis — *see* Mucopolysaccha-
      ridosis
    specified NEC E76.8
  glutamine E72.8
  glycine E72.50
  glycogen storage (hepatorenal) E74.09
  glycoprotein E77.9
    specified NEC E77.8
  glycosaminoglycan E76.9
    specified NEC E76.8
  in labor and delivery O75.89
  iron E83.10
  isoleucine E71.19
  leucine E71.19
  lipoid E78.9
  lipoprotein E78.9
    specified NEC E78.89
  magnesium E83.40
    hypermagnesemia E83.41
    hypomagnesemia E83.42
    other specified E83.49
  mineral E83.9
    specified NEC E83.89
  mitochondrial E88.40
    MELAS syndrome E88.41
    MERRF syndrome (myoclonic epilepsy associat-
      ed with ragged-red fibers) E88.42
    other specified E88.49
  ornithine E72.4
  phosphatases E83.30
  phosphorus E83.30
    acid phosphatase deficiency E83.39
    hypophosphatasia E83.39
    hypophosphatemia E83.39
      familial E83.31
    other specified E83.39
    pseudovitamin D deficiency E83.32
  plasma protein NEC E88.09
  porphyrin — *see* Porphyria
  postprocedural E89.89
    specified NEC E89.89
  purine E79.9
    specified NEC E79.8
  pyrimidine E79.9
    specified NEC E79.8
  pyruvate E74.4
  serine E72.8
  sodium E87.8
  specified NEC E88.89
  threonine E72.8
  valine E71.19
  zinc E83.2
methylmalonic acidemia E71.120
micturition NEC R39.19
  feeling of incomplete emptying R39.14
  hesitancy R39.11
  poor stream R39.12
  psychogenic F45.8
  split stream R39.13
  straining R39.16
  urgency R39.15
mitochondrial metabolism E88.40
mitral (valve) — *see* Endocarditis, mitral
mixed
  anxiety and depressive F41.8
  of scholastic skills (developmental) F81.89
  receptive expressive language F80.2

Disorder — *continued*
mood F39
  bipolar — *see* Disorder, bipolar
  depressive — *see* Disorder, depressive
  due to (secondary to)
    alcohol F10.94
    amphetamine F15.94
      in
        abuse F15.14
        dependence F15.24
    anxiolytic F13.94
      in
        abuse F13.14
        dependence F13.24
    cocaine F14.94
      in
        abuse F14.14
        dependence F14.24
    general medical condition F06.30
    hallucinogen F16.94
      in
        abuse F16.14
        dependence F16.24
    hypnotic F13.94
      in
        abuse F13.14
        dependence F13.24
    inhalant F18.94
      in
        abuse F18.14
        dependence F18.24
    opioid F11.94
      in
        abuse F11.14
        dependence F11.24
    phencyclidine (PCP) F16.94
      in
        abuse F16.14
        dependence F16.24
    physiological condition F06.30
      with
        depressive features F06.31
        major depressive-like episode F06.32
        manic features F06.33
        mixed features F06.34
    psychoactive substance NEC F19.94
      in
        abuse F19.14
        dependence F19.24
    sedative F13.94
      in
        abuse F13.14
        dependence F13.24
    volatile solvents F18.94
      in
        abuse F18.14
        dependence F18.24
  manic episode F30.9
    with psychotic symptoms F30.2
    without psychotic symptoms F30.10
      mild F30.11
      moderate F30.12
      severe F30.13
    in remission (full) F30.4
      partial F30.3
    specified type NEC F30.8
  organic F06.30
    right hemisphere F07.89
  persistent F34.9
    cyclothymia F34.0
    dysthymia F34.1
    specified type NEC F34.8
  recurrent F39
  right hemisphere organic F07.89
movement G25.9
  drug-induced G25.70
    akathisia G25.71
    specified NEC G25.79
  hysterical F44.4
  in diseases classified elsewhere — *see* category
    G26
  periodic limb G47.61
    sleep related G47.61
  sleep related NEC G47.69
  specified NEC G25.89
  stereotyped F98.4
  treatment-induced G25.9
multiple personality F44.81

☑ Additional Character Required — Refer to the Tabular List for Character Selection   ⩔ Subterms under main terms may continue to next column or page

Disorder — *continued*
- muscle M62.9
    - attachment, spine — *see* Enthesopathy, spinal
    - in trichinellosis — *see* Trichinellosis, with muscle disorder
    - psychogenic F45.8
    - specified type NEC M62.89
    - tone, newborn P94.9
        - specified NEC P94.8
- muscular
    - attachments (*see also* Enthesopathy)
        - spine — *see* Enthesopathy, spinal
    - urethra N36.44
- musculoskeletal system, soft tissue — *see* Disorder, soft tissue
- postprocedural M96.89
- psychogenic F45.8
- myoneural G70.9
    - due to lead G70.1
    - specified NEC G70.89
    - toxic G70.1
- myotonic NEC G71.19
- nail, in diseases classified elsewhere L62
- neck region NEC — *see* Dorsopathy, specified NEC
- nerve G58.9
    - abducent NEC — *see* Strabismus, paralytic, sixth nerve
    - accessory G52.8
    - acoustic — *see* subcategory H93.3 ☑
    - auditory — *see* subcategory H93.3 ☑
    - auriculotemporal G50.8
    - axillary G54.0
    - cerebral — *see* Disorder, nerve, cranial
    - cranial G52.9
        - eighth — *see* subcategory H93.3 ☑
        - eleventh G52.8
        - fifth G50.9
        - first G52.0
        - fourth NEC — *see* Strabismus, paralytic, fourth nerve
        - multiple G52.7
        - ninth G52.1
        - second NEC — *see* Disorder, nerve, optic
        - seventh NEC G51.8
        - sixth NEC — *see* Strabismus, paralytic, sixth nerve
        - specified NEC G52.8
        - tenth G52.2
        - third NEC — *see* Strabismus, paralytic, third nerve
        - twelfth G52.3
    - entrapment — *see* Neuropathy, entrapment
    - facial G51.9
        - specified NEC G51.8
    - femoral — *see* Lesion, nerve, femoral
    - glossopharyngeal NEC G52.1
    - hypoglossal G52.3
    - intercostal G58.0
    - lateral
        - cutaneous of thigh — *see* Mononeuropathy, lower limb, meralgia paresthetica
        - popliteal — *see* Lesion, nerve, popliteal
    - lower limb — *see* Mononeuropathy, lower limb
    - medial popliteal — *see* Lesion, nerve, popliteal, medial
    - median NEC — *see* Lesion, nerve, median
    - multiple G58.7
    - oculomotor NEC — *see* Strabismus, paralytic, third nerve
    - olfactory G52.0
    - optic NEC H47.09- ☑
        - hemorrhage into sheath — *see* Hemorrhage, optic nerve
        - ischemic H47.01- ☑
    - peroneal — *see* Lesion, nerve, popliteal
    - phrenic G58.8
    - plantar — *see* Lesion, nerve, plantar
    - pneumogastric G52.2
    - posterior tibial — *see* Syndrome, tarsal tunnel
    - radial — *see* Lesion, nerve, radial
    - recurrent laryngeal G52.2
    - root G54.9
        - cervical G54.2
        - lumbosacral G54.1
        - specified NEC G54.8
        - thoracic G54.3
    - sciatic NEC — *see* Lesion, nerve, sciatic

Disorder — *continued*
- nerve — *continued*
    - specified NEC G58.8
        - lower limb — *see* Mononeuropathy, lower limb, specified NEC
        - upper limb — *see* Mononeuropathy, upper limb, specified NEC
    - sympathetic G90.9
    - tibial — *see* Lesion, nerve, popliteal, medial
    - trigeminal G50.9
        - specified NEC G50.8
    - trochlear NEC — *see* Strabismus, paralytic, fourth nerve
    - ulnar — *see* Lesion, nerve, ulnar
    - upper limb — *see* Mononeuropathy, upper limb
    - vagus G52.2
- nervous system G98.8
    - autonomic (peripheral) G90.9
        - specified NEC G90.8
    - central G96.9
        - specified NEC G96.8
    - parasympathetic G90.9
    - specified NEC G98.8
    - sympathetic G90.9
    - vegetative G90.9
- neurohypophysis NEC E23.3
- neurological NEC R29.818
- neuromuscular G70.9
    - hereditary NEC G71.9
    - specified NEC G70.89
    - toxic G70.1
- neurotic F48.9
    - specified NEC F48.8
- neutrophil, polymorphonuclear D71
- nicotine use — *see* Dependence, drug, nicotine
- nightmare F51.5
- nose J34.9
    - specified NEC J34.89
- obsessive-compulsive F42
- odontogenesis NOS K00.9
- opioid use
    - with
        - opioid-induced psychotic disorder F11.959
            - with
                - delusions F11.950
                - hallucinations F11.951
        - due to drug abuse — *see* Abuse, drug, opioid
        - due to drug dependence — *see* Dependence, drug, opioid
- oppositional defiant F91.3
- optic
    - chiasm H47.49
        - due to
            - inflammatory disorder H47.41
            - neoplasm H47.42
            - vascular disorder H47.43
    - disc H47.39- ☑
        - coloboma — *see* Coloboma, optic disc
        - drusen — *see* Drusen, optic disc
        - pseudopapilledema — *see* Pseudopapilledema
    - radiations — *see* Disorder, visual, pathway
    - tracts — *see* Disorder, visual, pathway
- orbit H05.9
    - cyst — *see* Cyst, orbit
    - deformity — *see* Deformity, orbit
    - edema — *see* Edema, orbit
    - enophthalmos — *see* Enophthalmos
    - exophthalmos — *see* Exophthalmos
    - hemorrhage — *see* Hemorrhage, orbit
    - inflammation — *see* Inflammation, orbit
    - myopathy — *see* Myopathy, extraocular muscles
    - retained foreign body — *see* Foreign body, orbit, old
    - specified type NEC H05.89
- organic
    - anxiety F06.4
    - catatonic F06.1
    - delusional F06.2
    - dissociative F06.8
    - emotionally labile (asthenic) F06.8
    - mood (affective) F06.30
    - schizophrenia-like F06.2
- orgasmic (female) F52.31
    - male F52.32
- ornithine metabolism E72.4
- overanxious F41.1
    - of childhood F93.8

Disorder — *continued*
- pain
    - with related psychological factors F45.42
    - exclusively related to psychological factors F45.41
- pancreatic internal secretion E16.9
    - specified NEC E16.8
- panic F41.0
    - with agoraphobia F40.01
- papulosquamous L44.9
    - in diseases classified elsewhere L45
    - specified NEC L44.8
- paranoid F22
    - induced F24
    - shared F24
- parathyroid (gland) E21.5
    - specified NEC E21.4
- parietoalveolar NEC J84.09
- paroxysmal, mixed R56.9
- patella M22.9- ☑
    - chondromalacia — *see* Chondromalacia, patella
    - derangement NEC M22.3X- ☑
    - recurrent
        - dislocation — *see* Dislocation, patella, recurrent
        - subluxation — *see* Dislocation, patella, recurrent, incomplete
    - specified NEC M22.8X- ☑
- patellofemoral M22.2X- ☑
- pentose phosphate pathway with anemia D55.1
- perception, due to hallucinogens F16.983
    - in
        - abuse F16.183
        - dependence F16.283
- peripheral nervous system NEC G64
- peroxisomal E71.50
    - biogenesis
        - neonatal adrenoleukodystrophy E71.511
        - specified disorder NEC E71.518
        - Zellweger syndrome E71.510
    - rhizomelic chondrodysplasia punctata E71.540
    - specified form NEC E71.548
        - group 1 E71.518
        - group 2 E71.53
        - group 3 E71.542
    - X-linked adrenoleukodystrophy E71.529
        - adolescent E71.521
        - adrenomyeloneuropathy E71.522
        - childhood E71.520
        - specified form NEC E71.528
    - Zellweger-like syndrome E71.541
- persistent
    - (somatoform) pain F45.41
    - affective (mood) F34.9
- personality (*see also* Personality) F60.9
    - affective F34.0
    - aggressive F60.3
    - amoral F60.2
    - anankastic F60.5
    - antisocial F60.2
    - anxious F60.6
    - asocial F60.2
    - asthenic F60.7
    - avoidant F60.6
    - borderline F60.3
    - change (secondary) due to general medical condition F07.0
    - compulsive F60.5
    - cyclothymic F34.0
    - dependent (passive) F60.7
    - depressive F34.1
    - dissocial F60.2
    - emotional instability F60.3
    - expansive paranoid F60.0
    - explosive F60.3
    - following organic brain damage F07.9
    - histrionic F60.4
    - hyperthymic F34.0
    - hypothymic F34.1
    - hysterical F60.4
    - immature F60.89
    - inadequate F60.7
    - labile F60.3
    - mixed (nonspecific) F60.89
    - moral deficiency F60.2
    - narcissistic F60.81
    - negativistic F60.89
    - obsessional F60.5
    - obsessive (-compulsive) F60.5
    - organic F07.9

Disorder — *continued*
personality (*see also* Personality) — *continued*
  overconscientious F60.5
  paranoid F60.0
  passive (-dependent) F60.7
  passive-aggressive F60.89
  pathological NEC F60.9
  pseudosocial F60.2
  psychopathic F60.2
  schizoid F60.1
  schizotypal F21
  self-defeating F60.7
  specified NEC F60.89
  type A F60.5
  unstable (emotional) F60.3
pervasive, developmental F84.9
phobic anxiety, childhood F40.8
phosphate-losing tubular N25.0
pigmentation L81.9
  choroid, congenital Q14.3
  diminished melanin formation L81.6
  iron L81.8
  specified NEC L81.8
pinna (noninfective) H61.10- ☑
  deformity, acquired H61.11- ☑
  hematoma H61.12- ☑
  perichondritis — *see* Perichondritis, ear
  specified type NEC H61.19- ☑
pituitary gland E23.7
  iatrogenic (postprocedural) E89.3
  specified NEC E23.6
platelets D69.1
plexus G54.9
  specified NEC G54.8
polymorphonuclear neutrophils D71
porphyrin metabolism — *see* Porphyria
postconcussional F07.81
posthallucinogen perception F16.983
  in
    abuse F16.183
    dependence F16.283
postmenopausal N95.9
  specified NEC N95.8
postprocedural (postoperative) — *see* Complications, postprocedural
post-transplant lymphoproliferative D47.Z1 (*following* D47.4)
post-traumatic stress (PTSD) F43.10
  acute F43.11
  chronic F43.12
premenstrual dysphoric (PMDD) N94.3
prepuce N47.8
propionic acidemia E71.121
prostate N42.9
  specified NEC N42.89
psychogenic NOS (*see also* condition) F45.9
  anxiety F41.8
  appetite F50.9
  asthenic F48.8
  cardiovascular (system) F45.8
  compulsive F42
  cutaneous F54
  depressive F32.9
  digestive (system) F45.8
  dysmenorrheic F45.8
  dyspneic F45.8
  endocrine (system) F54
  eye NEC F45.8
  feeding — *see* Disorder, eating
  functional NEC F45.8
  gastric F45.8
  gastrointestinal (system) F45.8
  genitourinary (system) F45.8
  heart (function) (rhythm) NEC F45.8
  hyperventilatory F45.8
  hypochondriacal — *see* Disorder, hypochondriacal
  intestinal F45.8
  joint F45.8
  learning F81.9
  limb F45.8
  lymphatic (system) F45.8
  menstrual F45.8
  micturition F45.8
  monoplegic NEC F44.4
  motor F44.4
  muscle F45.8
  musculoskeletal F45.8
  neurocirculatory F45.8

Disorder — *continued*
psychogenic (*see also* condition) — *continued*
  obsessive F42
  occupational F48.8
  organ or part of body NEC F45.8
  paralytic NEC F44.4
  phobic F40.9
  physical NEC F45.8
  rectal F45.8
  respiratory (system) F45.8
  rheumatic F45.8
  sexual (function) F52.9
  skin (allergic) (eczematous) F54
  sleep F51.9
  specified part of body NEC F45.8
  stomach F45.8
psychological F99
  associated with
    disease classified elsewhere F54
    sexual
      development F66
      relationship F66
    uncertainty about gender identity F66
psychomotor NEC F44.4
  hysterical F44.4
psychoneurotic (*see also* Neurosis)
  mixed NEC F48.8
psychophysiologic — *see* Disorder, somatoform
psychosexual F65.9
  development F66
  identity of childhood F64.2
psychosomatic NOS — *see* Disorder, somatoform
  multiple F45.0
  undifferentiated F45.1
psychotic — *see* Psychosis
  transient (acute) F23
puberty E30.9
  specified NEC E30.8
pulmonary (valve) — *see* Endocarditis, pulmonary
purine metabolism E79.9
pyrimidine metabolism E79.9
pyruvate metabolism E74.4
reactive attachment (childhood) F94.1
reading R48.0
  developmental (specific) F81.0
receptive language F80.2
receptor, hormonal, peripheral (*see also* Syndrome, androgen insensitivity) E34.50
recurrent brief depressive F33.8
reflex R29.2
refraction H52.7
  aniseikonia H52.32
  anisometropia H52.31
  astigmatism — *see* Astigmatism
  hypermetropia — *see* Hypermetropia
  myopia — *see* Myopia
  presbyopia H52.4
  specified NEC H52.6
relationship F68.8
  due to sexual orientation F66
REM sleep behavior G47.52
renal function, impaired (tubular) N25.9
resonance R49.9
  specified NEC R49.8
respiratory function, impaired (*see also* Failure, respiration)
  postprocedural — *see* Complication, postoperative, respiratory system
  psychogenic F45.8
retina H35.9
  angioid streaks H35.33
  changes in vascular appearance H35.01- ☑
  degeneration — *see* Degeneration, retina
  dystrophy (hereditary) — *see* Dystrophy, retina
  edema H35.81
  hemorrhage — *see* Hemorrhage, retina
  ischemia H35.82
  macular degeneration — *see* Degeneration, macula
  microaneurysms H35.04- ☑
  microvascular abnormality NEC H35.09
  neovascularization — *see* Neovascularization, retina
  retinopathy — *see* Retinopathy
  separation of layers H35.70
    central serous chorioretinopathy H35.71- ☑
    pigment epithelium detachment (serous) H35.72- ☑
    hemorrhagic H35.73- ☑

Disorder — *continued*
retina — *continued*
  specified type NEC H35.89
  telangiectasis — *see* Telangiectasis, retina
  vasculitis — *see* Vasculitis, retina
retroperitoneal K68.9
right hemisphere organic affective F07.89
rumination (infant or child) F98.21
sacrum, sacrococcygeal NEC M53.3
schizoaffective F25.9
  bipolar type F25.0
  depressive type F25.1
  manic type F25.0
  mixed type F25.0
  specified NEC F25.8
schizoid of childhood F84.5
schizophreniform F20.81
  brief F23
schizotypal (personality) F21
secretion, thyrocalcitonin E07.0
seizure (*see also* Epilepsy) G40.909
  intractable G40.919
    with status epilepticus G40.911
semantic pragmatic F80.89
  with autism F84.0
sense of smell R43.1
  psychogenic F45.8
separation anxiety, of childhood F93.0
sexual
  arousal, female F52.22
  aversion F52.1
  function, psychogenic F52.9
  maturation F66
  nonorganic F52.9
  preference (*see also* Deviation, sexual) F65.9
    fetishistic transvestism F65.1
  relationship F66
shyness, of childhood and adolescence F40.10
sibling rivalry F93.8
sickle-cell (sickling) (homozygous) — *see* Disease, sickle-cell
  heterozygous D57.3
  specified type NEC D57.8- ☑
  trait D57.3
sinus (nasal) J34.9
  specified NEC J34.89
skin L98.9
  atrophic L90.9
    specified NEC L90.8
  granulomatous L92.9
    specified NEC L92.8
  hypertrophic L91.9
    specified NEC L91.8
  infiltrative NEC L98.6
  newborn P83.9
    specified NEC P83.8
  psychogenic (allergic) (eczematous) F54
sleep G47.9
  breathing-related — *see* Apnea, sleep
  circadian rhythm G47.20
    advance sleep phase type G47.22
    delayed sleep phase type G47.21
    due to
      alcohol
        abuse F10.182
        dependence F10.282
        use F10.982
      amphetamines
        abuse F15.182
        dependence F15.282
        use F15.982
      caffeine
        abuse F15.182
        dependence F15.282
        use F15.982
      cocaine
        abuse F14.182
        dependence F14.282
        use F14.982
      drug NEC
        abuse F19.182
        dependence F19.282
        use F19.982
      opioid
        abuse F11.182
        dependence F11.282
        use F11.982

☑ **Additional Character Required — Refer to the Tabular List for Character Selection**   ▽ Subterms under main terms may continue to next column or page

Disorder — *continued*
  sleep — *continued*
    circadian rhythm — *continued*
      due to — *continued*
        psychoactive substance NEC
          abuse F19.182
          dependence F19.282
          use F19.982
        sedative, hypnotic, or anxiolytic
          abuse F13.182
          dependence F13.282
          use F13.982
        stimulant NEC
          abuse F15.182
          dependence F15.282
          use F15.982
      free running type G47.24
      in conditions classified elsewhere G47.27
      irregular sleep wake type G47.23
      jet lag type G47.25
      shift work type G47.26
      specified NEC G47.29
    due to
      alcohol
        abuse F10.182
        dependence F10.282
        use F10.982
      amphetamine
        abuse F15.182
        dependence F15.282
        use F15.982
      anxiolytic
        abuse F13.182
        dependence F13.282
        use F13.982
      caffeine
        abuse F15.182
        dependence F15.282
        use F15.982
      cocaine
        abuse F14.182
        dependence F14.282
        use F14.982
      drug NEC
        abuse F19.182
        dependence F19.282
        use F19.982
      hypnotic
        abuse F13.182
        dependence F13.282
        use F13.982
      opioid
        abuse F11.182
        dependence F11.282
        use F11.982
      psychoactive substance NEC
        abuse F19.182
        dependence F19.282
        use F19.982
      sedative
        abuse F13.182
        dependence F13.282
        use F13.982
      stimulant NEC
        abuse F15.182
        dependence F15.282
        use F15.982
    emotional F51.9
    excessive somnolence — *see* Hypersomnia
    hypersomnia type — *see* Hypersomnia
    initiating or maintaining — *see* Insomnia
    nightmares F51.5
    nonorganic F51.9
      specified NEC F51.8
    parasomnia type G47.50
    specified NEC G47.8
    terrors F51.4
    walking F51.3
  sleep-wake pattern or schedule — *see* Disorder, sleep, circadian rhythm
  social
    anxiety of childhood F40.10
    functioning in childhood F94.9
      specified NEC F94.8
  soft tissue M79.9
    ankle M79.9
    due to use, overuse and pressure M70.90
      ankle M70.97- ☑

Disorder — *continued*
  soft tissue — *continued*
    due to use, overuse and pressure — *continued*
      bursitis — *see* Bursitis
      foot M70.97- ☑
      forearm M70.93- ☑
      hand M70.94- ☑
      lower leg M70.96- ☑
      multiple sites M70.99
      pelvic region M70.95- ☑
      shoulder region M70.91- ☑
      specified site NEC M70.98
      specified type NEC M70.80
        ankle M70.87- ☑
        foot M70.87- ☑
        forearm M70.83- ☑
        hand M70.84- ☑
        lower leg M70.86- ☑
        multiple sites M70.89
        pelvic region M70.85- ☑
        shoulder region M70.81- ☑
        specified site NEC M70.88
        thigh M70.85- ☑
        upper arm M70.82- ☑
      thigh M70.95- ☑
      upper arm M70.92- ☑
    foot M79.9
    forearm M79.9
    hand M79.9
    lower leg M79.9
    multiple sites M79.9
    occupational — *see* Disorder, soft tissue, due to use, overuse and pressure
    pelvic region M79.9
    shoulder region M79.9
    specified type NEC M79.89
    thigh M79.9
    upper arm M79.9
  somatization F45.0
  somatoform F45.9
    pain (persistent) F45.41
    somatization (multiple) (long-lasting) F45.0
    specified NEC F45.8
    undifferentiated F45.1
  somnolence, excessive — *see* Hypersomnia
  specific
    arithmetical F81.2
    developmental, of motor F82
    reading F81.0
    speech and language F80.9
    spelling F81.81
    written expression F81.81
  speech R47.9
    articulation (functional) (specific) F80.0
    developmental F80.9
    specified NEC R47.89
  spelling (specific) F81.81
  spine (*see also* Dorsopathy)
    ligamentous or muscular attachments, peripheral — *see* Enthesopathy, spinal
    specified NEC — *see* Dorsopathy, specified NEC
  stereotyped, habit or movement F98.4
  stomach (functional) — *see* Disorder, gastric
  stress F43.9
    post-traumatic F43.10
      acute F43.11
      chronic F43.12
  sulfur-bearing amino-acid metabolism E72.10
  sweat gland (eccrine) L74.9
    apocrine L75.9
      specified NEC L75.8
    specified NEC L74.8
  synovium M67.90
    acromioclavicular M67.91- ☑
    ankle M67.97- ☑
    elbow M67.92- ☑
    foot M67.97- ☑
    forearm M67.93- ☑
    hand M67.94- ☑
    hip M67.95- ☑
    knee M67.96- ☑
    multiple sites M67.99
    rupture — *see* Rupture, synovium
    shoulder M67.91- ☑
    specified type NEC M67.80
      acromioclavicular M67.81- ☑
      ankle M67.87-

Disorder — *continued*
  synovium — *continued*
    specified type — *continued*
      elbow M67.82- ☑
      foot M67.87- ☑
      hand M67.84- ☑
      hip M67.85- ☑
      knee M67.86- ☑
      multiple sites M67.89
      wrist M67.83- ☑
    synovitis — *see* Synovitis
    upper arm M67.92- ☑
    wrist M67.93- ☑
  temperature regulation, newborn P81.9
    specified NEC P81.8
  temporomandibular joint — *see* Anomaly, dentofacial, temporomandibular joint
  tendon M67.90
    acromioclavicular M67.91- ☑
    ankle M67.97- ☑
    contracture — *see* Contracture, tendon
    elbow M67.92- ☑
    foot M67.97- ☑
    forearm M67.93- ☑
    hand M67.94- ☑
    hip M67.95- ☑
    knee M67.96- ☑
    multiple sites M67.99
    rupture — *see* Rupture, tendon
    shoulder M67.91- ☑
    specified type NEC M67.80
      acromioclavicular M67.81- ☑
      ankle M67.87- ☑
      elbow M67.82- ☑
      foot M67.87- ☑
      hand M67.84- ☑
      hip M67.85- ☑
      knee M67.86- ☑
      multiple sites M67.89
      trunk M67.88
      wrist M67.83- ☑
    synovitis — *see* Synovitis
    tendinitis — *see* Tendinitis
    tenosynovitis — *see* Tenosynovitis
    trunk M67.98
    upper arm M67.92- ☑
    wrist M67.93- ☑
  thoracic root (nerve) NEC G54.3
  thyrocalcitonin hypersecretion E07.0
  thyroid (gland) E07.9
    function NEC, neonatal, transitory P72.2
    iodine-deficiency related E01.8
    specified NEC E07.89
  tic — *see* Tic
  tooth K08.9
    development K00.9
      specified NEC K00.8
    eruption K00.6
  Tourette's F95.2
  trance and possession F44.89
  tricuspid (valve) — *see* Endocarditis, tricuspid
  tryptophan metabolism E70.5
  tubular, phosphate-losing N25.0
  tubulo-interstitial (in)
    brucellosis A23.9 [N16]
    cystinosis E72.04
    diphtheria A36.84
    glycogen storage disease E74.00 [N16]
    leukemia NEC C95.9- ☑ [N16]
    lymphoma NEC C85.9- ☑ [N16]
    mixed cryoglobulinemia D89.1 [N16]
    multiple myeloma C90.0- ☑ [N16]
    Salmonella infection A02.25
    sarcoidosis D86.84
    sepsis A41.9 [N16]
      streptococcal A40.9 [N16]
    systemic lupus erythematosus M32.15
    toxoplasmosis B58.83
    transplant rejection T86.91 [N16]
    Wilson's disease E83.01 [N16]
  tubulo-renal function, impaired N25.9
    specified NEC N25.89
  tympanic membrane H73.9- ☑
    atrophy — *see* Atrophy, tympanic membrane
    infection — *see* Myringitis
    perforation — *see* Perforation, tympanum
    specified NEC H73.89- ☑

Disorder — Disorder

Disorder — *continued*
  unsocialized aggressive F91.1
  urea cycle metabolism E72.20
    argininemia E72.21
    argininosuccinic aciduria E72.22
    citrullinemia E72.23
    ornithine transcarbamylase deficiency E72.4
    other specified E72.29
  ureter (in) N28.9
    schistosomiasis B65.0 [N29]
    tuberculosis A18.11
  urethra N36.9
    specified NEC N36.8
  urinary system N39.9
    specified NEC N39.8
  valve, heart
    aortic — *see* Endocarditis, aortic
    mitral — *see* Endocarditis, mitral
    pulmonary — *see* Endocarditis, pulmonary
    rheumatic
      aortic — *see* Endocarditis, aortic, rheumatic
      mitral — *see* Endocarditis, mitral
      pulmonary — *see* Endocarditis, pulmonary, rheumatic
      tricuspid — *see* Endocarditis, tricuspid
    tricuspid — *see* Endocarditis, tricuspid
  vestibular function H81.9- ☑
    specified NEC — *see* subcategory H81.8 ☑
      in diseases classified elsewhere H82.- ☑
    vertigo — *see* Vertigo
  vision, binocular H53.30
    abnormal retinal correspondence H53.31
    diplopia H53.2
    fusion with defective stereopsis H53.32
    simultaneous perception H53.33
    suppression H53.34
  visual
    cortex
      blindness H47.619
        left brain H47.612
        right brain H47.611
      due to
        inflammatory disorder H47.629
          left brain H47.622
          right brain H47.621
        neoplasm H47.639
          left brain H47.632
          right brain H47.631
        vascular disorder H47.649
          left brain H47.642
          right brain H47.641
    pathway H47.9
      due to
        inflammatory disorder H47.51- ☑
        neoplasm H47.52- ☑
        vascular disorder H47.53- ☑
    optic chiasm — *see* Disorder, optic, chiasm
  vitreous body H43.9
    crystalline deposits — *see* Deposit, crystalline
    degeneration — *see* Degeneration, vitreous
    hemorrhage — *see* Hemorrhage, vitreous
    opacities — *see* Opacity, vitreous
    prolapse — *see* Prolapse, vitreous
    specified type NEC H43.89
  voice R49.9
    specified type NEC R49.8
  volatile solvent use
    due to drug abuse — *see* Abuse, drug, inhalant
    due to drug dependence — *see* Dependence, drug, inhalant
  white blood cells D72.9
    specified NEC D72.89
  withdrawing, child or adolescent F40.10
Disorientation R41.0
Displacement, displaced
  acquired traumatic of bone, cartilage, joint, tendon NEC — *see* Dislocation
  adrenal gland (congenital) Q89.1
  appendix, retrocecal (congenital) Q43.8
  auricle (congenital) Q17.4
  bladder (acquired) N32.89
    congenital Q64.19
  brachial plexus (congenital) Q07.8
  brain stem, caudal (congenital) Q04.8
  canaliculus (lacrimalis), congenital Q10.6
  cardia through esophageal hiatus (congenital) Q40.1
  cerebellum, caudal (congenital) Q04.8
  cervix — *see* Malposition, uterus

Displacement, displaced — *continued*
  colon (congenital) Q43.3
  device, implant or graft (*see also* Complications, by site and type, mechanical) T85.628 ☑
    arterial graft NEC — *see* Complication, cardiovascular device, mechanical, vascular
    breast (implant) T85.42 ☑
    catheter NEC T85.628 ☑
      dialysis (renal) T82.42 ☑
        intraperitoneal T85.621 ☑
      infusion NEC T82.524 ☑
        spinal (epidural) (subdural) T85.620 ☑
      urinary (indwelling) T83.028 ☑
        cystostomy T83.020 ☑
    electronic (electrode) (pulse generator) (stimulator) — *see* Complication, electronic stimulator
    fixation, internal (orthopedic) NEC — *see* Complication, fixation device, mechanical
    gastrointestinal — *see* Complications, prosthetic device, mechanical, gastrointestinal device
    genital NEC T83.428 ☑
      intrauterine contraceptive device T83.32 ☑
      penile prosthesis T83.420 ☑
    heart NEC — *see* Complication, cardiovascular device, mechanical
    joint prosthesis — *see* Complications, joint prosthesis, mechanical
    ocular — *see* Complications, prosthetic device, mechanical, ocular device
    orthopedic NEC — *see* Complication, orthopedic, device or graft, mechanical
    specified NEC T85.628 ☑
    urinary NEC (*see also* Complication, genitourinary, device, urinary, mechanical)
      graft T83.22 ☑
    vascular NEC — *see* Complication, cardiovascular device, mechanical
    ventricular intracranial shunt T85.02 ☑
  electronic stimulator
    bone T84.320 ☑
    cardiac — *see* Complications, cardiac device, electronic
    nervous system — *see* Complication, prosthetic device, mechanical, electronic nervous system stimulator
    urinary — *see* Complications, electronic stimulator, urinary
  esophageal mucosa into cardia of stomach, congenital Q39.8
  esophagus (acquired) K22.8
    congenital Q39.8
  eyeball (acquired) (lateral) (old) — *see* Displacement, globe
    congenital Q15.8
    current — *see* Avulsion, eye
  fallopian tube (acquired) N83.4
    congenital Q50.6
    opening (congenital) Q50.6
  gallbladder (congenital) Q44.1
  gastric mucosa (congenital) Q40.2
  globe (acquired) (old) (lateral) H05.21- ☑
    current — *see* Avulsion, eye
  heart (congenital) Q24.8
    acquired I51.89
  hymen (upward) (congenital) Q52.4
  intervertebral disc NEC
    with myelopathy — *see* Disorder, disc, with, myelopathy
    cervical, cervicothoracic (with) M50.20
      myelopathy — *see* Disorder, disc, cervical, with myelopathy
      neuritis, radiculitis or radiculopathy — *see* Disorder, disc, cervical, with neuritis
    due to trauma — *see* Dislocation, vertebra
    lumbar region M51.26
      with
        myelopathy M51.06
        neuritis, radiculitis, radiculopathy or sciatica M51.16
    lumbosacral region M51.27
      with
        neuritis, radiculitis, radiculopathy or sciatica M51.17
    sacrococcygeal region M53.3
    thoracic region M51.24
      with
        myelopathy M51.04

Displacement, displaced — *continued*
  intervertebral disc — *continued*
    thoracic region — *continued*
      with — *continued*
        neuritis, radiculitis, radiculopathy M51.14
      thoracolumbar region M51.25
        with
          myelopathy M51.05
          neuritis, radiculitis, radiculopathy M51.15
  intrauterine device T83.32 ☑
  kidney (acquired) N28.83
    congenital Q63.2
  lachrymal, lacrimal apparatus or duct (congenital) Q10.6
  lens, congenital Q12.1
  macula (congenital) Q14.1
  Meckel's diverticulum Q43.0
    malignant — *see* Table of Neoplasms, small intestine, malignant
  nail (congenital) Q84.6
    acquired L60.8
  opening of Wharton's duct in mouth Q38.4
  organ or site, congenital NEC — *see* Malposition, congenital
  ovary (acquired) N83.4
    congenital Q50.39
    free in peritoneal cavity (congenital) Q50.39
    into hernial sac N83.4
  oviduct (acquired) N83.4
    congenital Q50.6
  parathyroid (gland) E21.4
  parotid gland (congenital) Q38.4
  punctum lacrimale (congenital) Q10.6
  sacro-iliac (joint) (congenital) Q74.2
    current injury S33.2 ☑
    old — *see* subcategory M53.2 ☑
  salivary gland (any) (congenital) Q38.4
  spleen (congenital) Q89.09
  stomach, congenital Q40.2
  sublingual duct Q38.4
  tongue (downward) (congenital) Q38.3
  tooth, teeth, fully erupted M26.30
    horizontal M26.33
    vertical M26.34
  trachea (congenital) Q32.1
  ureter or ureteric opening or orifice (congenital) Q62.62
  uterine opening of oviducts or fallopian tubes Q50.6
  uterus, uterine — *see* Malposition, uterus
  ventricular septum Q21.0
    with rudimentary ventricle Q20.4
Disproportion
  between native and reconstructed breast N65.1
  fiber-type G71.2
Disruptio uteri — *see* Rupture, uterus
Disruption (of)
  ciliary body NEC H21.89
  closure of
    cornea T81.31 ☑
    craniotomy T81.32 ☑
    fascia (muscular) (superficial) T81.32 ☑
    internal organ or tissue T81.32 ☑
    laceration (external) (internal) T81.33 ☑
    ligament T81.32 ☑
    mucosa T81.31 ☑
    muscle or muscle flap T81.32 ☑
    ribs or rib cage T81.32 ☑
    skin and subcutaneous tissue (full-thickness) (superficial) T81.31 ☑
    skull T81.32 ☑
    sternum (sternotomy) T81.32 ☑
    tendon T81.32 ☑
    traumatic laceration (external) (internal) T81.33 ☑
  family Z63.8
    due to
      absence of family member due to military deployment Z63.31
      absence of family member NEC Z63.32
      alcoholism and drug addiction in family Z63.72
      bereavement Z63.4
      death (assumed) or disappearance of family member Z63.4
      divorce or separation Z63.5
      drug addiction in family Z63.72
      return of family member from military deployment (current or past conflict) Z63.71
      stressful life events NEC Z63.79
  iris NEC H21.89

☑ **Additional Character Required** — Refer to the Tabular List for Character Selection   ▽ Subterms under main terms may continue to next column or page

Disruption — *continued*
  ligament(s) (*see also* Sprain)
    knee
      current injury — *see* Dislocation, knee
      old (chronic) — *see* Derangement, knee, insta-
        bility
      spontaneous NEC — *see* Derangement, knee,
        disruption ligament
  ossicular chain — *see* Discontinuity, ossicles, ear
  pelvic ring (stable) S32.810 ☑
    unstable S32.811 ☑
  traumatic injury wound repair T81.33 ☑
  wound T81.30 ☑
    episiotomy O90.1
    operation T81.31 ☑
      cesarean O90.0
      external operation wound (superficial)
        T81.31 ☑
      internal operation wound (deep) T81.32 ☑
      perineal (obstetric) O90.1
    traumatic injury repair T81.33 ☑
Dissatisfaction with
  employment Z56.9
  school environment Z55.4
Dissecting — *see* condition
Dissection
  aorta I71.00
    abdominal I71.02
    thoracic I71.01
    thoracoabdominal I71.03
  artery
    carotid I77.71
    cerebral (nonruptured) I67.0
      ruptured — *see* Hemorrhage, intracranial,
        subarachnoid
    coronary I25.42
    iliac I77.72
    renal I77.73
    specified NEC I77.79
    vertebral I77.74
  traumatic — *see* Wound, open, by site
  vascular I99.8
  wound — *see* Wound, open
Disseminated — *see* condition
Dissociation
  auriculoventricular or atrioventricular (AV) (any de-
    gree) (isorhythmic) I45.89
    with heart block I44.2
  interference I45.89
Dissociative reaction, state F44.9
Dissolution, vertebra — *see* Osteoporosis
Distension, distention
  abdomen R14.0
  bladder N32.89
  cecum K63.89
  colon K63.89
  gallbladder K82.8
  intestine K63.89
  kidney N28.89
  liver K76.89
  seminal vesicle N50.8
  stomach K31.89
    acute K31.0
    psychogenic F45.8
  ureter — *see* Dilatation, ureter
  uterus N85.8
Distoma hepaticum infestation B66.3
Distomiasis B66.9
  bile passages B66.3
  hemic B65.9
  hepatic B66.3
    due to Clonorchis sinensis B66.1
  intestinal B66.5
  liver B66.3
    due to Clonorchis sinensis B66.1
  lung B66.4
  pulmonary B66.4
Distomolar (fourth molar) K00.1
Disto-occlusion (Division I) (Division II) M26.212
Distortion(s) (congenital)
  adrenal (gland) Q89.1
  arm NEC Q68.8
  bile duct or passage Q44.5
  bladder Q64.79
  brain Q04.9
  cervix (uteri) Q51.9
  chest (wall) Q67.8

Distortion(s) — *continued*
  chest (wall) Q67.8
    bones Q76.8
  clavicle Q74.0
  clitoris Q52.6
  coccyx Q76.49
  common duct Q44.5
  coronary Q24.5
  cystic duct Q44.5
  ear (auricle) (external) Q17.3
    inner Q16.5
    middle Q16.4
      ossicles Q16.3
  endocrine NEC Q89.2
  eustachian tube Q17.8
  eye (adnexa) Q15.8
  face bone(s) NEC Q75.8
  fallopian tube Q50.6
  femur NEC Q68.8
  fibula NEC Q68.8
  finger(s) Q68.1
  foot Q66.9
  genitalia, genital organ(s)
    female Q52.8
      external Q52.79
      internal NEC Q52.8
  gyri Q04.8
  hand bone(s) Q68.1
  heart (auricle) (ventricle) Q24.8
    valve (cusp) Q24.8
  hepatic duct Q44.5
  humerus NEC Q68.8
  hymen Q52.4
  intrafamilial communications Z63.8
  jaw NEC M26.89
  labium (majus) (minus) Q52.79
  leg NEC Q68.8
  lens Q12.8
  liver Q44.7
  lumbar spine Q76.49
    with disproportion O33.8
      causing obstructed labor O65.0
  lumbosacral (joint) (region) Q76.49
    kyphosis — *see* Kyphosis, congenital
    lordosis — *see* Lordosis, congenital
  nerve Q07.8
  nose Q30.8
  organ
    of Corti Q16.5
    or site not listed — *see* Anomaly, by site
  ossicles, ear Q16.3
  oviduct Q50.6
  pancreas Q45.3
  parathyroid (gland) Q89.2
  pituitary (gland) Q89.2
  radius NEC Q68.8
  sacroiliac joint Q74.2
  sacrum Q76.49
  scapula Q74.0
  shoulder girdle Q74.0
  skull bone(s) NEC Q75.8
    with
      anencephalus Q00.0
      encephalocele — *see* Encephalocele
      hydrocephalus Q03.9
        with spina bifida — *see* Spina bifida, with
          hydrocephalus
      microcephaly Q02
  spinal cord Q06.8
  spine Q76.49
    kyphosis — *see* Kyphosis, congenital
    lordosis — *see* Lordosis, congenital
  spleen Q89.09
  sternum NEC Q76.7
  thorax (wall) Q67.8
    bony Q76.8
  thymus (gland) Q89.2
  thyroid (gland) Q89.2
  tibia NEC Q68.8
  toe(s) Q66.9
  tongue Q38.3
  trachea (cartilage) Q32.1
  ulna NEC Q68.8
  ureter Q62.8
  urethra Q64.79
    causing obstruction Q64.39
  uterus Q51.9
  vagina Q52.4

Distortion(s) — *continued*
  vertebra Q76.49
    kyphosis — *see* Kyphosis, congenital
    lordosis — *see* Lordosis, congenital
  visual (*see also* Disturbance, vision)
    shape and size H53.15
  vulva Q52.79
  wrist (bones) (joint) Q68.8
Distress
  abdomen — *see* Pain, abdominal
  acute respiratory (adult) (child) J80
  epigastric R10.13
  fetal P84
    complicating pregnancy — *see* Stress, fetal
  gastrointestinal (functional) K30
    psychogenic F45.8
  intestinal (functional) NOS K59.9
    psychogenic F45.8
  maternal, during labor and delivery O75.0
  respiratory R06.00
    adult J80
    child J80
    newborn P22.9
      specified NEC P22.8
    orthopnea R06.01
    psychogenic F45.8
    shortness of breath R06.02
    specified type NEC R06.09
Distribution vessel, atypical Q27.9
  coronary artery Q24.5
  precerebral Q28.1
Districhiasis L68.8
Disturbance(s) (*see also* Disease)
  absorption K90.9
    calcium E58
    carbohydrate K90.4
    fat K90.4
      pancreatic K90.3
    protein K90.4
    starch K90.4
    vitamin — *see* Deficiency, vitamin
  acid-base equilibrium E87.8
    mixed E87.4
  activity and attention (with hyperkinesis) — *see* Disor-
    der, attention-deficit hyperactivity
  amino acid transport E72.00
  assimilation, food K90.9
  auditory nerve, except deafness — *see* subcategory
    H93.3 ☑
  behavior — *see* Disorder, conduct
  blood clotting (mechanism) (*see also* Defect, coagula-
    tion) D68.9
  cerebral
    nerve — *see* Disorder, nerve, cranial
    status, newborn P91.9
      specified NEC P91.8
  circulatory I99.9
  conduct (*see also* Disorder, conduct) F91.9
    adjustment reaction — *see* Disorder, adjustment
    compulsive F63.9
    disruptive F91.9
    hyperkinetic — *see* Disorder, attention-deficit hy-
      peractivity
    socialized F91.2
    specified NEC F91.8
    unsocialized F91.1
  coordination R27.8
  cranial nerve — *see* Disorder, nerve, cranial
  deep sensibility — *see* Disturbance, sensation
  digestive K30
    psychogenic F45.8
  electrolyte (*see also* Imbalance, electrolyte)
    newborn, transitory P74.4
      hyperammonemia P74.6
      potassium balance P74.3
      sodium balance P74.2
      specified type NEC P74.4
  emotions specific to childhood and adolescence F93.9
    with
      anxiety and fearfulness NEC F93.8
      elective mutism F94.0
      oppositional disorder F91.3
      sensitivity (withdrawal) F40.10
      shyness F40.10
      social withdrawal F40.10
    involving relationship problems F93.8
    mixed F93.8
    specified NEC F93.8

Disturbance(s) — *continued*
endocrine (gland) E34.9
    neonatal, transitory P72.9
        specified NEC P72.8
equilibrium R42
fructose metabolism E74.10
gait — *see* Gait
    hysterical F44.4
    psychogenic F44.4
gastrointestinal (functional) K30
    psychogenic F45.8
habit, child F98.9
hearing, except deafness and tinnitus — *see* Abnormal, auditory perception
heart, functional (conditions in I44-I50)
    due to presence of (cardiac) prosthesis I97.19- ☑
    postoperative I97.89
        cardiac surgery I97.19- ☑
hormones E34.9
innervation uterus (parasympathetic) (sympathetic) N85.8
keratinization NEC
    gingiva K05.10
        nonplaque induced K05.11
        plaque induced K05.10
    lip K13.0
    oral (mucosa) (soft tissue) K13.29
    tongue K13.29
learning (specific) — *see* Disorder, learning
memory — *see* Amnesia
    mild, following organic brain damage F06.8
mental F99
    associated with diseases classified elsewhere F54
metabolism E88.9
    with
        abortion — *see* Abortion, by type with other specified complication
        ectopic pregnancy O08.5
        molar pregnancy O08.5
    amino-acid E72.9
        aromatic E70.9
        branched-chain E71.2
        straight-chain E72.8
        sulfur-bearing E72.10
    ammonia E72.20
    arginine E72.21
    arginosuccinic acid E72.22
    carbohydrate E74.9
    cholesterol E78.9
    citrulline E72.23
    cystathionine E72.19
    general E88.9
    glutamine E72.8
    histidine E70.40
    homocystine E72.19
    hydroxylysine E72.3
    in labor or delivery O75.89
    iron E83.10
    lipoid E78.9
    lysine E72.3
    methionine E72.19
    neonatal, transitory P74.9
        calcium and magnesium P71.9
            specified type NEC P71.8
        carbohydrate metabolism P70.9
            specified type NEC P70.8
        specified NEC P74.8
    ornithine E72.4
    phosphate E83.39
    sodium NEC E87.8
    threonine E72.8
    tryptophan E70.5
    tyrosine E70.20
    urea cycle E72.20
motor R29.2
nervous, functional R45.0
neuromuscular mechanism (eye), due to syphilis A52.15
nutritional E63.9
    nail L60.3
ocular motion H51.9
    psychogenic F45.8
oculogyric H51.8
    psychogenic F45.8
oculomotor H51.9
    psychogenic F45.8
olfactory nerve R43.1
optic nerve NEC — *see* Disorder, nerve, optic

Disturbance(s) — *continued*
oral epithelium, including tongue NEC K13.29
perceptual due to
    alcohol withdrawal F10.232
    amphetamine intoxication F15.922
        in
            abuse F15.122
            dependence F15.222
    anxiolytic withdrawal F13.232
    cannabis intoxication (acute) F12.922
        in
            abuse F12.122
            dependence F12.222
    cocaine intoxication (acute) F14.922
        in
            abuse F14.122
            dependence F14.222
    hypnotic withdrawal F13.232
    opioid intoxication (acute) F11.922
        in
            abuse F11.122
            dependence F11.222
    phencyclidine intoxication (acute) F19.922
        in
            abuse F19.122
            dependence F19.222
    sedative withdrawal F13.232
personality (pattern) (trait) (*see also* Disorder, personality) F60.9
    following organic brain damage F07.9
polyglandular E31.9
    specified NEC E31.8
potassium balance, newborn P74.3
psychogenic F45.9
psychomotor F44.4
psychophysical visual H53.16
pupillary — *see* Anomaly, pupil, function
reflex R29.2
rhythm, heart I49.9
salivary secretion K11.7
sensation (cold) (heat) (localization) (tactile discrimination) (texture) (vibratory) NEC R20.9
    hysterical F44.6
    skin R20.9
        anesthesia R20.0
        hyperesthesia R20.3
        hypoesthesia R20.1
        paresthesia R20.2
        specified type NEC R20.8
    smell R43.9
        and taste (mixed) R43.8
        anosmia R43.0
        parosmia R43.1
        specified NEC R43.8
    taste R43.9
        and smell (mixed) R43.8
        parageusia R43.2
        specified NEC R43.8
sensory — *see* Disturbance, sensation
situational (transient) (*see also* Disorder, adjustment)
    acute F43.0
sleep G47.9
    nonorganic origin F51.9
smell — *see* Disturbance, sensation, smell
sociopathic F60.2
sodium balance, newborn P74.2
speech R47.9
    developmental F80.9
    specified NEC R47.89
stomach (functional) K31.9
sympathetic (nerve) G90.9
taste — *see* Disturbance, sensation, taste
temperature
    regulation, newborn P81.9
        specified NEC P81.8
    sense R20.8
        hysterical F44.6
tooth
    eruption K00.6
    formation K00.4
    structure, hereditary NEC K00.5
touch — *see* Disturbance, sensation
vascular I99.9
    arteriosclerotic — *see* Arteriosclerosis
vasomotor I73.9
vasospastic I73.9
vision, visual H53.9

Disturbance(s) — *continued*
vision, visual — *continued*
    following
        cerebral infarction I69.398
        cerebrovascular disease I69.998
            specified NEC I69.898
        intracerebral hemorrhage I69.198
        nontraumatic intracranial hemorrhage NEC I69.298
        specified disease NEC I69.898
        subarachnoid hemorrhage I69.098
    psychophysical H53.16
    specified NEC H53.8
    subjective H53.10
        day blindness H53.11
        discomfort H53.14- ☑
        distortions of shape and size H53.15
        loss
            sudden H53.13- ☑
            transient H53.12- ☑
        specified type NEC H53.19
voice R49.9
    psychogenic F44.4
    specified NEC R49.8
Diuresis R35.8
Diver's palsy, paralysis or squeeze T70.3 ☑
Diverticulitis (acute) K57.92
    bladder — *see* Cystitis
    ileum — *see* Diverticulitis, intestine, small
    intestine K57.92
        with
            abscess, perforation or peritonitis K57.80
                with bleeding K57.81
            bleeding K57.93
            congenital Q43.8
            large K57.32
                with
                    abscess, perforation or peritonitis K57.20
                        with bleeding K57.21
                    bleeding K57.33
                    small intestine K57.52
                        with
                            abscess, perforation or peritonitis K57.40
                                with bleeding K57.41
                            bleeding K57.53
            small K57.12
                with
                    abscess, perforation or peritonitis K57.00
                        with bleeding K57.01
                    bleeding K57.13
                    large intestine K57.52
                        with
                            abscess, perforation or peritonitis K57.40
                                with bleeding K57.41
                            bleeding K57.53
Diverticulosis K57.90
    with bleeding K57.91
    large intestine K57.30
        with
            bleeding K57.31
            small intestine K57.50
                with bleeding K57.51
    small intestine K57.10
        with
            bleeding K57.11
            large intestine K57.50
                with bleeding K57.51
Diverticulum, diverticula (multiple) K57.90
    appendix (noninflammatory) K38.2
    bladder (sphincter) N32.3
        congenital Q64.6
    bronchus (congenital) Q32.4
        acquired J98.09
    calyx, calyceal (kidney) N28.89
    cardia (stomach) K31.4
    cecum — *see* Diverticulosis, intestine, large
        congenital Q43.8
    colon — *see* Diverticulosis, intestine, large
        congenital Q43.8
    duodenum — *see* Diverticulosis, intestine, small
        congenital Q43.8
    epiphrenic (esophagus) K22.5
    esophagus (congenital) Q39.6
        acquired (epiphrenic) (pulsion) (traction) K22.5
    eustachian tube — *see* Disorder, eustachian tube, specified NEC

Diverticulum, diverticula — *continued*
  fallopian tube N83.8
  gastric K31.4
  heart (congenital) Q24.8
  ileum — *see* Diverticulosis, intestine, small
  jejunum — *see* Diverticulosis, intestine, small
  kidney (pelvis) (calyces) N28.89
    with calculus — *see* Calculus, kidney
  Meckel's (displaced) (hypertrophic) Q43.0
    malignant — *see* Table of Neoplasms, small intestine, malignant
  midthoracic K22.5
  organ or site, congenital NEC — *see* Distortion
  pericardium (congenital) (cyst) Q24.8
    acquired I31.8
  pharyngoesophageal (congenital) Q39.6
    acquired K22.5
  pharynx (congenital) Q38.7
  rectosigmoid — *see* Diverticulosis, intestine, large
    congenital Q43.8
  rectum — *see* Diverticulosis, intestine, large
  Rokitansky's K22.5
  seminal vesicle N50.8
  sigmoid — *see* Diverticulosis, intestine, large
    congenital Q43.8
  stomach (acquired) K31.4
    congenital Q40.2
  trachea (acquired) J39.8
  ureter (acquired) N28.89
    congenital Q62.8
  ureterovesical orifice N28.89
  urethra (acquired) N36.1
    congenital Q64.79
  ventricle, left (congenital) Q24.8
  vesical N32.3
    congenital Q64.6
  Zenker's (esophagus) K22.5
Division
  cervix uteri (acquired) N88.8
  glans penis Q55.69
  labia minora (congenital) Q52.79
  ligament (partial or complete) (current) (*see also* Sprain)
    with open wound — *see* Wound, open
  muscle (partial or complete) (current) (*see also* Injury, muscle)
    with open wound — *see* Wound, open
  nerve (traumatic) — *see* Injury, nerve
  spinal cord — *see* Injury, spinal cord, by region
  vein I87.8
Divorce, causing family disruption Z63.5
Dix-Hallpike neurolabyrinthitis — *see* Neuronitis, vestibular
Dizziness R42
  hysterical F44.89
  psychogenic F45.8
DMAC (disseminated mycobacterium avium-intracellulare complex) A31.2
DNR (do not resuscitate) Z66
Doan-Wiseman syndrome (primary splenic neutropenia) — *see* Agranulocytosis
Doehle-Heller aortitis A52.02
Dog bite — *see* Bite
Dohle body panmyelopathic syndrome D72.0
Dolichocephaly Q67.2
Dolichocolon Q43.8
Dolichostenomelia — *see* Syndrome, Marfan's
Donohue's syndrome E34.8
Donor (organ or tissue) Z52.9
  blood (whole) Z52.000
    autologous Z52.010
    specified component (lymphocytes) (platelets) NEC Z52.008
      autologous Z52.018
      specified donor NEC Z52.098
    specified donor NEC Z52.090
    stem cells Z52.001
      autologous Z52.011
      specified donor NEC Z52.091
  bone Z52.20
    autologous Z52.21
    marrow Z52.3
    specified type NEC Z52.29
  cornea Z52.5
  egg (Oocyte) Z52.819
    age 35 and over Z52.812
      anonymous recipient Z52.812
      designated recipient Z52.813

Donor — *continued*
  egg — *continued*
    under age 35 Z52.810
      anonymous recipient Z52.810
      designated recipient Z52.811
  kidney Z52.4
  liver Z52.6
  lung Z52.89
  lymphocyte — *see* Donor, blood, specified components NEC
  Oocyte — *see* Donor, egg
  platelets Z52.008
  potential, examination of Z00.5
  semen Z52.89
  skin Z52.10
    autologous Z52.11
    specified type NEC Z52.19
  specified organ or tissue NEC Z52.89
  sperm Z52.89
Donovanosis A58
Dorsalgia M54.9
  psychogenic F45.41
  specified NEC M54.89
Dorsopathy M53.9
  deforming M43.9
    specified NEC — *see* subcategory M43.8 ☑
  specified NEC M53.80
    cervical region M53.82
    cervicothoracic region M53.83
    lumbar region M53.86
    lumbosacral region M53.87
    occipito-atlanto-axial region M53.81
    sacrococcygeal region M53.88
    thoracic region M53.84
    thoracolumbar region M53.85
Double
  albumin E88.09
  aortic arch Q25.4
  auditory canal Q17.8
  auricle (heart) Q20.8
  bladder Q64.79
  cervix Q51.820
    with doubling of uterus (and vagina) Q51.10
      with obstruction Q51.11
  inlet ventricle Q20.4
  kidney with double pelvis (renal) Q63.0
  meatus urinarius Q64.75
  monster Q89.4
  outlet
    left ventricle Q20.2
    right ventricle Q20.1
  pelvis (renal) with double ureter Q62.5
  tongue Q38.3
  ureter (one or both sides) Q62.5
    with double pelvis (renal) Q62.5
  urethra Q64.74
  urinary meatus Q64.75
  uterus Q51.2
    with
      doubling of cervix (and vagina) Q51.10
        with obstruction Q51.11
      in pregnancy or childbirth O34.59- ☑
        causing obstructed labor O65.5
  vagina Q52.10
    with doubling of uterus (and cervix) Q51.10
      with obstruction Q51.11
  vision H53.2
  vulva Q52.79
Douglas' pouch, cul-de-sac — *see* condition
Down syndrome Q90.9
  meiotic nondisjunction Q90.0
  mitotic nondisjunction Q90.1
  mosaicism Q90.1
  translocation Q90.2
DPD (dihydropyrimidine dehydrogenase deficiency) E88.89
Dracontiasis B72
Dracunculiasis, dracunculosis B72
Dream state, hysterical F44.89
Drepanocytic anemia — *see* Disease, sickle-cell
Dresbach's syndrome (elliptocytosis) D58.1
Dreschlera (hawaiiensis) (infection) B43.8
Dressler's syndrome I24.1
Drift, ulnar — *see* Deformity, limb, specified type NEC, forearm

Drinking (alcohol)
  excessive, to excess NEC (without dependence) F10.10
    habitual (continual) (without remission) F10.20
      with remission F10.21
Drip, postnasal (chronic) R09.82
  due to
    allergic rhinitis — *see* Rhinitis, allergic
    common cold J00
    gastroesophageal reflux — *see* Reflux, gastroesophageal
    nasopharyngitis — *see* Nasopharyngitis
    other known condition — *code to* condition
    sinusitis — *see* Sinusitis
Droop
  facial R29.810
    cerebrovascular disease I69.992
      cerebral infarction I69.392
      intracerebral hemorrhage I69.192
      nontraumatic intracranial hemorrhage NEC I69.292
      specified disease NEC I69.892
      subarachnoid hemorrhage I69.092
Drop (in)
  attack NEC R55
  finger — *see* Deformity, finger
  foot — *see* Deformity, limb, foot, drop
  hematocrit (precipitous) R71.0
  hemoglobin R71.0
  toe — *see* Deformity, toe, specified NEC
  wrist — *see* Deformity, limb, wrist drop
Dropped heart beats I45.9
Dropsy, dropsical (*see also* Hydrops)
  abdomen R18.8
  brain — *see* Hydrocephalus
  cardiac, heart — *see* Failure, heart, congestive
  gangrenous — *see* Gangrene
  heart — *see* Failure, heart, congestive
  kidney — *see* Nephrosis
  lung — *see* Edema, lung
  newborn due to isoimmunization P56.0
  pericardium — *see* Pericarditis
Drowned, drowning (near) T75.1 ☑
Drowsiness R40.0
Drug
  abuse counseling and surveillance Z71.51
  addiction — *see* Dependence
  dependence — *see* Dependence
  habit — *see* Dependence
  harmful use — *see* Abuse, drug
  induced fever R50.2
  overdose — *see* Table of Drugs and Chemicals, by drug, poisoning
  poisoning — *see* Table of Drugs and Chemicals, by drug, poisoning
  resistant organism infection (*see also* Resistant, organism, to, drug) Z16.30
  therapy
    long term (current) (prophylactic) — *see* Therapy, drug long-term (current) (prophylactic)
    short term — *omit code*
  wrong substance given or taken in error — *see* Table of Drugs and Chemicals, by drug, poisoning
Drunkenness (without dependence) F10.129
  acute in alcoholism F10.229
  chronic (without remission) F10.20
    with remission F10.21
  pathological (without dependence) F10.129
    with dependence F10.229
  sleep F51.9
Drusen
  macula (degenerative) (retina) — *see* Degeneration, macula, drusen
  optic disc H47.32- ☑
Dry, dryness (*see also* condition)
  larynx J38.7
  mouth R68.2
    due to dehydration E86.0
  nose J34.89
  socket (teeth) M27.3
  throat J39.2
DSAP L56.5
Duane's syndrome H50.81- ☑
Dubin-Johnson disease or syndrome E80.6
Dubois' disease (thymus gland) A50.59 [E35]
Dubowitz' syndrome Q87.1
Duchenne-Aran muscular atrophy G12.21
Duchenne-Griesinger disease G71.0

Duchenne's
  disease or syndrome
    motor neuron disease G12.22
    muscular dystrophy G71.0
  locomotor ataxia (syphilitic) A52.11
  paralysis
    birth injury P14.0
    due to or associated with
      motor neuron disease G12.22
      muscular dystrophy G71.0
Ducrey's chancre A57
Duct, ductus — see condition
Duhring's disease (dermatitis herpetiformis) L13.0
Dullness, cardiac (decreased) (increased) R01.2
Dumb ague — see Malaria
Dumbness — see Aphasia
Dumdum fever B55.0
Dumping syndrome (postgastrectomy) K91.1
Duodenitis (nonspecific) (peptic) K29.80
  with bleeding K29.81
Duodenocholangitis — see Cholangitis
Duodenum, duodenal — see condition
Duplay's bursitis or periarthritis — see Tendinitis, calcific, shoulder
Duplication, duplex (see also Accessory)
  alimentary tract Q45.8
  anus Q43.4
  appendix (and cecum) Q43.4
  biliary duct (any) Q44.5
  bladder Q64.79
  cecum (and appendix) Q43.4
  cervix Q51.820
  chromosome NEC
    with complex rearrangements NEC Q92.5
    seen only at prometaphase Q92.8
  cystic duct Q44.5
  digestive organs Q45.8
  esophagus Q39.8
  frontonasal process Q75.8
  intestine (large) (small) Q43.4
  kidney Q63.0
  liver Q44.7
  pancreas Q45.3
  penis Q55.69
  respiratory organs NEC Q34.8
  salivary duct Q38.4
  spinal cord (incomplete) Q06.2
  stomach Q40.2
Dupré's disease (meningism) R29.1
Dupuytren's contraction or disease M72.0
Durand-Nicolas-Favre disease A55
Durotomy (inadvertent) (incidental) G97.41
Duroziez's disease (congenital mitral stenosis) Q23.2
Dutton's relapsing fever (West African) A68.1
Dwarfism E34.3
  achondroplastic Q77.4
  congenital E34.3
  constitutional E34.3
  hypochondroplastic Q77.4
  hypophyseal E23.0
  infantile E34.3
  Laron-type E34.3
  Lorain (-Levi) type E23.0
  metatropic Q77.8
  nephrotic-glycosuric (with hypophosphatemic rickets) E72.09
  nutritional E45
  pancreatic K86.8
  pituitary E23.0
  renal N25.0
  thanatophoric Q77.1
Dyke-Young anemia (secondary) (symptomatic) D59.1
Dysacusis — see Abnormal, auditory perception
Dysadrenocortism E27.9
  hyperfunction E27.0
Dysarthria R47.1
  following
    cerebral infarction I69.322
    cerebrovascular disease I69.922
      specified disease NEC I69.822
    intracerebral hemorrhage I69.122
    nontraumatic intracranial hemorrhage NEC I69.222
    subarachnoid hemorrhage I69.022
Dysautonomia (familial) G90.1
Dysbarism T70.3 ☑
Dysbasia R26.2
  angiosclerotica intermittens I73.9
  hysterical F44.4

Dysbasia — continued
  lordotica (progressiva) G24.1
  nonorganic origin F44.4
  psychogenic F44.4
Dysbetalipoproteinemia (familial) E78.2
Dyscalculia R48.8
  developmental F81.2
Dyschezia K59.00
Dyschondroplasia (with hemangiomata) Q78.4
Dyschromia (skin) L81.9
Dyscollagenosis M35.9
Dyscranio-pygo-phalangy Q87.0
Dyscrasia
  blood (with) D75.9
    antepartum hemorrhage — see Hemorrhage, antepartum, with coagulation defect
    intrapartum hemorrhage O67.0
    newborn P61.9
      specified type NEC P61.8
    puerperal, postpartum O72.3
  polyglandular, pluriglandular E31.9
Dysendocrinism E34.9
Dysentery, dysenteric (catarrhal) (diarrhea) (epidemic) (hemorrhagic) (infectious) (sporadic) (tropical) A09
  abscess, liver A06.4
  amebic (see also Amebiasis) A06.0
    with abscess — see Abscess, amebic
    acute A06.0
    chronic A06.1
  arthritis (see also category M01) A09
    bacillary (see also category M01) A03.9
  bacillary A03.9
    arthritis (see also category M01) A03.9
    Boyd A03.2
    Flexner A03.1
    Schmitz (-Stutzer) A03.0
    Shiga (-Kruse) A03.0
    Shigella A03.9
      boydii A03.2
      dysenteriae A03.0
      flexneri A03.1
      group A A03.0
      group B A03.1
      group C A03.2
      group D A03.3
      sonnei A03.3
      specified type NEC A03.8
    Sonne A03.3
    specified type NEC A03.8
  balantidial A07.0
  Balantidium coli A07.0
  Boyd's A03.2
  candidal B37.82
  Chilomastix A07.8
  Chinese A03.9
  coccidial A07.3
  Dientamoeba (fragilis) A07.8
  Embadomonas A07.8
  Entamoeba, entamebic — see Dysentery, amebic
  Flexner-Boyd A03.2
  Flexner's A03.1
  Giardia lamblia A07.1
  Hiss-Russell A03.1
  Lamblia A07.1
  leishmanial B55.0
  malarial — see Malaria
  metazoal B82.0
  monilial B37.82
  protozoal A07.9
  Salmonella A02.0
  schistosomal B65.1
  Schmitz (-Stutzer) A03.0
  Shiga (-Kruse) A03.0
  Shigella NOS — see Dysentery, bacillary
  Sonne A03.3
  strongyloidiasis B78.0
  trichomonal A07.8
  viral (see also Enteritis, viral) A08.4
Dysequilibrium R42
Dysesthesia R20.8
  hysterical F44.6
Dysfibrinogenemia (congenital) D68.2
Dysfunction
  adrenal E27.9
    hyperfunction E27.0
  autonomic
    due to alcohol G31.2
    somatoform F45.8

Dysfunction — continued
  bladder N31.9
    neurogenic NOS — see Dysfunction, bladder, neuromuscular
    neuromuscular NOS N31.9
      atonic (motor) (sensory) N31.2
      autonomous N31.2
      flaccid N31.2
      nonreflex N31.2
      reflex N31.1
      specified NEC N31.8
      uninhibited N31.0
  bleeding, uterus N93.8
  cerebral G93.89
  colon K59.9
    psychogenic F45.8
  colostomy K94.03
  cystic duct K82.8
  cystostomy (stoma) — see Complications, cystostomy
  ejaculatory N53.19
    anejaculatory orgasm N53.13
    painful N53.12
    premature F52.4
    retarded N53.11
  endocrine NOS E34.9
  endometrium N85.8
  enterostomy K94.13
  gallbladder K82.8
  gastrostomy (stoma) K94.23
  gland, glandular NOS E34.9
  heart I51.89
  hemoglobin D75.89
  hepatic K76.89
  hypophysis E23.7
  hypothalamic NEC E23.3
  ileostomy (stoma) K94.13
  jejunostomy (stoma) K94.13
  kidney — see Disease, renal
  labyrinthine — see subcategory H83.2 ☑
  left ventricular, following sudden emotional stress I51.81
  liver K76.89
  male — see Dysfunction, sexual, male
  orgasmic (female) F52.31
    male F52.32
  ovary E28.9
    specified NEC E28.8
  papillary muscle I51.89
  parathyroid E21.4
  physiological NEC R68.89
    psychogenic F59
  pineal gland E34.8
  pituitary (gland) E23.3
  platelets D69.1
  polyglandular E31.9
    specified NEC E31.8
  psychophysiologic F59
  psychosexual F52.9
    with
      dyspareunia F52.6
      premature ejaculation F52.4
      vaginismus F52.5
  pylorus K31.9
  rectum K59.9
    psychogenic F45.8
  reflex (sympathetic) — see Syndrome, pain, complex regional I
  segmental — see Dysfunction, somatic
  senile R54
  sexual (due to) R37
    alcohol F10.981
    amphetamine F15.981
      in
        abuse F15.181
        dependence F15.281
    anxiolytic F13.981
      in
        abuse F13.181
        dependence F13.281
    cocaine F14.981
      in
        abuse F14.181
        dependence F14.281
    excessive sexual drive F52.8
    failure of genital response (male) F52.21
      female F52.22
    female N94.9
      aversion F52.1

Dysfunction — *continued*
  sexual — *continued*
    female — *continued*
      dyspareunia N94.1
        psychogenic F52.6
      frigidity F52.22
      nymphomania F52.8
      orgasmic F52.31
      psychogenic F52.9
        aversion F52.1
        dyspareunia F52.6
        frigidity F52.22
        nymphomania F52.8
        orgasmic F52.31
        vaginismus F52.5
      vaginismus N94.2
        psychogenic F52.5
    hypnotic F13.981
      in
        abuse F13.181
        dependence F13.281
    inhibited orgasm (female) F52.31
      male F52.32
    lack
      of sexual enjoyment F52.1
      or loss of sexual desire F52.0
    male N53.9
      anejaculatory orgasm N53.13
      ejaculatory N53.19
        painful N53.12
        premature F52.4
        retarded N53.11
      erectile N52.9
        drug induced N52.2
        due to
          disease classified elsewhere N52.1
          drug N52.2
        postoperative (postprocedural) N52.39
        following
          prostatectomy N52.34
            radical N52.31
          radical cystectomy N52.32
          urethral surgery N52.33
        psychogenic F52.21
        specified cause NEC N52.8
        vasculogenic
          arterial insufficiency N52.01
            with corporo-venous occlusive N52.03
          corporo-venous occlusive N52.02
            with arterial insufficiency N52.03
      impotence — *see* Dysfunction, sexual, male, erectile
      psychogenic F52.9
        aversion F52.1
        erectile F52.21
        orgasmic F52.32
        premature ejaculation F52.4
        satyriasis F52.8
        specified type NEC F52.8
      specified type NEC N53.8
    nonorganic F52.9
      specified NEC F52.8
    opioid F11.981
      in
        abuse F11.181
        dependence F11.281
    orgasmic dysfunction (female) F52.31
      male F52.32
    premature ejaculation F52.4
    psychoactive substances NEC F19.981
      in
        abuse F19.181
        dependence F19.281
    psychogenic F52.9
    sedative F13.981
      in
        abuse F13.181
        dependence F13.281
    sexual aversion F52.1
    vaginismus (nonorganic) (psychogenic) F52.5
  sinoatrial node I49.5
  somatic M39.09
    abdomen M99.09
    acromioclavicular M99.07
    cervical region M99.01
    cervicothoracic M99.01
    costochondral M99.08

Dysfunction — *continued*
  somatic — *continued*
    costovertebral M99.08
    head region M99.00
    hip M99.05
    lower extremity M99.06
    lumbar region M99.03
    lumbosacral M99.03
    occipitocervical M99.00
    pelvic region M99.05
    pubic M99.05
    rib cage M99.08
    sacral region M99.04
    sacrococcygeal M99.04
    sacroiliac M99.04
    specified NEC M99.09
    sternochondral M99.08
    sternoclavicular M99.07
    thoracic region M99.02
    thoracolumbar M99.02
    upper extremity M99.07
  somatoform autonomic F45.8
  stomach K31.89
    psychogenic F45.8
  suprarenal E27.9
    hyperfunction E27.0
  symbolic R48.9
    specified type NEC R48.8
  temporomandibular (joint) M26.69
    joint-pain syndrome M26.62
  testicular (endocrine) E29.9
    specified NEC E29.8
  thymus E32.9
  thyroid E07.9
  ureterostomy (stoma) — *see* Complications, stoma, urinary tract
  urethrostomy (stoma) — *see* Complications, stoma, urinary tract
  uterus, complicating delivery O62.9
    hypertonic O62.4
    hypotonic O62.2
      primary O62.0
      secondary O62.1
  ventricular I51.9
    with congestive heart failure I50.9
    left, reversible, following sudden emotional stress I51.81

Dysgenesis
  gonadal (due to chromosomal anomaly) Q96.9
    pure Q99.1
  renal Q60.5
    bilateral Q60.4
    unilateral Q60.3
  reticular D72.0
  tidal platelet D69.3

Dysgerminoma
  specified site — *see* Neoplasm, malignant, by site
  unspecified site
    female C56.9
    male C62.90

Dysgeusia R43.2
Dysgraphia R27.8
Dyshidrosis, dysidrosis L30.1
Dyskaryotic cervical smear R87.619
Dyskeratosis L85.8
  cervix — *see* Dysplasia, cervix
  congenital Q82.8
  uterus NEC N85.8
Dyskinesia G24.9
  biliary (cystic duct or gallbladder) K82.8
  drug induced
    orofacial G24.01
  esophagus K22.4
  hysterical F44.4
  intestinal K59.8
  nonorganic origin F44.4
  orofacial (idiopathic) G24.4
    drug induced G24.01
  psychogenic F44.4
  subacute, drug induced G24.01
  tardive G24.01
    neuroleptic induced G24.01
  trachea J39.8
  tracheobronchial J98.09
Dyslalia (developmental) F80.0
Dyslexia R48.0
  developmental F81.0

Dyslipidemia E78.5
  depressed HDL cholesterol E78.6
  elevated fasting triglycerides E78.1
Dysmaturity (*see also* Light for dates)
  pulmonary (newborn) (Wilson-Mikity) P27.0
Dysmenorrhea (essential) (exfoliative) N94.6
  congestive (syndrome) N94.6
  primary N94.4
  psychogenic F45.8
  secondary N94.5
Dysmetabolic syndrome X E88.81
Dysmetria R27.8
Dysmorphism (due to)
  alcohol Q86.0
  exogenous cause NEC Q86.8
  hydantoin Q86.1
  warfarin Q86.2
Dysmorphophobia (nondelusional) F45.22
  delusional F22
Dysnomia R47.01
Dysorexia R63.0
  psychogenic F50.8
Dysostosis
  cleidocranial, cleidocranialis Q74.0
  craniofacial Q75.1
  Fairbank's (idiopathic familial generalized osteophytosis) Q78.9
  mandibulofacial (incomplete) Q75.4
  multiplex E76.01
  oculomandibular Q75.5
Dyspareunia (female) N94.1
  male N53.12
  nonorganic F52.6
  psychogenic F52.6
  secondary N94.1
Dyspepsia R10.13
  atonic K30
  functional (allergic) (congenital) (gastrointestinal) (occupational) (reflex) K30
  intestinal K59.8
  nervous F45.8
  neurotic F45.8
  psychogenic F45.8
Dysphagia R13.10
  cervical R13.19
  following
    cerebral infarction I69.391
    cerebrovascular disease I69.991
      specified NEC I69.891
    intracerebral hemorrhage I69.191
    nontraumatic intracranial hemorrhage NEC I69.291
    specified disease NEC I69.891
    subarachnoid hemorrhage I69.091
  functional (hysterical) F45.8
  hysterical F45.8
  nervous (hysterical) F45.8
  neurogenic R13.19
  oral phase R13.11
  oropharyngeal phase R13.12
  pharyneal phase R13.13
  pharyngoesophageal phase R13.14
  psychogenic F45.8
  sideropenic D50.1
  spastica K22.4
  specified NEC R13.19
Dysphagocytosis, congenital D71
Dysphasia R47.02
  developmental
    expressive type F80.1
    receptive type F80.2
  following
    cerebrovascular disease I69.921
      cerebral infarction I69.321
      intracerebral hemorrhage I69.121
      nontraumatic intracranial hemorrhage NEC I69.221
      specified disease NEC I69.821
      subarachnoid hemorrhage I69.021
Dysphonia R49.0
  functional F44.4
  hysterical F44.4
  psychogenic F44.4
  spastica J38.3
Dysphoria, postpartal O90.6
Dyspituitarism E23.3
Dysplasia (*see also* Anomaly)
  acetabular, congenital Q65.89
  alveolar capillary, with vein misalignment J84.843

Subterms under main terms may continue to next column or page   ☑ Additional Character Required — Refer to the Tabular List for Character Selection   119

Dysfunction — Dysplasia

Dysplasia — continued
anus (histologically confirmed) (mild) (moderate) K62.82
  severe D01.3
arrhythmogenic right ventricular I42.8
arterial, fibromuscular I77.3
asphyxiating thoracic (congenital) Q77.2
brain Q07.9
bronchopulmonary, perinatal P27.1
cervix (uteri) N87.9
  mild N87.0
  moderate N87.1
  severe D06.9
chondroectodermal Q77.6
colon D12.6
craniometaphyseal Q78.5
dentinal K00.5
diaphyseal, progressive Q78.3
dystrophic Q77.5
ectodermal (anhidrotic) (congenital) (hereditary) Q82.4
  hydrotic Q82.8
epithelial, uterine cervix — see Dysplasia, cervix
eye (congenital) Q11.2
fibrous
  bone NEC (monostotic) M85.00
    ankle M85.07- ☑
    foot M85.07- ☑
    forearm M85.03- ☑
    hand M85.04- ☑
    lower leg M85.06- ☑
    multiple site M85.09
    neck M85.08
    rib M85.08
    shoulder M85.01- ☑
    skull M85.08
    specified site NEC M85.08
    thigh M85.05- ☑
    toe M85.07- ☑
    upper arm M85.02- ☑
    vertebra M85.08
  diaphyseal, progressive Q78.3
  jaw M27.8
  polyostotic Q78.1
florid osseous (see also Cyst, calcifying odontogenic)
high grade, focal D12.6
hip, congenital Q65.89
joint, congenital Q74.8
kidney Q61.4
  multicystic Q61.4
leg Q74.2
lung, congenital (not associated with short gestation) Q33.6
mammary (gland) (benign) N60.9- ☑
  cyst (solitary) — see Cyst, breast
  cystic — see Mastopathy, cystic
  duct ectasia — see Ectasia, mammary duct
  fibroadenosis — see Fibroadenosis, breast
  fibrosclerosis — see Fibrosclerosis, breast
  specified type NEC N60.8- ☑
metaphyseal (Jansen's) (McKusick's) (Schmid's) Q78.5
muscle Q79.8
oculodentodigital Q87.0
periapical (cemental) (cemento-osseous) — see Cyst, calcifying odontogenic
periosteum — see Disorder, bone, specified type NEC
polyostotic fibrous Q78.1
prostate (see also Neoplasia, intraepithelial, prostate) N42.3
  severe D07.5
renal Q61.4
  multicystic Q61.4
retinal, congenital Q14.1
right ventricular, arrhythmogenic I42.8
septo-optic Q04.4
skin L98.8
spinal cord Q06.1
spondyloepiphyseal Q77.7
thymic, with immunodeficiency D82.1
vagina N89.3
  mild N89.0
  moderate N89.1
  severe NEC D07.2
vulva N90.3
  mild N90.0
  moderate N90.1
  severe NEC D07.1

Dyspnea (nocturnal) (paroxysmal) R06.00
asthmatic (bronchial) J45.909
  with
    bronchitis J45.909
      with
        exacerbation (acute) J45.901
        status asthmaticus J45.902
    chronic J44.9
    exacerbation (acute) J45.901
    status asthmaticus J45.902
  cardiac — see Failure, ventricular, left
cardiac — see Failure, ventricular, left
functional F45.8
hyperventilation R06.4
hysterical F45.8
newborn P28.89
orthopnea R06.01
psychogenic F45.8
shortness of breath R06.02
specified type NEC R06.09
Dyspraxia R27.8
developmental (syndrome) F82
Dysproteinemia E88.09
Dysreflexia, autonomic G90.4
Dysrhythmia
cardiac I49.9
  newborn
    bradycardia P29.12
    occurring before birth P03.819
      before onset of labor P03.810
      during labor P03.811
    tachycardia P29.11
  postoperative I97.89
cerebral or cortical — see Epilepsy
Dyssomnia — see Disorder, sleep
Dyssynergia
biliary K83.8
bladder sphincter N36.44
cerebellaris myoclonica (Hunt's ataxia) G11.1
Dysthymia F34.1
Dysthyroidism E07.9
Dystocia O66.9
affecting newborn P03.1
cervical (hypotonic) O62.2
  affecting newborn P03.6
  primary O62.0
  secondary O62.1
contraction ring O62.4
fetal O66.9
  abnormality NEC O66.3
  conjoined twins O66.3
  oversize O66.2
maternal O66.9
positional O64.9 ☑
shoulder (girdle) O66.0
  causing obstructed labor O66.0
uterine NEC O62.4
Dystonia G24.9
deformans progressiva G24.1
drug induced NEC G24.09
  acute G24.02
  specified NEC G24.09
familial G24.1
idiopathic G24.1
  familial G24.1
  nonfamilial G24.2
  orofacial G24.4
lenticularis G24.8
musculorum deformans G24.1
neuroleptic induced (acute) G24.02
orofacial (idiopathic) G24.4
oromandibular G24.4
  due to drug G24.01
specified NEC G24.8
torsion (familial) (idiopathic) G24.1
  acquired G24.8
  genetic G24.1
  symptomatic (nonfamilial) G24.2
Dystonic movements R25.8
Dystrophy, dystrophia
adiposogenital E23.6
Becker's type G71.0
cervical sympathetic G90.2
choroid (hereditary) H31.20
  central areolar H31.22
  choroideremia H31.21
  gyrate atrophy H31.23
  specified type NEC H31.29

Dystrophy, dystrophia — continued
cornea (hereditary) H18.50
  endothelial H18.51
  epithelial H18.52
  granular H18.53
  lattice H18.54
  macular H18.55
  specified type NEC H18.59
Duchenne's type G71.0
due to malnutrition E45
Erb's G71.0
Fuchs' H18.51
Gower's muscular G71.0
hair L67.8
infantile neuraxonal G31.89
Landouzy-Déjérine G71.0
Leyden-Möbius G71.0
muscular G71.0
  benign (Becker type) G71.0
  congenital (hereditary) (progressive) (with specific morphological abnormalities of the muscle fiber) G71.0
    myotonic G71.11
  distal G71.0
  Duchenne type G71.0
  Emery-Dreifuss G71.0
  Erb type G71.0
  facioscapulohumeral G71.0
  Gower's G71.0
  hereditary (progressive) G71.0
  Landouzy-Déjérine type G71.0
  limb-girdle G71.0
  myotonic G71.11
  progressive (hereditary) G71.0
    Charcot-Marie (-Tooth) type G60.0
  pseudohypertrophic (infantile) G71.0
  severe (Duchenne type) G71.0
myocardium, myocardial — see Degeneration, myocardial
nail L60.3
  congenital Q84.6
nutritional E45
ocular G71.0
oculocerebrorenal E72.03
oculopharyngeal G71.0
ovarian N83.8
polyglandular E31.8
reflex (neuromuscular) (sympathetic) — see Syndrome, pain, complex regional I
retinal (hereditary) H35.50
  in
    lipid storage disorders E75.6 [H36]
    systemic lipidoses E75.6 [H36]
  involving
    pigment epithelium H35.54
    sensory area H35.53
  pigmentary H35.52
  vitreoretinal H35.51
Salzmann's nodular — see Degeneration, cornea, nodular
scapuloperoneal G71.0
skin NEC L98.8
sympathetic (reflex) — see Syndrome, pain, complex regional I
  cervical G90.2
tapetoretinal H35.54
thoracic, asphyxiating Q77.2
unguium L60.3
  congenital Q84.6
vitreoretinal H35.51
vulva N90.4
yellow (liver) — see Failure, hepatic
Dysuria R30.0
psychogenic F45.8

E

Eales' disease H35.06- ☑
Ear (see also condition)
piercing Z41.3
tropical B36.8
wax (impacted) H61.20
  left H61.22
    with right H61.23
  right H61.21
    with left H61.23
Earache — see subcategory H92.0 ☑
Early satiety R68.81

Eaton-Lambert syndrome — *see* Syndrome, Lambert-Eaton
Eberth's disease (typhoid fever) A01.00
Ebola virus disease A98.4
Ebstein's anomaly or syndrome (heart) Q22.5
Eccentro-osteochondrodysplasia E76.29
Ecchondroma — *see* Neoplasm, bone, benign
Ecchondrosis D48.0
Ecchymosis R58
  conjunctiva — *see* Hemorrhage, conjunctiva
  eye (traumatic) — *see* Contusion, eyeball
  eyelid (traumatic) — *see* Contusion, eyelid
  newborn P54.5
  spontaneous R23.3
  traumatic — *see* Contusion
Echinococciasis — *see* Echinococcus
Echinococcosis — *see* Echinococcus
Echinococcus (infection) B67.90
  granulosus B67.4
    bone B67.2
    liver B67.0
    lung B67.1
    multiple sites B67.32
    specified site NEC B67.39
    thyroid B67.31 [E35]
  liver NOS B67.8
    granulosus B67.0
    multilocularis B67.5
  lung NEC B67.99
    granulosus B67.1
    multilocularis B67.69
  multilocularis B67.7
    liver B67.5
    multiple sites B67.61
    specified site NEC B67.69
  specified site NEC B67.99
    granulosus B67.39
    multilocularis B67.69
  thyroid NEC B67.99
    granulosus B67.31 [E35]
    multilocularis B67.69 [E35]
Echinorhynchiasis B83.8
Echinostomiasis B66.8
Echolalia R48.8
Echovirus, as cause of disease classified elsewhere B97.12
Eclampsia, eclamptic (coma) (convulsions) (delirium) (with hypertension) NEC O15.9
  during labor and delivery O15.1
  postpartum O15.2
  pregnancy O15.0- ☑
  puerperal O15.2
Economic circumstances affecting care Z59.9
Economo's disease A85.8
Ectasia, ectasis
  annuloaortic I35.8
  aorta I77.819
    with aneurysm — *see* Aneurysm, aorta
    abdominal I77.811
    thoracic I77.810
    thoracoabdominal I77.812
  breast — *see* Ectasia, mammary duct
  capillary I78.8
  cornea H18.71- ☑
  gastric antral vascular (GAVE) K31.819
    with hemorrhage K31.811
    without hemorrhage K31.819
  mammary duct N60.4- ☑
  salivary gland (duct) K11.8
  sclera — *see* Sclerectasia
Ecthyma L08.0
  contagiosum B08.02
  gangrenosum L08.0
  infectiosum B08.02
Ectocardia Q24.8
Ectodermal dysplasia (anhidrotic) Q82.4
Ectodermosis erosiva pluriorificialis L51.1
Ectopic, ectopia (congenital)
  abdominal viscera Q45.8
    due to defect in anterior abdominal wall Q79.59
  ACTH syndrome E24.3
  adrenal gland Q89.1
  anus Q43.5
  atrial beats I49.1
  beats I49.49
    atrial I49.1
    ventricular I49.3

Ectopic, ectopia — *continued*
  bladder Q64.10
  bone and cartilage in lung Q33.5
  brain Q04.8
  breast tissue Q83.8
  cardiac Q24.8
  cerebral Q04.8
  cordis Q24.8
  endometrium — *see* Endometriosis
  gastric mucosa Q40.2
  gestation — *see* Pregnancy, by site
  heart Q24.8
  hormone secretion NEC E34.2
  kidney (crossed) (pelvis) Q63.2
  lens, lentis Q12.1
  mole — *see* Pregnancy, by site
  organ or site NEC — *see* Malposition, congenital
  pancreas Q45.3
  pregnancy — *see* Pregnancy, ectopic
  pupil — *see* Abnormality, pupillary
  renal Q63.2
  sebaceous glands of mouth Q38.6
  spleen Q89.09
  testis Q53.00
    bilateral Q53.02
    unilateral Q53.01
  thyroid Q89.2
  tissue in lung Q33.5
  ureter Q62.63
  ventricular beats I49.3
  vesicae Q64.10
Ectromelia Q73.8
  lower limb — *see* Defect, reduction, limb, lower, specified type NEC
  upper limb — *see* Defect, reduction, limb, upper, specified type NEC
Ectropion H02.109
  cervix N86
    with cervicitis N72
  congenital Q10.1
  eyelid (paralytic) H02.109
    cicatricial H02.119
      left H02.116
        lower H02.115
        upper H02.114
      right H02.113
        lower H02.112
        upper H02.111
    congenital Q10.1
    left H02.106
      lower H02.105
      upper H02.104
    mechanical H02.129
      left H02.126
        lower H02.125
        upper H02.124
      right H02.123
        lower H02.122
        upper H02.121
    right H02.103
      lower H02.102
      upper H02.101
    senile H02.139
      left H02.136
        lower H02.135
        upper H02.134
      right H02.133
        lower H02.132
        upper H02.131
    spastic H02.149
      left H02.146
        lower H02.145
        upper H02.144
      right H02.143
        lower H02.142
        upper H02.141
  iris H21.89
  lip (acquired) K13.0
    congenital Q38.0
  urethra N36.8
  uvea H21.89
Eczema (acute) (chronic) (erythematous) (fissum) (rubrum) (squamous) (*see also* Dermatitis) L30.9
  contact — *see* Dermatitis, contact
  dyshydrotic L30.1
  external ear — *see* Otitis, externa, acute, eczematoid
  flexural L20.82
  herpeticum B00.0

Eczema — *continued*
  hypertrophicum L28.0
  hypostatic — *see* Varix, leg, with, inflammation
  impetiginous L01.1
  infantile (due to any substance) L20.83
    intertriginous L21.1
    seborrheic L21.1
  intertriginous NEC L30.4
    infantile L21.1
  intrinsic (allergic) L20.84
  lichenified NEC L28.0
  marginatum (hebrae) B35.6
  pustular L30.3
  stasis — *see* Varix, leg, with, inflammation
  vaccination, vaccinatum T88.1 ☑
  varicose — *see* Varix, leg, with, inflammation
Eczematid L30.2
Eddowes (-Spurway) **syndrome** Q78.0
Edema, edematous (infectious) (pitting) (toxic) R60.9
  with nephritis — *see* Nephrosis
  allergic T78.3 ☑
  amputation stump (surgical) (sequelae (late effect)) T87.89
  angioneurotic (allergic) (any site) (with urticaria) T78.3 ☑
    hereditary D84.1
  angiospastic I73.9
  Berlin's (traumatic) S05.8X- ☑
  brain (cytotoxic) (vasogenic) G93.6
    due to birth injury P11.0
    newborn (anoxia or hypoxia) P52.4
      birth injury P11.0
    traumatic — *see* Injury, intracranial, cerebral edema
  cardiac — *see* Failure, heart, congestive
  cardiovascular — *see* Failure, heart, congestive
  cerebral — *see* Edema, brain
  cerebrospinal — *see* Edema, brain
  cervix (uteri) (acute) N88.8
    puerperal, postpartum O90.89
  chronic hereditary Q82.0
  circumscribed, acute T78.3 ☑
    hereditary D84.1
  conjunctiva H11.42- ☑
  cornea H18.2- ☑
    idiopathic H18.22- ☑
    secondary H18.23- ☑
      due to contact lens H18.21- ☑
  due to
    lymphatic obstruction I89.0
    salt retention E87.0
  epiglottis — *see* Edema, glottis
  essential, acute T78.3 ☑
    hereditary D84.1
  extremities, lower — *see* Edema, legs
  eyelid NEC H02.849
    left H02.846
      lower H02.845
      upper H02.844
    right H02.843
      lower H02.842
      upper H02.841
  familial, hereditary Q82.0
  famine — *see* Malnutrition, severe
  generalized R60.1
  glottis, glottic, glottidis (obstructive) (passive) J38.4
    allergic T78.3 ☑
      hereditary D84.1
  heart — *see* Failure, heart, congestive
  heat T67.7 ☑
  hereditary Q82.0
  inanition — *see* Malnutrition, severe
  intracranial G93.6
  iris H21.89
  joint — *see* Effusion, joint
  larynx — *see* Edema, glottis
  legs R60.0
    due to venous obstruction I87.1
    hereditary Q82.0
  localized R60.0
    due to venous obstruction I87.1
  lower limbs — *see* Edema, legs
  lung J81.1
    with heart condition or failure — *see* Failure, ventricular, left
    acute J81.0
    chemical (acute) J68.1
      chronic J68.1

Edema, edematous — *continued*
  lung — *continued*
    chronic J81.1
      due to
        chemicals, gases, fumes or vapors (inhalation) J68.1
        external agent J70.9
          specified NEC J70.8
        radiation J70.1
      due to
        chemicals, fumes or vapors (inhalation) J68.1
        external agent J70.9
          specified NEC J70.8
        high altitude T70.29 ☑
        near drowning T75.1 ☑
        radiation J70.0
      meaning failure, left ventricle I50.1
  lymphatic I89.0
    due to mastectomy I97.2
  macula H35.81
    cystoid, following cataract surgery — *see* Complications, postprocedural, following cataract surgery
    diabetic — *see* Diabetes, by type, with, retinopathy, with macular edema
  malignant — *see* Gangrene, gas
  Milroy's Q82.0
  nasopharynx J39.2
  newborn P83.30
    hydrops fetalis — *see* Hydrops, fetalis
    specified NEC P83.39
  nutritional (*see also* Malnutrition, severe)
    with dyspigmentation, skin and hair E40
  optic disc or nerve — *see* Papilledema
  orbit H05.22- ☑
  pancreas K86.8
  papilla, optic — *see* Papilledema
  penis N48.89
  periodic T78.3 ☑
    hereditary D84.1
  pharynx J39.2
  pulmonary — *see* Edema, lung
  Quincke's T78.3 ☑
    hereditary D84.1
  renal — *see* Nephrosis
  retina H35.81
    diabetic — *see* Diabetes, by type, with, retinopathy, with macular edema
  salt E87.0
  scrotum N50.8
  seminal vesicle N50.8
  spermatic cord N50.8
  spinal (cord) (vascular) (nontraumatic) G95.19
  starvation — *see* Malnutrition, severe
  stasis — *see* Hypertension, venous, (chronic)
  subglottic — *see* Edema, glottis
  supraglottic — *see* Edema, glottis
  testis N44.8
  tunica vaginalis N50.8
  vas deferens N50.8
  vulva (acute) N90.89
Edentulism — *see* Absence, teeth, acquired
Edsall's disease T67.2 ☑
Educational handicap Z55.9
  specified NEC Z55.8
Edward's syndrome — *see* Trisomy, 18
Effect(s) (of) (from) — *see* Effect, adverse NEC
Effect, adverse
  abnormal gravitational (G) forces or states T75.81 ☑
  abuse — *see* Maltreatment
  air pressure T70.9 ☑
    specified NEC T70.8 ☑
  altitude (high) — *see* Effect, adverse, high altitude
  anesthesia (*see also* Anesthesia) T88.59 ☑
    in labor and delivery O74.9
    in pregnancy NEC O29.3- ☑
    local, toxic
      in labor and delivery O74.4
      postpartum, puerperal O89.3
    postpartum, puerperal O89.9
    specified NEC T88.59 ☑
      in labor and delivery O74.8
      postpartum, puerperal O89.8
    spinal and epidural T88.59 ☑
      headache T88.59 ☑
        in labor and delivery O74.5
        postpartum, puerperal O89.4

Effect, adverse — *continued*
  anesthesia (*see also* Anesthesia) — *continued*
    spinal and epidural — *continued*
      specified NEC
        in labor and delivery O74.6
        postpartum, puerperal O89.5
  antitoxin — *see* Complications, vaccination
  atmospheric pressure T70.9 ☑
    due to explosion T70.8 ☑
    high T70.3 ☑
    low — *see* Effect, adverse, high altitude
    specified effect NEC T70.8 ☑
  biological, correct substance properly administered — *see* Effect, adverse, drug
  blood (derivatives) (serum) (transfusion) — *see* Complications, transfusion
  chemical substance — *see* Table of Drugs and Chemicals
  cold (temperature) (weather) T69.9 ☑
    chilblains T69.1 ☑
    frostbite — *see* Frostbite
    specified effect NEC T69.8 ☑
  drugs and medicaments T88.7 ☑
    specified drug — *see* Table of Drugs and Chemicals, by drug, adverse effect
    specified effect — *code to* condition
  electric current, electricity (shock) T75.4 ☑
    burn — *see* Burn
  exertion (excessive) T73.3 ☑
  exposure — *see* Exposure
  external cause NEC T75.89 ☑
  foodstuffs T78.1 ☑
    allergic reaction — *see* Allergy, food
      causing anaphylaxis — *see* Shock, anaphylactic, due to food
    noxious — *see* Poisoning, food, noxious
  gases, fumes, or vapors T59.9- ☑
    specified agent — *see* Table of Drugs and Chemicals
  glue (airplane) sniffing
    due to drug abuse — *see* Abuse, drug, inhalant
    due to drug dependence — *see* Dependence, drug, inhalant
  heat — *see* Heat
  high altitude NEC T70.29 ☑
    anoxia T70.29 ☑
    on
      ears T70.0 ☑
      sinuses T70.1 ☑
    polycythemia D75.1
  high pressure fluids T70.4 ☑
  hot weather — *see* Heat
  hunger T73.0 ☑
  immersion, foot — *see* Immersion
  immunization — *see* Complications, vaccination
  immunological agents — *see* Complications, vaccination
  infrared (radiation) (rays) NOS T66 ☑
    dermatitis or eczema L59.8
  infusion — *see* Complications, infusion
  lack of care of infants — *see* Maltreatment, child
  lightning — *see* Lightning
  medical care T88.9 ☑
    specified NEC T88.8 ☑
  medicinal substance, correct, properly administered — *see* Effect, adverse, drug
  motion T75.3 ☑
  noise, on inner ear — *see* subcategory H83.3 ☑
  overheated places — *see* Heat
  psychosocial, of work environment Z56.5
  radiation (diagnostic) (infrared) (natural source) (therapeutic) (ultraviolet) (X-ray) NOS T66 ☑
    dermatitis or eczema — *see* Dermatitis, due to, radiation
    fibrosis of lung J70.1
    pneumonitis J70.0
    pulmonary manifestations
      acute J70.0
      chronic J70.1
    skin L59.9
  radioactive substance NOS
    dermatitis or eczema — *see* Radiodermatitis
  reduced temperature T69.9 ☑
    immersion foot or hand — *see* Immersion
    specified effect NEC T69.8 ☑
  serum NEC (*see also* Reaction, serum) T80.69 ☑

Effect, adverse — *continued*
  specified NEC T78.8 ☑
    external cause NEC T75.89 ☑
  strangulation — *see* Asphyxia, traumatic
  submersion T75.1 ☑
  thirst T73.1 ☑
  toxic — *see* Toxicity
  transfusion — *see* Complications, transfusion
  ultraviolet (radiation) (rays) NOS T66 ☑
    burn — *see* Burn
    dermatitis or eczema — *see* Dermatitis, due to, ultraviolet rays
      acute L56.8
  vaccine (any) — *see* Complications, vaccination
  vibration — *see* Vibration, adverse effects
  water pressure NEC T70.9 ☑
    specified NEC T70.8 ☑
  weightlessness T75.82 ☑
  whole blood — *see* Complications, transfusion
  work environment Z56.5
Effects, late — *see* Sequelae
Effluvium
  anagen L65.1
  telogen L65.0
Effort syndrome (psychogenic) F45.8
Effusion
  amniotic fluid — *see* Pregnancy, complicated by, premature rupture of membranes
  brain (serous) G93.6
  bronchial — *see* Bronchitis
  cerebral G93.6
  cerebrospinal (*see also* Meningitis)
    vessel G93.6
  chest — *see* Effusion, pleura
  chylous, chyliform (pleura) J94.0
  intracranial G93.6
  joint M25.40
    ankle M25.47- ☑
    elbow M25.42- ☑
    foot joint M25.47- ☑
    hand joint M25.44- ☑
    hip M25.45- ☑
    knee M25.46- ☑
    shoulder M25.41- ☑
    specified joint NEC M25.48
    wrist M25.43- ☑
  malignant pleural J91.0
  meninges — *see* Meningitis
  pericardium, pericardial (noninflammatory) I31.3
    acute — *see* Pericarditis, acute
  peritoneal (chronic) R18.8
  pleura, pleurisy, pleuritic, pleuropericardial J90
    chylous, chyliform J94.0
    due to systemic lupus erythematosis M32.13
    influenzal — *see* Influenza, with, respiratory manifestations NEC
    malignant J91.0
    newborn P28.89
    tuberculous NEC A15.6
      primary (progressive) A15.7
  spinal — *see* Meningitis
  thorax, thoracic — *see* Effusion, pleura
Egg shell nails L60.3
  congenital Q84.6
Egyptian splenomegaly B65.1
Ehlers-Danlos syndrome Q79.6
Ehrlichiosis A77.40
  due to
    E. chafeensis A77.41
    E. sennetsu A79.81
    specified organism NEC A77.49
Eichstedt's disease B36.0
Eisenmenger's
  complex or syndrome I27.89
  defect Q21.8
Ejaculation
  painful N53.12
  premature F52.4
  retarded N53.11
  retrograde N53.14
  semen, painful N53.12
    psychogenic F52.6
Ekbom's syndrome (restless legs) G25.81
Ekman's syndrome (brittle bones and blue sclera) Q78.0
Elastic skin Q82.8
  acquired L57.4

Elastofibroma — see Neoplasm, connective tissue, benign
Elastoma (juvenile) Q82.8
  Miescher's L87.2
Elastomyofibrosis I42.4
Elastosis
  actinic, solar L57.8
  atrophicans (senile) L57.4
  perforans serpiginosa L87.2
  senilis L57.4
Elbow — see condition
Electric current, electricity, effects (concussion) (fatal) (nonfatal) (shock) T75.4 ☑
  burn — see Burn
Electric feet syndrome E53.8
Electrocution T75.4 ☑
  from electroshock gun (taser) T75.4 ☑
Electrolyte imbalance E87.8
  with
    abortion — see Abortion by type, complicated by, electrolyte imbalance
    ectopic pregnancy O08.5
    molar pregnancy O08.5
Elephantiasis (nonfilarial) I89.0
  arabicum — see Infestation, filarial
  bancroftian B74.0
  congenital (any site) (hereditary) Q82.0
  due to
    Brugia (malayi) B74.1
      timori B74.2
    mastectomy I97.2
    Wuchereria (bancrofti) B74.0
  eyelid H02.859
    left H02.856
      lower H02.855
      upper H02.854
    right H02.853
      lower H02.852
      upper H02.851
  filarial, filariensis — see Infestation, filarial
  glandular I89.0
  graecorum A30.9
  lymphangiectatic I89.0
  lymphatic vessel I89.0
    due to mastectomy I97.2
  scrotum (nonfilarial) I89.0
  streptococcal I89.0
  surgical I97.89
    postmastectomy I97.2
  telangiectodes I89.0
  vulva (nonfilarial) N90.89
Elevated, elevation
  antibody titer R76.0
  basal metabolic rate R94.8
  blood pressure (see also Hypertension)
    reading (incidental) (isolated) (nonspecific), no diagnosis of hypertension R03.0
  blood sugar R73.9
  body temperature (of unknown origin) R50.9
  cancer antigen 125 [CA 125] R97.1
  carcinoembryonic antigen [CEA] R97.0
  cholesterol E78.0
    with high triglycerides E78.2
  conjugate, eye H51.0
  C-reactive protein (CRP) R79.82
  diaphragm, congenital Q79.1
  erythrocyte sedimentation rate R70.0
  fasting glucose R73.01
  fasting triglycerides E78.1
  finding on laboratory examination — see Findings, abnormal, inconclusive, without diagnosis, by type of exam
  GFR (glomerular filtration rate) — see Findings, abnormal, inconclusive, without diagnosis, by type of exam
  glucose tolerance (oral) R73.02
  immunoglobulin level R76.8
  indoleacetic acid R82.5
  lactic acid dehydrogenase (LDH) level R74.0
  leukocytes D72.829
  lipoprotein a level E78.8 ☑
  liver function
    study R94.5
    test R79.89
      alkaline phosphatase R74.8
      aminotransferase R74.0
      bilirubin R17
      hepatic enzyme R74.8

Elevated, elevation — continued
  liver function — continued
    test — continued
      lactate dehydrogenase R74.0
  lymphocytes D72.820
  prostate specific antigen [PSA] R97.2
  Rh titer — see Complication(s), transfusion, incompatibility reaction, Rh (factor)
  scapula, congenital Q74.0
  sedimentation rate R70.0
  SGOT R74.0
  SGPT R74.0
  transaminase level R74.0
  triglycerides E78.1
    with high cholesterol E78.2
  tumor associated antigens [TAA] NEC R97.8
  tumor specific antigens [TSA] NEC R97.8
  urine level of
    17-ketosteroids R82.5
    catecholamine R82.5
    indoleacetic acid R82.5
    steroids R82.5
    vanillylmandelic acid (VMA) R82.5
  venous pressure I87.8
  white blood cell count D72.829
    specified NEC D72.828
Elliptocytosis (congenital) (hereditary) D58.1
  Hb C (disease) D58.1
  hemoglobin disease D58.1
  sickle-cell (disease) D57.8- ☑
    trait D57.3
Ellison-Zollinger syndrome E16.4
Ellis-van Creveld syndrome (chondroectodermal dysplasia) Q77.6
Elongated, elongation (congenital) (see also Distortion)
  bone Q79.9
  cervix (uteri) Q51.828
    acquired N88.4
    hypertrophic N88.4
  colon Q43.8
  common bile duct Q44.5
  cystic duct Q44.5
  frenulum, penis Q55.69
  labia minora (acquired) N90.6
  ligamentum patellae Q74.1
  petiolus (epiglottidis) Q31.8
  tooth, teeth K00.2
  uvula Q38.6
Eltor cholera A00.1
Emaciation (due to malnutrition) E41
Embadomoniasis A07.8
Embedded tooth, teeth K01.0
  root only K08.3
Embolic — see condition
Embolism (multiple) (paradoxical) I74.9
  air (any site) (traumatic) T79.0 ☑
    following
      abortion — see Abortion by type complicated by embolism
      ectopic pregnancy O08.2
      infusion, therapeutic injection or transfusion T80.0 ☑
      molar pregnancy O08.2
      procedure NEC
        artery T81.719 ☑
          mesenteric T81.710 ☑
          renal T81.711 ☑
          specified NEC T81.718 ☑
        vein T81.72 ☑
    in pregnancy, childbirth or puerperium — see Embolism, obstetric
  amniotic fluid (pulmonary) (see also Embolism, obstetric)
    following
      abortion — see Abortion by type complicated by embolism
      ectopic pregnancy O08.2
      molar pregnancy O08.2
  aorta, aortic I74.10
    abdominal I74.09
      saddle I74.01
    bifurcation I74.09
    saddle I74.01
    thoracic I74.11
  artery I74.9
    auditory, internal I65.8
    basilar — see Occlusion, artery, basilar

Embolism — continued
  artery — continued
    carotid (common) (internal) — see Occlusion, artery, carotid
    cerebellar (anterior inferior) (posterior inferior) (superior) I66.3
    cerebral — see Occlusion, artery, cerebral
    choroidal (anterior) I66.8
    communicating posterior I66.8
    coronary (see also Infarct, myocardium)
      not resulting in infarction I24.0
    extremity I74.4
      lower I74.3
      upper I74.2
    hypophyseal I66.8
    iliac I74.5
    limb I74.4
      lower I74.3
      upper I74.2
    mesenteric (with gangrene) K55.0
    ophthalmic — see Occlusion, artery, retina
    peripheral I74.4
    pontine I66.8
    precerebral — see Occlusion, artery, precerebral
    pulmonary — see Embolism, pulmonary
    renal N28.0
    retinal — see Occlusion, artery, retina
    septic I76
    specified NEC I74.8
    vertebral — see Occlusion, artery, vertebral
  basilar (artery) I65.1
  blood clot
    following
      abortion — see Abortion by type complicated by embolism
      ectopic or molar pregnancy O08.2
    in pregnancy, childbirth or puerperium — see Embolism, obstetric
  brain (see also Occlusion, artery, cerebral)
    following
      abortion — see Abortion by type complicated by embolism
      ectopic or molar pregnancy O08.2
    puerperal, postpartum, childbirth — see Embolism, obstetric
  capillary I78.8
  cardiac (see also Infarct, myocardium)
    not resulting in infarction I24.0
  carotid (artery) (common) (internal) — see Occlusion, artery, carotid
  cavernous sinus (venous) — see Embolism, intracranial venous sinus
  cerebral — see Occlusion, artery, cerebral
  cholesterol — see Atheroembolism
  coronary (artery or vein) (systemic) — see Occlusion, coronary
  due to device, implant or graft (see also Complications, by site and type, specified NEC)
    arterial graft NEC T82.818 ☑
    breast (implant) T85.81 ☑
    catheter NEC T85.81 ☑
      dialysis (renal) T82.818 ☑
        intraperitoneal T85.81 ☑
      infusion NEC T82.818 ☑
        spinal (epidural) (subdural) T85.81 ☑
      urinary (indwelling) T83.81 ☑
    electronic (electrode) (pulse generator) (stimulator)
      bone T84.81 ☑
      cardiac T82.817 ☑
      nervous system (brain) (peripheral nerve) (spinal) T85.81 ☑
      urinary T83.81 ☑
    fixation, internal (orthopedic) NEC T84.81 ☑
    gastrointestinal (bile duct) (esophagus) T85.81 ☑
    genital NEC T83.81 ☑
    heart (graft) (valve) T82.817 ☑
    joint prosthesis T84.81 ☑
    ocular (corneal graft) (orbital implant) T85.81 ☑
    orthopedic (bone graft) NEC T86.838
    specified NEC T85.81 ☑
    urinary (graft) NEC T83.81 ☑
    vascular NEC T82.818 ☑
    ventricular intracranial shunt T85.81 ☑
  extremities
    lower — see Embolism, vein, lower extremity
      arterial I74.3
    upper I74.2

Embolism — *continued*
- eye H34.9
- fat (cerebral) (pulmonary) (systemic) T79.1 ☑
  - complicating delivery — *see* Embolism, obstetric
  - following
    - abortion — *see* Abortion by type complicated by embolism
    - ectopic or molar pregnancy O08.2
- following
  - abortion — *see* Abortion by type complicated by embolism
  - ectopic or molar pregnancy O08.2
  - infusion, therapeutic injection or transfusion air T80.0 ☑
- heart (fatty) (*see also* Infarct, myocardium)
  - not resulting in infarction I24.0
- hepatic (vein) I82.0
- in pregnancy, childbirth or puerperium — *see* Embolism, obstetric
- intestine (artery) (vein) (with gangrene) K55.0
- intracranial (*see also* Occlusion, artery, cerebral)
  - venous sinus (any) G08
    - nonpyogenic I67.6
- intraspinal venous sinuses or veins G08
  - nonpyogenic G95.19
- kidney (artery) N28.0
- lateral sinus (venous) — *see* Embolism, intracranial, venous sinus
- leg — *see* Embolism, vein, lower extremity
  - arterial I74.3
- longitudinal sinus (venous) — *see* Embolism, intracranial, venous sinus
- lung (massive) — *see* Embolism, pulmonary
- meninges I66.8
- mesenteric (artery) (vein) (with gangrene) K55.0
- obstetric (in) (pulmonary)
  - childbirth O88.82
    - air O88.02
    - amniotic fluid O88.12
    - blood clot O88.22
    - fat O88.82
    - pyemic O88.32
    - septic O88.32
    - specified type NEC O88.82
  - pregnancy O88.81- ☑
    - air O88.01- ☑
    - amniotic fluid O88.11- ☑
    - blood clot O88.21- ☑
    - fat O88.81- ☑
    - pyemic O88.31- ☑
    - septic O88.31- ☑
    - specified type NEC O88.81- ☑
  - puerperal O88.83
    - air O88.03
    - amniotic fluid O88.13
    - blood clot O88.23
    - fat O88.83
    - pyemic O88.33
    - septic O88.33
    - specified type NEC O88.83
- ophthalmic — *see* Occlusion, artery, retina
- penis N48.81
- peripheral artery NOS I74.4
- pituitary E23.6
- popliteal (artery) I74.3
- portal (vein) I81
- postoperative, postprocedural
  - artery T81.719 ☑
    - mesenteric T81.710 ☑
    - renal T81.711 ☑
    - specified NEC T81.718 ☑
  - vein T81.72 ☑
- precerebral artery — *see* Occlusion, artery, precerebral
- puerperal — *see* Embolism, obstetric
- pulmonary (acute) (artery) (vein) I26.99
  - with acute cor pulmonale I26.09
  - chronic I27.82
  - following
    - abortion — *see* Abortion by type complicated by embolism
    - ectopic or molar pregnancy O08.2
  - healed or old Z86.711
  - in pregnancy, childbirth or puerperium — *see* Embolism, obstetric
  - personal history of Z86.711
  - saddle I26.92
    - with acute cor pulmonale I26.02

Embolism — *continued*
- pulmonary — *continued*
  - septic I26.90
    - with acute cor pulmonale I26.01
  - pyemic (multiple) I76
    - following
      - abortion — *see* Abortion by type complicated by embolism
      - ectopic or molar pregnancy O08.2
    - Hemophilus influenzae A41.3
    - pneumococcal A40.3
      - with pneumonia J13
    - puerperal, postpartum, childbirth (any organism) — *see* Embolism, obstetric
    - specified organism NEC A41.89
    - staphylococcal A41.2
    - streptococcal A40.9
  - renal (artery) N28.0
    - vein I82.3
  - retina, retinal — *see* Occlusion, artery, retina
  - saddle
    - abdominal aorta I74.01
    - pulmonary artery I26.92
      - with acute cor pulmonale I26.02
  - septic (arterial) I76
    - complicating abortion — *see* Abortion, by type, complicated by, embolism
  - sinus — *see* Embolism, intracranial, venous sinus
  - soap complicating abortion — *see* Abortion, by type, complicated by, embolism
  - spinal cord G95.19
    - pyogenic origin G06.1
  - spleen, splenic (artery) I74.8
  - upper extremity I74.2
  - vein (acute) I82.90
    - antecubital I82.61- ☑
      - chronic I82.71- ☑
    - axillary I82.A1- ☑ (*following* I82.7)
      - chronic I82.A2- ☑ (*following* I82.7)
    - basilic I82.61- ☑
      - chronic I82.71- ☑
    - brachial I82.62- ☑
      - chronic I82.72- ☑
    - brachiocephalic (innominate) I82.290
      - chronic I82.291
    - cephalic I82.61- ☑
      - chronic I82.71- ☑
    - chronic I82.91
    - deep (DVT) I82.40- ☑
      - calf I82.4Z- ☑
        - chronic I82.5Z- ☑
      - lower leg I82.4Z- ☑
        - chronic I82.5Z- ☑
      - thigh I82.4Y- ☑
        - chronic I82.5Y- ☑
      - upper leg I82.4Y
        - chronic I82.5Y-
    - femoral I82.41- ☑
      - chronic I82.51- ☑
    - iliac (iliofemoral) I82.42- ☑
      - chronic I82.52- ☑
    - innominate I82.290
      - chronic I82.291
    - internal jugular I82.C1- ☑ (*following* I82.7)
      - chronic I82.C2- ☑ (*following* I82.7)
    - lower extremity
      - deep I82.40- ☑
        - chronic I82.50- ☑
        - specified NEC I82.49- ☑
          - chronic NEC I82.59- ☑
      - distal
        - deep I82.4Z- ☑
      - proximal
        - deep I82.4Y- ☑
          - chronic I82.5Y- ☑
      - superficial I82.81- ☑
    - popliteal I82.43- ☑
      - chronic I82.53- ☑
    - radial I82.62- ☑
      - chronic I82.72- ☑
    - renal I82.3
    - saphenous (greater) (lesser) I82.81- ☑
    - specified NEC I82.890
      - chronic NEC I82.891
    - subclavian I82.B1- ☑ (*following* I82.7)
      - chronic I82.B2- ☑ (*following* I82.7)

Embolism — *continued*
- vein — *continued*
  - thoracic NEC I82.290
    - chronic I82.291
  - tibial I82.44- ☑
    - chronic I82.54- ☑
  - ulnar I82.62- ☑
    - chronic I82.72- ☑
  - upper extremity I82.60- ☑
    - chronic I82.70- ☑
    - deep I82.62- ☑
      - chronic I82.72- ☑
    - superficial I82.61- ☑
      - chronic I82.71- ☑
  - vena cava
    - inferior (acute) I82.220
      - chronic I82.221
    - superior (acute) I82.210
      - chronic I82.211
  - venous sinus G08
  - vessels of brain — *see* Occlusion, artery, cerebral
- **Embolus** — *see* Embolism
- **Embryoma** (*see also* Neoplasm, uncertain behavior, by site)
  - benign — *see* Neoplasm, benign, by site
  - kidney C64.- ☑
  - liver C22.0
  - malignant (*see also* Neoplasm, malignant, by site)
    - kidney C64.- ☑
    - liver C22.0
    - testis C62.9- ☑
      - descended (scrotal) C62.1- ☑
      - undescended C62.0- ☑
  - testis C62.9- ☑
    - descended (scrotal) C62.1- ☑
    - undescended C62.0- ☑
- **Embryonic**
  - circulation Q28.9
  - heart Q28.9
  - vas deferens Q55.4
- **Embryopathia NOS** Q89.9
- **Embryotoxon** Q13.4
- **Emesis** — *see* Vomiting
- **Emotional lability** R45.86
- **Emotionality, pathological** F60.3
- **Emotogenic disease** — *see* Disorder, psychogenic
- **Emphysema** (atrophic) (bullous) (chronic) (interlobular) (lung) (obstructive) (pulmonary) (senile) (vesicular) J43.9
  - cellular tissue (traumatic) T79.7 ☑
    - surgical T81.82 ☑
  - centrilobular J43.2
  - compensatory J98.3
  - congenital (interstitial) P25.0
  - conjunctiva H11.89
  - connective tissue (traumatic) T79.7 ☑
    - surgical T81.82 ☑
  - due to chemicals, gases, fumes or vapors J68.4
  - eyelid(s) — *see* Disorder, eyelid, specified type NEC
    - surgical T81.82 ☑
    - traumatic T79.7 ☑
  - interstitial J98.2
    - congenital P25.0
    - perinatal period P25.0
  - laminated tissue T79.7 ☑
    - surgical T81.82 ☑
  - mediastinal J98.2
    - newborn P25.2
  - orbit, orbital — *see* Disorder, orbit, specified type NEC
  - panacinar J43.1
  - panlobular J43.1
  - specified NEC J43.8
  - subcutaneous (traumatic) T79.7 ☑
    - nontraumatic J98.2
    - postprocedural T81.82 ☑
    - surgical T81.82 ☑
  - surgical T81.82 ☑
  - thymus (gland) (congenital) E32.8
  - traumatic (subcutaneous) T79.7 ☑
  - unilateral J43.0
- **Empty nest syndrome** Z60.0
- **Empyema** (acute) (chest) (double) (pleura) (supradiaphragmatic) (thorax) J86.9
  - with fistula J86.0
  - accessory sinus (chronic) — *see* Sinusitis
  - antrum (chronic) — *see* Sinusitis, maxillary
  - brain (any part) — *see* Abscess, brain

Empyema — *continued*
  ethmoidal (chronic) (sinus) — *see* Sinusitis, ethmoidal
  extradural — *see* Abscess, extradural
  frontal (chronic) (sinus) — *see* Sinusitis, frontal
  gallbladder K81.0
  mastoid (process) (acute) — *see* Mastoiditis, acute
  maxilla, maxillary M27.2
    sinus (chronic) — *see* Sinusitis, maxillary
  nasal sinus (chronic) — *see* Sinusitis
  sinus (accessory) (chronic) (nasal) — *see* Sinusitis
  sphenoidal (sinus) (chronic) — *see* Sinusitis, sphe-
      noidal
  subarachnoid — *see* Abscess, extradural
  subdural — *see* Abscess, subdural
  tuberculous A15.6
  ureter — *see* Ureteritis
  ventricular — *see* Abscess, brain
En coup de sabre lesion L94.1
Enamel pearls K00.2
Enameloma K00.2
Enanthema, viral B09
Encephalitis (chronic) (hemorrhagic) (idiopathic)
      (nonepidemic) (spurious) (subacute) G04.90
  acute (*see also* Encephalitis, viral) A86
    disseminated G04.00
      infectious G04.01
      noninfectious G04.81
      postimmunization (postvaccination) G04.02
      postinfectious G04.01
    inclusion body A85.8
    necrotizing hemorrhagic G04.30
      postimmunization G04.32
      postinfectious G04.31
      specified NEC G04.39
  arboviral, arbovirus NEC A85.2
  arthropod-borne NEC (viral) A85.2
  Australian A83.4
  California (virus) A83.5
  Central European (tick-borne) A84.1
  Czechoslovakian A84.1
  Dawson's (inclusion body) A81.1
  diffuse sclerosing A81.1
  disseminated, acute G04.00
  due to
    cat scratch disease A28.1
    human immunodeficiency virus (HIV) disease
        B20 [G05.3]
    malaria — *see* Malaria
    rickettsiosis — *see* Rickettsiosis
    smallpox inoculation G04.02
    typhus — *see* Typhus
  Eastern equine A83.2
  endemic (viral) A86
  epidemic NEC (viral) A86
  equine (acute) (infectious) (viral) A83.9
    Eastern A83.2
    Venezuelan A92.2
    Western A83.1
  Far Eastern (tick-borne) A84.0
  following vaccination or other immunization proce-
      dure G04.02
  herpes zoster B02.0
  herpesviral B00.4
    due to herpesvirus 6 B10.01
    due to herpesvirus 7 B10.09
    specified NEC B10.09
  Ilheus (virus) A83.8
  in (due to)
    actinomycosis A42.82
    adenovirus A85.1
    African trypanosomiasis B56.9 [G05.3]
    Chagas' disease (chronic) B57.42
    cytomegalovirus B25.8
    enterovirus A85.0
    herpes (simplex) virus B00.4
      due to herpesvirus 6 B10.01
      due to herpesvirus 7 B10.09
      specified NEC B10.09
    infectious disease NEC B99 ☑ [G05.3]
    influenza — *see* Influenza, with, encephalopathy
    listeriosis A32.12
    measles B05.0
    mumps B26.2
    naegleriasis B60.2
    parasitic disease NEC B89 [G05.3]
    poliovirus A80.9 [G05.3]
    rubella B06.01

Encephalitis — *continued*
  in — *continued*
    syphilis
      congenital A50.42
      late A52.14
    systemic lupus erythematosus M32.19
    toxoplasmosis (acquired) B58.2
      congenital P37.1
    tuberculosis A17.82
    zoster B02.0
  inclusion body A81.1
  infectious (acute) (virus) NEC A86
  Japanese (B type) A83.0
  La Crosse A83.5
  lead — *see* Poisoning, lead
  lethargica (acute) (infectious) A85.8
  louping ill A84.8
  lupus erythematosus, systemic M32.19
  lymphatica A87.2
  Mengo A85.8
  meningococcal A39.81
  Murray Valley A83.4
  otitic NEC H66.40 [G05.3]
  parasitic NOS B71.9
  periaxial G37.0
  periaxialis (concentrica) (diffuse) G37.5
  postchickenpox B01.11
  postexanthematous NEC B09
  postimmunization G04.02
  postinfectious NEC G04.01
  postmeasles B05.0
  postvaccinal G04.02
  postvaricella B01.11
  postviral NEC A86
  Powassan A84.8
  Rasmussen G04.81
  Rio Bravo A85.8
  Russian
    autumnal A83.0
    spring-summer (taiga) A84.0
  saturnine — *see* Poisoning, lead
  specified NEC G04.81
  St. Louis A83.3
  subacute sclerosing A81.1
  summer A83.0
  suppurative G04.81
  tick-borne A84.9
  Torula, torular (cryptococcal) B45.1
  toxic NEC G92
  trichinosis B75 [G05.3]
  type
    B A83.0
    C A83.3
  van Bogaert's A81.1
  Venezuelan equine A92.2
  Vienna A85.8
  viral, virus A86
    arthropod-borne NEC A85.2
      mosquito-borne A83.9
        Australian X disease A83.4
        California virus A83.5
        Eastern equine A83.2
        Japanese (B type) A83.0
        Murray Valley A83.4
        specified NEC A83.8
        St. Louis A83.3
        type B A83.0
        type C A83.3
        Western equine A83.1
      tick-borne A84.9
        biundulant A84.1
        central European A84.1
        Czechoslovakian A84.1
        diphasic meningoencephalitis A84.1
        Far Eastern A84.0
        Russian spring-summer (taiga) A84.0
        specified NEC A84.8
    specified type NEC A85.8
  Western equine A83.1
Encephalocele Q01.9
  frontal Q01.0
  nasofrontal Q01.1
  occipital Q01.2
  specified NEC Q01.8
Encephalocystocele — *see* Encephalocele
Encephaloduroarteriomyosynangiosis (EDAMS) I67.5
Encephalomalacia (brain) (cerebellar) (cerebral) — *see*
  Softening, brain

Encephalomeningitis — *see* Meningoencephalitis
Encephalomeningocele — *see* Encephalocele
Encephalomeningomyelitis — *see* Meningoencephalitis
Encephalomyelitis (*see also* Encephalitis) G04.90
  acute disseminated G04.00
    infectious G04.01
    noninfectious G04.81
    postimmunization G04.02
    postinfectious G04.01
  acute necrotizing hemorrhagic G04.30
    postimmunization G04.32
    postinfectious G04.31
    specified NEC G04.39
  benign myalgic G93.3
  equine A83.9
    Eastern A83.2
    Venezuelan A92.2
    Western A83.1
  in diseases classified elsewhere G05.3
  myalgic, benign G93.3
  postchickenpox B01.11
  postinfectious NEC G04.01
  postmeasles B05.0
  postvaccinal G04.02
  postvaricella B01.11
  rubella B06.01
  specified NEC G04.81
  Venezuelan equine A92.2
Encephalomyelocele — *see* Encephalocele
Encephalomyelomeningitis — *see* Meningoencephalitis
Encephalomyelopathy G96.9
Encephalomyeloradiculitis (acute) G61.0
Encephalomyeloradiculoneuritis (acute) (Guillain-
  Barré) G61.0
Encephalomyeloradiculopathy G96.9
Encephalopathia hyperbilirubinemica, newborn
  P57.9
  due to isoimmunization (conditions in P55) P57.0
Encephalopathy (acute) G93.40
  acute necrotizing hemorrhagic G04.30
    postimmunization G04.32
    postinfectious G04.31
    specified NEC G04.39
  alcoholic G31.2
  anoxic — *see* Damage, brain, anoxic
  arteriosclerotic I67.2
  centrolobar progressive (Schilder) G37.0
  congenital Q07.9
  degenerative, in specified disease NEC G32.89
  demyelinating callosal G37.1
  due to
    drugs (*see also* Table of Drugs and Chemicals) G92
  hepatic — *see* Failure, hepatic
  hyperbilirubinemic, newborn P57.9
    due to isoimmunization (conditions in P55) P57.0
  hypertensive I67.4
  hypoglycemic E16.2
  hypoxic — *see* Damage, brain, anoxic
  hypoxic ischemic P91.60
    mild P91.61
    moderate P91.62
    severe P91.63
  in (due to) (with)
    birth injury P11.1
    hyperinsulinism E16.1 [G94]
    influenza — *see* Influenza, with, encephalopathy
    lack of vitamin (*see also* Deficiency, vitamin)
        E56.9 [G32.89]
    neoplastic disease (*see also* Neoplasm)
        D49.9 [G13.1]
    serum (*see also* Reaction, serum) T80.69 ☑
    syphilis A52.17
    trauma (postconcussional) F07.81
      current injury — *see* Injury, intracranial
    vaccination G04.02
  lead — *see* Poisoning, lead
  metabolic G93.41
    drug induced G92
    toxic G92
  myoclonic, early, symptomatic — *see* Epilepsy, gener-
      alized, specified NEC
  necrotizing, subacute (Leigh) G31.82
  pellagrous E52 [G32.89]
  portosystemic — *see* Failure, hepatic
  postcontusional F07.81
    current injury — *see* Injury, intracranial, diffuse

Index

Empyema — Encephalopathy

Encephalopathy — *continued*
  posthypoglycemic (coma) E16.1 [G94]
  postradiation G93.89
  saturnine — *see* Poisoning, lead
  septic G93.41
  specified NEC G93.49
  spongiform, subacute (viral) A81.09
  toxic G92
    metabolic G92
  traumatic (postconcussional) F07.81
    current injury — *see* Injury, intracranial
  vitamin B deficiency NEC E53.9 [G32.89]
    vitamin B1 E51.2
  Wernicke's E51.2
Encephalorrhagia — *see* Hemorrhage, intracranial, intracerebral
Encephalosis, posttraumatic F07.81
Enchondroma (*see also* Neoplasm, bone, benign)
Enchondromatosis (cartilaginous) (multiple) Q78.4
Encopresis R15.9
  functional F98.1
  nonorganic origin F98.1
  psychogenic F98.1
Encounter (with health service) (for) Z76.89
  adjustment and management (of)
    breast implant Z45.81 ☑
    implanted device NEC Z45.89
    myringotomy device (stent) (tube) Z45.82
  administrative purpose only Z02.9
    examination for
      adoption Z02.82
      armed forces Z02.3
      disability determination Z02.71
      driving license Z02.4
      employment Z02.1
      insurance Z02.6
      medical certificate NEC Z02.79
      paternity testing Z02.81
      residential institution admission Z02.2
      school admission Z02.0
      sports Z02.5
    specified reason NEC Z02.89
  aftercare — *see* Aftercare
  antenatal screening Z36
  assisted reproductive fertility procedure cycle Z31.83
  blood typing Z01.83
    Rh typing Z01.83
  breast augmentation or reduction Z41.1
  breast implant exchange (different material) (different size) Z45.81 ☑
  breast reconstruction following mastectomy Z42.1
  check-up — *see* Examination
  chemotherapy for neoplasm Z51.11
  colonoscopy, screening Z12.11
  counseling — *see* Counseling
  delivery, full-term, uncomplicated O80
    cesarean, without indication O82
  ear piercing Z41.3
  examination — *see* Examination
  expectant parent(s) (adoptive) pre-birth pediatrician visit Z76.81
  fertility preservation procedure (prior to cancer therapy) (prior to removal of gonads) Z31.84
  fitting (of) — *see* Fitting (and adjustment) (of)
  genetic
    counseling Z31.5
    testing — *see* Test, genetic
  hearing conservation and treatment Z01.12
  immunotherapy for neoplasm Z51.12
  in vitro fertilization cycle Z31.83
  instruction (in)
    child care (postpartal) (prenatal) Z32.3
    childbirth Z32.2
    natural family planning
      procreative Z31.61
      to avoid pregnancy Z30.02
  insulin pump titration Z46.81
  joint prosthesis insertion following prior explantation of joint prosthesis (staged procedure)
    hip Z47.32
    knee Z47.33
    shoulder Z47.31
  laboratory (as part of a general medical examination) Z00.00
    with abnormal findings Z00.01
  mental health services (for)
    abuse NEC
      perpetrator Z69.82

Encounter — *continued*
  mental health services — *continued*
    abuse — *continued*
      victim Z69.81
    child abuse
      nonparental
        perpetrator Z69.021
        victim Z69.020
      parental
        perpetrator Z69.011
        victim Z69.010
    spousal or partner abuse
      perpetrator Z69.12
      victim Z69.11
  observation (for) (ruled out)
    exposure to (suspected)
      anthrax Z03.810
      biological agent NEC Z03.818
  pediatrician visit, by expectant parent(s) (adoptive) Z76.81
  plastic and reconstructive surgery following medical procedure or healed injury NEC Z42.8
  pregnancy
    supervision of — *see* Pregnancy, supervision of
    test Z32.00
      result negative Z32.02
      result positive Z32.01
  radiation therapy (antineoplastic) Z51.0
  radiological (as part of a general medical examination) Z00.00
    with abnormal findings Z00.01
  reconstructive surgery following medical procedure or healed injury NEC Z42.8
  removal (of) (*see also* Removal)
    artificial
      arm Z44.00- ☑
        complete Z44.01- ☑
        partial Z44.02- ☑
      eye Z44.2- ☑
      leg Z44.10- ☑
        complete Z44.11- ☑
        partial Z44.12- ☑
    breast implant Z45.81 ☑
      tissue expander (without synchronous insertion of permanent implant) Z45.81 ☑
    device Z46.9
      specified NEC Z46.89
    external
      fixation device — *code to* fracture with seventh character D
      prosthesis, prosthetic device Z44.9
        breast Z44.3- ☑
        specified NEC Z44.8
    implanted device NEC Z45.89
    insulin pump Z46.81
    internal fixation device Z47.2
    myringotomy device (stent) (tube) Z45.82
    nervous system device NEC Z46.2
      brain neuropacemaker Z46.2
      visual substitution device Z46.2
        implanted Z45.31
    non-vascular catheter Z46.82
    orthodontic device Z46.4
    stent
      ureteral Z46.6
    urinary device Z46.6
  repeat cervical smear to confirm findings of recent normal smear following initial abnormal smear Z01.42
  respirator [ventilator] use during power failure Z99.12
  Rh typing Z01.83
  screening — *see* Screening
  specified NEC Z76.89
  sterilization Z30.2
  suspected condition, ruled out
    amniotic cavity and membrane Z03.71
    cervical shortening Z03.75
    fetal anomaly Z03.73
    fetal growth Z03.74
    maternal and fetal conditions NEC Z03.79
    oligohydramnios Z03.71
    placental problem Z03.72
    polyhydramnios Z03.71
  suspected exposure (to), ruled out
    anthrax Z03.810
    biological agents NEC Z03.818
  termination of pregnancy, elective Z33.2
  testing — *see* Test

Encounter — *continued*
  therapeutic drug level monitoring Z51.81
  titration, insulin pump Z46.81
  to determine fetal viability of pregnancy O36.80 ☑
  training
    insulin pump Z46.81
  X-ray of chest (as part of a general medical examination) Z00.00
    with abnormal findings Z00.01
Encystment — *see* Cyst
Endarteritis (bacterial, subacute) (infective) I77.6
  brain I67.7
  cerebral or cerebrospinal I67.7
  deformans — *see* Arteriosclerosis
  embolic — *see* Embolism
  obliterans (*see also* Arteriosclerosis)
    pulmonary I28.8
  pulmonary I28.8
  retina — *see* Vasculitis, retina
  senile — *see* Arteriosclerosis
  syphilitic A52.09
    brain or cerebral A52.04
    congenital A50.54 [I79.8]
  tuberculous A18.89
Endemic — *see* condition
Endocarditis (chronic) (marantic) (nonbacterial) (thrombotic) (valvular) I38
  with rheumatic fever (conditions in I00)
    active — *see* Endocarditis, acute, rheumatic
    inactive or quiescent (with chorea) I09.1
  acute or subacute I33.9
    infective I33.0
    rheumatic (aortic) (mitral) (pulmonary) (tricuspid) I01.1
      with chorea (acute) (rheumatic) (Sydenham's) I02.0
  aortic (heart) (nonrheumatic) (valve) I35.8
    with
      mitral disease I08.0
        with tricuspid (valve) disease I08.3
          active or acute I01.1
            with chorea (acute) (rheumatic) (Sydenham's) I02.0
        rheumatic fever (conditions in I00)
          active — *see* Endocarditis, acute, rheumatic
          inactive or quiescent (with chorea) I06.9
        tricuspid (valve) disease I08.2
          with mitral (valve) disease I08.3
    acute or subacute I33.9
    arteriosclerotic I35.8
    rheumatic I06.9
      with mitral disease I08.0
        with tricuspid (valve) disease I08.3
          active or acute I01.1
            with chorea (acute) (rheumatic) (Sydenham's) I02.0
      active or acute I01.1
        with chorea (acute) (rheumatic) (Sydenham's) I02.0
    specified NEC I06.8
    specified cause NEC I35.8
    syphilitic A52.03
  arteriosclerotic I38
  atypical verrucous (Libman-Sacks) M32.11
  bacterial (acute) (any valve) (subacute) I33.0
  candidal B37.6
  congenital Q24.8
  constrictive I33.0
  Coxiella burnetii A78 [I39]
  Coxsackie B33.21
  due to
    prosthetic cardiac valve T82.6 ☑
    Q fever A78 [I39]
    Serratia marcescens I33.0
    typhoid (fever) A01.02
  gonococcal A54.83
  infectious or infective (acute) (any valve) (subacute) I33.0
  lenta (acute) (any valve) (subacute) I33.0
  Libman-Sacks M32.11
  listerial A32.82
  Löffler's I42.3
  malignant (acute) (any valve) (subacute) I33.0
  meningococcal A39.51
  mitral (chronic) (double) (fibroid) (heart) (inactive) (valve) (with chorea) I05.9
    with
      aortic (valve) disease I08.0

Endocarditis — *continued*
  mitral — *continued*
    with — *continued*
      aortic disease — *continued*
        with tricuspid (valve) disease I08.3
          active or acute I01.1
            with chorea (acute) (rheumatic) (Sydenham's) I02.0
        rheumatic fever (conditions in I00)
          active — *see* Endocarditis, acute, rheumatic
          inactive or quiescent (with chorea) I05.9
        tricuspid (valve) disease I08.1
          with aortic (valve) disease I08.3
      active or acute I01.1
        with chorea (acute) (rheumatic) (Sydenham's) I02.0
      bacterial I33.0
      arteriosclerotic I34.8
      nonrheumatic I34.8
        acute or subacute I33.9
      specified NEC I05.8
  monilial B37.6
  multiple valves I08.9
    specified disorders I08.8
  mycotic (acute) (any valve) (subacute) I33.0
  pneumococcal (acute) (any valve) (subacute) I33.0
  pulmonary (chronic) (heart) (valve) I37.8
    with rheumatic fever (conditions in I00)
      active — *see* Endocarditis, acute, rheumatic
      inactive or quiescent (with chorea) I09.89
        with aortic, mitral or tricuspid disease I08.8
    acute or subacute I33.9
      rheumatic I01.1
        with chorea (acute) (rheumatic) (Sydenham's) I02.0
    arteriosclerotic I37.8
    congenital Q22.2
    rheumatic (chronic) (inactive) (with chorea) I09.89
      active or acute I01.1
        with chorea (acute) (rheumatic) (Sydenham's) I02.0
  syphilitic A52.03
  purulent (acute) (any valve) (subacute) I33.0
  Q fever A78 [I39]
  rheumatic (chronic) (inactive) (with chorea) I09.1
    active or acute (aortic) (mitral) (pulmonary) (tricuspid) I01.1
      with chorea (acute) (rheumatic) (Sydenham's) I02.0
  rheumatoid — *see* Rheumatoid, carditis
  septic (acute) (any valve) (subacute) I33.0
  streptococcal (acute) (any valve) (subacute) I33.0
  subacute — *see* Endocarditis, acute
  suppurative (acute) (any valve) (subacute) I33.0
  syphilitic A52.03
  toxic I33.9
  tricuspid (chronic) (heart) (inactive) (rheumatic) (valve) (with chorea) I07.9
    with
      aortic (valve) disease I08.2
        mitral (valve) disease I08.3
      mitral (valve) disease I08.1
        aortic (valve) disease I08.3
      rheumatic fever (conditions in I00)
        active — *see* Endocarditis, acute, rheumatic
        inactive or quiescent (with chorea) I07.8
    active or acute I01.1
      with chorea (acute) (rheumatic) (Sydenham's) I02.0
    arteriosclerotic I36.8
    nonrheumatic I36.8
      acute or subacute I33.9
    specified cause, except rheumatic I36.8
  tuberculous — *see* Tuberculosis, endocarditis
  typhoid A01.02
  ulcerative (acute) (any valve) (subacute) I33.0
  vegetative (acute) (any valve) (subacute) I33.0
  verrucous (atypical) (nonbacterial) (nonrheumatic) M32.11
Endocardium, endocardial (*see also* condition)
  cushion defect Q21.2
Endocervicitis (*see also* Cervicitis)
  due to intrauterine (contraceptive) device T83.6 ☑
  hyperplastic N72
Endocrine — *see* condition
Endocrinopathy, pluriglandular E31.9
Endodontic
  overfill M27.52

Endodontic — *continued*
  underfill M27.53
Endodontitis K04.0
Endomastoiditis — *see* Mastoiditis
Endometrioma N80.9
Endometriosis N80.9
  appendix N80.5
  bladder N80.8
  bowel N80.5
  broad ligament N80.3
  cervix N80.0
  colon N80.5
  cul-de-sac (Douglas') N80.3
  exocervix N80.0
  fallopian tube N80.2
  female genital organ NEC N80.8
  gallbladder N80.8
  in scar of skin N80.6
  internal N80.0
  intestine N80.5
  lung N80.8
  myometrium N80.0
  ovary N80.1
  parametrium N80.3
  pelvic peritoneum N80.3
  peritoneal (pelvic) N80.3
  rectovaginal septum N80.4
  rectum N80.5
  round ligament N80.3
  skin (scar) N80.6
  specified site NEC N80.8
  stromal D39.0
  umbilicus N80.8
  uterus (internal) N80.0
  vagina N80.4
  vulva N80.8
Endometritis (decidual) (nonspecific) (purulent) (senile) (atrophic) (suppurative) N71.9
  with ectopic pregnancy O08.0
  acute N71.0
  blenorrhagic (gonococcal) (acute) (chronic) A54.24
  cervix, cervical (with erosion or ectropion) (*see also* Cervicitis)
    hyperplastic N72
  chlamydial A56.11
  chronic N71.1
  following
    abortion — *see* Abortion by type complicated by genital infection
    ectopic or molar pregnancy O08.0
  gonococcal, gonorrheal (acute) (chronic) A54.24
  hyperplastic (*see also* Hyperplasia, endometrial) N85.00
    cervix N72
  puerperal, postpartum, childbirth O86.12
  subacute N71.0
  tuberculous A18.17
Endometrium — *see* condition
Endomyocardiopathy, South African I42.3
Endomyocarditis — *see* Endocarditis
Endomyofibrosis I42.3
Endomyometritis — *see* Endometritis
Endopericarditis — *see* Endocarditis
Endoperineuritis — *see* Disorder, nerve
Endophlebitis — *see* Phlebitis
Endophthalmia — *see* Endophthalmitis, purulent
Endophthalmitis (acute) (infective) (metastatic) (subacute) H44.009
  bleb associated (*see also* Bleb, inflamed (infected), postprocedural H59.4 ☑
  gonorrheal A54.39
  in (due to)
    cysticercosis B69.1
    onchocerciasis B73.01
    toxocariasis B83.0
  panuveitis — *see* Panuveitis
  parasitic H44.12- ☑
  purulent H44.00- ☑
    panophthalmitis — *see* Panophthalmitis
    vitreous abscess H44.02- ☑
  specified NEC H44.19
  sympathetic — *see* Uveitis, sympathetic
Endosalpingioma D28.2
Endosalpingiosis N94.89
Endosteitis — *see* Osteomyelitis
Endothelioma, bone — *see* Neoplasm, bone, malignant
Endotheliosis (hemorrhagic infectional) D69.8
Endotoxemia — code to condition

Endotrachelitis — *see* Cervicitis
Engelmann (-Camurati) **syndrome** Q78.3
English disease — *see* Rickets
Engman's disease L30.3
Engorgement
  breast N64.59
    newborn P83.4
    puerperal, postpartum O92.79
  lung (passive) — *see* Edema, lung
  pulmonary (passive) — *see* Edema, lung
  stomach K31.89
  venous, retina — *see* Occlusion, retina, vein, engorgement
Enlargement, enlarged (*see also* Hypertrophy)
  adenoids J35.2
    with tonsils J35.3
  alveolar ridge K08.8
    congenital — *see* Anomaly, alveolar
  apertures of diaphragm (congenital) Q79.1
  gingival K06.1
  heart, cardiac — *see* Hypertrophy, cardiac
  lacrimal gland, chronic H04.03- ☑
  liver — *see* Hypertrophy, liver
  lymph gland or node R59.9
    generalized R59.1
    localized R59.0
  orbit H05.34- ☑
  organ or site, congenital NEC — *see* Anomaly, by site
  parathyroid (gland) E21.0
  pituitary fossa R93.0
  prostate N40.0
    with lower urinary tract symptoms (LUTS) N40.1
    without lower urinary tract symtpoms (LUTS) N40.0
  sella turcica R93.0
  spleen — *see* Splenomegaly
  thymus (gland) (congenital) E32.0
  thyroid (gland) — *see* Goiter
  tongue K14.8
  tonsils J35.1
    with adenoids J35.3
  uterus N85.2
Enophthalmos H05.40- ☑
  due to
    orbital tissue atrophy H05.41- ☑
    trauma or surgery H05.42- ☑
Enostosis M27.8
Entamebic, entamebiasis — *see* Amebiasis
Entanglement
  umbilical cord(s) O69.2 ☑
    with compression O69.2 ☑
      without compression O69.82 ☑
    around neck (with compression) O69.1 ☑
      without compression O69.81 ☑
    of twins in monoamniotic sac O69.2 ☑
Enteralgia — *see* Pain, abdominal
Enteric — *see* condition
Enteritis (acute) (diarrheal) (hemorrhagic) (noninfective) (septic) K52.9
  adenovirus A08.2
  aertrycke infection A02.0
  allergic K52.2
  amebic (acute) A06.0
    with abscess — *see* Abscess, amebic
    chronic A06.1
      with abscess — *see* Abscess, amebic
      nondysenteric A06.2
    nondysenteric A06.2
  astrovirus A08.32
  bacillary NOS A03.9
  bacterial A04.9
    specified NEC A04.8
  calicivirus A08.31
  candidal B37.82
  Chilomastix A07.8
  choleriformis A00.1
  chronic (noninfectious) K52.9
    ulcerative — *see* Colitis, ulcerative
  cicatrizing (chronic) — *see* Enteritis, regional, small intestine
  Clostridium
    botulinum (food poisoning) A05.1
    difficile A04.7
  coccidial A07.3
  coxsackie virus A08.39
  dietetic K52.2
  drug-induced K52.1

Enteritis — *continued*
  due to
    astrovirus A08.32
    calicivirus A08.31
    coxsackie virus A08.39
    drugs K52.1
    echovirus A08.39
    enterovirus NEC A08.39
    food hypersensitivity K52.2
    infectious organism (bacterial) (viral) — *see* Enteritis, infectious
    torovirus A08.39
    Yersinia enterocolitica A04.6
  echovirus A08.39
  eltor A00.1
  enterovirus NEC A08.39
  eosinophilic K52.81
  epidemic (infectious) A09
  fulminant K55.0
  gangrenous — *see* Enteritis, infectious
  giardial A07.1
  infectious NOS A09
    due to
      adenovirus A08.2
      Aerobacter aerogenes A04.8
      Arizona (bacillus) A02.0
      bacteria NOS A04.9
        specified NEC A04.8
      Campylobacter A04.5
      Clostridium difficile A04.7
      Clostridium perfringens A04.8
      Enterobacter aerogenes A04.8
      enterovirus A08.39
      Escherichia coli A04.4
        enteroaggregative A04.4
        enterohemorrhagic A04.3
        enteroinvasive A04.2
        enteropathogenic A04.0
        enterotoxigenic A04.1
        specified NEC A04.4
      specified
        bacteria NEC A04.8
        virus NEC A08.39
      Staphylococcus A04.8
      virus NEC A08.4
        specified type NEC A08.39
      Yersinia enterocolitica A04.6
    specified organism NEC A08.8
  influenzal — *see* Influenza, with, digestive manifestations
  ischemic K55.9
    acute K55.0
    chronic K55.1
  microsporidial A07.8
  mucomembranous, myxomembranous — *see* Syndrome, irritable bowel
  mucous — *see* Syndrome, irritable bowel
  necroticans A05.2
  necrotizing of newborn — *see* Enterocolitis, necrotizing, in newborn
  neurogenic — *see* Syndrome, irritable bowel
  newborn necrotizing — *see* Enterocolitis, necrotizing, in newborn
  noninfectious K52.9
  norovirus A08.11
  parasitic NEC B82.9
  paratyphoid (fever) — *see* Fever, paratyphoid
  protozoal A07.9
    specified NEC A07.8
  radiation K52.0
  regional (of) K50.90
    with
      complication K50.919
        abscess K50.914
        fistula K50.913
        intestinal obstruction K50.912
        rectal bleeding K50.911
        specified complication NEC K50.918
    colon — *see* Enteritis, regional, large intestine
    duodenum — *see* Enteritis, regional, small intestine
    ileum — *see* Enteritis, regional, small intestine
    jejunum — *see* Enteritis, regional, small intestine
    large bowel — *see* Enteritis, regional, large intestine
    large intestine (colon) (rectum) K50.10
      with
        complication K50.119
          abscess K50.114

Enteritis — *continued*
  regional — *continued*
    large intestine — *continued*
      with — *continued*
        complication — *continued*
          fistula K50.113
          intestinal obstruction K50.112
          rectal bleeding K50.111
          small intestine (duodenum) (ileum) (jejunum) involvement K50.80
            with
              complication K50.819
                abscess K50.814
                fistula K50.813
                intestinal obstruction K50.812
                rectal bleeding K50.811
                specified complication NEC K50.818
        specified complication NEC K50.118
    rectum — *see* Enteritis, regional, large intestine
    small intestine (duodenum) (ileum) (jejunum) K50.00
      with
        complication K50.019
          abscess K50.014
          fistula K50.013
          intestinal obstruction K50.012
          large intestine (colon) (rectum) involvement K50.80
            with
              complication K50.819
                abscess K50.814
                fistula K50.813
                intestinal obstruction K50.812
                rectal bleeding K50.811
                specified complication NEC K50.818
          rectal bleeding K50.011
          specified complication NEC K50.018
  rotaviral A08.0
  Salmonella, salmonellosis (arizonae) (cholerae-suis) (enteritidis) (typhimurium) A02.0
  segmental — *see* Enteritis, regional
  septic A09
  Shigella — *see* Infection, Shigella
  small round structured NEC A08.19
  spasmodic, spastic — *see* Syndrome, irritable bowel
  staphylococcal A04.8
    due to food A05.0
  torovirus A08.39
  toxic NEC K52.1
    due to Clostridium difficile A04.7
  trichomonal A07.8
  tuberculous A18.32
  typhosa A01.00
  ulcerative (chronic) — *see* Colitis, ulcerative
  viral A08.4
    adenovirus A08.2
    enterovirus A08.39
    Rotavirus A08.0
    small round structured NEC A08.19
    specified NEC A08.39
    virus specified NEC A08.39
Enterobiasis B80
Enterobius vermicularis (infection) (infestation) B80
Enterocele (*see also* Hernia, abdomen)
  pelvic, pelvis (acquired) (congenital) N81.5
  vagina, vaginal (acquired) (congenital) NEC N81.5
Enterocolitis (*see also* Enteritis) K52.9
  due to Clostridium difficile A04.7
  fulminant ischemic K55.0
  granulomatous — *see* Enteritis, regional
  hemorrhagic (acute) K55.0
    chronic K55.1
  infectious NEC A09
  ischemic K55.9
  necrotizing
    due to Clostridium difficile A04.7
    in newborn P77.9
      stage 1 (without pneumatosis, without perforation) P77.1
      stage 2 (with pneumatosis, without perforation) P77.2
      stage 3 (with pneumatosis, with perforation) P77.3
  noninfectious K52.9
  newborn — *see* Enterocolitis, necrotizing, in newborn

Enterocolitis — *continued*
  pseudomembranous (newborn) A04.7
  radiation K52.0
    newborn — *see* Enterocolitis, necrotizing, in newborn
  ulcerative (chronic) — *see* Pancolitis, ulcerative (chronic)
Enterogastritis — *see* Enteritis
Enteropathy K63.9
  gluten-sensitive K90.0
  hemorrhagic, terminal K55.0
  protein-losing K90.4
Enteroperitonitis — *see* Peritonitis
Enteroptosis K63.4
Enterorrhagia K92.2
Enterospasm (*see also* Syndrome, irritable, bowel)
  psychogenic F45.8
Enterostenosis (*see also* Obstruction, intestine) K56.69
Enterostomy
  complication — *see* Complication, enterostomy
  status Z93.4
Enterovirus, as cause of disease classified elsewhere B97.10
  coxsackievirus B97.11
  echovirus B97.12
  other specified B97.19
Enthesopathy (peripheral) M77.9
  Achilles tendinitis — *see* Tendinitis, Achilles
  ankle and tarsus M77.9
    specified type NEC — *see* Enthesopathy, foot, specified type NEC
  anterior tibial syndrome M76.81- ☑
  calcaneal spur — *see* Spur, bone, calcaneal
  elbow region M77.8
    lateral epicondylitis — *see* Epicondylitis, lateral
    medial epicondylitis — *see* Epicondylitis, medial
  foot NEC M77.9
    metatarsalgia — *see* Metatarsalgia
    specified type NEC M77.5- ☑
  forearm M77.9
  gluteal tendinitis — *see* Tendinitis, gluteal
  hand M77.9
  hip — *see* Enthesopathy, lower limb, specified type NEC
  iliac crest spur — *see* Spur, bone, iliac crest
  iliotibial band syndrome — *see* Syndrome, iliotibial band
  knee — *see* Enthesopathy, lower limb, lower leg, specified type NEC
  lateral epicondylitis — *see* Epicondylitis, lateral
  lower limb (excluding foot) M76.9
    Achilles tendinitis — *see* Tendinitis, Achilles
    anterior tibial syndrome M76.81- ☑
    gluteal tendinitis — *see* Tendinitis, gluteal
    iliac crest spur — *see* Spur, bone, iliac crest
    iliotibial band syndrome — *see* Syndrome, iliotibial band
    patellar tendinitis — *see* Tendinitis, patellar
    pelvic region — *see* Enthesopathy, lower limb, specified type NEC
    peroneal tendinitis — *see* Tendinitis, peroneal
    posterior tibial syndrome M76.82- ☑
    psoas tendinitis — *see* Tendinitis, psoas
    shoulder M77.9
    specified type NEC M76.89- ☑
    tibial collateral bursitis — *see* Bursitis, tibial collateral
  medial epicondylitis — *see* Epicondylitis, medial
  metatarsalgia — *see* Metatarsalgia
  multiple sites M77.9
  patellar tendinitis — *see* Tendinitis, patellar
  pelvis M77.9
  periarthritis of wrist — *see* Periarthritis, wrist
  peroneal tendinitis — *see* Tendinitis, peroneal
  posterior tibial syndrome M76.82- ☑
  psoas tendinitis — *see* Tendinitis, psoas
  shoulder region — *see* Lesion, shoulder
  specified site NEC M77.9
  specified type NEC M77.8
  spinal M46.00
    cervical region M46.02
    cervicothoracic region M46.03
    lumbar region M46.06
    lumbosacral region M46.07
    multiple sites M46.09
    occipito-atlanto-axial region M46.01
    sacrococcygeal region M46.08

Enthesopathy — *continued*
  spinal — *continued*
    thoracic region M46.04
    thoracolumbar region M46.05
  tibial collateral bursitis — *see* Bursitis, tibial collateral
  upper arm M77.9
  wrist and carpus NEC M77.8
    calcaneal spur — *see* Spur, bone, calcaneal
    periarthritis of wrist — *see* Periarthritis, wrist
Entomophobia F40.218
Entomophthoromycosis B46.8
Entrance, air into vein — *see* Embolism, air
Entrapment, nerve — *see* Neuropathy, entrapment
Entropion (eyelid) (paralytic) H02.009
  cicatricial H02.019
    left H02.016
      lower H02.015
      upper H02.014
    right H02.013
      lower H02.012
      upper H02.011
  congenital Q10.2
  left H02.006
    lower H02.005
    upper H02.004
  mechanical H02.029
    left H02.026
      lower H02.025
      upper H02.024
    right H02.023
      lower H02.022
      upper H02.021
  right H02.003
    lower H02.002
    upper H02.001
  senile H02.039
    left H02.036
      lower H02.035
      upper H02.034
    right H02.033
      lower H02.032
      upper H02.031
  spastic H02.049
    left H02.046
      lower H02.045
      upper H02.044
    right H02.043
      lower H02.042
      upper H02.041
Enucleated eye (traumatic, current) S05.7- ☑
Enuresis R32
  functional F98.0
  habit disturbance F98.0
  nocturnal N39.44
    psychogenic F98.0
  nonorganic origin F98.0
  psychogenic F98.0
Eosinopenia — *see* Agranulocytosis
Eosinophilia (allergic) (hereditary) (idiopathic) (secondary) D72.1
  with
    angiolymphoid hyperplasia (ALHE) D18.01
  infiltrative J82
  Löffler's J82
  peritoneal — *see* Peritonitis, eosinophilic
  pulmonary NEC J82
  tropical (pulmonary) J82
Eosinophilia-myalgia syndrome M35.8
Ependymitis (acute) (cerebral) (chronic) (granular) — *see* Encephalomyelitis
Ependymoblastoma
  specified site — *see* Neoplasm, malignant, by site
  unspecified site C71.9
Ependymoma (epithelial) (malignant)
  anaplastic
    specified site — *see* Neoplasm, malignant, by site
    unspecified site C71.9
  benign
    specified site — *see* Neoplasm, benign, by site
    unspecified site D33.2
  myxopapillary D43.2
    specified site — *see* Neoplasm, uncertain behavior, by site
    unspecified site D43.2
  papillary D43.2
    specified site — *see* Neoplasm, uncertain behavior, by site
    unspecified site D43.2

Ependymoma — *continued*
  specified site — *see* Neoplasm, malignant, by site
  unspecified site C71.9
Ependymopathy G93.89
Ephelis, ephelides L81.2
Epiblepharon (congenital) Q10.3
Epicanthus, epicanthic fold (eyelid) (congenital) Q10.3
Epicondylitis (elbow)
  lateral M77.1- ☑
  medial M77.0- ☑
Epicystitis — *see* Cystitis
Epidemic — *see* condition
Epidermidalization, cervix — *see* Dysplasia, cervix
Epidermis, epidermal — *see* condition
Epidermodysplasia verruciformis B07.8
Epidermolysis
  bullosa (congenital) Q81.9
    acquired L12.30
      drug-induced L12.31
      specified cause NEC L12.35
    dystrophica Q81.2
    letalis Q81.1
    simplex Q81.0
    specified NEC Q81.8
  necroticans combustiformis L51.2
    due to drug — *see* Table of Drugs and Chemicals, by drug
Epidermophytid — *see* Dermatophytosis
Epidermophytosis (infected) — *see* Dermatophytosis
Epididymis — *see* condition
Epididymitis (acute) (nonvenereal) (recurrent) (residual) N45.1
  with orchitis N45.3
  blennorrhagic (gonococcal) A54.23
  caseous (tuberculous) A18.15
  chlamydial A56.19
  filarial (*see also* Infestation, filarial) B74.9 [N51]
  gonococcal A54.23
  syphilitic A52.76
  tuberculous A18.15
Epididymo-orchitis (*see also* Epididymitis) N45.3
Epidural — *see* condition
Epigastrium, epigastric — *see* condition
Epigastrocele — *see* Hernia, ventral
Epiglottis — *see* condition
Epiglottitis, epiglottiditis (acute) J05.10
  with obstruction J05.11
  chronic J37.0
Epignathus Q89.4
Epilepsia partialis continua (*see also* Kozhevnikof's epilepsy) G40.1- ☑
Epilepsy, epileptic, epilepsia (attack) (cerebral) (convulsion) (fit) (seizure) G40.909

> *Note: the following terms are to be considered equivalent to intractable: pharmacoresistant (pharmacologically resistant), treatment resistant, refractory (medically) and poorly controlled*

  with
    complex partial seizures — *see* Epilepsy, localization-related, symptomatic, with complex partial seizures
    grand mal seizures on awakening — *see* Epilepsy, generalized, specified NEC
    myoclonic absences — *see* Epilepsy, generalized, specified NEC
    myoclonic-astatic seizures — *see* Epilepsy, generalized, specified NEC
    simple partial seizures — *see* Epilepsy, localization-related, symptomatic, with simple partial seizures
  akinetic — *see* Epilepsy, generalized, specified NEC
  benign childhood with centrotemporal EEG spikes — *see* Epilepsy, localization-related, idiopathic
  benign myoclonic in infancy G40.80- ☑
  Bravais-jacksonian — *see* Epilepsy, localization-related, symptomatic, with simple partial seizures
  childhood
    with occipital EEG paroxysms — *see* Epilepsy, localization-related, idiopathic
    absence G40.A09 (*following* G40.3)
      intractable G40.A19 (*following* G40.3)
        with status epilepticus G40.A11 (*following* G40.3)
        without status epilepticus G40.A19 (*following* G40.3)

Epilepsy, epileptic, epilepsia — *continued*
  childhood — *continued*
    absence — *continued*
      not intractable G40.A09 (*following* G40.3)
        with status epilepticus G40.A01 (*following* G40.3)
        without status epilepticus G40.A09 (*following* G40.3)
  climacteric — *see* Epilepsy, specified NEC
  cysticercosis B69.0
  deterioration (mental) F06.8
  due to syphilis A52.19
  focal — *see* Epilepsy, localization-related, symptomatic, with simple partial seizures
  generalized
    idiopathic G40.309
      intractable G40.319
        with status epilepticus G40.311
        without status epilepticus G40.319
      not intractable G40.309
        with status epilepticus G40.301
        without status epilepticus G40.309
    specified NEC G40.409
      intractable G40.419
        with status epilepticus G40.411
        without status epilepticus G40.419
      not intractable G40.409
        with status epilepticus G40.401
        without status epilepticus G40.409
  impulsive petit mal — *see* Epilepsy, juvenile myoclonic
  intractable G40.919
    with status epilepticus G40.911
    without status epilepticus G40.919
  juvenile absence G40.A09 (*following* G40.3)
    intractable G40.A19 (*following* G40.3)
      with status epilepticus G40.A11 (*following* G40.3)
      without status epilepticus G40.A19 (*following* G40.3)
    not intractable G40.A09 (*following* G40.3)
      with status epilepticus G40.A01 (*following* G40.3)
      without status epilepticus G40.A09 (*following* G40.3)
  juvenile myoclonic G40.B09 (*following* G40.3)
    intractable G40.B19 (*following* G40.3)
      with status epilepticus G40.B11 (*following* G40.3)
      without status epilepticus G40.B19 (*following* G40.3)
    not intractable G40.B09 (*following* G40.3)
      with status epilepticus G40.B01 (*following* G40.3)
      without status epilepticus G40.B09 (*following* G40.3)
  localization-related (focal) (partial)
    idiopathic G40.009
      with seizures of localized onset G40.009
        intractable G40.019
          with status epilepticus G40.011
          without status epilepticus G40.019
        not intractable G40.009
          with status epilepticus G40.001
          without status epilepticus G40.009
    symptomatic
      with complex partial seizures G40.209
        intractable G40.219
          with status epilepticus G40.211
          without status epilepticus G40.219
        not intractable G40.209
          with status epilepticus G40.201
          without status epilepticus G40.209
      with simple partial seizures G40.109
        intractable G40.119
          with status epilepticus G40.111
          without status epilepticus G40.119
        not intractable G40.109
          with status epilepticus G40.101
          without status epilepticus G40.109
  myoclonus, myoclonic (progressive) — *see* Epilepsy, generalized, specified NEC
  not intractable G40.909
    with status epilepticus G40.901
    without status epilepticus G40.909
  on awakening — *see* Epilepsy, generalized, specified NEC
  parasitic NOS B71.9 [G94]

Epilepsy, epileptic, epilepsia — *continued*
partialis continua (*see also* Kozhevnikof's epilepsy)
  G40.1- ☑
peripheral — *see* Epilepsy, specified NEC
procursiva — *see* Epilepsy, localization-related,
  symptomatic, with simple partial seizures
progressive (familial) myoclonic — *see* Epilepsy, generalized, idiopathic
reflex — *see* Epilepsy, specified NEC
related to
  alcohol G40.509
    not intractable G40.509
      with status epilepticus G40.501
      without status epliepticus G40.509
  drugs G40.509
    not intractable G40.509
      with status epilepticus G40.501
      without status epliepticus G40.509
  external causes G40.509
    not intractable G40.509
      with status epilepticus G40.501
      without status epliepticus G40.509
  hormonal changes G40.509
    not intractable G40.509
      with status epilepticus G40.501
      without status epliepticus G40.509
  sleep deprivation G40.509
    not intractable G40.509
      with status epilepticus G40.501
      without status epliepticus G40.509
  stress G40.509
    not intractable G40.509
      with status epilepticus G40.501
      without status epliepticus G40.509
somatomotor — *see* Epilepsy, localization-related,
  symptomatic, with simple partial seizures
somatosensory — *see* Epilepsy, localization-related,
  symptomatic, with simple partial seizures
spasms G40.822
  intractable G40.824
    with status epilepticus G40.823
    without status epilepticus G40.824
  not intractable G40.822
    with status epilepticus G40.821
    without status epilepticus G40.822
specified NEC G40.802
  intractable G40.804
    with status epilepticus G40.803
    without status epilepticus G40.804
  not intractable G40.802
    with status epilepticus G40.801
    without status epilepticus G40.802
syndromes
  generalized
    idiopathic G40.309
      intractable G40.319
        with status epilepticus G40.311
        without status epilepticus G40.319
      not intractable G40.309
        with status epilepticus G40.301
        without status epilepticus G40.309
    specified NEC G40.409
      intractable G40.419
        with status epilepticus G40.411
        without status epilepticus G40.419
      not intractable G40.409
        with status epilepticus G40.401
        without status epilepticus G40.409
  localization-related (focal) (partial)
    idiopathic G40.009
      with seizures of localized onset G40.009
        intractable G40.019
          with status epilepticus G40.011
          without status epilepticus G40.019
        not intractable G40.009
          with status epilepticus G40.001
          without status epilepticus G40.009
    symptomatic
      with complex partial seizures G40.209
        intractable G40.219
          with status epilepticus G40.211
          without status epilepticus G40.219
        not intractable G40.209
          with status epilepticus G40.201
          without status epilepticus G40.209
      with simple partial seizures G40.109
        intractable G40.119
          with status epilepticus G40.111

Epilepsy, epileptic, epilepsia — *continued*
syndromes — *continued*
  localization-related — *continued*
    symptomatic — *continued*
      with simple partial seizures — *continued*
        intractable — *continued*
          without status epilepticus G40.119
        not intractable G40.109
          with status epilepticus G40.101
          without status epilepticus G40.109
  specified NEC G40.802
    intractable G40.804
      with status epilepticus G40.803
      without status epilepticus G40.804
    not intractable G40.802
      with status epilepticus G40.801
      without status epilepticus G40.802
tonic (-clonic) — *see* Epilepsy, generalized, specified
  NEC
twilight F05
uncinate (gyrus) — *see* Epilepsy, localization-related,
  symptomatic, with complex partial seizures
Unverricht (-Lundborg) (familial myoclonic) — *see*
  Epilepsy, generalized, idiopathic
visceral — *see* Epilepsy, specified NEC
visual — *see* Epilepsy, specified NEC
Epiloia Q85.1
Epimenorrhea N92.0
Epipharyngitis — *see* Nasopharyngitis
Epiphora H04.20- ☑
  due to
    excess lacrimation H04.21- ☑
    insufficient drainage H04.22- ☑
Epiphyseal arrest — *see* Arrest, epiphyseal
Epiphyseolysis, epiphysiolysis — *see* Osteochondropa-
  thy
Epiphysitis (*see also* Osteochondropathy)
  juvenile M92.9
  syphilitic (congenital) A50.02
Epiplocele — *see* Hernia, abdomen
Epiploitis — *see* Peritonitis
Epiplosarcomphalocele — *see* Hernia, umbilicus
Episcleritis (suppurative) H15.10- ☑
  in (due to)
    syphilis A52.71
    tuberculosis A18.51
  nodular H15.12- ☑
  periodica fugax H15.11- ☑
    angioneurotic — *see* Edema, angioneurotic
  syphilitic (late) A52.71
  tuberculous A18.51
Episode
  affective, mixed F39
  depersonalization (in neurotic state) F48.1
  depressive F32.9
    major F32.9
      mild F32.0
      moderate F32.1
      severe (without psychotic symptoms) F32.2
        with psychotic symptoms F32.3
    recurrent F33.9
      brief F33.8
    specified NEC F32.8
  hypomanic F30.8
  manic F30.9
    with
      psychotic symptoms F30.2
      remission (full) F30.4
        partial F30.3
    without psychotic symptoms F30.10
      mild F30.11
      moderate F30.12
      severe (without psychotic symptoms) F30.13
        with psychotic symptoms F30.2
    other specified F30.8
    recurrent F31.89
  psychotic F23
    organic F06.8
  schizophrenic (acute) NEC, brief F23
Epispadias (female) (male) Q64.0
Episplenitis D73.89
Epistaxis (multiple) R04.0
  hereditary I78.0
  vicarious menstruation N94.89
Epithelioma (malignant) (*see also* Neoplasm, malignant,
  by site)
  adenoides cysticum — *see* Neoplasm, skin, benign
  basal cell — *see* Neoplasm, skin, malignant

Epithelioma — *continued*
  benign — *see* Neoplasm, benign, by site
  Bowen's — *see* Neoplasm, skin, in situ
  calcifying, of Malherbe — *see* Neoplasm, skin, benign
  external site — *see* Neoplasm, skin, malignant
  intraepidermal, Jadassohn — *see* Neoplasm, skin, be-
    nign
  squamous cell — *see* Neoplasm, malignant, by site
Epitheliomatosis pigmented Q82.1
Epitheliopathy, multifocal placoid pigment
  H30.14- ☑
Epithelium, epithelial — *see* condition
Epituberculosis (with atelectasis) (allergic) A15.7
Eponychia Q84.6
Epstein's
  nephrosis or syndrome — *see* Nephrosis
  pearl K09.8
Epulis (gingiva) (fibrous) (giant cell) K06.8
Equinia A24.0
Equinovarus (congenital) (talipes) Q66.0
  acquired — *see* Deformity, limb, clubfoot
Equivalent
  convulsive (abdominal) — *see* Epilepsy, specified NEC
  epileptic (psychic) — *see* Epilepsy, localization-related,
    symptomatic, with complex partial seizures
Erb (-Duchenne) **paralysis** (birth injury) (newborn) P14.0
Erb-Goldflam disease or syndrome G70.00
  with exacerbation (acute) G70.01
  in crisis G70.01
Erb's
  disease G71.0
  palsy, paralysis (brachial) (birth) (newborn) P14.0
    spinal (spastic) syphilitic A52.17
  pseudohypertrophic muscular dystrophy G71.0
Erdheim's syndrome (acromegalic macrospondylitis)
  E22.0
Erection, painful (persistent) — *see* Priapism
Ergosterol deficiency (vitamin D) E55.9
  with
    adult osteomalacia M83.8
    rickets — *see* Rickets
Ergotism (*see also* Poisoning, food, noxious, plant)
  from ergot used as drug (migraine therapy) — *see*
    Table of Drugs and Chemicals
Erosio interdigitalis blastomycetica B37.2
Erosion
  artery I77.2
    without rupture I77.89
  bone — *see* Disorder, bone, density and structure,
    specified NEC
  bronchus J98.09
  cartilage (joint) — *see* Disorder, cartilage, specified
    type NEC
  cervix (uteri) (acquired) (chronic) (congenital) N86
    with cervicitis N72
  cornea (nontraumatic) — *see* Ulcer, cornea
    recurrent H18.83- ☑
    traumatic — *see* Abrasion, cornea
  dental (idiopathic) (occupational) (due to diet, drugs
    or vomiting) K03.2
  duodenum, postpyloric — *see* Ulcer, duodenum
  esophagus K22.10
    with bleeding K22.11
  gastric — *see* Ulcer, stomach
  gastrojejunal — *see* Ulcer, gastrojejunal
  implanted mesh — *see* Complications, mesh
  intestine K63.3
  lymphatic vessel I89.8
  pylorus, pyloric (ulcer) — *see* Ulcer, stomach
  spine, aneurysmal A52.09
  stomach — *see* Ulcer, stomach
  teeth (idiopathic) (occupational) (due to diet, drugs
    or vomiting) K03.2
  urethra N36.8
  uterus N85.8
Erotomania F52.8
Error
  metabolism, inborn — *see* Disorder, metabolism
  refractive — *see* Disorder, refraction
Eructation R14.2
  nervous or psychogenic F45.8
Eruption
  creeping B76.9
  drug (generalized) (taken internally) L27.0
    fixed L27.1
    in contact with skin — *see* Dermatitis, due to drugs
    localized L27.1

130

☑ Additional Character Required — Refer to the Tabular List for Character Selection   ▽ Subterms under main terms may continue to next column or page

Eruption — *continued*
- Hutchinson, summer L56.4
- Kaposi's varicelliform B00.0
- napkin L22
- polymorphous light (sun) L56.4
- recalcitrant pustular L13.8
- ringed R23.8
- skin (nonspecific) R21
  - creeping (meaning hookworm) B76.9
  - due to inoculation/vaccination (generalized) (*see also* Dermatitis, due to, vaccine) L27.0
    - localized L27.1
  - erysipeloid A26.0
  - feigned L98.1
  - Kaposi's varicelliform B00.0
  - lichenoid L28.0
  - meaning dermatitis — *see* Dermatitis
  - toxic NEC L53.0
- tooth, teeth, abnormal (incomplete) (late) (premature) (sequence) K00.6
- vesicular R23.8

Erysipelas (gangrenous) (infantile) (newborn) (phlegmonous) (suppurative) A46
- external ear A46 [H62.40]
- puerperal, postpartum O86.89

Erysipeloid A26.9
- cutaneous (Rosenbach's) A26.0
- disseminated A26.8
- sepsis A26.7
- specified NEC A26.8

Erythema, erythematous (infectional) (inflammation) L53.9
- ab igne L59.0
- annulare (centrifugum) (rheumaticum) L53.1
- arthriticum epidemicum A25.1
- brucellum — *see* Brucellosis
- chronic figurate NEC L53.3
- chronicum migrans (Borrelia burgdorferi) A69.20
- diaper L22
- due to
  - chemical NEC L53.0
    - in contact with skin L24.5
  - drug (internal use) — *see* Dermatitis, due to, drugs
- elevatum diutinum L95.1
- endemic E52
- epidemic, arthritic A25.1
- figuratum perstans L53.3
- gluteal L22
- heat — *code by site under* Burn, first degree
- ichthyosiforme congenitum bullous Q80.3
- in diseases classified elsewhere L54
- induratum (nontuberculous) L52
  - tuberculous A18.4
- infectiosum B08.3
- intertrigo L30.4
- iris L51.9
- marginatum L53.2
  - in (due to) acute rheumatic fever I00
- medicamentosum — *see* Dermatitis, due to, drugs
- migrans A26.0
  - chronicum A69.20
  - tongue K14.1
- multiforme (major) (minor) L51.9
  - bullous, bullosum L51.1
  - conjunctiva L51.1
  - nonbullous L51.0
  - pemphigoides L12.0
  - specified NEC L51.8
- napkin L22
- neonatorum P83.8
  - toxic P83.1
- nodosum L52
  - tuberculous A18.4
- palmar L53.8
- pernio T69.1 ☑
- rash, newborn P83.8
- scarlatiniform (recurrent) (exfoliative) L53.8
- solare L55.0
- specified NEC L53.8
- toxic, toxicum NEC L53.0
  - newborn P83.1
- tuberculous (primary) A18.4

Erythematous, erythematosus — *see* condition
Erythermalgia (primary) I73.81
Erythralgia I73.81
Erythrasma L08.1
Erythredema (polyneuropathy) — *see* Poisoning, mercury

Erythremia (acute) C94.0- ☑
- chronic D45
- secondary D75.1

Erythroblastopenia (*see also* Aplasia, red cell) D60.9
- congenital D61.01

Erythroblastophthisis D61.09
Erythroblastosis (fetalis) (newborn) P55.9
- due to
  - ABO (antibodies) (incompatibility) (isoimmunization) P55.1
  - Rh (antibodies) (incompatibility) (isoimmunization) P55.0

Erythrocyanosis (crurum) I73.89
Erythrocythemia — *see* Erythremia
Erythrocytosis (megalosplenic) (secondary) D75.1
- familial D75.0
- oval, hereditary — *see* Elliptocytosis
- secondary D75.1
- stress D75.1

Erythroderma (secondary) (*see also* Erythema) L53.9
- bullous ichthyosiform, congenital Q80.3
- desquamativum L21.1
- ichthyosiform, congenital (bullous) Q80.3
- neonatorum P83.8
- psoriaticum L40.8

Erythrodysesthesia, palmar plantar (PPE) L27.1
Erythrogenesis imperfecta D61.09
Erythroleukemia C94.0- ☑
Erythromelalgia I73.81
Erythrophagocytosis D75.89
Erythrophobia F40.298
Erythroplakia, oral epithelium, and tongue K13.29
Erythroplasia (Queyrat) D07.4
- specified site — *see* Neoplasm, skin, in situ
- unspecified site D07.4

Escherichia coli (E. coli), **as cause of disease classified elsewhere** B96.20
- non-O157 Shiga toxin-producing (with known O group) B96.22
- non-Shiga toxin-producing B96.29
- O157 B96.21
- O157 with confirmation of Shiga toxin when H antigen is unknown, or is not H7 B96.21
- O157:H- (nonmotile) with confirmation of Shiga toxin B96.21
- O157:H7 with or without confirmation of Shiga toxin-production B96.21
  - specified NEC B96.22
- Shiga toxin-producing (with unspecified O group) (STEC) B96.23
- specified NEC B96.29

Esophagismus K22.4
Esophagitis (acute) (alkaline) (chemical) (chronic) (infectional) (necrotic) (peptic) (postoperative) K20.9
- candidal B37.81
- due to gastrointestinal reflux disease K21.0
- eosinophilic K20.0
- reflux K21.0
- specified NEC K20.8
- tuberculous A18.83
- ulcerative K22.10
  - with bleeding K22.11

Esophagocele K22.5
Esophagomalacia K22.8
Esophagospasm K22.4
Esophagostenosis K22.2
Esophagostomiasis B81.8
Esophagotracheal — *see* condition
Esophagus — *see* condition
Esophoria H50.51
- convergence, excess H51.12
- divergence, insufficiency H51.8

Esotropia — *see* Strabismus, convergent concomitant
Espundia B55.2
Essential — *see* condition
Esthesioneuroblastoma C30.0
Esthesioneurocytoma C30.0
Esthesioneuroepithelioma C30.0
Esthiomene A55
Estivo-autumnal malaria (fever) B50.9
Estrangement (marital) Z63.5
- parent-child NEC Z62.890

Estriasis — *see* Myiasis
Ethanolism — *see* Alcoholism
Etherism — *see* Dependence, drug, inhalant
Ethmoid, ethmoidal — *see* condition

Ethmoiditis (chronic) (nonpurulent) (purulent) (*see also* Sinusitis, ethmoidal)
- influenzal — *see* Influenza, with, respiratory manifestations NEC
- Woakes' J33.1

Ethylism — *see* Alcoholism
Eulenburg's disease (congenital paramyotonia) G71.19
Eumycetoma B47.0
Eunuchoidism E29.1
- hypogonadotropic E23.0

European blastomycosis — *see* Cryptococcosis
Eustachian — *see* condition
Evaluation (for) (of)
- development state
  - adolescent Z00.3
  - period of
    - delayed growth in childhood Z00.70
      - with abnormal findings Z00.71
    - rapid growth in childhood Z00.2
  - puberty Z00.3
- growth and developmental state (period of rapid growth) Z00.2
- delayed growth Z00.70
  - with abnormal findings Z00.71
- mental health (status) Z00.8
  - requested by authority Z04.6
- period of
  - delayed growth in childhood Z00.70
    - with abnormal findings Z00.71
  - rapid growth in childhood Z00.2
- suspected condition — *see* Observation

Evans syndrome D69.41
Event, apparent life threatening in newborn and infant (ALTE) R68.13
Eventration (*see also* Hernia, ventral)
- colon into chest — *see* Hernia, diaphragm
- diaphragm (congenital) Q79.1

Eversion
- bladder N32.89
- cervix (uteri) N86
  - with cervicitis N72
- foot NEC (*see also* Deformity, valgus, ankle)
  - congenital Q66.6
- punctum lacrimale (postinfectional) (senile) H04.52- ☑
- ureter (meatus) N28.89
- urethra (meatus) N36.8
- uterus N81.4

Evidence
- cytologic
  - of malignancy on anal smear R85.614
  - of malignancy on cervical smear R87.614
  - of malignancy on vaginal smear R87.624

Evisceration
- birth injury P15.8
- traumatic NEC
  - eye — *see* Enucleated eye

Evulsion — *see* Avulsion
Ewing's sarcoma or tumor — *see* Neoplasm, bone, malignant
Examination (for) (following) (general) (of) (routine) Z00.00
- with abnormal findings Z00.01
- abuse, physical (alleged), ruled out
  - adult Z04.71
  - child Z04.72
- adolescent (development state) Z00.3
- alleged rape or sexual assault (victim), ruled out
  - adult Z04.41
  - child Z04.42
- allergy Z01.82
- annual (adult) (periodic) (physical) Z00.00
  - with abnormal findings Z00.01
  - gynecological Z01.419
    - with abnormal findings Z01.411
- antibody response Z01.84
- blood — *see* Examination, laboratory
- blood pressure Z01.30
  - with abnormal findings Z01.31
- cancer staging — *see* Neoplasm, malignant, by site
- cervical Papanicolaou smear Z12.4
  - as part of routine gynecological examination Z01.419
    - with abnormal findings Z01.411
- child (over 28 days old) Z00.129
  - with abnormal findings Z00.121
  - under 28 days old — *see* Newborn, examination
- clinical research control or normal comparison (control) (participant) Z00.6

Examination — *continued*
  contraceptive (drug) maintenance (routine) Z30.8
    device (intrauterine) Z30.431
  dental Z01.20
    with abnormal findings Z01.21
  developmental — *see* Examination, child
  donor (potential) Z00.5
  ear Z01.10
    with abnormal findings NEC Z01.118
  eye Z01.00
    with abnormal findings Z01.01
  following
    accident NEC Z04.3
      transport Z04.1
      work Z04.2
    assault, alleged, ruled out
      adult Z04.71
      child Z04.72
    motor vehicle accident Z04.1
    treatment (for) Z09
      combined NEC Z09
        fracture Z09
        malignant neoplasm Z08
      malignant neoplasm Z08
      mental disorder Z09
      specified condition NEC Z09
  follow-up (routine) (following) Z09
    chemotherapy NEC Z09
      malignant neoplasm Z08
    fracture Z09
    malignant neoplasm Z08
    postpartum Z39.2
    psychotherapy Z09
    radiotherapy NEC Z09
      malignant neoplasm Z08
    surgery NEC Z09
      malignant neoplasm Z08
  gynecological Z01.419
    with abnormal findings Z01.411
    for contraceptive maintenance Z30.8
  health — *see* Examination, medical
  hearing Z01.10
    with abnormal findings NEC Z01.118
    following failed hearing screening Z01.110
  immunity status testing Z01.84
  laboratory (as part of a general medical examination) Z00.00
    with abnormal findings Z00.01
    preprocedural Z01.812
  lactating mother Z39.1
  medical (adult) (for) (of) Z00.00
    with abnormal findings Z00.01
    administrative purpose only Z02.9
      specified NEC Z02.89
    admission to
      armed forces Z02.3
      old age home Z02.2
      prison Z02.89
      residential institution Z02.2
      school Z02.0
        following illness or medical treatment Z02.0
      summer camp Z02.89
    adoption Z02.82
    blood alcohol or drug level Z02.83
    camp (summer) Z02.89
    clinical research, normal subject (control) (participant) Z00.6
    control subject in clinical research (normal comparison) (participant) Z00.6
    donor (potential) Z00.5
    driving license Z02.4
    general (adult) Z00.00
      with abnormal findings Z00.01
    immigration Z02.89
    insurance purposes Z02.6
    marriage Z02.89
    medicolegal reasons NEC Z04.8
    naturalization Z02.89
    participation in sport Z02.5
    paternity testing Z02.81
    population survey Z00.8
    pre-employment Z02.1
    pre-operative — *see* Examination, pre-procedural
    pre-procedural
      cardiovascular Z01.810
      respiratory Z01.811
      specified NEC Z01.818

Examination — *continued*
  medical — *continued*
    preschool children
      for admission to school Z02.0
    prisoners
      for entrance into prison Z02.89
    recruitment for armed forces Z02.3
    specified NEC Z00.8
    sport competition Z02.5
  medicolegal reason NEC Z04.8
  newborn — *see* Newborn, examination
  pelvic (annual) (periodic) Z01.419
    with abnormal findings Z01.411
  period of rapid growth in childhood Z00.2
  periodic (adult) (annual) (routine) Z00.00
    with abnormal findings Z00.01
  physical (adult) (*see also* Examination, medical) Z00.00
    sports Z02.5
  postpartum
    immediately after delivery Z39.0
    routine follow-up Z39.2
  pre-chemotherapy (antineoplastic) Z01.818
  prenatal (normal pregnancy) (*see also* Pregnancy, normal) Z34.9- ☑
  pre-procedural (pre-operative)
    cardiovascular Z01.810
    laboratory Z01.812
    respiratory Z01.811
    specified NEC Z01.818
  prior to chemotherapy (antineoplastic) Z01.818
  psychiatric NEC Z00.8
    follow-up not needing further care Z09
    requested by authority Z04.6
  radiological (as part of a general medical examination) Z00.00
    with abnormal findings Z00.01
  repeat cervical smear to confirm findings of recent normal smear following initial abnormal smear Z01.42
  skin (hypersensitivity) Z01.82
  special (*see also* Examination, by type) Z01.89
    specified type NEC Z01.89
  specified type or reason NEC Z04.8
  teeth Z01.20
    with abnormal findings Z01.21
  urine — *see* Examination, laboratory
  vision Z01.00
    with abnormal findings Z01.01

Exanthem, exanthema (*see also* Rash)
  with enteroviral vesicular stomatitis B08.4
  Boston A88.0
  epidemic with meningitis A88.0 [G02]
  subitum B08.20
    due to human herpesvirus 6 B08.21
    due to human herpesvirus 7 B08.22
  viral, virus B09
    specified type NEC B08.8

Excess, excessive, excessively
  alcohol level in blood R78.0
  androgen (ovarian) E28.1
  attrition, tooth, teeth K03.0
  carotene, carotin (dietary) E67.1
  cold, effects of T69.9 ☑
    specified effect NEC T69.8 ☑
  convergence H51.12
  crying
    in child, adolescent, or adult R45.83
    in infant R68.11
  development, breast N62
  divergence H51.8
  drinking (alcohol) NEC (without dependence) F10.10
    habitual (continual) (without remission) F10.20
  eating R63.2
  estrogen E28.0
  fat (*see also* Obesity)
    in heart — *see* Degeneration, myocardial
    localized E65
  foreskin N47.8
  gas R14.0
  glucagon E16.3
  heat — *see* Heat
  intermaxillary vertical dimension of fully erupted teeth M26.37
  interocclusal distance of fully erupted teeth M26.37
  kalium E87.5
  large
    colon K59.3
      congenital Q43.8

Excess, excessive, excessively — *continued*
  large — *continued*
    infant P08.0
    organ or site, congenital NEC — *see* Anomaly, by site
  long
    organ or site, congenital NEC — *see* Anomaly, by site
  menstruation (with regular cycle) N92.0
    with irregular cycle N92.1
  napping Z72.821
  natrium E87.0
  number of teeth K00.1
  nutrient (dietary) NEC R63.2
  potassium (K) E87.5
  salivation K11.7
  secretion (*see also* Hypersecretion)
    milk O92.6
    sputum R09.3
    sweat R61
  sexual drive F52.8
  short
    organ or site, congenital NEC — *see* Anomaly, by site
    umbilical cord in labor or delivery O69.3 ☑
  skin, eyelid (acquired) — *see* Blepharochalasis
    congenital Q10.3
  sodium (Na) E87.0
  spacing of fully erupted teeth M26.32
  sputum R09.3
  sweating R61
  thirst R63.1
    due to deprivation of water T73.1 ☑
  tuberosity of jaw M26.07
  vitamin
    A (dietary) E67.0
      administered as drug (prolonged intake) — *see* Table of Drugs and Chemicals, vitamins, adverse effect
      overdose or wrong substance given or taken — *see* Table of Drugs and Chemicals, vitamins, poisoning
    D (dietary) E67.3
      administered as drug (prolonged intake) — *see* Table of Drugs and Chemicals, vitamins, adverse effect
      overdose or wrong substance given or taken — *see* Table of Drugs and Chemicals, vitamins, poisoning
  weight
    gain R63.5
    loss R63.4

Excitability, abnormal, under minor stress (personality disorder) F60.3

Excitation
  anomalous atrioventricular I45.6
  psychogenic F30.8
  reactive (from emotional stress, psychological trauma) F30.8

Excitement
  hypomanic F30.8
  manic F30.9
  mental, reactive (from emotional stress, psychological trauma) F30.8
  state, reactive (from emotional stress, psychological trauma) F30.8

Excoriation (traumatic) (*see also* Abrasion)
  neurotic L98.1

Exfoliation
  due to erythematous conditions according to extent of body surface involved L49.0
    less than 10 percent of body surface L49.0
    10-19 percent of body surface L49.1
    20-29 percent of body surface L49.2
    30-39 percent of body surface L49.3
    40-49 percent of body surface L49.4
    50-59 percent of body surface L49.5
    60-69 percent of body surface L49.6
    70-79 percent of body surface L49.7
    80-89 percent of body surface L49.8
    90-99 percent of body surface L49.9
  teeth, due to systemic causes K08.0

Exfoliative — *see* condition

Exhaustion, exhaustive (physical NEC) R53.83
  battle F43.0
  cardiac — *see* Failure, heart
  delirium F43.0

Exhaustion, exhaustive — *continued*
  due to
    cold T69.8 ☑
    excessive exertion T73.3 ☑
    exposure T73.2 ☑
    neurasthenia F48.8
  heart — *see* Failure, heart
  heat (*see also* Heat, exhaustion) T67.5 ☑
    due to
      salt depletion T67.4 ☑
      water depletion T67.3 ☑
  maternal, complicating delivery O75.81
  mental F48.8
  myocardium, myocardial — *see* Failure, heart
  nervous F48.8
  old age R54
  psychogenic F48.8
  psychosis F43.0
  senile R54
  vital NEC T73.0
Exhibitionism F65.2
Exocervicitis — *see* Cervicitis
Exomphalos Q79.2
  meaning hernia — *see* Hernia, umbilicus
Exophoria H50.52
  convergence, insufficiency H51.11
  divergence, excess H51.8
Exophthalmos H05.2- ☑
  congenital Q15.8
  constant NEC H05.24- ☑
  displacement, globe — *see* Displacement, globe
  due to thyrotoxicosis (hyperthyroidism) — *see* Hyperthyroidism, with, goiter (diffuse)
  dysthyroid — *see* Hyperthyroidism, with, goiter (diffuse)
  goiter — *see* Hyperthyroidism, with, goiter (diffuse)
  intermittent NEC H05.25- ☑
  malignant — *see* Hyperthyroidism, with, goiter (diffuse)
  orbital
    edema — *see* Edema, orbit
    hemorrhage — *see* Hemorrhage, orbit
  pulsating NEC H05.26- ☑
  thyrotoxic, thyrotropic — *see* Hyperthyroidism, with, goiter (diffuse)
Exostosis (*see also* Disorder, bone)
  cartilaginous — *see* Neoplasm, bone, benign
  congenital (multiple) Q78.6
  external ear canal H61.81- ☑
  gonococcal A54.49
  jaw (bone) M27.8
  multiple, congenital Q78.6
  orbit H05.35- ☑
  osteocartilaginous — *see* Neoplasm, bone, benign
  syphilitic A52.77
Exotropia — *see* Strabismus, divergent concomitant
Explanation of
  investigation finding Z71.2
  medication Z71.89
Exposure (to) (*see also* Contact, with) T75.89 ☑
  acariasis Z20.7
  AIDS virus Z20.6
  air pollution Z77.110
  algae and algae toxins Z77.121
  algae bloom Z77.121
  anthrax Z20.810
  aromatic amines Z77.020
  aromatic (hazardous) compounds NEC Z77.028
  aromatic dyes NOS Z77.028
  arsenic Z77.010
  asbestos Z77.090
  bacterial disease NEC Z20.818
  benzene Z77.021
  blue-green algae bloom Z77.121
  body fluids (potentially hazardous) Z77.21
  brown tide Z77.121
  chemicals (chiefly nonmedicinal) (hazardous) NEC Z77.098
  cholera Z20.09
  chromium compounds Z77.018
  cold, effects of T69.9
    specified effect NEC T69.8 ☑
  communicable disease Z20.9
    bacterial NEC Z20.818
    specified NEC Z20.89
    viral NEC Z20.828
  cyanobacteria bloom Z77.121

Exposure — *continued*
  disaster Z65.5
  discrimination Z60.5
  dyes Z77.098
  effects of T73.9 ☑
  environmental tobacco smoke (acute) (chronic) Z77.22
  Escherichia coli (E. coli) Z20.01
  exhaustion due to T73.2 ☑
  fiberglass — *see* Table of Drugs and Chemicals, fiberglass
  German measles Z20.4
  gonorrhea Z20.2
  hazardous metals NEC Z77.018
  hazardous substances NEC Z77.29
  hazards in the physical environment NEC Z77.128
  hazards to health NEC Z77.9
  human immunodeficiency virus (HIV) Z20.6
  human T-lymphotropic virus type-1 (HTLV-1) Z20.89
  implanted
    mesh — *see* Complications, mesh
    prosthetic materials NEC — *see* Complications, prosthetic materials NEC
  infestation (parasitic) NEC Z20.7
  intestinal infectious disease NEC Z20.09
    Escherichia coli (E. coli) Z20.01
  lead Z77.011
  meningococcus Z20.811
  mold (toxic) Z77.120
  nickel dust Z77.018
  noise Z77.122
  occupational
    air contaminants NEC Z57.39
    dust Z57.2
    environmental tobacco smoke Z57.31
    extreme temperature Z57.6
    noise Z57.0
    radiation Z57.1
    risk factors Z57.9
      specified NEC Z57.8
    toxic agents (gases) (liquids) (solids) (vapors) in agriculture Z57.4
    toxic agents (gases) (liquids) (solids) (vapors) in industry NEC Z57.5
    vibration Z57.7
  parasitic disease NEC Z20.7
  pediculosis Z20.7
  persecution Z60.5
  pfiesteria piscicida Z77.121
  poliomyelitis Z20.89
  pollution
    air Z77.110
    environmental NEC Z77.118
    soil Z77.112
    water Z77.111
  polycyclic aromatic hydrocarbons Z77.028
  prenatal (drugs) (toxic chemicals) — *see* Newborn, affected by (suspected to be), noxious substances transmitted via placenta or breast milk
  rabies Z20.3
  radiation, naturally occurring NEC Z77.123
  radon Z77.123
  red tide (Florida) Z77.121
  rubella Z20.4
  second hand tobacco smoke (acute) (chronic) Z77.22
    in the perinatal period P96.81
  sexually-transmitted disease Z20.2
  smallpox (laboratory) Z20.89
  syphilis Z20.2
  terrorism Z65.4
  torture Z65.4
  tuberculosis Z20.1
  uranium Z77.012
  varicella Z20.820
  venereal disease Z20.2
  viral disease NEC Z20.828
  war Z65.5
  water pollution Z77.111
Exsanguination — *see* Hemorrhage
Exstrophy
  abdominal contents Q45.8
  bladder Q64.10
    cloacal Q64.12
    specified type NEC Q64.19
    supravesical fissure Q64.11
Extensive — *see* condition
Extra (*see also* Accessory)
  marker chromosomes (normal individual) Q92.61
    in abnormal individual Q92.62

Extra — *continued*
  rib Q76.6
    cervical Q76.5
Extrasystoles (supraventricular) I49.49
  atrial I49.1
  auricular I49.1
  junctional I49.2
  ventricular I49.3
Extrauterine gestation or pregnancy — *see* Pregnancy, by site
Extravasation
  blood R58
  chyle into mesentery I89.8
  pelvicalyceal N13.8
  pyelosinus N13.8
  urine (from ureter) R39.0
  vesicant agent
    antineoplastic chemotherapy T80.810 ☑
    other agent NEC T80.818 ☑
Extremity — *see* condition, limb
Extrophy — *see* Exstrophy
Extroversion
  bladder Q64.19
  uterus N81.4
    complicating delivery O71.2
    postpartal (old) N81.4
Extruded tooth (teeth) M26.34
Extrusion
  breast implant (prosthetic) T85.42 ☑
  eye implant (globe) (ball) T85.328 ☑
  intervertebral disc — *see* Displacement, intervertebral disc
  ocular lens implant (prosthetic) — *see* Complications, intraocular lens
  vitreous — *see* Prolapse, vitreous
Exudate
  pleural — *see* Effusion, pleura
  retina H35.89
Exudative — *see* condition
Eye, eyeball, eyelid — *see* condition
Eyestrain — *see* Disturbance, vision, subjective
Eyeworm disease of Africa B74.3

F

Faber's syndrome (achlorhydric anemia) D50.9
Fabry (-Anderson) **disease** E75.21
Faciocephalalgia, autonomic (*see also* Neuropathy, peripheral, autonomic) G90.09
Factor(s)
  psychic, associated with diseases classified elsewhere F54
  psychological
    affecting physical conditions F54
    or behavioral
      affecting general medical condition F54
      associated with disorders or diseases classified elsewhere F54
Fahr disease (of brain) G23.8
Fahr Volhard disease (of kidney) I12.- ☑
Failure, failed
  abortion — *see* Abortion, attempted
  aortic (valve) I35.8
    rheumatic I06.8
  attempted abortion — *see* Abortion, attempted
  biventricular I50.9
  bone marrow — *see* Anemia, aplastic
  cardiac — *see* Failure, heart
  cardiorenal (chronic) I50.9
    hypertensive I13.2
  cardiorespiratory (*see also* Failure, heart) R09.2
  cardiovascular (chronic) — *see* Failure, heart
  cerebrovascular I67.9
  cervical dilatation in labor O62.0
  circulation, circulatory (peripheral) R57.9
    newborn P29.89
  compensation — *see* Disease, heart
  compliance with medical treatment or regimen — *see* Noncompliance
  congestive — *see* Failure, heart, congestive
  dental implant (endosseous) M27.69
    due to
      failure of dental prosthesis M27.63
      lack of attached gingiva M27.62
      occlusal trauma (poor prosthetic design) M27.62
      parafunctional habits M27.62

Failure, failed — *continued*
- dental implant — *continued*
  - due to — *continued*
    - periodontal infection (peri-implantitis) M27.62
    - poor oral hygiene M27.62
    - osseointegration M27.61
      - due to
        - complications of systemic disease M27.61
        - poor bone quality M27.61
      - iatrogenic M27.61
    - post-osseointegration
      - biological M27.62
        - due to complications of systemic disease M27.62
      - iatrogenic M27.62
      - mechanical M27.63
    - pre-integration M27.61
    - pre-osseointegration M27.61
    - specified NEC M27.69
- descent of head (at term) of pregnancy (mother) O32.4 ☑
- endosseous dental implant — *see* Failure, dental implant
- engagement of head (term of pregnancy) (mother) O32.4 ☑
- erection (penile) (*see also* Dysfunction, sexual, male, erectile) N52.9
  - nonorganic F52.21
- examination(s), anxiety concerning Z55.2
- expansion terminal respiratory units (newborn) (primary) P28.0
- forceps NOS (with subsequent cesarean delivery) O66.5
- gain weight (child over 28 days old) R62.51
  - adult R62.7
  - newborn P92.6
- genital response (male) F52.21
  - female F52.22
- heart (acute) (senile) (sudden) I50.9
  - with
    - acute pulmonary edema — *see* Failure, ventricular, left
    - decompensation — *see* Failure, heart, congestive
    - dilatation — *see* Disease, heart
  - arteriosclerotic I70.90
  - biventricular I50.9
  - combined left-right sided I50.9
  - compensated I50.9
  - complicating
    - anesthesia (general) (local) or other sedation
      - in labor and delivery O74.2
      - in pregnancy O29.12- ☑
      - postpartum, puerperal O89.1
    - delivery (cesarean) (instrumental) O75.4
  - congestive (compensated) (decompensated) I50.9
    - with rheumatic fever (conditions in I00)
      - active I01.8
      - inactive or quiescent (with chorea) I09.81
    - newborn P29.0
    - rheumatic (chronic) (inactive) (with chorea) I09.81
      - active or acute I01.8
        - with chorea I02.0
  - decompensated I50.9
  - degenerative — *see* Degeneration, myocardial
  - diastolic (congestive) I50.30
    - acute (congestive) I50.31
      - and (on) chronic (congestive) I50.33
    - chronic (congestive) I50.32
      - and (on) acute (congestive) I50.33
    - combined with systolic (congestive) I50.40
      - acute (congestive) I50.41
        - and (on) chronic (congestive) I50.43
      - chronic (congestive) I50.42
        - and (on) acute (congestive) I50.43
  - due to presence of cardiac prosthesis I97.13- ☑
  - following cardiac surgery I97.13- ☑
  - high output NOS I50.9
  - hypertensive — *see* Hypertension, heart
  - left (ventricular) — *see* Failure, ventricular, left
  - low output (syndrome) NOS I50.9
  - newborn P29.0
  - organic — *see* Disease, heart
  - peripartum O90.3
  - postprocedural I97.13- ☑
  - rheumatic (chronic) (inactive) I09.9
  - right (ventricular) (secondary to left heart failure) — *see* Failure, heart, congestive

Failure, failed — *continued*
- heart — *continued*
  - systolic (congestive) I50.20
    - acute (congestive) I50.21
      - and (on) chronic (congestive) I50.23
    - chronic (congestive) I50.22
      - and (on) acute (congestive) I50.23
    - combined with diastolic (congestive) I50.40
      - acute (congestive) I50.41
        - and (on) chronic (congestive) I50.43
      - chronic (congestive) I50.42
        - and (on) acute (congestive) I50.43
  - thyrotoxic (*see also* Thyrotoxicosis) E05.90 [I43]
    - with thyroid storm E05.91 [I43]
  - valvular — *see* Endocarditis
- hepatic K72.90
  - with coma K72.91
  - acute or subacute K72.00
    - with coma K72.01
    - due to drugs K71.10
      - with coma K71.11
  - alcoholic (acute) (chronic) (subacute) K70.40
    - with coma K70.41
  - chronic K72.10
    - with coma K72.11
    - due to drugs (acute) (subacute) (chronic) K71.10
      - with coma K71.11
  - due to drugs (acute) (subacute) (chronic) K71.10
    - with coma K71.11
  - postprocedural K91.82
- hepatorenal K76.7
- induction (of labor) O61.9
  - abortion — *see* Abortion, attempted
  - by
    - oxytocic drugs O61.0
    - prostaglandins O61.0
  - instrumental O61.1
  - mechanical O61.1
  - medical O61.0
  - specified NEC O61.8
  - surgical O61.1
- intubation during anesthesia T88.4 ☑
  - in pregnancy O29.6- ☑
  - labor and delivery O74.7
  - postpartum, puerperal O89.6
- involution, thymus (gland) E32.0
- kidney (*see also* Disease, kidney, chronic) N19
  - acute (*see also* Failure, renal, acute) N17.9
- lactation (complete) O92.3
  - partial O92.4
- Leydig's cell, adult E29.1
- liver — *see* Failure, hepatic
- menstruation at puberty N91.0
- mitral I05.8
- myocardial, myocardium (*see also* Failure, heart) I50.9
  - chronic (*see also* Failure, heart, congestive) I50.9
  - congestive (*see also* Failure, heart, congestive) I50.9
- orgasm (female) (psychogenic) F52.31
  - male F52.32
- ovarian (primary) E28.39
  - iatrogenic E89.40
    - asymptomatic E89.40
    - symptomatic E89.41
  - postprocedural (postablative) (postirradiation) (postsurgical) E89.40
    - asymptomatic E89.40
    - symptomatic E89.41
- ovulation causing infertility N97.0
- polyglandular, autoimmune E31.0
- prosthetic joint implant — *see* Complications, joint prosthesis, mechanical, breakdown, by site
- renal N19
  - with
    - tubular necrosis (acute) N17.0
  - acute N17.9
    - with
      - cortical necrosis N17.1
      - medullary necrosis N17.2
      - tubular necrosis N17.0
    - specified NEC N17.8
  - chronic N18.9
    - hypertensive — *see* Hypertension, kidney
  - congenital P96.0
  - end stage (chronic) N18.6
    - due to hypertension I12.0
  - following
    - abortion — *see* Abortion by type complicated by specified condition NEC

Failure, failed — *continued*
- renal — *continued*
  - following — *continued*
    - crushing T79.5 ☑
    - ectopic or molar pregnancy O08.4
    - labor and delivery (acute) O90.4
  - hypertensive — *see* Hypertension, kidney
  - postprocedural N99.0
- respiration, respiratory J96.90
  - with
    - hypercapnia J96.92
    - hypoxia J96.91
  - acute J96.00
    - with
      - hypercapnia J96.02
      - hypoxia J96.01
  - acute and (on) chronic J96.20
    - with
      - hypercapnia J96.22
      - hypoxia J96.21
  - center G93.89
  - chronic J96.10
    - with
      - hypercapnia J96.12
      - hypoxia J96.11
  - newborn P28.5
  - postprocedural (acute) J95.821
    - acute and chronic J95.822
- rotation
  - cecum Q43.3
  - colon Q43.3
  - intestine Q43.3
  - kidney Q63.2
- sedation (conscious) (moderate) during procedure T88.52 ☑
  - history of Z92.83
- segmentation (*see also* Fusion)
  - fingers — *see* Syndactylism, complex, fingers
  - vertebra Q76.49
    - with scoliosis Q76.3
- seminiferous tubule, adult E29.1
- senile (general) R54
- sexual arousal (male) F52.21
  - female F52.22
- testicular endocrine function E29.1
- to thrive (child over 28 days old) R62.51
  - adult R62.7
  - newborn P92.6
- transplant T86.92
  - bone T86.831
    - marrow T86.02
  - cornea T86.841
  - heart T86.22
    - with lung(s) T86.32
  - intestine T86.851
  - kidney T86.12
  - liver T86.42
  - lung(s) T86.811
    - with heart T86.32
  - pancreas T86.891
  - skin (allograft) (autograft) T86.821
  - specified organ or tissue NEC T86.891
  - stem cell (peripheral blood) (umbilical cord) T86.5
- trial of labor (with subsequent cesarean delivery) O66.40
  - following previous cesarean delivery O66.41
- tubal ligation N99.89
- urinary — *see* Disease, kidney, chronic
- vacuum extraction NOS (with subsequent cesarean delivery) O66.5
- vasectomy N99.89
- ventouse NOS (with subsequent cesarean delivery) O66.5
- ventricular (*see also* Failure, heart) I50.9
  - left I50.1
    - with rheumatic fever (conditions in I00)
      - active I01.8
        - with chorea I02.0
      - inactive or quiescent (with chorea) I09.81
      - rheumatic (chronic) (inactive) (with chorea) I09.81
        - active or acute I01.8
          - with chorea I02.0
  - right (*see also* Failure, heart, congestive) I50.9
- vital centers, newborn P91.8

Fainting (fit) R55

Fallen arches — *see* Deformity, limb, flat foot

Falling, falls (repeated) R29.6
  any organ or part — *see* Prolapse
Fallopian
  insufflation Z31.41
  tube — *see* condition
Fallot's
  pentalogy Q21.8
  tetrad or tetralogy Q21.3
  triad or trilogy Q22.3
False (*see also* condition)
  croup J38.5
  joint — *see* Nonunion, fracture
  labor (pains) O47.9
    at or after 37 completed weeks of gestation O47.1
    before 37 completed weeks of gestation O47.0- ☑
  passage, urethra (prostatic) N36.5
  pregnancy F45.8
Family, familial (*see also* condition)
  disruption Z63.8
    involving divorce or separation Z63.5
  Li-Fraumeni (syndrome) Z15.01
  planning advice Z30.09
  problem Z63.9
    specified NEC Z63.8
  retinoblastoma C69.2- ☑
Famine (effects of) T73.0 ☑
  edema — *see* Malnutrition, severe
Fanconi (-de Toni)(-Debré) **syndrome** E72.09
  with cystinosis E72.04
Fanconi's anemia (congenital pancytopenia) D61.09
Farber's disease or syndrome E75.29
Farcy A24.0
Farmer's
  lung J67.0
  skin L57.8
Farsightedness — *see* Hypermetropia
Fascia — *see* condition
Fasciculation R25.3
Fasciitis M72.9
  diffuse (eosinophilic) M35.4
  infective M72.8
    necrotizing M72.6
  necrotizing M72.6
  nodular M72.4
  perirenal (with ureteral obstruction) N13.5
    with infection N13.6
  plantar M72.2
  specified NEC M72.8
  traumatic (old) M72.8
    current — *code by* site under Sprain
Fascioliasis B66.3
Fasciolopsis, fasciolopsiasis (intestinal) B66.5
Fascioscapulohumeral myopathy G71.0
Fast pulse R00.0
Fat
  embolism — *see* Embolism, fat
  excessive (*see also* Obesity)
    in heart — *see* Degeneration, myocardial
  in stool R19.5
  localized (pad) E65
    heart — *see* Degeneration, myocardial
    knee M79.4
    retropatellar M79.4
  necrosis
    breast N64.1
    mesentery K65.4
    omentum K65.4
  pad E65
    knee M79.4
Fatigue R53.83
  auditory deafness — *see* Deafness
  chronic R53.82
  combat F43.0
  general R53.83
    psychogenic F48.8
  heat (transient) T67.6 ☑
  muscle M62.89
  myocardium — *see* Failure, heart
  neoplasm-related R53.0
  nervous, neurosis F48.8
  operational F48.8
  psychogenic (general) F48.8
  senile R54
  voice R49.8
Fatness — *see* Obesity
Fatty (*see also* condition)
  apron E65

Fatty — *continued*
  degeneration — *see* Degeneration, fatty
  heart (enlarged) — *see* Degeneration, myocardial
  liver NEC K76.0
    alcoholic K70.0
    nonalcoholic K76.0
  necrosis — *see* Degeneration, fatty
Fauces — *see* condition
Fauchard's disease (periodontitis) — *see* Periodontitis
Faucitis J02.9
Favism (anemia) D55.0
Favus — *see* Dermatophytosis
Fazio-Londe disease or syndrome G12.1
Fear complex or reaction F40.9
Fear of — *see* Phobia
Feared complaint unfounded Z71.1
Febris, febrile (*see also* Fever)
  flava (*see also* Fever, yellow) A95.9
  melitensis A23.0
  pestis — *see* Plague
  recurrens — *see* Fever, relapsing
  rubra A38.9
Fecal
  incontinence R15.9
  smearing R15.1
  soiling R15.1
  urgency R15.2
Fecalith (impaction) K56.41
  appendix K38.1
  congenital P76.8
Fede's disease K14.0
Feeble rapid pulse due to shock following injury
  T79.4 ☑
Feeble-minded F70
Feeding
  difficulties R63.3
  problem R63.3
    newborn P92.9
      specified NEC P92.8
    nonorganic (adult) — *see* Disorder, eating
Feeling (of)
  foreign body in throat R09.89
Feer's disease — *see* Poisoning, mercury
Feet — *see* condition
Feigned illness Z76.5
Feil-Klippel syndrome (brevicollis) Q76.1
Feinmesser's (hidrotic) **ectodermal dysplasia** Q82.4
Felinophobia F40.218
Felon (*see also* Cellulitis, digit)
  with lymphangitis — *see* Lymphangitis, acute, digit
Felty's syndrome M05.00
  ankle M05.07- ☑
  elbow M05.02- ☑
  foot joint M05.07- ☑
  hand joint M05.04- ☑
  hip M05.05- ☑
  knee M05.06- ☑
  multiple site M05.09
  shoulder M05.01- ☑
  vertebra — *see* Spondylitis, ankylosing
  wrist M05.03- ☑
Female genital cutting status — *see* Female genital
    mutilation status (FGM)
Female genital mutilation status (FGM) N90.810
  specified NEC N90.818
  type I (clitorectomy status) N90.811
  type II (clitorectomy with excision of labia minora sta-
    tus) N90.812
  type III (infibulation status) N90.813
  type IV N90.818
Femur, femoral — *see* condition
Fenestration, fenestrated (*see also* Imperfect, closure)
  aortico-pulmonary Q21.4
  cusps, heart valve NEC Q24.8
    pulmonary Q22.3
  pulmonic cusps Q22.3
Fernell's disease (aortic aneurysm) I71.9
Fertile eunuch syndrome E23.0
Fetid
  breath R19.6
  sweat L75.0
Fetishism F65.0
  transvestic F65.1
Fetus, fetal (*see also* condition)
  alcohol syndrome (dysmorphic) Q86.0
  compressus O31.0- ☑
  hydantoin syndrome Q86.1

Fetus, fetal — *continued*
  lung tissue P28.0
  papyraceous O31.0- ☑
Fever (inanition) (of unknown origin) (persistent) (with
    chills) (with rigor) R50.9
  abortus A23.1
  Aden (dengue) A90
  African tick-borne A68.1
  American
    mountain (tick) A93.2
    spotted A77.0
  aphthous B08.8
  arbovirus, arboviral A94
    hemorrhagic A94
    specified NEC A93.8
  Argentinian hemorrhagic A96.0
  Assam B55.0
  Australian Q A78
  Bangkok hemorrhagic A91
  Barmah forest A92.8
  Bartonella A44.0
  bilious, hemoglobinuric B50.8
  blackwater B50.8
  blister B00.1
  Bolivian hemorrhagic A96.1
  Bonvale dam T73.3 ☑
  boutonneuse A77.1
  brain — *see* Encephalitis
  Brazilian purpuric A48.4
  breakbone A90
  Bullis A77.0
  Bunyamwera A92.8
  Burdwan B55.0
  Bwamba A92.8
  Cameroon — *see* Malaria
  Canton A75.9
  catarrhal (acute) J00
    chronic J31.0
  cat-scratch A28.1
  Central Asian hemorrhagic A98.0
  cerebral — *see* Encephalitis
  cerebrospinal meningococcal A39.0
  Chagres B50.9
  Chandipura A92.8
  Changuinola A93.1
  Charcot's (biliary) (hepatic) (intermittent) — *see* Calcu-
    lus, bile duct
  Chikungunya (viral) (hemorrhagic) A92.0
  Chitral A93.1
  Colombo — *see* Fever, paratyphoid
  Colorado tick (virus) A93.2
  congestive (remittent) — *see* Malaria
  Congo virus A98.0
  continued malarial B50.9
  Corsican — *see* Malaria
  Crimean-Congo hemorrhagic A98.0
  Cyprus — *see* Brucellosis
  dandy A90
  deer fly — *see* Tularemia
  dengue (virus) A90
    hemorrhagic A91
    sandfly A93.1
  desert B38.0
  drug induced R50.2
  due to
    conditions classified elsewhere R50.81
    heat T67.0 ☑
  enteric A01.00
  enteroviral exanthematous (Boston exanthem) A88.0
  ephemeral (of unknown origin) R50.9
  epidemic hemorrhagic A98.5
  erysipelatous — *see* Erysipelas
  estivo-autumnal (malarial) B50.9
  famine A75.0
  five day A79.0
  following delivery O86.4
  Fort Bragg A27.89
  gastroenteric A01.00
  gastromalarial — *see* Malaria
  Gibraltar — *see* Brucellosis
  glandular — *see* Mononucleosis, infectious
  Guama (viral) A92.8
  Haverhill A25.1
  hay (allergic) J30.1
    with asthma (bronchial) J45.909
    with
      exacerbation (acute) J45.901
      status asthmaticus J45.902

Fever — *continued*
  hay — *continued*
    due to
      allergen other than pollen J30.89
      pollen, any plant or tree J30.1
  heat (effects) T67.0 ☑
  hematuric, bilious B50.8
  hemoglobinuric (malarial) (bilious) B50.8
  hemorrhagic (arthropod-borne) NOS A94
    with renal syndrome A98.5
    arenaviral A96.9
      specified NEC A96.8
    Argentinian A96.0
    Bangkok A91
    Bolivian A96.1
    Central Asian A98.0
    Chikungunya A92.0
    Crimean-Congo A98.0
    dengue (virus) A91
    epidemic A98.5
    Junin (virus) A96.0
    Korean A98.5
    Kyasanur forest A98.2
    Machupo (virus) A96.1
    mite-borne A93.8
    mosquito-borne A92.8
    Omsk A98.1
    Philippine A91
    Russian A98.5
    Singapore A91
    Southeast Asia A91
    Thailand A91
    tick-borne NEC A93.8
    viral A99
      specified NEC A98.8
  hepatic — *see* Cholecystitis
  herpetic — *see* Herpes
  icterohemorrhagic A27.0
  Indiana A93.8
  infective B99.9
    specified NEC B99.8
  intermittent (bilious) (*see also* Malaria)
    of unknown origin R50.9
    pernicious B50.9
  iodide R50.2
  Japanese river A75.3
  jungle (*see also* Malaria)
    yellow A95.0
  Junin (virus) hemorrhagic A96.0
  Katayama B65.2
  kedani A75.3
  Kenya (tick) A77.1
  Kew Garden A79.1
  Korean hemorrhagic A98.5
  Lassa A96.2
  Lone Star A77.0
  Machupo (virus) hemorrhagic A96.1
  malaria, malarial — *see* Malaria
  Malta A23.9
  Marseilles A77.1
  marsh — *see* Malaria
  Mayaro (viral) A92.8
  Mediterranean (*see also* Brucellosis) A23.9
    familial E85.0
    tick A77.1
  meningeal — *see* Meningitis
  Meuse A79.0
  Mexican A75.2
  mianeh A68.1
  miasmatic — *see* Malaria
  mosquito-borne (viral) A92.9
    hemorrhagic A92.8
  mountain (*see also* Brucellosis)
    meaning Rocky Mountain spotted fever A77.0
    tick (American) (Colorado) (viral) A93.2
  Mucambo (viral) A92.8
  mud A27.9
  Neapolitan — *see* Brucellosis
  neutropenic D70.9
  newborn P81.9
    environmental P81.0
  Nine-Mile A78
  non-exanthematous tick A93.2
  North Asian tick-borne A77.2
  Omsk hemorrhagic A98.1
  O'nyong-nyong (viral) A92.1
  Oropouche (viral) A93.0
  Oroya A44.0

Fever — *continued*
  paludal — *see* Malaria
  Panama (malarial) B50.9
  Pappataci A93.1
  paratyphoid A01.4
    A A01.1
    B A01.2
    C A01.3
  parrot A70
  periodic (Mediterranean) E85.0
  persistent (of unknown origin) R50.9
  petechial A39.0
  pharyngoconjunctival B30.2
  Philippine hemorrhagic A91
  phlebotomus A93.1
  Piry (virus) A93.8
  Pixuna (viral) A92.8
  Plasmodium ovale B53.0
  polioviral (nonparalytic) A80.4
  Pontiac A48.2
  postimmunization R50.83
  postoperative R50.82
    due to infection T81.4 ☑
  posttransfusion R50.84
  postvaccination R50.83
  presenting with conditions classified elsewhere R50.81
  pretibial A27.89
  puerperal O86.4
  Q A78
  quadrilateral A78
  quartan (malaria) B52.9
  Queensland (coastal) (tick) A77.3
  quintan A79.0
  rabbit — *see* Tularemia
  rat-bite A25.9
    due to
      Spirillum A25.0
      Streptobacillus moniliformis A25.1
  recurrent — *see* Fever, relapsing
  relapsing (Borrelia) A68.9
    Carter's (Asiatic) A68.1
    Dutton's (West African) A68.1
    Koch's A68.9
    louse-borne A68.0
    Novy's
      louse-borne A68.0
      tick-borne A68.1
    Obermeyer's (European) A68.0
    tick-borne A68.1
  remittent (bilious) (congestive) (gastric) — *see* Malaria
  rheumatic (active) (acute) (chronic) (subacute) I00
    with central nervous system involvement I02.9
    active with heart involvement — *see* category
      I01 ☑
    inactive or quiescent with
      cardiac hypertrophy I09.89
      carditis I09.9
      endocarditis I09.1
        aortic (valve) I06.9
          with mitral (valve) disease I08.0
        mitral (valve) I05.9
          with aortic (valve) disease I08.0
        pulmonary (valve) I09.89
        tricuspid (valve) I07.8
      heart disease NEC I09.89
      heart failure (congestive) (conditions in I50.9)
        I09.81
      left ventricular failure (conditions in I50.1)
        I09.81
      myocarditis, myocardial degeneration (condi-
        tions in I51.4) I09.0
      pancarditis I09.9
      pericarditis I09.2
  Rift Valley (viral) A92.4
  Rocky Mountain spotted A77.0
  rose J30.1
  Ross River B33.1
  Russian hemorrhagic A98.5
  San Joaquin (Valley) B38.0
  sandfly A93.1
  Sao Paulo A77.0
  scarlet A38.9
  seven day (leptospirosis) (autumnal) (Japanese) A27.89
    dengue A90
  shin-bone A79.0
  Singapore hemorrhagic A91
  solar A90
  Songo A98.5

Fever — *continued*
  sore B00.1
  South African tick-bite A68.1
  Southeast Asia hemorrhagic A91
  spinal — *see* Meningitis
  spirillary A25.0
  splenic — *see* Anthrax
  spotted A77.9
    American A77.0
    Brazilian A77.0
    cerebrospinal meningitis A39.0
    Colombian A77.0
    due to Rickettsia
      australis A77.3
      conorii A77.1
      rickettsii A77.0
      sibirica A77.2
      specified type NEC A77.8
    Ehrlichiosis A77.40
      due to
        E. chafeensis A77.41
        specified organism NEC A77.49
    Rocky Mountain A77.0
  steroid R50.2
  streptobacillary A25.1
  subtertian B50.9
  Sumatran mite A75.3
  sun A90
  swamp A27.9
  swine A02.8
  sylvatic, yellow A95.0
  Tahyna B33.8
  tertian — *see* Malaria, tertian
  Thailand hemorrhagic A91
  thermic T67.0 ☑
  three-day A93.1
  tick
    American mountain A93.2
    Colorado A93.2
    Kemerovo A93.8
    Mediterranean A77.1
    mountain A93.2
    nonexanthematous A93.2
    Quaranfil A93.8
  tick-bite NEC A93.8
  tick-borne (hemorrhagic) NEC A93.8
  trench A79.0
  tsutsugamushi A75.3
  typhogastric A01.00
  typhoid (abortive) (hemorrhagic) (intermittent) (ma-
    lignant) A01.00
    complicated by
      arthritis A01.04
      heart involvement A01.02
      meningitis A01.01
      osteomyelitis A01.05
      pneumonia A01.03
      specified NEC A01.09
  typhomalarial — *see* Malaria
  typhus — *see* Typhus (fever)
  undulant — *see* Brucellosis
  unknown origin R50.9
  uveoparotid D86.89
  valley B38.0
  Venezuelan equine A92.2
  vesicular stomatitis A93.8
  viral hemorrhagic — *see* Fever, hemorrhagic, by type
    of virus
  Volhynian A79.0
  Wesselsbron (viral) A92.8
  West
    African B50.8
    Nile (viral) A92.30
      with
        complications NEC A92.39
        cranial nerve disorders A92.32
        encephalitis A92.31
        encephalomyelitis A92.31
        neurologic manifestation NEC A92.32
        optic neuritis A92.32
        polyradiculitis A92.32
  Whitmore's — *see* Melioidosis
  Wolhynian A79.0
  worm B83.9
  yellow A95.9
    jungle A95.0
    sylvatic A95.0
    urban A95.1

☑ **Additional Character Required** — Refer to the Tabular List for Character Selection   ᵀᴬᴮ **Subterms under main terms may continue to next column or page**

Fever — *continued*
  Zika (viral) A92.8
Fibrillation
  atrial or auricular (established) I48.91
    chronic I48.2
    paroxysmal I48.0
    permanent I48.2
    persistent I48.1
  cardiac I49.8
  heart I49.8
  muscular M62.89
  ventricular I49.01
Fibrin
  ball or bodies, pleural (sac) J94.1
  chamber, anterior (eye) (gelatinous exudate) — *see* Iridocyclitis, acute
Fibrinogenolysis — *see* Fibrinolysis
Fibrinogenopenia D68.8
  acquired D65
  congenital D68.2
Fibrinolysis (hemorrhagic) (acquired) D65
  antepartum hemorrhage — *see* Hemorrhage, antepartum, with coagulation defect
  following
    abortion — *see* Abortion by type complicated by hemorrhage
    ectopic or molar pregnancy O08.1
  intrapartum O67.0
  newborn, transient P60
  postpartum O72.3
Fibrinopenia (hereditary) D68.2
  acquired D68.4
Fibrinopurulent — *see* condition
Fibrinous — *see* condition
Fibroadenoma
  cellular intracanalicular D24- ☑
  giant D24- ☑
  intracanalicular
    cellular D24- ☑
    giant D24- ☑
    specified site — *see* Neoplasm, benign, by site
    unspecified site D24- ☑
  juvenile D24- ☑
  pericanalicular
    specified site — *see* Neoplasm, benign, by site
    unspecified site D24- ☑
  phyllodes D24- ☑
  prostate D29.1
  specified site NEC — *see* Neoplasm, benign, by site
  unspecified site D24- ☑
Fibroadenosis, breast (chronic) (cystic) (diffuse) (periodic) (segmental) N60.2- ☑
Fibroangioma (*see also* Neoplasm, benign, by site)
  juvenile
    specified site — *see* Neoplasm, benign, by site
    unspecified site D10.6
Fibrochondrosarcoma — *see* Neoplasm, cartilage, malignant
Fibrocystic
  disease (*see also* Fibrosis, cystic)
    breast — *see* Mastopathy, cystic
    jaw M27.49
    kidney (congenital) Q61.8
    liver Q44.6
    pancreas E84.9
  kidney (congenital) Q61.8
Fibrodysplasia ossificans progressiva — *see* Myositis, ossificans, progressiva
Fibroelastosis (cordis) (endocardial) (endomyocardial) I42.4
Fibroid (tumor) (*see also* Neoplasm, connective tissue, benign)
  disease, lung (chronic) — *see* Fibrosis, lung
  heart (disease) — *see* Myocarditis
  in pregnancy or childbirth O34.1- ☑
    causing obstructed labor O65.5
  induration, lung (chronic) — *see* Fibrosis, lung
  lung — *see* Fibrosis, lung
  pneumonia (chronic) — *see* Fibrosis, lung
  uterus D25.9
Fibrolipoma — *see* Lipoma
Fibroliposarcoma — *see* Neoplasm, connective tissue, malignant
Fibroma (*see also* Neoplasm, connective tissue, benign)
  ameloblastic — *see* Cyst, calcifying odontogenic
  bone (nonossifying) — *see* Disorder, bone, specified type NEC

Fibroma — *continued*
  bone — *see* Disorder, bone, specified type — *continued*
    ossifying — *see* Neoplasm, bone, benign
  cementifying — *see* Neoplasm, bone, benign
  chondromyxoid — *see* Neoplasm, bone, benign
  desmoplastic — *see* Neoplasm, connective tissue, uncertain behavior
  durum — *see* Neoplasm, connective tissue, benign
  fascial — *see* Neoplasm, connective tissue, benign
  invasive — *see* Neoplasm, connective tissue, uncertain behavior
  molle — *see* Lipoma
  myxoid — *see* Neoplasm, connective tissue, benign
  nasopharynx, nasopharyngeal (juvenile) D10.6
  nonosteogenic (nonossifying) — *see* Dysplasia, fibrous
  odontogenic (central) — *see* Cyst, calcifying odontogenic
  ossifying — *see* Neoplasm, bone, benign
  periosteal — *see* Neoplasm, bone, benign
  soft — *see* Lipoma
Fibromatosis M72.9
  abdominal — *see* Neoplasm, connective tissue, uncertain behavior
  aggressive — *see* Neoplasm, connective tissue, uncertain behavior
  congenital generalized — *see* Neoplasm, connective tissue, uncertain behavior
  Dupuytren's M72.0
  gingival K06.1
  palmar (fascial) M72.0
  plantar (fascial) M72.2
  pseudosarcomatous (proliferative) (subcutaneous) M72.4
  retroperitoneal D48.3
  specified NEC M72.8
Fibromyalgia M79.7
Fibromyoma (*see also* Neoplasm, connective tissue, benign)
  uterus (corpus) (*see also* Leiomyoma, uterus)
    in pregnancy or childbirth — *see* Fibroid, in pregnancy or childbirth
      causing obstructed labor O65.5
Fibromyositis M79.7
Fibromyxolipoma D17.9
Fibromyxoma — *see* Neoplasm, connective tissue, benign
Fibromyxosarcoma — *see* Neoplasm, connective tissue, malignant
Fibro-odontoma, ameloblastic — *see* Cyst, calcifying odontogenic
Fibro-osteoma — *see* Neoplasm, bone, benign
Fibroplasia, retrolental H35.17- ☑
Fibropurulent — *see* condition
Fibrosarcoma (*see also* Neoplasm, connective tissue, malignant)
  ameloblastic C41.1
    upper jaw (bone) C41.0
  congenital — *see* Neoplasm, connective tissue, malignant
  fascial — *see* Neoplasm, connective tissue, malignant
  infantile — *see* Neoplasm, connective tissue, malignant
  odontogenic C41.1
    upper jaw (bone) C41.0
  periosteal — *see* Neoplasm, bone, malignant
Fibrosclerosis
  breast N60.3- ☑
  multifocal M35.5
  penis (corpora cavernosa) N48.6
Fibrosis, fibrotic
  adrenal (gland) E27.8
  amnion O41.8X- ☑
  anal papillae K62.89
  arteriocapillary — *see* Arteriosclerosis
  bladder N32.89
    interstitial — *see* Cystitis, chronic, interstitial
    localized submucosal — *see* Cystitis, chronic, interstitial
    panmural — *see* Cystitis, chronic, interstitial
  breast — *see* Fibrosclerosis, breast
  capillary (*see also* Arteriosclerosis) I70.90
    lung (chronic) — *see* Fibrosis, lung
  cardiac — *see* Myocarditis
  cervix N88.8
  chorion O41.8X- ☑
  corpus cavernosum (sclerosing) N48.6

Fibrosis, fibrotic — *continued*
  cystic (of pancreas) E84.9
    with
      distal intestinal obstruction syndrome E84.19
      fecal impaction E84.19
      intestinal manifestations NEC E84.19
      pulmonary manifestations E84.0
      specified manifestations NEC E84.8
  due to device, implant or graft (*see also* Complications, by site and type, specified NEC) T85.82 ☑
    arterial graft NEC T82.828 ☑
    breast (implant) T85.82 ☑
    catheter NEC T85.82 ☑
      dialysis (renal) T82.828 ☑
        intraperitoneal T85.82 ☑
      infusion NEC T82.828 ☑
        spinal (epidural) (subdural) T85.82 ☑
      urinary (indwelling) T83.82 ☑
    electronic (electrode) (pulse generator) (stimulator)
      bone T84.82 ☑
      cardiac T82.827 ☑
      nervous system (brain) (peripheral nerve) (spinal) T85.82 ☑
      urinary T83.82 ☑
    fixation, internal (orthopedic) NEC T84.82 ☑
    gastrointestinal (bile duct) (esophagus) T85.82 ☑
    genital NEC T83.82 ☑
    heart NEC T82.827 ☑
    joint prosthesis T84.82 ☑
    ocular (corneal graft) (orbital implant) NEC T85.82 ☑
    orthopedic NEC T84.82 ☑
    specified NEC T85.82 ☑
    urinary NEC T83.82 ☑
    vascular NEC T82.828 ☑
    ventricular intracranial shunt T85.82 ☑
  ejaculatory duct N50.8
  endocardium — *see* Endocarditis
  endomyocardial (tropical) I42.3
  epididymis N50.8
  eye muscle — *see* Strabismus, mechanical
  heart — *see* Myocarditis
  hepatic — *see* Fibrosis, liver
  hepatolienal (portal hypertension) K76.6
  hepatosplenic (portal hypertension) K76.6
  infrapatellar fat pad M79.4
  intrascrotal N50.8
  kidney N26.9
  liver K74.0
    with sclerosis K74.2
    alcoholic K70.2
  lung (atrophic) (chronic) (confluent) (massive) (perialveolar) (peribronchial) J84.10
    with
      anthracosilicosis J60
      anthracosis J60
      asbestosis J61
      bagassosis J67.1
      bauxite J63.1
      berylliosis J63.2
      byssinosis J66.0
      calcicosis J62.8
      chalicosis J62.8
      dust reticulation J64
      farmer's lung J67.0
      ganister disease J62.8
      graphite J63.3
      pneumoconiosis NOS J64
      siderosis J63.4
      silicosis J62.8
    capillary J84.10
    congenital P27.8
    diffuse (idiopathic) J84.10
      chemicals, gases, fumes or vapors (inhalation) J68.4
      interstitial J84.10
        acute J84.114
      talc J62.0
    following radiation J70.1
    idiopathic J84.112
    postinflammatory J84.10
    silicotic J62.8
    tuberculous — *see* Tuberculosis, pulmonary
  lymphatic gland I89.8
  median bar — *see* Hyperplasia, prostate
  mediastinum (idiopathic) J98.5
  meninges G96.19

Fibrosis, fibrotic — continued
myocardium, myocardial — see Myocarditis
ovary N83.8
oviduct N83.8
pancreas K86.8
penis NEC N48.6
pericardium I31.0
perineum, in pregnancy or childbirth O34.7- ☑
   causing obstructed labor O65.5
pleura J94.1
popliteal fat pad M79.4
prostate (chronic) — see Hyperplasia, prostate
pulmonary (see also Fibrosis, lung) J84.10
   congenital P27.8
   idiopathic J84.112
rectal sphincter K62.89
retroperitoneal, idiopathic (with ureteral obstruction) N13.5
   with infection N13.6
sclerosing mesenteric (idiopathic) K65.4
scrotum N50.8
seminal vesicle N50.8
senile R54
skin L90.5
spermatic cord N50.8
spleen D73.89
   in schistosomiasis (bilharziasis) B65.9 [D77]
subepidermal nodular — see Neoplasm, skin, benign
submucous (oral) (tongue) K13.5
testis N44.8
   chronic, due to syphilis A52.76
thymus (gland) E32.8
tongue, submucous K13.5
tunica vaginalis N50.8
uterus (non-neoplastic) N85.8
vagina N89.8
valve, heart — see Endocarditis
vas deferens N50.8
vein I87.8

Fibrositis (periarticular) M79.7
nodular, chronic (Jaccoud's) (rheumatoid) — see Arthropathy, postrheumatic, chronic

Fibrothorax J94.1

Fibrotic — see Fibrosis

Fibrous — see condition

Fibroxanthoma (see also Neoplasm, connective tissue, benign)
atypical — see Neoplasm, connective tissue, uncertain behavior
malignant — see Neoplasm, connective tissue, malignant

Fibroxanthosarcoma — see Neoplasm, connective tissue, malignant

Fiedler's
disease (icterohemorrhagic leptospirosis) A27.0
myocarditis (acute) I40.1

Fifth disease B08.3
venereal A55

Filaria, filarial, filariasis — see Infestation, filarial

Filatov's disease — see Mononucleosis, infectious

File-cutter's disease — see Poisoning, lead

Filling defect
biliary tract R93.2
bladder R93.4
duodenum R93.3
gallbladder R93.2
gastrointestinal tract R93.3
intestine R93.3
kidney R93.4
stomach R93.3
ureter R93.4

Fimbrial cyst Q50.4

Financial problem affecting care NOS Z59.9
bankruptcy Z59.8
foreclosure on loan Z59.8

Findings, abnormal, inconclusive, without diagnosis
(see also Abnormal)
17-ketosteroids, elevated R82.5
acetonuria R82.4
alcohol in blood R78.0
anisocytosis R71.8
antenatal screening of mother O28.9
   biochemical O28.1
   chromosomal O28.5
   cytological O28.2
   genetic O28.5
   hematological O28.0
   radiological O28.4

Findings, abnormal, inconclusive, without diagnosis — continued
antenatal screening of mother — continued
   specified NEC O28.8
   ultrasonic O28.3
antibody titer, elevated R76.0
anticardiolipin antibody R76.0
antiphosphatidylglycerol antibody R76.0
antiphosphatidylinositol antibody R76.0
antiphosphatidylserine antibody R76.0
antiphospholipid antibody R76.0
bacteriuria N39.0
bicarbonate E87.8
bile in urine R82.2
blood sugar R73.09
   high R73.9
   low (transient) E16.2
body fluid or substance, specified NEC R88.8
casts, urine R82.99
catecholamines R82.5
cells, urine R82.99
chloride E87.8
cholesterol E78.9
   high E78.0
      with high triglycerides E78.2
chyluria R82.0
cloudy
   dialysis effluent R88.0
   urine R82.90
creatinine clearance R94.4
crystals, urine R82.99
culture
   blood R78.81
   positive — see Positive, culture
echocardiogram R93.1
electrolyte level, urinary R82.99
function study NEC R94.8
   bladder R94.8
   endocrine NEC R94.7
      thyroid R94.6
   kidney R94.4
   liver R94.5
   pancreas R94.8
   placenta R94.8
   pulmonary R94.2
   spleen R94.8
gallbladder, nonvisualization R93.2
glucose (tolerance test) (non-fasting) R73.09
glycosuria R81
heart
   shadow R93.1
   sounds R01.2
hematinuria R82.3
hematocrit drop (precipitous) R71.0
hemoglobinuria R82.3
human papillomavirus (HPV) DNA test positive
   cervix
      high risk R87.810
      low risk R87.820
   vagina
      high risk R87.811
      low risk R87.821
in blood (of substance not normally found in blood) R78.9
   addictive drug NEC R78.4
   alcohol (excessive level) R78.0
   cocaine R78.2
   hallucinogen R78.3
   heavy metals (abnormal level) R78.79
   lead R78.71
   lithium (abnormal level) R78.89
   opiate drug R78.1
   psychotropic drug R78.5
   specified substance NEC R78.89
   steroid agent R78.6
indoleacetic acid, elevated R82.5
ketonuria R82.4
lactic acid dehydrogenase (LDH) R74.0
liver function test R79.89
mammogram NEC R92.8
   calcification (calculus) R92.1
   inconclusive result (due to dense breasts) R92.2
   microcalcification R92.0
mediastinal shift R93.8
melanin, urine R82.99
myoglobinuria R82.1
neonatal screening P09
nonvisualization of gallbladder R93.2

Findings, abnormal, inconclusive, without diagnosis — continued
odor of urine NOS R82.90
Papanicolaou cervix R87.619
   non-atypical endometrial cells R87.618
pneumoencephalogram R93.0
poikilocytosis R71.8
potassium (deficiency) E87.6
   excess E87.5
PPD R76.11
radiologic (X-ray) R93.8
   abdomen R93.5
   biliary tract R93.2
   breast R92.8
   gastrointestinal tract R93.3
   genitourinary organs R93.8
   head R93.0
   inconclusive due to excess body fat of patient R93.9
   intrathoracic organs NEC R93.1
   placenta R93.8
   retroperitoneum R93.5
   skin R93.8
   skull R93.0
   subcutaneous tissue R93.8
red blood cell (count) (morphology) (sickling) (volume) R71.8
scan NEC R94.8
   bladder R94.8
   bone R94.8
   kidney R94.4
   liver R93.2
   lung R94.2
   pancreas R94.8
   placental R94.8
   spleen R94.8
   thyroid R94.6
sedimentation rate, elevated R70.0
SGOT R74.0
SGPT R74.0
sodium (deficiency) E87.1
   excess E87.0
specified body fluid NEC R88.8
stress test R94.39
thyroid (function) (metabolic rate) (scan) (uptake) R94.6
transaminase (level) R74.0
triglycerides E78.9
   high E78.1
      with high cholesterol E78.2
tuberculin skin test (without active tuberculosis) R76.11
urine R82.90
   acetone R82.4
   bacteria N39.0
   bile R82.2
   casts or cells R82.99
   chyle R82.0
   culture positive R82.7
   glucose R81
   hemoglobin R82.3
   ketone R82.4
   sugar R81
vanillylmandelic acid (VMA), elevated R82.5
vectorcardiogram (VCG) R94.39
ventriculogram R93.0
white blood cell (count) (differential) (morphology) D72.9
xerography R92.8

Finger — see condition

Fire, Saint Anthony's — see Erysipelas

Fire-setting
pathological (compulsive) F63.1

Fish hook stomach K31.89

Fishmeal-worker's lung J67.8

Fissure, fissured
anus, anal K60.2
   acute K60.0
   chronic K60.1
   congenital Q43.8
ear, lobule, congenital Q17.8
epiglottis (congenital) Q31.8
larynx J38.7
   congenital Q31.8
lip K13.0
   congenital — see Cleft, lip
nipple N64.0
   associated with
      lactation O92.13

Fibrosis, fibrotic — Fissure, fissured

Fissure, fissured — *continued*
- nipple — *continued*
  - associated with — *continued*
    - pregnancy O92.11- ☑
    - puerperium O92.12
  - nose Q30.2
  - palate (congenital) — *see* Cleft, palate
  - skin R23.4
  - spine (congenital) (*see also* Spina bifida)
    - with hydrocephalus — *see* Spina bifida, by site, with hydrocephalus
  - tongue (acquired) K14.5
    - congenital Q38.3

Fistula (cutaneous) L98.8
- abdomen (wall) K63.2
  - bladder N32.2
  - intestine NEC K63.2
  - ureter N28.89
  - uterus N82.5
- abdominorectal K63.2
- abdominosigmoidal K63.2
- abdominothoracic J86.0
- abdominouterine N82.5
  - congenital Q51.7
- abdominovesical N32.2
- accessory sinuses — *see* Sinusitis
- actinomycotic — *see* Actinomycosis
- alveolar antrum — *see* Sinusitis, maxillary
- alveolar process K04.6
- anorectal K60.5
- antrobuccal — *see* Sinusitis, maxillary
- antrum — *see* Sinusitis, maxillary
- anus, anal (recurrent) (infectional) K60.3
  - congenital Q43.6
    - with absence, atresia and stenosis Q42.2
  - tuberculous A18.32
- aorta-duodenal I77.2
- appendix, appendicular K38.3
- arteriovenous (acquired) (nonruptured) I77.0
  - brain I67.1
    - congenital Q28.2
      - ruptured I60.8
    - ruptured I60.8
  - cerebral — *see* Fistula, arteriovenous, brain
  - congenital (peripheral) (*see also* Malformation, arteriovenous)
    - brain Q28.2
      - ruptured I60.8
    - coronary Q24.5
    - pulmonary Q25.72
  - coronary I25.41
    - congenital Q24.5
  - pulmonary I28.0
    - congenital Q25.72
  - surgically created (for dialysis) Z99.2
    - complication — *see* Complication, arteriovenous, fistula, surgically created
  - traumatic — *see* Injury, blood vessel
- artery I77.2
- aural (mastoid) — *see* Mastoiditis, chronic
- auricle (*see also* Disorder, pinna, specified type NEC)
  - congenital Q18.1
- Bartholin's gland N82.8
- bile duct (common) (hepatic) K83.3
  - with calculus, stones — *see* Calculus, bile duct
- biliary (tract) — *see* Fistula, bile duct
- bladder (sphincter) NEC (*see also* Fistula, vesico-) N32.2
  - into seminal vesicle N32.2
- bone (*see also* Disorder, bone, specified type NEC)
  - with osteomyelitis, chronic — *see* Osteomyelitis, chronic, with draining sinus
- brain G93.89
  - arteriovenous (acquired) I67.1
    - congenital Q28.2
- branchial (cleft) Q18.0
- branchiogenous Q18.0
- breast N61
  - puerperal, postpartum or gestational, due to mastitis (purulent) — *see* Mastitis, obstetric, purulent
- bronchial J86.0
- bronchocutaneous, bronchomediastinal, bronchopleural, bronchopleuromediastinal (infective) J86.0
  - tuberculous NEC A15.5
- bronchoesophageal J86.0
  - congenital Q39.2
    - with atresia of esophagus Q39.1
- bronchovisceral J86.0

Fistula — *continued*
- buccal cavity (infective) K12.2
- cecosigmoidal K63.2
- cecum K63.2
- cerebrospinal (fluid) G96.0
- cervical, lateral Q18.1
- cervicoaural Q18.1
- cervicosigmoidal N82.4
- cervicovesical N82.1
- cervix N82.8
- chest (wall) J86.0
- cholecystenteric — *see* Fistula, gallbladder
- cholecystocolic — *see* Fistula, gallbladder
- cholecystocolonic — *see* Fistula, gallbladder
- cholecystoduodenal — *see* Fistula, gallbladder
- cholecystogastric — *see* Fistula, gallbladder
- cholecystointestinal — *see* Fistula, gallbladder
- choledochoduodenal — *see* Fistula, bile duct
- cholocolic K82.3
- coccyx — *see* Sinus, pilonidal
- colon K63.2
- colostomy K94.09
- common duct — *see* Fistula, bile duct
- congenital, site not listed — *see* Anomaly, by site
- coronary, arteriovenous I25.41
  - congenital Q24.5
- costal region J86.0
- cul-de-sac, Douglas' N82.8
- cystic duct (*see also* Fistula, gallbladder)
  - congenital Q44.5
- dental K04.6
- diaphragm J86.0
- duodenum K31.6
- ear (external) (canal) — *see* Disorder, ear, external, specified type NEC
- enterocolic K63.2
- enterocutaneous K63.2
- enterouterine N82.4
  - congenital Q51.7
- enterovaginal N82.4
  - congenital Q52.2
  - large intestine N82.3
  - small intestine N82.2
- enterovesical N32.1
- epididymis N50.8
  - tuberculous A18.15
- esophagobronchial J86.0
  - congenital Q39.2
    - with atresia of esophagus Q39.1
- esophagocutaneous K22.8
- esophagopleural-cutaneous J86.0
- esophagotracheal J86.0
  - congenital Q39.2
    - with atresia of esophagus Q39.1
- esophagus K22.8
  - congenital Q39.2
    - with atresia of esophagus Q39.1
- ethmoid — *see* Sinusitis, ethmoidal
- eyeball (cornea) (sclera) — *see* Disorder, globe, hypotony
- eyelid H01.8
- fallopian tube, external N82.5
- fecal K63.2
  - congenital Q43.6
- from periapical abscess K04.6
- frontal sinus — *see* Sinusitis, frontal
- gallbladder K82.3
  - with calculus, cholelithiasis, stones — *see* Calculus, gallbladder
- gastric K31.6
- gastrocolic K31.6
  - congenital Q40.2
  - tuberculous A18.32
- gastroenterocolic K31.6
- gastroesophageal K31.6
- gastrojejunal K31.6
- gastrojejunocolic K31.6
- genital tract (female) N82.9
  - specified NEC N82.8
  - to intestine NEC N82.4
  - to skin N82.5
- hepatic artery-portal vein, congenital Q26.6
- hepatopleural J86.0
- hepatopulmonary J86.0
- ileorectal or ileosigmoidal K63.2
- ileovaginal N82.2
- ileovesical N32.1
- ileum K63.2

Fistula — *continued*
- in ano K60.3
  - tuberculous A18.32
- inner ear (labyrinth) — *see* subcategory H83.1 ☑
- intestine NEC K63.2
- intestinocolonic (abdominal) K63.2
- intestinoureteral N28.89
- intestinouterine N82.4
- intestinovaginal N82.4
  - large intestine N82.3
  - small intestine N82.2
- intestinovesical N32.1
- ischiorectal (fossa) K61.3
- jejunum K63.2
- joint M25.10
  - ankle M25.17- ☑
  - elbow M25.12- ☑
  - foot joint M25.17- ☑
  - hand joint M25.14- ☑
  - hip M25.15- ☑
  - knee M25.16- ☑
  - shoulder M25.11- ☑
  - specified joint NEC M25.18
  - tuberculous — *see* Tuberculosis, joint
  - vertebrae M25.18
  - wrist M25.13- ☑
- kidney N28.89
- labium (majus) (minus) N82.8
- labyrinth — *see* subcategory H83.1 ☑
- lacrimal (gland) (sac) H04.61- ☑
- lacrimonasal duct — *see* Fistula, lacrimal
- laryngotracheal, congenital Q34.8
- larynx J38.7
- lip K13.0
  - congenital Q38.0
- lumbar, tuberculous A18.01
- lung J86.0
- lymphatic I89.8
- mammary (gland) N61
- mastoid (process) (region) — *see* Mastoiditis, chronic
- maxillary J32.0
- medial, face and neck Q18.8
- mediastinal J86.0
- mediastinobronchial J86.0
- mediastinocutaneous J86.0
- middle ear — *see* subcategory H74.8 ☑
- mouth K12.2
- nasal J34.89
  - sinus — *see* Sinusitis
- nasopharynx J39.2
- nipple N64.0
- nose J34.89
- oral (cutaneous) K12.2
  - maxillary J32.0
  - nasal (with cleft palate) — *see* Cleft, palate
- orbit, orbital — *see* Disorder, orbit, specified type NEC
- oroantral J32.0
- oviduct, external N82.5
- palate (hard) M27.8
- pancreatic K86.8
- pancreaticoduodenal K86.8
- parotid (gland) K11.4
  - region K12.2
- penis N48.89
- perianal K60.3
- pericardium (pleura) (sac) — *see* Pericarditis
- pericecal K63.2
- perineorectal K60.4
- perineosigmoidal K63.2
- perineum, perineal (with urethral involvement) NEC N36.0
  - tuberculous A18.13
  - ureter N28.89
- perirectal K60.4
  - tuberculous A18.32
- peritoneum K65.9
- pharyngoesophageal J39.2
- pharynx J39.2
  - branchial cleft (congenital) Q18.0
- pilonidal (infected) (rectum) — *see* Sinus, pilonidal
- pleura, pleural, pleurocutaneous, pleuroperitoneal J86.0
  - tuberculous NEC A15.6
- pleuropericardial I31.8
- portal vein-hepatic artery, congenital Q26.6
- postauricular H70.81- ☑
- postoperative, persistent T81.83 ☑
  - specified site — *see* Fistula, by site

Fistula — *continued*
- preauricular (congenital) Q18.1
- prostate N42.89
- pulmonary J86.0
  - arteriovenous I28.0
    - congenital Q25.72
  - tuberculous — *see* Tuberculosis, pulmonary
- pulmonoperitoneal J86.0
- rectolabial N82.4
- rectosigmoid (intercommunicating) K63.2
- rectoureteral N28.89
- rectourethral N36.0
  - congenital Q64.73
- rectouterine N82.4
  - congenital Q51.7
- rectovaginal N82.3
  - congenital Q52.2
  - tuberculous A18.18
- rectovesical N32.1
  - congenital Q64.79
- rectovesicovaginal N82.3
- rectovulval N82.4
  - congenital Q52.79
- rectum (to skin) K60.4
  - congenital Q43.6
    - with absence, atresia and stenosis Q42.0
  - tuberculous A18.32
- renal N28.89
- retroauricular — *see* Fistula, postauricular
- salivary duct or gland (any) K11.4
  - congenital Q38.4
- scrotum (urinary) N50.8
  - tuberculous A18.15
- semicircular canals — *see* subcategory H83.1 ☑
- sigmoid K63.2
  - to bladder N32.1
- sinus — *see* Sinusitis
- skin L98.8
  - to genital tract (female) N82.5
- splenocolic D73.89
- stercoral K63.2
- stomach K31.6
- sublingual gland K11.4
- submandibular gland K11.4
- submaxillary (gland) K11.4
  - region K12.2
- thoracic J86.0
  - duct I89.8
- thoracoabdominal J86.0
- thoracogastric J86.0
- thoracointestinal J86.0
- thorax J86.0
- thyroglossal duct Q89.2
- thyroid E07.89
- trachea, congenital (external) (internal) Q32.1
- tracheoesophageal J86.0
  - congenital Q39.2
    - with atresia of esophagus Q39.1
  - following tracheostomy J95.04
- traumatic arteriovenous — *see* Injury, blood vessel, by site
- tuberculous — *code by* site under Tuberculosis
- typhoid A01.09
- umbilicourinary Q64.8
- urachus, congenital Q64.4
- ureter (persistent) N28.89
- ureteroabdominal N28.89
- ureterorectal N28.89
- ureterosigmoido-abdominal N28.89
- ureterovaginal N82.1
- ureterovesical N32.2
- urethra N36.0
  - congenital Q64.79
  - tuberculous A18.13
- urethroperineal N36.0
- urethroperineovesical N32.2
- urethrorectal N36.0
  - congenital Q64.73
- urethroscrotal N50.8
- urethrovaginal N82.1
- urethrovesical N32.2
- urinary (tract) (persistent) (recurrent) N36.0
- uteroabdominal N82.5
  - congenital Q51.7
- uteroenteric, uterointestinal N82.4
  - congenital Q51.7
- uterorectal N82.4
  - congenital Q51.7

Fistula — *continued*
- uteroureteric N82.1
- uterourethral Q51.7
- uterovaginal N82.8
- uterovesical N82.1
  - congenital Q51.7
- uterus N82.8
- vagina (postpartal) (wall) N82.8
- vaginocutaneous (postpartal) N82.5
- vaginointestinal NEC N82.4
  - large intestine N82.3
  - small intestine N82.2
- vaginoperineal N82.5
- vasocutaneous, congenital Q55.7
- vesical NEC N32.2
- vesicoabdominal N32.2
- vesicocervicovaginal N82.1
- vesicocolic N32.1
- vesicocutaneous N32.2
- vesicoenteric N32.1
- vesicointestinal N32.1
- vesicometrorectal N82.4
- vesicoperineal N32.2
- vesicorectal N32.1
  - congenital Q64.79
- vesicosigmoidal N32.1
- vesicosigmoidovaginal N82.3
- vesicoureteral N32.2
- vesicoureterovaginal N82.1
- vesicourethral N32.2
- vesicourethrorectal N32.1
- vesicouterine N82.1
  - congenital Q51.7
- vesicovaginal N82.0
- vulvorectal N82.4
  - congenital Q52.79

Fit R56.9
- epileptic — *see* Epilepsy
- fainting R55
- hysterical F44.5
- newborn P90

Fitting (and adjustment) (of)
- artificial
  - arm — *see* Admission, adjustment, artificial, arm
  - breast Z44.3 ☑
  - eye Z44.2 ☑
  - leg — *see* Admission, adjustment, artificial, leg
- automatic implantable cardiac defibrillator (with synchronous cardiac pacemaker) Z45.02
- brain neuropacemaker Z46.2
  - implanted Z45.42
- cardiac defibrillator — *see* Fitting (and adjustment) (of), automatic implantable cardiac defibrillator
- catheter, non-vascular Z46.82
- colostomy belt Z46.89
- contact lenses Z46.0
- cystostomy device Z46.6
- defibrillator, cardiac — *see* Fitting (and adjustment) (of), automatic implantable cardiac defibrillator
- dentures Z46.3
- device NOS Z46.9
  - abdominal Z46.89
  - gastrointestinal NEC Z46.59
  - implanted NEC Z45.89
  - nervous system Z46.2
    - implanted — *see* Admission, adjustment, device, implanted, nervous system
  - orthodontic Z46.4
  - orthoptic Z46.0
  - orthotic Z46.89
  - prosthetic (external) Z44.9
    - breast Z44.3 ☑
    - dental Z46.3
    - eye Z44.2 ☑
    - specified NEC Z44.8
  - specified NEC Z46.89
  - substitution
    - auditory Z46.2
      - implanted — *see* Admission, adjustment, device, implanted, hearing device
    - nervous system Z46.2
      - implanted — *see* Admission, adjustment, device, implanted, nervous system
    - visual Z46.2
      - implanted Z45.31
  - urinary Z46.6
- gastric lap band Z46.51
- gastrointestinal appliance NEC Z46.59

Fitting — *continued*
- glasses (reading) Z46.0
- hearing aid Z46.1
- ileostomy device Z46.89
- insulin pump Z46.81
- intestinal appliance NEC Z46.89
- myringotomy device (stent) (tube) Z45.82
- neuropacemaker Z46.2
  - implanted Z45.42
- non-vascular catheter Z46.82
- orthodontic device Z46.4
- orthopedic device (brace) (cast) (corset) (shoes) Z46.89
- pacemaker (cardiac) Z45.018
  - nervous system (brain) (peripheral nerve) (spinal cord) Z46.2
    - implanted Z45.42
  - pulse generator Z45.010
- portacath (port-a-cath) Z45.2
- prosthesis (external) Z44.9
  - arm — *see* Admission, adjustment, artificial, arm
  - breast Z44.3 ☑
  - dental Z46.3
  - eye Z44.2 ☑
  - leg — *see* Admission, adjustment, artificial, leg
  - specified NEC Z44.8
- spectacles Z46.0
- wheelchair Z46.89

Fitzhugh-Curtis syndrome
- due to
  - Chlamydia trachomatis A74.81
  - Neisseria gonorrhorea (gonococcal peritonitis) A54.85

Fitz's syndrome (acute hemorrhagic pancreatitis) K85.8

Fixation
- joint — *see* Ankylosis
- larynx J38.7
- stapes — *see* Ankylosis, ear ossicles
  - deafness — *see* Deafness, conductive
- uterus (acquired) — *see* Malposition, uterus
- vocal cord J38.3

Flabby ridge K06.8

Flaccid (*see also* condition)
- palate, congenital Q38.5

Flail
- chest S22.5 ☑
  - newborn (birth injury) P13.8
- joint (paralytic) M25.20
  - ankle M25.27- ☑
  - elbow M25.22- ☑
  - foot joint M25.27- ☑
  - hand joint M25.24- ☑
  - hip M25.25- ☑
  - knee M25.26- ☑
  - shoulder M25.21- ☑
  - specified joint NEC M25.28
  - wrist M25.23- ☑

Flajani's disease — *see* Hyperthyroidism, with, goiter (diffuse)

Flap, liver K71.3

Flashbacks (residual to hallucinogen use) F16.283

Flat
- chamber (eye) — *see* Disorder, globe, hypotony, flat anterior chamber
- chest, congenital Q67.8
- foot (acquired) (fixed type) (painful) (postural) (*see also* Deformity, limb, flat foot)
  - congenital (rigid) (spastic (everted)) Q66.5- ☑
  - rachitic sequelae (late effect) E64.3
- organ or site, congenital NEC — *see* Anomaly, by site
- pelvis M95.5
  - with disproportion (fetopelvic) O33.0
    - causing obstructed labor O65.0
  - congenital Q74.2

Flatau-Schilder disease G37.0

Flatback syndrome M40.30
- lumbar region M40.36
- lumbosacral region M40.37
- thoracolumbar region M40.35

Flattening
- head, femur M89.8X5
- hip — *see* Coxa, plana
- lip (congenital) Q18.8
- nose (congenital) Q67.4
  - acquired M95.0

Flatulence R14.3
- psychogenic F45.8

Flatus R14.3

☑ **Additional Character Required** — Refer to the Tabular List for Character Selection   ▽ Subterms under main terms may continue to next column or page

Flatus — *continued*
  vaginalis N89.8
Flax-dresser's disease J66.1
Flea bite — *see* Injury, bite, by site, superficial, insect
Flecks, glaucomatous (subcapsular) — *see* Cataract, complicated
Fleischer (-Kayser) **ring** (cornea) H18.04- ☑
Fleshy mole O02.0
Flexibilitas cerea — *see* Catalepsy
Flexion
  amputation stump (surgical) T87.89
  cervix — *see* Malposition, uterus
  contracture, joint — *see* Contraction, joint
  deformity, joint (*see also* Deformity, limb, flexion) M21.20
    hip, congenital Q65.89
  uterus (*see also* Malposition, uterus)
    lateral — *see* Lateroversion, uterus
Flexner-Boyd dysentery A03.2
Flexner's dysentery A03.1
Flexure — *see* Flexion
Flint murmur (aortic insufficiency) I35.1
Floater, vitreous — *see* Opacity, vitreous
Floating
  cartilage (joint) (*see also* Loose, body, joint)
    knee — *see* Derangement, knee, loose body
  gallbladder, congenital Q44.1
  kidney N28.89
    congenital Q63.8
  spleen D73.89
Flooding N92.0
Floor — *see* condition
Floppy
  baby syndrome (nonspecific) P94.2
  iris syndrome (intraoperative) (IFIS) H21.81
  nonrheumatic mitral valve syndrome I34.1
Flu (*see also* Influenza)
  avian (*see also* Influenza, due to, identified novel influenza A virus) J09.X2
  bird (*see also* Influenza, due to, identified novel influenza A virus) J09.X2
  intestinal NEC A08.4
  swine (viruses that normally cause infections in pigs) (*see also* Influenza, due to, identified novel influenza A virus) J09.X2
Fluctuating blood pressure I99.8
Fluid
  abdomen R18.8
  chest J94.8
  heart — *see* Failure, heart, congestive
  joint — *see* Effusion, joint
  loss (acute) E86.9
    with
      hypernatremia E87.0
      hyponatremia E87.1
  lung — *see* Edema, lung
  overload E87.70
    specified NEC E87.79
  peritoneal cavity R18.8
  pleural cavity J94.8
  retention R60.9
Flukes NEC (*see also* Infestation, fluke)
  blood NEC — *see* Schistosomiasis
  liver B66.3
Fluor (vaginalis) N89.8
  trichomonal or due to Trichomonas (vaginalis) A59.00
Fluorosis
  dental K00.3
  skeletal M85.10
    ankle M85.17- ☑
    foot M85.17- ☑
    forearm M85.13- ☑
    hand M85.14- ☑
    lower leg M85.16- ☑
    multiple site M85.19
    neck M85.18
    rib M85.18
    shoulder M85.11- ☑
    skull M85.18
    specified site NEC M85.18
    thigh M85.15- ☑
    toe M85.17- ☑
    upper arm M85.12- ☑
    vertebra M85.18
Flush syndrome E34.0
Flushing R23.2
  menopausal N95.1

Flutter
  atrial or auricular I48.92
    atypical I48.4
    type I I48.3
    type II I48.4
    typical I48.3
  heart I49.8
    atrial or auricular I48.92
      atypical I48.4
      type I I48.3
      type II I48.4
      typical I48.3
    ventricular I49.02
  ventricular I49.02
FNHTR (febrile nonhemolytic transfusion reaction) R50.84
Fochier's abscess — *code by* site under Abscess
Focus, Assmann's — *see* Tuberculosis, pulmonary
Fogo selvagem L10.3
Foix-Alajouanine syndrome G95.19
Fold, folds (anomalous) (*see also* Anomaly, by site)
  Descemet's membrane — *see* Change, corneal membrane, Descemet's, fold
  epicanthic Q10.3
  heart Q24.8
Folie à deux F24
Follicle
  cervix (nabothian) (ruptured) N88.8
  graafian, ruptured, with hemorrhage N83.0
  nabothian N88.8
Follicular — *see* condition
Folliculitis (superficial) L73.9
  abscedens et suffodiens L66.3
  cyst N83.0
  decalvans L66.2
  deep — *see* Furuncle, by site
  gonococcal (acute) (chronic) A54.01
  keloid, keloidalis L73.0
  pustular L01.02
  ulerythematosa reticulata L66.4
Folliculome lipidique
  specified site — *see* Neoplasm, benign, by site
  unspecified site
    female D27.9
    male D29.20
Følling's disease E70.0
Follow-up — *see* Examination, follow-up
Fong's syndrome (hereditary osteo-onychodysplasia) Q78.5
Food
  allergy L27.2
  asphyxia (from aspiration or inhalation) — *see* Foreign body, by site
  choked on — *see* Foreign body, by site
  deprivation T73.0 ☑
    specified kind of food NEC E63.8
  intoxication — *see* Poisoning, food
  lack of T73.0 ☑
  poisoning — *see* Poisoning, food
  rejection NEC — *see* Disorder, eating
  strangulation or suffocation — *see* Foreign body, by site
  toxemia — *see* Poisoning, food
Foot — *see* condition
Foramen ovale (nonclosure) (patent) (persistent) Q21.1
Forbes' glycogen storage disease E74.03
Fordyce-Fox disease L75.2
Fordyce's disease (mouth) Q38.6
Forearm — *see* condition
Foreign body
  with
    laceration — *see* Laceration, by site, with foreign body
    puncture wound — *see* Puncture, by site, with foreign body
  accidentally left following a procedure T81.509 ☑
    aspiration T81.506 ☑
      resulting in
        adhesions T81.516 ☑
        obstruction T81.526 ☑
        perforation T81.536 ☑
        specified complication NEC T81.596 ☑
    cardiac catheterization T81.505 ☑
      resulting in
        acute reaction T81.60 ☑
          aseptic peritonitis T81.61 ☑
          specified NEC T81.69 ☑
        adhesions T81.515 ☑

Foreign body — *continued*
  accidentally left following a procedure — *continued*
    cardiac catheterization — *continued*
      resulting in — *continued*
        obstruction T81.525 ☑
        perforation T81.535 ☑
        specified complication NEC T81.595 ☑
      causing
        acute reaction T81.60 ☑
          aseptic peritonitis T81.61 ☑
          specified complication NEC T81.69 ☑
        adhesions T81.519 ☑
        aseptic peritonitis T81.61 ☑
        obstruction T81.529 ☑
        perforation T81.539 ☑
        specified complication NEC T81.599 ☑
    endoscopy T81.504 ☑
      resulting in
        adhesions T81.514 ☑
        obstruction T81.524 ☑
        perforation T81.534 ☑
        specified complication NEC T81.594 ☑
    immunization T81.503 ☑
      resulting in
        adhesions T81.513 ☑
        obstruction T81.523 ☑
        perforation T81.533 ☑
        specified complication NEC T81.593 ☑
    infusion T81.501 ☑
      resulting in
        adhesions T81.511 ☑
        obstruction T81.521 ☑
        perforation T81.531 ☑
        specified complication NEC T81.591 ☑
    injection T81.503 ☑
      resulting in
        adhesions T81.513 ☑
        obstruction T81.523 ☑
        perforation T81.533 ☑
        specified complication NEC T81.593 ☑
    kidney dialysis T81.502 ☑
      resulting in
        adhesions T81.512 ☑
        obstruction T81.522 ☑
        perforation T81.532 ☑
        specified complication NEC T81.592 ☑
    packing removal T81.507 ☑
      resulting in
        acute reaction T81.60 ☑
          aseptic peritonitis T81.61 ☑
          specified NEC T81.69 ☑
        adhesions T81.517 ☑
        obstruction T81.527 ☑
        perforation T81.537 ☑
        specified complication NEC T81.597 ☑
    puncture T81.506 ☑
      resulting in
        adhesions T81.516 ☑
        obstruction T81.526 ☑
        perforation T81.536 ☑
        specified complication NEC T81.596 ☑
    specified procedure NEC T81.508 ☑
      resulting in
        acute reaction T81.60 ☑
          aseptic peritonitis T81.61 ☑
          specified NEC T81.69 ☑
        adhesions T81.518 ☑
        obstruction T81.528 ☑
        perforation T81.538 ☑
        specified complication NEC T81.598 ☑
    surgical operation T81.500 ☑
      resulting in
        acute reaction T81.60 ☑
          aseptic peritonitis T81.61 ☑
          specified NEC T81.69 ☑
        adhesions T81.510 ☑
        obstruction T81.520 ☑
        perforation T81.530 ☑
        specified complication NEC T81.590 ☑
    transfusion T81.501 ☑
      resulting in
        adhesions T81.511 ☑
        obstruction T81.521 ☑
        perforation T81.531 ☑
        specified complication NEC T81.591 ☑

Foreign body — *continued*
  alimentary tract T18.9 ☑
    anus T18.5 ☑
    colon T18.4 ☑
    esophagus — *see* Foreign body, esophagus
    mouth T18.0 ☑
    multiple sites T18.8 ☑
    rectosigmoid (junction) T18.5 ☑
    rectum T18.5 ☑
    small intestine T18.3 ☑
    specified site NEC T18.8 ☑
    stomach T18.2 ☑
  anterior chamber (eye) S05.5- ☑
  auditory canal — *see* Foreign body, entering through
      orifice, ear
  bronchus T17.50⊘ ☑
    causing
      asphyxiation T17.5⊘⊘ ☑
        food (bone) (seed) T17.52⊘ ☑
        gastric contents (vomitus) T17.51⊘ ☑
        specified type NEC T17.59⊘ ☑
      injury NEC T17.5⊘8 ☑
        food (bone) (seed) T17.528 ☑
        gastric contents (vomitus) T17.518 ☑
        specified type NEC T17.598 ☑
  canthus — *see* Foreign body, conjunctival sac
  ciliary body (eye) S05.5- ☑
  conjunctival sac T15.1- ☑
  cornea T15.0- ☑
  entering through orifice
    accessory sinus T17.0 ☑
    alimentary canal T18.9 ☑
      multiple parts T18.8 ☑
      specified part NEC T18.8 ☑
    alveolar process T18.0 ☑
    antrum (Highmore's) T17.0 ☑
    anus T18.5 ☑
    appendix T18.4 ☑
    auditory canal — *see* Foreign body, entering
        through orifice, ear
    auricle — *see* Foreign body, entering through ori-
        fice, ear
    bladder T19.1 ☑
    bronchioles — *see* Foreign body, respiratory tract,
        specified site NEC
    bronchus (main) — *see* Foreign body, bronchus
    buccal cavity T18.0 ☑
    canthus (inner) — *see* Foreign body, conjunctival
        sac
    cecum T18.4 ☑
    cervix (canal) (uteri) T19.3 ☑
    colon T18.4 ☑
    conjunctival sac — *see* Foreign body, conjunctival
        sac
    cornea — *see* Foreign body, cornea
    digestive organ or tract NOS T18.9 ☑
      multiple parts T18.8 ☑
      specified part NEC T18.8 ☑
    duodenum T18.3 ☑
    ear (external) T16.- ☑
    esophagus — *see* Foreign body, esophagus
    eye (external) NOS T15.9- ☑
      conjunctival sac — *see* Foreign body, conjunc-
          tival sac
      cornea — *see* Foreign body, cornea
      specified part NEC T15.8- ☑
    eyeball (*see also* Foreign body, entering through
        orifice, eye, specified part NEC)
      with penetrating wound — *see* Puncture, eye-
          ball
    eyelid (*see also* Foreign body, conjunctival sac)
        with
      laceration — *see* Laceration, eyelid, with
          foreign body
      puncture — *see* Puncture, eyelid, with for-
          eign body
      superficial injury — *see* Foreign body, super-
          ficial, eyelid
    gastrointestinal tract T18.9 ☑
      multiple parts T18.8 ☑
      specified part NEC T18.8 ☑
    genitourinary tract T19.9 ☑
      multiple parts T19.8 ☑
      specified part NEC T19.8 ☑
    globe — *see* Foreign body, entering through ori-
        fice, eyeball

Foreign body — *continued*
  entering through orifice — *continued*
    gum T18.0 ☑
    Highmore's antrum T17.0 ☑
    hypopharynx — *see* Foreign body, pharynx
    ileum T18.3 ☑
    intestine (small) T18.3 ☑
      large T18.4 ☑
    lacrimal apparatus (punctum) — *see* Foreign body,
        entering through orifice, eye, specified part
        NEC
    large intestine T18.4 ☑
    larynx — *see* Foreign body, larynx
    lung — *see* Foreign body, respiratory tract, speci-
        fied site NEC
    maxillary sinus T17.0 ☑
    mouth T18.0 ☑
    nasal sinus T17.0 ☑
    nasopharynx — *see* Foreign body, pharynx
    nose (passage) T17.1 ☑
    nostril T17.1 ☑
    oral cavity T18.0 ☑
    palate T18.0 ☑
    penis T19.4 ☑
    pharynx — *see* Foreign body, pharynx
    piriform sinus — *see* Foreign body, pharynx
    rectosigmoid (junction) T18.5 ☑
    rectum T18.5 ☑
    respiratory tract — *see* Foreign body, respiratory
        tract
    sinus (accessory) (frontal) (maxillary) (nasal)
        T17.0 ☑
    piriform — *see* Foreign body, pharynx
    small intestine T18.3 ☑
    stomach T18.2 ☑
    suffocation by — *see* Foreign body, by site
    tear ducts or glands — *see* Foreign body, entering
        through orifice, eye, specified part NEC
    throat — *see* Foreign body, pharynx
    tongue T18.0 ☑
    tonsil, tonsillar (fossa) — *see* Foreign body, pharynx
    trachea — *see* Foreign body, trachea
    ureter T19.8 ☑
    urethra T19.0 ☑
    uterus (any part) T19.3 ☑
    vagina T19.2 ☑
    vulva T19.2 ☑
  esophagus T18.10⊘ ☑
    causing
      injury NEC T18.10⊘ ☑
        food (bone) (seed) T18.12⊘ ☑
        gastric contents (vomitus) T18.11⊘ ☑
        specified type NEC T18.19⊘ ☑
      tracheal compression T18.10⊘ ☑
        food (bone) (seed) T18.12⊘ ☑
        gastric contents (vomitus) T18.11⊘ ☑
        specified type NEC T18.19⊘ ☑
  felling of, in throat R09.89
  fragment — *see* Retained, foreign body fragments
      (type of)
  genitourinary tract T19.9 ☑
    bladder T19.1 ☑
    multiple parts T19.8 ☑
    penis T19.4 ☑
    specified site NEC T19.8 ☑
    urethra T19.0 ☑
    uterus T19.3 ☑
      IUD Z97.5
    vagina T19.2 ☑
      contraceptive device Z97.5
    vulva T19.2 ☑
  granuloma (old) (soft tissue) (*see also* Granuloma,
      foreign body)
    skin L92.3
  in
    laceration — *see* Laceration, by site, with foreign
        body
    puncture wound — *see* Puncture, by site, with
        foreign body
    soft tissue (residual) M79.5
  inadvertently left in operation wound — *see* Foreign
      body, accidentally left during a procedure
  ingestion, ingested NOS T18.9 ☑
  inhalation or inspiration — *see* Foreign body, by site
  internal organ, not entering through a natural orifice
      — code as specific injury with foreign body

Foreign body — *continued*
  intraocular S05.5- ☑
    old, retained (nonmagnetic) H44.70- ☑
      anterior chamber H44.71- ☑
      ciliary body H44.72- ☑
      iris H44.72- ☑
      lens H44.73- ☑
      magnetic H44.60- ☑
        anterior chamber H44.61- ☑
        ciliary body H44.62- ☑
        iris H44.62- ☑
        lens H44.63- ☑
        posterior wall H44.64- ☑
        specified site NEC H44.69- ☑
        vitreous body H44.65- ☑
      posterior wall H44.74- ☑
      specified site NEC H44.79- ☑
      vitreous body H44.75- ☑
  iris — *see* Foreign body, intraocular
  lacrimal punctum — *see* Foreign body, entering
      through orifice, eye, specified part NEC
  larynx T17.30⊘ ☑
    causing
      asphyxiation T17.30⊘ ☑
        food (bone) (seed) T17.32⊘ ☑
        gastric contents (vomitus) T17.31⊘ ☑
        specified type NEC T17.39⊘ ☑
      injury NEC T17.30⊘ ☑
        food (bone) (seed) T17.328 ☑
        gastric contents (vomitus) T17.318 ☑
        specified type NEC T17.398 ☑
  lens — *see* Foreign body, intraocular
  ocular muscle S05.4- ☑
    old, retained — *see* Foreign body, orbit, old
  old or residual
    soft tissue (residual) M79.5
  operation wound, left accidentally — *see* Foreign
      body, accidentally left during a procedure
  orbit S05.4- ☑
    old, retained H05.5- ☑
  pharynx T17.20⊘ ☑
    causing
      asphyxiation T17.20⊘ ☑
        food (bone) (seed) T17.22⊘ ☑
        gastric contents (vomitus) T17.21⊘ ☑
        specified type NEC T17.29⊘ ☑
      injury NEC T17.20⊘ ☑
        food (bone) (seed) T17.228 ☑
        gastric contents (vomitus) T17.218 ☑
        specified type NEC T17.298 ☑
  respiratory tract T17.90⊘ ☑
    bronchioles — *see* Foreign body, respiratory tract,
        specified site NEC
    bronchus — *see* Foreign body, bronchus
    causing
      asphyxiation T17.90⊘ ☑
        food (bone) (seed) T17.92⊘ ☑
        gastric contents (vomitus) T17.91⊘ ☑
        specified type NEC T17.99⊘ ☑
      injury NEC T17.90⊘ ☑
        food (bone) (seed) T17.928 ☑
        gastric contents (vomitus) T17.918 ☑
        specified type NEC T17.998 ☑
    larynx — *see* Foreign body, larynx
    lung — *see* Foreign body, respiratory tract, speci-
        fied site NEC
    multiple parts — *see* Foreign body, respiratory
        tract, specified site NEC
    nasal sinus T17.0 ☑
    nasopharynx — *see* Foreign body, pharynx
    nose T17.1 ☑
    nostril T17.1 ☑
    pharynx — *see* Foreign body, pharynx
    specified site NEC T17.80⊘ ☑
      causing
        asphyxiation T17.80⊘ ☑
          food (bone) (seed) T17.82⊘ ☑
          gastric contents (vomitus) T17.81⊘ ☑
          specified type NEC T17.89⊘ ☑
        injury NEC T17.80⊘ ☑
          food (bone) (seed) T17.828 ☑
          gastric contents (vomitus) T17.818 ☑
          specified type NEC T17.898 ☑
    throat — *see* Foreign body, pharynx
    trachea — *see* Foreign body, trachea

☑ Additional Character Required — Refer to the Tabular List for Character Selection   ▽ Subterms under main terms may continue to next column or page

Foreign body — *continued*
retained (old) (nonmagnetic) (in)
anterior chamber (eye) — *see* Foreign body, intraocular, old, retained, anterior chamber
magnetic — *see* Foreign body, intraocular, old, retained, magnetic, anterior chamber
ciliary body — *see* Foreign body, intraocular, old, retained, ciliary body
magnetic — *see* Foreign body, intraocular, old, retained, magnetic, ciliary body
eyelid H02.819
left H02.816
lower H02.815
upper H02.814
right H02.813
lower H02.812
upper H02.811
fragments — *see* Retained, foreign body fragments (type of)
globe — *see* Foreign body, intraocular, old, retained
magnetic — *see* Foreign body, intraocular, old, retained, magnetic
intraocular — *see* Foreign body, intraocular, old, retained
magnetic — *see* Foreign body, intraocular, old, retained, magnetic
iris — *see* Foreign body, intraocular, old, retained, iris
magnetic — *see* Foreign body, intraocular, old, retained, magnetic, iris
lens — *see* Foreign body, intraocular, old, retained, lens
magnetic — *see* Foreign body, intraocular, old, retained, magnetic, lens
muscle — *see* Foreign body, retained, soft tissue
orbit — *see* Foreign body, orbit, old
posterior wall of globe — *see* Foreign body, intraocular, old, retained, posterior wall
magnetic — *see* Foreign body, intraocular, old, retained, magnetic, posterior wall
retrobulbar — *see* Foreign body, orbit, old, retrobulbar
soft tissue M79.5
vitreous — *see* Foreign body, intraocular, old, retained, vitreous body
magnetic — *see* Foreign body, intraocular, old, retained, magnetic, vitreous body
retina S05.5- ☑
superficial, without open wound
abdomen, abdominal (wall) S30.851 ☑
alveolar process S00.552 ☑
ankle S90.55- ☑
antecubital space — *see* Foreign body, superficial, forearm
anus S30.857 ☑
arm (upper) S40.85- ☑
auditory canal — *see* Foreign body, superficial, ear
auricle — *see* Foreign body, superficial, ear
axilla — *see* Foreign body, superficial, arm
back, lower S30.850 ☑
breast S20.15- ☑
brow S00.85 ☑
buttock S30.850 ☑
calf — *see* Foreign body, superficial, leg
canthus — *see* Foreign body, superficial, eyelid
cheek S00.85 ☑
internal S00.552 ☑
chest wall — *see* Foreign body, superficial, thorax
chin S00.85 ☑
clitoris S30.854 ☑
costal region — *see* Foreign body, superficial, thorax
digit(s)
foot — *see* Foreign body, superficial, toe
hand — *see* Foreign body, superficial, finger
ear S00.45- ☑
elbow S50.35- ☑
epididymis S30.853 ☑
epigastric region S30.851 ☑
epiglottis S10.15 ☑
esophagus, cervical S10.15 ☑
eyebrow — *see* Foreign body, superficial, eyelid
eyelid S00.25- ☑
face S00.85 ☑
finger(s) S60.459 ☑
index S60.45- ☑

Foreign body — *continued*
superficial, without open wound — *continued*
finger(s) — *continued*
little S60.45- ☑
middle S60.45- ☑
ring S60.45- ☑
flank S30.851 ☑
foot (except toe(s) alone) S90.85- ☑
toe — *see* Foreign body, superficial, toe
forearm S50.85- ☑
elbow only — *see* Foreign body, superficial, elbow
forehead S00.85 ☑
genital organs, external
female S30.856 ☑
male S30.855 ☑
groin S30.851 ☑
gum S00.552 ☑
hand S60.55- ☑
head S00.95 ☑
ear — *see* Foreign body, superficial, ear
eyelid — *see* Foreign body, superficial, eyelid
lip S00.551 ☑
nose S00.35 ☑
oral cavity S00.552 ☑
scalp S00.05 ☑
specified site NEC S00.85 ☑
heel — *see* Foreign body, superficial, foot
hip S70.25- ☑
inguinal region S30.851 ☑
interscapular region S20.459 ☑
jaw S00.85 ☑
knee S80.25- ☑
labium (majus) (minus) S30.854 ☑
larynx S10.15 ☑
leg (lower) S80.85- ☑
knee — *see* Foreign body, superficial, knee
upper — *see* Foreign body, superficial, thigh
lip S00.551 ☑
lower back S30.850 ☑
lumbar region S30.850 ☑
malar region S00.85 ☑
mammary — *see* Foreign body, superficial, breast
mastoid region S00.85 ☑
mouth S00.552 ☑
nail
finger — *see* Foreign body, superficial, finger
toe — *see* Foreign body, superficial, toe
nape S10.85 ☑
nasal S00.35 ☑
neck S10.95 ☑
specified site NEC S10.85 ☑
throat S10.15 ☑
nose S00.35 ☑
occipital region S00.05 ☑
oral cavity S00.552 ☑
orbital region — *see* Foreign body, superficial, eyelid
palate S00.552 ☑
palm — *see* Foreign body, superficial, hand
parietal region S00.05 ☑
pelvis S30.850 ☑
penis S30.852 ☑
perineum
female S30.854 ☑
male S30.850 ☑
periocular area — *see* Foreign body, superficial, eyelid
phalanges
finger — *see* Foreign body, superficial, finger
toe — *see* Foreign body, superficial, toe
pharynx S10.15 ☑
pinna — *see* Foreign body, superficial, ear
popliteal space — *see* Foreign body, superficial, knee
prepuce S30.852 ☑
pubic region S30.850 ☑
pudendum
female S30.856 ☑
male S30.855 ☑
sacral region S30.850 ☑
scalp S00.05 ☑
scapular region — *see* Foreign body, superficial, shoulder
scrotum S30.853 ☑
shin — *see* Foreign body, superficial, leg

Foreign body — *continued*
superficial, without open wound — *continued*
shoulder S40.25- ☑
sternal region S20.359 ☑
submaxillary region S00.85 ☑
submental region S00.85 ☑
subungual
finger(s) — *see* Foreign body, superficial, finger
toe(s) — *see* Foreign body, superficial, toe
supraclavicular fossa S10.85 ☑
supraorbital S00.85 ☑
temple S00.85 ☑
temporal region S00.85 ☑
testis S30.853 ☑
thigh S70.35- ☑
thorax, thoracic (wall) S20.95 ☑
back S20.45- ☑
front S20.35- ☑
throat S10.15 ☑
thumb S60.35- ☑
toe(s) (lesser) S90.456 ☑
great S90.45- ☑
tongue S00.552 ☑
trachea S10.15 ☑
tunica vaginalis S30.853 ☑
tympanum, tympanic membrane — *see* Foreign body, superficial, ear
uvula S00.552 ☑
vagina S30.854 ☑
vocal cords S10.15 ☑
vulva S30.854 ☑
wrist S60.85- ☑
swallowed T18.9 ☑
trachea T17.408 ☑
causing
asphyxiation T17.400 ☑
food (bone) (seed) T17.420 ☑
gastric contents (vomitus) T17.410 ☑
specified type NEC T17.490 ☑
injury NEC T17.408 ☑
food (bone) (seed) T17.428 ☑
gastric contents (vomitus) T17.418 ☑
specified type NEC T17.498 ☑
type of fragment — *see* Retained, foreign body fragments (type of)
vitreous (humor) S05.5- ☑
Forestier's disease (rhizomelic pseudopolyarthritis) M35.3
meaning ankylosing hyperostosis — *see* Hyperostosis, ankylosing
Formation
hyalin in cornea — *see* Degeneration, cornea
sequestrum in bone (due to infection) — *see* Osteomyelitis, chronic
valve
colon, congenital Q43.8
ureter (congenital) Q62.39
Formication R20.2
Fort Bragg fever A27.89
Fossa (*see also* condition)
pyriform — *see* condition
Foster-Kennedy syndrome H47.14- ☑
Fothergill's
disease (trigeminal neuralgia) (*see also* Neuralgia, trigeminal)
scarlatina anginosa A38.9
Foul breath R19.6
Foundling Z76.1
Fournier disease or gangrene N49.3
female N76.89
Fourth
cranial nerve — *see* condition
molar K00.1
Foville's (peduncular) **disease or syndrome** G46.3
Fox (-Fordyce) disease (apocrine miliaria) L75.2
Fracture, burst — *see* Fracture, traumatic, by site
Fracture, chronic — *see* Fracture, pathological
Fracture, insufficiency — *see* Fracture, pathologic, by site
Fracture, pathological (pathologic) (*see also* Fracture, traumatic) M84.40
ankle M84.47- ☑
carpus M84.44- ☑
clavicle M84.41- ☑
dental implant M27.63

Fracture, pathological — *continued*
dental restorative material K08.539
  with loss of material K08.531
  without loss of material K08.530
due to
  neoplastic disease NEC (*see also* Neoplasm)
    M84.50 ☑
    ankle M84.57- ☑
    carpus M84.54- ☑
    clavicle M84.51- ☑
    femur M84.55- ☑
    fibula M84.56- ☑
    finger M84.54- ☑
    hip M84.559 ☑
    humerus M84.52- ☑
    ilium M84.550 ☑
    ischium M84.550 ☑
    metacarpus M84.54- ☑
    metatarsus M84.57- ☑
    neck M84.58 ☑
    pelvis M84.550 ☑
    radius M84.53- ☑
    rib M84.58 ☑
    scapula M84.51- ☑
    skull M84.58 ☑
    specified site NEC M84.58 ☑
    tarsus M84.57- ☑
    tibia M84.56- ☑
    toe M84.57- ☑
    ulna M84.53- ☑
    vertebra M84.58 ☑
  osteoporosis M80.80 ☑
    disuse — *see* Osteoporosis, specified type NEC, with pathological fracture
    drug-induced — *see* Osteoporosis, drug induced, with pathological fracture
    idiopathic — *see* Osteoporosis, specified type NEC, with pathological fracture
    postmenopausal — *see* Osteoporosis, postmenopausal, with pathological fracture
    postoophorectomy — *see* Osteoporosis, postoophorectomy, with pathological fracture
    postsurgical malabsorption — *see* Osteoporosis, specified type NEC, with pathological fracture
    specified cause NEC — *see* Osteoporosis, specified type NEC, with pathological fracture
  specified disease NEC M84.60 ☑
    ankle M84.67- ☑
    carpus M84.64- ☑
    clavicle M84.61- ☑
    femur M84.65- ☑
    fibula M84.66- ☑
    finger M84.64- ☑
    hip M84.65- ☑
    humerus M84.62- ☑
    ilium M84.650 ☑
    ischium M84.650 ☑
    metacarpus M84.64- ☑
    metatarsus M84.67- ☑
    neck M84.68 ☑
    radius M84.63- ☑
    rib M84.68 ☑
    scapula M84.61- ☑
    skull M84.68 ☑
    tarsus M84.67- ☑
    tibia M84.66- ☑
    toe M84.67- ☑
    ulna M84.63- ☑
    vertebra M84.68 ☑
femur M84.45- ☑
fibula M84.46- ☑
finger M84.44- ☑
hip M84.459 ☑
humerus M84.42- ☑
ilium M84.454 ☑
ischium M84.454 ☑
joint prosthesis — *see* Complications, joint prosthesis, mechanical, breakdown, by site
  periprosthetic — *see* Complications, joint prosthesis, mechanical, periprosthesis, fracture, by site
metacarpus M84.44- ☑
metatarsus M84.47- ☑
neck M84.48 ☑

Fracture, pathological — *continued*
pelvis M84.454 ☑
radius M84.43- ☑
restorative material (dental) K08.539
  with loss of material K08.531
  without loss of material K08.530
rib M84.48 ☑
scapula M84.41- ☑
skull M84.48 ☑
tarsus M84.47- ☑
tibia M84.46- ☑
toe M84.47- ☑
ulna M84.43- ☑
vertebra M84.48 ☑
Fracture, traumatic (abduction) (adduction) (separation)
  (*see also* Fracture, pathological) T14.8
acetabulum S32.40- ☑
  column
    anterior (displaced) (iliopubic) S32.43- ☑
      nondisplaced S32.436 ☑
    posterior (displaced) (ilioischial) S32.443 ☑
      nondisplaced S32.44- ☑
  dome (displaced) S32.48- ☑
    nondisplaced S32.48 ☑
  specified NEC S32.49- ☑
  transverse (displaced) S32.45- ☑
    with associated posterior wall fracture (displaced) S32.46- ☑
      nondisplaced S32.46- ☑
    nondisplaced S32.45- ☑
  wall
    anterior (displaced) S32.41- ☑
      nondisplaced S32.41- ☑
    medial (displaced) S32.47- ☑
      nondisplaced S32.47- ☑
    posterior (displaced) S32.42- ☑
      with associated transverse fracture (displaced) S32.46- ☑
        nondisplaced S32.46- ☑
      nondisplaced S32.42- ☑
acromion — *see* Fracture, scapula, acromial process
ankle S82.899 ☑
  bimalleolar (displaced) S82.84- ☑
    nondisplaced S82.84- ☑
  lateral malleolus only (displaced) S82.6- ☑
    nondisplaced S82.6- ☑
  medial malleolus (displaced) S82.5- ☑
    associated with Maisonneuve's fracture — *see* Fracture, Maisonneuve's
    nondisplaced S82.5- ☑
  talus — *see* Fracture, tarsal, talus
  trimalleolar (displaced) S82.85- ☑
    nondisplaced S82.85- ☑
arm (upper) (*see also* Fracture, humerus, shaft)
  humerus — *see* Fracture, humerus
  radius — *see* Fracture, radius
  ulna — *see* Fracture, ulna
astragalus — *see* Fracture, tarsal, talus
atlas — *see* Fracture, neck, cervical vertebra, first
axis — *see* Fracture, neck, cervical vertebra, second
back — *see* Fracture, vertebra
Barton's — *see* Barton's fracture
base of skull — *see* Fracture, skull, base
basicervical (basal) (femoral) S72.0 ☑
Bennett's — *see* Bennett's fracture
bimalleolar — *see* Fracture, ankle, bimalleolar
blow-out S02.3 ☑
bone NEC T14.8
  birth injury P13.9
  following insertion of orthopedic implant, joint prosthesis or bone plate — *see* Fracture, following insertion of orthopedic implant, joint prosthesis or bone plate
  in (due to) neoplastic disease NEC — *see* Fracture, pathological, due to, neoplastic disease
  pathological (cause unknown) — *see* Fracture, pathological
breast bone — *see* Fracture, sternum
bucket handle (semilunar cartilage) — *see* Tear, meniscus
burst — *see* Fracture, traumatic, by site
calcaneus — *see* Fracture, tarsal, calcaneus
carpal bone(s) S62.10- ☑
  capitate (displaced) S62.13- ☑
    nondisplaced S62.13- ☑
  cuneiform — *see* Fracture, carpal bone, triquetrum

Fracture, traumatic — *continued*
carpal bone(s) — *continued*
  hamate (body) (displaced) S62.143 ☑
    hook process (displaced) S62.15- ☑
      nondisplaced S62.15- ☑
    nondisplaced S62.14- ☑
  larger multangular — *see* Fracture, carpal bones, trapezium
  lunate (displaced) S62.12- ☑
    nondisplaced S62.12- ☑
  navicular S62.00- ☑
    distal pole (displaced) S62.01- ☑
      nondisplaced S62.01- ☑
    middle third (displaced) S62.02- ☑
      nondisplaced S62.02- ☑
    proximal third (displaced) S62.03- ☑
      nondisplaced S62.03- ☑
    volar tuberosity — *see* Fracture, carpal bones, navicular, distal pole
  os magnum — *see* Fracture, carpal bones, capitate
  pisiform (displaced) S62.16- ☑
    nondisplaced S62.16- ☑
  semilunar — *see* Fracture, carpal bones, lunate
  smaller multangular — *see* Fracture, carpal bones, trapezoid
  trapezium (displaced) S62.17- ☑
    nondisplaced S62.17- ☑
  trapezoid (displaced) S62.18- ☑
    nondisplaced S62.18- ☑
  triquetrum (displaced) S62.11- ☑
    nondisplaced S62.11- ☑
  unciform — *see* Fracture, carpal bones, hamate
cervical — *see* Fracture, vertebra, cervical
clavicle S42.00- ☑
  acromial end (displaced) S42.03- ☑
    nondisplaced S42.03- ☑
  birth injury P13.4
  lateral end — *see* Fracture, clavicle, acromial end
  shaft (displaced) S42.02- ☑
    nondisplaced S42.02- ☑
  sternal end (anterior) (displaced) S42.01- ☑
    nondisplaced S42.01- ☑
    posterior S42.01- ☑
coccyx S32.2 ☑
collapsed — *see* Collapse, vertebra
collar bone — *see* Fracture, clavicle
Colles' — *see* Colles' fracture
compression, not due to trauma — *see* Collapse, vertebra
coronoid process — *see* Fracture, ulna, upper end, coronoid process
corpus cavernosum penis S39.840 ☑
costochondral cartilage S23.41 ☑
costochondral, costosternal junction — *see* Fracture, rib
cranium — *see* Fracture, skull
cricoid cartilage S12.8 ☑
cuboid (ankle) — *see* Fracture, tarsal, cuboid
cuneiform
  foot — *see* Fracture, tarsal, cuneiform
  wrist — *see* Fracture, carpal, triquetrum
delayed union — *see* Delay, union, fracture
dental restorative material K08.539
  with loss of material K08.531
  without loss of material K08.530
due to
  birth injury — *see* Birth, injury, fracture
  osteoporosis — *see* Osteoporosis, with fracture
Dupuytren's — *see* Fracture, ankle, lateral malleolus
elbow S42.40- ☑
ethmoid (bone) (sinus) — *see* Fracture, skull, base
face bone S02.92 ☑
fatigue (*see also* Fracture, stress)
  vertebra M48.40 ☑
    cervical region M48.42 ☑
    cervicothoracic region M48.43 ☑
    lumbar region M48.46 ☑
    lumbosacral region M48.47 ☑
    occipito-atlanto-axial region M48.41 ☑
    sacrococcygeal region M48.48 ☑
    thoracic region M48.44 ☑
    thoracolumbar region M48.45 ☑
femur, femoral S72.9- ☑
  basicervical (basal) S72.0 ☑
  birth injury P13.2
  capital epiphyseal S79.01- ☑

Fracture, traumatic — *continued*
femur, femoral — *continued*
   condyles, epicondyles — *see* Fracture, femur, lower end
   distal end — *see* Fracture, femur, lower end
   epiphysis
     head — *see* Fracture, femur, upper end, epiphysis
     lower — *see* Fracture, femur, lower end, epiphysis
     upper — *see* Fracture, femur, upper end, epiphysis
   following insertion of implant, prosthesis or plate M96.66- ☑
   head — *see* Fracture, femur, upper end, head
   intertrochanteric — *see* Fracture, femur, trochanteric
   intratrochanteric — *see* Fracture, femur, trochanteric
   lower end S72.40- ☑
     condyle (displaced) S72.41- ☑
       lateral (displaced) S72.42- ☑
         nondisplaced S72.42- ☑
       medial (displaced) S72.43- ☑
         nondisplaced S72.43- ☑
       nondisplaced S72.41- ☑
     epiphysis (displaced) S72.44- ☑
       nondisplaced S72.44- ☑
     physeal S79.10- ☑
       Salter-Harris
         Type I S79.11- ☑
         Type II S79.12- ☑
         Type III S79.13- ☑
         Type IV S79.14- ☑
       specified NEC S79.19- ☑
     specified NEC S72.49- ☑
     supracondylar (displaced) S72.45- ☑
       with intracondylar extension (displaced) S72.46- ☑
         nondisplaced S72.46- ☑
       nondisplaced S72.45- ☑
     torus S72.47- ☑
   neck — *see* Fracture, femur, upper end, neck
   petrochanteric — *see* Fracture, femur, trochanteric
   shaft (lower third) (middle third) (upper third) S72.30- ☑
     comminuted (displaced) S72.35- ☑
       nondisplaced S72.35- ☑
     oblique (displaced) S72.33- ☑
       nondisplaced S72.33- ☑
     segmental (displaced) S72.36- ☑
       nondisplaced S72.36- ☑
     specified NEC S72.39- ☑
     spiral (displaced) S72.34- ☑
       nondisplaced S72.34- ☑
     transverse (displaced) S72.32- ☑
       nondisplaced S72.32- ☑
   specified site NEC — *see* subcategory S72.8 ☑
   subcapital (displaced) S72.01- ☑
   subtrochanteric (region) (section) (displaced) S72.2- ☑
     nondisplaced S72.2- ☑
   transcervical — *see* Fracture, femur, upper end, neck
   transtrochanteric — *see* Fracture, femur, trochanteric
   trochanteric S72.10- ☑
     apophyseal (displaced) S72.13- ☑
       nondisplaced S72.13- ☑
     greater trochanter (displaced) S72.11- ☑
       nondisplaced S72.11- ☑
     intertrochanteric (displaced) S72.14- ☑
       nondisplaced S72.14- ☑
     lesser trochanter (displaced) S72.12- ☑
       nondisplaced S72.12- ☑
   upper end S72.00- ☑
     apophyseal (displaced) S72.13- ☑
       nondisplaced S72.13- ☑
     cervicotrochanteric — *see* Fracture, femur, upper, neck, base
     epiphysis (displaced) S72.02- ☑
       nondisplaced S72.02- ☑
     head S72.05- ☑
       articular (displaced) S72.06- ☑
         nondisplaced S72.06- ☑

Fracture, traumatic — *continued*
femur, femoral — *continued*
   upper end — *continued*
     head — *continued*
       specified NEC S72.09- ☑
     intertrochanteric (displaced) S72.14- ☑
       nondisplaced S72.14- ☑
     intracapsular S72.01- ☑
     midcervical (displaced) S72.03- ☑
       nondisplaced S72.03- ☑
     neck S72.00- ☑
       base (displaced) S72.04- ☑
         nondisplaced S72.04- ☑
       specified NEC S72.09- ☑
     pertrochanteric — *see* Fracture, femur, upper end, trochanteric
     physeal S79.00- ☑
       Salter-Harris type I S79.01- ☑
       specified NEC S79.09- ☑
     subcapital (displaced) S72.01- ☑
     subtrochanteric (displaced) S72.2- ☑
       nondisplaced S72.2- ☑
     transcervical — *see* Fracture, femur, upper end, midcervical
     trochanteric S72.10- ☑
       greater (displaced) S72.11- ☑
         nondisplaced S72.11- ☑
       lesser (displaced) S72.12- ☑
         nondisplaced S72.12- ☑
fibula (shaft) (styloid) S82.40- ☑
   comminuted (displaced) S82.45- ☑
     nondisplaced S82.45- ☑
   following insertion of implant, prosthesis or plate M96.67- ☑
   involving ankle or malleolus — *see* Fracture, fibula, lateral malleolus
   lateral malleolus (displaced) S82.6- ☑
     nondisplaced S82.6- ☑
   lower end
     physeal S89.30- ☑
       Salter-Harris
         Type I S89.31- ☑
         Type II S89.32- ☑
       specified NEC S89.39- ☑
     specified NEC S82.83- ☑
     torus S82.82- ☑
   oblique (displaced) S82.43- ☑
     nondisplaced S82.43- ☑
   segmental (displaced) S82.46- ☑
     nondisplaced S82.46- ☑
   specified NEC S82.49- ☑
   spiral (displaced) S82.44- ☑
     nondisplaced S82.44- ☑
   transverse (displaced) S82.42- ☑
     nondisplaced S82.42- ☑
   upper end
     physeal S89.20- ☑
       Salter-Harris
         Type I S89.21- ☑
         Type II S89.22- ☑
       specified NEC S89.29- ☑
     specified NEC S82.83- ☑
     torus S82.81- ☑
finger (except thumb) S62.60- ☑
   distal phalanx (displaced) S62.63- ☑
     nondisplaced S62.66- ☑
   index S62.60- ☑
     distal phalanx (displaced) S62.63- ☑
       nondisplaced S62.66- ☑
     medial phalanx (displaced) S62.62- ☑
       nondisplaced S62.65- ☑
     proximal phalanx (displaced) S62.61- ☑
       nondisplaced S62.64- ☑
   little S62.60- ☑
     distal phalanx (displaced) S62.63- ☑
       nondisplaced S62.66- ☑
     medial phalanx (displaced) S62.62- ☑
       nondisplaced S62.65- ☑
     proximal phalanx (displaced) S62.61- ☑
       nondisplaced S62.64- ☑
     medial phalanx (displaced) S62.62- ☑
       nondisplaced S62.65- ☑
   middle S62.60- ☑
     distal phalanx (displaced) S62.63- ☑
       nondisplaced S62.66- ☑

Fracture, traumatic — *continued*
finger — *continued*
   middle — *continued*
     medial phalanx (displaced) S62.62- ☑
       nondisplaced S62.65- ☑
     proximal phalanx (displaced) S62.61- ☑
       nondisplaced S62.64- ☑
   proximal phalanx (displaced) S62.61- ☑
     nondisplaced S62.64- ☑
   ring S62.60- ☑
     distal phalanx (displaced) S62.63- ☑
       nondisplaced S62.66- ☑
     medial phalanx (displaced) S62.62- ☑
       nondisplaced S62.65- ☑
     proximal phalanx (displaced) S62.61- ☑
       nondisplaced S62.64- ☑
   thumb — *see* Fracture, thumb
following insertion (intraoperative) (postoperative) of orthopedic implant, joint prosthesis or bone plate M96.69
   femur M96.66- ☑
   fibula M96.67- ☑
   humerus M96.62- ☑
   pelvis M96.65
   radius M96.63- ☑
   specified bone NEC M96.69
   tibia M96.67- ☑
   ulna M96.63- ☑
foot S92.90- ☑
   astragalus — *see* Fracture, tarsal, talus
   calcaneus — *see* Fracture, tarsal, calcaneus
   cuboid — *see* Fracture, tarsal, cuboid
   cuneiform — *see* Fracture, tarsal, cuneiform
   metatarsal — *see* Fracture, metatarsal
   navicular — *see* Fracture, tarsal, navicular
   talus — *see* Fracture, tarsal, talus
   tarsal — *see* Fracture, tarsal
   toe — *see* Fracture, toe
forearm S52.9- ☑
   radius — *see* Fracture, radius
   ulna — *see* Fracture, ulna
fossa (anterior) (middle) (posterior) S02.19 ☑
frontal (bone) (skull) S02.0 ☑
   sinus S02.19 ☑
glenoid (cavity) (scapula) — *see* Fracture, scapula, glenoid cavity
greenstick — *see* Fracture, by site
hallux — *see* Fracture, toe, great
hand S62.9- ☑
   carpal — *see* Fracture, carpal bone
   finger (except thumb) — *see* Fracture, finger
   metacarpal — *see* Fracture, metacarpal
   navicular (scaphoid) (hand) — *see* Fracture, carpal bone, navicular
   thumb — *see* Fracture, thumb
healed or old
   with complications — *code by* Nature of the complication
heel bone — *see* Fracture, tarsal, calcaneus
Hill-Sachs S42.29- ☑
hip — *see* Fracture, femur, neck
humerus S42.30- ☑
   anatomical neck — *see* Fracture, humerus, upper end
   articular process — *see* Fracture, humerus, lower end
   capitellum — *see* Fracture, humerus, lower end, condyle, lateral
   distal end — *see* Fracture, humerus, lower end
   epiphysis
     lower — *see* Fracture, humerus, lower end, physeal
     upper — *see* Fracture, humerus, upper end, physeal
   external condyle — *see* Fracture, humerus, lower end, condyle, lateral
   following insertion of implant, prosthesis or plate M96.62- ☑
   great tuberosity — *see* Fracture, humerus, upper end, greater tuberosity
   intercondylar — *see* Fracture, humerus, lower end
   internal epicondyle — *see* Fracture, humerus, lower end, epicondyle, medial
   lesser tuberosity — *see* Fracture, humerus, upper end, lesser tuberosity

Fracture, traumatic — *continued*
  humerus — *continued*
    lower end S42.40- ☑
      condyle
        lateral (displaced) S42.45- ☑
          nondisplaced S42.45- ☑
        medial (displaced) S42.46- ☑
          nondisplaced S42.46- ☑
      epicondyle
        lateral (displaced) S42.43- ☑
          nondisplaced S42.43- ☑
        medial (displaced) S42.44- ☑
          incarcerated S42.44- ☑
          nondisplaced S42.44- ☑
      physeal S49.10- ☑
        Salter-Harris
          Type I S49.11- ☑
          Type II S49.12- ☑
          Type III S49.13- ☑
          Type IV S49.14- ☑
        specified NEC S49.19- ☑
      specified NEC (displaced) S42.49- ☑
        nondisplaced S42.49- ☑
      supracondylar (simple) (displaced) S42.41- ☑
        comminuted (displaced) S42.42- ☑
          nondisplaced S42.42- ☑
        nondisplaced S42.41- ☑
      torus S42.48- ☑
      transcondylar (displaced) S42.47- ☑
        nondisplaced S42.47- ☑
    proximal end — *see* Fracture, humerus, upper end
    shaft S42.30- ☑
      comminuted (displaced) S42.35- ☑
        nondisplaced S42.35- ☑
      greenstick S42.31- ☑
      oblique (displaced) S42.33- ☑
        nondisplaced S42.33- ☑
      segmental (displaced) S42.36- ☑
        nondisplaced S42.36- ☑
      specified NEC S42.39- ☑
      spiral (displaced) S42.34- ☑
        nondisplaced S42.34- ☑
      transverse (displaced) S42.32- ☑
        nondisplaced S42.32- ☑
    supracondylar — *see* Fracture, humerus, lower end
    surgical neck — *see* Fracture, humerus, upper end, surgical neck
    trochlea — *see* Fracture, humerus, lower end, condyle, medial
    tuberosity — *see* Fracture, humerus, upper end
    upper end S42.20- ☑
      anatomical neck — *see* Fracture, humerus, upper end, specified NEC
      articular head — *see* Fracture, humerus, upper end, specified NEC
      epiphysis — *see* Fracture, humerus, upper end, physeal
      greater tuberosity (displaced) S42.25- ☑
        nondisplaced S42.25- ☑
      lesser tuberosity (displaced) S42.26- ☑
        nondisplaced S42.26- ☑
      physeal S49.00- ☑
        Salter-Harris
          Type I S49.01- ☑
          Type II S49.02- ☑
          Type III S49.03- ☑
          Type IV S49.04- ☑
        specified NEC S49.09- ☑
      specified NEC (displaced) S42.29- ☑
        nondisplaced S42.29- ☑
      surgical neck (displaced) S42.21- ☑
        four-part S42.24- ☑
        nondisplaced S42.21- ☑
        three-part S42.23- ☑
        two-part (displaced) S42.22- ☑
          nondisplaced S42.22- ☑
      torus S42.27- ☑
      transepiphyseal — *see* Fracture, humerus, upper end, physeal
  hyoid bone S12.8 ☑
  ilium S32.30- ☑
    with disruption of pelvic ring — *see* Disruption, pelvic ring
    avulsion (displaced) S32.31- ☑
      nondisplaced S32.31- ☑
    specified NEC S32.39- ☑

Fracture, traumatic — *continued*
  impaction, impacted — *code as* Fracture, by site
  innominate bone — *see* Fracture, ilium
  instep — *see* Fracture, foot
  ischium S32.60- ☑
    with disruption of pelvic ring — *see* Disruption, pelvic ring
    avulsion (displaced) S32.61- ☑
      nondisplaced S32.61- ☑
    specified NEC S32.69- ☑
  jaw (bone) (lower) — *see* Fracture, mandible
    upper — *see* Fracture, maxilla
  joint prosthesis — *see* Complications, joint prosthesis, mechanical, breakdown, by site
    periprosthetic — *see* Complications, joint prosthesis, mechanical, periprosthesis, fracture, by site
  knee cap — *see* Fracture, patella
  larynx S12.8 ☑
  late effects — *see* Sequelae, fracture
  leg (lower) S82.9- ☑
    ankle — *see* Fracture, ankle
    femur — *see* Fracture, femur
    fibula — *see* Fracture, fibula
    malleolus — *see* Fracture, ankle
    patella — *see* Fracture, patella
    specified site NEC S82.89- ☑
    tibia — *see* Fracture, tibia
  lumbar spine — *see* Fracture, vertebra, lumbar
  lumbosacral spine S32.9 ☑
  Maisonneuve's (displaced) S82.86- ☑
    nondisplaced S82.86- ☑
  malar bone (*see also* Fracture, maxilla) S02.400 ☑
  malleolus — *see* Fracture, ankle
  malunion — *see* Fracture, by site
  mandible (lower jaw (bone)) S02.609 ☑
    alveolus S02.67 ☑
    angle (of jaw) S02.65 ☑
    body, unspecified S02.600 ☑
    condylar process S02.61 ☑
    coronoid process S02.63 ☑
    ramus, unspecified S02.64 ☑
    specified site NEC S02.69 ☑
    subcondylar process S02.62 ☑
    symphysis S02.66 ☑
  manubrium (sterni) S22.21 ☑
    dissociation from sternum S22.23 ☑
  march — *see* Fracture, traumatic, stress, by site
  maxilla, maxillary (bone) (sinus) (superior) (upper jaw) S02.401 ☑
    alveolus S02.42 ☑
    inferior — *see* Fracture, mandible
    LeFort I S02.411 ☑
    LeFort II S02.412 ☑
    LeFort III S02.413 ☑
  metacarpal S62.309 ☑
    base (displaced) S62.319 ☑
      nondisplaced S62.349 ☑
    fifth S62.30- ☑
      base (displaced) S62.31- ☑
        nondisplaced S62.34- ☑
      neck (displaced) S62.33- ☑
        nondisplaced S62.36- ☑
      shaft (displaced) S62.32- ☑
        nondisplaced S62.35- ☑
      specified NEC S62.398 ☑
    first S62.20- ☑
      base NEC (displaced) S62.23- ☑
        nondisplaced S62.23- ☑
      Bennett's — *see* Bennett's fracture
      neck (displaced) S62.25- ☑
        nondisplaced S62.25- ☑
      shaft (displaced) S62.24- ☑
        nondisplaced S62.24- ☑
      specified NEC S62.29- ☑
    fourth S62.30- ☑
      base (displaced) S62.31- ☑
        nondisplaced S62.34- ☑
      neck (displaced) S62.33- ☑
        nondisplaced S62.36- ☑
      shaft (displaced) S62.32- ☑
        nondisplaced S62.35- ☑
      specified NEC S62.39- ☑
    neck (displaced) S62.33- ☑
      nondisplaced S62.36- ☑
    Rolando's — *see* Rolando's fracture

Fracture, traumatic — *continued*
  metacarpal — *continued*
    second S62.30- ☑
      base (displaced) S62.31- ☑
        nondisplaced S62.34- ☑
      neck (displaced) S62.33- ☑
        nondisplaced S62.36- ☑
      shaft (displaced) S62.32- ☑
        nondisplaced S62.35- ☑
      specified NEC S62.39- ☑
    shaft (displaced) S62.32- ☑
      nondisplaced S62.35- ☑
    specified NEC S62.399 ☑
    third S62.30- ☑
      base (displaced) S62.31- ☑
        nondisplaced S62.34- ☑
      neck (displaced) S62.33- ☑
        nondisplaced S62.36- ☑
      shaft (displaced) S62.32- ☑
        nondisplaced S62.35- ☑
      specified NEC S62.39- ☑
  metastatic — *see* Fracture, pathological, due to, neoplastic disease (*see also* Neoplasm)
  metatarsal bone S92.30- ☑
    fifth (displaced) S92.35- ☑
      nondisplaced S92.35- ☑
    first (displaced) S92.31- ☑
      nondisplaced S92.31- ☑
    fourth (displaced) S92.34- ☑
      nondisplaced S92.34- ☑
    second (displaced) S92.32- ☑
      nondisplaced S92.32- ☑
    third (displaced) S92.33- ☑
      nondisplaced S92.33- ☑
  Monteggia's — *see* Monteggia's fracture
  multiple
    hand (and wrist) NEC — *see* Fracture, by site
    ribs — *see* Fracture, rib, multiple
  nasal (bone(s)) S02.2 ☑
  navicular (scaphoid) (foot) (*see also* Fracture, tarsal, navicular)
    hand — *see* Fracture, carpal, navicular
  neck S12.9 ☑
    cervical vertebra S12.9 ☑
      fifth (displaced) S12.400 ☑
        nondisplaced S12.401 ☑
        specified type NEC (displaced) S12.490 ☑
          nondisplaced S12.491 ☑
      first (displaced) S12.000 ☑
        burst (stable) S12.01 ☑
          unstable S12.02 ☑
        lateral mass (displaced) S12.040 ☑
          nondisplaced S12.041 ☑
        nondisplaced S12.001 ☑
        posterior arch (displaced) S12.030 ☑
          nondisplaced S12.031 ☑
        specified type NEC (displaced) S12.090 ☑
          nondisplaced S12.091 ☑
      fourth (displaced) S12.300 ☑
        nondisplaced S12.301 ☑
        specified type NEC (displaced) S12.390 ☑
          nondisplaced S12.391 ☑
      second (displaced) S12.100 ☑
        dens (anterior) (displaced) (type II) S12.110 ☑
          nondisplaced S12.112 ☑
          posterior S12.111 ☑
        specified type NEC (displaced) S12.120 ☑
          nondisplaced S12.121 ☑
        nondisplaced S12.101 ☑
        specified type NEC (displaced) S12.190 ☑
          nondisplaced S12.191 ☑
      seventh (displaced) S12.600 ☑
        nondisplaced S12.601 ☑
        specified type NEC (displaced) S12.690 ☑
          displaced S12.691 ☑
      sixth (displaced) S12.500 ☑
        nondisplaced S12.501 ☑
        specified type NEC (displaced) S12.590 ☑
          displaced S12.591 ☑
      third (displaced) S12.200 ☑
        nondisplaced S12.201 ☑
        specified type NEC (displaced) S12.290 ☑
          displaced S12.291 ☑

☑ Additional Character Required — Refer to the Tabular List for Character Selection   ▽ Subterms under main terms may continue to next column or page

Fracture, traumatic — *continued*
  neck — *continued*
    hyoid bone S12.8 ☑
    larynx S12.8 ☑
    specified site NEC S12.8 ☑
    thyroid cartilage S12.8 ☑
    trachea S12.8 ☑
  neoplastic NEC — *see* Fracture, pathological, due to, neoplastic disease
  neural arch — *see* Fracture, vertebra
  newborn — *see* Birth, injury, fracture
  nontraumatic — *see* Fracture, pathological
  nonunion — *see* Nonunion, fracture
  nose, nasal (bone) (septum) S02.2 ☑
  occiput — *see* Fracture, skull, base, occiput
  odontoid process — *see* Fracture, neck, cervical vertebra, second
  olecranon (process) (ulna) — *see* Fracture, ulna, upper end, olecranon process
  orbit, orbital (bone) (region) S02.8 ☑
    floor (blow-out) S02.3 ☑
    roof S02.19 ☑
  os
    calcis — *see* Fracture, tarsal, calcaneus
    magnum — *see* Fracture, carpal, capitate
    pubis — *see* Fracture, pubis
  palate S02.8 ☑
  parietal bone (skull) S02.0 ☑
  patella S82.00- ☑
    comminuted (displaced) S82.04- ☑
      nondisplaced S82.04- ☑
    longitudinal (displaced) S82.02- ☑
      nondisplaced S82.02- ☑
    osteochondral (displaced) S82.01- ☑
      nondisplaced S82.01- ☑
    specified NEC S82.09- ☑
    transverse (displaced) S82.03- ☑
      nondisplaced S82.03- ☑
  pedicle (of vertebral arch) — *see* Fracture, vertebra
  pelvis, pelvic (bone) S32.9 ☑
    acetabulum — *see* Fracture, acetabulum
    circle — *see* Disruption, pelvic ring
    following insertion of implant, prosthesis or plate M96.65
    ilium — *see* Fracture, ilium
    ischium — *see* Fracture, ischium
    multiple
      with disruption of pelvic ring (circle) — *see* Disruption, pelvic ring
      without disruption of pelvic ring (circle) S32.82 ☑
    pubis — *see* Fracture, pubis
    sacrum — *see* Fracture, sacrum
    specified site NEC S32.89 ☑
  phalanx
    foot — *see* Fracture, toe
    hand — *see* Fracture, finger
  pisiform — *see* Fracture, carpal, pisiform
  pond — *see* Fracture, skull
  prosthetic device, internal — *see* Complications, prosthetic device, by site, mechanical
  pubis S32.50- ☑
    with disruption of pelvic ring — *see* Disruption, pelvic ring
    specified site NEC S32.59- ☑
    superior rim S32.51- ☑
  radius S52.9- ☑
    distal end — *see* Fracture, radius, lower end
    following insertion of implant, prosthesis or plate M96.63- ☑
    head — *see* Fracture, radius, upper end, head
    lower end S52.50- ☑
      Barton's — *see* Barton's fracture
      Colles' — *see* Colles' fracture
      extraarticular NEC S52.55- ☑
      intraarticular NEC S52.57- ☑
      physeal S59.20- ☑
        Salter-Harris
          Type I S59.21- ☑
          Type II S59.22- ☑
          Type III S59.23- ☑
          Type IV S59.24- ☑
        specified NEC S59.29- ☑
      Smith's — *see* Smith's fracture
      specified NEC S52.59- ☑

Fracture, traumatic — *continued*
  radius — *continued*
    lower end — *continued*
      styloid process (displaced) S52.51- ☑
        nondisplaced S52.51- ☑
      torus S52.52- ☑
    neck — *see* Fracture, radius, upper end
    proximal end — *see* Fracture, radius, upper end
    shaft S52.30- ☑
      bent bone S52.38- ☑
      comminuted (displaced) S52.35- ☑
        nondisplaced S52.35- ☑
      Galeazzi's — *see* Galeazzi's fracture
      greenstick S52.31- ☑
      oblique (displaced) S52.33- ☑
        nondisplaced S52.33- ☑
      segmental (displaced) S52.36- ☑
        nondisplaced S52.36- ☑
      specified NEC S52.39- ☑
      spiral (displaced) S52.34- ☑
        nondisplaced S52.34- ☑
      transverse (displaced) S52.32- ☑
        nondisplaced S52.32- ☑
    upper end S52.10- ☑
      head (displaced) S52.12- ☑
        nondisplaced S52.12- ☑
      neck (displaced) S52.13- ☑
        nondisplaced S52.13- ☑
      physeal S59.10- ☑
        Salter-Harris
          Type I S59.11- ☑
          Type II S59.12- ☑
          Type III S59.13- ☑
          Type IV S59.14- ☑
        specified NEC S59.19- ☑
      specified NEC S52.18- ☑
      torus S52.11- ☑
  ramus
    inferior or superior, pubis — *see* Fracture, pubis
    mandible — *see* Fracture, mandible
  restorative material (dental) K08.539
    with loss of material K08.531
    without loss of material K08.530
  rib S22.3- ☑
    with flail chest — *see* Flail, chest
    multiple S22.4- ☑
      with flail chest — *see* Flail, chest
  root, tooth — *see* Fracture, tooth
  sacrum S32.10 ☑
    specified NEC S32.19 ☑
    Type
      1 S32.14 ☑
      2 S32.15 ☑
      3 S32.16 ☑
      4 S32.17 ☑
    Zone
      I S32.119 ☑
        displaced (minimally) S32.111 ☑
          severely S32.112 ☑
        nondisplaced S32.110 ☑
      II S32.129 ☑
        displaced (minimally) S32.121 ☑
          severely S32.122 ☑
        nondisplaced S32.120 ☑
      III S32.139 ☑
        displaced (minimally) S32.131 ☑
          severely S32.132 ☑
        nondisplaced S32.130 ☑
  scaphoid (hand) (*see also* Fracture, carpal, navicular)
    foot — *see* Fracture, tarsal, navicular
  scapula S42.10- ☑
    acromial process (displaced) S42.12- ☑
      nondisplaced S42.12- ☑
    body (displaced) S42.11- ☑
      nondisplaced S42.11- ☑
    coracoid process (displaced) S42.13- ☑
      nondisplaced S42.13- ☑
    glenoid cavity (displaced) S42.14- ☑
      nondisplaced S42.14- ☑
    neck (displaced) S42.15- ☑
      nondisplaced S42.15- ☑
    specified NEC S42.19- ☑
  semilunar bone, wrist — *see* Fracture, carpal, lunate
  sequelae — *see* Sequelae, fracture
  sesamoid bone
    hand — *see* Fracture, carpal

Fracture, traumatic — *continued*
  sesamoid bone — *continued*
    other — *code by* site under Fracture
  shepherd's — *see* Fracture, tarsal, talus
  shoulder (girdle) S42.9- ☑
    blade — *see* Fracture, scapula
  sinus (ethmoid) (frontal) S02.19 ☑
  skull S02.91 ☑
    base S02.10 ☑
      occiput S02.119 ☑
        condyle S02.113 ☑
          type I S02.110 ☑
          type II S02.111 ☑
          type III S02.112 ☑
        specified NEC S02.118 ☑
      specified NEC S02.19 ☑
    birth injury P13.0
    frontal bone S02.0 ☑
    parietal bone S02.0 ☑
    specified site NEC S02.8 ☑
    temporal bone S02.19 ☑
    vault S02.0 ☑
  Smith's — *see* Smith's fracture
  sphenoid (bone) (sinus) S02.19 ☑
  spine — *see* Fracture, vertebra
  spinous process — *see* Fracture, vertebra
  spontaneous (cause unknown) — *see* Fracture, pathological
  stave (of thumb) — *see* Fracture, metacarpal, first
  sternum S22.20 ☑
    with flail chest — *see* Flail, chest
    body S22.22 ☑
    manubrium S22.21 ☑
    xiphoid (process) S22.24 ☑
  stress M84.30 ☑
    ankle M84.37- ☑
    carpus M84.34- ☑
    clavicle M84.31- ☑
    femoral neck M84.359 ☑
    femur M84.35- ☑
    fibula M84.36- ☑
    finger M84.34- ☑
    hip M84.359 ☑
    humerus M84.32- ☑
    ilium M84.350 ☑
    ischium M84.350 ☑
    metacarpus M84.34- ☑
    metatarsus M84.37- ☑
    neck — *see* Fracture, fatigue, vertebra
    pelvis M84.350 ☑
    radius M84.33- ☑
    rib M84.38 ☑
    scapula M84.31- ☑
    skull M84.38 ☑
    tarsus M84.37- ☑
    tibia M84.36- ☑
    toe M84.37- ☑
    ulna M84.33- ☑
    vertebra — *see* Fracture, fatigue, vertebra
  supracondylar, elbow — *see* Fracture, humerus, lower end, supracondylar
  symphysis pubis — *see* Fracture, pubis
  talus (ankle bone) — *see* Fracture, tarsal, talus
  tarsal bone(s) S92.20- ☑
    astragalus — *see* Fracture, tarsal, talus
    calcaneus S92.00- ☑
      anterior process (displaced) S92.02- ☑
        nondisplaced S92.02- ☑
      body (displaced) S92.01- ☑
        nondisplaced S92.01- ☑
      extraarticular NEC (displaced) S92.05- ☑
        nondisplaced S92.05- ☑
      intraarticular (displaced) S92.06- ☑
        nondisplaced S92.06- ☑
      tuberosity (displaced) S92.04- ☑
        avulsion (displaced) S92.03- ☑
          nondisplaced S92.03- ☑
        nondisplaced S92.04- ☑
    cuboid (displaced) S92.21- ☑
      nondisplaced S92.21- ☑
    cuneiform
      intermediate (displaced) S92.23- ☑
        nondisplaced S92.23- ☑
      lateral (displaced) S92.22- ☑
        nondisplaced S92.22- ☑

Fracture, traumatic — *continued*
tarsal bone(s) — *continued*
cuneiform — *continued*
medial (displaced) S92.24- ☑
nondisplaced S92.24- ☑
navicular (displaced) S92.25- ☑
nondisplaced S92.25- ☑
scaphoid — *see* Fracture, tarsal, navicular
talus S92.10- ☑
avulsion (displaced) S92.15- ☑
nondisplaced S92.15- ☑
body (displaced) S92.12- ☑
nondisplaced S92.12- ☑
dome (displaced) S92.14- ☑
nondisplaced S92.14- ☑
head (displaced) S92.12- ☑
nondisplaced S92.12- ☑
lateral process (displaced) S92.14- ☑
nondisplaced S92.14- ☑
neck (displaced) S92.11- ☑
nondisplaced S92.11- ☑
posterior process (displaced) S92.13- ☑
nondisplaced S92.13- ☑
specified NEC S92.19- ☑
temporal bone (styloid) S02.19 ☑
thorax (bony) S22.9 ☑
with flail chest — *see* Flail, chest
rib S22.3- ☑
multiple S22.4- ☑
with flail chest — *see* Flail, chest
sternum S22.20 ☑
body S22.22 ☑
manubrium S22.21 ☑
xiphoid process S22.24 ☑
vertebra (displaced) S22.009 ☑
burst (stable) S22.001 ☑
unstable S22.002 ☑
eighth S22.069 ☑
burst (stable) S22.061 ☑
unstable S22.062 ☑
specified type NEC S22.068 ☑
wedge compression S22.060 ☑
eleventh S22.089 ☑
burst (stable) S22.081 ☑
unstable S22.082 ☑
specified type NEC S22.088 ☑
wedge compression S22.080 ☑
fifth S22.059 ☑
burst (stable) S22.051 ☑
unstable S22.052 ☑
specified type NEC S22.058 ☑
wedge compression S22.050 ☑
first S22.019 ☑
burst (stable) S22.011 ☑
unstable S22.012 ☑
specified type NEC S22.018 ☑
wedge compression S22.010 ☑
fourth S22.049 ☑
burst (stable) S22.041 ☑
unstable S22.042 ☑
specified type NEC S22.048 ☑
wedge compression S22.040 ☑
ninth S22.079 ☑
burst (stable) S22.071 ☑
unstable S22.072 ☑
specified type NEC S22.078 ☑
wedge compression S22.070 ☑
nondisplaced S22.001 ☑
second S22.029 ☑
burst (stable) S22.021 ☑
unstable S22.022 ☑
specified type NEC S22.028 ☑
wedge compression S22.020 ☑
seventh S22.069 ☑
burst (stable) S22.061 ☑
unstable S22.062 ☑
specified type NEC S22.068 ☑
wedge compression S22.060 ☑
sixth S22.059 ☑
burst (stable) S22.051 ☑
unstable S22.052 ☑
specified type NEC S22.058 ☑
wedge compression S22.050 ☑
specified type NEC S22.008 ☑

Fracture, traumatic — *continued*
thorax — *continued*
vertebra — *continued*
tenth S22.079 ☑
burst (stable) S22.071 ☑
unstable S22.072 ☑
specified type NEC S22.078 ☑
wedge compression S22.070 ☑
third S22.039 ☑
burst (stable) S22.031 ☑
unstable S22.032 ☑
specified type NEC S22.038 ☑
wedge compression S22.030 ☑
twelfth S22.089 ☑
burst (stable) S22.081 ☑
unstable S22.082 ☑
specified type NEC S22.088 ☑
wedge compression S22.080 ☑
wedge compression S22.000 ☑
thumb S62.50- ☑
distal phalanx (displaced) S62.52- ☑
nondisplaced S62.52- ☑
proximal phalanx (displaced) S62.51- ☑
nondisplaced S62.51- ☑
thyroid cartilage S12.8 ☑
tibia (shaft) S82.20- ☑
comminuted (displaced) S82.25- ☑
nondisplaced S82.25- ☑
condyles — *see* Fracture, tibia, upper end
distal end — *see* Fracture, tibia, lower end
epiphysis
lower — *see* Fracture, tibia, lower end
upper — *see* Fracture, tibia, upper end
following insertion of implant, prosthesis or plate
M96.67-
head (involving knee joint) — *see* Fracture, tibia, upper end
intercondyloid eminence — *see* Fracture, tibia, upper end
involving ankle or malleolus — *see* Fracture, ankle, medial malleolus
lower end S82.30- ☑
physeal S89.10- ☑
Salter-Harris
Type I S89.11- ☑
Type II S89.12- ☑
Type III S89.13- ☑
Type IV S89.14- ☑
specified NEC S89.19- ☑
pilon (displaced) S82.87- ☑
nondisplaced S82.87- ☑
specified NEC S82.39- ☑
torus S82.31- ☑
malleolus — *see* Fracture, ankle, medial malleolus
oblique (displaced) S82.23- ☑
nondisplaced S82.23- ☑
pilon — *see* Fracture, tibia, lower end, pilon
proximal end — *see* Fracture, tibia, upper end
segmental (displaced) S82.26- ☑
nondisplaced S82.26- ☑
specified NEC S82.29- ☑
spine — *see* Fracture, upper end, spine
spiral (displaced) S82.24- ☑
nondisplaced S82.24- ☑
transverse (displaced) S82.22- ☑
nondisplaced S82.22- ☑
tuberosity — *see* Fracture, tibia, upper end, tuberosity
upper end S82.10- ☑
bicondylar (displaced) S82.14- ☑
nondisplaced S82.14- ☑
lateral condyle (displaced) S82.12- ☑
nondisplaced S82.12- ☑
medial condyle (displaced) S82.13- ☑
nondisplaced S82.13- ☑
physeal S89.00- ☑
Salter-Harris
Type I S89.01- ☑
Type II S89.02- ☑
Type III S89.03- ☑
Type IV S89.04- ☑
specified NEC S89.09- ☑
plateau — *see* Fracture, tibia, upper end, bicondylar
specified NEC S82.19- ☑
spine

Fracture, traumatic — *continued*
tibia — *continued*
upper end — *continued*
spine (displaced) S82.11- ☑
nondisplaced S82.11- ☑
torus S82.16- ☑
tuberosity (displaced) S82.15- ☑
nondisplaced S82.15- ☑
toe S92.91- ☑
great (displaced) S92.40- ☑
distal phalanx (displaced) S92.42- ☑
nondisplaced S92.42- ☑
nondisplaced S92.40- ☑
proximal phalanx (displaced) S92.41- ☑
nondisplaced S92.41- ☑
specified NEC S92.49- ☑
lesser (displaced) S92.50- ☑
distal phalanx (displaced) S92.53- ☑
nondisplaced S92.53- ☑
medial phalanx (displaced) S92.52- ☑
nondisplaced S92.52- ☑
nondisplaced S92.50- ☑
proximal phalanx (displaced) S92.51- ☑
nondisplaced S92.51- ☑
specified NEC S92.59- ☑
tooth (root) S02.5
trachea (cartilage) S12.8 ☑
transverse process — *see* Fracture, vertebra
trapezium or trapezoid bone — *see* Fracture, carpal
trimalleolar — *see* Fracture, ankle, trimalleolar
triquetrum (cuneiform of carpus) — *see* Fracture, carpal, triquetrum
trochanter — *see* Fracture, femur, trochanteric
tuberosity (external) — *code by* site under Fracture
ulna (shaft) S52.20- ☑
bent bone S52.28- ☑
coronoid process — *see* Fracture, ulna, upper end, coronoid process
distal end — *see* Fracture, ulna, lower end
following insertion of implant, prosthesis or plate M96.63- ☑
head S52.00- ☑
lower end S52.60- ☑
physeal S59.00- ☑
Salter-Harris
Type I S59.01- ☑
Type II S59.02- ☑
Type III S59.03- ☑
Type IV S59.04- ☑
specified NEC S59.09- ☑
specified NEC S52.69- ☑
styloid process (displaced) S52.61- ☑
nondisplaced S52.61- ☑
torus S52.62- ☑
proximal end — *see* Fracture, ulna, upper end
shaft S52.20- ☑
comminuted (displaced) S52.25- ☑
nondisplaced S52.25- ☑
greenstick S52.21- ☑
Monteggia's — *see* Monteggia's fracture
oblique (displaced) S52.23- ☑
nondisplaced S52.23- ☑
segmental (displaced) S52.26- ☑
nondisplaced S52.26- ☑
specified NEC S52.29- ☑
spiral (displaced) S52.24- ☑
nondisplaced S52.24- ☑
transverse (displaced) S52.22- ☑
nondisplaced S52.22- ☑
upper end S52.00- ☑
coronoid process (displaced) S52.04- ☑
nondisplaced S52.04- ☑
olecranon process (displaced) S52.02- ☑
with intraarticular extension S52.03- ☑
nondisplaced S52.02- ☑
with intraarticular extension S52.03- ☑
specified NEC S52.09- ☑
torus S52.01- ☑
unciform — *see* Fracture, carpal, hamate
vault of skull S02.0 ☑
vertebra, vertebral (arch) (body) (column) (neural arch) (pedicle) (spinous process) (transverse process)
atlas — *see* Fracture, neck, cervical vertebra, first
axis — *see* Fracture, neck, cervical vertebra, second

Fracture, traumatic — *continued*
  vertebra, vertebral — *continued*
    cervical (teardrop) S12.9 ☑
      axis — *see* Fracture, neck, cervical vertebra, second
      first (atlas) — *see* Fracture, neck, cervical vertebra, first
      second (axis) — *see* Fracture, neck, cervical vertebra, second
    chronic M84.48 ☑
    coccyx S32.2 ☑
    dorsal — *see* Fracture, thorax, vertebra
    lumbar S32.009 ☑
      burst (stable) S32.001 ☑
        unstable S32.002 ☑
      fifth S32.059 ☑
        burst (stable) S32.051 ☑
          unstable S32.052 ☑
        specified type NEC S32.058 ☑
        wedge compression S32.050 ☑
      first S32.019 ☑
        burst (stable) S32.011 ☑
          unstable S32.012 ☑
        specified type NEC S32.018 ☑
        wedge compression S32.010 ☑
      fourth S32.049 ☑
        burst (stable) S32.041 ☑
          unstable S32.042 ☑
        specified type NEC S32.048 ☑
        wedge compression S32.040 ☑
      second S32.029 ☑
        burst (stable) S32.021 ☑
          unstable S32.022 ☑
        specified type NEC S32.028 ☑
        wedge compression S32.020 ☑
      specified type NEC S32.008 ☑
      third S32.039 ☑
        burst (stable) S32.031 ☑
          unstable S32.032 ☑
        specified type NEC S32.038 ☑
        wedge compression S32.030 ☑
      wedge compression S32.000 ☑
    metastatic — *see* Collapse, vertebra, in, specified disease NEC (*see also* Neoplasm)
    newborn (birth injury) P11.5
    sacrum S32.10 ☑
      specified NEC S32.19 ☑
      Type
        1 S32.14 ☑
        2 S32.15 ☑
        3 S32.16 ☑
        4 S32.17 ☑
      Zone
        I S32.119 ☑
          displaced (minimally) S32.111 ☑
            severely S32.112 ☑
          nondisplaced S32.110 ☑
        II S32.129 ☑
          displaced (minimally) S32.121 ☑
            severely S32.122 ☑
          nondisplaced S32.120 ☑
        III S32.139 ☑
          displaced (minimally) S32.131 ☑
            severely S32.132 ☑
          nondisplaced S32.130 ☑
    thoracic — *see* Fracture, thorax, vertebra
    vertex S02.0 ☑
    vomer (bone) S02.2 ☑
    wrist S62.10- ☑
      carpal — *see* Fracture, carpal bone
      navicular (scaphoid) (hand) — *see* Fracture, carpal, navicular
    xiphisternum, xiphoid (process) S22.24 ☑
    zygoma S02.402 ☑
Fragile, fragility
  autosomal site Q95.5
  bone, congenital (with blue sclera) Q78.0
  capillary (hereditary) D69.8
  hair L67.8
  nails L60.3
  non-sex chromosome site Q95.5
  X chromosome Q99.2
Fragilitas
  crinium L67.8
  ossium (with blue sclerae) (hereditary) Q78.0
  unguium L60.3

Fragilitas — *continued*
  unguium L60.3
    congenital Q84.6
Fragments, cataract (lens), **following cataract surgery** H59.02- ☑
  retained foreign body — *see* Retained, foreign body fragments (type of)
Frailty (frail) R54
  mental R41.81
Frambesia, frambesial (tropica) (*see also* Yaws)
  initial lesion or ulcer A66.0
  primary A66.0
Frambeside
  gummatous A66.4
  of early yaws A66.2
Frambesioma A66.1
Franceschetti-Klein (-Wildervanck) **disease or syndrome** Q75.4
Francis' disease — *see* Tularemia
Franklin disease C88.2
Frank's essential thrombocytopenia D69.3
Fraser's syndrome Q87.0
Freckle(s) L81.2
  malignant melanoma in — *see* Melanoma
  melanotic (Hutchinson's) — *see* Melanoma, in situ
  retinal D49.81
Frederickson's hyperlipoproteinemia, type
  I and V E78.3
  IIA E78.0
  IIB and III E78.2
  IV E78.1
Freeman Sheldon syndrome Q87.0
Freezing (*see also* Effect, adverse, cold) T69.9 ☑
Freiberg's disease (infraction of metatarsal head or osteochondrosis) — *see* Osteochondrosis, juvenile, metatarsus
Frei's disease A55
Fremitus, friction, cardiac R01.2
Frenum, frenulum
  external os Q51.828
  tongue (shortening) (congenital) Q38.1
Frequency micturition (nocturnal) R35.0
  psychogenic F45.8
Frey's syndrome
  auriculotemporal G50.8
  hyperhidrosis L74.52
Friction
  burn — *see* Burn, by site
  fremitus, cardiac R01.2
  precordial R01.2
  sounds, chest R09.89
Friderichsen-Waterhouse syndrome or disease A39.1
Friedländer's B (bacillus) **NEC** (*see also* condition) A49.8
Friedreich's
  ataxia G11.1
  combined systemic disease G11.1
  facial hemihypertrophy Q67.4
  sclerosis (cerebellum) (spinal cord) G11.1
Frigidity F52.22
Fröhlich's syndrome E23.6
Frontal (*see also* condition)
  lobe syndrome F07.0
Frostbite (superficial) T33.90 ☑
  with
    partial thickness skin loss — *see* Frostbite (superficial), by site
    tissue necrosis T34.90 ☑
  abdominal wall T33.3 ☑
    with tissue necrosis T34.3 ☑
  ankle T33.81- ☑
    with tissue necrosis T34.81- ☑
  arm T33.4- ☑
    with tissue necrosis T34.4- ☑
    finger(s) — *see* Frostbite, finger
    hand — *see* Frostbite, hand
    wrist — *see* Frostbite, wrist
  ear T33.01- ☑
    with tissue necrosis T34.01- ☑
  face T33.09 ☑
    with tissue necrosis T34.09 ☑
  finger T33.53- ☑
    with tissue necrosis T34.53- ☑
  foot T33.82- ☑
    with tissue necrosis T34.82- ☑
  hand T33.52- ☑
    with tissue necrosis T34.52- ☑

Frostbite — *continued*
  head T33.09 ☑
    with tissue necrosis T34.09 ☑
    ear — *see* Frostbite, ear
    nose — *see* Frostbite, nose
  hip (and thigh) T33.6- ☑
    with tissue necrosis T34.6- ☑
  knee T33.7- ☑
    with tissue necrosis T34.7- ☑
  leg T33.9- ☑
    with tissue necrosis T34.9- ☑
    ankle — *see* Frostbite, ankle
    foot — *see* Frostbite, foot
    knee — *see* Frostbite, knee
    lower T33.7- ☑
      with tissue necrosis T34.7- ☑
    thigh — *see* Frostbite, hip
    toe — *see* Frostbite, toe
  limb
    lower T33.99 ☑
      with tissue necrosis T34.99 ☑
    upper — *see* Frostbite, arm
  neck T33.1 ☑
    with tissue necrosis T34.1 ☑
  nose T33.02 ☑
    with tissue necrosis T34.02 ☑
  pelvis T33.3 ☑
    with tissue necrosis T34.3 ☑
  specified site NEC T33.99 ☑
    with tissue necrosis T34.99 ☑
  thigh — *see* Frostbite, hip
  thorax T33.2 ☑
    with tissue necrosis T34.2 ☑
  toes T33.83- ☑
    with tissue necrosis T34.83- ☑
  trunk T33.99 ☑
    with tissue necrosis T34.99 ☑
  wrist T33.51- ☑
    with tissue necrosis T34.51- ☑
Frotteurism F65.81
Frozen (*see also* Effect, adverse, cold) T69.9 ☑
  pelvis (female) N94.89
    male K66.8
  shoulder — *see* Capsulitis, adhesive
Fructokinase deficiency E74.11
Fructose 1,6 diphosphatase deficiency E74.19
Fructosemia (benign) (essential) E74.12
Fructosuria (benign) (essential) E74.11
Fuchs'
  black spot (myopic) H44.2- ☑
  dystrophy (corneal endothelium) H18.51
  heterochromic cyclitis — *see* Cyclitis, Fuchs' heterochromic
Fucosidosis E77.1
Fugue R68.89
  dissociative F44.1
  hysterical (dissociative) F44.1
  postictal in epilepsy — *see* Epilepsy
  reaction to exceptional stress (transient) F43.0
Fulminant, fulminating — *see* condition
Functional (*see also* condition)
  bleeding (uterus) N93.8
Functioning, intellectual, borderline R41.83
Fundus — *see* condition
Fungemia NOS B49
Fungus, fungous
  cerebral G93.89
  disease NOS B49
  infection — *see* Infection, fungus
Funiculitis (acute) (chronic) (endemic) N49.1
  gonococcal (acute) (chronic) A54.23
  tuberculous A18.15
Funnel
  breast (acquired) M95.4
    congenital Q67.6
    sequelae (late effect) of rickets E64.3
  chest (acquired) M95.4
    congenital Q67.6
    sequelae (late effect) of rickets E64.3
  pelvis (acquired) M95.5
    with disproportion (fetopelvic) O33.3 ☑
      causing obstructed labor O65.3
    congenital Q74.2
FUO (fever of unknown origin) R50.9
Furfur L21.0
  microsporon B36.0

Furrier's lung J67.8
Furrowed K14.5
　nail(s) (transverse) L60.4
　　congenital Q84.6
　tongue K14.5
　　congenital Q38.3
Furuncle L02.92
　abdominal wall L02.221
　ankle — *see* Furuncle, lower limb
　antecubital space — *see* Furuncle, upper limb
　anus K61.0
　arm — *see* Furuncle, upper limb
　auditory canal, external — *see* Abscess, ear, external
　auricle (ear) — *see* Abscess, ear, external
　axilla (region) L02.42- ☑
　back (any part) L02.222
　breast N61
　buttock L02.32
　cheek (external) L02.02
　chest wall L02.223
　chin L02.02
　corpus cavernosum N48.21
　ear, external — *see* Abscess, ear, external
　external auditory canal — *see* Abscess, ear, external
　eyelid — *see* Abscess, eyelid
　face L02.02
　femoral (region) — *see* Furuncle, lower limb
　finger — *see* Furuncle, hand
　flank L02.221
　foot L02.62- ☑
　forehead L02.02
　gluteal (region) L02.32
　groin L02.224
　hand L02.52- ☑
　head L02.821
　　face L02.02
　hip — *see* Furuncle, lower limb
　kidney — *see* Abscess, kidney
　knee — *see* Furuncle, lower limb
　labium (majus) (minus) N76.4
　lacrimal
　　gland — *see* Dacryoadenitis
　　passages (duct) (sac) — *see* Inflammation, lacrimal, passages, acute
　leg (any part) — *see* Furuncle, lower limb
　lower limb L02.42- ☑
　malignant A22.0
　mouth K12.2
　navel L02.226

Furuncle — *continued*
　neck L02.12
　nose J34.0
　orbit, orbital — *see* Abscess, orbit
　palmar (space) — *see* Furuncle, hand
　partes posteriores L02.32
　pectoral region L02.223
　penis N48.21
　perineum L02.225
　pinna — *see* Abscess, ear, external
　popliteal — *see* Furuncle, lower limb
　prepatellar — *see* Furuncle, lower limb
　scalp L02.821
　seminal vesicle N49.0
　shoulder — *see* Furuncle, upper limb
　specified site NEC L02.828
　submandibular K12.2
　temple (region) L02.02
　thumb — *see* Furuncle, hand
　toe — *see* Furuncle, foot
　trunk L02.229
　　abdominal wall L02.221
　　back L02.222
　　chest wall L02.223
　　groin L02.224
　　perineum L02.225
　　umbilicus L02.226
　umbilicus L02.226
　upper limb L02.42- ☑
　vulva N76.4
Furunculosis — *see* Furuncle
Fused — *see* Fusion, fused
Fusion, fused (congenital)
　astragaloscaphoid Q74.2
　atria Q21.1
　auditory canal Q16.1
　auricles, heart Q21.1
　binocular with defective stereopsis H53.32
　bone Q79.8
　cervical spine M43.22
　choanal Q30.0
　commissure, mitral valve Q23.2
　cusps, heart valve NEC Q24.8
　　mitral Q23.2
　　pulmonary Q22.1
　　tricuspid Q22.4
　ear ossicles Q16.3
　fingers Q70.0 ☑
　hymen Q52.3

Fusion, fused — *continued*
　joint (acquired) (*see also* Ankylosis)
　　congenital Q74.8
　kidneys (incomplete) Q63.1
　labium (majus) (minus) Q52.5
　larynx and trachea Q34.8
　limb, congenital Q74.8
　　lower Q74.2
　　upper Q74.0
　lobes, lung Q33.8
　lumbosacral (acquired) M43.27
　　arthrodesis status Z98.1
　　congenital Q76.49
　　postprocedural status Z98.1
　nares, nose, nasal, nostril(s) Q30.0
　organ or site not listed — *see* Anomaly, by site
　ossicles Q79.9
　　auditory Q16.3
　pulmonic cusps Q22.1
　ribs Q76.6
　sacroiliac (joint) (acquired) M43.28
　　arthrodesis status Z98.1
　　congenital Q74.2
　　postprocedural status Z98.1
　spine (acquired) NEC M43.20
　　arthrodesis status Z98.1
　　cervical region M43.22
　　cervicothoracic region M43.23
　　congenital Q76.49
　　lumbar M43.26
　　lumbosacral region M43.27
　　occipito-atlanto-axial region M43.21
　　postoperative status Z98.1
　　sacrococcygeal region M43.28
　　thoracic region M43.24
　　thoracolumbar region M43.25
　sublingual duct with submaxillary duct at opening in mouth Q38.4
　testes Q55.1
　toes Q70.2- ☑
　tooth, teeth K00.2
　trachea and esophagus Q39.8
　twins Q89.4
　vagina Q52.4
　ventricles, heart Q21.0
　vertebra (arch) — *see* Fusion, spine
　vulva Q52.5
Fusospirillosis (mouth) (tongue) (tonsil) A69.1
Fussy baby R68.12

G

Gain in weight (abnormal) (excessive) (*see also* Weight, gain)
Gaisböck's disease (polycythemia hypertonica) D75.1
Gait abnormality R26.9
  ataxic R26.0
  falling R29.6
  hysterical (ataxic) (staggering) F44.4
  paralytic R26.1
  spastic R26.1
  specified type NEC R26.89
  staggering R26.0
  unsteadiness R26.81
  walking difficulty NEC R26.2
Galactocele (breast) N64.89
  puerperal, postpartum O92.79
Galactokinase deficiency E74.29
Galactophoritis N61
  gestational, puerperal, postpartum O91.2- ☑
Galactorrhea O92.6
  not associated with childbirth N64.3
Galactosemia (classic) (congenital) E74.21
Galactosuria E74.29
Galacturia R82.0
  schistosomiasis (bilharziasis) B65.0
Galeazzi's fracture S52.37- ☑
Galen's vein — *see* condition
Galeophobia F40.218
Gall duct — *see* condition
Gallbladder (*see also* condition)
  acute K81.0
Gallop rhythm R00.8
Gallstone (colic) (cystic duct) (gallbladder) (impacted) (multiple) (*see also* Calculus, gallbladder)
  with
    cholecystitis — *see* Calculus, gallbladder, with cholecystitis
  bile duct (common) (hepatic) — *see* Calculus, bile duct
  causing intestinal obstruction K56.3
  specified NEC K80.80
    with obstruction K80.81
Gambling Z72.6
  pathological (compulsive) F63.0
Gammopathy (of undetermined significance [MGUS]) D47.2
  associated with lymphoplasmacytic dyscrasia D47.2
  monoclonal D47.2
  polyclonal D89.0
Gamna's disease (siderotic splenomegaly) D73.1
Gamophobia F40.298
Gampsodactylia (congenital) Q66.7
Gamstorp's disease (adynamia episodica hereditaria) G72.3
Gandy-Nanta disease (siderotic splenomegaly) D73.1
Gang
  membership offenses Z72.810
Gangliocytoma D36.10
Ganglioglioma — *see* Neoplasm, uncertain behavior, by site
Ganglion (compound) (diffuse) (joint) (tendon (sheath)) M67.40
  ankle M67.47- ☑
  foot M67.47- ☑
  forearm M67.43- ☑
  hand M67.44- ☑
  lower leg M67.46- ☑
  multiple sites M67.49
  of yaws (early) (late) A66.6
  pelvic region M67.45- ☑
  periosteal — *see* Periostitis
  shoulder region M67.41- ☑
  specified site NEC M67.48
  thigh region M67.45- ☑
  tuberculous A18.09
  upper arm M67.42- ☑
  wrist M67.43- ☑
Ganglioneuroblastoma — *see* Neoplasm, nerve, malignant

Ganglioneuroma D36.10
  malignant — *see* Neoplasm, nerve, malignant
Ganglioneuromatosis D36.10
Ganglionitis
  fifth nerve — *see* Neuralgia, trigeminal
  gasserian (postherpetic) (postzoster) B02.21
  geniculate G51.1
    newborn (birth injury) P11.3
    postherpetic, postzoster B02.21
  herpes zoster B02.21
  postherpetic geniculate B02.21
Gangliosidosis E75.10
  GM1 E75.19
  GM2 E75.00
    other specified E75.09
    Sandhoff disease E75.01
    Tay-Sachs disease E75.02
  GM3 E75.19
  mucolipidosis IV E75.11
Gangosa A66.5
Gangrene, gangrenous (connective tissue) (dropsical) (dry) (moist) (skin) (ulcer) (*see also* Necrosis) I96
  with diabetes (mellitus) — *see* Diabetes, gangrene
  abdomen (wall) I96
  alveolar M27.3
  appendix K35.80
    with
      perforation or rupture K35.2
      peritoneal abscess K35.3
      peritonitis NEC K35.3
        generalized (with perforation or rupture) K35.2
        localized (with perforation or rupture) K35.3
  arteriosclerotic (general) (senile) — *see* Arteriosclerosis, extremities, with, gangrene
  auricle I96
  Bacillus welchii A48.0
  bladder (infectious) — *see* Cystitis, specified type NEC
  bowel, cecum, or colon — *see* Gangrene, intestine
  Clostridium perfringens or welchii A48.0
  cornea H18.89- ☑
  corpora cavernosa N48.29
    noninfective N48.89
  cutaneous, spreading I96
  decubital — *see* Ulcer, pressure, by site
  diabetic (any site) — *see* Diabetes, gangrene
  emphysematous — *see* Gangrene, gas
  epidemic — *see* Poisoning, food, noxious, plant
  epididymis (infectional) N45.1
  erysipelas — *see* Erysipelas
  extremity (lower) (upper) I96
  Fournier N49.3
    female N76.89
  fusospirochetal A69.0
  gallbladder — *see* Cholecystitis, acute
  gas (bacillus) A48.0
    following
      abortion — *see* Abortion by type complicated by infection
      ectopic or molar pregnancy O08.0
  glossitis K14.0
  hernia — *see* Hernia, by site, with gangrene
  intestine, intestinal (hemorrhagic) (massive) K55.0
    with
      mesenteric embolism K55.0
      obstruction — *see* Obstruction, intestine
  laryngitis J04.0
  limb (lower) (upper) I96
  lung J85.0
    spirochetal A69.8
  lymphangitis I89.1
  Meleney's (synergistic) — *see* Ulcer, skin
  mesentery K55.0
    with
      embolism K55.0
      intestinal obstruction — *see* Obstruction, intestine
  mouth A69.0
  ovary — *see* Oophoritis
  pancreas K85.9
  penis N48.29
    noninfective N48.89

Gangrene, gangrenous — *continued*
  perineum I96
  pharynx (*see also* Pharyngitis)
    Vincent's A69.1
  presenile I73.1
  progressive synergistic — *see* Ulcer, skin
  pulmonary J85.0
  pulpal (dental) K04.1
  quinsy J36
  Raynaud's (symmetric gangrene) I73.01
  retropharyngeal J39.2
  scrotum N49.3
    noninfective N50.8
  senile (atherosclerotic) — *see* Arteriosclerosis, extremities, with, gangrene
  spermatic cord N49.1
    noninfective N50.8
  spine I96
  spirochetal NEC A69.8
  spreading cutaneous I96
  stomatitis A69.0
  symmetrical I73.01
  testis (infectional) N45.2
    noninfective N44.8
  throat (*see also* Pharyngitis)
    diphtheritic A36.0
    Vincent's A69.1
  thyroid (gland) E07.89
  tooth (pulp) K04.1
  tuberculous NEC — *see* Tuberculosis
  tunica vaginalis N49.1
    noninfective N50.8
  umbilicus I96
  uterus — *see* Endometritis
  uvulitis K12.2
  vas deferens N49.1
    noninfective N50.8
  vulva N76.89
Ganister disease J62.8
Ganser's syndrome (hysterical) F44.89
Gardner-Diamond syndrome (autoerythrocyte sensitization) D69.2
Gargoylism E76.01
Garré's disease, osteitis (sclerosing), osteomyelitis — *see* Osteomyelitis, specified type NEC
Garrod's pad, knuckle M72.1
Gartner's duct
  cyst Q52.4
  persistent Q50.6
Gas R14.3
  asphyxiation, inhalation, poisoning, suffocation NEC — *see* Table of Drugs and Chemicals
  excessive R14.0
  gangrene A48.0
    following
      abortion — *see* Abortion by type complicated by infection
      ectopic or molar pregnancy O08.0
  on stomach R14.0
  pains R14.1
Gastralgia (*see also* Pain, abdominal)
Gastrectasis K31.0
  psychogenic F45.8
Gastric — *see* condition
Gastrinoma
  malignant
    pancreas C25.4
    specified site NEC — *see* Neoplasm, malignant, by site
    unspecified site C25.4
  specified site — *see* Neoplasm, uncertain behavior
  unspecified site D37.9
Gastritis (simple) K29.70
  with bleeding K29.71
  acute (erosive) K29.00
    with bleeding K29.01
  alcoholic K29.20
    with bleeding K29.21
  allergic K29.60
    with bleeding K29.61
  atrophic (chronic) K29.40
    with bleeding K29.41

Gastritis — *continued*
chronic (antral) (fundal) K29.50
  with bleeding K29.51
  atrophic K29.40
    with bleeding K29.41
  superficial K29.30
    with bleeding K29.31
dietary counseling and surveillance Z71.3
due to diet deficiency E63.9
eosinophilic K52.81
giant hypertrophic K29.60
  with bleeding K29.61
granulomatous K29.60
  with bleeding K29.61
hypertrophic (mucosa) K29.60
  with bleeding K29.61
nervous F54
spastic K29.60
  with bleeding K29.61
specified NEC K29.60
  with bleeding K29.61
superficial chronic K29.30
  with bleeding K29.31
tuberculous A18.83
viral NEC A08.4
Gastrocarcinoma — *see* Neoplasm, malignant, stomach
Gastrocolic — *see* condition
Gastrodisciasis, gastrodiscoidiasis B66.8
Gastroduodenitis K29.90
with bleeding K29.91
virus, viral A08.4
  specified type NEC A08.39
Gastrodynia — *see* Pain, abdominal
Gastroenteritis (acute) (chronic) (noninfectious) (*see also* Enteritis) K52.9
allergic K52.2
dietetic K52.2
drug-induced K52.1
due to
  Cryptosporidium A07.2
  drugs K52.1
  food poisoning — *see* Intoxication, foodborne
  radiation K52.0
eosinophilic K52.81
epidemic (infectious) A09
food hypersensitivity K52.2
infectious — *see* Enteritis, infectious
influenzal — *see* Influenza, with gastroenteritis
noninfectious K52.9
  specified NEC K52.89
rotaviral A08.0
Salmonella A02.0
toxic K52.1
viral NEC A08.4
  acute infectious A08.39
    type Norwalk A08.11
  infantile (acute) A08.39
  Norwalk agent A08.11
  rotaviral A08.0
  severe of infants A08.39
  specified type NEC A08.39
Gastroenteropathy (*see also* Gastroenteritis) K52.9
acute, due to Norovirus A08.11
acute, due to Norwalk agent A08.11
infectious A09
Gastroenteroptosis K63.4
Gastroesophageal laceration- hemorrhage syndrome K22.6
Gastrointestinal — *see* condition
Gastrojejunal — *see* condition
Gastrojejunitis (*see also* Enteritis) K52.9
Gastrojejunocolic — *see* condition
Gastroliths K31.89
Gastromalacia K31.89
Gastroparalysis K31.84
diabetic — *see* Diabetes, gastroparalysis
Gastroparesis K31.84
diabetic — *see* Diabetes, by type, with gastroparesis
Gastropathy K31.9
congestive portal K31.89
erythematous K29.70
exudative K90.89
portal hypertensive K31.89
Gastroptosis K31.89
Gastrorrhagia K92.2
psychogenic F45.8
Gastroschisis (congenital) Q79.3

Gastrospasm (neurogenic) (reflex) K31.89
neuritic F45.8
psychogenic F45.8
Gastrostaxis — *see* Gastritis, with bleeding
Gastrostenosis K31.89
Gastrostomy
attention to Z43.1
status Z93.1
Gastrosuccorrhea (continuous) (intermittent) K31.89
neurotic F45.8
psychogenic F45.8
Gatophobia F40.218
Gaucher's disease or splenomegaly (adult) (infantile) E75.22
Gee (-Herter)(-Thaysen) **disease** (nontropical sprue) K90.0
Gélineau's syndrome G47.419
with cataplexy G47.411
Gemination, tooth, teeth K00.2
Gemistocytoma
specified site — *see* Neoplasm, malignant, by site
unspecified site C71.9
General, generalized — *see* condition
Genetic
carrier (status)
  cystic fibrosis Z14.1
  hemophilia A (asymptomatic) Z14.01
    symptomatic Z14.02
  specified NEC Z14.8
susceptibility to disease NEC Z15.89
  malignant neoplasm Z15.09
    breast Z15.01
    endometrium Z15.04
    ovary Z15.02
    prostate Z15.03
    specified NEC Z15.09
  multiple endocrine neoplasia Z15.81
Genital — *see* condition
Genito-anorectal syndrome A55
Genitourinary system — *see* condition
Genu
congenital Q74.1
extrorsum (acquired) (*see also* Deformity, varus, knee)
  congenital Q74.1
  sequelae (late effect) of rickets E64.3
introrsum (acquired) (*see also* Deformity, valgus, knee)
  congenital Q74.1
  sequelae (late effect) of rickets E64.3
rachitic (old) E64.3
recurvatum (acquired) (*see also* Deformity, limb, specified type NEC, lower leg)
  congenital Q68.2
  sequelae (late effect) of rickets E64.3
valgum (acquired) (knock-knee) M21.06- ☑
  congenital Q74.1
  sequelae (late effect) of rickets E64.3
varum (acquired) (bowleg) M21.16- ☑
  congenital Q74.1
  sequelae (late effect) of rickets E64.3
Geographic tongue K14.1
Geophagia — *see* Pica
Geotrichosis B48.3
stomatitis B48.3
Gephyrophobia F40.242
Gerbode defect Q21.0
GERD (gastroesophageal reflux disease) K21.9
Gerhardt's
disease (erythromelalgia) I73.81
syndrome (vocal cord paralysis) J38.00
  bilateral J38.02
  unilateral J38.01
German measles (*see also* Rubella)
exposure to Z20.4
Germinoblastoma (diffuse) C85.9- ☑
follicular C82.9- ☑
Germinoma — *see* Neoplasm, malignant, by site
Gerontoxon — *see* Degeneration, cornea, senile
Gerstmann's syndrome R48.8
developmental F81.2
Gerstmann-Sträussler-Scheinker syndrome (GSS) A81.82
Gestation (period) (*see also* Pregnancy)
ectopic — *see* Pregnancy, by site
multiple O30.9- ☑
  greater than quadruplets — *see* Pregnancy, multiple (gestation), specified NEC
  specified NEC — *see* Pregnancy, multiple (gestation), specified NEC

Gestational
mammary abscess O91.11- ☑
purulent mastitis O91.11- ☑
subareolar abscess O91.11- ☑
Ghon tubercle, primary infection A15.7
Ghost
teeth K00.4
vessels (cornea) H16.41- ☑
Ghoul hand A66.3
Gianotti-Crosti disease L44.4
Giant
cell
  epulis K06.8
  peripheral granuloma K06.8
esophagus, congenital Q39.5
kidney, congenital Q63.3
urticaria T78.3 ☑
  hereditary D84.1
Giardiasis A07.1
Gibert's disease or pityriasis L42
Giddiness R42
hysterical F44.89
psychogenic F45.8
Gierke's disease (glycogenosis I) E74.01
Gigantism (cerebral) (hypophyseal) (pituitary) E22.0
constitutional E34.4
Gilbert's disease or syndrome E80.4
Gilchrist's disease B40.9
Gilford-Hutchinson disease E34.8
Gilles de la Tourette's disease or syndrome (motor-verbal tic) F95.2
Gingivitis K05.10
acute (catarrhal) K05.00
  necrotizing A69.1
  nonplaque induced K05.01
  plaque induced K05.00
chronic (desquamative) (hyperplastic) (simple marginal) (ulcerative) K05.10
  nonplaque induced K05.11
  plaque induced K05.10
expulsiva — *see* Periodontitis
necrotizing ulcerative (acute) A69.1
pellagrous E52
  acute necrotizing A69.1
Vincent's A69.1
Gingivoglossitis K14.0
Gingivopericementitis — *see* Periodontitis
Gingivosis — *see* Gingivitis, chronic
Gingivostomatitis K05.10
herpesviral B00.2
necrotizing ulcerative (acute) A69.1
Gland, glandular — *see* condition
Glanders A24.0
Glanzmann (-Naegeli) **disease or thrombasthenia** D69.1
Glasgow coma scale
total score
  3-8 R40.243
  9-12 R40.242
  13-15 R40.241
Glass-blower's disease (cataract) — *see* Cataract, specified NEC
Glaucoma H40.9
with
  increased episcleral venous pressure H40.81- ☑
  pseudoexfoliation of lens — *see* Glaucoma, open angle, primary, capsular
absolute H44.51- ☑
angle-closure (primary) H40.20- ☑
  acute (attack) (crisis) H40.21- ☑
  chronic H40.22- ☑
  intermittent H40.23- ☑
  residual stage H40.24- ☑
borderline H40.00- ☑
capsular (with pseudoexfoliation of lens) — *see* Glaucoma, open angle, primary, capsular
childhood Q15.0
closed angle — *see* Glaucoma, angle-closure
congenital Q15.0
corticosteroid-induced — *see* Glaucoma, secondary, drugs
hypersecretion H40.82- ☑
in (due to)
  amyloidosis E85.4 [H42]
  aniridia Q13.1 [H42]
  concussion of globe — *see* Glaucoma, secondary, trauma

☑ Additional Character Required — Refer to the Tabular List for Character Selection   ▽ Subterms under main terms may continue to next column or page

Glaucoma — *continued*
  in — *continued*
    dislocation of lens — *see* Glaucoma, secondary
    disorder of lens NEC — *see* Glaucoma, secondary
    drugs — *see* Glaucoma, secondary, drugs
    endocrine disease NOS E34.9 [H42]
    eye
      inflammation — *see* Glaucoma, secondary, inflammation
      trauma — *see* Glaucoma, secondary, trauma
    hypermature cataract — *see* Glaucoma, secondary
    iridocyclitis — *see* Glaucoma, secondary, inflammation
    lens disorder — *see* Glaucoma, secondary
    Lowe's syndrome E72.03 [H42]
    metabolic disease NOS E88.9 [H42]
    ocular disorders NEC — *see* Glaucoma, secondary
    onchocerciasis B73.02
    pupillary block — *see* Glaucoma, secondary
    retinal vein occlusion — *see* Glaucoma, secondary
    Rieger's anomaly Q13.81 [H42]
    rubeosis of iris — *see* Glaucoma, secondary
    tumor of globe — *see* Glaucoma, secondary
  infantile Q15.0
  low tension — *see* Glaucoma, open angle, primary, low-tension
  malignant H40.83- ☑
  narrow angle — *see* Glaucoma, angle-closure
  newborn Q15.0
  noncongestive (chronic) — *see* Glaucoma, open angle
  nonobstructive — *see* Glaucoma, open angle
  obstructive (*see also* Glaucoma, angle-closure)
    due to lens changes — *see* Glaucoma, secondary
  open angle H40.10- ☑
    primary H40.11- ☑
      capsular (with pseudoexfoliation of lens) H40.14- ☑
      low-tension H40.12- ☑
      pigmentary H40.13- ☑
      residual stage H40.15- ☑
  phacolytic — *see* Glaucoma, secondary
  pigmentary — *see* Glaucoma, open angle, primary, pigmentary
  postinfectious — *see* Glaucoma, secondary, inflammation
  secondary (to) H40.5- ☑
    drugs H40.6- ☑
    inflammation H40.4- ☑
    trauma H40.3- ☑
  simple (chronic) H40.11 ☑
  simplex H40.11 ☑
  specified type NEC H40.89
  suspect H40.00- ☑
  syphilitic A52.71
  traumatic (*see also* Glaucoma, secondary, trauma)
    newborn (birth injury) P15.3
  tuberculous A18.59
Glaucomatous flecks (subcapsular) — *see* Cataract, complicated
Glazed tongue K14.4
Gleet (gonococcal) A54.01
Glénard's disease K63.4
Glioblastoma (multiforme)
  with sarcomatous component
    specified site — *see* Neoplasm, malignant, by site
    unspecified site C71.9
  giant cell
    specified site — *see* Neoplasm, malignant, by site
    unspecified site C71.9
  specified site — *see* Neoplasm, malignant, by site
  unspecified site C71.9
Glioma (malignant)
  astrocytic
    specified site — *see* Neoplasm, malignant, by site
    unspecified site C71.9
  mixed
    specified site — *see* Neoplasm, malignant, by site
    unspecified site C71.9
  nose Q30.8
  specified site NEC — *see* Neoplasm, malignant, by site
  subependymal D43.2
    specified site — *see* Neoplasm, uncertain behavior, by site
    unspecified site D43.2
  unspecified site C71.9
Gliomatosis cerebri C71.0

Glioneuroma — *see* Neoplasm, uncertain behavior, by site
Gliosarcoma
  specified site — *see* Neoplasm, malignant, by site
  unspecified site C71.9
Gliosis (cerebral) G93.89
  spinal G95.89
Glisson's disease — *see* Rickets
Globinuria R82.3
Globus (hystericus) F45.8
Glomangioma D18.00
  intra-abdominal D18.03
  intracranial D18.02
  skin D18.01
  specified site NEC D18.09
Glomangiomyoma D18.00
  intra-abdominal D18.03
  intracranial D18.02
  skin D18.01
  specified site NEC D18.09
Glomangiosarcoma — *see* Neoplasm, connective tissue, malignant
Glomerular
  disease in syphilis A52.75
  nephritis — *see* Glomerulonephritis
Glomerulitis — *see* Glomerulonephritis
Glomerulonephritis (*see also* Nephritis) N05.9
  with
    edema — *see* Nephrosis
    minimal change N05.0
    minor glomerular abnormality N05.0
  acute N00.9
  chronic N03.9
  crescentic (diffuse) NEC (*see also* N00-N07 with fourth character .7) N05.7
  dense deposit (*see also* N00-N07 with fourth character .6) N05.6
  diffuse
    crescentic (*see also* N00-N07 with fourth character .7) N05.7
    endocapillary proliferative (*see also* N00-N07 with fourth character .4) N05.4
    membranous (*see also* N00-N07 with fourth character .2) N05.2
    mesangial proliferative (*see also* N00-N07 with fourth character .3) N05.3
    mesangiocapillary (*see also* N00-N07 with fourth character .5) N05.5
    sclerosing N05.8
  endocapillary proliferative (diffuse) NEC (*see also* N00-N07 with fourth character .4) N05.4
  extracapillary NEC (*see also* N00-N07 with fourth character .7) N05.7
  focal (and segmental) (*see also* N00-N07 with fourth character .1) N05.1
  hypocomplementemic — *see* Glomerulonephritis, membranoproliferative
  IgA — *see* Nephropathy, IgA
  immune complex (circulating) NEC N05.8
  in (due to)
    amyloidosis E85.4 [N08]
    bilharziasis B65.9 [N08]
    cryoglobulinemia D89.1 [N08]
    defibrination syndrome D65 [N08]
    diabetes mellitus — *see* Diabetes, glomerulosclerosis
    disseminated intravascular coagulation D65 [N08]
    Fabry (-Anderson) disease E75.21 [N08]
    Goodpasture's syndrome M31.0
    hemolytic-uremic syndrome D59.3
    Henoch (-Schönlein) purpura D69.0 [N08]
    lecithin cholesterol acyltransferase deficiency E78.6 [N08]
    microscopic polyangiitis M31.7 [N08]
    multiple myeloma C90.0- ☑ [N08]
    Plasmodium malariae B52.0
    schistosomiasis B65.9 [N08]
    sepsis A41.9 [N08]
      streptococcal A40- ☑ [N08]
    sickle-cell disorders D57.- ☑ [N08]
    strongyloidiasis B78.9 [N08]
    subacute bacterial endocarditis I33.0 [N08]
    syphilis (late) congenital A50.59 [N08]
    systemic lupus erythematosus M32.14
    thrombotic thrombocytopenic purpura M31.1 [N08]
    typhoid fever A01.09
    Waldenström macroglobulinemia C88.0 [N08]

Glomerulonephritis — *continued*
  in — *continued*
    Wegener's granulomatosis M31.31
  latent or quiescent N03.9
  lobular, lobulonodular — *see* Glomerulonephritis, membranoproliferative
  membranoproliferative (diffuse)(type 1 or 3) (*see also* N00-N07 with fourth character .5) N05.5
    dense deposit (type 2) NEC (*see also* N00-N07 with fourth character .6) N05.6
  membranous (diffuse) NEC (*see also* N00-N07 with fourth character .2) N05.2
  mesangial
    IgA/IgG — *see* Nephropathy, IgA
    proliferative (diffuse) NEC (*see also* N00-N07 with fourth character .3) N05.3
  mesangiocapillary (diffuse) NEC (*see also* N00-N07 with fourth character .5) N05.5
  necrotic, necrotizing NEC (*see also* N00- N07 with fourth character .8) N05.8
  nodular — *see* Glomerulonephritis, membranoproliferative
  poststreptococcal NEC N05.9
    acute N00.9
    chronic N03.9
    rapidly progressive N01.9
  proliferative NEC (*see also* N00-N07 with fourth character .8) N05.8
    diffuse (lupus) M32.14
  rapidly progressive N01.9
  sclerosing, diffuse N05.8
  specified pathology NEC (*see also* N00- N07 with fourth character .8) N05.8
  subacute N01.9
Glomerulopathy — *see* Glomerulonephritis
Glomerulosclerosis (*see also* Sclerosis, renal)
  intercapillary (nodular) (with diabetes) — *see* Diabetes, glomerulosclerosis
  intracapillary — *see* Diabetes, glomerulosclerosis
Glossagra K14.6
Glossalgia K14.6
Glossitis (chronic superficial) (gangrenous) (Moeller's) K14.0
  areata exfoliativa K14.1
  atrophic K14.4
  benign migratory K14.1
  cortical superficial, sclerotic K14.0
  Hunter's D51.0
  interstitial, sclerous K14.0
  median rhomboid K14.2
  pellagrous E52
  superficial, chronic K14.0
Glossocele K14.8
Glossodynia K14.6
  exfoliativa K14.4
Glossoncus K14.8
Glossopathy K14.9
Glossophytia K14.3
Glossoplegia K14.8
Glossoptosis K14.8
Glossopyrosis K14.6
Glossotrichia K14.3
Glossy skin L90.8
Glottis — *see* condition
Glottitis (*see also* Laryngitis) J04.0
Glucagonoma
  pancreas
    benign D13.7
    malignant C25.4
    uncertain behavior D37.8
  specified site NEC
    benign — *see* Neoplasm, benign, by site
    malignant — *see* Neoplasm, malignant, by site
    uncertain behavior — *see* Neoplasm, uncertain behavior, by site
  unspecified site
    benign D13.7
    malignant C25.4
    uncertain behavior D37.8
Glucoglycinuria E72.51
Glucose-galactose malabsorption E74.39
Glue
  ear — *see* Otitis, media, nonsuppurative, chronic, mucoid
  sniffing (airplane) — *see* Abuse, drug, inhalant
    dependence — *see* Dependence, drug, inhalant
Glutaric aciduria E72.3

Subterms under main terms may continue to next column or page
☑ Additional Character Required — Refer to the Tabular List for Character Selection
153

Index

Glycinemia — Gout, gouty

Glycinemia E72.51
Glycinuria (renal) (with ketosis) E72.09
Glycogen
  infiltration — *see* Disease, glycogen storage
  storage disease — *see* Disease, glycogen storage
Glycogenosis (diffuse) (generalized) (*see also* Disease,
    glycogen storage)
  cardiac E74.02 [I43]
  diabetic, secondary — *see* Diabetes, glycogenosis,
      secondary
  pulmonary interstitial J84.842
Glycopenia E16.2
Glycosuria R81
  renal E74.8
Gnathostoma spinigerum (infection) (infestation),
    gnathostomiasis (wandering swelling) B83.1
Goiter (plunging) (substernal) E04.9
  with
    hyperthyroidism (recurrent) — *see* Hyperthy-
        roidism, with, goiter
    thyrotoxicosis — *see* Hyperthyroidism, with, goiter
  adenomatous — *see* Goiter, nodular
  cancerous C73
  congenital (nontoxic) E03.0
    diffuse E03.0
    parenchymatous E03.0
    transitory, with normal functioning P72.0
  cystic E04.2
    due to iodine-deficiency E01.1
  due to
    enzyme defect in synthesis of thyroid hormone
        E07.1
    iodine-deficiency (endemic) E01.2
  dyshormonogenetic (familial) E07.1
  endemic (iodine-deficiency) E01.2
    diffuse E01.0
    multinodular E01.1
  exophthalmic — *see* Hyperthyroidism, with, goiter
  iodine-deficiency (endemic) E01.2
    diffuse E01.0
    multinodular E01.1
    nodular E01.1
  lingual Q89.2
  lymphadenoid E06.3
  malignant C73
  multinodular (cystic) (nontoxic) E04.2
    toxic or with hyperthyroidism E05.20
      with thyroid storm E05.21
  neonatal NEC P72.0
  nodular (nontoxic) (due to) E04.9
    with
      hyperthyroidism E05.20
        with thyroid storm E05.21
      thyrotoxicosis E05.20
        with thyroid storm E05.21
    endemic E01.1
    iodine-deficiency E01.1
    sporadic E04.9
    toxic E05.20
      with thyroid storm E05.21
  nontoxic E04.9
    diffuse (colloid) E04.0
    multinodular E04.2
    simple E04.0
    specified NEC E04.8
    uninodular E04.1
  simple E04.0
  toxic — *see* Hyperthyroidism, with, goiter
  uninodular (nontoxic) E04.1
    toxic or with hyperthyroidism E05.10
      with thyroid storm E05.11
Goiter-deafness syndrome E07.1
Goldberg syndrome Q89.8
Goldberg-Maxwell syndrome E34.51
Goldblatt's hypertension or kidney I70.1
Goldenhar (-Gorlin) **syndrome** Q87.0
Goldflam-Erb disease or syndrome G70.00
  with exacerbation (acute) G70.01
  in crisis G70.01
Goldscheider's disease Q81.8
Goldstein's disease (familial hemorrhagic telangiectasia)
    I78.0
Golfer's elbow — *see* Epicondylitis, medial
Gonadoblastoma
  specified site — *see* Neoplasm, uncertain behavior,
      by site
  unspecified site
    female D39.10

Gonadoblastoma — *continued*
  unspecified site — *continued*
    male D40.10
Gonecystitis — *see* Vesiculitis
Gongylonemiasis B83.8
Goniosynechiae — *see* Adhesions, iris, goniosynechiae
Gonococcemia A54.86
Gonococcus, gonococcal (disease) (infection) (*see also*
    condition) A54.9
  anus A54.6
  bursa, bursitis A54.49
  conjunctiva, conjunctivitis (neonatorum) A54.31
  endocardium A54.83
  eye A54.30
    conjunctivitis A54.31
    iridocyclitis A54.32
    keratitis A54.33
    newborn A54.31
    other specified A54.39
  fallopian tubes (acute) (chronic) A54.24
  genitourinary (organ) (system) (tract) (acute)
    lower A54.00
      with abscess (accessory gland) (periurethral)
          A54.1
    upper (*see also* condition) A54.29
  heart A54.83
  iridocyclitis A54.32
  joint A54.42
  lymphatic (gland) (node) A54.89
  meninges, meningitis A54.81
  musculoskeletal A54.40
    arthritis A54.42
    osteomyelitis A54.43
    other specified A54.49
    spondylopathy A54.41
  pelviperitonitis A54.24
  pelvis (acute) (chronic) A54.24
  pharynx A54.5
  proctitis A54.6
  pyosalpinx (acute) (chronic) A54.24
  rectum A54.6
  skin A54.89
  specified site NEC A54.89
  tendon sheath A54.49
  throat A54.5
  urethra (acute) (chronic) A54.01
    with abscess (accessory gland) (periurethral) A54.1
  vulva (acute) (chronic) A54.02
Gonocytoma
  specified site — *see* Neoplasm, uncertain behavior,
      by site
  unspecified site
    female D39.10
    male D40.10
Gonorrhea (acute) (chronic) A54.9
  Bartholin's gland (acute) (chronic) (purulent) A54.02
    with abscess (accessory gland) (periurethral) A54.1
  bladder A54.01
  cervix A54.03
  conjunctiva, conjunctivitis (neonatorum) A54.31
  contact Z20.2
  Cowper's gland (with abscess) A54.1
  exposure to Z20.2
  fallopian tube (acute) (chronic) A54.24
  kidney (acute) (chronic) A54.21
  lower genitourinary tract A54.00
    with abscess (accessory gland) (periurethral) A54.1
  ovary (acute) (chronic) A54.24
  pelvis (acute) (chronic) A54.24
    female pelvic inflammatory disease A54.24
  penis A54.09
  prostate (acute) (chronic) A54.22
  seminal vesicle (acute) (chronic) A54.23
  specified site not listed (*see also* Gonococcus) A54.89
  spermatic cord (acute) (chronic) A54.23
  urethra A54.01
    with abscess (accessory gland) (periurethral) A54.1
  vagina A54.02
  vas deferens (acute) (chronic) A54.23
  vulva A54.02
Goodall's disease A08.19
Goodpasture's syndrome M31.0
Gopalan's syndrome (burning feet) E53.0
Gorlin-Chaudry Moss syndrome Q87.0
Gottron's papules L94.4
Gougerot-Blum syndrome (pigmented purpuric
    lichenoid dermatitis) L81.7

Gougerot-Carteaud disease or syndrome (confluent
    reticulate papillomatosis) L83
Gougerot's syndrome (trisymptomatic) L81.7
Gouley's syndrome (constrictive pericarditis) I31.1
Goundou A66.6
Gout, chronic (*see also* Gout, gouty) M1A.9 ☑ (*following*
    M08)
  drug-induced M1A.20 ☑ (*following* M08)
    ankle M1A.27- ☑ (*following* M08)
    elbow M1A.22- ☑ (*following* M08)
    foot joint M1A.27- ☑ (*following* M08)
    hand joint M1A.24- ☑ (*following* M08)
    hip M1A.25- ☑ (*following* M08)
    knee M1A.26- ☑ (*following* M08)
    multiple site M1A.29- ☑ (*following* M08)
    shoulder M1A.21- ☑ (*following* M08)
    vertebrae M1A.28 ☑ (*following* M08)
    wrist M1A.23- ☑ (*following* M08)
  idiopathic M1A.00 ☑ (*following* M08)
    ankle M1A.07- ☑ (*following* M08)
    elbow M1A.02- ☑ (*following* M08)
    foot joint M1A.07- ☑ (*following* M08)
    hand joint M1A.04- ☑ (*following* M08)
    hip M1A.05- ☑ (*following* M08)
    knee M1A.06- ☑ (*following* M08)
    multiple site M1A.09 ☑ (*following* M08)
    shoulder M1A.01- ☑ (*following* M08)
    vertebrae M1A.08 ☑ (*following* M08)
    wrist M1A.03- ☑ (*following* M08)
  in (due to) renal impairment M1A.30 ☑ (*following*
      M08)
    ankle M1A.37- ☑ (*following* M08)
    elbow M1A.32- ☑ (*following* M08)
    foot joint M1A.37- ☑ (*following* M08)
    hand joint M1A.34- ☑ (*following* M08)
    hip M1A.35- ☑ (*following* M08)
    knee M1A.36- ☑ (*following* M08)
    multiple site M1A.39 ☑ (*following* M08)
    shoulder M1A.31- ☑ (*following* M08)
    vertebrae M1A.38 ☑ (*following* M08)
    wrist M1A.33- ☑ (*following* M08)
  lead-induced M1A.10 ☑ (*following* M08)
    ankle M1A.17- ☑ (*following* M08)
    elbow M1A.12- ☑ (*following* M08)
    foot joint M1A.17- ☑ (*following* M08)
    hand joint M1A.14- ☑ (*following* M08)
    hip M1A.15- ☑ (*following* M08)
    knee M1A.16- ☑ (*following* M08)
    multiple site M1A.19 ☑ (*following* M08)
    shoulder M1A.11- ☑ (*following* M08)
    vertebrae M1A.18 ☑ (*following* M08)
    wrist M1A.13- ☑ (*following* M08)
  primary — *see* Gout, chronic, idiopathic
  saturnine — *see* Gout, chronic, lead-induced
  secondary NEC M1A.40 ☑ (*following* M08)
    ankle M1A.47- ☑ (*following* M08)
    elbow M1A.42- ☑ (*following* M08)
    foot joint M1A.47- ☑ (*following* M08)
    hand joint M1A.44- ☑ (*following* M08)
    hip M1A.45- ☑ (*following* M08)
    knee M1A.46- ☑ (*following* M08)
    multiple site M1A.49 ☑ (*following* M08)
    shoulder M1A.41- ☑ (*following* M08)
    vertebrae M1A.48 ☑ (*following* M08)
    wrist M1A.43- ☑ (*following* M08)
  syphilitic (*see also* subcategory M14.8-) A52.77
  tophi M1A.9 ☑ (*following* M08)
Gout, gouty (acute) (attack) (flare) (*see also* Gout,
    chronic) M10.9
  drug-induced M10.20
    ankle M10.27- ☑
    elbow M10.22- ☑
    foot joint M10.27- ☑
    hand joint M10.24- ☑
    hip M10.25- ☑
    knee M10.26- ☑
    multiple site M10.29
    shoulder M10.21- ☑
    vertebrae M10.28
    wrist M10.23- ☑
  idiopathic M10.00
    ankle M10.07- ☑
    elbow M10.02- ☑
    foot joint M10.07- ☑
    hand joint M10.04- ☑
    hip M10.05- ☑

☑ **Additional Character Required** — Refer to the Tabular List for Character Selection   ☑ **Subterms under main terms may continue to next column or page**

Gout, gouty — *continued*
  idiopathic — *continued*
    knee M10.06- ☑
    multiple site M10.09
    shoulder M10.01- ☑
    vertebrae M10.08
    wrist M10.03- ☑
  in (due to) renal impairment M10.30
    ankle M10.37- ☑
    elbow M10.32- ☑
    foot joint M10.37- ☑
    hand joint M10.34- ☑
    hip M10.35- ☑
    knee M10.36- ☑
    multiple site M10.39
    shoulder M10.31- ☑
    vertebrae M10.38
    wrist M10.33- ☑
  lead-induced M10.10
    ankle M10.17- ☑
    elbow M10.12- ☑
    foot joint M10.17- ☑
    hand joint M10.14- ☑
    hip M10.15- ☑
    knee M10.16- ☑
    multiple site M10.19
    shoulder M10.11- ☑
    vertebrae M10.18
    wrist M10.13- ☑
  primary — *see* Gout, idiopathic
  saturnine — *see* Gout, lead-induced
  secondary NEC M10.40
    ankle M10.47- ☑
    elbow M10.42- ☑
    foot joint M10.47- ☑
    hand joint M10.44- ☑
    hip M10.45- ☑
    knee M10.46- ☑
    multiple site M10.49
    shoulder M10.41- ☑
    vertebrae M10.48
    wrist M10.43- ☑
  syphilitic (*see also* subcategory M14.8-) A52.77
  tophi — *see* Gout, chronic
Gower's
  muscular dystrophy G71.0
  syndrome (vasovagal attack) R55
Gradenigo's syndrome — *see* Otitis, media, suppurative, acute
Graefe's disease — *see* Strabismus, paralytic, ophthalmoplegia, progressive
Graft-versus-host disease D89.813
  acute D89.810
  acute on chronic D89.812
  chronic D89.811
Grain mite (itch) B88.0
Grainhandler's disease or lung J67.8
Grand mal — *see* Epilepsy, generalized, specified NEC
Grand multipara status only (not pregnant) Z64.1
  pregnant — *see* Pregnancy, complicated by, grand multiparity
Granite worker's lung J62.8
Granular (*see also* condition)
  inflammation, pharynx J31.2
  kidney (contracting) — *see* Sclerosis, renal
  liver K74.69
Granulation tissue (abnormal) (excessive) L92.9
  postmastoidectomy cavity — *see* Complications, postmastoidectomy, granulation
Granulocytopenia (primary) (malignant) — *see* Agranulocytosis
Granuloma L92.9
  abdomen K66.8
    from residual foreign body L92.3
    pyogenicum L98.0
  actinic L57.5
  annulare (perforating) L92.0
  apical K04.5
  aural — *see* Otitis, externa, specified NEC
  beryllium (skin) L92.3
  bone
    eosinophilic C96.6
    from residual foreign body — *see* Osteomyelitis, specified type NEC
    lung C96.6
  brain (any site) G06.0
    schistosomiasis B65.9 [G07]

Granuloma — *continued*
  canaliculus lacrimalis — *see* Granuloma, lacrimal
  candidal (cutaneous) B37.2
  cerebral (any site) G06.0
  coccidioidal (primary) (progressive) B38.7
    lung B38.1
    meninges B38.4
  colon K63.89
  conjunctiva H11.22- ☑
  dental K04.5
  ear, middle — *see* Cholesteatoma
  eosinophilic C96.6
    bone C96.6
    lung C96.6
    oral mucosa K13.4
    skin L92.2
  eyelid H01.8
  facial (e) L92.2
  foreign body (in soft tissue) NEC M60.20
    ankle M60.27- ☑
    foot M60.27- ☑
    forearm M60.23- ☑
    hand M60.24- ☑
    in operation wound — *see* Foreign body, accidentally left during a procedure
    lower leg M60.26- ☑
    pelvic region M60.25- ☑
    shoulder region M60.21- ☑
    skin L92.3
    specified site NEC M60.28
    subcutaneous tissue L92.3
    thigh M60.25- ☑
    upper arm M60.22- ☑
  gangraenescens M31.2
  genito-inguinale A58
  giant cell (central) (reparative) (jaw) M27.1
    gingiva (peripheral) K06.8
  gland (lymph) I88.8
  hepatic NEC K75.3
    in (due to)
      berylliosis J63.2 [K77]
      sarcoidosis D86.89
  Hodgkin C81.9 ☑
  ileum K63.89
  infectious B99.9
    specified NEC B99.8
  inguinale (Donovan) (venereal) A58
  intestine NEC K63.89
  intracranial (any site) G06.0
  intraspinal (any part) G06.1
  iridocyclitis — *see* Iridocyclitis, chronic
  jaw (bone) (central) M27.1
    reparative giant cell M27.1
  kidney (*see also* Infection, kidney) N15.8
  lacrimal H04.81- ☑
  larynx J38.7
  lethal midline (faciale(e)) M31.2
  liver NEC — *see* Granuloma, hepatic
  lung (infectious) (*see also* Fibrosis, lung)
    coccidioidal B38.1
    eosinophilic C96.6
  Majocchi's B35.8
  malignant (facial(e)) M31.2
  mandible (central) M27.1
  midline (lethal) M31.2
  monilial (cutaneous) B37.2
  nasal sinus — *see* Sinusitis
  operation wound T81.89 ☑
    foreign body — *see* Foreign body, accidentally left during a procedure
    stitch T81.89 ☑
    talc — *see* Foreign body, accidentally left during a procedure
  oral mucosa K13.4
  orbit, orbital H05.11- ☑
  paracoccidioidal B41.8
  penis, venereal A58
  periapical K04.5
  peritoneum K66.8
    due to ova of helminths NOS (*see also* Helminthiasis) B83.9 [K67]
  postmastoidectomy cavity — *see* Complications, postmastoidectomy, recurrent cholesteatoma
  prostate N42.89
  pudendi (ulcerating) A58
  pulp, internal (tooth) K03.3
  pyogenic, pyogenicum (of) (skin) L98.0
    gingiva K06.8

Granuloma — *continued*
  pyogenic, pyogenicum — *continued*
    maxillary alveolar ridge K04.5
    oral mucosa K13.4
  rectum K62.89
  reticulohistiocytic D76.3
  rubrum nasi L74.8
  Schistosoma — *see* Schistosomiasis
  septic (skin) L98.0
  silica (skin) L92.3
  sinus (accessory) (infective) (nasal) — *see* Sinusitis
  skin L92.9
    from residual foreign body L92.3
    pyogenicum L98.0
  spine
    syphilitic (epidural) A52.19
    tuberculous A18.01
  stitch (postoperative) T81.89 ☑
  suppurative (skin) L98.0
  swimming pool A31.1
  talc (*see also* Granuloma, foreign body)
    in operation wound — *see* Foreign body, accidentally left during a procedure
  telangiectaticum (skin) L98.0
  tracheostomy J95.09
  trichophyticum B35.8
  tropicum A66.4
  umbilicus L92.9
  urethra N36.8
  uveitis — *see* Iridocyclitis, chronic
  vagina A58
  venereum A58
  vocal cord J38.3
Granulomatosis L92.9
  lymphoid C83.8- ☑
  miliary (listerial) A32.89
  necrotizing, respiratory M31.30
  progressive septic D71
  specified NEC L92.8
  Wegener's M31.30
    with renal involvement M31.31
Granulomatous tissue (abnormal) (excessive) L92.9
Granulosis rubra nasi L74.8
Graphite fibrosis (of lung) J63.3
Graphospasm F48.8
  organic G25.89
Grating scapula M89.8X1
Gravel (urinary) — *see* Calculus, urinary
Graves' disease — *see* Hyperthyroidism, with, goiter
Gravis — *see* condition
Grawitz tumor C64.- ☑
Gray syndrome (newborn) P93.0
Grayness, hair (premature) L67.1
  congenital Q84.2
Green sickness D50.8
Greenfield's disease
  meaning
    concentric sclerosis (encephalitis periaxialis concentrica) G37.5
    metachromatic leukodystrophy E75.25
Greenstick fracture — code as Fracture, by site
Grey syndrome (newborn) P93.0
Grief F43.21
  prolonged F43.29
  reaction (*see also* Disorder, adjustment) F43.20
Griesinger's disease B76.9
Grinder's lung or pneumoconiosis J62.8
Grinding, teeth
  psychogenic F45.8
  sleep related G47.63
Grip
  Dabney's B33.0
  devil's B33.0
Grippe, grippal (*see also* Influenza)
  Balkan A78
  summer, of Italy A93.1
Grisel's disease M43.6
Groin — *see* condition
Grooved tongue K14.5
Ground itch B76.9
Grover's disease or syndrome L11.1
Growing pains, children R29.898
Growth (fungoid) (neoplastic) (new) (*see also* Neoplasm)
  adenoid (vegetative) J35.8
  benign — *see* Neoplasm, benign, by site
  malignant — *see* Neoplasm, malignant, by site
  rapid, childhood Z00.2

Growth — *continued*
  secondary — *see* Neoplasm, secondary, by site
Gruby's disease B35.Ø
Gubler-Millard paralysis or syndrome G46.3
Guerin-Stern syndrome Q74.3
Guidance, insufficient anterior (occlusal) M26.54
Guillain-Barré disease or syndrome G61.Ø
  sequelae G65.Ø
Guinea worms (infection) (infestation) B72
Guinon's disease (motor-verbal tic) F95.2
Gull's disease EØ3.4
Gum — *see* condition
Gumboil KØ4.7
  with sinus KØ4.6
Gumma (syphilitic) A52.79
  artery A52.Ø9
    cerebral A52.Ø4
  bone A52.77
    of yaws (late) A66.6
  brain A52.19
  cauda equina A52.19
  central nervous system A52.3
  ciliary body A52.71
  congenital A5Ø.59
  eyelid A52.71
  heart A52.Ø6
  intracranial A52.19
  iris A52.71
  kidney A52.75
  larynx A52.73
  leptomeninges A52.19
  liver A52.74
  meninges A52.19
  myocardium A52.Ø6
  nasopharynx A52.73
  neurosyphilitic A52.3
  nose A52.73
  orbit A52.71
  palate (soft) A52.79
  penis A52.76
  pericardium A52.Ø6
  pharynx A52.73
  pituitary A52.79
  scrofulous (tuberculous) A18.4
  skin A52.79
  specified site NEC A52.79
  spinal cord A52.19
  tongue A52.79
  tonsil A52.73
  trachea A52.73
  tuberculous A18.4
  ulcerative due to yaws A66.4
  ureter A52.75
  yaws A66.4
    bone A66.6
Gunn's syndrome QØ7.8
Gunshot wound (*see also* Wound, open)
  fracture — *code as* Fracture, by site
  internal organs — *see* Injury, by site
Gynandrism Q56.Ø
Gynandroblastoma
  specified site — *see* Neoplasm, uncertain behavior, by site
  unspecified site
    female D39.1Ø
    male D4Ø.1Ø
Gynecological examination (periodic) (routine) ZØ1.419
  with abnormal findings ZØ1.411
Gynecomastia N62
Gynephobia F4Ø.291
Gyrate scalp Q82.8

H

H (Hartnup's) **disease** E72.Ø2
Haas' disease or osteochondrosis (juvenile) (head of humerus) — *see* Osteochondrosis, juvenile, humerus
Habit, habituation
  bad sleep Z72.821
  chorea F95.8
  disturbance, child F98.9
  drug — *see* Dependence, drug
  irregular sleep Z72.821
  laxative F55.2
  spasm — *see* Tic
  tic — *see* Tic

Haemophilus (H.) **influenzae, as cause of disease classified elsewhere** B96.3
Haff disease — *see* Poisoning, mercury
Hageman's factor defect, deficiency or disease D68.2
Haglund's disease or osteochondrosis (juvenile) (os tibiale externum) — *see* Osteochondrosis, juvenile, tarsus
Hailey-Hailey disease Q82.8
Hair (*see also* condition)
  plucking F63.3
    in stereotyped movement disorder F98.4
  tourniquet syndrome (*see also* Constriction, external, by site)
    finger S6Ø.44- ✓
    penis S3Ø.842 ✓
    thumb S6Ø.34- ✓
    toe S9Ø.44- ✓
Hairball in stomach T18.2 ✓
Hair-pulling, pathological (compulsive) F63.3
Hairy black tongue K14.3
Half vertebra Q76.49
Halitosis R19.6
Hallerman-Streiff syndrome Q87.Ø
Hallervorden-Spatz disease G23.Ø
Hallopeau's acrodermatitis or disease L4Ø.2
Hallucination R44.3
  auditory R44.Ø
  gustatory R44.2
  olfactory R44.2
  specified NEC R44.2
  tactile R44.2
  visual R44.1
Hallucinosis (chronic) F28
  alcoholic (acute) F1Ø.951
    in
      abuse F1Ø.151
      dependence F1Ø.251
  drug-induced F19.951
    cannabis F12.951
    cocaine F14.951
    hallucinogen F16.151
    in
      abuse F19.151
        cannabis F12.151
        cocaine F14.151
        hallucinogen F16.151
        inhalant F18.151
        opioid F11.151
        sedative, anxiolytic or hypnotic F13.151
        stimulant NEC F15.151
      dependence F19.251
        cannabis F12.251
        cocaine F14.251
        hallucinogen F16.251
        inhalant F18.251
        opioid F11.251
        sedative, anxiolytic or hypnotic F13.251
        stimulant NEC F15.251
    inhalant F18.951
    opioid F11.951
    sedative, anxiolytic or hypnotic F13.951
    stimulant NEC F15.951
  organic FØ6.Ø
Hallux
  deformity (acquired) NEC M2Ø.5X- ✓
  limitus M2Ø.5X- ✓
  malleus (acquired) NEC M2Ø.3- ✓
  rigidus (acquired) M2Ø.2- ✓
    congenital Q74.2
    sequelae (late effect) of rickets E64.3
  valgus (acquired) M2Ø.1- ✓
    congenital Q66.6
  varus (acquired) M2Ø.3- ✓
    congenital Q66.3
Halo, visual H53.19
Hamartoma, hamartoblastoma Q85.9
  epithelial (gingival), odontogenic, central or peripheral — *see* Cyst, calcifying odontogenic
Hamartosis Q85.9
Hamman-Rich syndrome J84.114
Hammer toe (acquired) NEC (*see also* Deformity, toe, hammer toe)
  congenital Q66.89
  sequelae (late effect) of rickets E64.3
Hand — *see* condition
Hand-foot syndrome L27.1

Handicap, handicapped
  educational Z55.9
    specified NEC Z55.8
Hand-Schüller-Christian disease or syndrome C96.5
Hanging (asphyxia) (strangulation) (suffocation) — *see* Asphyxia, traumatic, due to mechanical threat
Hangnail (*see also* Cellulitis, digit)
  with lymphangitis — *see* Lymphangitis, acute, digit
Hangover (alcohol) F1Ø.129
Hanhart's syndrome Q87.Ø
Hanot-Chauffard (-Troisier) **syndrome** E83.19
Hanot's cirrhosis or disease K74.3
Hansen's disease — *see* Leprosy
Hantaan virus disease (Korean hemorrhagic fever) A98.5
Hantavirus disease (with renal manifestations) (Dobrava) (Puumala) (Seoul) A98.5
  with pulmonary manifestations (Andes) (Bayou) (Bermejo) (Black Creek Canal) (Choclo) (Juquitiba) (Laguna negra) (Lechiguanas) (New York) (Oran) (Sin nombre) B33.4
Happy puppet syndrome Q93.5
Harada's disease or syndrome H3Ø.81- ✓
Hardening
  artery — *see* Arteriosclerosis
  brain G93.89
Harelip (complete) (incomplete) — *see* Cleft, lip
Harlequin (newborn) Q8Ø.4
Harley's disease D59.6
Harmful use (of)
  alcohol F1Ø.1Ø
  anxiolytics — *see* Abuse, drug, sedative
  cannabinoids — *see* Abuse, drug, cannabis
  cocaine — *see* Abuse, drug, cocaine
  drug — *see* Abuse, drug
  hallucinogens — *see* Abuse, drug, hallucinogen
  hypnotics — *see* Abuse, drug, sedative
  opioids — *see* Abuse, drug, opioid
  PCP (phencyclidine) — *see* Abuse, drug, hallucinogen
  sedatives — *see* Abuse, drug, sedative
  stimulants NEC — *see* Abuse, drug, stimulant
Harris' lines — *see* Arrest, epiphyseal
Hartnup's disease E72.Ø2
Harvester's lung J67.Ø
Harvesting ovum for in vitro fertilization Z31.83
Hashimoto's disease or thyroiditis EØ6.3
Hashitoxicosis (transient) EØ6.3
Hassal-Henle bodies or warts (cornea) H18.49
Haut mal — *see* Epilepsy, generalized, specified NEC
Haverhill fever A25.1
Hay fever (*see also* Fever, hay) J3Ø.1
Hayem-Widal syndrome D59.8
Haygarth's nodes M15.8
Haymaker's lung J67.Ø
Hb (abnormal)
  Bart's disease D56.Ø
  disease — *see* Disease, hemoglobin
  trait — *see* Trait
Head — *see* condition
Headache R51
  allergic NEC G44.89
  associated with sexual activity G44.82
  chronic daily R51
  cluster G44.ØØ9
    chronic G44.Ø29
      intractable G44.Ø21
      not intractable G44.Ø29
    episodic G44.Ø19
      intractable G44.Ø11
      not intractable G44.Ø19
    intractable G44.ØØ1
    not intractable G44.ØØ9
  cough (primary) G44.83
  daily chronic R51
  drug-induced NEC G44.4Ø
    intractable G44.41
    not intractable G44.4Ø
  exertional (primary) G44.84
  histamine G44.ØØ9
    intractable G44.ØØ1
    not intractable G44.ØØ9
  hypnic G44.81
  lumbar puncture G97.1
  medication overuse G44.4Ø
    intractable G44.41
    not intractable G44.4Ø
  menstrual — *see* Migraine, menstrual
  migraine (type) (*see also* Migraine) G43.9Ø9

✓ **Additional Character Required** — Refer to the Tabular List for Character Selection   ▽ Subterms under main terms may continue to next column or page

Headache — *continued*
  nasal septum R51
  neuralgiform, short lasting unilateral, with conjunctival injection and tearing (SUNCT) G44.059
    intractable G44.051
    not intractable G44.059
  new daily persistent (NDPH) G44.52
  orgasmic G44.82
  periodic syndromes in adults and children G43.C0 (*following* G43.7)
    with refractory migraine G43.C1 (*following* G43.7)
    without refractory migraine G43.C0 (*following* G43.7)
    intractable G43.C1 (*following* G43.7)
    not intractable G43.C0 (*following* G43.7)
  postspinal puncture G97.1
  post-traumatic G44.309
    acute G44.319
      intractable G44.311
      not intractable G44.319
    chronic G44.329
      intractable G44.321
      not intractable G44.329
    intractable G44.301
    not intractable G44.309
  pre-menstrual — *see* Migraine, menstrual
  preorgasmic G44.82
  primary
    cough G44.83
    exertional G44.84
    stabbing G44.85
    thunderclap G44.53
  rebound G44.40
    intractable G44.41
    not intractable G44.40
  short lasting unilateral neuralgiform, with conjunctival injection and tearing (SUNCT) G44.059
    intractable G44.051
    not intractable G44.059
  specified syndrome NEC G44.89
  spinal and epidural anesthesia - induced T88.59 ☑
    in labor and delivery O74.5
    in pregnancy O29.4- ☑
    postpartum, puerperal O89.4
  spinal fluid loss (from puncture) G97.1
  stabbing (primary) G44.85
  tension (-type) G44.209
    chronic G44.229
      intractable G44.221
      not intractable G44.229
    episodic G44.219
      intractable G44.211
      not intractable G44.219
    intractable G44.201
    not intractable G44.209
  thunderclap (primary) G44.53
  vascular NEC G44.1
Healthy
  infant
    accompanying sick mother Z76.3
    receiving care Z76.2
  person accompanying sick person Z76.3
Hearing examination Z01.10
  with abnormal findings NEC Z01.118
  following failed hearing screening Z01.110
  for hearing conservation and treatment Z01.12
Heart — *see* condition
Heart beat
  abnormality R00.9
    specified NEC R00.8
  awareness R00.2
  rapid R00.0
  slow R00.1
Heartburn R12
  psychogenic F45.8
Heat (effects) T67.9 ☑
  apoplexy T67.0 ☑
  burn (*see also* Burn) L55.9
  collapse T67.1 ☑
  cramps T67.2 ☑
  dermatitis or eczema L59.0
  edema T67.7 ☑
  erythema — *code by site under* Burn, first degree
  excessive T67.9 ☑
    specified effect NEC T67.8 ☑
  exhaustion T67.5 ☑
    anhydrotic T67.3 ☑

Heat — *continued*
  exhaustion — *continued*
    due to
      salt (and water) depletion T67.4 ☑
      water depletion T67.3 ☑
        with salt depletion T67.4 ☑
  fatigue (transient) T67.6 ☑
  fever T67.0 ☑
  hyperpyrexia T67.0 ☑
  prickly L74.0
  prostration — *see* Heat, exhaustion
  pyrexia T67.0 ☑
  rash L74.0
  specified effect NEC T67.8 ☑
  stroke T67.0 ☑
  sunburn — *see* Sunburn
  syncope T67.1 ☑
Heavy-for-dates NEC (infant) (4000g to 4499g) P08.1
  exceptionally (4500g or more) P08.0
Hebephrenia, hebephrenic (schizophrenia) F20.1
Heberden's disease or nodes (with arthropathy) M15.1
Hebra's
  pityriasis L26
  prurigo L28.2
Heel — *see* condition
Heerfordt's disease D86.89
Hegglin's anomaly or syndrome D72.0
Heilmeyer-Schoner disease D45
Heine-Medin disease A80.9
Heinz body anemia, congenital D58.2
Heliophobia F40.228
Heller's disease or syndrome F84.3
HELLP syndrome (hemolysis, elevated liver enzymes and low platelet count) O14.2- ☑
Helminthiasis (*see also* Infestation, helminth)
  Ancylostoma B76.0
  intestinal B82.0
    mixed types (types classifiable to more than one of the titles B65.0-B81.3 and B81.8) B81.4
    specified type NEC B81.8
  mixed types (intestinal) (types classifiable to more than one of the titles B65.0-B81.3 and B81.8) B81.4
  Necator (americanus) B76.1
  specified type NEC B83.8
Heloma L84
Hemangioblastoma — *see* Neoplasm, connective tissue, uncertain behavior
  malignant — *see* Neoplasm, connective tissue, malignant
Hemangioendothelioma (*see also* Neoplasm, uncertain behavior, by site)
  benign D18.00
    intra-abdominal D18.03
    intracranial D18.02
    skin D18.01
    specified site NEC D18.09
  bone (diffuse) — *see* Neoplasm, bone, malignant
  epithelioid (*see also* Neoplasm, uncertain behavior, by site)
    malignant — *see* Neoplasm, malignant, by site
  malignant — *see* Neoplasm, connective tissue, malignant
Hemangiofibroma — *see* Neoplasm, benign, by site
Hemangiolipoma — *see* Lipoma
Hemangioma D18.00
  arteriovenous D18.00
    intra-abdominal D18.03
    intracranial D18.02
    skin D18.01
    specified site NEC D18.09
  capillary D18.00
    intra-abdominal D18.03
    intracranial D18.02
    skin D18.01
    specified site NEC D18.09
  cavernous D18.00
    intra-abdominal D18.03
    intracranial D18.02
    skin D18.01
    specified site NEC D18.09
  epithelioid D18.00
    intra-abdominal D18.03
    intracranial D18.02
    skin D18.01
    specified site NEC D18.09

Hemangioma — *continued*
  histiocytoid D18.00
    intra-abdominal D18.03
    intracranial D18.02
    skin D18.01
    specified site NEC D18.09
  infantile D18.00
    intra-abdominal D18.03
    intracranial D18.02
    skin D18.01
    specified site NEC D18.09
  intra-abdominal D18.03
  intracranial D18.02
  intramuscular D18.00
    intra-abdominal D18.03
    intracranial D18.02
    skin D18.01
    specified site NEC D18.09
  juvenile D18.00
  malignant — *see* Neoplasm, connective tissue, malignant
  plexiform D18.00
    intra-abdominal D18.03
    intracranial D18.02
    skin D18.01
    specified site NEC D18.09
  racemose D18.00
    intra-abdominal D18.03
    intracranial D18.02
    skin D18.01
    specified site NEC D18.09
  sclerosing — *see* Neoplasm, skin, benign
  simplex D18.00
    intra-abdominal D18.03
    intracranial D18.02
    skin D18.01
    specified site NEC D18.09
  skin D18.01
  specified site NEC D18.09
  venous D18.00
    intra-abdominal D18.03
    intracranial D18.02
    skin D18.01
    specified site NEC D18.09
  verrucous keratotic D18.00
    intra-abdominal D18.03
    intracranial D18.02
    skin D18.01
    specified site NEC D18.09
Hemangiomatosis (systemic) I78.8
  involving single site — *see* Hemangioma
Hemangiopericytoma (*see also* Neoplasm, connective tissue, uncertain behavior)
  benign — *see* Neoplasm, connective tissue, benign
  malignant — *see* Neoplasm, connective tissue, malignant
Hemangiosarcoma — *see* Neoplasm, connective tissue, malignant
Hemarthrosis (nontraumatic) M25.00
  ankle M25.07- ☑
  elbow M25.02- ☑
  foot joint M25.07- ☑
  hand joint M25.04- ☑
  hip M25.05- ☑
  in hemophilic arthropathy — *see* Arthropathy, hemophilic
  knee M25.06- ☑
  shoulder M25.01- ☑
  specified joint NEC M25.08
  traumatic — *see* Sprain, by site
  vertebrae M25.08
  wrist M25.03- ☑
Hematemesis K92.0
  with ulcer — *code by site under* Ulcer, with hemorrhage K27.4
  newborn, neonatal P54.0
    due to swallowed maternal blood P78.2
Hematidrosis L74.8
Hematinuria (*see also* Hemoglobinuria)
  malarial B50.8
Hematobilia K83.8
Hematocele
  female NEC N94.89
    with ectopic pregnancy O00.9
    ovary N83.8
  male N50.1
Hematochezia (*see also* Melena) K92.1

Hematochyluria (see also Infestation, filarial)
  schistosomiasis (bilharziasis) B65.0
Hematocolpos (with hematometra or hematosalpinx)
  N89.7
Hematocornea — see Pigmentation, cornea, stromal
Hematogenous — see condition
Hematoma (traumatic) (skin surface intact) (see also
  Contusion)
  with
    injury of internal organs — see Injury, by site
    open wound — see Wound, open
  amputation stump (surgical) (late) T87.89
  aorta, dissecting I71.00
    abdominal I71.02
    thoracic I71.01
    thoracoabdominal I71.03
  aortic intramural — see Dissection, aorta
  arterial (complicating trauma) — see Injury, blood
    vessel, by site
  auricle — see Contusion, ear
    nontraumatic — see Disorder, pinna, hematoma
  birth injury NEC P15.8
  brain (traumatic)
    with
      cerebral laceration or contusion (diffuse) — see
        Injury, intracranial, diffuse
        focal — see Injury, intracranial, focal
    cerebellar, traumatic S06.37- ☑
    intracerebral, traumatic — see Injury, intracranial,
      intracerebral hemorrhage
    newborn NEC P52.4
      birth injury P10.1
    nontraumatic — see Hemorrhage, intracranial
    subarachnoid, arachnoid, traumatic — see Injury,
      intracranial, subarachnoid hemorrhage
    subdural, traumatic — see Injury, intracranial,
      subdural hemorrhage
  breast (nontraumatic) N64.89
  broad ligament (nontraumatic) N83.7
    traumatic S37.892 ☑
  cerebellar, traumatic S06.37- ☑
  cerebral — see Hematoma, brain
  cerebrum S06.36- ☑
    left S06.35- ☑
    right S06.34- ☑
  cesarean delivery wound O90.2
  complicating delivery (perineal) (pelvic) (vagina) (vul-
    va) O71.7
  corpus cavernosum (nontraumatic) N48.89
  epididymis (nontraumatic) N50.1
  epidural (traumatic) — see Injury, intracranial, epidural
    hemorrhage
    spinal — see Injury, spinal cord, by region
  episiotomy O90.2
  face, birth injury P15.4
  genital organ NEC (nontraumatic)
    female (nonobstetric) N94.89
      traumatic S30.202 ☑
    male N50.1
      traumatic S30.201 ☑
  internal organs — see Injury, by site
  intracerebral, traumatic — see Injury, intracranial, in-
    tracerebral hemorrhage
  intraoperative — see Complications, intraoperative,
    hemorrhage
  labia (nontraumatic) (nonobstetric) N90.89
  liver (subcapsular) (nontraumatic) K76.89
    birth injury P15.0
  mediastinum — see Injury, intrathoracic
  mesosalpinx (nontraumatic) N83.7
    traumatic S37.898 ☑
  muscle — code by site under Contusion
  nontraumatic
    muscle M79.81
    soft tissue M79.81
  obstetrical surgical wound O90.2
  orbit, orbital (nontraumatic) (see also Hemorrhage,
    orbit)
    traumatic — see Contusion, orbit
  pelvis (female) (nontraumatic) (nonobstetric) N94.89
    obstetric O71.7
    traumatic — see Injury, by site
  penis (nontraumatic) N48.89
    birth injury P15.5
  perianal (nontraumatic) K64.5
  perineal S30.23 ☑
    complicating delivery O71.7

Hematoma — continued
  perirenal — see Injury, kidney
  pinna — see Contusion, ear
    nontraumatic — see Disorder, pinna, hematoma
  placenta O43.89- ☑
  postoperative (postprocedural) — see Complication,
    postprocedural, hemorrhage
  retroperitoneal (nontraumatic) K66.1
    traumatic S36.892 ☑
  scrotum, superficial S30.22 ☑
    birth injury P15.5
  seminal vesicle (nontraumatic) N50.1
    traumatic S37.892 ☑
  spermatic cord (traumatic) S37.892 ☑
    nontraumatic N50.1
  spinal (cord) (meninges) (see also Injury, spinal cord,
    by region)
    newborn (birth injury) P11.5
  spleen D73.5
    intraoperative — see Complications, intraoperative,
      hemorrhage, spleen
    postprocedural (postoperative) — see Complica-
      tions, postprocedural, hemorrhage, spleen
  sternocleidomastoid, birth injury P15.2
  sternomastoid, birth injury P15.2
  subarachnoid (traumatic) — see Injury, intracranial,
    subarachnoid hemorrhage
    newborn P52.5
      due to birth injury P10.3
    nontraumatic — see Hemorrhage, intracranial,
      subarachnoid
  subdural (traumatic) — see Injury, intracranial, subdu-
    ral hemorrhage
    newborn (localized) P52.8
      birth injury P10.0
    nontraumatic — see Hemorrhage, intracranial,
      subdural
  superficial, newborn P54.5
  testis (nontraumatic) N50.1
    birth injury P15.5
  tunica vaginalis (nontraumatic) N50.1
  umbilical cord, complicating delivery O69.5 ☑
  uterine ligament (broad) (nontraumatic) N83.7
    traumatic S37.892 ☑
  vagina (ruptured) (nontraumatic) N89.8
    complicating delivery O71.7
  vas deferens (nontraumatic) N50.1
    traumatic S37.892 ☑
  vitreous — see Hemorrhage, vitreous
  vulva (nontraumatic) (nonobstetric) N90.89
    complicating delivery O71.7
    newborn (birth injury) P15.5
Hematometra N85.7
  with hematocolpos N89.7
Hematomyelia (central) G95.19
  newborn (birth injury) P11.5
  traumatic T14.8
Hematomyelitis G04.90
Hematoperitoneum — see Hemoperitoneum
Hematophobia F40.230
Hematopneumothorax (see Hemothorax)
Hematopoiesis, cyclic D70.4
Hematoporphyria — see Porphyria
Hematorachis, hematorrhachis G95.19
  newborn (birth injury) P11.5
Hematosalpinx N83.6
  with
    hematocolpos N89.7
    hematometra N85.7
      with hematocolpos N89.7
  infectional — see Salpingitis
Hematospermia R36.1
Hematothorax (see Hemothorax)
Hematuria R31.9
  benign (familial) (of childhood) (see also Hematuria,
    idiopathic)
    essential microscopic R31.1
  due to sulphonamide, sulfonamide — see Table of
    Drugs and Chemicals, by drug
  endemic (see also Schistosomiasis) B65.0
  gross R31.0
  idiopathic N02.9
    with glomerular lesion
      crescentic (diffuse) glomerulonephritis N02.7
      dense deposit disease N02.6
      endocapillary proliferative glomerulonephritis
        N02.4

Hematuria — continued
  idiopathic — continued
    with glomerular lesion — continued
      focal and segmental hyalinosis or sclerosis
        N02.1
      membranoproliferative (diffuse) N02.5
      membranous (diffuse) N02.2
      mesangial proliferative (diffuse) N02.3
      mesangiocapillary (diffuse) N02.5
      minor abnormality N02.0
      proliferative NEC N02.8
      specified pathology NEC N02.8
  intermittent — see Hematuria, idiopathic
  malarial B50.8
  microscopic NEC R31.2
    benign essential R31.1
  paroxysmal (see also Hematuria, idiopathic)
    nocturnal D59.5
  persistent — see Hematuria, idiopathic
  recurrent — see Hematuria, idiopathic
  tropical (see also Schistosomiasis) B65.0
  tuberculous A18.13
Hemeralopia (day blindness) H53.11
  vitamin A deficiency E50.5
Hemi-akinesia R41.4
Hemianalgesia R20.0
Hemianencephaly Q00.0
Hemianesthesia R20.0
Hemianopia, hemianopsia (heteronymous) H53.47
  homonymous H53.46- ☑
  syphilitic A52.71
Hemiathetosis R25.8
Hemiatrophy R68.89
  cerebellar G31.9
  face, facial, progressive (Romberg) G51.8
  tongue K14.8
Hemiballism (us) G25.5
Hemicardia Q24.8
Hemicephalus, hemicephaly Q00.0
Hemichorea G25.5
Hemicolitis, left — see Colitis, left sided
Hemicrania
  congenital malformation Q00.0
  continua G44.51
  meaning migraine (see also Migraine) G43.909
  paroxysmal G44.039
    chronic G44.049
      intractable G44.041
      not intractable G44.049
    episodic G44.039
      intractable G44.031
      not intractable G44.039
    intractable G44.031
    not intractable G44.039
Hemidystrophy — see Hemiatrophy
Hemiectromelia Q73.8
Hemihypalgesia R20.8
Hemihypesthesia R20.1
Hemi-inattention R41.4
Hemimelia Q73.8
  lower limb — see Defect, reduction, lower limb, spec-
    ified type NEC
  upper limb — see Defect, reduction, upper limb,
    specified type NEC
Hemiparalysis — see Hemiplegia
Hemiparesis — see Hemiplegia
Hemiparesthesia R20.2
Hemiparkinsonism G20
Hemiplegia G81.9- ☑
  alternans facialis G83.89
  ascending NEC G81.90
    spinal G95.89
  congenital (cerebral) G80.8
    spastic G80.2
  embolic (current episode) I63.4- ☑
  flaccid G81.0- ☑
  following
    cerebrovascular disease I69.959
      cerebral infarction I69.35- ☑
      intracerebral hemorrhage I69.15- ☑
      nontraumatic intracranial hemorrhage NEC
        I69.25- ☑
      specified disease NEC I69.85- ☑
      stroke NOS I69.35- ☑
      subarachnoid hemorrhage I69.05- ☑
  hysterical F44.4

Hemiplegia — continued
  newborn NEC P91.8
    birth injury P11.9
  spastic G81.1- ☑
    congenital G80.2
  thrombotic (current episode) I63.3 ☑
Hemisection, spinal cord — see Injury, spinal cord, by
    region
Hemispasm (facial) R25.2
Hemisporosis B48.8
Hemitremor R25.1
Hemivertebra Q76.49
  failure of segmentation with scoliosis Q76.3
  fusion with scoliosis Q76.3
Hemochromatosis E83.119
  with refractory anemia D46.1
  due to repeated red blood cell transfusion E83.111
  hereditary (primary) E83.110
  primary E83.110
  specified NEC E83.118
Hemoglobin (see also condition)
  abnormal (disease) — see Disease, hemoglobin
  AS genotype D57.3
  Constant Spring D58.2
  E-beta thalassemia D56.5
  fetal, hereditary persistence (HPFH) D56.4
  H Constant Spring D56.0
  low NOS D64.9
  S (Hb S), heterozygous D57.3
Hemoglobinemia D59.9
  due to blood transfusion T80.89 ☑
  paroxysmal D59.6
    nocturnal D59.5
Hemoglobinopathy (mixed) D58.2
  with thalassemia D56.8
  sickle-cell D57.1
    with thalassemia D57.40
      with crisis (vasoocclusive pain) D57.419
        with
          acute chest syndrome D57.411
          splenic sequestration D57.412
      without crisis D57.40
Hemoglobinuria R82.3
  with anemia, hemolytic, acquired (chronic) NEC D59.6
  cold (agglutinin) (paroxysmal) (with Raynaud's syn-
      drome) D59.6
  due to exertion or hemolysis NEC D59.6
  intermittent D59.6
  malarial B50.8
  march D59.6
  nocturnal (paroxysmal) D59.5
  paroxysmal (cold) D59.6
    nocturnal D59.5
Hemolymphangioma D18.1
Hemolysis
  intravascular
    with
      abortion — see Abortion, by type, complicated
          by, hemorrhage
      ectopic or molar pregnancy O08.1
      hemorrhage
        antepartum — see Hemorrhage, antepar-
            tum, with coagulation defect
        intrapartum (see also Hemorrhage, compli-
            cating, delivery) O67.0
      postpartum O72.3
    neonatal (excessive) P58.9
      specified NEC P58.8
Hemolytic — see condition
Hemopericardium I31.2
  following acute myocardial infarction (current compli-
      cation) I23.0
  newborn P54.8
  traumatic — see Injury, heart, with hemopericardium
Hemoperitoneum K66.1
  infectional K65.9
  traumatic S36.899 ☑
    with open wound — see Wound, open, with pene-
        tration into peritoneal cavity
Hemophilia (classical) (familial) (hereditary) D66
  A D66
  acquired D68.311
  autoimmune D68.311
  B D67
  C D68.1
  calcipriva (see also Defect, coagulation) D68.4
  nonfamilial (see also Defect, coagulation) D68.4
  secondary D68.311

Hemophilia — continued
  vascular D68.0
Hemophthalmos H44.81- ☑
Hemopneumothorax (see also Hemothorax)
  traumatic S27.2 ☑
Hemoptysis R04.2
  newborn P26.9
  tuberculous — see Tuberculosis, pulmonary
Hemorrhage, hemorrhagic (concealed) R58
  abdomen R58
  accidental antepartum — see Hemorrhage, antepar-
      tum
  acute idiopathic pulmonary, in infants R04.81
  adenoid J35.8
  adrenal (capsule) (gland) E27.49
    medulla E27.8
    newborn P54.4
  after delivery — see Hemorrhage, postpartum
  alveolar
    lung, newborn P26.8
    process K08.8
  alveolus K08.8
  amputation stump (surgical) T87.89
  anemia (chronic) D50.0
    acute D62
  antepartum (with) O46.90
    with coagulation defect O46.00- ☑
      afibrinogenemia O46.01- ☑
      disseminated intravascular coagulation
          O46.02- ☑
      hypofibrinogenemia O46.01- ☑
      specified defect NEC O46.09- ☑
    before 20 weeks gestation O20.9
      specified type NEC O20.8
      threatened abortion O20.0
    due to
      abruptio placenta (see also Abruptio placentae)
          O45.9- ☑
      leiomyoma, uterus — see Hemorrhage, antepar-
          tum, specified cause NEC
      placenta previa O44.1- ☑
      specified cause NEC — see subcategory O46.8X- ☑
  anus (sphincter) K62.5
  apoplexy (stroke) — see Hemorrhage, intracranial, in-
      tracerebral
  arachnoid — see Hemorrhage, intracranial, subarach-
      noid
  artery R58
    brain — see Hemorrhage, intracranial, intracerebral
  basilar (ganglion) I61.0
  bladder N32.89
  bowel K92.2
    newborn P54.3
  brain (miliary) (nontraumatic) — see Hemorrhage, in-
      tracranial, intracerebral
    due to
      birth injury P10.1
      syphilis A52.05
    epidural or extradural (traumatic) — see Injury,
        intracranial, epidural hemorrhage
      newborn P52.4
        birth injury P10.1
    subarachnoid — see Hemorrhage, intracranial,
        subarachnoid
    subdural — see Hemorrhage, intracranial, subdural
  brainstem (nontraumatic) I61.3
    traumatic S06.38- ☑
  breast N64.59
  bronchial tube — see Hemorrhage, lung
  bronchopulmonary — see Hemorrhage, lung
  bronchus — see Hemorrhage, lung
  bulbar I61.5
  capillary I78.8
    primary D69.8
  cecum K92.2
  cerebellar, cerebellum (nontraumatic) I61.4
    newborn P52.6
    traumatic S06.37- ☑
  cerebral, cerebrum (see also Hemorrhage, intracranial,
      intracerebral)
    lobe I61.1
    newborn (anoxic) P52.4
      birth injury P10.1
  cerebromeningeal I61.8
  cerebrospinal — see Hemorrhage, intracranial, intrac-
      erebral
  cervix (uteri) (stump) NEC N88.8

Hemorrhage, hemorrhagic — continued
  chamber, anterior (eye) — see Hyphema
  childbirth — see Hemorrhage, complicating, delivery
  choroid H31.30- ☑
    expulsive H31.31- ☑
  ciliary body — see Hyphema
  cochlea — see subcategory H83.8 ☑
  colon K92.2
  complicating
    abortion — see Abortion, by type, complicated by,
        hemorrhage
    delivery O67.9
      associated with coagulation defect (afibrinogen-
          emia) (DIC) (hyperfibrinolysis) O67.0
      specified cause NEC O67.8
    surgical procedure — see Hemorrhage, intraoper-
        ative
  conjunctiva H11.3- ☑
    newborn P54.8
  cord, newborn (stump) P51.9
  corpus luteum (ruptured) cyst N83.1
  cortical (brain) I61.1
  cranial — see Hemorrhage, intracranial
  cutaneous R23.3
    due to autosensitivity, erythrocyte D69.2
    newborn P54.5
  delayed
    following ectopic or molar pregnancy O08.1
    postpartum O72.2
  diathesis (familial) D69.9
  disease D69.9
    newborn P53
    specified type NEC D69.8
  due to or associated with
    afibrinogenemia or other coagulation defect
        (conditions in categories D65- D69)
      antepartum — see Hemorrhage, antepartum,
          with coagulation defect
      intrapartum O67.0
    dental implant M27.61
    device, implant or graft (see also Complications,
        by site and type, specified NEC) T85.83 ☑
      arterial graft NEC T82.838 ☑
      breast T85.83 ☑
      catheter NEC T85.83 ☑
        dialysis (renal) T82.838 ☑
          intraperitoneal T85.83 ☑
        infusion NEC T82.838 ☑
          spinal (epidural) (subdural) T85.83 ☑
        urinary (indwelling) T83.83 ☑
      electronic (electrode) (pulse generator) (stimu-
          lator)
        bone T84.83 ☑
        cardiac T82.837 ☑
        nervous system (brain) (peripheral nerve)
            (spinal) T85.83 ☑
        urinary T83.83 ☑
      fixation, internal (orthopedic) NEC T84.83 ☑
      gastrointestinal (bile duct) (esophagus)
          T85.83 ☑
      genital NEC T83.83 ☑
      heart NEC T82.837 ☑
      joint prosthesis T84.83 ☑
      ocular (corneal graft) (orbital implant) NEC
          T85.83 ☑
      orthopedic NEC T84.83 ☑
        bone graft T86.838
      specified NEC T85.83 ☑
      urinary NEC T83.83 ☑
      vascular NEC T82.838 ☑
      ventricular intracranial shunt T85.83 ☑
  duodenum, duodenal K92.2
    ulcer — see Ulcer, duodenum, with hemorrhage
  dura mater — see Hemorrhage, intracranial, subdural
  endotracheal — see Hemorrhage, lung
  epicranial subaponeurotic (massive), birth injury P12.2
  epidural (traumatic) (see also Injury, intracranial,
      epidural hemorrhage)
    nontraumatic I62.1
  esophagus K22.8
    varix I85.01
      secondary I85.11
  excessive, following ectopic gestation (subsequent
      episode) O08.1
  extradural (traumatic) — see Injury, intracranial,
      epidural hemorrhage
    birth injury P10.8

Hemorrhage, hemorrhagic — *continued*
  extradural — *see* Injury, intracranial, epidural hemor-
      rhage — *continued*
    newborn (anoxic) (nontraumatic) P52.8
    nontraumatic I62.1
  eye NEC H57.8
    fundus — *see* Hemorrhage, retina
    lid — *see* Disorder, eyelid, specified type NEC
  fallopian tube N83.6
  fibrinogenolysis — *see* Fibrinolysis
  fibrinolytic (acquired) — *see* Fibrinolysis
  from
    ear (nontraumatic) — *see* Otorrhagia
    tracheostomy stoma J95.01
  fundus, eye — *see* Hemorrhage, retina
  funis — *see* Hemorrhage, umbilicus, cord
  gastric — *see* Hemorrhage, stomach
  gastroenteric K92.2
    newborn P54.3
  gastrointestinal (tract) K92.2
    newborn P54.3
  genital organ, male N50.1
  genitourinary (tract) NOS R31.9
  gingiva K06.8
  globe (eye) — *see* Hemophthalmos
  graafian follicle cyst (ruptured) N83.0
  gum K06.8
  heart I51.89
  hypopharyngeal (throat) R04.1
  intermenstrual (regular) N92.3
    irregular N92.1
  internal (organs) NEC R58
    capsule I61.0
    ear — *see* subcategory H83.8 ☑
    newborn P54.8
  intestine K92.2
    newborn P54.3
  intra-abdominal R58
  intra-alveolar (lung), newborn P26.8
  intracerebral (nontraumatic) — *see* Hemorrhage, in-
      tracranial, intracerebral
  intracranial (nontraumatic) I62.9
    birth injury P10.9
    epidural, nontraumatic I62.1
    extradural, nontraumatic I62.1
    intracerebral (nontraumatic) (in) I61.9
      brain stem I61.3
      cerebellum I61.4
      hemisphere I61.2
        cortical (superficial) I61.1
        subcortical (deep) I61.0
      intraoperative
        during a nervous system procedure G97.31
        during other procedure G97.32
      intraventricular I61.5
      multiple localized I61.6
      newborn P52.4
        birth injury P10.1
      postprocedural
        following a nervous system procedure
            G97.51
        following other procedure G97.52
      specified NEC I61.8
      superficial I61.1
      traumatic (diffuse) — *see* Injury, intracranial,
          diffuse
        focal — *see* Injury, intracranial, focal
    newborn P52.9
      specified NEC P52.8
    subarachnoid (nontraumatic) (from) I60.9
      intracranial (cerebral) artery I60.7
        anterior communicating I60.2- ☑
        basilar I60.4
        carotid siphon and bifurcation I60.0- ☑
        communicating I60.7
          anterior I60.2- ☑
          posterior I60.3- ☑
        middle cerebral I60.1- ☑
        posterior communicating I60.3- ☑
        specified artery NEC I60.6
        vertebral I60.5- ☑
      newborn P52.5
        birth injury P10.3
      specified NEC I60.8
      traumatic S06.6X- ☑
    subdural (nontraumatic) I62.00
      acute I62.01
      birth injury P10.0

Hemorrhage, hemorrhagic — *continued*
  intracranial — *continued*
    subdural — *continued*
      chronic I62.03
      newborn (anoxic) (hypoxic) P52.8
        birth injury P10.0
      spinal G95.19
      subacute I62.02
      traumatic — *see* Injury, intracranial, subdural
          hemorrhage
    traumatic — *see* Injury, intracranial, focal brain in-
        jury
  intramedullary NEC G95.19
  intraocular — *see* Hemophthalmos
  intraoperative, intraprocedural — *see* Complication,
      hemorrhage (hematoma), intraoperative (in-
      traprocedural), by site
  intrapartum — *see* Hemorrhage, complicating, deliv-
      ery
  intrapelvic
    female N94.89
    male K66.1
  intraperitoneal K66.1
  intrapontine I61.3
  intraprocedural — *see* Complication, hemorrhage
      (hematoma), intraoperative (intraprocedural),
      by site
  intrauterine N85.7
    complicating delivery (*see also* Hemorrhage, com-
        plicating, delivery) O67.9
    postpartum — *see* Hemorrhage, postpartum
  intraventricular I61.5
    newborn (nontraumatic) (*see also* Newborn, affect-
        ed by, hemorrhage) P52.3
      due to birth injury P10.2
      grade
        1 P52.0
        2 P52.1
        3 P52.21
        4 P52.22
  intravesical N32.89
  iris (postinfectional) (postinflammatory) (toxic) — *see*
      Hyphema
  joint (nontraumatic) — *see* Hemarthrosis
  kidney N28.89
  knee (joint) (nontraumatic) — *see* Hemarthrosis, knee
  labyrinth — *see* subcategory H83.8 ☑
  lenticular striate artery I61.0
  ligature, vessel — *see* Hemorrhage, postoperative
  liver K76.89
  lung R04.89
    newborn P26.9
      massive P26.1
      specified NEC P26.8
    tuberculous — *see* Tuberculosis, pulmonary
  massive umbilical, newborn P51.0
  mediastinum — *see* Hemorrhage, lung
  medulla I61.3
  membrane (brain) I60.8
    spinal cord — *see* Hemorrhage, spinal cord
  meninges, meningeal (brain) (middle) I60.8
    spinal cord — *see* Hemorrhage, spinal cord
  mesentery K66.1
  metritis — *see* Endometritis
  mouth K13.79
  mucous membrane NEC R58
    newborn P54.8
  muscle M62.89
  nail (subungual) L60.8
  nasal turbinate R04.0
    newborn P54.8
  navel, newborn P51.9
  newborn P54.9
    specified NEC P54.8
  nipple N64.59
  nose R04.0
    newborn P54.8
  omentum K66.1
  optic nerve (sheath) H47.02- ☑
  orbit, orbital H05.23- ☑
  ovary NEC N83.8
  oviduct N83.6
  pancreas K86.8
  parathyroid (gland) (spontaneous) E21.4
  parturition — *see* Hemorrhage, complicating, delivery
  penis N48.89
  pericardium, pericarditis I31.2
  peritoneum, peritoneal K66.1

Hemorrhage, hemorrhagic — *continued*
  peritonsillar tissue J35.8
    due to infection J36
  petechial R23.3
    due to autosensitivity, erythrocyte D69.2
  pituitary (gland) E23.6
  pleura — *see* Hemorrhage, lung
  polioencephalitis, superior E51.2
  polymyositis — *see* Polymyositis
  pons, pontine I61.3
  posterior fossa (nontraumatic) I61.8
    newborn P52.6
  postmenopausal N95.0
  postnasal R04.0
  postoperative — *see* Complications, postprocedural,
      hemorrhage, by site
  postpartum NEC (following delivery of placenta) O72.1
    delayed or secondary O72.2
    retained placenta O72.0
    third stage O72.0
  pregnancy — *see* Hemorrhage, antepartum
  preretinal — *see* Hemorrhage, retina
  prostate N42.1
  puerperal — *see* Hemorrhage, postpartum
    delayed or secondary O72.2
  pulmonary R04.89
    newborn P26.9
      massive P26.1
      specified NEC P26.8
    tuberculous — *see* Tuberculosis, pulmonary
  purpura (primary) D69.3
  rectum (sphincter) K62.5
    newborn P54.2
  recurring, following initial hemorrhage at time of injury
      T79.2 ☑
  renal N28.89
  respiratory passage or tract R04.9
    specified NEC R04.89
  retina, retinal (vessels) H35.6- ☑
    diabetic — *see* Diabetes, retinal, hemorrhage
  retroperitoneal R58
  scalp R58
  scrotum N50.1
  secondary (nontraumatic) R58
    following initial hemorrhage at time of injury
        T79.2 ☑
  seminal vesicle N50.1
  skin R23.3
    newborn P54.5
  slipped umbilical ligature P51.8
  spermatic cord N50.1
  spinal (cord) G95.19
    newborn (birth injury) P11.5
  spleen D73.5
    intraoperative — *see* Complications, intraoperative,
        hemorrhage, spleen
    postprocedural — *see* Complications, postproce-
        dural, hemorrhage, spleen
  stomach K92.2
    newborn P54.3
    ulcer — *see* Ulcer, stomach, with hemorrhage
  subarachnoid (nontraumatic) — *see* Hemorrhage, in-
      tracranial, subarachnoid
  subconjunctival (*see also* Hemorrhage, conjunctiva)
    birth injury P15.3
  subcortical (brain) I61.0
  subcutaneous R23.3
  subdiaphragmatic R58
  subdural (acute) (nontraumatic) — *see* Hemorrhage,
      intracranial, subdural
  subependymal
    newborn P52.0
      with intraventricular extension P52.1
        and intracerebral extension P52.22
  subgaleal P12.1
  subhyaloid — *see* Hemorrhage, retina
  subperiosteal — *see* Disorder, bone, specified type
      NEC
  subretinal — *see* Hemorrhage, retina
  subtentorial — *see* Hemorrhage, intracranial, subdural
  subungual L60.8
  suprarenal (capsule) (gland) E27.49
    newborn P54.4
  tentorium (traumatic) NEC — *see* Hemorrhage, brain
    newborn (birth injury) P10.4
  testis N50.1
  third stage (postpartum) O72.0
  thorax — *see* Hemorrhage, lung

☑ Additional Character Required — Refer to the Tabular List for Character Selection   ▽ Subterms under main terms may continue to next column or page

Hemorrhage, hemorrhagic — *continued*
  throat R04.1
  thymus (gland) E32.8
  thyroid (cyst) (gland) E07.89
  tongue K14.8
  tonsil J35.8
  trachea — *see* Hemorrhage, lung
  tracheobronchial R04.89
    newborn P26.0
  traumatic — *code to* specific injury
    cerebellar — *see* Hemorrhage, brain
    intracranial — *see* Hemorrhage, brain
    recurring or secondary (following initial hemor-
        rhage at time of injury) T79.2 ☑
  tuberculous NEC (*see also* Tuberculosis, pulmonary)
      A15.0
  tunica vaginalis N50.1
  ulcer — *code by* site under Ulcer, with hemorrhage
      K27.4
  umbilicus, umbilical
    cord
      after birth, newborn P51.9
      complicating delivery O69.5 ☑
    newborn P51.9
      massive P51.0
      slipped ligature P51.8
      stump P51.9
  urethra (idiopathic) N36.8
  uterus, uterine (abnormal) N93.9
    climacteric N92.4
    complicating delivery — *see* Hemorrhage, compli-
        cating, delivery
    dysfunctional or functional N93.8
    intermenstrual (regular) N92.3
      irregular N92.1
    postmenopausal N95.0
    postpartum — *see* Hemorrhage, postpartum
    preclimacteric or premenopausal N92.4
    prepubertal N93.8
    pubertal N92.2
  vagina (abnormal) N93.9
    newborn P54.6
  vas deferens N50.1
  vasa previa O69.4 ☑
  ventricular I61.5
  vesical N32.89
  viscera NEC R58
    newborn P54.8
  vitreous (humor) (intraocular) H43.1- ☑
  vulva N90.89
Hemorrhoids (bleeding) (without mention of degree)
    K64.9
  1st degree (grade/stage I) (without prolapse outside
      of anal canal) K64.0
  2nd degree (grade/stage II) (that prolapse with
      straining but retract spontaneously) K64.1
  3rd degree (grade/stage III) (that prolapse with
      straining and require manual replacement back
      inside anal canal) K64.2
  4th degree (grade/stage IV) (with prolapsed tissue that
      cannot be manually replaced) K64.3
  complicating
    pregnancy O22.4 ☑
    puerperium O87.2
  external K64.4
    with
      thrombosis K64.5
  internal (without mention of degree) K64.8
  prolapsed K64.8
  skin tags
    anus K64.4
    residual K64.4
  specified NEC K64.8
  strangulated (*see also* Hemorrhoids, by degree) K64.8
  thrombosed (*see also* Hemorrhoids, by degree) K64.5
  ulcerated (*see also* Hemorrhoids, by degree) K64.8
Hemosalpinx N83.6
  with
    hematocolpos N89.7
    hematometra N85.7
      with hematocolpos N89.7
Hemosiderosis (dietary) E83.19
  pulmonary, idiopathic E83.1- ☑ [J84.03]
  transfusion T80.89 ☑
Hemothorax (bacterial) (nontuberculous) J94.2
  newborn P54.8
  traumatic S27.1 ☑
    with pneumothorax S27.2 ☑

Hemothorax — *continued*
  tuberculous NEC A15.6
Henoch (-Schönlein) **disease or syndrome** (purpura)
      D69.0
Henpue, henpuye A66.6
Hepar lobatum (syphilitic) A52.74
Hepatalgia K76.89
Hepatitis K75.9
  acute B17.9
    with coma K72.01
    with hepatic failure — *see* Failure, hepatic
    alcoholic — *see* Hepatitis, alcoholic
    infectious B15.9
      with hepatic coma B15.0
    viral B17.9
  alcoholic (acute) (chronic) K70.10
    with ascites K70.11
  amebic — *see* Abscess, liver, amebic
  anicteric, (viral) — *see* Hepatitis, viral
  antigen-associated (HAA) — *see* Hepatitis, B
  Australia-antigen (positive) — *see* Hepatitis, B
  autoimmune K75.4
  B B19.10
    with hepatic coma B19.11
    acute B16.9
      with
        delta-agent (coinfection) (without hepatic
            coma) B16.1
          with hepatic coma B16.0
        hepatic coma (without delta-agent coinfec-
            tion) B16.2
    chronic B18.1
      with delta-agent B18.0
  bacterial NEC K75.89
  C (viral) B19.20
    with hepatic coma B19.21
    acute B17.10
      with hepatic coma B17.11
    chronic B18.2
  catarrhal (acute) B15.9
    with hepatic coma B15.0
  cholangiolitic K75.89
  cholestatic K75.89
  chronic K73.9
    active NEC K73.2
    lobular NEC K73.1
    persistent NEC K73.0
    specified NEC K73.8
  cytomegaloviral B25.1
  due to ethanol (acute) (chronic) — *see* Hepatitis, alco-
      holic
  epidemic B15.9
    with hepatic coma B15.0
  fulminant NEC (viral) — *see* Hepatitis, viral
  granulomatous NEC K75.3
  herpesviral B00.81
  history of
    B Z86.19
    C Z86.19
  homologous serum — *see* Hepatitis, viral, type B
  in (due to)
    mumps B26.81
    toxoplasmosis (acquired) B58.1
      congenital (active) P37.1 [K77]
  infectious, infective (acute) (chronic) (subacute) B15.9
    with hepatic coma B15.0
  inoculation — *see* Hepatitis, viral, type B
  interstitial (chronic) K74.69
  lupoid NEC K75.4
  malignant NEC (with hepatic failure) K72.90
    with coma K72.91
  neonatal (idiopathic) (toxic) P59.29
  neonatal giant cell P59.29
  newborn P59.29
  postimmunization — *see* Hepatitis, viral, type B
  post-transfusion — *see* Hepatitis, viral, type B
  reactive, nonspecific K75.2
  serum — *see* Hepatitis, viral, type B
  specified type NEC
    with hepatic failure — *see* Failure, hepatic
  syphilitic (late) A52.74
    congenital (early) A50.08 [K77]
      late A50.59 [K77]
    secondary A51.45
  toxic (*see also* Disease, liver, toxic) K71.6
  tuberculous A18.83
  viral, virus B19.9
    with hepatic coma B19.0

Hepatitis — *continued*
  viral, virus — *continued*
    acute B18.9
    chronic B18.9
      specified NEC B18.8
      type
        B B18.1
          with delta-agent B18.0
        C B18.2
    congenital P35.3
    coxsackie B33.8 [K77]
    cytomegalic inclusion B25.1
    in remission, any type — *code to* Hepatitis, chronic,
        by type
    non-A, non-B B17.8
    specified type NEC (with or without coma) B17.8
      type
        A B15.9
          with hepatic coma B15.0
        B B19.10
          with hepatic coma B19.11
          acute B16.9
            with
              delta-agent (coinfection) (without
                  hepatic coma) B16.1
                with hepatic coma B16.0
              hepatic coma (without delta-agent
                  coinfection) B16.2
          chronic B18.1
            with delta-agent B18.0
        C B19.20
          with hepatic coma B19.21
          acute B17.10
            with hepatic coma B17.11
          chronic B18.2
        E B17.2
    non-A, non-B B17.8
Hepatization lung (acute) — *see* Pneumonia, lobar
Hepatoblastoma C22.2
Hepatocarcinoma C22.0
Hepatocholangiocarcinoma C22.0
Hepatocholangioma, benign D13.4
Hepatocholangitis K75.89
Hepatolenticular degeneration E83.01
Hepatoma (malignant) C22.0
  benign D13.4
  embryonal C22.0
Hepatomegaly (*see also* Hypertrophy, liver)
  with splenomegaly R16.2
  congenital Q44.7
  in mononucleosis
    gammaherpesviral B27.09
    infectious specified NEC B27.89
Hepatoptosis K76.89
Hepatorenal syndrome following labor and delivery
    O90.4
Hepatosis K76.89
Hepatosplenomegaly R16.2
  hyperlipemic (Bürger-Grütz type) E78.3 [K77]
Hereditary — *see* condition
Heredodegeneration, macular — *see* Dystrophy, retina
Heredopathia atactica polyneuritiformis G60.1
Heredosyphilis — *see* Syphilis, congenital
Herlitz' syndrome Q81.1
Hermansky-Pudlak syndrome E70.331
Hermaphrodite, hermaphroditism (true) Q56.0
  46,XX with streak gonads Q99.1
  46,XX/46,XY Q99.0
  46,XY with streak gonads Q99.1
  chimera 46,XX/46,XY Q99.0
Hernia, hernial (acquired) (recurrent) K46.9
  with
    gangrene — *see* Hernia, by site, with, gangrene
    incarceration — *see* Hernia, by site, with, obstruc-
        tion
    irreducible — *see* Hernia, by site, with, obstruction
    obstruction — *see* Hernia, by site, with, obstruction
    strangulation — *see* Hernia, by site, with, obstruc-
        tion
  abdomen, abdominal K46.9
    with
      gangrene (and obstruction) K46.1
      obstruction K46.0
    femoral — *see* Hernia, femoral
    incisional — *see* Hernia, incisional
    inguinal — *see* Hernia, inguinal
    specified site NEC K45.8

Hernia, hernial — *continued*
   abdomen, abdominal — *continued*
      specified site — *continued*
         with
            gangrene (and obstruction) K45.1
            obstruction K45.0
         umbilical — *see* Hernia, umbilical
         wall — *see* Hernia, ventral
      appendix — *see* Hernia, abdomen
      bladder (mucosa) (sphincter)
         congenital (female) (male) Q79.51
         female — *see* Cystocele
         male N32.89
      brain, congenital — *see* Encephalocele
      cartilage, vertebra — *see* Displacement, intervertebral disc
      cerebral, congenital (*see also* Encephalocele)
         endaural Q01.8
      ciliary body (traumatic) S05.2- ☑
      colon — *see* Hernia, abdomen
      Cooper's — *see* Hernia, abdomen, specified site NEC
      crural — *see* Hernia, femoral
      diaphragm, diaphragmatic K44.9
         with
            gangrene (and obstruction) K44.1
            obstruction K44.0
         congenital Q79.0
      direct (inguinal) — *see* Hernia, inguinal
      diverticulum, intestine — *see* Hernia, abdomen
      double (inguinal) — *see* Hernia, inguinal, bilateral
      due to adhesions (with obstruction) K56.5
      epigastric (*see also* Hernia, ventral) K43.9
      esophageal hiatus — *see* Hernia, hiatal
      external (inguinal) — *see* Hernia, inguinal
      fallopian tube N83.4
      fascia M62.89
      femoral K41.90
         with
            gangrene (and obstruction) K41.40
               not specified as recurrent K41.40
               recurrent K41.41
            obstruction K41.30
               not specified as recurrent K41.30
               recurrent K41.31
         bilateral K41.20
            with
               gangrene (and obstruction) K41.10
                  not specified as recurrent K41.10
                  recurrent K41.11
               obstruction K41.00
                  not specified as recurrent K41.00
                  recurrent K41.01
            not specified as recurrent K41.20
            recurrent K41.21
         not specified as recurrent K41.90
         recurrent K41.91
         unilateral K41.90
            with
               gangrene (and obstruction) K41.40
                  not specified as recurrent K41.40
                  recurrent K41.41
               obstruction K41.30
                  not specified as recurrent K41.30
                  recurrent K41.31
            not specified as recurrent K41.90
            recurrent K41.91
      foramen magnum G93.5
         congenital Q01.8
      funicular (umbilical) (*see also* Hernia, umbilicus)
         spermatic (cord) — *see* Hernia, inguinal
      gastrointestinal tract — *see* Hernia, abdomen
      Hesselbach's — *see* Hernia, femoral, specified site NEC
      hiatal (esophageal) (sliding) K44.9
         with
            gangrene (and obstruction) K44.1
            obstruction K44.0
         congenital Q40.1
      hypogastric — *see* Hernia, ventral
      incarcerated (*see also* Hernia, by site, with obstruction)
         with gangrene — *see* Hernia, by site, with gangrene
      incisional K43.2
         with
            gangrene (and obstruction) K43.1
            obstruction K43.0
      indirect (inguinal) — *see* Hernia, inguinal
      inguinal (direct) (external) (funicular) (indirect) (internal) (oblique) (scrotal) (sliding) K40.90

Hernia, hernial — *continued*
   inguinal — *continued*
      with
         gangrene (and obstruction) K40.40
            not specified as recurrent K40.40
            recurrent K40.41
         obstruction K40.30
            not specified as recurrent K40.30
            recurrent K40.31
      bilateral K40.20
         with
            gangrene (and obstruction) K40.10
               not specified as recurrent K40.10
               recurrent K40.11
            obstruction K40.00
               not specified as recurrent K40.00
               recurrent K40.01
         not specified as recurrent K40.20
         recurrent K40.21
      not specified as recurrent K40.90
      recurrent K40.91
      unilateral K40.90
         with
            gangrene (and obstruction) K40.40
               not specified as recurrent K40.40
               recurrent K40.41
            obstruction K40.30
               not specified as recurrent K40.30
               recurrent K40.31
         not specified as recurrent K40.90
         recurrent K40.91
   internal (*see also* Hernia, abdomen)
      inguinal — *see* Hernia, inguinal
   interstitial — *see* Hernia, abdomen
   intervertebral cartilage or disc — *see* Displacement, intervertebral disc
   intestine, intestinal — *see* Hernia, by site
   intra-abdominal — *see* Hernia, abdomen
   iris (traumatic) S05.2- ☑
   irreducible (*see also* Hernia, by site, with obstruction)
      with gangrene — *see* Hernia, by site, with gangrene
   ischiatic — *see* Hernia, abdomen, specified site NEC
   ischiorectal — *see* Hernia, abdomen, specified site NEC
   lens (traumatic) S05.2- ☑
   linea (alba) (semilunaris) — *see* Hernia, ventral
   Littre's — *see* Hernia, abdomen
   lumbar — *see* Hernia, abdomen, specified site NEC
   lung (subcutaneous) J98.4
   mediastinum J98.5
   mesenteric (internal) — *see* Hernia, abdomen
   midline — *see* Hernia, ventral
   muscle (sheath) M62.89
   nucleus pulposus — *see* Displacement, intervertebral disc
   oblique (inguinal) — *see* Hernia, inguinal
   obstructive (*see also* Hernia, by site, with obstruction)
      with gangrene — *see* Hernia, by site, with gangrene
   obturator — *see* Hernia, abdomen, specified site NEC
   omental — *see* Hernia, abdomen
   ovary N83.4
   oviduct N83.4
   paraesophageal (*see also* Hernia, diaphragm)
      congenital Q40.1
   parastomal K43.5
      with
         gangrene (and obstruction) K43.4
         obstruction K43.3
   paraumbilical — *see* Hernia, umbilicus
   perineal — *see* Hernia, abdomen, specified site NEC
   Petit's — *see* Hernia, abdomen, specified site NEC
   postoperative — *see* Hernia, incisional
   pregnant uterus — *see* Abnormal, uterus in pregnancy or childbirth
   prevesical N32.89
   properitoneal — *see* Hernia, abdomen, specified site NEC
   pudendal — *see* Hernia, abdomen, specified site NEC
   rectovaginal N81.6
   retroperitoneal — *see* Hernia, abdomen, specified site NEC
   Richter's — *see* Hernia, abdomen, with obstruction
   Rieux's, Riex's — *see* Hernia, abdomen, specified site NEC

Hernia, hernial — *continued*
   sac condition (adhesion) (dropsy) (inflammation) (laceration) (suppuration) — *code by site under* Hernia
   sciatic — *see* Hernia, abdomen, specified site NEC
   scrotum, scrotal — *see* Hernia, inguinal
   sliding (inguinal) (*see also* Hernia, inguinal)
      hiatus — *see* Hernia, hiatal
   spigelian — *see* Hernia, ventral
   spinal — *see* Spina bifida
   strangulated (*see also* Hernia, by site, with obstruction)
      with gangrene — *see* Hernia, by site, with gangrene
   subxiphoid — *see* Hernia, ventral
   supra-umbilicus — *see* Hernia, ventral
   tendon — *see* Disorder, tendon, specified type NEC
   Treitz's (fossa) — *see* Hernia, abdomen, specified site NEC
   tunica vaginalis Q55.29
   umbilicus, umbilical K42.9
      with
         gangrene (and obstruction) K42.1
         obstruction K42.0
   ureter N28.89
   urethra, congenital Q64.79
   urinary meatus, congenital Q64.79
   uterus N81.4
      pregnant — *see* Abnormal, uterus in pregnancy or childbirth
   vaginal (anterior) (wall) — *see* Cystocele
   Velpeau's — *see* Hernia, femoral
   ventral K43.9
      with
         gangrene (and obstruction) K43.7
         obstruction K43.6
      incisional K43.2
         with
            gangrene (and obstruction) K43.1
            obstruction K43.0
         recurrent — *see* Hernia, incisional
      specified NEC K43.9
         with
            gangrene (and obstruction) K43.7
            obstruction K43.6
   vesical
      congenital (female) (male) Q79.51
      female — *see* Cystocele
      male N32.89
   vitreous (into wound) S05.2- ☑
      into anterior chamber — *see* Prolapse, vitreous
Herniation (*see also* Hernia)
   brain (stem) G93.5
   cerebral G93.5
   mediastinum J98.5
   nucleus pulposus — *see* Displacement, intervertebral disc
Herpangina B08.5
Herpes, herpesvirus, herpetic B00.9
   anogenital A60.9
      perianal skin A60.1
      rectum A60.1
      urogenital tract A60.00
         cervix A60.03
         male genital organ NEC A60.02
         penis A60.01
         specified site NEC A60.09
         vagina A60.04
         vulva A60.04
   blepharitis (zoster) B02.39
      simplex B00.59
   circinatus B35.4
      bullosus L12.0
   conjunctivitis (simplex) B00.53
      zoster B02.31
   cornea B02.33
   encephalitis B00.4
      due to herpesvirus 6 B10.01
      due to herpesvirus 7 B10.09
      specified NEC B10.09
   eye (zoster) B02.30
      simplex B00.50
   eyelid (zoster) B02.39
      simplex B00.59
   facialis B00.1
   febrilis B00.1
   geniculate ganglionitis B02.21
   genital, genitalis A60.00
      female A60.09

Herpes, herpesvirus, herpetic — *continued*
  genital, genitalis — *continued*
    male A60.02
  gestational, gestationis O26.4- ☑
  gingivostomatitis B00.2
  human B00.9
    1 — *see* Herpes, simplex
    2 — *see* Herpes, simplex
    3 — *see* Varicella
    4 — *see* Mononucleosis, Epstein-Barr (virus)
    5 — *see* Disease, cytomegalic inclusion (generalized)
    6
      encephalitis B10.01
      specified NEC B10.81
    7
      encephalitis B10.09
      specified NEC B10.82
    8 B10.89
  infection NEC B10.89
    Kaposi's sarcoma associated B10.89
  iridocyclitis (simplex) B00.51
    zoster B02.32
  iris (vesicular erythema multiforme) L51.9
  iritis (simplex) B00.51
  Kaposi's sarcoma associated B10.89
  keratitis (simplex) (dendritic) (disciform) (interstitial) B00.52
    zoster (interstitial) B02.33
  keratoconjunctivitis (simplex) B00.52
    zoster B02.33
  labialis B00.1
  lip B00.1
  meningitis (simplex) B00.3
    zoster B02.1
  ophthalmicus (zoster) NEC B02.30
    simplex B00.50
  penis A60.01
  perianal skin A60.1
  pharyngitis, pharyngotonsillitis B00.2
  rectum A60.1
  scrotum A60.02
  sepsis B00.7
  simplex B00.9
    complicated NEC B00.89
    congenital P35.2
    conjunctivitis B00.53
    external ear B00.1
    eyelid B00.59
    hepatitis B00.81
    keratitis (interstitial) B00.52
    myeitis B00.82
    specified complication NEC B00.89
    visceral B00.89
  stomatitis B00.2
  tonsurans B35.0
  visceral B00.89
  vulva A60.04
  whitlow B00.89
  zoster (*see also* condition) B02.9
    auricularis B02.21
    complicated NEC B02.8
    conjunctivitis B02.31
    disseminated B02.7
    encephalitis B02.0
    eye (lid) B02.39
    geniculate ganglionitis B02.21
    keratitis (interstitial) B02.33
    meningitis B02.1
    myelitis B02.24
    neuritis, neuralgia B02.29
    ophthalmicus NEC B02.30
    oticus B02.21
    polyneuropathy B02.23
    specified complication NEC B02.8
    trigeminal neuralgia B02.22
Herpesvirus (human) — *see* Herpes
Herpetophobia F40.218
Herrick's anemia — *see* Disease, sickle-cell
Hers' disease E74.09
Herter-Gee syndrome K90.0
Herxheimer's reaction R68.89
Hesitancy
  of micturition R39.11
  urinary R39.11
Hesselbach's hernia — *see* Hernia, femoral, specified site NEC

Heterochromia (congenital) Q13.2
  cataract — *see* Cataract, complicated
  cyclitis (Fuchs) — *see* Cyclitis, Fuchs' heterochromic
  hair L67.1
  iritis — *see* Cyclitis, Fuchs' heterochromic
  retained metallic foreign body (nonmagnetic) — *see* Foreign body, intraocular, old, retained
    magnetic — *see* Foreign body, intraocular, old, retained, magnetic
  uveitis — *see* Cyclitis, Fuchs' heterochromic
Heterophoria — *see* Strabismus, heterophoria
Heterophyes, heterophyiasis (small intestine) B66.8
Heterotopia, heterotopic (*see also* Malposition, congenital)
  cerebralis Q04.8
Heterotropia — *see* Strabismus
Heubner-Herter disease K90.0
Hexadactylism Q69.9
HGSIL (cytology finding) (high grade squamous intraepithelial lesion on cytologic smear) (Pap smear finding)
  anus R85.613
  cervix R87.613
    biopsy (histology) finding — *code to* CIN II or CIN III
  vagina R87.623
    biopsy (histology) finding — *code to* VAIN II or VAIN III
Hibernoma — *see* Lipoma
Hiccup, hiccough R06.6
  epidemic B33.0
  psychogenic F45.8
Hidden penis (congenital) Q55.64
  acquired N48.83
Hidradenitis (axillaris) (suppurative) L73.2
Hidradenoma (nodular) (*see also* Neoplasm, skin, benign)
  clear cell — *see* Neoplasm, skin, benign
  papillary — *see* Neoplasm, skin, benign
Hidrocystoma — *see* Neoplasm, skin, benign
High
  altitude effects T70.20 ☑
    anoxia T70.29 ☑
    on
      ears T70.0 ☑
      sinuses T70.1 ☑
    polycythemia D75.1
  arch
    foot Q66.7
    palate, congenital Q38.5
  arterial tension — *see* Hypertension
  basal metabolic rate R94.8
  blood pressure (*see also* Hypertension)
    borderline R03.0
    reading (incidental) (isolated) (nonspecific), without diagnosis of hypertension R03.0
  cholesterol E78.0
    with high triglycerides E78.2
  diaphragm (congenital) Q79.1
  expressed emotional level within family Z63.8
  head at term O32.4 ☑
  palate, congenital Q38.5
  risk
    infant NEC Z76.2
    sexual behavior (heterosexual) Z72.51
      bisexual Z72.53
      homosexual Z72.52
  temperature (of unknown origin) R50.9
  thoracic rib Q76.6
  triglycerides E78.1
    with high cholesterol E78.2
Hildenbrand's disease A75.0
Hilum — *see* condition
Hip — *see* condition
Hippel's disease Q85.8
Hippophobia F40.218
Hippus H57.09
Hirschsprung's disease or megacolon Q43.1
Hirsutism, hirsuties L68.0
Hirudiniasis
  external B88.3
  internal B83.4
Hiss-Russell dysentery A03.1
Histidinemia, histidinuria E70.41
Histiocytoma (*see also* Neoplasm, skin, benign)
  fibrous (*see also* Neoplasm, skin, benign)
    atypical — *see* Neoplasm, connective tissue, uncertain behavior

Histiocytoma — *continued*
  fibrous (*see also* Neoplasm, skin, benign) — *continued*
    malignant — *see* Neoplasm, connective tissue, malignant
Histiocytosis D76.3
  acute differentiated progressive C96.0
  Langerhans' cell NEC C96.6
    multifocal X
      multisystemic (disseminated) C96.0
      unisystemic C96.5
    pulmonary, adult (adult PLCH) J84.82
    unifocal (X) C96.6
  lipid, lipoid D76.3
    essential E75.29
  malignant C96.A (*following* C96.6)
  mononuclear phagocytes NEC D76.1
    Langerhans' cells C96.6
  non-Langerhans cell D76.3
  polyostotic sclerosing D76.3
  sinus, with massive lymphadenopathy D76.3
  syndrome NEC D76.3
  X NEC C96.6
    acute (progressive) C96.0
    chronic C96.6
    multifocal C96.5
    multisystemic C96.0
    unifocal C96.6
Histoplasmosis B39.9
  with pneumonia NEC B39.2
  African B39.5
  American — *see* Histoplasmosis, capsulati
  capsulati B39.4
    disseminated B39.3
    generalized B39.3
    pulmonary B39.2
      acute B39.0
      chronic B39.1
  Darling's B39.4
  duboisii B39.5
  lung NEC B39.2
History
  family (of) (*see also* History, personal (of))
    alcohol abuse Z81.1
    allergy NEC Z84.89
    anemia Z83.2
    arthritis Z82.61
    asthma Z82.5
    blindness Z82.1
    cardiac death (sudden) Z82.41
    carrier of genetic disease Z84.81
    chromosomal anomaly Z82.79
    chronic
      disabling disease NEC Z82.8
      lower respiratory disease Z82.5
    colonic polyps Z83.71
    congenital malformations and deformations Z82.79
      polycystic kidney Z82.71
    consanguinity Z84.3
    deafness Z82.2
    diabetes mellitus Z83.3
    disability NEC Z82.8
    disease or disorder (of)
      allergic NEC Z84.89
      behavioral NEC Z81.8
      blood and blood-forming organs Z83.2
      cardiovascular NEC Z82.49
      chronic disabling NEC Z82.8
      digestive Z83.79
      ear NEC Z83.52
      endocrine NEC Z83.49
      eye NEC Z83.518
        glaucoma Z83.511
      genitourinary NEC Z84.2
      glaucoma Z83.511
      hematological Z83.2
      immune mechanism Z83.2
      infectious NEC Z83.1
      ischemic heart Z82.49
      kidney Z84.1
      mental NEC Z81.8
      metabolic Z83.49
      musculoskeletal NEC Z82.69
      neurological NEC Z82.0
      nutritional Z83.49
      parasitic NEC Z83.1
      psychiatric NEC Z81.8
      respiratory NEC Z83.6

History — *continued*
family (*see also* History, personal) — *continued*
   disease or disorder — *continued*
      skin and subcutaneous tissue NEC Z84.0
      specified NEC Z84.89
     drug abuse NEC Z81.3
     epilepsy Z82.0
     genetic disease carrier Z84.81
     glaucoma Z83.511
     hearing loss Z82.2
     human immunodeficiency virus (HIV) infection Z83.0
     Huntington's chorea Z82.0
     intellectual disability Z81.0
     leukemia Z80.6
     malignant neoplasm (of) NOS Z80.9
       bladder Z80.52
       breast Z80.3
       bronchus Z80.1
       digestive organ Z80.0
       gastrointestinal tract Z80.0
       genital organ Z80.49
         ovary Z80.41
         prostate Z80.42
         specified organ NEC Z80.49
         testis Z80.43
       hematopoietic NEC Z80.7
       intrathoracic organ NEC Z80.2
       kidney Z80.51
       lung Z80.1
       lymphatic NEC Z80.7
       ovary Z80.41
       prostate Z80.42
       respiratory organ NEC Z80.2
       specified site NEC Z80.8
       testis Z80.43
       trachea Z80.1
       urinary organ or tract Z80.59
         bladder Z80.52
         kidney Z80.51
   mental
     disorder NEC Z81.8
   multiple endocrine neoplasia (MEN) syndrome Z83.41
   osteoporosis Z82.62
   polycystic kidney Z82.71
   polyps (colon) Z83.71
   psychiatric disorder Z81.8
   psychoactive substance abuse NEC Z81.3
   respiratory condition NEC Z83.6
     asthma and other lower respiratory conditions Z82.5
   self-harmful behavior Z81.8
   skin condition Z84.0
   specified condition NEC Z84.89
   stroke (cerebrovascular) Z82.3
   substance abuse NEC Z81.4
     alcohol Z81.1
     drug NEC Z81.3
     psychoactive NEC Z81.3
     tobacco Z81.2
   sudden cardiac death Z82.41
   tobacco abuse Z81.2
   violence, violent behavior Z81.8
   visual loss Z82.1
personal (of) (*see also* History, family (of))
   abuse
     adult Z91.419
       physical and sexual Z91.410
       psychological Z91.411
     childhood Z62.819
       physical Z62.810
       psychological Z62.811
       sexual Z62.810
   alcohol dependence F10.21
   allergy (to) Z88.9
     analgesic agent NEC Z88.6
     anesthetic Z88.4
     antibiotic agent NEC Z88.1
     anti-infective agent NEC Z88.3
     contrast media Z91.041
     drugs, medicaments and biological substances Z88.9
       specified NEC Z88.8
     food Z91.018
       additives Z91.02
       eggs Z91.012
       milk products Z91.011

History — *continued*
personal (*see also* History, family) — *continued*
   allergy — *continued*
     food — *continued*
       peanuts Z91.010
       seafood Z91.013
       specified food NEC Z91.018
     insect Z91.038
       bee Z91.030
     latex Z91.040
     medicinal agents Z88.9
       specified NEC Z88.8
     narcotic agent NEC Z88.5
     nonmedicinal agents Z91.048
     penicillin Z88.0
     serum Z88.7
     specified NEC Z91.09
     sulfonamides Z88.2
     vaccine Z88.7
   anaphylactic shock Z87.892
   anaphylaxis Z87.892
   behavioral disorders Z86.59
   benign carcinoid tumor Z86.012
   benign neoplasm Z86.018
     brain Z86.011
     carcinoid Z86.012
     colonic polyps Z86.010
   brain injury (traumatic) Z87.820
   breast implant removal Z98.86
   calculi, renal Z87.442
   cancer — *see* History, personal (of), malignant neoplasm (of)
   cardiac arrest (death), successfully resuscitated Z86.74
   cerebral infarction without residual deficit Z86.73
   cervical dysplasia Z87.410
   chemotherapy for neoplastic condition Z92.21
   childhood abuse — *see* History, personal (of), abuse
   cleft lip (corrected) Z87.730
   cleft palate (corrected) Z87.730
   collapsed vertebra (healed) Z87.311
     due to osteoporosis Z87.310
   combat and operational stress reaction Z86.51
   congenital malformation (corrected) Z87.798
     circulatory system (corrected) Z87.74
     digestive system (corrected) NEC Z87.738
     ear (corrected) Z87.720
     eye (corrected) Z87.721
     face and neck (corrected) Z87.790
     genitourinary system (corrected) NEC Z87.718
     heart (corrected) Z87.74
     integument (corrected) Z87.76
     limb(s) (corrected) Z87.76
     musculoskeletal system (corrected) Z87.76
     neck (corrected) Z87.790
     nervous system (corrected) NEC Z87.728
     respiratory system (corrected) Z87.75
     sense organs (corrected) NEC Z87.728
     specified NEC Z87.798
   contraception Z92.0
   deployment (military) Z91.82
   diabetic foot ulcer Z86.31
   disease or disorder (of) Z87.898
     anaphylaxis Z87.892
     blood and blood-forming organs Z86.2
     circulatory system Z86.79
       specified condition NEC Z86.79
     connective tissue Z87.39
     digestive system Z87.19
       colonic polyp Z86.010
       peptic ulcer disease Z87.11
       specified condition NEC Z87.19
     ear Z86.69
     endocrine Z86.39
       diabetic foot ulcer Z86.31
       gestational diabetes Z86.32
       specified type NEC Z86.39
     eye Z86.69
     genital (track) system NEC
       female Z87.42
       male Z87.438
     hematological Z86.2
     Hodgkin Z85.71
     immune mechanism Z86.2
     infectious Z86.19
       malaria Z86.13

History — *continued*
personal (*see also* History, family) — *continued*
   disease or disorder — *continued*
     infectious — *continued*
       Methicillin resistant Staphylococcus aureus (MRSA) Z86.14
       poliomyelitis Z86.12
       specified NEC Z86.19
       tuberculosis Z86.11
     mental NEC Z86.59
     metabolic Z86.39
       diabetic foot ulcer Z86.31
       gestational diabetes Z86.32
       specified type NEC Z86.39
     musculoskeletal NEC Z87.39
     nervous system Z86.69
     nutritional Z86.39
     parasitic Z86.19
     respiratory system NEC Z87.09
     sense organs Z86.69
     skin Z87.2
     specified site or type NEC Z87.898
     subcutaneous tissue Z87.2
     trophoblastic Z87.59
     urinary system NEC Z87.448
   drug dependence — *see* Dependence, drug, by type, in remission
   drug therapy
     antineoplastic chemotherapy Z92.21
     estrogen Z92.23
     immunosupression Z92.25
     inhaled steroids Z92.240
     monoclonal drug Z92.22
     specified NEC Z92.29
     steroid Z92.241
     systemic steroids Z92.241
   dysplasia
     cervical Z87.410
     prostatic Z87.430
     vaginal Z87.411
     vulvar Z87.412
   embolism (venous) Z86.718
     pulmonary Z86.711
   encephalitis Z86.61
   estrogen therapy Z92.23
   extracorporeal membrane oxygenation (ECMO) Z92.81
   failed conscious sedation Z92.83
   failed moderate sedation Z92.83
   fall, falling Z91.81
   fracture (healed)
     fatigue Z87.312
     fragility Z87.310
     osteoporosis Z87.310
     pathological NEC Z87.311
     stress Z87.312
     traumatic Z87.81
   gestational diabetes Z86.32
   hepatitis
     B Z86.19
     C Z86.19
   Hodgkin disease Z85.71
   hyperthermia, malignant Z88.4
   hypospadias (corrected) Z87.710
   hysterectomy Z90.710
   immunosupression therapy Z92.25
   in situ neoplasm
     breast Z86.000
     cervix uteri Z86.001
     specified NEC Z86.008
   in utero procedure during pregnancy Z98.870
   in utero procedure while a fetus Z98.871
   infection NEC Z86.19
     central nervous system Z86.61
     Methicillin resistant Staphylococcus aureus (MRSA) Z86.14
     urinary (recurrent) (tract) Z87.440
   injury NEC Z87.828
   irradiation Z92.3
   kidney stones Z87.442
   leukemia Z85.6
   lymphoma (non-Hodgkin) Z85.72
   malignant melanoma (skin) Z85.820
   malignant neoplasm (of) Z85.9
     accessory sinuses Z85.22
     anus NEC Z85.048
       carcinoid Z85.040
     bladder Z85.51

History — continued
  personal (see also History, family) — continued
    malignant neoplasm — continued
      bone Z85.830
      brain Z85.841
      breast Z85.3
      bronchus NEC Z85.118
        carcinoid Z85.110
      carcinoid — see History, personal (of), malig-
          nant neoplasm, by site, carcinioid
      cervix Z85.41
      colon NEC Z85.038
        carcinoid Z85.030
      digestive organ Z85.00
        specified NEC Z85.09
      endocrine gland NEC Z85.858
      epididymis Z85.48
      esophagus Z85.01
      eye Z85.840
      gastrointestinal tract — see History, malignant
          neoplasm, digestive organ
      genital organ
        female Z85.40
          specified NEC Z85.44
        male Z85.45
          specified NEC Z85.49
      hematopoietic NEC Z85.79
      intrathoracic organ Z85.20
      kidney NEC Z85.528
        carcinoid Z85.520
      large intestine NEC Z85.038
        carcinoid Z85.030
      larynx Z85.21
      liver Z85.05
      lung NEC Z85.118
        carcinoid Z85.110
      mediastinum Z85.29
      Merkel cell Z85.821
      middle ear Z85.22
      nasal cavities Z85.22
      nervous system NEC Z85.848
      oral cavity Z85.819
        specified site NEC Z85.818
      ovary Z85.43
      pancreas Z85.07
      pelvis Z85.53
      pharynx Z85.819
        specified site NEC Z85.818
      pleura Z85.29
      prostate Z85.46
      rectosigmoid junction NEC Z85.048
        carcinoid Z85.040
      rectum NEC Z85.048
        carcinoid Z85.040
      respiratory organ Z85.20
      sinuses, accessory Z85.22
      skin NEC Z85.828
        melanoma Z85.820
        Merkel cell Z85.821
      small intestine NEC Z85.068
        carcinoid Z85.060
      soft tissue Z85.831
      specified site NEC Z85.89
      stomach NEC Z85.028
        carcinoid Z85.020
      testis Z85.47
      thymus NEC Z85.238
        carcinoid Z85.230
      thyroid Z85.850
      tongue Z85.810
      trachea Z85.12
      urinary organ or tract Z85.50
        specified NEC Z85.59
      uterus Z85.42
    maltreatment Z91.89
    medical treatment NEC Z92.89
    melanoma (malignant) (skin) Z85.820
    meningitis Z86.61
    mental disorder Z86.59
    Merkel cell carcinoma (skin) Z85.821
    Methicillin resistant Staphylococcus aureus (MRSA)
        Z86.14
    military deployment Z91.82
    military war, peacekeeping and humanitarian de-
        ployment (current or past conflict) Z91.82
    myocardial infarction (old) I25.2
    neglect (in)
      adult Z91.412

History — continued
  personal (see also History, family) — continued
    neglect — continued
      childhood Z62.812
    neoplasm
      benign Z86.018
        brain Z86.011
        colon polyp Z86.010
      in situ
        breast Z86.000
        cervix uteri Z86.001
        specified NEC Z86.008
      malignant — see History of, malignant neo-
          plasm
      uncertain behavior Z86.03
    nephrotic syndrome Z87.441
    nicotine dependence Z87.891
    noncompliance with medical treatment or regimen
        — see Noncompliance
    nutritional deficiency Z86.39
    obstetric complications Z87.59
      childbirth Z87.59
      pregnancy Z87.59
      pre-term labor Z87.51
      puerperium Z87.59
    osteoporosis fractures Z87.31 ☑
    parasuicide (attempt) Z91.5
    physical trauma NEC Z87.828
      self-harm or suicide attempt Z91.5
    pneumonia (recurrent) Z87.01
    poisoning NEC Z91.89
      self-harm or suicide attempt Z91.5
    poor personal hygiene Z91.89
    preterm labor Z87.51
    procedure during pregnancy Z98.870
    procedure while a fetus Z98.871
    prolonged reversible ischemic neurologic deficit
        (PRIND) Z86.73
    prostatic dysplasia Z87.430
    psychological
      abuse
        adult Z91.411
        child Z62.811
      trauma, specified NEC Z91.49
    radiation therapy Z92.3
    removal
      implant
        breast Z98.86
    renal calculi Z87.442
    respiratory condition NEC Z87.09
    retained foreign body fully removed Z87.821
    risk factors NEC Z91.89
    self-harm Z91.5
    self-poisoning attempt Z91.5
    sex reassignment Z87.890
    sleep-wake cycle problem Z72.821
    specified NEC Z87.898
    steroid therapy (systemic) Z92.241
      inhaled Z92.240
    stroke without residual deficits Z86.73
    substance abuse NEC F10-F19 with fifth character
        1
    sudden cardiac arrest Z86.74
    sudden cardiac death successfully resuscitated
        Z86.74
    suicide attempt Z91.5
    surgery NEC Z98.89
      sex reassignment Z87.890
      transplant — see Transplant
    thrombophlebitis Z86.72
    thrombosis (venous) Z86.718
      pulmonary Z86.711
    tobacco dependence Z87.891
    transient ischemic attack (TIA) without residual
        deficits Z86.73
    trauma (physical) NEC Z87.828
      psychological NEC Z91.49
      self-harm Z91.5
    traumatic brain injury Z87.820
    unhealthy sleep-wake cycle Z72.821
    urinary calculi Z87.442
    urinary (recurrent) (tract) infection(s) Z87.440
    vaginal dysplasia Z87.411
    venous thrombosis or embolism Z86.718
      pulmonary Z86.711
    vulvar dysplasia Z87.412
His-Werner disease A79.0

HIV (see also Human, immunodeficiency virus) B20
  laboratory evidence (nonconclusive) R75
  nonconclusive test (in infants) R75
  positive, seropositive Z21
Hives (bold) — see Urticaria
Hoarseness R49.0
Hobo Z59.0
Hodgkin disease — see Lymphoma, Hodgkin
Hodgson's disease I71.2
  ruptured I71.1
Hoffa-Kastert disease E88.89
Hoffa's disease E88.89
Hoffmann-Bouveret syndrome I47.9
Hoffmann's syndrome E03.9 [G73.7]
Hole (round)
  macula H35.34- ☑
  retina (without detachment) — see Break, retina,
      round hole
    with detachment — see Detachment, retina, with
        retinal, break
Holiday relief care Z75.5
Hollenhorst's plaque — see Occlusion, artery, retina
Hollow foot (congenital) Q66.7
  acquired — see Deformity, limb, foot, specified NEC
Holoprosencephaly Q04.2
Holt-Oram syndrome Q87.2
Homelessness Z59.0
Homesickness — see Disorder, adjustment
Homocystinemia, homocystinuria E72.11
Homogentisate 1,2-dioxygenase deficiency E70.29
Homologous serum hepatitis (prophylactic) (therapeu-
    tic) — see Hepatitis, viral, type B
Honeycomb lung J98.4
  congenital Q33.0
Hooded
  clitoris Q52.6
  penis Q55.69
Hookworm (anemia) (disease) (infection) (infestation)
    B76.9
  specified NEC B76.8
Hordeolum (eyelid) (externum) (recurrent) H00.019
  internum H00.029
    left H00.026
      lower H00.025
      upper H00.024
    right H00.023
      lower H00.022
      upper H00.021
  left H00.016
    lower H00.015
    upper H00.014
  right H00.013
    lower H00.012
    upper H00.011
Horn
  cutaneous L85.8
  nail L60.2
    congenital Q84.6
Horner (-Claude Bernard) **syndrome** G90.2
  traumatic — see Injury, nerve, cervical sympathetic
Horseshoe kidney (congenital) Q63.1
Horton's headache or neuralgia G44.099
  intractable G44.091
  not intractable G44.099
Hospital hopper syndrome — see Disorder, factitious
Hospitalism in children — see Disorder, adjustment
Hostility R45.5
  towards child Z62.3
Hot flashes
  menopausal N95.1
Hourglass (contracture) (see also Contraction, hourglass)
  stomach K31.89
    congenital Q40.2
    stricture K31.2
Household, housing circumstance affecting care
    Z59.9
  specified NEC Z59.8
Housemaid's knee — see Bursitis, prepatellar
Hudson (-Stähli) **line** (cornea) — see Pigmentation,
    cornea, anterior
Human
  bite (open wound) (see also Bite)
    intact skin surface — see Bite, superficial
  herpesvirus — see Herpes
  immunodeficiency virus (HIV) disease (infection) B20
    asymptomatic status Z21
    contact Z20.6

Human — *continued*
immunodeficiency virus disease — *continued*
counseling Z71.7
dementia B20 [F02.80]
with behavioral disturbance B20 [F02.81]
exposure to Z20.6
laboratory evidence R75
type-2 (HIV 2) as cause of disease classified elsewhere B97.35
papillomavirus (HPV)
DNA test positive
high risk
cervix R87.810
vagina R87.811
low risk
cervix R87.820
vagina R87.821
screening for Z11.51
T-cell lymphotropic virus
type-1 (HTLV-I) infection B33.3
as cause of disease classified elsewhere B97.33
carrier Z22.6
type-2 (HTLV-II) as cause of disease classified elsewhere B97.34
Humidifier lung or pneumonitis J67.7
Humiliation (experience) **in childhood** Z62.898
Humpback (acquired) — *see* Kyphosis
Hunchback (acquired) — *see* Kyphosis
Hunger T73.0 ☑
air, psychogenic F45.8
Hungry bone syndrome E83.81
Hunner's ulcer — *see* Cystitis, chronic, interstitial
Hunter's
glossitis D51.0
syndrome E76.1
Huntington's disease or chorea G10
with dementia G10 [F02.80]
with behavioral disturbance G10 [F02.81]
Hunt's
disease or syndrome (herpetic geniculate ganglionitis) B02.21
dyssynergia cerebellaris myoclonica G11.1
neuralgia B02.21
Hurler (-Scheie) **disease or syndrome** E76.02
Hurst's disease G36.1
Hurthle cell
adenocarcinoma C73
adenoma D34
carcinoma C73
tumor D34
Hutchinson-Boeck disease or syndrome — *see* Sarcoidosis
Hutchinson-Gilford disease or syndrome E34.8
Hutchinson's
disease, meaning
angioma serpiginosum L81.7
pompholyx (cheiropompholyx) L30.1
prurigo estivalis L56.4
summer eruption or summer prurigo L56.4
melanotic freckle — *see* Melanoma, in situ
malignant melanoma in — *see* Melanoma
teeth or incisors (congenital syphilis) A50.52
triad (congenital syphilis) A50.53
Hyalin plaque, sclera, senile H15.89
Hyaline membrane (disease) (lung) (pulmonary) (newborn) P22.0
Hyalinosis
cutis (et mucosae) E78.89
focal and segmental (glomerular) (*see also* N00-N07 with fourth character .1) N05.1
Hyalitis, hyalosis, asteroid (*see also* Deposit, crystalline)
syphilitic (late) A52.71
Hydatid
cyst or tumor — *see* Echinococcus
mole — *see* Hydatidiform mole
Morgagni
female Q50.5
male (epididymal) Q55.4
testicular Q55.29
Hydatidiform mole (benign) (complicating pregnancy) (delivered) (undelivered) O01.9
classical O01.0
complete O01.0
incomplete O01.1
invasive D39.2
malignant D39.2
partial O01.1
Hydatidosis — *see* Echinococcus

Hydradenitis (axillaris) (suppurative) L73.2
Hydradenoma — *see* Hidradenoma
Hydramnios O40.- ☑
Hydrancephaly, hydranencephaly Q04.3
with spina bifida — *see* Spina bifida, with hydrocephalus
Hydrargyrism NEC — *see* Poisoning, mercury
Hydrarthrosis (*see also* Effusion, joint)
gonococcal A54.42
intermittent M12.40
ankle M12.47- ☑
elbow M12.42- ☑
foot joint M12.47- ☑
hand joint M12.44- ☑
hip M12.45- ☑
knee M12.46- ☑
multiple site M12.49
shoulder M12.41- ☑
specified joint NEC M12.48
wrist M12.43- ☑
of yaws (early) (late) (*see also* subcategory M14.8-) A66.6
syphilitic (late) A52.77
congenital A50.55 [M12.80]
Hydremia D64.89
Hydrencephalocele (congenital) — *see* Encephalocele
Hydrencephalomeningocele (congenital) — *see* Encephalocele
Hydroa R23.8
aestivale L56.4
vacciniforme L56.4
Hydroadenitis (axillaris) (suppurative) L73.2
Hydrocalycosis — *see* Hydronephrosis
Hydrocele (spermatic cord) (testis) (tunica vaginalis) N43.3
canal of Nuck N94.89
communicating N43.2
congenital P83.5
congenital P83.5
encysted N43.0
female NEC N94.89
infected N43.1
newborn P83.5
round ligament N94.89
specified NEC N43.2
spinalis — *see* Spina bifida
vulva N90.89
Hydrocephalus (acquired) (external) (internal) (malignant) (recurrent) G91.9
aqueduct Sylvius stricture Q03.0
causing disproportion O33.6 ☑
with obstructed labor O66.3
communicating G91.0
congenital (external) (internal) Q03.9
with spina bifida Q05.4
cervical Q05.0
dorsal Q05.1
lumbar Q05.2
lumbosacral Q05.2
sacral Q05.3
thoracic Q05.1
thoracolumbar Q05.1
specified NEC Q03.8
due to toxoplasmosis (congenital) P37.1
foramen Magendie block (acquired) G91.1
congenital (*see also* Hydrocephalus, congenital) Q03.1
in (due to)
infectious disease NEC B89 [G91.4]
neoplastic disease NEC (*see also* Neoplasm) G91.4
parasitic disease B89 [G91.4]
newborn Q03.9
with spina bifida — *see* Spina bifida, with hydrocephalus
noncommunicating G91.1
normal pressure G91.2
secondary G91.0
obstructive G91.1
otitic G93.2
post-traumatic NEC G91.3
secondary G91.4
post-traumatic G91.3
specified NEC G91.8
syphilitic, congenital A50.49
Hydrocolpos (congenital) N89.8
Hydrocystoma — *see* Neoplasm, skin, benign
Hydroencephalocele (congenital) — *see* Encephalocele

Hydroencephalomeningocele (congenital) — *see* Encephalocele
Hydrohematopneumothorax — *see* Hemothorax
Hydromeningitis — *see* Meningitis
Hydromeningocele (spinal) (*see also* Spina bifida)
cranial — *see* Encephalocele
Hydrometra N85.8
Hydrometrocolpos N89.8
Hydromicrocephaly Q02
Hydromphalos (since birth) Q45.8
Hydromyelia Q06.4
Hydromyelocele — *see* Spina bifida
Hydronephrosis (atrophic) (early) (functionless) (intermittent) (primary) (secondary) NEC N13.30
with
infection N13.6
obstruction (by) (of)
renal calculus N13.2
with infection N13.6
ureteral NEC N13.1
with infection N13.6
calculus N13.2
with infection N13.6
ureteropelvic junction (congenital) Q62.0
with infection N13.6
ureteral stricture NEC N13.1
with infection N13.6
congenital Q62.0
specified type NEC N13.39
tuberculous A18.11
Hydropericarditis — *see* Pericarditis
Hydropericardium — *see* Pericarditis
Hydroperitoneum R18.8
Hydrophobia — *see* Rabies
Hydrophthalmos Q15.0
Hydropneumohemothorax — *see* Hemothorax
Hydropneumopericarditis — *see* Pericarditis
Hydropneumopericardium — *see* Pericarditis
Hydropneumothorax J94.8
traumatic — *see* Injury, intrathoracic, lung
tuberculous NEC A15.6
Hydrops R60.9
abdominis R18.8
articulorum intermittens — *see* Hydrarthrosis, intermittent
cardiac — *see* Failure, heart, congestive
causing obstructed labor (mother) O66.3
endolymphatic H81.0- ☑
fetal — *see* Pregnancy, complicated by, hydrops, fetalis
fetalis P83.2
due to
ABO isoimmunization P56.0
alpha thalassemia D56.0
hemolytic disease P56.90
specified NEC P56.99
isoimmunization (ABO) (Rh) P56.0
other specified nonhemolytic disease NEC P83.2
Rh incompatibility P56.0
during pregnancy — *see* Pregnancy, complicated by, hydrops, fetalis
gallbladder K82.1
joint — *see* Effusion, joint
labyrinth H81.0- ☑
newborn (idiopathic) P83.2
due to
ABO isoimmunization P56.0
alpha thalassemia D56.0
hemolytic disease P56.90
specified NEC P56.99
isoimmunization (ABO) (Rh) P56.0
Rh incompatibility P56.0
nutritional — *see* Malnutrition, severe
pericardium — *see* Pericarditis
pleura — *see* Hydrothorax
spermatic cord — *see* Hydrocele
Hydropyonephrosis N13.6
Hydrorachis Q06.4
Hydrorrhea (nasal) J34.89
pregnancy — *see* Rupture, membranes, premature
Hydrosadenitis (axillaris) (suppurative) L73.2
Hydrosalpinx (fallopian tube) (follicularis) N70.11
Hydrothorax (double) (pleura) J94.8
chylous (nonfilarial) I89.8
filarial (*see also* Infestation, filarial) B74.9 [J91.8]
traumatic — *see* Injury, intrathoracic
tuberculous NEC (non primary) A15.6

☑ **Additional Character Required** — **Refer to the Tabular List for Character Selection** ▽ **Subterms under main terms may continue to next column or page**

Hydroureter (*see also* Hydronephrosis) N13.4
  with infection N13.6
  congenital Q62.39
Hydroureteronephrosis — *see* Hydronephrosis
Hydrourethra N36.8
Hydroxykynureninuria E70.8
Hydroxylysinemia E72.3
Hydroxyprolinemia E72.59
Hygiene, sleep
  abuse Z72.821
  inadequate Z72.821
  poor Z72.821
Hygroma (congenital) (cystic) D18.1
  praepatellare, prepatellar — *see* Bursitis, prepatellar
Hymen — *see* condition
Hymenolepis, hymenolepiasis (diminuta) (infection) (infestation) (nana) B71.0
Hypalgesia R20.8
Hyperacidity (gastric) K31.89
  psychogenic F45.8
Hyperactive, hyperactivity F90.9
  basal cell, uterine cervix — *see* Dysplasia, cervix
  bowel sounds R19.12
  cervix epithelial (basal) — *see* Dysplasia, cervix
  child F90.9
    attention deficit — *see* Disorder, attention-deficit hyperactivity
  detrusor muscle N32.81
  gastrointestinal K31.89
    psychogenic F45.8
  nasal mucous membrane J34.3
  stomach K31.89
  thyroid (gland) — *see* Hyperthyroidism
Hyperacusis H93.23- ☑
Hyperadrenalism E27.5
Hyperadrenocorticism E24.9
  congenital E25.0
  iatrogenic E24.2
    correct substance properly administered — *see* Table of Drugs and Chemicals, by drug, adverse effect
    overdose or wrong substance given or taken — *see* Table of Drugs and Chemicals, by drug, poisoning
  not associated with Cushing's syndrome E27.0
  pituitary-dependent E24.0
Hyperaldosteronism E26.9
  familial (type I) E26.02
  glucocorticoid-remediable E26.02
  primary (due to (bilateral) adrenal hyperplasia) E26.09
  primary NEC E26.09
  secondary E26.1
  specified NEC E26.89
Hyperalgesia R20.8
Hyperalimentation R63.2
  carotene, carotin E67.1
  specified NEC E67.8
  vitamin
    A E67.0
    D E67.3
Hyperaminoaciduria
  arginine E72.21
  cystine E72.01
  lysine E72.3
  ornithine E72.4
Hyperammonemia (congenital) E72.20
Hyperazotemia — *see* Uremia
Hyperbetalipoproteinemia (familial) E78.0
  with prebetalipoproteinemia E78.2
Hyperbilirubinemia
  constitutional E80.6
  familial conjugated E80.6
  neonatal (transient) — *see* Jaundice, newborn
Hypercalcemia, hypocalciuric, familial E83.52
Hypercalciuria, idiopathic E83.52
Hypercapnia R06.89
  newborn P84
Hypercarotenemia, hypercarotinemia (dietary) E67.1
Hypercementosis K03.4
Hyperchloremia E87.8
Hyperchlorhydria K31.89
  neurotic F45.8
  psychogenic F45.8
Hypercholesterinemia — *see* Hypercholesterolemia
Hypercholesterolemia (essential) (familial) (hereditary) (primary) (pure) E78.0
  with hyperglyceridemia, endogenous E78.2

Hypercholesterolemia — *continued*
  dietary counseling and surveillance Z71.3
Hyperchylia gastrica, psychogenic F45.8
Hyperchylomicronemia (familial) (primary) E78.3
  with hyperbetalipoproteinemia E78.3
Hypercoagulable (state) D68.59
  activated protein C resistance D68.51
  antithrombin (III) deficiency D68.59
  factor V Leiden mutation D68.51
  primary NEC D68.59
  protein C deficiency D68.59
  protein S deficiency D68.59
  prothrombin gene mutation D68.52
  secondary D68.69
  specified NEC D68.69
Hypercoagulation (state) D68.59
Hypercorticalism, pituitary-dependent E24.0
Hypercorticosolism — *see* Cushing's, syndrome
Hypercorticosteronism E24.2
  correct substance properly administered — *see* Table of Drugs and Chemicals, by drug, adverse effect
  overdose or wrong substance given or taken — *see* Table of Drugs and Chemicals, by drug, poisoning
Hypercortisonism E24.2
  correct substance properly administered — *see* Table of Drugs and Chemicals, by drug, adverse effect
  overdose or wrong substance given or taken — *see* Table of Drugs and Chemicals, by drug, poisoning
Hyperekplexia Q89.8
Hyperelectrolytemia E87.8
Hyperemesis R11.10
  with nausea R11.2
  gravidarum (mild) O21.0
    with
      carbohydrate depletion O21.1
      dehydration O21.1
      electrolyte imbalance O21.1
      metabolic disturbance O21.1
    severe (with metabolic disturbance) O21.1
  projectile R11.12
  psychogenic F45.8
Hyperemia (acute) (passive) R68.89
  anal mucosa K62.89
  bladder N32.89
  cerebral I67.89
  conjunctiva H11.43- ☑
  ear internal, acute — *see* subcategory H83.0 ☑
  enteric K59.8
  eye — *see* Hyperemia, conjunctiva
  eyelid (active) (passive) — *see* Disorder, eyelid, specified type NEC
  intestine K59.8
  iris — *see* Disorder, iris, vascular
  kidney N28.89
  labyrinth — *see* subcategory H83.0 ☑
  liver (active) K76.89
  lung (passive) — *see* Edema, lung
  pulmonary (passive) — *see* Edema, lung
  renal N28.89
  retina H35.89
  stomach K31.89
Hyperesthesia (body surface) R20.3
  larynx (reflex) J38.7
    hysterical F44.89
  pharynx (reflex) J39.2
    hysterical F44.89
Hyperestrogenism (drug-induced) (iatrogenic) E28.0
Hyperexplexia Q89.8
Hyperfibrinolysis — *see* Fibrinolysis
Hyperfructosemia E74.19
Hyperfunction
  adrenal cortex, not associated with Cushing's syndrome E27.0
    medulla E27.5
      adrenomedullary E27.5
    virilism E25.9
      congenital E25.0
  ovarian E28.8
  pancreas K86.8
  parathyroid (gland) E21.3
  pituitary (gland) (anterior) E22.9
    specified NEC E22.8
  polyglandular E31.1
  testicular E29.0

Hypergammaglobulinemia D89.2
  polyclonal D89.0
  Waldenström D89.0
Hypergastrinemia E16.4
Hyperglobulinemia R77.1
Hyperglycemia, hyperglycemic (transient) R73.9
  coma — *see* Diabetes, by type, with coma
  postpancreatectomy E89.1
Hyperglyceridemia (endogenous) (essential) (familial) (hereditary) (pure) E78.1
  mixed E78.3
Hyperglycinemia (non-ketotic) E72.51
Hypergonadism
  ovarian E28.8
  testicular (primary) (infantile) E29.0
Hyperheparinemia D68.32
Hyperhidrosis, hyperidrosis R61
  focal
    primary L74.519
      axilla L74.510
      face L74.511
      palms L74.512
      soles L74.513
    secondary L74.52
  generalized R61
  localized
    primary L74.519
      axilla L74.510
      face L74.511
      palms L74.512
      soles L74.513
    secondary L74.52
  psychogenic F45.8
  secondary R61
    focal L74.52
Hyperhistidinemia E70.41
Hyperhomocysteinemia E72.11
Hyperhydroxyprolinemia E72.59
Hyperinsulinism (functional) E16.1
  with
    coma (hypoglycemic) E15
    encephalopathy E16.1 [G94]
  ectopic E16.1
  therapeutic misadventure (from administration of insulin) — *see* subcategory T38.3 ☑
Hyperkalemia E87.5
Hyperkeratosis (*see also* Keratosis) L85.9
  cervix N88.0
  due to yaws (early) (late) (palmar or plantar) A66.3
  follicularis Q82.8
    penetrans (in cutem) L87.0
  palmoplantaris climacterica L85.1
  pinta A67.1
  senile (with pruritus) L57.0
  universalis congenita Q80.8
  vocal cord J38.3
  vulva N90.4
Hyperkinesia, hyperkinetic (disease) (reaction) (syndrome) (childhood) (adolescence) (*see also* Disorder, attention-deficit hyperactivity)
  heart I51.89
Hyperleucine-isoleucinemia E71.19
Hyperlipemia, hyperlipidemia E78.5
  combined E78.2
    familial E78.4
  group
    A E78.0
    B E78.1
    C E78.2
    D E78.3
  mixed E78.2
  specified NEC E78.4
Hyperlipidosis E75.6
  hereditary NEC E75.5
Hyperlipoproteinemia E78.5
  Fredrickson's type
    I E78.3
    IIa E78.0
    IIb E78.2
    III E78.2
    IV E78.1
    V E78.3
  low-density-lipoprotein-type (LDL) E78.0
  very-low-density-lipoprotein-type (VLDL) E78.1
Hyperlucent lung, unilateral J43.0
Hyperlysinemia E72.3
Hypermagnesemia E83.41
  neonatal P71.8

Hypermenorrhea N92.0
Hypermethioninemia E72.19
Hypermetropia (congenital) H52.0- ☑
Hypermobility, hypermotility
  cecum — see Syndrome, irritable bowel
  coccyx — see subcategory M53.2 ☑
  colon — see Syndrome, irritable bowel
    psychogenic F45.8
  ileum K58.9
  intestine (see also Syndrome, irritable bowel) K58.9
    psychogenic F45.8
  meniscus (knee) — see Derangement, knee, meniscus
  scapula — see Instability, joint, shoulder
  stomach K31.89
    psychogenic F45.8
  syndrome M35.7
  urethra N36.41
    with intrinsic sphincter deficiency N36.43
Hypernasality R49.21
Hypernatremia E87.0
Hypernephroma C64.- ☑
Hyperopia — see Hypermetropia
Hyperorexia nervosa F50.2
Hyperornithinemia E72.4
Hyperosmia R43.1
Hyperosmolality E87.0
Hyperostosis (monomelic) (see also Disorder, bone, density and structure, specified NEC)
  ankylosing (spine) M48.10
    cervical region M48.12
    cervicothoracic region M48.13
    lumbar region M48.16
    lumbosacral region M48.17
    multiple sites M48.19
    occipito-atlanto-axial region M48.11
    sacrococcygeal region M48.18
    thoracic region M48.14
    thoracolumbar region M48.15
  cortical (skull) M85.2
    infantile M89.8X- ☑
  frontal, internal of skull M85.2
  interna frontalis M85.2
  skeletal, diffuse idiopathic — see Hyperostosis, ankylosing
  skull M85.2
    congenital Q75.8
  vertebral, ankylosing — see Hyperostosis, ankylosing
Hyperovarism E28.8
Hyperoxaluria (primary) E72.53
Hyperparathyroidism E21.3
  primary E21.0
  secondary (renal) N25.81
    non-renal E21.1
  specified NEC E21.2
  tertiary E21.2
Hyperpathia R20.8
Hyperperistalsis R19.2
  psychogenic F45.8
Hyperpermeability, capillary I78.8
Hyperphagia R63.2
Hyperphenylalaninemia NEC E70.1
Hyperphoria (alternating) H50.53
Hyperphosphatemia E83.39
Hyperpiesis, hyperpiesia — see Hypertension
Hyperpigmentation (see also Pigmentation)
  melanin NEC L81.4
  postinflammatory L81.0
Hyperpinealism E34.8
Hyperpituitarism E22.9
Hyperplasia, hyperplastic
  adenoids J35.2
  adrenal (capsule) (cortex) (gland) E27.8
    with
      sexual precocity (male) E25.9
        congenital E25.0
      virilism, adrenal E25.9
        congenital E25.0
      virilization (female) E25.9
        congenital E25.0
    congenital E25.0
      salt-losing E25.0
  adrenomedullary E27.5
  angiolymphoid, eosinophilia (ALHE) D18.01
  appendix (lymphoid) K38.0
  artery, fibromuscular I77.3
  bone (see also Hypertrophy, bone)
    marrow D75.89

Hyperplasia, hyperplastic — continued
  breast (see also Hypertrophy, breast)
    ductal (atypical) N60.9- ☑
  C-cell, thyroid E07.0
  cementation (tooth) (teeth) K03.4
  cervical gland R59.0
  cervix (uteri) (basal cell) (endometrium) (polypoid) (see also Dysplasia, cervix)
    congenital Q51.828
  clitoris, congenital Q52.6
  denture K06.2
  endocervicitis N72
  endometrium, endometrial (adenomatous) (benign) (cystic) (glandular) (glandular-cystic) (polypoid) N85.00
    with atypia N85.02
    cervix — see Dysplasia, cervix
    complex (without atypia) N85.01
    simple (without atypia) N85.01
  epithelial L85.9
    focal, oral, including tongue K13.29
    nipple N62
    skin L85.9
    tongue K13.29
    vaginal wall N89.3
  erythroid D75.89
  fibromuscular of artery (carotid) (renal) I77.3
  genital
    female NEC N94.89
    male N50.8
  gingiva K06.1
  glandularis cystica uteri (interstitialis) (see also Hyperplasia, endometrial) N85.00
  gum K06.1
  hymen, congenital Q52.4
  irritative, edentulous (alveolar) K06.2
  jaw M26.09
    alveolar M26.79
    lower M26.03
      alveolar M26.72
    upper M26.01
      alveolar M26.71
  kidney (congenital) Q63.3
  labia N90.6
    epithelial N90.3
  liver (congenital) Q44.7
    nodular, focal K76.89
  lymph gland or node R59.9
  mandible, mandibular M26.03
    alveolar M26.72
    unilateral condylar M27.8
  maxilla, maxillary M26.01
    alveolar M26.71
  myometrium, myometrial N85.2
  neuroendocrine cell, of infancy J84.841
  nose
    lymphoid J34.89
    polypoid J33.9
  oral mucosa (irritative) K13.6
  organ or site, congenital NEC — see Anomaly, by site
  ovary N83.8
  palate, papillary (irritative) K13.6
  pancreatic islet cells E16.9
    alpha E16.8
      with excess
        gastrin E16.4
        glucagon E16.3
    beta E16.1
  parathyroid (gland) E21.0
  pharynx (lymphoid) J39.2
  prostate (adenofibromatous) (nodular) N40.0
    with lower urinary tract symptoms (LUTS) N40.1
    without lower urinary tract symtpoms (LUTS) N40.0
  renal artery I77.89
  reticulo-endothelial (cell) D75.89
  salivary gland (any) K11.1
  Schimmelbusch's — see Mastopathy, cystic
  suprarenal capsule (gland) E27.8
  thymus (gland) (persistent) E32.0
  thyroid (gland) — see Goiter
  tonsils (faucial) (infective) (lingual) (lymphoid) J35.1
    with adenoids J35.3
  unilateral condylar M27.8
  uterus, uterine N85.2
    endometrium (glandular) (see also Hyperplasia, endometrial) N85.00
  vulva N90.6
    epithelial N90.3

Hyperpnea — see Hyperventilation
Hyperpotassemia E87.5
Hyperprebetalipoproteinemia (familial) E78.1
Hyperprolactinemia E22.1
Hyperprolinemia (type I) (type II) E72.59
Hyperproteinemia E88.09
Hyperprothrombinemia, causing coagulation factor deficiency D68.4
Hyperpyrexia R50.9
  heat (effects) T67.0 ☑
  malignant, due to anesthetic T88.3 ☑
  rheumatic — see Fever, rheumatic
  unknown origin R50.9
Hyper-reflexia R29.2
Hypersalivation K11.7
Hypersecretion
  ACTH (not associated with Cushing's syndrome) E27.0
    pituitary E24.0
  adrenaline E27.5
  adrenomedullary E27.5
  androgen (testicular) E29.0
    ovarian (drug-induced) (iatrogenic) E28.1
  calcitonin E07.0
  catecholamine E27.5
  corticoadrenal E24.9
  cortisol E24.9
  epinephrine E27.5
  estrogen E28.0
  gastric K31.89
    psychogenic F45.8
  gastrin E16.4
  glucagon E16.3
  hormone(s)
    ACTH (not associated with Cushing's syndrome) E27.0
      pituitary E24.0
    antidiuretic E22.2
    growth E22.0
    intestinal NEC E34.1
    ovarian androgen E28.1
    pituitary E22.9
    testicular E29.0
    thyroid stimulating E05.80
      with thyroid storm E05.81
  insulin — see Hyperinsulinism
  lacrimal glands — see Epiphora
  medulloadrenal E27.5
  milk O92.6
  ovarian androgens E28.1
  salivary gland (any) K11.7
  thyrocalcitonin E07.0
  upper respiratory J39.8
Hypersegmentation, leukocytic, hereditary D72.0
Hypersensitive, hypersensitiveness, hypersensitivity (see also Allergy)
  carotid sinus G90.01
  colon — see Irritable, colon
  drug T88.7 ☑
  gastrointestinal K52.2
    psychogenic F45.8
  labyrinth — see subcategory H83.2 ☑
  pain R20.8
  pneumonitis — see Pneumonitis, allergic
  reaction T78.40 ☑
    upper respiratory tract NEC J39.3
Hypersomnia (organic) G47.10
  due to
    alcohol
      abuse F10.182
      dependence F10.282
      use F10.982
    amphetamines
      abuse F15.182
      dependence F15.282
      use F15.982
    caffeine
      abuse F15.182
      dependence F15.282
      use F15.982
    cocaine
      abuse F14.182
      dependence F14.282
      use F14.982
    drug NEC
      abuse F19.182
      dependence F19.282
      use F19.982
    medical condition G47.14

☑ Additional Character Required — Refer to the Tabular List for Character Selection   Subterms under main terms may continue to next column or page

Hypersomnia — *continued*
due to — *continued*
mental disorder F51.13
opioid
abuse F11.182
dependence F11.282
use F11.982
psychoactive substance NEC
abuse F19.182
dependence F19.282
use F19.982
sedative, hypnotic, or anxiolytic
abuse F13.182
dependence F13.282
use F13.982
stimulant NEC
abuse F15.182
dependence F15.282
use F15.982
idiopathic G47.11
with long sleep time G47.11
without long sleep time G47.12
menstrual related G47.13
nonorganic origin F51.11
specified NEC F51.19
not due to a substance or known physiological condition F51.11
specified NEC F51.19
primary F51.11
recurrent G47.13
specified NEC G47.19
Hypersplenia, hypersplenism D73.1
Hyperstimulation, ovaries (associated with induced ovulation) N98.1
Hypersusceptibility — *see* Allergy
Hypertelorism (ocular) (orbital) Q75.2
Hypertension, hypertensive (accelerated) (benign) (essential) (idiopathic) (malignant) (systemic) I10
with
heart involvement (conditions in I51.4 - I51.9 due to hypertension) — *see* Hypertension, heart
kidney involvement — *see* Hypertension, kidney
benign, intracranial G93.2
borderline R03.0
cardiorenal (disease) I13.10
with heart failure I13.0
with stage 1 through stage 4 chronic kidney disease I13.0
with stage 5 or end stage renal disease I13.2
without heart failure I13.10
with stage 1 through stage 4 chronic kidney disease I13.10
with stage 5 or end stage renal disease I13.11
cardiovascular
disease (arteriosclerotic) (sclerotic) — *see* Hypertension, heart
renal (disease) — *see* Hypertension, cardiorenal
chronic venous — *see* Hypertension, venous (chronic)
complicating
childbirth (labor) O10.92
with
heart disease O10.12
with renal disease O10.32
renal disease O10.22
with heart disease O10.32
essential O10.02
secondary O10.42
pregnancy O16.- ☑
with edema (*see also* Pre-eclampsia) O14.9- ☑
gestational (pregnancy induced) (transient) (without proteinuria) O13.- ☑
with proteinuria O14.9- ☑
mild pre-eclampsia O14.0- ☑
moderate pre-eclampsia O14.0- ☑
severe pre-eclampsia O14.1- ☑
with hemolysis, elevated liver enzymes and low platelet count (HELLP) O14.2- ☑
pre-existing O10.91- ☑
with
heart disease O10.11- ☑
with renal disease O10.31- ☑
pre-eclampsia O11.- ☑
renal disease O10.21- ☑
with heart disease O10.31- ☑
essential O10.01- ☑
secondary O10.41- ☑

Hypertension, hypertensive — *continued*
complicating — *continued*
puerperium, pre-existing O10.93
with
heart disease O10.13
with renal disease O10.33
renal disease O10.23
with heart disease O10.33
essential O10.03
pregnancy-induced O13.9
secondary O10.43
due to
endocrine disorders I15.2
pheochromocytoma I15.2
renal disorders NEC I15.1
arterial I15.0
renovascular disorders I15.0
specified disease NEC I15.8
encephalopathy I67.4
gestational (without significant proteinuria) (pregnancy-induced) (transient) O13.- ☑
with significant proteinuria — *see* Pre-eclampsia
Goldblatt's I70.1
heart (disease) (conditions in I51.4-I51.9 due to hypertension) I11.9
with
heart failure (congestive) I11.0
kidney disease (chronic) — *see* Hypertension, cardiorenal
intracranial (benign) G93.2
kidney I12.9
with
heart disease — *see* Hypertension, cardiorenal
stage 1 through stage 4 chronic kidney disease I12.9
stage 5 chronic kidney disease (CKD) or end stage renal disease (ESRD) I12.0
lesser circulation I27.0
newborn P29.2
pulmonary (persistent) P29.3
ocular H40.05- ☑
pancreatic duct — *code to* underlying condition
with chronic pancreatitis K86.1
portal (due to chronic liver disease) (idiopathic) K76.6
gastropathy K31.89
in (due to) schistosomiasis (bilharziasis) B65.9 [K77]
postoperative I97.3
psychogenic F45.8
pulmonary (artery) (secondary) NEC I27.2
with
cor pulmonale (chronic) I27.2
acute I26.09
right heart ventricular strain/failure I27.2
acute I26.09
of newborn (persistent) P29.3
primary (idiopathic) I27.0
renal — *see* Hypertension, kidney
renovascular I15.0
secondary NEC I15.9
due to
endocrine disorders I15.2
pheochromocytoma I15.2
renal disorders NEC I15.1
arterial I15.0
renovascular disorders I15.0
specified NEC I15.8
venous (chronic)
due to
deep vein thrombosis — *see* Syndrome, postthrombotic
idiopathic I87.309
with
inflammation I87.32- ☑
with ulcer I87.33- ☑
specified complication NEC I87.39- ☑
ulcer I87.31- ☑
with inflammation I87.33- ☑
asymptomatic I87.30- ☑
Hypertensive urgency — *see* Hypertension
Hyperthecosis ovary E28.8
Hyperthermia (of unknown origin) (*see also* Hyperpyrexia)
malignant, due to anesthesia T88.3 ☑
newborn P81.9
environmental P81.0
Hyperthyroid (recurrent) — *see* Hyperthyroidism

Hyperthyroidism (latent) (pre-adult) (recurrent) E05.90
with
goiter (diffuse) E05.00
with thyroid storm E05.01
nodular (multinodular) E05.20
with thyroid storm E05.21
uninodular E05.10
with thyroid storm E05.11
storm E05.91
due to ectopic thyroid tissue E05.30
with thyroid storm E05.31
neonatal, transitory P72.1
specified NEC E05.80
with thyroid storm E05.81
Hypertony, hypertonia, hypertonicity
bladder N31.8
congenital P94.1
stomach K31.89
psychogenic F45.8
uterus, uterine (contractions) (complicating delivery) O62.4
Hypertrichosis L68.9
congenital Q84.2
eyelid H02.869
left H02.866
lower H02.865
upper H02.864
right H02.863
lower H02.862
upper H02.861
lanuginosa Q84.2
acquired L68.1
localized L68.2
specified NEC L68.8
Hypertriglyceridemia, essential E78.1
Hypertrophy, hypertrophic
adenofibromatous, prostate — *see* Enlargement, enlarged, prostate
adenoids (infective) J35.2
with tonsils J35.3
adrenal cortex E27.8
alveolar process or ridge — *see* Anomaly, alveolar
anal papillae K62.89
artery I77.89
congenital NEC Q27.8
digestive system Q27.8
lower limb Q27.8
specified site NEC Q27.8
upper limb Q27.8
auricular — *see* Hypertrophy, cardiac
Bartholin's gland N75.8
bile duct (common) (hepatic) K83.8
bladder (sphincter) (trigone) N32.89
bone M89.30
carpus M89.34- ☑
clavicle M89.31- ☑
femur M89.35- ☑
fibula M89.36- ☑
finger M89.34- ☑
humerus M89.32- ☑
ilium M89.359
ischium M89.359
metacarpus M89.34- ☑
metatarsus M89.37- ☑
multiple sites M89.39
neck M89.38
radius M89.33- ☑
rib M89.38
scapula M89.31- ☑
skull M89.38
tarsus M89.37- ☑
tibia M89.36- ☑
toe M89.37- ☑
ulna M89.33- ☑
vertebra M89.38
brain G93.89
breast N62
cystic — *see* Mastopathy, cystic
newborn P83.4
pubertal, massive N62
puerperal, postpartum — *see* Disorder, breast, specified type NEC
senile (parenchymatous) N62
cardiac (chronic) (idiopathic) I51.7
with rheumatic fever (conditions in I00)
active I01.8
inactive or quiescent (with chorea) I09.89
congenital NEC Q24.8

Hypertrophy, hypertrophic — *continued*
cardiac — *continued*
fatty — *see* Degeneration, myocardial
hypertensive — *see* Hypertension, heart
rheumatic (with chorea) I09.89
active or acute I01.8
with chorea I02.0
valve — *see* Endocarditis
cartilage — *see* Disorder, cartilage, specified type NEC
cecum — *see* Megacolon
cervix (uteri) N88.8
congenital Q51.828
elongation N88.4
clitoris (cirrhotic) N90.89
congenital Q52.6
colon (*see also* Megacolon)
congenital Q43.2
conjunctiva, lymphoid H11.89
corpora cavernosa N48.89
cystic duct K82.8
duodenum K31.89
endometrium (glandular) (*see also* Hyperplasia, endometrial) N85.00
cervix N88.8
epididymis N50.8
esophageal hiatus (congenital) Q79.1
with hernia — *see* Hernia, hiatal
eyelid — *see* Disorder, eyelid, specified type NEC
fat pad E65
knee (infrapatellar) (popliteal) (prepatellar)
(retropatellar) M79.4
foot (congenital) Q74.2
frenulum, frenum (tongue) K14.8
lip K13.0
gallbladder K82.8
gastric mucosa K29.60
with bleeding K29.61
gland, glandular R59.9
generalized R59.1
localized R59.0
gum (mucous membrane) K06.1
heart (idiopathic) (*see also* Hypertrophy, cardiac)
valve (*see also* Endocarditis) I38
hemifacial Q67.4
hepatic — *see* Hypertrophy, liver
hiatus (esophageal) Q79.1
hilus gland R59.0
hymen, congenital Q52.4
ileum K63.89
intestine NEC K63.89
jejunum K63.89
kidney (compensatory) N28.81
congenital Q63.3
labium (majus) (minus) N90.6
ligament — *see* Disorder, ligament
lingual tonsil (infective) J35.1
with adenoids J35.3
lip K13.0
congenital Q18.6
liver R16.0
acute K76.89
cirrhotic — *see* Cirrhosis, liver
congenital Q44.7
fatty — *see* Fatty, liver
lymph, lymphatic gland R59.9
generalized R59.1
localized R59.0
tuberculous — *see* Tuberculosis, lymph gland
mammary gland — *see* Hypertrophy, breast
Meckel's diverticulum (congenital) Q43.0
malignant — *see* Table of Neoplasms, small intestine, malignant
median bar — *see* Hyperplasia, prostate
meibomian gland — *see* Chalazion
meniscus, knee, congenital Q74.1
metatarsal head — *see* Hypertrophy, bone, metatarsus
metatarsus — *see* Hypertrophy, bone, metatarsus
mucous membrane
alveolar ridge K06.2
gum K06.1
nose (turbinate) J34.3
muscle M62.89
muscular coat, artery I77.89
myocardium (*see also* Hypertrophy, cardiac)
idiopathic I42.2
myometrium N85.2
nail L60.2
congenital Q84.5

Hypertrophy, hypertrophic — *continued*
nasal J34.89
alae J34.89
bone J34.89
cartilage J34.89
mucous membrane (septum) J34.3
sinus J34.89
turbinate J34.3
nasopharynx, lymphoid (infectional) (tissue) (wall)
J35.2
nipple N62
organ or site, congenital NEC — *see* Anomaly, by site
ovary N83.8
palate (hard) M27.8
soft K13.79
pancreas, congenital Q45.3
parathyroid (gland) E21.0
parotid gland K11.1
penis N48.89
pharyngeal tonsil J35.2
pharynx J39.2
lymphoid (infectional) (tissue) (wall) J35.2
pituitary (anterior) (fossa) (gland) E23.6
prepuce (congenital) N47.8
female N90.89
prostate — *see* Enlargement, enlarged, prostate
congenital Q55.4
pseudomuscular G71.0
pylorus (adult) (muscle) (sphincter) K31.1
congenital or infantile Q40.0
rectal, rectum (sphincter) K62.89
rhinitis (turbinate) J31.0
salivary gland (any) K11.1
congenital Q38.4
scaphoid (tarsal) — *see* Hypertrophy, bone, tarsus
scar L91.0
scrotum N50.8
seminal vesicle N50.8
sigmoid — *see* Megacolon
skin L91.9
specified NEC L91.8
spermatic cord N50.8
spleen — *see* Splenomegaly
spondylitis — *see* Spondylosis
stomach K31.89
sublingual gland K11.1
submandibular gland K11.1
suprarenal cortex (gland) E27.8
synovial NEC M67.20
acromioclavicular M67.21- ☑
ankle M67.27- ☑
elbow M67.22- ☑
foot M67.27- ☑
hand M67.24- ☑
hip M67.25- ☑
knee M67.26- ☑
multiple sites M67.29
specified site NEC M67.28
wrist M67.23- ☑
tendon — *see* Disorder, tendon, specified type NEC
testis N44.8
congenital Q55.29
thymic, thymus (gland) (congenital) E32.0
thyroid (gland) — *see* Goiter
toe (congenital) Q74.2
acquired (*see also* Deformity, toe, specified NEC)
tongue K14.8
congenital Q38.2
papillae (foliate) K14.3
tonsils (faucial) (infective) (lingual) (lymphoid) J35.1
with adenoids J35.3
tunica vaginalis N50.8
ureter N28.89
urethra N36.8
uterus N85.2
neck (with elongation) N88.4
puerperal O90.89
uvula K13.79
vagina N89.8
vas deferens N50.8
vein I87.8
ventricle, ventricular (heart) (*see also* Hypertrophy,
cardiac)
congenital Q24.8
in tetralogy of Fallot Q21.3
verumontanum N36.8
vocal cord J38.3

Hypertrophy, hypertrophic — *continued*
vulva N90.6
stasis (nonfilarial) N90.6
Hypertropia H50.2- ☑
Hypertyrosinemia E70.21
Hyperuricemia (asymptomatic) E79.0
Hypervalinemia E71.19
Hyperventilation (tetany) R06.4
hysterical F45.8
psychogenic F45.8
syndrome F45.8
Hypervitaminosis (dietary) NEC E67.8
A E67.0
administered as drug (prolonged intake) — *see*
Table of Drugs and Chemicals, vitamins, adverse effect
overdose or wrong substance given or taken —
see Table of Drugs and Chemicals, vitamins,
poisoning
B6 E67.2
D E67.3
administered as drug (prolonged intake) — *see*
Table of Drugs and Chemicals, vitamins, adverse effect
overdose or wrong substance given or taken —
see Table of Drugs and Chemicals, vitamins,
poisoning
K E67.8
administered as drug (prolonged intake) — *see*
Table of Drugs and Chemicals, vitamins, adverse effect
overdose or wrong substance given or taken —
see Table of Drugs and Chemicals, vitamins,
poisoning
Hypervolemia E87.70
specified NEC E87.79
Hypesthesia R20.1
cornea — *see* Anesthesia, cornea
Hyphema H21.0- ☑
traumatic S05.1- ☑
Hypoacidity, gastric K31.89
psychogenic F45.8
Hypoadrenalism, hypoadrenia E27.40
primary E27.1
tuberculous A18.7
Hypoadrenocorticism E27.40
pituitary E23.0
primary E27.1
Hypoalbuminemia E88.09
Hypoaldosteronism E27.40
Hypoalphalipoproteinemia E78.6
Hypobarism T70.29 ☑
Hypobaropathy T70.29 ☑
Hypobetalipoproteinemia (familial) E78.6
Hypocalcemia E83.51
dietary E58
neonatal P71.1
due to cow's milk P71.0
phosphate-loading (newborn) P71.1
Hypochloremia E87.8
Hypochlorhydria K31.89
neurotic F45.8
psychogenic F45.8
Hypochondria, hypochondriac, hypochondriasis
(reaction) F45.21
sleep F51.03
Hypochondrogenesis Q77.0
Hypochondroplasia Q77.4
Hypochromasia, blood cells D50.8
Hypodontia — *see* Anodontia
Hypoeosinophilia D72.89
Hypoesthesia R20.1
Hypofibrinogenemia D68.8
acquired D65
congenital (hereditary) D68.2
Hypofunction
adrenocortical E27.40
drug-induced E27.3
postprocedural E89.6
primary E27.1
adrenomedullary, postprocedural E89.6
cerebral R29.818
corticoadrenal NEC E27.40
intestinal K59.8
labyrinth — *see* subcategory H83.2 ☑
ovary E28.39
pituitary (gland) (anterior) E23.0

☑ **Additional Character Required — Refer to the Tabular List for Character Selection**   🔻 **Subterms under main terms may continue to next column or page**

Hypofunction — *continued*
  testicular E29.1
    postprocedural (postsurgical) (postirradiation) (iatrogenic) E89.5
Hypogalactia O92.4
Hypogammaglobulinemia (*see also* Agammaglobulinemia) D80.1
  hereditary D80.0
  nonfamilial D80.1
  transient, of infancy D80.7
Hypogenitalism (congenital) — *see* Hypogonadism
Hypoglossia Q38.3
Hypoglycemia (spontaneous) E16.2
  coma E15
    diabetic — *see* Diabetes, coma
  diabetic — *see* Diabetes, hypoglycemia
  dietary counseling and surveillance Z71.3
  drug-induced E16.0
    with coma (nondiabetic) E15
  due to insulin E16.0
    with coma (nondiabetic) E15
    therapeutic misadventure — *see* subcategory T38.3 ☑
  functional, nonhyperinsulinemic E16.1
  iatrogenic E16.0
    with coma (nondiabetic) E15
  in infant of diabetic mother P70.1
    gestational diabetes P70.0
  infantile E16.1
  leucine-induced E71.19
  neonatal (transitory) P70.4
    iatrogenic P70.3
  reactive (not drug-induced) E16.1
  transitory neonatal P70.4
Hypogonadism
  female E28.39
  hypogonadotropic E23.0
  male E29.1
  ovarian (primary) E28.39
  pituitary E23.0
  testicular (primary) E29.1
Hypohidrosis, hypoidrosis L74.4
Hypoinsulinemia, postprocedural E89.1
Hypokalemia E87.6
Hypoleukocytosis — *see* Agranulocytosis
Hypolipoproteinemia (alpha) (beta) E78.6
Hypomagnesemia E83.42
  neonatal P71.2
Hypomania, hypomanic reaction F30.8
Hypomenorrhea — *see* Oligomenorrhea
Hypometabolism R63.8
Hypomotility
  gastrointestinal (tract) K31.89
    psychogenic F45.8
  intestine K59.8
    psychogenic F45.8
  stomach K31.89
    psychogenic F45.8
Hyponasality R49.22
Hyponatremia E87.1
Hypo-osmolality E87.1
Hypo-ovarianism, hypo-ovarism E28.39
Hypoparathyroidism E20.9
  familial E20.8
  idiopathic E20.0
  neonatal, transitory P71.4
  postprocedural E89.2
  specified NEC E20.8
Hypoperfusion (in)
  newborn P96.89
Hypopharyngitis — *see* Laryngopharyngitis
Hypophoria H50.53
Hypophosphatemia, hypophosphatasia (acquired) (congenital) (renal) E83.39
  familial E83.31
Hypophyseal, hypophysis (*see also* condition)
  dwarfism E23.0
  gigantism E22.0
Hypopiesis — *see* Hypotension
Hypopinealism E34.8
Hypopituitarism (juvenile) E23.0
  drug-induced E23.1
  due to
    hypophysectomy E89.3
    radiotherapy E89.3
  iatrogenic NEC E23.1
  postirradiation E89.3

Hypopituitarism — *continued*
  postpartum E23.0
  postprocedural E89.3
Hypoplasia, hypoplastic
  adrenal (gland), congenital Q89.1
  alimentary tract, congenital Q45.8
    upper Q40.8
  anus, anal (canal) Q42.3
    with fistula Q42.2
  aorta, aortic Q25.4
    ascending, in hypoplastic left heart syndrome Q23.4
    valve Q23.1
      in hypoplastic left heart syndrome Q23.4
  areola, congenital Q83.8
  arm (congenital) — *see* Defect, reduction, upper limb
  artery (peripheral) Q27.8
    brain (congenital) Q28.3
    coronary Q24.5
    digestive system Q27.8
    lower limb Q27.8
    pulmonary Q25.79
      functional, unilateral J43.0
    retinal (congenital) Q14.1
    specified site NEC Q27.8
    umbilical Q27.0
    upper limb Q27.8
  auditory canal Q17.8
    causing impairment of hearing Q16.9
  biliary duct or passage Q44.5
  bone NOS Q79.9
    face Q75.8
    marrow D61.9
      megakaryocytic D69.49
    skull — *see* Hypoplasia, skull
  brain Q02
    gyri Q04.3
    part of Q04.3
  breast (areola) N64.82
  bronchus Q32.4
  cardiac Q24.8
  carpus — *see* Defect, reduction, upper limb, specified type NEC
  cartilage hair Q78.5
  cecum Q42.8
  cementum K00.4
  cephalic Q02
  cerebellum Q04.3
  cervix (uteri), congenital Q51.821
  clavicle (congenital) Q74.0
  coccyx Q76.49
  colon Q42.9
    specified NEC Q42.8
  corpus callosum Q04.0
  cricoid cartilage Q31.2
  digestive organ(s) or tract NEC Q45.8
    upper (congenital) Q40.8
  ear (auricle) (lobe) Q17.2
    middle Q16.4
  enamel of teeth (neonatal) (postnatal) (prenatal) K00.4
  endocrine (gland) NEC Q89.2
  endometrium N85.8
  epididymis (congenital) Q55.4
  epiglottis Q31.2
  erythroid, congenital D61.01
  esophagus (congenital) Q39.8
  eustachian tube Q17.8
  eye Q11.2
  eyelid (congenital) Q10.3
  face Q18.8
    bone(s) Q75.8
  femur (congenital) — *see* Defect, reduction, lower limb, specified type NEC
  fibula (congenital) — *see* Defect, reduction, lower limb, specified type NEC
  finger (congenital) — *see* Defect, reduction, upper limb, specified type NEC
  focal dermal Q82.8
  foot — *see* Defect, reduction, lower limb, specified type NEC
  gallbladder Q44.0
  genitalia, genital organ(s)
    female, congenital Q52.8
      external Q52.79
      internal NEC Q52.8
    in adiposogenital dystrophy E23.6
  glottis Q31.2
  hair Q84.2

Hypoplasia, hypoplastic — *continued*
  hand (congenital) — *see* Defect, reduction, upper limb, specified type NEC
  heart Q24.8
  humerus (congenital) — *see* Defect, reduction, upper limb, specified type NEC
  intestine (small) Q41.9
    large Q42.9
      specified NEC Q42.8
  jaw M26.09
    alveolar M26.79
    lower M26.04
      alveolar M26.74
    upper M26.02
      alveolar M26.73
  kidney(s) Q60.5
    bilateral Q60.4
    unilateral Q60.3
  labium (majus) (minus), congenital Q52.79
  larynx Q31.2
  left heart syndrome Q23.4
  leg (congenital) — *see* Defect, reduction, lower limb
  limb Q73.8
    lower (congenital) — *see* Defect, reduction, lower limb
    upper (congenital) — *see* Defect, reduction, upper limb
  liver Q44.7
  lung (lobe) (not associated with short gestation) Q33.6
    associated with immaturity, low birth weight, prematurity, or short gestation P28.0
  mammary (areola), congenital Q83.8
  mandible, mandibular M26.04
    alveolar M26.74
    unilateral condylar M27.8
  maxillary M26.02
    alveolar M26.73
  medullary D61.9
  megakaryocytic D69.49
  metacarpus — *see* Defect, reduction, upper limb, specified type NEC
  metatarsus — *see* Defect, reduction, lower limb, specified type NEC
  muscle Q79.8
  nail(s) Q84.6
  nose, nasal Q30.1
  optic nerve H47.03- ☑
  osseous meatus (ear) Q17.8
  ovary, congenital Q50.39
  pancreas Q45.0
  parathyroid (gland) Q89.2
  parotid gland Q38.4
  patella Q74.1
  pelvis, pelvic girdle Q74.2
  penis (congenital) Q55.62
  peripheral vascular system Q27.8
    digestive system Q27.8
    lower limb Q27.8
    specified site NEC Q27.8
    upper limb Q27.8
  pituitary (gland) (congenital) Q89.2
  pulmonary (not associated with short gestation) Q33.6
    artery, functional J43.0
    associated with short gestation P28.0
  radioulnar — *see* Defect, reduction, upper limb, specified type NEC
  radius — *see* Defect, reduction, upper limb
  rectum Q42.1
    with fistula Q42.0
  respiratory system NEC Q34.8
  rib Q76.6
  right heart syndrome Q22.6
  sacrum Q76.49
  scapula Q74.0
  scrotum Q55.1
  shoulder girdle Q74.0
  skin Q82.8
  skull (bone) Q75.8
    with
      anencephaly Q00.0
      encephalocele — *see* Encephalocele
      hydrocephalus Q03.9
        with spina bifida — *see* Spina bifida, by site, with hydrocephalus
      microcephaly Q02
  spinal (cord) (ventral horn cell) Q06.1
  spine Q76.49
  sternum Q76.7

Hypoplasia, hypoplastic — *continued*
- tarsus — *see* Defect, reduction, lower limb, specified type NEC
- testis Q55.1
- thymic, with immunodeficiency D82.1
- thymus (gland) Q89.2
  - with immunodeficiency D82.1
- thyroid (gland) E03.1
  - cartilage Q31.2
- tibiofibular (congenital) — *see* Defect, reduction, lower limb, specified type NEC
- toe — *see* Defect, reduction, lower limb, specified type NEC
- tongue Q38.3
- Turner's K00.4
- ulna (congenital) — *see* Defect, reduction, upper limb
- umbilical artery Q27.0
- unilateral condylar M27.8
- ureter Q62.8
- uterus, congenital Q51.811
- vagina Q52.4
- vascular NEC peripheral Q27.8
  - brain Q28.3
  - digestive system Q27.8
  - lower limb Q27.8
  - specified site NEC Q27.8
  - upper limb Q27.8
- vein(s) (peripheral) Q27.8
  - brain Q28.3
  - digestive system Q27.8
  - great Q26.8
  - lower limb Q27.8
  - specified site NEC Q27.8
  - upper limb Q27.8
- vena cava (inferior) (superior) Q26.8
- vertebra Q76.49
- vulva, congenital Q52.79
- zonule (ciliary) Q12.8

Hypopotassemia E87.6
Hypoproconvertinemia, congenital (hereditary) D68.2
Hypoproteinemia E77.8
Hypoprothrombinemia (congenital) (hereditary) (idiopathic) D68.2
- acquired D68.4
- newborn, transient P61.6

Hypoptyalism K11.7
Hypopyon (eye) (anterior chamber) — *see* Iridocyclitis, acute, hypopyon
Hypopyrexia R68.0
Hyporeflexia R29.2
Hyposecretion
- ACTH E23.0
- antidiuretic hormone E23.2
- ovary E28.39
- salivary gland (any) K11.7
- vasopressin E23.2

Hyposegmentation, leukocytic, hereditary D72.0
Hyposiderinemia D50.9
Hypospadias Q54.9
- balanic Q54.0
- coronal Q54.0
- glandular Q54.0
- penile Q54.1
- penoscrotal Q54.2
- perineal Q54.3
- specified NEC Q54.8

Hypospermatogenesis — *see* Oligospermia
Hyposplenism D73.0
Hypostasis pulmonary, passive — *see* Edema, lung
Hypostatic — *see* condition
Hyposthenuria N28.89
Hypotension (arterial) (constitutional) I95.9
- chronic I95.89
- drug-induced I95.2
- due to (of) hemodialysis I95.3
- iatrogenic I95.89
- idiopathic (permanent) I95.0
- intracranial, following ventricular shunting (ventriculostomy) G97.2
- intra-dialytic I95.3
- maternal, syndrome (following labor and delivery) O26.5- ☑
- neurogenic, orthostatic G90.3
- orthostatic (chronic) I95.1
  - due to drugs I95.2
  - neurogenic G90.3
- postoperative I95.81
- postural I95.1

Hypotension — *continued*
- specified NEC I95.89
Hypothermia (accidental) T68 ☑
- due to anesthesia, anesthetic T88.51 ☑
- low environmental temperature T68 ☑
- neonatal P80.9
  - environmental (mild) NEC P80.8
  - mild P80.8
  - severe (chronic) (cold injury syndrome) P80.0
  - specified NEC P80.8
- not associated with low environmental temperature R68.0
Hypothyroidism (acquired) E03.9
- congenital (without goiter) E03.1
  - with goiter (diffuse) E03.0
- due to
  - exogenous substance NEC E03.2
  - iodine-deficiency, acquired E01.8
    - subclinical E02
  - irradiation therapy E89.0
  - medicament NEC E03.2
  - P-aminosalicylic acid (PAS) E03.2
  - phenylbutazone E03.2
  - resorcinol E03.2
  - sulfonamide E03.2
  - surgery E89.0
  - thiourea group drugs E03.2
- iatrogenic NEC E03.2
- iodine-deficiency (acquired) E01.8
  - congenital — *see* Syndrome, iodine- deficiency, congenital
  - subclinical E02
- neonatal, transitory P72.2
- postinfectious E03.3
- postirradiation E89.0
- postprocedural E89.0
- postsurgical E89.0
- specified NEC E03.8
- subclinical, iodine-deficiency related E02
Hypotonia, hypotonicity, hypotony
- bladder N31.2
- congenital (benign) P94.2
- eye — *see* Disorder, globe, hypotony
Hypotrichosis — *see* Alopecia
Hypotropia H50.2- ☑
Hypoventilation R06.89
- congenital central alveolar G47.35
- sleep related
  - idiopathic nonobstructive alveolar G47.34
  - in conditions classified elsewhere G47.36
Hypovitaminosis — *see* Deficiency, vitamin
Hypovolemia E86.1
- surgical shock T81.19 ☑
- traumatic (shock) T79.4 ☑
Hypoxemia R09.02
- newborn P84
- sleep related, in conditions classified elsewhere G47.36
Hypoxia (see also Anoxia) R09.02
- cerebral, during a procedure NEC G97.81
  - postprocedural NEC G97.82
- intrauterine P84
- myocardial — *see* Insufficiency, coronary
- newborn P84
- sleep-related G47.34
Hypsarrhythmia — *see* Epilepsy, generalized, specified NEC
Hysteralgia, pregnant uterus O26.89- ☑
Hysteria, hysterical (conversion) (dissociative state) F44.9
- anxiety F41.8
- convulsions F44.5
- psychosis, acute F44.9
Hysteroepilepsy F44.5

I

Ichthyoparasitism due to Vandellia cirrhosa B88.8
Ichthyosis (congenital) Q80.9
- acquired L85.0
- fetalis Q80.4
- hystrix Q80.8
- lamellar Q80.2
- lingual K13.29
- palmaris and plantaris Q82.8
- simplex Q80.0
- vera Q80.8
- vulgaris Q80.0

Ichthyosis — *continued*
- X-linked Q80.1
Ichthyotoxism — *see* Poisoning, fish
- bacterial — *see* Intoxication, foodborne
Icteroanemia, hemolytic (acquired) D59.9
- congenital — *see* Spherocytosis
Icterus (see also Jaundice)
- conjunctiva R17
- gravis, newborn P55.0
- hematogenous (acquired) D59.9
- hemolytic (acquired) D59.9
  - congenital — *see* Spherocytosis
- hemorrhagic (acute) (leptospiral) (spirochetal) A27.0
  - newborn P53
- infectious B15.9
  - with hepatic coma B15.0
  - leptospiral A27.0
  - spirochetal A27.0
- neonatorum — *see* Jaundice, newborn
- newborn P59.9
- spirochetal A27.0
Ictus solaris, solis T67.0 ☑
Id reaction (due to bacteria) L30.2
Ideation
- homicidal R45.850
- suicidal R45.851
Identity disorder (child) F64.9
- gender role F64.2
- psychosexual F64.2
Idioglossia F80.0
Idiopathic — *see* condition
Idiot, idiocy (congenital) F73
- amaurotic (Bielschowsky(-Jansky)) (family) (infantile (late)) (juvenile (late)) (Vogt-Spielmeyer) E75.4
- microcephalic Q02
IgE asthma J45.909
IIAC (idiopathic infantile arterial calcification) Q28.8
Ileitis (chronic) (noninfectious) (see also Enteritis) K52.9
- backwash — *see* Pancolitis, ulcerative (chronic)
- infectious A09
- regional (ulcerative) — *see* Enteritis, regional, small intestine
- segmental — *see* Enteritis, regional
- terminal (ulcerative) — *see* Enteritis, regional, small intestine
Ileocolitis (see also Enteritis) K52.9
- infectious A09
- regional — *see* Enteritis, regional
Ileostomy
- attention to Z43.2
- malfunctioning K94.13
- status Z93.2
  - with complication — *see* Complications, enterostomy
Ileotyphus — *see* Typhoid
Ileum — *see* condition
Ileus (bowel) (colon) (inhibitory) (intestine) K56.7
- adynamic K56.0
- due to gallstone (in intestine) K56.3
- duodenal (chronic) K31.5
- gallstone K56.3
- mechanical NEC K56.69
- meconium P76.0
  - in cystic fibrosis E84.11
  - meaning meconium plug (without cystic fibrosis) P76.0
- myxedema K59.8
- neurogenic K56.0
  - Hirschsprung's disease or megacolon Q43.1
- newborn
  - due to meconium P76.0
    - in cystic fibrosis E84.11
    - meaning meconium plug (without cystic fibrosis) P76.0
  - transitory P76.1
- obstructive K56.69
- paralytic K56.0
Iliac — *see* condition
Iliotibial band syndrome M76.3- ☑
Illiteracy Z55.0
Illness (see also Disease) R69
- manic-depressive — *see* Disorder, bipolar
Imbalance R26.89
- autonomic G90.8
- constituents of food intake E63.1
- electrolyte E87.8

Imbalance — *continued*
  electrolyte — *continued*
    with
      abortion — *see* Abortion by type, complicated by, electrolyte imbalance
      molar pregnancy O08.5
    due to hyperemesis gravidarum O21.1
    following ectopic or molar pregnancy O08.5
    neonatal, transitory NEC P74.4
      potassium P74.3
      sodium P74.2
  endocrine E34.9
  eye muscle NOS H50.9
  hormone E34.9
  hysterical F44.4
  labyrinth — *see* subcategory H83.2 ☑
  posture R29.3
  protein-energy — *see* Malnutrition
  sympathetic G90.8
Imbecile, imbecility (I.Q. 35-49) F71
Imbedding, intrauterine device T83.39 ☑
Imbibition, cholesterol (gallbladder) K82.4
Imbrication, teeth,, fully erupted M26.30
Imerslund (-Gräsbeck) **syndrome** D51.1
Immature (*see also* Immaturity)
  birth (less than 37 completed weeks) — *see* Preterm, newborn
    extremely (less than 28 completed weeks) — *see* Immaturity, extreme
  personality F60.89
Immaturity (less than 37 completed weeks) (*see also* Preterm, newborn)
  extreme of newborn (less than 28 completed weeks of gestation) (less than 196 completed days of gestation) (unspecified weeks of gestation) P07.20
    gestational age
      less than 23 completed weeks P07.21
      23 completed weeks (23 weeks, 0 days through 23 weeks, 6 days) P07.22
      24 completed weeks (24 weeks, 0 days through 24 weeks, 6 days) P07.23
      25 completed weeks (25 weeks, 0 days through 25 weeks, 6 days) P07.24
      26 completed weeks (26 weeks, 0 days through 26 weeks, 6 days) P07.25
      27 completed weeks (27 weeks, 0 days through 27 weeks, 6 days) P07.26
  fetus or infant light-for-dates — *see* Light-for-dates
  lung, newborn P28.0
  organ or site NEC — *see* Hypoplasia
  pulmonary, newborn P28.0
  reaction F60.89
  sexual (female) (male), after puberty E30.0
Immersion T75.1 ☑
  foot T69.02- ☑
  hand T69.01- ☑
Immobile, immobility
  complete, due to severe physical disability or frailty R53.2
  intestine K59.8
  syndrome (paraplegic) M62.3
Immune reconstitution (inflammatory) syndrome [IRIS] D89.3
Immunization (*see also* Vaccination)
  ABO — *see* Incompatibility, ABO
    in newborn P55.1
  complication — *see* Complications, vaccination
  encounter for Z23
  not done (not carried out) Z28.9
    because (of)
      acute illness of patient Z28.01
      allergy to vaccine (or component) Z28.04
      caregiver refusal Z28.82
      chronic illness of patient Z28.02
      contraindication NEC Z28.09
      group pressure Z28.1
      guardian refusal Z28.82
      immune compromised state of patient Z28.03
      parent refusal Z28.82
      patient had disease being vaccinated against Z28.81
      patient refusal Z28.21
      patient's belief Z28.1
      religious beliefs of patient Z28.1
      specified reason NEC Z28.89
        of patient Z28.29
      unspecified patient reason Z28.20

Immunization — *continued*
  Rh factor
    affecting management of pregnancy NEC O36.09- ☑
      anti-D antibody O36.01- ☑
    from transfusion — *see* Complication(s), transfusion, incompatibility reaction, Rh (factor)
Immunocytoma C83.0- ☑
Immunodeficiency D84.9
  with
    adenosine-deaminase deficiency D81.3
    antibody defects D80.9
      specified type NEC D80.8
    hyperimmunoglobulinemia D80.6
    increased immunoglobulin M (IgM) D80.5
    major defect D82.9
      specified type NEC D82.8
    partial albinism D82.8
    short-limbed stature D82.2
    thrombocytopenia and eczema D82.0
  antibody with
    hyperimmunoglobulinemia D80.6
    near-normal immunoglobulins D80.6
  autosomal recessive, Swiss type D80.0
  combined D81.9
    biotin-dependent carboxylase D81.819
      biotinidase D81.810
      holocarboxylase synthetase D81.818
      specified type NEC D81.818
    severe (SCID) D81.9
      with
        low or normal B-cell numbers D81.2
        low T- and B-cell numbers D81.1
        reticular dysgenesis D81.0
    specified type NEC D81.89
  common variable D83.9
    with
      abnormalities of B-cell numbers and function D83.0
      autoantibodies to B- or T-cells D83.2
      immunoregulatory T-cell disorders D83.1
    specified type NEC D83.8
  following hereditary defective response to Epstein-Barr virus (EBV) D82.3
  selective, immunoglobulin
    A (IgA) D80.2
    G (IgG) (subclasses) D80.3
    M (IgM) D80.4
  severe combined (SCID) D81.9
  specified type NEC D84.8
  X-linked, with increased IgM D80.5
Immunotherapy (encounter for)
  antineoplastic Z51.12
Impaction, impacted
  bowel, colon, rectum (*see also* Impaction, fecal) K56.49
    by gallstone K56.3
  calculus — *see* Calculus
  cerumen (ear) (external) H61.2- ☑
  cuspid — *see* Impaction, tooth
  dental (same or adjacent tooth) K01.1
  fecal, feces K56.41
  fracture — *see* Fracture, by site
  gallbladder — *see* Calculus, gallbladder
  gallstone(s) — *see* Calculus, gallbladder
    bile duct (common) (hepatic) — *see* Calculus, bile duct
    cystic duct — *see* Calculus, gallbladder
    in intestine, with obstruction (any part) K56.3
  intestine (calculous) NEC (*see also* Impaction, fecal) K56.49
    gallstone, with ileus K56.3
  intrauterine device (IUD) T83.39 ☑
  molar — *see* Impaction, tooth
  shoulder, causing obstructed labor O66.0
  tooth, teeth K01.1
  turbinate J34.89
Impaired, impairment (function)
  auditory discrimination — *see* Abnormal, auditory perception
  cognitive, mild, so stated G31.84
  dual sensory Z73.82
  fasting glucose R73.01
  glucose tolerance (oral) R73.02
  hearing — *see* Deafness
  heart — *see* Disease, heart
  kidney N28.9
    disorder resulting from N25.9
      specified NEC N25.89

Impaired, impairment — *continued*
  liver K72.90
    with coma K72.91
  mastication K08.8
  mild cognitive, so stated G31.84
  mobility
    ear ossicles — *see* Ankylosis, ear ossicles
    requiring care provider Z74.09
  myocardium, myocardial — *see* Insufficiency, myocardial
  rectal sphincter R19.8
  renal (acute) (chronic) N28.9
    disorder resulting from N25.9
      specified NEC N25.89
  vision NEC H54.7
    both eyes H54.3
Impediment, speech R47.9
  psychogenic (childhood) F98.8
  slurring R47.81
  specified NEC R47.89
Impending
  coronary syndrome I20.0
  delirium tremens F10.239
  myocardial infarction I20.0
Imperception auditory (acquired) (*see also* Deafness)
  congenital H93.25
Imperfect
  aeration, lung (newborn) NEC — *see* Atelectasis
  closure (congenital)
    alimentary tract NEC Q45.8
      lower Q43.8
      upper Q40.8
    atrioventricular ostium Q21.2
    atrium (secundum) Q21.1
    branchial cleft or sinus Q18.0
    choroid Q14.3
    cricoid cartilage Q31.8
    cusps, heart valve NEC Q24.8
      pulmonary Q22.3
    ductus
      arteriosus Q25.0
      Botalli Q25.0
    ear drum (causing impairment of hearing) Q16.4
    esophagus with communication to bronchus or trachea Q39.1
    eyelid Q10.3
    foramen
      botalli Q21.1
      ovale Q21.1
    genitalia, genital organ(s) or system
      female Q52.8
        external Q52.79
        internal NEC Q52.8
      male Q55.8
    glottis Q31.8
    interatrial ostium or septum Q21.1
    interauricular ostium or septum Q21.1
    interventricular ostium or septum Q21.0
    larynx Q31.8
    lip — *see* Cleft, lip
    nasal septum Q30.3
    nose Q30.2
    omphalomesenteric duct Q43.0
    optic nerve entry Q14.2
    organ or site not listed — *see* Anomaly, by site
    ostium
      interatrial Q21.1
      interauricular Q21.1
      interventricular Q21.0
    palate — *see* Cleft, palate
    preauricular sinus Q18.1
    retina Q14.1
    roof of orbit Q75.8
    sclera Q13.5
    septum
      aorticopulmonary Q21.4
      atrial (secundum) Q21.1
      between aorta and pulmonary artery Q21.4
      heart Q21.9
      interatrial (secundum) Q21.1
      interauricular (secundum) Q21.1
      interventricular Q21.0
        in tetralogy of Fallot Q21.3
      nasal Q30.3
      ventricular Q21.0
        with pulmonary stenosis or atresia, dextraposition of aorta, and hypertrophy of right ventricle Q21.3

Imperfect — *continued*
  closure — *continued*
    septum — *continued*
      ventricular — *continued*
        in tetralogy of Fallot Q21.3
      skull Q75.0
        with
          anencephaly Q00.0
          encephalocele — *see* Encephalocele
          hydrocephalus Q03.9
            with spina bifida — *see* Spina bifida, by
              site, with hydrocephalus
          microcephaly Q02
      spine (with meningocele) — *see* Spina bifida
      trachea Q32.1
      tympanic membrane (causing impairment of
        hearing) Q16.4
      uterus Q51.818
      vitelline duct Q43.0
  erection — *see* Dysfunction, sexual, male, erectile
  fusion — *see* Imperfect, closure
  inflation, lung (newborn) — *see* Atelectasis
  posture R29.3
  rotation, intestine Q43.3
  septum, ventricular Q21.0
Imperfectly descended testis — *see* Cryptorchid
Imperforate (congenital) (*see also* Atresia)
  anus Q42.3
    with fistula Q42.2
  cervix (uteri) Q51.828
  esophagus Q39.0
    with tracheoesophageal fistula Q39.1
  hymen Q52.3
  jejunum Q41.1
  pharynx Q38.8
  rectum Q42.1
    with fistula Q42.0
  urethra Q64.39
  vagina Q52.4
Impervious (congenital) (*see also* Atresia)
  anus Q42.3
    with fistula Q42.2
  bile duct Q44.2
  esophagus Q39.0
    with tracheoesophageal fistula Q39.1
  intestine (small) Q41.9
    large Q42.9
      specified NEC Q42.8
  rectum Q42.1
    with fistula Q42.0
  ureter — *see* Atresia, ureter
  urethra Q64.39
Impetiginization of dermatoses L01.1
Impetigo (any organism) (any site) (circinate) (contagiosa) (simplex) (vulgaris) L01.00
  Bockhart's L01.02
  bullous, bullosa L01.03
  external ear L01.00 [H62.40]
  follicularis L01.02
  furfuracea L30.5
  herpetiformis L40.1
    nonobstetrical L40.1
  neonatorum L01.03
  nonbullous L01.01
  specified type NEC L01.09
  ulcerative L01.09
Impingement (on teeth)
  soft tissue
    anterior M26.81
    posterior M26.82
Implant, endometrial N80.9
Implantation
  anomalous — *see* Anomaly, by site
    ureter Q62.63
  cyst
    external area or site (skin) NEC L72.0
    iris — *see* Cyst, iris, implantation
    vagina N89.8
    vulva N90.7
  dermoid (cyst) — *see* Implantation, cyst
Impotence (sexual) N52.9
  counseling Z70.1
  organic origin (*see also* Dysfunction, sexual, male,
    erectile) N52.9
  psychogenic F52.21
Impression, basilar Q75.8
Imprisonment, anxiety concerning Z65.1
Improper care (child) (newborn) — *see* Maltreatment

Improperly tied umbilical cord (causing hemorrhage) P51.8
Impulsiveness (impulsive) R45.87
Inability to swallow — *see* Aphagia
Inaccessible, inaccessibility
  health care NEC Z75.3
    due to
      waiting period Z75.2
        for admission to facility elsewhere Z75.1
  other helping agencies Z75.4
Inactive — *see* condition
Inadequate, inadequacy
  aesthetics of dental restoration K08.56
  biologic, constitutional, functional, or social F60.7
  development
    child R62.50
    genitalia
      after puberty NEC E30.0
      congenital
        female Q52.8
          external Q52.79
          internal Q52.8
        male Q55.8
    lungs Q33.6
      associated with short gestation P28.0
    organ or site not listed — *see* Anomaly, by site
  diet (causing nutritional deficiency) E63.9
  eating habits Z72.4
  environment, household Z59.1
  family support Z63.8
  food (supply) NEC Z59.4
    hunger effects T73.0 ☑
  functional F60.7
  household care, due to
    family member
      handicapped or ill Z74.2
      on vacation Z75.5
      temporarily away from home Z74.2
    technical defects in home Z59.1
    temporary absence from home of person rendering
      care Z74.2
  housing (heating) (space) Z59.1
  income (financial) Z59.6
  intrafamilial communication Z63.8
  material resources Z59.9
  mental — *see* Disability, intellectual
  parental supervision or control of child Z62.0
  personality F60.7
  pulmonary
    function R06.89
      newborn P28.5
    ventilation, newborn P28.5
  sample of cytologic smear
    anus R85.615
    cervix R87.615
    vagina R87.625
  social F60.7
    insurance Z59.7
    skills NEC Z73.4
  supervision of child by parent Z62.0
  teaching affecting education Z55.8
  welfare support Z59.7
Inanition R64
  with edema — *see* Malnutrition, severe
  due to
    deprivation of food T73.0 ☑
    malnutrition — *see* Malnutrition
  fever R50.9
Inappropriate
  change in quantitative human chorionic gonadotropin
    (hCG) in early pregnancy O02.81
  diet or eating habits Z72.4
  level of quantitative human chorionic gonadotropin
    (hCG) for gestational age in early pregnancy
    O02.81
  secretion
    antidiuretic hormone (ADH) (excessive) E22.2
      deficiency E23.2
    pituitary (posterior) E22.2
Inattention at or after birth — *see* Neglect
Incarceration, incarcerated
  enterocele K46.0
    gangrenous K46.1
  epiplocele K46.0
    gangrenous K46.1
  exophthalmos K42.0
    gangrenous K42.1

Incarceration, incarcerated — *continued*
  hernia (*see also* Hernia, by site, with
    obstruction)
    with gangrene — *see* Hernia, by site, with gangrene
  iris, in wound — *see* Injury, eye, laceration, with prolapse
  lens, in wound — *see* Injury, eye, laceration, with
    prolapse
  omphalocele K42.0
  prison, anxiety concerning Z65.1
  rupture — *see* Hernia, by site
  sarcoepiplocele K46.0
    gangrenous K46.1
  sarcoepiplomphalocele K42.0
    with gangrene K42.1
  uterus N85.8
    gravid O34.51- ☑
      causing obstructed labor O65.5
Incised wound
  external — *see* Laceration
  internal organs — *see* Injury, by site
Incision, incisional
  hernia K43.2
    with
      gangrene (and obstruction) K43.1
      obstruction K43.0
  surgical, complication — *see* Complications, surgical
    procedure
  traumatic
    external — *see* Laceration
    internal organs — *see* Injury, by site
Inclusion
  azurophilic leukocytic D72.0
  blennorrhea (neonatal) (newborn) P39.1
  gallbladder in liver (congenital) Q44.1
Incompatibility
  ABO
    affecting management of pregnancy O36.11- ☑
      anti-A sensitization O36.11- ☑
      anti-B sensitization O36.19- ☑
      specified NEC O36.19- ☑
    infusion or transfusion reaction — *see* Complication(s), transfusion, incompatibility reaction,
      ABO
    newborn P55.1
  blood (group) (Duffy) (K(ell)) (Kidd) (Lewis) (M) (S) NEC
    affecting management of pregnancy O36.11- ☑
      anti-A sensitization O36.11- ☑
      anti-B sensitization O36.19- ☑
    infusion or transfusion reaction T80.89 ☑
    newborn P55.8
  divorce or estrangement Z63.5
  Rh (blood group) (factor) Z31.82
    affecting management of pregnancy NEC
      O36.09- ☑
      anti-D antibody O36.01- ☑
    infusion or transfusion reaction — *see* Complication(s), transfusion, incompatibility reaction,
      Rh (factor)
    newborn P55.0
  rhesus — *see* Incompatibility, Rh
Incompetency, incompetent, incompetence
  annular
    aortic (valve) — *see* Insufficiency, aortic
    mitral (valve) I34.0
    pulmonary valve (heart) I37.1
  aortic (valve) — *see* Insufficiency, aortic
  cardiac valve — *see* Endocarditis
  cervix, cervical (os) N88.3
    in pregnancy O34.3- ☑
  chronotropic I45.89
    with
      autonomic dysfunction G90.8
      ischemic heart disease I25.89
      left ventricular dysfunction I51.89
      sinus node dysfunction I49.8
  esophagogastric (junction) (sphincter) K22.0
  mitral (valve) — *see* Insufficiency, mitral
  pelvic fundus N81.89
  pubocervical tissue N81.82
  pulmonary valve (heart) I37.1
    congenital Q22.3
  rectovaginal tissue N81.83
  tricuspid (annular) (valve) — *see* Insufficiency, tricuspid
  valvular — *see* Endocarditis
    congenital Q24.8

Incompetency, incompetent, incompetence — *continued*
　vein, venous (saphenous) (varicose) — *see* Varix, leg
Incomplete (*see also* condition)
　bladder, emptying R33.9
　defecation R15.0
　expansion lungs (newborn) NEC — *see* Atelectasis
　rotation, intestine Q43.3
Inconclusive
　diagnostic imaging due to excess body fat of patient R93.9
　findings on diagnostic imaging of breast NEC R92.8
　mammogram (due to dense breasts) R92.2
Incontinence R32
　anal sphincter R15.9
　feces R15.9
　　nonorganic origin F98.1
　overflow N39.490
　psychogenic F45.8
　rectal R15.9
　reflex N39.498
　stress (female) (male) N39.3
　　and urge N39.46
　urethral sphincter R32
　urge N39.41
　　and stress (female) (male) N39.46
　urine (urinary) R32
　　continuous N39.45
　　due to cognitive impairment, or severe physical disability or immobility R39.81
　　functional R39.81
　　mixed (stress and urge) N39.46
　　nocturnal N39.44
　　nonorganic origin F98.0
　　overflow N39.490
　　post dribbling N39.43
　　reflex N39.498
　　specified NEC N39.498
　　stress (female) (male) N39.3
　　　and urge N39.46
　　total N39.498
　　unaware N39.42
　　urge N39.41
　　　and stress (female) (male) N39.46
Incontinentia pigmenti Q82.3
Incoordinate, incoordination
　esophageal-pharyngeal (newborn) — *see* Dysphagia
　muscular R27.8
　uterus (action) (contractions) (complicating delivery) O62.4
Increase, increased
　abnormal, in development R63.8
　androgens (ovarian) E28.1
　anticoagulants (antithrombin) (anti-VIIIa) (anti-IXa) (anti-Xa) (anti-XIa) — *see* Circulating anticoagulants
　cold sense R20.8
　estrogen E28.0
　function
　　adrenal
　　　cortex — *see* Cushing's, syndrome
　　　medulla E27.5
　　pituitary (gland) (anterior) (lobe) E22.9
　　　posterior E22.2
　heat sense R20.8
　intracranial pressure (benign) G93.2
　permeability, capillaries I78.8
　pressure, intracranial G93.2
　secretion
　　gastrin E16.4
　　glucagon E16.3
　　pancreas, endocrine E16.9
　　　growth hormone-releasing hormone E16.8
　　　pancreatic polypeptide E16.8
　　　somatostatin E16.8
　　　vasoactive-intestinal polypeptide E16.8
　sphericity, lens Q12.4
　splenic activity D73.1
　venous pressure I87.8
　portal K76.6
Increta placenta O43.22- ☑
Incrustation, cornea, foreign body (lead)(zinc) — *see* Foreign body, cornea
Incyclophoria H50.54
Incyclotropia — *see* Cyclotropia
Indeterminate sex Q56.4
India rubber skin Q82.8

Indigestion (acid) (bilious) (functional) K30
　catarrhal K31.89
　due to decomposed food NOS A05.9
　nervous F45.8
　psychogenic F45.8
Indirect — *see* condition
Induratio penis plastica N48.6
Induration, indurated
　brain G93.89
　breast (fibrous) N64.51
　　puerperal, postpartum O92.29
　broad ligament N83.8
　chancre
　　anus A51.1
　　congenital A50.07
　　extragenital NEC A51.2
　corpora cavernosa (penis) (plastic) N48.6
　liver (chronic) K76.89
　lung (black) (chronic) (fibroid) (*see also* Fibrosis, lung) J84.10
　　essential brown J84.03
　penile (plastic) N48.6
　phlebitic — *see* Phlebitis
　skin R23.4
Inebriety (without dependence) — *see* Alcohol, intoxication
Inefficiency, kidney N28.9
Inelasticity, skin R23.4
Inequality, leg (length) (acquired) (*see also* Deformity, limb, unequal length)
　congenital — *see* Defect, reduction, lower limb
　lower leg — *see* Deformity, limb, unequal length
Inertia
　bladder (neurogenic) N31.2
　stomach K31.89
　　psychogenic F45.8
　uterus, uterine during labor O62.2
　　during latent phase of labor O62.0
　　primary O62.0
　　secondary O62.1
　vesical (neurogenic) N31.2
Infancy, infantile, infantilism (*see also* condition)
　celiac K90.0
　genitalia, genitals (after puberty) E30.0
　Herter's (nontropical sprue) K90.0
　intestinal K90.0
　Lorain E23.0
　pancreatic K86.8
　pelvis M95.5
　　with disproportion (fetopelvic) O33.1
　　　causing obstructed labor O65.1
　pituitary E23.0
　renal N25.0
　uterus — *see* Infantile, genitalia
Infant(s) (*see also* Infancy)
　excessive crying R68.11
　irritable child R68.12
　lack of care — *see* Neglect
　liveborn (singleton) Z38.2
　　born in hospital Z38.00
　　　by cesarean Z38.01
　　born outside hospital Z38.1
　　multiple NEC Z38.8
　　　born in hospital Z38.68
　　　　by cesarean Z38.69
　　　born outside hospital Z38.7
　　quadruplet Z38.8
　　　born in hospital Z38.63
　　　　by cesarean Z38.64
　　　born outside hospital Z38.7
　　quintuplet Z38.8
　　　born in hospital Z38.65
　　　　by cesarean Z38.66
　　　born outside hospital Z38.7
　　triplet Z38.8
　　　born in hospital Z38.61
　　　　by cesarean Z38.62
　　　born outside hospital Z38.7
　　twin Z38.5
　　　born in hospital Z38.30
　　　　by cesarean Z38.31
　　　born outside hospital Z38.4
　of diabetic mother (syndrome of) P70.1
　　gestational diabetes P70.0
Infantile (*see also* condition)
　genitalia, genitals E30.0
　os, uterine E30.0
　penis E30.0

Infantile — *continued*
　testis E29.1
　uterus E30.0
Infantilism — *see* Infancy
Infarct, infarction
　adrenal (capsule) (gland) E27.49
　appendices epiploicae K55.0
　bowel K55.0
　brain (stem) — *see* Infarct, cerebral
　breast N64.89
　brewer's (kidney) N28.0
　cardiac — *see* Infarct, myocardium
　cerebellar — *see* Infarct, cerebral
　cerebral (*see also* Occlusion, artery cerebral or precerebral, with infarction) I63.9
　　aborted I63.9
　　cortical I63.9
　　due to
　　　cerebral venous thrombosis, nonpyogenic I63.6
　　　embolism
　　　　cerebral arteries I63.4- ☑
　　　　precerebral arteries I63.1- ☑
　　　occlusion NEC
　　　　cerebral arteries I63.5- ☑
　　　　precerebral arteries I63.2- ☑
　　　stenosis NEC
　　　　cerebral arteries I63.5- ☑
　　　　precerebral arteries I63.2- ☑
　　　thrombosis
　　　　cerebral artery I63.3- ☑
　　　　precerebral artery I63.0- ☑
　　intraoperative
　　　during cardiac surgery I97.810
　　　during other surgery I97.811
　　postprocedural
　　　following cardiac surgery I97.820
　　　following other surgery I97.821
　　specified NEC I63.8
　colon (acute) (agnogenic) (embolic) (hemorrhagic) (nonocclusive) (nonthrombotic) (occlusive) (segmental) (thrombotic) (with gangrene) K55.0
　coronary artery — *see* Infarct, myocardium
　embolic — *see* Embolism
　fallopian tube N83.8
　gallbladder K82.8
　heart — *see* Infarct, myocardium
　hepatic K76.3
　hypophysis (anterior lobe) E23.6
　impending (myocardium) I20.0
　intestine (acute) (agnogenic) (embolic) (hemorrhagic) (nonocclusive) (nonthrombotic) (occlusive) (thrombotic) (with gangrene) K55.0
　kidney N28.0
　liver K76.3
　lung (embolic) (thrombotic) — *see* Embolism, pulmonary
　lymph node I89.8
　mesentery, mesenteric (embolic) (thrombotic) (with gangrene) K55.2
　muscle (ischemic) M62.20
　　ankle M62.27- ☑
　　foot M62.27- ☑
　　forearm M62.23- ☑
　　hand M62.24- ☑
　　lower leg M62.26- ☑
　　pelvic region M62.25- ☑
　　shoulder region M62.21- ☑
　　specified site NEC M62.28
　　thigh M62.25- ☑
　　upper arm M62.22- ☑
　myocardium, myocardial (acute) (with stated duration of 4 weeks or less) I21.3
　　diagnosed on ECG, but presenting no symptoms I25.2
　　healed or old I25.2
　　intraoperative
　　　during cardiac surgery I97.790
　　　during other surgery I97.791
　　non-Q wave I21.4
　　non-ST elevation (NSTEMI) I21.4
　　　subsequent I22.2
　　nontransmural I21.4
　　past (diagnosed on ECG or other investigation, but currently presenting no symptoms) I25.2
　　postprocedural
　　　following cardiac surgery I97.190
　　　following other surgery I97.191
　　Q wave (see also, Infarct, myocardium, by site) I21.3

Infarct, infarction — *continued*
  myocardium, myocardial — *continued*
    ST elevation (STEMI) I21.3
      anterior (anteroapical) (anterolateral) (anteroseptal) (Q wave) (wall) I21.09
        subsequent I22.0
      inferior (diaphragmatic) (inferolateral) (inferoposterior) (wall) NEC I21.19
        subsequent I22.1
      inferoposterior transmural (Q wave) I21.11
      involving
        coronary artery of anterior wall NEC I21.09
        coronary artery of inferior wall NEC I21.19
        diagonal coronary artery I21.02
        left anterior descending coronary artery I21.02
        left circumflex coronary artery I21.21
        left main coronary artery I21.01
        oblique marginal coronary artery I21.21
        right coronary artery I21.11
      lateral (apical-lateral) (basal-lateral) (high) I21.29
        subsequent I22.8
      posterior (posterobasal) (posterolateral) (posteroseptal) (true) I21.29
        subsequent I22.8
      septal I21.29
        subsequent I22.8
      specified NEC I21.29
        subsequent I22.8
      subsequent I22.9
    subsequent (recurrent) (reinfarction) I22.9
      anterior (anteroapical) (anterolateral) (anteroseptal) (wall) I22.0
      diaphragmatic (wall) I22.1
      inferior (diaphragmatic) (inferolateral) (inferoposterior) (wall) I22.1
      lateral (apical-lateral) (basal-lateral) (high) I22.8
      non-ST elevation (NSTEMI) I22.2
      posterior (posterobasal) (posterolateral) (posteroseptal) (true) I22.8
      septal I22.8
      specified NEC I22.8
      ST elevation I22.9
        anterior (anteroapical) (anterolateral) (anteroseptal) (wall) I22.0
        inferior (diaphragmatic) (inferolateral) (inferoposterior) (wall) I22.1
        specified NEC I22.8
      subendocardial I22.2
      transmural I22.9
        anterior (anteroapical) (anterolateral) (anteroseptal) (wall) I22.0
        diaphragmatic (wall) I22.1
        inferior (diaphragmatic) (inferolateral) (inferoposterior) (wall) I22.1
        lateral (apical-lateral) (basal-lateral) (high) I22.8
        posterior (posterobasal) (posterolateral) (posteroseptal) (true) I22.8
        specified NEC I22.8
    syphilitic A52.06
    transmural I21.3
      anterior (anteroapical) (anterolateral) (anteroseptal) (Q wave) (wall) NEC I21.09
      inferior (diaphragmatic) (inferolateral) (inferoposterior) (Q wave) (wall) NEC I21.19
      inferoposterior (Q wave) I21.11
      lateral (apical-lateral) (basal-lateral) (high) NEC I21.29
      posterior (posterobasal) (posterolateral) (posteroseptal) (true) NEC I21.29
      septal NEC I21.29
      specified NEC I21.29
  nontransmural I21.4
  omentum K55.0
  ovary N83.8
  pancreas K86.8
  papillary muscle — *see* Infarct, myocardium
  parathyroid gland E21.4
  pituitary (gland) E23.6
  placenta O43.81- ☑
  prostate N42.89
  pulmonary (artery) (vein) (hemorrhagic) — *see* Embolism, pulmonary
  renal (embolic) (thrombotic) N28.0
  retina, retinal (artery) — *see* Occlusion, artery, retina
  spinal (cord) (acute) (embolic) (nonembolic) G95.11

Infarct, infarction — *continued*
  spleen D73.5
    embolic or thrombotic I74.8
  subendocardial (acute) (nontransmural) I21.4
  suprarenal (capsule) (gland) E27.49
  testis N50.1
  thrombotic (*see also* Thrombosis)
    artery, arterial — *see* Embolism
  thyroid (gland) E07.89
  ventricle (heart) — *see* Infarct, myocardium
Infecting — *see* condition
Infection, infected, infective (opportunistic) B99.9
  with
    drug resistant organism — *see* Resistance (to), drug (*see also* specific organism)
    lymphangitis — *see* Lymphangitis
    organ dysfunction (acute) R65.20
      with septic shock R65.21
  abscess (skin) — *code by* site under Abscess
  Absidia — *see* Mucormycosis
  Acanthamoeba — *see* Acanthamebiasis
  Acanthocheilonema (perstans) (streptocerca) B74.4
  accessory sinus (chronic) — *see* Sinusitis
  achorion — *see* Dermatophytosis
  Acremonium falciforme B47.0
  acromioclavicular M00.9
  Actinobacillus (actinomycetem-comitans) A28.8
    mallei A24.0
    muris A25.1
  Actinomadura B47.1
  Actinomyces (israelii) (*see also* Actinomycosis) A42.9
  Actinomycetales — *see* Actinomycosis
  actinomycotic NOS — *see* Actinomycosis
  adenoid (and tonsil) J03.90
    chronic J35.02
  adenovirus NEC
    as cause of disease classified elsewhere B97.0
    unspecified nature or site B34.0
  aerogenes capsulatus A48.0
  aertrycke — *see* Infection, salmonella
  alimentary canal NOS — *see* Enteritis, infectious
  Allescheria boydii B48.2
  Alternaria B48.8
  alveolus, alveolar (process) K04.7
  Ameba, amebic (histolytica) — *see* Amebiasis
  amniotic fluid, sac or cavity O41.10- ☑
    chorioamnionitis O41.12- ☑
    placentitis O41.14- ☑
  amputation stump (surgical) — *see* Complication, amputation stump, infection
  Ancylostoma (duodenalis) B76.0
  Anisakiasis, Anisakis larvae B81.0
  anthrax — *see* Anthrax
  antrum (chronic) — *see* Sinusitis, maxillary
  anus, anal (papillae) (sphincter) K62.89
  arbovirus (arbor virus) A94
    specified type NEC A93.8
  artificial insemination N98.0
  Ascaris lumbricoides — *see* Ascariasis
  Ascomycetes B47.0
  Aspergillus (flavus) (fumigatus) (terreus) — *see* Aspergillosis
  atypical
    acid-fast (bacilli) — *see* Mycobacterium, atypical
    mycobacteria — *see* Mycobacterium, atypical
    virus A81.9
      specified type NEC A81.89
  auditory meatus (external) — *see* Otitis, externa, infective
  auricle (ear) — *see* Otitis, externa, infective
  axillary gland (lymph) L04.2
  Bacillus A49.9
    abortus A23.1
    anthracis — *see* Anthrax
    Ducrey's (any location) A57
    Flexner's A03.1
    Friedländer's NEC A49.8
    gas (gangrene) A48.0
    mallei A24.0
    melitensis A23.0
    paratyphoid, paratyphosus A01.4
      A A01.1
      B A01.2
      C A01.3
    Shiga (-Kruse) A03.0
    suipestifer — *see* Infection, salmonella
    swimming pool A31.1

Infection, infected, infective — *continued*
  Bacillus — *continued*
    typhosa A01.00
    welchii — *see* Gangrene, gas
  bacterial NOS A49.9
    as cause of disease classified elsewhere B96.89
      Bacteroides fragilis [B. fragilis] B96.6
      Clostridium perfringens [C. perfringens] B96.7
      Enterobacter sakazakii B96.89
      Enterococcus B95.2
      Escherichia coli [E. coli] (*see also* Escherichia coli) B96.20
      Helicobacter pylori [H.pylori] B96.81
      Hemophilus influenzae [H. influenzae] B96.3
      Klebsiella pneumoniae [K. pneumoniae] B96.1
      Mycoplasma pneumoniae [M. pneumoniae] B96.0
      Proteus (mirabilis) (morganii) B96.4
      Pseudomonas (aeruginosa) (mallei) (pseudomallei) B96.5
      Staphylococcus B95.8
        aureus (methicillin susceptible) (MSSA) B95.61
        methicillin resistant (MRSA) B95.62
        specified NEC B95.7
      Streptococcus B95.5
        group A B95.0
        group B B95.1
        pneumoniae B95.3
        specified NEC B95.4
      Vibrio vulnificus B96.82
    specified NEC A48.8
  Bacterium
    paratyphosum A01.4
      A A01.1
      B A01.2
      C A01.3
    typhosum A01.00
  Bacteroides NEC A49.8
    fragilis, as cause of disease classified elsewhere B96.6
  Balantidium coli A07.0
  Bartholin's gland N75.8
  Basidiobolus B46.8
  bile duct (common) (hepatic) — *see* Cholangitis
  bladder — *see* Cystitis
  Blastomyces, blastomycotic (*see also* Blastomycosis)
    brasiliensis — *see* Paracoccidioidomycosis
    dermatitidis — *see* Blastomycosis
    European — *see* Cryptococcosis
    Loboi B48.0
    North American B40.9
    South American — *see* Paracoccidioidomycosis
  bleb, postprocedure — *see* Blebitis
  bone — *see* Osteomyelitis
  Bordetella — *see* Whooping cough
  Borrelia bergdorfi A69.20
  brain (*see also* Encephalitis) G04.90
    membranes — *see* Meningitis
    septic G06.0
      meninges — *see* Meningitis, bacterial
  branchial cyst Q18.0
  breast — *see* Mastitis
  bronchus — *see* Bronchitis
  Brucella A23.9
    abortus A23.1
    canis A23.3
    melitensis A23.0
    mixed A23.8
    specified NEC A23.8
    suis A23.2
  Brugia (malayi) B74.1
    timori B74.2
  bursa — *see* Bursitis, infective
  buttocks (skin) L08.9
  Campylobacter, intestinal A04.5
    as cause of disease classified elsewhere B96.81
  Candida (albicans) (tropicalis) — *see* Candidiasis
  candiru B88.8
  Capillaria (intestinal) B81.1
    hepatica B83.8
    philippinensis B81.1
  cartilage — *see* Disorder, cartilage, specified type NEC
  cat liver fluke B66.0
  catheter-related bloodstream (CRBSI) T80.211 ☑
  cellulitis — *code by* site under Cellulitis
  central line-associated T80.219 ☑
    bloodstream (CLABSI) T80.211 ☑

Infection, infected, infective — *continued*
  central line-associated — *continued*
    specified NEC T80.218 ☑
  Cephalosporium falciforme B47.0
  cerebrospinal — *see* Meningitis
  cervical gland (lymph) L04.0
  cervix — *see* Cervicitis
  cesarean delivery wound (puerperal) O86.0
  cestodes — *see* Infestation, cestodes
  chest J22
  Chilomastix (intestinal) A07.8
  Chlamydia, chlamydial A74.9
    anus A56.3
    genitourinary tract A56.2
      lower A56.00
        specified NEC A56.19
    lymphogranuloma A55
    pharynx A56.4
    psittaci A70
    rectum A56.3
    sexually transmitted NEC A56.8
  cholera — *see* Cholera
  Cladosporium
    bantianum (brain abscess) B43.1
    carrionii B43.0
    castellanii B36.1
    trichoides (brain abscess) B43.1
    werneckii B36.1
  Clonorchis (sinensis) (liver) B66.1
  Clostridium NEC
    bifermentans A48.0
    botulinum (food poisoning) A05.1
      infant A48.51
      wound A48.52
    difficile
      as cause of disease classified elsewhere B96.89
      foodborne (disease) A04.7
      gas gangrene A48.0
      necrotizing enterocolitis A04.7
      sepsis A41.4
    gas-forming NEC A48.0
    histolyticum A48.0
    novyi, causing gas gangrene A48.0
    oedematiens A48.0
    perfringens
      as cause of disease classified elsewhere B96.7
      due to food A05.2
      foodborne (disease) A05.2
      gas gangrene A48.0
      sepsis A41.4
    septicum, causing gas gangrene A48.0
    sordellii, causing gas gangrene A48.0
    welchii
      as cause of disease classified elsewhere B96.7
      foodborne (disease) A05.2
      gas gangrene A48.0
      necrotizing enteritis A05.2
      sepsis A41.4
  Coccidioides (immitis) — *see* Coccidioidomycosis
  colon — *see* Enteritis, infectious
  colostomy K94.02
  common duct — *see* Cholangitis
  congenital P39.9
    Candida (albicans) P37.5
    cytomegalovirus P35.1
    hepatitis, viral P35.3
    herpes simplex P35.2
    infectious or parasitic disease P37.9
      specified NEC P37.8
    listeriosis (disseminated) P37.2
    malaria NEC P37.4
      falciparum P37.3
    Plasmodium falciparum P37.3
    poliomyelitis P35.8
    rubella P35.0
    skin P39.4
    toxoplasmosis (acute) (subacute) (chronic) P37.1
    tuberculosis P37.0
    urinary (tract) P39.3
    vaccinia P35.8
    virus P35.9
      specified type NEC P35.8
  Conidiobolus B46.8
  coronavirus NEC B34.2
    as cause of disease classified elsewhere B97.29
    severe acute respiratory syndrome (SARS associated) B97.21
  corpus luteum — *see* Salpingo-oophoritis

Infection, infected, infective — *continued*
  Corynebacterium diphtheriae — *see* Diphtheria
  cotia virus B08.8
  Coxiella burnetii A78
  coxsackie — *see* Coxsackie
  Cryptococcus neoformans — *see* Cryptococcosis
  Cryptosporidium A07.2
  Cunninghamella — *see* Mucormycosis
  cyst — *see* Cyst
  cystic duct (*see also* Cholecystitis) K81.9
  Cysticercus cellulosae — *see* Cysticercosis
  cytomegalovirus, cytomegaloviral B25.9
    congenital P35.1
    maternal, maternal care for (suspected) damage to fetus O35.3 ☑
    mononucleosis B27.10
      with
        complication NEC B27.19
        meningitis B27.12
        polyneuropathy B27.11
  delta-agent (acute), in hepatitis B carrier B17.0
  dental (pulpal origin) K04.7
  Deuteromycetes B47.0
  Dicrocoelium dendriticum B66.2
  Dipetalonema (perstans) (streptocerca) B74.4
  diphtherial — *see* Diphtheria
  Diphyllobothrium (adult) (latum) (pacificum) B70.0
    larval B70.1
  Diplogonoporus (grandis) B71.8
  Dipylidium caninum B67.4
  Dirofilaria B74.8
  Dracunculus medinensis B72
  Drechslera (hawaiiensis) B43.8
  Ducrey Haemophilus (any location) A57
  due to or resulting from
    artificial insemination N98.0
    central venous catheter T80.219 ☑
      bloodstream T80.211 ☑
      exit or insertion site T80.212 ☑
      localized T80.212 ☑
      port or reservoir T80.212 ☑
      specified NEC T80.218 ☑
      tunnel T80.212 ☑
    device, implant or graft (*see also* Complications, by site and type, infection or inflammation) T85.79 ☑
      arterial graft NEC T82.7 ☑
      breast (implant) T85.79 ☑
      catheter NEC T85.79 ☑
        dialysis (renal) T82.7 ☑
          intraperitoneal T85.71 ☑
        infusion NEC T82.7 ☑
          spinal (epidural) (subdural) T85.79 ☑
        urinary (indwelling) T83.51 ☑
      electronic (electrode) (pulse generator) (stimulator)
        bone T84.7 ☑
        cardiac T82.7 ☑
        nervous system (brain) (peripheral nerve) (spinal) T85.79 ☑
        urinary T83.59 ☑
      fixation, internal (orthopedic) NEC — *see* Complication, fixation device, infection
      gastrointestinal (bile duct) (esophagus) T85.79 ☑
      genital NEC T83.6 ☑
      heart NEC T82.7 ☑
        valve (prosthesis) T82.6 ☑
          graft T82.7 ☑
      joint prosthesis — *see* Complication, joint prosthesis, infection
      ocular (corneal graft) (orbital implant) NEC T85.79 ☑
      orthopedic NEC T84.7 ☑
      specified NEC T85.79 ☑
      urinary NEC T83.59 ☑
      vascular NEC T82.7 ☑
      ventricular intracranial shunt T85.79 ☑
    Hickman catheter T80.219 ☑
      bloodstream T80.211 ☑
      localized T80.212 ☑
      specified NEC T80.218 ☑
    immunization or vaccination T88.0 ☑
    infusion, injection or transfusion NEC T80.29 ☑
    injury NEC — *code by* site under Wound, open

Infection, infected, infective — *continued*
  due to or resulting from — *continued*
    peripherally inserted central catheter (PICC) T80.219 ☑
      bloodstream T80.211 ☑
      localized T80.212 ☑
      specified NEC T80.218 ☑
    portacath (port-a-cath) T80.219 ☑
      bloodstream T80.211 ☑
      localized T80.212 ☑
      specified NEC T80.218 ☑
    surgery T81.4 ☑
    triple lumen catheter T80.219 ☑
      bloodstream T80.211 ☑
      localized T80.212 ☑
      specified NEC T80.218 ☑
    umbilical venous catheter T80.219 ☑
      bloodstream T80.211 ☑
      localized T80.212 ☑
      specified NEC T80.218 ☑
  during labor NEC O75.3
  ear (middle) (*see also* Otitis media)
    external — *see* Otitis, externa, infective
    inner — *see* subcategory H83.0 ☑
  Eberthella typhosa A01.00
  Echinococcus — *see* Echinococcus
  echovirus
    as cause of disease classified elsewhere B97.12
    unspecified nature or site B34.1
  endocardium I33.0
  endocervix — *see* Cervicitis
  Entamoeba — *see* Amebiasis
  enteric — *see* Enteritis, infectious
  Enterobacter sakazakii B96.89
  Enterobius vermicularis B80
  enterostomy K94.12
  enterovirus B34.1
    as cause of disease classified elsewhere B97.10
      coxsackievirus B97.11
      echovirus B97.12
      specified NEC B97.19
  Entomophthora B46.8
  Epidermophyton — *see* Dermatophytosis
  epididymis — *see* Epididymitis
  episiotomy (puerperal) O86.0
  Erysipelothrix (insidiosa) (rhusiopathiae) — *see* Erysipeloid
  erythema infectiosum B08.3
  Escherichia (E.) coli NEC A49.8
    as cause of disease classified elsewhere (*see also* Escherichia coli) B96.20
    congenital P39.8
      sepsis P36.4
    generalized A41.51
    intestinal — *see* Enteritis, infectious, due to, Escherichia coli
  ethmoidal (chronic) (sinus) — *see* Sinusitis, ethmoidal
  eustachian tube (ear) — *see* Salpingitis, eustachian
  external auditory canal (meatus) NEC — *see* Otitis, externa, infective
  eye (purulent) — *see* Endophthalmitis, purulent
  eyelid — *see* Inflammation, eyelid
  fallopian tube — *see* Salpingo-oophoritis
  Fasciola (gigantica) (hepatica) (indica) B66.3
  Fasciolopsis (buski) B66.5
  filarial — *see* Infestation, filarial
  finger (skin) L08.9
    nail L03.01-
      fungus B35.1
  fish tapeworm B70.0
    larval B70.1
  flagellate, intestinal A07.9
  fluke — *see* Infestation, fluke
  focal
    teeth (pulpal origin) K04.7
    tonsils J35.01
  Fonsecaea (compactum) (pedrosoi) B43.0
  food — *see* Intoxication, foodborne
  foot (skin) L08.9
    dermatophytic fungus B35.3
  Francisella tularensis — *see* Tularemia
  frontal (sinus) (chronic) — *see* Sinusitis, frontal
  fungus NOS B49
    beard B35.0
    dermatophyte — *see* Dermatophytosis
    foot B35.3
    groin B35.6

Infection, infected, infective — *continued*
  fungus — *continued*
    hand B35.2
    nail B35.1
    pathogenic to compromised host only B48.8
    perianal (area) B35.6
    scalp B35.0
    skin B36.9
      foot B35.3
      hand B35.2
      toenails B35.1
  Fusarium B48.8
  gallbladder — *see* Cholecystitis
  gas bacillus — *see* Gangrene, gas
  gastrointestinal — *see* Enteritis, infectious
  generalized NEC — *see* Sepsis
  genital organ or tract
    female — *see* Disease, pelvis, inflammatory
    male N49.9
      multiple sites N49.8
      specified NEC N49.8
  Ghon tubercle, primary A15.7
  Giardia lamblia A07.1
  gingiva (chronic) K05.10
    acute K05.00
      nonplaque induced K05.01
      plaque induced K05.00
    nonplaque induced K05.11
    plaque induced K05.10
  glanders A24.0
  glenosporopsis B48.0
  Gnathostoma (spinigerum) B83.1
  Gongylonema B83.8
  gonococcal — *see* Gonococcus
  gram-negative bacilli NOS A49.9
  guinea worm B72
  gum (chronic) K05.10
    acute K05.00
      nonplaque induced K05.01
      plaque induced K05.00
    nonplaque induced K05.11
    plaque induced K05.10
  Haemophilus — *see* Infection, Hemophilus
  heart — *see* Carditis
  Helicobacter pylori A04.8
    as cause of disease classified elsewhere B96.81
  helminths B83.9
    intestinal B82.0
      mixed (types classifiable to more than one of
        the titles B65.0-B81.3 and B81.8) B81.4
      specified type NEC B81.8
    specified type NEC B83.8
  Hemophilus
    aegyptius, systemic A48.4
    ducrey (any location) A57
    generalized A41.3
    influenzae NEC A49.2
      as cause of disease classified elsewhere B96.3
  herpes (simplex) (*see also* Herpes)
    congenital P35.2
    disseminated B00.7
    zoster B02.9
  herpesvirus, herpesviral — *see* Herpes
  Heterophyes (heterophyes) B66.8
  hip (joint) NEC M00.9
    due to internal joint prosthesis
      left T84.52 ☑
      right T84.51 ☑
    skin NEC L08.9
  Histoplasma — *see* Histoplasmosis
    American B39.4
    capsulatum B39.4
  hookworm B76.9
  human
    papilloma virus A63.0
    T-cell lymphotropic virus type-1 (HTLV-1) B33.3
  hydrocele N43.0
  Hymenolepis B71.0
  hypopharynx — *see* Pharyngitis
  inguinal (lymph) glands L04.1
    due to soft chancre A57
  intervertebral disc, pyogenic M46.30
    cervical region M46.32
    cervicothoracic region M46.33
    lumbar region M46.36
    lumbosacral region M46.37
    multiple sites M46.39
    occipito-atlanto-axial region M46.31

Infection, infected, infective — *continued*
  intervertebral disc, pyogenic — *continued*
    sacrococcygeal region M46.38
    thoracic region M46.34
    thoracolumbar region M46.35
  intestine, intestinal — *see* Enteritis, infectious
    specified NEC A08.8
  intra-amniotic affecting newborn NEC P39.2
  Isospora belli or hominis A07.3
  Japanese B encephalitis A83.0
  jaw (bone) (lower) (upper) M27.2
  joint NEC M00.9
    due to internal joint prosthesis T84.50 ☑
  kidney (cortex) (hematogenous) N15.9
    with calculus N20.0
      with hydronephrosis N13.6
    following ectopic gestation O08.83
    pelvis and ureter (cystic) N28.85
    puerperal (postpartum) O86.21
    specified NEC N15.8
  Klebsiella (K.) pneumoniae NEC A49.8
    as cause of disease classified elsewhere B96.1
  knee (joint) NEC M00.9
    due to internal joint prosthesis
      left T84.54 ☑
      right T84.53 ☑
    joint M00.9
    skin L08.9
  Koch's — *see* Tuberculosis
  labia (majora) (minora) (acute) — *see* Vulvitis
  lacrimal
    gland — *see* Dacryoadenitis
    passages (duct) (sac) — *see* Inflammation, lacrimal,
      passages
  lancet fluke B66.2
  larynx NEC J38.7
  leg (skin) NOS L08.9
  Legionella pneumophila A48.1
    nonpneumonic A48.2
  Leishmania (*see also* Leishmaniasis)
    aethiopica B55.1
    braziliensis B55.2
    chagasi B55.0
    donovani B55.0
    infantum B55.0
    major B55.1
    mexicana B55.1
    tropica B55.1
  lentivirus, as cause of disease classified elsewhere
    B97.31
  Leptosphaeria senegalensis B47.0
  Leptospira interrogans A27.9
    autumnalis A27.89
    canicola A27.89
    hebdomadis A27.89
    icterohaemorrhagiae A27.0
    pomona A27.89
    specified type NEC A27.89
  leptospirochetal NEC — *see* Leptospirosis
  Listeria monocytogenes (*see also* Listeriosis)
    congenital P37.2
  Loa loa B74.3
    with conjunctival infestation B74.3
    eyelid B74.3
  Loboa loboi B48.0
  local, skin (staphylococcal) (streptococcal) L08.9
    abscess — *code by* site under Abscess
    cellulitis — *code by* site under Cellulitis
    specified NEC L08.89
    ulcer — *see* Ulcer, skin
  Loefflerella mallei A24.0
  lung (*see also* Pneumonia) J18.9
    atypical Mycobacterium A31.0
    spirochetal A69.8
    tuberculous — *see* Tuberculosis, pulmonary
    virus — *see* Pneumonia, viral
  lymph gland (*see also* Lymphadenitis, acute)
    mesenteric I88.0
  lymphoid tissue, base of tongue or posterior pharynx,
    NEC (chronic) J35.03
  Madurella (grisea) (mycetomii) B47.0
  major
    following ectopic or molar pregnancy O08.0
    puerperal, postpartum, childbirth O85
  Malassezia furfur B36.0
  Malleomyces
    mallei A24.0
    pseudomallei (whitmori) — *see* Melioidosis

Infection, infected, infective — *continued*
  mammary gland N61
  Mansonella (ozzardi) (perstans) (streptocerca) B74.4
  mastoid — *see* Mastoiditis
  maxilla, maxillary M27.2
    sinus (chronic) — *see* Sinusitis, maxillary
  mediastinum J98.5
  Medina (worm) B72
  meibomian cyst or gland — *see* Hordeolum
  meninges — *see* Meningitis, bacterial
  meningococcal (*see also* condition) A39.9
    adrenals A39.1
    brain A39.81
    cerebrospinal A39.0
    conjunctiva A39.89
    endocardium A39.51
    heart A39.50
      endocardium A39.51
      myocardium A39.52
      pericardium A39.53
    joint A39.83
    meninges A39.0
    meningococcemia A39.4
      acute A39.2
      chronic A39.3
    myocardium A39.52
    pericardium A39.53
    retrobulbar neuritis A39.82
    specified site NEC A39.89
  mesenteric lymph nodes or glands NEC I88.0
  Metagonimus B66.8
  metatarsophalangeal M00.9
  methicillin
    resistant Staphylococcus aureus (MRSA) A49.02
    susceptible Staphylococcus aureus (MSSA) A49.01
  Microsporum, microsporic — *see* Dermatophytosis
  mixed flora (bacterial) NEC A49.8
  Monilia — *see* Candidiasis
  Monosporium apiospermum B48.2
  mouth, parasitic B37.0
  Mucor — *see* Mucormycosis
  muscle NEC — *see* Myositis, infective
  mycelium NOS B49
  mycetoma B47.9
    actinomycotic NEC B47.1
    mycotic NEC B47.0
  Mycobacterium, mycobacterial — *see* Mycobacterium
  Mycoplasma NEC A49.3
    pneumoniae, as cause of disease classified else-
      where B96.0
  mycotic NOS B49
    pathogenic to compromised host only B48.8
    skin NOS B36.9
  myocardium NEC I40.0
  nail (chronic)
    with lymphangitis — *see* Lymphangitis, acute,
      digit
    finger L03.01- ☑
      fungus B35.1
    ingrowing L60.0
    toe L03.03- ☑
      fungus B35.1
  nasal sinus (chronic) — *see* Sinusitis
  nasopharynx — *see* Nasopharyngitis
  navel L08.82
  Necator americanus B76.1
  Neisseria — *see* Gonococcus
  Neotestudina rosatii B47.0
  newborn P39.9
    intra-amniotic NEC P39.2
    skin P39.4
    specified type NEC P39.8
  nipple N61
    associated with
      lactation O91.03
      pregnancy O91.01- ☑
      puerperium O91.02
  Nocardia — *see* Nocardiosis
  obstetrical surgical wound (puerperal) O86.0
  Oesophagostomum (apiostomum) B81.8
  Oestrus ovis — *see* Myiasis
  Oidium albicans B37.9
  Onchocerca (volvulus) — *see* Onchocerciasis
  oncovirus, as cause of disease classified elsewhere
    B97.32
  operation wound T81.4 ☑
  Opisthorchis (felineus) (viverrini) B66.0
  orbit, orbital — *see* Inflammation, orbit

Infection, infected, infective — *continued*
orthopoxvirus NEC B08.09
ovary — *see* Salpingo-oophoritis
Oxyuris vermicularis B80
pancreas (acute) K85.9
  abscess — *see* Pancreatitis, acute
  specified NEC K85.8
papillomavirus, as cause of disease classified elsewhere
  B97.7
papovavirus NEC B34.4
Paracoccidioides brasiliensis — *see* Paracoccidioidomycosis
Paragonimus (westermani) B66.4
parainfluenza virus B34.8
parameningococcus NOS A39.9
parapoxvirus B08.60
  specified NEC B08.69
parasitic B89
Parastrongylus
  cantonensis B83.2
  costaricensis B81.3
  paratyphoid A01.4
    Type A A01.1
    Type B A01.2
    Type C A01.3
paraurethral ducts N34.2
parotid gland — *see* Sialoadenitis
parvovirus NEC B34.3
  as cause of disease classified elsewhere B97.6
Pasteurella NEC A28.0
  multocida A28.0
  pestis — *see* Plague
  pseudotuberculosis A28.0
  septica (cat bite) (dog bite) A28.0
  tularensis — *see* Tularemia
pelvic, female — *see* Disease, pelvis, inflammatory
Penicillium (marneffei) B48.4
penis (glans) (retention) NEC N48.29
periapical K04.5
peridental, periodontal K05.20
  generalized K05.22
  localized K05.21
perinatal period P39.9
  specified type NEC P39.8
perineal repair (puerperal) O86.0
periorbital — *see* Inflammation, orbit
perirectal K62.89
perirenal — *see* Infection, kidney
peritoneal — *see* Peritonitis
periureteral N28.89
Petriellidium boydii B48.2
pharynx (*see also* Pharyngitis)
  coxsackievirus B08.5
  posterior, lymphoid (chronic) J35.03
Phialophora
  gougerotii (subcutaneous abscess or cyst) B43.2
  jeanselmei (subcutaneous abscess or cyst) B43.2
  verrucosa (skin) B43.0
Piedraia hortae B36.3
pinta A67.9
  intermediate A67.1
  late A67.2
  mixed A67.3
  primary A67.0
pinworm B80
pityrosporum furfur B36.0
pleuro-pneumonia-like organism (PPLO) NEC A49.3
  as cause of disease classified elsewhere B96.0
pneumococcus, pneumococcal NEC A49.1
  as cause of disease classified elsewhere B95.3
  generalized (purulent) A40.3
    with pneumonia J13
Pneumocystis carinii (pneumonia) B59
Pneumocystis jiroveci (pneumonia) B59
port or reservoir T80.212 ☑
postoperative T81.4 ☑
postoperative wound T81.4 ☑
postprocedural T81.4 ☑
postvaccinal T88.0 ☑
prepuce NEC N47.7
  with penile inflammation N47.6
prion — *see* Disease, prion, central nervous system
prostate (capsule) — *see* Prostatitis
Proteus (mirabilis) (morganii) (vulgaris) NEC A49.8
  as cause of disease classified elsewhere B96.4
protozoal NEC B64
  intestinal A07.9
    specified NEC A07.8

Infection, infected, infective — *continued*
protozoal — *continued*
  specified NEC B60.8
Pseudoallescheria boydii B48.2
Pseudomonas NEC A49.8
  as cause of disease classified elsewhere B96.5
  mallei A24.0
  pneumonia J15.1
  pseudomallei — *see* Melioidosis
puerperal O86.4
  genitourinary tract NEC O86.89
  major or generalized O85
  minor O86.4
  specified NEC O86.89
pulmonary — *see* Infection, lung
purulent — *see* Abscess
Pyrenochaeta romeroi B47.0
Q fever A78
rectum (sphincter) K62.89
renal (*see also* Infection, kidney)
  pelvis and ureter (cystic) N28.85
reovirus, as cause of disease classified elsewhere B97.5
respiratory (tract) NEC J98.8
  acute J22
  chronic J98.8
  influenzal (upper) (acute) — *see* Influenza, with,
    respiratory manifestations NEC
  lower (acute) J22
    chronic — *see* Bronchitis, chronic
  rhinovirus J00
  syncytial virus, as cause of disease classified else-
    where B97.4
  upper (acute) NOS J06.9
    chronic J39.8
    streptococcal J06.9
    viral NOS J06.9
resulting from
  presence of internal prosthesis, implant, graft —
    see Complications, by site and type, infection
retortamoniasis A07.8
retroperitoneal NEC K68.9
retrovirus B33.3
  as cause of disease classified elsewhere B97.30
    human
      immunodeficiency, type 2 (HIV 2) B97.35
      T-cell lymphotropic
        type I (HTLV-I) B97.33
        type II (HTLV-II) B97.34
    lentivirus B97.31
    oncovirus B97.32
    specified NEC B97.39
Rhinosporidium (seeberi) B48.1
rhinovirus
  as cause of disease classified elsewhere B97.89
  unspecified nature or site B34.8
Rhizopus — *see* Mucormycosis
rickettsial NOS A79.9
roundworm (large) NEC B82.0
  Ascariasis (*see also* Ascariasis) B77.9
rubella — *see* Rubella
Saccharomyces — *see* Candidiasis
salivary duct or gland (any) — *see* Sialoadenitis
Salmonella (aertrycke) (arizonae) (callinarum)
  (cholerae-suis) (enteritidis) (suipestifer) (typhimurium) A02.9
  with
    (gastro)enteritis A02.0
    sepsis A02.1
    specified manifestation NEC A02.8
  due to food (poisoning) A02.9
  hirschfeldii A01.3
  localized A02.20
    arthritis A02.23
    meningitis A02.21
    osteomyelitis A02.24
    pneumonia A02.22
    pyelonephritis A02.25
    specified NEC A02.29
  paratyphi A01.4
    A A01.1
    B A01.2
    C A01.3
  schottmuelleri A01.2
  typhi, typhosa — *see* Typhoid
Sarcocystis A07.8
scabies B86
Schistosoma — *see* Infestation, Schistosoma
scrotum (acute) NEC N49.2

Infection, infected, infective — *continued*
seminal vesicle — *see* Vesiculitis
septic
  localized, skin — *see* Abscess
sheep liver fluke B66.3
Shigella A03.9
  boydii A03.2
  dysenteriae A03.0
  flexneri A03.1
  group
    A A03.0
    B A03.1
    C A03.2
    D A03.3
  Schmitz (-Stutzer) A03.0
  schmitzii A03.0
  shigae A03.0
  sonnei A03.3
  specified NEC A03.8
shoulder (joint) NEC M00.9
  due to internal joint prosthesis T84.59 ☑
  skin NEC L08.9
sinus (accessory) (chronic) (nasal) (*see also* Sinusitis)
  pilonidal — *see* Sinus, pilonidal
  skin NEC L08.89
Skene's duct or gland — *see* Urethritis
skin (local) (staphylococcal) (streptococcal) L08.9
  abscess — *code by* site under Abscess
  cellulitis — *code by* site under Cellulitis
  due to fungus B36.9
    specified type NEC B36.8
  mycotic B36.9
    specified type NEC B36.8
  newborn P39.4
  ulcer — *see* Ulcer, skin
slow virus A81.9
  specified NEC A81.89
Sparganum (mansoni) (proliferum) (baxteri) B70.1
specific (*see also* Syphilis)
  to perinatal period — *see* Infection, congenital
specified NEC B99.8
spermatic cord NEC N49.1
sphenoidal (sinus) — *see* Sinusitis, sphenoidal
spinal cord NOS (*see also* Myelitis) G04.91
  abscess G06.1
  meninges — *see* Meningitis
  streptococcal G04.89
Spirillum A25.0
spirochetal NOS A69.9
  lung A69.8
  specified NEC A69.8
Spirometra larvae B70.1
spleen D73.89
Sporotrichum, Sporothrix (schenckii) — *see* Sporotrichosis
staphylococcal, unspecified site
  as cause of disease classified elsewhere B95.8
    aureus (methicillin susceptible) (MSSA) B95.61
      methicillin resistant (MRSA) B95.62
    specified NEC B95.7
  aureus (methicillin susceptible) (MSSA) A49.01
    methicillin resistant (MRSA) A49.02
  food poisoning A05.0
  generalized (purulent) A41.2
  pneumonia — *see* Pneumonia, staphylococcal
Stellantchasmus falcatus B66.8
streptobacillus moniliformis A25.1
streptococcal NEC A49.1
  as cause of disease classified elsewhere B95.5
  B genitourinary complicating
    childbirth O98.82
    pregnancy O98.81- ☑
    puerperium O98.83
  congenital
    sepsis P36.10
      group B P36.0
      specified NEC P36.19
  generalized (purulent) A40.9
Streptomyces B47.1
Strongyloides (stercoralis) — *see* Strongyloidiasis
stump (amputation) (surgical) — *see* Complication,
  amputation stump, infection
subcutaneous tissue, local L08.9
suipestifer — *see* Infection, salmonella
swimming pool bacillus A31.1
Taenia — *see* Infestation, Taenia
Taeniarhynchus saginatus B68.1
tapeworm — *see* Infestation, tapeworm

Infection, infected, infective — *continued*
tendon (sheath) — *see* Tenosynovitis, infective NEC
Ternidens diminutus B81.8
testis — *see* Orchitis
threadworm B80
throat — *see* Pharyngitis
thyroglossal duct K14.8
toe (skin) L08.9
  cellulitis L03.03- ☑
    fungus B35.1
  nail L03.03- ☑
    fungus B35.1
tongue NEC K14.0
  parasitic B37.0
tonsil (and adenoid) (faucial) (lingual) (pharyngeal) —
  see Tonsillitis
tooth, teeth K04.7
  periapical K04.7
  peridental, periodontal K05.20
    generalized K05.22
    localized K05.21
  pulp K04.0
  socket M27.3
TORCH — *see* Infection, congenital
  without active infection P00.2
Torula histolytica — *see* Cryptococcosis
Toxocara (canis) (cati) (felis) B83.0
Toxoplasma gondii — *see* Toxoplasma
trachea, chronic J42
trematode NEC — *see* Infestation, fluke
trench fever A79.0
Treponema pallidum — *see* Syphilis
Trichinella (spiralis) B75
Trichomonas A59.9
  cervix A59.09
  intestine A07.8
  prostate A59.02
  specified site NEC A59.8
  urethra A59.03
  urogenitalis A59.00
  vagina A59.01
  vulva A59.01
Trichophyton, trichophytic — *see* Dermatophytosis
Trichosporon (beigelii) cutaneum B36.2
Trichostrongylus B81.2
Trichuris (trichiura) B79
Trombicula (irritans) B88.0
Trypanosoma
  brucei
    gambiense B56.0
    rhodesiense B56.1
  cruzi — *see* Chagas' disease
  tubal — *see* Salpingo-oophoritis
tuberculous NEC — *see* Tuberculosis
tubo-ovarian — *see* Salpingo-oophoritis
tunica vaginalis N49.1
tunnel T80.212 ☑
tympanic membrane NEC — *see* Myringitis
typhoid (abortive) (ambulant) (bacillus) — *see* Typhoid
typhus A75.9
  flea-borne A75.2
  mite-borne A75.3
  recrudescent A75.1
  tick-borne A77.9
    African A77.1
    North Asian A77.2
umbilicus L08.82
ureter N28.86
urethra — *see* Urethritis
urinary (tract) N39.0
  bladder — *see* Cystitis
  complicating
    pregnancy O23.4- ☑
      specified type NEC O23.3- ☑
  kidney — *see* Infection, kidney
  newborn P39.3
  puerperal (postpartum) O86.20
  tuberculous A18.13
  urethra — *see* Urethritis
uterus, uterine — *see* Endometritis
vaccination T88.0 ☑
vaccinia not from vaccination B08.011
vagina (acute) — *see* Vaginitis
varicella B01.9
varicose veins — *see* Varix
vas deferens NEC N49.1
vesical — *see* Cystitis

Infection, infected, infective — *continued*
Vibrio
  cholerae A00.0
    El Tor A00.1
  parahaemolyticus (food poisoning) A05.3
  vulnificus
    as cause of disease classified elsewhere B96.82
    foodborne intoxication A05.5
Vincent's (gum) (mouth) (tonsil) A69.1
virus, viral NOS B34.9
  adenovirus
    as cause of disease classified elsewhere B97.0
    unspecified nature or site B34.0
  arborvirus, arbovirus arthropod-borne A94
  as cause of disease classified elsewhere B97.89
    adenovirus B97.0
    coronavirus B97.29
      SARS-associated B97.21
    coxsackievirus B97.11
    echovirus B97.12
    enterovirus B97.10
      coxsackievirus B97.11
      echovirus B97.12
      specified NEC B97.19
    human
      immunodeficiency, type 2 (HIV 2) B97.35
      metapneumovirus B97.81
      T-cell lymphotropic
        type I (HTLV-I) B97.33
        type II (HTLV-II) B97.34
    papillomavirus B97.7
    parvovirus B97.6
    reovirus B97.5
    respiratory syncytial B97.4
    retrovirus B97.30
      human
        immunodeficiency, type 2 (HIV 2) B97.35
        T-cell lymphotropic,
          type I (HTLV-I) B97.33
          type II (HTLV-II) B97.34
      lentivirus B97.31
      oncovirus B97.32
      specified NEC B97.39
    specified NEC B97.89
  central nervous system A89
    atypical A81.9
      specified NEC A81.89
    enterovirus NEC A88.8
      meningitis A87.0
    slow virus A81.9
      specified NEC A81.89
    specified NEC A88.8
  chest J98.8
  cotia B08.8
  coxsackie (*see also* Infection, coxsackie) B34.1
    as cause of disease classified elsewhere B97.11
  ECHO
    as cause of disease classified elsewhere B97.12
    unspecified nature or site B34.1
  encephalitis, tick-borne A84.9
  enterovirus, as cause of disease classified elsewhere
    B97.10
    coxsackievirus B97.11
    echovirus B97.12
    specified NEC B97.19
  exanthem NOS B09
  human metapneumovirus as cause of disease
    classified elsewhere B97.81
  human papilloma as cause of disease classified
    elsewhere B97.7
  intestine — *see* Enteritis, viral
  respiratory syncytial
    as cause of disease classified elsewhere B97.4
    bronchopneumonia J12.1
    common cold syndrome J00
    nasopharyngitis (acute) J00
  rhinovirus
    as cause of disease classified elsewhere B97.89
    unspecified nature or site B34.8
  slow A81.9
    specified NEC A81.89
  specified type NEC B33.8
    as cause of disease classified elsewhere B97.89
    unspecified nature or site B34.8
  unspecified nature or site B34.9
  West Nile — *see* Virus, West Nile
  vulva (acute) — *see* Vulvitis
  West Nile — *see* Virus, West Nile

Infection, infected, infective — *continued*
whipworm B79
worms B83.9
  specified type NEC B83.8
Wuchereria (bancrofti) B74.0
  malayi B74.1
yatapoxvirus B08.70
  specified NEC B08.79
yeast (*see also* Candidiasis) B37.9
yellow fever — *see* Fever, yellow
Yersinia
  enterocolitica (intestinal) A04.6
  pestis — *see* Plague
  pseudotuberculosis A28.2
Zeis' gland — *see* Hordeolum
zoonotic bacterial NOS A28.9
Zopfia senegalensis B47.0
Infective, infectious — *see* condition
Infertility
  female N97.9
    age-related N97.8
    associated with
      anovulation N97.0
      cervical (mucus) disease or anomaly N88.3
      congenital anomaly
        cervix N88.3
        fallopian tube N97.1
        uterus N97.2
        vagina N97.8
      dysmucorrhea N88.3
      fallopian tube disease or anomaly N97.1
      pituitary-hypothalamic origin E23.0
      specified origin NEC N97.8
      Stein-Leventhal syndrome E28.2
      uterine disease or anomaly N97.2
      vaginal disease or anomaly N97.8
    due to
      cervical anomaly N88.3
      fallopian tube anomaly N97.1
      ovarian failure E28.39
      Stein-Leventhal syndrome E28.2
      uterine anomaly N97.2
      vaginal anomaly N97.8
    nonimplantation N97.2
    origin
      cervical N88.3
      tubal (block) (occlusion) (stenosis) N97.1
      uterine N97.2
      vaginal N97.8
  male N46.9
    azoospermia N46.01
      extratesticular cause N46.029
        drug therapy N46.021
        efferent duct obstruction N46.023
        infection N46.022
        radiation N46.024
        specified cause NEC N46.029
        systemic disease N46.025
    oligospermia N46.11
      extratesticular cause N46.129
        drug therapy N46.121
        efferent duct obstruction N46.123
        infection N46.122
        radiation N46.124
        specified cause NEC N46.129
        systemic disease N46.125
    specified type NEC N46.8
Infestation B88.9
Acanthocheilonema (perstans) (streptocerca) B74.4
Acariasis B88.0
  demodex folliculorum B88.0
  sarcoptes scabiei B86
  trombiculae B88.0
Agamofilaria streptocerca B74.4
Ancylostoma, ankylostoma (braziliense) (caninum)
  (ceylanicum) (duodenale) B76.0
  americanum B76.1
  new world B76.1
Anisakis larvae, anisakiasis B81.0
arthropod NEC B88.2
Ascaris lumbricoides — *see* Ascariasis
Balantidium coli A07.0
beef tapeworm B68.1
Bothriocephalus (latus) B70.0
  larval B70.1
broad tapeworm B70.0
  larval B70.1
Brugia (malayi) B74.1

Infestation — *continued*
 Brugia (malayi) B74.1
  timori B74.2
 candiru B88.8
 Capillaria
  hepatica B83.8
  philippinensis B81.1
 cat liver fluke B66.0
 cestodes B71.9
  diphyllobothrium — *see* Infestation, diphyllobothrium
  dipylidiasis B71.1
  hymenolepiasis B71.0
  specified type NEC B71.8
 chigger B88.0
 chigo, chigoe B88.1
 Clonorchis (sinensis) (liver) B66.1
 coccidial A07.3
 crab-lice B85.3
 Cysticercus cellulosae — *see* Cysticercosis
 Demodex (folliculorum) B88.0
 Dermanyssus gallinae B88.0
 Dermatobia (hominis) — *see* Myiasis
 Dibothriocephalus (latus) B70.0
  larval B70.1
 Dicrocoelium dendriticum B66.2
 Diphyllobothrium (adult) (latum) (intestinal) (pacificum) B70.0
  larval B70.1
 Diplogonoporus (grandis) B71.8
 Dipylidium caninum B67.4
 Distoma hepaticum B66.3
 dog tapeworm B67.4
 Dracunculus medinensis B72
 dragon worm B72
 dwarf tapeworm B71.0
 Echinococcus — *see* Echinococcus
 Echinostomum ilocanum B66.8
 Entamoeba (histolytica) — *see* Infection, Ameba
 Enterobius vermicularis B80
 eyelid
  in (due to)
   leishmaniasis B55.1
   loiasis B74.3
   onchocerciasis B73.09
   phthiriasis B85.3
  parasitic NOS B89
 eyeworm B74.3
 Fasciola (gigantica) (hepatica) (indica) B66.3
 Fasciolopsis (buski) (intestine) B66.5
 filarial B74.9
  bancroftian B74.0
  conjunctiva B74.9
  due to
   Acanthocheilonema (perstans) (streptocerca) B74.4
   Brugia (malayi) B74.1
    timori B74.2
   Dracunculus medinensis B72
   guinea worm B72
   loa loa B74.3
   Mansonella (ozzardi) (perstans) (streptocerca) B74.4
   Onchocerca volvulus B73.00
    eye B73.00
    eyelid B73.09
   Wuchereria (bancrofti) B74.0
  Malayan B74.1
  ozzardi B74.4
  specified type NEC B74.8
 fish tapeworm B70.0
  larval B70.1
 fluke B66.9
  blood NOS — *see* Schistosomiasis
  cat liver B66.0
  intestinal B66.5
  lancet B66.2
  liver (sheep) B66.3
   cat B66.0
   Chinese B66.1
   due to clonorchiasis B66.1
   oriental B66.1
  lung (oriental) B66.4
  sheep liver B66.3
  specified type NEC B66.8
 fly larvae — *see* Myiasis
 Gasterophilus (intestinalis) — *see* Myiasis
 Gastrodiscoides hominis B66.8

Infestation — *continued*
 Giardia lamblia A07.1
 Gnathostoma (spinigerum) B83.1
 Gongylonema B83.8
 guinea worm B72
 helminth B83.9
  angiostrongyliasis B83.2
   intestinal B81.3
  gnathostomiasis B83.1
  hirudiniasis, internal B83.4
  intestinal B82.0
   angiostrongyliasis B81.3
   anisakiasis B81.0
   ascariasis — *see* Ascariasis
   capillariasis B81.1
   cysticercosis — *see* Cysticercosis
   diphyllobothriasis — *see* Infestation, diphyllobothriasis
   dracunculiasis B72
   echinococcus — *see* Echinococcosis
   enterobiasis B80
   filariasis — *see* Infestation, filarial
   fluke — *see* Infestation, fluke
   hookworm — *see* Infestation, hookworm
   mixed (types classifiable to more than one of the titles B65.0-B81.3 and B81.8) B81.4
   onchocerciasis — *see* Onchocerciasis
   schistosomiasis — *see* Infestation, schistosoma
   specified
    cestode NEC — *see* Infestation, cestode type NEC B81.8
   strongyloidiasis — *see* Strongyloidiasis
   taenia — *see* Infestation, taenia
   trichinellosis B75
   trichostrongyliasis B81.2
   trichuriasis B79
  specified type NEC B83.8
  syngamiasis B83.3
  visceral larva migrans B83.0
 Heterophyes (heterophyes) B66.8
 hookworm B76.9
  ancylostomiasis B76.0
  necatoriasis B76.1
  specified type NEC B76.8
 Hymenolepis (diminuta) (nana) B71.0
 intestinal NEC B82.9
 leeches (aquatic) (land) — *see* Hirudiniasis
 Leishmania — *see* Leishmaniasis
 lice, louse — *see* Infestation, Pediculus
 Linguatula B88.8
 Liponyssoides sanguineus B88.0
 Loa loa B74.3
  conjunctival B74.3
  eyelid B74.3
 louse — *see* Infestation, Pediculus
 maggots — *see* Myiasis
 Mansonella (ozzardi) (perstans) (streptocerca) B74.4
 Medina (worm) B72
 Metagonimus (yokogawai) B66.8
 microfilaria streptocerca — *see* Onchocerciasis
  eye B73.00
  eyelid B73.09
 mites B88.9
  scabic B86
 Monilia (albicans) — *see* Candidiasis
 mouth B37.0
 Necator americanus B76.1
 nematode NEC (intestinal) B82.0
  Ancylostoma B76.0
  conjunctiva NEC B83.9
  Enterobius vermicularis B80
  Gnathostoma spinigerum B83.1
  physaloptera B80
  specified NEC B81.8
  trichostrongylus B81.2
  trichuris (trichuria) B79
 Oesophagostomum (apiostomum) B81.8
 Oestrus ovis (*see also* Myiasis) B87.9
 Onchocerca (volvulus) — *see* Onchocerciasis
 Opisthorchis (felineus) (viverrini) B66.0
 orbit, parasitic NOS B89
 Oxyuris vermicularis B80
 Paragonimus (westermani) B66.4
 parasite, parasitic B89
  eyelid B89
  intestinal NOS B82.9
  mouth B37.0
  skin B88.9

Infestation — *continued*
 parasite, parasitic — *continued*
  tongue B37.0
 Parastrongylus
  cantonensis B83.2
  costaricensis B81.3
 Pediculus B85.2
  body B85.1
  capitis (humanus) (any site) B85.0
  corporis (humanus) (any site) B85.1
  head B85.0
  mixed (classifiable to more than one of the titles B85.0 - B85.3) B85.4
  pubis (any site) B85.3
 Pentastoma B88.8
 Phthirus (pubis) (any site) B85.3
  with any infestation classifiable to B85.0 - B85.2 B85.4
 pinworm B80
 pork tapeworm (adult) B68.0
 protozoal NEC B64
  intestinal A07.9
   specified NEC A07.8
  specified NEC B60.8
 pubic, louse B85.3
 rat tapeworm B71.0
 red bug B88.0
 roundworm (large) NEC B82.0
  Ascariasis (*see also* Ascariasis) B77.9
 sandflea B88.1
 Sarcoptes scabiei B86
 scabies B86
 Schistosoma B65.9
  bovis B65.8
  cercariae B65.3
  haematobium B65.0
  intercalatum B65.8
  japonicum B65.2
  mansoni B65.1
  mattheei B65.8
  mekongi B65.8
  specified type NEC B65.8
  spindale B65.8
 screw worms — *see* Myiasis
 skin NOS B88.9
 Sparganum (mansoni) (proliferum) (baxteri) B70.1
  larval B70.1
 specified type NEC B88.8
 Spirometra larvae B70.1
 Stellantchasmus falcatus B66.8
 Strongyloides stercoralis — *see* Strongyloidiasis
 Taenia B68.9
  diminuta B71.0
  echinococcus — *see* Echinococcus
  mediocanellata B68.1
  nana B71.0
  saginata B68.1
  solium (intestinal form) B68.0
   larval form — *see* Cysticercosis
 Taeniarhynchus saginatus B68.1
 tapeworm B71.9
  beef B68.1
  broad B70.0
   larval B70.1
  dog B67.4
  dwarf B71.0
  fish B70.0
   larval B70.1
  pork B68.0
  rat B71.0
 Ternidens diminutus B81.8
 Tetranychus molestissimus B88.0
 threadworm B80
 tongue B37.0
 Toxocara (canis) (cati) (felis) B83.0
 trematode(s) NEC — *see* Infestation, fluke
 Trichinella (spiralis) B75
 Trichocephalus B79
 Trichomonas — *see* Trichomoniasis
 Trichostrongylus B81.2
 Trichuris (trichiura) B79
 Trombicula (irritans) B88.0
 Tunga penetrans B88.1
 Uncinaria americana B76.1
 Vandellia cirrhosa B88.8
 whipworm B79
 worms B83.9
  intestinal B82.0

Infestation — *continued*
  Wuchereria (bancrofti) B74.0
Infiltrate, infiltration
  amyloid (generalized) (localized) — *see* Amyloidosis
  calcareous NEC R89.7
    localized — *see* Degeneration, by site
  calcium salt R89.7
  cardiac
    fatty — *see* Degeneration, myocardial
    glycogenic E74.02 [I43]
  corneal — *see* Edema, cornea
  eyelid — *see* Inflammation, eyelid
  glycogen, glycogenic — *see* Disease, glycogen storage
  heart, cardiac
    fatty — *see* Degeneration, myocardial
    glycogenic E74.02 [I43]
  inflammatory in vitreous H43.89
  kidney N28.89
  leukemic — *see* Leukemia
  liver K76.89
    fatty — *see* Fatty, liver NEC
    glycogen (*see also* Disease, glycogen storage) E74.03 [K77]
  lung R91.8
    eosinophilic J82
  lymphatic (*see also* Leukemia, lymphatic) C91.9- ☑
    gland I88.9
  muscle, fatty M62.89
  myocardium, myocardial
    fatty — *see* Degeneration, myocardial
    glycogenic E74.02 [I43]
  on chest x-ray R91.8
  pulmonary R91.8
    with eosinophilia J82
  skin (lymphocytic) L98.6
  thymus (gland) (fatty) E32.8
  urine R39.0
  vesicant agent
    antineoplastic chemotherapy T80.810 ☑
    other agent NEC T80.818 ☑
  vitreous body H43.89
Infirmity R68.89
  senile R54
Inflammation, inflamed, inflammatory (with exudation)
  abducent (nerve) — *see* Strabismus, paralytic, sixth nerve
  accessory sinus (chronic) — *see* Sinusitis
  adrenal (gland) E27.8
  alveoli, teeth M27.3
    scorbutic E54
  anal canal, anus K62.89
  antrum (chronic) — *see* Sinusitis, maxillary
  appendix — *see* Appendicitis
  arachnoid — *see* Meningitis
  areola N61
    puerperal, postpartum or gestational — *see* Infection, nipple
  areolar tissue NOS L08.9
  artery — *see* Arteritis
  auditory meatus (external) — *see* Otitis, externa
  Bartholin's gland N75.8
  bile duct (common) (hepatic) or passage — *see* Cholangitis
  bladder — *see* Cystitis
  bone — *see* Osteomyelitis
  brain (*see also* Encephalitis)
    membrane — *see* Meningitis
  breast N61
    puerperal, postpartum, gestational — *see* Mastitis, obstetric
  broad ligament — *see* Disease, pelvis, inflammatory
  bronchi — *see* Bronchitis
  catarrhal J00
  cecum — *see* Appendicitis
  cerebral (*see also* Encephalitis)
    membrane — *see* Meningitis
  cerebrospinal
    meningococcal A39.0
  cervix (uteri) — *see* Cervicitis
  chest J98.8
  chorioretinal H30.9- ☑
    cyclitis — *see* Cyclitis
    disseminated H30.10- ☑
      generalized H30.13- ☑
      peripheral H30.12- ☑
      posterior pole H30.11- ☑

Inflammation, inflamed, inflammatory — *continued*
  chorioretinal — *continued*
    epitheliopathy — *see* Epitheliopathy
    focal H30.00- ☑
      juxtapapillary H30.01- ☑
      macular H30.04- ☑
      paramacular — *see* Inflammation, chorioretinal, focal, macular
      peripheral H30.03- ☑
      posterior pole H30.02- ☑
    specified type NEC H30.89- ☑
  choroid — *see* Inflammation, chorioretinal
  chronic, postmastoidectomy cavity — *see* Complications, postmastoidectomy, inflammation
  colon — *see* Enteritis
  connective tissue (diffuse) NEC — *see* Disorder, soft tissue, specified type NEC
  cornea — *see* Keratitis
  corpora cavernosa N48.29
  cranial nerve — *see* Disorder, nerve, cranial
  Douglas' cul-de-sac or pouch (chronic) N73.0
  due to device, implant or graft (*see also* Complications, by site and type, infection or inflammation)
    arterial graft T82.7 ☑
    breast (implant) T85.79 ☑
    catheter T85.79 ☑
      dialysis (renal) T82.7 ☑
        intraperitoneal T85.71 ☑
      infusion T82.7 ☑
        spinal (epidural) (subdural) T85.79 ☑
      urinary (indwelling) T83.51 ☑
    electronic (electrode) (pulse generator) (stimulator)
      bone T84.7 ☑
      cardiac T82.7 ☑
      nervous system (brain) (peripheral nerve) (spinal) T85.79 ☑
      urinary T83.59 ☑
    fixation, internal (orthopedic) NEC — *see* Complication, fixation device, infection
    gastrointestinal (bile duct) (esophagus) T85.79 ☑
    genital NEC T83.6 ☑
    heart NEC T82.7 ☑
      valve (prosthesis) T82.6 ☑
      graft T82.7 ☑
    joint prosthesis — *see* Complication, joint prosthesis, infection
    ocular (corneal graft) (orbital implant) NEC T85.79 ☑
    orthopedic NEC T84.7 ☑
    specified NEC T85.79 ☑
    urinary NEC T83.59 ☑
    vascular NEC T82.7 ☑
    ventricular intracranial shunt T85.79 ☑
  duodenum K29.80
    with bleeding K29.81
  dura mater — *see* Meningitis
  ear (middle) (*see also* Otitis, media)
    external — *see* Otitis, externa
    inner — *see* subcategory H83.0 ☑
  epididymis — *see* Epididymitis
  esophagus K20.9
  ethmoidal (sinus) (chronic) — *see* Sinusitis, ethmoidal
  eustachian tube (catarrhal) — *see* Salpingitis, eustachian
  eyelid H01.9
    abscess — *see* Abscess, eyelid
    blepharitis — *see* Blepharitis
    chalazion — *see* Chalazion
    dermatosis (noninfectious) — *see* Dermatosis, eyelid
    hordeolum — *see* Hordeolum
    specified NEC H01.8
  fallopian tube — *see* Salpingo-oophoritis
  fascia — *see* Myositis
  follicular, pharynx J31.2
  frontal (sinus) (chronic) — *see* Sinusitis, frontal
  gallbladder — *see* Cholecystitis
  gastric — *see* Gastritis
  gastrointestinal — *see* Enteritis
  genital organ (internal) (diffuse)
    female — *see* Disease, pelvis, inflammatory
    male N49.9
      multiple sites N49.8
      specified NEC N49.8
  gland (lymph) — *see* Lymphadenitis

Inflammation, inflamed, inflammatory — *continued*
  glottis — *see* Laryngitis
  granular, pharynx J31.2
  gum K05.10
    nonplaque induced K05.11
    plaque induced K05.10
  heart — *see* Carditis
  hepatic duct — *see* Cholangitis
  ileoanal (internal) pouch K91.850
  ileum (*see also* Enteritis)
    regional or terminal — *see* Enteritis, regional
  intestinal pouch K91.850
  intestine (any part) — *see* Enteritis
  jaw (acute) (bone) (chronic) (lower) (suppurative) (upper) M27.2
  joint NEC — *see* Arthritis
    sacroiliac M46.1
  kidney — *see* Nephritis
  knee (joint) M13.169
    tuberculous A18.02
  labium (majus) (minus) — *see* Vulvitis
  lacrimal
    gland — *see* Dacryoadenitis
    passages (duct) (sac) (*see also* Dacryocystitis)
      canaliculitis — *see* Canaliculitis, lacrimal
  larynx — *see* Laryngitis
  leg NOS L08.9
  lip K13.0
  liver (capsule) (*see also* Hepatitis)
    chronic K73.9
    suppurative K75.0
  lung (acute) (*see also* Pneumonia)
    chronic J98.4
  lymph gland or node — *see* Lymphadenitis
  lymphatic vessel — *see* Lymphangitis
  maxilla, maxillary M27.2
    sinus (chronic) — *see* Sinusitis, maxillary
  membranes of brain or spinal cord — *see* Meningitis
  meninges — *see* Meningitis
  mouth K12.1
  muscle — *see* Myositis
  myocardium — *see* Myocarditis
  nasal sinus (chronic) — *see* Sinusitis
  nasopharynx — *see* Nasopharyngitis
  navel L08.82
  nerve NEC — *see* Neuralgia
  nipple N61
    puerperal, postpartum or gestational — *see* Infection, nipple
  nose — *see* Rhinitis
  oculomotor (nerve) — *see* Strabismus, paralytic, third nerve
  optic nerve — *see* Neuritis, optic
  orbit (chronic) H05.10
    acute H05.00
      abscess — *see* Abscess, orbit
      cellulitis — *see* Cellulitis, orbit
      osteomyelitis — *see* Osteomyelitis, orbit
      periostitis — *see* Periostitis, orbital
      tenonitis — *see* Tenonitis, eye
    granuloma — *see* Granuloma, orbit
    myositis — *see* Myositis, orbital
  ovary — *see* Salpingo-oophoritis
  oviduct — *see* Salpingo-oophoritis
  pancreas (acute) — *see* Pancreatitis
  parametrium N73.0
  parotid region L08.9
  pelvis, female — *see* Disease, pelvis, inflammatory
  penis (corpora cavernosa) N48.29
  perianal K62.89
  pericardium — *see* Pericarditis
  perineum (female) (male) L08.9
  perirectal K62.89
  peritoneum — *see* Peritonitis
  periuterine — *see* Disease, pelvis, inflammatory
  perivesical — *see* Cystitis
  petrous bone (acute) (chronic) — *see* Petrositis
  pharynx (acute) — *see* Pharyngitis
  pia mater — *see* Meningitis
  pleura — *see* Pleurisy
  polyp, colon (*see also* Polyp, colon, inflammatory) K51.40
  prostate (*see also* Prostatitis)
    specified type NEC N41.8
  rectosigmoid — *see* Rectosigmoiditis
  rectum (*see also* Proctitis) K62.89

Inflammation, inflamed, inflammatory — *continued*
  respiratory, upper (*see also* Infection, respiratory, upper) J06.9
    acute, due to radiation J70.0
    chronic, due to external agent — *see* condition, respiratory, chronic, due to
    due to
      chemicals, gases, fumes or vapors (inhalation) J68.2
      radiation J70.1
  retina — *see* Chorioretinitis
  retrocecal — *see* Appendicitis
  retroperitoneal — *see* Peritonitis
  salivary duct or gland (any) (suppurative) — *see* Sialoadenitis
  scorbutic, alveoli, teeth E54
  scrotum N49.2
  seminal vesicle — *see* Vesiculitis
  sigmoid — *see* Enteritis
  sinus — *see* Sinusitis
  Skene's duct or gland — *see* Urethritis
  skin L08.9
  spermatic cord N49.1
  sphenoidal (sinus) — *see* Sinusitis, sphenoidal
  spinal
    cord — *see* Encephalitis
    membrane — *see* Meningitis
    nerve — *see* Disorder, nerve
  spine — *see* Spondylopathy, inflammatory
  spleen (capsule) D73.89
  stomach — *see* Gastritis
  subcutaneous tissue L08.9
  suprarenal (gland) E27.8
  synovial — *see* Tenosynovitis
  tendon (sheath) NEC — *see* Tenosynovitis
  testis — *see* Orchitis
  throat (acute) — *see* Pharyngitis
  thymus (gland) E32.8
  thyroid (gland) — *see* Thyroiditis
  tongue K14.0
  tonsil — *see* Tonsillitis
  trachea — *see* Tracheitis
  trochlear (nerve) — *see* Strabismus, paralytic, fourth nerve
  tubal — *see* Salpingo-oophoritis
  tuberculous NEC — *see* Tuberculosis
  tubo-ovarian — *see* Salpingo-oophoritis
  tunica vaginalis N49.1
  tympanic membrane — *see* Tympanitis
  umbilicus, umbilical L08.82
  uterine ligament — *see* Disease, pelvis, inflammatory
  uterus (catarrhal) — *see* Endometritis
  uveal tract (anterior) NOS (*see also* Iridocyclitis)
    posterior — *see* Chorioretinitis
  vagina — *see* Vaginitis
  vas deferens N49.1
  vein (*see also* Phlebitis)
    intracranial or intraspinal (septic) G08
    thrombotic I80.9
      leg — *see* Phlebitis, leg
      lower extremity — *see* Phlebitis, leg
  vocal cord J38.3
  vulva — *see* Vulvitis
  Wharton's duct (suppurative) — *see* Sialoadenitis
Inflation, lung, imperfect (newborn) — *see* Atelectasis
Influenza (bronchial) (epidemic) (respiratory (upper)) (unidentified influenza virus) J11.1
  with
    digestive manifestations J11.2
    encephalopathy J11.81
    enteritis J11.2
    gastroenteritis J11.2
    gastrointestinal manifestations J11.2
    laryngitis J11.1
    myocarditis J11.82
    otitis media J11.83
    pharyngitis J11.1
    pneumonia J11.00
      specified type J11.08
    respiratory manifestations NEC J11.1
    specified manifestation NEC J11.89
  A/H5N1 (*see also* Influenza, due to, identified novel influenza A virus) J09.X2
  avian (*see also* Influenza, due to, identified novel influenza A virus) J09.X2

Influenza — *continued*
  bird (*see also* Influenza, due to, identified novel influenza A virus) J09.X2
  due to
    avian (*see also* Influenza, due to, identified novel influenza A virus) J09.X2
    identified influenza virus NEC J10.1
      with
        digestive manifestations J10.2
        encephalopathy J10.81
        enteritis J10.2
        gastroenteritis J10.2
        gastrointestinal manifestations J10.2
        laryngitis J10.1
        myocarditis J10.82
        otitis media J10.83
        pharyngitis J10.1
        pneumonia (unspecified type) J10.00
          with same identified influenza virus J10.01
          specified type NEC J10.08
        respiratory manifestations NEC J10.1
        specified manifestation NEC J10.89
    identified novel influenza A virus J09.X2
      with
        digestive manifestations J09.X3
        encephalopathy J09.X9
        enteritis J09.X3
        gastroenteritis J09.X3
        gastrointestinal manifestations J09.X3
        laryngitis J09.X2
        myocarditis J09.X9
        otitis media J09.X9
        pharyngitis J09.X2
        pneumonia J09.X1
        respiratory manifestations NEC J09.X2
        specified manifestation NEC J09.X9
        upper respiratory symptoms J09.X2
  novel (2009) H1N1 influenza (*see also* Influenza, due to, identified influenza virus NEC) J10.1
  novel influenza A/H1N1 (*see also* Influenza, due to, identified influenza virus NEC) J10.1
  of other animal origin, not bird or swine (*see also* Influenza, due to, identified novel influenza A virus) J09.X2
  swine (viruses that normally cause infections in pigs) (*see also* Influenza, due to, identified novel influenza A virus) J09.X2
Influenzal — *see* Influenza
Influenza-like disease — *see* Influenza
Infraction, Freiberg's (metatarsal head) — *see* Osteochondrosis, juvenile, metatarsus
Infraeruption of tooth (teeth) M26.34
Infusion complication, misadventure, or reaction — *see* Complications, infusion
Ingestion
  chemical — *see* Table of Drugs and Chemicals, by substance, poisoning
  drug or medicament
    correct substance properly administered — *see* Table of Drugs and Chemicals, by drug, adverse effect
    overdose or wrong substance given or taken — *see* Table of Drugs and Chemicals, by drug, poisoning
  foreign body — *see* Foreign body, alimentary tract
  tularemia A21.3
Ingrowing
  hair (beard) L73.1
  nail (finger) (toe) L60.0
Inguinal (*see also* condition)
  testicle Q53.9
    bilateral Q53.21
    unilateral Q53.11
Inhalation
  anthrax A22.1
  flame T27.3
  food or foreign body — *see* Foreign body, by site
  gases, fumes, or vapors NEC T59.9-
    specified agent — *see* Table of Drugs and Chemicals, by substance
  liquid or vomitus — *see* Asphyxia
  meconium (newborn) P24.00
    with
      with respiratory symptoms P24.01
      pneumonia (pneumonitis) P24.01
  mucus — *see* Asphyxia, mucus

Inhalation — *continued*
  oil or gasoline (causing suffocation) — *see* Foreign body, by site
  smoke J70.5
    due to chemicals, gases, fumes and vapors J68.9
  steam — *see* Toxicity, vapors
  stomach contents or secretions — *see* Foreign body, by site
    due to anesthesia (general) (local) or other sedation T88.59 ☑
      in labor and delivery O74.0
      in pregnancy O29.01- ☑
      postpartum, puerperal O89.01
Inhibition, orgasm
  female F52.31
  male F52.32
Inhibitor, systemic lupus erythematosus (presence of) D68.62
Iniencephalus, iniencephaly Q00.2
Injection, traumatic jet (air) (industrial) (water) (paint or dye) T70.4 ☑
Injury (*see also* specified injury type) T14.90
  abdomen, abdominal S39.91 ☑
    blood vessel — *see* Injury, blood vessel, abdomen
    cavity — *see* Injury, intra-abdominal
    contusion S30.1 ☑
    internal — *see* Injury, intra-abdominal
    intra-abdominal organ — *see* Injury, intra-abdominal
    nerve — *see* Injury, nerve, abdomen
    open — *see* Wound, open, abdomen
    specified NEC S39.81 ☑
    superficial — *see* Injury, superficial, abdomen
  Achilles tendon S86.00- ☑
    laceration S86.02- ☑
    specified type NEC S86.09- ☑
    strain S86.01- ☑
  acoustic, resulting in deafness — *see* Injury, nerve, acoustic
  adrenal (gland) S37.819 ☑
    contusion S37.812 ☑
    laceration S37.813 ☑
    specified type NEC S37.818 ☑
  alveolar (process) S09.93 ☑
  ankle S99.91- ☑
    contusion — *see* Contusion, ankle
    dislocation — *see* Dislocation, ankle
    fracture — *see* Fracture, ankle
    nerve — *see* Injury, nerve, ankle
    open — *see* Wound, open, ankle
    specified type NEC S99.81- ☑
    sprain — *see* Sprain, ankle
    superficial — *see* Injury, superficial, ankle
  anterior chamber, eye — *see* Injury, eye, specified site NEC
  anus — *see* Injury, abdomen
  aorta (thoracic) S25.00 ☑
    abdominal S35.00 ☑
      laceration (minor) (superficial) S35.01 ☑
        major S35.02 ☑
      specified type NEC S35.09 ☑
    laceration (minor) (superficial) S25.01 ☑
      major S25.02 ☑
    specified type NEC S25.09 ☑
  arm (upper) S49.9- ☑
    blood vessel — *see* Injury, blood vessel, arm
    contusion — *see* Contusion, arm, upper
    fracture — *see* Fracture, humerus
    lower — *see* Injury, forearm
    muscle — *see* Injury, muscle, shoulder
    nerve — *see* Injury, nerve, arm
    open — *see* Wound, open, arm
    specified type NEC S49.8- ☑
    superficial — *see* Injury, superficial, arm
  artery (complicating trauma) (*see also* Injury, blood vessel, by site)
    cerebral or meningeal — *see* Injury, intracranial
  auditory canal (external) (meatus) S09.91 ☑
  auricle, auris, ear S09.91 ☑
  axilla — *see* Injury, shoulder
  back — *see* Injury, back, lower
  bile duct S36.13 ☑
  birth (*see also* Birth, injury) P15.9
  bladder (sphincter) S37.20 ☑
    at delivery O71.5
    contusion S37.22 ☑

Injury — *continued*
  bladder — *continued*
    laceration S37.23 ☑
    obstetrical trauma O71.5
    specified type NEC S37.29 ☑
  blast (air) (hydraulic) (immersion) (underwater) NEC T14.8
    acoustic nerve trauma — *see* Injury, nerve, acoustic
    bladder — *see* Injury, bladder
    brain — *see* Concussion
    colon — *see* Injury, intestine, large
    ear (primary) S09.31- ☑
      secondary S09.39- ☑
    generalized T70.8 ☑
    lung — *see* Injury, intrathoracic, lung
    multiple body organs T70.8 ☑
    peritoneum S36.81 ☑
    rectum S36.61 ☑
    retroperitoneum S36.898 ☑
    small intestine S36.419 ☑
      duodenum S36.410 ☑
      specified site NEC S36.418 ☑
    specified
      intra-abdominal organ NEC S36.898 ☑
      pelvic organ NEC S37.899 ☑
  blood vessel NEC T14.8
    abdomen S35.9 ☑
      aorta — *see* Injury, aorta, abdominal
      celiac artery — *see* Injury, blood vessel, celiac artery
      iliac vessel — *see* Injury, blood vessel, iliac
      laceration S35.91
      mesenteric vessel — *see* Injury, mesenteric
      portal vein — *see* Injury, blood vessel, portal vein
      renal vessel — *see* Injury, blood vessel, renal
      specified vessel NEC S35.8X- ☑
      splenic vessel — *see* Injury, blood vessel, splenic
      vena cava — *see* Injury, vena cava, inferior
    ankle — *see* Injury, blood vessel, foot
    aorta (abdominal) (thoracic) — *see* Injury, aorta
    arm (upper) NEC S45.90- ☑
      forearm — *see* Injury, blood vessel, forearm
      laceration S45.91- ☑
      specified
        site NEC S45.80- ☑
          laceration S45.81- ☑
          specified type NEC S45.89- ☑
        type NEC S45.99- ☑
      superficial vein S45.30- ☑
        laceration S45.31- ☑
        specified type NEC S45.39- ☑
    axillary
      artery S45.00- ☑
        laceration S45.01- ☑
        specified type NEC S45.09- ☑
      vein S45.20- ☑
        laceration S45.21- ☑
        specified type NEC S45.29- ☑
    azygos vein — *see* Injury, blood vessel, thoracic, specified site NEC
    brachial
      artery S45.10- ☑
        laceration S45.11- ☑
        specified type NEC S45.19- ☑
      vein S45.20- ☑
        laceration S45.219 ☑
        specified type NEC S45.29- ☑
    carotid artery (common) (external) (internal, extracranial) S15.00- ☑
      internal, intracranial S06.8- ☑
      laceration (minor) (superficial) S15.01- ☑
        major S15.02- ☑
      specified type NEC S15.09- ☑
    celiac artery S35.219 ☑
      branch S35.299 ☑
        laceration (minor) (superficial) S35.291 ☑
          major S35.292 ☑
        specified NEC S35.298 ☑
      laceration (minor) (superficial) S35.211 ☑
        major S35.212 ☑
      specified type NEC S35.218 ☑
    cerebral — *see* Injury, intracranial
    deep plantar — *see* Injury, blood vessel, plantar artery

Injury — *continued*
  blood vessel — *continued*
    digital (hand) — *see* Injury, blood vessel, finger
    dorsal
      artery (foot) S95.00- ☑
        laceration S95.01- ☑
        specified type NEC S95.09- ☑
      vein (foot) S95.20- ☑
        laceration S95.21- ☑
        specified type NEC S95.29- ☑
    due to accidental laceration during procedure — *see* Laceration, accidental complicating surgery
    extremity — *see* Injury, blood vessel, limb
    femoral
      artery (common) (superficial) S75.00- ☑
        laceration (minor) (superficial) S75.01- ☑
          major S75.02- ☑
        specified type NEC S75.09- ☑
      vein (hip level) (thigh level) S75.10- ☑
        laceration (minor) (superficial) S75.11- ☑
          major S75.12- ☑
        specified type NEC S75.19- ☑
    finger S65.50- ☑
      index S65.50- ☑
        laceration S65.51- ☑
        specified type NEC S65.59- ☑
      laceration S65.51- ☑
      little S65.50- ☑
        laceration S65.51- ☑
        specified type NEC S65.59- ☑
      middle S65.50- ☑
        laceration S65.51- ☑
        specified type NEC S65.59- ☑
      specified type NEC S65.59- ☑
      thumb — *see* Injury, blood vessel, thumb
    foot S95.90- ☑
      dorsal
        artery — *see* Injury, blood vessel, dorsal, artery
        vein — *see* Injury, blood vessel, dorsal, vein
      laceration S95.91- ☑
      plantar artery — *see* Injury, blood vessel, plantar artery
      specified
        site NEC S95.80- ☑
          laceration S95.81- ☑
          specified type NEC S95.89- ☑
        specified type NEC S95.99- ☑
    forearm S55.90- ☑
      laceration S55.91- ☑
      radial artery — *see* Injury, blood vessel, radial artery
      specified
        site NEC S55.80- ☑
          laceration S55.81- ☑
          specified type NEC S55.89- ☑
        type NEC S55.99- ☑
      ulnar artery — *see* Injury, blood vessel, ulnar artery
      vein S55.20- ☑
        laceration S55.21- ☑
        specified type NEC S55.29- ☑
    gastric
      artery — *see* Injury, mesenteric, artery, branch
      vein — *see* Injury, blood vessel, abdomen
    gastroduodenal artery — *see* Injury, mesenteric, artery, branch
    greater saphenous vein (lower leg level) S85.30- ☑
      hip (and thigh) level S75.20- ☑
        laceration (minor) (superficial) S75.21- ☑
          major S75.22- ☑
        specified type NEC S75.29- ☑
      laceration S85.31- ☑
      specified type NEC S85.39- ☑
    hand (level) S65.90- ☑
      finger — *see* Injury, blood vessel, finger
      laceration S65.91- ☑
      palmar arch — *see* Injury, blood vessel, palmar arch
      radial artery — *see* Injury, blood vessel, radial artery, hand
      specified
        site NEC S65.80- ☑
          laceration S65.81- ☑
          specified type NEC S65.89- ☑

Injury — *continued*
  blood vessel — *continued*
    hand — *continued*
      specified — *continued*
        type NEC S65.99- ☑
      thumb — *see* Injury, blood vessel, thumb
      ulnar artery — *see* Injury, blood vessel, ulnar artery, hand
    head S09.0 ☑
      intracranial — *see* Injury, intracranial
      multiple S09.0 ☑
    hepatic
      artery — *see* Injury, mesenteric, artery
      vein — *see* Injury, vena cava, inferior
    hip S75.90- ☑
      femoral artery — *see* Injury, blood vessel, femoral, artery
      femoral vein — *see* Injury, blood vessel, femoral, vein
      greater saphenous vein — *see* Injury, blood vessel, greater saphenous, hip level
      laceration S75.91- ☑
      specified
        site NEC S75.80- ☑
          laceration S75.81- ☑
          specified type NEC S75.89- ☑
        type NEC S75.99- ☑
    hypogastric (artery) (vein) — *see* Injury, blood vessel, iliac
    iliac S35.5- ☑
      artery S35.51- ☑
      specified vessel NEC S35.5- ☑
      uterine vessel — *see* Injury, blood vessel, uterine
      vein S35.51- ☑
    innominate — *see* Injury, blood vessel, thoracic, innominate
    intercostal (artery) (vein) — *see* Injury, blood vessel, thoracic, intercostal
    jugular vein (external) S15.20- ☑
      internal S15.30- ☑
        laceration (minor) (superficial) S15.31- ☑
          major S15.32- ☑
        specified type NEC S15.39- ☑
      laceration (minor) (superficial) S15.21- ☑
        major S15.22- ☑
      specified type NEC S15.29- ☑
    leg (level) (lower) S85.90- ☑
      greater saphenous — *see* Injury, blood vessel, greater saphenous
      laceration S85.91- ☑
      lesser saphenous — *see* Injury, blood vessel, lesser saphenous
      peroneal artery — *see* Injury, blood vessel, peroneal artery
      popliteal
        artery — *see* Injury, blood vessel, popliteal, artery
        vein — *see* Injury, blood vessel, popliteal, vein
      specified
        site NEC S85.80- ☑
          laceration S85.81- ☑
          specified type NEC S85.89- ☑
        type NEC S85.99- ☑
      thigh — *see* Injury, blood vessel, hip
      tibial artery — *see* Injury, blood vessel, tibial artery
    lesser saphenous vein (lower leg level) S85.40- ☑
      laceration S85.41- ☑
      specified type NEC S85.49- ☑
    limb
      lower — *see* Injury, blood vessel, leg
      upper — *see* Injury, blood vessel, arm
    lower back — *see* Injury, blood vessel, abdomen
      specified NEC — *see* Injury, blood vessel, abdomen, specified, site NEC
    mammary (artery) (vein) — *see* Injury, blood vessel, thoracic, specified site NEC
    mesenteric (inferior) (superior)
      artery — *see* Injury, mesenteric, artery
      vein — *see* Injury, blood vessel, mesenteric, vein
    neck S15.9 ☑
      specified site NEC S15.8 ☑
    ovarian (artery) (vein) — *see* subcategory S35.8 ☑

☑ **Additional Character Required** — Refer to the Tabular List for Character Selection   ▽ Subterms under main terms may continue to next column or page

Injury — *continued*
　eyelid S09.93 ☑
　　abrasion — *see* Abrasion, eyelid
　　contusion — *see* Contusion, eyelid
　　open — *see* Wound, open, eyelid
　face S09.93 ☑
　fallopian tube S37.509 ☑
　　bilateral S37.502 ☑
　　　blast injury S37.512 ☑
　　　contusion S37.522 ☑
　　　laceration S37.532 ☑
　　　specified type NEC S37.592 ☑
　　blast injury (primary) S37.519 ☑
　　　bilateral S37.512 ☑
　　　secondary — *see* Injury, fallopian tube, specified type NEC
　　　unilateral S37.511 ☑
　　contusion S37.529 ☑
　　　bilateral S37.522 ☑
　　　unilateral S37.521 ☑
　　laceration S37.539 ☑
　　　bilateral S37.532 ☑
　　　unilateral S37.531 ☑
　　specified type NEC S37.599 ☑
　　　bilateral S37.592 ☑
　　　unilateral S37.591 ☑
　　unilateral S37.501 ☑
　　　blast injury S37.511 ☑
　　　contusion S37.521 ☑
　　　laceration S37.531 ☑
　　　specified type NEC S37.591 ☑
　fascia — *see* Injury, muscle
　fifth cranial nerve (trigeminal) — *see* Injury, nerve, trigeminal
　finger (nail) S69.9- ☑
　　blood vessel — *see* Injury, blood vessel, finger
　　contusion — *see* Contusion, finger
　　dislocation — *see* Dislocation, finger
　　fracture — *see* Fracture, finger
　　muscle — *see* Injury, muscle, finger
　　nerve — *see* Injury, nerve, digital, finger
　　open — *see* Wound, open, finger
　　specified NEC S69.8- ☑
　　sprain — *see* Sprain, finger
　　superficial — *see* Injury, superficial, finger
　first cranial nerve (olfactory) — *see* Injury, nerve, olfactory
　flank — *see* Injury, abdomen
　foot S99.92- ☑
　　blood vessel — *see* Injury, blood vessel, foot
　　contusion — *see* Contusion, foot
　　dislocation — *see* Dislocation, foot
　　fracture — *see* Fracture, foot
　　muscle — *see* Injury, muscle, foot
　　open — *see* Wound, open, foot
　　specified type NEC S99.82- ☑
　　sprain — *see* Sprain, foot
　　superficial — *see* Injury, superficial, foot
　forceps NOS P15.9
　forearm S59.91- ☑
　　blood vessel — *see* Injury, blood vessel, forearm
　　contusion — *see* Contusion, forearm
　　fracture — *see* Fracture, forearm
　　muscle — *see* Injury, muscle, forearm
　　nerve — *see* Injury, nerve, forearm
　　open — *see* Wound, open, forearm
　　specified NEC S59.81- ☑
　　superficial — *see* Injury, superficial, forearm
　forehead S09.90 ☑
　fourth cranial nerve (trochlear) — *see* Injury, nerve, trochlear
　gallbladder S36.129 ☑
　　contusion S36.122 ☑
　　laceration S36.123 ☑
　　specified NEC S36.128 ☑
　ganglion
　　celiac, coeliac — *see* Injury, nerve, lumbosacral, sympathetic
　　gasserian — *see* Injury, nerve, trigeminal
　　stellate — *see* Injury, nerve, thorax, sympathetic
　　thoracic sympathetic — *see* Injury, nerve, thorax, sympathetic
　gasserian ganglion — *see* Injury, nerve, trigeminal
　gastric artery — *see* Injury, blood vessel, celiac artery, branch

Injury — *continued*
　gastroduodenal artery — *see* Injury, blood vessel, celiac artery, branch
　gastrointestinal tract — *see* Injury, intra-abdominal
　　with open wound into abdominal cavity — *see* Wound, open, with penetration into peritoneal cavity
　　colon — *see* Injury, intestine, large
　　rectum — *see* Injury, intestine, large, rectum
　　　with open wound into abdominal cavity S36.61 ☑
　　small intestine — *see* Injury, intestine, small
　　specified site NEC — *see* Injury, intra-abdominal, specified, site NEC
　　stomach — *see* Injury, stomach
　genital organ(s)
　　external S39.94 ☑
　　　specified NEC S39.848 ☑
　　internal S37.90 ☑
　　　fallopian tube — *see* Injury, fallopian tube
　　　ovary — *see* Injury, ovary
　　　prostate — *see* Injury, prostate
　　　seminal vesicle — *see* Injury, pelvis, organ, specified site NEC
　　　uterus — *see* Injury, uterus
　　　vas deferens — *see* Injury, pelvis, organ, specified site NEC
　　obstetrical trauma O71.9
　gland
　　lacrimal laceration — *see* Injury, eye, specified site NEC
　　salivary S09.90 ☑
　　thyroid NEC S19.84 ☑
　globe (eye) S05.90 ☑
　　specified NEC S05.8X- ☑
　groin — *see* Injury, abdomen
　gum S09.90 ☑
　hand S69.9- ☑
　　blood vessel — *see* Injury, blood vessel, hand
　　contusion — *see* Contusion, hand
　　fracture — *see* Fracture, hand
　　muscle — *see* Injury, muscle, hand
　　nerve — *see* Injury, nerve, hand
　　open — *see* Wound, open, hand
　　specified NEC S69.8- ☑
　　sprain — *see* Sprain, hand
　　superficial — *see* Injury, superficial, hand
　head S09.90 ☑
　　with loss of consciousness S06.9- ☑
　　specified NEC S09.8 ☑
　heart S26.90 ☑
　　with hemopericardium S26.00 ☑
　　　contusion S26.01 ☑
　　　laceration (mild) S26.020 ☑
　　　　major S26.022 ☑
　　　　moderate S26.021 ☑
　　　specified type NEC S26.09 ☑
　　without hemopericardium S26.10 ☑
　　　contusion S26.11 ☑
　　　laceration S26.12 ☑
　　　specified type NEC S26.19 ☑
　　contusion S26.91 ☑
　　laceration S26.92 ☑
　　specified type NEC S26.99 ☑
　heel — *see* Injury, foot
　hepatic
　　artery — *see* Injury, blood vessel, celiac artery, branch
　　duct — *see* Injury, liver
　　vein — *see* Injury, vena cava, inferior
　hip S79.91- ☑
　　blood vessel — *see* Injury, blood vessel, hip
　　contusion — *see* Contusion, hip
　　dislocation — *see* Dislocation, hip
　　fracture — *see* Fracture, femur, neck
　　muscle — *see* Injury, muscle, hip
　　nerve — *see* Injury, nerve, hip
　　open — *see* Wound, open, hip
　　specified NEC S79.81- ☑
　　sprain — *see* Sprain, hip
　　superficial — *see* Injury, superficial, hip
　hymen S39.94 ☑
　hypogastric
　　blood vessel — *see* Injury, blood vessel, iliac
　　plexus — *see* Injury, nerve, lumbosacral, sympathetic

Injury — *continued*
　ileum — *see* Injury, intestine, small
　iliac region S39.91 ☑
　instrumental (during surgery) — *see* Laceration, accidental complicating surgery
　　birth injury — *see* Birth, injury
　　nonsurgical — *see* Injury, by site
　　obstetrical O71.9
　　　bladder O71.5
　　　cervix O71.3
　　　high vaginal O71.4
　　　perineal NOS O70.9
　　　urethra O71.5
　　　uterus O71.5
　　　　with rupture or perforation O71.1
　internal T14.8
　　aorta — *see* Injury, aorta
　　bladder (sphincter) — *see* Injury, bladder
　　　with
　　　　ectopic or molar pregnancy O08.6
　　　　following ectopic or molar pregnancy O08.6
　　　　obstetrical trauma O71.5
　　bronchus, bronchi — *see* Injury, intrathoracic, bronchus
　　cecum — *see* Injury, intestine, large
　　cervix (uteri) (*see also* Injury, uterus)
　　　with ectopic or molar pregnancy O08.6
　　　following ectopic or molar pregnancy O08.6
　　　obstetrical trauma O71.3
　　chest — *see* Injury, intrathoracic
　　gastrointestinal tract — *see* Injury, intra-abdominal
　　heart — *see* Injury, heart
　　intestine NEC — *see* Injury, intestine
　　intrauterine — *see* Injury, uterus
　　mesentery — *see* Injury, intra-abdominal, specified, site NEC
　　pelvis, pelvic (organ) S37.90 ☑
　　　following ectopic or molar pregnancy (subsequent episode) O08.6
　　　obstetrical trauma NEC O71.5
　　　　rupture or perforation O71.1
　　　specified NEC S39.83 ☑
　　rectum — *see* Injury, intestine, large, rectum
　　stomach — *see* Injury, stomach
　　ureter — *see* Injury, ureter
　　urethra (sphincter) following ectopic or molar pregnancy O08.6
　　uterus — *see* Injury, uterus
　interscapular area — *see* Injury, thorax
　intestine
　　large S36.509 ☑
　　　ascending (right) S36.500 ☑
　　　　blast injury (primary) S36.510 ☑
　　　　　secondary S36.590 ☑
　　　　contusion S36.520 ☑
　　　　laceration S36.530 ☑
　　　　specified type NEC S36.590 ☑
　　　blast injury (primary) S36.519 ☑
　　　　ascending (right) S36.510 ☑
　　　　descending (left) S36.512 ☑
　　　　rectum S36.61 ☑
　　　　sigmoid S36.513 ☑
　　　　specified site NEC S36.518 ☑
　　　　transverse S36.511 ☑
　　　contusion S36.529 ☑
　　　　ascending (right) S36.520 ☑
　　　　descending (left) S36.522 ☑
　　　　rectum S36.62 ☑
　　　　sigmoid S36.523 ☑
　　　　specified site NEC S36.528 ☑
　　　　transverse S36.521 ☑
　　　descending (left) S36.502 ☑
　　　　blast injury (primary) S36.512 ☑
　　　　　secondary S36.592 ☑
　　　　contusion S36.522 ☑
　　　　laceration S36.532 ☑
　　　　specified type NEC S36.592 ☑
　　　laceration S36.539 ☑
　　　　ascending (right) S36.530 ☑
　　　　descending (left) S36.532 ☑
　　　　rectum S36.63 ☑
　　　　sigmoid S36.533 ☑
　　　　specified site NEC S36.538 ☑
　　　　transverse S36.531 ☑
　　　rectum S36.60 ☑
　　　　blast injury (primary) S36.61 ☑

☑ Additional Character Required — Refer to the Tabular List for Character Selection　　🔽 Subterms under main terms may continue to next column or page

Injury — continued
　intestine — continued
　　large — continued
　　　rectum — continued
　　　　blast injury — continued
　　　　　secondary S36.69 ☑
　　　　contusion S36.62 ☑
　　　　laceration S36.63 ☑
　　　　specified type NEC S36.69 ☑
　　　sigmoid S36.503 ☑
　　　　blast injury (primary) S36.513 ☑
　　　　　secondary S36.593 ☑
　　　　contusion S36.523 ☑
　　　　laceration S36.533 ☑
　　　　specified type NEC S36.593 ☑
　　　specified
　　　　site NEC S36.508 ☑
　　　　　blast injury (primary) S36.518 ☑
　　　　　　secondary S36.598 ☑
　　　　　contusion S36.528 ☑
　　　　　laceration S36.538 ☑
　　　　　specified type NEC S36.598 ☑
　　　　type NEC S36.599 ☑
　　　　　ascending (right) S36.590 ☑
　　　　　descending (left) S36.592 ☑
　　　　　rectum S36.69 ☑
　　　　　sigmoid S36.593 ☑
　　　　　specified site NEC S36.598 ☑
　　　　　transverse S36.591 ☑
　　　transverse S36.501 ☑
　　　　blast injury (primary) S36.511 ☑
　　　　　secondary S36.591 ☑
　　　　contusion S36.521 ☑
　　　　laceration S36.531 ☑
　　　　specified type NEC S36.591 ☑
　　small S36.409 ☑
　　　blast injury (primary) S36.419 ☑
　　　　duodenum S36.410 ☑
　　　　secondary S36.499 ☑
　　　　　duodenum S36.490 ☑
　　　　　specified site NEC S36.498 ☑
　　　　specified site NEC S36.418 ☑
　　　contusion S36.429 ☑
　　　　duodenum S36.420 ☑
　　　　specified site NEC S36.428 ☑
　　　duodenum S36.400 ☑
　　　　blast injury (primary) S36.410 ☑
　　　　　secondary S36.490 ☑
　　　　contusion S36.420 ☑
　　　　laceration S36.430 ☑
　　　　specified NEC S36.490 ☑
　　　laceration S36.439 ☑
　　　　duodenum S36.430 ☑
　　　　specified site NEC S36.438 ☑
　　　specified
　　　　site NEC S36.408 ☑
　　　　type NEC S36.499 ☑
　　　　　duodenum S36.490 ☑
　　　　　specified site NEC S36.498 ☑
　intra-abdominal S36.90 ☑
　　adrenal gland — see Injury, adrenal gland
　　bladder — see Injury, bladder
　　colon — see Injury, intestine, large
　　contusion S36.92 ☑
　　fallopian tube — see Injury, fallopian tube
　　gallbladder — see Injury, gallbladder
　　intestine — see Injury, intestine
　　kidney — see Injury, kidney
　　laceration S36.93 ☑
　　liver — see Injury, liver
　　ovary — see Injury, ovary
　　pancreas — see Injury, pancreas
　　pelvic NOS S37.90 ☑
　　peritoneum — see Injury, intra-abdominal, speci-
　　　fied, site NEC
　　prostate — see Injury, prostate
　　rectum — see Injury, intestine, large, rectum
　　retroperitoneum — see Injury, intra-abdominal,
　　　specified, site NEC
　　seminal vesicle — see Injury, pelvis, organ, speci-
　　　fied site NEC
　　small intestine — see Injury, intestine, small

Injury — continued
　intra-abdominal — continued
　　specified
　　　pelvic S37.90 ☑
　　　　specified
　　　　　site NEC S37.899 ☑
　　　　　　specified type NEC S37.898 ☑
　　　　　type NEC S37.99 ☑
　　　site NEC S36.899 ☑
　　　　contusion S36.892 ☑
　　　　laceration S36.893 ☑
　　　　specified type NEC S36.898 ☑
　　　type NEC S36.99 ☑
　　spleen — see Injury, spleen
　　stomach — see Injury, stomach
　　ureter — see Injury, ureter
　　urethra — see Injury, urethra
　　uterus — see Injury, uterus
　　vas deferens — see Injury, pelvis, organ, specified
　　　site NEC
　intracranial (traumatic) S06.9- ☑
　　cerebellar hemorrhage, traumatic — see Injury,
　　　intracranial, focal
　　cerebral edema, traumatic S06.1X- ☑
　　　diffuse S06.1X- ☑
　　　focal S06.1X- ☑
　　diffuse (axonal) S06.2X- ☑
　　epidural hemorrhage (traumatic) S06.4X- ☑
　　focal brain injury S06.30- ☑
　　　contusion — see Contusion, cerebral
　　　laceration — see Laceration, cerebral
　　　intracerebral hemorrhage, traumatic S06.36- ☑
　　　　left side S06.35- ☑
　　　　right side S06.34- ☑
　　subarachnoid hemorrhage, traumatic S06.6X- ☑
　　subdural hemorrhage, traumatic S06.5X- ☑
　intraocular — see Injury, eyeball, penetrating
　intrathoracic S27.9 ☑
　　bronchus S27.409 ☑
　　　bilateral S27.402 ☑
　　　blast injury (primary) S27.419 ☑
　　　　bilateral S27.412 ☑
　　　　secondary — see Injury, intrathoracic,
　　　　　bronchus, specified type NEC
　　　　unilateral S27.411 ☑
　　　contusion S27.429 ☑
　　　　bilateral S27.422 ☑
　　　　unilateral S27.421 ☑
　　　laceration S27.439 ☑
　　　　bilateral S27.432 ☑
　　　　unilateral S27.431 ☑
　　　specified type NEC S27.499 ☑
　　　　bilateral S27.492 ☑
　　　　unilateral S27.491 ☑
　　　unilateral S27.401 ☑
　　diaphragm S27.809 ☑
　　　contusion S27.802 ☑
　　　laceration S27.803 ☑
　　　specified type NEC S27.808 ☑
　　esophagus (thoracic) S27.819 ☑
　　　contusion S27.812 ☑
　　　laceration S27.813 ☑
　　　specified type NEC S27.818 ☑
　　heart — see Injury, heart
　　hemopneumothorax S27.2 ☑
　　hemothorax S27.1 ☑
　　lung S27.309 ☑
　　　aspiration J69.0
　　　bilateral S27.302 ☑
　　　blast injury (primary) S27.319 ☑
　　　　bilateral S27.312 ☑
　　　　secondary — see Injury, intrathoracic, lung,
　　　　　specified type NEC
　　　　unilateral S27.311 ☑
　　　contusion S27.329 ☑
　　　　bilateral S27.322 ☑
　　　　unilateral S27.321 ☑
　　　laceration S27.339 ☑
　　　　bilateral S27.332 ☑
　　　　unilateral S27.331 ☑
　　　specified type NEC S27.399 ☑
　　　　bilateral S27.392 ☑
　　　　unilateral S27.391 ☑
　　　unilateral S27.301 ☑
　　pleura S27.60 ☑
　　　laceration S27.63 ☑

Injury — continued
　intrathoracic — continued
　　pleura — continued
　　　specified type NEC S27.69 ☑
　　pneumothorax S27.0 ☑
　　specified organ NEC S27.899 ☑
　　　contusion S27.892 ☑
　　　laceration S27.893 ☑
　　　specified type NEC S27.898 ☑
　　thoracic duct — see Injury, intrathoracic, specified
　　　organ NEC
　　thymus gland — see Injury, intrathoracic, specified
　　　organ NEC
　　trachea, thoracic S27.50 ☑
　　　blast (primary) S27.51 ☑
　　　contusion S27.52 ☑
　　　laceration S27.53 ☑
　　　specified type NEC S27.59 ☑
　iris — see Injury, eye, specified site NEC
　　penetrating — see Injury, eyeball, penetrating
　jaw S09.93 ☑
　jejunum — see Injury, intestine, small
　joint NOS T14.8
　　old or residual — see Disorder, joint, specified type
　　　NEC
　kidney S37.00- ☑
　　acute (nontraumatic) N17.9
　　contusion — see Contusion, kidney
　　laceration — see Laceration, kidney
　　specified NEC S37.09- ☑
　knee S89.9- ☑
　　contusion — see Contusion, knee
　　dislocation — see Dislocation, knee
　　meniscus (lateral) (medial) — see Sprain, knee,
　　　specified site NEC
　　　old injury or tear — see Derangement, knee,
　　　　meniscus, due to old injury
　　open — see Wound, open, knee
　　specified NEC S89.8- ☑
　　sprain — see Sprain, knee
　　superficial — see Injury, superficial, knee
　labium (majus) (minus) S39.94 ☑
　labyrinth, ear S09.30- ☑
　lacrimal apparatus, duct, gland, or sac — see Injury,
　　eye, specified site NEC
　larynx NEC S19.81 ☑
　leg (lower) S89.9- ☑
　　blood vessel — see Injury, blood vessel, leg
　　contusion — see Contusion, leg
　　fracture — see Fracture, leg
　　muscle — see Injury, muscle, leg
　　nerve — see Injury, nerve, leg
　　open — see Wound, open, leg
　　specified NEC S89.8- ☑
　　superficial — see Injury, superficial, leg
　lens, eye — see Injury, eye, specified site NEC
　　penetrating — see Injury, eyeball, penetrating
　limb NEC T14.8
　lip S09.93 ☑
　liver S36.119 ☑
　　contusion S36.112 ☑
　　laceration S36.113 ☑
　　　major (stellate) S36.116 ☑
　　　minor S36.114 ☑
　　　moderate S36.115 ☑
　　specified NEC S36.118 ☑
　lower back S39.92 ☑
　　specified NEC S39.82 ☑
　lumbar, lumbosacral (region) S39.92 ☑
　　plexus — see Injury, lumbosacral plexus
　lumbosacral plexus S34.4 ☑
　lung (see also Injury, intrathoracic, lung)
　　aspiration J69.0
　　transfusion-related (TRALI) J95.84
　lymphatic thoracic duct — see Injury, intrathoracic,
　　specified organ NEC
　malar region S09.93 ☑
　mastoid region S09.90 ☑
　maxilla S09.93 ☑
　mediastinum — see Injury, intrathoracic, specified
　　organ NEC
　membrane, brain — see Injury, intracranial
　meningeal artery — see Injury, intracranial, subdural
　　hemorrhage
　meninges (cerebral) — see Injury, intracranial

☟ Subterms under main terms may continue to next column or page　　　☑ Additional Character Required — Refer to the Tabular List for Character Selection　　　**187**

Injury — Injury

Injury — *continued*
  mesenteric
    artery
      branch S35.299 ☑
        laceration (minor) (superficial) S35.291 ☑
          major S35.292 ☑
        specified NEC S35.298 ☑
      inferior S35.239 ☑
        laceration (minor) (superficial) S35.231 ☑
          major S35.232 ☑
        specified NEC S35.238 ☑
      superior S35.229 ☑
        laceration (minor) (superficial) S35.221 ☑
          major S35.222 ☑
        specified NEC S35.228 ☑
    plexus (inferior) (superior) — *see* Injury, nerve, lumbosacral, sympathetic
    vein
      inferior S35.349 ☑
        laceration S35.341 ☑
        specified NEC S35.348 ☑
      superior S35.339 ☑
        laceration S35.331 ☑
        specified NEC S35.338 ☑
  mesentery — *see* Injury, intra-abdominal, specified site NEC
  mesosalpinx — *see* Injury, pelvic organ, specified site NEC
  middle ear S09.30- ☑
  midthoracic region NOS S29.9 ☑
  mouth S09.93 ☑
  multiple NOS T07
  muscle (and fascia) (and tendon)
    abdomen S39.001 ☑
      laceration S39.021 ☑
      specified type NEC S39.091 ☑
      strain S39.011 ☑
    abductor
      thumb, forearm level — *see* Injury, muscle, thumb, abductor
    adductor
      thigh S76.20- ☑
        laceration S76.22- ☑
        specified type NEC S76.29- ☑
        strain S76.21- ☑
    ankle — *see* Injury, muscle, foot
    anterior muscle group, at leg level (lower) S86.20- ☑
      laceration S86.22- ☑
      specified type NEC S86.29- ☑
      strain S86.21- ☑
    arm (upper) — *see* Injury, muscle, shoulder
    biceps (parts NEC) S46.20- ☑
      laceration S46.22- ☑
      long head S46.10- ☑
        laceration S46.12- ☑
        specified type NEC S46.19- ☑
        strain S46.11- ☑
      specified type NEC S46.29- ☑
      strain S46.21- ☑
    extensor
      finger(s) (other than thumb) — *see* Injury, muscle, finger by site, extensor
      forearm level, specified NEC — *see* Injury, muscle, forearm, extensor
      thumb — *see* Injury, muscle, thumb, extensor
      toe (large) (ankle level) (foot level) — *see* Injury, muscle, toe, extensor
    finger
      extensor (forearm level) S56.40- ☑
        hand level S66.309 ☑
          laceration S66.329 ☑
          specified type NEC S66.399 ☑
          strain S66.319 ☑
        laceration S56.429 ☑
        specified type NEC S56.499 ☑
        strain S56.419 ☑
      flexor (forearm level) S56.10- ☑
        hand level S66.109 ☑
          laceration S66.129 ☑
          specified type NEC S66.199 ☑
          strain S66.119 ☑
        laceration S56.129 ☑
        specified type NEC S56.199 ☑
        strain S56.119 ☑

Injury — *continued*
  muscle — *continued*
    finger — *continued*
      index
        extensor (forearm level)
          hand level S66.308 ☑
            laceration S66.32- ☑
            specified type NEC S66.39- ☑
            strain S66.31- ☑
          specified type NEC S56.492- ☑
        flexor (forearm level)
          hand level S66.108 ☑
            laceration S66.12- ☑
            specified type NEC S66.19- ☑
            strain S66.11- ☑
          specified type NEC S56.19- ☑
          strain S56.11- ☑
        intrinsic S66.50- ☑
          laceration S66.52- ☑
          specified type NEC S66.59- ☑
          strain S66.51- ☑
      intrinsic S66.509 ☑
        laceration S66.529 ☑
        specified type NEC S66.599 ☑
        strain S66.519 ☑
      little
        extensor (forearm level)
          hand level S66.30- ☑
            laceration S66.32- ☑
            specified type NEC S66.39- ☑
            strain S66.31- ☑
          laceration S56.42- ☑
          specified type NEC S56.49- ☑
          strain S56.41- ☑
        flexor (forearm level)
          hand level S66.10- ☑
            laceration S66.12- ☑
            specified type NEC S66.19- ☑
            strain S66.11- ☑
          laceration S56.12- ☑
          specified type NEC S56.19- ☑
          strain S56.11- ☑
        intrinsic S66.50- ☑
          laceration S66.52- ☑
          specified type NEC S66.59- ☑
          strain S66.51- ☑
      middle
        extensor (forearm level)
          hand level S66.30- ☑
            laceration S66.32- ☑
            specified type NEC S66.39- ☑
            strain S66.31- ☑
          laceration S56.42- ☑
          specified type NEC S56.49- ☑
          strain S56.41- ☑
        flexor (forearm level)
          hand level S66.10- ☑
            laceration S66.12- ☑
            specified type NEC S66.19- ☑
            strain S66.11- ☑
          laceration S56.12- ☑
          specified type NEC S56.19- ☑
          strain S56.11- ☑
        intrinsic S66.50- ☑
          laceration S66.52- ☑
          specified type NEC S66.59- ☑
          strain S66.51- ☑
      ring
        extensor (forearm level)
          hand level S66.30- ☑
            laceration S66.32- ☑
            specified type NEC S66.39- ☑
            strain S66.31- ☑
          laceration S56.42- ☑
          specified type NEC S56.49- ☑
          strain S56.41- ☑
        flexor (forearm level)
          hand level S66.10- ☑
            laceration S66.12- ☑
            specified type NEC S66.19- ☑
            strain S66.11- ☑
          laceration S56.12- ☑
          specified type NEC S56.19- ☑
          strain S56.11- ☑
        intrinsic S66.50- ☑
          laceration S66.52- ☑

Injury — *continued*
  muscle — *continued*
    finger — *continued*
      ring — *continued*
        intrinsic — *continued*
          specified type NEC S66.59- ☑
          strain S66.51- ☑
    flexor
      finger(s) (other than thumb) — *see* Injury, muscle, finger
      forearm level, specified NEC — *see* Injury, muscle, forearm, flexor
      thumb — *see* Injury, muscle, thumb, flexor
      toe (long) (ankle level) (foot level) — *see* Injury, muscle, toe, flexor
    foot S96.90- ☑
      intrinsic S96.20- ☑
        laceration S96.22- ☑
        specified type NEC S96.29- ☑
        strain S96.21- ☑
      laceration S96.92- ☑
      long extensor, toe — *see* Injury, muscle, toe, extensor
      long flexor, toe — *see* Injury, muscle, toe, flexor
      specified
        site NEC S96.80- ☑
          laceration S96.82- ☑
          specified type NEC S96.89- ☑
          strain S96.81- ☑
        type S96.99- ☑
      strain S96.91- ☑
    forearm (level) S56.90- ☑
      extensor S56.50- ☑
        laceration S56.52- ☑
        specified type NEC S56.59- ☑
        strain S56.51- ☑
      flexor S56.20- ☑
        laceration S56.22- ☑
        specified type NEC S56.29- ☑
        strain S56.21- ☑
      laceration S56.92- ☑
      specified S56.99- ☑
        site NEC S56.80- ☑
          laceration S56.82- ☑
          strain S56.81- ☑
          type NEC S56.89- ☑
      strain S56.91- ☑
    hand (level) S66.90- ☑
      laceration S66.92- ☑
      specified
        site NEC S66.80- ☑
          laceration S66.82- ☑
          specified type NEC S66.89- ☑
          strain S66.81- ☑
          type NEC S66.99- ☑
      strain S66.91- ☑
    head S09.10 ☑
      laceration S09.12 ☑
      specified type NEC S09.19 ☑
      strain S09.11 ☑
    hip NEC S76.00- ☑
      laceration S76.02- ☑
      specified type NEC S76.09- ☑
      strain S76.01- ☑
    intrinsic
      ankle and foot level — *see* Injury, muscle, foot, intrinsic
      finger (other than thumb) — *see* Injury, muscle, finger by site, intrinsic
      foot (level) — *see* Injury, muscle, foot, intrinsic
      thumb — *see* Injury, muscle, thumb, intrinsic
    leg (level) (lower) S86.90- ☑
      Achilles tendon — *see* Injury, Achilles tendon
      anterior muscle group — *see* Injury, muscle, anterior muscle group
      laceration S86.92- ☑
      peroneal muscle group — *see* Injury, muscle, peroneal muscle group
      posterior muscle group — *see* Injury, muscle, posterior muscle group, leg level
      specified
        site NEC S86.80- ☑
          laceration S86.82- ☑
          specified type NEC S86.89- ☑
          strain S86.81- ☑
          type NEC S86.99- ☑

☑ Additional Character Required — Refer to the Tabular List for Character Selection   ⬙ Subterms under main terms may continue to next column or page

Injury — *continued*
　muscle — *continued*
　　leg — *continued*
　　　strain S86.91- ☑
　　long
　　　extensor toe, at ankle and foot level — *see* In-
　　　　jury, muscle, toe, extensor
　　　flexor, toe, at ankle and foot level — *see* Injury,
　　　　muscle, toe, flexor
　　　head, biceps — *see* Injury, muscle, biceps, long
　　　　head
　　lower back S39.002 ☑
　　　laceration S39.022 ☑
　　　specified type NEC S39.092 ☑
　　　strain S39.012 ☑
　　neck (level) S16.9 ☑
　　　laceration S16.2 ☑
　　　specified type NEC S16.8 ☑
　　　strain S16.1 ☑
　　pelvis S39.003 ☑
　　　laceration S39.023 ☑
　　　specified type NEC S39.093 ☑
　　　strain S39.013 ☑
　　peroneal muscle group, at leg level (lower)
　　　S86.30- ☑
　　　laceration S86.32- ☑
　　　specified type NEC S86.39- ☑
　　　strain S86.31- ☑
　　posterior muscle (group)
　　　leg level (lower) S86.10- ☑
　　　　laceration S86.12- ☑
　　　　specified type NEC S86.19- ☑
　　　　strain S86.11- ☑
　　　thigh level S76.30- ☑
　　　　laceration S76.32- ☑
　　　　specified type NEC S76.39- ☑
　　　　strain S76.31- ☑
　　quadriceps (thigh) S76.10- ☑
　　　laceration S76.12- ☑
　　　specified type NEC S76.19- ☑
　　　strain S76.11- ☑
　　shoulder S46.90- ☑
　　　laceration S46.92- ☑
　　　rotator cuff — *see* Injury, rotator cuff
　　　specified site NEC S46.80- ☑
　　　　laceration S46.82- ☑
　　　　specified type NEC S46.89- ☑
　　　　strain S46.81- ☑
　　　specified type NEC S46.99- ☑
　　　strain S46.91- ☑
　　thigh NEC (level) S76.90- ☑
　　　adductor — *see* Injury, muscle, adductor, thigh
　　　laceration S76.92- ☑
　　　posterior muscle (group) — *see* Injury, muscle,
　　　　posterior muscle, thigh level
　　　quadriceps — *see* Injury, muscle, quadriceps
　　　specified
　　　　site NEC S76.80- ☑
　　　　　laceration S76.82- ☑
　　　　　specified type NEC S76.89- ☑
　　　　　strain S76.81- ☑
　　　　type NEC S76.99- ☑
　　　strain S76.91- ☑
　　thorax (level) S29.009 ☑
　　　back wall S29.002 ☑
　　　front wall S29.001 ☑
　　　laceration S29.029 ☑
　　　　back wall S29.022 ☑
　　　　front wall S29.021 ☑
　　　specified type NEC S29.099 ☑
　　　　back wall S29.092 ☑
　　　　front wall S29.091 ☑
　　　strain S29.019 ☑
　　　　back wall S29.012 ☑
　　　　front wall S29.011 ☑
　　thumb
　　　abductor (forearm level) S56.30- ☑
　　　　laceration S56.32- ☑
　　　　specified type NEC S56.39- ☑
　　　　strain S56.31- ☑
　　　extensor (forearm level) S56.30- ☑
　　　　hand level S66.20- ☑
　　　　　laceration S66.22- ☑
　　　　　specified type NEC S66.29- ☑
　　　　　strain S66.21- ☑
　　　　laceration S56.32- ☑

Injury — *continued*
　muscle — *continued*
　　thumb — *continued*
　　　extensor — *continued*
　　　　specified type NEC S56.39- ☑
　　　　strain S56.31- ☑
　　　flexor (forearm level) S56.00- ☑
　　　　hand level S66.00- ☑
　　　　　laceration S66.02- ☑
　　　　　specified type NEC S66.09- ☑
　　　　　strain S66.01- ☑
　　　　laceration S56.02- ☑
　　　　specified type NEC S56.09- ☑
　　　　strain S56.01- ☑
　　　　wrist level — *see* Injury, muscle, thumb,
　　　　　flexor, hand level
　　　intrinsic S66.40- ☑
　　　　laceration S66.42- ☑
　　　　specified type NEC S66.49- ☑
　　　　strain S66.41- ☑
　　toe (*see also* Injury, muscle, foot)
　　　extensor, long S96.10- ☑
　　　　laceration S96.12- ☑
　　　　specified type NEC S96.19- ☑
　　　　strain S96.11- ☑
　　　flexor, long S96.00- ☑
　　　　laceration S96.02- ☑
　　　　specified type NEC S96.09- ☑
　　　　strain S96.01- ☑
　　triceps S46.30- ☑
　　　laceration S46.32- ☑
　　　specified type NEC S46.39- ☑
　　　strain S46.31- ☑
　　wrist (and hand) level — *see* Injury, muscle, hand
　musculocutaneous nerve — *see* Injury, nerve, muscu-
　　locutaneous
　myocardium — *see* Injury, heart
　nape — *see* Injury, neck
　nasal (septum) (sinus) S09.92 ☑
　nasopharynx S09.92 ☑
　neck S19.9 ☑
　　specified NEC S19.80 ☑
　　　specified site NEC S19.89 ☑
　nerve NEC T14.8
　　abdomen S34.9 ☑
　　　peripheral S34.6 ☑
　　　specified site NEC S34.8 ☑
　　abducens S04.4- ☑
　　　contusion S04.4- ☑
　　　laceration S04.4- ☑
　　　specified type NEC S04.4- ☑
　　abducent — *see* Injury, nerve, abducens
　　accessory S04.7- ☑
　　　contusion S04.7- ☑
　　　laceration S04.7- ☑
　　　specified type NEC S04.7- ☑
　　acoustic S04.6- ☑
　　　contusion S04.6- ☑
　　　laceration S04.6- ☑
　　　specified type NEC S04.6- ☑
　　ankle S94.9- ☑
　　　cutaneous sensory S94.3- ☑
　　　specified site NEC — *see* subcategory S94.8 ☑
　　anterior crural, femoral — *see* Injury, nerve, femoral
　　arm (upper) S44.9- ☑
　　　axillary — *see* Injury, nerve, axillary
　　　cutaneous — *see* Injury, nerve, cutaneous, arm
　　　median — *see* Injury, nerve, median, upper arm
　　　musculocutaneous — *see* Injury, nerve, muscu-
　　　　locutaneous
　　　radial — *see* Injury, nerve, radial, upper arm
　　　specified site NEC — *see* subcategory S44.8 ☑
　　　ulnar — *see* Injury, nerve, ulnar, arm
　　auditory — *see* Injury, nerve, acoustic
　　axillary S44.3- ☑
　　brachial plexus — *see* Injury, brachial plexus
　　cervical sympathetic S14.5 ☑
　　cranial S04.9 ☑
　　　contusion S04.9 ☑
　　　eighth (acoustic or auditory) — *see* Injury,
　　　　nerve, acoustic
　　　eleventh (accessory) — *see* Injury, nerve, acces-
　　　　sory
　　　fifth (trigeminal) — *see* Injury, nerve, trigeminal
　　　first (olfactory) — *see* Injury, nerve, olfactory
　　　fourth (trochlear) — *see* Injury, nerve, trochlear

Injury — *continued*
　nerve — *continued*
　　cranial — *continued*
　　　laceration S04.9 ☑
　　　ninth (glossopharyngeal) — *see* Injury, nerve,
　　　　glossopharyngeal
　　　second (optic) — *see* Injury, nerve, optic
　　　seventh (facial) — *see* Injury, nerve, facial
　　　sixth (abducent) — *see* Injury, nerve, abducens
　　　specified
　　　　nerve NEC S04.89- ☑
　　　　　contusion S04.89- ☑
　　　　　laceration S04.89- ☑
　　　　　specified type NEC S04.89- ☑
　　　　type NEC S04.9 ☑
　　　tenth (pneumogastric or vagus) — *see* Injury,
　　　　nerve, vagus
　　　third (oculomotor) — *see* Injury, nerve, oculo-
　　　　motor
　　　twelfth (hypoglossal) — *see* Injury, nerve, hy-
　　　　poglossal
　　cutaneous sensory
　　　ankle (level) S94.3- ☑
　　　arm (upper) (level) S44.5- ☑
　　　foot (level) — *see* Injury, nerve, cutaneous
　　　　sensory, ankle
　　　forearm (level) S54.3- ☑
　　　hip (level) S74.2- ☑
　　　leg (lower level) S84.2- ☑
　　　shoulder (level) — *see* Injury, nerve, cutaneous
　　　　sensory, arm
　　　thigh (level) — *see* Injury, nerve, cutaneous
　　　　sensory, hip
　　deep peroneal — *see* Injury, nerve, peroneal, foot
　　digital
　　　finger S64.4- ☑
　　　　index S64.49- ☑
　　　　little S64.49- ☑
　　　　middle S64.49- ☑
　　　　ring S64.49- ☑
　　　thumb S64.3- ☑
　　　toe — *see* Injury, nerve, ankle, specified site
　　　　NEC
　　eighth cranial (acoustic or auditory) — *see* Injury,
　　　nerve, acoustic
　　eleventh cranial (accessory) — *see* Injury, nerve,
　　　accessory
　　facial S04.5- ☑
　　　contusion S04.5- ☑
　　　laceration S04.5- ☑
　　　newborn P11.3
　　　specified type NEC S04.5- ☑
　　femoral (hip level) (thigh level) S74.1- ☑
　　fifth cranial (trigeminal) — *see* Injury, nerve,
　　　trigeminal
　　finger (digital) — *see* Injury, nerve, digital, finger
　　first cranial (olfactory) — *see* Injury, nerve, olfactory
　　foot S94.9- ☑
　　　cutaneous sensory S94.3- ☑
　　　deep peroneal S94.2- ☑
　　　lateral plantar S94.0- ☑
　　　medial plantar S94.1- ☑
　　　specified site NEC — *see* subcategory S94.8 ☑
　　forearm (level) S54.9- ☑
　　　cutaneous sensory — *see* Injury, nerve, cuta-
　　　　neous sensory, forearm
　　　median — *see* Injury, nerve, median
　　　radial — *see* Injury, nerve, radial
　　　specified site NEC — *see* subcategory S54.8 ☑
　　　ulnar — *see* Injury, nerve, ulnar
　　fourth cranial (trochlear) — *see* Injury, nerve,
　　　trochlear
　　glossopharyngeal S04.89- ☑
　　　specified type NEC S04.89- ☑
　　hand S64.9- ☑
　　　median — *see* Injury, nerve, median, hand
　　　radial — *see* Injury, nerve, radial, hand
　　　specified NEC — *see* subcategory S64.8 ☑
　　　ulnar — *see* Injury, nerve, ulnar, hand
　　hip (level) S74.9- ☑
　　　cutaneous sensory — *see* Injury, nerve, cuta-
　　　　neous sensory, hip
　　　femoral — *see* Injury, nerve, femoral
　　　sciatic — *see* Injury, nerve, sciatic
　　　specified site NEC — *see* subcategory S74.8 ☑

Injury — *continued*
  nerve — *continued*
    hypoglossal S04.89- ☑
      specified type NEC S04.89- ☑
    lateral plantar S94.0- ☑
    leg (lower) S84.9- ☑
      cutaneous sensory — *see* Injury, nerve, cutaneous sensory, leg
      peroneal — *see* Injury, nerve, peroneal
      specified site NEC — *see* subcategory S84.8 ☑
      tibial — *see* Injury, nerve, tibial
      upper — *see* Injury, nerve, thigh
    lower
      back — *see* Injury, nerve, abdomen, specified site NEC
        peripheral — *see* Injury, nerve, abdomen, peripheral
      limb — *see* Injury, nerve, leg
    lumbar plexus — *see* Injury, nerve, lumbosacral, sympathetic
    lumbar spinal — *see* Injury, nerve, spinal, lumbar
    lumbosacral
      plexus — *see* Injury, nerve, lumbosacral, sympathetic
      sympathetic S34.5 ☑
    medial plantar S94.1- ☑
    median (forearm level) S54.1- ☑
      hand (level) S64.1- ☑
      upper arm (level) S44.1- ☑
      wrist (level) — *see* Injury, nerve, median, hand
    musculocutaneous S44.4- ☑
    musculospiral (upper arm level) — *see* Injury, nerve, radial, upper arm
    neck S14.9 ☑
      peripheral S14.4 ☑
      specified site NEC S14.8 ☑
      sympathetic S14.5 ☑
    ninth cranial (glossopharyngeal) — *see* Injury, nerve, glossopharyngeal
    oculomotor S04.1- ☑
      contusion S04.1- ☑
      laceration S04.1- ☑
      specified type NEC S04.1- ☑
    olfactory S04.81- ☑
      specified type NEC S04.81- ☑
    optic S04.01- ☑
      contusion S04.01- ☑
      laceration S04.01- ☑
      specified type NEC S04.01- ☑
    pelvic girdle — *see* Injury, nerve, hip
    pelvis — *see* Injury, nerve, abdomen, specified site NEC
      peripheral — *see* Injury, nerve, abdomen, peripheral
    peripheral NEC T14.8
      abdomen — *see* Injury, nerve, abdomen, peripheral
      lower back — *see* Injury, nerve, abdomen, peripheral
      neck — *see* Injury, nerve, neck, peripheral
      pelvis — *see* Injury, nerve, abdomen, peripheral
      specified NEC T14.8
    peroneal (lower leg level) S84.1- ☑
      foot S94.2- ☑
    plexus
      brachial — *see* Injury, brachial plexus
      celiac, coeliac — *see* Injury, nerve, lumbosacral, sympathetic
      mesenteric, inferior — *see* Injury, nerve, lumbosacral, sympathetic
      sacral — *see* Injury, lumbosacral plexus
      spinal
        brachial — *see* Injury, brachial plexus
        lumbosacral — *see* Injury, lumbosacral plexus
    pneumogastric — *see* Injury, nerve, vagus
    radial (forearm level) S54.2- ☑
      hand (level) S64.2- ☑
      upper arm (level) S44.2- ☑
      wrist (level) — *see* Injury, nerve, radial, hand
    root — *see* Injury, nerve, spinal, root
    sacral plexus — *see* Injury, lumbosacral plexus
    sacral spinal — *see* Injury, nerve, spinal, sacral
    sciatic (hip level) (thigh level) S74.0- ☑
    second cranial (optic) — *see* Injury, nerve, optic
    seventh cranial (facial) — *see* Injury, nerve, facial

Injury — *continued*
  nerve — *continued*
    shoulder — *see* Injury, nerve, arm
    sixth cranial (abducent) — *see* Injury, nerve, abducens
    spinal
      plexus — *see* Injury, nerve, plexus, spinal
      root
        cervical S14.2 ☑
        dorsal S24.2 ☑
        lumbar S34.21 ☑
        sacral S34.22 ☑
        thoracic — *see* Injury, nerve, spinal, root, dorsal
    splanchnic — *see* Injury, nerve, lumbosacral, sympathetic
    sympathetic NEC — *see* Injury, nerve, lumbosacral, sympathetic
      cervical — *see* Injury, nerve, cervical sympathetic
    tenth cranial (pneumogastric or vagus) — *see* Injury, nerve, vagus
    thigh (level) — *see* Injury, nerve, hip
      cutaneous sensory — *see* Injury, nerve, cutaneous sensory, hip
      femoral — *see* Injury, nerve, femoral
      sciatic — *see* Injury, nerve, sciatic
      specified NEC — *see* Injury, nerve, hip
    third cranial (oculomotor) — *see* Injury, nerve, oculomotor
    thorax S24.9 ☑
      peripheral S24.3 ☑
      specified site NEC S24.8 ☑
      sympathetic S24.4 ☑
    thumb, digital — *see* Injury, nerve, digital, thumb
    tibial (lower leg level) (posterior) S84.0- ☑
    toe — *see* Injury, nerve, ankle
    trigeminal S04.3- ☑
      contusion S04.3- ☑
      laceration S04.3- ☑
      specified type NEC S04.3- ☑
    trochlear S04.2- ☑
      contusion S04.2- ☑
      laceration S04.2- ☑
      specified type NEC S04.2- ☑
    twelfth cranial (hypoglossal) — *see* Injury, nerve, hypoglossal
    ulnar (forearm level) S54.0- ☑
      arm (upper) (level) S44.0- ☑
      hand (level) S64.0- ☑
      wrist (level) — *see* Injury, nerve, ulnar, hand
    vagus S04.89- ☑
      specified type NEC S04.89- ☑
    wrist (level) — *see* Injury, nerve, hand
  ninth cranial nerve (glossopharyngeal) — *see* Injury, nerve, glossopharyngeal
  nose (septum) S09.92 ☑
  obstetrical O71.9
    specified NEC O71.89
  occipital (region) (scalp) S09.90 ☑
    lobe — *see* Injury, intracranial
  optic chiasm S04.02 ☑
  optic radiation S04.03- ☑
  optic tract and pathways S04.03- ☑
  orbit, orbital (region) — *see* Injury, eye
    penetrating (with foreign body) — *see* Injury, eye, orbit, penetrating
    specified NEC — *see* Injury, eye, specified site NEC
  ovary, ovarian S37.409 ☑
    bilateral S37.402 ☑
      contusion S37.422 ☑
      laceration S37.432 ☑
      specified type NEC S37.492 ☑
    blood vessel — *see* Injury, blood vessel, ovarian
    contusion S37.429 ☑
      bilateral S37.422 ☑
      unilateral S37.421 ☑
    laceration S37.439 ☑
      bilateral S37.432 ☑
      unilateral S37.431 ☑
    specified type NEC S37.499 ☑
      bilateral S37.492 ☑
      unilateral S37.491 ☑
    unilateral S37.401 ☑
      contusion S37.421 ☑
      laceration S37.431 ☑

Injury — *continued*
  ovary, ovarian — *continued*
    unilateral — *continued*
      specified type NEC S37.491 ☑
  palate (hard) (soft) S09.93 ☑
  pancreas S36.209 ☑
    body S36.201 ☑
      contusion S36.221 ☑
      laceration S36.231 ☑
        major S36.261 ☑
        minor S36.241 ☑
        moderate S36.251 ☑
      specified type NEC S36.291 ☑
    contusion S36.229 ☑
    head S36.200 ☑
      contusion S36.220 ☑
      laceration S36.230 ☑
        major S36.260 ☑
        minor S36.240 ☑
        moderate S36.250 ☑
      specified type NEC S36.290 ☑
    laceration S36.239 ☑
      major S36.269 ☑
      minor S36.249 ☑
      moderate S36.259 ☑
    specified type NEC S36.299 ☑
    tail S36.202 ☑
      contusion S36.222 ☑
      laceration S36.232 ☑
        major S36.262 ☑
        minor S36.242 ☑
        moderate S36.252 ☑
      specified type NEC S36.292 ☑
  parietal (region) (scalp) S09.90 ☑
    lobe — *see* Injury, intracranial
  patellar ligament (tendon) S76.10- ☑
    laceration S76.12- ☑
    specified NEC S76.19- ☑
    strain S76.11- ☑
  pelvis, pelvic (floor) S39.93 ☑
    complicating delivery O70.1
    joint or ligament, complicating delivery O71.6
    organ S37.90 ☑
      with ectopic or molar pregnancy O08.6
      complication of abortion — *see* Abortion
      contusion S37.92 ☑
      following ectopic or molar pregnancy O08.6
      laceration S37.93 ☑
      obstetrical trauma NEC O71.5
      specified
        site NEC S37.899 ☑
          contusion S37.892 ☑
          laceration S37.893 ☑
          specified type NEC S37.898 ☑
        type NEC S37.99 ☑
    specified NEC S39.83 ☑
  penis S39.94 ☑
  perineum S39.94 ☑
  peritoneum S36.81 ☑
    laceration S36.893 ☑
  periurethral tissue — *see* Injury, urethra
    complicating delivery O71.82
  phalanges
    foot — *see* Injury, foot
    hand — *see* Injury, hand
  pharynx NEC S19.85 ☑
  pleura — *see* Injury, intrathoracic, pleura
  plexus
    brachial — *see* Injury, brachial plexus
    cardiac — *see* Injury, nerve, thorax, sympathetic
    celiac, coeliac — *see* Injury, nerve, lumbosacral, sympathetic
    esophageal — *see* Injury, nerve, thorax, sympathetic
    hypogastric — *see* Injury, nerve, lumbosacral, sympathetic
    lumbar, lumbosacral — *see* Injury, lumbosacral plexus
    mesenteric — *see* Injury, nerve, lumbosacral, sympathetic
    pulmonary — *see* Injury, nerve, thorax, sympathetic
  postcardiac surgery (syndrome) I97.0
  prepuce S39.94 ☑
  prostate S37.829 ☑
    contusion S37.822 ☑

☑ **Additional Character Required** — Refer to the Tabular List for Character Selection   ▽ **Subterms under main terms may continue to next column or page**

Injury — *continued*
  prostate — *continued*
    laceration S37.823 ☑
    specified type NEC S37.828 ☑
  pubic region S39.94 ☑
  pudendum S39.94 ☑
  pulmonary plexus — *see* Injury, nerve, thorax, sympathetic
  rectovaginal septum NEC S39.83 ☑
  rectum — *see* Injury, intestine, large, rectum
  retina — *see* Injury, eye, specified site NEC
    penetrating — *see* Injury, eyeball, penetrating
  retroperitoneal — *see* Injury, intra-abdominal, specified site NEC
  rotator cuff (muscle(s)) (tendon(s)) S46.00- ☑
    laceration S46.02- ☑
    specified type NEC S46.09- ☑
    strain S46.01- ☑
  round ligament — *see* Injury, pelvic organ, specified site NEC
  sacral plexus — *see* Injury, lumbosacral plexus
  salivary duct or gland S09.93 ☑
  scalp S09.90 ☑
    newborn (birth injury) P12.9
      due to monitoring (electrode) (sampling incision) P12.4
      specified NEC P12.89
        caput succedaneum P12.81
  scapular region — *see* Injury, shoulder
  sclera — *see* Injury, eye, specified site NEC
    penetrating — *see* Injury, eyeball, penetrating
  scrotum S39.94 ☑
  second cranial nerve (optic) — *see* Injury, nerve, optic
  seminal vesicle — *see* Injury, pelvic organ, specified site NEC
  seventh cranial nerve (facial) — *see* Injury, nerve, facial
  shoulder S49.9- ☑
    blood vessel — *see* Injury, blood vessel, arm
    contusion — *see* Contusion, shoulder
    dislocation — *see* Dislocation, shoulder
    fracture — *see* Fracture, shoulder
    muscle — *see* Injury, muscle, shoulder
    nerve — *see* Injury, nerve, shoulder
    open — *see* Wound, open, shoulder
    specified type NEC S49.8- ☑
    sprain — *see* Sprain, shoulder girdle
    superficial — *see* Injury, superficial, shoulder
  sinus
    cavernous — *see* Injury, intracranial
    nasal S09.92 ☑
  sixth cranial nerve (abducent) — *see* Injury, nerve, abducens
  skeleton, birth injury P13.9
    specified part NEC P13.8
  skin NEC T14.8
    surface intact — *see* Injury, superficial
  skull NEC S09.90 ☑
  specified NEC T14.8
  spermatic cord (pelvic region) S37.898 ☑
    scrotal region S39.848 ☑
  spinal (cord)
    cervical (neck) S14.109 ☑
      anterior cord syndrome S14.139 ☑
        C1 level S14.131 ☑
        C2 level S14.132 ☑
        C3 level S14.133 ☑
        C4 level S14.134 ☑
        C5 level S14.135 ☑
        C6 level S14.136 ☑
        C7 level S14.137 ☑
        C8 level S14.138 ☑
      Brown-Séquard syndrome S14.149 ☑
        C1 level S14.141 ☑
        C2 level S14.142 ☑
        C3 level S14.143 ☑
        C4 level S14.144 ☑
        C5 level S14.145 ☑
        C6 level S14.146 ☑
        C7 level S14.147 ☑
        C8 level S14.148 ☑
      C1 level S14.101 ☑
      C2 level S14.102 ☑
      C3 level S14.103 ☑
      C4 level S14.104 ☑
      C5 level S14.105 ☑
      C6 level S14.106 ☑

Injury — *continued*
  spinal — *continued*
    cervical — *continued*
      C7 level S14.107 ☑
      C8 level S14.108 ☑
      central cord syndrome S14.129 ☑
        C1 level S14.121 ☑
        C2 level S14.122 ☑
        C3 level S14.123 ☑
        C4 level S14.124 ☑
        C5 level S14.125 ☑
        C6 level S14.126 ☑
        C7 level S14.127 ☑
        C8 level S14.128 ☑
      complete lesion S14.119 ☑
        C1 level S14.111 ☑
        C2 level S14.112 ☑
        C3 level S14.113 ☑
        C4 level S14.114 ☑
        C5 level S14.115 ☑
        C6 level S14.116 ☑
        C7 level S14.117 ☑
        C8 level S14.118 ☑
      concussion S14.0 ☑
      edema S14.0 ☑
      incomplete lesion specified NEC S14.159 ☑
        C1 level S14.151 ☑
        C2 level S14.152 ☑
        C3 level S14.153 ☑
        C4 level S14.154 ☑
        C5 level S14.155 ☑
        C6 level S14.156 ☑
        C7 level S14.157 ☑
        C8 level S14.158 ☑
      posterior cord syndrome S14.159 ☑
        C1 level S14.151 ☑
        C2 level S14.152 ☑
        C3 level S14.153 ☑
        C4 level S14.154 ☑
        C5 level S14.155 ☑
        C6 level S14.156 ☑
        C7 level S14.157 ☑
        C8 level S14.158 ☑
    dorsal — *see* Injury, spinal, thoracic
    lumbar S34.109 ☑
      complete lesion S34.119 ☑
        L1 level S34.111 ☑
        L2 level S34.112 ☑
        L3 level S34.113 ☑
        L4 level S34.114 ☑
        L5 level S34.115 ☑
      concussion S34.01 ☑
      edema S34.01 ☑
      incomplete lesion S34.129 ☑
        L1 level S34.121 ☑
        L2 level S34.122 ☑
        L3 level S34.123 ☑
        L4 level S34.124 ☑
        L5 level S34.125 ☑
      L1 level S34.101 ☑
      L2 level S34.102 ☑
      L3 level S34.103 ☑
      L4 level S34.104 ☑
      L5 level S34.105 ☑
    nerve root NEC
      cervical — *see* Injury, nerve, spinal, root, cervical
      dorsal — *see* Injury, nerve, spinal, root, dorsal
      lumbar S34.21 ☑
      sacral S34.22 ☑
      thoracic — *see* Injury, nerve, spinal, root, dorsal
    plexus
      brachial — *see* Injury, brachial plexus
      lumbosacral — *see* Injury, lumbosacral plexus
    sacral S34.139 ☑
      complete lesion S34.131 ☑
      incomplete lesion S34.132 ☑
    thoracic S24.109 ☑
      anterior cord syndrome S24.139 ☑
        T1 level S24.131 ☑
        T2-T6 level S24.132 ☑
        T7-T10 level S24.133 ☑
        T11-T12 level S24.134 ☑
      Brown-Séquard syndrome S24.149 ☑
        T1 level S24.141 ☑

Injury — *continued*
  spinal — *continued*
    thoracic — *continued*
      Brown-Séquard syndrome — *continued*
        T2-T6 level S24.142 ☑
        T7-T10 level S24.143 ☑
        T11-T12 level S24.144 ☑
      complete lesion S24.119 ☑
        T1 level S24.111 ☑
        T2-T6 level S24.112 ☑
        T7-T10 level S24.113 ☑
        T11-T12 level S24.114 ☑
      concussion S24.0 ☑
      edema S24.0 ☑
      incomplete lesion specified NEC S24.159 ☑
        T1 level S24.151 ☑
        T2-T6 level S24.152 ☑
        T7-T10 level S24.153 ☑
        T11-T12 level S24.154 ☑
      posterior cord syndrome S24.159 ☑
        T1 level S24.151 ☑
        T2-T6 level S24.152 ☑
        T7-T10 level S24.153 ☑
        T11-T12 level S24.154 ☑
      T1 level S24.101 ☑
      T2-T6 level S24.102 ☑
      T7-T10 level S24.103 ☑
      T11-T12 level S24.104 ☑
  splanchnic nerve — *see* Injury, nerve, lumbosacral, sympathetic
  spleen S36.00 ☑
    contusion S36.029 ☑
      major S36.021 ☑
      minor S36.020 ☑
    laceration S36.039 ☑
      major (massive) (stellate) S36.032 ☑
      moderate S36.031 ☑
      superficial (capsular) (minor) S36.030 ☑
    specified type NEC S36.09 ☑
  splenic artery — *see* Injury, blood vessel, celiac artery, branch
  stellate ganglion — *see* Injury, nerve, thorax, sympathetic
  sternal region S29.9 ☑
  stomach S36.30 ☑
    contusion S36.32 ☑
    laceration S36.33 ☑
    specified type NEC S36.39 ☑
  subconjunctival — *see* Injury, eye, conjunctiva
  subcutaneous NEC T14.8
  submaxillary region S09.93 ☑
  submental region S09.93 ☑
  subungual
    fingers — *see* Injury, hand
    toes — *see* Injury, foot
  superficial NEC T14.8
    abdomen, abdominal (wall) S30.92 ☑
      abrasion S30.811 ☑
      bite S30.871 ☑
        insect S30.861 ☑
      contusion S30.1 ☑
      external constriction S30.841 ☑
      foreign body S30.851 ☑
    abrasion — *see* Abrasion, by site
    adnexa, eye NEC — *see* Injury, eye, specified site NEC
    alveolar process — *see* Injury, superficial, oral cavity
    ankle S90.91- ☑
      abrasion — *see* Abrasion, ankle
      bite — *see* Bite, ankle
      blister — *see* Blister, ankle
      contusion — *see* Contusion, ankle
      external constriction — *see* Constriction, external, ankle
      foreign body — *see* Foreign body, superficial, ankle
    anus S30.98 ☑
    arm (upper) S40.92- ☑
      abrasion — *see* Abrasion, arm
      bite — *see* Bite, superficial, arm
      blister — *see* Blister, arm (upper)
      contusion — *see* Contusion, arm
      external constriction — *see* Constriction, external, arm

▽ **Subterms under main terms may continue to next column or page**   ☑ **Additional Character Required — Refer to the Tabular List for Character Selection**   **191**

Injury — Injury

Injury — *continued*
  superficial — *continued*
    arm — *continued*
      foreign body — *see* Foreign body, superficial, arm
      auditory canal (external) (meatus) — *see* Injury, superficial, ear
      auricle — *see* Injury, superficial, ear
      axilla — *see* Injury, superficial, arm
      back (*see also* Injury, superficial, thorax, back)
        lower S30.91 ☑
          abrasion S30.810 ☑
          contusion S30.0 ☑
          external constriction S30.840 ☑
          superficial
            bite NEC S30.870 ☑
              insect S30.860 ☑
            foreign body S30.850 ☑
      bite NEC — *see* Bite, superficial NEC, by site
      blister — *see* Blister, by site
      breast S20.10- ☑
        abrasion — *see* Abrasion, breast
        bite — *see* Bite, superficial, breast
        contusion — *see* Contusion, breast
        external constriction — *see* Constriction, external, breast
        foreign body — *see* Foreign body, superficial, breast
      brow — *see* Injury, superficial, head, specified NEC
      buttock S30.91 ☑
      calf — *see* Injury, superficial, leg
      canthus, eye — *see* Injury, superficial, periocular area
      cheek (external) — *see* Injury, superficial, head, specified NEC
        internal — *see* Injury, superficial, oral cavity
      chest wall — *see* Injury, superficial, thorax
      chin — *see* Injury, superficial, head NEC
      clitoris S30.95 ☑
      conjunctiva — *see* Injury, eye, conjunctiva
        with foreign body (in conjunctival sac) — *see* Foreign body, conjunctival sac
      contusion — *see* Contusion, by site
      costal region — *see* Injury, superficial, thorax
      digit(s)
        hand — *see* Injury, superficial, finger
      ear (auricle) (canal) (external) S00.40- ☑
        abrasion — *see* Abrasion, ear
        bite — *see* Bite, superficial, ear
        contusion — *see* Contusion, ear
        external constriction — *see* Constriction, external, ear
        foreign body — *see* Foreign body, superficial, ear
      elbow S50.90- ☑
        abrasion — *see* Abrasion, elbow
        bite — *see* Bite, superficial, elbow
        blister — *see* Blister, elbow
        contusion — *see* Contusion, elbow
        external constriction — *see* Constriction, external, elbow
        foreign body — *see* Foreign body, superficial, elbow
      epididymis S30.94 ☑
      epigastric region S30.92 ☑
      epiglottis — *see* Injury, superficial, throat
      esophagus
        cervical — *see* Injury, superficial, throat
      external constriction — *see* Constriction, external, by site
      extremity NEC T14.8
      eyeball NEC — *see* Injury, eye, specified site NEC
      eyebrow — *see* Injury, superficial, periocular area
      eyelid S00.20- ☑
        abrasion — *see* Abrasion, eyelid
        bite — *see* Bite, superficial, eyelid
        contusion — *see* Contusion, eyelid
        external constriction — *see* Constriction, external, eyelid
        foreign body — *see* Foreign body, superficial, eyelid
      face NEC — *see* Injury, superficial, head, specified NEC
      finger(s) S60.949 ☑
        abrasion — *see* Abrasion, finger
        bite — *see* Bite, superficial, finger

Injury — *continued*
  superficial — *continued*
    finger(s) — *continued*
      blister — *see* Blister, finger
      contusion — *see* Contusion, finger
      external constriction — *see* Constriction, external, finger
      foreign body — *see* Foreign body, superficial, finger
      index S60.94- ☑
      insect bite — *see* Bite, by site, superficial, insect
      little S60.94- ☑
      middle S60.94- ☑
      ring S60.94- ☑
    flank S30.92 ☑
    foot S90.92- ☑
      abrasion — *see* Abrasion, foot
      bite — *see* Bite, foot
      blister — *see* Blister, foot
      contusion — *see* Contusion, foot
      external constriction — *see* Constriction, external, foot
      foreign body — *see* Foreign body, superficial, foot
    forearm S50.91- ☑
      abrasion — *see* Abrasion, forearm
      bite — *see* Bite, forearm, superficial
      blister — *see* Blister, forearm
      contusion — *see* Contusion, forearm
      elbow only — *see* Injury, superficial, elbow
      external constriction — *see* Constriction, external, forearm
      foreign body — *see* Foreign body, superficial, forearm
    forehead — *see* Injury, superficial, head NEC
    foreign body — *see* Foreign body, superficial
    genital organs, external
      female S30.97 ☑
      male S30.96 ☑
    globe (eye) — *see* Injury, eye, specified site NEC
    groin S30.92 ☑
    gum — *see* Injury, superficial, oral cavity
    hand S60.92- ☑
      abrasion — *see* Abrasion, hand
      bite — *see* Bite, superficial, hand
      contusion — *see* Contusion, hand
      external constriction — *see* Constriction, external, hand
      foreign body — *see* Foreign body, superficial, hand
    head S00.90 ☑
      ear — *see* Injury, superficial, ear
      eyelid — *see* Injury, superficial, eyelid
      nose S00.30 ☑
      oral cavity S00.502 ☑
      scalp S00.00 ☑
      specified site NEC S00.80 ☑
    heel — *see* Injury, superficial, foot
    hip S70.91- ☑
      abrasion — *see* Abrasion, hip
      bite — *see* Bite, superficial, hip
      blister — *see* Blister, hip
      contusion — *see* Contusion, hip
      external constriction — *see* Constriction, external, hip
      foreign body — *see* Foreign body, superficial, hip
    iliac region — *see* Injury, superficial, abdomen
    inguinal region — *see* Injury, superficial, abdomen
    insect bite — *see* Bite, by site, superficial, insect
    interscapular region — *see* Injury, superficial, thorax, back
    jaw — *see* Injury, superficial, head, specified NEC
    knee S80.91- ☑
      abrasion — *see* Abrasion, knee
      bite — *see* Bite, superficial, knee
      blister — *see* Blister, knee
      contusion — *see* Contusion, knee
      external constriction — *see* Constriction, external, knee
      foreign body — *see* Foreign body, superficial, knee
    labium (majus) (minus) S30.95 ☑
    lacrimal (apparatus) (gland) (sac) — *see* Injury, eye, specified site NEC
    larynx — *see* Injury, superficial, throat

Injury — *continued*
  superficial — *continued*
    leg (lower) S80.92- ☑
      abrasion — *see* Abrasion, leg
      bite — *see* Bite, superficial, leg
      contusion — *see* Contusion, leg
      external constriction — *see* Constriction, external, leg
      foreign body — *see* Foreign body, superficial, leg
      knee — *see* Injury, superficial, knee
    limb NEC T14.8
    lip S00.501 ☑
    lower back S30.91 ☑
    lumbar region S30.91 ☑
    malar region — *see* Injury, superficial, head, specified NEC
    mammary — *see* Injury, superficial, breast
    mastoid region — *see* Injury, superficial, head, specified NEC
    mouth — *see* Injury, superficial, oral cavity
    muscle NEC T14.8
    nail NEC T14.8
      finger — *see* Injury, superficial, finger
      toe — *see* Injury, superficial, toe
    nasal (septum) — *see* Injury, superficial, nose
    neck S10.90 ☑
      specified site NEC S10.80 ☑
    nose (septum) S00.30 ☑
    occipital region — *see* Injury, superficial, scalp
    oral cavity S00.502 ☑
    orbital region — *see* Injury, superficial, periocular area
    palate — *see* Injury, superficial, oral cavity
    palm — *see* Injury, superficial, hand
    parietal region — *see* Injury, superficial, scalp
    pelvis S30.91 ☑
      girdle — *see* Injury, superficial, hip
    penis S30.93 ☑
    perineum
      female S30.95 ☑
      male S30.91 ☑
    periocular area S00.20- ☑
      abrasion — *see* Abrasion, eyelid
      bite — *see* Bite, superficial, eyelid
      contusion — *see* Contusion, eyelid
      external constriction — *see* Constriction, external, eyelid
      foreign body — *see* Foreign body, superficial, eyelid
    phalanges
      finger — *see* Injury, superficial, finger
      toe — *see* Injury, superficial, toe
    pharynx — *see* Injury, superficial, throat
    pinna — *see* Injury, superficial, ear
    popliteal space — *see* Injury, superficial, knee
    prepuce S30.93 ☑
    pubic region S30.91 ☑
    pudendum
      female S30.97 ☑
      male S30.96 ☑
    sacral region S30.91 ☑
    scalp S00.00 ☑
    scapular region — *see* Injury, superficial, shoulder
    sclera — *see* Injury, eye, specified site NEC
    scrotum S30.94 ☑
    shin — *see* Injury, superficial, leg
    shoulder S40.91- ☑
      abrasion — *see* Abrasion, shoulder
      bite — *see* Bite, superficial, shoulder
      blister — *see* Blister, shoulder
      contusion — *see* Contusion, shoulder
      external constriction — *see* Constriction, external, shoulder
      foreign body — *see* Foreign body, superficial, shoulder
    skin NEC T14.8
    sternal region — *see* Injury, superficial, thorax, front
    subconjunctival — *see* Injury, eye, specified site NEC
    subcutaneous NEC T14.8
    submaxillary region — *see* Injury, superficial, head, specified NEC
    submental region — *see* Injury, superficial, head, specified NEC

☑ **Additional Character Required — Refer to the Tabular List for Character Selection**   🔺 **Subterms under main terms may continue to next column or page**

Injury — *continued*
  superficial — *continued*
    subungual
      finger(s) — *see* Injury, superficial, finger
      toe(s) — *see* Injury, superficial, toe
    supraclavicular fossa — *see* Injury, superficial, neck
    supraorbital — *see* Injury, superficial, head, specified NEC
    temple — *see* Injury, superficial, head, specified NEC
    temporal region — *see* Injury, superficial, head, specified NEC
    testis S30.94 ☑
    thigh S70.92- ☑
      abrasion — *see* Abrasion, thigh
      bite — *see* Bite, superficial, thigh
      blister — *see* Blister, thigh
      contusion — *see* Contusion, thigh
      external constriction — *see* Constriction, external, thigh
      foreign body — *see* Foreign body, superficial, thigh
    thorax, thoracic (wall) S20.90 ☑
      abrasion — *see* Abrasion, thorax
      back S20.40- ☑
      bite — *see* Bite, thorax, superficial
      blister — *see* Blister, thorax
      contusion — *see* Contusion, thorax
      external constriction — *see* Constriction, external, thorax
      foreign body — *see* Foreign body, superficial, thorax
      front S20.30- ☑
    throat S10.10 ☑
      abrasion S10.11 ☑
      bite S10.17 ☑
        insect S10.16 ☑
      blister S10.12 ☑
      contusion S10.0 ☑
      external constriction S10.14 ☑
      foreign body S10.15 ☑
    thumb S60.93- ☑
      abrasion — *see* Abrasion, thumb
      bite — *see* Bite, superficial, thumb
      blister — *see* Blister, thumb
      contusion — *see* Contusion, thumb
      external constriction — *see* Constriction, external, thumb
      foreign body — *see* Foreign body, superficial, thumb
      insect bite — *see* Bite, by site, superficial, insect
      specified type NEC S60.39 ☑
    toe(s) S90.93- ☑
      abrasion — *see* Abrasion, toe
      bite — *see* Bite, toe
      blister — *see* Blister, toe
      contusion — *see* Contusion, toe
      external constriction — *see* Constriction, external, toe
      foreign body — *see* Foreign body, superficial, toe
      great S90.93- ☑
    tongue — *see* Injury, superficial, oral cavity
    tooth, teeth — *see* Injury, superficial, oral cavity
    trachea S10.10 ☑
    tunica vaginalis S30.94 ☑
    tympanum, tympanic membrane — *see* Injury, superficial, ear
    uvula — *see* Injury, superficial, oral cavity
    vagina S30.95 ☑
    vocal cords — *see* Injury, superficial, throat
    vulva S30.95 ☑
    wrist S60.91- ☑
  supraclavicular region — *see* Injury, neck
  supraorbital S09.93 ☑
  suprarenal gland (multiple) — *see* Injury, adrenal
  surgical complication (external or internal site) — *see* Laceration, accidental complicating surgery
  temple S09.90 ☑
  temporal region S09.90 ☑
  tendon (*see also* Injury, muscle, by site)
    abdomen — *see* Injury, muscle, abdomen
    Achilles — *see* Injury, Achilles tendon
    lower back — *see* Injury, muscle, lower back
    pelvic organs — *see* Injury, muscle, pelvis

Injury — *continued*
  tenth cranial nerve (pneumogastric or vagus) — *see* Injury, nerve, vagus
  testis S39.94 ☑
  thigh S79.92- ☑
    blood vessel — *see* Injury, blood vessel, hip
    contusion — *see* Contusion, thigh
    fracture — *see* Fracture, femur
    muscle — *see* Injury, muscle, thigh
    nerve — *see* Injury, nerve, thigh
    open — *see* Wound, open, thigh
    specified NEC S79.82- ☑
    superficial — *see* Injury, superficial, thigh
  third cranial nerve (oculomotor) — *see* Injury, nerve, oculomotor
  thorax, thoracic S29.9 ☑
    blood vessel — *see* Injury, blood vessel, thorax
    cavity — *see* Injury, intrathoracic
    dislocation — *see* Dislocation, thorax
    external (wall) S29.9 ☑
      contusion — *see* Contusion, thorax
      nerve — *see* Injury, nerve, thorax
      open — *see* Wound, open, thorax
      specified NEC S29.8 ☑
      sprain — *see* Sprain, thorax
      superficial — *see* Injury, superficial, thorax
    fracture — *see* Fracture, thorax
    internal — *see* Injury, intrathoracic
    intrathoracic organ — *see* Injury, intrathoracic
    sympathetic ganglion — *see* Injury, nerve, thorax, sympathetic
  throat (*see also* Injury, neck) S19.9 ☑
  thumb S69.9- ☑
    blood vessel — *see* Injury, blood vessel, thumb
    contusion — *see* Contusion, thumb
    dislocation — *see* Dislocation, thumb
    fracture — *see* Fracture, thumb
    muscle — *see* Injury, muscle, thumb
    nerve — *see* Injury, nerve, digital, thumb
    open — *see* Wound, open, thumb
    specified NEC S69.8- ☑
    sprain — *see* Sprain, thumb
    superficial — *see* Injury, superficial, thumb
  thymus (gland) — *see* Injury, intrathoracic, specified organ NEC
  thyroid (gland) NEC S19.84 ☑
  toe S99.92- ☑
    contusion — *see* Contusion, toe
    dislocation — *see* Dislocation, toe
    fracture — *see* Fracture, toe
    muscle — *see* Injury, muscle, toe
    open — *see* Wound, open, toe
    specified type NEC S99.82- ☑
    sprain — *see* Sprain, toe
    superficial — *see* Injury, superficial, toe
  tongue S09.93 ☑
  tonsil S09.93 ☑
  tooth S09.93 ☑
  trachea (cervical) NEC S19.82 ☑
    thoracic — *see* Injury, intrathoracic, trachea, thoracic
  transfusion-related acute lung (TRALI) J95.84
  tunica vaginalis S39.94 ☑
  twelfth cranial nerve (hypoglossal) — *see* Injury, nerve, hypoglossal
  ureter S37.10 ☑
    contusion S37.12 ☑
    laceration S37.13 ☑
    specified type NEC S37.19 ☑
  urethra (sphincter) S37.30 ☑
    at delivery O71.5
    contusion S37.32 ☑
    laceration S37.33 ☑
    specified type NEC S37.39 ☑
  urinary organ S37.90 ☑
    contusion S37.92 ☑
    laceration S37.93 ☑
    specified
      site NEC S37.899 ☑
        contusion S37.892 ☑
        laceration S37.893 ☑
        specified type NEC S37.898 ☑
      type NEC S37.99 ☑
  uterus, uterine S37.60 ☑
    with ectopic or molar pregnancy O08.6
    blood vessel — *see* Injury, blood vessel, iliac

Injury — *continued*
  uterus, uterine — *continued*
    contusion S37.62 ☑
    laceration S37.63 ☑
      cervix at delivery O71.3
    rupture associated with obstetrics — *see* Rupture, uterus
    specified type NEC S37.69 ☑
  uvula S09.93 ☑
  vagina S39.93 ☑
    abrasion S30.814 ☑
    bite S31.45 ☑
      insect S30.864 ☑
      superficial NEC S30.874 ☑
    contusion S30.23 ☑
    crush S38.03 ☑
    during delivery — *see* Laceration, vagina, during delivery
    external constriction S30.844 ☑
    insect bite S30.864 ☑
    laceration S31.41 ☑
      with foreign body S31.42 ☑
    open wound S31.40 ☑
    puncture S31.43 ☑
      with foreign body S31.44 ☑
    superficial S30.95 ☑
      foreign body S30.854 ☑
  vas deferens — *see* Injury, pelvic organ, specified site NEC
  vascular NEC T14.8
  vein — *see* Injury, blood vessel
  vena cava (superior) S25.20 ☑
    inferior S35.10 ☑
      laceration (minor) (superficial) S35.11 ☑
        major S35.12 ☑
      specified type NEC S35.19 ☑
    laceration (minor) (superficial) S25.21 ☑
      major S25.22 ☑
    specified type NEC S25.29 ☑
  vesical (sphincter) — *see* Injury, bladder
  visual cortex S04.04- ☑
  vitreous (humor) S05.90 ☑
    specified NEC S05.8X- ☑
  vocal cord NEC S19.83 ☑
  vulva S39.94 ☑
    abrasion S30.814 ☑
    bite S31.45 ☑
      insect S30.864 ☑
      superficial NEC S30.874 ☑
    contusion S30.23 ☑
    crush S38.03 ☑
    during delivery — *see* Laceration, perineum, female, during delivery
    external constriction S30.844 ☑
    insect bite S30.864 ☑
    laceration S31.41 ☑
      with foreign body S31.42 ☑
    open wound S31.40 ☑
    puncture S31.43 ☑
      with foreign body S31.44 ☑
    superficial S30.95 ☑
      foreign body S30.854 ☑
  whiplash (cervical spine) S13.4 ☑
  wrist S69.9- ☑
    blood vessel — *see* Injury, blood vessel, hand
    contusion — *see* Contusion, wrist
    dislocation — *see* Dislocation, wrist
    fracture — *see* Fracture, wrist
    muscle — *see* Injury, muscle, hand
    nerve — *see* Injury, nerve, hand
    open — *see* Wound, open, wrist
    specified NEC S69.8- ☑
    sprain — *see* Sprain, wrist
    superficial — *see* Injury, superficial, wrist
Inoculation (*see also* Vaccination)
  complication or reaction — *see* Complications, vaccination
Insanity, insane (*see also* Psychosis)
  adolescent — *see* Schizophrenia
  confusional F28
    acute or subacute F05
  delusional F22
  senile F03 ☑
Insect
  bite — *see* Bite, by site, superficial, insect

Insect — *continued*
  venomous, poisoning NEC (by) — *see* Venom, arthropod
Insensitivity
  adrenocorticotropin hormone (ACTH) E27.49
  androgen E34.50
    complete E34.51
    partial E34.52
Insertion
  cord (umbilical) lateral or velamentous O43.12- ☑
  intrauterine contraceptive device (encounter for) — *see* Intrauterine contraceptive device
Insolation (sunstroke) T67.0 ☑
Insomnia (organic) G47.00
  without objective findings F51.02
  adjustment F51.02
  adjustment disorder F51.02
  behavioral, of childhood Z73.819
    combined type Z73.812
    limit setting type Z73.811
    sleep-onset association type Z73.810
  childhood Z73.819
  chronic F51.04
    somatized tension F51.04
  conditioned F51.04
  due to
    alcohol
      abuse F10.182
      dependence F10.282
      use F10.982
    amphetamines
      abuse F15.182
      dependence F15.282
      use F15.982
    anxiety disorder F51.05
    caffeine
      abuse F15.182
      dependence F15.282
      use F15.982
    cocaine
      abuse F14.182
      dependence F14.282
      use F14.982
    depression F51.05
    drug NEC
      abuse F19.182
      dependence F19.282
      use F19.982
    medical condition G47.01
    mental disorder NEC F51.05
    opioid
      abuse F11.182
      dependence F11.282
      use F11.982
    psychoactive substance NEC
      abuse F19.182
      dependence F19.182
      use F19.982
    sedative, hypnotic, or anxiolytic
      abuse F13.182
      dependence F13.282
      use F13.982
    stimulant NEC
      abuse F15.182
      dependence F15.282
      use F15.982
  fatal familial (FFI) A81.83
  idiopathic F51.01
  learned F51.3
  nonorganic origin F51.01
  not due to a substance or known physiological condition F51.01
    specified NEC F51.09
  paradoxical F51.03
  primary F51.01
  psychiatric F51.05
  psychophysiologic F51.04
  related to psychopathology F51.05
  short-term F51.02
  specified NEC G47.09
  stress-related F51.02
  transient F51.02
Inspiration
  food or foreign body — *see* Foreign body, by site
  mucus — *see* Asphyxia, mucus
Inspissated bile syndrome (newborn) P59.1
Instability
  emotional (excessive) F60.3

Instability — *continued*
  joint (post-traumatic) M25.30
    ankle M25.37- ☑
    due to old ligament injury — *see* Disorder, ligament
    elbow M25.32- ☑
    flail — *see* Flail, joint
    foot M25.37- ☑
    hand M25.34- ☑
    hip M25.35- ☑
    knee M25.36- ☑
    lumbosacral — *see* subcategory M53.2 ☑
    prosthesis — *see* Complications, joint prosthesis, mechanical, displacement, by site
    sacroiliac — *see* subcategory M53.2 ☑
    secondary to
      old ligament injury — *see* Disorder, ligament
      removal of joint prosthesis M96.89
    shoulder (region) M25.31- ☑
    spine — *see* subcategory M53.2 ☑
    wrist M25.33- ☑
  knee (chronic) M23.5- ☑
  lumbosacral — *see* subcategory M53.2 ☑
  nervous F48.8
  personality (emotional) F60.3
  spine — *see* Instability, joint, spine
  vasomotor R55
Institutional syndrome (childhood) F94.2
Institutionalization, affecting child Z62.22
  disinhibited attachment F94.2
Insufficiency, insufficient
  accommodation, old age H52.4
  adrenal (gland) E27.40
    primary E27.1
  adrenocortical E27.40
    drug-induced E27.3
    iatrogenic E27.3
    primary E27.1
  anterior (occlusal) guidance M26.54
  anus K62.89
  aortic (valve) I35.1
    with
      mitral (valve) disease I08.0
        with tricuspid (valve) disease I08.3
      stenosis I35.2
      tricuspid (valve) disease I08.2
        with mitral (valve) disease I08.3
    congenital Q23.1
    rheumatic I06.1
      with
        mitral (valve) disease I08.0
          with tricuspid (valve) disease I08.3
        stenosis I06.2
          with mitral (valve) disease I08.0
            with tricuspid (valve) disease I08.3
        tricuspid (valve) disease I08.2
          with mitral (valve) disease I08.3
    specified cause NEC I35.1
    syphilitic A52.03
  arterial I77.1
    basilar G45.0
    carotid (hemispheric) G45.1
    cerebral I67.81
    coronary (acute or subacute) I24.8
    mesenteric K55.1
    peripheral I73.9
    precerebral (multiple) (bilateral) G45.2
    vertebral G45.0
  arteriovenous I99.8
  biliary K83.8
  cardiac (*see also* Insufficiency, myocardial)
    due to presence of (cardiac) prosthesis I97.11- ☑
    postprocedural I97.11- ☑
  cardiorenal, hypertensive I13.2
  cardiovascular — *see* Disease, cardiovascular
  cerebrovascular (acute) I67.81
    with transient focal neurological signs and symptoms G45.8
  circulatory NEC I99.8
    newborn P29.89
  convergence H51.11
  coronary (acute or subacute) I24.8
    chronic or with a stated duration of over 4 weeks I25.89
  corticoadrenal E27.40
    primary E27.1
  dietary E63.9
  divergence H51.8

Insufficiency, insufficient — *continued*
  food T73.0 ☑
  gastroesophageal K22.8
  gonadal
    ovary E28.39
    testis E29.1
  heart (*see also* Insufficiency, myocardial)
    newborn P29.0
    valve — *see* Endocarditis
  hepatic — *see* Failure, hepatic
  idiopathic autonomic G90.09
  interocclusal distance of fully erupted teeth (ridge) M26.36
  kidney N28.9
    acute N28.9
    chronic N18.9
  lacrimal (secretion) H04.12- ☑
    passages — *see* Stenosis, lacrimal
  liver — *see* Failure, hepatic
  lung — *see* Insufficiency, pulmonary
  mental (congenital) — *see* Disability, intellectual
  mesenteric K55.1
  mitral (valve) I34.0
    with
      aortic valve disease I08.0
        with tricuspid (valve) disease I08.3
      obstruction or stenosis I05.2
        with aortic valve disease I08.0
      tricuspid (valve) disease I08.1
        with aortic (valve) disease I08.3
    congenital Q23.3
    rheumatic I05.1
      with
        aortic valve disease I08.0
          with tricuspid (valve) disease I08.3
        obstruction or stenosis I05.2
          with aortic valve disease I08.0
            with tricuspid (valve) disease I08.3
        tricuspid (valve) disease I08.1
          with aortic (valve) disease I08.3
      active or acute I01.1
        with chorea, rheumatic (Sydenham's) I02.0
    specified cause, except rheumatic I34.0
  muscle (*see also* Disease, muscle)
    heart — *see* Insufficiency, myocardial
    ocular NEC H50.9
  myocardial, myocardium (with arteriosclerosis) I50.9
    with
      rheumatic fever (conditions in I00) I09.0
        active, acute or subacute I01.2
          with chorea I02.0
        inactive or quiescent (with chorea) I09.0
    congenital Q24.8
    hypertensive — *see* Hypertension, heart
    newborn P29.0
    rheumatic I09.0
      active, acute, or subacute I01.2
    syphilitic A52.06
  nourishment T73.0 ☑
  pancreatic K86.8
  parathyroid (gland) E20.9
  peripheral vascular (arterial) I73.9
  pituitary E23.0
  placental (mother) O36.51- ☑
  platelets D69.6
  prenatal care affecting management of pregnancy O09.3- ☑
  progressive pluriglandular E31.0
  pulmonary J98.4
    acute, following surgery (nonthoracic) J95.2
      thoracic J95.1
    chronic, following surgery J95.3
    following
      shock J98.4
      trauma J98.4
    newborn P28.5
    valve I37.1
      with stenosis I37.2
      congenital Q22.2
      rheumatic I09.89
        with aortic, mitral or tricuspid (valve) disease I08.8
  pyloric K31.89
  renal (acute) N28.9
    chronic N18.9
  respiratory R06.89
    newborn P28.5
  rotation — *see* Malrotation

☑ **Additional Character Required** — Refer to the Tabular List for Character Selection
▽ Subterms under main terms may continue to next column or page

Insufficiency, insufficient — continued
  sleep syndrome F51.12
  social insurance Z59.7
  suprarenal E27.40
    primary E27.1
  tarso-orbital fascia, congenital Q10.3
  testis E29.1
  thyroid (gland) (acquired) E03.9
    congenital E03.1
  tricuspid (valve) (rheumatic) I07.1
    with
      aortic (valve) disease I08.2
        with mitral (valve) disease I08.3
      mitral (valve) disease I08.1
        with aortic (valve) disease I08.3
      obstruction or stenosis I07.2
        with aortic (valve) disease I08.2
          with mitral (valve) disease I08.3
    congenital Q22.8
    nonrheumatic I36.1
      with stenosis I36.2
  urethral sphincter R32
  valve, valvular (heart) — see Endocarditis
    congenital Q24.8
  vascular I99.8
    intestine K55.9
      acute K55.0
    mesenteric K55.1
    peripheral I73.9
    renal — see Hypertension, kidney
  velopharyngeal
    acquired K13.79
    congenital Q38.8
  venous (chronic) (peripheral) I87.2
  ventricular — see Insufficiency, myocardial
  welfare support Z59.7
Insufflation, fallopian Z31.41
Insular — see condition
Insulinoma
  pancreas
    benign D13.7
    malignant C25.4
    uncertain behavior D37.8
  specified site
    benign — see Neoplasm, by site, benign
    malignant — see Neoplasm, by site, malignant
    uncertain behavior — see Neoplasm, by site, uncertain behavior
  unspecified site
    benign D13.7
    malignant C25.4
    uncertain behavior D37.8
Insuloma — see Insulinoma
Interference
  balancing side M26.56
  non-working side M26.56
Intermenstrual — see condition
Intermittent — see condition
Internal — see condition
Interrogation
  cardiac defibrillator (automatic) (implantable) Z45.02
  cardiac pacemaker Z45.018
  cardiac (event) (loop) recorder Z45.09
  infusion pump (implanted) (intrathecal) Z45.1
  neurostimulator Z46.2
Interruption
  bundle of His I44.30
  phase-shift, sleep cycle — see Disorder, sleep, circadian rhythm
  sleep phase-shift, or 24 hour sleep-wake cycle — see Disorder, sleep, circadian rhythm
Interstitial — see condition
Intertrigo L30.4
  labialis K13.0
Intervertebral disc — see condition
Intestine, intestinal — see condition
Intolerance
  carbohydrate K90.4
  disaccharide, hereditary E73.0
  fat NEC K90.4
    pancreatic K90.3
  food K90.4
    dietary counseling and surveillance Z71.3
  fructose E74.10
    hereditary E74.12
  glucose (-galactose) E74.39
  gluten K90.0

Intolerance — continued
  lactose E73.9
    specified NEC E73.8
  lysine E72.3
  milk NEC K90.4
    lactose E73.9
  protein K90.4
  starch NEC K90.4
  sucrose (-isomaltose) E74.31
Intoxicated NEC (without dependence) — see Alcohol, intoxication
Intoxication
  acid E87.2
  alcoholic (acute) (without dependence) — see Alcohol, intoxication
  alimentary canal K52.1
  amphetamine (without dependence) — see Abuse, drug, stimulant, with intoxication
    with dependence — see Dependence, drug, stimulant, with intoxication
  anxiolytic (acute) (without dependence) — see Abuse, drug, sedative, with intoxication
    with dependence — see Dependence, drug, sedative, with intoxication
  caffeine (acute) (without dependence) — see Abuse, drug, stimulant, with intoxication
    with dependence — see Dependence, drug, stimulant, with intoxication
  cannabinoids (acute) (without dependence) — see Abuse, drug, cannabis, with intoxication
    with dependence — see Dependence, drug, cannabis, with intoxication
  chemical — see Table of Drugs and Chemicals
    via placenta or breast milk — see - Absorption, chemical, through placenta
  cocaine (acute) (without dependence) — see Abuse, drug, cocaine, with intoxication
    with dependence — see Dependence, drug, cocaine, with intoxication
  drug
    acute (without dependence) — see Abuse, drug, by type with intoxication
      with dependence — see Dependence, drug, by type with intoxication
    addictive
      via placenta or breast milk — see Absorption, drug, addictive, through placenta
    newborn P93.8
      gray baby syndrome P93.0
    overdose or wrong substance given or taken — see Table of Drugs and Chemicals, by drug, poisoning
  enteric K52.1
  foodborne A05.9
    bacterial A05.9
    classical (Clostridium botulinum) A05.1
    due to
      Bacillus cereus A05.4
      bacterium A05.9
        specified NEC A05.8
      Clostridium
        botulinum A05.1
        perfringens A05.2
        welchii A05.2
      Salmonella A02.9
        with
          (gastro)enteritis A02.0
          localized infection(s) A02.20
            arthritis A02.23
            meningitis A02.21
            osteomyelitis A02.24
            pneumonia A02.22
            pyelonephritis A02.25
            specified NEC A02.29
          sepsis A02.1
          specified manifestation NEC A02.8
      Staphylococcus A05.0
      Vibrio
        parahaemolyticus A05.3
        vulnificus A05.5
    enterotoxin, staphylococcal A05.0
    noxious — see Poisoning, food, noxious
  gastrointestinal K52.1
  hallucinogenic (without dependence) — see Abuse, drug, hallucinogen, with intoxication
    with dependence — see Dependence, drug, hallucinogen, with intoxication

Intoxication — continued
  hypnotic (acute) (without dependence) — see Abuse, drug, sedative, with intoxication
    with dependence — see Dependence, drug, sedative, with intoxication
  inhalant (acute) (without dependence) — see Abuse, drug, inhalant, with intoxication
    with dependence — see Dependence, drug, inhalant, with intoxication
  meaning
    inebriation — see category F10 ☑
    poisoning — see Table of Drugs and Chemicals
  methyl alcohol (acute) (without dependence) — see Alcohol, intoxication
  opioid (acute) (without dependence) — see Abuse, drug, opioid, with intoxication
    with dependence — see Dependence, drug, opioid, with intoxication
  pathologic NEC (without dependence) — see Alcohol, intoxication
  phencyclidine (without dependence) — see Abuse, drug, psychoactive NEC, with intoxication
    with dependence — see Dependence, drug, psychoactive NEC, with intoxication
  potassium (K) E87.5
  psychoactive substance NEC (without dependence) — see Abuse, drug, psychoactive NEC, with intoxication
    with dependence — see Dependence, drug, psychoactive NEC, with intoxication
  sedative (acute) (without dependence) — see Abuse, drug, sedative, with intoxication
    with dependence — see Dependence, drug, sedative, with intoxication
  serum (see also Reaction, serum) T80.69 ☑
  uremic — see Uremia
  volatile solvents (acute) (without dependence) — see Abuse, drug, inhalant, with intoxication
    with dependence — see Dependence, drug, inhalant, with intoxication
  water E87.79
Intracranial — see condition
Intrahepatic gallbladder Q44.1
Intraligamentous — see condition
Intrathoracic (see also condition)
  kidney Q63.2
Intrauterine contraceptive device
  checking Z30.431
  in situ Z97.5
  insertion Z30.430
    immediately following removal Z30.433
  management Z30.431
  reinsertion Z30.433
  removal Z30.432
  replacement Z30.433
  retention in pregnancy O26.3- ☑
Intraventricular — see condition
Intrinsic deformity — see Deformity
Intubation, difficult or failed T88.4 ☑
Intumescence, lens (eye) (cataract) — see Cataract
Intussusception (bowel) (colon) (enteric) (ileocecal) (ileocolic) (intestine) (rectum) K56.1
  appendix K38.8
  congenital Q43.8
  ureter (with obstruction) N13.5
Invagination (bowel, colon, intestine or rectum) K56.1
Inversion
  albumin-globulin (A-G) ratio E88.09
  bladder N32.89
  cecum — see Intussusception
  cervix N88.8
  chromosome in normal individual Q95.1
  circadian rhythm — see Disorder, sleep, circadian rhythm
  nipple N64.59
    congenital Q83.8
    gestational — see Retraction, nipple
    puerperal, postpartum — see Retraction, nipple
  nyctohemeral rhythm — see Disorder, sleep, circadian rhythm
  optic papilla Q14.2
  organ or site, congenital NEC — see Anomaly, by site
  sleep rhythm — see Disorder, sleep, circadian rhythm
  testis (congenital) Q55.29
  uterus (chronic) (postinfectional) (postpartal, old) N85.5
    postpartum O71.2

Inversion — *continued*
    vagina (posthysterectomy) N99.3
    ventricular Q20.5
Investigation (*see also* Examination) Z04.9
    clinical research subject (control) (normal comparison)
        (participant) Z00.6
Involuntary movement, abnormal R25.9
Involution, involutional (*see also* condition)
    breast, cystic — *see* Dysplasia, mammary, specified
        type NEC
    depression (single episode) F32.8
        recurrent episode F33.9
    melancholia (recurrent episode) (single episode) F32.8
    ovary, senile — *see* Atrophy, ovary
    thymus failure E32.8
I.Q.
    under 20 F73
    20-34 F72
    35-49 F71
    50-69 F70
IRDS (type I) P22.0
    type II P22.1
Irideremia Q13.1
Iridis rubeosis — *see* Disorder, iris, vascular
Iridochoroiditis (panuveitis) — *see* Panuveitis
Iridocyclitis H20.9
    acute H20.0- ☑
        hypopyon H20.05- ☑
        primary H20.01- ☑
        recurrent H20.02- ☑
        secondary (noninfectious) H20.04- ☑
            infectious H20.03- ☑
    chronic H20.1- ☑
    due to allergy — *see* Iridocyclitis, acute, secondary
    endogenous — *see* Iridocyclitis, acute, primary
    Fuchs' — *see* Cyclitis, Fuchs' heterochromic
    gonococcal A54.32
    granulomatous — *see* Iridocyclitis, chronic
    herpes, herpetic (simplex) B00.51
        zoster B02.32
    hypopyon — *see* Iridocyclitis, acute, hypopyon
    in (due to)
        ankylosing spondylitis M45.9
        gonococcal infection A54.32
        herpes (simplex) virus B00.51
            zoster B02.32
        infectious disease NOS B99 ☑
        parasitic disease NOS B89 [H22]
        sarcoidosis D86.83
        syphilis A51.43
        tuberculosis A18.54
        zoster B02.32
    lens-induced H20.2- ☑
    nongranulomatous — *see* Iridocyclitis, acute
    recurrent — *see* Iridocyclitis, acute, recurrent
    rheumatic — *see* Iridocyclitis, chronic
    subacute — *see* Iridocyclitis, acute
    sympathetic — *see* Uveitis, sympathetic
    syphilitic (secondary) A51.43
    tuberculous (chronic) A18.54
    Vogt-Koyanagi H20.82- ☑
Iridocyclochoroiditis (panuveitis) — *see* Panuveitis
Iridodialysis H21.53- ☑
Iridodonesis H21.89
Iridoplegia (complete) (partial) (reflex) H57.09
Iridoschisis H21.25- ☑
Iris (*see also* condition)
    bombé — *see* Membrane, pupillary
Iritis (*see also* Iridocyclitis)
    chronic — *see* Iridocyclitis, chronic
    diabetic — *see* E08-E13 with .39
    due to
        herpes simplex B00.51
        leprosy A30.9 [H22]
    gonococcal A54.32
    gouty M10.9
    granulomatous — *see* Iridocyclitis, chronic
    lens induced — *see* Iridocyclitis, lens-induced
    papulosa (syphilitic) A52.71
    rheumatic — *see* Iridocyclitis, chronic
    syphilitic (secondary) A51.43
        congenital (early) A50.01
        late A52.71
    tuberculous A18.54
Iron — *see* condition
Iron-miner's lung J63.4
Irradiated enamel (tooth, teeth) K03.89

Irradiation effects, adverse T66 ☑
Irreducible, irreducibility — *see* condition
Irregular, irregularity
    action, heart I49.9
    alveolar process K08.8
    bleeding N92.6
    breathing R06.89
    contour of cornea (acquired) — *see* Deformity, cornea
        congenital Q13.4
    contour, reconstructed breast N65.0
    dentin (in pulp) K04.3
    eye movements H55.89
        nystagmus — *see* Nystagmus
        saccadic H55.81
    labor O62.2
    menstruation (cause unknown) N92.6
    periods N92.6
    prostate N42.9
    pupil — *see* Abnormality, pupillary
    reconstructed breast N65.0
    respiratory R06.89
    septum (nasal) J34.2
    shape, organ or site, congenital NEC — *see* Distortion
    sleep-wake pattern (rhythm) G47.23
Irritable, irritability R45.4
    bladder N32.89
    bowel (syndrome) K58.9
        with diarrhea K58.0
        psychogenic F45.8
    bronchial — *see* Bronchitis
    cerebral, in newborn P91.3
    colon K58.9
        with diarrhea K58.0
        psychogenic F45.8
    duodenum K59.8
    heart (psychogenic) F45.8
    hip — *see* Derangement, joint, specified type NEC, hip
    ileum K59.8
    infant R68.12
    jejunum K59.8
    rectum K59.8
    stomach K31.89
        psychogenic F45.8
    sympathetic G90.8
    urethra N36.8
Irritation
    anus K62.89
    axillary nerve G54.0
    bladder N32.89
    brachial plexus G54.0
    bronchial — *see* Bronchitis
    cervical plexus G54.2
    cervix — *see* Cervicitis
    choroid, sympathetic — *see* Endophthalmitis
    cranial nerve — *see* Disorder, nerve, cranial
    gastric K31.89
        psychogenic F45.8
    globe, sympathetic — *see* Uveitis, sympathetic
    labyrinth — *see* subcategory H83.2 ☑
    lumbosacral plexus G54.1
    meninges (traumatic) — *see* Injury, intracranial
        nontraumatic — *see* Meningismus
    nerve — *see* Disorder, nerve
    nervous R45.0
    penis N48.89
    perineum NEC L29.3
    peripheral autonomic nervous system G90.8
    peritoneum — *see* Peritonitis
    pharynx J39.2
    plantar nerve — *see* Lesion, nerve, plantar
    spinal (cord) (traumatic) (*see also* Injury, spinal cord,
        by region)
        nerve G58.9
            root NEC — *see* Radiculopathy
        nontraumatic — *see* Myelopathy
    stomach K31.89
        psychogenic F45.8
    sympathetic nerve NEC G90.8
    ulnar nerve — *see* Lesion, nerve, ulnar
    vagina N89.8
Ischemia, ischemic I99.8
    bowel (transient)
        acute K55.0
        chronic K55.1
        due to mesenteric artery insufficiency K55.1
    brain — *see* Ischemia, cerebral
    cardiac (see Disease, heart, ischemic)
    cardiomyopathy I25.5

Ischemia, ischemic — *continued*
    cerebral (chronic) (generalized) I67.82
        arteriosclerotic I67.2
        intermittent G45.9
        newborn P91.0
        recurrent focal G45.8
        transient G45.9
    colon chronic (due to mesenteric artery insufficiency)
        K55.1
    coronary — *see* Disease, heart, ischemic
    demand (coronary) (*see also* Angina) I24.8
    heart (chronic or with a stated duration of over 4
        weeks) I25.9
        acute or with a stated duration of 4 weeks or less
            I24.9
        subacute I24.9
    infarction, muscle — *see* Infarct, muscle
    intestine (large) (small) (transient) K55.9
        acute K55.0
        chronic K55.1
        due to mesenteric artery insufficiency K55.1
    kidney N28.0
    mesenteric, acute K55.0
    muscle, traumatic T79.6 ☑
    myocardium, myocardial (chronic or with a stated
        duration of over 4 weeks) I25.9
        acute, without myocardial infarction I24.0
        silent (asymptomatic) I25.6
        transient of newborn P29.4
    renal N28.0
    retina, retinal — *see* Occlusion, artery, retina
    small bowel
        acute K55.0
        chronic K55.1
        due to mesenteric artery insufficiency K55.1
    spinal cord G95.11
    subendocardial — *see* Insufficiency, coronary
    supply (coronary) (*see also* Angina) I25.9
        due to vasospasm I20.1
Ischial spine — *see* condition
Ischialgia — *see* Sciatica
Ischiopagus Q89.4
Ischium, ischial — *see* condition
Ischuria R34
Iselin's disease or osteochondrosis — *see* Osteochon-
    drosis, juvenile, metatarsus
Islands of
    parotid tissue in
        lymph nodes Q38.6
        neck structures Q38.6
    submaxillary glands in
        fascia Q38.6
        lymph nodes Q38.6
        neck muscles Q38.6
Islet cell tumor, pancreas D13.7
Isoimmunization NEC (*see also* Incompatibility)
    affecting management of pregnancy (ABO) (with hy-
        drops fetalis) O36.11- ☑
        anti-A sensitization O36.11- ☑
        anti-B sensitization O36.19- ☑
        anti-c sensitization O36.09- ☑
        anti-C sensitization O36.09- ☑
        anti-E sensitization O36.09- ☑
        anti-e sensitization O36.09- ☑
        Rh NEC O36.09- ☑
            anti-D antibody O36.01- ☑
        specified NEC O36.19- ☑
    newborn P55.9
        with
            hydrops fetalis P56.0
            kernicterus P57.0
        ABO (blood groups) P55.1
        Rhesus (Rh) factor P55.0
        specified type NEC P55.8
Isolation, isolated
    dwelling Z59.8
    family Z63.79
    social Z60.4
Isoleucinosis E71.19
Isomerism atrial appendages (with asplenia or
    polysplenia) Q20.6
Isosporiasis, isosporosis A07.3
Isovaleric acidemia E71.110
Issue of
    medical certificate Z02.79
        for disability determination Z02.71

  ☑ **Additional Character Required** — **Refer to the Tabular List for Character Selection**   ▽ **Subterms under main terms may continue to next column or page**

Issue of — *continued*
repeat prescription (appliance) (glasses) (medicinal substance, medicament, medicine) Z76.0
contraception — *see* Contraception
Itch, itching (*see also* Pruritus)
baker's L23.6
barber's B35.0
bricklayer's L24.5
cheese B88.0
clam digger's B65.3
coolie B76.9
copra B88.0
dew B76.9
dhobi B35.6
filarial — *see* Infestation, filarial
grain B88.0
grocer's B88.0
ground B76.9
harvest B88.0
jock B35.6
Malabar B35.5
beard B35.0
foot B35.3
scalp B35.0
meaning scabies B86
Norwegian B86
perianal L29.0
poultrymen's B88.0
sarcoptic B86
scabies B86
scrub B88.0
straw B88.0
swimmer's B65.3
water B76.9
winter L29.8
Ivemark's syndrome (asplenia with congenital heart disease) Q89.01
Ivory bones Q78.2
Ixodiasis NEC B88.8

J

Jaccoud's syndrome — *see* Arthropathy, postrheumatic, chronic
Jackson's
membrane Q43.3
paralysis or syndrome G83.89
veil Q43.3
Jacquet's dermatitis (diaper dermatitis) L22
Jadassohn-Pellizari's disease or anetoderma L90.2
Jadassohn's
blue nevus — *see* Nevus
intraepidermal epithelioma — *see* Neoplasm, skin, benign
Jaffe-Lichtenstein (-Uehlinger) **syndrome** — *see* Dysplasia, fibrous, bone NEC
Jakob-Creutzfeldt disease or syndrome — *see* Creutzfeldt-Jakob disease or syndrome
Jaksch-Luzet disease D64.89
Jamaican
neuropathy G92
paraplegic tropical ataxic-spastic syndrome G92
Janet's disease F48.8
Janiceps Q89.4
Jansky-Bielschowsky amaurotic idiocy E75.4
Japanese
B-type encephalitis A83.0
river fever A75.3
Jaundice (yellow) R17
acholuric (familial) (splenomegalic) (*see also* Spherocytosis)
acquired D59.8
breast-milk (inhibitor) P59.3
catarrhal (acute) B15.9
with hepatic coma B15.0
cholestatic (benign) R17
due to or associated with
delayed conjugation P59.8
associated with (due to) preterm delivery P59.0
preterm delivery P59.0
epidemic (catarrhal) B15.9
with hepatic coma B15.0
leptospiral A27.0
spirochetal A27.0
familial nonhemolytic (congenital) (Gilbert) E80.4
Crigler-Najjar E80.5
febrile (acute) B15.9
with hepatic coma B15.0

Jaundice — *continued*
febrile — *continued*
leptospiral A27.0
spirochetal A27.0
hematogenous D59.9
hemolytic (acquired) D59.9
congenital — *see* Spherocytosis
hemorrhagic (acute) (leptospiral) (spirochetal) A27.0
infectious (acute) (subacute) B15.9
with hepatic coma B15.0
leptospiral A27.0
spirochetal A27.0
leptospiral (hemorrhagic) A27.0
malignant (without coma) K72.90
with coma K72.91
neonatal — *see* Jaundice, newborn
newborn P59.9
due to or associated with
ABO
antibodies P55.1
incompatibility, maternal/fetal P55.1
isoimmunization P55.1
absence or deficiency of enzyme system for bilirubin conjugation (congenital) P59.8
bleeding P58.1
breast milk inhibitors to conjugation P59.3
associated with preterm delivery P59.0
bruising P58.0
Crigler-Najjar syndrome E80.5
delayed conjugation P59.8
associated with preterm delivery P59.0
drugs or toxins
given to newborn P58.42
transmitted from mother P58.41
excessive hemolysis P58.9
due to
bleeding P58.1
bruising P58.0
drugs or toxins
given to newborn P58.42
transmitted from mother P58.41
infection P58.2
polycythemia P58.3
swallowed maternal blood P58.5
specified type NEC P58.8
galactosemia E74.21
Gilbert syndrome E80.4
hemolytic disease P55.9
ABO isoimmunization P55.1
Rh isoimmunization P55.0
specified NEC P55.8
hepatocellular damage P59.20
specified NEC P59.29
hereditary hemolytic anemia P58.8
hypothyroidism, congenital E03.1
incompatibility, maternal/fetal NOS P55.9
infection P58.2
inspissated bile syndrome P59.1
isoimmunization NOS P55.9
mucoviscidosis E84.9
polycythemia P58.3
preterm delivery P59.0
Rh
antibodies P55.0
incompatibility, maternal/fetal P55.0
isoimmunization P55.0
specified cause NEC P59.8
swallowed maternal blood P58.5
spherocytosis (congenital) D58.0
nonhemolytic congenital familial (Gilbert) E80.4
nuclear, newborn (*see also* Kernicterus of newborn) P57.9
obstructive (*see also* Obstruction, bile duct) K83.1
post-immunization — *see* Hepatitis, viral, type, B
post-transfusion — *see* Hepatitis, viral, type, B
regurgitation (*see also* Obstruction, bile duct) K83.1
serum (homologous) (prophylactic) (therapeutic) — *see* Hepatitis, viral, type, B
spirochetal (hemorrhagic) A27.0
symptomatic R17
newborn P59.9
Jaw — *see* condition
Jaw-winking phenomenon or syndrome Q07.8
Jealousy
alcoholic F10.988
childhood F93.8
sibling F93.8
Jejunitis — *see* Enteritis

Jejunostomy status Z93.4
Jejunum, jejunal — *see* condition
Jensen's disease — *see* Inflammation, chorioretinal, focal, juxtapapillary
Jerks, myoclonic G25.3
Jervell-Lange-Nielsen syndrome I45.81
Jeune's disease Q77.2
Jigger disease B88.1
Job's syndrome (chronic granulomatous disease) D71
Joint (*see also* condition)
mice — *see* Loose, body, joint
knee M23.4- ☑
Jordan's anomaly or syndrome D72.0
Joseph-Diamond-Blackfan anemia (congenital hypoplastic) D61.01
Jungle yellow fever A95.0
Jüngling's disease — *see* Sarcoidosis
Juvenile — *see* condition

K

Kahler's disease C90.0- ☑
Kakke E51.11
Kala-azar B55.0
Kallmann's syndrome E23.0
Kanner's syndrome (autism) — *see* Psychosis, childhood
Kaposi's
dermatosis (xeroderma pigmentosum) Q82.1
lichen ruber L44.0
acuminatus L44.0
sarcoma
colon C46.4
connective tissue C46.1
gastrointestinal organ C46.4
lung C46.5- ☑
lymph node (multiple) C46.3
palate (hard) (soft) C46.2
rectum C46.4
skin (multiple sites) C46.0
specified site NEC C46.7
stomach C46.4
unspecified site C46.9
varicelliform eruption B00.0
vaccinia T88.1 ☑
Kartagener's syndrome or triad (sinusitis, bronchiectasis, situs inversus) Q89.3
Karyotype
with abnormality except iso (Xq) Q96.2
45,X Q96.0
46,X
iso (Xq) Q96.1
46,XX Q98.3
with streak gonads Q50.32
hermaphrodite (true) Q99.1
male Q98.3
46,XY
with streak gonads Q56.1
female Q97.3
hermaphrodite (true) Q99.1
47,XXX Q97.0
47,XXY Q98.0
47,XYY Q98.5
Kaschin-Beck disease — *see* Disease, Kaschin-Beck
Katayama's disease or fever B65.2
Kawasaki's syndrome M30.3
Kayser-Fleischer ring (cornea) (pseudosclerosis) H18.04- ☑
Kaznelson's syndrome (congenital hypoplastic anemia) D61.01
Kearns-Sayre syndrome H49.81- ☑
Kedani fever A75.3
Kelis L91.0
Kelly (-Patterson) **syndrome** (sideropenic dysphagia) D50.1
Keloid, cheloid L91.0
acne L73.0
Addison's L94.0
cornea — *see* Opacity, cornea
Hawkin's L91.0
scar L91.0
Keloma L91.0
Kenya fever A77.1
Keratectasia (*see also* Ectasia, cornea)
congenital Q13.4
Keratinization of alveolar ridge mucosa
excessive K13.23
minimal K13.22

Keratinized residual ridge mucosa
  excessive K13.23
  minimal K13.22
Keratitis (nodular) (nonulcerative) (simple) (zonular) H16.9
  with ulceration (central) (marginal) (perforated) (ring) — see Ulcer, cornea
  actinic — see Photokeratitis
  arborescens (herpes simplex) B00.52
  areolar H16.11- ☑
  bullosa H16.8
  deep H16.309
    specified type NEC H16.399
  dendritic (a) (herpes simplex) B00.52
  disciform (is) (herpes simplex) B00.52
    varicella B01.81
  filamentary H16.12- ☑
  gonococcal (congenital or prenatal) A54.33
  herpes, herpetic (simplex) B00.52
    zoster B02.33
  in (due to)
    acanthamebiasis B60.13
    adenovirus B30.0
    exanthema (see also Exanthem) B09
    herpes (simplex) virus B00.52
    measles B05.81
    syphilis A50.31
    tuberculosis A18.52
    zoster B02.33
  interstitial (nonsyphilitic) H16.30- ☑
    diffuse H16.32- ☑
    herpes, herpetic (simplex) B00.52
      zoster B02.33
    sclerosing H16.33- ☑
    specified type NEC H16.39- ☑
    syphilitic (congenital) (late) A50.31
    tuberculous A18.52
  macular H16.11- ☑
  nummular H16.11- ☑
  oyster shuckers' H16.8
  parenchymatous — see Keratitis, interstitial
  petrificans H16.8
  postmeasles B05.81
  punctata
    leprosa A30.9 [H16.14-] ☑
    syphilitic (profunda) A50.31
  punctate H16.14- ☑
  purulent H16.8
  rosacea L71.8
  sclerosing H16.33- ☑
  specified type NEC H16.8
  stellate H16.11- ☑
  striate H16.11- ☑
  superficial H16.10- ☑
    with conjunctivitis — see Keratoconjunctivitis
    due to light — see Photokeratitis
  suppurative H16.8
  syphilitic (congenital) (prenatal) A50.31
  trachomatous A71.1
    sequelae B94.0
  tuberculous A18.52
  vesicular H16.8
  xerotic (see also Keratomalacia) H16.8
    vitamin A deficiency E50.4
Keratoacanthoma L85.8
Keratocele — see Descemetocele
Keratoconjunctivitis H16.20- ☑
  Acanthamoeba B60.13
  adenoviral B30.0
  epidemic B30.0
  exposure H16.21- ☑
  herpes, herpetic (simplex) B00.52
    zoster B02.33
  in exanthema (see also Exanthem) B09
  infectious B30.0
  lagophthalmic — see Keratoconjunctivitis, specified type NEC
  neurotrophic H16.23- ☑
  phlyctenular H16.25- ☑
  postmeasles B05.81
  shipyard B30.0
  sicca (Sjogren's) M35.0- ☑
    not Sjogren's H16.22- ☑
  specified type NEC H16.29- ☑
  tuberculous (phlyctenular) A18.52
  vernal H16.26- ☑
Keratoconus H18.60- ☑

Keratoconus H18.60- ☑
  congenital Q13.4
  stable H18.61- ☑
  unstable H18.62- ☑
Keratocyst (dental) (odontogenic) — see Cyst, calcifying odontogenic
Keratoderma, keratodermia (congenital) (palmaris et plantaris) (symmetrical) Q82.8
  acquired L85.1
    in diseases classified elsewhere L86
  climactericum L85.1
  gonococcal A54.89
  gonorrheal A54.89
  punctata L85.2
  Reiter's — see Reiter's disease
Keratodermatocele — see Descemetocele
Keratoglobus H18.79 ☑
  congenital Q15.8
    with glaucoma Q15.0
Keratohemia — see Pigmentation, cornea, stromal
Keratoiritis (see also Iridocyclitis)
  syphilitic A50.39
  tuberculous A18.54
Keratoma L57.0
  palmaris and plantaris hereditarium Q82.8
  senile L57.0
Keratomalacia H18.44- ☑
  vitamin A deficiency E50.4
Keratomegaly Q13.4
Keratomycosis B49
  nigrans, nigricans (palmaris) B36.1
Keratopathy H18.9
  band H18.42- ☑
  bullous (aphakic), following cataract surgery H59.01- ☑
  bullous H18.1- ☑
Keratoscleritis, tuberculous A18.52
Keratosis L57.0
  actinic L57.0
  arsenical L85.8
  congenital, specified NEC Q80.8
  female genital NEC N94.89
  follicularis Q82.8
    acquired L11.0
    congenita Q82.8
    et parafollicularis in cutem penetrans L87.0
    spinulosa (decalvans) Q82.8
    vitamin A deficiency E50.8
  gonococcal A54.89
  male genital (external) N50.8
  nigricans L83
  obturans, external ear (canal) — see Cholesteatoma, external ear
  palmaris et plantaris (inherited) (symmetrical) Q82.8
    acquired L85.1
  penile N48.89
  pharynx J39.2
  pilaris, acquired L85.8
  punctata (palmaris et plantaris) L85.2
  scrotal N50.8
  seborrheic L82.1
    inflamed L82.0
  senile L57.0
  solar L57.0
  tonsillaris J35.8
  vagina N89.4
  vegetans Q82.8
  vitamin A deficiency E50.8
  vocal cord J38.3
Kerato-uveitis — see Iridocyclitis
Kerion (celsi) B35.0
Kernicterus of newborn (not due to isoimmunization) P57.9
  due to isoimmunization (conditions in P55.0-P55.9) P57.0
  specified type NEC P57.8
Kerunoparalysis T75.09 ☑
Keshan disease E59
Ketoacidosis E87.2
  diabetic — see Diabetes, by type, with ketoacidosis
Ketonuria R82.4
Ketosis NEC E88.89
  diabetic — see Diabetes, by type, with with ketoacidosis
Kew Garden fever A79.1
Kidney — see condition

Kienböck's disease (see also Osteochondrosis, juvenile, hand, carpal lunate)
  adult M93.1
Kimmelstiel (-Wilson) **disease** — see Diabetes, Kimmelstiel (-Wilson) disease
Kink, kinking
  artery I77.1
  hair (acquired) L67.8
  ileum or intestine — see Obstruction, intestine
  Lane's — see Obstruction, intestine
  organ or site, congenital NEC — see Anomaly, by site
  ureter (pelvic junction) N13.5
    with
      hydronephrosis N13.1
        with infection N13.6
      pyelonephritis (chronic) N11.1
    congenital Q62.39
  vein(s) I87.8
    caval I87.1
    peripheral I87.1
Kinnier Wilson's disease (hepatolenticular degeneration) E83.01
Kissing spine M48.20
  cervical region M48.22
  cervicothoracic region M48.23
  lumbar region M48.26
  lumbosacral region M48.27
  occipito-atlanto-axial region M48.21
  thoracic region M48.24
  thoracolumbar region M48.25
Klatskin's tumor C22.1
Klauder's disease A26.8
Klebs' disease (see also Glomerulonephritis) N05- ☑
Klebsiella (K.) **pneumoniae, as cause of disease classified elsewhere** B96.1
Klein (e)-**Levin syndrome** G47.13
Kleptomania F63.2
Klinefelter's syndrome Q98.4
  karyotype 47,XXY Q98.0
  male with more than two X chromosomes Q98.1
Klippel-Feil deficiency, disease, or syndrome (brevicollis) Q76.1
Klippel's disease I67.2
Klippel-Trenaunay (-Weber) **syndrome** Q87.2
Klumpke (-Déjerine) **palsy, paralysis** (birth) (newborn) P14.1
Knee — see condition
Knock knee (acquired) M21.06- ☑
  congenital Q74.1
Knot(s)
  intestinal, syndrome (volvulus) K56.2
  surfer S89.8- ☑
  umbilical cord (true) O69.2 ☑
Knotting (of)
  hair L67.8
  intestine K56.2
Knuckle pad (Garrod's) M72.1
Koch's
  infection — see Tuberculosis
  relapsing fever A68.9
Koch-Weeks' conjunctivitis — see Conjunctivitis, acute, mucopurulent
Köebner's syndrome Q81.8
Köenig's disease (osteochondritis dissecans) — see Osteochondritis, dissecans
Köhler-Pellegrini-Steida disease or syndrome (calcification, knee joint) — see Bursitis, tibial collateral
Köhler's disease
  patellar — see Osteochondrosis, juvenile, patella
  tarsal navicular — see Osteochondrosis, juvenile, tarsus
Koilonychia L60.3
  congenital Q84.6
Kojevnikov's, epilepsy — see Kozhevnikof's epilepsy
Koplik's spots B05.9
Kopp's asthma E32.8
Korsakoff's (Wernicke) **disease, psychosis or syndrome** (alcoholic) F10.96
  with dependence F10.26
  drug-induced
    due to drug abuse — see Abuse, drug, by type, with amnestic disorder
    due to drug dependence — see Dependence, drug, by type, with amnestic disorder
  nonalcoholic F04
Korsakov's disease, psychosis or syndrome — see Korsakoff's disease

Korsakow's disease, psychosis or syndrome — *see* Korsakoff's disease
Kostmann's disease or syndrome (infantile genetic agranulocytosis) — *see* Agranulocytosis
Kozhevnikof's epilepsy G40.109
   intractable G40.119
     with status epilepticus G40.111
     without status epilepticus G40.119
   not intractable G40.109
     with status epilepticus G40.101
     without status epilepticus G40.109
Krabbe's
   disease E75.23
   syndrome, congenital muscle hypoplasia Q79.8
Kraepelin-Morel disease — *see* Schizophrenia
Kraft-Weber-Dimitri disease Q85.8
Kraurosis
   ani K62.89
   penis N48.0
   vagina N89.8
   vulva N90.4
Kreotoxism A05.9
Krukenberg's
   spindle — *see* Pigmentation, cornea, posterior
   tumor C79.6- ☑
Kufs' disease E75.4
Kugelberg-Welander disease G12.1
Kuhnt-Junius degeneration (*see also* Degeneration, macula) H35.32
Kümmell's disease or spondylitis — *see* Spondylopathy, traumatic
Kupffer cell sarcoma C22.3
Kuru A81.81
Kussmaul's
   disease M30.0
   respiration E87.2
     in diabetic acidosis — *see* Diabetes, by type, with ketoacidosis
Kwashiorkor E40
   marasmic, marasmus type E42
Kyasanur Forest disease A98.2
Kyphoscoliosis, kyphoscoliotic (acquired) (*see also* Scoliosis) M41.9
   congenital Q67.5
   heart (disease) I27.1
   sequelae of rickets E64.3
   tuberculous A18.01
Kyphosis, kyphotic (acquired) M40.209
   cervical region M40.202
   cervicothoracic region M40.203
   congenital Q76.419
     cervical region Q76.412
     cervicothoracic region Q76.413
     occipito-atlanto-axial region Q76.411
     thoracic region Q76.414
     thoracolumbar region Q76.415
   Morquio-Brailsford type (spinal) (*see also* subcategory M49.8) E76.219
   postlaminectomy M96.3
   postradiation therapy M96.2
   postural (adolescent) M40.00
     cervicothoracic region M40.03
     thoracic region M40.04
     thoracolumbar region M40.05
   secondary NEC M40.10
     cervical region M40.12
     cervicothoracic region M40.13
     thoracic region M40.14
     thoracolumbar region M40.15
   sequelae of rickets E64.3
   specified type NEC M40.299
     cervical region M40.292
     cervicothoracic region M40.293
     thoracic region M40.294
     thoracolumbar region M40.295
   syphilitic, congenital A50.56
   thoracic region M40.204
   thoracolumbar region M40.205
   tuberculous A18.01
Kyrle disease L87.0

L

Labia, labium — *see* condition
Labile
   blood pressure R09.89
   vasomotor system I73.9

Labioglossal paralysis G12.29
Labium leporinum — *see* Cleft, lip
Labor — *see* Delivery
Labored breathing — *see* Hyperventilation
Labyrinthitis (circumscribed) (destructive) (diffuse) (inner ear) (latent) (purulent) (suppurative) (*see also* subcategory) H83.0 ☑
   syphilitic A52.79
Laceration
   with abortion — *see* Abortion, by type, complicated by laceration of pelvic organs
   abdomen, abdominal
     wall S31.119 ☑
       with
         foreign body S31.129 ☑
         penetration into peritoneal cavity S31.619 ☑
           with foreign body S31.629 ☑
       epigastric region S31.112 ☑
         with
           foreign body S31.122 ☑
           penetration into peritoneal cavity S31.612 ☑
             with foreign body S31.622 ☑
       left
         lower quadrant S31.114 ☑
           with
             foreign body S31.124 ☑
             penetration into peritoneal cavity S31.614 ☑
               with foreign body S31.624 ☑
         upper quadrant S31.111 ☑
           with
             foreign body S31.121 ☑
             penetration into peritoneal cavity S31.611 ☑
               with foreign body S31.621 ☑
       periumbilic region S31.115 ☑
         with
           foreign body S31.125 ☑
           penetration into peritoneal cavity S31.615 ☑
             with foreign body S31.625 ☑
       right
         lower quadrant S31.113 ☑
           with
             foreign body S31.123 ☑
             penetration into peritoneal cavity S31.613 ☑
               with foreign body S31.623 ☑
         upper quadrant S31.110 ☑
           with
             foreign body S31.120 ☑
             penetration into peritoneal cavity S31.610 ☑
               with foreign body S31.620 ☑
   accidental, complicating surgery — *see* Complications, surgical, accidental puncture or laceration
   Achilles tendon S86.02- ☑
   adrenal gland S37.813 ☑
   alveolar (process) — *see* Laceration, oral cavity
   ankle S91.01- ☑
     with
       foreign body S91.02- ☑
   antecubital space — *see* Laceration, elbow
   anus (sphincter) S31.831 ☑
     with
       ectopic or molar pregnancy O08.6
       foreign body S31.832 ☑
     complicating delivery — *see* Delivery, complicated, by, laceration, anus (sphincter)
     following ectopic or molar pregnancy O08.6
     nontraumatic, nonpuerperal — *see* Fissure, anus
   arm (upper) S41.11- ☑
     with foreign body S41.12- ☑
     lower — *see* Laceration, forearm
   auditory canal (external) (meatus) — *see* Laceration, ear
   auricle, ear — *see* Laceration, ear
   axilla — *see* Laceration, arm
   back (*see also* Laceration, thorax, back)
     lower S31.010 ☑
       with
         foreign body S31.020 ☑
         with penetration into retroperitoneal space S31.021 ☑

Laceration — *continued*
   back (*see also* Laceration, thorax, back) — *continued*
     lower — *continued*
       with — *continued*
         penetration into retroperitoneal space S31.011 ☑
   bile duct S36.13 ☑
   bladder S37.23 ☑
     with ectopic or molar pregnancy O08.6
     following ectopic or molar pregnancy O08.6
     obstetrical trauma O71.5
   blood vessel — *see* Injury, blood vessel
   bowel (*see also* Laceration, intestine)
     with ectopic or molar pregnancy O08.6
     complicating abortion — *see* Abortion, by type, complicated by, specified condition NEC
     following ectopic or molar pregnancy O08.6
     obstetrical trauma O71.5
   brain (any part) (cortex) (diffuse) (membrane) (*see also* Injury, intracranial, diffuse)
     during birth P10.8
       with hemorrhage P10.1
     focal — *see* Injury, intracranial, focal brain injury
   brainstem S06.38- ☑
   breast S21.01- ☑
     with foreign body S21.02- ☑
   broad ligament S37.893 ☑
     with ectopic or molar pregnancy O08.6
     following ectopic or molar pregnancy O08.6
     laceration syndrome N83.8
     obstetrical trauma O71.6
     syndrome (laceration) N83.8
   buttock S31.801 ☑
     with foreign body S31.802 ☑
     left S31.821 ☑
       with foreign body S31.822 ☑
     right S31.811 ☑
       with foreign body S31.812 ☑
   calf — *see* Laceration, leg
   canaliculus lacrimalis — *see* Laceration, eyelid
   canthus, eye — *see* Laceration, eyelid
   capsule, joint — *see* Sprain
   causing eversion of cervix uteri (old) N86
   central (perineal), complicating delivery O70.9
   cerebellum, traumatic S06.37- ☑
   cerebral S06.33- ☑
     during birth P10.8
       with hemorrhage P10.1
     left side S06.32- ☑
     right side S06.31- ☑
   cervix (uteri)
     with ectopic or molar pregnancy O08.6
     following ectopic or molar pregnancy O08.6
     nonpuerperal, nontraumatic N88.1
     obstetrical trauma (current) O71.3
     old (postpartal) N88.1
     traumatic S37.63 ☑
   cheek (external) S01.41- ☑
     with foreign body S01.42- ☑
     internal — *see* Laceration, oral cavity
   chest wall — *see* Laceration, thorax
   chin — *see* Laceration, head, specified site NEC
   chordae tendinae NEC I51.1
     concurrent with acute myocardial infarction — *see* Infarct, myocardium
     following acute myocardial infarction (current complication) I23.4
   clitoris — *see* Laceration, vulva
   colon — *see* Laceration, intestine, large, colon
   common bile duct S36.13 ☑
   cortex (cerebral) — *see* Injury, intracranial, diffuse
   costal region — *see* Laceration, thorax
   cystic duct S36.13 ☑
   diaphragm S27.803 ☑
   digit(s)
     foot — *see* Laceration, toe
     hand — *see* Laceration, finger
   duodenum S36.430 ☑
   ear (canal) (external) S01.31- ☑
     with foreign body S01.32- ☑
     drum S09.2- ☑
   elbow S51.01- ☑
     with
       foreign body S51.02- ☑
   epididymis — *see* Laceration, testis

Laceration — *continued*
  epigastric region — *see* Laceration, abdomen, wall,
      epigastric region
  esophagus K22.8
    traumatic
      cervical S11.21 ☑
        with foreign body S11.22 ☑
      thoracic S27.813 ☑
  eye (ball) S05.3-
    with prolapse or loss of intraocular tissue S05.2- ☑
    penetrating S05.6- ☑
  eyebrow — *see* Laceration, eyelid
  eyelid S01.11- ☑
    with foreign body S01.12- ☑
  face NEC — *see* Laceration, head, specified site NEC
  fallopian tube S37.539 ☑
    bilateral S37.532 ☑
    unilateral S37.531 ☑
  finger(s) S61.219 ☑
    with
      damage to nail S61.319 ☑
        with
          foreign body S61.329 ☑
      foreign body S61.229 ☑
    index S61.218 ☑
      with
        damage to nail S61.318 ☑
          with
            foreign body S61.328 ☑
        foreign body S61.228 ☑
      left S61.211 ☑
        with
          damage to nail S61.311 ☑
            with
              foreign body S61.321 ☑
          foreign body S61.221 ☑
      right S61.210 ☑
        with
          damage to nail S61.310 ☑
            with
              foreign body S61.320 ☑
          foreign body S61.220 ☑
    little S61.218 ☑
      with
        damage to nail S61.318 ☑
          with
            foreign body S61.328 ☑
        foreign body S61.228 ☑
      left S61.217 ☑
        with
          damage to nail S61.317 ☑
            with
              foreign body S61.327 ☑
          foreign body S61.227 ☑
      right S61.216 ☑
        with
          damage to nail S61.316 ☑
            with
              foreign body S61.326 ☑
          foreign body S61.226 ☑
    middle S61.218 ☑
      with
        damage to nail S61.318 ☑
          with
            foreign body S61.328 ☑
        foreign body S61.228 ☑
      left S61.213 ☑
        with
          damage to nail S61.313 ☑
            with
              foreign body S61.323 ☑
          foreign body S61.223 ☑
      right S61.212 ☑
        with
          damage to nail S61.312 ☑
            with
              foreign body S61.322 ☑
          foreign body S61.222 ☑
    ring S61.218 ☑
      with
        damage to nail S61.318 ☑
          with
            foreign body S61.328 ☑
        foreign body S61.228 ☑

Laceration — *continued*
  finger(s) — *continued*
    ring — *continued*
      left S61.215 ☑
        with
          damage to nail S61.315 ☑
            with
              foreign body S61.325 ☑
          foreign body S61.225 ☑
      right S61.214 ☑
        with
          damage to nail S61.314 ☑
            with
              foreign body S61.324 ☑
          foreign body S61.224 ☑
  flank S31.119 ☑
    with foreign body S31.129 ☑
  foot (except toe(s) alone) S91.319 ☑
    with foreign body S91.329 ☑
    left S91.312 ☑
      with foreign body S91.322 ☑
    right S91.311 ☑
      with foreign body S91.321 ☑
    toe — *see* Laceration, toe
  forearm S51.819 ☑
    with
      foreign body S51.829 ☑
    elbow only — *see* Laceration, elbow
    left S51.812 ☑
      with
        foreign body S51.822 ☑
    right S51.811 ☑
      with
        foreign body S51.821 ☑
  forehead S01.81 ☑
    with foreign body S01.82 ☑
  fourchette O70.0
    with ectopic or molar pregnancy O08.6
    complicating delivery O70.0
    following ectopic or molar pregnancy O08.6
  gallbladder S36.123 ☑
  genital organs, external
    female S31.512 ☑
      with foreign body S31.522 ☑
      vagina — *see* Laceration, vagina
      vulva — *see* Laceration, vulva
    male S31.511 ☑
      with foreign body S31.521 ☑
      penis — *see* Laceration, penis
      scrotum — *see* Laceration, scrotum
      testis — *see* Laceration, testis
  groin — *see* Laceration, abdomen, wall
  gum — *see* Laceration, oral cavity
  hand S61.419 ☑
    with
      foreign body S61.429 ☑
    finger — *see* Laceration, finger
    left S61.412 ☑
      with
        foreign body S61.422 ☑
    right S61.411 ☑
      with
        foreign body S61.421 ☑
    thumb — *see* Laceration, thumb
  head S01.91 ☑
    with foreign body S01.92 ☑
    cheek — *see* Laceration, cheek
    ear — *see* Laceration, ear
    eyelid — *see* Laceration, eyelid
    lip — *see* Laceration, lip
    nose — *see* Laceration, nose
    oral cavity — *see* Laceration, oral cavity
    scalp S01.01 ☑
      with foreign body S01.02 ☑
    specified site NEC S01.81 ☑
      with foreign body S01.82 ☑
    temporomandibular area — *see* Laceration, cheek
  heart — *see* Injury, heart, laceration
  heel — *see* Laceration, foot
  hepatic duct S36.13 ☑
  hip S71.019 ☑
    with foreign body S71.029 ☑
    left S71.012 ☑
      with foreign body S71.022 ☑
    right S71.011 ☑
      with foreign body S71.021 ☑

Laceration — *continued*
  hymen — *see* Laceration, vagina
  hypochondrium — *see* Laceration, abdomen, wall
  hypogastric region — *see* Laceration, abdomen, wall
  ileum S36.438 ☑
  inguinal region — *see* Laceration, abdomen, wall
  instep — *see* Laceration, foot
  internal organ — *see* Injury, by site
  interscapular region — *see* Laceration, thorax, back
  intestine
    large
      colon S36.539 ☑
        ascending S36.530 ☑
        descending S36.532 ☑
        sigmoid S36.533 ☑
        specified site NEC S36.538 ☑
      rectum S36.63 ☑
        transverse S36.531 ☑
    small S36.439 ☑
      duodenum S36.430 ☑
      specified site NEC S36.438 ☑
  intra-abdominal organ S36.93 ☑
    intestine — *see* Laceration, intestine
    liver — *see* Laceration, liver
    pancreas — *see* Laceration, pancreas
    peritoneum S36.81 ☑
    specified site NEC S36.893 ☑
    spleen — *see* Laceration, spleen
    stomach — *see* Laceration, stomach
  intracranial NEC (*see also* Injury, intracranial, diffuse)
    birth injury P10.9
  jaw — *see* Laceration, head, specified site NEC
  jejunum S36.438 ☑
  joint capsule — *see* Sprain, by site
  kidney S37.03-
    major (greater than 3 cm) (massive) (stellate)
        S37.06- ☑
    minor (less than 1 cm) S37.04- ☑
    moderate (1 to 3 cm) S37.05- ☑
      multiple S37.06- ☑
  knee S81.01- ☑
    with foreign body S81.02- ☑
  labium (majus) (minus) — *see* Laceration, vulva
  lacrimal duct — *see* Laceration, eyelid
  large intestine — *see* Laceration, intestine, large
  larynx S11.011 ☑
    with foreign body S11.012 ☑
  leg (lower) S81.819 ☑
    with foreign body S81.829 ☑
    foot — *see* Laceration, foot
    knee — *see* Laceration, knee
    left S81.812 ☑
      with foreign body S81.822 ☑
    right S81.811 ☑
      with foreign body S81.821 ☑
    upper — *see* Laceration, thigh
  ligament — *see* Sprain
  lip S01.511 ☑
    with foreign body S01.521 ☑
  liver S36.113 ☑
    major (stellate) S36.116 ☑
    minor S36.114 ☑
    moderate S36.115 ☑
  loin — *see* Laceration, abdomen, wall
  lower back — *see* Laceration, back, lower
  lumbar region — *see* Laceration, back, lower
  lung S27.339 ☑
    bilateral S27.332 ☑
    unilateral S27.331 ☑
  malar region — *see* Laceration, head, specified site
      NEC
  mammary — *see* Laceration, breast
  mastoid region — *see* Laceration, head, specified site
      NEC
  meninges — *see* Injury, intracranial, diffuse
  meniscus — *see* Tear, meniscus
  mesentery S36.893 ☑
  mesosalpinx S37.893 ☑
  mouth — *see* Laceration, oral cavity
  muscle — *see* Injury, muscle, by site, laceration
  nail
    finger — *see* Laceration, finger, with damage to
        nail
    toe — *see* Laceration, toe, with damage to nail
  nasal (septum) (sinus) — *see* Laceration, nose

☑ **Additional Character Required** — Refer to the Tabular List for Character Selection

▽ Subterms under main terms may continue to next column or page

Laceration — *continued*
- nasopharynx — *see* Laceration, head, specified site NEC
- neck S11.91 ☑
  - with foreign body S11.92 ☑
  - involving
    - cervical esophagus S11.21 ☑
      - with foreign body S11.22 ☑
    - larynx — *see* Laceration, larynx
    - pharynx — *see* Laceration, pharynx
    - thyroid gland — *see* Laceration, thyroid gland
    - trachea — *see* Laceration, trachea
    - specified site NEC S11.81 ☑
      - with foreign body S11.82 ☑
- nerve — *see* Injury, nerve
- nose (septum) (sinus) S01.21 ☑
  - with foreign body S01.22 ☑
- ocular NOS S05.3- ☑
  - adnexa NOS S01.11- ☑
- oral cavity S01.512 ☑
  - with foreign body S01.522 ☑
- orbit (eye) — *see* Wound, open, ocular, orbit
- ovary S37.439 ☑
  - bilateral S37.432 ☑
  - unilateral S37.431 ☑
- palate — *see* Laceration, oral cavity
- palm — *see* Laceration, hand
- pancreas S36.239 ☑
- pelvic S31.010 ☑
  - with
    - foreign body S31.020 ☑
      - penetration into retroperitoneal cavity S31.021 ☑
    - penetration into retroperitoneal cavity S31.011 ☑
  - floor (*see also* Laceration, back, lower)
    - with ectopic or molar pregnancy O08.6
    - complicating delivery O70.1
    - following ectopic or molar pregnancy O08.6
    - old (postpartal) N81.89
  - organ S37.93 ☑
- penis S31.21 ☑
  - with foreign body S31.22 ☑
- perineum
  - female S31.41 ☑
    - with
      - ectopic or molar pregnancy O08.6
      - foreign body S31.42 ☑
    - during delivery O70.9
      - first degree O70.0
      - fourth degree O70.3
      - second degree O70.1
      - third degree O70.2
    - old (postpartal) N81.89
    - postpartal N81.89
    - secondary (postpartal) O90.1
  - male S31.119 ☑
    - with foreign body S31.129 ☑
- periocular area (with or without lacrimal passages) — *see* Laceration, eyelid
- peritoneum S36.893 ☑
- periumbilic region — *see* Laceration, abdomen, wall, periumbilic
- periurethral tissue — *see* Laceration, urethra
- phalanges
  - finger — *see* Laceration, finger
  - toe — *see* Laceration, toe
- pharynx S11.21 ☑
  - with foreign body S11.22 ☑
- pinna — *see* Laceration, ear
- popliteal space — *see* Laceration, knee
- prepuce — *see* Laceration, penis
- prostate S37.823 ☑
- pubic region S31.119 ☑
  - with foreign body S31.129 ☑
- pudendum — *see* Laceration, genital organs, external
- rectovaginal septum — *see* Laceration, vagina
- rectum S36.63 ☑
- retroperitoneum S36.893 ☑
- round ligament S37.893 ☑
- sacral region — *see* Laceration, back, lower
- sacroiliac region — *see* Laceration, back, lower
- salivary gland — *see* Laceration, oral cavity
- scalp S01.01 ☑
  - with foreign body S01.02 ☑
- scapular region — *see* Laceration, shoulder

Laceration — *continued*
- scrotum S31.31 ☑
  - with foreign body S31.32 ☑
- seminal vesicle S37.893 ☑
- shin — *see* Laceration, leg
- shoulder S41.019 ☑
  - with foreign body S41.029 ☑
  - left S41.012 ☑
    - with foreign body S41.022 ☑
  - right S41.011 ☑
    - with foreign body S41.021 ☑
- small intestine — *see* Laceration, intestine, small
- spermatic cord — *see* Laceration, testis
- spinal cord (meninges) (*see also* Injury, spinal cord, by region)
  - due to injury at birth P11.5
  - newborn (birth injury) P11.5
- spleen S36.039 ☑
  - major (massive) (stellate) S36.032 ☑
  - moderate S36.031 ☑
  - superficial (minor) S36.030 ☑
- sternal region — *see* Laceration, thorax, front
- stomach S36.33 ☑
- submaxillary region — *see* Laceration, head, specified site NEC
- submental region — *see* Laceration, head, specified site NEC
- subungual
  - finger(s) — *see* Laceration, finger, with damage to nail
  - toe(s) — *see* Laceration, toe, with damage to nail
- suprarenal gland — *see* Laceration, adrenal gland
- temple, temporal region — *see* Laceration, head, specified site NEC
- temporomandibular area — *see* Laceration, cheek
- tendon — *see* Injury, muscle, by site, laceration
  - Achilles S86.02- ☑
- tentorium cerebelli — *see* Injury, intracranial, diffuse
- testis S31.31 ☑
  - with foreign body S31.32 ☑
- thigh S71.11- ☑
  - with foreign body S71.12- ☑
- thorax, thoracic (wall) S21.91 ☑
  - with foreign body S21.92 ☑
    - back S21.22- ☑
      - with penetration into thoracic cavity S21.42- ☑
    - front S21.12- ☑
      - with penetration into thoracic cavity S21.32- ☑
  - back S21.21- ☑
    - with
      - foreign body S21.22- ☑
        - with penetration into thoracic cavity S21.42- ☑
      - penetration into thoracic cavity S21.41- ☑
  - breast — *see* Laceration, breast
  - front S21.11- ☑
    - with
      - foreign body S21.12- ☑
        - with penetration into thoracic cavity S21.32- ☑
      - penetration into thoracic cavity S21.31- ☑
- thumb S61.019 ☑
  - with
    - damage to nail S61.119 ☑
      - with
        - foreign body S61.129 ☑
    - foreign body S61.029 ☑
  - left S61.012 ☑
    - with
      - damage to nail S61.112 ☑
        - with
          - foreign body S61.122 ☑
      - foreign body S61.022 ☑
  - right S61.011 ☑
    - with
      - damage to nail S61.111 ☑
        - with
          - foreign body S61.121 ☑
      - foreign body S61.021 ☑
- thyroid gland S11.11 ☑
  - with foreign body S11.12 ☑

Laceration — *continued*
- toe(s) S91.119 ☑
  - with
    - damage to nail S91.219 ☑
      - with
        - foreign body S91.229 ☑
    - foreign body S91.129 ☑
  - great S91.113 ☑
    - with
      - damage to nail S91.213 ☑
        - with
          - foreign body S91.223 ☑
      - foreign body S91.123 ☑
    - left S91.112 ☑
      - with
        - damage to nail S91.212 ☑
          - with
            - foreign body S91.222 ☑
        - foreign body S91.122 ☑
    - right S91.111 ☑
      - with
        - damage to nail S91.211 ☑
          - with
            - foreign body S91.221 ☑
        - foreign body S91.121 ☑
  - lesser S91.116 ☑
    - with
      - damage to nail S91.216 ☑
        - with
          - foreign body S91.226 ☑
      - foreign body S91.126 ☑
    - left S91.115 ☑
      - with
        - damage to nail S91.215 ☑
          - with
            - foreign body S91.225 ☑
        - foreign body S91.125 ☑
    - right S91.114 ☑
      - with
        - damage to nail S91.214 ☑
          - with
            - foreign body S91.224 ☑
        - foreign body S91.124 ☑
- tongue — *see* Laceration, oral cavity
- trachea S11.021 ☑
  - with foreign body S11.022 ☑
- tunica vaginalis — *see* Laceration, testis
- tympanum, tympanic membrane — *see* Laceration, ear, drum
- umbilical region S31.115 ☑
  - with foreign body S31.125 ☑
- ureter S37.13 ☑
- urethra S37.33 ☑
  - with or following ectopic or molar pregnancy O08.6
  - obstetrical trauma O71.5
- urinary organ NEC S37.893 ☑
- uterus S37.63 ☑
  - with ectopic or molar pregnancy O08.6
  - following ectopic or molar pregnancy O08.6
  - nonpuerperal, nontraumatic N85.8
  - obstetrical trauma NEC O71.81
  - old (postpartal) N85.8
- uvula — *see* Laceration, oral cavity
- vagina S31.41 ☑
  - with
    - ectopic or molar pregnancy O08.6
    - foreign body S31.42 ☑
  - during delivery O71.4
    - with perineal laceration — *see* Laceration, perineum, female, during delivery
  - following ectopic or molar pregnancy O08.6
  - nonpuerperal, nontraumatic N89.8
  - old (postpartal) N89.8
- vas deferens S37.893 ☑
- vesical — *see* Laceration, bladder
- vocal cords S11.031 ☑
  - with foreign body S11.032 ☑
- vulva S31.41 ☑
  - with
    - ectopic or molar pregnancy O08.6
    - foreign body S31.42 ☑
  - complicating delivery O70.0
  - following ectopic or molar pregnancy O08.6
  - nonpuerperal, nontraumatic N90.89
  - old (postpartal) N90.89

Laceration — *continued*
wrist S61.519 ☑
with
foreign body S61.529 ☑
left S61.512 ☑
with
foreign body S61.522 ☑
right S61.511 ☑
with
foreign body S61.521 ☑
Lack of
achievement in school Z55.3
adequate
food Z59.4
intermaxillary vertical dimension of fully erupted teeth M26.36
sleep Z72.820
appetite (see Anorexia) R63.0
awareness R41.9
care
in home Z74.2
of infant (at or after birth) T76.02 ☑
confirmed T74.02 ☑
cognitive functions R41.9
coordination R27.9
ataxia R27.0
specified type NEC R27.8
development (physiological) R62.50
failure to thrive (child over 28 days old) R62.51
adult R62.7
newborn P92.6
short stature R62.52
specified type NEC R62.59
energy R53.83
financial resources Z59.6
food T73.0 ☑
growth R62.52
heating Z59.1
housing (permanent) (temporary) Z59.0
adequate Z59.1
learning experiences in childhood Z62.898
leisure time (affecting life-style) Z73.2
material resources Z59.9
memory (*see also* Amnesia)
mild, following organic brain damage F06.8
ovulation N97.0
parental supervision or control of child Z62.0
person able to render necessary care Z74.2
physical exercise Z72.3
play experience in childhood Z62.898
posterior occlusal support M26.57
relaxation (affecting life-style) Z73.2
sexual
desire F52.0
enjoyment F52.1
shelter Z59.0
sleep (adequate) Z72.820
supervision of child by parent Z62.0
support, posterior occlusal M26.57
water T73.1 ☑
Lacrimal — *see* condition
Lacrimation, abnormal — *see* Epiphora
Lacrimonasal duct — *see* condition
Lactation, lactating (breast) (puerperal, postpartum)
associated
cracked nipple O92.13
retracted nipple O92.03
defective O92.4
disorder NEC O92.79
excessive O92.6
failed (complete) O92.3
partial O92.4
mastitis NEC — *see* Mastitis, obstetric
mother (care and/or examination) Z39.1
nonpuerperal N64.3
Lacticemia, excessive E87.2
Lacunar skull Q75.8
Laennec's cirrhosis K74.69
alcoholic K70.30
with ascites K70.31
Lafora's disease — *see* Epilepsy, generalized, idiopathic
Lag, lid (nervous) — *see* Retraction, lid
Lagophthalmos (eyelid) (nervous) H02.209
cicatricial H02.219
left H02.216
lower H02.215
upper H02.214

Lagophthalmos — *continued*
cicatricial — *continued*
right H02.213
lower H02.212
upper H02.211
keratoconjunctivitis — *see* Keratoconjunctivitis
left H02.206
lower H02.205
upper H02.204
mechanical H02.229
left H02.226
lower H02.225
upper H02.224
right H02.223
lower H02.222
upper H02.221
paralytic H02.239
left H02.236
lower H02.235
upper H02.234
right H02.233
lower H02.232
upper H02.231
right H02.203
lower H02.202
upper H02.201
Laki-Lorand factor deficiency — *see* Defect, coagulation, specified type NEC
Lalling F80.0
Lambert-Eaton syndrome — *see* Syndrome, Lambert-Eaton
Lambliasis, lambliosis A07.1
Landau-Kleffner syndrome — *see* Epilepsy, specified NEC
Landouzy-Déjérine dystrophy or facioscapulohumeral atrophy G71.0
Landouzy's disease (icterohemorrhagic leptospirosis) A27.0
Landry-Guillain-Barré, syndrome or paralysis G61.0
Landry's disease or paralysis G61.0
Lane's
band Q43.3
kink — *see* Obstruction, intestine
syndrome K90.2
Langdon Down syndrome — *see* Trisomy, 21
Lapsed immunization schedule status Z28.3
Large
baby (regardless of gestational age) (4000g to 4499g) P08.1
ear, congenital Q17.1
physiological cup Q14.2
stature R68.89
Large-for-dates NEC (infant) (4000g to 4499g) P08.1
affecting management of pregnancy O36.6- ☑
exceptionally (4500g or more) P08.0
Larsen-Johansson disease or osteochondrosis — *see* Osteochondrosis, juvenile, patella
Larsen's syndrome (flattened facies and multiple congenital dislocations) Q74.8
Larva migrans
cutaneous B76.9
Ancylostoma B76.0
visceral B83.0
Laryngeal — *see* condition
Laryngismus (stridulus) J38.5
congenital P28.89
diphtheritic A36.2
Laryngitis (acute) (edematous) (fibrinous) (infective) (infiltrative) (malignant) (membranous) (phlegmonous) (pneumococcal) (pseudomembranous) (septic) (subglottic) (suppurative) (ulcerative) J04.0
with
influenza, flu, or grippe — *see* Influenza, with, laryngitis
tracheitis (acute) — *see* Laryngotracheitis
atrophic J37.0
catarrhal J37.0
chronic J37.0
with tracheitis (chronic) J37.1
diphtheritic A36.2
due to external agent — *see* Inflammation, respiratory, upper, due to
H. influenzae J04.0
Hemophilus influenzae J04.0
hypertrophic J37.0
influenzal — *see* Influenza, with, respiratory manifestations NEC
obstructive J05.0

Laryngitis — *continued*
sicca J37.0
spasmodic J05.0
acute J04.0
streptococcal J04.0
stridulous J05.0
syphilitic (late) A52.73
congenital A50.59 [J99]
early A50.03 [J99]
tuberculous A15.5
Vincent's A69.1
Laryngocele (congenital) (ventricular) Q31.3
Laryngofissure J38.7
congenital Q31.8
Laryngomalacia (congenital) Q31.5
Laryngopharyngitis (acute) J06.0
chronic J37.0
due to external agent — *see* Inflammation, respiratory, upper, due to
Laryngoplegia J38.00
bilateral J38.02
unilateral J38.01
Laryngoptosis J38.7
Laryngospasm J38.5
Laryngostenosis J38.6
Laryngotracheitis (acute) (Infectional) (infective) (viral) J04.2
atrophic J37.1
catarrhal J37.1
chronic J37.1
diphtheritic A36.2
due to external agent — *see* Inflammation, respiratory, upper, due to
Hemophilus influenzae J04.2
hypertrophic J37.1
influenzal — *see* Influenza, with, respiratory manifestations NEC
pachydermic J38.7
sicca J37.1
spasmodic J38.5
acute J05.0
streptococcal J04.2
stridulous J38.5
syphilitic (late) A52.73
congenital A50.59 [J99]
early A50.03 [J99]
tuberculous A15.5
Vincent's A69.1
Laryngotracheobronchitis — *see* Bronchitis
Larynx, laryngeal — *see* condition
Lassa fever A96.2
Lassitude — *see* Weakness
Late
talker R62.0
walker R62.0
Late effect(s) — *see* Sequelae
Latent — *see* condition
Laterocession — *see* Lateroversion
Lateroflexion — *see* Lateroversion
Lateroversion
cervix — *see* Lateroversion, uterus
uterus, uterine (cervix) (postinfectional) (postpartal, old) N85.4
congenital Q51.818
in pregnancy or childbirth O34.59- ☑
Lathyrism — *see* Poisoning, food, noxious, plant
Launois' syndrome (pituitary gigantism) E22.0
Launois-Bensaude adenolipomatosis E88.89
Laurence-Moon (-Bardet)-**Biedl syndrome** Q87.89
Lax, laxity (*see also* Relaxation)
ligament (ous) (*see also* Disorder, ligament)
familial M35.7
knee — *see* Derangement, knee
skin (acquired) L57.4
congenital Q82.8
Laxative habit F55.2
Lazy leukocyte syndrome D70.8
Lead miner's lung J63.6
Leak, leakage
air NEC J93.82
postprocedural J95.812
amniotic fluid — *see* Rupture, membranes, premature
blood (microscopic), fetal, into maternal circulation
affecting management of pregnancy — *see* Pregnancy, complicated by
cerebrospinal fluid G96.0
from spinal (lumbar) puncture G97.0

Leak, leakage — *continued*
  device, implant or graft (*see also* Complications, by
    site and type, mechanical)
    arterial graft NEC — *see* Complication, cardiovas-
      cular device, mechanical, vascular
    breast (implant) T85.43 ☑
    catheter NEC T85.638 ☑
      dialysis (renal) T82.43 ☑
        intraperitoneal T85.631 ☑
      infusion NEC T82.534 ☑
        spinal (epidural) (subdural) T85.630 ☑
      urinary, indwelling T83.038 ☑
        cystostomy T83.030 ☑
    gastrointestinal — *see* Complications, prosthetic
      device, mechanical, gastrointestinal device
    genital NEC T83.498 ☑
      penile prosthesis T83.490 ☑
    heart NEC — *see* Complication, cardiovascular de-
      vice, mechanical
    joint prosthesis — *see* Complications, joint prosthe-
      sis, mechanical, specified NEC, by site
    ocular NEC — *see* Complications, prosthetic device,
      mechanical, ocular device
    orthopedic NEC — *see* Complication, orthopedic,
      device, mechanical
    persistent air J93.82
    specified NEC T85.638 ☑
    urinary NEC (*see also* Complication, genitourinary,
      device, urinary, mechanical)
      graft T83.23 ☑
    vascular NEC — *see* Complication, cardiovascular
      device, mechanical
    ventricular intracranial shunt T85.03 ☑
  urine — *see* Incontinence
Leaky heart — *see* Endocarditis
Learning defect (specific) F81.9
Leather bottle stomach C16.9
Leber's
  congenital amaurosis H35.50
  optic atrophy (hereditary) H47.22
Lederer's anemia D59.1
Leeches (external) — *see* Hirudiniasis
Leg — *see* condition
Legg (-Calvé)-**Perthes disease, syndrome or osteo-
  chondrosis** M91.1- ☑
Legionellosis A48.1
  nonpneumonic A48.2
Legionnaires'
  disease A48.1
    nonpneumonic A48.2
    pneumonia A48.1
Leigh's disease G31.82
Leiner's disease L21.1
Leiofibromyoma — *see* Leiomyoma
Leiomyoblastoma — *see* Neoplasm, connective tissue,
  benign
Leiomyofibroma (*see also* Neoplasm, connective tissue,
  benign)
  uterus (cervix) (corpus) D25.9
Leiomyoma (*see also* Neoplasm, connective tissue, benign)
  bizarre — *see* Neoplasm, connective tissue, benign
  cellular — *see* Neoplasm, connective tissue, benign
  epithelioid — *see* Neoplasm, connective tissue, benign
  uterus (cervix) (corpus) D25.9
    intramural D25.1
    submucous D25.0
    subserosal D25.2
  vascular — *see* Neoplasm, connective tissue, benign
Leiomyoma, leiomyomatosis (intravascular) — *see*
  Neoplasm, connective tissue, uncertain behavior
Leiomyosarcoma (*see also* Neoplasm, connective tissue,
  malignant)
  epithelioid — *see* Neoplasm, connective tissue, malig-
    nant
  myxoid — *see* Neoplasm, connective tissue, malignant
Leishmaniasis B55.9
  American (mucocutaneous) B55.2
    cutaneous B55.1
  Asian Desert B55.1
  Brazilian B55.2
  cutaneous (any type) B55.1
  dermal (*see also* Leishmaniasis, cutaneous)
    post-kala-azar B55.0
  eyelid B55.1
  infantile B55.0
  Mediterranean B55.0

Leishmaniasis — *continued*
  mucocutaneous (American) (New World) B55.2
  naso-oral B55.2
  nasopharyngeal B55.2
  old world B55.1
  tegumentaria diffusa B55.1
  visceral B55.0
Leishmanoid, dermal (*see also* Leishmaniasis, cutaneous)
  post-kala-azar B55.0
Lenegre's disease I44.2
Lengthening, leg — *see* Deformity, limb, unequal length
Lennert's lymphoma — *see* Lymphoma, Lennert's
Lennox-Gastaut syndrome G40.812
  intractable G40.814
    with status epilepticus G40.813
    without status epilepticus G40.814
  not intractable G40.812
    with status epilepticus G40.811
    without status epilepticus G40.812
Lens — *see* condition
Lenticonus (anterior) (posterior) (congenital) Q12.8
Lenticular degeneration, progressive E83.01
Lentiglobus (posterior) (congenital) Q12.8
Lentigo (congenital) L81.4
  maligna (*see also* Melanoma, in situ)
    melanoma — *see* Melanoma
Lentivirus, as cause of disease classified elsewhere
  B97.31
Leontiasis
  ossium M85.2
  syphilitic (late) A52.78
    congenital A50.59
Lepothrix A48.8
Lepra — *see* Leprosy
Leprechaunism E34.8
Leprosy A30.- ☑
  with muscle disorder A30.9 [M63.80]
    ankle A30.9 [M63.87-] ☑
    foot A30.9 [M63.87-] ☑
    forearm A30.9 [M63.83-] ☑
    hand A30.9 [M63.84-] ☑
    lower leg A30.9 [M63.86-] ☑
    multiple sites A30.9 [M63.89]
    pelvic region A30.9 [M63.85-] ☑
    shoulder region A30.9 [M63.81-] ☑
    specified site NEC A30.9 [M63.88]
    thigh A30.9 [M63.85-] ☑
    upper arm A30.9 [M63.82-] ☑
  anesthetic A30.9
  BB A30.3
  BL A30.4
  borderline (infiltrated) (neuritic) A30.3
    lepromatous A30.4
    tuberculoid A30.2
  BT A30.2
  dimorphous (infiltrated) (neuritic) A30.3
  I A30.0
  indeterminate (macular) (neuritic) A30.0
  lepromatous (diffuse) (infiltrated) (macular) (neuritic)
    (nodular) A30.5
  LL A30.5
  macular (early) (neuritic) (simple) A30.9
  maculoanesthetic A30.9
  mixed A30.3
  neural A30.9
  nodular A30.5
  primary neuritic A30.3
  specified type NEC A30.8
  TT A30.1
  tuberculoid (major) (minor) A30.1
Leptocytosis, hereditary D56.9
Leptomeningitis (chronic) (circumscribed) (hemorrhagic)
  (nonsuppurative) — *see* Meningitis
Leptomeningopathy G96.19
Leptospiral — *see* condition
Leptospirochetal — *see* condition
Leptospirosis A27.9
  canicola A27.89
  due to Leptospira interrogans serovar icterohaemor-
    rhagiae A27.0
  icterohemorrhagica A27.0
  pomona A27.89
  Weil's disease A27.0
Leptus dermatitis B88.0
Leriche's syndrome (aortic bifurcation occlusion) I74.09
Leri's pleonosteosis Q78.8

Leri-Weill syndrome Q77.8
Lermoyez' syndrome — *see* Vertigo, peripheral NEC
Lesch-Nyhan syndrome E79.1
Leser-Trélat disease L82.1
  inflamed L82.0
Lesion(s) (nontraumatic)
  abducens nerve — *see* Strabismus, paralytic, sixth
    nerve
  alveolar process K08.9
  angiocentric immunoproliferative D47.Z9 (*following*
    D47.4)
  anorectal K62.9
  aortic (valve) I35.9
  auditory nerve — *see* subcategory H93.3 ☑
  basal ganglion G25.9
  bile duct — *see* Disease, bile duct
  biomechanical M99.9
    specified type NEC M99.89
      abdomen M99.89
      acromioclavicular M99.87
      cervical region M99.81
      cervicothoracic M99.81
      costochondral M99.88
      costovertebral M99.88
      head region M99.80
      hip M99.85
      lower extremity M99.86
      lumbar region M99.83
      lumbosacral M99.83
      occipitocervical M99.80
      pelvic region M99.85
      pubic M99.85
      rib cage M99.88
      sacral region M99.84
      sacrococcygeal M99.84
      sacroiliac M99.84
      specified NEC M99.89
      sternochondral M99.88
      sternoclavicular M99.87
      thoracic region M99.82
      thoracolumbar M99.82
      upper extremity M99.87
  bladder N32.9
  bone — *see* Disorder, bone
  brachial plexus G54.0
  brain G93.9
    congenital Q04.9
    vascular I67.9
      degenerative I67.9
      hypertensive I67.4
  buccal cavity K13.79
  calcified — *see* Calcification
  canthus — *see* Disorder, eyelid
  carate — *see* Pinta, lesions
  cardia K22.9
  cardiac (*see also* Disease, heart) I51.9
    congenital Q24.9
    valvular — *see* Endocarditis
  cauda equina G83.4
  cecum K63.9
  cerebral — *see* Lesion, brain
  cerebrovascular I67.9
    degenerative I67.9
    hypertensive I67.4
  cervical (nerve) root NEC G54.2
  chiasmal — *see* Disorder, optic, chiasm
  chorda tympani G51.8
  coin, lung R91.1
  colon K63.9
  congenital — *see* Anomaly, by site
  conjunctiva H11.9
  conus medullaris — *see* Injury, conus medullaris
  coronary artery — *see* Ischemia, heart
  cranial nerve G52.9
    eighth — *see* Disorder, ear
    eleventh G52.9
    fifth G50.9
    first G52.0
    fourth — *see* Strabismus, paralytic, fourth nerve
    seventh G51.9
    sixth — *see* Strabismus, paralytic, sixth nerve
    tenth G52.2
    twelfth G52.3
  cystic — *see* Cyst
  degenerative — *see* Degeneration
  duodenum K31.9
  edentulous (alveolar) ridge, associated with trauma,
    due to traumatic occlusion K06.2

Lesion(s) — *continued*
en coup de sabre L94.1
eyelid — *see* Disorder, eyelid
gasserian ganglion G50.8
gastric K31.9
gastroduodenal K31.9
gastrointestinal K63.9
gingiva, associated with trauma K06.2
glomerular
focal and segmental (*see also* N00-N07 with fourth character .1) N05.1
minimal change (*see also* N00-N07 with fourth character .0) N05.0
heart (organic) — *see* Disease, heart
hyperchromic, due to pinta (carate) A67.1
hyperkeratotic — *see* Hyperkeratosis
hypothalamic E23.7
ileocecal K63.9
ileum K63.9
iliohypogastric nerve G57.8- ☑
inflammatory — *see* Inflammation
intestine K63.9
intracerebral — *see* Lesion, brain
intrachiasmal (optic) — *see* Disorder, optic, chiasm
intracranial, space-occupying R90.0
joint — *see* Disorder, joint
sacroiliac (old) M53.3
keratotic — *see* Keratosis
kidney — *see* Disease, renal
laryngeal nerve (recurrent) G52.2
lip K13.0
liver K76.9
lumbosacral
plexus G54.1
root (nerve) NEC G54.4
lung (coin) R91.1
maxillary sinus J32.0
mitral I05.9
Morel-Lavallée — *see* Hematoma, by site
motor cortex NEC G93.89
mouth K13.79
nerve G58.9
femoral G57.2- ☑
median G56.1- ☑
carpal tunnel syndrome — *see* Syndrome, carpal tunnel
plantar G57.6- ☑
popliteal (lateral) G57.3- ☑
medial G57.4- ☑
radial G56.3- ☑
sciatic G57.0- ☑
spinal — *see* Injury, nerve, spinal
ulnar G56.2- ☑
nervous system, congenital Q07.9
nonallopathic — *see* Lesion, biomechanical
nose (internal) J34.89
obstructive — *see* Obstruction
obturator nerve G57.8- ☑
oral mucosa K13.70
organ or site NEC — *see* Disease, by site
osteolytic — *see* Osteolysis
peptic K27.9
periodontal, due to traumatic occlusion K05.5
pharynx J39.2
pigment, pigmented (skin) L81.9
pinta — *see* Pinta, lesions
polypoid — *see* Polyp
prechiasmal (optic) — *see* Disorder, optic, chiasm
primary (*see also* Syphilis, primary) A51.0
carate A67.0
pinta A67.0
yaws A66.0
pulmonary J98.4
valve I37.9
pylorus K31.9
rectosigmoid K63.9
retina, retinal H35.9
sacroiliac (joint) (old) M53.3
salivary gland K11.9
benign lymphoepithelial K11.8
saphenous nerve G57.8- ☑
sciatic nerve G57.0- ☑
secondary — *see* Syphilis, secondary
shoulder (region) M75.9- ☑
specified NEC M75.8- ☑
sigmoid K63.9
sinus (accessory) (nasal) J34.89

Lesion(s) — *continued*
skin L98.9
suppurative L08.0
SLAP S43.43- ☑
spinal cord G95.9
congenital Q06.9
spleen D73.89
stomach K31.9
superior glenoid labrum S43.43- ☑
syphilitic — *see* Syphilis
tertiary — *see* Syphilis, tertiary
thoracic root (nerve) NEC G54.3
tonsillar fossa J35.9
tooth, teeth K08.9
white spot
chewing surface K02.51
pit and fissure surface K02.51
smooth surface K02.61
traumatic — *see* specific type of injury by site
tricuspid (valve) I07.9
nonrheumatic I36.9
trigeminal nerve G50.9
ulcerated or ulcerative — *see* Ulcer, skin
uterus N85.9
vagus nerve G52.2
valvular — *see* Endocarditis
vascular I99.9
affecting central nervous system I67.9
following trauma NEC T14.8
umbilical cord, complicating delivery O69.5 ☑
warty — *see* Verruca
white spot (tooth)
chewing surface K02.51
pit and fissure surface K02.51
smooth surface K02.61
Lethargic — *see* condition
Lethargy R53.83
Letterer-Siwe's disease C96.0
Leukemia, leukemic C95.9- ☑
acute basophilic C94.8- ☑
acute bilineal C95.0- ☑
acute erythroid C94.0- ☑
acute lymphoblastic C91.0- ☑
acute megakaryoblastic C94.2- ☑
acute megakaryocytic C94.2- ☑
acute mixed lineage C95.0- ☑
acute monoblastic (monoblastic/monocytic) C93.0- ☑
acute monocytic (monoblastic/monocytic) C93.0- ☑
acute myeloblastic (minimal differentiation) (with maturation) C92.0- ☑
acute myeloid
with
11q23-abnormality C92.6- ☑
dysplasia of remaining hematopoesis and/or myelodysplastic disease in its history C92.A- ☑ (*following* C92.6)
multilineage dysplasia C92.A- ☑ (*following* C92.6)
variation of MLL-gene C92.6- ☑
M6 (a)(b) C94.0- ☑
M7 C94.2- ☑
acute myelomonocytic C92.5- ☑
acute promyelocytic C92.4- ☑
adult T-cell (HTLV-1-associated) (acute variant) (chronic variant) (lymphomatoid variant) (smouldering variant) C91.5- ☑
aggressive NK-cell C94.8- ☑
AML (1/ETO) (M0) (M1) (M2) (without a FAB classification) C92.0- ☑
AML M3 C92.4- ☑
AML M4 (Eo with inv(16) or t(16;16)) C92.5- ☑
AML M5 C93.0- ☑
AML M5a C93.0- ☑
AML M5b C93.0- ☑
AML Me with t (15;17) and variants C92.4- ☑
atypical chronic myeloid, BCR/ABL-negative C92.2- ☑
biphenotypic acute C95.0- ☑
blast cell C95.0- ☑
Burkitt-type, mature B-cell C91.A- ☑ (*following* C91.6)
chronic lymphocytic, of B-cell type C91.1- ☑
chronic monocytic C93.1- ☑
chronic myelogenous (Philadelphia chromosome (Ph1) positive) (t(9;22)) (q34;q11) (with crisis of blast cells) C92.1- ☑
chronic myeloid, BCR/ABL-positive C92.1- ☑
atypical, BCR/ABL-negative C92.2- ☑
chronic myelomonocytic C93.1- ☑

Leukemia, leukemic — *continued*
chronic neutrophilic D47.1
CMML (-1) (-2) (with eosinophilia) C93.1- ☑
granulocytic (*see also* Category C92) C92.9- ☑
hairy cell C91.4- ☑
juvenile myelomonocytic C93.3- ☑
lymphoid C91.9- ☑
specified NEC C91.Z- ☑ (*following* C91.6)
mast cell C94.3- ☑
mature B-cell, Burkitt-type C91.A- ☑ (*following* C91.6)
monocytic (subacute) C93.9- ☑
specified NEC C93.Z- ☑ (*following* C93.3)
myelogenous (*see also* Category C92) C92.9- ☑
myeloid C92.9- ☑
specified NEC C92.Z- ☑ (*following* C92.6)
plasma cell C90.1- ☑
plasmacytic C90.1- ☑
prolymphocytic
of B-cell type C91.3- ☑
of T-cell type C91.6- ☑
specified NEC C94.8- ☑
stem cell, of unclear lineage C95.0- ☑
subacute lymphocytic C91.9- ☑
T-cell large granular lymphocytic C91.Z- ☑ (*following* C91.6)
unspecified cell type C95.9- ☑
acute C95.0- ☑
chronic C95.1- ☑
Leukemoid reaction (*see also* Reaction, leukemoid) D72.823
Leukoaraiosis (hypertensive) I67.81
Leukoariosis — *see* Leukoaraiosis
Leukocoria — *see* Disorder, globe, degenerated condition, leucocoria
Leukocytopenia D72.819
Leukocytosis D72.829
eosinophilic D72.1
Leukoderma, leukodermia NEC L81.5
syphilitic A51.39
late A52.79
Leukodystrophy E75.29
Leukoedema, oral epithelium K13.29
Leukoencephalitis G04.81
acute (subacute) hemorrhagic G36.1
postimmunization or postvaccinal G04.02
postinfectious G04.01
subacute sclerosing A81.1
van Bogaert's (sclerosing) A81.1
Leukoencephalopathy (*see also* Encephalopathy) G93.49
Binswanger's I67.3
heroin vapor G92
metachromatic E75.25
multifocal (progressive) A81.2
postimmunization and postvaccinal G04.02
progressive multifocal A81.2
reversible, posterior G93.6
van Bogaert's (sclerosing) A81.1
vascular, progressive I67.3
Leukoerythroblastosis D75.9
Leukokeratosis (*see also* Leukoplakia)
mouth K13.21
nicotina palati K13.24
oral mucosa K13.21
tongue K13.21
vocal cord J38.3
Leukokraurosis vulva (e) N90.4
Leukoma (cornea) (*see also* Opacity, cornea)
adherent H17.0- ☑
interfering with central vision — *see* Opacity, cornea, central
Leukomalacia, cerebral, newborn P91.2
periventricular P91.2
Leukomelanopathy, hereditary D72.0
Leukonychia (punctata) (striata) L60.8
congenital Q84.4
Leukopathia unguium L60.8
congenital Q84.4
Leukopenia D72.819
basophilic D72.818
chemotherapy (cancer) induced D70.1
congenital D70.0
cyclic D70.0
drug induced NEC D70.2
due to cytoreductive cancer chemotherapy D70.1
eosinophilic D72.818
familial D70.0

☑ **Additional Character Required** — Refer to the Tabular List for Character Selection   Subterms under main terms may continue to next column or page

Leukopenia — continued
- infantile genetic D70.0
- malignant D70.9
- periodic D70.0
- transitory neonatal P61.5

Leukopenic — see condition

Leukoplakia
- anus K62.89
- bladder (postinfectional) N32.89
- buccal K13.21
- cervix (uteri) N88.0
- esophagus K22.8
- gingiva K13.21
- hairy (oral mucosa) (tongue) K13.3
- kidney (pelvis) N28.89
- larynx J38.7
- lip K13.21
- mouth K13.21
- oral epithelium, including tongue (mucosa) K13.21
- palate K13.21
- pelvis (kidney) N28.89
- penis (infectional) N48.0
- rectum K62.89
- syphilitic (late) A52.79
- tongue K13.21
- ureter (postinfectional) N28.89
- urethra (postinfectional) N36.8
- uterus N85.8
- vagina N89.4
- vocal cord J38.3
- vulva N90.4

Leukorrhea N89.8
- due to Trichomonas (vaginalis) A59.00
- trichomonal A59.00

Leukosarcoma C85.9- ☑

Levocardia (isolated) Q24.1
- with situs inversus Q89.3

Levotransposition Q20.5

Lev's disease or syndrome (acquired complete heart block) I44.2

Levulosuria — see Fructosuria

Levurid L30.2

Lewy body (ies) (dementia) (disease) G31.83

Leyden-Moebius dystrophy G71.0

Leydig cell
- carcinoma
  - specified site — see Neoplasm, malignant, by site
  - unspecified site
    - female C56.9
    - male C62.9- ☑
- tumor
  - benign
    - specified site — see Neoplasm, benign, by site
    - unspecified site
      - female D27.- ☑
      - male D29.2- ☑
  - malignant
    - specified site — see Neoplasm, malignant, by site
    - unspecified site
      - female C56.-
      - male C62.9- ☑
  - specified site — see Neoplasm, uncertain behavior, by site
  - unspecified site
    - female D39.1- ☑
    - male D40.1- ☑

Leydig-Sertoli cell tumor
- specified site — see Neoplasm, benign, by site
- unspecified site
  - female D27.- ☑
  - male D29.2- ☑

LGSIL (Low grade squamous intraepithelial lesion on cytologic smear of)
- anus R85.612
- cervix R87.612
- vagina R87.622

Liar, pathologic F60.2

Libido
- decreased R68.82

Libman-Sacks disease M32.11

Lice (infestation) B85.2
- body (Pediculus corporis) B85.1
- crab B85.3
- head (Pediculus capitis) B85.0
- mixed (classifiable to more than one of the titles B85.0-B85.3) B85.4

Lice — continued
- pubic (Phthirus pubis) B85.3

Lichen L28.0
- albus L90.0
  - penis N48.0
  - vulva N90.4
- amyloidosis E85.4 [L99]
- atrophicus L90.0
  - penis N48.0
  - vulva N90.4
- congenital Q82.8
- myxedematosus L98.5
- nitidus L44.1
- pilaris Q82.8
  - acquired L85.8
- planopilaris L66.1
- planus (chronicus) L43.9
  - annularis L43.8
  - bullous L43.1
  - follicular L66.1
  - hypertrophic L43.0
  - moniliformis L44.3
  - of Wilson L43.9
  - specified NEC L43.8
  - subacute (active) L43.3
  - tropicus L43.3
- ruber
  - acuminatus L44.0
  - moniliformis L44.3
  - planus L43.9
- sclerosus (et atrophicus) L90.0
  - penis N48.0
  - vulva N90.4
- scrofulosus (primary) (tuberculous) A18.4
- simplex (chronicus) (circumscriptus) L28.0
- striatus L44.2
- urticatus L28.2

Lichenification L28.0

Lichenoides tuberculosis (primary) A18.4

Lichtheim's disease or syndrome — see Degeneration, combined

Lien migrans D73.89

Ligament — see condition

Light
- for gestational age — see Light for dates
- headedness R42

Light-for-dates (infant) P05.00
- with weight of
  - 1000-1249 grams P05.04
  - 1250-1499 grams P05.05
  - 1500-1749 grams P05.06
  - 1750-1999 grams P05.07
  - 2000-2499 grams P05.08
  - 499 grams or less P05.01
  - 500-749 grams P05.02
  - 750-999 grams P05.03
- affecting management of pregnancy O36.59- ☑
- and small-for-dates — see Small for dates

Lightning (effects) (stroke) (struck by) T75.00 ☑
- burn — see Burn
- foot E53.8
- shock T75.01 ☑
- specified effect NEC T75.09 ☑

Lightwood-Albright syndrome N25.89

Lightwood's disease or syndrome (renal tubular acidosis) N25.89

Lignac (-de Toni) (-Fanconi) (-Debré) **disease or syndrome** E72.09
- with cystinosis E72.04

Ligneous thyroiditis E06.5

Likoff's syndrome I20.8

Limb — see condition

Limbic epilepsy personality syndrome F07.0

Limitation, limited
- activities due to disability Z73.6
- cardiac reserve — see Disease, heart
- eye muscle duction, traumatic — see Strabismus, mechanical
- mandibular range of motion M26.52

Lindau (-von Hippel) **disease** Q85.8

Line(s)
- Beau's L60.4
- Harris' — see Arrest, epiphyseal
- Hudson's (cornea) — see Pigmentation, cornea, anterior
- Stähli's (cornea) — see Pigmentation, cornea, anterior

Linea corneae senilis — see Change, cornea, senile

Lingua
- geographica K14.1
- nigra (villosa) K14.3
- plicata K14.5
- tylosis K13.29

Lingual — see condition

Linguatulosis B88.8

Linitis (gastric) **plastica** C16.9

Lip — see condition

Lipedema — see Edema

Lipemia (see also Hyperlipidemia)
- retina, retinalis E78.3

Lipidosis E75.6
- cerebral (infantile) (juvenile) (late) E75.4
- cerebroretinal E75.4
- cerebroside E75.22
- cholesterol (cerebral) E75.5
- glycolipid E75.21
- hepatosplenomegalic E78.3
- sphingomyelin — see Niemann-Pick disease or syndrome
- sulfatide E75.29

Lipoadenoma — see Neoplasm, benign, by site

Lipoblastoma — see Lipoma

Lipoblastomatosis — see Lipoma

Lipochondrodystrophy E76.01

Lipochrome histiocytosis (familial) D71

Lipodermatosclerosis — see Varix, leg, with, inflammation
- ulcerated — see Varix, leg, with, ulcer, with inflammation by site

Lipodystrophia progressiva E88.1

Lipodystrophy (progressive) E88.1
- insulin E88.1
- intestinal K90.81
- mesenteric K65.4

Lipofibroma — see Lipoma

Lipofuscinosis, neuronal (with ceroidosis) E75.4

Lipogranuloma, sclerosing L92.8

Lipogranulomatosis E78.89

Lipoid (see also condition)
- histiocytosis D76.3
  - essential E75.29
- nephrosis N04.9
- proteinosis of Urbach E78.89

Lipoidemia — see Hyperlipidemia

Lipoidosis — see Lipidosis

Lipoma D17.9
- fetal D17.9
  - fat cell D17.9
- infiltrating D17.9
- intramuscular D17.9
- pleomorphic D17.9
- site classification
  - arms (skin) (subcutaneous) D17.2- ☑
  - connective tissue D17.30
    - intra-abdominal D17.5
    - intrathoracic D17.4
    - peritoneum D17.79
    - retroperitoneum D17.79
    - specified site NEC D17.39
    - spermatic cord D17.6
  - face (skin) (subcutaneous) D17.0
  - genitourinary organ NEC D17.72
  - head (skin) (subcutaneous) D17.0
  - intra-abdominal D17.5
  - intrathoracic D17.4
  - kidney D17.71
  - legs (skin) (subcutaneous) D17.2- ☑
  - neck (skin) (subcutaneous) D17.0
  - peritoneum D17.79
  - retroperitoneum D17.79
  - skin D17.30
    - specified site NEC D17.39
  - specified site NEC D17.79
  - spermatic cord D17.6
  - subcutaneous D17.30
    - specified site NEC D17.39
  - trunk (skin) (subcutaneous) D17.1
  - unspecified D17.9
- spindle cell D17.9

Lipomatosis E88.2
- dolorosa (Dercum) E88.2
- fetal — see Lipoma
- Launois-Bensaude E88.89

Lipomyoma — see Lipoma

Lipomyxoma — see Lipoma

Lipomyxosarcoma — see Neoplasm, connective tissue, malignant
Lipoprotein metabolism disorder E78.9
Lipoproteinemia E78.5
  broad-beta E78.2
  floating-beta E78.2
  hyper-pre-beta E78.1
Liposarcoma (see also Neoplasm, connective tissue, malignant)
  dedifferentiated — see Neoplasm, connective tissue, malignant
  differentiated type — see Neoplasm, connective tissue, malignant
  embryonal — see Neoplasm, connective tissue, malignant
  mixed type — see Neoplasm, connective tissue, malignant
  myxoid — see Neoplasm, connective tissue, malignant
  pleomorphic — see Neoplasm, connective tissue, malignant
  round cell — see Neoplasm, connective tissue, malignant
  well differentiated type — see Neoplasm, connective tissue, malignant
Liposynovitis prepatellaris E88.89
Lipping, cervix N86
Lipschütz disease or ulcer N76.6
Lipuria R82.0
  schistosomiasis (bilharziasis) B65.0
Lisping F80.0
Lissauer's paralysis A52.17
Lissencephalia, lissencephaly Q04.3
Listeriosis, listerellosis A32.9
  congenital (disseminated) P37.2
  cutaneous A32.0
  neonatal, newborn (disseminated) P37.2
  oculoglandular A32.81
  specified NEC A32.89
Lithemia E79.0
Lithiasis — see Calculus
Lithosis J62.8
Lithuria R82.99
Litigation, anxiety concerning Z65.3
Little leaguer's elbow — see Epicondylitis, medial
Little's disease G80.9
Littre's
  gland — see condition
  hernia — see Hernia, abdomen
Littritis — see Urethritis
Livedo (annularis) (racemosa) (reticularis) R23.1
Liver — see condition
Living alone (problems with) Z60.2
  with handicapped person Z74.2
Lloyd's syndrome — see Adenomatosis, endocrine
Loa loa, loaiasis, loasis B74.3
Lobar — see condition
Lobomycosis B48.0
Lobo's disease B48.0
Lobotomy syndrome F07.0
Lobstein (-Ekman) **disease or syndrome** Q78.0
Lobster-claw hand Q71.6- ☑
Lobulation (congenital) (see also Anomaly, by site)
  kidney, Q63.1
  liver, abnormal Q44.7
  spleen Q89.09
Lobule, lobular — see condition
Local, localized — see condition
Locked twins causing obstructed labor O66.1
Locked-in state G83.5
Locking
  joint — see Derangement, joint, specified type NEC
  knee — see Derangement, knee
Lockjaw — see Tetanus
Löffler's
  endocarditis I42.3
  eosinophilia J82
  pneumonia J82
  syndrome (eosinophilic pneumonitis) J82
Loiasis (with conjunctival infestation) (eyelid) B74.3
Lone Star fever A77.0
Long
  labor O63.9
    first stage O63.0
    second stage O63.1
  QT syndrome I45.81
Longitudinal stripes or grooves, nails L60.8
  congenital Q84.6

Long-term (current) (prophylactic) **drug therapy** (use of)
  agents affecting estrogen receptors and estrogen levels NEC Z79.818
  anastrozole (Arimidex) Z79.811
  antibiotics Z79.2
    short-term use — omit code
  anticoagulants Z79.01
  anti-inflammatory, non-steroidal (NSAID) Z79.1
  antiplatelet Z79.02
  antithrombotics Z79.02
  aromatase inhibitors Z79.811
  aspirin Z79.82
  birth control pill or patch Z79.3
  bisphosphonates Z79.83
  contraceptive, oral Z79.3
  drug, specified NEC Z79.899
  estrogen receptor downregulators Z79.818
  Evista Z79.810
  exemestane (Aromasin) Z79.811
  Fareston Z79.810
  fulvestrant (Faslodex) Z79.818
  gonadotropin-releasing hormone (GnRH) agonist Z79.818
  goserelin acetate (Zoladex) Z79.818
  hormone replacement (postmenopausal) Z79.890
  insulin Z79.4
  letrozole (Femara) Z79.811
  leuprolide acetate (leuprorelin) (Lupron) Z79.818
  megestrol acetate (Megace) Z79.818
  methadone for pain management Z79.891
  Nolvadex Z79.810
  non-steroidal anti-inflammatories (NSAID) Z79.1
  opiate analgesic Z79.891
  oral contraceptive Z79.3
  raloxifene (Evista) Z79.810
  selective estrogen receptor modulators (SERMs) Z79.810
  steroids
    inhaled Z79.51
    systemic Z79.52
  tamoxifen (Nolvadex) Z79.810
  toremifene (Fareston) Z79.810
Loop
  intestine — see Volvulus
  vascular on papilla (optic) Q14.2
Loose (see also condition)
  body
    joint M24.00
      ankle M24.07- ☑
      elbow M24.02- ☑
      hand M24.04- ☑
      hip M24.05- ☑
      knee M23.4- ☑
      shoulder (region) M24.01- ☑
      specified site NEC M24.08
      toe M24.07- ☑
      vertebra M24.08
      wrist M24.03- ☑
    knee M23.4- ☑
    sheath, tendon — see Disorder, tendon, specified type NEC
  cartilage — see Loose, body, joint
  tooth, teeth K08.8
Loosening
  aseptic
    joint prosthesis — see Complications, joint prosthesis, mechanical, loosening, by site
  epiphysis — see Osteochondropathy
  mechanical
    joint prosthesis — see Complications, joint prosthesis, mechanical, loosening, by site
Looser-Milkman (-Debray) **syndrome** M83.8
Lop ear (deformity) Q17.3
Lorain (-Levi) **short stature syndrome** E23.0
Lordosis M40.50
  acquired — see Lordosis, specified type NEC
  congenital Q76.429
    lumbar region Q76.426
    lumbosacral region Q76.427
    sacral region Q76.428
    sacrococcygeal region Q76.428
    thoracolumbar region Q76.425
  lumbar region M40.56
  lumbosacral region M40.57
  postsurgical M96.4
  postural — see Lordosis, specified type NEC
  rachitic (late effect) (sequelae) E64.3

Lordosis — continued
  sequelae of rickets E64.3
  specified type NEC M40.40
    lumbar region M40.46
    lumbosacral region M40.47
    thoracolumbar region M40.45
  thoracolumbar region M40.55
  tuberculous A18.01
Loss (of)
  appetite (see Anorexia) R63.0
    hysterical F50.8
    nonorganic origin F50.8
    psychogenic F50.8
  blood — see Hemorrhage
  consciousness, transient R55
    traumatic — see Injury, intracranial
  control, sphincter, rectum R15.9
    nonorganic origin F98.1
  elasticity, skin R23.4
  family (member) in childhood Z62.898
  fluid (acute) E86.9
    with
      hypernatremia E87.0
      hyponatremia E87.1
  function of labyrinth — see subcategory H83.2 ☑
  hair, nonscarring — see Alopecia
  hearing (see also Deafness)
    central NOS H90.5
    neural NOS H90.5
    perceptive NOS H90.5
    sensorineural NOS H90.5
    sensory NOS H90.5
  height R29.890
  limb or member, traumatic, current — see Amputation, traumatic
  love relationship in childhood Z62.898
  memory (see also Amnesia)
    mild, following organic brain damage F06.8
  mind — see Psychosis
  occlusal vertical dimension of fully erupted teeth M26.37
  organ or part — see Absence, by site, acquired
  ossicles, ear (partial) H74.32- ☑
  parent in childhood Z63.4
  pregnancy, recurrent N96
    without current pregnancy N96
    care in current pregnancy O26.2- ☑
  recurrent pregnancy — see Loss, pregnancy, recurrent
  self-esteem, in childhood Z62.898
  sense of
    smell — see Disturbance, sensation, smell
    taste — see Disturbance, sensation, taste
    touch R20.8
  sensory R44.9
    dissociative F44.6
  sexual desire F52.0
  sight (acquired) (complete) (congenital) — see Blindness
  substance of
    bone — see Disorder, bone, density and structure, specified NEC
    cartilage — see Disorder, cartilage, specified type NEC
      auricle (ear) — see Disorder, pinna, specified type NEC
    vitreous (humor) H15.89
  tooth, teeth — see Absence, teeth, acquired
  vision, visual H54.7
    both eyes H54.3
    one eye H54.60
      left (normal vision on right) H54.62
      right (normal vision on left) H54.61
    specified as blindness — see Blindness
    subjective
      sudden H53.13- ☑
      transient H53.12- ☑
  vitreous — see Prolapse, vitreous
  voice — see Aphonia
  weight (abnormal) (cause unknown) R63.4
Louis-Bar syndrome (ataxia-telangiectasia) G11.3
Louping ill (encephalitis) A84.8
Louse, lousiness — see Lice
Low
  achiever, school Z55.3
  back syndrome M54.5
  basal metabolic rate R94.8
  birthweight (2499 grams or less) P07.10

☑ **Additional Character Required** — Refer to the Tabular List for Character Selection   ▽ **Subterms under main terms may continue to next column or page**

Low — *continued*
  birthweight — *continued*
    with weight of
      1000-1249 grams P07.14
      1250-1499 grams P07.15
      1500-1749 grams P07.16
      1750-1999 grams P07.17
      2000-2499 grams P07.18
    extreme (999 grams or less) P07.00
      with weight of
        499 grams or less P07.01
        500-749 grams P07.02
        750-999 grams P07.03
    for gestational age — *see* Light for dates
  blood pressure (*see also* Hypotension)
    reading (incidental) (isolated) (nonspecific) R03.1
  cardiac reserve — *see* Disease, heart
  function (*see also* Hypofunction)
    kidney N28.9
  hematocrit D64.9
  hemoglobin D64.9
  income Z59.6
  level of literacy Z55.0
  lying
    kidney N28.89
    organ or site, congenital — *see* Malposition, congenital
  output syndrome (cardiac) — *see* Failure, heart
  platelets (blood) — *see* Thrombocytopenia
  reserve, kidney N28.89
  salt syndrome E87.1
  self esteem R45.81
  set ears Q17.4
  vision H54.2
    one eye (other eye normal) H54.50
      left (normal vision on right) H54.52
      other eye blind — *see* Blindness
      right (normal vision on left) H54.51
Low-density-lipoprotein-type (LDL) **hyperlipoproteinemia** E78.0
Lowe's syndrome E72.03
Lown-Ganong-Levine syndrome I45.6
LSD reaction (acute) (without dependence) F16.90
  with dependence F16.20
L-shaped kidney Q63.8
Ludwig's angina or disease K12.2
Lues (venerea), **luetic** — *see* Syphilis
Luetscher's syndrome (dehydration) E86.0
Lumbago, lumbalgia M54.5
  with sciatica M54.4- ☑
    due to intervertebral disc disorder M51.17
    due to displacement, intervertebral disc M51.27
      with sciatica M51.17
Lumbar — *see* condition
Lumbarization, vertebra, congenital Q76.49
Lumbermen's itch B88.0
Lump — *see* Mass
Lunacy — *see* Psychosis
Lung — *see* condition
Lupoid (miliary) **of Boeck** D86.3
Lupus
  anticoagulant D68.62
    with
      hemorrhagic disorder D68.312
      hypercoagulable state D68.62
      finding without diagnosis R76.0
  discoid (local) L93.0
  erythematosus (discoid) (local) L93.0
    disseminated — *see* Lupus, erythematosus, systemic
    eyelid H01.129
      left H01.126
        lower H01.125
        upper H01.124
      right H01.123
        lower H01.122
        upper H01.121
    profundus L93.2
    specified NEC L93.2
    subacute cutaneous L93.1
    systemic M32.9
      with organ or system involvement M32.10
        endocarditis M32.11
        lung M32.13
        pericarditis M32.12
        renal (glomerular) M32.14
          tubulo-interstitial M32.15
        specified organ or system NEC M32.19

Lupus — *continued*
  erythematosus — *continued*
    systemic — *continued*
      drug-induced M32.0
      inhibitor (presence of) D68.62
        with
          hemorrhagic disorder D68.312
          hypercoagulable state D68.62
        finding without diagnosis R76.0
      specified NEC M32.8
  exedens A18.4
  hydralazine M32.0
    correct substance properly administered — *see* Table of Drugs and Chemicals, by drug, adverse effect
    overdose or wrong substance given or taken — *see* Table of Drugs and Chemicals, by drug, poisoning
  nephritis (chronic) M32.14
  nontuberculous, not disseminated L93.0
  panniculitis L93.2
  pernio (Besnier) D86.3
  systemic — *see* Lupus, erythematosus, systemic
  tuberculous A18.4
    eyelid A18.4
  vulgaris A18.4
    eyelid A18.4
Luteinoma D27.- ☑
Lutembacher's disease or syndrome (atrial septal defect with mitral stenosis) Q21.1
Luteoma D27.- ☑
Lutz (-Splendore-de Almeida) **disease** — *see* Paracoccidioidomycosis
Luxation (*see also* Dislocation)
  eyeball (nontraumatic) — *see* Luxation, globe
    birth injury P15.3
  globe, nontraumatic H44.82- ☑
  lacrimal gland — *see* Dislocation, lacrimal gland
  lens (old) (partial) (spontaneous)
    congenital Q12.1
    syphilitic A50.39
Lycanthropy F22
Lyell's syndrome L51.2
  due to drug L51.2
    correct substance properly administered — *see* Table of Drugs and Chemicals, by drug, adverse effect
    overdose or wrong substance given or taken — *see* Table of Drugs and Chemicals, by drug, poisoning
Lyme disease A69.20
Lymph
  gland or node — *see* condition
  scrotum — *see* Infestation, filarial
Lymphadenitis I88.9
  with ectopic or molar pregnancy O08.0
  acute L04.9
    axilla L04.2
    face L04.0
    head L04.0
    hip L04.3
    limb
      lower L04.3
      upper L04.2
    neck L04.0
    shoulder L04.2
    specified site NEC L04.8
    trunk L04.1
  anthracosis (occupational) J60
  any site, except mesenteric I88.9
    chronic I88.1
    subacute I88.1
  breast
    gestational — *see* Mastitis, obstetric
    puerperal, postpartum (nonpurulent) O91.22
  chancroidal (congenital) A57
  chronic I88.1
    mesenteric I88.0
  due to
    Brugia (malayi) B74.1
      timori B74.2
    chlamydial lymphogranuloma A55
    diphtheria (toxin) A36.89
    lymphogranuloma venereum A55
    Wuchereria bancrofti B74.0
  following ectopic or molar pregnancy O08.0
  gonorrheal A54.89
  infective — *see* Lymphadenitis, acute

Lymphadenitis — *continued*
  mesenteric (acute) (chronic) (nonspecific) (subacute) I88.0
    due to Salmonella typhi A01.09
    tuberculous A18.39
  mycobacterial A31.8
  purulent — *see* Lymphadenitis, acute
  pyogenic — *see* Lymphadenitis, acute
  regional, nonbacterial I88.8
  septic — *see* Lymphadenitis, acute
  subacute, unspecified site I88.1
  suppurative — *see* Lymphadenitis, acute
  syphilitic (early) (secondary) A51.49
    late A52.79
  tuberculous — *see* Tuberculosis, lymph gland
  venereal (chlamydial) A55
Lymphadenoid goiter E06.3
Lymphadenopathy (generalized) R59.1
  angioimmunoblastic, with dysproteinemia (AILD) C86.5
  due to toxoplasmosis (acquired) B58.89
    congenital (acute) (subacute) (chronic) P37.1
  localized R59.0
  syphilitic (early) (secondary) A51.49
Lymphadenosis R59.1
Lymphangiectasis I89.0
  conjunctiva H11.89
  postinfectional I89.0
  scrotum I89.0
Lymphangiectatic elephantiasis, nonfilarial I89.0
Lymphangioendothelioma D18.1
  malignant — *see* Neoplasm, connective tissue, malignant
Lymphangioleiomyomatosis J84.81
Lymphangioma D18.1
  capillary D18.1
  cavernous D18.1
  cystic D18.1
  malignant — *see* Neoplasm, connective tissue, malignant
Lymphangiomyoma D18.1
Lymphangiomyomatosis J84.81
Lymphangiosarcoma — *see* Neoplasm, connective tissue, malignant
Lymphangitis I89.1
  with
    abscess — *code by* site under Abscess
    cellulitis — *code by* site under Cellulitis
    ectopic or molar pregnancy O08.0
  acute L03.91
    abdominal wall L03.321
    ankle — *see* Lymphangitis, acute, lower limb
    arm — *see* Lymphangitis, acute, upper limb
    auricle (ear) — *see* Lymphangitis, acute, ear
    axilla L03.12- ☑
    back (any part) L03.322
    buttock L03.327
    cervical (meaning neck) L03.222
    cheek (external) L03.212
    chest wall L03.323
    digit
      finger — *see* Lymphangitis, acute, finger
      toe — *see* Lymphangitis, acute, toe
    ear (external) H60.1- ☑
    external auditory canal — *see* Lymphangitis, acute, ear
    eyelid — *see* Abscess, eyelid
    face NEC L03.212
    finger (intrathecal) (periosteal) (subcutaneous) (subcuticular) L03.02- ☑
    foot — *see* Lymphangitis, acute, lower limb
    gluteal (region) L03.327
    groin L03.324
    hand — *see* Lymphangitis, acute, upper limb
    head NEC L03.891
      face (any part, except ear, eye and nose) L03.212
    heel — *see* Lymphangitis, acute, lower limb
    hip — *see* Lymphangitis, acute, lower limb
    jaw (region) L03.212
    knee — *see* Lymphangitis, acute, lower limb
    leg — *see* Lymphangitis, acute, lower limb
    lower limb L03.12- ☑
      toe — *see* Lymphangitis, acute, toe
    navel L03.326
    neck (region) L03.222
    orbit, orbital — *see* Cellulitis, orbit

Lymphangitis — *continued*
  acute — *continued*
    pectoral (region) L03.323
    perineal, perineum L03.325
    scalp (any part) L03.891
    shoulder — *see* Lymphangitis, acute, upper limb
    specified site NEC L03.898
    thigh — *see* Lymphangitis, acute, lower limb
    thumb (intrathecal) (periosteal) (subcutaneous)
        (subcuticular) — *see* Lymphangitis, acute,
        finger
    toe (intrathecal) (periosteal) (subcutaneous) (sub-
        cuticular) L03.04- ☑
    trunk L03.329
      abdominal wall L03.321
      back (any part) L03.322
      buttock L03.327
      chest wall L03.323
      groin L03.324
      perineal, perineum L03.325
      umbilicus L03.326
    umbilicus L03.326
    upper limb L03.12- ☑
      axilla — *see* Lymphangitis, acute, axilla
      finger — *see* Lymphangitis, acute, finger
      thumb — *see* Lymphangitis, acute, finger
    wrist — *see* Lymphangitis, acute, upper limb
  breast
    gestational — *see* Mastitis, obstetric
  chancroidal A57
  chronic (any site) I89.1
  due to
    Brugia (malayi) B74.1
      timori B74.2
    Wuchereria bancrofti B74.0
  following ectopic or molar pregnancy O08.89
  penis
    acute N48.29
    gonococcal (acute) (chronic) A54.09
  puerperal, postpartum, childbirth O86.89
  strumous, tuberculous A18.2
  subacute (any site) I89.1
  tuberculous — *see* Tuberculosis, lymph gland
Lymphatic (vessel) — *see* condition
Lymphatism E32.8
Lymphectasia I89.0
Lymphedema (acquired) (*see also* Elephantiasis)
  congenital Q82.0
  hereditary (chronic) (idiopathic) Q82.0
  postmastectomy I97.2
  praecox I89.0
  secondary I89.0
  surgical NEC I97.89
    postmastectomy (syndrome) I97.2
Lymphoblastic — *see* condition
Lymphoblastoma (diffuse) — *see* Lymphoma, lym-
    phoblastic (diffuse)
  giant follicular — *see* Lymphoma, lymphoblastic (dif-
    fuse)
  macrofollicular — *see* Lymphoma, lymphoblastic
    (diffuse)
Lymphocele I89.8
Lymphocytic
  chorioencephalitis (acute) (serous) A87.2
  choriomeningitis (acute) (serous) A87.2
  meningoencephalitis A87.2
Lymphocytoma, benign cutis L98.8
Lymphocytopenia D72.810
Lymphocytosis (symptomatic) D72.820
  infectious (acute) B33.8
Lymphoepithelioma — *see* Neoplasm, malignant, by
    site
Lymphogranuloma (malignant) (*see also* Lymphoma,
    Hodgkin)
  chlamydial A55
  inguinale A55
  venereum (any site) (chlamydial) (with stricture of
    rectum) A55
Lymphogranulomatosis (malignant) (*see also* Lym-
    phoma, Hodgkin)
  benign (Boeck's sarcoid) (Schaumann's) D86.1
Lymphohistiocytosis, hemophagocytic (familial) D76.1
Lymphoid — *see* condition
Lymphoma (of) (malignant) C85.90
  adult T-cell (HTLV-1-associated) (acute variant)
    (chronic variant) (lymphomatoid variant)
    (smouldering variant) C91.5- ☑

Lymphoma — *continued*
  anaplastic large cell
    ALK-negative C84.7- ☑
    ALK-positive C84.6- ☑
    CD30-positive C84.6- ☑
    primary cutaneous C86.6
  angioimmunoblastic T-cell C86.5
  BALT C88.4
  B-cell C85.1- ☑
  blastic NK-cell C86.4
  B-precursor C83.5- ☑
  bronchial-associated lymphoid tissue [BALT-lym-
    phoma] C88.4
  Burkitt (atypical) C83.7- ☑
  Burkitt-like C83.7- ☑
  centrocytic C83.1- ☑
  cutaneous follicle center C82.6- ☑
  cutaneous T-cell C84.A- ☑ (*following* C84.7)
  diffuse follicle center C82.5- ☑
  diffuse large cell C83.3- ☑
    anaplastic C83.3- ☑
    B-cell C83.3- ☑
    CD30-positive C83.3- ☑
    centroblastic C83.3- ☑
    immunoblastic C83.3- ☑
    plasmablastic C83.3- ☑
    subtype not specified C83.3- ☑
    T-cell rich C83.3- ☑
  enteropathy-type (associated) (intestinal) T-cell C86.2
  extranodal marginal zone B-cell lymphoma of mucosa-
    associated lymphoid tissue [MALT-lymphoma]
    C88.4
  extranodal NK/T-cell, nasal type C86.0
  follicular C82.9- ☑
    grade
      I C82.0- ☑
      II C82.1- ☑
      III C82.2- ☑
      IIIa C82.3- ☑
      IIIb C82.4- ☑
    specified NEC C82.8- ☑
  hepatosplenic T-cell (alpha-beta) (gamma-delta) C86.1
  histiocytic C85.9- ☑
    true C96.A (*following* C96.6)
  Hodgkin C81.9
    classical C81.7- ☑
      lymphocyte depleted C81.3- ☑
      lymphocyte-rich C81.4- ☑
      mixed cellularity C81.2- ☑
      nodular sclerosis C81.1- ☑
      specified NEC C81.7- ☑
    lymphocyte depleted classical C81.3- ☑
    lymphocyte-rich classical C81.4- ☑
    mixed cellularity classical C81.2- ☑
    nodular
      lymphocyte predominant C81.0- ☑
      sclerosis classical C81.1- ☑
  intravascular large B-cell C83.8- ☑
  Lennert's C84.4- ☑
  lymphoblastic (diffuse) C83.5- ☑
  lymphoblastic B-cell C83.5- ☑
  lymphoblastic T-cell C83.5- ☑
  lymphoepithelioid C84.4- ☑
  lymphoplasmacytic C83.0- ☑
    with IgM-production C88.0
  MALT C88.4
  mantle cell C83.1- ☑
  mature T-cell NEC C84.4- ☑
  mature T/NK-cell C84.9- ☑
    specified NEC C84.Z- ☑ (*following* C84.7)
  mediastinal (thymic) large B-cell C85.2- ☑
  Mediterranean C88.3
  mucosa-associated lymphoid tissue [MALT-lymphoma]
    C88.4
  NK/T cell C84.9- ☑
  nodal marginal zone C83.0- ☑
  non-follicular (diffuse) C83.9- ☑
    specified NEC C83.8- ☑
  non-Hodgkin (*see also* Lymphoma, by type) C85.9- ☑
    specified NEC C85.8- ☑
  non-leukemic variant of B-CLL C83.0- ☑
  peripheral T-cell, not classified C84.4- ☑
  primary cutaneous
    anaplastic large cell C86.6
    CD30-positive large T-cell C86.6
  primary effusion B-cell C83.8- ☑

Lymphoma — *continued*
  SALT C88.4
  skin-associated lymphoid tissue [SALT-lymphoma]
    C88.4
  small cell B-cell C83.0- ☑
  splenic marginal zone C83.0- ☑
  subcutaneous panniculitis-like T-cell C86.3
  T-precursor C83.5- ☑
  true histiocytic C96.A (*following* C96.6)
Lymphomatosis — *see* Lymphoma
Lymphopathia venereum, veneris A55
Lymphopenia D72.810
Lymphoplasmacytic leukemia — *see* Leukemia,
    chronic lymphocytic, B-cell type
Lymphoproliferation, X-linked disease D82.3
Lymphoreticulosis, benign (of inoculation) A28.1
Lymphorrhea I89.8
Lymphosarcoma (diffuse) (*see also* Lymphoma)
    C85.9- ☑
Lymphostasis I89.8
Lypemania — *see* Melancholia
Lysine and hydroxylysine metabolism disorder E72.3
Lyssa — *see* Rabies

M

Macacus ear Q17.3
Maceration, wet feet, tropical (syndrome) T69.02- ☑
MacLeod's syndrome J43.0
Macrocephalia, macrocephaly Q75.3
Macrocheilia, macrochilia (congenital) Q18.6
Macrocolon (*see also* Megacolon) Q43.1
Macrocornea Q15.8
  with glaucoma Q15.0
Macrocytic — *see* condition
Macrocytosis D75.89
Macrodactylia, macrodactylism (fingers) (thumbs)
    Q74.0
  toes Q74.2
Macrodontia K00.2
Macrogenia M26.05
Macrogenitosomia (adrenal) (male) (praecox) E25.9
  congenital E25.0
Macroglobulinemia (idiopathic) (primary) C88.0
  monoclonal (essential) D47.2
  Waldenström C88.0
Macroglossia (congenital) Q38.2
  acquired K14.8
Macrognathia, macrognathism (congenital)
    (mandibular) (maxillary) M26.09
Macrogyria (congenital) Q04.8
Macrohydrocephalus — *see* Hydrocephalus
Macromastia — *see* Hypertrophy, breast
Macrophthalmos Q11.3
  in congenital glaucoma Q15.0
Macropsia H53.15
Macrosigmoid K59.3
  congenital Q43.2
Macrospondylitis , acromegalic E22.0
Macrostomia (congenital) Q18.4
Macrotia (external ear) (congenital) Q17.1
Macula
  cornea, corneal — *see* Opacity, cornea
  degeneration (atrophic) (exudative) (senile) (*see also*
    Degeneration, macula)
  hereditary — *see* Dystrophy, retina
Maculae ceruleae B85.1
Maculopathy, toxic — *see* Degeneration, macula, toxic
Madarosis (eyelid) H02.729
  left H02.726
    lower H02.725
    upper H02.724
  right H02.723
    lower H02.722
    upper H02.721
Madelung's
  deformity (radius) Q74.0
  disease
    radial deformity Q74.0
    symmetrical lipomas, neck E88.89
Madness — *see* Psychosis
Madura
  foot B47.9
    actinomycotic B47.1
    mycotic B47.0
Maduromycosis B47.0
Maffucci's syndrome Q78.4

☑ **Additional Character Required** — Refer to the Tabular List for Character Selection   ▽ **Subterms under main terms may continue to next column or page**

Magnesium metabolism disorder — *see* Disorder, metabolism, magnesium
Main en griffe (acquired) (*see also* Deformity, limb, clawhand)
    congenital Q74.0
Maintenance (encounter for)
    antineoplastic chemotherapy Z51.11
    antineoplastic radiation therapy Z51.0
    methadone F11.20
Majocchi's
    disease L81.7
    granuloma B35.8
Major — *see* condition
Mal de los pintos — *see* Pinta
Mal de mer T75.3 ☑
Malabar itch (any site) B35.5
Malabsorption K90.9
    calcium K90.89
    carbohydrate K90.4
    disaccharide E73.9
    fat K90.4
    galactose E74.20
    glucose (-galactose) E74.39
    intestinal K90.9
        specified NEC K90.89
    isomaltose E74.31
    lactose E73.9
    methionine E72.19
    monosaccharide E74.39
    postgastrectomy K91.2
    postsurgical K91.2
    protein K90.4
    starch K90.4
    sucrose E74.39
    syndrome K90.9
        postsurgical K91.2
Malacia, bone (adult) M83.9
    juvenile — *see* Rickets
Malacoplakia
    bladder N32.89
    pelvis (kidney) N28.89
    ureter N28.89
    urethra N36.8
Malacosteon, juvenile — *see* Rickets
Maladaptation — *see* Maladjustment
Maladie de Roger Q21.0
Maladjustment
    conjugal Z63.0
        involving divorce or estrangement Z63.5
    educational Z55.4
    family Z63.9
    marital Z63.0
        involving divorce or estrangement Z63.5
    occupational NEC Z56.89
    simple, adult — *see* Disorder, adjustment
    situational — *see* Disorder, adjustment
    social Z60.9
        due to
            acculturation difficulty Z60.3
            discrimination and persecution (perceived) Z60.5
            exclusion and isolation Z60.4
            life-cycle (phase of life) transition Z60.0
            rejection Z60.4
            specified reason NEC Z60.8
Malaise R53.81
Malakoplakia — *see* Malacoplakia
Malaria, malarial (fever) B54
    with
        blackwater fever B50.8
            hemoglobinuric (bilious) B50.8
        hemoglobinuria B50.8
    accidentally induced (therapeutically) — *code by type under Malaria*
    algid B50.9
    cerebral B50.0 [G94]
    clinically diagnosed (without parasitological confirmation) B54
    congenital NEC P37.4
        falciparum P37.3
    congestion, congestive B54
    continued (fever) B50.9
    estivo-autumnal B50.9
    falciparum B50.9
        with complications NEC B50.8
            cerebral B50.0 [G94]
        severe B50.8
    hemorrhagic B54

Malaria, malarial — *continued*
    malariae B52.9
        with
            complications NEC B52.8
            glomerular disorder B52.0
    malignant (tertian) — *see* Malaria, falciparum
    mixed infections — *code to first listed type in B50-B53*
    ovale B53.0
    parasitologically confirmed NEC B53.8
    pernicious, acute — *see* Malaria, falciparum
    Plasmodium (P.)
        falciparum NEC — *see* Malaria, falciparum
        malariae NEC B52.9
            with Plasmodium
                falciparum (and or vivax) — *see* Malaria, falciparum
                vivax (*see also* Malaria, vivax)
                    and falciparum — *see* Malaria, falciparum
        ovale B53.0
            with Plasmodium malariae (*see also* Malaria, malariae)
            and vivax (*see also* Malaria, vivax)
                and falciparum — *see* Malaria, falciparum
        simian B53.1
            with Plasmodium malariae (*see also* Malaria, malariae)
            and vivax (*see also* Malaria, vivax)
                and falciparum — *see* Malaria, falciparum
        vivax NEC B51.9
            with Plasmodium falciparum — *see* Malaria, falciparum
    quartan — *see* Malaria, malariae
    quotidian — *see* Malaria, falciparum
    recurrent B54
    remittent B54
    specified type NEC (parasitologically confirmed) B53.8
    spleen B54
    subtertian (fever) — *see* Malaria, falciparum
    tertian (benign) (*see also* Malaria, vivax)
        malignant B50.9
    tropical B50.9
    typhoid B54
    vivax B51.9
        with
            complications NEC B51.8
            ruptured spleen B51.0
Malassez's disease (cystic) N50.8
Malassimilation K90.9
Maldescent, testis Q53.9
    bilateral Q53.20
        abdominal Q53.21
        perineal Q53.22
    unilateral Q53.10
        abdominal Q53.11
        perineal Q53.12
Maldevelopment (*see also* Anomaly)
    brain Q07.9
    colon Q43.9
    hip Q74.2
        congenital dislocation Q65.2
            bilateral Q65.1
            unilateral Q65.0- ☑
    mastoid process Q75.8
    middle ear Q16.4
        except ossicles Q16.4
        ossicles Q16.3
    ossicles Q16.3
    spine Q76.49
    toe Q74.2
Male type pelvis Q74.2
    with disproportion (fetopelvic) O33.3 ☑
        causing obstructed labor O65.3
Malformation (congenital) (*see also* Anomaly)
    adrenal gland Q89.1
    affecting multiple systems with skeletal changes NEC Q87.5
    alimentary tract Q45.9
        specified type NEC Q45.8
        upper Q40.9
            specified type NEC Q40.8
    aorta Q25.9
        atresia Q25.2
        coarctation (preductal) (postductal) Q25.1
        patent ductus arteriosus Q25.0
        specified type NEC Q25.4

Malformation — *continued*
    aorta — *continued*
        stenosis (supravalvular) Q25.3
    aortic valve Q23.9
        specified NEC Q23.8
    arteriovenous, aneurysmatic (congenital) Q27.30
        brain Q28.2
        cerebral Q28.2
        peripheral Q27.30
            digestive system Q27.33
            lower limb Q27.32
            other specified site Q27.39
            renal vessel Q27.34
            upper limb Q27.31
        precerebral vessels (nonruptured) Q28.0
    auricle
        ear (congenital) Q17.3
            acquired H61.119
                left H61.112
                    with right H61.113
                right H61.111
                    with left H61.113
    bile duct Q44.5
    bladder Q64.79
        aplasia Q64.5
        diverticulum Q64.6
        exstrophy — *see* Exstrophy, bladder
        neck obstruction Q64.31
    bone Q79.9
        face Q75.9
            specified type NEC Q75.8
        skull Q75.9
            specified type NEC Q75.8
    brain (multiple) Q04.9
        arteriovenous Q28.2
        specified type NEC Q04.8
    branchial cleft Q18.2
    breast Q83.9
        specified type NEC Q83.8
    broad ligament Q50.6
    bronchus Q32.4
    bursa Q79.9
    cardiac
        chambers Q20.9
            specified type NEC Q20.8
        septum Q21.9
            specified type NEC Q21.8
    cerebral Q04.9
        vessels Q28.3
    cervix uteri Q51.9
        specified type NEC Q51.828
    Chiari
        Type I G93.5
        Type II Q07.01
    choroid (congenital) Q14.3
        plexus Q07.8
    circulatory system Q28.9
    cochlea Q16.5
    cornea Q13.4
    coronary vessels Q24.5
    corpus callosum (congenital) Q04.0
    diaphragm Q79.1
    digestive system NEC, specified type NEC Q45.8
    dura Q07.9
        brain Q04.9
        spinal Q06.9
    ear Q17.9
        causing impairment of hearing Q16.9
        external Q17.9
            accessory auricle Q17.0
            causing impairment of hearing Q16.9
                absence of
                    auditory canal Q16.1
                    auricle Q16.0
            macrotia Q17.1
            microtia Q17.2
            misplacement Q17.4
            misshapen NEC Q17.3
            prominence Q17.5
            specified type NEC Q17.8
        inner Q16.5
        middle Q16.4
            absence of eustachian tube Q16.2
            ossicles (fusion) Q16.3
        ossicles Q16.3
        specified type NEC Q17.8
    epididymis Q55.4

Malformation — continued
  esophagus Q39.9
    specified type NEC Q39.8
  eye Q15.9
    lid Q10.3
    specified NEC Q15.8
  fallopian tube Q50.6
  genital organ — see Anomaly, genitalia
  great
    artery Q25.9
      aorta — see Malformation, aorta
      pulmonary artery — see Malformation, pul-
        monary, artery
      specified type NEC Q25.8
    vein Q26.9
      anomalous
        portal venous connection Q26.5
        pulmonary venous connection Q26.4
          partial Q26.3
          total Q26.2
      persistent left superior vena cava Q26.1
      portal vein-hepatic artery fistula Q26.6
      specified type NEC Q26.8
      vena cava stenosis, congenital Q26.0
  gum Q38.6
  hair Q84.2
  heart Q24.9
    specified type NEC Q24.8
  integument Q84.9
    specified type NEC Q84.8
  internal ear Q16.5
  intestine Q43.9
    specified type NEC Q43.8
  iris Q13.2
  joint Q74.9
    ankle Q74.2
    lumbosacral Q76.49
    sacroiliac Q74.2
    specified type NEC Q74.8
  kidney Q63.9
    accessory Q63.0
    giant Q63.3
    horseshoe Q63.1
    hydronephrosis Q62.0
    malposition Q63.2
    specified type NEC Q63.8
  lacrimal apparatus Q10.6
  lingual Q38.3
  lip Q38.0
  liver Q44.7
  lung Q33.9
  meninges or membrane (congenital) Q07.9
    cerebral Q04.8
    spinal (cord) Q06.9
  middle ear Q16.4
    ossicles Q16.3
  mitral valve Q23.9
    specified NEC Q23.8
  Mondini's (congenital) (malformation, cochlea) Q16.5
  mouth (congenital) Q38.6
  multiple types NEC Q89.7
  musculoskeletal system Q79.9
  myocardium Q24.8
  nail Q84.6
  nervous system (central) Q07.9
  nose Q30.9
    specified type NEC Q30.8
  optic disc Q14.2
  orbit Q10.7
  ovary Q50.39
  palate Q38.5
  parathyroid gland Q89.2
  pelvic organs or tissues NEC
    in pregnancy or childbirth O34.8- ☑
      causing obstructed labor O65.5
  penis Q55.69
    aplasia Q55.5
    curvature (lateral) Q55.61
    hypoplasia Q55.62
  pericardium Q24.8
  peripheral vascular system Q27.9
    specified type NEC Q27.8
  pharynx Q38.8
  precerebral vessels Q28.1
  prostate Q55.4
  pulmonary
    arteriovenous Q25.72

Malformation — continued
  pulmonary — continued
    artery Q25.9
      atresia Q25.5
      specified type NEC Q25.79
      stenosis Q25.6
    valve Q22.3
  renal artery Q27.2
  respiratory system Q34.9
  retina Q14.1
  scrotum — see Malformation, testis and scrotum
  seminal vesicles Q55.4
  sense organs NEC Q07.9
  skin Q82.9
  specified NEC Q89.8
  spinal
    cord Q06.9
    nerve root Q07.8
  spine Q76.49
    kyphosis — see Kyphosis, congenital
    lordosis — see Lordosis, congenital
  spleen Q89.09
  stomach Q40.3
    specified type NEC Q40.2
  teeth, tooth K00.9
  tendon Q79.9
  testis and scrotum Q55.20
    aplasia Q55.0
    hypoplasia Q55.1
    polyorchism Q55.21
    retractile testis Q55.22
    scrotal transposition Q55.23
    specified NEC Q55.29
  thorax, bony Q76.9
  throat Q38.8
  thyroid gland Q89.2
  tongue (congenital) Q38.3
    hypertrophy Q38.2
    tie Q38.1
  trachea Q32.1
  tricuspid valve Q22.9
    specified type NEC Q22.8
  umbilical cord NEC (complicating delivery) O69.89 ☑
  umbilicus Q89.9
  ureter Q62.8
    agenesis Q62.4
    duplication Q62.5
    malposition — see Malposition, congenital, ureter
    obstructive defect — see Defect, obstructive, ureter
    vesico-uretero-renal reflux Q62.7
  urethra Q64.79
    aplasia Q64.5
    duplication Q64.74
    posterior valves Q64.2
    prolapse Q64.71
    stricture Q64.32
  urinary system Q64.9
  uterus Q51.9
    specified type NEC Q51.818
  vagina Q52.4
  vas deferens Q55.4
    atresia Q55.3
  vascular system, peripheral Q27.9
  venous — see Anomaly, vein(s)
  vulva Q52.70
Malfunction (see also Dysfunction)
  cardiac electronic device T82.119 ☑
    electrode T82.110 ☑
    pulse generator T82.111 ☑
    specified type NEC T82.118 ☑
  catheter device NEC T85.618 ☑
    cystostomy T83.010 ☑
    dialysis (renal) (vascular) T82.41 ☑
      intraperitoneal T85.611 ☑
    infusion NEC T82.514 ☑
      spinal (epidural) (subdural) T85.610 ☑
    urinary, indwelling T83.018 ☑
  colostomy K94.03
    valve K94.03
  cystostomy (stoma) N99.512
    catheter T83.010 ☑
  enteric stoma K94.13
  enterostomy K94.13
  esophagostomy K94.33
  gastroenteric K31.89
  gastrostomy K94.23
  ileostomy K94.13
    valve K94.13

Malfunction — continued
  jejunostomy K94.13
  pacemaker — see Malfunction, cardiac electronic de-
    vice
  prosthetic device, internal — see Complications,
    prosthetic device, by site, mechanical
  tracheostomy J95.03
  urinary device NEC — see Complication, genitourinary,
    device, urinary, mechanical
  valve
    colostomy K94.03
    heart T82.09 ☑
    ileostomy K94.13
  vascular graft or shunt NEC — see Complication, car-
    diovascular device, mechanical, vascular
  ventricular (communicating shunt) T85.01 ☑
Malherbe's tumor — see Neoplasm, skin, benign
Malibu disease L98.8
Malignancy (see also Neoplasm, malignant, by site)
  unspecified site (primary) C80.1
Malignant — see condition
Malingerer, malingering Z76.5
Mallet finger (acquired) — see Deformity, finger, mallet
  finger
  congenital Q74.0
  sequelae of rickets E64.3
Malleus A24.0
Mallory's bodies R89.7
Mallory-Weiss syndrome K22.6
Malnutrition E46
  degree
    first E44.1
      mild (protein) E44.1
      moderate (protein) E44.0
    second E44.0
      severe (protein-energy) E43
        intermediate form E42
          with
            kwashiorkor (and marasmus) E42
            marasmus E41
    third E43
  following gastrointestinal surgery K91.2
  intrauterine
    light-for-dates — see Light for dates
    small-for-dates — see Small for dates
  lack of care, or neglect (child) (infant) T76.02 ☑
    confirmed T74.02 ☑
  malignant E40
  protein E46
    calorie E46
      mild E44.1
      moderate E44.0
      severe E43
        intermediate form E42
          with
            kwashiorkor (and marasmus) E42
            marasmus E41
    energy E46
      mild E44.1
      moderate E44.0
      severe E43
        intermediate form E42
          with
            kwashiorkor (and marasmus) E42
            marasmus E41
  severe (protein-energy) E43
    with
      kwashiorkor (and marasmus) E42
      marasmus E41
Malocclusion (teeth) M26.4
  Angle's M26.219
    class I M26.211
    class II M26.212
    class III M26.213
  due to
    abnormal swallowing M26.59
    mouth breathing M26.59
    tongue, lip or finger habits M26.59
  temporomandibular (joint) M26.69
Malposition
  cervix — see Malposition, uterus
  congenital
    adrenal (gland) Q89.1
    alimentary tract Q45.8
      lower Q43.8
      upper Q40.8
    aorta Q25.4
    appendix Q43.8

☑ **Additional Character Required — Refer to the Tabular List for Character Selection**   ▽ **Subterms under main terms may continue to next column or page**

Malposition — *continued*
  congenital — *continued*
    arterial trunk Q20.0
    artery (peripheral) Q27.8
      coronary Q24.5
      digestive system Q27.8
      lower limb Q27.8
      pulmonary Q25.79
      specified site NEC Q27.8
      upper limb Q27.8
    auditory canal Q17.8
      causing impairment of hearing Q16.9
    auricle (ear) Q17.4
      causing impairment of hearing Q16.9
      cervical Q18.2
    biliary duct or passage Q44.5
    bladder (mucosa) — *see* Exstrophy, bladder
    brachial plexus Q07.8
    brain tissue Q04.8
    breast Q83.8
    bronchus Q32.4
    cecum Q43.8
    clavicle Q74.0
    colon Q43.8
    digestive organ or tract NEC Q45.8
      lower Q43.8
      upper Q40.8
    ear (auricle) (external) Q17.4
      ossicles Q16.3
    endocrine (gland) NEC Q89.2
    epiglottis Q31.8
    eustachian tube Q17.8
    eye Q15.8
    facial features Q18.8
    fallopian tube Q50.6
    finger(s) Q68.1
      supernumerary Q69.0
    foot Q66.9
    gallbladder Q44.1
    gastrointestinal tract Q45.8
    genitalia, genital organ(s) or tract
      female Q52.8
        external Q52.79
        internal NEC Q52.8
      male Q55.8
    glottis Q31.8
    hand Q68.1
    heart Q24.8
      dextrocardia Q24.0
        with complete transposition of viscera Q89.3
    hepatic duct Q44.5
    hip (joint) Q65.89
    intestine (large) (small) Q43.8
      with anomalous adhesions, fixation or malrotation Q43.3
    joint NEC Q68.8
    kidney Q63.2
    larynx Q31.8
    limb Q68.8
      lower Q68.8
      upper Q68.8
    liver Q44.7
    lung (lobe) Q33.8
    nail(s) Q84.6
    nerve Q07.8
    nervous system NEC Q07.8
    nose, nasal (septum) Q30.8
    organ or site not listed — *see* Anomaly, by site
    ovary Q50.39
    pancreas Q45.3
    parathyroid (gland) Q89.2
    patella Q74.1
    peripheral vascular system Q27.8
    pituitary (gland) Q89.2
    respiratory organ or system NEC Q34.8
    rib (cage) Q76.6
      supernumerary in cervical region Q76.5
    scapula Q74.0
    shoulder Q74.0
    spinal cord Q06.8
    spleen Q89.09
    sternum NEC Q76.7
    stomach Q40.2
    symphysis pubis Q74.2
    thymus (gland) Q89.2
    thyroid (gland) (tissue) Q89.2
      cartilage Q31.8

Malposition — *continued*
  congenital — *continued*
    toe(s) Q66.9
      supernumerary Q69.2
    tongue Q38.3
    trachea Q32.1
    ureter Q62.60
      deviation Q62.61
      displacement Q62.62
      ectopia Q62.63
      specified type NEC Q62.69
    uterus Q51.818
    vein(s) (peripheral) Q27.8
      great Q26.8
    vena cava (inferior) (superior) Q26.8
  device, implant or graft (*see also* Complications, by site and type, mechanical) T85.628 ☑
    arterial graft NEC — *see* Complication, cardiovascular device, mechanical, vascular
    breast (implant) T85.42 ☑
    catheter NEC T85.628 ☑
      cystostomy T83.020 ☑
      dialysis (renal) T82.42 ☑
        intraperitoneal T85.621 ☑
      infusion NEC T82.524 ☑
        spinal (epidural) (subdural) T85.620 ☑
      urinary, indwelling T83.028 ☑
    electronic (electrode) (pulse generator) (stimulator)
      bone T84.320 ☑
      cardiac T82.129 ☑
        electrode T82.120 ☑
        pulse generator T82.121 ☑
        specified type NEC T82.128 ☑
      nervous system — *see* Complication, prosthetic device, mechanical, electronic nervous system stimulator
      urinary — *see* Complication, genitourinary, device, urinary, mechanical
    fixation, internal (orthopedic) NEC — *see* Complication, fixation device, mechanical
    gastrointestinal — *see* Complications, prosthetic device, mechanical, gastrointestinal device
    genital NEC T83.428 ☑
      intrauterine contraceptive device T83.32 ☑
      penile prosthesis T83.420 ☑
    heart NEC — *see* Complication, cardiovascular device, mechanical
    joint prosthesis — *see* Complication, joint prosthesis, mechanical
    ocular NEC — *see* Complications, prosthetic device, mechanical, ocular device
    orthopedic NEC — *see* Complication, orthopedic, device, mechanical
    specified NEC T85.628 ☑
    urinary NEC (*see also* Complication, genitourinary, device, urinary, mechanical)
      graft T83.22 ☑
    vascular NEC — *see* Complication, cardiovascular device, mechanical
    ventricular intracranial shunt T85.02 ☑
  fetus — *see* Pregnancy, complicated by (management affected by), presentation, fetal
  gallbladder K82.8
  gastrointestinal tract, congenital Q45.8
  heart, congenital NEC Q24.8
  joint prosthesis — *see* Complications, joint prosthesis, mechanical, displacement, by site
  stomach K31.89
    congenital Q40.2
  tooth, teeth, fully erupted M26.30
  uterus (acute) (acquired) (adherent) (asymptomatic) (postinfectional) (postpartal, old) N85.4
    anteflexion or anteversion N85.4
      congenital Q51.818
    flexion N85.4
      lateral — *see* Lateroversion, uterus
    inversion N85.5
    lateral (flexion) (version) — *see* Lateroversion, uterus
      in pregnancy or childbirth — *see* subcategory O34.5 ☑
    retroflexion or retroversion — *see* Retroversion, uterus
Malposture R29.3
Malrotation
  cecum Q43.3
  colon Q43.3

Malrotation — *continued*
  intestine Q43.3
  kidney Q63.2
Malta fever — *see* Brucellosis
Maltreatment
  adult
    abandonment
      confirmed T74.01 ☑
      suspected T76.01 ☑
    confirmed T74.91 ☑
    history of Z91.419
    neglect
      confirmed T74.01 ☑
      suspected T76.01 ☑
    physical abuse
      confirmed T74.11 ☑
      suspected T76.11 ☑
    psychological abuse
      confirmed T74.31 ☑
      history of Z91.411
      suspected T76.31 ☑
    sexual abuse
      confirmed T74.21 ☑
      suspected T76.21 ☑
    suspected T76.91 ☑
  child
    abandonment
      confirmed T74.02 ☑
      suspected T76.02 ☑
    confirmed T74.92 ☑
    history of — *see* History, personal (of), abuse
    neglect
      confirmed T74.02 ☑
      history of — *see* History, personal (of), abuse
      suspected T76.02 ☑
    physical abuse
      confirmed T74.12 ☑
      history of — *see* History, personal (of), abuse
      suspected T76.12 ☑
    psychological abuse
      confirmed T74.32 ☑
      history of — *see* History, personal (of), abuse
      suspected T76.32 ☑
    sexual abuse
      confirmed T74.22 ☑
      history of — *see* History, personal (of), abuse
      suspected T76.22 ☑
    suspected T76.92 ☑
  personal history of Z91.89
Maltworker's lung J67.4
Malunion, fracture — *see* Fracture, by site
Mammillitis N61
  puerperal, postpartum O91.02
Mammitis — *see* Mastitis
Mammogram (examination) Z12.39
  routine Z12.31
Mammoplasia N62
Management (of)
  bone conduction hearing device (implanted) Z45.320
  cardiac pacemaker NEC Z45.018
  cerebrospinal fluid drainage device Z45.41
  cochlear device (implanted) Z45.321
  contraceptive Z30.9
    specified NEC Z30.8
  implanted device Z45.9
    specified NEC Z45.89
  infusion pump Z45.1
  procreative Z31.9
    male factor infertility in female Z31.81
    specified NEC Z31.89
  prosthesis (external) (*see also* Fitting) Z44.9
    implanted Z45.9
      specified NEC Z45.89
  renal dialysis catheter Z49.01
  vascular access device Z45.2
Mangled — *see* specified injury by site
Mania (monopolar) (*see also* Disorder, mood, manic episode)
  with psychotic symptoms F30.2
  without psychotic symptoms F30.10
    mild F30.11
    moderate F30.12
    severe F30.13
  Bell's F30.8
  chronic (recurrent) F31.89
  hysterical F44.89
  puerperal F30.8

Mania — continued
   recurrent F31.89
Manic-depressive insanity, psychosis, or syndrome — see Disorder, bipolar
Mannosidosis E77.1
Mansonelliasis, mansonellosis B74.4
Manson's
   disease B65.1
   schistosomiasis B65.1
Manual — see condition
Maple-bark-stripper's lung (disease) J67.6
Maple-syrup-urine disease E71.0
Marable's syndrome (celiac artery compression) I77.4
Marasmus E41
   due to malnutrition E41
   intestinal E41
   nutritional E41
   senile R54
   tuberculous NEC — see Tuberculosis
Marble
   bones Q78.2
   skin R23.8
Marburg virus disease A98.3
March
   fracture — see Fracture, traumatic, stress, by site
   hemoglobinuria D59.6
Marchesani (-Weill) **syndrome** Q87.0
Marchiafava (-Bignami) **syndrome or disease** G37.1
Marchiafava-Micheli syndrome D59.5
Marcus Gunn's syndrome Q07.8
Marfan's syndrome — see Syndrome, Marfan's
Marie-Bamberger disease — see Osteoarthropathy, hypertrophic, specified NEC
Marie-Charcot-Tooth neuropathic muscular atrophy G60.0
Marie's
   cerebellar ataxia (late-onset) G11.2
   disease or syndrome (acromegaly) E22.0
Marie-Strümpell arthritis, disease or spondylitis — see Spondylitis, ankylosing
Marion's disease (bladder neck obstruction) N32.0
Marital conflict Z63.0
Mark
   port wine Q82.5
   raspberry Q82.5
   strawberry Q82.5
   stretch L90.6
   tattoo L81.8
Marker heterochromatin — see Extra, marker chromosomes
Maroteaux-Lamy syndrome (mild) (severe) E76.29
Marrow (bone)
   arrest D61.9
   poor function D75.89
Marseilles fever A77.1
Marsh fever — see Malaria
Marshall's (hidrotic) **ectodermal dysplasia** Q82.4
Marsh's disease (exophthalmic goiter) E05.00
   with storm E05.01
Masculinization (female) **with adrenal hyperplasia** E25.9
   congenital E25.0
Masculinovoblastoma D27.- ☑
Masochism (sexual) F65.51
Mason's lung J62.8
Mass
   abdominal R19.00
      epigastric R19.06
      generalized R19.07
      left lower quadrant R19.04
      left upper quadrant R19.02
      periumbilic R19.05
      right lower quadrant R19.03
      right upper quadrant R19.01
      specified site NEC R19.09
   breast N63
   chest R22.2
   cystic — see Cyst
   ear H93.8- ☑
   head R22.0
   intra-abdominal (diffuse) (generalized) — see Mass, abdominal
   kidney N28.89
   liver R16.0
   localized (skin) R22.9
      chest R22.2
      head R22.0

Mass — continued
   localized — continued
      limb
         lower R22.4- ☑
         upper R22.3- ☑
      neck R22.1
      trunk R22.2
   lung R91.8
   malignant — see Neoplasm, malignant, by site
   neck R22.1
   pelvic (diffuse) (generalized) — see Mass, abdominal
   specified organ NEC — see Disease, by site
   splenic R16.1
   substernal thyroid — see Goiter
   superficial (localized) R22.9
   umbilical (diffuse) (generalized) R19.09
Massive — see condition
Mast cell
   disease, systemic tissue D47.0
   leukemia C94.3- ☑
   sarcoma C96.2
   tumor D47.0
      malignant C96.2
Mastalgia N64.4
Masters-Allen syndrome N83.8
Mastitis (acute) (diffuse) (nonpuerperal) (subacute) N61
   chronic (cystic) — see Mastopathy, cystic
   cystic (Schimmelbusch's type) — see Mastopathy, cystic
   fibrocystic — see Mastopathy, cystic
   infective N61
      newborn P39.0
   interstitial, gestational or puerperal — see Mastitis, obstetric
   neonatal (noninfective) P83.4
      infective P39.0
   obstetric (interstitial) (nonpurulent)
      associated with
         lactation O91.23
         pregnancy O91.21- ☑
         puerperium O91.22
      purulent
         associated with
            lactation O91.13
            pregnancy O91.11- ☑
            puerperium O91.12
   periductal — see Ectasia, mammary duct
   phlegmonous — see Mastopathy, cystic
   plasma cell — see Ectasia, mammary duct
Mastocytoma D47.0
   malignant C96.2
Mastocytosis Q82.2
   aggressive systemic C96.2
   indolent systemic D47.0
   malignant C96.2
   systemic, associated with clonal hematopoetic non-mast-cell disease (SM-AHNMD) D47.0
Mastodynia N64.4
Mastoid — see condition
Mastoidalgia — see subcategory H92.0 ☑
Mastoiditis (coalescent) (hemorrhagic) (suppurative) H70.9- ☑
   acute, subacute H70.00- ☑
      complicated NEC H70.09- ☑
      subperiosteal H70.01- ☑
   chronic (necrotic) (recurrent) H70.1- ☑
   in (due to)
      infectious disease NEC B99 ☑ [H75.0-] ☑
      parasitic disease NEC B89 [H75.0-] ☑
      tuberculosis A18.03
   petrositis — see Petrositis
   postauricular fistula — see Fistula, postauricular
   specified NEC H70.89- ☑
   tuberculous A18.03
Mastopathy, mastopathia N64.9
   chronica cystica — see Mastopathy, cystic
   cystic (chronic) (diffuse) N60.1- ☑
      with epithelial proliferation N60.3- ☑
   diffuse cystic — see Mastopathy, cystic
   estrogenic, oestrogenica N64.89
   ovarian origin N64.89
Mastoplasia, mastoplastia N62
Masturbation (excessive) F98.8
Maternal care (for) — see Pregnancy (complicated by) (management affected by)
Matheiu's disease (leptospiral jaundice) A27.0

Mauclaire's disease or osteochondrosis — see Osteochondrosis, juvenile, hand, metacarpal
Maxcy's disease A75.2
Maxilla, maxillary — see condition
May (-Hegglin) **anomaly or syndrome** D72.0
McArdle (-Schmid)(-Pearson) **disease** (glycogen storage) E74.04
McCune-Albright syndrome Q78.1
McQuarrie's syndrome (idiopathic familial hypoglycemia) E16.2
Meadow's syndrome Q86.1
Measles (black) (hemorrhagic) (suppressed) B05.9
   with
      complications NEC B05.89
      encephalitis B05.0
      intestinal complications B05.4
      keratitis (keratoconjunctivitis) B05.81
      meningitis B05.1
      otitis media B05.3
      pneumonia B05.2
   French — see Rubella
   German — see Rubella
   Liberty — see Rubella
Meatitis, urethral — see Urethritis
Meatus, meatal — see condition
Meat-wrappers' asthma J68.9
Meckel-Gruber syndrome Q61.9
Meckel's diverticulitis, diverticulum (displaced) (hypertrophic) Q43.0
   malignant — see Table of Neoplasms, small intestine, malignant
Meconium
   ileus, newborn P76.0
      in cystic fibrosis E84.11
      meaning meconium plug (without cystic fibrosis) P76.0
   obstruction, newborn P76.0
      due to fecaliths P76.0
      in mucoviscidosis E84.11
   peritonitis P78.0
   plug syndrome (newborn) NEC P76.0
Median (see also condition)
   arcuate ligament syndrome I77.4
   bar (prostate) (vesical orifice) — see Hyperplasia, prostate
   rhomboid glossitis K14.2
Mediastinal shift R93.8
Mediastinitis (acute) (chronic) J98.5
   syphilitic A52.73
   tuberculous A15.8
Mediastinopericarditis (see also Pericarditis)
   acute I30.9
   adhesive I31.0
   chronic I31.8
   rheumatic I09.2
Mediastinum, mediastinal — see condition
Medicine poisoning — see Table of Drugs and Chemicals, by drug, poisoning
Mediterranean
   fever — see Brucellosis
      familial E85.0
      tick A77.1
   kala-azar B55.0
   leishmaniasis B55.0
   tick fever A77.1
Medulla — see condition
Medullary cystic kidney Q61.5
Medullated fibers
   optic (nerve) Q14.8
   retina Q14.1
Medulloblastoma
   desmoplastic C71.6
   specified site — see Neoplasm, malignant, by site
   unspecified site C71.6
Medulloepithelioma (see also Neoplasm, malignant, by site)
   teratoid — see Neoplasm, malignant, by site
Medullomyoblastoma
   specified site — see Neoplasm, malignant, by site
   unspecified site C71.6
Meekeren-Ehlers-Danlos syndrome Q79.6
Megacolon (acquired) (functional) (not Hirschsprung's disease) (in) K59.3
   Chagas' disease B57.32
   congenital, congenitum (aganglionic) Q43.1
   Hirschsprung's (disease) Q43.1

☑ Additional Character Required — Refer to the Tabular List for Character Selection   Subterms under main terms may continue to next column or page

Megacolon — *continued*
  toxic NEC K59.3
    due to Clostridium difficile A04.7
Megaesophagus (functional) K22.0
  congenital Q39.5
  in (due to) Chagas' disease B57.31
Megalencephaly Q04.5
Megalerythema (epidemic) B08.3
Megaloappendix Q43.8
Megalocephalus, megalocephaly NEC Q75.3
Megalocornea Q15.8
  with glaucoma Q15.0
Megalocytic anemia D53.1
Megalodactylia (fingers) (thumbs) (congenital) Q74.0
  toes Q74.2
Megaloduodenum Q43.8
Megaloesophagus (functional) K22.0
  congenital Q39.5
Megalogastria (acquired) K31.89
  congenital Q40.2
Megalophthalmos Q11.3
Megalopsia H53.15
Megalosplenia — *see* Splenomegaly
Megaloureter N28.82
  congenital Q62.2
Megarectum K62.89
Megasigmoid K59.3
  congenital Q43.2
Megaureter N28.82
  congenital Q62.2
Megavitamin-B6 syndrome E67.2
Megrim — *see* Migraine
Meibomian
  cyst, infected — *see* Hordeolum
  gland — *see* condition
  sty, stye — *see* Hordeolum
Meibomitis — *see* Hordeolum
Meige-Milroy disease (chronic hereditary edema) Q82.0
Meige's syndrome Q82.0
Melalgia, nutritional E53.8
Melancholia F32.9
  climacteric (single episode) F32.8
    recurrent episode F33.9
  hypochondriac F45.29
  intermittent (single episode) F32.8
    recurrent episode F33.9
  involutional (single episode) F32.8
    recurrent episode F33.9
  menopausal (single episode) F32.8
    recurrent episode F33.9
  puerperal F32.8
  reactive (emotional stress or trauma) F32.3
  recurrent F33.9
  senile F03 ☑
  stuporous (single episode) F32.8
    recurrent episode F33.9
Melanemia R79.89
Melanoameloblastoma — *see* Neoplasm, bone, benign
Melanoblastoma — *see* Melanoma
Melanocarcinoma — *see* Melanoma
Melanocytoma, eyeball D31.4- ☑
Melanocytosis, neurocutaneous Q82.8
Melanoderma, melanodermia L81.4
Melanodontia, infantile K03.89
Melanodontoclasia K03.89
Melanoepithelioma — *see* Melanoma
Melanoma (malignant) C43.9
  acral lentiginous, malignant — *see* Melanoma, skin, by site
  amelanotic — *see* Melanoma, skin, by site
  balloon cell — *see* Melanoma, skin, by site
  benign — *see* Nevus
  desmoplastic, malignant — *see* Melanoma, skin, by site
  epithelioid cell — *see* Melanoma, skin, by site
    with spindle cell, mixed — *see* Melanoma, skin, by site
  in
    giant pigmented nevus — *see* Melanoma, skin, by site
    Hutchinson's melanotic freckle — *see* Melanoma, skin, by site
    junctional nevus — *see* Melanoma, skin, by site
    precancerous melanosis — *see* Melanoma, skin, by site
  in situ D03.9
    abdominal wall D03.59

Melanoma — *continued*
  in situ — *continued*
    ala nasi D03.39
    ankle D03.7- ☑
    anus, anal (margin) (skin) D03.51
    arm D03.6- ☑
    auditory canal D03.2- ☑
    auricle (ear) D03.2- ☑
    auricular canal (external) D03.2- ☑
    axilla, axillary fold D03.59
    back D03.59
    breast D03.52
    brow D03.39
    buttock D03.59
    canthus (eye) D03.1- ☑
    cheek (external) D03.39
    chest wall D03.59
    chin D03.39
    choroid D03.8
    conjunctiva D03.8
    ear (external) D03.2- ☑
    external meatus (ear) D03.2- ☑
    eye D03.8
    eyebrow D03.39
    eyelid (lower) (upper) D03.1- ☑
    face D03.30
      specified NEC D03.39
    female genital organ (external) NEC D03.8
    finger D03.6- ☑
    flank D03.59
    foot D03.7- ☑
    forearm D03.6- ☑
    forehead D03.39
    foreskin D03.8
    gluteal region D03.59
    groin D03.59
    hand D03.6- ☑
    heel D03.7- ☑
    helix D03.2- ☑
    hip D03.7- ☑
    interscapular region D03.59
    iris D03.8
    jaw D03.39
    knee D03.7- ☑
    labium (majus) (minus) D03.8
    lacrimal gland D03.8
    leg D03.7- ☑
    lip (lower) (upper) D03.0
    lower limb NEC D03.7- ☑
    male genital organ (external) NEC D03.8
    nail D03.9
      finger D03.6- ☑
      toe D03.7- ☑
    neck D03.4
    nose (external) D03.39
    orbit D03.8
    penis D03.8
    perianal skin D03.51
    perineum D03.51
    pinna D03.2- ☑
    popliteal fossa or space D03.7- ☑
    prepuce D03.8
    pudendum D03.8
    retina D03.8
    retrobulbar D03.8
    scalp D03.4
    scrotum D03.8
    shoulder D03.6- ☑
    specified site NEC D03.8
    submammary fold D03.52
    temple D03.39
    thigh D03.7- ☑
    toe D03.7- ☑
    trunk NEC D03.59
    umbilicus D03.59
    upper limb NEC D03.6- ☑
    vulva D03.8
  juvenile — *see* Nevus
  malignant, of soft parts except skin — *see* Neoplasm, connective tissue, malignant
  metastatic
    breast C79.81
    genital organ C79.82
    specified site NEC C79.89
  neurotropic, malignant — *see* Melanoma, skin, by site
  nodular — *see* Melanoma, skin, by site
  regressing, malignant — *see* Melanoma, skin, by site

Melanoma — *continued*
  skin C43.9
    abdominal wall C43.59
    ala nasi C43.31
    ankle C43.7- ☑
    anus, anal (skin) C43.51
    arm C43.6- ☑
    auditory canal (external) C43.2- ☑
    auricle (ear) C43.2- ☑
    auricular canal (external) C43.2- ☑
    axilla, axillary fold C43.59
    back C43.59
    breast (female) (male) C43.52
    brow C43.39
    buttock C43.59
    canthus (eye) C43.1- ☑
    cheek (external) C43.39
    chest wall C43.59
    chin C43.39
    ear (external) C43.2- ☑
    elbow C43.6- ☑
    external meatus (ear) C43.2- ☑
    eyebrow C43.39
    eyelid (lower) (upper) C43.1- ☑
    face C43.30
      specified NEC C43.39
    female genital organ (external) NEC C51.9
    finger C43.6- ☑
    flank C43.59
    foot C43.7- ☑
    forearm C43.6- ☑
    forehead C43.39
    foreskin C60.0
    glabella C43.39
    gluteal region C43.59
    groin C43.59
    hand C43.6- ☑
    heel C43.7- ☑
    helix C43.2- ☑
    hip C43.7- ☑
    interscapular region C43.59
    jaw (external) C43.39
    knee C43.7- ☑
    labium C51.9
      majus C51.0
      minus C51.1
    leg C43.7- ☑
    lip (lower) (upper) C43.0
    lower limb NEC C43.7- ☑
    male genital organ (external) NEC C63.9
    nail
      finger C43.6- ☑
      toe C43.7- ☑
    nasolabial groove C43.39
    nates C43.59
    neck C43.4
    nose (external) C43.31
    overlapping site C43.8
    palpebra C43.1- ☑
    penis C60.9
    perianal skin C43.51
    perineum C43.51
    pinna C43.2- ☑
    popliteal fossa or space C43.7- ☑
    prepuce C60.0
    pudendum C51.9
    scalp C43.4
    scrotum C63.2
    shoulder C43.6- ☑
    skin NEC C43.9
    submammary fold C43.52
    temple C43.39
    thigh C43.7- ☑
    toe C43.7- ☑
    trunk NEC C43.59
    umbilicus C43.59
    upper limb NEC C43.6- ☑
    vulva C51.9
      overlapping sites C51.8
  spindle cell
    with epithelioid, mixed — *see* Melanoma, skin, by site
    type A C69.4- ☑
    type B C69.4- ☑
  superficial spreading — *see* Melanoma, skin, by site
Melanosarcoma (*see also* Melanoma)
  epithelioid cell — *see* Melanoma

▽ Subterms under main terms may continue to next column or page   ☑ **Additional Character Required** — **Refer to the Tabular List for Character Selection**

Melanosis L81.4
addisonian E27.1
tuberculous A18.7
adrenal E27.1
colon K63.89
conjunctiva — see Pigmentation, conjunctiva
congenital Q13.89
cornea (presenile) (senile) (see also Pigmentation,
cornea)
congenital Q13.4
eye NEC H57.8
congenital Q15.8
lenticularis progressiva Q82.1
liver K76.89
precancerous (see also Melanoma, in situ)
malignant melanoma in — see Melanoma
Riehl's L81.4
sclera H15.89
congenital Q13.89
suprarenal E27.1
tar L81.4
toxic L81.4
Melanuria R82.99
MELAS syndrome E88.41
Melasma L81.1
adrenal (gland) E27.1
suprarenal (gland) E27.1
Melena K92.1
with ulcer — code by site under Ulcer, with hemorrhage K27.4
due to swallowed maternal blood P78.2
newborn, neonatal P54.1
due to swallowed maternal blood P78.2
Meleney's
gangrene (cutaneous) — see Ulcer, skin
ulcer (chronic undermining) — see Ulcer, skin
Melioidosis A24.9
acute A24.1
chronic A24.2
fulminating A24.1
pneumonia A24.1
pulmonary (chronic) A24.2
acute A24.1
subacute A24.2
sepsis A24.1
specified NEC A24.3
subacute A24.2
Melitensis, febris A23.0
Melkersson (-Rosenthal) **syndrome** G51.2
Mellitus, diabetes — see Diabetes
Melorheostosis (bone) — see Disorder, bone, density
and structure, specified NEC
Meloschisis Q18.4
Melotia Q17.4
Membrana
capsularis lentis posterior Q13.89
epipapillaris Q14.2
Membranacea placenta O43.19- ☑
Membranaceous uterus N85.8
Membrane(s), membranous (see also condition)
cyclitic — see Membrane, pupillary
folds, congenital — see Web
Jackson's Q43.3
over face of newborn P28.9
premature rupture — see Rupture, membranes, premature
pupillary H21.4- ☑
persistent Q13.89
retained (with hemorrhage) (complicating delivery)
O72.2
without hemorrhage O73.1
secondary cataract — see Cataract, secondary
unruptured (causing asphyxia) — see Asphyxia, newborn
vitreous — see Opacity, vitreous, membranes and
strands
Membranitis — see Chorioamnionitis
Memory disturbance, lack or loss (see also Amnesia)
mild, following organic brain damage F06.8
Menadione deficiency E56.1
Menarche
delayed E30.0
precocious E30.1
Mendacity, pathologic F60.2
Mendelson's syndrome (due to anesthesia) J95.4
in labor and delivery O74.0
in pregnancy O29.01- ☑

Mendelson's syndrome — continued
obstetric O74.0
postpartum, puerperal O89.01
Ménétrier's disease or syndrome K29.60
with bleeding K29.61
Ménière's disease, syndrome or vertigo H81.0- ☑
Meninges, meningeal — see condition
Meningioma (see also Neoplasm, meninges, benign)
angioblastic — see Neoplasm, meninges, benign
angiomatous — see Neoplasm, meninges, benign
endotheliomatous — see Neoplasm, meninges, benign
fibroblastic — see Neoplasm, meninges, benign
fibrous — see Neoplasm, meninges, benign
hemangioblastic — see Neoplasm, meninges, benign
hemangiopericytic — see Neoplasm, meninges, benign
malignant — see Neoplasm, meninges, malignant
meningiothelial — see Neoplasm, meninges, benign
meningotheliomatous — see Neoplasm, meninges,
benign
mixed — see Neoplasm, meninges, benign
multiple — see Neoplasm, meninges, uncertain behavior
papillary — see Neoplasm, meninges, uncertain behavior
psammomatous — see Neoplasm, meninges, benign
syncytial — see Neoplasm, meninges, benign
transitional — see Neoplasm, meninges, benign
Meningiomatosis (diffuse) — see Neoplasm, meninges,
uncertain behavior
Meningism — see Meningismus
Meningismus (infectional) (pneumococcal) R29.1
due to serum or vaccine R29.1
influenzal — see Influenza, with, manifestations NEC
Meningitis (basal) (basic) (brain) (cerebral) (cervical)
(congestive) (diffuse) (hemorrhagic) (infantile)
(membranous) (metastatic) (nonspecific) (pontine)
(progressive) (simple) (spinal) (subacute) (sympathetic) (toxic) G03.9
abacterial G03.0
actinomycotic A42.81
adenoviral A87.1
arbovirus A87.8
aseptic (acute) G03.0
bacterial G00.9
Escherichia coli (E. coli) G00.8
Friedländer (bacillus) G00.8
gram-negative G00.9
H. influenzae G00.0
Klebsiella G00.8
pneumococcal G00.1
specified organism NEC G00.8
staphylococcal G00.3
streptococcal (acute) G00.2
benign recurrent (Mollaret) G03.2
candidal B37.5
caseous (tuberculous) A17.0
cerebrospinal A39.0
chronic NEC G03.1
clear cerebrospinal fluid NEC G03.0
coxsackievirus A87.0
cryptococcal B45.1
diplococcal (gram positive) A39.0
echovirus A87.0
enteroviral A87.0
eosinophilic B83.2
epidemic NEC A39.0
Escherichia coli (E. coli) G00.8
fibrinopurulent G00.9
specified organism NEC G00.8
Friedländer (bacillus) G00.8
gonococcal A54.81
gram-negative cocci G00.9
gram-positive cocci G00.9
H. influenzae G00.0
Haemophilus (influenzae) G00.0
in (due to)
adenovirus A87.1
African trypanosomiasis B56.9 [G02]
anthrax A22.8
bacterial disease NEC A48.8 [G01]
Chagas' disease (chronic) B57.41
chickenpox B01.0
coccidioidomycosis B38.4
Diplococcus pneumoniae G00.1
enterovirus A87.0
herpes (simplex) virus B00.3
zoster B02.1

Meningitis — continued
in — continued
infectious mononucleosis B27.92
leptospirosis A27.81
Listeria monocytogenes A32.11
Lyme disease A69.21
measles B05.1
mumps (virus) B26.1
neurosyphilis (late) A52.13
parasitic disease NEC B89 [G02]
poliovirus A80.9 [G02]
preventive immunization, inoculation or vaccination G03.8
rubella B06.02
Salmonella infection A02.21
specified cause NEC G03.8
typhoid fever A01.01
varicella B01.0
viral disease NEC A87.8
whooping cough A37.90
zoster B02.1
infectious G00.9
influenzal (H. influenzae) G00.0
Klebsiella G00.8
leptospiral (aseptic) A27.81
lymphocytic (acute) (benign) (serous) A87.2
meningococcal A39.0
Mima polymorpha G00.8
Mollaret (benign recurrent) G03.2
monilial B37.5
mycotic NEC B49 [G02]
Neisseria A39.0
nonbacterial G03.0
nonpyogenic NEC G03.0
ossificans G96.19
pneumococcal G00.1
poliovirus A80.9 [G02]
postmeasles B05.1
purulent G00.9
specified organism NEC G00.8
pyogenic G00.9
specified organism NEC G00.8
Salmonella (arizonae) (Cholerae-Suis) (enteritidis) (typhimurium) A02.21
septic G00.9
specified organism NEC G00.8
serosa circumscripta NEC G03.0
serous NEC G93.2
specified organism NEC G00.8
sporotrichosis B42.81
staphylococcal G00.3
sterile G03.0
streptococcal (acute) G00.2
suppurative G00.9
specified organism NEC G00.8
syphilitic (late) (tertiary) A52.13
acute A51.41
congenital A50.41
secondary A51.41
Torula histolytica (cryptococcal) B45.1
traumatic (complication of injury) T79.8 ☑
tuberculous A17.0
typhoid A01.01
viral NEC A87.9
Yersinia pestis A20.3
Meningocele (spinal) (see also Spina bifida)
with hydrocephalus — see Spina bifida, by site, with
hydrocephalus
acquired (traumatic) G96.19
cerebral — see Encephalocele
Meningocerebritis — see Meningoencephalitis
Meningococcemia A39.4
acute A39.2
chronic A39.3
Meningococcus, meningococcal (see also condition)
A39.9
adrenalitis, hemorrhagic A39.1
carrier (suspected) of Z22.31
meningitis (cerebrospinal) A39.0
Meningoencephalitis (see also Encephalitis) G04.90
acute NEC (see also Encephalitis, viral) A86
bacterial NEC G04.2
California A83.5
diphasic A84.1
eosinophilic B83.2
epidemic A39.81
herpesviral, herpetic B00.4
due to herpesvirus 6 B10.01

☑ **Additional Character Required** — Refer to the Tabular List for Character Selection   ▽ **Subterms under main terms may continue to next column or page**

Meningoencephalitis — *continued*
  herpesviral, herpetic — *continued*
    due to herpesvirus 7 B10.09
    specified NEC B10.09
  in (due to)
    blastomycosis NEC B40.81
    diseases classified elsewhere G05.3
    free-living amebae B60.2
    H. influenzae G00.0
    Hemophilus influenzae (H .influenzae) G04.2
    herpes B00.4
      due to herpesvirus 6 B10.01
      due to herpesvirus 7 B10.09
      specified NEC B10.09
    Lyme disease A69.22
    mercury — *see* subcategory T56.1 ☑
    mumps B26.2
    Naegleria (amebae) (organisms) (fowleri) B60.2
    Parastrongylus cantonensis B83.2
    toxoplasmosis (acquired) B58.2
      congenital P37.1
  infectious (acute) (viral) A86
  influenzal (H. influenzae) G04.2
  Listeria monocytogenes A32.12
  lymphocytic (serous) A87.2
  mumps B26.2
  parasitic NEC B89 [G05.3]
  pneumococcal G00.1
  primary amebic B60.2
  specific (syphilitic) A52.14
  specified organism NEC G04.81
  staphylococcal G04.2
  streptococcal G04.2
  syphilitic A52.14
  toxic NEC G92
    due to mercury — *see* subcategory T56.1 ☑
  tuberculous A17.82
  virus NEC A86
Meningoencephalocele (*see also* Encephalocele)
  syphilitic A52.19
    congenital A50.49
Meningoencephalomyelitis (*see also* Meningoen-cephalitis)
  acute NEC (viral) A86
    disseminated G04.00
      postimmunization or postvaccination G04.02
      postinfectious G04.01
  due to
    actinomycosis A42.82
    Torula B45.1
    Toxoplasma or toxoplasmosis (acquired) B58.2
      congenital P37.1
  postimmunization or postvaccination G04.02
Meningoencephalomyelopathy G96.9
Meningoencephalopathy G96.9
Meningomyelitis (*see also* Meningoencephalitis)
  bacterial NEC G04.2
  blastomycotic NEC B40.81
  cryptococcal B45.1
  in diseases classified elsewhere G05.4
  meningococcal A39.81
  syphilitic A52.14
  tuberculous A17.82
Meningomyelocele (*see also* Spina bifida)
  syphilitic A52.19
Meningomyeloneuritis — *see* Meningoencephalitis
Meningoradiculitis — *see* Meningitis
Meningovascular — *see* condition
Menkes' disease or syndrome E83.09
  meaning maple-syrup-urine disease E71.0
Menometrorrhagia N92.1
Menopause, menopausal (asymptomatic) (state) Z78.0
  arthritis (any site) NEC — *see* Arthritis, specified form NEC
  bleeding N92.4
  depression (single episode) F32.8
    agitated (single episode) F32.2
      recurrent episode F33.9
    psychotic (single episode) F32.8
      recurrent episode F33.9
    recurrent episode F33.9
  melancholia (single episode) F32.8
    recurrent episode F33.9
  paranoid state F22
  premature E28.319
    asymptomatic E28.319
      postirradiation E89.40
      postsurgical E89.40

Menopause, menopausal — *continued*
  premature — *continued*
    symptomatic E28.310
      postirradiation E89.41
      postsurgical E89.41
  psychosis NEC F28
  symptomatic N95.1
  toxic polyarthritis NEC — *see* Arthritis, specified form NEC
Menorrhagia (primary) N92.0
  climacteric N92.4
    menopausal N92.4
  menopausal N92.4
  postclimacteric N95.0
  postmenopausal N95.0
  preclimacteric or premenopausal N92.4
  pubertal (menses retained) N92.2
Menostaxis N92.0
Menses, retention N94.89
Menstrual — *see* Menstruation
Menstruation
  absent — *see* Amenorrhea
  anovulatory N97.0
  cycle, irregular N92.6
  delayed N91.0
  disorder N93.9
    psychogenic F45.8
  during pregnancy O20.8
  excessive (with regular cycle) N92.0
    with irregular cycle N92.1
    at puberty N92.2
  frequent N92.0
  infrequent — *see* Oligomenorrhea
  irregular N92.6
    specified NEC N92.5
  latent N92.5
  membranous N92.5
  painful (*see also* Dysmenorrhea) N94.6
    primary N94.4
    psychogenic F45.8
    secondary N94.5
  passage of clots N92.0
  precocious E30.1
  protracted N92.5
  rare — *see* Oligomenorrhea
  retained N94.89
  retrograde N92.5
  scanty — *see* Oligomenorrhea
  suppression N94.89
  vicarious (nasal) N94.89
Mental (*see also* condition)
  deficiency — *see* Disability, intellectual
  deterioration — *see* Psychosis
  disorder — *see* Disorder, mental
  exhaustion F48.8
  insufficiency (congenital) — *see* Disability, intellectual
  observation without need for further medical care Z03.89
  retardation — *see* Disability, intellectual
  subnormality — *see* Disability, intellectuall
  upset — *see* Disorder, mental
Meralgia paresthetica G57.1- ☑
Mercurial — *see* condition
Mercurialism — *see* subcategory T56.1 ☑
Merkel cell tumor — *see* Carcinoma, Merkel cell
Merocele — *see* Hernia, femoral
Meromelia
  lower limb — *see* Defect, reduction, lower limb
    intercalary
      femur — *see* Defect, reduction, lower limb, specified type NEC
        tibiofibular (complete) (incomplete) — *see* Defect, reduction, lower limb
    upper limb — *see* Defect, reduction, upper limb
      intercalary, humeral, radioulnar — *see* Agenesis, arm, with hand present
MERRF syndrome (myoclonic epilepsy associated with ragged-red fiber) E88.42
Merzbacher-Pelizaeus disease E75.29
Mesaortitis — *see* Aortitis
Mesarteritis — *see* Arteritis
Mesencephalitis — *see* Encephalitis
Mesenchymoma (*see also* Neoplasm, connective tissue, uncertain behavior)
  benign — *see* Neoplasm, connective tissue, benign
  malignant — *see* Neoplasm, connective tissue, malig-nant

Mesenteritis
  retractile K65.4
  sclerosing K65.4
Mesentery, mesenteric — *see* condition
Mesiodens, mesiodentes K00.1
Mesio-occlusion M26.213
Mesocolon — *see* condition
Mesonephroma (malignant) — *see* Neoplasm, malig-nant, by site
  benign — *see* Neoplasm, benign, by site
Mesophlebitis — *see* Phlebitis
Mesostromal dysgenesia Q13.89
Mesothelioma (malignant) C45.9
  benign
    mesentery D19.1
    mesocolon D19.1
    omentum D19.1
    peritoneum D19.1
    pleura D19.0
    specified site NEC D19.7
    unspecified site D19.9
  biphasic C45.9
    benign
      mesentery D19.1
      mesocolon D19.1
      omentum D19.1
      peritoneum D19.1
      pleura D19.0
      specified site NEC D19.7
      unspecified site D19.9
  cystic D48.4
  epithelioid C45.9
    benign
      mesentery D19.1
      mesocolon D19.1
      omentum D19.1
      peritoneum D19.1
      pleura D19.0
      specified site NEC D19.7
      unspecified site D19.9
  fibrous C45.9
    benign
      mesentery D19.1
      mesocolon D19.1
      omentum D19.1
      peritoneum D19.1
      pleura D19.0
      specified site NEC D19.7
      unspecified site D19.9
  site classification
    liver C45.7
    lung C45.7
    mediastinum C45.7
    mesentery C45.1
    mesocolon C45.1
    omentum C45.1
    pericardium C45.2
    peritoneum C45.1
    pleura C45.0
      parietal C45.0
    retroperitoneum C45.7
    specified site NEC C45.7
    unspecified C45.9
Metabolic syndrome E88.81
Metagonimiasis B66.8
Metagonimus infestation (intestine) B66.8
Metal
  pigmentation L81.8
  polisher's disease J62.8
Metamorphopsia H53.15
Metaplasia
  apocrine (breast) — *see* Dysplasia, mammary, specified type NEC
  cervix (squamous) — *see* Dysplasia, cervix
  endometrium (squamous) (uterus) N85.8
  esophagus
  kidney (pelvis) (squamous) N28.89
  myelogenous D73.1
  myeloid (agnogenic) (megakaryocytic) D73.1
  spleen D73.1
  squamous cell, bladder N32.89
Metastasis, metastatic
  abscess — *see* Abscess
  calcification E83.59
  cancer
    from specified site — *see* Neoplasm, malignant, by site

Metastasis, metastatic — *continued*
   cancer — *continued*
      to specified site — *see* Neoplasm, secondary, by site
   deposits (in) — *see* Neoplasm, secondary, by site
   disease (*see also* Neoplasm, secondary, by site) C79.9
   spread (to) — *see* Neoplasm, secondary, by site
Metastrongyliasis B83.8
Metatarsalgia M77.4- ☑
   anterior G57.6- ☑
   Morton's G57.6- ☑
Metatarsus, metatarsal (*see also* condition)
   valgus (abductus), congenital Q66.6
   varus (adductus) (congenital) Q66.2
Methadone use F11.20
Methemoglobinemia D74.9
   acquired (with sulfhemoglobinemia) D74.8
   congenital D74.0
   enzymatic (congenital) D74.0
   Hb M disease D74.0
   hereditary D74.0
   toxic D74.8
Methemoglobinuria — *see* Hemoglobinuria
Methioninemia E72.19
Methylmalonic acidemia E71.120
Metritis (catarrhal) (hemorrhagic) (septic) (suppurative)
      (*see also* Endometritis)
   cervical — *see* Cervicitis
Metropathia hemorrhagica N93.8
Metroperitonitis — *see* Peritonitis, pelvic, female
Metrorrhagia N92.1
   climacteric N92.4
   menopausal N92.4
   postpartum NEC (atonic) (following delivery of placenta) O72.1
      delayed or secondary O72.2
   preclimacteric or premenopausal N92.4
   psychogenic F45.8
Metrorrhexis — *see* Rupture, uterus
Metrosalpingitis N70.91
Metrostaxis N93.8
Metrovaginitis — *see* Endometritis
Meyer-Schwickerath and Weyers syndrome Q87.0
Meynert's amentia (nonalcoholic) F04
   alcoholic F10.96
      with dependence F10.26
Mibelli's disease (porokeratosis) Q82.8
Mice, joint — *see* Loose, body, joint
   knee M23.4- ☑
Micrencephalon, micrencephaly Q02
Microalbuminuria R80.9
Microaneurysm, retinal (*see also* Disorder, retina, microaneurysms)
   diabetic — *see* E08-E13 with .31
Microangiopathy (peripheral) I73.9
   thrombotic M31.1
Microcalcifications, breast R92.0
Microcephalus, microcephalic, microcephaly Q02
   due to toxoplasmosis (congenital) P37.1
Microcheilia Q18.7
Microcolon (congenital) Q43.8
Microcornea (congenital) Q13.4
Microcytic — *see* condition
Microdeletions NEC Q93.88
Microdontia K00.2
Microdrepanocytosis D57.40
   with crisis (vasoocclusive pain) D57.419
      with
         acute chest syndrome D57.411
         splenic sequestration D57.412
Microembolism
   atherothrombotic — *see* Atheroembolism
   retinal — *see* Occlusion, artery, retina
Microencephalon Q02
Microfilaria streptocerca infestation — *see* Onchocerciasis
Microgastria (congenital) Q40.2
Microgenia M26.06
Microgenitalia, congenital
   female Q52.8
   male Q55.8
Microglioma — *see* Lymphoma, non-Hodgkin, specified NEC
Microglossia (congenital) Q38.3
Micrognathia, micrognathism (congenital)
   (mandibular) (maxillary) M26.09
Microgyria (congenital) Q04.3

Microinfarct of heart — *see* Insufficiency, coronary
Microlentia (congenital) Q12.8
Microlithiasis, alveolar, pulmonary J84.02
Micromastia N64.82
Micromyelia (congenital) Q06.8
Micropenis Q55.62
Microphakia (congenital) Q12.8
Microphthalmos, microphthalmia (congenital) Q11.2
   due to toxoplasmosis P37.1
Micropsia H53.15
Microscopic polyangiitis (polyarteritis) M31.7
Microsporidiosis B60.8
   intestinal A07.8
Microsporon furfur infestation B36.0
Microsporosis (*see also* Dermatophytosis)
   nigra B36.1
Microstomia (congenital) Q18.5
Microtia (congenital) (external ear) Q17.2
Microtropia H50.40
Microvillus inclusion disease (MVD) (MVID) Q43.8
Micturition
   disorder NEC R39.19
      psychogenic F45.8
   frequency R35.0
      psychogenic F45.8
   hesitancy R39.11
   incomplete emptying R39.14
   nocturnal R35.1
   painful R30.9
      dysuria R30.0
      psychogenic F45.8
      tenesmus R30.1
   poor stream R39.12
   split stream R39.13
   straining R39.16
   urgency R39.15
Mid plane — *see* condition
Middle
   ear — *see* condition
   lobe (right) syndrome J98.19
Miescher's elastoma L87.2
Mietens' syndrome Q87.2
Migraine (idiopathic) G43.909
   with aura (acute-onset) (prolonged) (typical) (without headache) G43.109
      with refractory migraine G43.119
         with status migrainosus G43.111
         without status migrainosus G43.119
      without mention of refractory migraine G43.109
         with status migrainosus G43.101
         without status migrainosus G43.109
      intractable G43.119
         with status migrainosus G43.111
         without status migrainosus G43.119
      not intractable G43.109
         with status migrainosus G43.101
         without status migrainosus G43.109
      persistent G43.509
         with cerebral infarction G43.609
            with refractory migraine G43.619
               with status migrainosus G43.611
               without status migrainosus G43.619
            without refractory migraine G43.609
               with status migrainosus G43.601
               without status migrainosus G43.609
            intractable G43.619
               with status migrainosus G43.611
               without status migrainosus G43.619
            not intractable G43.609
               with status migrainosus G43.601
               without status migrainosus G43.609
         without cerebral infarction G43.509
            with refractory migraine G43.519
               with status migrainosus G43.511
               without status migrainosus G43.519
            without refractory migraine G43.509
               with status migrainosus G43.501
               without status migrainosus G43.509
            intractable G43.519
               with status migrainosus G43.511
               without status migrainosus G43.519
            not intractable G43.509
               with status migrainosus G43.501
               without status migrainosus G43.509
   with refractory migraine G43.919
      with status migrainosus G43.911
      without status migrainosus G43.919

Migraine — *continued*
   without aura G43.009
      with refractory migraine G43.019
         with status migrainosus G43.011
         without status migrainosus G43.019
      without mention of refractory migraine G43.009
         with status migrainosus G43.001
         without status migrainosus G43.009
      chronic G43.709
         with refractory migraine G43.719
            with status migrainosus G43.711
            without status migrainosus G43.719
         without refractory migraine G43.709
            with status migrainosus G43.701
            without status migrainosus G43.709
         intractable
            with status migrainosus G43.711
            without status migrainosus G43.719
         not intractable
            with status migrainosus G43.701
            without status migrainosus G43.709
      intractable
         with status migrainosus G43.011
         without status migrainosus G43.019
      not intractable
         with status migrainosus G43.001
         without status migrainosus G43.009
   without refractory migraine G43.909
      with status migrainosus G43.901
      without status migrainosus G43.919
   abdominal G43.D0 (*following* G43.7)
      with refractory migraine G43.D1 (*following* G43.7)
      without refractory migraine G43.D0 (*following* G43.7)
      intractable G43.D1 (*following* G43.7)
      not intractable G43.D0 (*following* G43.7)
   basilar — *see* Migraine, with aura
   classical — *see* Migraine, with aura
   common — *see* Migraine, without aura
   complicated G43.109
   equivalents — *see* Migraine, with aura
   familiar — *see* Migraine, hemiplegic
   hemiplegic G43.409
      with refractory migraine G43.419
         with status migrainosus G43.411
         without status migrainosus G43.419
      without refractory migraine G43.409
         with status migrainosus G43.401
         without status migrainosus G43.409
      intractable G43.419
         with status migrainosus G43.411
         without status migrainosus G43.419
      not intractable G43.409
         with status migrainosus G43.401
         without status migrainosus G43.409
   intractable G43.919
      with status migrainosus G43.911
      without status migrainosus G43.919
   menstrual G43.829
      with refractory migraine G43.839
         with status migrainosus G43.831
         without status migrainosus G43.839
      without refractory migraine G43.829
         with status migrainosus G43.821
         without status migrainosus G43.829
      intractable G43.839
         with status migrainosus G43.831
         without status migrainosus G43.839
      not intractable 4G43.829
         with status migrainosus G43.821
         without status migrainosus G43.829
   menstrually related — *see* Migraine, menstrual
   not intractable G43.909
      with status migrainosus G43.901
      without status migrainosus G43.919
   ophthalmoplegic G43.B0 (*following* G43.7)
      with refractory migraine G43.B1 (*following* G43.7)
      without refractory migraine G43.B0 (*following* G43.7)
      intractable G43.B1 (*following* G43.7)
      not intractable G43.B0 (*following* G43.7)
   persistent aura (with, without) cerebral infarction — *see* Migraine, with aura, persistent
   preceded or accompanied by transient focal neurological phenomena — *see* Migraine, with aura
   pre-menstrual — *see* Migraine, menstrual
   pure menstrual — *see* Migraine, menstrual
   retinal — *see* Migraine, with aura

☑ **Additional Character Required** — Refer to the Tabular List for Character Selection   ▽ **Subterms under main terms may continue to next column or page**

Migraine — continued
  specified NEC G43.809
    intractable G43.819
      with status migrainosus G43.811
      without status migrainosus G43.819
    not intractable G43.809
      with status migrainosus G43.801
      without status migrainosus G43.809
  sporadic — see Migraine, hemiplegic
  transformed — see Migraine, without aura, chronic
  triggered seizures — see Migraine, with aura
Migrant, social Z59.0
Migration, anxiety concerning Z60.3
Migratory, migrating (see also condition)
  person Z59.0
  testis Q55.29
Mikity-Wilson disease or syndrome P27.0
Mikulicz' disease or syndrome K11.8
Miliaria L74.3
  alba L74.1
  apocrine L75.2
  crystallina L74.1
  profunda L74.2
  rubra L74.0
  tropicalis L74.2
Miliary — see condition
Milium L72.0
  colloid L57.8
Milk
  crust L21.0
  excessive secretion O92.6
  poisoning — see Poisoning, food, noxious
  retention O92.79
  sickness — see Poisoning, food, noxious
  spots I31.0
Milk-alkali disease or syndrome E83.52
Milk-leg (deep vessels) (nonpuerperal) — see Embolism, vein, lower extremity
  complicating pregnancy O22.3- ☑
  puerperal, postpartum, childbirth O87.1
Milkman's disease or syndrome M83.8
Milky urine — see Chyluria
Millard-Gubler (-Foville) **paralysis or syndrome** G46.3
Millar's asthma J38.5
Miller Fisher syndrome G61.0
Mills' disease — see Hemiplegia
Millstone maker's pneumoconiosis J62.8
Milroy's disease (chronic hereditary edema) Q82.0
Minamata disease T26.1- ☑
Miners' asthma or lung J60
Minkowski-Chauffard syndrome — see Spherocytosis
Minor — see condition
Minor's disease (hematomyelia) G95.19
Minot's disease (hemorrhagic disease), newborn P53
Minot-von Willebrand-Jurgens disease or syndrome (angiohemophilia) D68.0
Minus (and plus) **hand** (intrinsic) — see Deformity, limb, specified type NEC, forearm
Miosis (pupil) H57.03
Mirizzi's syndrome (hepatic duct stenosis) K83.1
Mirror writing F81.0
Misadventure (of) (prophylactic) (therapeutic) (see also Complications) T88.9 ☑
  administration of insulin (by accident) — see subcategory T38.3 ☑
  infusion — see Complications, infusion
  local applications (of fomentations, plasters, etc.) T88.9 ☑
    burn or scald — see Burn
    specified NEC T88.8 ☑
  medical care (early) (late) T88.9 ☑
    adverse effect of drugs or chemicals — see Table of Drugs and Chemicals
    burn or scald — see Burn
    specified NEC T88.8 ☑
  specified NEC T88.8 ☑
  surgical procedure (early) (late) — see Complications, surgical procedure
  transfusion — see Complications, transfusion
  vaccination or other immunological procedure — see Complications, vaccination
Miscarriage O03.9
Misdirection, aqueous H40.83- ☑
Misperception, sleep state F51.02
Misplaced, misplacement
  ear Q17.4

Misplaced, misplacement — continued
  kidney (acquired) N28.89
    congenital Q63.2
  organ or site, congenital NEC — see Malposition, congenital
Missed
  abortion O02.1
  delivery O36.4 ☑
Missing — see Absence
Misuse of drugs F19.99
Mitchell's disease (erythromelalgia) I73.81
Mite(s) (infestation) B88.9
  diarrhea B88.0
  grain (itch) B88.0
  hair follicle (itch) B88.0
  in sputum B88.0
Mitral — see condition
Mittelschmerz N94.0
Mixed — see condition
MNGIE (Mitochondrial Neurogastrointestinal Encephalopathy) **syndrome** E88.49
Mobile, mobility
  cecum Q43.3
  excessive — see Hypermobility
  gallbladder, congenital Q44.1
  kidney N28.89
  organ or site, congenital NEC — see Malposition, congenital
Mobitz heart block (atrioventricular) I44.1
Moebius, Möbius
  disease (ophthalmoplegic migraine) — see Migraine, ophthalmoplegic
  syndrome Q87.0
    congenital oculofacial paralysis (with other anomalies) Q87.0
    ophthalmoplegic migraine — see Migraine, ophthalmoplegic
Moeller's glossitis K14.0
Mohr's syndrome (Types I and II) Q87.0
Mola destruens D39.2
Molar pregnancy O02.0
Molarization of premolars K00.2
Molding, head (during birth) — omit code
Mole (pigmented) (see also Nevus)
  blood O02.0
  Breus' O02.0
  cancerous — see Melanoma
  carneous O02.0
  destructive D39.2
  fleshy O02.0
  hydatid, hydatidiform (benign) (complicating pregnancy) (delivered) (undelivered) O01.9
    classical O01.0
    complete O01.0
    incomplete O01.1
    invasive D39.2
    malignant D39.2
    partial O01.1
  intrauterine O02.0
  invasive (hydatidiform) D39.2
  malignant
    meaning
      malignant hydatidiform mole D39.2
      melanoma — see Melanoma
  nonhydatidiform O02.0
  nonpigmented — see Nevus
  pregnancy NEC O02.0
  skin — see Nevus
  tubal O00.1
  vesicular — see Mole, hydatidiform
Molimen, molimina (menstrual) N94.3
Molluscum contagiosum (epitheliale) B08.1
Mönckeberg's arteriosclerosis, disease, or sclerosis — see Arteriosclerosis, extremities
Mondini's malformation (cochlea) Q16.5
Mondor's disease I80.8
Monge's disease T70.29 ☑
Monilethrix (congenital) Q84.1
Moniliasis (see also Candidiasis) B37.9
  neonatal P37.5
Monitoring (encounter for)
  therapeutic drug level Z51.81
Monkey malaria B53.1
Monkeypox B04
Monoarthritis M13.10
  ankle M13.17- ☑
  elbow M13.12- ☑

Monoarthritis — continued
  foot joint M13.17- ☑
  hand joint M13.14- ☑
  hip M13.15- ☑
  knee M13.16- ☑
  shoulder M13.11- ☑
  wrist M13.13- ☑
Monoblastic — see condition
Monochromat (ism), monochromatopsia (acquired) (congenital) H53.51
Monocytic — see condition
Monocytopenia D72.818
Monocytosis (symptomatic) D72.821
Monomania — see Psychosis
Mononeuritis G58.9
  cranial nerve — see Disorder, nerve, cranial
  femoral nerve G57.2- ☑
  lateral
    cutaneous nerve of thigh G57.1- ☑
    popliteal nerve G57.3- ☑
  lower limb G57.9- ☑
    specified nerve NEC G57.8- ☑
  medial popliteal nerve G57.4- ☑
  median nerve G56.1- ☑
  multiplex G58.7
  plantar nerve G57.6- ☑
  posterior tibial nerve G57.5- ☑
  radial nerve G56.3- ☑
  sciatic nerve G57.0- ☑
  specified NEC G58.8
  tibial nerve G57.4- ☑
  ulnar nerve G56.2- ☑
  upper limb G56.9- ☑
    specified nerve NEC G56.8- ☑
  vestibular — see subcategory H93.3 ☑
Mononeuropathy G58.9
  carpal tunnel syndrome — see Syndrome, carpal tunnel
  diabetic NEC — see E08-E13 with .41
  femoral nerve — see Lesion, nerve, femoral
  ilioinguinal nerve G57.8- ☑
  in diseases classified elsewhere — see category G59
  intercostal G58.0
  lower limb G57.9- ☑
    causalgia — see Causalgia, lower limb
    femoral nerve — see Lesion, nerve, femoral
    meralgia paresthetica G57.1- ☑
    plantar nerve — see Lesion, nerve, plantar
    popliteal nerve — see Lesion, nerve, popliteal
    sciatic nerve — see Lesion, nerve, sciatic
    specified NEC G57.8- ☑
    tarsal tunnel syndrome — see Syndrome, tarsal tunnel
  median nerve — see Lesion, nerve, median
  multiplex G58.7
  obturator nerve G57.8- ☑
  popliteal nerve — see Lesion, nerve, popliteal
  radial nerve — see Lesion, nerve, radial
  saphenous nerve G57.8- ☑
  specified NEC G58.8
  tarsal tunnel syndrome — see Syndrome, tarsal tunnel
  tuberculous A17.83
  ulnar nerve — see Lesion, nerve, ulnar
  upper limb G56.9- ☑
    carpal tunnel syndrome — see Syndrome, carpal tunnel
    causalgia — see Causalgia
    median nerve — see Lesion, nerve, median
    radial nerve — see Lesion, nerve, radial
    specified site NEC G56.8- ☑
    ulnar nerve — see Lesion, nerve, ulnar
Mononucleosis, infectious B27.90
  with
    complication NEC B27.99
    meningitis B27.92
    polyneuropathy B27.91
  cytomegaloviral B27.10
    with
      complication NEC B27.19
      meningitis B27.12
      polyneuropathy B27.11
  Epstein-Barr (virus) B27.00
    with
      complication NEC B27.09
      meningitis B27.02
      polyneuropathy B27.01

Mononucleosis, infectious — continued
  gammaherpesviral B27.00
    with
      complication NEC B27.09
      meningitis B27.02
      polyneuropathy B27.01
    specified NEC B27.80
      with
        complication NEC B27.89
        meningitis B27.82
        polyneuropathy B27.81
Monoplegia G83.3- ☑
  congenital (cerebral) G80.8
    spastic G80.1
  embolic (current episode) I63.4 ☑
  following
    cerebrovascular disease
      cerebral infarction
        lower limb I69.34- ☑
        upper limb I69.33- ☑
      intracerebral hemorrhage
        lower limb I69.14- ☑
        upper limb I69.13- ☑
      lower limb I69.94- ☑
      nontraumatic intracranial hemorrhage NEC
        lower limb I69.24- ☑
        upper limb I69.23- ☑
      specified disease NEC
        lower limb I69.84- ☑
        upper limb I69.83- ☑
      stroke NOS
        lower limb I69.34- ☑
        upper limb I69.33- ☑
      subarachnoid hemorrhage
        lower limb I69.04- ☑
        lower limb I69.03- ☑
      upper limb I69.93- ☑
  hysterical (transient) F44.4
  lower limb G83.1- ☑
  psychogenic (conversion reaction) F44.4
  thrombotic (current episode) I63.3 ☑
  transient R29.818
  upper limb G83.2- ☑
Monorchism, monorchidism Q55.0
Monosomy (see also Deletion, chromosome) Q93.9
  specified NEC Q93.89
  whole chromosome
    meiotic nondisjunction Q93.0
    mitotic nondisjunction Q93.1
    mosaicism Q93.1
  X Q96.9
Monster, monstrosity (single) Q89.7
  acephalic Q00.0
  twin Q89.4
Monteggia's fracture (-dislocation) S52.27- ☑
Mooren's ulcer (cornea) — see Ulcer, cornea, Mooren's
Moore's syndrome — see Epilepsy, specified NEC
Mooser-Neill reaction A75.2
Mooser's bodies A75.2
Morbidity not stated or unknown R69
Morbilli — see Measles
Morbus (see also Disease)
  angelicus, anglorum E55.0
  Beigel B36.2
  caducus — see Epilepsy
  celiacus K90.0
  comitialis — see Epilepsy
  cordis (see also Disease, heart) I51.9
    valvulorum — see Endocarditis
  coxae senilis M16.9
    tuberculous A18.02
  hemorrhagicus neonatorum P53
  maculosus neonatorum P54.5
Morel (-Stewart)(-Morgagni) **syndrome** M85.2
Morel-Kraepelin disease — see Schizophrenia
Morel-Moore syndrome M85.2
Morgagni's
  cyst, organ, hydatid, or appendage
    female Q50.5
    male (epididymal) Q55.4
      testicular Q55.29
  syndrome M85.2
Morgagni-Stewart-Morel syndrome M85.2
Morgagni-Stokes-Adams syndrome I45.9
Morgagni-Turner (-Albright) **syndrome** Q96.9
Moria F07.0
Moron (I.Q. 50-69) F70

Morphea L94.0
Morphinism (without remission) F11.20
  with remission F11.21
Morphinomania (without remission) F11.20
  with remission F11.21
Morquio (-Ullrich)(-Brailsford) **disease or syndrome** —
  see Mucopolysaccharidosis
Mortification (dry) (moist) — see Gangrene
Morton's metatarsalgia (neuralgia)(neuroma) (syn-
  drome) G57.6- ☑
Morvan's disease or syndrome G60.8
Mosaicism, mosaic (autosomal) (chromosomal)
  45,X/46,XX Q96.3
  45,X/other cell lines NEC with abnormal sex chromo-
    some Q96.4
  sex chromosome
    female Q97.8
    lines with various numbers of X chromosomes
      Q97.2
    male Q98.7
  XY Q96.3
Moschowitz' disease M31.1
Mother yaw A66.0
Motion sickness (from travel, any vehicle) (from round-
  abouts or swings) T75.3 ☑
Mottled, mottling, teeth (enamel) (endemic) (nonen-
  demic) K00.3
Mounier-Kuhn syndrome Q32.4
  with bronchiectasis J47.9
    exacerbation (acute) J47.1
    lower respiratory infection J47.0
  acquired J98.09
    with bronchiectasis J47.9
      with
        exacerbation (acute) J47.1
        lower respiratory infection J47.0
Mountain
  sickness T70.29 ☑
    with polycythemia , acquired (acute) D75.1
  tick fever A93.2
Mouse, joint — see Loose, body, joint
  knee M23.4- ☑
Mouth — see condition
Movable
  coccyx — see subcategory M53.2 ☑
  kidney N28.89
    congenital Q63.8
  spleen D73.89
Movements, dystonic R25.8
Moyamoya disease I67.5
MRSA (Methicillin resistant Staphylococcus aureus)
  infection A49.02
    as the cause of diseases classified elsewhere B95.62
  sepsis A41.02
MSSA (Methicillin susceptible Staphylococcus aureus)
  infection A49.01
    as the cause of diseases classified elsewhere B95.61
  sepsis A41.01
Mucha-Habermann disease L41.0
Mucinosis (cutaneous) (focal) (papular) (skin) L98.5
  oral K13.79
Mucocele
  appendix K38.8
  buccal cavity K13.79
  gallbladder K82.1
  lacrimal sac, chronic H04.43- ☑
  nasal sinus J34.1
  nose J34.1
  salivary gland (any) K11.6
  sinus (accessory) (nasal) J34.1
  turbinate (bone) (middle) (nasal) J34.1
  uterus N85.8
Mucolipidosis
  I E77.1
  II, III E77.0
  IV E75.11
Mucopolysaccharidosis E76.3
  beta-gluduronidase deficiency E76.29
  cardiopathy E76.3 [I52]
  Hunter's syndrome E76.1
  Hurler's syndrome E76.01
  Hurler-Scheie syndrome E76.02
  Maroteaux-Lamy syndrome E76.29
  Morquio syndrome E76.219
    A E76.210
    B E76.211
    classic E76.210

Mucopolysaccharidosis — continued
  Sanfilippo syndrome E76.22
  Scheie's syndrome E76.03
  specified NEC E76.29
  type
    I
      Hurler's syndrome E76.01
      Hurler-Scheie syndrome E76.02
      Scheie's syndrome E76.03
    II E76.1
    III E76.22
    IV E76.219
    IVA E76.210
    IVB E76.211
    VI E76.29
    VII E76.29
Mucormycosis B46.5
  cutaneous B46.3
  disseminated B46.4
  gastrointestinal B46.2
  generalized B46.4
  pulmonary B46.0
  rhinocerebral B46.1
  skin B46.3
  subcutaneous B46.3
Mucositis (ulcerative) K12.30
  due to drugs NEC K12.32
  gastrointestinal K92.81
  mouth (oral) (oropharyngeal) K12.30
    due to antineoplastic therapy K12.31
    due to drugs NEC K12.32
    due to radiation K12.33
    specified NEC K12.39
    viral K12.39
  nasal J34.81
  oral cavity — see Mucositis, mouth
  oral soft tissues — see Mucositis, mouth
  vagina and vulva N76.81
Mucositis necroticans agranulocytica — see Agranulocytosis
Mucous (see also condition)
  patches (syphilitic) A51.39
    congenital A50.07
Mucoviscidosis E84.9
  with meconium obstruction E84.11
Mucus
  asphyxia or suffocation — see Asphyxia, mucus
  in stool R19.5
  plug — see Asphyxia, mucus
Muguet B37.0
Mulberry molars (congenital syphilis) A50.52
Müllerian mixed tumor
  specified site — see Neoplasm, malignant, by site
  unspecified site C54.9
Multicystic kidney (development) Q61.4
Multiparity (grand) Z64.1
  affecting management of pregnancy, labor and deliv-
    ery (supervision only) O09.4- ☑
  requiring contraceptive management — see Contra-
    ception
Multipartita placenta O43.19- ☑
Multiple, multiplex (see also condition)
  digits (congenital) Q69.9
  endocrine neoplasia — see Neoplasia, endocrine,
    multiple (MEN)
  personality F44.81
Mumps B26.9
  arthritis B26.85
  complication NEC B26.89
  encephalitis B26.2
  hepatitis B26.81
  meningitis (aseptic) B26.1
  meningoencephalitis B26.2
  myocarditis B26.82
  oophoritis B26.89
  orchitis B26.0
  pancreatitis B26.3
  polyneuropathy B26.84
Mumu (see also Infestation, filarial) B74.9 [N51]
Münchhausen's syndrome — see Disorder, factitious
Münchmeyer's syndrome — see Myositis, ossificans,
  progressiva
Mural — see condition
Murmur (cardiac) (heart) (organic) R01.1
  abdominal R19.15
  aortic (valve) — see Endocarditis, aortic
  benign R01.0
  diastolic — see Endocarditis

☑ **Additional Character Required** — Refer to the Tabular List for Character Selection   ▽ **Subterms under main terms may continue to next column or page**

Murmur — *continued*
  Flint I35.1
  functional R01.0
  Graham Steell I37.1
  innocent R01.0
  mitral (valve) — *see* Insufficiency, mitral
  nonorganic R01.0
  presystolic, mitral — *see* Insufficiency, mitral
  pulmonic (valve) I37.8
  systolic (valvular) — *see* Endocarditis
  tricuspid (valve) I07.9
  valvular — *see* Endocarditis
Murri's disease (intermittent hemoglobinuria) D59.6
Muscle, muscular (*see also* condition)
  carnitine (palmityltransferase) deficiency E71.314
Musculoneuralgia — *see* Neuralgia
Mushrooming hip — *see* Derangement, joint, specified
    NEC, hip
Mushroom-workers' (pickers') disease or lung J67.5
Mutation(s)
  factor V Leiden D68.51
  prothrombin gene D68.52
  surfactant, of lung J84.83
Mutism (*see also* Aphasia)
  deaf (acquired) (congenital) NEC H91.3
  elective (adjustment reaction) (childhood) F94.0
  hysterical F44.4
  selective (childhood) F94.0
MVD (microvillus inclusion disease) Q43.8
MVID (microvillus inclusion disease) Q43.8
Myalgia M79.1
  epidemic (cervical) B33.0
  traumatic NEC T14.8
Myasthenia G70.9
  congenital G70.2
  cordis — *see* Failure, heart
  developmental G70.2
  gravis G70.00
    with exacerbation (acute) G70.01
    in crisis G70.01
    neonatal, transient P94.0
    pseudoparalytica G70.00
      with exacerbation (acute) G70.01
      in crisis G70.01
  stomach, psychogenic F45.8
  syndrome
    in
      diabetes mellitus — *see* E08-E13 with .44
      neoplastic disease (*see also* Neoplasm)
        D49.9 [G73.3]
      pernicious anemia D51.0 [G73.3]
      thyrotoxicosis E05.90 [G73.3]
        with thyroid storm E05.91 [G73.3]
Myasthenic M62.81
Mycelium infection B49
Mycetismus — *see* Poisoning, food, noxious, mushroom
Mycetoma B47.9
  actinomycotic B47.1
  bone (mycotic) B47.9 [M90.80]
  eumycotic B47.0
  foot B47.9
    actinomycotic B47.1
    mycotic B47.0
  madurae NEC B47.9
    mycotic B47.0
  maduromycotic B47.0
  mycotic B47.0
  nocardial B47.1
Mycobacteriosis — *see* Mycobacterium
Mycobacterium, mycobacterial (infection) A31.9
  anonymous A31.9
  atypical A31.9
    cutaneous A31.1
    pulmonary A31.0
      tuberculous — *see* Tuberculosis, pulmonary
    specified site NEC A31.8
  avium (intracellulare complex) A31.0
  balnei A31.1
  Battey A31.0
  chelonei A31.8
  cutaneous A31.1
  extrapulmonary systemic A31.8
  fortuitum A31.8
  intracellulare (Battey bacillus) A31.0
  kakaferifu A31.8
  kansasii (yellow bacillus) A31.0
  kasongo A31.8
  leprae (*see also* Leprosy) A30.9

Mycobacterium, mycobacterial — *continued*
  luciflavum A31.1
  marinum (M. balnei) A31.1
  nonspecific — *see* Mycobacterium, atypical
  pulmonary (atypical) A31.0
    tuberculous — *see* Tuberculosis, pulmonary
  scrofulaceum A31.8
  simiae A31.8
  systemic, extrapulmonary A31.8
  szulgai A31.8
  terrae A31.8
  triviale A31.8
  tuberculosis (human, bovine) — *see* Tuberculosis
  ulcerans A31.1
  xenopi A31.8
Mycoplasma (M.) pneumoniae, as cause of disease classified elsewhere B96.0
Mycosis, mycotic B49
  cutaneous NEC B36.9
  ear B36.8
  fungoides (extranodal) (solid organ) C84.0- ☑
  mouth B37.0
  nails B35.1
  opportunistic B48.8
  skin NEC B36.9
  specified NEC B48.8
  stomatitis B37.0
  vagina, vaginitis (candidal) B37.3
Mydriasis (pupil) H57.04
Myelatelia Q06.1
Myelinolysis, pontine, central G37.2
Myelitis (acute) (ascending) (childhood) (chronic) (descending) (diffuse) (disseminated) (idiopathic) (pressure) (progressive) (spinal cord) (subacute) (*see also* Encephalitis) G04.91
  herpes simplex B00.82
  herpes zoster B02.24
  in diseases classified elsewhere G05.4
  necrotizing, subacute G37.4
  optic neuritis in G36.0
  postchickenpox B01.12
  postherpetic B02.24
  postimmunization G04.02
  postinfectious NEC G04.89
  postvaccinal G04.02
  specified NEC G04.89
  syphilitic (transverse) A52.14
  toxic G92
  transverse (in demyelinating diseases of central nervous system) G37.3
  tuberculous A17.82
  varicella B01.12
Myeloblastic — *see* condition
Myeloblastoma
  granular cell (*see also* Neoplasm, connective tissue)
    malignant — *see* Neoplasm, connective tissue, malignant
    tongue D10.1
Myelocele — *see* Spina bifida
Myelocystocele — *see* Spina bifida
Myelocytic — *see* condition
Myelodysplasia D46.9
  specified NEC D46.Z (*following* D46.4)
  spinal cord (congenital) Q06.1
Myelodysplastic syndrome D46.9
  with
    5q deletion D46.C (*following* D46.2)
    isolated del (5q) chromosomal abnormality D46.C
      (*following* D46.2)
    specified NEC D46.Z (*following* D46.4)
Myeloencephalitis — *see* Encephalitis
Myelofibrosis D75.81
  with myeloid metaplasia D47.4
  acute C94.4- ☑
  idiopathic (chronic) D47.4
  primary D47.1
  secondary D75.81
    in myeloproliferative disease D47.4
Myelogenous — *see* condition
Myeloid — *see* condition
Myelokathexis D70.9
Myeloleukodystrophy E75.29
Myelolipoma — *see* Lipoma
Myeloma (multiple) C90.0- ☑
  monostotic C90.3 ☑
    plasma cell C90.0- ☑
  plasma cell C90.0- ☑

Myeloma — *continued*
  solitary (*see also* Plasmacytoma, solitary) C90.3- ☑
Myelomalacia G95.89
Myelomatosis C90.0- ☑
Myelomeningitis — *see* Meningoencephalitis
Myelomeningocele (spinal cord) — *see* Spina bifida
Myelo-osteo-musculodysplasia hereditaria Q79.8
Myelopathic
  anemia D64.89
  muscle atrophy — *see* Atrophy, muscle, spinal
  pain syndrome G89.0
Myelopathy (spinal cord) G95.9
  drug-induced G95.89
  in (due to)
    degeneration or displacement, intervertebral disc
      NEC — *see* Disorder, disc, with, myelopathy
    infection — *see* Encephalitis
    intervertebral disc disorder (*see also* Disorder, disc, with, myelopathy)
    mercury — *see* subcategory T56.1 ☑
    neoplastic disease (*see also* Neoplasm)
      D49.9 [G99.2]
    pernicious anemia D51.0 [G99.2]
    spondylosis — *see* Spondylosis, with myelopathy NEC
  necrotic (subacute) (vascular) G95.19
  radiation-induced G95.89
  spondylogenic NEC — *see* Spondylosis, with myelopathy NEC
  toxic G95.89
  transverse, acute G37.3
  vascular G95.19
  vitamin B12 E53.8 [G32.0]
Myelophthisis D61.82
Myeloradiculitis G04.91
Myeloradiculodysplasia (spinal) Q06.1
Myelosarcoma C92.3- ☑
Myelosclerosis D75.89
  with myeloid metaplasia D47.4
  disseminated, of nervous system G35
  megakaryocytic D47.4
    with myeloid metaplasia D47.4
Myelosis
  acute C92.0- ☑
  aleukemic C92.9- ☑
  chronic D47.1
  erythremic (acute) C94.0- ☑
  megakaryocytic C94.2- ☑
  nonleukemic D72.828
  subacute C92.9- ☑
Myiasis (cavernous) B87.9
  aural B87.4
  creeping B87.0
  cutaneous B87.0
  dermal B87.0
  ear (external) (middle) B87.4
  eye B87.2
  genitourinary B87.81
  intestinal B87.82
  laryngeal B87.3
  nasopharyngeal B87.3
  ocular B87.2
  orbit B87.2
  skin B87.0
  specified site NEC B87.89
  traumatic B87.1
  wound B87.1
Myoadenoma, prostate — *see* Hyperplasia, prostate
Myoblastoma
  granular cell (*see also* Neoplasm, connective tissue, benign)
    malignant — *see* Neoplasm, connective tissue, malignant
    tongue D10.1
Myocardial — *see* condition
Myocardiopathy (congestive) (constrictive) (familial) (hypertrophic nonobstructive) (idiopathic) (infiltrative) (obstructive) (primary) (restrictive) (sporadic) (*see also* Cardiomyopathy) I42.9
  alcoholic I42.6
  cobalt-beer I42.6
  glycogen storage E74.02 [I43]
  hypertrophic obstructive I42.1
  in (due to)
    beriberi E51.12
    cardiac glycogenosis E74.02 [I43]
    Friedreich's ataxia G11.1 [I43]

Myocardiopathy — *continued*
in — *continued*
    myotonia atrophica G71.11 [I43]
    progressive muscular dystrophy G71.0 [I43]
  obscure (African) I42.8
  secondary I42.9
  thyrotoxic E05.90 [I43]
    with storm E05.91 [I43]
  toxic NEC I42.7
Myocarditis (with arteriosclerosis)(chronic)(fibroid) (interstitial) (old) (progressive) (senile) I51.4
  with
    rheumatic fever (conditions in I00) I09.0
      active — *see* Myocarditis, acute, rheumatic
      inactive or quiescent (with chorea) I09.0
  active I40.9
    rheumatic I01.2
      with chorea (acute) (rheumatic) (Sydenham's) I02.0
  acute or subacute (interstitial) I40.9
    due to
      streptococcus (beta-hemolytic) I01.2
    idiopathic I40.1
    rheumatic I01.2
      with chorea (acute) (rheumatic) (Sydenham's) I02.0
    specified NEC I40.8
  aseptic of newborn B33.22
  bacterial (acute) I40.0
  Coxsackie (virus) B33.22
  diphtheritic A36.81
  eosinophilic I40.1
  epidemic of newborn (Coxsackie) B33.22
  Fiedler's (acute) (isolated) I40.1
  giant cell (acute) (subacute) I40.1
  gonococcal A54.83
  granulomatous (idiopathic) (isolated) (nonspecific) I40.1
  hypertensive — *see* Hypertension, heart
  idiopathic (granulomatous) I40.1
  in (due to)
    diphtheria A36.81
    epidemic louse-borne typhus A75.0 [I41]
    Lyme disease A69.29
    sarcoidosis D86.85
    scarlet fever A38.1
    toxoplasmosis (acquired) B58.81
    typhoid A01.02
    typhus NEC A75.9 [I41]
  infective I40.0
  influenzal — *see* Influenza, with, myocarditis
  isolated (acute) I40.1
  meningococcal A39.52
  mumps B26.82
  nonrheumatic, active I40.9
  parenchymatous I40.9
  pneumococcal I40.0
  rheumatic (chronic) (inactive) (with chorea) I09.0
    active or acute I01.2
      with chorea (acute) (rheumatic) (Sydenham's) I02.0
  rheumatoid — *see* Rheumatoid, carditis
  septic I40.0
  staphylococcal I40.0
  suppurative I40.0
  syphilitic (chronic) A52.06
  toxic I40.8
    rheumatic — *see* Myocarditis, acute, rheumatic
  tuberculous A18.84
  typhoid A01.02
  valvular — *see* Endocarditis
  virus, viral I40.0
    of newborn (Coxsackie) B33.22
Myocardium, myocardial — *see* condition
Myocardosis — *see* Cardiomyopathy
Myoclonus, myoclonic, myoclonia (familial) (essential) (multifocal) (simplex) G25.3
  drug-induced G25.3
  epilepsy (*see also* Epilepsy, generalized, specified NEC) G40.4- ☑
    familial (progressive) G25.3
  epileptica G40.409
    with status epilepticus G40.401
  facial G51.3
  familial progressive G25.3
  Friedreich's G25.3
  jerks G25.3
  massive G25.3

Myoclonus, myoclonic, myoclonia — *continued*
  palatal G25.3
  pharyngeal G25.3
Myocytolysis I51.5
Myodiastasis — *see* Diastasis, muscle
Myoendocarditis — *see* Endocarditis
Myoepithelioma — *see* Neoplasm, benign, by site
Myofasciitis (acute) — *see* Myositis
Myofibroma (*see also* Neoplasm, connective tissue, benign)
  uterus (cervix) (corpus) — *see* Leiomyoma
Myofibromatosis D48.1
  infantile Q89.8
Myofibrosis M62.89
  heart — *see* Myocarditis
  scapulohumeral — *see* Lesion, shoulder, specified NEC
Myofibrositis M79.7
  scapulohumeral — *see* Lesion, shoulder, specified NEC
Myoglobulinuria, myoglobinuria (primary) R82.1
Myokymia, facial G51.4
Myolipoma — *see* Lipoma
Myoma (*see also* Neoplasm, connective tissue, benign)
  malignant — *see* Neoplasm, connective tissue, malignant
  prostate D29.1
  uterus (cervix) (corpus) — *see* Leiomyoma
Myomalacia M62.89
Myometritis — *see* Endometritis
Myometrium — *see* condition
Myonecrosis, clostridial A48.0
Myopathy G72.9
  acute
    necrotizing G72.81
    quadriplegic G72.81
  alcoholic G72.1
  benign congenital G71.2
  central core G71.2
  centronuclear G71.2
  congenital (benign) G71.2
  critical illness G72.81
  distal G71.0
  drug-induced G72.0
  endocrine NEC E34.9 [G73.7]
  extraocular muscles H05.82- ☑
  facioscapulohumeral G71.0
  hereditary G71.9
    specified NEC G71.8
  immune NEC G72.49
  in (due to)
    Addison's disease E27.1 [G73.7]
    alcohol G72.1
    amyloidosis E85.0 [G73.7]
    cretinism E00.9 [G73.7]
    Cushing's syndrome E24.9 [G73.7]
    drugs G72.0
    endocrine disease NEC E34.9 [G73.7]
    giant cell arteritis M31.6 [G73.7]
    glycogen storage disease E74.00 [G73.7]
    hyperadrenocorticism E24.9 [G73.7]
    hyperparathyroidism NEC E21.3 [G73.7]
    hypoparathyroidism E20.9 [G73.7]
    hypopituitarism E23.0 [G73.7]
    hypothyroidism E03.9 [G73.7]
    infectious disease NEC B99 ☑ [G73.7]
    lipid storage disease E75.6 [G73.7]
    metabolic disease NEC E88.9 [G73.7]
    myxedema E03.9 [G73.7]
    parasitic disease NEC B89 [G73.7]
    polyarteritis nodosa M30.0 [G73.7]
    rheumatoid arthritis — *see* Rheumatoid, myopathy
    sarcoidosis D86.87
    scleroderma M34.82
    sicca syndrome M35.03
    Sjögren's syndrome M35.03
    systemic lupus erythematosus M32.19
    thyrotoxicosis (hyperthyroidism) E05.90 [G73.7]
      with thyroid storm E05.91 [G73.7]
    toxic agent NEC G72.2
  inflammatory NEC G72.49
  intensive care (ICU) G72.81
  limb-girdle G71.0
  mitochondrial NEC G71.3
  myotubular G71.2
  mytonic, proximal (PROMM) G71.11
  nemaline G71.2
  ocular G71.0
  oculopharyngeal G71.0
  of critical illness G72.81

Myopathy — *continued*
  primary G71.9
    specified NEC G71.8
  progressive NEC G72.89
  proximal myotonic (PROMM) G71.11
  rod G71.2
  scapulohumeral G71.0
  specified NEC G72.89
  toxic G72.2
Myopericarditis (*see also* Pericarditis)
  chronic rheumatic I09.2
Myopia (axial) (congenital) H52.1- ☑
  degenerative (malignant) H44.2- ☑
  malignant H44.2- ☑
  pernicious H44.2- ☑
  progressive high (degenerative) H44.2- ☑
Myosarcoma — *see* Neoplasm, connective tissue, malignant
Myosis (pupil) H57.03
  stromal (endolymphatic) D39.0
Myositis M60.9
  clostridial A48.0
  due to posture — *see* Myositis, specified type NEC
  epidemic B33.0
  fibrosa or fibrous (chronic), Volkmann's T79.6 ☑
  foreign body granuloma — *see* Granuloma, foreign body
  in (due to)
    bilharziasis B65.9 [M63.8-] ☑
    cysticercosis B69.81
    leprosy A30.9 [M63.8-] ☑
    mycosis B49 [M63.8-] ☑
    sarcoidosis D86.87
    schistosomiasis B65.9 [M63.8-] ☑
    syphilis
      late A52.78
      secondary A51.49
    toxoplasmosis (acquired) B58.82
    trichinellosis B75 [M63.8-] ☑
    tuberculosis A18.09
  inclusion body [IBM] G72.41
  infective M60.009
    arm M60.002
      left M60.001
      right M60.000
    leg M60.005
      left M60.004
      right M60.003
    lower limb M60.005
      ankle M60.07- ☑
      foot M60.07- ☑
      lower leg M60.06- ☑
      thigh M60.05- ☑
      toe M60.07- ☑
    multiple sites M60.09
    specified site NEC M60.08
    upper limb M60.002
      finger M60.04- ☑
      forearm M60.03- ☑
      hand M60.04- ☑
      shoulder region M60.01- ☑
      upper arm M60.02- ☑
  interstitial M60.10
    ankle M60.17- ☑
    foot M60.17- ☑
    forearm M60.13- ☑
    hand M60.14- ☑
    lower leg M60.16- ☑
    multiple sites M60.19
    shoulder region M60.11- ☑
    specified site NEC M60.18
    thigh M60.15- ☑
    upper arm M60.12- ☑
  mycotic B49 [M63.8-] ☑
  orbital, chronic H05.12- ☑
  ossificans or ossifying (circumscripta) (*see also* Ossification, muscle, specified NEC)
    in (due to)
      burns M61.30
        ankle M61.37- ☑
        foot M61.37- ☑
        forearm M61.33- ☑
        hand M61.34- ☑
        lower leg M61.36- ☑
        multiple sites M61.39
        pelvic region M61.35- ☑
        shoulder region M61.31- ☑

Myositis — *continued*
  ossificans or ossifying (*see also* Ossification, muscle, specified) — *continued*
    in — *continued*
      burns — *continued*
        specified site NEC M61.38
        thigh M61.35- ☑
        upper arm M61.32- ☑
      quadriplegia or paraplegia M61.20
        ankle M61.27- ☑
        foot M61.27- ☑
        forearm M61.23- ☑
        hand M61.24- ☑
        lower leg M61.26- ☑
        multiple sites M61.29
        pelvic region M61.25- ☑
        shoulder region M61.21- ☑
        specified site NEC M61.28
        thigh M61.25- ☑
        upper arm M61.22- ☑
    progressiva M61.10
      ankle M61.17- ☑
      finger M61.14- ☑
      foot M61.17- ☑
      forearm M61.13- ☑
      hand M61.14- ☑
      lower leg M61.16- ☑
      multiple sites M61.19
      pelvic region M61.15- ☑
      shoulder region M61.11- ☑
      specified site NEC M61.18
      thigh M61.15- ☑
      toe M61.17- ☑
      upper arm M61.12- ☑
    traumatica M61.00
      ankle M61.07- ☑
      foot M61.07- ☑
      forearm M61.03- ☑
      hand M61.04- ☑

Myositis — *continued*
  ossificans or ossifying (*see also* Ossification, muscle, specified) — *continued*
    traumatica — *continued*
      lower leg M61.06- ☑
      multiple sites M61.09
      pelvic region M61.05- ☑
      shoulder region M61.01- ☑
      specified site NEC M61.08
      thigh M61.05- ☑
      upper arm M61.02- ☑
  purulent — *see* Myositis, infective
  specified type NEC M60.80
    ankle M60.87- ☑
    foot M60.87- ☑
    forearm M60.83- ☑
    hand M60.84- ☑
    lower leg M60.86- ☑
    multiple sites M60.89
    pelvic region M60.85- ☑
    shoulder region M60.81- ☑
    specified site NEC M60.88
    thigh M60.85- ☑
    upper arm M60.82- ☑
  suppurative — *see* Myositis, infective
  traumatic (old) — *see* Myositis, specified type NEC
Myospasia impulsiva F95.2
Myotonia (acquisita) (intermittens) M62.89
  atrophica G71.11
  chondrodystrophic G71.13
  congenita (acetazolamide responsive) (dominant) (recessive) G71.12
  drug-induced G71.14
  dystrophica G71.11
  fluctuans G71.19
  levior G71.12
  permanens G71.19
  symptomatic G71.19

Myotonic pupil — *see* Anomaly, pupil, function, tonic pupil
Myriapodiasis B88.2
Myringitis H73.2- ☑
  with otitis media — *see* Otitis, media
  acute H73.00- ☑
    bullous H73.01- ☑
    specified NEC H73.09- ☑
  bullous — *see* Myringitis, acute, bullous
  chronic H73.1- ☑
Mysophobia F40.228
Mytilotoxism — *see* Poisoning, fish
Myxadenitis labialis K13.0
Myxedema (adult) (idiocy) (infantile) (juvenile) (*see also* Hypothyroidism) E03.9
  circumscribed E05.90
    with storm E05.91
  coma E03.5
  congenital E00.1
  cutis L98.5
  localized (pretibial) E05.90
    with storm E05.91
  papular L98.5
Myxochondrosarcoma — *see* Neoplasm, cartilage, malignant
Myxofibroma — *see* Neoplasm, connective tissue, benign
  odontogenic — *see* Cyst, calcifying odontogenic
Myxofibrosarcoma — *see* Neoplasm, connective tissue, malignant
Myxolipoma D17.9
Myxoliposarcoma — *see* Neoplasm, connective tissue, malignant
Myxoma (*see also* Neoplasm, connective tissue, benign)
  nerve sheath — *see* Neoplasm, nerve, benign
  odontogenic — *see* Cyst, calcifying odontogenic
Myxosarcoma — *see* Neoplasm, connective tissue, malignant

N

Naegeli's
  disease Q82.8
  leukemia, monocytic C93.1- ☑
Naegleriasis (with meningoencephalitis) B60.2
Naffziger's syndrome G54.0
Naga sore — see Ulcer, skin
Nägele's pelvis M95.5
  with disproportion (fetopelvic) O33.0
    causing obstructed labor O65.0
Nail (see also condition)
  biting F98.8
  patella syndrome Q87.2
Nanism, nanosomia — see Dwarfism
Nanophyetiasis B66.8
Nanukayami A27.89
Napkin rash L22
Narcolepsy G47.419
  with cataplexy G47.411
  in conditions classified elsewhere G47.429
    with cataplexy G47.421
Narcosis R06.89
Narcotism — see Dependence
NARP (Neuropathy, Ataxia and Retinitis pigmentosa)
  syndrome E88.49
Narrow
  anterior chamber angle H40.03- ☑
  pelvis — see Contraction, pelvis
Narrowing (see also Stenosis)
  artery I77.1
    auditory, internal I65.8
    basilar — see Occlusion, artery, basilar
    carotid — see Occlusion, artery, carotid
    cerebellar — see Occlusion, artery, cerebellar
    cerebral — see Occlusion artery, cerebral
    choroidal — see Occlusion, artery, cerebral, specified NEC
    communicating posterior — see Occlusion, artery, cerebral, specified NEC
    coronary (see also Disease, heart, ischemic, atherosclerotic)
      congenital Q24.5
        syphilitic A50.54 [I52]
      due to syphilis NEC A52.06
    hypophyseal — see Occlusion, artery, cerebral, specified NEC
    pontine — see Occlusion, artery, cerebral, specified NEC
    precerebral — see Occlusion, artery, precerebral
    vertebral — see Occlusion, artery, vertebral
  auditory canal (external) — see Stenosis, external ear canal
  eustachian tube — see Obstruction, eustachian tube
  eyelid — see Disorder, eyelid function
  larynx J38.6
  mesenteric artery K55.0
  palate M26.89
  palpebral fissure — see Disorder, eyelid function
  ureter N13.5
    with infection N13.6
  urethra — see Stricture, urethra
Narrowness, abnormal, eyelid Q10.3
Nasal — see condition
Nasolachrymal, nasolacrimal — see condition
Nasopharyngeal (see also condition)
  pituitary gland Q89.2
  torticollis M43.6
Nasopharyngitis (acute) (infective) (streptococcal) (subacute) J00
  chronic (suppurative) (ulcerative) J31.1
Nasopharynx, nasopharyngeal — see condition
Natal tooth, teeth K00.6
Nausea (without vomiting) R11.0
  with vomiting R11.2
  gravidarum — see Hyperemesis, gravidarum
  marina T75.3 ☑
  navalis T75.3 ☑
Navel — see condition
Neapolitan fever — see Brucellosis

Near drowning T75.1 ☑
Nearsightedness — see Myopia
Near-syncope R55
Nebula, cornea — see Opacity, cornea
Necator americanus infestation B76.1
Necatoriasis B76.1
Neck — see condition
Necrobiosis R68.89
  lipoidica NEC L92.1
    with diabetes — see E08-E13 with .620
Necrolysis, toxic epidermal L51.2
  due to drug
    correct substance properly administered — see Table of Drugs and Chemicals, by drug, adverse effect
    overdose or wrong substance given or taken — see Table of Drugs and Chemicals, by drug, poisoning
Necrophilia F65.89
Necrosis, necrotic (ischemic) (see also Gangrene)
  adrenal (capsule) (gland) E27.49
  amputation stump (surgical) (late) T87.50
    arm T87.5- ☑
    leg T87.5- ☑
  antrum J32.0
  aorta (hyaline) (see also Aneurysm, aorta)
    cystic medial — see Dissection, aorta
  artery I77.5
  bladder (aseptic) (sphincter) N32.89
  bone (see also Osteonecrosis) M87.9
    aseptic or avascular — see Osteonecrosis
      idiopathic M87.00
    ethmoid J32.2
    jaw M27.2
    tuberculous — see Tuberculosis, bone
  brain I67.89
  breast (aseptic) (fat) (segmental) N64.1
  bronchus J98.09
  central nervous system NEC I67.89
  cerebellar I67.89
  cerebral I67.89
  colon K55.0
  cornea H18.40
  cortical (acute) (renal) N17.1
  cystic medial (aorta) — see Dissection, aorta
  dental pulp K04.1
  esophagus K22.8
  ethmoid (bone) J32.2
  eyelid — see Disorder, eyelid, degenerative
  fat, fatty (generalized) (see also Disorder, soft tissue, specified type NEC)
    abdominal wall K65.4
    breast (aseptic) (segmental) N64.1
    localized — see Degeneration, by site, fatty
    mesentery K65.4
    omentum K65.4
    pancreas K86.8
    peritoneum K65.4
    skin (subcutaneous), newborn P83.0
    subcutaneous, due to birth injury P15.6
  gallbladder — see Cholecystitis, acute
  heart — see Infarct, myocardium
  hip, aseptic or avascular — see Osteonecrosis, by type, femur
  intestine (acute) (hemorrhagic) (massive) K55.0
  jaw M27.2
  kidney (bilateral) N28.0
    acute N17.9
    cortical (acute) (bilateral) N17.1
      with ectopic or molar pregnancy O08.4
    medullary (bilateral) (in acute renal failure) (papillary) N17.2
    papillary (bilateral) (in acute renal failure) N17.2
    tubular N17.0
      with ectopic or molar pregnancy O08.4
      complicating
        abortion — see Abortion, by type, complicated by, tubular necrosis
        ectopic or molar pregnancy O08.4
        pregnancy — see Pregnancy, complicated by, diseases of, specified type or system NEC

Necrosis, necrotic — continued
  kidney — continued
    tubular — continued
      following ectopic or molar pregnancy O08.4
      traumatic T79.5 ☑
  larynx J38.7
  liver (with hepatic failure) (cell) — see Failure, hepatic
    hemorrhagic, central K76.2
  lung J85.0
  lymphatic gland — see Lymphadenitis, acute
  mammary gland (fat) (segmental) N64.1
  mastoid (chronic) — see Mastoiditis, chronic
  medullary (acute) (renal) N17.2
  mesentery K55.0
    fat K65.4
  mitral valve — see Insufficiency, mitral
  myocardium, myocardial — see Infarct, myocardium
  nose J34.0
  omentum (with mesenteric infarction) K55.0
    fat K65.4
  orbit, orbital — see Osteomyelitis, orbit
  ossicles, ear — see Abnormal, ear ossicles
  ovary N70.92
  pancreas (aseptic) (duct) (fat) K86.8
    acute (infective) — see Pancreatitis, acute
    infective — see Pancreatitis, acute
  papillary (acute) (renal) N17.2
  perineum N90.89
  peritoneum (with mesenteric infarction) K55.0
    fat K65.4
  pharynx J02.9
    in granulocytopenia — see Neutropenia
    Vincent's A69.1
  phosphorus — see subcategory T54.2 ☑
  pituitary (gland) (postpartum) (Sheehan) E23.0
  pressure — see Ulcer, pressure, by site
  pulmonary J85.0
  pulp (dental) K04.1
  radiation — see Necrosis, by site
  radium — see Necrosis, by site
  renal — see Necrosis, kidney
  sclera H15.89
  scrotum N50.8
  skin or subcutaneous tissue NEC I96
  spine, spinal (column) (see also Osteonecrosis, by type, vertebra)
    cord G95.19
  spleen D73.5
  stomach K31.89
  stomatitis (ulcerative) A69.0
  subcutaneous fat, newborn P83.8
  subendocardial (acute) I21.4
    chronic I25.89
  suprarenal (capsule) (gland) E27.49
  testis N50.8
  thymus (gland) E32.8
  tonsil J35.8
  trachea J39.8
  tuberculous NEC — see Tuberculosis
  tubular (acute) (anoxic) (renal) (toxic) N17.0
    postprocedural N99.0
  vagina N89.8
  vertebra (see also Osteonecrosis, by type, vertebra)
    tuberculous A18.01
  vulva N90.89
  X-ray — see Necrosis, by site
Necrospermia — see Infertility, male
Need (for)
  care provider because (of)
    assistance with personal care Z74.1
    continuous supervision required Z74.3
    impaired mobility Z74.09
    no other household member able to render care Z74.2
    specified reason NEC Z74.8
  immunization — see Vaccination
  vaccination — see Vaccination
Neglect
  adult
    confirmed T74.01 ☑
    history of Z91.412
    suspected T76.01 ☑

Neglect — *continued*
  child (childhood)
    confirmed T74.02 ☑
    history of Z62.812
    suspected T76.02 ☑
  emotional, in childhood Z62.898
  hemispatial R41.4
  left-sided R41.4
  sensory R41.4
  visuospatial R41.4
Neisserian infection NEC — *see* Gonococcus
Nelaton's syndrome G60.8
Nelson's syndrome E24.1
Nematodiasis (intestinal) B82.0
  Ancylostoma B76.0
Neonatal (*see also* Newborn)
  acne L70.4
  bradycardia P29.12
  screening, abnormal findings on P09
  tachycardia P29.11
  tooth, teeth K00.6
Neonatorum — *see* condition
Neoplasia
  endocrine, multiple (MEN) E31.20
    type I E31.21
    type IIA E31.22
    type IIB E31.23
  intraepithelial (histologically confirmed)
    anal (AIN) (histologically confirmed) K62.82
      grade I K62.82
      grade II K62.82
      severe D01.3
    cervical glandular (histologically confirmed) D06.9
    cervix (uteri) (CIN) (histologically confirmed) N87.9
      glandular D06.9
      grade I N87.0
      grade II N87.1
      grade III (severe dysplasia) (*see also* Carcinoma, cervix uteri, in situ) D06.9
    prostate (histologically confirmed) (PIN I) (PIN II) N42.3
      grade I N42.3
      grade II N42.3
      severe D07.5
    vagina (histologically confirmed) (VAIN) N89.3
      grade I N89.0
      grade II N89.1
      grade III (severe dysplasia) D07.2
    vulva (histologically confirmed) (VIN) N90.3
      grade I N90.0
      grade II N90.1
      grade III (severe dysplasia) D07.1
Neoplasm, neoplastic (*see also* Table of Neoplasms)
  lipomatous, benign — *see* Lipoma
Neovascularization
  ciliary body — *see* Disorder, iris, vascular
  cornea H16.40- ☑
    deep H16.44- ☑
    ghost vessels — *see* Ghost, vessels
    localized H16.43- ☑
    pannus — *see* Pannus
  iris — *see* Disorder, iris, vascular
  retina H35.05- ☑
Nephralgia N23
Nephritis, nephritic (albuminuric) (azotemic) (congenital) (disseminated) (epithelial) (familial) (focal) (granulomatous) (hemorrhagic) (infantile) (nonsuppurative, excretory) (uremic) N05.9
  with
    dense deposit disease N05.6
    diffuse
      crescentic glomerulonephritis N05.7
      endocapillary proliferative glomerulonephritis N05.4
      membranous glomerulonephritis N05.2
      mesangial proliferative glomerulonephritis N05.3
      mesangiocapillary glomerulonephritis N05.5
    edema — *see* Nephrosis
    focal and segmental glomerular lesions N05.1
    foot process disease N04.9
    glomerular lesion
      diffuse sclerosing N05.8
      hypocomplementemic — *see* Nephritis, membranoproliferative
      IgA — *see* Nephropathy, IgA
      lobular, lobulonodular — *see* Nephritis, membranoproliferative

Nephritis, nephritic — *continued*
  with — *continued*
    glomerular lesion — *continued*
      nodular — *see* Nephritis, membranoproliferative
    lesion of
      glomerulonephritis, proliferative N05.8
      renal necrosis N05.9
    minor glomerular abnormality N05.0
    specified morphological changes NEC N05.8
  acute N00.9
    with
      dense deposit disease N00.6
      diffuse
        crescentic glomerulonephritis N00.7
        endocapillary proliferative glomerulonephritis N00.4
        membranous glomerulonephritis N00.2
        mesangial proliferative glomerulonephritis N00.3
        mesangiocapillary glomerulonephritis N00.5
      focal and segmental glomerular lesions N00.1
      minor glomerular abnormality N00.0
      specified morphological changes NEC N00.8
  amyloid E85.4 [N08]
  antiglomerular basement membrane (anti-GBM) antibody NEC
    in Goodpasture's syndrome M31.0
  antitubular basement membrane (tubulo-interstitial) NEC N12
    toxic — *see* Nephropathy, toxic
  arteriolar — *see* Hypertension, kidney
  arteriosclerotic — *see* Hypertension, kidney
  ascending — *see* Nephritis, tubulo-interstitial
  atrophic N03.9
  Balkan (endemic) N15.0
  calculous, calculus — *see* Calculus, kidney
  cardiac — *see* Hypertension, kidney
  cardiovascular — *see* Hypertension, kidney
  chronic N03.9
    with
      dense deposit disease N03.6
      diffuse
        crescentic glomerulonephritis N03.7
        endocapillary proliferative glomerulonephritis N03.4
        membranous glomerulonephritis N03.2
        mesangial proliferative glomerulonephritis N03.3
        mesangiocapillary glomerulonephritis N03.5
      focal and segmental glomerular lesions N03.1
      minor glomerular abnormality N03.0
      specified morphological changes NEC N03.8
    arteriosclerotic — *see* Hypertension, kidney
  cirrhotic N26.9
  complicating pregnancy O26.83- ☑
  croupous N00.9
  degenerative — *see* Nephrosis
  diffuse sclerosing N05.8
  due to
    diabetes mellitus — *see* E08-E13 with .21
    subacute bacterial endocarditis I33.0
    systemic lupus erythematosus (chronic) M32.14
    typhoid fever A01.09
  gonococcal (acute) (chronic) A54.21
  hypocomplementemic — *see* Nephritis, membranoproliferative
  IgA — *see* Nephropathy, IgA
  immune complex (circulating) NEC N05.8
  infective — *see* Nephritis, tubulo-interstitial
  interstitial — *see* Nephritis, tubulo-interstitial
  lead N14.3
  membranoproliferative (diffuse) (type 1 or 3) (*see also* N00-N07 with fourth character .5) N05.5
    type 2 (*see also* N00-N07 with fourth character .6) N05.6
  minimal change N05.0
  necrotic, necrotizing NEC (*see also* N00-N07 with fourth character .8) N05.8
  nephrotic — *see* Nephrosis
  nodular — *see* Nephritis, membranoproliferative
  polycystic Q61.3
    adult type Q61.2
    autosomal
      dominant Q61.2
      recessive NEC Q61.19
    childhood type NEC Q61.19
    infantile type NEC Q61.19

Nephritis, nephritic — *continued*
  poststreptococcal N05.9
    acute N00.9
    chronic N03.9
    rapidly progressive N01.9
  proliferative NEC (*see also* N00-N07 with fourth character .8) N05.8
  purulent — *see* Nephritis, tubulo-interstitial
  rapidly progressive N01.9
    with
      dense deposit disease N01.6
      diffuse
        crescentic glomerulonephritis N01.7
        endocapillary proliferative glomerulonephritis N01.4
        membranous glomerulonephritis N01.2
        mesangial proliferative glomerulonephritis N01.3
        mesangiocapillary glomerulonephritis N01.5
      focal and segmental glomerular lesions N01.1
      minor glomerular abnormality N01.0
      specified morphological changes NEC N01.8
  salt losing or wasting NEC N28.89
  saturnine N14.3
  sclerosing, diffuse N05.8
  septic — *see* Nephritis, tubulo-interstitial
  specified pathology NEC (*see also* N00-N07 with fourth character .8) N05.8
  subacute N01.9
  suppurative — *see* Nephritis, tubulo-interstitial
  syphilitic (late) A52.75
    congenital A50.59 [N08]
    early (secondary) A51.44
  toxic — *see* Nephropathy, toxic
  tubal, tubular — *see* Nephritis, tubulo-interstitial
  tuberculous A18.11
  tubulo-interstitial (in) N12
    acute (infectious) N10
    chronic (infectious) N11.9
      nonobstructive N11.8
        reflux-associated N11.0
      obstructive N11.1
      specified NEC N11.8
    due to
      brucellosis A23.9 [N16]
      cryoglobulinemia D89.1 [N16]
      glycogen storage disease E74.00 [N16]
    Sjögren's syndrome M35.04
  vascular — *see* Hypertension, kidney
  war N00.9
Nephroblastoma (epithelial) (mesenchymal) C64- ☑
Nephrocalcinosis E83.59 [N29]
Nephrocystitis, pustular — *see* Nephritis, tubulo-interstitial
Nephrolithiasis (congenital) (pelvis) (recurrent) (*see also* Calculus, kidney)
Nephroma C64- ☑
  mesoblastic D41.0- ☑
Nephronephritis — *see* Nephrosis
Nephronophthisis Q61.5
Nephropathia epidemica A98.5
Nephropathy (*see also* Nephritis) N28.9
  with
    edema — *see* Nephrosis
    glomerular lesion — *see* Glomerulonephritis
  amyloid, hereditary E85.0
  analgesic N14.0
    with medullary necrosis, acute N17.2
  Balkan (endemic) N15.0
  chemical — *see* Nephropathy, toxic
  diabetic — *see* E08-E13 with .21
  drug-induced N14.2
    specified NEC N14.1
  focal and segmental hyalinosis or sclerosis N02.1
  heavy metal-induced N14.3
  hereditary NEC N07.9
    with
      dense deposit disease N07.6
      diffuse
        crescentic glomerulonephritis N07.7
        endocapillary proliferative glomerulonephritis N07.4
        membranous glomerulonephritis N07.2
        mesangial proliferative glomerulonephritis N07.3
        mesangiocapillary glomerulonephritis N07.5
      focal and segmental glomerular lesions N07.1
      minor glomerular abnormality N07.0

⬇ Subterms under main terms may continue to next column or page   ☑ Additional Character Required — Refer to the Tabular List for Character Selection

Nephropathy — *continued*
  hereditary — *continued*
    with — *continued*
      specified morphological changes NEC N07.8
  hypercalcemic N25.89
  hypertensive — *see* Hypertension, kidney
  hypokalemic (vacuolar) N25.89
  IgA N02.8
    with glomerular lesion N02.9
      focal and segmental hyalinosis or sclerosis
          N02.1
      membranoproliferative (diffuse) N02.5
      membranous (diffuse) N02.2
      mesangial proliferative N02.3
      mesangiocapillary (diffuse) N02.5
      proliferative NEC N02.8
      specified pathology NEC N02.8
  lead N14.3
  membranoproliferative (diffuse) N02.5
  membranous (diffuse) N02.2
  mesangial (IgA/IgG) — *see* Nephropathy, IgA
    proliferative (diffuse) N02.3
  mesangiocapillary (diffuse) N02.5
  obstructive N13.8
  phenacetin N17.2
  phosphate-losing N25.0
  potassium depletion N25.89
  pregnancy-related O26.83- ☑
  proliferative NEC (*see also* N00-N07 with fourth character .8) N05.8
  protein-losing N25.89
  saturnine N14.3
  sickle-cell D57.- ☑ [N08]
  toxic NEC N14.4
    due to
      drugs N14.2
        analgesic N14.0
        specified NEC N14.1
      heavy metals N14.3
  vasomotor N17.0
  water-losing N25.89
Nephroptosis N28.83
Nephropyosis — *see* Abscess, kidney
Nephrorrhagia N28.89
Nephrosclerosis (arteriolar)(arteriosclerotic) (chronic)
    (hyaline) (*see also* Hypertension, kidney)
  hyperplastic — *see* Hypertension, kidney
  senile N26.9
Nephrosis, nephrotic (Epstein's) (syndrome) (congenital)
    N04.9
  with
    foot process disease N04.9
    glomerular lesion N04.1
    hypocomplementemic N04.5
  acute N04.9
  anoxic — *see* Nephrosis, tubular
  chemical — *see* Nephrosis, tubular
  cholemic K76.7
  diabetic — *see* E08-E13 with .21
  Finnish type (congenital) Q89.8
  hemoglobin N10
  hemoglobinuric — *see* Nephrosis, tubular
  in
    amyloidosis E85.4 [N08]
    diabetes mellitus — *see* E08-E13 with .21
    epidemic hemorrhagic fever A98.5
    malaria (malariae) B52.0
  ischemic — *see* Nephrosis, tubular
  lipoid N04.9
  lower nephron — *see* Nephrosis, tubular
  malarial (malariae) B52.0
  minimal change N04.0
  myoglobin N10
  necrotizing — *see* Nephrosis, tubular
  osmotic (sucrose) N25.89
  radiation N04.9
  syphilitic (late) A52.75
  toxic — *see* Nephrosis, tubular
  tubular (acute) N17.0
    postprocedural N99.0
    radiation N04.9
Nephrosonephritis, hemorrhagic (endemic) A98.5
Nephrostomy
  attention to Z43.6
  status Z93.6
Nerve (*see also* condition)
  injury — *see* Injury, nerve, by body site
Nerves R45.0

Nervous (*see also* condition) R45.0
  heart F45.8
  stomach F45.8
  tension R45.0
Nervousness R45.0
Nesidioblastoma
  pancreas D13.7
  specified site NEC — *see* Neoplasm, benign, by site
  unspecified site D13.7
Nettleship's syndrome Q82.2
Neumann's disease or syndrome L10.1
Neuralgia, neuralgic (acute) M79.2
  accessory (nerve) G52.8
  acoustic (nerve) — *see* subcategory H93.3 ☑
  auditory (nerve) — *see* subcategory H93.3 ☑
  ciliary G44.009
    intractable G44.001
    not intractable G44.009
  cranial
    nerve (*see also* Disorder, nerve, cranial)
      fifth or trigeminal — *see* Neuralgia, trigeminal
    postherpetic, postzoster B02.29
  ear — *see* subcategory H92.0 ☑
  facialis vera G51.1
  Fothergill's — *see* Neuralgia, trigeminal
  glossopharyngeal (nerve) G52.1
  Horton's G44.099
    intractable G44.091
    not intractable G44.099
  Hunt's B02.21
  hypoglossal (nerve) G52.3
  infraorbital — *see* Neuralgia, trigeminal
  malarial — *see* Malaria
  migrainous G44.009
    intractable G44.001
    not intractable G44.009
  Morton's G57.6- ☑
  nerve, cranial — *see* Disorder, nerve, cranial
  nose G52.0
  occipital M54.81
  olfactory G52.0
  penis N48.9
  perineum R10.2
  postherpetic NEC B02.29
    trigeminal B02.22
  pubic region R10.2
  scrotum R10.2
  Sluder's G44.89
  specified nerve NEC G58.8
  spermatic cord R10.2
  sphenopalatine (ganglion) G90.09
  trifacial — *see* Neuralgia, trigeminal
  trigeminal G50.0
    postherpetic, postzoster B02.22
  vagus (nerve) G52.2
  writer's F48.8
    organic G25.89
Neurapraxia — *see* Injury, nerve
Neurasthenia F48.8
  cardiac F45.8
  gastric F45.8
  heart F45.8
Neurilemmoma (*see also* Neoplasm, nerve, benign)
  acoustic (nerve) D33.3
  malignant (*see also* Neoplasm, nerve, malignant)
    acoustic (nerve) C72.4- ☑
Neurilemmosarcoma — *see* Neoplasm, nerve, malignant
Neurinoma — *see* Neoplasm, nerve, benign
Neurinomatosis — *see* Neoplasm, nerve, uncertain behavior
Neuritis (rheumatoid) M79.2
  abducens (nerve) — *see* Strabismus, paralytic, sixth nerve
  accessory (nerve) G52.8
  acoustic (nerve) (*see also* subcategory) H93.3 ☑
    in (due to)
      infectious disease NEC B99 ☑ [H94.0-] ☑
      parasitic disease NEC B89 [H94.0-] ☑
      syphilitic A52.15
  alcoholic G62.1
    with psychosis — *see* Psychosis, alcoholic
  amyloid, any site E85.4 [G63]
  auditory (nerve) — *see* subcategory H93.3 ☑
  brachial — *see* Radiculopathy
    due to displacement, intervertebral disc — *see*
        Disorder, disc, cervical, with neuritis

Neuritis — *continued*
  cranial nerve
    due to Lyme disease A69.22
    eighth or acoustic or auditory — *see* subcategory
        H93.3 ☑
    eleventh or accessory G52.8
    fifth or trigeminal G51.0
    first or olfactory G52.0
    fourth or trochlear — *see* Strabismus, paralytic,
        fourth nerve
    second or optic — *see* Neuritis, optic
    seventh or facial G51.8
      newborn (birth injury) P11.3
    sixth or abducent — *see* Strabismus, paralytic, sixth
        nerve
    tenth or vagus G52.2
    third or oculomotor — *see* Strabismus, paralytic,
        third nerve
    twelfth or hypoglossal G52.3
  Déjérine-Sottas G60.0
  diabetic (mononeuropathy) — *see* E08-E13 with .41
    polyneuropathy — *see* E08-E13 with .42
  due to
    beriberi E51.11
    displacement, prolapse or rupture, intervertebral
        disc — *see* Disorder, disc, with, radiculopathy
    herniation, nucleus pulposus M51.9 [G55]
  endemic E51.11
  facial G51.8
    newborn (birth injury) P11.3
  general — *see* Polyneuropathy
  geniculate ganglion G51.1
    due to herpes (zoster) B02.21
  gouty M10.00 [G63]
  hypoglossal (nerve) G52.3
  ilioinguinal (nerve) G57.9- ☑
  infectious (multiple) NEC G61.0
  interstitial hypertrophic progressive G60.0
  lumbar M54.16
  lumbosacral M54.17
  multiple (*see also* Polyneuropathy)
    endemic E51.11
    infective, acute G61.0
  multiplex endemica E51.11
  nerve root — *see* Radiculopathy
  oculomotor (nerve) — *see* Strabismus, paralytic, third
      nerve
  olfactory nerve G52.0
  optic (nerve) (hereditary) (sympathetic) H46.9
    with demyelination G36.0
    in myelitis G36.0
    nutritional H46.2
    papillitis — *see* Papillitis, optic
    retrobulbar H46.1- ☑
    specified type NEC H46.8
    toxic H46.3
  peripheral (nerve) G62.9
    multiple — *see* Polyneuropathy
    single — *see* Mononeuritis
  pneumogastric (nerve) G52.2
  postherpetic, postzoster B02.29
  progressive hypertrophic interstitial G60.0
  retrobulbar (*see also* Neuritis, optic, retrobulbar)
    in (due to)
      late syphilis A52.15
      meningococcal infection A39.82
    meningococcal A39.82
    syphilitic A52.15
  sciatic (nerve) (*see also* Sciatica)
    due to displacement of intervertebral disc — *see*
        Disorder, disc, with, radiculopathy
  serum (*see also* Reaction, serum) T80.69 ☑
  shoulder-girdle G54.5
  specified nerve NEC G58.8
  spinal (nerve) root — *see* Radiculopathy
  syphilitic A52.15
  thenar (median) G56.1- ☑
  thoracic M54.14
  toxic NEC G62.2
  trochlear (nerve) — *see* Strabismus, paralytic, fourth
      nerve
  vagus (nerve) G52.2
Neuroastrocytoma — *see* Neoplasm, uncertain behavior, by site
Neuroavitaminosis E56.9 [G99.8]
Neuroblastoma
  olfactory C30.0
  specified site — *see* Neoplasm, malignant, by site

☑ **Additional Character Required** — Refer to the Tabular List for Character Selection   ▽ **Subterms under main terms may continue to next column or page**

Neuroblastoma — *continued*
  unspecified site C74.90
Neurochorioretinitis — *see* Chorioretinitis
Neurocirculatory asthenia F45.8
Neurocysticercosis B69.0
Neurocytoma — *see* Neoplasm, benign, by site
Neurodermatitis (circumscribed) (circumscripta) (local) L28.0
  atopic L20.81
  diffuse (Brocq) L20.81
  disseminated L20.81
Neuroencephalomyelopathy, optic G36.0
Neuroepithelioma (*see also* Neoplasm, malignant, by site)
  olfactory C30.0
Neurofibroma (*see also* Neoplasm, nerve, benign)
  melanotic — *see* Neoplasm, nerve, benign
  multiple — *see* Neurofibromatosis
  plexiform — *see* Neoplasm, nerve, benign
Neurofibromatosis (multiple) (nonmalignant) Q85.00
  acoustic Q85.02
  malignant — *see* Neoplasm, nerve, malignant
  specified NEC Q85.09
  type 1 (von Recklinghausen) Q85.01
  type 2 Q85.02
Neurofibrosarcoma — *see* Neoplasm, nerve, malignant
Neurogenic (*see also* condition)
  bladder (*see also* Dysfunction, bladder, neuromuscular) N31.9
    cauda equina syndrome G83.4
  bowel NEC K59.2
  heart F45.8
Neuroglioma — *see* Neoplasm, uncertain behavior, by site
Neurolabyrinthitis (of Dix and Hallpike) — *see* Neuronitis, vestibular
Neurolathyrism — *see* Poisoning, food, noxious, plant
Neuroleprosy A30.9
Neuroma (*see also* Neoplasm, nerve, benign)
  acoustic (nerve) D33.3
  amputation (stump) (traumatic) (surgical complication) (late) T87.3- ☑
    arm T87.3- ☑
    leg T87.3- ☑
  digital (toe) G57.6- ☑
  interdigital (toe) G58.8
    lower limb G57.8- ☑
    upper limb G56.8- ☑
  intermetatarsal G57.8- ☑
  Morton's G57.6- ☑
  nonneoplastic
    arm G56.9- ☑
    leg G57.9- ☑
    lower extremity G57.9- ☑
    upper extremity G56.9- ☑
  optic (nerve) D33.3
  plantar G57.6- ☑
  plexiform — *see* Neoplasm, nerve, benign
  surgical (nonneoplastic)
    arm G56.9- ☑
    leg G57.9- ☑
    lower extremity G57.9- ☑
    upper extremity G56.9- ☑
Neuromyalgia — *see* Neuralgia
Neuromyasthenia (epidemic) (postinfectious) G93.3
Neuromyelitis G36.9
  ascending G61.0
  optica G36.0
Neuromyopathy G70.9
  paraneoplastic D49.9 [G13.0]
Neuromyotonia (Isaacs) G71.19
Neuronevus — *see* Nevus
Neuronitis G58.9
  ascending (acute) G57.2- ☑
  vestibular H81.2- ☑
Neuroparalytic — *see* condition
Neuropathy, neuropathic G62.9
  acute motor G62.81
  alcoholic G62.1
    with psychosis — *see* Psychosis, alcoholic
  arm G56.9- ☑
  autonomic, peripheral — *see* Neuropathy, peripheral, autonomic
  axillary G56.9- ☑
  bladder N31.9
    atonic (motor) (sensory) N31.2
    autonomous N31.2

Neuropathy, neuropathic — *continued*
  bladder — *continued*
    flaccid N31.2
    nonreflex N31.2
    reflex N31.1
    uninhibited N31.0
  brachial plexus G54.0
  cervical plexus G54.2
  chronic
    progressive segmentally demyelinating G62.89
    relapsing demyelinating G62.89
  Déjérine-Sottas G60.0
  diabetic — *see* E08-E13 with .40
    mononeuropathy — *see* E08-E13 with .41
    polyneuropathy — *see* E08-E13 with .42
  entrapment G58.9
    iliohypogastric nerve G57.8- ☑
    ilioinguinal nerve G57.8- ☑
    lateral cutaneous nerve of thigh G57.1- ☑
    median nerve G56.0- ☑
    obturator nerve G57.8- ☑
    peroneal nerve G57.3- ☑
    posterior tibial nerve G57.5- ☑
    saphenous nerve G57.8- ☑
    ulnar nerve G56.2- ☑
  facial nerve G51.9
  hereditary G60.9
    motor and sensory (types I-IV) G60.0
    sensory G60.8
    specified NEC G60.8
  hypertrophic G60.0
    Charcot-Marie-Tooth G60.0
    Déjérine-Sottas G60.0
    interstitial progressive G60.0
    of infancy G60.0
    Refsum G60.1
  idiopathic G60.9
    progressive G60.3
    specified NEC G60.8
  in association with hereditary ataxia G60.2
  intercostal G58.0
  ischemic — *see* Disorder, nerve
  Jamaica (ginger) G62.2
  leg NEC G57.9- ☑
  lower extremity G57.9- ☑
  lumbar plexus G54.1
  median nerve G56.1- ☑
  motor and sensory (*see also* Polyneuropathy)
    hereditary (types I-IV) G60.0
  multiple (acute) (chronic) — *see* Polyneuropathy
  optic (nerve) (*see also* Neuritis, optic)
    ischemic H47.01- ☑
  paraneoplastic (sensorial) (Denny Brown) D49.9 [G13.0]
  peripheral (nerve) (*see also* Polyneuropathy) G62.9
    autonomic G90.9
      idiopathic G90.09
      in (due to)
        amyloidosis E85.4 [G99.0]
        diabetes mellitus — *see* E08-E13 with .43
        endocrine disease NEC E34.9 [G99.0]
        gout M10.00 [G99.0]
        hyperthyroidism E05.90 [G99.0]
          with thyroid storm E05.91 [G99.0]
        metabolic disease NEC E88.9 [G99.0]
    idiopathic G60.9
      progressive G60.3
    in (due to)
      antitetanus serum G62.0
      arsenic G62.2
      drugs NEC G62.0
      lead G62.2
      organophosphate compounds G62.2
      toxic agent NEC G62.2
  plantar nerves G57.6- ☑
  progressive
    hypertrophic interstitial G60.0
    inflammatory G62.81
  radicular NEC — *see* Radiculopathy
  sacral plexus G54.1
  sciatic G57.0- ☑
  serum G61.1
  toxic NEC G62.2
  trigeminal sensory G50.8
  ulnar nerve G56.2- ☑
  uremic N18.9 [G63]
  vitamin B12 E53.8 [G63]
    with anemia (pernicious) D51.0 [G63]
      due to dietary deficiency D51.3 [G63]

Neurophthisis (*see also* Disorder, nerve)
  peripheral, diabetic — *see* E08-E13 with .42
Neuroretinitis — *see* Chorioretinitis
Neuroretinopathy, hereditary optic H47.22
Neurosarcoma — *see* Neoplasm, nerve, malignant
Neurosclerosis — *see* Disorder, nerve
Neurosis, neurotic F48.9
  anankastic F42
  anxiety (state) F41.1
    panic type F41.0
  asthenic F48.8
  bladder F45.8
  cardiac (reflex) F45.8
  cardiovascular F45.8
  character F60.9
  colon F45.8
  compensation F68.1 ☑
  compulsive, compulsion F42
  conversion F44.9
  craft F48.8
  cutaneous F45.8
  depersonalization F48.1
  depressive (reaction) (type) F34.1
  environmental F48.8
  excoriation L98.1
  fatigue F48.8
  functional — *see* Disorder, somatoform
  gastric F45.8
  gastrointestinal F45.8
  heart F45.8
  hypochondriacal F45.21
  hysterical F44.9
  incoordination F45.8
    larynx F45.8
    vocal cord F45.8
  intestine F45.8
  larynx (sensory) F45.8
    hysterical F44.4
  mixed NEC F48.8
  musculoskeletal F45.8
  obsessional F42
  obsessive-compulsive F42
  occupational F48.8
  ocular NEC F45.8
  organ — *see* Disorder, somatoform
  pharynx F45.8
  phobic F40.9
  posttraumatic (situational) F43.10
    acute F43.11
    chronic F43.12
  psychasthenic (type) F48.8
  railroad F48.8
  rectum F45.8
  respiratory F45.8
  rumination F45.8
  sexual F65.9
  situational F48.8
  social F40.10
    generalized F40.11
  specified type NEC F48.8
  state F48.9
    with depersonalization episode F48.1
  stomach F45.8
  traumatic F43.10
    acute F43.11
    chronic F43.12
  vasomotor F45.8
  visceral F45.8
  war F48.8
Neurospongioblastosis diffusa Q85.1
Neurosyphilis (arrested) (early) (gumma) (late) (latent) (recurrent) (relapse) A52.3
  with ataxia (cerebellar) (locomotor) (spastic) (spinal) A52.19
  aneurysm (cerebral) A52.05
  arachnoid (adhesive) A52.13
  arteritis (any artery) (cerebral) A52.04
  asymptomatic A52.2
  congenital A50.40
  dura (mater) A52.13
  general paresis A52.17
  hemorrhagic A52.05
  juvenile (asymptomatic) (meningeal) A50.40
  leptomeninges (aseptic) A52.13
  meningeal, meninges (adhesive) A52.13
  meningitis A52.13
  meningovascular (diffuse) A52.13
  optic atrophy A52.15

Neurosyphilis — continued
   parenchymatous (degenerative) A52.19
   paresis, paretic A52.17
      juvenile A50.45
   remission in (sustained) A52.3
   serological (without symptoms) A52.2
   specified nature or site NEC A52.19
   tabes, tabetic (dorsalis) A52.11
      juvenile A50.45
   taboparesis A52.17
      juvenile A50.45
   thrombosis (cerebral) A52.05
   vascular (cerebral) NEC A52.05
Neurothekeoma — see Neoplasm, nerve, benign
Neurotic — see Neurosis
Neurotoxemia — see Toxemia
Neutroclusion M26.211
Neutropenia, neutropenic (chronic) (genetic) (idiopathic) (immune) (infantile) (malignant) (pernicious) (splenic) D70.9
   congenital (primary) D70.0
   cyclic D70.4
   cytoreductive cancer chemotherapy sequela D70.1
   drug-induced D70.2
      due to cytoreductive cancer chemotherapy D70.1
   due to infection D70.3
   fever D70.9
   neonatal, transitory (isoimmune) (maternal transfer) P61.5
   periodic D70.4
   secondary (cyclic) (periodic) (splenic) D70.4
      drug-induced D70.2
         due to cytoreductive cancer chemotherapy D70.1
   toxic D70.8
Neutrophilia, hereditary giant D72.0
Nevocarcinoma — see Melanoma
Nevus D22.9
   achromic — see Neoplasm, skin, benign
   amelanotic — see Neoplasm, skin, benign
   angiomatous D18.00
      intra-abdominal D18.03
      intracranial D18.02
      skin D18.01
      specified site NEC D18.09
   araneus I78.1
   balloon cell — see Neoplasm, skin, benign
   bathing trunk D48.5
   blue — see Neoplasm, skin, benign
      cellular — see Neoplasm, skin, benign
      giant — see Neoplasm, skin, benign
      Jadassohn's — see Neoplasm, skin, benign
      malignant — see Melanoma
   capillary D18.00
      intra-abdominal D18.03
      intracranial D18.02
      skin D18.01
      specified site NEC D18.09
   cavernous D18.00
      intra-abdominal D18.03
      intracranial D18.02
      skin D18.01
      specified site NEC D18.09
   cellular — see Neoplasm, skin, benign
      blue — see Neoplasm, skin, benign
   choroid D31.3- ☑
   comedonicus Q82.5
   conjunctiva D31.0- ☑
   dermal — see Neoplasm, skin, benign
      with epidermal nevus — see Neoplasm, skin, benign
   dysplastic — see Neoplasm, skin, benign
   eye D31.9- ☑
   flammeus Q82.5
   hemangiomatous D18.00
      intra-abdominal D18.03
      intracranial D18.02
      skin D18.01
      specified site NEC D18.09
   iris D31.4- ☑
   lacrimal gland D31.5- ☑
   lymphatic D18.1
   magnocellular
      specified site — see Neoplasm, benign, by site
      unspecified site D31.40
   malignant — see Melanoma
   meaning hemangioma D18.00
      intra-abdominal D18.03

Nevus — continued
   meaning hemangioma — continued
      intracranial D18.02
      skin D18.01
      specified site NEC D18.09
   mouth (mucosa) D10.30
      specified site NEC D10.39
      white sponge Q38.6
   multiplex Q85.1
   non-neoplastic I78.1
   oral mucosa D10.30
      specified site NEC D10.39
      white sponge Q38.6
   orbit D31.6- ☑
   pigmented
      giant (see also Neoplasm, skin, uncertain behavior) D48.5
         malignant melanoma in — see Melanoma
   portwine Q82.5
   retina D31.2- ☑
   retrobulbar D31.6- ☑
   sanguineous Q82.5
   senile I78.1
   skin D22.9
      abdominal wall D22.5
      ala nasi D22.39
      ankle D22.7- ☑
      anus, anal D22.5
      arm D22.6- ☑
      auditory canal (external) D22.2- ☑
      auricle (ear) D22.2- ☑
      auricular canal (external) D22.2- ☑
      axilla, axillary fold D22.5
      back D22.5
      breast D22.5
      brow D22.39
      buttock D22.5
      canthus (eye) D22.1- ☑
      cheek (external) D22.39
      chest wall D22.5
      chin D22.39
      ear (external) D22.2- ☑
      external meatus (ear) D22.2- ☑
      eyebrow D22.39
      eyelid (lower) (upper) D22.1- ☑
      face D22.30
         specified NEC D22.39
      female genital organ (external) NEC D28.0
      finger D22.6- ☑
      flank D22.5
      foot D22.7- ☑
      forearm D22.6- ☑
      forehead D22.39
      foreskin D29.0
      genital organ (external) NEC
         female D28.0
         male D29.9
      gluteal region D22.5
      groin D22.5
      hand D22.6- ☑
      heel D22.7- ☑
      helix D22.2- ☑
      hip D22.7- ☑
      interscapular region D22.5
      jaw D22.39
      knee D22.7- ☑
      labium (majus) (minus) D28.0
      leg D22.7- ☑
      lip (lower) (upper) D22.0
      lower limb D22.7- ☑
      male genital organ (external) D29.9
      nail D22.9
         finger D22.6- ☑
         toe D22.7- ☑
      nasolabial groove D22.39
      nates D22.5
      neck D22.4
      nose (external) D22.39
      palpebra D22.1- ☑
      penis D29.0
      perianal skin D22.5
      perineum D22.5
      pinna D22.2- ☑
      popliteal fossa or space D22.7- ☑
      prepuce D29.0
      pudendum D28.0
      scalp D22.4

Nevus — continued
   skin — continued
      scrotum D29.4
      shoulder D22.6- ☑
      submammary fold D22.5
      temple D22.39
      thigh D22.7- ☑
      toe D22.7- ☑
      trunk NEC D22.5
      umbilicus D22.5
      upper limb D22.6- ☑
      vulva D28.0
   specified site NEC — see Neoplasm, by site, benign
   spider I78.1
   stellar I78.1
   strawberry Q82.5
   Sutton's — see Neoplasm, skin, benign
   unius lateris Q82.5
   Unna's Q82.5
   vascular Q82.5
   verrucous Q82.5
Newborn (infant) (liveborn) (singleton) Z38.2
   abstinence syndrome P96.1
   acne L70.4
   affected by (suspected to be)
      abnormalities of membranes P02.9
         specified NEC P02.8
      abruptio placenta P02.1
      amino-acid metabolic disorder, transitory P74.8
      amniocentesis (while in utero) P00.6
      amnionitis P02.7
      apparent life threatening event (ALTE) R68.13
      bleeding (into)
         cerebral cortex P52.22
         germinal matrix P52.0
         ventricles P52.1
      breech delivery P03.0
      cardiac arrest P29.81
      cardiomyopathy I42.8
         congenital I42.4
      cerebral ischemia P91.0
      Cesarean delivery P03.4
      chemotherapy agents P04.1
      chorioamnionitis P02.7
      cocaine (crack) P04.41
      complications of labor and delivery P03.9
         specified NEC P03.89
      compression of umbilical cord NEC P02.5
      contracted pelvis P03.1
      delivery P03.9
         Cesarean P03.4
         forceps P03.2
         vacuum extractor P03.3
      entanglement (knot) in umbilical cord P02.5
      environmental chemicals P04.6
      fetal (intrauterine)
         growth retardation P05.9
         malnutrition not light or small for gestational age P05.2
      forceps delivery P03.2
      heart rate abnormalities
         bradycardia P29.12
         intrauterine P03.819
            before onset of labor P03.810
            during labor P03.811
         tachycardia P29.11
      hemorrhage (antepartum) P02.1
         cerebellar (nontraumatic) P52.6
         intracerebral (nontraumatic) P52.4
         intracranial (nontraumatic) P52.9
            specified NEC P52.8
         intraventricular (nontraumatic) P52.3
            grade 1 P52.0
            grade 2 P52.1
            grade 3 P52.21
            grade 4 P52.22
         posterior fossa (nontraumatic) P52.6
         subarachnoid (nontraumatic) P52.5
         subependymal P52.0
           with intracerebral extension P52.22
           with intraventricular extension P52.21
              with enlargment of ventricles P52.21
           without intraventricular extension P52.0
      hypoxic ischemic encephalopathy [HIE] P91.60
         mild P91.61
         moderate P91.62
         severe P91.63
      induction of labor P03.89

☑ **Additional Character Required** — Refer to the Tabular List for Character Selection   ▽ **Subterms under main terms may continue to next column or page**

Newborn — *continued*
  affected by — *continued*
    intestinal perforation P78.0
    intrauterine (fetal) blood loss P50.9
      due to (from)
        cut end of co-twin cord P50.5
        hemorrhage into
          co-twin P50.3
          maternal circulation P50.4
        placenta P50.2
        ruptured cord blood P50.1
        vasa previa P50.0
      specified NEC P50.8
    intrauterine (fetal) hemorrhage P50.9
    intrauterine (in utero) procedure P96.5
    malpresentation (malposition) NEC P03.1
    maternal (complication of) (use of)
      alcohol P04.3
      analgesia (maternal) P04.0
      anesthesia (maternal) P04.0
      blood loss P02.1
      circulatory disease P00.3
      condition P00.9
        specified NEC P00.89
      delivery P03.9
        Cesarean P03.4
        forceps P03.2
        vacuum extractor P03.3
      diabetes mellitus (pre-existing) P70.1
      disorder P00.9
        specified NEC P00.89
      drugs (addictive) (illegal) NEC P04.49
      ectopic pregnancy P01.4
      gestational diabetes P70.0
      hemorrhage P02.1
      hypertensive disorder P00.0
      incompetent cervix P01.0
      infectious disease P00.2
      injury P00.5
      labor and delivery P03.9
      malpresentation before labor P01.7
      maternal death P01.6
      medical procedure P00.7
      medication P04.1
      multiple pregnancy P01.5
      nutritional disorder P00.4
      oligohydramnios P01.2
      parasitic disease P00.2
      periodontal disease P00.81
      placenta previa P02.0
      polyhydramnios P01.3
      precipitate delivery P03.5
      pregnancy P01.9
        specified P01.8
      premature rupture of membranes P01.1
      renal disease P00.1
      respiratory disease P00.3
      surgical procedure P00.6
      urinary tract disease P00.1
      uterine contraction (abnormal) P03.6
    meconium peritonitis P78.0
    medication (legal) (maternal use) (prescribed) P04.1
    membrane abnormalities P02.9
      specified NEC P02.8
    membranitis P02.7
    methamphetamine(s) P04.49
    mixed metabolic and respiratory acidosis P84
    neonatal abstinence syndrome P96.1
    noxious substances transmitted via placenta or
      breast milk P04.9
      specified NEC P04.8
    nutritional supplements P04.5
    placenta previa P02.0
    placental
      abnormality (functional) (morphological)
        P02.20
        specified NEC P02.29
      dysfunction P02.29
      infarction P02.29
      insufficiency P02.29
      separation NEC P02.1
      transfusion syndromes P02.3
    placentitis P02.7
    precipitate delivery P03.5
    prolapsed cord P02.4
    respiratory arrest P28.81
    slow intrauterine growth P05.9
    tobacco P04.2

Newborn — *continued*
  affected by — *continued*
    twin to twin transplacental transfusion P02.3
    umbilical cord (tightly) around neck P02.5
    umbilical cord condition P02.60
      short cord P02.69
      specified NEC P02.69
    uterine contractions (abnormal) P03.6
    vasa previa P02.69
      from intrauterine blood loss P50.0
  apnea P28.3
    obstructive P28.4
    primary P28.3
    specified P28.4
  born in hospital Z38.00
    by cesarean Z38.01
  born outside hospital Z38.1
  breast buds P96.89
  breast engorgement P83.4
  check-up — *see* Newborn, examination
  convulsion P90
  dehydration P74.1
  examination
    8 to 28 days old Z00.111
    under 8 days old Z00.110
  fever P81.9
    environmentally-induced P81.0
  hyperbilirubinemia P59.9
    of prematurity P59.0
  hypernatremia P74.2
  hyponatremia P74.2
  infection P39.9
    candidal P37.5
    specified NEC P39.8
    urinary tract P39.3
  jaundice P59.8
    due to
      breast milk inhibitor P59.3
      hepatocellular damage P59.20
        specified NEC P59.29
      preterm delivery P59.0
    of prematurity P59.0
    specified NEC P59.8
  late metabolic acidosis P74.0
  mastitis P39.0
    infective P39.0
    noninfective P83.4
  multiple born NEC Z38.8
    born in hospital Z38.68
      by cesarean Z38.69
    born outside hospital Z38.7
  omphalitis P38.9
    with mild hemorrhage P38.1
    without hemorrhage P38.9
  post-term P08.21
  prolonged gestation (over 42 completed weeks)
    P08.22
  quadruplet Z38.8
    born in hospital Z38.63
      by cesarean Z38.64
    born outside hospital Z38.7
  quintuplet Z38.8
    born in hospital Z38.65
      by cesarean Z38.66
    born outside hospital Z38.7
  seizure P90
  sepsis (congenital) P36.9
    due to
      anaerobes NEC P36.5
      Escherichia coli P36.4
      Staphylococcus P36.30
        aureus P36.2
        specified NEC P36.39
      Streptococcus P36.10
        group B P36.0
        specified NEC P36.19
    specified NEC P36.8
  triplet Z38.8
    born in hospital Z38.61
      by cesarean Z38.62
    born outside hospital Z38.7
  twin Z38.5
    born in hospital Z38.30
      by cesarean Z38.31
    born outside hospital Z38.4
  vomiting P92.09
    bilious P92.01
  weight check Z00.111

Newcastle conjunctivitis or disease B30.8
Nezelof's syndrome (pure alymphocytosis) D81.4
Niacin (amide) **deficiency** E52
Nicolas (-Durand)-**Favre disease** A55
Nicotine — *see* Tobacco
Nicotinic acid deficiency E52
Niemann-Pick disease or syndrome E75.249
  specified NEC E75.248
  type
    A E75.240
    B E75.241
    C E75.242
    D E75.243
Night
  blindness — *see* Blindness, night
  sweats R61
  terrors (child) F51.4
Nightmares (REM sleep type) F51.5
Nipple — *see* condition
Nisbet's chancre A57
Nishimoto (-Takeuchi) **disease** I67.5
Nitritoid crisis or reaction — *see* Crisis, nitritoid
Nitrosohemoglobinemia D74.8
Njovera A65
Nocardiosis, nocardiasis A43.9
  cutaneous A43.1
  lung A43.0
  pneumonia A43.0
  pulmonary A43.0
  specified site NEC A43.8
Nocturia R35.1
  psychogenic F45.8
Nocturnal — *see* condition
Nodal rhythm I49.8
Node(s) (*see also* Nodule)
  Bouchard's (with arthropathy) M15.2
  Haygarth's M15.8
  Heberden's (with arthropathy) M15.1
  larynx J38.7
  lymph — *see* condition
  milker's B08.03
  Osler's I33.0
  Schmorl's — *see* Schmorl's disease
  singer's J38.2
  teacher's J38.2
  tuberculous — *see* Tuberculosis, lymph gland
  vocal cord J38.2
Nodule(s), **nodular**
  actinomycotic — *see* Actinomycosis
  breast NEC N63
  colloid (cystic), thyroid E04.1
  cutaneous — *see* Swelling, localized
  endometrial (stromal) D26.1
  Haygarth's M15.8
  inflammatory — *see* Inflammation
  juxta-articular
    syphilitic A52.77
    yaws A66.7
  larynx J38.7
  lung, solitary (subsegmental branch of the bronchial
    tree) R91.1
    multiple R91.8
  milker's B08.03
  prostate N40.2
    with lower urinary tract symptoms (LUTS) N40.3
    without lower urinary tract symptoms (LUTS) N40.2
  pulmonary, solitary (subsegmental branch of the
    bronchial tree) R91.1
  retrocardiac R09.89
  rheumatoid M06.30
    ankle M06.37- ☑
    elbow M06.32- ☑
    foot joint M06.37- ☑
    hand joint M06.34- ☑
    hip M06.35- ☑
    knee M06.36- ☑
    multiple site M06.39
    shoulder M06.31- ☑
    vertebra M06.38
    wrist M06.33- ☑
  scrotum (inflammatory) N49.2
  singer's J38.2
  solitary, lung (subsegmental branch of the bronchial
    tree) R91.1
    multiple R91.8
  subcutaneous — *see* Swelling, localized
  teacher's J38.2

Nodule(s), nodular — *continued*
  thyroid (cold) (gland) (nontoxic) E04.1
    with thyrotoxicosis E05.20
      with thyroid storm E05.21
    toxic or with hyperthyroidism E05.20
      with thyroid storm E05.21
  vocal cord J38.2
Noma (gangrenous) (hospital) (infective) A69.0
  auricle I96
  mouth A69.0
  pudendi N76.89
  vulvae N76.89
Nomad, nomadism Z59.0
Nonautoimmune hemolytic anemia D59.4
  drug-induced D59.2
Nonclosure (*see also* Imperfect, closure)
  ductus arteriosus (Botallo's) Q25.0
  foramen
    botalli Q21.1
    ovale Q21.1
Noncompliance Z91.19
  with
    dialysis Z91.15
    dietary regimen Z91.11
    medical treatment Z91.19
    medication regimen NEC Z91.14
      underdosing (*see also* Table of Drugs and
        Chemicals, categories T36-T50, with final
        character 6) Z91.14
        intentional NEC Z91.128
          due to financial hardship of patient
            Z91.120
        unintentional NEC Z91.138
          due to patient's age related debility
            Z91.130
    renal dialysis Z91.15
Nondescent (congenital) (*see also* Malposition, congenital)
  cecum Q43.3
  colon Q43.3
  testicle Q53.9
    bilateral Q53.20
      abdominal Q53.21
      perineal Q53.22
    unilateral Q53.10
      abdominal Q53.11
      perineal Q53.12
Nondevelopment
  brain Q02
    part of Q04.3
  heart Q24.8
  organ or site, congenital NEC — *see* Hypoplasia
Nonengagement
  head NEC O32.4 ☑
    in labor, causing obstructed labor O64.8 ☑
Nonexanthematous tick fever A93.2
Nonexpansion, lung (newborn) P28.0
Nonfunctioning
  cystic duct (*see also* Disease, gallbladder) K82.8
  gallbladder (*see also* Disease, gallbladder) K82.8
  kidney N28.9
  labyrinth — *see* subcategory H83.2 ☑
Non-Hodgkin lymphoma NEC — *see* Lymphoma, non-Hodgkin
Nonimplantation, ovum N97.2
Noninsufflation, fallopian tube N97.1
Non-ketotic hyperglycinemia E72.51
Nonne-Milroy syndrome Q82.0
Nonovulation N97.0
Nonpatent fallopian tube N97.1
Nonpneumatization, lung NEC P28.0
Nonrotation — *see* Malrotation
Nonsecretion, urine — *see* Anuria
Nonunion
  fracture — *see* Fracture, by site
  organ or site, congenital NEC — *see* Imperfect, closure
  symphysis pubis, congenital Q74.2
Nonvisualization, gallbladder R93.2
Nonvital, nonvitalized tooth K04.99
Non-working side interference M26.56
Noonan's syndrome Q87.1
Normocytic anemia (infectional) due to blood loss
  (chronic) D50.0
  acute D62
Norrie's disease (congenital) Q15.8
North American blastomycosis B40.9
Norwegian itch B86

Nose, nasal — *see* condition
Nosebleed R04.0
Nose-picking F98.8
Nosomania F45.21
Nosophobia F45.22
Nostalgia F43.20
Notch of iris Q13.2
Notching nose, congenital (tip) Q30.2
Nothnagel's
  syndrome — *see* Strabismus, paralytic, third nerve
  vasomotor acroparesthesia I73.89
Novy's relapsing fever A68.9
  louse-borne A68.0
  tick-borne A68.1
Noxious
  foodstuffs, poisoning by — *see* Poisoning, food, noxious, plant
  substances transmitted through placenta or breast
    milk P04.9
Nucleus pulposus — *see* condition
Numbness R20.0
Nuns' knee — *see* Bursitis, prepatellar
Nursemaid's elbow S53.03- ☑
Nutcracker esophagus K22.4
Nutmeg liver K76.1
Nutrient element deficiency E61.9
  specified NEC E61.8
Nutrition deficient or insufficient (*see also* Malnutrition) E46
  due to
    insufficient food T73.0 ☑
    lack of
      care (child) T76.02 ☑
        adult T76.01 ☑
      food T73.0 ☑
Nutritional stunting E45
Nyctalopia (night blindness) — *see* Blindness, night
Nycturia R35.1
  psychogenic F45.8
Nymphomania F52.8
Nystagmus H55.00
  benign paroxysmal — *see* Vertigo, benign paroxysmal
  central positional H81.4- ☑
  congenital H55.01
  dissociated H55.04
  latent H55.02
  miners' H55.09
  positional
    benign paroxysmal H81.4- ☑
    central H81.4- ☑
  specified form NEC H55.09
  visual deprivation H55.03

O

Obermeyer's relapsing fever (European) A68.0
Obesity E66.9
  with alveolar hyperventilation E66.2
  adrenal E27.8
  complicating
    childbirth O99.214
    pregnancy O99.21- ☑
    puerperium O99.215
  constitutional E66.8
  dietary counseling and surveillance Z71.3
  drug-induced E66.1
  due to
    drug E66.1
    excess calories E66.09
      morbid E66.01
      severe E66.01
  endocrine E66.8
  endogenous E66.8
  familial E66.8
  glandular E66.8
  hypothyroid — *see* Hypothyroidism
  morbid E66.01
    with alveolar hypoventilation E66.2
    due to excess calories E66.01
  nutritional E66.09
  pituitary E23.6
  severe E66.01
  specified type NEC E66.8
Oblique — *see* condition
Obliteration
  appendix (lumen) K38.8
  artery I77.1

Obliteration — *continued*
  bile duct (noncalculous) K83.1
  common duct (noncalculous) K83.1
  cystic duct — *see* Obstruction, gallbladder
  disease, arteriolar I77.1
  endometrium N85.8
  eye, anterior chamber — *see* Disorder, globe, hypotony
  fallopian tube N97.1
  lymphatic vessel I89.0
    due to mastectomy I97.2
  organ or site, congenital NEC — *see* Atresia, by site
  ureter N13.5
    with infection N13.6
  urethra — *see* Stricture, urethra
  vein I87.8
  vestibule (oral) K08.8
Observation (following) (for) (without need for further
  medical care) Z04.9
  accident NEC Z04.3
    at work Z04.2
    transport Z04.1
  adverse effect of drug Z03.6
  alleged rape or sexual assault (victim), ruled out
    adult Z04.41
    child Z04.42
  criminal assault Z04.8
  development state
    adolescent Z00.3
    period of rapid growth in childhood Z00.2
    puberty Z00.3
  disease, specified NEC Z03.89
  following work accident Z04.2
  growth and development state — *see* Observation,
    development state
  injuries (accidental) NEC (*see also* Observation, accident)
  newborn (for suspected condition, ruled out) — *see* -
    Newborn, affected by (suspected to be), maternal (complication of) (use of)
  postpartum
    immediately after delivery Z39.0
    routine follow-up Z39.2
  pregnancy (normal) (without complication) Z34.9- ☑
    high risk O09.9- ☑
  suicide attempt, alleged NEC Z03.89
    self-poisoning Z03.6
  suspected, ruled out (*see also* Suspected condition,
    ruled out)
    abuse, physical
      adult Z04.71
      child Z04.72
    accident at work Z04.2
    adult battering victim Z04.71
    child battering victim Z04.72
    condition NEC Z03.89
      newborn — *see* Newborn, affected by (suspected to be), maternal (complication of) (use of)
    drug poisoning or adverse effect Z03.6
    exposure (to)
      anthrax Z03.810
      biological agent NEC Z03.818
    inflicted injury NEC Z04.8
    suicide attempt, alleged Z03.89
      self-poisoning Z03.6
    toxic effects from ingested substance (drug) (poison) Z03.6
  toxic effects from ingested substance (drug) (poison)
    Z03.6
Obsession, obsessional state F42
Obsessive-compulsive neurosis or reaction F42
Obstetric embolism, septic — *see* Embolism, obstetric,
  septic
Obstetrical trauma (complicating delivery) O71.9
  with or following ectopic or molar pregnancy O08.6
  specified type NEC O71.89
Obstipation — *see* Constipation
Obstruction, obstructed, obstructive
  airway J98.8
    with
      allergic alveolitis J67.9
      asthma J45.909
        with
          exacerbation (acute) J45.901
          status asthmaticus J45.902
      bronchiectasis J47.9

☑ **Additional Character Required** — **Refer to the Tabular List for Character Selection**   ▽ **Subterms under main terms may continue to next column or page**

Obstruction, obstructed, obstructive — *continued*
airway — *continued*
  with
    bronchiectasis — *continued*
      with — *continued*
        exacerbation (acute) J47.1
        lower respiratory infection J47.0
    bronchitis (chronic) J44.9
    emphysema J43.9
    chronic J44.9
      with
        allergic alveolitis — *see* Pneumonitis, hyper-
          sensitivity
        bronchiectasis J47.9
          with
            exacerbation (acute) J47.1
            lower respiratory infection J47.0
  due to
    foreign body — *see* Foreign body, by site,
      causing asphyxia
    inhalation of fumes or vapors J68.9
  laryngospasm J38.5
ampulla of Vater K83.1
aortic (heart) (valve) — *see* Stenosis, aortic
aortoiliac I74.09
aqueduct of Sylvius G91.1
  congenital Q03.0
    with spina bifida — *see* Spina bifida, by site,
      with hydrocephalus
Arnold-Chiari — *see* Arnold-Chiari disease
artery (*see also* Embolism, artery) I74.9
  basilar (complete) (partial) — *see* Occlusion, artery,
    basilar
  carotid (complete) (partial) — *see* Occlusion, artery,
    carotid
  cerebellar — *see* Occlusion, artery, cerebellar
  cerebral (anterior) (middle) (posterior) — *see* Oc-
    clusion, artery, cerebral
  precerebral — *see* Occlusion, artery, precerebral
  renal N28.0
  retinal NEC — *see* Occlusion, artery, retina
  vertebral (complete) (partial) — *see* Occlusion,
    artery, vertebral
band (intestinal) K56.69
bile duct or passage (common) (hepatic) (noncalculous) K83.1
  with calculus K80.51
  congenital (causing jaundice) Q44.3
biliary (duct) (tract) K83.1
  gallbladder K82.0
bladder-neck (acquired) N32.0
  congenital Q64.31
  due to hyperplasia (hypertrophy) of prostate —
    see Hyperplasia, prostate
bowel — *see* Obstruction, intestine
bronchus J98.09
canal, ear — *see* Stenosis, external ear canal
cardia K22.2
caval veins (inferior) (superior) I87.1
cecum — *see* Obstruction, intestine
circulatory I99.8
colon — *see* Obstruction, intestine
common duct (noncalculous) K83.1
coronary (artery) — *see* Occlusion, coronary
cystic duct (*see also* Obstruction, gallbladder)
  with calculus K80.21
device, implant or graft (*see also* Complications, by
  site and type, mechanical) T85.698 ☑
  arterial graft NEC — *see* Complication, cardiovas-
    cular device, mechanical, vascular
  catheter NEC T85.628 ☑
    cystostomy T83.090 ☑
    dialysis (renal) T82.49 ☑
      intraperitoneal T85.691 ☑
    infusion NEC T82.594 ☑
      spinal (epidural) (subdural) T85.690 ☑
    urinary, indwelling T83.098 ☑
    due to infection T85.79 ☑
  gastrointestinal — *see* Complications, prosthetic
    device, mechanical, gastrointestinal device
  genital NEC T83.498 ☑
    intrauterine contraceptive device T83.39 ☑
    penile prosthesis T83.490 ☑
  heart NEC — *see* Complication, cardiovascular de-
    vice, mechanical
  joint prosthesis — *see* Complications, joint prosthe-
    sis, mechanical, specified NEC, by site

Obstruction, obstructed, obstructive — *continued*
device, implant or graft (*see also* Complications, by site
  and type, mechanical) — *continued*
  orthopedic NEC — *see* Complication, orthopedic,
    device, mechanical
  specified NEC T85.628 ☑
  urinary NEC (*see also* Complication, genitourinary,
    device, urinary, mechanical)
    graft T83.29 ☑
  vascular NEC — *see* Complication, cardiovascular
    device, mechanical
  ventricular intracranial shunt T85.09 ☑
  due to foreign body accidentally left in operative
    wound T81.529 ☑
duodenum K31.5
ejaculatory duct N50.8
esophagus K22.2
eustachian tube (complete) (partial) H68.10- ☑
  cartilagenous (extrinsic) H68.13- ☑
    intrinsic H68.12- ☑
  osseous H68.11- ☑
fallopian tube (bilateral) N97.1
fecal K56.41
  with hernia — *see* Hernia, by site, with obstruction
foramen of Monro (congenital) Q03.8
  with spina bifida — *see* Spina bifida, by site, with
    hydrocephalus
foreign body — *see* Foreign body
gallbladder K82.0
  with calculus, stones K80.21
  congenital Q44.1
gastric outlet K31.1
gastrointestinal — *see* Obstruction, intestine
hepatic K76.89
  duct (noncalculous) K83.1
ileum — *see* Obstruction, intestine
iliofemoral (artery) I74.5
intestine K56.60
  with
    adhesions (intestinal) (peritoneal) K56.5
  adynamic K56.0
  by gallstone K56.3
  congenital (small) Q41.9
    large Q42.9
      specified part NEC Q42.8
  neurogenic K56.0
    Hirschsprung's disease or megacolon Q43.1
  newborn P76.9
    due to
      fecaliths P76.8
      inspissated milk P76.2
      meconium (plug) P76.0
        in mucoviscidosis E84.11
    specified NEC P76.8
  postoperative K91.3
  reflex K56.0
  specified NEC K56.69
  volvulus K56.2
intracardiac ball valve prosthesis T82.09 ☑
jejunum — *see* Obstruction, intestine
joint prosthesis — *see* Complications, joint prosthesis,
  mechanical, specified NEC, by site
kidney (calices) N28.89
labor — *see* Delivery
lacrimal (passages) (duct)
  by
    dacryolith — *see* Dacryolith
    stenosis — *see* Stenosis, lacrimal
  congenital Q10.5
  neonatal H04.53- ☑
lacrimonasal duct — *see* Obstruction, lacrimal
lacteal, with steatorrhea K90.2
laryngitis — *see* Laryngitis
larynx NEC J38.6
  congenital Q31.8
lung J98.4
  disease, chronic J44.9
lymphatic I89.0
meconium (plug)
  newborn P76.0
    due to fecaliths P76.0
    in mucoviscidosis E84.11
mitral — *see* Stenosis, mitral
nasal J34.89
nasolacrimal duct (*see also* Obstruction, lacrimal)
  congenital Q10.5
nasopharynx J39.2
nose J34.89

Obstruction, obstructed, obstructive — *continued*
organ or site, congenital NEC — *see* Atresia, by site
pancreatic duct K86.8
parotid duct or gland K11.8
pelviureteral junction N13.5
  congenital Q62.39
pharynx J39.2
portal (circulation) (vein) I81
prostate (*see also* Hyperplasia, prostate)
  valve (urinary) N32.0
pulmonary valve (heart) I37.0
pyelonephritis (chronic) N11.1
pylorus
  adult K31.1
  congenital or infantile Q40.0
rectosigmoid — *see* Obstruction, intestine
rectum K62.4
renal N28.89
  outflow N13.8
  pelvis, congenital Q62.39
respiratory J98.8
  chronic J44.9
retinal (vessels) H34.9
salivary duct (any) K11.8
  with calculus K11.5
sigmoid — *see* Obstruction, intestine
sinus (accessory) (nasal) J34.89
Stensen's duct K11.8
stomach NEC K31.89
  acute K31.0
  congenital Q40.2
  due to pylorospasm K31.3
submandibular duct K11.8
submaxillary gland K11.8
  with calculus K11.5
thoracic duct I89.0
thrombotic — *see* Thrombosis
trachea J39.8
tracheostomy airway J95.03
tricuspid (valve) — *see* Stenosis, tricuspid
upper respiratory, congenital Q34.8
ureter (functional) (pelvic junction) NEC N13.5
  with
    hydronephrosis N13.1
      with infection N13.6
    pyelonephritis (chronic) N11.1
  congenital Q62.39
  due to calculus — *see* Calculus, ureter
urethra NEC N36.8
  congenital Q64.39
urinary (moderate) N13.9
  due to hyperplasia (hypertrophy) of prostate —
    see Hyperplasia, prostate
  organ or tract (lower) N13.9
  prostatic valve N32.0
  specified NEC N13.8
uropathy N13.9
uterus N85.8
vagina N89.5
valvular — *see* Endocarditis
vein, venous I87.1
  caval (inferior) (superior) I87.1
  thrombotic — *see* Thrombosis
vena cava (inferior) (superior) I87.1
vesical NEC N32.0
vesicourethral orifice N32.0
  congenital Q64.31
vessel NEC I99.8
Obturator — *see* condition
Occlusal wear, teeth K03.0
Occlusio pupillae — *see* Membrane, pupillary
Occlusion, occluded
anus K62.4
  congenital Q42.3
    with fistula Q42.2
aortoiliac (chronic) I74.09
aqueduct of Sylvius G91.1
  congenital Q03.0
    with spina bifida — *see* Spina bifida, by site,
      with hydrocephalus
artery (*see also* Embolism, artery) I74.9
  auditory, internal I65.8
  basilar I65.1
    with
      infarction I63.22
      due to
        embolism I63.12
        thrombosis I63.02

Obstruction, obstructed, obstructive — Occlusion, occluded

Occlusion, occluded — continued
  artery (see also Embolism, artery) — continued
    brain or cerebral I66.9
      with infarction (due to) I63.5 ☑
        embolism I63.4 ☑
        thrombosis I63.3 ☑
    carotid I65.2- ☑
      with
        infarction I63.23- ☑
          due to
            embolism I63.13- ☑
            thrombosis I63.03- ☑
    cerebellar (anterior inferior) (posterior inferior)
      (superior) I66.3
      with infarction I63.54- ☑
        due to
          embolism I63.44- ☑
          thrombosis I63.34- ☑
    cerebral I66.9
      with infarction I63.50
        due to
          embolism I63.40
            specified NEC I63.49
          thrombosis I63.30
            specified NEC I63.39
      anterior I66.1- ☑
        with infarction I63.52- ☑
          due to
            embolism I63.42- ☑
            thrombosis I63.32- ☑
      middle I66.0- ☑
        with infarction I63.51- ☑
          due to
            embolism I63.41- ☑
            thrombosis I63.31- ☑
      posterior I66.2- ☑
        with infarction I63.53- ☑
          due to
            embolism I63.43- ☑
            thrombosis I63.33- ☑
      specified NEC I66.8
        with infarction I63.59
          due to
            embolism I63.4 ☑
            thrombosis I63.3 ☑
    choroidal (anterior) — see Occlusion, artery, pre-
      cerebral, specified NEC
    communicating posterior — see Occlusion, artery,
      cerebral, specified NEC
    complete
      coronary I25.82
      extremities I70.92
    coronary (acute) (thrombotic) (without myocardial
      infarction) I24.0
      with myocardial infarction — see Infarction,
        myocardium
      chronic total I25.82
      complete I25.82
      healed or old I25.2
      total (chronic) I25.82
    hypophyseal — see Occlusion, artery, precerebral,
      specified NEC
    iliac I74.5
    lower extremities due to stenosis or stricture I77.1
    mesenteric (embolic) (thrombotic) K55.0
    perforating — see Occlusion, artery, cerebral,
      specified NEC
    peripheral I77.9
      thrombotic or embolic I74.4
    pontine — see Occlusion, artery, cerebral, specified
      NEC
    precerebral I65.9
      with infarction I63.20
        due to
          embolism I63.10
            specified NEC I63.19
          thrombosis I63.00
            specified NEC I63.09
        specified NEC I63.29
      basilar — see Occlusion, artery, basilar
      carotid — see Occlusion, artery, carotid
      puerperal O88.23
      specified NEC I65.8
        with infarction I63.29
          due to
            embolism I63.19
            thrombosis I63.00

Occlusion, occluded — continued
  artery (see also Embolism, artery) — continued
    precerebral — continued
      vertebral — see Occlusion, artery, vertebral
    renal N28.0
    retinal
      branch H34.23- ☑
      central H34.1- ☑
      partial H34.21- ☑
      transient H34.0- ☑
    spinal — see Occlusion, artery, precerebral, verte-
      bral
    total (chronic)
      coronary I25.82
      extremities I70.92
    vertebral I65.0- ☑
      with
        infarction I63.21- ☑
          due to
            embolism I63.11- ☑
            thrombosis I63.01- ☑
  basilar artery — see Occlusion, artery, basilar
  bile duct (common) (hepatic) (noncalculous) K83.1
  bowel — see Obstruction, intestine
  carotid (artery) (common) (internal) — see Occlusion,
    artery, carotid
  centric (of teeth) M26.59
    maximum intercuspation discrepancy M26.55
  cerebellar (artery) — see Occlusion, artery, cerebellar
  cerebral (artery) — see Occlusion, artery, cerebral
  cerebrovascular (see also Occlusion, artery, cerebral)
    with infarction I63.5 ☑
  cervical canal — see Stricture, cervix
  cervix (uteri) — see Stricture, cervix
  choanal Q30.0
  choroidal (artery) — see Occlusion, artery, precerebral,
    specified NEC
  colon — see Obstruction, intestine
  communicating posterior artery — see Occlusion,
    artery, precerebral, specified NEC
  coronary (artery) (vein) (thrombotic) (see also Infarct,
    myocardium)
    chronic total I25.82
    healed or old I25.2
    not resulting in infarction I24.0
    total (chronic) I25.82
  cystic duct — see Obstruction, gallbladder
  embolic — see Embolism
  fallopian tube N97.1
    congenital Q50.6
  gallbladder (see also Obstruction, gallbladder)
    congenital (causing jaundice) Q44.1
  gingiva, traumatic K06.2
  hymen N89.6
    congenital Q52.3
  hypophyseal (artery) — see Occlusion, artery, precere-
    bral, specified NEC
  iliac artery I74.5
  intestine — see Obstruction, intestine
  lacrimal passages — see Obstruction, lacrimal
  lung J98.4
  lymph or lymphatic channel I89.0
  mammary duct N64.89
  mesenteric artery (embolic) (thrombotic) K55.0
  nose J34.89
    congenital Q30.0
  organ or site, congenital NEC — see Atresia, by site
  oviduct N97.1
    congenital Q50.6
  peripheral arteries
    due to stricture or stenosis I77.1
    upper extremity I74.2
  pontine (artery) — see Occlusion, artery, precerebral,
    specified NEC
  posterior lingual, of mandibular teeth M26.29
  precerebral artery — see Occlusion, artery, precerebral
  punctum lacrimale — see Obstruction, lacrimal
  pupil — see Membrane, pupillary
  pylorus, adult (see also Stricture, pylorus) K31.1
  renal artery N28.0
  retina, retinal
    artery — see Occlusion, artery, retinal
    vein (central) H34.81- ☑
      engorgement H34.82- ☑
      tributary H34.83- ☑
    vessels H34.9

Occlusion, occluded — continued
  spinal artery — see Occlusion, artery, precerebral,
    vertebral
  teeth (mandibular) (posterior lingual) M26.29
  thoracic duct I89.0
  thrombotic — see Thrombosis, artery
  traumatic
    edentulous (alveolar) ridge K06.2
    gingiva K06.2
    periodontal K05.5
  tubal N97.1
  ureter (complete) (partial) N13.5
    congenital Q62.10
  ureteropelvic junction N13.5
    congenital Q62.11
  ureterovesical orifice N13.5
    congenital Q62.12
  urethra — see Stricture, urethra
  uterus N85.8
  vagina N89.5
  vascular NEC I99.8
  vein — see Thrombosis
    retinal — see Occlusion, retinal, vein
  vena cava (inferior) (superior) — see Embolism, vena
    cava
  ventricle (brain) NEC G91.1
  vertebral (artery) — see Occlusion, artery, vertebral
  vessel (blood) I99.8
  vulva N90.5

Occult
  blood in feces (stools) R19.5

Occupational
  problems NEC Z56.89

Ochlophobia — see Agoraphobia

Ochronosis (endogenous) E70.29

Ocular muscle — see condition

Oculogyric crisis or disturbance H51.8
  psychogenic F45.8

Oculomotor syndrome H51.9

Oculopathy
  syphilitic NEC A52.71
    congenital
      early A50.01
      late A50.30
    early (secondary) A51.43
    late A52.71

Oddi's sphincter spasm K83.4

Odontalgia K08.8

Odontoameloblastoma — see Cyst, calcifying odontogenic

Odontoclasia K03.89

Odontodysplasia, regional K00.4

Odontogenesis imperfecta K00.5

Odontoma (ameloblastic) (complex) (compound) (fi-
  broameloblastic) — see Cyst, calcifying odontogenic

Odontomyelitis (closed) (open) K04.0

Odontorrhagia K08.8

Odontosarcoma, ameloblastic C41.1
  upper jaw (bone) C41.0

Oestriasis — see Myiasis

Oguchi's disease H53.63

Ohara's disease — see Tularemia

Oidiomycosis — see Candidiasis

Oidium albicans infection — see Candidiasis

Old age (without mention of debility) R54
  dementia F03 ☑

Old (previous) **myocardial infarction** I25.2

Olfactory — see condition

Oligemia — see Anemia

Oligoastrocytoma
  specified site — see Neoplasm, malignant, by site
  unspecified site C71.9

Oligocythemia D64.9

Oligodendroblastoma
  specified site — see Neoplasm, malignant
  unspecified site C71.9

Oligodendroglioma
  anaplastic type
    specified site — see Neoplasm, malignant, by site
    unspecified site C71.9
  specified site — see Neoplasm, malignant, by site
  unspecified site C71.9

Oligodontia — see Anodontia

Oligoencephalon Q02

Oligohidrosis L74.4

Oligohydramnios O41.0- ☑

Oligohydrosis L74.4

☑ **Additional Character Required** — Refer to the Tabular List for Character Selection

▽ Subterms under main terms may continue to next column or page

Oligomenorrhea N91.5
   primary N91.3
   secondary N91.4
Oligophrenia (*see also* Disability, intellectual)
   phenylpyruvic E70.0
Oligospermia N46.11
   due to
      drug therapy N46.121
      efferent duct obstruction N46.123
      infection N46.122
      radiation N46.124
      specified cause NEC N46.129
      systemic disease N46.125
Oligotrichia — *see* Alopecia
Oliguria R34
   postprocedural N99.0
   with, complicating or following ectopic or molar
      pregnancy O08.4
Ollier's disease Q78.4
Omenotocele — *see* Hernia, abdomen, specified site
   NEC
Omentitis — *see* Peritonitis
Omentum, omental — *see* condition
Omphalitis (congenital) (newborn) P38.9
   with mild hemorrhage P38.1
   without hemorrhage P38.9
   not of newborn L08.82
   tetanus A33
Omphalocele Q79.2
Omphalomesenteric duct, persistent Q43.0
Omphalorrhagia, newborn P51.9
Omsk hemorrhagic fever A98.1
Onanism (excessive) F98.8
Onchocerciasis, onchocercosis B73.1
   with
      eye disease B73.00
         endophthalmitis B73.01
         eyelid B73.09
         glaucoma B73.02
         specified NEC B73.09
   eyelid B73.09
   eye NEC B73.00
Oncocytoma — *see* Neoplasm, benign, by site
Oncovirus, as cause of disease classified elsewhere
   B97.32
Ondine's curse — *see* Apnea, sleep
Oneirophrenia F23
Onychauxis L60.2
   congenital Q84.5
Onychia (*see also* Cellulitis, digit)
   with lymphangitis — *see* Lymphangitis, acute, digit
   candidal B37.2
   dermatophytic B35.1
Onychitis (*see also* Cellulitis, digit)
   with lymphangitis — *see* Lymphangitis, acute, digit
Onychocryptosis L60.0
Onychodystrophy L60.3
   congenital Q84.6
Onychogryphosis, onychogryposis L60.2
Onycholysis L60.1
Onychomadesis L60.8
Onychomalacia L60.3
Onychomycosis (finger) (toe) B35.1
Onycho-osteodysplasia Q79.8
Onychophagia F98.8
Onychophosis L60.8
Onychoptosis L60.8
Onychorrhexis L60.3
   congenital Q84.6
Onychoschizia L60.3
Onyxis (finger) (toe) L60.0
Onyxitis (*see also* Cellulitis, digit)
   with lymphangitis — *see* Lymphangitis, acute, digit
Oophoritis (cystic) (infectional) (interstitial) N70.92
   with salpingitis N70.93
   acute N70.02
      with salpingitis N70.03
   chronic N70.12
      with salpingitis N70.13
   complicating abortion — *see* Abortion, by type, complicated by, oophoritis
Oophorocele N83.4
Opacity, opacities
   cornea H17.- ☑
      central H17.1- ☑
      congenital Q13.3
      degenerative — *see* Degeneration, cornea

Opacity, opacities — *continued*
   cornea — *continued*
      hereditary — *see* Dystrophy, cornea
      inflammatory — *see* Keratitis
      minor H17.81- ☑
      peripheral H17.82- ☑
      sequelae of trachoma (healed) B94.0
      specified NEC H17.89
   enamel (teeth) (fluoride) (nonfluoride) K00.3
   lens — *see* Cataract
   snowball — *see* Deposit, crystalline
   vitreous (humor) NEC H43.39- ☑
      congenital Q14.0
      membranes and strands H43.31- ☑
Opalescent dentin (hereditary) K00.5
Open, opening
   abnormal, organ or site, congenital — *see* Imperfect, closure
   angle with
      borderline
         findings
            high risk H40.02- ☑
            low risk H40.01- ☑
         intraocular pressure H40.00- ☑
      cupping of discs H40.01- ☑
      glaucoma (primary) — *see* Glaucoma, open angle
   bite
      anterior M26.220
      posterior M26.221
   false — *see* Imperfect, closure
   margin on tooth restoration K08.51
   restoration margins of tooth K08.51
   wound — *see* Wound, open
Operational fatigue F48.8
Operative — *see* condition
Operculitis — *see* Periodontitis
Operculum — *see* Break, retina
Ophiasis L63.2
Ophthalmia (*see also* Conjunctivitis) H10.9
   actinic rays — *see* Photokeratitis
   allergic (acute) — *see* Conjunctivitis, acute, atopic
   blennorrhagic (gonococcal) (neonatorum) A54.31
   diphtheritic A36.86
   Egyptian A71.1
   electrica — *see* Photokeratitis
   gonococcal (neonatorum) A54.31
   metastatic — *see* Endophthalmitis, purulent
   migraine — *see* Migraine, ophthalmoplegic
   neonatorum, newborn P39.1
      gonococcal A54.31
   nodosa H16.24- ☑
   purulent — *see* Conjunctivitis, acute, mucopurulent
   spring — *see* Conjunctivitis, acute, atopic
   sympathetic — *see* Uveitis, sympathetic
Ophthalmitis — *see* Ophthalmia
Ophthalmocele (congenital) Q15.8
Ophthalmoneuromyelitis G36.0
Ophthalmoplegia (*see also* Strabismus, paralytic)
   anterior internuclear — *see* Ophthalmoplegia, internuclear
   ataxia-areflexia G61.0
   diabetic — *see* E08-E13 with .39
   exophthalmic E05.00
      with thyroid storm E05.01
   external H49.88- ☑
      progressive H49.4- ☑
         with pigmentary retinopathy — *see* Kearns-Sayre syndrome
      total H49.3- ☑
   internal (complete) (total) H52.51- ☑
   internuclear H51.2- ☑
   migraine — *see* Migraine, ophthalmoplegic
   Parinaud's H49.88- ☑
   progressive external — *see* Ophthalmoplegia, external, progressive
   supranuclear, progressive G23.1
   total (external) — *see* Ophthalmoplegia, external, total
Opioid(s)
   abuse — *see* Abuse, drug, opioids
   dependence — *see* Dependence, drug, opioids
Opisthognathism M26.09
Opisthorchiasis (felineus) (viverrini) B66.0
Opitz' disease D73.2
Opiumism — *see* Dependence, drug, opioid
Oppenheim's disease G70.2
Oppenheim-Urbach disease (necrobiosis lipoidica diabeticorum) — *see* E08-E13 with .620

Optic nerve — *see* condition
Orbit — *see* condition
Orchioblastoma C62.9- ☑
Orchitis (gangrenous) (nonspecific) (septic) (suppurative)
   N45.2
   blennorrhagic (gonococcal) (acute) (chronic) A54.23
   chlamydial A56.19
   filarial (*see also* Infestation, filarial) B74.9 [N51]
   gonococcal (acute) (chronic) A54.23
   mumps B26.0
   syphilitic A52.76
   tuberculous A18.15
Orf (virus disease) B08.02
Organic (*see also* condition)
   brain syndrome F09
   heart — *see* Disease, heart
   mental disorder F09
   psychosis F09
Orgasm
   anejaculatory N53.13
Oriental
   bilharziasis B65.2
   schistosomiasis B65.2
Orifice — *see* condition
Origin of both great vessels from right ventricle
   Q20.1
Ormond's disease (with ureteral obstruction) N13.5
   with infection N13.6
Ornithine metabolism disorder E72.4
Ornithinemia (Type I) (Type II) E72.4
Ornithosis A70
Orotaciduria, oroticaciduria (congenital) (hereditary)
   (pyrimidine deficiency) E79.8
   anemia D53.0
Orthodontics
   adjustment Z46.4
   fitting Z46.4
Orthopnea R06.01
Orthopoxvirus B08.09
   specified NEC B08.09
Os, uterus — *see* condition
Osgood-Schlatter disease or osteochondrosis — *see*
   Osteochondrosis, juvenile, tibia
Osler (-Weber)-**Rendu disease** I78.0
Osler's nodes I33.0
Osmidrosis L75.0
Osseous — *see* condition
Ossification
   artery — *see* Arteriosclerosis
   auricle (ear) — *see* Disorder, pinna, specified type NEC
   bronchial J98.09
   cardiac — *see* Degeneration, myocardial
   cartilage (senile) — *see* Disorder, cartilage, specified type NEC
   coronary (artery) — *see* Disease, heart, ischemic, atherosclerotic
   diaphragm J98.6
   ear, middle — *see* Otosclerosis
   falx cerebri G96.19
   fontanel, premature Q75.0
   heart (*see also* Degeneration, myocardial)
      valve — *see* Endocarditis
   larynx J38.7
   ligament — *see* Disorder, tendon, specified type NEC
      posterior longitudinal — *see* Spondylopathy, specified NEC
   meninges (cerebral) (spinal) G96.19
   multiple, eccentric centers — *see* Disorder, bone, development or growth
   muscle (*see also* Calcification, muscle)
      due to burns — *see* Myositis, ossificans, in, burns
      paralytic — *see* Myositis, ossificans, in, quadriplegia
      progressive — *see* Myositis, ossificans, progressiva
      specified NEC M61.50
         ankle M61.57- ☑
         foot M61.57- ☑
         forearm M61.53- ☑
         hand M61.54- ☑
         lower leg M61.56- ☑
         multiple sites M61.59
         pelvic region M61.55- ☑
         shoulder region M61.51- ☑
         specified site NEC M61.58
         thigh M61.55- ☑
         upper arm M61.52- ☑
      traumatic — *see* Myositis, ossificans, traumatica

Ossification — *continued*
  myocardium, myocardial — *see* Degeneration, myocardial
  penis N48.89
  periarticular — *see* Disorder, joint, specified type NEC
  pinna — *see* Disorder, pinna, specified type NEC
  rider's bone — *see* Ossification, muscle, specified NEC
  sclera H15.89
  subperiosteal, post-traumatic M89.8X- ☑
  tendon — *see* Disorder, tendon, specified type NEC
  trachea J39.8
  tympanic membrane — *see* Disorder, tympanic membrane, specified NEC
  vitreous (humor) — *see* Deposit, crystalline
Osteitis (*see also* Osteomyelitis)
  alveolar M27.3
  condensans M85.30
    ankle M85.37- ☑
    foot M85.37- ☑
    forearm M85.33- ☑
    hand M85.34- ☑
    lower leg M85.36- ☑
    multiple site M85.39
    neck M85.38
    rib M85.38
    shoulder M85.31- ☑
    skull M85.38
    specified site NEC M85.38
    thigh M85.35- ☑
    toe M85.37- ☑
    upper arm M85.32- ☑
    vertebra M85.38
  deformans M88.9
    in (due to)
      malignant neoplasm of bone C41.9 [M90.60]
      neoplastic disease (*see also* Neoplasm) D49.9 [M90.60]
        carpus D49.9 [M90.64-] ☑
        clavicle D49.9 [M90.61-] ☑
        femur D49.9 [M90.65-] ☑
        fibula D49.9 [M90.66-] ☑
        finger D49.9 [M90.64-] ☑
        humerus D49.9 [M90.62-] ☑
        ilium D49.9 [M90.65-] ☑
        ischium D49.9 [M90.65-] ☑
        metacarpus D49.9 [M90.64-] ☑
        metatarsus D49.9 [M90.67-] ☑
        multiple sites D49.9 [M90.69]
        neck D49.9 [M90.68]
        radius D49.9 [M90.63-] ☑
        rib D49.9 [M90.68]
        scapula D49.9 [M90.61-] ☑
        skull D49.9 [M90.68]
        tarsus D49.9 [M90.67-] ☑
        tibia D49.9 [M90.66-] ☑
        toe D49.9 [M90.67-] ☑
        ulna D49.9 [M90.63-] ☑
        vertebra D49.9 [M90.68]
    skull M88.0
    specified NEC — *see* Paget's disease, bone, by site
    vertebra M88.1
  due to yaws A66.6
  fibrosa NEC — *see* Cyst, bone, by site
    circumscripta — *see* Dysplasia, fibrous, bone NEC
    cystica (generalisata) E21.0
    disseminata Q78.1
    osteoplastica E21.0
  fragilitans Q78.0
  Garr's (sclerosing) — *see* Osteomyelitis, specified type NEC
  jaw (acute) (chronic) (lower) (suppurative) (upper) M27.2
  parathyroid E21.0
  petrous bone (acute) (chronic) — *see* Petrositis
  sclerotic, nonsuppurative — *see* Osteomyelitis, specified type NEC
  tuberculosa A18.09
    cystica D86.89
    multiplex cystoides D86.89
Osteoarthritis M19.90
  ankle M19.07- ☑
  elbow M19.02- ☑
  foot joint M19.07- ☑
  generalized M15.9
    erosive M15.4
    primary M15.0
    specified NEC M15.8

Osteoarthritis — *continued*
  hand joint M19.04- ☑
    first carpometacarpal joint M18.9
  hip M16.1- ☑
    bilateral M16.0
    due to hip dysplasia (unilateral) M16.3- ☑
      bilateral M16.2
  interphalangeal
    distal (Heberden) M15.1
    proximal (Bouchard) M15.2
  knee M17.9
    bilateral M17.0
  post-traumatic NEC M19.92
    ankle M19.17- ☑
    elbow M19.12- ☑
    foot joint M19.17- ☑
    hand joint M19.14- ☑
      first carpometacarpal joint M18.3- ☑
        bilateral M18.2
    hip M16.5- ☑
      bilateral M16.4
    knee M17.3- ☑
      bilateral M17.2
    shoulder M19.11- ☑
    wrist M19.13- ☑
  primary M19.91
    ankle M19.07- ☑
    elbow M19.02- ☑
    foot joint M19.07- ☑
    hand joint M19.04- ☑
      first carpometacarpal joint M18.1- ☑
        bilateral M18.0
    hip M16.1- ☑
      bilateral M16.0
    knee M17.1- ☑
      bilateral M17.0
    shoulder M19.01- ☑
    spine — *see* Spondylosis
    wrist M19.03- ☑
  secondary M19.93
    ankle M19.27- ☑
    elbow M19.22- ☑
    foot joint M19.27- ☑
    hand joint M19.24- ☑
      first carpometacarpal joint M18.5- ☑
        bilateral M18.4
    hip M16.7
      bilateral M16.6
    knee M17.5
      bilateral M17.4
    multiple M15.3
    shoulder M19.21- ☑
    spine — *see* Spondylosis
    wrist M19.23- ☑
  shoulder M19.01- ☑
  spine — *see* Spondylosis
  wrist M19.03- ☑
Osteoarthropathy (hypertrophic) M19.90
  ankle — *see* Osteoarthritis, primary, ankle
  elbow — *see* Osteoarthritis, primary, elbow
  foot joint — *see* Osteoarthritis, primary, foot
  hand joint — *see* Osteoarthritis, primary, hand joint
  knee joint — *see* Osteoarthritis, primary, knee
  multiple site — *see* Osteoarthritis, primary, multiple joint
  pulmonary (*see also* Osteoarthropathy, specified type NEC)
    hypertrophic — *see* Osteoarthropathy, hypertrophic, specified type NEC
  secondary — *see* Osteoarthropathy, specified type NEC
  secondary hypertrophic — *see* Osteoarthropathy, specified type NEC
  shoulder — *see* Osteoarthritis, primary, shoulder
  specified joint NEC — *see* Osteoarthritis, primary, specified joint NEC
  specified type NEC M89.40
    carpus M89.44- ☑
    clavicle M89.41- ☑
    femur M89.45- ☑
    fibula M89.46- ☑
    finger M89.44- ☑
    humerus M89.42- ☑
    ilium M89.459
    ischium M89.459
    metacarpus M89.44- ☑

Osteoarthropathy — *continued*
  specified type — *continued*
    metatarsus M89.47- ☑
    multiple sites M89.49
    neck M89.48
    radius M89.43- ☑
    rib M89.48
    scapula M89.41- ☑
    skull M89.48
    tarsus M89.47- ☑
    tibia M89.46- ☑
    toe M89.47- ☑
    ulna M89.43- ☑
    vertebra M89.48
  spine — *see* Spondylosis
  wrist — *see* Osteoarthritis, primary, wrist
Osteoarthrosis (degenerative) (hypertrophic) (joint) (*see also* Osteoarthritis)
  deformans alkaptonurica E70.29 [M36.8]
  erosive M15.4
  generalized M15.9
    primary M15.0
  polyarticular M15.9
  spine — *see* Spondylosis
Osteoblastoma — *see* Neoplasm, bone, benign
  aggressive — *see* Neoplasm, bone, uncertain behavior
Osteochondritis (*see also* Osteochondropathy, by site)
  Brailsford's — *see* Osteochondrosis, juvenile, radius
  dissecans M93.20
    ankle M93.27- ☑
    elbow M93.22- ☑
    foot M93.27- ☑
    hand M93.24- ☑
    hip M93.25- ☑
    knee M93.26- ☑
    multiple sites M93.29
    shoulder M93.21- ☑
    specified site NEC M93.28
    wrist M93.23- ☑
  juvenile M92.9
    patellar — *see* Osteochondrosis, juvenile, patella
  syphilitic (congenital) (early) A50.02 [M90.80]
    ankle A50.02 [M90.87-] ☑
    elbow A50.02 [M90.82-] ☑
    foot A50.02 [M90.87-] ☑
    forearm A50.02 [M90.83-] ☑
    hand A50.02 [M90.84-] ☑
    hip A50.02 [M90.85-] ☑
    knee A50.02 [M90.86-] ☑
    multiple sites A50.02 [M90.89]
    shoulder joint A50.02 [M90.81-] ☑
    specified site NEC A50.02 [M90.88]
Osteochondroarthrosis deformans endemica — *see* Disease, Kaschin-Beck
Osteochondrodysplasia Q78.9
  with defects of growth of tubular bones and spine Q77.9
  specified NEC Q77.8
  specified NEC Q78.8
Osteochondrodystrophy E78.9
Osteochondrolysis — *see* Osteochondritis, dissecans
Osteochondroma — *see* Neoplasm, bone, benign
Osteochondromatosis D48.0
  syndrome Q78.4
Osteochondromyxosarcoma — *see* Neoplasm, bone, malignant
Osteochondropathy M93.90
  ankle M93.97- ☑
  elbow M93.92- ☑
  foot M93.97- ☑
  hand M93.94- ☑
  hip M93.95- ☑
  Kienböck's disease of adults M93.1
  knee M93.96- ☑
  multiple joints M93.99
  osteochondritis dissecans — *see* Osteochondritis, dissecans
  osteochondrosis — *see* Osteochondrosis
  shoulder region M93.91- ☑
  slipped upper femoral epiphysis — *see* Slipped, epiphysis, upper femoral
  specified joint NEC M93.98
  specified type NEC M93.80
    ankle M93.87- ☑
    elbow M93.82- ☑
    foot M93.87- ☑

☑ **Additional Character Required** — Refer to the Tabular List for Character Selection   ⬇ **Subterms under main terms may continue to next column or page**

Osteochondropathy — *continued*
  specified type — *continued*
    hand M93.84- ☑
    hip M93.85- ☑
    knee M93.86- ☑
    multiple joints M93.89
    shoulder region M93.81- ☑
    specified joint NEC M93.88
    wrist M93.83- ☑
  syphilitic, congenital
    early A50.02 [M90.80]
    late A50.56 [M90.80]
  wrist M93.93- ☑
Osteochondrosarcoma — *see* Neoplasm, bone, malignant
Osteochondrosis (*see also* Osteochondropathy, by site)
  acetabulum (juvenile) M91.0
  adult — *see* Osteochondropathy, specified type NEC, by site
  astragalus (juvenile) — *see* Osteochondrosis, juvenile, tarsus
  Blount's — *see* Osteochondrosis, juvenile, tibia
  Buchanan's M91.0
  Burns' — *see* Osteochondrosis, juvenile, ulna
  calcaneus (juvenile) — *see* Osteochondrosis, juvenile, tarsus
  capitular epiphysis (femur) (juvenile) — *see* Legg-Calvé-Perthes disease
  carpal (juvenile) (lunate) (scaphoid) — *see* Osteochondrosis, juvenile, hand, carpal lunate
    adult M93.1
  coxae juvenilis — *see* Legg-Calvé-Perthes disease
  deformans juvenilis, coxae — *see* Legg-Calvé-Perthes disease
  Diaz's — *see* Osteochondrosis, juvenile, tarsus
  dissecans (knee) (shoulder) — *see* Osteochondritis, dissecans
  femoral capital epiphysis (juvenile) — *see* Legg-Calvé-Perthes disease
  femur (head), juvenile — *see* Legg-Calvé-Perthes disease
  fibula (juvenile) — *see* Osteochondrosis, juvenile, fibula
  foot NEC (juvenile) M92.8
  Freiberg's — *see* Osteochondrosis, juvenile, metatarsus
  Haas' (juvenile) — *see* Osteochondrosis, juvenile, humerus
  Haglund's — *see* Osteochondrosis, juvenile, tarsus
  hip (juvenile) — *see* Legg-Calvé-Perthes disease
  humerus (capitulum) (head) (juvenile) — *see* Osteochondrosis, juvenile, humerus
  ilium, iliac crest (juvenile) M91.0
  ischiopubic synchondrosis M91.0
  Iselin's — *see* Osteochondrosis, juvenile, metatarsus
  juvenile, juvenilis M92.9
    after congenital dislocation of hip reduction — *see* Osteochondrosis, juvenile, hip, specified NEC
    arm — *see* Osteochondrosis, juvenile, upper limb NEC
    capitular epiphysis (femur) — *see* Legg-Calvé-Perthes disease
    clavicle, sternal epiphysis — *see* Osteochondrosis, juvenile, upper limb NEC
    coxae — *see* Legg-Calvé-Perthes disease
    deformans M92.9
    fibula M92.5- ☑
    foot NEC M92.8
    hand M92.20- ☑
      carpal lunate M92.21- ☑
      metacarpal head M92.22- ☑
      specified site NEC M92.29- ☑
    head of femur — *see* Legg-Calvé-Perthes disease
    hip and pelvis M91.9- ☑
      coxa plana — *see* Coxa, plana
      femoral head — *see* Legg-Calvé-Perthes disease
      pelvis M91.0
      pseudocoxalgia — *see* Pseudocoxalgia
      specified NEC M91.8- ☑
    humerus M92.0- ☑
    limb
      lower NEC M92.8
      upper NEC — *see* Osteochondrosis, juvenile, upper limb NEC
    medial cuneiform bone — *see* Osteochondrosis, juvenile, tarsus
    metatarsus M92.7- ☑
    patella M92.4- ☑

Osteochondrosis — *continued*
  juvenile, juvenilis — *continued*
    radius M92.1- ☑
    specified site NEC M92.8
    spine M42.00
      cervical region M42.02
      cervicothoracic region M42.03
      lumbar region M42.06
      lumbosacral region M42.07
      multiple sites M42.09
      occipito-atlanto-axial region M42.01
      sacrococcygeal region M42.08
      thoracic region M42.04
      thoracolumbar region M42.05
    tarsus M92.6- ☑
    tibia M92.5- ☑
    ulna M92.1- ☑
    upper limb NEC M92.3- ☑
    vertebra (body) (epiphyseal plates) (Calvé's) (Scheuermann's) — *see* Osteochondrosis, juvenile, spine
  Kienböck's — *see* Osteochondrosis, juvenile, hand, carpal lunate
    adult M93.1
  Köhler's
    patellar — *see* Osteochondrosis, juvenile, patella
    tarsal navicular — *see* Osteochondrosis, juvenile, tarsus
  Legg-Perthes (-Calvé)(-Waldenström) — *see* Legg-Calvé-Perthes disease
  limb
    lower NEC (juvenile) M92.8
    upper NEC (juvenile) — *see* Osteochondrosis, juvenile, upper limb NEC
  lunate bone (carpal) (juvenile) (*see also* Osteochondrosis, juvenile, hand, carpal lunate)
    adult M93.1
  Mauclaire's — *see* Osteochondrosis, juvenile, hand, metacarpal
  metacarpal (head) (juvenile) — *see* Osteochondrosis, juvenile, hand, metacarpal
  metatarsus (fifth) (head) (juvenile) (second) — *see* Osteochondrosis, juvenile, metatarsus
  navicular (juvenile) — *see* Osteochondrosis, juvenile, tarsus
  os
    calcis (juvenile) — *see* Osteochondrosis, juvenile, tarsus
    tibiale externum (juvenile) — *see* Osteochondrosis, juvenile, tarsus
  Osgood-Schlatter — *see* Osteochondrosis, juvenile, tibia
  Panner's — *see* Osteochondrosis, juvenile, humerus
  patellar center (juvenile) (primary) (secondary) — *see* Osteochondrosis, juvenile, patella
  pelvis (juvenile) M91.0
  Pierson's M91.0
  radius (head) (juvenile) — *see* Osteochondrosis, juvenile, radius
  Scheuermann's — *see* Osteochondrosis, juvenile, spine
  Sever's — *see* Osteochondrosis, juvenile, tarsus
  Sinding-Larsen — *see* Osteochondrosis, juvenile, patella
  spine M42.9
    adult M42.10
      cervical region M42.12
      cervicothoracic region M42.13
      lumbar region M42.16
      lumbosacral region M42.17
      multiple sites M42.19
      occipito-atlanto-axial region M42.11
      sacrococcygeal region M42.18
      thoracic region M42.14
      thoracolumbar region M42.15
    juvenile — *see* Osteochondrosis, juvenile, spine
  symphysis pubis (juvenile) M91.0
  syphilitic (congenital) A50.02
  talus (juvenile) — *see* Osteochondrosis, juvenile, tarsus
  tarsus (navicular) (juvenile) — *see* Osteochondrosis, juvenile, tarsus
  tibia (proximal) (tubercle) (juvenile) — *see* Osteochondrosis, juvenile, tibia
  tuberculous — *see* Tuberculosis, bone
  ulna (lower) (juvenile) — *see* Osteochondrosis, juvenile, ulna
  van Neck's M91.0
  vertebral — *see* Osteochondrosis, spine

Osteoclastoma D48.0
  malignant — *see* Neoplasm, bone, malignant
Osteodynia — *see* Disorder, bone, specified type NEC
Osteodystrophy Q78.9
  azotemic N25.0
  congenital Q78.9
  parathyroid, secondary E21.1
  renal N25.0
Osteofibroma — *see* Neoplasm, bone, benign
Osteofibrosarcoma — *see* Neoplasm, bone, malignant
Osteogenesis imperfecta Q78.0
Osteogenic — *see* condition
Osteolysis M89.50
  carpus M89.54- ☑
  clavicle M89.51- ☑
  femur M89.55- ☑
  fibula M89.56- ☑
  finger M89.54- ☑
  humerus M89.52- ☑
  ilium M89.559
  ischium M89.559
  joint prosthesis (periprosthetic) — *see* Complications, joint prosthesis, mechanical, periprosthetic, osteolysis, by site
  metacarpus M89.54- ☑
  metatarsus M89.57- ☑
  multiple sites M89.59
  neck M89.58
  periprosthetic — *see* Complications, joint prosthesis, mechanical, periprosthetic, osteolysis, by site
  radius M89.53- ☑
  rib M89.58
  scapula M89.51- ☑
  skull M89.58
  tarsus M89.57- ☑
  tibia M89.56- ☑
  toe M89.57- ☑
  ulna M89.53- ☑
  vertebra M89.58
Osteoma (*see also* Neoplasm, bone, benign)
  osteoid (*see also* Neoplasm, bone, benign)
    giant — *see* Neoplasm, bone, benign
Osteomalacia M83.9
  adult M83.9
    drug-induced NEC M83.5
    due to
      malabsorption (postsurgical) M83.2
      malnutrition M83.3
    specified NEC M83.8
  aluminium-induced M83.4
  infantile — *see* Rickets
  juvenile — *see* Rickets
  oncogenic E83.89
  pelvis M83.8
  puerperal M83.0
  senile M83.1
  vitamin-D-resistant in adults E83.31 [M90.8-] ☑
    carpus E83.31 [M90.84-] ☑
    clavicle E83.31 [M90.81-] ☑
    femur E83.31 [M90.85-] ☑
    fibula E83.31 [M90.86-] ☑
    finger E83.31 [M90.84-] ☑
    humerus E83.31 [M90.82-] ☑
    ilium E83.31 [M90.859]
    ischium E83.31 [M90.859]
    metacarpus E83.31 [M90.84-] ☑
    metatarsus E83.31 [M90.87-] ☑
    multiple sites E83.31 [M90.89]
    neck E83.31 [M90.88]
    radius E83.31 [M90.83-] ☑
    rib E83.31 [M90.88]
    scapula E83.31 [M90.819]
    skull E83.31 [M90.88]
    tarsus E83.31 [M90.879]
    tibia E83.31 [M90.869]
    toe E83.31 [M90.879]
    ulna E83.31 [M90.839]
    vertebra E83.31 [M90.88]
Osteomyelitis (general) (infective) (localized) (neonatal) (purulent) (septic) (staphylococcal) (streptococcal) (suppurative) (with periostitis) M86.9
  acute M86.10
    carpus M86.14- ☑
    clavicle M86.11- ☑
    femur M86.15- ☑
    fibula M86.16- ☑
    finger M86.14- ☑

Osteomyelitis — *continued*
  acute — *continued*
    hematogenous M86.00
      carpus M86.04- ✔
      clavicle M86.01- ✔
      femur M86.05- ✔
      fibula M86.06- ✔
      finger M86.04- ✔
      humerus M86.02- ✔
      ilium M86.059
      ischium M86.059
      mandible M27.2
      metacarpus M86.04- ✔
      metatarsus M86.07- ✔
      multiple sites M86.09
      neck M86.08
      orbit H05.02- ✔
      petrous bone — *see* Petrositis
      radius M86.03- ✔
      rib M86.08
      scapula M86.01- ✔
      skull M86.08
      tarsus M86.07- ✔
      tibia M86.06- ✔
      toe M86.07- ✔
      ulna M86.03- ✔
      vertebra — *see* Osteomyelitis, vertebra
    humerus M86.12- ✔
    ilium M86.159
    ischium M86.159
    mandible M27.2
    metacarpus M86.14- ✔
    metatarsus M86.17- ✔
    multiple sites M86.19
    neck M86.18
    orbit H05.02- ✔
    petrous bone — *see* Petrositis
    radius M86.13- ✔
    rib M86.18
    scapula M86.11- ✔
    skull M86.18
    tarsus M86.17- ✔
    tibia M86.16- ✔
    toe M86.17- ✔
    ulna M86.13- ✔
    vertebra — *see* Osteomyelitis, vertebra
  chronic (or old) M86.60
    with draining sinus M86.40
      carpus M86.44- ✔
      clavicle M86.41- ✔
      femur M86.45- ✔
      fibula M86.46- ✔
      finger M86.44- ✔
      humerus M86.42- ✔
      ilium M86.459
      ischium M86.459
      mandible M27.2
      metacarpus M86.44- ✔
      metatarsus M86.47- ✔
      multiple sites M86.49
      neck M86.48
      orbit H05.02- ✔
      petrous bone — *see* Petrositis
      radius M86.43- ✔
      rib M86.48
      scapula M86.41- ✔
      skull M86.48
      tarsus M86.47- ✔
      tibia M86.46- ✔
      toe M86.47- ✔
      ulna M86.43- ✔
      vertebra — *see* Osteomyelitis, vertebra
    carpus M86.64- ✔
    clavicle M86.61- ✔
    femur M86.65- ✔
    fibula M86.66- ✔
    finger M86.64- ✔
    hematogenous NEC M86.50
      carpus M86.54- ✔
      clavicle M86.51- ✔
      femur M86.55- ✔
      fibula M86.56- ✔
      finger M86.54- ✔
      humerus M86.52- ✔
      ilium M86.559
      ischium M86.559

Osteomyelitis — *continued*
  chronic — *continued*
    hematogenous — *continued*
      mandible M27.2
      metacarpus M86.54- ✔
      metatarsus M86.57- ✔
      multifocal M86.30
        carpus M86.34- ✔
        clavicle M86.31- ✔
        femur M86.35- ✔
        fibula M86.36- ✔
        finger M86.34- ✔
        humerus M86.32- ✔
        ilium M86.359
        ischium M86.359
        metacarpus M86.34- ✔
        metatarsus M86.37- ✔
        multiple sites M86.39
        neck M86.38
        radius M86.33- ✔
        rib M86.38
        scapula M86.31- ✔
        skull M86.38
        tarsus M86.37- ✔
        tibia M86.36- ✔
        toe M86.37- ✔
        ulna M86.33- ✔
        vertebra — *see* Osteomyelitis, vertebra
      multiple sites M86.59
      neck M86.58
      orbit H05.02- ✔
      petrous bone — *see* Petrositis
      radius M86.53- ✔
      rib M86.58
      scapula M86.51- ✔
      skull M86.58
      tarsus M86.57- ✔
      tibia M86.56- ✔
      toe M86.57- ✔
      ulna M86.53- ✔
      vertebra — *see* Osteomyelitis, vertebra
    humerus M86.62- ✔
    ilium M86.659
    ischium M86.659
    mandible M27.2
    metacarpus M86.64- ✔
    metatarsus M86.67- ✔
    multifocal — *see* Osteomyelitis, chronic, hematogenous, multifocal
    multiple sites M86.69
    neck M86.68
    orbit H05.02- ✔
    petrous bone — *see* Petrositis
    radius M86.63- ✔
    rib M86.68
    scapula M86.61- ✔
    skull M86.68
    tarsus M86.67- ✔
    tibia M86.66- ✔
    toe M86.67- ✔
    ulna M86.63- ✔
    vertebra — *see* Osteomyelitis, vertebra
  echinococcal B67.2
  Garr's — *see* Osteomyelitis, specified type NEC
  jaw (acute) (chronic) (lower) (neonatal) (suppurative) (upper) M27.2
  nonsuppurating — *see* Osteomyelitis, specified type NEC
  orbit H05.02- ✔
  petrous bone — *see* Petrositis
  Salmonella (arizonae) (cholerae-suis) (enteritidis) (typhimurium) A02.24
  sclerosing, nonsuppurative — *see* Osteomyelitis, specified type NEC
  specified type NEC (*see also* subcategory) M86.8X- ✔
    mandible M27.2
    orbit H05.02- ✔
    petrous bone — *see* Petrositis
    vertebra — *see* Osteomyelitis, vertebra
  subacute M86.20
    carpus M86.24- ✔
    clavicle M86.21- ✔
    femur M86.25- ✔
    fibula M86.26- ✔
    finger M86.24- ✔
    humerus M86.22- ✔

Osteomyelitis — *continued*
  subacute — *continued*
    mandible M27.2
    metacarpus M86.24- ✔
    metatarsus M86.27- ✔
    multiple sites M86.29
    neck M86.28
    orbit H05.02- ✔
    petrous bone — *see* Petrositis
    radius M86.23- ✔
    rib M86.28
    scapula M86.21- ✔
    skull M86.28
    tarsus M86.27- ✔
    tibia M86.26- ✔
    toe M86.27- ✔
    ulna M86.23- ✔
    vertebra — *see* Osteomyelitis, vertebra
  syphilitic A52.77
    congenital (early) A50.02 [M90.80]
  tuberculous — *see* Tuberculosis, bone
  typhoid A01.05
  vertebra M46.20
    cervical region M46.22
    cervicothoracic region M46.23
    lumbar region M46.26
    lumbosacral region M46.27
    occipito-atlanto-axial region M46.21
    sacrococcygeal region M46.28
    thoracic region M46.24
    thoracolumbar region M46.25
Osteomyelofibrosis D75.89
Osteomyelosclerosis D75.89
Osteonecrosis M87.9
  due to
    drugs — *see* Osteonecrosis, secondary, due to, drugs
    trauma — *see* Osteonecrosis, secondary, due to, trauma
  idiopathic aseptic M87.00
    ankle M87.07- ✔
    carpus M87.03- ✔
    clavicle M87.01- ✔
    femur M87.05- ✔
    fibula M87.06- ✔
    finger M87.04- ✔
    humerus M87.02- ✔
    ilium M87.050
    ischium M87.050
    metacarpus M87.04- ✔
    metatarsus M87.07- ✔
    multiple sites M87.09
    neck M87.08
    pelvis M87.050
    radius M87.03- ✔
    rib M87.08
    scapula M87.01- ✔
    skull M87.08
    tarsus M87.07- ✔
    tibia M87.06- ✔
    toe M87.07- ✔
    ulna M87.03- ✔
    vertebra M87.08
  secondary NEC M87.30
    carpus M87.33- ✔
    clavicle M87.31- ✔
    due to
      drugs M87.10
        carpus M87.13- ✔
        clavicle M87.11- ✔
        femur M87.15- ✔
        fibula M87.16- ✔
        finger M87.14- ✔
        humerus M87.12- ✔
        ilium M87.159
        ischium M87.159
        jaw M87.180
        metacarpus M87.14- ✔
        metatarsus M87.17- ✔
        multiple sites M87.19
        neck M87.18 ✔
        radius M87.13- ✔
        rib M87.18
        scapula M87.11- ✔
        skull M87.18
        tarsus M87.17- ✔
        tibia M87.16- ✔

✔ **Additional Character Required** — Refer to the Tabular List for Character Selection   ▽ **Subterms under main terms may continue to next column or page**

Osteonecrosis — *continued*
secondary — *continued*
  due to — *continued*
    drugs — *continued*
      toe M87.17- ☑
      ulna M87.13- ☑
      vertebra M87.18 ☑
     hemoglobinopathy NEC D58.2 [M90.50]
      carpus D58.2 [M90.54-] ☑
      clavicle D58.2 [M90.51-] ☑
      femur D58.2 [M90.55-] ☑
      fibula D58.2 [M90.56-] ☑
      finger D58.2 [M90.54-] ☑
      humerus D58.2 [M90.52-] ☑
      ilium D58.2 [M90.55-] ☑
      ischium D58.2 [M90.55-] ☑
      metacarpus D58.2 [M90.54-] ☑
      metatarsus D58.2 [M90.57-] ☑
      multiple sites D58.2 [M90.58]
      neck D58.2 [M90.58]
      radius D58.2 [M90.53-] ☑
      rib D58.2 [M90.58]
      scapula D58.2 [M90.51-] ☑
      skull D58.2 [M90.58]
      tarsus D58.2 [M90.57-] ☑
      tibia D58.2 [M90.56-] ☑
      toe D58.2 [M90.57-] ☑
      ulna D58.2 [M90.53-] ☑
      vertebra D58.2 [M90.58]
    trauma (previous) M87.20
     carpus M87.23- ☑
     clavicle M87.21- ☑
     femur M87.25- ☑
     fibula M87.26- ☑
     finger M87.24- ☑
     humerus M87.22- ☑
     ilium M87.25- ☑
     ischium M87.25- ☑
     metacarpus M87.24- ☑
     metatarsus M87.27- ☑
     multiple sites M87.29
     neck M87.28
     radius M87.23- ☑
     rib M87.28
     scapula M87.21- ☑
     skull M87.28
     tarsus M87.27- ☑
     tibia M87.26- ☑
     toe M87.27- ☑
     ulna M87.23- ☑
     vertebra M87.28
  femur M87.35- ☑
  fibula M87.36- ☑
  finger M87.34- ☑
  humerus M87.32- ☑
  ilium M87.350
  in
    caisson disease T70.3 ☑ [M90.50]
     carpus T70.3 ☑ [M90.54-] ☑
     clavicle T70.3 ☑ [M90.51-] ☑
     femur T70.3 ☑ [M90.55-] ☑
     fibula T70.3 ☑ [M90.56-] ☑
     finger T70.3 ☑ [M90.54-] ☑
     humerus T70.3 ☑ [M90.52-] ☑
     ilium T70.3 ☑ [M90.55-] ☑
     ischium T70.3 ☑ [M90.55-] ☑
     metacarpus T70.3 ☑ [M90.54-] ☑
     metatarsus T70.3 ☑ [M90.57-] ☑
     multiple sites T70.3 ☑ [M90.59]
     neck T70.3 ☑ [M90.58]
     radius T70.3 ☑ [M90.53-] ☑
     rib T70.3 ☑ [M90.58]
     scapula T70.3 ☑ [M90.51-] ☑
     skull T70.3 ☑ [M90.58]
     tarsus T70.3 ☑ [M90.57-] ☑
     tibia T70.3 ☑ [M90.56-] ☑
     toe T70.3 ☑ [M90.57-] ☑
     ulna T70.3 ☑ [M90.53-] ☑
     vertebra T70.3 ☑ [M90.58]
  ischium M87.350
  metacarpus M87.34- ☑
  metatarsus M87.37- ☑
  multiple site M87.39
  neck M87.38
  radius M87.33- ☑
  rib M87.38

Osteonecrosis — *continued*
secondary — *continued*
  scapula M87.319
  skull M87.38
  tarsus M87.379
  tibia M87.366
  toe M87.379
  ulna M87.33- ☑
  vertebra M87.38
 specified type NEC M87.80
  carpus M87.83- ☑
  clavicle M87.81- ☑
  femur M87.85- ☑
  fibula M87.86- ☑
  finger M87.84- ☑
  humerus M87.82- ☑
  ilium M87.85- ☑
  ischium M87.85- ☑
  metacarpus M87.84- ☑
  metatarsus M87.87- ☑
  multiple sites M87.89
  neck M87.88
  radius M87.83- ☑
  rib M87.88
  scapula M87.81- ☑
  skull M87.88
  tarsus M87.87- ☑
  tibia M87.86- ☑
  toe M87.87- ☑
  ulna M87.83- ☑
  vertebra M87.88

Osteo-onycho-arthro-dysplasia Q79.8
Osteo-onychodysplasia, hereditary Q79.8
Osteopathia condensans disseminata Q78.8
Osteopathy (*see also* Osteomyelitis, Osteonecrosis, Osteoporosis)
 after poliomyelitis M89.60
  carpus M89.64- ☑
  clavicle M89.61- ☑
  femur M89.65- ☑
  fibula M89.66- ☑
  finger M89.64- ☑
  humerus M89.62- ☑
  ilium M89.659
  ischium M89.659
  metacarpus M89.64- ☑
  metatarsus M89.67- ☑
  multiple sites M89.69
  neck M89.68
  radius M89.63- ☑
  rib M89.68
  scapula M89.61- ☑
  skull M89.68
  tarsus M89.67- ☑
  tibia M89.66- ☑
  toe M89.67- ☑
  ulna M89.63- ☑
  vertebra M89.68
 in (due to)
  renal osteodystrophy N25.0
  specified diseases classified elsewhere — *see* subcategory M90.8 ☑
Osteopenia M85.8- ☑
 borderline M85.8- ☑
Osteoperiostitis — *see* Osteomyelitis, specified type NEC
Osteopetrosis (familial) Q78.2
Osteophyte M25.70
 ankle M25.77- ☑
 elbow M25.72- ☑
 foot joint M25.77- ☑
 hand joint M25.74- ☑
 hip M25.75- ☑
 knee M25.76- ☑
 shoulder M25.71- ☑
 spine M25.78
 vertebrae M25.78
 wrist M25.73- ☑
Osteopoikilosis Q78.8
Osteoporosis (female) (male) M81.0
 with current pathological fracture M80.00 ☑
 age-related M81.0
  with current pathologic fracture M80.00 ☑
   carpus M80.04- ☑
   clavicle M80.01- ☑
   fibula M80.06- ☑

Osteoporosis — *continued*
age-related — *continued*
  with current pathologic fracture — *continued*
   finger M80.04- ☑
   humerus M80.02- ☑
   ilium M80.05- ☑
   ischium M80.05- ☑
   metacarpus M80.04- ☑
   metatarsus M80.07- ☑
   pelvis M80.05- ☑
   radius M80.03- ☑
   scapula M80.01- ☑
   tarsus M80.07- ☑
   tibia M80.06- ☑
   toe M80.07- ☑
   ulna M80.03- ☑
   vertebra M80.08 ☑
 disuse M81.8
  with current pathological fracture M80.80 ☑
   carpus M80.84- ☑
   clavicle M80.81- ☑
   fibula M80.86- ☑
   finger M80.84- ☑
   humerus M80.82- ☑
   ilium M80.85- ☑
   ischium M80.85- ☑
   metacarpus M80.84- ☑
   metatarsus M80.87- ☑
   pelvis M80.85- ☑
   radius M80.83- ☑
   scapula M80.81- ☑
   tarsus M80.87- ☑
   tibia M80.86- ☑
   toe M80.87- ☑
   ulna M80.83- ☑
   vertebra M80.88 ☑
 drug-induced — *see* Osteoporosis, specified type NEC
 idiopathic — *see* Osteoporosis, specified type NEC
 involutional — *see* Osteoporosis, age-related
 Lequesne M81.6
 localized M81.6
 postmenopausal M81.0
  with pathological fracture M80.00 ☑
   carpus M80.04- ☑
   clavicle M80.01- ☑
   fibula M80.06- ☑
   finger M80.04- ☑
   humerus M80.02- ☑
   ilium M80.05- ☑
   ischium M80.05- ☑
   metacarpus M80.04- ☑
   metatarsus M80.07- ☑
   pelvis M80.05- ☑
   radius M80.03- ☑
   scapula M80.01- ☑
   tarsus M80.07- ☑
   tibia M80.06- ☑
   toe M80.07- ☑
   ulna M80.03- ☑
   vertebra M80.08 ☑
 postoophorectomy — *see* Osteoporosis, specified type NEC
 postsurgical malabsorption — *see* Osteoporosis, specified type NEC
 post-traumatic — *see* Osteoporosis, specified type NEC
 senile — *see* Osteoporosis, age-related
 specified type NEC M81.8
  with pathological fracture M80.80 ☑
   carpus M80.84- ☑
   clavicle M80.81- ☑
   fibula M80.86- ☑
   finger M80.84- ☑
   humerus M80.82- ☑
   ilium M80.85- ☑
   ischium M80.85- ☑
   metacarpus M80.84- ☑
   metatarsus M80.87- ☑
   pelvis M80.85- ☑
   radius M80.83- ☑
   scapula M80.81- ☑
   tarsus M80.87- ☑
   tibia M80.86- ☑
   toe M80.87- ☑
   ulna M80.83- ☑
   vertebra M80.88 ☑

Osteopsathyrosis (idiopathica) Q78.0
Osteoradionecrosis, jaw (acute) (chronic) (lower)
    (suppurative) (upper) M27.2
Osteosarcoma (any form) — see Neoplasm, bone, malig-
    nant
Osteosclerosis Q78.2
    acquired M85.8- ☑
    congenita Q77.4
    fragilitas (generalisata) Q78.2
    myelofibrosis D75.81
Osteosclerotic anemia D64.89
Osteosis
    cutis L94.2
    renal fibrocystic N25.0
Österreicher-Turner syndrome Q87.2
Ostium
    atrioventriculare commune Q21.2
    primum (arteriosum) (defect) (persistent) Q21.2
    secundum (arteriosum) (defect) (patent) (persistent)
        Q21.1
Ostrum-Furst syndrome Q75.8
Otalgia H92.0 ☑
Otitis (acute) H66.90
    with effusion (see also Otitis, media, nonsuppurative)
        purulent — see Otitis, media, suppurative
    adhesive — see subcategory H74.1 ☑
    chronic (see also Otitis, media, chronic)
        with effusion (see also Otitis, media, nonsuppura-
            tive, chronic)
    externa H60.9- ☑
        abscess — see Abscess, ear, external
        acute (noninfective) H60.50- ☑
            actinic H60.51- ☑
            chemical H60.52- ☑
            contact H60.53- ☑
            eczematoid H60.54- ☑
            infective — see Otitis, externa, infective
            reactive H60.55- ☑
            specified NEC H60.59- ☑
        cellulitis — see Cellulitis, ear
        chronic H60.6- ☑
        diffuse — see Otitis, externa, infective, diffuse
        hemorrhagic — see Otitis, externa, infective,
            hemorrhagic
        in (due to)
            aspergillosis B44.89
            candidiasis B37.84
            erysipelas A46 [H62.40]
            herpes (simplex) virus infection B00.1
                zoster B02.8
            impetigo L01.00 [H62.40]
            infectious disease NEC B99 ☑ [H62.4-] ☑
            mycosis NEC B36.9 [H62.40]
            parasitic disease NEC B89 [H62.40]
            viral disease NEC B34.9 [H62.40]
            zoster B02.8
        infective NEC H60.39- ☑
            abscess — see Abscess, ear, external
            cellulitis — see Cellulitis, ear
            diffuse H60.31- ☑
            hemorrhagic H60.32- ☑
            swimmer's ear — see Swimmer's, ear
        malignant H60.2- ☑
        mycotic B36.9 [H62.40]
        necrotizing — see Otitis, externa, malignant
        Pseudomonas aeruginosa — see Otitis, externa,
            malignant
        reactive — see Otitis, externa, acute, reactive
        specified NEC — see subcategory H60.8 ☑
        tropical B36.8
    insidiosa — see Otosclerosis
    interna H83.0 ☑
    media (hemorrhagic) (staphylococcal) (streptococcal)
        H66.9- ☑
        with effusion (nonpurulent) — see Otitis, media,
            nonsuppurative
        acute, subacute H66.90
            allergic — see Otitis, media, nonsuppurative,
                acute, allergic
            exudative — see Otitis, media, nonsuppurative,
                acute
            mucoid — see Otitis, media, nonsuppurative,
                acute
            necrotizing (see also Otitis, media, suppurative,
                acute)
                in
                    measles B05.3

Otitis — continued
    media — continued
        acute, subacute — continued
            necrotizing (see also Otitis, media, suppurative,
                acute) — continued
                in — continued
                    scarlet fever A38.0
            nonsuppurative NEC — see Otitis, media, non-
                suppurative, acute
            purulent — see Otitis, media, suppurative,
                acute
            sanguinous — see Otitis, media, nonsuppura-
                tive, acute
            secretory — see Otitis, media, nonsuppurative,
                acute, serous
            seromucinous — see Otitis, media, nonsuppu-
                rative, acute
            serous — see Otitis, media, nonsuppurative,
                acute, serous
            suppurative — see Otitis, media, suppurative,
                acute
        allergic — see Otitis, media, nonsuppurative
        catarrhal — see Otitis, media, nonsuppurative
        chronic H66.90
            with effusion (nonpurulent) — see Otitis, media,
                nonsuppurative, chronic
            allergic — see Otitis, media, nonsuppurative,
                chronic, allergic
            benign suppurative — see Otitis, media, suppu-
                rative, chronic, tubotympanic
            catarrhal — see Otitis, media, nonsuppurative,
                chronic, serous
            exudative — see Otitis, media, nonsuppurative,
                chronic
            mucinous — see Otitis, media, nonsuppurative,
                chronic, mucoid
            mucoid — see Otitis, media, nonsuppurative,
                chronic, mucoid
            nonsuppurative NEC — see Otitis, media, non-
                suppurative, chronic
            purulent — see Otitis, media, suppurative,
                chronic
            secretory — see Otitis, media, nonsuppurative,
                chronic, mucoid
            seromucinous — see Otitis, media, nonsuppu-
                rative, chronic
            serous — see Otitis, media, nonsuppurative,
                chronic, serous
            suppurative — see Otitis, media, suppurative,
                chronic
            transudative — see Otitis, media, nonsuppura-
                tive, chronic, mucoid
        exudative — see Otitis, media, nonsuppurative
        in (due to) (with)
            influenza — see Influenza, with, otitis media
            measles B05.3
            scarlet fever A38.0
            tuberculosis A18.6
            viral disease NEC B34.- ☑ [H67.-] ☑
        mucoid — see Otitis, media, nonsuppurative
        nonsuppurative H65.9- ☑
            acute or subacute NEC H65.19- ☑
                allergic H65.11- ☑
                    recurrent H65.11- ☑
                recurrent H65.19- ☑
                secretory — see Otitis, media, nonsuppura-
                    tive, serous
                serous H65.0- ☑
                    recurrent H65.0- ☑
            chronic H65.49- ☑
                allergic H65.41- ☑
                mucoid H65.3- ☑
                serous H65.2- ☑
        postmeasles B05.3
        purulent — see Otitis, media, suppurative
        secretory — see Otitis, media, nonsuppurative
        seromucinous — see Otitis, media, nonsuppurative
        serous — see Otitis, media, nonsuppurative
        suppurative H66.4- ☑
            acute H66.00- ☑
                with rupture of ear drum H66.01- ☑
                recurrent H66.00- ☑
                    with rupture of ear drum H66.01- ☑
            chronic (see also subcategory) H66.3 ☑
                atticoantral H66.2- ☑
                benign — see Otitis, media, suppurative,
                    chronic, tubotympanic

Otitis — continued
    media — continued
        suppurative — continued
            chronic (see also subcategory) — continued
                tubotympanic H66.1- ☑
            transudative — see Otitis, media, nonsuppurative
            tuberculous A18.6
Otocephaly Q18.2
Otolith syndrome — see subcategory H81.8 ☑
Otomycosis (diffuse) NEC B36.9 [H62.40]
    in
        aspergillosis B44.89
        candidiasis B37.84
        moniliasis B37.84
Otoporosis — see Otosclerosis
Otorrhagia (nontraumatic) H92.2- ☑
    traumatic — code by Type of injury
Otorrhea H92.1- ☑
    cerebrospinal G96.0
Otosclerosis (general) H80.9- ☑
    cochlear (endosteal) H80.2- ☑
    involving
        otic capsule — see Otosclerosis, cochlear
        oval window
            nonobliterative H80.0- ☑
            obliterative H80.1- ☑
        round window — see Otosclerosis, cochlear
    nonobliterative — see Otosclerosis, involving, oval
        window, nonobliterative
    obliterative — see Otosclerosis, involving, oval win-
        dow, obliterative
    specified NEC H80.8- ☑
Otospongiosis — see Otosclerosis
Otto's disease or pelvis M24.7
Outcome of delivery Z37.9
    multiple births Z37.9
        all liveborn Z37.50
            quadruplets Z37.52
            quintuplets Z37.53
            sextuplets Z37.54
            specified number NEC Z37.59
            triplets Z37.51
        all stillborn Z37.7
        some liveborn Z37.60
            quadruplets Z37.62
            quintuplets Z37.63
            sextuplets Z37.64
            specified number NEC Z37.69
            triplets Z37.61
    single NEC Z37.9
        liveborn Z37.0
        stillborn Z37.1
    twins NEC Z37.9
        both liveborn Z37.2
        both stillborn Z37.4
        one liveborn, one stillborn Z37.3
Outlet — see condition
Ovalocytosis (congenital) (hereditary) — see Elliptocyto-
    sis
Ovarian — see Condition
Ovariocele N83.4
Ovaritis (cystic) — see Oophoritis
Ovary, ovarian (see also condition)
    resistant syndrome E28.39
    vein syndrome N13.8
Overactive (see also Hyperfunction)
    adrenal cortex NEC E27.0
    bladder N32.81
    hypothalamus E23.3
    thyroid — see Hyperthyroidism
Overactivity R46.3
    child — see Disorder, attention-deficit hyperactivity
Overbite (deep) (excessive) (horizontal) (vertical) M26.29
Overbreathing — see Hyperventilation
Overconscientious personality F60.5
Overdevelopment — see Hypertrophy
Overdistension — see Distension
Overdose, overdosage (drug) — see Table of Drugs and
    Chemicals, by drug, poisoning
Overeating R63.2
    nonorganic origin F50.8
    psychogenic F50.8
Overexertion (effects) (exhaustion) T73.3 ☑
Overexposure (effects) T73.9 ☑
    exhaustion T73.2 ☑
Overfeeding — see Overeating
    newborn P92.4

Overfill, endodontic M27.52
Overgrowth, bone — *see* Hypertrophy, bone
Overhanging of dental restorative material (unrepairable) K08.52
Overheated (places) (effects) — *see* Heat
Overjet (excessive horizontal) M26.23
Overlaid, overlying (suffocation) — *see* Asphyxia, traumatic, due to mechanical threat
Overlap, excessive horizontal (teeth) M26.23
Overlapping toe (acquired) (*see also* Deformity, toe, specified NEC)
   congenital (fifth toe) Q66.89
Overload
   circulatory, due to transfusion (blood) (blood components) (TACO) E87.71
   fluid E87.70
      due to transfusion (blood) (blood components) E87.71
      specified NEC E87.79
   iron, due to repeated red blood cell transfusions E83.111
   potassium (K) E87.5
   sodium (Na) E87.0
Overnutrition — *see* Hyperalimentation
Overproduction (*see also* Hypersecretion)
   ACTH E27.0
   catecholamine E27.5
   growth hormone E22.0
Overprotection, child by parent Z62.1
Overriding
   aorta Q25.4
   finger (acquired) — *see* Deformity, finger
      congenital Q68.1
   toe (acquired) (*see also* Deformity, toe, specified NEC)
      congenital Q66.89
Overstrained R53.83
   heart — *see* Hypertrophy, cardiac
Overuse, muscle NEC M70.8- ☑
Overweight E66.3
Overworked R53.83
Oviduct — *see* condition
Ovotestis Q56.0
Ovulation (cycle)
   failure or lack of N97.0
   pain N94.0
Ovum — *see* condition
Owren's disease or syndrome (parahemophilia) D68.2
Ox heart — *see* Hypertrophy, cardiac
Oxalosis E72.53
Oxaluria E72.53
Oxycephaly, oxycephalic Q75.0
   syphilitic, congenital A50.02
Oxyuriasis B80
Oxyuris vermicularis (infestation) B80
Ozena J31.0

P

Pachyderma, pachydermia L85.9
   larynx (verrucosa) J38.7
Pachydermatocele (congenital) Q82.8
Pachydermoperiostosis (*see also* Osteoarthropathy, hypertrophic, specified type NEC)
   clubbed nail M89.40 [L62]
Pachygyria Q04.3
Pachymeningitis (adhesive) (basal) (brain) (cervical) (chronic)(circumscribed) (external) (fibrous) (hemorrhagic) (hypertrophic) (internal) (purulent) (spinal) (suppurative) — *see* Meningitis
Pachyonychia (congenital) Q84.5
Pacinian tumor — *see* Neoplasm, skin, benign
Pad, knuckle or Garrod's M72.1
Paget's disease
   with infiltrating duct carcinoma — *see* Neoplasm, breast, malignant
   bone M88.9
      carpus M88.84- ☑
      clavicle M88.81- ☑
      femur M88.85- ☑
      fibula M88.86- ☑
      finger M88.84- ☑
      humerus M88.82- ☑
      ilium M88.85- ☑
      in neoplastic disease — *see* Osteitis, deformans, in neoplastic disease
      ischium M88.85- ☑
      metacarpus M88.84- ☑

Paget's disease — *continued*
   bone — *continued*
      metatarsus M88.87- ☑
      multiple sites M88.89
      neck M88.88
      radius M88.83- ☑
      rib M88.88
      scapula M88.81- ☑
      skull M88.0
      tarsus M88.87- ☑
      tibia M88.86- ☑
      toe M88.87- ☑
      ulna M88.83- ☑
      vertebra M88.88
   breast (female) C50.01- ☑
      male C50.02- ☑
   extramammary (*see also* Neoplasm, skin, malignant)
      anus C21.0
      margin C44.590
      skin C44.590
   intraductal carcinoma — *see* Neoplasm, breast, malignant
   malignant — *see* Neoplasm, skin, malignant
      breast (female) C50.01- ☑
      male C50.02- ☑
      unspecified site (female) C50.01- ☑
      male C50.02- ☑
   mammary — *see* Paget's disease, breast
   nipple — *see* Paget's disease, breast
   osteitis deformans — *see* Paget's disease, bone
Paget-Schroetter syndrome I82.890
Pain(s) (*see also* Painful) R52
   abdominal R10.9
      colic R10.83
      generalized R10.84
         with acute abdomen R10.0
      lower R10.30
         left quadrant R10.32
         pelvic or perineal R10.2
         periumbilical R10.33
         right quadrant R10.31
      rebound — *see* Tenderness, abdominal, rebound
      severe with abdominal rigidity R10.0
      tenderness — *see* Tenderness, abdominal
      upper R10.10
         epigastric R10.13
         left quadrant R10.12
         right quadrant R10.11
   acute R52
      due to trauma G89.11
      neoplasm related G89.3
      postprocedural NEC G89.18
      post-thoracotomy G89.12
      specified by site — *code to* Pain, by site
   adnexa (uteri) R10.2
   anginoid — *see* Pain, precordial
   anus K62.89
   arm — *see* Pain, limb, upper
   axillary (axilla) M79.62- ☑
   back (postural) M54.9
   bladder R39.89
      associated with micturition — *see* Micturition, painful
   bone — *see* Disorder, bone, specified type NEC
   breast N64.4
   broad ligament R10.2
   cancer associated (acute) (chronic) G89.3
   cecum — *see* Pain, abdominal
   cervicobrachial M53.1
   chest (central) R07.9
      anterior wall R07.89
      atypical R07.89
      ischemic I20.9
      musculoskeletal R07.89
      non-cardiac R07.89
      on breathing R07.1
      pleurodynia R07.81
      precordial R07.2
      wall (anterior) R07.89
   chronic G89.29
      associated with significant psychosocial dysfunction G89.4
      due to trauma G89.21
      neoplasm related G89.3
      postoperative NEC G89.28
      postprocedural NEC G89.28
      post-thoracotomy G89.22

Pain(s) — *continued*
   chronic — *continued*
      specified NEC G89.29
   coccyx M53.3
   colon — *see* Pain, abdominal
   coronary — *see* Angina
   costochondral R07.1
   diaphragm R07.1
   due to cancer G89.3
   due to device, implant or graft (*see also* Complications, by site and type, specified NEC) T85.84 ☑
      arterial graft NEC T82.848 ☑
      breast (implant) T85.84 ☑
      catheter NEC T85.84 ☑
         dialysis (renal) T82.848 ☑
            intraperitoneal T85.84 ☑
         infusion NEC T82.848 ☑
            spinal (epidural) (subdural) T85.84 ☑
         urinary (indwelling) T83.84 ☑
      electronic (electrode) (pulse generator) (stimulator)
         bone T84.84 ☑
         cardiac T82.847 ☑
         nervous system (brain) (peripheral nerve) (spinal) T85.84 ☑
         urinary T83.84 ☑
      fixation, internal (orthopedic) NEC T84.84 ☑
      gastrointestinal (bile duct) (esophagus) T85.84 ☑
      genital NEC T83.84 ☑
      heart NEC T82.847 ☑
      infusion NEC T85.84 ☑
      joint prosthesis T84.84 ☑
      ocular (corneal graft) (orbital implant) NEC T85.84 ☑
      orthopedic NEC T84.84 ☑
      specified NEC T85.84 ☑
      urinary NEC T83.84 ☑
      vascular NEC T82.848 ☑
      ventricular intracranial shunt T85.84 ☑
   due to malignancy (primary) (secondary) G89.3
   ear — *see* subcategory H92.0 ☑
   epigastric, epigastrium R10.13
   eye — *see* Pain, ocular
   face, facial R51
      atypical G50.1
   female genital organs NEC N94.89
   finger — *see* Pain, limb, upper
   flank — *see* Pain, abdominal
   foot — *see* Pain, limb, lower
   gallbladder K82.9
   gas (intestinal) R14.1
   gastric — *see* Pain, abdominal
   generalized NOS R52
   genital organ
      female N94.89
      male N50.8
   groin — *see* Pain, abdominal, lower
   hand — *see* Pain, limb, upper
   head — *see* Headache
   heart — *see* Pain, precordial
   infra-orbital — *see* Neuralgia, trigeminal
   intercostal R07.82
   intermenstrual N94.0
   jaw R68.84
   joint M25.50
      ankle M25.57- ☑
      elbow M25.52- ☑
      finger M79.64- ☑
      foot M79.67- ☑
      hand M79.64- ☑
      hip M25.55- ☑
      knee M25.56- ☑
      shoulder M25.51- ☑
      toe M79.67- ☑
      wrist M25.53- ☑
   kidney N23
   laryngeal R07.0
   leg — *see* Pain, limb, lower
   limb M79.609
      lower M79.60- ☑
         foot M79.67- ☑
         lower leg M79.66- ☑
         thigh M79.65- ☑
         toe M79.67- ☑
      upper M79.60- ☑
         axilla M79.62- ☑
         finger M79.64- ☑

Pain(s) — continued
  limb — continued
    upper — continued
      forearm M79.63- ☑
      hand M79.64- ☑
      upper arm M79.62- ☑
  loin M54.5
  low back M54.5
  lumbar region M54.5
  mandibular R68.84
  mastoid — see subcategory H92.0 ☑
  maxilla R68.84
  menstrual (see also Dysmenorrhea) N94.6
  metacarpophalangeal (joint) — see Pain, joint, hand
  metatarsophalangeal (joint) — see Pain, joint, foot
  mouth K13.79
  muscle — see Myalgia
  musculoskeletal (see also Pain, by site) M79.1
  myofascial M79.1
  nasal J34.89
  nasopharynx J39.2
  neck NEC M54.2
  nerve NEC — see Neuralgia
  neuromuscular — see Neuralgia
  nose J34.89
  ocular H57.1- ☑
  ophthalmic — see Pain, ocular
  orbital region — see Pain, ocular
  ovary N94.89
  over heart — see Pain, precordial
  ovulation N94.0
  pelvic (female) R10.2
  penis N48.89
  pericardial — see Pain, precordial
  perineal, perineum R10.2
  pharynx J39.2
  pleura, pleural, pleuritic R07.81
  postoperative NOS G89.18
  postprocedural NOS G89.18
  post-thoracotomy G89.12
  precordial (region) R07.2
  premenstrual N94.3
  psychogenic (persistent) (any site) F45.41
  radicular (spinal) — see Radiculopathy
  rectum K62.89
  respiration R07.1
  retrosternal R07.2
  rheumatoid, muscular — see Myalgia
  rib R07.81
  root (spinal) — see Radiculopathy
  round ligament (stretch) R10.2
  sacroiliac M53.3
  sciatic — see Sciatica
  scrotum N50.8
  seminal vesicle N50.8
  shoulder M25.51- ☑
  spermatic cord N50.8
  spinal root — see Radiculopathy
  spine M54.9
    cervical M54.2
    low back M54.5
      with sciatica M54.4- ☑
    thoracic M54.6
  stomach — see Pain, abdominal
  substernal R07.2
  temporomandibular (joint) M26.62
  testis N50.8
  thoracic spine M54.6
    with radicular and visceral pain M54.14
  throat R07.0
  tibia — see Pain, limb, lower
  toe — see Pain, limb, lower
  tongue K14.6
  tooth K08.8
  trigeminal — see Neuralgia, trigeminal
  tumor associated G89.3
  ureter N23
  urinary (organ) (system) N23
  uterus NEC N94.89
  vagina R10.2
  vertebrogenic (syndrome) M54.89
  vesical R39.89
    associated with micturition — see Micturition,
      painful
  vulva R10.2
Painful (see also Pain)
  coitus
    female N94.1

Painful — continued
  coitus — continued
    male N53.12
      psychogenic F52.6
  ejaculation (semen) N53.12
    psychogenic F52.6
  erection — see Priapism
  feet syndrome E53.8
  joint replacement (hip) (knee) T84.84 ☑
  menstruation — see Dysmenorrhea
    psychogenic F45.8
  micturition — see Micturition, painful
  respiration R07.1
  scar NEC L90.5
  wire sutures T81.89 ☑
Painter's colic — see subcategory T56.0 ☑
Palate — see condition
Palatoplegia K13.79
Palatoschisis — see Cleft, palate
Palilalia R48.8
Palliative care Z51.5
Pallor R23.1
  optic disc, temporal — see Atrophy, optic
Palmar (see also condition)
  fascia — see condition
Palpable
  cecum K63.89
  kidney N28.89
  ovary N83.8
  prostate N42.9
  spleen — see Splenomegaly
Palpitations (heart) R00.2
  psychogenic F45.8
Palsy (see also Paralysis) G83.9
  atrophic diffuse (progressive) G12.22
  Bell's (see also Palsy, facial)
    newborn P11.3
  brachial plexus NEC G54.0
    newborn (birth injury) P14.3
  brain — see Palsy, cerebral
  bulbar (progressive) (chronic) G12.22
    of childhood (Fazio-Londe) G12.1
    pseudo NEC G12.29
    supranuclear (progressive) G23.1
  cerebral (congenital) G80.9
    ataxic G80.4
    athetoid G80.3
    choreathetoid G80.3
    diplegic G80.8
      spastic G80.1
    dyskinetic G80.3
      athetoid G80.3
      choreathetoid G80.3
      distonic G80.3
    dystonic G80.3
    hemiplegic G80.8
      spastic G80.2
    mixed G80.8
    monoplegic G80.8
      spastic G80.1
    paraplegic G80.8
      spastic G80.1
    quadriplegic G80.8
      spastic G80.0
    spastic G80.1
      diplegic G80.1
      hemiplegic G80.2
      monoplegic G80.1
      quadriplegic G80.0
      specified NEC G80.1
      tetrapelgic G80.0
    specified NEC G80.8
    syphilitic A52.12
      congenital A50.49
    tetraplegic G80.8
      spastic G80.0
  cranial nerve (see also Disorder, nerve, cranial)
    multiple G52.7
      in
        infectious disease B99 ☑ [G53]
        neoplastic disease (see also Neoplasm)
          D49.9 [G53]
        parasitic disease B89 [G53]
        sarcoidosis D86.82
  creeping G12.22
  diver's T70.3 ☑
  Erb's P14.0

Palsy — continued
  facial G51.0
    newborn (birth injury) P11.3
  glossopharyngeal G52.1
  Klumpke (-Déjérine) P14.1
  lead — see subcategory T56.0 ☑
  median nerve (tardy) G56.1- ☑
  nerve G58.9
    specified NEC G58.8
  peroneal nerve (acute) (tardy) G57.3- ☑
  progressive supranuclear G23.1
  pseudobulbar NEC G12.29
  radial nerve (acute) G56.3- ☑
  seventh nerve (see also Palsy, facial)
    newborn P11.3
  shaking — see Parkinsonism
  spastic (cerebral) (spinal) G80.1
  ulnar nerve (tardy) G56.2- ☑
  wasting G12.29
Paludism — see Malaria
Panangiitis M30.0
Panaritis, panaritium (see also Cellulitis, digit)
  with lymphangitis — see Lymphangitis, acute, digit
Panarteritis nodosa M30.0
  brain or cerebral I67.7
Pancake heart R93.1
  with cor pulmonale (chronic) I27.81
Pancarditis (acute) (chronic) I51.89
  rheumatic I09.89
    active or acute I01.8
Pancoast's syndrome or tumor C34.1- ☑
Pancolitis, ulcerative (chronic) K51.00
  with
    abscess K51.014
    complication K51.019
    fistula K51.013
    obstruction K51.012
    rectal bleeding K51.011
    specified complication NEC K51.018
Pancreas, pancreatic — see condition
Pancreatitis (annular) (apoplectic) (calcareous) (edematous) (hemorrhagic) (malignant) (recurrent) (subacute) (suppurative) K85.9
  acute K85.9
    alcohol induced K85.2
    biliary K85.1
    drug induced K85.3
    gallstone K85.1
    idiopathic K85.0
    specified NEC K85.8
  chronic (infectious) K86.1
    alcohol-induced K86.0
    recurrent K86.1
    relapsing K86.1
  cystic (chronic) K86.1
  cytomegaloviral B25.2
  fibrous (chronic) K86.1
  gallstone K85.1
  gangrenous K85.8
  interstitial (chronic) K86.1
    acute K85.8
  mumps B26.3
  recurrent (chronic) K86.1
  relapsing, chronic K86.1
  syphilitic A52.74
Pancreatoblastoma — see Neoplasm, pancreas, malignant
Pancreolithiasis K86.8
Pancytolysis D75.89
Pancytopenia (acquired) D61.818
  with
    malformations D61.09
    myelodysplastic syndrome — see Syndrome,
      myelodysplastic
  antineoplastic chemotherapy induced D61.810
  congenital D61.09
  drug-induced NEC D61.811
Panencephalitis, subacute, sclerosing A81.1
Panhematopenia D61.9
  congenital D61.09
  constitutional D61.09
  splenic, primary D73.1
Panhemocytopenia D61.9
  congenital D61.09
  constitutional D61.09
Panhypogonadism E29.1
Panhypopituitarism E23.0
  prepubertal E23.0

☑ **Additional Character Required** — Refer to the Tabular List for Character Selection   ▽ Subterms under main terms may continue to next column or page

Panic (attack) (state) F41.Ø
   reaction to exceptional stress (transient) F43.Ø
Panmyelopathy, familial, constitutional D61.09
Panmyelophthisis D61.82
   congenital D61.09
Panmyelosis (acute) (with myelofibrosis) C94.4- ☑
Panner's disease — see Osteochondrosis, juvenile,
   humerus
Panneuritis endemica E51.11
Panniculitis (nodular) (nonsuppurative) M79.3
   back M54.ØØ
      cervical region M54.Ø2
      cervicothoracic region M54.Ø3
      lumbar region M54.Ø6
      lumbosacral region M54.Ø7
      multiple sites M54.Ø9
      occipito-atlanto-axial region M54.Ø1
      sacrococcygeal region M54.Ø8
      thoracic region M54.Ø4
      thoracolumbar region M54.Ø5
   lupus L93.2
   mesenteric K65.4
   neck M54.Ø2
      cervicothoracic region M54.Ø3
      occipito-atlanto-axial region M54.Ø1
   relapsing M35.6
Panniculus adiposus (abdominal) E65
Pannus (allergic) (cornea) (degenerativus) (keratic)
   H16.42- ☑
   abdominal (symptomatic) E65
   trachomatosus, trachomatous (active) A71.1
Panophthalmitis H44.Ø1- ☑
Pansinusitis (chronic) (hyperplastic) (nonpurulent) (purulent) J32.4
   acute JØ1.4Ø
      recurrent JØ1.41
   tuberculous A15.8
Panuveitis (sympathetic) H44.11- ☑
Panvalvular disease IØ8.9
   specified NEC IØ8.8
Papanicolaou smear, cervix Z12.4
   as part of routine gynecological examination ZØ1.419
      with abnormal findings ZØ1.411
   for suspected neoplasm Z12.4
   nonspecific abnormal finding R87.619
   routine ZØ1.419
      with abnormal findings ZØ1.411
Papilledema (choked disc) H47.1Ø
   associated with
      decreased ocular pressure H47.12
      increased intracranial pressure H47.11
      retinal disorder H47.13
   Foster-Kennedy syndrome H47.14- ☑
Papillitis H46.ØØ
   anus K62.89
   chronic lingual K14.4
   necrotizing, kidney N17.2
   optic H46.Ø- ☑
   rectum K62.89
   renal, necrotizing N17.2
   tongue K14.Ø
Papilloma (see also Neoplasm, benign, by site)
   acuminatum (female) (male) (anogenital) A63.Ø
   benign pinta (primary) A67.Ø
   bladder (urinary) (transitional cell) D41.4
   choroid plexus (lateral ventricle) (third ventricle) D33.Ø
      anaplastic C71.5
      fourth ventricle D33.1
      malignant C71.5
   renal pelvis (transitional cell) D41.1- ☑
      benign D3Ø.1- ☑
   Schneiderian
      specified site — see Neoplasm, benign, by site
      unspecified site D14.Ø
   serous surface
      borderline malignancy
         specified site — see Neoplasm, uncertain be-
            havior, by site
         unspecified site D39.1Ø
      specified site — see Neoplasm, benign, by site
      unspecified site D27.9
   transitional (cell)
      bladder (urinary) D41.4
      inverted type — see Neoplasm, uncertain behavior,
         by site
      renal pelvis D41.1- ☑
      ureter D41.2- ☑

Papilloma — continued
   ureter (transitional cell) D41.2- ☑
      benign D3Ø.2- ☑
   urothelial — see Neoplasm, uncertain behavior, by
      site
   villous — see Neoplasm, uncertain behavior, by site
      adenocarcinoma in — see Neoplasm, malignant,
         by site
      in situ — see Neoplasm, in situ
   yaws, plantar or palmar A66.1
Papillomata, multiple, of yaws A66.1
Papillomatosis (see also Neoplasm, benign, by site)
   confluent and reticulated L83
   cystic, breast — see Mastopathy, cystic
   ductal, breast — see Mastopathy, cystic
   intraductal (diffuse) — see Neoplasm, benign, by site
   subareolar duct D24- ☑
Papillomavirus, as cause of disease classified elsewhere B97.7
Papillon-Léage and Psaume syndrome Q87.Ø
Papule(s) R23.8
   carate (primary) A67.Ø
   fibrous, of nose D22.39
   Gottron's L94.4
   pinta (primary) A67.Ø
Papulosis
   lymphomatoid C86.6
   malignant I77.89
Papyraceous fetus O31.Ø- ☑
Para-albuminemia E88.Ø9
Paracephalus Q89.7
Parachute mitral valve Q23.2
Paracoccidioidomycosis B41.9
   disseminated B41.7
   generalized B41.7
   mucocutaneous-lymphangitic B41.8
   pulmonary B41.Ø
   specified NEC B41.8
   visceral B41.8
Paradentosis KØ5.4
Paraffinoma T88.8 ☑
Paraganglioma D44.7
   adrenal D35.Ø- ☑
      malignant C74.1- ☑
   aortic body D44.7
      malignant C75.5
   carotid body D44.6
      malignant C75.4
   chromaffin (see also Neoplasm, benign, by site)
      malignant — see Neoplasm, malignant, by site
   extra-adrenal D44.7
      malignant C75.5
         specified site — see Neoplasm, malignant, by
            site
         unspecified site C75.5
      specified site — see Neoplasm, uncertain behavior,
         by site
      unspecified site D44.7
   gangliocytic D13.2
      specified site — see Neoplasm, benign, by site
      unspecified site D13.2
   glomus jugulare D44.7
      malignant C75.5
   jugular D44.7
   malignant C75.5
      specified site — see Neoplasm, malignant, by site
      unspecified site C75.5
   nonchromaffin D44.7
      malignant C75.5
         specified site — see Neoplasm, malignant, by
            site
         unspecified site C75.5
      specified site — see Neoplasm, uncertain behavior,
         by site
      unspecified site D44.7
   parasympathetic D44.7
      specified site — see Neoplasm, uncertain behavior,
         by site
      unspecified site D44.7
   specified site — see Neoplasm, uncertain behavior,
      by site
   sympathetic D44.7
      specified site — see Neoplasm, uncertain behavior,
         by site
      unspecified site D44.7
   unspecified site D44.7

Parageusia R43.2
   psychogenic F45.8
Paragonimiasis B66.4
Paragranuloma, Hodgkin — see Lymphoma, Hodgkin,
   classical, specified NEC
Parahemophilia (see also Defect, coagulation) D68.2
Parakeratosis R23.4
   variegata L41.Ø
Paralysis, paralytic (complete) (incomplete) G83.9
   with
      syphilis A52.17
   abducens, abducent (nerve) — see Strabismus, para-
      lytic, sixth nerve
   abductor, lower extremity G57.9- ☑
   accessory nerve G52.8
   accommodation (see also Paresis, of accommodation)
      hysterical F44.89
   acoustic nerve (except Deafness) H93.3 ☑
   agitans (see also Parkinsonism) G2Ø
      arteriosclerotic G21.4
   alternating (oculomotor) G83.89
   amyotrophic G12.21
   ankle G57.9- ☑
   anus (sphincter) K62.89
   arm — see Monoplegia, upper limb
   ascending (spinal), acute G61.Ø
   association G12.29
   asthenic bulbar G7Ø.ØØ
      with exacerbation (acute) G7Ø.Ø1
      in crisis G7Ø.Ø1
   ataxic (hereditary) G11.9
      general (syphilitic) A52.17
   atrophic G58.9
      infantile, acute — see Poliomyelitis, paralytic
      progressive G12.22
      spinal (acute) — see Poliomyelitis, paralytic
   axillary G54.Ø
   Babinski-Nageotte's G83.89
   Bell's G51.Ø
      newborn P11.3
   Benedikt's G46.3
   birth injury P14.9
      spinal cord P11.5
   bladder (neurogenic) (sphincter) N31.2
   bowel, colon or intestine K56.Ø
   brachial plexus G54.Ø
      birth injury P14.3
      newborn (birth injury) P14.3
   brain G83.9
      diplegia G83.Ø
      triplegia G83.89
   bronchial J98.Ø9
   Brown-Séquard G83.81
   bulbar (chronic) (progressive) G12.22
      infantile — see Poliomyelitis, paralytic
      poliomyelitic — see Poliomyelitis, paralytic
      pseudo G12.29
   bulbospinal G7Ø.ØØ
      with exacerbation (acute) G7Ø.Ø1
      in crisis G7Ø.Ø1
   cardiac (see also Failure, heart) I5Ø.9
   cerebrocerebellar, diplegic G8Ø.1
   cervical
      plexus G54.2
      sympathetic G9Ø.Ø9
   Céstan-Chenais G46.3
   Charcot-Marie-Tooth type G6Ø.Ø
   Clark's G8Ø.9
   colon K56.Ø
   compressed air T7Ø.3 ☑
   compression
      arm G56.9- ☑
      leg G57.9- ☑
      lower extremity G57.9- ☑
      upper extremity G56.9- ☑
   congenital (cerebral) — see Palsy, cerebral
   conjugate movement (gaze) (of eye) H51.Ø
      cortical (nuclear) (supranuclear) H51.Ø
   cordis — see Failure, heart
   cranial or cerebral nerve G52.9
   creeping G12.22
   crossed leg G83.89
   crutch — see Injury, brachial plexus
   deglutition R13.Ø
      hysterical F44.4
   dementia A52.17
   descending (spinal) NEC G12.29

Paralysis, paralytic — *continued*
diaphragm (flaccid) J98.6
  due to accidental dissection of phrenic nerve during procedure — *see* Puncture, accidental complicating surgery
digestive organs NEC K59.8
diplegic — *see* Diplegia
divergence (nuclear) H51.8
diver's T70.3 ☑
Duchenne's
  birth injury P14.0
  due to or associated with
    motor neuron disease G12.22
    muscular dystrophy G71.0
due to intracranial or spinal birth injury — *see* Palsy, cerebral
embolic (current episode) I63.4 ☑
Erb (-Duchenne) (birth) (newborn) P14.0
Erb's syphilitic spastic spinal A52.17
esophagus K22.8
eye muscle (extrinsic) H49.9
  intrinsic (*see also* Paresis, of accommodation)
facial (nerve) G51.0
  birth injury P11.3
  congenital P11.3
  following operation NEC — *see* Puncture, accidental complicating surgery
  newborn (birth injury) P11.3
familial (recurrent) (periodic) G72.3
  spastic G11.4
fauces J39.2
finger G56.9- ☑
gait R26.1
gastric nerve (nondiabetic) G52.2
gaze, conjugate H51.0
general (progressive) (syphilitic) A52.17
  juvenile A50.45
glottis J38.00
  bilateral J38.02
  unilateral J38.01
gluteal G54.1
Gubler (-Millard) G46.3
hand — *see* Monoplegia, upper limb
heart — *see* Arrest, cardiac
hemiplegic — *see* Hemiplegia
hyperkalemic periodic (familial) G72.3
hypoglossal (nerve) G52.3
hypokalemic periodic G72.3
hysterical F44.4
ileus K56.0
infantile (*see also* Poliomyelitis, paralytic) A80.30
  bulbar — *see* Poliomyelitis, paralytic
  cerebral — *see* Palsy, cerebral
  spastic — *see* Palsy, cerebral, spastic
infective — *see* Poliomyelitis, paralytic
inferior nuclear G83.9
internuclear — *see* Ophthalmoplegia, internuclear
intestine K56.0
iris H57.09
  due to diphtheria (toxin) A36.89
ischemic, Volkmann's (complicating trauma) T79.6 ☑
Jackson's G83.89
jake — *see* Poisoning, food, noxious, plant
Jamaica ginger (jake) G62.2
juvenile general A50.45
Klumpke (-Déjérine) (birth) (newborn) P14.1
labioglossal (laryngeal) (pharyngeal) G12.29
Landry's G61.0
laryngeal nerve (recurrent) (superior) (unilateral) J38.00
  bilateral J38.02
  unilateral J38.01
larynx J38.00
  bilateral J38.02
  due to diphtheria (toxin) A36.2
  unilateral J38.01
lateral G12.21
lead T56.0 ☑
left side — *see* Hemiplegia
leg G83.1- ☑
  both — *see* Paraplegia
  crossed G83.89
  hysterical F44.4
  psychogenic F44.4
  transient or transitory R29.818
    traumatic NEC — *see* Injury, nerve, leg
levator palpebrae superioris — *see* Blepharoptosis, paralytic
limb — *see* Monoplegia

Paralysis, paralytic — *continued*
lip K13.0
Lissauer's A52.17
lower limb — *see* Monoplegia, lower limb
  both — *see* Paraplegia
lung J98.4
median nerve G56.1- ☑
medullary (tegmental) G83.89
mesencephalic NEC G83.89
  tegmental G83.89
middle alternating G83.89
Millard-Gubler-Foville G46.3
monoplegic — *see* Monoplegia
motor G83.9
muscle, muscular NEC G72.89
  due to nerve lesion G58.9
  eye (extrinsic) H49.9
    intrinsic — *see* Paresis, of accommodation
    oblique — *see* Strabismus, paralytic, fourth nerve
  iris sphincter H21.9
  ischemic (Volkmann's) (complicating trauma) T79.6 ☑
  progressive G12.21
  pseudohypertrophic G71.0
musculocutaneous nerve G56.9- ☑
musculospiral G56.9- ☑
nerve (*see also* Disorder, nerve)
  abducent — *see* Strabismus, paralytic, sixth nerve
  accessory G52.8
  auditory (except Deafness) H93.3 ☑
  birth injury P14.9
  cranial or cerebral G52.9
  facial G51.0
    birth injury P11.3
    congenital P11.3
    newborn (birth injury) P11.3
  fourth or trochlear — *see* Strabismus, paralytic, fourth nerve
  newborn (birth injury) P14.9
  oculomotor — *see* Strabismus, paralytic, third nerve
  phrenic (birth injury) P14.2
  radial G56.3- ☑
  seventh or facial G51.0
    newborn (birth injury) P11.3
  sixth or abducent — *see* Strabismus, paralytic, sixth nerve
  syphilitic A52.15
  third or oculomotor — *see* Strabismus, paralytic, third nerve
  trigeminal G50.9
  trochlear — *see* Strabismus, paralytic, fourth nerve
  ulnar G56.2- ☑
normokalemic periodic G72.3
ocular H49.9
  alternating G83.89
oculofacial, congenital (Moebius) Q87.0
oculomotor (external bilateral) (nerve) — *see* Strabismus, paralytic, third nerve
palate (soft) K13.79
paratrigeminal G50.9
periodic (familial) (hyperkalemic) (hypokalemic) (myotonic) (normokalemic) (potassium sensitive) (secondary) G72.3
peripheral autonomic nervous system — *see* Neuropathy, peripheral, autonomic
peroneal (nerve) G57.3- ☑
pharynx J39.2
phrenic nerve G56.8- ☑
plantar nerve(s) G57.6- ☑
pneumogastric nerve G52.2
poliomyelitis (current) — *see* Poliomyelitis, paralytic
popliteal nerve G57.3- ☑
postepileptic transitory G83.84
progressive (atrophic) (bulbar) (spinal) G12.22
  general A52.17
  infantile acute — *see* Poliomyelitis, paralytic
  supranuclear G23.1
pseudobulbar G12.29
pseudohypertrophic (muscle) G71.0
psychogenic F44.4
quadriceps G57.9- ☑
quadriplegic — *see* Tetraplegia
radial nerve G56.3- ☑
rectus muscle (eye) H49.9
recurrent isolated sleep G47.53

Paralysis, paralytic — *continued*
respiratory (muscle) (system) (tract) R06.81
  center NEC G93.89
  congenital P28.89
  newborn P28.89
right side — *see* Hemiplegia
saturnine T56.0 ☑
sciatic nerve G57.0- ☑
senile G83.9
shaking — *see* Parkinsonism
shoulder G56.9- ☑
sleep, recurrent isolated G47.53
spastic G83.9
  cerebral — *see* Palsy, cerebral, spastic
  congenital (cerebral) — *see* Palsy, cerebral, spastic
  familial G11.4
  hereditary G11.4
  quadriplegic G80.0
  syphilitic (spinal) A52.17
sphincter, bladder — *see* Paralysis, bladder
spinal (cord) G83.9
  accessory nerve G52.8
  acute — *see* Poliomyelitis, paralytic
  ascending acute G61.0
  atrophic (acute) (*see also* Poliomyelitis, paralytic)
    spastic, syphilitic A52.17
  congenital NEC — *see* Palsy, cerebral
  hereditary G95.89
  infantile — *see* Poliomyelitis, paralytic
  progressive G12.21
  sequelae NEC G83.89
sternomastoid G52.8
stomach K31.84
  diabetic — *see* Diabetes, by type, with gastroparesis
  nerve G52.2
    diabetic — *see* Diabetes, by type, with gastroparesis
stroke — *see* Infarct, brain
subcapsularis G56.8- ☑
supranuclear (progressive) G23.1
sympathetic G90.8
  cervical G90.09
  nervous system — *see* Neuropathy, peripheral, autonomic
syndrome G83.9
  specified NEC G83.89
syphilitic spastic spinal (Erb's) A52.17
thigh G57.9- ☑
throat J39.2
  diphtheritic A36.0
  muscle J39.2
thrombotic (current episode) I63.3 ☑
thumb G56.9- ☑
tick — *see* Toxicity, venom, arthropod, specified NEC
Todd's (postepileptic transitory paralysis) G83.84
toe G57.6- ☑
tongue K14.8
transient R29.5
  arm or leg NEC R29.818
  traumatic NEC — *see* Injury, nerve
trapezius G52.8
traumatic, transient NEC — *see* Injury, nerve
trembling — *see* Parkinsonism
triceps brachii G56.9- ☑
trigeminal nerve G50.9
trochlear (nerve) — *see* Strabismus, paralytic, fourth nerve
ulnar nerve G56.2- ☑
upper limb — *see* Monoplegia, upper limb
uremic N18.9 [G99.8]
uveoparotitic D86.89
uvula K13.79
  postdiphtheritic A36.0
vagus nerve G52.2
vasomotor NEC G90.8
velum palati K13.79
vesical — *see* Paralysis, bladder
vestibular nerve (except Vertigo) H93.3 ☑
vocal cords J38.00
  bilateral J38.02
  unilateral J38.01
Volkmann's (complicating trauma) T79.6 ☑
wasting G12.29
Weber's G46.3
wrist G56.9- ☑
Paramedial urethrovesical orifice Q64.79

Paramenia N92.6
Parametritis (see also Disease, pelvis, inflammatory) N73.2
  acute N73.0
  complicating abortion — see Abortion, by type, complicated by, parametritis
Parametrium, parametric — see condition
Paramnesia — see Amnesia
Paramolar K00.1
Paramyloidosis E85.8
Paramyoclonus multiplex G25.3
Paramyotonia (congenita) G71.19
Parangi — see Yaws
Paranoia (querulans) F22
  senile F03 ☑
Paranoid
  dementia (senile) F03 ☑
    praecox — see Schizophrenia
  personality F60.0
  psychosis (climacteric) (involutional) (menopausal) F22
    psychogenic (acute) F23
    senile F03 ☑
  reaction (acute) F23
    chronic F22
  schizophrenia F20.0
  state (climacteric) (involutional) (menopausal) (simple) F22
    senile F03 ☑
  tendencies F60.0
  traits F60.0
  trends F60.0
  type, psychopathic personality F60.0
Paraparesis — see Paraplegia
Paraphasia R47.02
Paraphilia F65.9
Paraphimosis (congenital) N47.2
  chancroidal A57
Paraphrenia, paraphrenic (late) F22
  schizophrenia F20.0
Paraplegia (lower) G82.20
  ataxic — see Degeneration, combined, spinal cord
  complete G82.21
  congenital (cerebral) G80.8
    spastic G80.1
  familial spastic G11.4
  functional (hysterical) F44.4
  hereditary, spastic G11.4
  hysterical F44.4
  incomplete G82.22
  Pott's A18.01
  psychogenic F44.4
  spastic
    Erb's spinal, syphilitic A52.17
    hereditary G11.4
    tropical G04.1
  syphilitic (spastic) A52.17
  tropical spastic G04.1
Parapoxvirus B08.60
  specified NEC B08.69
Paraproteinemia D89.2
  benign (familial) D89.2
  monoclonal D47.2
  secondary to malignant disease D47.2
Parapsoriasis L41.9
  en plaques L41.4
  guttata L41.1
  large plaque L41.4
  retiform, retiformis L41.5
  small plaque L41.3
  specified NEC L41.8
  varioliformis (acuta) L41.0
Parasitic (see also condition)
  disease NEC B89
  stomatitis B37.0
  sycosis (beard) (scalp) B35.0
  twin Q89.4
Parasitism B89
  intestinal B82.9
  skin B88.9
  specified — see Infestation
Parasitophobia F40.218
Parasomnia G47.50
  due to
    alcohol
      abuse F10.182
      dependence F10.282

Parasomnia — continued
  due to — continued
    alcohol — continued
      use F10.982
    amphetamines
      abuse F15.182
      dependence F15.282
      use F15.982
    caffeine
      abuse F15.182
      dependence F15.282
      use F15.982
    cocaine
      abuse F14.182
      dependence F14.282
      use F14.982
    drug NEC
      abuse F19.182
      dependence F19.282
      use F19.982
    opioid
      abuse F11.182
      dependence F11.282
      use F11.982
    psychoactive substance NEC
      abuse F19.182
      dependence F19.282
      use F19.982
    sedative, hypnotic, or anxiolytic
      abuse F13.182
      dependence F13.282
      use F13.982
    stimulant NEC
      abuse F15.182
      dependence F15.282
      use F15.982
  in conditions classified elsewhere G47.54
  nonorganic origin F51.8
  organic G47.50
  specified NEC G47.59
Paraspadias Q54.9
Paraspasmus facialis G51.8
Parasuicide (attempt)
  history of (personal) Z91.5
    in family Z81.8
Parathyroid gland — see condition
Parathyroid tetany E20.9
Paratrachoma A74.0
Paratyphilitis — see Appendicitis
Paratyphoid (fever) — see Fever, paratyphoid
Paratyphus — see Fever, paratyphoid
Paraurethral duct Q64.79
  nonorganic origin F51.5
Paraurethritis (see also Urethritis)
  gonococcal (acute) (chronic) (with abscess) A54.1
Paravaccinia NEC B08.04
Paravaginitis — see Vaginitis
Parencephalitis (see also Encephalitis)
  sequelae G09
Parent-child conflict — see Conflict, parent-child
  estrangement NEC Z62.890
Paresis (see also Paralysis)
  accommodation — see Paresis, of accommodation
  Bernhardt's G57.1- ☑
  bladder (sphincter) (see also Paralysis, bladder)
    tabetic A52.17
  bowel, colon or intestine K56.0
  extrinsic muscle, eye H49.9
  general (progressive) (syphilitic) A52.17
    juvenile A50.45
  heart — see Failure, heart
  insane (syphilitic) A52.17
  juvenile (general) A50.45
  of accommodation H52.52- ☑
  peripheral progressive (idiopathic) G60.3
  pseudohypertrophic G71.0
  senile G83.9
  syphilitic (general) A52.17
    congenital A50.45
  vesical NEC N31.2
Paresthesia (see also Disturbance, sensation)
  Bernhardt G57.1- ☑
Paretic — see condition
Parinaud's
  conjunctivitis H10.89
  oculoglandular syndrome H10.89
  ophthalmoplegia H49.88- ☑

Parkinsonism (idiopathic) (primary) G20
  with neurogenic orthostatic hypotension (symptomatic) G90.3
  arteriosclerotic G21.4
  dementia G31.83 [F02.80]
    with behavioral disturbance G31.83 [F02.81]
  due to
    drugs NEC G21.19
      neuroleptic G21.11
  neuroleptic induced G21.11
  postencephalitic G21.3
  secondary G21.9
    due to
      arteriosclerosis G21.4
      drugs NEC G21.19
        neuroleptic G21.11
      encephalitis G21.3
      external agents NEC G21.2
      syphilis A52.19
    specified NEC G21.8
  syphilitic A52.19
  treatment-induced NEC G21.19
  vascular G21.4
Parkinson's disease, syndrome or tremor — see Parkinsonism
Parodontitis — see Periodontitis
Parodontosis K05.4
Paronychia (see also Cellulitis, digit)
  with lymphangitis — see Lymphangitis, acute, digit
  candidal (chronic) B37.2
  tuberculous (primary) A18.4
Parorexia (psychogenic) F50.8
Parosmia R43.1
  psychogenic F45.8
Parotid gland — see condition
Parotitis, parotiditis (allergic)(nonspecific toxic) (purulent) (septic) (suppurative) (see also Sialoadenitis)
  epidemic — see Mumps
  infectious — see Mumps
  postoperative K91.89
  surgical K91.89
Parrot fever A70
Parrot's disease (early congenital syphilitic pseudoparalysis) A50.02
Parry-Romberg syndrome G51.8
Parry's disease or syndrome E05.00
  with thyroid storm E05.01
Pars planitis — see Cyclitis
Parsonage (-Aldren)-**Turner syndrome** G54.5
Parson's disease (exophthalmic goiter) E05.00
  with thyroid storm E05.01
Particolored infant Q82.8
Parturition — see Delivery
Parulis K04.7
  with sinus K04.6
Parvovirus, as cause of disease classified elsewhere B97.6
Pasini and Pierini's atrophoderma L90.3
Passage
  false, urethra N36.5
  meconium (newborn) during delivery P03.82
  of sounds or bougies — see Attention to, artificial, opening
Passive — see condition
  smoking Z77.22
Pasteurella septica A28.0
Pasteurellosis — see Infection, Pasteurella
PAT (paroxysmal atrial tachycardia) I47.1
Patau's syndrome — see Trisomy, 13
Patches
  mucous (syphilitic) A51.39
    congenital A50.07
  smokers' (mouth) K13.24
Patellar — see condition
Patent (see also Imperfect, closure)
  canal of Nuck Q52.4
  cervix N88.3
  ductus arteriosus or Botallo's Q25.0
  foramen
    botalli Q21.1
    ovale Q21.1
  interauricular septum Q21.1
  interventricular septum Q21.0
  omphalomesenteric duct Q43.0
  os (uteri) — see Patent, cervix
  ostium secundum Q21.1
  urachus Q64.4

Patent — *continued*
vitelline duct Q43.0
Paterson (-Brown)(-Kelly) **syndrome or web** D50.1
Pathologic, pathological (*see also* condition)
asphyxia R09.01
fire-setting F63.1
gambling F63.0
ovum O02.0
resorption, tooth K03.3
stealing F63.2
Pathology (of) — *see* Disease
periradicular, associated with previous endodontic
treatment NEC M27.59
Pattern, sleep-wake, irregular G47.23
Patulous (*see also* Imperfect, closure (congenital))
alimentary tract Q45.8
lower Q43.8
upper Q40.8
eustachian tube H69.0- ☑
Pause, sinoatrial I49.5
Paxton's disease B36.2
Pearl(s)
enamel K00.2
Epstein's K09.8
Pearl-worker's disease — *see* Osteomyelitis, specified
type NEC
Pectenosis K62.4
Pectoral — *see* condition
Pectus
carinatum (congenital) Q67.7
acquired M95.4
rachitic sequelae (late effect) E64.3
excavatum (congenital) Q67.6
acquired M95.4
rachitic sequelae (late effect) E64.3
recurvatum (congenital) Q67.6
Pedatrophia E41
Pederosis F65.4
Pediculosis (infestation) B85.2
capitis (head-louse) (any site) B85.0
corporis (body-louse) (any site) B85.1
eyelid B85.0
mixed (classifiable to more than one of the titles B85.0-
B85.3) B85.4
pubis (pubic louse) (any site) B85.3
vestimenti B85.1
vulvae B85.3
Pediculus (infestation) — *see* Pediculosis
Pedophilia F65.4
Peg-shaped teeth K00.2
Pelade — *see* Alopecia, areata
Pelger-Huët anomaly or syndrome D72.0
Peliosis (rheumatica) D69.0
hepatis K76.4
with toxic liver disease K71.8
Pelizaeus-Merzbacher disease E75.29
Pellagra (alcoholic) (with polyneuropathy) E52
**Pellagra-cerebellar-ataxia-renal aminoaciduria
syndrome** E72.02
Pellegrini (-Stieda) **disease or syndrome** — *see* Bursitis,
tibial collateral
Pellizzi's syndrome E34.8
Pel's crisis A52.11
Pelvic (*see also* condition)
examination (periodic) (routine) Z01.419
with abnormal findings Z01.411
kidney, congenital Q63.2
Pelviolithiasis — *see* Calculus, kidney
Pelviperitonitis (*see also* Peritonitis, pelvic)
gonococcal A54.24
puerperal O85
Pelvis — *see* condition or type
Pemphigoid L12.9
benign, mucous membrane L12.1
bullous L12.0
cicatricial L12.1
juvenile L12.2
ocular L12.1
specified NEC L12.8
Pemphigus L10.9
benign familial (chronic) Q82.8
Brazilian L10.3
circinatus L13.0
conjunctiva L12.1
drug-induced L10.5
erythematosus L10.4
foliaceous L10.2

Pemphigus — *continued*
gangrenous — *see* Gangrene
neonatorum L01.03
ocular L12.1
paraneoplastic L10.81
specified NEC L10.89
syphilitic (congenital) A50.06
vegetans L10.1
vulgaris L10.0
wildfire L10.3
Pendred's syndrome E07.1
Pendulous
abdomen, in pregnancy — *see* Pregnancy, complicated by, abnormal, pelvic organs or tissues NEC
breast N64.89
Penetrating wound (*see also* Puncture)
with internal injury — *see* Injury, by site
eyeball — *see* Puncture, eyeball
orbit (with or without foreign body) — *see* Puncture,
orbit
uterus by instrument with or following ectopic or
molar pregnancy O08.6
Penicillosis B48.4
Penis — *see* condition
Penitis N48.29
Pentalogy of Fallot Q21.8
Pentasomy X syndrome Q97.1
Pentosuria (essential) E74.8
Peregrinating patient — *see* Disorder, factitious
Perforation, perforated (nontraumatic) (of)
accidental during procedure (blood vessel) (nerve)
(organ) — *see* Complication, accidental puncture or laceration
antrum — *see* Sinusitis, maxillary
appendix K35.2
atrial septum, multiple Q21.1
attic, ear — *see* Perforation, tympanum, attic
bile duct (common) (hepatic) K83.2
cystic K82.2
bladder (urinary)
with or following ectopic or molar pregnancy O08.6
obstetrical trauma O71.5
traumatic S37.29 ☑
at delivery O71.5
bowel K63.1
with or following ectopic or molar pregnancy O08.6
newborn P78.0
obstetrical trauma O71.5
traumatic — *see* Laceration, intestine
broad ligament N83.8
with or following ectopic or molar pregnancy O08.6
obstetrical trauma O71.6
by
device, implant or graft (*see also* Complications,
by site and type, mechanical) T85.628 ☑
arterial graft NEC — *see* Complication, cardiovascular device, mechanical, vascular
breast (implant) T85.49 ☑
catheter NEC T85.698 ☑
cystostomy T83.090 ☑
dialysis (renal) T82.49 ☑
intraperitoneal T85.691 ☑
infusion NEC T82.594 ☑
spinal (epidural) (subdural) T85.690 ☑
electronic (electrode) (pulse generator) (stimulator)
bone T84.390 ☑
cardiac T82.199 ☑
electrode T82.190 ☑
pulse generator T82.191 ☑
specified type NEC T82.198 ☑
nervous system — *see* Complication, prosthetic device, mechanical, electronic
nervous system stimulator
urinary — *see* Complication, genitourinary,
device, urinary, mechanical
fixation, internal (orthopedic) NEC — *see*
Complication, fixation device, mechanical
gastrointestinal — *see* Complications, prosthetic device, mechanical, gastrointestinal
device
genital NEC T83.498 ☑
intrauterine contraceptive device T83.39 ☑
penile prosthesis T83.490 ☑
heart NEC — *see* Complication, cardiovascular
device, mechanical

Perforation, perforated — *continued*
by — *continued*
device, implant or graft (*see also* Complications, by
site and type, mechanical) — *continued*
joint prosthesis — *see* Complications, joint
prosthesis, mechanical, specified NEC, by
site
ocular NEC — *see* Complications, prosthetic
device, mechanical, ocular device
orthopedic NEC — *see* Complication, orthopedic, device, mechanical
specified NEC T85.628 ☑
urinary, indwelling T83.098 ☑
urinary NEC (*see also* Complication, genitourinary, device, urinary, mechanical)
graft T83.29 ☑
vascular NEC — *see* Complication, cardiovascular device, mechanical
ventricular intracranial shunt T85.09 ☑
foreign body left accidentally in operative wound
T81.539 ☑
instrument (any) during a procedure, accidental
— *see* Puncture, accidental complicating
surgery
cecum K35.2
cervix (uteri) N88.8
with or following ectopic or molar pregnancy O08.6
obstetrical trauma O71.3
colon K63.1
newborn P78.0
obstetrical trauma O71.5
traumatic — *see* Laceration, intestine, large
common duct (bile) K83.2
cornea (due to ulceration) — *see* Ulcer, cornea, perforated
cystic duct K82.2
diverticulum (intestine) K57.80
with bleeding K57.81
large intestine K57.20
with
bleeding K57.21
small intestine K57.40
with bleeding K57.41
small intestine K57.00
with
bleeding K57.01
large intestine K57.40
with bleeding K57.41
ear drum — *see* Perforation, tympanum
esophagus K22.3
ethmoidal sinus — *see* Sinusitis, ethmoidal
frontal sinus — *see* Sinusitis, frontal
gallbladder K82.2
heart valve — *see* Endocarditis
ileum K63.1
newborn P78.0
obstetrical trauma O71.5
traumatic — *see* Laceration, intestine, small
instrumental, surgical (accidental) (blood vessel)
(nerve) (organ) — *see* Puncture, accidental
complicating surgery
intestine NEC K63.1
with ectopic or molar pregnancy O08.6
newborn P78.0
obstetrical trauma O71.5
traumatic — *see* Laceration, intestine
ulcerative NEC K63.1
newborn P78.0
jejunum, jejunal K63.1
obstetrical trauma O71.5
traumatic — *see* Laceration, intestine, small
ulcer — *see* Ulcer, gastrojejunal, with perforation
joint prosthesis — *see* Complications, joint prosthesis,
mechanical, specified NEC, by site
mastoid (antrum) (cell) — *see* Disorder, mastoid,
specified NEC
maxillary sinus — *see* Sinusitis, maxillary
membrana tympani — *see* Perforation, tympanum
nasal
septum J34.89
congenital Q30.3
syphilitic A52.73
sinus J34.89
congenital Q30.8
due to sinusitis — *see* Sinusitis
palate (*see also* Cleft, palate) Q35.9
syphilitic A52.79

Perforation, perforated — *continued*
palatine vault (*see also* Cleft, palate, hard) Q35.1
  syphilitic A52.79
    congenital A50.59
pars flaccida (ear drum) — *see* Perforation, tympanum, attic
pelvic
  floor S31.030 ☑
    with
      ectopic or molar pregnancy O08.6
      penetration into retroperitoneal space S31.031 ☑
      retained foreign body S31.040 ☑
        with penetration into retroperitoneal space S31.041 ☑
    following ectopic or molar pregnancy O08.6
    obstetrical trauma O70.1
  organ S37.99 ☑
    adrenal gland S37.818 ☑
    bladder — *see* Perforation, bladder
    fallopian tube S37.599 ☑
      bilateral S37.592 ☑
      unilateral S37.591 ☑
    kidney S37.09- ☑
    obstetrical trauma O71.5
    ovary S37.499 ☑
      bilateral S37.492 ☑
      unilateral S37.491 ☑
    prostate S37.828 ☑
    specified organ NEC S37.898 ☑
    ureter — *see* Perforation, ureter
    urethra — *see* Perforation, urethra
    uterus — *see* Perforation, uterus
perineum — *see* Laceration, perineum
pharynx J39.2
rectum K63.1
  newborn P78.0
  obstetrical trauma O71.5
  traumatic S36.63 ☑
root canal space due to endodontic treatment M27.51
sigmoid K63.1
  newborn P78.0
  obstetrical trauma O71.5
  traumatic S36.533 ☑
sinus (accessory) (chronic) (nasal) J34.89
sphenoidal sinus — *see* Sinusitis, sphenoidal
surgical (accidental) (by instrument) (blood vessel) (nerve) (organ) — *see* Puncture, accidental complicating surgery
traumatic
  external — *see* Puncture
  eye — *see* Puncture, eyeball
  internal organ — *see* Injury, by site
tympanum, tympanic (membrane) (persistent post-traumatic) (postinflammatory) H72.9- ☑
  attic H72.1- ☑
    multiple — *see* Perforation, tympanum, multiple
    total — *see* Perforation, tympanum, total
  central H72.0- ☑
    multiple — *see* Perforation, tympanum, multiple
    total — *see* Perforation, tympanum, total
  marginal NEC — *see* subcategory H72.2 ☑
  multiple H72.81- ☑
  pars flaccida — *see* Perforation, tympanum, attic
  total H72.82- ☑
  traumatic, current episode S09.2- ☑
typhoid, gastrointestinal — *see* Typhoid
ulcer — *see* Ulcer, by site, with perforation
ureter N28.89
  traumatic S37.19 ☑
urethra N36.8
  with ectopic or molar pregnancy O08.6
  following ectopic or molar pregnancy O08.6
  obstetrical trauma O71.5
  traumatic S37.39 ☑
    at delivery O71.5
uterus
  with ectopic or molar pregnancy O08.6
  by intrauterine contraceptive device T83.39 ☑
  following ectopic or molar pregnancy O08.6
  obstetrical trauma O71.1
  traumatic S37.69 ☑
    obstetric O71.1
uvula K13.79
  syphilitic A52.79

Perforation, perforated — *continued*
vagina O71.4
  obstetrical trauma O71.4
  other trauma — *see* Puncture, vagina
Periadenitis mucosa necrotica recurrens K12.0
Periappendicitis (acute) — *see* Appendicitis
Periarteritis nodosa (disseminated) (infectious) (necrotizing) M30.0
Periarthritis (joint) (*see also* Enthesopathy)
  Duplay's M75.0- ☑
  gonococcal A54.42
  humeroscapularis — *see* Capsulitis, adhesive
  scapulohumeral — *see* Capsulitis, adhesive
  shoulder — *see* Capsulitis, adhesive
  wrist M77.2- ☑
Periarthrosis (angioneural) — *see* Enthesopathy
Pericapsulitis, adhesive (shoulder) — *see* Capsulitis, adhesive
Pericarditis (with decompensation) (with effusion) I31.9
  with rheumatic fever (conditions in I00)
    active — *see* Pericarditis, rheumatic
    inactive or quiescent I09.2
  acute (hemorrhagic) (nonrheumatic) (Sicca) I30.9
    with chorea (acute) (rheumatic) (Sydenham's) I02.0
    benign I30.8
    nonspecific I30.0
    rheumatic I01.0
      with chorea (acute) (Sydenham's) I02.0
  adhesive or adherent (chronic) (external) (internal) I31.0
    acute — *see* Pericarditis, acute
    rheumatic I09.2
  bacterial (acute) (subacute) (with serous or seropurulent effusion) I30.1
  calcareous I31.1
  cholesterol (chronic) I31.8
    acute I30.9
  chronic (nonrheumatic) I31.9
    rheumatic I09.2
  constrictive (chronic) I31.1
  coxsackie B33.23
  fibrinocaseous (tuberculous) A18.84
  fibrinopurulent I30.1
  fibrinous I30.8
  fibrous I31.0
  gonococcal A54.83
  idiopathic I30.0
  in systemic lupus erythematosus M32.12
  infective I30.1
  meningococcal A39.53
  neoplastic (chronic) I31.8
    acute I30.9
  obliterans, obliterating I31.0
  plastic I31.0
  pneumococcal I30.1
  postinfarction I24.1
  purulent I30.1
  rheumatic (active) (acute) (with effusion) (with pneumonia) I01.0
    with chorea (acute) (rheumatic) (Sydenham's) I02.0
    chronic or inactive (with chorea) I09.2
  rheumatoid — *see* Rheumatoid, carditis
  septic I30.1
  serofibrinous I30.8
  staphylococcal I30.1
  streptococcal I30.1
  suppurative I30.1
  syphilitic A52.06
  tuberculous A18.84
  uremic N18.9 [I32]
  viral I30.8
Pericardium, pericardial — *see* condition
Pericellulitis — *see* Cellulitis
Pericementitis (chronic) (suppurative) (*see also* Periodontitis)
  acute K05.20
    generalized K05.22
    localized K05.21
Perichondritis
  auricle — *see* Perichondritis, ear
  bronchus J98.09
  ear (external) H61.00- ☑
    acute H61.01- ☑
    chronic H61.02- ☑
    external auditory canal — *see* Perichondritis, ear
  larynx J38.7
    syphilitic A52.73
    typhoid A01.09

Perichondritis — *continued*
  nose J34.89
  pinna — *see* Perichondritis, ear
  trachea J39.8
Periclasia K05.4
Pericoronitis — *see* Periodontitis
Pericystitis N30.90
  with hematuria N30.91
Peridiverticulitis (intestine) K57.92
  cecum — *see* Diverticulitis, intestine, large
  colon — *see* Diverticulitis, intestine, large
  duodenum — *see* Diverticulitis, intestine, small
  intestine — *see* Diverticulitis, intestine
  jejunum — *see* Diverticulitis, intestine, small
  rectosigmoid — *see* Diverticulitis, intestine, large
  rectum — *see* Diverticulitis, intestine, large
  sigmoid — *see* Diverticulitis, intestine, large
Periendocarditis — *see* Endocarditis
Periepididymitis N45.1
Perifolliculitis L01.02
  abscedens, caput, scalp L66.3
  capitis, abscedens (et suffodiens) L66.3
  superficial pustular L01.02
Perihepatitis K65.8
Perilabyrinthitis (acute) — *see* subcategory H83.0 ☑
Perimeningitis — *see* Meningitis
Perimetritis — *see* Endometritis
Perimetrosalpingitis — *see* Salpingo-oophoritis
Perineocele N81.81
Perinephric, perinephritic — *see* condition
Perinephritis (*see also* Infection, kidney)
  purulent — *see* Abscess, kidney
Perineum, perineal — *see* condition
Perineuritis NEC — *see* Neuralgia
Periodic — *see* condition
Periodontitis (chronic) (complex) (compound) (local) (simplex) K05.30
  acute K05.20
    generalized K05.22
    localized K05.21
  apical K04.5
    acute (pulpal origin) K04.4
  generalized K05.32
  localized K05.31
Periodontoclasia K05.4
Periodontosis (juvenile) K05.4
Periods (*see also* Menstruation)
  heavy N92.0
  irregular N92.6
  shortened intervals (irregular) N92.1
Perionychia (*see also* Cellulitis, digit)
  with lymphangitis — *see* Lymphangitis, acute, digit
Perioophoritis — *see* Salpingo-oophoritis
Periorchitis N45.2
Periosteum, periosteal — *see* condition
Periostitis (albuminosa) (circumscribed) (diffuse) (infective) (monomelic) (*see also* Osteomyelitis)
  alveolar M27.3
  alveolodental M27.3
  dental M27.3
  gonorrheal A54.43
  jaw (lower) (upper) M27.2
  orbit H05.03- ☑
  syphilitic A52.77
    congenital (early) A50.02 [M90.80]
    secondary A51.46
  tuberculous — *see* Tuberculosis, bone
  yaws (hypertrophic) (early) (late) A66.6 [M90.80]
Periostosis (hyperplastic) (*see also* Disorder, bone, specified type NEC)
  with osteomyelitis — *see* Osteomyelitis, specified type NEC
Peripartum
  cardiomyopathy O90.3
Periphlebitis — *see* Phlebitis
Periproctitis K62.89
Periprostatitis — *see* Prostatitis
Perirectal — *see* condition
Perirenal — *see* condition
Perisalpingitis — *see* Salpingo-oophoritis
Perisplenitis (infectional) D73.89
Peristalsis, visible or reversed R19.2
Peritendinitis — *see* Enthesopathy
Peritoneum, peritoneal — *see* condition
Peritonitis (adhesive) (bacterial) (fibrinous) (hemorrhagic) (idiopathic) (localized) (perforative) (primary) (with adhesions) (with effusion) K65.9

Peritonitis — *continued*
  with or following
    abscess K65.1
    appendicitis K35.2
      with perforation or rupture K35.2
      generalized K35.2
      localized K35.3
    diverticular disease (intestine) K57.80
      with bleeding K57.81
    ectopic or molar pregnancy O08.0
    large intestine K57.20
      with
        bleeding K57.21
        small intestine K57.40
          with bleeding K57.41
    small intestine K57.00
      with
        bleeding K57.01
        large intestine K57.40
          with bleeding K57.41
  acute (generalized) K65.0
  aseptic T81.61 ☑
  bile, biliary K65.3
  chemical T81.61 ☑
  chlamydial A74.81
  chronic proliferative K65.8
  complicating abortion — *see* Abortion, by type, complicated by, pelvic peritonitis
  congenital P78.1
  diaphragmatic K65.0
  diffuse K65.0
  diphtheritic A36.89
  disseminated K65.0
  due to
    bile K65.3
    foreign
      body or object accidentally left during a procedure (instrument) (sponge) (swab) T81.599 ☑
      substance accidentally left during a procedure (chemical) (powder) (talc) T81.61 ☑
    talc T81.61 ☑
    urine K65.8
  eosinophilic K65.8
    acute K65.0
  fibrocaseous (tuberculous) A18.31
  fibropurulent K65.0
  following ectopic or molar pregnancy O08.0
  general (ized) K65.0
  gonococcal A54.85
  meconium (newborn) P78.0
  neonatal P78.1
    meconium P78.0
  pancreatic K65.0
  paroxysmal, familial E85.0
    benign E85.0
  pelvic
    female N73.5
      acute N73.3
      chronic N73.4
        with adhesions N73.6
    male K65.0
  periodic, familial E85.0
  proliferative, chronic K65.8
  puerperal, postpartum, childbirth O85
  purulent K65.0
  septic K65.0
  specified NEC K65.8
  spontaneous bacterial K65.2
  subdiaphragmatic K65.0
  subphrenic K65.0
  suppurative K65.0
  syphilitic A52.74
    congenital (early) A50.08 [K67]
  talc T81.61 ☑
  tuberculous A18.31
  urine K65.8
Peritonsillar — *see* condition
Peritonsillitis J36
Perityphlitis K37
Periureteritis N28.89
Periurethral — *see* condition
Periurethritis (gangrenous) — *see* Urethritis
Periuterine — *see* condition
Perivaginitis — *see* Vaginitis
Perivasculitis, retinal H35.06- ☑
Perivasitis (chronic) N49.1
Perivesiculitis (seminal) — *see* Vesiculitis

Perlèche NEC K13.0
  due to
    candidiasis B37.83
    moniliasis B37.83
    riboflavin deficiency E53.0
    vitamin B2 (riboflavin) deficiency E53.0
Pernicious — *see* condition
Pernio, perniosis T69.1 ☑
Perpetrator (of abuse) — *see* Index to External Causes of Injury, Perpetrator
Persecution
  delusion F22
  social Z60.5
Perseveration (tonic) R48.8
Persistence, persistent (congenital)
  anal membrane Q42.3
    with fistula Q42.2
  arteria stapedia Q16.3
  atrioventricular canal Q21.2
  branchial cleft Q18.0
  bulbus cordis in left ventricle Q21.8
  canal of Cloquet Q14.0
  capsule (opaque) Q12.8
  cilioretinal artery or vein Q14.8
  cloaca Q43.7
  communication — *see* Fistula, congenital
  convolutions
    aortic arch Q25.4
    fallopian tube Q50.6
    oviduct Q50.6
    uterine tube Q50.6
  double aortic arch Q25.4
  ductus arteriosus (Botalli) Q25.0
  fetal
    circulation P29.3
    form of cervix (uteri) Q51.828
    hemoglobin, hereditary (HPFH) D56.4
  foramen
    Botalli Q21.1
    ovale Q21.1
  Gartner's duct Q52.4
  hemoglobin, fetal (hereditary) (HPFH) D56.4
  hyaloid
    artery (generally incomplete) Q14.0
    system Q14.8
  hymen, in pregnancy or childbirth — *see* Pregnancy, complicated by, abnormal, vulva
  lanugo Q84.2
  left
    posterior cardinal vein Q26.8
    root with right arch of aorta Q25.4
    superior vena cava Q26.1
  Meckel's diverticulum Q43.0
    malignant — *see* Table of Neoplasms, small intestine, malignant
  mucosal disease (middle ear) — *see* Otitis, media, suppurative, chronic, tubotympanic
  nail(s), anomalous Q84.6
  omphalomesenteric duct Q43.0
  organ or site not listed — *see* Anomaly, by site
  ostium
    atrioventriculare commune Q21.2
    primum Q21.2
    secundum Q21.1
  ovarian rests in fallopian tube Q50.6
  pancreatic tissue in intestinal tract Q43.8
  primary (deciduous)
    teeth K00.6
    vitreous hyperplasia Q14.0
  pupillary membrane Q13.89
  rhesus (Rh) titer — *see* Complication(s), transfusion, incompatibility reaction, Rh (factor)
  right aortic arch Q25.4
  sinus
    urogenitalis
      female Q52.8
      male Q55.8
    venosus with imperfect incorporation in right auricle Q26.8
  thymus (gland) (hyperplasia) E32.0
  thyroglossal duct Q89.2
  thyrolingual duct Q89.2
  truncus arteriosus or communis Q20.0
  tunica vasculosa lentis Q12.2
  umbilical sinus Q64.4
  urachus Q64.4
  vitelline duct Q43.0

Person (with)
  admitted for clinical research, as a control subject (normal comparison) (participant) Z00.6
  awaiting admission to adequate facility elsewhere Z75.1
  concern (normal) about sick person in family Z63.6
  consulting on behalf of another Z71.0
  feigning illness Z76.5
  living (in)
    without
      adequate housing (heating) (space) Z59.1
      housing (permanent) (temporary) Z59.0
      person able to render necessary care Z74.2
      shelter Z59.0
    alone Z60.2
    boarding school Z59.3
    residential institution Z59.3
  on waiting list Z75.1
  sick or handicapped in family Z63.6
Personality (disorder) F60.9
  accentuation of traits (type A pattern) Z73.1
  affective F34.0
  aggressive F60.3
  amoral F60.2
  anacastic, anankastic F60.5
  antisocial F60.2
  anxious F60.6
  asocial F60.2
  asthenic F60.7
  avoidant F60.6
  borderline F60.3
  change due to organic condition (enduring) F07.0
  compulsive F60.5
  cycloid F34.0
  cyclothymic F34.0
  dependent F60.7
  depressive F34.1
  dissocial F60.2
  dual F44.81
  eccentric F60.89
  emotionally unstable F60.3
  expansive paranoid F60.0
  explosive F60.3
  fanatic F60.0
  haltlose type F60.89
  histrionic F60.4
  hyperthymic F34.0
  hypothymic F34.1
  hysterical F60.4
  immature F60.89
  inadequate F60.7
  labile (emotional) F60.3
  mixed (nonspecific) F60.81
  morally defective F60.2
  multiple F44.81
  narcissistic F60.81
  obsessional F60.5
  obsessive (-compulsive) F60.5
  organic F07.0
  overconscientious F60.5
  paranoid F60.0
  passive (-dependent) F60.7
  passive-aggressive F60.89
  pathologic F60.9
  pattern defect or disturbance F60.9
  pseudopsychopathic (organic) F07.0
  pseudoretarded (organic) F07.0
  psychoinfantile F60.4
  psychoneurotic NEC F60.89
  psychopathic F60.2
  querulant F60.0
  sadistic F60.89
  schizoid F60.1
  self-defeating F60.7
  sensitive paranoid F60.0
  sociopathic (amoral) (antisocial) (asocial) (dissocial) F60.2
  specified NEC F60.89
  type A Z73.1
  unstable (emotional) F60.3
Perthes' disease — *see* Legg-Calvé-Perthes disease
Pertussis (*see also* Whooping cough) A37.90
Perversion, perverted
  appetite F50.8
    psychogenic F50.8
  function
    pituitary gland E23.2
      posterior lobe E22.2

Perversion, perverted — *continued*
 sense of smell and taste R43.8
  psychogenic F45.8
 sexual — *see* Deviation, sexual
Pervious, congenital (*see also* Imperfect, closure)
 ductus arteriosus Q25.0
Pes (congenital) (*see also* Talipes)
 acquired (*see also* Deformity, limb, foot, specified NEC)
  planus — *see* Deformity, limb, flat foot
 adductus Q66.89
 cavus Q66.7
 deformity NEC, acquired — *see* Deformity, limb, foot, specified NEC
 planus (acquired) (any degree) (*see also* Deformity, limb, flat foot)
  rachitic sequelae (late effect) E64.3
 valgus Q66.6
Pest, pestis — *see* Plague
Petechia, petechiae R23.3
 newborn P54.5
Petechial typhus A75.9
Peter's anomaly Q13.4
Petit mal seizure — *see* Epilepsy, generalized, specified NEC
Petit's hernia — *see* Hernia, abdomen, specified site NEC
Petrellidosis B48.2
Petrositis H70.20- ☑
 acute H70.21- ☑
 chronic H70.22- ☑
Peutz-Jeghers disease or syndrome Q85.8
Peyronie's disease N48.6
Pfeiffer's disease — *see* Mononucleosis, infectious
Phagedena (dry) (moist) (sloughing) (*see also* Gangrene)
 geometric L88
 penis N48.29
 tropical — *see* Ulcer, skin
 vulva N76.6
Phagedenic — *see* condition
Phakoma H35.89
Phakomatosis (*see also* specific eponymous syndromes) Q85.9
 Bourneville's Q85.1
 specified NEC Q85.8
Phantom limb syndrome (without pain) G54.7
 with pain G54.6
Pharyngeal pouch syndrome D82.1
Pharyngitis (acute) (catarrhal) (gangrenous) (infective) (malignant) (membranous) (phlegmonous) (pseudomembranous) (simple) (subacute) (suppurative) (ulcerative) (viral) J02.9
 with influenza, flu, or grippe — *see* Influenza, with, pharyngitis
 aphthous B08.5
 atrophic J31.2
 chlamydial A56.4
 chronic (atrophic) (granular) (hypertrophic) J31.2
 coxsackievirus B08.5
 diphtheritic A36.0
 enteroviral vesicular B08.5
 follicular (chronic) J31.2
 fusospirochetal A69.1
 gonococcal A54.5
 granular (chronic) J31.2
 herpesviral B00.2
 hypertrophic J31.2
 infectional, chronic J31.2
 influenzal — *see* Influenza, with, respiratory manifestations NEC
 lymphonodular, acute (enteroviral) B08.8
 pneumococcal J02.8
 purulent J02.9
 putrid J02.9
 septic J02.0
 sicca J31.2
 specified organism NEC J02.8
 staphylococcal J02.8
 streptococcal J02.0
 syphilitic, congenital (early) A50.03
 tuberculous A15.8
 vesicular, enteroviral B08.5
 viral NEC J02.8
Pharyngoconjunctivitis, viral B30.2
Pharyngolaryngitis (acute) J06.0
 chronic J37.0
Pharyngoplegia J39.2
Pharyngotonsillitis, herpesviral B00.2

Pharyngotracheitis, chronic J42
Pharynx, pharyngeal — *see* condition
Phenomenon
 Arthus' — *see* Arthus' phenomenon
 jaw-winking Q07.8
 lupus erythematosus (LE) cell M32.9
 Raynaud's (secondary) I73.00
  with gangrene I73.01
 vasomotor R55
 vasospastic I73.9
 vasovagal R55
 Wenckebach's I44.1
Phenylketonuria E70.1
 classical E70.0
 maternal E70.1
Pheochromoblastoma
 specified site — *see* Neoplasm, malignant, by site
 unspecified site C74.10
Pheochromocytoma
 malignant
  specified site — *see* Neoplasm, malignant, by site
  unspecified site C74.10
 specified site — *see* Neoplasm, benign, by site
 unspecified site D35.00
Pheohyphomycosis — *see* Chromomycosis
Pheomycosis — *see* Chromomycosis
Phimosis (congenital) (due to infection) N47.1
 chancroidal A57
Phlebectasia (*see also* Varix)
 congenital Q27.4
Phlebitis (infective) (pyemic) (septic) (suppurative) I80.9
 antepartum — *see* Thrombophlebitis, antepartum
 blue — *see* Phlebitis, leg, deep
 breast, superficial I80.8
 cavernous (venous) sinus — *see* Phlebitis, intracranial (venous) sinus
 cerebral (venous) sinus — *see* Phlebitis, intracranial (venous) sinus
 chest wall, superficial I80.8
 cranial (venous) sinus — *see* Phlebitis, intracranial (venous) sinus
 deep (vessels) — *see* Phlebitis, leg, deep
 due to implanted device — *see* Complications, by site and type, specified NEC
 during or resulting from a procedure T81.72 ☑
 femoral vein (superficial) I80.1- ☑
 femoropopliteal vein I80.0- ☑
 gestational — *see* Phlebopathy, gestational
 hepatic veins I80.8
 iliofemoral — *see* Phlebitis, femoral vein
 intracranial (venous) sinus (any) G08
  nonpyogenic I67.6
 intraspinal venous sinuses and veins G08
  nonpyogenic G95.19
 lateral (venous) sinus — *see* Phlebitis, intracranial (venous) sinus
 leg I80.3
  antepartum — *see* Thrombophlebitis, antepartum
  deep (vessels) NEC I80.20- ☑
   iliac I80.21- ☑
   popliteal vein I80.22- ☑
   specified vessel NEC I80.29- ☑
   tibial vein I80.23- ☑
  femoral vein (superficial) I80.1- ☑
  superficial (vessels) I80.0- ☑
 longitudinal sinus — *see* Phlebitis, intracranial (venous) sinus
 lower limb — *see* Phlebitis, leg
 migrans, migrating (superficial) I82.1
 pelvic
  with ectopic or molar pregnancy O08.0
  following ectopic or molar pregnancy O08.0
  puerperal, postpartum O87.1
 popliteal vein — *see* Phlebitis, leg, deep, popliteal
 portal (vein) K75.1
 postoperative T81.72 ☑
 pregnancy — *see* Thrombophlebitis, antepartum
 puerperal, postpartum, childbirth O87.0
  deep O87.1
  pelvic O87.1
  superficial O87.0
 retina — *see* Vasculitis, retina
 saphenous (accessory) (great) (long) (small) — *see* Phlebitis, leg, superficial
 sinus (meninges) — *see* Phlebitis, intracranial (venous) sinus
 specified site NEC I80.8

Phlebitis — *continued*
 syphilitic A52.09
 tibial vein — *see* Phlebitis, leg, deep, tibial
 ulcerative I80.9
  leg — *see* Phlebitis, leg
 umbilicus I80.8
 uterus (septic) — *see* Endometritis
 varicose (leg) (lower limb) — *see* Varix, leg, with, inflammation
Phlebofibrosis I87.8
Phleboliths I87.8
Phlebopathy,
 gestational O22.9- ☑
 puerperal O87.9
Phlebosclerosis I87.8
Phlebothrombosis (*see also* Thrombosis)
 antepartum — *see* Thrombophlebitis, antepartum
 pregnancy — *see* Thrombophlebitis, antepartum
 puerperal — *see* Thrombophlebitis, puerperal
Phlebotomus fever A93.1
Phlegmasia
 alba dolens O87.1
  nonpuerperal — *see* Phlebitis, femoral vein
 cerulea dolens — *see* Phlebitis, leg, deep
Phlegmon — *see* Abscess
Phlegmonous — *see* condition
Phlyctenulosis (allergic) (keratoconjunctivitis) (nontuberculous) (*see also* Keratoconjunctivitis)
 cornea — *see* Keratoconjunctivitis
 tuberculous A18.52
Phobia, phobic F40.9
 animal F40.218
  spiders F40.210
 examination F40.298
 reaction F40.9
 simple F40.298
 social F40.10
  generalized F40.11
 specific (isolated) F40.298
  animal F40.218
   spiders F40.210
  blood F40.230
  injection F40.231
  injury F40.233
  men F40.290
  natural environment F40.228
   thunderstorms F40.220
  situational F40.248
   bridges F40.242
   closed in spaces F40.240
   flying F40.243
   heights F40.241
  specified focus NEC F40.298
  transfusion F40.231
  women F40.291
 specified NEC F40.8
  medical care NEC F40.232
 state F40.9
Phocas' disease — *see* Mastopathy, cystic
Phocomelia Q73.1
 lower limb — *see* Agenesis, leg, with foot present
 upper limb — *see* Agenesis, arm, with hand present
Phoria H50.50
Phosphate-losing tubular disorder N25.0
Phosphatemia E83.39
Phosphaturia E83.39
Photodermatitis (sun) L56.8
 chronic L57.8
 due to drug L56.8
 light other than sun L59.8
Photokeratitis H16.13- ☑
Photophobia H53.14- ☑
Photophthalmia — *see* Photokeratitis
Photopsia H53.19
Photoretinitis — *see* Retinopathy, solar
Photosensitivity, photosensitization (sun) skin L56.8
 light other than sun L59.8
Phrenitis — *see* Encephalitis
Phrynoderma (vitamin A deficiency) E50.8
Phthiriasis (pubis) B85.3
 with any infestation classifiable to B85.0-B85.2 B85.4
Phthirus infestation — *see* Phthiriasis
Phthisis (*see also* Tuberculosis)
 bulbi (infectional) — *see* Disorder, globe, degenerated condition, atrophy
 eyeball (due to infection) — *see* Disorder, globe, degenerated condition, atrophy

Phycomycosis — see Zygomycosis
Physalopteriasis B81.8
Physical restraint status Z78.1
Phytobezoar T18.9 ☑
    intestine T18.3 ☑
    stomach T18.2 ☑
Pian — see Yaws
Pianoma A66.1
Pica F50.8
    in adults F50.8
    infant or child F98.3
Picking, nose F98.8
Pick-Niemann disease — see Niemann-Pick disease or
    syndrome
Pick's
    cerebral atrophy G31.01 [F02.80]
        with behavioral disturbance G31.01 [F02.81]
    disease or syndrome (brain) G31.01 [F02.80]
        with behavioral disturbance G31.01 [F02.81]
Pickwickian syndrome E66.2
Piebaldism E70.39
Piedra (beard) (scalp) B36.8
    black B36.3
    white B36.2
Pierre Robin deformity or syndrome Q87.0
Pierson's disease or osteochondrosis M91.0
Pig-bel A05.2
Pigeon
    breast or chest (acquired) M95.4
        congenital Q67.7
        rachitic sequelae (late effect) E64.3
    breeder's disease or lung J67.2
    fancier's disease or lung J67.2
    toe — see Deformity, toe, specified NEC
Pigmentation (abnormal) (anomaly) L81.9
    conjunctiva H11.13- ☑
    cornea (anterior) H18.01- ☑
        posterior H18.05- ☑
        stromal H18.06- ☑
    diminished melanin formation NEC L81.6
    iron L81.8
    lids, congenital Q82.8
    limbus corneae — see Pigmentation, cornea
    metals L81.8
    optic papilla, congenital Q14.2
    retina, congenital (grouped) (nevoid) Q14.1
    scrotum, congenital Q82.8
    tattoo L81.8
Piles (see also Hemorrhoids) K64.9
Pili
    annulati or torti (congenital) Q84.1
    incarnati L73.1
Pill roller hand (intrinsic) — see Parkinsonism
Pilomatrixoma — see Neoplasm, skin, benign
    malignant — see Neoplasm, skin, malignant
Pilonidal — see condition
Pimple R23.8
Pinched nerve — see Neuropathy, entrapment
Pindborg tumor — see Cyst, calcifying odontogenic
Pineal body or gland — see condition
Pinealoblastoma C75.3
Pinealoma D44.5
    malignant C75.3
Pineoblastoma C75.3
Pineocytoma D44.5
Pinguecula H11.15- ☑
Pingueculitis H10.81- ☑
Pinhole meatus (see also Stricture, urethra) N35.9
Pink
    disease — see subcategory T56.1 ☑
    eye — see Conjunctivitis, acute, mucopurulent
Pinkus' disease (lichen nitidus) L44.1
Pinpoint
    meatus — see Stricture, urethra
    os (uteri) — see Stricture, cervix
Pins and needles R20.2
Pinta A67.9
    cardiovascular lesions A67.2
    chancre (primary) A67.0
    erythematous plaques A67.1
    hyperchromic lesions A67.1
    hyperkeratosis A67.1
    lesions A67.9
        cardiovascular A67.2
        hyperchromic A67.1
        intermediate A67.1
        late A67.2

Pinta — continued
    lesions — continued
        mixed A67.3
        primary A67.0
        skin (achromic) (cicatricial) (dyschromic) A67.2
            hyperchromic A67.1
            mixed (achromic and hyperchromic) A67.3
    papule (primary) A67.0
    skin lesions (achromic) (cicatricial) (dyschromic) A67.2
        hyperchromic A67.1
        mixed (achromic and hyperchromic) A67.3
    vitiligo A67.2
Pintids A67.1
Pinworm (disease) (infection) (infestation) B80
Piroplasmosis B60.0
Pistol wound — see Gunshot wound
Pitchers' elbow — see Derangement, joint, specified
    type NEC, elbow
Pithecoid pelvis Q74.2
    with disproportion (fetopelvic) O33.0
        causing obstructed labor O65.0
Pithiatism F48.8
Pitted — see Pitting
Pitting (see also Edema) R60.9
    lip R60.0
    nail L60.8
    teeth K00.4
Pituitary gland — see condition
Pituitary-snuff-taker's disease J67.8
Pityriasis (capitis) L21.0
    alba L30.5
    circinata (et maculata) L42
    furfuracea L21.0
    Hebra's L26
    lichenoides L41.0
        chronica L41.1
        et varioliformis (acuta) L41.0
    maculata (et circinata) L30.5
    nigra B36.1
    pilaris, Hebra's L44.0
    rosea L42
    rotunda L44.8
    rubra (Hebra) pilaris L44.0
    simplex L30.5
    specified type NEC L30.5
    streptogenes L30.5
    versicolor (scrotal) B36.0
Placenta, placental — see Pregnancy, complicated by
    (care of) (management affected by), specified con-
    dition
Placentitis O41.14- ☑
Plagiocephaly Q67.3
Plague A20.9
    abortive A20.8
    ambulatory A20.8
    asymptomatic A20.8
    bubonic A20.0
    cellulocutaneous A20.1
    cutaneobubonic A20.1
    lymphatic gland A20.0
    meningitis A20.3
    pharyngeal A20.8
    pneumonic (primary) (secondary) A20.2
    pulmonary, pulmonic A20.2
    septicemic A20.7
    tonsillar A20.8
        septicemic A20.7
Planning, family
    contraception Z30.9
    procreation Z31.69
Plaque(s)
    artery, arterial — see Arteriosclerosis
    calcareous — see Calcification
    coronary, lipid rich I25.83
    epicardial I31.8
    erythematous, of pinta A67.1
    Hollenhorst's — see Occlusion, artery, retina
    lipid rich, coronary I25.83
    pleural (without asbestos) J92.9
        with asbestos J92.0
    tongue K13.29
Plasmacytoma C90.3- ☑
    extramedullary C90.2- ☑
    medullary C90.0- ☑
    solitary C90.3- ☑
Plasmacytopenia D72.818
Plasmacytosis D72.822
Plaster ulcer — see Ulcer, pressure, by site

Plateau iris syndrome (post-iridectomy) (postprocedu-
    ral) (without glaucoma) H21.82
    with glaucoma H40.22- ☑
Platybasia Q75.8
Platyonychia (congenital) Q84.6
    acquired L60.8
Platypelloid pelvis M95.5
    with disproportion (fetopelvic) O33.0
        causing obstructed labor O65.0
    congenital Q74.2
Platyspondylisis Q76.49
Plaut (-Vincent) **disease** (see also Vincent's) A69.1
Plethora R23.2
    newborn P61.1
Pleura, pleural — see condition
Pleuralgia R07.81
Pleurisy (acute) (adhesive) (chronic) (costal) (diaphrag-
    matic) (double) (dry) (fibrinous) (fibrous) (interlobar)
    (latent) (plastic) (primary) (residual) (sicca) (sterile)
    (subacute) (unresolved) R09.1
    with
        adherent pleura J86.0
        effusion J90
            chylous, chyliform J94.0
            tuberculous (non primary) A15.6
                primary (progressive) A15.7
        tuberculosis — see Pleurisy, tuberculous (non pri-
            mary)
    encysted — see Pleurisy, with effusion
    exudative — see Pleurisy, with effusion
    fibrinopurulent, fibropurulent — see Pyothorax
    hemorrhagic — see Hemothorax
    pneumococcal J90
    purulent — see Pyothorax
    septic — see Pyothorax
    serofibrinous — see Pleurisy, with effusion
    seropurulent — see Pyothorax
    serous — see Pleurisy, with effusion
    staphylococcal J86.9
    streptococcal J90
    suppurative — see Pyothorax
    traumatic (post) (current) — see Injury, intrathoracic,
        pleura
    tuberculous (with effusion) (non primary) A15.6
        primary (progressive) A15.7
Pleuritis sicca — see Pleurisy
Pleurobronchopneumonia — see Pneumonia, broncho-
Pleurodynia R07.81
    epidemic B33.0
    viral B33.0
Pleuropericarditis (see also Pericarditis)
    acute I30.9
Pleuropneumonia (acute) (bilateral) (double) (septic)
    (see also Pneumonia) J18.8
    chronic — see Fibrosis, lung
Pleuro-pneumonia-like-organism (PPLO), as cause of
    disease classified elsewhere B96.0
Pleurorrhea — see Pleurisy, with effusion
Plexitis, brachial G54.0
Plica
    polonica B85.0
    syndrome, knee M67.5- ☑
    tonsil J35.8
Plicated tongue K14.5
Plug
    bronchus NEC J98.09
    meconium (newborn) NEC syndrome P76.0
    mucus — see Asphyxia, mucus
Plumbism — see subcategory T56.0 ☑
Plummer's disease E05.20
    with thyroid storm E05.21
Plummer-Vinson syndrome D50.1
Pluricarential syndrome of infancy E40
Plus (and minus) **hand** (intrinsic) — see Deformity, limb,
    specified type NEC, forearm
Pneumathemia — see Air, embolism
Pneumatic hammer (drill) syndrome T75.21 ☑
Pneumatocele (lung) J98.4
    intracranial G93.89
    tension J44.9
Pneumatosis
    cystoides intestinalis K63.89
    intestinalis K63.89
    peritonei K66.8
Pneumaturia R39.89
Pneumoblastoma — see Neoplasm, lung, malignant
Pneumocephalus G93.89

☑ **Additional Character Required** — Refer to the Tabular List for Character Selection   ▽ **Subterms under main terms may continue to next column or page**

Pneumococcemia A40.3
Pneumococcus, pneumococcal — *see* condition
Pneumoconiosis (due to) (inhalation of) J64
   with tuberculosis (any type in A15) J65
   aluminum J63.0
   asbestos J61
   bagasse, bagassosis J67.1
   bauxite J63.1
   beryllium J63.2
   coal miners' (simple) J60
   coalworkers' (simple) J60
   collier's J60
   cotton dust J66.0
   diatomite (diatomaceous earth) J62.8
   dust
      inorganic NEC J63.6
      lime J62.8
      marble J62.8
      organic NEC J66.8
   fumes or vapors (from silo) J68.9
   graphite J63.3
   grinder's J62.8
   kaolin J62.8
   mica J62.8
   millstone maker's J62.8
   mineral fibers NEC J61
   miner's J60
   moldy hay J67.0
   potter's J62.8
   rheumatoid — *see* Rheumatoid, lung
   sandblaster's J62.8
   silica, silicate NEC J62.8
      with carbon J60
   stonemason's J62.8
   talc (dust) J62.0
Pneumocystis carinii pneumonia B59
Pneumocystis jiroveci (pneumonia) B59
Pneumocystosis (with pneumonia) B59
Pneumohemopericardium I31.2
Pneumohemothorax J94.2
   traumatic S27.2 ☑
Pneumohydropericardium — *see* Pericarditis
Pneumohydrothorax — *see* Hydrothorax
Pneumomediastinum J98.2
   congenital or perinatal P25.2
Pneumomycosis B49 [J99]
Pneumonia (acute) (double) (migratory) (purulent)
      (septic) (unresolved) J18.9
   with
      influenza — *see* Influenza, with, pneumonia
      lung abscess J85.1
         due to specified organism — *see* Pneumonia,
            in (due to)
   adenoviral J12.0
   adynamic J18.2
   alba A50.04
   allergic (eosinophilic) J82
   alveolar — *see* Pneumonia, lobar
   anaerobes J15.8
   anthrax A22.1
   apex, apical — *see* Pneumonia, lobar
   Ascaris B77.81
   aspiration J69.0
      due to
         aspiration of microorganisms
            bacterial J15.9
            viral J12.9
         food (regurgitated) J69.0
         gastric secretions J69.0
         milk (regurgitated) J69.0
         oils, essences J69.1
         solids, liquids NEC J69.8
         vomitus J69.0
      newborn P24.81
         amniotic fluid (clear) P24.11
         blood P24.21
         food (regurgitated) P24.31
         liquor (amnii) P24.11
         meconium P24.01
         milk P24.31
         mucus P24.11
         specified NEC P24.81
         stomach contents P24.31
      postprocedural J95.4
   atypical NEC J18.9
   bacillus J15.9
      specified NEC J15.8

Pneumonia — *continued*
   bacterial J15.9
      specified NEC J15.8
   Bacteroides (fragilis) (oralis) (melaninogenicus) J15.8
   basal, basic, basilar — *see* Pneumonia, by type
   bronchiolitis obliterans organized (BOOP) J84.89
   broncho-, bronchial (confluent) (croupous) (diffuse)
      (disseminated) (hemorrhagic) (involving lobes)
      (lobar) (terminal) J18.0
      allergic (eosinophilic) J82
      aspiration — *see* Pneumonia, aspiration
      bacterial J15.9
         specified NEC J15.8
      chronic — *see* Fibrosis, lung
      diplococcal J13
      Eaton's agent J15.7
      Escherichia coli (E. coli) J15.5
      Friedländer's bacillus J15.0
      Hemophilus influenzae J14
      hypostatic J18.2
      inhalation (*see also* Pneumonia, aspiration)
         due to fumes or vapors (chemical) J68.0
         of oils or essences J69.1
      Klebsiella (pneumoniae) J15.0
      lipid, lipoid J69.1
         endogenous J84.89
      Mycoplasma (pneumoniae) J15.7
      pleuro-pneumonia-like-organisms (PPLO) J15.7
      pneumococcal J13
      Proteus J15.6
      Pseudomonas J15.1
      Serratia marcescens J15.6
      specified organism NEC J16.8
      staphylococcal — *see* Pneumonia, staphylococcal
      streptococcal NEC J15.4
         group B J15.3
         pneumoniae J13
      viral, virus — *see* Pneumonia, viral
   Butyrivibrio (fibriosolvens) J15.8
   Candida B37.1
   caseous — *see* Tuberculosis, pulmonary
   catarrhal — *see* Pneumonia, broncho
   chlamydial J16.0
      congenital P23.1
   cholesterol J84.89
   cirrhotic (chronic) — *see* Fibrosis, lung
   Clostridium (haemolyticum) (novyi) J15.8
   confluent — *see* Pneumonia, broncho
   congenital (infective) P23.9
      due to
         bacterium NEC P23.6
         Chlamydia P23.1
         Escherichia coli P23.4
         Haemophilus influenzae P23.6
         infective organism NEC P23.8
         Klebsiella pneumoniae P23.6
         Mycoplasma P23.6
         Pseudomonas P23.5
         Staphylococcus P23.2
         Streptococcus (except group B) P23.6
          group B P23.3
         viral agent P23.0
      specified NEC P23.8
   croupous — *see* Pneumonia, lobar
   cryptogenic organizing J84.116
   cytomegalic inclusion B25.0
   cytomegaloviral B25.0
   deglutition — *see* Pneumonia, aspiration
   desquamative interstitial J84.117
   diffuse — *see* Pneumonia, broncho
   diplococcal, diplococcus (broncho-) (lobar) J13
   disseminated (focal) — *see* Pneumonia, broncho
   Eaton's agent J15.7
   embolic, embolism — *see* Embolism, pulmonary
   Enterobacter J15.6
   eosinophilic J82
   Escherichia coli (E. coli) J15.5
   Eubacterium J15.8
   fibrinous — *see* Pneumonia, lobar
   fibroid, fibrous (chronic) — *see* Fibrosis, lung
   Friedländer's bacillus J15.0
   Fusobacterium (nucleatum) J15.8
   gangrenous J85.0
   giant cell (measles) B05.2
   gonococcal A54.84
   gram-negative bacteria NEC J15.6
      anaerobic J15.8
   Hemophilus influenzae (broncho) (lobar) J14

Pneumonia — *continued*
   human metapneumovirus J12.3
   hypostatic (broncho) (lobar) J18.2
   in (due to)
      actinomycosis A42.0
      adenovirus J12.0
      anthrax A22.1
      ascariasis B77.81
      aspergillosis B44.9
      Bacillus anthracis A22.1
      Bacterium anitratum J15.6
      candidiasis B37.1
      chickenpox B01.2
      Chlamydia J16.0
         neonatal P23.1
      coccidioidomycosis B38.2
         acute B38.0
         chronic B38.1
      cytomegalovirus disease B25.0
      Diplococcus (pneumoniae) J13
      Eaton's agent J15.7
      Enterobacter J15.6
      Escherichia coli (E. coli) J15.5
      Friedländer's bacillus J15.0
      fumes and vapors (chemical) (inhalation) J68.0
      gonorrhea A54.84
      Hemophilus influenzae (H. influenzae) J14
      Herellea J15.6
      histoplasmosis B39.2
         acute B39.0
         chronic B39.1
      human metapneumovirus J12.3
      Klebsiella (pneumoniae) J15.0
      measles B05.2
      Mycoplasma (pneumoniae) J15.7
      nocardiosis, nocardiasis A43.0
      ornithosis A70
      parainfluenza virus J12.2
      pleuro-pneumonia-like-organism (PPLO) J15.7
      pneumococcus J13
      pneumocystosis (Pneumocystis carinii) (Pneumo-
         cystis jiroveci) B59
      Proteus J15.6
      Pseudomonas NEC J15.1
         pseudomallei A24.1
      psittacosis A70
      Q fever A78
      respiratory syncytial virus J12.1
      rheumatic fever I00 [J17]
      rubella B06.81
      Salmonella (infection) A02.22
         typhi A01.03
      schistosomiasis B65.9 [J17]
      Serratia marcescens J15.6
      specified
         bacterium NEC J15.8
         organism NEC J16.8
      spirochetal NEC A69.8
      Staphylococcus J15.20
         aureus (methicillin susceptible) (MSSA) J15.211
            methicillin resistant (MRSA) J15.212
         specified NEC J15.29
      Streptococcus J15.4
         group B J15.3
         pneumoniae J13
         specified NEC J15.4
      toxoplasmosis B58.3
      tularemia A21.2
      typhoid (fever) A01.03
      varicella B01.2
      virus — *see* Pneumonia, viral
      whooping cough A37.91
         due to
            Bordetella parapertussis A37.11
            Bordetella pertussis A37.01
            specified NEC A37.81
      Yersinia pestis A20.2
   inhalation of food or vomit — *see* Pneumonia, aspira-
      tion
   interstitial J84.9
      chronic J84.111
      desquamative J84.117
      due to
         collagen vascular disease J84.17
         known underlying cause J84.17
      idiopathic NOS J84.111
      in disease classified elsewhere J84.17

Pneumonia — *continued*
  interstitial — *continued*
    lymphocytic (due to collagen vascular disease) (in diseases classified elsewhere) J84.17
    lymphoid J84.2
    non-specific J84.89
      due to
        collagen vascular disease J84.17
        known underlying cause J84.17
      idiopathic J84.113
      in diseases classified elsewhere J84.17
    plasma cell B59
    pseudomonas J15.1
    usual J84.112
      due to collagen vascular disease J84.17
      idiopathic J84.112
      in diseases classified elsewhere J84.17
  Klebsiella (pneumoniae) J15.0
  lipid, lipoid (exogenous) J69.1
    endogenous J84.89
  lobar (disseminated) (double) (interstitial) J18.1
    bacterial J15.9
      specified NEC J15.8
    chronic — *see* Fibrosis, lung
    Escherichia coli (E. coli) J15.5
    Friedländer's bacillus J15.0
    Hemophilus influenzae J14
    hypostatic J18.2
    Klebsiella (pneumoniae) J15.0
    pneumococcal J13
    Proteus J15.6
    Pseudomonas J15.1
    specified organism NEC J16.8
    staphylococcal — *see* Pneumonia, staphylococcal
    streptococcal NEC J15.4
    Streptococcus pneumoniae J13
    viral, virus — *see* Pneumonia, viral
  lobular — *see* Pneumonia, broncho
  Löffler's J82
  lymphoid interstitial J84.2
  massive — *see* Pneumonia, lobar
  meconium P24.01
  MSSA (methicillin susceptible Staphylococcus aureus) J15.211
  multilobar — *see* Pneumonia, by type
  Mycoplasma (pneumoniae) J15.7
  necrotic J85.0
  neonatal P23.9
    aspiration — *see* Aspiration, by substance, with pneumonia
  nitrogen dioxide J68.9
  organizing J84.89
    due to
      collagen vascular disease J84.17
      known underlying cause J84.17
    in diseases classified elsewhere J84.17
  orthostatic J18.2
  parainfluenza virus J12.2
  parenchymatous — *see* Fibrosis, lung
  passive J18.2
  patchy — *see* Pneumonia, broncho
  Peptococcus J15.8
  Peptostreptococcus J15.8
  plasma cell (of infants) B59
  pleurolobar — *see* Pneumonia, lobar
  pleuro-pneumonia-like organism (PPLO) J15.7
  pneumococcal (broncho) (lobar) J13
  Pneumocystis (carinii) (jiroveci) B59
  postinfectional NEC B99 ☑ [J17]
  postmeasles B05.2
  Proteus J15.6
  Pseudomonas J15.1
  psittacosis A70
  radiation J70.0
  respiratory syncytial virus J12.1
  resulting from a procedure J95.89
  rheumatic I00 [J17]
  Salmonella (arizonae) (cholerae-suis) (enteritidis) (typhimurium) A02.22
    typhi A01.03
    typhoid fever A01.03
  SARS-associated coronavirus J12.81
  segmented, segmental — *see* Pneumonia, broncho-
  Serratia marcescens J15.6
  specified NEC J18.8
    bacterium NEC J15.8
    organism NEC J16.8
    virus NEC J12.89

Pneumonia — *continued*
  spirochetal NEC A69.8
  staphylococcal (broncho) (lobar) J15.20
    aureus (methicillin susceptible) (MSSA) J15.211
      methicillin resistant (MRSA) J15.212
    specified NEC J15.29
  static, stasis J18.2
  streptococcal NEC (broncho) (lobar) J15.4
    group
      A J15.4
      B J15.3
      specified NEC J15.4
  Streptococcus pneumoniae J13
  syphilitic, congenital (early) A50.04
  traumatic (complication) (early) (secondary) T79.8 ☑
  tuberculous (any) — *see* Tuberculosis, pulmonary
  tularemic A21.2
  varicella B01.2
  Veillonella J15.8
  ventilator associated J95.851
  viral, virus (broncho) (interstitial) (lobar) J12.9
    adenoviral J12.0
    congenital P23.0
    human metapneumovirus J12.3
    parainfluenza J12.2
    respiratory syncytial J12.1
    SARS-associated coronavirus J12.81
    specified NEC J12.89
  white (congenital) A50.04
Pneumonic — *see* condition
Pneumonitis (acute) (primary) (*see also* Pneumonia)
  air-conditioner J67.7
  allergic (due to) J67.9
    organic dust NEC J67.8
    red cedar dust J67.8
    sequoiosis J67.8
    wood dust J67.8
  aspiration J69.0
    due to
      anesthesia J95.4
        during
          labor and delivery O74.0
          pregnancy O29.01- ☑
          puerperium O89.01
      fumes or gases J68.0
    obstetric O74.0
  chemical (due to gases, fumes or vapors) (inhalation) J68.0
    due to anesthesia J95.4
  cholesterol J84.89
  chronic — *see* Fibrosis, lung
  congenital rubella P35.0
  crack (cocaine) J68.0
  due to
    beryllium J68.0
    cadmium J68.0
    crack (cocaine) J68.0
    detergent J69.8
    fluorocarbon-polymer J68.0
    food, vomit (aspiration) J69.0
    fumes or vapors J68.0
    gases, fumes or vapors (inhalation) J68.0
    inhalation
      blood J69.8
      essences J69.1
      food (regurgitated), milk, vomit J69.0
      oils, essences J69.1
      saliva J69.0
      solids, liquids NEC J69.8
    manganese J68.0
    nitrogen dioxide J68.0
    oils, essences J69.1
    solids, liquids NEC J69.8
    toxoplasmosis (acquired) B58.3
      congenital P37.1
    vanadium J68.0
    ventilator J95.851
  eosinophilic J82
  hypersensitivity J67.9
    air conditioner lung J67.7
    bagassosis J67.1
    bird fancier's lung J67.2
    farmer's lung J67.0
    maltworker's lung J67.4
    maple bark-stripper's lung J67.6
    mushroom worker's lung J67.5
    specified organic dust NEC J67.8
    suberosis J67.3

Pneumonitis — *continued*
  interstitial (chronic) J84.89
    acute J84.114
    lymphoid J84.2
    non-specific J84.89
      idiopathic J84.113
  lymphoid, interstitial J84.2
  meconium P24.01
  postanesthetic J95.4
    correct substance properly administered — *see* Table of Drugs and Chemicals, by drug, adverse effect
    in labor and delivery O74.0
    in pregnancy O29.01- ☑
    obstetric O74.0
    overdose or wrong substance given or taken (by accident) — *see* Table of Drugs and Chemicals, by drug, poisoning
  postpartum, puerperal O89.01
  postoperative J95.4
    obstetric O74.0
  radiation J70.0
  rubella, congenital P35.0
  ventilation (air-conditioning) J67.7
  ventilator associated J95.851
  wood-dust J67.8
Pneumoconiosis — *see* Pneumoconiosis
Pneumoparotid K11.8
Pneumopathy NEC J98.4
  alveolar J84.09
  due to organic dust NEC J66.8
  parietoalveolar J84.09
Pneumopericarditis (*see also* Pericarditis)
  acute I30.9
Pneumopericardium (*see also* Pericarditis)
  congenital P25.3
  newborn P25.3
  traumatic (post) — *see* Injury, heart
Pneumophagia (psychogenic) F45.8
Pneumopleurisy, pneumopleuritis (*see also* Pneumonia) J18.8
Pneumopyopericardium I30.1
Pneumopyothorax — *see* Pyopneumothorax
  with fistula J86.0
Pneumorrhagia (*see also* Hemorrhage, lung)
  tuberculous — *see* Tuberculosis, pulmonary
Pneumothorax NOS J93.9
  acute J93.83
  chronic J93.81
  congenital P25.1
  perinatal period P25.1
  postprocedural J95.811
  specified NEC J93.83
  spontaneous NOS J93.83
    newborn P25.1
    primary J93.11
    secondary J93.12
    tension J93.0
  tense valvular, infectional J93.0
  tension (spontaneous) J93.0
  traumatic S27.0 ☑
    with hemothorax S27.2 ☑
  tuberculous — *see* Tuberculosis, pulmonary
Podagra (*see also* Gout) M10.9
Podencephalus Q01.9
Poikilocytosis R71.8
Poikiloderma L81.6
  Civatte's L57.3
  congenital Q82.8
  vasculare atrophicans L94.5
Poikilodermatomyositis M33.10
  with
    myopathy M33.12
    respiratory involvement M33.11
    specified organ involvement NEC M33.19
Pointed ear (congenital) Q17.3
Poison ivy, oak, sumac or other plant dermatitis (allergic) (contact) L23.7
Poisoning (acute) (*see also* Table of Drugs and Chemicals)
  algae and toxins T65.82- ☑
  Bacillus B (aertrycke) (cholerae (suis)) (paratyphosus) (suipestifer) A02.9
    botulinus A05.1
  bacterial toxins A05.9
  berries, noxious — *see* Poisoning, food, noxious, berries
  botulism A05.1
  ciguatera fish T61.0- ☑

☑ **Additional Character Required** — **Refer to the Tabular List for Character Selection** ▽ **Subterms under main terms may continue to next column or page**

Poisoning — *continued*
Clostridium botulinum A05.1
death-cap (Amanita phalloides) (Amanita verna) —
   see Poisoning, food, noxious, mushrooms
drug — *see* Table of Drugs and Chemicals, by drug,
   poisoning
epidemic, fish (noxious) — *see* Poisoning, seafood
   bacterial A05.9
fava bean D55.0
fish (noxious) T61.9- ☑
   bacterial — *see* Intoxication, foodborne, by agent
   ciguatera fish — *see* Poisoning, ciguatera fish
   scombroid fish — *see* Poisoning, scombroid fish
   specified type NEC T61.77- ☑
food (acute) (diseased) (infected) (noxious) NEC
   T62.9- ☑
   bacterial — *see* Intoxication, foodborne, by agent
   due to
      Bacillus (aertrycke) (choleraesuis) (paratypho-
         sus) (suipestifer) A02.9
         botulinus A05.1
      Clostridium (perfringens) (Welchii) A05.2
      salmonella (aertrycke) (callinarum) (choleraesu-
         is) (enteritidis) (paratyphi) (suipestifer)
         A02.9
         with
            gastroenteritis A02.0
            sepsis A02.1
      staphylococcus A05.0
      Vibrio
         parahaemolyticus A05.3
         vulnificus A05.5
   noxious or naturally toxic T62.9- ☑
      berries — *see* subcategory T62.1 ☑
      fish — *see* Poisoning, seafood
      mushrooms — *see* subcategory T62.0X ☑
      plants NEC — *see* subcategory T62.2X ☑
      seafood — *see* Poisoning, seafood
      specified NEC — *see* subcategory T62.8X ☑
ichthyotoxism — *see* Poisoning, seafood
kreotoxism, food A05.9
latex T65.81- ☑
lead T56.0- ☑
mushroom — *see* Poisoning, food, noxious, mushroom
mussels (*see also* Poisoning, shellfish)
   bacterial — *see* Intoxication, foodborne, by agent
nicotine (tobacco) T65.2- ☑
noxious foodstuffs — *see* Poisoning, food, noxious
plants, noxious — *see* Poisoning, food, noxious, plants
   NEC
ptomaine — *see* Poisoning, food
radiation J70.0
Salmonella (arizonae) (cholerae-suis) (enteritidis) (typhimurium) A02.9
scombroid fish T61.1- ☑
seafood (noxious) T61.9- ☑
   bacterial — *see* Intoxication, foodborne, by agent
   fish — *see* Poisoning, fish
   shellfish — *see* Poisoning, shellfish
   specified NEC — *see* subcategory T61.8X ☑
shellfish (amnesic) (azaspiracid) (diarrheic) (neurotoxic)
   (noxious) (paralytic) T61.78- ☑
   bacterial — *see* Intoxication, foodborne, by agent
   ciguatera mollusk — *see* Poisoning, ciguatera fish
specified substance NEC T65.891 ☑
Staphylococcus, food A05.0
tobacco (nicotine) T65.2- ☑
water E87.79
Poker spine — *see* Spondylitis, ankylosing
Poland syndrome Q79.8
Polioencephalitis (acute) (bulbar) A80.9
inferior G12.22
influenzal — *see* Influenza, with, encephalopathy
superior hemorrhagic (acute) (Wernicke's) E51.2
   Wernicke's E51.2
Polioencephalomyelitis (acute) (anterior) A80.9
with beriberi E51.2
Polioencephalopathy, superior hemorrhagic E51.2
with
   beriberi E51.11
   pellagra E52
Poliomeningoencephalitis — *see* Meningoencephalitis
Poliomyelitis (acute) (anterior) (epidemic) A80.9
with paralysis (bulbar) — *see* Poliomyelitis, paralytic
abortive A80.4
ascending (progressive) — *see* Poliomyelitis, paralytic
bulbar (paralytic) — *see* Poliomyelitis, paralytic

Poliomyelitis — *continued*
congenital P35.8
nonepidemic A80.9
nonparalytic A80.4
paralytic A80.30
   specified NEC A80.39
   vaccine-associated A80.0
   wild virus
      imported A80.1
      indigenous A80.2
spinal, acute A80.9
Poliosis (eyebrow) (eyelashes) L67.1
circumscripta, acquired L67.1
Pollakiuria R35.0
psychogenic F45.8
Pollinosis J30.1
Pollitzer's disease L73.2
Polyadenitis (*see also* Lymphadenitis)
malignant A20.0
Polyalgia M79.89
Polyangiitis M30.0
microscopic M31.7
overlap syndrome M30.8
Polyarteritis
microscopic M31.7
nodosa M30.0
   with lung involvement M30.1
   juvenile M30.2
   related condition NEC M30.8
Polyarthralgia — *see* Pain, joint
Polyarthritis, polyarthropathy (*see also* Arthritis) M13.0
due to or associated with other specified conditions
   — *see* Arthritis
epidemic (Australian) (with exanthema) B33.1
infective — *see* Arthritis, pyogenic or pyemic
inflammatory M06.4
juvenile (chronic) (seronegative) M08.3
migratory — *see* Fever, rheumatic
rheumatic, acute — *see* Fever, rheumatic
Polyarthrosis M15.9
post-traumatic M15.3
primary M15.0
specified NEC M15.8
Polycarential syndrome of infancy E40
Polychondritis (atrophic) (chronic) (*see also* Disorder,
cartilage, specified type NEC)
relapsing M94.1
Polycoria Q13.2
Polycystic (disease)
degeneration, kidney Q61.3
   autosomal dominant (adult type) Q61.2
   autosomal recessive (infantile type) NEC Q61.19
kidney Q61.3
   autosomal
      dominant Q61.2
      recessive NEC Q61.19
   autosomal dominant (adult type) Q61.2
   autosomal recessive (childhood type) NEC Q61.19
   infantile type NEC Q61.19
liver Q44.6
lung J98.4
   congenital Q33.0
ovary, ovaries E28.2
spleen Q89.09
Polycythemia (secondary) D75.1
acquired D75.1
benign (familial) D75.0
due to
   donor twin P61.1
   erythropoietin D75.1
   fall in plasma volume D75.1
   high altitude D75.1
   maternal-fetal transfusion P61.1
   stress D75.1
emotional D75.1
erythropoietin D75.1
familial (benign) D75.0
Gaisböck's (hypertonica) D75.1
high altitude D75.1
hypertonica D75.1
hypoxemic D75.1
neonatorum P61.1
nephrogenous D75.1
relative D75.1
secondary D75.1
spurious D75.1
stress D75.1
vera D45

Polycytosis cryptogenica D75.1
Polydactylism, polydactyly Q69.9
toes Q69.2
Polydipsia R63.1
Polydystrophy, pseudo-Hurler E77.0
Polyembryoma — *see* Neoplasm, malignant, by site
Polyglandular
deficiency E31.0
dyscrasia E31.9
dysfunction E31.9
syndrome E31.8
Polyhydramnios O40.- ☑
Polymastia Q83.1
Polymenorrhea N92.0
Polymyalgia M35.3
arteritica, giant cell M31.5
rheumatica M35.3
   with giant cell arteritis M31.5
Polymyositis (acute) (chronic) (hemorrhagic) M33.20
with
   myopathy M33.22
   respiratory involvement M33.21
   skin involvement — *see* Dermatopolymyositis
   specified organ involvement NEC M33.29
ossificans (generalisata) (progressiva) — *see* Myositis,
   ossificans, progressiva
Polyneuritis, polyneuritic (*see also* Polyneuropathy)
acute (post-)infective G61.0
alcoholic G62.1
cranialis G52.7
demyelinating, chronic inflammatory (CIDP) G61.81
diabetic — *see* Diabetes, polyneuropathy
diphtheritic A36.83
due to lack of vitamin NEC E56.9 [G63]
endemic E51.11
erythredema — *see* subcategory T56.1 ☑
febrile, acute G61.0
hereditary ataxic G60.1
idiopathic, acute G61.0
infective (acute) G61.0
inflammatory, chronic demyelinating (CIDP) G61.81
nutritional E63.9 [G63]
postinfective (acute) G61.0
specified NEC G62.89
Polyneuropathy (peripheral) G62.9
alcoholic G62.1
amyloid (Portuguese) E85.1 [G63]
arsenical G62.2
critical illness G62.81
demyelinating, chronic inflammatory (CIDP) G61.81
diabetic — *see* Diabetes, polyneuropathy
drug-induced G62.0
hereditary G60.9
   specified NEC G60.8
idiopathic G60.9
   progressive G60.3
in (due to)
   alcohol G62.1
      sequelae G65.2
   amyloidosis, familial (Portuguese) E85.1 [G63]
   antitetanus serum G61.1
   arsenic G62.2
      sequelae G65.2
   avitaminosis NEC E56.9 [G63]
   beriberi E51.11
   collagen vascular disease NEC M35.9 [G63]
   deficiency (of)
      B (-complex) vitamins E53.9 [G63]
      vitamin B6 E53.1 [G63]
   diabetes — *see* Diabetes, polyneuropathy
   diphtheria A36.83
   drug or medicament G62.0
      correct substance properly administered — *see*
         Table of Drugs and Chemicals, by drug,
         adverse effect
      overdose or wrong substance given or taken
         — *see* Table of Drugs and Chemicals, by
         drug, poisoning
   endocrine disease NEC E34.9 [G63]
   herpes zoster B02.23
   hypoglycemia E16.2 [G63]
   infectious
      disease NEC B99 ☑ [G63]
      mononucleosis B27.91
   lack of vitamin NEC E56.9 [G63]
   lead G62.2
      sequelae G65.2
   leprosy A30.9 [G63]

Polyneuropathy — continued
in — continued
Lyme disease A69.22
metabolic disease NEC E88.9 [G63]
microscopic polyangiitis M31.7 [G63]
mumps B26.84
neoplastic disease (see also Neoplasm) D49.9 [G63]
nutritional deficiency NEC E63.9 [G63]
organophosphate compounds G62.2
sequelae G65.2
parasitic disease NEC B89 [G63]
pellagra E52 [G63]
polyarteritis nodosa M30.0
porphyria E80.20 [G63]
radiation G62.82
rheumatoid arthritis — see Rheumatoid, polyneuropathy
sarcoidosis D86.89
serum G61.1
syphilis (late) A52.15
congenital A50.43
systemic
connective tissue disorder M35.9 [G63]
lupus erythematosus M32.19
toxic agent NEC G62.2
sequelae G65.2
triorthocresyl phosphate G62.2
sequelae G65.2
tuberculosis A17.89
uremia N18.9 [G63]
vitamin B12 deficiency E53.8 [G63]
with anemia (pernicious) D51.0 [G63]
due to dietary deficiency D51.3 [G63]
zoster B02.23
inflammatory G61.9
chronic demyelinating (CIDP) G61.81
sequelae G65.1
specified NEC G61.89
lead G62.2
sequelae G65.2
nutritional NEC E63.9 [G63]
postherpetic (zoster) B02.23
progressive G60.3
radiation-induced G62.82
sensory (hereditary) (idiopathic) G60.8
specified NEC G62.89
syphilitic (late) A52.15
congenital A50.43
Polyopia H53.8
Polyorchism, polyorchidism Q55.21
Polyosteoarthritis (see also Osteoarthritis, generalized) M15.9
post-traumatic M15.3
specified NEC M15.8
Polyostotic fibrous dysplasia Q78.1
Polyotia Q17.0
Polyp, polypus
accessory sinus J33.8
adenocarcinoma in — see Neoplasm, malignant, by site
adenocarcinoma in situ in — see Neoplasm, in situ, by site
adenoid tissue J33.0
adenomatous (see also Neoplasm, benign, by site)
adenocarcinoma in — see Neoplasm, malignant, by site
adenocarcinoma in situ in — see Neoplasm, in situ, by site
carcinoma in — see Neoplasm, malignant, by site
carcinoma in situ in — see Neoplasm, in situ, by site
multiple — see Neoplasm, benign
adenocarcinoma in — see Neoplasm, malignant, by site
adenocarcinoma in situ in — see Neoplasm, in situ, by site
antrum J33.8
anus, anal (canal) K62.0
Bartholin's gland N84.3
bladder D41.4
carcinoma in — see Neoplasm, malignant, by site
carcinoma in situ in — see Neoplasm, in situ, by site
cecum D12.0
cervix (uteri) N84.1
in pregnancy or childbirth — see Pregnancy, complicated by, abnormal, cervix
mucous N84.1
nonneoplastic N84.1

Polyp, polypus — continued
choanal J33.0
cholesterol K82.4
clitoris N84.3
colon K63.5
adenomatous D12.6
ascending D12.2
cecum D12.0
descending D12.4
inflammatory K51.40
with
abscess K51.414
complication K51.419
specified NEC K51.418
fistula K51.413
intestinal obstruction K51.412
rectal bleeding K51.411
sigmoid D12.5
transverse D12.3
corpus uteri N84.0
dental K04.0
duodenum K31.7
ear (middle) H74.4- ✅
endometrium N84.0
ethmoidal (sinus) J33.8
fallopian tube N84.8
female genital tract N84.9
specified NEC N84.8
frontal (sinus) J33.8
gallbladder K82.4
gingiva, gum K06.8
labia, labium (majus) (minus) N84.3
larynx (mucous) J38.1
adenomatous D14.1
malignant — see Neoplasm, malignant, by site
maxillary (sinus) J33.8
middle ear — see Polyp, ear (middle)
myometrium N84.0
nares
anterior J33.9
posterior J33.0
nasal (mucous) J33.9
cavity J33.0
septum J33.0
nasopharyngeal J33.0
nose (mucous) J33.9
oviduct N84.8
pharynx J39.2
placenta O90.89
prostate — see Enlargement, enlarged, prostate
pudenda, pudendum N84.3
pulpal (dental) K04.0
rectum (nonadenomatous) K62.1
adenomatous — see Polyp, adenomatous
septum (nasal) J33.0
sinus (accessory) (ethmoidal) (frontal) (maxillary) (sphenoidal) J33.8
sphenoidal (sinus) J33.8
stomach K31.7
adenomatous D13.1
tube, fallopian N84.8
turbinate, mucous membrane J33.8
umbilical, newborn P83.6
ureter N28.89
urethra N36.2
uterus (body) (corpus) (mucous) N84.0
cervix N84.1
in pregnancy or childbirth — see Pregnancy, complicated by, tumor, uterus
vagina N84.2
vocal cord (mucous) J38.1
vulva N84.3
Polyphagia R63.2
Polyploidy Q92.7
Polypoid — see condition
Polyposis (see also Polyp)
coli (adenomatous) D12.6
adenocarcinoma in C18.9
adenocarcinoma in situ in — see Neoplasm, in situ, by site
carcinoma in C18.9
colon (adenomatous) D12.6
familial D12.6
adenocarcinoma in situ in — see Neoplasm, in situ, by site
intestinal (adenomatous) D12.6
malignant lymphomatous C83.1- ✅

Polyposis — continued
multiple, adenomatous (see also Neoplasm, benign) D36.9
Polyradiculitis — see Polyneuropathy
Polyradiculoneuropathy (acute) (postinfective) (segmentally demyelinating) G61.0
Polyserositis
due to pericarditis I31.1
pericardial I31.1
periodic, familial E85.0
tuberculous A19.9
acute A19.1
chronic A19.8
Polysplenia syndrome Q89.09
Polysyndactyly (see also Syndactylism, syndactyly) Q70.4
Polytrichia L68.3
Polyunguia Q84.6
Polyuria R35.8
nocturnal R35.1
psychogenic F45.8
Pompe's disease (glycogen storage) E74.02
Pompholyx L30.1
Poncet's disease (tuberculous rheumatism) A18.09
Pond fracture — see Fracture, skull
Ponos B55.0
Pons, pontine — see condition
Poor
aesthetic of existing restoration of tooth K08.56
contractions, labor O62.2
gingival margin to tooth restoration K08.51
personal hygiene R46.0
prenatal care, affecting management of pregnancy — see Pregnancy, complicated by, insufficient, prenatal care
sucking reflex (newborn) R29.2
urinary stream R39.12
vision NEC H54.7
Poradenitis, nostras inguinalis or venerea A55
Porencephaly (congenital) (developmental) (true) Q04.6
acquired G93.0
nondevelopmental G93.0
traumatic (post) F07.89
Porocephaliasis B88.8
Porokeratosis Q82.8
Poroma, eccrine — see Neoplasm, skin, benign
Porphyria (South African) E80.20
acquired E80.20
acute intermittent (hepatic) (Swedish) E80.21
cutanea tarda (hereditary) (symptomatic) E80.1
due to drugs E80.20
correct substance properly administered — see Table of Drugs and Chemicals, by drug, adverse effect
overdose or wrong substance given or taken — see Table of Drugs and Chemicals, by drug, poisoning
erythropoietic (congenital) (hereditary) E80.0
hepatocutaneous type E80.1
secondary E80.20
toxic NEC E80.20
variegata E80.20
Porphyrinuria — see Porphyria
Porphyruria — see Porphyria
Port wine nevus, mark, or stain Q82.5
Portal — see condition
Posadas-Wernicke disease B38.9
Positive
culture (nonspecific)
blood R78.81
bronchial washings R84.5
cerebrospinal fluid R83.5
cervix uteri R87.5
nasal secretions R84.5
nipple discharge R89.5
nose R84.5
staphylococcus (Methicillin susceptible) Z22.321
Methicillin resistant Z22.322
peritoneal fluid R85.5
pleural fluid R84.5
prostatic secretions R86.5
saliva R85.5
seminal fluid R86.5
sputum R84.5
synovial fluid R89.5
throat scrapings R84.5
urine R82.7
vagina R87.5
vulva R87.5

✅ Additional Character Required — Refer to the Tabular List for Character Selection · Subterms under main terms may continue to next column or page

Positive — *continued*
  culture — *continued*
    wound secretions R89.5
   PPD (skin test) R76.11
   serology for syphilis A53.0
    with signs or symptoms — *code as* Syphilis, by site
     and stage
    false R76.8
   skin test, tuberculin (without active tuberculosis)
    R76.11
   test, human immunodeficiency virus (HIV) R75
   VDRL A53.0
    with signs or symptoms — *code by* site and stage
     under Syphilis A53.9
   Wassermann reaction A53.0
Postcardiotomy syndrome I97.0
Postcaval ureter Q62.62
Postcholecystectomy syndrome K91.5
Postclimacteric bleeding N95.0
Postcommissurotomy syndrome I97.0
Postconcussional syndrome F07.81
Postcontusional syndrome F07.81
Postcricoid region — *see* condition
Post-dates (40-42 weeks) (pregnancy) (mother) O48.0
  more than 42 weeks gestation O48.1
Postencephalitic syndrome F07.89
Posterior — *see* condition
Posterolateral sclerosis (spinal cord) — *see* Degeneration, combined
Postexanthematous — *see* condition
Postfebrile — *see* condition
Postgastrectomy dumping syndrome K91.1
Posthemiplegic chorea — *see* Monoplegia
Posthemorrhagic anemia (chronic) D50.0
  acute D62
  newborn P61.3
Postherpetic neuralgia (zoster) B02.29
  trigeminal B02.22
Posthitis N47.7
Postimmunization complication or reaction — *see* Complications, vaccination
Postinfectious — *see* condition
Postlaminectomy syndrome NEC M96.1
Postleukotomy syndrome F07.0
Postmastectomy lymphedema (syndrome) I97.2
Postmaturity, postmature (over 42 weeks)
  maternal (over 42 weeks gestation) O48.1
  newborn P08.22
Postmeasles complication NEC (*see also* condition)
  B05.89
Postmenopausal
  endometrium (atrophic) N95.8
   suppurative (*see also* Endometritis) N71.9
  osteoporosis — *see* Osteoporosis, postmenopausal
Postnasal drip R09.82
  due to
   allergic rhinitis — *see* Rhinitis, allergic
   common cold J00
   gastroesophageal reflux — *see* Reflux, gastroesophageal
   nasopharyngitis — *see* Nasopharyngitis
   other known condition — *code to* condition
   sinusitis — *see* Sinusitis
Postnatal — *see* condition
Postoperative (postprocedural) — *see* Complication, postoperative
  pneumothorax, therapeutic Z98.3
  state NEC Z98.89
Postpancreatectomy hyperglycemia E89.1
Postpartum — *see* Puerperal
Postphlebitic syndrome — *see* Syndrome, postthrombotic
Postpolio (myelitic) **syndrome** G14
Postpoliomyelitic (*see also* condition)
  osteopathy — *see* Osteopathy, after poliomyelitis
Postprocedural (*see also* Postoperative)
  hypoinsulinemia E89.1
Postschizophrenic depression F32.8
Postsurgery status (*see also* Status (post))
  pneumothorax, therapeutic Z98.3
Post-term (40-42 weeks) (pregnancy) (mother) O48.0
  infant P08.21
  more than 42 weeks gestation (mother) O48.1
Post-traumatic brain syndrome, nonpsychotic F07.81
Post-typhoid abscess A01.09
Postures, hysterical F44.2

Postvaccinal reaction or complication — *see* Complications, vaccination
Postvalvulotomy syndrome I97.0
Potain's
  disease (pulmonary edema) — *see* Edema, lung
  syndrome (gastrectasis with dyspepsia) K31.0
Potter's
  asthma J62.8
  facies Q60.6
  lung J62.8
  syndrome (with renal agenesis) Q60.6
Pott's
  curvature (spinal) A18.01
  disease or paraplegia A18.01
  spinal curvature A18.01
  tumor, puffy — *see* Osteomyelitis, specified type NEC
Pouch
  bronchus Q32.4
  Douglas' — *see* condition
  esophagus, esophageal, congenital Q39.6
   acquired K22.5
  gastric K31.4
  Hartmann's K82.8
  pharynx, pharyngeal (congenital) Q38.7
Pouchitis K91.850
Poultrymen's itch B88.0
Poverty NEC Z59.6
  extreme Z59.5
Poxvirus NEC B08.8
Prader-Willi syndrome Q87.1
Preauricular appendage or tag Q17.0
Prebetalipoproteinemia (acquired) (essential) (familial) (hereditary) (primary) (secondary) E78.1
  with chylomicronemia E78.3
Precipitate labor or delivery O62.3
Preclimacteric bleeding (menorrhagia) N92.4
Precocious
  adrenarche E30.1
  menarche E30.1
  menstruation E30.1
  pubarche E30.1
  puberty E30.1
   central E22.8
  sexual development NEC E30.1
  thelarche E30.8
Precocity, sexual (constitutional) (cryptogenic) (female) (idiopathic) (male) E30.1
  with adrenal hyperplasia E25.9
   congenital E25.0
Precordial pain R07.2
Predeciduous teeth K00.2
Prediabetes, prediabetic R73.09
  complicating
   pregnancy — *see* Pregnancy, complicated by, diseases of, specified type or system NEC
   puerperium O99.89
Predislocation status of hip at birth Q65.6
Pre-eclampsia O14.9- ☑
  with pre-existing hypertension — *see* Hypertension, complicating pregnancy, pre-existing, with, pre-eclampsia
  mild O14.0- ☑
  moderate O14.0- ☑
  severe O14.1- ☑
   with hemolysis, elevated liver enzymes and low platelet count (HELLP) O14.2- ☑
Pre-eruptive color change, teeth, tooth K00.8
Pre-excitation atrioventricular conduction I45.6
Preglaucoma H40.00- ☑
Pregnancy (single) (uterine) (*see also* Delivery and Puerperal)

> Note: The Tabular must be reviewed for assignment of appropriate seventh character for multiple gestation codes in Chapter 15

> Note: The Tabular must be reviewed for assignment of the appropriate character indicating the trimester of the pregnancy

  abdominal (ectopic) O00.0
   with viable fetus O36.7- ☑
  ampullar O00.1
  biochemical O02.81
  broad ligament O00.8
  cervical O00.8
  chemical O02.81

Pregnancy — *continued*
  complicated by (care of) (management affected by)
   abnormal, abnormality
    cervix O34.4- ☑
     causing obstructed labor O65.5
    cord (umbilical) O69.9 ☑
    findings on antenatal screening of mother O28.9
     biochemical O28.1
     chromosomal O28.5
     cytological O28.2
     genetic O28.5
     hematological O28.0
     radiological O28.4
     specified NEC O28.8
     ultrasonic O28.3
    glucose (tolerance) NEC O99.810
    pelvic organs O34.9- ☑
     specified NEC O34.8- ☑
      causing obstructed labor O65.5
    pelvis (bony) (major) NEC O33.0
    perineum O34.7- ☑
    position
     placenta O44.1- ☑
      without hemorrhage O44.0- ☑
     uterus O34.59- ☑
    uterus O34.59- ☑
     causing obstructed labor O65.5
     congenital O34.0- ☑
    vagina O34.6- ☑
     causing obstructed labor O65.5
    vulva O34.7- ☑
     causing obstructed labor O65.5
   abruptio placentae — *see* Abruptio placentae
   abscess or cellulitis
    bladder O23.1- ☑
    breast O91.11- ☑
    genital organ or tract O23.9- ☑
   abuse
    physical O9A.31 ☑ (*following* O99)
    psychological O9A.51 ☑ (*following* O99)
    sexual O9A.41 ☑ (*following* O99)
   adverse effect anesthesia O29.9- ☑
    aspiration pneumonitis O29.01- ☑
    cardiac arrest O29.11- ☑
    cardiac complication NEC O29.19- ☑
    cardiac failure O29.12- ☑
    central nervous system complication NEC O29.29- ☑
    cerebral anoxia O29.21- ☑
    failed or difficult intubation O29.6- ☑
    inhalation of stomach contents or secretions NOS O29.01- ☑
    local, toxic reaction O29.3X ☑
    Mendelson's syndrome O29.01- ☑
    pressure collapse of lung O29.02- ☑
    pulmonary complications NEC O29.09- ☑
    specified NEC O29.8X- ☑
    spinal and epidural type NEC O29.5X ☑
     induced headache O29.4- ☑
   albuminuria O12.1- ☑
   alcohol use O99.31- ☑
   amnionitis O41.12- ☑
   anaphylactoid syndrome of pregnancy O88.01- ☑
   anemia (conditions in D50-D64) (pre-existing) O99.01- ☑
    complicating the puerperium O99.03
   antepartum hemorrhage O46.9- ☑
    with coagulation defect — *see* Hemorrhage, antepartum, with coagulation defect
    specified NEC O46.8X- ☑
   appendicitis O99.61- ☑
   atrophy (yellow) (acute) liver (subacute) O26.61- ☑
   bariatric surgery status O99.84- ☑
   bicornis or bicornuate uterus O34.59- ☑
   biliary tract problems O26.61- ☑
   breech presentation O32.1 ☑
   cardiovascular diseases (conditions in I00-I09, I20-I52, I70-I99) O99.41- ☑
   cerebrovascular disorders (conditions in I60-I69) O99.41- ☑
   cervical shortening O26.87- ☑
   cervicitis O23.51- ☑
   chloasma (gravidarum) O26.89- ☑
   cholecystitis O99.61- ☑
   cholestasis (intrahepatic) O26.61- ☑

Pregnancy — *continued*
complicated by — *continued*
  chorioamnionitis O41.12- ☑
  circulatory system disorder (conditions in I00-I09, I20-I99, O99.41-)
  compound presentation O32.6 ☑
  conjoined twins O30.02- ☑
  connective system disorders (conditions in M00-M99) O99.89
  contracted pelvis (general) O33.1
    inlet O33.2
    outlet O33.3 ☑
  convulsions (eclamptic) (uremic) (*see also* Eclampsia) O15.9
  cracked nipple O92.11- ☑
  cystitis O23.1- ☑
  cystocele O34.8- ☑
  death of fetus (near term) O36.4 ☑
    early pregnancy O02.1
    of one fetus or more in multiple gestation O31.2- ☑
  deciduitis O41.14- ☑
  decreased fetal movement O36.81- ☑
  dental problems O99.61- ☑
  diabetes (mellitus) O24.91- ☑
    gestational (pregnancy induced) — *see* Diabetes, gestational
    pre-existing O24.31- ☑
      specified NEC O24.81- ☑
      type 1 O24.01- ☑
      type 2 O24.11- ☑
  digestive system disorders (conditions in K00-K93) O99.61- ☑
  diseases of — *see* Pregnancy, complicated by, specified body system disease
    biliary tract O26.61- ☑
    blood NEC (conditions in D65-D77) O99.11- ☑
    liver O26.61- ☑
    specified NEC O99.89
  disorders of — *see* Pregnancy, complicated by, specified body system disorder
    amniotic fluid and membranes O41.9- ☑
      specified NEC O41.8X- ☑
    biliary tract O26.61- ☑
    ear and mastoid process (conditions in H60-H95) O99.89
    eye and adnexa (conditions in H00-H59) O99.89
    liver O26.61- ☑
    skin (conditions in L00-L99) O99.71- ☑
    specified NEC O99.89
  displacement, uterus NEC O34.59- ☑
    causing obstructed labor O65.5
  disproportion (due to) O33.9
    fetal deformities NEC O33.7
    generally contracted pelvis O33.1
    hydrocephalic fetus O33.6 ☑
    inlet contraction of pelvis O33.2
    mixed maternal and fetal origin O33.4 ☑
    specified NEC O33.8
  double uterus O34.59- ☑
    causing obstructed labor O65.5
  drug use (conditions in F11-F19) O99.32- ☑
  eclampsia, eclamptic (coma) (convulsions) (delirium) (nephritis) (uremia) (*see also* Eclampsia) O15.-
  ectopic pregnancy — *see* Pregnancy, ectopic
  edema O12.0- ☑
    with
      gestational hypertension, mild (*see also* Preeclampsia) O14.0- ☑
      proteinuria O12.2- ☑
  effusion, amniotic fluid — *see* Pregnancy, complicated by, premature rupture of membranes
  elderly
    multigravida O09.52- ☑
    primigravida O09.51- ☑
  embolism (*see also* Embolism, obstetric, pregnancy) O88.- ☑
  endocrine diseases NEC O99.28- ☑
  endometritis O86.12
  excessive weight gain O26.0- ☑
  exhaustion O26.81- ☑
    during labor and delivery O75.81
  face presentation O32.3 ☑
  failed induction of labor O61.9
    instrumental O61.1
    mechanical O61.1

Pregnancy — *continued*
complicated by — *continued*
  failed induction of labor — *continued*
    medical O61.0
    specified NEC O61.8
    surgical O61.1
  failed or difficult intubation for anesthesia O29.6- ☑
  false labor (pains) O47.9
    at or after 37 completed weeks of pregnancy O47.1
    before 37 completed weeks of pregnancy O47.0- ☑
  fatigue O26.81- ☑
    during labor and delivery O75.81
  fatty metamorphosis of liver O26.61- ☑
  female genital mutilation O34.8- ☑ [N90.81-] ☑
  fetal (maternal care for)
    abnormality or damage O35.9 ☑
      acid-base balance O68
      specified type NEC O35.8 ☑
    acidemia O68
    acidosis O68
    alkalosis O68
    anemia and thrombocytopenia O36.82- ☑
    anencephaly O35.0 ☑
    chromosomal abnormality (conditions in Q90-Q99) O35.1 ☑
    conjoined twins O30.02- ☑
    damage from
      amniocentesis O35.7 ☑
      biopsy procedures O35.7 ☑
      drug addiction O35.5 ☑
      hematological investigation O35.7 ☑
      intrauterine contraceptive device O35.7 ☑
      maternal
        alcohol addiction O35.4 ☑
        cytomegalovirus infection O35.3 ☑
        disease NEC O35.8 ☑
        drug addiction O35.5 ☑
        listeriosis O35.8 ☑
        rubella O35.3 ☑
        toxoplasmosis O35.8 ☑
        viral infection O35.3 ☑
      medical procedure NEC O35.7 ☑
      radiation O35.6 ☑
    death (near term) O36.4 ☑
      early pregnancy O02.1
    decreased movement O36.81- ☑
    disproportion due to deformity (fetal) O33.7
    excessive growth (large for dates) O36.6- ☑
    growth retardation O36.59- ☑
      light for dates O36.59- ☑
      small for dates O36.59- ☑
    heart rate irregularity (bradycardia) (decelerations) (tachycardia) O76
    hereditary disease O35.2 ☑
    hydrocephalus O35.0 ☑
    intrauterine death O36.4 ☑
    poor growth O36.59- ☑
      light for dates O36.59- ☑
      small for dates O36.59- ☑
    problem O36.9- ☑
      specified NEC O36.89- ☑
    reduction (elective) O31.3- ☑
    selective termination O31.3- ☑
    spina bifida O35.0 ☑
    thrombocytopenia O36.82- ☑
  fibroid (tumor) (uterus) O34.1- ☑
  fissure of nipple O92.11- ☑
  gallstones O99.61- ☑
  gastric banding status O99.84- ☑
  gastric bypass status O99.84- ☑
  genital herpes (asymptomatic) (history of) (inactive) O98.51- ☑
  genital tract infection O23.9- ☑
  glomerular diseases (conditions in N00-N07) O26.83- ☑
    with hypertension, pre-existing — *see* Hypertension, complicating, pregnancy, pre-existing, with, renal disease
  gonorrhea O98.21- ☑
  grand multiparity O09.4 ☑
  habitual aborter — *see* Pregnancy, complicated by, recurrent pregnancy loss

Pregnancy — *continued*
complicated by — *continued*
  HELLP syndrome (hemolysis, elevated liver enzymes and low platelet count) O14.2- ☑
  hemorrhage
    antepartum — *see* Hemorrhage, antepartum
    before 20 completed weeks gestation O20.9
      specified NEC O20.8
    due to premature separation, placenta (*see also* Abruptio placentae) O45.9- ☑
    early O20.9
      specified NEC O20.8
    threatened abortion O20.0
  hemorrhoids O22.4- ☑
  hepatitis (viral) O98.41- ☑
  herniation of uterus O34.59- ☑
  high
    head at term O32.4 ☑
    risk — *see* Supervision (of) (for), high-risk
  history of in utero procedure during previous pregnancy O09.82- ☑
  HIV O98.71- ☑
  human immunodeficiency virus (HIV) disease O98.71- ☑
  hydatidiform mole (*see also* Mole, hydatidiform) O01.9
  hydramnios O40.- ☑
  hydrocephalic fetus (disproportion) O33.6 ☑
  hydrops
    amnii O40.- ☑
    fetalis O36.2- ☑
      associated with isoimmunization (*see also* Pregnancy, complicated by, isoimmunization) O36.11- ☑
  hydrorrhea O42.90
  hyperemesis (gravidarum) (mild) (*see also* Hyperemesis, gravidarum) O21.0
  hypertension — *see* Hypertension, complicating pregnancy
  hypertensive
    heart and renal disease, pre-existing — *see* Hypertension, complicating, pregnancy, pre-existing, with, heart disease, with renal disease
    heart disease, pre-existing — *see* Hypertension, complicating, pregnancy, pre-existing, with heart disease
    renal disease, pre-existing — *see* Hypertension, complicating, pregnancy, pre-existing, with, renal disease
  hypotension O26.5- ☑
  immune disorders NEC (conditions in D80-D89) O99.11- ☑
  incarceration, uterus O34.51- ☑
  incompetent cervix O34.3- ☑
  inconclusive fetal viability O36.80 ☑
  infection(s) O98.91- ☑
    amniotic fluid or sac O41.10- ☑
    bladder O23.1- ☑
    carrier state NEC O99.830
      streptococcus B O99.820
    genital organ or tract O23.9- ☑
      specified NEC O23.59- ☑
    genitourinary tract O23.9- ☑
    gonorrhea O98.21- ☑
    hepatitis (viral) O98.41- ☑
    HIV O98.71- ☑
    human immunodeficiency virus (HIV) O98.71- ☑
    kidney O23.0- ☑
    nipple O91.01- ☑
    parasitic disease O98.91- ☑
      specified NEC O98.81- ☑
    protozoal disease O98.61- ☑
    sexually transmitted NEC O98.31- ☑
    specified type NEC O98.81- ☑
    syphilis O98.11- ☑
    tuberculosis O98.01- ☑
    urethra O23.2- ☑
    urinary (tract) O23.4- ☑
      specified NEC O23.3- ☑
    viral disease O98.51- ☑
  injury or poisoning (conditions in S00-T88) O9A.21- ☑ (*following* O99)
  due to abuse
    physical O9A.31- ☑ (*following* O99)

☑ **Additional Character Required** — Refer to the Tabular List for Character Selection   ▽ Subterms under main terms may continue to next column or page

Pregnancy — *continued*
  complicated by — *continued*
    injury or poisoning — *continued*
      due to abuse — *continued*
        psychological O9A.51- ☑ (*following* O99)
        sexual O9A.41- ☑ (*following* O99)
    insufficient
      prenatal care O09.3- ☑
      weight gain O26.1- ☑
    insulin resistance O26.89 ☑
    intrauterine fetal death (near term) O36.4 ☑
      early pregnancy O02.1
      multiple gestation (one fetus or more)
        O31.2- ☑
    isoimmunization O36.11- ☑
      anti-A sensitization O36.11- ☑
      anti-B sensitization O36.19- ☑
      Rh O36.09- ☑
        anti-D antibody O36.01- ☑
      specified NEC O36.19- ☑
    laceration of uterus NEC O71.81
    malformation
      placenta, placental (vessel) O43.10- ☑
        specified NEC O43.19- ☑
      uterus (congenital) O34.0- ☑
    malnutrition (conditions in E40-E46) O25.1- ☑
    maternal hypotension syndrome O26.5- ☑
    mental disorders (conditions in F01-F09, F20-F99)
      O99.34- ☑
      alcohol use O99.31- ☑
      drug use O99.32- ☑
      smoking O99.33- ☑
    mentum presentation O32.3 ☑
    metabolic disorders O99.28- ☑
    missed
      abortion O02.1
      delivery O36.4 ☑
    multiple gestations O30.9- ☑
      conjoined twins O30.02- ☑
      quadruplet — *see* Pregnancy, quadruplet
      specified complication NEC O31.8X- ☑
      specified number of multiples NEC — *see*
        Pregnancy, multiple (gestation), specified
        NEC
      triplet — *see* Pregnancy, triplet
      twin — *see* Pregnancy, twin
    musculoskeletal condition (conditions is M00-M99)
      O99.89
    necrosis, liver (conditions in K72) O26.61- ☑
    neoplasm
      benign
        cervix O34.4- ☑
        corpus uteri O34.1- ☑
        uterus O34.1- ☑
      malignant O9A.11- ☑ (*following* O99)
    nephropathy NEC O26.83- ☑
    nervous system condition (conditions in G00-G99)
      O99.35- ☑
    nutritional diseases NEC O99.28- ☑
    obesity (pre-existing) O99.21- ☑
    obesity surgery status O99.84- ☑
    oblique lie or presentation O32.2 ☑
    older mother — *see* Pregnancy, complicated by,
      elderly
    oligohydramnios O41.0- ☑
      with premature rupture of membranes (*see also*
        Pregnancy, complicated by, premature
        rupture of membranes) O42.- ☑
    onset (spontaneous) of labor after 37 completed
      weeks of gestation but before 39 completed
      weeks gestation, with delivery by (planned)
      cesarean section O75.82
    oophoritis O23.52- ☑
    overdose, drug (*see also* Table of Drugs and
      Chemicals, by drug, poisoning) O9A.21- ☑
      (*following* O99)
    oversize fetus O33.5 ☑
    papyraceous fetus O31.0- ☑
    pelvic inflammatory disease O99.89
    periodontal disease O99.61- ☑
    peripheral neuritis O26.82- ☑
    peritoneal (pelvic) adhesions O99.89
    phlebitis O22.9- ☑
    phlebopathy O22.9- ☑
    phlebothrombosis (superficial) O22.2- ☑
      deep O22.3- ☑

Pregnancy — *continued*
  complicated by — *continued*
    placenta accreta O43.21- ☑
    placenta increta O43.22- ☑
    placenta percreta O43.23- ☑
    placenta previa O44.1- ☑
      without hemorrhage O44.0- ☑
    placental disorder O43.9- ☑
      specified NEC O43.89- ☑
    placental dysfunction O43.89- ☑
    placental infarction O43.81- ☑
    placental insufficiency O36.51- ☑
    placental transfusion syndromes
      fetomaternal O43.01- ☑
      fetus to fetus O43.02- ☑
      maternofetal O43.01- ☑
    placentitis O41.14- ☑
    pneumonia O99.51- ☑
    poisoning (*see also* Table of Drugs and Chemicals)
      O9A.21 ☑ (*following* O99)
    polyhydramnios O40- ☑
    polymorphic eruption of pregnancy O26.86
    poor obstetric history NEC O09.29- ☑
    postmaturity (post-term) (40 to 42 weeks) O48.0
      more than 42 completed weeks gestation
        (prolonged) O48.1
    pre-eclampsia O14.9- ☑
      mild O14.0- ☑
      moderate O14.0- ☑
      severe O14.1- ☑
        with hemolysis, elevated liver enzymes and
          low platelet count (HELLP) O14.2- ☑
    premature labor — *see* Pregnancy, complicated
      by, preterm labor
    premature rupture of membranes O42.90
      with onset of labor
        after 24 hours O42.10
          after 37 weeks gestation O42.12
          pre-term (before 37 completed weeks
            of gestation) O42.11- ☑
        within 24 hours O42.00
          after 37 weeks gestation O42.02
          pre-term (before 37 completed weeks
            of gestation) O42.01- ☑
      after 37 weeks gestation O42.92
      full-term O42.92
      pre-term (before 37 completed weeks of gesta-
        tion) O42.91- ☑
    premature separation of placenta (*see also* Abrup-
      tio placentae) O45.9- ☑
    presentation, fetal — *see* Delivery, complicated
      by, malposition
    preterm delivery O60.10 ☑
    preterm labor
      with delivery O60.10 ☑
        preterm O60.10 ☑
        term O60.20 ☑
      without delivery O60.00
        second trimester O60.02
        third trimester O60.03
      second trimester
        with preterm delivery
          second trimester O60.12 ☑
          third trimester O60.13 ☑
        with term delivery O60.22 ☑
        without delivery O60.02
      third trimester
        with term delivery O60.23 ☑
        with third trimester preterm delivery
          O60.14 ☑
        without delivery O60.03
    previous history of — *see* Pregnancy, supervision
      of, high-risk
    prolapse, uterus O34.52- ☑
    proteinuria (gestational) O12.1- ☑
      with edema O12.2- ☑
    pruritic urticarial papules and plaques of pregnancy
      (PUPPP) O26.86
    pruritus (neurogenic) O26.89- ☑
    psychosis or psychoneurosis (puerperal) F53
    ptyalism O26.89- ☑
    PUPPP (pruritic urticarial papules and plaques of
      pregnancy) O26.86
    pyelitis O23.0- ☑
    recurrent pregnancy loss O26.2- ☑

Pregnancy — *continued*
  complicated by — *continued*
    renal disease or failure NEC O26.83- ☑
      with secondary hypertension, pre-existing —
        see Hypertension, complicating, pregnan-
        cy, pre-existing, secondary
      hypertensive, pre-existing — *see* Hypertension,
        complicating, pregnancy, pre-existing,
        with, renal disease
    respiratory condition (conditions in J00-J99)
      O99.51- ☑
    retained, retention
      dead ovum O02.0
      intrauterine contraceptive device O26.3- ☑
    retroversion, uterus O34.53- ☑
    Rh immunization, incompatibility or sensitization
      NEC O36.09- ☑
      anti-D antibody O36.01- ☑
    rupture
      amnion (premature) (*see also* Pregnancy, com-
        plicated by, premature rupture of mem-
        branes) O42- ☑
      membranes (premature) (*see also* Pregnancy,
        complicated by, premature rupture of
        membranes) O42- ☑
      uterus (during labor) O71.1
        before onset of labor O71.0- ☑
    salivation (excessive) O26.89- ☑
    salpingitis O23.52- ☑
    salpingo-oophoritis O23.52- ☑
    sepsis (conditions in A40, A41) O98.81- ☑
    size date discrepancy (uterine) O26.84- ☑
    skin condition (conditions in L00-L99) O99.71- ☑
    smoking (tobacco) O99.33- ☑
    social problem O09.7- ☑
    specified condition NEC O26.89- ☑
    spotting O26.85- ☑
    streptococcus B carrier state O99.820
    subluxation of symphysis (pubis) O26.71- ☑
    syphilis (conditions in A50-A53) O98.11- ☑
    threatened
      abortion O20.0
      labor O47.9
        at or after 37 completed weeks of gestation
          O47.1
        before 37 completed weeks of gestation
          O47.0- ☑
    thrombophlebitis (superficial) O22.2- ☑
    thrombosis O22.9- ☑
      cerebral venous O22.5- ☑
      cerebrovenous sinus O22.5- ☑
      deep O22.3- ☑
    torsion of uterus O34.59- ☑
    toxemia O14.9- ☑
    transverse lie or presentation O32.2 ☑
    tuberculosis (conditions in A15-A19) O98.01- ☑
    tumor (benign)
      cervix O34.4- ☑
      malignant O9A.11- ☑ (*following* O99)
      uterus O34.1- ☑
    unstable lie O32.0 ☑
    upper respiratory infection O99.51- ☑
    urethritis O23.2- ☑
    uterine size date discrepancy O26.84- ☑
    vaginitis or vulvitis O23.59- ☑
    varicose veins (lower extremities) O22.0- ☑
      genitals O22.1- ☑
      legs O22.0- ☑
      perineal O22.1- ☑
      vaginal or vulval O22.1- ☑
    venereal disease NEC (conditions in A63.8)
      O98.31- ☑
    venous disorders O22.9- ☑
      specified NEC O22.8X- ☑
    very young mother — *see* Pregnancy, complicated
      by, young mother
    viral diseases (conditions in A80-B09, B25-B34)
      O98.51- ☑
    vomiting O21.9
      due to diseases classified elsewhere O21.8
      hyperemesis gravidarum (mild) (*see also* Hyper-
        emesis, gravidarum) O21.0
      late (occurring after 20 weeks of gestation)
        O21.2
    young mother
      multigravida O09.62- ☑

Pregnancy — Pregnancy

Pregnancy — *continued*
  complicated by — *continued*
    young mother — *continued*
      primigravida O09.61- ☑
  complicated NOS O26.9- ☑
  concealed O09.3- ☑
  continuing following
    elective fetal reduction of one or more fetus O31.3- ☑
    intrauterine death of one or more fetus O31.2- ☑
    spontaneous abortion of one or more fetus O31.1- ☑
  cornual O00.8
  ectopic (ruptured) O00.9
    abdominal O00.0
      with viable fetus O36.7- ☑
    cervical O00.8
    complicated (by) O08.9
      afibrinogenemia O08.1
      cardiac arrest O08.81
      chemical damage of pelvic organ(s) O08.6
      circulatory collapse O08.3
      defibrination syndrome O08.1
      electrolyte imbalance O08.5
      embolism (amniotic fluid) (blood clot) (pulmonary) (septic) O08.2
      endometritis O08.0
      genital tract and pelvic infection O08.0
      hemorrhage (delayed) (excessive) O08.1
      infection
        genital tract or pelvic O08.0
        kidney O08.83
        urinary tract O08.3
      intravascular coagulation O08.1
      laceration of pelvic organ(s) O08.6
      metabolic disorder O08.5
      oliguria O08.4
      oophoritis O08.0
      parametritis O08.0
      pelvic peritonitis O08.0
      perforation of pelvic organ(s) O08.6
      renal failure or shutdown O08.4
      salpingitis or salpingo-oophoritis O08.0
      sepsis O08.82
      shock O08.83
        septic O08.82
      specified condition NEC O08.89
      tubular necrosis (renal) O08.4
      uremia O08.4
      urinary infection O08.83
      venous complication NEC O08.7
        embolism O08.2
    cornual O00.8
    intraligamentous O00.8
    mural O00.8
    ovarian O00.2
    specified site NEC O00.8
    tubal (ruptured) O00.1
  examination (normal) Z34.9- ☑
    first Z34.0- ☑
    high-risk — *see* Pregnancy, supervision of, high-risk
    specified Z34.8- ☑
  extrauterine — *see* Pregnancy, ectopic
  fallopian O00.1
  false F45.8
  hidden O09.3- ☑
  high-risk — *see* Pregnancy, supervision of, high-risk
  incidental finding Z33.1
  interstitial O00.8
  intraligamentous O00.8
  intramural O00.8
  intraperitoneal O00.0
  isthmian O00.1
  mesometric (mural) O00.8
  molar NEC O02.0
    complicated (by) O08.9
      afibrinogenemia O08.1
      cardiac arrest O08.81
      chemical damage of pelvic organ(s) O08.6
      circulatory collapse O08.3
      defibrination syndrome O08.1
      electrolyte imbalance O08.5
      embolism (amniotic fluid) (blood clot) (pulmonary) (septic) O08.2
      endometritis O08.0
      genital tract and pelvic infection O08.0
      hemorrhage (delayed) (excessive) O08.1

Pregnancy — *continued*
  molar — *continued*
    complicated — *continued*
      infection
        genital tract or pelvic O08.0
        kidney O08.83
        urinary tract O08.83
      intravascular coagulation O08.1
      laceration of pelvic organ(s) O08.6
      metabolic disorder O08.5
      oliguria O08.4
      oophoritis O08.0
      parametritis O08.0
      pelvic peritonitis O08.0
      perforation of pelvic organ(s) O08.6
      renal failure or shutdown O08.4
      salpingitis or salpingo-oophoritis O08.0
      sepsis O08.82
      shock O08.3
        septic O08.82
      specified condition NEC O08.89
      tubular necrosis (renal) O08.4
      uremia O08.4
      urinary infection O08.83
      venous complication NEC O08.7
        embolism O08.2
    hydatidiform (*see also* Mole, hydatidiform) O01.9
  multiple (gestation) O30.9- ☑
    greater than quadruplets — *see* Pregnancy, multiple (gestation), specified NEC
    specified NEC O30.80- ☑
      with
        two or more monoamniotic fetuses O30.82- ☑
        two or more monochorionic fetuses O30.81- ☑
      two or more monoamniotic fetuses O30.82- ☑
      two or more monochorionic fetuses O30.81- ☑
      unable to determine number of placenta and number of amniotic sacs O30.89- ☑
      unspecified number of placenta and unspecified number of amniotic sacs O30.80- ☑
  mural O00.8
  normal (supervision of) Z34.9- ☑
    first Z34.0- ☑
    high-risk — *see* Pregnancy, supervision of, high-risk
    specified Z34.8- ☑
  ovarian O00.2
  postmature (40 to 42 weeks) O48.0
    more than 42 weeks gestation O48.1
  post-term (40 to 42 weeks) O48.0
  prenatal care only Z34.9- ☑
    first Z34.0- ☑
    high-risk — *see* Pregnancy, supervision of, high-risk
    specified Z34.8- ☑
  prolonged (more than 42 weeks gestation) O48.1
  quadruplet O30.20- ☑
    with
      two or more monoamniotic fetuses O30.22- ☑
      two or more monochorionic fetuses O30.21- ☑
    two or more monoamniotic fetuses O30.22- ☑
    two or more monochorionic fetuses O30.21- ☑
    unable to determine number of placenta and number of amniotic sacs O30.29- ☑
    unspecified number of placenta and unspecified number of amniotic sacs O30.20- ☑
  quintuplet — *see* Pregnancy, multiple (gestation), specified NEC
  sextuplet — *see* Pregnancy, multiple (gestation), specified NEC
  supervision of
    concealed pregnancy O09.3- ☑
    elderly mother
      multigravida O09.52- ☑
      primigravida O09.51- ☑
    hidden pregnancy O09.3- ☑
    high-risk O09.9- ☑
      due to (history of)
        ectopic pregnancy O09.1- ☑
        elderly — *see* Pregnancy, supervision, elderly mother
        grand multiparity O09.4 ☑
        in utero procedure during previous pregnancy O09.82- ☑
        in vitro fertilization O09.81- ☑

Pregnancy — *continued*
  supervision of — *continued*
    high-risk — *continued*
      due to — *continued*
        infertility O09.0- ☑
        insufficient prenatal care O09.3- ☑
        molar pregnancy O09.1- ☑
        multiple previous pregnancies O09.4- ☑
        older mother — *see* Pregnancy, supervision of, elderly mother
        poor reproductive or obstetric history NEC O09.29- ☑
        pre-term labor O09.21- ☑
        previous
          neonatal death O09.29- ☑
          social problems O09.7- ☑
        specified NEC O09.89- ☑
        very young mother — *see* Pregnancy, supervision, young mother
      resulting from in vitro fertilization O09.81- ☑
    normal Z34.9- ☑
      first Z34.0- ☑
      specified NEC Z34.8- ☑
    young mother
      multigravida O09.62- ☑
      primigravida O09.61- ☑
  triplet O30.10- ☑
    with
      two or more monoamniotic fetuses O30.12- ☑
      two or more monochrorionic fetuses O30.11- ☑
    two or more monoamniotic fetuses O30.12- ☑
    two or more monochrorionic fetuses O30.11- ☑
    unable to determine number of placenta and number of amniotic sacs O30.19- ☑
    unspecified number of placenta and unspecified number of amniotic sacs O30.10- ☑
  tubal (with abortion) (with rupture) O00.1
  twin O30.00- ☑
    conjoined O30.02- ☑
    dichorionic/diamniotic (two placenta, two amniotic sacs) O30.04- ☑
    monochorionic/diamniotic (one placenta, two amniotic sacs) O30.03- ☑
    monochorionic/monoamniotic (one placenta, one amniotic sac) O30.01- ☑
    unable to determine number of placenta and number of amniotic sacs O30.09- ☑
    unspecified number of placenta and unspecified number of amniotic sacs O30.00- ☑
  unwanted Z64.0
  weeks of gestation
    8 weeks Z3A.08 (*following* Z36)
    9 weeks Z3A.09 (*following* Z36)
    10 weeks Z3A.10 (*following* Z36)
    11 weeks Z3A.11 (*following* Z36)
    12 weeks Z3A.12 (*following* Z36)
    13 weeks Z3A.13 (*following* Z36)
    14 weeks Z3A.14 (*following* Z36)
    15 weeks Z3A.15 (*following* Z36)
    16 weeks Z3A.16 (*following* Z36)
    17 weeks Z3A.17 (*following* Z36)
    18 weeks Z3A.18 (*following* Z36)
    19 weeks Z3A.19 (*following* Z36)
    20 weeks Z3A.20 (*following* Z36)
    21 weeks Z3A.21 (*following* Z36)
    22 weeks Z3A.22 (*following* Z36)
    23 weeks Z3A.23 (*following* Z36)
    24 weeks Z3A.24 (*following* Z36)
    25 weeks Z3A.25 (*following* Z36)
    26 weeks Z3A.26 (*following* Z36)
    27 weeks Z3A.27 (*following* Z36)
    28 weeks Z3A.28 (*following* Z36)
    29 weeks Z3A.29 (*following* Z36)
    30 weeks Z3A.30 (*following* Z36)
    31 weeks Z3A.31 (*following* Z36)
    32 weeks Z3A.32 (*following* Z36)
    33 weeks Z3A.33 (*following* Z36)
    34 weeks Z3A.34 (*following* Z36)
    35 weeks Z3A.35 (*following* Z36)
    36 weeks Z3A.36 (*following* Z36)
    37 weeks Z3A.37 (*following* Z36)
    38 weeks Z3A.38 (*following* Z36)
    39 weeks Z3A.39 (*following* Z36)
    40 weeks Z3A.40 (*following* Z36)
    41 weeks Z3A.41 (*following* Z36)
    42 weeks Z3A.42 (*following* Z36)

Pregnancy — *continued*
  weeks of gestation — *continued*
    greater than 42 weeks Z3A.49 (*following* Z36)
    less than 8 weeks Z3A.01 (*following* Z36)
    not specified Z3A.00 (*following* Z36)
Preiser's disease — *see* Osteonecrosis, secondary, due to, trauma, metacarpus
Pre-kwashiorkor — *see* Malnutrition, severe
Preleukemia (syndrome) D46.9
Preluxation, hip, congenital Q65.6
Premature (*see also* condition)
  adrenarche E27.0
  aging E34.8
  beats I49.40
    atrial I49.1
    auricular I49.1
    supraventricular I49.1
  birth NEC — *see* Preterm, newborn
  closure, foramen ovale Q21.8
  contraction
    atrial I49.1
    atrioventricular I49.2
    auricular I49.1
    auriculoventricular I49.49
    heart (extrasystole) I49.49
    junctional I49.2
    ventricular I49.3
  delivery (*see also* Pregnancy, complicated by, preterm labor) O60.10 ☑
  ejaculation F52.4
  infant NEC — *see* Preterm, newborn
    light-for-dates — *see* Light for dates
  labor — *see* Pregnancy, complicated by, preterm labor
  lungs P28.0
  menopause E28.319
    asymptomatic E28.319
    symptomatic E28.310
  newborn
    less than 37 completed weeks — *see* Preterm, newborn
    extreme (less than 28 completed weeks) — *see* Immaturity, extreme
  puberty E30.1
  rupture membranes or amnion — *see* Pregnancy, complicated by, premature rupture of membranes
  senility E34.8
  thelarche E30.8
  ventricular systole I49.3
Prematurity NEC (less than 37 completed weeks) — *see* Preterm, newborn
  extreme (less than 28 completed weeks) — *see* Immaturity, extreme
Premenstrual
  dysphoric disorder (PMDD) N94.3
  tension (syndrome) N94.3
Premolarization, cuspids K00.2
Prenatal
  care, normal pregnancy — *see* Pregnancy, normal
  screening of mother Z36
  teeth K00.6
Preparatory care for subsequent treatment NEC
  for dialysis Z49.01
    peritoneal Z49.02
Prepartum — *see* condition
Preponderance, left or right ventricular I51.7
Prepuce — *see* condition
PRES (posterior reversible encephalopathy syndrome) I67.83
Presbycardia R54
Presbycusis, presbyacusia H91.1- ☑
Presbyesophagus K22.8
Presbyophrenia F03 ☑
Presbyopia H52.4
Prescription of contraceptives (initial) Z30.019
  emergency (postcoital) Z30.012
  implantable subdermal Z30.019
  injectable Z30.013
  intrauterine contraceptive device Z30.014
  pills Z30.011
  postcoital (emergency) Z30.012
  repeat Z30.40
    implantable subdermal Z30.49
    injectable Z30.42
    pills Z30.41
    specified type NEC Z30.49
  specified type NEC Z30.018

Presence (of)
  ankle-joint implant (functional) (prosthesis) Z96.66- ☑
  aortocoronary (bypass) graft Z95.1
  arterial-venous shunt (dialysis) Z99.2
  artificial
    eye (globe) Z97.0
    heart (fully implantable) (mechanical) Z95.812
      valve Z95.2
    larynx Z96.3
    lens (intraocular) Z96.1
    limb (complete) (partial) Z97.1- ☑
      arm Z97.1- ☑
        bilateral Z97.15
      leg Z97.1- ☑
        bilateral Z97.16
  audiological implant (functional) Z96.29
  bladder implant (functional) Z96.0
  bone
    conduction hearing device Z96.29
    implant (functional) NEC Z96.7
    joint (prosthesis) — *see* Presence, joint implant
  cardiac
    defibrillator (functional) (with synchronous cardiac pacemaker) Z95.810
    implant or graft Z95.9
      specified type NEC Z95.818
    pacemaker Z95.0
  cerebrospinal fluid drainage device Z98.2
  cochlear implant (functional) Z96.21
  contact lens (es) Z97.3
  coronary artery graft or prosthesis Z95.5
  CSF shunt Z98.2
  dental prosthesis device Z97.2
  dentures Z97.2
  device (external) NEC Z97.8
    cardiac NEC Z95.818
    heart assist Z95.811
    implanted (functional) Z96.9
      specified NEC Z96.89
    prosthetic Z97.8
  ear implant Z96.20
    cochlear implant Z96.21
    myringotomy tube Z96.22
    specified type NEC Z96.29
  elbow-joint implant (functional) (prosthesis) Z96.62- ☑
  endocrine implant (functional) NEC Z96.49
  eustachian tube stent or device (functional) Z96.29
  external hearing-aid or device Z97.4
  finger-joint implant (functional) (prosthetic) Z96.69- ☑
  functional implant Z96.9
    specified NEC Z96.89
  graft
    cardiac NEC Z95.818
    vascular NEC Z95.828
  hearing-aid or device (external) Z97.4
    implant (bone) (cochlear) (functional) Z96.21
  heart assist device Z95.811
  heart valve implant (functional) Z95.2
    prosthetic Z95.2
    specified type NEC Z95.4
    xenogenic Z95.3
  hip-joint implant (functional) (prosthesis) Z96.64- ☑
  implanted device (artificial) (functional) (prosthetic) Z96.9
    automatic cardiac defibrillator (with synchronous cardiac pacemaker) Z95.810
    cardiac pacemaker Z95.0
    cochlear Z96.21
    dental Z96.5
    heart Z95.812
    heart valve Z95.2
      prosthetic Z95.2
      specified NEC Z95.4
      xenogenic Z95.3
    insulin pump Z96.41
    intraocular lens Z96.1
    joint Z96.60
      ankle Z96.66- ☑
      elbow Z96.62- ☑
      finger Z96.69- ☑
      hip Z96.64- ☑
      knee Z96.65- ☑
      shoulder Z96.61- ☑
      specified NEC Z96.698
      wrist Z96.63- ☑
    larynx Z96.3
    myringotomy tube Z96.22

Presence — *continued*
  implanted device — *continued*
    otological Z96.20
      cochlear Z96.21
      eustachian stent Z96.29
      myringotomy Z96.22
      specified NEC Z96.29
      stapes Z96.29
    skin Z96.81
    skull plate Z96.7
    specified NEC Z96.89
    urogenital Z96.0
  insulin pump (functional) Z96.41
  intestinal bypass or anastomosis Z98.0
  intraocular lens (functional) Z96.1
  intrauterine contraceptive device (IUD) Z97.5
  intravascular implant (functional) (prosthetic) NEC Z95.9
    coronary artery Z95.5
    defibrillator (with synchronous cardiac pacemaker) Z95.810
    peripheral vessel (with angioplasty) Z95.820
  joint implant (prosthetic) (any) Z96.60
    ankle — *see* Presence, ankle joint implant
    elbow — *see* Presence, elbow joint implant
    finger — *see* Presence, finger joint implant
    hip — *see* Presence, hip joint implant
    knee — *see* Presence, knee joint implant
    shoulder — *see* Presence, shoulder joint implant
    specified joint NEC Z96.698
    wrist — *see* Presence, wrist joint implant
  knee-joint implant (functional) (prosthesis) Z96.65- ☑
  laryngeal implant (functional) Z96.3
  mandibular implant (dental) Z96.5
  myringotomy tube(s) Z96.22
  orthopedic-joint implant (prosthetic) (any) — *see* Presence, joint implant
  otological implant (functional) Z96.29
  shoulder-joint implant (functional) (prosthesis) Z96.61- ☑
  skull-plate implant Z96.7
  spectacles Z97.3
  stapes implant (functional) Z96.29
  systemic lupus erythematosus [SLE] inhibitor D68.62
  tendon implant (functional) (graft) Z96.7
  tooth root(s) implant Z96.5
  ureteral stent Z96.0
  urethral stent Z96.0
  urogenital implant (functional) Z96.0
  vascular implant or device Z95.9
    access port device Z95.828
    specified type NEC Z95.828
  wrist-joint implant (functional) (prosthesis) Z96.63- ☑
Presenile (*see also* condition)
  dementia F03 ☑
  premature aging E34.8
Presentation, fetal — *see* Delivery, complicated by, malposition
Prespondylolisthesis (congenital) Q76.2
Pressure
  area, skin — *see* Ulcer, pressure, by site
  brachial plexus G54.0
  brain G93.5
    injury at birth NEC P11.1
  cerebral — *see* Pressure, brain
  chest R07.89
  cone, tentorial G93.5
  hyposystolic (*see also* Hypotension)
    incidental reading, without diagnosis of hypotension R03.1
  increased
    intracranial (benign) G93.2
      injury at birth P11.0
    intraocular H40.05- ☑
  lumbosacral plexus G54.1
  mediastinum J98.5
  necrosis (chronic) — *see* Ulcer, pressure, by site
  parental, inappropriate (excessive) Z62.6
  sore (chronic) — *see* Ulcer, pressure, by site
  spinal cord G95.20
  ulcer (chronic) — *see* Ulcer, pressure, by site
  venous, increased I87.8
Pre-syncope R55
Preterm
  delivery (*see also* Pregnancy, complicated by, preterm labor) O60.10 ☑
  labor — *see* Pregnancy, complicated by, preterm labor

Preterm — *continued*
newborn (infant) P07.30
gestational age
28 completed weeks (28 weeks, 0 days through 28 weeks, 6 days) P07.31
29 completed weeks (29 weeks, 0 days through 29 weeks, 6 days) P07.32
30 completed weeks (30 weeks, 0 days through 30 weeks, 6 days) P07.33
31 completed weeks (31 weeks, 0 days through 31 weeks, 6 days) P07.34
32 completed weeks (32 weeks, 0 days through 32 weeks, 6 days) P07.35
33 completed weeks (33 weeks, 0 days through 33 weeks, 6 days) P07.36
34 completed weeks (34 weeks, 0 days through 34 weeks, 6 days) P07.37
35 completed weeks (35 weeks, 0 days through 35 weeks, 6 days) P07.38
36 completed weeks (36 weeks, 0 days through 36 weeks, 6 days) P07.39
Previa
placenta (low) (marginal) (partial) (total) (with hemorrhage) O44.1- ☑
without hemorrhage O44.0- ☑
vasa O69.4 ☑
Priapism N48.30
due to
disease classified elsewhere N48.32
drug N48.33
specified cause NEC N48.39
trauma N48.31
Prickling sensation (skin) R20.2
Prickly heat L74.0
Primary — *see* condition
Primigravida
elderly, affecting management of pregnancy, labor and delivery (supervision only) — *see* Pregnancy, complicated by, elderly, primigravida
older, affecting management of pregnancy, labor and delivery (supervision only) — *see* Pregnancy, complicated by, elderly, primigravida
very young, affecting management of pregnancy, labor and delivery (supervision only) — *see* Pregnancy, complicated by, young mother, primigravida
Primipara
elderly, affecting management of pregnancy, labor and delivery (supervision only) — *see* Pregnancy, complicated by, elderly, primigravida
older, affecting management of pregnancy, labor and delivery (supervision only) — *see* Pregnancy, complicated by, elderly, primigravida
very young, affecting management of pregnancy, labor and delivery (supervision only) — *see* Pregnancy, complicated by, young mother, primigravida
Primus varus (bilateral) Q66.2
PRIND (Prolonged reversible ischemic neurologic deficit) I63.9
Pringle's disease (tuberous sclerosis) Q85.1
Prinzmetal angina I20.1
Prizefighter ear — *see* Cauliflower ear
Problem (with) (related to)
academic Z55.8
acculturation Z60.3
adjustment (to)
change of job Z56.1
life-cycle transition Z60.0
pension Z60.0
retirement Z60.0
adopted child Z62.821
alcoholism in family Z63.72
atypical parenting situation Z62.9
bankruptcy Z59.8
behavioral (adult) F69
drug seeking Z72.89
birth of sibling affecting child Z62.898
care (of)
provider dependency Z74.9
specified NEC Z74.8
sick or handicapped person in family or household Z63.6
child
abuse (affecting the child) — *see* Maltreatment, child
custody or support proceedings Z65.3
in care of non-parental family member Z62.21
in foster care Z62.21
in welfare custody Z62.21

Problem — *continued*
child — *continued*
living in orphanage or group home Z62.22
child-rearing Z62.9
specified NEC Z62.898
communication (developmental) F80.9
conflict or discord (with)
boss Z56.4
classmates Z55.4
counselor Z64.4
employer Z56.4
family Z63.9
specified NEC Z63.8
probation officer Z64.4
social worker Z64.4
teachers Z55.4
workmates Z56.4
conviction in legal proceedings Z65.0
with imprisonment Z65.1
counselor Z64.4
creditors Z59.8
digestive K92.9
drug addict in family Z63.72
ear — *see* Disorder, ear
economic Z59.9
affecting care Z59.9
specified NEC Z59.8
education Z55.9
specified NEC Z55.8
employment Z56.9
change of job Z56.1
discord Z56.4
environment Z56.5
sexual harassment Z56.81
specified NEC Z56.89
stressful schedule Z56.3
stress NEC Z56.6
threat of job loss Z56.2
unemployment Z56.0
enuresis, child F98.0
eye H57.9
failed examinations (school) Z55.2
falling Z91.81
family (*see also* Disruption, family) Z63.9
specified NEC Z63.8
feeding (elderly) (infant) R63.3
newborn P92.9
breast P92.5
overfeeding P92.4
slow P92.2
specified NEC P92.8
underfeeding P92.3
nonorganic F50.8
finance Z59.9
specified NEC Z59.8
foreclosure on loan Z59.8
foster child Z62.822
frightening experience(s) in childhood Z62.898
genital NEC
female N94.9
male N50.9
health care Z75.9
specified NEC Z75.8
hearing — *see* Deafness
homelessness Z59.0
housing Z59.9
inadequate Z59.1
isolated Z59.8
specified NEC Z59.8
identity (of childhood) F93.8
illegitimate pregnancy (unwanted) Z64.0
illiteracy Z55.0
impaired mobility Z74.09
imprisonment or incarceration Z65.1
inadequate teaching affecting education Z55.8
inappropriate (excessive) parental pressure Z62.6
influencing health status NEC Z78.9
in-law Z63.1
institutionalization, affecting child Z62.22
intrafamilial communication Z63.8
jealousy, child F93.8
landlord Z59.2
language (developmental) F80.9
learning (developmental) F81.9
legal Z65.3
conviction without imprisonment Z65.0
imprisonment Z65.1
release from prison Z65.2

Problem — *continued*
life-management Z73.9
specified NEC Z73.89
life-style Z72.9
gambling Z72.6
high-risk sexual behavior (heterosexual) Z72.51
bisexual Z72.53
homosexual Z72.52
inappropriate eating habits Z72.4
self-damaging behavior NEC Z72.89
specified NEC Z72.89
tobacco use Z72.0
literacy Z55.9
low level Z55.0
specified NEC Z55.8
living alone Z60.2
lodgers Z59.2
loss of love relationship in childhood Z62.898
marital Z63.0
involving
divorce Z63.5
estrangement Z63.5
gender identity F66
mastication K08.8
medical
care, within family Z63.6
facilities Z75.9
specified NEC Z75.8
mental F48.9
multiparity Z64.1
negative life events in childhood Z62.9
altered pattern of family relationships Z62.898
frightening experience Z62.898
loss of
love relationship Z62.898
self-esteem Z62.898
physical abuse (alleged) — *see* Maltreatment, child
removal from home Z62.29
specified event NEC Z62.898
neighbor Z59.2
neurological NEC R29.818
new step-parent affecting child Z62.898
none (feared complaint unfounded) Z71.1
occupational NEC Z56.89
parent-child — *see* Conflict, parent-child
personal hygiene Z91.89
personality F69
phase-of-life transition, adjustment Z60.0
presence of sick or disabled person in family or household Z63.79
needing care Z63.6
primary support group (family) Z63.9
specified NEC Z63.8
probation officer Z64.4
psychiatric F99
psychosexual (development) F66
psychosocial Z65.9
specified NEC Z65.8
relationship Z63.9
childhood F93.8
release from prison Z65.2
removal from home affecting child Z62.29
seeking and accepting known hazardous and harmful
behavioral or psychological interventions Z65.8
chemical, nutritional or physical interventions Z65.8
sexual function (nonorganic) F52.9
sight H54.7
sleep disorder, child F51.9
smell — *see* Disturbance, sensation, smell
social
environment Z60.9
specified NEC Z60.8
exclusion and rejection Z60.4
worker Z64.4
speech R47.9
developmental F80.9
specified NEC R47.89
swallowing — *see* Dysphagia
taste — *see* Disturbance, sensation, taste
tic, child F95.0
underachievement in school Z55.3
unemployment Z56.0
threatened Z56.2
unwanted pregnancy Z64.0
upbringing Z62.9
specified NEC Z62.898
urinary N39.9
voice production R47.89

☑ **Additional Character Required — Refer to the Tabular List for Character Selection**   ▽ Subterms under main terms may continue to next column or page

Problem — *continued*
work schedule (stressful) Z56.3
Procedure (surgical)
for purpose other than remedying health state Z41.9
specified NEC Z41.8
not done Z53.9
because of
administrative reasons Z53.8
contraindication Z53.09
smoking Z53.01
patient's decision Z53.20
for reasons of belief or group pressure Z53.1
left against medical advice (AMA) Z53.21
specified reason NEC Z53.29
specified reason NEC Z53.8
Procidentia (uteri) N81.3
Proctalgia K62.89
fugax K59.4
spasmodic K59.4
Proctitis K62.89
amebic (acute) A06.0
chlamydial A56.3
gonococcal A54.6
granulomatous — *see* Enteritis, regional, large intestine
herpetic A60.1
radiation K62.7
tuberculous A18.32
ulcerative (chronic) K51.20
with
complication K51.219
abscess K51.214
fistula K51.213
obstruction K51.212
rectal bleeding K51.211
specified NEC K51.218
Proctocele
female (without uterine prolapse) N81.6
with uterine prolapse N81.2
complete N81.3
male K62.3
Proctocolitis, mucosal — *see* Rectosigmoiditis, ulcerative
Proctoptosis K62.3
Proctorrhagia K62.5
Proctosigmoiditis K63.89
ulcerative (chronic) — *see* Rectosigmoiditis, ulcerative
Proctospasm K59.4
psychogenic F45.8
Profichet's disease — *see* Disorder, soft tissue, specified type NEC
Progeria E34.8
Prognathism (mandibular) (maxillary) M26.19
Progonoma (melanotic) — *see* Neoplasm, benign, by site
Progressive — *see* condition
Prolactinoma
specified site — *see* Neoplasm, benign, by site
unspecified site D35.2
Prolapse, prolapsed
anus, anal (canal) (sphincter) K62.2
arm or hand O32.2 ☑
causing obstructed labor O64.4 ☑
bladder (mucosa) (sphincter) (acquired)
congenital Q79.4
female — *see* Cystocele
male N32.89
breast implant (prosthetic) T85.49 ☑
cecostomy K94.09
cecum K63.4
cervix, cervical (hypertrophied) N81.2
anterior lip, obstructing labor O65.5
congenital Q51.828
postpartal, old N81.2
stump N81.85
ciliary body (traumatic) — *see* Laceration, eye(ball), with prolapse or loss of interocular tissue
colon (pedunculated) K63.4
colostomy K94.09
disc (intervertebral) — *see* Displacement, intervertebral disc
eye implant (orbital) T85.398 ☑
lens (ocular) — *see* Complications, intraocular lens
fallopian tube N83.4
gastric (mucosa) K31.89
genital, female N81.9
specified NEC N81.89
globe, nontraumatic — *see* Luxation, globe

Prolapse, prolapsed — *continued*
ileostomy bud K94.19
intervertebral disc — *see* Displacement, intervertebral disc
intestine (small) K63.4
iris (traumatic) — *see* Laceration, eye(ball), with prolapse or loss of interocular tissue
nontraumatic H21.89
kidney N28.83
congenital Q63.2
laryngeal muscles or ventricle J38.7
meatus urinarius N36.8
mitral (valve) I34.1
ocular lens implant — *see* Complications, intraocular lens
organ or site, congenital NEC — *see* Malposition, congenital
ovary N83.4
pelvic floor, female N81.89
perineum, female N81.89
rectum (mucosa) (sphincter) K62.3
due to trichuris trichuria B79
spleen D73.89
stomach K31.89
umbilical cord
complicating delivery O69.0 ☑
urachus, congenital Q64.4
ureter N28.89
with obstruction N13.5
with infection N13.6
ureterovesical orifice N28.89
urethra (acquired) (infected) (mucosa) N36.8
congenital Q64.71
urinary meatus N36.8
congenital Q64.72
uterovaginal N81.4
complete N81.3
incomplete N81.2
uterus (with prolapse of vagina) N81.4
complete N81.3
congenital Q51.818
first degree N81.2
in pregnancy or childbirth — *see* Pregnancy, complicated by, abnormal, uterus
incomplete N81.2
postpartal (old) N81.4
second degree N81.2
third degree N81.3
uveal (traumatic) — *see* Laceration, eye(ball), with prolapse or loss of interocular tissue
vagina (anterior) (wall) — *see* Cystocele
with prolapse of uterus N81.4
complete N81.3
incomplete N81.2
posterior wall N81.6
posthysterectomy N99.3
vitreous (humor) H43.0- ☑
in wound — *see* Laceration, eye(ball), with prolapse or loss of interocular tissue
womb — *see* Prolapse, uterus
Prolapsus, female N81.9
specified NEC N81.89
Proliferation(s)
primary cutaneous CD30-positive large T-cell C86.6
Proliferative — *see* condition
Prolonged, prolongation (of)
bleeding (time) (idiopathic) R79.1
coagulation (time) R79.1
gestation (over 42 completed weeks)
mother O48.1
newborn P08.22
interval I44.0
labor O63.9
first stage O63.0
second stage O63.1
partial thromboplastin time (PTT) R79.1
pregnancy (more than 42 weeks gestation) O48.1
prothrombin time R79.1
QT interval I45.81
uterine contractions in labor O62.4
Prominence, prominent
auricle (congenital) (ear) Q17.5
ischial spine or sacral promontory
with disproportion (fetopelvic) O33.0
causing obstructed labor O65.0
nose (congenital) acquired M95.0
Promiscuity — *see* High, risk, sexual behavior

Pronation
ankle — *see* Deformity, limb, foot, specified NEC
foot (*see also* Deformity, limb, foot, specified NEC)
congenital Q74.2
Prophylactic
administration of
antibiotics, long-term Z79.2
short-term use — *omit code*
drug (*see also* Long-term (current) drug therapy (use of)) Z79.899
medication Z79.899
organ removal (for neoplasia management) Z40.00
breast Z40.01
ovary Z40.02
specified site NEC Z40.09
surgery Z40.9
for risk factors related to malignant neoplasm — *see* Prophylactic, organ removal
specified NEC Z40.8
vaccination Z23
Propionic acidemia E71.121
Proptosis (ocular) (*see also* Exophthalmos)
thyroid — *see* Hyperthyroidism, with goiter
Prosecution, anxiety concerning Z65.3
Prosopagnosia R48.3
Prosoacdynia N42.81
Prostate, prostatic — *see* condition
Prostatism — *see* Hyperplasia, prostate
Prostatitis (congestive) (suppurative) (with cystitis) N41.9
acute N41.0
cavitary N41.8
chronic N41.1
diverticular N41.8
due to Trichomonas (vaginalis) A59.02
fibrous N41.1
gonococcal (acute) (chronic) A54.22
granulomatous N41.4
hypertrophic N41.1
subacute N41.1
trichomonal A59.02
tuberculous A18.14
Prostatocystitis N41.3
Prostatorrhea N42.89
Prostatosis N42.82
Prostration R53.83
heat (*see also* Heat, exhaustion)
anhydrotic T67.3 ☑
due to
salt (and water) depletion T67.4 ☑
water depletion T67.3 ☑
nervous F48.8
senile R54
Protanomaly (anomalous trichromat) H53.54
Protanopia (complete) (incomplete) H53.54
Protection (against) (from) — *see* Prophylactic
Protein
deficiency NEC — *see* Malnutrition
malnutrition — *see* Malnutrition
sickness (*see also* Reaction, serum) T80.69 ☑
Proteinemia R77.9
Proteinosis
alveolar (pulmonary) J84.01
lipid or lipoid (of Urbach) E78.89
Proteinuria R80.9
Bence Jones R80.3
complicating pregnancy — *see* Proteinuria, gestational
gestational O12.1- ☑
with edema O12.2- ☑
idiopathic R80.0
isolated R80.0
with glomerular lesion N06.9
dense deposit disease N06.6
diffuse
crescentic glomerulonephritis N06.7
endocapillary proliferative glomerulonephritis N06.4
mesangiocapillary glomerulonephritis N06.5
focal and segmental hyalinosis or sclerosis N06.1
membranous (diffuse) N06.2
mesangial proliferative (diffuse) N06.3
minimal change N06.0
specified pathology NEC N06.8
orthostatic R80.2
with glomerular lesion — *see* Proteinuria, isolated, with glomerular lesion

Proteinuria — *continued*
  persistent R80.1
    with glomerular lesion — *see* Proteinuria, isolated, with glomerular lesion
  postural R80.2
    with glomerular lesion — *see* Proteinuria, isolated, with glomerular lesion
  pre-eclamptic — *see* Pre-eclampsia
  specified type NEC R80.8
Proteolysis, pathologic D65
Proteus (mirabilis) (morganii), **as cause of disease classified elsewhere** B96.4
Prothrombin gene mutation D68.52
Protoporphyria, erythropoietic E80.0
Protozoal (*see also* condition)
  disease B64
    specified NEC B60.8
Protrusion, protrusio
  acetabuli M24.7
  acetabulum (into pelvis) M24.7
  device, implant or graft (*see also* Complications, by site and type, mechanical) T85.698 ☑
    arterial graft NEC — *see* Complication, cardiovascular device, mechanical, vascular
    breast (implant) T85.49 ☑
    catheter NEC T85.698 ☑
      cystostomy T83.090 ☑
      dialysis (renal) T82.49 ☑
        intraperitoneal T85.691 ☑
      infusion NEC T82.594 ☑
        spinal (epidural) (subdural) T85.690 ☑
      urinary, indwelling T83.098 ☑
    electronic (electrode) (pulse generator) (stimulator)
      bone T84.390 ☑
      nervous system — *see* Complication, prosthetic device, mechanical, electronic nervous system stimulator
    fixation, internal (orthopedic) NEC — *see* Complication, fixation device, mechanical
    gastrointestinal — *see* Complications, prosthetic device, mechanical, gastrointestinal device
    genital NEC T83.498 ☑
      intrauterine contraceptive device T83.39 ☑
      penile prosthesis T83.490 ☑
    heart NEC — *see* Complication, cardiovascular device, mechanical
    joint prosthesis — *see* Complications, joint prosthesis, mechanical, specified NEC, by site
    ocular NEC — *see* Complications, prosthetic device, mechanical, ocular device
    orthopedic NEC — *see* Complication, orthopedic, device, mechanical
    specified NEC T85.628 ☑
    urinary NEC (*see also* Complication, genitourinary, device, urinary, mechanical)
      graft T83.29 ☑
    vascular NEC — *see* Complication, cardiovascular device, mechanical
    ventricular intracranial shunt T85.09 ☑
  intervertebral disc — *see* Displacement, intervertebral disc
  joint prosthesis — *see* Complications, joint prosthesis, mechanical, specified NEC, by site
  nucleus pulposus — *see* Displacement, intervertebral disc
Prune belly (syndrome) Q79.4
Prurigo (ferox) (gravis) (Hebrae) (Hebra's) (mitis) (simplex) L28.2
  Besnier's L20.0
  estivalis L56.4
  nodularis L28.1
  psychogenic F45.8
Pruritus, pruritic (essential) L29.9
  ani, anus L29.0
    psychogenic F45.8
  anogenital L29.3
    psychogenic F45.8
  due to onchocerca volvulus B73.1
  gravidarum — *see* Pregnancy, complicated by, specified pregnancy-related condition NEC
  hiemalis L29.8
  neurogenic (any site) F45.8
  perianal L29.0
  psychogenic (any site) F45.8
  scroti, scrotum L29.1
    psychogenic F45.8
  senile, senilis L29.8

Pruritus, pruritic — *continued*
  specified NEC L29.8
    psychogenic F45.8
  Trichomonas A59.9
  vulva, vulvae L29.2
    psychogenic F45.8
Pseudarthrosis, pseudoarthrosis (bone) — *see* Nonunion, fracture
  clavicle, congenital Q74.0
  joint, following fusion or arthrodesis M96.0
Pseudoaneurysm — *see* Aneurysm
Pseudoangina (pectoris) — *see* Angina
Pseudoangioma I81
Pseudoarteriosus Q28.8
Pseudoarthrosis — *see* Pseudarthrosis
Pseudobulbar affect (PBA) F48.2
Pseudochromhidrosis L67.8
Pseudocirrhosis, liver, pericardial I31.1
Pseudocowpox B08.03
Pseudocoxalgia M91.3- ☑
Pseudo-Cushing's syndrome, alcohol-induced E24.4
Pseudocyesis F45.8
Pseudocyst
  lung J98.4
  pancreas K86.3
  retina — *see* Cyst, retina
Pseudoelephantiasis neuroarthritica Q82.0
Pseudoexfoliation, capsule (lens) — *see* Cataract, specified NEC
Pseudofolliculitis barbae L73.1
Pseudoglioma H44.89
Pseudohemophilia (Bernuth's) (hereditary) (type B) D68.0
  Type A D69.8
  vascular D69.8
Pseudohermaphroditism Q56.3
  adrenal E25.8
  female Q56.2
    with adrenocortical disorder E25.8
    without adrenocortical disorder Q56.2
    adrenal, congenital E25.0
  male Q56.1
    with
      5-alpha-reductase deficiency E29.1
      adrenocortical disorder E25.8
      androgen resistance E34.51
      cleft scrotum Q56.1
      feminizing testis E34.51
    without gonadal disorder Q56.1
    adrenal E25.8
Pseudo-Hurler's polydystrophy E77.0
Pseudohydrocephalus G93.2
Pseudohypertrophic muscular dystrophy (Erb's) G71.0
Pseudohypertrophy, muscle G71.0
Pseudohypoparathyroidism E20.1
Pseudoinsomnia F51.03
Pseudoleukemia, infantile D64.89
Pseudomembranous — *see* condition
Pseudomeningocele (cerebral) (infective) (post-traumatic) G96.19
  postprocedural (spinal) G97.82
Pseudomenses (newborn) P54.6
Pseudomenstruation (newborn) P54.6
Pseudomonas
  aeruginosa, as cause of disease classified elsewhere B96.5
  mallei infection A24.0
    as cause of disease classified elsewhere B96.5
    pseudomallei, as cause of disease classified elsewhere B96.5
Pseudomyotonia G71.19
Pseudomyxoma peritonei C78.6
Pseudoneuritis, optic (nerve) (disc) (papilla), **congenital** Q14.2
Pseudo-obstruction intestine (acute) (chronic) (idiopathic) (intermittent secondary) (primary) K59.8
Pseudopapilledema H47.33- ☑
  congenital Q14.2
Pseudoparalysis
  arm or leg R29.818
  atonic, congenital P94.2
Pseudopelade L66.0
Pseudophakia Z96.1
Pseudopolyarthritis, rhizomelic M35.3
Pseudopolycythemia D75.1
Pseudopseudohypoparathyroidism E20.1

Pseudopterygium H11.81- ☑
Pseudoptosis (eyelid) — *see* Blepharochalasis
Pseudopuberty, precocious
  female heterosexual E25.8
  male isosexual E25.8
Pseudorickets (renal) N25.0
Pseudorubella B08.20
Pseudosclerema, newborn P83.8
Pseudosclerosis (brain)
  Jakob's — *see* Creutzfeldt-Jakob disease or syndrome of Westphal (Strümpell) E83.01
  spastic — *see* Creutzfeldt-Jakob disease or syndrome
Pseudotetanus — *see* Convulsions
Pseudotetany R29.0
  hysterical F44.5
Pseudotruncus arteriosus Q25.4
Pseudotuberculosis A28.2
  enterocolitis A04.8
  pasteurella (infection) A28.0
Pseudotumor
  cerebri G93.2
  orbital H05.11 ☑
Pseudoxanthoma elasticum Q82.8
Psilosis (sprue) (tropical) K90.1
  nontropical K90.0
Psittacosis A70
Psoitis M60.88
Psoriasis L40.9
  arthropathic L40.50
    arthritis mutilans L40.52
    distal interphalangeal L40.51
    juvenile L40.54
    other specified L40.59
    spondylitis L40.53
  buccal K13.29
  flexural L40.8
  guttate L40.4
  mouth K13.29
  nummular L40.0
  plaque L40.0
  psychogenic F54
  pustular (generalized) L40.1
    palmaris et plantaris L40.3
  specified NEC L40.8
  vulgaris L40.0
Psychasthenia F48.8
Psychiatric disorder or problem F99
Psychogenic (*see also* condition)
  factors associated with physical conditions F54
Psychological and behavioral factors affecting medical condition F59
Psychoneurosis, psychoneurotic (*see also* Neurosis)
  anxiety (state) F41.1
  depersonalization F48.1
  hypochondriacal F45.21
  hysteria F44.9
  neurasthenic F48.8
  personality NEC F60.89
Psychopathy, psychopathic
  affectionless F94.2
  autistic F84.5
  constitution, post-traumatic F07.81
  personality — *see* Disorder, personality
  sexual — *see* Deviation, sexual
  state F60.2
Psychosexual identity disorder of childhood F64.2
Psychosis, psychotic F29
  acute (transient) F23
    hysterical F44.9
  affective — *see* Disorder, mood
  alcoholic F10.959
    with
      abuse F10.159
      anxiety disorder F10.980
        with
          abuse F10.180
          dependence F10.280
      delirium tremens F10.231
      delusions F10.950
        with
          abuse F10.150
          dependence F10.250
      dementia F10.97
        with dependence F10.27
      dependence F10.259

Psychosis, psychotic — *continued*
  alcoholic — *continued*
    with — *continued*
      hallucinosis F10.951
        with
          abuse F10.151
          dependence F10.251
      mood disorder F10.94
        with
          abuse F10.14
          dependence F10.24
      paranoia F10.950
        with
          abuse F10.150
          dependence F10.250
      persisting amnesia F10.96
        with dependence F10.26
    amnestic confabulatory F10.96
      with dependence F10.26
    delirium tremens F10.231
    Korsakoff's, Korsakov's, Korsakow's F10.26
    paranoid type F10.950
      with
        abuse F10.150
        dependence F10.250
  anergastic — *see* Psychosis, organic
  arteriosclerotic (simple type) (uncomplicated) F01.50
    with behavioral disturbance F01.51
  childhood F84.0
    atypical F84.8
  climacteric — *see* Psychosis, involutional
  confusional F29
    acute or subacute F05
    reactive F23
  cycloid F23
  depressive — *see* Disorder, depressive
  disintegrative (childhood) F84.3
  drug-induced — *see* F11-F19 with .X59
    paranoid and hallucinatory states — *see* F11-F19
      with .X50 or .X51
  due to or associated with
    addiction, drug — *see* F11-F19 with .X59
    dependence
      alcohol F10.259
      drug — *see* F11-F19 with .X59
    epilepsy F06.8
    Huntington's chorea F06.8
    ischemia, cerebrovascular (generalized) F06.8
    multiple sclerosis F06.8
    physical disease F06.8
    presenile dementia F03 ☑
    senile dementia F03 ☑
    vascular disease (arteriosclerotic) (cerebral) F01.50
      with behavioral disturbance F01.51
  epileptic F06.8
  episode F23
    due to or associated with physical condition F06.8
  exhaustive F43.0
  hallucinatory, chronic F28
  hypomanic F30.8
  hysterical (acute) F44.9
  induced F24
  infantile F84.0
    atypical F84.8
  infective (acute) (subacute) F05
  involutional F28
    depressive — *see* Disorder, depressive
    melancholic — *see* Disorder, depressive
    paranoid (state) F22
  Korsakoff's, Korsakov's, Korsakow's (nonalcoholic) F04
    alcoholic F10.96
      in dependence F10.26
    induced by other psychoactive substance — *see*
      categories F11-F19 with .X5X
  mania, manic (single episode) F30.2
    recurrent type F31.89
  manic-depressive — *see* Disorder, mood
  menopausal — *see* Psychosis, involutional
  mixed schizophrenic and affective F25.8
  multi-infarct (cerebrovascular) F01.50
    with behavioral disturbance F01.51
  nonorganic F29
    specified NEC F28
  organic F09
    due to or associated with
      arteriosclerosis (cerebral) — *see* Psychosis, ar-
        teriosclerotic

Psychosis, psychotic — *continued*
  organic — *continued*
    due to or associated with — *continued*
      cerebrovascular disease, arteriosclerotic — *see*
        Psychosis, arteriosclerotic
      childbirth — *see* Psychosis, puerperal
      Creutzfeldt-Jakob disease or syndrome — *see*
        Creutzfeldt-Jakob disease or syndrome
      dependence, alcohol F10.259
      disease
        alcoholic liver F10.259
        brain, arteriosclerotic — *see* Psychosis, arte-
          riosclerotic
        cerebrovascular F01.50
          with behavioral disturbance F01.51
        Creutzfeldt-Jakob — *see* Creutzfeldt-Jakob
          disease or syndrome
        endocrine or metabolic F06.8
          acute or subacute F05
        liver, alcoholic F10.259
      epilepsy transient (acute) F05
      infection
        brain (intracranial) F06.8
          acute or subacute F05
      intoxication
        alcoholic (acute) F10.259
        drug F11-F19 with .X59
      ischemia, cerebrovascular (generalized) — *see*
        Psychosis, arteriosclerotic
      puerperium — *see* Psychosis, puerperal
      trauma, brain (birth) (from electric current)
        (surgical) F06.8
        acute or subacute F05
    infective F06.8
      acute or subacute F05
    post-traumatic F06.8
      acute or subacute F05
  paranoiac F22
  paranoid (climacteric) (involutional) (menopausal) F22
    psychogenic (acute) F23
    schizophrenic F20.0
    senile F03 ☑
  postpartum F53
  presbyophrenic (type) F03 ☑
  presenile F03 ☑
  psychogenic (paranoid) F23
    depressive F32.3
  puerperal F53
    specified type — *see* Psychosis, by type
  reactive (brief) (transient) (emotional stress) (psycho-
    logical trauma) F23
    depressive F32.3
      recurrent F33.3
    excitative type F30.8
  schizoaffective F25.9
    depressive type F25.1
    manic type F25.0
  schizophrenia, schizophrenic — *see* Schizophrenia
  schizophrenia-like, in epilepsy F06.2
  schizophreniform F20.81
    affective type F25.9
    brief F23
    confusional type F23
    depressive type F25.1
    manic type F25.0
    mixed type F25.0
  senile NEC F03 ☑
    depressed or paranoid type F03 ☑
    simple deterioration F03 ☑
    specified type — *code to* condition
  shared F24
  situational (reactive) F23
  symbiotic (childhood) F84.3
  symptomatic F09
Psychosomatic — *see* Disorder, psychosomatic
Psychosyndrome, organic F07.9
**Psychotic episode due to or associated with physical
  condition** F06.8
Pterygium (eye) H11.00- ☑
  amyloid H11.01- ☑
  central H11.02- ☑
  colli Q18.3
  double H11.03- ☑
  peripheral
    progressive H11.05- ☑
    stationary H11.04- ☑
  recurrent H11.06- ☑

Ptilosis (eyelid) — *see* Madarosis
Ptomaine (poisoning) — *see* Poisoning, food
Ptosis (*see also* Blepharoptosis)
  adiposa (false) — *see* Blepharoptosis
  breast N64.81
  cecum K63.4
  colon K63.4
  congenital (eyelid) Q10.0
    specified site NEC — *see* Anomaly, by site
  eyelid — *see* Blepharoptosis
    congenital Q10.0
  gastric K31.89
  intestine K63.4
  kidney N28.83
  liver K76.89
  renal N28.83
  splanchnic K63.4
  spleen D73.89
  stomach K31.89
  viscera K63.4
PTP D69.51
Ptyalism (periodic) K11.7
  hysterical F45.8
  pregnancy — *see* Pregnancy, complicated by, specified
    pregnancy-related condition NEC
  psychogenic F45.8
Ptyalolithiasis K11.5
Pubarche, precocious E30.1
Pubertas praecox E30.1
Puberty (development state) Z00.3
  bleeding (excessive) N92.2
  delayed E30.0
  precocious (constitutional) (cryptogenic) (idiopathic)
    E30.1
    central E22.8
    due to
      ovarian hyperfunction E28.1
        estrogen E28.0
      testicular hyperfunction E29.0
  premature E30.1
    due to
      adrenal cortical hyperfunction E25.8
      pineal tumor E34.8
      pituitary (anterior) hyperfunction E22.8
Puckering, macula — *see* Degeneration, macula, puckering
Pudenda, pudendum — *see* condition
Puente's disease (simple glandular cheilitis) K13.0
Puerperal, puerperium (complicated by, complications)
  abnormal glucose (tolerance test) O99.815
  abscess
    areola O91.02
      associated with lactation O91.03
    Bartholin's gland O86.19
    breast O91.12
      associated with lactation O91.13
    cervix (uteri) O86.11
    genital organ NEC O86.19
    kidney O86.21
    mammary O91.12
      associated with lactation O91.13
    nipple O91.02
      associated with lactation O91.03
    peritoneum O85
    subareolar O91.12
      associated with lactation O91.13
    urinary tract — *see* Puerperal, infection, urinary
    uterus O86.12
    vagina (wall) O86.13
    vaginorectal O86.13
    vulvovaginal gland O86.13
  adnexitis O86.19
  afibrinogenemia, or other coagulation defect O72.3
  albuminuria (acute) (subacute) — *see* Proteinuria,
    gestational
  alcohol use O99.315
  anemia O90.81
    pre-existing (pre-pregnancy) O99.03
  anesthetic death O89.8
  apoplexy O99.43
  bariatric surgery status O99.845
  blood disorder NEC O99.13
  blood dyscrasia O72.3
  cardiomyopathy O90.3
  cerebrovascular disorder (conditions in I60-I69) O99.43
  cervicitis O86.11
  circulatory system disorder O99.43
  coagulopathy (any) O72.3

Puerperal, puerperium — *continued*
 complications O90.9
  specified NEC O90.89
 convulsions — *see* Eclampsia
 cystitis O86.22
 cystopyelitis O86.29
 delirium NEC F05
 diabetes O24.93
  gestational — *see* Puerperal, gestational diabetes
  pre-existing O24.33
   specified NEC O24.83
   type 1 O24.03
   type 2 O24.13
 digestive system disorder O99.63
 disease O90.9
  breast NEC O92.29
  cerebrovascular (acute) O99.43
  nonobstetric NEC O99.89
  tubo-ovarian O86.19
  Valsuani's O99.03
 disorder O90.9
  biliary tract O26.63
  lactation O92.70
  liver O26.63
  nonobstetric NEC O99.89
 disruption
  cesarean wound O90.0
  episiotomy wound O90.1
  perineal laceration wound O90.1
 drug use O99.325
 eclampsia (with pre-existing hypertension) O15.2
 embolism (pulmonary) (blood clot) — *see* Embolism, obstetric, puerperal
 endocrine, nutritional or metabolic disease NEC O99.285
 endophlebitis — *see* Puerperal, phlebitis
 endotrachelitis O86.11
 failure
  lactation (complete) O92.3
   partial O92.4
  renal, acute O90.4
 fever (of unknown origin) O86.4
  septic O85
 fissure, nipple O92.12
  associated with lactation O92.13
 fistula
  breast (due to mastitis) O91.12
   associated with lactation O91.13
  nipple O91.02
   associated with lactation O91.03
 galactophoritis O91.22
  associated with lactation O91.23
 galactorrhea O92.6
 gastric banding status O99.845
 gastric bypass status O99.845
 gastrointestinal disease NEC O99.63
 gestational diabetes O24.439
  diet controlled O24.430
  insulin (and diet) controlled O24.434
 gonorrhea O98.23
 hematoma, subdural O99.43
 hemiplegia, cerebral O99.355
  due to cerbrovascular disorder O99.43
 hemorrhage O72.1
  brain O99.43
  bulbar O99.43
  cerebellar O99.43
  cerebral O99.43
  cortical O99.43
  delayed or secondary O72.2
  extradural O99.43
  internal capsule O99.43
  intracranial O99.43
  intrapontine O99.43
  meningeal O99.43
  pontine O99.43
  retained placenta O72.0
  subarachnoid O99.43
  subcortical O99.43
  subdural O99.43
  third stage O72.0
  uterine, delayed O72.2
  ventricular O99.43
 hemorrhoids O87.2
 hepatorenal syndrome O90.4
 hypertension — *see* Hypertension, complicating, puerperium
 hypertrophy, breast O92.29

Puerperal, puerperium — *continued*
 induration breast (fibrous) O92.29
 infection O86.4
  cervix O86.11
  generalized O85
  genital tract NEC O86.19
   obstetric surgical wound O86.0
  kidney (bacillus coli) O86.21
  maternal O98.93
   carrier state NEC O99.835
   gonorrhea O98.23
   human immunodeficiency virus (HIV) O98.73
   protozoal O98.63
   sexually transmitted NEC O98.33
   specified NEC O98.83
   streptococcus B carrier state O99.825
   syphilis O98.13
   tuberculosis O98.03
   viral hepatitis O98.43
   viral NEC O98.53
  nipple O91.02
   associated with lactation O91.03
  peritoneum O85
  renal O86.21
  specified NEC O86.89
  urinary (asymptomatic) (tract) NEC O86.20
   bladder O86.22
   kidney O86.21
   specified site NEC O86.29
   urethra O86.22
  vagina O86.13
  vein — *see* Puerperal, phlebitis
 ischemia, cerebral O99.43
 lymphangitis O86.89
  breast O91.22
   associated with lactation O91.23
 malignancy O9A.13 (*following* O99)
 malnutrition O25.3
 mammillitis O91.02
  associated with lactation O91.03
 mammitis O91.22
  associated with lactation O91.23
 mania F30.8
 mastitis O91.22
  associated with lactation O91.23
  purulent O91.12
   associated with lactation O91.13
 melancholia — *see* Disorder, depressive
 mental disorder NEC O99.345
 metroperitonitis O85
 metrorrhagia — *see* Hemorrhage, postpartum
 metrosalpingitis O86.19
 metrovaginitis O86.13
 milk leg O87.1
 monoplegia, cerebral O99.43
 mood disturbance O90.6
 necrosis, liver (acute) (subacute) (conditions in subcategory K72.0) O26.63
  with renal failure O90.4
 nervous system disorder O99.355
 obesity (pre-existing prior to pregnancy) O99.215
 obesity surgery status O99.845
 occlusion, precerebral artery O99.43
 paralysis
  bladder (sphincter) O90.89
  cerebral O99.43
 paralytic stroke O99.43
 parametritis O85
 paravaginitis O86.13
 pelviperitonitis O85
 perimetritis O86.12
 perimetrosalpingitis O86.19
 perinephritis O86.21
 periphlebitis — *see* Puerperal phlebitis
 peritoneal infection O85
 peritonitis (pelvic) O85
 perivaginitis O86.13
 phlebitis O87.0
  deep O87.1
  pelvic O87.1
  superficial O87.0
 phlebothrombosis, deep O87.1
 phlegmasia alba dolens O87.1
 placental polyp O90.89
 pneumonia, embolic — *see* Embolism, obstetric, puerperal
 pre-eclampsia — *see* Pre-eclampsia
 psychosis F53

Puerperal, puerperium — *continued*
 pyelitis O86.21
 pyelocystitis O86.29
 pyelonephritis O86.21
 pyelonephrosis O86.21
 pyemia O85
 pyocystitis O86.29
 pyohemia O85
 pyometra O86.12
 pyonephritis O86.21
 pyosalpingitis O86.19
 pyrexia (of unknown origin) O86.4
 renal
  disease NEC O90.89
  failure O90.4
 respiratory disease NEC O99.53
 retention
  decidua — *see* Retention, decidua
  placenta O72.0
  secundines — *see* Retention, secundines
 retrated nipple O92.02
 salpingo-ovaritis O86.19
 salpingoperitonitis O85
 secondary perineal tear O90.1
 sepsis (pelvic) O85
 sepsis O85
 septic thrombophlebitis O86.81
 skin disorder NEC O99.73
 specified condition NEC O99.89
 stroke O99.43
 subinvolution (uterus) O90.89
 subluxation of symphysis (pubis) O26.73
 suppuration — *see* Puerperal, abscess
 tetanus A34
 thelitis O91.02
  associated with lactation O91.03
 thrombocytopenia O72.3
 thrombophlebitis (superficial) O87.0
  deep O87.1
  pelvic O87.1
  septic O86.81
 thrombosis (venous) — *see* Thrombosis, puerperal
 thyroiditis O90.5
 toxemia (eclamptic) (pre-eclamptic) (with convulsions) O15.2
 trauma, non-obstetric O9A.23 (*following* O99)
  caused by abuse (physical) (suspected) O9A.33 (*following* O99)
   confirmed O9A.33 (*following* O99)
   psychological (suspected) O9A.53 (*following* O99)
    confirmed O9A.53 (*following* O99)
   sexual (suspected) O9A.43 (*following* O99)
    confirmed O9A.43 (*following* O99)
 uremia (due to renal failure) O90.4
 urethritis O86.22
 vaginitis O86.13
 varicose veins (legs) O87.4
  vulva or perineum O87.8
 venous O87.9
 vulvitis O86.19
 vulvovaginitis O86.13
 white leg O87.1
Puerperium — *see* Puerperal
Pulmolithiasis J98.4
Pulmonary — *see* condition
Pulpitis (acute) (anachoretic) (chronic) (hyperplastic) (irreversible) (putrescent) (reversible) (suppurative) (ulcerative) K04.0
Pulpless tooth K04.99
Pulse
 alternating R00.8
 bigeminal R00.8
 fast R00.0
 feeble, rapid due to shock following injury T79.4 ☑
 rapid R00.0
 weak R09.89
Pulsus alternans or trigeminus R00.8
Punch drunk F07.81
Punctum lacrimale occlusion — *see* Obstruction, lacrimal
Puncture
 abdomen, abdominal
  wall S31.139 ☑
   with
    foreign body S31.149 ☑

☑ **Additional Character Required — Refer to the Tabular List for Character Selection**   ☒ Subterms under main terms may continue to next column or page

Puncture — *continued*
  abdomen, abdominal — *continued*
    wall — *continued*
      with — *continued*
        penetration into peritoneal cavity
          S31.639 ☑
          with foreign body S31.649 ☑
      epigastric region S31.132 ☑
        with
          foreign body S31.142 ☑
          penetration into peritoneal cavity
            S31.632 ☑
            with foreign body S31.642 ☑
      left
        lower quadrant S31.134 ☑
          with
            foreign body S31.144 ☑
            penetration into peritoneal cavity
              S31.634 ☑
              with foreign body S31.644 ☑
        upper quadrant S31.131 ☑
          with
            foreign body S31.141 ☑
            penetration into peritoneal cavity
              S31.631 ☑
              with foreign body S31.641 ☑
      periumbilic region S31.135 ☑
        with
          foreign body S31.145 ☑
          penetration into peritoneal cavity
            S31.635 ☑
            with foreign body S31.645 ☑
      right
        lower quadrant S31.133 ☑
          with
            foreign body S31.143 ☑
            penetration into peritoneal cavity
              S31.633 ☑
              with foreign body S31.643 ☑
        upper quadrant S31.130 ☑
          with
            foreign body S31.140 ☑
            penetration into peritoneal cavity
              S31.630 ☑
              with foreign body S31.640 ☑
  accidental, complicating surgery — *see* Complication,
    accidental puncture or laceration
  alveolar (process) — *see* Puncture, oral cavity
  ankle S91.039 ☑
    with
      foreign body S91.049 ☑
    left S91.032 ☑
      with
        foreign body S91.042 ☑
    right S91.031 ☑
      with
        foreign body S91.041 ☑
  anus S31.833 ☑
    with foreign body S31.834 ☑
  arm (upper) S41.139 ☑
    with foreign body S41.149 ☑
    left S41.132 ☑
      with foreign body S41.142 ☑
    lower — *see* Puncture, forearm
    right S41.131 ☑
      with foreign body S41.141 ☑
  auditory canal (external) (meatus) — *see* Puncture,
    ear
  auricle, ear — *see* Puncture, ear
  axilla — *see* Puncture, arm
  back (*see also* Puncture, thorax, back)
    lower S31.030 ☑
      with
        foreign body S31.040 ☑
          with penetration into retroperitoneal
            space S31.041 ☑
        penetration into retroperitoneal space
          S31.031 ☑
  bladder (traumatic) S37.29 ☑
    nontraumatic N32.89
  breast S21.039 ☑
    with foreign body S21.049 ☑
    left S21.032 ☑
      with foreign body S21.042 ☑
    right S21.031 ☑
      with foreign body S21.041 ☑

Puncture — *continued*
  buttock S31.803 ☑
    with foreign body S31.804 ☑
    left S31.823 ☑
      with foreign body S31.824 ☑
    right S31.813 ☑
      with foreign body S31.814 ☑
  by
    device, implant or graft — *see* Complications, by
      site and type, mechanical
    foreign body left accidentally in operative wound
      T81.539 ☑
    instrument (any) during a procedure, accidental
      — *see* Puncture, accidental complicating
      surgery
  calf — *see* Puncture, leg
  canaliculus lacrimalis — *see* Puncture, eyelid
  canthus, eye — *see* Puncture, eyelid
  cervical esophagus S11.23 ☑
    with foreign body S11.24 ☑
  cheek (external) S01.439 ☑
    with foreign body S01.449 ☑
    internal — *see* Puncture, oral cavity
    left S01.432 ☑
      with foreign body S01.442 ☑
    right S01.431 ☑
      with foreign body S01.441 ☑
  chest wall — *see* Puncture, thorax
  chin — *see* Puncture, head, specified site NEC
  clitoris — *see* Puncture, vulva
  costal region — *see* Puncture, thorax
  digit(s)
    foot — *see* Puncture, toe
    hand — *see* Puncture, finger
  ear (canal) (external) S01.339 ☑
    with foreign body S01.349 ☑
    drum S09.2- ☑
    left S01.332 ☑
      with foreign body S01.342 ☑
    right S01.331 ☑
      with foreign body S01.341 ☑
  elbow S51.039 ☑
    with
      foreign body S51.049 ☑
    left S51.032 ☑
      with
        foreign body S51.042 ☑
    right S51.031 ☑
      with
        foreign body S51.041 ☑
  epididymis — *see* Puncture, testis
  epigastric region — *see* Puncture, abdomen, wall,
    epigastric
  epiglottis S11.83 ☑
    with foreign body S11.84 ☑
  esophagus
    cervical S11.23 ☑
      with foreign body S11.24 ☑
    thoracic S27.818 ☑
  eyeball S05.6- ☑
    with foreign body S05.5- ☑
  eyebrow — *see* Puncture, eyelid
  eyelid S01.13- ☑
    with foreign body S01.14- ☑
    left S01.132 ☑
      with foreign body S01.142 ☑
    right S01.131 ☑
      with foreign body S01.141 ☑
  face NEC — *see* Puncture, head, specified site NEC
  finger(s) S61.239 ☑
    with
      damage to nail S61.339 ☑
        with
          foreign body S61.349 ☑
      foreign body S61.249 ☑
    index S61.238 ☑
      with
        damage to nail S61.338 ☑
          with
            foreign body S61.348 ☑
        foreign body S61.248 ☑
      left S61.231 ☑
        with
          damage to nail S61.331 ☑
            with
              foreign body S61.341 ☑

Puncture — *continued*
  finger(s) — *continued*
    index — *continued*
      left — *continued*
        with — *continued*
          foreign body S61.241 ☑
      right S61.230 ☑
        with
          damage to nail S61.330 ☑
            with
              foreign body S61.340 ☑
          foreign body S61.240 ☑
    little S61.238 ☑
      with
        damage to nail S61.338 ☑
          with
            foreign body S61.348 ☑
        foreign body S61.248 ☑
      left S61.237 ☑
        with
          damage to nail S61.337 ☑
            with
              foreign body S61.347 ☑
          foreign body S61.247 ☑
      right S61.236 ☑
        with
          damage to nail S61.336 ☑
            with
              foreign body S61.346 ☑
          foreign body S61.246 ☑
    middle S61.238 ☑
      with
        damage to nail S61.338 ☑
          with
            foreign body S61.348 ☑
        foreign body S61.248 ☑
      left S61.233 ☑
        with
          damage to nail S61.333 ☑
            with
              foreign body S61.343 ☑
          foreign body S61.243 ☑
      right S61.232 ☑
        with
          damage to nail S61.332 ☑
            with
              foreign body S61.342 ☑
          foreign body S61.242 ☑
    ring S61.238 ☑
      with
        damage to nail S61.338 ☑
          with
            foreign body S61.348 ☑
        foreign body S61.248 ☑
      left S61.235 ☑
        with
          damage to nail S61.335 ☑
            with
              foreign body S61.345 ☑
          foreign body S61.245 ☑
      right S61.234 ☑
        with
          damage to nail S61.334 ☑
            with
              foreign body S61.344 ☑
          foreign body S61.244 ☑
  flank S31.139 ☑
    with foreign body S31.149 ☑
  foot (except toe(s) alone) S91.339 ☑
    with foreign body S91.349 ☑
    left S91.332 ☑
      with foreign body S91.342 ☑
    right S91.331 ☑
      with foreign body S91.341 ☑
    toe — *see* Puncture, toe
  forearm S51.839 ☑
    with
      foreign body S51.849 ☑
    elbow only — *see* Puncture, elbow
    left S51.832 ☑
      with
        foreign body S51.842 ☑
    right S51.831 ☑
      with
        foreign body S51.841 ☑
  forehead — *see* Puncture, head, specified site NEC

Puncture — *continued*
genital organs, external
female S31.532 ☑
with foreign body S31.542 ☑
vagina — *see* Puncture, vagina
vulva — *see* Puncture, vulva
male S31.531 ☑
with foreign body S31.541 ☑
penis — *see* Puncture, penis
scrotum — *see* Puncture, scrotum
testis — *see* Puncture, testis
groin — *see* Puncture, abdomen, wall
gum — *see* Puncture, oral cavity
hand S61.439 ☑
with
foreign body S61.449 ☑
finger — *see* Puncture, finger
left S61.432 ☑
with
foreign body S61.442 ☑
right S61.431 ☑
with
foreign body S61.441 ☑
thumb — *see* Puncture, thumb
head S01.93 ☑
with foreign body S01.94 ☑
cheek — *see* Puncture, cheek
ear — *see* Puncture, ear
eyelid — *see* Puncture, eyelid
lip — *see* Puncture, oral cavity
nose — *see* Puncture, nose
oral cavity — *see* Puncture, oral cavity
scalp S01.03 ☑
with foreign body S01.04 ☑
specified site NEC S01.83 ☑
with foreign body S01.84 ☑
temporomandibular area — *see* Puncture, cheek
heart S26.99 ☑
with hemopericardium S26.09 ☑
without hemopericardium S26.19 ☑
heel — *see* Puncture, foot
hip S71.039 ☑
with foreign body S71.049 ☑
left S71.032 ☑
with foreign body S71.042 ☑
right S71.031 ☑
with foreign body S71.041 ☑
hymen — *see* Puncture, vagina
hypochondrium — *see* Puncture, abdomen, wall
hypogastric region — *see* Puncture, abdomen, wall
inguinal region — *see* Puncture, abdomen, wall
instep — *see* Puncture, foot
internal organs — *see* Injury, by site
interscapular region — *see* Puncture, thorax, back
intestine
large
colon S36.599 ☑
ascending S36.590 ☑
descending S36.592 ☑
sigmoid S36.593 ☑
specified site NEC S36.598 ☑
transverse S36.591 ☑
rectum S36.69 ☑
small S36.499 ☑
duodenum S36.490 ☑
specified site NEC S36.498 ☑
intra-abdominal organ S36.99 ☑
gallbladder S36.128 ☑
intestine — *see* Puncture, intestine
liver S36.118 ☑
pancreas — *see* Puncture, pancreas
peritoneum S36.81 ☑
specified site NEC S36.898 ☑
spleen S36.09 ☑
stomach S36.39 ☑
jaw — *see* Puncture, head, specified site NEC
knee S81.039 ☑
with foreign body S81.049 ☑
left S81.032 ☑
with foreign body S81.042 ☑
right S81.031 ☑
with foreign body S81.041 ☑
labium (majus) (minus) — *see* Puncture, vulva
lacrimal duct — *see* Puncture, eyelid
larynx S11.013 ☑
with foreign body S11.014 ☑

Puncture — *continued*
leg (lower) S81.839 ☑
with foreign body S81.849 ☑
foot — *see* Puncture, foot
knee — *see* Puncture, knee
left S81.832 ☑
with foreign body S81.842 ☑
right S81.831 ☑
with foreign body S81.841 ☑
upper — *see* Puncture, thigh
lip S01.531 ☑
with foreign body S01.541 ☑
loin — *see* Puncture, abdomen, wall
lower back — *see* Puncture, back, lower
lumbar region — *see* Puncture, back, lower
malar region — *see* Puncture, head, specified site NEC
mammary — *see* Puncture, breast
mastoid region — *see* Puncture, head, specified site NEC
mouth — *see* Puncture, oral cavity
nail
finger — *see* Puncture, finger, with damage to nail
toe — *see* Puncture, toe, with damage to nail
nasal (septum) (sinus) — *see* Puncture, nose
nasopharynx — *see* Puncture, head, specified site NEC
neck S11.93 ☑
with foreign body S11.94 ☑
involving
cervical esophagus — *see* Puncture, cervical esophagus
larynx — *see* Puncture, larynx
pharynx — *see* Puncture, pharynx
thyroid gland — *see* Puncture, thyroid gland
trachea — *see* Puncture, trachea
specified site NEC S11.83 ☑
with foreign body S11.84 ☑
nose (septum) (sinus) S01.23 ☑
with foreign body S01.24 ☑
ocular — *see* Puncture, eyeball
oral cavity S01.532 ☑
with foreign body S01.542 ☑
orbit S05.4- ☑
palate — *see* Puncture, oral cavity
palm — *see* Puncture, hand
pancreas S36.299 ☑
body S36.291 ☑
head S36.290 ☑
tail S36.292 ☑
pelvis — *see* Puncture, back, lower
penis S31.23 ☑
with foreign body S31.24 ☑
perineum
female S31.43 ☑
with foreign body S31.44 ☑
male S31.139 ☑
with foreign body S31.149 ☑
periocular area (with or without lacrimal passages) — *see* Puncture, eyelid
phalanges
finger — *see* Puncture, finger
toe — *see* Puncture, toe
pharynx S11.23 ☑
with foreign body S11.24 ☑
pinna — *see* Puncture, ear
popliteal space — *see* Puncture, knee
prepuce — *see* Puncture, penis
pubic region S31.139 ☑
with foreign body S31.149 ☑
pudendum — *see* Puncture, genital organs, external
rectovaginal septum — *see* Puncture, vagina
sacral region — *see* Puncture, back, lower
sacroiliac region — *see* Puncture, back, lower
salivary gland — *see* Puncture, oral cavity
scalp S01.03 ☑
with foreign body S01.04 ☑
scapular region — *see* Puncture, shoulder
scrotum S31.33 ☑
with foreign body S31.34 ☑
shin — *see* Puncture, leg
shoulder S41.039 ☑
with foreign body S41.049 ☑
left S41.032 ☑
with foreign body S41.042 ☑
right S41.031 ☑
with foreign body S41.041 ☑
spermatic cord — *see* Puncture, testis

Puncture — *continued*
sternal region — *see* Puncture, thorax, front
submaxillary region — *see* Puncture, head, specified site NEC
submental region — *see* Puncture, head, specified site NEC
subungual
finger(s) — *see* Puncture, finger, with damage to nail
toe — *see* Puncture, toe, with damage to nail
supraclavicular fossa — *see* Puncture, neck, specified site NEC
temple, temporal region — *see* Puncture, head, specified site NEC
temporomandibular area — *see* Puncture, cheek
testis S31.33 ☑
with foreign body S31.34 ☑
thigh S71.139 ☑
with foreign body S71.149 ☑
left S71.132 ☑
with foreign body S71.142 ☑
right S71.131 ☑
with foreign body S71.141 ☑
thorax, thoracic (wall) S21.93 ☑
with foreign body S21.94 ☑
back S21.23- ☑
with
foreign body S21.24- ☑
with penetration S21.44 ☑
penetration S21.43 ☑
breast — *see* Puncture, breast
front S21.13- ☑
with
foreign body S21.14- ☑
with penetration S21.34 ☑
penetration S21.33 ☑
throat — *see* Puncture, neck
thumb S61.039 ☑
with
damage to nail S61.139 ☑
with
foreign body S61.149 ☑
foreign body S61.049 ☑
left S61.032 ☑
with
damage to nail S61.132 ☑
with
foreign body S61.142 ☑
foreign body S61.042 ☑
right S61.031 ☑
with
damage to nail S61.131 ☑
with
foreign body S61.141 ☑
foreign body S61.041 ☑
thyroid gland S11.13 ☑
with foreign body S11.14 ☑
toe(s) S91.139 ☑
with
damage to nail S91.239 ☑
with
foreign body S91.249 ☑
foreign body S91.149 ☑
great S91.133 ☑
with
damage to nail S91.233 ☑
with
foreign body S91.243 ☑
foreign body S91.143 ☑
left S91.132 ☑
with
damage to nail S91.232 ☑
with
foreign body S91.242 ☑
foreign body S91.142 ☑
right S91.131 ☑
with
damage to nail S91.231 ☑
with
foreign body S91.241 ☑
foreign body S91.141 ☑
lesser S91.136 ☑
with
damage to nail S91.236 ☑
with
foreign body S91.246 ☑

☑ **Additional Character Required — Refer to the Tabular List for Character Selection**   ▽ **Subterms under main terms may continue to next column or page**

Puncture — *continued*
  toe(s) — *continued*
    lesser — *continued*
      with — *continued*
        foreign body S91.146 ☑
      left S91.135 ☑
        with
          damage to nail S91.235 ☑
            with
              foreign body S91.245 ☑
          foreign body S91.145 ☑
      right S91.134 ☑
        with
          damage to nail S91.234 ☑
            with
              foreign body S91.244 ☑
          foreign body S91.144 ☑
  tongue — *see* Puncture, oral cavity
  trachea S11.023 ☑
    with foreign body S11.024 ☑
  tunica vaginalis — *see* Puncture, testis
  tympanum, tympanic membrane S09.2- ☑
  umbilical region S31.135 ☑
    with foreign body S31.145 ☑
  uvula — *see* Puncture, oral cavity
  vagina S31.43 ☑
    with foreign body S31.44 ☑
  vocal cords S11.033 ☑
    with foreign body S11.034 ☑
  vulva S31.43 ☑
    with foreign body S31.44 ☑
  wrist S61.539 ☑
    with
      foreign body S61.549 ☑
    left S61.532 ☑
      with
        foreign body S61.542 ☑
    right S61.531 ☑
      with
        foreign body S61.541 ☑
PUO (pyrexia of unknown origin) R50.9
Pupillary membrane (persistent) Q13.89
Pupillotonia — *see* Anomaly, pupil, function, tonic pupil
Purpura D69.2
  abdominal D69.0
  allergic D69.0
  anaphylactoid D69.0
  annularis telangiectodes L81.7
  arthritic D69.0
  autoerythrocyte sensitization D69.2
  autoimmune D69.0
  bacterial D69.0
  Bateman's (senile) D69.2
  capillary fragility (hereditary) (idiopathic) D69.8
  cryoglobulinemic D89.1
  Devil's pinches D69.2
  fibrinolytic — *see* Fibrinolysis
  fulminans, fulminous D65
  gangrenous D65
  hemorrhagic, hemorrhagica D69.3
    not due to thrombocytopenia D69.0
  Henoch (-Schönlein) (allergic) D69.0
  hypergammaglobulinemic (benign) (Waldenström) D89.0
  idiopathic (thrombocytopenic) D69.3
    nonthrombocytopenic D69.0
  immune thrombocytopenic D69.3
  infectious D69.0
  malignant D69.0
  neonatorum P54.5
  nervosa D69.0
  newborn P54.5
  nonthrombocytopenic D69.2
    hemorrhagic D69.0
    idiopathic D69.0
  nonthrombopenic D69.2
  peliosis rheumatica D69.0
  posttransfusion (post-transfusion) (from (fresh) whole blood or blood products) D69.51
  primary D69.49
  red cell membrane sensitivity D69.2
  rheumatica D69.0
  Schönlein (-Henoch) (allergic) D69.0
  scorbutic E54 [D77]
  senile D69.2
  simplex D69.2
  symptomatica D69.0

Purpura — *continued*
  telangiectasia annularis L81.7
  thrombocytopenic D69.49
    congenital D69.42
    hemorrhagic D69.3
    hereditary D69.42
    idiopathic D69.3
    immune D69.3
    neonatal, transitory P61.0
    thrombotic M31.1
  thrombohemolytic — *see* Fibrinolysis
  thrombolytic — *see* Fibrinolysis
  thrombopenic D69.49
  thrombotic, thrombocytopenic M31.1
  toxic D69.0
  vascular D69.0
  visceral symptoms D69.0
Purpuric spots R23.3
Purulent — *see* condition
Pus
  in
    stool R19.5
    urine N39.0
  tube (rupture) — *see* Salpingo-oophoritis
Pustular rash L08.0
Pustule (nonmalignant) L08.9
  malignant A22.0
Pustulosis palmaris et plantaris L40.3
Putnam (-Dana) **disease or syndrome** — *see* Degeneration, combined
Putrescent pulp (dental) K04.1
Pyarthritis, pyarthrosis — *see* Arthritis, pyogenic or pyemic
  tuberculous — *see* Tuberculosis, joint
Pyelectasis — *see* Hydronephrosis
Pyelitis (congenital) (uremic) (*see also* Pyelonephritis)
  with
    calculus — *see* category N20 ☑
      with hydronephrosis N13.2
    contracted kidney N11.9
  acute N10
  chronic N11.9
    with calculus — *see* category N20 ☑
      with hydronephrosis N13.2
  cystica N28.84
  puerperal (postpartum) O86.21
  tuberculous A18.11
Pyelocystitis — *see* Pyelonephritis
Pyelonephritis (*see also* Nephritis, tubulo-interstitial)
  with
    calculus — *see* category N20 ☑
      with hydronephrosis N13.2
    contracted kidney N11.9
  acute N10
  calculous — *see* category N20 ☑
    with hydronephrosis N13.2
  chronic N11.9
    with calculus — *see* category N20 ☑
      with hydronephrosis N13.2
    associated with ureteral obstruction or stricture N11.1
    nonobstructive N11.8
      with reflux (vesicoureteral) N11.0
    obstructive N11.1
    specified NEC N11.8
  in (due to)
    brucellosis A23.9 [N16]
    cryoglobulinemia (mixed) D89.1 [N16]
    cystinosis E72.04
    diphtheria A36.84
    glycogen storage disease E74.09 [N16]
    leukemia NEC C95.9- ☑ [N16]
    lymphoma NEC C85.90 [N16]
    multiple myeloma C90.0- ☑ [N16]
    obstruction N11.1
    Salmonella infection A02.25
    sarcoidosis D86.84
    sepsis A41.9 [N16]
    Sjögren's disease M35.04
    toxoplasmosis B58.83
    transplant rejection T86.91 [N16]
    Wilson's disease E83.01 [N16]
  nonobstructive N12
    with reflux (vesicoureteral) N11.0
    chronic N11.8
  syphilitic A52.75
Pyelonephrosis (obstructive) N11.1
  chronic N11.9

Pyelophlebitis I80.8
Pyeloureteritis cystica N28.85
Pyemia, pyemic (fever) (infection) (purulent) (*see also* Sepsis)
  joint — *see* Arthritis, pyogenic or pyemic
  liver K75.1
  pneumococcal A40.3
  portal K75.1
  postvaccinal T88.0 ☑
  puerperal, postpartum, childbirth O85
  specified organism NEC A41.89
  tuberculous — *see* Tuberculosis, miliary
Pygopagus Q89.4
Pyknoepilepsy (idiopathic) — *see* Pyknolepsy
Pyknolepsy G40.A09 (*following* G40.3)
  intractable G40.A19 (*following* G40.3)
    with status epilepticus G40.A11 (*following* G40.3)
    without status epilepticus G40.A19 (*following* G40.3)
  not intractable G40.A09 (*following* G40.3)
    with status epilepticus G40.A01 (*following* G40.3)
    without status epilepticus G40.A09 (*following* G40.3)
Pylephlebitis K75.1
Pyle's syndrome Q78.5
Pylethrombophlebitis K75.1
Pylethrombosis K75.1
Pyloritis K29.90
  with bleeding K29.91
Pylorospasm (reflex) **NEC** K31.3
  congenital or infantile Q40.0
  neurotic F45.8
  newborn Q40.0
  psychogenic F45.8
Pylorus, pyloric — *see* condition
Pyoarthrosis — *see* Arthritis, pyogenic or pyemic
Pyocele
  mastoid — *see* Mastoiditis, acute
  sinus (accessory) — *see* Sinusitis
  turbinate (bone) J32.9
  urethra (*see also* Urethritis) N34.0
Pyocolpos — *see* Vaginitis
Pyocystitis N30.80
  with hematuria N30.81
Pyoderma, pyodermia L08.0
  gangrenosum L88
  newborn P39.4
  phagedenic L88
  vegetans L08.81
Pyodermatitis L08.0
  vegetans L08.81
Pyogenic — *see* condition
Pyohydronephrosis N13.6
Pyometra, pyometrium, pyometritis — *see* Endometritis
Pyomyositis (tropical) — *see* Myositis, infective
Pyonephritis N12
Pyonephrosis N13.6
  tuberculous A18.11
Pyo-oophoritis — *see* Salpingo-oophoritis
Pyo-ovarium — *see* Salpingo-oophoritis
Pyopericarditis, pyopericardium I30.1
Pyophlebitis — *see* Phlebitis
Pyopneumopericardium I30.1
Pyopneumothorax (infective) J86.9
  with fistula J86.0
  tuberculous NEC A15.6
Pyosalpinx, pyosalpingitis (*see also* Salpingo-oophoritis)
Pyothorax J86.9
  with fistula J86.0
  tuberculous NEC A15.6
Pyoureter N28.89
  tuberculous A18.11
Pyramidopallidonigral syndrome G20
Pyrexia (of unknown origin) R50.9
  atmospheric T67.0 ☑
  during labor NEC O75.2
  heat T67.0 ☑
  newborn P81.9
    environmentally-induced P81.0
  persistent R50.9
  puerperal O86.4
Pyroglobulinemia NEC E88.09
Pyromania F63.1
Pyrosis R12
Pyuria (bacterial) N39.0

Q

Q fever A78
  with pneumonia A78
Quadricuspid aortic valve Q23.8
Quadrilateral fever A78
Quadriparesis — *see* Quadriplegia
  meaning muscle weakness M62.81
Quadriplegia G82.50
  complete
    C1-C4 level G82.51
    C5-C7 level G82.53
  congenital (cerebral) (spinal) G80.8
    spastic G80.0
  embolic (current episode) I63.4 ☑
  functional R53.2
  incomplete
    C1-C4 level G82.52
    C5-C7 level G82.54
  thrombotic (current episode) I63.3 ☑
  traumatic — *code to* injury with seventh character S
    current episode — *see* Injury, spinal (cord), cervical
Quadruplet, pregnancy — *see* Pregnancy, quadruplet
Quarrelsomeness F60.3
Queensland fever A77.3
Quervain's disease M65.4
  thyroid E06.1
Queyrat's erythroplasia D07.4
  penis D07.4
  specified site — *see* Neoplasm, skin, in situ
  unspecified site D07.4
Quincke's disease or edema T78.3 ☑
  hereditary D84.1
Quinsy (gangrenous) J36
Quintan fever A79.0
Quintuplet, pregnancy — *see* Pregnancy, quintuplet

R

Rabbit fever — *see* Tularemia
Rabies A82.9
  contact Z20.3
  exposure to Z20.3
  inoculation reaction — *see* Complications, vaccination
  sylvatic A82.0
  urban A82.1
Rachischisis — *see* Spina bifida
Rachitic (*see also* condition)
  deformities of spine (late effect) (sequelae) E64.3
  pelvis (late effect) (sequelae) E64.3
    with disproportion (fetopelvic) O33.0
      causing obstructed labor O65.0
Rachitis, rachitism (acute) (tarda) (*see also* Rickets)
  renalis N25.0
  sequelae E64.3
Radial nerve — *see* condition
Radiation
  burn — *see* Burn
  effects NOS T66 ☑
  sickness NOS T66 ☑
  therapy, encounter for Z51.0
Radiculitis (pressure) (vertebrogenic) — *see* Radiculopathy
Radiculomyelitis (*see also* Encephalitis)
  toxic, due to
    Clostridium tetani A35
    Corynebacterium diphtheriae A36.82
Radiculopathy M54.10
  cervical region M54.12
  cervicothoracic region M54.13
  due to
    disc disorder
      C3 M50.11
      C4 M50.11
      C5 M50.12
      C6 M50.12
      C7 M50.12
      C8 M50.13
    displacement of intervertebral disc — *see* Disorder, disc, with, radiculopathy
  leg M54.1- ☑
  lumbar region M54.16
  lumbosacral region M54.17
  occipito-atlanto-axial region M54.11
  postherpetic B02.29
  sacrococcygeal region M54.18

Radiculopathy — *continued*
  syphilitic A52.11
  thoracic region (with visceral pain) M54.14
  thoracolumbar region M54.15
Radiodermal burns (acute, chronic, or occupational) — *see* Burn
Radiodermatitis L58.9
  acute L58.0
  chronic L58.1
Radiotherapy session Z51.0
Rage, meaning rabies — *see* Rabies
Ragpicker's disease A22.1
Ragsorter's disease A22.1
Raillietiniasis B71.8
Railroad neurosis F48.8
Railway spine F48.8
Raised (*see also* Elevated)
  antibody titer R76.0
Rake teeth, tooth M26.39
Rales R09.89
Ramifying renal pelvis Q63.8
Ramsay-Hunt disease or syndrome (*see also* Hunt's disease) B02.21
  meaning dyssynergia cerebellaris myoclonica G11.1
Ranula K11.6
  congenital Q38.4
Rape
  adult
    confirmed T74.21 ☑
    suspected T76.21 ☑
  alleged, observation or examination, ruled out
    adult Z04.41
    child Z04.42
  child
    confirmed T74.22 ☑
    suspected T76.22 ☑
Rapid
  feeble pulse, due to shock, following injury T79.4 ☑
  heart (beat) R00.0
    psychogenic F45.8
  second stage (delivery) O62.3
  time-zone change syndrome — *see* Disorder, sleep, circadian rhythm, psychogenic
Rarefaction, bone — *see* Disorder, bone, density and structure, specified NEC
Rash (toxic) R21
  canker A38.9
  diaper L22
  drug (internal use) L27.0
    contact (*see also* Dermatitis, due to, drugs, external) L25.1
  following immunization T88.1 ☑
  food — *see* Dermatitis, due to, food
  heat L74.0
  napkin (psoriasiform) L22
  nettle — *see* Urticaria
  pustular L08.0
  rose R21
    epidemic B06.9
  scarlet A38.9
  serum (*see also* Reaction, serum) T80.69 ☑
  wandering tongue K14.1
Rasmussen aneurysm — *see* Tuberculosis, pulmonary
Rasmussen encephalitis G04.81
Rat-bite fever A25.9
  due to Streptobacillus moniliformis A25.1
  spirochetal (morsus muris) A25.0
Rathke's pouch tumor D44.3
Raymond (-Céstan) **syndrome** I65.8
Raynaud's disease, phenomenon or syndrome (secondary) I73.00
  with gangrene (symmetric) I73.01
RDS (newborn) (type I) P22.0
  type II P22.1
Reaction (*see also* Disorder)
  adaptation — *see* Disorder, adjustment
  adjustment (anxiety) (conduct disorder) (depressiveness) (distress) — *see* Disorder, adjustment
    with
      mutism, elective (child) (adolescent) F94.0
  adverse
    food (any) (ingested) NEC T78.1 ☑
      anaphylactic — *see* Shock, anaphylactic, due to food
  affective — *see* Disorder, mood
  allergic — *see* Allergy
  anaphylactic — *see* Shock, anaphylactic

Reaction — *continued*
  anaphylactoid — *see* Shock, anaphylactic
  anesthesia — *see* Anesthesia, complication
  antitoxin (prophylactic) (therapeutic) — *see* Complications, vaccination
  anxiety F41.1
  Arthus — *see* Arthus' phenomenon
  asthenic F48.8
  combat and operational stress F43.0
  compulsive F42
  conversion F44.9
  crisis, acute F43.0
  deoxyribonuclease (DNA) (DNase) hypersensitivity D69.2
  depressive (single episode) F32.9
    affective (single episode) F31.4
      recurrent episode F33.9
    neurotic F34.1
    psychoneurotic F34.1
    psychotic F32.3
    recurrent — *see* Disorder, depressive, recurrent
  dissociative F44.9
  drug NEC T88.7 ☑
    addictive — *see* Dependence, drug
      transmitted via placenta or breast milk — *see* Absorption, drug, addictive, through placenta
    allergic — *see* Allergy, drug
    lichenoid L43.2
    newborn P93.8
      gray baby syndrome P93.0
    overdose or poisoning (by accident) — *see* Table of Drugs and Chemicals, by drug, poisoning
    photoallergic L56.1
    phototoxic L56.0
    withdrawal — *see* Dependence, by drug, with, withdrawal
      infant of dependent mother P96.1
      newborn P96.1
    wrong substance given or taken (by accident) — *see* Table of Drugs and Chemicals, by drug, poisoning
  fear F40.9
    child (abnormal) F93.8
  febrile nonhemolytic transfusion (FNHTR) R50.84
  fluid loss, cerebrospinal G97.1
  foreign
    body NEC — *see* Granuloma, foreign body
      in operative wound (inadvertently left) — *see* Foreign body, accidentally left during a procedure
    substance accidentally left during a procedure (chemical) (powder) (talc) T81.60 ☑
      aseptic peritonitis T81.61 ☑
      body or object (instrument) (sponge) (swab) — *see* Foreign body, accidentally left during a procedure
      specified reaction NEC T81.69 ☑
  grief — *see* Disorder, adjustment
  Herxheimer's R68.89
  hyperkinetic — *see* Hyperkinesia
  hypochondriacal F45.20
  hypoglycemic, due to insulin E16.0
    with coma (diabetic) — *see* Diabetes, coma nondiabetic E15
    therapeutic misadventure — *see* subcategory T38.3 ☑
  hypomanic F30.8
  hysterical F44.9
  immunization — *see* Complications, vaccination
  incompatibility
    ABO blood group (infusion) (transfusion) — *see* Complication(s), transfusion, incompatibility reaction, ABO
    delayed serologic T80.39 ☑
    minor blood group (Duffy) (E) (K(ell)) (Kidd) (Lewis) (M) (N) (P) (S) T80.89 ☑
    Rh (factor) (infusion) (transfusion) — *see* Complication(s), transfusion, incompatibility reaction, Rh (factor)
  inflammatory — *see* Infection
  infusion — *see* Complications, infusion
  inoculation (immune serum) — *see* Complications, vaccination
  insulin T38.3- ☑
  involutional psychotic — *see* Disorder, depressive

☑ **Additional Character Required** — Refer to the Tabular List for Character Selection   ⬇ **Subterms under main terms may continue to next column or page**

Reaction — *continued*
  leukemoid D72.823
    basophilic D72.823
    lymphocytic D72.823
    monocytic D72.823
    myelocytic D72.823
    neutrophilic D72.823
  LSD (acute)
    due to drug abuse — *see* Abuse, drug, hallucinogen
    due to drug dependence — *see* Dependence, drug, hallucinogen
  lumbar puncture G97.1
  manic-depressive — *see* Disorder, bipolar
  neurasthenic F48.8
  neurogenic — *see* Neurosis
  neurotic F48.9
  neurotic-depressive F34.1
  nitritoid — *see* Crisis, nitritoid
  nonspecific
    to
      cell mediated immunity measurement of gamma interferon antigen response without active tuberculosis R76.12
      QuantiFERON-TB test (QFT) without active tuberculosis R76.12
      tuberculin test (*see also* Reaction, tuberculin skin test) R76.11
  obsessive-compulsive F42
  organic, acute or subacute — *see* Delirium
  paranoid (acute) F23
    chronic F22
    senile F03 ☑
  passive dependency F60.7
  phobic F40.9
  post-traumatic stress, uncomplicated Z73.3
  psychogenic F99
  psychoneurotic (*see also* Neurosis)
    compulsive F42
    depersonalization F48.1
    depressive F34.1
    hypochondriacal F45.20
    neurasthenic F48.8
    obsessive F42
  psychophysiologic — *see* Disorder, somatoform
  psychosomatic — *see* Disorder, somatoform
  psychotic — *see* Psychosis
  scarlet fever toxin — *see* Complications, vaccination
  schizophrenic F23
    acute (brief) (undifferentiated) F23
    latent F21
    undifferentiated (acute) (brief) F23
  serological for syphilis — *see* Serology for syphilis
  serum T80.69 ☑
    anaphylactic (immediate) (*see also* Shock, anaphylactic) T80.59 ☑
    specified reaction NEC
      due to
        administration of blood and blood products T80.61 ☑
        immunization T80.62 ☑
        serum specified NEC T80.69 ☑
        vaccination T80.62 ☑
  situational — *see* Disorder, adjustment
  somatization — *see* Disorder, somatoform
  spinal puncture G97.1
  stress (severe) F43.9
    acute (agitation) ("daze") (disorientation) (disturbance of consciousness) (flight reaction) (fugue) F43.0
    specified NEC F43.8
  surgical procedure — *see* Complications, surgical procedure
  tetanus antitoxin — *see* Complications, vaccination
  toxic, to local anesthesia T81.89 ☑
    in labor and delivery O74.4
    in pregnancy O29.3X- ☑
    postpartum, puerperal O89.3
  toxin-antitoxin — *see* Complications, vaccination
  transfusion (blood) (bone marrow) (lymphocytes) (allergic) — *see* Complications, transfusion
  tuberculin skin test, abnormal R76.11
  vaccination (any) — *see* Complications, vaccination
  withdrawing, child or adolescent F93.8
Reactive airway disease — *see* Asthma
Reactive depression — *see* Reaction, depressive

Rearrangement
  chromosomal
    balanced (in) Q95.9
      abnormal individual (autosomal) Q95.2
        non-sex (autosomal) chromosomes Q95.2
        sex/non-sex chromosomes Q95.3
      specified NEC Q95.8
Recalcitrant patient — *see* Noncompliance
Recanalization, thrombus — *see* Thrombosis
Recession, receding
  chamber angle (eye) H21.55- ☑
  chin M26.09
  gingival (generalized) (localized) (postinfective) (postoperative) K06.0
Recklinghausen disease Q85.01
  bones E21.0
Reclus' disease (cystic) — *see* Mastopathy, cystic
Recrudescent typhus (fever) A75.1
Recruitment, auditory H93.21- ☑
Rectalgia K62.89
Rectitis K62.89
Rectocele
  female (without uterine prolapse) N81.6
    with uterine prolapse N81.4
      incomplete N81.2
  in pregnancy — *see* Pregnancy, complicated by, abnormal, pelvic organs or tissues NEC
  male K62.3
Rectosigmoid junction — *see* condition
Rectosigmoiditis K63.89
  ulcerative (chronic) K51.30
    with
      complication K51.319
        abscess K51.314
        fistula K51.313
        obstruction K51.312
        rectal bleeding K51.311
        specified NEC K51.318
Rectourethral — *see* condition
Rectovaginal — *see* condition
Rectovesical — *see* condition
Rectum, rectal — *see* condition
Recurrent — *see* condition
  pregnancy loss — *see* Loss (of), pregnancy, recurrent
Red bugs B88.0
Red tide (*see also* Table of Drugs and Chemicals) T65.82- ☑
Red-cedar lung or pneumonitis J67.8
Reduced
  mobility Z74.09
  ventilatory or vital capacity R94.2
Redundant, redundancy
  anus (congenital) Q43.8
  clitoris N90.89
  colon (congenital) Q43.8
  foreskin (congenital) N47.8
  intestine (congenital) Q43.8
  labia N90.6
  organ or site, congenital NEC — *see* Accessory
  panniculus (abdominal) E65
  prepuce (congenital) N47.8
  pylorus K31.89
  rectum (congenital) Q43.8
  scrotum N50.8
  sigmoid (congenital) Q43.8
  skin (of face) L57.4
    eyelids — *see* Blepharochalasis
  stomach K31.89
Reduplication — *see* Duplication
Reflex R29.2
  hyperactive gag J39.2
  pupillary, abnormal — *see* Anomaly, pupil, function
  vasoconstriction I73.9
  vasovagal R55
Reflux K21.9
  acid K21.9
  esophageal K21.9
    with esophagitis K21.0
    newborn P78.83
  gastroesophageal K21.9
    with esophagitis K21.0
  mitral — *see* Insufficiency, mitral
  ureteral — *see* Reflux, vesicoureteral

Reflux — *continued*
  vesicoureteral (with scarring) N13.70
    with
      nephropathy N13.729
        with hydroureter N13.739
          bilateral N13.732
          unilateral N13.731
        without hydroureter N13.729
          bilateral N13.722
          unilateral N13.721
        bilateral N13.722
        unilateral N13.721
      pyelonephritis (chronic) N11.0
    without nephropathy N13.71
    congenital Q62.7
Reforming, artificial openings — *see* Attention to, artificial, opening
Refractive error — *see* Disorder, refraction
Refsum's disease or syndrome G60.1
Refusal of
  food, psychogenic F50.8
  treatment (because of) Z53.20
    left against medical advice (AMA) Z53.21
    patient's decision NEC Z53.29
    reasons of belief or group pressure Z53.1
Regional — *see* condition
Regurgitation R11.10
  aortic (valve) — *see* Insufficiency, aortic
  food (*see also* Vomiting)
    with reswallowing — *see* Rumination
    newborn P92.1
  gastric contents — *see* Vomiting
  heart — *see* Endocarditis
  mitral (valve) — *see* Insufficiency, mitral
    congenital Q23.3
  myocardial — *see* Endocarditis
  pulmonary (valve) (heart) I37.1
    congenital Q22.2
    syphilitic A52.03
  tricuspid — *see* Insufficiency, tricuspid
  valve, valvular — *see* Endocarditis
    congenital Q24.8
  vesicoureteral — *see* Reflux, vesicoureteral
Reichmann's disease or syndrome K31.89
Reifenstein syndrome E34.52
Reinsertion, contraceptive device Z30.433
Reiter's disease, syndrome, or urethritis M02.30
  ankle M02.37- ☑
  elbow M02.32- ☑
  foot joint M02.37- ☑
  hand joint M02.34- ☑
  hip M02.35- ☑
  knee M02.36- ☑
  multiple site M02.39
  shoulder M02.31- ☑
  vertebra M02.38
  wrist M02.33- ☑
Rejection
  food, psychogenic F50.8
  transplant T86.91
    bone T86.830
      marrow T86.01
    cornea T86.840
    heart T86.21
      with lung(s) T86.31
    intestine T86.850
    kidney T86.11
    liver T86.41
    lung(s) T86.810
      with heart T86.31
    organ (immune or nonimmune cause) T86.91
    pancreas T86.890
    skin (allograft) (autograft) T86.820
    specified NEC T86.890
    stem cell (peripheral blood) (umbilical cord) T86.5
Relapsing fever A68.9
  Carter's (Asiatic) A68.1
  Dutton's (West African) A68.1
  Koch's A68.9
  louse-borne (epidemic) A68.0
  Novy's (American) A68.1
  Obermeyers's (European) A68.0
  Spirillum A68.9
  tick-borne (endemic) A68.1
Relationship
  occlusal
    open anterior M26.220

Relationship — *continued*
  occlusal — *continued*
    open posterior M26.221
Relaxation
  anus (sphincter) K62.89
    psychogenic F45.8
  arch (foot) (*see also* Deformity, limb, flat foot)
  back ligaments — *see* Instability, joint, spine
  bladder (sphincter) N31.2
  cardioesophageal K21.9
  cervix — *see* Incompetency, cervix
  diaphragm J98.6
  joint (capsule) (ligament) (paralytic) — *see* Flail, joint
    congenital NEC Q74.8
  lumbosacral (joint) — *see* subcategory M53.2 ☑
  pelvic floor N81.89
  perineum N81.89
  posture R29.3
  rectum (sphincter) K62.89
  sacroiliac (joint) — *see* subcategory M53.2 ☑
  scrotum N50.8
  urethra (sphincter) N36.44
  vesical N31.2
Release from prison, anxiety concerning Z65.2
Remains
  canal of Cloquet Q14.0
  capsule (opaque) Q14.8
Remittent fever (malarial) B54
Remnant
  canal of Cloquet Q14.0
  capsule (opaque) Q14.8
  cervix, cervical stump (acquired) (postoperative) N88.8
  cystic duct, postcholecystectomy K91.5
  fingernail L60.8
    congenital Q84.6
  meniscus, knee — *see* Derangement, knee, meniscus, specified NEC
  thyroglossal duct Q89.2
  tonsil J35.8
    infected (chronic) J35.01
  urachus Q64.4
Removal (from) (of)
  artificial
    arm Z44.00- ☑
      complete Z44.01- ☑
      partial Z44.02- ☑
    eye Z44.2- ☑
    leg Z44.10- ☑
      complete Z44.11- ☑
      partial Z44.12- ☑
  breast implant Z45.81 ☑
  cardiac pulse generator (battery) (end-of-life) Z45.010
  catheter (urinary) (indwelling) Z46.6
    from artificial opening — *see* Attention to, artificial, opening
    non-vascular Z46.82
    vascular NEC Z45.2
  device Z46.9
    contraceptive Z30.432
    implanted NEC Z45.89
    specified NEC Z46.89
  drains Z48.03
  dressing (nonsurgical) Z48.00
    surgical Z48.01
  external
    fixation device — *code to* fracture with seventh character D
    prosthesis, prosthetic device Z44.9
      breast Z44.3- ☑
      specified NEC Z44.8
  home in childhood (to foster home or institution) Z62.29
  ileostomy Z43.2
  insulin pump Z46.81
  myringotomy device (stent) (tube) Z45.82
  nervous system device NEC Z46.2
    brain neuropacemaker Z46.2
    visual substitution device Z46.2
      implanted Z45.31
  non-vascular catheter Z46.82
  organ, prophylactic (for neoplasia management) — *see* Prophylactic, organ removal
  orthodontic device Z46.4
  staples Z48.02
  stent
    ureteral Z46.6
  suture Z48.02
  urinary device Z46.6

Removal — *continued*
  vascular access device or catheter Z45.2
Ren
  arcuatus Q63.1
  mobile, mobilis N28.89
    congenital Q63.8
  unguliformis Q63.1
Renal — *see* condition
Rendu-Osler-Weber disease or syndrome I78.0
Reninoma D41.0- ☑
Renon-Delille syndrome E23.3
Reovirus, as cause of disease classified elsewhere B97.5
Repeated falls NEC R29.6
Replaced chromosome by dicentric ring Q93.2
Replacement by artificial or mechanical device or prosthesis of
  bladder Z96.0
  blood vessel NEC Z95.828
  bone NEC Z96.7
  cochlea Z96.21
  coronary artery Z95.5
  eustachian tube Z96.29
  eye globe Z97.0
  heart Z95.812
    valve Z95.2
      prosthetic Z95.2
      specified NEC Z95.4
      xenogenic Z95.3
  intestine Z96.89
  joint Z96.60
    hip — *see* Presence, hip joint implant
    knee — *see* Presence, knee joint implant
    specified site NEC Z96.698
  larynx Z96.3
  lens Z96.1
  limb(s) — *see* Presence, artificial, limb
  mandible NEC (for tooth root implant(s)) Z96.5
  organ NEC Z96.89
  peripheral vessel NEC Z95.828
  stapes Z96.29
  teeth Z97.2
  tendon Z96.7
  tissue NEC Z96.89
  tooth root(s) Z96.5
  vessel NEC Z95.828
    coronary (artery) Z95.5
Request for expert evidence Z04.8
Reserve, decreased or low
  cardiac — *see* Disease, heart
  kidney N28.89
Residual (*see also* condition)
  ovary syndrome N99.83
  state, schizophrenic F20.5
  urine R39.19
Resistance, resistant (to)
  activated protein C D68.51
  complicating pregnancy O26.89 ☑
  insulin E88.81
  organism(s)
    to
      drug
        aminoglycosides Z16.29
        amoxicillin Z16.11
        ampicillin Z16.11
        antibiotic(s) Z16.20
          multiple Z16.24
          specified NEC Z16.29
        antifungal Z16.32
        antimicrobial (single) Z16.30
          multiple Z16.35
          specified NEC Z16.39
        antimycbacterial (single) Z16.341
          multiple Z16.342
        antiparasitic Z16.31
        antiviral Z16.33
        beta lactam antibiotics Z16.10
          specified NEC Z16.19
        cephalosporins Z16.19
        extended beta lactamase (ESBL) Z16.12
        fluoroquinolones Z16.23
        macrolides Z16.29
        methicillin — *see* MRSA
        multiple drugs (MDRO) Z16.24
          antibiotics Z16.24
        penicillins Z16.11
        quinine (and related compounds) Z16.31
        quinolones Z16.23

Resistance, resistant — *continued*
  organism(s) — *continued*
    to — *continued*
      drug — *continued*
        sulfonamides Z16.29
        tetracyclines Z16.29
        tuberculostatics (single) Z16.341
          multiple Z16.342
        vancomycin Z16.21
          related antibiotics Z16.22
  thyroid hormone E07.89
Resorption
  dental (roots) K03.3
    alveoli M26.79
  teeth (external) (internal) (pathological) (roots) K03.3
Respiration
  Cheyne-Stokes R06.3
  decreased due to shock, following injury T79.4 ☑
  disorder of, psychogenic F45.8
  insufficient, or poor R06.89
    newborn P28.5
  painful R07.1
  sighing, psychogenic F45.8
Respiratory (*see also* condition)
  distress syndrome (newborn) (type I) P22.0
    type II P22.1
  syncytial virus, as cause of disease classified elsewhere B97.4
Respite care Z75.5
Response (drug)
  photoallergic L56.1
  phototoxic L56.0
Restless legs (syndrome) G25.81
Restlessness R45.1
Restoration (of)
  dental
    aesthetically inadequate or displeasing K08.56
    defective K08.50
      specified NEC K08.59
    failure of marginal integrity K08.51
    failure of periodontal anatomical intergrity K08.54
  organ continuity from previous sterilization (tuboplasty) (vasoplasty) Z31.0
    aftercare Z31.42
  tooth (existing)
    contours biologically incompatible with oral health K08.54
    open margins K08.51
    overhanging K08.52
    poor aesthetic K08.56
    poor gingival margins K08.51
  unsatisfactory, of tooth K08.50
    specified NEC K08.59
Restorative material (dental)
  allergy to K08.55
  fractured K08.539
    with loss of material K08.531
    without loss of material K08.530
  unrepairable overhanging of K08.52
Restriction of housing space Z59.1
Rests, ovarian, in fallopian tube Q50.6
Restzustand (schizophrenic) F20.5
Retained (*see also* Retention)
  cholelithiasis following cholecystectomy K91.86
  foreign body fragments (type of) Z18.9
    acrylics Z18.2
    animal quill(s) or spines Z18.31
    cement Z18.83
    concrete Z18.83
    crystalline Z18.83
    depleted isotope Z18.09
    depleted uranium Z18.01
    diethylhexylphthalates Z18.2
    glass Z18.81
    isocyanate Z18.2
    magnetic metal Z18.11
    metal Z18.10
    nonmagnectic metal Z18.12
    nontherapeutic radioactive Z18.09
    organic NEC Z18.39
    plastic Z18.2
    quill(s) (animal) Z18.31
    radioactive (nontherapeutic) NEC Z18.09
    specified NEC Z18.89
    spine(s) (animal) Z18.31
    stone Z18.83
    tooth (teeth) Z18.32
    wood Z18.33

☑ **Additional Character Required — Refer to the Tabular List for Character Selection**　　🔻 **Subterms under main terms may continue to next column or page**

Retained — *continued*
  fragments (type of) Z18.9
    acrylics Z18.2
    animal quill(s) or spines Z18.31
    cement Z18.83
    concrete Z18.83
    crystalline Z18.83
    depleted isotope Z18.09
    depleted uranium Z18.01
    diethylhexylphthalates Z18.2
    glass Z18.81
    isocyanate Z18.2
    magnetic metal Z18.11
    metal Z18.10
    nonmagnectic metal Z18.12
    nontherapeutic radioactive Z18.09
    organic NEC Z18.39
    plastic Z18.2
    quill(s) (animal) Z18.31
    radioactive (nontherapeutic) NEC Z18.09
    specified NEC Z18.89
    spine(s) (animal) Z18.31
    stone Z18.83
    tooth (teeth) Z18.32
    wood Z18.33
  gallstones, following cholecystectomy K91.86
Retardation
  development, developmental, specific — *see* Disorder, developmental
  endochondral bone growth — *see* Disorder, bone, development or growth
  growth R62.50
    due to malnutrition E45
  mental — *see* Disability, intellectual
  motor function, specific F82
  physical (child) R62.52
    due to malnutrition E45
  reading (specific) F81.0
  spelling (specific) (without reading disorder) F81.81
Retching — *see* Vomiting
Retention (*see also* Retained)
  bladder — *see* Retention, urine
  carbon dioxide E87.2
  cholelithiasis following cholecystectomy K91.86
  cyst — *see* Cyst
  dead
    fetus (at or near term) (mother) O36.4 ☑
      early fetal death O02.1
    ovum O02.0
  decidua (fragments) (following delivery) (with hemorrhage) O72.2
    without hemorrhage O73.1
  deciduous tooth K00.6
  dental root K08.3
  fecal — *see* Constipation
  fetus
    dead O36.4 ☑
      early O02.1
  fluid R60.9
  foreign body (*see also* Foreign body, retained)
    current trauma — *code as* Foreign body, by site or type
  gallstones, following cholecystectomy K91.86
  gastric K31.89
  intrauterine contraceptive device, in pregnancy — *see* Pregnancy, complicated by, retention, intrauterine device
  membranes (complicating delivery) (with hemorrhage) O72.2
    with abortion — *see* Abortion, by type
    without hemorrhage O73.1
  meniscus — *see* Derangement, meniscus
  menses N94.89
  milk (puerperal, postpartum) O92.79
  nitrogen, extrarenal R39.2
  ovary syndrome N99.83
  placenta (total) (with hemorrhage) O72.0
    without hemorrhage O73.0
    portions or fragments (with hemorrhage) O72.2
      without hemorrhage O73.1
  products of conception
    early pregnancy (dead fetus) O02.1
    following
      delivery (with hemorrhage) O72.2
        without hemorrhage O73.1
  secundines (following delivery) (with hemorrhage) O72.0
    without hemorrhage O73.0

Retention — *continued*
  secundines — *continued*
    complicating puerperium (delayed hemorrhage) O72.2
    partial O72.2
      without hemorrhage O73.1
  smegma, clitoris N90.89
  urine R33.9
    drug-induced R33.0
    due to hyperplasia (hypertrophy) of prostate — *see* Hyperplasia, prostate
    organic R33.8
      drug-induced R33.0
    psychogenic F45.8
    specified NEC R33.8
  water (in tissues) — *see* Edema
Reticulation, dust — *see* Pneumoconiosis
Reticulocytosis R70.1
Reticuloendotheliosis
  acute infantile C96.0
  leukemic C91.4- ☑
  malignant C96.9
  nonlipid C96.0
Reticulohistiocytoma (giant-cell) D76.3
Reticuloid, actinic L57.1
Reticulosis (skin)
  acute of infancy C96.0
  hemophagocytic, familial D76.1
  histiocytic medullary C96.9
  lipomelanotic I89.8
  malignant (midline) C86.0
  nonlipid C96.0
  polymorphic C83.8- ☑
  Sézary — *see* Sézary disease
Retina, retinal (*see also* condition)
  dark area D49.81
Retinitis (*see also* Inflammation, chorioretinal)
  albuminurica N18.9 [H32]
  diabetic — *see* Diabetes, retinitis
  disciformis — *see* Degeneration, macula
  focal — *see* Inflammation, chorioretinal, focal
  gravidarum — *see* Pregnancy, complicated by, specified pregnancy-related condition NEC
  juxtapapillaris — *see* Inflammation, chorioretinal, focal, juxtapapillary
  luetic — *see* Retinitis, syphilitic
  pigmentosa H35.52
  proliferans — *see* Disorder, globe, degenerative, specified type NEC
  proliferating — *see* Disorder, globe, degenerative, specified type NEC
  renal N18.9 [H32]
  syphilitic (early) (secondary) A51.43
    central, recurrent A52.71
    congenital (early) A50.01 [H32]
    late A52.71
  tuberculous A18.53
Retinoblastoma C69.2- ☑
  differentiated C69.2- ☑
  undifferentiated C69.2- ☑
Retinochoroiditis (*see also* Inflammation, chorioretinal)
  disseminated — *see* Inflammation, chorioretinal, disseminated
    syphilitic A52.71
  focal — *see* Inflammation, chorioretinal
  juxtapapillaris — *see* Inflammation, chorioretinal, focal, juxtapapillary
Retinopathy (background) H35.00
  arteriosclerotic I70.8 [H35.0-] ☑
  atherosclerotic I70.8 [H35.0-] ☑
  central serous — *see* Chorioretinopathy, central serous
  Coats H35.02- ☑
  diabetic — *see* Diabetes, retinopathy
  exudative H35.02- ☑
  hypertensive H35.03- ☑
  in (due to)
    diabetes — *see* Diabetes, retinopathy
    sickle-cell disorders D57.- ☑ [H36]
  of prematurity H35.10- ☑
    stage 0 H35.11- ☑
    stage 1 H35.12- ☑
    stage 2 H35.13- ☑
    stage 3 H35.14- ☑
    stage 4 H35.15- ☑
    stage 5 H35.16- ☑
  pigmentary, congenital — *see* Dystrophy, retina

Retinopathy — *continued*
  proliferative NEC H35.2- ☑
    diabetic — *see* Diabetes, retinopathy, proliferative
  sickle-cell D57.- ☑ [H36]
  solar H31.02- ☑
Retinoschisis H33.10- ☑
  congenital Q14.1
  specified type NEC H33.19- ☑
Retortamoniasis A07.8
Retractile testis Q55.22
Retraction
  cervix — *see* Retroversion, uterus
  drum (membrane) — *see* Disorder, tympanic membrane, specified NEC
  finger — *see* Deformity, finger
  lid H02.539
    left H02.536
      lower H02.535
      upper H02.534
    right H02.533
      lower H02.532
      upper H02.531
  lung J98.4
  mediastinum J98.5
  nipple N64.53
    associated with
      lactation O92.03
      pregnancy O92.01- ☑
      puerperium O92.02
    congenital Q83.8
  palmar fascia M72.0
  pleura — *see* Pleurisy
  ring, uterus (Bandl's) (pathological) O62.4
  sternum (congenital) Q76.7
    acquired M95.4
  uterus — *see* Retroversion, uterus
  valve (heart) — *see* Endocarditis
Retrobulbar — *see* condition
Retrocecal — *see* condition
Retrocession — *see* Retroversion
Retrodisplacement — *see* Retroversion
Retroflection, retroflexion — *see* Retroversion
Retrognathia, retrognathism (mandibular) (maxillary) M26.19
Retrograde menstruation N92.5
Retroperineal — *see* condition
Retroperitoneal — *see* condition
Retroperitonitis K68.9
Retropharyngeal — *see* condition
Retroplacental — *see* condition
Retroposition — *see* Retroversion
Retroprosthetic membrane T85.398 ☑
Retrosternal thyroid (congenital) Q89.2
Retroversion, retroverted
  cervix — *see* Retroversion, uterus
  female NEC — *see* Retroversion, uterus
  iris H21.89
  testis (congenital) Q55.29
  uterus (acquired) (acute) (any degree) (asymptomatic) (cervix) (postinfectional) (postpartal, old) N85.4
    congenital Q51.818
    in pregnancy O34.53- ☑
Retrovirus, as cause of disease classified elsewhere B97.30
  human
    immunodeficiency, type 2 (HIV 2) B97.35
    T-cell lymphotropic
      type I (HTLV-I) B97.33
      type II (HTLV-II) B97.34
  lentivirus B97.31
  oncovirus B97.32
  specified NEC B97.39
Retrusion, premaxilla (developmental) M26.09
Rett's disease or syndrome F84.2
Reverse peristalsis R19.2
Reye's syndrome G93.7
Rh (factor)
  hemolytic disease (newborn) P55.0
  incompatibility, immunization or sensitization
    affecting management of pregnancy NEC O36.09- ☑
      anti-D antibody O36.01- ☑
    newborn P55.0
    transfusion reaction — *see* Complication(s), transfusion, incompatibility reaction, Rh (factor)
  negative mother affecting newborn P55.0

Rh — *continued*
  titer elevated — *see* Complication(s), transfusion, incompatibility reaction, Rh (factor)
  transfusion reaction — *see* Complication(s), transfusion, incompatibility reaction, Rh (factor)
Rhabdomyolysis (idiopathic) NEC M62.82
  traumatic T79.6 ☑
Rhabdomyoma (*see also* Neoplasm, connective tissue, benign)
  adult — *see* Neoplasm, connective tissue, benign
  fetal — *see* Neoplasm, connective tissue, benign
  glycogenic — *see* Neoplasm, connective tissue, benign
Rhabdomyosarcoma (any type) — *see* Neoplasm, connective tissue, malignant
Rhabdosarcoma — *see* Rhabdomyosarcoma
Rhesus (factor) **incompatibility** — *see* Rh, incompatibility
Rheumatic (acute) (subacute) (chronic)
  adherent pericardium I09.2
  coronary arteritis I01.9
  degeneration, myocardium I09.0
  fever (acute) — *see* Fever, rheumatic
  heart — *see* Disease, heart, rheumatic
  myocardial degeneration — *see* Degeneration, myocardium
  myocarditis (chronic) (inactive) (with chorea) I09.0
    with chorea (acute) (rheumatic) (Sydenham's) I02.0
    active or acute I01.2
  pancarditis, acute I01.8
    with chorea (acute (rheumatic) Sydenham's) I02.0
  pericarditis (active) (acute) (with effusion) (with pneumonia) I01.0
    with chorea (acute) (rheumatic) (Sydenham's) I02.0
    chronic or inactive I09.2
  pneumonia I00 [J17]
  torticollis M43.6
  typhoid fever A01.09
Rheumatism (articular) (neuralgic) (nonarticular) M79.0
  gout — *see* Arthritis, rheumatoid
  intercostal, meaning Tietze's disease M94.0
  palindromic (any site) M12.30
    ankle M12.37- ☑
    elbow M12.32- ☑
    foot joint M12.37- ☑
    hand joint M12.34- ☑
    hip M12.35- ☑
    knee M12.36- ☑
    multiple site M12.39
    shoulder M12.31- ☑
    specified joint NEC M12.38
    vertebrae M12.38
    wrist M12.33- ☑
  sciatic M54.4- ☑
Rheumatoid (*see also* condition)
  arthritis (*see also* Arthritis, rheumatoid)
    with involvement of organs NEC M05.60
      ankle M05.67- ☑
      elbow M05.62- ☑
      foot joint M05.67- ☑
      hand joint M05.64- ☑
      hip M05.65- ☑
      knee M05.66- ☑
      multiple site M05.69
      shoulder M05.61- ☑
      vertebra — *see* Spondylitis, ankylosing
      wrist M05.63- ☑
    seronegative — *see* Arthritis, rheumatoid, seronegative
    seropositive — *see* Arthritis, rheumatoid, seropositive
  carditis M05.30
    ankle M05.37- ☑
    elbow M05.32- ☑
    foot joint M05.37- ☑
    hand joint M05.34- ☑
    hip M05.35- ☑
    knee M05.36- ☑
    multiple site M05.39
    shoulder M05.31- ☑
    vertebra — *see* Spondylitis, ankylosing
    wrist M05.33- ☑
  endocarditis — *see* Rheumatoid, carditis
  lung (disease) M05.10
    ankle M05.17- ☑
    elbow M05.12- ☑
    foot joint M05.17- ☑
    hand joint M05.14- ☑

Rheumatoid — *continued*
  lung — *continued*
    hip M05.15- ☑
    knee M05.16- ☑
    multiple site M05.19
    shoulder M05.11- ☑
    vertebra — *see* Spondylitis, ankylosing
    wrist M05.13- ☑
  myocarditis — *see* Rheumatoid, carditis
  myopathy M05.40
    ankle M05.47- ☑
    elbow M05.42- ☑
    foot joint M05.47- ☑
    hand joint M05.44- ☑
    hip M05.45- ☑
    knee M05.46- ☑
    multiple site M05.49
    shoulder M05.41- ☑
    vertebra — *see* Spondylitis, ankylosing
    wrist M05.43- ☑
  pericarditis — *see* Rheumatoid, carditis
  polyarthritis — *see* Arthritis, rheumatoid
  polyneuropathy M05.50
    ankle M05.57- ☑
    elbow M05.52- ☑
    foot joint M05.57- ☑
    hand joint M05.54- ☑
    hip M05.55- ☑
    knee M05.56- ☑
    multiple site M05.59
    shoulder M05.51- ☑
    vertebra — *see* Spondylitis, ankylosing
    wrist M05.53- ☑
  vasculitis M05.20
    ankle M05.27- ☑
    elbow M05.22- ☑
    foot joint M05.27- ☑
    hand joint M05.24- ☑
    hip M05.25- ☑
    knee M05.26- ☑
    multiple site M05.29
    shoulder M05.21- ☑
    vertebra — *see* Spondylitis, ankylosing
    wrist M05.23- ☑
Rhinitis (atrophic) (catarrhal) (chronic) (croupous) (fibrinous) (granulomatous) (hyperplastic) (hypertrophic) (membranous) (obstructive) (purulent) (suppurative) (ulcerative) J31.0
  with
    sore throat — *see* Nasopharyngitis
  acute J00
  allergic J30.9
    with asthma J45.909
      with
        exacerbation (acute) J45.901
        status asthmaticus J45.902
      due to
        food J30.5
        pollen J30.1
      nonseasonal J30.89
      perennial J30.89
      seasonal NEC J30.2
      specified NEC J30.89
  infective J00
  pneumococcal J00
  syphilitic A52.73
    congenital A50.05 [J99]
  tuberculous A15.8
  vasomotor J30.0
Rhinoantritis (chronic) — *see* Sinusitis, maxillary
Rhinodacryolith — *see* Dacryolith
Rhinolith (nasal sinus) J34.89
Rhinomegaly J34.89
Rhinopharyngitis (acute) (subacute) (*see also* Nasopharyngitis)
  chronic J31.1
  destructive ulcerating A66.5
  mutilans A66.5
Rhinophyma L71.1
Rhinorrhea J34.89
  cerebrospinal (fluid) G96.0
  paroxysmal — *see* Rhinitis, allergic
  spasmodic — *see* Rhinitis, allergic
Rhinosalpingitis — *see* Salpingitis, eustachian
Rhinoscleroma A48.8
Rhinosporidiosis B48.1
Rhinovirus infection NEC B34.8

Rhizomelic chondrodysplasia punctata E71.540
Rhythm
  atrioventricular nodal I49.8
  disorder I49.9
    coronary sinus I49.8
    ectopic I49.8
    nodal I49.8
  escape I49.9
  heart, abnormal I49.9
  idioventricular I44.2
  nodal I49.8
  sleep, inversion G47.2- ☑
    nonorganic origin — *see* Disorder, sleep, circadian rhythm, psychogenic
Rhytidosis facialis L98.8
Rib (*see also* condition)
  cervical Q76.5
Riboflavin deficiency E53.0
Rice bodies (*see also* Loose, body, joint)
  knee M23.4- ☑
Richter syndrome — *see* Leukemia, chronic lymphocytic, B-cell type
Richter's hernia — *see* Hernia, abdomen, with obstruction
Ricinism — *see* Poisoning, food, noxious, plant
Rickets (active) (acute) (adolescent) (chest wall) (congenital) (current) (infantile) (intestinal) E55.0
  adult — *see* Osteomalacia
  celiac K90.0
  hypophosphatemic with nephrotic-glycosuric dwarfism E72.09
  inactive E64.3
  kidney N25.0
  renal N25.0
  sequelae, any E64.3
  vitamin-D-resistant E83.31 [M90.80]
Rickettsial disease A79.9
  specified type NEC A79.89
Rickettsialpox (Rickettsia akari) A79.1
Rickettsiosis A79.9
  due to
    Ehrlichia sennetsu A79.81
    Rickettsia akari (rickettsialpox) A79.1
  specified type NEC A79.89
  tick-borne A77.9
  vesicular A79.1
Rider's bone — *see* Ossification, muscle, specified NEC
Ridge, alveolus (*see also* condition)
  flabby K06.8
Ridged ear, congenital Q17.3
Riedel's
  lobe, liver Q44.7
  struma, thyroiditis or disease E06.5
Rieger's anomaly or syndrome Q13.81
Riehl's melanosis L81.4
Rietti-Greppi-Micheli anemia D56.9
Rieux's hernia — *see* Hernia, abdomen, specified site NEC
Riga (-Fede) **disease** K14.0
Riggs' disease — *see* Periodontitis
Right middle lobe syndrome J98.11
Rigid, rigidity (*see also* condition)
  abdominal R19.30
    with severe abdominal pain R10.0
    epigastric R19.36
    generalized R19.37
    left lower quadrant R19.34
    left upper quadrant R19.32
    periumbilic R19.35
    right lower quadrant R19.33
    right upper quadrant R19.31
  articular, multiple, congenital Q68.8
  cervix (uteri) in pregnancy — *see* Pregnancy, complicated by, abnormal, cervix
  hymen (acquired) (congenital) N89.6
  nuchal R29.1
  pelvic floor in pregnancy — *see* Pregnancy, complicated by, abnormal, pelvic organs or tissues NEC
  perineum or vulva in pregnancy — *see* Pregnancy, complicated by, abnormal, vulva
  spine — *see* Dorsopathy, specified NEC
  vagina in pregnancy — *see* Pregnancy, complicated by, abnormal, vagina
Rigors R68.89
  with fever R50.9
Riley-Day syndrome G90.1
RIND (reversible ischemic neurologic deficit) I63.9

☑ Additional Character Required — Refer to the Tabular List for Character Selection   ▽ Subterms under main terms may continue to next column or page

Ring(s)

- aorta (vascular) Q25.4
- Bandl's O62.4
- contraction, complicating delivery O62.4
- esophageal, lower (muscular) K22.2
- Fleischer's (cornea) H18.04- ☑
- hymenal, tight (acquired) (congenital) N89.6
- Kayser-Fleischer (cornea) H18.04- ☑
- retraction, uterus, pathological O62.4
- Schatzki's (esophagus) (lower) K22.2
  - congenital Q39.3
- Soemmerring's — see Cataract, secondary
- vascular (congenital) Q25.8
  - aorta Q25.4

Ringed hair (congenital) Q84.1

Ringworm B35.9
- beard B35.0
- black dot B35.0
- body B35.4
- Burmese B35.5
- corporeal B35.4
- foot B35.3
- groin B35.6
- hand B35.2
- honeycomb B35.0
- nails B35.1
- perianal (area) B35.6
- scalp B35.0
- specified NEC B35.8
- Tokelau B35.5

Rise, venous pressure I87.8

Risk, suicidal
- meaning personal history of attempted suicide Z91.5
- meaning suicidal ideation — see Ideation, suicidal

Ritter's disease L00

Rivalry, sibling Z62.891

Rivalta's disease A42.2

River blindness B73.01

Robert's pelvis Q74.2
- with disproportion (fetopelvic) O33.0
  - causing obstructed labor O65.0

Robin (-Pierre) **syndrome** Q87.0

Robinow-Silvermann-Smith syndrome Q87.1

Robinson's (hidrotic) **ectodermal dysplasia or syndrome** Q82.4

Robles' disease B73.01

Rocky Mountain (spotted) **fever** A77.0

Roetheln — see Rubella

Roger's disease Q21.0

Rokitansky-Aschoff sinuses (gallbladder) K82.8

Rolando's fracture (displaced) S62.22- ☑
- nondisplaced S62.22- ☑

Romano-Ward (prolonged QT interval) **syndrome** I45.81

Romberg's disease or syndrome G51.8

Roof, mouth — see condition

Rosacea L71.9
- acne L71.9
- keratitis L71.8
- specified NEC L71.8

Rosary, rachitic E55.0

Rose
- cold J30.1
- fever J30.1
- rash R21
  - epidemic B06.9

Rosenbach's erysipeloid A26.0

Rosenthal's disease or syndrome D68.1

Roseola B09
- infantum B08.20
  - due to human herpesvirus 6 B08.21
  - due to human herpesvirus 7 B08.22

Ross River disease or fever B33.1

Rossbach's disease K31.89
- psychogenic F45.8

Rostan's asthma (cardiac) — see Failure, ventricular, left

Rotation
- anomalous, incomplete or insufficient, intestine Q43.3
- cecum (congenital) Q43.3
- colon (congenital) Q43.3
- spine, incomplete or insufficient — see Dorsopathy, deforming, specified NEC
- tooth, teeth, fully erupted M26.35
- vertebra, incomplete or insufficient — see Dorsopathy, deforming, specified NEC

Rotes Quérol disease or syndrome — see Hyperostosis, ankylosing

Roth (-Bernhardt) **disease or syndrome** — see Meralgia paraesthetica

Rothmund (-Thomson) **syndrome** Q82.8

Rotor's disease or syndrome E80.6

Round
- back (with wedging of vertebrae) — see Kyphosis
  - sequelae (late effect) of rickets E64.3
- worms (large) (infestation) NEC B82.0
  - Ascariasis (see also Ascariasis) B77.9

Roussy-Lévy syndrome G60.0

Rubella (German measles) B06.9
- complication NEC B06.09
  - neurological B06.00
- congenital P35.0
- contact Z20.4
- exposure to Z20.4
- maternal
  - care for (suspected) damage to fetus O35.3 ☑
    - manifest rubella in infant P35.0
  - suspected damage to fetus affecting management of pregnancy O35.3 ☑
- specified complications NEC B06.89

Rubeola (meaning measles) — see Measles
- meaning rubella — see Rubella

Rubeosis, iris — see Disorder, iris, vascular

Rubinstein-Taybi syndrome Q87.2

Rudimentary (congenital) (see also Agenesis)
- arm — see Defect, reduction, upper limb
- bone Q79.9
- cervix uteri Q51.828
- eye Q11.2
- lobule of ear Q17.3
- patella Q74.1
- respiratory organs in thoracopagus Q89.4
- tracheal bronchus Q32.4
- uterus Q51.818
  - in male Q56.1
- vagina Q52.0

Ruled out condition — see Observation, suspected

Rumination R11.10
- with nausea R11.2
- disorder of infancy F98.21
- neurotic F42
- newborn P92.1
- obsessional F42
- psychogenic F42

Runeberg's disease D51.0

Runny nose R09.89

Rupia (syphilitic) A51.39
- congenital A50.06
- tertiary A52.79

Rupture, ruptured
- abscess (spontaneous) — code by site under Abscess
- aneurysm — see Aneurysm
- anus (sphincter) — see Laceration, anus
- aorta, aortic I71.8
  - abdominal I71.3
  - arch I71.1
  - ascending I71.1
  - descending I71.8
    - abdominal I71.3
    - thoracic I71.1
  - syphilitic A52.01
  - thoracoabdominal I71.5
  - thorax, thoracic I71.1
  - transverse I71.1
  - traumatic — see Injury, aorta, laceration, major
  - valve or cusp (see also Endocarditis, aortic) I35.8
- appendix (with peritonitis) K35.2
- arteriovenous fistula, brain I60.8
- artery I77.2
  - brain — see Hemorrhage, intracranial, intracerebral
  - coronary — see Infarct, myocardium
  - heart — see Infarct, myocardium
  - pulmonary I28.8
  - traumatic (complication) — see Injury, blood vessel
- bile duct (common) (hepatic) K83.2
  - cystic K82.2
- bladder (sphincter) (nontraumatic) (spontaneous) N32.89
  - following ectopic or molar pregnancy O08.6
  - obstetrical trauma O71.5
  - traumatic S37.29 ☑
- blood vessel (see also Hemorrhage)
  - brain — see Hemorrhage, intracranial, intracerebral
  - heart — see Infarct, myocardium

Rupture, ruptured — continued
- blood vessel (see also Hemorrhage) — continued
  - traumatic (complication) — see Injury, blood vessel, laceration, major, by site
- bone — see Fracture
- bowel (nontraumatic) K63.1
- brain
  - aneurysm (congenital) (see also Hemorrhage, intracranial, subarachnoid)
    - syphilitic A52.05
  - hemorrhagic — see Hemorrhage, intracranial, intracerebral
- capillaries I78.8
- cardiac (auricle) (ventricle) (wall) I23.3
  - with hemopericardium I23.0
  - infectional I40.9
  - traumatic — see Injury, heart
- cartilage (articular) (current) (see also Sprain)
  - knee S83.3- ☑
  - semilunar — see Tear, meniscus
- cecum (with peritonitis) K65.0
  - with peritoneal abscess K35.3
  - traumatic S36.598 ☑
- celiac artery, traumatic — see Injury, blood vessel, celiac artery, laceration, major
- cerebral aneurysm (congenital) (see Hemorrhage, intracranial, subarachnoid)
- cervix (uteri)
  - with ectopic or molar pregnancy O08.6
  - following ectopic or molar pregnancy O08.6
  - obstetrical trauma O71.3
  - traumatic S37.69 ☑
- chordae tendineae NEC I51.1
  - concurrent with acute myocardial infarction — see Infarct, myocardium
  - following acute myocardial infarction (current complication) I23.4
- choroid (direct) (indirect) (traumatic) H31.32- ☑
- circle of Willis I60.6
- colon (nontraumatic) K63.1
  - traumatic — see Injury, intestine, large
- cornea (traumatic) — see Injury, eye, laceration
- coronary (artery) (thrombotic) — see Infarct, myocardium
- corpus luteum (infected) (ovary) N83.1
- cyst — see Cyst
- cystic duct K82.2
- Descemet's membrane — see Change, corneal membrane, Descemet's, rupture
  - traumatic — see Injury, eye, laceration
- diaphragm, traumatic — see Injury, intrathoracic, diaphragm
- disc — see Rupture, intervertebral disc
- diverticulum (intestine) K57.80
  - with bleeding K57.81
    - bladder N32.3
    - large intestine K57.20
      - with
        - bleeding K57.21
        - small intestine K57.40
          - with bleeding K57.41
    - small intestine K57.00
      - with
        - bleeding K57.01
        - large intestine K57.40
          - with bleeding K57.41
- duodenal stump K31.89
- ear drum (nontraumatic) (see also Perforation, tympanum)
  - traumatic S09.2- ☑
    - due to blast injury — see Injury, blast, ear
- esophagus K22.3
- eye (without prolapse or loss of intraocular tissue) — see Injury, eye, laceration
- fallopian tube NEC (nonobstetric) (nontraumatic) N83.8
  - due to pregnancy O00.1
- fontanel P13.1
- gallbladder K82.2
  - traumatic S36.128 ☑
- gastric (see also Rupture, stomach)
  - vessel K92.2
- globe (eye) (traumatic) — see Injury, eye, laceration
- graafian follicle (hematoma) N83.0
- heart — see Rupture, cardiac
- hymen (nontraumatic) (nonintentional) N89.8
- internal organ, traumatic — see Injury, by site

Rupture, ruptured — continued
  intervertebral disc — see Displacement, intervertebral disc
    traumatic — see Rupture, traumatic, intervertebral disc
  intestine NEC (nontraumatic) K63.1
    traumatic — see Injury, intestine
  iris (see also Abnormality, pupillary)
    traumatic — see Injury, eye, laceration
  joint capsule, traumatic — see Sprain
  kidney (traumatic) S37.06- ☑
    birth injury P15.8
    nontraumatic N28.89
  lacrimal duct (traumatic) — see Injury, eye, specified site NEC
  lens (cataract) (traumatic) — see Cataract, traumatic
  ligament, traumatic — see Rupture, traumatic, ligament, by site
  liver S36.116 ☑
    birth injury P15.0
  lymphatic vessel I89.8
  marginal sinus (placental) (with hemorrhage) — see Hemorrhage, antepartum, specified cause NEC
  membrana tympani (nontraumatic) — see Perforation, tympanum
  membranes (spontaneous)
    artificial
      delayed delivery following O75.5
    delayed delivery following — see Pregnancy, complicated by, premature rupture of membranes
  meningeal artery I60.8
  meniscus (knee) (see also Tear, meniscus)
    old — see Derangement, meniscus
    site other than knee — code as Sprain
  mesenteric artery, traumatic — see Injury, mesenteric, artery, laceration, major
  mesentery (nontraumatic) K66.8
    traumatic — see Injury, intra-abdominal, specified, site NEC
  mitral (valve) I34.8
  muscle (traumatic) (see also Strain)
    diastasis — see Diastasis, muscle
    nontraumatic M62.10
      ankle M62.17- ☑
      foot M62.17- ☑
      forearm M62.13- ☑
      hand M62.14- ☑
      lower leg M62.16- ☑
      pelvic region M62.15- ☑
      shoulder region M62.11- ☑
      specified site NEC M62.18
      thigh M62.15- ☑
      upper arm M62.12- ☑
    traumatic — see Strain, by site
  musculotendinous junction NEC, nontraumatic — see Rupture, tendon, spontaneous
  mycotic aneurysm causing cerebral hemorrhage — see Hemorrhage, intracranial, subarachnoid
  myocardium, myocardial — see Rupture, cardiac
    traumatic — see Injury, heart
  nontraumatic, meaning hernia — see Hernia
  obstructed — see Hernia, by site, obstructed
  operation wound — see Disruption, wound, operation
  ovary, ovarian N83.8
    corpus luteum cyst N83.1
    follicle (graafian) N83.0
  oviduct (nonobstetric) (nontraumatic) N83.8
    due to pregnancy O00.1
  pancreas (nontraumatic) K86.8
    traumatic S36.299 ☑
  papillary muscle NEC I51.2
    following acute myocardial infarction (current complication) I23.5
  pelvic
    floor, complicating delivery O70.1
    organ NEC, obstetrical trauma O71.5
  perineum (nonobstetric) (nontraumatic) N90.89
    complicating delivery — see Delivery, complicated, by, laceration, anus (sphincter)
  postoperative wound — see Disruption, wound, operation
  prostate (traumatic) S37.828 ☑
  pulmonary
    artery I28.8
    valve (heart) I37.8
    vein I28.8

Rupture, ruptured — continued
  pulmonary — continued
    vessel I28.8
  pus tube — see Salpingitis
  pyosalpinx — see Salpingitis
  rectum (nontraumatic) K63.1
    traumatic S36.69 ☑
  retina, retinal (traumatic) (without detachment) (see also Break, retina)
    with detachment — see Detachment, retina, with retinal, break
  rotator cuff (nontraumatic) M75.10- ☑
    complete M75.12- ☑
    incomplete M75.11- ☑
  sclera — see Injury, eye, laceration
  sigmoid (nontraumatic) K63.1
    traumatic S36.593 ☑
  spinal cord (see also Injury, spinal cord, by region)
    due to injury at birth P11.5
    newborn (birth injury) P11.5
  spleen (traumatic) S36.09 ☑
    birth injury P15.1
    congenital (birth injury) P15.1
    due to P. vivax malaria B51.0
    nontraumatic D73.5
    spontaneous D73.5
  splenic vein R58
    traumatic — see Injury, blood vessel, splenic vein
  stomach (nontraumatic) (spontaneous) K31.89
    traumatic S36.39 ☑
  supraspinatus (complete) (incomplete) (nontraumatic) — see Tear, rotator cuff
  symphysis pubis
    obstetric O71.6
    traumatic S33.4 ☑
  synovium (cyst) M66.10
    ankle M66.17- ☑
    elbow M66.12- ☑
    finger M66.14- ☑
    foot M66.17- ☑
    forearm M66.13- ☑
    hand M66.14- ☑
    pelvic region M66.15- ☑
    shoulder region M66.11- ☑
    specified site NEC M66.18
    thigh M66.15- ☑
    toe M66.17- ☑
    upper arm M66.12- ☑
    wrist M66.13- ☑
  tendon (traumatic) — see Strain
    nontraumatic (spontaneous) M66.9
      ankle M66.87- ☑
      extensor M66.20
        ankle M66.27- ☑
        foot M66.27- ☑
        forearm M66.23- ☑
        hand M66.24- ☑
        lower leg M66.26- ☑
        multiple sites M66.29
        pelvic region M66.25- ☑
        shoulder region M66.21- ☑
        specified site NEC M66.28
        thigh M66.25- ☑
        upper arm M66.22- ☑
      flexor M66.30
        ankle M66.37- ☑
        foot M66.37- ☑
        forearm M66.33- ☑
        hand M66.34- ☑
        lower leg M66.36- ☑
        multiple sites M66.39
        pelvic region M66.35- ☑
        shoulder region M66.31- ☑
        specified site NEC M66.38
        thigh M66.35- ☑
        upper arm M66.32- ☑
      foot M66.87- ☑
      forearm M66.83- ☑
      hand M66.84- ☑
      lower leg M66.86- ☑
      multiple sites M66.89
      pelvic region M66.85- ☑
      shoulder region M66.81- ☑
      specified
        site NEC M66.88
        tendon M66.80

Rupture, ruptured — continued
  tendon — see Strain — continued
    nontraumatic — continued
      thigh M66.85- ☑
      upper arm M66.82- ☑
  thoracic duct I89.8
  tonsil J35.8
  traumatic
    aorta — see Injury, aorta, laceration, major
    diaphragm — see Injury, intrathoracic, diaphragm
    external site — see Wound, open, by site
    eye — see Injury, eye, laceration
    internal organ — see Injury, by site
    intervertebral disc
      cervical S13.0 ☑
      lumbar S33.0 ☑
      thoracic S23.0 ☑
    kidney S37.06- ☑
    ligament (see also Sprain)
      ankle — see Sprain, ankle
      carpus — see Rupture, traumatic, ligament, wrist
      collateral (hand) — see Rupture, traumatic, ligament, finger, collateral
      finger (metacarpophalangeal) (interphalangeal) S63.40- ☑
        collateral S63.41- ☑
          index S63.41- ☑
          little S63.41- ☑
          middle S63.41- ☑
          ring S63.41- ☑
        index S63.40- ☑
        little S63.40- ☑
        middle S63.40- ☑
        palmar S63.42- ☑
          index S63.42- ☑
          little S63.42- ☑
          middle S63.42- ☑
          ring S63.42- ☑
        ring S63.40- ☑
        specified site NEC S63.499 ☑
          index S63.49- ☑
          little S63.49- ☑
          middle S63.49- ☑
          ring S63.49- ☑
        volar plate S63.43- ☑
          index S63.43- ☑
          little S63.43- ☑
          middle S63.43- ☑
          ring S63.43- ☑
      foot — see Sprain, foot
      radial collateral S53.2- ☑
      radiocarpal — see Rupture, traumatic, ligament, wrist, radiocarpal
      ulnar collateral S53.3- ☑
      ulnocarpal — see Rupture, traumatic, ligament, wrist, ulnocarpal
      wrist S63.30- ☑
        collateral S63.31- ☑
        radiocarpal S63.32- ☑
        specified site NEC S63.39- ☑
        ulnocarpal (palmar) S63.33- ☑
    liver S36.116 ☑
    membrana tympani — see Rupture, ear drum, traumatic
    muscle or tendon — see Strain
    myocardium — see Injury, heart
    pancreas S36.299 ☑
    rectum S36.69 ☑
    sigmoid S36.593 ☑
    spleen S36.09 ☑
    stomach S36.39 ☑
    symphysis pubis S33.4 ☑
    tympanum, tympanic (membrane) — see Rupture, ear drum, traumatic
    ureter S37.19 ☑
    uterus S37.69 ☑
    vagina — see Injury, vagina
    vena cava — see Injury, vena cava, laceration, major
  tricuspid (heart) (valve) I07.8
  tube, tubal (nonobstetric) (nontraumatic) N83.8
    abscess — see Salpingitis
    due to pregnancy O00.1

☑ Additional Character Required — Refer to the Tabular List for Character Selection   ▽ Subterms under main terms may continue to next column or page

Rupture, ruptured — *continued*
  tympanum, tympanic (membrane) (nontraumatic)
    (*see also* Perforation, tympanic membrane)
      H72.9- ☑
    traumatic — *see* Rupture, ear drum, traumatic
  umbilical cord, complicating delivery O69.89 ☑
  ureter (traumatic) S37.19 ☑
    nontraumatic N28.89
  urethra (nontraumatic) N36.8
    with ectopic or molar pregnancy O08.6
    following ectopic or molar pregnancy O08.6
    obstetrical trauma O71.5
    traumatic S37.39 ☑
  uterosacral ligament (nonobstetric) (nontraumatic)
    N83.8
  uterus (traumatic) S37.69 ☑
    before labor O71.0- ☑
    during or after labor O71.1
    nonpuerperal, nontraumatic N85.8
    pregnant (during labor) O71.1
      before labor O71.0- ☑
  vagina — *see* Injury, vagina
  valve, valvular (heart) — *see* Endocarditis
  varicose vein — *see* Varix
  varix — *see* Varix
  vena cava R58
    traumatic — *see* Injury, vena cava, laceration, major
  vesical (urinary) N32.89
  vessel (blood) R58
    pulmonary I28.8
    traumatic — *see* Injury, blood vessel
  viscus R19.8
  vulva complicating delivery O70.0
Russell-Silver syndrome Q87.1
Russian spring-summer type encephalitis A84.0
Rust's disease (tuberculous cervical spondylitis) A18.01
Ruvalcaba-Myhre-Smith syndrome E71.440
Rytand-Lipsitch syndrome I44.2

S

Saber, sabre shin or tibia (syphilitic) A50.56 [M90.8-] ☑
Sac lacrimal — *see* condition
Saccharomyces infection B37.9
Saccharopinuria E72.3
Saccular — *see* condition
Sacculation
  aorta (nonsyphilitic) — *see* Aneurysm, aorta
  bladder N32.3
  intralaryngeal (congenital) (ventricular) Q31.3
  larynx (congenital) (ventricular) Q31.3
  organ or site, congenital — *see* Distortion
  pregnant uterus — *see* Pregnancy, complicated by,
    abnormal, uterus
  ureter N28.89
  urethra N36.1
  vesical N32.3
Sachs' amaurotic familial idiocy or disease E75.02
Sachs-Tay disease E75.02
Sacks-Libman disease M32.11
Sacralgia M53.3
Sacralization Q76.49
Sacrodynia M53.3
Sacroiliac joint — *see* condition
Sacroiliitis NEC M46.1
Sacrum — *see* condition
Saddle
  back — *see* Lordosis
  embolus
    abdominal aorta I74.01
    pulmonary artery I26.92
      with acute cor pulmonale I26.02
  injury — *code to* condition
  nose M95.0
    due to syphilis A50.57
Sadism (sexual) F65.52
Sadness, postpartal O90.6
Sadomasochism F65.50
Saemisch's ulcer (cornea) — *see* Ulcer, cornea, central
Sahib disease B55.0
Sailors' skin L57.8
Saint
  Anthony's fire — *see* Erysipelas
  triad — *see* Hernia, diaphragm
  Vitus' dance — *see* Chorea, Sydenham's
Salaam
  attack(s) — *see* Epilepsy, spasms

Salaam — *continued*
  tic R25.8
Salicylism
  abuse F55.8
  overdose or wrong substance given — *see* Table of
    Drugs and Chemicals, by drug, poisoning
Salivary duct or gland — *see* condition
Salivation, excessive K11.7
Salmonella — *see* Infection, Salmonella
Salmonellosis A02.0
Salpingitis (catarrhal) (fallopian tube) (nodular) (pseud-
  ofollicular) (purulent) (septic) N70.91
  with oophoritis N70.93
  acute N70.01
    with oophoritis N70.03
  chlamydial A56.11
  chronic N70.11
    with oophoritis N70.13
  complicating abortion — *see* Abortion, by type, com-
    plicated by, salpingitis
  ear — *see* Salpingitis, eustachian
  eustachian (tube) H68.00- ☑
    acute H68.01- ☑
    chronic H68.02- ☑
  follicularis N70.11
    with oophoritis N70.13
  gonococcal (acute) (chronic) A54.24
  interstitial, chronic N70.11
    with oophoritis N70.13
  isthmica nodosa N70.11
    with oophoritis N70.13
  specific (gonococcal) (acute) (chronic) A54.24
  tuberculous (acute) (chronic) A18.17
  venereal (gonococcal) (acute) (chronic) A54.24
Salpingocele N83.4
Salpingo-oophoritis (catarrhal) (purulent) (ruptured)
  (septic) (suppurative) N70.93
  acute N70.03
    with ectopic or molar pregnancy O08.0
    following ectopic or molar pregnancy O08.0
    gonococcal A54.24
  chronic N70.13
  following ectopic or molar pregnancy O08.0
  gonococcal (acute) (chronic) A54.24
  puerperal O86.19
  specific (gonococcal) (acute) (chronic) A54.24
  subacute N70.03
  tuberculous (acute) (chronic) A18.17
  venereal (gonococcal) (acute) (chronic) A54.24
Salpingo-ovaritis — *see* Salpingo-oophoritis
Salpingoperitonitis — *see* Salpingo-oophoritis
Salzmann's nodular dystrophy — *see* Degeneration,
  cornea, nodular
Sampson's cyst or tumor N80.1
San Joaquin (Valley) **fever** B38.0
Sandblaster's asthma, lung or pneumoconiosis J62.8
Sander's disease (paranoia) F22
Sandfly fever A93.1
Sandhoff's disease E75.01
Sanfilippo (Type B) (Type C) (Type D) **syndrome** E76.22
Sanger-Brown ataxia G11.2
Sao Paulo fever or typhus A77.0
Saponification, mesenteric K65.8
Sarcocele (benign)
  syphilitic A52.76
    congenital A50.59
Sarcocystosis A07.8
Sarcoepiplocele — *see* Hernia
Sarcoepiplomphalocele Q79.2
Sarcoid (*see also* Sarcoidosis)
  arthropathy D86.86
  Boeck's D86.9
  Darier-Roussy D86.3
  iridocyclitis D86.83
  meningitis D86.81
  myocarditis D86.85
  myositis D86.87
  pyelonephritis D86.84
  Spiegler-Fendt L08.89
Sarcoidosis D86.9
  with
    cranial nerve palsies D86.82
    hepatic granuloma D86.89
    polyarthritis D86.86
    tubulo-interstitial nephropathy D86.84
  combined sites NEC D86.89

Sarcoidosis — *continued*
  lung D86.0
    and lymph nodes D86.2
  lymph nodes D86.1
    and lung D86.2
  meninges D86.81
  skin D86.3
  specified type NEC D86.89
Sarcoma (of) (*see also* Neoplasm, connective tissue, malignant)
  alveolar soft part — *see* Neoplasm, connective tissue,
    malignant
  ameloblastic C41.1
    upper jaw (bone) C41.0
  botryoid — *see* Neoplasm, connective tissue, malig-
    nant
  botryoides — *see* Neoplasm, connective tissue, malig-
    nant
  cerebellar C71.6
    circumscribed (arachnoidal) C71.6
  circumscribed (arachnoidal) cerebellar C71.6
  clear cell (*see also* Neoplasm, connective tissue, malig-
    nant)
    kidney C64.- ☑
  dendritic cells (accessory cells) C96.4
  embryonal — *see* Neoplasm, connective tissue, malig-
    nant
  endometrial (stromal) C54.1
    isthmus C54.0
  epithelioid (cell) — *see* Neoplasm, connective tissue,
    malignant
  Ewing's — *see* Neoplasm, bone, malignant
  follicular dendritic cell C96.4
  germinoblastic (diffuse) — *see* Lymphoma, diffuse
    large cell
    follicular — *see* Lymphoma, follicular, specified
      NEC
  giant cell (except of bone) (*see also* Neoplasm, connec-
    tive tissue, malignant)
    bone — *see* Neoplasm, bone, malignant
  glomoid — *see* Neoplasm, connective tissue, malig-
    nant
  granulocytic C92.3- ☑
  hemangioendothelial — *see* Neoplasm, connective
    tissue, malignant
  hemorrhagic, multiple — *see* Sarcoma, Kaposi's
  histiocytic C96.A (*following* C96.6)
  Hodgkin — *see* Lymphoma, Hodgkin
  immunoblastic (diffuse) — *see* Lymphoma, diffuse
    large cell
  interdigitating dendritic cell C96.4
  Kaposi's
    colon C46.4
    connective tissue C46.1
    gastrointestinal organ C46.4
    lung C46.5- ☑
    lymph node(s) C46.3
    palate (hard) (soft) C46.2
    rectum C46.4
    skin C46.0
    specified site NEC C46.7
    stomach C46.4
    unspecified site C46.9
  Kupffer cell C22.3
  Langerhans cell C96.4
  leptomeningeal — *see* Neoplasm, meninges, malig-
    nant
  liver NEC C22.4
  lymphangioendothelial — *see* Neoplasm, connective
    tissue, malignant
  lymphoblastic — *see* Lymphoma, lymphoblastic (dif-
    fuse)
  lymphocytic — *see* Lymphoma, small cell B-cell
  mast cell C96.2
  melanotic — *see* Melanoma
  meningeal — *see* Neoplasm, meninges, malignant
  meningothelial — *see* Neoplasm, meninges, malignant
  mesenchymal (*see also* Neoplasm, connective tissue,
    malignant)
    mixed — *see* Neoplasm, connective tissue, malig-
      nant
  mesothelial — *see* Mesothelioma
  monstrocellular
    specified site — *see* Neoplasm, malignant, by site
    unspecified site C71.9
  myeloid C92.3- ☑
  neurogenic — *see* Neoplasm, nerve, malignant

Sarcoma — *continued*
  odontogenic C41.1
    upper jaw (bone) C41.Ø
  osteoblastic — *see* Neoplasm, bone, malignant
  osteogenic (*see also* Neoplasm, bone, malignant)
    juxtacortical — *see* Neoplasm, bone, malignant
    periosteal — *see* Neoplasm, bone, malignant
  periosteal (*see also* Neoplasm, bone, malignant)
    osteogenic — *see* Neoplasm, bone, malignant
  pleomorphic cell — *see* Neoplasm, connective tissue, malignant
  reticulum cell (diffuse) — *see* Lymphoma, diffuse large cell
    nodular — *see* Lymphoma, follicular
    pleomorphic cell type — *see* Lymphoma, diffuse large cell
  rhabdoid — *see* Neoplasm, malignant, by site
  round cell — *see* Neoplasm, connective tissue, malignant
  small cell — *see* Neoplasm, connective tissue, malignant
  soft tissue — *see* Neoplasm, connective tissue, malignant
  spindle cell — *see* Neoplasm, connective tissue, malignant
  stromal (endometrial) C54.1
    isthmus C54.Ø
  synovial (*see also* Neoplasm, connective tissue, malignant)
    biphasic — *see* Neoplasm, connective tissue, malignant
    epithelioid cell — *see* Neoplasm, connective tissue, malignant
    spindle cell — *see* Neoplasm, connective tissue, malignant
Sarcomatosis
  meningeal — *see* Neoplasm, meninges, malignant
  specified site NEC — *see* Neoplasm, connective tissue, malignant
  unspecified site C8Ø.1
Sarcosinemia E72.59
Sarcosporidiosis (intestinal) AØ7.8
Satiety, early R68.81
Saturnine — *see* condition
Saturnism
  overdose or wrong substance given or taken — *see* Table of Drugs and Chemicals, by drug, poisoning
Satyriasis F52.8
Sauriasis — *see* Ichthyosis
SBE (subacute bacterial endocarditis) I33.Ø
Scabies (any site) B86
Scabs R23.4
Scaglietti-Dagnini syndrome E22.Ø
Scald — *see* Burn
Scalenus anticus (anterior) **syndrome** G54.Ø
Scales R23.4
Scaling, skin R23.4
Scalp — *see* condition
Scapegoating affecting child Z62.3
Scaphocephaly Q75.Ø
Scapulalgia M89.8X1
Scapulohumeral myopathy G71.Ø
Scar, scarring (*see also* Cicatrix) L9Ø.5
  adherent L9Ø.5
  atrophic L9Ø.5
  cervix
    in pregnancy or childbirth — *see* Pregnancy, complicated by, abnormal cervix
  cheloid L91.Ø
  chorioretinal H31.ØØ- ☑
    posterior pole macula H31.Ø1- ☑
    postsurgical H59.81- ☑
    solar retinopathy H31.Ø2- ☑
    specified type NEC H31.Ø9- ☑
  choroid — *see* Scar, chorioretinal
  conjunctiva H11.24- ☑
  cornea H17.9
    xerophthalmic (*see also* Opacity, cornea)
      vitamin A deficiency E5Ø.6
  duodenum, obstructive K31.5
  hypertrophic L91.Ø
  keloid L91.Ø
  labia N9Ø.89
  lung (base) J98.4
  macula — *see* Scar, chorioretinal, posterior pole
  muscle M62.89

Scar, scarring — *continued*
  myocardium, myocardial I25.2
  painful L9Ø.5
  posterior pole (eye) — *see* Scar, chorioretinal, posterior pole
  retina — *see* Scar, chorioretinal
  trachea J39.8
  uterus N85.8
    in pregnancy O34.29
  vagina N89.8
    postoperative N99.2
  vulva N9Ø.89
Scarabiasis B88.2
Scarlatina (anginosa) (maligna) (ulcerosa) A38.9
  myocarditis (acute) A38.1
    old — *see* Myocarditis
  otitis media A38.Ø
Scarlet fever (albuminuria) (angina) A38.9
Schamberg's disease (progressive pigmentary dermatosis) L81.7
Schatzki's ring (acquired) (esophagus) (lower) K22.2
  congenital Q39.3
Schaufenster krankheit I2Ø.8
Schaumann's
  benign lymphogranulomatosis D86.1
  disease or syndrome — *see* Sarcoidosis
Scheie's syndrome E76.Ø3
Schenck's disease B42.1
Scheuermann's disease or osteochondrosis — *see* Osteochondrosis, juvenile, spine
Schilder (-Flatau) **disease** G37.Ø
Schilling-type monocytic leukemia C93.Ø- ☑
Schimmelbusch's disease, cystic mastitis, or hyperplasia — *see* Mastopathy, cystic
Schistosoma infestation — *see* Infestation, Schistosoma
Schistosomiasis B65.9
  with muscle disorder B65.9 [M63.8Ø]
    ankle B65.9 [M63.87-] ☑
    foot B65.9 [M63.87-] ☑
    forearm B65.9 [M63.83-] ☑
    hand B65.9 [M63.84-] ☑
    lower leg B65.9 [M63.86-] ☑
    multiple sites B65.9 [M63.89]
    pelvic region B65.9 [M63.85-] ☑
    shoulder region B65.9 [M63.81-] ☑
    specified site NEC B65.9 [M63.88]
    thigh B65.9 [M63.85-] ☑
    upper arm B65.9 [M63.82-] ☑
  Asiatic B65.2
  bladder B65.Ø
  chestermani B65.8
  colon B65.1
  cutaneous B65.3
  due to
    S. haematobium B65.Ø
    S. japonicum B65.2
    S. mansoni B65.1
    S. mattheii B65.8
  Eastern B65.2
  genitourinary tract B65.Ø
  intestinal B65.1
  lung NEC B65.9 [J99]
    pneumonia B65.9 [J17]
  Manson's (intestinal) B65.1
  oriental B65.2
  pulmonary NEC B65.9 [J99]
    pneumonia B65.9
  Schistosoma
    haematobium B65.Ø
    japonicum B65.2
    mansoni B65.1
  specified type NEC B65.8
  urinary B65.Ø
  vesical B65.Ø
Schizencephaly QØ4.6
Schizoaffective psychosis F25.9
Schizodontia KØØ.2
Schizoid personality F6Ø.1
Schizophrenia, schizophrenic F2Ø.9
  acute (brief) (undifferentiated) F23
  atypical (form) F2Ø.3
  borderline F21
  catalepsy F2Ø.2
  catatonic (type) (excited) (withdrawn) F2Ø.2
  cenesthopathic, cenesthesiopathic F2Ø.89
  childhood type F84.5
  chronic undifferentiated F2Ø.5

Schizophrenia, schizophrenic — *continued*
  cyclic F25.Ø
  disorganized (type) F2Ø.1
  flexibilitas cerea F2Ø.2
  hebephrenic (type) F2Ø.1
  incipient F21
  latent F21
  negative type F2Ø.5
  paranoid (type) F2Ø.Ø
  paraphrenic F2Ø.Ø
  post-psychotic depression F32.8
  prepsychotic F21
  prodromal F21
  pseudoneurotic F21
  pseudopsychopathic F21
  reaction F23
  residual (state) (type) F2Ø.5
  restzustand F2Ø.5
  schizoaffective (type) — *see* Psychosis, schizoaffective
  simple (type) F2Ø.89
  simplex F2Ø.89
  specified type NEC F2Ø.89
  stupor F2Ø.2
  syndrome of childhood F84.5
  undifferentiated (type) F2Ø.3
    chronic F2Ø.5
Schizothymia (persistent) F6Ø.1
Schlatter-Osgood disease or osteochondrosis — *see* Osteochondrosis, juvenile, tibia
Schlatter's tibia — *see* Osteochondrosis, juvenile, tibia
Schmidt's syndrome (polyglandular, autoimmune) E31.Ø
Schmincke's carcinoma or tumor — *see* Neoplasm, nasopharynx, malignant
Schmitz (-Stutzer) **dysentery** AØ3.Ø
Schmorl's disease or nodes
  lumbar region M51.46
  lumbosacral region M51.47
  sacrococcygeal region M53.3
  thoracic region M51.44
  thoracolumbar region M51.45
Schneiderian
  papilloma — *see* Neoplasm, nasopharynx, benign
    specified site — *see* Neoplasm, benign, by site
    unspecified site D14.Ø
  specified site — *see* Neoplasm, malignant, by site
    unspecified site C3Ø.Ø
Scholte's syndrome (malignant carcinoid) E34.Ø
Scholz (-Bielchowsky-Henneberg) **disease or syndrome** E75.25
Schönlein (-Henoch) disease or purpura (primary) (rheumatic) D69.Ø
Schottmuller's disease AØ1.4
Schroeder's syndrome (endocrine hypertensive) E27.Ø
Schüller-Christian disease or syndrome C96.5
Schultze's type acroparesthesia, simple I73.89
Schultz's disease or syndrome — *see* Agranulocytosis
Schwalbe-Ziehen-Oppenheim disease G24.1
Schwannoma (*see also* Neoplasm, nerve, benign)
  malignant (*see also* Neoplasm, nerve, malignant)
    with rhabdomyoblastic differentiation — *see* Neoplasm, nerve, malignant
  melanocytic — *see* Neoplasm, nerve, benign
  pigmented — *see* Neoplasm, nerve, benign
Schwannomatosis Q85.Ø3
Schwartz (-Jampel) **syndrome** G71.13
Schwartz-Bartter syndrome E22.2
Schweniger-Buzzi anetoderma L9Ø.1
Sciatic — *see* condition
Sciatica (infective)
  with lumbago M54.4- ☑
    due to intervertebral disc disorder — *see* Disorder, disc, with, radiculopathy
  due to displacement of intervertebral disc (with lumbago) — *see* Disorder, disc, with, radiculopathy
  wallet M54.3- ☑
Scimitar syndrome Q26.8
Sclera — *see* condition
Sclerectasia H15.84- ☑
Scleredema
  adultorum — *see* Sclerosis, systemic
  Buschke's — *see* Sclerosis, systemic
  newborn P83.Ø
Sclerema (adiposum) (edematosum) (neonatorum) (newborn) P83.Ø
  adultorum — *see* Sclerosis, systemic
Scleriasis — *see* Scleroderma

☑ **Additional Character Required** — Refer to the Tabular List for Character Selection   ▽ **Subterms under main terms may continue to next column or page**

Scleritis H15.00- ☑
  with corneal involvement H15.04- ☑
  anterior H15.01- ☑
  brawny H15.02- ☑
  in (due to) zoster B02.34
  posterior H15.03- ☑
  specified type NEC H15.09- ☑
  syphilitic A52.71
  tuberculous (nodular) A18.51
Sclerochoroiditis H31.8
Scleroconjunctivitis — *see* Scleritis
Sclerocystic ovary syndrome E28.2
Sclerodactyly, sclerodactylia L94.3
Scleroderma, sclerodermia (acrosclerotic) (diffuse)
    (generalized) (progressive) (pulmonary) (*see also*
    Sclerosis, systemic) M34.9
  circumscribed L94.0
  linear L94.1
  localized L94.0
  newborn P83.8
  systemic M34.9
Sclerokeratitis H16.8
  tuberculous A18.52
Scleroma nasi A48.8
Scleromalacia (perforans) H15.05- ☑
Scleromyxedema L98.5
Sclérose en plaques G35
Sclerosis, sclerotic
  adrenal (gland) E27.8
  Alzheimer's — *see* Disease, Alzheimer's
  amyotrophic (lateral) G12.21
  aorta, aortic I70.0
    valve — *see* Endocarditis, aortic
  artery, arterial, arteriolar, arteriovascular — *see* Arte-
    riosclerosis
  ascending multiple G35
  brain (generalized) (lobular) G37.9
    artery, arterial I67.2
    diffuse G37.0
    disseminated G35
    insular G35
    Krabbe's E75.23
    miliary G35
    multiple G35
    presenile (Alzheimer's) — *see* Disease, Alzheimer's,
      early onset
    senile (arteriosclerotic) I67.2
    stem, multiple G35
    tuberous Q85.1
  bulbar, multiple G35
  bundle of His I44.39
  cardiac — *see* Disease, heart, ischemic, atherosclerotic
  cardiorenal — *see* Hypertension, cardiorenal
  cardiovascular (*see also* Disease, cardiovascular)
    renal — *see* Hypertension, cardiorenal
  cerebellar — *see* Sclerosis, brain
  cerebral — *see* Sclerosis, brain
  cerebrospinal (disseminated) (multiple) G35
  cerebrovascular I67.2
  choroid — *see* Degeneration, choroid
  combined (spinal cord) (*see also* Degeneration, com-
    bined)
    multiple G35
  concentric (Balo) G37.5
  cornea — *see* Opacity, cornea
  coronary (artery) I25.10
    with angina pectoris — *see* Arteriosclerosis, coro-
      nary (artery),
  corpus cavernosum
    female N90.89
    male N48.6
  diffuse (brain) (spinal cord) G37.0
  disseminated G35
  dorsal G35
  dorsolateral (spinal cord) — *see* Degeneration, com-
    bined
  endometrium N85.5
  extrapyramidal G25.9
  eye, nuclear (senile) — *see* Cataract, senile, nuclear
  focal and segmental (glomerular) (*see also* N00-N07
    with fourth character .1) N05.1
  Friedreich's (spinal cord) G11.1
  funicular (spermatic cord) N50.8
  general (vascular) — *see* Arteriosclerosis
  gland (lymphatic) I89.8
  hepatic K74.1
    alcoholic K70.2

Sclerosis, sclerotic — *continued*
  hereditary
    cerebellar G11.9
    spinal (Friedreich's ataxia) G11.1
  hippocampal G93.81
  insular G35
  kidney — *see* Sclerosis, renal
  larynx J38.7
  lateral (amyotrophic) (descending) (primary) (spinal)
    G12.21
  lens, senile nuclear — *see* Cataract, senile, nuclear
  liver K74.1
    with fibrosis K74.2
      alcoholic K70.2
    alcoholic K70.2
    cardiac K76.1
  lung — *see* Fibrosis, lung
  mastoid — *see* Mastoiditis, chronic
  mesial temporal G93.81
  mitral I05.8
  Mönckeberg's (medial) — *see* Arteriosclerosis, extrem-
    ities
  multiple (brain stem) (cerebral) (generalized) (spinal
    cord) G35
  myocardium, myocardial — *see* Disease, heart, is-
    chemic, atherosclerotic
  nuclear (senile), eye — *see* Cataract, senile, nuclear
  ovary N83.8
  pancreas K86.8
  penis N48.6
  peripheral arteries — *see* Arteriosclerosis, extremities
  plaques G35
  pluriglandular E31.8
  polyglandular E31.8
  posterolateral (spinal cord) — *see* Degeneration,
    combined
  presenile (Alzheimer's) — *see* Disease, Alzheimer's,
    early onset
  primary, lateral G12.29
  progressive, systemic M34.0
  pulmonary — *see* Fibrosis, lung
    artery I27.0
    valve (heart) — *see* Endocarditis, pulmonary
  renal N26.9
    with
      cystine storage disease E72.09
      hypertensive heart disease (conditions in I11)
        — *see* Hypertension, cardiorenal
      arteriolar (hyaline) (hyperplastic) — *see* Hyperten-
        sion, kidney
  retina (senile) (vascular) H35.00
  senile (vascular) — *see* Arteriosclerosis
  spinal (cord) (progressive) G95.89
    ascending G61.0
    combined (*see also* Degeneration, combined)
      multiple G35
      syphilitic A52.11
    disseminated G35
    dorsolateral — *see* Degeneration, combined
    hereditary (Friedreich's) (mixed form) G11.1
    lateral (amyotrophic) G12.21
    multiple G35
    posterior (syphilitic) A52.11
  stomach K31.89
  subendocardial, congenital I42.4
  systemic M34.9
    with
      lung involvement M34.81
      myopathy M34.82
      polyneuropathy M34.83
    drug-induced M34.2
    due to chemicals NEC M34.2
    progressive M34.0
    specified NEC M34.89
  temporal (mesial) G93.81
  tricuspid (heart) (valve) I07.8
  tuberous (brain) Q85.1
  tympanic membrane — *see* Disorder, tympanic
    membrane, specified NEC
  valve, valvular (heart) — *see* Endocarditis
  vascular — *see* Arteriosclerosis
  vein I87.8
Scoliosis (acquired) (postural) M41.9
  adolescent (idiopathic) — *see* Scoliosis, idiopathic,
    juvenile
  congenital Q67.5
    due to bony malformation Q76.3
    failure of segmentation (hemivertebra) Q76.3

Scoliosis — *continued*
  congenital — *continued*
    hemivertebra fusion Q76.3
    postural Q67.5
  idiopathic M41.20
    adolescent M41.129
      cervical region M41.122
      cervicothoracic region M41.123
      lumbar region M41.126
      lumbosacral region M41.127
      thoracic region M41.124
      thoracolumbar region M41.125
    cervical region M41.22
    cervicothoracic region M41.23
    infantile M41.00
      cervical region M41.02
      cervicothoracic region M41.03
      lumbar region M41.06
      lumbosacral region M41.07
      sacrococcygeal region M41.08
      thoracic region M41.04
      thoracolumbar region M41.05
    juvenile M41.119
      cervical region M41.112
      cervicothoracic region M41.113
      lumbar region M41.116
      lumbosacral region M41.117
      thoracic region M41.114
      thoracolumbar region M41.115
    lumbar region M41.26
    lumbosacral region M41.27
    thoracic region M41.24
    thoracolumbar region M41.25
  neuromuscular M41.40
    cervical region M41.42
    cervicothoracic region M41.43
    lumbar region M41.46
    lumbosacral region M41.47
    occipito-atlanto-axial region M41.41
    thoracic region M41.44
    thoracolumbar region M41.45
  paralytic — *see* Scoliosis, neuromuscular
  postradiation therapy M96.5
  rachitic (late effect or sequelae) E64.3 [M49.80]
    cervical region E64.3 [M49.82]
    cervicothoracic region E64.3 [M49.83]
    lumbar region E64.3 [M49.86]
    lumbosacral region E64.3 [M49.87]
    multiple sites E64.3 [M49.89]
    occipito-atlanto-axial region E64.3 [M49.81]
    sacrococcygeal region E64.3 [M49.88]
    thoracic region E64.3 [M49.84]
    thoracolumbar region E64.3 [M49.85]
  sciatic M54.4- ☑
  secondary (to) NEC M41.50
    cerebral palsy, Friedreich's ataxia, poliomyelitis,
      neuromuscular disorders — *see* Scoliosis,
      neuromuscular
    cervical region M41.52
    cervicothoracic region M41.53
    lumbar region M41.56
    lumbosacral region M41.57
    thoracic region M41.54
    thoracolumbar region M41.55
  specified form NEC M41.80
    cervical region M41.82
    cervicothoracic region M41.83
    lumbar region M41.86
    lumbosacral region M41.87
    thoracic region M41.84
    thoracolumbar region M41.85
  thoracogenic M41.30
    thoracic region M41.34
    thoracolumbar region M41.35
  tuberculous A18.01
Scoliotic pelvis
  with disproportion (fetopelvic) O33.0
    causing obstructed labor O65.0
Scorbutus, scorbutic (*see also* Scurvy)
  anemia D53.2
Scotoma (arcuate) (Bjerrum) (central) (ring) (*see also*
    Defect, visual field, localized, scotoma)
  scintillating H53.19
Scratch — *see* Abrasion
Scratchy throat R09.89
Screening (for) Z13.9
  alcoholism Z13.89
  anemia Z13.0

Screening — *continued*
anomaly, congenital Z13.89
antenatal, of mother Z36
arterial hypertension Z13.6
arthropod-borne viral disease NEC Z11.59
bacteriuria, asymptomatic Z13.89
behavioral disorder Z13.89
brain injury, traumatic Z13.850
bronchitis, chronic Z13.83
brucellosis Z11.2
cardiovascular disorder Z13.6
cataract Z13.5
chlamydial diseases Z11.8
cholera Z11.0
chromosomal abnormalities (nonprocreative) NEC
　　Z13.79
colonoscopy Z12.11
congenital
　dislocation of hip Z13.89
　eye disorder Z13.5
　malformation or deformation Z13.89
contamination NEC Z13.88
cystic fibrosis Z13.228
dengue fever Z11.59
dental disorder Z13.84
depression Z13.89
developmental handicap Z13.4
　in early childhood Z13.4
diabetes mellitus Z13.1
diphtheria Z11.2
disability, intellectual Z13.4
disease or disorder Z13.9
　bacterial NEC Z11.2
　　intestinal infectious Z11.0
　　respiratory tuberculosis Z11.1
　blood or blood-forming organ Z13.0
　cardiovascular Z13.6
　Chagas' Z11.6
　chlamydial Z11.8
　dental Z13.89
　developmental Z13.4
　digestive tract NEC Z13.818
　　lower GI Z13.811
　　upper GI Z13.810
　ear Z13.5
　endocrine Z13.29
　eye Z13.5
　genitourinary Z13.89
　heart Z13.6
　human immunodeficiency virus (HIV) infection
　　　Z11.4
　immunity Z13.0
　infection
　　intestinal Z11.0
　　　specified NEC Z11.6
　infectious Z11.9
　mental Z13.89
　metabolic Z13.228
　neurological Z13.89
　nutritional Z13.21
　　metabolic Z13.228
　　　lipoid disorders Z13.220
　protozoal Z11.6
　　intestinal Z11.0
　respiratory Z13.83
　rheumatic Z13.828
　rickettsial Z11.8
　sexually-transmitted NEC Z11.3
　　human immunodeficiency virus (HIV) Z11.4
　sickle-cell (trait) Z13.0
　skin Z13.89
　specified NEC Z13.89
　spirochetal Z11.8
　thyroid Z13.29
　vascular Z13.6
　venereal Z11.3
　viral NEC Z11.59
　　human immunodeficiency virus (HIV) Z11.4
　　intestinal Z11.0
elevated titer Z13.89
emphysema Z13.83
encephalitis, viral (mosquito- or tick-borne) Z11.59
exposure to contaminants (toxic) Z13.88
fever
　dengue Z11.59
　hemorrhagic Z11.59
　yellow Z11.59
filariasis Z11.6

Screening — *continued*
galactosemia Z13.228
gastrointestinal condition Z13.818
genetic (nonprocreative) - for procreative manage-
　　ment — *see* Testing, genetic, for procreative
　　management
　disease carrier status (nonprocreative) Z13.71
　specified NEC (nonprocreative) Z13.79
genitourinary condition Z13.89
glaucoma Z13.5
gonorrhea Z11.3
gout Z13.89
helminthiasis (intestinal) Z11.6
hematopoietic malignancy Z12.89
hemoglobinopathies NEC Z13.0
hemorrhagic fever Z11.59
Hodgkin disease Z12.89
human immunodeficiency virus (HIV) Z11.4
human papillomavirus Z11.51
hypertension Z13.6
immunity disorders Z13.0
infection
　mycotic Z11.8
　parasitic Z11.8
ingestion of radioactive substance Z13.88
intellectual disability Z13.4
intestinal
　helminthiasis Z11.6
　infectious disease Z11.0
leishmaniasis Z11.6
leprosy Z11.2
leptospirosis Z11.8
leukemia Z12.89
lymphoma Z12.89
malaria Z11.6
malnutrition Z13.29
　metabolic Z13.228
　nutritional Z13.21
measles Z11.59
mental disorder Z13.89
metabolic errors, inborn Z13.228
multiphasic Z13.89
musculoskeletal disorder Z13.828
　osteoporosis Z13.820
mycoses Z11.8
myocardial infarction (acute) Z13.6
neoplasm (malignant) (of) Z12.9
　bladder Z12.6
　blood Z12.89
　breast Z12.39
　　routine mammogram Z12.31
　cervix Z12.4
　colon Z12.11
　genitourinary organs NEC Z12.79
　　bladder Z12.6
　　cervix Z12.4
　　ovary Z12.73
　　prostate Z12.5
　　testis Z12.71
　　vagina Z12.72
　hematopoietic system Z12.89
　intestinal tract Z12.10
　　colon Z12.11
　　rectum Z12.12
　　small intestine Z12.13
　lung Z12.2
　lymph (glands) Z12.89
　nervous system Z12.82
　oral cavity Z12.81
　prostate Z12.5
　rectum Z12.12
　respiratory organs Z12.2
　skin Z12.83
　small intestine Z12.13
　specified site NEC Z12.89
　stomach Z12.0
nephropathy Z13.89
nervous system disorders NEC Z13.858
neurological condition Z13.89
osteoporosis Z13.820
parasitic infestation Z11.9
　specified NEC Z11.8
phenylketonuria Z13.228
plague Z11.2
poisoning (chemical) (heavy metal) Z13.88
poliomyelitis Z11.59
postnatal, chromosomal abnormalities Z13.89
prenatal, of mother Z36

Screening — *continued*
protozoal disease Z11.6
　intestinal Z11.0
pulmonary tuberculosis Z11.1
radiation exposure Z13.88
respiratory condition Z13.83
respiratory tuberculosis Z11.1
rheumatoid arthritis Z13.828
rubella Z11.59
schistosomiasis Z11.6
sexually-transmitted disease NEC Z11.3
　human immunodeficiency virus (HIV) Z11.4
sickle-cell disease or trait Z13.0
skin condition Z13.89
sleeping sickness Z11.6
special Z13.9
　specified NEC Z13.89
syphilis Z11.3
tetanus Z11.2
trachoma Z11.8
traumatic brain injury Z13.850
trypanosomiasis Z11.6
tuberculosis, respiratory Z11.1
venereal disease Z11.3
viral encephalitis (mosquito- or tick-borne) Z11.59
whooping cough Z11.2
worms, intestinal Z11.6
yaws Z11.8
yellow fever Z11.59
Scrofula, scrofulosis (tuberculosis of cervical lymph
　　glands) A18.2
Scrofulide (primary) (tuberculous) A18.4
Scrofuloderma, scrofulodermia (any site) (primary)
　　A18.4
Scrofulosus lichen (primary) (tuberculous) A18.4
Scrofulous — *see* condition
Scrotal tongue K14.5
Scrotum — *see* condition
Scurvy, scorbutic E54
　anemia D53.2
　gum E54
　infantile E54
　rickets E55.0 [M90.80]
Sealpox B08.62
Seasickness T75.3 ☑
Seatworm (infection) (infestation) B80
Sebaceous (*see also* condition)
　cyst — *see* Cyst, sebaceous
Seborrhea, seborrheic L21.9
　capillitii R23.8
　capitis L21.0
　dermatitis L21.9
　　infantile L21.1
　eczema L21.9
　　infantile L21.1
　sicca L21.0
Seckel's syndrome Q87.1
Seclusion, pupil — *see* Membrane, pupillary
Second hand tobacco smoke exposure (acute)
　　(chronic) Z77.22
　in the perinatal period P96.81
Secondary
　dentin (in pulp) K04.3
　neoplasm, secondaries — *see* Table of Neoplasms,
　　secondary
Secretion
　antidiuretic hormone, inappropriate E22.2
　catecholamine, by pheochromocytoma E27.5
　hormone
　　antidiuretic, inappropriate (syndrome) E22.2
　　by
　　　carcinoid tumor E34.0
　　　pheochromocytoma E27.5
　　ectopic NEC E34.2
　urinary
　　excessive R35.8
　　suppression R34
Section
　nerve, traumatic — *see* Injury, nerve
Segmentation, incomplete (congenital) (*see also* Fu-
　　sion)
　bone NEC Q78.8
　lumbosacral (joint) (vertebra) Q76.49
Seitelberger's syndrome (infantile neuraxonal dystro-
　　phy) G31.89
Seizure(s) (*see also* Convulsions) R56.9
　akinetic — *see* Epilepsy, generalized, specified NEC
　atonic — *see* Epilepsy, generalized, specified NEC

Seizure(s) — *continued*
  autonomic (hysterical) F44.5
  convulsive — *see* Convulsions
  cortical (focal) (motor) — *see* Epilepsy, localization-
      related, symptomatic, with simple partial
      seizures
  disorder (*see also* Epilepsy) G40.909
  due to stroke — *see* Sequelae (of), disease, cerebrovas-
      cular, by type, specified NEC
  epileptic — *see* Epilepsy
  febrile (simple) R56.00
      with status epilepticus G40.901
      complex (atypical) (complicated) R56.01
          with status epilepticus G40.901
  grand mal G40.409
      intractable G40.419
          with status epilepticus G40.411
          without status epilepticus G40.419
      not intractable G40.409
          with status epilepticus G40.401
          without status epilepticus G40.409
  heart — *see* Disease, heart
  hysterical F44.5
  intractable G40.919
      with status epilepticus G40.911
  Jacksonian (focal) (motor type) (sensory type) — *see*
      Epilepsy, localization-related, symptomatic, with
      simple partial seizures
  newborn P90
  nonspecific epileptic
      atonic — *see* Epilepsy, generalized, specified NEC
      clonic — *see* Epilepsy, generalized, specified NEC
      myoclonic — *see* Epilepsy, generalized, specified
          NEC
      tonic — *see* Epilepsy, generalized, specified NEC
      tonic-clonic — *see* Epilepsy, generalized, specified
          NEC
  partial, developing into secondarily generalized
      seizures
      complex — *see* Epilepsy, localization-related,
          symptomatic, with complex partial seizures
      simple — *see* Epilepsy, localization-related, symp-
          tomatic, with simple partial seizures
  petit mal G40.409
      intractable G40.419
          with status epilepticus G40.411
          without status epilepticus G40.419
      not intractable G40.409
          with status epilepticus G40.401
          without status epilepticus G40.409
  post traumatic R56.1
  recurrent G40.909
  specified NEC G40.89
  uncinate — *see* Epilepsy, localization-related, symp-
      tomatic, with complex partial seizures
Selenium deficiency, dietary E59
Self-damaging behavior (life-style) Z72.89
Self-harm (attempted)
  history (personal) Z91.5
      in family Z81.8
Self-mutilation (attempted)
  history (personal) Z91.5
      in family Z81.8
Self-poisoning
  history (personal) Z91.5
      in family Z81.8
  observation following (alleged) attempt Z03.6
Semicoma R40.1
Seminal vesiculitis N49.0
Seminoma C62.9- ☑
  specified site — *see* Neoplasm, malignant, by site
Senear-Usher disease or syndrome L10.4
Senectus R54
Senescence (without mention of psychosis) R54
Senile, senility (*see also* condition) R41.81
  with
      acute confusional state F05
      mental changes NOS F03 ☑
      psychosis NEC — *see* Psychosis, senile
  asthenia R54
  cervix (atrophic) N88.8
  debility R54
  endometrium (atrophic) N85.8
  fallopian tube (atrophic) — *see* Atrophy, fallopian tube
  heart (failure) R54
  ovary (atrophic) — *see* Atrophy, ovary
  premature E34.8

Senile, senility — *continued*
  vagina, vaginitis (atrophic) N95.2
  wart L82.1
Sensation
  burning (skin) R20.8
      tongue K14.6
  loss of R20.8
  prickling (skin) R20.2
  tingling (skin) R20.2
Sense loss
  smell — *see* Disturbance, sensation, smell
  taste — *see* Disturbance, sensation, taste
  touch R20.8
Sensibility disturbance (cortical) (deep) (vibratory)
      R20.9
Sensitive, sensitivity (*see also* Allergy)
  carotid sinus G90.01
  child (excessive) F93.8
  cold, autoimmune D59.1
  dentin K03.89
  latex Z91.040
  methemoglobin D74.8
  tuberculin, without clinical or radiological symptoms
      R76.11
  visual
      glare H53.71
      impaired contrast H53.72
Sensitiver Beziehungswahn F22
Sensitization, auto-erythrocytic D69.2
Separation
  anxiety, abnormal (of childhood) F93.0
  apophysis, traumatic — *code as* Fracture, by site
  choroid — *see* Detachment, choroid
  epiphysis, epiphyseal
      nontraumatic (*see also* Osteochondropathy, speci-
          fied type NEC)
      upper femoral — *see* Slipped, epiphysis, upper
          femoral
      traumatic — *code as* Fracture, by site
  fracture — *see* Fracture
  infundibulum cardiac from right ventricle by a partition
      Q24.3
  joint (traumatic) (current) — *code by* site under Dislo-
      cation
  pubic bone, obstetrical trauma O71.6
  retina, retinal — *see* Detachment, retina
  symphysis pubis, obstetrical trauma O71.6
  tracheal ring, incomplete, congenital Q32.1
Sepsis (generalized) (unspecified organism) A41.9
  with
      organ dysfunction (acute) (multiple) R65.20
          with septic shock R65.21
  actinomycotic A42.7
  adrenal hemorrhage syndrome (meningococcal) A39.1
  anaerobic A41.4
  Bacillus anthracis A22.7
  Brucella (*see also* Brucellosis) A23.9
  candidal B37.7
  cryptogenic A41.9
  due to device, implant or graft T85.79 ☑
      arterial graft NEC T82.7 ☑
      breast (implant) T85.79 ☑
      catheter NEC T85.79 ☑
          dialysis (renal) T82.7 ☑
              intraperitoneal T85.71 ☑
          infusion NEC T82.7 ☑
              spinal (epidural) (subdural) T85.79 ☑
          urinary (indwelling) T83.51 ☑
      ectopic or molar pregnancy O08.82
      electronic (electrode) (pulse generator) (stimulator)
          bone T84.7 ☑
          cardiac T82.7 ☑
          nervous system (brain) (peripheral nerve)
              (spinal) T85.79 ☑
          urinary T83.59 ☑
      fixation, internal (orthopedic) — *see* Complication,
          fixation device, infection
      gastrointestinal (bile duct) (esophagus) T85.79 ☑
      genital T83.6 ☑
      heart NEC T82.7 ☑
          valve (prosthesis) T82.6 ☑
              graft T82.7 ☑
      joint prosthesis — *see* Complication, joint prosthe-
          sis, infection
      ocular (corneal graft) (orbital implant) T85.79 ☑
      orthopedic NEC T84.7 ☑

Sepsis — *continued*
  due to device, implant or graft — *continued*
      orthopedic — *continued*
          fixation device, internal — *see* Complication,
              fixation device, infection
          specified NEC T85.79 ☑
          vascular T82.7 ☑
          ventricular intracranial shunt T85.79 ☑
  during labor O75.3
  Enterococcus A41.81
  Erysipelothrix (rhusiopathiae) (erysipeloid) A26.7
  Escherichia coli (E. coli) A41.5 ☑
  extraintestinal yersiniosis A28.2
  following
      abortion (subsequent episode) O08.0
          current episode — *see* Abortion
      ectopic or molar pregnancy O08.82
      immunization T88.0 ☑
      infusion, therapeutic injection or transfusion NEC
          T80.29 ☑
  gangrenous A41.9
  gonococcal A54.86
  Gram-negative (organism) A41.5 ☑
      anaerobic A41.4
  Haemophilus influenzae A41.3
  herpesviral B00.7
  intra-abdominal K65.1
  intraocular — *see* Endophthalmitis, purulent
  Listeria monocytogenes A32.7
  localized — *code to* specific localized infection
      in operation wound T81.4 ☑
      skin — *see* Abscess
  malleus A24.0
  melioidosis A24.1
  meningeal — *see* Meningitis
  meningococcal A39.4
      acute A39.2
      chronic A39.3
  MSSA (Methicillin susceptible Staphylococcus aureus)
      A41.01
  newborn P36.9
      due to
          anaerobes NEC P36.5
          Escherichia coli P36.4
          Staphylococcus P36.30
              aureus P36.2
              specified NEC P36.39
          Streptococcus P36.10
              group B P36.0
              specified NEC P36.19
          specified NEC P36.8
  Pasteurella multocida A28.0
  pelvic, puerperal, postpartum, childbirth O85
  pneumococcal A40.3
  postprocedural T81.4 ☑
  puerperal, postpartum, childbirth (pelvic) O85
  Salmonella (arizonae) (cholerae-suis) (enteritidis) (ty-
      phimurium) A02.1
  severe R65.20
      with septic shock R65.21
  Shigella (*see also* Dysentery, bacillary) A03.9
  skin, localized — *see* Abscess
  specified organism NEC A41.89
  Staphylococcus, staphylococcal A41.2
      aureus (methicillin susceptible) (MSSA) A41.01
          methicillin resistant (MRSA) A41.02
      coagulase-negative A41.1
      specified NEC A41.1
  Streptococcus, streptococcal A40.9
      agalactiae A40.1
      group
          A A40.0
          B A40.1
          D A41.81
      neonatal P36.10
          group B P36.0
          specified NEC P36.19
      pneumoniae A40.3
      pyogenes A40.0
      specified NEC A40.8
  tracheostomy stoma J95.02
  tularemic A21.7
  umbilical, umbilical cord (newborn) — *see* Sepsis,
      newborn
  Yersinia pestis A20.7
Septate — *see* Septum

Septic — see condition
- arm — see Cellulitis, upper limb
  - with lymphangitis — see Lymphangitis, acute, upper limb
- embolus — see Embolism
- finger — see Cellulitis, digit
  - with lymphangitis — see Lymphangitis, acute, digit
- foot — see Cellulitis, lower limb
  - with lymphangitis — see Lymphangitis, acute, lower limb
- gallbladder (acute) K81.Ø
- hand — see Cellulitis, upper limb
  - with lymphangitis — see Lymphangitis, acute, upper limb
- joint — see Arthritis, pyogenic or pyemic
- leg — see Cellulitis, lower limb
  - with lymphangitis — see Lymphangitis, acute, lower limb
- nail (see also Cellulitis, digit)
  - with lymphangitis — see Lymphangitis, acute, digit
- sore (see also Abscess)
  - throat J02.Ø
    - streptococcal J02.Ø
- spleen (acute) D73.89
- teeth, tooth (pulpal origin) KØ4.4
- throat — see Pharyngitis
- thrombus — see Thrombosis
- toe — see Cellulitis, digit
  - with lymphangitis — see Lymphangitis, acute, digit
- tonsils, chronic J35.Ø1
  - with adenoiditis J35.Ø3
- uterus — see Endometritis

Septicemia A41.9
- meaning sepsis — see Sepsis

Septum, septate (congenital) (see also Anomaly, by site)
- anal Q42.3
  - with fistula Q42.2
- aqueduct of Sylvius QØ3.Ø
  - with spina bifida — see Spina bifida, by site, with hydrocephalus
- uterus (complete) (partial) Q51.2
- vagina Q52.1Ø
  - in pregnancy — see Pregnancy, complicated by, abnormal vagina
    - causing obstructed labor O65.5
  - longitudinal (with or without obstruction) Q52.12
  - transverse Q52.11

Sequelae (of) (see also condition)
- abscess, intracranial or intraspinal (conditions in GØ6) GØ9
- amputation — code to injury with seventh character S
- burn and corrosion — code to injury with seventh character S
- calcium deficiency E64.8
- cerebrovascular disease — see Sequelae, disease, cerebrovascular
- childbirth O94
- contusion — code to injury with seventh character S
- corrosion — see Sequelae, burn and corrosion
- crushing injury — code to injury with seventh character S
- disease
  - cerebrovascular I69.9Ø
    - alteration of sensation I69.998
    - aphasia I69.92Ø
    - apraxia I69.99Ø
    - ataxia I69.993
    - cognitive deficits I69.91
    - disturbance of vision I69.998
    - dysarthria I69.922
    - dysphagia I69.991
    - dysphasia I69.921
    - facial droop I69.992
    - facial weakness I69.992
    - fluency disorder I69.923
    - hemiplegia I69.95- ☑
    - hemorrhage
      - intracerebral — see Sequelae, hemorrhage, intracerebral
      - intracranial, nontraumatic NEC — see Sequelae, hemorrhage, intracranial, nontraumatic

Sequelae — continued
- disease — continued
  - cerebrovascular — continued
    - hemorrhage — continued
      - subarachnoid — see Sequelae, hemorrhage, subarachnoid
    - language deficit I69.928
    - monoplegia
      - lower limb I69.84- ☑
      - upper limb I69.93- ☑
    - paralytic syndrome I69.96- ☑
    - specified effect NEC I69.998
    - specified type NEC I69.8Ø
      - alteration of sensation I69.898
      - aphasia I69.82Ø
      - apraxia I69.89Ø
      - ataxia I69.893
      - cognitive deficits I69.81
      - disturbance of vision I69.898
      - dysarthria I69.822
      - dysphagia I69.891
      - dysphasia I69.821
      - facial droop I69.892
      - facial weakness I69.892
      - fluency disorder I69.823
      - hemiplegia I69.85- ☑
      - language deficit I69.828
      - monoplegia
        - lower limb I69.84- ☑
        - upper limb I69.83- ☑
      - paralytic syndrome I69.86- ☑
      - specified effect NEC I69.898
    - speech deficit I69.928
      - speech deficit I69.828
    - stroke NOS — see Sequelae, stroke NOS
- dislocation — code to injury with seventh character S
- encephalitis or encephalomyelitis (conditions in GØ4) GØ9
  - in infectious disease NEC B94.8
  - viral B94.1
- external cause — code to injury with seventh character S
- foreign body entering natural orifice — code to injury with seventh character S
- fracture — code to injury with seventh character S
- frostbite — code to injury with seventh character S
- Hansen's disease B92
- hemorrhage
  - intracerebral I69.1Ø
    - alteration of sensation I69.198
    - aphasia I69.12Ø
    - apraxia I69.19Ø
    - ataxia I69.193
    - cognitive deficits I69.11
    - disturbance of vision I69.198
    - dysarthria I69.122
    - dysphagia I69.191
    - dysphasia I69.121
    - facial droop I69.192
    - facial weakness I69.192
    - fluency disorder I69.123
    - hemiplegia I69.15- ☑
    - language deficit NEC I69.128
    - monoplegia
      - lower limb I69.14- ☑
      - upper limb I69.13- ☑
    - paralytic syndrome I69.16- ☑
    - specified effect NEC I69.198
    - speech deficit NEC I69.128
  - intracranial, nontraumatic NEC I69.2Ø
    - alteration of sensation I69.298
    - aphasia I69.22Ø
    - apraxia I69.29Ø
    - ataxia I69.293
    - cognitive deficits I69.21
    - disturbance of vision I69.298
    - dysarthria I69.222
    - dysphagia I69.291
    - dysphasia I69.221
    - facial droop I69.292
    - facial weakness I69.292
    - fluency disorder I69.223
    - hemiplegia I69.25- ☑
    - language deficit NEC I69.228
    - monoplegia
      - lower limb I69.24- ☑
      - upper limb I69.23- ☑
    - paralytic syndrome I69.26- ☑

Sequelae — continued
- hemorrhage — continued
  - intracranial, nontraumatic — continued
    - specified effect NEC I69.298
    - speech deficit NEC I69.228
  - subarachnoid I69.ØØ
    - alteration of sensation I69.Ø98
    - aphasia I69.Ø2Ø
    - apraxia I69.Ø9Ø
    - ataxia I69.Ø93
    - cognitive deficits I69.Ø1
    - disturbance of vision I69.Ø98
    - dysarthria I69.Ø22
    - dysphagia I69.Ø91
    - dysphasia I69.Ø21
    - facial droop I69.Ø92
    - facial weakness I69.Ø92
    - fluency disorder I69.Ø23
    - hemiplegia I69.Ø5- ☑
    - language deficit NEC I69.Ø28
    - monoplegia
      - lower limb I69.Ø4- ☑
      - upper limb I69.Ø3- ☑
    - paralytic syndrome I69.Ø6- ☑
    - specified effect NEC I69.Ø98
    - speech deficit NEC I69.Ø28
- hepatitis, viral B94.2
- hyperalimentation E68
- infarction
  - cerebral I69.3Ø
    - alteration of sensation I69.398
    - aphasia I69.32Ø
    - apraxia I69.39Ø
    - ataxia I69.393
    - cognitive deficits I69.31
    - disturbance of vision I69.398
    - dysarthria I69.322
    - dysphagia I69.391
    - dysphasia I69.321
    - facial droop I69.392
    - facial weakness I69.392
    - fluency disorder I69.323
    - hemiplegia I69.35- ☑
    - language deficit NEC I69.328
    - monoplegia
      - lower limb I69.34- ☑
      - upper limb I69.33- ☑
    - paralytic syndrome I69.36- ☑
    - specified effect NEC I69.398
    - speech deficit NEC I69.328
- infection, pyogenic, intracranial or intraspinal GØ9
- infectious disease B94.9
  - specified NEC B94.8
- injury — code to injury with seventh character S
- leprosy B92
- meningitis
  - bacterial (conditions in GØØ) GØ9
  - other or unspecified cause (conditions in GØ3) GØ9
- muscle (and tendon) injury — code to injury with seventh character S
- myelitis — see Sequelae, encephalitis
- niacin deficiency E64.8
- nutritional deficiency E64.9
  - specified NEC E64.8
- obstetrical condition O94
- parasitic disease B94.9
- phlebitis or thrombophlebitis of intracranial or intraspinal venous sinuses and veins (conditions in GØ8) GØ9
- poisoning — code to poisoning with seventh character S
  - nonmedicinal substance — see Sequelae, toxic effect, nonmedicinal substance
- poliomyelitis (acute) B91
- pregnancy O94
- protein-energy malnutrition E64.Ø
- puerperium O94
- rickets E64.3
- selenium deficiency E64.8
- sprain and strain — code to injury with seventh character S
- stroke NOS I69.3Ø
  - alteration in sensation I69.398
  - aphasia I69.32Ø
  - apraxia I69.39Ø
  - ataxia I69.393
  - cognitive deficits I69.31
  - disturbance of vision I69.398

276

☑ Additional Character Required — Refer to the Tabular List for Character Selection   Subterms under main terms may continue to next column or page

Sequelae — continued
  stroke — continued
    dysarthria I69.322
    dysphagia I69.391
    dysphasia I69.321
    facial droop I69.392
    facial weakness I69.392
    hemiplegia I69.35- ☑
    language deficit NEC I69.328
    monoplegia
      lower limb I69.34- ☑
      upper limb I69.33- ☑
    paralytic syndrome I69.36- ☑
    specified effect NEC I69.398
    speech deficit NEC I69.328
  tendon and muscle injury — code to injury with seventh character S
  thiamine deficiency E64.8
  trachoma B94.0
  tuberculosis B90.9
    bones and joints B90.2
    central nervous system B90.0
    genitourinary B90.1
    pulmonary (respiratory) B90.9
    specified organs NEC B90.8
  viral
    encephalitis B94.1
    hepatitis B94.2
  vitamin deficiency NEC E64.8
    A E64.1
    B E64.8
    C E64.2
  wound, open — code to injury with seventh character S
Sequestration (see also Sequestrum)
  lung, congenital Q33.2
Sequestrum
  bone — see Osteomyelitis, chronic
  dental M27.2
  jaw bone M27.2
  orbit — see Osteomyelitis, orbit
  sinus (accessory) (nasal) — see Sinusitis
Sequoiosis lung or pneumonitis J67.8
Serology for syphilis
  doubtful
    with signs or symptoms — code by site and stage under Syphilis
    follow-up of latent syphilis — see Syphilis, latent
  negative, with signs or symptoms — code by site and stage under Syphilis
  positive A53.0
    with signs or symptoms — code by site and stage under Syphilis
  reactivated A53.0
Seroma (see also Hematoma)
  traumatic, secondary and recurrent T79.2 ☑
Seropurulent — see condition
Serositis, multiple K65.8
  pericardial I31.1
  peritoneal K65.8
Serous — see condition
Sertoli cell
  adenoma
    specified site — see Neoplasm, benign, by site
    unspecified site
      female D27.9
      male D29.20
  carcinoma
    specified site — see Neoplasm, malignant, by site
    unspecified site (male) C62.9- ☑
      female C56.9
  tumor
    with lipid storage
      specified site — see Neoplasm, benign, by site
      unspecified site
        female D27.9
        male D29.20
    specified site — see Neoplasm, benign, by site
    unspecified site
      female D27.9
      male D29.20
Sertoli-Leydig cell tumor — see Neoplasm, benign, by site
  specified site — see Neoplasm, benign, by site
  unspecified site
    female D27.9
    male D29.20

Serum
  allergy, allergic reaction (see also Reaction, serum) T80.69 ☑
    shock (see also Shock, anaphylactic) T80.59 ☑
  arthritis (see also Reaction, serum) T80.69 ☑
  complication or reaction NEC (see also Reaction, serum) T80.69 ☑
  disease NEC (see also Reaction, serum) T80.69 ☑
  hepatitis (see also Hepatitis, viral, type B)
    carrier (suspected) of Z22.51
  intoxication (see also Reaction, serum) T80.69 ☑
  neuritis (see also Reaction, serum) T80.69 ☑
  neuropathy G61.1
  poisoning NEC (see also Reaction, serum) T80.69 ☑
  rash NEC (see also Reaction, serum) T80.69 ☑
  reaction NEC (see also Reaction, serum) T80.69 ☑
  sickness NEC (see also Reaction, serum) T80.69 ☑
  urticaria (see also Reaction, serum) T80.69 ☑
Sesamoiditis M25.8- ☑
Severe sepsis R65.20
  with septic shock R65.21
Sever's disease or osteochondrosis — see Osteochondrosis, juvenile, tarsus
Sex
  chromosome mosaics Q97.8
    lines with various numbers of X chromosomes Q97.2
  education Z70.8
  reassignment surgery status Z87.890
Sextuplet pregnancy — see Pregnancy, sextuplet
Sexual
  function, disorder of (psychogenic) F52.9
  immaturity (female) (male) E30.0
  impotence (psychogenic) organic origin NEC — see Dysfunction, sexual, male
  precocity (constitutional) (cryptogenic)(female) (idiopathic) (male) E30.1
Sexuality, pathologic — see Deviation, sexual
Sézary disease C84.1- ☑
Shadow, lung R91.8
Shaking palsy or paralysis — see Parkinsonism
Shallowness, acetabulum — see Derangement, joint, specified type NEC, hip
Shaver's disease J63.1
Sheath (tendon) — see condition
Sheathing, retinal vessels H35.01- ☑
Shedding
  nail L60.8
  premature, primary (deciduous) teeth K00.6
Sheehan's disease or syndrome E23.0
Shelf, rectal K62.89
Shell teeth K00.5
Shellshock (current) F43.0
  lasting state — see Disorder, post-traumatic stress
Shield kidney Q63.1
Shift
  auditory threshold (temporary) H93.24- ☑
  mediastinal R93.8
Shifting sleep-work schedule (affecting sleep) G47.26
Shiga (-Kruse) **dysentery** A03.0
Shiga's bacillus A03.0
Shigella (dysentery) — see Dysentery, bacillary
Shigellosis A03.9
  Group A A03.0
  Group B A03.1
  Group C A03.2
  Group D A03.3
Shin splints S86.89- ☑
Shingles — see Herpes, zoster
Shipyard disease or eye B30.0
Shirodkar suture, in pregnancy — see Pregnancy, complicated by, incompetent cervix
Shock R57.9
  with ectopic or molar pregnancy O08.3
  adrenal (cortical) (Addisonian) E27.2
  adverse food reaction (anaphylactic) — see Shock, anaphylactic, due to food
  allergic — see Shock, anaphylactic
  anaphylactic T78.2
    chemical — see Table of Drugs and Chemicals
    due to drug or medicinal substance
      correct substance properly administered T88.6 ☑
      overdose or wrong substance given or taken (by accident) — see Table of Drugs and Chemicals, by drug, poisoning

Shock — continued
  anaphylactic — continued
    due to food (nonpoisonous) T78.00 ☑
      additives T78.06 ☑
      dairy products T78.07 ☑
      eggs T78.08 ☑
      fish T78.03 ☑
        shellfish T78.02 ☑
      fruit T78.04 ☑
      milk T78.07 ☑
      nuts T78.05 ☑
        peanuts T78.01 ☑
      peanuts T78.01 ☑
      seeds T78.05 ☑
      specified type NEC T78.09 ☑
      vegetable T78.04 ☑
    following sting(s) — see Venom
    immunization T80.52 ☑
    serum T80.59 ☑
      blood and blood products T80.51 ☑
      immunization T80.52 ☑
      specified NEC T80.59 ☑
      vaccination T80.52 ☑
  anaphylactoid — see Shock, anaphylactic
  anesthetic
    correct substance properly administered T88.2 ☑
    overdose or wrong substance given or taken — see Table of Drugs and Chemicals, by drug, poisoning
    specified anesthetic — see Table of Drugs and Chemicals, by drug, poisoning
  cardiogenic R57.0
  chemical substance — see Table of Drugs and Chemicals
  complicating ectopic or molar pregnancy O08.3
  culture — see Disorder, adjustment
  drug
    due to correct substance properly administered T88.6 ☑
    overdose or wrong substance given or taken (by accident) — see Table of Drugs and Chemicals, by drug, poisoning
  during or after labor and delivery O75.1
  electric T75.4 ☑
    (taser) T75.4 ☑
  endotoxic R65.21
    postprocedural (during or resulting from a procedure, not elsewhere classified) T81.12 ☑
  following
    ectopic or molar pregnancy O08.3
    injury (immediate) (delayed) T79.4 ☑
    labor and delivery O75.1
  food (anaphylactic) — see Shock, anaphylactic, due to food
  from electroshock gun (taser) T75.4 ☑
  gram-negative R65.21
    postprocedural (during or resulting from a procedure, not elsewhere classified) T81.12 ☑
  hematologic R57.8
  hemorrhagic
    surgery (intraoperative) (postoperative) T81.19 ☑
    trauma T79.4 ☑
  hypovolemic R57.1
    surgical T81.19 ☑
    traumatic T79.4 ☑
  insulin E15
    therapeutic misadventure — see subcategory T38.3 ☑
  kidney N17.0
    traumatic (following crushing) T79.5 ☑
  lightning T75.01 ☑
  lung J80
  obstetric O75.1
    with ectopic or molar pregnancy O08.3
    following ectopic or molar pregnancy O08.3
  pleural (surgical) T81.19 ☑
    due to trauma T79.4 ☑
  postprocedural (postoperative) T81.10 ☑
    with ectopic or molar pregnancy O08.3
    cardiogenic T81.11 ☑
    endotoxic T81.12 ☑
    following ectopic or molar pregnancy O08.3
    gram-negative T81.12 ☑
    hypovolemic T81.19 ☑
    septic T81.12 ☑
    specified type NEC T81.19 ☑

Shock — *continued*
- psychic F43.0
- septic (due to severe sepsis) R65.21
- specified NEC R57.8
- surgical T81.10 ☑
- taser gun (taser) T75.4 ☑
- therapeutic misadventure NEC T81.10 ☑
- thyroxin
  - overdose or wrong substance given or taken — *see* Table of Drugs and Chemicals, by drug, poisoning
- toxic, syndrome A48.3
- transfusion — *see* Complications, transfusion
- traumatic (immediate) (delayed) T79.4 ☑

Shoemaker's chest M95.4
Short, shortening, shortness
- arm (acquired) (*see also* Deformity, limb, unequal length)
  - congenital Q71.81- ☑
    - forearm — *see* Deformity, limb, unequal length
- bowel syndrome K91.2
- breath R06.02
- cervical (complicating pregnancy) O26.87- ☑
  - non-gravid uterus N88.3
- common bile duct, congenital Q44.5
- cord (umbilical), complicating delivery O69.3 ☑
- cystic duct, congenital Q44.5
- esophagus (congenital) Q39.8
- femur (acquired) — *see* Deformity, limb, unequal length, femur
  - congenital — *see* Defect, reduction, lower limb, longitudinal, femur
- frenum, frenulum, linguae (congenital) Q38.1
- hip (acquired) (*see also* Deformity, limb, unequal length)
  - congenital Q65.89
- leg (acquired) (*see also* Deformity, limb, unequal length)
  - congenital Q72.81- ☑
  - lower leg (*see also* Deformity, limb, unequal length)
- limbed stature, with immunodeficiency D82.2
- lower limb (acquired) (*see also* Deformity, limb, unequal length)
  - congenital Q72.81- ☑
- organ or site, congenital NEC — *see* Distortion
- palate, congenital Q38.5
- radius (acquired) (*see also* Deformity, limb, unequal length)
  - congenital — *see* Defect, reduction, upper limb, longitudinal, radius
- rib syndrome Q77.2
- stature (child) (hereditary) (idiopathic) NEC R62.52
  - constitutional E34.3
  - due to endocrine disorder E34.3
  - Laron-type E34.3
- tendon (*see also* Contraction, tendon)
  - with contracture of joint — *see* Contraction, joint
  - Achilles (acquired) M67.0- ☑
    - congenital Q66.89
    - congenital Q79.8
- thigh (acquired) (*see also* Deformity, limb, unequal length, femur)
  - congenital — *see* Defect, reduction, lower limb, longitudinal, femur
- tibialis anterior (tendon) — *see* Contraction, tendon
- umbilical cord
  - complicating delivery O69.3 ☑
- upper limb, congenital — *see* Defect, reduction, upper limb, specified type NEC
- urethra N36.8
- uvula, congenital Q38.5
- vagina (congenital) Q52.4

Shortsightedness — *see* Myopia
Shoshin (acute fulminating beriberi) E51.11
Shoulder — *see* condition
Shovel-shaped incisors K00.2
Shower, thromboembolic — *see* Embolism
Shunt
- arterial-venous (dialysis) Z99.2
- arteriovenous, pulmonary (acquired) I28.0
  - congenital Q25.72
- cerebral ventricle (communicating) in situ Z98.2
- surgical, prosthetic, with complications — *see* Complications, cardiovascular, device or implant

Shutdown, renal N28.9
Shy-Drager syndrome G90.3

Sialadenitis, sialadenosis (any gland) (chronic) (periodic) (suppurative) — *see* Sialoadenitis
Sialectasia K11.8
Sialidosis E77.1
Sialitis, silitis (any gland) (chronic) (suppurative) — *see* Sialoadenitis
Sialoadenitis (any gland) (periodic) (suppurative) K11.20
- acute K11.21
  - recurrent K11.22
- chronic K11.23
Sialoadenopathy K11.9
Sialoangitis — *see* Sialoadenitis
Sialodochitis (fibrinosa) — *see* Sialoadenitis
Sialodocholithiasis K11.5
Sialolithiasis K11.5
Sialometaplasia, necrotizing K11.8
Sialorrhea (*see also* Ptyalism)
- periodic — *see* Sialoadenitis
Sialosis K11.7
Siamese twin Q89.4
Sibling rivalry Z62.891
Sicard's syndrome G52.7
Sicca syndrome M35.00
- with
  - keratoconjunctivitis M35.01
  - lung involvement M35.02
  - myopathy M35.03
  - renal tubulo-interstitial disorders M35.04
- specified organ involvement NEC M35.09
Sick R69
- or handicapped person in family Z63.79
  - needing care at home Z63.6
- sinus (syndrome) I49.5
Sick-euthyroid syndrome E07.81
Sickle-cell
- anemia — *see* Disease, sickle-cell
- trait D57.3
Sicklemia (*see also* Disease, sickle-cell)
- trait D57.3
Sickness
- air (travel) T75.3 ☑
- airplane T75.3 ☑
- alpine T70.29 ☑
- altitude T70.20 ☑
- Andes T70.29 ☑
- aviator's T70.29 ☑
- balloon T70.29 ☑
- car T75.3 ☑
- compressed air T70.3 ☑
- decompression T70.3 ☑
- green D50.8
- milk — *see* Poisoning, food, noxious
- motion T75.3 ☑
- mountain T70.29 ☑
  - acute D75.1
- protein (*see also* Reaction, serum) T80.69 ☑
- radiation T66 ☑
- roundabout (motion) T75.3 ☑
- sea T75.3 ☑
- serum NEC (*see also* Reaction, serum) T80.69 ☑
- sleeping (African) B56.9
  - by Trypanosoma B56.9
    - brucei
      - gambiense B56.0
      - rhodesiense B56.1
    - East African B56.1
    - Gambian B56.0
    - Rhodesian B56.1
    - West African B56.0
- swing (motion) T75.3 ☑
- train (railway) (travel) T75.3 ☑
- travel (any vehicle) T75.3 ☑
Sideropenia — *see* Anemia, iron deficiency
Siderosilicosis J62.8
Siderosis (lung) J63.4
- eye (globe) — *see* Disorder, globe, degenerative, siderosis
Siemens' syndrome (ectodermal dysplasia) Q82.8
Sighing R06.89
- psychogenic F45.8
Sigmoid (*see also* condition)
- flexure — *see* condition
- kidney Q63.1
Sigmoiditis (*see also* Enteritis) K52.9
- infectious A09
- noninfectious K52.9
Silfversköld's syndrome Q78.9

Silicosiderosis J62.8
Silicosis, silicotic (simple) (complicated) J62.8
- with tuberculosis J65
Silicotuberculosis J65
Silo-fillers' disease J68.8
- bronchitis J68.0
- pneumonitis J68.0
- pulmonary edema J68.1
Silver's syndrome Q87.1
Simian malaria B53.1
Simmonds' cachexia or disease E23.0
Simons' disease or syndrome (progressive lipodystrophy) E88.1
Simple, simplex — *see* condition
Simulation, conscious (of illness) Z76.5
Simultanagnosia (asimultagnosia) R48.3
Sin Nombre virus disease (Hantavirus) (cardio)-pulmonary syndrome) B33.4
Sinding-Larsen disease or osteochondrosis — *see* Osteochondrosis, juvenile, patella
Singapore hemorrhagic fever A91
Singer's node or nodule J38.2
Single
- atrium Q21.2
- coronary artery Q24.5
- umbilical artery Q27.0
- ventricle Q20.4
Singultus R06.6
- epidemicus B33.0
Sinus (*see also* Fistula)
- abdominal K63.89
- arrest I45.5
- arrhythmia I49.8
- bradycardia R00.1
- branchial cleft (internal) (external) Q18.0
- coccygeal — *see* Sinus, pilonidal
- dental K04.6
- dermal (congenital) Q06.8
  - with abscess Q06.8
  - coccygeal, pilonidal — *see* Sinus, coccygeal
- infected, skin NEC L08.89
- marginal, ruptured or bleeding — *see* Hemorrhage, antepartum, specified cause NEC
- medial, face and neck Q18.8
- pause I45.5
- pericranii Q01.9
- pilonidal (infected) (rectum) L05.92
  - with abscess L05.02
- preauricular Q18.1
- rectovaginal N82.3
- Rokitansky-Aschoff (gallbladder) K82.8
- sacrococcygeal (dermoid) (infected) — *see* Sinus, pilonidal
- tachycardia R00.0
  - paroxysmal I47.1
- tarsi syndrome M25.57- ☑
- testis N50.8
- tract (postinfective) — *see* Fistula
- urachus Q64.4
Sinusitis (accessory) (chronic) (hyperplastic) (nasal) (nonpurulent) (purulent) J32.9
- acute J01.90
  - ethmoidal J01.20
    - recurrent J01.21
  - frontal J01.10
    - recurrent J01.11
  - involving more than one sinus, other than pansinusitis J01.80
    - recurrent J01.81
  - maxillary J01.00
    - recurrent J01.01
  - pansinusitis J01.40
    - recurrent J01.41
  - recurrent J01.91
  - specified NEC J01.80
    - recurrent J01.81
  - sphenoidal J01.30
    - recurrent J01.31
- allergic — *see* Rhinitis, allergic
- due to high altitude T70.1 ☑
- ethmoidal J32.2
  - acute J01.20
    - recurrent J01.21
- frontal J32.1
  - acute J01.10
    - recurrent J01.11
- influenzal — *see* Influenza, with, respiratory manifestations NEC

☑ Additional Character Required — Refer to the Tabular List for Character Selection   ▽ Subterms under main terms may continue to next column or page

Sinusitis — *continued*
  involving more than one sinus but not pansinusitis
      J32.8
    acute J01.80
      recurrent J01.81
  maxillary J32.0
    acute J01.00
      recurrent J01.01
  sphenoidal J32.3
    acute J01.30
      recurrent J01.31
  tuberculous, any sinus A15.8
Sinusitis-bronchiectasis-situs inversus (syndrome)
    (triad) Q89.3
Sipple's syndrome E31.22
Sirenomelia (syndrome) Q87.2
Siriasis T67.0 ☑
Sirkari's disease B55.0
Siti A65
Situation, psychiatric F99
Situational
  disturbance (transient) — *see* Disorder, adjustment
    acute F43.0
  maladjustment — *see* Disorder, adjustment
  reaction — *see* Disorder, adjustment
    acute F43.0
Situs inversus or transversus (abdominalis) (thoracis)
    Q89.3
Sixth disease B08.20
  due to human herpesvirus 6 B08.21
  due to human herpesvirus 7 B08.22
Sjögren-Larsson syndrome Q87.1
Sjögren's syndrome or disease — *see* Sicca syndrome
Skeletal — *see* condition
Skene's gland — *see* condition
Skenitis — *see* Urethritis
Skerljevo A65
Skevas-Zerfus disease — *see* Toxicity, venom, marine
    animal, sea anemone
Skin (*see also* condition)
  clammy R23.1
  donor — *see* Donor, skin
  hidebound M35.9
Slate-dressers' or slate-miners' lung J62.8
Sleep
  apnea — *see* Apnea, sleep
  deprivation Z72.820
  disorder or disturbance G47.9
      child F51.9
      nonorganic origin F51.9
      specified NEC G47.8
  disturbance G47.9
      nonorganic origin F51.9
  drunkenness F51.9
  rhythm inversion G47.2- ☑
  terrors F51.4
  walking F51.3
      hysterical F44.89
Sleep hygiene
  abuse Z72.821
  inadequate Z72.821
  poor Z72.821
Sleeping sickness — *see* Sickness, sleeping
Sleeplessness — *see* Insomnia
  menopausal N95.1
Sleep-wake schedule disorder G47.20
Slim disease (in HIV infection) B20
Slipped, slipping
  epiphysis (traumatic) (*see also* Osteochondropathy,
      specified type NEC)
    capital femoral (traumatic)
      acute (on chronic) S79.01- ☑
    current traumatic — *code as* Fracture, by site
    upper femoral (nontraumatic) M93.00- ☑
      acute M93.01- ☑
        on chronic M93.03- ☑
      chronic M93.02- ☑
  intervertebral disc — *see* Displacement, intervertebral
      disc
  ligature, umbilical P51.8
  patella — *see* Disorder, patella, derangement NEC
  rib M89.8X8
  sacroiliac joint — *see* subcategory M53.2 ☑
  tendon — *see* Disorder, tendon
  ulnar nerve, nontraumatic — *see* Lesion, nerve, ulnar
  vertebra NEC — *see* Spondylolisthesis
Slocumb's syndrome E27.0

Sloughing (multiple) (phagedena) (skin) (*see also* Gan-
    grene)
  abscess — *see* Abscess
  appendix K38.8
  fascia — *see* Disorder, soft tissue, specified type NEC
  scrotum N50.8
  tendon — *see* Disorder, tendon
  transplanted organ — *see* Rejection, transplant
  ulcer — *see* Ulcer, skin
Slow
  feeding, newborn P92.2
  flow syndrome, coronary I20.8
  heart (beat) R00.1
Slowing, urinary stream R39.19
Sluder's neuralgia (syndrome) G44.89
Slurred, slurring speech R47.81
Small (ness)
  for gestational age — *see* Small for dates
  introitus, vagina N89.6
  kidney (unknown cause) N27.9
    bilateral N27.1
    unilateral N27.0
  ovary (congenital) Q50.39
  pelvis
    with disproportion (fetopelvic) O33.1
      causing obstructed labor O65.1
  uterus N85.8
  white kidney N03.9
Small-and-light-for-dates — *see* Small for dates
Small-for-dates (infant) P05.10
  with weight of
    1000-1249 grams P05.14
    1250-1499 grams P05.15
    1500-1749 grams P05.16
    1750-1999 grams P05.17
    2000-2499 grams P05.18
    499 grams or less P05.11
    500-749 grams P05.12
    750-999 grams P05.13
Smallpox B03
Smearing, fecal R15.1
Smith-Lemli-Opitz syndrome E78.72
Smith's fracture S52.54- ☑
Smoker — *see* Dependence, drug, nicotine
Smoker's
  bronchitis J41.0
  cough J41.0
  palate K13.24
  throat J31.2
  tongue K13.24
Smoking
  passive Z77.22
Smothering spells R06.81
Snaggle teeth, tooth M26.39
Snapping
  finger — *see* Trigger finger
  hip — *see* Derangement, joint, specified type NEC, hip
    involving the iliotibial band M76.3- ☑
  knee — *see* Derangement, knee
    involving the iliotibial band M76.3- ☑
Sneddon-Wilkinson disease or syndrome (sub-corneal
    pustular dermatosis) L13.1
Sneezing (intractable) R06.7
Sniffing
  cocaine
    abuse — *see* Abuse, drug, cocaine
    dependence — *see* Dependence, drug, cocaine
  gasoline
    abuse — *see* Abuse, drug, inhalant
    dependence — *see* Dependence, drug, inhalant
  glue (airplane)
    abuse — *see* Abuse, drug, inhalant
    drug dependence — *see* Dependence, drug, in-
      halant
Sniffles
  newborn P28.89
Snoring R06.83
Snow blindness — *see* Photokeratitis
Snuffles (non-syphilitic) R06.5
  newborn P28.89
  syphilitic (infant) A50.05 [J99]
Social
  exclusion Z60.4
    due to discrimination or persecution (perceived)
      Z60.5
  migrant Z59.0
    acculturation difficulty Z60.3

Social — *continued*
  rejection Z60.4
    due to discrimination or persecution Z60.5
  role conflict NEC Z73.5
  skills inadequacy NEC Z73.4
  transplantation Z60.3
Sodoku A25.0
Soemmerring's ring — *see* Cataract, secondary
Soft (*see also* condition)
  nails L60.3
Softening
  bone — *see* Osteomalacia
  brain (necrotic) (progressive) G93.89
    congenital Q04.8
    embolic I63.4 ☑
    hemorrhagic — *see* Hemorrhage, intracranial, in-
      tracerebral
    occlusive I63.5 ☑
    thrombotic I63.3 ☑
  cartilage M94.2- ☑
    patella M22.4- ☑
  cerebellar — *see* Softening, brain
  cerebral — *see* Softening, brain
  cerebrospinal — *see* Softening, brain
  myocardial, heart — *see* Degeneration, myocardial
  spinal cord G95.89
  stomach K31.89
Soldier's
  heart F45.8
  patches I31.0
Solitary
  cyst, kidney N28.1
  kidney, congenital Q60.0
Solvent abuse — *see* Abuse, drug, inhalant
  dependence — *see* Dependence, drug, inhalant
Somatization reaction, somatic reaction — *see* Disor-
    der, somatoform
Somnambulism F51.3
  hysterical F44.89
Somnolence R40.0
  nonorganic origin F51.11
Sonne dysentery A03.3
Soor B37.0
Sore
  bed — *see* Ulcer, pressure, by site
  chiclero B55.1
  Delhi B55.1
  desert — *see* Ulcer, skin
  eye H57.1- ☑
  Lahore B55.1
  mouth K13.79
    canker K12.0
  muscle M79.1
  Naga — *see* Ulcer, skin
  of skin — *see* Ulcer, skin
  oriental B55.1
  pressure — *see* Ulcer, pressure, by site
  skin L98.9
  soft A57
  throat (acute) (*see also* Pharyngitis)
    with influenza, flu, or grippe — *see* Influenza, with,
      respiratory manifestations NEC
    chronic J31.2
    coxsackie (virus) B08.5
    diphtheritic A36.0
    herpesviral B00.2
    influenzal — *see* Influenza, with, respiratory mani-
      festations NEC
    septic J02.0
    streptococcal (ulcerative) J02.0
    viral NEC J02.8
      coxsackie B08.5
  tropical — *see* Ulcer, skin
  veldt — *see* Ulcer, skin
Soto's syndrome (cerebral gigantism) Q87.3
South African cardiomyopathy syndrome I42.8
Southeast Asian hemorrhagic fever A91
Spacing
  abnormal, tooth, teeth, fully erupted M26.30
  excessive, tooth, fully erupted M26.32
Spade-like hand (congenital) Q68.1
Spading nail L60.8
  congenital Q84.6
Spanish collar N47.1
Sparganosis B70.1
Spasm(s), **spastic, spasticity** (*see also* condition) R25.2
  accommodation — *see* Spasm, of accommodation

Spasm(s), spastic, spasticity — *continued*
- ampulla of Vater K83.4
- anus, ani (sphincter) (reflex) K59.4
  - psychogenic F45.8
- artery I73.9
  - cerebral G45.9
- Bell's G51.3
- bladder (sphincter, external or internal) N32.89
  - psychogenic F45.8
- bronchus, bronchiole J98.01
- cardia K22.0
- cardiac I20.1
- carpopedal — *see* Tetany
- cerebral (arteries) (vascular) G45.9
- cervix, complicating delivery O62.4
- ciliary body (of accommodation) — *see* Spasm, of accommodation
- colon K58.9
  - with diarrhea K58.0
  - psychogenic F45.8
- common duct K83.8
- compulsive — *see* Tic
- conjugate H51.8
- coronary (artery) I20.1
- diaphragm (reflex) R06.6
  - epidemic B33.0
  - psychogenic F45.8
- duodenum K59.8
- epidemic diaphragmatic (transient) B33.0
- esophagus (diffuse) K22.4
  - psychogenic F45.8
- facial G51.3
- fallopian tube N83.8
- gastrointestinal (tract) K31.89
  - psychogenic F45.8
- glottis J38.5
  - hysterical F44.4
  - psychogenic F45.8
    - conversion reaction F44.4
  - reflex through recurrent laryngeal nerve J38.5
- habit — *see* Tic
- heart I20.1
- hemifacial (clonic) G51.3
- hourglass — *see* Contraction, hourglass
- hysterical F44.4
- infantile — *see* Epilepsy, spasms
- inferior oblique, eye H51.8
- intestinal (*see also* Syndrome, irritable bowel) K58.9
  - psychogenic F45.8
- larynx, laryngeal J38.5
  - hysterical F44.4
  - psychogenic F45.8
    - conversion reaction F44.4
- levator palpebrae superioris — *see* Disorder, eyelid function
- muscle NEC M62.838
  - back M62.830
- nerve, trigeminal G51.0
- nervous F45.8
- nodding F98.4
- occupational F48.8
- oculogyric H51.8
  - psychogenic F45.8
- of accommodation H52.53- ☑
- ophthalmic artery — *see* Occlusion, artery, retina
- perineal, female N94.89
- peroneo-extensor (*see also* Deformity, limb, flat foot)
- pharynx (reflex) J39.2
  - hysterical F45.8
  - psychogenic F45.8
- psychogenic F45.8
- pylorus NEC K31.3
  - adult hypertrophic K31.89
  - congenital or infantile Q40.0
  - psychogenic F45.8
- rectum (sphincter) K59.4
  - psychogenic F45.8
- retinal (artery) — *see* Occlusion, artery, retina
- sigmoid (*see also* Syndrome, irritable bowel) K58.9
  - psychogenic F45.8
- sphincter of Oddi K83.4
- stomach K31.89
  - neurotic F45.8
- throat J39.2
  - hysterical F45.8
  - psychogenic F45.8
- tic F95.9
  - chronic F95.1

Spasm(s), spastic, spasticity — *continued*
- tic — *continued*
  - transient of childhood F95.0
- tongue K14.8
- torsion (progressive) G24.1
- trigeminal nerve — *see* Neuralgia, trigeminal
- ureter N13.5
- urethra (sphincter) N35.9
- uterus N85.8
  - complicating labor O62.4
- vagina N94.2
  - psychogenic F52.5
- vascular I73.9
- vasomotor I73.9
- vein NEC I87.8
- viscera — *see* Pain, abdominal

Spasmodic — *see* condition
Spasmophilia — *see* Tetany
Spasmus nutans F98.4
Spastic, spasticity (*see also* Spasm)
- child (cerebral) (congenital) (paralysis) G80.1

Speaker's throat R49.8
Specific, specified — *see* condition
Speech
- defect, disorder, disturbance, impediment R47.9
  - psychogenic, in childhood and adolescence F98.8
  - slurring R47.81
  - specified NEC R47.89

Spencer's disease A08.19
Spens' syndrome (syncope with heart block) I45.9
Sperm counts (fertility testing) Z31.41
- postvasectomy Z30.8
- reversal Z31.42

Spermatic cord — *see* condition
Spermatocele N43.40
- congenital Q55.4
- multiple N43.42
- single N43.41

Spermatocystitis N49.0
Spermatocytoma C62.9- ☑
- specified site — *see* Neoplasm, malignant, by site

Spermatorrhea N50.8
Sphacelus — *see* Gangrene
Sphenoidal — *see* condition
Sphenoiditis (chronic) — *see* Sinusitis, sphenoidal
Sphenopalatine ganglion neuralgia G90.09
Sphericity, increased, lens (congenital) Q12.4
Spherocytosis (congenital) (familial) (hereditary) D58.0
- hemoglobin disease D58.0
- sickle-cell (disease) D57.8- ☑

Spherophakia Q12.4
Sphincter — *see* condition
Sphincteritis, sphincter of Oddi — *see* Cholangitis
Sphingolipidosis E75.3
- specified NEC E75.29

Sphingomyelinosis E75.3
Spicule tooth K00.2
Spider
- bite — *see* Toxicity, venom, spider
- fingers — *see* Syndrome, Marfan's
- nevus I78.1
- toes — *see* Syndrome, Marfan's
- vascular I78.1

Spiegler-Fendt
- benign lymphocytoma L98.8
- sarcoid L08.89

Spielmeyer-Vogt disease E75.4
Spina bifida (aperta) Q05.9
- with hydrocephalus NEC Q05.4
- cervical Q05.5
  - with hydrocephalus Q05.0
- dorsal Q05.6
  - with hydrocephalus Q05.1
- lumbar Q05.7
  - with hydrocephalus Q05.2
- lumbosacral Q05.7
  - with hydrocephalus Q05.2
- occulta Q76.0
- sacral Q05.8
  - with hydrocephalus Q05.3
- thoracic Q05.6
  - with hydrocephalus Q05.1
- thoracolumbar Q05.6
  - with hydrocephalus Q05.1

Spindle, Krukenberg's — *see* Pigmentation, cornea, posterior
Spine, spinal — *see* condition

Spiradenoma (eccrine) — *see* Neoplasm, skin, benign
Spirillosis A25.0
Spirillum
- minus A25.0
- obermeieri infection A68.0

Spirochetal — *see* condition
Spirochetosis A69.9
- arthritic, arthritica A69.9
- bronchopulmonary A69.8
- icterohemorrhagic A27.0
- lung A69.8

Spirometrosis B70.1
Spitting blood — *see* Hemoptysis
Splanchnoptosis K63.4
Spleen, splenic — *see* condition
Splenectasis — *see* Splenomegaly
Splenitis (interstitial) (malignant) (nonspecific) D73.89
- malarial (*see also* Malaria) B54 [D77]
- tuberculous A18.85

Splenocele D73.89
Splenomegaly, splenomegalia (Bengal) (cryptogenic) (idiopathic) (tropical) R16.1
- with hepatomegaly R16.2
- cirrhotic D73.2
- congenital Q89.09
- congestive, chronic D73.2
- Egyptian B65.1
- Gaucher's E75.22
- malarial (*see also* Malaria) B54 [D77]
- neutropenic D73.81
- Niemann-Pick — *see* Niemann-Pick disease or syndrome
- siderotic D73.2
- syphilitic A52.79
  - congenital (early) A50.08 [D77]

Splenopathy D73.9
Splenoptosis D73.89
Splenosis D73.89
Splinter — *see* Foreign body, superficial, by site
Split, splitting
- foot Q72.7- ☑
- heart sounds R01.2
- lip, congenital — *see* Cleft, lip
- nails L60.3
- urinary stream R39.13

Spondylarthrosis — *see* Spondylosis
Spondylitis (chronic) (*see also* Spondylopathy, inflammatory)
- ankylopoietica — *see* Spondylitis, ankylosing
- ankylosing (chronic) M45.9
  - with lung involvement M45.9 [J99]
  - cervical region M45.2
  - cervicothoracic region M45.3
  - juvenile M08.1
  - lumbar region M45.6
  - lumbosacral region M45.7
  - multiple sites M45.0
  - occipito-atlanto-axial region M45.1
  - sacrococcygeal region M45.8
  - thoracic region M45.4
  - thoracolumbar region M45.5
- atrophic (ligamentous) — *see* Spondylitis, ankylosing
- deformans (chronic) — *see* Spondylosis
- gonococcal A54.41
- gouty M10.08
- in (due to)
  - brucellosis A23.9 [M49.80]
    - cervical region A23.9 [M49.82]
    - cervicothoracic region A23.9 [M49.83]
    - lumbar region A23.9 [M49.86]
    - lumbosacral region A23.9 [M49.87]
    - multiple sites A23.9 [M49.89]
    - occipito-atlanto-axial region A23.9 [M49.81]
    - sacrococcygeal region A23.9 [M49.88]
    - thoracic region A23.9 [M49.84]
    - thoracolumbar region A23.9 [M49.85]
  - enterobacteria (*see also* subcategory M49.8) A04.9
  - tuberculosis A18.01
- infectious NEC — *see* Spondylopathy, infective
- juvenile ankylosing (chronic) M08.1
- Kümmell's — *see* Spondylopathy, traumatic
- Marie-Strümpell — *see* Spondylitis, ankylosing
- muscularis — *see* Spondylopathy, specified NEC
- psoriatic L40.53
- rheumatoid — *see* Spondylitis, ankylosing
- rhizomelica — *see* Spondylitis, ankylosing
- sacroiliac NEC M46.1

☑ **Additional Character Required** — Refer to the Tabular List for Character Selection   🔻 **Subterms under main terms may continue to next column or page**

Spondylitis — *continued*
    senescent, senile — *see* Spondylosis
    traumatic (chronic) or post-traumatic — *see* Spondylopathy, traumatic
    tuberculous A18.01
    typhosa A01.05
Spondylolisthesis (acquired) (degenerative) M43.10
    with disproportion (fetopelvic) O33.0
        causing obstructed labor O65.0
    cervical region M43.12
    cervicothoracic region M43.13
    congenital Q76.2
    lumbar region M43.16
    lumbosacral region M43.17
    multiple sites M43.19
    occipito-atlanto-axial region M43.11
    sacrococcygeal region M43.18
    thoracic region M43.14
    thoracolumbar region M43.15
    traumatic (old) M43.10
        acute
            fifth cervical (displaced) S12.430 ☑
                nondisplaced S12.431 ☑
                specified type NEC (displaced) S12.450 ☑
                    nondisplaced S12.451 ☑
                type III S12.44 ☑
            fourth cervical (displaced) S12.330 ☑
                nondisplaced S12.331 ☑
                specified type NEC (displaced) S12.350 ☑
                    nondisplaced S12.351 ☑
                type III S12.34 ☑
            second cervical (displaced) S12.130 ☑
                nondisplaced S12.131 ☑
                specified type NEC (displaced) S12.150 ☑
                    nondisplaced S12.151 ☑
                type III S12.14 ☑
            seventh cervical (displaced) S12.630 ☑
                nondisplaced S12.631 ☑
                specified type NEC (displaced) S12.650 ☑
                    nondisplaced S12.651 ☑
                type III S12.64 ☑
            sixth cervical (displaced) S12.530 ☑
                nondisplaced S12.531 ☑
                specified type NEC (displaced) S12.550 ☑
                    nondisplaced S12.551 ☑
                type III S12.54 ☑
            third cervical (displaced) S12.230 ☑
                nondisplaced S12.231 ☑
                specified type NEC (displaced) S12.250 ☑
                    nondisplaced S12.251 ☑
                type III S12.24 ☑
Spondylolysis (acquired) M43.00
    cervical region M43.02
    cervicothoracic region M43.03
    congenital Q76.2
    lumbar region M43.06
    lumbosacral region M43.07
        with disproportion (fetopelvic) O33.0
            causing obstructed labor O65.8
    multiple sites M43.09
    occipito-atlanto-axial region M43.01
    sacrococcygeal region M43.08
    thoracic region M43.04
    thoracolumbar region M43.05
Spondylopathy M48.9
    infective NEC M46.50
        cervical region M46.52
        cervicothoracic region M46.53
        lumbar region M46.56
        lumbosacral region M46.57
        multiple sites M46.59
        occipito-atlanto-axial region M46.51
        sacrococcygeal region M46.58
        thoracic region M46.54
        thoracolumbar region M46.55
    inflammatory M46.90
        cervical region M46.92
        cervicothoracic region M46.93
        lumbar region M46.96
        lumbosacral region M46.97
        multiple sites M46.99
        occipito-atlanto-axial region M46.91
        sacrococcygeal region M46.98
        specified type NEC M46.80
            cervical region M46.82
            cervicothoracic region M46.83
            lumbar region M46.86

Spondylopathy — *continued*
    inflammatory — *continued*
        specified type — *continued*
            lumbosacral region M46.87
            multiple sites M46.89
            occipito-atlanto-axial region M46.81
            sacrococcygeal region M46.88
            thoracic region M46.84
            thoracolumbar region M46.85
        thoracic region M46.94
        thoracolumbar region M46.95
    neuropathic, in
        syringomyelia and syringobulbia G95.0
        tabes dorsalis A52.11
    specified NEC — *see* subcategory M48.8 ☑
    traumatic M48.30
        cervical region M48.32
        cervicothoracic region M48.33
        lumbar region M48.36
        lumbosacral region M48.37
        occipito-atlanto-axial region M48.31
        sacrococcygeal region M48.38
        thoracic region M48.34
        thoracolumbar region M48.35
Spondylosis M47.9
    with
        disproportion (fetopelvic) O33.0
            causing obstructed labor O65.0
        myelopathy NEC M47.10
            cervical region M47.12
            cervicothoracic region M47.13
            lumbar region M47.16
            occipito-atlanto-axial region M47.11
            thoracic region M47.14
            thoracolumbar region M47.15
        radiculopathy M47.20
            cervical region M47.22
            cervicothoracic region M47.23
            lumbar region M47.26
            lumbosacral region M47.27
            occipito-atlanto-axial region M47.21
            sacrococcygeal region M47.28
            thoracic region M47.24
            thoracolumbar region M47.25
    without myelopathy or radiculopathy M47.819
        cervical region M47.812
        cervicothoracic region M47.813
        lumbar region M47.816
        lumbosacral region M47.817
        occipito-atlanto-axial region M47.811
        sacrococcygeal region M47.818
        thoracic region M47.814
        thoracolumbar region M47.815
    specified NEC M47.899
        cervical region M47.892
        cervicothoracic region M47.893
        lumbar region M47.896
        lumbosacral region M47.897
        occipito-atlanto-axial region M47.891
        sacrococcygeal region M47.898
        thoracic region M47.894
        thoracolumbar region M47.895
    traumatic — *see* Spondylopathy, traumatic
Sponge
    inadvertently left in operation wound — *see* Foreign body, accidentally left during a procedure
    kidney (medullary) Q61.5
Sponge-diver's disease — *see* Toxicity, venom, marine animal, sea anemone
Spongioblastoma (any type) — *see* Neoplasm, malignant, by site
    specified site — *see* Neoplasm, malignant, by site
    unspecified site C71.9
Spongioneuroblastoma — *see* Neoplasm, malignant, by site
Spontaneous (*see also* condition)
    fracture (cause unknown) — *see* Fracture, pathological
Spoon nail L60.3
    congenital Q84.6
Sporadic — *see* condition
Sporothrix schenckii infection — *see* Sporotrichosis
Sporotrichosis B42.9
    arthritis B42.82
    disseminated B42.7
    generalized B42.7
    lymphocutaneous (fixed) (progressive) B42.1
    pulmonary B42.0
    specified NEC B42.89

Spots, spotting (in) (of)
    Bitot's (*see also* Pigmentation, conjunctiva)
        in the young child E50.1
            vitamin A deficiency E50.1
    café, au lait L81.3
    Cayenne pepper I78.1
    cotton wool, retina — *see* Occlusion, artery, retina
    de Morgan's (senile angiomas) I78.1
    Fuchs' black (myopic) H44.2- ☑
    intermenstrual (regular) N92.0
        irregular N92.1
    Koplik's B05.9
    liver L81.4
    pregnancy O26.85- ☑
    purpuric R23.3
    ruby I78.1
Spotted fever — *see* Fever, spotted N92.3
Sprain (joint) (ligament)
    acromioclavicular joint or ligament S43.5- ☑
    ankle S93.40- ☑
        calcaneofibular ligament S93.41- ☑
        deltoid ligament S93.42- ☑
        internal collateral ligament — *see* Sprain, ankle, specified ligament NEC
        specified ligament NEC S93.49- ☑
        talofibular ligament — *see* Sprain, ankle, specified ligament NEC
        tibiofibular ligament S93.43- ☑
    anterior longitudinal, cervical S13.4 ☑
    atlas, atlanto-axial, atlanto-occipital S13.4 ☑
    breast bone — *see* Sprain, sternum
    calcaneofibular — *see* Sprain, ankle
    carpal — *see* Sprain, wrist
    carpometacarpal — *see* Sprain, hand, specified site NEC
    cartilage
        costal S23.41 ☑
        semilunar (knee) — *see* Sprain, knee, specified site NEC
            with current tear — *see* Tear, meniscus
        thyroid region S13.5 ☑
        xiphoid — *see* Sprain, sternum
    cervical, cervicodorsal, cervicothoracic S13.4 ☑
    chondrosternal S23.421 ☑
    coracoclavicular S43.8- ☑
    coracohumeral S43.41- ☑
    coronary, knee — *see* Sprain, knee, specified site NEC
    costal cartilage S23.41 ☑
    cricoarytenoid articulation or ligament S13.5 ☑
    cricothyroid articulation S13.5 ☑
    cruciate, knee — *see* Sprain, knee, cruciate
    deltoid, ankle — *see* Sprain, ankle
    dorsal (spine) S23.3 ☑
    elbow S53.40- ☑
        radial collateral ligament S53.43- ☑
        radiohumeral S53.41- ☑
        rupture
            radial collateral ligament — *see* Rupture, traumatic, ligament, radial collateral
            ulnar collateral ligament — *see* Rupture, traumatic, ligament, ulnar collateral
        specified type NEC S53.49- ☑
        ulnar collateral ligament S53.44- ☑
        ulnohumeral S53.42- ☑
    femur, head — *see* Sprain, hip
    fibular collateral, knee — *see* Sprain, knee, collateral
    fibulocalcaneal — *see* Sprain, ankle
    finger(s) S63.61- ☑
        index S63.61- ☑
        interphalangeal (joint) S63.63- ☑
            index S63.63- ☑
            little S63.63- ☑
            middle S63.63- ☑
            ring S63.63- ☑
        little S63.61- ☑
        metacarpophalangeal (joint) S63.65- ☑
        middle S63.61- ☑
        ring S63.61- ☑
        specified site NEC S63.69- ☑
            index S63.69- ☑
            little S63.69- ☑
            middle S63.69- ☑
            ring S63.69- ☑
    foot S93.60- ☑
        specified ligament NEC S93.69- ☑
        tarsal ligament S93.61- ☑

Sprain — *continued*
  foot — *continued*
    tarsometatarsal ligament S93.62- ☑
    toe — *see* Sprain, toe
  hand S63.9- ☑
    finger — *see* Sprain, finger
    specified site NEC — *see* subcategory S63.8 ☑
    thumb — *see* Sprain, thumb
  head S03.9 ☑
  hip S73.10- ☑
    iliofemoral ligament S73.11- ☑
    ischiocapsular (ligament) S73.12- ☑
    specified NEC S73.19- ☑
  iliofemoral — *see* Sprain, hip
  innominate
    acetabulum — *see* Sprain, hip
    sacral junction S33.6 ☑
  internal
    collateral, ankle — *see* Sprain, ankle
    semilunar cartilage — *see* Sprain, knee, specified
      site NEC
  interphalangeal
    finger — *see* Sprain, finger, interphalangeal (joint)
    toe — *see* Sprain, toe, interphalangeal joint
  ischiocapsular — *see* Sprain, hip
  ischiofemoral — *see* Sprain, hip
  jaw (articular disc) (cartilage) (meniscus) S03.4 ☑
    old M26.69
  knee S83.9- ☑
    collateral ligament S83.40- ☑
      lateral (fibular) S83.42- ☑
      medial (tibial) S83.41- ☑
    cruciate ligament S83.50- ☑
      anterior S83.51- ☑
      posterior S83.52- ☑
    lateral (fibular) collateral ligament S83.42- ☑
    medial (tibial) collateral ligament S83.41- ☑
    patellar ligament S76.11- ☑
    specified site NEC S83.8X- ☑
    superior tibiofibular joint (ligament) S83.6- ☑
  lateral collateral, knee — *see* Sprain, knee, collateral
  lumbar (spine) S33.5 ☑
  lumbosacral S33.9 ☑
  mandible (articular disc) S03.4 ☑
    old M26.69
  medial collateral, knee — *see* Sprain, knee, collateral
  meniscus
    jaw S03.4 ☑
      old M26.69
    knee — *see* Sprain, knee, specified site NEC
      with current tear — *see* Tear, meniscus
        old — *see* Derangement, knee, meniscus,
          due to old tear
    mandible S03.4 ☑
      old M26.69
  metacarpal (distal) (proximal) — *see* Sprain, hand,
    specified site NEC
  metacarpophalangeal — *see* Sprain, finger, metacar-
    pophalangeal (joint)
  metatarsophalangeal — *see* Sprain, toe, metatarsopha-
    langeal joint
  midcarpal — *see* Sprain, hand, specified site NEC
  midtarsal — *see* Sprain, foot, specified site NEC
  neck S13.9 ☑
    anterior longitudinal cervical ligament S13.4 ☑
    atlanto-axial joint S13.4 ☑
    atlanto-occipital joint S13.4 ☑
    cervical spine S13.4 ☑
    cricoarytenoid ligament S13.5 ☑
    cricothyroid ligament S13.5 ☑
    specified site NEC S13.8 ☑
    thyroid region (cartilage) S13.5 ☑
  nose S03.8 ☑
  orbicular, hip — *see* Sprain, hip
  patella — *see* Sprain, knee, specified site NEC
  patellar ligament S76.11- ☑
  pelvis NEC S33.8 ☑
  phalanx
    finger — *see* Sprain, finger
    toe — *see* Sprain, toe
  pubofemoral — *see* Sprain, hip
  radiocarpal — *see* Sprain, wrist
  radiohumeral — *see* Sprain, elbow
  radius, collateral — *see* Rupture, traumatic, ligament,
    radial collateral
  rib (cage) S23.41 ☑

Sprain — *continued*
  rotator cuff (capsule) S43.42- ☑
  sacroiliac (region)
    chronic or old — *see* subcategory M53.2 ☑
    joint S33.6 ☑
  scaphoid (hand) — *see* Sprain, hand, specified site
    NEC
  scapula (r) — *see* Sprain, shoulder girdle, specified site
    NEC
  semilunar cartilage (knee) — *see* Sprain, knee, speci-
    fied site NEC
    with current tear — *see* Tear, meniscus
      old — *see* Derangement, knee, meniscus, due
        to old tear
  shoulder joint S43.40- ☑
    acromioclavicular joint (ligament) — *see* Sprain,
      acromioclavicular joint
    blade — *see* Sprain, shoulder, girdle, specified site
      NEC
    coracoclavicular joint (ligament) — *see* Sprain,
      coracoclavicular joint
    coracohumeral ligament — *see* Sprain, coraco-
      humeral joint
    girdle S43.9- ☑
      specified site NEC S43.8- ☑
    rotator cuff — *see* Sprain, rotator cuff
    specified site NEC S43.49- ☑
    sternoclavicular joint (ligament) — *see* Sprain,
      sternoclavicular joint
  spine
    cervical S13.4 ☑
    lumbar S33.5 ☑
    thoracic S23.3 ☑
  sternoclavicular joint S43.6- ☑
  sternum S23.429 ☑
    chondrosternal joint S23.421 ☑
    specified site NEC S23.428 ☑
    sternoclavicular (joint) (ligament) S23.420 ☑
  symphysis
    jaw S03.4 ☑
      old M26.69
    mandibular S03.4 ☑
      old M26.69
  talofibular — *see* Sprain, ankle
  tarsal — *see* Sprain, foot, specified site NEC
  tarsometatarsal — *see* Sprain, foot, specified site NEC
  temporomandibular S03.4 ☑
    old M26.69
  thorax S23.9 ☑
    ribs S23.41 ☑
    specified site NEC S23.8 ☑
    spine S23.3 ☑
    sternum — *see* Sprain, sternum
  thumb S63.60- ☑
    interphalangeal (joint) S63.62- ☑
    metacarpophalangeal (joint) S63.64- ☑
    specified site NEC S63.68- ☑
  thyroid cartilage or region S13.5 ☑
  tibia (proximal end) — *see* Sprain, knee, specified site
    NEC
  tibial collateral, knee — *see* Sprain, knee, collateral
  tibiofibular
    distal — *see* Sprain, ankle
    superior — *see* Sprain, knee, specified site NEC
  toe(s) S93.50- ☑
    great S93.50- ☑
    interphalangeal joint S93.51- ☑
      great S93.51- ☑
      lesser S93.51- ☑
    lesser S93.50- ☑
    metatarsophalangeal joint S93.52- ☑
      great S93.52- ☑
      lesser S93.52- ☑
  ulna, collateral — *see* Rupture, traumatic, ligament,
    ulnar collateral
  ulnohumeral — *see* Sprain, elbow
  wrist S63.50- ☑
    carpal S63.51- ☑
    radiocarpal S63.52- ☑
    specified site NEC S63.59- ☑
  xiphoid cartilage — *see* Sprain, sternum
Sprengel's deformity (congenital) Q74.0
Sprue (tropical) K90.1
  celiac K90.0
  idiopathic K90.0
  meaning thrush B37.0

Sprue — *continued*
  nontropical K90.0
Spur, bone (*see also* Enthesopathy)
  calcaneal M77.3- ☑
  iliac crest M76.2- ☑
  nose (septum) J34.89
Spurway's syndrome Q78.0
Sputum
  abnormal (amount) (color) (odor) (purulent) R09.3
  blood-stained R04.2
  excessive (cause unknown) R09.3
Squamous (*see also* condition)
  epithelium in
    cervical canal (congenital) Q51.828
    uterine mucosa (congenital) Q51.818
Squashed nose M95.0
  congenital Q67.4
Squeeze, diver's T70.3 ☑
Squint (*see also* Strabismus)
  accommodative — *see* Strabismus, convergent con-
    comitant
St. Hubert's disease A82.9
Stab (*see also* Laceration)
  internal organs — *see* Injury, by site
Stafne's cyst or cavity M27.0
Staggering gait R26.0
  hysterical F44.4
Staghorn calculus — *see* Calculus, kidney
Stähli's line (cornea) (pigment) — *see* Pigmentation,
  cornea, anterior
Stain, staining
  meconium (newborn) P96.83
  port wine Q82.5
  tooth, teeth (hard tissues) (extrinsic) K03.6
    due to
      accretions K03.6
      deposits (betel) (black) (green) (materia alba)
        (orange) (soft) (tobacco) K03.6
      metals (copper) (silver) K03.7
      nicotine K03.6
      pulpal bleeding K03.7
      tobacco K03.6
    intrinsic K00.8
Stammering (*see also* Disorder, fluency) F80.81
Standstill
  auricular I45.5
  cardiac — *see* Arrest, cardiac
  sinoatrial I45.5
  ventricular — *see* Arrest, cardiac
Stannosis J63.5
Stanton's disease — *see* Melioidosis
Staphylitis (acute) (catarrhal) (chronic) (gangrenous)
  (membranous) (suppurative) (ulcerative) K12.2
Staphylococcal scalded skin syndrome L00
Staphylococcemia A41.2
Staphylococcus, staphylococcal (*see also* condition)
  as cause of disease classified elsewhere B95.8
    aureus (methicillin susceptible) (MSSA) B95.61
      methicillin resistant (MRSA) B95.62
  specified NEC, as cause of disease classified elsewhere
    B95.7
Staphyloma (sclera)
  cornea H18.72- ☑
  equatorial H15.81- ☑
  localized (anterior) H15.82- ☑
  posticum H15.83- ☑
  ring H15.85- ☑
Stargardt's disease — *see* Dystrophy, retina
Starvation (inanition) (due to lack of food) T73.0 ☑
  edema — *see* Malnutrition, severe
Stasis
  bile (noncalculous) K83.1
  bronchus J98.09
    with infection — *see* Bronchitis
  cardiac — *see* Failure, heart, congestive
  cecum K59.8
  colon K59.8
  dermatitis — *see* Varix, leg, with, inflammation
  duodenal K31.5
  eczema — *see* Varix, leg, with, inflammation
  edema — *see* Hypertension, venous (chronic), idiopath-
    ic
  foot T69.0- ☑
  ileocecal coil K59.8
  ileum K59.8
  intestinal K59.8
  jejunum K59.8

☑ **Additional Character Required — Refer to the Tabular List for Character Selection**   ▧ **Subterms under main terms may continue to next column or page**

Stasis — *continued*
  kidney N19
  liver (cirrhotic) K76.1
  lymphatic I89.8
  pneumonia J18.2
  pulmonary — *see* Edema, lung
  rectal K59.8
  renal N19
    tubular N17.0
  ulcer — *see* Varix, leg, with, ulcer
    without varicose veins I87.2
  urine — *see* Retention, urine
  venous I87.8
State (of)
  affective and paranoid, mixed, organic psychotic F06.8
  agitated R45.1
    acute reaction to stress F43.0
  anxiety (neurotic) F41.1
  apprehension F41.1
  burn-out Z73.0
  climacteric, female Z78.0
    symptomatic N95.1
  compulsive F42
    mixed with obsessional thoughts F42
  confusional (psychogenic) F44.89
    acute (*see also* Delirium)
      with
        arteriosclerotic dementia F01.50
          with behavioral disturbance F01.51
        senility or dementia F05
      alcoholic F10.231
    epileptic F05
    reactive (from emotional stress, psychological
      trauma) F44.89
    subacute — *see* Delirium
  convulsive — *see* Convulsions
  crisis F43.0
  depressive F32.9
    neurotic F34.1
  dissociative F44.9
  emotional shock (stress) R45.7
  hypercoagulation — *see* Hypercoagulable
  locked-in G83.5
  menopausal Z78.0
    symptomatic N95.1
  neurotic F48.9
    with depersonalization F48.1
  obsessional F42
  oneiroid (schizophrenia-like) F23
  organic
    hallucinatory (nonalcoholic) F06.0
    paranoid (-hallucinatory) F06.2
  panic F41.0
  paranoid F22
    climacteric F22
    involutional F22
    menopausal F22
    organic F06.2
    senile F03 ☑
    simple F22
  persistent vegetative R40.3
  phobic F40.9
  postleukotomy F07.0
  pregnant, incidental Z33.1
  psychogenic, twilight F44.89
  psychopathic (constitutional) F60.2
  psychotic, organic (*see also* Psychosis, organic)
    mixed paranoid and affective F06.8
    senile or presenile F03 ☑
    transient NEC F06.8
      with
        depression F06.31
        hallucinations F06.0
  residual schizophrenic F20.5
  restlessness R45.1
  stress (emotional) R45.7
  tension (mental) F48.9
    specified NEC F48.8
  transient organic psychotic NEC F06.8
    depressive type F06.31
    hallucinatory type F06.30
  twilight
    epileptic F05
    psychogenic F44.89
  vegetative, persistent R40.3
  vital exhaustion Z73.0
  withdrawal, — *see* Withdrawal, state

Status (post) (*see also* Presence (of))
  absence, epileptic — *see* Epilepsy, by type, with status
    epilepticus
  administration of tPA (rtPA) in a different facility
    within the last 24 hours prior to admission to
    current facility Z92.82
  adrenalectomy (unilateral) (bilateral) E89.6
  anastomosis Z98.0
  anginosus I20.9
  angioplasty (peripheral) Z98.62
    with implant Z95.820
    coronary artery Z98.61
      with implant Z95.5
  aortocoronary bypass Z95.1
  arthrodesis Z98.1
  artificial opening (of) Z93.9
    gastrointestinal tract Z93.4
    specified NEC Z93.8
    urinary tract Z93.6
    vagina Z93.8
  asthmaticus — *see* Asthma, by type, with status asth-
    maticus
  awaiting organ transplant Z76.82
  bariatric surgery Z98.84
  bed confinement Z74.01
  bleb, filtering (vitreous), after glaucoma surgery Z98.83
  breast implant Z98.82
    removal Z98.86
  cataract extraction Z98.4- ☑
  cholecystectomy Z90.49
  clitorectomy N90.811
    with excision of labia minora N90.812
  colectomy (complete) (partial) Z90.49
  colonization — *see* Carrier (suspected) of
  colostomy Z93.3
  convulsivus idiopathicus — *see* Epilepsy, by type, with
    status epilepticus
  coronary artery angioplasty — *see* Status, angioplasty,
    coronary artery
  cystectomy (urinary bladder) Z90.6
  cystostomy Z93.50
    appendico-vesicostomy Z93.52
    cutaneous Z93.51
    specified NEC Z93.59
  delinquent immunization Z28.3
  dental Z98.818
    crown Z98.811
    fillings Z98.811
    restoration Z98.811
    sealant Z98.810
    specified NEC Z98.818
  deployment (current) (military) Z56.82
  dialysis (hemodialysis) (peritoneal) Z99.2
  do not resuscitate (DNR) Z66
  donor — *see* Donor
  embedded fragments — *see* Retained, foreign body
    fragments (type of)
  embedded splinter — *see* Retained, foreign body
    fragments (type of)
  enterostomy Z93.4
  epileptic, epilepticus (*see also* Epilepsy, by type, with
    status epilepticus) G40.901
  estrogen receptor
    negative Z17.1
    positive Z17.0
  female genital cutting — *see* Female genital mutilation
    status
  female genital mutilation — *see* Female genital muti-
    lation status
  filtering (vitreous) bleb after glaucoma surgery Z98.83
  gastrectomy (complete) (partial) Z90.3
  gastric banding Z98.84
  gastric bypass for obesity Z98.84
  gastrostomy Z93.1
  human immunodeficiency virus (HIV) infection,
    asymptomatic Z21
  hysterectomy (complete) (total) Z90.710
    partial (with remaining cervial stump) Z90.711
  ileostomy Z93.2
  implant
    breast Z98.82
  infibulation N90.813
  intestinal bypass Z98.0
  jejunostomy Z93.4
  lapsed immunization schedule Z28.3
  laryngectomy Z90.02
  lymphaticus E32.8
  marmoratus G80.3

Status — *continued*
  mastectomy (unilateral) (bilateral) Z90.1- ☑
  military deployment status (current) Z56.82
    in theater or in support of military war, peacekeep-
      ing and humanitarian operations Z56.82
  nephrectomy (unilateral) (bilateral) Z90.5
  nephrostomy Z93.6
  obesity surgery Z98.84
  oophorectomy
    bilateral Z90.722
    unilateral Z90.721
  organ replacement
    by artificial or mechanical device or prosthesis of
      artery Z95.828
      bladder Z96.0
      blood vessel Z95.828
      breast Z97.8
      eye globe Z97.0
      heart Z95.812
        valve Z95.2
      intestine Z97.8
      joint Z96.60
        hip — *see* Presence, hip joint implant
        knee — *see* Presence, knee joint implant
        specified site NEC Z96.698
      kidney Z97.8
      larynx Z96.3
      lens Z96.1
      limbs — *see* Presence, artificial, limb
      liver Z97.8
      lung Z97.8
      pancreas Z97.8
    by organ transplant (heterologous)(homologous)
      — *see* Transplant
  pacemaker
    brain Z96.89
    cardiac Z95.0
    specified NEC Z96.89
  pancreatectomy Z90.410
    complete Z90.410
    partial Z90.411
    total Z90.410
  physical restraint Z78.1
  pneumonectomy (complete) (partial) Z90.2
  pneumothorax, therapeutic Z98.3
  postcommotio cerebri F07.81
  postoperative (postprocedural) NEC Z98.89
    breast implant Z98.82
    dental Z98.818
      crown Z98.811
      fillings Z98.811
      restoration Z98.811
      sealant Z98.810
      specified NEC Z98.818
    pneumothorax, therapeutic Z98.3
  postpartum (routine follow-up) Z39.2
    care immediately after delivery Z39.0
  postsurgical (postprocedural) NEC Z98.89
    pneumothorax, therapeutic Z98.3
  pregnancy, incidental Z33.1
  prosthesis coronary angioplasty Z95.5
  pseudophakia Z96.1
  renal dialysis (hemodialysis) (peritoneal) Z99.2
  retained foreign body — *see* Retained, foreign body
    fragments (type of)
  reversed jejunal transposition (for bypass) Z98.0
  salpingo-oophorectomy
    bilateral Z90.722
    unilateral Z90.721
  sex reassignment surgery status Z87.890
  shunt
    arteriovenous (for dialysis) Z99.2
    cerebrospinal fluid Z98.2
    ventricular (communicating) (for drainage) Z98.2
  splenectomy Z90.81
  thymicolymphaticus E32.8
  thymicus E32.8
  thymolymphaticus E32.8
  thyroidectomy (hypothyroidism) E89.0
  tooth (teeth) extraction (*see also* Absence, teeth, ac-
    quired) K08.409
  tPA (rtPA) administration in a different facility within
    the last 24 hours prior to admission to current
    facility Z92.82
  tracheostomy Z93.0
  transplant — *see* Transplant
    organ removed Z98.85
  tubal ligation Z98.51

Status — *continued*
underimmunization Z28.3
ureterostomy Z93.6
urethrostomy Z93.6
vagina, artificial Z93.8
vasectomy Z98.52
wheelchair confinement Z99.3
Stealing
child problem F91.8
in company with others Z72.810
pathological (compulsive) F63.2
Steam burn — *see* Burn
Steatocystoma multiplex L72.2
Steatohepatitis (nonalcoholic) (NASH) K75.81
Steatoma L72.3
eyelid (cystic) — *see* Dermatosis, eyelid
infected — *see* Hordeolum
Steatorrhea (chronic) K90.4
with lacteal obstruction K90.2
idiopathic (adult) (infantile) K90.0
pancreatic K90.3
primary K90.0
tropical K90.1
Steatosis E88.89
heart — *see* Degeneration, myocardial
kidney N28.89
liver NEC K76.0
Steele-Richardson-Olszewski disease or syndrome
G23.1
Steinbrocker's syndrome G90.8
Steinert's disease G71.11
Stein-Leventhal syndrome E28.2
Stein's syndrome E28.2
STEMI (*see also* Infarct, myocardium, ST elevation) I21.3
Stenocardia I20.8
Stenocephaly Q75.8
Stenosis, stenotic (cicatricial) (*see also* Stricture)
ampulla of Vater K83.1
anus, anal (canal) (sphincter) K62.4
and rectum K62.4
congenital Q42.3
with fistula Q42.2
aorta (ascending) (supraventricular) (congenital) Q25.3
arteriosclerotic I70.0
calcified I70.0
aortic (valve) I35.0
with insufficiency I35.2
congenital Q23.0
rheumatic I06.0
with
incompetency, insufficiency or regurgitation
I06.2
with mitral (valve) disease I08.0
with tricuspid (valve) disease I08.3
mitral (valve) disease I08.0
with tricuspid (valve) disease I08.3
tricuspid (valve) disease I08.2
with mitral (valve) disease I08.3
specified cause NEC I35.0
syphilitic A52.03
aqueduct of Sylvius (congenital) Q03.0
with spina bifida — *see* Spina bifida, by site, with
hydrocephalus
acquired G91.1
artery NEC (*see also* Arteriosclerosis) I77.1
celiac I77.4
cerebral — *see* Occlusion, artery, cerebral
extremities — *see* Arteriosclerosis, extremities
precerebral — *see* Occlusion, artery, precerebral
pulmonary (congenital) Q25.6
acquired I28.8
renal I70.1
bile duct (common) (hepatic) K83.1
congenital Q44.3
bladder-neck (acquired) N32.0
congenital Q64.31
brain G93.89
bronchus J98.09
congenital Q32.3
syphilitic A52.72
cardia (stomach) K22.2
congenital Q39.3
cardiovascular — *see* Disease, cardiovascular
caudal M48.08
cervix, cervical (canal) N88.2
congenital Q51.828
in pregnancy or childbirth — *see* Pregnancy,
complicated by, abnormal cervix

Stenosis, stenotic — *continued*
colon (*see also* Obstruction, intestine)
congenital Q42.9
specified NEC Q42.8
colostomy K94.03
common (bile) duct K83.1
congenital Q44.3
coronary (artery) — *see* Disease, heart, ischemic,
atherosclerotic
cystic duct — *see* Obstruction, gallbladder
due to presence of device, implant or graft (*see also*
Complications, by site and type, specified NEC)
T85.85 ☑
arterial graft NEC T82.858 ☑
breast (implant) T85.85 ☑
catheter T85.85 ☑
dialysis (renal) T82.858 ☑
intraperitoneal T85.85 ☑
infusion NEC T82.858 ☑
spinal (epidural) (subdural) T85.85 ☑
urinary (indwelling) T83.85 ☑
fixation, internal (orthopedic) NEC T84.85 ☑
gastrointestinal (bile duct) (esophagus) T85.85 ☑
genital NEC T83.85 ☑
heart NEC T82.857 ☑
joint prosthesis T84.85 ☑
ocular (corneal graft) (orbital implant) NEC
T85.85 ☑
orthopedic NEC T84.85 ☑
specified NEC T85.85 ☑
urinary NEC T83.85 ☑
vascular NEC T82.858 ☑
ventricular intracranial shunt T85.85 ☑
duodenum K31.5
congenital Q41.0
ejaculatory duct NEC N50.8
endocervical os — *see* Stenosis, cervix
enterostomy K94.13
esophagus K22.2
congenital Q39.3
syphilitic A52.79
congenital A50.59 [K23]
eustachian tube — *see* Obstruction, eustachian tube
external ear canal (acquired) H61.30- ☑
congenital Q16.1
due to
inflammation H61.32- ☑
trauma H61.31- ☑
postprocedural H95.81- ☑
specified cause NEC H61.39- ☑
gallbladder — *see* Obstruction, gallbladder
glottis J38.6
heart valve (congenital) Q24.8
aortic Q23.0
mitral Q23.2
pulmonary Q22.1
tricuspid Q22.4
hepatic duct K83.1
hymen N89.6
hypertrophic subaortic (idiopathic) I42.1
ileum K56.69
congenital Q41.2
infundibulum cardia Q24.3
intervertebral foramina (*see also* Lesion, biomechanical, specified NEC)
connective tissue M99.79
abdomen M99.79
cervical region M99.71
cervicothoracic M99.71
head region M99.70
lumbar region M99.73
lumbosacral M99.73
occipitocervical M99.70
sacral region M99.74
sacrococcygeal M99.74
sacroiliac M99.74
specified NEC M99.79
thoracic region M99.72
thoracolumbar M99.72
disc M99.79
abdomen M99.79
cervical region M99.71
cervicothoracic M99.71
head region M99.70
lower extremity M99.76
lumbar region M99.73
lumbosacral M99.73

Stenosis, stenotic — *continued*
intervertebral foramina (*see also* Lesion, biomechanical,
specified) — *continued*
disc — *continued*
occipitocervical M99.70
pelvic M99.75
rib cage M99.78
sacral region M99.74
sacrococcygeal M99.74
sacroiliac M99.74
specified NEC M99.79
thoracic region M99.72
thoracolumbar M99.72
upper extremity M99.77
osseous M99.69
abdomen M99.69
cervical region M99.61
cervicothoracic M99.61
head region M99.60
lower extremity M99.66
lumbar region M99.63
lumbosacral M99.63
occipitocervical M99.60
pelvic M99.65
rib cage M99.68
sacral region M99.64
sacrococcygeal M99.64
sacroiliac M99.64
specified NEC M99.69
thoracic region M99.62
thoracolumbar M99.62
upper extremity M99.67
subluxation — *see* Stenosis, intervertebral foramina, osseous
intestine (*see also* Obstruction, intestine)
congenital (small) Q41.9
large Q42.9
specified NEC Q42.8
specified NEC Q41.8
jejunum K56.69
congenital Q41.1
lacrimal (passage)
canaliculi H04.54- ☑
congenital Q10.5
duct H04.55- ☑
punctum H04.56- ☑
sac H04.57- ☑
lacrimonasal duct — *see* Stenosis, lacrimal, duct
congenital Q10.5
larynx J38.6
congenital NEC Q31.8
subglottic Q31.1
syphilitic A52.73
congenital A50.59 [J99]
mitral (chronic) (inactive) (valve) I05.0
with
aortic valve disease I08.0
incompetency, insufficiency or regurgitation
I05.2
active or acute I01.1
with rheumatic or Sydenham's chorea I02.0
congenital Q23.2
specified cause, except rheumatic I34.2
syphilitic A52.03
myocardium, myocardial (*see also* Degeneration, myocardial)
hypertrophic subaortic (idiopathic) I42.1
nares (anterior) (posterior) J34.89
congenital Q30.0
nasal duct (*see also* Stenosis, lacrimal, duct)
congenital Q10.5
nasolacrimal duct (*see also* Stenosis, lacrimal, duct)
congenital Q10.5
neural canal (*see also* Lesion, biomechanical, specified
NEC)
connective tissue M99.49
abdomen M99.49
cervical region M99.41
cervicothoracic M99.41
head region M99.40
lower extremity M99.46
lumbar region M99.43
lumbosacral M99.43
occipitocervical M99.40
pelvic M99.45
rib cage M99.48
sacral region M99.44
sacrococcygeal M99.44

☑ **Additional Character Required** — Refer to the Tabular List for Character Selection   ▽ Subterms under main terms may continue to next column or page

Stenosis, stenotic — *continued*
- neural canal (*see also* Lesion, biomechanical, specified) — *continued*
    - connective tissue — *continued*
        - sacroiliac M99.44
        - specified NEC M99.49
        - thoracic region M99.42
        - thoracolumbar M99.42
        - upper extremity M99.47
    - intervertebral disc M99.59
        - abdomen M99.59
        - cervical region M99.51
        - cervicothoracic M99.51
        - head region M99.50
        - lower extremity M99.56
        - lumbar region M99.53
        - lumbosacral M99.53
        - occipitocervical M99.50
        - pelvic M99.55
        - rib cage M99.58
        - sacral region M99.54
        - sacrococcygeal M99.54
        - sacroiliac M99.54
        - specified NEC M99.59
        - thoracic region M99.52
        - thoracolumbar M99.52
        - upper extremity M99.57
    - osseous M99.39
        - abdomen M99.39
        - cervical region M99.31
        - cervicothoracic M99.31
        - head region M99.30
        - lower extremity M99.36
        - lumbar region M99.33
        - lumbosacral M99.33
        - occipitocervical M99.30
        - pelvic M99.35
        - rib cage M99.38
        - sacral region M99.34
        - sacrococcygeal M99.34
        - sacroiliac M99.34
        - specified NEC M99.39
        - thoracic region M99.32
        - thoracolumbar M99.32
        - upper extremity M99.37
    - subluxation M99.29
        - cervical region M99.21
        - cervicothoracic M99.21
        - head region M99.20
        - lower extremity M99.26
        - lumbar region M99.23
        - lumbosacral M99.23
        - occipitocervical M99.20
        - pelvic M99.25
        - rib cage M99.28
        - sacral region M99.24
        - sacrococcygeal M99.24
        - sacroiliac M99.24
        - specified NEC M99.29
        - thoracic region M99.22
        - thoracolumbar M99.22
        - upper extremity M99.27
- organ or site, congenital NEC — *see* Atresia, by site
- papilla of Vater K83.1
- pulmonary (artery) (congenital) Q25.6
    - with ventricular septal defect, transposition of aorta, and hypertrophy of right ventricle Q21.3
    - acquired I28.8
    - in tetralogy of Fallot Q21.3
    - infundibular Q24.3
    - subvalvular Q24.3
    - supravalvular Q25.6
    - valve I37.0
        - with insufficiency I37.2
        - congenital Q22.1
        - rheumatic I09.89
            - with aortic, mitral or tricuspid (valve) disease I08.8
    - vein, acquired I28.8
    - vessel NEC I28.8
- pulmonic (congenital) Q22.1
    - infundibular Q24.3
    - subvalvular Q24.3
- pylorus (hypertrophic) (acquired) K31.1
    - adult K31.1
    - congenital Q40.0
    - infantile Q40.0

Stenosis, stenotic — *continued*
- rectum (sphincter) — *see* Stricture, rectum
- renal artery I70.1
    - congenital Q27.1
- salivary duct (any) K11.8
- sphincter of Oddi K83.1
- spinal M48.00
    - cervical region M48.02
    - cervicothoracic region M48.03
    - lumbar region M48.06
    - lumbosacral region M48.07
    - occipito-atlanto-axial region M48.01
    - sacrococcygeal region M48.08
    - thoracic region M48.04
    - thoracolumbar region M48.05
- stomach, hourglass K31.2
- subaortic (congenital) Q24.4
    - hypertrophic (idiopathic) I42.1
- subglottic J38.6
    - congenital Q31.1
    - postprocedural J95.5
- trachea J39.8
    - congenital Q32.1
    - syphilitic A52.73
    - tuberculous NEC A15.5
- tracheostomy J95.03
- tricuspid (valve) I07.0
    - with
        - aortic (valve) disease I08.2
        - incompetency, insufficiency or regurgitation I07.2
            - with aortic (valve) disease I08.2
                - with mitral (valve) disease I08.3
        - mitral (valve) disease I08.1
            - with aortic (valve) disease I08.3
    - congenital Q22.4
    - nonrheumatic I36.0
        - with insufficiency I36.2
- tubal N97.1
- ureter — *see* Atresia, ureter
- ureteropelvic junction, congenital Q62.11
- ureterovesical orifice, congenital Q62.12
- urethra (valve) (*see also* Stricture, urethra)
    - congenital Q64.32
- urinary meatus, congenital Q64.33
- vagina N89.5
    - congenital Q52.4
    - in pregnancy — *see* Pregnancy, complicated by, abnormal vagina
        - causing obstructed labor O65.5
- valve (cardiac) (heart) (*see also* Endocarditis) I38
    - congenital Q24.8
        - aortic Q23.0
        - mitral Q23.2
        - pulmonary Q22.1
        - tricuspid Q22.4
- vena cava (inferior) (superior) I87.1
    - congenital Q26.0
- vesicourethral orifice Q64.31
- vulva N90.5

Stent jail T82.897 ☑
Stercolith (impaction) K56.41
- appendix K38.1
Stercoraceous, stercoral ulcer K63.3
- anus or rectum K62.6
Stereotypies NEC F98.4
Sterility — *see* Infertility
Sterilization — *see* Encounter (for), sterilization
Sternalgia — *see* Angina
Sternopagus Q89.4
Sternum bifidum Q76.7
Steroid
- effects (adverse) (adrenocortical) (iatrogenic)
    - cushingoid E24.2
        - correct substance properly administered — *see* Table of Drugs and Chemicals, by drug, adverse effect
        - overdose or wrong substance given or taken — *see* Table of Drugs and Chemicals, by drug, poisoning
    - diabetes — *see* subcategory E09 ☑
        - correct substance properly administered — *see* Table of Drugs and Chemicals, by drug, adverse effect
        - overdose or wrong substance given or taken — *see* Table of Drugs and Chemicals, by drug, poisoning
    - fever R50.2

Steroid — *continued*
- effects — *continued*
    - insufficiency E27.3
        - correct substance properly administered — *see* Table of Drugs and Chemicals, by drug, adverse effect
        - overdose or wrong substance given or taken — *see* Table of Drugs and Chemicals, by drug, poisoning
- responder H40.04- ☑
Stevens-Johnson disease or syndrome L51.1
- toxic epidermal necrolysis overlap L51.3
Stewart-Morel syndrome M85.2
Sticker's disease B08.3
Sticky eye — *see* Conjunctivitis, acute, mucopurulent
Stieda's disease — *see* Bursitis, tibial collateral
Stiff neck — *see* Torticollis
Stiff-man syndrome G25.82
Stiffness, joint NEC M25.60
- ankle M25.67- ☑
- ankylosis — *see* Ankylosis, joint
- contracture — *see* Contraction, joint
- elbow M25.62- ☑
- foot M25.67- ☑
- hand M25.64- ☑
- hip M25.65- ☑
- knee M25.66- ☑
- shoulder M25.61- ☑
- wrist M25.63- ☑
Stigmata congenital syphilis A50.59
Stillbirth P95
Still-Felty syndrome — *see* Felty's syndrome
Still's disease or syndrome (juvenile) M08.20
- adult-onset M06.1
- ankle M08.27- ☑
- elbow M08.22- ☑
- foot joint M08.27- ☑
- hand joint M08.24- ☑
- hip M08.25- ☑
- knee M08.26- ☑
- multiple site M08.29
- shoulder M08.21- ☑
- vertebra M08.28
- wrist M08.23- ☑
Stimulation, ovary E28.1
Sting (venomous) (with allergic or anaphylactic shock) — *see* Table of Drugs and Chemicals, by animal or substance, poisoning
Stippled epiphyses Q78.8
Stitch
- abscess T81.4 ☑
- burst (in operation wound) — *see* Disruption, wound, operation
Stokes' disease E05.00
- with thyroid storm E05.01
Stokes-Adams disease or syndrome I45.9
Stokvis (-Talma) **disease** D74.8
Stoma malfunction
- colostomy K94.03
- enterostomy K94.13
- gastrostomy K94.23
- ileostomy K94.13
- tracheostomy J95.03
Stomach — *see* condition
Stomatitis (denture) (ulcerative) K12.1
- angular K13.0
    - due to dietary or vitamin deficiency E53.0
- aphthous K12.0
- bovine B08.61
- candidal B37.0
- catarrhal K12.1
- diphtheritic A36.89
- due to
    - dietary deficiency E53.0
    - thrush B37.0
    - vitamin deficiency
        - B group NEC E53.9
        - B2 (riboflavin) E53.0
- epidemic B08.8
- epizootic B08.8
- follicular K12.1
- gangrenous A69.0
- Geotrichum B48.3
- herpesviral, herpetic B00.2
- herpetiformis K12.0
- malignant K12.1
- membranous acute K12.1

Stomatitis — continued
- monilial B37.Ø
- mycotic B37.Ø
- necrotizing ulcerative A69.Ø
- parasitic B37.Ø
- septic K12.1
- spirochetal A69.1
- suppurative (acute) K12.2
- ulceromembranous A69.1
- vesicular K12.1
  - with exanthem (enteroviral) BØ8.4
  - virus disease A93.8
- Vincent's A69.1

Stomatocytosis D58.8
Stomatomycosis B37.Ø
Stomatorrhagia K13.79
Stone(s) (see also Calculus)
- bladder (diverticulum) N21.Ø
- cystine E72.Ø9
- heart syndrome I5Ø.1
- kidney N2Ø.Ø
- prostate N42.Ø
- pulpal (dental) KØ4.2
- renal N2Ø.Ø
- salivary gland or duct (any) K11.5
- urethra (impacted) N21.1
- urinary (duct) (impacted) (passage) N2Ø.9
  - bladder (diverticulum) N21.Ø
  - lower tract N21.9
  - specified NEC N21.8
- xanthine E79.8 [N22]

Stonecutter's lung J62.8
Stonemason's asthma, disease, lung or pneumoconiosis J62.8
Stoppage
- heart — see Arrest, cardiac
- urine — see Retention, urine

Storm, thyroid — see Thyrotoxicosis
Strabismus (congenital) (nonparalytic) H5Ø.9
- concomitant H5Ø.4Ø
  - convergent — see Strabismus, convergent concomitant
  - divergent — see Strabismus, divergent concomitant
- convergent concomitant H5Ø.ØØ
  - accommodative component H5Ø.43
  - alternating H5Ø.Ø5
    - with
      - A pattern H5Ø.Ø6
      - specified nonconcomitances NEC H5Ø.Ø8
      - V pattern H5Ø.Ø7
  - monocular H5Ø.Ø1- ☑
    - with
      - A pattern H5Ø.Ø2- ☑
      - specified nonconcomitances NEC H5Ø.Ø4- ☑
      - V pattern H5Ø.Ø3- ☑
    - intermittent H5Ø.31- ☑
      - alternating H5Ø.32
- cyclotropia H5Ø.1- ☑
- divergent concomitant H5Ø.1Ø
  - alternating H5Ø.15
    - with
      - A pattern H5Ø.16
      - specified nonconcomitances NEC H5Ø.18
      - V pattern H5Ø.17
  - monocular H5Ø.11- ☑
    - with
      - A pattern H5Ø.12- ☑
      - specified nonconcomitances NEC H5Ø.14- ☑
      - V pattern H5Ø.13- ☑
    - intermittent H5Ø.33 ☑
      - alternating H5Ø.34
- Duane's syndrome H5Ø.81- ☑
- due to adhesions, scars H5Ø.69
- heterophoria H5Ø.5Ø
  - alternating H5Ø.55
  - cyclophoria H5Ø.54
  - esophoria H5Ø.51
  - exophoria H5Ø.52
  - vertical H5Ø.53
- heterotropia H5Ø.4Ø
  - intermittent H5Ø.3Ø
- hypertropia H5Ø.2- ☑
- hypotropia — see Hypertropia
- latent H5Ø.5Ø
- mechanical H5Ø.6Ø
  - Brown's sheath syndrome H5Ø.61- ☑

Strabismus — continued
- mechanical — continued
  - specified type NEC H5Ø.69
- monofixation syndrome H5Ø.42
- paralytic H49.9
  - abducens nerve H49.2- ☑
  - fourth nerve H49.1- ☑
  - Kearns-Sayre syndrome H49.81- ☑
  - ophthalmoplegia (external)
    - progressive H49.4- ☑
      - with pigmentary retinopathy H49.81- ☑
    - total H49.3- ☑
  - sixth nerve H49.2- ☑
  - specified type NEC H49.88- ☑
  - third nerve H49.Ø- ☑
  - trochlear nerve H49.1- ☑
- specified type NEC H5Ø.89
- vertical H5Ø.2- ☑

Strain
- back S39.Ø12 ☑
- cervical S16.1 ☑
- eye NEC — see Disturbance, vision, subjective
- heart — see Disease, heart
- low back S39.Ø12 ☑
- mental NOS Z73.3
  - work-related Z56.6
- muscle (tendon) — see Injury, muscle, by site, strain
- neck S16.1 ☑
- physical NOS Z73.3
  - work-related Z56.6
- postural (see also Disorder, soft tissue, due to use)
- psychological NEC Z73.3
- tendon — see Injury, muscle, by site, strain

Straining, on urination R39.16
Strand, vitreous — see Opacity, vitreous, membranes and strands
Strangulation, strangulated (see also Asphyxia, traumatic)
- appendix K38.8
- bladder-neck N32.Ø
- bowel or colon K56.2
- food or foreign body — see Foreign body, by site
- hemorrhoids — see Hemorrhoids, with complication
- hernia (see also Hernia, by site, with obstruction)
  - with gangrene — see Hernia, by site, with gangrene
- intestine (large) (small) K56.2
  - with hernia (see also Hernia, by site, with obstruction)
    - with gangrene — see Hernia, by site, with gangrene
- mesentery K56.2
- mucus — see Asphyxia, mucus
- omentum K56.2
- organ or site, congenital NEC — see Atresia, by site
- ovary — see Torsion, ovary
- penis N48.89
  - foreign body T19.4 ☑
- rupture — see Hernia, by site, with obstruction
- stomach due to hernia (see also Hernia, by site, with obstruction)
  - with gangrene — see Hernia, by site, with gangrene
- vesicourethral orifice N32.Ø

Strangury R3Ø.Ø
Straw itch B88.Ø
Strawberry
- gallbladder K82.4
- mark Q82.5
- tongue (red) (white) K14.3

Streak(s)
- macula, angioid H35.33
- ovarian Q5Ø.32

Strephosymbolia F81.Ø
- secondary to organic lesion R48.8

Streptobacillary fever A25.1
Streptobacillosis A25.1
Streptobacillus moniliformis A25.1
Streptococcus, streptococcal (see also condition)
- as cause of disease classified elsewhere B95.5
- group
  - A, as cause of disease classified elsewhere B95.Ø
  - B, as cause of disease classified elsewhere B95.1
  - D, as cause of disease classified elsewhere B95.2
- pneumoniae, as cause of disease classified elsewhere B95.3

Streptococcus, streptococcal — continued
- specified NEC, as cause of disease classified elsewhere B95.4

Streptomycosis B47.1
Streptotrichosis A48.8
Stress F43.9
- family — see Disruption, family
- fetal P84
  - complicating pregnancy O77.9
    - due to drug administration O77.1
- mental NEC Z73.3
  - work-related Z56.6
- physical NEC Z73.3
  - work-related Z56.6
- polycythemia D75.1
- reaction (see also Reaction, stress) F43.9
- work schedule Z56.3

Stretching, nerve — see Injury, nerve
Striae albicantes, atrophicae or distensae (cutis) L9Ø.6
Stricture (see also Stenosis)
- ampulla of Vater K83.1
- anus (sphincter) K62.4
  - congenital Q42.3
    - with fistula Q42.2
  - infantile Q42.3
    - with fistula Q42.2
- aorta (ascending) (congenital) Q25.3
  - arteriosclerotic I7Ø.Ø
  - calcified I7Ø.Ø
  - supravalvular, congenital Q25.3
- aortic (valve) — see Stenosis, aortic
- aqueduct of Sylvius (congenital) QØ3.Ø
  - with spina bifida — see Spina bifida, by site, with hydrocephalus
  - acquired G91.1
- artery I77.1
  - basilar — see Occlusion, artery, basilar
  - carotid — see Occlusion, artery, carotid
  - celiac I77.4
  - congenital (peripheral) Q27.8
    - cerebral Q28.3
    - coronary Q24.5
    - digestive system Q27.8
    - lower limb Q27.8
    - retinal Q14.1
    - specified site NEC Q27.8
    - umbilical Q27.Ø
    - upper limb Q27.8
  - coronary — see Disease, heart, ischemic, atherosclerotic
    - congenital Q24.5
  - precerebral — see Occlusion, artery, precerebral
  - pulmonary (congenital) Q25.6
    - acquired I28.8
  - renal I7Ø.1
  - vertebral — see Occlusion, artery, vertebral
- auditory canal (external) (congenital)
  - acquired — see Stenosis, external ear canal
- bile duct (common) (hepatic) K83.1
  - congenital Q44.3
  - postoperative K91.89
- bladder N32.89
  - neck N32.Ø
- bowel — see Obstruction, intestine
- brain G93.89
- bronchus J98.Ø9
  - congenital Q32.3
  - syphilitic A52.72
- cardia (stomach) K22.2
  - congenital Q39.3
- cardiac (see also Disease, heart)
  - orifice (stomach) K22.2
- cecum — see Obstruction, intestine
- cervix, cervical (canal) N88.2
  - congenital Q51.828
  - in pregnancy — see Pregnancy, complicated by, abnormal cervix
    - causing obstructed labor O65.5
- colon (see also Obstruction, intestine)
  - congenital Q42.9
    - specified NEC Q42.8
- colostomy K94.Ø3
- common (bile) duct K83.1
- coronary — see Disease, heart, ischemic, atherosclerotic
- cystic duct — see Obstruction, gallbladder
- digestive organs NEC, congenital Q45.8

Index

Stricture — Strümpell-Westphal pseudosclerosis

Stuart deficiency disease (factor X) D68.2
Stuart-Prower factor deficiency (factor X) D68.2
Student's elbow — *see* Bursitis, elbow, olecranon
Stump — *see* Amputation
Stunting, nutritional E45
Stupor (catatonic) R40.1
  depressive F32.8
  dissociative F44.2
  manic F30.2
  manic-depressive F31.89
  psychogenic (anergic) F44.2
  reaction to exceptional stress (transient) F43.0
Sturge (-Weber) (-Dimitri) (-Kalischer) **disease or syndrome** Q85.8
Stuttering F80.81
  adult onset F98.5
  childhood onset F80.81
  following cerebrovascular disease — *see* Disorder, fluency. following cerebrovascular disease
  in conditions classified elsewhere R47.82
Sty, stye (external) (internal) (meibomian) (zeisian) — *see* Hordeolum
Subacidity, gastric K31.89
  psychogenic F45.8
Subacute — *see* condition
Subarachnoid — *see* condition
Subcortical — *see* condition
Subcostal syndrome, nerve compression — *see* Mononeuropathy, upper limb, specified site NEC
Subcutaneous, subcuticular — *see* condition
Subdural — *see* condition
Subendocardium — *see* condition
Subependymoma
  specified site — *see* Neoplasm, uncertain behavior, by site
  unspecified site D43.2
Suberosis J67.3
Subglossitis — *see* Glossitis
Subhemophilia D66
Subinvolution
  breast (postlactational) (postpuerperal) N64.89
  puerperal O90.89
  uterus (chronic) (nonpuerperal) N85.3
    puerperal O90.89
Sublingual — *see* condition
Sublinguitis — *see* Sialoadenitis
Subluxatable hip Q65.6
Subluxation (*see also* Dislocation)
  acromioclavicular S43.11- ☑
  ankle S93.0- ☑
  atlantoaxial, recurrent M43.4
    with myelopathy M43.3
  carpometacarpal (joint) NEC S63.05- ☑
    thumb S63.04- ☑
  complex, vertebral — *see* Complex, subluxation
  congenital (*see also* Malposition, congenital)
    hip — *see* Dislocation, hip, congenital, partial
    joint (excluding hip)
      lower limb Q68.8
      shoulder Q68.8
      upper limb Q68.8
  elbow (traumatic) S53.10- ☑
    anterior S53.11- ☑
    lateral S53.14- ☑
    medial S53.13- ☑
    posterior S53.12- ☑
    specified type NEC S53.19- ☑
  finger S63.20- ☑
    index S63.20- ☑
    interphalangeal S63.22- ☑
      distal S63.24- ☑
        index S63.24- ☑
        little S63.24- ☑
        middle S63.24- ☑
        ring S63.24- ☑
      index S63.22- ☑
      little S63.22- ☑
      middle S63.22- ☑
      proximal S63.23- ☑
        index S63.23- ☑
        little S63.23- ☑
        middle S63.23- ☑
        ring S63.23- ☑
      ring S63.22- ☑
    little S63.20- ☑

Subluxation — *continued*
  finger — *continued*
    metacarpophalangeal S63.21- ☑
      index S63.21- ☑
      little S63.21- ☑
      middle S63.21- ☑
      ring S63.21- ☑
    middle S63.20- ☑
    ring S63.20- ☑
  foot S93.30- ☑
    specified site NEC S93.33- ☑
    tarsal joint S93.31- ☑
    tarsometatarsal joint S93.32- ☑
    toe — *see* Subluxation, toe
  hip S73.00- ☑
    anterior S73.03- ☑
      obturator S73.02- ☑
    central S73.04- ☑
    posterior S73.01- ☑
  interphalangeal (joint)
    finger S63.22- ☑
      distal joint S63.24- ☑
        index S63.24- ☑
        little S63.24- ☑
        middle S63.24- ☑
        ring S63.24- ☑
      index S63.22- ☑
      little S63.22- ☑
      middle S63.22- ☑
      proximal joint S63.23- ☑
        index S63.23- ☑
        little S63.23- ☑
        middle S63.23- ☑
        ring S63.23- ☑
      ring S63.22- ☑
    thumb S63.12- ☑
      distal joint S63.14- ☑
      proximal joint S63.13- ☑
    toe S93.13- ☑
      great S93.13- ☑
      lesser S93.13- ☑
  joint prosthesis — *see* Complications, joint prosthesis, mechanical, displacement, by site
  knee S83.10- ☑
    cap — *see* Subluxation, patella
    patella — *see* Subluxation, patella
    proximal tibia
      anteriorly S83.11- ☑
      laterally S83.14- ☑
      medially S83.13- ☑
      posteriorly S83.12- ☑
    specified type NEC S83.19- ☑
  lens — *see* Dislocation, lens, partial
  ligament, traumatic — *see* Sprain, by site
  metacarpal (bone)
    proximal end S63.06- ☑
  metacarpophalangeal (joint)
    finger S63.21- ☑
      index S63.21- ☑
      little S63.21- ☑
      middle S63.21- ☑
      ring S63.21- ☑
    thumb S63.11- ☑
  metatarsophalangeal joint S93.14- ☑
    great toe S93.14- ☑
    lesser toe S93.14- ☑
  midcarpal (joint) S63.03- ☑
  patella S83.00- ☑
    lateral S83.01- ☑
    recurrent (nontraumatic) — *see* Dislocation, patella, recurrent, incomplete
    specified type NEC S83.09- ☑
  pathological — *see* Dislocation, pathological
  radial head S53.00- ☑
    anterior S53.01- ☑
    nursemaid's elbow S53.03- ☑
    posterior S53.02- ☑
    specified type NEC S53.09- ☑
  radiocarpal (joint) S63.02- ☑
  radioulnar (joint)
    distal S63.01- ☑
    proximal — *see* Subluxation, elbow
  shoulder
    congenital Q68.8
    girdle S43.30- ☑
      scapula S43.31- ☑

Subluxation — *continued*
  shoulder — *continued*
    girdle — *continued*
      specified site NEC S43.39- ☑
    traumatic S43.00- ☑
      anterior S43.01- ☑
      inferior S43.03- ☑
      posterior S43.02- ☑
      specified type NEC S43.08- ☑
  sternoclavicular (joint) S43.20- ☑
    anterior S43.21- ☑
    posterior S43.22- ☑
  symphysis (pubis)
  thumb S63.103 ☑
    interphalangeal joint — *see* Subluxation, interphalangeal (joint), thumb
    metacarpophalangeal joint — *see* Subluxation, metacarpophalangeal (joint), thumb
  toe(s) S93.10- ☑
    great S93.10- ☑
      interphalangeal joint S93.13- ☑
      metatarsophalangeal joint S93.14- ☑
    interphalangeal joint S93.13- ☑
    lesser S93.10- ☑
      interphalangeal joint S93.13- ☑
      metatarsophalangeal joint S93.14- ☑
    metatarsophalangeal joint S93.149 ☑
  ulna
    distal end S63.07- ☑
    proximal end — *see* Subluxation, elbow
  ulnohumeral joint — *see* Subluxation, elbow
  vertebral
    recurrent NEC — *see* subcategory M43.5 ☑
    traumatic
      cervical S13.100 ☑
        atlantoaxial joint S13.120 ☑
        atlantooccipital joint S13.110 ☑
        atloidoccipital joint S13.110 ☑
        joint between
          C0 and C1 S13.110 ☑
          C1 and C2 S13.120 ☑
          C2 and C3 S13.130 ☑
          C3 and C4 S13.140 ☑
          C4 and C5 S13.150 ☑
          C5 and C6 S13.160 ☑
          C6 and C7 S13.170 ☑
          C7 and T1 S13.180 ☑
        occipitoatloid joint S13.110 ☑
      lumbar S33.100 ☑
        joint between
          L1 and L2 S33.110 ☑
          L2 and L3 S33.120 ☑
          L3 and L4 S33.130 ☑
          L4 and L5 S33.140 ☑
      thoracic S23.100 ☑
        joint between
          T1 and T2 S23.110 ☑
          T2 and T3 S23.120 ☑
          T3 and T4 S23.122 ☑
          T4 and T5 S23.130 ☑
          T5 and T6 S23.132 ☑
          T6 and T7 S23.140 ☑
          T7 and T8 S23.142 ☑
          T8 and T9 S23.150 ☑
          T9 and T10 S23.152 ☑
          T10 and T11 S23.160 ☑
          T11 and T12 S23.162 ☑
          T12 and L1 S23.170 ☑
  wrist (carpal bone) S63.00- ☑
    carpometacarpal joint — *see* Subluxation, carpometacarpal (joint)
    distal radioulnar joint — *see* Subluxation, radioulnar (joint), distal
    metacarpal bone, proximal — *see* Subluxation, metacarpal (bone), proximal end
    midcarpal — *see* Subluxation, midcarpal (joint)
    radiocarpal joint — *see* Subluxation, radiocarpal (joint)
    recurrent — *see* Dislocation, recurrent, wrist
    specified site NEC S63.09- ☑
    ulna — *see* Subluxation, ulna, distal end
Submaxillary — *see* condition
Submersion (fatal) (nonfatal) T75.1 ☑
Submucous — *see* condition
Subnormal, subnormality
  accommodation (old age) H52.4

Subnormal, subnormality — *continued*
mental — *see* Disability, intellectual
temperature (accidental) T68 ☑
Subphrenic — *see* condition
Subscapular nerve — *see* condition
Subseptus uterus Q51.2
Subsiding appendicitis K36
Substernal thyroid E04.9
congenital Q89.2
Substitution disorder F44.9
Subtentorial — *see* condition
Subthyroidism (acquired) (*see also* Hypothyroidism)
congenital E03.1
Succenturiate placenta O43.19- ☑
Sucking thumb, child (excessive) F98.8
Sudamen, sudamina L74.1
Sudanese kala-azar B55.0
Sudden
hearing loss — *see* Deafness, sudden
heart failure — *see* Failure, heart
Sudeck's atrophy, disease, or syndrome — *see* Algoneurodystrophy
Suffocation — *see* Asphyxia, traumatic
Sugar
blood
high (transient) R73.9
low (transient) E16.2
in urine R81
Suicide, suicidal (attempted) T14.91
by poisoning — *see* Table of Drugs and Chemicals
history of (personal) Z91.5
in family Z81.8
ideation — *see* Ideation, suicidal
risk
meaning personal history of attempted suicide
Z91.5
meaning suicidal ideation — *see* Ideation, suicidal
tendencies
meaning personal history of attempted suicide
Z91.5
meaning suicidal ideation — *see* Ideation, suicidal
trauma — *see* nature of injury by site
Suipestifer infection — *see* Infection, salmonella
Sulfhemoglobinemia, sulphemoglobinemia (acquired) (with methemoglobinemia) D74.8
Sumatran mite fever A75.3
Summer — *see* condition
Sunburn L55.9
first degree L55.0
second degree L55.1
third degree L55.2
SUNCT (short lasting unilateral neuralgiform headache
with conjunctival injection and tearing) G44.059
intractable G44.051
not intractable G44.059
Sunken acetabulum — *see* Derangement, joint, specified type NEC, hip
Sunstroke T67.0 ☑
Superfecundation — *see* Pregnancy, multiple
Superfetation — *see* Pregnancy, multiple
Superinvolution (uterus) N85.8
Supernumerary (congenital)
aortic cusps Q23.8
auditory ossicles Q16.3
bone Q79.8
breast Q83.1
carpal bones Q74.0
cusps, heart valve NEC Q24.8
aortic Q23.8
mitral Q23.2
pulmonary Q22.3
digit(s) Q69.9
ear (lobule) Q17.0
fallopian tube Q50.6
finger Q69.0
hymen Q52.4
kidney Q63.0
lacrimonasal duct Q10.6
lobule (ear) Q17.0
mitral cusps Q23.2
muscle Q79.8
nipple(s) Q83.3
organ or site not listed — *see* Accessory
ossicles, auditory Q16.3
ovary Q50.31
oviduct Q50.6
pulmonary, pulmonic cusps Q22.3

Supernumerary — *continued*
rib Q76.6
cervical or first (syndrome) Q76.5
roots (of teeth) K00.2
spleen Q89.09
tarsal bones Q74.2
teeth K00.1
testis Q55.29
thumb Q69.1
toe Q69.2
uterus Q51.2
vagina Q52.1 ☑
vertebra Q76.49
Supervision (of)
contraceptive — *see* Prescription, contraceptives
dietary (for) Z71.3
allergy (food) Z71.3
colitis Z71.3
diabetes mellitus Z71.3
food allergy or intolerance Z71.3
gastritis Z71.3
hypercholesterolemia Z71.3
hypoglycemia Z71.3
intolerance (food) Z71.3
obesity Z71.3
specified NEC Z71.3
healthy infant or child Z76.2
foundling Z76.1
high-risk pregnancy — *see* Pregnancy, complicated
by, high, risk
lactation Z39.1
pregnancy — *see* Pregnancy, supervision of
Supplemental teeth K00.1
Suppression
binocular vision H53.34
lactation O92.5
menstruation N94.89
ovarian secretion E28.39
renal N28.9
urine, urinary secretion R34
Suppuration, suppurative (*see also* condition)
accessory sinus (chronic) — *see* Sinusitis
adrenal gland
antrum (chronic) — *see* Sinusitis, maxillary
bladder — *see* Cystitis
brain G06.0
sequelae G09
breast N61
puerperal, postpartum or gestational — *see* Mastitis, obstetric, purulent
dental periosteum M27.3
ear (middle) (*see also* Otitis, media)
external NEC — *see* Otitis, externa, infective
internal — *see* subcategory H83.0 ☑
ethmoidal (chronic) (sinus) — *see* Sinusitis, ethmoidal
fallopian tube — *see* Salpingo-oophoritis
frontal (chronic) (sinus) — *see* Sinusitis, frontal
gallbladder (acute) K81.0
gum K05.20
generalized K05.22
localized K05.21
intracranial G06.0
joint — *see* Arthritis, pyogenic or pyemic
labyrinthine — *see* subcategory H83.0 ☑
lung — *see* Abscess, lung
mammary gland N61
puerperal, postpartum O91.12
associated with lactation O91.13
maxilla, maxillary M27.2
sinus (chronic) — *see* Sinusitis, maxillary
muscle — *see* Myositis, infective
nasal sinus (chronic) — *see* Sinusitis
pancreas, acute K85.8
parotid gland — *see* Sialoadenitis
pelvis, pelvic
female — *see* Disease, pelvis, inflammatory
male K65.0
pericranial — *see* Osteomyelitis
salivary duct or gland (any) — *see* Sialoadenitis
sinus (accessory) (chronic) (nasal) — *see* Sinusitis
sphenoidal sinus (chronic) — *see* Sinusitis, sphenoidal
thymus (gland) E32.1
thyroid (gland) E06.0
tonsil — *see* Tonsillitis
uterus — *see* Endometritis
Supraeruption of tooth (teeth) M26.34

Supraglottitis J04.30
with obstruction J04.31
Suprarenal (gland) — *see* condition
Suprascapular nerve — *see* condition
Suprasellar — *see* condition
Surfer's knots or nodules S89.8- ☑
Surgical
emphysema T81.82 ☑
procedures, complication or misadventure — *see*
Complications, surgical procedures
shock T81.10 ☑
Surveillance (of) (for) (*see also* Observation)
alcohol abuse Z71.41
contraceptive — *see* Prescription, contraceptives
dietary Z71.3
drug abuse Z71.51
Susceptibility to disease, genetic Z15.89
malignant neoplasm Z15.09
breast Z15.01
endometrium Z15.04
ovary Z15.02
prostate Z15.03
specified NEC Z15.09
multiple endocrine neoplasia Z15.81
Suspected condition, ruled out (*see also* Observation,
suspected)
amniotic cavity and membrane Z03.71
cervical shortening Z03.75
fetal anomaly Z03.73
fetal growth Z03.74
maternal and fetal conditions NEC Z03.79
oligohydramnios Z03.71
placental problem Z03.72
polyhydramnios Z03.71
Suspended uterus
in pregnancy or childbirth — *see* Pregnancy, complicated by, abnormal uterus
Sutton's nevus D22.9
Suture
burst (in operation wound) T81.31 ☑
external operation wound T81.31 ☑
internal operation wound T81.32 ☑
inadvertently left in operation wound — *see* Foreign
body, accidentally left during a procedure
removal Z48.02
Swab inadvertently left in operation wound — *see*
Foreign body, accidentally left during a procedure
Swallowed, swallowing
difficulty — *see* Dysphagia
foreign body — *see* Foreign body, alimentary tract
Swan-neck deformity (finger) — *see* Deformity, finger,
swan-neck
Swearing, compulsive F42
in Gilles de la Tourette's syndrome F95.2
Sweat, sweats
fetid L75.0
night R61
Sweating, excessive R61
Sweeley-Klionsky disease E75.21
Sweet's disease or dermatosis L98.2
Swelling (of) R60.9
abdomen, abdominal (not referable to any particular
organ) — *see* Mass, abdominal
ankle — *see* Effusion, joint, ankle
arm M79.89
forearm M79.89
breast N63
Calabar B74.3
cervical gland R59.0
chest, localized R22.2
ear H93.8- ☑
extremity (lower) (upper) — *see* Disorder, soft tissue,
specified type NEC
finger M79.89
foot M79.89
glands R59.9
generalized R59.1
localized R59.0
hand M79.89
head (localized) R22.0
inflammatory — *see* Inflammation
intra-abdominal — *see* Mass, abdominal
joint — *see* Effusion, joint
leg M79.89
lower M79.89
limb — *see* Disorder, soft tissue, specified type NEC

Swelling — *continued*
localized (skin) R22.9
chest R22.2
head R22.0
limb
lower — *see* Mass, localized, limb, lower
upper — *see* Mass, localized, limb, upper
neck R22.1
trunk R22.2
neck (localized) R22.1
pelvic — *see* Mass, abdominal
scrotum N50.8
splenic — *see* Splenomegaly
testis N50.8
toe M79.89
umbilical R19.09
wandering, due to Gnathostoma (spinigerum) B83.1
white — *see* Tuberculosis, arthritis
Swift (-Feer) **disease**
overdose or wrong substance given or taken — *see* Table of Drugs and Chemicals, by drug, poisoning
Swimmer's
cramp T75.1 ☑
ear H60.33- ☑
itch B65.3
Swimming in the head R42
Swollen — *see* Swelling
Swyer syndrome Q99.1
Sycosis L73.8
barbae (not parasitic) L73.8
contagiosa (mycotic) B35.0
lupoides L73.8
mycotic B35.0
parasitic B35.0
vulgaris L73.8
Sydenham's chorea — *see* Chorea, Sydenham's
Sylvatic yellow fever A95.0
Sylvest's disease B33.0
Symblepharon H11.23- ☑
congenital Q10.3
Symond's syndrome G93.2
Sympathetic — *see* condition
Sympatheticotonia G90.8
Sympathicoblastoma
specified site — *see* Neoplasm, malignant, by site
unspecified site C74.90
Sympathogonioma — *see* Sympathicoblastoma
Symphalangy (fingers) (toes) Q70.9
Symptoms NEC R68.89
breast NEC N64.59
development NEC R63.8
factitious, self-induced — *see* Disorder, factitious
genital organs, female R10.2
involving
abdomen NEC R19.8
appearance NEC R46.89
awareness R41.9
altered mental status R41.82
amnesia — *see* Amnesia
borderline intellectual functioning R41.83
coma — *see* Coma
disorientation R41.0
neurologic neglect syndrome R41.4
senile cognitive decline R41.81
specified symptom NEC R41.89
behavior NEC R46.89
cardiovascular system NEC R09.89
chest NEC R09.89
circulatory system NEC R09.89
cognitive functions R41.9
altered mental status R41.82
amnesia — *see* Amnesia
borderline intellectual functioning R41.83
coma — *see* Coma
disorientation R41.0
neurologic neglect syndrome R41.4
senile cognitive decline R41.81
specified symptom NEC R41.89
development NEC R62.50
digestive system NEC R19.8
emotional state NEC R45.89
emotional lability R45.86
food and fluid intake R63.8
general perceptions and sensations R44.9
specified NEC R44.8
musculoskeletal system R29.91

Symptoms — *continued*
involving — *continued*
musculoskeletal system R29.91
specified NEC R29.898
nervous system R29.90
specified NEC R29.818
pelvis NEC R19.8
respiratory system NEC R09.89
skin and integument R23.9
urinary system R39.9
menopausal N95.1
metabolism NEC R63.8
neurotic F48.8
of infancy R68.19
pelvis NEC, female R10.2
skin and integument NEC R23.9
subcutaneous tissue NEC R23.9
Sympus Q74.2
Syncephalus Q89.4
Synchondrosis
abnormal (congenital) Q78.8
ischiopubic M91.0
Synchysis (scintillans) (senile) (vitreous body) H43.89
Syncope (near) (pre-) R55
anginosa I20.8
bradycardia R00.1
cardiac R55
carotid sinus G90.01
due to spinal (lumbar) puncture G97.1
heart R55
heat T67.1 ☑
laryngeal R05
psychogenic F48.8
tussive R05
vasoconstriction R55
vasodepressor R55
vasomotor R55
vasovagal R55
Syndactylism, syndactyly Q70.9
complex (with synostosis)
fingers Q70.0- ☑
toes Q70.2- ☑
simple (without synostosis)
fingers Q70.1- ☑
toes Q70.3- ☑
Syndrome (*see also* Disease)
48,XXXX Q97.1
49,XXXXX Q97.1
5q minus NOS D46.C (*following* D46.2)
abdominal
acute R10.0
muscle deficiency Q79.4
abnormal innervation H02.519
left H02.516
lower H02.515
upper H02.514
right H02.513
lower H02.512
upper H02.511
abstinence, neonatal P96.1
acid pulmonary aspiration, obstetric O74.0
acquired immunodeficiency — *see* Human, immunodeficiency virus (HIV) disease
acute abdominal R10.0
acute respiratory distress (adult) (child) J80
Adair-Dighton Q78.0
Adams-Stokes (-Morgagni) I45.9
adiposogenital E23.6
adrenal
hemorrhage (meningococcal) A39.1
meningococcic A39.1
adrenocortical — *see* Cushing's, syndrome
adrenogenital E25.9
congenital, associated with enzyme deficiency E25.0
afferent loop NEC K91.89
Alagille's Q44.7
alcohol withdrawal (without convulsions) — *see* Dependence, alcohol, with, withdrawal
Alder's D72.0
Aldrich (-Wiskott) D82.0
alien hand R41.4
Alport Q87.81
alveolar hypoventilation E66.2
alveolocapillary block J84.10
amnesic, amnestic (confabulatory) (due to) — *see* Disorder, amnesic
amyostatic (Wilson's disease) E83.01

Syndrome — *continued*
androgen insensitivity E34.50
complete E34.51
partial E34.52
androgen resistance (*see also* Syndrome, androgen insensitivity) E34.50
Angelman Q93.5
anginal — *see* Angina
ankyloglossia superior Q38.1
anterior
chest wall R07.89
cord G83.82
spinal artery G95.19
compression M47.019
cervical region M47.012
cervicothoracic region M47.013
lumbar region M47.016
occipito-atlanto-axial region M47.011
thoracic region M47.014
thoracolumbar region M47.015
tibial M76.81- ☑
antibody deficiency D80.9
agammaglobulinemic D80.1
hereditary D80.0
congenital D80.0
hypogammaglobulinemic D80.1
hereditary D80.0
anticardiolipin (-antibody) D68.61
antiphospholipid (-antibody) D68.61
aortic
arch M31.4
bifurcation I74.09
aortomesenteric duodenum occlusion K31.5
apical ballooning (transient left ventricular) I51.81
arcuate ligament I77.4
argentaffin, argintaffinoma E34.0
Arnold-Chiari — *see* Arnold-Chiari disease
Arrillaga-Ayerza I27.0
Asherman's N85.6
aspiration, of newborn — *see* Aspiration, by substance, with pneumonia
meconium P24.01
ataxia-telangiectasia G11.3
auriculotemporal G50.8
autoerythrocyte sensitization (Gardner-Diamond) D69.2
autoimmune lymphoproliferative [ALPS] D89.82
autoimmune polyglandular E31.0
autosomal — *see* Abnormal, autosomes
Avellis' G46.8
Ayerza (-Arrillaga) I27.0
Babinski-Nageotte G83.89
Bakwin-Krida Q79.8
bare lymphocyte D81.6
Barré-Guillain G61.0
Barré-Liéou M53.0
Barrett's — *see* Barrett's, esophagus
Barsony-Polgar K22.4
Bársony-Teschendorf K22.4
Barth E78.71
Bartter's E26.81
basal cell nevus Q87.89
Basedow's E05.00
with thyroid storm E05.01
basilar artery G45.0
Batten-Steinert G71.11
battered
baby or child — *see* Maltreatment, child, physical abuse
spouse — *see* Maltreatment, adult, physical abuse
Beals Q87.40
Beau's I51.5
Beck's I65.8
Benedikt's G46.3
Béquez César (-Steinbrinck-Chédiak-Higashi) E70.330
Bernhardt-Roth — *see* Meralgia paresthetica
Bernheim's I50.9
big spleen D73.1
bilateral polycystic ovarian E28.2
Bing-Horton's — *see* Horton's headache
Birt-Hogg-Dube syndrome Q87.89
Björck (-Thorsen) E34.0
black
lung J60
widow spider bite — *see* Toxicity, venom, spider, black widow
Blackfan-Diamond D61.01

☑ Additional Character Required — Refer to the Tabular List for Character Selection ▽ Subterms under main terms may continue to next column or page

Syndrome — continued
blind loop K90.2
  congenital Q43.8
  postsurgical K91.2
blue sclera Q78.0
blue toe I75.02- ☑
Boder-Sedgewick G11.3
Boerhaave's K22.3
Borjeson Forssman Lehmann Q89.8
Bouillaud's I01.9
Bourneville (-Pringle) Q85.1
Bouveret (-Hoffman) I47.9
brachial plexus G54.0
bradycardia-tachycardia I49.5
brain (nonpsychotic) F09
  with psychosis, psychotic reaction F09
  acute or subacute — see Delirium
  congenital — see Disability, intellectual
  organic F09
    post-traumatic (nonpsychotic) F07.81
      psychotic F09
    personality change F07.0
    postcontusional F07.81
    post-traumatic, nonpsychotic F09
    psycho-organic F09
    psychotic F06.8
brain stem stroke G46.3
Brandt's (acrodermatitis enteropathica) E83.2
broad ligament laceration N83.8
Brock's J98.11
bronze baby P83.8
Brown-Sequard G83.81
bubbly lung P27.0
Buchem's M85.2
Budd-Chiari I82.0
bulbar (progressive) G12.22
Bürger-Grütz E78.3
Burke's K86.8
Burnett's (milk-alkali) E83.52
burning feet E53.9
Bywaters' T79.5 ☑
Call-Fleming I67.841
carbohydrate-deficient glycoprotein (CDGS) E77.8
carcinogenic thrombophlebitis I82.1
carcinoid E34.0
cardiac asthma I50.1
cardiacos negros I27.0
cardiofaciocutaneous Q87.89
cardiopulmonary-obesity E66.2
cardiorenal — see Hypertension, cardiorenal
cardiorespiratory distress (idiopathic), newborn P22.0
cardiovascular renal — see Hypertension, cardiorenal
carotid
  artery (hemispheric) (internal) G45.1
  body G90.01
  sinus G90.01
carpal tunnel G56.0- ☑
Cassidy (-Scholte) E34.0
cat cry Q93.4
cat eye Q92.8
cauda equina G83.4
causalgia — see Causalgia
celiac K90.0
  artery compression I77.4
  axis I77.4
central pain G89.0
cerebellar
  hereditary G11.9
  stroke G46.4
cerebellomedullary malformation — see Spina bifida
cerebral
  artery
    anterior G46.1
    middle G46.0
    posterior G46.2
  gigantism E22.0
cervical (root) M53.1
  disc — see Disorder, disc, cervical, with neuritis
  fusion Q76.1
  posterior, sympathicus M53.0
  rib Q76.5
  sympathetic paralysis G90.2
cervicobrachial (diffuse) M53.1
cervicocranial M53.0
cervicodorsal outlet G54.2
cervicothoracic outlet G54.0
Céstan (-Raymond) I65.8

Syndrome — continued
Charcot's (angina cruris) (intermittent claudication) I73.9
Charcot-Weiss-Baker G90.09
CHARGE Q89.8
Chédiak-Higashi (-Steinbrinck) E70.330
chest wall R07.1
Chiari's (hepatic vein thrombosis) I82.0
Chilaiditi's Q43.3
child maltreatment — see Maltreatment, child
chondrocostal junction M94.0
chondroectodermal dysplasia Q77.6
chromosome 4 short arm deletion Q93.3
chromosome 5 short arm deletion Q93.4
chronic
  pain G89.4
    personality F68.8
Clarke-Hadfield K86.8
Clerambault's automatism G93.89
Clouston's (hidrotic ectodermal dysplasia) Q82.4
clumsiness, clumsy child F82
cluster headache G44.009
  intractable G44.001
  not intractable G44.009
Coffin-Lowry Q89.8
cold injury (newborn) P80.0
combined immunity deficiency D81.9
compartment (deep) (posterior) (traumatic) T79.A0 ☑ (following T79.7)
  abdomen T79.A3 ☑ (following T79.7)
  lower extremity (hip, buttock, thigh, leg, foot, toes) T79.A2 ☑ (following T79.7)
  nontraumatic
    abdomen M79.A3 (following M79.7)
    lower extremity (hip, buttock, thigh, leg, foot, toes) M79.A2- ☑ (following M79.7)
    specified site NEC M79.A9 (following M79.7)
    upper extremity (shoulder, arm, forearm, wrist, hand, fingers) M79.A1- ☑ (following M79.7)
  postprocedural — see Syndrome, compartment, nontraumatic
  specified site NEC T79.A9 ☑ (following T79.7)
  upper extremity (shoulder, arm, forearm, wrist, hand, fingers) T79.A1 ☑ (following T79.7)
complex regional pain — see Syndrome, pain, complex regional
compression T79.5 ☑
  anterior spinal — see Syndrome, anterior, spinal artery, compression
  cauda equina G83.4
  celiac artery I77.4
  vertebral artery M47.029
    cervical region M47.022
    occipito-atlanto-axial region M47.021
concussion F07.81
congenital
  affecting multiple systems NEC Q87.89
  central alveolar hypoventilation G47.35
  facial diplegia Q87.0
  muscular hypertrophy-cerebral Q87.89
  oculo-auriculovertebral Q87.0
  oculofacial diplegia (Moebius) Q87.0
  rubella (manifest) P35.0
congestion-fibrosis (pelvic), female N94.89
congestive dysmenorrhea N94.6
connective tissue M35.9
  overlap NEC M35.1
Conn's E26.01
conus medullaris G95.81
cord
  anterior G83.82
  posterior G83.83
coronary
  acute NEC I24.9
  insufficiency or intermediate I20.0
  slow flow I20.8
Costen's (complex) M26.69
costochondral junction M94.0
costoclavicular G54.0
costovertebral E22.0
Cowden Q85.8
craniovertebral M53.0
Creutzfeldt-Jakob — see Creutzfeldt-Jakob disease or syndrome
crib death R99
cricopharyngeal — see Dysphagia
cri-du-chat Q93.4

Syndrome — continued
croup J05.0
CRPS I — see Syndrome, pain, complex regional I
crush T79.5 ☑
cryptophthalmos Q87.0
cubital tunnel — see Lesion, nerve, ulnar
Curschmann (-Batten) (-Steinert) G71.11
Cushing's E24.9
  alcohol-induced E24.4
  drug-induced E24.2
  due to
    alcohol
    drugs E24.2
    ectopic ACTH E24.3
    overproduction of pituitary ACTH E24.0
  overdose or wrong substance given or taken — see Table of Drugs and Chemicals, by drug, poisoning
  pituitary-dependent E24.0
  specified type NEC E24.8
cystic duct stump K91.5
Dana-Putnam D51.0
Danbolt (-Cross) (acrodermatitis enteropathica) E83.2
Dandy-Walker Q03.1
  with spina bifida Q07.01
Danlos' Q79.8
De Quervain E34.51
de Toni-Fanconi (-Debré) E72.09
  with cystinosis E72.04
defibrination (see also Fibrinolysis)
  with
    antepartum hemorrhage — see Hemorrhage, antepartum, with coagulation defect
    intrapartum hemorrhage — see Hemorrhage, complicating, delivery
  newborn P60
  postpartum O72.3
Degos' I77.89
Déjérine-Roussy G89.0
delayed sleep phase G47.21
demyelinating G37.9
dependence — see F10-F19 with fourth character .2
depersonalization (-derealization) F48.1
di George's D82.1
diabetes mellitus in newborn infant P70.2
diabetes mellitus-hypertension-nephrosis — see Diabetes, nephrosis
diabetes-nephrosis — see Diabetes, nephrosis
diabetic amyotrophy — see Diabetes, amyotrophy
Diamond-Blackfan D61.01
Diamond-Gardener D69.2
DIC (diffuse or disseminated intravascular coagulopathy) D65
Dighton's Q78.0
disequilibrium E87.8
Döhle body-panmyelopathic D72.0
dorsolateral medullary G46.4
double athetosis G80.3
Down (see also Down syndrome) Q90.9
Dresbach's (elliptocytosis) D58.1
Dressler's (postmyocardial infarction) I24.1
  postcardiotomy I97.0
drug withdrawal, infant of dependent mother P96.1
dry eye H04.12- ☑
due to abnormality
  chromosomal Q99.9
    sex
      female phenotype Q97.9
      male phenotype Q98.9
    specified NEC Q99.8
dumping (postgastrectomy) K91.1
  nonsurgical K31.89
Dupré's (meningism) R29.1
dysmetabolic X E88.81
dyspraxia, developmental F82
Eagle-Barrett Q79.4
Eaton-Lambert — see Syndrome, Lambert-Eaton
Ebstein's Q22.5
ectopic ACTH E24.3
eczema-thrombocytopenia D82.0
Eddowes' Q78.0
effort (psychogenic) F45.8
Ehlers-Danlos Q79.6
Eisenmenger's I27.89
Ekman's Q78.0
electric feet E53.8
Ellis-van Creveld Q77.6
empty nest Z60.0

Syndrome — *continued*
endocrine-hypertensive E27.0
entrapment — *see* Neuropathy, entrapment
eosinophilia-myalgia M35.8
epileptic (*see also* Epilepsy, by type)
    absence G40.A09 (*following* G40.3)
        intractable G40.A19 (*following* G40.3)
            with status epilepticus G40.A11 (*following* G40.3)
            without status epilepticus G40.A19 (*following* G40.3)
        not intractable G40.A09 (*following* G40.3)
            with status epilepticus G40.A01 (*following* G40.3)
            without status epilepticus G40.A09 (*following* G40.3)
Erdheim-Chester (ECD) E88.89
Erdheim's E22.0
erythrocyte fragmentation D59.4
Evans D69.41
exhaustion F48.8
extrapyramidal G25.9
    specified NEC G25.89
eye retraction — *see* Strabismus
eyelid-malar-mandible Q87.0
Faber's D50.9
facial pain, paroxysmal G50.0
Fallot's Q21.3
familial eczema-thrombocytopenia (Wiskott-Aldrich) D82.0
Fanconi (-de Toni) (-Debré) E72.09
    with cystinosis E72.04
Fanconi's (anemia) (congenital pancytopenia) D61.09
fatigue
    chronic R53.82
    psychogenic F48.8
faulty bowel habit K59.3
Feil-Klippel (brevicollis) Q76.1
Felty's — *see* Felty's syndrome
fertile eunuch E23.0
fetal
    alcohol (dysmorphic) Q86.0
    hydantoin Q86.1
Fiedler's I40.1
first arch Q87.0
fish odor E72.8
Fisher's G61.0
Fitzhugh-Curtis
    due to
        Chlamydia trachomatis A74.81
        Neisseria gonorrhorea (gonococcal peritonitis) A54.85
Fitz's K85.8
Flajani (-Basedow) E05.00
    with thyroid storm E05.01
flatback — *see* Flatback syndrome
floppy
    baby P94.2
    iris (intraoeprative) (IFIS) H21.81
    mitral valve I34.1
flush E34.0
Foix-Alajouanine G95.19
Fong's Q79.8
foramen magnum G93.5
Foster-Kennedy H47.14- ☑
Foville's (peduncular) G46.3
fragile X Q99.2
Franceschetti Q75.4
Frey's
    auriculotemporal G50.8
    hyperhidrosis L74.52
Friderichsen-Waterhouse A39.1
Froin's G95.89
frontal lobe F07.0
Fukuhara E88.49
functional
    bowel K59.9
    prepubertal castrate E29.1
Gaisböck's D75.1
ganglion (basal ganglia brain) G25.9
    geniculi G51.1
Gardner-Diamond D69.2
gastroesophageal
    junction K22.0
    laceration-hemorrhage K22.6
gastrojejunal loop obstruction K91.89
Gee-Herter-Heubner K90.0

Syndrome — *continued*
Gelineau's G47.419
    with cataplexy G47.411
genito-anorectal A55
Gerstmann-Sträussler-Scheinker (GSS) A81.82
Gianotti-Crosti L44.4
giant platelet (Bernard-Soulier) D69.1
Gilles de la Tourette's F95.2
goiter-deafness E07.1
Goldberg Q89.8
Goldberg-Maxwell E34.51
Good's D83.8
Gopalan' (burning feet) E53.8
Gorlin's Q87.89
Gougerot-Blum L81.7
Gouley's I31.1
Gower's R55
gray or grey (newborn) P93.0
    platelet D69.1
Gubler-Millard G46.3
Guillain-Barré (-Strohl) G61.0
gustatory sweating G50.8
Hadfield-Clarke K86.8
hair tourniquet — *see* Constriction, external, by site
Hamman's J98.19
hand-foot L27.1
hand-shoulder G90.8
hantavirus (cardio)-pulmonary (HPS) (HCPS) B33.4
happy puppet Q93.5
Harada's H30.81- ☑
Hayem-Faber D50.9
headache NEC G44.89
    complicated NEC G44.59
Heberden's I20.8
Hedinger's E34.0
Hegglin's D72.0
HELLP (hemolysis, elevated liver enzymes and low platelet count) O14.2- ☑
hemolytic-uremic D59.3
hemophagocytic, infection-associated D76.2
Henoch-Schönlein D69.0
hepatic flexure K59.8
hepatopulmonary K76.81
hepatorenal K76.7
    following delivery O90.4
    postoperative or postprocedural K91.83
    postpartum, puerperal O90.4
hepatourologic K76.7
Herter (-Gee) (nontropical sprue) K90.0
Heubner-Herter K90.0
Heyd's K76.7
Hilger's G90.09
histamine-like (fish poisoning) — *see* Poisoning, fish
histiocytic D76.3
histiocytosis NEC D76.3
HIV infection, acute B20
Hoffmann-Werdnig G12.0
Hollander-Simons E88.1
Hoppe-Goldflam G70.00
    with exacerbation (acute) G70.01
    in crisis G70.01
Horner's G90.2
hungry bone E83.81
hunterian glossitis D51.0
Hutchinson's triad A50.53
hyperabduction G54.0
hyperammonemia-hyperornithinemia-homocitrullinemia E72.4
hypereosinophilic (idiopathic) D72.1
hyperimmunoglobulin E (IgE) D82.4
hyperkalemic E87.5
hyperkinetic — *see* Hyperkinesia
hypermobility M35.7
hypernatremia E87.0
hyperosmolarity E87.0
hyperperfusion G97.82
hypersplenic D73.1
hypertransfusion, newborn P61.1
hyperventilation F45.8
hyperviscosity (of serum)
    polycythemic D75.1
    sclerothymic D58.8
hypoglycemic (familial) (neonatal) E16.2
hypokalemic E87.6
hyponatremic E87.1
hypopituitarism E23.0
hypoplastic left-heart Q23.4
hypopotassemia E87.6

Syndrome — *continued*
hyposmolality E87.1
hypotension, maternal O26.5- ☑
hypothenar hammer I73.89
ICF (intravascular coagulation-fibrinolysis) D65
idiopathic
    cardiorespiratory distress, newborn P22.0
    nephrotic (infantile) N04.9
iliotibial band M76.3- ☑
immobility, immobilization (paraplegic) M62.3
immune reconstitution D89.3
immune reconstitution inflammatory [IRIS] D89.3
immunity deficiency, combined D81.9
immunodeficiency
    acquired — *see* Human, immunodeficiency virus (HIV) disease
    combined D81.9
impending coronary I20.0
impingement, shoulder M75.4- ☑
inappropriate secretion of antidiuretic hormone E22.2
infant
    gestational diabetes P70.0
    of diabetic mother P70.1
infantilism (pituitary) E23.0
inferior vena cava I87.1
inspissated bile (newborn) P59.1
institutional (childhood) F94.2
insufficient sleep F51.12
intermediate coronary (artery) I20.0
interspinous ligament — *see* Spondylopathy, specified NEC
intestinal
    carcinoid E34.0
    knot K56.2
intravascular coagulation-fibrinolysis (ICF) D65
iodine-deficiency, congenital E00.9
    type
        mixed E00.2
        myxedematous E00.1
        neurological E00.0
IRDS (idiopathic respiratory distress, newborn) P22.0
irritable
    bowel K58.9
        with diarrhea K58.0
        psychogenic F45.8
    heart (psychogenic) F45.8
    weakness F48.8
ischemic bowel (transient) K55.9
    chronic K55.1
    due to mesenteric artery insufficiency K55.1
IVC (intravascular coagulopathy) D65
Ivemark's Q89.01
Jaccoud's — *see* Arthropathy, postrheumatic, chronic
Jackson's G83.89
Jakob-Creutzfeldt — *see* Creutzfeldt-Jakob disease or syndrome
jaw-winking Q07.8
Jervell-Lange-Nielsen I45.81
jet lag G47.25
Job's D71
Joseph-Diamond-Blackfan D61.01
jugular foramen G52.7
Kabuki Q89.8
Kanner's (autism) F84.0
Kartagener's Q89.3
Kelly's D50.1
Kimmelstein-Wilson — *see* Diabetes, specified type, with Kimmelstein-Wilson disease
Klein (e)-Levine G47.13
Klippel-Feil (brevicollis) Q76.1
Köhler-Pellegrini-Steida — *see* Bursitis, tibial collateral
König's K59.8
Korsakoff (-Wernicke) (nonalcoholic) F04
    alcoholic F10.26
Kostmann's D70.0
Krabbe's congenital muscle hypoplasia Q79.8
labyrinthine — *see* subcategory H83.2 ☑
lacunar NEC G46.7
Lambert-Eaton G70.80
    in
        neoplastic disease G73.1
        specified disease NEC G70.81
Landau-Kleffner — *see* Epilepsy, specified NEC
Larsen's Q74.8
lateral
    cutaneous nerve of thigh G57.1- ☑
    medullary G46.4
Launois' E22.0

Syndrome — *continued*
  lazy
    leukocyte D70.8
    posture M62.3
  Lemiere I80.8
  Lennox-Gastaut G40.812
    intractable G40.814
      with status epilepticus G40.813
      without status epilepticus G40.814
    not intractable G40.812
      with status epilepticus G40.811
      without status epilepticus G40.812
  lenticular, progressive E83.01
  Leopold-Levi's E05.90
  Lev's I44.2
  Lichtheim's D51.0
  Li-Fraumeni Z15.01
  Lightwood's N25.89
  Lignac (de Toni) (-Fanconi) (-Debré) E72.09
    with cystinosis E72.04
  Likoff's I20.8
  limbic epilepsy personality F07.0
  liver-kidney K76.7
  lobotomy F07.0
  Loffler's J82
  long arm 18 or 21 deletion Q93.89
  long QT I45.81
  Louis-Barré G11.3
  low
    atmospheric pressure T70.29 ☑
    back M54.5
    output (cardiac) I50.9
  lower radicular, newborn (birth injury) P14.8
  Luetscher's (dehydration) E86.0
  Lupus anticoagulant D68.62
  Lutembacher's Q21.1
  macrophage activation D76.1
    due to infection D76.2
  magnesium-deficiency R29.0
  Mal de Debarquement R42
  malabsorption K90.9
    postsurgical K91.2
  malformation, congenital, due to
    alcohol Q86.0
    exogenous cause NEC Q86.8
    hydantoin Q86.1
    warfarin Q86.2
  malignant
    carcinoid E34.0
    neuroleptic G21.0
  Mallory-Weiss K22.6
  mandibulofacial dysostosis Q75.4
  manic-depressive — *see* Disorder, bipolar, affective
  maple-syrup-urine E71.0
  Marable's I77.4
  Marfan's Q87.40
    with
      cardiovascular manifestations Q87.418
        aortic dilation Q87.410
      ocular manifestations Q87.42
      skeletal manifestations Q87.43
  Marie's (acromegaly) E22.0
  maternal hypotension — *see* Syndrome, hypotension, maternal
  May (-Hegglin) D72.0
  McArdle (-Schmidt) (-Pearson) E74.04
  McQuarrie's E16.2
  meconium plug (newborn) P76.0
  median arcuate ligament I77.4
  Meekeren-Ehlers-Danlos Q79.6
  megavitamin-B6 E67.2
  Meige G24.4
  MELAS E88.41
  Mendelson's O74.0
  MERRF (myoclonic epilepsy associated with ragged-red fibers) E88.42
  mesenteric
    artery (superior) K55.1
    vascular insufficiency K55.1
  metabolic E88.81
  metastatic carcinoid E34.0
  micrognathia-glossoptosis Q87.0
  midbrain NEC G93.89
  middle lobe (lung) J98.19
  middle radicular G54.0
  migraine (*see also* Migraine) G43.909
  Mikulicz' K11.8
  milk-alkali E83.52

Syndrome — *continued*
  Millard-Gubler G46.3
  Miller-Dieker Q93.88
  Miller-Fisher G61.0
  Minkowski-Chauffard D58.0
  Mirizzi's K83.1
  MNGIE (Mitochondrial Neurogastrointestinal Encephalopathy) E88.49
  Möbius, ophthalmoplegic migraine — *see* Migraine, ophthalmoplegic
  monofixation H50.42
  Morel-Moore M85.2
  Morel-Morgagni M85.2
  Morgagni (-Morel) (-Stewart) M85.2
  Morgagni-Adams-Stokes I45.9
  Mounier-Kuhn Q32.4
    with bronchiectasis J47.9
      with
        exacerbation (acute) J47.1
        lower respiratory infection J47.0
    acquired J98.09
      with bronchiectasis J47.9
        with
          exacerbation (acute) J47.1
          lower respiratory infection J47.0
  mucocutaneous lymph node (acute febrile) (MCLS) M30.3
  multiple endocrine neoplasia (MEN) — *see* Neoplasia, endocrine, multiple (MEN)
  multiple operations — *see* Disorder, factitious
  myasthenic G70.9
    in
      diabetes mellitus — *see* Diabetes, amyotrophy
      endocrine disease NEC E34.9 [G73.3]
      neoplastic disease (*see also* Neoplasm) D49.9 [G73.3]
        thyrotoxicosis (hyperthyroidism) E05.90 [G73.3]
          with thyroid storm E05.91 [G73.3]
  myelodysplastic D46.9
    with
      5q deletion D46.C (*following* D46.2)
      isolated del (5q) chromosomal abnormality D46.C (*following* D46.2)
    lesions, low grade D46.20
    specified NEC D46.Z (*following* D46.4)
  myelopathic pain G89.0
  myeloproliferative (chronic) D47.1
  myofascial pain M79.1
  Naffziger's G54.0
  nail patella Q87.2
  NARP (Neuropathy, Ataxia and Retinitis pigmentosa) E88.49
  neonatal abstinence P96.1
  nephritic (*see also* Nephritis)
    with edema — *see* Nephrosis
    acute N00.9
    chronic N03.9
    rapidly progressive N01.9
  nephrotic (congenital) (*see also* Nephrosis) N04.9
    with
      dense deposit disease N04.6
      diffuse
        crescentic glomerulonephritis N04.7
        endocapillary proliferative glomerulonephritis N04.4
        membranous glomerulonephritis N04.2
        mesangial proliferative glomerulonephritis N04.3
        mesangiocapillary glomerulonephritis N04.5
      focal and segmental glomerular lesions N04.1
      minor glomerular abnormality N04.0
      specified morphological changes NEC N04.8
    diabetic — *see* Diabetes, nephrosis
  neurologic neglect R41.4
  Nezelof's D81.4
  Nonne-Milroy-Meige Q82.0
  Nothnagel's vasomotor acroparesthesia I73.89
  oculomotor H51.9
  ophthalmoplegia-cerebellar ataxia — *see* Strabismus, paralytic, third nerve
  oral-facial-digital Q87.0
  organic
    affective F06.30
    amnesic (not alcohol- or drug-induced) F04
    brain F09
    depressive F06.31
    hallucinosis F06.0
    personality F07.0

Syndrome — *continued*
  Ormond's N13.5
  oro-facial-digital Q87.0
  os trigonum Q68.8
  Osler-Weber-Rendu I78.0
  osteoporosis-osteomalacia M83.8
  Osterreicher-Turner Q79.8
  otolith — *see* subcategory H81.8 ☑
  oto-palatal-digital Q87.0
  outlet (thoracic) G54.0
  ovary
    polycystic E28.2
    resistant E28.39
    sclerocystic E28.2
  Owren's D68.2
  Paget-Schroetter I82.890
  pain (*see also* Pain)
    complex regional I G90.50
      lower limb G90.52- ☑
        specified site NEC G90.59
      upper limb G90.51- ☑
    complex regional II — *see* Causalgia
  painful
    bruising D69.2
    feet E53.8
    prostate N42.81
  paralysis agitans — *see* Parkinsonism
  paralytic G83.9
    specified NEC G83.89
  Parinaud's H51.0
  parkinsonian — *see* Parkinsonism
  Parkinson's — *see* Parkinsonism
  paroxysmal facial pain G50.0
  Parry's E05.00
    with thyroid storm E05.01
  Parsonage (-Aldren)-Turner G54.5
  patella clunk M25.86- ☑
  Paterson (-Brown) (-Kelly) D50.1
  pectoral girdle I77.89
  pectoralis minor I77.89
  Pelger-Huet D72.0
  pellagra-cerebellar ataxia-renal aminoaciduria E72.02
  pellagroid E52
  Pellegrini-Stieda — *see* Bursitis, tibial collateral
  pelvic congestion-fibrosis, female N94.89
  penta X Q97.1
  peptic ulcer — *see* Ulcer, peptic
  perabduction I77.89
  periodic headache, in adults and children — *see* Headache, periodic syndromes in adults and children
  periurethral fibrosis N13.5
  phantom limb (without pain) G54.7
    with pain G54.6
  pharyngeal pouch D82.1
  Pick's (heart) (liver) I31.1
  Pickwickian E66.2
  PIE (pulmonary infiltration with eosinophilia) J82
  pigmentary pallidal degeneration (progressive) G23.0
  pineal E34.8
  pituitary E22.0
  placental transfusion — *see* Pregnancy, complicated by, placental transfusion syndromes
  plantar fascia M72.2
  plateau iris (post-iridectomy) (postprocedural) H21.82
  Plummer-Vinson D50.1
  pluricarential of infancy E40
  plurideficiency E40
  pluriglandular (compensatory) E31.8
    autoimmune E31.0
  pneumatic hammer T75.21 ☑
  polyangiitis overlap M30.8
  polycarential of infancy E40
  polyglandular E31.8
    autoimmune E31.0
  polysplenia Q89.09
  pontine NEC G93.89
  popliteal
    artery entrapment I77.89
    web Q87.89
  post chemoembolization — *code to* associated conditions
  postcardiac injury
    postcardiotomy I97.0
    postmyocardial infarction I24.1
  postcardiotomy I97.0
  postcholecystectomy K91.5
  postcommissurotomy I97.0

Syndrome — *continued*
- postconcussional F07.81
- postcontusional F07.81
- postencephalitic F07.89
- posterior
  - cervical sympathetic M53.0
  - cord G83.83
  - fossa compression G93.5
  - reversible encephalopathy (PRES) I67.83
- postgastrectomy (dumping) K91.1
- postgastric surgery K91.1
- postinfarction I24.1
- postlaminectomy NEC M96.1
- postleukotomy F07.0
- postmastectomy lymphedema I97.2
- postmyocardial infarction I24.1
- postoperative NEC T81.9 ☑
  - blind loop K90.2
- postpartum panhypopituitary (Sheehan) E23.0
- postpolio (myelitic) G14
- postthrombotic I87.009
  - with
    - inflammation I87.02- ☑
      - with ulcer I87.03- ☑
    - specified complication NEC I87.09- ☑
    - ulcer I87.01- ☑
      - with inflammation I87.03- ☑
  - asymptomatic I87.00- ☑
- postvagotomy K91.1
- postvalvulotomy I97.0
- postviral NEC G93.3
  - fatigue G93.3
- Potain's K31.0
- potassium intoxication E87.5
- precerebral artery (multiple) (bilateral) G45.2
- preinfarction I20.0
- preleukemic D46.9
- premature senility E34.8
- premenstrual dysphoric N94.3
- premenstrual tension N94.3
- Prinzmetal-Massumi R07.1
- prune belly Q79.4
- pseudo -Turner's Q87.1
- pseudocarpal tunnel (sublimis) — *see* Syndrome, carpal tunnel
- pseudoparalytica G70.00
  - with exacerbation (acute) G70.01
  - in crisis G70.01
- psycho-organic (nonpsychotic severity) F07.9
  - acute or subacute F05
  - depressive type F06.31
  - hallucinatory type F06.0
  - nonpsychotic severity F07.0
  - specified NEC F07.89
- pulmonary
  - arteriosclerosis I27.0
  - dysmaturity (Wilson-Mikity) P27.0
  - hypoperfusion (idiopathic) P22.0
  - renal (hemorrhagic) (Goodpasture's) M31.0
- pure
  - motor lacunar G46.5
  - sensory lacunar G46.6
- Putnam-Dana D51.0
- pyramidopallidonigral G20
- pyriformis — *see* Lesion, nerve, sciatic
- QT interval prolongation I45.81
- radicular NEC — *see* Radiculopathy
  - upper limbs, newborn (birth injury) P14.3
- rapid time-zone change G47.25
- Rasmussen G04.81
- Raymond (-Céstan) I65.8
- Raynaud's I73.00
  - with gangrene I73.01
- RDS (respiratory distress syndrome, newborn) P22.0
- reactive airways dysfunction J68.3
- Refsum's G60.1
- Reifenstein E34.52
- renal glomerulohyalinosis-diabetic — *see* Diabetes, nephrosis
- Rendu-Osler-Weber I78.0
- residual ovary N99.83
- resistant ovary E28.39
- respiratory
  - distress
    - acute J80
      - adult J80
      - child J80

Syndrome — *continued*
- respiratory — *continued*
  - distress — *continued*
    - newborn (idiopathic) (type I) P22.0
      - type II P22.1
- restless legs G25.81
- retinoblastoma (familial) C69.2 ☑
- retroperitoneal fibrosis N13.5
- retroviral seroconversion (acute) Z21
- Reye's G93.7
- Richter — *see* Leukemia, chronic lymphocytic, B-cell type
- Ridley's I50.1
- right
  - heart, hypoplastic Q22.6
  - ventricular obstruction — *see* Failure, heart, congestive
- Romano-Ward (prolonged QT interval) I45.81
- rotator cuff, shoulder (*see also* Tear, rotator cuff) M75.10- ☑
- Rotes Quérol — *see* Hyperostosis, ankylosing
- Roth — *see* Meralgia paresthetica
- rubella (congenital) P35.0
- Ruvalcaba-Myhre-Smith E71.440
- Rytand-Lipsitch I44.2
- salt
  - depletion E87.1
    - due to heat NEC T67.8 ☑
      - causing heat exhaustion or prostration T67.4 ☑
  - low E87.1
- salt-losing N28.89
- Scaglietti-Dagnini E22.0
- scalenus anticus (anterior) G54.0
- scapulocostal — *see* Mononeuropathy, upper limb, specified site NEC
- scapuloperoneal G71.0
- schizophrenic, of childhood NEC F84.5
- Schnitzler D47.2
- Scholte's E34.0
- Schroeder's E27.0
- Schüller-Christian C96.5
- Schwachman's — *see* Syndrome, Shwachman's
- Schwartz (-Jampel) G71.13
- Schwartz-Bartter E22.2
- scimitar Q26.8
- sclerocystic ovary E28.2
- Seitelberger's G31.89
- septicemic adrenal hemorrhage A39.1
- seroconversion, retroviral (acute) Z21
- serous meningitis G93.2
- severe acute respiratory (SARS) J12.81
- shaken infant T74.4 ☑
- shock (traumatic) T79.4 ☑
  - kidney N17.0
    - following crush injury T79.5 ☑
  - toxic A48.3
- shock-lung J80
- Shone's — *code to* specific anomalies
- short
  - bowel K91.2
  - rib Q77.2
- shoulder-hand — *see* Algoneurodystrophy
- Shwachman's D70.4
- sicca — *see* Sicca syndrome
- sick
  - cell E87.1
  - sinus I49.5
- sick-euthyroid E07.81
- sideropenic D50.1
- Siemens' ectodermal dysplasia Q82.4
- Silfverskiöld's Q78.9
- Simons' E88.1
- sinus tarsi M25.57- ☑
- sinusitis-bronchiectasis-situs inversus Q89.3
- Sipple's E31.22
- sirenomelia Q87.2
- Slocumb's E27.0
- slow flow, coronary I20.8
- Sluder's G44.89
- Smith-Magenis Q93.88
- Sneddon-Wilkinson L13.1
- Sotos' E22.0
- South African cardiomyopathy I42.8
- spasmodic
  - upward movement, eyes H51.8
  - winking F95.8
- Spen's I45.9

Syndrome — *continued*
- splenic
  - agenesis Q89.01
  - flexure K59.8
  - neutropenia D73.81
- Spurway's Q78.0
- staphylococcal scalded skin L00
- Stein-Leventhal E28.2
- Stein's E28.2
- Stevens-Johnson syndrome L51.1
  - toxic epidermal necrolysis overlap L51.3
- Stewart-Morel M85.2
- Stickler Q89.8
- stiff baby Q89.8
- stiff man G25.82
- Still-Felty — *see* Felty's syndrome
- Stokes (-Adams) I45.9
- stone heart I50.1
- straight back, congenital Q76.49
- subclavian steal G45.8
- subcoracoid-pectoralis minor G54.0
- subcostal nerve compression I77.89
- subphrenic interposition Q43.3
- superior
  - cerebellar artery I63.8
  - mesenteric artery K55.1
  - semi-circular canal dehiscence H83.8X- ☑
  - vena cava I87.1
- supine hypotensive (maternal) — *see* Syndrome, hypotension, maternal
- suprarenal cortical E27.0
- supraspinatus (*see also* Tear, rotator cuff) M75.10- ☑
- Susac G93.49
- swallowed blood P78.2
- sweat retention L74.0
- Swyer Q99.1
- Symond's G93.2
- sympathetic
  - cervical paralysis G90.2
  - pelvic, female N94.89
- systemic inflammatory response (SIRS), of non-infectious origin (without organ dysfunction) R65.10
  - with acute organ dysfunction R65.11
- tachycardia-bradycardia I49.5
- takotsubo I51.81
- TAR (thrombocytopenia with absent radius) Q87.2
- tarsal tunnel G57.5- ☑
- teething K00.7
- tegmental G93.89
- telangiectasic-pigmentation-cataract Q82.8
- temporal pyramidal apex — *see* Otitis, media, suppurative, acute
- temporomandibular joint-pain-dysfunction M26.62
- Terry's H44.2- ☑
- testicular feminization (*see also* Syndrome, androgen insensitivity) E34.51
- thalamic pain (hyperesthetic) G89.0
- thoracic outlet (compression) G54.0
- Thorson-Björck E34.0
- thrombocytopenia with absent radius (TAR) Q87.2
- thyroid-adrenocortical insufficiency E31.0
- tibial
  - anterior M76.81- ☑
  - posterior M76.82- ☑
- Tietze's M94.0
- time-zone (rapid) G47.25
- Toni-Fanconi E72.09
  - with cystinosis E72.04
- Touraine's Q79.8
- tourniquet — *see* Constriction, external, by site
- toxic shock A48.3
- transient left ventricular apical ballooning I51.81
- traumatic vasospastic T75.22 ☑
- Treacher Collins Q75.4
- triple X, female Q97.0
- trisomy Q92.9
  - 13 Q91.7
    - meiotic nondisjunction Q91.4
    - mitotic nondisjunction Q91.5
    - mosaicism Q91.5
    - translocation Q91.6
  - 18 Q91.3
    - meiotic nondisjunction Q91.0
    - mitotic nondisjunction Q91.1
    - mosaicism Q91.1
    - translocation Q91.2
  - 20 (q)(p) Q92.8

Syndrome — continued
  trisomy — continued
    21 Q90.9
      meiotic nondisjunction Q90.0
      mitotic nondisjunction Q90.1
      mosaicism Q90.1
      translocation Q90.2
    22 Q92.8
  tropical wet feet T69.0- ☑
  Trousseau's I82.1
  tumor lysis (following antineoplastic chemotherapy)
      (spontaneous) NEC E88.3
  Twiddler's (due to)
    automatic implantable defibrillator T82.198 ☑
    cardiac pacemaker T82.198 ☑
  Unverricht (-Lundborg) — see Epilepsy, generalized,
      idiopathic
  upward gaze H51.8
  uremia, chronic (see also Disease, kidney, chronic)
      N18.9
  urethral N34.3
  urethro-oculo-articular — see Reiter's disease
  urohepatic K76.7
  vago-hypoglossal G52.7
  van Buchem's M85.2
  van der Hoeve's Q78.0
  vascular NEC in cerebrovascular disease G46.8
  vasoconstriction, reversible cerebrovascular I67.841
  vasomotor I73.9
  vasospastic (traumatic) T75.22 ☑
  vasovagal R55
  VATER Q87.2
  velo-cardio-facial Q93.81
  vena cava (inferior) (superior) (obstruction) I87.1
  vertebral
    artery G45.0
      compression — see Syndrome, anterior, spinal
          artery, compression
    steal G45.0
  vertebro-basilar artery G45.0
  vertebrogenic (pain) M54.89
  vertiginous — see Disorder, vestibular function
  Vinson-Plummer D50.1
  virus B34.9
  visceral larva migrans B83.0
  visual disorientation H53.8
  vitamin B6 deficiency E53.1
  vitreal corneal H59.01- ☑
  vitreous (touch) H59.01- ☑
  Vogt-Koyanagi H20.82- ☑
  Volkmann's T79.6 ☑
  von Schroetter's I82.890
  von Willebrand (-Jürgen) D68.0
  Waldenström-Kjellberg D50.1
  Wallenberg's G46.3
  water retention E87.79
  Waterhouse (-Friderichsen) A39.1
  Weber-Gubler G46.3
  Weber-Leyden G46.3
  Weber's G46.3
  Wegener's M31.30
    with
      kidney involvement M31.31
      lung involvement M31.30
        with kidney involvement M31.31
  Weingarten's (tropical eosinophilia) J82
  Weiss-Baker G90.09
  Werdnig-Hoffman G12.0
  Wermer's E31.21
  Werner's E34.8
  Wernicke-Korsakoff (nonalcoholic) F04
    alcoholic F10.26
  Westphal-Strümpell E83.01
  West's — see Epilepsy, spasms
  wet
    feet (maceration) (tropical) T69.0- ☑
    lung, newborn P22.1
  whiplash S13.4 ☑
  whistling face Q87.0
  Wilkie's K55.1
  Wilkinson-Sneddon L13.1
  Willebrand (-Jürgens) D68.0
  Wilson's (hepatolenticular degeneration) E83.01
  Wiskott-Aldrich D82.0
  withdrawal — see Withdrawal, state
    drug
      infant of dependent mother P96.1
      therapeutic use, newborn P96.2

Syndrome — continued
  Woakes' (ethmoiditis) J33.1
  Wright's (hyperabduction) I77.89
  X I20.9
  XXXX Q97.1
  XXXXX Q97.1
  XXXXY Q98.1
  XXY Q98.0
  yellow nail L60.5
  Zahorsky's B08.5
  Zellweger syndrome E71.510
  Zellweger-like syndrome E71.541
Synechia (anterior) (iris) (posterior) (pupil) (see also Ad-
    hesions, iris)
  intra-uterine (traumatic) N85.6
Synesthesia R20.8
Syngamiasis, syngamosis B83.3
Synodontia K00.2
Synorchidism, synorchism Q55.1
Synostosis (congenital) Q78.8
  astragalo-scaphoid Q74.2
  radioulnar Q74.0
Synovial sarcoma — see Neoplasm, connective tissue,
    malignant
Synovioma (malignant) (see also Neoplasm, connective
    tissue, malignant)
  benign — see Neoplasm, connective tissue, benign
Synoviosarcoma — see Neoplasm, connective tissue,
    malignant
Synovitis (see also Tenosynovitis)
  crepitant
    hand M70.0- ☑
    wrist M70.03- ☑
  gonococcal A54.49
  gouty — see Gout, idiopathic
  in (due to)
    crystals M65.8- ☑
    gonorrhea A54.49
    syphilis (late) A52.78
    use, overuse, pressure — see Disorder, soft tissue,
        due to use
  infective NEC — see Tenosynovitis, infective NEC
  specified NEC — see Tenosynovitis, specified type NEC
  syphilitic A52.78
    congenital (early) A50.02
  toxic — see Synovitis, transient
  transient M67.3- ☑
    ankle M67.37- ☑
    elbow M67.32- ☑
    foot joint M67.37- ☑
    hand joint M67.34- ☑
    hip M67.35- ☑
    knee M67.36- ☑
    multiple site M67.39
    pelvic region M67.35- ☑
    shoulder M67.31- ☑
    specified joint NEC M67.38
    wrist M67.33- ☑
  traumatic, current — see Sprain
  tuberculous — see Tuberculosis, synovitis
  villonodular (pigmented) M12.2- ☑
    ankle M12.27- ☑
    elbow M12.22- ☑
    foot joint M12.27- ☑
    hand joint M12.24- ☑
    hip M12.25- ☑
    knee M12.26- ☑
    multiple site M12.29
    pelvic region M12.25- ☑
    shoulder M12.21- ☑
    specified joint NEC M12.28
    vertebrae M12.28
    wrist M12.23- ☑
Syphilid A51.39
  congenital A50.06
  newborn A50.06
  tubercular (late) A52.79
Syphilis, syphilitic (acquired) A53.9
  abdomen (late) A52.79
  acoustic nerve A52.15
  adenopathy (secondary) A51.49
  adrenal (gland) (with cortical hypofunction) A52.79
  age under 2 years NOS (see also Syphilis, congenital,
      early)
    acquired A51.9
  alopecia (secondary) A51.32
  anemia (late) A52.79 [D63.8]

Syphilis, syphilitic — continued
  aneurysm (aorta) (ruptured) A52.01
    central nervous system A52.05
    congenital A50.54 [I79.0]
  anus (late) A52.74
    primary A51.1
    secondary A51.39
  aorta (arch) (abdominal) (thoracic) A52.02
    aneurysm A52.01
  aortic (insufficiency) (regurgitation) (stenosis) A52.03
    aneurysm A52.01
  arachnoid (adhesive) (cerebral) (spinal) A52.13
  asymptomatic — see Syphilis, latent
  ataxia (locomotor) A52.11
  atrophoderma maculatum A51.39
  auricular fibrillation A52.06
  bladder (late) A52.76
  bone A52.77
    secondary A51.46
  brain A52.17
  breast (late) A52.79
  bronchus (late) A52.72
  bubo (primary) A51.0
  bulbar palsy A52.19
  bursa (late) A52.78
  cardiac decompensation A52.06
  cardiovascular A52.00
  central nervous system (late) (recurrent) (relapse)
      (tertiary) A52.3
    with
      ataxia A52.11
      general paralysis A52.17
        juvenile A50.45
      paresis (general) A52.17
        juvenile A50.45
      tabes (dorsalis) A52.11
        juvenile A50.45
      taboparesis A52.17
        juvenile A50.45
    aneurysm A52.05
    congenital A50.40
    juvenile A50.40
    remission in (sustained) A52.3
    serology doubtful, negative, or positive A52.3
    specified nature or site NEC A52.19
    vascular A52.05
  cerebral A52.17
    meningovascular A52.13
    nerves (multiple palsies) A52.15
    sclerosis A52.17
    thrombosis A52.05
  cerebrospinal (tabetic type) A52.12
  cerebrovascular A52.05
  cervix (late) A52.76
  chancre (multiple) A51.0
    extragenital A51.2
    Rollet's A51.0
  Charcot's joint A52.16
  chorioretinitis A51.43
    congenital A50.01
    late A52.71
    prenatal A50.01
  choroiditis — see Syphilitic chorioretinitis
  choroidoretinitis — see Syphilitic chorioretinitis
  ciliary body (secondary) A51.43
    late A52.71
  colon (late) A52.74
  combined spinal sclerosis A52.11
  condyloma (latum) A51.31
  congenital A50.9
    with
      paresis (general) A50.45
      tabes (dorsalis) A50.45
      taboparesis A50.45
    early, or less than 2 years after birth NEC A50.2
      with manifestations — see Syphilis, congenital,
          early, symptomatic
      latent (without manifestations) A50.1
        negative spinal fluid test A50.1
        serology positive A50.1
      symptomatic A50.09
        cutaneous A50.06
        mucocutaneous A50.07
        oculopathy A50.01
        osteochondropathy A50.02
        pharyngitis A50.03
        pneumonia A50.04
        rhinitis A50.05

Syphilis, syphilitic — *continued*
congenital — *continued*
early, or less than 2 years after birth — *continued*
symptomatic — *continued*
visceral A50.08
chorioretinitis, choroiditis A50.01 [H32]
interstitial keratitis A50.31
juvenile neurosyphilis A50.45
late, or 2 years or more after birth NEC A50.7
chorioretinitis, choroiditis A50.32
interstitial keratitis A50.31
juvenile neurosyphilis A50.45
latent (without manifestations) A50.6
negative spinal fluid test A50.6
serology positive A50.6
symptomatic or with manifestations NEC A50.59
arthropathy A50.55
cardiovascular A50.54
Clutton's joints A50.51
Hutchinson's teeth A50.52
Hutchinson's triad A50.53
osteochondropathy A50.56
saddle nose A50.57
conjugal A53.9
tabes A52.11
conjunctiva (late) A52.71
contact Z20.2
cord bladder A52.19
cornea, late A52.71
coronary (artery) (sclerosis) A52.06
coryza, congenital A50.05
cranial nerve A52.15
multiple palsies A52.15
cutaneous — *see* Syphilis, skin
dacryocystitis (late) A52.71
degeneration, spinal cord A52.12
dementia paralytica A52.17
juvenilis A50.45
destruction of bone A52.77
dilatation, aorta A52.01
due to blood transfusion A53.9
dura mater A52.13
ear A52.79
inner A52.79
nerve (eighth) A52.15
neurorecurrence A52.15
early A51.9
cardiovascular A52.00
central nervous system A52.3
latent (without manifestations) (less than 2 years after infection) A51.5
negative spinal fluid test A51.5
serological relapse after treatment A51.5
serology positive A51.5
relapse (treated, untreated) A51.9
skin A51.39
symptomatic A51.9
extragenital chancre A51.2
primary, except extragenital chancre A51.0
secondary (*see also* Syphilis, secondary) A51.39
relapse (treated, untreated) A51.49
ulcer A51.39
eighth nerve (neuritis) A52.15
endemic A65
endocarditis A52.03
aortic A52.03
pulmonary A52.03
epididymis (late) A52.76
epiglottis (late) A52.73
epiphysitis (congenital) (early) A50.02
episcleritis (late) A52.71
esophagus A52.79
eustachian tube A52.73
exposure to Z20.2
eye A52.71
eyelid (late) (with gumma) A52.71
fallopian tube (late) A52.76
fracture A52.77
gallbladder (late) A52.74
gastric (polyposis) (late) A52.74
general A53.9
paralysis A52.17
juvenile A50.45
genital (primary) A51.0
glaucoma A52.71

Syphilis, syphilitic — *continued*
gumma NEC A52.79
cardiovascular system A52.00
central nervous system A52.3
congenital A50.59
heart (block) (decompensation) (disease) (failure) A52.06 [I52]
valve NEC A52.03
hemianesthesia A52.19
hemianopsia A52.71
hemiparesis A52.17
hemiplegia A52.17
hepatic artery A52.09
hepatis A52.74
hepatomegaly, congenital A50.08
hereditaria tarda — *see* Syphilis, congenital, late
hereditary — *see* Syphilis, congenital
Hutchinson's teeth A50.52
hyalitis A52.71
inactive — *see* Syphilis, latent
infantum — *see* Syphilis, congenital
inherited — *see* Syphilis, congenital
internal ear A52.79
intestine (late) A52.74
iris, iritis (secondary) A51.43
late A52.71
joint (late) A52.77
keratitis (congenital) (interstitial) (late) A50.31
kidney (late) A52.75
lacrimal passages (late) A52.71
larynx (late) A52.73
late A52.9
cardiovascular A52.00
central nervous system A52.3
kidney A52.75
latent or 2 years or more after infection (without manifestations) A52.8
negative spinal fluid test A52.8
serology positive A52.8
paresis A52.17
specified site NEC A52.79
symptomatic or with manifestations A52.79
tabes A52.11
latent A53.0
with signs or symptoms — *code by* site and stage under Syphilis
early, or less than 2 years after infection A51.5
central nervous system A52.2
date of infection unspecified A53.0
follow-up of latent syphilis A53.0
date of infection unspecified A53.0
late, or 2 years or more after infection A52.8
late, or 2 years or more after infection A52.8
positive serology (only finding) A53.0
early, or less than 2 years after infection A51.5
date of infection unspecified A53.0
late, or 2 years or more after infection A52.8
lens (late) A52.71
leukoderma A51.39
late A52.79
lienitis A52.79
lip A51.39
chancre (primary) A51.2
late A52.79
Lissauer's paralysis A52.17
liver A52.74
locomotor ataxia A52.11
lung A52.72
lymph gland (early) (secondary) A51.49
late A52.79
lymphadenitis (secondary) A51.49
macular atrophy of skin A51.39
striated A52.79
mediastinum (late) A52.73
meninges (adhesive) (brain) (spinal cord) A52.13
meningitis A52.13
acute (secondary) A51.41
congenital A50.41
meningoencephalitis A52.14
meningovascular A52.13
congenital A50.41
mesarteritis A52.09
brain A52.04
middle ear A52.77
mitral stenosis A52.03
monoplegia A52.17
mouth (secondary) A51.39
late A52.79

Syphilis, syphilitic — *continued*
mucocutaneous (secondary) A51.39
late A52.79
mucous
membrane (secondary) A51.39
late A52.79
patches A51.39
congenital A50.07
mulberry molars A50.52
muscle A52.78
myocardium A52.06
nasal sinus (late) A52.73
neonatorum — *see* Syphilis, congenital
nephrotic syndrome (secondary) A51.44
nerve palsy (any cranial nerve) A52.15
multiple A52.15
nervous system, central A52.3
neuritis A52.15
acoustic A52.15
neurorecidive of retina A52.19
neuroretinitis A52.19
newborn — *see* Syphilis, congenital
nodular superficial (late) A52.79
nonvenereal A65
nose (late) A52.73
saddle back deformity A50.57
occlusive arterial disease A52.09
oculopathy A52.71
ophthalmic (late) A52.71
optic nerve (atrophy) (neuritis) (papilla) A52.15
orbit (late) A52.71
organic A53.9
osseous (late) A52.77
osteochondritis (congenital) (early) A50.02 [M90.80]
osteoporosis A52.77
ovary (late) A52.76
oviduct (late) A52.76
palate (late) A52.79
pancreas (late) A52.74
paralysis A52.17
general A52.17
juvenile A50.45
paresis (general) A52.17
juvenile A50.45
paresthesia A52.19
Parkinson's disease or syndrome A52.19
paroxysmal tachycardia A52.06
pemphigus (congenital) A50.06
penis (chancre) A51.0
late A52.76
pericardium A52.06
perichondritis, larynx (late) A52.73
periosteum (late) A52.77
congenital (early) A50.02 [M90.80]
early (secondary) A51.46
peripheral nerve A52.79
petrous bone (late) A52.77
pharynx (late) A52.73
secondary A51.39
pituitary (gland) A52.79
pleura (late) A52.73
pneumonia, white A50.04
pontine lesion A52.17
portal vein A52.09
primary A51.0
anal A51.1
and secondary — *see* Syphilis, secondary
central nervous system A52.3
extragenital chancre NEC A51.2
fingers A51.2
genital A51.0
lip A51.2
specified site NEC A51.2
tonsils A51.2
prostate (late) A52.76
ptosis (eyelid) A52.71
pulmonary (late) A52.72
artery A52.09
pyelonephritis (late) A52.75
recently acquired, symptomatic A51.9
rectum (late) A52.74
respiratory tract (late) A52.73
retina, late A52.71
retrobulbar neuritis A52.15
salpingitis A52.76
sclera (late) A52.71
sclerosis
cerebral A52.17

☑ **Additional Character Required** — **Refer to the Tabular List for Character Selection**   ▽ **Subterms under main terms may continue to next column or page**

Syphilis, syphilitic — *continued*
  sclerosis — *continued*
    coronary A52.06
    multiple A52.11
  scotoma (central) A52.71
  scrotum (late) A52.76
  secondary (and primary) A51.49
    adenopathy A51.49
    anus A51.39
    bone A51.46
    chorioretinitis, choroiditis A51.43
    hepatitis A51.45
    liver A51.45
    lymphadenitis A51.49
    meningitis (acute) A51.41
    mouth A51.39
    mucous membranes A51.39
    periosteum, periostitis A51.46
    pharynx A51.39
    relapse (treated, untreated) A51.49
    skin A51.39
    specified form NEC A51.49
    tonsil A51.39
    ulcer A51.39
    viscera NEC A51.49
    vulva A51.39
  seminal vesicle (late) A52.76
  seronegative with signs or symptoms — *code by* site and stage under Syphilis
  seropositive
    with signs or symptoms — *code by* site and stage under Syphilis
    follow-up of latent syphilis — *see* Syphilis, latent
    only finding — *see* Syphilis, latent
  seventh nerve (paralysis) A52.15
  sinus, sinusitis (late) A52.73
  skeletal system A52.77
  skin (with ulceration) (early) (secondary) A51.39
    late or tertiary A52.79
  small intestine A52.74
  spastic spinal paralysis A52.17
  spermatic cord (late) A52.76
  spinal (cord) A52.12

Syphilis, syphilitic — *continued*
  spleen A52.79
  splenomegaly A52.79
  spondylitis A52.77
  staphyloma A52.71
  stigmata (congenital) A50.59
  stomach A52.74
  synovium A52.78
  tabes dorsalis (late) A52.11
    juvenile A50.45
  tabetic type A52.11
    juvenile A50.45
  taboparesis A52.17
    juvenile A50.45
  tachycardia A52.06
  tendon (late) A52.78
  tertiary A52.9
    with symptoms NEC A52.79
    cardiovascular A52.00
    central nervous system A52.3
    multiple NEC A52.79
    specified site NEC A52.79
  testis A52.76
  thorax A52.73
  throat A52.73
  thymus (gland) (late) A52.79
  thyroid (late) A52.79
  tongue (late) A52.79
  tonsil (lingual) (late) A52.73
    primary A51.2
    secondary A51.39
  trachea (late) A52.73
  tunica vaginalis (late) A52.76
  ulcer (any site) (early) (secondary) A51.39
    late A52.79
    perforating A52.79
      foot A52.11
  urethra (late) A52.76
  urogenital (late) A52.76
  uterus (late) A52.76
  uveal tract (secondary) A51.43
    late A52.71

Syphilis, syphilitic — *continued*
  uveitis (secondary) A51.43
    late A52.71
  uvula (late) (perforated) A52.79
  vagina A51.0
    late A52.76
  valvulitis NEC A52.03
  vascular A52.00
    brain (cerebral) A52.05
  ventriculi A52.74
  vesicae urinariae (late) A52.76
  viscera (abdominal) (late) A52.74
    secondary A51.49
  vitreous (opacities) (late) A52.71
    hemorrhage A52.71
  vulva A51.0
    late A52.76
    secondary A51.39
Syphiloma A52.79
  cardiovascular system A52.00
  central nervous system A52.3
  circulatory system A52.00
  congenital A50.59
Syphilophobia F45.29
Syringadenoma (*see also* Neoplasm, skin, benign)
  papillary — *see* Neoplasm, skin, benign
Syringobulbia G95.0
Syringocystadenoma — *see* Neoplasm, skin, benign
  papillary — *see* Neoplasm, skin, benign
Syringoma (*see also* Neoplasm, skin, benign)
  chondroid — *see* Neoplasm, skin, benign
Syringomyelia G95.0
Syringomyelitis — *see* Encephalitis
Syringomyelocele — *see* Spina bifida
Syringopontia G95.0
System, systemic (*see also* condition)
  disease, combined — *see* Degeneration, combined
  inflammatory response syndrome (SIRS) of non-infectious origin (without organ dysfunction) R65.10
    with acute organ dysfunction R65.11
  lupus erythematosus M32.9
    inhibitor present D68.62

T

Tabacism, tabacosis, tabagism (*see also* Poisoning, tobacco)
  meaning dependence (without remission) F17.200
    with
      disorder F17.299
        remission F17.211
        specified disorder NEC F17.298
        withdrawal F17.203
Tabardillo A75.9
  flea-borne A75.2
  louse-borne A75.0
Tabes, tabetic A52.10
  with
    central nervous system syphilis A52.10
    Charcot's joint A52.16
    cord bladder A52.19
    crisis, viscera (any) A52.19
    paralysis, general A52.17
    paresis (general) A52.17
    perforating ulcer (foot) A52.19
  arthropathy (Charcot) A52.16
  bladder A52.19
  bone A52.11
  cerebrospinal A52.12
  congenital A50.45
  conjugal A52.10
  dorsalis A52.11
    juvenile A50.49
  juvenile A50.49
  latent A52.19
  mesenterica A18.39
  paralysis, insane, general A52.17
  spasmodic A52.17
  syphilis (cerebrospinal) A52.12
Taboparalysis A52.17
Taboparesis (remission) A52.17
  juvenile A50.45
TAC (trigeminal autonomic cephalgia) **NEC** G44.099
  intractable G44.091
  not intractable G44.099
Tache noir S60.22- ☑
Tachyalimentation K91.2
Tachyarrhythmia, tachyrhythmia — *see* Tachycardia
Tachycardia R00.0
  atrial (paroxysmal) I47.1
  auricular I47.1
  AV nodal re-entry (re-entrant) I47.1
  junctional (paroxysmal) I47.1
  newborn P29.11
  nodal (paroxysmal) I47.1
  non-paroxysmal AV nodal I45.89
  paroxysmal (sustained) (nonsustained) I47.9
    with sinus bradycardia I49.5
    atrial (PAT) I47.1
    atrioventricular (AV) (re-entrant) I47.1
      psychogenic F54
    junctional I47.1
      ectopic I47.1
    nodal I47.1
    psychogenic (atrial) (supraventricular) (ventricular) F54
    supraventricular (sustained) I47.1
      psychogenic F54
    ventricular I47.2
      psychogenic F54
  psychogenic F45.8
  sick sinus I49.5
  sinoauricular NOS R00.0
    paroxysmal I47.1
  sinus [sinusal] NOS R00.0
    paroxysmal I47.1
  supraventricular I47.1
  ventricular (paroxysmal) (sustained) I47.2
    psychogenic F54
Tachygastria K31.89
Tachypnea R06.82
  hysterical F45.8
  newborn (idiopathic) (transitory) P22.1
  psychogenic F45.8
  transitory, of newborn P22.1

TACO (transfusion associated circulatory overload) E87.71
Taenia (infection) (infestation) B68.9
  diminuta B71.0
  echinococcal infestation B67.90
  mediocanellata B68.1
  nana B71.0
  saginata B68.1
  solium (intestinal form) B68.0
    larval form — *see* Cysticercosis
Taeniasis (intestine) — *see* Taenia
Tag (hypertrophied skin) (infected) L91.8
  adenoid J35.8
  anus K64.4
  hemorrhoidal K64.4
  hymen N89.8
  perineal N90.89
  preauricular Q17.0
  sentinel K64.4
  skin L91.8
    accessory (congenital) Q82.8
    anus K64.4
    congenital Q82.8
    preauricular Q17.0
  tonsil J35.8
  urethra, urethral N36.8
  vulva N90.89
Tahyna fever B33.8
Takahara's disease E80.3
Takayasu's disease or syndrome M31.4
Talcosis (pulmonary) J62.0
Talipes (congenital) Q66.89
  acquired, planus — *see* Deformity, limb, flat foot
  asymmetric Q66.89
  calcaneovalgus Q66.4
  calcaneovarus Q66.1
  calcaneus Q66.89
  cavus Q66.7
  equinovalgus Q66.6
  equinovarus Q66.0
  equinus Q66.89
  percavus Q66.7
  planovalgus Q66.6
  planus (acquired) (any degree) (*see also* Deformity, limb, flat foot)
    congenital Q66.5- ☑
    due to rickets (sequelae) E64.3
  valgus Q66.6
  varus Q66.3
Tall stature, constitutional E34.4
Talma's disease M62.89
Talon noir S90.3- ☑
  hand S60.22- ☑
  heel S90.3- ☑
  toe S90.1- ☑
Tamponade, heart I31.4
Tanapox (virus disease) B08.71
Tangier disease E78.6
Tantrum, child problem F91.8
Tapeworm (infection) (infestation) — *see* Infestation, tapeworm
Tapia's syndrome G52.7
TAR (thrombocytopenia with absent radius) **syndrome** Q87.2
Tarral-Besnier disease L44.0
Tarsal tunnel syndrome — *see* Syndrome, tarsal tunnel
Tarsalgia — *see* Pain, limb, lower
Tarsitis (eyelid) H01.8
  syphilitic A52.71
  tuberculous A18.4
Tartar (teeth) (dental calculus) K03.6
Tattoo (mark) L81.8
Tauri's disease E74.09
Taurodontism K00.2
Taussig-Bing syndrome Q20.1
Taybi's syndrome Q87.2
Tay-Sachs amaurotic familial idiocy or disease E75.02
TBI (traumatic brain injury) — *see* category S06 ☑
Teacher's node or nodule J38.2
Tear, torn (traumatic) (*see also* Laceration)
  with abortion — *see* Abortion
  annular fibrosis M51.35
  anus, anal (sphincter) S31.831 ☑

Tear, torn — *continued*
  anus, anal — *continued*
    complicating delivery
      with third degree perineal laceration O70.2
        with mucosa O70.3
      without third degree perineal laceration O70.4
    nontraumatic (healed) (old) K62.81
  articular cartilage, old — *see* Derangement, joint, articular cartilage, by site
  bladder
    with ectopic or molar pregnancy O08.6
    following ectopic or molar pregnancy O08.6
    obstetrical O71.5
    traumatic — *see* Injury, bladder
  bowel
    with ectopic or molar pregnancy O08.6
    following ectopic or molar pregnancy O08.6
    obstetrical trauma O71.5
  broad ligament
    with ectopic or molar pregnancy O08.6
    following ectopic or molar pregnancy O08.6
    obstetrical trauma O71.6
  bucket handle (knee) (meniscus) — *see* Tear, meniscus
  capsule, joint — *see* Sprain
  cartilage (*see also* Sprain)
    articular, old — *see* Derangement, joint, articular cartilage, by site
  cervix
    with ectopic or molar pregnancy O08.6
    following ectopic or molar pregnancy O08.6
    obstetrical trauma (current) O71.3
    old N88.1
    traumatic — *see* Injury, uterus
  dural G97.41
    nontraumatic G96.11
  internal organ — *see* Injury, by site
  knee cartilage
    articular (current) S83.3- ☑
    old — *see* Derangement, knee, meniscus, due to old tear
  ligament — *see* Sprain
  meniscus (knee) (current injury) S83.209 ☑
    bucket-handle S83.20- ☑
    lateral
      bucket-handle S83.25- ☑
      complex S83.27- ☑
      peripheral S83.26- ☑
      specified type NEC S83.28- ☑
    medial
      bucket-handle S83.21- ☑
      complex S83.23- ☑
      peripheral S83.22- ☑
      specified type NEC S83.24- ☑
    old — *see* Derangement, knee, meniscus, due to old tear
    site other than knee — *code as* Sprain
    specified type NEC S83.20- ☑
  muscle — *see* Strain
  pelvic
    floor, complicating delivery O70.1
    organ NEC, obstetrical trauma O71.5
      with ectopic or molar pregnancy O08.6
      following ectopic or molar pregnancy O08.6
  perineal, secondary O90.1
  periurethral tissue, obstetrical trauma O71.82
    with ectopic or molar pregnancy O08.6
    following ectopic or molar pregnancy O08.6
  rectovaginal septum — *see* Laceration, vagina
  retina, retinal (without detachment) (horseshoe) (*see also* Break, retina, horseshoe)
    with detachment — *see* Detachment, retina, with retinal, break
  rotator cuff (nontraumatic) M75.10- ☑
    complete M75.12- ☑
    incomplete M75.11- ☑
    traumatic S46.01- ☑
    capsule S43.42- ☑
  semilunar cartilage, knee — *see* Tear, meniscus
  supraspinatus (complete) (incomplete) (nontraumatic) (*see also* Tear, rotator cuff) M75.10- ☑
  tendon — *see* Strain
  tentorial, at birth P10.4

☑ **Additional Character Required** — Refer to the Tabular List for Character Selection   ▽ Subterms under main terms may continue to next column or page

Tear, torn — *continued*
  umbilical cord
    complicating delivery O69.89 ☑
  urethra
    with ectopic or molar pregnancy O08.6
    following ectopic or molar pregnancy O08.6
    obstetrical trauma O71.5
  uterus — *see* Injury, uterus
  vagina — *see* Laceration, vagina
  vessel, from catheter — *see* Puncture, accidental complicating surgery
  vulva, complicating delivery O70.0
Tear-stone — *see* Dacryolith
Teeth (*see also* condition)
  grinding
    psychogenic F45.8
    sleep related G47.63
Teething (syndrome) K00.7
Telangiectasia, telangiectasis (verrucous) I78.1
  ataxic (cerebellar) (Louis-Bar) G11.3
  familial I78.0
  hemorrhagic, hereditary (congenital) (senile) I78.0
  hereditary, hemorrhagic (congenital) (senile) I78.0
  juxtafoveal H35.07- ☑
  macular H35.07- ☑
  parafoveal H35.07- ☑
  retinal (idiopathic) (juxtafoveal) (macular) (parafoveal) H35.07- ☑
  spider I78.1
Telephone scatologia F65.89
Telescoped bowel or intestine K56.1
  congenital Q43.8
Temperature
  body, high (of unknown origin) R50.9
  cold, trauma from T69.9 ☑
    newborn P80.0
    specified effect NEC T69.8 ☑
Temple — *see* condition
Temporal — *see* condition
Temporomandibular joint pain-dysfunction syndrome M26.62
Temporosphenoidal — *see* condition
Tendency
  bleeding — *see* Defect, coagulation
  suicide
    meaning personal history of attempted suicide Z91.5
    meaning suicidal ideation — *see* Ideation, suicidal
  to fall R29.6
Tenderness, abdominal R10.819
  epigastric R10.816
  generalized R10.817
  left lower quadrant R10.814
  left upper quadrant R10.812
  periumbilic R10.815
  rebound R10.829
    epigastric R10.826
    generalized R10.827
    left lower quadrant R10.824
    left upper quadrant R10.822
    periumbilic R10.825
    right lower quadrant R10.823
    right upper quadrant R10.821
  right lower quadrant R10.813
  right upper quadrant R10.811
Tendinitis, tendonitis (*see also* Enthesopathy)
  Achilles M76.6- ☑
  adhesive — *see* Tenosynovitis, specified type NEC
    shoulder — *see* Capsulitis, adhesive
  bicipital M75.2- ☑
  calcific M65.2- ☑
    ankle M65.27- ☑
    foot M65.27- ☑
    forearm M65.23- ☑
    hand M65.24- ☑
    lower leg M65.26- ☑
    multiple sites M65.29
    pelvic region M65.25- ☑
    shoulder M75.3- ☑
    specified site NEC M65.28
    thigh M65.25- ☑
    upper arm M65.22- ☑
  due to use, overuse, pressure (*see also* Disorder, soft tissue, due to use)
    specified NEC — *see* Disorder, soft tissue, due to use, specified NEC
  gluteal M76.0- ☑

Tendinitis, tendonitis — *continued*
  patellar M76.5- ☑
  peroneal M76.7- ☑
  psoas M76.1- ☑
  tibial (posterior) M76.82- ☑
    anterior M76.81- ☑
  trochanteric — *see* Bursitis, hip, trochanteric
Tendon — *see* condition
Tendosynovitis — *see* Tenosynovitis
Tenesmus (rectal) R19.8
  vesical R30.1
Tennis elbow — *see* Epicondylitis, lateral
Tenonitis (*see also* Tenosynovitis)
  eye (capsule) H05.04- ☑
Tenontosynovitis — *see* Tenosynovitis
Tenontothecitis — *see* Tenosynovitis
Tenophyte — *see* Disorder, synovium, specified type NEC
Tenosynovitis (*see also* Synovitis) M65.9
  adhesive — *see* Tenosynovitis, specified type NEC
    shoulder — *see* Capsulitis, adhesive
  bicipital (calcifying) — *see* Tendinitis, bicipital
  gonococcal A54.49
  in (due to)
    crystals M65.8- ☑
    gonorrhea A54.49
    syphilis (late) A52.78
    use, overuse, pressure (*see also* Disorder, soft tissue, due to use)
      specified NEC — *see* Disorder, soft tissue, due to use, specified NEC
  infective NEC M65.1- ☑
    ankle M65.17- ☑
    foot M65.17- ☑
    forearm M65.13- ☑
    hand M65.14- ☑
    lower leg M65.16- ☑
    multiple sites M65.19
    pelvic region M65.15- ☑
    shoulder region M65.11- ☑
    specified site NEC M65.18
    thigh M65.15- ☑
    upper arm M65.12- ☑
  radial styloid M65.4
  shoulder region M65.81- ☑
    adhesive — *see* Capsulitis, adhesive
  specified type NEC M65.88
    ankle M65.87- ☑
    foot M65.87- ☑
    forearm M65.83- ☑
    hand M65.84- ☑
    lower leg M65.86- ☑
    multiple sites M65.89
    pelvic region M65.85- ☑
    shoulder region M65.81- ☑
    specified site NEC M65.88
    thigh M65.85- ☑
    upper arm M65.82- ☑
  tuberculous — *see* Tuberculosis, tenosynovitis
Tenovaginitis — *see* Tenosynovitis
Tension
  arterial, high (*see also* Hypertension)
    without diagnosis of hypertension R03.0
  headache G44.209
    intractable G44.201
    not intractable G44.209
  nervous R45.0
  pneumothorax J93.0
  premenstrual N94.3
  state (mental) F48.9
Tentorium — *see* condition
Teratencephalus Q89.8
Teratism Q89.7
Teratoblastoma (malignant) — *see* Neoplasm, malignant, by site
Teratocarcinoma (*see also* Neoplasm, malignant, by site)
  liver C22.7
Teratoma (solid) (*see also* Neoplasm, uncertain behavior, by site)
  with embryonal carcinoma, mixed — *see* Neoplasm, malignant, by site
  with malignant transformation — *see* Neoplasm, malignant, by site
  adult (cystic) — *see* Neoplasm, benign, by site
  benign — *see* Neoplasm, benign, by site

Teratoma — *continued*
  combined with choriocarcinoma — *see* Neoplasm, malignant, by site
  cystic (adult) — *see* Neoplasm, benign, by site
  differentiated — *see* Neoplasm, benign, by site
  embryonal (*see also* Neoplasm, malignant, by site)
    liver C22.7
  immature — *see* Neoplasm, malignant, by site
  liver C22.7
    adult, benign, cystic, differentiated type or mature D13.4
  malignant (*see also* Neoplasm, malignant, by site)
    anaplastic — *see* Neoplasm, malignant, by site
    intermediate — *see* Neoplasm, malignant, by site
      specified site — *see* Neoplasm, malignant, by site
      unspecified site C62.90
    undifferentiated — *see* Neoplasm, malignant, by site
  mature — *see* Neoplasm, uncertain behavior, by site
    malignant — *see* Neoplasm, by site, malignant, by site
  ovary D27.- ☑
    embryonal, immature or malignant C56- ☑
  solid — *see* Neoplasm, uncertain behavior, by site
  testis C62.9- ☑
    adult, benign, cystic, differentiated type or mature D29.2- ☑
    scrotal C62.1- ☑
    undescended C62.0- ☑
Termination
  anomalous (*see also* Malposition, congenital)
    right pulmonary vein Q26.3
  pregnancy, elective Z33.2
Ternidens diminutus infestation B81.8
Ternidensiasis B81.8
Terror(s) night (child) F51.4
Terrorism, victim of Z65.4
Terry's syndrome H44.2- ☑
Tertiary — *see* condition
Test, tests, testing (for)
  adequacy (for dialysis)
    hemodialysis Z49.31
    peritoneal Z49.32
  blood pressure Z01.30
    abnormal reading — *see* Blood, pressure
  blood typing Z01.83
    Rh typing Z01.83
  blood-alcohol Z04.8
    positive — *see* Findings, abnormal, in blood
  blood-drug Z04.8
    positive — *see* Findings, abnormal, in blood
  cardiac pulse generator (battery) Z45.010
  fertility Z31.41
  genetic
    disease carrier status for procreative management
      female Z31.430
      male Z31.440
    male partner of patient with recurrent pregnancy loss Z31.441
    procreative management NEC
      female Z31.438
      male Z31.448
  hearing Z01.10
    with abnormal findings NEC Z01.118
  HIV (human immunodeficiency virus)
    nonconclusive (in infants) R75
    positive Z21
    seropositive Z21
  immunity status Z01.84
  intelligence NEC Z01.89
  laboratory (as part of a general medical examination) Z00.00
    with abnormal finding Z00.01
    for medicolegal reason NEC Z04.8
  male partner of patient with recurrent pregnancy loss Z31.441
  Mantoux (for tuberculosis) Z11.1
    abnormal result R76.11
  pregnancy, positive first pregnancy — *see* Pregnancy, normal, first
  procreative Z31.49
    fertility Z31.41
  skin, diagnostic
    allergy Z01.82
      special screening examination — *see* Screening, by name of disease

Test, tests, testing — *continued*
- skin, diagnostic — *continued*
  - Mantoux Z11.1
  - tuberculin Z11.1
  - specified NEC Z01.89
- tuberculin Z11.1
  - abnormal result R76.11
- vision Z01.00
  - with abnormal findings Z01.01
- Wassermann Z11.3
  - positive — *see* Serology for syphilis, positive

Testicle, testicular, testis (*see also* condition)
- feminization syndrome (*see also* Syndrome, androgen insensitivity) E34.51
- migrans Q55.29

Tetanus, tetanic (cephalic) (convulsions) A35
- with
  - abortion A34
  - ectopic or molar pregnancy O08.0
- following ectopic or molar pregnancy O08.0
- inoculation reaction (due to serum) — *see* Complications, vaccination
- neonatorum A33
- obstetrical A34
- puerperal, postpartum, childbirth A34

Tetany (due to) R29.0
- alkalosis E87.3
- associated with rickets E55.0
- convulsions R29.0
  - hysterical F44.5
- functional (hysterical) F44.5
- hyperkinetic R29.0
  - hysterical F44.5
- hyperpnea R06.4
  - hysterical F44.5
  - psychogenic F45.8
- hyperventilation (*see also* Hyperventilation) R06.4
  - hysterical F44.5
- neonatal (without calcium or magnesium deficiency) P71.3
- parathyroid (gland) E20.9
- parathyroprival E89.2
- post- (para)thyroidectomy E89.2
- postoperative E89.2
- pseudotetany R29.0
- psychogenic (conversion reaction) F44.5

Tetralogy of Fallot Q21.3
Tetraplegia (chronic) (*see also* Quadriplegia) G82.50
Thailand hemorrhagic fever A91
Thalassanemia — *see* Thalassemia
Thalassemia (anemia) (disease) D56.9
- with other hemoglobinopathy D56.8
- alpha (major) (severe) (triple gene defect) D56.0
  - minor D56.3
  - silent carrier D56.3
  - trait D56.3
- beta (severe) D56.1
  - homozygous D56.1
  - major D56.1
  - minor D56.3
  - trait D56.3
- delta-beta (homozygous) D56.2
  - minor D56.3
  - trait D56.3
- dominant D56.8
- hemoglobin
  - C D56.8
  - E-beta D56.5
- intermedia D56.1
- major D56.1
- minor D56.3
- mixed D56.8
- sickle-cell — *see* Disease, sickle-cell, thalassemia
- specified type NEC D56.8
- trait D56.3
- variants D56.8

Thanatophoric dwarfism or short stature Q77.1
Thaysen-Gee disease (nontropical sprue) K90.0
Thaysen's disease K90.0
Thecoma D27- ☑
- luteinized D27- ☑
- malignant C56- ☑
Thelarche, premature E30.8
Thelaziasis B83.8
Thelitis N61
- puerperal, postpartum or gestational — *see* Infection, nipple
Therapeutic — *see* condition

Therapy
- drug, long-term (current) (prophylactic)
  - agents affecting estrogen receptors and estrogen levels NEC Z79.818
  - anastrozole (Arimidex) Z79.811
  - antibiotics Z79.2
    - short-term use — *omit code*
  - anticoagulants Z79.01
  - anti-inflammatory Z79.1
  - antiplatelet Z79.02
  - antithrombotics Z79.02
  - aromatase inhibitors Z79.811
  - aspirin Z79.82
  - birth control pill or patch Z79.3
  - bisphosphonates Z79.83
  - contraceptive, oral Z79.3
  - drug, specified NEC Z79.899
  - estrogen receptor downregulators Z79.818
  - Evista Z79.810
  - exemestane (Aromasin) Z79.811
  - Fareston Z79.810
  - fulvestrant (Faslodex) Z79.818
  - gonadotropin-releasing hormone (GnRH) agonist Z79.818
  - goserelin acetate (Zoladex) Z79.818
  - hormone replacement (postmenopausal) Z79.890
  - insulin Z79.4
  - letrozole (Femara) Z79.811
  - leuprolide acetate (leuprorelin) (Lupron) Z79.818
  - megestrol acetate (Megace) Z79.818
  - methadone
    - for pain management Z79.891
    - maintenance therapy F11.20
  - Nolvadex Z79.810
  - opiate analgesic Z79.891
  - oral contraceptive Z79.3
  - raloxifene (Evista) Z79.810
  - selective estrogen receptor modulators (SERMs) Z79.810
  - short term — *omit code*
  - steroids
    - inhaled Z79.51
    - systemic Z79.52
  - tamoxifen (Nolvadex) Z79.810
  - toremifene (Fareston) Z79.810
Thermic — *see* condition
Thermography (abnormal) (*see also* Abnormal, diagnostic imaging) R93.8
- breast R92.8
Thermoplegia T67.0 ☑
Thesaurismosis, glycogen — *see* Disease, glycogen storage
Thiamin deficiency E51.9
- specified NEC E51.8
Thiaminic deficiency with beriberi E51.11
Thibierge-Weissenbach syndrome — *see* Sclerosis, systemic
Thickening
- bone — *see* Hypertrophy, bone
- breast N64.59
- endometrium R93.8
- epidermal L85.9
  - specified NEC L85.8
- hymen N89.6
- larynx J38.7
- nail L60.2
  - congenital Q84.5
- periosteal — *see* Hypertrophy, bone
- pleura J92.9
  - with asbestos J92.0
- skin R23.4
- subepiglottic J38.7
- tongue K14.8
- valve, heart — *see* Endocarditis
Thigh — *see* condition
Thinning vertebra — *see* Spondylopathy, specified NEC
Thirst, excessive R63.1
- due to deprivation of water T73.1 ☑
Thomsen disease G71.12
Thoracic (*see also* condition)
- kidney Q63.2
- outlet syndrome G54.0
Thoracogastroschisis (congenital) Q79.8
Thoracopagus Q89.4
Thorax — *see* condition
Thorn's syndrome N28.89
Thorson-Björck syndrome E34.0
Threadworm (infection) (infestation) B80

Threatened
- abortion O20.0
  - with subsequent abortion O03.9
- job loss, anxiety concerning Z56.2
- labor (without delivery) O47.9
  - after 37 completed weeks of gestation O47.1
  - before 37 completed weeks of gestation O47.0- ☑
- loss of job, anxiety concerning Z56.2
- miscarriage O20.0
- unemployment, anxiety concerning Z56.2
Three-day fever A93.1
Threshers' lung J67.0
Thrix annulata (congenital) Q84.1
Throat — *see* condition
Thrombasthenia (Glanzmann) (hemorrhagic) (hereditary) D69.1
Thromboangiitis I73.1
- obliterans (general) I73.1
  - cerebral I67.89
  - vessels
    - brain I67.89
    - spinal cord I67.89
Thromboarteritis — *see* Arteritis
Thromboasthenia (Glanzmann) (hemorrhagic) (hereditary) D69.1
Thrombocytasthenia (Glanzmann) D69.1
Thrombocythemia (essential) (hemorrhagic) (idiopathic) (primary) D47.3
Thrombocytopathy (dystrophic) (granulopenic) D69.1
Thrombocytopenia, thrombocytopenic D69.6
- with absent radius (TAR) Q87.2
- congenital D69.42
- dilutional D69.59
- due to
  - (massive) blood transfusion D69.59
  - drugs D69.59
  - extracorporeal circulation of blood D69.59
  - platelet alloimmunization D69.59
- essential D69.3
- heparin induced (HIT) D75.82
- hereditary D69.42
- idiopathic D69.3
- neonatal, transitory P61.0
  - due to
    - exchange transfusion P61.0
    - idiopathic maternal thrombocytopenia P61.0
    - isoimmunization P61.0
- primary NEC D69.49
  - idiopathic D69.3
- puerperal, postpartum O72.3
- secondary D69.59
- transient neonatal P61.0
Thrombocytosis, essential D47.3
- primary D47.3
Thromboembolism — *see* Embolism
Thrombopathy (Bernard-Soulier) D69.1
- constitutional D68.0
- Willebrand-Jurgens D68.0
Thrombopenia — *see* Thrombocytopenia
Thrombophilia D68.59
- primary NEC D68.59
- secondary NEC D68.69
- specified NEC D68.69
Thrombophlebitis I80.9
- antepartum O22.2- ☑
  - deep O22.3- ☑
  - superficial O22.2- ☑
- cavernous (venous) sinus G08
  - complicating pregnancy O22.5- ☑
  - nonpyogenic I67.6
- cerebral (sinus) (vein) G08
  - nonpyogenic I67.6
  - sequelae G09
- due to implanted device — *see* Complications, by site and type, specified NEC
- during or resulting from a procedure NEC T81.72 ☑
- femoral vein (superficial) I80.1- ☑
- femoropopliteal vein I80.0- ☑
- hepatic (vein) I80.8
- idiopathic, recurrent I82.1
- iliofemoral I80.1- ☑
- intracranial venous sinus (any) G08
  - nonpyogenic I67.6
  - sequelae G09
- intraspinal venous sinuses and veins G08
  - nonpyogenic G95.19
- lateral (venous) sinus G08
  - nonpyogenic I67.6

Thrombophlebitis — *continued*
leg I80.299
  superficial I80.0- ☑
longitudinal (venous) sinus G08
  nonpyogenic I67.6
lower extremity I80.299
migrans, migrating I82.1
pelvic
  with ectopic or molar pregnancy O08.0
  following ectopic or molar pregnancy O08.0
  puerperal O87.1
popliteal vein — *see* Phlebitis, leg, deep, popliteal
portal (vein) K75.1
postoperative T81.72 ☑
pregnancy — *see* Thrombophlebitis, antepartum
puerperal, postpartum, childbirth O87.0
  deep O87.1
  pelvic O87.1
  septic O86.81
  superficial O87.0
saphenous (greater) (lesser) I80.0- ☑
sinus (intracranial) G08
  nonpyogenic I67.6
specified site NEC I80.8
tibial vein I80.23- ☑

Thrombosis, thrombotic (bland) (multiple) (progressive)
  (silent) (vessel) I82.90
anal K64.5
antepartum — *see* Thrombophlebitis, antepartum
aorta, aortic I74.10
  abdominal I74.09
    saddle I74.01
  bifurcation I74.09
  saddle I74.01
  specified site NEC I74.19
  terminal I74.09
  thoracic I74.11
  valve — *see* Endocarditis, aortic
apoplexy I63.3 ☑
artery, arteries (postinfectional) I74.9
  auditory, internal — *see* Occlusion, artery, precerebral, specified NEC
  basilar — *see* Occlusion, artery, basilar
  carotid (common) (internal) — *see* Occlusion, artery, carotid
  cerebellar (anterior inferior) (posterior inferior) (superior) — *see* Occlusion, artery, cerebellar
  cerebral — *see* Occlusion, artery, cerebral
  choroidal (anterior) — *see* Occlusion, artery, cerebral, specified NEC
  communicating, posterior — *see* Occlusion, artery, cerebral, specified NEC
  coronary (*see also* Infarct, myocardium)
    not resulting in infarction I24.0
  hepatic I74.8
  hypophyseal — *see* Occlusion, artery, cerebral, specified NEC
  iliac I74.5
  limb I74.4
    lower I74.3
    upper I74.2
  meningeal, anterior or posterior — *see* Occlusion, artery, cerebral, specified NEC
  mesenteric (with gangrene) K55.0
  ophthalmic — *see* Occlusion, artery, retina
  pontine — *see* Occlusion, artery, cerebral, specified NEC
  precerebral — *see* Occlusion, artery, precerebral
  pulmonary (iatrogenic) — *see* Embolism, pulmonary
  renal N28.0
  retinal — *see* Occlusion, artery, retina
  spinal, anterior or posterior G95.11
  traumatic NEC T14.8
  vertebral — *see* Occlusion, artery, vertebral
atrium, auricular (*see also* Infarct, myocardium)
  following acute myocardial infarction (current complication) I23.6
  not resulting in infarction I24.0
basilar (artery) — *see* Occlusion, artery, basilar
brain (artery) (stem) (*see also* Occlusion, artery, cerebral)
  due to syphilis A52.05
  puerperal O99.43
  sinus — *see* Thrombosis, intracranial venous sinus
capillary I78.8

Thrombosis, thrombotic — *continued*
cardiac (*see also* Infarct, myocardium)
  not resulting in infarction I24.0
  valve — *see* Endocarditis
carotid (artery) (common) (internal) — *see* Occlusion, artery, carotid
cavernous (venous) sinus — *see* Thrombosis, intracranial venous sinus
cerebellar artery (anterior inferior) (posterior inferior) (superior) I66.3
cerebral (artery) — *see* Occlusion, artery, cerebral
cerebrovenous sinus (*see also* Thrombosis, intracranial venous sinus)
  puerperium O87.3
chronic I82.91
coronary (artery) (vein) (*see also* Infarct, myocardium)
  not resulting in infarction I24.0
corpus cavernosum N48.89
cortical I66.9
deep — *see* Embolism, vein, lower extremity
due to device, implant or graft (*see also* Complications, by site and type, specified NEC) T85.86 ☑
  arterial graft NEC T82.868 ☑
  breast (implant) T85.86 ☑
  catheter NEC T85.86 ☑
    dialysis (renal) T82.868 ☑
      intraperitoneal T85.86 ☑
    infusion NEC T82.868 ☑
      spinal (epidural) (subdural) T85.86 ☑
    urinary (indwelling) T83.86 ☑
  electronic (electrode) (pulse generator) (stimulator)
    bone T84.86 ☑
    cardiac T82.867 ☑
    nervous system (brain) (peripheral nerve) (spinal) T85.86 ☑
    urinary T83.86 ☑
  fixation, internal (orthopedic) NEC T84.86 ☑
  gastrointestinal (bile duct) (esophagus) T85.86 ☑
  genital NEC T83.86 ☑
  heart T82.867 ☑
  joint prosthesis T84.86 ☑
  ocular (corneal graft) (orbital implant) NEC T85.86 ☑
  orthopedic NEC T84.86 ☑
  specified NEC T85.86 ☑
  urinary NEC T83.86 ☑
  vascular NEC T82.868 ☑
  ventricular intracranial shunt T85.86 ☑
during the puerperium — *see* Thrombosis, puerperal
endocardial (*see also* Infarct, myocardium)
  not resulting in infarction I24.0
eye — *see* Occlusion, retina
genital organ
  female NEC N94.89
    pregnancy — *see* Thrombophlebitis, antepartum
  male N50.1
gestational — *see* Phlebopathy, gestational
heart (chamber) (*see also* Infarct, myocardium)
  not resulting in infarction I24.0
hepatic (vein) I82.0
  artery I74.8
history (of) Z86.718
intestine (with gangrene) K55.0
intracardiac NEC (apical) (atrial) (auricular) (ventricular) (old) I51.3
intracranial (arterial) I66.9
  venous sinus (any) G08
    nonpyogenic origin I67.6
    puerperium O87.3
intramural (*see also* Infarct, myocardium)
  not resulting in infarction I24.0
intraspinal venous sinuses and veins G08
  nonpyogenic G95.19
kidney (artery) N28.0
lateral (venous) sinus — *see* Thrombosis, intracranial venous sinus
leg — *see* Thrombosis, vein, lower extremity
  arterial I74.3
liver (venous) I82.0
  artery I74.8
  portal vein I81
longitudinal (venous) sinus — *see* Thrombosis, intracranial venous sinus
lower limb — *see* Thrombosis, vein, lower extremity
lung (iatrogenic) (postoperative) — *see* Embolism, pulmonary

Thrombosis, thrombotic — *continued*
meninges (brain) (arterial) I66.8
mesenteric (artery) (with gangrene) K55.0
  vein (inferior) (superior) I81
mitral I34.8
mural (*see also* Infarct, myocardium)
  due to syphilis A52.06
  not resulting in infarction I24.0
omentum (with gangrene) K55.0
ophthalmic — *see* Occlusion, retina
pampiniform plexus (male) N50.1
parietal (*see also* Infarct, myocardium)
  not resulting in infarction I24.0
penis, superficial vein N48.81
perianal venous K64.5
peripheral arteries I74.4
  upper I74.2
personal history (of) Z86.718
portal I81
  due to syphilis A52.09
puerperal, postpartum O87.0
  brain (artery) O99.43
    venous (sinus) O87.3
  cardiac O99.43
  cerebral (artery) O99.43
    venous (sinus) O87.3
  superficial O87.0
pulmonary (artery) (iatrogenic) (postoperative) (vein) — *see* Embolism, pulmonary
renal (artery) N28.0
  vein I82.3
resulting from presence of device, implant or graft — *see* Complications, by site and type, specified NEC
retina, retinal — *see* Occlusion, retina
scrotum N50.1
seminal vesicle N50.1
sigmoid (venous) sinus — *see* Thrombosis, intracranial venous sinus
sinus, intracranial (any) — *see* Thrombosis, intracranial venous sinus
specified site NEC I82.890
  chronic I82.891
spermatic cord N50.1
spinal cord (arterial) G95.11
  due to syphilis A52.09
  pyogenic origin G06.1
spleen, splenic D73.5
  artery I74.8
testis N50.1
traumatic NEC T14.8
tricuspid I07.8
tumor — *see* Neoplasm, unspecified behavior, by site
tunica vaginalis N50.1
umbilical cord (vessels), complicating delivery O69.5 ☑
vas deferens N50.1
vein (acute) I82.90
  antecubital I82.61- ☑
    chronic I82.71- ☑
  axillary I82.A1- ☑ (*following* I82.7)
    chronic I82.A2- ☑ (*following* I82.7)
  basilic I82.61- ☑
    chronic I82.71- ☑
  brachial I82.62- ☑
    chronic I82.72- ☑
  brachiocephalic (innominate) I82.290
    chronic I82.291
  cephalic I82.61- ☑
    chronic I82.71- ☑
  cerebral, nonpyogenic I67.6
  chronic I82.91
  deep (DVT) I82.40- ☑
    calf I82.4Z- ☑
      chronic I82.5Z- ☑
    lower leg I82.4Z- ☑
      chronic I82.5Z- ☑
    thigh I82.4Y- ☑
      chronic I82.5Y- ☑
    upper leg I82.4Y ☑
      chronic I82.5y--
  femoral I82.41- ☑
    chronic I82.51- ☑
  iliac (iliofemoral) I82.42- ☑
    chronic I82.52- ☑
  innominate I82.290
    chronic I82.291

Thrombosis, thrombotic — *continued*
  vein — *continued*
    internal jugular I82.C1- ☑ *(following* I82.7)
      chronic I82.C2- ☑ *(following* I82.7)
    lower extremity
      deep I82.40- ☑
        chronic I82.50- ☑
          specified NEC I82.49- ☑
            chronic NEC I82.59- ☑
      distal
        deep I82.4Z- ☑
      proximal
        deep I82.4Y- ☑
          chronic I82.5Y- ☑
      superficial I82.81- ☑
    perianal K64.5
    popliteal I82.43- ☑
      chronic I82.53- ☑
    radial I82.62- ☑
      chronic I82.72- ☑
    renal I82.3
    saphenous (greater) (lesser) I82.81- ☑
    specified NEC I82.890
      chronic NEC I82.891
    subclavian I82.B1- ☑ *(following* I82.7)
      chronic I82.B2- ☑ *(following* I82.7)
    thoracic NEC I82.290
      chronic I82.291
    tibial I82.44- ☑
      chronic I82.54- ☑
    ulnar I82.62- ☑
      chronic I82.72- ☑
    upper extremity I82.60- ☑
      chronic I82.70- ☑
      deep I82.62- ☑
        chronic I82.72- ☑
      superficial I82.61- ☑
        chronic I82.71- ☑
  vena cava
    inferior I82.220
      chronic I82.221
    superior I82.210
      chronic I82.211
  venous, perianal K64.5
  ventricle *(see also* Infarct, myocardium)
    following acute myocardial infarction (current complication) I23.6
    not resulting in infarction I24.0
Thrombus — *see* Thrombosis
Thrush *(see also* Candidiasis)
  newborn P37.5
  oral B37.0
  vaginal B37.3
Thumb *(see also* condition)
  sucking (child problem) F98.8
Thymitis E32.8
Thymoma (benign) D15.0
  malignant C37
Thymus, thymic (gland) — *see* condition
Thyrocele — *see* Goiter
Thyroglossal *(see also* condition)
  cyst Q89.2
  duct, persistent Q89.2
Thyroid (gland) (body) *(see also* condition)
  hormone resistance E07.89
  lingual Q89.2
  nodule (cystic) (nontoxic) (single) E04.1
Thyroiditis E06.9
  acute (nonsuppurative) (pyogenic) (suppurative) E06.0
  autoimmune E06.3
  chronic (nonspecific) (sclerosing) E06.5
    with thyrotoxicosis, transient E06.2
    fibrous E06.5
    lymphadenoid E06.3
    lymphocytic E06.3
    lymphoid E06.3
  de Quervain's E06.1
  drug-induced E06.4
  fibrous (chronic) E06.5
  giant-cell (follicular) E06.1
  granulomatous (de Quervain) (subacute) E06.1
  Hashimoto's (struma lymphomatosa) E06.3
  iatrogenic E06.4
  ligneous E06.5
  lymphocytic (chronic) E06.3
  lymphoid E06.3
  lymphomatous E06.3

Thyroiditis — *continued*
  nonsuppurative E06.1
  postpartum, puerperal O90.5
  pseudotuberculous E06.1
  pyogenic E06.0
  radiation E06.4
  Riedel's E06.5
  subacute (granulomatous) E06.1
  suppurative E06.0
  tuberculous A18.81
  viral E06.1
  woody E06.5
Thyrolingual duct, persistent Q89.2
Thyromegaly E01.0
Thyrotoxic
  crisis — *see* Thyrotoxicosis
  heart disease or failure *(see also* Thyrotoxicosis) E05.90 [I43]
    with thyroid storm E05.91 [I43]
  storm — *see* Thyrotoxicosis
Thyrotoxicosis (recurrent) E05.90
  with
    goiter (diffuse) E05.00
      with thyroid storm E05.01
      adenomatous uninodular E05.10
        with thyroid storm E05.11
      multinodular E05.20
        with thyroid storm E05.21
      nodular E05.20
        with thyroid storm E05.21
      uninodular E05.10
        with thyroid storm E05.11
    infiltrative
      dermopathy E05.00
        with thyroid storm E05.01
      ophthalmopathy E05.00
        with thyroid storm E05.01
    single thyroid nodule E05.10
      with thyroid storm E05.11
    thyroid storm E05.91
  due to
    ectopic thyroid nodule or tissue E05.30
      with thyroid storm E05.31
    ingestion of (excessive) thyroid material E05.40
      with thyroid storm E05.41
    overproduction of thyroid-stimulating hormone E05.80
      with thyroid storm E05.81
    specified cause NEC E05.80
      with thyroid storm E05.81
  factitia E05.40
    with thyroid storm E05.41
  heart E05.90 [I43]
    with thyroid storm E05.91 [I43]
    failure E05.90 [I43]
  neonatal (transient) P72.1
  transient with chronic thyroiditis E06.2
Tibia vara — *see* Osteochondrosis, juvenile, tibia
Tic (disorder) F95.9
  breathing F95.8
  child problem F95.0
  compulsive F95.1
  de la Tourette F95.2
  degenerative (generalized) (localized) G25.69
    facial G25.69
  disorder
    chronic
      motor F95.1
      vocal F95.1
    combined vocal and multiple motor F95.2
    transient F95.0
  douloureux G50.0
    atypical G50.1
    postherpetic, postzoster B02.22
  drug-induced G25.61
  eyelid F95.8
  habit F95.9
    chronic F95.1
    transient of childhood F95.0
  lid, transient of childhood F95.0
  motor-verbal F95.2
  occupational F48.8
  orbicularis F95.8
    transient of childhood F95.0
  organic origin G25.69
  postchoreic G25.69
  psychogenic, compulsive F95.1
  salaam R25.8

Tic — *continued*
  spasm (motor or vocal) F95.9
    chronic F95.1
    transient of childhood F95.0
  specified NEC F95.8
Tick-borne — *see* condition
Tietze's disease or syndrome M94.0
Tight, tightness
  anus K62.89
  chest R07.89
  fascia (lata) M62.89
  foreskin (congenital) N47.1
  hymen, hymenal ring N89.6
  introitus (acquired) (congenital) N89.6
  rectal sphincter K62.89
  tendon — *see* Short, tendon
  urethral sphincter N35.9
Tilting vertebra — *see* Dorsopathy, deforming, specified NEC
Timidity, child F93.8
Tinea (intersecta) (tarsi) B35.9
  amiantacea L44.8
  asbestina B35.0
  barbae B35.0
  beard B35.0
  black dot B35.0
  blanca B36.2
  capitis B35.0
  corporis B35.4
  cruris B35.6
  flava B36.0
  foot B35.3
  furfuracea B36.0
  imbricata (Tokelau) B35.5
  kerion B35.0
  manuum B35.2
  microsporic — *see* Dermatophytosis
  nigra B36.1
  nodosa — *see* Piedra
  pedis B35.3
  scalp B35.0
  specified site NEC B35.8
  sycosis B35.0
  tonsurans B35.0
  trichophytic — *see* Dermatophytosis
  unguium B35.1
  versicolor B36.0
Tingling sensation (skin) R20.2
Tin-miner's lung J63.5
Tinnitus (audible) (aurium) (subjective) — *see* subcategory H93.1 ☑
Tipped tooth (teeth) M26.33
Tipping
  pelvis M95.5
    with disproportion (fetopelvic) O33.0
      causing obstructed labor O65.0
  tooth (teeth), fully erupted M26.33
Tiredness R53.83
Tissue — *see* condition
Tobacco (nicotine)
  dependence — *see* Dependence, drug, nicotine
  harmful use Z72.0
  heart — *see* Tobacco, toxic effect
  maternal use, affecting newborn P04.2
  toxic effect — *see* Table of Drugs and Chemicals, by substance, poisoning
    chewing tobacco — *see* Table of Drugs and Chemicals, by substance, poisoning
    cigarettes — *see* Table of Drugs and Chemicals, by substance, poisoning
  use Z72.0
    complicating
      childbirth O99.334
      pregnancy O99.33- ☑
      puerperium O99.335
    counseling and surveillance Z71.6
  withdrawal state — *see* Dependence, drug, nicotine
Tocopherol deficiency E56.0
Todd's
  cirrhosis K74.3
  paralysis (postepileptic) (transitory) G83.84
Toe — *see* condition
Toilet, artificial opening — *see* Attention to, artificial, opening
Tokelau (ringworm) B35.5
Tollwut — *see* Rabies
Tommaselli's disease R31.9

Tommaselli's disease — *continued*
  correct substance properly administered — *see* Table of Drugs and Chemicals, by drug, adverse effect
  overdose or wrong substance given or taken — *see* Table of Drugs and Chemicals, by drug, poisoning
Tongue (*see also* condition)
  tie Q38.1
Tonic pupil — *see* Anomaly, pupil, function, tonic pupil
Toni-Fanconi syndrome (cystinosis) E72.09
  with cystinosis E72.04
Tonsil — *see* condition
Tonsillitis (acute) (catarrhal) (croupous) (follicular) (gangrenous) (infective) (lacunar) (lingual) (malignant) (membranous) (parenchymatous) (phlegmonous) (pseudomembranous) (purulent) (septic) (subacute) (suppurative) (toxic) (ulcerative) (vesicular) (viral) J03.90
  chronic J35.01
    with adenoiditis J35.03
  diphtheritic A36.0
  hypertrophic J35.01
    with adenoiditis J35.03
  recurrent J03.91
  specified organism NEC J03.80
    recurrent J03.81
  staphylococcal J03.80
    recurrent J03.81
  streptococcal J03.00
    recurrent J03.01
  tuberculous A15.8
  Vincent's A69.1
Tooth, teeth — *see* condition
Toothache K08.8
Topagnosis R20.8
Tophi — *see* Gout, chronic
TORCH infection — *see* Infection, congenital
  without active infection P00.2
Torn — *see* Tear
Tornwaldt's cyst or disease J39.2
Torsion
  accessory tube — *see* Torsion, fallopian tube
  adnexa (female) — *see* Torsion, fallopian tube
  aorta, acquired I77.1
  appendix epididymis N44.04
  appendix testis N44.03
  bile duct (common) (hepatic) K83.8
    congenital Q44.5
  bowel, colon or intestine K56.2
  cervix — *see* Malposition, uterus
  cystic duct K82.8
  dystonia — *see* Dystonia, torsion
  epididymis (appendix) N44.04
  fallopian tube N83.52
    with ovary N83.53
  gallbladder K82.8
    congenital Q44.1
  hydatid of Morgagni
    female N83.52
    male N44.03
  kidney (pedicle) (leading to infarction) N28.0
  Meckel's diverticulum (congenital) Q43.0
    malignant — *see* Table of Neoplasms, small intestine, malignant
  mesentery K56.2
  omentum K56.2
  organ or site, congenital NEC — *see* Anomaly, by site
  ovary (pedicle) N83.51
    with fallopian tube N83.53
    congenital Q50.2
  oviduct — *see* Torsion, fallopian tube
  penis (acquired) N48.82
    congenital Q55.63
  spasm — *see* Dystonia, torsion
  spermatic cord N44.02
    extravaginal N44.01
    intravaginal N44.02
  spleen D73.5
  testis, testicle N44.00
    appendix N44.03
  tibia — *see* Deformity, limb, specified type NEC, lower leg
  uterus — *see* Malposition, uterus
Torticollis (intermittent) (spastic) M43.6
  congenital (sternomastoid) Q68.0
  due to birth injury P15.8
  hysterical F44.4
  ocular R29.891

Torticollis — *continued*
  psychogenic F45.8
    conversion reaction F44.4
  rheumatic M43.6
  rheumatoid M06.88
  spasmodic G24.3
  traumatic, current S13.4 ☑
Tortipelvis G24.1
Tortuous
  artery I77.1
  organ or site, congenital NEC — *see* Distortion
  retinal vessel, congenital Q14.1
  ureter N13.8
  urethra N36.8
  vein — *see* Varix
Torture, victim of Z65.4
Torula, torular (histolytica) (infection) — *see* Cryptococcosis
Torulosis — *see* Cryptococcosis
Torus (mandibularis) (palatinus) M27.0
  fracture — *see* Fracture, by site, torus
Touraine's syndrome Q79.8
Tourette's syndrome F95.2
Tourniquet syndrome — *see* Constriction, external, by site
Tower skull Q75.0
  with exophthalmos Q87.0
Toxemia R68.89
  bacterial — *see* Sepsis
  burn — *see* Burn
  eclamptic (with pre-existing hypertension) — *see* Eclampsia
  erysipelatous — *see* Erysipelas
  fatigue R68.89
  food — *see* Poisoning, food
  gastrointestinal K52.1
  intestinal K52.1
  kidney — *see* Uremia
  malarial — *see* Malaria
  myocardial — *see* Myocarditis, toxic
  of pregnancy — *see* Pre-eclampsia
  pre-eclamptic — *see* Pre-eclampsia
  small intestine K52.1
  staphylococcal, due to food A05.0
  stasis R68.89
  uremic — *see* Uremia
  urinary — *see* Uremia
Toxemica cerebropathia psychica (nonalcoholic) F04
  alcoholic — *see* Alcohol, amnestic disorder
Toxic (poisoning) (*see also* condition) T65.91 ☑
  effect — *see* Table of Drugs and Chemicals, by substance, poisoning
  shock syndrome A48.3
  thyroid (gland) — *see* Thyrotoxicosis
Toxicemia — *see* Toxemia
Toxicity — *see* Table of Drugs and Chemicals, by substance, poisoning
  fava bean D55.0
  food, noxious — *see* Poisoning, food
  from drug or nonmedicinal substance — *see* Table of Drugs and Chemicals, by drug
Toxicosis (*see also* Toxemia)
  capillary, hemorrhagic D69.0
Toxinfection, gastrointestinal K52.1
Toxocariasis B83.0
Toxoplasma, toxoplasmosis (acquired) B58.9
  with
    hepatitis B58.1
    meningoencephalitis B58.2
    ocular involvement B58.00
    other organ involvement B58.89
    pneumonia, pneumonitis B58.3
  congenital (acute) (subacute) (chronic) P37.1
  maternal, manifest toxoplasmosis in infant (acute) (subacute) (chronic) P37.1
tPA (rtPA) **administration in a different facility within the last 24 hours prior to admission to current facility** Z92.82
Trabeculation, bladder N32.89
Trachea — *see* condition
Tracheitis (catarrhal) (infantile) (membranous) (plastic) (septal) (suppurative) (viral) J04.10
  with
    bronchitis (15 years of age and above) J40
      acute or subacute — *see* Bronchitis, acute
      chronic J42
      tuberculous NEC A15.5

Tracheitis — *continued*
  with — *continued*
    bronchitis — *continued*
      under 15 years of age J20.9
    laryngitis (acute) J04.2
      chronic J37.1
      tuberculous NEC A15.5
  acute J04.10
    with obstruction J04.11
  chronic J42
    with
      bronchitis (chronic) J42
      laryngitis (chronic) J37.1
  diphtheritic (membranous) A36.89
  due to external agent — *see* Inflammation, respiratory, upper, due to
  syphilitic A52.73
  tuberculous A15.5
Trachelitis (nonvenereal) — *see* Cervicitis
Tracheobronchial — *see* condition
Tracheobronchitis (15 years of age and above) (*see also* Bronchitis)
  due to
    Bordetella bronchiseptica A37.80
      with pneumonia A37.81
    Francisella tularensis A21.8
Tracheobronchomegaly Q32.4
  with bronchiectasis J47.9
    with
      exacerbation (acute) J47.1
      lower respiratory infection J47.0
  acquired J98.09
    with bronchiectasis J47.9
      with
        exacerbation (acute) J47.1
        lower respiratory infection J47.0
Tracheobronchopneumonitis — *see* Pneumonia, broncho-
Tracheocele (external) (internal) J39.8
  congenital Q32.1
Tracheomalacia J39.8
  congenital Q32.0
Tracheopharyngitis (acute) J06.9
  chronic J42
  due to external agent — *see* Inflammation, respiratory, upper, due to
Tracheostenosis J39.8
Tracheostomy
  complication — *see* Complication, tracheostomy
  status Z93.0
    attention to Z43.0
    malfunctioning J95.03
Trachoma, trachomatous A71.9
  active (stage) A71.1
  contraction of conjunctiva A71.1
  dubium A71.0
  healed or sequelae B94.0
  initial (stage) A71.0
  pannus A71.1
  Türck's J37.0
Traction, vitreomacular H43.82- ☑
Train sickness T75.3 ☑
Trait(s)
  Hb-S D57.3
  hemoglobin
    abnormal NEC D58.2
      with thalassemia D56.3
    C — *see* Disease, hemoglobin C
    S (Hb-S) D57.3
  Lepore D56.3
  personality, accentuated Z73.1
  sickle-cell D57.3
    with elliptocytosis or spherocytosis D57.3
  type A personality Z73.1
Tramp Z59.0
Trance R41.89
  hysterical F44.89
Transaminasemia R74.0
Transection
  abdomen (partial) S38.3 ☑
  aorta (incomplete) (*see also* Injury, aorta)
    complete — *see* Injury, aorta, laceration, major
  carotid artery (incomplete) (*see also* Injury, blood vessel, carotid, laceration)
    complete — *see* Injury, blood vessel, carotid, laceration, major
  celiac artery (incomplete) S35.211 ☑

Transection — *continued*
  celiac artery — *continued*
    branch (incomplete) S35.291 ☑
      complete S35.292 ☑
    complete S35.212 ☑
  innominate
    artery (incomplete) (*see also* Injury, blood vessel,
      thoracic, innominate, artery, laceration)
      complete — *see* Injury, blood vessel, thoracic,
        innominate, artery, laceration, major
    vein (incomplete) (*see also* Injury, blood vessel,
      thoracic, innominate, vein, laceration)
      complete — *see* Injury, blood vessel, thoracic,
        innominate, vein, laceration, major
  jugular vein (external) (incomplete) (*see also* Injury,
    blood vessel, jugular vein, laceration)
    complete — *see* Injury, blood vessel, jugular vein,
      laceration, major
    internal (incomplete) (*see also* Injury, blood vessel,
      jugular vein, internal, laceration)
      complete — *see* Injury, blood vessel, jugular
        vein, internal, laceration, major
  mesenteric artery (incomplete) (*see also* Injury,
    mesenteric, artery, laceration)
    complete — *see* Injury, mesenteric artery, lacera-
      tion, major
  pulmonary vessel (incomplete) (*see also* Injury, blood
    vessel, thoracic, pulmonary, laceration)
    complete — *see* Injury, blood vessel, thoracic,
      pulmonary, laceration, major
  subclavian — *see* Transection, innominate
  vena cava (incomplete) (*see also* Injury, vena cava)
    complete — *see* Injury, vena cava, laceration, major
  vertebral artery (incomplete) (*see also* Injury, blood
    vessel, vertebral, laceration)
    complete — *see* Injury, blood vessel, vertebral,
      laceration, major
Transfusion
  associated (red blood cell) hemochromatosis E83.111
  blood
    ABO incompatible — *see* Complication(s), transfu-
      sion, incompatibility reaction, ABO
    minor blood group (Duffy) (E) (K(ell)) (Kidd) (Lewis)
      (M) (N) (P) (S) T80.89 ☑
    reaction or complication — *see* Complications,
      transfusion
  fetomaternal (mother) — *see* Pregnancy, complicated
    by, placenta, transfusion syndrome
  maternofetal (mother) — *see* Pregnancy, complicated
    by, placenta, transfusion syndrome
  placental (syndrome) (mother) — *see* Pregnancy,
    complicated by, placenta, transfusion syndrome
  reaction (adverse) — *see* Complications, transfusion
  related acute lung injury (TRALI) J95.84
  twin-to-twin — *see* Pregnancy, complicated by, pla-
    centa, transfusion syndrome, fetus to fetus
Transient (meaning homeless) (*see also* condition) Z59.0
Translocation
  balanced autosomal Q95.9
    in normal individual Q95.0
  chromosomes NEC Q99.8
    balanced and insertion in normal individual Q95.0
  Down syndrome Q90.2
  trisomy
    13 Q91.6
    18 Q91.2
    21 Q90.2
Translucency, iris — *see* Degeneration, iris
**Transmission of chemical substances through the
  placenta** — *see* Absorption, chemical, through
  placenta
Transparency, lung, unilateral J43.0
Transplant (ed) (status) Z94.9
  awaiting organ Z76.82
  bone Z94.6
    marrow Z94.81
  candidate Z76.82
  complication — *see* Complication, transplant
  cornea Z94.7
  heart Z94.1
    and lung(s) Z94.3
    valve Z95.2
      prosthetic Z95.2
      specified NEC Z95.4
      xenogenic Z95.3
  intestine Z94.82
  kidney Z94.0

Transplant — *continued*
  liver Z94.4
  lung(s) Z94.2
    and heart Z94.3
  organ (failure) (infection) (rejection) Z94.9
    removal status Z98.85
  pancreas Z94.83
  skin Z94.5
  social Z60.3
  specified organ or tissue NEC Z94.89
  stem cells Z94.84
  tissue Z94.9
Transplants, ovarian, endometrial N80.1
Transposed — *see* Transposition
Transposition (congenital) (*see also* Malposition, congenital)
  abdominal viscera Q89.3
  aorta (dextra) Q20.3
  appendix Q43.8
  colon Q43.8
  corrected Q20.5
  great vessels (complete) (partial) Q20.3
  heart Q24.0
    with complete transposition of viscera Q89.3
  intestine (large) (small) Q43.8
  reversed jejunal (for bypass) (status) Z98.0
  scrotum Q55.23
  stomach Q40.2
    with general transposition of viscera Q89.3
  tooth, teeth, fully erupted M26.30
  vessels, great (complete) (partial) Q20.3
  viscera (abdominal) (thoracic) Q89.3
Transsexualism F64.1
Transverse (*see also* condition)
  arrest (deep), in labor O64.0 ☑
  lie (mother) O32.2 ☑
    causing obstructed labor O64.8 ☑
Transvestism, transvestitism (dual-role) F64.1
  fetishistic F65.1
Trapped placenta (with hemorrhage) O72.0
  without hemorrhage O73.0
Trauma, traumatism (*see also* Injury)
  acoustic — *see* subcategory H83.3 ☑
  birth — *see* Birth, injury
  complicating ectopic or molar pregnancy O08.6
  during delivery O71.9
  following ectopic or molar pregnancy O08.6
  obstetric O71.9
    specified NEC O71.89
Traumatic (*see also* condition)
  brain injury — *see* category S06 ☑
Treacher Collins syndrome Q75.4
Treitz's hernia — *see* Hernia, abdomen, specified site
  NEC
Trematode infestation — *see* Infestation, fluke
Trematodiasis — *see* Infestation, fluke
Trembling paralysis — *see* Parkinsonism
Tremor(s) R25.1
  drug induced G25.1
  essential (benign) G25.0
  familial G25.0
  hereditary G25.0
  hysterical F44.4
  intention G25.2
  medication induced postural G25.1
  mercurial — *see* subcategory T56.1 ☑
  Parkinson's — *see* Parkinsonism
  psychogenic (conversion reaction) F44.4
  senilis R54
  specified type NEC G25.2
Trench
  fever A79.0
  foot — *see* Immersion, foot
  mouth A69.1
Treponema pallidum infection — *see* Syphilis
Treponematosis
  due to
    T. pallidum — *see* Syphilis
    T. pertenue — *see* Yaws
Triad
  Hutchinson's (congenital syphilis) A50.53
  Kartagener's Q89.3
  Saint's — *see* Hernia, diaphragm
Trichiasis (eyelid) H02.059
  with entropion — *see* Entropion
  left H02.056
    lower H02.055

Trichiasis — *continued*
  left — *continued*
    upper H02.054
  right H02.053
    lower H02.052
    upper H02.051
Trichinella spiralis (infection) (infestation) B75
Trichinellosis, trichiniasis, trichinelliasis, trichinosis
  B75
  with muscle disorder B75 [M63.80]
    ankle B75 [M63.87-] ☑
    foot B75 [M63.87-] ☑
    forearm B75 [M63.83-] ☑
    hand B75 [M63.84-] ☑
    lower leg B75 [M63.86-] ☑
    multiple sites B75 [M63.89]
    pelvic region B75 [M63.85-] ☑
    shoulder region B75 [M63.81-] ☑
    specified site NEC B75 [M63.88]
    thigh B75 [M63.85-] ☑
    upper arm B75 [M63.82-] ☑
Trichobezoar T18.9 ☑
  intestine T18.3 ☑
  stomach T18.2 ☑
Trichocephaliasis, trichocephalosis B79
Trichocephalus infestation B79
Trichoclasis L67.8
Trichoepithelioma (*see also* Neoplasm, skin, benign)
  malignant — *see* Neoplasm, skin, malignant
Trichofolliculoma — *see* Neoplasm, skin, benign
Tricholemmoma — *see* Neoplasm, skin, benign
Trichomoniasis A59.9
  bladder A59.03
  cervix A59.09
  intestinal A07.8
  prostate A59.02
  seminal vesicles A59.09
  specified site NEC A59.8
  urethra A59.03
  urogenitalis A59.00
  vagina A59.01
  vulva A59.01
Trichomycosis
  axillaris A48.8
  nodosa, nodularis B36.8
Trichonodosis L67.8
Trichophytid, trichophyton infection — *see* Dermato-
  phytosis
Trichophytobezoar T18.9 ☑
  intestine T18.3 ☑
  stomach T18.2 ☑
Trichophytosis — *see* Dermatophytosis
Trichoptilosis L67.8
Trichorrhexis (nodosa) (invaginata) L67.0
Trichosis axillaris A48.8
Trichosporosis nodosa B36.2
Trichostasis spinulosa (congenital) Q84.1
Trichostrongyliasis, trichostrongylosis (small intes-
  tine) B81.2
Trichostrongylus infection B81.2
Trichotillomania F63.3
Trichromat, trichromatopsia, anomalous (congenital)
  H53.55
Trichuriasis B79
Trichuris trichiura (infection) (infestation) (any site) B79
Tricuspid (valve) — *see* condition
Trifid (*see also* Accessory)
  kidney (pelvis) Q63.8
  tongue Q38.3
Trigeminal neuralgia — *see* Neuralgia, trigeminal
Trigeminy R00.8
Trigger finger (acquired) M65.30
  congenital Q74.0
  index finger M65.32- ☑
  little finger M65.35- ☑
  middle finger M65.33- ☑
  ring finger M65.34- ☑
  thumb M65.31- ☑
Trigonitis (bladder) (chronic) (pseudomembranous)
  N30.30
  with hematuria N30.31
Trigonocephaly Q75.0
Trilocular heart — *see* Cor triloculare
Trimethylaminuria E72.52
Tripartite placenta O43.19- ☑
Triphalangeal thumb Q74.0

☑ Additional Character Required — Refer to the Tabular List for Character Selection   ▽ Subterms under main terms may continue to next column or page

Index

Tuberculosis, tubercular, tuberculous — Tuberculosis, tubercular, tuberculous

Tuberculosis, tubercular, tuberculous — *continued*
ear — *continued*
    skin (primary) A18.4
elbow A18.02
emphysema — *see* Tuberculosis, pulmonary
empyema A15.6
encephalitis A17.82
endarteritis A18.89
endocarditis A18.84
    aortic A18.84
    mitral A18.84
    pulmonary A18.84
    tricuspid A18.84
endocrine glands NEC A18.82
endometrium A18.17
enteric, enterica, enteritis A18.32
enterocolitis A18.32
epididymis, epididymitis A18.15
epidural abscess (cerebral) (spinal) A17.81
epiglottis A15.5
episcleritis A18.51
erythema (induratum) (nodosum) (primary) A18.4
esophagus A18.83
eustachian tube A18.6
exposure (to) Z20.1
exudative — *see* Tuberculosis, pulmonary
eye A18.50
eyelid (primary) (lupus) A18.4
fallopian tube (acute) (chronic) A18.17
fascia A18.09
fauces A15.8
female pelvic inflammatory disease A18.17
finger A18.03
first infection A15.7
gallbladder A18.83
ganglion A18.09
gastritis A18.83
gastrocolic fistula A18.32
gastroenteritis A18.32
gastrointestinal tract A18.32
general, generalized — *see* Tuberculosis, miliary
genital organs A18.10
genitourinary A18.10
genu A18.02
glandula suprarenalis A18.7
glandular, general A18.2
glottis A15.5
grinder's J65
gum A18.83
hand A18.03
heart A18.84
hematogenous — *see* Tuberculosis, miliary
hemoptysis — *see* Tuberculosis, pulmonary
hemorrhage NEC — *see* Tuberculosis, pulmonary
hemothorax A15.6
hepatitis A18.83
hilar lymph nodes A15.4
    primary (progressive) A15.7
hip (joint) (disease) (bone) A18.02
hydropneumothorax A15.6
hydrothorax A15.6
hypoadrenalism A18.7
hypopharynx A15.8
ileocecal (hyperplastic) A18.32
ileocolitis A18.32
ileum A18.32
iliac spine (superior) A18.03
immunological findings only A15.7
indurativa (primary) A18.4
infantile A15.7
infection A15.9
    without clinical manifestations A15.7
infraclavicular gland A18.2
inguinal gland A18.2
inguinalis A18.2
intestine (any part) A18.32
iridocyclitis A18.54
iris, iritis A18.54
ischiorectal A18.32
jaw A18.03
jejunum A18.32
joint A18.02
    vertebral A18.01
keratitis (interstitial) A18.52
keratoconjunctivitis A18.52
kidney A18.11
knee (joint) A18.02
kyphosis, kyphoscoliosis A18.01

Tuberculosis, tubercular, tuberculous — *continued*
laryngitis A15.5
larynx A15.5
latent R76.11
leptomeninges, leptomeningitis (cerebral) (spinal)
    A17.0
lichenoides (primary) A18.4
linguae A18.83
lip A18.83
liver A18.83
lordosis A18.01
lung — *see* Tuberculosis, pulmonary
lupus vulgaris A18.4
lymph gland or node (peripheral) A18.2
    abdomen A18.39
    bronchial A15.4
        primary (progressive) A15.7
    cervical A18.2
    hilar A15.4
        primary (progressive) A15.7
    intrathoracic A15.4
        primary (progressive) A15.7
    mediastinal A15.4
        primary (progressive) A15.7
    mesenteric A18.39
    retroperitoneal A18.39
    tracheobronchial A15.4
        primary (progressive) A15.7
lymphadenitis — *see* Tuberculosis, lymph gland
lymphangitis — *see* Tuberculosis, lymph gland
lymphatic (gland) (vessel) — *see* Tuberculosis, lymph
    gland
mammary gland A18.89
marasmus A15.9
mastoiditis A18.03
mediastinal lymph gland or node A15.4
    primary (progressive) A15.7
mediastinitis A15.8
    primary (progressive) A15.7
mediastinum A15.8
    primary (progressive) A15.7
medulla A17.81
melanosis, Addisonian A18.7
meninges, meningitis (basilar) (cerebral) (cere-
    brospinal) (spinal) A17.0
meningoencephalitis A17.82
mesentery, mesenteric (gland or node) A18.39
miliary A19.9
    acute A19.2
        multiple sites A19.1
        single specified site A19.0
    chronic A19.8
    specified NEC A19.8
millstone makers' J65
miner's J65
molder's J65
mouth A18.83
multiple A19.9
    acute A19.1
    chronic A19.8
muscle A18.09
myelitis A17.82
myocardium, myocarditis A18.84
nasal (passage) (sinus) A15.8
nasopharynx A15.8
neck gland A18.2
nephritis A18.11
nerve (mononeuropathy) A17.83
nervous system A17.9
nose (septum) A15.8
ocular A18.50
omentum A18.31
oophoritis (acute) (chronic) A18.17
optic (nerve trunk) (papilla) A18.59
orbit A18.59
orchitis A18.15
organ, specified NEC A18.89
osseous — *see* Tuberculosis, bone
osteitis — *see* Tuberculosis, bone
osteomyelitis — *see* Tuberculosis, bone
otitis media A18.6
ovary, ovaritis (acute) (chronic) A18.17
oviduct (acute) (chronic) A18.17
pachymeningitis A17.0
palate (soft) A18.83
pancreas A18.83
papulonecrotic (a) (primary) A18.4
parathyroid glands A18.82

Tuberculosis, tubercular, tuberculous — *continued*
paronychia (primary) A18.4
parotid gland or region A18.83
pelvis (bony) A18.03
penis A18.15
peribronchitis A15.5
pericardium, pericarditis A18.84
perichondritis, larynx A15.5
periostitis — *see* Tuberculosis, bone
perirectal fistula A18.32
peritoneum NEC A18.31
peritonitis A18.31
pharynx, pharyngitis A15.8
phlyctenulosis (keratoconjunctivitis) A18.52
phthisis NEC — *see* Tuberculosis, pulmonary
pituitary gland A18.82
pleura, pleural, pleurisy, pleuritis (fibrinous) (oblitera-
    tive) (purulent) (simple plastic) (with effusion)
    A15.6
    primary (progressive) A15.7
pneumonia, pneumonic — *see* Tuberculosis, pul-
    monary
pneumothorax (spontaneous) (tense valvular) — *see*
    Tuberculosis, pulmonary
polyneuropathy A17.89
polyserositis A19.9
    acute A19.1
    chronic A19.8
potter's J65
prepuce A18.15
primary (complex) A15.7
proctitis A18.32
prostate, prostatitis A18.14
pulmonalis — *see* Tuberculosis, pulmonary
pulmonary (cavitated) (fibrotic) (infiltrative) (nodular)
    A15.0
    childhood type or first infection A15.7
    primary (complex) A15.7
pyelitis A18.11
pyelonephritis A18.11
pyemia — *see* Tuberculosis, miliary
pyonephrosis A18.11
pyopneumothorax A15.6
pyothorax A15.6
rectum (fistula) (with abscess) A18.32
reinfection stage — *see* Tuberculosis, pulmonary
renal A18.11
renis A18.11
respiratory A15.9
    primary A15.7
    specified site NEC A15.8
retina, retinitis A18.53
retroperitoneal (lymph gland or node) A18.39
rheumatism NEC A18.09
rhinitis A15.8
sacroiliac (joint) A18.01
sacrum A18.01
salivary gland A18.83
salpingitis (acute) (chronic) A18.17
sandblaster's J65
sclera A18.51
scoliosis A18.01
scrofulous A18.2
scrotum A18.15
seminal tract or vesicle A18.15
senile A15.9
septic — *see* Tuberculosis, miliary
shoulder (joint) A18.02
    blade A18.03
sigmoid A18.32
sinus (any nasal) A15.8
    bone A18.03
    epididymis A18.15
skeletal NEC A18.03
skin (any site) (primary) A18.4
small intestine A18.32
soft palate A18.83
spermatic cord A18.15
spine, spinal (column) A18.01
    cord A17.81
    medulla A17.81
    membrane A17.0
    meninges A17.0
spleen, splenitis A18.85
spondylitis A18.01
sternoclavicular joint A18.02
stomach A18.83
stonemason's J65

☑ **Additional Character Required** — Refer to the Tabular List for Character Selection   ▽ Subterms under main terms may continue to next column or page

Tuberculosis, tubercular, tuberculous — *continued*
  subcutaneous tissue (cellular) (primary) A18.4
  subcutis (primary) A18.4
  subdeltoid bursa A18.83
  submaxillary (region) A18.83
  supraclavicular gland A18.2
  suprarenal (capsule) (gland) A18.7
  swelling, joint (*see also* category M01) (*see also* Tuberculosis, joint) A18.02
  symphysis pubis A18.02
  synovitis A18.09
    articular A18.02
    spine or vertebra A18.01
  systemic — *see* Tuberculosis, miliary
  tarsitis A18.4
  tendon (sheath) — *see* Tuberculosis, tenosynovitis
  tenosynovitis A18.09
    spine or vertebra A18.01
  testis A18.15
  throat A15.8
  thymus gland A18.82
  thyroid gland A18.81
  tongue A18.83
  tonsil, tonsillitis A15.8
  trachea, tracheal A15.5
    lymph gland or node A15.4
      primary (progressive) A15.7
  tracheobronchial A15.5
    lymph gland or node A15.4
      primary (progressive) A15.7
  tubal (acute) (chronic) A18.17
  tunica vaginalis A18.15
  ulcer (skin) (primary) A18.4
    bowel or intestine A18.32
    specified NEC — *see* Tuberculosis, by site
  unspecified site A15.9
  ureter A18.11
  urethra, urethral (gland) A18.13
  urinary organ or tract A18.13
  uterus A18.17
  uveal tract A18.54
  uvula A18.83
  vagina A18.18
  vas deferens A18.15
  verruca, verrucosa (cutis) (primary) A18.4
  vertebra (column) A18.01
  vesiculitis A18.15
  vulva A18.18
  wrist (joint) A18.02
Tuberculum
  Carabelli — *see* Excludes Note at K00.2
  occlusal — *see* Excludes Note at K00.2
  paramolare K00.2
Tuberosity, enitre maxillary M26.07
Tuberous sclerosis (brain) Q85.1
Tubo-ovarian — *see* condition
Tuboplasty, after previous sterilization Z31.0
  aftercare Z31.42
Tubotympanitis, catarrhal (chronic) — *see* Otitis, media, nonsuppurative, chronic, serous
Tularemia A21.9
  with
    conjunctivitis A21.1
    pneumonia A21.2
  abdominal A21.3
  bronchopneumonic A21.2
  conjunctivitis A21.1
  cryptogenic A21.3
  enteric A21.3
  gastrointestinal A21.3
  generalized A21.7
  ingestion A21.3
  intestinal A21.3
  oculoglandular A21.1
  ophthalmic A21.1
  pneumonia (any), pneumonic A21.2
  pulmonary A21.2
  sepsis A21.7
  specified NEC A21.8
  typhoidal A21.7
  ulceroglandular A21.0
Tularensis conjunctivitis A21.1
Tumefaction (*see also* Swelling)
  liver — *see* Hypertrophy, liver
Tumor (*see also* Neoplasm, unspecified behavior, by site)
  acinar cell — *see* Neoplasm, uncertain behavior, by site

Tumor — *continued*
  acinic cell — *see* Neoplasm, uncertain behavior, by site
  adenocarcinoid — *see* Neoplasm, malignant, by site
  adenomatoid (*see also* Neoplasm, benign, by site)
    odontogenic — *see* Cyst, calcifying odontogenic
  adnexal (skin) — *see* Neoplasm, skin, benign, by site
  adrenal
    cortical (benign) D35.0- ☑
      malignant C74.0- ☑
    rest — *see* Neoplasm, benign, by site
  alpha-cell
    malignant
      pancreas C25.4
      specified site NEC — *see* Neoplasm, malignant, by site
      unspecified site C25.4
    pancreas D13.7
    specified site NEC — *see* Neoplasm, benign, by site
    unspecified site D13.7
  aneurysmal — *see* Aneurysm
  aortic body D44.7
    malignant C75.5
  Askin's — *see* Neoplasm, connective tissue, malignant
  basal cell (*see also* Neoplasm, skin, uncertain behavior) D48.5
  Bednar — *see* Neoplasm, skin, malignant
  benign (unclassified) — *see* Neoplasm, benign, by site
  beta-cell
    malignant
      pancreas C25.4
      specified site NEC — *see* Neoplasm, malignant, by site
      unspecified site C25.4
    pancreas D13.7
    specified site NEC — *see* Neoplasm, benign, by site
    unspecified site D13.7
  Brenner D27.9
    borderline malignancy D39.1- ☑
    malignant C56- ☑
    proliferating D39.1- ☑
  bronchial alveolar, intravascular D38.1
  Brooke's — *see* Neoplasm, skin, benign
  brown fat — *see* Lipoma
  Burkitt — *see* Lymphoma, Burkitt
  calcifying epithelial odontogenic — *see* Cyst, calcifying odontogenic
  carcinoid
    benign D3A.00 (*following* D36)
      appendix D3A.020 (*following* D36)
      ascending colon D3A.022 (*following* D36)
      bronchus (lung) D3A.090 (*following* D36)
      cecum D3A.021 (*following* D36)
      colon D3A.029 (*following* D36)
      descending colon D3A.024 (*following* D36)
      duodenum D3A.010 (*following* D36)
      foregut NOS D3A.094 (*following* D36)
      hindgut NOS D3A.096 (*following* D36)
      ileum D3A.012 (*following* D36)
      jejunum D3A.011 (*following* D36)
      kidney D3A.093 (*following* D36)
      large intestine D3A.029 (*following* D36)
      lung (bronchus) D3A.090 (*following* D36)
      midgut NOS D3A.095 (*following* D36)
      rectum D3A.026 (*following* D36)
      sigmoid colon D3A.025 (*following* D36)
      small intestine D3A.019 (*following* D36)
      specified NEC D3A.098 (*following* D36)
      stomach D3A.092 (*following* D36)
      thymus D3A.091 (*following* D36)
      transverse colon D3A.023 (*following* D36)
    malignant C7A.00 (*following* C75)
      appendix C7A.020 (*following* C75)
      ascending colon C7A.022 (*following* C75)
      bronchus (lung) C7A.090 (*following* C75)
      cecum C7A.021 (*following* C75)
      colon C7A.029 (*following* C75)
      descending colon C7A.024 (*following* C75)
      duodenum C7A.010 (*following* C75)
      foregut NOS C7A.094 (*following* C75)
      hindgut NOS C7A.096 (*following* C75)
      ileum C7A.012 (*following* C75)
      jejunum C7A.011 (*following* C75)
      kidney C7A.093 (*following* C75)
      large intestine C7A.029 (*following* C75)
      lung (bronchus) C7A.090 (*following* C75)
      midgut NOS C7A.095 (*following* C75)
      rectum C7A.026 (*following* C75)

Tumor — *continued*
  carcinoid — *continued*
    malignant — *continued*
      sigmoid colon C7A.025 (*following* C75)
      small intestine C7A.019 (*following* C75)
      specified NEC C7A.098 (*following* C75)
      stomach C7A.092 (*following* C75)
      thymus C7A.091 (*following* C75)
      transverse colon C7A.023 (*following* C75)
      mesentary metastasis C7B.04 (*following* C75)
      secondary C7B.00 (*following* C75)
        bone C7B.03 (*following* C75)
        distant lymph nodes C7B.01 (*following* C75)
        liver C7B.02 (*following* C75)
        peritoneum C7B.04 (*following* C75)
        specified NEC C7B.09 (*following* C75)
  carotid body D44.6
    malignant C75.4
  cells (*see also* Neoplasm, unspecified behavior, by site)
    benign — *see* Neoplasm, benign, by site
    malignant — *see* Neoplasm, malignant, by site
    uncertain whether benign or malignant — *see* Neoplasm, uncertain behavior, by site
  cervix, in pregnancy or childbirth — *see* Pregnancy, complicated by, tumor, cervix
  chondromatous giant cell — *see* Neoplasm, bone, benign
  chromaffin (*see also* Neoplasm, benign, by site)
    malignant — *see* Neoplasm, malignant, by site
  Cock's peculiar L72.3
  Codman's — *see* Neoplasm, bone, benign
  dentigerous, mixed — *see* Cyst, calcifying odontogenic
  dermoid — *see* Neoplasm, benign, by site
    with malignant transformation C56- ☑
  desmoid (extra-abdominal) (*see also* Neoplasm, connective tissue, uncertain behavior)
    abdominal — *see* Neoplasm, connective tissue, uncertain behavior
  embolus — *see* Neoplasm, secondary, by site
  embryonal (mixed) (*see also* Neoplasm, uncertain behavior, by site)
    liver C22.7
  endodermal sinus
    specified site — *see* Neoplasm, malignant, by site
    unspecified site
      female C56.- ☑
      male C62.90
  epithelial
    benign — *see* Neoplasm, benign, by site
    malignant — *see* Neoplasm, malignant, by site
  Ewing's — *see* Neoplasm, bone, malignant, by site
  fatty — *see* Lipoma
  fibroid — *see* Leiomyoma
  G cell
    malignant
      pancreas C25.4
      specified site NEC — *see* Neoplasm, malignant, by site
      unspecified site C25.4
    specified site — *see* Neoplasm, uncertain behavior, by site
    unspecified site D37.8
  germ cell (*see also* Neoplasm, malignant, by site)
    mixed — *see* Neoplasm, malignant, by site
  ghost cell, odontogenic — *see* Cyst, calcifying odontogenic
  giant cell (*see also* Neoplasm, uncertain behavior, by site)
    bone D48.0
      malignant — *see* Neoplasm, bone, malignant
      chondromatous — *see* Neoplasm, bone, benign
    malignant — *see* Neoplasm, malignant, by site
    soft parts — *see* Neoplasm, connective tissue, uncertain behavior
      malignant — *see* Neoplasm, connective tissue, malignant
  glomus D18.00
    intra-abdominal D18.03
    intracranial D18.02
    jugulare D44.7
      malignant C75.5
    skin D18.01
    specified site NEC D18.09
  gonadal stromal — *see* Neoplasm, uncertain behavior, by site

Tumor — continued
  granular cell (see also Neoplasm, connective tissue, benign)
    malignant — see Neoplasm, connective tissue, malignant
  granulosa cell D39.1- ☑
    juvenile D39.1-
    malignant C56- ☑
  granulosa cell-theca cell D39.1- ☑
    malignant C56- ☑
  Grawitz's C64- ☑
  hemorrhoidal — see Hemorrhoids
  hilar cell D27- ☑
  hilus cell D27- ☑
  Hurthle cell (benign) D34
    malignant C73
  hydatid — see Echinococcus
  hypernephroid (see also Neoplasm, uncertain behavior, by site)
  interstitial cell (see also Neoplasm, uncertain behavior, by site)
    benign — see Neoplasm, benign, by site
    malignant — see Neoplasm, malignant, by site
  intravascular bronchial alveolar D38.1
  islet cell — see Neoplasm, benign, by site
    malignant — see Neoplasm, malignant, by site
      pancreas C25.4
      specified site NEC — see Neoplasm, malignant, by site
      unspecified site C25.4
    pancreas D13.7
    specified site NEC — see Neoplasm, benign, by site
    unspecified site D13.7
  juxtaglomerular D41.0- ☑
  Klatskin's C22.1
  Krukenberg's C79.6- ☑
  Leydig cell — see Neoplasm, uncertain behavior, by site
    benign — see Neoplasm, benign, by site
      specified site — see Neoplasm, benign, by site
      unspecified site
        female D27.9
        male D29.20
    malignant — see Neoplasm, malignant, by site
      specified site — see Neoplasm, malignant, by site
      unspecified site
        female C56.9
        male C62.90
    specified site — see Neoplasm, uncertain behavior, by site
    unspecified site
      female D39.10
      male D40.10
  lipid cell, ovary D27- ☑
  lipoid cell, ovary D27- ☑
  malignant (see also Neoplasm, malignant, by site) C80.1
    fusiform cell (type) C80.1
    giant cell (type) C80.1
    localized, plasma cell — see Plasmacytoma, solitary
    mixed NEC C80.1
    small cell (type) C80.1
    spindle cell (type) C80.1
    unclassified C80.1
  mast cell D47.0
    malignant C96.2
  melanotic, neuroectodermal — see Neoplasm, benign, by site
  Merkel cell — see Carcinoma, Merkel cell
  mesenchymal
    malignant — see Neoplasm, connective tissue, malignant
    mixed — see Neoplasm, connective tissue, uncertain behavior
  mesodermal, mixed (see also Neoplasm, malignant, by site)
    liver C22.4
  mesonephric (see also Neoplasm, uncertain behavior, by site)
    malignant — see Neoplasm, malignant, by site
  metastatic
    from specified site — see Neoplasm, malignant, by site
    of specified site — see Neoplasm, malignant, by site

Tumor — continued
  metastatic — continued
    to specified site — see Neoplasm, secondary, by site
  mixed NEC (see also Neoplasm, benign, by site)
    malignant — see Neoplasm, malignant, by site
  mucinous of low malignant potential
    specified site — see Neoplasm, malignant, by site
    unspecified site C56.9
  mucocarcinoid
    specified site — see Neoplasm, malignant, by site
    unspecified site C18.1
  mucoepidermoid — see Neoplasm, uncertain behavior, by site
  Müllerian, mixed
    specified site — see Neoplasm, malignant, by site
    unspecified site C54.9
  myoepithelial — see Neoplasm, benign, by site
  neuroectodermal (peripheral) — see Neoplasm, malignant, by site
    primitive
      specified site — see Neoplasm, malignant, by site
      unspecified site C71.9
  neuroendocrine D3A.8 (following D36)
    malignant poorly differentiated C7A.1 (following C75)
    secondary NEC C7B.8 (following C75)
    specified NEC C7A.8 (following C75)
  neurogenic olfactory C30.0
  nonencapsulated sclerosing C73
  odontogenic (adenomatoid) (benign) (calcifying epithelial) (keratocystic) (squamous) — see Cyst, calcifying odontogenic
    malignant C41.1
      upper jaw (bone) C41.0
  ovarian stromal D39.1- ☑
  ovary, in pregnancy — see Pregnancy, complicated by
  pacinian — see Neoplasm, skin, benign
  Pancoast's — see Pancoast's syndrome
  papillary (see also Papilloma)
    cystic D37.9
    mucinous of low malignant potential C56- ☑
      specified site — see Neoplasm, malignant, by site
      unspecified site C56.9
    serous of low malignant potential
      specified site — see Neoplasm, malignant, by site
      unspecified site C56.9
  pelvic, in pregnancy or childbirth — see Pregnancy, complicated by
  phantom F45.8
  phyllodes D48.6- ☑
    benign D24- ☑
    malignant — see Neoplasm, breast, malignant
  Pindborg — see Cyst, calcifying odontogenic
  placental site trophoblastic D39.2
  plasma cell (malignant) (localized) — see Plasmacytoma, solitary
  polyvesicular vitelline
    specified site — see Neoplasm, malignant, by site
    unspecified site
      female C56.9
      male C62.90
  Pott's puffy — see Osteomyelitis, specified NEC
  Rathke's pouch D44.3
  retinal anlage — see Neoplasm, benign, by site
  salivary gland type, mixed — see Neoplasm, salivary gland, benign
    malignant — see Neoplasm, salivary gland, malignant
  Sampson's N80.1
  Schmincke's — see Neoplasm, nasopharynx, malignant
  sclerosing stromal D27- ☑
  sebaceous — see Cyst, sebaceous
  secondary — see Neoplasm, secondary, by site
    carcinoid C7B.00 (following C75)
      bone C7B.03 (following C75)
      distant lymph nodes C7B.01 (following C75)
      liver C7B.02 (following C75)
      peritoneum C7B.04 (following C75)
      specified NEC C7B.09 (following C75)
      neuroendocrine NEC C7B.8 (following C75)
    serous of low malignant potential
      specified site — see Neoplasm, malignant, by site

Tumor — continued
  serous of low malignant potential — continued
    unspecified site C56.9
  Sertoli cell — see Neoplasm, benign, by site
    with lipid storage
      specified site — see Neoplasm, benign, by site
      unspecified site
        female D27.9
        male D29.20
    specified site — see Neoplasm, benign, by site
    unspecified site
      female D27.9
      male D29.20
  Sertoli-Leydig cell — see Neoplasm, benign, by site
    specified site — see Neoplasm, benign, by site
    unspecified site
      female D27.9
      male D29.20
  sex cord (-stromal) — see Neoplasm, uncertain behavior, by site
    with annular tubules D39.1- ☑
  skin appendage — see Neoplasm, skin, benign
  smooth muscle — see Neoplasm, connective tissue, uncertain behavior
  soft tissue
    benign — see Neoplasm, connective tissue, benign
    malignant — see Neoplasm, connective tissue, malignant
  sternomastoid (congenital) Q68.0
  stromal
    endometrial D39.0
    gastric D48.1
      benign D21.4
      malignant C16.9
      uncertain behavior D48.1
    gastrointestinal
      benign D21.4
      malignant C49.4
      uncertain behavior D48.1
    intestine
      benign D21.4
      malignant C49.4
      uncertain behavior D48.1
    ovarian D39.1- ☑
    stomach
      benign D21.4
      malignant C16.9
      uncertain behavior D48.1
  sweat gland (see also Neoplasm, skin, uncertain behavior)
    benign — see Neoplasm, skin, benign
    malignant — see Neoplasm, skin, malignant
  syphilitic, brain A52.17
  testicular D40.10
  testicular stromal D40.1- ☑
  theca cell D27.- ☑
  theca cell-granulosa cell D39.1- ☑
  Triton, malignant — see Neoplasm, nerve, malignant
  trophoblastic, placental site D39.2
  turban D23.4
  uterus (body), in pregnancy or childbirth — see Pregnancy, complicated by, tumor, uterus
  vagina, in pregnancy or childbirth — see Pregnancy, complicated by
  varicose — see Varix
  von Recklinghausen's — see Neurofibromatosis
  vulva or perineum, in pregnancy or childbirth — see Pregnancy, complicated by
    causing obstructed labor O65.5
  Warthin's — see Neoplasm, salivary gland, benign
  Wilms' C64- ☑
  yolk sac — see Neoplasm, malignant, by site
    specified site — see Neoplasm, malignant, by site
    unspecified site
      female C56.9
      male C62.90
Tumor lysis syndrome (following antineoplastic chemotherapy) (spontaneous) NEC E88.3
Tumorlet — see Neoplasm, uncertain behavior, by site
Tungiasis B88.1
Tunica vasculosa lentis Q12.2
Turban tumor D23.4
Türck's trachoma J37.0
Turner-Kieser syndrome Q79.8
Turner-like syndrome Q87.1
Turner's
  hypoplasia (tooth) K00.4

☑ **Additional Character Required — Refer to the Tabular List for Character Selection**   ▽ Subterms under main terms may continue to next column or page

Turner's — *continued*
  syndrome Q96.9
    specified NEC Q96.8
  tooth K00.4
Turner-Ullrich syndrome Q96.9
Tussis convulsiva — *see* Whooping cough
Twiddler's syndrome (due to)
  automatic implantable defibrillatorT82.198
  cardiac pacemaker T82.198 ☑
Twilight state
  epileptic F05
  psychogenic F44.89
Twin (newborn) (*see also* Newborn, twin)
  conjoined Q89.4
  pregnancy — *see* Pregnancy, twin, conjoined
Twinning, teeth K00.2
Twist, twisted
  bowel, colon or intestine K56.2
  hair (congenital) Q84.1
  mesentery K56.2
  omentum K56.2
  organ or site, congenital NEC — *see* Anomaly, by site
  ovarian pedicle — *see* Torsion, ovary
Twitching R25.3
Tylosis (acquired) L84
  buccalis K13.29
  linguae K13.29
  palmaris et plantaris (congenital) (inherited) Q82.8
    acquired L85.1
Tympanism R14.0
Tympanites (abdominal) (intestinal) R14.0
Tympanitis — *see* Myringitis
Tympanosclerosis H74.0 ☑
Tympanum — *see* condition
Tympany
  abdomen R14.0
  chest R09.89
Type A behavior pattern Z73.1
Typhlitis — *see* Appendicitis
Typhoenteritis — *see* Typhoid
Typhoid (abortive) (ambulant) (any site) (clinical) (fever) (hemorrhagic) (infection) (intermittent) (malignant) (rheumatic) (Widal negative) A01.00
  with pneumonia A01.03
  abdominal A01.09
  arthritis A01.04
  carrier (suspected) of Z22.0
  cholecystitis (current) A01.09
  endocarditis A01.02
  heart involvement A01.02
  inoculation reaction — *see* Complications, vaccination
  meningitis A01.01
  mesenteric lymph nodes A01.09
  myocarditis A01.02
  osteomyelitis A01.05
  perichondritis, larynx A01.09
  pneumonia A01.03
  specified NEC A01.09
  spine A01.05
  ulcer (perforating) A01.09
Typhomalaria (fever) — *see* Malaria
Typhomania A01.00
Typhoperitonitis A01.09
Typhus (fever) A75.9
  abdominal, abdominalis — *see* Typhoid
  African tick A77.1
  amarillic A95.9
  brain A75.9 [G94]
  cerebral A75.9 [G94]
  classical A75.0
  due to Rickettsia
    prowazekii A75.0
      recrudescent A75.1
    tsutsugamushi A75.3
    typhi A75.2
  endemic (flea-borne) A75.2
  epidemic (louse-borne) A75.0
  exanthematicus SAI A75.0
    brillii SAI A75.1
    mexicanus SAI A75.2
    typhus murinus A75.2
  exanthematic NEC A75.0
  flea-borne A75.2
  India tick A77.1
  Kenya (tick) A77.1
  louse-borne A75.0
  Mexican A75.2
  mite-borne A75.3

Typhus — *continued*
  murine A75.2
  North Asian tick-borne A77.2
  petechial A75.9
  Queensland tick A77.3
  rat A75.2
  recrudescent A75.1
  recurrens — *see* Fever, relapsing
  Sao Paulo A77.0
  scrub (China) (India) (Malaysia) (New Guinea) A75.3
  shop (of Malaysia) A75.2
  Siberian tick A77.2
  tick-borne A77.9
  tropical (mite-borne) A75.3
Tyrosinemia E70.21
  newborn, transitory P74.5
Tyrosinosis E70.21
Tyrosinuria E70.29

U

Uhl's anomaly or disease Q24.8
Ulcer, ulcerated, ulcerating, ulceration, ulcerative
  alveolar process M27.3
  amebic (intestine) A06.1
    skin A06.7
  anastomotic — *see* Ulcer, gastrojejunal
  anorectal K62.6
  antral — *see* Ulcer, stomach
  anus (sphincter) (solitary) K62.6
  aorta — *see* Aneurysm
  aphthous (oral) (recurrent) K12.0
    genital organ(s)
      female N76.6
      male N50.8
  artery I77.2
  atrophic — *see* Ulcer, skin
    decubitus — *see* Ulcer, pressure, by site
  back L98.429
    with
      bone necrosis L98.424
      exposed fat layer L98.422
      muscle necrosis L98.423
      skin breakdown only L98.421
  Barrett's (esophagus) K22.10
    with bleeding K22.11
  bile duct (common) (hepatic) K83.8
  bladder (solitary) (sphincter) NEC N32.89
    bilharzial B65.9 [N33]
    in schistosomiasis (bilharzial) B65.9 [N33]
    submucosal — *see* Cystitis, interstitial
    tuberculous A18.12
  bleeding K27.4
  bone — *see* Osteomyelitis, specified type NEC
  bowel — *see* Ulcer, intestine
  breast N61
  bronchus J98.09
  buccal (cavity) (traumatic) K12.1
  Buruli A31.1
  buttock L98.419
    with
      bone necrosis L98.414
      exposed fat layer L98.412
      muscle necrosis L98.413
      skin breakdown only L98.411
  cancerous — *see* Neoplasm, malignant, by site
  cardia K22.10
    with bleeding K22.11
  cardioesophageal (peptic) K22.10
    with bleeding K22.11
  cecum — *see* Ulcer, intestine
  cervix (uteri) (decubitus) (trophic) N86
    with cervicitis N72
  chancroidal A57
  chiclero B55.1
  chronic (cause unknown) — *see* Ulcer, skin
  Cochin-China B55.1
  colon — *see* Ulcer, intestine
  conjunctiva H11.89
  cornea H16.00- ☑
    with hypopyon H16.03- ☑
    central H16.01- ☑
    dendritic (herpes simplex) B00.52
    marginal H16.04- ☑
    Mooren's H16.05- ☑
    mycotic H16.06- ☑
    perforated H16.07- ☑

Ulcer, ulcerated, ulcerating, ulceration, ulcerative
  — *continued*
  cornea — *continued*
    ring H16.02- ☑
    tuberculous (phlyctenular) A18.52
  corpus cavernosum (chronic) N48.5
  crural — *see* Ulcer, lower limb
  Curling's — *see* Ulcer, peptic, acute
  Cushing's — *see* Ulcer, peptic, acute
  cystic duct K82.8
  cystitis (interstitial) — *see* Cystitis, interstitial
  decubitus — *see* Ulcer, pressure, by site
  dendritic, cornea (herpes simplex) B00.52
  diabetes, diabetic — *see* Diabetes, ulcer
  Dieulafoy's K25.0
  due to
    infection NEC — *see* Ulcer, skin
    radiation NEC L59.8
    trophic disturbance (any region) — *see* Ulcer, skin
    X-ray L58.1
  duodenum, duodenal (eroded) (peptic) K26.9
    with
      hemorrhage K26.4
        and perforation K26.6
      perforation K26.5
    acute K26.3
      with
        hemorrhage K26.0
          and perforation K26.2
        perforation K26.1
    chronic K26.7
      with
        hemorrhage K26.4
          and perforation K26.6
        perforation K26.5
  dysenteric A09
  elusive — *see* Cystitis, interstitial
  endocarditis (acute) (chronic) (subacute) I28.8
  epiglottis J38.7
  esophagus (peptic) K22.10
    with bleeding K22.11
    due to
      aspirin K22.10
        with bleeding K22.11
      gastrointestinal reflux disease K21.0
      ingestion of chemical or medicament K22.10
        with bleeding K22.11
      fungal K22.10
        with bleeding K22.11
      infective K22.10
        with bleeding K22.11
    varicose — *see* Varix, esophagus
  eyelid (region) H01.8
  fauces J39.2
  Fenwick (-Hunner) (solitary) — *see* Cystitis, interstitial
  fistulous — *see* Ulcer, skin
  foot (indolent) (trophic) — *see* Ulcer, lower limb
  frambesial, initial A66.0
  frenum (tongue) K14.0
  gallbladder or duct K82.8
  gangrenous — *see* Gangrene
  gastric — *see* Ulcer, stomach
  gastrocolic — *see* Ulcer, gastrojejunal
  gastroduodenal — *see* Ulcer, peptic
  gastroesophageal — *see* Ulcer, stomach
  gastrointestinal — *see* Ulcer, gastrojejunal
  gastrojejunal (peptic) K28.9
    with
      hemorrhage K28.4
        and perforation K28.6
      perforation K28.5
    acute K28.3
      with
        hemorrhage K28.0
          and perforation K28.2
        perforation K28.1
    chronic K28.7
      with
        hemorrhage K28.4
          and perforation K28.6
        perforation K28.5
  gastrojejunocolic — *see* Ulcer, gastrojejunal
  gingiva K06.8
  gingivitis K05.10
    nonplaque induced K05.11
    plaque induced K05.10
  glottis J38.7
  granuloma of pudenda A58

Ulcer, ulcerated, ulcerating, ulceration, ulcerative
 — *continued*
gum K06.8
gumma, due to yaws A66.4
heel — *see* Ulcer, lower limb
hemorrhoid (*see also* Hemorrhoids, by degree) K64.8
Hunner's — *see* Cystitis, interstitial
hypopharynx J39.2
hypopyon (chronic) (subacute) — *see* Ulcer, cornea, with hypopyon
hypostaticum — *see* Ulcer, varicose
ileum — *see* Ulcer, intestine
intestine, intestinal K63.3
    with perforation K63.1
    amebic A06.1
    duodenal — *see* Ulcer, duodenum
    granulocytopenic (with hemorrhage) — *see* Neutropenia
    marginal — *see* Ulcer, gastrojejunal
    perforating K63.1
        newborn P78.0
    primary, small intestine K63.3
    rectum K62.6
    stercoraceous, stercoral K63.3
    tuberculous A18.32
    typhoid (fever) — *see* Typhoid
    varicose I86.8
jejunum, jejunal — *see* Ulcer, gastrojejunal
keratitis — *see* Ulcer, cornea
knee — *see* Ulcer, lower limb
labium (majus) (minus) N76.6
laryngitis — *see* Laryngitis
larynx (aphthous) (contact) J38.7
    diphtheritic A36.2
leg — *see* Ulcer, lower limb
lip K13.0
Lipschütz's N76.6
lower limb (atrophic) (chronic) (neurogenic) (perforating) (pyogenic) (trophic) (tropical) L97.909
    with
        bone necrosis L97.904
        exposed fat layer L97.902
        muscle necrosis L97.903
        skin breakdown only L97.901
    ankle L97.309
        with
            bone necrosis L97.304
            exposed fat layer L97.302
            muscle necrosis L97.303
            skin breakdown only L97.301
        left L97.329
            with
                bone necrosis L97.324
                exposed fat layer L97.322
                muscle necrosis L97.323
                skin breakdown only L97.321
        right L97.319
            with
                bone necrosis L97.314
                exposed fat layer L97.312
                muscle necrosis L97.313
                skin breakdown only L97.311
    calf L97.209
        with
            bone necrosis L97.204
            exposed fat layer L97.202
            muscle necrosis L97.203
            skin breakdown only L97.201
        left L97.229
            with
                bone necrosis L97.224
                exposed fat layer L97.222
                muscle necrosis L97.223
                skin breakdown only L97.221
        right L97.219
            with
                bone necrosis L97.214
                exposed fat layer L97.212
                muscle necrosis L97.213
                skin breakdown only L97.211
    decubitus — *see* Ulcer, pressure, by site
    foot specified NEC L97.509
        with
            bone necrosis L97.504
            exposed fat layer L97.502
            muscle necrosis L97.503
            skin breakdown only L97.501
        left L97.529

Ulcer, ulcerated, ulcerating, ulceration, ulcerative
 — *continued*
lower limb — *continued*
    foot specified — *continued*
        left — *continued*
            with
                bone necrosis L97.524
                exposed fat layer L97.522
                muscle necrosis L97.523
                skin breakdown only L97.521
        right L97.519
            with
                bone necrosis L97.514
                exposed fat layer L97.512
                muscle necrosis L97.513
                skin breakdown only L97.511
    heel L97.409
        with
            bone necrosis L97.404
            exposed fat layer L97.402
            muscle necrosis L97.403
            skin breakdown only L97.401
        left L97.429
            with
                bone necrosis L97.424
                exposed fat layer L97.422
                muscle necrosis L97.423
                skin breakdown only L97.421
        right L97.419
            with
                bone necrosis L97.414
                exposed fat layer L97.412
                muscle necrosis L97.413
                skin breakdown only L97.411
    left L97.929
        with
            bone necrosis L97.924
            exposed fat layer L97.922
            muscle necrosis L97.923
            skin breakdown only L97.921
    leprous A30.1
    lower leg NOS L97.909
        with
            bone necrosis L97.904
            exposed fat layer L97.902
            muscle necrosis L97.903
            skin breakdown only L97.901
        left L97.929
            with
                bone necrosis L97.924
                exposed fat layer L97.922
                muscle necrosis L97.923
                skin breakdown only L97.921
        right L97.919
            with
                bone necrosis L97.914
                exposed fat layer L97.912
                muscle necrosis L97.913
                skin breakdown only L97.911
    specified site NEC L97.809
        with
            bone necrosis L97.804
            exposed fat layer L97.802
            muscle necrosis L97.803
            skin breakdown only L97.801
        left L97.829
            with
                bone necrosis L97.824
                exposed fat layer L97.822
                muscle necrosis L97.823
                skin breakdown only L97.821
        right L97.819
            with
                bone necrosis L97.814
                exposed fat layer L97.812
                muscle necrosis L97.813
                skin breakdown only L97.811
    midfoot L97.409
        with
            bone necrosis L97.404
            exposed fat layer L97.402
            muscle necrosis L97.403
            skin breakdown only L97.401
        left L97.429
            with
                bone necrosis L97.424
                exposed fat layer L97.422
                muscle necrosis L97.423

Ulcer, ulcerated, ulcerating, ulceration, ulcerative
 — *continued*
lower limb — *continued*
    midfoot — *continued*
        left — *continued*
            with — *continued*
                skin breakdown only L97.421
            right L97.419
                with
                    bone necrosis L97.414
                    exposed fat layer L97.412
                    muscle necrosis L97.413
                    skin breakdown only L97.411
        right L97.919
            with
                bone necrosis L97.914
                exposed fat layer L97.912
                muscle necrosis L97.913
                skin breakdown only L97.911
    syphilitic A52.19
    thigh L97.109
        with
            bone necrosis L97.104
            exposed fat layer L97.102
            muscle necrosis L97.103
            skin breakdown only L97.101
        left L97.129
            with
                bone necrosis L97.124
                exposed fat layer L97.122
                muscle necrosis L97.123
                skin breakdown only L97.121
        right L97.119
            with
                bone necrosis L97.114
                exposed fat layer L97.112
                muscle necrosis L97.113
                skin breakdown only L97.111
    toe L97.509
        with
            bone necrosis L97.504
            exposed fat layer L97.502
            muscle necrosis L97.503
            skin breakdown only L97.501
        left L97.529
            with
                bone necrosis L97.524
                exposed fat layer L97.522
                muscle necrosis L97.523
                skin breakdown only L97.521
        right L97.519
            with
                bone necrosis L97.514
                exposed fat layer L97.512
                muscle necrosis L97.513
                skin breakdown only L97.511
    varicose — *see* Varix, leg, with, ulcer
luetic — *see* Ulcer, syphilitic
lung J98.4
    tuberculous — *see* Tuberculosis, pulmonary
malignant — *see* Neoplasm, malignant, by site
marginal NEC — *see* Ulcer, gastrojejunal
meatus (urinarius) N34.2
Meckel's diverticulum Q43.0
    malignant — *see* Table of Neoplasms, small intestine, malignant
Meleney's (chronic undermining) — *see* Ulcer, skin
Mooren's (cornea) — *see* Ulcer, cornea, Mooren's
mycobacterial (skin) A31.1
nasopharynx J39.2
neck, uterus N86
neurogenic NEC — *see* Ulcer, skin
nose, nasal (passage) (infective) (septum) J34.0
    skin — *see* Ulcer, skin
    spirochetal A69.8
    varicose (bleeding) I86.8
oral mucosa (traumatic) K12.1
palate (soft) K12.1
penis (chronic) N48.5
peptic (site unspecified) K27.9
    with
        hemorrhage K27.4
            and perforation K27.6
        perforation K27.5
    acute K27.3
        with
            hemorrhage K27.0
                and perforation K27.2

Ulcer, ulcerated, ulcerating, ulceration, ulcerative
— *continued*
  peptic — *continued*
    acute — *continued*
      with — *continued*
        perforation K27.1
      chronic K27.7
        with
          hemorrhage K27.4
            and perforation K27.6
          perforation K27.5
      esophagus K22.10
        with bleeding K22.11
      newborn P78.82
    perforating K27.5
    skin — *see* Ulcer, skin
  peritonsillar J35.8
  phagedenic (tropical) — *see* Ulcer, skin
  pharynx J39.2
  phlebitis — *see* Phlebitis
  plaster — *see* Ulcer, pressure, by site
  popliteal space — *see* Ulcer, lower limb
  postpyloric — *see* Ulcer, duodenum
  prepuce N47.7
  prepyloric — *see* Ulcer, stomach
  pressure (pressure area) L89.9- ☑
    ankle L89.5- ☑
    back L89.1- ☑
    buttock L89.3- ☑
    coccyx L89.15- ☑
    contiguous site of back, buttock, hip L89.4- ☑
    elbow L89.0- ☑
    face L89.81- ☑
    head L89.81- ☑
    heel L89.6- ☑
    hip L89.2- ☑
    sacral region (tailbone) L89.15- ☑
    specified site NEC L89.89- ☑
    stage 1 (healing) (pre-ulcer skin changes limited
        to persistent focal edema)
      ankle L89.5- ☑
      back L89.1- ☑
      buttock L89.3- ☑
      coccyx L89.15- ☑
      contiguous site of back, buttock, hip L89.4- ☑
      elbow L89.0- ☑
      face L89.81- ☑
      head L89.81- ☑
      heel L89.6- ☑
      hip L89.2- ☑
      sacral region (tailbone) L89.15- ☑
      specified site NEC L89.89- ☑
    stage 2 (healing) (abrasion, blister, partial thickness
        skin loss involving epidermis and/or dermis)
      ankle L89.5- ☑
      back L89.1- ☑
      buttock L89.3- ☑
      coccyx L89.15- ☑
      contiguous site of back, buttock, hip L89.4- ☑
      elbow L89.0- ☑
      face L89.81- ☑
      head L89.81- ☑
      heel L89.6- ☑
      hip L89.2- ☑
      sacral region (tailbone) L89.15- ☑
      specified site NEC L89.89- ☑
    stage 3 (healing) (full thickness skin loss involving
        damage or necrosis of subcutaneous tissue)
      ankle L89.5- ☑
      back L89.1- ☑
      buttock L89.3- ☑
      coccyx L89.15- ☑
      contiguous site of back, buttock, hip L89.4- ☑
      elbow L89.0- ☑
      face L89.81- ☑
      head L89.81- ☑
      heel L89.6- ☑
      hip L89.2- ☑
      sacral region (tailbone) L89.15- ☑
      specified site NEC L89.89- ☑
    stage 4 (healing) (necrosis of soft tissues through
        to underlying muscle, tendon, or bone)
      ankle L89.5- ☑
      back L89.1- ☑
      buttock L89.3- ☑
      coccyx L89.15- ☑

Ulcer, ulcerated, ulcerating, ulceration, ulcerative
— *continued*
  pressure — *continued*
    stage 4 — *continued*
      contiguous site of back, buttock, hip L89.4- ☑
      elbow L89.0- ☑
      face L89.81- ☑
      head L89.81- ☑
      heel L89.6- ☑
      hip L89.2- ☑
      sacral region (tailbone) L89.15- ☑
      specified site NEC L89.89- ☑
    unspecified stage
      ankle L89.5- ☑
      back L89.1- ☑
      buttock L89.3- ☑
      coccyx L89.15- ☑
      contiguous site of back, buttock, hip L89.4- ☑
      elbow L89.0- ☑
      face L89.81- ☑
      head L89.81- ☑
      heel L89.6- ☑
      hip L89.2- ☑
      sacral region (tailbone) L89.15- ☑
      specified site NEC L89.89- ☑
    unstageable
      ankle L89.5- ☑
      back L89.1- ☑
      buttock L89.3- ☑
      coccyx L89.15- ☑
      contiguous site of back, buttock, hip L89.4- ☑
      elbow L89.0- ☑
      face L89.81- ☑
      head L89.81- ☑
      heel L89.6- ☑
      hip L89.2- ☑
      sacral region (tailbone) L89.15- ☑
      specified site NEC L89.89- ☑
  primary of intestine K63.3
    with perforation K63.1
  prostate N41.9
  pyloric — *see* Ulcer, stomach
  rectosigmoid K63.3
    with perforation K63.1
  rectum (sphincter) (solitary) K62.6
    stercoraceous, stercoral K62.6
  retina — *see* Inflammation, chorioretinal
  rodent (*see also* Neoplasm, skin, malignant)
  sclera — *see* Scleritis
  scrofulous (tuberculous) A18.2
  scrotum N50.8
    tuberculous A18.15
    varicose I86.1
  seminal vesicle N50.8
  sigmoid — *see* Ulcer, intestine
  skin (atrophic) (chronic) (neurogenic) (non-healing)
      (perforating) (pyogenic) (trophic) (tropical)
      L98.499
    with gangrene — *see* Gangrene
    amebic A06.7
    back — *see* Ulcer, back
    buttock — *see* Ulcer, buttock
    decubitus — *see* Ulcer, pressure
    lower limb — *see* Ulcer, lower limb
    mycobacterial A31.1
    specified site NEC L98.499
      with
        bone necrosis L98.494
        exposed fat layer L98.492
        muscle necrosis L98.493
        skin breakdown only L98.491
    tuberculous (primary) A18.4
    varicose — *see* Ulcer, varicose
  sloughing — *see* Ulcer, skin
  solitary, anus or rectum (sphincter) K62.6
  sore throat J02.9
    streptococcal J02.0
  spermatic cord N50.8
  spine (tuberculous) A18.01
  stasis (venous) — *see* Varix, leg, with, ulcer
    without varicose veins I87.2
  stercoraceous, stercoral K63.3
    with perforation K63.1
    anus or rectum K62.6
  stoma, stomal — *see* Ulcer, gastrojejunal
  stomach (eroded) (peptic) (round) K25.9
    with

Ulcer, ulcerated, ulcerating, ulceration, ulcerative
— *continued*
  stomach — *continued*
    with — *continued*
      hemorrhage K25.4
        and perforation K25.6
      perforation K25.5
    acute K25.3
      with
        hemorrhage K25.0
          and perforation K25.2
        perforation K25.1
    chronic K25.7
      with
        hemorrhage K25.4
          and perforation K25.6
        perforation K25.5
  stomal — *see* Ulcer, gastrojejunal
  stomatitis K12.1
  stress — *see* Ulcer, peptic
  strumous (tuberculous) A18.2
  submucosal, bladder — *see* Cystitis, interstitial
  syphilitic (any site) (early) (secondary) A51.39
    late A52.79
      perforating A52.79
        foot A52.11
  testis N50.8
  thigh — *see* Ulcer, lower limb
  throat J39.2
    diphtheritic A36.0
  toe — *see* Ulcer, lower limb
  tongue (traumatic) K14.0
  tonsil J35.8
    diphtheritic A36.0
  trachea J39.8
  trophic — *see* Ulcer, skin
  tropical — *see* Ulcer, skin
  tuberculous — *see* Tuberculosis, ulcer
  tunica vaginalis N50.8
  turbinate J34.89
  typhoid (perforating) — *see* Typhoid
  unspecified site — *see* Ulcer, skin
  urethra (meatus) — *see* Urethritis
  uterus N85.8
    cervix N86
      with cervicitis N72
    neck N86
      with cervicitis N72
  vagina N76.5
    in Behçet's disease M35.2 [N77.0]
    pessary N89.8
  valve, heart I33.0
  varicose (lower limb, any part) (*see also* Varix, leg, with,
      ulcer)
    broad ligament I86.2
    esophagus — *see* Varix, esophagus
    inflamed or infected — *see* Varix, leg, with ulcer,
        with inflammation
    nasal septum I86.8
    perineum I86.3
    scrotum I86.1
    specified site NEC I86.8
    sublingual I86.0
    vulva I86.3
  vas deferens N50.8
  vulva (acute) (infectional) N76.6
    in (due to)
      Behçet's disease M35.2 [N77.0]
      herpesviral (herpes simplex) infection A60.04
      tuberculosis A18.18
  vulvobuccal, recurring N76.6
  X-ray L58.1
  yaws A66.4
Ulcerosa scarlatina A38.8
Ulcus (*see also* Ulcer)
  cutis tuberculosum A18.4
  duodeni — *see* Ulcer, duodenum
  durum (syphilitic) A51.0
    extragenital A51.2
  gastrojejunale — *see* Ulcer, gastrojejunal
  hypostaticum — *see* Ulcer, varicose
  molle (cutis) (skin) A57
  serpens corneae — *see* Ulcer, cornea, central
  ventriculi — *see* Ulcer, stomach
Ulegyria Q04.8
Ulerythema
  ophryogenes, congenital Q84.2
  sycosiforme L73.8

Ullrich (-Bonnevie)(-Turner) **syndrome** Q87.1
Ullrich-Feichtiger syndrome Q87.0
Ulnar — *see* condition
Ulorrhagia, ulorrhea K06.8
Umbilicus, umbilical — *see* condition
Unacceptable
 contours of tooth K08.54
 morphology of tooth K08.54
Unavailability (of)
 bed at medical facility Z75.1
 health service-related agencies Z75.4
 medical facilities (at) Z75.3
  due to
   investigation by social service agency Z75.2
   lack of services at home Z75.0
   remoteness from facility Z75.3
   waiting list Z75.1
  home Z75.0
  outpatient clinic Z75.3
 schooling Z55.1
 social service agencies Z75.4
Uncinaria americana infestation B76.1
Uncinariasis B76.9
Uncongenial work Z56.5
Unconscious (ness) — *see* Coma
Under observation — *see* Observation
Underachievement in school Z55.3
Underdevelopment (*see also* Undeveloped)
 nose Q30.1
 sexual E30.0
Underdosing (*see also* Table of Drugs and Chemicals,
  categories T36-T50, with final character 6) Z91.14
 intentional NEC Z91.128
  due to financial hardship of patient Z91.120
 unintentional NEC Z91.138
  due to patient's age related debility Z91.130
Underfeeding, newborn P92.3
Underfill, endodontic M27.53
Underimmunization status Z28.3
Undernourishment — *see* Malnutrition
Undernutrition — *see* Malnutrition
Underweight R63.6
 for gestational age — *see* Light for dates
Underwood's disease P83.0
Undescended (*see also* Malposition, congenital)
 cecum Q43.3
 colon Q43.3
 testicle — *see* Cryptorchid
Undeveloped, undevelopment (*see also* Hypoplasia)
 brain (congenital) Q02
 cerebral (congenital) Q02
 heart Q24.8
 lung Q33.6
 testis E29.1
 uterus E30.0
Undiagnosed (disease) R69
Undulant fever — *see* Brucellosis
Unemployment, anxiety concerning Z56.0
 threatened Z56.2
Unequal length (acquired) (limb) (*see also* Deformity,
  limb, unequal length)
 leg (*see also* Deformity, limb, unequal length)
  congenital Q72.9- ☑
Unextracted dental root K08.3
Unguis incarnatus L60.0
Unhappiness R45.2
Unicornate uterus Q51.4
Unilateral (*see also* condition)
 development, breast N64.89
 organ or site, congenital NEC — *see* Agenesis, by site
Unilocular heart Q20.8
Union, abnormal (*see also* Fusion)
 larynx and trachea Q34.8
Universal mesentery Q43.3
**Unrepairable overhanging of dental restorative
  materials** K08.52
Unsatisfactory
 restoration of tooth K08.50
  specified NEC K08.59
 sample of cytologic smear
  anus R85.615
  cervix R87.615
  vagina R87.625
 surroundings Z59.1
  work Z56.5
Unsoundness of mind — *see* Psychosis

Unstable
 back NEC — *see* Instability, joint, spine
 hip (congenital) Q65.6
  acquired — *see* Derangement, joint, specified type
   NEC, hip
 joint — *see* Instability, joint
  secondary to removal of joint prosthesis M96.89
 lie (mother) O32.0 ☑
 lumbosacral joint (congenital)
  acquired — *see* subcategory M53.2 ☑
 sacroiliac — *see* subcategory M53.2 ☑
 spine NEC — *see* Instability, joint, spine
Unsteadiness on feet R26.81
Untruthfulness, child problem F91.8
Unverricht (-Lundborg) **disease or epilepsy** — *see*
  Epilepsy, generalized, idiopathic
Unwanted pregnancy Z64.0
Upbringing, institutional Z62.22
 away from parents NEC Z62.29
 in care of non-parental family member Z62.21
 in foster care Z62.21
 in orphanage or group home Z62.22
 in welfare custody Z62.21
Upper respiratory — *see* condition
Upset
 gastric K30
 gastrointestinal K30
  psychogenic F45.8
 intestinal (large) (small) K59.9
  psychogenic F45.8
 menstruation N93.9
 mental F48.9
 stomach K30
  psychogenic F45.8
Urachus (*see also* condition)
 patent or persistent Q64.4
Urbach-Oppenheim disease (necrobiosis lipoidica diabeticorum) — *see* E08-E13 with .620
Urbach's lipoid proteinosis E78.89
Urbach-Wiethe disease E78.89
Urban yellow fever A95.1
Urea
 blood, high — *see* Uremia
 cycle metabolism disorder — *see* Disorder, urea cycle
  metabolism
Uremia, uremic N19
 with
  ectopic or molar pregnancy O08.4
  polyneuropathy N18.9 [G63]
 chronic (*see also* Disease, kidney, chronic) N18.9
  due to hypertension — *see* Hypertensive, kidney
 complicating
  ectopic or molar pregnancy O08.4
 congenital P96.0
 extrarenal R39.2
 following ectopic or molar pregnancy O08.4
 newborn P96.0
 prerenal R39.2
Ureter, ureteral — *see* condition
Ureteralgia N23
Ureterectasis — *see* Hydroureter
Ureteritis N28.89
 cystica N28.86
 due to calculus N20.1
  with calculus, kidney N20.2
   with hydronephrosis N13.2
 gonococcal (acute) (chronic) A54.21
 nonspecific N28.89
Ureterocele N28.89
 congenital (orthotopic) Q62.31
  ectopic Q62.32
Ureterolith, ureterolithiasis — *see* Calculus, ureter
Ureterostomy
 attention to Z43.6
 status Z93.6
Urethra, urethral — *see* condition
Urethralgia R39.89
Urethritis (anterior) (posterior) N34.2
 calculous N21.1
 candidal B37.41
 chlamydial A56.01
 diplococcal (gonococcal) A54.01
  with abscess (accessory gland) (periurethral) A54.1
 gonococcal A54.01
  with abscess (accessory gland) (periurethral) A54.1
 nongonococcal N34.1
  Reiter's — *see* Reiter's disease

Urethritis — *continued*
 nonspecific N34.1
 nonvenereal N34.1
 postmenopausal N34.2
 puerperal O86.22
 Reiter's — *see* Reiter's disease
 specified NEC N34.2
 trichomonal or due to Trichomonas (vaginalis) A59.03
Urethrocele N81.0
 with
  cystocele — *see* Cystocele
  prolapse of uterus — *see* Prolapse, uterus
Urethrolithiasis (with colic or infection) N21.1
Urethrorectal — *see* condition
Urethrorrhagia N36.8
Urethrorrhea R36.9
Urethrostomy
 attention to Z43.6
 status Z93.6
Urethrotrigonitis — *see* Trigonitis
Urethrovaginal — *see* condition
Urgency
 fecal R15.2
 hypertensive — *see* Hypertension
 urinary N39.41
Urhidrosis, uridrosis L74.8
Uric acid in blood (increased) E79.0
Uricacidemia (asymptomatic) E79.0
Uricemia (asymptomatic) E79.0
Uricosuria R82.99
Urinary — *see* condition
Urination
 frequent R35.0
 painful R30.9
Urine
 blood in — *see* Hematuria
 discharge, excessive R35.8
 enuresis, nonorganic origin F98.0
 extravasation R39.0
 frequency R35.0
 incontinence R32
  nonorganic origin F98.0
 intermittent stream R39.19
 pus in N39.0
 retention or stasis R33.9
  organic R33.8
   drug-induced R33.0
  psychogenic F45.8
 secretion
  deficient R34
  excessive R35.8
  frequency R35.0
 stream
  intermittent R39.19
  slowing R39.19
  splitting R39.13
  weak R39.12
Urinemia — *see* Uremia
Urinoma, urethra N36.8
Uroarthritis, infectious (Reiter's) — *see* Reiter's disease
Urodialysis R34
Urolithiasis — *see* Calculus, urinary
Uronephrosis — *see* Hydronephrosis
Uropathy N39.9
 obstructive N13.9
  specified NEC N13.8
 reflux N13.9
  specified NEC N13.8
 vesicoureteral reflux-associated — *see* Reflux, vesicoureteral
Urosepsis — *code to* condition
Urticaria L50.9
 with angioneurotic edema T78.3 ☑
  hereditary D84.1
 allergic L50.0
 cholinergic L50.5
 chronic L50.8
 cold, familial L50.2
 contact L50.6
 dermatographic L50.3
 due to
  cold or heat L50.2
  drugs L50.0
  food L50.0
  inhalants L50.0
  plants L50.6
 serum (*see also* Reaction, serum) T80.69 ☑

Urticaria — *continued*
　factitial L50.3
　giant T78.3 ☑
　　hereditary D84.1
　gigantea T78.3 ☑
　idiopathic L50.1
　larynx T78.3 ☑
　　hereditary D84.1
　neonatorum P83.8
　nonallergic L50.1
　papulosa (Hebra) L28.2
　pigmentosa Q82.2
　recurrent periodic L50.8
　serum (*see also* Reaction, serum) T80.69 ☑
　solar L56.3
　specified type NEC L50.8
　thermal (cold) (heat) L50.2
　vibratory L50.4
　xanthelasmoidea Q82.2
Use (of)
　alcohol F10.99
　　with sleep disorder F10.982
　　harmful — *see* Abuse, alcohol
　amphetamines — *see* Use, stimulant NEC
　caffeine — *see* Use, stimulant NEC
　cannabis F12.90
　　with
　　　anxiety disorder F12.980
　　　intoxication F12.929
　　　　with
　　　　　delirium F12.921
　　　　　perceptual disturbance F12.922
　　　　uncomplicated F12.920
　　　other specified disorder F12.988
　　　psychosis F12.959
　　　　delusions F12.950
　　　　hallucinations F12.951
　　　unspecified disorder F12.99
　cocaine F14.90
　　with
　　　anxiety disorder F14.980
　　　intoxication F14.929
　　　　with
　　　　　delirium F14.921
　　　　　perceptual disturbance F14.922
　　　　uncomplicated F14.920
　　　other specified disorder F14.988
　　　psychosis F14.959
　　　　delusions F14.950
　　　　hallucinations F14.951
　　　sexual dysfunction F14.981
　　　sleep disorder F14.982
　　　unspecified disorder F14.99
　　harmful — *see* Abuse, drug, cocaine
　drug(s) NEC F19.90
　　with sleep disorder F19.982
　　harmful — *see* Abuse, drug, by type
　hallucinogen NEC F16.90
　　with
　　　anxiety disorder F16.980
　　　intoxication F16.929
　　　　with
　　　　　delirium F16.921
　　　　uncomplicated F16.920
　　　mood disorder F16.94
　　　other specified disorder F16.988
　　　perception disorder (flashbacks) F16.983
　　　psychosis F16.959
　　　　delusions F16.950
　　　　hallucinations F16.951
　　　unspecified disorder F16.99
　　harmful — *see* Abuse, drug, hallucinogen NEC
　inhalants F18.90
　　with
　　　anxiety disorder F18.980
　　　intoxication F18.929
　　　　with delirium F18.921
　　　　uncomplicated F18.920
　　　mood disorder F18.94
　　　other specified disorder F18.988
　　　persisting dementia F18.97
　　　psychosis F18.959
　　　　delusions F18.950
　　　　hallucinations F18.951
　　　unspecified disorder F18.99
　　harmful — *see* Abuse, drug, inhalant
　methadone F11.20

Use — *continued*
　nonprescribed drugs F19.90
　　harmful — *see* Abuse, non-psychoactive substance
　opioid F11.90
　　with
　　　disorder F11.99
　　　　mood F11.94
　　　　sleep F11.982
　　　　specified type NEC F11.988
　　　intoxication F11.929
　　　　with
　　　　　delirium F11.921
　　　　　perceptual disturbance F11.922
　　　　uncomplicated F11.920
　　　withdrawal F11.93
　　harmful — *see* Abuse, drug, opioid
　patent medicines F19.90
　　harmful — *see* Abuse, non-psychoactive substance
　psychoactive drug NEC F19.90
　　with
　　　anxiety disorder F19.980
　　　intoxication F19.929
　　　　with
　　　　　delirium F19.921
　　　　　perceptual disturbance F19.922
　　　　uncomplicated F19.920
　　　mood disorder F19.94
　　　other specified disorder F19.988
　　　persisting
　　　　amnestic disorder F19.96
　　　　dementia F19.97
　　　psychosis F19.959
　　　　delusions F19.950
　　　　hallucinations F19.951
　　　sexual dysfunction F19.981
　　　sleep disorder F19.982
　　　unspecified disorder F19.99
　　　withdrawal F19.939
　　　　with
　　　　　delirium F19.931
　　　　　perceptual disturbance F19.932
　　　　uncomplicated F19.930
　　harmful — *see* Abuse, drug NEC, psychoactive NEC
　sedative, hypnotic, or anxiolytic F13.90
　　with
　　　anxiety disorder F13.980
　　　intoxication F13.929
　　　　with
　　　　　delirium F13.921
　　　　uncomplicated F13.920
　　　other specified disorder F13.988
　　　persisting
　　　　amnestic disorder F13.96
　　　　dementia F13.97
　　　psychosis F13.959
　　　　delusions F13.950
　　　　hallucinations F13.951
　　　sexual dysfunction F13.981
　　　sleep disorder F13.982
　　　unspecified disorder F13.99
　　harmful — *see* Abuse, drug, sedative, hypnotic, or
　　　anxiolytic
　stimulant NEC F15.90
　　with
　　　anxiety disorder F15.980
　　　intoxication F15.929
　　　　with
　　　　　delirium F15.921
　　　　　perceptual disturbance F15.922
　　　　uncomplicated F15.920
　　　mood disorder F15.94
　　　other specified disorder F15.988
　　　psychosis F15.959
　　　　delusions F15.950
　　　　hallucinations F15.951
　　　sexual dysfunction F15.981
　　　sleep disorder F15.982
　　　unspecified disorder F15.99
　　　withdrawal F15.93
　　harmful — *see* Abuse, drug, stimulant NEC
　tobacco Z72.0
　　with dependence — *see* Dependence, drug, nicotine
　volatile solvents (*see also* Use, inhalant) F18.90
　　harmful — *see* Abuse, drug, inhalant
Usher-Senear disease or syndrome L10.4
Uta B55.1
Uteromegaly N85.2

Uterovaginal — *see* condition
Uterovesical — *see* condition
Uveal — *see* condition
Uveitis (anterior) (*see also* Iridocyclitis)
　acute — *see* Iridocyclitis, acute
　chronic — *see* Iridocyclitis, chronic
　due to toxoplasmosis (acquired) B58.09
　　congenital P37.1
　granulomatous — *see* Iridocyclitis, chronic
　heterochromic — *see* Cyclitis, Fuchs' heterochromic
　lens-induced — *see* Iridocyclitis, lens-induced
　posterior — *see* Chorioretinitis
　sympathetic H44.13- ☑
　syphilitic (secondary) A51.43
　　congenital (early) A50.01
　　late A52.71
　tuberculous A18.54
Uveoencephalitis — *see* Inflammation, chorioretinal
Uveokeratitis — *see* Iridocyclitis
Uveoparotitis D86.89
Uvula — *see* condition
Uvulitis (acute) (catarrhal) (chronic) (membranous)
　(suppurative) (ulcerative) K12.2

V

Vaccination (prophylactic)
　complication or reaction — *see* Complications, vaccination
　delayed Z28.9
　encounter for Z23
　not done — *see* Immunization, not done, because of)
Vaccinia (generalized) (localized) T88.1 ☑
　without vaccination B08.011
　congenital P35.8
Vacuum, in sinus (accessory) (nasal) J34.89
Vagabond, vagabondage Z59.0
Vagabond's disease B85.1
Vagina, vaginal — *see* condition
Vaginalitis (tunica) (testis) N49.1
Vaginismus (reflex) N94.2
　functional F52.5
　nonorganic F52.5
　psychogenic F52.5
　secondary N94.2
Vaginitis (acute) (circumscribed) (diffuse) (emphysematous) (nonvenereal) (ulcerative) N76.0
　with ectopic or molar pregnancy O08.0
　amebic A06.82
　atrophic, postmenopausal N95.2
　bacterial N76.0
　blennorrhagic (gonococcal) A54.02
　candidal B37.3
　chlamydial A56.02
　chronic N76.1
　due to Trichomonas (vaginalis) A59.01
　following ectopic or molar pregnancy O08.0
　gonococcal A54.02
　　with abscess (accessory gland) (periurethral) A54.1
　granuloma A58
　in (due to)
　　candidiasis B37.3
　　herpesviral (herpes simplex) infection A60.04
　　pinworm infection B80 [N77.1]
　monilial B37.3
　mycotic (candidal) B37.3
　postmenopausal atrophic N95.2
　puerperal (postpartum) O86.13
　senile (atrophic) N95.2
　subacute or chronic N76.1
　syphilitic (early) A51.0
　　late A52.76
　trichomonal A59.01
　tuberculous A18.18
Vaginosis — *see* Vaginitis
Vagotonia G52.2
Vagrancy Z59.0
VAIN — *see* Neoplasia, intraepithelial, vagina
Vallecula — *see* condition
Valley fever B38.0
Valsuani's disease — *see* Anemia, obstetric
Valve, valvular (formation) (*see also* condition)
　cerebral ventricle (communicating) in situ Z98.2
　cervix, internal os Q51.828
　congenital NEC — *see* Atresia, by site
　ureter (pelvic junction) (vesical orifice) Q62.39
　urethra (congenital) (posterior) Q64.2

Valvulitis (chronic) — *see* Endocarditis
Valvulopathy — *see* Endocarditis
Van Bogaert's leukoencephalopathy (sclerosing) (subacute) A81.1
Van Bogaert-Scherer-Epstein disease or syndrome E75.5
Van Buchem's syndrome M85.2
Van Creveld-von Gierke disease E74.01
Van der Hoeve (-de Kleyn) **syndrome** Q78.0
Van der Woude's syndrome Q38.0
Van Neck's disease or osteochondrosis M91.0
Vanishing lung J44.9
Vapor asphyxia or suffocation T59.9 ☑
   specified agent — *see* Table of Drugs and Chemicals
Variance, lethal ball, prosthetic heart valve T82.09 ☑
Variants, thalassemic D56.8
Variations in hair color L67.1
Varicella B01.9
   with
      complications NEC B01.89
      encephalitis B01.11
      encephalomyelitis B01.11
      meningitis B01.0
      myelitis B01.12
      pneumonia B01.2
   congenital P35.8
Varices — *see* Varix
Varicocele (scrotum) (thrombosed) I86.1
   ovary I86.2
   perineum I86.3
   spermatic cord (ulcerated) I86.1
Varicose
   aneurysm (ruptured) I77.0
   dermatitis — *see* Varix, leg, with, inflammation
   eczema — *see* Varix, leg, with, inflammation
   phlebitis — *see* Varix, with, inflammation
   tumor — *see* Varix
   ulcer (lower limb, any part) (*see also* Varix, leg, with, ulcer)
      anus (*see also* Hemorrhoids) K64.8
      esophagus — *see* Varix, esophagus
      inflamed or infected — *see* Varix, leg, with ulcer, with inflammation
      nasal septum I86.8
      perineum I86.3
      scrotum I86.1
      specified site NEC I86.8
   vein — *see* Varix
   vessel — *see* Varix, leg
Varicosis, varicosities, varicosity — *see* Varix
Variola (major) (minor) B03
Varioloid B03
Varix (lower limb) (ruptured) I83.90
   with
      edema I83.899
      inflammation I83.10
         with ulcer (venous) I83.209
      pain I83.819
      specified complication NEC I83.899
      stasis dermatitis I83.10
         with ulcer (venous) I83.209
      swelling I83.899
      ulcer I83.009
         with inflammation I83.209
   aneurysmal I77.0
   asymptomatic I83.9- ☑
   bladder I86.2
   broad ligament I86.2
   complicating
      childbirth (lower extremity) O87.4
         anus or rectum O87.2
         genital (vagina, vulva or perineum) O87.8
      pregnancy (lower extremity) O22.0- ☑
         anus or rectum O22.4- ☑
         genital (vagina, vulva or perineum) O22.1- ☑
      puerperium (lower extremity) O87.4
         anus or rectum O87.2
         genital (vagina, vulva, perineum) O87.8
   congenital (any site) Q27.8
   esophagus (idiopathic) (primary) (ulcerated) I85.00
      bleeding I85.01
      congenital Q27.8
      in (due to)
         alcoholic liver disease I85.10
            bleeding I85.11
         cirrhosis of liver I85.10
            bleeding I85.11

Varix — *continued*
   esophagus — *continued*
      in — *continued*
         portal hypertension I85.10
            bleeding I85.11
         schistosomiasis I85.10
            bleeding I85.11
         toxic liver disease I85.10
            bleeding I85.11
      secondary I85.10
         bleeding I85.11
   gastric I86.4
   inflamed or infected I83.10
      ulcerated I83.209
   labia (majora) I86.3
   leg (asymptomatic) I83.90
      with
         edema I83.899
         inflammation I83.10
            with ulcer — *see* Varix, leg, with, ulcer, with inflammation by site
         pain I83.819
         specified complication NEC I83.899
         swelling I83.899
         ulcer I83.009
            with inflammation I83.209
            ankle I83.003
               with inflammation I83.203
            calf I83.002
               with inflammation I83.202
            foot NEC I83.005
               with inflammation I83.205
            heel I83.004
               with inflammation I83.204
            lower leg NEC I83.008
               with inflammation I83.208
            midfoot I83.004
               with inflammation I83.204
            thigh I83.001
               with inflammation I83.201
      bilateral (asymptomatic) I83.93
         with
            edema I83.893
            pain I83.813
            specified complication NEC I83.893
            swelling I83.893
            ulcer I83.009
               with inflammation I83.209
      left (asymptomatic) I83.92
         with
            edema I83.892
            inflammation I83.12
               with ulcer — *see* Varix, leg, with, ulcer, with inflammation by site
            pain I83.812
            specified complication NEC I83.892
            swelling I83.892
            ulcer I83.029
               with inflammation I83.229
               ankle I83.023
                  with inflammation I83.223
               calf I83.022
                  with inflammation I83.222
               foot NEC I83.025
                  with inflammation I83.225
               heel I83.024
                  with inflammation I83.224
               lower leg NEC I83.028
                  with inflammation I83.228
               midfoot I83.024
                  with inflammation I83.224
               thigh I83.021
                  with inflammation I83.221
      right (asymptomatic) I83.91
         with
            edema I83.891
            inflammation I83.11
               with ulcer — *see* Varix, leg, with, ulcer, with inflammation by site
            pain I83.811
            specified complication NEC I83.891
            swelling I83.891
            ulcer I83.019
               with inflammation I83.219
               ankle I83.013
                  with inflammation I83.213
               calf I83.012
                  with inflammation I83.212

Varix — *continued*
   leg — *continued*
      right — *continued*
         with — *continued*
            ulcer — *continued*
               foot NEC I83.015
                  with inflammation I83.215
               heel I83.014
                  with inflammation I83.214
               lower leg NEC I83.018
                  with inflammation I83.218
               midfoot I83.014
                  with inflammation I83.214
               thigh I83.011
                  with inflammation I83.211
   nasal septum I86.8
   orbit I86.8
      congenital Q27.8
   ovary I86.2
   papillary I78.1
   pelvis I86.2
   perineum I86.3
   pharynx I86.8
   placenta O43.89- ☑
   renal papilla I86.8
   retina H35.09
   scrotum (ulcerated) I86.1
   sigmoid colon I86.8
   specified site NEC I86.8
   spinal (cord) (vessels) I86.8
   spleen, splenic (vein) (with phlebolith) I86.8
   stomach I86.4
   sublingual I86.0
   ulcerated I83.009
      inflamed or infected I83.209
   uterine ligament I86.2
   vagina I86.8
   vocal cord I86.8
   vulva I86.3
Vas deferens — *see* condition
Vas deferentitis N49.1
Vasa previa O69.4 ☑
   hemorrhage from, affecting newborn P50.0
Vascular (*see also* condition)
   loop on optic papilla Q14.2
   spasm I73.9
   spider I78.1
Vascularization, cornea — *see* Neovascularization, cornea
Vasculitis I77.6
   allergic D69.0
   cryoglobulinemic D89.1
   disseminated I77.6
   hypocomplementemic M31.8
   kidney I77.89
   livedoid L95.0
   nodular L95.8
   retina H35.06- ☑
   rheumatic — *see* Fever, rheumatic
   rheumatoid — *see* Rheumatoid, vasculitis
   skin (limited to) L95.9
      specified NEC L95.8
Vasculopathy, necrotizing M31.9
   cardiac allograft T86.290
   specified NEC M31.8
Vasitis (nodosa) N49.1
   tuberculous A18.15
Vasodilation I73.9
Vasomotor — *see* condition
Vasoplasty, after previous sterilization Z31.0
   aftercare Z31.42
Vasospasm (vasoconstriction) I73.9
   cerebral (cerebrovascular) (artery) I67.848
      reversible I67.841
   coronary I20.1
   nerve
      arm — *see* Mononeuropathy, upper limb
      brachial plexus G54.0
      cervical plexus G54.2
      leg — *see* Mononeuropathy, lower limb
   peripheral NOS I73.9
   retina (artery) — *see* Occlusion, artery, retina
Vasospastic — *see* condition
Vasovagal attack (paroxysmal) R55
   psychogenic F45.8
VATER syndrome Q87.2
Vater's ampulla — *see* condition

☑ Additional Character Required — Refer to the Tabular List for Character Selection   ▽ Subterms under main terms may continue to next column or page

Vegetation, vegetative
  adenoid (nasal fossa) J35.8
  endocarditis (acute) (any valve) (subacute) I33.0
  heart (mycotic) (valve) I33.0
Veil
  Jackson's Q43.3
Vein, venous — *see* condition
Veldt sore — *see* Ulcer, skin
Velpeau's hernia — *see* Hernia, femoral
Venereal
  bubo A55
  disease A64
  granuloma inguinale A58
  lymphogranuloma (Durand-Nicolas-Favre) A55
Venofibrosis I87.8
Venom, venomous — *see* Table of Drugs and Chemicals, by animal or substance, poisoning
Venous — *see* condition
Ventilator lung, newborn P27.8
Ventral — *see* condition
Ventricle, ventricular (*see also* condition)
  escape I49.3
  inversion Q20.5
Ventriculitis (cerebral) (*see also* Encephalitis) G04.90
Ventriculostomy status Z98.2
Vernet's syndrome G52.7
Verneuil's disease (syphilitic bursitis) A52.78
Verruca (due to HPV) (filiformis) (simplex) (viral) (vulgaris) B07.9
  acuminata A63.0
  necrogenica (primary) (tuberculosa) A18.4
  plana B07.8
  plantaris B07.0
  seborrheica L82.1
    inflamed L82.0
  senile (seborrheic) L82.1
    inflamed L82.0
  tuberculosa (primary) A18.4
  venereal A63.0
Verrucosities — *see* Verruca
Verruga peruana, peruviana A44.1
Version
  with extraction
  cervix — *see* Malposition, uterus
  uterus (postinfectional) (postpartal, old) — *see* Malposition, uterus
Vertebra, vertebral — *see* condition
Vertical talus (congenital) Q66.80
  left foot Q66.82
  right foot Q66.81
Vertigo R42
  auditory — *see* Vertigo, aural
  aural H81.31- ☑
  benign paroxysmal (positional) H81.1- ☑
  central (origin) H81.4- ☑
  cerebral H81.4- ☑
  Dix and Hallpike (epidemic) — *see* Neuronitis, vestibular
  due to infrasound T75.23 ☑
  epidemic A88.1
    Dix and Hallpike — *see* Neuronitis, vestibular
    Pedersen's — *see* Neuronitis, vestibular
    vestibular neuronitis — *see* Neuronitis, vestibular
  hysterical F44.89
  infrasound T75.23 ☑
  labyrinthine — *see* subcategory H81.0 ☑
  laryngeal R05
  malignant positional H81.4- ☑
  Ménière's — *see* subcategory H81.0 ☑
  menopausal N95.1
  otogenic — *see* Vertigo, aural
  paroxysmal positional, benign — *see* Vertigo, benign paroxysmal
  Pedersen's (epidemic) — *see* Neuronitis, vestibular
  peripheral NEC H81.39- ☑
  positional
    benign paroxysmal — *see* Vertigo, benign paroxysmal
    malignant H81.4- ☑
Very-low-density-lipoprotein-type (VLDL) **hyperlipoproteinemia** E78.1
Vesania — *see* Psychosis
Vesical — *see* condition
Vesicle
  cutaneous R23.8
  seminal — *see* condition
  skin R23.8

Vesicocolic — *see* condition
Vesicoperineal — *see* condition
Vesicorectal — *see* condition
Vesicourethrorectal — *see* condition
Vesicovaginal — *see* condition
Vesicular — *see* condition
Vesiculitis (seminal) N49.0
  amebic A06.82
  gonorrheal (acute) (chronic) A54.23
  trichomonal A59.09
  tuberculous A18.15
Vestibulitis (ear) (*see also* subcategory) H83.0 ☑
  nose (external) J34.89
  vulvar N94.810
Vestibulopathy , acute peripheral (recurrent) — *see* Neuronitis, vestibular
Vestige, vestigial (*see also* Persistence)
  branchial Q18.0
  structures in vitreous Q14.0
Vibration
  adverse effects T75.20 ☑
    pneumatic hammer syndrome T75.21 ☑
    specified effect NEC T75.29 ☑
    vasospastic syndrome T75.22 ☑
    vertigo from infrasound T75.23 ☑
  exposure (occupational) Z57.7
  vertigo T75.23 ☑
Vibriosis A28.9
Victim (of)
  crime Z65.4
  disaster Z65.5
  terrorism Z65.4
  torture Z65.4
  war Z65.5
Vidal's disease L28.0
Villaret's syndrome G52.7
Villous — *see* condition
VIN — *see* Neoplasia, intraepithelial, vulva
Vincent's infection (angina) (gingivitis) A69.1
  stomatitis NEC A69.1
Vinson-Plummer syndrome D50.1
Violence, physical R45.6
Viosterol deficiency — *see* Deficiency, calciferol
Vipoma — *see* Neoplasm, malignant, by site
Viremia B34.9
Virilism (adrenal) E25.9
  congenital E25.0
Virilization (female) (suprarenal) E25.9
  congenital E25.0
  isosexual E28.2
Virulent bubo A57
Virus, viral (*see also* condition)
  as cause of disease classified elsewhere B97.89
  cytomegalovirus B25.9
  human immunodeficiency (HIV) — *see* Human, immunodeficiency virus (HIV) disease
  infection — *see* Infection, virus
  specified NEC B34.8
  swine influenza (viruses that normally cause infections in pigs) (*see also* Influenza, due to, identified novel influenza A virus) J09.X2
  West Nile (fever) A92.30
    with
      complications NEC A92.39
      cranial nerve disorders A92.32
      encephalitis A92.31
      encephalomyelitis A92.31
      neurologic manifestation NEC A92.32
      optic neuritis A92.32
      polyradiculitis A92.32
Viscera, visceral — *see* condition
Visceroptosis K63.4
Visible peristalsis R19.2
Vision, visual
  binocular, suppression H53.34
  blurred, blurring H53.8
    hysterical F44.6
  defect, defective NEC H54.7
  disorientation (syndrome) H53.8
  disturbance H53.9
    hysterical F44.6
  double H53.2
  examination Z01.00
    with abnormal findings Z01.01
  field, limitation (defect) — *see* Defect, visual field
  hallucinations R44.1
  halos H53.19

Vision, visual — *continued*
  loss — *see* Loss, vision
    sudden — *see* Disturbance, vision, subjective, loss, sudden
  low (both eyes) — *see* Low, vision
  perception, simultaneous without fusion H53.33
Vitality, lack or want of R53.83
  newborn P96.89
Vitamin deficiency — *see* Deficiency, vitamin
Vitelline duct, persistent Q43.0
Vitiligo L80
  eyelid H02.739
    left H02.736
      lower H02.735
      upper H02.734
    right H02.733
      lower H02.732
      upper H02.731
  pinta A67.2
  vulva N90.89
Vitreal corneal syndrome H59.01- ☑
Vitreoretinopathy, proliferative (*see also* Retinopathy, proliferative)
  with retinal detachment — *see* Detachment, retina, traction
Vitreous (*see also* condition)
  touch syndrome — *see* Complication, postprocedural, following cataract surgery
Vocal cord — *see* condition
Vogt-Koyanagi syndrome H20.82- ☑
Vogt's disease or syndrome G80.3
Vogt-Spielmeyer amaurotic idiocy or disease E75.4
Voice
  change R49.9
    specified NEC R49.8
  loss — *see* Aphonia
Volhynian fever A79.0
Volkmann's ischemic contracture or paralysis (complicating trauma) T79.6 ☑
Volvulus (bowel) (colon) (duodenum) (intestine) K56.2
  with perforation K56.2
  congenital Q43.8
  fallopian tube — *see* Torsion, fallopian tube
  oviduct — *see* Torsion, fallopian tube
  stomach (due to absence of gastrocolic ligament) K31.89
Vomiting R11.10
  with nausea R11.2
  without nausea R11.11
  asphyxia — *see* Foreign body, by site, causing asphyxia, gastric contents
  bilious (cause unknown) R11.14
    following gastro-intestinal surgery K91.0
    in newborn P92.01
  blood — *see* Hematemesis
  causing asphyxia, choking, or suffocation — *see* Foreign body, by site
  cyclical G43.A0 (*following* G43.7)
    with refractory migraine G43.A1 (*following* G43.7)
    without refractory migraine G43.A0 (*following* G43.7)
    intractable G43.A1 (*following* G43.7)
    not intractable G43.A0 (*following* G43.7)
    psychogenic F50.8
  fecal mater R11.13
  following gastrointestinal surgery K91.0
    psychogenic F50.8
  functional K31.89
  hysterical F50.8
  nervous F50.8
  neurotic F50.8
  newborn NEC P92.09
    bilious P92.01
  periodic R11.10
    psychogenic F50.8
  projectile R11.12
  psychogenic F50.8
  uremic — *see* Uremia
Vomito negro — *see* Fever, yellow
Von Bezold's abscess — *see* Mastoiditis, acute
Von Economo-Cruchet disease A85.8
Von Eulenburg's disease G71.19
Von Gierke's disease E74.01
Von Hippel (-Lindau) **disease or syndrome** Q85.8
Von Jaksch's anemia or disease D64.89

Von Recklinghausen
- disease (neurofibromatosis) Q85.01
  - bones E21.0
Von Schroetter's syndrome I82.890
Von Willebrand (-Jurgens)(-Minot) **disease or syndrome** D68.0
Von Zumbusch's disease L40.1
Voyeurism F65.3
Vrolik's disease Q78.0
Vulva — *see* condition
Vulvismus N94.2
Vulvitis (acute) (allergic) (atrophic) (hypertrophic) (intertriginous) (senile) N76.2
- with ectopic or molar pregnancy O08.0
- adhesive, congenital Q52.79
- blennorrhagic (gonococcal) A54.02
- candidal B37.3
- chlamydial A56.02
- due to Haemophilus ducreyi A57
- following ectopic or molar pregnancy O08.0
- gonococcal A54.02
  - with abscess (accessory gland) (periurethral) A54.1
- herpesviral A60.04
- leukoplakic N90.4
- monilial B37.3
- puerperal (postpartum) O86.19
- subacute or chronic N76.3
- syphilitic (early) A51.0
  - late A52.76
- trichomonal A59.01
- tuberculous A18.18
Vulvodynia N94.819
- specified NEC N94.818
Vulvorectal — *see* condition
Vulvovaginitis (acute) — *see* Vaginitis

W

Waiting list, person on Z75.1
- for organ transplant Z76.82
- undergoing social agency investigation Z75.2
Waldenström
- hypergammaglobulinemia D89.0
- syndrome or macroglobulinemia C88.0
Waldenström-Kjellberg syndrome D50.1
Walking
- difficulty R26.2
  - psychogenic F44.4
- sleep F51.3
  - hysterical F44.89
Wall, abdominal — *see* condition
Wallenberg's disease or syndrome G46.3
Wallgren's disease I87.8
Wandering
- gallbladder, congenital Q44.1
- in diseases classified elsewhere Z91.83
- kidney, congenital Q63.8
- organ or site, congenital NEC — *see* Malposition, congenital, by site
- pacemaker (heart) I49.8
- spleen D73.89
War neurosis F48.8
Wart (due to HPV) (filiform) (infectious) (viral) B07.9
- anogenital region (venereal) A63.0
- common B07.8
- external genital organs (venereal) A63.0
- flat B07.8
- Hassal-Henle's (of cornea) H18.49
- Peruvian A44.1
- plantar B07.0
- prosector (tuberculous) A18.4
- seborrheic L82.1
  - inflamed L82.0
- senile (seborrheic) L82.1
  - inflamed L82.0
- tuberculous A18.4
- venereal A63.0
Warthin's tumor — *see* Neoplasm, salivary gland, benign
Wassilieff's disease A27.0
Wasting
- disease R64
  - due to malnutrition E41
- extreme (due to malnutrition) E41
- muscle NEC — *see* Atrophy, muscle
Water
- clefts (senile cataract) — *see* Cataract, senile, incipient
- deprivation of T73.1 ☑

Water — *continued*
- intoxication E87.79
- itch B76.9
- lack of T73.1 ☑
- loading E87.70
- on
  - brain — *see* Hydrocephalus
  - chest J94.8
- poisoning E87.79
Waterbrash R12
Waterhouse (-Friderichsen) **syndrome or disease** (meningococcal) A39.1
Water-losing nephritis N25.89
Watermelon stomach K31.819
- with hemorrhage K31.811
- without hemorrhage K31.819
Watsoniasis B66.8
Wax in ear — *see* Impaction, cerumen
Weak, weakening, weakness (generalized) R53.1
- arches (acquired) (*see also* Deformity, limb, flat foot)
- bladder (sphincter) R32
- facial R29.810
  - following
    - cerebrovascular disease I69.992
      - cerebral infarction I69.392
      - intracerebral hemorrhage I69.192
      - nontraumatic intracranial hemorrhage NEC I69.292
      - specified disease NEC I69.892
      - stroke I69.392
      - subarachnoid hemorrhage I69.092
- foot (double) — *see* Weak, arches
- heart, cardiac — *see* Failure, heart
- mind F70
- muscle M62.81
- myocardium — *see* Failure, heart
- newborn P96.89
- pelvic fundus N81.89
- pubocervical tissue N81.82
- rectovaginal tissue N81.83
- senile R54
- urinary stream R39.12
- valvular — *see* Endocarditis
Wear, worn (with normal or routine use)
- articular bearing surface of internal joint prosthesis — *see* Complications, joint prosthesis, mechanical, wear of articular bearing surfaces, by site
- device, implant or graft — *see* Complications, by site, mechanical complication
- tooth, teeth (approximal) (hard tissues) (interproximal) (occlusal) K03.0
Weather, weathered
- effects of
  - cold T69.9 ☑
    - specified effect NEC T69.8 ☑
  - hot — *see* Heat
- skin L57.8
Weaver's syndrome Q87.3
Web, webbed (congenital)
- duodenal Q43.8
- esophagus Q39.4
- fingers Q70.1- ☑
- larynx (glottic) (subglottic) Q31.0
- neck (pterygium colli) Q18.3
- Paterson-Kelly D50.1
- popliteal syndrome Q87.89
- toes Q70.3- ☑
Weber-Christian disease M35.6
Weber-Cockayne syndrome (epidermolysis bullosa) Q81.8
Weber-Gubler syndrome G46.3
Weber-Leyden syndrome G46.3
Weber-Osler syndrome I78.0
Weber's paralysis or syndrome G46.3
Wedge-shaped or wedging vertebra — *see* Collapse, vertebra NEC
Wegener's granulomatosis or syndrome M31.30
- with
  - kidney involvement M31.31
  - lung involvement M31.30
    - with kidney involvement M31.31
Wegner's disease A50.02
Weight
- 1000-2499 grams at birth (low) — *see* Low, birthweight
- 999 grams or less at birth (extremely low) — *see* Low, birthweight, extreme

Weight — *continued*
- gain (abnormal) (excessive) R63.5
  - in pregnancy — *see* Pregnancy, complicated by, excessive weight gain
  - low — *see* Pregnancy, complicated by, insufficient, weight gain
- loss (abnormal) (cause unknown) R63.4
Weightlessness (effect of) T75.82 ☑
Weil (I)-**Marchesani syndrome** Q87.1
Weil's disease A27.0
Weingarten's syndrome J82
Weir Mitchell's disease I73.81
Weiss-Baker syndrome G90.09
Wells' disease L98.3
Wen — *see* Cyst, sebaceous
Wenckebach's block or phenomenon I44.1
Werdnig-Hoffmann syndrome (muscular atrophy) G12.0
Werlhof's disease D69.3
Wermer's disease or syndrome E31.21
Werner-His disease A79.0
Werner's disease or syndrome E34.8
Wernicke-Korsakoff's syndrome or psychosis (alcoholic) F10.96
- with dependence F10.26
- drug-induced
  - due to drug abuse — *see* Abuse, drug, by type, with amnestic disorder
  - due to drug dependence — *see* Dependence, drug, by type, with amnestic disorder
- nonalcoholic F04
Wernicke-Posadas disease B38.9
Wernicke's
- developmental aphasia F80.2
- disease or syndrome E51.2
- encephalopathy E51.2
- polioencephalitis, superior E51.2
West African fever B50.8
Westphal-Strümpell syndrome E83.01
West's syndrome — *see* Epilepsy, spasms
Wet
- feet, tropical (maceration) (syndrome) — *see* Immersion, foot
- lung (syndrome), newborn P22.1
Wharton's duct — *see* condition
Wheal — *see* Urticaria
Wheezing R06.2
Whiplash injury S13.4 ☑
Whipple's disease (*see also* subcategory M14.8-) K90.81
Whipworm (disease) (infection) (infestation) B79
Whistling face Q87.0
White (*see also* condition)
- kidney, small N03.9
- leg, puerperal, postpartum, childbirth O87.1
- mouth B37.0
- patches of mouth K13.29
- spot lesions, teeth
  - chewing surface K02.51
  - pit and fissure surface K02.51
  - smooth surface K02.61
Whitehead L70.0
Whitlow (*see also* Cellulitis, digit)
- with lymphangitis — *see* Lymphangitis, acute, digit
- herpesviral B00.89
Whitmore's disease or fever — *see* Melioidosis
Whooping cough A37.90
- with pneumonia A37.91
  - due to Bordetella
    - bronchiseptica A37.81
    - parapertussis A37.11
    - pertussis A37.01
  - specified organism NEC A37.81
- due to
  - Bordetella
    - bronchiseptica A37.80
      - with pneumonia A37.81
    - parapertussis A37.10
      - with pneumonia A37.11
    - pertussis A37.00
      - with pneumonia A37.01
    - specified NEC A37.80
      - with pneumonia A37.81
Wichman's asthma J38.5
Wide cranial sutures, newborn P96.3
Widening aorta — *see* Ectasia, aorta
- with aneurysm — *see* Aneurysm, aorta
Wilkie's disease or syndrome K55.1

Wilkinson-Sneddon disease or syndrome L13.1
Willebrand (-Jürgens) **thrombopathy** D68.0
Willige-Hunt disease or syndrome G23.1
Wilms' tumor C64- ☑
Wilson-Mikity syndrome P27.0
Wilson's
  disease or syndrome E83.01
  hepatolenticular degeneration E83.01
  lichen ruber L43.9
Window (see also Imperfect, closure)
  aorticopulmonary Q21.4
Winter — see condition
Wiskott-Aldrich syndrome D82.0
Withdrawal state (see also Dependence, drug by type,
  with withdrawal)
  newborn
    correct therapeutic substance properly adminis-
      tered P96.2
    infant of dependent mother P96.1
  therapeutic substance, neonatal P96.2
Witts' anemia D50.8
Witzelsucht F07.0
Woakes' ethmoiditis or syndrome J33.1
Wolff-Hirschorn syndrome Q93.3
Wolff-Parkinson-White syndrome I45.6
Wolhynian fever A79.0
Wolman's disease E75.5
Wood lung or pneumonitis J67.8
Woolly, wooly hair (congenital) (nevus) Q84.1
Woolsorter's disease A22.1
Word
  blindness (congenital) (developmental) F81.0
  deafness (congenital) (developmental) H93.25
Worm(s) (infection) (infestation) (see also Infestation,
  helminth)
  guinea B72
  in intestine NEC B82.0
Worm-eaten soles A66.3
Worn out — see Exhaustion
  cardiac
    defibrillator (with synchronous cardiace pacemak-
      er) Z45.02
    pacemaker
      battery Z45.010
      lead Z45.018
  device, implant or graft — see Complications, by site,
    mechanical
Worried well Z71.1
Worries R45.82
Wound, open
  abdomen, abdominal
    wall S31.109 ☑
      with penetration into peritoneal cavity
        S31.609 ☑
      bite — see Bite, abdomen, wall
      epigastric region S31.102 ☑
        with penetration into peritoneal cavity
          S31.602 ☑
        bite — see Bite, abdomen, wall, epigastric
          region
        laceration — see Laceration, abdomen, wall,
          epigastric region
        puncture — see Puncture, abdomen, wall,
          epigastric region
      laceration — see Laceration, abdomen, wall
      left
        lower quadrant S31.104 ☑
          with penetration into peritoneal cavity
            S31.604 ☑
          bite — see Bite, abdomen, wall, left,
            lower quadrant
          laceration — see Laceration, abdomen,
            wall, left, lower quadrant
          puncture — see Puncture, abdomen,
            wall, left, lower quadrant
        upper quadrant S31.101 ☑
          with penetration into peritoneal cavity
            S31.601 ☑
          bite — see Bite, abdomen, wall, left, up-
            per quadrant
          laceration — see Laceration, abdomen,
            wall, left, upper quadrant
          puncture — see Puncture, abdomen,
            wall, left, upper quadrant
      periumbilic region S31.105 ☑
        with penetration into peritoneal cavity
          S31.605 ☑

Wound, open — continued
  abdomen, abdominal — continued
    wall — continued
      periumbilic region — continued
        bite — see Bite, abdomen, wall, periumbilic
          region
        laceration — see Laceration, abdomen, wall,
          periumbilic region
        puncture — see Puncture, abdomen, wall,
          periumbilic region
      puncture — see Puncture, abdomen, wall
      right
        lower quadrant S31.103 ☑
          with penetration into peritoneal cavity
            S31.603 ☑
          bite — see Bite, abdomen, wall, right,
            lower quadrant
          laceration — see Laceration, abdomen,
            wall, right, lower quadrant
          puncture — see Puncture, abdomen,
            wall, right, lower quadrant
        upper quadrant S31.100 ☑
          with penetration into peritoneal cavity
            S31.600 ☑
          bite — see Bite, abdomen, wall, right,
            upper quadrant
          laceration — see Laceration, abdomen,
            wall, right, upper quadrant
          puncture — see Puncture, abdomen,
            wall, right, upper quadrant
  alveolar (process) — see Wound, open, oral cavity
  ankle S91.00- ☑
    bite — see Bite, ankle
    laceration — see Laceration, ankle
    puncture — see Puncture, ankle
  antecubital space — see Wound, open, elbow
  anterior chamber, eye — see Wound, open, ocular
  anus S31.839 ☑
    bite S31.835 ☑
    laceration — see Laceration, anus
    puncture — see Puncture, anus
  arm (upper) S41.10- ☑
    with amputation — see Amputation, traumatic,
      arm
    bite — see Bite, arm
    forearm — see Wound, open, forearm
    laceration — see Laceration, arm
    puncture — see Puncture, arm
  auditory canal (external) (meatus) — see Wound, open,
    ear
  auricle, ear — see Wound, open, ear
  axilla — see Wound, open, arm
  back (see also Wound, open, thorax, back)
    lower S31.000 ☑
      with penetration into retroperitoneal space
        S31.001 ☑
      bite — see Bite, back, lower
      laceration — see Laceration, back, lower
      puncture — see Puncture, back, lower
  bite — see Bite
  blood vessel — see Injury, blood vessel
  breast S21.00- ☑
    with amputation — see Amputation, traumatic,
      breast
    bite — see Bite, breast
    laceration — see Laceration, breast
    puncture — see Puncture, breast
  buttock S31.809 ☑
    bite — see Bite, buttock
    laceration — see Laceration, buttock
    left S31.829 ☑
    puncture — see Puncture, buttock
    right S31.819 ☑
  calf — see Wound, open, leg
  canaliculus lacrimalis — see Wound, open, eyelid
  canthus, eye — see Wound, open, eyelid
  cervical esophagus S11.20 ☑
    bite S11.25 ☑
    laceration — see Laceration, esophagus, traumatic,
      cervical
    puncture — see Puncture, cervical esophagus
  cheek (external) S01.40- ☑
    bite — see Bite, cheek
    internal — see Wound, open, oral cavity
    laceration — see Laceration, cheek
    puncture — see Puncture, cheek

Wound, open — continued
  chest wall — see Wound, open, thorax
  chin — see Wound, open, head, specified site NEC
  choroid — see Wound, open, ocular
  ciliary body (eye) — see Wound, open, ocular
  clitoris S31.40 ☑
    with amputation — see Amputation, traumatic,
      clitoris
    bite S31.45 ☑
    laceration — see Laceration, vulva
    puncture — see Puncture, vulva
  conjunctiva — see Wound, open, ocular
  cornea — see Wound, open, ocular
  costal region — see Wound, open, thorax
  Descemet's membrane — see Wound, open, ocular
  digit(s)
    foot — see Wound, open, toe
    hand — see Wound, open, finger
  ear (canal) (external) S01.30- ☑
    with amputation — see Amputation, traumatic,
      ear
    bite — see Bite, ear
    drum S09.2- ☑
    laceration — see Laceration, ear
    puncture — see Puncture, ear
  elbow S51.00- ☑
    bite — see Bite, elbow
    laceration — see Laceration, elbow
    puncture — see Puncture, elbow
  epididymis — see Wound, open, testis
  epigastric region S31.102 ☑
    with penetration into peritoneal cavity S31.602 ☑
    bite — see Bite, abdomen, wall, epigastric region
    laceration — see Laceration, abdomen, wall, epi-
      gastric region
    puncture — see Puncture, abdomen, wall, epigas-
      tric region
  epiglottis — see Wound, open, neck, specified site
    NEC
  esophagus (thoracic) S27.819 ☑
    cervical — see Wound, open, cervical esophagus
    laceration S27.813 ☑
    specified type NEC S27.818 ☑
  eye — see Wound, open, ocular
  eyeball — see Wound, open, ocular
  eyebrow — see Wound, open, eyelid
  eyelid S01.10- ☑
    bite — see Bite, eyelid
    laceration — see Laceration, eyelid
    puncture — see Puncture, eyelid
  face NEC — see Wound, open, head, specified site NEC
  finger(s) S61.209 ☑
    with
      amputation — see Amputation, traumatic, fin-
        ger
      damage to nail S61.309 ☑
    bite — see Bite, finger
    index S61.208 ☑
      with
        damage to nail S61.308 ☑
      left S61.201 ☑
        with
          damage to nail S61.301 ☑
      right S61.200 ☑
        with
          damage to nail S61.300 ☑
    laceration — see Laceration, finger
    little S61.208 ☑
      with
        damage to nail S61.308 ☑
      left S61.207 ☑
        with damage to nail S61.307 ☑
      right S61.206 ☑
        with damage to nail S61.306 ☑
    middle S61.208 ☑
      with
        damage to nail S61.308 ☑
      left S61.203 ☑
        with damage to nail S61.303 ☑
      right S61.202 ☑
        with damage to nail S61.302 ☑
    puncture — see Puncture, finger
    ring S61.208 ☑
      with
        damage to nail S61.308 ☑

Index

Wilkinson-Sneddon disease or syndrome — Wound, open

Wound, open — *continued*
  finger(s) — *continued*
    ring — *continued*
      left S61.205 ☑
        with damage to nail S61.305 ☑
      right S61.204 ☑
        with damage to nail S61.304 ☑
  flank — *see* Wound, open, abdomen, wall
  foot (except toe(s) alone) S91.30- ☑
    with amputation — *see* Amputation, traumatic, foot
    bite — *see* Bite, foot
    laceration — *see* Laceration, foot
    puncture — *see* Puncture, foot
    toe — *see* Wound, open, toe
  forearm S51.80- ☑
    with
      amputation — *see* Amputation, traumatic, forearm
    bite — *see* Bite, forearm
    elbow only — *see* Wound, open, elbow
    laceration — *see* Laceration, forearm
    puncture — *see* Puncture, forearm
  forehead — *see* Wound, open, head, specified site NEC
  genital organs, external
    with amputation — *see* Amputation, traumatic, genital organs
    bite — *see* Bite, genital organ
    female S31.502 ☑
      vagina S31.40 ☑
      vulva S31.40 ☑
    laceration — *see* Laceration, genital organ
    male S31.501 ☑
      penis S31.20 ☑
      scrotum S31.30 ☑
      testes S31.30 ☑
    puncture — *see* Puncture, genital organ
  globe (eye) — *see* Wound, open, ocular
  groin — *see* Wound, open, abdomen, wall
  gum — *see* Wound, open, oral cavity
  hand S61.40- ☑
    with
      amputation — *see* Amputation, traumatic, hand
    bite — *see* Bite, hand
    finger(s) — *see* Wound, open, finger
    laceration — *see* Laceration, hand
    puncture — *see* Puncture, hand
    thumb — *see* Wound, open, thumb
  head S01.90 ☑
    bite — *see* Bite, head
    cheek — *see* Wound, open, cheek
    ear — *see* Wound, open, ear
    eyelid — *see* Wound, open, eyelid
    laceration — *see* Laceration, head
    lip — *see* Wound, open, lip
    nose S01.20 ☑
    oral cavity — *see* Wound, open, oral cavity
    puncture — *see* Puncture, head
    scalp — *see* Wound, open, scalp
    specified site NEC S01.80 ☑
    temporomandibular area — *see* Wound, open, cheek
  heel — *see* Wound, open, foot
  hip S71.00- ☑
    with amputation — *see* Amputation, traumatic, hip
    bite — *see* Bite, hip
    laceration — *see* Laceration, hip
    puncture — *see* Puncture, hip
  hymen S31.40 ☑
    bite — *see* Bite, vulva
    laceration — *see* Laceration, vagina
    puncture — *see* Puncture, vagina
  hypochondrium S31.109 ☑
    bite — *see* Bite, hypochondrium
    laceration — *see* Laceration, hypochondrium
    puncture — *see* Puncture, hypochondrium
  hypogastric region S31.109 ☑
    bite — *see* Bite, hypogastric region
    laceration — *see* Laceration, hypogastric region
    puncture — *see* Puncture, hypogastric region
  iliac (region) — *see* Wound, open, inguinal region
  inguinal region S31.109 ☑
    bite — *see* Bite, abdomen, wall, lower quadrant
    laceration — *see* Laceration, inguinal region

Wound, open — *continued*
  inguinal region — *continued*
    puncture — *see* Puncture, inguinal region
  instep — *see* Wound, open, foot
  interscapular region — *see* Wound, open, thorax, back
  intraocular — *see* Wound, open, ocular
  iris — *see* Wound, open, ocular
  jaw — *see* Wound, open, head, specified site NEC
  knee S81.00- ☑
    bite — *see* Bite, knee
    laceration — *see* Laceration, knee
    puncture — *see* Puncture, knee
  labium (majus) (minus) — *see* Wound, open, vulva
  laceration — *see* Laceration, by site
  lacrimal duct — *see* Wound, open, eyelid
  larynx S11.019 ☑
    bite — *see* Bite, larynx
    laceration — *see* Laceration, larynx
    puncture — *see* Puncture, larynx
  left
    lower quadrant S31.104 ☑
      with penetration into peritoneal cavity S31.604 ☑
      bite — *see* Bite, abdomen, wall, left, lower quadrant
      laceration — *see* Laceration, abdomen, wall, left, lower quadrant
      puncture — *see* Puncture, abdomen, wall, left, lower quadrant
    upper quadrant S31.101 ☑
      with penetration into peritoneal cavity S31.601 ☑
      bite — *see* Bite, abdomen, wall, left, upper quadrant
      laceration — *see* Laceration, abdomen, wall, left, upper quadrant
      puncture — *see* Puncture, abdomen, wall, left, upper quadrant
  leg (lower) S81.80- ☑
    with amputation — *see* Amputation, traumatic, leg
    ankle — *see* Wound, open, ankle
    bite — *see* Bite, leg
    foot — *see* Wound, open, foot
    knee — *see* Wound, open, knee
    laceration — *see* Laceration, leg
    puncture — *see* Puncture, leg
    toe — *see* Wound, open, toe
    upper — *see* Wound, open, thigh
  lip S01.501 ☑
    bite — *see* Bite, lip
    laceration — *see* Laceration, lip
    puncture — *see* Puncture, lip
  loin S31.109 ☑
    bite — *see* Bite, abdomen, wall
    laceration — *see* Laceration, loin
    puncture — *see* Puncture, loin
  lower back — *see* Wound, open, back, lower
  lumbar region — *see* Wound, open, back, lower
  malar region — *see* Wound, open, head, specified site NEC
  mammary — *see* Wound, open, breast
  mastoid region — *see* Wound, open, head, specified site NEC
  mouth — *see* Wound, open, oral cavity
  nail
    finger — *see* Wound, open, finger, with damage to nail
    toe — *see* Wound, open, toe, with damage to nail
  nape (neck) — *see* Wound, open, neck
  nasal (septum) (sinus) — *see* Wound, open, nose
  nasopharynx — *see* Wound, open, head, specified site NEC
  neck S11.90 ☑
    bite — *see* Bite, neck
    involving
      cervical esophagus S11.20 ☑
      larynx — *see* Wound, open, larynx
      pharynx S11.20 ☑
      thyroid S11.10 ☑
      trachea (cervical) S11.029 ☑
        bite — *see* Bite, trachea
        laceration S11.021 ☑
          with foreign body S11.022 ☑
        puncture S11.023 ☑
          with foreign body S11.024 ☑

Wound, open — *continued*
  neck — *continued*
    laceration — *see* Laceration, neck
    puncture — *see* Puncture, neck
    specified site NEC S11.80 ☑
      specified type NEC S11.89 ☑
  nose (septum) (sinus) S01.20 ☑
    with amputation — *see* Amputation, traumatic, nose
    bite — *see* Bite, nose
    laceration — *see* Laceration, nose
    puncture — *see* Puncture, nose
  ocular S05.90 ☑
    avulsion (traumatic enucleation) S05.7- ☑
    eyeball S05.6- ☑
      with foreign body S05.5- ☑
    eyelid — *see* Wound, open, eyelid
    laceration and rupture S05.3- ☑
      with prolapse or loss of intraocular tissue S05.2- ☑
    orbit (penetrating) (with or without foreign body) S05.4- ☑
    periocular area — *see* Wound, open, eyelid
    specified NEC S05.8X- ☑
  oral cavity S01.502 ☑
    bite S01.552 ☑
    laceration — *see* Laceration, oral cavity
    puncture — *see* Puncture, oral cavity
  orbit — *see* Wound, open, ocular, orbit
  palate — *see* Wound, open, oral cavity
  palm — *see* Wound, open, hand
  pelvis, pelvic (*see also* Wound, open, back, lower)
    girdle — *see* Wound, open, hip
  penetrating — *see* Puncture, by site
  penis S31.20 ☑
    with amputation — *see* Amputation, traumatic, penis
    bite S31.25 ☑
    laceration — *see* Laceration, penis
    puncture — *see* Puncture, penis
  perineum
    bite — *see* Bite, perineum
    female S31.502 ☑
    laceration — *see* Laceration, perineum
    male S31.501 ☑
    puncture — *see* Puncture, perineum
  periocular area (with or without lacrimal passages) — *see* Wound, open, eyelid
  periumbilic region S31.105 ☑
    with penetration into peritoneal cavity S31.605 ☑
    bite — *see* Bite, abdomen, wall, periumbilic region
    laceration — *see* Laceration, abdomen, wall, periumbilic region
    puncture — *see* Puncture, abdomen, wall, periumbilic region
  phalanges
    finger — *see* Wound, open, finger
    toe — *see* Wound, open, toe
  pharynx S11.20 ☑
  pinna — *see* Wound, open, ear
  popliteal space — *see* Wound, open, knee
  prepuce — *see* Wound, open, penis
  pubic region — *see* Wound, open, back, lower
  pudendum — *see* Wound, open, genital organs, external
  puncture wound — *see* Puncture
  rectovaginal septum — *see* Wound, open, vagina
  right
    lower quadrant S31.103 ☑
      with penetration into peritoneal cavity S31.603 ☑
      bite — *see* Bite, abdomen, wall, right, lower quadrant
      laceration — *see* Laceration, abdomen, wall, right, lower quadrant
      puncture — *see* Puncture, abdomen, wall, right, lower quadrant
    upper quadrant S31.100 ☑
      with penetration into peritoneal cavity S31.600 ☑
      bite — *see* Bite, abdomen, wall, right, upper quadrant
      laceration — *see* Laceration, abdomen, wall, right, upper quadrant
      puncture — *see* Puncture, abdomen, wall, right, upper quadrant

☑ **Additional Character Required — Refer to the Tabular List for Character Selection** ▽ Subterms under main terms may continue to next column or page

Wound, open — *continued*
  sacral region — *see* Wound, open, back, lower
  sacroiliac region — *see* Wound, open, back, lower
  salivary gland — *see* Wound, open, oral cavity
  scalp S01.00 ☑
    bite S01.05 ☑
    laceration — *see* Laceration, scalp
    puncture — *see* Puncture, scalp
  scalpel, newborn (birth injury) P15.8
  scapular region — *see* Wound, open, shoulder
  sclera — *see* Wound, open, ocular
  scrotum S31.30 ☑
    with amputation — *see* Amputation, traumatic, scrotum
    bite S31.35 ☑
    laceration — *see* Laceration, scrotum
    puncture — *see* Puncture, scrotum
  shin — *see* Wound, open, leg
  shoulder S41.00- ☑
    with amputation — *see* Amputation, traumatic, arm
    bite — *see* Bite, shoulder
    laceration — *see* Laceration, shoulder
    puncture — *see* Puncture, shoulder
  skin NOS T14.8
  spermatic cord — *see* Wound, open, testis
  sternal region — *see* Wound, open, thorax, front wall
  submaxillary region — *see* Wound, open, head, specified site NEC
  submental region — *see* Wound, open, head, specified site NEC
  subungual
    finger(s) — *see* Wound, open, finger
    toe(s) — *see* Wound, open, toe
  supraclavicular region — *see* Wound, open, neck, specified site NEC
  temple, temporal region — *see* Wound, open, head, specified site NEC
  temporomandibular area — *see* Wound, open, cheek
  testis S31.30 ☑
    with amputation — *see* Amputation, traumatic, testes
    bite S31.35 ☑
    laceration — *see* Laceration, testis
    puncture — *see* Puncture, testis
  thigh S71.10- ☑
    with amputation — *see* Amputation, traumatic, hip
    bite — *see* Bite, thigh
    laceration — *see* Laceration, thigh
    puncture — *see* Puncture, thigh
  thorax, thoracic (wall) S21.90 ☑
    back S21.20-
      with penetration S21.40 ☑
    bite — *see* Bite, thorax
    breast — *see* Wound, open, breast
    front S21.10-
      with penetration S21.30 ☑
    laceration — *see* Laceration, thorax
    puncture — *see* Puncture, thorax
  throat — *see* Wound, open, neck
  thumb S61.009 ☑
    with
      amputation — *see* Amputation, traumatic, thumb
      damage to nail S61.109 ☑
    bite — *see* Bite, thumb
    laceration — *see* Laceration, thumb
    left S61.002 ☑
      with
        damage to nail S61.102 ☑
    puncture — *see* Puncture, thumb
    right S61.001 ☑
      with
        damage to nail S61.101 ☑
  thyroid (gland) — *see* Wound, open, neck, thyroid
  toe(s) S91.109 ☑
    with
      amputation — *see* Amputation, traumatic, toe
      damage to nail S91.209 ☑
    bite — *see* Bite, toe
    great S91.103 ☑
      with
        damage to nail S91.203 ☑

Wound, open — *continued*
  toe(s) — *continued*
    great — *continued*
      left S91.102 ☑
        with
          damage to nail S91.202 ☑
      right S91.101 ☑
        with
          damage to nail S91.201 ☑
      laceration — *see* Laceration, toe
    lesser S91.106 ☑
      with
        damage to nail S91.206 ☑
      left S91.105 ☑
        with
          damage to nail S91.205 ☑
      right S91.104 ☑
        with
          damage to nail S91.204 ☑
    puncture — *see* Puncture, toe
  tongue — *see* Wound, open, oral cavity
  trachea (cervical region) — *see* Wound, open, neck, trachea
  tunica vaginalis — *see* Wound, open, testis
  tympanum, tympanic membrane S09.2- ☑
    laceration — *see* Laceration, ear, drum
    puncture — *see* Puncture, tympanum
  umbilical region — *see* Wound, open, abdomen, wall, periumbilic region
  uvula — *see* Wound, open, oral cavity
  vagina S31.40 ☑
    bite S31.45 ☑
    laceration — *see* Laceration, vagina
    puncture — *see* Puncture, vagina
  vitreous (humor) — *see* Wound, open, ocular
  vocal cord S11.039 ☑
    bite — *see* Bite, vocal cord
    laceration S11.031 ☑
      with foreign body S11.032 ☑
    puncture S11.033 ☑
      with foreign body S11.034 ☑
  vulva S31.40 ☑
    with amputation — *see* Amputation, traumatic, vulva
    bite S31.45 ☑
    laceration — *see* Laceration, vulva
    puncture — *see* Puncture, vulva
  wrist S61.50- ☑
    bite — *see* Bite, wrist
    laceration — *see* Laceration, wrist
    puncture — *see* Puncture, wrist
Wound, superficial — *see* Injury (*see also* specified injury type)
Wright's syndrome G54.0
Wrist — *see* condition
Wrong drug (by accident) (given in error) — *see* Table of Drugs and Chemicals, by drug, poisoning
Wry neck — *see* Torticollis
Wuchereria (bancrofti) **infestation** B74.0
Wuchereriasis B74.0
Wuchernde Struma Langhans C73

X

Xanthelasma (eyelid) (palpebrarum) H02.60
  left H02.66
    lower H02.65
    upper H02.64
  right H02.63
    lower H02.62
    upper H02.61
Xanthelasmatosis (essential) E78.2
Xanthinuria, hereditary E79.8
Xanthoastrocytoma
  specified site — *see* Neoplasm, malignant, by site
  unspecified site C71.9
Xanthofibroma — *see* Neoplasm, connective tissue, benign
Xanthogranuloma D76.3
Xanthoma(s), xanthomatosis (primary) (familial) (hereditary) E75.5
  with
    hyperlipoproteinemia
      Type I E78.3
      Type III E78.2
      Type IV E78.1

Xanthoma(s), xanthomatosis — *continued*
  with — *continued*
    hyperlipoproteinemia — *continued*
      Type V E78.3
  bone (generalisata) C96.5
  cerebrotendinous E75.5
  cutaneotendinous E75.5
  disseminatum (skin) E78.2
  eruptive E78.2
  hypercholesterinemic E78.0
  hypercholesterolemic E78.0
  hyperlipidemic E78.5
  joint E75.5
  multiple (skin) E78.2
  tendon (sheath) E75.5
  tuberosum E78.2
  tuberous E78.2
  tubo-eruptive E78.2
  verrucous, oral mucosa K13.4
Xanthosis R23.8
Xenophobia F40.10
Xeroderma (*see also* Ichthyosis)
  acquired L85.0
  eyelid H01.149
    left H01.146
      lower H01.145
      upper H01.144
    right H01.143
      lower H01.142
      upper H01.141
  pigmentosum Q82.1
  vitamin A deficiency E50.8
Xerophthalmia (vitamin A deficiency) E50.7
  unrelated to vitamin A deficiency — *see* Keratoconjunctivitis
Xerosis
  conjunctiva H11.14- ☑
    with Bitot's spots (*see also* Pigmentation, conjunctiva)
      vitamin A deficiency E50.1
      vitamin A deficiency E50.0
  cornea H18.89- ☑
    with ulceration — *see* Ulcer, cornea
      vitamin A deficiency E50.3
      vitamin A deficiency E50.2
  cutis L85.3
  skin L85.3
Xerostomia K11.7
Xiphopagus Q89.4
XO syndrome Q96.9
X-ray (of)
  abnormal findings — *see* Abnormal, diagnostic imaging
  breast (mammogram) (routine) Z12.31
  chest
    routine (as part of a general medical examination) Z00.00
      with abnormal findings Z00.01
    routine (as part of a general medical examination) Z00.00
      with abnormal findings Z00.01
XXXXY syndrome Q98.1
XXY syndrome Q98.0

Y

Yaba pox (virus disease) B08.72
Yatapoxvirus B08.70
  specified NEC B08.79
Yawning R06.89
  psychogenic F45.8
Yaws A66.9
  cutaneous, less than five years after infection A66.2
  bone lesions A66.6
  butter A66.1
  chancre A66.0
  early (cutaneous) (macular) (maculopapular) (micropapular) (papular) A66.2
    frambeside A66.2
    skin lesions NEC A66.2
  eyelid A66.2
  ganglion A66.6
  gangosis, gangosa A66.5
  gumma, gummata A66.4
    bone A66.6
  gummatous
    frambeside A66.4
    osteitis A66.6

▽ Subterms under main terms may continue to next column or page   ☑ Additional Character Required — Refer to the Tabular List for Character Selection

Wound, open — Yaws

319

Yaws — *continued*
  gummatous — *continued*
    periostitis A66.6
  hydrarthrosis (*see also* subcategory M14.8-) A66.6
  hyperkeratosis (early) (late) A66.3
  initial lesions A66.0
  joint lesions (*see also* subcategory M14.8-) A66.6
  juxta-articular nodules A66.7
  late nodular (ulcerated) A66.4
  latent (without clinical manifestations) (with positive
    serology) A66.8
  mother A66.0
  mucosal A66.7
  multiple papillomata A66.1
  nodular, late (ulcerated) A66.4
  osteitis A66.6
  papilloma, plantar or palmar A66.1
  periostitis (hypertrophic) A66.6

Yaws — *continued*
  specified NEC A66.7
  ulcers A66.4
  wet crab A66.1
Yeast infection (*see also* Candidiasis) B37.9
Yellow
  atrophy (liver) — *see* Failure, hepatic
  fever — *see* Fever, yellow
  jack — *see* Fever, yellow
  jaundice — *see* Jaundice
  nail syndrome L60.5
Yersiniosis (*see also* Infection, Yersinia)
  extraintestinal A28.2
  intestinal A04.6

Z

Zahorsky's syndrome (herpangina) B08.5

Zellweger's syndrome Q87.89
Zenker's diverticulum (esophagus) K22.5
Ziehen-Oppenheim disease G24.1
Zieve's syndrome K70.0
Zinc
  deficiency, dietary E60
  metabolism disorder E83.2
Zollinger-Ellison syndrome E16.4
Zona — *see* Herpes, zoster
Zoophobia F40.218
Zoster (herpes) — *see* Herpes, zoster
Zygomycosis B46.9
  specified NEC B46.8
Zymotic — *see* condition

☑ **Additional Character Required** — **Refer to the Tabular List for Character Selection**   ▽ **Subterms under main terms may continue to next column or page**

ICD-10-CM Neoplasm Table

Note: The list below gives the code number for neoplasms by anatomical site. For each site there are six possible code numbers according to whether the neoplasm in question is malignant, benign, in situ, of uncertain behavior, or of unspecified nature. The description of the neoplasm will often indicate which of the six columns is appropriate; e.g., malignant melanoma of skin, benign fibroadenoma of breast, carcinoma in situ of cervix uteri. Where such descriptors are not present, the remainder of the Index should be consulted where guidance is given to the appropriate column for each morphological (histological) variety listed; e.g., Mesonephroma – see Neoplasm, malignant; Embryoma (see also Neoplasm, uncertain behavior); Disease, Bowen's – see Neoplasm, skin, in situ. However, the guidance in the Index can be overridden if one of the descriptors mentioned above is present; e.g., malignant adenoma of colon is coded to C18.9 and not to D12.6 as the adjective "malignant" overrides the Index entry "Adenoma (see also Neoplasm, benign)." Codes listed with a dash -, following the code have a required 5th character for laterality. The tabular list must be reviewed for the complete code.

	Malignant Primary	Malignant Secondary	Ca in situ	Benign	Uncertain	Unspecified Behavior
Neoplasm, neoplastic	C80.1	C79.9	D09.9	D36.9	D48.9	D49.9
abdomen,						
abdominal	C76.2	C79.8-✓	D09.8	D36.7	D48.7	D49.89
cavity	C76.2	C79.8-✓	D09.8	D36.7	D48.7	D49.89
organ	C76.2	C79.8-✓	D09.8	D36.7	D48.7	D49.89
viscera	C76.2	C79.8-✓	D09.8	D36.7	D48.7	D49.89
wall — *see also* Neoplasm, abdomen, wall,						
skin	C44.509	C79.2	D04.5	D23.5	D48.5	D49.2
connective tissue	C49.4	C79.8-✓	—	D21.4	D48.1	D49.2
skin	C44.509	—	—	—	—	—
basal cell carcinoma	C44.519	—	—	—	—	—
specified type NEC	C44.599	—	—	—	—	—
squamous cell carcinoma	C44.529	—	—	—	—	—
abdominopelvic	C76.8	C79.8-✓	—	D36.7	D48.7	D49.89
accessory sinus — *see* Neoplasm, sinus						
acoustic nerve	C72.4-✓	C79.49	—	D33.3	D43.3	D49.7
adenoid (pharynx) (tissue)	C11.1	C79.89	D00.08	D10.6	D37.05	D49.0
adipose tissue — *see also* Neoplasm, connective tissue	C49.4	C79.89	—	D21.9	D48.1	D49.2
adnexa (uterine)	C57.4	C79.89	D07.39	D28.7	D39.8	D49.5
adrenal	C74.9-✓	C79.7-✓	D09.3	D35.0-✓	D44.1-✓	D49.7
capsule	C74.9-✓	C79.7-✓	D09.3	D35.0-✓	D44.1-✓	D49.7
cortex	C74.0-✓	C79.7-✓	D09.3	D35.0-✓	D44.1-✓	D49.7
gland	C74.9-✓	C79.7-✓	D09.3	D35.0-✓	D44.1-✓	D49.7
medulla	C74.1-✓	C79.7-✓	D09.3	D35.0-✓	D44.1-✓	D49.7
ala nasi (external) — *see also* Neoplasm, skin, nose	C44.301	C79.2	D04.39	D23.39	D48.5	D49.2
alimentary canal or tract NEC	C26.9	C78.80	D01.9	D13.9	D37.9	D49.0
alveolar	C03.9	C79.89	D00.03	D10.39	D37.09	D49.0
mucosa	C03.9	C79.89	D00.03	D10.39	D37.09	D49.0
lower	C03.1	C79.89	D00.03	D10.39	D37.09	D49.0
upper	C03.0	C79.89	D00.03	D10.39	D37.09	D49.0
ridge or process	C41.1	C79.51	—	D16.5	D48.0	D49.2
carcinoma	C03.9	C79.8-✓	—	—	—	—
lower	C03.1	C79.8-✓	—	—	—	—
upper	C03.0	C79.8-✓	—	—	—	—
lower	C41.1	C79.51	—	D16.5	D48.0	D49.2
mucosa	C03.9	C79.89	D00.03	D10.39	D37.09	D49.0
lower	C03.1	C79.89	D00.03	D10.39	D37.09	D49.0
upper	C03.0	C79.89	D00.03	D10.39	D37.09	D49.0
upper	C41.0	C79.51	—	D16.4	D48.0	D49.2
sulcus	C06.1	C79.89	D00.02	D10.39	D37.09	D49.0
alveolus	C03.9	C79.89	D00.03	D10.39	D37.09	D49.0
lower	C03.1	C79.89	D00.03	D10.39	D37.09	D49.0
upper	C03.0	C79.89	D00.03	D10.39	D37.09	D49.0
ampulla of Vater	C24.1	C78.89	D01.5	D13.5	D37.6	D49.0
ankle NEC	C76.5-✓	C79.89	D04.7-✓	D36.7	D48.7	D49.89

	Malignant Primary	Malignant Secondary	Ca in situ	Benign	Uncertain	Unspecified Behavior
Neoplasm, neoplastic — *continued*						
anorectum, anorectal (junction)	C21.8	C78.5	D01.3	D12.9	D37.8	D49.0
antecubital fossa or space	C76.4-✓	C79.89	D04.6-✓	D36.7	D48.7	D49.89
antrum (Highmore) (maxillary)	C31.0	C78.39	D02.3	D14.0	D38.5	D49.1
pyloric	C16.3	C78.89	D00.2	D13.1	D37.1	D49.0
tympanicum	C30.1	C78.39	D02.3	D14.0	D38.5	D49.1
anus, anal	C21.0	C78.5	D01.3	D12.9	D37.8	D49.0
canal	C21.1	C78.5	D01.3	D12.9	D37.8	D49.0
cloacogenic zone	C21.2	C78.5	D01.3	D12.9	D37.8	D49.0
margin — *see also* Neoplasm, anus, skin	C44.500	C79.2	D04.5	D23.5	D48.5	D49.2
overlapping lesion with rectosigmoid junction or rectum	C21.8	—	—	—	—	—
skin	C44.500	C79.2	D04.5	D23.5	D48.5	D49.2
basal cell carcinoma	C44.510	—	—	—	—	—
specified type NEC	C44.590	—	—	—	—	—
squamous cell carcinoma	C44.520	—	—	—	—	—
sphincter	C21.1	C78.5	D01.3	D12.9	D37.8	D49.0
aorta (thoracic)	C49.3	C79.89	—	D21.3	D48.1	D49.2
abdominal	C49.4	C79.89	—	D21.4	D48.1	D49.2
aortic body	C75.5	C79.89	—	D35.6	D44.7	D49.7
aponeurosis	C49.9	C79.89	—	D21.9	D48.1	D49.2
palmar	C49.1-✓	C79.89	—	D21.1-✓	D48.1	D49.2
plantar	C49.2-✓	C79.89	—	D21.2-✓	D48.1	D49.2
appendix	C18.1	C78.5	D01.0	D12.1	D37.3	D49.0
arachnoid	C70.9	C79.49	—	D32.9	D42.9	D49.7
cerebral	C70.0	C79.32	—	D32.0	D42.0	D49.7
spinal	C70.1	C79.49	—	D32.1	D42.1	D49.7
areola	C50.0-✓	C79.81	D05-✓	D24-✓	D48.6-✓	D49.3
arm NEC	C76.4-✓	C79.89	D04.6-✓	D36.7	D48.7	D49.89
artery — *see* Neoplasm, connective tissue						
aryepiglottic fold	C13.1	C79.89	D00.08	D10.7	D37.05	D49.0
hypopharyngeal aspect	C13.1	C79.89	D00.08	D10.7	D37.05	D49.0
laryngeal aspect	C32.1	C78.39	D02.0	D14.1	D38.0	D49.1
marginal zone	C13.1	C79.89	D00.08	D10.7	D37.05	D49.0
arytenoid (cartilage)	C32.3	C78.39	D02.0	D14.1	D38.0	D49.1
fold — *see* Neoplasm, aryepiglottic						
associated with transplanted organ	C80.2	—	—	—	—	—
atlas	C41.2	C79.51	—	D16.6	D48.0	D49.2
atrium, cardiac	C38.0	C79.89	—	D15.1	D48.7	D49.89
auditory						
canal (external) (skin) A81	C44.20-✓	C79.2	D04.2-✓	D23.2-✓	D48.5	D49.2
internal	C30.1	C78.39	D02.3	D14.0	D38.5	D49.1
nerve	C72.4-✓	C79.49	—	D33.3	D43.3	D49.7
tube	C30.1	C78.39	D02.3	D14.0	D38.5	D49.1
opening	C11.2	C79.89	D00.08	D10.6	D37.05	D49.0
auricle, ear — *see also* Neoplasm, skin, ear	C44.20-✓	C79.2	D04.2-✓	D23.2-✓	D48.5	D49.2
auricular canal (external) — *see also* Neoplasm, skin, ear	C44.20-✓	C79.2	D04.2-✓	D23.2-✓	D48.5	D49.2
internal	C30.1	C78.39	D02.3	D14.0	D38.5	D49.2
autonomic nerve or nervous system NEC (see Neoplasm, nerve, peripheral)						
axilla, axillary	C76.1	C79.89	D09.8	D36.7	D48.7	D49.89
fold — *see also* Neoplasm, skin, trunk	C44.509	C79.2	D04.5	D23.5	D48.5	D49.2
back NEC	C76.8	C79.89	D04.5	D36.7	D48.7	D49.89

Neoplasm, neoplastic — *continued*	Malignant Primary	Malignant Secondary	Ca in situ	Benign	Uncertain	Unspecified Behavior
Bartholin's gland	C51.0	C79.82	D07.1	D28.0	D39.8	D49.5
basal ganglia	C71.0	C79.31	—	D33.0	D43.0	D49.6
basis pedunculi	C71.7	C79.31	—	D33.1	D43.1	D49.6
bile or biliary (tract)	C24.9	C78.89	D01.5	D13.5	D37.6	D49.0
canaliculi (biliferi) (intrahepatic)	C22.1	C78.7	D01.5	D13.4	D37.6	D49.0
canals, interlobular	C22.1	C78.89	D01.5	D13.4	D37.6	D49.0
duct or passage (common) (cystic) (extrahepatic)	C24.0	C78.89	D01.5	D13.5	D37.6	D49.0
interlobular	C22.1	C78.89	D01.5	D13.4	D37.6	D49.0
intrahepatic	C22.1	C78.7	D01.5	D13.4	D37.6	D49.0
and extrahepatic	C24.8	C78.89	D01.5	D13.5	D37.6	D49.0
bladder (urinary)	C67.9	C79.11	D09.0	D30.3	D41.4	D49.4
dome	C67.1	C79.11	D09.0	D30.3	D41.4	D49.4
neck	C67.5	C79.11	D09.0	D30.3	D41.4	D49.4
orifice	C67.9	C79.11	D09.0	D30.3	D41.4	D49.4
ureteric	C67.6	C79.11	D09.0	D30.3	D41.4	D49.4
urethral	C67.5	C79.11	D09.0	D30.3	D41.4	D49.4
overlapping lesion	C67.8	—	—	—	—	—
sphincter	C67.8	C79.11	D09.0	D30.3	D41.4	D49.4
trigone	C67.0	C79.11	D09.0	D30.3	D41.4	D49.4
urachus	C67.7	C79.11	D09.0	D30.3	D41.4	D49.4
wall	C67.9	C79.11	D09.0	D30.3	D41.4	D49.4
anterior	C67.3	C79.11	D09.0	D30.3	D41.4	D49.4
lateral	C67.2	C79.11	D09.0	D30.3	D41.4	D49.4
posterior	C67.4	C79.11	D09.0	D30.3	D41.4	D49.4
blood vessel — *see* Neoplasm, connective tissue						
bone (periosteum)	C41.9	C79.51	—	D16.9	D48.0	D49.2
acetabulum	C41.4	C79.51	—	D16.8	D48.0	D49.2
ankle	C40.3-☑	C79.51	—	D16.3-☑	—	—
arm NEC	C40.0-☑	C79.51	—	D16.0-☑	—	—
astragalus	C40.3-☑	C79.51	—	D16.3-☑	—	—
atlas	C41.2	C79.51	—	D16.6	D48.0	D49.2
axis	C41.2	C79.51	—	D16.6	D48.0	D49.2
back NEC	C41.2	C79.51	—	D16.6	D48.0	D49.2
calcaneus	C40.3-☑	C79.51	—	D16.3-☑	—	—
calvarium	C41.0	C79.51	—	D16.4	D48.0	D49.2
carpus (any)	C40.1-☑	C79.51	—	D16.1-☑	—	—
cartilage NEC	C41.9	C79.51	—	D16.9	D48.0	D49.2
clavicle	C41.3	C79.51	—	D16.7	D48.0	D49.2
clivus	C41.0	C79.51	—	D16.4	D48.0	D49.2
coccygeal vertebra	C41.4	C79.51	—	D16.8	D48.0	D49.2
coccyx	C41.4	C79.51	—	D16.8	D48.0	D49.2
costal cartilage	C41.3	C79.51	—	D16.7	D48.0	D49.2
costovertebral joint	C41.3	C79.51	—	D16.7	D48.0	D49.2
cranial	C41.0	C79.51	—	D16.4	D48.0	D49.2
cuboid	C40.3-☑	C79.51	—	D16.3-☑	—	—
cuneiform	C41.9	C79.51	—	D16.9	D48.0	D49.2
elbow	C40.0-☑	C79.51	—	D16.0-☑	—	—
ethmoid (labyrinth)	C41.0	C79.51	—	D16.4	D48.0	D49.2
face	C41.0	C79.51	—	D16.4	D48.0	D49.2
femur (any part)	C40.2-☑	C79.51	—	D16.2-☑	—	—
fibula (any part)	C40.2-☑	C79.51	—	D16.2-☑	—	—
finger (any)	C40.1-☑	C79.51	—	D16.1-☑	—	—
foot	C40.3-☑	C79.51	—	D16.3-☑	—	—
forearm	C40.0-☑	C79.51	—	D16.0-☑	—	—
frontal	C41.0	C79.51	—	D16.4	D48.0	D49.2
hand	C40.1-☑	C79.51	—	D16.1-☑	—	—
heel	C40.3-☑	C79.51	—	D16.3-☑	—	—
hip	C41.4	C79.51	—	D16.8	D48.0	D49.2
humerus (any part)	C40.0-☑	C79.51	—	D16.0-☑	—	—
hyoid	C41.0	C79.51	—	D16.4	D48.0	D49.2
ilium	C41.4	C79.51	—	D16.8	D48.0	D49.2
innominate	C41.4	C79.51	—	D16.8	D48.0	D49.2
intervertebral cartilage or disc	C41.2	C79.51	—	D16.6	D48.0	D49.2
ischium	C41.4	C79.51	—	D16.8	D48.0	D49.2
jaw (lower)	C41.1	C79.51	—	D16.5	D48.0	D49.2
knee	C40.2-☑	C79.51	—	D16.2-☑	—	—
leg NEC	C40.2-☑	C79.51	—	D16.2-☑	—	—
limb NEC	C40.9-☑	C79.51	—	D16.9	—	—

Neoplasm, neoplastic — *continued*	Malignant Primary	Malignant Secondary	Ca in situ	Benign	Uncertain	Unspecified Behavior
bone — *continued*						
limb — *continued*						
lower (long bones)	C40.2-☑	C79.51	—	D16.2-☑	—	—
short bones	C40.3-☑	C79.51	—	D16.3-☑	—	—
upper (long bones)	C40.0-☑	C79.51	—	D16.0-☑	—	—
short bones	C40.1-☑	C79.51	—	D16.1-☑	—	—
malar	C41.0	C79.51	—	D16.4	D48.0	D49.2
mandible	C41.1	C79.51	—	D16.5	D48.0	D49.2
marrow NEC (any bone)	C96.9	C79.52	—	—	D47.9	D49.89
mastoid	C41.0	C79.51	—	D16.4	D48.0	D49.2
maxilla, maxillary (superior)	C41.0	C79.51	—	D16.4	D48.0	D49.2
inferior	C41.1	C79.51	—	D16.5	D48.0	D49.2
metacarpus (any)	C40.1-☑	C79.51	—	D16.1-☑	—	—
metatarsus (any)	C40.3-☑	C79.51	—	D16.3-☑	—	—
navicular						
ankle	C40.3-☑	C79.51	—	—	—	—
hand	C40.1-☑	C79.51	—	—	—	—
nose, nasal	C41.0	C79.51	—	D16.4	D48.0	D49.2
occipital	C41.0	C79.51	—	D16.4	D48.0	D49.2
orbit	C41.0	C79.51	—	D16.4	D48.0	D49.2
overlapping sites	C40.8-☑	—	—	—	—	—
parietal	C41.0	C79.51	—	D16.4	D48.0	D49.2
patella	C40.2-☑	C79.51	—	—	—	—
pelvic	C41.4	C79.51	—	D16.8	D48.0	D49.2
phalanges						
foot	C40.3-☑	C79.51	—	—	—	—
hand	C40.1-☑	C79.51	—	—	—	—
pubic	C41.4	C79.51	—	D16.8	D48.0	D49.2
radius (any part)	C40.0-☑	C79.51	—	D16.0-☑	—	—
rib	C41.3	C79.51	—	D16.7	D48.0	D49.2
sacral vertebra	C41.4	C79.51	—	D16.8	D48.0	D49.2
sacrum	C41.4	C79.51	—	D16.8	D48.0	D49.2
scaphoid						
of ankle	C40.3-☑	C79.51	—	—	—	—
of hand	C40.1-☑	C79.51	—	—	—	—
scapula (any part)	C40.0-☑	C79.51	—	D16.0-☑	—	—
sella turcica	C41.0	C79.51	—	D16.4	D48.0	D49.2
shoulder	C40.0-☑	C79.51	—	D16.0-☑	—	—
skull	C41.0	C79.51	—	D16.4	D48.0	D49.2
sphenoid	C41.0	C79.51	—	D16.4	D48.0	D49.2
spine, spinal (column)	C41.2	C79.51	—	D16.6	D48.0	D49.2
coccyx	C41.4	C79.51	—	D16.8	D48.0	D49.2
sacrum	C41.4	C79.51	—	D16.8	D48.0	D49.2
sternum	C41.3	C79.51	—	D16.7	D48.0	D49.2
tarsus (any)	C40.3-☑	C79.51	—	—	—	—
temporal	C41.0	C79.51	—	D16.4	D48.0	D49.2
thumb	C40.1-☑	C79.51	—	—	—	—
tibia (any part)	C40.2-☑	C79.51	—	—	—	—
toe (any)	C40.3-☑	C79.51	—	—	—	—
trapezium	C40.1-☑	C79.51	—	—	—	—
trapezoid	C40.1-☑	C79.51	—	—	—	—
turbinate	C41.0	C79.51	—	D16.4	D48.0	D49.2
ulna (any part)	C40.0-☑	C79.51	—	D16.0-☑	—	—
unciform	C40.1-☑	C79.51	—	—	—	—
vertebra (column)	C41.2	C79.51	—	D16.6	D48.0	D49.2
coccyx	C41.4	C79.51	—	D16.8	D48.0	D49.2
sacrum	C41.4	C79.51	—	D16.8	D48.0	D49.2
vomer	C41.0	C79.51	—	D16.4	D48.0	D49.2
wrist	C40.1-☑	C79.51	—	—	—	—
xiphoid process	C41.3	C79.51	—	D16.7	D48.0	D49.2
zygomatic	C41.0	C79.51	—	D16.4	D48.0	D49.2
book-leaf (mouth) — *ventral surface of tongue and floor of mouth*	C06.89	C79.89	D00.00	D10.39	D37.09	D49.0
bowel — *see* Neoplasm, intestine						
brachial plexus	C47.1-☑	C79.89	—	D36.12	D48.2	D49.2
brain NEC	C71.9	C79.31	—	D33.2	D43.2	D49.6
basal ganglia	C71.0	C79.31	—	D33.0	D43.0	D49.6
cerebellopontine angle	C71.6	C79.31	—	D33.1	D43.1	D49.6
cerebellum NOS	C71.6	C79.31	—	D33.1	D43.1	D49.6
cerebrum	C71.0	C79.31	—	D33.0	D43.0	D49.6

☑ Additional Character Required — Refer to the Tabular List for Character Selection ▽ Subterms under main terms may continue to next column or page

	Malignant Primary	Malignant Secondary	Ca in situ	Benign	Uncertain	Unspecified Behavior
Neoplasm, neoplastic — *continued*						
brain — *continued*						
choroid plexus	C71.7	C79.31	—	D33.1	D43.1	D49.6
corpus callosum	C71.8	C79.31	—	D33.2	D43.2	D49.6
corpus striatum	C71.0	C79.31	—	D33.0	D43.0	D49.6
cortex (cerebral)	C71.0	C79.31	—	D33.0	D43.0	D49.6
frontal lobe	C71.1	C79.31	—	D33.0	D43.0	D49.6
globus pallidus	C71.0	C79.31	—	D33.0	D43.0	D49.6
hippocampus	C71.2	C79.31	—	D33.0	D43.0	D49.6
hypothalamus	C71.0	C79.31	—	D33.0	D43.0	D49.6
internal capsule	C71.0	C79.31	—	D33.0	D43.0	D49.6
medulla oblongata	C71.7	C79.31	—	D33.1	D43.1	D49.6
meninges	C70.0	C79.32	—	D32.0	D42.0	D49.7
midbrain	C71.7	C79.31	—	D33.1	D43.1	D49.6
occipital lobe	C71.4	C79.31	—	D33.0	D43.0	D49.6
overlapping lesion	C71.8	C79.31	—	—	—	—
parietal lobe	C71.3	C79.31	—	D33.0	D43.0	D49.6
peduncle	C71.7	C79.31	—	D33.1	D43.1	D49.6
pons	C71.7	C79.31	—	D33.1	D43.1	D49.6
stem	C71.7	C79.31	—	D33.1	D43.1	D49.6
tapetum	C71.8	C79.31	—	D33.2	D43.2	D49.6
temporal lobe	C71.2	C79.31	—	D33.0	D43.0	D49.6
thalamus	C71.0	C79.31	—	D33.0	D43.0	D49.6
uncus	C71.2	C79.31	—	D33.0	D43.0	D49.6
ventricle (floor)	C71.5	C79.31	—	D33.0	D43.0	D49.6
fourth	C71.7	C79.31	—	D33.1	D43.1	D49.6
branchial (cleft) (cyst) (vestiges)	C10.4	C79.89	D00.08	D10.5	D37.05	D49.0
breast (connective tissue) (glandular tissue) (soft parts)	C50.9-☑	C79.81	D05.-☑	D24.-☑	D48.6-☑	D49.3
areola	C50.0-☑	C79.81	D05.-☑	D24.-☑	D48.6-☑	D49.3
axillary tail	C50.6-☑	C79.81	D05.-☑	D24.-☑	D48.6-☑	D49.3
central portion	C50.1-☑	C79.81	D05.-☑	D24.-☑	D48.6-☑	D49.3
inner	C50.8-☑	C79.81	D05.-☑	D24.-☑	D48.6-☑	D49.3
lower	C50.8-☑	C79.81	D05.-☑	D24.-☑	D48.6-☑	D49.3
lower-inner quadrant	C50.3-☑	C79.81	D05.-☑	D24.-☑	D48.6-☑	D49.3
lower-outer quadrant	C50.5-☑	C79.81	D05.-☑	D24.-☑	D48.6-☑	D49.3
mastectomy site (skin) — *see also Neoplasm, breast, skin*	C44.501	C79.2	—	—	—	—
specified as breast tissue	C50.8-☑	C79.81	—	—	—	—
midline	C50.8-☑	C79.81	D05.-☑	D24.-☑	D48.6-☑	D49.3
nipple	C50.0-☑	C79.81	D05.-☑	D24.-☑	D48.6-☑	D49.3
outer	C50.8-☑	C79.81	D05.-☑	D24.-☑	D48.6-☑	D49.3
overlapping lesion	C50.8-☑	—	—	—	—	—
skin	C44.501	C79.2	D04.5	D23.5	D48.5	D49.2
basal cell carcinoma	C44.511	—	—	—	—	—
specified type NEC	C44.591	—	—	—	—	—
squamous cell carcinoma	C44.521	—	—	—	—	—
tail (axillary)	C50.6-☑	C79.81	D05.-☑	D24.-☑	D48.6-☑	D49.3
upper	C50.8-☑	C79.81	D05.-☑	D24.-☑	D48.6-☑	D49.3
upper-inner quadrant	C50.2-☑	C79.81	D05.-☑	D24.-☑	D48.6-☑	D49.3
upper-outer quadrant	C50.4-☑	C79.81	D05.-☑	D24.-☑	D48.6-☑	D49.3
broad ligament	C57.1-☑	C79.82	D07.39	D28.2	D39.8	D49.5
bronchiogenic, bronchogenic (lung)	C34.9-☑	C78.0-☑	D02.2-☑	D14.3-☑	D38.1	D49.1
bronchiole	C34.9-☑	C78.0-☑	D02.2-☑	D14.3-☑	D38.1	D49.1
bronchus	C34.9-☑	C78.0-☑	D02.2-☑	D14.3-☑	D38.1	D49.1
carina	C34.0-☑	C78.0-☑	D02.2-☑	D14.3-☑	D38.1	D49.1
lower lobe of lung	C34.3-☑	C78.0-☑	D02.2-☑	D14.3-☑	D38.1	D49.1
main	C34.0-☑	C78.0-☑	D02.2-☑	D14.3-☑	D38.1	D49.1
middle lobe of lung	C34.2	C78.0-☑	D02.21	D14.31	D38.1	D49.1
overlapping lesion	C34.8-☑	—	—	—	—	—
upper lobe of lung	C34.1-☑	C78.0-☑	D02.2-☑	D14.3-☑	D38.1	D49.1
brow	C44.309	C79.2	D04.39	D23.39	D48.5	D49.2
basal cell carcinoma	C44.319	—	—	—	—	—
specified type NEC	C44.399	—	—	—	—	—

	Malignant Primary	Malignant Secondary	Ca in situ	Benign	Uncertain	Unspecified Behavior
Neoplasm, neoplastic — *continued*						
brow — *continued*						
squamous cell carcinoma	C44.329	—	—	—	—	—
buccal (cavity)	C06.9	C79.89	D00.00	D10.39	D37.09	D49.0
commissure	C06.0	C79.89	D00.02	D10.39	D37.09	D49.0
groove (lower) (upper)	C06.1	C79.89	D00.02	D10.39	D37.09	D49.0
mucosa	C06.0	C79.89	D00.02	D10.39	D37.09	D49.0
sulcus (lower) (upper)	C06.1	C79.89	D00.02	D10.39	D37.09	D49.0
bulbourethral gland	C68.0	C79.19	D09.19	D30.4	D41.3	D49.5
bursa — *see Neoplasm, connective tissue*						
buttock NEC	C76.3	C79.89	D04.5	D36.7	D48.7	D49.89
calf	C76.5-☑	C79.89	D04.7-☑	D36.7	D48.7	D49.89
calvarium	C41.0	C79.51	—	D16.4	D48.0	D49.2
calyx, renal	C65.-☑	C79.0-☑	D09.19	D30.1-☑	D41.1-☑	D49.5
canal						
anal	C21.1	C78.5	D01.3	D12.9	D37.8	D49.0
auditory (external) — *see also Neoplasm, skin, ear*	C44.20-☑	C79.2	D04.2-☑	D23.2-☑	D48.5	D49.2
auricular (external) — *see also Neoplasm, skin, ear*	C44.20-☑	C79.2	D04.2-☑	D23.2-☑	D48.5	D49.2
canaliculi, biliary (biliferi) (intrahepatic)	C22.1	C78.7	D01.5	D13.4	D37.6	D49.0
canthus (eye) (inner) (outer)	C44.10-☑	C79.2	D04.1-☑	D23.1-☑	D48.5	D49.2
basal cell carcinoma	C44.11-☑	—	—	—	—	—
specified type NEC	C44.19-☑	—	—	—	—	—
squamous cell carcinoma	C44.12-☑	—	—	—	—	—
capillary — *see Neoplasm, connective tissue*						
caput coli	C18.0	C78.5	D01.0	D12.0	D37.4	D49.0
carcinoid — *see Tumor, carcinoid*						
cardia (gastric)	C16.0	C78.89	D00.2	D13.1	D37.1	D49.0
cardiac orifice (stomach)	C16.0	C78.89	D00.2	D13.1	D37.1	D49.0
cardio-esophageal junction	C16.0	C78.89	D00.2	D13.1	D37.1	D49.0
cardio-esophagus	C16.0	C78.89	D00.2	D13.1	D37.1	D49.0
carina (bronchus)	C34.0-☑	C78.0-☑	D02.2-☑	D14.3-☑	D38.1	D49.1
carotid (artery)	C49.0	C79.89	—	D21.0	D48.1	D49.2
body	C75.4	C79.89	—	D35.5	D44.6	D49.7
carpus (any bone)	C40.1-☑	C79.51	—	D16.1-☑	—	—
cartilage (articular) (joint) NEC — *see also Neoplasm, bone*	C41.9	C79.51	—	D16.9	D48.0	D49.2
arytenoid	C32.3	C78.39	D02.0	D14.1	D38.0	D49.1
auricular	C49.0	C79.89	—	D21.0	D48.1	D49.2
bronchi	C34.0-☑	C78.39	—	D14.3-☑	D38.1	D49.1
costal	C41.3	C79.51	—	D16.7	D48.0	D49.2
cricoid	C32.3	C78.39	D02.0	D14.1	D38.0	D49.1
cuneiform	C32.3	C78.39	D02.0	D14.1	D38.0	D49.1
ear (external)	C49.0	C79.89	—	D21.0	D48.1	D49.2
ensiform	C41.3	C79.51	—	D16.7	D48.0	D49.2
epiglottis	C32.1	C78.39	D02.0	D14.1	D38.0	D49.1
anterior surface	C10.1	C79.89	D00.08	D10.5	D37.05	D49.0
eyelid	C49.0	C79.89	—	D21.0	D48.1	D49.2
intervertebral	C41.2	C79.51	—	D16.6	D48.0	D49.2
larynx, laryngeal	C32.3	C78.39	D02.0	D14.1	D38.0	D49.1
nose, nasal	C30.0	C78.39	D02.3	D14.0	D38.5	D49.1
pinna	C49.0	C79.89	—	D21.0	D48.1	D49.2
rib	C41.3	C79.51	—	D16.7	D48.0	D49.2
semilunar (knee)	C40.2-☑	C79.51	—	D16.2-☑	D48.0	D49.2
thyroid	C32.3	C78.39	D02.0	D14.1	D38.0	D49.1
trachea	C33	C78.39	D02.1	D14.2	D38.1	D49.1
cauda equina	C72.1	C79.49	—	D33.4	D43.4	D49.7
cavity						
buccal	C06.9	C79.89	D00.00	D10.30	D37.09	D49.0
nasal	C30.0	C78.39	D02.3	D14.0	D38.5	D49.1
oral	C06.9	C79.89	D00.00	D10.30	D37.09	D49.0
peritoneal	C48.2	C78.6	—	D20.1	D48.4	D49.0
tympanic	C30.1	C78.39	D02.3	D14.0	D38.5	D49.1
cecum	C18.0	C78.5	D01.0	D12.0	D37.4	D49.0

Neoplasm, neoplastic — continued	Malignant Primary	Malignant Secondary	Ca in situ	Benign	Uncertain	Unspecified Behavior
central nervous system	C72.9	C79.40	—	—	—	—
cerebellopontine (angle)	C71.6	C79.31	—	D33.1	D43.1	D49.6
cerebellum, cerebellar	C71.6	C79.31	—	D33.1	D43.1	D49.6
cerebrum, cerebral (cortex) (hemisphere) (white matter)	C71.0	C79.31	—	D33.0	D43.0	D49.6
meninges	C70.0	C79.32	—	D32.0	D42.0	D49.7
peduncle	C71.7	C79.31	—	D33.1	D43.1	D49.6
ventricle	C71.5	C79.31	—	D33.0	D43.0	D49.6
fourth	C71.7	C79.31	—	D33.1	D43.1	D49.6
cervical region	C76.0	C79.89	D09.8	D36.7	D48.7	D49.89
cervix (cervical) (uteri) (uterus)	C53.9	C79.82	D06.9	D26.0	D39.0	D49.5
canal	C53.0	C79.82	D06.0	D26.0	D39.0	D49.5
endocervix (canal) (gland)	C53.0	C79.82	D06.0	D26.0	D39.0	D49.5
exocervix	C53.1	C79.82	D06.1	D26.0	D39.0	D49.5
external os	C53.1	C79.82	D06.1	D26.0	D39.0	D49.5
internal os	C53.0	C79.82	D06.0	D26.0	D39.0	D49.5
nabothian gland	C53.0	C79.82	D06.0	D26.0	D39.0	D49.5
overlapping lesion	C53.8	—	—	—	—	—
squamocolumnar junction	C53.8	C79.82	D06.7	D26.0	D39.0	D49.5
stump	C53.8	C79.82	D06.7	D26.0	D39.0	D49.5
cheek	C76.0	C79.89	D09.8	D36.7	D48.7	D49.89
external	C44.309	C79.2	D04.39	D23.39	D48.5	D49.2
basal cell carcinoma	C44.319	—	—	—	—	—
specified type NEC	C44.399	—	—	—	—	—
squamous cell carcinoma	C44.329	—	—	—	—	—
inner aspect	C06.0	C79.89	D00.02	D10.39	D37.09	D49.0
internal	C06.0	C79.89	D00.02	D10.39	D37.09	D49.0
mucosa	C06.0	C79.89	D00.02	D10.39	D37.09	D49.0
chest (wall) NEC	C76.1	C79.89	D09.8	D36.7	D48.7	D49.89
chiasma opticum	C72.3-☑	C79.49	—	D33.3	D43.3	D49.7
chin	C44.309	C79.2	D04.39	D23.39	D48.5	D49.2
basal cell carcinoma	C44.319	—	—	—	—	—
specified type NEC	C44.399	—	—	—	—	—
squamous cell carcinoma	C44.329	—	—	—	—	—
choana	C11.3	C79.89	D00.08	D10.6	D37.05	D49.0
cholangiole	C22.1	C78.89	D01.5	D13.4	D37.6	D49.0
choledochal duct	C24.0	C78.89	D01.5	D13.5	D37.6	D49.0
choroid	C69.3-☑	C79.49	D09.2-☑	D31.3-☑	D48.7	D49.81
plexus	C71.5	C79.31	—	D33.0	D43.0	D49.6
ciliary body	C69.4-☑	C79.49	D09.2-☑	D31.4-☑	D48.7	D49.89
clavicle	C41.3	C79.51	—	D16.7	D48.0	D49.2
clitoris	C51.2	C79.82	D07.1	D28.0	D39.8	D49.5
clivus	C41.0	C79.51	—	D16.4	D48.0	D49.2
cloacogenic zone	C21.2	C78.5	D01.3	D12.9	D37.8	D49.0
coccygeal						
body or glomus	C49.5	C79.89	—	D21.5	D48.1	D49.2
vertebra	C41.4	C79.51	—	D16.8	D48.0	D49.2
coccyx	C41.4	C79.51	—	D16.8	D48.0	D49.2
colon — see also Neoplasm, intestine, large	C18.9	C78.5	—	—	—	—
with rectum	C19	C78.5	D01.1	D12.7	D37.5	D49.0
columnella — see also Neoplasm, skin, face	C44.390	C79.2	D04.39	D23.39	D48.5	D49.2
column, spinal — see Neoplasm, spine						
commissure						
labial, lip	C00.6	C79.89	D00.01	D10.39	D37.01	D49.0
laryngeal	C32.0	C78.39	D02.0	D14.1	D38.0	D49.1
common (bile) duct	C24.0	C78.89	D01.5	D13.5	D37.6	D49.0
concha — see also Neoplasm, skin, ear	C44.20-☑	C79.2	D04.2-☑	D23.2-☑	D48.5	D49.2
nose	C30.0	C78.39	D02.3	D14.0	D38.5	D49.1
conjunctiva	C69.0-☑	C79.49	D09.2-☑	D31.0-☑	D48.7	D49.89

Neoplasm, neoplastic — continued	Malignant Primary	Malignant Secondary	Ca in situ	Benign	Uncertain	Unspecified Behavior
connective tissue NEC	C49.9	C79.89	—	D21.9	D48.1	D49.2

Note: For neoplasms of connective tissue (blood vessel, bursa, fascia, ligament, muscle, peripheral nerves, sympathetic and parasympathetic nerves and ganglia, synovia, tendon, etc.) or of morphological types that indicate connective tissue, code according to the list under "Neoplasm, connective tissue". For sites that do not appear in this list, code to neoplasm of that site; e.g., fibrosarcoma, pancreas (C25.9)

Note: Morphological types that indicate connective tissue appear in their proper place in the alphabetic index with the instruction "see Neoplasm, connective tissue ...."

	Malignant Primary	Malignant Secondary	Ca in situ	Benign	Uncertain	Unspecified Behavior
abdomen	C49.4	C79.89	—	D21.4	D48.1	D49.2
abdominal wall	C49.4	C79.89	—	D21.4	D48.1	D49.2
ankle	C49.2-☑	C79.89	—	D21.2-☑	D48.1	D49.2
antecubital fossa or space	C49.1-☑	C79.89	—	D21.1-☑	D48.1	D49.2
arm	C49.1-☑	C79.89	—	D21.1-☑	D48.1	D49.2
auricle (ear)	C49.0	C79.89	—	D21.0	D48.1	D49.2
axilla	C49.3	C79.89	—	D21.3	D48.1	D49.2
back	C49.6	C79.89	—	D21.6	D48.1	D49.2
breast — see Neoplasm, breast						
buttock	C49.5	C79.89	—	D21.5	D48.1	D49.2
calf	C49.2-☑	C79.89	—	D21.2-☑	D48.1	D49.2
cervical region	C49.0	C79.89	—	D21.0	D48.1	D49.2
cheek	C49.0	C79.89	—	D21.0	D48.1	D49.2
chest (wall)	C49.3	C79.89	—	D21.3	D48.1	D49.2
chin	C49.0	C79.89	—	D21.0	D48.1	D49.2
diaphragm	C49.3	C79.89	—	D21.3	D48.1	D49.2
ear (external)	C49.0	C79.89	—	D21.0	D48.1	D49.2
elbow	C49.1-☑	C79.89	—	D21.1-☑	D48.1	D49.2
extrarectal	C49.5	C79.89	—	D21.5	D48.1	D49.2
extremity	C49.9	C79.89	—	D21.9	D48.1	D49.2
lower	C49.2-☑	C79.89	—	D21.2-☑	D48.1	D49.2
upper	C49.1-☑	C79.89	—	D21.1-☑	D48.1	D49.2
eyelid	C49.0	C79.89	—	D21.0	D48.1	D49.2
face	C49.0	C79.89	—	D21.0	D48.1	D49.2
finger	C49.1-☑	C79.89	—	D21.1-☑	D48.1	D49.2
flank	C49.6	C79.89	—	D21.6	D48.1	D49.2
foot	C49.2-☑	C79.89	—	D21.2-☑	D48.1	D49.2
forearm	C49.1-☑	C79.89	—	D21.1-☑	D48.1	D49.2
forehead	C49.0	C79.89	—	D21.0	D48.1	D49.2
gastric	C49.4	C79.89	—	D21.4	D48.1	D49.2
gastrointestinal	C49.4	C79.89	—	D21.4	D48.1	D49.2
gluteal region	C49.5	C79.89	—	D21.5	D48.1	D49.2
great vessels NEC	C49.3	C79.89	—	D21.3	D48.1	D49.2
groin	C49.5	C79.89	—	D21.5	D48.1	D49.2
hand	C49.1-☑	C79.89	—	D21.1-☑	D48.1	D49.2
head	C49.0	C79.89	—	D21.0	D48.1	D49.2
heel	C49.2-☑	C79.89	—	D21.2-☑	D48.1	D49.2
hip	C49.2-☑	C79.89	—	D21.2-☑	D48.1	D49.2
hypochondrium	C49.4	C79.89	—	D21.4	D48.1	D49.2
iliopsoas muscle	C49.5	C79.89	—	D21.5	D48.1	D49.2
infraclavicular region	C49.3	C79.89	—	D21.3	D48.1	D49.2
inguinal (canal) (region)	C49.5	C79.89	—	D21.5	D48.1	D49.2
intestinal	C49.4	C79.89	—	D21.4	D48.1	D49.2
intrathoracic	C49.3	C79.89	—	D21.3	D48.1	D49.2
ischiorectal fossa	C49.5	C79.89	—	D21.5	D48.1	D49.2
jaw	C03.9	C79.89	D00.03	D10.39	D48.1	D49.0
knee	C49.2-☑	C79.89	—	D21.2-☑	D48.1	D49.2
leg	C49.2-☑	C79.89	—	D21.2-☑	D48.1	D49.2
limb NEC	C49.9	C79.89	—	D21.9	D48.1	D49.2
lower	C49.2-☑	C79.89	—	D21.2-☑	D48.1	D49.2
upper	C49.1-☑	C79.89	—	D21.1-☑	D48.1	D49.2
nates	C49.5	C79.89	—	D21.5	D48.1	D49.2
neck	C49.0	C79.89	—	D21.0	D48.1	D49.2
orbit	C69.6-☑	C79.49	D09.2-☑	D31.6-☑	D48.1	D49.89
overlapping lesion	C49.8	—	—	—	—	—
pararectal	C49.5	C79.89	—	D21.5	D48.1	D49.2
para-urethral	C49.5	C79.89	—	D21.5	D48.1	D49.2
paravaginal	C49.5	C79.89	—	D21.5	D48.1	D49.2
pelvis (floor)	C49.5	C79.89	—	D21.5	D48.1	D49.2
pelvo-abdominal	C49.8	C79.89	—	D21.6	D48.1	D49.2
perineum	C49.5	C79.89	—	D21.5	D48.1	D49.2
perirectal (tissue)	C49.5	C79.89	—	D21.5	D48.1	D49.2

Neoplasm, neoplastic — *continued*

	Malignant Primary	Malignant Secondary	Ca in situ	Benign	Uncertain	Unspecified Behavior
connective tissue — *continued*						
periurethral (tissue)	C49.5	C79.89	—	D21.5	D48.1	D49.2
popliteal fossa or space	C49.2-☑	C79.89	—	D21.2-☑	D48.1	D49.2
presacral	C49.5	C79.89	—	D21.5	D48.1	D49.2
psoas muscle	C49.4	C79.89	—	D21.4	D48.1	D49.2
pterygoid fossa	C49.0	C79.89	—	D21.0	D48.1	D49.2
rectovaginal septum or wall	C49.5	C79.89	—	D21.5	D48.1	D49.2
rectovesical	C49.5	C79.89	—	D21.5	D48.1	D49.2
retroperitoneum	C48.0	C78.6	—	D20.0	D48.3	D49.0
sacrococcygeal region	C49.5	C79.89	—	D21.5	D48.1	D49.2
scalp	C49.0	C79.89	—	D21.0	D48.1	D49.2
scapular region	C49.3	C79.89	—	D21.3	D48.1	D49.2
shoulder	C49.1-☑	C79.89	—	D21.1-☑	D48.1	D49.2
skin (dermis) NEC — *see also* Neoplasm, skin, by site	C44.90	C79.2	D04.9	D23.9	D48.5	D49.2
stomach	C49.4	C79.89	—	D21.4	D48.1	D49.2
submental	C49.0	C79.89	—	D21.0	D48.1	D49.2
supraclavicular region	C49.0	C79.89	—	D21.0	D48.1	D49.2
temple	C49.0	C79.89	—	D21.0	D48.1	D49.2
temporal region	C49.0	C79.89	—	D21.0	D48.1	D49.2
thigh	C49.2-☑	C79.89	—	D21.2-☑	D48.1	D49.2
thoracic (duct) (wall)	C49.3	C79.89	—	D21.3	D48.1	D49.2
thorax	C49.3	C79.89	—	D21.3	D48.1	D49.2
thumb	C49.1-☑	C79.89	—	D21.1-☑	D48.1	D49.2
toe	C49.2-☑	C79.89	—	D21.2-☑	D48.1	D49.2
trunk	C49.6	C79.89	—	D21.6	D48.1	D49.2
umbilicus	C49.4	C79.89	—	D21.4	D48.1	D49.2
vesicorectal	C49.5	C79.89	—	D21.5	D48.1	D49.2
wrist	C49.1-☑	C79.89	—	D21.1-☑	D48.1	D49.2
conus medullaris	C72.0	C79.49	—	D33.4	D43.4	D49.7
cord (true) (vocal)	C32.0	C78.39	D02.0	D14.1	D38.0	D49.1
false	C32.1	C78.39	D02.0	D14.1	D38.0	D49.1
spermatic	C63.1-☑	C79.82	D07.69	D29.8	D40.8	D49.5
spinal (cervical) (lumbar) (thoracic)	C72.0	C79.49	—	D33.4	D43.4	D49.7
cornea (limbus)	C69.1-☑	C79.49	D09.2-☑	D31.1-☑	D48.7	D49.89
corpus						
albicans	C56.-☑	C79.6-☑	D07.39	D27.-☑	D39.1-☑	D49.5
callosum, brain	C71.0	C79.31	—	D33.2	D43.2	D49.6
cavernosum	C60.2	C79.82	D07.4	D29.0	D40.8	D49.5
gastric	C16.2	C78.89	D00.2	D13.1	D37.1	D49.0
overlapping sites	C54.8	—	—	—	—	—
penis	C60.2	C79.82	D07.4	D29.0	D40.8	D49.5
striatum, cerebrum	C71.0	C79.31	—	D33.0	D43.0	D49.6
uteri	C54.9	C79.82	D07.0	D26.1	D39.0	D49.5
isthmus	C54.0	C79.82	D07.0	D26.1	D39.0	D49.5
cortex						
adrenal	C74.0-☑	C79.7-☑	D09.3	D35.0-☑	D44.1-☑	D49.7
cerebral	C71.0	C79.31	—	D33.0	D43.0	D49.6
costal cartilage	C41.3	C79.51	—	D16.7	D48.0	D49.2
costovertebral joint	C41.3	C79.51	—	D16.7	D48.0	D49.2
Cowper's gland	C68.0	C79.19	D09.19	D30.4	D41.3	D49.5
cranial (fossa, any)	C71.9	C79.31	—	D33.2	D43.2	D49.6
meninges	C70.0	C79.32	—	D32.0	D42.0	D49.7
nerve	C72.50	C79.49	—	D33.3	D43.3	D49.7
specified NEC	C72.59	C79.49	—	D33.3	D43.3	D49.7
craniobuccal pouch	C75.2	C79.89	D09.3	D35.2	D44.3	D49.7
craniopharyngeal (duct) (pouch)	C75.2	C79.89	D09.3	D35.3	D44.4	D49.7
cricoid	C13.0	C79.89	D00.08	D10.7	D37.05	D49.0
cartilage	C32.3	C78.39	D02.0	D14.1	D38.0	D49.1
cricopharynx	C13.0	C79.89	D00.08	D10.7	D37.05	D49.0
crypt of Morgagni	C21.8	C78.5	D01.3	D12.9	D37.8	D49.0
crystalline lens	C69.4-☑	C79.49	D09.2-☑	D31.4-☑	D48.7	D49.89
cul-de-sac (Douglas')	C48.1	C78.6	—	D20.1	D48.4	D49.0
cuneiform cartilage	C32.3	C78.39	D02.0	D14.1	D38.0	D49.1
cutaneous — *see* Neoplasm, skin						
cutis — *see* Neoplasm, skin						

Neoplasm, neoplastic — *continued*

	Malignant Primary	Malignant Secondary	Ca in situ	Benign	Uncertain	Unspecified Behavior
cystic (bile) duct (common)	C24.0	C78.89	D01.5	D13.5	D37.6	D49.0
dermis — *see* Neoplasm, skin						
diaphragm	C49.3	C79.89	—	D21.3	D48.1	D49.2
digestive organs, system, tube, or tract NEC	C26.9	C78.89	D01.9	D13.9	D37.9	D49.0
disc, intervertebral	C41.2	C79.51	—	D16.6	D48.0	D49.2
disease, generalized	C80.0	—	—	—	—	—
disseminated	C80.0	—	—	—	—	—
Douglas' cul-de-sac or pouch	C48.1	C78.6	—	D20.1	D48.4	D49.0
duodenojejunal junction	C17.8	C78.4	D01.49	D13.39	D37.2	D49.0
duodenum	C17.0	C78.4	D01.49	D13.2	D37.2	D49.0
dura (cranial) (mater)	C70.9	C79.49	—	D32.9	D42.9	D49.7
cerebral	C70.0	C79.32	—	D32.0	D42.0	D49.7
spinal	C70.1	C79.49	—	D32.1	D42.1	D49.7
ear (external) — *see also* Neoplasm, skin, ear	C44.20-☑	C79.2	D04.2-☑	D23.2-☑	D48.5	D49.2
auricle or auris — *see also* Neoplasm, skin, ear	C44.20-☑	C79.2	D04.2-☑	D23.2-☑	D48.5	D49.2
canal, external — *see also* Neoplasm, skin, ear	C44.20-☑	C79.2	D04.2-☑	D23.2-☑	D48.5	D49.2
cartilage	C49.0	C79.89	—	D21.0	D48.1	D49.2
external meatus — *see also* Neoplasm, skin, ear	C44.20-☑	C79.2	D04.2-☑	D23.2-☑	D48.5	D49.2
inner	C30.1	C78.39	D02.3	D14.0	D38.5	D49.1
lobule — *see also* Neoplasm, skin, ear	C44.20-☑	C79.2	D04.2-☑	D23.2-☑	D48.5	D49.2
middle	C30.1	C78.39	D02.3	D14.0	D38.5	D49.1
overlapping lesion with accessory sinuses	C31.8	—	—	—	—	—
skin	C44.20-☑	C79.2	D04.2-☑	D23.2-☑	D48.5	D49.2
basal cell carcinoma	C44.21-☑	—	—	—	—	—
specified type NEC	C44.29-☑	—	—	—	—	—
squamous cell carcinoma	C44.22-☑	—	—	—	—	—
earlobe	C44.20-☑	C79.2	D04.2-☑	D23.2-☑	D48.5	D49.2
basal cell carcinoma	C44.21-☑	—	—	—	—	—
specified type NEC	C44.29-☑	—	—	—	—	—
squamous cell carcinoma	C44.22-☑	—	—	—	—	—
ejaculatory duct	C63.7	C79.82	D07.69	D29.8	D40.8	D49.5
elbow NEC	C76.4-☑	C79.89	D04.6-☑	D36.7	D48.7	D49.89
endocardium	C38.0	C79.89	—	D15.1	D48.7	D49.89
endocervix (canal) (gland)	C53.0	C79.82	D06.0	D26.0	D39.0	D49.5
endocrine gland NEC	C75.9	C79.89	D09.3	D35.9	D44.9	D49.7
pluriglandular	C75.8	C79.89	D09.3	D35.7	D44.9	D49.7
endometrium (gland) (stroma)	C54.1	C79.82	D07.0	D26.1	D39.0	D49.5
ensiform cartilage	C41.3	C79.51	—	D16.7	D48.0	D49.2
enteric — *see* Neoplasm, intestine						
ependyma (brain)	C71.5	C79.31	—	D33.0	D43.0	D49.6
fourth ventricle	C71.7	C79.31	—	D33.1	D43.1	D49.6
epicardium	C38.0	C79.89	—	D15.1	D48.7	D49.89
epididymis	C63.0-☑	C79.82	D07.69	D29.3-☑	D40.8	D49.5
epidural	C72.9	C79.49	—	D33.9	D43.9	D49.7
epiglottis	C32.1	C78.39	D02.0	D14.1	D38.0	D49.1
anterior aspect or surface	C10.1	C79.89	D00.08	D10.5	D37.05	D49.0
cartilage	C32.3	C78.39	D02.0	D14.1	D38.0	D49.1
free border (margin)	C10.1	C79.89	D00.08	D10.5	D37.05	D49.0
junctional region	C10.8	C79.89	D00.08	D10.5	D37.05	D49.0
posterior (laryngeal) surface	C32.1	C78.39	D02.0	D14.1	D38.0	D49.1

Neoplasm, neoplastic — continued	Malignant Primary	Malignant Secondary	Ca in situ	Benign	Uncertain	Unspecified Behavior
epiglottis — *continued*						
suprahyoid portion	C32.1	C78.39	D02.0	D14.1	D38.0	D49.1
esophagogastric junction	C16.0	C78.89	D00.2	D13.1	D37.1	D49.0
esophagus	C15.9	C78.89	D00.1	D13.0	D37.8	D49.0
abdominal	C15.5	C78.89	D00.1	D13.0	D37.8	D49.0
cervical	C15.3	C78.89	D00.1	D13.0	D37.8	D49.0
distal (third)	C15.5	C78.89	D00.1	D13.0	D37.8	D49.0
lower (third)	C15.5	C78.89	D00.1	D13.0	D37.8	D49.0
middle (third)	C15.4	C78.89	D00.1	D13.0	D37.8	D49.0
overlapping lesion	C15.8	—	—	—	—	—
proximal (third)	C15.3	C78.89	D00.1	D13.0	D37.8	D49.0
thoracic	C15.4	C78.89	D00.1	D13.0	D37.8	D49.0
upper (third)	C15.3	C78.89	D00.1	D13.0	D37.8	D49.0
ethmoid (sinus)	C31.1	C78.39	D02.3	D14.0	D38.5	D49.1
bone or labyrinth	C41.0	C79.51	—	D16.4	D48.0	D49.2
eustachian tube	C30.1	C78.39	D02.3	D14.0	D38.5	D49.1
exocervix	C53.1	C79.82	D06.1	D26.0	D39.0	D49.5
external						
meatus (ear) — *see also* Neoplasm, skin, ear	C44.20-☑	C79.2	D04.2-☑	D23.2-☑	D48.5	D49.2
os, cervix uteri	C53.1	C79.82	D06.1	D26.0	D39.0	D49.5
extradural	C72.9	C79.49	—	D33.9	D43.9	D49.7
extrahepatic (bile) duct	C24.0	C78.89	D01.5	D13.5	D37.6	D49.0
overlapping lesion with gallbladder	C24.8	—	—	—	—	—
extraocular muscle	C69.6-☑	C79.49	D09.2-☑	D31.6-☑	D48.7	D49.89
extrarectal	C76.3	C79.89	D09.8	D36.7	D48.7	D49.89
extremity	C76.8	C79.89	D04.8	D36.7	D48.7	D49.89
lower	C76.5-☑	C79.89	D04.7-☑	D36.7	D48.7	D49.89
upper	C76.4-☑	C79.89	D04.6-☑	D36.7	D48.7	D49.89
eyeball	C69.9-☑	C79.49	D09.2-☑	D31.9-☑	D48.7	D49.89
eyebrow	C44.309	C79.2	D04.39	D23.39	D48.5	D49.2
basal cell carcinoma	C44.319	—	—	—	—	—
specified type NEC	C44.399	—	—	—	—	—
squamous cell carcinoma	C44.329	—	—	—	—	—
eyelid (lower) (skin) (upper)	C44.10-☑	—	—	—	—	—
basal cell carcinoma	C44.11-☑	—	—	—	—	—
cartilage	C49.0	C79.89	—	D21.0	D48.1	D49.2
specified type NEC	C44.19-☑	—	—	—	—	—
squamous cell carcinoma	C44.12-☑	—	—	—	—	—
eye NEC	C69.9-☑	C79.49	D09.2-☑	D31.9-☑	D48.7	D49.89
overlapping sites	C69.8-☑	—	—	—	—	—
face NEC	C76.0	C79.89	D04.39	D36.7	D48.7	D49.89
fallopian tube (accessory)	C57.0-☑	C79.82	D07.39	D28.2	D39.8	D49.5
falx (cerebella) (cerebri)	C70.0	C79.32	—	D32.0	D42.0	D49.7
fascia — *see also* Neoplasm, connective tissue						
palmar	C49.1-☑	C79.89	—	D21.1-☑	D48.1	D49.2
plantar	C49.2-☑	C79.89	—	D21.2-☑	D48.1	D49.2
fatty tissue — *see* Neoplasm, connective tissue						
fauces, faucial NEC	C10.9	C79.89	D00.08	D10.5	D37.05	D49.0
pillars	C09.1	C79.89	D00.08	D10.5	D37.05	D49.0
tonsil	C09.9	C79.89	D00.08	D10.4	D37.05	D49.0
femur (any part)	C40.2-☑	—	—	D16.2-☑	—	—
fetal membrane	C58	C79.82	D07.0	D26.7	D39.2	D49.5
fibrous tissue — *see* Neoplasm, connective tissue						
fibula (any part)	C40.2-☑	C79.51	—	D16.2-☑	—	—
filum terminale	C72.0	C79.49	—	D33.4	D43.4	D49.7
finger NEC	C76.4-☑	C79.89	D04.6-☑	D36.7	D48.7	D49.89
flank NEC	C76.8	C79.89	D04.5	D36.7	D48.7	D49.89
follicle, nabothian	C53.0	C79.82	D06.0	D26.0	D39.0	D49.5
foot NEC	C76.5-☑	C79.89	D04.7-☑	D36.7	D48.7	D49.89
forearm NEC	C76.4-☑	C79.89	D04.6-☑	D36.7	D48.7	D49.89
forehead (skin)	C44.309	C79.2	D04.39	D23.39	D48.5	D49.2

Neoplasm, neoplastic — continued	Malignant Primary	Malignant Secondary	Ca in situ	Benign	Uncertain	Unspecified Behavior
forehead — *continued*						
basal cell carcinoma	C44.319	—	—	—	—	—
specified type NEC	C44.399					
squamous cell carcinoma	C44.329	—	—	—	—	—
foreskin	C60.0	C79.82	D07.4	D29.0	D40.8	D49.5
fornix						
pharyngeal	C11.3	C79.89	D00.08	D10.6	D37.05	D49.0
vagina	C52	C79.82	D07.2	D28.1	D39.8	D49.5
fossa (of)						
anterior (cranial)	C71.9	C79.31	—	D33.2	D43.2	D49.6
cranial	C71.9	C79.31	—	D33.2	D43.2	D49.6
ischiorectal	C76.3	C79.89	D09.8	D36.7	D48.7	D49.89
middle (cranial)	C71.9	C79.31	—	D33.2	D43.2	D49.6
piriform	C12	C79.89	D00.08	D10.7	D37.05	D49.0
pituitary	C75.1	C79.89	D09.3	D35.2	D44.3	D49.7
posterior (cranial)	C71.9	C79.31	—	D33.2	D43.2	D49.6
pterygoid	C49.0	C79.89	—	D21.0	D48.1	D49.2
pyriform	C12	C79.89	D00.08	D10.7	D37.05	D49.0
Rosenmuller	C11.2	C79.89	D00.08	D10.6	D37.05	D49.0
tonsillar	C09.0	C79.89	D00.08	D10.5	D37.05	D49.0
fourchette	C51.9	C79.82	D07.1	D28.0	D39.8	D49.5
frenulum						
labii — *see* Neoplasm, lip, internal						
linguae	C02.2	C79.89	D00.07	D10.1	D37.02	D49.0
frontal						
bone	C41.0	C79.51	—	D16.4	D48.0	D49.2
lobe, brain	C71.1	C79.31	—	D33.0	D43.0	D49.6
pole	C71.1	C79.31	—	D33.0	D43.0	D49.6
sinus	C31.2	C78.39	D02.3	D14.0	D38.5	D49.1
fundus						
stomach	C16.1	C78.89	D00.2	D13.1	D37.1	D49.0
uterus	C54.3	C79.82	D07.0	D26.1	D39.0	D49.5
gallbladder	C23	C78.89	D01.5	D13.5	D37.6	D49.0
overlapping lesion with extrahepatic bile ducts	C24.8	—	—	—	—	—
gall duct (extrahepatic)	C24.0	C78.89	D01.5	D13.5	D37.6	D49.0
intrahepatic	C22.1	C78.7	D01.5	D13.4	D37.6	D49.0
ganglia — *see also* Neoplasm, nerve, peripheral	C47.9	C79.89	—	D36.10	D48.2	D49.2
basal	C71.0	C79.31	—	D33.0	D43.0	D49.6
cranial nerve	C72.50	C79.49	—	D33.3	D43.3	D49.7
Gartner's duct	C52	C79.82	D07.2	D28.1	D39.8	D49.5
gastric — *see* Neoplasm, stomach						
gastrocolic	C26.9	C78.89	D01.9	D13.9	D37.9	D49.0
gastroesophageal junction	C16.0	C78.89	D00.2	D13.1	D37.1	D49.0
gastrointestinal (tract) NEC	C26.9	C78.89	D01.9	D13.9	D37.9	D49.0
generalized	C80.0	—	—	—	—	—
genital organ or tract						
female NEC	C57.9	C79.82	D07.30	D28.9	D39.9	D49.5
overlapping lesion	C57.8	—	—	—	—	—
specified site NEC	C57.7	C79.82	D07.39	D28.7	D39.8	D49.5
male NEC	C63.9	C79.82	D07.60	D29.9	D40.9	D49.5
overlapping lesion	C63.8	—	—	—	—	—
specified site NEC	C63.7	C79.82	D07.69	D29.8	D40.8	D49.5
genitourinary tract						
female	C57.9	C79.82	D07.30	D28.9	D39.9	D49.5
male	C63.9	C79.82	D07.60	D29.9	D40.9	D49.5
gingiva (alveolar) (marginal)	C03.9	C79.89	D00.03	D10.39	D37.09	D49.0
lower	C03.1	C79.89	D00.03	D10.39	D37.09	D49.0
mandibular	C03.1	C79.89	D00.03	D10.39	D37.09	D49.0
maxillary	C03.0	C79.89	D00.03	D10.39	D37.09	D49.0
upper	C03.0	C79.89	D00.03	D10.39	D37.09	D49.0
gland, glandular (lymphatic) (system) — *see also* Neoplasm, lymph gland						
endocrine NEC	C75.9	C79.89	D09.3	D35.9	D44.9	D49.7

☑ **Additional Character Required — Refer to the Tabular List for Character Selection**   ▽ Subterms under main terms may continue to next column or page

Neoplasm, neoplastic — continued	Malignant Primary	Malignant Secondary	Ca in situ	Benign	Uncertain	Unspecified Behavior
gland, glandular — *see also* Neoplasm, lymph gland — *continued*						
salivary — *see* Neoplasm, salivary gland						
glans penis	C60.1	C79.82	D07.4	D29.0	D40.8	D49.5
globus pallidus	C71.0	C79.31	—	D33.0	D43.0	D49.6
glomus						
coccygeal	C49.5	C79.89	—	D21.5	D48.1	D49.2
jugularis	C75.5	C79.89	—	D35.6	D44.7	D49.7
glosso-epiglottic fold(s)	C10.1	C79.89	D00.08	D10.5	D37.05	D49.0
glossopalatine fold	C09.1	C79.89	D00.08	D10.5	D37.05	D49.0
glossopharyngeal sulcus	C09.0	C79.89	D00.08	D10.5	D37.05	D49.0
glottis	C32.0	C78.39	D02.0	D14.1	D38.0	D49.1
gluteal region	C76.3	C79.89	D04.5	D36.7	D48.7	D49.89
great vessels NEC	C49.3	C79.89	—	D21.3	D48.1	D49.2
groin NEC	C76.3	C79.89	D04.5	D36.7	D48.7	D49.89
gum	C03.9	C79.89	D00.03	D10.39	D37.09	D49.0
lower	C03.1	C79.89	D00.03	D10.39	D37.09	D49.0
upper	C03.0	C79.89	D00.03	D10.39	D37.09	D49.0
hand NEC	C76.4-✓	C79.89	D04.6-✓	D36.7	D48.7	D49.89
head NEC	C76.0	C79.89	D04.4	D36.7	D48.7	D49.89
heart	C38.0	C79.89	—	D15.1	D48.7	D49.89
heel NEC	C76.5-✓	C79.89	D04.7-✓	D36.7	D48.7	D49.89
helix — *see also* Neoplasm, skin, ear	C44.20-✓	C79.2	D04.2-✓	D23.2-✓	D48.5	D49.2
hematopoietic, hemopoietic tissue NEC	C96.9	—	—	—	—	—
specified NEC	C96.Z	—	—	—	—	—
hemisphere, cerebral	C71.0	C79.31	—	D33.0	D43.0	D49.6
hemorrhoidal zone	C21.1	C78.5	D01.3	D12.9	D37.8	D49.0
hepatic — *see also* Index to disease, by histology	C22.9	C78.7	D01.5	D13.4	D37.6	D49.0
duct (bile)	C24.0	C78.89	D01.5	D13.5	D37.6	D49.0
flexure (colon)	C18.3	C78.5	D01.0	D12.3	D37.4	D49.0
primary	C22.8	C78.7	D01.5	D13.4	D37.6	D49.0
hepatobiliary	C24.9	C78.89	D01.5	D13.5	D37.6	D49.0
hepatoblastoma	C22.2	C78.7	D01.5	D13.4	D37.6	D49.0
hepatoma	C22.0	C78.7	D01.5	D13.4	D37.6	D49.0
hilus of lung	C34.0-✓	C78.0-✓	D02.2-✓	D14.3-✓	D38.1	D49.1
hippocampus, brain	C71.2	C79.31	—	D33.0	D43.0	D49.6
hip NEC	C76.5-✓	C79.89	D04.7-✓	D36.7	D48.7	D49.89
humerus (any part)	C40.0-✓	C79.51	—	D16.0-✓	—	—
hymen	C52	C79.82	D07.2	D28.1	D39.8	D49.5
hypopharynx, hypopharyngeal NEC	C13.9	C79.89	D00.08	D10.7	D37.05	D49.0
overlapping lesion	C13.8	—	—	—	—	—
postcricoid region	C13.0	C79.89	D00.08	D10.7	D37.05	D49.0
posterior wall	C13.2	C79.89	D00.08	D10.7	D37.05	D49.0
pyriform fossa (sinus)	C12	C79.89	D00.08	D10.7	D37.05	D49.0
hypophysis	C75.1	C79.89	D09.3	D35.2	D44.3	D49.7
hypothalamus	C71.0	C79.31	—	D33.0	D43.0	D49.6
ileocecum, ileocecal (coil) (junction) (valve)	C18.0	C78.5	D01.0	D12.0	D37.4	D49.0
ileum	C17.2	C78.4	D01.49	D13.39	D37.2	D49.0
ilium	C41.4	C79.51	—	D16.8	D48.0	D49.2
immunoproliferative NEC	C88.9	—	—	—	—	—
infraclavicular (region)	C76.1	C79.89	D04.5	D36.7	D48.7	D49.89
inguinal (region)	C76.3	C79.89	D04.5	D36.7	D48.7	D49.89
insula	C71.0	C79.31	—	D33.0	D43.0	D49.6
insular tissue (pancreas)	C25.4	C78.89	D01.7	D13.7	D37.8	D49.0
brain	C71.0	C79.31	—	D33.0	D43.0	D49.6
interarytenoid fold	C13.1	C78.39	D00.08	D10.7	D37.05	D49.0
hypopharyngeal aspect	C13.1	C79.89	D00.08	D10.7	D37.05	D49.0
laryngeal aspect	C32.1	C78.39	D02.0	D14.1	D38.0	D49.1
marginal zone	C13.1	C79.89	D00.08	D10.7	D37.05	D49.0
interdental papillae	C03.9	C79.89	D00.03	D10.39	D37.09	D49.0

Neoplasm, neoplastic — continued	Malignant Primary	Malignant Secondary	Ca in situ	Benign	Uncertain	Unspecified Behavior
interdental papillae — *continued*						
lower	C03.1	C79.89	D00.03	D10.39	D37.09	D49.0
upper	C03.0	C79.89	D00.03	D10.39	D37.09	D49.0
internal						
capsule	C71.0	C79.31	—	D33.0	D43.0	D49.6
os (cervix)	C53.0	C79.82	D06.0	D26.0	D39.0	D49.5
intervertebral cartilage or disc	C41.2	C79.51	—	D16.6	D48.0	D49.2
intestine, intestinal	C26.0	C78.80	D01.40	D13.9	D37.8	D49.0
large	C18.9	C78.5	D01.0	D12.6	D37.4	D49.0
appendix	C18.1	C78.5	D01.0	D12.1	D37.3	D49.0
caput coli	C18.0	C78.5	D01.0	D12.0	D37.4	D49.0
cecum	C18.0	C78.5	D01.0	D12.0	D37.4	D49.0
colon	C18.9	C78.5	D01.0	D12.6	D37.4	D49.0
and rectum	C19	C78.5	D01.1	D12.7	D37.5	D49.0
ascending	C18.2	C78.5	D01.0	D12.2	D37.4	D49.0
caput	C18.0	C78.5	D01.0	D12.0	D37.4	D49.0
descending	C18.6	C78.5	D01.0	D12.4	D37.4	D49.0
distal	C18.6	C78.5	D01.0	D12.4	D37.4	D49.0
left	C18.6	C78.5	D01.0	D12.4	D37.4	D49.0
overlapping lesion	C18.8	—	—	—	—	—
pelvic	C18.7	C78.5	D01.0	D12.5	D37.4	D49.0
right	C18.2	C78.5	D01.0	D12.2	D37.4	D49.0
sigmoid (flexure)	C18.7	C78.5	D01.0	D12.5	D37.4	D49.0
transverse	C18.4	C78.5	D01.0	D12.3	D37.4	D49.0
hepatic flexure	C18.3	C78.5	D01.0	D12.3	D37.4	D49.0
ileocecum, ileocecal (coil) (valve)	C18.0	C78.5	D01.0	D12.0	D37.4	D49.0
overlapping lesion	C18.8	—	—	—	—	—
sigmoid flexure (lower) (upper)	C18.7	C78.5	D01.0	D12.5	D37.4	D49.0
splenic flexure	C18.5	C78.5	D01.0	D12.3	D37.4	D49.0
small	C17.9	C78.4	D01.40	D13.30	D37.2	D49.0
duodenum	C17.0	C78.4	D01.49	D13.2	D37.2	D49.0
ileum	C17.2	C78.4	D01.49	D13.39	D37.2	D49.0
jejunum	C17.1	C78.4	D01.49	D13.39	D37.2	D49.0
overlapping lesion	C17.8	—	—	—	—	—
tract NEC	C26.0	C78.89	D01.40	D13.9	D37.8	D49.0
intra-abdominal	C76.2	C79.89	D09.8	D36.7	D48.7	D49.89
intracranial NEC	C71.9	C79.31	—	D33.2	D43.2	D49.6
intrahepatic (bile) duct	C22.1	C78.7	D01.5	D13.4	D37.6	D49.0
intraocular	C69.9-✓	C79.49	D09.2-✓	D31.9-✓	D48.7	D49.89
intraorbital	C69.6-✓	C79.49	D09.2-✓	D31.6-✓	D48.7	D49.89
intrasellar	C75.1	C79.89	D09.3	D35.2	D44.3	D49.7
intrathoracic (cavity) (organs)	C76.1	C79.89	D09.8	D15.9	D48.7	D49.89
specified NEC	C76.1	C79.89	D09.8	D15.7	—	—
iris	C69.4-✓	C79.49	D09.2-✓	D31.4-✓	D48.7	D49.89
ischiorectal (fossa)	C76.3	C79.89	D09.8	D36.7	D48.7	D49.89
ischium	C41.4	C79.51	—	D16.8	D48.0	D49.2
island of Reil	C71.0	C79.31	—	D33.0	D43.0	D49.6
islands or islets of Langerhans	C25.4	C78.89	D01.7	D13.7	D37.8	D49.0
isthmus uteri	C54.0	C79.82	D07.0	D26.1	D39.0	D49.5
jaw	C76.0	C79.89	D09.8	D36.7	D48.7	D49.89
bone	C41.1	C79.51	—	D16.5	D48.0	D49.2
lower	C41.1	C79.51	—	D16.5	—	—
upper	C41.0	C79.51	—	D16.4	—	—
carcinoma (any type) (lower) (upper)	C76.0	C79.89		—	—	—
skin — *see also* Neoplasm, skin, face	C44.309	C79.2	D04.39	D23.39	D48.5	D49.2
soft tissues	C03.9	C79.89	D00.03	D10.39	D37.09	D49.0
lower	C03.1	C79.89	D00.03	D10.39	D37.09	D49.0
upper	C03.0	C79.89	D00.03	D10.39	D37.09	D49.0
jejunum	C17.1	C78.4	D01.49	D13.39	D37.2	D49.0
joint NEC — *see also* Neoplasm, bone	C41.9	C79.51	—	D16.9	D48.0	D49.2
acromioclavicular	C40.0-✓	C79.51	—	D16.0-✓	—	—

Neoplasm, neoplastic — continued	Malignant Primary	Malignant Secondary	Ca in situ	Benign	Uncertain	Unspecified Behavior
joint — see also Neoplasm, bone — continued						
bursa or synovial membrane — see Neoplasm, connective tissue						
costovertebral	C41.3	C79.51	—	D16.7	D48.0	D49.2
sternocostal	C41.3	C79.51	—	D16.7	D48.0	D49.2
temporomandibular	C41.1	C79.51	—	D16.5	D48.0	D49.2
junction						
anorectal	C21.8	C78.5	D01.3	D12.9	D37.8	D49.0
cardioesophageal	C16.0	C78.89	D00.2	D13.1	D37.1	D49.0
esophagogastric	C16.0	C78.89	D00.2	D13.1	D37.1	D49.0
gastroesophageal	C16.0	C78.89	D00.2	D13.1	D37.1	D49.0
hard and soft palate	C05.9	C79.89	D00.00	D10.39	D37.09	D49.0
ileocecal	C18.0	C78.5	D01.0	D12.0	D37.4	D49.0
pelvirectal	C19	C78.5	D01.1	D12.7	D37.5	D49.0
pelviureteric	C65.-☑	C79.0-☑	D09.19	D30.1-☑	D41.1-☑	D49.5
rectosigmoid	C19	C78.5	D01.1	D12.7	D37.5	D49.0
squamocolumnar, of cervix	C53.8	C79.82	D06.7	D26.0	D39.0	D49.5
Kaposi's sarcoma — see Kaposi's, sarcoma						
kidney (parenchymal)	C64.-☑	C79.0-☑	D09.19	D30.0-☑	D41.0-☑	D49.5
calyx	C65.-☑	C79.0-☑	D09.19	D30.1-☑	D41.1-☑	D49.5
hilus	C65.-☑	C79.0-☑	D09.19	D30.1-☑	D41.1-☑	D49.5
pelvis	C65.-☑	C79.0-☑	D09.19	D30.1-☑	D41.1-☑	D49.5
knee NEC	C76.5-☑	C79.89	D04.7-☑	D36.7	D48.7	D49.89
labia (skin)	C51.9	C79.82	D07.1	D28.0	D39.8	D49.5
majora	C51.0	C79.82	D07.1	D28.0	D39.8	D49.5
minora	C51.1	C79.82	D07.1	D28.0	D39.8	D49.5
labial — see also Neoplasm, lip	C00.9	C79.89	D00.01	D10.0	D37.01	D49.0
sulcus (lower)	C06.1	C79.89	D00.02	D10.39	D37.09	D49.0
(upper)						
labium (skin)	C51.9	C79.82	D07.1	D28.0	D39.8	D49.5
majus	C51.0	C79.82	D07.1	D28.0	D39.8	D49.5
minus	C51.1	C79.82	D07.1	D28.0	D39.8	D49.5
lacrimal						
canaliculi	C69.5-☑	C79.49	D09.2-☑	D31.5-☑	D48.7	D49.89
duct (nasal)	C69.5-☑	C79.49	D09.2-☑	D31.5-☑	D48.7	D49.89
gland	C69.5-☑	C79.49	D09.2-☑	D31.5-☑	D48.7	D49.89
punctum	C69.5-☑	C79.49	D09.2-☑	D31.5-☑	D48.7	D49.89
sac	C69.5-☑	C79.49	D09.2-☑	D31.5-☑	D48.7	D49.89
Langerhans, islands or islets	C25.4	C78.89	D01.7	D13.7	D37.8	D49.0
laryngopharynx	C13.9	C79.89	D00.08	D10.7	D37.05	D49.0
larynx, laryngeal NEC	C32.9	C78.39	D02.0	D14.1	D38.0	D49.1
aryepiglottic fold	C32.1	C78.39	D02.0	D14.1	D38.0	D49.1
cartilage (arytenoid) (cricoid) (cuneiform) (thyroid)	C32.3	C78.39	D02.0	D14.1	D38.0	D49.1
commissure (anterior) (posterior)	C32.0	C78.39	D02.0	D14.1	D38.0	D49.1
extrinsic NEC	C32.1	C78.39	D02.0	D14.1	D38.0	D49.1
meaning hypopharynx	C13.9	C79.89	D00.08	D10.7	D37.05	D49.0
interarytenoid fold	C32.1	C78.39	D02.0	D14.1	D38.0	D49.1
intrinsic	C32.0	C78.39	D02.0	D14.1	D38.0	D49.1
overlapping lesion	C32.8	—	—	—	—	—
ventricular band	C32.1	C78.39	D02.0	D14.1	D38.0	D49.1
leg NEC	C76.5-☑	C79.89	D04.7-☑	D36.7	D48.7	D49.89
lens, crystalline	C69.4-☑	C79.49	D09.2-☑	D31.4-☑	D48.7	D49.89
lid (lower) (upper)	C44.10-☑	C79.2	D04.1-☑	D23.1-☑	D48.5	D49.2
basal cell carcinoma	C44.11-☑	—	—	—	—	—
specified type NEC	C44.19-☑	—	—	—	—	—
squamous cell carcinoma	C44.12-☑	—	—	—	—	—
ligament — see also Neoplasm, connective tissue						

Neoplasm, neoplastic — continued	Malignant Primary	Malignant Secondary	Ca in situ	Benign	Uncertain	Unspecified Behavior
ligament — see also Neoplasm, connective tissue — continued						
broad	C57.1-☑	C79.82	D07.39	D28.2	D39.8	D49.5
Mackenrodt's	C57.7	C79.82	D07.39	D28.7	D39.8	D49.5
non-uterine — see Neoplasm, connective tissue						
round	C57.2-☑	C79.82	—	D28.2	D39.8	D49.5
sacro-uterine	C57.3	C79.82	—	D28.2	D39.8	D49.5
uterine	C57.3	C79.82	—	D28.2	D39.8	D49.5
utero-ovarian	C57.7	C79.82	D07.39	D28.2	D39.8	D49.5
uterosacral	C57.3	C79.82	—	D28.2	D39.8	D49.5
limb	C76.8	C79.89	D04.8	D36.7	D48.7	D49.89
lower	C76.5-☑	C79.89	D04.7-☑	D36.7	D48.7	D49.89
upper	C76.4-☑	C79.89	D04.6-☑	D36.7	D48.7	D49.89
limbus of cornea	C69.1-☑	C79.49	D09.2-☑	D31.1-☑	D48.7	D49.89
lingual NEC — see also Neoplasm, tongue	C02.9	C79.89	D00.07	D10.1	D37.02	D49.0
lingula, lung	C34.1-☑	C78.0-☑	D02.2-☑	D14.3-☑	D38.1	D49.1
lip	C00.9	C79.89	D00.01	D10.0	D37.01	D49.0
buccal aspect — see Neoplasm, lip, internal						
commissure	C00.6	C79.89	D00.01	D10.0	D37.01	D49.0
external	C00.2	C79.89	D00.01	D10.0	D37.01	D49.0
lower	C00.1	C79.89	D00.01	D10.0	D37.01	D49.0
upper	C00.0	C79.89	D00.01	D10.0	D37.01	D49.0
frenulum — see Neoplasm, lip, internal						
inner aspect — see Neoplasm, lip, internal						
internal	C00.5	C79.89	D00.01	D10.0	D37.01	D49.0
lower	C00.4	C79.89	D00.01	D10.0	D37.01	D49.0
upper	C00.3	C79.89	D00.01	D10.0	D37.01	D49.0
lipstick area	C00.2	C79.89	D00.01	D10.0	D37.01	D49.0
lower	C00.1	C79.89	D00.01	D10.0	D37.01	D49.0
upper	C00.0	C79.89	D00.01	D10.0	D37.01	D49.0
lower	C00.1	C79.89	D00.01	D10.0	D37.01	D49.0
internal	C00.4	C79.89	D00.01	D10.0	D37.01	D49.0
mucosa — see Neoplasm, lip, internal						
oral aspect — see Neoplasm, lip, internal						
overlapping lesion	C00.8	—	—			
with oral cavity or pharynx	C14.8	—	—			
skin (commissure) (lower) (upper)	C44.00	C79.2	D04.0	D23.0	D48.5	D49.2
basal cell carcinoma	C44.01	—	—			
specified type NEC	C44.09	—	—			
squamous cell carcinoma	C44.02	—	—			
upper	C00.0	C79.89	D00.01	D10.0	D37.01	D49.0
internal	C00.3	C79.89	D00.01	D10.0	D37.01	D49.0
vermilion border	C00.2	C79.89	D00.01	D10.0	D37.01	D49.0
lower	C00.1	C79.89	D00.01	D10.0	D37.01	D49.0
upper	C00.0	C79.89	D00.01	D10.0	D37.01	D49.0
lipomatous — see Lipoma, by site						
liver — see also Index to disease, by histology	C22.9	C78.7	D01.5	D13.4	D37.6	D49.0
primary	C22.8	C78.7	D01.5	D13.4	D37.6	D49.0
lumbosacral plexus	C47.5	C79.89	—	D36.16	D48.2	D49.2
lung	C34.9-☑	C78.0-☑	D02.2-☑	D14.3-☑	D38.1	D49.1
azygos lobe	C34.1-☑	C78.0-☑	D02.2-☑	D14.3-☑	D38.1	D49.1
carina	C34.0-☑	C78.0-☑	D02.2-☑	D14.3-☑	D38.1	D49.1
hilus	C34.0-☑	C78.0-☑	D02.2-☑	D14.3-☑	D38.1	D49.1
lingula	C34.1-☑	C78.0-☑	D02.2-☑	D14.3-☑	D38.1	D49.1
lobe NEC	C34.9-☑	C78.0-☑	D02.2-☑	D14.3-☑	D38.1	D49.1
lower lobe	C34.3-☑	C78.0-☑	D02.2-☑	D14.3-☑	D38.1	D49.1

☑ Additional Character Required — Refer to the Tabular List for Character Selection   🔺 Subterms under main terms may continue to next column or page

Neoplasm, neoplastic — continued	Malignant Primary	Malignant Secondary	Ca in situ	Benign	Uncertain	Unspecified Behavior
lung — continued						
main bronchus	C34.0-✓	C78.0-✓	D02.2-✓	D14.3-✓	D38.1	D49.1
mesothelioma — see Mesothelioma						
middle lobe	C34.2	C78.0-✓	D02.21	D14.31	D38.1	D49.1
overlapping lesion	C34.8-✓	—	—	—	—	—
upper lobe	C34.1-✓	C78.0-✓	D02.2-✓	D14.3-✓	D38.1	D49.1
lymph, lymphatic channel						
NEC	C49.9	C79.89	—	D21.9	D48.1	D49.2
gland (secondary)		C77.9	—	D36.0	D48.7	D49.89
abdominal	—	C77.2	—	D36.0	D48.7	D49.89
aortic	—	C77.2	—	D36.0	D48.7	D49.89
arm	—	C77.3	—	D36.0	D48.7	D49.89
auricular (anterior) (posterior)	—	C77.0	—	D36.0	D48.7	D49.89
axilla, axillary	—	C77.3	—	D36.0	D48.7	D49.89
brachial	—	C77.3	—	D36.0	D48.7	D49.89
bronchial	—	C77.1	—	D36.0	D48.7	D49.89
bronchopulmonary	—	C77.1	—	D36.0	D48.7	D49.89
celiac	—	C77.2	—	D36.0	D48.7	D49.89
cervical	—	C77.0	—	D36.0	D48.7	D49.89
cervicofacial	—	C77.0	—	D36.0	D48.7	D49.89
Cloquet	—	C77.4	—	D36.0	D48.7	D49.89
colic	—	C77.2	—	D36.0	D48.7	D49.89
common duct	—	C77.2	—	D36.0	D48.7	D49.89
cubital	—	C77.3	—	D36.0	D48.7	D49.89
diaphragmatic	—	C77.1	—	D36.0	D48.7	D49.89
epigastric, inferior	—	C77.1	—	D36.0	D48.7	D49.89
epitrochlear	—	C77.3	—	D36.0	D48.7	D49.89
esophageal	—	C77.1	—	D36.0	D48.7	D49.89
face	—	C77.0	—	D36.0	D48.7	D49.89
femoral	—	C77.4	—	D36.0	D48.7	D49.89
gastric	—	C77.2	—	D36.0	D48.7	D49.89
groin	—	C77.4	—	D36.0	D48.7	D49.89
head	—	C77.0	—	D36.0	D48.7	D49.89
hepatic	—	C77.2	—	D36.0	D48.7	D49.89
hilar (pulmonary)	—	C77.1	—	D36.0	D48.7	D49.89
splenic	—	C77.2	—	D36.0	D48.7	D49.89
hypogastric	—	C77.5	—	D36.0	D48.7	D49.89
ileocolic	—	C77.2	—	D36.0	D48.7	D49.89
iliac	—	C77.5	—	D36.0	D48.7	D49.89
infraclavicular	—	C77.3	—	D36.0	D48.7	D49.89
inguina, inguinal	—	C77.4	—	D36.0	D48.7	D49.89
innominate	—	C77.1	—	D36.0	D48.7	D49.89
intercostal	—	C77.1	—	D36.0	D48.7	D49.89
intestinal	—	C77.2	—	D36.0	D48.7	D49.89
intrabdominal	—	C77.2	—	D36.0	D48.7	D49.89
intrapelvic	—	C77.5	—	D36.0	D48.7	D49.89
intrathoracic	—	C77.1	—	D36.0	D48.7	D49.89
jugular	—	C77.0	—	D36.0	D48.7	D49.89
leg	—	C77.4	—	D36.0	D48.7	D49.89
limb						
lower	—	C77.4	—	D36.0	D48.7	D49.89
upper	—	C77.3	—	D36.0	D48.7	D49.89
lower limb	—	C77.4	—	D36.0	D48.7	D49.89
lumbar	—	C77.2	—	D36.0	D48.7	D49.89
mandibular	—	C77.0	—	D36.0	D48.7	D49.89
mediastinal	—	C77.1	—	D36.0	D48.7	D49.89
mesenteric (inferior) (superior)	—	C77.2	—	D36.0	D48.7	D49.89
midcolic	—	C77.2	—	D36.0	D48.7	D49.89
multiple sites in categories C77.0-C77.5	—	C77.8	—	D36.0	D48.7	D49.89
neck	—	C77.0	—	D36.0	D48.7	D49.89
obturator	—	C77.5	—	D36.0	D48.7	D49.89
occipital	—	C77.0	—	D36.0	D48.7	D49.89
pancreatic	—	C77.2	—	D36.0	D48.7	D49.89
para-aortic	—	C77.2	—	D36.0	D48.7	D49.89
paracervical	—	C77.5	—	D36.0	D48.7	D49.89
parametrial	—	C77.5	—	D36.0	D48.7	D49.89
parasternal	—	C77.1	—	D36.0	D48.7	D49.89
parotid	—	C77.0	—	D36.0	D48.7	D49.89
pectoral	—	C77.3	—	D36.0	D48.7	D49.89
pelvic	—	C77.5	—	D36.0	D48.7	D49.89
peri-aortic	—	C77.2	—	D36.0	D48.7	D49.89
peripancreatic	—	C77.2	—	D36.0	D48.7	D49.89
popliteal	—	C77.4	—	D36.0	D48.7	D49.89
porta hepatis	—	C77.2	—	D36.0	D48.7	D49.89

Neoplasm, neoplastic — continued	Malignant Primary	Malignant Secondary	Ca in situ	Benign	Uncertain	Unspecified Behavior
lymph, lymphatic channel — continued						
gland — continued						
portal	—	C77.2	—	D36.0	D48.7	D49.89
preauricular	—	C77.0	—	D36.0	D48.7	D49.89
prelaryngeal	—	C77.0	—	D36.0	D48.7	D49.89
presymphysial	—	C77.5	—	D36.0	D48.7	D49.89
pretracheal	—	C77.0	—	D36.0	D48.7	D49.89
primary (any site) NEC	C96.9	—	—	—	—	—
pulmonary (hiler)	—	C77.1	—	D36.0	D48.7	D49.89
pyloric	—	C77.2	—	D36.0	D48.7	D49.89
retroperitoneal	—	C77.2	—	D36.0	D48.7	D49.89
retropharyngeal	—	C77.0	—	D36.0	D48.7	D49.89
Rosenmuller's	—	C77.4	—	D36.0	D48.7	D49.89
sacral	—	C77.5	—	D36.0	D48.7	D49.89
scalene	—	C77.0	—	D36.0	D48.7	D49.89
site NEC	—	C77.9	—	D36.0	D48.7	D49.89
splenic (hilar)	—	C77.2	—	D36.0	D48.7	D49.89
subclavicular	—	C77.3	—	D36.0	D48.7	D49.89
subinguinal	—	C77.4	—	D36.0	D48.7	D49.89
sublingual	—	C77.0	—	D36.0	D48.7	D49.89
submandibular	—	C77.0	—	D36.0	D48.7	D49.89
submaxillary	—	C77.0	—	D36.0	D48.7	D49.89
submental	—	C77.0	—	D36.0	D48.7	D49.89
subscapular	—	C77.3	—	D36.0	D48.7	D49.89
supraclavicular	—	C77.0	—	D36.0	D48.7	D49.89
thoracic	—	C77.1	—	D36.0	D48.7	D49.89
tibial	—	C77.4	—	D36.0	D48.7	D49.89
tracheal	—	C77.1	—	D36.0	D48.7	D49.89
tracheobronchial	—	C77.1	—	D36.0	D48.7	D49.89
upper limb	—	C77.3	—	D36.0	D48.7	D49.89
Virchow's	—	C77.0	—	D36.0	D48.7	D49.89
node — see also Neoplasm, lymph gland						
primary NEC	C96.9	—	—	—	—	—
vessel — see also Neoplasm, connective						
tissue	C49.9	C79.89	—	D21.9	D48.1	D49.2
Mackenrodt's ligament	C57.7	C79.82	D07.39	D28.7	D39.8	D49.5
malar	C41.0	C79.51	—	D16.4	D48.0	D49.2
region — see Neoplasm, cheek						
mammary gland — see Neoplasm, breast						
mandible	C41.1	C79.51	—	D16.5	D48.0	D49.2
alveolar mucosa (carcinoma)	C03.1	C79.89	D00.03	D10.39	D37.09	D49.0
ridge or process	C41.1	C79.51	—	D16.5	D48.0	D49.2
marrow (bone) NEC	C96.9	C79.52	—	—	D47.9	D49.89
mastectomy site (skin) — see also Neoplasm, breast, skin	C44.501	C79.2	—	—	—	—
specified as breast tissue	C50.8-✓	C79.81	—	—	—	—
mastoid (air cells) (antrum) (cavity)	C30.1	C78.39	D02.3	D14.0	D38.5	D49.1
bone or process	C41.0	C79.51	—	D16.4	D48.0	D49.2
maxilla, maxillary (superior)	C41.0	C79.51	—	D16.4	D48.0	D49.2
alveolar mucosa	C03.0	C79.89	D00.03	D10.39	D37.09	D49.0
ridge or process (carcinoma)	C41.0	C79.51	—	D16.4	D48.0	D49.2
antrum	C31.0	C78.39	D02.3	D14.0	D38.5	D49.1
carcinoma	C03.0	C79.51	—	—	—	—
inferior — see Neoplasm, mandible						
sinus	C31.0	C78.39	D02.3	D14.0	D38.5	D49.1
meatus external (ear) — see also Neoplasm, skin, ear	C44.20-✓	C79.2	D04.2-✓	D23.2-✓	D48.5	D49.2
Meckel diverticulum, malignant	C17.3	C78.4	D01.49	D13.39	D37.2	D49.0

Neoplasm, neoplastic — *continued*

	Malignant Primary	Malignant Secondary	Ca in situ	Benign	Uncertain	Unspecified Behavior
mediastinum,						
mediastinal	C38.3	C78.1	—	D15.2	D38.3	D49.89
anterior	C38.1	C78.1	—	D15.2	D38.3	D49.89
posterior	C38.2	C78.1	—	D15.2	D38.3	D49.89
medulla						
adrenal	C74.1-☑	C79.7-☑	D09.3	D35.0-☑	D44.1-☑	D49.7
oblongata	C71.7	C79.31	—	D33.1	D43.1	D49.6
meibomian gland	C44.10-☑	C79.2	D04.1-☑	D23.1-☑	D48.5	D49.2
basal cell carcinoma	C44.11-☑	—	—	—	—	—
specified type NEC	C44.19-☑	—	—	—	—	—
squamous cell carcinoma	C44.12-☑	—	—	—	—	—
melanoma — *see* Melanoma						
meninges	C70.9	C79.49	—	D32.9	D42.9	D49.7
brain	C70.0	C79.32	—	D32.0	D42.0	D49.7
cerebral	C70.0	C79.32	—	D32.0	D42.0	D49.7
crainial	C70.0	C79.32	—	D32.0	D42.0	D49.7
intracranial	C70.0	C79.32	—	D32.0	D42.0	D49.7
spinal (cord)	C70.1	C79.49	—	D32.1	D42.1	D49.7
meniscus, knee joint (lateral) (medial)	C40.2-☑	C79.51	—	D16.2-☑	D48.0	D49.2
Merkel cell — *see* Carcinoma, Merkel cell						
mesentery, mesenteric	C48.1	C78.6	—	D20.1	D48.4	D49.0
mesoappendix	C48.1	C78.6	—	D20.1	D48.4	D49.0
mesocolon	C48.1	C78.6	—	D20.1	D48.4	D49.0
mesopharynx — *see* Neoplasm, oropharynx						
mesosalpinx	C57.1-☑	C79.82	D07.39	D28.2	D39.8	D49.5
mesothelial tissue — *see* Mesothelioma						
mesothelioma — *see* Mesothelioma						
mesovarium	C57.1-☑	C79.82	D07.39	D28.2	D39.8	D49.5
metacarpus (any bone)	C40.1-☑	C79.51	—	D16.1-☑	—	—
metastatic NEC — *see also* Neoplasm, by site, secondary	—	C79.9	—	—	—	—
metatarsus (any bone)	C40.3-☑	C79.51	—	D16.3-☑	—	—
midbrain	C71.7	C79.31	—	D33.1	D43.1	D49.6
milk duct — *see* Neoplasm, breast						
mons						
pubis	C51.9	C79.82	D07.1	D28.0	D39.8	D49.5
veneris	C51.9	C79.82	D07.1	D28.0	D39.8	D49.5
motor tract	C72.9	C79.49	—	D33.9	D43.9	D49.7
brain	C71.9	C79.31	—	D33.2	D43.2	D49.6
cauda equina	C72.1	C79.49	—	D33.4	D43.4	D49.7
spinal	C72.0	C79.49	—	D33.4	D43.4	D49.7
mouth	C06.9	C79.89	D00.00	D10.30	D37.09	D49.0
book-leaf	C06.89	C79.89	—	—	—	—
floor	C04.9	C79.89	D00.06	D10.2	D37.09	D49.0
anterior portion	C04.0	C79.89	D00.06	D10.2	D37.09	D49.0
lateral portion	C04.1	C79.89	D00.06	D10.2	D37.09	D49.0
overlapping lesion	C04.8	—	—	—	—	—
overlapping NEC	C06.80	—	—	—	—	—
roof	C05.9	C79.89	D00.00	D10.39	D37.09	D49.0
specified part NEC	C06.89	C79.89	D00.00	D10.39	D37.09	D49.0
vestibule	C06.1	C79.89	D00.00	D10.39	D37.09	D49.0
mucosa						
alveolar (ridge or process)	C03.9	C79.89	D00.03	D10.39	D37.09	D49.0
lower	C03.1	C79.89	D00.03	D10.39	D37.09	D49.0
upper	C03.0	C79.89	D00.03	D10.39	D37.09	D49.0
buccal	C06.0	C79.89	D00.02	D10.39	D37.09	D49.0
cheek	C06.0	C79.89	D00.02	D10.39	D37.09	D49.0
lip — *see* Neoplasm, lip, internal						
nasal	C30.0	C78.39	D02.3	D14.0	D38.5	D49.1
oral	C06.0	C79.89	D00.02	D10.39	D37.09	D49.0
Mullerian duct						
female	C57.7	C79.82	D07.39	D28.7	D39.8	D49.5
male	C63.7	C79.82	D07.69	D29.8	D40.8	D49.5

Neoplasm, neoplastic — *continued*

	Malignant Primary	Malignant Secondary	Ca in situ	Benign	Uncertain	Unspecified Behavior
muscle — *see also* Neoplasm, connective tissue						
extraocular	C69.6-☑	C79.49	D09.2-☑	D31.6-☑	D48.7	D49.89
myocardium	C38.0	C79.89	—	D15.1	D48.7	D49.89
myometrium	C54.2	C79.82	D07.0	D26.1	D39.0	D49.5
myopericardium	C38.0	C79.89	—	D15.1	D48.7	D49.89
nabothian gland (follicle)	C53.0	C79.82	D06.0	D26.0	D39.0	D49.5
nail — *see also* Neoplasm, skin, limb						
finger — *see also* Neoplasm, skin, limb, upper	C44.60-☑	C79.2	D04.6-☑	D23.6-☑	D48.5	D49.2
toe — *see also* Neoplasm, skin, limb, lower	C44.70-☑	C79.2	D04.7-☑	D23.7-☑	D48.5	D49.2
nares, naris (anterior) (posterior)	C30.0	C78.39	D02.3	D14.0	D38.5	D49.1
nasal — *see* Neoplasm, nose						
nasolabial groove — *see also* Neoplasm, skin, face	C44.309	C79.2	D04.39	D23.39	D48.5	D49.2
nasolacrimal duct	C69.5-☑	C79.49	D09.2-☑	D31.5-☑	D48.7	D49.89
nasopharynx, nasopharyngeal	C11.9	C79.89	D00.08	D10.6	D37.05	D49.0
floor	C11.3	C79.89	D00.08	D10.6	D37.05	D49.0
overlapping lesion	C11.8	—	—	—	—	—
roof	C11.0	C79.89	D00.08	D10.6	D37.05	D49.0
wall	C11.9	C79.89	D00.08	D10.6	D37.05	D49.0
anterior	C11.3	C79.89	D00.08	D10.6	D37.05	D49.0
lateral	C11.2	C79.89	D00.08	D10.6	D37.05	D49.0
posterior	C11.1	C79.89	D00.08	D10.6	D37.05	D49.0
superior	C11.0	C79.89	D00.08	D10.6	D37.05	D49.0
nates — *see also* Neoplasm, skin, trunk	C44.509	C79.2	D04.5	D23.5	D48.5	D49.2
neck NEC	C76.0	C79.89	D09.8	D36.7	D48.7	D49.89
skin	C44.40	—	—	—	—	—
basal cell carcinoma	C44.41	—	—	—	—	—
specified type NEC	C44.49	—	—	—	—	—
squamous cell carcinoma	C44.42	—	—	—	—	—
nerve (ganglion)	C47.9	C79.89	—	D36.10	D48.2	D49.2
abducens	C72.59	C79.49	—	D33.3	D43.3	D49.7
accessory (spinal)	C72.59	C79.49	—	D33.3	D43.3	D49.7
acoustic	C72.4-☑	C79.49	—	D33.3	D43.3	D49.7
auditory	C72.4-☑	C79.49	—	D33.3	D43.3	D49.7
autonomic NEC — *see also* Neoplasm, nerve, peripheral	C47.9	C79.89	—	D36.10	D48.2	D49.2
brachial	C47.1-☑	C79.89	—	D36.12	D48.2	D49.2
cranial	C72.50	C79.49	—	D33.3	D43.3	D49.7
specified NEC	C72.59	C79.49	—	D33.3	D43.3	D49.7
facial	C72.59	C79.49	—	D33.3	D43.3	D49.7
femoral	C47.2-☑	C79.89	—	D36.13	D48.2	D49.2
ganglion NEC — *see also* Neoplasm, nerve, peripheral	C47.9	C79.89	—	D36.10	D48.2	D49.2
glossopharyngeal	C72.59	C79.49	—	D33.3	D43.3	D49.7
hypoglossal	C72.59	C79.49	—	D33.3	D43.3	D49.7
intercostal	C47.3	C79.89	—	D36.14	D48.2	D49.2
lumbar	C47.6	C79.89	—	D36.17	D48.2	D49.2
median	C47.1-☑	C79.89	—	D36.12	D48.2	D49.2
obturator	C47.2-☑	C79.89	—	D36.13	D48.2	D49.2
oculomotor	C72.59	C79.49	—	D33.3	D43.3	D49.7
olfactory	C47.2-☑	C79.49	—	D33.3	D43.3	D49.7
optic	C72.3-☑	C79.49	—	D33.3	D43.3	D49.7
parasympathetic NEC	C47.9	C79.89	—	D36.10	D48.2	D49.2
peripheral NEC	C47.9	C79.89	—	D36.10	D48.2	D49.2
abdomen	C47.4	C79.89	—	D36.15	D48.2	D49.2
abdominal wall	C47.4	C79.89	—	D36.15	D48.2	D49.2
ankle	C47.2-☑	C79.89	—	D36.13	D48.2	D49.2

☑ Additional Character Required — Refer to the Tabular List for Character Selection   ▽ Subterms under main terms may continue to next column or page

Neoplasm, neoplastic — continued
nerve — continued
peripheral — continued

	Malignant Primary	Malignant Secondary	Ca in situ	Benign	Uncertain	Unspecified Behavior
antecubital fossa or space	C47.1-☑	C79.89	—	D36.12	D48.2	D49.2
arm	C47.1-☑	C79.89	—	D36.12	D48.2	D49.2
auricle (ear)	C47.0	C79.89	—	D36.11	D48.2	D49.2
axilla	C47.3	C79.89	—	D36.12	D48.2	D49.2
back	C47.6	C79.89	—	D36.17	D48.2	D49.2
buttock	C47.5	C79.89	—	D36.16	D48.2	D49.2
calf	C47.2-☑	C79.89	—	D36.13	D48.2	D49.2
cervical region	C47.0	C79.89	—	D36.11	D48.2	D49.2
cheek	C47.0	C79.89	—	D36.11	D48.2	D49.2
chest (wall)	C47.3	C79.89	—	D36.14	D48.2	D49.2
chin	C47.0	C79.89	—	D36.11	D48.2	D49.2
ear (external)	C47.0	C79.89	—	D36.11	D48.2	D49.2
elbow	C47.1-☑	C79.89	—	D36.12	D48.2	D49.2
extrarectal	C47.5	C79.89	—	D36.16	D48.2	D49.2
extremity	C47.9	C79.89	—	D36.10	D48.2	D49.2
lower	C47.2-☑	C79.89	—	D36.13	D48.2	D49.2
upper	C47.1-☑	C79.89	—	D36.12	D48.2	D49.2
eyelid	C47.0	C79.89	—	D36.11	D48.2	D49.2
face	C47.0	C79.89	—	D36.11	D48.2	D49.2
finger	C47.1-☑	C79.89	—	D36.12	D48.2	D49.2
flank	C47.6	C79.89	—	D36.17	D48.2	D49.2
foot	C47.2-☑	C79.89	—	D36.13	D48.2	D49.2
forearm	C47.1-☑	C79.89	—	D36.12	D48.2	D49.2
forehead	C47.0	C79.89	—	D36.11	D48.2	D49.2
gluteal region	C47.5	C79.89	—	D36.16	D48.2	D49.2
groin	C47.5	C79.89	—	D36.16	D48.2	D49.2
hand	C47.1-☑	C79.89	—	D36.12	D48.2	D49.2
head	C47.0	C79.89	—	D36.11	D48.2	D49.2
heel	C47.2-☑	C79.89	—	D36.13	D48.2	D49.2
hip	C47.2-☑	C79.89	—	D36.13	D48.2	D49.2
infraclavicular region	C47.3	C79.89	—	D36.14	D48.2	D49.2
inguinal (canal) (region)	C47.5	C79.89	—	D36.16	D48.2	D49.2
intrathoracic	C47.3	C79.89	—	D36.14	D48.2	D49.2
ischiorectal fossa	C47.5	C79.89	—	D36.16	D48.2	D49.2
knee	C47.2-☑	C79.89	—	D36.13	D48.2	D49.2
leg	C47.2-☑	C79.89	—	D36.13	D48.2	D49.2
limb NEC	C47.9	C79.89	—	D36.10	D48.2	D49.2
lower	C47.2-☑	C79.89	—	D36.13	D48.2	D49.2
upper	C47.1-☑	C79.89	—	D36.12	D48.2	D49.2
nates	C47.5	C79.89	—	D36.16	D48.2	D49.2
neck	C47.0	C79.89	—	D36.11	D48.2	D49.2
orbit	C69.6-☑	C79.49	—	D31.6-☑	D48.7	D49.2
pararectal	C47.5	C79.89	—	D36.16	D48.2	D49.2
paraurethral	C47.5	C79.89	—	D36.16	D48.2	D49.2
paravaginal	C47.5	C79.89	—	D36.16	D48.2	D49.2
pelvis (floor)	C47.5	C79.89	—	D36.16	D48.2	D49.2
pelvoabdominal	C47.8	C79.89	—	D36.17	D48.2	D49.2
perineum	C47.5	C79.89	—	D36.16	D48.2	D49.2
perirectal (tissue)	C47.5	C79.89	—	D36.16	D48.2	D49.2
periurethral (tissue)	C47.5	C79.89	—	D36.16	D48.2	D49.2
popliteal fossa or space	C47.2-☑	C79.89	—	D36.13	D48.2	D49.2
presacral	C47.5	C79.89	—	D36.16	D48.2	D49.2
pterygoid fossa	C47.0	C79.89	—	D36.11	D48.2	D49.2
rectovaginal septum or wall	C47.5	C79.89	—	D36.16	D48.2	D49.2
rectovesical	C47.5	C79.89	—	D36.16	D48.2	
sacrococcygeal region	C47.5	C79.89	—	D36.16	D48.2	D49.2
scalp	C47.0	C79.89	—	D36.11	D48.2	D49.2
scapular region	C47.3	C79.89	—	D36.14	D48.2	D49.2
shoulder	C47.1-☑	C79.89	—	D36.12	D48.2	D49.2
submental	C47.0	C79.89	—	D36.11	D48.2	D49.2
supraclavicular region	C47.0	C79.89	—	D36.11	D48.2	D49.2
temple	C47.0	C79.89	—	D36.11	D48.2	D49.2
temporal region	C47.0	C79.89	—	D36.11	D48.2	D49.2
thigh	C47.2-☑	C79.89	—	D36.13	D48.2	D49.2
thoracic (duct) (wall)	C47.3	C79.89	—	D36.14	D48.2	D49.2
thorax	C47.3	C79.89	—	D36.14	D48.2	D49.2
thumb	C47.1-☑	C79.89	—	D36.12	D48.2	D49.2

Neoplasm, neoplastic — continued
nerve — continued
peripheral — continued

	Malignant Primary	Malignant Secondary	Ca in situ	Benign	Uncertain	Unspecified Behavior
toe	C47.2-☑	C79.89	—	D36.13	D48.2	D49.2
trunk	C47.6	C79.89	—	D36.17	D48.2	D49.2
umbilicus	C47.4	C79.89	—	D36.15	D48.2	D49.2
vesicorectal	C47.5	C79.89	—	D36.16	D48.2	D49.2
wrist	C47.1-☑	C79.89	—	D36.12	D48.2	D49.2
radial	C47.1-☑	C79.89	—	D36.12	D48.2	D49.2
sacral	C47.5	C79.89	—	D36.16	D48.2	D49.2
sciatic	C47.2-☑	C79.89	—	D36.13	D48.2	D49.2
spinal NEC	C47.9	C79.89	—	D36.10	D48.2	D49.2
accessory	C72.59	C79.49	—	D33.3	D43.3	D49.7
sympathetic NEC — see also Neoplasm, nerve, peripheral	C47.9	C79.89	—	D36.10	D48.2	D49.2
trigeminal	C72.59	C79.49	—	D33.3	D43.3	D49.7
trochlear	C72.59	C79.49	—	D33.3	D43.3	D49.7
ulnar	C47.1-☑	C79.89	—	D36.12	D48.2	D49.2
vagus	C72.59	C79.49	—	D33.3	D43.3	D49.7
nervous system (central)	C72.9	C79.40	—	D33.9	D43.9	D49.7
autonomic — see Neoplasm, nerve, peripheral						
parasympathetic — see Neoplasm, nerve, peripheral						
specified site NEC	—	C79.49	—	D33.7	D43.8	—
sympathetic — see Neoplasm, nerve, peripheral						
nevus — see Nevus						
nipple	C50.0-☑	C79.81	D05.-☑	D24.-☑	—	—
nose, nasal	C76.0	C79.89	D09.8	D36.7	D48.7	D49.89
ala (external) (nasi) — see also Neoplasm, nose, skin	C44.301	C79.2	D04.39	D23.39	D48.5	D49.2
bone	C41.0	C79.51	—	D16.4	D48.0	D49.2
cartilage	C30.0	C78.39	D02.3	D14.0	D38.5	D49.1
cavity	C30.0	C78.39	D02.3	D14.0	D38.5	D49.1
choana	C11.3	C79.89	D00.08	D10.6	D37.05	D49.0
external (skin) — see also Neoplasm, nose, skin	C44.301	C79.2	D04.39	D23.39	D48.5	D49.2
fossa	C30.0	C78.39	D02.3	D14.0	D38.5	D49.1
internal	C30.0	C78.39	D02.3	D14.0	D38.5	D49.1
mucosa	C30.0	C78.39	D02.3	D14.0	D38.5	D49.1
septum	C30.0	C78.39	D02.3	D14.0	D38.5	D49.1
posterior margin	C11.3	C79.89	D00.08	D10.6	D37.05	D49.0
sinus — see Neoplasm, sinus						
skin	C44.301	C79.2	D04.39	D23.39	D48.5	D49.2
basal cell carcinoma	C44.311	—	—	—	—	—
specified type NEC	C44.391	—	—	—	—	—
squamous cell carcinoma	C44.321	—	—	—	—	—
turbinate (mucosa)	C30.0	C78.39	D02.3	D14.0	D38.5	D49.1
bone	C41.0	C79.51	—	D16.4	D48.0	D49.2
vestibule	C30.0	C78.39	D02.3	D14.0	D38.5	D49.1
nostril	C30.0	C78.39	D02.3	D14.0	D38.5	D49.1
nucleus pulposus	C41.2	C79.51	—	D16.6	D48.0	D49.2
occipital bone	C41.0	C79.51	—	D16.4	D48.0	D49.2
lobe or pole, brain	C71.4	C79.31	—	D33.0	D43.0	D49.6
odontogenic — see Neoplasm, jaw bone						
olfactory nerve or bulb	C72.2-☑	C79.49	—	D33.3	D43.3	D49.7
olive (brain)	C71.7	C79.31	—	D33.1	D43.1	D49.6
omentum	C48.1	C78.6	—	D20.1	D48.4	D49.0
operculum (brain)	C71.0	C79.31	—	D33.0	D43.0	D49.6
optic nerve, chiasm, or tract	C72.3-☑	C79.49	—	D33.3	D43.3	D49.7
oral (cavity)	C06.9	C79.89	D00.00	D10.30	D37.09	D49.0
ill-defined	C14.8	C79.89	D00.00	D10.30	D37.09	D49.0
mucosa	C06.0	C79.89	D00.02	D10.39	D37.09	D49.0

Neoplasm, neoplastic — continued	Malignant Primary	Malignant Secondary	Ca in situ	Benign	Uncertain	Unspecified Behavior
orbit	C69.6-✓	C79.49	D09.2-✓	D31.6-✓	D48.7	D49.89
autonomic nerve	C69.6-✓	C79.49	—	D31.6-✓	D48.7	D49.2
bone	C41.0	C79.51	—	D16.4	D48.0	D49.2
eye	C69.6-✓	C79.49	D09.2-✓	D31.6-✓	D48.7	D49.89
peripheral nerves	C69.6-✓	C79.49	—	D31.6-✓	D48.7	D49.2
soft parts	C69.6-✓	C79.49	D09.2-✓	D31.6-✓	D48.7	D49.89
organ of Zuckerkandl	C75.5	C79.89	—	D35.6	D44.7	D49.7
oropharynx	C10.9	C79.89	D00.08	D10.5	D37.05	D49.0
branchial cleft (vestige)	C10.4	C79.89	D00.08	D10.5	D37.05	D49.0
junctional region	C10.8	C79.89	D00.08	D10.5	D37.05	D49.0
lateral wall	C10.2	C79.89	D00.08	D10.5	D37.05	D49.0
overlapping lesion	C10.8	—	—	—	—	—
pillars or fauces	C09.1	C79.89	D00.08	D10.5	D37.05	D49.0
posterior wall	C10.3	C79.89	D00.08	D10.5	D37.05	D49.0
vallecula	C10.0	C79.89	D00.08	D10.5	D37.05	D49.0
os						
external	C53.1	C79.82	D06.1	D26.0	D39.0	D49.5
internal	C53.0	C79.82	D06.0	D26.0	D39.0	D49.5
ovary	C56.-✓	C79.6-✓	D07.39	D27.-✓	D39.1-✓	D49.5
oviduct	C57.0-✓	C79.82	D07.39	D28.2	D39.8	D49.5
palate	C05.9	C79.89	D00.00	D10.39	D37.09	D49.0
hard	C05.0	C79.89	D00.05	D10.39	D37.09	D49.0
junction of hard and soft palate	C05.9	C79.89	D00.00	D10.39	D37.09	D49.0
overlapping lesions	C05.8	—	—	—	—	—
soft	C05.1	C79.89	D00.04	D10.39	D37.09	D49.0
nasopharyngeal surface	C11.3	C79.89	D00.08	D10.6	D37.05	D49.0
posterior surface	C11.3	C79.89	D00.08	D10.6	D37.05	D49.0
superior surface	C11.3	C79.89	D00.08	D10.6	D37.05	D49.0
palatoglossal arch	C09.1	C79.89	D00.00	D10.5	D37.09	D49.0
palatopharyngeal arch	C09.1	C79.89	D00.00	D10.5	D37.09	D49.0
pallium	C71.0	C79.31	—	D33.0	D43.0	D49.6
palpebra	C44.10-✓	C79.2	D04.1-✓	D23.1-✓	D48.5	D49.2
basal cell carcinoma	C44.11-✓	—	—	—	—	—
specified type NEC	C44.19-✓	—	—	—	—	—
squamous cell carcinoma	C44.12-✓	—	—	—	—	—
pancreas	C25.9	C78.89	D01.7	D13.6	D37.8	D49.0
body	C25.1	C78.89	D01.7	D13.6	D37.8	D49.0
duct (of Santorini) (of Wirsung)	C25.3	C78.89	D01.7	D13.6	D37.8	D49.0
ectopic tissue	C25.7	C78.89	—	D13.6	D37.8	D49.0
head	C25.0	C78.89	D01.7	D13.6	D37.8	D49.0
islet cells	C25.4	C78.89	D01.7	D13.7	D37.8	D49.0
neck	C25.7	C78.89	D01.7	D13.6	D37.8	D49.0
overlapping lesion	C25.8	—	—	—	—	—
tail	C25.2	C78.89	D01.7	D13.6	D37.8	D49.0
para-aortic body	C75.5	C79.89	—	D35.6	D44.7	D49.7
paraganglion NEC	C75.5	C79.89	—	D35.6	D44.7	D49.7
parametrium	C57.3	C79.82	—	D28.2	D39.8	D49.5
paranephric	C48.0	C78.6	—	D20.0	D48.3	D49.0
pararectal	C76.3	C79.89	—	D36.7	D48.7	D49.89
parasagittal (region)	C76.0	C79.89	D09.8	D36.7	D48.7	D49.89
parasellar	C72.9	C79.49	—	D33.9	D43.8	D49.7
parathyroid (gland)	C75.0	C79.89	D09.3	D35.1	D44.2	D49.7
paraurethral	C76.3	C79.89	—	D36.7	D48.7	D49.89
gland	C68.1	C79.19	D09.19	D30.8	D41.8	D49.5
paravaginal	C76.3	C79.89	—	D36.7	D48.7	D49.89
parenchyma, kidney	C64.-✓	C79.0-✓	D09.19	D30.0-✓	D41.0-✓	D49.5
parietal						
bone	C41.0	C79.51	—	D16.4	D48.0	D49.2
lobe, brain	C71.3	C79.31	—	D33.0	D43.0	D49.6
paroophoron	C57.1-✓	C79.82	D07.39	D28.2	D39.8	D49.5
parotid (duct) (gland)	C07	C79.89	D00.00	D11.0	D37.030	D49.0
parovarium	C57.1-✓	C79.82	D07.39	D28.2	D39.8	D49.5
patella	C40.20	C79.51	—			
peduncle, cerebral	C71.7	C79.31	—	D33.1	D43.1	D49.6
pelvirectal junction	C19	C78.5	D01.1	D12.7	D37.5	D49.0
pelvis, pelvic	C76.3	C79.89	D09.8	D36.7	D48.7	D49.89
bone	C41.4	C79.51	—	D16.8	D48.0	D49.2
floor	C76.3	C79.89	D09.8	D36.7	D48.7	D49.89
renal	C65.-✓	C79.0-✓	D09.19	D30.1-✓	D41.1-✓	D49.5
viscera	C76.3	C79.89	D09.8	D36.7	D48.7	D49.89

Neoplasm, neoplastic — continued	Malignant Primary	Malignant Secondary	Ca in situ	Benign	Uncertain	Unspecified Behavior
pelvis, pelvic — continued						
wall	C76.3	C79.89	D09.8	D36.7	D48.7	D49.89
pelvo-abdominal	C76.8	C79.89	D09.8	D36.7	D48.7	D49.89
penis	C60.9	C79.82	D07.4	D29.0	D40.8	D49.5
body	C60.2	C79.82	D07.4	D29.0	D40.8	D49.5
corpus (cavernosum)	C60.2	C79.82	D07.4	D29.0	D40.8	D49.5
glans	C60.1	C79.82	D07.4	D29.0	D40.8	D49.5
overlapping sites	C60.8	—	—	—	—	—
skin NEC	C60.9	C79.82	D07.4	D29.0	D40.8	D49.5
periadrenal (tissue)	C48.0	C78.6	—	D20.0	D48.3	D49.0
perianal (skin) — see also Neoplasm, anus, skin	C44.500	C79.2	D04.5	D23.5	D48.5	D49.2
pericardium	C38.0	C79.89	—	D15.1	D48.7	D49.89
perinephric	C48.0	C78.6	—	D20.0	D48.3	D49.0
perineum	C76.3	C79.89	D09.8	D36.7	D48.7	D49.89
periodontal tissue NEC	C03.9	C79.89	D00.03	D10.39	D37.09	D49.0
periosteum — see Neoplasm, bone						
peripancreatic	C48.0	C78.6	—	D20.0	D48.3	D49.0
peripheral nerve NEC	C47.9	C79.89	—	D36.10	D48.2	D49.2
perirectal (tissue)	C76.3	C79.89	—	D36.7	D48.7	D49.89
perirenal (tissue)	C48.0	C78.6	—	D20.0	D48.3	D49.0
peritoneum, peritoneal (cavity)	C48.2	C78.6	—	D20.1	D48.4	D49.0
benign mesothelial tissue — see Mesothelioma, benign						
overlapping lesion with digestive organs	C48.8	—	—	—	—	—
	C26.9	—		—	—	—
parietal	C48.1	C78.6	—	D20.1	D48.4	D49.0
pelvic	C48.1	C78.6	—	D20.1	D48.4	D49.0
specified part NEC	C48.1	C78.6	—	D20.1	D48.4	D49.0
peritonsillar (tissue)	C76.0	C79.89	D09.8	D36.7	D48.7	D49.89
periurethral tissue	C76.3	C79.89	—	D36.7	D48.7	D49.89
phalanges						
foot	C40.3-✓	C79.51	—	D16.3-✓	—	—
hand	C40.1-✓	C79.51	—	D16.1-✓	—	—
pharynx, pharyngeal	C14.0	C79.89	D00.08	D10.9	D37.05	D49.0
bursa	C11.1	C79.89	D00.08	D10.6	D37.05	D49.0
fornix	C11.3	C79.89	D00.08	D10.6	D37.05	D49.0
recess	C11.2	C79.89	D00.08	D10.6	D37.05	D49.0
region	C14.0	C79.89	D00.08	D10.9	D37.05	D49.0
tonsil	C11.1	C79.89	D00.08	D10.6	D37.05	D49.0
wall (lateral) (posterior)	C14.0	C79.89	D00.08	D10.9	D37.05	D49.0
pia mater	C70.9	C79.40	—	D32.9	D42.9	D49.7
cerebral	C70.0	C79.32	—	D32.0	D42.0	D49.7
cranial	C70.0	C79.32	—	D32.0	D42.0	D49.7
spinal	C70.1	C79.49	—	D32.1	D42.1	D49.7
pillars of fauces	C09.1	C79.89	D00.08	D10.5	D37.05	D49.0
pineal (body) (gland)	C75.3	C79.89	D09.3	D35.4	D44.5	D49.7
pinna (ear) NEC — see also Neoplasm, skin, ear	C44.20-✓	C79.2	D04.2-✓	D23.2-✓	D48.5	D49.2
piriform fossa or sinus	C12	C79.89	D00.08	D10.7	D37.05	D49.0
pituitary (body) (fossa) (gland) (lobe)	C75.1	C79.89	D09.3	D35.2	D44.3	D49.7
placenta	C58	C79.82	D07.0	D26.7	D39.2	D49.5
pleura, pleural (cavity)	C38.4	C78.2	—	D19.0	D38.2	D49.1
overlapping lesion with heart or mediastinum	C38.8	—	—	—	—	—
parietal	C38.4	C78.2	—	D19.0	D38.2	D49.1
visceral	C38.4	C78.2	—	D19.0	D38.2	D49.1
plexus						
brachial	C47.1-✓	C79.89	—	D36.12	D48.2	D49.2
cervical	C47.0	C79.89	—	D36.11	D48.2	D49.2
choroid	C71.5	C79.31	—	D33.0	D43.0	D49.6
lumbosacral	C47.5	C79.89	—	D36.16	D48.2	D49.2
sacral	C47.5	C79.89	—	D36.16	D48.2	D49.2
pluriendocrine	C75.8	C79.89	D09.3	D35.7	D44.9	D49.7

✓ Additional Character Required — Refer to the Tabular List for Character Selection   Ⓦ Subterms under main terms may continue to next column or page

Neoplasm, neoplastic — continued

	Malignant Primary	Malignant Secondary	Ca in situ	Benign	Uncertain	Unspecified Behavior
pole						
frontal	C71.1	C79.31	—	D33.0	D43.0	D49.6
occipital	C71.4	C79.31	—	D33.0	D43.0	D49.6
pons (varolii)	C71.7	C79.31	—	D33.1	D43.1	D49.6
popliteal fossa or space	C76.5-☑	C79.89	D04.7-☑	D36.7	D48.7	D49.89
postcricoid (region)	C13.0	C79.89	D00.08	D10.7	D37.05	D49.0
posterior fossa (cranial)	C71.9	C79.31	—	D33.2	D43.2	D49.6
postnasal space	C11.9	C79.89	D00.08	D10.6	D37.05	D49.0
prepuce	C60.0	C79.82	D07.4	D29.0	D40.8	D49.5
prepylorus	C16.4	C78.89	D00.2	D13.1	D37.1	D49.0
presacral (region)	C76.3	C79.89	—	D36.7	D48.7	D49.89
prostate (gland)	C61	C79.82	D07.5	D29.1	D40.0	D49.5
utricle	C68.0	C79.19	D09.19	D30.4	D41.3	D49.5
pterygoid fossa	C49.0	C79.89	—	D21.0	D48.1	D49.2
pubic bone	C41.4	C79.51	—	D16.8	D48.0	D49.2
pudenda, pudendum (femaie)	C51.9	C79.82	D07.1	D28.0	D39.8	D49.5
pulmonary — see also Neoplasm, lung	C34.9-☑	C78.0-☑	D02.2-☑	D14.3-☑	D38.1	D49.1
putamen	C71.0	C79.31	—	D33.0	D43.0	D49.6
pyloric						
antrum	C16.3	C78.89	D00.2	D13.1	D37.1	D49.0
canal	C16.4	C78.89	D00.2	D13.1	D37.1	D49.0
pylorus	C16.4	C78.89	D00.2	D13.1	D37.1	D49.0
pyramid (brain)	C71.7	C79.31	—	D33.1	D43.1	D49.6
pyriform fossa or sinus	C12	C79.89	D00.08	D10.7	D37.05	D49.0
radius (any part)	C40.0-☑	C79.51	—	D16.0-☑	—	—
Rathke's pouch	C75.1	C79.89	D09.3	D35.2	D44.3	D49.7
rectosigmoid (junction)	C19	C78.5	D01.1	D12.7	D37.5	D49.0
overlapping lesion with anus or rectum	C21.8	—	—	—	—	—
rectouterine pouch	C48.1	C78.6	—	D20.1	D48.4	D49.0
rectovaginal septum or wall	C76.3	C79.89	D09.8	D36.7	D48.7	D49.89
rectovesical septum	C76.3	C79.89	D09.8	D36.7	D48.7	D49.89
rectum (ampulla)	C20	C78.5	D01.2	D12.8	D37.5	D49.0
and colon	C19	C78.5	D01.1	D12.7	D37.5	D49.0
overlapping lesion with anus or rectosigmoid junction	C21.8	—	—	—	—	—
renal	C64.-☑	C79.0-☑	D09.19	D30.0-☑	D41.0-☑	D49.5
calyx	C65.-☑	C79.0-☑	D09.19	D30.1-☑	D41.1-☑	D49.5
hilus	C65.-☑	C79.0-☑	D09.19	D30.1-☑	D41.1-☑	D49.5
parenchyma	C64.-☑	C79.0-☑	D09.19	D30.0-☑	D41.0-☑	D49.5
pelvis	C65.-☑	C79.0-☑	D09.19	D30.1-☑	D41.1-☑	D49.5
respiratory						
organs or system NEC	C39.9	C78.30	D02.4	D14.4	D38.6	D49.1
tract NEC	C39.9	C78.30	D02.4	D14.4	D38.5	D49.1
upper	C39.0	C78.30	D02.4	D14.4	D38.5	D49.1
retina	C69.2-☑	C79.49	D09.2-☑	D31.2-☑	D48.7	D49.81
retrobulbar	C69.6-☑	C79.49	—	D31.6-☑	D48.7	D49.89
retrocecal	C48.0	C78.6	—	D20.0	D48.3	D49.0
retromolar (area) (triangle) (trigone)	C06.2	C79.89	D00.00	D10.39	D37.09	D49.0
retro-orbital	C76.0	C79.89	D09.8	D36.7	D48.7	D49.89
retroperitoneal (space) (tissue)	C48.0	C78.6	—	D20.0	D48.3	D49.0
retroperitoneum	C48.0	C78.6	—	D20.0	D48.3	D49.0
retropharyngeal	C14.0	C79.89	D00.08	D10.9	D37.05	D49.0
retrovesical (septum)	C76.3	C79.89	D09.8	D36.7	D48.7	D49.89
rhinencephalon	C71.0	C79.31	—	D33.0	D43.0	D49.6
rib	C41.3	C79.51	—	D16.7	D48.0	D49.2
Rosenmuller's fossa	C11.2	C79.89	D00.08	D10.6	D37.05	D49.0
round ligament	C57.2☑	C79.82	—	D28.2	D39.8	D49.5
sacrococcyx, sacrococcygeal region	C41.4	C79.51	—	D16.8	D48.0	D49.2
	C76.3	C79.89	D09.8	D36.7	D48.7	D49.89
sacrouterine ligament	C57.3	C79.82	—	D28.2	D39.8	D49.5
sacrum, sacral (vertebra)	C41.4	C79.51	—	D16.8	D48.0	D49.2

Neoplasm, neoplastic — continued

	Malignant Primary	Malignant Secondary	Ca in situ	Benign	Uncertain	Unspecified Behavior
salivary gland or duct (major)	C08.9	C79.89	D00.00	D11.9	D37.039	D49.0
minor NEC	C06.9	C79.89	D00.00	D10.39	D37.04	D49.0
overlapping lesion	C08.9	—	—	—	—	—
parotid	C07	C79.89	D00.00	D11.0	D37.030	D49.0
pluriglandular	C08.9	C79.89	D00.00	D11.9	D37.039	D49.0
sublingual	C08.1	C79.89	D00.00	D11.7	D37.031	D49.0
submandibular	C08.0	C79.89	D00.00	D11.7	D37.032	D49.0
submaxillary	C08.0	C79.89	D00.00	D11.7	D37.032	D49.0
salpinx (uterine)	C57.0-☑	C79.82	D07.39	D28.2	D39.8	D49.5
Santorini's duct	C25.3	C78.89	D01.7	D13.6	D37.8	D49.0
scalp	C44.40	C79.2	D04.4	D23.4	D48.5	D49.2
basal cell carcinoma	C44.41	—	—	—	—	—
specified type NEC	C44.49	—	—	—	—	—
squamous cell carcinoma	C44.42	—	—	—	—	—
scapula (any part)	C40.0-☑	C79.51	—	D16.0-☑	—	—
scapular region	C76.1	C79.89	D09.8	D36.7	D48.7	D49.89
scar NEC — see also Neoplasm, skin, by site	C44.90	C79.2	D04.9	D23.9	D48.5	D49.2
sciatic nerve	C47.2-☑	C79.89	—	D36.13	D48.2	D49.2
sclera	C69.4-☑	C79.49	D09.2-☑	D31.4-☑	D48.7	D49.89
scrotum (skin)	C63.2	C79.82	D07.61	D29.4	D40.8	D49.5
sebaceous gland — see Neoplasm, skin						
sella turcica	C75.1	C79.89	D09.3	D35.2	D44.3	D49.7
bone	C41.0	C79.51	—	D16.4	D48.0	D49.2
semilunar cartilage (knee)	C40.2-☑	C79.51	—	D16.2-☑	D48.0	D49.2
seminal vesicle	C63.7	C79.82	D07.69	D29.8	D40.8	D49.5
septum						
nasal	C30.0	C78.39	D02.3	D14.0	D38.5	D49.1
posterior margin	C11.3	C79.89	D00.08	D10.6	D37.05	D49.0
rectovaginal	C76.3	C79.89	D09.8	D36.7	D48.7	D49.89
rectovesical	C76.3	C79.89	D09.8	D36.7	D48.7	D49.89
urethrovaginal	C57.9	C79.82	D07.30	D28.9	D39.9	D49.5
vesicovaginal	C57.9	C79.82	D07.30	D28.9	D39.9	D49.5
shoulder NEC	C76.4-☑	C79.89	D04.6-☑	D36.7	D48.7	D49.89
sigmoid flexure (lower) (upper)	C18.7	C78.5	D01.0	D12.5	D37.4	D49.0
sinus (accessory)	C31.9	C78.39	D02.3	D14.0	D38.5	D49.1
bone (any)	C41.0	C79.51	—	D16.4	D48.0	D49.2
ethmoidal	C31.1	C78.39	D02.3	D14.0	D38.5	D49.1
frontal	C31.2	C78.39	D02.3	D14.0	D38.5	D49.1
maxillary	C31.0	C78.39	D02.3	D14.0	D38.5	D49.1
nasal, paranasal NEC	C31.9	C78.39	D02.3	D14.0	D38.5	D49.1
overlapping lesion	C31.8	—	—	—	—	—
pyriform	C12	C79.89	D00.08	D10.7	D37.05	D49.0
sphenoid	C31.3	C78.39	D02.3	D14.0	D38.5	D49.1
skeleton, skeletal NEC	C41.9	C79.51	—	D16.9	D48.0	D49.2
Skene's gland	C68.1	C79.19	D09.19	D30.8	D41.8	D49.5
skin NOS	C44.90	C79.2	D04.9	D23.9	D48.5	D49.2
abdominal wall	C44.509	C79.2	D04.5	D23.5	D48.5	D49.2
basal cell carcinoma	C44.519	—	—	—	—	—
specified type NEC	C44.599	—	—	—	—	—
squamous cell carcinoma	C44.529	—	—	—	—	—
ala nasi — see also Neoplasm, nose, skin	C44.301	C79.2	D04.39	D23.39	D48.5	D49.2
ankle — see also Neoplasm, skin, limb, lower	C44.70-☑	C79.2	D04.7-☑	D23.7-☑	D48.5	D49.2
antecubital space — see also Neoplasm, skin, limb, upper	C44.60-☑	C79.2	D04.6-☑	D23.6-☑	D48.5	D49.2
anus	C44.500	C79.2	D04.5	D23.5	D48.5	D49.2
basal cell carcinoma	C44.510	—	—	—	—	—
specified type NEC	C44.590	—	—	—	—	—
squamous cell carcinoma	C44.520	—	—	—	—	—

Neoplasm, neoplastic — continued
skin — continued

	Malignant Primary	Malignant Secondary	Ca in situ	Benign	Uncertain	Unspecified Behavior
arm — see also Neoplasm, skin, limb, upper	C44.60-✓	C79.2	D04.6-✓	D23.6-✓	D48.5	D49.2
auditory canal (external) — see also Neoplasm, skin, ear	C44.20-✓	C79.2	D04.2-✓	D23.2-✓	D48.5	D49.2
auricle (ear) — see also Neoplasm, skin, ear	C44.20-✓	C79.2	D04.2-✓	D23.2-✓	D48.5	D49.2
auricular canal (external) — see also Neoplasm, skin, ear	C44.20-✓	C79.2	D04.2-✓	D23.2-✓	D48.5	D49.2
axilla, axillary fold — see also Neoplasm, skin, trunk	C44.509	C79.2	D04.5	D23.5	D48.5	D49.2
back — see also Neoplasm, skin, trunk	C44.509	C79.2	D04.5	D23.5	D48.5	D49.2
basal cell carcinoma	C44.91	—	—	—	—	—
breast	C44.501	C79.2	D04.5	D23.5	D48.5	D49.2
basal cell carcinoma	C44.511	—	—	—	—	—
specified type NEC	C44.591	—	—	—	—	—
squamous cell carcinoma	C44.521	—	—	—	—	—
brow — see also Neoplasm, skin, face	C44.309	C79.2	D04.39	D23.39	D48.5	D49.2
buttock — see also Neoplasm, skin, trunk	C44.509	C79.2	D04.5	D23.5	D48.5	D49.2
calf — see also Neoplasm, skin, limb, lower	C44.70-✓	C79.2	D04.7-✓	D23.7-✓	D48.5	D49.2
canthus (eye) (inner) (outer)	C44.10-✓	C79.2	D04.1-✓	D23.1-✓	D48.5	D49.2
basal cell carcinoma	C44.11-✓	—	—	—	—	—
specified type NEC	C44.19-✓	—	—	—	—	—
squamous cell carcinoma	C44.12-✓	—	—	—	—	—
cervical region — see also Neoplasm, skin, neck	C44.40	C79.2	D04.4	D23.4	D48.5	D49.2
cheek (external) — see also Neoplasm, skin, face	C44.309	C79.2	D04.39	D23.39	D48.5	D49.2
chest (wall) — see also Neoplasm, skin, trunk	C44.509	C79.2	D04.5	D23.5	D48.5	D49.2
chin — see also Neoplasm, skin, face	C44.309	C79.2	D04.39	D23.39	D48.5	D49.2
clavicular area — see also Neoplasm, skin, trunk	C44.509	C79.2	D04.5	D23.5	D48.5	D49.2
clitoris	C51.2	C79.82	D07.1	D28.0	D39.8	D49.5
columnella — see also Neoplasm, skin, face	C44.309	C79.2	D04.39	D23.39	D48.5	D49.2
concha — see also Neoplasm, skin, ear	C44.20-✓	C79.2	D04.2-✓	D23.2-✓	D48.5	D49.2
ear (external)	C44.20-✓	C79.2	D04.2-✓	D23.2-✓	D48.5	D49.2
basal cell carcinoma	C44.21-✓	—	—	—	—	—
specified type NEC	C44.29-✓	—	—	—	—	—
squamous cell carcinoma	C44.22-✓	—	—	—	—	—
elbow — see also Neoplasm, skin, limb, upper	C44.60-✓	C79.2	D04.6-✓	D23.6-✓	D48.5	D49.2

Neoplasm, neoplastic — continued
skin — continued

	Malignant Primary	Malignant Secondary	Ca in situ	Benign	Uncertain	Unspecified Behavior
eyebrow — see also Neoplasm, skin, face	C44.309	C79.2	D04.39	D23.39	D48.5	D49.2
eyelid	C44.10-✓	C79.2	D04.1-✓	D23.1-✓	D48.5	D49.2
basal cell carcinoma	C44.11-✓	—	—	—	—	—
specified type NEC	C44.19-✓	—	—	—	—	—
squamous cell carcinoma	C44.12-✓	—	—	—	—	—
face NOS	C44.300	C79.2	D04.30	D23.30	D48.5	D49.2
basal cell carcinoma	C44.310	—	—	—	—	—
specified type NEC	C44.390	—	—	—	—	—
squamous cell carcinoma	C44.320	—	—	—	—	—
female genital organs (external)	C51.9	C79.82	D07.1	D28.0	D39.8	D49.5
clitoris	C51.2	C79.82	D07.1	D28.0	D39.8	D49.5
labium NEC	C51.9	C79.82	D07.1	D28.0	D39.8	D49.5
majus	C51.0	C79.82	D07.1	D28.0	D39.8	D49.5
minus	C51.1	C79.82	D07.1	D28.0	D39.8	D49.5
pudendum	C51.9	C79.82	D07.1	D28.0	D39.8	D49.5
vulva	C51.9	C79.82	D07.1	D28.0	D39.8	D49.5
finger — see also Neoplasm, skin, limb, upper	C44.60-✓	C79.2	D04.6-✓	D23.6-✓	D48.5	D49.2
flank — see also Neoplasm, skin, trunk	C44.509	C79.2	D04.5	D23.5	D48.5	D49.2
foot — see also Neoplasm, skin, limb, lower	C44.70-✓	C79.2	D04.7-✓	D23.7-✓	D48.5	D49.2
forearm — see also Neoplasm, skin, limb, upper	C44.60-✓	C79.2	D04.6-✓	D23.6-✓	D48.5	D49.2
forehead — see also Neoplasm, skin, face	C44.309	C79.2	D04.39	D23.39	D48.5	D49.2
glabella — see also Neoplasm, skin, face	C44.309	C79.2	D04.39	D23.39	D48.5	D49.2
gluteal region — see also Neoplasm, skin, trunk	C44.509	C79.2	D04.5	D23.5	D48.5	D49.2
groin — see also Neoplasm, skin, trunk	C44.509	C79.2	D04.5	D23.5	D48.5	D49.2
hand — see also Neoplasm, skin, limb, upper	C44.60-✓	C79.2	D04.6-✓	D23.6-✓	D48.5	D49.2
head NEC — see also Neoplasm, skin, scalp	C44.40	C79.2	D04.4	D23.4	D48.5	D49.2
heel — see also Neoplasm, skin, limb, lower	C44.70-✓	C79.2	D04.7-✓	D23.7-✓	D48.5	D49.2
helix — see also Neoplasm, skin, ear	C44.20-✓	C79.2	D04.2-✓	D23.2-✓	D48.5	D49.2
hip — see also Neoplasm, skin, limb, lower	C44.70-✓	C79.2	D04.7-✓	D23.7-✓	D48.5	D49.2
infraclavicular region — see also Neoplasm, skin, trunk	C44.509	C79.2	D04.5	D23.5	D48.5	D49.2
inguinal region — see also Neoplasm, skin, trunk	C44.509	C79.2	D04.5	D23.5	D48.5	D49.2
jaw — see also Neoplasm, skin, face	C44.309	C79.2	D04.39	D23.39	D48.5	D49.2
Kaposi's sarcoma — see Kaposi's, sarcoma, skin						
knee — see also Neoplasm, skin, limb, lower	C44.70-✓	C79.2	D04.7-✓	D23.7-✓	D48.5	D49.2

✓ Additional Character Required — Refer to the Tabular List for Character Selection   ▽ Subterms under main terms may continue to next column or page

Neoplasm, neoplastic — continued	Malignant Primary	Malignant Secondary	Ca in situ	Benign	Uncertain	Unspecified Behavior
skin — continued						
labia						
majora	C51.0	C79.82	D07.1	D28.0	D39.8	D49.5
minora	C51.1	C79.82	D07.1	D28.0	D39.8	D49.5
leg — see also Neoplasm, skin, limb, lower	C44.70-☑	C79.2	D04.7-☑	D23.7-☑	D48.5	D49.2
lid (lower) (upper)	C44.10-☑	C79.2	D04.1-☑	D23.1-☑	D48.5	D49.2
basal cell carcinoma	C44.11-☑	—	—	—	—	—
specified type NEC	C44.19-☑	—	—	—	—	—
squamous cell carcinoma	C44.12-☑	—	—	—	—	—
limb NEC	C44.90	C79.2	D04.9	D23.9	D48.5	D49.2
basal cell carcinoma	C44.91	—	—	—	—	—
lower	C44.70-☑	C79.2	D04.7-☑	D23.7-☑	D48.5	D49.2
basal cell carcinoma	C44.71-☑	—	—	—	—	—
specified type NEC	C44.79-☑	—	—	—	—	—
squamous cell carcinoma	C44.72-☑	—	—	—	—	—
upper	C44.60-☑	C79.2	D04.6-☑	D23.6-☑	D48.5	D49.2
basal cell carcinoma	C44.61-☑	—	—	—	—	—
specified type NEC	C44.69-☑	—	—	—	—	—
squamous cell carcinoma	C44.62-☑	—	—	—	—	—
lip (lower) (upper)	C44.00	C79.2	D04.0	D23.0	D48.5	D49.2
basal cell carcinoma	C44.01	—	—	—	—	—
specified type NEC	C44.09	—	—	—	—	—
squamous cell carcinoma	C44.02	—	—	—	—	—
male genital organs	C63.9	C79.82	D07.60	D29.9	D40.8	D49.5
penis	C60.9	C79.82	D07.4	D29.0	D40.8	D49.5
prepuce	C60.0	C79.82	D07.4	D29.0	D40.8	D49.5
scrotum	C63.2	C79.82	D07.61	D29.4	D40.8	D49.5
mastectomy site (skin) — see also Neoplasm, skin,						
breast	C44.501	C79.2	—	—	—	—
specified as breast tissue	C50.8-☑	C79.81	—	—	—	—
meatus, acoustic (external) — see also Neoplasm, skin,						
ear	C44.20-☑	C79.2	D04.2-☑	D23.2-☑	D48.5	D49.2
melanotic — see Melanoma						
Merkel cell — see Carcinoma, Merkel cell						
nates — see also Neoplasm, skin,						
trunk	C44.509	C79.2	D04.5	D23.5	D48.5	D49.2
neck	C44.40	C79.2	D04.4	D23.4	D48.5	D49.2
basal cell carcinoma	C44.41	—	—	—	—	—
specified type NEC	C44.49	—	—	—	—	—
squamous cell carcinoma	C44.42	—	—	—	—	—
nevus — see Nevus, skin						
nose (external) — see also Neoplasm, nose, skin	C44.301	C79.2	D04.39	D23.39	D48.5	D49.2
overlapping lesion	C44.80	—	—	—	—	—
basal cell carcinoma	C44.81	—	—	—	—	—
specified type NEC	C44.89	—	—	—	—	—
squamous cell carcinoma	C44.82	—	—	—	—	—
palm — see also Neoplasm, skin, limb, upper	C44.60-☑	C79.2	D04.6-☑	D23.6-☑	D48.5	D49.2
palpebra	C44.10-☑	C79.2	D04.1-☑	D23.1-☑	D48.5	D49.2
basal cell carcinoma	C44.11-☑	—	—	—	—	—
specified type NEC	C44.19-☑	—	—	—	—	—
squamous cell carcinoma	C44.12-☑	—	—	—	—	—
penis NEC	C60.9	C79.82	D07.4	D29.0	D40.8	D49.5
perianal — see also Neoplasm, skin, anus	C44.500	C79.82	D04.5	D23.5	D48.5	D49.2
perineum — see also Neoplasm, skin, anus	C44.500	C79.2	D04.5	D23.5	D48.5	D49.2
pinna — see also Neoplasm, skin, ear	C44.20-☑	C79.2	D04.2-☑	D23.2-☑	D48.5	D49.2
plantar — see also Neoplasm, skin, limb, lower	C44.70-☑	C79.2	D04.7-☑	D23.7-☑	D48.5	D49.2
popliteal fossa or space — see also Neoplasm, skin, limb, lower	C44.70-☑	C79.2	D04.7-☑	D23.7-☑	D48.5	D49.2
prepuce	C60.0	C79.82	D07.4	D29.0	D40.8	D49.5
pubes — see also Neoplasm, skin, trunk	C44.509	C79.2	D04.5	D23.5	D48.5	D49.2
sacrococcygeal region — see also Neoplasm, skin, trunk	C44.509	C79.2	D04.5	D23.5	D48.5	D49.2
scalp	C44.40	C79.2	D04.4	D23.4	D48.5	D49.2
basal cell carcinoma	C44.41	—	—	—	—	—
specified type NEC	C44.49	—	—	—	—	—
squamous cell carcinoma	C44.42	—	—	—	—	—
scapular region — see also Neoplasm, skin, trunk	C44.509	C79.2	D04.5	D23.5	D48.5	D49.2
scrotum	C63.2	C79.82	D07.61	D29.4	D40.8	D49.5
shoulder — see also Neoplasm, skin, limb, upper	C44.60-☑	C79.2	D04.6-☑	D23.6-☑	D48.5	D49.2
sole (foot) — see also Neoplasm, skin, limb, lower	C44.70-☑	C79.2	D04.7-☑	D23.7-☑	D48.5	D49.2
specified sites NEC	C44.80	C79.2	D04.8	D23.9	D48.5	D49.2
basal cell carcinoma	C44.81	—	—	—	—	—
specified type NEC	C44.89	—	—	—	—	—
squamous cell carcinoma	C44.82	—	—	—	—	—
specified type NEC	C44.99	—	—	—	—	—
squamous cell carcinoma	C44.92	—	—	—	—	—
submammary fold — see also Neoplasm, skin, trunk	C44.509	C79.2	D04.5	D23.5	D48.5	D49.2
supraclavicular region — see also Neoplasm, skin, neck	C44.40	C79.2	D04.4	D23.4	D48.5	D49.2
temple — see also Neoplasm, skin, face	C44.309	C79.2	D04.39	D23.39	D48.5	D49.2
thigh — see also Neoplasm, skin, limb, lower	C44.70-☑	C79.2	D04.7-☑	D23.7-☑	D48.5	D49.2
thoracic wall — see also Neoplasm, skin, trunk	C44.509	C79.2	D04.5	D23.5	D48.5	D49.2

Neoplasm, neoplastic — continued	Malignant Primary	Malignant Secondary	Ca in situ	Benign	Uncertain	Unspecified Behavior
skin — continued						
thumb — see also Neoplasm, skin, limb, upper	C44.60-☑	C79.2	D04.6-☑	D23.6-☑	D48.5	D49.2
toe — see also Neoplasm, skin, limb, lower	C44.70-☑	C79.2	D04.7-☑	D23.7-☑	D48.5	D49.2
tragus — see also Neoplasm, skin, ear	C44.20-☑	C79.2	D04.2-☑	D23.2-☑	D48.5	D49.2
trunk	C44.509	C79.2	D04.5	D23.5	D48.5	D49.2
basal cell carcinoma	C44.519	—	—	—	—	—
specified type NEC	C44.599	—	—	—	—	—
squamous cell carcinoma	C44.529	—	—	—	—	—
umbilicus — see also Neoplasm, skin, trunk	C44.509	C79.2	D04.5	D23.5	D48.5	D49.2
vulva	C51.9	C79.82	D07.1	D28.0	D39.8	D49.5
overlapping lesion	C51.8	—	—	—	—	—
wrist — see also Neoplasm, skin, limb, upper	C44.60-☑	C79.2	D04.6-☑	D23.6-☑	D48.5	D49.2
skull	C41.0	C79.51	—	D16.4	D48.0	D49.2
soft parts or tissues — see Neoplasm, connective tissue						
specified site NEC	C76.8	C79.89	D09.8	D36.7	D48.7	D49.89
spermatic cord	C63.1-☑	C79.82	D07.69	D29.8	D40.8	D49.5
sphenoid	C31.3	C78.39	D02.3	D14.0	D38.5	D49.1
bone	C41.0	C79.51	—	D16.4	D48.0	D49.2
sinus	C31.3	C78.39	D02.3	D14.0	D38.5	D49.1
sphincter						
anal	C21.1	C78.5	D01.3	D12.9	D37.8	D49.0
of Oddi	C24.0	C78.89	D01.5	D13.5	D37.6	D49.0
spine, spinal (column)	C41.2	C79.51	—	D16.6	D48.0	D49.2
bulb	C71.7	C79.31	—	D33.1	D43.1	D49.6
coccyx	C41.4	C79.51	—	D16.8	D48.0	D49.2
cord (cervical) (lumbar) (sacral) (thoracic)	C72.0	C79.49	—	D33.4	D43.4	D49.7
dura mater	C70.1	C79.49	—	D32.1	D42.1	D49.7
lumbosacral	C41.2	C79.51	—	D16.6	D48.0	D49.2
marrow NEC	C96.9	C79.52	—	—	D47.9	D49.89
membrane	C70.1	C79.49	—	D32.1	D42.1	D49.7
meninges	C70.1	C79.49	—	D32.1	D42.1	D49.7
nerve (root)	C47.9	C79.89	—	D36.10	D48.2	D49.2
pia mater	C70.1	C79.49	—	D32.1	D42.1	D49.7
root	C47.9	C79.89	—	D36.10	D48.2	D49.2
sacrum	C41.4	C79.51	—	D16.8	D48.0	D49.2
spleen, splenic NEC	C26.1	C78.89	D01.7	D13.9	D37.8	D49.0
flexure (colon)	C18.5	C78.5	D01.0	D12.3	D37.4	D49.0
stem, brain	C71.7	C79.31	—	D33.1	D43.1	D49.6
Stensen's duct	C07	C79.89	D00.00	D11.0	D37.030	D49.0
sternum	C41.3	C79.51	—	D16.7	D48.0	D49.2
stomach	C16.9	C78.89	D00.2	D13.1	D37.1	D49.0
antrum (pyloric)	C16.3	C78.89	D00.2	D13.1	D37.1	D49.0
body	C16.2	C78.89	D00.2	D13.1	D37.1	D49.0
cardia	C16.0	C78.89	D00.2	D13.1	D37.1	D49.0
cardiac orifice	C16.0	C78.89	D00.2	D13.1	D37.1	D49.0
corpus	C16.2	C78.89	D00.2	D13.1	D37.1	D49.0
fundus	C16.1	C78.89	D00.2	D13.1	D37.1	D49.0
greater curvature NEC	C16.6	C78.89	D00.2	D13.1	D37.1	D49.0
lesser curvature NEC	C16.5	C78.89	D00.2	D13.1	D37.1	D49.0
overlapping lesion	C16.8	—	—	—	—	—
prepylorus	C16.4	C78.89	D00.2	D13.1	D37.1	D49.0
pylorus	C16.4	C78.89	D00.2	D13.1	D37.1	D49.0
wall NEC	C16.9	C78.89	D00.2	D13.1	D37.1	D49.0
anterior NEC	C16.8	C78.89	D00.2	D13.1	D37.1	D49.0
posterior NEC	C16.8	C78.89	D00.2	D13.1	D37.1	D49.0
stroma, endometrial	C54.1	C79.82	D07.0	D26.1	D39.0	D49.5
stump, cervical	C53.8	C79.82	D06.7	D26.0	D39.0	D49.5

Neoplasm, neoplastic — continued	Malignant Primary	Malignant Secondary	Ca in situ	Benign	Uncertain	Unspecified Behavior
subcutaneous (nodule) (tissue) NEC — see Neoplasm, connective tissue						
subdural	C70.9	C79.32	—	D32.9	D42.9	D49.7
subglottis, subglottic	C32.2	C78.39	D02.0	D14.1	D38.0	D49.1
sublingual	C04.9	C79.89	D00.06	D10.2	D37.09	D49.0
gland or duct	C08.1	C79.89	D00.00	D11.7	D37.031	D49.0
submandibular gland	C08.0	C79.89	D00.00	D11.7	D37.032	D49.0
submaxillary gland or duct	C08.0	C79.89	D00.00	D11.7	D37.032	D49.0
submental	C76.0	C79.89	D09.8	D36.7	D48.7	D49.89
subpleural	C34.9-☑	C78.0-☑	D02.2-☑	D14.3-☑	D38.1	D49.1
substernal	C38.1	C78.1	—	D15.2	D38.3	D49.89
sudoriferous, sudoriparous gland, site unspecified	C44.90	C79.2	D04.9	D23.9	D48.5	D49.2
specified site — see Neoplasm, skin						
supraclavicular region	C76.0	C79.89	D09.8	D36.7	D48.7	D49.89
supraglottis	C32.1	C78.39	D02.0	D14.1	D38.0	D49.1
suprarenal	C74.9-☑	C79.7-☑	D09.3	D35.0-☑	D44.1-☑	D49.7
capsule	C74.9-☑	C79.7-☑	D09.3	D35.0-☑	D44.1-☑	D49.7
cortex	C74.0-☑	C79.7-☑	D09.3	D35.0-☑	D44.1-☑	D49.7
gland	C74.9-☑	C79.7-☑	D09.3	D35.0-☑	D44.1-☑	D49.7
medulla	C74.1-☑	C79.7-☑	D09.3	D35.0-☑	D44.1-☑	D49.7
suprasellar (region)	C71.9	C79.31	—	D33.2	D43.2	D49.6
supratentorial (brain) NEC	C71.0	C79.31	—	D33.0	D43.0	D49.6
sweat gland (apocrine) (eccrine), site unspecified	C44.90	C79.2	D04.9	D23.9	D48.5	D49.2
specified site — see Neoplasm, skin						
sympathetic nerve or nervous system NEC	C47.9	C79.89	—	D36.10	D48.2	D49.2
symphysis pubis	C41.4	C79.51	—	D16.8	D48.0	D49.2
synovial membrane — see Neoplasm, connective tissue						
tapetum, brain	C71.8	C79.31	—	D33.2	D43.2	D49.6
tarsus (any bone)	C40.3-☑	C79.51	—	D16.3-☑	—	—
temple (skin) — see also Neoplasm, skin, face	C44.309	C79.2	D04.39	D23.39	D48.5	D49.2
temporal						
bone	C41.0	C79.51	—	D16.4	D48.0	D49.2
lobe or pole	C71.2	C79.31	—	D33.0	D43.0	D49.6
region	C76.0	C79.89	D09.8	D36.7	D48.7	D49.89
skin — see also Neoplasm, skin, face	C44.309	C79.2	D04.39	D23.39	D48.5	D49.2
tendon (sheath) — see Neoplasm, connective tissue						
tentorium (cerebelli)	C70.0	C79.32	—	D32.0	D42.0	D49.7
testis, testes	C62.9-☑	C79.82	D07.69	D29.2-☑	D40.1-☑	D49.5
descended	C62.1-☑	C79.82	D07.69	D29.2-☑	D40.1-☑	D49.5
ectopic	C62.0-☑	C79.82	D07.69	D29.2-☑	D40.1-☑	D49.5
retained	C62.0-☑	C79.82	D07.69	D29.2-☑	D40.1-☑	D49.5
scrotal	C62.1-☑	C79.82	D07.69	D29.2-☑	D40.1-☑	D49.5
undescended	C62.0-☑	C79.82	D07.69	D29.2-☑	D40.1-☑	D49.5
unspecified whether descended or undescended	C62.9-☑	C79.82	D07.69	D29.2-☑	D40.1-☑	D49.5
thalamus	C71.0	C79.31	—	D33.0	D43.0	D49.6
thigh NEC	C76.5-☑	C79.89	D04.7-☑	D36.7	D48.7	D49.89
thorax, thoracic (cavity) (organs NEC)	C76.1	C79.89	D09.8	D36.7	D48.7	D49.89
duct	C49.3	C79.89	—	D21.3	D48.1	D49.2
wall NEC	C76.1	C79.89	D09.8	D36.7	D48.7	D49.89
throat	C14.0	C79.89	D00.08	D10.9	D37.05	D49.0
thumb NEC	C76.4-☑	C79.89	D04.6-☑	D36.7	D48.7	D49.89
thymus (gland)	C37	C79.89	D09.3	D15.0	D38.4	D49.89
thyroglossal duct	C73	C79.89	D09.3	D34	D44.0	D49.7

Neoplasm, neoplastic — continued	Malignant Primary	Malignant Secondary	Ca in situ	Benign	Uncertain	Unspecified Behavior
thyroid (gland)	C73	C79.89	D09.3	D34	D44.0	D49.7
cartilage	C32.3	C78.39	D02.0	D14.1	D38.0	D49.1
tibia (any part)	C40.2-☑	C79.51	—	D16.2-☑	—	—
toe NEC	C76.5-☑	C79.89	D04.7-☑	D36.7	D48.7	D49.89
tongue	C02.9	C79.89	D00.07	D10.1	D37.02	D49.0
anterior (two-thirds) NEC	C02.3	C79.89	D00.07	D10.1	D37.02	D49.0
dorsal surface	C02.0	C79.89	D00.07	D10.1	D37.02	D49.0
ventral surface	C02.2	C79.89	D00.07	D10.1	D37.02	D49.0
base (dorsal surface)	C01	C79.89	D00.07	D10.1	D37.02	D49.0
border (lateral)	C02.1	C79.89	D00.07	D10.1	D37.02	D49.0
dorsal surface NEC	C02.0	C79.89	D00.07	D10.1	D37.02	D49.0
fixed part NEC	C01	C79.89	D00.07	D10.1	D37.02	D49.0
foreamen cecum	C02.0	C79.89	D00.07	D10.1	D37.02	D49.0
frenulum linguae	C02.2	C79.89	D00.07	D10.1	D37.02	D49.0
junctional zone	C02.8	C79.89	D00.07	D10.1	D37.02	D49.0
margin (lateral)	C02.1	C79.89	D00.07	D10.1	D37.02	D49.0
midline NEC	C02.0	C79.89	D00.07	D10.1	D37.02	D49.0
mobile part NEC	C02.3	C79.89	D00.07	D10.1	D37.02	D49.0
overlapping lesion	C02.8	—	—	—	—	—
posterior (third)	C01	C79.89	D00.07	D10.1	D37.02	D49.0
root	C01	C79.89	D00.07	D10.1	D37.02	D49.0
surface (dorsal)	C02.0	C79.89	D00.07	D10.1	D37.02	D49.0
base	C01	C79.89	D00.07	D10.1	D37.02	D49.0
ventral	C02.2	C79.89	D00.07	D10.1	D37.02	D49.0
tip	C02.1	C79.89	D00.07	D10.1	D37.02	D49.0
tonsil	C02.4	C79.89	D00.07	D10.1	D37.02	D49.0
tonsil	C09.9	C79.89	D00.08	D10.4	D37.05	D49.0
fauces, faucial	C09.9	C79.89	D00.08	D10.4	D37.05	D49.0
lingual	C02.4	C79.89	D00.07	D10.1	D37.02	D49.0
overlapping sites	C09.8	—	—	—	—	—
palatine	C09.9	C79.89	D00.08	D10.4	D37.05	D49.0
pharyngeal	C11.1	C79.89	D00.08	D10.6	D37.05	D49.0
pillar (anterior) (posterior)	C09.1	C79.89	D00.08	D10.5	D37.05	D49.0
tonsillar fossa	C09.0	C79.89	D00.08	D10.5	D37.05	D49.0
tooth socket NEC	C03.9	C79.89	D00.03	D10.39	D37.09	D49.0
trachea (cartilage) (mucosa)	C33	C78.39	D02.1	D14.2	D38.1	D49.1
overlapping lesion with bronchus or lung	C34.8-☑	—	—	—	—	—
tracheobronchial	C34.8-☑	C78.39	D02.1	D14.2	D38.1	D49.1
overlapping lesion with lung	C34.8-☑	—	—	—	—	—
tragus — see also Neoplasm, skin, ear	C44.20-☑	C79.2	D04.2-☑	D23.2-☑	D48.5	D49.2
trunk NEC	C76.8	C79.89	D04.5	D36.7	D48.7	D49.89
tubo-ovarian	C57.8	C79.82	D07.39	D28.7	D39.8	D49.5
tunica vaginalis	C63.7	C79.82	D07.69	D29.8	D40.8	D49.5
turbinate (bone)	C41.0	C79.51	—	D16.4	D48.0	D49.2
nasal	C30.0	C78.39	D02.3	D14.0	D38.5	D49.1
tympanic cavity	C30.1	C78.39	D02.3	D14.0	D38.5	D49.1
ulna (any part)	C40.0-☑	C79.51	—	D16.0-☑	—	—
umbilicus, umbilical — see also Neoplasm, skin, trunk	C44.509	C79.2	D04.5	D23.5	D48.5	D49.2
uncus, brain	C71.2	C79.31	—	D33.0	D43.0	D49.6
unknown site or unspecified	C80.1	C79.9	D09.9	D36.9	D48.9	D49.9
urachus	C67.7	C79.11	D09.0	D30.3	D41.4	D49.4
ureter-bladder (junction)	C67.6	C79.11	D09.0	D30.3	D41.4	D49.4
ureter, ureteral	C66.-☑	C79.19	D09.19	D30.2-☑	D41.2-☑	D49.5
orifice (bladder)	C67.6	C79.11	D09.0	D30.3	D41.4	D49.4
urethra, urethral (gland)	C68.0	C79.19	D09.19	D30.4	D41.3	D49.5
orifice, internal	C67.5	C79.11	D09.0	D30.3	D41.4	D49.4
urethrovaginal (septum)	C57.9	C79.82	D07.30	D28.9	D39.8	D49.5
urinary organ or system	C68.9	C79.10	D09.10	D30.9	D41.9	D49.5
bladder — see Neoplasm, bladder						
overlapping lesion	C68.8	—	—	—	—	—
specified sites NEC	C68.8	C79.19	D09.19	D30.8	D41.8	D49.5
utero-ovarian	C57.8	C79.82	D07.39	D28.7	D39.8	D49.5
ligament	C57.1-☑	C79.82	D07.39	D28.2	D39.8	D49.5
uterosacral ligament	C57.3	C79.82	—	D28.2	D39.8	D49.5

Neoplasm, neoplastic — continued	Malignant Primary	Malignant Secondary	Ca in situ	Benign	Uncertain	Unspecified Behavior
uterus, uteri, uterine	C55	C79.82	D07.0	D26.9	D39.0	D49.5
adnexa NEC	C57.4	C79.82	D07.39	D28.7	D39.8	D49.5
body	C54.9	C79.82	D07.0	D26.1	D39.0	D49.5
cervix	C53.9	C79.82	D06.9	D26.0	D39.0	D49.5
cornu	C54.9	C79.82	D07.0	D26.1	D39.0	D49.5
corpus	C54.9	C79.82	D07.0	D26.1	D39.0	D49.5
endocervix (canal) (gland)	C53.0	C79.82	D06.0	D26.0	D39.0	D49.5
endometrium	C54.1	C79.82	D07.0	D26.1	D39.0	D49.5
exocervix	C53.1	C79.82	D06.1	D26.0	D39.0	D49.5
external os	C53.1	C79.82	D06.1	D26.0	D39.0	D49.5
fundus	C54.3	C79.82	D07.0	D26.1	D39.0	D49.5
internal os	C53.0	C79.82	D06.0	D26.0	D39.0	D49.5
isthmus	C54.0	C79.82	D07.0	D26.1	D39.0	D49.5
ligament	C57.3	C79.82	—	D28.2	D39.8	D49.5
broad	C57.1-☑	C79.82	D07.39	D28.2	D39.8	D49.5
round	C57.2-☑	C79.82	—	D28.2	D39.8	D49.5
lower segment	C54.0	C79.82	D07.0	D26.1	D39.0	D49.5
myometrium	C54.2	C79.82	D07.0	D26.1	D39.0	D49.5
overlapping sites	C54.8	—	—	—	—	—
squamocolumnar junction	C53.8	C79.82	D06.7	D26.0	D39.0	D49.5
tube	C57.0-☑	C79.82	D07.39	D28.2	D39.8	D49.5
utricle, prostatic	C68.0	C79.19	D09.19	D30.4	D41.3	D49.5
uveal tract	C69.4-☑	C79.49	D09.2-☑	D31.4-☑	D48.7	D49.89
uvula	C05.2	C79.89	D00.04	D10.39	D37.09	D49.0
vagina, vaginal (fornix) (vault) (wall)	C52	C79.82	D07.2	D28.1	D39.8	D49.5
vaginovesical	C57.9	C79.82	D07.30	D28.9	D39.9	D49.5
septum	C57.9	C79.82	D07.30	D28.9	D39.9	D49.5
vallecula (epigiottis)	C10.0	C79.89	D00.08	D10.5	D37.05	D49.0
vascular — see Neoplasm, connective tissue						
vas deferens	C63.1-☑	C79.82	D07.69	D29.8	D40.8	D49.5
Vater's ampulla	C24.1	C78.89	D01.5	D13.5	D37.6	D49.0
vein, venous — see Neoplasm, connective tissue						
vena cava (abdominal) (inferior)	C49.4	C79.89	—	D21.4	D48.1	D49.2
superior	C49.3	C79.89	—	D21.3	D48.1	D49.2
ventricle (cerebral) (floor) (lateral) (third)	C71.5	C79.31	—	D33.0	D43.0	D49.6
cardiac (left) (right)	C38.0	C79.89	—	D15.1	D48.7	D49.89
fourth	C71.7	C79.31	—	D33.1	D43.1	D49.6
ventricular band of larynx	C32.1	C78.39	D02.0	D14.1	D38.0	D49.1
ventriculus — see Neoplasm, stomach						
vermillion border — see Neoplasm, lip						
vermis, cerebellum	C71.6	C79.31	—	D33.1	D43.1	D49.6
vertebra (column)	C41.2	C79.51	—	D16.6	D48.0	D49.2
coccyx	C41.4	C79.51	—	D16.8	D48.0	D49.2
marrow NEC	C96.9	C79.52	—	—	D47.9	D49.89
sacrum	C41.4	C79.51	—	D16.8	D48.0	D49.2
vesical — see Neoplasm, bladder						
vesicle, seminal	C63.7	C79.82	D07.69	D29.8	D40.8	D49.5
vesicocervical tissue	C57.9	C79.82	D07.30	D28.9	D39.9	D49.5
vesicorectal	C76.3	C79.82	D09.8	D36.7	D48.7	D49.89
vesicovaginal	C57.9	C79.82	D07.30	D28.9	D39.9	D49.5
septum	C57.9	C79.82	D07.30	D28.9	D39.8	D49.5
vessel (blood) — see Neoplasm, connective tissue						
vestibular gland, greater	C51.0	C79.82	D07.1	D28.0	D39.8	D49.5
vestibule						
mouth	C06.1	C79.89	D00.00	D10.39	D37.09	D49.0
nose	C30.0	C78.39	D02.3	D14.0	D38.5	D49.1
Virchow's gland	C77.0	C77.0	—	D36.0	D48.7	D49.89
viscera NEC	C76.8	C79.89	D09.8	D36.7	D48.7	D49.89
vocal cords (true)	C32.0	C78.39	D02.0	D14.1	D38.0	D49.1
false	C32.1	C78.39	D02.0	D14.1	D38.0	D49.1
vomer	C41.0	C79.51	—	D16.4	D48.0	D49.2
vulva	C51.9	C79.82	D07.1	D28.0	D39.8	D49.5
vulvovaginal gland	C51.0	C79.82	D07.1	D28.0	D39.8	D49.5
Waldeyer's ring	C14.2	C79.89	D00.08	D10.9	D37.05	D49.0
Wharton's duct	C08.0	C79.89	D00.00	D11.7	D37.032	D49.0

	Malignant Primary	Malignant Secondary	Ca in situ	Benign	Uncertain	Unspecified Behavior
Neoplasm, neoplastic — *continued*						
white matter (central) (cerebral)	C71.Ø	C79.31	—	D33.Ø	D43.Ø	D49.6
windpipe	C33	C78.39	DØ2.1	D14.2	D38.1	D49.1
Wirsung's duct	C25.3	C78.89	DØ1.7	D13.6	D37.8	D49.Ø
wolffian (body) (duct)						
female	C57.7	C79.82	DØ7.39	D28.7	D39.8	D49.5
male	C63.7	C79.82	DØ7.69	D29.8	D4Ø.8	D49.5
womb — *see* Neoplasm, uterus						
wrist NEC	C76.4-☑	C79.89	DØ4.6-☑	D36.7	D48.7	D49.89
xiphoid process	C41.3	C79.51	—	D16.7	D48.Ø	D49.2
Zuckerkandl organ	C75.5	C79.89	—	D35.6	D44.7	D49.7

ICD-10-CM Table of Drugs and Chemicals

Substance	Poisoning, Accidental (unintentional)	Poisoning, Intentional Self-harm	Poisoning, Assault	Poisoning, Undetermined	Adverse Effect	Under-dosing
14-Hydroxydihydromorphinone	T40.2X1	T40.2X2	T40.2X3	T40.2X4	T40.2X5	T40.2X6
1-Propanol	T51.3X1	T51.3X2	T51.3X3	T51.3X4	—	—
2,3,7,8-Tetrachlorodibenzo-p-dioxin	T53.7X1	T53.7X2	T53.7X3	T53.7X4	—	—
2,4,5-T (trichlorophenoxyacetic acid)	T60.1X1	T60.1X2	T60.1X3	T60.1X4	—	—
2,4,5-Trichlorophenoxyacetic acid	T60.3X1	T60.3X2	T60.3X3	T60.3X4	—	—
2,4-D (dichlorophenoxyacetic acid)	T60.3X1	T60.3X2	T60.3X3	T60.3X4	—	—
2,4-Toluene diisocyanate	T65.0X1	T65.0X2	T65.0X3	T65.0X4	—	—
2-Deoxy-5-fluorouridine	T45.1X1	T45.1X2	T45.1X3	T45.1X4	T45.1X5	T45.1X6
2-Ethoxyethanol	T52.3X1	T52.3X2	T52.3X3	T52.3X4	—	—
2-Methoxyethanol	T52.3X1	T52.3X2	T52.3X3	T52.3X4	—	—
2-Propanol	T51.2X1	T51.2X2	T51.2X3	T51.2X4	—	—
4-Aminobutyric acid	T43.8X1	T43.8X2	T43.8X3	T43.8X4	T43.8X5	T43.8X6
4-Aminophenol derivatives	T39.1X1	T39.1X2	T39.1X3	T39.1X4	T39.1X5	T39.1X6
5-Deoxy-5-fluorouridine	T45.1X1	T45.1X2	T45.1X3	T45.1X4	T45.1X5	T45.1X6
5-Methoxypsoralen (5-MOP)	T50.991	T50.992	T50.993	T50.994	T50.995	T50.996
8-Aminoquinoline drugs	T37.2X1	T37.2X2	T37.2X3	T37.2X4	T37.2X5	T37.2X6
8-Methoxypsoralen (8-MOP)	T50.991	T50.992	T50.993	T50.994	T50.995	T50.996
ABOB	T37.5X1	T37.5X2	T37.5X3	T37.5X4	T37.5X5	T37.5X6
Abrine	T62.2X1	T62.2X2	T62.2X3	T62.2X4	—	—
Abrus (seed)	T62.2X1	T62.2X2	T62.2X3	T62.2X4	—	—
Absinthe	T51.0X1	T51.0X2	T51.0X3	T51.0X4	—	—
beverage	T51.0X1	T51.0X2	T51.0X3	T51.0X4	—	—
Acaricide	T60.8X1	T60.8X2	T60.8X3	T60.8X4	—	—
Acebutolol	T44.7X1	T44.7X2	T44.7X3	T44.7X4	T44.7X5	T44.7X6
Acecarbromal	T42.6X1	T42.6X2	T42.6X3	T42.6X4	T42.6X5	T42.6X6
Aceclidine	T44.1X1	T44.1X2	T44.1X3	T44.1X4	T44.1X5	T44.1X6
Acedapsone	T37.0X1	T37.0X2	T37.0X3	T37.0X4	T37.0X5	T37.0X6
Acefylline piperazine	T48.6X1	T48.6X2	T48.6X3	T48.6X4	T48.6X5	T48.6X6
Acemorphan	T40.2X1	T40.2X2	T40.2X3	T40.2X4	T40.2X5	T40.2X6
Acenocoumarin	T45.511	T45.512	T45.513	T45.514	T45.515	T45.516
Acenocoumarol	T45.511	T45.512	T45.513	T45.514	T45.515	T45.516
Acepifylline	T48.6X1	T48.6X2	T48.6X3	T48.6X4	T48.6X5	T48.6X6
Acepromazine	T43.3X1	T43.3X2	T43.3X3	T43.3X4	T43.3X5	T43.3X6
Acesulfamethoxypyridazine	T37.0X1	T37.0X2	T37.0X3	T37.0X4	T37.0X5	T37.0X6
Acetal	T52.8X1	T52.8X2	T52.8X3	T52.8X4	—	—
Acetaldehyde (vapor)	T52.8X1	T52.8X2	T52.8X3	T52.8X4	—	—
liquid	T65.891	T65.892	T65.893	T65.894	—	—
Acetaminophen	T39.1X1	T39.1X2	T39.1X3	T39.1X4	T39.1X5	T39.1X6
Acetaminosalol	T39.1X1	T39.1X2	T39.1X3	T39.1X4	T39.1X5	T39.1X6
Acetanilide	T39.1X1	T39.1X2	T39.1X3	T39.1X4	T39.1X5	T39.1X6
Acetarsol	T37.3X1	T37.3X2	T37.3X3	T37.3X4	T37.3X5	T37.3X6
Acetazolamide	T50.2X1	T50.2X2	T50.2X3	T50.2X4	T50.2X5	T50.2X6
Acetiamine	T45.2X1	T45.2X2	T45.2X3	T45.2X4	T45.2X5	T45.2X6
Acetic						
acid	T54.2X1	T54.2X2	T54.2X3	T54.2X4	—	—
with sodium acetate (ointment)	T49.3X1	T49.3X2	T49.3X3	T49.3X4	T49.3X5	T49.3X6
ester (solvent)(vapor)	T52.8X1	T52.8X2	T52.8X3	T52.8X4	—	—
irrigating solution	T50.3X1	T50.3X2	T50.3X3	T50.3X4	T50.3X5	T50.3X6
medicinal (lotion)	T49.2X1	T49.2X2	T49.2X3	T49.2X4	T49.2X5	T49.2X6
anhydride	T65.891	T65.892	T65.893	T65.894	—	—
ether (vapor)	T52.8X1	T52.8X2	T52.8X3	T52.8X4	—	—
Acetohexamide	T38.3X1	T38.3X2	T38.3X3	T38.3X4	T38.3X5	T38.3X6
Acetohydroxamic acid	T50.991	T50.992	T50.993	T50.994	T50.995	T50.996
Acetomenaphthone	T45.7X1	T45.7X2	T45.7X3	T45.7X4	T45.7X5	T45.7X6
Acetomorphine	T40.1X1	T40.1X2	T40.1X3	T40.1X4	—	—
Acetone (oils)	T52.4X1	T52.4X2	T52.4X3	T52.4X4	—	—
chlorinated	T52.4X1	T52.4X2	T52.4X3	T52.4X4	—	—
vapor	T52.4X1	T52.4X2	T52.4X3	T52.4X4	—	—
Acetonitrile	T52.8X1	T52.8X2	T52.8X3	T52.8X4	—	—
Acetophenazine	T43.3X1	T43.3X2	T43.3X3	T43.3X4	T43.3X5	T43.3X6
Acetophenetedin	T39.1X1	T39.1X2	T39.1X3	T39.1X4	T39.1X5	T39.1X6
Acetophenone	T52.4X1	T52.4X2	T52.4X3	T52.4X4	—	—
Acetorphine	T40.2X1	T40.2X2	T40.2X3	T40.2X4	—	—
Acetosulfone (sodium)	T37.1X1	T37.1X2	T37.1X3	T37.1X4	T37.1X5	T37.1X6
Acetrizoate (sodium)	T50.8X1	T50.8X2	T50.8X3	T50.8X4	T50.8X5	T50.8X6
Acetrizoic acid	T50.8X1	T50.8X2	T50.8X3	T50.8X4	T50.8X5	T50.8X6
Acetyl						
bromide	T53.6X1	T53.6X2	T53.6X3	T53.6X4	—	—
chloride	T53.6X1	T53.6X2	T53.6X3	T53.6X4	—	—
Acetylcarbromal	T42.6X1	T42.6X2	T42.6X3	T42.6X4	T42.6X5	T42.6X6

Substance	Poisoning, Accidental (unintentional)	Poisoning, Intentional Self-harm	Poisoning, Assault	Poisoning, Undetermined	Adverse Effect	Under-dosing
Acetylcholine						
chloride	T44.1X1	T44.1X2	T44.1X3	T44.1X4	T44.1X5	T44.1X6
derivative	T44.1X1	T44.1X2	T44.1X3	T44.1X4	T44.1X5	T44.1X6
Acetylcysteine	T48.4X1	T48.4X2	T48.4X3	T48.4X4	T48.4X5	T48.4X6
Acetyldigitoxin	T46.0X1	T46.0X2	T46.0X3	T46.0X4	T46.0X5	T46.0X6
Acetyldigoxin	T46.0X1	T46.0X2	T46.0X3	T46.0X4	T46.0X5	T46.0X6
Acetyldihydrocodeine	T40.2X1	T40.2X2	T40.2X3	T40.2X4	—	—
Acetyldihydrocodeinone	T40.2X1	T40.2X2	T40.2X3	T40.2X4	—	—
Acetylene (gas)	T59.891	T59.892	T59.893	T59.894	—	—
dichloride	T53.6X1	T53.6X2	T53.6X3	T53.6X4	—	—
incomplete combustion of	T58.11	T58.12	T58.13	T58.14	—	—
industrial	T59.891	T59.892	T59.893	T59.894	—	—
tetrachloride	T53.6X1	T53.6X2	T53.6X3	T53.6X4	—	—
vapor	T53.6X1	T53.6X2	T53.6X3	T53.6X4	—	—
Acetylpheneturide	T42.6X1	T42.6X2	T42.6X3	T42.6X4	T42.6X5	T42.6X6
Acetylphenylhydrazine	T39.8X1	T39.8X2	T39.8X3	T39.8X4	T39.8X5	T39.8X6
Acetylsalicylic acid (salts)	T39.011	T39.012	T39.013	T39.014	T39.015	T39.016
enteric coated	T39.011	T39.012	T39.013	T39.014	T39.015	T39.016
Acetylsulfamethoxypyridazine	T37.0X1	T37.0X2	T37.0X3	T37.0X4	T37.0X5	T37.0X6
Achromycin	T36.4X1	T36.4X2	T36.4X3	T36.4X4	T36.4X5	T36.4X6
ophthalmic preparation	T49.5X1	T49.5X2	T49.5X3	T49.5X4	T49.5X5	T49.5X6
topical NEC	T49.0X1	T49.0X2	T49.0X3	T49.0X4	T49.0X5	T49.0X6
Aciclovir	T37.5X1	T37.5X2	T37.5X3	T37.5X4	T37.5X5	T37.5X6
Acidifying agent NEC	T50.901	T50.902	T50.903	T50.904	T50.905	T50.906
Acid (corrosive) NEC	T54.2X1	T54.2X2	T54.2X3	T54.2X4	—	—
Acipimox	T46.6X1	T46.6X2	T46.6X3	T46.6X4	T46.6X5	T46.6X6
Acitretin	T50.991	T50.992	T50.993	T50.994	T50.995	T50.996
Aclarubicin	T45.1X1	T45.1X2	T45.1X3	T45.1X4	T45.1X5	T45.1X6
Aclatonium napadisilate	T48.1X1	T48.1X2	T48.1X3	T48.1X4	T48.1X5	T48.1X6
Aconite (wild)	T46.991	T46.992	T46.993	T46.994	T46.995	T46.996
Aconitine	T46.991	T46.992	T46.993	T46.994	T46.995	T46.996
Aconitum ferox	T46.991	T46.992	T46.993	T46.994	T46.995	T46.996
Acridine	T65.6X1	T65.6X2	T65.6X3	T65.6X4	—	—
vapor	T59.891	T59.892	T59.893	T59.894	—	—
Acriflavine	T37.91	T37.92	T37.93	T37.94	T37.95	T37.96
Acriflavinium chloride	T49.0X1	T49.0X2	T49.0X3	T49.0X4	T49.0X5	T49.0X6
Acrinol	T49.0X1	T49.0X2	T49.0X3	T49.0X4	T49.0X5	T49.0X6
Acrisorcin	T49.0X1	T49.0X2	T49.0X3	T49.0X4	T49.0X5	T49.0X6
Acrivastine	T45.0X1	T45.0X2	T45.0X3	T45.0X4	T45.0X5	T45.0X6
Acrolein (gas)	T59.891	T59.892	T59.893	T59.894	—	—
liquid	T54.1X1	T54.1X2	T54.1X3	T54.1X4	—	—
Acrylamide	T65.891	T65.892	T65.893	T65.894	—	—
Acrylic resin	T49.3X1	T49.3X2	T49.3X3	T49.3X4	T49.3X5	T49.3X6
Acrylonitrile	T65.891	T65.892	T65.893	T65.894	—	—
Actaea spicata	T62.2X1	T62.2X2	T62.2X3	T62.2X4	—	—
berry	T62.1X1	T62.1X2	T62.1X3	T62.1X4	—	—
Acterol	T37.3X1	T37.3X2	T37.3X3	T37.3X4	T37.3X5	T37.3X6
ACTH	T38.811	T38.812	T38.813	T38.814	T38.815	T38.816
Actinomycin C	T45.1X1	T45.1X2	T45.1X3	T45.1X4	T45.1X5	T45.1X6
Actinomycin D	T45.1X1	T45.1X2	T45.1X3	T45.1X4	T45.1X5	T45.1X6
Activated charcoal — see also Charcoal, medicinal	T47.6X1	T47.6X2	T47.6X3	T47.6X4	T47.6X5	T47.6X6
Acyclovir	T37.5X1	T37.5X2	T37.5X3	T37.5X4	T37.5X5	T37.5X6
Adenine	T45.2X1	T45.2X2	T45.2X3	T45.2X4	T45.2X5	T45.2X6
arabinoside	T37.5X1	T37.5X2	T37.5X3	T37.5X4	T37.5X5	T37.5X6
Adenosine (phosphate)	T46.2X1	T46.2X2	T46.2X3	T46.2X4	T46.2X5	T46.2X6
ADH	T38.891	T38.892	T38.893	T38.894	T38.895	T38.896
Adhesive NEC	T65.891	T65.892	T65.893	T65.894	—	—
Adicillin	T36.0X1	T36.0X2	T36.0X3	T36.0X4	T36.0X5	T36.0X6
Adiphenine	T44.3X1	T44.3X2	T44.3X3	T44.3X4	T44.3X5	T44.3X6
Adipiodone	T50.8X1	T50.8X2	T50.8X3	T50.8X4	T50.8X5	T50.8X6
Adjunct, pharmaceutical	T50.901	T50.902	T50.903	T50.904	T50.905	T50.906
Adrenal (extract, cortex or medulla) (glucocorticoids) (hormones) (mineralocorticoids)	T38.0X1	T38.0X2	T38.0X3	T38.0X4	T38.0X5	T38.0X6
ENT agent	T49.6X1	T49.6X2	T49.6X3	T49.6X4	T49.6X5	T49.6X6
ophthalmic preparation	T49.5X1	T49.5X2	T49.5X3	T49.5X4	T49.5X5	T49.5X6
topical NEC	T49.0X1	T49.0X2	T49.0X3	T49.0X4	T49.0X5	T49.0X6
Adrenalin — see Adrenaline						
Adrenaline	T44.5X1	T44.5X2	T44.5X3	T44.5X4	T44.5X5	T44.5X6
Adrenergic NEC	T44.901	T44.902	T44.903	T44.904	T44.905	T44.906
blocking agent NEC	T44.8X1	T44.8X2	T44.8X3	T44.8X4	T44.8X5	T44.8X6
beta, heart	T44.7X1	T44.7X2	T44.7X3	T44.7X4	T44.7X5	T44.7X6
specified NEC	T44.991	T44.992	T44.993	T44.994	T44.995	T44.996
Adrenochrome						
derivative	T46.991	T46.992	T46.993	T46.994	T46.995	T46.996

Substance	Poisoning, Accidental (unintentional)	Poisoning, Intentional Self-harm	Poisoning, Assault	Poisoning, Undetermined	Adverse Effect	Under-dosing
Adrenochrome — *continued*						
(mono) semicarbazone	T46.991	T46.992	T46.993	T46.994	T46.995	T46.996
Adrenocorticotrophic hormone	T38.811	T38.812	T38.813	T38.814	T38.815	T38.816
Adrenocorticotrophin	T38.811	T38.812	T38.813	T38.814	T38.815	T38.816
Adriamycin	T45.1X1	T45.1X2	T45.1X3	T45.1X4	T45.1X5	T45.1X6
Aerosol spray NEC	T65.91	T65.92	T65.93	T65.94	—	—
Aerosporin	T36.8X1	T36.8X2	T36.8X3	T36.8X4	T36.8X5	T36.8X6
ENT agent	T49.6X1	T49.6X2	T49.6X3	T49.6X4	T49.6X5	T49.6X6
ophthalmic preparation	T49.5X1	T49.5X2	T49.5X3	T49.5X4	T49.5X5	T49.5X6
topical NEC	T49.0X1	T49.0X2	T49.0X3	T49.0X4	T49.0X5	T49.0X6
Aethusa cynapium	T62.2X1	T62.2X2	T62.2X3	T62.2X4	—	—
Afghanistan black	T40.7X1	T40.7X2	T40.7X3	T40.7X4	T40.7X5	T40.7X6
Aflatoxin	T64.01	T64.02	T64.03	T64.04	—	—
Afloqualone	T42.8X1	T42.8X2	T42.8X3	T42.8X4	T42.8X5	T42.8X6
African boxwood	T62.2X1	T62.2X2	T62.2X3	T62.2X4	—	—
Agar	T47.4X1	T47.4X2	T47.4X3	T47.4X4	T47.4X5	T47.4X6
Agonist						
predominantly						
alpha-adrenoreceptor	T44.4X1	T44.4X2	T44.4X3	T44.4X4	T44.4X5	T44.4X6
beta-adrenoreceptor	T44.5X1	T44.5X2	T44.5X3	T44.5X4	T44.5X5	T44.5X6
Agricultural agent NEC	T65.91	T65.92	T65.93	T65.94	—	—
Agrypnal	T42.3X1	T42.3X2	T42.3X3	T42.3X4	T42.3X5	T42.3X6
AHLG	T50.Z11	T50.Z12	T50.Z13	T50.Z14	T50.Z15	T50.Z16
Air contaminant(s), source/type NOS	T65.91	T65.92	T65.93	T65.94	—	—
Ajmaline	T46.2X1	T46.2X2	T46.2X3	T46.2X4	T46.2X5	T46.2X6
Akee	T62.1X1	T62.1X2	T62.1X3	T62.1X4	—	—
Akrinol	T49.0X1	T49.0X2	T49.0X3	T49.0X4	T49.0X5	T49.0X6
Akritoin	T37.8X1	T37.8X2	T37.8X3	T37.8X4	T37.8X5	T37.8X6
Alacepril	T46.4X1	T46.4X2	T46.4X3	T46.4X4	T46.4X5	T46.4X6
Alantolactone	T37.4X1	T37.4X2	T37.4X3	T37.4X4	T37.4X5	T37.4X6
Albamycin	T36.8X1	T36.8X2	T36.8X3	T36.8X4	T36.8X5	T36.8X6
Albendazole	T37.4X1	T37.4X2	T37.4X3	T37.4X4	T37.4X5	T37.4X6
Albumin						
bovine	T45.8X1	T45.8X2	T45.8X3	T45.8X4	T45.8X5	T45.8X6
human serum	T45.8X1	T45.8X2	T45.8X3	T45.8X4	T45.8X5	T45.8X6
salt-poor	T45.8X1	T45.8X2	T45.8X3	T45.8X4	T45.8X5	T45.8X6
normal human serum	T45.8X1	T45.8X2	T45.8X3	T45.8X4	T45.8X5	T45.8X6
Albuterol	T48.6X1	T48.6X2	T48.6X3	T48.6X4	T48.6X5	T48.6X6
Albutoin	T42.0X1	T42.0X2	T42.0X3	T42.0X4	T42.0X5	T42.0X6
Alclometasone	T49.0X1	T49.0X2	T49.0X3	T49.0X4	T49.0X5	T49.0X6
Alcohol	T51.91	T51.92	T51.93	T51.94	—	—
absolute	T51.0X1	T51.0X2	T51.0X3	T51.0X4	—	—
beverage	T51.0X1	T51.0X2	T51.0X3	T51.0X4	—	—
allyl	T51.8X1	T51.8X2	T51.8X3	T51.8X4	—	—
amyl	T51.3X1	T51.3X2	T51.3X3	T51.3X4	—	—
antifreeze	T51.1X1	T51.1X2	T51.1X3	T51.1X4	—	—
beverage	T51.0X1	T51.0X2	T51.0X3	T51.0X4	—	—
butyl	T51.3X1	T51.3X2	T51.3X3	T51.3X4	—	—
dehydrated	T51.0X1	T51.0X2	T51.0X3	T51.0X4	—	—
beverage	T51.0X1	T51.0X2	T51.0X3	T51.0X4	—	—
denatured	T51.0X1	T51.0X2	T51.0X3	T51.0X4	—	—
deterrent NEC	T50.6X1	T50.6X2	T50.6X3	T50.6X4	T50.6X5	T50.6X6
diagnostic (gastric function)	T50.8X1	T50.8X2	T50.8X3	T50.8X4	T50.8X5	T50.8X6
ethyl	T51.0X1	T51.0X2	T51.0X3	T51.0X4	—	—
beverage	T51.0X1	T51.0X2	T51.0X3	T51.0X4	—	—
grain	T51.0X1	T51.0X2	T51.0X3	T51.0X4	—	—
beverage	T51.0X1	T51.0X2	T51.0X3	T51.0X4	—	—
industrial	T51.0X1	T51.0X2	T51.0X3	T51.0X4	—	—
isopropyl	T51.2X1	T51.2X2	T51.2X3	T51.2X4	—	—
methyl	T51.1X1	T51.1X2	T51.1X3	T51.1X4	—	—
preparation for consumption	T51.0X1	T51.0X2	T51.0X3	T51.0X4	—	—
propyl	T51.3X1	T51.3X2	T51.3X3	T51.3X4	—	—
secondary	T51.2X1	T51.2X2	T51.2X3	T51.2X4	—	—
radiator	T51.1X1	T51.1X2	T51.1X3	T51.1X4	—	—
rubbing	T51.2X1	T51.2X2	T51.2X3	T51.2X4	—	—
specified type NEC	T51.8X1	T51.8X2	T51.8X3	T51.8X4	—	—
surgical	T51.0X1	T51.0X2	T51.0X3	T51.0X4	—	—
vapor (from any type of Alcohol)	T59.891	T59.892	T59.893	T59.894	—	—
wood	T51.1X1	T51.1X2	T51.1X3	T51.1X4	—	—
Alcuronium (chloride)	T48.1X1	T48.1X2	T48.1X3	T48.1X4	T48.1X5	T48.1X6
Aldactone	T50.0X1	T50.0X2	T50.0X3	T50.0X4	T50.0X5	T50.0X6
Aldesulfone sodium	T37.1X1	T37.1X2	T37.1X3	T37.1X4	T37.1X5	T37.1X6
Aldicarb	T60.0X1	T60.0X2	T60.0X3	T60.0X4	—	—
Aldomet	T46.5X1	T46.5X2	T46.5X3	T46.5X4	T46.5X5	T46.5X6
Aldosterone	T50.0X1	T50.0X2	T50.0X3	T50.0X4	T50.0X5	T50.0X6
Aldrin (dust)	T60.1X1	T60.1X2	T60.1X3	T60.1X4	—	—
Aleve — *see* Naproxen						
Alexitol sodium	T47.1X1	T47.1X2	T47.1X3	T47.1X4	T47.1X5	T47.1X6

Substance	Poisoning, Accidental (unintentional)	Poisoning, Intentional Self-harm	Poisoning, Assault	Poisoning, Undetermined	Adverse Effect	Under-dosing
Alfacalcidol	T45.2X1	T45.2X2	T45.2X3	T45.2X4	T45.2X5	T45.2X6
Alfadolone	T41.1X1	T41.1X2	T41.1X3	T41.1X4	T41.1X5	T41.1X6
Alfaxalone	T41.1X1	T41.1X2	T41.1X3	T41.1X4	T41.1X5	T41.1X6
Alfentanil	T40.4X1	T40.4X2	T40.4X3	T40.4X4	T40.4X5	T40.4X6
Alfuzosin (hydrochloride)	T44.8X1	T44.8X2	T44.8X3	T44.8X4	T44.8X5	T44.8X6
Algae (harmful) (toxin)	T65.821	T65.822	T65.823	T65.824	—	—
Algeldrate	T47.1X1	T47.1X2	T47.1X3	T47.1X4	T47.1X5	T47.1X6
Algin	T47.8X1	T47.8X2	T47.8X3	T47.8X4	T47.8X5	T47.8X6
Alglucerase	T45.3X1	T45.3X2	T45.3X3	T45.3X4	T45.3X5	T45.3X6
Alidase	T45.3X1	T45.3X2	T45.3X3	T45.3X4	T45.3X5	T45.3X6
Alimemazine	T43.3X1	T43.3X2	T43.3X3	T43.3X4	T43.3X5	T43.3X6
Aliphatic thiocyanates	T65.0X1	T65.0X2	T65.0X3	T65.0X4	—	—
Alizapride	T45.0X1	T45.0X2	T45.0X3	T45.0X4	T45.0X5	T45.0X6
Alkali (caustic)	T54.3X1	T54.3X2	T54.3X3	T54.3X4	—	—
Alkaline antiseptic solution (aromatic)	T49.6X1	T49.6X2	T49.6X3	T49.6X4	T49.6X5	T49.6X6
Alkalinizing agents (medicinal)	T50.901	T50.902	T50.903	T50.904	T50.905	T50.906
Alkalizing agent NEC	T50.901	T50.902	T50.903	T50.904	T50.905	T50.906
Alka-seltzer	T39.011	T39.012	T39.013	T39.014	T39.015	T39.016
Alkavervir	T46.5X1	T46.5X2	T46.5X3	T46.5X4	T46.5X5	T46.5X6
Alkonium (bromide)	T49.0X1	T49.0X2	T49.0X3	T49.0X4	T49.0X5	T49.0X6
Alkylating drug NEC	T45.1X1	T45.1X2	T45.1X3	T45.1X4	T45.1X5	T45.1X6
antimyeloproliferative	T45.1X1	T45.1X2	T45.1X3	T45.1X4	T45.1X5	T45.1X6
lymphatic	T45.1X1	T45.1X2	T45.1X3	T45.1X4	T45.1X5	T45.1X6
Alkylisocyanate	T65.0X1	T65.0X2	T65.0X3	T65.0X4	—	—
Allantoin	T49.4X1	T49.4X2	T49.4X3	T49.4X4	T49.4X5	T49.4X6
Allegron	T43.011	T43.012	T43.013	T43.014	T43.015	T43.016
Allethrin	T49.0X1	T49.0X2	T49.0X3	T49.0X4	T49.0X5	T49.0X6
Allobarbital	T42.3X1	T42.3X2	T42.3X3	T42.3X4	T42.3X5	T42.3X6
Allopurinol	T50.4X1	T50.4X2	T50.4X3	T50.4X4	T50.4X5	T50.4X6
Allyl						
alcohol	T51.8X1	T51.8X2	T51.8X3	T51.8X4	—	—
disulfide	T46.6X1	T46.6X2	T46.6X3	T46.6X4	T46.6X5	T46.6X6
Allylestrenol	T38.5X1	T38.5X2	T38.5X3	T38.5X4	T38.5X5	T38.5X6
Allylisopropylacetylurea	T42.6X1	T42.6X2	T42.6X3	T42.6X4	T42.6X5	T42.6X6
Allylisopropylmalonylurea	T42.3X1	T42.3X2	T42.3X3	T42.3X4	T42.3X5	T42.3X6
Allylthiourea	T49.3X1	T49.3X2	T49.3X3	T49.3X4	T49.3X5	T49.3X6
Allyltribromide	T42.6X1	T42.6X2	T42.6X3	T42.6X4	T42.6X5	T42.6X6
Allypropymal	T42.3X1	T42.3X2	T42.3X3	T42.3X4	T42.3X5	T42.3X6
Almagate	T47.1X1	T47.1X2	T47.1X3	T47.1X4	T47.1X5	T47.1X6
Almasilate	T47.1X1	T47.1X2	T47.1X3	T47.1X4	T47.1X5	T47.1X6
Almitrine	T50.7X1	T50.7X2	T50.7X3	T50.7X4	T50.7X5	T50.7X6
Aloes	T47.2X1	T47.2X2	T47.2X3	T47.2X4	T47.2X5	T47.2X6
Aloglutamol	T47.1X1	T47.1X2	T47.1X3	T47.1X4	T47.1X5	T47.1X6
Aloin	T47.2X1	T47.2X2	T47.2X3	T47.2X4	T47.2X5	T47.2X6
Aloxidone	T42.2X1	T42.2X2	T42.2X3	T42.2X4	T42.2X5	T42.2X6
Alpha						
acetyldigoxin	T46.0X1	T46.0X2	T46.0X3	T46.0X4	T46.0X5	T46.0X6
adrenergic blocking drug	T44.6X1	T44.6X2	T44.6X3	T44.6X4	T44.6X5	T44.6X6
amylase	T45.3X1	T45.3X2	T45.3X3	T45.3X4	T45.3X5	T45.3X6
tocoferol (acetate)	T45.2X1	T45.2X2	T45.2X3	T45.2X4	T45.2X5	T45.2X6
tocopherol	T45.2X1	T45.2X2	T45.2X3	T45.2X4	T45.2X5	T45.2X6
Alphadolone	T41.1X1	T41.1X2	T41.1X3	T41.1X4	T41.1X5	T41.1X6
Alphaprodine	T40.4X1	T40.4X2	T40.4X3	T40.4X4	T40.4X5	T40.4X6
Alphaxalone	T41.1X1	T41.1X2	T41.1X3	T41.1X4	T41.1X5	T41.1X6
Alprazolam	T42.4X1	T42.4X2	T42.4X3	T42.4X4	T42.4X5	T42.4X6
Alprenolol	T44.7X1	T44.7X2	T44.7X3	T44.7X4	T44.7X5	T44.7X6
Alprostadil	T46.7X1	T46.7X2	T46.7X3	T46.7X4	T46.7X5	T46.7X6
Alsactide	T38.811	T38.812	T38.813	T38.814	T38.815	T38.816
Alseroxylon	T46.5X1	T46.5X2	T46.5X3	T46.5X4	T46.5X5	T46.5X6
Alteplase	T45.611	T45.612	T45.613	T45.614	T45.615	T45.616
Altizide	T50.2X1	T50.2X2	T50.2X3	T50.2X4	T50.2X5	T50.2X6
Altretamine	T45.1X1	T45.1X2	T45.1X3	T45.1X4	T45.1X5	T45.1X6
Alum (medicinal)	T49.4X1	T49.4X2	T49.4X3	T49.4X4	T49.4X5	T49.4X6
nonmedicinal (ammonium) (potassium)	T56.891	T56.892	T56.893	T56.894	—	—
Aluminium, aluminum						
acetate	T49.2X1	T49.2X2	T49.2X3	T49.2X4	T49.2X5	T49.2X6
solution	T49.0X1	T49.0X2	T49.0X3	T49.0X4	T49.0X5	T49.0X6
aspirin	T39.011	T39.012	T39.013	T39.014	T39.015	T39.016
bis (acetylsalicylate)	T39.011	T39.012	T39.013	T39.014	T39.015	T39.016
carbonate (gel, basic)	T47.1X1	T47.1X2	T47.1X3	T47.1X4	T47.1X5	T47.1X6
chlorhydroxide-complex	T47.1X1	T47.1X2	T47.1X3	T47.1X4	T47.1X5	T47.1X6
chloride	T49.2X1	T49.2X2	T49.2X3	T49.2X4	T49.2X5	T49.2X6
clofibrate	T46.6X1	T46.6X2	T46.6X3	T46.6X4	T46.6X5	T46.6X6
diacetate	T49.2X1	T49.2X2	T49.2X3	T49.2X4	T49.2X5	T49.2X6
glycinate	T47.1X1	T47.1X2	T47.1X3	T47.1X4	T47.1X5	T47.1X6
hydroxide (gel)	T47.1X1	T47.1X2	T47.1X3	T47.1X4	T47.1X5	T47.1X6
hydroxide-magnesium carb. gel	T47.1X1	T47.1X2	T47.1X3	T47.1X4	T47.1X5	T47.1X6
magnesium silicate	T47.1X1	T47.1X2	T47.1X3	T47.1X4	T47.1X5	T47.1X6
nicotinate	T46.7X1	T46.7X2	T46.7X3	T46.7X4	T46.7X5	T46.7X6

340

Additional Character May Be Required — Refer to the Tabular List for Character Selection   ▼ Subterms under main terms may continue to next column or page

Substance	Poisoning, Accidental (unintentional)	Poisoning, Intentional Self-harm	Poisoning, Assault	Poisoning, Undetermined	Adverse Effect	Under-dosing
Aluminium, aluminum — *continued*						
ointment (surgical) (topical)	T49.3X1	T49.3X2	T49.3X3	T49.3X4	T49.3X5	T49.3X6
phosphate	T47.1X1	T47.1X2	T47.1X3	T47.1X4	T47.1X5	T47.1X6
salicylate	T39.091	T39.092	T39.093	T39.094	T39.095	T39.096
silicate	T47.1X1	T47.1X2	T47.1X3	T47.1X4	T47.1X5	T47.1X6
sodium silicate	T47.1X1	T47.1X2	T47.1X3	T47.1X4	T47.1X5	T47.1X6
subacetate	T49.2X1	T49.2X2	T49.2X3	T49.2X4	T49.2X5	T49.2X6
sulfate	T49.0X1	T49.0X2	T49.0X3	T49.0X4	T49.0X5	T49.0X6
tannate	T47.6X1	T47.6X2	T47.6X3	T47.6X4	T47.6X5	T47.6X6
topical NEC	T49.3X1	T49.3X2	T49.3X3	T49.3X4	T49.3X5	T49.3X6
Alurate	T42.3X1	T42.3X2	T42.3X3	T42.3X4	T42.3X5	T42.3X6
Alverine	T44.3X1	T44.3X2	T44.3X3	T44.3X4	T44.3X5	T44.3X6
Alvodine	T40.2X1	T40.2X2	T40.2X3	T40.2X4	T40.2X5	T40.2X6
Amanita phalloides	T62.0X1	T62.0X2	T62.0X3	T62.0X4	—	—
Amanitine	T62.0X1	T62.0X2	T62.0X3	T62.0X4	—	—
Amantadine	T42.8X1	T42.8X2	T42.8X3	T42.8X4	T42.8X5	T42.8X6
Ambazone	T49.6X1	T49.6X2	T49.6X3	T49.6X4	T49.6X5	T49.6X6
Ambenonium (chloride)	T44.0X1	T44.0X2	T44.0X3	T44.0X4	T44.0X5	T44.0X6
Ambroxol	T48.4X1	T48.4X2	T48.4X3	T48.4X4	T48.4X5	T48.4X6
Ambuphylline	T48.6X1	T48.6X2	T48.6X3	T48.6X4	T48.6X5	T48.6X6
Ambutonium bromide	T44.3X1	T44.3X2	T44.3X3	T44.3X4	T44.3X5	T44.3X6
Amcinonide	T49.0X1	T49.0X2	T49.0X3	T49.0X4	T49.0X5	T49.0X6
Amdinocilline	T36.0X1	T36.0X2	T36.0X3	T36.0X4	T36.0X5	T36.0X6
Ametazole	T50.8X1	T50.8X2	T50.8X3	T50.8X4	T50.8X5	T50.8X6
Amethocaine	T41.3X1	T41.3X2	T41.3X3	T41.3X4	T41.3X5	T41.3X6
regional	T41.3X1	T41.3X2	T41.3X3	T41.3X4	T41.3X5	T41.3X6
spinal	T41.3X1	T41.3X2	T41.3X3	T41.3X4	T41.3X5	T41.3X6
Amethopterin	T45.1X1	T45.1X2	T45.1X3	T45.1X4	T45.1X5	T45.1X6
Amezinium metilsulfate	T44.991	T44.992	T44.993	T44.994	T44.995	T44.996
Amfebutamone	T43.291	T43.292	T43.293	T43.294	T43.295	T43.296
Amfepramone	T50.5X1	T50.5X2	T50.5X3	T50.5X4	T50.5X5	T50.5X6
Amfetamine	T43.621	T43.622	T43.623	T43.624	T43.625	T43.626
Amfetaminil	T43.621	T43.622	T43.623	T43.624	T43.625	T43.626
Amfomycin	T36.8X1	T36.8X2	T36.8X3	T36.8X4	T36.8X5	T36.8X6
Amidefrine mesilate	T48.5X1	T48.5X2	T48.5X3	T48.5X4	T48.5X5	T48.5X6
Amidone	T40.3X1	T40.3X2	T40.3X3	T40.3X4	T40.3X5	T40.3X6
Amidopyrine	T39.2X1	T39.2X2	T39.2X3	T39.2X4	T39.2X5	T39.2X6
Amidotrizoate	T50.8X1	T50.8X2	T50.8X3	T50.8X4	T50.8X5	T50.8X6
Amiflamine	T43.1X1	T43.1X2	T43.1X3	T43.1X4	T43.1X5	T43.1X6
Amikacin	T36.5X1	T36.5X2	T36.5X3	T36.5X4	T36.5X5	T36.5X6
Amikhelline	T46.3X1	T46.3X2	T46.3X3	T46.3X4	T46.3X5	T46.3X6
Amiloride	T50.2X1	T50.2X2	T50.2X3	T50.2X4	T50.2X5	T50.2X6
Aminacrine	T49.0X1	T49.0X2	T49.0X3	T49.0X4	T49.0X5	T49.0X6
Amineptine	T43.011	T43.012	T43.013	T43.014	T43.015	T43.016
Aminitrozole	T37.3X1	T37.3X2	T37.3X3	T37.3X4	T37.3X5	T37.3X6
Aminoacetic acid (derivatives)	T50.3X1	T50.3X2	T50.3X3	T50.3X4	T50.3X5	T50.3X6
Amino acids	T50.3X1	T50.3X2	T50.3X3	T50.3X4	T50.3X5	T50.3X6
Aminoacridine	T49.0X1	T49.0X2	T49.0X3	T49.0X4	T49.0X5	T49.0X6
Aminobenzoic acid (-p)	T49.3X1	T49.3X2	T49.3X3	T49.3X4	T49.3X5	T49.3X6
Aminocaproic acid	T45.621	T45.622	T45.623	T45.624	T45.625	T45.626
Aminoethylisothiourium	T45.8X1	T45.8X2	T45.8X3	T45.8X4	T45.8X5	T45.8X6
Aminofenazone	T39.2X1	T39.2X2	T39.2X3	T39.2X4	T39.2X5	T39.2X6
Aminoglutethimide	T45.1X1	T45.1X2	T45.1X3	T45.1X4	T45.1X5	T45.1X6
Aminohippuric acid	T50.8X1	T50.8X2	T50.8X3	T50.8X4	T50.8X5	T50.8X6
Aminomethylbenzoic acid	T45.691	T45.692	T45.693	T45.694	T45.695	T45.696
Aminometradine	T50.2X1	T50.2X2	T50.2X3	T50.2X4	T50.2X5	T50.2X6
Aminopentamide	T44.3X1	T44.3X2	T44.3X3	T44.3X4	T44.3X5	T44.3X6
Aminophenazone	T39.2X1	T39.2X2	T39.2X3	T39.2X4	T39.2X5	T39.2X6
Aminophenol	T54.0X1	T54.0X2	T54.0X3	T54.0X4	—	—
Aminophenylpyridone	T43.591	T43.592	T43.593	T43.594	T43.595	T43.596
Aminophylline	T48.6X1	T48.6X2	T48.6X3	T48.6X4	T48.6X5	T48.6X6
Aminopterin sodium	T45.1X1	T45.1X2	T45.1X3	T45.1X4	T45.1X5	T45.1X6
Aminopyrine	T39.2X1	T39.2X2	T39.2X3	T39.2X4	T39.2X5	T39.2X6
Aminorex	T50.5X1	T50.5X2	T50.5X3	T50.5X4	T50.5X5	T50.5X6
Aminosalicylic acid	T37.1X1	T37.1X2	T37.1X3	T37.1X4	T37.1X5	T37.1X6
Aminosalylum	T37.1X1	T37.1X2	T37.1X3	T37.1X4	T37.1X5	T37.1X6
Amiodarone	T46.2X1	T46.2X2	T46.2X3	T46.2X4	T46.2X5	T46.2X6
Amiphenazole	T50.7X1	T50.7X2	T50.7X3	T50.7X4	T50.7X5	T50.7X6
Amiquinsin	T46.5X1	T46.5X2	T46.5X3	T46.5X4	T46.5X5	T46.5X6
Amisometradine	T50.2X1	T50.2X2	T50.2X3	T50.2X4	T50.2X5	T50.2X6
Amisulpride	T43.591	T43.592	T43.593	T43.594	T43.595	T43.596
Amitriptyline	T43.011	T43.012	T43.013	T43.014	T43.015	T43.016
Amitriptylinoxide	T43.011	T43.012	T43.013	T43.014	T43.015	T43.016
Amlexanox	T48.6X1	T48.6X2	T48.6X3	T48.6X4	T48.6X5	T48.6X6
Ammonia (fumes) (gas) (vapor)	T59.891	T59.892	T59.893	T59.894	—	—
aromatic spirit	T48.991	T48.992	T48.993	T48.994	T48.995	T48.996
liquid (household)	T54.3X1	T54.3X2	T54.3X3	T54.3X4	—	—
Ammoniated mercury	T49.0X1	T49.0X2	T49.0X3	T49.0X4	T49.0X5	T49.0X6
Ammonium						
acid tartrate	T49.5X1	T49.5X2	T49.5X3	T49.5X4	T49.5X5	T49.5X6
Ammonium — *continued*						
bromide	T42.6X1	T42.6X2	T42.6X3	T42.6X4	T42.6X5	T42.6X6
carbonate	T54.3X1	T54.3X2	T54.3X3	T54.3X4	—	—
chloride	T50.991	T50.992	T50.993	T50.994	T50.995	T50.996
expectorant	T48.4X1	T48.4X2	T48.4X3	T48.4X4	T48.4X5	T48.4X6
compounds (household) NEC	T54.3X1	T54.3X2	T54.3X3	T54.3X4	—	—
fumes (any usage)	T59.891	T59.892	T59.893	T59.894	—	—
industrial	T54.3X1	T54.3X2	T54.3X3	T54.3X4	—	—
ichthyosulronate	T49.4X1	T49.4X2	T49.4X3	T49.4X4	T49.4X5	T49.4X6
mandelate	T37.91	T37.92	T37.93	T37.94	T37.95	T37.96
sulfamate	T60.3X1	T60.3X2	T60.3X3	T60.3X4	—	—
sulfonate resin	T47.8X1	T47.8X2	T47.8X3	T47.8X4	T47.8X5	T47.8X6
Amobarbital (sodium)	T42.3X1	T42.3X2	T42.3X3	T42.3X4	T42.3X5	T42.3X6
Amodiaquine	T37.2X1	T37.2X2	T37.2X3	T37.2X4	T37.2X5	T37.2X6
Amopyroquin (e)	T37.2X1	T37.2X2	T37.2X3	T37.2X4	T37.2X5	T37.2X6
Amoxapine	T43.011	T43.012	T43.013	T43.014	T43.015	T43.016
Amoxicillin	T36.0X1	T36.0X2	T36.0X3	T36.0X4	T36.0X5	T36.0X6
Amperozide	T43.591	T43.592	T43.593	T43.594	T43.595	T43.596
Amphenidone	T43.591	T43.592	T43.593	T43.594	T43.595	T43.596
Amphetamine NEC	T43.621	T43.622	T43.623	T43.624	T43.625	T43.626
Amphomycin	T36.8X1	T36.8X2	T36.8X3	T36.8X4	T36.8X5	T36.8X6
Amphotalide	T37.4X1	T37.4X2	T37.4X3	T37.4X4	T37.4X5	T37.4X6
Amphotericin B	T36.7X1	T36.7X2	T36.7X3	T36.7X4	T36.7X5	T36.7X6
topical	T49.0X1	T49.0X2	T49.0X3	T49.0X4	T49.0X5	T49.0X6
Ampicillin	T36.0X1	T36.0X2	T36.0X3	T36.0X4	T36.0X5	T36.0X6
Amprotropine	T44.3X1	T44.3X2	T44.3X3	T44.3X4	T44.3X5	T44.3X6
Amsacrine	T45.1X1	T45.1X2	T45.1X3	T45.1X4	T45.1X5	T45.1X6
Amygdaline	T62.2X1	T62.2X2	T62.2X3	T62.2X4	—	—
Amyl						
acetate	T52.8X1	T52.8X2	T52.8X3	T52.8X4	—	—
vapor	T59.891	T59.892	T59.893	T59.894	—	—
alcohol	T51.3X1	T51.3X2	T51.3X3	T51.3X4	—	—
chloride	T53.6X1	T53.6X2	T53.6X3	T53.6X4	—	—
formate	T52.8X1	T52.8X2	T52.8X3	T52.8X4	—	—
nitrite	T46.3X1	T46.3X2	T46.3X3	T46.3X4	T46.3X5	T46.3X6
propionate	T65.891	T65.892	T65.893	T65.894	—	—
Amylase	T47.5X1	T47.5X2	T47.5X3	T47.5X4	T47.5X5	T47.5X6
Amyleine, regional	T41.3X1	T41.3X2	T41.3X3	T41.3X4	T41.3X5	T41.3X6
Amylene						
dichloride	T53.6X1	T53.6X2	T53.6X3	T53.6X4	—	—
hydrate	T51.3X1	T51.3X2	T51.3X3	T51.3X4	—	—
Amylmetacresol	T49.6X1	T49.6X2	T49.6X3	T49.6X4	T49.6X5	T49.6X6
Amylobarbitone	T42.3X1	T42.3X2	T42.3X3	T42.3X4	T42.3X5	T42.3X6
Amylocaine, regional	T41.3X1	T41.3X2	T41.3X3	T41.3X4	T41.3X5	T41.3X6
infiltration (subcutaneous)	T41.3X1	T41.3X2	T41.3X3	T41.3X4	T41.3X5	T41.3X6
nerve block (peripheral) (plexus)	T41.3X1	T41.3X2	T41.3X3	T41.3X4	T41.3X5	T41.3X6
spinal	T41.3X1	T41.3X2	T41.3X3	T41.3X4	T41.3X5	T41.3X6
topical (surface)	T41.3X1	T41.3X2	T41.3X3	T41.3X4	T41.3X5	T41.3X6
Amylopectin	T47.6X1	T47.6X2	T47.6X3	T47.6X4	T47.6X5	T47.6X6
Amytal (sodium)	T42.3X1	T42.3X2	T42.3X3	T42.3X4	T42.3X5	T42.3X6
Anabolic steroid	T38.7X1	T38.7X2	T38.7X3	T38.7X4	T38.7X5	T38.7X6
Analeptic NEC	T50.7X1	T50.7X2	T50.7X3	T50.7X4	T50.7X5	T50.7X6
Analgesic	T39.91	T39.92	T39.93	T39.94	T39.95	T39.96
anti-inflammatory NEC	T39.91	T39.92	T39.93	T39.94	T39.95	T39.96
propionic acid derivative	T39.311	T39.312	T39.313	T39.314	T39.315	T39.316
antirheumatic NEC	T39.4X1	T39.4X2	T39.4X3	T39.4X4	T39.4X5	T39.4X6
aromatic NEC	T39.1X1	T39.1X2	T39.1X3	T39.1X4	T39.1X5	T39.1X6
narcotic NEC	T40.601	T40.602	T40.603	T40.604	T40.605	T40.606
combination	T40.601	T40.602	T40.603	T40.604	T40.605	T40.606
obstetric	T40.601	T40.602	T40.603	T40.604	T40.605	T40.606
non-narcotic NEC	T39.91	T39.92	T39.93	T39.94	T39.95	T39.96
combination	T39.91	T39.92	T39.93	T39.94	T39.95	T39.96
pyrazole	T39.2X1	T39.2X2	T39.2X3	T39.2X4	T39.2X5	T39.2X6
specified NEC	T39.8X1	T39.8X2	T39.8X3	T39.8X4	T39.8X5	T39.8X6
Analgin	T39.2X1	T39.2X2	T39.2X3	T39.2X4	T39.2X5	T39.2X6
Anamirta cocculus	T62.1X1	T62.1X2	T62.1X3	T62.1X4	—	—
Ancillin	T36.0X1	T36.0X2	T36.0X3	T36.0X4	T36.0X5	T36.0X6
Ancrod	T45.691	T45.692	T45.693	T45.694	T45.695	T45.696
Androgen	T38.7X1	T38.7X2	T38.7X3	T38.7X4	T38.7X5	T38.7X6
Androgen-estrogen mixture	T38.7X1	T38.7X2	T38.7X3	T38.7X4	T38.7X5	T38.7X6
Androstalone	T38.7X1	T38.7X2	T38.7X3	T38.7X4	T38.7X5	T38.7X6
Androstanolone	T38.7X1	T38.7X2	T38.7X3	T38.7X4	T38.7X5	T38.7X6
Androsterone	T38.7X1	T38.7X2	T38.7X3	T38.7X4	T38.7X5	T38.7X6
Anemone pulsatilla	T62.2X1	T62.2X2	T62.2X3	T62.2X4	—	—
Anesthesia						
caudal	T41.3X1	T41.3X2	T41.3X3	T41.3X4	T41.3X5	T41.3X6
endotracheal	T41.0X1	T41.0X2	T41.0X3	T41.0X4	T41.0X5	T41.0X6
epidural	T41.3X1	T41.3X2	T41.3X3	T41.3X4	T41.3X5	T41.3X6
inhalation	T41.0X1	T41.0X2	T41.0X3	T41.0X4	T41.0X5	T41.0X6
local	T41.3X1	T41.3X2	T41.3X3	T41.3X4	T41.3X5	T41.3X6

Table of Drugs and Chemicals

Anesthesia — Antifreeze

Substance	Poisoning, Accidental (unintentional)	Poisoning, Intentional Self-harm	Poisoning, Assault	Poisoning, Undetermined	Adverse Effect	Under-dosing
Anesthesia — continued						
mucosal	T41.3X1	T41.3X2	T41.3X3	T41.3X4	T41.3X5	T41.3X6
muscle relaxation	T48.1X1	T48.1X2	T48.1X3	T48.1X4	T48.1X5	T48.1X6
nerve blocking	T41.3X1	T41.3X2	T41.3X3	T41.3X4	T41.3X5	T41.3X6
plexus blocking	T41.3X1	T41.3X2	T41.3X3	T41.3X4	T41.3X5	T41.3X6
potentiated	T41.201	T41.202	T41.203	T41.204	T41.205	T41.206
rectal	T41.201	T41.202	T41.203	T41.204	T41.205	T41.206
general	T41.201	T41.202	T41.203	T41.204	T41.205	T41.206
local	T41.3X1	T41.3X2	T41.3X3	T41.3X4	T41.3X5	T41.3X6
regional	T41.3X1	T41.3X2	T41.3X3	T41.3X4	T41.3X5	T41.3X6
surface	T41.3X1	T41.3X2	T41.3X3	T41.3X4	T41.3X5	T41.3X6
Anesthetic NEC — *see also*	T41.41	T41.42	T41.43	T41.44	T41.45	T41.46
Anesthesia						
with muscle relaxant	T41.201	T41.202	T41.203	T41.204	T41.205	T41.206
general	T41.201	T41.202	T41.203	T41.204	T41.205	T41.206
local	T41.3X1	T41.3X2	T41.3X3	T41.3X4	T41.3X5	T41.3X6
gaseous NEC	T41.0X1	T41.0X2	T41.0X3	T41.0X4	T41.0X5	T41.0X6
general NEC	T41.201	T41.202	T41.203	T41.204	T41.205	T41.206
halogenated hydrocarbon derivatives NEC	T41.0X1	T41.0X2	T41.0X3	T41.0X4	T41.0X5	T41.0X6
infiltration NEC	T41.3X1	T41.3X2	T41.3X3	T41.3X4	T41.3X5	T41.3X6
intravenous NEC	T41.1X1	T41.1X2	T41.1X3	T41.1X4	T41.1X5	T41.1X6
local NEC	T41.3X1	T41.3X2	T41.3X3	T41.3X4	T41.3X5	T41.3X6
rectal	T41.201	T41.202	T41.203	T41.204	T41.205	T41.206
general	T41.201	T41.202	T41.203	T41.204	T41.205	T41.206
local	T41.3X1	T41.3X2	T41.3X3	T41.3X4	T41.3X5	T41.3X6
regional NEC	T41.3X1	T41.3X2	T41.3X3	T41.3X4	T41.3X5	T41.3X6
spinal NEC	T41.3X1	T41.3X2	T41.3X3	T41.3X4	T41.3X5	T41.3X6
thiobarbiturate	T41.1X1	T41.1X2	T41.1X3	T41.1X4	T41.1X5	T41.1X6
topical	T41.3X1	T41.3X2	T41.3X3	T41.3X4	T41.3X5	T41.3X6
Aneurine	T45.2X1	T45.2X2	T45.2X3	T45.2X4	T45.2X5	T45.2X6
Angio-Conray	T50.8X1	T50.8X2	T50.8X3	T50.8X4	T50.8X5	T50.8X6
Angiotensin	T44.5X1	T44.5X2	T44.5X3	T44.5X4	T44.5X5	T44.5X6
Angiotensinamide	T44.991	T44.992	T44.993	T44.994	T44.995	T44.996
Anhydrohydroxy-progesterone	T38.5X1	T38.5X2	T38.5X3	T38.5X4	T38.5X5	T38.5X6
Anhydron	T50.2X1	T50.2X2	T50.2X3	T50.2X4	T50.2X5	T50.2X6
Anileridine	T40.4X1	T40.4X2	T40.4X3	T40.4X4	T40.4X5	T40.4X6
Aniline (dye) (liquid)	T65.3X1	T65.3X2	T65.3X3	T65.3X4	—	—
analgesic	T39.1X1	T39.1X2	T39.1X3	T39.1X4	T39.1X5	T39.1X6
derivatives, therapeutic NEC	T39.1X1	T39.1X2	T39.1X3	T39.1X4	T39.1X5	T39.1X6
vapor	T65.3X1	T65.3X2	T65.3X3	T65.3X4	—	—
Aniscoropine	T44.3X1	T44.3X2	T44.3X3	T44.3X4	T44.3X5	T44.3X6
Anise oil	T47.5X1	T47.5X2	T47.5X3	T47.5X4	T47.5X5	T47.5X6
Anisidine	T65.3X1	T65.3X2	T65.3X3	T65.3X4	—	—
Anisindione	T45.511	T45.512	T45.513	T45.514	T45.515	T45.516
Anisotropine methyl-bromide	T44.3X1	T44.3X2	T44.3X3	T44.3X4	T44.3X5	T44.3X6
Anistreplase	T45.611	T45.612	T45.613	T45.614	T45.615	T45.616
Anorexiant (central)	T50.5X1	T50.5X2	T50.5X3	T50.5X4	T50.5X5	T50.5X6
Anorexic agents	T50.5X1	T50.5X2	T50.5X3	T50.5X4	T50.5X5	T50.5X6
Ansamycin	T36.6X1	T36.6X2	T36.6X3	T36.6X4	T36.6X5	T36.6X6
Ant (bite) (sting)	T63.421	T63.422	T63.423	T63.424	—	—
Antabuse	T50.6X1	T50.6X2	T50.6X3	T50.6X4	T50.6X5	T50.6X6
Antacid NEC	T47.1X1	T47.1X2	T47.1X3	T47.1X4	T47.1X5	T47.1X6
Antagonist						
Aldosterone	T50.0X1	T50.0X2	T50.0X3	T50.0X4	T50.0X5	T50.0X6
alpha-adrenoreceptor	T44.6X1	T44.6X2	T44.6X3	T44.6X4	T44.6X5	T44.6X6
anticoagulant	T45.7X1	T45.7X2	T45.7X3	T45.7X4	T45.7X5	T45.7X6
beta-adrenoreceptor	T44.7X1	T44.7X2	T44.7X3	T44.7X4	T44.7X5	T44.7X6
extrapyramidal NEC	T44.3X1	T44.3X2	T44.3X3	T44.3X4	T44.3X5	T44.3X6
folic acid	T45.1X1	T45.1X2	T45.1X3	T45.1X4	T45.1X5	T45.1X6
H2 receptor	T47.0X1	T47.0X2	T47.0X3	T47.0X4	T47.0X5	T47.0X6
heavy metal	T45.8X1	T45.8X2	T45.8X3	T45.8X4	T45.8X5	T45.8X6
narcotic analgesic	T50.7X1	T50.7X2	T50.7X3	T50.7X4	T50.7X5	T50.7X6
opiate	T50.7X1	T50.7X2	T50.7X3	T50.7X4	T50.7X5	T50.7X6
pyrimidine	T45.1X1	T45.1X2	T45.1X3	T45.1X4	T45.1X5	T45.1X6
serotonin	T46.5X1	T46.5X2	T46.5X3	T46.5X4	T46.5X5	T46.5X6
Antazolin(e)	T45.0X1	T45.0X2	T45.0X3	T45.0X4	T45.0X5	T45.0X6
Anterior pituitary hormone NEC	T38.811	T38.812	T38.813	T38.814	T38.815	T38.816
Anthelmintic NEC	T37.4X1	T37.4X2	T37.4X3	T37.4X4	T37.4X5	T37.4X6
Anthiolimine	T37.4X1	T37.4X2	T37.4X3	T37.4X4	T37.4X5	T37.4X6
Anthralin	T49.4X1	T49.4X2	T49.4X3	T49.4X4	T49.4X5	T49.4X6
Anthramycin	T45.1X1	T45.1X2	T45.1X3	T45.1X4	T45.1X5	T45.1X6
Antiadrenergic NEC	T44.8X1	T44.8X2	T44.8X3	T44.8X4	T44.8X5	T44.8X6
Antiallergic NEC	T45.0X1	T45.0X2	T45.0X3	T45.0X4	T45.0X5	T45.0X6
Antiandrogen NEC	T38.6X1	T38.6X2	T38.6X3	T38.6X4	T38.6X5	T38.6X6
Anti-anemic (drug) (preparation)	T45.8X1	T45.8X2	T45.8X3	T45.8X4	T45.8X5	T45.8X6
Antianxiety drug NEC	T43.501	T43.502	T43.503	T43.504	T43.505	T43.506
Antiaris toxicaria	T65.891	T65.892	T65.893	T65.894	—	—
Antiarteriosclerotic drug	T46.6X1	T46.6X2	T46.6X3	T46.6X4	T46.6X5	T46.6X6

Substance	Poisoning, Accidental (unintentional)	Poisoning, Intentional Self-harm	Poisoning, Assault	Poisoning, Undetermined	Adverse Effect	Under-dosing
Antiasthmatic drug NEC	T48.6X1	T48.6X2	T48.6X3	T48.6X4	T48.6X5	T48.6X6
Antibiotic NEC	T36.91	T36.92	T36.93	T36.94	T36.95	T36.96
aminoglycoside	T36.5X1	T36.5X2	T36.5X3	T36.5X4	T36.5X5	T36.5X6
anticancer	T45.1X1	T45.1X2	T45.1X3	T45.1X4	T45.1X5	T45.1X6
antifungal	T36.7X1	T36.7X2	T36.7X3	T36.7X4	T36.7X5	T36.7X6
antimycobacterial	T36.5X1	T36.5X2	T36.5X3	T36.5X4	T36.5X5	T36.5X6
antineoplastic	T45.1X1	T45.1X2	T45.1X3	T45.1X4	T45.1X5	T45.1X6
b-lactam NEC	T36.1X1	T36.1X2	T36.1X3	T36.1X4	T36.1X5	T36.1X6
cephalosporin (group)	T36.1X1	T36.1X2	T36.1X3	T36.1X4	T36.1X5	T36.1X6
chloramphenicol (group)	T36.2X1	T36.2X2	T36.2X3	T36.2X4	T36.2X5	T36.2X6
ENT	T49.6X1	T49.6X2	T49.6X3	T49.6X4	T49.6X5	T49.6X6
eye	T49.5X1	T49.5X2	T49.5X3	T49.5X4	T49.5X5	T49.5X6
fungicidal (local)	T49.0X1	T49.0X2	T49.0X3	T49.0X4	T49.0X5	T49.0X6
intestinal	T36.8X1	T36.8X2	T36.8X3	T36.8X4	T36.8X5	T36.8X6
local	T49.0X1	T49.0X2	T49.0X3	T49.0X4	T49.0X5	T49.0X6
macrolides	T36.3X1	T36.3X2	T36.3X3	T36.3X4	T36.3X5	T36.3X6
polypeptide	T36.8X1	T36.8X2	T36.8X3	T36.8X4	T36.8X5	T36.8X6
specified NEC	T36.8X1	T36.8X2	T36.8X3	T36.8X4	T36.8X5	T36.8X6
tetracycline (group)	T36.4X1	T36.4X2	T36.4X3	T36.4X4	T36.4X5	T36.4X6
throat	T49.6X1	T49.6X2	T49.6X3	T49.6X4	T49.6X5	T49.6X6
Anticancer agents NEC	T45.1X1	T45.1X2	T45.1X3	T45.1X4	T45.1X5	T45.1X6
Anticholesterolemic drug NEC	T46.6X1	T46.6X2	T46.6X3	T46.6X4	T46.6X5	T46.6X6
Anticholinergic NEC	T44.3X1	T44.3X2	T44.3X3	T44.3X4	T44.3X5	T44.3X6
Anticholinesterase	T44.0X1	T44.0X2	T44.0X3	T44.0X4	T44.0X5	T44.0X6
organophosphorus						
insecticide	T60.0X1	T60.0X2	T60.0X3	T60.0X4	—	—
nerve gas	T59.891	T59.892	T59.893	T59.894	—	—
reversible	T44.0X1	T44.0X2	T44.0X3	T44.0X4	T44.0X5	T44.0X6
ophthalmological	T49.5X1	T49.5X2	T49.5X3	T49.5X4	T49.5X5	T49.5X6
Anticoagulant NEC	T45.511	T45.512	T45.513	T45.514	T45.515	T45.516
Antagonist	T45.7X1	T45.7X2	T45.7X3	T45.7X4	T45.7X5	T45.7X6
Anti-common-cold drug NEC	T48.5X1	T48.5X2	T48.5X3	T48.5X4	T48.5X5	T48.5X6
Anticonvulsant	T42.71	T42.72	T42.73	T42.74	T42.75	T42.76
barbiturate	T42.3X1	T42.3X2	T42.3X3	T42.3X4	T42.3X5	T42.3X6
combination (with barbiturate)	T42.3X1	T42.3X2	T42.3X3	T42.3X4	T42.3X5	T42.3X6
hydantoin	T42.0X1	T42.0X2	T42.0X3	T42.0X4	T42.0X5	T42.0X6
hypnotic NEC	T42.6X1	T42.6X2	T42.6X3	T42.6X4	T42.6X5	T42.6X6
oxazolidinedione	T42.2X1	T42.2X2	T42.2X3	T42.2X4	T42.2X5	T42.2X6
pyrimidinedione	T42.6X1	T42.6X2	T42.6X3	T42.6X4	T42.6X5	T42.6X6
specified NEC	T42.6X1	T42.6X2	T42.6X3	T42.6X4	T42.6X5	T42.6X6
succinimide	T42.2X1	T42.2X2	T42.2X3	T42.2X4	T42.2X5	T42.2X6
Antidepressant	T43.201	T43.202	T43.203	T43.204	T43.205	T43.206
monoamine oxidase inhibitor	T43.1X1	T43.1X2	T43.1X3	T43.1X4	T43.1X5	T43.1X6
selective serotonin norepinephrine reuptake inhibitor	T43.211	T43.212	T43.213	T43.214	T43.215	T43.216
selective serotonin reuptake inhibitor	T43.221	T43.222	T43.223	T43.224	T43.225	T43.226
specified NEC	T43.291	T43.292	T43.293	T43.294	T43.295	T43.296
tetracyclic	T43.021	T43.022	T43.023	T43.024	T43.025	T43.026
triazolopyridine	T43.211	T43.212	T43.213	T43.214	T43.215	T43.216
tricyclic	T43.011	T43.012	T43.013	T43.014	T43.015	T43.016
Antidiabetic NEC	T38.3X1	T38.3X2	T38.3X3	T38.3X4	T38.3X5	T38.3X6
biguanide	T38.3X1	T38.3X2	T38.3X3	T38.3X4	T38.3X5	T38.3X6
and sulfonyl combined	T38.3X1	T38.3X2	T38.3X3	T38.3X4	T38.3X5	T38.3X6
combined	T38.3X1	T38.3X2	T38.3X3	T38.3X4	T38.3X5	T38.3X6
sulfonylurea	T38.3X1	T38.3X2	T38.3X3	T38.3X4	T38.3X5	T38.3X6
Antidiarrheal drug NEC	T47.6X1	T47.6X2	T47.6X3	T47.6X4	T47.6X5	T47.6X6
absorbent	T47.6X1	T47.6X2	T47.6X3	T47.6X4	T47.6X5	T47.6X6
Anti-D immunoglobulin (human)	T50.Z11	T50.Z12	T50.Z13	T50.Z14	T50.Z15	T50.Z16
Antidiphtheria serum	T50.Z11	T50.Z12	T50.Z13	T50.Z14	T50.Z15	T50.Z16
Antidiuretic hormone	T38.891	T38.892	T38.893	T38.894	T38.895	T38.896
Antidote NEC	T50.6X1	T50.6X2	T50.6X3	T50.6X4	T50.6X5	T50.6X6
heavy metal	T45.8X1	T45.8X2	T45.8X3	T45.8X4	T45.8X5	T45.8X6
Antidysrhythmic NEC	T46.2X1	T46.2X2	T46.2X3	T46.2X4	T46.2X5	T46.2X6
Antiemetic drug	T45.0X1	T45.0X2	T45.0X3	T45.0X4	T45.0X5	T45.0X6
Antiepilepsy agent	T42.71	T42.72	T42.73	T42.74	T42.75	T42.76
combination	T42.5X1	T42.5X2	T42.5X3	T42.5X4	T42.5X5	T42.5X6
mixed	T42.5X1	T42.5X2	T42.5X3	T42.5X4	T42.5X5	T42.5X6
specified, NEC	T42.6X1	T42.6X2	T42.6X3	T42.6X4	T42.6X5	T42.6X6
Antiestrogen NEC	T38.6X1	T38.6X2	T38.6X3	T38.6X4	T38.6X5	T38.6X6
Antifertility pill	T38.4X1	T38.4X2	T38.4X3	T38.4X4	T38.4X5	T38.4X6
Antifibrinolytic drug	T45.621	T45.622	T45.623	T45.624	T45.625	T45.626
Antifilarial drug	T37.4X1	T37.4X2	T37.4X3	T37.4X4	T37.4X5	T37.4X6
Antiflatulent	T47.5X1	T47.5X2	T47.5X3	T47.5X4	T47.5X5	T47.5X6
Antifreeze	T65.91	T65.92	T65.93	T65.94	—	—
alcohol	T51.1X1	T51.1X2	T51.1X3	T51.1X4	—	—
ethylene glycol	T51.8X1	T51.8X2	T51.8X3	T51.8X4	—	—

Table of Drugs and Chemicals

Substance	Poisoning, Accidental (unintentional)	Poisoning, Intentional Self-harm	Poisoning, Assault	Poisoning, Undetermined	Adverse Effect	Under-dosing
Antifungal						
antibiotic (systemic)	T36.7X1	T36.7X2	T36.7X3	T36.7X4	T36.7X5	T36.7X6
anti-infective NEC	T37.91	T37.92	T37.93	T37.94	T37.95	T37.96
disinfectant, local	T49.0X1	T49.0X2	T49.0X3	T49.0X4	T49.0X5	T49.0X6
nonmedicinal (spray)	T60.3X1	T60.3X2	T60.3X3	T60.3X4	—	—
topical	T49.0X1	T49.0X2	T49.0X3	T49.0X4	T49.0X5	T49.0X6
Anti-gastric-secretion drug NEC	T47.1X1	T47.1X2	T47.1X3	T47.1X4	T47.1X5	T47.1X6
Antigonadotrophin NEC	T38.6X1	T38.6X2	T38.6X3	T38.6X4	T38.6X5	T38.6X6
Antihallucinogen	T43.501	T43.502	T43.503	T43.504	T43.505	T43.506
Antihelmintics	T37.4X1	T37.4X2	T37.4X3	T37.4X4	T37.4X5	T37.4X6
Antihemophilic						
factor	T45.8X1	T45.8X2	T45.8X3	T45.8X4	T45.8X5	T45.8X6
fraction	T45.8X1	T45.8X2	T45.8X3	T45.8X4	T45.8X5	T45.8X6
globulin concentrate	T45.7X1	T45.7X2	T45.7X3	T45.7X4	T45.7X5	T45.7X6
human plasma	T45.8X1	T45.8X2	T45.8X3	T45.8X4	T45.8X5	T45.8X6
plasma, dried	T45.7X1	T45.7X2	T45.7X3	T45.7X4	T45.7X5	T45.7X6
Antihemorrhoidal preparation	T49.2X1	T49.2X2	T49.2X3	T49.2X4	T49.2X5	T49.2X6
Antiheparin drug	T45.7X1	T45.7X2	T45.7X3	T45.7X4	T45.7X5	T45.7X6
Antihistamine	T45.0X1	T45.0X2	T45.0X3	T45.0X4	T45.0X5	T45.0X6
Antihookworm drug	T37.4X1	T37.4X2	T37.4X3	T37.4X4	T37.4X5	T37.4X6
Anti-human lymphocytic globulin	T50.Z11	T50.Z12	T50.Z13	T50.Z14	T50.Z15	T50.Z16
Antihyperlipidemic drug	T46.6X1	T46.6X2	T46.6X3	T46.6X4	T46.6X5	T46.6X6
Antihypertensive drug NEC	T46.5X1	T46.5X2	T46.5X3	T46.5X4	T46.5X5	T46.5X6
Anti-infective NEC	T37.91	T37.92	T37.93	T37.94	T37.95	T37.96
anthelmintic	T37.4X1	T37.4X2	T37.4X3	T37.4X4	T37.4X5	T37.4X6
antibiotics	T36.91	T36.92	T36.93	T36.94	T36.95	T36.96
specified NEC	T36.8X1	T36.8X2	T36.8X3	T36.8X4	T36.8X5	T36.8X6
antimalarial	T37.2X1	T37.2X2	T37.2X3	T37.2X4	T37.2X5	T37.2X6
antimycobacterial NEC	T37.1X1	T37.1X2	T37.1X3	T37.1X4	T37.1X5	T37.1X6
antibiotics	T36.5X1	T36.5X2	T36.5X3	T36.5X4	T36.5X5	T36.5X6
antiprotozoal NEC	T37.3X1	T37.3X2	T37.3X3	T37.3X4	T37.3X5	T37.3X6
blood	T37.2X1	T37.2X2	T37.2X3	T37.2X4	T37.2X5	T37.2X6
antiviral	T37.5X1	T37.5X2	T37.5X3	T37.5X4	T37.5X5	T37.5X6
arsenical	T37.8X1	T37.8X2	T37.8X3	T37.8X4	T37.8X5	T37.8X6
bismuth, local	T49.0X1	T49.0X2	T49.0X3	T49.0X4	T49.0X5	T49.0X6
ENT	T49.6X1	T49.6X2	T49.6X3	T49.6X4	T49.6X5	T49.6X6
eye NEC	T49.5X1	T49.5X2	T49.5X3	T49.5X4	T49.5X5	T49.5X6
heavy metals NEC	T37.8X1	T37.8X2	T37.8X3	T37.8X4	T37.8X5	T37.8X6
local NEC	T49.0X1	T49.0X2	T49.0X3	T49.0X4	T49.0X5	T49.0X6
specified NEC	T49.0X1	T49.0X2	T49.0X3	T49.0X4	T49.0X5	T49.0X6
mixed	T37.91	T37.92	T37.93	T37.94	T37.95	T37.96
ophthalmic preparation	T49.5X1	T49.5X2	T49.5X3	T49.5X4	T49.5X5	T49.5X6
topical NEC	T49.0X1	T49.0X2	T49.0X3	T49.0X4	T49.0X5	T49.0X6
Anti-inflammatory drug NEC	T39.391	T39.392	T39.393	T39.394	T39.395	T39.396
local	T49.0X1	T49.0X2	T49.0X3	T49.0X4	T49.0X5	T49.0X6
nonsteroidal NEC	T39.391	T39.392	T39.393	T39.394	T39.395	T39.396
propionic acid derivative	T39.311	T39.312	T39.313	T39.314	T39.315	T39.316
specified NEC	T39.391	T39.392	T39.393	T39.394	T39.395	T39.396
Antikaluretic	T50.3X1	T50.3X2	T50.3X3	T50.3X4	T50.3X5	T50.3X6
Antiknock (tetraethyl lead)	T56.0X1	T56.0X2	T56.0X3	T56.0X4	—	—
Antilipemic drug NEC	T46.6X1	T46.6X2	T46.6X3	T46.6X4	T46.6X5	T46.6X6
Antimalarial	T37.2X1	T37.2X2	T37.2X3	T37.2X4	T37.2X5	T37.2X6
prophylactic NEC	T37.2X1	T37.2X2	T37.2X3	T37.2X4	T37.2X5	T37.2X6
pyrimidine derivative	T37.2X1	T37.2X2	T37.2X3	T37.2X4	T37.2X5	T37.2X6
Antimetabolite	T45.1X1	T45.1X2	T45.1X3	T45.1X4	T45.1X5	T45.1X6
Antimitotic agent	T45.1X1	T45.1X2	T45.1X3	T45.1X4	T45.1X5	T45.1X6
Antimony (compounds) (vapor) NEC	T56.891	T56.892	T56.893	T56.894	—	—
anti-infectives	T37.8X1	T37.8X2	T37.8X3	T37.8X4	T37.8X5	T37.8X6
dimercaptosuccinate	T37.3X1	T37.3X2	T37.3X3	T37.3X4	T37.3X5	T37.3X6
hydride	T56.891	T56.892	T56.893	T56.894	—	—
pesticide (vapor)	T60.8X1	T60.8X2	T60.8X3	T60.8X4	—	—
potassium (sodium)	T37.8X1	T37.8X2	T37.8X3	T37.8X4	T37.8X5	T37.8X6
tartrate						
sodium	T37.3X1	T37.3X2	T37.3X3	T37.3X4	T37.3X5	T37.3X6
dimercaptosuccinate						
tartrated	T37.8X1	T37.8X2	T37.8X3	T37.8X4	T37.8X5	T37.8X6
Antimuscarinic NEC	T44.3X1	T44.3X2	T44.3X3	T44.3X4	T44.3X5	T44.3X6
Antimycobacterial drug NEC	T37.1X1	T37.1X2	T37.1X3	T37.1X4	T37.1X5	T37.1X6
antibiotics	T36.5X1	T36.5X2	T36.5X3	T36.5X4	T36.5X5	T36.5X6
combination	T37.1X1	T37.1X2	T37.1X3	T37.1X4	T37.1X5	T37.1X6
Antinausea drug	T45.0X1	T45.0X2	T45.0X3	T45.0X4	T45.0X5	T45.0X6
Antinematode drug	T37.4X1	T37.4X2	T37.4X3	T37.4X4	T37.4X5	T37.4X6
Antineoplastic NEC	T45.1X1	T45.1X2	T45.1X3	T45.1X4	T45.1X5	T45.1X6
alkaloidal	T45.1X1	T45.1X2	T45.1X3	T45.1X4	T45.1X5	T45.1X6
antibiotics	T45.1X1	T45.1X2	T45.1X3	T45.1X4	T45.1X5	T45.1X6
combination	T45.1X1	T45.1X2	T45.1X3	T45.1X4	T45.1X5	T45.1X6
estrogen	T38.5X1	T38.5X2	T38.5X3	T38.5X4	T38.5X5	T38.5X6

Substance	Poisoning, Accidental (unintentional)	Poisoning, Intentional Self-harm	Poisoning, Assault	Poisoning, Undetermined	Adverse Effect	Under-dosing
Antineoplastic — *continued*						
steroid	T38.7X1	T38.7X2	T38.7X3	T38.7X4	T38.7X5	T38.7X6
Antiparasitic drug (systemic)	T37.91	T37.92	T37.93	T37.94	T37.95	T37.96
local	T49.0X1	T49.0X2	T49.0X3	T49.0X4	T49.0X5	T49.0X6
specified NEC	T37.8X1	T37.8X2	T37.8X3	T37.8X4	T37.8X5	T37.8X6
Antiparkinsonism drug NEC	T42.8X1	T42.8X2	T42.8X3	T42.8X4	T42.8X5	T42.8X6
Antiperspirant NEC	T49.2X1	T49.2X2	T49.2X3	T49.2X4	T49.2X5	T49.2X6
Antiphlogistic NEC	T39.4X1	T39.4X2	T39.4X3	T39.4X4	T39.4X5	T39.4X6
Antiplatyhelmintic drug	T37.4X1	T37.4X2	T37.4X3	T37.4X4	T37.4X5	T37.4X6
Antiprotozoal drug NEC	T37.3X1	T37.3X2	T37.3X3	T37.3X4	T37.3X5	T37.3X6
blood	T37.2X1	T37.2X2	T37.2X3	T37.2X4	T37.2X5	T37.2X6
local	T49.0X1	T49.0X2	T49.0X3	T49.0X4	T49.0X5	T49.0X6
Antipruritic drug NEC	T49.1X1	T49.1X2	T49.1X3	T49.1X4	T49.1X5	T49.1X6
Antipsychotic drug	T43.501	T43.502	T43.503	T43.504	T43.505	T43.506
specified NEC	T43.591	T43.592	T43.593	T43.594	T43.595	T43.596
Antipyretic	T39.91	T39.92	T39.93	T39.94	T39.95	T39.96
specified NEC	T39.8X1	T39.8X2	T39.8X3	T39.8X4	T39.8X5	T39.8X6
Antipyrine	T39.2X1	T39.2X2	T39.2X3	T39.2X4	T39.2X5	T39.2X6
Antirabies hyperimmune serum	T50.Z11	T50.Z12	T50.Z13	T50.Z14	T50.Z15	T50.Z16
Antirheumatic NEC	T39.4X1	T39.4X2	T39.4X3	T39.4X4	T39.4X5	T39.4X6
Antirigidity drug NEC	T42.8X1	T42.8X2	T42.8X3	T42.8X4	T42.8X5	T42.8X6
Antischistosomal drug	T37.4X1	T37.4X2	T37.4X3	T37.4X4	T37.4X5	T37.4X6
Antiscorpion sera	T50.Z11	T50.Z12	T50.Z13	T50.Z14	T50.Z15	T50.Z16
Antiseborrheics	T49.4X1	T49.4X2	T49.4X3	T49.4X4	T49.4X5	T49.4X6
Antiseptics (external) (medicinal)	T49.0X1	T49.0X2	T49.0X3	T49.0X4	T49.0X5	T49.0X6
Antistine	T45.0X1	T45.0X2	T45.0X3	T45.0X4	T45.0X5	T45.0X6
Antitapeworm drug	T37.4X1	T37.4X2	T37.4X3	T37.4X4	T37.4X5	T37.4X6
Antitetanus immunoglobulin	T50.Z11	T50.Z12	T50.Z13	T50.Z14	T50.Z15	T50.Z16
Antithyroid drug NEC	T38.2X1	T38.2X2	T38.2X3	T38.2X4	T38.2X5	T38.2X6
Antitoxin	T50.Z11	T50.Z12	T50.Z13	T50.Z14	T50.Z15	T50.Z16
diphtheria	T50.Z11	T50.Z12	T50.Z13	T50.Z14	T50.Z15	T50.Z16
gas gangrene	T50.Z11	T50.Z12	T50.Z13	T50.Z14	T50.Z15	T50.Z16
tetanus	T50.Z11	T50.Z12	T50.Z13	T50.Z14	T50.Z15	T50.Z16
Antitrichomonal drug	T37.3X1	T37.3X2	T37.3X3	T37.3X4	T37.3X5	T37.3X6
Antituberculars	T37.1X1	T37.1X2	T37.1X3	T37.1X4	T37.1X5	T37.1X6
antibiotics	T36.5X1	T36.5X2	T36.5X3	T36.5X4	T36.5X5	T36.5X6
Antitussive NEC	T48.3X1	T48.3X2	T48.3X3	T48.3X4	T48.3X5	T48.3X6
codeine mixture	T40.2X1	T40.2X2	T40.2X3	T40.2X4	T40.2X5	T40.2X6
opiate	T40.2X1	T40.2X2	T40.2X3	T40.2X4	T40.2X5	T40.2X6
Antivaricose drug	T46.8X1	T46.8X2	T46.8X3	T46.8X4	T46.8X5	T46.8X6
Antivenin, antivenom (sera)	T50.Z11	T50.Z12	T50.Z13	T50.Z14	T50.Z15	T50.Z16
crotaline	T50.Z11	T50.Z12	T50.Z13	T50.Z14	T50.Z15	T50.Z16
spider bite	T50.Z11	T50.Z12	T50.Z13	T50.Z14	T50.Z15	T50.Z16
Antivertigo drug	T45.0X1	T45.0X2	T45.0X3	T45.0X4	T45.0X5	T45.0X6
Antiviral drug NEC	T37.5X1	T37.5X2	T37.5X3	T37.5X4	T37.5X5	T37.5X6
eye	T49.5X1	T49.5X2	T49.5X3	T49.5X4	T49.5X5	T49.5X6
Antiwhipworm drug	T37.4X1	T37.4X2	T37.4X3	T37.4X4	T37.4X5	T37.4X6
Ant poison — *see* Insecticide						
Antrol — *see also* by specific chemical substance	T60.91	T60.92	T60.93	T60.94	—	—
fungicide	T60.91	T60.92	T60.93	T60.94	—	—
ANTU (alpha naphthylthiourea)	T60.4X1	T60.4X2	T60.4X3	T60.4X4	—	—
Apalcillin	T36.0X1	T36.0X2	T36.0X3	T36.0X4	T36.0X5	T36.0X6
APC	T48.5X1	T48.5X2	T48.5X3	T48.5X4	T48.5X5	T48.5X6
Aplonidine	T44.4X1	T44.4X2	T44.4X3	T44.4X4	T44.4X5	T44.4X6
Apomorphine	T47.7X1	T47.7X2	T47.7X3	T47.7X4	T47.7X5	T47.7X6
Appetite depressants, central	T50.5X1	T50.5X2	T50.5X3	T50.5X4	T50.5X5	T50.5X6
Apraclonidine (hydrochloride)	T44.4X1	T44.4X2	T44.4X3	T44.4X4	T44.4X5	T44.4X6
Apresoline	T46.5X1	T46.5X2	T46.5X3	T46.5X4	T46.5X5	T46.5X6
Aprindine	T46.2X1	T46.2X2	T46.2X3	T46.2X4	T46.2X5	T46.2X6
Aprobarbital	T42.3X1	T42.3X2	T42.3X3	T42.3X4	T42.3X5	T42.3X6
Apronalide	T42.6X1	T42.6X2	T42.6X3	T42.6X4	T42.6X5	T42.6X6
Aprotinin	T45.621	T45.622	T45.623	T45.624	T45.625	T45.626
Aptocaine	T41.3X1	T41.3X2	T41.3X3	T41.3X4	T41.3X5	T41.3X6
Aqua fortis	T54.2X1	T54.2X2	T54.2X3	T54.2X4	—	—
Ara-A	T37.5X1	T37.5X2	T37.5X3	T37.5X4	T37.5X5	T37.5X6
Ara-C	T45.1X1	T45.1X2	T45.1X3	T45.1X4	T45.1X5	T45.1X6
Arachis oil	T49.3X1	T49.3X2	T49.3X3	T49.3X4	T49.3X5	T49.3X6
cathartic	T47.4X1	T47.4X2	T47.4X3	T47.4X4	T47.4X5	T47.4X6
Aralen	T37.2X1	T37.2X2	T37.2X3	T37.2X4	T37.2X5	T37.2X6
Arecoline	T44.1X1	T44.1X2	T44.1X3	T44.1X4	T44.1X5	T44.1X6
Arginine	T50.991	T50.992	T50.993	T50.994	T50.995	T50.996
glutamate	T50.991	T50.992	T50.993	T50.994	T50.995	T50.996
Argyrol	T49.0X1	T49.0X2	T49.0X3	T49.0X4	T49.0X5	T49.0X6
ENT agent	T49.6X1	T49.6X2	T49.6X3	T49.6X4	T49.6X5	T49.6X6

Antifungal — Argyrol

Substance	Poisoning, Accidental (unintentional)	Poisoning, Intentional Self-harm	Poisoning, Assault	Poisoning, Undetermined	Adverse Effect	Under-dosing
Argyrol — continued						
ophthalmic preparation	T49.5X1	T49.5X2	T49.5X3	T49.5X4	T49.5X5	T49.5X6
Aristocort	T38.0X1	T38.0X2	T38.0X3	T38.0X4	T38.0X5	T38.0X6
ENT agent	T49.6X1	T49.6X2	T49.6X3	T49.6X4	T49.6X5	T49.6X6
ophthalmic preparation	T49.5X1	T49.5X2	T49.5X3	T49.5X4	T49.5X5	T49.5X6
topical NEC	T49.0X1	T49.0X2	T49.0X3	T49.0X4	T49.0X5	T49.0X6
Aromatics, corrosive	T54.1X1	T54.1X2	T54.1X3	T54.1X4	—	—
disinfectants	T54.1X1	T54.1X2	T54.1X3	T54.1X4	—	—
Arsenate of lead	T57.0X1	T57.0X2	T57.0X3	T57.0X4	—	—
herbicide	T57.0X1	T57.0X2	T57.0X3	T57.0X4	—	—
Arsenic, arsenicals (compounds) (dust) (vapor) NEC	T57.0X1	T57.0X2	T57.0X3	T57.0X4	—	—
anti-infectives	T37.8X1	T37.8X2	T37.8X3	T37.8X4	T37.8X5	T37.8X6
pesticide (dust) (fumes)	T57.0X1	T57.0X2	T57.0X3	T57.0X4	—	—
Arsine (gas)	T57.0X1	T57.0X2	T57.0X3	T57.0X4	—	—
Arsphenamine (silver)	T37.8X1	T37.8X2	T37.8X3	T37.8X4	T37.8X5	T37.8X6
Arsthinol	T37.3X1	T37.3X2	T37.3X3	T37.3X4	T37.3X5	T37.3X6
Artane	T44.3X1	T44.3X2	T44.3X3	T44.3X4	T44.3X5	T44.3X6
Arthropod (venomous) NEC	T63.481	T63.482	T63.483	T63.484	—	—
Articaine	T41.3X1	T41.3X2	T41.3X3	T41.3X4	T41.3X5	T41.3X6
Asbestos	T57.8X1	T57.8X2	T57.8X3	T57.8X4	—	—
Ascaridole	T37.4X1	T37.4X2	T37.4X3	T37.4X4	T37.4X5	T37.4X6
Ascorbic acid	T45.2X1	T45.2X2	T45.2X3	T45.2X4	T45.2X5	T45.2X6
Asiaticoside	T49.0X1	T49.0X2	T49.0X3	T49.0X4	T49.0X5	T49.0X6
Asparaginase	T45.1X1	T45.1X2	T45.1X3	T45.1X4	T45.1X5	T45.1X6
Aspidium (oleoresin)	T37.4X1	T37.4X2	T37.4X3	T37.4X4	T37.4X5	T37.4X6
Aspirin (aluminum) (soluble)	T39.011	T39.012	T39.013	T39.014	T39.015	T39.016
Aspoxicillin	T36.0X1	T36.0X2	T36.0X3	T36.0X4	T36.0X5	T36.0X6
Astemizole	T45.0X1	T45.0X2	T45.0X3	T45.0X4	T45.0X5	T45.0X6
Astringent (local)	T49.2X1	T49.2X2	T49.2X3	T49.2X4	T49.2X5	T49.2X6
specified NEC	T49.2X1	T49.2X2	T49.2X3	T49.2X4	T49.2X5	T49.2X6
Astromicin	T36.5X1	T36.5X2	T36.5X3	T36.5X4	T36.5X5	T36.5X6
Ataractic drug NEC	T43.501	T43.502	T43.503	T43.504	T43.505	T43.506
Atenolol	T44.7X1	T44.7X2	T44.7X3	T44.7X4	T44.7X5	T44.7X6
Atonia drug, intestinal	T47.4X1	T47.4X2	T47.4X3	T47.4X4	T47.4X5	T47.4X6
Atophan	T50.4X1	T50.4X2	T50.4X3	T50.4X4	T50.4X5	T50.4X6
Atracurium besilate	T48.1X1	T48.1X2	T48.1X3	T48.1X4	T48.1X5	T48.1X6
Atropine	T44.3X1	T44.3X2	T44.3X3	T44.3X4	T44.3X5	T44.3X6
derivative	T44.3X1	T44.3X2	T44.3X3	T44.3X4	T44.3X5	T44.3X6
methonitrate	T44.3X1	T44.3X2	T44.3X3	T44.3X4	T44.3X5	T44.3X6
Attapulgite	T47.6X1	T47.6X2	T47.6X3	T47.6X4	T47.6X5	T47.6X6
Auramine	T65.891	T65.892	T65.893	T65.894	—	—
dye	T65.6X1	T65.6X2	T65.6X3	T65.6X4	—	—
fungicide	T60.3X1	T60.3X2	T60.3X3	T60.3X4	—	—
Auranofin	T39.4X1	T39.4X2	T39.4X3	T39.4X4	T39.4X5	T39.4X6
Aurantiin	T46.991	T46.992	T46.993	T46.994	T46.995	T46.996
Aureomycin	T36.4X1	T36.4X2	T36.4X3	T36.4X4	T36.4X5	T36.4X6
ophthalmic preparation	T49.5X1	T49.5X2	T49.5X3	T49.5X4	T49.5X5	T49.5X6
topical NEC	T49.0X1	T49.0X2	T49.0X3	T49.0X4	T49.0X5	T49.0X6
Aurothioglucose	T39.4X1	T39.4X2	T39.4X3	T39.4X4	T39.4X5	T39.4X6
Aurothioglycanide	T39.4X1	T39.4X2	T39.4X3	T39.4X4	T39.4X5	T39.4X6
Aurothiomalate sodium	T39.4X1	T39.4X2	T39.4X3	T39.4X4	T39.4X5	T39.4X6
Aurotioprol	T39.4X1	T39.4X2	T39.4X3	T39.4X4	T39.4X5	T39.4X6
Automobile fuel	T52.0X1	T52.0X2	T52.0X3	T52.0X4	—	—
Autonomic nervous system agent NEC	T44.901	T44.902	T44.903	T44.904	T44.905	T44.906
Avlosulfon	T37.1X1	T37.1X2	T37.1X3	T37.1X4	T37.1X5	T37.1X6
Avomine	T42.6X1	T42.6X2	T42.6X3	T42.6X4	T42.6X5	T42.6X6
Axerophthol	T45.2X1	T45.2X2	T45.2X3	T45.2X4	T45.2X5	T45.2X6
Azacitidine	T45.1X1	T45.1X2	T45.1X3	T45.1X4	T45.1X5	T45.1X6
Azacyclonol	T43.591	T43.592	T43.593	T43.594	T43.595	T43.596
Azadirachta	T60.2X1	T60.2X2	T60.2X3	T60.2X4	—	—
Azanidazole	T37.3X1	T37.3X2	T37.3X3	T37.3X4	T37.3X5	T37.3X6
Azapetine	T46.7X1	T46.7X2	T46.7X3	T46.7X4	T46.7X5	T46.7X6
Azapropazone	T39.2X1	T39.2X2	T39.2X3	T39.2X4	T39.2X5	T39.2X6
Azaribine	T45.1X1	T45.1X2	T45.1X3	T45.1X4	T45.1X5	T45.1X6
Azaserine	T45.1X1	T45.1X2	T45.1X3	T45.1X4	T45.1X5	T45.1X6
Azatadine	T45.0X1	T45.0X2	T45.0X3	T45.0X4	T45.0X5	T45.0X6
Azatepa	T45.1X1	T45.1X2	T45.1X3	T45.1X4	T45.1X5	T45.1X6
Azathioprine	T45.1X1	T45.1X2	T45.1X3	T45.1X4	T45.1X5	T45.1X6
Azelaic acid	T49.0X1	T49.0X2	T49.0X3	T49.0X4	T49.0X5	T49.0X6
Azelastine	T45.0X1	T45.0X2	T45.0X3	T45.0X4	T45.0X5	T45.0X6
Azidocillin	T36.0X1	T36.0X2	T36.0X3	T36.0X4	T36.0X5	T36.0X6
Azidothymidine	T37.5X1	T37.5X2	T37.5X3	T37.5X4	T37.5X5	T37.5X6
Azinphos (ethyl) (methyl)	T60.0X1	T60.0X2	T60.0X3	T60.0X4	—	—
Aziridine (chelating)	T54.1X1	T54.1X2	T54.1X3	T54.1X4	—	—
Azithromycin	T36.3X1	T36.3X2	T36.3X3	T36.3X4	T36.3X5	T36.3X6
Azlocillin	T36.0X1	T36.0X2	T36.0X3	T36.0X4	T36.0X5	T36.0X6
Azobenzene smoke	T65.3X1	T65.3X2	T65.3X3	T65.3X4	—	—
acaricide	T60.8X1	T60.8X2	T60.8X3	T60.8X4	—	—
Azosulfamide	T37.0X1	T37.0X2	T37.0X3	T37.0X4	T37.0X5	T37.0X6
AZT	T37.5X1	T37.5X2	T37.5X3	T37.5X4	T37.5X5	T37.5X6
Aztreonam	T36.1X1	T36.1X2	T36.1X3	T36.1X4	T36.1X5	T36.1X6

Substance	Poisoning, Accidental (unintentional)	Poisoning, Intentional Self-harm	Poisoning, Assault	Poisoning, Undetermined	Adverse Effect	Under-dosing
Azulfidine	T37.0X1	T37.0X2	T37.0X3	T37.0X4	T37.0X5	T37.0X6
Azuresin	T50.8X1	T50.8X2	T50.8X3	T50.8X4	T50.8X5	T50.8X6
b-acetyldigoxin	T46.0X1	T46.0X2	T46.0X3	T46.0X4	T46.0X5	T46.0X6
P-Acetamidophenol	T39.1X1	T39.1X2	T39.1X3	T39.1X4	T39.1X5	T39.1X6
Bacampicillin	T36.0X1	T36.0X2	T36.0X3	T36.0X4	T36.0X5	T36.0X6
Bacillus						
lactobacillus	T47.8X1	T47.8X2	T47.8X3	T47.8X4	T47.8X5	T47.8X6
subtilis	T47.6X1	T47.6X2	T47.6X3	T47.6X4	T47.6X5	T47.6X6
Bacimycin	T49.0X1	T49.0X2	T49.0X3	T49.0X4	T49.0X5	T49.0X6
ophthalmic preparation	T49.5X1	T49.5X2	T49.5X3	T49.5X4	T49.5X5	T49.5X6
Bacitracin zinc	T49.0X1	T49.0X2	T49.0X3	T49.0X4	T49.0X5	T49.0X6
with neomycin	T49.0X1	T49.0X2	T49.0X3	T49.0X4	T49.0X5	T49.0X6
ENT agent	T49.6X1	T49.6X2	T49.6X3	T49.6X4	T49.6X5	T49.6X6
ophthalmic preparation	T49.5X1	T49.5X2	T49.5X3	T49.5X4	T49.5X5	T49.5X6
topical NEC	T49.0X1	T49.0X2	T49.0X3	T49.0X4	T49.0X5	T49.0X6
Baclofen	T42.8X1	T42.8X2	T42.8X3	T42.8X4	T42.8X5	T42.8X6
Baking soda	T50.991	T50.992	T50.993	T50.994	T50.995	T50.996
BAL	T45.8X1	T45.8X2	T45.8X3	T45.8X4	T45.8X5	T45.8X6
Bambuterol	T48.6X1	T48.6X2	T48.6X3	T48.6X4	T48.6X5	T48.6X6
Bamethan (sulfate)	T46.7X1	T46.7X2	T46.7X3	T46.7X4	T46.7X5	T46.7X6
Bamifylline	T48.6X1	T48.6X2	T48.6X3	T48.6X4	T48.6X5	T48.6X6
Bamipine	T45.0X1	T45.0X2	T45.0X3	T45.0X4	T45.0X5	T45.0X6
Baneberry — see Actaea spicata						
Banewort — see Belladonna						
Barbenyl	T42.3X1	T42.3X2	T42.3X3	T42.3X4	T42.3X5	T42.3X6
Barbexaclone	T42.6X1	T42.6X2	T42.6X3	T42.6X4	T42.6X5	T42.6X6
Barbital	T42.3X1	T42.3X2	T42.3X3	T42.3X4	T42.3X5	T42.3X6
sodium	T42.3X1	T42.3X2	T42.3X3	T42.3X4	T42.3X5	T42.3X6
Barbitone	T42.3X1	T42.3X2	T42.3X3	T42.3X4	T42.3X5	T42.3X6
Barbiturate NEC	T42.3X1	T42.3X2	T42.3X3	T42.3X4	T42.3X5	T42.3X6
with tranquilizer	T42.3X1	T42.3X2	T42.3X3	T42.3X4	T42.3X5	T42.3X6
anesthetic (intravenous)	T41.1X1	T41.1X2	T41.1X3	T41.1X4	T41.1X5	T41.1X6
Barium (carbonate) (chloride) (sulfite)	T57.8X1	T57.8X2	T57.8X3	T57.8X4	—	—
diagnostic agent	T50.8X1	T50.8X2	T50.8X3	T50.8X4	T50.8X5	T50.8X6
pesticide	T60.4X1	T60.4X2	T60.4X3	T60.4X4	—	—
rodenticide	T60.4X1	T60.4X2	T60.4X3	T60.4X4	—	—
sulfate (medicinal)	T50.8X1	T50.8X2	T50.8X3	T50.8X4	T50.8X5	T50.8X6
Barrier cream	T49.3X1	T49.3X2	T49.3X3	T49.3X4	T49.3X5	T49.3X6
Basic fuchsin	T49.0X1	T49.0X2	T49.0X3	T49.0X4	T49.0X5	T49.0X6
Battery acid or fluid	T54.2X1	T54.2X2	T54.2X3	T54.2X4	—	—
Bay rum	T51.8X1	T51.8X2	T51.8X3	T51.8X4	—	—
b-benzalbutyramide	T46.6X1	T46.6X2	T46.6X3	T46.6X4	T46.6X5	T46.6X6
BCG (vaccine)	T50.A91	T50.A92	T50.A93	T50.A94	T50.A95	T50.A96
BCNU	T45.1X1	T45.1X2	T45.1X3	T45.1X4	T45.1X5	T45.1X6
Bearsfoot	T62.2X1	T62.2X2	T62.2X3	T62.2X4	—	—
Beclamide	T42.6X1	T42.6X2	T42.6X3	T42.6X4	T42.6X5	T42.6X6
Beclomethasone	T44.5X1	T44.5X2	T44.5X3	T44.5X4	T44.5X5	T44.5X6
Bee (sting) (venom)	T63.441	T63.442	T63.443	T63.444	—	—
Befunolol	T49.5X1	T49.5X2	T49.5X3	T49.5X4	T49.5X5	T49.5X6
Bekanamycin	T36.5X1	T36.5X2	T36.5X3	T36.5X4	T36.5X5	T36.5X6
Belladonna — see also Nightshade						
alkaloids	T44.3X1	T44.3X2	T44.3X3	T44.3X4	T44.3X5	T44.3X6
extract	T44.3X1	T44.3X2	T44.3X3	T44.3X4	T44.3X5	T44.3X6
herb	T44.3X1	T44.3X2	T44.3X3	T44.3X4	T44.3X5	T44.3X6
Bemegride	T50.7X1	T50.7X2	T50.7X3	T50.7X4	T50.7X5	T50.7X6
Benactyzine	T44.3X1	T44.3X2	T44.3X3	T44.3X4	T44.3X5	T44.3X6
Benadryl	T45.0X1	T45.0X2	T45.0X3	T45.0X4	T45.0X5	T45.0X6
Benaprizine	T44.3X1	T44.3X2	T44.3X3	T44.3X4	T44.3X5	T44.3X6
Benazepril	T46.4X1	T46.4X2	T46.4X3	T46.4X4	T46.4X5	T46.4X6
Bencyclane	T46.7X1	T46.7X2	T46.7X3	T46.7X4	T46.7X5	T46.7X6
Bendazol	T46.3X1	T46.3X2	T46.3X3	T46.3X4	T46.3X5	T46.3X6
Bendrofluazide	T50.2X1	T50.2X2	T50.2X3	T50.2X4	T50.2X5	T50.2X6
Bendroflumethiazide	T50.2X1	T50.2X2	T50.2X3	T50.2X4	T50.2X5	T50.2X6
Benemid	T50.4X1	T50.4X2	T50.4X3	T50.4X4	T50.4X5	T50.4X6
Benethamine penicillin	T36.0X1	T36.0X2	T36.0X3	T36.0X4	T36.0X5	T36.0X6
Benexate	T47.1X1	T47.1X2	T47.1X3	T47.1X4	T47.1X5	T47.1X6
Benfluorex	T46.6X1	T46.6X2	T46.6X3	T46.6X4	T46.6X5	T46.6X6
Benfotiamine	T45.2X1	T45.2X2	T45.2X3	T45.2X4	T45.2X5	T45.2X6
Benisone	T49.0X1	T49.0X2	T49.0X3	T49.0X4	T49.0X5	T49.0X6
Benomyl	T60.0X1	T60.0X2	T60.0X3	T60.0X4	—	—
Benoquin	T49.8X1	T49.8X2	T49.8X3	T49.8X4	T49.8X5	T49.8X6
Benoxinate	T41.3X1	T41.3X2	T41.3X3	T41.3X4	T41.3X5	T41.3X6
Benperidol	T43.4X1	T43.4X2	T43.4X3	T43.4X4	T43.4X5	T43.4X6
Benproperine	T48.3X1	T48.3X2	T48.3X3	T48.3X4	T48.3X5	T48.3X6
Benserazide	T42.8X1	T42.8X2	T42.8X3	T42.8X4	T42.8X5	T42.8X6
Bentazepam	T42.4X1	T42.4X2	T42.4X3	T42.4X4	T42.4X5	T42.4X6
Bentiromide	T50.8X1	T50.8X2	T50.8X3	T50.8X4	T50.8X5	T50.8X6
Bentonite	T49.3X1	T49.3X2	T49.3X3	T49.3X4	T49.3X5	T49.3X6
Benzalbutyramide	T46.6X1	T46.6X2	T46.6X3	T46.6X4	T46.6X5	T46.6X6
Benzalkonium (chloride)	T49.0X1	T49.0X2	T49.0X3	T49.0X4	T49.0X5	T49.0X6
ophthalmic preparation	T49.5X1	T49.5X2	T49.5X3	T49.5X4	T49.5X5	T49.5X6

Substance	Poisoning, Accidental (unintentional)	Poisoning, Intentional Self-harm	Poisoning, Assault	Poisoning, Undetermined	Adverse Effect	Under-dosing
Benzamidosalicylate (calcium)	T37.1X1	T37.1X2	T37.1X3	T37.1X4	T37.1X5	T37.1X6
Benzamine	T41.3X1	T41.3X2	T41.3X3	T41.3X4	T41.3X5	T41.3X6
lactate	T49.1X1	T49.1X2	T49.1X3	T49.1X4	T49.1X5	T49.1X6
Benzamphetamine	T50.5X1	T50.5X2	T50.5X3	T50.5X4	T50.5X5	T50.5X6
Benzapril hydrochloride	T46.5X1	T46.5X2	T46.5X3	T46.5X4	T46.5X5	T46.5X6
Benzathine benzylpenicillin	T36.0X1	T36.0X2	T36.0X3	T36.0X4	T36.0X5	T36.0X6
Benzathine penicillin	T36.0X1	T36.0X2	T36.0X3	T36.0X4	T36.0X5	T36.0X6
Benzatropine	T42.8X1	T42.8X2	T42.8X3	T42.8X4	T42.8X5	T42.8X6
Benzbromarone	T50.4X1	T50.4X2	T50.4X3	T50.4X4	T50.4X5	T50.4X6
Benzcarbimine	T45.1X1	T45.1X2	T45.1X3	T45.1X4	T45.1X5	T45.1X6
Benzedrex	T44.991	T44.992	T44.993	T44.994	T44.995	T44.996
Benzedrine (amphetamine)	T43.621	T43.622	T43.623	T43.624	T43.625	T43.626
Benzenamine	T65.3X1	T65.3X2	T65.3X3	T65.3X4	—	—
Benzene	T52.1X1	T52.1X2	T52.1X3	T52.1X4	—	—
homologues (acetyl) (dimethyl) (methyl) (solvent)	T52.2X1	T52.2X2	T52.2X3	T52.2X4	—	—
Benzethonium (chloride)	T49.0X1	T49.0X2	T49.0X3	T49.0X4	T49.0X5	T49.0X6
Benzfetamine	T50.5X1	T50.5X2	T50.5X3	T50.5X4	T50.5X5	T50.5X6
Benzhexol	T44.3X1	T44.3X2	T44.3X3	T44.3X4	T44.3X5	T44.3X6
Benzhydramine (chloride)	T45.0X1	T45.0X2	T45.0X3	T45.0X4	T45.0X5	T45.0X6
Benzidine	T65.891	T65.892	T65.893	T65.894	—	—
Benzilonium bromide	T44.3X1	T44.3X2	T44.3X3	T44.3X4	T44.3X5	T44.3X6
Benzimidazole	T60.3X1	T60.3X2	T60.3X3	T60.3X4	—	—
Benzin (e) — see Ligroin						
Benziodarone	T46.3X1	T46.3X2	T46.3X3	T46.3X4	T46.3X5	T46.3X6
Benznidazole	T37.3X1	T37.3X2	T37.3X3	T37.3X4	T37.3X5	T37.3X6
Benzocaine	T41.3X1	T41.3X2	T41.3X3	T41.3X4	T41.3X5	T41.3X6
Benzodiapin	T42.4X1	T42.4X2	T42.4X3	T42.4X4	T42.4X5	T42.4X6
Benzodiazepine NEC	T42.4X1	T42.4X2	T42.4X3	T42.4X4	T42.4X5	T42.4X6
Benzoic acid	T49.0X1	T49.0X2	T49.0X3	T49.0X4	T49.0X5	T49.0X6
with salicylic acid	T49.0X1	T49.0X2	T49.0X3	T49.0X4	T49.0X5	T49.0X6
Benzoin (tincture)	T48.5X1	T48.5X2	T48.5X3	T48.5X4	T48.5X5	T48.5X6
Benzol (benzene)	T52.1X1	T52.1X2	T52.1X3	T52.1X4	—	—
vapor	T52.0X1	T52.0X2	T52.0X3	T52.0X4	—	—
Benzomorphan	T40.2X1	T40.2X2	T40.2X3	T40.2X4	T40.2X5	T40.2X6
Benzonatate	T48.3X1	T48.3X2	T48.3X3	T48.3X4	T48.3X5	T48.3X6
Benzophenones	T49.3X1	T49.3X2	T49.3X3	T49.3X4	T49.3X5	T49.3X6
Benzopyrone	T46.991	T46.992	T46.993	T46.994	T46.995	T46.996
Benzothiadiazides	T50.2X1	T50.2X2	T50.2X3	T50.2X4	T50.2X5	T50.2X6
Benzoxonium chloride	T49.0X1	T49.0X2	T49.0X3	T49.0X4	T49.0X5	T49.0X6
Benzoylpas calcium	T37.1X1	T37.1X2	T37.1X3	T37.1X4	T37.1X5	T37.1X6
Benzoyl peroxide	T49.0X1	T49.0X2	T49.0X3	T49.0X4	T49.0X5	T49.0X6
Benzperidin	T43.591	T43.592	T43.593	T43.594	T43.595	T43.596
Benzperidol	T43.591	T43.592	T43.593	T43.594	T43.595	T43.596
Benzphetamine	T50.5X1	T50.5X2	T50.5X3	T50.5X4	T50.5X5	T50.5X6
Benzpyrinium bromide	T44.1X1	T44.1X2	T44.1X3	T44.1X4	T44.1X5	T44.1X6
Benzquinamide	T45.0X1	T45.0X2	T45.0X3	T45.0X4	T45.0X5	T45.0X6
Benzthiazide	T50.2X1	T50.2X2	T50.2X3	T50.2X4	T50.2X5	T50.2X6
Benztropine						
anticholinergic	T44.3X1	T44.3X2	T44.3X3	T44.3X4	T44.3X5	T44.3X6
antiparkinson	T42.8X1	T42.8X2	T42.8X3	T42.8X4	T42.8X5	T42.8X6
Benzydamine	T49.0X1	T49.0X2	T49.0X3	T49.0X4	T49.0X5	T49.0X6
Benzyl						
acetate	T52.8X1	T52.8X2	T52.8X3	T52.8X4	—	—
alcohol	T49.0X1	T49.0X2	T49.0X3	T49.0X4	T49.0X5	T49.0X6
benzoate	T49.0X1	T49.0X2	T49.0X3	T49.0X4	T49.0X5	T49.0X6
Benzoic acid	T49.0X1	T49.0X2	T49.0X3	T49.0X4	T49.0X5	T49.0X6
morphine	T40.2X1	T40.2X2	T40.2X3	T40.2X4	—	—
nicotinate	T46.6X1	T46.6X2	T46.6X3	T46.6X4	T46.6X5	T46.6X6
penicillin	T36.0X1	T36.0X2	T36.0X3	T36.0X4	T36.0X5	T36.0X6
Benzylhydrochlorthiazide	T50.2X1	T50.2X2	T50.2X3	T50.2X4	T50.2X5	T50.2X6
Benzylpenicillin	T36.0X1	T36.0X2	T36.0X3	T36.0X4	T36.0X5	T36.0X6
Benzylthiouracil	T38.2X1	T38.2X2	T38.2X3	T38.2X4	T38.2X5	T38.2X6
Bephenium hydroxynaphthoate	T37.4X1	T37.4X2	T37.4X3	T37.4X4	T37.4X5	T37.4X6
Bepridil	T46.1X1	T46.1X2	T46.1X3	T46.1X4	T46.1X5	T46.1X6
Bergamot oil	T65.891	T65.892	T65.893	T65.894	—	—
Bergapten	T50.991	T50.992	T50.993	T50.994	T50.995	T50.996
Berries, poisonous	T62.1X1	T62.1X2	T62.1X3	T62.1X4	—	—
Beryllium (compounds)	T56.7X1	T56.7X2	T56.7X3	T56.7X4	—	—
beta adrenergic blocking agent, heart	T44.7X1	T44.7X2	T44.7X3	T44.7X4	T44.7X5	T44.7X6
Betacarotene	T45.2X1	T45.2X2	T45.2X3	T45.2X4	T45.2X5	T45.2X6
Beta-Chlor	T42.6X1	T42.6X2	T42.6X3	T42.6X4	T42.6X5	T42.6X6
Betahistine	T46.7X1	T46.7X2	T46.7X3	T46.7X4	T46.7X5	T46.7X6
Betaine	T47.5X1	T47.5X2	T47.5X3	T47.5X4	T47.5X5	T47.5X6
Betamethasone	T49.0X1	T49.0X2	T49.0X3	T49.0X4	T49.0X5	T49.0X6
topical	T49.0X1	T49.0X2	T49.0X3	T49.0X4	T49.0X5	T49.0X6
Betamicin	T36.8X1	T36.8X2	T36.8X4	T36.8X4	T36.8X5	T36.8X6
Betanidine	T46.5X1	T46.5X2	T46.5X3	T46.5X4	T46.5X5	T46.5X6
Betaxolol	T44.7X1	T44.7X2	T44.7X3	T44.7X4	T44.7X5	T44.7X6
Betazole	T50.8X1	T50.8X2	T50.8X3	T50.8X4	T50.8X5	T50.8X6
Bethanechol	T44.1X1	T44.1X2	T44.1X3	T44.1X4	T44.1X5	T44.1X6
chloride	T44.1X1	T44.1X2	T44.1X3	T44.1X4	T44.1X5	T44.1X6
Bethanidine	T46.5X1	T46.5X2	T46.5X3	T46.5X4	T46.5X5	T46.5X6
Betoxycaine	T41.3X1	T41.3X2	T41.3X3	T41.3X4	T41.3X5	T41.3X6
Betula oil	T49.3X1	T49.3X2	T49.3X3	T49.3X4	T49.3X5	T49.3X6
Bevantolol	T44.7X1	T44.7X2	T44.7X3	T44.7X4	T44.7X5	T44.7X6
Bevonium metilsulfate	T44.3X1	T44.3X2	T44.3X3	T44.3X4	T44.3X5	T44.3X6
Bezafibrate	T46.6X1	T46.6X2	T46.6X3	T46.6X4	T46.6X5	T46.6X6
Bezitramide	T40.4X1	T40.4X2	T40.4X3	T40.4X4	T40.4X5	T40.4X6
BHA	T50.991	T50.992	T50.993	T50.994	T50.995	T50.996
Bhang	T40.7X1	T40.7X2	T40.7X3	T40.7X4	T40.7X5	T40.7X6
BHC (medicinal)	T49.0X1	T49.0X2	T49.0X3	T49.0X4	T49.0X5	T49.0X6
nonmedicinal (vapor)	T53.6X1	T53.6X2	T53.6X3	T53.6X4	—	—
Bialamicol	T37.3X1	T37.3X2	T37.3X3	T37.3X4	T37.3X5	T37.3X6
Bibenzonium bromide	T48.3X1	T48.3X2	T48.3X3	T48.3X4	T48.3X5	T48.3X6
Bibrocathol	T49.5X1	T49.5X2	T49.5X3	T49.5X4	T49.5X5	T49.5X6
Bichloride of mercury — see Mercury, chloride						
Bichromates (calcium) (potassium) (sodium) (crystals)	T57.8X1	T57.8X2	T57.8X3	T57.8X4		
fumes	T56.2X1	T56.2X2	T56.2X3	T56.2X4		
Biclotymol	T49.6X1	T49.6X2	T49.6X3	T49.6X4	T49.6X5	T49.6X6
Bicucculine	T50.7X1	T50.7X2	T50.7X3	T50.7X4	T50.7X5	T50.7X6
Bifemelane	T43.291	T43.292	T43.293	T43.294	T43.295	T43.296
Biguanide derivatives, oral	T38.3X1	T38.3X2	T38.3X3	T38.3X4	T38.3X5	T38.3X6
Bile salts	T47.5X1	T47.5X2	T47.5X3	T47.5X4	T47.5X5	T47.5X6
Biligrafin	T50.8X1	T50.8X2	T50.8X3	T50.8X4	T50.8X5	T50.8X6
Bilopaque	T50.8X1	T50.8X2	T50.8X3	T50.8X4	T50.8X5	T50.8X6
Binifibrate	T46.6X1	T46.6X2	T46.6X3	T46.6X4	T46.6X5	T46.6X6
Binitrobenzol	T65.3X1	T65.3X2	T65.3X3	T65.3X4	—	—
Bioflavonoid(s)	T46.991	T46.992	T46.993	T46.994	T46.995	T46.996
Biological substance NEC	T50.901	T50.902	T50.903	T50.904	T50.905	T50.906
Biotin	T45.2X1	T45.2X2	T45.2X3	T45.2X4	T45.2X5	T45.2X6
Biperiden	T44.3X1	T44.3X2	T44.3X3	T44.3X4	T44.3X5	T44.3X6
Bisacodyl	T47.2X1	T47.2X2	T47.2X3	T47.2X4	T47.2X5	T47.2X6
Bisbentiamine	T45.2X1	T45.2X2	T45.2X3	T45.2X4	T45.2X5	T45.2X6
Bisbutiamine	T45.2X1	T45.2X2	T45.2X3	T45.2X4	T45.2X5	T45.2X6
Bisdequalinium (salts) (diacetate)	T49.6X1	T49.6X2	T49.6X3	T49.6X4	T49.6X5	T49.6X6
Bishydroxycoumarin	T45.511	T45.512	T45.513	T45.514	T45.515	T45.516
Bismarsen	T37.8X1	T37.8X2	T37.8X3	T37.8X4	T37.8X5	T37.8X6
Bismuth salts	T47.6X1	T47.6X2	T47.6X3	T47.6X4	T47.6X5	T47.6X6
aluminate	T47.1X1	T47.1X2	T47.1X3	T47.1X4	T47.1X5	T47.1X6
anti-infectives	T37.8X1	T37.8X2	T37.8X3	T37.8X4	T37.8X5	T37.8X6
formic iodide	T49.0X1	T49.0X2	T49.0X3	T49.0X4	T49.0X5	T49.0X6
glycolylarsenate	T49.0X1	T49.0X2	T49.0X3	T49.0X4	T49.0X5	T49.0X6
nonmedicinal (compounds) NEC	T65.91	T65.92	T65.93	T65.94	—	—
subcarbonate	T47.6X1	T47.6X2	T47.6X3	T47.6X4	T47.6X5	T47.6X6
subsalicylate	T37.8X1	T37.8X2	T37.8X3	T37.8X4	T37.8X5	T37.8X6
sulfarsphenamine	T37.8X1	T37.8X2	T37.8X3	T37.8X4	T37.8X5	T37.8X6
Bisoprolol	T44.7X1	T44.7X2	T44.7X3	T44.7X4	T44.7X5	T44.7X6
Bisoxatin	T47.2X1	T47.2X2	T47.2X3	T47.2X4	T47.2X5	T47.2X6
Bisulepin (hydrochloride)	T45.0X1	T45.0X2	T45.0X3	T45.0X4	T45.0X5	T45.0X6
Bithionol	T37.8X1	T37.8X2	T37.8X3	T37.8X4	T37.8X5	T37.8X6
anthelminthic	T37.4X1	T37.4X2	T37.4X3	T37.4X4	T37.4X5	T37.4X6
Bitolterol	T48.6X1	T48.6X2	T48.6X3	T48.6X4	T48.6X5	T48.6X6
Bitoscanate	T37.4X1	T37.4X2	T37.4X3	T37.4X4	T37.4X5	T37.4X6
Bitter almond oil	T62.8X1	T62.8X2	T62.8X3	T62.8X4	—	—
Bittersweet	T62.2X1	T62.2X2	T62.2X3	T62.2X4	—	—
Black						
flag	T60.91	T60.92	T60.93	T60.94	—	—
henbane	T62.2X1	T62.2X2	T62.2X3	T62.2X4	—	—
leaf (40)	T60.91	T60.92	T60.93	T60.94	—	—
widow spider (bite)	T63.311	T63.312	T63.313	T63.314	—	—
antivenin	T50.Z11	T50.Z12	T50.Z13	T50.Z14	T50.Z15	T50.Z16
Blast furnace gas (carbon monoxide from)	T58.8X1	T58.8X2	T58.8X3	T58.8X4	—	—
Bleach	T54.91	T54.92	T54.93	T54.94	—	—
Bleaching agent (medicinal)	T49.4X1	T49.4X2	T49.4X3	T49.4X4	T49.4X5	T49.4X6
Bleomycin	T45.1X1	T45.1X2	T45.1X3	T45.1X4	T45.1X5	T45.1X6
Blockain	T41.3X1	T41.3X2	T41.3X3	T41.3X4	T41.3X5	T41.3X6
infiltration (subcutaneous)	T41.3X1	T41.3X2	T41.3X3	T41.3X4	T41.3X5	T41.3X6
nerve block (peripheral) (plexus)	T41.3X1	T41.3X2	T41.3X3	T41.3X4	T41.3X5	T41.3X6
topical (surface)	T41.3X1	T41.3X2	T41.3X3	T41.3X4	T41.3X5	T41.3X6
Blockers, calcium channel	T46.1X1	T46.1X2	T46.1X3	T46.1X4	T46.1X5	T46.1X6
Blood (derivatives) (natural) (plasma) (whole)	T45.8X1	T45.8X2	T45.8X3	T45.8X4	T45.8X5	T45.8X6
dried	T45.8X1	T45.8X2	T45.8X3	T45.8X4	T45.8X5	T45.8X6
drug affecting NEC	T45.91	T45.92	T45.93	T45.94	T45.95	T45.96

Table of Drugs and Chemicals

Benzamidosalicylate — Blood

Table of Drugs and Chemicals

Substance	Poisoning, Accidental (unintentional)	Poisoning, Intentional Self-harm	Poisoning, Assault	Poisoning, Undetermined	Adverse Effect	Under-dosing
Blood — continued						
expander NEC	T45.8X1	T45.8X2	T45.8X3	T45.8X4	T45.8X5	T45.8X6
fraction NEC	T45.8X1	T45.8X2	T45.8X3	T45.8X4	T45.8X5	T45.8X6
substitute (macromolecular)	T45.8X1	T45.8X2	T45.8X3	T45.8X4	T45.8X5	T45.8X6
Blue velvet	T40.2X1	T40.2X2	T40.2X3	T40.2X4	—	—
Bone meal	T62.8X1	T62.8X2	T62.8X3	T62.8X4	—	—
Bonine	T45.0X1	T45.0X2	T45.0X3	T45.0X4	T45.0X5	T45.0X6
Bopindolol	T44.7X1	T44.7X2	T44.7X3	T44.7X4	T44.7X5	T44.7X6
Boracic acid	T49.0X1	T49.0X2	T49.0X3	T49.0X4	T49.0X5	T49.0X6
ENT agent	T49.6X1	T49.6X2	T49.6X3	T49.6X4	T49.6X5	T49.6X6
ophthalmic preparation	T49.5X1	T49.5X2	T49.5X3	T49.5X4	T49.5X5	T49.5X6
Borane complex	T57.8X1	T57.8X2	T57.8X3	T57.8X4	—	—
Borate(s)	T57.8X1	T57.8X2	T57.8X3	T57.8X4	—	—
buffer	T50.991	T50.992	T50.993	T50.994	T50.995	T50.996
cleanser	T54.91	T54.92	T54.93	T54.94	—	—
sodium	T57.8X1	T57.8X2	T57.8X3	T57.8X4	—	—
Borax (cleanser)	T54.91	T54.92	T54.93	T54.94	—	—
Bordeaux mixture	T60.3X1	T60.3X2	T60.3X3	T60.3X4	—	—
Boric acid	T49.0X1	T49.0X2	T49.0X3	T49.0X4	T49.0X5	T49.0X6
ENT agent	T49.6X1	T49.6X2	T49.6X3	T49.6X4	T49.6X5	T49.6X6
ophthalmic preparation	T49.5X1	T49.5X2	T49.5X3	T49.5X4	T49.5X5	T49.5X6
Bornaprine	T44.3X1	T44.3X2	T44.3X3	T44.3X4	T44.3X5	T44.3X6
Boron	T57.8X1	T57.8X2	T57.8X3	T57.8X4	—	—
hydride NEC	T57.8X1	T57.8X2	T57.8X3	T57.8X4	—	—
fumes or gas	T57.8X1	T57.8X2	T57.8X3	T57.8X4	—	—
trifluoride	T59.891	T59.892	T59.893	T59.894	—	—
Botox	T48.291	T48.292	T48.293	T48.294	T48.295	T48.296
Botulinus anti-toxin (type A, B)	T50.Z11	T50.Z12	T50.Z13	T50.Z14	T50.Z15	T50.Z16
Brake fluid vapor	T59.891	T59.892	T59.893	T59.894	—	—
Brallobarbital	T42.3X1	T42.3X2	T42.3X3	T42.3X4	T42.3X5	T42.3X6
Bran (wheat)	T47.4X1	T47.4X2	T47.4X3	T47.4X4	T47.4X5	T47.4X6
Brass (fumes)	T56.891	T56.892	T56.893	T56.894	—	—
Brasso	T52.0X1	T52.0X2	T52.0X3	T52.0X4	—	—
Bretylium tosilate	T46.2X1	T46.2X2	T46.2X3	T46.2X4	T46.2X5	T46.2X6
Brevital (sodium)	T41.1X1	T41.1X2	T41.1X3	T41.1X4	T41.1X5	T41.1X6
Brinase	T45.3X1	T45.3X2	T45.3X3	T45.3X4	T45.3X5	T45.3X6
British antilewisite	T45.8X1	T45.8X2	T45.8X3	T45.8X4	T45.8X5	T45.8X6
Brodifacoum	T60.4X1	T60.4X2	T60.4X3	T60.4X4	—	—
Bromal (hydrate)	T42.6X1	T42.6X2	T42.6X3	T42.6X4	T42.6X5	T42.6X6
Bromazepam	T42.4X1	T42.4X2	T42.4X3	T42.4X4	T42.4X5	T42.4X6
Bromazine	T45.0X1	T45.0X2	T45.0X3	T45.0X4	T45.0X5	T45.0X6
Brombenzylcyanide	T59.3X1	T59.3X2	T59.3X3	T59.3X4	—	—
Bromelains	T45.3X1	T45.3X2	T45.3X3	T45.3X4	T45.3X5	T45.3X6
Bromethalin	T60.4X1	T60.4X2	T60.4X3	T60.4X4	—	—
Bromhexine	T48.4X1	T48.4X2	T48.4X3	T48.4X4	T48.4X5	T48.4X6
Bromide salts	T42.6X1	T42.6X2	T42.6X3	T42.6X4	T42.6X5	T42.6X6
Bromindione	T45.511	T45.512	T45.513	T45.514	T45.515	T45.516
Bromine						
compounds (medicinal)	T42.6X1	T42.6X2	T42.6X3	T42.6X4	T42.6X5	T42.6X6
sedative	T42.6X1	T42.6X2	T42.6X3	T42.6X4	T42.6X5	T42.6X6
vapor	T59.891	T59.892	T59.893	T59.894	—	—
Bromisoval	T42.6X1	T42.6X2	T42.6X3	T42.6X4	T42.6X5	T42.6X6
Bromisovalum	T42.6X1	T42.6X2	T42.6X3	T42.6X4	T42.6X5	T42.6X6
Bromobenzylcyanide	T59.3X1	T59.3X2	T59.3X3	T59.3X4	—	—
Bromochlorosalicylani-lide	T49.0X1	T49.0X2	T49.0X3	T49.0X4	T49.0X5	T49.0X6
Bromocriptine	T42.8X1	T42.8X2	T42.8X3	T42.8X4	T42.8X5	T42.8X6
Bromodiphenhydramine	T45.0X1	T45.0X2	T45.0X3	T45.0X4	T45.0X5	T45.0X6
Bromoform	T42.6X1	T42.6X2	T42.6X3	T42.6X4	T42.6X5	T42.6X6
Bromophenol blue reagent	T50.991	T50.992	T50.993	T50.994	T50.995	T50.996
Bromopride	T47.8X1	T47.8X2	T47.8X3	T47.8X4	T47.8X5	T47.8X6
Bromosalicylchloranitide	T49.0X1	T49.0X2	T49.0X3	T49.0X4	T49.0X5	T49.0X6
Bromosalicylhydroxamic acid	T37.1X1	T37.1X2	T37.1X3	T37.1X4	T37.1X5	T37.1X6
Bromo-seltzer	T39.1X1	T39.1X2	T39.1X3	T39.1X4	T39.1X5	T39.1X6
Bromoxynil	T60.3X1	T60.3X2	T60.3X3	T60.3X4	—	—
Bromperidol	T43.4X1	T43.4X2	T43.4X3	T43.4X4	T43.4X5	T43.4X6
Brompheniramine	T45.0X1	T45.0X2	T45.0X3	T45.0X4	T45.0X5	T45.0X6
Bromsulfophthalein	T50.8X1	T50.8X2	T50.8X3	T50.8X4	T50.8X5	T50.8X6
Bromural	T42.6X1	T42.6X2	T42.6X3	T42.6X4	T42.6X5	T42.6X6
Bromvaletone	T42.6X1	T42.6X2	T42.6X3	T42.6X4	T42.6X5	T42.6X6
Bronchodilator NEC	T48.6X1	T48.6X2	T48.6X3	T48.6X4	T48.6X5	T48.6X6
Brotizolam	T42.4X1	T42.4X2	T42.4X3	T42.4X4	T42.4X5	T42.4X6
Brovincamine	T46.7X1	T46.7X2	T46.7X3	T46.7X4	T46.7X5	T46.7X6
Brown recluse spider (bite) (venom)	T63.331	T63.332	T63.333	T63.334	—	—
Brown spider (bite) (venom)	T63.391	T63.392	T63.393	T63.394	—	—
Broxaterol	T48.6X1	T48.6X2	T48.6X3	T48.6X4	T48.6X5	T48.6X6
Broxuridine	T45.1X1	T45.1X2	T45.1X3	T45.1X4	T45.1X5	T45.1X6
Broxyquinoline	T37.8X1	T37.8X2	T37.8X3	T37.8X4	T37.8X5	T37.8X6
Bruceine	T48.291	T48.292	T48.293	T48.294	T48.295	T48.296
Brucia	T62.2X1	T62.2X2	T62.2X3	T62.2X4	—	—

Substance	Poisoning, Accidental (unintentional)	Poisoning, Intentional Self-harm	Poisoning, Assault	Poisoning, Undetermined	Adverse Effect	Under-dosing
Brucine	T65.1X1	T65.1X2	T65.1X3	T65.1X4	—	—
Brunswick green — see Copper						
Bruten — see Ibuprofen						
Bryonia	T47.2X1	T47.2X2	T47.2X3	T47.2X4	T47.2X5	T47.2X6
Buclizine	T45.0X1	T45.0X2	T45.0X3	T45.0X4	T45.0X5	T45.0X6
Buclosamide	T49.0X1	T49.0X2	T49.0X3	T49.0X4	T49.0X5	T49.0X6
Budesonide	T44.5X1	T44.5X2	T44.5X3	T44.5X4	T44.5X5	T44.5X6
Budralazine	T46.5X1	T46.5X2	T46.5X3	T46.5X4	T46.5X5	T46.5X6
Bufferin	T39.011	T39.012	T39.013	T39.014	T39.015	T39.016
Buflomedil	T46.7X1	T46.7X2	T46.7X3	T46.7X4	T46.7X5	T46.7X6
Buformin	T38.3X1	T38.3X2	T38.3X3	T38.3X4	T38.3X5	T38.3X6
Bufotenine	T40.991	T40.992	T40.993	T40.994	—	—
Bufrolin	T48.6X1	T48.6X2	T48.6X3	T48.6X4	T48.6X5	T48.6X6
Bufylline	T48.6X1	T48.6X2	T48.6X3	T48.6X4	T48.6X5	T48.6X6
Bulk filler	T50.5X1	T50.5X2	T50.5X3	T50.5X4	T50.5X5	T50.5X6
cathartic	T47.4X1	T47.4X2	T47.4X3	T47.4X4	T47.4X5	T47.4X6
Bumetanide	T50.1X1	T50.1X2	T50.1X3	T50.1X4	T50.1X5	T50.1X6
Bunaftine	T46.2X1	T46.2X2	T46.2X3	T46.2X4	T46.2X5	T46.2X6
Bunamiodyl	T50.8X1	T50.8X2	T50.8X3	T50.8X4	T50.8X5	T50.8X6
Bunazosin	T44.6X1	T44.6X2	T44.6X3	T44.6X4	T44.6X5	T44.6X6
Bunitrolol	T44.7X1	T44.7X2	T44.7X3	T44.7X4	T44.7X5	T44.7X6
Buphenine	T46.7X1	T46.7X2	T46.7X3	T46.7X4	T46.7X5	T46.7X6
Bupivacaine	T41.3X1	T41.3X2	T41.3X3	T41.3X4	T41.3X5	T41.3X6
infiltration (subcutaneous)	T41.3X1	T41.3X2	T41.3X3	T41.3X4	T41.3X5	T41.3X6
nerve block (peripheral) (plexus)	T41.3X1	T41.3X2	T41.3X3	T41.3X4	T41.3X5	T41.3X6
spinal	T41.3X1	T41.3X2	T41.3X3	T41.3X4	T41.3X5	T41.3X6
Bupranolol	T44.7X1	T44.7X2	T44.7X3	T44.7X4	T44.7X5	T44.7X6
Buprenorphine	T40.4X1	T40.4X2	T40.4X3	T40.4X4	T40.4X5	T40.4X6
Bupropion	T43.291	T43.292	T43.293	T43.294	T43.295	T43.296
Burimamide	T47.1X1	T47.1X2	T47.1X3	T47.1X4	T47.1X5	T47.1X6
Buserelin	T38.891	T38.892	T38.893	T38.894	T38.895	T38.896
Buspirone	T43.591	T43.592	T43.593	T43.594	T43.595	T43.596
Busulfan, busulphan	T45.1X1	T45.1X2	T45.1X3	T45.1X4	T45.1X5	T45.1X6
Butabarbital (sodium)	T42.3X1	T42.3X2	T42.3X3	T42.3X4	T42.3X5	T42.3X6
Butabarbitone	T42.3X1	T42.3X2	T42.3X3	T42.3X4	T42.3X5	T42.3X6
Butabarpal	T42.3X1	T42.3X2	T42.3X3	T42.3X4	T42.3X5	T42.3X6
Butacaine	T41.3X1	T41.3X2	T41.3X3	T41.3X4	T41.3X5	T41.3X6
Butalamine	T46.7X1	T46.7X2	T46.7X3	T46.7X4	T46.7X5	T46.7X6
Butalbital	T42.3X1	T42.3X2	T42.3X3	T42.3X4	T42.3X5	T42.3X6
Butallylonal	T42.3X1	T42.3X2	T42.3X3	T42.3X4	T42.3X5	T42.3X6
Butamben	T41.3X1	T41.3X2	T41.3X3	T41.3X4	T41.3X5	T41.3X6
Butamirate	T48.3X1	T48.3X2	T48.3X3	T48.3X4	T48.3X5	T48.3X6
Butane (distributed in mobile container)	T59.891	T59.892	T59.893	T59.894	—	—
distributed through pipes	T59.891	T59.892	T59.893	T59.894	—	—
incomplete combustion	T58.11	T58.12	T58.13	T58.14	—	—
Butanilicaine	T41.3X1	T41.3X2	T41.3X3	T41.3X4	T41.3X5	T41.3X6
Butanol	T51.3X1	T51.3X2	T51.3X3	T51.3X4	—	—
Butanone, 2-butanone	T52.4X1	T52.4X2	T52.4X3	T52.4X4	—	—
Butantrone	T49.4X1	T49.4X2	T49.4X3	T49.4X4	T49.4X5	T49.4X6
Butaperazine	T43.3X1	T43.3X2	T43.3X3	T43.3X4	T43.3X5	T43.3X6
Butazolidin	T39.2X1	T39.2X2	T39.2X3	T39.2X4	T39.2X5	T39.2X6
Butetamate	T48.6X1	T48.6X2	T48.6X3	T48.6X4	T48.6X5	T48.6X6
Butethal	T42.3X1	T42.3X2	T42.3X3	T42.3X4	T42.3X5	T42.3X6
Butethamate	T44.3X1	T44.3X2	T44.3X3	T44.3X4	T44.3X5	T44.3X6
Buthalitone (sodium)	T41.1X1	T41.1X2	T41.1X3	T41.1X4	T41.1X5	T41.1X6
Butisol (sodium)	T42.3X1	T42.3X2	T42.3X3	T42.3X4	T42.3X5	T42.3X6
Butizide	T50.2X1	T50.2X2	T50.2X3	T50.2X4	T50.2X5	T50.2X6
Butobarbital	T42.3X1	T42.3X2	T42.3X3	T42.3X4	T42.3X5	T42.3X6
sodium	T42.3X1	T42.3X2	T42.3X3	T42.3X4	T42.3X5	T42.3X6
Butobarbitone	T42.3X1	T42.3X2	T42.3X3	T42.3X4	T42.3X5	T42.3X6
Butoconazole (nitrate)	T49.0X1	T49.0X2	T49.0X3	T49.0X4	T49.0X5	T49.0X6
Butorphanol	T40.4X1	T40.4X2	T40.4X3	T40.4X4	T40.4X5	T40.4X6
Butriptyline	T43.011	T43.012	T43.013	T43.014	T43.015	T43.016
Butropium bromide	T44.3X1	T44.3X2	T44.3X3	T44.3X4	T44.3X5	
Buttercups	T62.2X1	T62.2X2	T62.2X3	T62.2X4	—	—
Butter of antimony — see Antimony						
Butyl						
acetate (secondary)	T52.8X1	T52.8X2	T52.8X3	T52.8X4	—	—
alcohol	T51.3X1	T51.3X2	T51.3X3	T51.3X4	—	—
aminobenzoate	T41.3X1	T41.3X2	T41.3X3	T41.3X4	T41.3X5	T41.3X6
butyrate	T52.8X1	T52.8X2	T52.8X3	T52.8X4	—	—
carbinol	T51.3X1	T51.3X2	T51.3X3	T51.3X4	—	—
carbitol	T52.3X1	T52.3X2	T52.3X3	T52.3X4	—	—
cellosolve	T52.3X1	T52.3X2	T52.3X3	T52.3X4	—	—
chloral (hydrate)	T42.6X1	T42.6X2	T42.6X3	T42.6X4	T42.6X5	T42.6X6
formate	T52.8X1	T52.8X2	T52.8X3	T52.8X4	—	—
lactate	T52.8X1	T52.8X2	T52.8X3	T52.8X4	—	—
propionate	T52.8X1	T52.8X2	T52.8X3	T52.8X4	—	—
scopolamine bromide	T44.3X1	T44.3X2	T44.3X3	T44.3X4	T44.3X5	T44.3X6
thiobarbital sodium	T41.1X1	T41.1X2	T41.1X3	T41.1X4	T41.1X5	T41.1X6

Substance	Poisoning, Accidental (unintentional)	Poisoning, Intentional Self-harm	Poisoning, Assault	Poisoning, Undetermined	Adverse Effect	Under-dosing
Butylated hydroxanisole	T50.991	T50.992	T50.993	T50.994	T50.995	T50.996
Butylchloral hydrate	T42.6X1	T42.6X2	T42.6X3	T42.6X4	T42.6X5	T42.6X6
Butyltoluene	T52.2X1	T52.2X2	T52.2X3	T52.2X4	—	—
Butyn	T41.3X1	T41.3X2	T41.3X3	T41.3X4	T41.3X5	T41.3X6
Butyrophenone (-based tranquilizers)	T43.4X1	T43.4X2	T43.4X3	T43.4X4	T43.4X5	T43.4X6
Cabergoline	T42.8X1	T42.8X2	T42.8X3	T42.8X4	T42.8X5	T42.8X6
Cacodyl, cacodylic acid	T57.0X1	T57.0X2	T57.0X3	T57.0X4	—	—
Cactinomycin	T45.1X1	T45.1X2	T45.1X3	T45.1X4	T45.1X5	T45.1X6
Cade oil	T49.4X1	T49.4X2	T49.4X3	T49.4X4	T49.4X5	T49.4X6
Cadexomer iodine	T49.0X1	T49.0X2	T49.0X3	T49.0X4	T49.0X5	T49.0X6
Cadmium (chloride) (fumes) (oxide)	T56.3X1	T56.3X2	T56.3X3	T56.3X4	—	—
sulfide (medicinal) NEC	T49.4X1	T49.4X2	T49.4X3	T49.4X4	T49.4X5	T49.4X6
Cadralazine	T46.5X1	T46.5X2	T46.5X3	T46.5X4	T46.5X5	T46.5X6
Caffeine	T43.611	T43.612	T43.613	T43.614	T43.615	T43.616
Calabar bean	T62.2X1	T62.2X2	T62.2X3	T62.2X4	—	—
Caladium seguinum	T62.2X1	T62.2X2	T62.2X3	T62.2X4	—	—
Calamine (lotion)	T49.3X1	T49.3X2	T49.3X3	T49.3X4	T49.3X5	T49.3X6
Calcifediol	T45.2X1	T45.2X2	T45.2X3	T45.2X4	T45.2X5	T45.2X6
Calciferol	T45.2X1	T45.2X2	T45.2X3	T45.2X4	T45.2X5	T45.2X6
Calcitonin	T50.991	T50.992	T50.993	T50.994	T50.995	T50.996
Calcitriol	T45.2X1	T45.2X2	T45.2X3	T45.2X4	T45.2X5	T45.2X6
Calcium	T50.3X1	T50.3X2	T50.3X3	T50.3X4	T50.3X5	T50.3X6
actylsalicylate	T39.011	T39.012	T39.013	T39.014	T39.015	T39.016
benzamidosalicylate	T37.1X1	T37.1X2	T37.1X3	T37.1X4	T37.1X5	T37.1X6
bromide	T42.6X1	T42.6X2	T42.6X3	T42.6X4	T42.6X5	T42.6X6
bromolactobionate	T42.6X1	T42.6X2	T42.6X3	T42.6X4	T42.6X5	T42.6X6
carbaspirin	T39.011	T39.012	T39.013	T39.014	T39.015	T39.016
carbimide	T50.6X1	T50.6X2	T50.6X3	T50.6X4	T50.6X5	T50.6X6
carbonate	T47.1X1	T47.1X2	T47.1X3	T47.1X4	T47.1X5	T47.1X6
chloride	T50.991	T50.992	T50.993	T50.994	T50.995	T50.996
anhydrous	T50.991	T50.992	T50.993	T50.994	T50.995	T50.996
cyanide	T57.8X1	T57.8X2	T57.8X3	T57.8X4	—	—
dioctyl sulfosuccinate	T47.4X1	T47.4X2	T47.4X3	T47.4X4	T47.4X5	T47.4X6
disodium edathamil	T45.8X1	T45.8X2	T45.8X3	T45.8X4	T45.8X5	T45.8X6
disodium edetate	T45.8X1	T45.8X2	T45.8X3	T45.8X4	T45.8X5	T45.8X6
dobesilate	T46.991	T46.992	T46.993	T46.994	T46.995	T46.996
EDTA	T45.8X1	T45.8X2	T45.8X3	T45.8X4	T45.8X5	T45.8X6
ferrous citrate	T45.4X1	T45.4X2	T45.4X3	T45.4X4	T45.4X5	T45.4X6
folinate	T45.8X1	T45.8X2	T45.8X3	T45.8X4	T45.8X5	T45.8X6
glubionate	T50.3X1	T50.3X2	T50.3X3	T50.3X4	T50.3X5	T50.3X6
gluconate	T50.3X1	T50.3X2	T50.3X3	T50.3X4	T50.3X5	T50.3X6
gluconogalactogluconate	T50.3X1	T50.3X2	T50.3X3	T50.3X4	T50.3X5	T50.3X6
hydrate, hydroxide	T54.3X1	T54.3X2	T54.3X3	T54.3X4	—	—
hypochlorite	T54.3X1	T54.3X2	T54.3X3	T54.3X4	—	—
iodide	T48.4X1	T48.4X2	T48.4X3	T48.4X4	T48.4X5	T48.4X6
ipodate	T50.8X1	T50.8X2	T50.8X3	T50.8X4	T50.8X5	T50.8X6
lactate	T50.3X1	T50.3X2	T50.3X3	T50.3X4	T50.3X5	T50.3X6
leucovorin	T45.8X1	T45.8X2	T45.8X3	T45.8X4	T45.8X5	T45.8X6
mandelate	T37.91	T37.92	T37.93	T37.94	T37.95	T37.96
oxide	T54.3X1	T54.3X2	T54.3X3	T54.3X4	—	—
pantothenate	T45.2X1	T45.2X2	T45.2X3	T45.2X4	T45.2X5	T45.2X6
phosphate	T50.3X1	T50.3X2	T50.3X3	T50.3X4	T50.3X5	T50.3X6
salicylate	T39.091	T39.092	T39.093	T39.094	T39.095	T39.096
salts	T50.3X1	T50.3X2	T50.3X3	T50.3X4	T50.3X5	T50.3X6
Calculus-dissolving drug	T50.991	T50.992	T50.993	T50.994	T50.995	T50.996
Calomel	T49.0X1	T49.0X2	T49.0X3	T49.0X4	T49.0X5	T49.0X6
Caloric agent	T50.3X1	T50.3X2	T50.3X3	T50.3X4	T50.3X5	T50.3X6
Calusterone	T38.7X1	T38.7X2	T38.7X3	T38.7X4	T38.7X5	T38.7X6
Camazepam	T42.4X1	T42.4X2	T42.4X3	T42.4X4	T42.4X5	T42.4X6
Camomile	T49.0X1	T49.0X2	T49.0X3	T49.0X4	T49.0X5	T49.0X6
Camoquin	T37.2X1	T37.2X2	T37.2X3	T37.2X4	T37.2X5	T37.2X6
Camphor						
insecticide	T60.2X1	T60.2X2	T60.2X3	T60.2X4	—	—
medicinal	T49.8X1	T49.8X2	T49.8X3	T49.8X4	T49.8X5	T49.8X6
Camylofin	T44.3X1	T44.3X2	T44.3X3	T44.3X4	T44.3X5	T44.3X6
Cancer chemotherapy drug regimen	T45.1X1	T45.1X2	T45.1X3	T45.1X4	T45.1X5	T45.1X6
Candeptin	T49.0X1	T49.0X2	T49.0X3	T49.0X4	T49.0X5	T49.0X6
Candicidin	T49.0X1	T49.0X2	T49.0X3	T49.0X4	T49.0X5	T49.0X6
Cannabinol	T40.7X1	T40.7X2	T40.7X3	T40.7X4	T40.7X5	T40.7X6
Cannabis (derivatives)	T40.7X1	T40.7X2	T40.7X3	T40.7X4	T40.7X5	T40.7X6
Canned heat	T51.1X1	T51.1X2	T51.1X3	T51.1X4	—	—
Canrenoic acid	T50.0X1	T50.0X2	T50.0X3	T50.0X4	T50.0X5	T50.0X6
Canrenone	T50.0X1	T50.0X2	T50.0X3	T50.0X4	T50.0X5	T50.0X6
Cantharides, cantharidin, cantharis	T49.8X1	T49.8X2	T49.8X3	T49.8X4	T49.8X5	T49.8X6
Canthaxanthin	T50.991	T50.992	T50.993	T50.994	T50.995	T50.996
Capillary-active drug NEC	T46.901	T46.902	T46.903	T46.904	T46.905	T46.906
Capreomycin	T36.8X1	T36.8X2	T36.8X3	T36.8X4	T36.8X5	T36.8X6
Capsicum	T49.4X1	T49.4X2	T49.4X3	T49.4X4	T49.4X5	T49.4X6
Captafol	T60.3X1	T60.3X2	T60.3X3	T60.3X4	—	—
Captan	T60.3X1	T60.3X2	T60.3X3	T60.3X4	—	—
Captodiame, captodiamine	T43.591	T43.592	T43.593	T43.594	T43.595	T43.596
Captopril	T46.4X1	T46.4X2	T46.4X3	T46.4X4	T46.4X5	T46.4X6
Caramiphen	T44.3X1	T44.3X2	T44.3X3	T44.3X4	T44.3X5	T44.3X6
Carazolol	T44.7X1	T44.7X2	T44.7X3	T44.7X4	T44.7X5	T44.7X6
Carbachol	T44.1X1	T44.1X2	T44.1X3	T44.1X4	T44.1X5	T44.1X6
Carbacrylamine (resin)	T50.3X1	T50.3X2	T50.3X3	T50.3X4	T50.3X5	T50.3X6
Carbamate (insecticide)	T60.0X1	T60.0X2	T60.0X3	T60.0X4	—	—
Carbamate (sedative)	T42.6X1	T42.6X2	T42.6X3	T42.6X4	T42.6X5	T42.6X6
herbicide	T60.0X1	T60.0X2	T60.0X3	T60.0X4	—	—
insecticide	T60.0X1	T60.0X2	T60.0X3	T60.0X4	—	—
Carbamazepine	T42.1X1	T42.1X2	T42.1X3	T42.1X4	T42.1X5	T42.1X6
Carbamide	T47.3X1	T47.3X2	T47.3X3	T47.3X4	T47.3X5	T47.3X6
peroxide	T49.0X1	T49.0X2	T49.0X3	T49.0X4	T49.0X5	T49.0X6
topical	T49.8X1	T49.8X2	T49.8X3	T49.8X4	T49.8X5	T49.8X6
Carbamylcholine chloride	T44.1X1	T44.1X2	T44.1X3	T44.1X4	T44.1X5	T44.1X6
Carbaril	T60.0X1	T60.0X2	T60.0X3	T60.0X4	—	—
Carbarsone	T37.3X1	T37.3X2	T37.3X3	T37.3X4	T37.3X5	T37.3X6
Carbaryl	T60.0X1	T60.0X2	T60.0X3	T60.0X4	—	—
Carbaspirin	T39.011	T39.012	T39.013	T39.014	T39.015	T39.016
Carbazochrome (salicylate) (sodium sulfonate)	T49.4X1	T49.4X2	T49.4X3	T49.4X4	T49.4X5	T49.4X6
Carbenicillin	T36.0X1	T36.0X2	T36.0X3	T36.0X4	T36.0X5	T36.0X6
Carbenoxolone	T47.1X1	T47.1X2	T47.1X3	T47.1X4	T47.1X5	T47.1X6
Carbetapentane	T48.3X1	T48.3X2	T48.3X3	T48.3X4	T48.3X5	T48.3X6
Carbethyl salicylate	T39.091	T39.092	T39.093	T39.094	T39.095	T39.096
Carbidopa (with levodopa)	T42.8X1	T42.8X2	T42.8X3	T42.8X4	T42.8X5	T42.8X6
Carbimazole	T38.2X1	T38.2X2	T38.2X3	T38.2X4	T38.2X5	T38.2X6
Carbinol	T51.1X1	T51.1X2	T51.1X3	T51.1X4	—	—
Carbinoxamine	T45.0X1	T45.0X2	T45.0X3	T45.0X4	T45.0X5	T45.0X6
Carbiphene	T39.8X1	T39.8X2	T39.8X3	T39.8X4	T39.8X5	T39.8X6
Carbitol	T52.3X1	T52.3X2	T52.3X3	T52.3X4	—	—
Carbocaine	T41.3X1	T41.3X2	T41.3X3	T41.3X4	T41.3X5	T41.3X6
infiltration (subcutaneous)	T41.3X1	T41.3X2	T41.3X3	T41.3X4	T41.3X5	T41.3X6
nerve block (peripheral) (plexus)	T41.3X1	T41.3X2	T41.3X3	T41.3X4	T41.3X5	T41.3X6
topical (surface)	T41.3X1	T41.3X2	T41.3X3	T41.3X4	T41.3X5	T41.3X6
Carbocisteine	T48.4X1	T48.4X2	T48.4X3	T48.4X4	T48.4X5	T48.4X6
Carbocromen	T46.3X1	T46.3X2	T46.3X3	T46.3X4	T46.3X5	T46.3X6
Carbol fuchsin	T49.0X1	T49.0X2	T49.0X3	T49.0X4	T49.0X5	T49.0X6
Carbolic acid — see also Phenol	T54.0X1	T54.0X2	T54.0X3	T54.0X4	—	—
Carbolonium (bromide)	T48.1X1	T48.1X2	T48.1X3	T48.1X4	T48.1X5	T48.1X6
Carbo medicinalis	T47.6X1	T47.6X2	T47.6X3	T47.6X4	T47.6X5	T47.6X6
Carbomycin	T36.8X1	T36.8X2	T36.8X3	T36.8X4	T36.8X5	T36.8X6
Carbon						
bisulfide (liquid)	T65.4X1	T65.4X2	T65.4X3	T65.4X4	—	—
vapor	T65.4X1	T65.4X2	T65.4X3	T65.4X4	—	—
dioxide (gas)	T59.7X1	T59.7X2	T59.7X3	T59.7X4	—	—
medicinal	T41.5X1	T41.5X2	T41.5X3	T41.5X4	T41.5X5	T41.5X6
nonmedicinal	T59.7X1	T59.7X2	T59.7X3	T59.7X4	—	—
snow	T49.4X1	T49.4X2	T49.4X3	T49.4X4	T49.4X5	T49.4X6
disulfide (liquid)	T65.4X1	T65.4X2	T65.4X3	T65.4X4	—	—
vapor	T65.4X1	T65.4X2	T65.4X3	T65.4X4	—	—
monoxide (from incomplete combustion)	T58.91	T58.92	T58.93	T58.94	—	—
blast furnace gas	T58.8X1	T58.8X2	T58.8X3	T58.8X4	—	—
butane (distributed in mobile container)	T58.11	T58.12	T58.13	T58.14	—	—
distributed through pipes	T58.11	T58.12	T58.13	T58.14	—	—
charcoal fumes	T58.2X1	T58.2X2	T58.2X3	T58.2X4	—	—
coal	T58.2X1	T58.2X2	T58.2X3	T58.2X4	—	—
coke (in domestic stoves, fireplaces)	T58.2X1	T58.2X2	T58.2X3	T58.2X4	—	—
exhaust gas (motor) not in transit	T58.01	T58.02	T58.03	T58.04	—	—
combustion engine, any not in watercraft	T58.01	T58.02	T58.03	T58.04	—	—
farm tractor, not in transit	T58.01	T58.02	T58.03	T58.04	—	—
gas engine	T58.01	T58.02	T58.03	T58.04	—	—
motor pump	T58.01	T58.02	T58.03	T58.04	—	—
motor vehicle, not in transit	T58.01	T58.02	T58.03	T58.04	—	—
fuel (in domestic use)	T58.2X1	T58.2X2	T58.2X3	T58.2X4	—	—
gas (piped)	T58.11	T58.12	T58.13	T58.14	—	—
in mobile container	T58.11	T58.12	T58.13	T58.14	—	—
piped (natural)	T58.11	T58.12	T58.13	T58.14	—	—
utility	T58.11	T58.12	T58.13	T58.14	—	—
in mobile container	T58.11	T58.12	T58.13	T58.14	—	—
gas (piped)	T58.11	T58.12	T58.13	T58.14	—	—
illuminating gas	T58.11	T58.12	T58.13	T58.14	—	—

Substance	Poisoning, Accidental (unintentional)	Poisoning, Intentional Self-harm	Poisoning, Assault	Poisoning, Undetermined	Adverse Effect	Under-dosing
Carbon — *continued*						
monoxide — *continued*						
industrial fuels or gases, any	T58.8X1	T58.8X2	T58.8X3	T58.8X4	—	—
kerosene (in domestic stoves, fireplaces)	T58.2X1	T58.2X2	T58.2X3	T58.2X4	—	—
kiln gas or vapor	T58.8X1	T58.8X2	T58.8X3	T58.8X4	—	—
motor exhaust gas, not in transit	T58.Ø1	T58.Ø2	T58.Ø3	T58.Ø4	—	—
piped gas (manufactured) (natural)	T58.11	T58.12	T58.13	T58.14	—	—
producer gas	T58.8X1	T58.8X2	T58.8X3	T58.8X4	—	—
propane (distributed in mobile container)	T58.11	T58.12	T58.13	T58.14	—	—
distributed through pipes	T58.11	T58.12	T58.13	T58.14	—	—
solid (in domestic stoves, fireplaces)	T58.2X1	T58.2X2	T58.2X3	T58.2X4	—	—
specified source NEC	T58.8X1	T58.8X2	T58.8X3	T58.8X4	—	—
stove gas	T58.11	T58.12	T58.13	T58.14	—	—
piped	T58.11	T58.12	T58.13	T58.14	—	—
utility gas	T58.11	T58.12	T58.13	T58.14	—	—
piped	T58.11	T58.12	T58.13	T58.14	—	—
water gas	T58.11	T58.12	T58.13	T58.14	—	—
wood (in domestic stoves, fireplaces)	T58.2X1	T58.2X2	T58.2X3	T58.2X4	—	—
tetrachloride (vapor) NEC	T53.ØX1	T53.ØX2	T53.ØX3	T53.ØX4	—	—
liquid (cleansing agent) NEC	T53.ØX1	T53.ØX2	T53.ØX3	T53.ØX4	—	—
solvent	T53.ØX1	T53.ØX2	T53.ØX3	T53.ØX4	—	—
Carbonic acid gas	T59.7X1	T59.7X2	T59.7X3	T59.7X4	—	—
anhydrase inhibitor NEC	T5Ø.2X1	T5Ø.2X2	T5Ø.2X3	T5Ø.2X4	T5Ø.2X5	T5Ø.2X6
Carbophenothion	T6Ø.ØX1	T6Ø.ØX2	T6Ø.ØX3	T6Ø.ØX4	—	—
Carboplatin	T45.1X1	T45.1X2	T45.1X3	T45.1X4	T45.1X5	T45.1X6
Carboprost	T48.ØX1	T48.ØX2	T48.ØX3	T48.ØX4	T48.ØX5	T48.ØX6
Carboquone	T45.1X1	T45.1X2	T45.1X3	T45.1X4	T45.1X5	T45.1X6
Carbowax	T49.3X1	T49.3X2	T49.3X3	T49.3X4	T49.3X5	T49.3X6
Carboxymethylcellulose	T47.4X1	T47.4X2	T47.4X3	T47.4X4	T47.4X5	T47.4X6
Carbrital	T42.3X1	T42.3X2	T42.3X3	T42.3X4	T42.3X5	T42.3X6
Carbromal	T42.6X1	T42.6X2	T42.6X3	T42.6X4	T42.6X5	T42.6X6
Carbutamide	T38.3X1	T38.3X2	T38.3X3	T38.3X4	T38.3X5	T38.3X6
Carbuterol	T48.6X1	T48.6X2	T48.6X3	T48.6X4	T48.6X5	T48.6X6
Cardiac						
depressants	T46.2X1	T46.2X2	T46.2X3	T46.2X4	T46.2X5	T46.2X6
rhythm regulator	T46.2X1	T46.2X2	T46.2X3	T46.2X4	T46.2X5	T46.2X6
specified NEC	T46.2X1	T46.2X2	T46.2X3	T46.2X4	T46.2X5	T46.2X6
Cardiografin	T5Ø.8X1	T5Ø.8X2	T5Ø.8X3	T5Ø.8X4	T5Ø.8X5	T5Ø.8X6
Cardiogreen	T5Ø.8X1	T5Ø.8X2	T5Ø.8X3	T5Ø.8X4	T5Ø.8X5	T5Ø.8X6
Cardiotonic (glycoside) **NEC**	T46.ØX1	T46.ØX2	T46.ØX3	T46.ØX4	T46.ØX5	T46.ØX6
Cardiovascular drug NEC	T46.9Ø1	T46.9Ø2	T46.9Ø3	T46.9Ø4	T46.9Ø5	T46.9Ø6
Cardrase	T5Ø.2X1	T5Ø.2X2	T5Ø.2X3	T5Ø.2X4	T5Ø.2X5	T5Ø.2X6
Carfecillin	T36.ØX1	T36.ØX2	T36.ØX3	T36.ØX4	T36.ØX5	T36.ØX6
Carfenazine	T43.3X1	T43.3X2	T43.3X3	T43.3X4	T43.3X5	T43.3X6
Carfusin	T49.ØX1	T49.ØX2	T49.ØX3	T49.ØX4	T49.ØX5	T49.ØX6
Carindacillin	T36.ØX1	T36.ØX2	T36.ØX3	T36.ØX4	T36.ØX5	T36.ØX6
Carisoprodol	T42.8X1	T42.8X2	T42.8X3	T42.8X4	T42.8X5	T42.8X6
Carmellose	T47.4X1	T47.4X2	T47.4X3	T47.4X4	T47.4X5	T47.4X6
Carminative	T47.5X1	T47.5X2	T47.5X3	T47.5X4	T47.5X5	T47.5X6
Carmofur	T45.1X1	T45.1X2	T45.1X3	T45.1X4	T45.1X5	T45.1X6
Carmustine	T45.1X1	T45.1X2	T45.1X3	T45.1X4	T45.1X5	T45.1X6
Carotene	T45.2X1	T45.2X2	T45.2X3	T45.2X4	T45.2X5	T45.2X6
Carphenazine	T43.3X1	T43.3X2	T43.3X3	T43.3X4	T43.3X5	T43.3X6
Carpipramine	T42.4X1	T42.4X2	T42.4X3	T42.4X4	T42.4X5	T42.4X6
Carprofen	T39.311	T39.312	T39.313	T39.314	T39.315	T39.316
Carpronium chloride	T44.3X1	T44.3X2	T44.3X3	T44.3X4	T44.3X5	T44.3X6
Carrageenan	T47.8X1	T47.8X2	T47.8X3	T47.8X4	T47.8X5	T47.8X6
Carteolol	T44.7X1	T44.7X2	T44.7X3	T44.7X4	T44.7X5	T44.7X6
Carter's Little Pills	T47.2X1	T47.2X2	T47.2X3	T47.2X4	T47.2X5	T47.2X6
Cascara (sagrada)	T47.2X1	T47.2X2	T47.2X3	T47.2X4	T47.2X5	T47.2X6
Cassava	T62.2X1	T62.2X2	T62.2X3	T62.2X4	—	—
Castellani's paint	T49.ØX1	T49.ØX2	T49.ØX3	T49.ØX4	T49.ØX5	T49.ØX6
Castor						
bean	T62.2X1	T62.2X2	T62.2X3	T62.2X4	—	—
oil	T47.2X1	T47.2X2	T47.2X3	T47.2X4	T47.2X5	T47.2X6
Catalase	T45.3X1	T45.3X2	T45.3X3	T45.3X4	T45.3X5	T45.3X6
Caterpillar (sting)	T63.431	T63.432	T63.433	T63.434	—	—
Catha (edulis) (tea)	T43.691	T43.692	T43.693	T43.694	—	—
Cathartic NEC	T47.4X1	T47.4X2	T47.4X3	T47.4X4	T47.4X5	T47.4X6
anthracene derivative	T47.2X1	T47.2X2	T47.2X3	T47.2X4	T47.2X5	T47.2X6
bulk	T47.4X1	T47.4X2	T47.4X3	T47.4X4	T47.4X5	T47.4X6
contact	T47.2X1	T47.2X2	T47.2X3	T47.2X4	T47.2X5	T47.2X6
emollient NEC	T47.4X1	T47.4X2	T47.4X3	T47.4X4	T47.4X5	T47.4X6
irritant NEC	T47.2X1	T47.2X2	T47.2X3	T47.2X4	T47.2X5	T47.2X6

Substance	Poisoning, Accidental (unintentional)	Poisoning, Intentional Self-harm	Poisoning, Assault	Poisoning, Undetermined	Adverse Effect	Under-dosing
Cathartic — *continued*						
mucilage	T47.4X1	T47.4X2	T47.4X3	T47.4X4	T47.4X5	T47.4X6
saline	T47.3X1	T47.3X2	T47.3X3	T47.3X4	T47.3X5	T47.3X6
vegetable	T47.2X1	T47.2X2	T47.2X3	T47.2X4	T47.2X5	T47.2X6
Cathine	T5Ø.5X1	T5Ø.5X2	T5Ø.5X3	T5Ø.5X4	T5Ø.5X5	T5Ø.5X6
Cathomycin	T36.8X1	T36.8X2	T36.8X3	T36.8X4	T36.8X5	T36.8X6
Cation exchange resin	T5Ø.3X1	T5Ø.3X2	T5Ø.3X3	T5Ø.3X4	T5Ø.3X5	T5Ø.3X6
Caustic(s) NEC	T54.91	T54.92	T54.93	T54.94	—	—
alkali	T54.3X1	T54.3X2	T54.3X3	T54.3X4	—	—
hydroxide	T54.3X1	T54.3X2	T54.3X3	T54.3X4	—	—
potash	T54.3X1	T54.3X2	T54.3X3	T54.3X4	—	—
soda	T54.3X1	T54.3X2	T54.3X3	T54.3X4	—	—
specified NEC	T54.91	T54.92	T54.93	T54.94	—	—
Ceepryn	T49.ØX1	T49.ØX2	T49.ØX3	T49.ØX4	T49.ØX5	T49.ØX6
ENT agent	T49.6X1	T49.6X2	T49.6X3	T49.6X4	T49.6X5	T49.6X6
lozenges	T49.6X1	T49.6X2	T49.6X3	T49.6X4	T49.6X5	T49.6X6
Cefacetrile	T36.1X1	T36.1X2	T36.1X3	T36.1X4	T36.1X5	T36.1X6
Cefaclor	T36.1X1	T36.1X2	T36.1X3	T36.1X4	T36.1X5	T36.1X6
Cefadroxil	T36.1X1	T36.1X2	T36.1X3	T36.1X4	T36.1X5	T36.1X6
Cefalexin	T36.1X1	T36.1X2	T36.1X3	T36.1X4	T36.1X5	T36.1X6
Cefaloglycin	T36.1X1	T36.1X2	T36.1X3	T36.1X4	T36.1X5	T36.1X6
Cefaloridine	T36.1X1	T36.1X2	T36.1X3	T36.1X4	T36.1X5	T36.1X6
Cefalosporins	T36.1X1	T36.1X2	T36.1X3	T36.1X4	T36.1X5	T36.1X6
Cefalotin	T36.1X1	T36.1X2	T36.1X3	T36.1X4	T36.1X5	T36.1X6
Cefamandole	T36.1X1	T36.1X2	T36.1X3	T36.1X4	T36.1X5	T36.1X6
Cefamycin antibiotic	T36.1X1	T36.1X2	T36.1X3	T36.1X4	T36.1X5	T36.1X6
Cefapirin	T36.1X1	T36.1X2	T36.1X3	T36.1X4	T36.1X5	T36.1X6
Cefatrizine	T36.1X1	T36.1X2	T36.1X3	T36.1X4	T36.1X5	T36.1X6
Cefazedone	T36.1X1	T36.1X2	T36.1X3	T36.1X4	T36.1X5	T36.1X6
Cefazolin	T36.1X1	T36.1X2	T36.1X3	T36.1X4	T36.1X5	T36.1X6
Cefbuperazone	T36.1X1	T36.1X2	T36.1X3	T36.1X4	T36.1X5	T36.1X6
Cefetamet	T36.1X1	T36.1X2	T36.1X3	T36.1X4	T36.1X5	T36.1X6
Cefixime	T36.1X1	T36.1X2	T36.1X3	T36.1X4	T36.1X5	T36.1X6
Cefmenoxime	T36.1X1	T36.1X2	T36.1X3	T36.1X4	T36.1X5	T36.1X6
Cefmetazole	T36.1X1	T36.1X2	T36.1X3	T36.1X4	T36.1X5	T36.1X6
Cefminox	T36.1X1	T36.1X2	T36.1X3	T36.1X4	T36.1X5	T36.1X6
Cefonicid	T36.1X1	T36.1X2	T36.1X3	T36.1X4	T36.1X5	T36.1X6
Cefoperazone	T36.1X1	T36.1X2	T36.1X3	T36.1X4	T36.1X5	T36.1X6
Ceforanide	T36.1X1	T36.1X2	T36.1X3	T36.1X4	T36.1X5	T36.1X6
Cefotaxime	T36.1X1	T36.1X2	T36.1X3	T36.1X4	T36.1X5	T36.1X6
Cefotetan	T36.1X1	T36.1X2	T36.1X3	T36.1X4	T36.1X5	T36.1X6
Cefotiam	T36.1X1	T36.1X2	T36.1X3	T36.1X4	T36.1X5	T36.1X6
Cefoxitin	T36.1X1	T36.1X2	T36.1X3	T36.1X4	T36.1X5	T36.1X6
Cefpimizole	T36.1X1	T36.1X2	T36.1X3	T36.1X4	T36.1X5	T36.1X6
Cefpiramide	T36.1X1	T36.1X2	T36.1X3	T36.1X4	T36.1X5	T36.1X6
Cefradine	T36.1X1	T36.1X2	T36.1X3	T36.1X4	T36.1X5	T36.1X6
Cefroxadine	T36.1X1	T36.1X2	T36.1X3	T36.1X4	T36.1X5	T36.1X6
Cefsulodin	T36.1X1	T36.1X2	T36.1X3	T36.1X4	T36.1X5	T36.1X6
Ceftazidime	T36.1X1	T36.1X2	T36.1X3	T36.1X4	T36.1X5	T36.1X6
Cefteram	T36.1X1	T36.1X2	T36.1X3	T36.1X4	T36.1X5	T36.1X6
Ceftezole	T36.1X1	T36.1X2	T36.1X3	T36.1X4	T36.1X5	T36.1X6
Ceftizoxime	T36.1X1	T36.1X2	T36.1X3	T36.1X4	T36.1X5	T36.1X6
Ceftriaxone	T36.1X1	T36.1X2	T36.1X3	T36.1X4	T36.1X5	T36.1X6
Cefuroxime	T36.1X1	T36.1X2	T36.1X3	T36.1X4	T36.1X5	T36.1X6
Cefuzonam	T36.1X1	T36.1X2	T36.1X3	T36.1X4	T36.1X5	T36.1X6
Celestone	T38.ØX1	T38.ØX2	T38.ØX3	T38.ØX4	T38.ØX5	T38.ØX6
topical	T49.ØX1	T49.ØX2	T49.ØX3	T49.ØX4	T49.ØX5	T49.ØX6
Celiprolol	T44.7X1	T44.7X2	T44.7X3	T44.7X4	T44.7X5	T44.7X6
Cellosolve	T52.91	T52.92	T52.93	T52.94	—	—
Cell stimulants and proliferants	T49.8X1	T49.8X2	T49.8X3	T49.8X4	T49.8X5	T49.8X6
Cellulose						
cathartic	T47.4X1	T47.4X2	T47.4X3	T47.4X4	T47.4X5	T47.4X6
hydroxyethyl	T47.4X1	T47.4X2	T47.4X3	T47.4X4	T47.4X5	T47.4X6
nitrates (topical)	T49.3X1	T49.3X2	T49.3X3	T49.3X4	T49.3X5	T49.3X6
oxidized	T49.4X1	T49.4X2	T49.4X3	T49.4X4	T49.4X5	T49.4X6
Centipede (bite)	T63.411	T63.412	T63.413	T63.414	—	—
Central nervous system						
depressants	T42.71	T42.72	T42.73	T42.74	T42.75	T42.76
anesthetic (general) NEC	T41.2Ø1	T41.2Ø2	T41.2Ø3	T41.2Ø4	T41.2Ø5	T41.2Ø6
gases NEC	T41.ØX1	T41.ØX2	T41.ØX3	T41.ØX4	T41.ØX5	T41.ØX6
intravenous	T41.1X1	T41.1X2	T41.1X3	T41.1X4	T41.1X5	T41.1X6
barbiturates	T42.3X1	T42.3X2	T42.3X3	T42.3X4	T42.3X5	T42.3X6
benzodiazepines	T42.4X1	T42.4X2	T42.4X3	T42.4X4	T42.4X5	T42.4X6
bromides	T42.6X1	T42.6X2	T42.6X3	T42.6X4	T42.6X5	T42.6X6
cannabis sativa	T4Ø.7X1	T4Ø.7X2	T4Ø.7X3	T4Ø.7X4	T4Ø.7X5	T4Ø.7X6
chloral hydrate	T42.6X1	T42.6X2	T42.6X3	T42.6X4	T42.6X5	T42.6X6
ethanol	T51.ØX1	T51.ØX2	T51.ØX3	T51.ØX4	—	—
hallucinogenics	T4Ø.9Ø1	T4Ø.9Ø2	T4Ø.9Ø3	T4Ø.9Ø4	T4Ø.9Ø5	T4Ø.9Ø6
hypnotics	T42.71	T42.72	T42.73	T42.74	T42.75	T42.76
specified NEC	T42.6X1	T42.6X2	T42.6X3	T42.6X4	T42.6X5	T42.6X6
muscle relaxants	T42.8X1	T42.8X2	T42.8X3	T42.8X4	T42.8X5	T42.8X6
paraldehyde	T42.6X1	T42.6X2	T42.6X3	T42.6X4	T42.6X5	T42.6X6

Additional Character May Be Required — Refer to the Tabular List for Character Selection ▽ Subterms under main terms may continue to next column or page

Substance	Poisoning, Accidental (unintentional)	Poisoning, Intentional Self-harm	Poisoning, Assault	Poisoning, Undetermined	Adverse Effect	Under-dosing
Central nervous system — *continued*						
depressants — *continued*						
sedatives;	T42.71	T42.72	T42.73	T42.74	T42.75	T42.76
sedative-hypnotics						
mixed NEC	T42.6X1	T42.6X2	T42.6X3	T42.6X4	T42.6X5	T42.6X6
specified NEC	T42.6X1	T42.6X2	T42.6X3	T42.6X4	T42.6X5	T42.6X6
muscle-tone depressants	T42.8X1	T42.8X2	T42.8X3	T42.8X4	T42.8X5	T42.8X6
stimulants	T43.601	T43.602	T43.603	T43.604	T43.605	T43.606
amphetamines	T43.621	T43.622	T43.623	T43.624	T43.625	T43.626
analeptics	T50.7X1	T50.7X2	T50.7X3	T50.7X4	T50.7X5	T50.7X6
antidepressants	T43.201	T43.202	T43.203	T43.204	T43.205	T43.206
opiate antagonists	T50.7X1	T50.7X2	T50.7X3	T50.7X4	T50.7X5	T50.7X6
specified NEC	T43.691	T43.692	T43.693	T43.694	T43.695	T43.696
Cephalexin	T36.1X1	T36.1X2	T36.1X3	T36.1X4	T36.1X5	T36.1X6
Cephaloglycin	T36.1X1	T36.1X2	T36.1X3	T36.1X4	T36.1X5	T36.1X6
Cephaloridine	T36.1X1	T36.1X2	T36.1X3	T36.1X4	T36.1X5	T36.1X6
Cephalosporins	T36.1X1	T36.1X2	T36.1X3	T36.1X4	T36.1X5	T36.1X6
N (adicillin)	T36.0X1	T36.0X2	T36.0X3	T36.0X4	T36.0X5	T36.0X6
Cephalothin	T36.1X1	T36.1X2	T36.1X3	T36.1X4	T36.1X5	T36.1X6
Cephalotin	T36.1X1	T36.1X2	T36.1X3	T36.1X4	T36.1X5	T36.1X6
Cephradine	T36.1X1	T36.1X2	T36.1X3	T36.1X4	T36.1X5	T36.1X6
Cerbera (odallam)	T62.2X1	T62.2X2	T62.2X3	T62.2X4	—	—
Cerberin	T46.0X1	T46.0X2	T46.0X3	T46.0X4	T46.0X5	T46.0X6
Cerebral stimulants	T43.601	T43.602	T43.603	T43.604	T43.605	T43.606
psychotherapeutic	T43.601	T43.602	T43.603	T43.604	T43.605	T43.606
specified NEC	T43.691	T43.692	T43.693	T43.694	T43.695	T43.696
Cerium oxalate	T45.0X1	T45.0X2	T45.0X3	T45.0X4	T45.0X5	T45.0X6
Cerous oxalate	T45.0X1	T45.0X2	T45.0X3	T45.0X4	T45.0X5	T45.0X6
Ceruletide	T50.8X1	T50.8X2	T50.8X3	T50.8X4	T50.8X5	T50.8X6
Cetalkonium (chloride)	T49.0X1	T49.0X2	T49.0X3	T49.0X4	T49.0X5	T49.0X6
Cethexonium chloride	T49.0X1	T49.0X2	T49.0X3	T49.0X4	T49.0X5	T49.0X6
Cetiedil	T46.7X1	T46.7X2	T46.7X3	T46.7X4	T46.7X5	T46.7X6
Cetirizine	T45.0X1	T45.0X2	T45.0X3	T45.0X4	T45.0X5	T45.0X6
Cetomacrogol	T50.991	T50.992	T50.993	T50.994	T50.995	T50.996
Cetotiamine	T45.2X1	T45.2X2	T45.2X3	T45.2X4	T45.2X5	T45.2X6
Cetoxime	T45.0X1	T45.0X2	T45.0X3	T45.0X4	T45.0X5	T45.0X6
Cetraxate	T47.1X1	T47.1X2	T47.1X3	T47.1X4	T47.1X5	T47.1X6
Cetrimide	T49.0X1	T49.0X2	T49.0X3	T49.0X4	T49.0X5	T49.0X6
Cetrimonium (bromide)	T49.0X1	T49.0X2	T49.0X3	T49.0X4	T49.0X5	T49.0X6
Cetylpyridinium chloride	T49.0X1	T49.0X2	T49.0X3	T49.0X4	T49.0X5	T49.0X6
ENT agent	T49.6X1	T49.6X2	T49.6X3	T49.6X4	T49.6X5	T49.6X6
lozenges	T49.6X1	T49.6X2	T49.6X3	T49.6X4	T49.6X5	T49.6X6
Cevadilla — *see* Sabadilla						
Cevitamic acid	T45.2X1	T45.2X2	T45.2X3	T45.2X4	T45.2X5	T45.2X6
Chalk, precipitated	T47.1X1	T47.1X2	T47.1X3	T47.1X4	T47.1X5	T47.1X6
Chamomile	T49.0X1	T49.0X2	T49.0X3	T49.0X4	T49.0X5	T49.0X6
Ch'an su	T46.0X1	T46.0X2	T46.0X3	T46.0X4	T46.0X5	T46.0X6
Charcoal	T47.6X1	T47.6X2	T47.6X3	T47.6X4	T47.6X5	T47.6X6
activated — *see also* Charcoal, medicinal	T47.6X1	T47.6X2	T47.6X3	T47.6X4	T47.6X5	T47.6X6
fumes (Carbon monoxide)	T58.2X1	T58.2X2	T58.2X3	T58.2X4	—	—
industrial	T58.8X1	T58.8X2	T58.8X3	T58.8X4	—	—
medicinal (activated)	T47.6X1	T47.6X2	T47.6X3	T47.6X4	T47.6X5	T47.6X6
antidiarrheal	T47.6X1	T47.6X2	T47.6X3	T47.6X4	T47.6X5	T47.6X6
poison control	T47.8X1	T47.8X2	T47.8X3	T47.8X4	T47.8X5	T47.8X6
specified use other than for diarrhea	T47.8X1	T47.8X2	T47.8X3	T47.8X4	T47.8X5	T47.8X6
topical	T49.8X1	T49.8X2	T49.8X3	T49.8X4	T49.8X5	T49.8X6
Chaulmosulfone	T37.1X1	T37.1X2	T37.1X3	T37.1X4	T37.1X5	T37.1X6
Chelating agent NEC	T50.6X1	T50.6X2	T50.6X3	T50.6X4	T50.6X5	T50.6X6
Chelidonium majus	T62.2X1	T62.2X2	T62.2X3	T62.2X4	—	—
Chemical substance NEC	T65.91	T65.92	T65.93	T65.94	—	—
Chenodeoxycholic acid	T47.5X1	T47.5X2	T47.5X3	T47.5X4	T47.5X5	T47.5X6
Chenodiol	T47.5X1	T47.5X2	T47.5X3	T47.5X4	T47.5X5	T47.5X6
Chenopodium	T37.4X1	T37.4X2	T37.4X3	T37.4X4	T37.4X5	T37.4X6
Cherry laurel	T62.2X1	T62.2X2	T62.2X3	T62.2X4	—	—
Chinidin (e)	T46.2X1	T46.2X2	T46.2X3	T46.2X4	T46.2X5	T46.2X6
Chiniofon	T37.8X1	T37.8X2	T37.8X3	T37.8X4	T37.8X5	T37.8X6
Chlophedianol	T48.3X1	T48.3X2	T48.3X3	T48.3X4	T48.3X5	T48.3X6
Chloral	T42.6X1	T42.6X2	T42.6X3	T42.6X4	T42.6X5	T42.6X6
derivative	T42.6X1	T42.6X2	T42.6X3	T42.6X4	T42.6X5	T42.6X6
hydrate	T42.6X1	T42.6X2	T42.6X3	T42.6X4	T42.6X5	T42.6X6
Chloralamide	T42.6X1	T42.6X2	T42.6X3	T42.6X4	T42.6X5	T42.6X6
Chloralodol	T42.6X1	T42.6X2	T42.6X3	T42.6X4	T42.6X5	T42.6X6
Chloralose	T60.4X1	T60.4X2	T60.4X3	T60.4X4	—	—
Chlorambucil	T45.1X1	T45.1X2	T45.1X3	T45.1X4	T45.1X5	T45.1X6
Chloramine	T57.8X1	T57.8X2	T57.8X3	T57.8X4	—	—
T	T49.0X1	T49.0X2	T49.0X3	T49.0X4	T49.0X5	T49.0X6
topical	T49.0X1	T49.0X2	T49.0X3	T49.0X4	T49.0X5	T49.0X6
Chloramphenicol	T36.2X1	T36.2X2	T36.2X3	T36.2X4	T36.2X5	T36.2X6
ENT agent	T49.6X1	T49.6X2	T49.6X3	T49.6X4	T49.6X5	T49.6X6
ophthalmic preparation	T49.5X1	T49.5X2	T49.5X3	T49.5X4	T49.5X5	T49.5X6

Substance	Poisoning, Accidental (unintentional)	Poisoning, Intentional Self-harm	Poisoning, Assault	Poisoning, Undetermined	Adverse Effect	Under-dosing
Chloramphenicol — *continued*						
topical NEC	T49.0X1	T49.0X2	T49.0X3	T49.0X4	T49.0X5	T49.0X6
Chlorate (potassium) (sodium)	T60.3X1	T60.3X2	T60.3X3	T60.3X4	—	—
NEC						
herbicide	T60.3X1	T60.3X2	T60.3X3	T60.3X4	—	—
Chlorazanil	T50.2X1	T50.2X2	T50.2X3	T50.2X4	T50.2X5	T50.2X6
Chlorbenzene, chlorbenzol	T53.7X1	T53.7X2	T53.7X3	T53.7X4	—	—
Chlorbenzoxamine	T44.3X1	T44.3X2	T44.3X3	T44.3X4	T44.3X5	T44.3X6
Chlorbutol	T42.6X1	T42.6X2	T42.6X3	T42.6X4	T42.6X5	T42.6X6
Chlorcyclizine	T45.0X1	T45.0X2	T45.0X3	T45.0X4	T45.0X5	T45.0X6
Chlordan (e) (dust)	T60.1X1	T60.1X2	T60.1X3	T60.1X4	—	—
Chlordantoin	T49.0X1	T49.0X2	T49.0X3	T49.0X4	T49.0X5	T49.0X6
Chlordiazepoxide	T42.4X1	T42.4X2	T42.4X3	T42.4X4	T42.4X5	T42.4X6
Chlordiethyl benzamide	T49.3X1	T49.3X2	T49.3X3	T49.3X4	T49.3X5	T49.3X6
Chloresium	T49.8X1	T49.8X2	T49.8X3	T49.8X4	T49.8X5	T49.8X6
Chlorethiazol	T42.6X1	T42.6X2	T42.6X3	T42.6X4	T42.6X5	T42.6X6
Chlorethyl — *see* Ethyl chloride						
Chloretone	T42.6X1	T42.6X2	T42.6X3	T42.6X4	T42.6X5	T42.6X6
Chlorex	T53.6X1	T53.6X2	T53.6X3	T53.6X4	—	—
insecticide	T60.1X1	T60.1X2	T60.1X3	T60.1X4	—	—
Chlorfenvinphos	T60.0X1	T60.0X2	T60.0X3	T60.0X4	—	—
Chlorhexadol	T42.6X1	T42.6X2	T42.6X3	T42.6X4	T42.6X5	T42.6X6
Chlorhexamide	T45.1X1	T45.1X2	T45.1X3	T45.1X4	T45.1X5	T45.1X6
Chlorhexidine	T49.0X1	T49.0X2	T49.0X3	T49.0X4	T49.0X5	T49.0X6
Chlorhydroxyquinolin	T49.0X1	T49.0X2	T49.0X3	T49.0X4	T49.0X5	T49.0X6
Chloride of lime (bleach)	T54.3X1	T54.3X2	T54.3X3	T54.3X4	—	—
Chlorimipramine	T43.011	T43.012	T43.013	T43.014	T43.015	T43.016
Chlorinated						
camphene	T53.6X1	T53.6X2	T53.6X3	T53.6X4	—	—
diphenyl	T53.7X1	T53.7X2	T53.7X3	T53.7X4	—	—
hydrocarbons NEC	T53.91	T53.92	T53.93	T53.94	—	—
solvents	T53.91	T53.92	T53.93	T53.94	—	—
lime (bleach)	T54.3X1	T54.3X2	T54.3X3	T54.3X4	—	—
and boric acid solution	T49.0X1	T49.0X2	T49.0X3	T49.0X4	T49.0X5	T49.0X6
naphthalene (insecticide)	T60.1X1	T60.1X2	T60.1X3	T60.1X4	—	—
industrial (non-pesticide)	T53.7X1	T53.7X2	T53.7X3	T53.7X4	—	—
pesticide NEC	T60.8X1	T60.8X2	T60.8X3	T60.8X4	—	—
soda — *see also* sodium hypochlorite						
solution	T49.0X1	T49.0X2	T49.0X3	T49.0X4	T49.0X5	T49.0X6
Chlorine (fumes) (gas)	T59.4X1	T59.4X2	T59.4X3	T59.4X4	—	—
bleach	T54.3X1	T54.3X2	T54.3X3	T54.3X4	—	—
compound gas NEC	T59.4X1	T59.4X2	T59.4X3	T59.4X4	—	—
disinfectant	T59.4X1	T59.4X2	T59.4X3	T59.4X4	—	—
releasing agents NEC	T59.4X1	T59.4X2	T59.4X3	T59.4X4	—	—
Chlorisondamine chloride	T46.991	T46.992	T46.993	T46.994	T46.995	T46.996
Chlormadinone	T38.5X1	T38.5X2	T38.5X3	T38.5X4	T38.5X5	T38.5X6
Chlormephos	T60.0X1	T60.0X2	T60.0X3	T60.0X4	—	—
Chlormerodrin	T50.2X1	T50.2X2	T50.2X3	T50.2X4	T50.2X5	T50.2X6
Chlormethiazole	T42.6X1	T42.6X2	T42.6X3	T42.6X4	T42.6X5	T42.6X6
Chlormethine	T45.1X1	T45.1X2	T45.1X3	T45.1X4	T45.1X5	T45.1X6
Chlormethylenecycline	T36.4X1	T36.4X2	T36.4X3	T36.4X4	T36.4X5	T36.4X6
Chlormezanone	T42.6X1	T42.6X2	T42.6X3	T42.6X4	T42.6X5	T42.6X6
Chloroacetic acid	T60.3X1	T60.3X2	T60.3X3	T60.3X4	—	—
Chloroacetone	T59.3X1	T59.3X2	T59.3X3	T59.3X4	—	—
Chloroacetophenone	T59.3X1	T59.3X2	T59.3X3	T59.3X4	—	—
Chloroaniline	T53.7X1	T53.7X2	T53.7X3	T53.7X4	—	—
Chlorobenzene, chlorobenzol	T53.7X1	T53.7X2	T53.7X3	T53.7X4	—	—
Chlorobromomethane (fire extinguisher)	T53.6X1	T53.6X2	T53.6X3	T53.6X4	—	—
Chlorobutanol	T49.0X1	T49.0X2	T49.0X3	T49.0X4	T49.0X5	T49.0X6
Chlorocresol	T49.0X1	T49.0X2	T49.0X3	T49.0X4	T49.0X5	T49.0X6
Chlorodehydromethyltestosterone	T38.7X1	T38.7X2	T38.7X3	T38.7X4	T38.7X5	T38.7X6
Chlorodinitrobenzene	T53.7X1	T53.7X2	T53.7X3	T53.7X4	—	—
dust or vapor	T53.7X1	T53.7X2	T53.7X3	T53.7X4	—	—
Chlorodiphenyl	T53.7X1	T53.7X2	T53.7X3	T53.7X4	—	—
Chloroethane — *see* Ethyl chloride						
Chloroethylene	T53.6X1	T53.6X2	T53.6X3	T53.6X4	—	—
Chlorofluorocarbons	T53.5X1	T53.5X2	T53.5X3	T53.5X4	—	—
Chloroform (fumes) (vapor)	T53.1X1	T53.1X2	T53.1X3	T53.1X4	—	—
anesthetic	T41.0X1	T41.0X2	T41.0X3	T41.0X4	T41.0X5	T41.0X6
solvent	T53.1X1	T53.1X2	T53.1X3	T53.1X4	—	—
water, concentrated	T41.0X1	T41.0X2	T41.0X3	T41.0X4	T41.0X5	T41.0X6
Chloroguanide	T37.2X1	T37.2X2	T37.2X3	T37.2X4	T37.2X5	T37.2X6
Chloromycetin	T36.2X1	T36.2X2	T36.2X3	T36.2X4	T36.2X5	T36.2X6
ENT agent	T49.6X1	T49.6X2	T49.6X3	T49.6X4	T49.6X5	T49.6X6
ophthalmic preparation	T49.5X1	T49.5X2	T49.5X3	T49.5X4	T49.5X5	T49.5X6
otic solution	T49.6X1	T49.6X2	T49.6X3	T49.6X4	T49.6X5	T49.6X6
topical NEC	T49.0X1	T49.0X2	T49.0X3	T49.0X4	T49.0X5	T49.0X6
Chloronitrobenzene	T53.7X1	T53.7X2	T53.7X3	T53.7X4	—	—
dust or vapor	T53.7X1	T53.7X2	T53.7X3	T53.7X4	—	—

Table of Drugs and Chemicals

Substance	Poisoning, Accidental (unintentional)	Poisoning, Intentional Self-harm	Poisoning, Assault	Poisoning, Undetermined	Adverse Effect	Under-dosing
Chlorophacinone	T60.4X1	T60.4X2	T60.4X3	T60.4X4	—	—
Chlorophenol	T53.7X1	T53.7X2	T53.7X3	T53.7X4	—	—
Chlorophenothane	T60.1X1	T60.1X2	T60.1X3	T60.1X4	—	—
Chlorophyll	T50.991	T50.992	T50.993	T50.994	T50.995	T50.996
Chloropicrin (fumes)	T53.6X1	T53.6X2	T53.6X3	T53.6X4	—	—
fumigant	T60.8X1	T60.8X2	T60.8X3	T60.8X4	—	—
fungicide	T60.3X1	T60.3X2	T60.3X3	T60.3X4	—	—
pesticide	T60.8X1	T60.8X2	T60.8X3	T60.8X4	—	—
Chloroprocaine	T41.3X1	T41.3X2	T41.3X3	T41.3X4	T41.3X5	T41.3X6
infiltration (subcutaneous)	T41.3X1	T41.3X2	T41.3X3	T41.3X4	T41.3X5	T41.3X6
nerve block (peripheral) (plexus)	T41.3X1	T41.3X2	T41.3X3	T41.3X4	T41.3X5	T41.3X6
spinal	T41.3X1	T41.3X2	T41.3X3	T41.3X4	T41.3X5	T41.3X6
Chloroptic	T49.5X1	T49.5X2	T49.5X3	T49.5X4	T49.5X5	T49.5X6
Chloropurine	T45.1X1	T45.1X2	T45.1X3	T45.1X4	T45.1X5	T45.1X6
Chloropyramine	T45.0X1	T45.0X2	T45.0X3	T45.0X4	T45.0X5	T45.0X6
Chloropyrifos	T60.0X1	T60.0X2	T60.0X3	T60.0X4	—	—
Chloropyrilene	T45.0X1	T45.0X2	T45.0X3	T45.0X4	T45.0X5	T45.0X6
Chloroquine	T37.2X1	T37.2X2	T37.2X3	T37.2X4	T37.2X5	T37.2X6
Chlorothalonil	T60.3X1	T60.3X2	T60.3X3	T60.3X4	—	—
Chlorothen	T45.0X1	T45.0X2	T45.0X3	T45.0X4	T45.0X5	T45.0X6
Chlorothiazide	T50.2X1	T50.2X2	T50.2X3	T50.2X4	T50.2X5	T50.2X6
Chlorothymol	T49.4X1	T49.4X2	T49.4X3	T49.4X4	T49.4X5	T49.4X6
Chlorotrianisene	T38.5X1	T38.5X2	T38.5X3	T38.5X4	T38.5X5	T38.5X6
Chlorovinyldichloroarsine, not in war	T57.0X1	T57.0X2	T57.0X3	T57.0X4	—	—
Chloroxine	T49.4X1	T49.4X2	T49.4X3	T49.4X4	T49.4X5	T49.4X6
Chloroxylenol	T49.0X1	T49.0X2	T49.0X3	T49.0X4	T49.0X5	T49.0X6
Chlorphenamine	T45.0X1	T45.0X2	T45.0X3	T45.0X4	T45.0X5	T45.0X6
Chlorphenesin	T42.8X1	T42.8X2	T42.8X3	T42.8X4	T42.8X5	T42.8X6
topical (antifungal)	T49.0X1	T49.0X2	T49.0X3	T49.0X4	T49.0X5	T49.0X6
Chlorpheniramine	T45.0X1	T45.0X2	T45.0X3	T45.0X4	T45.0X5	T45.0X6
Chlorphenoxamine	T45.0X1	T45.0X2	T45.0X3	T45.0X4	T45.0X5	T45.0X6
Chlorphentermine	T50.5X1	T50.5X2	T50.5X3	T50.5X4	T50.5X5	T50.5X6
Chlorprocaine — see Chloroprocaine						
Chlorproguanil	T37.2X1	T37.2X2	T37.2X3	T37.2X4	T37.2X5	T37.2X6
Chlorpromazine	T43.3X1	T43.3X2	T43.3X3	T43.3X4	T43.3X5	T43.3X6
Chlorpropamide	T38.3X1	T38.3X2	T38.3X3	T38.3X4	T38.3X5	T38.3X6
Chlorprothixene	T43.4X1	T43.4X2	T43.4X3	T43.4X4	T43.4X5	T43.4X6
Chlorquinaldol	T49.0X1	T49.0X2	T49.0X3	T49.0X4	T49.0X5	T49.0X6
Chlorquinol	T49.0X1	T49.0X2	T49.0X3	T49.0X4	T49.0X5	T49.0X6
Chlortalidone	T50.2X1	T50.2X2	T50.2X3	T50.2X4	T50.2X5	T50.2X6
Chlortetracycline	T36.4X1	T36.4X2	T36.4X3	T36.4X4	T36.4X5	T36.4X6
Chlorthalidone	T50.2X1	T50.2X2	T50.2X3	T50.2X4	T50.2X5	T50.2X6
Chlorthion	T60.0X1	T60.0X2	T60.0X3	T60.0X4	—	—
Chlorthiophos	T60.0X1	T60.0X2	T60.0X3	T60.0X4	—	—
Chlortrianisene	T38.5X1	T38.5X2	T38.5X3	T38.5X4	T38.5X5	T38.5X6
Chlor-Trimeton	T45.0X1	T45.0X2	T45.0X3	T45.0X4	T45.0X5	T45.0X6
Chlorzoxazone	T42.8X1	T42.8X2	T42.8X3	T42.8X4	T42.8X5	T42.8X6
Choke damp	T59.7X1	T59.7X2	T59.7X3	T59.7X4	—	—
Cholagogues	T47.5X1	T47.5X2	T47.5X3	T47.5X4	T47.5X5	T47.5X6
Cholebrine	T50.8X1	T50.8X2	T50.8X3	T50.8X4	T50.8X5	T50.8X6
Cholecalciferol	T45.2X1	T45.2X2	T45.2X3	T45.2X4	T45.2X5	T45.2X6
Cholecystokinin	T50.8X1	T50.8X2	T50.8X3	T50.8X4	T50.8X5	T50.8X6
Cholera vaccine	T50.A91	T50.A92	T50.A93	T50.A94	T50.A95	T50.A96
Choleretic	T47.5X1	T47.5X2	T47.5X3	T47.5X4	T47.5X5	T47.5X6
Cholesterol-lowering agents	T46.6X1	T46.6X2	T46.6X3	T46.6X4	T46.6X5	T46.6X6
Cholestyramine (resin)	T46.6X1	T46.6X2	T46.6X3	T46.6X4	T46.6X5	T46.6X6
Cholic acid	T47.5X1	T47.5X2	T47.5X3	T47.5X4	T47.5X5	T47.5X6
Choline	T48.6X1	T48.6X2	T48.6X3	T48.6X4	T48.6X5	T48.6X6
chloride	T50.991	T50.992	T50.993	T50.994	T50.995	T50.996
dihydrogen citrate	T50.991	T50.992	T50.993	T50.994	T50.995	T50.996
salicylate	T39.091	T39.092	T39.093	T39.094	T39.095	T39.096
theophyllinate	T48.6X1	T48.6X2	T48.6X3	T48.6X4	T48.6X5	T48.6X6
Cholinergic (drug) NEC	T44.1X1	T44.1X2	T44.1X3	T44.1X4	T44.1X5	T44.1X6
muscle tone enhancer	T44.1X1	T44.1X2	T44.1X3	T44.1X4	T44.1X5	T44.1X6
organophosphorus	T44.0X1	T44.0X2	T44.0X3	T44.0X4	T44.0X5	T44.0X6
insecticide	T60.0X1	T60.0X2	T60.0X3	T60.0X4	—	—
nerve gas	T59.891	T59.892	T59.893	T59.894	—	—
trimethyl ammonium propanediol	T44.1X1	T44.1X2	T44.1X3	T44.1X4	T44.1X5	T44.1X6
Cholinesterase reactivator	T50.6X1	T50.6X2	T50.6X3	T50.6X4	T50.6X5	T50.6X6
Cholografin	T50.8X1	T50.8X2	T50.8X3	T50.8X4	T50.8X5	T50.8X6
Chorionic gonadotropin	T38.891	T38.892	T38.893	T38.894	T38.895	T38.896
Chromate	T56.2X1	T56.2X2	T56.2X3	T56.2X4	—	—
dust or mist	T56.2X1	T56.2X2	T56.2X3	T56.2X4	—	—
lead — see also lead	T56.0X1	T56.0X2	T56.0X3	T56.0X4	—	—
paint	T56.0X1	T56.0X2	T56.0X3	T56.0X4	—	—
Chromic						
acid	T56.2X1	T56.2X2	T56.2X3	T56.2X4	—	—
dust or mist	T56.2X1	T56.2X2	T56.2X3	T56.2X4	—	—
Chromic — continued						
phosphate 32P	T45.1X1	T45.1X2	T45.1X3	T45.1X4	T45.1X5	T45.1X6
Chromium	T56.2X1	T56.2X2	T56.2X3	T56.2X4	—	—
compounds — see Chromate						
sesquioxide	T50.8X1	T50.8X2	T50.8X3	T50.8X4	T50.8X5	T50.8X6
Chromomycin A3	T45.1X1	T45.1X2	T45.1X3	T45.1X4	T45.1X5	T45.1X6
Chromonar	T46.3X1	T46.3X2	T46.3X3	T46.3X4	T46.3X5	T46.3X6
Chromyl chloride	T56.2X1	T56.2X2	T56.2X3	T56.2X4	—	—
Chrysarobin	T49.4X1	T49.4X2	T49.4X3	T49.4X4	T49.4X5	T49.4X6
Chrysazin	T47.2X1	T47.2X2	T47.2X3	T47.2X4	T47.2X5	T47.2X6
Chymar	T45.3X1	T45.3X2	T45.3X3	T45.3X4	T45.3X5	T45.3X6
ophthalmic preparation	T49.5X1	T49.5X2	T49.5X3	T49.5X4	T49.5X5	T49.5X6
Chymopapain	T45.3X1	T45.3X2	T45.3X3	T45.3X4	T45.3X5	T45.3X6
Chymotrypsin	T45.3X1	T45.3X2	T45.3X3	T45.3X4	T45.3X5	T45.3X6
ophthalmic preparation	T49.5X1	T49.5X2	T49.5X3	T49.5X4	T49.5X5	T49.5X6
Cianidanol	T50.991	T50.992	T50.993	T50.994	T50.995	T50.996
Cianopramine	T43.011	T43.012	T43.013	T43.014	T43.015	T43.016
Cibenzoline	T46.2X1	T46.2X2	T46.2X3	T46.2X4	T46.2X5	T46.2X6
Ciclacillin	T36.0X1	T36.0X2	T36.0X3	T36.0X4	T36.0X5	T36.0X6
Ciclobarbital — see Hexobarbital						
Ciclonicate	T46.7X1	T46.7X2	T46.7X3	T46.7X4	T46.7X5	T46.7X6
Ciclopirox (olamine)	T49.0X1	T49.0X2	T49.0X3	T49.0X4	T49.0X5	T49.0X6
Ciclosporin	T45.1X1	T45.1X2	T45.1X3	T45.1X4	T45.1X5	T45.1X6
Cicuta maculata or virosa	T62.2X1	T62.2X2	T62.2X3	T62.2X4	—	—
Cicutoxin	T62.2X1	T62.2X2	T62.2X3	T62.2X4	—	—
Cigarette lighter fluid	T52.0X1	T52.0X2	T52.0X3	T52.0X4	—	—
Cigarettes (tobacco)	T65.221	T65.222	T65.223	T65.224	—	—
Ciguatoxin	T61.01	T61.02	T61.03	T61.04	—	—
Cilazapril	T46.4X1	T46.4X2	T46.4X3	T46.4X4	T46.4X5	T46.4X6
Cimetidine	T47.0X1	T47.0X2	T47.0X3	T47.0X4	T47.0X5	T47.0X6
Cimetropium bromide	T44.3X1	T44.3X2	T44.3X3	T44.3X4	T44.3X5	T44.3X6
Cinchocaine	T41.3X1	T41.3X2	T41.3X3	T41.3X4	T41.3X5	T41.3X6
topical (surface)	T41.3X1	T41.3X2	T41.3X3	T41.3X4	T41.3X5	T41.3X6
Cinchona	T37.2X1	T37.2X2	T37.2X3	T37.2X4	T37.2X5	T37.2X6
Cinchonine alkaloids	T37.2X1	T37.2X2	T37.2X3	T37.2X4	T37.2X5	T37.2X6
Cinchophen	T50.4X1	T50.4X2	T50.4X3	T50.4X4	T50.4X5	T50.4X6
Cinepazide	T46.7X1	T46.7X2	T46.7X3	T46.7X4	T46.7X5	T46.7X6
Cinnamedrine	T48.5X1	T48.5X2	T48.5X3	T48.5X4	T48.5X5	T48.5X6
Cinnarizine	T45.0X1	T45.0X2	T45.0X3	T45.0X4	T45.0X5	T45.0X6
Cinoxacin	T37.8X1	T37.8X2	T37.8X3	T37.8X4	T37.8X5	T37.8X6
Ciprofibrate	T46.6X1	T46.6X2	T46.6X3	T46.6X4	T46.6X5	T46.6X6
Ciprofloxacin	T36.8X1	T36.8X2	T36.8X3	T36.8X4	T36.8X5	T36.8X6
Cisapride	T47.8X1	T47.8X2	T47.8X3	T47.8X4	T47.8X5	T47.8X6
Cisplatin	T45.1X1	T45.1X2	T45.1X3	T45.1X4	T45.1X5	T45.1X6
Citalopram	T43.221	T43.222	T43.223	T43.224	T43.225	T43.226
Citanest	T41.3X1	T41.3X2	T41.3X3	T41.3X4	T41.3X5	T41.3X6
infiltration (subcutaneous)	T41.3X1	T41.3X2	T41.3X3	T41.3X4	T41.3X5	T41.3X6
nerve block (peripheral) (plexus)	T41.3X1	T41.3X2	T41.3X3	T41.3X4	T41.3X5	T41.3X6
Citric acid	T47.5X1	T47.5X2	T47.5X3	T47.5X4	T47.5X5	T47.5X6
Citrovorum (factor)	T45.8X1	T45.8X2	T45.8X3	T45.8X4	T45.8X5	T45.8X6
Claviceps purpurea	T62.2X1	T62.2X2	T62.2X3	T62.2X4	—	—
Clavulanic acid	T36.1X1	T36.1X2	T36.1X3	T36.1X4	T36.1X5	T36.1X6
Cleaner, cleansing agent, type not specified	T65.891	T65.892	T65.893	T65.894	—	—
of paint or varnish	T52.91	T52.92	T52.93	T52.94	—	—
specified type NEC	T65.891	T65.892	T65.893	T65.894	—	—
Clebopride	T47.8X1	T47.8X2	T47.8X3	T47.8X4	T47.8X5	T47.8X6
Clefamide	T37.3X1	T37.3X2	T37.3X3	T37.3X4	T37.3X5	T37.3X6
Clemastine	T45.0X1	T45.0X2	T45.0X3	T45.0X4	T45.0X5	T45.0X6
Clematis vitalba	T62.2X1	T62.2X2	T62.2X3	T62.2X4	—	—
Clemizole	T45.0X1	T45.0X2	T45.0X3	T45.0X4	T45.0X5	T45.0X6
penicillin	T36.0X1	T36.0X2	T36.0X3	T36.0X4	T36.0X5	T36.0X6
Clenbuterol	T48.6X1	T48.6X2	T48.6X3	T48.6X4	T48.6X5	T48.6X6
Clidinium bromide	T44.3X1	T44.3X2	T44.3X3	T44.3X4	T44.3X5	T44.3X6
Clindamycin	T36.8X1	T36.8X2	T36.8X3	T36.8X4	T36.8X5	T36.8X6
Clinofibrate	T46.6X1	T46.6X2	T46.6X3	T46.6X4	T46.6X5	T46.6X6
Clioquinol	T37.8X1	T37.8X2	T37.8X3	T37.8X4	T37.8X5	T37.8X6
Cliradon	T40.2X1	T40.2X2	T40.2X3	T40.2X4	—	—
Clobazam	T42.4X1	T42.4X2	T42.4X3	T42.4X4	T42.4X5	T42.4X6
Clobenzorex	T50.5X1	T50.5X2	T50.5X3	T50.5X4	T50.5X5	T50.5X6
Clobetasol	T49.0X1	T49.0X2	T49.0X3	T49.0X4	T49.0X5	T49.0X6
Clobetasone	T49.0X1	T49.0X2	T49.0X3	T49.0X4	T49.0X5	T49.0X6
Clobutinol	T48.3X1	T48.3X2	T48.3X3	T48.3X4	T48.3X5	T48.3X6
Clocortolone	T38.0X1	T38.0X2	T38.0X3	T38.0X4	T38.0X5	T38.0X6
Clodantoin	T49.0X1	T49.0X2	T49.0X3	T49.0X4	T49.0X5	T49.0X6
Clodronic acid	T50.991	T50.992	T50.993	T50.994	T50.995	T50.996
Clofazimine	T37.1X1	T37.1X2	T37.1X3	T37.1X4	T37.1X5	T37.1X6
Clofedanol	T48.3X1	T48.3X2	T48.3X3	T48.3X4	T48.3X5	T48.3X6
Clofenamide	T50.2X1	T50.2X2	T50.2X3	T50.2X4	T50.2X5	T50.2X6
Clofenotane	T49.0X1	T49.0X2	T49.0X3	T49.0X4	T49.0X5	T49.0X6
Clofezone	T39.2X1	T39.2X2	T39.2X3	T39.2X4	T39.2X5	T39.2X6
Clofibrate	T46.6X1	T46.6X2	T46.6X3	T46.6X4	T46.6X5	T46.6X6

Chlorophacinone — Clofibrate

Substance	Poisoning, Accidental (unintentional)	Poisoning, Intentional Self-harm	Poisoning, Assault	Poisoning, Undetermined	Adverse Effect	Under-dosing
Clofibride	T46.6X1	T46.6X2	T46.6X3	T46.6X4	T46.6X5	T46.6X6
Cloforex	T50.5X1	T50.5X2	T50.5X3	T50.5X4	T50.5X5	T50.5X6
Clomethiazole	T42.6X1	T42.6X2	T42.6X3	T42.6X4	T42.6X5	T42.6X6
Clometocillin	T36.0X1	T36.0X2	T36.0X3	T36.0X4	T36.0X5	T36.0X6
Clomifene	T38.5X1	T38.5X2	T38.5X3	T38.5X4	T38.5X5	T38.5X6
Clomiphene	T38.5X1	T38.5X2	T38.5X3	T38.5X4	T38.5X5	T38.5X6
Clomipramine	T43.011	T43.012	T43.013	T43.014	T43.015	T43.016
Clomocycline	T36.4X1	T36.4X2	T36.4X3	T36.4X4	T36.4X5	T36.4X6
Clonazepam	T42.4X1	T42.4X2	T42.4X3	T42.4X4	T42.4X5	T42.4X6
Clonidine	T46.5X1	T46.5X2	T46.5X3	T46.5X4	T46.5X5	T46.5X6
Clonixin	T39.8X1	T39.8X2	T39.8X3	T39.8X4	T39.8X5	T39.8X6
Clopamide	T50.2X1	T50.2X2	T50.2X3	T50.2X4	T50.2X5	T50.2X6
Clopenthixol	T43.4X1	T43.4X2	T43.4X3	T43.4X4	T43.4X5	T43.4X6
Cloperastine	T48.3X1	T48.3X2	T48.3X3	T48.3X4	T48.3X5	T48.3X6
Clophedianol	T48.3X1	T48.3X2	T48.3X3	T48.3X4	T48.3X5	T48.3X6
Cloponone	T36.2X1	T36.2X2	T36.2X3	T36.2X4	T36.2X5	T36.2X6
Cloprednol	T38.0X1	T38.0X2	T38.0X3	T38.0X4	T38.0X5	T38.0X6
Cloral betaine	T42.6X1	T42.6X2	T42.6X3	T42.6X4	T42.6X5	T42.6X6
Cloramfenicol	T36.2X1	T36.2X2	T36.2X3	T36.2X4	T36.2X5	T36.2X6
Clorazepate (dipotassium)	T42.4X1	T42.4X2	T42.4X3	T42.4X4	T42.4X5	T42.4X6
Clorexolone	T50.2X1	T50.2X2	T50.2X3	T50.2X4	T50.2X5	T50.2X6
Clorfenamine	T45.0X1	T45.0X2	T45.0X3	T45.0X4	T45.0X5	T45.0X6
Clorgiline	T43.1X1	T43.1X2	T43.1X3	T43.1X4	T43.1X5	T43.1X6
Clorotepine	T44.3X1	T44.3X2	T44.3X3	T44.3X4	T44.3X5	T44.3X6
Clorox (bleach)	T54.91	T54.92	T54.93	T54.94	—	—
Clorprenaline	T48.6X1	T48.6X2	T48.6X3	T48.6X4	T48.6X5	T48.6X6
Clortermine	T50.5X1	T50.5X2	T50.5X3	T50.5X4	T50.5X5	T50.5X6
Clotiapine	T43.591	T43.592	T43.593	T43.594	T43.595	T43.596
Clotiazepam	T42.4X1	T42.4X2	T42.4X3	T42.4X4	T42.4X5	T42.4X6
Clotibric acid	T46.6X1	T46.6X2	T46.6X3	T46.6X4	T46.6X5	T46.6X6
Clotrimazole	T49.0X1	T49.0X2	T49.0X3	T49.0X4	T49.0X5	T49.0X6
Cloxacillin	T36.0X1	T36.0X2	T36.0X3	T36.0X4	T36.0X5	T36.0X6
Cloxazolam	T42.4X1	T42.4X2	T42.4X3	T42.4X4	T42.4X5	T42.4X6
Cloxiquine	T49.0X1	T49.0X2	T49.0X3	T49.0X4	T49.0X5	T49.0X6
Clozapine	T42.4X1	T42.4X2	T42.4X3	T42.4X4	T42.4X5	T42.4X6
Coagulant NEC	T45.7X1	T45.7X2	T45.7X3	T45.7X4	T45.7X5	T45.7X6
Coal (carbon monoxide from) — see also Carbon, monoxide, coal	T58.2X1	T58.2X2	T58.2X3	T58.2X4	—	—
oil — see Kerosene						
tar	T49.1X1	T49.1X2	T49.1X3	T49.1X4	T49.1X5	T49.1X6
fumes	T59.891	T59.892	T59.893	T59.894	—	—
medicinal (ointment)	T49.4X1	T49.4X2	T49.4X3	T49.4X4	T49.4X5	T49.4X6
analgesics NEC	T39.2X1	T39.2X2	T39.2X3	T39.2X4	T39.2X5	T39.2X6
naphtha (solvent)	T52.0X1	T52.0X2	T52.0X3	T52.0X4	—	—
Cobalamine	T45.2X1	T45.2X2	T45.2X3	T45.2X4	T45.2X5	T45.2X6
Cobalt (nonmedicinal) (fumes) (industrial)	T56.891	T56.892	T56.893	T56.894	—	—
medicinal (trace) (chloride)	T45.8X1	T45.8X2	T45.8X3	T45.8X4	T45.8X5	T45.8X6
Cobra (venom)	T63.041	T63.042	T63.043	T63.044		
Coca (leaf)	T40.5X1	T40.5X2	T40.5X3	T40.5X4	T40.5X5	T40.5X6
Cocaine	T40.5X1	T40.5X2	T40.5X3	T40.5X4	T40.5X5	T40.5X6
topical anesthetic	T41.3X1	T41.3X2	T41.3X3	T41.3X4	T41.3X5	T41.3X6
Cocarboxylase	T45.3X1	T45.3X2	T45.3X3	T45.3X4	T45.3X5	T45.3X6
Coccidioidin	T50.8X1	T50.8X2	T50.8X3	T50.8X4	T50.8X5	T50.8X6
Cocculus indicus	T62.1X1	T62.1X2	T62.1X3	T62.1X4	—	—
Cochineal	T65.6X1	T65.6X2	T65.6X3	T65.6X4	—	—
medicinal products	T50.991	T50.992	T50.993	T50.994	T50.995	T50.996
Codeine	T40.2X1	T40.2X2	T40.2X3	T40.2X4	T40.2X5	T40.2X6
Cod-liver oil	T45.2X1	T45.2X2	T45.2X3	T45.2X4	T45.2X5	T45.2X6
Coenzyme A	T50.991	T50.992	T50.993	T50.994	T50.995	T50.996
Coffee	T62.8X1	T62.8X2	T62.8X3	T62.8X4	—	—
Cogalactoisomerase	T50.991	T50.992	T50.993	T50.994	T50.995	T50.996
Cogentin	T44.3X1	T44.3X2	T44.3X3	T44.3X4	T44.3X5	T44.3X6
Coke fumes or gas (carbon monoxide)	T58.2X1	T58.2X2	T58.2X3	T58.2X4	—	—
industrial use	T58.8X1	T58.8X2	T58.8X3	T58.8X4	—	—
Colace	T47.4X1	T47.4X2	T47.4X3	T47.4X4	T47.4X5	T47.4X6
Colaspase	T45.1X1	T45.1X2	T45.1X3	T45.1X4	T45.1X5	T45.1X6
Colchicine	T50.4X1	T50.4X2	T50.4X3	T50.4X4	T50.4X5	T50.4X6
Colchicum	T62.2X1	T62.2X2	T62.2X3	T62.2X4	—	—
Cold cream	T49.3X1	T49.3X2	T49.3X3	T49.3X4	T49.3X5	T49.3X6
Colecalciferol	T45.2X1	T45.2X2	T45.2X3	T45.2X4	T45.2X5	T45.2X6
Colestipol	T46.6X1	T46.6X2	T46.6X3	T46.6X4	T46.6X5	T46.6X6
Colestyramine	T46.6X1	T46.6X2	T46.6X3	T46.6X4	T46.6X5	T46.6X6
Colimycin	T36.8X1	T36.8X2	T36.8X3	T36.8X4	T36.8X5	T36.8X6
Colistimethate	T36.8X1	T36.8X2	T36.8X3	T36.8X4	T36.8X5	T36.8X6
Colistin	T36.8X1	T36.8X2	T36.8X3	T36.8X4	T36.8X5	T36.8X6
sulfate (eye preparation)	T49.5X1	T49.5X2	T49.5X3	T49.5X4	T49.5X5	T49.5X6
Collagen	T50.991	T50.992	T50.993	T50.994	T50.995	T50.996
Collagenase	T49.4X1	T49.4X2	T49.4X3	T49.4X4	T49.4X5	T49.4X6
Collodion	T49.3X1	T49.3X2	T49.3X3	T49.3X4	T49.3X5	T49.3X6
Colocynth	T47.2X1	T47.2X2	T47.2X3	T47.2X4	T47.2X5	T47.2X6

Substance	Poisoning, Accidental (unintentional)	Poisoning, Intentional Self-harm	Poisoning, Assault	Poisoning, Undetermined	Adverse Effect	Under-dosing
Colophony adhesive	T49.3X1	T49.3X2	T49.3X3	T49.3X4	T49.3X5	T49.3X6
Colorant — see also Dye	T50.991	T50.992	T50.993	T50.994	T50.995	T50.996
Coloring matter — see Dye(s)						
Combustion gas (after combustion) — see Carbon, monoxide						
prior to combustion	T59.891	T59.892	T59.893	T59.894	—	—
Compazine	T43.3X1	T43.3X2	T43.3X3	T43.3X4	T43.3X5	T43.3X6
Compound						
1080 (sodium fluoroacetate)	T60.4X1	T60.4X2	T60.4X3	T60.4X4	—	—
269 (endrin)	T60.1X1	T60.1X2	T60.1X3	T60.1X4	—	—
3422 (parathion)	T60.0X1	T60.0X2	T60.0X3	T60.0X4	—	—
3911 (phorate)	T60.0X1	T60.0X2	T60.0X3	T60.0X4	—	—
3956 (toxaphene)	T60.1X1	T60.1X2	T60.1X3	T60.1X4	—	—
4049 (malathion)	T60.0X1	T60.0X2	T60.0X3	T60.0X4	—	—
4069 (malathion)	T60.0X1	T60.0X2	T60.0X3	T60.0X4	—	—
4124 (dicapthon)	T60.0X1	T60.0X2	T60.0X3	T60.0X4	—	—
42 (warfarin)	T60.4X1	T60.4X2	T60.4X3	T60.4X4	—	—
497 (dieldrin)	T60.1X1	T60.1X2	T60.1X3	T60.1X4	—	—
E (cortisone)	T38.0X1	T38.0X2	T38.0X3	T38.0X4	T38.0X5	T38.0X6
F (hydrocortisone)	T38.0X1	T38.0X2	T38.0X3	T38.0X4	T38.0X5	T38.0X6
Congener, anabolic	T38.7X1	T38.7X2	T38.7X3	T38.7X4	T38.7X5	T38.7X6
Congo red	T50.8X1	T50.8X2	T50.8X3	T50.8X4	T50.8X5	T50.8X6
Coniine, conine	T62.2X1	T62.2X2	T62.2X3	T62.2X4		
Conium (maculatum)	T62.2X1	T62.2X2	T62.2X3	T62.2X4		
Conjugated estrogenic substances	T38.5X1	T38.5X2	T38.5X3	T38.5X4	T38.5X5	T38.5X6
Contac	T48.5X1	T48.5X2	T48.5X3	T48.5X4	T48.5X5	T48.5X6
Contact lens solution	T49.5X1	T49.5X2	T49.5X3	T49.5X4	T49.5X5	T49.5X6
Contraceptive (oral)	T38.4X1	T38.4X2	T38.4X3	T38.4X4	T38.4X5	T38.4X6
vaginal	T49.8X1	T49.8X2	T49.8X3	T49.8X4	T49.8X5	T49.8X6
Contrast medium, radiography	T50.8X1	T50.8X2	T50.8X3	T50.8X4	T50.8X5	T50.8X6
Convallaria glycosides	T46.0X1	T46.0X2	T46.0X3	T46.0X4	T46.0X5	T46.0X6
Convallaria majalis	T62.2X1	T62.2X2	T62.2X3	T62.2X4		
berry	T62.1X1	T62.1X2	T62.1X3	T62.1X4		
Copperhead snake (bite) (venom)	T63.061	T63.062	T63.063	T63.064		
Copper (dust) (fumes) (nonmedicinal) NEC	T56.4X1	T56.4X2	T56.4X3	T56.4X4		
arsenate, arsenite	T57.0X1	T57.0X2	T57.0X3	T57.0X4	—	—
insecticide	T60.2X1	T60.2X2	T60.2X3	T60.2X4	—	—
emetic	T47.7X1	T47.7X2	T47.7X3	T47.7X4	T47.7X5	T47.7X6
fungicide	T60.3X1	T60.3X2	T60.3X3	T60.3X4	—	—
gluconate	T49.0X1	T49.0X2	T49.0X3	T49.0X4	T49.0X5	T49.0X6
insecticide	T60.2X1	T60.2X2	T60.2X3	T60.2X4	—	—
medicinal (trace)	T45.8X1	T45.8X2	T45.8X3	T45.8X4	T45.8X5	T45.8X6
oleate	T49.0X1	T49.0X2	T49.0X3	T49.0X4	T49.0X5	T49.0X6
sulfate	T56.4X1	T56.4X2	T56.4X3	T56.4X4		
cupric	T56.4X1	T56.4X2	T56.4X3	T56.4X4		
fungicide	T60.3X1	T60.3X2	T60.3X3	T60.3X4		
medicinal						
ear	T49.6X1	T49.6X2	T49.6X3	T49.6X4	T49.6X5	T49.6X6
emetic	T47.7X1	T47.7X2	T47.7X3	T47.7X4	T47.7X5	T47.7X6
eye	T49.5X1	T49.5X2	T49.5X3	T49.5X4	T49.5X5	T49.5X6
cuprous	T56.4X1	T56.4X2	T56.4X3	T56.4X4		
fungicide	T60.3X1	T60.3X2	T60.3X3	T60.3X4		
medicinal						
ear	T49.6X1	T49.6X2	T49.6X3	T49.6X4	T49.6X5	T49.6X6
emetic	T47.7X1	T47.7X2	T47.7X3	T47.7X4	T47.7X5	T47.7X6
eye	T49.5X1	T49.5X2	T49.5X3	T49.5X4	T49.5X5	T49.5X6
Coral (sting)	T63.691	T63.692	T63.693	T63.694		
snake (bite) (venom)	T63.021	T63.022	T63.023	T63.024		
Corbadrine	T49.6X1	T49.6X2	T49.6X3	T49.6X4	T49.6X5	T49.6X6
Cordite	T65.891	T65.892	T65.893	T65.894		
vapor	T59.891	T59.892	T59.893	T59.894		
Cordran	T49.0X1	T49.0X2	T49.0X3	T49.0X4	T49.0X5	T49.0X6
Corn cures	T49.4X1	T49.4X2	T49.4X3	T49.4X4	T49.4X5	T49.4X6
Cornhusker's lotion	T49.3X1	T49.3X2	T49.3X3	T49.3X4	T49.3X5	T49.3X6
Corn starch	T49.3X1	T49.3X2	T49.3X3	T49.3X4	T49.3X5	T49.3X6
Coronary vasodilator NEC	T46.3X1	T46.3X2	T46.3X3	T46.3X4	T46.3X5	T46.3X6
Corrosive NEC	T54.91	T54.92	T54.93	T54.94	—	—
acid NEC	T54.2X1	T54.2X2	T54.2X3	T54.2X4	—	—
aromatics	T54.1X1	T54.1X2	T54.1X3	T54.1X4	—	—
disinfectant	T54.1X1	T54.1X2	T54.1X3	T54.1X4	—	—
fumes NEC	T54.91	T54.92	T54.93	T54.94	—	—
specified NEC	T54.91	T54.92	T54.93	T54.94	—	—
sublimate	T56.1X1	T56.1X2	T56.1X3	T56.1X4	—	—
Cortate	T38.0X1	T38.0X2	T38.0X3	T38.0X4	T38.0X5	T38.0X6
Cort-Dome	T38.0X1	T38.0X2	T38.0X3	T38.0X4	T38.0X5	T38.0X6
ENT agent	T49.6X1	T49.6X2	T49.6X3	T49.6X4	T49.6X5	T49.6X6
ophthalmic preparation	T49.5X1	T49.5X2	T49.5X3	T49.5X4	T49.5X5	T49.5X6

Clofibride — Cort-Dome

Table of Drugs and Chemicals

Cort-Dome — Dantron

Substance	Poisoning, Accidental (unintentional)	Poisoning, Intentional Self-harm	Poisoning, Assault	Poisoning, Undetermined	Adverse Effect	Under-dosing
Cort-Dome — continued						
topical NEC	T49.0X1	T49.0X2	T49.0X3	T49.0X4	T49.0X5	T49.0X6
Cortef	T38.0X1	T38.0X2	T38.0X3	T38.0X4	T38.0X5	T38.0X6
ENT agent	T49.6X1	T49.6X2	T49.6X3	T49.6X4	T49.6X5	T49.6X6
ophthalmic preparation	T49.5X1	T49.5X2	T49.5X3	T49.5X4	T49.5X5	T49.5X6
topical NEC	T49.0X1	T49.0X2	T49.0X3	T49.0X4	T49.0X5	T49.0X6
Corticosteroid	T38.0X1	T38.0X2	T38.0X3	T38.0X4	T38.0X5	T38.0X6
ENT agent	T49.6X1	T49.6X2	T49.6X3	T49.6X4	T49.6X5	T49.6X6
mineral	T50.0X1	T50.0X2	T50.0X3	T50.0X4	T50.0X5	T50.0X6
ophthalmic	T49.5X1	T49.5X2	T49.5X3	T49.5X4	T49.5X5	T49.5X6
topical NEC	T49.0X1	T49.0X2	T49.0X3	T49.0X4	T49.0X5	T49.0X6
Corticotropin	T38.811	T38.812	T38.813	T38.814	T38.815	T38.816
Cortisol	T49.0X1	T49.0X2	T49.0X3	T49.0X4	T49.0X5	T49.0X6
ENT agent	T49.6X1	T49.6X2	T49.6X3	T49.6X4	T49.6X5	T49.6X6
ophthalmic preparation	T49.5X1	T49.5X2	T49.5X3	T49.5X4	T49.5X5	T49.5X6
topical NEC	T49.0X1	T49.0X2	T49.0X3	T49.0X4	T49.0X5	T49.0X6
Cortisone (acetate)	T38.0X1	T38.0X2	T38.0X3	T38.0X4	T38.0X5	T38.0X6
ENT agent	T49.6X1	T49.6X2	T49.6X3	T49.6X4	T49.6X5	T49.6X6
ophthalmic preparation	T49.5X1	T49.5X2	T49.5X3	T49.5X4	T49.5X5	T49.5X6
topical NEC	T49.0X1	T49.0X2	T49.0X3	T49.0X4	T49.0X5	T49.0X6
Cortivazol	T38.0X1	T38.0X2	T38.0X3	T38.0X4	T38.0X5	T38.0X6
Cortogen	T38.0X1	T38.0X2	T38.0X3	T38.0X4	T38.0X5	T38.0X6
ENT agent	T49.6X1	T49.6X2	T49.6X3	T49.6X4	T49.6X5	T49.6X6
ophthalmic preparation	T49.5X1	T49.5X2	T49.5X3	T49.5X4	T49.5X5	T49.5X6
Cortone	T38.0X1	T38.0X2	T38.0X3	T38.0X4	T38.0X5	T38.0X6
ENT agent	T49.6X1	T49.6X2	T49.6X3	T49.6X4	T49.6X5	T49.6X6
ophthalmic preparation	T49.5X1	T49.5X2	T49.5X3	T49.5X4	T49.5X5	T49.5X6
Cortril	T38.0X1	T38.0X2	T38.0X3	T38.0X4	T38.0X5	T38.0X6
ENT agent	T49.6X1	T49.6X2	T49.6X3	T49.6X4	T49.6X5	T49.6X6
ophthalmic preparation	T49.5X1	T49.5X2	T49.5X3	T49.5X4	T49.5X5	T49.5X6
topical NEC	T49.0X1	T49.0X2	T49.0X3	T49.0X4	T49.0X5	T49.0X6
Corynebacterium parvum	T45.1X1	T45.1X2	T45.1X3	T45.1X4	T45.1X5	T45.1X6
Cosmetic preparation	T49.8X1	T49.8X2	T49.8X3	T49.8X4	T49.8X5	T49.8X6
Cosmetics	T49.8X1	T49.8X2	T49.8X3	T49.8X4	T49.8X5	T49.8X6
Cosyntropin	T38.811	T38.812	T38.813	T38.814	T38.815	T38.816
Cotarnine	T45.7X1	T45.7X2	T45.7X3	T45.7X4	T45.7X5	T45.7X6
Co-trimoxazole	T36.8X1	T36.8X2	T36.8X3	T36.8X4	T36.8X5	T36.8X6
Cottonseed oil	T49.3X1	T49.3X2	T49.3X3	T49.3X4	T49.3X5	T49.3X6
Cough mixture (syrup)	T48.4X1	T48.4X2	T48.4X3	T48.4X4	T48.4X5	T48.4X6
containing opiates	T40.2X1	T40.2X2	T40.2X3	T40.2X4	T40.2X5	T40.2X6
expectorants	T48.4X1	T48.4X2	T48.4X3	T48.4X4	T48.4X5	T48.4X6
Coumadin	T45.511	T45.512	T45.513	T45.514	T45.515	T45.516
rodenticide	T60.4X1	T60.4X2	T60.4X3	T60.4X4	—	—
Coumaphos	T60.0X1	T60.0X2	T60.0X3	T60.0X4	—	—
Coumarin	T45.511	T45.512	T45.513	T45.514	T45.515	T45.516
Coumetarol	T45.511	T45.512	T45.513	T45.514	T45.515	T45.516
Cowbane	T62.2X1	T62.2X2	T62.2X3	T62.2X4	—	—
Cozyme	T45.2X1	T45.2X2	T45.2X3	T45.2X4	T45.2X5	T45.2X6
Crack	T40.5X1	T40.5X2	T40.5X3	T40.5X4	—	—
Crataegus extract	T46.0X1	T46.0X2	T46.0X3	T46.0X4	T46.0X5	T46.0X6
Creolin	T54.1X1	T54.1X2	T54.1X3	T54.1X4	—	—
disinfectant	T54.1X1	T54.1X2	T54.1X3	T54.1X4	—	—
Creosol (compound)	T49.0X1	T49.0X2	T49.0X3	T49.0X4	T49.0X5	T49.0X6
Creosote (coal tar) (beechwood)	T49.0X1	T49.0X2	T49.0X3	T49.0X4	T49.0X5	T49.0X6
medicinal (expectorant)	T48.4X1	T48.4X2	T48.4X3	T48.4X4	T48.4X5	T48.4X6
syrup	T48.4X1	T48.4X2	T48.4X3	T48.4X4	T48.4X5	T48.4X6
Cresol(s)	T49.0X1	T49.0X2	T49.0X3	T49.0X4	T49.0X5	T49.0X6
and soap solution	T49.0X1	T49.0X2	T49.0X3	T49.0X4	T49.0X5	T49.0X6
Cresyl acetate	T49.0X1	T49.0X2	T49.0X3	T49.0X4	T49.0X5	T49.0X6
Cresylic acid	T49.0X1	T49.0X2	T49.0X3	T49.0X4	T49.0X5	T49.0X6
Crimidine	T60.4X1	T60.4X2	T60.4X3	T60.4X4	—	—
Croconazole	T37.8X1	T37.8X2	T37.8X3	T37.8X4	T37.8X5	T37.8X6
Cromoglicic acid	T48.6X1	T48.6X2	T48.6X3	T48.6X4	T48.6X5	T48.6X6
Cromolyn	T48.6X1	T48.6X2	T48.6X3	T48.6X4	T48.6X5	T48.6X6
Cromonar	T46.3X1	T46.3X2	T46.3X3	T46.3X4	T46.3X5	T46.3X6
Cropropamide	T39.8X1	T39.8X2	T39.8X3	T39.8X4	T39.8X5	T39.8X6
with crotethamide	T50.7X1	T50.7X2	T50.7X3	T50.7X4	T50.7X5	T50.7X6
Crotamiton	T49.0X1	T49.0X2	T49.0X3	T49.0X4	T49.0X5	T49.0X6
Crotethamide	T39.8X1	T39.8X2	T39.8X3	T39.8X4	T39.8X5	T39.8X6
with cropropamide	T50.7X1	T50.7X2	T50.7X3	T50.7X4	T50.7X5	T50.7X6
Croton (oil)	T47.2X1	T47.2X2	T47.2X3	T47.2X4	T47.2X5	T47.2X6
chloral	T42.6X1	T42.6X2	T42.6X3	T42.6X4	T42.6X5	T42.6X6
Crude oil	T52.0X1	T52.0X2	T52.0X3	T52.0X4	—	—
Cryogenine	T39.8X1	T39.8X2	T39.8X3	T39.8X4	T39.8X5	T39.8X6
Cryolite (vapor)	T60.1X1	T60.1X2	T60.1X3	T60.1X4	—	—
insecticide	T60.1X1	T60.1X2	T60.1X3	T60.1X4	—	—
Cryptenamine (tannates)	T46.5X1	T46.5X2	T46.5X3	T46.5X4	T46.5X5	T46.5X6
Crystal violet	T49.0X1	T49.0X2	T49.0X3	T49.0X4	T49.0X5	T49.0X6
Cuckoopint	T62.2X1	T62.2X2	T62.2X3	T62.2X4	—	—
Cumetharol	T45.511	T45.512	T45.513	T45.514	T45.515	T45.516
Cupric						
acetate	T60.3X1	T60.3X2	T60.3X3	T60.3X4	—	—
Cupric — continued						
acetoarsenite	T57.0X1	T57.0X2	T57.0X3	T57.0X4	—	—
arsenate	T57.0X1	T57.0X2	T57.0X3	T57.0X4	—	—
gluconate	T49.0X1	T49.0X2	T49.0X3	T49.0X4	T49.0X5	T49.0X6
oleate	T49.0X1	T49.0X2	T49.0X3	T49.0X4	T49.0X5	T49.0X6
sulfate	T56.4X1	T56.4X2	T56.4X3	T56.4X4	—	—
Cuprous sulfate — see also Copper sulfate	T56.4X1	T56.4X2	T56.4X3	T56.4X4	—	—
Curare, curarine	T48.1X1	T48.1X2	T48.1X3	T48.1X4	T48.1X5	T48.1X6
Cyamemazine	T43.3X1	T43.3X2	T43.3X3	T43.3X4	T43.3X5	T43.3X6
Cyamopsis tetragonoloba	T46.6X1	T46.6X2	T46.6X3	T46.6X4	T46.6X5	T46.6X6
Cyanacetyl hydrazide	T37.1X1	T37.1X2	T37.1X3	T37.1X4	T37.1X5	T37.1X6
Cyanic acid (gas)	T59.891	T59.892	T59.893	T59.894	—	—
Cyanide(s) (compounds) (potassium) (sodium) NEC	T65.0X1	T65.0X2	T65.0X3	T65.0X4	—	—
dust or gas (inhalation) NEC	T57.3X1	T57.3X2	T57.3X3	T57.3X4	—	—
fumigant	T65.0X1	T65.0X2	T65.0X3	T65.0X4	—	—
hydrogen	T57.3X1	T57.3X2	T57.3X3	T57.3X4	—	—
mercuric — see Mercury						
pesticide (dust) (fumes)	T65.0X1	T65.0X2	T65.0X3	T65.0X4	—	—
Cyanoacrylate adhesive	T49.3X1	T49.3X2	T49.3X3	T49.3X4	T49.3X5	T49.3X6
Cyanocobalamin	T45.8X1	T45.8X2	T45.8X3	T45.8X4	T45.8X5	T45.8X6
Cyanogen (chloride) (gas) NEC	T59.891	T59.892	T59.893	T59.894	—	—
Cyclacillin	T36.0X1	T36.0X2	T36.0X3	T36.0X4	T36.0X5	T36.0X6
Cyclaine	T41.3X1	T41.3X2	T41.3X3	T41.3X4	T41.3X5	T41.3X6
Cyclamate	T50.991	T50.992	T50.993	T50.994	T50.995	T50.996
Cyclamen europaeum	T62.2X1	T62.2X2	T62.2X3	T62.2X4	—	—
Cyclandelate	T46.7X1	T46.7X2	T46.7X3	T46.7X4	T46.7X5	T46.7X6
Cyclazocine	T50.7X1	T50.7X2	T50.7X3	T50.7X4	T50.7X5	T50.7X6
Cyclizine	T45.0X1	T45.0X2	T45.0X3	T45.0X4	T45.0X5	T45.0X6
Cyclobarbital	T42.3X1	T42.3X2	T42.3X3	T42.3X4	T42.3X5	T42.3X6
Cyclobarbitone	T42.3X1	T42.3X2	T42.3X3	T42.3X4	T42.3X5	T42.3X6
Cyclobenzaprine	T48.1X1	T48.1X2	T48.1X3	T48.1X4	T48.1X5	T48.1X6
Cyclodrine	T44.3X1	T44.3X2	T44.3X3	T44.3X4	T44.3X5	T44.3X6
Cycloguanil embonate	T37.2X1	T37.2X2	T37.2X3	T37.2X4	T37.2X5	T37.2X6
Cyclohexane	T52.8X1	T52.8X2	T52.8X3	T52.8X4	—	—
Cyclohexanol	T51.8X1	T51.8X2	T51.8X3	T51.8X4	—	—
Cyclohexanone	T52.4X1	T52.4X2	T52.4X3	T52.4X4	—	—
Cycloheximide	T60.3X1	T60.3X2	T60.3X3	T60.3X4	—	—
Cyclohexyl acetate	T52.8X1	T52.8X2	T52.8X3	T52.8X4	—	—
Cycloleucin	T45.1X1	T45.1X2	T45.1X3	T45.1X4	T45.1X5	T45.1X6
Cyclomethycaine	T41.3X1	T41.3X2	T41.3X3	T41.3X4	T41.3X5	T41.3X6
Cyclopentamine	T44.4X1	T44.4X2	T44.4X3	T44.4X4	T44.4X5	T44.4X6
Cyclopenthiazide	T50.2X1	T50.2X2	T50.2X3	T50.2X4	T50.2X5	T50.2X6
Cyclopentolate	T44.3X1	T44.3X2	T44.3X3	T44.3X4	T44.3X5	T44.3X6
Cyclophosphamide	T45.1X1	T45.1X2	T45.1X3	T45.1X4	T45.1X5	T45.1X6
Cycloplegic drug	T49.5X1	T49.5X2	T49.5X3	T49.5X4	T49.5X5	T49.5X6
Cyclopropane	T41.291	T41.292	T41.293	T41.294	T41.295	T41.296
Cyclopyrabital	T39.8X1	T39.8X2	T39.8X3	T39.8X4	T39.8X5	T39.8X6
Cycloserine	T37.1X1	T37.1X2	T37.1X3	T37.1X4	T37.1X5	T37.1X6
Cyclosporin	T45.1X1	T45.1X2	T45.1X3	T45.1X4	T45.1X5	T45.1X6
Cyclothiazide	T50.2X1	T50.2X2	T50.2X3	T50.2X4	T50.2X5	T50.2X6
Cycrimine	T44.3X1	T44.3X2	T44.3X3	T44.3X4	T44.3X5	T44.3X6
Cyhalothrin	T60.1X1	T60.1X2	T60.1X3	T60.1X4	—	—
Cymarin	T46.0X1	T46.0X2	T46.0X3	T46.0X4	T46.0X5	T46.0X6
Cypermethrin	T60.1X1	T60.1X2	T60.1X3	T60.1X4	—	—
Cyphenothrin	T60.2X1	T60.2X2	T60.2X3	T60.2X4	—	—
Cyproheptadine	T45.0X1	T45.0X2	T45.0X3	T45.0X4	T45.0X5	T45.0X6
Cyproterone	T38.6X1	T38.6X2	T38.6X3	T38.6X4	T38.6X5	T38.6X6
Cysteamine	T50.6X1	T50.6X2	T50.6X3	T50.6X4	T50.6X5	T50.6X6
Cytarabine	T45.1X1	T45.1X2	T45.1X3	T45.1X4	T45.1X5	T45.1X6
Cytisus						
laburnum	T62.2X1	T62.2X2	T62.2X3	T62.2X4	—	—
scoparius	T62.2X1	T62.2X2	T62.2X3	T62.2X4	—	—
Cytochrome C	T47.5X1	T47.5X2	T47.5X3	T47.5X4	T47.5X5	T47.5X6
Cytomel	T38.1X1	T38.1X2	T38.1X3	T38.1X4	T38.1X5	T38.1X6
Cytosine arabinoside	T45.1X1	T45.1X2	T45.1X3	T45.1X4	T45.1X5	T45.1X6
Cytoxan	T45.1X1	T45.1X2	T45.1X3	T45.1X4	T45.1X5	T45.1X6
Cytozyme	T45.7X1	T45.7X2	T45.7X3	T45.7X4	T45.7X5	T45.7X6
S-Carboxymethylcysteine	T48.4X1	T48.4X2	T48.4X3	T48.4X4	T48.4X5	T48.4X6
Dacarbazine	T45.1X1	T45.1X2	T45.1X3	T45.1X4	T45.1X5	T45.1X6
Dactinomycin	T45.1X1	T45.1X2	T45.1X3	T45.1X4	T45.1X5	T45.1X6
DADPS	T37.1X1	T37.1X2	T37.1X3	T37.1X4	T37.1X5	T37.1X6
Dakin's solution	T49.0X1	T49.0X2	T49.0X3	T49.0X4	T49.0X5	T49.0X6
Dalapon (sodium)	T60.3X1	T60.3X2	T60.3X3	T60.3X4	—	—
Dalmane	T42.4X1	T42.4X2	T42.4X3	T42.4X4	T42.4X5	T42.4X6
Danazol	T38.6X1	T38.6X2	T38.6X3	T38.6X4	T38.6X5	T38.6X6
Danilone	T45.511	T45.512	T45.513	T45.514	T45.515	T45.516
Danthron	T47.2X1	T47.2X2	T47.2X3	T47.2X4	T47.2X5	T47.2X6
Dantrolene	T42.8X1	T42.8X2	T42.8X3	T42.8X4	T42.8X5	T42.8X6
Dantron	T47.2X1	T47.2X2	T47.2X3	T47.2X4	T47.2X5	T47.2X6

Substance	Poisoning, Accidental (unintentional)	Poisoning, Intentional Self-harm	Poisoning, Assault	Poisoning, Undetermined	Adverse Effect	Under-dosing
Daphne (gnidium) (mezereum)	T62.2X1	T62.2X2	T62.2X3	T62.2X4	—	—
berry	T62.1X1	T62.1X2	T62.1X3	T62.1X4	—	—
Dapsone	T37.1X1	T37.1X2	T37.1X3	T37.1X4	T37.1X5	T37.1X6
Daraprim	T37.2X1	T37.2X2	T37.2X3	T37.2X4	T37.2X5	T37.2X6
Darnel	T62.2X1	T62.2X2	T62.2X3	T62.2X4	—	—
Darvon	T39.8X1	T39.8X2	T39.8X3	T39.8X4	T39.8X5	T39.8X6
Daunomycin	T45.1X1	T45.1X2	T45.1X3	T45.1X4	T45.1X5	T45.1X6
Daunorubicin	T45.1X1	T45.1X2	T45.1X3	T45.1X4	T45.1X5	T45.1X6
DBI	T38.3X1	T38.3X2	T38.3X3	T38.3X4	T38.3X5	T38.3X6
D-Con	T60.91	T60.92	T60.93	T60.94	—	—
insecticide	T60.2X1	T60.2X2	T60.2X3	T60.2X4	—	—
rodenticide	T60.4X1	T60.4X2	T60.4X3	T60.4X4	—	—
DDAVP	T38.891	T38.892	T38.893	T38.894	T38.895	T38.896
DDE (bis(chlorophenyl)-dichloroethylene)	T60.2X1	T60.2X2	T60.2X3	T60.2X4	—	—
DDS	T37.1X1	T37.1X2	T37.1X3	T37.1X4	T37.1X5	T37.1X6
DDT (dust)	T60.1X1	T60.1X2	T60.1X3	T60.1X4	—	—
Deadly nightshade — see also Belladonna						
berry	T62.1X1	T62.1X2	T62.1X3	T62.1X4	—	—
Deamino-D-arginine vasopressin	T38.891	T38.892	T38.893	T38.894	T38.895	T38.896
Deanol (aceglumate)	T50.991	T50.992	T50.993	T50.994	T50.995	T50.996
Debrisoquine	T46.5X1	T46.5X2	T46.5X3	T46.5X4	T46.5X5	T46.5X6
Decaborane	T57.8X1	T57.8X2	T57.8X3	T57.8X4	—	—
fumes	T59.891	T59.892	T59.893	T59.894	—	—
Decadron	T38.0X1	T38.0X2	T38.0X3	T38.0X4	T38.0X5	T38.0X6
ENT agent	T49.6X1	T49.6X2	T49.6X3	T49.6X4	T49.6X5	T49.6X6
ophthalmic preparation	T49.5X1	T49.5X2	T49.5X3	T49.5X4	T49.5X5	T49.5X6
topical NEC	T49.0X1	T49.0X2	T49.0X3	T49.0X4	T49.0X5	T49.0X6
Decahydronaphthalene	T52.8X1	T52.8X2	T52.8X3	T52.8X4	—	—
Decalin	T52.8X1	T52.8X2	T52.8X3	T52.8X4	—	—
Decamethonium (bromide)	T48.1X1	T48.1X2	T48.1X3	T48.1X4	T48.1X5	T48.1X6
Decholin	T47.5X1	T47.5X2	T47.5X3	T47.5X4	T47.5X5	T47.5X6
Declomycin	T36.4X1	T36.4X2	T36.4X3	T36.4X4	T36.4X5	T36.4X6
Decongestant, nasal (mucosa)	T48.5X1	T48.5X2	T48.5X3	T48.5X4	T48.5X5	T48.5X6
combination	T48.5X1	T48.5X2	T48.5X3	T48.5X4	T48.5X5	T48.5X6
Deet	T60.8X1	T60.8X2	T60.8X3	T60.8X4	—	—
Deferoxamine	T45.8X1	T45.8X2	T45.8X3	T45.8X4	T45.8X5	T45.8X6
Deflazacort	T38.0X1	T38.0X2	T38.0X3	T38.0X4	T38.0X5	T38.0X6
Deglycyrrhizinized extract of licorice	T48.4X1	T48.4X2	T48.4X3	T48.4X4	T48.4X5	T48.4X6
Dehydrocholic acid	T47.5X1	T47.5X2	T47.5X3	T47.5X4	T47.5X5	T47.5X6
Dehydroemetine	T37.3X1	T37.3X2	T37.3X3	T37.3X4	T37.3X5	T37.3X6
Dekalin	T52.8X1	T52.8X2	T52.8X3	T52.8X4	—	—
Delalutin	T38.5X1	T38.5X2	T38.5X3	T38.5X4	T38.5X5	T38.5X6
Delorazepam	T42.4X1	T42.4X2	T42.4X3	T42.4X4	T42.4X5	T42.4X6
Delphinium	T62.2X1	T62.2X2	T62.2X3	T62.2X4		
Deltamethrin	T60.1X1	T60.1X2	T60.1X3	T60.1X4	—	—
Deltasone	T38.0X1	T38.0X2	T38.0X3	T38.0X4	T38.0X5	T38.0X6
Deltra	T38.0X1	T38.0X2	T38.0X3	T38.0X4	T38.0X5	T38.0X6
Delvinal	T42.3X1	T42.3X2	T42.3X3	T42.3X4	T42.3X5	T42.3X6
Demecarium (bromide)	T49.5X1	T49.5X2	T49.5X3	T49.5X4	T49.5X5	T49.5X6
Demeclocycline	T36.4X1	T36.4X2	T36.4X3	T36.4X4	T36.4X5	T36.4X6
Demecolcine	T45.1X1	T45.1X2	T45.1X3	T45.1X4	T45.1X5	T45.1X6
Demegestone	T38.5X1	T38.5X2	T38.5X3	T38.5X4	T38.5X5	T38.5X6
Demelanizing agents	T49.8X1	T49.8X2	T49.8X3	T49.8X4	T49.8X5	T49.8X6
Demephion -O and -S	T60.0X1	T60.0X2	T60.0X3	T60.0X4	—	—
Demerol	T40.2X1	T40.2X2	T40.2X3	T40.2X4	T40.2X5	T40.2X6
Demethylchlortetracycline	T36.4X1	T36.4X2	T36.4X3	T36.4X4	T36.4X5	T36.4X6
Demethyltetracycline	T36.4X1	T36.4X2	T36.4X3	T36.4X4	T36.4X5	T36.4X6
Demeton -O and -S	T60.0X1	T60.0X2	T60.0X3	T60.0X4	—	—
Demulcent (external)	T49.3X1	T49.3X2	T49.3X3	T49.3X4	T49.3X5	T49.3X6
specified NEC	T49.3X1	T49.3X2	T49.3X3	T49.3X4	T49.3X5	T49.3X6
Demulen	T38.4X1	T38.4X2	T38.4X3	T38.4X4	T38.4X5	T38.4X6
Denatured alcohol	T51.0X1	T51.0X2	T51.0X3	T51.0X4	—	—
Dendrid	T49.5X1	T49.5X2	T49.5X3	T49.5X4	T49.5X5	T49.5X6
Dental drug, topical application NEC	T49.7X1	T49.7X2	T49.7X3	T49.7X4	T49.7X5	T49.7X6
Dentifrice	T49.7X1	T49.7X2	T49.7X3	T49.7X4	T49.7X5	T49.7X6
Deodorant spray (feminine hygiene)	T49.8X1	T49.8X2	T49.8X3	T49.8X4	T49.8X5	T49.8X6
Deoxycortone	T50.0X1	T50.0X2	T50.0X3	T50.0X4	T50.0X5	T50.0X6
Deoxyribonuclease (pancreatic)	T45.3X1	T45.3X2	T45.3X3	T45.3X4	T45.3X5	T45.3X6
Depilatory	T49.4X1	T49.4X2	T49.4X3	T49.4X4	T49.4X5	T49.4X6
Deprenalin	T42.8X1	T42.8X2	T42.8X3	T42.8X4	T42.8X5	T42.8X6
Deprenyl	T42.8X1	T42.8X2	T42.8X3	T42.8X4	T42.8X5	T42.8X6
Depressant						
appetite (central)	T50.5X1	T50.5X2	T50.5X3	T50.5X4	T50.5X5	T50.5X6
cardiac	T46.2X1	T46.2X2	T46.2X3	T46.2X4	T46.2X5	T46.2X6

Substance	Poisoning, Accidental (unintentional)	Poisoning, Intentional Self-harm	Poisoning, Assault	Poisoning, Undetermined	Adverse Effect	Under-dosing
Depressant — continued						
central nervous system (anesthetic) — see also	T42.71	T42.72	T42.73	T42.74	T42.75	T42.76
Central nervous system, depressants						
general anesthetic	T41.201	T41.202	T41.203	T41.204	T41.205	T41.206
muscle tone	T42.8X1	T42.8X2	T42.8X3	T42.8X4	T42.8X5	T42.8X6
muscle tone, central	T42.8X1	T42.8X2	T42.8X3	T42.8X4	T42.8X5	T42.8X6
psychotherapeutic	T43.501	T43.502	T43.503	T43.504	T43.505	T43.506
Depressant, appetite	T50.5X1	T50.5X2	T50.5X3	T50.5X4	T50.5X5	T50.5X6
Deptropine	T45.0X1	T45.0X2	T45.0X3	T45.0X4	T45.0X5	T45.0X6
Dequalinium (chloride)	T49.0X1	T49.0X2	T49.0X3	T49.0X4	T49.0X5	T49.0X6
Derris root	T60.2X1	T60.2X2	T60.2X3	T60.2X4	—	—
Deserpidine	T46.5X1	T46.5X2	T46.5X3	T46.5X4	T46.5X5	T46.5X6
Desferrioxamine	T45.8X1	T45.8X2	T45.8X3	T45.8X4	T45.8X5	T45.8X6
Desipramine	T43.011	T43.012	T43.013	T43.014	T43.015	T43.016
Deslanoside	T46.0X1	T46.0X2	T46.0X3	T46.0X4	T46.0X5	T46.0X6
Desloughing agent	T49.4X1	T49.4X2	T49.4X3	T49.4X4	T49.4X5	T49.4X6
Desmethylimipramine	T43.011	T43.012	T43.013	T43.014	T43.015	T43.016
Desmopressin	T38.891	T38.892	T38.893	T38.894	T38.895	T38.896
Desocodeine	T40.2X1	T40.2X2	T40.2X3	T40.2X4	T40.2X5	T40.2X6
Desogestrel	T38.5X1	T38.5X2	T38.5X3	T38.5X4	T38.5X5	T38.5X6
Desomorphine	T40.2X1	T40.2X2	T40.2X3	T40.2X4	—	—
Desonide	T49.0X1	T49.0X2	T49.0X3	T49.0X4	T49.0X5	T49.0X6
Desoximetasone	T49.0X1	T49.0X2	T49.0X3	T49.0X4	T49.0X5	T49.0X6
Desoxycorticosteroid	T50.0X1	T50.0X2	T50.0X3	T50.0X4	T50.0X5	T50.0X6
Desoxycortone	T50.0X1	T50.0X2	T50.0X3	T50.0X4	T50.0X5	T50.0X6
Desoxyephedrine	T43.621	T43.622	T43.623	T43.624	T43.625	T43.626
Detaxtran	T46.6X1	T46.6X2	T46.6X3	T46.6X4	T46.6X5	T46.6X6
Detergent	T49.2X1	T49.2X2	T49.2X3	T49.2X4	T49.2X5	T49.2X6
external medication	T49.2X1	T49.2X2	T49.2X3	T49.2X4	T49.2X5	T49.2X6
local	T49.2X1	T49.2X2	T49.2X3	T49.2X4	T49.2X5	T49.2X6
medicinal	T49.2X1	T49.2X2	T49.2X3	T49.2X4	T49.2X5	T49.2X6
nonmedicinal	T55.1X1	T55.1X2	T55.1X3	T55.1X4	—	—
specified NEC	T55.1X1	T55.1X2	T55.1X3	T55.1X4	—	—
Deterrent, alcohol	T50.6X1	T50.6X2	T50.6X3	T50.6X4	T50.6X5	T50.6X6
Detoxifying agent	T50.6X1	T50.6X2	T50.6X3	T50.6X4	T50.6X5	T50.6X6
Detrothyronine	T38.1X1	T38.1X2	T38.1X3	T38.1X4	T38.1X5	T38.1X6
Dettol (external medication)	T49.0X1	T49.0X2	T49.0X3	T49.0X4	T49.0X5	T49.0X6
Dexamethasone	T38.0X1	T38.0X2	T38.0X3	T38.0X4	T38.0X5	T38.0X6
ENT agent	T49.6X1	T49.6X2	T49.6X3	T49.6X4	T49.6X5	T49.6X6
ophthalmic preparation	T49.5X1	T49.5X2	T49.5X3	T49.5X4	T49.5X5	T49.5X6
topical NEC	T49.0X1	T49.0X2	T49.0X3	T49.0X4	T49.0X5	T49.0X6
Dexamfetamine	T43.621	T43.622	T43.623	T43.624	T43.625	T43.626
Dexamphetamine	T43.621	T43.622	T43.623	T43.624	T43.625	T43.626
Dexbrompheniramine	T45.0X1	T45.0X2	T45.0X3	T45.0X4	T45.0X5	T45.0X6
Dexchlorpheniramine	T45.0X1	T45.0X2	T45.0X3	T45.0X4	T45.0X5	T45.0X6
Dexedrine	T43.621	T43.622	T43.623	T43.624	T43.625	T43.626
Dexetimide	T44.3X1	T44.3X2	T44.3X3	T44.3X4	T44.3X5	T44.3X6
Dexfenfluramine	T50.5X1	T50.5X2	T50.5X3	T50.5X4	T50.5X5	T50.5X6
Dexpanthenol	T45.2X1	T45.2X2	T45.2X3	T45.2X4	T45.2X5	T45.2X6
Dextran (40) (70) (150)	T45.8X1	T45.8X2	T45.8X3	T45.8X4	T45.8X5	T45.8X6
Dextriferron	T45.4X1	T45.4X2	T45.4X3	T45.4X4	T45.4X5	T45.4X6
Dextroamphetamine	T43.621	T43.622	T43.623	T43.624	T43.625	T43.626
Dextro calcium pantothenate	T45.2X1	T45.2X2	T45.2X3	T45.2X4	T45.2X5	T45.2X6
Dextromethorphan	T48.3X1	T48.3X2	T48.3X3	T48.3X4	T48.3X5	T48.3X6
Dextromoramide	T40.4X1	T40.4X2	T40.4X3	T40.4X4	—	—
topical	T49.8X1	T49.8X2	T49.8X3	T49.8X4	T49.8X5	T49.8X6
Dextro pantothenyl alcohol	T45.2X1	T45.2X2	T45.2X3	T45.2X4	T45.2X5	T45.2X6
Dextropropoxyphene	T40.4X1	T40.4X2	T40.4X3	T40.4X4	T40.4X5	T40.4X6
Dextrorphan	T40.2X1	T40.2X2	T40.2X3	T40.2X4	T40.2X5	T40.2X6
Dextrose	T50.3X1	T50.3X2	T50.3X3	T50.3X4	T50.3X5	T50.3X6
concentrated solution, intravenous	T46.8X1	T46.8X2	T46.8X3	T46.8X4	T46.8X5	T46.8X6
Dextrothyroxin	T38.1X1	T38.1X2	T38.1X3	T38.1X4	T38.1X5	T38.1X6
Dextrothyroxine sodium	T38.1X1	T38.1X2	T38.1X3	T38.1X4	T38.1X5	T38.1X6
DFP	T44.0X1	T44.0X2	T44.0X3	T44.0X4	T44.0X5	T44.0X6
DHE	T37.3X1	T37.3X2	T37.3X3	T37.3X4	T37.3X5	T37.3X6
45	T46.5X1	T46.5X2	T46.5X3	T46.5X4	T46.5X5	T46.5X6
Diabinese	T38.3X1	T38.3X2	T38.3X3	T38.3X4	T38.3X5	T38.3X6
Diacetone alcohol	T52.4X1	T52.4X2	T52.4X3	T52.4X4	—	—
Diacetyl monoxime	T50.991	T50.992	T50.993	T50.994	—	—
Diacetylmorphine	T40.1X1	T40.1X2	T40.1X3	T40.1X4	—	—
Diachylon plaster	T49.4X1	T49.4X2	T49.4X3	T49.4X4	T49.4X5	T49.4X6
Diaethylstilboestrolum	T38.5X1	T38.5X2	T38.5X3	T38.5X4	T38.5X5	T38.5X6
Diagnostic agent NEC	T50.8X1	T50.8X2	T50.8X3	T50.8X4	T50.8X5	T50.8X6
Dial (soap)	T49.2X1	T49.2X2	T49.2X3	T49.2X4	T49.2X5	T49.2X6
sedative	T42.3X1	T42.3X2	T42.3X3	T42.3X4	T42.3X5	T42.3X6
Dialkyl carbonate	T52.91	T52.92	T52.93	T52.94	—	—
Diallylbarbituric acid	T42.3X1	T42.3X2	T42.3X3	T42.3X4	T42.3X5	T42.3X6
Diallymal	T42.3X1	T42.3X2	T42.3X3	T42.3X4	T42.3X5	T42.3X6

Table of Drugs and Chemicals

Daphne — Diallymal

Substance	Poisoning, Accidental (unintentional)	Poisoning, Intentional Self-harm	Poisoning, Assault	Poisoning, Undetermined	Adverse Effect	Under-dosing
Dialysis solution (intraperitoneal)	T50.3X1	T50.3X2	T50.3X3	T50.3X4	T50.3X5	T50.3X6
Diaminodiphenylsulfone	T37.1X1	T37.1X2	T37.1X3	T37.1X4	T37.1X5	T37.1X6
Diamorphine	T40.1X1	T40.1X2	T40.1X3	T40.1X4	—	—
Diamox	T50.2X1	T50.2X2	T50.2X3	T50.2X4	T50.2X5	T50.2X6
Diamthazole	T49.0X1	T49.0X2	T49.0X3	T49.0X4	T49.0X5	T49.0X6
Dianthone	T47.2X1	T47.2X2	T47.2X3	T47.2X4	T47.2X5	T47.2X6
Diaphenylsulfone	T37.0X1	T37.0X2	T37.0X3	T37.0X4	T37.0X5	T37.0X6
Diasone (sodium)	T37.1X1	T37.1X2	T37.1X3	T37.1X4	T37.1X5	T37.1X6
Diastase	T47.5X1	T47.5X2	T47.5X3	T47.5X4	T47.5X5	T47.5X6
Diatrizoate	T50.8X1	T50.8X2	T50.8X3	T50.8X4	T50.8X5	T50.8X6
Diazepam	T42.4X1	T42.4X2	T42.4X3	T42.4X4	T42.4X5	T42.4X6
Diazinon	T60.0X1	T60.0X2	T60.0X3	T60.0X4	—	—
Diazomethane (gas)	T59.891	T59.892	T59.893	T59.894	—	—
Diazoxide	T46.5X1	T46.5X2	T46.5X3	T46.5X4	T46.5X5	T46.5X6
Dibekacin	T36.5X1	T36.5X2	T36.5X3	T36.5X4	T36.5X5	T36.5X6
Dibenamine	T44.6X1	T44.6X2	T44.6X3	T44.6X4	T44.6X5	T44.6X6
Dibenzepin	T43.011	T43.012	T43.013	T43.014	T43.015	T43.016
Dibenzheptropine	T45.0X1	T45.0X2	T45.0X3	T45.0X4	T45.0X5	T45.0X6
Dibenzyline	T44.6X1	T44.6X2	T44.6X3	T44.6X4	T44.6X5	T44.6X6
Diborane (gas)	T59.891	T59.892	T59.893	T59.894	—	—
Dibromochloropropane	T60.8X1	T60.8X2	T60.8X3	T60.8X4	—	—
Dibromodulcitol	T45.1X1	T45.1X2	T45.1X3	T45.1X4	T45.1X5	T45.1X6
Dibromoethane	T53.6X1	T53.6X2	T53.6X3	T53.6X4	—	—
Dibromomannitol	T45.1X1	T45.1X2	T45.1X3	T45.1X4	T45.1X5	T45.1X6
Dibromopropamidine isethionate	T49.0X1	T49.0X2	T49.0X3	T49.0X4	T49.0X5	T49.0X6
Dibrompropamidine	T49.0X1	T49.0X2	T49.0X3	T49.0X4	T49.0X5	T49.0X6
Dibucaine	T41.3X1	T41.3X2	T41.3X3	T41.3X4	T41.3X5	T41.3X6
topical (surface)	T41.3X1	T41.3X2	T41.3X3	T41.3X4	T41.3X5	T41.3X6
Dibunate sodium	T48.3X1	T48.3X2	T48.3X3	T48.3X4	T48.3X5	T48.3X6
Dibutoline sulfate	T44.3X1	T44.3X2	T44.3X3	T44.3X4	T44.3X5	T44.3X6
Dicamba	T60.3X1	T60.3X2	T60.3X3	T60.3X4	—	—
Dicapthon	T60.0X1	T60.0X2	T60.0X3	T60.0X4	—	—
Dichlobenil	T60.3X1	T60.3X2	T60.3X3	T60.3X4	—	—
Dichlone	T60.3X1	T60.3X2	T60.3X3	T60.3X4	—	—
Dichloralphenozone	T42.6X1	T42.6X2	T42.6X3	T42.6X4	T42.6X5	T42.6X6
Dichlorbenzidine	T65.3X1	T65.3X2	T65.3X3	T65.3X4	—	—
Dichlorhydrin	T52.8X1	T52.8X2	T52.8X3	T52.8X4	—	—
Dichlorhydroxyquinoline	T37.8X1	T37.8X2	T37.8X3	T37.8X4	T37.8X5	T37.8X6
Dichlorobenzene	T53.7X1	T53.7X2	T53.7X3	T53.7X4	—	—
Dichlorobenzyl alcohol	T49.6X1	T49.6X2	T49.6X3	T49.6X4	T49.6X5	T49.6X6
Dichlorodifluoromethane	T53.5X1	T53.5X2	T53.5X3	T53.5X4	—	—
Dichloroethane	T52.8X1	T52.8X2	T52.8X3	T52.8X4	—	—
Dichloroethylene	T53.6X1	T53.6X2	T53.6X3	T53.6X4	—	—
Dichloroethyl sulfide, not in war	T59.891	T59.892	T59.893	T59.894	—	—
Dichloroformoxine, not in war	T59.891	T59.892	T59.893	T59.894	—	—
Dichlorohydrin, alpha-dichlorohydrin	T52.8X1	T52.8X2	T52.8X3	T52.8X4	—	—
Dichloromethane (solvent)	T53.4X1	T53.4X2	T53.4X3	T53.4X4	—	—
vapor	T53.4X1	T53.4X2	T53.4X3	T53.4X4	—	—
Dichloronaphthoquinone	T60.3X1	T60.3X2	T60.3X3	T60.3X4	—	—
Dichlorophen	T37.4X1	T37.4X2	T37.4X3	T37.4X4	T37.4X5	T37.4X6
Dichloropropene	T60.3X1	T60.3X2	T60.3X3	T60.3X4	—	—
Dichloropropionic acid	T60.3X1	T60.3X2	T60.3X3	T60.3X4	—	—
Dichlorphenamide	T50.2X1	T50.2X2	T50.2X3	T50.2X4	T50.2X5	T50.2X6
Dichlorvos	T60.0X1	T60.0X2	T60.0X3	T60.0X4	—	—
Diclofenac	T39.391	T39.392	T39.393	T39.394	T39.395	T39.396
Diclofenamide	T50.2X1	T50.2X2	T50.2X3	T50.2X4	T50.2X5	T50.2X6
Diclofensine	T43.291	T43.292	T43.293	T43.294	T43.295	T43.296
Diclonixine	T39.8X1	T39.8X2	T39.8X3	T39.8X4	T39.8X5	T39.8X6
Dicloxacillin	T36.0X1	T36.0X2	T36.0X3	T36.0X4	T36.0X5	T36.0X6
Dicophane	T49.0X1	T49.0X2	T49.0X3	T49.0X4	T49.0X5	T49.0X6
Dicoumarol, dicoumarin, dicumarol	T45.511	T45.512	T45.513	T45.514	T45.515	T45.516
Dicrotophos	T60.0X1	T60.0X2	T60.0X3	T60.0X4	—	—
Dicyanogen (gas)	T65.0X1	T65.0X2	T65.0X3	T65.0X4	—	—
Dicyclomine	T44.3X1	T44.3X2	T44.3X3	T44.3X4	T44.3X5	T44.3X6
Dicycloverine	T44.3X1	T44.3X2	T44.3X3	T44.3X4	T44.3X5	T44.3X6
Dideoxycytidine	T37.5X1	T37.5X2	T37.5X3	T37.5X4	T37.5X5	T37.5X6
Dideoxyinosine	T37.5X1	T37.5X2	T37.5X3	T37.5X4	T37.5X5	T37.5X6
Dieldrin (vapor)	T60.1X1	T60.1X2	T60.1X3	T60.1X4	—	—
Diemal	T42.3X1	T42.3X2	T42.3X3	T42.3X4	T42.3X5	T42.3X6
Dienestrol	T38.5X1	T38.5X2	T38.5X3	T38.5X4	T38.5X5	T38.5X6
Dienoestrol	T38.5X1	T38.5X2	T38.5X3	T38.5X4	T38.5X5	T38.5X6
Dietetic drug NEC	T50.901	T50.902	T50.903	T50.904	T50.905	T50.906
Diethazine	T42.8X1	T42.8X2	T42.8X3	T42.8X4	T42.8X5	T42.8X6
Diethyl						
barbituric acid	T42.3X1	T42.3X2	T42.3X3	T42.3X4	T42.3X5	T42.3X6
carbamazine	T37.4X1	T37.4X2	T37.4X3	T37.4X4	T37.4X5	T37.4X6
carbinol	T51.3X1	T51.3X2	T51.3X3	T51.3X4	—	—
Diethyl — continued						
carbonate	T52.8X1	T52.8X2	T52.8X3	T52.8X4	—	—
ether (vapor) — see also ether	T41.0X1	T41.0X2	T41.0X3	T41.0X4	T41.0X5	T41.0X6
oxide	T52.8X1	T52.8X2	T52.8X3	T52.8X4	—	—
propion	T50.5X1	T50.5X2	T50.5X3	T50.5X4	T50.5X5	T50.5X6
stilbestrol	T38.5X1	T38.5X2	T38.5X3	T38.5X4	T38.5X5	T38.5X6
toluamide (nonmedicinal)	T60.8X1	T60.8X2	T60.8X3	T60.8X4	—	—
medicinal	T49.3X1	T49.3X2	T49.3X3	T49.3X4	T49.3X5	T49.3X6
Diethylcarbamazine	T37.4X1	T37.4X2	T37.4X3	T37.4X4	T37.4X5	T37.4X6
Diethylene						
dioxide	T52.8X1	T52.8X2	T52.8X3	T52.8X4	—	—
glycol (monoacetate) (monobutyl ether) (monoethyl ether)	T52.3X1	T52.3X2	T52.3X3	T52.3X4	—	—
Diethylhexylphthalate	T65.891	T65.892	T65.893	T65.894	—	—
Diethylpropion	T50.5X1	T50.5X2	T50.5X3	T50.5X4	T50.5X5	T50.5X6
Diethylstilbestrol	T38.5X1	T38.5X2	T38.5X3	T38.5X4	T38.5X5	T38.5X6
Diethylstilboestrol	T38.5X1	T38.5X2	T38.5X3	T38.5X4	T38.5X5	T38.5X6
Diethylsulfone-diethylmethane	T42.6X1	T42.6X2	T42.6X3	T42.6X4	T42.6X5	T42.6X6
Diethyltoluamide	T49.0X1	T49.0X2	T49.0X3	T49.0X4	T49.0X5	T49.0X6
Diethyltryptamine (DET)	T40.991	T40.992	T40.993	T40.994	—	—
Difebarbamate	T42.3X1	T42.3X2	T42.3X3	T42.3X4	T42.3X5	T42.3X6
Difencloxazine	T40.2X1	T40.2X2	T40.2X3	T40.2X4	T40.2X5	T40.2X6
Difenidol	T45.0X1	T45.0X2	T45.0X3	T45.0X4	T45.0X5	T45.0X6
Difenoxin	T47.6X1	T47.6X2	T47.6X3	T47.6X4	T47.6X5	T47.6X6
Difetarsone	T37.3X1	T37.3X2	T37.3X3	T37.3X4	T37.3X5	T37.3X6
Diffusin	T45.3X1	T45.3X2	T45.3X3	T45.3X4	T45.3X5	T45.3X6
Diflorasone	T49.0X1	T49.0X2	T49.0X3	T49.0X4	T49.0X5	T49.0X6
Diflos	T44.0X1	T44.0X2	T44.0X3	T44.0X4	T44.0X5	T44.0X6
Diflubenzuron	T60.1X1	T60.1X2	T60.1X3	T60.1X4	—	—
Diflucortolone	T49.0X1	T49.0X2	T49.0X3	T49.0X4	T49.0X5	T49.0X6
Diflunisal	T39.091	T39.092	T39.093	T39.094	T39.095	T39.096
Difluoromethyldopa	T42.8X1	T42.8X2	T42.8X3	T42.8X4	T42.8X5	T42.8X6
Difluorophate	T44.0X1	T44.0X2	T44.0X3	T44.0X4	T44.0X5	T44.0X6
Digestant NEC	T47.5X1	T47.5X2	T47.5X3	T47.5X4	T47.5X5	T47.5X6
Digitalin (e)	T46.0X1	T46.0X2	T46.0X3	T46.0X4	T46.0X5	T46.0X6
Digitalis (leaf)(glycoside)	T46.0X1	T46.0X2	T46.0X3	T46.0X4	T46.0X5	T46.0X6
lanata	T46.0X1	T46.0X2	T46.0X3	T46.0X4	T46.0X5	T46.0X6
purpurea	T46.0X1	T46.0X2	T46.0X3	T46.0X4	T46.0X5	T46.0X6
Digitoxin	T46.0X1	T46.0X2	T46.0X3	T46.0X4	T46.0X5	T46.0X6
Digitoxose	T46.0X1	T46.0X2	T46.0X3	T46.0X4	T46.0X5	T46.0X6
Digoxin	T46.0X1	T46.0X2	T46.0X3	T46.0X4	T46.0X5	T46.0X6
Digoxine	T46.0X1	T46.0X2	T46.0X3	T46.0X4	T46.0X5	T46.0X6
Dihydralazine	T46.5X1	T46.5X2	T46.5X3	T46.5X4	T46.5X5	T46.5X6
Dihydrazine	T46.5X1	T46.5X2	T46.5X3	T46.5X4	T46.5X5	T46.5X6
Dihydrocodeine	T40.2X1	T40.2X2	T40.2X3	T40.2X4	T40.2X5	T40.2X6
Dihydrocodeinone	T40.2X1	T40.2X2	T40.2X3	T40.2X4	T40.2X5	T40.2X6
Dihydroergocornine	T46.7X1	T46.7X2	T46.7X3	T46.7X4	T46.7X5	T46.7X6
Dihydroergocristine (mesilate)	T46.7X1	T46.7X2	T46.7X3	T46.7X4	T46.7X5	T46.7X6
Dihydroergokryptine	T46.7X1	T46.7X2	T46.7X3	T46.7X4	T46.7X5	T46.7X6
Dihydroergotamine	T46.5X1	T46.5X2	T46.5X3	T46.5X4	T46.5X5	T46.5X6
Dihydroergotoxine	T46.7X1	T46.7X2	T46.7X3	T46.7X4	T46.7X5	T46.7X6
mesilate	T46.7X1	T46.7X2	T46.7X3	T46.7X4	T46.7X5	T46.7X6
Dihydrohydroxycodeinone	T40.2X1	T40.2X2	T40.2X3	T40.2X4	T40.2X5	T40.2X6
Dihydrohydroxymorphinone	T40.2X1	T40.2X2	T40.2X3	T40.2X4	T40.2X5	T40.2X6
Dihydroisocodeine	T40.2X1	T40.2X2	T40.2X3	T40.2X4	T40.2X5	T40.2X6
Dihydromorphine	T40.2X1	T40.2X2	T40.2X3	T40.2X4	—	—
Dihydromorphinone	T40.2X1	T40.2X2	T40.2X3	T40.2X4	T40.2X5	T40.2X6
Dihydrostreptomycin	T36.5X1	T36.5X2	T36.5X3	T36.5X4	T36.5X5	T36.5X6
Dihydrotachysterol	T45.2X1	T45.2X2	T45.2X3	T45.2X4	T45.2X5	T45.2X6
Dihydroxyaluminum aminoacetate	T47.1X1	T47.1X2	T47.1X3	T47.1X4	T47.1X5	T47.1X6
Dihydroxyaluminum sodium carbonate	T47.1X1	T47.1X2	T47.1X3	T47.1X4	T47.1X5	T47.1X6
Dihydroxyanthraquinone	T47.2X1	T47.2X2	T47.2X3	T47.2X4	T47.2X5	T47.2X6
Dihydroxycodeinone	T40.2X1	T40.2X2	T40.2X3	T40.2X4	T40.2X5	T40.2X6
Dihydroxypropyl theophylline	T50.2X1	T50.2X2	T50.2X3	T50.2X4	T50.2X5	T50.2X6
Diiodohydroxyquin	T37.8X1	T37.8X2	T37.8X3	T37.8X4	T37.8X5	T37.8X6
topical	T49.0X1	T49.0X2	T49.0X3	T49.0X4	T49.0X5	T49.0X6
Diiodohydroxyquinoline	T37.8X1	T37.8X2	T37.8X3	T37.8X4	T37.8X5	T37.8X6
Diiodotyrosine	T38.2X1	T38.2X2	T38.2X3	T38.2X4	T38.2X5	T38.2X6
Diisopromine	T44.3X1	T44.3X2	T44.3X3	T44.3X4	T44.3X5	T44.3X6
Diisopropylamine	T46.3X1	T46.3X2	T46.3X3	T46.3X4	T46.3X5	T46.3X6
Diisopropylfluorophosphonate	T44.0X1	T44.0X2	T44.0X3	T44.0X4	T44.0X5	T44.0X6
Dilantin	T42.0X1	T42.0X2	T42.0X3	T42.0X4	T42.0X5	T42.0X6
Dilaudid	T40.2X1	T40.2X2	T40.2X3	T40.2X4	T40.2X5	T40.2X6
Dilazep	T46.3X1	T46.3X2	T46.3X3	T46.3X4	T46.3X5	T46.3X6
Dill	T47.5X1	T47.5X2	T47.5X3	T47.5X4	T47.5X5	T47.5X6
Diloxanide	T37.3X1	T37.3X2	T37.3X3	T37.3X4	T37.3X5	T37.3X6
Diltiazem	T46.1X1	T46.1X2	T46.1X3	T46.1X4	T46.1X5	T46.1X6

Additional Character May Be Required — Refer to the Tabular List for Character Selection   ▽ Subterms under main terms may continue to next column or page

Substance	Poisoning, Accidental (unintentional)	Poisoning, Intentional Self-harm	Poisoning, Assault	Poisoning, Undetermined	Adverse Effect	Under-dosing
Dimazole	T49.0X1	T49.0X2	T49.0X3	T49.0X4	T49.0X5	T49.0X6
Dimefline	T50.7X1	T50.7X2	T50.7X3	T50.7X4	T50.7X5	T50.7X6
Dimefox	T60.0X1	T60.0X2	T60.0X3	T60.0X4	—	—
Dimemorfan	T48.3X1	T48.3X2	T48.3X3	T48.3X4	T48.3X5	T48.3X6
Dimenhydrinate	T45.0X1	T45.0X2	T45.0X3	T45.0X4	T45.0X5	T45.0X6
Dimercaprol (British anti-lewisite)	T45.8X1	T45.8X2	T45.8X3	T45.8X4	T45.8X5	T45.8X6
Dimercaptopropanol	T45.8X1	T45.8X2	T45.8X3	T45.8X4	T45.8X5	T45.8X6
Dimestrol	T38.5X1	T38.5X2	T38.5X3	T38.5X4	T38.5X5	T38.5X6
Dimetane	T45.0X1	T45.0X2	T45.0X3	T45.0X4	T45.0X5	T45.0X6
Dimethicone	T47.1X1	T47.1X2	T47.1X3	T47.1X4	T47.1X5	T47.1X6
Dimethindene	T45.0X1	T45.0X2	T45.0X3	T45.0X4	T45.0X5	T45.0X6
Dimethisoquin	T49.1X1	T49.1X2	T49.1X3	T49.1X4	T49.1X5	T49.1X6
Dimethisterone	T38.5X1	T38.5X2	T38.5X3	T38.5X4	T38.5X5	T38.5X6
Dimethoate	T60.0X1	T60.0X2	T60.0X3	T60.0X4	—	—
Dimethocaine	T41.3X1	T41.3X2	T41.3X3	T41.3X4	T41.3X5	T41.3X6
Dimethoxanate	T48.3X1	T48.3X2	T48.3X3	T48.3X4	T48.3X5	T48.3X6
Dimethyl						
arsine, arsinic acid	T57.0X1	T57.0X2	T57.0X3	T57.0X4	—	—
carbinol	T51.2X1	T51.2X2	T51.2X3	T51.2X4	—	—
carbonate	T52.8X1	T52.8X2	T52.8X3	T52.8X4	—	—
diguanide	T38.3X1	T38.3X2	T38.3X3	T38.3X4	T38.3X5	T38.3X6
ketone	T52.4X1	T52.4X2	T52.4X3	T52.4X4	—	—
vapor	T52.4X1	T52.4X2	T52.4X3	T52.4X4	—	—
meperidine	T40.2X1	T40.2X2	T40.2X3	T40.2X4	T40.2X5	T40.2X6
parathion	T60.0X1	T60.0X2	T60.0X3	T60.0X4	—	—
phthlate	T49.3X1	T49.3X2	T49.3X3	T49.3X4	T49.3X5	T49.3X6
polysiloxane	T47.8X1	T47.8X2	T47.8X3	T47.8X4	T47.8X5	T47.8X6
sulfate (fumes)	T59.891	T59.892	T59.893	T59.894	—	—
liquid	T65.891	T65.892	T65.893	T65.894	—	—
sulfoxide (nonmedicinal)	T52.8X1	T52.8X2	T52.8X3	T52.8X4	—	—
medicinal	T49.4X1	T49.4X2	T49.4X3	T49.4X4	T49.4X5	T49.4X6
tryptamine	T40.991	T40.992	T40.993	T40.994	—	—
tubocurarine	T48.1X1	T48.1X2	T48.1X3	T48.1X4	T48.1X5	T48.1X6
Dimethylamine sulfate	T49.4X1	T49.4X2	T49.4X3	T49.4X4	T49.4X5	T49.4X6
Dimethylformamide	T52.8X1	T52.8X2	T52.8X3	T52.8X4	—	—
Dimethyltubocurarinium chloride	T48.1X1	T48.1X2	T48.1X3	T48.1X4	T48.1X5	T48.1X6
Dimeticone	T47.1X1	T47.1X2	T47.1X3	T47.1X4	T47.1X5	T47.1X6
Dimetilan	T60.0X1	T60.0X2	T60.0X3	T60.0X4	—	—
Dimetindene	T45.0X1	T45.0X2	T45.0X3	T45.0X4	T45.0X5	T45.0X6
Dimetotiazine	T43.3X1	T43.3X2	T43.3X3	T43.3X4	T43.3X5	T43.3X6
Dimorpholamine	T50.7X1	T50.7X2	T50.7X3	T50.7X4	T50.7X5	T50.7X6
Dimoxyline	T46.3X1	T46.3X2	T46.3X3	T46.3X4	T46.3X5	T46.3X6
Dinitrobenzene	T65.3X1	T65.3X2	T65.3X3	T65.3X4	—	—
vapor	T59.891	T59.892	T59.893	T59.894	—	—
Dinitrobenzol	T65.3X1	T65.3X2	T65.3X3	T65.3X4	—	—
vapor	T59.891	T59.892	T59.893	T59.894	—	—
Dinitrobutylphenol	T65.3X1	T65.3X2	T65.3X3	T65.3X4	—	—
Dinitro (-ortho-)cresol (pesticide) (spray)	T65.3X1	T65.3X2	T65.3X3	T65.3X4	—	—
Dinitrocyclohexylphenol	T65.3X1	T65.3X2	T65.3X3	T65.3X4	—	—
Dinitrophenol	T65.3X1	T65.3X2	T65.3X3	T65.3X4	—	—
Dinoprost	T48.0X1	T48.0X2	T48.0X3	T48.0X4	T48.0X5	T48.0X6
Dinoprostone	T48.0X1	T48.0X2	T48.0X3	T48.0X4	T48.0X5	T48.0X6
Dinoseb	T60.3X1	T60.3X2	T60.3X3	T60.3X4	—	—
Dioctyl sulfosuccinate (calcium) (sodium)	T47.4X1	T47.4X2	T47.4X3	T47.4X4	T47.4X5	T47.4X6
Diodone	T50.8X1	T50.8X2	T50.8X3	T50.8X4	T50.8X5	T50.8X6
Diodoquin	T37.8X1	T37.8X2	T37.8X3	T37.8X4	T37.8X5	T37.8X6
Dionin	T40.2X1	T40.2X2	T40.2X3	T40.2X4	T40.2X5	T40.2X6
Diosmin	T46.991	T46.992	T46.993	T46.994	T46.995	T46.996
Dioxane	T52.8X1	T52.8X2	T52.8X3	T52.8X4	—	—
Dioxathion	T60.0X1	T60.0X2	T60.0X3	T60.0X4	—	—
Dioxin	T53.7X1	T53.7X2	T53.7X3	T53.7X4	—	—
Dioxopromethazine	T43.3X1	T43.3X2	T43.3X3	T43.3X4	T43.3X5	T43.3X6
Dioxyline	T46.3X1	T46.3X2	T46.3X3	T46.3X4	T46.3X5	T46.3X6
Dipentene	T52.8X1	T52.8X2	T52.8X3	T52.8X4	—	—
Diperodon	T41.3X1	T41.3X2	T41.3X3	T41.3X4	T41.3X5	T41.3X6
Diphacinone	T60.4X1	T60.4X2	T60.4X3	T60.4X4	—	—
Diphemanil	T44.3X1	T44.3X2	T44.3X3	T44.3X4	T44.3X5	T44.3X6
metilsulfate	T44.3X1	T44.3X2	T44.3X3	T44.3X4	T44.3X5	T44.3X6
Diphenadione	T45.511	T45.512	T45.513	T45.514	T45.515	T45.516
rodenticide	T60.4X1	T60.4X2	T60.4X3	T60.4X4	—	—
Diphenhydramine	T45.0X1	T45.0X2	T45.0X3	T45.0X4	T45.0X5	T45.0X6
Diphenidol	T45.0X1	T45.0X2	T45.0X3	T45.0X4	T45.0X5	T45.0X6
Diphenoxylate	T47.6X1	T47.6X2	T47.6X3	T47.6X4	T47.6X5	T47.6X6
Diphenylamine	T65.3X1	T65.3X2	T65.3X3	T65.3X4	—	—
Diphenylbutazone	T39.2X1	T39.2X2	T39.2X3	T39.2X4	T39.2X5	T39.2X6
Diphenylchloroarsine, not in war	T57.0X1	T57.0X2	T57.0X3	T57.0X4	—	—
Diphenylhydantoin	T42.0X1	T42.0X2	T42.0X3	T42.0X4	T42.0X5	T42.0X6
Diphenylmethane dye	T52.1X1	T52.1X2	T52.1X3	T52.1X4	—	—

Substance	Poisoning, Accidental (unintentional)	Poisoning, Intentional Self-harm	Poisoning, Assault	Poisoning, Undetermined	Adverse Effect	Under-dosing
Diphenylpyraline	T45.0X1	T45.0X2	T45.0X3	T45.0X4	T45.0X5	T45.0X6
Diphtheria						
antitoxin	T50.Z11	T50.Z12	T50.Z13	T50.Z14	T50.Z15	T50.Z16
toxoid	T50.A91	T50.A92	T50.A93	T50.A94	T50.A95	T50.A96
with tetanus toxoid	T50.A21	T50.A22	T50.A23	T50.A24	T50.A25	T50.A26
with pertussis component	T50.A11	T50.A12	T50.A13	T50.A14	T50.A15	T50.A16
vaccine	T50.A91	T50.A92	T50.A93	T50.A94	T50.A95	T50.A96
combination						
without pertussis	T50.A21	T50.A22	T50.A23	T50.A24	T50.A25	T50.A26
including pertussis	T50.A11	T50.A12	T50.A13	T50.A14	T50.A15	T50.A16
Diphylline	T50.2X1	T50.2X2	T50.2X3	T50.2X4	T50.2X5	T50.2X6
Dipipanone	T40.4X1	T40.4X2	T40.4X3	T40.4X4	—	—
Dipivefrine	T49.5X1	T49.5X2	T49.5X3	T49.5X4	T49.5X5	T49.5X6
Diplovax	T50.B91	T50.B92	T50.B93	T50.B94	T50.B95	T50.B96
Diprophylline	T50.2X1	T50.2X2	T50.2X3	T50.2X4	T50.2X5	T50.2X6
Dipropyline	T48.291	T48.292	T48.293	T48.294	T48.295	T48.296
Dipyridamole	T46.3X1	T46.3X2	T46.3X3	T46.3X4	T46.3X5	T46.3X6
Dipyrone	T39.2X1	T39.2X2	T39.2X3	T39.2X4	T39.2X5	T39.2X6
Diquat (dibromide)	T60.3X1	T60.3X2	T60.3X3	T60.3X4	—	—
Disinfectant	T65.891	T65.892	T65.893	T65.894	—	—
alkaline	T54.3X1	T54.3X2	T54.3X3	T54.3X4	—	—
aromatic	T54.1X1	T54.1X2	T54.1X3	T54.1X4	—	—
intestinal	T37.8X1	T37.8X2	T37.8X3	T37.8X4	T37.8X5	T37.8X6
Disipal	T42.8X1	T42.8X2	T42.8X3	T42.8X4	T42.8X5	T42.8X6
Disodium edetate	T50.6X1	T50.6X2	T50.6X3	T50.6X4	T50.6X5	T50.6X6
Disoprofol	T41.291	T41.292	T41.293	T41.294	T41.295	T41.296
Disopyramide	T46.2X1	T46.2X2	T46.2X3	T46.2X4	T46.2X5	T46.2X6
Distigmine (bromide)	T44.0X1	T44.0X2	T44.0X3	T44.0X4	T44.0X5	T44.0X6
Disulfamide	T50.2X1	T50.2X2	T50.2X3	T50.2X4	T50.2X5	T50.2X6
Disulfanilamide	T37.0X1	T37.0X2	T37.0X3	T37.0X4	T37.0X5	T37.0X6
Disulfiram	T50.6X1	T50.6X2	T50.6X3	T50.6X4	T50.6X5	T50.6X6
Disulfoton	T60.0X1	T60.0X2	T60.0X3	T60.0X4	—	—
Dithiazanine iodide	T37.4X1	T37.4X2	T37.4X3	T37.4X4	T37.4X5	T37.4X6
Dithiocarbamate	T60.0X1	T60.0X2	T60.0X3	T60.0X4	—	—
Dithranol	T49.4X1	T49.4X2	T49.4X3	T49.4X4	T49.4X5	T49.4X6
Diucardin	T50.2X1	T50.2X2	T50.2X3	T50.2X4	T50.2X5	T50.2X6
Diupres	T50.2X1	T50.2X2	T50.2X3	T50.2X4	T50.2X5	T50.2X6
Diuretic NEC	T50.2X1	T50.2X2	T50.2X3	T50.2X4	T50.2X5	T50.2X6
benzothiadiazine	T50.2X1	T50.2X2	T50.2X3	T50.2X4	T50.2X5	T50.2X6
carbonic acid anhydrase inhibitors	T50.2X1	T50.2X2	T50.2X3	T50.2X4	T50.2X5	T50.2X6
furfuryl NEC	T50.2X1	T50.2X2	T50.2X3	T50.2X4	T50.2X5	T50.2X6
loop (high-ceiling)	T50.1X1	T50.1X2	T50.1X3	T50.1X4	T50.1X5	T50.1X6
mercurial NEC	T50.2X1	T50.2X2	T50.2X3	T50.2X4	T50.2X5	T50.2X6
osmotic	T50.2X1	T50.2X2	T50.2X3	T50.2X4	T50.2X5	T50.2X6
purine NEC	T50.2X1	T50.2X2	T50.2X3	T50.2X4	T50.2X5	T50.2X6
saluretic NEC	T50.2X1	T50.2X2	T50.2X3	T50.2X4	T50.2X5	T50.2X6
sulfonamide	T50.2X1	T50.2X2	T50.2X3	T50.2X4	T50.2X5	T50.2X6
thiazide NEC	T50.2X1	T50.2X2	T50.2X3	T50.2X4	T50.2X5	T50.2X6
xanthine	T50.2X1	T50.2X2	T50.2X3	T50.2X4	T50.2X5	T50.2X6
Diurgin	T50.2X1	T50.2X2	T50.2X3	T50.2X4	T50.2X5	T50.2X6
Diuril	T50.2X1	T50.2X2	T50.2X3	T50.2X4	T50.2X5	T50.2X6
Diuron	T60.3X1	T60.3X2	T60.3X3	T60.3X4	—	—
Divalproex	T42.6X1	T42.6X2	T42.6X3	T42.6X4	T42.6X5	T42.6X6
Divinyl ether	T41.0X1	T41.0X2	T41.0X3	T41.0X4	T41.0X5	T41.0X6
Dixanthogen	T49.0X1	T49.0X2	T49.0X3	T49.0X4	T49.0X5	T49.0X6
Dixyrazine	T43.3X1	T43.3X2	T43.3X3	T43.3X4	T43.3X5	T43.3X6
D-lysergic acid diethylamide	T40.8X1	T40.8X2	T40.8X3	T40.8X4	—	—
DMCT	T36.4X1	T36.4X2	T36.4X3	T36.4X4	T36.4X5	T36.4X6
DMSO — see Dimethyl sulfoxide						
DNBP	T60.3X1	T60.3X2	T60.3X3	T60.3X4	—	—
DNOC	T65.3X1	T65.3X2	T65.3X3	T65.3X4	—	—
Dobutamine	T44.5X1	T44.5X2	T44.5X3	T44.5X4	T44.5X5	T44.5X6
DOCA	T38.0X1	T38.0X2	T38.0X3	T38.0X4	T38.0X5	T38.0X6
Docusate sodium	T47.4X1	T47.4X2	T47.4X3	T47.4X4	T47.4X5	T47.4X6
Dodicin	T49.0X1	T49.0X2	T49.0X3	T49.0X4	T49.0X5	T49.0X6
Dofamium chloride	T49.0X1	T49.0X2	T49.0X3	T49.0X4	T49.0X5	T49.0X6
Dolophine	T40.3X1	T40.3X2	T40.3X3	T40.3X4	T40.3X5	T40.3X6
Doloxene	T39.8X1	T39.8X2	T39.8X3	T39.8X4	T39.8X5	T39.8X6
Domestic gas (after combustion) — see Gas, utility						
prior to combustion	T59.891	T59.892	T59.893	T59.894	—	—
Domiodol	T48.4X1	T48.4X2	T48.4X3	T48.4X4	T48.4X5	T48.4X6
Domiphen (bromide)	T49.0X1	T49.0X2	T49.0X3	T49.0X4	T49.0X5	T49.0X6
Domperidone	T45.0X1	T45.0X2	T45.0X3	T45.0X4	T45.0X5	T45.0X6
Dopa	T42.8X1	T42.8X2	T42.8X3	T42.8X4	T42.8X5	T42.8X6
Dopamine	T44.991	T44.992	T44.993	T44.994	T44.995	T44.996
Doriden	T42.6X1	T42.6X2	T42.6X3	T42.6X4	T42.6X5	T42.6X6
Dormiral	T42.3X1	T42.3X2	T42.3X3	T42.3X4	T42.3X5	T42.3X6
Dormison	T42.6X1	T42.6X2	T42.6X3	T42.6X4	T42.6X5	T42.6X6
Dornase	T48.4X1	T48.4X2	T48.4X3	T48.4X4	T48.4X5	T48.4X6

▽ Subterms under main terms may continue to next column or page   Additional Character May Be Required — Refer to the Tabular List for Character Selection

Substance	Poisoning, Accidental (unintentional)	Poisoning, Intentional Self-harm	Poisoning, Assault	Poisoning, Undetermined	Adverse Effect	Under-dosing
Dorsacaine	T41.3X1	T41.3X2	T41.3X3	T41.3X4	T41.3X5	T41.3X6
Dosulepin	T43.011	T43.012	T43.013	T43.014	T43.015	T43.016
Dothiepin	T43.011	T43.012	T43.013	T43.014	T43.015	T43.016
Doxantrazole	T48.6X1	T48.6X2	T48.6X3	T48.6X4	T48.6X5	T48.6X6
Doxapram	T50.7X1	T50.7X2	T50.7X3	T50.7X4	T50.7X5	T50.7X6
Doxazosin	T44.6X1	T44.6X2	T44.6X3	T44.6X4	T44.6X5	T44.6X6
Doxepin	T43.011	T43.012	T43.013	T43.014	T43.015	T43.016
Doxifluridine	T45.1X1	T45.1X2	T45.1X3	T45.1X4	T45.1X5	T45.1X6
Doxorubicin	T45.1X1	T45.1X2	T45.1X3	T45.1X4	T45.1X5	T45.1X6
Doxycycline	T36.4X1	T36.4X2	T36.4X3	T36.4X4	T36.4X5	T36.4X6
Doxylamine	T45.0X1	T45.0X2	T45.0X3	T45.0X4	T45.0X5	T45.0X6
Dramamine	T45.0X1	T45.0X2	T45.0X3	T45.0X4	T45.0X5	T45.0X6
Drano (drain cleaner)	T54.3X1	T54.3X2	T54.3X3	T54.3X4	—	—
Dressing, live pulp	T49.7X1	T49.7X2	T49.7X3	T49.7X4	T49.7X5	T49.7X6
Drocode	T40.2X1	T40.2X2	T40.2X3	T40.2X4	T40.2X5	T40.2X6
Dromoran	T40.2X1	T40.2X2	T40.2X3	T40.2X4	T40.2X5	T40.2X6
Dromostanolone	T38.7X1	T38.7X2	T38.7X3	T38.7X4	T38.7X5	T38.7X6
Dronabinol	T40.7X1	T40.7X2	T40.7X3	T40.7X4	T40.7X5	T40.7X6
Droperidol	T43.591	T43.592	T43.593	T43.594	T43.595	T43.596
Dropropizine	T48.3X1	T48.3X2	T48.3X3	T48.3X4	T48.3X5	T48.3X6
Drostanolone	T38.7X1	T38.7X2	T38.7X3	T38.7X4	T38.7X5	T38.7X6
Drotaverine	T44.3X1	T44.3X2	T44.3X3	T44.3X4	T44.3X5	T44.3X6
Drotrecogin alfa	T45.511	T45.512	T45.513	T45.514	T45.515	T45.516
Drug NEC	T50.901	T50.902	T50.903	T50.904	T50.905	T50.906
specified NEC	T50.991	T50.992	T50.993	T50.994	T50.995	T50.996
DTIC	T45.1X1	T45.1X2	T45.1X3	T45.1X4	T45.1X5	T45.1X6
Duboisine	T44.3X1	T44.3X2	T44.3X3	T44.3X4	T44.3X5	T44.3X6
Dulcolax	T47.2X1	T47.2X2	T47.2X3	T47.2X4	T47.2X5	T47.2X6
Duponol (C) (EP)	T49.2X1	T49.2X2	T49.2X3	T49.2X4	T49.2X5	T49.2X6
Durabolin	T38.7X1	T38.7X2	T38.7X3	T38.7X4	T38.7X5	T38.7X6
Dyclone	T41.3X1	T41.3X2	T41.3X3	T41.3X4	T41.3X5	T41.3X6
Dyclonine	T41.3X1	T41.3X2	T41.3X3	T41.3X4	T41.3X5	T41.3X6
Dydrogesterone	T38.5X1	T38.5X2	T38.5X3	T38.5X4	T38.5X5	T38.5X6
Dye NEC	T65.6X1	T65.6X2	T65.6X3	T65.6X4	—	—
antiseptic	T49.0X1	T49.0X2	T49.0X3	T49.0X4	T49.0X5	T49.0X6
diagnostic agents	T50.8X1	T50.8X2	T50.8X3	T50.8X4	T50.8X5	T50.8X6
pharmaceutical NEC	T50.901	T50.902	T50.903	T50.904	T50.905	T50.906
Dyflos	T44.0X1	T44.0X2	T44.0X3	T44.0X4	T44.0X5	T44.0X6
Dymelor	T38.3X1	T38.3X2	T38.3X3	T38.3X4	T38.3X5	T38.3X6
Dynamite	T65.3X1	T65.3X2	T65.3X3	T65.3X4	—	—
fumes	T59.891	T59.892	T59.893	T59.894	—	—
Dyphylline	T44.3X1	T44.3X2	T44.3X3	T44.3X4	T44.3X5	T44.3X6
b-eucaine	T49.1X1	T49.1X2	T49.1X3	T49.1X4	T49.1X5	T49.1X6
Ear drug NEC	T49.6X1	T49.6X2	T49.6X3	T49.6X4	T49.6X5	T49.6X6
Ear preparations	T49.6X1	T49.6X2	T49.6X3	T49.6X4	T49.6X5	T49.6X6
Echothiophate, echothiopate, ecothiopate	T49.5X1	T49.5X2	T49.5X3	T49.5X4	T49.5X5	T49.5X6
Econazole	T49.0X1	T49.0X2	T49.0X3	T49.0X4	T49.0X5	T49.0X6
Ecothiopate iodide	T49.5X1	T49.5X2	T49.5X3	T49.5X4	T49.5X5	T49.5X6
Ecstasy	T43.621	T43.622	T43.623	T43.624	T43.625	T43.626
Ectylurea	T42.6X1	T42.6X2	T42.6X3	T42.6X4	T42.6X5	T42.6X6
Edathamil disodium	T45.8X1	T45.8X2	T45.8X3	T45.8X4	T45.8X5	T45.8X6
Edecrin	T50.1X1	T50.1X2	T50.1X3	T50.1X4	T50.1X5	T50.1X6
Edetate, disodium (calcium)	T45.8X1	T45.8X2	T45.8X3	T45.8X4	T45.8X5	T45.8X6
Edoxudine	T49.5X1	T49.5X2	T49.5X3	T49.5X4	T49.5X5	T49.5X6
Edrophonium	T44.0X1	T44.0X2	T44.0X3	T44.0X4	T44.0X5	T44.0X6
chloride	T44.0X1	T44.0X2	T44.0X3	T44.0X4	T44.0X5	T44.0X6
EDTA	T50.6X1	T50.6X2	T50.6X3	T50.6X4	T50.6X5	T50.6X6
Eflornithine	T37.2X1	T37.2X2	T37.2X3	T37.2X4	T37.2X5	T37.2X6
Efloxate	T46.3X1	T46.3X2	T46.3X3	T46.3X4	T46.3X5	T46.3X6
Elase	T49.8X1	T49.8X2	T49.8X3	T49.8X4	T49.8X5	T49.8X6
Elastase	T47.5X1	T47.5X2	T47.5X3	T47.5X4	T47.5X5	T47.5X6
Elaterium	T47.2X1	T47.2X2	T47.2X3	T47.2X4	T47.2X5	T47.2X6
Elcatonin	T50.991	T50.992	T50.993	T50.994	T50.995	T50.996
Elder	T62.2X1	T62.2X2	T62.2X3	T62.2X4	—	—
berry, (unripe)	T62.1X1	T62.1X2	T62.1X3	T62.1X4	—	—
Electrolyte balance drug	T50.3X1	T50.3X2	T50.3X3	T50.3X4	T50.3X5	T50.3X6
Electrolytes NEC	T50.3X1	T50.3X2	T50.3X3	T50.3X4	T50.3X5	T50.3X6
Electrolytic agent NEC	T50.3X1	T50.3X2	T50.3X3	T50.3X4	T50.3X5	T50.3X6
Elemental diet	T50.901	T50.902	T50.903	T50.904	T50.905	T50.906
Elliptinium acetate	T45.1X1	T45.1X2	T45.1X3	T45.1X4	T45.1X5	T45.1X6
Embramine	T45.0X1	T45.0X2	T45.0X3	T45.0X4	T45.0X5	T45.0X6
Emepronium (salts)	T44.3X1	T44.3X2	T44.3X3	T44.3X4	T44.3X5	T44.3X6
bromide	T44.3X1	T44.3X2	T44.3X3	T44.3X4	T44.3X5	T44.3X6
Emetic NEC	T47.7X1	T47.7X2	T47.7X3	T47.7X4	T47.7X5	T47.7X6
Emetine	T37.3X1	T37.3X2	T37.3X3	T37.3X4	T37.3X5	T37.3X6
Emollient NEC	T49.3X1	T49.3X2	T49.3X3	T49.3X4	T49.3X5	T49.3X6
Emorfazone	T39.8X1	T39.8X2	T39.8X3	T39.8X4	T39.8X5	T39.8X6
Emylcamate	T43.591	T43.592	T43.593	T43.594	T43.595	T43.596
Enalapril	T46.4X1	T46.4X2	T46.4X3	T46.4X4	T46.4X5	T46.4X6
Enalaprilat	T46.4X1	T46.4X2	T46.4X3	T46.4X4	T46.4X5	T46.4X6
Encainide	T46.2X1	T46.2X2	T46.2X3	T46.2X4	T46.2X5	T46.2X6
Endocaine	T41.3X1	T41.3X2	T41.3X3	T41.3X4	T41.3X5	T41.3X6
Endosulfan	T60.2X1	T60.2X2	T60.2X3	T60.2X4	—	—
Endothall	T60.3X1	T60.3X2	T60.3X3	T60.3X4	—	—
Endralazine	T46.5X1	T46.5X2	T46.5X3	T46.5X4	T46.5X5	T46.5X6
Endrin	T60.1X1	T60.1X2	T60.1X3	T60.1X4	—	—
Enflurane	T41.0X1	T41.0X2	T41.0X3	T41.0X4	T41.0X5	T41.0X6
Enhexymal	T42.3X1	T42.3X2	T42.3X3	T42.3X4	T42.3X5	T42.3X6
Enocitabine	T45.1X1	T45.1X2	T45.1X3	T45.1X4	T45.1X5	T45.1X6
Enovid	T38.4X1	T38.4X2	T38.4X3	T38.4X4	T38.4X5	T38.4X6
Enoxacin	T36.8X1	T36.8X2	T36.8X3	T36.8X4	T36.8X5	T36.8X6
Enoxaparin (sodium)	T45.511	T45.512	T45.513	T45.514	T45.515	T45.516
Enpiprazole	T43.591	T43.592	T43.593	T43.594	T43.595	T43.596
Enprofylline	T48.6X1	T48.6X2	T48.6X3	T48.6X4	T48.6X5	T48.6X6
Enprostil	T47.1X1	T47.1X2	T47.1X3	T47.1X4	T47.1X5	T47.1X6
Enterogastrone	T38.891	T38.892	T38.893	T38.894	T38.895	T38.896
ENT preparations (anti-infectives)	T49.6X1	T49.6X2	T49.6X3	T49.6X4	T49.6X5	T49.6X6
Enviomycin	T36.8X1	T36.8X2	T36.8X3	T36.8X4	T36.8X5	T36.8X6
Enzodase	T45.3X1	T45.3X2	T45.3X3	T45.3X4	T45.3X5	T45.3X6
Enzyme NEC	T45.3X1	T45.3X2	T45.3X3	T45.3X4	T45.3X5	T45.3X6
depolymerizing	T49.8X1	T49.8X2	T49.8X3	T49.8X4	T49.8X5	T49.8X6
fibrolytic	T45.3X1	T45.3X2	T45.3X3	T45.3X4	T45.3X5	T45.3X6
gastric	T47.5X1	T47.5X2	T47.5X3	T47.5X4	T47.5X5	T47.5X6
intestinal	T47.5X1	T47.5X2	T47.5X3	T47.5X4	T47.5X5	T47.5X6
local action	T49.4X1	T49.4X2	T49.4X3	T49.4X4	T49.4X5	T49.4X6
proteolytic	T49.4X1	T49.4X2	T49.4X3	T49.4X4	T49.4X5	T49.4X6
thrombolytic	T45.3X1	T45.3X2	T45.3X3	T45.3X4	T45.3X5	T45.3X6
EPAB	T41.3X1	T41.3X2	T41.3X3	T41.3X4	T41.3X5	T41.3X6
Epanutin	T42.0X1	T42.0X2	T42.0X3	T42.0X4	T42.0X5	T42.0X6
Ephedra	T44.991	T44.992	T44.993	T44.994	T44.995	T44.996
Ephedrine	T44.991	T44.992	T44.993	T44.994	T44.995	T44.996
Epichlorhydrin, epichlorohydrin	T52.8X1	T52.8X2	T52.8X3	T52.8X4	—	—
Epicillin	T36.0X1	T36.0X2	T36.0X3	T36.0X4	T36.0X5	T36.0X6
Epiestriol	T38.5X1	T38.5X2	T38.5X3	T38.5X4	T38.5X5	T38.5X6
Epilim — see Sodium valproate						
Epimestrol	T38.5X1	T38.5X2	T38.5X3	T38.5X4	T38.5X5	T38.5X6
Epinephrine	T44.5X1	T44.5X2	T44.5X3	T44.5X4	T44.5X5	T44.5X6
Epirubicin	T45.1X1	T45.1X2	T45.1X3	T45.1X4	T45.1X5	T45.1X6
Epitiostanol	T38.7X1	T38.7X2	T38.7X3	T38.7X4	T38.7X5	T38.7X6
Epitizide	T50.2X1	T50.2X2	T50.2X3	T50.2X4	T50.2X5	T50.2X6
EPN	T60.0X1	T60.0X2	T60.0X3	T60.0X4	—	—
EPO	T45.8X1	T45.8X2	T45.8X3	T45.8X4	T45.8X5	T45.8X6
Epoetin alpha	T45.8X1	T45.8X2	T45.8X3	T45.8X4	T45.8X5	T45.8X6
Epomediol	T50.991	T50.992	T50.993	T50.994	T50.995	T50.996
Epoprostenol	T45.521	T45.522	T45.523	T45.524	T45.525	T45.526
Epoxy resin	T65.891	T65.892	T65.893	T65.894	—	—
Eprazinone	T48.4X1	T48.4X2	T48.4X3	T48.4X4	T48.4X5	T48.4X6
Epsilon aminocaproic acid	T45.621	T45.622	T45.623	T45.624	T45.625	T45.626
Epsom salt	T47.3X1	T47.3X2	T47.3X3	T47.3X4	T47.3X5	T47.3X6
Eptazocine	T40.4X1	T40.4X2	T40.4X3	T40.4X4	T40.4X5	T40.4X6
Equanil	T43.591	T43.592	T43.593	T43.594	T43.595	T43.596
Equisetum	T62.2X1	T62.2X2	T62.2X3	T62.2X4	—	—
diuretic	T50.2X1	T50.2X2	T50.2X3	T50.2X4	T50.2X5	T50.2X6
Ergobasine	T48.0X1	T48.0X2	T48.0X3	T48.0X4	T48.0X5	T48.0X6
Ergocalciferol	T45.2X1	T45.2X2	T45.2X3	T45.2X4	T45.2X5	T45.2X6
Ergoloid mesylates	T46.7X1	T46.7X2	T46.7X3	T46.7X4	T46.7X5	T46.7X6
Ergometrine	T48.0X1	T48.0X2	T48.0X3	T48.0X4	T48.0X5	T48.0X6
Ergonovine	T48.0X1	T48.0X2	T48.0X3	T48.0X4	T48.0X5	T48.0X6
Ergotamine	T46.5X1	T46.5X2	T46.5X3	T46.5X4	T46.5X5	T46.5X6
Ergotocine	T48.0X1	T48.0X2	T48.0X3	T48.0X4	T48.0X5	T48.0X6
Ergotrate	T48.0X1	T48.0X2	T48.0X3	T48.0X4	T48.0X5	T48.0X6
Ergot NEC	T64.81	T64.82	T64.83	T64.84	—	—
derivative	T48.0X1	T48.0X2	T48.0X3	T48.0X4	T48.0X5	T48.0X6
medicinal (alkaloids)	T48.0X1	T48.0X2	T48.0X3	T48.0X4	T48.0X5	T48.0X6
prepared	T48.0X1	T48.0X2	T48.0X3	T48.0X4	T48.0X5	T48.0X6
Eritrityl tetranitrate	T46.3X1	T46.3X2	T46.3X3	T46.3X4	T46.3X5	T46.3X6
Erythrityl tetranitrate	T46.3X1	T46.3X2	T46.3X3	T46.3X4	T46.3X5	T46.3X6
Erythrol tetranitrate	T46.3X1	T46.3X2	T46.3X3	T46.3X4	T46.3X5	T46.3X6
Erythromycin (salts)	T36.3X1	T36.3X2	T36.3X3	T36.3X4	T36.3X5	T36.3X6
ophthalmic preparation	T49.5X1	T49.5X2	T49.5X3	T49.5X4	T49.5X5	T49.5X6
topical NEC	T49.0X1	T49.0X2	T49.0X3	T49.0X4	T49.0X5	T49.0X6
Erythropoietin	T45.8X1	T45.8X2	T45.8X3	T45.8X4	T45.8X5	T45.8X6
human	T45.8X1	T45.8X2	T45.8X3	T45.8X4	T45.8X5	T45.8X6
Escin	T46.991	T46.992	T46.993	T46.994	T46.995	T46.996
Esculin	T45.2X1	T45.2X2	T45.2X3	T45.2X4	T45.2X5	T45.2X6
Esculoside	T45.2X1	T45.2X2	T45.2X3	T45.2X4	T45.2X5	T45.2X6
ESDT (ether-soluble tar distillate)	T49.1X1	T49.1X2	T49.1X3	T49.1X4	T49.1X5	T49.1X6
Eserine	T49.5X1	T49.5X2	T49.5X3	T49.5X4	T49.5X5	T49.5X6
Esflurbiprofen	T39.311	T39.312	T39.313	T39.314	T39.315	T39.316
Eskabarb	T42.3X1	T42.3X2	T42.3X3	T42.3X4	T42.3X5	T42.3X6
Eskalith	T43.8X1	T43.8X2	T43.8X3	T43.8X4	T43.8X5	T43.8X6
Esmolol	T44.7X1	T44.7X2	T44.7X3	T44.7X4	T44.7X5	T44.7X6

Additional Character May Be Required — Refer to the Tabular List for Character Selection ▽ Subterms under main terms may continue to next column or page

Substance	Poisoning, Accidental (unintentional)	Poisoning, Intentional Self-harm	Poisoning, Assault	Poisoning, Undetermined	Adverse Effect	Under-dosing
Estanozolol	T38.7X1	T38.7X2	T38.7X3	T38.7X4	T38.7X5	T38.7X6
Estazolam	T42.4X1	T42.4X2	T42.4X3	T42.4X4	T42.4X5	T42.4X6
Estradiol	T38.5X1	T38.5X2	T38.5X3	T38.5X4	T38.5X5	T38.5X6
with testosterone	T38.7X1	T38.7X2	T38.7X3	T38.7X4	T38.7X5	T38.7X6
benzoate	T38.5X1	T38.5X2	T38.5X3	T38.5X4	T38.5X5	T38.5X6
Estramustine	T45.1X1	T45.1X2	T45.1X3	T45.1X4	T45.1X5	T45.1X6
Estriol	T38.5X1	T38.5X2	T38.5X3	T38.5X4	T38.5X5	T38.5X6
Estrogen	T38.5X1	T38.5X2	T38.5X3	T38.5X4	T38.5X5	T38.5X6
with progesterone	T38.5X1	T38.5X2	T38.5X3	T38.5X4	T38.5X5	T38.5X6
conjugated	T38.5X1	T38.5X2	T38.5X3	T38.5X4	T38.5X5	T38.5X6
Estrone	T38.5X1	T38.5X2	T38.5X3	T38.5X4	T38.5X5	T38.5X6
Estropipate	T38.5X1	T38.5X2	T38.5X3	T38.5X4	T38.5X5	T38.5X6
Etacrynate sodium	T50.1X1	T50.1X2	T50.1X3	T50.1X4	T50.1X5	T50.1X6
Etacrynic acid	T50.1X1	T50.1X2	T50.1X3	T50.1X4	T50.1X5	T50.1X6
Etafedrine	T48.6X1	T48.6X2	T48.6X3	T48.6X4	T48.6X5	T48.6X6
Etafenone	T46.3X1	T46.3X2	T46.3X3	T46.3X4	T46.3X5	T46.3X6
Etambutol	T37.1X1	T37.1X2	T37.1X3	T37.1X4	T37.1X5	T37.1X6
Etamiphyllin	T48.6X1	T48.6X2	T48.6X3	T48.6X4	T48.6X5	T48.6X6
Etamivan	T50.7X1	T50.7X2	T50.7X3	T50.7X4	T50.7X5	T50.7X6
Etamsylate	T45.7X1	T45.7X2	T45.7X3	T45.7X4	T45.7X5	T45.7X6
Etebenecid	T50.4X1	T50.4X2	T50.4X3	T50.4X4	T50.4X5	T50.4X6
Ethacridine	T49.0X1	T49.0X2	T49.0X3	T49.0X4	T49.0X5	T49.0X6
Ethacrynic acid	T50.1X1	T50.1X2	T50.1X3	T50.1X4	T50.1X5	T50.1X6
Ethadione	T42.2X1	T42.2X2	T42.2X3	T42.2X4	T42.2X5	T42.2X6
Ethambutol	T37.1X1	T37.1X2	T37.1X3	T37.1X4	T37.1X5	T37.1X6
Ethamide	T50.2X1	T50.2X2	T50.2X3	T50.2X4	T50.2X5	T50.2X6
Ethamivan	T50.7X1	T50.7X2	T50.7X3	T50.7X4	T50.7X5	T50.7X6
Ethamsylate	T45.7X1	T45.7X2	T45.7X3	T45.7X4	T45.7X5	T45.7X6
Ethanol	T51.0X1	T51.0X2	T51.0X3	T51.0X4	—	—
beverage	T51.0X1	T51.0X2	T51.0X3	T51.0X4	—	—
Ethanolamine oleate	T46.8X1	T46.8X2	T46.8X3	T46.8X4	T46.8X5	T46.8X6
Ethaverine	T44.3X1	T44.3X2	T44.3X3	T44.3X4	T44.3X5	T44.3X6
Ethchlorvynol	T42.6X1	T42.6X2	T42.6X3	T42.6X4	T42.6X5	T42.6X6
Ethebenecid	T50.4X1	T50.4X2	T50.4X3	T50.4X4	T50.4X5	T50.4X6
Ether (vapor)	T41.0X1	T41.0X2	T41.0X3	T41.0X4	T41.0X5	T41.0X6
anesthetic	T41.0X1	T41.0X2	T41.0X3	T41.0X4	T41.0X5	T41.0X6
divinyl	T41.0X1	T41.0X2	T41.0X3	T41.0X4	T41.0X5	T41.0X6
ethyl (medicinal)	T41.0X1	T41.0X2	T41.0X3	T41.0X4	T41.0X5	T41.0X6
nonmedicinal	T52.8X1	T52.8X2	T52.8X3	T52.8X4	—	—
petroleum — see Ligroin						
solvent	T52.8X1	T52.8X2	T52.8X3	T52.8X4	—	—
Ethiazide	T50.2X1	T50.2X2	T50.2X3	T50.2X4	T50.2X5	T50.2X6
Ethidium chloride (vapor)	T59.891	T59.892	T59.893	T59.894		
Ethinamate	T42.6X1	T42.6X2	T42.6X3	T42.6X4	T42.6X5	T42.6X6
Ethinylestradiol, ethinyloestradiol	T38.5X1	T38.5X2	T38.5X3	T38.5X4	T38.5X5	T38.5X6
with						
levonorgestrel	T38.4X1	T38.4X2	T38.4X3	T38.4X4	T38.4X5	T38.4X6
norethisterone	T38.4X1	T38.4X2	T38.4X3	T38.4X4	T38.4X5	T38.4X6
Ethiodized oil (131 I)	T50.8X1	T50.8X2	T50.8X3	T50.8X4	T50.8X5	T50.8X6
Ethion	T60.0X1	T60.0X2	T60.0X3	T60.0X4	—	—
Ethionamide	T37.1X1	T37.1X2	T37.1X3	T37.1X4	T37.1X5	T37.1X6
Ethioniamide	T37.1X1	T37.1X2	T37.1X3	T37.1X4	T37.1X5	T37.1X6
Ethisterone	T38.5X1	T38.5X2	T38.5X3	T38.5X4	T38.5X5	T38.5X6
Ethobral	T42.3X1	T42.3X2	T42.3X3	T42.3X4	T42.3X5	T42.3X6
Ethocaine (infiltration)	T41.3X1	T41.3X2	T41.3X3	T41.3X4	T41.3X5	T41.3X6
(topical)						
nerve block (peripheral) (plexus)	T41.3X1	T41.3X2	T41.3X3	T41.3X4	T41.3X5	T41.3X6
spinal	T41.3X1	T41.3X2	T41.3X3	T41.3X4	T41.3X5	T41.3X6
Ethoheptazine	T40.4X1	T40.4X2	T40.4X3	T40.4X4	T40.4X5	T40.4X6
Ethopropazine	T44.3X1	T44.3X2	T44.3X3	T44.3X4	T44.3X5	T44.3X6
Ethosuximide	T42.2X1	T42.2X2	T42.2X3	T42.2X4	T42.2X5	T42.2X6
Ethotoin	T42.0X1	T42.0X2	T42.0X3	T42.0X4	T42.0X5	T42.0X6
Ethoxazene	T37.91	T37.92	T37.93	T37.94	T37.95	T37.96
Ethoxazorutoside	T46.991	T46.992	T46.993	T46.994	T46.995	T46.996
Ethoxzolamide	T50.2X1	T50.2X2	T50.2X3	T50.2X4	T50.2X5	T50.2X6
Ethyl						
acetate	T52.8X1	T52.8X2	T52.8X3	T52.8X4	—	—
alcohol	T51.0X1	T51.0X2	T51.0X3	T51.0X4	—	—
beverage	T51.0X1	T51.0X2	T51.0X3	T51.0X4	—	—
aldehyde (vapor)	T59.891	T59.892	T59.893	T59.894	—	—
liquid	T52.8X1	T52.8X2	T52.8X3	T52.8X4	—	—
aminobenzoate	T41.3X1	T41.3X2	T41.3X3	T41.3X4	T41.3X5	T41.3X6
aminophenothiazine	T43.3X1	T43.3X2	T43.3X3	T43.3X4	T43.3X5	T43.3X6
benzoate	T52.8X1	T52.8X2	T52.8X3	T52.8X4	—	—
biscoumacetate	T45.511	T45.512	T45.513	T45.514	T45.515	T45.516
bromide (anesthetic)	T41.0X1	T41.0X2	T41.0X3	T41.0X4	T41.0X5	T41.0X6
carbamate	T45.1X1	T45.1X2	T45.1X3	T45.1X4	T45.1X5	T45.1X6
carbinol	T51.3X1	T51.3X2	T51.3X3	T51.3X4	—	—
carbonate	T52.8X1	T52.8X2	T52.8X3	T52.8X4	—	—
chaulmoograte	T37.1X1	T37.1X2	T37.1X3	T37.1X4	T37.1X5	T37.1X6
chloride (anesthetic)	T41.0X1	T41.0X2	T41.0X3	T41.0X4	T41.0X5	T41.0X6

Substance	Poisoning, Accidental (unintentional)	Poisoning, Intentional Self-harm	Poisoning, Assault	Poisoning, Undetermined	Adverse Effect	Under-dosing
Ethyl — continued						
chloride — continued						
anesthetic (local)	T41.3X1	T41.3X2	T41.3X3	T41.3X4	T41.3X5	T41.3X6
inhaled	T41.0X1	T41.0X2	T41.0X3	T41.0X4	T41.0X5	T41.0X6
local	T49.4X1	T49.4X2	T49.4X3	T49.4X4	T49.4X5	T49.4X6
solvent	T53.6X1	T53.6X2	T53.6X3	T53.6X4	—	—
dibunate	T48.3X1	T48.3X2	T48.3X3	T48.3X4	T48.3X5	T48.3X6
dichloroarsine (vapor)	T57.0X1	T57.0X2	T57.0X3	T57.0X4	—	—
estranol	T38.7X1	T38.7X2	T38.7X3	T38.7X4	T38.7X5	T38.7X6
ether — see also ether	T52.8X1	T52.8X2	T52.8X3	T52.8X4		
formate NEC (solvent)	T52.0X1	T52.0X2	T52.0X3	T52.0X4	—	—
fumarate	T49.4X1	T49.4X2	T49.4X3	T49.4X4	T49.4X5	T49.4X6
hydroxyisobutyrate NEC (solvent)	T52.8X1	T52.8X2	T52.8X3	T52.8X4	—	—
iodoacetate	T59.3X1	T59.3X2	T59.3X3	T59.3X4		
lactate NEC (solvent)	T52.8X1	T52.8X2	T52.8X3	T52.8X4	—	—
loflazepate	T42.4X1	T42.4X2	T42.4X3	T42.4X4	T42.4X5	T42.4X6
mercuric chloride	T56.1X1	T56.1X2	T56.1X3	T56.1X4	—	—
methylcarbinol	T51.8X1	T51.8X2	T51.8X3	T51.8X4	—	—
morphine	T40.2X1	T40.2X2	T40.2X3	T40.2X4	T40.2X5	T40.2X6
noradrenaline	T48.6X1	T48.6X2	T48.6X3	T48.6X4	T48.6X5	T48.6X6
oxybutyrate NEC (solvent)	T52.8X1	T52.8X2	T52.8X3	T52.8X4	—	—
Ethylene (gas)	T59.891	T59.892	T59.893	T59.894		
anesthetic (general)	T41.0X1	T41.0X2	T41.0X3	T41.0X4	T41.0X5	T41.0X6
chlorohydrin	T52.8X1	T52.8X2	T52.8X3	T52.8X4		
vapor	T53.6X1	T53.6X2	T53.6X3	T53.6X4		
dichloride	T52.8X1	T52.8X2	T52.8X3	T52.8X4		
vapor	T53.6X1	T53.6X2	T53.6X3	T53.6X4		
dinitrate	T52.3X1	T52.3X2	T52.3X3	T52.3X4		
glycol(s)	T52.8X1	T52.8X2	T52.8X3	T52.8X4		
dinitrate	T52.3X1	T52.3X2	T52.3X3	T52.3X4		
monobutyl ether	T52.3X1	T52.3X2	T52.3X3	T52.3X4		
imine	T54.1X1	T54.1X2	T54.1X3	T54.1X4		
oxide (fumigant) (nonmedicinal)	T59.891	T59.892	T59.893	T59.894		
medicinal	T49.0X1	T49.0X2	T49.0X3	T49.0X4	T49.0X5	T49.0X6
Ethylenediaminetetra-acetic acid	T50.6X1	T50.6X2	T50.6X3	T50.6X4	T50.6X5	T50.6X6
Ethylenediamine theophylline	T48.6X1	T48.6X2	T48.6X3	T48.6X4	T48.6X5	T48.6X6
Ethylenedinitrilotetra-acetate	T50.6X1	T50.6X2	T50.6X3	T50.6X4	T50.6X5	T50.6X6
Ethylestrenol	T38.7X1	T38.7X2	T38.7X3	T38.7X4	T38.7X5	T38.7X6
Ethylhydroxycellulose	T47.4X1	T47.4X2	T47.4X3	T47.4X4	T47.4X5	T47.4X6
Ethylidene						
chloride NEC	T53.6X1	T53.6X2	T53.6X3	T53.6X4	—	—
diacetate	T60.3X1	T60.3X2	T60.3X3	T60.3X4	—	—
dicoumarin	T45.511	T45.512	T45.513	T45.514	T45.515	T45.516
dicoumarol	T45.511	T45.512	T45.513	T45.514	T45.515	T45.516
diethyl ether	T52.0X1	T52.0X2	T52.0X3	T52.0X4	—	—
Ethylmorphine	T40.2X1	T40.2X2	T40.2X3	T40.2X4	T40.2X5	T40.2X6
Ethylnorepinephrine	T48.6X1	T48.6X2	T48.6X3	T48.6X4	T48.6X5	T48.6X6
Ethylparachlorophen-oxyisobutyrate	T46.6X1	T46.6X2	T46.6X3	T46.6X4	T46.6X5	T46.6X6
Ethynodiol	T38.4X1	T38.4X2	T38.4X3	T38.4X4	T38.4X5	T38.4X6
with mestranol diacetate	T38.4X1	T38.4X2	T38.4X3	T38.4X4	T38.4X5	T38.4X6
Etidocaine	T41.3X1	T41.3X2	T41.3X3	T41.3X4	T41.3X5	T41.3X6
infiltration (subcutaneous)	T41.3X1	T41.3X2	T41.3X3	T41.3X4	T41.3X5	T41.3X6
nerve (peripheral) (plexus)	T41.3X1	T41.3X2	T41.3X3	T41.3X4	T41.3X5	T41.3X6
Etidronate	T50.991	T50.992	T50.993	T50.994	T50.995	T50.996
Etidronic acid (disodium salt)	T50.991	T50.992	T50.993	T50.994	T50.995	T50.996
Etifoxine	T42.6X1	T42.6X2	T42.6X3	T42.6X4	T42.6X5	T42.6X6
Etilefrine	T44.4X1	T44.4X2	T44.4X3	T44.4X4	T44.4X5	T44.4X6
Etilfen	T42.3X1	T42.3X2	T42.3X3	T42.3X4	T42.3X5	T42.3X6
Etinodiol	T38.4X1	T38.4X2	T38.4X3	T38.4X4	T38.4X5	T38.4X6
Etiroxate	T46.6X1	T46.6X2	T46.6X3	T46.6X4	T46.6X5	T46.6X6
Etizolam	T42.4X1	T42.4X2	T42.4X3	T42.4X4	T42.4X5	T42.4X6
Etodolac	T39.391	T39.392	T39.393	T39.394	T39.395	T39.396
Etofamide	T37.3X1	T37.3X2	T37.3X3	T37.3X4	T37.3X5	T37.3X6
Etofibrate	T46.6X1	T46.6X2	T46.6X3	T46.6X4	T46.6X5	T46.6X6
Etofylline	T46.7X1	T46.7X2	T46.7X3	T46.7X4	T46.7X5	T46.7X6
clofibrate	T46.6X1	T46.6X2	T46.6X3	T46.6X4	T46.6X5	T46.6X6
Etoglucid	T45.1X1	T45.1X2	T45.1X3	T45.1X4	T45.1X5	T45.1X6
Etomidate	T41.1X1	T41.1X2	T41.1X3	T41.1X4	T41.1X5	T41.1X6
Etomide	T39.8X1	T39.8X2	T39.8X3	T39.8X4	T39.8X5	T39.8X6
Etomidoline	T44.3X1	T44.3X2	T44.3X3	T44.3X4	T44.3X5	T44.3X6
Etoposide	T45.1X1	T45.1X2	T45.1X3	T45.1X4	T45.1X5	T45.1X6
Etorphine	T40.2X1	T40.2X2	T40.2X3	T40.2X4	T40.2X5	T40.2X6
Etoval	T42.3X1	T42.3X2	T42.3X3	T42.3X4	T42.3X5	T42.3X6
Etozolin	T50.1X1	T50.1X2	T50.1X3	T50.1X4	T50.1X5	T50.1X6
Etretinate	T50.991	T50.992	T50.993	T50.994	T50.995	T50.996
Etryptamine	T43.691	T43.692	T43.693	T43.694	T43.695	T43.696
Etybenzatropine	T44.3X1	T44.3X2	T44.3X3	T44.3X4	T44.3X5	T44.3X6

Substance	Poisoning, Accidental (unintentional)	Poisoning, Intentional Self-harm	Poisoning, Assault	Poisoning, Undetermined	Adverse Effect	Under-dosing
Etynodiol	T38.4X1	T38.4X2	T38.4X3	T38.4X4	T38.4X5	T38.4X6
Eucaine	T41.3X1	T41.3X2	T41.3X3	T41.3X4	T41.3X5	T41.3X6
Eucalyptus oil	T49.7X1	T49.7X2	T49.7X3	T49.7X4	T49.7X5	T49.7X6
Eucatropine	T49.5X1	T49.5X2	T49.5X3	T49.5X4	T49.5X5	T49.5X6
Eucodal	T40.2X1	T40.2X2	T40.2X3	T40.2X4	T40.2X5	T40.2X6
Euneryl	T42.3X1	T42.3X2	T42.3X3	T42.3X4	T42.3X5	T42.3X6
Euphthalmine	T44.3X1	T44.3X2	T44.3X3	T44.3X4	T44.3X5	T44.3X6
Eurax	T49.0X1	T49.0X2	T49.0X3	T49.0X4	T49.0X5	T49.0X6
Euresol	T49.4X1	T49.4X2	T49.4X3	T49.4X4	T49.4X5	T49.4X6
Euthroid	T38.1X1	T38.1X2	T38.1X3	T38.1X4	T38.1X5	T38.1X6
Evans blue	T50.8X1	T50.8X2	T50.8X3	T50.8X4	T50.8X5	T50.8X6
Evipal	T42.3X1	T42.3X2	T42.3X3	T42.3X4	T42.3X5	T42.3X6
sodium	T41.1X1	T41.1X2	T41.1X3	T41.1X4	T41.1X5	T41.1X6
Evipan	T42.3X1	T42.3X2	T42.3X3	T42.3X4	T42.3X5	T42.3X6
sodium	T41.1X1	T41.1X2	T41.1X3	T41.1X4	T41.1X5	T41.1X6
Exalamide	T49.0X1	T49.0X2	T49.0X3	T49.0X4	T49.0X5	T49.0X6
Exalgin	T39.1X1	T39.1X2	T39.1X3	T39.1X4	T39.1X5	T39.1X6
Excipients, pharmaceutical	T50.901	T50.902	T50.903	T50.904	T50.905	T50.906
Exhaust gas (engine) (motor vehicle)	T58.01	T58.02	T58.03	T58.04	—	—
Ex-Lax (phenolphthalein)	T47.2X1	T47.2X2	T47.2X3	T47.2X4	T47.2X5	T47.2X6
Expectorant NEC	T48.4X1	T48.4X2	T48.4X3	T48.4X4	T48.4X5	T48.4X6
Extended insulin zinc suspension	T38.3X1	T38.3X2	T38.3X3	T38.3X4	T38.3X5	T38.3X6
External medications (skin) (mucous membrane)	T49.91	T49.92	T49.93	T49.94	T49.95	T49.96
dental agent	T49.7X1	T49.7X2	T49.7X3	T49.7X4	T49.7X5	T49.7X6
ENT agent	T49.6X1	T49.6X2	T49.6X3	T49.6X4	T49.6X5	T49.6X6
ophthalmic preparation	T49.5X1	T49.5X2	T49.5X3	T49.5X4	T49.5X5	T49.5X6
specified NEC	T49.8X1	T49.8X2	T49.8X3	T49.8X4	T49.8X5	T49.8X6
Extrapyramidal antagonist NEC	T44.3X1	T44.3X2	T44.3X3	T44.3X4	T44.3X5	T44.3X6
Eye agents (anti-infective)	T49.5X1	T49.5X2	T49.5X3	T49.5X4	T49.5X5	T49.5X6
Eye drug NEC	T49.5X1	T49.5X2	T49.5X3	T49.5X4	T49.5X5	T49.5X6
FAC (fluorouracil + doxorubicin + cyclophosphamide)	T45.1X1	T45.1X2	T45.1X3	T45.1X4	T45.1X5	T45.1X6
Factor						
I (fibrinogen)	T45.8X1	T45.8X2	T45.8X3	T45.8X4	T45.8X5	T45.8X6
III (thromboplastin)	T45.8X1	T45.8X2	T45.8X3	T45.8X4	T45.8X5	T45.8X6
IX complex	T45.7X1	T45.7X2	T45.7X3	T45.7X4	T45.7X5	T45.7X6
human	T45.8X1	T45.8X2	T45.8X3	T45.8X4	T45.8X5	T45.8X6
VIII (antihemophilic Factor) (concentrate)	T45.8X1	T45.8X2	T45.8X3	T45.8X4	T45.8X5	T45.8X6
Famotidine	T47.0X1	T47.0X2	T47.0X3	T47.0X4	T47.0X5	T47.0X6
Fat suspension, intravenous	T50.991	T50.992	T50.993	T50.994	T50.995	T50.996
Fazadinium bromide	T48.1X1	T48.1X2	T48.1X3	T48.1X4	T48.1X5	T48.1X6
Febarbamate	T42.3X1	T42.3X2	T42.3X3	T42.3X4	T42.3X5	T42.3X6
Fecal softener	T47.4X1	T47.4X2	T47.4X3	T47.4X4	T47.4X5	T47.4X6
Fedrilate	T48.3X1	T48.3X2	T48.3X3	T48.3X4	T48.3X5	T48.3X6
Felodipine	T46.1X1	T46.1X2	T46.1X3	T46.1X4	T46.1X5	T46.1X6
Felypressin	T38.891	T38.892	T38.893	T38.894	T38.895	T38.896
Femoxetine	T43.221	T43.222	T43.223	T43.224	T43.225	T43.226
Fenalcomine	T46.3X1	T46.3X2	T46.3X3	T46.3X4	T46.3X5	T46.3X6
Fenamisal	T37.1X1	T37.1X2	T37.1X3	T37.1X4	T37.1X5	T37.1X6
Fenazone	T39.2X1	T39.2X2	T39.2X3	T39.2X4	T39.2X5	T39.2X6
Fenbendazole	T37.4X1	T37.4X2	T37.4X3	T37.4X4	T37.4X5	T37.4X6
Fenbutrazate	T50.5X1	T50.5X2	T50.5X3	T50.5X4	T50.5X5	T50.5X6
Fencamfamine	T43.691	T43.692	T43.693	T43.694	T43.695	T43.696
Fendiline	T46.1X1	T46.1X2	T46.1X3	T46.1X4	T46.1X5	T46.1X6
Fenetylline	T43.691	T43.692	T43.693	T43.694	T43.695	T43.696
Fenflumizole	T39.391	T39.392	T39.393	T39.394	T39.395	T39.396
Fenfluramine	T50.5X1	T50.5X2	T50.5X3	T50.5X4	T50.5X5	T50.5X6
Fenobarbital	T42.3X1	T42.3X2	T42.3X3	T42.3X4	T42.3X5	T42.3X6
Fenofibrate	T46.6X1	T46.6X2	T46.6X3	T46.6X4	T46.6X5	T46.6X6
Fenoprofen	T39.311	T39.312	T39.313	T39.314	T39.315	T39.316
Fenoterol	T48.6X1	T48.6X2	T48.6X3	T48.6X4	T48.6X5	T48.6X6
Fenoverine	T44.3X1	T44.3X2	T44.3X3	T44.3X4	T44.3X5	T44.3X6
Fenoxazoline	T48.5X1	T48.5X2	T48.5X3	T48.5X4	T48.5X5	T48.5X6
Fenproporex	T50.5X1	T50.5X2	T50.5X3	T50.5X4	T50.5X5	T50.5X6
Fenquizone	T50.2X1	T50.2X2	T50.2X3	T50.2X4	T50.2X5	T50.2X6
Fentanyl	T40.4X1	T40.4X2	T40.4X3	T40.4X4	T40.4X5	T40.4X6
Fentazin	T43.3X1	T43.3X2	T43.3X3	T43.3X4	T43.3X5	T43.3X6
Fenthion	T60.0X1	T60.0X2	T60.0X3	T60.0X4	—	—
Fenticlor	T49.0X1	T49.0X2	T49.0X3	T49.0X4	T49.0X5	T49.0X6
Fenylbutazone	T39.2X1	T39.2X2	T39.2X3	T39.2X4	T39.2X5	T39.2X6
Feprazone	T39.2X1	T39.2X2	T39.2X3	T39.2X4	T39.2X5	T39.2X6
Fer de lance (bite) (venom)	T63.061	T63.062	T63.063	T63.064	—	—
Ferric — see also Iron						
chloride	T45.4X1	T45.4X2	T45.4X3	T45.4X4	T45.4X5	T45.4X6
citrate	T45.4X1	T45.4X2	T45.4X3	T45.4X4	T45.4X5	T45.4X6
hydroxide						
colloidal	T45.4X1	T45.4X2	T45.4X3	T45.4X4	T45.4X5	T45.4X6

Substance	Poisoning, Accidental (unintentional)	Poisoning, Intentional Self-harm	Poisoning, Assault	Poisoning, Undetermined	Adverse Effect	Under-dosing
Ferric — see also Iron — continued						
hydroxide — continued						
polymaltose	T45.4X1	T45.4X2	T45.4X3	T45.4X4	T45.4X5	T45.4X6
pyrophosphate	T45.4X1	T45.4X2	T45.4X3	T45.4X4	T45.4X5	T45.4X6
Ferritin	T45.4X1	T45.4X2	T45.4X3	T45.4X4	T45.4X5	T45.4X6
Ferrocholinate	T45.4X1	T45.4X2	T45.4X3	T45.4X4	T45.4X5	T45.4X6
Ferrodextrane	T45.4X1	T45.4X2	T45.4X3	T45.4X4	T45.4X5	T45.4X6
Ferropolimaler	T45.4X1	T45.4X2	T45.4X3	T45.4X4	T45.4X5	T45.4X6
Ferrous — see also Iron						
phosphate	T45.4X1	T45.4X2	T45.4X3	T45.4X4	T45.4X5	T45.4X6
salt	T45.4X1	T45.4X2	T45.4X3	T45.4X4	T45.4X5	T45.4X6
with folic acid	T45.4X1	T45.4X2	T45.4X3	T45.4X4	T45.4X5	T45.4X6
Ferrous fumerate, gluconate, lactate, salt NEC, sulfate (medicinal)	T45.4X1	T45.4X2	T45.4X3	T45.4X4	T45.4X5	T45.4X6
Ferrovanadium (fumes)	T59.891	T59.892	T59.893	T59.894	—	—
Ferrum — see Iron						
Fertilizers NEC	T65.891	T65.892	T65.893	T65.894	—	—
with herbicide mixture	T60.3X1	T60.3X2	T60.3X3	T60.3X4	—	—
Fetoxilate	T47.6X1	T47.6X2	T47.6X3	T47.6X4	T47.6X5	T47.6X6
Fiber, dietary	T47.4X1	T47.4X2	T47.4X3	T47.4X4	T47.4X5	T47.4X6
Fiberglass	T65.831	T65.832	T65.833	T65.834	—	—
Fibrinogen (human)	T45.8X1	T45.8X2	T45.8X3	T45.8X4	T45.8X5	T45.8X6
Fibrinolysin (human)	T45.691	T45.692	T45.693	T45.694	T45.695	T45.696
Fibrinolysis						
affecting drug	T45.601	T45.602	T45.603	T45.604	T45.605	T45.606
inhibitor NEC	T45.621	T45.622	T45.623	T45.624	T45.625	T45.626
Fibrinolytic drug	T45.611	T45.612	T45.613	T45.614	T45.615	T45.616
Filix mas	T37.4X1	T37.4X2	T37.4X3	T37.4X4	T37.4X5	T37.4X6
Filtering cream	T49.3X1	T49.3X2	T49.3X3	T49.3X4	T49.3X5	T49.3X6
Fiorinal	T39.011	T39.012	T39.013	T39.014	T39.015	T39.016
Firedamp	T59.891	T59.892	T59.893	T59.894	—	—
Fish, noxious, nonbacterial	T61.91	T61.92	T61.93	T61.94	—	—
ciguatera	T61.01	T61.02	T61.03	T61.04	—	—
scombroid	T61.11	T61.12	T61.13	T61.14	—	—
shell	T61.781	T61.782	T61.783	T61.784	—	—
specified NEC	T61.771	T61.772	T61.773	T61.774	—	—
Flagyl	T37.3X1	T37.3X2	T37.3X3	T37.3X4	T37.3X5	T37.3X6
Flavine adenine dinucleotide	T45.2X1	T45.2X2	T45.2X3	T45.2X4	T45.2X5	T45.2X6
Flavodic acid	T46.991	T46.992	T46.993	T46.994	T46.995	T46.996
Flavoxate	T44.3X1	T44.3X2	T44.3X3	T44.3X4	T44.3X5	T44.3X6
Flaxedil	T48.1X1	T48.1X2	T48.1X3	T48.1X4	T48.1X5	T48.1X6
Flaxseed (medicinal)	T49.3X1	T49.3X2	T49.3X3	T49.3X4	T49.3X5	T49.3X6
Flecainide	T46.2X1	T46.2X2	T46.2X3	T46.2X4	T46.2X5	T46.2X6
Fleroxacin	T36.8X1	T36.8X2	T36.8X3	T36.8X4	T36.8X5	T36.8X6
Floctafenine	T39.8X1	T39.8X2	T39.8X3	T39.8X4	T39.8X5	T39.8X6
Flomax	T44.6X1	T44.6X2	T44.6X3	T44.6X4	T44.6X5	T44.6X6
Flomoxef	T36.1X1	T36.1X2	T36.1X3	T36.1X4	T36.1X5	T36.1X6
Flopropione	T44.3X1	T44.3X2	T44.3X3	T44.3X4	T44.3X5	T44.3X6
Florantyrone	T47.5X1	T47.5X2	T47.5X3	T47.5X4	T47.5X5	T47.5X6
Floraquin	T37.8X1	T37.8X2	T37.8X3	T37.8X4	T37.8X5	T37.8X6
Florinef	T38.0X1	T38.0X2	T38.0X3	T38.0X4	T38.0X5	T38.0X6
ENT agent	T49.6X1	T49.6X2	T49.6X3	T49.6X4	T49.6X5	T49.6X6
ophthalmic preparation	T49.5X1	T49.5X2	T49.5X3	T49.5X4	T49.5X5	T49.5X6
topical NEC	T49.0X1	T49.0X2	T49.0X3	T49.0X4	T49.0X5	T49.0X6
Flowers of sulfur	T49.4X1	T49.4X2	T49.4X3	T49.4X4	T49.4X5	T49.4X6
Floxuridine	T45.1X1	T45.1X2	T45.1X3	T45.1X4	T45.1X5	T45.1X6
Fluanisone	T43.4X1	T43.4X2	T43.4X3	T43.4X4	T43.4X5	T43.4X6
Flubendazole	T37.4X1	T37.4X2	T37.4X3	T37.4X4	T37.4X5	T37.4X6
Fluclorolone acetonide	T49.0X1	T49.0X2	T49.0X3	T49.0X4	T49.0X5	T49.0X6
Flucloxacillin	T36.0X1	T36.0X2	T36.0X3	T36.0X4	T36.0X5	T36.0X6
Fluconazole	T37.8X1	T37.8X2	T37.8X3	T37.8X4	T37.8X5	T37.8X6
Flucytosine	T37.8X1	T37.8X2	T37.8X3	T37.8X4	T37.8X5	T37.8X6
Fludeoxyglucose (18F)	T50.8X1	T50.8X2	T50.8X3	T50.8X4	T50.8X5	T50.8X6
Fludiazepam	T42.4X1	T42.4X2	T42.4X3	T42.4X4	T42.4X5	T42.4X6
Fludrocortisone	T50.0X1	T50.0X2	T50.0X3	T50.0X4	T50.0X5	T50.0X6
ENT agent	T49.6X1	T49.6X2	T49.6X3	T49.6X4	T49.6X5	T49.6X6
ophthalmic preparation	T49.5X1	T49.5X2	T49.5X3	T49.5X4	T49.5X5	T49.5X6
topical NEC	T49.0X1	T49.0X2	T49.0X3	T49.0X4	T49.0X5	T49.0X6
Fludroxycortide	T49.0X1	T49.0X2	T49.0X3	T49.0X4	T49.0X5	T49.0X6
Flufenamic acid	T39.391	T39.392	T39.393	T39.394	T39.395	T39.396
Fluindione	T45.511	T45.512	T45.513	T45.514	T45.515	T45.516
Flumequine	T37.8X1	T37.8X2	T37.8X3	T37.8X4	T37.8X5	T37.8X6
Flumethasone	T49.0X1	T49.0X2	T49.0X3	T49.0X4	T49.0X5	T49.0X6
Flumethiazide	T50.2X1	T50.2X2	T50.2X3	T50.2X4	T50.2X5	T50.2X6
Flumidin	T37.5X1	T37.5X2	T37.5X3	T37.5X4	T37.5X5	T37.5X6
Flunarizine	T46.7X1	T46.7X2	T46.7X3	T46.7X4	T46.7X5	T46.7X6
Flunidazole	T37.8X1	T37.8X2	T37.8X3	T37.8X4	T37.8X5	T37.8X6
Flunisolide	T48.6X1	T48.6X2	T48.6X3	T48.6X4	T48.6X5	T48.6X6
Flunitrazepam	T42.4X1	T42.4X2	T42.4X3	T42.4X4	T42.4X5	T42.4X6
Fluocinolone (acetonide)	T49.0X1	T49.0X2	T49.0X3	T49.0X4	T49.0X5	T49.0X6
Fluocinonide	T49.0X1	T49.0X2	T49.0X3	T49.0X4	T49.0X5	T49.0X6

Additional Character May Be Required — Refer to the Tabular List for Character Selection   ▽ Subterms under main terms may continue to next column or page

Substance	Poisoning, Accidental (unintentional)	Poisoning, Intentional Self-harm	Poisoning, Assault	Poisoning, Undetermined	Adverse Effect	Under-dosing
Fluocortin (butyl)	T49.0X1	T49.0X2	T49.0X3	T49.0X4	T49.0X5	T49.0X6
Fluocortolone	T49.0X1	T49.0X2	T49.0X3	T49.0X4	T49.0X5	T49.0X6
Fluohydrocortisone	T38.0X1	T38.0X2	T38.0X3	T38.0X4	T38.0X5	T38.0X6
ENT agent	T49.6X1	T49.6X2	T49.6X3	T49.6X4	T49.6X5	T49.6X6
ophthalmic preparation	T49.5X1	T49.5X2	T49.5X3	T49.5X4	T49.5X5	T49.5X6
topical NEC	T49.0X1	T49.0X2	T49.0X3	T49.0X4	T49.0X5	T49.0X6
Fluonid	T49.0X1	T49.0X2	T49.0X3	T49.0X4	T49.0X5	T49.0X6
Fluopromazine	T43.3X1	T43.3X2	T43.3X3	T43.3X4	T43.3X5	T43.3X6
Fluoracetate	T60.8X1	T60.8X2	T60.8X3	T60.8X4	—	—
Fluorescein	T50.8X1	T50.8X2	T50.8X3	T50.8X4	T50.8X5	T50.8X6
Fluorhydrocortisone	T50.0X1	T50.0X2	T50.0X3	T50.0X4	T50.0X5	T50.0X6
Fluoride (nonmedicinal) (pesticide) (sodium) **NEC**	T60.8X1	T60.8X2	T60.8X3	T60.8X4	—	—
hydrogen — *see* Hydrofluoric acid						
medicinal NEC	T50.991	T50.992	T50.993	T50.994	T50.995	T50.996
dental use	T49.7X1	T49.7X2	T49.7X3	T49.7X4	T49.7X5	T49.7X6
not pesticide NEC	T54.91	T54.92	T54.93	T54.94		
stannous	T49.7X1	T49.7X2	T49.7X3	T49.7X4	T49.7X5	T49.7X6
Fluorinated corticosteroids	T38.0X1	T38.0X2	T38.0X3	T38.0X4	T38.0X5	T38.0X6
Fluorine (gas)	T59.5X1	T59.5X2	T59.5X3	T59.5X4	—	—
salt — *see* Fluoride(s)						
Fluoristan	T49.7X1	T49.7X2	T49.7X3	T49.7X4	T49.7X5	T49.7X6
Fluormetholone	T49.0X1	T49.0X2	T49.0X3	T49.0X4	T49.0X5	T49.0X6
Fluoroacetate	T60.8X1	T60.8X2	T60.8X3	T60.8X4	—	—
Fluorocarbon monomer	T53.6X1	T53.6X2	T53.6X3	T53.6X4	—	—
Fluorocytosine	T37.8X1	T37.8X2	T37.8X3	T37.8X4	T37.8X5	T37.8X6
Fluorodeoxyuridine	T45.1X1	T45.1X2	T45.1X3	T45.1X4	T45.1X5	T45.1X6
Fluorometholone	T49.0X1	T49.0X2	T49.0X3	T49.0X4	T49.0X5	T49.0X6
ophthalmic preparation	T49.5X1	T49.5X2	T49.5X3	T49.5X4	T49.5X5	T49.5X6
Fluorophosphate insecticide	T60.0X1	T60.0X2	T60.0X3	T60.0X4	—	—
Fluorosol	T46.3X1	T46.3X2	T46.3X3	T46.3X4	T46.3X5	T46.3X6
Fluorouracil	T45.1X1	T45.1X2	T45.1X3	T45.1X4	T45.1X5	T45.1X6
Fluorphenylalanine	T49.5X1	T49.5X2	T49.5X3	T49.5X4	T49.5X5	T49.5X6
Fluothane	T41.0X1	T41.0X2	T41.0X3	T41.0X4	T41.0X5	T41.0X6
Fluoxetine	T43.221	T43.222	T43.223	T43.224	T43.225	T43.226
Fluoxymesterone	T38.7X1	T38.7X2	T38.7X3	T38.7X4	T38.7X5	T38.7X6
Flupenthixol	T43.4X1	T43.4X2	T43.4X3	T43.4X4	T43.4X5	T43.4X6
Flupentixol	T43.4X1	T43.4X2	T43.4X3	T43.4X4	T43.4X5	T43.4X6
Fluphenazine	T43.3X1	T43.3X2	T43.3X3	T43.3X4	T43.3X5	T43.3X6
Fluprednidene	T49.0X1	T49.0X2	T49.0X3	T49.0X4	T49.0X5	T49.0X6
Fluprednisolone	T38.0X1	T38.0X2	T38.0X3	T38.0X4	T38.0X5	T38.0X6
Fluradoline	T39.8X1	T39.8X2	T39.8X3	T39.8X4	T39.8X5	T39.8X6
Flurandrenolide	T49.0X1	T49.0X2	T49.0X3	T49.0X4	T49.0X5	T49.0X6
Flurandrenolone	T49.0X1	T49.0X2	T49.0X3	T49.0X4	T49.0X5	T49.0X6
Flurazepam	T42.4X1	T42.4X2	T42.4X3	T42.4X4	T42.4X5	T42.4X6
Flurbiprofen	T39.311	T39.312	T39.313	T39.314	T39.315	T39.316
Flurobate	T49.0X1	T49.0X2	T49.0X3	T49.0X4	T49.0X5	T49.0X6
Fluroxene	T41.0X1	T41.0X2	T41.0X3	T41.0X4	T41.0X5	T41.0X6
Fluspirilene	T43.591	T43.592	T43.593	T43.594	T43.595	T43.596
Flutamide	T38.6X1	T38.6X2	T38.6X3	T38.6X4	T38.6X5	T38.6X6
Flutazolam	T42.4X1	T42.4X2	T42.4X3	T42.4X4	T42.4X5	T42.4X6
Fluticasone propionate	T49.1X1	T49.1X2	T49.1X3	T49.1X4	T49.1X5	T49.1X6
Flutoprazepam	T42.4X1	T42.4X2	T42.4X3	T42.4X4	T42.4X5	T42.4X6
Flutropium bromide	T48.6X1	T48.6X2	T48.6X3	T48.6X4	T48.6X5	T48.6X6
Fluvoxamine	T43.221	T43.222	T43.223	T43.224	T43.225	T43.226
Folacin	T45.8X1	T45.8X2	T45.8X3	T45.8X4	T45.8X5	T45.8X6
Folic acid	T45.8X1	T45.8X2	T45.8X3	T45.8X4	T45.8X5	T45.8X6
with ferrous salt	T45.2X1	T45.2X2	T45.2X3	T45.2X4	T45.2X5	T45.2X6
antagonist	T45.1X1	T45.1X2	T45.1X3	T45.1X4	T45.1X5	T45.1X6
Folinic acid	T45.8X1	T45.8X2	T45.8X3	T45.8X4	T45.8X5	T45.8X6
Folium stramoniae	T48.6X1	T48.6X2	T48.6X3	T48.6X4	T48.6X5	T48.6X6
Follicle-stimulating hormone, human	T38.811	T38.812	T38.813	T38.814	T38.815	T38.816
Folpet	T60.3X1	T60.3X2	T60.3X3	T60.3X4	—	—
Fominoben	T48.3X1	T48.3X2	T48.3X3	T48.3X4	T48.3X5	T48.3X6
Food, foodstuffs, noxious, nonbacterial, NEC	T62.91	T62.92	T62.93	T62.94	—	—
berries	T62.1X1	T62.1X2	T62.1X3	T62.1X4	—	—
fish — *see also* Fish	T61.91	T61.92	T61.93	T61.94	—	—
mushrooms	T62.0X1	T62.0X2	T62.0X3	T62.0X4	—	—
plants	T62.2X1	T62.2X2	T62.2X3	T62.2X4	—	—
seafood	T61.91	T61.92	T61.93	T61.94	—	—
specified NEC	T61.8X1	T61.8X2	T61.8X3	T61.8X4	—	—
seeds	T62.2X1	T62.2X2	T62.2X3	T62.2X4	—	—
shellfish	T61.781	T61.782	T61.783	T61.784	—	—
specified NEC	T62.8X1	T62.8X2	T62.8X3	T62.8X4	—	—
Fool's parsley	T62.2X1	T62.2X2	T62.2X3	T62.2X4	—	—
Formaldehyde (solution), gas or vapor	T59.2X1	T59.2X2	T59.2X3	T59.2X4	—	—
fungicide	T60.3X1	T60.3X2	T60.3X3	T60.3X4	—	—
Formalin	T59.2X1	T59.2X2	T59.2X3	T59.2X4	—	—
fungicide	T60.3X1	T60.3X2	T60.3X3	T60.3X4	—	—
vapor	T59.2X1	T59.2X2	T59.2X3	T59.2X4	—	—
Formic acid	T54.2X1	T54.2X2	T54.2X3	T54.2X4	—	—
vapor	T59.891	T59.892	T59.893	T59.894	—	—
Foscarnet sodium	T37.5X1	T37.5X2	T37.5X3	T37.5X4	T37.5X5	T37.5X6
Fosfestrol	T38.5X1	T38.5X2	T38.5X3	T38.5X4	T38.5X5	T38.5X6
Fosfomycin	T36.8X1	T36.8X2	T36.8X3	T36.8X4	T36.8X5	T36.8X6
Fosfonet sodium	T37.5X1	T37.5X2	T37.5X3	T37.5X4	T37.5X5	T37.5X6
Fosinopril	T46.4X1	T46.4X2	T46.4X3	T46.4X4	T46.4X5	T46.4X6
sodium	T46.4X1	T46.4X2	T46.4X3	T46.4X4	T46.4X5	T46.4X6
Fowler's solution	T57.0X1	T57.0X2	T57.0X3	T57.0X4	—	—
Foxglove	T62.2X1	T62.2X2	T62.2X3	T62.2X4	—	—
Framycetin	T36.5X1	T36.5X2	T36.5X3	T36.5X4	T36.5X5	T36.5X6
Frangula	T47.2X1	T47.2X2	T47.2X3	T47.2X4	T47.2X5	T47.2X6
extract	T47.2X1	T47.2X2	T47.2X3	T47.2X4	T47.2X5	T47.2X6
Frei antigen	T50.8X1	T50.8X2	T50.8X3	T50.8X4	T50.8X5	T50.8X6
Freon	T53.5X1	T53.5X2	T53.5X3	T53.5X4	—	—
Fructose	T50.3X1	T50.3X2	T50.3X3	T50.3X4	T50.3X5	T50.3X6
Frusemide	T50.1X1	T50.1X2	T50.1X3	T50.1X4	T50.1X5	T50.1X6
FSH	T38.811	T38.812	T38.813	T38.814	T38.815	T38.816
Ftorafur	T45.1X1	T45.1X2	T45.1X3	T45.1X4	T45.1X5	T45.1X6
Fuel						
automobile	T52.0X1	T52.0X2	T52.0X3	T52.0X4	—	—
exhaust gas, not in transit	T58.01	T58.02	T58.03	T58.04		
vapor NEC	T52.0X1	T52.0X2	T52.0X3	T52.0X4	—	—
gas (domestic use) — *see also* Carbon, monoxide, fuel, utility	T59.891	T59.892	T59.893	T59.894	—	—
utility	T59.891	T59.892	T59.893	T59.894	—	—
incomplete combustion of — *see* Carbon, monoxide, fuel, utility						
in mobile container	T59.891	T59.892	T59.893	T59.894	—	—
piped (natural)	T59.891	T59.892	T59.893	T59.894	—	—
industrial, incomplete combustion	T58.8X1	T58.8X2	T58.8X3	T58.8X4	—	—
Fugillin	T36.8X1	T36.8X2	T36.8X3	T36.8X4	T36.8X5	T36.8X6
Fulminate of mercury	T56.1X1	T56.1X2	T56.1X3	T56.1X4	—	—
Fulvicin	T36.7X1	T36.7X2	T36.7X3	T36.7X4	T36.7X5	T36.7X6
Fumadil	T36.8X1	T36.8X2	T36.8X3	T36.8X4	T36.8X5	T36.8X6
Fumagillin	T36.8X1	T36.8X2	T36.8X3	T36.8X4	T36.8X5	T36.8X6
Fumaric acid	T49.4X1	T49.4X2	T49.4X3	T49.4X4	T49.4X5	T49.4X6
Fumes (from)	T59.91	T59.92	T59.93	T59.94	—	—
carbon monoxide — *see* Carbon, monoxide						
charcoal (domestic use) — *see* Charcoal, fumes						
chloroform — *see* Chloroform						
coke (in domestic stoves, fireplaces) — *see* Coke fumes						
corrosive NEC	T54.91	T54.92	T54.93	T54.94	—	—
ether — *see* ether						
freons	T53.5X1	T53.5X2	T53.5X3	T53.5X4	—	—
hydrocarbons	T59.891	T59.892	T59.893	T59.894	—	—
petroleum (liquefied)	T59.891	T59.892	T59.893	T59.894	—	—
distributed through pipes (pure or mixed with air)	T59.891	T59.892	T59.893	T59.894		
lead — *see* lead						
metal — *see* Metals, or the specified metal						
nitrogen dioxide	T59.0X1	T59.0X2	T59.0X3	T59.0X4	—	—
pesticides — *see* Pesticides						
petroleum (liquefied)	T59.891	T59.892	T59.893	T59.894	—	—
distributed through pipes (pure or mixed with air)	T59.891	T59.892	T59.893	T59.894		
polyester	T59.891	T59.892	T59.893	T59.894	—	—
specified source NEC — *see also* substance specified	T59.891	T59.892	T59.893	T59.894		
sulfur dioxide	T59.1X1	T59.1X2	T59.1X3	T59.1X4	—	—
Fumigant NEC	T60.91	T60.92	T60.93	T60.94	—	—
Fungicide NEC (nonmedicinal)	T60.3X1	T60.3X2	T60.3X3	T60.3X4	—	—
Fungi, noxious, used as food	T62.0X1	T62.0X2	T62.0X3	T62.0X4	—	—
Fungizone	T36.7X1	T36.7X2	T36.7X3	T36.7X4	T36.7X5	T36.7X6
topical	T49.0X1	T49.0X2	T49.0X3	T49.0X4	T49.0X5	T49.0X6
Furacin	T49.0X1	T49.0X2	T49.0X3	T49.0X4	T49.0X5	T49.0X6
Furadantin	T37.91	T37.92	T37.93	T37.94	T37.95	T37.96
Furazolidone	T37.8X1	T37.8X2	T37.8X3	T37.8X4	T37.8X5	T37.8X6

Substance	Poisoning, Accidental (unintentional)	Poisoning, Intentional Self-harm	Poisoning, Assault	Poisoning, Undetermined	Adverse Effect	Under-dosing
Furazolium chloride	T49.0X1	T49.0X2	T49.0X3	T49.0X4	T49.0X5	T49.0X6
Furfural	T52.8X1	T52.8X2	T52.8X3	T52.8X4	—	—
Furnace (coal burning) (domestic), gas from	T58.2X1	T58.2X2	T58.2X3	T58.2X4	—	—
industrial	T58.8X1	T58.8X2	T58.8X3	T58.8X4	—	—
Furniture polish	T65.891	T65.892	T65.893	T65.894	—	—
Furosemide	T50.1X1	T50.1X2	T50.1X3	T50.1X4	T50.1X5	T50.1X6
Furoxone	T37.91	T37.92	T37.93	T37.94	T37.95	T37.96
Fursultiamine	T45.2X1	T45.2X2	T45.2X3	T45.2X4	T45.2X5	T45.2X6
Fusafungine	T36.8X1	T36.8X2	T36.8X3	T36.8X4	T36.8X5	T36.8X6
Fusel oil (any) (amyl) (butyl) (propyl), vapor	T51.3X1	T51.3X2	T51.3X3	T51.3X4	—	—
Fusidate (ethanolamine) (sodium)	T36.8X1	T36.8X2	T36.8X3	T36.8X4	T36.8X5	T36.8X6
Fusidic acid	T36.8X1	T36.8X2	T36.8X3	T36.8X4	T36.8X5	T36.8X6
Fytic acid, nonasodium	T50.6X1	T50.6X2	T50.6X3	T50.6X4	T50.6X5	T50.6X6
b-Galactosidase	T47.5X1	T47.5X2	T47.5X3	T47.5X4	T47.5X5	T47.5X6
GABA	T43.8X1	T43.8X2	T43.8X3	T43.8X4	T43.8X5	T43.8X6
Gadopentetic acid	T50.8X1	T50.8X2	T50.8X3	T50.8X4	T50.8X5	T50.8X6
Galactose	T50.3X1	T50.3X2	T50.3X3	T50.3X4	T50.3X5	T50.3X6
Galantamine	T44.0X1	T44.0X2	T44.0X3	T44.0X4	T44.0X5	T44.0X6
Gallamine (triethiodide)	T48.1X1	T48.1X2	T48.1X3	T48.1X4	T48.1X5	T48.1X6
Gallium citrate	T50.991	T50.992	T50.993	T50.994	T50.995	T50.996
Gallopamil	T46.1X1	T46.1X2	T46.1X3	T46.1X4	T46.1X5	T46.1X6
Gamboge	T47.2X1	T47.2X2	T47.2X3	T47.2X4	T47.2X5	T47.2X6
Gamimune	T50.Z11	T50.Z12	T50.Z13	T50.Z14	T50.Z15	T50.Z16
Gamma-aminobutyric acid	T43.8X1	T43.8X2	T43.8X3	T43.8X4	T43.8X5	T43.8X6
Gamma-benzene hexachloride (medicinal)	T49.0X1	T49.0X2	T49.0X3	T49.0X4	T49.0X5	T49.0X6
nonmedicinal, vapor	T53.6X1	T53.6X2	T53.6X3	T53.6X4	—	—
Gamma-BHC (medicinal) — *see also* Gamma-benzene hexachloride	T49.0X1	T49.0X2	T49.0X3	T49.0X4	T49.0X5	T49.0X6
Gamma globulin	T50.Z11	T50.Z12	T50.Z13	T50.Z14	T50.Z15	T50.Z16
Gamulin	T50.Z11	T50.Z12	T50.Z13	T50.Z14	T50.Z15	T50.Z16
Ganciclovir (sodium)	T37.5X1	T37.5X2	T37.5X3	T37.5X4	T37.5X5	T37.5X6
Ganglionic blocking drug NEC	T44.2X1	T44.2X2	T44.2X3	T44.2X4	T44.2X5	T44.2X6
specified NEC	T44.2X1	T44.2X2	T44.2X3	T44.2X4	T44.2X5	T44.2X6
Ganja	T40.7X1	T40.7X2	T40.7X3	T40.7X4	T40.7X5	T40.7X6
Garamycin	T36.5X1	T36.5X2	T36.5X3	T36.5X4	T36.5X5	T36.5X6
ophthalmic preparation	T49.5X1	T49.5X2	T49.5X3	T49.5X4	T49.5X5	T49.5X6
topical NEC	T49.0X1	T49.0X2	T49.0X3	T49.0X4	T49.0X5	T49.0X6
Gardenal	T42.3X1	T42.3X2	T42.3X3	T42.3X4	T42.3X5	T42.3X6
Gardepanyl	T42.3X1	T42.3X2	T42.3X3	T42.3X4	T42.3X5	T42.3X6
Gas	T59.91	T59.92	T59.93	T59.94	—	—
acetylene	T59.891	T59.892	T59.893	T59.894	—	—
incomplete combustion of	T58.11	T58.12	T58.13	T58.14	—	—
air contaminants, source or type not specified	T59.91	T59.92	T59.93	T59.94	—	—
anesthetic	T41.0X1	T41.0X2	T41.0X3	T41.0X4	T41.0X5	T41.0X6
blast furnace	T58.8X1	T58.8X2	T58.8X3	T58.8X4	—	—
butane — *see* butane						
carbon monoxide — *see* Carbon, monoxide						
chlorine	T59.4X1	T59.4X2	T59.4X3	T59.4X4	—	—
coal	T58.2X1	T58.2X2	T58.2X3	T58.2X4	—	—
cyanide	T57.3X1	T57.3X2	T57.3X3	T57.3X4	—	—
dicyanogen	T65.0X1	T65.0X2	T65.0X3	T65.0X4	—	—
domestic — *see* Domestic gas						
exhaust	T58.01	T58.02	T58.03	T58.04	—	—
from utility (for cooking, heating, or lighting) (after combustion) — *see* Carbon, monoxide, fuel, utility						
prior to combustion	T59.891	T59.892	T59.893	T59.894	—	—
from wood- or coal-burning stove or fireplace	T58.2X1	T58.2X2	T58.2X3	T58.2X4	—	—
fuel (domestic use) (after combustion) — *see also* Carbon, monoxide, fuel						
industrial use	T58.8X1	T58.8X2	T58.8X3	T58.8X4	—	—
prior to combustion	T59.891	T59.892	T59.893	T59.894	—	—
utility	T59.891	T59.892	T59.893	T59.894	—	—
incomplete combustion of — *see* Carbon, monoxide, fuel, utility						
in mobile container	T59.891	T59.892	T59.893	T59.894	—	—
piped (natural)	T59.891	T59.892	T59.893	T59.894	—	—
garage	T58.01	T58.02	T58.03	T58.04	—	—
Gas — *continued*						
hydrocarbon NEC	T59.891	T59.892	T59.893	T59.894	—	—
incomplete combustion of — *see* Carbon, monoxide, fuel, utility						
liquefied — *see* butane						
piped	T59.891	T59.892	T59.893	T59.894	—	—
hydrocyanic acid	T65.0X1	T65.0X2	T65.0X3	T65.0X4	—	—
illuminating (after combustion)	T58.11	T58.12	T58.13	T58.14	—	—
prior to combustion	T59.891	T59.892	T59.893	T59.894	—	—
incomplete combustion, any — *see* Carbon, monoxide						
kiln	T58.8X1	T58.8X2	T58.8X3	T58.8X4	—	—
lacrimogenic	T59.3X1	T59.3X2	T59.3X3	T59.3X4	—	—
liquefied petroleum — *see* butane						
marsh	T59.891	T59.892	T59.893	T59.894	—	—
motor exhaust, not in transit	T58.01	T58.02	T58.03	T58.04	—	—
mustard, not in war	T59.891	T59.892	T59.893	T59.894	—	—
natural	T59.891	T59.892	T59.893	T59.894	—	—
nerve, not in war	T59.91	T59.92	T59.93	T59.94	—	—
oil	T52.0X1	T52.0X2	T52.0X3	T52.0X4	—	—
petroleum (liquefied) (distributed in mobile containers)	T59.891	T59.892	T59.893	T59.894	—	—
piped (pure or mixed with air)	T59.891	T59.892	T59.893	T59.894	—	—
piped (manufactured) (natural) NEC	T59.891	T59.892	T59.893	T59.894	—	—
producer	T58.8X1	T58.8X2	T58.8X3	T58.8X4	—	—
propane — *see* propane						
refrigerant (chlorofluoro-carbon)	T53.5X1	T53.5X2	T53.5X3	T53.5X4	—	—
not chlorofluoro-carbon	T59.891	T59.892	T59.893	T59.894	—	—
sewer	T59.91	T59.92	T59.93	T59.94	—	—
specified source NEC	T59.91	T59.92	T59.93	T59.94	—	—
stove (after combustion)	T58.11	T58.12	T58.13	T58.14	—	—
prior to combustion	T59.891	T59.892	T59.893	T59.894	—	—
tear	T59.3X1	T59.3X2	T59.3X3	T59.3X4	—	—
therapeutic	T41.5X1	T41.5X2	T41.5X3	T41.5X4	T41.5X5	T41.5X6
utility (for cooking, heating, or lighting) (piped) NEC	T59.891	T59.892	T59.893	T59.894	—	—
incomplete combustion of — *see* Carbon, monoxide, fuel, utilty						
in mobile container	T59.891	T59.892	T59.893	T59.894	—	—
piped (natural)	T59.891	T59.892	T59.893	T59.894	—	—
water	T58.11	T58.12	T58.13	T58.14	—	—
incomplete combustion of — *see* Carbon, monoxide, fuel, utility						
Gaseous substance — *see* Gas						
Gasoline	T52.0X1	T52.0X2	T52.0X3	T52.0X4	—	—
vapor	T52.0X1	T52.0X2	T52.0X3	T52.0X4	—	—
Gastric enzymes	T47.5X1	T47.5X2	T47.5X3	T47.5X4	T47.5X5	T47.5X6
Gastrografin	T50.8X1	T50.8X2	T50.8X3	T50.8X4	T50.8X5	T50.8X6
Gastrointestinal drug	T47.91	T47.92	T47.93	T47.94	T47.95	T47.96
biological	T47.8X1	T47.8X2	T47.8X3	T47.8X4	T47.8X5	T47.8X6
specified NEC	T47.8X1	T47.8X2	T47.8X3	T47.8X4	T47.8X5	T47.8X6
Gaultheria procumbens	T62.2X1	T62.2X2	T62.2X3	T62.2X4	—	—
Gefarnate	T44.3X1	T44.3X2	T44.3X3	T44.3X4	T44.3X5	T44.3X6
Gelatin (intravenous)	T45.8X1	T45.8X2	T45.8X3	T45.8X4	T45.8X5	T45.8X6
absorbable (sponge)	T45.7X1	T45.7X2	T45.7X3	T45.7X4	T45.7X5	T45.7X6
Gelfilm	T49.8X1	T49.8X2	T49.8X3	T49.8X4	T49.8X5	T49.8X6
Gelfoam	T45.7X1	T45.7X2	T45.7X3	T45.7X4	T45.7X5	T45.7X6
Gelsemine	T50.991	T50.992	T50.993	T50.994	T50.995	T50.996
Gelsemium (sempervirens)	T62.2X1	T62.2X2	T62.2X3	T62.2X4	—	—
Gemeprost	T48.0X1	T48.0X2	T48.0X3	T48.0X4	T48.0X5	T48.0X6
Gemfibrozil	T46.6X1	T46.6X2	T46.6X3	T46.6X4	T46.6X5	T46.6X6
Gemonil	T42.3X1	T42.3X2	T42.3X3	T42.3X4	T42.3X5	T42.3X6
Gentamicin	T36.5X1	T36.5X2	T36.5X3	T36.5X4	T36.5X5	T36.5X6
ophthalmic preparation	T49.5X1	T49.5X2	T49.5X3	T49.5X4	T49.5X5	T49.5X6
topical NEC	T49.0X1	T49.0X2	T49.0X3	T49.0X4	T49.0X5	T49.0X6
Gentian	T47.5X1	T47.5X2	T47.5X3	T47.5X4	T47.5X5	T47.5X6
violet	T49.0X1	T49.0X2	T49.0X3	T49.0X4	T49.0X5	T49.0X6
Gepefrine	T44.4X1	T44.4X2	T44.4X3	T44.4X4	T44.4X5	T44.4X6
Gestonorone caproate	T38.5X1	T38.5X2	T38.5X3	T38.5X4	T38.5X5	T38.5X6
Gexane	T49.0X1	T49.0X2	T49.0X3	T49.0X4	T49.0X5	T49.0X6
Gila monster (venom)	T63.111	T63.112	T63.113	T63.114	—	—
Ginger	T47.5X1	T47.5X2	T47.5X3	T47.5X4	T47.5X5	T47.5X6
Jamaica — *see* Jamaica, ginger						

Substance	Poisoning, Accidental (unintentional)	Poisoning, Intentional Self-harm	Poisoning, Assault	Poisoning, Undetermined	Adverse Effect	Under-dosing
Gitalin	T46.0X1	T46.0X2	T46.0X3	T46.0X4	T46.0X5	T46.0X6
amorphous	T46.0X1	T46.0X2	T46.0X3	T46.0X4	T46.0X5	T46.0X6
Gitaloxin	T46.0X1	T46.0X2	T46.0X3	T46.0X4	T46.0X5	T46.0X6
Gitoxin	T46.0X1	T46.0X2	T46.0X3	T46.0X4	T46.0X5	T46.0X6
Glafenine	T39.8X1	T39.8X2	T39.8X3	T39.8X4	T39.8X5	T39.8X6
Glandular extract (medicinal) NEC	T50.Z91	T50.Z92	T50.Z93	T50.Z94	T50.Z95	T50.Z96
Glaucarubin	T37.3X1	T37.3X2	T37.3X3	T37.3X4	T37.3X5	T37.3X6
Glibenclamide	T38.3X1	T38.3X2	T38.3X3	T38.3X4	T38.3X5	T38.3X6
Glibornuride	T38.3X1	T38.3X2	T38.3X3	T38.3X4	T38.3X5	T38.3X6
Gliclazide	T38.3X1	T38.3X2	T38.3X3	T38.3X4	T38.3X5	T38.3X6
Glimidine	T38.3X1	T38.3X2	T38.3X3	T38.3X4	T38.3X5	T38.3X6
Glipizide	T38.3X1	T38.3X2	T38.3X3	T38.3X4	T38.3X5	T38.3X6
Gliquidone	T38.3X1	T38.3X2	T38.3X3	T38.3X4	T38.3X5	T38.3X6
Glisolamide	T38.3X1	T38.3X2	T38.3X3	T38.3X4	T38.3X5	T38.3X6
Glisoxepide	T38.3X1	T38.3X2	T38.3X3	T38.3X4	T38.3X5	T38.3X6
Globin zinc insulin	T38.3X1	T38.3X2	T38.3X3	T38.3X4	T38.3X5	T38.3X6
Globulin						
antilymphocytic	T50.Z11	T50.Z12	T50.Z13	T50.Z14	T50.Z15	T50.Z16
antirhesus	T50.Z11	T50.Z12	T50.Z13	T50.Z14	T50.Z15	T50.Z16
antivenin	T50.Z11	T50.Z12	T50.Z13	T50.Z14	T50.Z15	T50.Z16
antiviral	T50.Z11	T50.Z12	T50.Z13	T50.Z14	T50.Z15	T50.Z16
Glucagon	T38.3X1	T38.3X2	T38.3X3	T38.3X4	T38.3X5	T38.3X6
Glucocorticoids	T38.0X1	T38.0X2	T38.0X3	T38.0X4	T38.0X5	T38.0X6
Glucocorticosteroid	T38.0X1	T38.0X2	T38.0X3	T38.0X4	T38.0X5	T38.0X6
Gluconic acid	T50.991	T50.992	T50.993	T50.994	T50.995	T50.996
Glucosamine sulfate	T39.4X1	T39.4X2	T39.4X3	T39.4X4	T39.4X5	T39.4X6
Glucose	T50.3X1	T50.3X2	T50.3X3	T50.3X4	T50.3X5	T50.3X6
with sodium chloride	T50.3X1	T50.3X2	T50.3X3	T50.3X4	T50.3X5	T50.3X6
Glucosulfone sodium	T37.1X1	T37.1X2	T37.1X3	T37.1X4	T37.1X5	T37.1X6
Glucurolactone	T47.8X1	T47.8X2	T47.8X3	T47.8X4	T47.8X5	T47.8X6
Glue NEC	T52.8X1	T52.8X2	T52.8X3	T52.8X4	—	—
Glutamic acid	T47.5X1	T47.5X2	T47.5X3	T47.5X4	T47.5X5	T47.5X6
Glutaral (medicinal)	T49.0X1	T49.0X2	T49.0X3	T49.0X4	T49.0X5	T49.0X6
nonmedicinal	T65.891	T65.892	T65.893	T65.894	—	—
Glutaraldehyde (nonmedicinal)	T65.891	T65.892	T65.893	T65.894	—	—
medicinal	T49.0X1	T49.0X2	T49.0X3	T49.0X4	T49.0X5	T49.0X6
Glutathione	T50.6X1	T50.6X2	T50.6X3	T50.6X4	T50.6X5	T50.6X6
Glutethimide	T42.6X1	T42.6X2	T42.6X3	T42.6X4	T42.6X5	T42.6X6
Glyburide	T38.3X1	T38.3X2	T38.3X3	T38.3X4	T38.3X5	T38.3X6
Glycerin	T47.4X1	T47.4X2	T47.4X3	T47.4X4	T47.4X5	T47.4X6
Glycerol	T47.4X1	T47.4X2	T47.4X3	T47.4X4	T47.4X5	T47.4X6
borax	T49.6X1	T49.6X2	T49.6X3	T49.6X4	T49.6X5	T49.6X6
intravenous	T50.3X1	T50.3X2	T50.3X3	T50.3X4	T50.3X5	T50.3X6
iodinated	T48.4X1	T48.4X2	T48.4X3	T48.4X4	T48.4X5	T48.4X6
Glycerophosphate	T50.991	T50.992	T50.993	T50.994	T50.995	T50.996
Glyceryl						
gualacolate	T48.4X1	T48.4X2	T48.4X3	T48.4X4	T48.4X5	T48.4X6
nitrate	T46.3X1	T46.3X2	T46.3X3	T46.3X4	T46.3X5	T46.3X6
triacetate (topical)	T49.0X1	T49.0X2	T49.0X3	T49.0X4	T49.0X5	T49.0X6
trinitrate	T46.3X1	T46.3X2	T46.3X3	T46.3X4	T46.3X5	T46.3X6
Glycine	T50.3X1	T50.3X2	T50.3X3	T50.3X4	T50.3X5	T50.3X6
Glyclopyramide	T38.3X1	T38.3X2	T38.3X3	T38.3X4	T38.3X5	T38.3X6
Glycobiarsol	T37.3X1	T37.3X2	T37.3X3	T37.3X4	T37.3X5	T37.3X6
Glycols (ether)	T52.3X1	T52.3X2	T52.3X3	T52.3X4	—	—
Glyconiazide	T37.1X1	T37.1X2	T37.1X3	T37.1X4	T37.1X5	T37.1X6
Glycopyrrolate	T44.3X1	T44.3X2	T44.3X3	T44.3X4	T44.3X5	T44.3X6
Glycopyrronium	T44.3X1	T44.3X2	T44.3X3	T44.3X4	T44.3X5	T44.3X6
bromide	T44.3X1	T44.3X2	T44.3X3	T44.3X4	T44.3X5	T44.3X6
Glycoside, cardiac (stimulant)	T46.0X1	T46.0X2	T46.0X3	T46.0X4	T46.0X5	T46.0X6
Glycyclamide	T38.3X1	T38.3X2	T38.3X3	T38.3X4	T38.3X5	T38.3X6
Glycyrrhiza extract	T48.4X1	T48.4X2	T48.4X3	T48.4X4	T48.4X5	T48.4X6
Glycyrrhizic acid	T48.4X1	T48.4X2	T48.4X3	T48.4X4	T48.4X5	T48.4X6
Glycyrrhizinate potassium	T48.4X1	T48.4X2	T48.4X3	T48.4X4	T48.4X5	T48.4X6
Glymidine sodium	T38.3X1	T38.3X2	T38.3X3	T38.3X4	T38.3X5	T38.3X6
Glyphosate	T60.3X1	T60.3X2	T60.3X3	T60.3X4	—	—
Glyphylline	T48.6X1	T48.6X2	T48.6X3	T48.6X4	T48.6X5	T48.6X6
Gold						
colloidal (I98Au)	T45.1X1	T45.1X2	T45.1X3	T45.1X4	T45.1X5	T45.1X6
salts	T39.4X1	T39.4X2	T39.4X3	T39.4X4	T39.4X5	T39.4X6
Golden sulfide of antimony	T56.891	T56.892	T56.893	T56.894	—	—
Goldylocks	T62.2X1	T62.2X2	T62.2X3	T62.2X4	—	—
Gonadal tissue extract	T38.901	T38.902	T38.903	T38.904	T38.905	T38.906
female	T38.5X1	T38.5X2	T38.5X3	T38.5X4	T38.5X5	T38.5X6
male	T38.7X1	T38.7X2	T38.7X3	T38.7X4	T38.7X5	T38.7X6
Gonadorelin	T38.891	T38.892	T38.893	T38.894	T38.895	T38.896
Gonadotropin	T38.891	T38.892	T38.893	T38.894	T38.895	T38.896
chorionic	T38.891	T38.892	T38.893	T38.894	T38.895	T38.896
pituitary	T38.811	T38.812	T38.813	T38.814	T38.815	T38.816
Goserelin	T45.1X1	T45.1X2	T45.1X3	T45.1X4	T45.1X5	T45.1X6
Grain alcohol	T51.0X1	T51.0X2	T51.0X3	T51.0X4	—	—
Gramicidin	T49.0X1	T49.0X2	T49.0X3	T49.0X4	T49.0X5	T49.0X6
Granisetron	T45.0X1	T45.0X2	T45.0X3	T45.0X4	T45.0X5	T45.0X6
Gratiola officinalis	T62.2X1	T62.2X2	T62.2X3	T62.2X4	—	—
Grease	T65.891	T65.892	T65.893	T65.894	—	—
Green hellebore	T62.2X1	T62.2X2	T62.2X3	T62.2X4	—	—
Green soap	T49.2X1	T49.2X2	T49.2X3	T49.2X4	T49.2X5	T49.2X6
Grifulvin	T36.7X1	T36.7X2	T36.7X3	T36.7X4	T36.7X5	T36.7X6
Griseofulvin	T36.7X1	T36.7X2	T36.7X3	T36.7X4	T36.7X5	T36.7X6
Growth hormone	T38.811	T38.812	T38.813	T38.814	T38.815	T38.816
Guaiacol derivatives	T48.4X1	T48.4X2	T48.4X3	T48.4X4	T48.4X5	T48.4X6
Guaiac reagent	T50.991	T50.992	T50.993	T50.994	T50.995	T50.996
Guaifenesin	T48.4X1	T48.4X2	T48.4X3	T48.4X4	T48.4X5	T48.4X6
Guaimesal	T48.4X1	T48.4X2	T48.4X3	T48.4X4	T48.4X5	T48.4X6
Guaiphenesin	T48.4X1	T48.4X2	T48.4X3	T48.4X4	T48.4X5	T48.4X6
Guamecycline	T36.4X1	T36.4X2	T36.4X3	T36.4X4	T36.4X5	T36.4X6
Guanabenz	T46.5X1	T46.5X2	T46.5X3	T46.5X4	T46.5X5	T46.5X6
Guanacline	T46.5X1	T46.5X2	T46.5X3	T46.5X4	T46.5X5	T46.5X6
Guanadrel	T46.5X1	T46.5X2	T46.5X3	T46.5X4	T46.5X5	T46.5X6
Guanatol	T37.2X1	T37.2X2	T37.2X3	T37.2X4	T37.2X5	T37.2X6
Guanethidine	T46.5X1	T46.5X2	T46.5X3	T46.5X4	T46.5X5	T46.5X6
Guanfacine	T46.5X1	T46.5X2	T46.5X3	T46.5X4	T46.5X5	T46.5X6
Guano	T65.891	T65.892	T65.893	T65.894	—	—
Guanochlor	T46.5X1	T46.5X2	T46.5X3	T46.5X4	T46.5X5	T46.5X6
Guanoclor	T46.5X1	T46.5X2	T46.5X3	T46.5X4	T46.5X5	T46.5X6
Guanoctine	T46.5X1	T46.5X2	T46.5X3	T46.5X4	T46.5X5	T46.5X6
Guanoxabenz	T46.5X1	T46.5X2	T46.5X3	T46.5X4	T46.5X5	T46.5X6
Guanoxan	T46.5X1	T46.5X2	T46.5X3	T46.5X4	T46.5X5	T46.5X6
Guar gum (medicinal)	T46.6X1	T46.6X2	T46.6X3	T46.6X4	T46.6X5	T46.6X6
Hachimycin	T36.7X1	T36.7X2	T36.7X3	T36.7X4	T36.7X5	T36.7X6
Hair						
dye	T49.4X1	T49.4X2	T49.4X3	T49.4X4	T49.4X5	T49.4X6
preparation NEC	T49.4X1	T49.4X2	T49.4X3	T49.4X4	T49.4X5	T49.4X6
Halazepam	T42.4X1	T42.4X2	T42.4X3	T42.4X4	T42.4X5	T42.4X6
Halcinolone	T49.0X1	T49.0X2	T49.0X3	T49.0X4	T49.0X5	T49.0X6
Halcinonide	T49.0X1	T49.0X2	T49.0X3	T49.0X4	T49.0X5	T49.0X6
Halethazole	T49.0X1	T49.0X2	T49.0X3	T49.0X4	T49.0X5	T49.0X6
Hallucinogen NEC	T40.901	T40.902	T40.903	T40.904	T40.905	T40.906
Halofantrine	T37.2X1	T37.2X2	T37.2X3	T37.2X4	T37.2X5	T37.2X6
Halofenate	T46.6X1	T46.6X2	T46.6X3	T46.6X4	T46.6X5	T46.6X6
Halometasone	T49.0X1	T49.0X2	T49.0X3	T49.0X4	T49.0X5	T49.0X6
Haloperidol	T43.4X1	T43.4X2	T43.4X3	T43.4X4	T43.4X5	T43.4X6
Haloprogin	T49.0X1	T49.0X2	T49.0X3	T49.0X4	T49.0X5	T49.0X6
Halotex	T49.0X1	T49.0X2	T49.0X3	T49.0X4	T49.0X5	T49.0X6
Halothane	T41.0X1	T41.0X2	T41.0X3	T41.0X4	T41.0X5	T41.0X6
Haloxazolam	T42.4X1	T42.4X2	T42.4X3	T42.4X4	T42.4X5	T42.4X6
Halquinols	T49.0X1	T49.0X2	T49.0X3	T49.0X4	T49.0X5	T49.0X6
Hamamelis	T49.2X1	T49.2X2	T49.2X3	T49.2X4	T49.2X5	T49.2X6
Haptendextran	T45.8X1	T45.8X2	T45.8X3	T45.8X4	T45.8X5	T45.8X6
Harmonyl	T46.5X1	T46.5X2	T46.5X3	T46.5X4	T46.5X5	T46.5X6
Hartmann's solution	T50.3X1	T50.3X2	T50.3X3	T50.3X4	T50.3X5	T50.3X6
Hashish	T40.7X1	T40.7X2	T40.7X3	T40.7X4	T40.7X5	T40.7X6
Hawaiian Woodrose seeds	T40.991	T40.992	T40.993	T40.994	—	—
HCB	T60.3X1	T60.3X2	T60.3X3	T60.3X4	—	—
HCH	T53.6X1	T53.6X2	T53.6X3	T53.6X4	—	—
medicinal	T49.0X1	T49.0X2	T49.0X3	T49.0X4	T49.0X5	T49.0X6
HCN	T57.3X1	T57.3X2	T57.3X3	T57.3X4	—	—
Headache cures, drugs, powders NEC	T50.901	T50.902	T50.903	T50.904	T50.905	T50.906
Heavenly Blue (morning glory)	T40.991	T40.992	T40.993	T40.994	—	—
Heavy metal antidote	T45.8X1	T45.8X2	T45.8X3	T45.8X4	T45.8X5	T45.8X6
Hedaquinium	T49.0X1	T49.0X2	T49.0X3	T49.0X4	T49.0X5	T49.0X6
Hedge hyssop	T62.2X1	T62.2X2	T62.2X3	T62.2X4	—	—
Heet	T49.8X1	T49.8X2	T49.8X3	T49.8X4	T49.8X5	T49.8X6
Helenin	T37.4X1	T37.4X2	T37.4X3	T37.4X4	T37.4X5	T37.4X6
Helium (nonmedicinal) NEC	T59.891	T59.892	T59.893	T59.894	—	—
medicinal	T48.991	T48.992	T48.993	T48.994	T48.995	T48.996
Helebore (black) (green) (white)	T62.2X1	T62.2X2	T62.2X3	T62.2X4	—	—
Hematin	T45.8X1	T45.8X2	T45.8X3	T45.8X4	T45.8X5	T45.8X6
Hematinic preparation	T45.8X1	T45.8X2	T45.8X3	T45.8X4	T45.8X5	T45.8X6
Hematological agent	T45.91	T45.92	T45.93	T45.94	T45.95	T45.96
specified NEC	T45.8X1	T45.8X2	T45.8X3	T45.8X4	T45.8X5	T45.8X6
Hemlock	T62.2X1	T62.2X2	T62.2X3	T62.2X4	—	—
Hemostatic	T45.621	T45.622	T45.623	T45.624	T45.625	T45.626
drug, systemic	T45.621	T45.622	T45.623	T45.624	T45.625	T45.626
Hemostyptic	T49.4X1	T49.4X2	T49.4X3	T49.4X4	T49.4X5	T49.4X6
Henbane	T62.2X1	T62.2X2	T62.2X3	T62.2X4	—	—
Heparin (sodium)	T45.511	T45.512	T45.513	T45.514	T45.515	T45.516
action reverser	T45.7X1	T45.7X2	T45.7X3	T45.7X4	T45.7X5	T45.7X6
Heparin-fraction	T45.511	T45.512	T45.513	T45.514	T45.515	T45.516
Heparinoid (systemic)	T45.511	T45.512	T45.513	T45.514	T45.515	T45.516

▼ Subterms under main terms may continue to next column or page   Additional Character May Be Required — Refer to the Tabular List for Character Selection   361

Gitalin — Heparinoid

Substance	Poisoning, Accidental (unintentional)	Poisoning, Intentional Self-harm	Poisoning, Assault	Poisoning, Undetermined	Adverse Effect	Under-dosing
Hepatic secretion stimulant	T47.8X1	T47.8X2	T47.8X3	T47.8X4	T47.8X5	T47.8X6
Hepatitis B						
immune globulin	T50.Z11	T50.Z12	T50.Z13	T50.Z14	T50.Z15	T50.Z16
vaccine	T50.B91	T50.B92	T50.B93	T50.B94	T50.B95	T50.B96
Hepronicate	T46.7X1	T46.7X2	T46.7X3	T46.7X4	T46.7X5	T46.7X6
Heptabarb	T42.3X1	T42.3X2	T42.3X3	T42.3X4	T42.3X5	T42.3X6
Heptabarbital	T42.3X1	T42.3X2	T42.3X3	T42.3X4	T42.3X5	T42.3X6
Heptabarbitone	T42.3X1	T42.3X2	T42.3X3	T42.3X4	T42.3X5	T42.3X6
Heptachlor	T60.1X1	T60.1X2	T60.1X3	T60.1X4	—	—
Heptalgin	T40.2X1	T40.2X2	T40.2X3	T40.2X4	T40.2X5	T40.2X6
Heptaminol	T46.3X1	T46.3X2	T46.3X3	T46.3X4	T46.3X5	T46.3X6
Herbicide NEC	T60.3X1	T60.3X2	T60.3X3	T60.3X4	—	—
Heroin	T40.1X1	T40.1X2	T40.1X3	T40.1X4	—	—
Herplex	T49.5X1	T49.5X2	T49.5X3	T49.5X4	T49.5X5	T49.5X6
HES	T45.8X1	T45.8X2	T45.8X3	T45.8X4	T45.8X5	T45.8X6
Hesperidin	T46.991	T46.992	T46.993	T46.994	T46.995	T46.996
Hetacillin	T36.0X1	T36.0X2	T36.0X3	T36.0X4	T36.0X5	T36.0X6
Hetastarch	T45.8X1	T45.8X2	T45.8X3	T45.8X4	T45.8X5	T45.8X6
HETP	T60.0X1	T60.0X2	T60.0X3	T60.0X4	—	—
Hexachlorobenzene (vapor)	T60.3X1	T60.3X2	T60.3X3	T60.3X4	—	—
Hexachlorocyclohexane	T53.6X1	T53.6X2	T53.6X3	T53.6X4	—	—
Hexachlorophene	T49.0X1	T49.0X2	T49.0X3	T49.0X4	T49.0X5	T49.0X6
Hexadiline	T46.3X1	T46.3X2	T46.3X3	T46.3X4	T46.3X5	T46.3X6
Hexadimethrine (bromide)	T45.7X1	T45.7X2	T45.7X3	T45.7X4	T45.7X5	T45.7X6
Hexadylamine	T46.3X1	T46.3X2	T46.3X3	T46.3X4	T46.3X5	T46.3X6
Hexaethyl tetraphosphate	T60.0X1	T60.0X2	T60.0X3	T60.0X4	—	—
Hexafluorenium bromide	T48.1X1	T48.1X2	T48.1X3	T48.1X4	T48.1X5	T48.1X6
Hexafluronium (bromide)	T48.1X1	T48.1X2	T48.1X3	T48.1X4	T48.1X5	T48.1X6
Hexa-germ	T49.2X1	T49.2X2	T49.2X3	T49.2X4	T49.2X5	T49.2X6
Hexahydrobenzol	T52.8X1	T52.8X2	T52.8X3	T52.8X4	—	—
Hexahydrocresol(s)	T51.8X1	T51.8X2	T51.8X3	T51.8X4	—	—
arsenide	T57.0X1	T57.0X2	T57.0X3	T57.0X4	—	—
arseniurated	T57.0X1	T57.0X2	T57.0X3	T57.0X4	—	—
cyanide	T57.3X1	T57.3X2	T57.3X3	T57.3X4	—	—
gas	T59.891	T59.892	T59.893	T59.894	—	—
Fluoride (liquid)	T57.8X1	T57.8X2	T57.8X3	T57.8X4	—	—
vapor	T59.891	T59.892	T59.893	T59.894	—	—
phophorated	T60.0X1	T60.0X2	T60.0X3	T60.0X4	—	—
sulfate	T57.8X1	T57.8X2	T57.8X3	T57.8X4	—	—
sulfide (gas)	T59.6X1	T59.6X2	T59.6X3	T59.6X4	—	—
arseniurated	T57.0X1	T57.0X2	T57.0X3	T57.0X4	—	—
sulfurated	T57.8X1	T57.8X2	T57.8X3	T57.8X4	—	—
Hexahydrophenol	T51.8X1	T51.8X2	T51.8X3	T51.8X4	—	—
Hexalen	T51.8X1	T51.8X2	T51.8X3	T51.8X4	—	—
Hexamethonium bromide	T44.2X1	T44.2X2	T44.2X3	T44.2X4	T44.2X5	T44.2X6
Hexamethylene	T52.8X1	T52.8X2	T52.8X3	T52.8X4	—	—
Hexamethylmelamine	T45.1X1	T45.1X2	T45.1X3	T45.1X4	T45.1X5	T45.1X6
Hexamidine	T49.0X1	T49.0X2	T49.0X3	T49.0X4	T49.0X5	T49.0X6
Hexamine (mandelate)	T37.8X1	T37.8X2	T37.8X3	T37.8X4	T37.8X5	T37.8X6
Hexanone, 2-hexanone	T52.4X1	T52.4X2	T52.4X3	T52.4X4	—	—
Hexanuorenium	T48.1X1	T48.1X2	T48.1X3	T48.1X4	T48.1X5	T48.1X6
Hexapropymate	T42.6X1	T42.6X2	T42.6X3	T42.6X4	T42.6X5	T42.6X6
Hexasonium iodide	T44.3X1	T44.3X2	T44.3X3	T44.3X4	T44.3X5	T44.3X6
Hexcarbacholine bromide	T48.1X1	T48.1X2	T48.1X3	T48.1X4	T48.1X5	T48.1X6
Hexemal	T42.3X1	T42.3X2	T42.3X3	T42.3X4	T42.3X5	T42.3X6
Hexestrol	T38.5X1	T38.5X2	T38.5X3	T38.5X4	T38.5X5	T38.5X6
Hexethal (sodium)	T42.3X1	T42.3X2	T42.3X3	T42.3X4	T42.3X5	T42.3X6
Hexetidine	T37.8X1	T37.8X2	T37.8X3	T37.8X4	T37.8X5	T37.8X6
Hexobarbital	T42.3X1	T42.3X2	T42.3X3	T42.3X4	T42.3X5	T42.3X6
rectal	T41.291	T41.292	T41.293	T41.294	T41.295	T41.296
sodium	T41.1X1	T41.1X2	T41.1X3	T41.1X4	T41.1X5	T41.1X6
Hexobendine	T46.3X1	T46.3X2	T46.3X3	T46.3X4	T46.3X5	T46.3X6
Hexocyclium	T44.3X1	T44.3X2	T44.3X3	T44.3X4	T44.3X5	T44.3X6
metilsulfate	T44.3X1	T44.3X2	T44.3X3	T44.3X4	T44.3X5	T44.3X6
Hexoestrol	T38.5X1	T38.5X2	T38.5X3	T38.5X4	T38.5X5	T38.5X6
Hexone	T52.4X1	T52.4X2	T52.4X3	T52.4X4	—	—
Hexoprenaline	T48.6X1	T48.6X2	T48.6X3	T48.6X4	T48.6X5	T48.6X6
Hexylcaine	T41.3X1	T41.3X2	T41.3X3	T41.3X4	T41.3X5	T41.3X6
Hexylresorcinol	T52.2X1	T52.2X2	T52.2X3	T52.2X4	—	—
HGH (human growth hormone)	T38.811	T38.812	T38.813	T38.814	T38.815	T38.816
Hinkle's pills	T47.2X1	T47.2X2	T47.2X3	T47.2X4	T47.2X5	T47.2X6
Histalog	T50.8X1	T50.8X2	T50.8X3	T50.8X4	T50.8X5	T50.8X6
Histamine (phosphate)	T50.8X1	T50.8X2	T50.8X3	T50.8X4	T50.8X5	T50.8X6
Histoplasmin	T50.8X1	T50.8X2	T50.8X3	T50.8X4	T50.8X5	T50.8X6
Holly berries	T62.2X1	T62.2X2	T62.2X3	T62.2X4	—	—
Homatropine	T44.3X1	T44.3X2	T44.3X3	T44.3X4	T44.3X5	T44.3X6
methylbromide	T44.3X1	T44.3X2	T44.3X3	T44.3X4	T44.3X5	T44.3X6
Homochlorcyclizine	T45.0X1	T45.0X2	T45.0X3	T45.0X4	T45.0X5	T45.0X6
Homosalate	T49.3X1	T49.3X2	T49.3X3	T49.3X4	T49.3X5	T49.3X6
Homo-tet	T50.Z11	T50.Z12	T50.Z13	T50.Z14	T50.Z15	T50.Z16

Substance	Poisoning, Accidental (unintentional)	Poisoning, Intentional Self-harm	Poisoning, Assault	Poisoning, Undetermined	Adverse Effect	Under-dosing
Hormone	T38.801	T38.802	T38.803	T38.804	T38.805	T38.806
adrenal cortical steroids	T38.0X1	T38.0X2	T38.0X3	T38.0X4	T38.0X5	T38.0X6
androgenic	T38.7X1	T38.7X2	T38.7X3	T38.7X4	T38.7X5	T38.7X6
anterior pituitary NEC	T38.811	T38.812	T38.813	T38.814	T38.815	T38.816
antidiabetic agents	T38.3X1	T38.3X2	T38.3X3	T38.3X4	T38.3X5	T38.3X6
antidiuretic	T38.891	T38.892	T38.893	T38.894	T38.895	T38.896
cancer therapy	T45.1X1	T45.1X2	T45.1X3	T45.1X4	T45.1X5	T45.1X6
follicle stimulating	T38.811	T38.812	T38.813	T38.814	T38.815	T38.816
gonadotropic	T38.891	T38.892	T38.893	T38.894	T38.895	T38.896
pituitary	T38.811	T38.812	T38.813	T38.814	T38.815	T38.816
growth	T38.811	T38.812	T38.813	T38.814	T38.815	T38.816
luteinizing	T38.811	T38.812	T38.813	T38.814	T38.815	T38.816
ovarian	T38.5X1	T38.5X2	T38.5X3	T38.5X4	T38.5X5	T38.5X6
oxytocic	T48.0X1	T48.0X2	T48.0X3	T48.0X4	T48.0X5	T48.0X6
parathyroid (derivatives)	T50.991	T50.992	T50.993	T50.994	T50.995	T50.996
pituitary (posterior) NEC	T38.891	T38.892	T38.893	T38.894	T38.895	T38.896
anterior	T38.811	T38.812	T38.813	T38.814	T38.815	T38.816
specified, NEC	T38.891	T38.892	T38.893	T38.894	T38.895	T38.896
thyroid	T38.1X1	T38.1X2	T38.1X3	T38.1X4	T38.1X5	T38.1X6
Hornet (sting)	T63.451	T63.452	T63.453	T63.454	—	—
Horse anti-human lymphocytic serum	T50.Z11	T50.Z12	T50.Z13	T50.Z14	T50.Z15	T50.Z16
Horticulture agent NEC	T65.91	T65.92	T65.93	T65.94	—	—
with pesticide	T60.91	T60.92	T60.93	T60.94	—	—
Human						
albumin	T45.8X1	T45.8X2	T45.8X3	T45.8X4	T45.8X5	T45.8X6
growth hormone (HGH)	T38.811	T38.812	T38.813	T38.814	T38.815	T38.816
immune serum	T50.Z11	T50.Z12	T50.Z13	T50.Z14	T50.Z15	T50.Z16
Hyaluronidase	T45.3X1	T45.3X2	T45.3X3	T45.3X4	T45.3X5	T45.3X6
Hyazyme	T45.3X1	T45.3X2	T45.3X3	T45.3X4	T45.3X5	T45.3X6
Hycodan	T40.2X1	T40.2X2	T40.2X3	T40.2X4	T40.2X5	T40.2X6
Hydantoin derivative NEC	T42.0X1	T42.0X2	T42.0X3	T42.0X4	T42.0X5	T42.0X6
Hydeltra	T38.0X1	T38.0X2	T38.0X3	T38.0X4	T38.0X5	T38.0X6
Hydergine	T44.6X1	T44.6X2	T44.6X3	T44.6X4	T44.6X5	T44.6X6
Hydrabamine penicillin	T36.0X1	T36.0X2	T36.0X3	T36.0X4	T36.0X5	T36.0X6
Hydralazine	T46.5X1	T46.5X2	T46.5X3	T46.5X4	T46.5X5	T46.5X6
Hydrargaphen	T49.0X1	T49.0X2	T49.0X3	T49.0X4	T49.0X5	T49.0X6
Hydrargyri aminochloridum	T49.0X1	T49.0X2	T49.0X3	T49.0X4	T49.0X5	T49.0X6
Hydrastine	T48.291	T48.292	T48.293	T48.294	T48.295	T48.296
Hydrazine	T54.1X1	T54.1X2	T54.1X3	T54.1X4	—	—
monoamine oxidase inhibitors	T43.1X1	T43.1X2	T43.1X3	T43.1X4	T43.1X5	T43.1X6
Hydrazoic acid, azides	T54.2X1	T54.2X2	T54.2X3	T54.2X4	—	—
Hydriodic acid	T48.4X1	T48.4X2	T48.4X3	T48.4X4	T48.4X5	T48.4X6
Hydrocarbon gas	T59.891	T59.892	T59.893	T59.894	—	—
incomplete combustion of — see Carbon, monoxide, fuel, utility						
liquefied (mobile container)	T59.891	T59.892	T59.893	T59.894	—	—
piped (natural)	T59.891	T59.892	T59.893	T59.894	—	—
Hydrochloric acid (liquid)	T54.2X1	T54.2X2	T54.2X3	T54.2X4	—	—
medicinal (digestant)	T47.5X1	T47.5X2	T47.5X3	T47.5X4	T47.5X5	T47.5X6
vapor	T59.891	T59.892	T59.893	T59.894	—	—
Hydrochlorothiazide	T50.2X1	T50.2X2	T50.2X3	T50.2X4	T50.2X5	T50.2X6
Hydrocodone	T40.2X1	T40.2X2	T40.2X3	T40.2X4	T40.2X5	T40.2X6
Hydrocortisone (derivatives)	T49.0X1	T49.0X2	T49.0X3	T49.0X4	T49.0X5	T49.0X6
aceponate	T49.0X1	T49.0X2	T49.0X3	T49.0X4	T49.0X5	T49.0X6
ENT agent	T49.6X1	T49.6X2	T49.6X3	T49.6X4	T49.6X5	T49.6X6
ophthalmic preparation	T49.5X1	T49.5X2	T49.5X3	T49.5X4	T49.5X5	T49.5X6
topical NEC	T49.0X1	T49.0X2	T49.0X3	T49.0X4	T49.0X5	T49.0X6
Hydrocortone	T38.0X1	T38.0X2	T38.0X3	T38.0X4	T38.0X5	T38.0X6
ENT agent	T49.6X1	T49.6X2	T49.6X3	T49.6X4	T49.6X5	T49.6X6
ophthalmic preparation	T49.5X1	T49.5X2	T49.5X3	T49.5X4	T49.5X5	T49.5X6
topical NEC	T49.0X1	T49.0X2	T49.0X3	T49.0X4	T49.0X5	T49.0X6
Hydrocyanic acid (liquid)	T57.3X1	T57.3X2	T57.3X3	T57.3X4	—	—
gas	T65.0X1	T65.0X2	T65.0X3	T65.0X4	—	—
Hydroflumethiazide	T50.2X1	T50.2X2	T50.2X3	T50.2X4	T50.2X5	T50.2X6
Hydrofluoric acid (liquid)	T54.2X1	T54.2X2	T54.2X3	T54.2X4	—	—
vapor	T59.891	T59.892	T59.893	T59.894	—	—
Hydrogen	T59.891	T59.892	T59.893	T59.894	—	—
arsenide	T57.0X1	T57.0X2	T57.0X3	T57.0X4	—	—
arseniureted	T57.0X1	T57.0X2	T57.0X3	T57.0X4	—	—
chloride	T57.8X1	T57.8X2	T57.8X3	T57.8X4	—	—
cyanide (salts)	T57.3X1	T57.3X2	T57.3X3	T57.3X4	—	—
gas	T57.3X1	T57.3X2	T57.3X3	T57.3X4	—	—
Fluoride	T59.5X1	T59.5X2	T59.5X3	T59.5X4	—	—
vapor	T59.5X1	T59.5X2	T59.5X3	T59.5X4	—	—
peroxide	T49.0X1	T49.0X2	T49.0X3	T49.0X4	T49.0X5	T49.0X6
phosphureted	T57.1X1	T57.1X2	T57.1X3	T57.1X4	—	—
sulfide	T59.6X1	T59.6X2	T59.6X3	T59.6X4	—	—
arseniureted	T57.0X1	T57.0X2	T57.0X3	T57.0X4	—	—
sulfureted	T59.6X1	T59.6X2	T59.6X3	T59.6X4	—	—

Additional Character May Be Required — Refer to the Tabular List for Character Selection   Subterms under main terms may continue to next column or page

Substance	Poisoning, Accidental (unintentional)	Poisoning, Intentional Self-harm	Poisoning, Assault	Poisoning, Undetermined	Adverse Effect	Under-dosing
Hydromethylpyridine	T46.7X1	T46.7X2	T46.7X3	T46.7X4	T46.7X5	T46.7X6
Hydromorphinol	T40.2X1	T40.2X2	T40.2X3	T40.2X4	—	—
Hydromorphinone	T40.2X1	T40.2X2	T40.2X3	T40.2X4	T40.2X5	T40.2X6
Hydromorphone	T40.2X1	T40.2X2	T40.2X3	T40.2X4	T40.2X5	T40.2X6
Hydromox	T50.2X1	T50.2X2	T50.2X3	T50.2X4	T50.2X5	T50.2X6
Hydrophilic lotion	T49.3X1	T49.3X2	T49.3X3	T49.3X4	T49.3X5	T49.3X6
Hydroquinidine	T46.2X1	T46.2X2	T46.2X3	T46.2X4	T46.2X5	T46.2X6
Hydroquinone	T52.2X1	T52.2X2	T52.2X3	T52.2X4	—	—
vapor	T59.891	T59.892	T59.893	T59.894	—	—
Hydrosulfuric acid (gas)	T59.6X1	T59.6X2	T59.6X3	T59.6X4	—	—
Hydrotalcite	T47.1X1	T47.1X2	T47.1X3	T47.1X4	T47.1X5	T47.1X6
Hydrous wool fat	T49.3X1	T49.3X2	T49.3X3	T49.3X4	T49.3X5	T49.3X6
Hydroxide, caustic	T54.3X1	T54.3X2	T54.3X3	T54.3X4	—	—
Hydroxocobalamin	T45.8X1	T45.8X2	T45.8X3	T45.8X4	T45.8X5	T45.8X6
Hydroxyamphetamine	T49.5X1	T49.5X2	T49.5X3	T49.5X4	T49.5X5	T49.5X6
Hydroxycarbamide	T45.1X1	T45.1X2	T45.1X3	T45.1X4	T45.1X5	T45.1X6
Hydroxychloroquine	T37.8X1	T37.8X2	T37.8X3	T37.8X4	T37.8X5	T37.8X6
Hydroxydihydrocodeinone	T40.2X1	T40.2X2	T40.2X3	T40.2X4	T40.2X5	T40.2X6
Hydroxyestrone	T38.5X1	T38.5X2	T38.5X3	T38.5X4	T38.5X5	T38.5X6
Hydroxyethyl starch	T45.8X1	T45.8X2	T45.8X3	T45.8X4	T45.8X5	T45.8X6
Hydroxymethylpentanone	T52.4X1	T52.4X2	T52.4X3	T52.4X4	—	—
Hydroxyphenamate	T43.591	T43.592	T43.593	T43.594	T43.595	T43.596
Hydroxyphenylbutazone	T39.2X1	T39.2X2	T39.2X3	T39.2X4	T39.2X5	T39.2X6
Hydroxyprogesterone	T38.5X1	T38.5X2	T38.5X3	T38.5X4	T38.5X5	T38.5X6
caproate	T38.5X1	T38.5X2	T38.5X3	T38.5X4	T38.5X5	T38.5X6
Hydroxyquinoline (derivatives) NEC	T37.8X1	T37.8X2	T37.8X3	T37.8X4	T37.8X5	T37.8X6
Hydroxystilbamidine	T37.3X1	T37.3X2	T37.3X3	T37.3X4	T37.3X5	T37.3X6
Hydroxytoluene (nonmedicinal)	T54.0X1	T54.0X2	T54.0X3	T54.0X4	—	—
medicinal	T49.0X1	T49.0X2	T49.0X3	T49.0X4	T49.0X5	T49.0X6
Hydroxyurea	T45.1X1	T45.1X2	T45.1X3	T45.1X4	T45.1X5	T45.1X6
Hydroxyzine	T43.591	T43.592	T43.593	T43.594	T43.595	T43.596
Hyoscine	T44.3X1	T44.3X2	T44.3X3	T44.3X4	T44.3X5	T44.3X6
Hyoscyamine	T44.3X1	T44.3X2	T44.3X3	T44.3X4	T44.3X5	T44.3X6
Hyoscyamus	T44.3X1	T44.3X2	T44.3X3	T44.3X4	T44.3X5	T44.3X6
dry extract	T44.3X1	T44.3X2	T44.3X3	T44.3X4	T44.3X5	T44.3X6
Hypaque	T50.8X1	T50.8X2	T50.8X3	T50.8X4	T50.8X5	T50.8X6
Hypertussis	T50.Z11	T50.Z12	T50.Z13	T50.Z14	T50.Z15	T50.Z16
Hypnotic	T42.71	T42.72	T42.73	T42.74	T42.75	T42.76
anticonvulsant	T42.71	T42.72	T42.73	T42.74	T42.75	T42.76
specified NEC	T42.6X1	T42.6X2	T42.6X3	T42.6X4	T42.6X5	T42.6X6
Hypochlorite	T49.0X1	T49.0X2	T49.0X3	T49.0X4	T49.0X5	T49.0X6
Hypophysis, posterior	T38.891	T38.892	T38.893	T38.894	T38.895	T38.896
Hypotensive NEC	T46.5X1	T46.5X2	T46.5X3	T46.5X4	T46.5X5	T46.5X6
Hypromellose	T49.5X1	T49.5X2	T49.5X3	T49.5X4	T49.5X5	T49.5X6
Ibacitabine	T37.5X1	T37.5X2	T37.5X3	T37.5X4	T37.5X5	T37.5X6
Ibopamine	T44.991	T44.992	T44.993	T44.994	T44.995	T44.996
Ibufenac	T39.311	T39.312	T39.313	T39.314	T39.315	T39.316
Ibuprofen	T39.311	T39.312	T39.313	T39.314	T39.315	T39.316
Ibuproxam	T39.311	T39.312	T39.313	T39.314	T39.315	T39.316
Ibuterol	T48.6X1	T48.6X2	T48.6X3	T48.6X4	T48.6X5	T48.6X6
Ichthammol	T49.0X1	T49.0X2	T49.0X3	T49.0X4	T49.0X5	T49.0X6
Ichthyol	T49.4X1	T49.4X2	T49.4X3	T49.4X4	T49.4X5	T49.4X6
Idarubicin	T45.1X1	T45.1X2	T45.1X3	T45.1X4	T45.1X5	T45.1X6
Idrocilamide	T42.8X1	T42.8X2	T42.8X3	T42.8X4	T42.8X5	T42.8X6
Ifenprodil	T46.7X1	T46.7X2	T46.7X3	T46.7X4	T46.7X5	T46.7X6
Ifosfamide	T45.1X1	T45.1X2	T45.1X3	T45.1X4	T45.1X5	T45.1X6
Iletin	T38.3X1	T38.3X2	T38.3X3	T38.3X4	T38.3X5	T38.3X6
Ilex	T62.2X1	T62.2X2	T62.2X3	T62.2X4	—	—
Illuminating gas (after combustion)	T58.11	T58.12	T58.13	T58.14	—	—
prior to combustion	T59.891	T59.892	T59.893	T59.894	—	—
Ilopan	T45.2X1	T45.2X2	T45.2X3	T45.2X4	T45.2X5	T45.2X6
Iloprost	T46.7X1	T46.7X2	T46.7X3	T46.7X4	T46.7X5	T46.7X6
Ilotycin	T36.3X1	T36.3X2	T36.3X3	T36.3X4	T36.3X5	T36.3X6
ophthalmic preparation	T49.5X1	T49.5X2	T49.5X3	T49.5X4	T49.5X5	T49.5X6
topical NEC	T49.0X1	T49.0X2	T49.0X3	T49.0X4	T49.0X5	T49.0X6
Imidazole-4-carboxamide	T45.1X1	T45.1X2	T45.1X3	T45.1X4	T45.1X5	T45.1X6
Iminostilbene	T42.1X1	T42.1X2	T42.1X3	T42.1X4	T42.1X5	T42.1X6
Imipenem	T36.0X1	T36.0X2	T36.0X3	T36.0X4	T36.0X5	T36.0X6
Imipramine	T43.011	T43.012	T43.013	T43.014	T43.015	T43.016
Immu-G	T50.Z11	T50.Z12	T50.Z13	T50.Z14	T50.Z15	T50.Z16
Immuglobin	T50.Z11	T50.Z12	T50.Z13	T50.Z14	T50.Z15	T50.Z16
Immune						
globulin	T50.Z11	T50.Z12	T50.Z13	T50.Z14	T50.Z15	T50.Z16
serum globulin	T50.Z11	T50.Z12	T50.Z13	T50.Z14	T50.Z15	T50.Z16
Immunoglobin human	T50.Z11	T50.Z12	T50.Z13	T50.Z14	T50.Z15	T50.Z16
(intravenous) (normal)						
unmodified	T50.Z11	T50.Z12	T50.Z13	T50.Z14	T50.Z15	T50.Z16
Immunosuppressive drug	T45.1X1	T45.1X2	T45.1X3	T45.1X4	T45.1X5	T45.1X6
Immu-tetanus	T50.Z11	T50.Z12	T50.Z13	T50.Z14	T50.Z15	T50.Z16
Indalpine	T43.221	T43.222	T43.223	T43.224	T43.225	T43.226

Substance	Poisoning, Accidental (unintentional)	Poisoning, Intentional Self-harm	Poisoning, Assault	Poisoning, Undetermined	Adverse Effect	Under-dosing
Indanazoline	T48.5X1	T48.5X2	T48.5X3	T48.5X4	T48.5X5	T48.5X6
Indandione (derivatives)	T45.511	T45.512	T45.513	T45.514	T45.515	T45.516
Indapamide	T46.5X1	T46.5X2	T46.5X3	T46.5X4	T46.5X5	T46.5X6
Indendione (derivatives)	T45.511	T45.512	T45.513	T45.514	T45.515	T45.516
Indenolol	T44.7X1	T44.7X2	T44.7X3	T44.7X4	T44.7X5	T44.7X6
Inderal	T44.7X1	T44.7X2	T44.7X3	T44.7X4	T44.7X5	T44.7X6
Indian						
hemp	T40.7X1	T40.7X2	T40.7X3	T40.7X4	T40.7X5	T40.7X6
tobacco	T62.2X1	T62.2X2	T62.2X3	T62.2X4	—	—
Indigo carmine	T50.8X1	T50.8X2	T50.8X3	T50.8X4	T50.8X5	T50.8X6
Indobufen	T45.521	T45.522	T45.523	T45.524	T45.525	T45.526
Indocin	T39.2X1	T39.2X2	T39.2X3	T39.2X4	T39.2X5	T39.2X6
Indocyanine green	T50.8X1	T50.8X2	T50.8X3	T50.8X4	T50.8X5	T50.8X6
Indometacin	T39.391	T39.392	T39.393	T39.394	T39.395	T39.396
Indomethacin	T39.391	T39.392	T39.393	T39.394	T39.395	T39.396
farnesil	T39.4X1	T39.4X2	T39.4X3	T39.4X4	T39.4X5	T39.4X6
Indoramin	T44.6X1	T44.6X2	T44.6X3	T44.6X4	T44.6X5	T44.6X6
Industrial						
alcohol	T51.0X1	T51.0X2	T51.0X3	T51.0X4	—	—
fumes	T59.891	T59.892	T59.893	T59.894	—	—
solvents (fumes) (vapors)	T52.91	T52.92	T52.93	T52.94	—	—
Influenza vaccine	T50.B91	T50.B92	T50.B93	T50.B94	T50.B95	T50.B96
Ingested substance NEC	T65.91	T65.92	T65.93	T65.94	—	—
INH	T37.1X1	T37.1X2	T37.1X3	T37.1X4	T37.1X5	T37.1X6
Inhalation, gas (noxious) — see Gas						
Inhibitor						
angiotensin-converting enzyme	T46.4X1	T46.4X2	T46.4X3	T46.4X4	T46.4X5	T46.4X6
carbonic anhydrase	T50.2X1	T50.2X2	T50.2X3	T50.2X4	T50.2X5	T50.2X6
fibrinolysis	T45.621	T45.622	T45.623	T45.624	T45.625	T45.626
monoamine oxidase NEC	T43.1X1	T43.1X2	T43.1X3	T43.1X4	T43.1X5	T43.1X6
hydrazine	T43.1X1	T43.1X2	T43.1X3	T43.1X4	T43.1X5	T43.1X6
postsynaptic	T43.8X1	T43.8X2	T43.8X3	T43.8X4	T43.8X5	T43.8X6
prothrombin synthesis	T45.511	T45.512	T45.513	T45.514	T45.515	T45.516
Ink	T65.891	T65.892	T65.893	T65.894	—	—
Inorganic substance NEC	T57.91	T57.92	T57.93	T57.94	—	—
Inosine pranobex	T37.5X1	T37.5X2	T37.5X3	T37.5X4	T37.5X5	T37.5X6
Inositol	T50.991	T50.992	T50.993	T50.994	T50.995	T50.996
nicotinate	T46.7X1	T46.7X2	T46.7X3	T46.7X4	T46.7X5	T46.7X6
Inproquone	T45.1X1	T45.1X2	T45.1X3	T45.1X4	T45.1X5	T45.1X6
Insecticide NEC	T60.91	T60.92	T60.93	T60.94	—	—
carbamate	T60.0X1	T60.0X2	T60.0X3	T60.0X4	—	—
chlorinated	T60.1X1	T60.1X2	T60.1X3	T60.1X4	—	—
mixed	T60.91	T60.92	T60.93	T60.94	—	—
organochlorine	T60.1X1	T60.1X2	T60.1X3	T60.1X4	—	—
organophosphorus	T60.0X1	T60.0X2	T60.0X3	T60.0X4	—	—
Insect (sting), venomous	T63.481	T63.482	T63.483	T63.484	—	—
ant	T63.421	T63.422	T63.423	T63.424	—	—
bee	T63.441	T63.442	T63.443	T63.444	—	—
caterpillar	T63.431	T63.432	T63.433	T63.434	—	—
hornet	T63.451	T63.452	T63.453	T63.454	—	—
wasp	T63.461	T63.462	T63.463	T63.464	—	—
Insular tissue extract	T38.3X1	T38.3X2	T38.3X3	T38.3X4	T38.3X5	T38.3X6
Insulin (amorphous) (globin) (isophane) (Lente) (NPH) (Semilente) (Ultralente)	T38.3X1	T38.3X2	T38.3X3	T38.3X4	T38.3X5	T38.3X6
defalan	T38.3X1	T38.3X2	T38.3X3	T38.3X4	T38.3X5	T38.3X6
human	T38.3X1	T38.3X2	T38.3X3	T38.3X4	T38.3X5	T38.3X6
injection, soluble	T38.3X1	T38.3X2	T38.3X3	T38.3X4	T38.3X5	T38.3X6
biphasic	T38.3X1	T38.3X2	T38.3X3	T38.3X4	T38.3X5	T38.3X6
intermediate acting	T38.3X1	T38.3X2	T38.3X3	T38.3X4	T38.3X5	T38.3X6
protamine zinc	T38.3X1	T38.3X2	T38.3X3	T38.3X4	T38.3X5	T38.3X6
slow acting	T38.3X1	T38.3X2	T38.3X3	T38.3X4	T38.3X5	T38.3X6
zinc						
protamine injection	T38.3X1	T38.3X2	T38.3X3	T38.3X4	T38.3X5	T38.3X6
suspension (amorphous) (crystalline)	T38.3X1	T38.3X2	T38.3X3	T38.3X4	T38.3X5	T38.3X6
Interferon (alpha) (beta) (gamma)	T37.5X1	T37.5X2	T37.5X3	T37.5X4	T37.5X5	T37.5X6
Intestinal motility control drug	T47.6X1	T47.6X2	T47.6X3	T47.6X4	T47.6X5	T47.6X6
biological	T47.8X1	T47.8X2	T47.8X3	T47.8X4	T47.8X5	T47.8X6
Intranarcon	T41.1X1	T41.1X2	T41.1X3	T41.1X4	T41.1X5	T41.1X6
Intravenous						
amino acids	T50.991	T50.992	T50.993	T50.994	T50.995	T50.996
fat suspension	T50.991	T50.992	T50.993	T50.994	T50.995	T50.996
Inulin	T50.8X1	T50.8X2	T50.8X3	T50.8X4	T50.8X5	T50.8X6
Invert sugar	T50.3X1	T50.3X2	T50.3X3	T50.3X4	T50.3X5	T50.3X6
Inza — see Naproxen						
Iobenzamic acid	T50.8X1	T50.8X2	T50.8X3	T50.8X4	T50.8X5	T50.8X6
Iocarmic acid	T50.8X1	T50.8X2	T50.8X3	T50.8X4	T50.8X5	T50.8X6
Iocetamic acid	T50.8X1	T50.8X2	T50.8X3	T50.8X4	T50.8X5	T50.8X6

Substance	Poisoning, Accidental (unintentional)	Poisoning, Intentional Self-harm	Poisoning, Assault	Poisoning, Undetermined	Adverse Effect	Under-dosing
Iodamide	T50.8X1	T50.8X2	T50.8X3	T50.8X4	T50.8X5	T50.8X6
Iodide NEC — *see also* Iodine	T49.0X1	T49.0X2	T49.0X3	T49.0X4	T49.0X5	T49.0X6
mercury (ointment)	T49.0X1	T49.0X2	T49.0X3	T49.0X4	T49.0X5	T49.0X6
methylate	T49.0X1	T49.0X2	T49.0X3	T49.0X4	T49.0X5	T49.0X6
potassium (expectorant) NEC	T48.4X1	T48.4X2	T48.4X3	T48.4X4	T48.4X5	T48.4X6
Iodinated						
contrast medium	T50.8X1	T50.8X2	T50.8X3	T50.8X4	T50.8X5	T50.8X6
glycerol	T48.4X1	T48.4X2	T48.4X3	T48.4X4	T48.4X5	T48.4X6
human serum albumin (131I)	T50.8X1	T50.8X2	T50.8X3	T50.8X4	T50.8X5	T50.8X6
Iodine (antiseptic, external) (tincture) **NEC**	T49.0X1	T49.0X2	T49.0X3	T49.0X4	T49.0X5	T49.0X6
125 — *see also* Radiation sickness, and Exposure to radioactivce isotopes						
therapeutic	T50.991	T50.992	T50.993	T50.994	T50.995	T50.996
131 — *see also* Radiation sickness, and Exposure to radioactivce isotopes	T50.8X1	T50.8X2	T50.8X3	T50.8X4	T50.8X5	T50.8X6
therapeutic	T38.2X1	T38.2X2	T38.2X3	T38.2X4	T38.2X5	T38.2X6
diagnostic	T50.8X1	T50.8X2	T50.8X3	T50.8X4	T50.8X5	T50.8X6
for thyroid conditions (antithyroid)	T38.2X1	T38.2X2	T38.2X3	T38.2X4	T38.2X5	T38.2X6
solution	T49.0X1	T49.0X2	T49.0X3	T49.0X4	T49.0X5	T49.0X6
vapor	T59.891	T59.892	T59.893	T59.894	—	—
Iodipamide	T50.8X1	T50.8X2	T50.8X3	T50.8X4	T50.8X5	T50.8X6
Iodized (poppy seed) oil	T50.8X1	T50.8X2	T50.8X3	T50.8X4	T50.8X5	T50.8X6
Iodobismitol	T37.8X1	T37.8X2	T37.8X3	T37.8X4	T37.8X5	T37.8X6
Iodochlorhydroxyquin	T37.8X1	T37.8X2	T37.8X3	T37.8X4	T37.8X5	T37.8X6
topical	T49.0X1	T49.0X2	T49.0X3	T49.0X4	T49.0X5	T49.0X6
Iodochlorhydroxyquinoline	T37.8X1	T37.8X2	T37.8X3	T37.8X4	T37.8X5	T37.8X6
Iodocholesterol (131I)	T50.8X1	T50.8X2	T50.8X3	T50.8X4	T50.8X5	T50.8X6
Iodoform	T49.0X1	T49.0X2	T49.0X3	T49.0X4	T49.0X5	T49.0X6
Iodohippuric acid	T50.8X1	T50.8X2	T50.8X3	T50.8X4	T50.8X5	T50.8X6
Iodopanoic acid	T50.8X1	T50.8X2	T50.8X3	T50.8X4	T50.8X5	T50.8X6
Iodophthalein (sodium)	T50.8X1	T50.8X2	T50.8X3	T50.8X4	T50.8X5	T50.8X6
Iodopyracet	T50.8X1	T50.8X2	T50.8X3	T50.8X4	T50.8X5	T50.8X6
Iodoquinol	T37.8X1	T37.8X2	T37.8X3	T37.8X4	T37.8X5	T37.8X6
Iodoxamic acid	T50.8X1	T50.8X2	T50.8X3	T50.8X4	T50.8X5	T50.8X6
Iofendylate	T50.8X1	T50.8X2	T50.8X3	T50.8X4	T50.8X5	T50.8X6
Ioglycamic acid	T50.8X1	T50.8X2	T50.8X3	T50.8X4	T50.8X5	T50.8X6
Iohexol	T50.8X1	T50.8X2	T50.8X3	T50.8X4	T50.8X5	T50.8X6
Ion exchange resin						
anion	T47.8X1	T47.8X2	T47.8X3	T47.8X4	T47.8X5	T47.8X6
cation	T50.3X1	T50.3X2	T50.3X3	T50.3X4	T50.3X5	T50.3X6
cholestyramine	T46.6X1	T46.6X2	T46.6X3	T46.6X4	T46.6X5	T46.6X6
intestinal	T47.8X1	T47.8X2	T47.8X3	T47.8X4	T47.8X5	T47.8X6
Iopamidol	T50.8X1	T50.8X2	T50.8X3	T50.8X4	T50.8X5	T50.8X6
Iopanoic acid	T50.8X1	T50.8X2	T50.8X3	T50.8X4	T50.8X5	T50.8X6
Iophenoic acid	T50.8X1	T50.8X2	T50.8X3	T50.8X4	T50.8X5	T50.8X6
Iopodate, sodium	T50.8X1	T50.8X2	T50.8X3	T50.8X4	T50.8X5	T50.8X6
Iopodic acid	T50.8X1	T50.8X2	T50.8X3	T50.8X4	T50.8X5	T50.8X6
Iopromide	T50.8X1	T50.8X2	T50.8X3	T50.8X4	T50.8X5	T50.8X6
Iopydol	T50.8X1	T50.8X2	T50.8X3	T50.8X4	T50.8X5	T50.8X6
Iotalamic acid	T50.8X1	T50.8X2	T50.8X3	T50.8X4	T50.8X5	T50.8X6
Iothalamate	T50.8X1	T50.8X2	T50.8X3	T50.8X4	T50.8X5	T50.8X6
Iothiouracil	T38.2X1	T38.2X2	T38.2X3	T38.2X4	T38.2X5	T38.2X6
Iotrol	T50.8X1	T50.8X2	T50.8X3	T50.8X4	T50.8X5	T50.8X6
Iotrolan	T50.8X1	T50.8X2	T50.8X3	T50.8X4	T50.8X5	T50.8X6
Iotroxate	T50.8X1	T50.8X2	T50.8X3	T50.8X4	T50.8X5	T50.8X6
Iotroxic acid	T50.8X1	T50.8X2	T50.8X3	T50.8X4	T50.8X5	T50.8X6
Ioversol	T50.8X1	T50.8X2	T50.8X3	T50.8X4	T50.8X5	T50.8X6
Ioxaglate	T50.8X1	T50.8X2	T50.8X3	T50.8X4	T50.8X5	T50.8X6
Ioxaglic acid	T50.8X1	T50.8X2	T50.8X3	T50.8X4	T50.8X5	T50.8X6
Ioxitalamic acid	T50.8X1	T50.8X2	T50.8X3	T50.8X4	T50.8X5	T50.8X6
Ipecac	T47.7X1	T47.7X2	T47.7X3	T47.7X4	T47.7X5	T47.7X6
Ipecacuanha	T48.4X1	T48.4X2	T48.4X3	T48.4X4	T48.4X5	T48.4X6
Ipodate, calcium	T50.8X1	T50.8X2	T50.8X3	T50.8X4	T50.8X5	T50.8X6
Ipral	T42.3X1	T42.3X2	T42.3X3	T42.3X4	T42.3X5	T42.3X6
Ipratropium (bromide)	T48.6X1	T48.6X2	T48.6X3	T48.6X4	T48.6X5	T48.6X6
Ipriflavone	T46.3X1	T46.3X2	T46.3X3	T46.3X4	T46.3X5	T46.3X6
Iprindole	T43.011	T43.012	T43.013	T43.014	T43.015	T43.016
Iproclozide	T43.1X1	T43.1X2	T43.1X3	T43.1X4	T43.1X5	T43.1X6
Iprofenin	T50.8X1	T50.8X2	T50.8X3	T50.8X4	T50.8X5	T50.8X6
Iproheptine	T49.2X1	T49.2X2	T49.2X3	T49.2X4	T49.2X5	T49.2X6
Iproniazid	T43.1X1	T43.1X2	T43.1X3	T43.1X4	T43.1X5	T43.1X6
Iproplatin	T45.1X1	T45.1X2	T45.1X3	T45.1X4	T45.1X5	T45.1X6
Iproveratril	T46.1X1	T46.1X2	T46.1X3	T46.1X4	T46.1X5	T46.1X6
Iron (compounds) (medicinal) **NEC**	T45.4X1	T45.4X2	T45.4X3	T45.4X4	T45.4X5	T45.4X6
ammonium	T45.4X1	T45.4X2	T45.4X3	T45.4X4	T45.4X5	T45.4X6
dextran injection	T45.4X1	T45.4X2	T45.4X3	T45.4X4	T45.4X5	T45.4X6

Substance	Poisoning, Accidental (unintentional)	Poisoning, Intentional Self-harm	Poisoning, Assault	Poisoning, Undetermined	Adverse Effect	Under-dosing
Iron (compounds) (medicinal) **NEC** — *continued*						
nonmedicinal	T56.891	T56.892	T56.893	T56.894	—	—
salts	T45.4X1	T45.4X2	T45.4X3	T45.4X4	T45.4X5	T45.4X6
sorbitex	T45.4X1	T45.4X2	T45.4X3	T45.4X4	T45.4X5	T45.4X6
sorbitol citric acid complex	T45.4X1	T45.4X2	T45.4X3	T45.4X4	T45.4X5	T45.4X6
Irrigating fluid (vaginal)	T49.8X1	T49.8X2	T49.8X3	T49.8X4	T49.8X5	T49.8X6
eye	T49.5X1	T49.5X2	T49.5X3	T49.5X4	T49.5X5	T49.5X6
Isepamicin	T36.5X1	T36.5X2	T36.5X3	T36.5X4	T36.5X5	T36.5X6
Isoaminile (citrate)	T48.3X1	T48.3X2	T48.3X3	T48.3X4	T48.3X5	T48.3X6
Isoamyl nitrite	T46.3X1	T46.3X2	T46.3X3	T46.3X4	T46.3X5	T46.3X6
Isobenzan	T60.1X1	T60.1X2	T60.1X3	T60.1X4	—	—
Isobutyl acetate	T52.8X1	T52.8X2	T52.8X3	T52.8X4	—	—
Isocarboxazid	T43.1X1	T43.1X2	T43.1X3	T43.1X4	T43.1X5	T43.1X6
Isoconazole	T49.0X1	T49.0X2	T49.0X3	T49.0X4	T49.0X5	T49.0X6
Isocyanate	T65.0X1	T65.0X2	T65.0X3	T65.0X4	—	—
Isoephedrine	T44.991	T44.992	T44.993	T44.994	T44.995	T44.996
Isoetarine	T48.6X1	T48.6X2	T48.6X3	T48.6X4	T48.6X5	T48.6X6
Isoethadione	T42.2X1	T42.2X2	T42.2X3	T42.2X4	T42.2X5	T42.2X6
Isoetharine	T44.5X1	T44.5X2	T44.5X3	T44.5X4	T44.5X5	T44.5X6
Isoflurane	T41.0X1	T41.0X2	T41.0X3	T41.0X4	T41.0X5	T41.0X6
Isoflurophate	T44.0X1	T44.0X2	T44.0X3	T44.0X4	T44.0X5	T44.0X6
Isomaltose, ferric complex	T45.4X1	T45.4X2	T45.4X3	T45.4X4	T45.4X5	T45.4X6
Isometheptene	T44.3X1	T44.3X2	T44.3X3	T44.3X4	T44.3X5	T44.3X6
Isoniazid	T37.1X1	T37.1X2	T37.1X3	T37.1X4	T37.1X5	T37.1X6
with						
rifampicin	T36.6X1	T36.6X2	T36.6X3	T36.6X4	T36.6X5	T36.6X6
thioacetazone	T37.1X1	T37.1X2	T37.1X3	T37.1X4	T37.1X5	T37.1X6
Isonicotinic acid hydrazide	T37.1X1	T37.1X2	T37.1X3	T37.1X4	T37.1X5	T37.1X6
Isonipecaine	T40.4X1	T40.4X2	T40.4X3	T40.4X4	T40.4X5	T40.4X6
Isopentaquine	T37.2X1	T37.2X2	T37.2X3	T37.2X4	T37.2X5	T37.2X6
Isophane insulin	T38.3X1	T38.3X2	T38.3X3	T38.3X4	T38.3X5	T38.3X6
Isophorone	T65.891	T65.892	T65.893	T65.894	—	—
Isophosphamide	T45.1X1	T45.1X2	T45.1X3	T45.1X4	T45.1X5	T45.1X6
Isopregnenone	T38.5X1	T38.5X2	T38.5X3	T38.5X4	T38.5X5	T38.5X6
Isoprenaline	T48.6X1	T48.6X2	T48.6X3	T48.6X4	T48.6X5	T48.6X6
Isopromethazine	T43.3X1	T43.3X2	T43.3X3	T43.3X4	T43.3X5	T43.3X6
Isopropamide	T44.3X1	T44.3X2	T44.3X3	T44.3X4	T44.3X5	T44.3X6
iodide	T44.3X1	T44.3X2	T44.3X3	T44.3X4	T44.3X5	T44.3X6
Isopropanol	T51.2X1	T51.2X2	T51.2X3	T51.2X4	—	—
Isopropyl						
acetate	T52.8X1	T52.8X2	T52.8X3	T52.8X4	—	—
alcohol	T51.2X1	T51.2X2	T51.2X3	T51.2X4	—	—
medicinal	T49.4X1	T49.4X2	T49.4X3	T49.4X4	T49.4X5	T49.4X6
ether	T52.8X1	T52.8X2	T52.8X3	T52.8X4	—	—
Isopropylaminophenazone	T39.2X1	T39.2X2	T39.2X3	T39.2X4	T39.2X5	T39.2X6
Isoproterenol	T48.6X1	T48.6X2	T48.6X3	T48.6X4	T48.6X5	T48.6X6
Isosorbide dinitrate	T46.3X1	T46.3X2	T46.3X3	T46.3X4	T46.3X5	T46.3X6
Isothipendyl	T45.0X1	T45.0X2	T45.0X3	T45.0X4	T45.0X5	T45.0X6
Isotretinoin	T50.991	T50.992	T50.993	T50.994	T50.995	T50.996
Isoxazolyl penicillin	T36.0X1	T36.0X2	T36.0X3	T36.0X4	T36.0X5	T36.0X6
Isoxicam	T39.391	T39.392	T39.393	T39.394	T39.395	T39.396
Isoxsuprine	T46.7X1	T46.7X2	T46.7X3	T46.7X4	T46.7X5	T46.7X6
Ispagula	T47.4X1	T47.4X2	T47.4X3	T47.4X4	T47.4X5	T47.4X6
husk	T47.4X1	T47.4X2	T47.4X3	T47.4X4	T47.4X5	T47.4X6
Isradipine	T46.1X1	T46.1X2	T46.1X3	T46.1X4	T46.1X5	T46.1X6
I-thyroxine sodium	T38.1X1	T38.1X2	T38.1X3	T38.1X4	T38.1X5	T38.1X6
Itraconazole	T37.8X1	T37.8X2	T37.8X3	T37.8X4	T37.8X5	T37.8X6
Itramin tosilate	T46.3X1	T46.3X2	T46.3X3	T46.3X4	T46.3X5	T46.3X6
Ivermectin	T37.4X1	T37.4X2	T37.4X3	T37.4X4	T37.4X5	T37.4X6
Izoniazid	T37.1X1	T37.1X2	T37.1X3	T37.1X4	T37.1X5	T37.1X6
with thioacetazone	T37.1X1	T37.1X2	T37.1X3	T37.1X4	T37.1X5	T37.1X6
Jalap	T47.2X1	T47.2X2	T47.2X3	T47.2X4	T47.2X5	T47.2X6
Jamaica						
dogwood (bark)	T39.8X1	T39.8X2	T39.8X3	T39.8X4	T39.8X5	T39.8X6
ginger	T65.891	T65.892	T65.893	T65.894	—	—
root	T62.2X1	T62.2X2	T62.2X3	T62.2X4	—	—
Jatropha	T62.2X1	T62.2X2	T62.2X3	T62.2X4	—	—
curcas	T62.2X1	T62.2X2	T62.2X3	T62.2X4	—	—
Jectofer	T45.4X1	T45.4X2	T45.4X3	T45.4X4	T45.4X5	T45.4X6
Jellyfish (sting)	T63.621	T63.622	T63.623	T63.624	—	—
Jequirity (bean)	T62.2X1	T62.2X2	T62.2X3	T62.2X4	—	—
Jimson weed (stramonium)	T62.2X1	T62.2X2	T62.2X3	T62.2X4	—	—
seeds	T62.2X1	T62.2X2	T62.2X3	T62.2X4	—	—
Josamycin	T36.3X1	T36.3X2	T36.3X3	T36.3X4	T36.3X5	T36.3X6
Juniper tar	T49.1X1	T49.1X2	T49.1X3	T49.1X4	T49.1X5	T49.1X6
Kallidinogenase	T46.7X1	T46.7X2	T46.7X3	T46.7X4	T46.7X5	T46.7X6
Kallikrein	T46.7X1	T46.7X2	T46.7X3	T46.7X4	T46.7X5	T46.7X6
Kanamycin	T36.5X1	T36.5X2	T36.5X3	T36.5X4	T36.5X5	T36.5X6
Kantrex	T36.5X1	T36.5X2	T36.5X3	T36.5X4	T36.5X5	T36.5X6
Kaolin	T47.6X1	T47.6X2	T47.6X3	T47.6X4	T47.6X5	T47.6X6
light	T47.6X1	T47.6X2	T47.6X3	T47.6X4	T47.6X5	T47.6X6
Karaya (gum)	T47.4X1	T47.4X2	T47.4X3	T47.4X4	T47.4X5	T47.4X6

Substance	Poisoning, Accidental (unintentional)	Poisoning, Intentional Self-harm	Poisoning, Assault	Poisoning, Undetermined	Adverse Effect	Under-dosing
Kebuzone	T39.2X1	T39.2X2	T39.2X3	T39.2X4	T39.2X5	T39.2X6
Kelevan	T60.1X1	T60.1X2	T60.1X3	T60.1X4	—	—
Kemithal	T41.1X1	T41.1X2	T41.1X3	T41.1X4	T41.1X5	T41.1X6
Kenacort	T38.0X1	T38.0X2	T38.0X3	T38.0X4	T38.0X5	T38.0X6
Keratolytic drug NEC	T49.4X1	T49.4X2	T49.4X3	T49.4X4	T49.4X5	T49.4X6
anthracene	T49.4X1	T49.4X2	T49.4X3	T49.4X4	T49.4X5	T49.4X6
Keratoplastic NEC	T49.4X1	T49.4X2	T49.4X3	T49.4X4	T49.4X5	T49.4X6
Kerosene, kerosine (fuel) (solvent) NEC	T52.0X1	T52.0X2	T52.0X3	T52.0X4	—	—
insecticide	T52.0X1	T52.0X2	T52.0X3	T52.0X4	—	—
vapor	T52.0X1	T52.0X2	T52.0X3	T52.0X4	—	—
Ketamine	T41.291	T41.292	T41.293	T41.294	T41.295	T41.296
Ketazolam	T42.4X1	T42.4X2	T42.4X3	T42.4X4	T42.4X5	T42.4X6
Ketazon	T39.2X1	T39.2X2	T39.2X3	T39.2X4	T39.2X5	T39.2X6
Ketobemidone	T40.4X1	T40.4X2	T40.4X3	T40.4X4	—	—
Ketoconazole	T49.0X1	T49.0X2	T49.0X3	T49.0X4	T49.0X5	T49.0X6
Ketols	T52.4X1	T52.4X2	T52.4X3	T52.4X4	—	—
Ketone oils	T52.4X1	T52.4X2	T52.4X3	T52.4X4	—	—
Ketoprofen	T39.311	T39.312	T39.313	T39.314	T39.315	T39.316
Ketorolac	T39.8X1	T39.8X2	T39.8X3	T39.8X4	T39.8X5	T39.8X6
Ketotifen	T45.0X1	T45.0X2	T45.0X3	T45.0X4	T45.0X5	T45.0X6
Khat	T43.691	T43.692	T43.693	T43.694	—	—
Khellin	T46.3X1	T46.3X2	T46.3X3	T46.3X4	T46.3X5	T46.3X6
Khelloside	T46.3X1	T46.3X2	T46.3X3	T46.3X4	T46.3X5	T46.3X6
Kiln gas or vapor (carbon monoxide)	T58.8X1	T58.8X2	T58.8X3	T58.8X4	—	—
Kitasamycin	T36.3X1	T36.3X2	T36.3X3	T36.3X4	T36.3X5	T36.3X6
Konsyl	T47.4X1	T47.4X2	T47.4X3	T47.4X4	T47.4X5	T47.4X6
Kosam seed	T62.2X1	T62.2X2	T62.2X3	T62.2X4	—	—
Krait (venom)	T63.091	T63.092	T63.093	T63.094	—	—
Kwell (insecticide)	T60.1X1	T60.1X2	T60.1X3	T60.1X4	—	—
anti-infective (topical)	T49.0X1	T49.0X2	T49.0X3	T49.0X4	T49.0X5	T49.0X6
Labetalol	T44.8X1	T44.8X2	T44.8X3	T44.8X4	T44.8X5	T44.8X6
Laburnum (seeds)	T62.2X1	T62.2X2	T62.2X3	T62.2X4	—	—
leaves	T62.2X1	T62.2X2	T62.2X3	T62.2X4	—	—
Lachesine	T49.5X1	T49.5X2	T49.5X3	T49.5X4	T49.5X5	T49.5X6
Lacidipine	T46.5X1	T46.5X2	T46.5X3	T46.5X4	T46.5X5	T46.5X6
Lacquer	T65.6X1	T65.6X2	T65.6X3	T65.6X4	—	—
Lacrimogenic gas	T59.3X1	T59.3X2	T59.3X3	T59.3X4	—	—
Lactated potassic saline	T50.3X1	T50.3X2	T50.3X3	T50.3X4	T50.3X5	T50.3X6
Lactic acid	T49.8X1	T49.8X2	T49.8X3	T49.8X4	T49.8X5	T49.8X6
Lactobacillus						
acidophilus	T47.6X1	T47.6X2	T47.6X3	T47.6X4	T47.6X5	T47.6X6
compound	T47.6X1	T47.6X2	T47.6X3	T47.6X4	T47.6X5	T47.6X6
bifidus, lyophilized	T47.6X1	T47.6X2	T47.6X3	T47.6X4	T47.6X5	T47.6X6
bulgaricus	T47.6X1	T47.6X2	T47.6X3	T47.6X4	T47.6X5	T47.6X6
sporogenes	T47.6X1	T47.6X2	T47.6X3	T47.6X4	T47.6X5	T47.6X6
Lactoflavin	T45.2X1	T45.2X2	T45.2X3	T45.2X4	T45.2X5	T45.2X6
Lactose (as excipient)	T50.901	T50.902	T50.903	T50.904	T50.905	T50.906
Lactuca (virosa) (extract)	T42.6X1	T42.6X2	T42.6X3	T42.6X4	T42.6X5	T42.6X6
Lactucarium	T42.6X1	T42.6X2	T42.6X3	T42.6X4	T42.6X5	T42.6X6
Lactulose	T47.3X1	T47.3X2	T47.3X3	T47.3X4	T47.3X5	T47.3X6
Laevo — see Levo-						
Lanatosides	T46.0X1	T46.0X2	T46.0X3	T46.0X4	T46.0X5	T46.0X6
Lanolin	T49.3X1	T49.3X2	T49.3X3	T49.3X4	T49.3X5	T49.3X6
Largactil	T43.3X1	T43.3X2	T43.3X3	T43.3X4	T43.3X5	T43.3X6
Larkspur	T62.2X1	T62.2X2	T62.2X3	T62.2X4	—	—
Laroxyl	T43.011	T43.012	T43.013	T43.014	T43.015	T43.016
Lasix	T50.1X1	T50.1X2	T50.1X3	T50.1X4	T50.1X5	T50.1X6
Lassar's paste	T49.4X1	T49.4X2	T49.4X3	T49.4X4	T49.4X5	T49.4X6
Latamoxef	T36.1X1	T36.1X2	T36.1X3	T36.1X4	T36.1X5	T36.1X6
Latex	T65.811	T65.812	T65.813	T65.814	—	—
Lathyrus (seed)	T62.2X1	T62.2X2	T62.2X3	T62.2X4	—	—
Laudanum	T40.0X1	T40.0X2	T40.0X3	T40.0X4	T40.0X5	T40.0X6
Laudexium	T48.1X1	T48.1X2	T48.1X3	T48.1X4	T48.1X5	T48.1X6
Laughing gas	T41.0X1	T41.0X2	T41.0X3	T41.0X4	T41.0X5	T41.0X6
Laurel, black or cherry	T62.2X1	T62.2X2	T62.2X3	T62.2X4	—	—
Laurolinium	T49.0X1	T49.0X2	T49.0X3	T49.0X4	T49.0X5	T49.0X6
Lauryl sulfoacetate	T49.2X1	T49.2X2	T49.2X3	T49.2X4	T49.2X5	T49.2X6
Laxative NEC	T47.4X1	T47.4X2	T47.4X3	T47.4X4	T47.4X5	T47.4X6
osmotic	T47.3X1	T47.3X2	T47.3X3	T47.3X4	T47.3X5	T47.3X6
saline	T47.3X1	T47.3X2	T47.3X3	T47.3X4	T47.3X5	T47.3X6
stimulant	T47.2X1	T47.2X2	T47.2X3	T47.2X4	T47.2X5	T47.2X6
L-dopa	T42.8X1	T42.8X2	T42.8X3	T42.8X4	T42.8X5	T42.8X6
Lead (dust) (fumes) (vapor) NEC	T56.0X1	T56.0X2	T56.0X3	T56.0X4	—	—
acetate	T49.2X1	T49.2X2	T49.2X3	T49.2X4	T49.2X5	T49.2X6
alkyl (fuel additive)	T56.0X1	T56.0X2	T56.0X3	T56.0X4	—	—
anti-infectives	T37.8X1	T37.8X2	T37.8X3	T37.8X4	T37.8X5	T37.8X6
antiknock compound (tetraethyl)	T56.0X1	T56.0X2	T56.0X3	T56.0X4	—	—

Substance	Poisoning, Accidental (unintentional)	Poisoning, Intentional Self-harm	Poisoning, Assault	Poisoning, Undetermined	Adverse Effect	Under-dosing
Lead (dust) (fumes) (vapor) NEC						
— continued						
arsenate, arsenite (dust)(herbicide) (insecticide) (vapor)	T57.0X1	T57.0X2	T57.0X3	T57.0X4	—	—
carbonate	T56.0X1	T56.0X2	T56.0X3	T56.0X4	—	—
paint	T56.0X1	T56.0X2	T56.0X3	T56.0X4	—	—
chromate	T56.0X1	T56.0X2	T56.0X3	T56.0X4	—	—
paint	T56.0X1	T56.0X2	T56.0X3	T56.0X4	—	—
dioxide	T56.0X1	T56.0X2	T56.0X3	T56.0X4	—	—
inorganic	T56.0X1	T56.0X2	T56.0X3	T56.0X4	—	—
iodide	T56.0X1	T56.0X2	T56.0X3	T56.0X4	—	—
pigment (paint)	T56.0X1	T56.0X2	T56.0X3	T56.0X4	—	—
monoxide (dust)	T56.0X1	T56.0X2	T56.0X3	T56.0X4	—	—
paint	T56.0X1	T56.0X2	T56.0X3	T56.0X4	—	—
organic	T56.0X1	T56.0X2	T56.0X3	T56.0X4	—	—
oxide	T56.0X1	T56.0X2	T56.0X3	T56.0X4	—	—
paint	T56.0X1	T56.0X2	T56.0X3	T56.0X4	—	—
paint	T56.0X1	T56.0X2	T56.0X3	T56.0X4	—	—
salts	T56.0X1	T56.0X2	T56.0X3	T56.0X4	—	—
specified compound NEC	T56.0X1	T56.0X2	T56.0X3	T56.0X4	—	—
tetra-ethyl	T56.0X1	T56.0X2	T56.0X3	T56.0X4	—	—
Lebanese red	T40.7X1	T40.7X2	T40.7X3	T40.7X4	T40.7X5	T40.7X6
Lefetamine	T39.8X1	T39.8X2	T39.8X3	T39.8X4	T39.8X5	T39.8X6
Lenperone	T43.4X1	T43.4X2	T43.4X3	T43.4X4	T43.4X5	T43.4X6
Lente lietin (insulin)	T38.3X1	T38.3X2	T38.3X3	T38.3X4	T38.3X5	T38.3X6
Leptazol	T50.7X1	T50.7X2	T50.7X3	T50.7X4	T50.7X5	T50.7X6
Leptophos	T60.0X1	T60.0X2	T60.0X3	T60.0X4	—	—
Leritine	T40.2X1	T40.2X2	T40.2X3	T40.2X4	T40.2X5	T40.2X6
Letosteine	T48.4X1	T48.4X2	T48.4X3	T48.4X4	T48.4X5	T48.4X6
Letter	T38.1X1	T38.1X2	T38.1X3	T38.1X4	T38.1X5	T38.1X6
Lettuce opium	T42.6X1	T42.6X2	T42.6X3	T42.6X4	T42.6X5	T42.6X6
Leucinocaine	T41.3X1	T41.3X2	T41.3X3	T41.3X4	T41.3X5	T41.3X6
Leucocianidol	T46.991	T46.992	T46.993	T46.994	T46.995	T46.996
Leucovorin (factor)	T45.8X1	T45.8X2	T45.8X3	T45.8X4	T45.8X5	T45.8X6
Leukeran	T45.1X1	T45.1X2	T45.1X3	T45.1X4	T45.1X5	T45.1X6
Leuprolide	T38.891	T38.892	T38.893	T38.894	T38.895	T38.896
Levalbuterol	T48.6X1	T48.6X2	T48.6X3	T48.6X4	T48.6X5	T48.6X6
Levallorphan	T50.7X1	T50.7X2	T50.7X3	T50.7X4	T50.7X5	T50.7X6
Levamisole	T37.4X1	T37.4X2	T37.4X3	T37.4X4	T37.4X5	T37.4X6
Levanil	T42.6X1	T42.6X2	T42.6X3	T42.6X4	T42.6X5	T42.6X6
Levarterenol	T44.4X1	T44.4X2	T44.4X3	T44.4X4	T44.4X5	T44.4X6
Levdropropizine	T48.3X1	T48.3X2	T48.3X3	T48.3X4	T48.3X5	T48.3X6
Levobunolol	T49.5X1	T49.5X2	T49.5X3	T49.5X4	T49.5X5	T49.5X6
Levocabastine (hydrochloride)	T45.0X1	T45.0X2	T45.0X3	T45.0X4	T45.0X5	T45.0X6
Levocarnitine	T50.991	T50.992	T50.993	T50.994	T50.995	T50.996
Levodopa	T42.8X1	T42.8X2	T42.8X3	T42.8X4	T42.8X5	T42.8X6
with carbidopa	T42.8X1	T42.8X2	T42.8X3	T42.8X4	T42.8X5	T42.8X6
Levo-dromoran	T40.2X1	T40.2X2	T40.2X3	T40.2X4	T40.2X5	T40.2X6
Levoglutamide	T50.991	T50.992	T50.993	T50.994	T50.995	T50.996
Levoid	T38.1X1	T38.1X2	T38.1X3	T38.1X4	T38.1X5	T38.1X6
Levo-isomethadone	T40.3X1	T40.3X2	T40.3X3	T40.3X4	T40.3X5	T40.3X6
Levomepromazine	T43.3X1	T43.3X2	T43.3X3	T43.3X4	T43.3X5	T43.3X6
Levonordefrin	T49.6X1	T49.6X2	T49.6X3	T49.6X4	T49.6X5	T49.6X6
Levonorgestrel	T38.4X1	T38.4X2	T38.4X3	T38.4X4	T38.4X5	T38.4X6
with ethinylestradiol	T38.5X1	T38.5X2	T38.5X3	T38.5X4	T38.5X5	T38.5X6
Levopromazine	T43.3X1	T43.3X2	T43.3X3	T43.3X4	T43.3X5	T43.3X6
Levoprome	T42.6X1	T42.6X2	T42.6X3	T42.6X4	T42.6X5	T42.6X6
Levopropoxyphene	T40.4X1	T40.4X2	T40.4X3	T40.4X4	T40.4X5	T40.4X6
Levopropylhexedrine	T50.5X1	T50.5X2	T50.5X3	T50.5X4	T50.5X5	T50.5X6
Levoproxyphylline	T48.6X1	T48.6X2	T48.6X3	T48.6X4	T48.6X5	T48.6X6
Levorphanol	T40.4X1	T40.4X2	T40.4X3	T40.4X4	T40.4X5	T40.4X6
Levothyroxine	T38.1X1	T38.1X2	T38.1X3	T38.1X4	T38.1X5	T38.1X6
sodium	T38.1X1	T38.1X2	T38.1X3	T38.1X4	T38.1X5	T38.1X6
Levsin	T44.3X1	T44.3X2	T44.3X3	T44.3X4	T44.3X5	T44.3X6
Levulose	T50.3X1	T50.3X2	T50.3X3	T50.3X4	T50.3X5	T50.3X6
Lewisite (gas), not in war	T57.0X1	T57.0X2	T57.0X3	T57.0X4	—	—
Librium	T42.4X1	T42.4X2	T42.4X3	T42.4X4	T42.4X5	T42.4X6
Lidex	T49.0X1	T49.0X2	T49.0X3	T49.0X4	T49.0X5	T49.0X6
Lidocaine	T41.3X1	T41.3X2	T41.3X3	T41.3X4	T41.3X5	T41.3X6
regional	T41.3X1	T41.3X2	T41.3X3	T41.3X4	T41.3X5	T41.3X6
spinal	T41.3X1	T41.3X2	T41.3X3	T41.3X4	T41.3X5	T41.3X6
Lidofenin	T50.8X1	T50.8X2	T50.8X3	T50.8X4	T50.8X5	T50.8X6
Lidoflazine	T46.1X1	T46.1X2	T46.1X3	T46.1X4	T46.1X5	T46.1X6
Lighter fluid	T52.0X1	T52.0X2	T52.0X3	T52.0X4	—	—
Lignin hemicellulose	T47.6X1	T47.6X2	T47.6X3	T47.6X4	T47.6X5	T47.6X6
Lignocaine	T41.3X1	T41.3X2	T41.3X3	T41.3X4	T41.3X5	T41.3X6
regional	T41.3X1	T41.3X2	T41.3X3	T41.3X4	T41.3X5	T41.3X6
spinal	T41.3X1	T41.3X2	T41.3X3	T41.3X4	T41.3X5	T41.3X6
Ligroin (e) (solvent)	T52.0X1	T52.0X2	T52.0X3	T52.0X4	—	—
vapor	T59.891	T59.892	T59.893	T59.894	—	—
Ligustrum vulgare	T62.2X1	T62.2X2	T62.2X3	T62.2X4	—	—

Substance	Poisoning, Accidental (unintentional)	Poisoning, Intentional Self-harm	Poisoning, Assault	Poisoning, Undetermined	Adverse Effect	Under-dosing
Lily of the valley	T62.2X1	T62.2X2	T62.2X3	T62.2X4	—	—
Lime (chloride)	T54.3X1	T54.3X2	T54.3X3	T54.3X4	—	—
Limonene	T52.8X1	T52.8X2	T52.8X3	T52.8X4	—	—
Lincomycin	T36.8X1	T36.8X2	T36.8X3	T36.8X4	T36.8X5	T36.8X6
Lindane (insecticide) (nonmedicinal) (vapor)	T53.6X1	T53.6X2	T53.6X3	T53.6X4	—	—
medicinal	T49.0X1	T49.0X2	T49.0X3	T49.0X4	T49.0X5	T49.0X6
Liniments NEC	T49.91	T49.92	T49.93	T49.94	T49.95	T49.96
Linoleic acid	T46.6X1	T46.6X2	T46.6X3	T46.6X4	T46.6X5	T46.6X6
Linolenic acid	T46.6X1	T46.6X2	T46.6X3	T46.6X4	T46.6X5	T46.6X6
Linseed	T47.4X1	T47.4X2	T47.4X3	T47.4X4	T47.4X5	T47.4X6
Liothyronine	T38.1X1	T38.1X2	T38.1X3	T38.1X4	T38.1X5	T38.1X6
Liotrix	T38.1X1	T38.1X2	T38.1X3	T38.1X4	T38.1X5	T38.1X6
Lipancreatin	T47.5X1	T47.5X2	T47.5X3	T47.5X4	T47.5X5	T47.5X6
Lipo-alprostadil	T46.7X1	T46.7X2	T46.7X3	T46.7X4	T46.7X5	T46.7X6
Lipo-Lutin	T38.5X1	T38.5X2	T38.5X3	T38.5X4	T38.5X5	T38.5X6
Lipotropic drug NEC	T50.901	T50.902	T50.903	T50.904	T50.905	T50.906
Liquefied petroleum gases	T59.891	T59.892	T59.893	T59.894	—	—
piped (pure or mixed with air)	T59.891	T59.892	T59.893	T59.894	—	—
Liquid						
paraffin	T47.4X1	T47.4X2	T47.4X3	T47.4X4	T47.4X5	T47.4X6
petrolatum	T47.4X1	T47.4X2	T47.4X3	T47.4X4	T47.4X5	T47.4X6
topical	T49.3X1	T49.3X2	T49.3X3	T49.3X4	T49.3X5	T49.3X6
specified NEC	T65.891	T65.892	T65.893	T65.894	—	—
substance	T65.91	T65.92	T65.93	T65.94	—	—
Liquor creosolis compositus	T65.891	T65.892	T65.893	T65.894	—	—
Liquorice	T48.4X1	T48.4X2	T48.4X3	T48.4X4	T48.4X5	T48.4X6
extract	T47.8X1	T47.8X2	T47.8X3	T47.8X4	T47.8X5	T47.8X6
Lisinopril	T46.4X1	T46.4X2	T46.4X3	T46.4X4	T46.4X5	T46.4X6
Lisuride	T42.8X1	T42.8X2	T42.8X3	T42.8X4	T42.8X5	T42.8X6
Lithane	T43.8X1	T43.8X2	T43.8X3	T43.8X4	T43.8X5	T43.8X6
Lithium	T56.891	T56.892	T56.893	T56.894	—	—
gluconate	T43.591	T43.592	T43.593	T43.594	T43.595	T43.596
salts (carbonate)	T43.591	T43.592	T43.593	T43.594	T43.595	T43.596
Lithonate	T43.8X1	T43.8X2	T43.8X3	T43.8X4	T43.8X5	T43.8X6
Liver						
extract	T45.8X1	T45.8X2	T45.8X3	T45.8X4	T45.8X5	T45.8X6
for parenteral use	T45.8X1	T45.8X2	T45.8X3	T45.8X4	T45.8X5	T45.8X6
fraction 1	T45.8X1	T45.8X2	T45.8X3	T45.8X4	T45.8X5	T45.8X6
hydrolysate	T45.8X1	T45.8X2	T45.8X3	T45.8X4	T45.8X5	T45.8X6
Lizard (bite) (venom)	T63.121	T63.122	T63.123	T63.124	—	—
LMD	T45.8X1	T45.8X2	T45.8X3	T45.8X4	T45.8X5	T45.8X6
Lobelia	T62.2X1	T62.2X2	T62.2X3	T62.2X4	—	—
Lobeline	T50.7X1	T50.7X2	T50.7X3	T50.7X4	T50.7X5	T50.7X6
Local action drug NEC	T49.8X1	T49.8X2	T49.8X3	T49.8X4	T49.8X5	T49.8X6
Locorten	T49.0X1	T49.0X2	T49.0X3	T49.0X4	T49.0X5	T49.0X6
Lofepramine	T43.011	T43.012	T43.013	T43.014	T43.015	T43.016
Lolium temulentum	T62.2X1	T62.2X2	T62.2X3	T62.2X4	—	—
Lomotil	T47.6X1	T47.6X2	T47.6X3	T47.6X4	T47.6X5	T47.6X6
Lomustine	T45.1X1	T45.1X2	T45.1X3	T45.1X4	T45.1X5	T45.1X6
Lonidamine	T45.1X1	T45.1X2	T45.1X3	T45.1X4	T45.1X5	T45.1X6
Loperamide	T47.6X1	T47.6X2	T47.6X3	T47.6X4	T47.6X5	T47.6X6
Loprazolam	T42.4X1	T42.4X2	T42.4X3	T42.4X4	T42.4X5	T42.4X6
Lorajmine	T46.2X1	T46.2X2	T46.2X3	T46.2X4	T46.2X5	T46.2X6
Loratidine	T45.0X1	T45.0X2	T45.0X3	T45.0X4	T45.0X5	T45.0X6
Lorazepam	T42.4X1	T42.4X2	T42.4X3	T42.4X4	T42.4X5	T42.4X6
Lorcainide	T46.2X1	T46.2X2	T46.2X3	T46.2X4	T46.2X5	T46.2X6
Lormetazepam	T42.4X1	T42.4X2	T42.4X3	T42.4X4	T42.4X5	T42.4X6
Lotions NEC	T49.91	T49.92	T49.93	T49.94	T49.95	T49.96
Lotusate	T42.3X1	T42.3X2	T42.3X3	T42.3X4	T42.3X5	T42.3X6
Lovastatin	T46.6X1	T46.6X2	T46.6X3	T46.6X4	T46.6X5	T46.6X6
Lowila	T49.2X1	T49.2X2	T49.2X3	T49.2X4	T49.2X5	T49.2X6
Loxapine	T43.591	T43.592	T43.593	T43.594	T43.595	T43.596
Lozenges (throat)	T49.6X1	T49.6X2	T49.6X3	T49.6X4	T49.6X5	T49.6X6
LSD	T40.8X1	T40.8X2	T40.8X3	T40.8X4	—	—
L-Tryptophan — see amino acid						
Lubricant, eye	T49.5X1	T49.5X2	T49.5X3	T49.5X4	T49.5X5	T49.5X6
Lubricating oil NEC	T52.0X1	T52.0X2	T52.0X3	T52.0X4	—	—
Lucanthone	T37.4X1	T37.4X2	T37.4X3	T37.4X4	T37.4X5	T37.4X6
Luminal	T42.3X1	T42.3X2	T42.3X3	T42.3X4	T42.3X5	T42.3X6
Lung irritant (gas) NEC	T59.91	T59.92	T59.93	T59.94	—	—
Luteinizing hormone	T38.811	T38.812	T38.813	T38.814	T38.815	T38.816
Lutocylol	T38.5X1	T38.5X2	T38.5X3	T38.5X4	T38.5X5	T38.5X6
Lutromone	T38.5X1	T38.5X2	T38.5X3	T38.5X4	T38.5X5	T38.5X6
Lututrin	T48.291	T48.292	T48.293	T48.294	T48.295	T48.296
Lye (concentrated)	T54.3X1	T54.3X2	T54.3X3	T54.3X4	—	—
Lygranum (skin test)	T50.8X1	T50.8X2	T50.8X3	T50.8X4	T50.8X5	T50.8X6
Lymecycline	T36.4X1	T36.4X2	T36.4X3	T36.4X4	T36.4X5	T36.4X6
Lymphogranuloma venereum antigen	T50.8X1	T50.8X2	T50.8X3	T50.8X4	T50.8X5	T50.8X6
Lynestrenol	T38.4X1	T38.4X2	T38.4X3	T38.4X4	T38.4X5	T38.4X6
Lyovac Sodium Edecrin	T50.1X1	T50.1X2	T50.1X3	T50.1X4	T50.1X5	T50.1X6
Lypressin	T38.891	T38.892	T38.893	T38.894	T38.895	T38.896
Lysergic acid diethylamide	T40.8X1	T40.8X2	T40.8X3	T40.8X4	—	—
Lysergide	T40.8X1	T40.8X2	T40.8X3	T40.8X4	—	—
Lysine vasopressin	T38.891	T38.892	T38.893	T38.894	T38.895	T38.896
Lysol	T54.1X1	T54.1X2	T54.1X3	T54.1X4	—	—
Lysozyme	T49.0X1	T49.0X2	T49.0X3	T49.0X4	T49.0X5	T49.0X6
Lytta (vitatta)	T49.8X1	T49.8X2	T49.8X3	T49.8X4	T49.8X5	T49.8X6
Mace	T59.3X1	T59.3X2	T59.3X3	T59.3X4	—	—
Macrogol	T50.991	T50.992	T50.993	T50.994	T50.995	T50.996
Macrolide						
anabolic drug	T38.7X1	T38.7X2	T38.7X3	T38.7X4	T38.7X5	T38.7X6
antibiotic	T36.3X1	T36.3X2	T36.3X3	T36.3X4	T36.3X5	T36.3X6
Mafenide	T49.0X1	T49.0X2	T49.0X3	T49.0X4	T49.0X5	T49.0X6
Magaldrate	T47.1X1	T47.1X2	T47.1X3	T47.1X4	T47.1X5	T47.1X6
Magic mushroom	T40.991	T40.992	T40.993	T40.994	—	—
Magnamycin	T36.8X1	T36.8X2	T36.8X3	T36.8X4	T36.8X5	T36.8X6
Magnesia magma	T47.1X1	T47.1X2	T47.1X3	T47.1X4	T47.1X5	T47.1X6
Magnesium NEC	T56.891	T56.892	T56.893	T56.894	—	—
carbonate	T47.1X1	T47.1X2	T47.1X3	T47.1X4	T47.1X5	T47.1X6
citrate	T47.4X1	T47.4X2	T47.4X3	T47.4X4	T47.4X5	T47.4X6
hydroxide	T47.1X1	T47.1X2	T47.1X3	T47.1X4	T47.1X5	T47.1X6
oxide	T47.1X1	T47.1X2	T47.1X3	T47.1X4	T47.1X5	T47.1X6
peroxide	T49.0X1	T49.0X2	T49.0X3	T49.0X4	T49.0X5	T49.0X6
salicylate	T39.091	T39.092	T39.093	T39.094	T39.095	T39.096
silicofluoride	T50.3X1	T50.3X2	T50.3X3	T50.3X4	T50.3X5	T50.3X6
sulfate	T47.4X1	T47.4X2	T47.4X3	T47.4X4	T47.4X5	T47.4X6
thiosulfate	T45.0X1	T45.0X2	T45.0X3	T45.0X4	T45.0X5	T45.0X6
trisilicate	T47.1X1	T47.1X2	T47.1X3	T47.1X4	T47.1X5	T47.1X6
Malathion (medicinal)	T49.0X1	T49.0X2	T49.0X3	T49.0X4	T49.0X5	T49.0X6
insecticide	T60.0X1	T60.0X2	T60.0X3	T60.0X4	—	—
Male fern extract	T37.4X1	T37.4X2	T37.4X3	T37.4X4	T37.4X5	T37.4X6
M-AMSA	T45.1X1	T45.1X2	T45.1X3	T45.1X4	T45.1X5	T45.1X6
Mandelic acid	T37.8X1	T37.8X2	T37.8X3	T37.8X4	T37.8X5	T37.8X6
Manganese (dioxide) (salts)	T57.2X1	T57.2X2	T57.2X3	T57.2X4	—	—
medicinal	T50.991	T50.992	T50.993	T50.994	T50.995	T50.996
Mannitol	T47.3X1	T47.3X2	T47.3X3	T47.3X4	T47.3X5	T47.3X6
hexanitrate	T46.3X1	T46.3X2	T46.3X3	T46.3X4	T46.3X5	T46.3X6
Mannomustine	T45.1X1	T45.1X2	T45.1X3	T45.1X4	T45.1X5	T45.1X6
MAO inhibitors	T43.1X1	T43.1X2	T43.1X3	T43.1X4	T43.1X5	T43.1X6
Mapharsen	T37.8X1	T37.8X2	T37.8X3	T37.8X4	T37.8X5	T37.8X6
Maphenide	T49.0X1	T49.0X2	T49.0X3	T49.0X4	T49.0X5	T49.0X6
Maprotiline	T43.021	T43.022	T43.023	T43.024	T43.025	T43.026
Marcaine	T41.3X1	T41.3X2	T41.3X3	T41.3X4	T41.3X5	T41.3X6
infiltration (subcutaneous)	T41.3X1	T41.3X2	T41.3X3	T41.3X4	T41.3X5	T41.3X6
nerve block (peripheral) (plexus)	T41.3X1	T41.3X2	T41.3X3	T41.3X4	T41.3X5	T41.3X6
Marezine	T45.0X1	T45.0X2	T45.0X3	T45.0X4	T45.0X5	T45.0X6
Marihuana	T40.7X1	T40.7X2	T40.7X3	T40.7X4	T40.7X5	T40.7X6
Marijuana	T40.7X1	T40.7X2	T40.7X3	T40.7X4	T40.7X5	T40.7X6
Marine (sting)	T63.691	T63.692	T63.693	T63.694	—	—
animals (sting)	T63.691	T63.692	T63.693	T63.694	—	—
plants (sting)	T63.711	T63.712	T63.713	T63.714	—	—
Marplan	T43.1X1	T43.1X2	T43.1X3	T43.1X4	T43.1X5	T43.1X6
Marsh gas	T59.891	T59.892	T59.893	T59.894	—	—
Marsilid	T43.1X1	T43.1X2	T43.1X3	T43.1X4	T43.1X5	T43.1X6
Matulane	T45.1X1	T45.1X2	T45.1X3	T45.1X4	T45.1X5	T45.1X6
Mazindol	T50.5X1	T50.5X2	T50.5X3	T50.5X4	T50.5X5	T50.5X6
MCPA	T60.3X1	T60.3X2	T60.3X3	T60.3X4	—	—
MDMA	T43.621	T43.622	T43.623	T43.624	T43.625	T43.626
Meadow saffron	T62.2X1	T62.2X2	T62.2X3	T62.2X4	—	—
Measles virus vaccine (attenuated)	T50.B91	T50.B92	T50.B93	T50.B94	T50.B95	T50.B96
Meat, noxious	T62.8X1	T62.8X2	T62.8X3	T62.8X4	—	—
Meballymal	T42.3X1	T42.3X2	T42.3X3	T42.3X4	T42.3X5	T42.3X6
Mebanazine	T43.1X1	T43.1X2	T43.1X3	T43.1X4	T43.1X5	T43.1X6
Mebaral	T42.3X1	T42.3X2	T42.3X3	T42.3X4	T42.3X5	T42.3X6
Mebendazole	T37.4X1	T37.4X2	T37.4X3	T37.4X4	T37.4X5	T37.4X6
Mebeverine	T44.3X1	T44.3X2	T44.3X3	T44.3X4	T44.3X5	T44.3X6
Mebhydrolin	T45.0X1	T45.0X2	T45.0X3	T45.0X4	T45.0X5	T45.0X6
Mebumal	T42.3X1	T42.3X2	T42.3X3	T42.3X4	T42.3X5	T42.3X6
Mebutamate	T43.591	T43.592	T43.593	T43.594	T43.595	T43.596
Mecamylamine	T44.2X1	T44.2X2	T44.2X3	T44.2X4	T44.2X5	T44.2X6
Mechlorethamine	T45.1X1	T45.1X2	T45.1X3	T45.1X4	T45.1X5	T45.1X6
Mecillinam	T36.0X1	T36.0X2	T36.0X3	T36.0X4	T36.0X5	T36.0X6
Meclizine (hydrochloride)	T45.0X1	T45.0X2	T45.0X3	T45.0X4	T45.0X5	T45.0X6
Meclocycline	T36.4X1	T36.4X2	T36.4X3	T36.4X4	T36.4X5	T36.4X6
Meclofenamate	T39.391	T39.392	T39.393	T39.394	T39.395	T39.396
Meclofenamic acid	T39.391	T39.392	T39.393	T39.394	T39.395	T39.396
Meclofenoxate	T43.691	T43.692	T43.693	T43.694	T43.695	T43.696
Meclozine	T45.0X1	T45.0X2	T45.0X3	T45.0X4	T45.0X5	T45.0X6
Mecobalamin	T45.8X1	T45.8X2	T45.8X3	T45.8X4	T45.8X5	T45.8X6
Mecoprop	T60.3X1	T60.3X2	T60.3X3	T60.3X4	—	—

Additional Character May Be Required — Refer to the Tabular List for Character Selection   ▽ Subterms under main terms may continue to next column or page

Table of Drugs and Chemicals

Substance	Poisoning, Accidental (unintentional)	Poisoning, Intentional Self-harm	Poisoning, Assault	Poisoning, Undetermined	Adverse Effect	Underdosing
Mecrilate	T49.3X1	T49.3X2	T49.3X3	T49.3X4	T49.3X5	T49.3X6
Mecysteine	T48.4X1	T48.4X2	T48.4X3	T48.4X4	T48.4X5	T48.4X6
Medazepam	T42.4X1	T42.4X2	T42.4X3	T42.4X4	T42.4X5	T42.4X6
Medicament NEC	T50.901	T50.902	T50.903	T50.904	T50.905	T50.906
Medinal	T42.3X1	T42.3X2	T42.3X3	T42.3X4	T42.3X5	T42.3X6
Medomin	T42.3X1	T42.3X2	T42.3X3	T42.3X4	T42.3X5	T42.3X6
Medrogestone	T38.5X1	T38.5X2	T38.5X3	T38.5X4	T38.5X5	T38.5X6
Medroxalol	T44.8X1	T44.8X2	T44.8X3	T44.8X4	T44.8X5	T44.8X6
Medroxyprogesterone acetate (depot)	T38.5X1	T38.5X2	T38.5X3	T38.5X4	T38.5X5	T38.5X6
Medrysone	T49.0X1	T49.0X2	T49.0X3	T49.0X4	T49.0X5	T49.0X6
Mefenamic acid	T39.391	T39.392	T39.393	T39.394	T39.395	T39.396
Mefenorex	T50.5X1	T50.5X2	T50.5X3	T50.5X4	T50.5X5	T50.5X6
Mefloquine	T37.2X1	T37.2X2	T37.2X3	T37.2X4	T37.2X5	T37.2X6
Mefruside	T50.2X1	T50.2X2	T50.2X3	T50.2X4	T50.2X5	T50.2X6
Megahallucinogen	T40.901	T40.902	T40.903	T40.904	T40.905	T40.906
Megestrol	T38.5X1	T38.5X2	T38.5X3	T38.5X4	T38.5X5	T38.5X6
Meglumine						
antimoniate	T37.8X1	T37.8X2	T37.8X3	T37.8X4	T37.8X5	T37.8X6
diatrizoate	T50.8X1	T50.8X2	T50.8X3	T50.8X4	T50.8X5	T50.8X6
iodipamide	T50.8X1	T50.8X2	T50.8X3	T50.8X4	T50.8X5	T50.8X6
iotroxate	T50.8X1	T50.8X2	T50.8X3	T50.8X4	T50.8X5	T50.8X6
MEK (methyl ethyl ketone)	T52.4X1	T52.4X2	T52.4X3	T52.4X4	—	—
Meladinin	T49.3X1	T49.3X2	T49.3X3	T49.3X4	T49.3X5	T49.3X6
Meladrazine	T44.3X1	T44.3X2	T44.3X3	T44.3X4	T44.3X5	T44.3X6
Melaleuca alternifolia oil	T49.0X1	T49.0X2	T49.0X3	T49.0X4	T49.0X5	T49.0X6
Melanizing agents	T49.3X1	T49.3X2	T49.3X3	T49.3X4	T49.3X5	T49.3X6
Melanocyte-stimulating hormone	T38.891	T38.892	T38.893	T38.894	T38.895	T38.896
Melarsonyl potassium	T37.3X1	T37.3X2	T37.3X3	T37.3X4	T37.3X5	T37.3X6
Melarsoprol	T37.3X1	T37.3X2	T37.3X3	T37.3X4	T37.3X5	T37.3X6
Melia azedarach	T62.2X1	T62.2X2	T62.2X3	T62.2X4		
Melitracen	T43.011	T43.012	T43.013	T43.014	T43.015	T43.016
Mellaril	T43.3X1	T43.3X2	T43.3X3	T43.3X4	T43.3X5	T43.3X6
Meloxine	T49.3X1	T49.3X2	T49.3X3	T49.3X4	T49.3X5	T49.3X6
Melperone	T43.4X1	T43.4X2	T43.4X3	T43.4X4	T43.4X5	T43.4X6
Melphalan	T45.1X1	T45.1X2	T45.1X3	T45.1X4	T45.1X5	T45.1X6
Memantine	T43.8X1	T43.8X2	T43.8X3	T43.8X4	T43.8X5	T43.8X6
Menadiol	T45.7X1	T45.7X2	T45.7X3	T45.7X4	T45.7X5	T45.7X6
sodium sulfate	T45.7X1	T45.7X2	T45.7X3	T45.7X4	T45.7X5	T45.7X6
Menadione	T45.7X1	T45.7X2	T45.7X3	T45.7X4	T45.7X5	T45.7X6
sodium bisulfite	T45.7X1	T45.7X2	T45.7X3	T45.7X4	T45.7X5	T45.7X6
Menaphthone	T45.7X1	T45.7X2	T45.7X3	T45.7X4	T45.7X5	T45.7X6
Menaquinone	T45.7X1	T45.7X2	T45.7X3	T45.7X4	T45.7X5	T45.7X6
Menatetrenone	T45.7X1	T45.7X2	T45.7X3	T45.7X4	T45.7X5	T45.7X6
Meningococcal vaccine	T50.A91	T50.A92	T50.A93	T50.A94	T50.A95	T50.A96
Menningovax (-AC) (-C)	T50.A91	T50.A92	T50.A93	T50.A94	T50.A95	T50.A96
Menotropins	T38.811	T38.812	T38.813	T38.814	T38.815	T38.816
Menthol	T48.5X1	T48.5X2	T48.5X3	T48.5X4	T48.5X5	T48.5X6
Mepacrine	T37.2X1	T37.2X2	T37.2X3	T37.2X4	T37.2X5	T37.2X6
Meparfynol	T42.6X1	T42.6X2	T42.6X3	T42.6X4	T42.6X5	T42.6X6
Mepartricin	T36.7X1	T36.7X2	T36.7X3	T36.7X4	T36.7X5	T36.7X6
Mepazine	T43.3X1	T43.3X2	T43.3X3	T43.3X4	T43.3X5	T43.3X6
Mepenzolate	T44.3X1	T44.3X2	T44.3X3	T44.3X4	T44.3X5	T44.3X6
bromide	T44.3X1	T44.3X2	T44.3X3	T44.3X4	T44.3X5	T44.3X6
Meperidine	T40.4X1	T40.4X2	T40.4X3	T40.4X4	T40.4X5	T40.4X6
Mephebarbital	T42.3X1	T42.3X2	T42.3X3	T42.3X4	T42.3X5	T42.3X6
Mephenamin (e)	T42.8X1	T42.8X2	T42.8X3	T42.8X4	T42.8X5	T42.8X6
Mephenesin	T42.8X1	T42.8X2	T42.8X3	T42.8X4	T42.8X5	T42.8X6
Mephenhydramine	T45.0X1	T45.0X2	T45.0X3	T45.0X4	T45.0X5	T45.0X6
Mephenoxalone	T42.8X1	T42.8X2	T42.8X3	T42.8X4	T42.8X5	T42.8X6
Mephentermine	T44.991	T44.992	T44.993	T44.994	T44.995	T44.996
Mephenytoin	T42.0X1	T42.0X2	T42.0X3	T42.0X4	T42.0X5	T42.0X6
with phenobarbital	T42.3X1	T42.3X2	T42.3X3	T42.3X4	T42.3X5	T42.3X6
Mephobarbital	T42.3X1	T42.3X2	T42.3X3	T42.3X4	T42.3X5	T42.3X6
Mephosfolan	T60.0X1	T60.0X2	T60.0X3	T60.0X4	—	—
Mepindolol	T44.7X1	T44.7X2	T44.7X3	T44.7X4	T44.7X5	T44.7X6
Mepiperphenidol	T44.3X1	T44.3X2	T44.3X3	T44.3X4	T44.3X5	T44.3X6
Mepitiostane	T38.7X1	T38.7X2	T38.7X3	T38.7X4	T38.7X5	T38.7X6
Mepivacaine	T41.3X1	T41.3X2	T41.3X3	T41.3X4	T41.3X5	T41.3X6
epidural	T41.3X1	T41.3X2	T41.3X3	T41.3X4	T41.3X5	T41.3X6
Meprednisone	T38.0X1	T38.0X2	T38.0X3	T38.0X4	T38.0X5	T38.0X6
Meprobam	T43.591	T43.592	T43.593	T43.594	T43.595	T43.596
Meprobamate	T43.591	T43.592	T43.593	T43.594	T43.595	T43.596
Meproscillarin	T46.0X1	T46.0X2	T46.0X3	T46.0X4	T46.0X5	T46.0X6
Meprylcaine	T41.3X1	T41.3X2	T41.3X3	T41.3X4	T41.3X5	T41.3X6
Meptazinol	T39.8X1	T39.8X2	T39.8X3	T39.8X4	T39.8X5	T39.8X6
Mepyramine	T45.0X1	T45.0X2	T45.0X3	T45.0X4	T45.0X5	T45.0X6
Mequitazine	T43.3X1	T43.3X2	T43.3X3	T43.3X4	T43.3X5	T43.3X6
Meralluride	T50.2X1	T50.2X2	T50.2X3	T50.2X4	T50.2X5	T50.2X6
Merbaphen	T50.2X1	T50.2X2	T50.2X3	T50.2X4	T50.2X5	T50.2X6
Merbromin	T49.0X1	T49.0X2	T49.0X3	T49.0X4	T49.0X5	T49.0X6
Mercaptobenzothiazole salts	T49.0X1	T49.0X2	T49.0X3	T49.0X4	T49.0X5	T49.0X6
Mercaptomerin	T50.2X1	T50.2X2	T50.2X3	T50.2X4	T50.2X5	T50.2X6
Mercaptopurine	T45.1X1	T45.1X2	T45.1X3	T45.1X4	T45.1X5	T45.1X6
Mercumatilin	T50.2X1	T50.2X2	T50.2X3	T50.2X4	T50.2X5	T50.2X6
Mercuramide	T50.2X1	T50.2X2	T50.2X3	T50.2X4	T50.2X5	T50.2X6
Mercurochrome	T49.0X1	T49.0X2	T49.0X3	T49.0X4	T49.0X5	T49.0X6
Mercurophylline	T50.2X1	T50.2X2	T50.2X3	T50.2X4	T50.2X5	T50.2X6
Mercury, mercurial, mercuric, mercurous (compounds) (cyanide) (fumes) (nonmedicinal) (vapor) NEC	T56.1X1	T56.1X2	T56.1X3	T56.1X4	—	—
ammoniated	T49.0X1	T49.0X2	T49.0X3	T49.0X4	T49.0X5	T49.0X6
anti-infective						
local	T49.0X1	T49.0X2	T49.0X3	T49.0X4	T49.0X5	T49.0X6
systemic	T37.8X1	T37.8X2	T37.8X3	T37.8X4	T37.8X5	T37.8X6
topical	T49.0X1	T49.0X2	T49.0X3	T49.0X4	T49.0X5	T49.0X6
chloride (ammoniated)	T49.0X1	T49.0X2	T49.0X3	T49.0X4	T49.0X5	T49.0X6
fungicide	T56.1X1	T56.1X2	T56.1X3	T56.1X4	—	—
diuretic NEC	T50.2X1	T50.2X2	T50.2X3	T50.2X4	T50.2X5	T50.2X6
fungicide	T56.1X1	T56.1X2	T56.1X3	T56.1X4	—	—
organic (fungicide)	T56.1X1	T56.1X2	T56.1X3	T56.1X4	—	—
oxide, yellow	T49.0X1	T49.0X2	T49.0X3	T49.0X4	T49.0X5	T49.0X6
Mersalyl	T50.2X1	T50.2X2	T50.2X3	T50.2X4	T50.2X5	T50.2X6
Merthiolate	T49.0X1	T49.0X2	T49.0X3	T49.0X4	T49.0X5	T49.0X6
ophthalmic preparation	T49.5X1	T49.5X2	T49.5X3	T49.5X4	T49.5X5	T49.5X6
Meruvax	T50.B91	T50.B92	T50.B93	T50.B94	T50.B95	T50.B96
Mesalazine	T47.8X1	T47.8X2	T47.8X3	T47.8X4	T47.8X5	T47.8X6
Mescal buttons	T40.991	T40.992	T40.993	T40.994	—	—
Mescaline	T40.991	T40.992	T40.993	T40.994	—	—
Mesna	T48.4X1	T48.4X2	T48.4X3	T48.4X4	T48.4X5	T48.4X6
Mesoglycan	T46.6X1	T46.6X2	T46.6X3	T46.6X4	T46.6X5	T46.6X6
Mesoridazine	T43.3X1	T43.3X2	T43.3X3	T43.3X4	T43.3X5	T43.3X6
Mestanolone	T38.7X1	T38.7X2	T38.7X3	T38.7X4	T38.7X5	T38.7X6
Mesterolone	T38.7X1	T38.7X2	T38.7X3	T38.7X4	T38.7X5	T38.7X6
Mestranol	T38.5X1	T38.5X2	T38.5X3	T38.5X4	T38.5X5	T38.5X6
Mesulergine	T42.8X1	T42.8X2	T42.8X3	T42.8X4	T42.8X5	T42.8X6
Mesulfen	T49.0X1	T49.0X2	T49.0X3	T49.0X4	T49.0X5	T49.0X6
Mesuximide	T42.2X1	T42.2X2	T42.2X3	T42.2X4	T42.2X5	T42.2X6
Metabutethamine	T41.3X1	T41.3X2	T41.3X3	T41.3X4	T41.3X5	T41.3X6
Metactesylacetate	T49.0X1	T49.0X2	T49.0X3	T49.0X4	T49.0X5	T49.0X6
Metacycline	T36.4X1	T36.4X2	T36.4X3	T36.4X4	T36.4X5	T36.4X6
Metaldehyde (snail killer) NEC	T60.8X1	T60.8X2	T60.8X3	T60.8X4	—	—
Metals (heavy) (nonmedicinal)	T56.91	T56.92	T56.93	T56.94	—	—
dust, fumes, or vapor NEC	T56.91	T56.92	T56.93	T56.94	—	—
light NEC	T56.91	T56.92	T56.93	T56.94	—	—
dust, fumes, or vapor NEC	T56.91	T56.92	T56.93	T56.94	—	—
specified NEC	T56.891	T56.892	T56.893	T56.894	—	—
thallium	T56.811	T56.812	T56.813	T56.814	—	—
Metamfetamine	T43.621	T43.622	T43.623	T43.624	T43.625	T43.626
Metamizole sodium	T39.2X1	T39.2X2	T39.2X3	T39.2X4	T39.2X5	T39.2X6
Metampicillin	T36.0X1	T36.0X2	T36.0X3	T36.0X4	T36.0X5	T36.0X6
Metamucil	T47.4X1	T47.4X2	T47.4X3	T47.4X4	T47.4X5	T47.4X6
Metandienone	T38.7X1	T38.7X2	T38.7X3	T38.7X4	T38.7X5	T38.7X6
Metandrostenolone	T38.7X1	T38.7X2	T38.7X3	T38.7X4	T38.7X5	T38.7X6
Metaphen	T49.0X1	T49.0X2	T49.0X3	T49.0X4	T49.0X5	T49.0X6
Metaphos	T60.0X1	T60.0X2	T60.0X3	T60.0X4	—	—
Metapramine	T43.011	T43.012	T43.013	T43.014	T43.015	T43.016
Metaproterenol	T48.291	T48.292	T48.293	T48.294	T48.295	T48.296
Metaraminol	T44.4X1	T44.4X2	T44.4X3	T44.4X4	T44.4X5	T44.4X6
Metaxalone	T42.8X1	T42.8X2	T42.8X3	T42.8X4	T42.8X5	T42.8X6
Metenolone	T38.7X1	T38.7X2	T38.7X3	T38.7X4	T38.7X5	T38.7X6
Metergoline	T42.8X1	T42.8X2	T42.8X3	T42.8X4	T42.8X5	T42.8X6
Metescufylline	T46.991	T46.992	T46.993	T46.994	T46.995	T46.996
Metetoin	T42.0X1	T42.0X2	T42.0X3	T42.0X4	T42.0X5	T42.0X6
Metformin	T38.3X1	T38.3X2	T38.3X3	T38.3X4	T38.3X5	T38.3X6
Methacholine	T44.1X1	T44.1X2	T44.1X3	T44.1X4	T44.1X5	T44.1X6
Methacycline	T36.4X1	T36.4X2	T36.4X3	T36.4X4	T36.4X5	T36.4X6
Methadone	T40.3X1	T40.3X2	T40.3X3	T40.3X4	T40.3X5	T40.3X6
Methallenestril	T38.5X1	T38.5X2	T38.5X3	T38.5X4	T38.5X5	T38.5X6
Methallenoestril	T38.5X1	T38.5X2	T38.5X3	T38.5X4	T38.5X5	T38.5X6
Methamphetamine	T43.621	T43.622	T43.623	T43.624	T43.625	T43.626
Methampyrone	T39.2X1	T39.2X2	T39.2X3	T39.2X4	T39.2X5	T39.2X6
Methandienone	T38.7X1	T38.7X2	T38.7X3	T38.7X4	T38.7X5	T38.7X6
Methandriol	T38.7X1	T38.7X2	T38.7X3	T38.7X4	T38.7X5	T38.7X6
Methandrostenolone	T38.7X1	T38.7X2	T38.7X3	T38.7X4	T38.7X5	T38.7X6
Methane	T59.891	T59.892	T59.893	T59.894	—	—
Methanethiol	T59.891	T59.892	T59.893	T59.894	—	—
Methaniazide	T37.1X1	T37.1X2	T37.1X3	T37.1X4	T37.1X5	T37.1X6
Methanol (vapor)	T51.1X1	T51.1X2	T51.1X3	T51.1X4		

Substance	Poisoning, Accidental (unintentional)	Poisoning, Intentional Self-harm	Poisoning, Assault	Poisoning, Undetermined	Adverse Effect	Underdosing
Methantheline	T44.3X1	T44.3X2	T44.3X3	T44.3X4	T44.3X5	T44.3X6
Methanthelinium bromide	T44.3X1	T44.3X2	T44.3X3	T44.3X4	T44.3X5	T44.3X6
Methaphenilene	T45.0X1	T45.0X2	T45.0X3	T45.0X4	T45.0X5	T45.0X6
Methapyrilene	T45.0X1	T45.0X2	T45.0X3	T45.0X4	T45.0X5	T45.0X6
Methaqualone (compound)	T42.6X1	T42.6X2	T42.6X3	T42.6X4	T42.6X5	T42.6X6
Metharbital	T42.3X1	T42.3X2	T42.3X3	T42.3X4	T42.3X5	T42.3X6
Methazolamide	T50.2X1	T50.2X2	T50.2X3	T50.2X4	T50.2X5	T50.2X6
Methdilazine	T43.3X1	T43.3X2	T43.3X3	T43.3X4	T43.3X5	T43.3X6
Methedrine	T43.621	T43.622	T43.623	T43.624	T43.625	T43.626
Methenamine (mandelate)	T37.8X1	T37.8X2	T37.8X3	T37.8X4	T37.8X5	T37.8X6
Methenolone	T38.7X1	T38.7X2	T38.7X3	T38.7X4	T38.7X5	T38.7X6
Methergine	T48.0X1	T48.0X2	T48.0X3	T48.0X4	T48.0X5	T48.0X6
Methetoin	T42.0X1	T42.0X2	T42.0X3	T42.0X4	T42.0X5	T42.0X6
Methiacil	T38.2X1	T38.2X2	T38.2X3	T38.2X4	T38.2X5	T38.2X6
Methicillin	T36.0X1	T36.0X2	T36.0X3	T36.0X4	T36.0X5	T36.0X6
Methimazole	T38.2X1	T38.2X2	T38.2X3	T38.2X4	T38.2X5	T38.2X6
Methiodal sodium	T50.8X1	T50.8X2	T50.8X3	T50.8X4	T50.8X5	T50.8X6
Methionine	T50.991	T50.992	T50.993	T50.994	T50.995	T50.996
Methisazone	T37.5X1	T37.5X2	T37.5X3	T37.5X4	T37.5X5	T37.5X6
Methisoprinol	T37.5X1	T37.5X2	T37.5X3	T37.5X4	T37.5X5	T37.5X6
Methitural	T42.3X1	T42.3X2	T42.3X3	T42.3X4	T42.3X5	T42.3X6
Methixene	T44.3X1	T44.3X2	T44.3X3	T44.3X4	T44.3X5	T44.3X6
Methobarbital, methobarbitone	T42.3X1	T42.3X2	T42.3X3	T42.3X4	T42.3X5	T42.3X6
Methocarbamol	T42.8X1	T42.8X2	T42.8X3	T42.8X4	T42.8X5	T42.8X6
skeletal muscle relaxant	T48.1X1	T48.1X2	T48.1X3	T48.1X4	T48.1X5	T48.1X6
Methohexital	T41.1X1	T41.1X2	T41.1X3	T41.1X4	T41.1X5	T41.1X6
Methohexitone	T41.1X1	T41.1X2	T41.1X3	T41.1X4	T41.1X5	T41.1X6
Methoin	T42.0X1	T42.0X2	T42.0X3	T42.0X4	T42.0X5	T42.0X6
Methopholine	T39.8X1	T39.8X2	T39.8X3	T39.8X4	T39.8X5	T39.8X6
Methopromazine	T43.3X1	T43.3X2	T43.3X3	T43.3X4	T43.3X5	T43.3X6
Methorate	T48.3X1	T48.3X2	T48.3X3	T48.3X4	T48.3X5	T48.3X6
Methoserpidine	T46.5X1	T46.5X2	T46.5X3	T46.5X4	T46.5X5	T46.5X6
Methotrexate	T45.1X1	T45.1X2	T45.1X3	T45.1X4	T45.1X5	T45.1X6
Methotrimeprazine	T43.3X1	T43.3X2	T43.3X3	T43.3X4	T43.3X5	T43.3X6
Methoxa-Dome	T49.3X1	T49.3X2	T49.3X3	T49.3X4	T49.3X5	T49.3X6
Methoxamine	T44.4X1	T44.4X2	T44.4X3	T44.4X4	T44.4X5	T44.4X6
Methoxsalen	T50.991	T50.992	T50.993	T50.994	T50.995	T50.996
Methoxyaniline	T65.3X1	T65.3X2	T65.3X3	T65.3X4	—	—
Methoxybenzyl penicillin	T36.0X1	T36.0X2	T36.0X3	T36.0X4	T36.0X5	T36.0X6
Methoxychlor	T53.7X1	T53.7X2	T53.7X3	T53.7X4	—	—
Methoxy-DDT	T53.7X1	T53.7X2	T53.7X3	T53.7X4	—	—
Methoxyflurane	T41.0X1	T41.0X2	T41.0X3	T41.0X4	T41.0X5	T41.0X6
Methoxyphenamine	T48.6X1	T48.6X2	T48.6X3	T48.6X4	T48.6X5	T48.6X6
Methoxypromazine	T43.3X1	T43.3X2	T43.3X3	T43.3X4	T43.3X5	T43.3X6
Methscopolamine bromide	T44.3X1	T44.3X2	T44.3X3	T44.3X4	T44.3X5	T44.3X6
Methsuximide	T42.2X1	T42.2X2	T42.2X3	T42.2X4	T42.2X5	T42.2X6
Methyclothiazide	T50.2X1	T50.2X2	T50.2X3	T50.2X4	T50.2X5	T50.2X6
Methyl						
acetate	T52.4X1	T52.4X2	T52.4X3	T52.4X4	—	—
acetone	T52.4X1	T52.4X2	T52.4X3	T52.4X4	—	—
acrylate	T65.891	T65.892	T65.893	T65.894	—	—
alcohol	T51.1X1	T51.1X2	T51.1X3	T51.1X4	—	—
aminophenol	T65.3X1	T65.3X2	T65.3X3	T65.3X4	—	—
amphetamine	T43.621	T43.622	T43.623	T43.624	T43.625	T43.626
androstanolone	T38.7X1	T38.7X2	T38.7X3	T38.7X4	T38.7X5	T38.7X6
atropine	T44.3X1	T44.3X2	T44.3X3	T44.3X4	T44.3X5	T44.3X6
benzene	T52.2X1	T52.2X2	T52.2X3	T52.2X4	—	—
benzoate	T52.8X1	T52.8X2	T52.8X3	T52.8X4	—	—
benzol	T52.2X1	T52.2X2	T52.2X3	T52.2X4	—	—
bromide (gas)	T59.891	T59.892	T59.893	T59.894	—	—
fumigant	T60.8X1	T60.8X2	T60.8X3	T60.8X4	—	—
butanol	T51.3X1	T51.3X2	T51.3X3	T51.3X4	—	—
carbinol	T51.1X1	T51.1X2	T51.1X3	T51.1X4	—	—
carbonate	T52.8X1	T52.8X2	T52.8X3	T52.8X4	—	—
CCNU	T45.1X1	T45.1X2	T45.1X3	T45.1X4	T45.1X5	T45.1X6
cellosolve	T52.91	T52.92	T52.93	T52.94	—	—
cellulose	T47.4X1	T47.4X2	T47.4X3	T47.4X4	T47.4X5	T47.4X6
chloride (gas)	T59.891	T59.892	T59.893	T59.894	—	—
chloroformate	T59.3X1	T59.3X2	T59.3X3	T59.3X4	—	—
cyclohexane	T52.8X1	T52.8X2	T52.8X3	T52.8X4	—	—
cyclohexanol	T51.8X1	T51.8X2	T51.8X3	T51.8X4	—	—
cyclohexanone	T52.8X1	T52.8X2	T52.8X3	T52.8X4	—	—
cyclohexyl acetate	T52.8X1	T52.8X2	T52.8X3	T52.8X4	—	—
demeton	T60.0X1	T60.0X2	T60.0X3	T60.0X4	—	—
dihydromorphinone	T40.2X1	T40.2X2	T40.2X3	T40.2X4	T40.2X5	T40.2X6
ergometrine	T48.0X1	T48.0X2	T48.0X3	T48.0X4	T48.0X5	T48.0X6
ergonovine	T48.0X1	T48.0X2	T48.0X3	T48.0X4	T48.0X5	T48.0X6
ethyl ketone	T52.4X1	T52.4X2	T52.4X3	T52.4X4	—	—
glucamine antimonate	T37.8X1	T37.8X2	T37.8X3	T37.8X4	T37.8X5	T37.8X6
hydrazine	T65.891	T65.892	T65.893	T65.894	—	—
iodide	T65.891	T65.892	T65.893	T65.894	—	—
isobutyl ketone	T52.4X1	T52.4X2	T52.4X3	T52.4X4	—	—

Substance	Poisoning, Accidental (unintentional)	Poisoning, Intentional Self-harm	Poisoning, Assault	Poisoning, Undetermined	Adverse Effect	Underdosing
Methyl — continued						
isothiocyanate	T60.3X1	T60.3X2	T60.3X3	T60.3X4	—	—
mercaptan	T59.891	T59.892	T59.893	T59.894	—	—
morphine NEC	T40.2X1	T40.2X2	T40.2X3	T40.2X4	T40.2X5	T40.2X6
nicotinate	T49.4X1	T49.4X2	T49.4X3	T49.4X4	T49.4X5	T49.4X6
paraben	T49.0X1	T49.0X2	T49.0X3	T49.0X4	T49.0X5	T49.0X6
parafynol	T42.6X1	T42.6X2	T42.6X3	T42.6X4	T42.6X5	T42.6X6
parathion	T60.0X1	T60.0X2	T60.0X3	T60.0X4	—	—
peridol	T43.4X1	T43.4X2	T43.4X3	T43.4X4	T43.4X5	T43.4X6
phenidate	T43.631	T43.632	T43.633	T43.634	T43.635	T43.636
prednisolone	T38.0X1	T38.0X2	T38.0X3	T38.0X4	T38.0X5	T38.0X6
ENT agent	T49.6X1	T49.6X2	T49.6X3	T49.6X4	T49.6X5	T49.6X6
ophthalmic preparation	T49.5X1	T49.5X2	T49.5X3	T49.5X4	T49.5X5	T49.5X6
topical NEC	T49.0X1	T49.0X2	T49.0X3	T49.0X4	T49.0X5	T49.0X6
propylcarbinol	T51.3X1	T51.3X2	T51.3X3	T51.3X4	—	—
rosaniline NEC	T49.0X1	T49.0X2	T49.0X3	T49.0X4	T49.0X5	T49.0X6
salicylate	T49.2X1	T49.2X2	T49.2X3	T49.2X4	T49.2X5	T49.2X6
sulfate (fumes)	T59.891	T59.892	T59.893	T59.894	—	—
liquid	T52.8X1	T52.8X2	T52.8X3	T52.8X4	—	—
sulfonal	T42.6X1	T42.6X2	T42.6X3	T42.6X4	T42.6X5	T42.6X6
testosterone	T38.7X1	T38.7X2	T38.7X3	T38.7X4	T38.7X5	T38.7X6
thiouracil	T38.2X1	T38.2X2	T38.2X3	T38.2X4	T38.2X5	T38.2X6
Methylamphetamine	T43.621	T43.622	T43.623	T43.624	T43.625	T43.626
Methylated spirit	T51.1X1	T51.1X2	T51.1X3	T51.1X4	—	—
Methylatropine nitrate	T44.3X1	T44.3X2	T44.3X3	T44.3X4	T44.3X5	T44.3X6
Methylbenactyzium bromide	T44.3X1	T44.3X2	T44.3X3	T44.3X4	T44.3X5	T44.3X6
Methylbenzethonium chloride	T49.0X1	T49.0X2	T49.0X3	T49.0X4	T49.0X5	T49.0X6
Methylcellulose	T47.4X1	T47.4X2	T47.4X3	T47.4X4	T47.4X5	T47.4X6
laxative	T47.4X1	T47.4X2	T47.4X3	T47.4X4	T47.4X5	T47.4X6
Methylchlorophenoxyacetic acid	T60.3X1	T60.3X2	T60.3X3	T60.3X4	—	—
Methyldopa	T46.5X1	T46.5X2	T46.5X3	T46.5X4	T46.5X5	T46.5X6
Methyldopate	T46.5X1	T46.5X2	T46.5X3	T46.5X4	T46.5X5	T46.5X6
Methylene						
blue	T50.6X1	T50.6X2	T50.6X3	T50.6X4	T50.6X5	T50.6X6
chloride or dichloride (solvent) NEC	T53.4X1	T53.4X2	T53.4X3	T53.4X4	—	—
Methylenedioxyamphetamine	T43.621	T43.622	T43.623	T43.624	T43.625	T43.626
Methylenedioxymethamphetamine	T43.621	T43.622	T43.623	T43.624	T43.625	T43.626
Methylergometrine	T48.0X1	T48.0X2	T48.0X3	T48.0X4	T48.0X5	T48.0X6
Methylergonovine	T48.0X1	T48.0X2	T48.0X3	T48.0X4	T48.0X5	T48.0X6
Methylestrenolone	T38.5X1	T38.5X2	T38.5X3	T38.5X4	T38.5X5	T38.5X6
Methylethyl cellulose	T50.991	T50.992	T50.993	T50.994	T50.995	T50.996
Methylhexabital	T42.3X1	T42.3X2	T42.3X3	T42.3X4	T42.3X5	T42.3X6
Methylmorphine	T40.2X1	T40.2X2	T40.2X3	T40.2X4	T40.2X5	T40.2X6
Methylparaben (ophthalmic)	T49.5X1	T49.5X2	T49.5X3	T49.5X4	T49.5X5	T49.5X6
Methylparafynol	T42.6X1	T42.6X2	T42.6X3	T42.6X4	T42.6X5	T42.6X6
Methylpentynol, methylpenthynol	T42.6X1	T42.6X2	T42.6X3	T42.6X4	T42.6X5	T42.6X6
Methylphenidate	T43.631	T43.632	T43.633	T43.634	T43.635	T43.636
Methylphenobarbital	T42.3X1	T42.3X2	T42.3X3	T42.3X4	T42.3X5	T42.3X6
Methylpolysiloxane	T47.1X1	T47.1X2	T47.1X3	T47.1X4	T47.1X5	T47.1X6
Methylprednisolone — see Methyl, prednisolone						
Methylrosaniline	T49.0X1	T49.0X2	T49.0X3	T49.0X4	T49.0X5	T49.0X6
Methylrosanilinium chloride	T49.0X1	T49.0X2	T49.0X3	T49.0X4	T49.0X5	T49.0X6
Methyltestosterone	T38.7X1	T38.7X2	T38.7X3	T38.7X4	T38.7X5	T38.7X6
Methylthionine chloride	T50.6X1	T50.6X2	T50.6X3	T50.6X4	T50.6X5	T50.6X6
Methylthioninium chloride	T50.6X1	T50.6X2	T50.6X3	T50.6X4	T50.6X5	T50.6X6
Methylthiouracil	T38.2X1	T38.2X2	T38.2X3	T38.2X4	T38.2X5	T38.2X6
Methyprylon	T42.6X1	T42.6X2	T42.6X3	T42.6X4	T42.6X5	T42.6X6
Methysergide	T46.5X1	T46.5X2	T46.5X3	T46.5X4	T46.5X5	T46.5X6
Metiamide	T47.1X1	T47.1X2	T47.1X3	T47.1X4	T47.1X5	T47.1X6
Meticillin	T36.0X1	T36.0X2	T36.0X3	T36.0X4	T36.0X5	T36.0X6
Meticrane	T50.2X1	T50.2X2	T50.2X3	T50.2X4	T50.2X5	T50.2X6
Metildigoxin	T46.0X1	T46.0X2	T46.0X3	T46.0X4	T46.0X5	T46.0X6
Metipranolol	T49.5X1	T49.5X2	T49.5X3	T49.5X4	T49.5X5	T49.5X6
Metirosine	T46.5X1	T46.5X2	T46.5X3	T46.5X4	T46.5X5	T46.5X6
Metisazone	T37.5X1	T37.5X2	T37.5X3	T37.5X4	T37.5X5	T37.5X6
Metixene	T44.3X1	T44.3X2	T44.3X3	T44.3X4	T44.3X5	T44.3X6
Metizoline	T48.5X1	T48.5X2	T48.5X3	T48.5X4	T48.5X5	T48.5X6
Metoclopramide	T45.0X1	T45.0X2	T45.0X3	T45.0X4	T45.0X5	T45.0X6
Metofenazate	T43.3X1	T43.3X2	T43.3X3	T43.3X4	T43.3X5	T43.3X6
Metofoline	T39.8X1	T39.8X2	T39.8X3	T39.8X4	T39.8X5	T39.8X6
Metolazone	T50.2X1	T50.2X2	T50.2X3	T50.2X4	T50.2X5	T50.2X6
Metopon	T40.2X1	T40.2X2	T40.2X3	T40.2X4	T40.2X5	T40.2X6
Metoprine	T45.1X1	T45.1X2	T45.1X3	T45.1X4	T45.1X5	T45.1X6
Metoprolol	T44.7X1	T44.7X2	T44.7X3	T44.7X4	T44.7X5	T44.7X6
Metrifonate	T60.0X1	T60.0X2	T60.0X3	T60.0X4	—	—

Additional Character May Be Required — Refer to the Tabular List for Character Selection

▽ Subterms under main terms may continue to next column or page

Substance	Poisoning, Accidental (unintentional)	Poisoning, Intentional Self-harm	Poisoning, Assault	Poisoning, Undetermined	Adverse Effect	Under-dosing
Metrizamide	T50.8X1	T50.8X2	T50.8X3	T50.8X4	T50.8X5	T50.8X6
Metrizoic acid	T50.8X1	T50.8X2	T50.8X3	T50.8X4	T50.8X5	T50.8X6
Metronidazole	T37.8X1	T37.8X2	T37.8X3	T37.8X4	T37.8X5	T37.8X6
Metycaine	T41.3X1	T41.3X2	T41.3X3	T41.3X4	T41.3X5	T41.3X6
infiltration (subcutaneous)	T41.3X1	T41.3X2	T41.3X3	T41.3X4	T41.3X5	T41.3X6
nerve block (peripheral) (plexus)	T41.3X1	T41.3X2	T41.3X3	T41.3X4	T41.3X5	T41.3X6
topical (surface)	T41.3X1	T41.3X2	T41.3X3	T41.3X4	T41.3X5	T41.3X6
Metyrapone	T50.8X1	T50.8X2	T50.8X3	T50.8X4	T50.8X5	T50.8X6
Mevinphos	T60.0X1	T60.0X2	T60.0X3	T60.0X4	—	—
Mexazolam	T42.4X1	T42.4X2	T42.4X3	T42.4X4	T42.4X5	T42.4X6
Mexenone	T49.3X1	T49.3X2	T49.3X3	T49.3X4	T49.3X5	T49.3X6
Mexiletine	T46.2X1	T46.2X2	T46.2X3	T46.2X4	T46.2X5	T46.2X6
Mezereon	T62.2X1	T62.2X2	T62.2X3	T62.2X4	—	—
berries	T62.1X1	T62.1X2	T62.1X3	T62.1X4	—	—
Mezlocillin	T36.0X1	T36.0X2	T36.0X3	T36.0X4	T36.0X5	T36.0X6
Mianserin	T43.021	T43.022	T43.023	T43.024	T43.025	T43.026
Micatin	T49.0X1	T49.0X2	T49.0X3	T49.0X4	T49.0X5	T49.0X6
Miconazole	T49.0X1	T49.0X2	T49.0X3	T49.0X4	T49.0X5	T49.0X6
Micronomicin	T36.5X1	T36.5X2	T36.5X3	T36.5X4	T36.5X5	T36.5X6
Midazolam	T42.4X1	T42.4X2	T42.4X3	T42.4X4	T42.4X5	T42.4X6
Midecamycin	T36.3X1	T36.3X2	T36.3X3	T36.3X4	T36.3X5	T36.3X6
Mifepristone	T38.6X1	T38.6X2	T38.6X3	T38.6X4	T38.6X5	T38.6X6
Milk of magnesia	T47.1X1	T47.1X2	T47.1X3	T47.1X4	T47.1X5	T47.1X6
Millipede (tropical) (venomous)	T63.411	T63.412	T63.413	T63.414	—	—
Miltown	T43.591	T43.592	T43.593	T43.594	T43.595	T43.596
Milverine	T44.3X1	T44.3X2	T44.3X3	T44.3X4	T44.3X5	T44.3X6
Minaprine	T43.291	T43.292	T43.293	T43.294	T43.295	T43.296
Minaxolone	T41.291	T41.292	T41.293	T41.294	T41.295	T41.296
Mineral						
acids	T54.2X1	T54.2X2	T54.2X3	T54.2X4	—	—
oil (laxative)(medicinal)	T47.4X1	T47.4X2	T47.4X3	T47.4X4	T47.4X5	T47.4X6
emulsion	T47.2X1	T47.2X2	T47.2X3	T47.2X4	T47.2X5	T47.2X6
nonmedicinal	T52.0X1	T52.0X2	T52.0X3	T52.0X4	—	—
topical	T49.3X1	T49.3X2	T49.3X3	T49.3X4	T49.3X5	T49.3X6
salt NEC	T50.3X1	T50.3X2	T50.3X3	T50.3X4	T50.3X5	T50.3X6
spirits	T52.0X1	T52.0X2	T52.0X3	T52.0X4	—	—
Mineralocorticosteroid	T50.0X1	T50.0X2	T50.0X3	T50.0X4	T50.0X5	T50.0X6
Minocycline	T36.4X1	T36.4X2	T36.4X3	T36.4X4	T36.4X5	T36.4X6
Minoxidil	T46.7X1	T46.7X2	T46.7X3	T46.7X4	T46.7X5	T46.7X6
Miokamycin	T36.3X1	T36.3X2	T36.3X3	T36.3X4	T36.3X5	T36.3X6
Miotic drug	T49.5X1	T49.5X2	T49.5X3	T49.5X4	T49.5X5	T49.5X6
Mipafox	T60.0X1	T60.0X2	T60.0X3	T60.0X4	—	—
Mirex	T60.1X1	T60.1X2	T60.1X3	T60.1X4	—	—
Mirtazapine	T43.021	T43.022	T43.023	T43.024	T43.025	T43.026
Misonidazole	T37.3X1	T37.3X2	T37.3X3	T37.3X4	T37.3X5	T37.3X6
Misoprostol	T47.1X1	T47.1X2	T47.1X3	T47.1X4	T47.1X5	T47.1X6
Mithramycin	T45.1X1	T45.1X2	T45.1X3	T45.1X4	T45.1X5	T45.1X6
Mitobronitol	T45.1X1	T45.1X2	T45.1X3	T45.1X4	T45.1X5	T45.1X6
Mitoguazone	T45.1X1	T45.1X2	T45.1X3	T45.1X4	T45.1X5	T45.1X6
Mitolactol	T45.1X1	T45.1X2	T45.1X3	T45.1X4	T45.1X5	T45.1X6
Mitomycin	T45.1X1	T45.1X2	T45.1X3	T45.1X4	T45.1X5	T45.1X6
Mitopodozide	T45.1X1	T45.1X2	T45.1X3	T45.1X4	T45.1X5	T45.1X6
Mitotane	T45.1X1	T45.1X2	T45.1X3	T45.1X4	T45.1X5	T45.1X6
Mitoxantrone	T45.1X1	T45.1X2	T45.1X3	T45.1X4	T45.1X5	T45.1X6
Mivacurium chloride	T48.1X1	T48.1X2	T48.1X3	T48.1X4	T48.1X5	T48.1X6
Miyari bacteria	T47.6X1	T47.6X2	T47.6X3	T47.6X4	T47.6X5	T47.6X6
Moclobemide	T43.1X1	T43.1X2	T43.1X3	T43.1X4	T43.1X5	T43.1X6
Moderil	T46.5X1	T46.5X2	T46.5X3	T46.5X4	T46.5X5	T46.5X6
Mofebutazone	T39.2X1	T39.2X2	T39.2X3	T39.2X4	T39.2X5	T39.2X6
Mogadon — see Nitrazepam						
Molindone	T43.591	T43.592	T43.593	T43.594	T43.595	T43.596
Molsidomine	T46.3X1	T46.3X2	T46.3X3	T46.3X4	T46.3X5	T46.3X6
Mometasone	T49.0X1	T49.0X2	T49.0X3	T49.0X4	T49.0X5	T49.0X6
Monistat	T49.0X1	T49.0X2	T49.0X3	T49.0X4	T49.0X5	T49.0X6
Monkshood	T62.2X1	T62.2X2	T62.2X3	T62.2X4	—	—
Monoamine oxidase inhibitor NEC	T43.1X1	T43.1X2	T43.1X3	T43.1X4	T43.1X5	T43.1X6
hydrazine	T43.1X1	T43.1X2	T43.1X3	T43.1X4	T43.1X5	T43.1X6
Monobenzone	T49.4X1	T49.4X2	T49.4X3	T49.4X4	T49.4X5	T49.4X6
Monochloroacetic acid	T60.3X1	T60.3X2	T60.3X3	T60.3X4	—	—
Monochlorobenzene	T53.7X1	T53.7X2	T53.7X3	T53.7X4	—	—
Monoethanolamine	T46.8X1	T46.8X2	T46.8X3	T46.8X4	T46.8X5	T46.8X6
oleate	T46.8X1	T46.8X2	T46.8X3	T46.8X4	T46.8X5	T46.8X6
Monooctanoin	T50.991	T50.992	T50.993	T50.994	T50.995	T50.996
Monophenylbutazone	T39.2X1	T39.2X2	T39.2X3	T39.2X4	T39.2X5	T39.2X6
Monosodium glutamate	T65.891	T65.892	T65.893	T65.894	—	—
Monosulfiram	T49.0X1	T49.0X2	T49.0X3	T49.0X4	T49.0X5	T49.0X6
Monoxide, carbon — see Carbon, monoxide						
Monoxidine hydrochloride	T46.1X1	T46.1X2	T46.1X3	T46.1X4	T46.1X5	T46.1X6
Monuron	T60.3X1	T60.3X2	T60.3X3	T60.3X4	—	—
Moperone	T43.4X1	T43.4X2	T43.4X3	T43.4X4	T43.4X5	T43.4X6
Mopidamol	T45.1X1	T45.1X2	T45.1X3	T45.1X4	T45.1X5	T45.1X6
MOPP (mechloreth-amine + vincristine + prednisone + procarba-zine)	T45.1X1	T45.1X2	T45.1X3	T45.1X4	T45.1X5	T45.1X6
Morfin	T40.2X1	T40.2X2	T40.2X3	T40.2X4	T40.2X5	T40.2X6
Morinamide	T37.1X1	T37.1X2	T37.1X3	T37.1X4	T37.1X5	T37.1X6
Morning glory seeds	T40.991	T40.992	T40.993	T40.994	—	—
Moroxydine	T37.5X1	T37.5X2	T37.5X3	T37.5X4	T37.5X5	T37.5X6
Morphazinamide	T37.1X1	T37.1X2	T37.1X3	T37.1X4	T37.1X5	T37.1X6
Morphine	T40.2X1	T40.2X2	T40.2X3	T40.2X4	T40.2X5	T40.2X6
antagonist	T50.7X1	T50.7X2	T50.7X3	T50.7X4	T50.7X5	T50.7X6
Morpholinylethylmorphine	T40.2X1	T40.2X2	T40.2X3	T40.2X4	—	—
Morsuximide	T42.2X1	T42.2X2	T42.2X3	T42.2X4	T42.2X5	T42.2X6
Mosapramine	T43.591	T43.592	T43.593	T43.594	T43.595	T43.596
Moth balls — see also Pesticides	T60.2X1	T60.2X2	T60.2X3	T60.2X4	—	—
naphthalene	T60.2X1	T60.2X2	T60.2X3	T60.2X4	—	—
paradichlorobenzene	T60.1X1	T60.1X2	T60.1X3	T60.1X4	—	—
Motor exhaust gas	T58.01	T58.02	T58.03	T58.04	—	—
Mouthwash (antiseptic) (zinc chloride)	T49.6X1	T49.6X2	T49.6X3	T49.6X4	T49.6X5	T49.6X6
Moxastine	T45.0X1	T45.0X2	T45.0X3	T45.0X4	T45.0X5	T45.0X6
Moxaverine	T44.3X1	T44.3X2	T44.3X3	T44.3X4	T44.3X5	T44.3X6
Moxisylyte	T46.7X1	T46.7X2	T46.7X3	T46.7X4	T46.7X5	T46.7X6
Mucilage, plant	T47.4X1	T47.4X2	T47.4X3	T47.4X4	T47.4X5	T47.4X6
Mucolytic drug	T48.4X1	T48.4X2	T48.4X3	T48.4X4	T48.4X5	T48.4X6
Mucomyst	T48.4X1	T48.4X2	T48.4X3	T48.4X4	T48.4X5	T48.4X6
Mucous membrane agents (external)	T49.91	T49.92	T49.93	T49.94	T49.95	T49.96
specified NEC	T49.8X1	T49.8X2	T49.8X3	T49.8X4	T49.8X5	T49.8X6
Mumps						
immune globulin (human)	T50.Z11	T50.Z12	T50.Z13	T50.Z14	T50.Z15	T50.Z16
skin test antigen	T50.8X1	T50.8X2	T50.8X3	T50.8X4	T50.8X5	T50.8X6
vaccine	T50.B91	T50.B92	T50.B93	T50.B94	T50.B95	T50.B96
Mumpsvax	T50.B91	T50.B92	T50.B93	T50.B94	T50.B95	T50.B96
Mupirocin	T49.0X1	T49.0X2	T49.0X3	T49.0X4	T49.0X5	T49.0X6
Muriatic acid — see Hydrochloric acid						
Muromonab-CD3	T45.1X1	T45.1X2	T45.1X3	T45.1X4	T45.1X5	T45.1X6
Muscle-action drug NEC	T48.201	T48.202	T48.203	T48.204	T48.205	T48.206
Muscle affecting agents NEC	T48.201	T48.202	T48.203	T48.204	T48.205	T48.206
oxytocic	T48.0X1	T48.0X2	T48.0X3	T48.0X4	T48.0X5	T48.0X6
relaxants	T48.201	T48.202	T48.203	T48.204	T48.205	T48.206
central nervous system	T42.8X1	T42.8X2	T42.8X3	T42.8X4	T42.8X5	T42.8X6
skeletal	T48.1X1	T48.1X2	T48.1X3	T48.1X4	T48.1X5	T48.1X6
smooth	T44.3X1	T44.3X2	T44.3X3	T44.3X4	T44.3X5	T44.3X6
Muscle relaxant — see Relaxant, muscle						
Muscle-tone depressant, central NEC	T42.8X1	T42.8X2	T42.8X3	T42.8X4	T42.8X5	T42.8X6
specified NEC	T42.8X1	T42.8X2	T42.8X3	T42.8X4	T42.8X5	T42.8X6
Mushroom, noxious	T62.0X1	T62.0X2	T62.0X3	T62.0X4	—	—
Mussel, noxious	T61.781	T61.782	T61.783	T61.784	—	—
Mustard (emetic)	T47.7X1	T47.7X2	T47.7X3	T47.7X4	T47.7X5	T47.7X6
black	T47.7X1	T47.7X2	T47.7X3	T47.7X4	T47.7X5	T47.7X6
gas, not in war	T59.91	T59.92	T59.93	T59.94	—	—
nitrogen	T45.1X1	T45.1X2	T45.1X3	T45.1X4	T45.1X5	T45.1X6
Mustine	T45.1X1	T45.1X2	T45.1X3	T45.1X4	T45.1X5	T45.1X6
M-vac	T45.1X1	T45.1X2	T45.1X3	T45.1X4	T45.1X5	T45.1X6
Mycifradin	T36.5X1	T36.5X2	T36.5X3	T36.5X4	T36.5X5	T36.5X6
topical	T49.0X1	T49.0X2	T49.0X3	T49.0X4	T49.0X5	T49.0X6
Mycitracin	T36.8X1	T36.8X2	T36.8X3	T36.8X4	T36.8X5	T36.8X6
ophthalmic preparation	T49.5X1	T49.5X2	T49.5X3	T49.5X4	T49.5X5	T49.5X6
Mycostatin	T36.7X1	T36.7X2	T36.7X3	T36.7X4	T36.7X5	T36.7X6
topical	T49.0X1	T49.0X2	T49.0X3	T49.0X4	T49.0X5	T49.0X6
Mycotoxins	T64.81	T64.82	T64.83	T64.84	—	—
aflatoxin	T64.01	T64.02	T64.03	T64.04	—	—
specified NEC	T64.81	T64.82	T64.83	T64.84	—	—
Mydriacyl	T44.3X1	T44.3X2	T44.3X3	T44.3X4	T44.3X5	T44.3X6
Mydriatic drug	T49.5X1	T49.5X2	T49.5X3	T49.5X4	T49.5X5	T49.5X6
Myelobromal	T45.1X1	T45.1X2	T45.1X3	T45.1X4	T45.1X5	T45.1X6
Myleran	T45.1X1	T45.1X2	T45.1X3	T45.1X4	T45.1X5	T45.1X6
Myochrysin (e)	T39.2X1	T39.2X2	T39.2X3	T39.2X4	T39.2X5	T39.2X6
Myoneural blocking agents	T48.1X1	T48.1X2	T48.1X3	T48.1X4	T48.1X5	T48.1X6
Myralact	T49.0X1	T49.0X2	T49.0X3	T49.0X4	T49.0X5	T49.0X6
Myristica fragrans	T62.2X1	T62.2X2	T62.2X3	T62.2X4	—	—
Myristicin	T65.891	T65.892	T65.893	T65.894	—	—
Mysoline	T42.3X1	T42.3X2	T42.3X3	T42.3X4	T42.3X5	T42.3X6
Nabilone	T40.7X1	T40.7X2	T40.7X3	T40.7X4	T40.7X5	T40.7X6
Nabumetone	T39.391	T39.392	T39.393	T39.394	T39.395	T39.396
Nadolol	T44.7X1	T44.7X2	T44.7X3	T44.7X4	T44.7X5	T44.7X6

Table of Drugs and Chemicals

Nafcillin — Nitronaphthalene

Substance	Poisoning, Accidental (unintentional)	Poisoning, Intentional Self-harm	Poisoning, Assault	Poisoning, Undetermined	Adverse Effect	Under-dosing
Nafcillin	T36.0X1	T36.0X2	T36.0X3	T36.0X4	T36.0X5	T36.0X6
Nafoxidine	T38.6X1	T38.6X2	T38.6X3	T38.6X4	T38.6X5	T38.6X6
Naftazone	T46.991	T46.992	T46.993	T46.994	T46.995	T46.996
Naftidrofuryl (oxalate)	T46.7X1	T46.7X2	T46.7X3	T46.7X4	T46.7X5	T46.7X6
Naftifine	T49.0X1	T49.0X2	T49.0X3	T49.0X4	T49.0X5	T49.0X6
Nail polish remover	T52.91	T52.92	T52.93	T52.94		
Nalbuphine	T40.4X1	T40.4X2	T40.4X3	T40.4X4	T40.4X5	T40.4X6
Naled	T60.0X1	T60.0X2	T60.0X3	T60.0X4		
Nalidixic acid	T37.8X1	T37.8X2	T37.8X3	T37.8X4	T37.8X5	T37.8X6
Nalorphine	T50.7X1	T50.7X2	T50.7X3	T50.7X4	T50.7X5	T50.7X6
Naloxone	T50.7X1	T50.7X2	T50.7X3	T50.7X4	T50.7X5	T50.7X6
Naltrexone	T50.7X1	T50.7X2	T50.7X3	T50.7X4	T50.7X5	T50.7X6
Namenda	T43.8X1	T43.8X2	T43.8X3	T43.8X4	T43.8X5	T43.8X6
Nandrolone	T38.7X1	T38.7X2	T38.7X3	T38.7X4	T38.7X5	T38.7X6
Naphazoline	T48.5X1	T48.5X2	T48.5X3	T48.5X4	T48.5X5	T48.5X6
Naphtha (painters') (petroleum)	T52.0X1	T52.0X2	T52.0X3	T52.0X4	—	—
solvent	T52.0X1	T52.0X2	T52.0X3	T52.0X4	—	—
vapor	T52.0X1	T52.0X2	T52.0X3	T52.0X4	—	—
Naphthalene	T60.2X1	T60.2X2	T60.2X3	T60.2X4	—	—
(non-chlorinated)						
chlorinated	T60.1X1	T60.1X2	T60.1X3	T60.1X4	—	—
vapor	T60.1X1	T60.1X2	T60.1X3	T60.1X4	—	—
insecticide or moth repellent	T60.2X1	T60.2X2	T60.2X3	T60.2X4	—	—
chlorinated	T60.1X1	T60.1X2	T60.1X3	T60.1X4	—	—
vapor	T60.2X1	T60.2X2	T60.2X3	T60.2X4	—	—
chlorinated	T60.1X1	T60.1X2	T60.1X3	T60.1X4	—	—
Naphthol	T65.891	T65.892	T65.893	T65.894	—	—
Naphthylamine	T65.891	T65.892	T65.893	T65.894	—	—
Naphthylthiourea (ANTU)	T60.4X1	T60.4X2	T60.4X3	T60.4X4	—	—
Naprosyn — see Naproxen						
Naproxen	T39.311	T39.312	T39.313	T39.314	T39.315	T39.316
Narcotic (drug)	T40.601	T40.602	T40.603	T40.604	T40.605	T40.606
analgesic NEC	T40.601	T40.602	T40.603	T40.604	T40.605	T40.606
antagonist	T50.7X1	T50.7X2	T50.7X3	T50.7X4	T50.7X5	T50.7X6
specified NEC	T40.691	T40.692	T40.693	T40.694	T40.695	T40.696
synthetic	T40.4X1	T40.4X2	T40.4X3	T40.4X4	T40.4X5	T40.4X6
Narcotine	T48.3X1	T48.3X2	T48.3X3	T48.3X4	T48.3X5	T48.3X6
Nardil	T43.1X1	T43.1X2	T43.1X3	T43.1X4	T43.1X5	T43.1X6
Nasal drug NEC	T49.6X1	T49.6X2	T49.6X3	T49.6X4	T49.6X5	T49.6X6
Natamycin	T49.0X1	T49.0X2	T49.0X3	T49.0X4	T49.0X5	T49.0X6
Natrium cyanide — see Cyanide(s)						
Natural						
blood (product)	T45.8X1	T45.8X2	T45.8X3	T45.8X4	T45.8X5	T45.8X6
gas (piped)	T59.891	T59.892	T59.893	T59.894	—	—
incomplete combustion	T58.11	T58.12	T58.13	T58.14	—	—
Nealbarbital	T42.3X1	T42.3X2	T42.3X3	T42.3X4	T42.3X5	T42.3X6
Nectadon	T48.3X1	T48.3X2	T48.3X3	T48.3X4	T48.3X5	T48.3X6
Nedocromil	T48.6X1	T48.6X2	T48.6X3	T48.6X4	T48.6X5	T48.6X6
Nefopam	T39.8X1	T39.8X2	T39.8X3	T39.8X4	T39.8X5	T39.8X6
Nematocyst (sting)	T63.691	T63.692	T63.693	T63.694	—	—
Nembutal	T42.3X1	T42.3X2	T42.3X3	T42.3X4	T42.3X5	T42.3X6
Nemonapride	T43.591	T43.592	T43.593	T43.594	T43.595	T43.596
Neoarsphenamine	T37.8X1	T37.8X2	T37.8X3	T37.8X4	T37.8X5	T37.8X6
Neocinchophen	T50.4X1	T50.4X2	T50.4X3	T50.4X4	T50.4X5	T50.4X6
Neomycin (derivatives)	T36.5X1	T36.5X2	T36.5X3	T36.5X4	T36.5X5	T36.5X6
with						
bacitracin	T49.0X1	T49.0X2	T49.0X3	T49.0X4	T49.0X5	T49.0X6
neostigmine	T44.0X1	T44.0X2	T44.0X3	T44.0X4	T44.0X5	T44.0X6
ENT agent	T49.6X1	T49.6X2	T49.6X3	T49.6X4	T49.6X5	T49.6X6
ophthalmic preparation	T49.5X1	T49.5X2	T49.5X3	T49.5X4	T49.5X5	T49.5X6
topical NEC	T49.0X1	T49.0X2	T49.0X3	T49.0X4	T49.0X5	T49.0X6
Neonal	T42.3X1	T42.3X2	T42.3X3	T42.3X4	T42.3X5	T42.3X6
Neoprontosil	T37.0X1	T37.0X2	T37.0X3	T37.0X4	T37.0X5	T37.0X6
Neosalvarsan	T37.8X1	T37.8X2	T37.8X3	T37.8X4	T37.8X5	T37.8X6
Neosilversalvarsan	T37.8X1	T37.8X2	T37.8X3	T37.8X4	T37.8X5	T37.8X6
Neosporin	T36.8X1	T36.8X2	T36.8X3	T36.8X4	T36.8X5	T36.8X6
ENT agent	T49.6X1	T49.6X2	T49.6X3	T49.6X4	T49.6X5	T49.6X6
opthalmic preparation	T49.5X1	T49.5X2	T49.5X3	T49.5X4	T49.5X5	T49.5X6
topical NEC	T49.0X1	T49.0X2	T49.0X3	T49.0X4	T49.0X5	T49.0X6
Neostigmine bromide	T44.0X1	T44.0X2	T44.0X3	T44.0X4	T44.0X5	T44.0X6
Neraval	T42.3X1	T42.3X2	T42.3X3	T42.3X4	T42.3X5	T42.3X6
Neravan	T42.3X1	T42.3X2	T42.3X3	T42.3X4	T42.3X5	T42.3X6
Nerium oleander	T62.2X1	T62.2X2	T62.2X3	T62.2X4	—	—
Nerve gas, not in war	T59.91	T59.92	T59.93	T59.94	—	—
Nesacaine	T41.3X1	T41.3X2	T41.3X3	T41.3X4	T41.3X5	T41.3X6
infiltration (subcutaneous)	T41.3X1	T41.3X2	T41.3X3	T41.3X4	T41.3X5	T41.3X6
nerve block (peripheral) (plexus)	T41.3X1	T41.3X2	T41.3X3	T41.3X4	T41.3X5	T41.3X6
Netilmicin	T36.5X1	T36.5X2	T36.5X3	T36.5X4	T36.5X5	T36.5X6
Neurobarb	T42.3X1	T42.3X2	T42.3X3	T42.3X4	T42.3X5	T42.3X6
Neuroleptic drug NEC	T43.501	T43.502	T43.503	T43.504	T43.505	T43.506
Neuromuscular blocking drug	T48.1X1	T48.1X2	T48.1X3	T48.1X4	T48.1X5	T48.1X6
Neutral insulin injection	T38.3X1	T38.3X2	T38.3X3	T38.3X4	T38.3X5	T38.3X6
Neutral spirits	T51.0X1	T51.0X2	T51.0X3	T51.0X4		
beverage	T51.0X1	T51.0X2	T51.0X3	T51.0X4		
Niacin	T46.7X1	T46.7X2	T46.7X3	T46.7X4	T46.7X5	T46.7X6
Niacinamide	T45.2X1	T45.2X2	T45.2X3	T45.2X4	T45.2X5	T45.2X6
Nialamide	T43.1X1	T43.1X2	T43.1X3	T43.1X4	T43.1X5	T43.1X6
Niaprazine	T42.6X1	T42.6X2	T42.6X3	T42.6X4	T42.6X5	T42.6X6
Nicametate	T46.7X1	T46.7X2	T46.7X3	T46.7X4	T46.7X5	T46.7X6
Nicardipine	T46.1X1	T46.1X2	T46.1X3	T46.1X4	T46.1X5	T46.1X6
Nicergoline	T46.7X1	T46.7X2	T46.7X3	T46.7X4	T46.7X5	T46.7X6
Nickel (carbonyl) (tetra-carbonyl) (fumes) (vapor)	T56.891	T56.892	T56.893	T56.894	—	—
Nickelocene	T56.891	T56.892	T56.893	T56.894	—	—
Niclosamide	T37.4X1	T37.4X2	T37.4X3	T37.4X4	T37.4X5	T37.4X6
Nicofuranose	T46.7X1	T46.7X2	T46.7X3	T46.7X4	T46.7X5	T46.7X6
Nicomorphine	T40.2X1	T40.2X2	T40.2X3	T40.2X4		
Nicorandil	T46.3X1	T46.3X2	T46.3X3	T46.3X4	T46.3X5	T46.3X6
Nicotiana (plant)	T62.2X1	T62.2X2	T62.2X3	T62.2X4		
Nicotinamide	T45.2X1	T45.2X2	T45.2X3	T45.2X4	T45.2X5	T45.2X6
Nicotine (insecticide) (spray) (sulfate) NEC	T60.2X1	T60.2X2	T60.2X3	T60.2X4		
from tobacco	T65.291	T65.292	T65.293	T65.294		
cigarettes	T65.221	T65.222	T65.223	T65.224		
not insecticide	T65.291	T65.292	T65.293	T65.294		
Nicotinic acid	T46.7X1	T46.7X2	T46.7X3	T46.7X4	T46.7X5	T46.7X6
Nicotinyl alcohol	T46.7X1	T46.7X2	T46.7X3	T46.7X4	T46.7X5	T46.7X6
Nicoumalone	T45.511	T45.512	T45.513	T45.514	T45.515	T45.516
Nifedipine	T46.1X1	T46.1X2	T46.1X3	T46.1X4	T46.1X5	T46.1X6
Nifenazone	T39.2X1	T39.2X2	T39.2X3	T39.2X4	T39.2X5	T39.2X6
Nifuraldezone	T37.91	T37.92	T37.93	T37.94	T37.95	T37.96
Nifuratel	T37.8X1	T37.8X2	T37.8X3	T37.8X4	T37.8X5	T37.8X6
Nifurtimox	T37.3X1	T37.3X2	T37.3X3	T37.3X4	T37.3X5	T37.3X6
Nifurtoinol	T37.8X1	T37.8X2	T37.8X3	T37.8X4	T37.8X5	T37.8X6
Nightshade, deadly (solanum) — see also Belladonna	T62.2X1	T62.2X2	T62.2X3	T62.2X4	—	—
berry	T62.1X1	T62.1X2	T62.1X3	T62.1X4	—	—
Nikethamide	T50.7X1	T50.7X2	T50.7X3	T50.7X4	T50.7X5	T50.7X6
Nilstat	T36.7X1	T36.7X2	T36.7X3	T36.7X4	T36.7X5	T36.7X6
topical	T49.0X1	T49.0X2	T49.0X3	T49.0X4	T49.0X5	T49.0X6
Nilutamide	T38.6X1	T38.6X2	T38.6X3	T38.6X4	T38.6X5	T38.6X6
Nimesulide	T39.391	T39.392	T39.393	T39.394	T39.395	T39.396
Nimetazepam	T42.4X1	T42.4X2	T42.4X3	T42.4X4	T42.4X5	T42.4X6
Nimodipine	T46.1X1	T46.1X2	T46.1X3	T46.1X4	T46.1X5	T46.1X6
Nimorazole	T37.3X1	T37.3X2	T37.3X3	T37.3X4	T37.3X5	T37.3X6
Nimustine	T45.1X1	T45.1X2	T45.1X3	T45.1X4	T45.1X5	T45.1X6
Niridazole	T37.4X1	T37.4X2	T37.4X3	T37.4X4	T37.4X5	T37.4X6
Nisentil	T40.2X1	T40.2X2	T40.2X3	T40.2X4	T40.2X5	T40.2X6
Nisoldipine	T46.1X1	T46.1X2	T46.1X3	T46.1X4	T46.1X5	T46.1X6
Nitramine	T65.3X1	T65.3X2	T65.3X3	T65.3X4	—	—
Nitrate, organic	T46.3X1	T46.3X2	T46.3X3	T46.3X4	T46.3X5	T46.3X6
Nitrazepam	T42.4X1	T42.4X2	T42.4X3	T42.4X4	T42.4X5	T42.4X6
Nitrefazole	T50.6X1	T50.6X2	T50.6X3	T50.6X4	T50.6X5	T50.6X6
Nitrendipine	T46.1X1	T46.1X2	T46.1X3	T46.1X4	T46.1X5	T46.1X6
Nitric						
acid (liquid)	T54.2X1	T54.2X2	T54.2X3	T54.2X4	—	—
vapor	T59.891	T59.892	T59.893	T59.894	—	—
oxide (gas)	T59.0X1	T59.0X2	T59.0X3	T59.0X4	—	—
Nitrimidazine	T37.3X1	T37.3X2	T37.3X3	T37.3X4	T37.3X5	T37.3X6
Nitrite, amyl (medicinal) (vapor)	T46.3X1	T46.3X2	T46.3X3	T46.3X4	T46.3X5	T46.3X6
Nitroaniline	T65.3X1	T65.3X2	T65.3X3	T65.3X4	—	—
vapor	T59.891	T59.892	T59.893	T59.894	—	—
Nitrobenzene, nitrobenzol	T65.3X1	T65.3X2	T65.3X3	T65.3X4	—	—
vapor	T65.3X1	T65.3X2	T65.3X3	T65.3X4	—	—
Nitrocellulose	T65.891	T65.892	T65.893	T65.894	—	—
lacquer	T65.891	T65.892	T65.893	T65.894	—	—
Nitrodiphenyl	T65.3X1	T65.3X2	T65.3X3	T65.3X4	—	—
Nitrofural	T49.0X1	T49.0X2	T49.0X3	T49.0X4	T49.0X5	T49.0X6
Nitrofurantoin	T37.8X1	T37.8X2	T37.8X3	T37.8X4	T37.8X5	T37.8X6
Nitrofurazone	T49.0X1	T49.0X2	T49.0X3	T49.0X4	T49.0X5	T49.0X6
Nitrogen	T59.0X1	T59.0X2	T59.0X3	T59.0X4	—	—
mustard	T45.1X1	T45.1X2	T45.1X3	T45.1X4	T45.1X5	T45.1X6
Nitroglycerin, nitroglycerol (medicinal)	T46.3X1	T46.3X2	T46.3X3	T46.3X4	T46.3X5	T46.3X6
nonmedicinal	T65.5X1	T65.5X2	T65.5X3	T65.5X4	—	—
fumes	T65.5X1	T65.5X2	T65.5X3	T65.5X4	—	—
Nitroglycol	T52.3X1	T52.3X2	T52.3X3	T52.3X4	—	—
Nitrohydrochloric acid	T54.2X1	T54.2X2	T54.2X3	T54.2X4	—	—
Nitromersol	T49.0X1	T49.0X2	T49.0X3	T49.0X4	T49.0X5	T49.0X6
Nitronaphthalene	T65.891	T65.892	T65.893	T65.894		

Additional Character May Be Required — Refer to the Tabular List for Character Selection ▽ Subterms under main terms may continue to next column or page

Substance	Poisoning, Accidental (unintentional)	Poisoning, Intentional Self-harm	Poisoning, Assault	Poisoning, Undetermined	Adverse Effect	Under-dosing
Nitrophenol	T54.0X1	T54.0X2	T54.0X3	T54.0X4	—	—
Nitropropane	T52.8X1	T52.8X2	T52.8X3	T52.8X4	—	—
Nitroprusside	T46.5X1	T46.5X2	T46.5X3	T46.5X4	T46.5X5	T46.5X6
Nitrosodimethylamine	T65.3X1	T65.3X2	T65.3X3	T65.3X4	—	—
Nitrothiazol	T37.4X1	T37.4X2	T37.4X3	T37.4X4	T37.4X5	T37.4X6
Nitrotoluene, nitrotoluol	T65.3X1	T65.3X2	T65.3X3	T65.3X4	—	—
vapor	T65.3X1	T65.3X2	T65.3X3	T65.3X4	—	—
Nitrous						
acid (liquid)	T54.2X1	T54.2X2	T54.2X3	T54.2X4	—	—
fumes	T59.891	T59.892	T59.893	T59.894	—	—
ether spirit	T46.3X1	T46.3X2	T46.3X3	T46.3X4	T46.3X5	T46.3X6
oxide	T41.0X1	T41.0X2	T41.0X3	T41.0X4	T41.0X5	T41.0X6
Nitroxoline	T37.8X1	T37.8X2	T37.8X3	T37.8X4	T37.8X5	T37.8X6
Nitrozone	T49.0X1	T49.0X2	T49.0X3	T49.0X4	T49.0X5	T49.0X6
Nizatidine	T47.0X1	T47.0X2	T47.0X3	T47.0X4	T47.0X5	T47.0X6
Nizofenone	T43.8X1	T43.8X2	T43.8X3	T43.8X4	T43.8X5	T43.8X6
Noctec	T42.6X1	T42.6X2	T42.6X3	T42.6X4	T42.6X5	T42.6X6
Noludar	T42.6X1	T42.6X2	T42.6X3	T42.6X4	T42.6X5	T42.6X6
Nomegestrol	T38.5X1	T38.5X2	T38.5X3	T38.5X4	T38.5X5	T38.5X6
Nomifensine	T43.291	T43.292	T43.293	T43.294	T43.295	T43.296
Nonoxinol	T49.8X1	T49.8X2	T49.8X3	T49.8X4	T49.8X5	T49.8X6
Nonylphenoxy	T49.8X1	T49.8X2	T49.8X3	T49.8X4	T49.8X5	T49.8X6
(polyethoxyethanol)						
Noptil	T42.3X1	T42.3X2	T42.3X3	T42.3X4	T42.3X5	T42.3X6
Noradrenaline	T44.4X1	T44.4X2	T44.4X3	T44.4X4	T44.4X5	T44.4X6
Noramidopyrine	T39.2X1	T39.2X2	T39.2X3	T39.2X4	T39.2X5	T39.2X6
methanesulfonate sodium	T39.2X1	T39.2X2	T39.2X3	T39.2X4	T39.2X5	T39.2X6
Norbormide	T60.4X1	T60.4X2	T60.4X3	T60.4X4	—	—
Nordazepam	T42.4X1	T42.4X2	T42.4X3	T42.4X4	T42.4X5	T42.4X6
Norepinephrine	T44.4X1	T44.4X2	T44.4X3	T44.4X4	T44.4X5	T44.4X6
Norethandrolone	T38.7X1	T38.7X2	T38.7X3	T38.7X4	T38.7X5	T38.7X6
Norethindrone	T38.4X1	T38.4X2	T38.4X3	T38.4X4	T38.4X5	T38.4X6
Norethisterone (acetate)	T38.4X1	T38.4X2	T38.4X3	T38.4X4	T38.4X5	T38.4X6
(enantate)						
with ethinylestradiol	T38.5X1	T38.5X2	T38.5X3	T38.5X4	T38.5X5	T38.5X6
Noretynodrel	T38.5X1	T38.5X2	T38.5X3	T38.5X4	T38.5X5	T38.5X6
Norfenefrine	T44.4X1	T44.4X2	T44.4X3	T44.4X4	T44.4X5	T44.4X6
Norfloxacin	T36.8X1	T36.8X2	T36.8X3	T36.8X4	T36.8X5	T36.8X6
Norgestrel	T38.4X1	T38.4X2	T38.4X3	T38.4X4	T38.4X5	T38.4X6
Norgestrienone	T38.4X1	T38.4X2	T38.4X3	T38.4X4	T38.4X5	T38.4X6
Norlestrin	T38.4X1	T38.4X2	T38.4X3	T38.4X4	T38.4X5	T38.4X6
Norlutin	T38.4X1	T38.4X2	T38.4X3	T38.4X4	T38.4X5	T38.4X6
Normal serum albumin (human),	T45.8X1	T45.8X2	T45.8X3	T45.8X4	T45.8X5	T45.8X6
salt-poor						
Normethandrone	T38.5X1	T38.5X2	T38.5X3	T38.5X4	T38.5X5	T38.5X6
Normison — *see*						
Benzodiazepines						
Normorphine	T40.2X1	T40.2X2	T40.2X3	T40.2X4	—	—
Norpseudoephedrine	T50.5X1	T50.5X2	T50.5X3	T50.5X4	T50.5X5	T50.5X6
Nortestosterone	T38.7X1	T38.7X2	T38.7X3	T38.7X4	T38.7X5	T38.7X6
(furanpropionate)						
Nortriptyline	T43.011	T43.012	T43.013	T43.014	T43.015	T43.016
Noscapine	T48.3X1	T48.3X2	T48.3X3	T48.3X4	T48.3X5	T48.3X6
Nose preparations	T49.6X1	T49.6X2	T49.6X3	T49.6X4	T49.6X5	T49.6X6
Novobiocin	T36.5X1	T36.5X2	T36.5X3	T36.5X4	T36.5X5	T36.5X6
Novocain (infiltration)	T41.3X1	T41.3X2	T41.3X3	T41.3X4	T41.3X5	T41.3X6
(topical)						
nerve block (peripheral)	T41.3X1	T41.3X2	T41.3X3	T41.3X4	T41.3X5	T41.3X6
(plexus)						
spinal	T41.3X1	T41.3X2	T41.3X3	T41.3X4	T41.3X5	T41.3X6
Noxious foodstuff	T62.91	T62.92	T62.93	T62.94		
specified NEC	T62.8X1	T62.8X2	T62.8X3	T62.8X4	—	—
Noxiptiline	T43.011	T43.012	T43.013	T43.014	T43.015	T43.016
Noxytiolin	T49.0X1	T49.0X2	T49.0X3	T49.0X4	T49.0X5	T49.0X6
NPH Iletin (insulin)	T38.3X1	T38.3X2	T38.3X3	T38.3X4	T38.3X5	T38.3X6
Numorphan	T40.2X1	T40.2X2	T40.2X3	T40.2X4	T40.2X5	T40.2X6
Nunol	T42.3X1	T42.3X2	T42.3X3	T42.3X4	T42.3X5	T42.3X6
Nupercaine (spinal	T41.3X1	T41.3X2	T41.3X3	T41.3X4	T41.3X5	T41.3X6
anesthetic)						
topical (surface)	T41.3X1	T41.3X2	T41.3X3	T41.3X4	T41.3X5	T41.3X6
Nutmeg oil (liniment)	T49.3X1	T49.3X2	T49.3X3	T49.3X4	T49.3X5	T49.3X6
Nutritional supplement	T50.901	T50.902	T50.903	T50.904	T50.905	T50.906
Nux vomica	T65.1X1	T65.1X2	T65.1X3	T65.1X4	—	—
Nydrazid	T37.1X1	T37.1X2	T37.1X3	T37.1X4	T37.1X5	T37.1X6
Nylidrin	T46.7X1	T46.7X2	T46.7X3	T46.7X4	T46.7X5	T46.7X6
Nystatin	T36.7X1	T36.7X2	T36.7X3	T36.7X4	T36.7X5	T36.7X6
topical	T49.0X1	T49.0X2	T49.0X3	T49.0X4	T49.0X5	T49.0X6
Nytol	T45.0X1	T45.0X2	T45.0X3	T45.0X4	T45.0X5	T45.0X6
Obidoxime chloride	T50.6X1	T50.6X2	T50.6X3	T50.6X4	T50.6X5	T50.6X6
Octafonium (chloride)	T49.3X1	T49.3X2	T49.3X3	T49.3X4	T49.3X5	T49.3X6
Octamethyl	T60.0X1	T60.0X2	T60.0X3	T60.0X4	—	—
pyrophosphoramide						
Octanoin	T50.991	T50.992	T50.993	T50.994	T50.995	T50.996
Octatropine	T44.3X1	T44.3X2	T44.3X3	T44.3X4	T44.3X5	T44.3X6
methylbromide						
Octotiamine	T45.2X1	T45.2X2	T45.2X3	T45.2X4	T45.2X5	T45.2X6
Octoxinol (9)	T49.8X1	T49.8X2	T49.8X3	T49.8X4	T49.8X5	T49.8X6
Octreotide	T38.991	T38.992	T38.993	T38.994	T38.995	T38.996
Octyl nitrite	T46.3X1	T46.3X2	T46.3X3	T46.3X4	T46.3X5	T46.3X6
Oestradiol	T38.5X1	T38.5X2	T38.5X3	T38.5X4	T38.5X5	T38.5X6
Oestriol	T38.5X1	T38.5X2	T38.5X3	T38.5X4	T38.5X5	T38.5X6
Oestrogen	T38.5X1	T38.5X2	T38.5X3	T38.5X4	T38.5X5	T38.5X6
Oestrone	T38.5X1	T38.5X2	T38.5X3	T38.5X4	T38.5X5	T38.5X6
Ofloxacin	T36.8X1	T36.8X2	T36.8X3	T36.8X4	T36.8X5	T36.8X6
Oil (of)	T65.891	T65.892	T65.893	T65.894	—	—
bitter almond	T62.8X1	T62.8X2	T62.8X3	T62.8X4	—	—
cloves	T49.7X1	T49.7X2	T49.7X3	T49.7X4	T49.7X5	T49.7X6
colors	T65.6X1	T65.6X2	T65.6X3	T65.6X4	—	—
fumes	T59.891	T59.892	T59.893	T59.894	—	—
lubricating	T52.0X1	T52.0X2	T52.0X3	T52.0X4	—	—
Niobe	T52.8X1	T52.8X2	T52.8X3	T52.8X4	—	—
vitriol (liquid)	T54.2X1	T54.2X2	T54.2X3	T54.2X4	—	—
fumes	T54.2X1	T54.2X2	T54.2X3	T54.2X4	—	—
wintergreen (bitter) NEC	T49.3X1	T49.3X2	T49.3X3	T49.3X4	T49.3X5	T49.3X6
Oily preparation (for skin)	T49.3X1	T49.3X2	T49.3X3	T49.3X4	T49.3X5	T49.3X6
Ointment NEC	T49.3X1	T49.3X2	T49.3X3	T49.3X4	T49.3X5	T49.3X6
Olanzapine	T43.591	T43.592	T43.593	T43.594	T43.595	T43.596
Oleander	T62.2X1	T62.2X2	T62.2X3	T62.2X4	—	—
Oleandomycin	T36.3X1	T36.3X2	T36.3X3	T36.3X4	T36.3X5	T36.3X6
Oleandrin	T46.0X1	T46.0X2	T46.0X3	T46.0X4	T46.0X5	T46.0X6
Oleic acid	T46.6X1	T46.6X2	T46.6X3	T46.6X4	T46.6X5	T46.6X6
Oleovitamin A	T45.2X1	T45.2X2	T45.2X3	T45.2X4	T45.2X5	T45.2X6
Oleum ricini	T47.2X1	T47.2X2	T47.2X3	T47.2X4	T47.2X5	T47.2X6
Olive oil (medicinal) **NEC**	T47.4X1	T47.4X2	T47.4X3	T47.4X4	T47.4X5	T47.4X6
Olivomycin	T45.1X1	T45.1X2	T45.1X3	T45.1X4	T45.1X5	T45.1X6
Olsalazine	T47.8X1	T47.8X2	T47.8X3	T47.8X4	T47.8X5	T47.8X6
Omeprazole	T47.1X1	T47.1X2	T47.1X3	T47.1X4	T47.1X5	T47.1X6
OMPA	T60.0X1	T60.0X2	T60.0X3	T60.0X4	—	—
Oncovin	T45.1X1	T45.1X2	T45.1X3	T45.1X4	T45.1X5	T45.1X6
Ondansetron	T45.0X1	T45.0X2	T45.0X3	T45.0X4	T45.0X5	T45.0X6
Ophthaine	T41.3X1	T41.3X2	T41.3X3	T41.3X4	T41.3X5	T41.3X6
Ophthetic	T41.3X1	T41.3X2	T41.3X3	T41.3X4	T41.3X5	T41.3X6
Opiate NEC	T40.601	T40.602	T40.603	T40.604	T40.605	T40.606
antagonists	T50.7X1	T50.7X2	T50.7X3	T50.7X4	T50.7X5	T50.7X6
Opioid NEC	T40.2X1	T40.2X2	T40.2X3	T40.2X4	T40.2X5	T40.2X6
Opipramol	T43.011	T43.012	T43.013	T43.014	T43.015	T43.016
Opium alkaloids (total)	T40.0X1	T40.0X2	T40.0X3	T40.0X4	T40.0X5	T40.0X6
standardized powdered	T40.0X1	T40.0X2	T40.0X3	T40.0X4	T40.0X5	T40.0X6
tincture (camphorated)	T40.0X1	T40.0X2	T40.0X3	T40.0X4	T40.0X5	T40.0X6
Oracon	T38.4X1	T38.4X2	T38.4X3	T38.4X4	T38.4X5	T38.4X6
Oragrafin	T50.8X1	T50.8X2	T50.8X3	T50.8X4	T50.8X5	T50.8X6
Oral contraceptives	T38.4X1	T38.4X2	T38.4X3	T38.4X4	T38.4X5	T38.4X6
Oral rehydration salts	T50.3X1	T50.3X2	T50.3X3	T50.3X4	T50.3X5	T50.3X6
Orazamide	T50.991	T50.992	T50.993	T50.994	T50.995	T50.996
Orciprenaline	T48.291	T48.292	T48.293	T48.294	T48.295	T48.296
Organidin	T48.4X1	T48.4X2	T48.4X3	T48.4X4	T48.4X5	T48.4X6
Organonitrate NEC	T46.3X1	T46.3X2	T46.3X3	T46.3X4	T46.3X5	T46.3X6
Organophosphates	T60.0X1	T60.0X2	T60.0X3	T60.0X4	—	—
Orimune	T50.B91	T50.B92	T50.B93	T50.B94	T50.B95	T50.B96
Orinase	T38.3X1	T38.3X2	T38.3X3	T38.3X4	T38.3X5	T38.3X6
Ormeloxifene	T38.6X1	T38.6X2	T38.6X3	T38.6X4	T38.6X5	T38.6X6
Ornidazole	T37.3X1	T37.3X2	T37.3X3	T37.3X4	T37.3X5	T37.3X6
Ornithine aspartate	T50.991	T50.992	T50.993	T50.994	T50.995	T50.996
Ornoprostil	T47.1X1	T47.1X2	T47.1X3	T47.1X4	T47.1X5	T47.1X6
Orphenadrine	T42.8X1	T42.8X2	T42.8X3	T42.8X4	T42.8X5	T42.8X6
(hydrochloride)						
Ortal (sodium)	T42.3X1	T42.3X2	T42.3X3	T42.3X4	T42.3X5	T42.3X6
Orthoboric acid	T49.0X1	T49.0X2	T49.0X3	T49.0X4	T49.0X5	T49.0X6
ENT agent	T49.6X1	T49.6X2	T49.6X3	T49.6X4	T49.6X5	T49.6X6
ophthalmic preparation	T49.5X1	T49.5X2	T49.5X3	T49.5X4	T49.5X5	T49.5X6
Orthocaine	T41.3X1	T41.3X2	T41.3X3	T41.3X4	T41.3X5	T41.3X6
Orthodichlorobenzene	T53.7X1	T53.7X2	T53.7X3	T53.7X4	—	—
Ortho-Novum	T38.4X1	T38.4X2	T38.4X3	T38.4X4	T38.4X5	T38.4X6
Orthotolidine (reagent)	T54.2X1	T54.2X2	T54.2X3	T54.2X4	—	—
Osmic acid (liquid)	T54.2X1	T54.2X2	T54.2X3	T54.2X4	—	—
fumes	T54.2X1	T54.2X2	T54.2X3	T54.2X4	—	—
Osmotic diuretics	T50.2X1	T50.2X2	T50.2X3	T50.2X4	T50.2X5	T50.2X6
Otilonium bromide	T44.3X1	T44.3X2	T44.3X3	T44.3X4	T44.3X5	T44.3X6
Otorhinolaryngological drug NEC	T49.6X1	T49.6X2	T49.6X3	T49.6X4	T49.6X5	T49.6X6
Ouabain (e)	T46.0X1	T46.0X2	T46.0X3	T46.0X4	T46.0X5	T46.0X6
Ovarian						
hormone	T38.5X1	T38.5X2	T38.5X3	T38.5X4	T38.5X5	T38.5X6
stimulant	T38.5X1	T38.5X2	T38.5X3	T38.5X4	T38.5X5	T38.5X6
Ovral	T38.4X1	T38.4X2	T38.4X3	T38.4X4	T38.4X5	T38.4X6
Ovulen	T38.4X1	T38.4X2	T38.4X3	T38.4X4	T38.4X5	T38.4X6

Table of Drugs and Chemicals

Oxacillin — Penicilloyl polylysine

Substance	Poisoning, Accidental (unintentional)	Poisoning, Intentional Self-harm	Poisoning, Assault	Poisoning, Undetermined	Adverse Effect	Underdosing
Oxacillin	T36.0X1	T36.0X2	T36.0X3	T36.0X4	T36.0X5	T36.0X6
Oxalic acid	T54.2X1	T54.2X2	T54.2X3	T54.2X4	—	—
ammonium salt	T50.991	T50.992	T50.993	T50.994	T50.995	T50.996
Oxamniquine	T37.4X1	T37.4X2	T37.4X3	T37.4X4	T37.4X5	T37.4X6
Oxanamide	T43.591	T43.592	T43.593	T43.594	T43.595	T43.596
Oxandrolone	T38.7X1	T38.7X2	T38.7X3	T38.7X4	T38.7X5	T38.7X6
Oxantel	T37.4X1	T37.4X2	T37.4X3	T37.4X4	T37.4X5	T37.4X6
Oxapium iodide	T44.3X1	T44.3X2	T44.3X3	T44.3X4	T44.3X5	T44.3X6
Oxaprotiline	T43.021	T43.022	T43.023	T43.024	T43.025	T43.026
Oxaprozin	T39.311	T39.312	T39.313	T39.314	T39.315	T39.316
Oxatomide	T45.0X1	T45.0X2	T45.0X3	T45.0X4	T45.0X5	T45.0X6
Oxazepam	T42.4X1	T42.4X2	T42.4X3	T42.4X4	T42.4X5	T42.4X6
Oxazimedrine	T50.5X1	T50.5X2	T50.5X3	T50.5X4	T50.5X5	T50.5X6
Oxazolam	T42.4X1	T42.4X2	T42.4X3	T42.4X4	T42.4X5	T42.4X6
Oxazolidine derivatives	T42.2X1	T42.2X2	T42.2X3	T42.2X4	T42.2X5	T42.2X6
Oxazolidinedione (derivative)	T42.2X1	T42.2X2	T42.2X3	T42.2X4	T42.2X5	T42.2X6
Ox bile extract	T47.5X1	T47.5X2	T47.5X3	T47.5X4	T47.5X5	T47.5X6
Oxcarbazepine	T42.1X1	T42.1X2	T42.1X3	T42.1X4	T42.1X5	T42.1X6
Oxedrine	T44.4X1	T44.4X2	T44.4X3	T44.4X4	T44.4X5	T44.4X6
Oxeladin (citrate)	T48.3X1	T48.3X2	T48.3X3	T48.3X4	T48.3X5	T48.3X6
Oxendolone	T38.5X1	T38.5X2	T38.5X3	T38.5X4	T38.5X5	T38.5X6
Oxetacaine	T41.3X1	T41.3X2	T41.3X3	T41.3X4	T41.3X5	T41.3X6
Oxethazine	T41.3X1	T41.3X2	T41.3X3	T41.3X4	T41.3X5	T41.3X6
Oxetorone	T39.8X1	T39.8X2	T39.8X3	T39.8X4	T39.8X5	T39.8X6
Oxiconazole	T49.0X1	T49.0X2	T49.0X3	T49.0X4	T49.0X5	T49.0X6
Oxidizing agent NEC	T54.91	T54.92	T54.93	T54.94	—	—
Oxipurinol	T50.4X1	T50.4X2	T50.4X3	T50.4X4	T50.4X5	T50.4X6
Oxitriptan	T43.291	T43.292	T43.293	T43.294	T43.295	T43.296
Oxitropium bromide	T48.6X1	T48.6X2	T48.6X3	T48.6X4	T48.6X5	T48.6X6
Oxodipine	T46.1X1	T46.1X2	T46.1X3	T46.1X4	T46.1X5	T46.1X6
Oxolamine	T48.3X1	T48.3X2	T48.3X3	T48.3X4	T48.3X5	T48.3X6
Oxolinic acid	T37.8X1	T37.8X2	T37.8X3	T37.8X4	T37.8X5	T37.8X6
Oxomemazine	T43.3X1	T43.3X2	T43.3X3	T43.3X4	T43.3X5	T43.3X6
Oxophenarsine	T37.3X1	T37.3X2	T37.3X3	T37.3X4	T37.3X5	T37.3X6
Oxprenolol	T44.7X1	T44.7X2	T44.7X3	T44.7X4	T44.7X5	T44.7X6
Oxsoralen	T49.3X1	T49.3X2	T49.3X3	T49.3X4	T49.3X5	T49.3X6
Oxtriphylline	T48.6X1	T48.6X2	T48.6X3	T48.6X4	T48.6X5	T48.6X6
Oxybate sodium	T41.291	T41.292	T41.293	T41.294	T41.295	T41.296
Oxybuprocaine	T41.3X1	T41.3X2	T41.3X3	T41.3X4	T41.3X5	T41.3X6
Oxybutynin	T44.3X1	T44.3X2	T44.3X3	T44.3X4	T44.3X5	T44.3X6
Oxychlorosene	T49.0X1	T49.0X2	T49.0X3	T49.0X4	T49.0X5	T49.0X6
Oxycodone	T40.2X1	T40.2X2	T40.2X3	T40.2X4	T40.2X5	T40.2X6
Oxyfedrine	T46.3X1	T46.3X2	T46.3X3	T46.3X4	T46.3X5	T46.3X6
Oxygen	T41.5X1	T41.5X2	T41.5X3	T41.5X4	T41.5X5	T41.5X6
Oxylone	T49.0X1	T49.0X2	T49.0X3	T49.0X4	T49.0X5	T49.0X6
ophthalmic preparation	T49.5X1	T49.5X2	T49.5X3	T49.5X4	T49.5X5	T49.5X6
Oxymesterone	T38.7X1	T38.7X2	T38.7X3	T38.7X4	T38.7X5	T38.7X6
Oxymetazoline	T48.5X1	T48.5X2	T48.5X3	T48.5X4	T48.5X5	T48.5X6
Oxymetholone	T38.7X1	T38.7X2	T38.7X3	T38.7X4	T38.7X5	T38.7X6
Oxymorphone	T40.2X1	T40.2X2	T40.2X3	T40.2X4	T40.2X5	T40.2X6
Oxypertine	T43.591	T43.592	T43.593	T43.594	T43.595	T43.596
Oxyphenbutazone	T39.2X1	T39.2X2	T39.2X3	T39.2X4	T39.2X5	T39.2X6
Oxyphencyclimine	T44.3X1	T44.3X2	T44.3X3	T44.3X4	T44.3X5	T44.3X6
Oxyphenisatine	T47.2X1	T47.2X2	T47.2X3	T47.2X4	T47.2X5	T47.2X6
Oxyphenonium bromide	T44.3X1	T44.3X2	T44.3X3	T44.3X4	T44.3X5	T44.3X6
Oxypolygelatin	T45.8X1	T45.8X2	T45.8X3	T45.8X4	T45.8X5	T45.8X6
Oxyquinoline (derivatives)	T37.8X1	T37.8X2	T37.8X3	T37.8X4	T37.8X5	T37.8X6
Oxytetracycline	T36.4X1	T36.4X2	T36.4X3	T36.4X4	T36.4X5	T36.4X6
Oxytocic drug NEC	T48.0X1	T48.0X2	T48.0X3	T48.0X4	T48.0X5	T48.0X6
Oxytocin (synthetic)	T48.0X1	T48.0X2	T48.0X3	T48.0X4	T48.0X5	T48.0X6
Ozone	T59.891	T59.892	T59.893	T59.894	—	—
PABA	T49.3X1	T49.3X2	T49.3X3	T49.3X4	T49.3X5	T49.3X6
Packed red cells	T45.8X1	T45.8X2	T45.8X3	T45.8X4	T45.8X5	T45.8X6
Padimate	T49.3X1	T49.3X2	T49.3X3	T49.3X4	T49.3X5	T49.3X6
Paint NEC	T65.6X1	T65.6X2	T65.6X3	T65.6X4	—	—
cleaner	T52.91	T52.92	T52.93	T52.94	—	—
fumes NEC	T59.891	T59.892	T59.893	T59.894	—	—
lead (fumes)	T56.0X1	T56.0X2	T56.0X3	T56.0X4	—	—
solvent NEC	T52.8X1	T52.8X2	T52.8X3	T52.8X4	—	—
stripper	T52.8X1	T52.8X2	T52.8X3	T52.8X4	—	—
Palfium	T40.2X1	T40.2X2	T40.2X3	T40.2X4	—	—
Palm kernel oil	T50.991	T50.992	T50.993	T50.994	T50.995	T50.996
Paludrine	T37.2X1	T37.2X2	T37.2X3	T37.2X4	T37.2X5	T37.2X6
PAM (pralidoxime)	T50.6X1	T50.6X2	T50.6X3	T50.6X4	T50.6X5	T50.6X6
Pamaquine (naphthoute)	T37.2X1	T37.2X2	T37.2X3	T37.2X4	T37.2X5	T37.2X6
Panadol	T39.1X1	T39.1X2	T39.1X3	T39.1X4	T39.1X5	T39.1X6
Pancreatic						
digestive secretion stimulant	T47.8X1	T47.8X2	T47.8X3	T47.8X4	T47.8X5	T47.8X6
dornase	T45.3X1	T45.3X2	T45.3X3	T45.3X4	T45.3X5	T45.3X6
Pancreatin	T47.5X1	T47.5X2	T47.5X3	T47.5X4	T47.5X5	T47.5X6
Pancrelipase	T47.5X1	T47.5X2	T47.5X3	T47.5X4	T47.5X5	T47.5X6

Substance	Poisoning, Accidental (unintentional)	Poisoning, Intentional Self-harm	Poisoning, Assault	Poisoning, Undetermined	Adverse Effect	Underdosing
Pancuronium (bromide)	T48.1X1	T48.1X2	T48.1X3	T48.1X4	T48.1X5	T48.1X6
Pangamic acid	T45.2X1	T45.2X2	T45.2X3	T45.2X4	T45.2X5	T45.2X6
Panthenol	T45.2X1	T45.2X2	T45.2X3	T45.2X4	T45.2X5	T45.2X6
topical	T49.8X1	T49.8X2	T49.8X3	T49.8X4	T49.8X5	T49.8X6
Pantopon	T40.0X1	T40.0X2	T40.0X3	T40.0X4	T40.0X5	T40.0X6
Pantothenic acid	T45.2X1	T45.2X2	T45.2X3	T45.2X4	T45.2X5	T45.2X6
Panwarfin	T45.511	T45.512	T45.513	T45.514	T45.515	T45.516
Papain	T47.5X1	T47.5X2	T47.5X3	T47.5X4	T47.5X5	T47.5X6
digestant	T47.5X1	T47.5X2	T47.5X3	T47.5X4	T47.5X5	T47.5X6
Papaveretum	T40.0X1	T40.0X2	T40.0X3	T40.0X4	T40.0X5	T40.0X6
Papaverine	T44.3X1	T44.3X2	T44.3X3	T44.3X4	T44.3X5	T44.3X6
Para-acetamidophenol	T39.1X1	T39.1X2	T39.1X3	T39.1X4	T39.1X5	T39.1X6
Para-aminobenzoic acid	T49.3X1	T49.3X2	T49.3X3	T49.3X4	T49.3X5	T49.3X6
Para-aminophenol derivatives	T39.1X1	T39.1X2	T39.1X3	T39.1X4	T39.1X5	T39.1X6
Para-aminosalicylic acid	T37.1X1	T37.1X2	T37.1X3	T37.1X4	T37.1X5	T37.1X6
Paracetaldehyde	T42.6X1	T42.6X2	T42.6X3	T42.6X4	T42.6X5	T42.6X6
Paracetamol	T39.1X1	T39.1X2	T39.1X3	T39.1X4	T39.1X5	T39.1X6
Parachlorophenol (camphorated)	T49.0X1	T49.0X2	T49.0X3	T49.0X4	T49.0X5	T49.0X6
Paracodin	T40.2X1	T40.2X2	T40.2X3	T40.2X4	T40.2X5	T40.2X6
Paradione	T42.2X1	T42.2X2	T42.2X3	T42.2X4	T42.2X5	T42.2X6
Paraffin(s) (wax)	T52.0X1	T52.0X2	T52.0X3	T52.0X4	—	—
liquid (medicinal)	T47.4X1	T47.4X2	T47.4X3	T47.4X4	T47.4X5	T47.4X6
nonmedicinal	T52.0X1	T52.0X2	T52.0X3	T52.0X4	—	—
Paraformaldehyde	T60.3X1	T60.3X2	T60.3X3	T60.3X4	—	—
Paraldehyde	T42.6X1	T42.6X2	T42.6X3	T42.6X4	T42.6X5	T42.6X6
Paramethadione	T42.2X1	T42.2X2	T42.2X3	T42.2X4	T42.2X5	T42.2X6
Paramethasone	T38.0X1	T38.0X2	T38.0X3	T38.0X4	T38.0X5	T38.0X6
acetate	T49.0X1	T49.0X2	T49.0X3	T49.0X4	T49.0X5	T49.0X6
Paraoxon	T60.0X1	T60.0X2	T60.0X3	T60.0X4	—	—
Paraquat	T60.3X1	T60.3X2	T60.3X3	T60.3X4	—	—
Parasympatholytic NEC	T44.3X1	T44.3X2	T44.3X3	T44.3X4	T44.3X5	T44.3X6
Parasympathomimetic drug NEC	T44.1X1	T44.1X2	T44.1X3	T44.1X4	T44.1X5	T44.1X6
Parathion	T60.0X1	T60.0X2	T60.0X3	T60.0X4	—	—
Parathormone	T50.991	T50.992	T50.993	T50.994	T50.995	T50.996
Parathyroid extract	T50.991	T50.992	T50.993	T50.994	T50.995	T50.996
Paratyphoid vaccine	T50.A91	T50.A92	T50.A93	T50.A94	T50.A95	T50.A96
Paredrine	T44.4X1	T44.4X2	T44.4X3	T44.4X4	T44.4X5	T44.4X6
Paregoric	T40.0X1	T40.0X2	T40.0X3	T40.0X4	T40.0X5	T40.0X6
Pargyline	T46.5X1	T46.5X2	T46.5X3	T46.5X4	T46.5X5	T46.5X6
Paris green	T57.0X1	T57.0X2	T57.0X3	T57.0X4	—	—
insecticide	T57.0X1	T57.0X2	T57.0X3	T57.0X4	—	—
Parnate	T43.1X1	T43.1X2	T43.1X3	T43.1X4	T43.1X5	T43.1X6
Paromomycin	T36.5X1	T36.5X2	T36.5X3	T36.5X4	T36.5X5	T36.5X6
Paroxypropione	T45.1X1	T45.1X2	T45.1X3	T45.1X4	T45.1X5	T45.1X6
Parzone	T40.2X1	T40.2X2	T40.2X3	T40.2X4	T40.2X5	T40.2X6
PAS	T37.1X1	T37.1X2	T37.1X3	T37.1X4	T37.1X5	T37.1X6
Pasiniazid	T37.1X1	T37.1X2	T37.1X3	T37.1X4	T37.1X5	T37.1X6
PBB (polybrominated biphenyls)	T65.891	T65.892	T65.893	T65.894	—	—
PCB	T65.891	T65.892	T65.893	T65.894	—	—
PCP						
meaning pentachlorophenol	T60.1X1	T60.1X2	T60.1X3	T60.1X4	—	—
fungicide	T60.3X1	T60.3X2	T60.3X3	T60.3X4	—	—
herbicide	T60.3X1	T60.3X2	T60.3X3	T60.3X4	—	—
insecticide	T60.1X1	T60.1X2	T60.1X3	T60.1X4	—	—
meaning phencyclidine	T40.991	T40.992	T40.993	T40.994	—	—
Peach kernel oil (emulsion)	T47.4X1	T47.4X2	T47.4X3	T47.4X4	T47.4X5	T47.4X6
Peanut oil (emulsion) NEC	T47.4X1	T47.4X2	T47.4X3	T47.4X4	T47.4X5	T47.4X6
topical	T49.3X1	T49.3X2	T49.3X3	T49.3X4	T49.3X5	T49.3X6
Pearly Gates (morning glory seeds)	T40.991	T40.992	T40.993	T40.994	—	—
Pecazine	T43.3X1	T43.3X2	T43.3X3	T43.3X4	T43.3X5	T43.3X6
Pectin	T47.6X1	T47.6X2	T47.6X3	T47.6X4	T47.6X5	T47.6X6
Pefloxacin	T37.8X1	T37.8X2	T37.8X3	T37.8X4	T37.8X5	T37.8X6
Pegademase, bovine	T50.Z91	T50.Z92	T50.Z93	T50.Z94	T50.Z95	T50.Z96
Pelletierine tannate	T37.4X1	T37.4X2	T37.4X3	T37.4X4	T37.4X5	T37.4X6
Pemirolast (potassium)	T48.6X1	T48.6X2	T48.6X3	T48.6X4	T48.6X5	T48.6X6
Pemoline	T50.7X1	T50.7X2	T50.7X3	T50.7X4	T50.7X5	T50.7X6
Pempidine	T44.2X1	T44.2X2	T44.2X3	T44.2X4	T44.2X5	T44.2X6
Penamecillin	T36.0X1	T36.0X2	T36.0X3	T36.0X4	T36.0X5	T36.0X6
Penbutolol	T44.7X1	T44.7X2	T44.7X3	T44.7X4	T44.7X5	T44.7X6
Penethamate	T36.0X1	T36.0X2	T36.0X3	T36.0X4	T36.0X5	T36.0X6
Penfluridol	T43.591	T43.592	T43.593	T43.594	T43.595	T43.596
Penflutizide	T50.2X1	T50.2X2	T50.2X3	T50.2X4	T50.2X5	T50.2X6
Pengitoxin	T46.0X1	T46.0X2	T46.0X3	T46.0X4	T46.0X5	T46.0X6
Penicillamine	T50.6X1	T50.6X2	T50.6X3	T50.6X4	T50.6X5	T50.6X6
Penicillin (any)	T36.0X1	T36.0X2	T36.0X3	T36.0X4	T36.0X5	T36.0X6
Penicillinase	T45.3X1	T45.3X2	T45.3X3	T45.3X4	T45.3X5	T45.3X6
Penicilloyl polylysine	T50.8X1	T50.8X2	T50.8X3	T50.8X4	T50.8X5	T50.8X6

Additional Character May Be Required — Refer to the Tabular List for Character Selection

▽ Subterms under main terms may continue to next column or page

Substance	Poisoning, Accidental (unintentional)	Poisoning, Intentional Self-harm	Poisoning, Assault	Poisoning, Undetermined	Adverse Effect	Under-dosing
Penimepicycline	T36.4X1	T36.4X2	T36.4X3	T36.4X4	T36.4X5	T36.4X6
Pentachloroethane	T53.6X1	T53.6X2	T53.6X3	T53.6X4	—	—
Pentachloronaphthalene	T53.7X1	T53.7X2	T53.7X3	T53.7X4	—	—
Pentachlorophenol	T60.1X1	T60.1X2	T60.1X3	T60.1X4	—	—
(pesticide)						
fungicide	T60.3X1	T60.3X2	T60.3X3	T60.3X4	—	—
herbicide	T60.3X1	T60.3X2	T60.3X3	T60.3X4	—	—
insecticide	T60.1X1	T60.1X2	T60.1X3	T60.1X4	—	—
Pentaerythritol	T46.3X1	T46.3X2	T46.3X3	T46.3X4	T46.3X5	T46.3X6
chloral	T42.6X1	T42.6X2	T42.6X3	T42.6X4	T42.6X5	T42.6X6
tetranitrate NEC	T46.3X1	T46.3X2	T46.3X3	T46.3X4	T46.3X5	T46.3X6
Pentaerythrityl tetranitrate	T46.3X1	T46.3X2	T46.3X3	T46.3X4	T46.3X5	T46.3X6
Pentagastrin	T50.8X1	T50.8X2	T50.8X3	T50.8X4	T50.8X5	T50.8X6
Pentalin	T53.6X1	T53.6X2	T53.6X3	T53.6X4	—	—
Pentamethonium bromide	T44.2X1	T44.2X2	T44.2X3	T44.2X4	T44.2X5	T44.2X6
Pentamidine	T37.3X1	T37.3X2	T37.3X3	T37.3X4	T37.3X5	T37.3X6
Pentanol	T51.3X1	T51.3X2	T51.3X3	T51.3X4	—	—
Pentapyrrolinium (bitartrate)	T44.2X1	T44.2X2	T44.2X3	T44.2X4	T44.2X5	T44.2X6
Pentaquine	T37.2X1	T37.2X2	T37.2X3	T37.2X4	T37.2X5	T37.2X6
Pentazocine	T40.4X1	T40.4X2	T40.4X3	T40.4X4	T40.4X5	T40.4X6
Pentetrazole	T50.7X1	T50.7X2	T50.7X3	T50.7X4	T50.7X5	T50.7X6
Penthienate bromide	T44.3X1	T44.3X2	T44.3X3	T44.3X4	T44.3X5	T44.3X6
Pentifylline	T46.7X1	T46.7X2	T46.7X3	T46.7X4	T46.7X5	T46.7X6
Pentobarbital	T42.3X1	T42.3X2	T42.3X3	T42.3X4	T42.3X5	T42.3X6
sodium	T42.3X1	T42.3X2	T42.3X3	T42.3X4	T42.3X5	T42.3X6
Pentobarbitone	T42.3X1	T42.3X2	T42.3X3	T42.3X4	T42.3X5	T42.3X6
Pentolonium tartrate	T44.2X1	T44.2X2	T44.2X3	T44.2X4	T44.2X5	T44.2X6
Pentosan polysulfate (sodium)	T39.8X1	T39.8X2	T39.8X3	T39.8X4	T39.8X5	T39.8X6
Pentostatin	T45.1X1	T45.1X2	T45.1X3	T45.1X4	T45.1X5	T45.1X6
Pentothal	T41.1X1	T41.1X2	T41.1X3	T41.1X4	T41.1X5	T41.1X6
Pentoxifylline	T46.7X1	T46.7X2	T46.7X3	T46.7X4	T46.7X5	T46.7X6
Pentoxyverine	T48.3X1	T48.3X2	T48.3X3	T48.3X4	T48.3X5	T48.3X6
Pentrinat	T46.3X1	T46.3X2	T46.3X3	T46.3X4	T46.3X5	T46.3X6
Pentylenetetrazole	T50.7X1	T50.7X2	T50.7X3	T50.7X4	T50.7X5	T50.7X6
Pentylsalicylamide	T37.1X1	T37.1X2	T37.1X3	T37.1X4	T37.1X5	T37.1X6
Pentymal	T42.3X1	T42.3X2	T42.3X3	T42.3X4	T42.3X5	T42.3X6
Peplomycin	T45.1X1	T45.1X2	T45.1X3	T45.1X4	T45.1X5	T45.1X6
Peppermint (oil)	T47.5X1	T47.5X2	T47.5X3	T47.5X4	T47.5X5	T47.5X6
Pepsin	T47.5X1	T47.5X2	T47.5X3	T47.5X4	T47.5X5	T47.5X6
digestant	T47.5X1	T47.5X2	T47.5X3	T47.5X4	T47.5X5	T47.5X6
Pepstatin	T47.1X1	T47.1X2	T47.1X3	T47.1X4	T47.1X5	T47.1X6
Peptavlon	T50.8X1	T50.8X2	T50.8X3	T50.8X4	T50.8X5	T50.8X6
Perazine	T43.3X1	T43.3X2	T43.3X3	T43.3X4	T43.3X5	T43.3X6
Percaine (spinal)	T41.3X1	T41.3X2	T41.3X3	T41.3X4	T41.3X5	T41.3X6
topical (surface)	T41.3X1	T41.3X2	T41.3X3	T41.3X4	T41.3X5	T41.3X6
Perchloroethylene	T53.3X1	T53.3X2	T53.3X3	T53.3X4	—	—
medicinal	T37.4X1	T37.4X2	T37.4X3	T37.4X4	T37.4X5	T37.4X6
vapor	T53.3X1	T53.3X2	T53.3X3	T53.3X4	—	—
Percodan	T40.2X1	T40.2X2	T40.2X3	T40.2X4	T40.2X5	T40.2X6
Percogesic — see also acetaminophen	T45.0X1	T45.0X2	T45.0X3	T45.0X4	T45.0X5	T45.0X6
Percorten	T38.0X1	T38.0X2	T38.0X3	T38.0X4	T38.0X5	T38.0X6
Pergolide	T42.8X1	T42.8X2	T42.8X3	T42.8X4	T42.8X5	T42.8X6
Pergonal	T38.811	T38.812	T38.813	T38.814	T38.815	T38.816
Perhexilene	T46.3X1	T46.3X2	T46.3X3	T46.3X4	T46.3X5	T46.3X6
Perhexiline (maleate)	T45.0X1	T45.0X2	T45.0X3	T45.0X4	T45.0X5	T45.0X6
Periactin	T43.3X1	T43.3X2	T43.3X3	T43.3X4	T43.3X5	T43.3X6
Periciazine	T42.6X1	T42.6X2	T42.6X3	T42.6X4	T42.6X5	T42.6X6
Periclor	T46.4X1	T46.4X2	T46.4X3	T46.4X4	T46.4X5	T46.4X6
Perindopril	T39.8X1	T39.8X2	T39.8X3	T39.8X4	T39.8X5	T39.8X6
Perisoxal	T50.3X1	T50.3X2	T50.3X3	T50.3X4	T50.3X5	T50.3X6
Peritoneal dialysis solution	T46.3X1	T46.3X2	T46.3X3	T46.3X4	T46.3X5	T46.3X6
Peritrate	T42.4X1	T42.4X2	T42.4X3	T42.4X4	T42.4X5	T42.4X6
Perlapine	T65.891	T65.892	T65.893	T65.894	—	—
Permanganate	T60.1X1	T60.1X2	T60.1X3	T60.1X4	—	—
Permethrin	T42.3X1	T42.3X2	T42.3X3	T42.3X4	T42.3X5	T42.3X6
Pernocton	T42.3X1	T42.3X2	T42.3X3	T42.3X4	T42.3X5	T42.3X6
Pernoston	T40.2X1	T40.2X2	T40.2X3	T40.2X4	—	—
Peronine	T43.3X1	T43.3X2	T43.3X3	T43.3X4	T43.3X5	T43.3X6
Perphenazine	T43.011	T43.012	T43.013	T43.014	T43.015	T43.016
Pertofrane						
Pertussis						
immune serum (human)	T50.Z11	T50.Z12	T50.Z13	T50.Z14	T50.Z15	T50.Z16
vaccine (with diphtheria toxoid)	T50.A11	T50.A12	T50.A13	T50.A14	T50.A15	T50.A16
(with tetanus toxoid)						
Peruvian balsam	T49.0X1	T49.0X2	T49.0X3	T49.0X4	T49.0X5	T49.0X6
Peruvoside	T46.0X1	T46.0X2	T46.0X3	T46.0X4	T46.0X5	T46.0X6
Pesticide (dust) (fumes) (vapor)	T60.91	T60.92	T60.93	T60.94	—	—
NEC						
arsenic	T57.0X1	T57.0X2	T57.0X3	T57.0X4	—	—
Pesticide (dust) (fumes) (vapor) NEC — continued						
chlorinated	T60.1X1	T60.1X2	T60.1X3	T60.1X4	—	—
cyanide	T65.0X1	T65.0X2	T65.0X3	T65.0X4	—	—
kerosene	T52.0X1	T52.0X2	T52.0X3	T52.0X4	—	—
mixture (of compounds)	T60.91	T60.92	T60.93	T60.94	—	—
naphthalene	T60.2X1	T60.2X2	T60.2X3	T60.2X4	—	—
organochlorine (compounds)	T60.1X1	T60.1X2	T60.1X3	T60.1X4	—	—
petroleum (distillate) (products) NEC	T60.8X1	T60.8X2	T60.8X3	T60.8X4	—	—
specified ingredient NEC	T60.8X1	T60.8X2	T60.8X3	T60.8X4	—	—
strychnine	T65.1X1	T65.1X2	T65.1X3	T65.1X4	—	—
thallium	T60.4X1	T60.4X2	T60.4X3	T60.4X4	—	—
Pethidine	T40.4X1	T40.4X2	T40.4X3	T40.4X4	T40.4X5	T40.4X6
Petrichloral	T42.6X1	T42.6X2	T42.6X3	T42.6X4	T42.6X5	T42.6X6
Petrol	T52.0X1	T52.0X2	T52.0X3	T52.0X4	—	—
vapor	T52.0X1	T52.0X2	T52.0X3	T52.0X4	—	—
Petrolatum	T49.3X1	T49.3X2	T49.3X3	T49.3X4	T49.3X5	T49.3X6
hydrophilic	T49.3X1	T49.3X2	T49.3X3	T49.3X4	T49.3X5	T49.3X6
liquid	T47.4X1	T47.4X2	T47.4X3	T47.4X4	T47.4X5	T47.4X6
topical	T49.3X1	T49.3X2	T49.3X3	T49.3X4	T49.3X5	T49.3X6
nonmedicinal	T52.0X1	T52.0X2	T52.0X3	T52.0X4	—	—
red veterinary	T49.3X1	T49.3X2	T49.3X3	T49.3X4	T49.3X5	T49.3X6
white	T49.3X1	T49.3X2	T49.3X3	T49.3X4	T49.3X5	T49.3X6
Petroleum (products) NEC	T52.0X1	T52.0X2	T52.0X3	T52.0X4	—	—
benzine(s) — see Ligroin						
ether — see Ligroin						
jelly — see Petrolatum						
naphtha — see Ligroin						
pesticide	T60.8X1	T60.8X2	T60.8X3	T60.8X4	—	—
solids	T52.0X1	T52.0X2	T52.0X3	T52.0X4	—	—
solvents	T52.0X1	T52.0X2	T52.0X3	T52.0X4	—	—
vapor	T52.0X1	T52.0X2	T52.0X3	T52.0X4	—	—
Peyote	T40.991	T40.992	T40.993	T40.994	—	—
Phanodorm, phanodorn	T42.3X1	T42.3X2	T42.3X3	T42.3X4	T42.3X5	T42.3X6
Phanquinone	T37.3X1	T37.3X2	T37.3X3	T37.3X4	T37.3X5	T37.3X6
Phanquone	T37.3X1	T37.3X2	T37.3X3	T37.3X4	T37.3X5	T37.3X6
Pharmaceutical						
adjunct NEC	T50.901	T50.902	T50.903	T50.904	T50.905	T50.906
excipient NEC	T50.901	T50.902	T50.903	T50.904	T50.905	T50.906
sweetener	T50.901	T50.902	T50.903	T50.904	T50.905	T50.906
viscous agent	T50.901	T50.902	T50.903	T50.904	T50.905	T50.906
Phemitone	T42.3X1	T42.3X2	T42.3X3	T42.3X4	T42.3X5	T42.3X6
Phenacaine	T41.3X1	T41.3X2	T41.3X3	T41.3X4	T41.3X5	T41.3X6
Phenacemide	T42.6X1	T42.6X2	T42.6X3	T42.6X4	T42.6X5	T42.6X6
Phenacetin	T39.1X1	T39.1X2	T39.1X3	T39.1X4	T39.1X5	T39.1X6
Phenadoxone	T40.2X1	T40.2X2	T40.2X3	T40.2X4	—	—
Phenaglycodol	T43.591	T43.592	T43.593	T43.594	T43.595	T43.596
Phenantoin	T42.0X1	T42.0X2	T42.0X3	T42.0X4	T42.0X5	T42.0X6
Phenaphthazine reagent	T50.991	T50.992	T50.993	T50.994	T50.995	T50.996
Phenazocine	T40.4X1	T40.4X2	T40.4X3	T40.4X4	T40.4X5	T40.4X6
Phenazone	T39.2X1	T39.2X2	T39.2X3	T39.2X4	T39.2X5	T39.2X6
Phenazopyridine	T39.8X1	T39.8X2	T39.8X3	T39.8X4	T39.8X5	T39.8X6
Phenbenicillin	T36.0X1	T36.0X2	T36.0X3	T36.0X4	T36.0X5	T36.0X6
Phenbutrazate	T50.5X1	T50.5X2	T50.5X3	T50.5X4	T50.5X5	T50.5X6
Phencyclidine	T40.991	T40.992	T40.993	T40.994	T40.995	T40.996
Phendimetrazine	T50.5X1	T50.5X2	T50.5X3	T50.5X4	T50.5X5	T50.5X6
Phenelzine	T43.1X1	T43.1X2	T43.1X3	T43.1X4	T43.1X5	T43.1X6
Phenemal	T42.3X1	T42.3X2	T42.3X3	T42.3X4	T42.3X5	T42.3X6
Phenergan	T42.6X1	T42.6X2	T42.6X3	T42.6X4	T42.6X5	T42.6X6
Pheneticillin	T36.0X1	T36.0X2	T36.0X3	T36.0X4	T36.0X5	T36.0X6
Pheneturide	T42.6X1	T42.6X2	T42.6X3	T42.6X4	T42.6X5	T42.6X6
Phenformin	T38.3X1	T38.3X2	T38.3X3	T38.3X4	T38.3X5	T38.3X6
Phenglutarimide	T44.3X1	T44.3X2	T44.3X3	T44.3X4	T44.3X5	T44.3X6
Phenicarbazide	T39.8X1	T39.8X2	T39.8X3	T39.8X4	T39.8X5	T39.8X6
Phenindamine	T45.0X1	T45.0X2	T45.0X3	T45.0X4	T45.0X5	T45.0X6
Phenindione	T45.511	T45.512	T45.513	T45.514	T45.515	T45.516
Pheniprazine	T43.1X1	T43.1X2	T43.1X3	T43.1X4	T43.1X5	T43.1X6
Pheniramine	T45.0X1	T45.0X2	T45.0X3	T45.0X4	T45.0X5	T45.0X6
Phenisatin	T47.2X1	T47.2X2	T47.2X3	T47.2X4	T47.2X5	T47.2X6
Phenmetrazine	T50.5X1	T50.5X2	T50.5X3	T50.5X4	T50.5X5	T50.5X6
Phenobal	T42.3X1	T42.3X2	T42.3X3	T42.3X4	T42.3X5	T42.3X6
Phenobarbital	T42.3X1	T42.3X2	T42.3X3	T42.3X4	T42.3X5	T42.3X6
with						
mephenytoin	T42.3X1	T42.3X2	T42.3X3	T42.3X4	T42.3X5	T42.3X6
phenytoin	T42.3X1	T42.3X2	T42.3X3	T42.3X4	T42.3X5	T42.3X6
sodium	T42.3X1	T42.3X2	T42.3X3	T42.3X4	T42.3X5	T42.3X6
Phenobarbitone	T42.3X1	T42.3X2	T42.3X3	T42.3X4	T42.3X5	T42.3X6
Phenobutiodil	T50.8X1	T50.8X2	T50.8X3	T50.8X4	T50.8X5	T50.8X6
Phenoctide	T49.0X1	T49.0X2	T49.0X3	T49.0X4	T49.0X5	T49.0X6
Phenol	T49.0X1	T49.0X2	T49.0X3	T49.0X4	T49.0X5	T49.0X6
disinfectant	T54.0X1	T54.0X2	T54.0X3	T54.0X4	—	—

Table of Drugs and Chemicals

Penimepicycline — Phenol

Table of Drugs and Chemicals

Substance	Poisoning, Accidental (unintentional)	Poisoning, Intentional Self-harm	Poisoning, Assault	Poisoning, Undetermined	Adverse Effect	Under-dosing
Phenol — *continued*						
in oil injection	T46.8X1	T46.8X2	T46.8X3	T46.8X4	T46.8X5	T46.8X6
medicinal	T49.1X1	T49.1X2	T49.1X3	T49.1X4	T49.1X5	T49.1X6
nonmedicinal NEC	T54.0X1	T54.0X2	T54.0X3	T54.0X4	—	—
pesticide	T60.8X1	T60.8X2	T60.8X3	T60.8X4	—	—
red	T50.8X1	T50.8X2	T50.8X3	T50.8X4	T50.8X5	T50.8X6
Phenolic preparation	T49.1X1	T49.1X2	T49.1X3	T49.1X4	T49.1X5	T49.1X6
Phenolphthalein	T47.2X1	T47.2X2	T47.2X3	T47.2X4	T47.2X5	T47.2X6
Phenolsulfonphthalein	T50.8X1	T50.8X2	T50.8X3	T50.8X4	T50.8X5	T50.8X6
Phenomorphan	T40.2X1	T40.2X2	T40.2X3	T40.2X4	—	—
Phenonyl	T42.3X1	T42.3X2	T42.3X3	T42.3X4	T42.3X5	T42.3X6
Phenoperidine	T40.4X1	T40.4X2	T40.4X3	T40.4X4	—	—
Phenopyrazone	T46.991	T46.992	T46.993	T46.994	T46.995	T46.996
Phenoquin	T50.4X1	T50.4X2	T50.4X3	T50.4X4	T50.4X5	T50.4X6
Phenothiazine (psychotropic) NEC	T43.3X1	T43.3X2	T43.3X3	T43.3X4	T43.3X5	T43.3X6
insecticide	T60.2X1	T60.2X2	T60.2X3	T60.2X4	—	—
Phenothrin	T49.0X1	T49.0X2	T49.0X3	T49.0X4	T49.0X5	T49.0X6
Phenoxybenzamine	T46.7X1	T46.7X2	T46.7X3	T46.7X4	T46.7X5	T46.7X6
Phenoxyethanol	T49.0X1	T49.0X2	T49.0X3	T49.0X4	T49.0X5	T49.0X6
Phenoxymethyl penicillin	T36.0X1	T36.0X2	T36.0X3	T36.0X4	T36.0X5	T36.0X6
Phenprobamate	T42.8X1	T42.8X2	T42.8X3	T42.8X4	T42.8X5	T42.8X6
Phenprocoumon	T45.511	T45.512	T45.513	T45.514	T45.515	T45.516
Phensuximide	T42.2X1	T42.2X2	T42.2X3	T42.2X4	T42.2X5	T42.2X6
Phentermine	T50.5X1	T50.5X2	T50.5X3	T50.5X4	T50.5X5	T50.5X6
Phenthicillin	T36.0X1	T36.0X2	T36.0X3	T36.0X4	T36.0X5	T36.0X6
Phentolamine	T46.7X1	T46.7X2	T46.7X3	T46.7X4	T46.7X5	T46.7X6
Phenyl						
butazone	T39.2X1	T39.2X2	T39.2X3	T39.2X4	T39.2X5	T39.2X6
enediamine	T65.3X1	T65.3X2	T65.3X3	T65.3X4	—	—
hydrazine	T65.3X1	T65.3X2	T65.3X3	T65.3X4	—	—
antineoplastic	T45.1X1	T45.1X2	T45.1X3	T45.1X4	T45.1X5	T45.1X6
mercuric compounds — see Mercury						
salicylate	T49.3X1	T49.3X2	T49.3X3	T49.3X4	T49.3X5	T49.3X6
Phenylalanine mustard	T45.1X1	T45.1X2	T45.1X3	T45.1X4	T45.1X5	T45.1X6
Phenylbutazone	T39.2X1	T39.2X2	T39.2X3	T39.2X4	T39.2X5	T39.2X6
Phenylenediamine	T65.3X1	T65.3X2	T65.3X3	T65.3X4	—	—
Phenylephrine	T44.4X1	T44.4X2	T44.4X3	T44.4X4	T44.4X5	T44.4X6
Phenylethylbiguanide	T38.3X1	T38.3X2	T38.3X3	T38.3X4	T38.3X5	T38.3X6
Phenylmercuric						
acetate	T49.0X1	T49.0X2	T49.0X3	T49.0X4	T49.0X5	T49.0X6
borate	T49.0X1	T49.0X2	T49.0X3	T49.0X4	T49.0X5	T49.0X6
nitrate	T49.0X1	T49.0X2	T49.0X3	T49.0X4	T49.0X5	T49.0X6
Phenylmethylbarbitone	T42.3X1	T42.3X2	T42.3X3	T42.3X4	T42.3X5	T42.3X6
Phenylpropanol	T47.5X1	T47.5X2	T47.5X3	T47.5X4	T47.5X5	T47.5X6
Phenylpropanolamine	T44.991	T44.992	T44.993	T44.994	T44.995	T44.996
Phenylsulfthion	T60.0X1	T60.0X2	T60.0X3	T60.0X4	—	—
Phenyltoloxamine	T45.0X1	T45.0X2	T45.0X3	T45.0X4	T45.0X5	T45.0X6
Phenyramidol, phenyramidon	T39.8X1	T39.8X2	T39.8X3	T39.8X4	T39.8X5	T39.8X6
Phenytoin	T42.0X1	T42.0X2	T42.0X3	T42.0X4	T42.0X5	T42.0X6
with Phenobarbital	T42.3X1	T42.3X2	T42.3X3	T42.3X4	T42.3X5	T42.3X6
pHisoHex	T49.2X1	T49.2X2	T49.2X3	T49.2X4	T49.2X5	T49.2X6
Pholcodine	T48.3X1	T48.3X2	T48.3X3	T48.3X4	T48.3X5	T48.3X6
Pholedrine	T46.991	T46.992	T46.993	T46.994	T46.995	T46.996
Phorate	T60.0X1	T60.0X2	T60.0X3	T60.0X4	—	—
Phosdrin	T60.0X1	T60.0X2	T60.0X3	T60.0X4	—	—
Phosfolan	T60.0X1	T60.0X2	T60.0X3	T60.0X4	—	—
Phosgene (gas)	T59.891	T59.892	T59.893	T59.894	—	—
Phosphamidon	T60.0X1	T60.0X2	T60.0X3	T60.0X4	—	—
Phosphate	T65.891	T65.892	T65.893	T65.894	—	—
laxative	T47.4X1	T47.4X2	T47.4X3	T47.4X4	T47.4X5	T47.4X6
organic	T60.0X1	T60.0X2	T60.0X3	T60.0X4	—	—
solvent	T52.91	T52.92	T52.93	T52.94	—	—
tricresyl	T65.891	T65.892	T65.893	T65.894	—	—
Phosphine	T57.1X1	T57.1X2	T57.1X3	T57.1X4	—	—
fumigant	T57.1X1	T57.1X2	T57.1X3	T57.1X4	—	—
Phospholine	T49.5X1	T49.5X2	T49.5X3	T49.5X4	T49.5X5	T49.5X6
Phosphoric acid	T54.2X1	T54.2X2	T54.2X3	T54.2X4	—	—
Phosphorus (compound) NEC	T57.1X1	T57.1X2	T57.1X3	T57.1X4	—	—
pesticide	T60.0X1	T60.0X2	T60.0X3	T60.0X4	—	—
Phthalates	T65.891	T65.892	T65.893	T65.894	—	—
Phthalic anhydride	T65.891	T65.892	T65.893	T65.894	—	—
Phthalimidoglutarimide	T42.6X1	T42.6X2	T42.6X3	T42.6X4	T42.6X5	T42.6X6
Phthalylsulfathiazole	T37.0X1	T37.0X2	T37.0X3	T37.0X4	T37.0X5	T37.0X6
Phylloquinone	T45.7X1	T45.7X2	T45.7X3	T45.7X4	T45.7X5	T45.7X6
Physeptone	T40.3X1	T40.3X2	T40.3X3	T40.3X4	T40.3X5	T40.3X6
Physostigma venenosum	T62.2X1	T62.2X2	T62.2X3	T62.2X4	—	—
Physostigmine	T49.5X1	T49.5X2	T49.5X3	T49.5X4	T49.5X5	T49.5X6
Phytolacca decandra	T62.2X1	T62.2X2	T62.2X3	T62.2X4	—	—
berries	T62.1X1	T62.1X2	T62.1X3	T62.1X4	—	—

Substance	Poisoning, Accidental (unintentional)	Poisoning, Intentional Self-harm	Poisoning, Assault	Poisoning, Undetermined	Adverse Effect	Under-dosing
Phytomenadione	T45.7X1	T45.7X2	T45.7X3	T45.7X4	T45.7X5	T45.7X6
Phytonadione	T45.7X1	T45.7X2	T45.7X3	T45.7X4	T45.7X5	T45.7X6
Picoperine	T48.3X1	T48.3X2	T48.3X3	T48.3X4	T48.3X5	T48.3X6
Picosulfate (sodium)	T47.2X1	T47.2X2	T47.2X3	T47.2X4	T47.2X5	T47.2X6
Picric (acid)	T54.2X1	T54.2X2	T54.2X3	T54.2X4	—	—
Picrotoxin	T50.7X1	T50.7X2	T50.7X3	T50.7X4	T50.7X5	T50.7X6
Piketoprofen	T49.0X1	T49.0X2	T49.0X3	T49.0X4	T49.0X5	T49.0X6
Pilocarpine	T44.1X1	T44.1X2	T44.1X3	T44.1X4	T44.1X5	T44.1X6
Pilocarpus (jaborandi) extract	T44.1X1	T44.1X2	T44.1X3	T44.1X4	T44.1X5	T44.1X6
Pilsicainide (hydrochloride)	T46.2X1	T46.2X2	T46.2X3	T46.2X4	T46.2X5	T46.2X6
Pimaricin	T36.7X1	T36.7X2	T36.7X3	T36.7X4	T36.7X5	T36.7X6
Pimeclone	T50.7X1	T50.7X2	T50.7X3	T50.7X4	T50.7X5	T50.7X6
Pimelic ketone	T52.8X1	T52.8X2	T52.8X3	T52.8X4	—	—
Pimethixene	T45.0X1	T45.0X2	T45.0X3	T45.0X4	T45.0X5	T45.0X6
Piminodine	T40.2X1	T40.2X2	T40.2X3	T40.2X4	T40.2X5	T40.2X6
Pimozide	T43.591	T43.592	T43.593	T43.594	T43.595	T43.596
Pinacidil	T46.5X1	T46.5X2	T46.5X3	T46.5X4	T46.5X5	T46.5X6
Pinaverium bromide	T44.3X1	T44.3X2	T44.3X3	T44.3X4	T44.3X5	T44.3X6
Pinazepam	T42.4X1	T42.4X2	T42.4X3	T42.4X4	T42.4X5	T42.4X6
Pindolol	T44.7X1	T44.7X2	T44.7X3	T44.7X4	T44.7X5	T44.7X6
Pindone	T60.4X1	T60.4X2	T60.4X3	T60.4X4	—	—
Pine oil (disinfectant)	T65.891	T65.892	T65.893	T65.894	—	—
Pinkroot	T37.4X1	T37.4X2	T37.4X3	T37.4X4	T37.4X5	T37.4X6
Pipadone	T40.2X1	T40.2X2	T40.2X3	T40.2X4	—	—
Pipamazine	T45.0X1	T45.0X2	T45.0X3	T45.0X4	T45.0X5	T45.0X6
Pipamperone	T43.4X1	T43.4X2	T43.4X3	T43.4X4	T43.4X5	T43.4X6
Pipazetate	T48.3X1	T48.3X2	T48.3X3	T48.3X4	T48.3X5	T48.3X6
Pipemidic acid	T37.8X1	T37.8X2	T37.8X3	T37.8X4	T37.8X5	T37.8X6
Pipenzolate bromide	T44.3X1	T44.3X2	T44.3X3	T44.3X4	T44.3X5	T44.3X6
Piperacetazine	T43.3X1	T43.3X2	T43.3X3	T43.3X4	T43.3X5	T43.3X6
Piperacillin	T36.0X1	T36.0X2	T36.0X3	T36.0X4	T36.0X5	T36.0X6
Piperazine	T37.4X1	T37.4X2	T37.4X3	T37.4X4	T37.4X5	T37.4X6
estrone sulfate	T38.5X1	T38.5X2	T38.5X3	T38.5X4	T38.5X5	T38.5X6
Piper cubeba	T62.2X1	T62.2X2	T62.2X3	T62.2X4	—	—
Piperidione	T48.3X1	T48.3X2	T48.3X3	T48.3X4	T48.3X5	T48.3X6
Piperidolate	T44.3X1	T44.3X2	T44.3X3	T44.3X4	T44.3X5	T44.3X6
Piperocaine	T41.3X1	T41.3X2	T41.3X3	T41.3X4	T41.3X5	T41.3X6
infiltration (subcutaneous)	T41.3X1	T41.3X2	T41.3X3	T41.3X4	T41.3X5	T41.3X6
nerve block (peripheral) (plexus)	T41.3X1	T41.3X2	T41.3X3	T41.3X4	T41.3X5	T41.3X6
topical (surface)	T41.3X1	T41.3X2	T41.3X3	T41.3X4	T41.3X5	T41.3X6
Piperonyl butoxide	T60.8X1	T60.8X2	T60.8X3	T60.8X4	—	—
Pipethanate	T44.3X1	T44.3X2	T44.3X3	T44.3X4	T44.3X5	T44.3X6
Pipobroman	T45.1X1	T45.1X2	T45.1X3	T45.1X4	T45.1X5	T45.1X6
Pipotiazine	T43.3X1	T43.3X2	T43.3X3	T43.3X4	T43.3X5	T43.3X6
Pipoxizine	T45.0X1	T45.0X2	T45.0X3	T45.0X4	T45.0X5	T45.0X6
Pipradrol	T43.691	T43.692	T43.693	T43.694	T43.695	T43.696
Piprinhydrinate	T45.0X1	T45.0X2	T45.0X3	T45.0X4	T45.0X5	T45.0X6
Pirarubicin	T45.1X1	T45.1X2	T45.1X3	T45.1X4	T45.1X5	T45.1X6
Pirazinamide	T37.1X1	T37.1X2	T37.1X3	T37.1X4	T37.1X5	T37.1X6
Pirbuterol	T48.6X1	T48.6X2	T48.6X3	T48.6X4	T48.6X5	T48.6X6
Pirenzepine	T47.1X1	T47.1X2	T47.1X3	T47.1X4	T47.1X5	T47.1X6
Piretanide	T50.1X1	T50.1X2	T50.1X3	T50.1X4	T50.1X5	T50.1X6
Piribedil	T42.8X1	T42.8X2	T42.8X3	T42.8X4	T42.8X5	T42.8X6
Piridoxilate	T46.3X1	T46.3X2	T46.3X3	T46.3X4	T46.3X5	T46.3X6
Piritramide	T40.4X1	T40.4X2	T40.4X3	T40.4X4	—	—
Piromidic acid	T37.8X1	T37.8X2	T37.8X3	T37.8X4	T37.8X5	T37.8X6
Piroxicam	T39.391	T39.392	T39.393	T39.394	T39.395	T39.396
beta-cyclodextrin complex	T39.8X1	T39.8X2	T39.8X3	T39.8X4	T39.8X5	T39.8X6
Pirozadil	T46.6X1	T46.6X2	T46.6X3	T46.6X4	T46.6X5	T46.6X6
Piscidia (bark) (erythrina)	T39.8X1	T39.8X2	T39.8X3	T39.8X4	T39.8X5	T39.8X6
Pitch	T65.891	T65.892	T65.893	T65.894	—	—
Pitkin's solution	T41.3X1	T41.3X2	T41.3X3	T41.3X4	T41.3X5	T41.3X6
Pitocin	T48.0X1	T48.0X2	T48.0X3	T48.0X4	T48.0X5	T48.0X6
Pitressin (tannate)	T38.891	T38.892	T38.893	T38.894	T38.895	T38.896
Pituitary extracts (posterior)	T38.891	T38.892	T38.893	T38.894	T38.895	T38.896
anterior	T38.811	T38.812	T38.813	T38.814	T38.815	T38.816
Pituitrin	T38.891	T38.892	T38.893	T38.894	T38.895	T38.896
Pivampicillin	T36.0X1	T36.0X2	T36.0X3	T36.0X4	T36.0X5	T36.0X6
Pivmecillinam	T36.0X1	T36.0X2	T36.0X3	T36.0X4	T36.0X5	T36.0X6
Placental hormone	T38.891	T38.892	T38.893	T38.894	T38.895	T38.896
Placidyl	T42.6X1	T42.6X2	T42.6X3	T42.6X4	T42.6X5	T42.6X6
Plague vaccine	T50.A91	T50.A92	T50.A93	T50.A94	T50.A95	T50.A96
Plant						
food or fertilizer NEC	T65.891	T65.892	T65.893	T65.894	—	—
containing herbicide	T60.3X1	T60.3X2	T60.3X3	T60.3X4	—	—
noxious, used as food	T62.2X1	T62.2X2	T62.2X3	T62.2X4	—	—
berries	T62.1X1	T62.1X2	T62.1X3	T62.1X4	—	—
seeds	T62.2X1	T62.2X2	T62.2X3	T62.2X4	—	—
specified type NEC	T62.2X1	T62.2X2	T62.2X3	T62.2X4	—	—
Plasma	T45.8X1	T45.8X2	T45.8X3	T45.8X4	T45.8X5	T45.8X6
expander NEC	T45.8X1	T45.8X2	T45.8X3	T45.8X4	T45.8X5	T45.8X6

Additional Character May Be Required — Refer to the Tabular List for Character Selection

▽ Subterms under main terms may continue to next column or page

Phenol — Plasma

Substance	Poisoning, Accidental (unintentional)	Poisoning, Intentional Self-harm	Poisoning, Assault	Poisoning, Undetermined	Adverse Effect	Under-dosing
Plasma — continued						
protein fraction (human)	T45.8X1	T45.8X2	T45.8X3	T45.8X4	T45.8X5	T45.8X6
Plasmanate	T45.8X1	T45.8X2	T45.8X3	T45.8X4	T45.8X5	T45.8X6
Plasminogen (tissue)	T45.611	T45.612	T45.613	T45.614	T45.615	T45.616
activator						
Plaster dressing	T49.3X1	T49.3X2	T49.3X3	T49.3X4	T49.3X5	T49.3X6
Plastic dressing	T49.3X1	T49.3X2	T49.3X3	T49.3X4	T49.3X5	T49.3X6
Plegicil	T43.3X1	T43.3X2	T43.3X3	T43.3X4	T43.3X5	T43.3X6
Plicamycin	T45.1X1	T45.1X2	T45.1X3	T45.1X4	T45.1X5	T45.1X6
Podophyllotoxin	T49.8X1	T49.8X2	T49.8X3	T49.8X4	T49.8X5	T49.8X6
Podophyllum (resin)	T49.4X1	T49.4X2	T49.4X3	T49.4X4	T49.4X5	T49.4X6
Poisonous berries	T62.1X1	T62.1X2	T62.1X3	T62.1X4	—	—
Poison NEC	T65.91	T65.92	T65.93	T65.94	—	—
Pokeweed (any part)	T62.2X1	T62.2X2	T62.2X3	T62.2X4	—	—
Poldine metilsulfate	T44.3X1	T44.3X2	T44.3X3	T44.3X4	T44.3X5	T44.3X6
Polidexide (sulfate)	T46.6X1	T46.6X2	T46.6X3	T46.6X4	T46.6X5	T46.6X6
Polidocanol	T46.8X1	T46.8X2	T46.8X3	T46.8X4	T46.8X5	T46.8X6
Poliomyelitis vaccine	T50.B91	T50.B92	T50.B93	T50.B94	T50.B95	T50.B96
Polish (car) (floor) (furniture)	T65.891	T65.892	T65.893	T65.894	—	—
(metal) (porcelain) (silver)						
abrasive	T65.891	T65.892	T65.893	T65.894	—	—
porcelain	T65.891	T65.892	T65.893	T65.894	—	—
Poloxalkol	T47.4X1	T47.4X2	T47.4X3	T47.4X4	T47.4X5	T47.4X6
Poloxamer	T47.4X1	T47.4X2	T47.4X3	T47.4X4	T47.4X5	T47.4X6
Polyaminostyrene resins	T50.3X1	T50.3X2	T50.3X3	T50.3X4	T50.3X5	T50.3X6
Polycarbophil	T47.4X1	T47.4X2	T47.4X3	T47.4X4	T47.4X5	T47.4X6
Polychlorinated biphenyl	T65.891	T65.892	T65.893	T65.894	—	—
Polycycline	T36.4X1	T36.4X2	T36.4X3	T36.4X4	T36.4X5	T36.4X6
Polyester fumes	T59.891	T59.892	T59.893	T59.894	—	—
Polyester resin hardener	T52.91	T52.92	T52.93	T52.94	—	—
fumes	T59.891	T59.892	T59.893	T59.894	—	—
Polyestradiol phosphate	T38.5X1	T38.5X2	T38.5X3	T38.5X4	T38.5X5	T38.5X6
Polyethanolamine alkyl sulfate	T49.2X1	T49.2X2	T49.2X3	T49.2X4	T49.2X5	T49.2X6
Polyethylene adhesive	T49.3X1	T49.3X2	T49.3X3	T49.3X4	T49.3X5	T49.3X6
Polyferose	T45.4X1	T45.4X2	T45.4X3	T45.4X4	T45.4X5	T45.4X6
Polygeline	T45.8X1	T45.8X2	T45.8X3	T45.8X4	T45.8X5	T45.8X6
Polymyxin	T36.8X1	T36.8X2	T36.8X3	T36.8X4	T36.8X5	T36.8X6
B	T36.8X1	T36.8X2	T36.8X3	T36.8X4	T36.8X5	T36.8X6
ENT agent	T49.6X1	T49.6X2	T49.6X3	T49.6X4	T49.6X5	T49.6X6
ophthalmic preparation	T49.5X1	T49.5X2	T49.5X3	T49.5X4	T49.5X5	T49.5X6
topical NEC	T49.0X1	T49.0X2	T49.0X3	T49.0X4	T49.0X5	T49.0X6
E sulfate (eye preparation)	T49.5X1	T49.5X2	T49.5X3	T49.5X4	T49.5X5	T49.5X6
Polynoxylin	T49.0X1	T49.0X2	T49.0X3	T49.0X4	T49.0X5	T49.0X6
Polyoestradiol phosphate	T38.5X1	T38.5X2	T38.5X3	T38.5X4	T38.5X5	T38.5X6
Polyoxymethyleneurea	T49.0X1	T49.0X2	T49.0X3	T49.0X4	T49.0X5	T49.0X6
Polysilane	T47.8X1	T47.8X2	T47.8X3	T47.8X4	T47.8X5	T47.8X6
Polytetrafluoroethylene (inhaled)	T59.891	T59.892	T59.893	T59.894	—	—
Polythiazide	T50.2X1	T50.2X2	T50.2X3	T50.2X4	T50.2X5	T50.2X6
Polyvidone	T45.8X1	T45.8X2	T45.8X3	T45.8X4	T45.8X5	T45.8X6
Polyvinylpyrrolidone	T45.8X1	T45.8X2	T45.8X3	T45.8X4	T45.8X5	T45.8X6
Pontocaine (hydrochloride) (infiltration) (topical)	T41.3X1	T41.3X2	T41.3X3	T41.3X4	T41.3X5	T41.3X6
nerve block (peripheral) (plexus)	T41.3X1	T41.3X2	T41.3X3	T41.3X4	T41.3X5	T41.3X6
spinal	T41.3X1	T41.3X2	T41.3X3	T41.3X4	T41.3X5	T41.3X6
Porfiromycin	T45.1X1	T45.1X2	T45.1X3	T45.1X4	T45.1X5	T45.1X6
Posterior pituitary hormone NEC	T38.891	T38.892	T38.893	T38.894	T38.895	T38.896
Pot	T40.7X1	T40.7X2	T40.7X3	T40.7X4	T40.7X5	T40.7X6
Potash (caustic)	T54.3X1	T54.3X2	T54.3X3	T54.3X4	—	—
Potassic saline injection (lactated)	T50.3X1	T50.3X2	T50.3X3	T50.3X4	T50.3X5	T50.3X6
Potassium-removing resin	T50.3X1	T50.3X2	T50.3X3	T50.3X4	T50.3X5	T50.3X6
Potassium-retaining drug	T50.3X1	T50.3X2	T50.3X3	T50.3X4	T50.3X5	T50.3X6
Potassium (salts) NEC	T50.3X1	T50.3X2	T50.3X3	T50.3X4	T50.3X5	T50.3X6
aminobenzoate	T45.8X1	T45.8X2	T45.8X3	T45.8X4	T45.8X5	T45.8X6
aminosalicylate	T37.1X1	T37.1X2	T37.1X3	T37.1X4	T37.1X5	T37.1X6
antimony ' tartrate'	T37.8X1	T37.8X2	T37.8X3	T37.8X4	T37.8X5	T37.8X6
arsenite (solution)	T57.0X1	T57.0X2	T57.0X3	T57.0X4	—	—
bichromate	T56.2X1	T56.2X2	T56.2X3	T56.2X4	—	—
bisulfate	T47.3X1	T47.3X2	T47.3X3	T47.3X4	T47.3X5	T47.3X6
bromide	T42.6X1	T42.6X2	T42.6X3	T42.6X4	T42.6X5	T42.6X6
canrenoate	T50.0X1	T50.0X2	T50.0X3	T50.0X4	T50.0X5	T50.0X6
carbonate	T54.3X1	T54.3X2	T54.3X3	T54.3X4	—	—
chlorate NEC	T65.891	T65.892	T65.893	T65.894	—	—
chloride	T50.3X1	T50.3X2	T50.3X3	T50.3X4	T50.3X5	T50.3X6
citrate	T50.991	T50.992	T50.993	T50.994	T50.995	T50.996
cyanide	T65.0X1	T65.0X2	T65.0X3	T65.0X4	—	—
ferric hexacyanoferrate (medicinal)	T50.6X1	T50.6X2	T50.6X3	T50.6X4	T50.6X5	T50.6X6
nonmedicinal	T65.891	T65.892	T65.893	T65.894	—	—

Substance	Poisoning, Accidental (unintentional)	Poisoning, Intentional Self-harm	Poisoning, Assault	Poisoning, Undetermined	Adverse Effect	Under-dosing
Potassium (salts) NEC — continued						
Fluoride	T57.8X1	T57.8X2	T57.8X3	T57.8X4	—	—
glucaldrate	T47.1X1	T47.1X2	T47.1X3	T47.1X4	T47.1X5	T47.1X6
hydroxide	T54.3X1	T54.3X2	T54.3X3	T54.3X4	—	—
iodate	T49.0X1	T49.0X2	T49.0X3	T49.0X4	T49.0X5	T49.0X6
iodide	T48.4X1	T48.4X2	T48.4X3	T48.4X4	T48.4X5	T48.4X6
nitrate	T57.8X1	T57.8X2	T57.8X3	T57.8X4	—	—
oxalate	T65.891	T65.892	T65.893	T65.894	—	—
perchlorate (nonmedicinal) NEC	T65.891	T65.892	T65.893	T65.894	—	—
antithyroid	T38.2X1	T38.2X2	T38.2X3	T38.2X4	T38.2X5	T38.2X6
medicinal	T38.2X1	T38.2X2	T38.2X3	T38.2X4	T38.2X5	T38.2X6
Permanganate (nonmedicinal)	T65.891	T65.892	T65.893	T65.894	—	—
medicinal	T49.0X1	T49.0X2	T49.0X3	T49.0X4	T49.0X5	T49.0X6
sulfate	T47.2X1	T47.2X2	T47.2X3	T47.2X4	T47.2X5	T47.2X6
Povidone	T45.8X1	T45.8X2	T45.8X3	T45.8X4	T45.8X5	T45.8X6
iodine	T49.0X1	T49.0X2	T49.0X3	T49.0X4	T49.0X5	T49.0X6
Practolol	T44.7X1	T44.7X2	T44.7X3	T44.7X4	T44.7X5	T44.7X6
Prajmalium bitartrate	T46.2X1	T46.2X2	T46.2X3	T46.2X4	T46.2X5	T46.2X6
Pralidoxime (iodide)	T50.6X1	T50.6X2	T50.6X3	T50.6X4	T50.6X5	T50.6X6
chloride	T50.6X1	T50.6X2	T50.6X3	T50.6X4	T50.6X5	T50.6X6
Pramiverine	T44.3X1	T44.3X2	T44.3X3	T44.3X4	T44.3X5	T44.3X6
Pramocaine	T49.1X1	T49.1X2	T49.1X3	T49.1X4	T49.1X5	T49.1X6
Pramoxine	T49.1X1	T49.1X2	T49.1X3	T49.1X4	T49.1X5	T49.1X6
Prasterone	T38.7X1	T38.7X2	T38.7X3	T38.7X4	T38.7X5	T38.7X6
Pravastatin	T46.6X1	T46.6X2	T46.6X3	T46.6X4	T46.6X5	T46.6X6
Prazepam	T42.4X1	T42.4X2	T42.4X3	T42.4X4	T42.4X5	T42.4X6
Praziquantel	T37.4X1	T37.4X2	T37.4X3	T37.4X4	T37.4X5	T37.4X6
Prazitone	T43.291	T43.292	T43.293	T43.294	T43.295	T43.296
Prazosin	T44.6X1	T44.6X2	T44.6X3	T44.6X4	T44.6X5	T44.6X6
Prednicarbate	T49.0X1	T49.0X2	T49.0X3	T49.0X4	T49.0X5	T49.0X6
Prednimustine	T45.1X1	T45.1X2	T45.1X3	T45.1X4	T45.1X5	T45.1X6
Prednisolone	T38.0X1	T38.0X2	T38.0X3	T38.0X4	T38.0X5	T38.0X6
ENT agent	T49.6X1	T49.6X2	T49.6X3	T49.6X4	T49.6X5	T49.6X6
ophthalmic preparation	T49.5X1	T49.5X2	T49.5X3	T49.5X4	T49.5X5	T49.5X6
steaglate	T49.0X1	T49.0X2	T49.0X3	T49.0X4	T49.0X5	T49.0X6
topical NEC	T49.0X1	T49.0X2	T49.0X3	T49.0X4	T49.0X5	T49.0X6
Prednisone	T38.0X1	T38.0X2	T38.0X3	T38.0X4	T38.0X5	T38.0X6
Prednylidene	T38.0X1	T38.0X2	T38.0X3	T38.0X4	T38.0X5	T38.0X6
Pregnandiol	T38.5X1	T38.5X2	T38.5X3	T38.5X4	T38.5X5	T38.5X6
Pregneninolone	T38.5X1	T38.5X2	T38.5X3	T38.5X4	T38.5X5	T38.5X6
Preludin	T43.691	T43.692	T43.693	T43.694	T43.695	T43.696
Premarin	T38.5X1	T38.5X2	T38.5X3	T38.5X4	T38.5X5	T38.5X6
Premedication anesthetic	T41.201	T41.202	T41.203	T41.204	T41.205	T41.206
Prenalterol	T44.5X1	T44.5X2	T44.5X3	T44.5X4	T44.5X5	T44.5X6
Prenoxdiazine	T48.3X1	T48.3X2	T48.3X3	T48.3X4	T48.3X5	T48.3X6
Prenylamine	T46.3X1	T46.3X2	T46.3X3	T46.3X4	T46.3X5	T46.3X6
Preparation H	T49.8X1	T49.8X2	T49.8X3	T49.8X4	T49.8X5	T49.8X6
Preparation, local	T49.4X1	T49.4X2	T49.4X3	T49.4X4	T49.4X5	T49.4X6
Preservative (nonmedicinal)	T65.891	T65.892	T65.893	T65.894	—	—
medicinal	T50.901	T50.902	T50.903	T50.904	T50.905	T50.906
wood	T60.91	T60.92	T60.93	T60.94	—	—
Prethcamide	T50.7X1	T50.7X2	T50.7X3	T50.7X4	T50.7X5	T50.7X6
Pride of China	T62.2X1	T62.2X2	T62.2X3	T62.2X4	—	—
Pridinol	T44.3X1	T44.3X2	T44.3X3	T44.3X4	T44.3X5	T44.3X6
Prifinium bromide	T44.3X1	T44.3X2	T44.3X3	T44.3X4	T44.3X5	T44.3X6
Prilocaine	T41.3X1	T41.3X2	T41.3X3	T41.3X4	T41.3X5	T41.3X6
infiltration (subcutaneous)	T41.3X1	T41.3X2	T41.3X3	T41.3X4	T41.3X5	T41.3X6
nerve block (peripheral) (plexus)	T41.3X1	T41.3X2	T41.3X3	T41.3X4	T41.3X5	T41.3X6
regional	T41.3X1	T41.3X2	T41.3X3	T41.3X4	T41.3X5	T41.3X6
Primaquine	T37.2X1	T37.2X2	T37.2X3	T37.2X4	T37.2X5	T37.2X6
Primidone	T42.6X1	T42.6X2	T42.6X3	T42.6X4	T42.6X5	T42.6X6
Primula (veris)	T62.2X1	T62.2X2	T62.2X3	T62.2X4	—	—
Prinadol	T40.2X1	T40.2X2	T40.2X3	T40.2X4	T40.2X5	T40.2X6
Priscol, Priscoline	T44.6X1	T44.6X2	T44.6X3	T44.6X4	T44.6X5	T44.6X6
Pristinamycin	T36.3X1	T36.3X2	T36.3X3	T36.3X4	T36.3X5	T36.3X6
Privet	T62.2X1	T62.2X2	T62.2X3	T62.2X4	—	—
berries	T62.1X1	T62.1X2	T62.1X3	T62.1X4	—	—
Privine	T44.4X1	T44.4X2	T44.4X3	T44.4X4	T44.4X5	T44.4X6
Pro-Banthine	T44.3X1	T44.3X2	T44.3X3	T44.3X4	T44.3X5	T44.3X6
Probarbital	T42.3X1	T42.3X2	T42.3X3	T42.3X4	T42.3X5	T42.3X6
Probenecid	T50.4X1	T50.4X2	T50.4X3	T50.4X4	T50.4X5	T50.4X6
Probucol	T46.6X1	T46.6X2	T46.6X3	T46.6X4	T46.6X5	T46.6X6
Procainamide	T46.2X1	T46.2X2	T46.2X3	T46.2X4	T46.2X5	T46.2X6
Procaine	T41.3X1	T41.3X2	T41.3X3	T41.3X4	T41.3X5	T41.3X6
benzylpenicillin	T36.0X1	T36.0X2	T36.0X3	T36.0X4	T36.0X5	T36.0X6
nerve block (peripheral) (plexus)	T41.3X1	T41.3X2	T41.3X3	T41.3X4	T41.3X5	T41.3X6
penicillin G	T36.0X1	T36.0X2	T36.0X3	T36.0X4	T36.0X5	T36.0X6
regional	T41.3X1	T41.3X2	T41.3X3	T41.3X4	T41.3X5	T41.3X6

Substance	Poisoning, Accidental (unintentional)	Poisoning, Intentional Self-harm	Poisoning, Assault	Poisoning, Undetermined	Adverse Effect	Under-dosing
Procaine — continued						
spinal	T41.3X1	T41.3X2	T41.3X3	T41.3X4	T41.3X5	T41.3X6
Procalmidol	T43.591	T43.592	T43.593	T43.594	T43.595	T43.596
Procarbazine	T45.1X1	T45.1X2	T45.1X3	T45.1X4	T45.1X5	T45.1X6
Procaterol	T44.5X1	T44.5X2	T44.5X3	T44.5X4	T44.5X5	T44.5X6
Prochlorperazine	T43.3X1	T43.3X2	T43.3X3	T43.3X4	T43.3X5	T43.3X6
Procyclidine	T44.3X1	T44.3X2	T44.3X3	T44.3X4	T44.3X5	T44.3X6
Producer gas	T58.8X1	T58.8X2	T58.8X3	T58.8X4	—	—
Profadol	T40.4X1	T40.4X2	T40.4X3	T40.4X4	T40.4X5	T40.4X6
Profenamine	T44.3X1	T44.3X2	T44.3X3	T44.3X4	T44.3X5	T44.3X6
Profenil	T44.3X1	T44.3X2	T44.3X3	T44.3X4	T44.3X5	T44.3X6
Proflavine	T49.0X1	T49.0X2	T49.0X3	T49.0X4	T49.0X5	T49.0X6
Progabide	T42.6X1	T42.6X2	T42.6X3	T42.6X4	T42.6X5	T42.6X6
Progesterone	T38.5X1	T38.5X2	T38.5X3	T38.5X4	T38.5X5	T38.5X6
Progestin	T38.5X1	T38.5X2	T38.5X3	T38.5X4	T38.5X5	T38.5X6
oral contraceptive	T38.4X1	T38.4X2	T38.4X3	T38.4X4	T38.4X5	T38.4X6
Progestogen NEC	T38.5X1	T38.5X2	T38.5X3	T38.5X4	T38.5X5	T38.5X6
Progestone	T38.5X1	T38.5X2	T38.5X3	T38.5X4	T38.5X5	T38.5X6
Proglumide	T47.1X1	T47.1X2	T47.1X3	T47.1X4	T47.1X5	T47.1X6
Proguanil	T37.2X1	T37.2X2	T37.2X3	T37.2X4	T37.2X5	T37.2X6
Prolactin	T38.811	T38.812	T38.813	T38.814	T38.815	T38.816
Prolintane	T43.691	T43.692	T43.693	T43.694	T43.695	T43.696
Proloid	T38.1X1	T38.1X2	T38.1X3	T38.1X4	T38.1X5	T38.1X6
Proluton	T38.5X1	T38.5X2	T38.5X3	T38.5X4	T38.5X5	T38.5X6
Promacetin	T37.1X1	T37.1X2	T37.1X3	T37.1X4	T37.1X5	T37.1X6
Promazine	T43.3X1	T43.3X2	T43.3X3	T43.3X4	T43.3X5	T43.3X6
Promedol	T40.2X1	T40.2X2	T40.2X3	T40.2X4	—	—
Promegestone	T38.5X1	T38.5X2	T38.5X3	T38.5X4	T38.5X5	T38.5X6
Promethazine (teoclate)	T43.3X1	T43.3X2	T43.3X3	T43.3X4	T43.3X5	T43.3X6
Promin	T37.1X1	T37.1X2	T37.1X3	T37.1X4	T37.1X5	T37.1X6
Pronase	T45.3X1	T45.3X2	T45.3X3	T45.3X4	T45.3X5	T45.3X6
Pronestyl (hydrochloride)	T46.2X1	T46.2X2	T46.2X3	T46.2X4	T46.2X5	T46.2X6
Pronetalol	T44.7X1	T44.7X2	T44.7X3	T44.7X4	T44.7X5	T44.7X6
Prontosil	T37.0X1	T37.0X2	T37.0X3	T37.0X4	T37.0X5	T37.0X6
Propachlor	T60.3X1	T60.3X2	T60.3X3	T60.3X4		
Propafenone	T46.2X1	T46.2X2	T46.2X3	T46.2X4	T46.2X5	T46.2X6
Propallylonal	T42.3X1	T42.3X2	T42.3X3	T42.3X4	T42.3X5	T42.3X6
Propamidine	T49.0X1	T49.0X2	T49.0X3	T49.0X4	T49.0X5	T49.0X6
Propane (distributed in mobile container)	T59.891	T59.892	T59.893	T59.894		
distributed through pipes	T59.891	T59.892	T59.893	T59.894	—	—
incomplete combustion	T58.11	T58.12	T58.13	T58.14	—	—
Propanidid	T41.291	T41.292	T41.293	T41.294	T41.295	T41.296
Propanil	T60.3X1	T60.3X2	T60.3X3	T60.3X4	—	—
Propantheline	T44.3X1	T44.3X2	T44.3X3	T44.3X4	T44.3X5	T44.3X6
bromide	T44.3X1	T44.3X2	T44.3X3	T44.3X4	T44.3X5	T44.3X6
Proparacaine	T41.3X1	T41.3X2	T41.3X3	T41.3X4	T41.3X5	T41.3X6
Propatylnitrate	T46.3X1	T46.3X2	T46.3X3	T46.3X4	T46.3X5	T46.3X6
Propicillin	T36.0X1	T36.0X2	T36.0X3	T36.0X4	T36.0X5	T36.0X6
Propiolactone	T49.0X1	T49.0X2	T49.0X3	T49.0X4	T49.0X5	T49.0X6
Propiomazine	T45.0X1	T45.0X2	T45.0X3	T45.0X4	T45.0X5	T45.0X6
Propionaidehyde (medicinal)	T42.6X1	T42.6X2	T42.6X3	T42.6X4	T42.6X5	T42.6X6
Propionate (calcium) (sodium)	T49.0X1	T49.0X2	T49.0X3	T49.0X4	T49.0X5	T49.0X6
Propion gel	T49.0X1	T49.0X2	T49.0X3	T49.0X4	T49.0X5	T49.0X6
Propitocaine	T41.3X1	T41.3X2	T41.3X3	T41.3X4	T41.3X5	T41.3X6
infiltration (subcutaneous)	T41.3X1	T41.3X2	T41.3X3	T41.3X4	T41.3X5	T41.3X6
nerve block (peripheral) (plexus)	T41.3X1	T41.3X2	T41.3X3	T41.3X4	T41.3X5	T41.3X6
Propofol	T41.291	T41.292	T41.293	T41.294	T41.295	T41.296
Propoxur	T60.0X1	T60.0X2	T60.0X3	T60.0X4	—	—
Propoxycaine	T41.3X1	T41.3X2	T41.3X3	T41.3X4	T41.3X5	T41.3X6
infiltration (subcutaneous)	T41.3X1	T41.3X2	T41.3X3	T41.3X4	T41.3X5	T41.3X6
nerve block (peripheral) (plexus)	T41.3X1	T41.3X2	T41.3X3	T41.3X4	T41.3X5	T41.3X6
topical (surface)	T41.3X1	T41.3X2	T41.3X3	T41.3X4	T41.3X5	T41.3X6
Propoxyphene	T40.4X1	T40.4X2	T40.4X3	T40.4X4	T40.4X5	T40.4X6
Propranolol	T44.7X1	T44.7X2	T44.7X3	T44.7X4	T44.7X5	T44.7X6
Propyl						
alcohol	T51.3X1	T51.3X2	T51.3X3	T51.3X4	—	—
carbinol	T51.3X1	T51.3X2	T51.3X3	T51.3X4	—	—
hexadrine	T44.4X1	T44.4X2	T44.4X3	T44.4X4	T44.4X5	T44.4X6
iodone	T50.8X1	T50.8X2	T50.8X3	T50.8X4	T50.8X5	T50.8X6
thiouracil	T38.2X1	T38.2X2	T38.2X3	T38.2X4	T38.2X5	T38.2X6
Propylaminophenothiazine	T43.3X1	T43.3X2	T43.3X3	T43.3X4	T43.3X5	T43.3X6
Propylene	T59.891	T59.892	T59.893	T59.894	—	—
Propylhexedrine	T48.5X1	T48.5X2	T48.5X3	T48.5X4	T48.5X5	T48.5X6
Propyliodone	T50.8X1	T50.8X2	T50.8X3	T50.8X4	T50.8X5	T50.8X6
Propylparaben (ophthalmic)	T49.5X1	T49.5X2	T49.5X3	T49.5X4	T49.5X5	T49.5X6
Propylthiouracil	T38.2X1	T38.2X2	T38.2X3	T38.2X4	T38.2X5	T38.2X6
Propyphenazone	T39.2X1	T39.2X2	T39.2X3	T39.2X4	T39.2X5	T39.2X6
Proquazone	T39.391	T39.392	T39.393	T39.394	T39.395	T39.396
Proscillaridin	T46.0X1	T46.0X2	T46.0X3	T46.0X4	T46.0X5	T46.0X6
Prostacyclin	T45.521	T45.522	T45.523	T45.524	T45.525	T45.526
Prostaglandin (I2)	T45.521	T45.522	T45.523	T45.524	T45.525	T45.526
E1	T46.7X1	T46.7X2	T46.7X3	T46.7X4	T46.7X5	T46.7X6
E2	T48.0X1	T48.0X2	T48.0X3	T48.0X4	T48.0X5	T48.0X6
F2 alpha	T48.0X1	T48.0X2	T48.0X3	T48.0X4	T48.0X5	T48.0X6
Prostigmin	T44.0X1	T44.0X2	T44.0X3	T44.0X4	T44.0X5	T44.0X6
Prosultiamine	T45.2X1	T45.2X2	T45.2X3	T45.2X4	T45.2X5	T45.2X6
Protamine sulfate	T45.7X1	T45.7X2	T45.7X3	T45.7X4	T45.7X5	T45.7X6
zinc insulin	T38.3X1	T38.3X2	T38.3X3	T38.3X4	T38.3X5	T38.3X6
Protease	T47.5X1	T47.5X2	T47.5X3	T47.5X4	T47.5X5	T47.5X6
Protectant, skin NEC	T49.3X1	T49.3X2	T49.3X3	T49.3X4	T49.3X5	T49.3X6
Protein hydrolysate	T50.991	T50.992	T50.993	T50.994	T50.995	T50.996
Prothiaden — see Dothiepin hydrochloride						
Prothionamide	T37.1X1	T37.1X2	T37.1X3	T37.1X4	T37.1X5	T37.1X6
Prothipendyl	T43.591	T43.592	T43.593	T43.594	T43.595	T43.596
Prothoate	T60.0X1	T60.0X2	T60.0X3	T60.0X4	—	—
Prothrombin						
activator	T45.7X1	T45.7X2	T45.7X3	T45.7X4	T45.7X5	T45.7X6
synthesis inhibitor	T45.511	T45.512	T45.513	T45.514	T45.515	T45.516
Protionamide	T37.1X1	T37.1X2	T37.1X3	T37.1X4	T37.1X5	T37.1X6
Protirelin	T38.891	T38.892	T38.893	T38.894	T38.895	T38.896
Protokylol	T48.6X1	T48.6X2	T48.6X3	T48.6X4	T48.6X5	T48.6X6
Protopam	T50.6X1	T50.6X2	T50.6X3	T50.6X4	T50.6X5	T50.6X6
Protoveratrine(s) (A) (B)	T46.5X1	T46.5X2	T46.5X3	T46.5X4	T46.5X5	T46.5X6
Protriptyline	T43.011	T43.012	T43.013	T43.014	T43.015	T43.016
Provera	T38.5X1	T38.5X2	T38.5X3	T38.5X4	T38.5X5	T38.5X6
Provitamin A	T45.2X1	T45.2X2	T45.2X3	T45.2X4	T45.2X5	T45.2X6
Proxibarbal	T42.3X1	T42.3X2	T42.3X3	T42.3X4	T42.3X5	T42.3X6
Proxymetacaine	T41.3X1	T41.3X2	T41.3X3	T41.3X4	T41.3X5	T41.3X6
Proxyphylline	T48.6X1	T48.6X2	T48.6X3	T48.6X4	T48.6X5	T48.6X6
Prozac — see Fluoxetine hydrochloride						
Prunus						
laurocerasus	T62.2X1	T62.2X2	T62.2X3	T62.2X4	—	—
virginiana	T62.2X1	T62.2X2	T62.2X3	T62.2X4	—	—
Prussian blue						
commercial	T65.891	T65.892	T65.893	T65.894	—	—
therapeutic	T50.6X1	T50.6X2	T50.6X3	T50.6X4	T50.6X5	T50.6X6
Prussic acid	T65.0X1	T65.0X2	T65.0X3	T65.0X4	—	—
vapor	T57.3X1	T57.3X2	T57.3X3	T57.3X4	—	—
Pseudoephedrine	T44.991	T44.992	T44.993	T44.994	T44.995	T44.996
Psilocin	T40.991	T40.992	T40.993	T40.994	—	—
Psilocybin	T40.991	T40.992	T40.993	T40.994	—	—
Psilocybine	T40.991	T40.992	T40.993	T40.994	—	—
Psoralene (nonmedicinal)	T65.891	T65.892	T65.893	T65.894	—	—
Psoralens (medicinal)	T50.991	T50.992	T50.993	T50.994	T50.995	T50.996
PSP (phenolsulfonphthalein)	T50.8X1	T50.8X2	T50.8X3	T50.8X4	T50.8X5	T50.8X6
Psychodysleptic drug NEC	T40.901	T40.902	T40.903	T40.904	T40.905	T40.906
Psychostimulant	T43.601	T43.602	T43.603	T43.604	T43.605	T43.606
amphetamine	T43.621	T43.622	T43.623	T43.624	T43.625	T43.626
caffeine	T43.611	T43.612	T43.613	T43.614	T43.615	T43.616
methylphenidate	T43.631	T43.632	T43.633	T43.634	T43.635	T43.636
specified NEC	T43.691	T43.692	T43.693	T43.694	T43.695	T43.696
Psychotherapeutic drug NEC	T43.91	T43.92	T43.93	T43.94	T43.95	T43.96
antidepressants — see also Antidepressant	T43.201	T43.202	T43.203	T43.204	T43.205	T43.206
specified NEC	T43.8X1	T43.8X2	T43.8X3	T43.8X4	T43.8X5	T43.8X6
tranquilizers NEC	T43.501	T43.502	T43.503	T43.504	T43.505	T43.506
Psychotomimetic agents	T40.901	T40.902	T40.903	T40.904	T40.905	T40.906
Psychotropic drug NEC	T43.91	T43.92	T43.93	T43.94	T43.95	T43.96
specified NEC	T43.8X1	T43.8X2	T43.8X3	T43.8X4	T43.8X5	T43.8X6
Psyllium hydrophilic mucilloid	T47.4X1	T47.4X2	T47.4X3	T47.4X4	T47.4X5	T47.4X6
Pteroylglutamic acid	T45.8X1	T45.8X2	T45.8X3	T45.8X4	T45.8X5	T45.8X6
Pteroyltriglutamate	T45.1X1	T45.1X2	T45.1X3	T45.1X4	T45.1X5	T45.1X6
PTFE — see Polytetrafluoroethylene						
Pulp						
devitalizing paste	T49.7X1	T49.7X2	T49.7X3	T49.7X4	T49.7X5	T49.7X6
dressing	T49.7X1	T49.7X2	T49.7X3	T49.7X4	T49.7X5	T49.7X6
Pulsatilla	T62.2X1	T62.2X2	T62.2X3	T62.2X4	—	—
Pumpkin seed extract	T37.4X1	T37.4X2	T37.4X3	T37.4X4	T37.4X5	T37.4X6
Purex (bleach)	T54.91	T54.92	T54.93	T54.94		
Purgative NEC — see also Cathartic	T47.4X1	T47.4X2	T47.4X3	T47.4X4	T47.4X5	T47.4X6
Purine analogue (antineoplastic)	T45.1X1	T45.1X2	T45.1X3	T45.1X4	T45.1X5	T45.1X6
Purine diuretics	T50.2X1	T50.2X2	T50.2X3	T50.2X4	T50.2X5	T50.2X6
Purinethol	T45.1X1	T45.1X2	T45.1X3	T45.1X4	T45.1X5	T45.1X6
PVP	T45.8X1	T45.8X2	T45.8X3	T45.8X4	T45.8X5	T45.8X6

Substance	Poisoning, Accidental (unintentional)	Poisoning, Intentional Self-harm	Poisoning, Assault	Poisoning, Undetermined	Adverse Effect	Under-dosing
Pyrabital	T39.8X1	T39.8X2	T39.8X3	T39.8X4	T39.8X5	T39.8X6
Pyramidon	T39.2X1	T39.2X2	T39.2X3	T39.2X4	T39.2X5	T39.2X6
Pyrantel	T37.4X1	T37.4X2	T37.4X3	T37.4X4	T37.4X5	T37.4X6
Pyrathiazine	T45.0X1	T45.0X2	T45.0X3	T45.0X4	T45.0X5	T45.0X6
Pyrazinamide	T37.1X1	T37.1X2	T37.1X3	T37.1X4	T37.1X5	T37.1X6
Pyrazinoic acid (amide)	T37.1X1	T37.1X2	T37.1X3	T37.1X4	T37.1X5	T37.1X6
Pyrazole (derivatives)	T39.2X1	T39.2X2	T39.2X3	T39.2X4	T39.2X5	T39.2X6
Pyrazolone analgesic NEC	T39.2X1	T39.2X2	T39.2X3	T39.2X4	T39.2X5	T39.2X6
Pyrethrin, pyrethrum (nonmedicinal)	T60.2X1	T60.2X2	T60.2X3	T60.2X4	—	—
Pyrethrum extract	T49.0X1	T49.0X2	T49.0X3	T49.0X4	T49.0X5	T49.0X6
Pyribenzamine	T45.0X1	T45.0X2	T45.0X3	T45.0X4	T45.0X5	T45.0X6
Pyridine	T52.8X1	T52.8X2	T52.8X3	T52.8X4		
aldoxime methiodide	T50.6X1	T50.6X2	T50.6X3	T50.6X4	T50.6X5	T50.6X6
aldoxime methyl chloride	T50.6X1	T50.6X2	T50.6X3	T50.6X4	T50.6X5	T50.6X6
vapor	T59.891	T59.892	T59.893	T59.894	—	—
Pyridium	T39.8X1	T39.8X2	T39.8X3	T39.8X4	T39.8X5	T39.8X6
Pyridostigmine bromide	T44.0X1	T44.0X2	T44.0X3	T44.0X4	T44.0X5	T44.0X6
Pyridoxal phosphate	T45.2X1	T45.2X2	T45.2X3	T45.2X4	T45.2X5	T45.2X6
Pyridoxine	T45.2X1	T45.2X2	T45.2X3	T45.2X4	T45.2X5	T45.2X6
Pyrilamine	T45.0X1	T45.0X2	T45.0X3	T45.0X4	T45.0X5	T45.0X6
Pyrimethamine	T37.2X1	T37.2X2	T37.2X3	T37.2X4	T37.2X5	T37.2X6
with sulfadoxine	T37.2X1	T37.2X2	T37.2X3	T37.2X4	T37.2X5	T37.2X6
Pyrimidine antagonist	T45.1X1	T45.1X2	T45.1X3	T45.1X4	T45.1X5	T45.1X6
Pyriminil	T60.4X1	T60.4X2	T60.4X3	T60.4X4	—	—
Pyrithione zinc	T49.4X1	T49.4X2	T49.4X3	T49.4X4	T49.4X5	T49.4X6
Pyrithyldione	T42.6X1	T42.6X2	T42.6X3	T42.6X4	T42.6X5	T42.6X6
Pyrogallic acid	T49.0X1	T49.0X2	T49.0X3	T49.0X4	T49.0X5	T49.0X6
Pyrogallol	T49.0X1	T49.0X2	T49.0X3	T49.0X4	T49.0X5	T49.0X6
Pyroxylin	T49.3X1	T49.3X2	T49.3X3	T49.3X4	T49.3X5	T49.3X6
Pyrrobutamine	T45.0X1	T45.0X2	T45.0X3	T45.0X4	T45.0X5	T45.0X6
Pyrrolizidine alkaloids	T62.8X1	T62.8X2	T62.8X3	T62.8X4	—	—
Pyrvinium chloride	T37.4X1	T37.4X2	T37.4X3	T37.4X4	T37.4X5	T37.4X6
PZI	T38.3X1	T38.3X2	T38.3X3	T38.3X4	T38.3X5	T38.3X6
Quaalude	T42.6X1	T42.6X2	T42.6X3	T42.6X4	T42.6X5	T42.6X6
Quarternary ammonium						
anti-infective	T49.0X1	T49.0X2	T49.0X3	T49.0X4	T49.0X5	T49.0X6
ganglion blocking	T44.2X1	T44.2X2	T44.2X3	T44.2X4	T44.2X5	T44.2X6
parasympatholytic	T44.3X1	T44.3X2	T44.3X3	T44.3X4	T44.3X5	T44.3X6
Quazepam	T42.4X1	T42.4X2	T42.4X3	T42.4X4	T42.4X5	T42.4X6
Quicklime	T54.3X1	T54.3X2	T54.3X3	T54.3X4	—	—
Quillaja extract	T48.4X1	T48.4X2	T48.4X3	T48.4X4	T48.4X5	T48.4X6
Quinacrine	T37.2X1	T37.2X2	T37.2X3	T37.2X4	T37.2X5	T37.2X6
Quinaglute	T46.2X1	T46.2X2	T46.2X3	T46.2X4	T46.2X5	T46.2X6
Quinalbarbital	T42.3X1	T42.3X2	T42.3X3	T42.3X4	T42.3X5	T42.3X6
Quinalbarbitone sodium	T42.3X1	T42.3X2	T42.3X3	T42.3X4	T42.3X5	T42.3X6
Quinalphos	T60.0X1	T60.0X2	T60.0X3	T60.0X4	—	—
Quinapril	T46.4X1	T46.4X2	T46.4X3	T46.4X4	T46.4X5	T46.4X6
Quinestradiol	T38.5X1	T38.5X2	T38.5X3	T38.5X4	T38.5X5	T38.5X6
Quinestradol	T38.5X1	T38.5X2	T38.5X3	T38.5X4	T38.5X5	T38.5X6
Quinestrol	T38.5X1	T38.5X2	T38.5X3	T38.5X4	T38.5X5	T38.5X6
Quinethazone	T50.2X1	T50.2X2	T50.2X3	T50.2X4	T50.2X5	T50.2X6
Quingestanol	T38.4X1	T38.4X2	T38.4X3	T38.4X4	T38.4X5	T38.4X6
Quinidine	T46.2X1	T46.2X2	T46.2X3	T46.2X4	T46.2X5	T46.2X6
Quinine	T37.2X1	T37.2X2	T37.2X3	T37.2X4	T37.2X5	T37.2X6
Quiniobine	T37.8X1	T37.8X2	T37.8X3	T37.8X4	T37.8X5	T37.8X6
Quinisocaine	T49.1X1	T49.1X2	T49.1X3	T49.1X4	T49.1X5	T49.1X6
Quinocide	T37.2X1	T37.2X2	T37.2X3	T37.2X4	T37.2X5	T37.2X6
Quinoline (derivatives) NEC	T37.8X1	T37.8X2	T37.8X3	T37.8X4	T37.8X5	T37.8X6
Quinupramine	T43.011	T43.012	T43.013	T43.014	T43.015	T43.016
Quotane	T41.3X1	T41.3X2	T41.3X3	T41.3X4	T41.3X5	T41.3X6
Rabies						
immune globulin (human)	T50.Z11	T50.Z12	T50.Z13	T50.Z14	T50.Z15	T50.Z16
vaccine	T50.B91	T50.B92	T50.B93	T50.B94	T50.B95	T50.B96
Racemoramide	T40.2X1	T40.2X2	T40.2X3	T40.2X4	—	—
Racemorphan	T40.2X1	T40.2X2	T40.2X3	T40.2X4	T40.2X5	T40.2X6
Racepinefrin	T44.5X1	T44.5X2	T44.5X3	T44.5X4	T44.5X5	T44.5X6
Raclopride	T43.591	T43.592	T43.593	T43.594	T43.595	T43.596
Radiator alcohol	T51.1X1	T51.1X2	T51.1X3	T51.1X4	—	—
Radioactive drug NEC	T50.8X1	T50.8X2	T50.8X3	T50.8X4	T50.8X5	T50.8X6
Radio-opaque (drugs) (materials)	T50.8X1	T50.8X2	T50.8X3	T50.8X4	T50.8X5	T50.8X6
Ramifenazone	T39.2X1	T39.2X2	T39.2X3	T39.2X4	T39.2X5	T39.2X6
Ramipril	T46.4X1	T46.4X2	T46.4X3	T46.4X4	T46.4X5	T46.4X6
Ranitidine	T47.0X1	T47.0X2	T47.0X3	T47.0X4	T47.0X5	T47.0X6
Ranunculus	T62.2X1	T62.2X2	T62.2X3	T62.2X4	—	—
Rat poison NEC	T60.4X1	T60.4X2	T60.4X3	T60.4X4	—	—
Rattlesnake (venom)	T63.011	T63.012	T63.013	T63.014	—	—
Raubasine	T46.7X1	T46.7X2	T46.7X3	T46.7X4	T46.7X5	T46.7X6
Raudixin	T46.5X1	T46.5X2	T46.5X3	T46.5X4	T46.5X5	T46.5X6
Rautensin	T46.5X1	T46.5X2	T46.5X3	T46.5X4	T46.5X5	T46.5X6
Rautina	T46.5X1	T46.5X2	T46.5X3	T46.5X4	T46.5X5	T46.5X6
Rautotal	T46.5X1	T46.5X2	T46.5X3	T46.5X4	T46.5X5	T46.5X6

Substance	Poisoning, Accidental (unintentional)	Poisoning, Intentional Self-harm	Poisoning, Assault	Poisoning, Undetermined	Adverse Effect	Under-dosing
Rauwiloid	T46.5X1	T46.5X2	T46.5X3	T46.5X4	T46.5X5	T46.5X6
Rauwoldin	T46.5X1	T46.5X2	T46.5X3	T46.5X4	T46.5X5	T46.5X6
Rauwolfia (alkaloids)	T46.5X1	T46.5X2	T46.5X3	T46.5X4	T46.5X5	T46.5X6
Razoxane	T45.1X1	T45.1X2	T45.1X3	T45.1X4	T45.1X5	T45.1X6
Realgar	T57.0X1	T57.0X2	T57.0X3	T57.0X4	—	—
Recombinant (R) — see specific protein						
Red blood cells, packed	T45.8X1	T45.8X2	T45.8X3	T45.8X4	T45.8X5	T45.8X6
Red squill (scilliroside)	T60.4X1	T60.4X2	T60.4X3	T60.4X4	—	—
Reducing agent, industrial NEC	T65.891	T65.892	T65.893	T65.894		
Refrigerant gas (chlorofluorocarbon)	T53.5X1	T53.5X2	T53.5X3	T53.5X4	—	—
not chlorofluorocarbon	T59.891	T59.892	T59.893	T59.894	—	—
Regroton	T50.2X1	T50.2X2	T50.2X3	T50.2X4	T50.2X5	T50.2X6
Rehydration salts (oral)	T50.3X1	T50.3X2	T50.3X3	T50.3X4	T50.3X5	T50.3X6
Rela	T42.8X1	T42.8X2	T42.8X3	T42.8X4	T42.8X5	T42.8X6
Relaxant, muscle						
anesthetic	T48.1X1	T48.1X2	T48.1X3	T48.1X4	T48.1X5	T48.1X6
central nervous system	T42.8X1	T42.8X2	T42.8X3	T42.8X4	T42.8X5	T42.8X6
skeletal NEC	T48.1X1	T48.1X2	T48.1X3	T48.1X4	T48.1X5	T48.1X6
smooth NEC	T44.3X1	T44.3X2	T44.3X3	T44.3X4	T44.3X5	T44.3X6
Remoxipride	T43.591	T43.592	T43.593	T43.594	T43.595	T43.596
Renese	T50.2X1	T50.2X2	T50.2X3	T50.2X4	T50.2X5	T50.2X6
Renografin	T50.8X1	T50.8X2	T50.8X3	T50.8X4	T50.8X5	T50.8X6
Replacement solution	T50.3X1	T50.3X2	T50.3X3	T50.3X4	T50.3X5	T50.3X6
Reproterol	T48.6X1	T48.6X2	T48.6X3	T48.6X4	T48.6X5	T48.6X6
Rescinnamine	T46.5X1	T46.5X2	T46.5X3	T46.5X4	T46.5X5	T46.5X6
Reserpin (e)	T46.5X1	T46.5X2	T46.5X3	T46.5X4	T46.5X5	T46.5X6
Resorcin, resorcinol (nonmedicinal)	T65.891	T65.892	T65.893	T65.894	—	—
medicinal	T49.4X1	T49.4X2	T49.4X3	T49.4X4	T49.4X5	T49.4X6
Respaire	T48.4X1	T48.4X2	T48.4X3	T48.4X4	T48.4X5	T48.4X6
Respiratory drug NEC	T48.901	T48.902	T48.903	T48.904	T48.905	T48.906
antiasthmatic NEC	T48.6X1	T48.6X2	T48.6X3	T48.6X4	T48.6X5	T48.6X6
anti-common-cold NEC	T48.5X1	T48.5X2	T48.5X3	T48.5X4	T48.5X5	T48.5X6
expectorant NEC	T48.4X1	T48.4X2	T48.4X3	T48.4X4	T48.4X5	T48.4X6
stimulant	T48.901	T48.902	T48.903	T48.904	T48.905	T48.906
Retinoic acid	T49.0X1	T49.0X2	T49.0X3	T49.0X4	T49.0X5	T49.0X6
Retinol	T45.2X1	T45.2X2	T45.2X3	T45.2X4	T45.2X5	T45.2X6
Rh (D) immune globulin (human)	T50.Z11	T50.Z12	T50.Z13	T50.Z14	T50.Z15	T50.Z16
Rhodine	T39.011	T39.012	T39.013	T39.014	T39.015	T39.016
RhoGAM	T50.Z11	T50.Z12	T50.Z13	T50.Z14	T50.Z15	T50.Z16
Rhubarb						
dry extract	T47.2X1	T47.2X2	T47.2X3	T47.2X4	T47.2X5	T47.2X6
tincture, compound	T47.2X1	T47.2X2	T47.2X3	T47.2X4	T47.2X5	T47.2X6
Ribavirin	T37.5X1	T37.5X2	T37.5X3	T37.5X4	T37.5X5	T37.5X6
Riboflavin	T45.2X1	T45.2X2	T45.2X3	T45.2X4	T45.2X5	T45.2X6
Ribostamycin	T36.5X1	T36.5X2	T36.5X3	T36.5X4	T36.5X5	T36.5X6
Ricin	T62.2X1	T62.2X2	T62.2X3	T62.2X4	—	—
Ricinus communis	T62.2X1	T62.2X2	T62.2X3	T62.2X4	—	—
Rickettsial vaccine NEC	T50.A91	T50.A92	T50.A93	T50.A94	T50.A95	T50.A96
Rifabutin	T36.6X1	T36.6X2	T36.6X3	T36.6X4	T36.6X5	T36.6X6
Rifamide	T36.6X1	T36.6X2	T36.6X3	T36.6X4	T36.6X5	T36.6X6
Rifampicin	T36.6X1	T36.6X2	T36.6X3	T36.6X4	T36.6X5	T36.6X6
with isoniazid	T37.1X1	T37.1X2	T37.1X3	T37.1X4	T37.1X5	T37.1X6
Rifampin	T36.6X1	T36.6X2	T36.6X3	T36.6X4	T36.6X5	T36.6X6
Rifamycin	T36.6X1	T36.6X2	T36.6X3	T36.6X4	T36.6X5	T36.6X6
Rifaximin	T36.6X1	T36.6X2	T36.6X3	T36.6X4	T36.6X5	T36.6X6
Rimantadine	T37.5X1	T37.5X2	T37.5X3	T37.5X4	T37.5X5	T37.5X6
Rimazolium metilsulfate	T39.8X1	T39.8X2	T39.8X3	T39.8X4	T39.8X5	T39.8X6
Rimifon	T37.1X1	T37.1X2	T37.1X3	T37.1X4	T37.1X5	T37.1X6
Rimiterol	T48.6X1	T48.6X2	T48.6X3	T48.6X4	T48.6X5	T48.6X6
Ringer (lactate) solution	T50.3X1	T50.3X2	T50.3X3	T50.3X4	T50.3X5	T50.3X6
Ristocetin	T36.8X1	T36.8X2	T36.8X3	T36.8X4	T36.8X5	T36.8X6
Ritalin	T43.631	T43.632	T43.633	T43.634	T43.635	T43.636
Ritodrine	T44.5X1	T44.5X2	T44.5X3	T44.5X4	T44.5X5	T44.5X6
Roach killer — see Insecticide						
Rociverine	T44.3X1	T44.3X2	T44.3X3	T44.3X4	T44.3X5	T44.3X6
Rocky Mountain spotted fever vaccine	T50.A91	T50.A92	T50.A93	T50.A94	T50.A95	T50.A96
Rodenticide NEC	T60.4X1	T60.4X2	T60.4X3	T60.4X4	—	—
Rohypnol	T42.4X1	T42.4X2	T42.4X3	T42.4X4	T42.4X5	T42.4X6
Rokitamycin	T36.3X1	T36.3X2	T36.3X3	T36.3X4	T36.3X5	T36.3X6
Rolaids	T47.1X1	T47.1X2	T47.1X3	T47.1X4	T47.1X5	T47.1X6
Rolitetracycline	T36.4X1	T36.4X2	T36.4X3	T36.4X4	T36.4X5	T36.4X6
Romilar	T48.3X1	T48.3X2	T48.3X3	T48.3X4	T48.3X5	T48.3X6
Ronifibrate	T46.6X1	T46.6X2	T46.6X3	T46.6X4	T46.6X5	T46.6X6
Rosaprostol	T47.1X1	T47.1X2	T47.1X3	T47.1X4	T47.1X5	T47.1X6
Rose bengal sodium (131I)	T50.8X1	T50.8X2	T50.8X3	T50.8X4	T50.8X5	T50.8X6
Rose water ointment	T49.3X1	T49.3X2	T49.3X3	T49.3X4	T49.3X5	T49.3X6
Rosoxacin	T37.8X1	T37.8X2	T37.8X3	T37.8X4	T37.8X5	T37.8X6

Substance	Poisoning, Accidental (unintentional)	Poisoning, Intentional Self-harm	Poisoning, Assault	Poisoning, Undetermined	Adverse Effect	Under-dosing
Rotenone	T60.2X1	T60.2X2	T60.2X3	T60.2X4	—	—
Rotoxamine	T45.0X1	T45.0X2	T45.0X3	T45.0X4	T45.0X5	T45.0X6
Rough-on-rats	T60.4X1	T60.4X2	T60.4X3	T60.4X4	—	—
Roxatidine	T47.0X1	T47.0X2	T47.0X3	T47.0X4	T47.0X5	T47.0X6
Roxithromycin	T36.3X1	T36.3X2	T36.3X3	T36.3X4	T36.3X5	T36.3X6
Rt-PA	T45.611	T45.612	T45.613	T45.614	T45.615	T45.616
Rubbing alcohol	T51.2X1	T51.2X2	T51.2X3	T51.2X4	—	—
Rubefacient	T49.4X1	T49.4X2	T49.4X3	T49.4X4	T49.4X5	T49.4X6
Rubella vaccine	T50.B91	T50.B92	T50.B93	T50.B94	T50.B95	T50.B96
Rubeola vaccine	T50.B91	T50.B92	T50.B93	T50.B94	T50.B95	T50.B96
Rubidium chloride Rb82	T50.8X1	T50.8X2	T50.8X3	T50.8X4	T50.8X5	T50.8X6
Rubidomycin	T45.1X1	T45.1X2	T45.1X3	T45.1X4	T45.1X5	T45.1X6
Rue	T62.2X1	T62.2X2	T62.2X3	T62.2X4	—	—
Rufocromomycin	T45.1X1	T45.1X2	T45.1X3	T45.1X4	T45.1X5	T45.1X6
Russel's viper venin	T45.7X1	T45.7X2	T45.7X3	T45.7X4	T45.7X5	T45.7X6
Ruta (graveolens)	T62.2X1	T62.2X2	T62.2X3	T62.2X4	—	—
Rutinum	T46.991	T46.992	T46.993	T46.994	T46.995	T46.996
Rutoside	T46.991	T46.992	T46.993	T46.994	T46.995	T46.996
b-sitosterol(s)	T46.6X1	T46.6X2	T46.6X3	T46.6X4	T46.6X5	T46.6X6
Sabadilla (plant)	T62.2X1	T62.2X2	T62.2X3	T62.2X4	—	—
pesticide	T60.2X1	T60.2X2	T60.2X3	T60.2X4	—	—
Saccharated iron oxide	T45.8X1	T45.8X2	T45.8X3	T45.8X4	T45.8X5	T45.8X6
Saccharin	T50.901	T50.902	T50.903	T50.904	T50.905	T50.906
Saccharomyces boulardii	T47.6X1	T47.6X2	T47.6X3	T47.6X4	T47.6X5	T47.6X6
Safflower oil	T46.6X1	T46.6X2	T46.6X3	T46.6X4	T46.6X5	T46.6X6
Safrazine	T43.1X1	T43.1X2	T43.1X3	T43.1X4	T43.1X5	T43.1X6
Salazosulfapyridine	T37.0X1	T37.0X2	T37.0X3	T37.0X4	T37.0X5	T37.0X6
Salbutamol	T48.6X1	T48.6X2	T48.6X3	T48.6X4	T48.6X5	T48.6X6
Salicylamide	T39.091	T39.092	T39.093	T39.094	T39.095	T39.096
Salicylate NEC	T39.091	T39.092	T39.093	T39.094	T39.095	T39.096
methyl	T49.3X1	T49.3X2	T49.3X3	T49.3X4	T49.3X5	T49.3X6
theobromine calcium	T50.2X1	T50.2X2	T50.2X3	T50.2X4	T50.2X5	T50.2X6
Salicylazosulfapyridine	T37.0X1	T37.0X2	T37.0X3	T37.0X4	T37.0X5	T37.0X6
Salicylhydroxamic acid	T49.0X1	T49.0X2	T49.0X3	T49.0X4	T49.0X5	T49.0X6
Salicylic acid	T49.4X1	T49.4X2	T49.4X3	T49.4X4	T49.4X5	T49.4X6
with benzoic acid	T49.4X1	T49.4X2	T49.4X3	T49.4X4	T49.4X5	T49.4X6
congeners	T39.091	T39.092	T39.093	T39.094	T39.095	T39.096
derivative	T39.091	T39.092	T39.093	T39.094	T39.095	T39.096
salts	T39.091	T39.092	T39.093	T39.094	T39.095	T39.096
Salinazid	T37.1X1	T37.1X2	T37.1X3	T37.1X4	T37.1X5	T37.1X6
Salmeterol	T48.6X1	T48.6X2	T48.6X3	T48.6X4	T48.6X5	T48.6X6
Salol	T49.3X1	T49.3X2	T49.3X3	T49.3X4	T49.3X5	T49.3X6
Salsalate	T39.091	T39.092	T39.093	T39.094	T39.095	T39.096
Salt-replacing drug	T50.901	T50.902	T50.903	T50.904	T50.905	T50.906
Salt-retaining mineralocorticoid	T50.0X1	T50.0X2	T50.0X3	T50.0X4	T50.0X5	T50.0X6
Salt substitute	T50.901	T50.902	T50.903	T50.904	T50.905	T50.906
Saluretic NEC	T50.2X1	T50.2X2	T50.2X3	T50.2X4	T50.2X5	T50.2X6
Saluron	T50.2X1	T50.2X2	T50.2X3	T50.2X4	T50.2X5	T50.2X6
Salvarsan 606 (neosilver) (silver)	T37.8X1	T37.8X2	T37.8X3	T37.8X4	T37.8X5	T37.8X6
Sambucus canadensis	T62.2X1	T62.2X2	T62.2X3	T62.2X4	—	—
berry	T62.1X1	T62.1X2	T62.1X3	T62.1X4	—	—
Sandril	T46.5X1	T46.5X2	T46.5X3	T46.5X4	T46.5X5	T46.5X6
Sanguinaria canadensis	T62.2X1	T62.2X2	T62.2X3	T62.2X4	—	—
Saniflush (cleaner)	T54.2X1	T54.2X2	T54.2X3	T54.2X4	—	—
Santonin	T37.4X1	T37.4X2	T37.4X3	T37.4X4	T37.4X5	T37.4X6
Santyl	T49.8X1	T49.8X2	T49.8X3	T49.8X4	T49.8X5	T49.8X6
Saralasin	T46.5X1	T46.5X2	T46.5X3	T46.5X4	T46.5X5	T46.5X6
Sarcolysin	T45.1X1	T45.1X2	T45.1X3	T45.1X4	T45.1X5	T45.1X6
Sarkomycin	T45.1X1	T45.1X2	T45.1X3	T45.1X4	T45.1X5	T45.1X6
Saroten	T43.011	T43.012	T43.013	T43.014	T43.015	T43.016
Saturnine — see Lead						
Savin (oil)	T49.4X1	T49.4X2	T49.4X3	T49.4X4	T49.4X5	T49.4X6
Scammony	T47.2X1	T47.2X2	T47.2X3	T47.2X4	T47.2X5	T47.2X6
Scarlet red	T49.8X1	T49.8X2	T49.8X3	T49.8X4	T49.8X5	T49.8X6
Scheele's green	T57.0X1	T57.0X2	T57.0X3	T57.0X4	—	—
insecticide	T57.0X1	T57.0X2	T57.0X3	T57.0X4	—	—
Schizontozide (blood)	T37.2X1	T37.2X2	T37.2X3	T37.2X4	T37.2X5	T37.2X6
(tissue)						
Schradan	T60.0X1	T60.0X2	T60.0X3	T60.0X4	—	—
Schweinfurth green	T57.0X1	T57.0X2	T57.0X3	T57.0X4	—	—
insecticide	T57.0X1	T57.0X2	T57.0X3	T57.0X4	—	—
Scilla, rat poison	T60.4X1	T60.4X2	T60.4X3	T60.4X4	—	—
Scillaren	T60.4X1	T60.4X2	T60.4X3	T60.4X4	—	—
Sclerosing agent	T46.8X1	T46.8X2	T46.8X3	T46.8X4	T46.8X5	T46.8X6
Scombrotoxin	T61.11	T61.12	T61.13	T61.14	—	—
Scopolamine	T44.3X1	T44.3X2	T44.3X3	T44.3X4	T44.3X5	T44.3X6
Scopolia extract	T44.3X1	T44.3X2	T44.3X3	T44.3X4	T44.3X5	T44.3X6
Scouring powder	T65.891	T65.892	T65.893	T65.894	—	—
Sea						
anemone (sting)	T63.631	T63.632	T63.633	T63.634	—	—
cucumber (sting)	T63.691	T63.692	T63.693	T63.694	—	—

Substance	Poisoning, Accidental (unintentional)	Poisoning, Intentional Self-harm	Poisoning, Assault	Poisoning, Undetermined	Adverse Effect	Under-dosing
Sea — continued						
snake (bite) (venom)	T63.091	T63.092	T63.093	T63.094	—	—
urchin spine (puncture)	T63.691	T63.692	T63.693	T63.694	—	—
Seafood	T61.91	T61.92	T61.93	T61.94	—	—
specified NEC	T61.8X1	T61.8X2	T61.8X3	T61.8X4	—	—
Secbutabarbital	T42.3X1	T42.3X2	T42.3X3	T42.3X4	T42.3X5	T42.3X6
Secbutabarbitone	T42.3X1	T42.3X2	T42.3X3	T42.3X4	T42.3X5	T42.3X6
Secnidazole	T37.3X1	T37.3X2	T37.3X3	T37.3X4	T37.3X5	T37.3X6
Secobarbital	T42.3X1	T42.3X2	T42.3X3	T42.3X4	T42.3X5	T42.3X6
Seconal	T42.3X1	T42.3X2	T42.3X3	T42.3X4	T42.3X5	T42.3X6
Secretin	T50.8X1	T50.8X2	T50.8X3	T50.8X4	T50.8X5	T50.8X6
Sedative NEC	T42.71	T42.72	T42.73	T42.74	T42.75	T42.76
mixed NEC	T42.6X1	T42.6X2	T42.6X3	T42.6X4	T42.6X5	T42.6X6
Sedormid	T42.6X1	T42.6X2	T42.6X3	T42.6X4	T42.6X5	T42.6X6
Seed disinfectant or dressing	T60.8X1	T60.8X2	T60.8X3	T60.8X4	—	—
Seeds (poisonous)	T62.2X1	T62.2X2	T62.2X3	T62.2X4	—	—
Selegiline	T42.8X1	T42.8X2	T42.8X3	T42.8X4	T42.8X5	T42.8X6
Selenium NEC	T56.891	T56.892	T56.893	T56.894	—	—
disulfide or sulfide	T49.4X1	T49.4X2	T49.4X3	T49.4X4	T49.4X5	T49.4X6
fumes	T59.891	T59.892	T59.893	T59.894	—	—
sulfide	T49.4X1	T49.4X2	T49.4X3	T49.4X4	T49.4X5	T49.4X6
Selenomethionine (75Se)	T50.8X1	T50.8X2	T50.8X3	T50.8X4	T50.8X5	T50.8X6
Selsun	T49.4X1	T49.4X2	T49.4X3	T49.4X4	T49.4X5	T49.4X6
Semustine	T45.1X1	T45.1X2	T45.1X3	T45.1X4	T45.1X5	T45.1X6
Senega syrup	T48.4X1	T48.4X2	T48.4X3	T48.4X4	T48.4X5	T48.4X6
Senna	T47.2X1	T47.2X2	T47.2X3	T47.2X4	T47.2X5	T47.2X6
Sennoside A+B	T47.2X1	T47.2X2	T47.2X3	T47.2X4	T47.2X5	T47.2X6
Septisol	T49.2X1	T49.2X2	T49.2X3	T49.2X4	T49.2X5	T49.2X6
Seractide	T38.811	T38.812	T38.813	T38.814	T38.815	T38.816
Serax	T42.4X1	T42.4X2	T42.4X3	T42.4X4	T42.4X5	T42.4X6
Serenesil	T42.6X1	T42.6X2	T42.6X3	T42.6X4	T42.6X5	T42.6X6
Serenium (hydrochloride)	T37.91	T37.92	T37.93	T37.94	T37.95	T37.96
Serepax — see Oxazepam						
Sermorelin	T38.891	T38.892	T38.893	T38.894	T38.895	T38.896
Sernyl	T41.1X1	T41.1X2	T41.1X3	T41.1X4	T41.1X5	T41.1X6
Serotonin	T50.991	T50.992	T50.993	T50.994	T50.995	T50.996
Serpasil	T46.5X1	T46.5X2	T46.5X3	T46.5X4	T46.5X5	T46.5X6
Serrapeptase	T45.3X1	T45.3X2	T45.3X3	T45.3X4	T45.3X5	T45.3X6
Serum						
antibotulinus	T50.Z11	T50.Z12	T50.Z13	T50.Z14	T50.Z15	T50.Z16
anticytotoxic	T50.Z11	T50.Z12	T50.Z13	T50.Z14	T50.Z15	T50.Z16
antidiphtheria	T50.Z11	T50.Z12	T50.Z13	T50.Z14	T50.Z15	T50.Z16
antimeningococcus	T50.Z11	T50.Z12	T50.Z13	T50.Z14	T50.Z15	T50.Z16
anti-Rh	T50.Z11	T50.Z12	T50.Z13	T50.Z14	T50.Z15	T50.Z16
anti-snake-bite	T50.Z11	T50.Z12	T50.Z13	T50.Z14	T50.Z15	T50.Z16
antitetanic	T50.Z11	T50.Z12	T50.Z13	T50.Z14	T50.Z15	T50.Z16
antitoxic	T50.Z11	T50.Z12	T50.Z13	T50.Z14	T50.Z15	T50.Z16
complement (inhibitor)	T45.8X1	T45.8X2	T45.8X3	T45.8X4	T45.8X5	T45.8X6
convalescent	T50.Z11	T50.Z12	T50.Z13	T50.Z14	T50.Z15	T50.Z16
hemolytic complement	T45.8X1	T45.8X2	T45.8X3	T45.8X4	T45.8X5	T45.8X6
immune (human)	T50.Z11	T50.Z12	T50.Z13	T50.Z14	T50.Z15	T50.Z16
protective NEC	T50.Z11	T50.Z12	T50.Z13	T50.Z14	T50.Z15	T50.Z16
Setastine	T45.0X1	T45.0X2	T45.0X3	T45.0X4	T45.0X5	T45.0X6
Setoperone	T43.591	T43.592	T43.593	T43.594	T43.595	T43.596
Sewer gas	T59.91	T59.92	T59.93	T59.94	—	—
Shampoo	T55.0X1	T55.0X2	T55.0X3	T55.0X4	—	—
Shellfish, noxious, nonbacterial	T61.781	T61.782	T61.783	T61.784	—	—
Sildenafil	T46.7X1	T46.7X2	T46.7X3	T46.7X4	T46.7X5	T46.7X6
Silibinin	T50.991	T50.992	T50.993	T50.994	T50.995	T50.996
Silicone NEC	T65.891	T65.892	T65.893	T65.894	—	—
medicinal	T49.3X1	T49.3X2	T49.3X3	T49.3X4	T49.3X5	T49.3X6
Silvadene	T49.0X1	T49.0X2	T49.0X3	T49.0X4	T49.0X5	T49.0X6
Silver	T49.0X1	T49.0X2	T49.0X3	T49.0X4	T49.0X5	T49.0X6
anti-infectives	T49.0X1	T49.0X2	T49.0X3	T49.0X4	T49.0X5	T49.0X6
arsphenamine	T37.8X1	T37.8X2	T37.8X3	T37.8X4	T37.8X5	T37.8X6
colloidal	T49.0X1	T49.0X2	T49.0X3	T49.0X4	T49.0X5	T49.0X6
nitrate	T49.0X1	T49.0X2	T49.0X3	T49.0X4	T49.0X5	T49.0X6
ophthalmic preparation	T49.5X1	T49.5X2	T49.5X3	T49.5X4	T49.5X5	T49.5X6
toughened (keratolytic)	T49.4X1	T49.4X2	T49.4X3	T49.4X4	T49.4X5	T49.4X6
nonmedicinal (dust)	T56.891	T56.892	T56.893	T56.894	—	—
protein	T49.5X1	T49.5X2	T49.5X3	T49.5X4	T49.5X5	T49.5X6
salvarsan	T37.8X1	T37.8X2	T37.8X3	T37.8X4	T37.8X5	T37.8X6
sulfadiazine	T49.0X1	T49.0X2	T49.0X3	T49.0X4	T49.0X5	T49.0X6
Silymarin	T50.991	T50.992	T50.993	T50.994	T50.995	T50.996
Simaldrate	T47.1X1	T47.1X2	T47.1X3	T47.1X4	T47.1X5	T47.1X6
Simazine	T60.3X1	T60.3X2	T60.3X3	T60.3X4	—	—
Simethicone	T47.1X1	T47.1X2	T47.1X3	T47.1X4	T47.1X5	T47.1X6
Simfibrate	T46.6X1	T46.6X2	T46.6X3	T46.6X4	T46.6X5	T46.6X6
Simvastatin	T46.6X1	T46.6X2	T46.6X3	T46.6X4	T46.6X5	T46.6X6
Sincalide	T50.8X1	T50.8X2	T50.8X3	T50.8X4	T50.8X5	T50.8X6
Sinequan	T43.011	T43.012	T43.013	T43.014	T43.015	T43.016

Table of Drugs and Chemicals — Singoserp — Solasulfone

Substance	Poisoning, Accidental (unintentional)	Poisoning, Intentional Self-harm	Poisoning, Assault	Poisoning, Undetermined	Adverse Effect	Under-dosing
Singoserp	T46.5X1	T46.5X2	T46.5X3	T46.5X4	T46.5X5	T46.5X6
Sintrom	T45.511	T45.512	T45.513	T45.514	T45.515	T45.516
Sisomicin	T36.5X1	T36.5X2	T36.5X3	T36.5X4	T36.5X5	T36.5X6
Sitosterols	T46.6X1	T46.6X2	T46.6X3	T46.6X4	T46.6X5	T46.6X6
Skeletal muscle relaxants	T48.1X1	T48.1X2	T48.1X3	T48.1X4	T48.1X5	T48.1X6
Skin						
agents (external)	T49.91	T49.92	T49.93	T49.94	T49.95	T49.96
specified NEC	T49.8X1	T49.8X2	T49.8X3	T49.8X4	T49.8X5	T49.8X6
test antigen	T50.8X1	T50.8X2	T50.8X3	T50.8X4	T50.8X5	T50.8X6
Sleep-eze	T45.0X1	T45.0X2	T45.0X3	T45.0X4	T45.0X5	T45.0X6
Sleeping draught, pill	T42.71	T42.72	T42.73	T42.74	T42.75	T42.76
Smallpox vaccine	T50.B11	T50.B12	T50.B13	T50.B14	T50.B15	T50.B16
Smelter fumes NEC	T56.91	T56.92	T56.93	T56.94	—	—
Smog	T59.1X1	T59.1X2	T59.1X3	T59.1X4	—	—
Smoke NEC	T59.811	T59.812	T59.813	T59.814	—	—
Smooth muscle relaxant	T44.3X1	T44.3X2	T44.3X3	T44.3X4	T44.3X5	T44.3X6
Snail killer NEC	T60.8X1	T60.8X2	T60.8X3	T60.8X4	—	—
Snake venom or bite	T63.001	T63.002	T63.003	T63.004	—	—
hemocoagulase	T45.7X1	T45.7X2	T45.7X3	T45.7X4	T45.7X5	T45.7X6
Snuff	T65.211	T65.212	T65.213	T65.214	—	—
Soap (powder) (product)	T55.0X1	T55.0X2	T55.0X3	T55.0X4	—	—
enema	T47.4X1	T47.4X2	T47.4X3	T47.4X4	T47.4X5	T47.4X6
medicinal, soft	T49.2X1	T49.2X2	T49.2X3	T49.2X4	T49.2X5	T49.2X6
superfatted	T49.2X1	T49.2X2	T49.2X3	T49.2X4	T49.2X5	T49.2X6
Sobrerol	T48.4X1	T48.4X2	T48.4X3	T48.4X4	T48.4X5	T48.4X6
Soda (caustic)	T54.3X1	T54.3X2	T54.3X3	T54.3X4	—	—
bicarb	T47.1X1	T47.1X2	T47.1X3	T47.1X4	T47.1X5	T47.1X6
chlorinated — see Sodium, hypochlorite						
Sodium						
acetosulfone	T37.1X1	T37.1X2	T37.1X3	T37.1X4	T37.1X5	T37.1X6
acetrizoate	T50.8X1	T50.8X2	T50.8X3	T50.8X4	T50.8X5	T50.8X6
acid phosphate	T50.3X1	T50.3X2	T50.3X3	T50.3X4	T50.3X5	T50.3X6
alginate	T47.8X1	T47.8X2	T47.8X3	T47.8X4	T47.8X5	T47.8X6
amidotrizoate	T50.8X1	T50.8X2	T50.8X3	T50.8X4	T50.8X5	T50.8X6
aminopterin	T45.1X1	T45.1X2	T45.1X3	T45.1X4	T45.1X5	T45.1X6
amylosulfate	T47.8X1	T47.8X2	T47.8X3	T47.8X4	T47.8X5	T47.8X6
amytal	T42.3X1	T42.3X2	T42.3X3	T42.3X4	T42.3X5	T42.3X6
antimony gluconate	T37.3X1	T37.3X2	T37.3X3	T37.3X4	T37.3X5	T37.3X6
arsenate	T57.0X1	T57.0X2	T57.0X3	T57.0X4	—	—
aurothiomalate	T39.4X1	T39.4X2	T39.4X3	T39.4X4	T39.4X5	T39.4X6
aurothiosulfate	T39.4X1	T39.4X2	T39.4X3	T39.4X4	T39.4X5	T39.4X6
barbiturate	T42.3X1	T42.3X2	T42.3X3	T42.3X4	T42.3X5	T42.3X6
basic phosphate	T47.4X1	T47.4X2	T47.4X3	T47.4X4	T47.4X5	T47.4X6
bicarbonate	T47.1X1	T47.1X2	T47.1X3	T47.1X4	T47.1X5	T47.1X6
bichromate	T57.8X1	T57.8X2	T57.8X3	T57.8X4	—	—
biphosphate	T50.3X1	T50.3X2	T50.3X3	T50.3X4	T50.3X5	T50.3X6
bisulfate	T65.891	T65.892	T65.893	T65.894	—	—
borate						
cleanser	T57.8X1	T57.8X2	T57.8X3	T57.8X4	—	—
eye	T49.5X1	T49.5X2	T49.5X3	T49.5X4	T49.5X5	T49.5X6
therapeutic	T49.8X1	T49.8X2	T49.8X3	T49.8X4	T49.8X5	T49.8X6
bromide	T42.6X1	T42.6X2	T42.6X3	T42.6X4	T42.6X5	T42.6X6
cacodylate (nonmedicinal) NEC	T50.8X1	T50.8X2	T50.8X3	T50.8X4	T50.8X5	T50.8X6
anti-infective	T37.8X1	T37.8X2	T37.8X3	T37.8X4	T37.8X5	T37.8X6
herbicide	T60.3X1	T60.3X2	T60.3X3	T60.3X4	—	—
calcium edetate	T45.8X1	T45.8X2	T45.8X3	T45.8X4	T45.8X5	T45.8X6
carbonate NEC	T54.3X1	T54.3X2	T54.3X3	T54.3X4	—	—
chlorate NEC	T65.891	T65.892	T65.893	T65.894	—	—
herbicide	T54.91	T54.92	T54.93	T54.94	—	—
chloride	T50.3X1	T50.3X2	T50.3X3	T50.3X4	T50.3X5	T50.3X6
with glucose	T50.3X1	T50.3X2	T50.3X3	T50.3X4	T50.3X5	T50.3X6
chromate	T65.891	T65.892	T65.893	T65.894	—	—
citrate	T50.991	T50.992	T50.993	T50.994	T50.995	T50.996
cromoglicate	T48.6X1	T48.6X2	T48.6X3	T48.6X4	T48.6X5	T48.6X6
cyanide	T65.0X1	T65.0X2	T65.0X3	T65.0X4	—	—
cyclamate	T50.3X1	T50.3X2	T50.3X3	T50.3X4	T50.3X5	T50.3X6
dehydrocholate	T45.8X1	T45.8X2	T45.8X3	T45.8X4	T45.8X5	T45.8X6
diatrizoate	T50.8X1	T50.8X2	T50.8X3	T50.8X4	T50.8X5	T50.8X6
dibunate	T48.4X1	T48.4X2	T48.4X3	T48.4X4	T48.4X5	T48.4X6
dioctyl sulfosuccinate	T47.4X1	T47.4X2	T47.4X3	T47.4X4	T47.4X5	T47.4X6
dipantoyl ferrate	T45.8X1	T45.8X2	T45.8X3	T45.8X4	T45.8X5	T45.8X6
edetate	T45.8X1	T45.8X2	T45.8X3	T45.8X4	T45.8X5	T45.8X6
ethacrynate	T50.1X1	T50.1X2	T50.1X3	T50.1X4	T50.1X5	T50.1X6
feredetate	T45.8X1	T45.8X2	T45.8X3	T45.8X4	T45.8X5	T45.8X6
Fluoride — see Fluoride						
fluoroacetate (dust) (pesticide)	T60.4X1	T60.4X2	T60.4X3	T60.4X4	—	—
free salt	T50.3X1	T50.3X2	T50.3X3	T50.3X4	T50.3X5	T50.3X6
fusidate	T36.8X1	T36.8X2	T36.8X3	T36.8X4	T36.8X5	T36.8X6
glucaldrate	T47.1X1	T47.1X2	T47.1X3	T47.1X4	T47.1X5	T47.1X6
glucosulfone	T37.1X1	T37.1X2	T37.1X3	T37.1X4	T37.1X5	T37.1X6

Substance	Poisoning, Accidental (unintentional)	Poisoning, Intentional Self-harm	Poisoning, Assault	Poisoning, Undetermined	Adverse Effect	Under-dosing
Sodium — continued						
glutamate	T45.8X1	T45.8X2	T45.8X3	T45.8X4	T45.8X5	T45.8X6
hydrogen carbonate	T50.3X1	T50.3X2	T50.3X3	T50.3X4	T50.3X5	T50.3X6
hydroxide	T54.3X1	T54.3X2	T54.3X3	T54.3X4	—	—
hypochlorite (bleach) NEC	T54.3X1	T54.3X2	T54.3X3	T54.3X4	—	—
disinfectant	T54.3X1	T54.3X2	T54.3X3	T54.3X4	—	—
medicinal (anti-infective) (external)	T49.0X1	T49.0X2	T49.0X3	T49.0X4	T49.0X5	T49.0X6
vapor	T54.3X1	T54.3X2	T54.3X3	T54.3X4	—	—
hyposulfite	T49.0X1	T49.0X2	T49.0X3	T49.0X4	T49.0X5	T49.0X6
indigotin disulfonate	T50.8X1	T50.8X2	T50.8X3	T50.8X4	T50.8X5	T50.8X6
iodide	T50.991	T50.992	T50.993	T50.994	T50.995	T50.996
I-131	T50.8X1	T50.8X2	T50.8X3	T50.8X4	T50.8X5	T50.8X6
therapeutic	T38.2X1	T38.2X2	T38.2X3	T38.2X4	T38.2X5	T38.2X6
iodohippurate (131I)	T50.8X1	T50.8X2	T50.8X3	T50.8X4	T50.8X5	T50.8X6
iopodate	T50.8X1	T50.8X2	T50.8X3	T50.8X4	T50.8X5	T50.8X6
iothalamate	T50.8X1	T50.8X2	T50.8X3	T50.8X4	T50.8X5	T50.8X6
iron edetate	T45.4X1	T45.4X2	T45.4X3	T45.4X4	T45.4X5	T45.4X6
lactate (compound solution)	T45.8X1	T45.8X2	T45.8X3	T45.8X4	T45.8X5	T45.8X6
lauryl (sulfate)	T49.2X1	T49.2X2	T49.2X3	T49.2X4	T49.2X5	T49.2X6
L-triiodothyronine	T38.1X1	T38.1X2	T38.1X3	T38.1X4	T38.1X5	T38.1X6
magnesium citrate	T50.991	T50.992	T50.993	T50.994	T50.995	T50.996
mersalate	T50.2X1	T50.2X2	T50.2X3	T50.2X4	T50.2X5	T50.2X6
metasilicate	T65.891	T65.892	T65.893	T65.894	—	—
metrizoate	T50.8X1	T50.8X2	T50.8X3	T50.8X4	T50.8X5	T50.8X6
monofluoroacetate (pesticide)	T60.1X1	T60.1X2	T60.1X3	T60.1X4	—	—
morrhuate	T46.8X1	T46.8X2	T46.8X3	T46.8X4	T46.8X5	T46.8X6
nafcillin	T36.0X1	T36.0X2	T36.0X3	T36.0X4	T36.0X5	T36.0X6
nitrate (oxidizing agent)	T65.891	T65.892	T65.893	T65.894	—	—
nitrite	T50.6X1	T50.6X2	T50.6X3	T50.6X4	T50.6X5	T50.6X6
nitroferricyanide	T46.5X1	T46.5X2	T46.5X3	T46.5X4	T46.5X5	T46.5X6
nitroprusside	T46.5X1	T46.5X2	T46.5X3	T46.5X4	T46.5X5	T46.5X6
oxalate	T65.891	T65.892	T65.893	T65.894	—	—
oxide/peroxide	T65.891	T65.892	T65.893	T65.894	—	—
oxybate	T41.291	T41.292	T41.293	T41.294	T41.295	T41.296
para-aminohippurate	T50.8X1	T50.8X2	T50.8X3	T50.8X4	T50.8X5	T50.8X6
perborate (nonmedicinal) NEC	T65.891	T65.892	T65.893	T65.894	—	—
medicinal	T49.0X1	T49.0X2	T49.0X3	T49.0X4	T49.0X5	T49.0X6
soap	T55.0X1	T55.0X2	T55.0X3	T55.0X4	—	—
percarbonate — see Sodium, perborate						
pertechnetate Tc99m	T50.8X1	T50.8X2	T50.8X3	T50.8X4	T50.8X5	T50.8X6
phosphate						
cellulose	T45.8X1	T45.8X2	T45.8X3	T45.8X4	T45.8X5	T45.8X6
dibasic	T47.2X1	T47.2X2	T47.2X3	T47.2X4	T47.2X5	T47.2X6
monobasic	T47.2X1	T47.2X2	T47.2X3	T47.2X4	T47.2X5	T47.2X6
phytate	T50.6X1	T50.6X2	T50.6X3	T50.6X4	T50.6X5	T50.6X6
picosulfate	T47.2X1	T47.2X2	T47.2X3	T47.2X4	T47.2X5	T47.2X6
polyhydroxyaluminium monocarbonate	T47.1X1	T47.1X2	T47.1X3	T47.1X4	T47.1X5	T47.1X6
polystyrene sulfonate	T50.3X1	T50.3X2	T50.3X3	T50.3X4	T50.3X5	T50.3X6
propionate	T49.0X1	T49.0X2	T49.0X3	T49.0X4	T49.0X5	T49.0X6
propyl hydroxybenzoate	T50.991	T50.992	T50.993	T50.994	T50.995	T50.996
psylliate	T46.8X1	T46.8X2	T46.8X3	T46.8X4	T46.8X5	T46.8X6
removing resins	T50.3X1	T50.3X2	T50.3X3	T50.3X4	T50.3X5	T50.3X6
salicylate	T39.091	T39.092	T39.093	T39.094	T39.095	T39.096
salt NEC	T50.3X1	T50.3X2	T50.3X3	T50.3X4	T50.3X5	T50.3X6
selenate	T60.2X1	T60.2X2	T60.2X3	T60.2X4	—	—
stibogluconate	T37.3X1	T37.3X2	T37.3X3	T37.3X4	T37.3X5	T37.3X6
sulfate	T47.4X1	T47.4X2	T47.4X3	T47.4X4	T47.4X5	T47.4X6
sulfoxone	T37.1X1	T37.1X2	T37.1X3	T37.1X4	T37.1X5	T37.1X6
tetradecyl sulfate	T46.8X1	T46.8X2	T46.8X3	T46.8X4	T46.8X5	T46.8X6
thiopental	T41.1X1	T41.1X2	T41.1X3	T41.1X4	T41.1X5	T41.1X6
thiosalicylate	T39.091	T39.092	T39.093	T39.094	T39.095	T39.096
thiosulfate	T50.6X1	T50.6X2	T50.6X3	T50.6X4	T50.6X5	T50.6X6
tolbutamide	T38.3X1	T38.3X2	T38.3X3	T38.3X4	T38.3X5	T38.3X6
(L)-triiodothyronine	T38.1X1	T38.1X2	T38.1X3	T38.1X4	T38.1X5	T38.1X6
tyropanoate	T50.8X1	T50.8X2	T50.8X3	T50.8X4	T50.8X5	T50.8X6
valproate	T42.6X1	T42.6X2	T42.6X3	T42.6X4	T42.6X5	T42.6X6
versenate	T50.6X1	T50.6X2	T50.6X3	T50.6X4	T50.6X5	T50.6X6
Sodium-free salt	T50.901	T50.902	T50.903	T50.904	T50.905	T50.906
Sodium-removing resin	T50.3X1	T50.3X2	T50.3X3	T50.3X4	T50.3X5	T50.3X6
Soft soap	T55.0X1	T55.0X2	T55.0X3	T55.0X4	—	—
Solanine	T62.2X1	T62.2X2	T62.2X3	T62.2X4	—	—
berries	T62.1X1	T62.1X2	T62.1X3	T62.1X4	—	—
Solanum dulcamara	T62.2X1	T62.2X2	T62.2X3	T62.2X4	—	—
berries	T62.1X1	T62.1X2	T62.1X3	T62.1X4	—	—
Solapsone	T37.1X1	T37.1X2	T37.1X3	T37.1X4	T37.1X5	T37.1X6
Solar lotion	T49.3X1	T49.3X2	T49.3X3	T49.3X4	T49.3X5	T49.3X6
Solasulfone	T37.1X1	T37.1X2	T37.1X3	T37.1X4	T37.1X5	T37.1X6

Substance	Poisoning, Accidental (unintentional)	Poisoning, Intentional Self-harm	Poisoning, Assault	Poisoning, Undetermined	Adverse Effect	Under-dosing
Soldering fluid	T65.891	T65.892	T65.893	T65.894	—	—
Solid substance	T65.91	T65.92	T65.93	T65.94	—	—
specified NEC	T65.891	T65.892	T65.893	T65.894	—	—
Solvent, industrial NEC	T52.91	T52.92	T52.93	T52.94	—	—
naphtha	T52.0X1	T52.0X2	T52.0X3	T52.0X4	—	—
petroleum	T52.0X1	T52.0X2	T52.0X3	T52.0X4	—	—
specified NEC	T52.8X1	T52.8X2	T52.8X3	T52.8X4	—	—
Soma	T42.8X1	T42.8X2	T42.8X3	T42.8X4	T42.8X5	T42.8X6
Somatorelin	T38.891	T38.892	T38.893	T38.894	T38.895	T38.896
Somatostatin	T38.991	T38.992	T38.993	T38.994	T38.995	T38.996
Somatotropin	T38.811	T38.812	T38.813	T38.814	T38.815	T38.816
Somatrem	T38.811	T38.812	T38.813	T38.814	T38.815	T38.816
Somatropin	T38.811	T38.812	T38.813	T38.814	T38.815	T38.816
Sominex	T45.0X1	T45.0X2	T45.0X3	T45.0X4	T45.0X5	T45.0X6
Somnos	T42.6X1	T42.6X2	T42.6X3	T42.6X4	T42.6X5	T42.6X6
Somonal	T42.3X1	T42.3X2	T42.3X3	T42.3X4	T42.3X5	T42.3X6
Soneryl	T42.3X1	T42.3X2	T42.3X3	T42.3X4	T42.3X5	T42.3X6
Soothing syrup	T50.901	T50.902	T50.903	T50.904	T50.905	T50.906
Sopor	T42.6X1	T42.6X2	T42.6X3	T42.6X4	T42.6X5	T42.6X6
Soporific	T42.71	T42.72	T42.73	T42.74	T42.75	T42.76
Soporific drug	T42.71	T42.72	T42.73	T42.74	T42.75	T42.76
specified type NEC	T42.6X1	T42.6X2	T42.6X3	T42.6X4	T42.6X5	T42.6X6
Sorbide nitrate	T46.3X1	T46.3X2	T46.3X3	T46.3X4	T46.3X5	T46.3X6
Sorbitol	T47.4X1	T47.4X2	T47.4X3	T47.4X4	T47.4X5	T47.4X6
Sotalol	T44.7X1	T44.7X2	T44.7X3	T44.7X4	T44.7X5	T44.7X6
Sotradecol	T46.8X1	T46.8X2	T46.8X3	T46.8X4	T46.8X5	T46.8X6
Soysterol	T46.6X1	T46.6X2	T46.6X3	T46.6X4	T46.6X5	T46.6X6
Spacoline	T44.3X1	T44.3X2	T44.3X3	T44.3X4	T44.3X5	T44.3X6
Spanish fly	T49.8X1	T49.8X2	T49.8X3	T49.8X4	T49.8X5	T49.8X6
Sparine	T43.3X1	T43.3X2	T43.3X3	T43.3X4	T43.3X5	T43.3X6
Sparteine	T48.0X1	T48.0X2	T48.0X3	T48.0X4	T48.0X5	T48.0X6
Spasmolytic						
anticholinergics	T44.3X1	T44.3X2	T44.3X3	T44.3X4	T44.3X5	T44.3X6
autonomic	T44.3X1	T44.3X2	T44.3X3	T44.3X4	T44.3X5	T44.3X6
bronchial NEC	T48.6X1	T48.6X2	T48.6X3	T48.6X4	T48.6X5	T48.6X6
quaternary ammonium	T44.3X1	T44.3X2	T44.3X3	T44.3X4	T44.3X5	T44.3X6
skeletal muscle NEC	T48.1X1	T48.1X2	T48.1X3	T48.1X4	T48.1X5	T48.1X6
Spectinomycin	T36.5X1	T36.5X2	T36.5X3	T36.5X4	T36.5X5	T36.5X6
Speed	T43.621	T43.622	T43.623	T43.624	T43.625	T43.626
Spermicide	T49.8X1	T49.8X2	T49.8X3	T49.8X4	T49.8X5	T49.8X6
Spider (bite) (venom)	T63.391	T63.392	T63.393	T63.394		
antivenin	T50.Z11	T50.Z12	T50.Z13	T50.Z14	T50.Z15	T50.Z16
Spigelia (root)	T37.4X1	T37.4X2	T37.4X3	T37.4X4	T37.4X5	T37.4X6
Spindle inactivator	T50.4X1	T50.4X2	T50.4X3	T50.4X4	T50.4X5	T50.4X6
Spiperone	T43.4X1	T43.4X2	T43.4X3	T43.4X4	T43.4X5	T43.4X6
Spiramycin	T36.3X1	T36.3X2	T36.3X3	T36.3X4	T36.3X5	T36.3X6
Spirapril	T46.4X1	T46.4X2	T46.4X3	T46.4X4	T46.4X5	T46.4X6
Spirilene	T43.591	T43.592	T43.593	T43.594	T43.595	T43.596
Spirit(s) (neutral) NEC	T51.0X1	T51.0X2	T51.0X3	T51.0X4	—	—
beverage	T51.0X1	T51.0X2	T51.0X3	T51.0X4	—	—
industrial	T51.0X1	T51.0X2	T51.0X3	T51.0X4	—	—
mineral	T52.0X1	T52.0X2	T52.0X3	T52.0X4	—	—
of salt — see Hydrochloric acid						
surgical	T51.0X1	T51.0X2	T51.0X3	T51.0X4	—	—
Spironolactone	T50.0X1	T50.0X2	T50.0X3	T50.0X4	T50.0X5	T50.0X6
Spiroperidol	T43.4X1	T43.4X2	T43.4X3	T43.4X4	T43.4X5	T43.4X6
Sponge, absorbable	T45.7X1	T45.7X2	T45.7X3	T45.7X4	T45.7X5	T45.7X6
(gelatin)						
Sporostacin	T49.0X1	T49.0X2	T49.0X3	T49.0X4	T49.0X5	T49.0X6
Spray (aerosol)	T65.91	T65.92	T65.93	T65.94	—	—
cosmetic	T65.891	T65.892	T65.893	T65.894	—	—
medicinal NEC	T50.901	T50.902	T50.903	T50.904	T50.905	T50.906
pesticides — see Pesticides						
specified content — see specific substance						
Spurge flax	T62.2X1	T62.2X2	T62.2X3	T62.2X4	—	—
Spurges	T62.2X1	T62.2X2	T62.2X3	T62.2X4	—	—
Sputum viscosity-lowering drug	T48.4X1	T48.4X2	T48.4X3	T48.4X4	T48.4X5	T48.4X6
Squill	T46.0X1	T46.0X2	T46.0X3	T46.0X4	T46.0X5	T46.0X6
rat poison	T60.4X1	T60.4X2	T60.4X3	T60.4X4	—	—
Squirting cucumber (cathartic)	T47.2X1	T47.2X2	T47.2X3	T47.2X4	T47.2X5	T47.2X6
Stains	T65.6X1	T65.6X2	T65.6X3	T65.6X4	—	—
Stannous fluoride	T49.7X1	T49.7X2	T49.7X3	T49.7X4	T49.7X5	T49.7X6
Stanolone	T38.7X1	T38.7X2	T38.7X3	T38.7X4	T38.7X5	T38.7X6
Stanozolol	T38.7X1	T38.7X2	T38.7X3	T38.7X4	T38.7X5	T38.7X6
Staphisagria or stavesacre (pediculicide)	T49.0X1	T49.0X2	T49.0X3	T49.0X4	T49.0X5	T49.0X6
Starch	T50.901	T50.902	T50.903	T50.904	T50.905	T50.906
Stelazine	T43.3X1	T43.3X2	T43.3X3	T43.3X4	T43.3X5	T43.3X6
Stemetil	T43.3X1	T43.3X2	T43.3X3	T43.3X4	T43.3X5	T43.3X6
Stepronin	T48.4X1	T48.4X2	T48.4X3	T48.4X4	T48.4X5	T48.4X6
Sterculia	T47.4X1	T47.4X2	T47.4X3	T47.4X4	T47.4X5	T47.4X6
Sternutator gas	T59.891	T59.892	T59.893	T59.894	—	—
Steroid	T38.0X1	T38.0X2	T38.0X3	T38.0X4	T38.0X5	T38.0X6
anabolic	T38.7X1	T38.7X2	T38.7X3	T38.7X4	T38.7X5	T38.7X6
androgenic	T38.7X1	T38.7X2	T38.7X3	T38.7X4	T38.7X5	T38.7X6
antineoplastic, hormone	T38.7X1	T38.7X2	T38.7X3	T38.7X4	T38.7X5	T38.7X6
estrogen	T38.5X1	T38.5X2	T38.5X3	T38.5X4	T38.5X5	T38.5X6
ENT agent	T49.6X1	T49.6X2	T49.6X3	T49.6X4	T49.6X5	T49.6X6
ophthalmic preparation	T49.5X1	T49.5X2	T49.5X3	T49.5X4	T49.5X5	T49.5X6
topical NEC	T49.0X1	T49.0X2	T49.0X3	T49.0X4	T49.0X5	T49.0X6
Stibine	T56.891	T56.892	T56.893	T56.894		
Stibogluconate	T37.3X1	T37.3X2	T37.3X3	T37.3X4	T37.3X5	T37.3X6
Stibophen	T37.4X1	T37.4X2	T37.4X3	T37.4X4	T37.4X5	T37.4X6
Stilbamidine (isetionate)	T37.3X1	T37.3X2	T37.3X3	T37.3X4	T37.3X5	T37.3X6
Stilbestrol	T38.5X1	T38.5X2	T38.5X3	T38.5X4	T38.5X5	T38.5X6
Stilboestrol	T38.5X1	T38.5X2	T38.5X3	T38.5X4	T38.5X5	T38.5X6
Stimulant						
central nervous system — see also Psychostimulant	T43.601	T43.602	T43.603	T43.604	T43.605	T43.606
analeptics	T50.7X1	T50.7X2	T50.7X3	T50.7X4	T50.7X5	T50.7X6
opiate antagonist	T50.7X1	T50.7X2	T50.7X3	T50.7X4	T50.7X5	T50.7X6
psychotherapeutic NEC — see also Psychotherapeutic drug	T43.601	T43.602	T43.603	T43.604	T43.605	T43.606
specified NEC	T43.691	T43.692	T43.693	T43.694	T43.695	T43.696
respiratory	T48.901	T48.902	T48.903	T48.904	T48.905	T48.906
Stone-dissolving drug	T50.901	T50.902	T50.903	T50.904	T50.905	T50.906
Storage battery (cells) (acid)	T54.2X1	T54.2X2	T54.2X3	T54.2X4		
Stovaine	T41.3X1	T41.3X2	T41.3X3	T41.3X4	T41.3X5	T41.3X6
infiltration (subcutaneous)	T41.3X1	T41.3X2	T41.3X3	T41.3X4	T41.3X5	T41.3X6
nerve block (peripheral) (plexus)	T41.3X1	T41.3X2	T41.3X3	T41.3X4	T41.3X5	T41.3X6
spinal	T41.3X1	T41.3X2	T41.3X3	T41.3X4	T41.3X5	T41.3X6
topical (surface)	T41.3X1	T41.3X2	T41.3X3	T41.3X4	T41.3X5	T41.3X6
Stovarsal	T37.8X1	T37.8X2	T37.8X3	T37.8X4	T37.8X5	T37.8X6
Stove gas — see Gas, stove						
Stoxil	T49.5X1	T49.5X2	T49.5X3	T49.5X4	T49.5X5	T49.5X6
Stramonium	T48.6X1	T48.6X2	T48.6X3	T48.6X4	T48.6X5	T48.6X6
natural state	T62.2X1	T62.2X2	T62.2X3	T62.2X4	—	—
Streptodornase	T45.3X1	T45.3X2	T45.3X3	T45.3X4	T45.3X5	T45.3X6
Streptoduocin	T36.5X1	T36.5X2	T36.5X3	T36.5X4	T36.5X5	T36.5X6
Streptokinase	T45.611	T45.612	T45.613	T45.614	T45.615	T45.616
Streptomycin (derivative)	T36.5X1	T36.5X2	T36.5X3	T36.5X4	T36.5X5	T36.5X6
Streptonivicin	T36.5X1	T36.5X2	T36.5X3	T36.5X4	T36.5X5	T36.5X6
Streptovarycin	T36.5X1	T36.5X2	T36.5X3	T36.5X4	T36.5X5	T36.5X6
Streptozocin	T45.1X1	T45.1X2	T45.1X3	T45.1X4	T45.1X5	T45.1X6
Streptozotocin	T45.1X1	T45.1X2	T45.1X3	T45.1X4	T45.1X5	T45.1X6
Stripper (paint) (solvent)	T52.8X1	T52.8X2	T52.8X3	T52.8X4	—	—
Strobane	T60.1X1	T60.1X2	T60.1X3	T60.1X4	—	—
Strofantina	T46.0X1	T46.0X2	T46.0X3	T46.0X4	T46.0X5	T46.0X6
Strophanthin (g) (k)	T46.0X1	T46.0X2	T46.0X3	T46.0X4	T46.0X5	T46.0X6
Strophanthus	T46.0X1	T46.0X2	T46.0X3	T46.0X4	T46.0X5	T46.0X6
Strophantin	T46.0X1	T46.0X2	T46.0X3	T46.0X4	T46.0X5	T46.0X6
Strophantin-g	T46.0X1	T46.0X2	T46.0X3	T46.0X4	T46.0X5	T46.0X6
Strychnine (nonmedicinal) (pesticide) (salts)	T65.1X1	T65.1X2	T65.1X3	T65.1X4	—	—
medicinal	T48.291	T48.292	T48.293	T48.294	T48.295	T48.296
Strychnos (ignatii) — see Strychnine						
Styramate	T42.8X1	T42.8X2	T42.8X3	T42.8X4	T42.8X5	T42.8X6
Styrene	T65.891	T65.892	T65.893	T65.894	—	—
Succinimide, antiepileptic or anticonvulsant	T42.2X1	T42.2X2	T42.2X3	T42.2X4	T42.2X5	T42.2X6
mercuric — see Mercury						
Succinylcholine	T48.1X1	T48.1X2	T48.1X3	T48.1X4	T48.1X5	T48.1X6
Succinylsulfathiazole	T37.0X1	T37.0X2	T37.0X3	T37.0X4	T37.0X5	T37.0X6
Sucralfate	T47.1X1	T47.1X2	T47.1X3	T47.1X4	T47.1X5	T47.1X6
Sucrose	T50.3X1	T50.3X2	T50.3X3	T50.3X4	T50.3X5	T50.3X6
Sufentanil	T40.4X1	T40.4X2	T40.4X3	T40.4X4	T40.4X5	T40.4X6
Sulbactam	T36.0X1	T36.0X2	T36.0X3	T36.0X4	T36.0X5	T36.0X6
Sulbenicillin	T36.0X1	T36.0X2	T36.0X3	T36.0X4	T36.0X5	T36.0X6
Sulbentine	T49.0X1	T49.0X2	T49.0X3	T49.0X4	T49.0X5	T49.0X6
Sulfacetamide	T49.0X1	T49.0X2	T49.0X3	T49.0X4	T49.0X5	T49.0X6
ophthalmic preparation	T49.5X1	T49.5X2	T49.5X3	T49.5X4	T49.5X5	T49.5X6
Sulfachlorpyridazine	T37.0X1	T37.0X2	T37.0X3	T37.0X4	T37.0X5	T37.0X6
Sulfacitine	T37.0X1	T37.0X2	T37.0X3	T37.0X4	T37.0X5	T37.0X6
Sulfadiasulfone sodium	T37.0X1	T37.0X2	T37.0X3	T37.0X4	T37.0X5	T37.0X6
Sulfadiazine	T37.0X1	T37.0X2	T37.0X3	T37.0X4	T37.0X5	T37.0X6
silver (topical)	T49.0X1	T49.0X2	T49.0X3	T49.0X4	T49.0X5	T49.0X6
Sulfadimethoxine	T37.0X1	T37.0X2	T37.0X3	T37.0X4	T37.0X5	T37.0X6
Sulfadimidine	T37.0X1	T37.0X2	T37.0X3	T37.0X4	T37.0X5	T37.0X6
Sulfadoxine	T37.0X1	T37.0X2	T37.0X3	T37.0X4	T37.0X5	T37.0X6
with pyrimethamine	T37.2X1	T37.2X2	T37.2X3	T37.2X4	T37.2X5	T37.2X6

Additional Character May Be Required — Refer to the Tabular List for Character Selection   ▽ Subterms under main terms may continue to next column or page

Substance	Poisoning, Accidental (unintentional)	Poisoning, Intentional Self-harm	Poisoning, Assault	Poisoning, Undetermined	Adverse Effect	Under-dosing
Sulfaethidole	T37.0X1	T37.0X2	T37.0X3	T37.0X4	T37.0X5	T37.0X6
Sulfafurazole	T37.0X1	T37.0X2	T37.0X3	T37.0X4	T37.0X5	T37.0X6
Sulfaguanidine	T37.0X1	T37.0X2	T37.0X3	T37.0X4	T37.0X5	T37.0X6
Sulfalene	T37.0X1	T37.0X2	T37.0X3	T37.0X4	T37.0X5	T37.0X6
Sulfaloxate	T37.0X1	T37.0X2	T37.0X3	T37.0X4	T37.0X5	T37.0X6
Sulfaloxic acid	T37.0X1	T37.0X2	T37.0X3	T37.0X4	T37.0X5	T37.0X6
Sulfamazone	T39.2X1	T39.2X2	T39.2X3	T39.2X4	T39.2X5	T39.2X6
Sulfamerazine	T37.0X1	T37.0X2	T37.0X3	T37.0X4	T37.0X5	T37.0X6
Sulfameter	T37.0X1	T37.0X2	T37.0X3	T37.0X4	T37.0X5	T37.0X6
Sulfamethazine	T37.0X1	T37.0X2	T37.0X3	T37.0X4	T37.0X5	T37.0X6
Sulfamethizole	T37.0X1	T37.0X2	T37.0X3	T37.0X4	T37.0X5	T37.0X6
Sulfamethoxazole	T37.0X1	T37.0X2	T37.0X3	T37.0X4	T37.0X5	T37.0X6
with trimethoprim	T36.8X1	T36.8X2	T36.8X3	T36.8X4	T36.8X5	T36.8X6
Sulfamethoxydiazine	T37.0X1	T37.0X2	T37.0X3	T37.0X4	T37.0X5	T37.0X6
Sulfamethoxypyridazine	T37.0X1	T37.0X2	T37.0X3	T37.0X4	T37.0X5	T37.0X6
Sulfamethylthiazole	T37.0X1	T37.0X2	T37.0X3	T37.0X4	T37.0X5	T37.0X6
Sulfametoxydiazine	T37.0X1	T37.0X2	T37.0X3	T37.0X4	T37.0X5	T37.0X6
Sulfamidopyrine	T39.2X1	T39.2X2	T39.2X3	T39.2X4	T39.2X5	T39.2X6
Sulfamonomethoxine	T37.0X1	T37.0X2	T37.0X3	T37.0X4	T37.0X5	T37.0X6
Sulfamoxole	T37.0X1	T37.0X2	T37.0X3	T37.0X4	T37.0X5	T37.0X6
Sulfamylon	T49.0X1	T49.0X2	T49.0X3	T49.0X4	T49.0X5	T49.0X6
Sulfan blue (diagnostic dye)	T50.8X1	T50.8X2	T50.8X3	T50.8X4	T50.8X5	T50.8X6
Sulfanilamide	T37.0X1	T37.0X2	T37.0X3	T37.0X4	T37.0X5	T37.0X6
Sulfanilylguanidine	T37.0X1	T37.0X2	T37.0X3	T37.0X4	T37.0X5	T37.0X6
Sulfaperin	T37.0X1	T37.0X2	T37.0X3	T37.0X4	T37.0X5	T37.0X6
Sulfaphenazole	T37.0X1	T37.0X2	T37.0X3	T37.0X4	T37.0X5	T37.0X6
Sulfaphenylthiazole	T37.0X1	T37.0X2	T37.0X3	T37.0X4	T37.0X5	T37.0X6
Sulfaproxyline	T39.2X1	T39.2X2	T39.2X3	T39.2X4	T39.2X5	T39.2X6
Sulfapyridine	T37.0X1	T37.0X2	T37.0X3	T37.0X4	T37.0X5	T37.0X6
Sulfapyrimidine	T37.0X1	T37.0X2	T37.0X3	T37.0X4	T37.0X5	T37.0X6
Sulfarsphenamine	T37.8X1	T37.8X2	T37.8X3	T37.8X4	T37.8X5	T37.8X6
Sulfasalazine	T37.0X1	T37.0X2	T37.0X3	T37.0X4	T37.0X5	T37.0X6
Sulfasuxidine	T37.0X1	T37.0X2	T37.0X3	T37.0X4	T37.0X5	T37.0X6
Sulfasymazine	T37.0X1	T37.0X2	T37.0X3	T37.0X4	T37.0X5	T37.0X6
Sulfated amylopectin	T47.8X1	T47.8X2	T47.8X3	T47.8X4	T47.8X5	T47.8X6
Sulfathiazole	T37.0X1	T37.0X2	T37.0X3	T37.0X4	T37.0X5	T37.0X6
Sulfatostearate	T49.2X1	T49.2X2	T49.2X3	T49.2X4	T49.2X5	T49.2X6
Sulfinpyrazone	T50.4X1	T50.4X2	T50.4X3	T50.4X4	T50.4X5	T50.4X6
Sulfiram	T49.0X1	T49.0X2	T49.0X3	T49.0X4	T49.0X5	T49.0X6
Sulfisomidine	T37.0X1	T37.0X2	T37.0X3	T37.0X4	T37.0X5	T37.0X6
Sulfisoxazole	T37.0X1	T37.0X2	T37.0X3	T37.0X4	T37.0X5	T37.0X6
ophthalmic preparation	T49.5X1	T49.5X2	T49.5X3	T49.5X4	T49.5X5	T49.5X6
Sulfobromophthalein (sodium)	T50.8X1	T50.8X2	T50.8X3	T50.8X4	T50.8X5	T50.8X6
Sulfobromphthalein	T50.8X1	T50.8X2	T50.8X3	T50.8X4	T50.8X5	T50.8X6
Sulfogaiacol	T48.4X1	T48.4X2	T48.4X3	T48.4X4	T48.4X5	T48.4X6
Sulfomyxin	T36.8X1	T36.8X2	T36.8X3	T36.8X4	T36.8X5	T36.8X6
Sulfonal	T42.6X1	T42.6X2	T42.6X3	T42.6X4	T42.6X5	T42.6X6
Sulfonamide NEC	T37.0X1	T37.0X2	T37.0X3	T37.0X4	T37.0X5	T37.0X6
eye	T49.5X1	T49.5X2	T49.5X3	T49.5X4	T49.5X5	T49.5X6
Sulfonazide	T37.1X1	T37.1X2	T37.1X3	T37.1X4	T37.1X5	T37.1X6
Sulfones	T37.1X1	T37.1X2	T37.1X3	T37.1X4	T37.1X5	T37.1X6
Sulfonethylmethane	T42.6X1	T42.6X2	T42.6X3	T42.6X4	T42.6X5	T42.6X6
Sulfonmethane	T42.6X1	T42.6X2	T42.6X3	T42.6X4	T42.6X5	T42.6X6
Sulfonphthal, sulfonphthol	T50.8X1	T50.8X2	T50.8X3	T50.8X4	T50.8X5	T50.8X6
Sulfonylurea derivatives, oral	T38.3X1	T38.3X2	T38.3X3	T38.3X4	T38.3X5	T38.3X6
Sulforidazine	T43.3X1	T43.3X2	T43.3X3	T43.3X4	T43.3X5	T43.3X6
Sulfoxone	T37.1X1	T37.1X2	T37.1X3	T37.1X4	T37.1X5	T37.1X6
Sulfuric acid	T54.2X1	T54.2X2	T54.2X3	T54.2X4	—	—
Sulfur, sulfurated, sulfuric, sulfurous, sulfuryl (compounds NEC) (medicinal)	T49.4X1	T49.4X2	T49.4X3	T49.4X4	T49.4X5	T49.4X6
acid	T54.2X1	T54.2X2	T54.2X3	T54.2X4	—	—
dioxide (gas)	T59.1X1	T59.1X2	T59.1X3	T59.1X4	—	—
ether — see Ether(s)						
hydrogen	T59.6X1	T59.6X2	T59.6X3	T59.6X4	—	—
medicinal (keratolytic) (ointment) NEC	T49.4X1	T49.4X2	T49.4X3	T49.4X4	T49.4X5	T49.4X6
ointment	T49.0X1	T49.0X2	T49.0X3	T49.0X4	T49.0X5	T49.0X6
pesticide (vapor)	T60.91	T60.92	T60.93	T60.94	—	—
vapor NEC	T59.891	T59.892	T59.893	T59.894	—	—
Sulglicotide	T47.1X1	T47.1X2	T47.1X3	T47.1X4	T47.1X5	T47.1X6
Sulindac	T39.391	T39.392	T39.393	T39.394	T39.395	T39.396
Sulisatin	T47.2X1	T47.2X2	T47.2X3	T47.2X4	T47.2X5	T47.2X6
Sulisobenzone	T49.3X1	T49.3X2	T49.3X3	T49.3X4	T49.3X5	T49.3X6
Sulkowitch's reagent	T50.8X1	T50.8X2	T50.8X3	T50.8X4	T50.8X5	T50.8X6
Sulmetozine	T44.3X1	T44.3X2	T44.3X3	T44.3X4	T44.3X5	T44.3X6
Suloctidil	T46.7X1	T46.7X2	T46.7X3	T46.7X4	T46.7X5	T46.7X6
Sulph- — see also Sulf-						
Sulphadiazine	T37.0X1	T37.0X2	T37.0X3	T37.0X4	T37.0X5	T37.0X6
Sulphadimethoxine	T37.0X1	T37.0X2	T37.0X3	T37.0X4	T37.0X5	T37.0X6
Sulphadimidine	T37.0X1	T37.0X2	T37.0X3	T37.0X4	T37.0X5	T37.0X6
Sulphadione	T37.1X1	T37.1X2	T37.1X3	T37.1X4	T37.1X5	T37.1X6
Sulphafurazole	T37.0X1	T37.0X2	T37.0X3	T37.0X4	T37.0X5	T37.0X6
Sulphamethizole	T37.0X1	T37.0X2	T37.0X3	T37.0X4	T37.0X5	T37.0X6
Sulphamethoxazole	T37.0X1	T37.0X2	T37.0X3	T37.0X4	T37.0X5	T37.0X6
Sulphan blue	T50.8X1	T50.8X2	T50.8X3	T50.8X4	T50.8X5	T50.8X6
Sulphaphenazole	T37.0X1	T37.0X2	T37.0X3	T37.0X4	T37.0X5	T37.0X6
Sulphapyridine	T37.0X1	T37.0X2	T37.0X3	T37.0X4	T37.0X5	T37.0X6
Sulphasalazine	T37.0X1	T37.0X2	T37.0X3	T37.0X4	T37.0X5	T37.0X6
Sulphinpyrazone	T50.4X1	T50.4X2	T50.4X3	T50.4X4	T50.4X5	T50.4X6
Sulpiride	T43.591	T43.592	T43.593	T43.594	T43.595	T43.596
Sulprostone	T48.0X1	T48.0X2	T48.0X3	T48.0X4	T48.0X5	T48.0X6
Sulpyrine	T39.2X1	T39.2X2	T39.2X3	T39.2X4	T39.2X5	T39.2X6
Sultamicillin	T36.0X1	T36.0X2	T36.0X3	T36.0X4	T36.0X5	T36.0X6
Sulthiame	T42.6X1	T42.6X2	T42.6X3	T42.6X4	T42.6X5	T42.6X6
Sultiame	T42.6X1	T42.6X2	T42.6X3	T42.6X4	T42.6X5	T42.6X6
Sultopride	T43.591	T43.592	T43.593	T43.594	T43.595	T43.596
Sumatriptan	T39.8X1	T39.8X2	T39.8X3	T39.8X4	T39.8X5	T39.8X6
Sunflower seed oil	T46.6X1	T46.6X2	T46.6X3	T46.6X4	T46.6X5	T46.6X6
Superinone	T48.4X1	T48.4X2	T48.4X3	T48.4X4	T48.4X5	T48.4X6
Suprofen	T39.311	T39.312	T39.313	T39.314	T39.315	T39.316
Suramin (sodium)	T37.4X1	T37.4X2	T37.4X3	T37.4X4	T37.4X5	T37.4X6
Surfacaine	T41.3X1	T41.3X2	T41.3X3	T41.3X4	T41.3X5	T41.3X6
Surital	T41.1X1	T41.1X2	T41.1X3	T41.1X4	T41.1X5	T41.1X6
Sutilains	T45.3X1	T45.3X2	T45.3X3	T45.3X4	T45.3X5	T45.3X6
Suxamethonium (chloride)	T48.1X1	T48.1X2	T48.1X3	T48.1X4	T48.1X5	T48.1X6
Suxethonium (chloride)	T48.1X1	T48.1X2	T48.1X3	T48.1X4	T48.1X5	T48.1X6
Suxibuzone	T39.2X1	T39.2X2	T39.2X3	T39.2X4	T39.2X5	T39.2X6
Sweetener	T50.901	T50.902	T50.903	T50.904	T50.905	T50.906
Sweet niter spirit	T46.3X1	T46.3X2	T46.3X3	T46.3X4	T46.3X5	T46.3X6
Sweet oil (birch)	T49.3X1	T49.3X2	T49.3X3	T49.3X4	T49.3X5	T49.3X6
Sym-dichloroethyl ether	T53.6X1	T53.6X2	T53.6X3	T53.6X4	—	—
Sympatholytic NEC	T44.8X1	T44.8X2	T44.8X3	T44.8X4	T44.8X5	T44.8X6
haloalkylamine	T44.8X1	T44.8X2	T44.8X3	T44.8X4	T44.8X5	T44.8X6
Sympathomimetic NEC	T44.901	T44.902	T44.903	T44.904	T44.905	T44.906
anti-common-cold	T48.5X1	T48.5X2	T48.5X3	T48.5X4	T48.5X5	T48.5X6
bronchodilator	T48.6X1	T48.6X2	T48.6X3	T48.6X4	T48.6X5	T48.6X6
specified NEC	T44.991	T44.992	T44.993	T44.994	T44.995	T44.996
Synagis	T50.B91	T50.B92	T50.B93	T50.B94	T50.B95	T50.B96
Synalar	T49.0X1	T49.0X2	T49.0X3	T49.0X4	T49.0X5	T49.0X6
Synthroid	T38.1X1	T38.1X2	T38.1X3	T38.1X4	T38.1X5	T38.1X6
Syntocinon	T48.0X1	T48.0X2	T48.0X3	T48.0X4	T48.0X5	T48.0X6
Syrosingopine	T46.5X1	T46.5X2	T46.5X3	T46.5X4	T46.5X5	T46.5X6
Systemic drug	T45.91	T45.92	T45.93	T45.94	T45.95	T45.96
specified NEC	T45.8X1	T45.8X2	T45.8X3	T45.8X4	T45.8X5	T45.8X6
Tablets — see also specified substance	T50.901	T50.902	T50.903	T50.904	T50.905	T50.906
Tace	T38.5X1	T38.5X2	T38.5X3	T38.5X4	T38.5X5	T38.5X6
Tacrine	T44.0X1	T44.0X2	T44.0X3	T44.0X4	T44.0X5	T44.0X6
Tadalafil	T46.7X1	T46.7X2	T46.7X3	T46.7X4	T46.7X5	T46.7X6
Talampicillin	T36.0X1	T36.0X2	T36.0X3	T36.0X4	T36.0X5	T36.0X6
Talbutal	T42.3X1	T42.3X2	T42.3X3	T42.3X4	T42.3X5	T42.3X6
Talc powder	T49.3X1	T49.3X2	T49.3X3	T49.3X4	T49.3X5	T49.3X6
Talcum	T49.3X1	T49.3X2	T49.3X3	T49.3X4	T49.3X5	T49.3X6
Taleranol	T38.6X1	T38.6X2	T38.6X3	T38.6X4	T38.6X5	T38.6X6
Tamoxifen	T38.6X1	T38.6X2	T38.6X3	T38.6X4	T38.6X5	T38.6X6
Tamsulosin	T44.6X1	T44.6X2	T44.6X3	T44.6X4	T44.6X5	T44.6X6
Tandearil, tanderil	T39.2X1	T39.2X2	T39.2X3	T39.2X4	T39.2X5	T39.2X6
Tannic acid	T49.2X1	T49.2X2	T49.2X3	T49.2X4	T49.2X5	T49.2X6
medicinal (astringent)	T49.2X1	T49.2X2	T49.2X3	T49.2X4	T49.2X5	T49.2X6
Tannin — see Tannic acid						
Tansy	T62.2X1	T62.2X2	T62.2X3	T62.2X4	—	—
TAO	T36.3X1	T36.3X2	T36.3X3	T36.3X4	T36.3X5	T36.3X6
Tapazole	T38.2X1	T38.2X2	T38.2X3	T38.2X4	T38.2X5	T38.2X6
Taractan	T43.591	T43.592	T43.593	T43.594	T43.595	T43.596
Tarantula (venomous)	T63.321	T63.322	T63.323	T63.324	—	—
Tartar emetic	T37.8X1	T37.8X2	T37.8X3	T37.8X4	T37.8X5	T37.8X6
Tartaric acid	T65.891	T65.892	T65.893	T65.894	—	—
Tartrated antimony (anti-infective)	T37.8X1	T37.8X2	T37.8X3	T37.8X4	T37.8X5	T37.8X6
Tartrate, laxative	T47.4X1	T47.4X2	T47.4X3	T47.4X4	T47.4X5	T47.4X6
Tar NEC	T52.0X1	T52.0X2	T52.0X3	T52.0X4	—	—
camphor	T60.1X1	T60.1X2	T60.1X3	T60.1X4	—	—
distillate	T49.1X1	T49.1X2	T49.1X3	T49.1X4	T49.1X5	T49.1X6
fumes	T59.891	T59.892	T59.893	T59.894	—	—
medicinal	T49.1X1	T49.1X2	T49.1X3	T49.1X4	T49.1X5	T49.1X6
ointment	T49.1X1	T49.1X2	T49.1X3	T49.1X4	T49.1X5	T49.1X6
Tauromustine	T45.1X1	T45.1X2	T45.1X3	T45.1X4	T45.1X5	T45.1X6
TCA — see Trichloroacetic acid						
TCDD	T53.7X1	T53.7X2	T53.7X3	T53.7X4	—	—
TDI (vapor)	T65.0X1	T65.0X2	T65.0X3	T65.0X4	—	—
Tear						
gas	T59.3X1	T59.3X2	T59.3X3	T59.3X4	—	—

Table of Drugs and Chemicals

Sulfaethidole — Tear

Table of Drugs and Chemicals

Substance	Poisoning, Accidental (unintentional)	Poisoning, Intentional Self-harm	Poisoning, Assault	Poisoning, Undetermined	Adverse Effect	Under-dosing
Tear — continued						
solution	T49.5X1	T49.5X2	T49.5X3	T49.5X4	T49.5X5	T49.5X6
Teclothiazide	T50.2X1	T50.2X2	T50.2X3	T50.2X4	T50.2X5	T50.2X6
Teclozan	T37.3X1	T37.3X2	T37.3X3	T37.3X4	T37.3X5	T37.3X6
Tegafur	T45.1X1	T45.1X2	T45.1X3	T45.1X4	T45.1X5	T45.1X6
Tegretol	T42.1X1	T42.1X2	T42.1X3	T42.1X4	T42.1X5	T42.1X6
Teicoplanin	T36.8X1	T36.8X2	T36.8X3	T36.8X4	T36.8X5	T36.8X6
Telepaque	T50.8X1	T50.8X2	T50.8X3	T50.8X4	T50.8X5	T50.8X6
Tellurium	T56.891	T56.892	T56.893	T56.894	—	—
fumes	T56.891	T56.892	T56.893	T56.894	—	—
TEM	T45.1X1	T45.1X2	T45.1X3	T45.1X4	T45.1X5	T45.1X6
Temazepam	T42.4X1	T42.4X2	T42.4X3	T42.4X4	T42.4X5	T42.4X6
Temocillin	T36.0X1	T36.0X2	T36.0X3	T36.0X4	T36.0X5	T36.0X6
Tenamfetamine	T43.621	T43.622	T43.623	T43.624	T43.625	T43.626
Teniposide	T45.1X1	T45.1X2	T45.1X3	T45.1X4	T45.1X5	T45.1X6
Tenitramine	T46.3X1	T46.3X2	T46.3X3	T46.3X4	T46.3X5	T46.3X6
Tenoglicin	T48.4X1	T48.4X2	T48.4X3	T48.4X4	T48.4X5	T48.4X6
Tenonitrozole	T37.3X1	T37.3X2	T37.3X3	T37.3X4	T37.3X5	T37.3X6
Tenoxicam	T39.391	T39.392	T39.393	T39.394	T39.395	T39.396
TEPA	T45.1X1	T45.1X2	T45.1X3	T45.1X4	T45.1X5	T45.1X6
TEPP	T60.0X1	T60.0X2	T60.0X3	T60.0X4	—	—
Teprotide	T46.5X1	T46.5X2	T46.5X3	T46.5X4	T46.5X5	T46.5X6
Terazosin	T44.6X1	T44.6X2	T44.6X3	T44.6X4	T44.6X5	T44.6X6
Terbufos	T60.0X1	T60.0X2	T60.0X3	T60.0X4	—	—
Terbutaline	T48.6X1	T48.6X2	T48.6X3	T48.6X4	T48.6X5	T48.6X6
Terconazole	T49.0X1	T49.0X2	T49.0X3	T49.0X4	T49.0X5	T49.0X6
Terfenadine	T45.0X1	T45.0X2	T45.0X3	T45.0X4	T45.0X5	T45.0X6
Teriparatide (acetate)	T50.991	T50.992	T50.993	T50.994	T50.995	T50.996
Terizidone	T37.1X1	T37.1X2	T37.1X3	T37.1X4	T37.1X5	T37.1X6
Terlipressin	T38.891	T38.892	T38.893	T38.894	T38.895	T38.896
Terodiline	T46.3X1	T46.3X2	T46.3X3	T46.3X4	T46.3X5	T46.3X6
Teroxalene	T37.4X1	T37.4X2	T37.4X3	T37.4X4	T37.4X5	T37.4X6
Terpin (cis) hydrate	T48.4X1	T48.4X2	T48.4X3	T48.4X4	T48.4X5	T48.4X6
Terramycin	T36.4X1	T36.4X2	T36.4X3	T36.4X4	T36.4X5	T36.4X6
Tertatolol	T44.7X1	T44.7X2	T44.7X3	T44.7X4	T44.7X5	T44.7X6
Tessalon	T48.3X1	T48.3X2	T48.3X3	T48.3X4	T48.3X5	T48.3X6
Testolactone	T38.7X1	T38.7X2	T38.7X3	T38.7X4	T38.7X5	T38.7X6
Testosterone	T38.7X1	T38.7X2	T38.7X3	T38.7X4	T38.7X5	T38.7X6
Tetanus toxoid or vaccine	T50.A91	T50.A92	T50.A93	T50.A94	T50.A95	T50.A96
antitoxin	T50.Z11	T50.Z12	T50.Z13	T50.Z14	T50.Z15	T50.Z16
immune globulin (human)	T50.Z11	T50.Z12	T50.Z13	T50.Z14	T50.Z15	T50.Z16
toxoid	T50.A91	T50.A92	T50.A93	T50.A94	T50.A95	T50.A96
with diphtheria toxoid	T50.A21	T50.A22	T50.A23	T50.A24	T50.A25	T50.A26
with pertussis	T50.A11	T50.A12	T50.A13	T50.A14	T50.A15	T50.A16
Tetrabenazine	T43.591	T43.592	T43.593	T43.594	T43.595	T43.596
Tetracaine	T41.3X1	T41.3X2	T41.3X3	T41.3X4	T41.3X5	T41.3X6
nerve block (peripheral) (plexus)	T41.3X1	T41.3X2	T41.3X3	T41.3X4	T41.3X5	T41.3X6
regional	T41.3X1	T41.3X2	T41.3X3	T41.3X4	T41.3X5	T41.3X6
spinal	T41.3X1	T41.3X2	T41.3X3	T41.3X4	T41.3X5	T41.3X6
Tetrachlorethylene — see Tetrachloroethylene						
Tetrachlormethiazide	T50.2X1	T50.2X2	T50.2X3	T50.2X4	T50.2X5	T50.2X6
Tetrachloroethane	T53.6X1	T53.6X2	T53.6X3	T53.6X4	—	—
vapor	T53.6X1	T53.6X2	T53.6X3	T53.6X4	—	—
paint or varnish	T53.6X1	T53.6X2	T53.6X3	T53.6X4	—	—
Tetrachloroethylene (liquid)	T53.3X1	T53.3X2	T53.3X3	T53.3X4	—	—
medicinal	T37.4X1	T37.4X2	T37.4X3	T37.4X4	T37.4X5	T37.4X6
vapor	T53.3X1	T53.3X2	T53.3X3	T53.3X4	—	—
Tetrachloromethane — see Carbon tetrachloride						
Tetracosactide	T38.811	T38.812	T38.813	T38.814	T38.815	T38.816
Tetracosactrin	T38.811	T38.812	T38.813	T38.814	T38.815	T38.816
Tetracycline	T36.4X1	T36.4X2	T36.4X3	T36.4X4	T36.4X5	T36.4X6
ophthalmic preparation	T49.5X1	T49.5X2	T49.5X3	T49.5X4	T49.5X5	T49.5X6
topical NEC	T49.0X1	T49.0X2	T49.0X3	T49.0X4	T49.0X5	T49.0X6
Tetradifon	T60.8X1	T60.8X2	T60.8X3	T60.8X4	—	—
Tetradotoxin	T61.771	T61.772	T61.773	T61.774	—	—
Tetraethyl						
lead	T56.0X1	T56.0X2	T56.0X3	T56.0X4	—	—
pyrophosphate	T60.0X1	T60.0X2	T60.0X3	T60.0X4	—	—
Tetraethylammonium chloride	T44.2X1	T44.2X2	T44.2X3	T44.2X4	T44.2X5	T44.2X6
Tetraethylthiuram disulfide	T50.6X1	T50.6X2	T50.6X3	T50.6X4	T50.6X5	T50.6X6
Tetrahydroaminoacridine	T44.0X1	T44.0X2	T44.0X3	T44.0X4	T44.0X5	T44.0X6
Tetrahydrocannabinol	T40.7X1	T40.7X2	T40.7X3	T40.7X4	T40.7X5	T40.7X6
Tetrahydrofuran	T52.8X1	T52.8X2	T52.8X3	T52.8X4	—	—
Tetrahydronaphthalene	T52.8X1	T52.8X2	T52.8X3	T52.8X4	—	—
Tetrahydrozoline	T49.5X1	T49.5X2	T49.5X3	T49.5X4	T49.5X5	T49.5X6
Tetralin	T52.8X1	T52.8X2	T52.8X3	T52.8X4	—	—
Tetramethrin	T60.2X1	T60.2X2	T60.2X3	T60.2X4	—	—
Tetramethylthiuram (disulfide) NEC	T60.3X1	T60.3X2	T60.3X3	T60.3X4	—	—
medicinal	T49.0X1	T49.0X2	T49.0X3	T49.0X4	T49.0X5	T49.0X6
Tetramisole	T37.4X1	T37.4X2	T37.4X3	T37.4X4	T37.4X5	T37.4X6
Tetranicotinoyl fructose	T46.7X1	T46.7X2	T46.7X3	T46.7X4	T46.7X5	T46.7X6
Tetrazepam	T42.4X1	T42.4X2	T42.4X3	T42.4X4	T42.4X5	T42.4X6
Tetronal	T42.6X1	T42.6X2	T42.6X3	T42.6X4	T42.6X5	T42.6X6
Tetryl	T65.3X1	T65.3X2	T65.3X3	T65.3X4	—	—
Tetrylammonium chloride	T44.2X1	T44.2X2	T44.2X3	T44.2X4	T44.2X5	T44.2X6
Tetryzoline	T49.5X1	T49.5X2	T49.5X3	T49.5X4	T49.5X5	T49.5X6
Thalidomide	T45.1X1	T45.1X2	T45.1X3	T45.1X4	T45.1X5	T45.1X6
Thallium (compounds) (dust) NEC	T56.811	T56.812	T56.813	T56.814	—	—
pesticide	T60.4X1	T60.4X2	T60.4X3	T60.4X4	—	—
THC	T40.7X1	T40.7X2	T40.7X3	T40.7X4	T40.7X5	T40.7X6
Thebacon	T40.2X1	T40.2X2	T40.2X3	T40.2X4	T40.2X5	T40.2X6
Thebaine	T40.2X1	T40.2X2	T40.2X3	T40.2X4	T40.2X5	T40.2X6
Thenoic acid	T49.6X1	T49.6X2	T49.6X3	T49.6X4	T49.6X5	T49.6X6
Thenyldiamine	T45.0X1	T45.0X2	T45.0X3	T45.0X4	T45.0X5	T45.0X6
Theobromine (calcium salicylate)	T48.6X1	T48.6X2	T48.6X3	T48.6X4	T48.6X5	T48.6X6
sodium salicylate	T48.6X1	T48.6X2	T48.6X3	T48.6X4	T48.6X5	T48.6X6
Theophyllamine	T48.6X1	T48.6X2	T48.6X3	T48.6X4	T48.6X5	T48.6X6
Theophylline	T48.6X1	T48.6X2	T48.6X3	T48.6X4	T48.6X5	T48.6X6
aminobenzoic acid	T48.6X1	T48.6X2	T48.6X3	T48.6X4	T48.6X5	T48.6X6
ethylenediamine	T48.6X1	T48.6X2	T48.6X3	T48.6X4	T48.6X5	T48.6X6
piperazine p-amino-benzoate	T48.6X1	T48.6X2	T48.6X3	T48.6X4	T48.6X5	T48.6X6
Thiabendazole	T37.4X1	T37.4X2	T37.4X3	T37.4X4	T37.4X5	T37.4X6
Thialbarbital	T41.1X1	T41.1X2	T41.1X3	T41.1X4	T41.1X5	T41.1X6
Thiamazole	T38.2X1	T38.2X2	T38.2X3	T38.2X4	T38.2X5	T38.2X6
Thiambutosine	T37.1X1	T37.1X2	T37.1X3	T37.1X4	T37.1X5	T37.1X6
Thiamine	T45.2X1	T45.2X2	T45.2X3	T45.2X4	T45.2X5	T45.2X6
Thiamphenicol	T36.2X1	T36.2X2	T36.2X3	T36.2X4	T36.2X5	T36.2X6
Thiamylal	T41.1X1	T41.1X2	T41.1X3	T41.1X4	T41.1X5	T41.1X6
sodium	T41.1X1	T41.1X2	T41.1X3	T41.1X4	T41.1X5	T41.1X6
Thiazesim	T43.291	T43.292	T43.293	T43.294	T43.295	T43.296
Thiazides (diuretics)	T50.2X1	T50.2X2	T50.2X3	T50.2X4	T50.2X5	T50.2X6
Thiazinamium metilsulfate	T43.3X1	T43.3X2	T43.3X3	T43.3X4	T43.3X5	T43.3X6
Thiethylperazine	T43.3X1	T43.3X2	T43.3X3	T43.3X4	T43.3X5	T43.3X6
Thimerosal	T49.0X1	T49.0X2	T49.0X3	T49.0X4	T49.0X5	T49.0X6
ophthalmic preparation	T49.5X1	T49.5X2	T49.5X3	T49.5X4	T49.5X5	T49.5X6
Thioacetazone	T37.1X1	T37.1X2	T37.1X3	T37.1X4	T37.1X5	T37.1X6
with isoniazid	T37.1X1	T37.1X2	T37.1X3	T37.1X4	T37.1X5	T37.1X6
Thiobarbital sodium	T41.1X1	T41.1X2	T41.1X3	T41.1X4	T41.1X5	T41.1X6
Thiobarbiturate anesthetic	T41.1X1	T41.1X2	T41.1X3	T41.1X4	T41.1X5	T41.1X6
Thiobismol	T37.8X1	T37.8X2	T37.8X3	T37.8X4	T37.8X5	T37.8X6
Thiobutabarbital sodium	T41.1X1	T41.1X2	T41.1X3	T41.1X4	T41.1X5	T41.1X6
Thiocarbamate (insecticide)	T60.0X1	T60.0X2	T60.0X3	T60.0X4	—	—
Thiocarbamide	T38.2X1	T38.2X2	T38.2X3	T38.2X4	T38.2X5	T38.2X6
Thiocarbarsone	T37.8X1	T37.8X2	T37.8X3	T37.8X4	T37.8X5	T37.8X6
Thiocarlide	T37.1X1	T37.1X2	T37.1X3	T37.1X4	T37.1X5	T37.1X6
Thioctamide	T50.991	T50.992	T50.993	T50.994	T50.995	T50.996
Thioctic acid	T50.991	T50.992	T50.993	T50.994	T50.995	T50.996
Thiofos	T60.0X1	T60.0X2	T60.0X3	T60.0X4	—	—
Thioglycolate	T49.4X1	T49.4X2	T49.4X3	T49.4X4	T49.4X5	T49.4X6
Thioglycolic acid	T65.891	T65.892	T65.893	T65.894	—	—
Thioguanine	T45.1X1	T45.1X2	T45.1X3	T45.1X4	T45.1X5	T45.1X6
Thiomercaptomerin	T50.2X1	T50.2X2	T50.2X3	T50.2X4	T50.2X5	T50.2X6
Thiomerin	T50.2X1	T50.2X2	T50.2X3	T50.2X4	T50.2X5	T50.2X6
Thiomersal	T49.0X1	T49.0X2	T49.0X3	T49.0X4	T49.0X5	T49.0X6
Thionazin	T60.0X1	T60.0X2	T60.0X3	T60.0X4	—	—
Thiopental (sodium)	T41.1X1	T41.1X2	T41.1X3	T41.1X4	T41.1X5	T41.1X6
Thiopentone (sodium)	T41.1X1	T41.1X2	T41.1X3	T41.1X4	T41.1X5	T41.1X6
Thiopropazate	T43.3X1	T43.3X2	T43.3X3	T43.3X4	T43.3X5	T43.3X6
Thioproperazine	T43.3X1	T43.3X2	T43.3X3	T43.3X4	T43.3X5	T43.3X6
Thioridazine	T43.3X1	T43.3X2	T43.3X3	T43.3X4	T43.3X5	T43.3X6
Thiosinamine	T49.3X1	T49.3X2	T49.3X3	T49.3X4	T49.3X5	T49.3X6
Thiotepa	T45.1X1	T45.1X2	T45.1X3	T45.1X4	T45.1X5	T45.1X6
Thiothixene	T43.4X1	T43.4X2	T43.4X3	T43.4X4	T43.4X5	T43.4X6
Thiouracil (benzyl) (methyl) (propyl)	T38.2X1	T38.2X2	T38.2X3	T38.2X4	T38.2X5	T38.2X6
Thiourea	T38.2X1	T38.2X2	T38.2X3	T38.2X4	T38.2X5	T38.2X6
Thiphenamil	T44.3X1	T44.3X2	T44.3X3	T44.3X4	T44.3X5	T44.3X6
Thiram	T60.3X1	T60.3X2	T60.3X3	T60.3X4	—	—
medicinal	T49.2X1	T49.2X2	T49.2X3	T49.2X4	T49.2X5	T49.2X6
Thonzylamine (systemic)	T45.0X1	T45.0X2	T45.0X3	T45.0X4	T45.0X5	T45.0X6
mucosal decongestant	T48.5X1	T48.5X2	T48.5X3	T48.5X4	T48.5X5	T48.5X6
Thorazine	T43.3X1	T43.3X2	T43.3X3	T43.3X4	T43.3X5	T43.3X6
Thorium dioxide suspension	T50.8X1	T50.8X2	T50.8X3	T50.8X4	T50.8X5	T50.8X6
Thornapple	T62.2X1	T62.2X2	T62.2X3	T62.2X4	—	—
Throat drug NEC	T49.6X1	T49.6X2	T49.6X3	T49.6X4	T49.6X5	T49.6X6

Tear — Throat drug NEC

Substance	Poisoning, Accidental (unintentional)	Poisoning, Intentional Self-harm	Poisoning, Assault	Poisoning, Undetermined	Adverse Effect	Under-dosing
Thrombin	T45.7X1	T45.7X2	T45.7X3	T45.7X4	T45.7X5	T45.7X6
Thrombolysin	T45.611	T45.612	T45.613	T45.614	T45.615	T45.616
Thromboplastin	T45.7X1	T45.7X2	T45.7X3	T45.7X4	T45.7X5	T45.7X6
Thurfyl nicotinate	T46.7X1	T46.7X2	T46.7X3	T46.7X4	T46.7X5	T46.7X6
Thymol	T49.0X1	T49.0X2	T49.0X3	T49.0X4	T49.0X5	T49.0X6
Thymopentin	T37.5X1	T37.5X2	T37.5X3	T37.5X4	T37.5X5	T37.5X6
Thymoxamine	T46.7X1	T46.7X2	T46.7X3	T46.7X4	T46.7X5	T46.7X6
Thymus extract	T38.891	T38.892	T38.893	T38.894	T38.895	T38.896
Thyreotrophic hormone	T38.811	T38.812	T38.813	T38.814	T38.815	T38.816
Thyroglobulin	T38.1X1	T38.1X2	T38.1X3	T38.1X4	T38.1X5	T38.1X6
Thyroid (hormone)	T38.1X1	T38.1X2	T38.1X3	T38.1X4	T38.1X5	T38.1X6
Thyrolar	T38.1X1	T38.1X2	T38.1X3	T38.1X4	T38.1X5	T38.1X6
Thyrotrophin	T38.811	T38.812	T38.813	T38.814	T38.815	T38.816
Thyrotropic hormone	T38.811	T38.812	T38.813	T38.814	T38.815	T38.816
Thyroxine	T38.1X1	T38.1X2	T38.1X3	T38.1X4	T38.1X5	T38.1X6
Tiabendazole	T37.4X1	T37.4X2	T37.4X3	T37.4X4	T37.4X5	T37.4X6
Tiamizide	T50.2X1	T50.2X2	T50.2X3	T50.2X4	T50.2X5	T50.2X6
Tianeptine	T43.291	T43.292	T43.293	T43.294	T43.295	T43.296
Tiapamil	T46.1X1	T46.1X2	T46.1X3	T46.1X4	T46.1X5	T46.1X6
Tiapride	T43.591	T43.592	T43.593	T43.594	T43.595	T43.596
Tiaprofenic acid	T39.311	T39.312	T39.313	T39.314	T39.315	T39.316
Tiaramide	T39.8X1	T39.8X2	T39.8X3	T39.8X4	T39.8X5	T39.8X6
Ticarcillin	T36.0X1	T36.0X2	T36.0X3	T36.0X4	T36.0X5	T36.0X6
Ticlatone	T49.0X1	T49.0X2	T49.0X3	T49.0X4	T49.0X5	T49.0X6
Ticlopidine	T45.521	T45.522	T45.523	T45.524	T45.525	T45.526
Ticrynafen	T50.1X1	T50.1X2	T50.1X3	T50.1X4	T50.1X5	T50.1X6
Tidiacic	T50.991	T50.992	T50.993	T50.994	T50.995	T50.996
Tiemonium	T44.3X1	T44.3X2	T44.3X3	T44.3X4	T44.3X5	T44.3X6
iodide	T44.3X1	T44.3X2	T44.3X3	T44.3X4	T44.3X5	T44.3X6
Tienilic acid	T50.1X1	T50.1X2	T50.1X3	T50.1X4	T50.1X5	T50.1X6
Tifenamil	T44.3X1	T44.3X2	T44.3X3	T44.3X4	T44.3X5	T44.3X6
Tigan	T45.0X1	T45.0X2	T45.0X3	T45.0X4	T45.0X5	T45.0X6
Tigloidine	T44.3X1	T44.3X2	T44.3X3	T44.3X4	T44.3X5	T44.3X6
Tilactase	T47.5X1	T47.5X2	T47.5X3	T47.5X4	T47.5X5	T47.5X6
Tiletamine	T41.291	T41.292	T41.293	T41.294	T41.295	T41.296
Tilidine	T40.4X1	T40.4X2	T40.4X3	T40.4X4	—	—
Timepidium bromide	T44.3X1	T44.3X2	T44.3X3	T44.3X4	T44.3X5	T44.3X6
Timiperone	T43.4X1	T43.4X2	T43.4X3	T43.4X4	T43.4X5	T43.4X6
Timolol	T44.7X1	T44.7X2	T44.7X3	T44.7X4	T44.7X5	T44.7X6
Tincture, iodine — see Iodine						
Tindal	T43.3X1	T43.3X2	T43.3X3	T43.3X4	T43.3X5	T43.3X6
Tinidazole	T37.3X1	T37.3X2	T37.3X3	T37.3X4	T37.3X5	T37.3X6
Tinoridine	T39.8X1	T39.8X2	T39.8X3	T39.8X4	T39.8X5	T39.8X6
Tin (chloride) (dust) (oxide) NEC	T56.6X1	T56.6X2	T56.6X3	T56.6X4	—	—
anti-infectives	T37.8X1	T37.8X2	T37.8X3	T37.8X4	T37.8X5	T37.8X6
Tiocarlide	T37.1X1	T37.1X2	T37.1X3	T37.1X4	T37.1X5	T37.1X6
Tioclomarol	T45.511	T45.512	T45.513	T45.514	T45.515	T45.516
Tioconazole	T49.0X1	T49.0X2	T49.0X3	T49.0X4	T49.0X5	T49.0X6
Tioguanine	T45.1X1	T45.1X2	T45.1X3	T45.1X4	T45.1X5	T45.1X6
Tiopronin	T50.991	T50.992	T50.993	T50.994	T50.995	T50.996
Tiotixene	T43.4X1	T43.4X2	T43.4X3	T43.4X4	T43.4X5	T43.4X6
Tioxolone	T49.4X1	T49.4X2	T49.4X3	T49.4X4	T49.4X5	T49.4X6
Tipepidine	T48.3X1	T48.3X2	T48.3X3	T48.3X4	T48.3X5	T48.3X6
Tiquizium bromide	T44.3X1	T44.3X2	T44.3X3	T44.3X4	T44.3X5	T44.3X6
Tiratricol	T38.1X1	T38.1X2	T38.1X3	T38.1X4	T38.1X5	T38.1X6
Tisopurine	T50.4X1	T50.4X2	T50.4X3	T50.4X4	T50.4X5	T50.4X6
Titanium (compounds)	T56.891	T56.892	T56.893	T56.894	—	—
(vapor)						
dioxide	T49.3X1	T49.3X2	T49.3X3	T49.3X4	T49.3X5	T49.3X6
ointment	T49.3X1	T49.3X2	T49.3X3	T49.3X4	T49.3X5	T49.3X6
oxide	T49.3X1	T49.3X2	T49.3X3	T49.3X4	T49.3X5	T49.3X6
tetrachloride	T56.891	T56.892	T56.893	T56.894	—	—
Titanocene	T56.891	T56.892	T56.893	T56.894	—	—
Titroid	T38.1X1	T38.1X2	T38.1X3	T38.1X4	T38.1X5	T38.1X6
Tizanidine	T42.8X1	T42.8X2	T42.8X3	T42.8X4	T42.8X5	T42.8X6
TMTD	T60.3X1	T60.3X2	T60.3X3	T60.3X4	—	—
TNT (fumes)	T65.3X1	T65.3X2	T65.3X3	T65.3X4	—	—
Toadstool	T62.0X1	T62.0X2	T62.0X3	T62.0X4	—	—
Tobacco NEC	T65.291	T65.292	T65.293	T65.294	—	—
cigarettes	T65.221	T65.222	T65.223	T65.224	—	—
Indian	T62.2X1	T62.2X2	T62.2X3	T62.2X4	—	—
smoke, second-hand	T65.221	T65.222	T65.223	T65.224	—	—
Tobramycin	T36.5X1	T36.5X2	T36.5X3	T36.5X4	T36.5X5	T36.5X6
Tocainide	T46.2X1	T46.2X2	T46.2X3	T46.2X4	T46.2X5	T46.2X6
Tocoferol	T45.2X1	T45.2X2	T45.2X3	T45.2X4	T45.2X5	T45.2X6
Tocopherol	T45.2X1	T45.2X2	T45.2X3	T45.2X4	T45.2X5	T45.2X6
acetate	T45.2X1	T45.2X2	T45.2X3	T45.2X4	T45.2X5	T45.2X6
Tocosamine	T48.0X1	T48.0X2	T48.0X3	T48.0X4	T48.0X5	T48.0X6
Todralazine	T46.5X1	T46.5X2	T46.5X3	T46.5X4	T46.5X5	T46.5X6
Tofisopam	T42.4X1	T42.4X2	T42.4X3	T42.4X4	T42.4X5	T42.4X6
Tofranil	T43.011	T43.012	T43.013	T43.014	T43.015	T43.016
Toilet deodorizer	T65.891	T65.892	T65.893	T65.894	—	—

Substance	Poisoning, Accidental (unintentional)	Poisoning, Intentional Self-harm	Poisoning, Assault	Poisoning, Undetermined	Adverse Effect	Under-dosing
Tolamolol	T44.7X1	T44.7X2	T44.7X3	T44.7X4	T44.7X5	T44.7X6
Tolazamide	T38.3X1	T38.3X2	T38.3X3	T38.3X4	T38.3X5	T38.3X6
Tolazoline	T46.7X1	T46.7X2	T46.7X3	T46.7X4	T46.7X5	T46.7X6
Tolbutamide (sodium)	T38.3X1	T38.3X2	T38.3X3	T38.3X4	T38.3X5	T38.3X6
Tolciclate	T49.0X1	T49.0X2	T49.0X3	T49.0X4	T49.0X5	T49.0X6
Tolmetin	T39.391	T39.392	T39.393	T39.394	T39.395	T39.396
Tolnaftate	T49.0X1	T49.0X2	T49.0X3	T49.0X4	T49.0X5	T49.0X6
Tolonidine	T46.5X1	T46.5X2	T46.5X3	T46.5X4	T46.5X5	T46.5X6
Toloxatone	T42.6X1	T42.6X2	T42.6X3	T42.6X4	T42.6X5	T42.6X6
Tolperisone	T44.3X1	T44.3X2	T44.3X3	T44.3X4	T44.3X5	T44.3X6
Tolserol	T42.8X1	T42.8X2	T42.8X3	T42.8X4	T42.8X5	T42.8X6
Toluene (liquid)	T52.2X1	T52.2X2	T52.2X3	T52.2X4	—	—
diisocyanate	T65.0X1	T65.0X2	T65.0X3	T65.0X4	—	—
Toluidine	T65.891	T65.892	T65.893	T65.894	—	—
vapor	T59.891	T59.892	T59.893	T59.894	—	—
Toluol (liquid)	T52.2X1	T52.2X2	T52.2X3	T52.2X4	—	—
vapor	T52.2X1	T52.2X2	T52.2X3	T52.2X4	—	—
Toluylenediamine	T65.3X1	T65.3X2	T65.3X3	T65.3X4	—	—
Tolylene-2,4-diisocyanate	T65.0X1	T65.0X2	T65.0X3	T65.0X4	—	—
Tonic NEC	T50.901	T50.902	T50.903	T50.904	T50.905	T50.906
Topical action drug NEC	T49.91	T49.92	T49.93	T49.94	T49.95	T49.96
ear, nose or throat	T49.6X1	T49.6X2	T49.6X3	T49.6X4	T49.6X5	T49.6X6
eye	T49.5X1	T49.5X2	T49.5X3	T49.5X4	T49.5X5	T49.5X6
skin	T49.91	T49.92	T49.93	T49.94	T49.95	T49.96
specified NEC	T49.8X1	T49.8X2	T49.8X3	T49.8X4	T49.8X5	T49.8X6
Toquizine	T44.3X1	T44.3X2	T44.3X3	T44.3X4	T44.3X5	T44.3X6
Toremifene	T38.6X1	T38.6X2	T38.6X3	T38.6X4	T38.6X5	T38.6X6
Tosylchloramide sodium	T49.8X1	T49.8X2	T49.8X3	T49.8X4	T49.8X5	T49.8X6
Toxaphene (dust) (spray)	T60.1X1	T60.1X2	T60.1X3	T60.1X4	—	—
Toxin, diphtheria (Schick Test)	T50.8X1	T50.8X2	T50.8X3	T50.8X4	T50.8X5	T50.8X6
Toxoid						
combined	T50.A21	T50.A22	T50.A23	T50.A24	T50.A25	T50.A26
diphtheria	T50.A91	T50.A92	T50.A93	T50.A94	T50.A95	T50.A96
tetanus	T50.A91	T50.A92	T50.A93	T50.A94	T50.A95	T50.A96
Trace element NEC	T45.8X1	T45.8X2	T45.8X3	T45.8X4	T45.8X5	T45.8X6
Tractor fuel NEC	T52.0X1	T52.0X2	T52.0X3	T52.0X4	—	—
Tragacanth	T50.991	T50.992	T50.993	T50.994	T50.995	T50.996
Tramadol	T40.4X1	T40.4X2	T40.4X3	T40.4X4	T40.4X5	T40.4X6
Tramazoline	T48.5X1	T48.5X2	T48.5X3	T48.5X4	T48.5X5	T48.5X6
Tranexamic acid	T45.621	T45.622	T45.623	T45.624	T45.625	T45.626
Tranilast	T45.0X1	T45.0X2	T45.0X3	T45.0X4	T45.0X5	T45.0X6
Tranquilizer NEC	T43.501	T43.502	T43.503	T43.504	T43.505	T43.506
with hypnotic or sedative	T42.6X1	T42.6X2	T42.6X3	T42.6X4	T42.6X5	T42.6X6
benzodiazepine NEC	T42.4X1	T42.4X2	T42.4X3	T42.4X4	T42.4X5	T42.4X6
butyrophenone NEC	T43.4X1	T43.4X2	T43.4X3	T43.4X4	T43.4X5	T43.4X6
carbamate	T43.591	T43.592	T43.593	T43.594	T43.595	T43.596
dimethylamine	T43.3X1	T43.3X2	T43.3X3	T43.3X4	T43.3X5	T43.3X6
ethylamine	T43.3X1	T43.3X2	T43.3X3	T43.3X4	T43.3X5	T43.3X6
hydroxyzine	T43.591	T43.592	T43.593	T43.594	T43.595	T43.596
major NEC	T43.501	T43.502	T43.503	T43.504	T43.505	T43.506
penothiazine NEC	T43.3X1	T43.3X2	T43.3X3	T43.3X4	T43.3X5	T43.3X6
phenothiazine-based	T43.3X1	T43.3X2	T43.3X3	T43.3X4	T43.3X5	T43.3X6
piperazine NEC	T43.3X1	T43.3X2	T43.3X3	T43.3X4	T43.3X5	T43.3X6
piperidine	T43.3X1	T43.3X2	T43.3X3	T43.3X4	T43.3X5	T43.3X6
propylamine	T43.3X1	T43.3X2	T43.3X3	T43.3X4	T43.3X5	T43.3X6
specified NEC	T43.591	T43.592	T43.593	T43.594	T43.595	T43.596
thioxanthene NEC	T43.591	T43.592	T43.593	T43.594	T43.595	T43.596
Tranxene	T42.4X1	T42.4X2	T42.4X3	T42.4X4	T42.4X5	T42.4X6
Tranylcypromine	T43.1X1	T43.1X2	T43.1X3	T43.1X4	T43.1X5	T43.1X6
Trapidil	T46.3X1	T46.3X2	T46.3X3	T46.3X4	T46.3X5	T46.3X6
Trasentine	T44.3X1	T44.3X2	T44.3X3	T44.3X4	T44.3X5	T44.3X6
Travert	T50.3X1	T50.3X2	T50.3X3	T50.3X4	T50.3X5	T50.3X6
Trazodone	T43.211	T43.212	T43.213	T43.214	T43.215	T43.216
Trecator	T37.1X1	T37.1X2	T37.1X3	T37.1X4	T37.1X5	T37.1X6
Treosulfan	T45.1X1	T45.1X2	T45.1X3	T45.1X4	T45.1X5	T45.1X6
Tretamine	T45.1X1	T45.1X2	T45.1X3	T45.1X4	T45.1X5	T45.1X6
Tretinoin	T49.0X1	T49.0X2	T49.0X3	T49.0X4	T49.0X5	T49.0X6
Tretoquinol	T48.6X1	T48.6X2	T48.6X3	T48.6X4	T48.6X5	T48.6X6
Triacetin	T49.0X1	T49.0X2	T49.0X3	T49.0X4	T49.0X5	T49.0X6
Triacetoxyanthracene	T49.4X1	T49.4X2	T49.4X3	T49.4X4	T49.4X5	T49.4X6
Triacetyloleandomycin	T36.3X1	T36.3X2	T36.3X3	T36.3X4	T36.3X5	T36.3X6
Triamcinolone	T49.0X1	T49.0X2	T49.0X3	T49.0X4	T49.0X5	T49.0X6
ENT agent	T49.6X1	T49.6X2	T49.6X3	T49.6X4	T49.6X5	T49.6X6
hexacetonide	T49.0X1	T49.0X2	T49.0X3	T49.0X4	T49.0X5	T49.0X6
ophthalmic preparation	T49.5X1	T49.5X2	T49.5X3	T49.5X4	T49.5X5	T49.5X6
topical NEC	T49.0X1	T49.0X2	T49.0X3	T49.0X4	T49.0X5	T49.0X6
Triampyzine	T44.3X1	T44.3X2	T44.3X3	T44.3X4	T44.3X5	T44.3X6
Triamterene	T50.2X1	T50.2X2	T50.2X3	T50.2X4	T50.2X5	T50.2X6
Triazine (herbicide)	T60.3X1	T60.3X2	T60.3X3	T60.3X4	—	—
Triaziquone	T45.1X1	T45.1X2	T45.1X3	T45.1X4	T45.1X5	T45.1X6
Triazolam	T42.4X1	T42.4X2	T42.4X3	T42.4X4	T42.4X5	T42.4X6
Triazole (herbicide)	T60.3X1	T60.3X2	T60.3X3	T60.3X4	—	—

Table of Drugs and Chemicals

Substance	Poisoning, Accidental (unintentional)	Poisoning, Intentional Self-harm	Poisoning, Assault	Poisoning, Undetermined	Adverse Effect	Under-dosing
Tribenoside	T46.991	T46.992	T46.993	T46.994	T46.995	T46.996
Tribromacetaldehyde	T42.6X1	T42.6X2	T42.6X3	T42.6X4	T42.6X5	T42.6X6
Tribromoethanol, rectal	T41.291	T41.292	T41.293	T41.294	T41.295	T41.296
Tribromomethane	T42.6X1	T42.6X2	T42.6X3	T42.6X4	T42.6X5	T42.6X6
Trichlorethane	T53.2X1	T53.2X2	T53.2X3	T53.2X4	—	—
Trichlorethylene	T53.2X1	T53.2X2	T53.2X3	T53.2X4	—	—
Trichlorfon	T60.0X1	T60.0X2	T60.0X3	T60.0X4	—	—
Trichlormethiazide	T50.2X1	T50.2X2	T50.2X3	T50.2X4	T50.2X5	T50.2X6
Trichlormethine	T45.1X1	T45.1X2	T45.1X3	T45.1X4	T45.1X5	T45.1X6
Trichloroacetic acid, Trichloracetic acid	T54.2X1	T54.2X2	T54.2X3	T54.2X4	—	—
medicinal	T49.4X1	T49.4X2	T49.4X3	T49.4X4	T49.4X5	T49.4X6
Trichloroethane	T53.2X1	T53.2X2	T53.2X3	T53.2X4	—	—
Trichloroethanol	T42.6X1	T42.6X2	T42.6X3	T42.6X4	T42.6X5	T42.6X6
Trichloroethylene (liquid) (vapor)	T53.2X1	T53.2X2	T53.2X3	T53.2X4	—	—
anesthetic (gas)	T41.0X1	T41.0X2	T41.0X3	T41.0X4	T41.0X5	T41.0X6
vapor NEC	T53.2X1	T53.2X2	T53.2X3	T53.2X4	—	—
Trichloroethyl phosphate	T42.6X1	T42.6X2	T42.6X3	T42.6X4	T42.6X5	T42.6X6
Trichlorofluoromethane NEC	T53.5X1	T53.5X2	T53.5X3	T53.5X4	—	—
Trichloronate	T60.0X1	T60.0X2	T60.0X3	T60.0X4	—	—
Trichloropropane	T53.6X1	T53.6X2	T53.6X3	T53.6X4	—	—
Trichlorotriethylamine	T45.1X1	T45.1X2	T45.1X3	T45.1X4	T45.1X5	T45.1X6
Trichomonacides NEC	T37.3X1	T37.3X2	T37.3X3	T37.3X4	T37.3X5	T37.3X6
Trichomycin	T36.7X1	T36.7X2	T36.7X3	T36.7X4	T36.7X5	T36.7X6
Triclobisonium chloride	T49.0X1	T49.0X2	T49.0X3	T49.0X4	T49.0X5	T49.0X6
Triclocarban	T49.0X1	T49.0X2	T49.0X3	T49.0X4	T49.0X5	T49.0X6
Triclofos	T42.6X1	T42.6X2	T42.6X3	T42.6X4	T42.6X5	T42.6X6
Triclosan	T49.0X1	T49.0X2	T49.0X3	T49.0X4	T49.0X5	T49.0X6
Tricresyl phosphate	T65.891	T65.892	T65.893	T65.894	—	—
solvent	T52.91	T52.92	T52.93	T52.94	—	—
Tricyclamol chloride	T44.3X1	T44.3X2	T44.3X3	T44.3X4	T44.3X5	T44.3X6
Tridesilon	T49.0X1	T49.0X2	T49.0X3	T49.0X4	T49.0X5	T49.0X6
Tridihexethyl iodide	T44.3X1	T44.3X2	T44.3X3	T44.3X4	T44.3X5	T44.3X6
Tridione	T42.2X1	T42.2X2	T42.2X3	T42.2X4	T42.2X5	T42.2X6
Trientine	T45.8X1	T45.8X2	T45.8X3	T45.8X4	T45.8X5	T45.8X6
Triethanolamine NEC	T54.3X1	T54.3X2	T54.3X3	T54.3X4	—	—
detergent	T54.3X1	T54.3X2	T54.3X3	T54.3X4	—	—
trinitrate (biphosphate)	T46.3X1	T46.3X2	T46.3X3	T46.3X4	T46.3X5	T46.3X6
Triethanomelamine	T45.1X1	T45.1X2	T45.1X3	T45.1X4	T45.1X5	T45.1X6
Triethylenemelamine	T45.1X1	T45.1X2	T45.1X3	T45.1X4	T45.1X5	T45.1X6
Triethylenephosphoramide	T45.1X1	T45.1X2	T45.1X3	T45.1X4	T45.1X5	T45.1X6
Triethylenethiophosphoramide	T45.1X1	T45.1X2	T45.1X3	T45.1X4	T45.1X5	T45.1X6
Trifluoperazine	T43.3X1	T43.3X2	T43.3X3	T43.3X4	T43.3X5	T43.3X6
Trifluoroethyl vinyl ether	T41.0X1	T41.0X2	T41.0X3	T41.0X4	T41.0X5	T41.0X6
Trifluperidol	T43.4X1	T43.4X2	T43.4X3	T43.4X4	T43.4X5	T43.4X6
Triflupromazine	T43.3X1	T43.3X2	T43.3X3	T43.3X4	T43.3X5	T43.3X6
Trifluridine	T37.5X1	T37.5X2	T37.5X3	T37.5X4	T37.5X5	T37.5X6
Triflusal	T45.521	T45.522	T45.523	T45.524	T45.525	T45.526
Trihexyphenidyl	T44.3X1	T44.3X2	T44.3X3	T44.3X4	T44.3X5	T44.3X6
Triiodothyronine	T38.1X1	T38.1X2	T38.1X3	T38.1X4	T38.1X5	T38.1X6
Trilene	T41.0X1	T41.0X2	T41.0X3	T41.0X4	T41.0X5	T41.0X6
Trilostane	T38.991	T38.992	T38.993	T38.994	T38.995	T38.996
Trimebutine	T44.3X1	T44.3X2	T44.3X3	T44.3X4	T44.3X5	T44.3X6
Trimecaine	T41.3X1	T41.3X2	T41.3X3	T41.3X4	T41.3X5	T41.3X6
Trimeprazine (tartrate)	T44.3X1	T44.3X2	T44.3X3	T44.3X4	T44.3X5	T44.3X6
Trimetaphan camsilate	T44.2X1	T44.2X2	T44.2X3	T44.2X4	T44.2X5	T44.2X6
Trimetazidine	T46.7X1	T46.7X2	T46.7X3	T46.7X4	T46.7X5	T46.7X6
Trimethadione	T42.2X1	T42.2X2	T42.2X3	T42.2X4	T42.2X5	T42.2X6
Trimethaphan	T44.2X1	T44.2X2	T44.2X3	T44.2X4	T44.2X5	T44.2X6
Trimethidinium	T44.2X1	T44.2X2	T44.2X3	T44.2X4	T44.2X5	T44.2X6
Trimethobenzamide	T45.0X1	T45.0X2	T45.0X3	T45.0X4	T45.0X5	T45.0X6
Trimethoprim	T37.8X1	T37.8X2	T37.8X3	T37.8X4	T37.8X5	T37.8X6
with sulfamethoxazole	T36.8X1	T36.8X2	T36.8X3	T36.8X4	T36.8X5	T36.8X6
Trimethylcarbinol	T51.3X1	T51.3X2	T51.3X3	T51.3X4	—	—
Trimethylpsoralen	T49.3X1	T49.3X2	T49.3X3	T49.3X4	T49.3X5	T49.3X6
Trimeton	T45.0X1	T45.0X2	T45.0X3	T45.0X4	T45.0X5	T45.0X6
Trimetrexate	T45.1X1	T45.1X2	T45.1X3	T45.1X4	T45.1X5	T45.1X6
Trimipramine	T43.011	T43.012	T43.013	T43.014	T43.015	T43.016
Trimustine	T45.1X1	T45.1X2	T45.1X3	T45.1X4	T45.1X5	T45.1X6
Trinitrine	T46.3X1	T46.3X2	T46.3X3	T46.3X4	T46.3X5	T46.3X6
Trinitrobenzol	T65.3X1	T65.3X2	T65.3X3	T65.3X4	—	—
Trinitrophenol	T65.3X1	T65.3X2	T65.3X3	T65.3X4	—	—
Trinitrotoluene (fumes)	T65.3X1	T65.3X2	T65.3X3	T65.3X4	—	—
Trional	T42.6X1	T42.6X2	T42.6X3	T42.6X4	T42.6X5	T42.6X6
Triorthocresyl phosphate	T65.891	T65.892	T65.893	T65.894	—	—
Trioxide of arsenic	T57.0X1	T57.0X2	T57.0X3	T57.0X4	—	—
Trioxysalen	T49.4X1	T49.4X2	T49.4X3	T49.4X4	T49.4X5	T49.4X6
Tripamide	T50.2X1	T50.2X2	T50.2X3	T50.2X4	T50.2X5	T50.2X6
Triparanol	T46.6X1	T46.6X2	T46.6X3	T46.6X4	T46.6X5	T46.6X6
Tripelennamine	T45.0X1	T45.0X2	T45.0X3	T45.0X4	T45.0X5	T45.0X6
Triperiden	T44.3X1	T44.3X2	T44.3X3	T44.3X4	T44.3X5	T44.3X6
Triperidol	T43.4X1	T43.4X2	T43.4X3	T43.4X4	T43.4X5	T43.4X6
Triphenylphosphate	T65.891	T65.892	T65.893	T65.894	—	—
Triple						
bromides	T42.6X1	T42.6X2	T42.6X3	T42.6X4	T42.6X5	T42.6X6
carbonate	T47.1X1	T47.1X2	T47.1X3	T47.1X4	T47.1X5	T47.1X6
vaccine						
DPT	T50.A11	T50.A12	T50.A13	T50.A14	T50.A15	T50.A16
including pertussis	T50.A11	T50.A12	T50.A13	T50.A14	T50.A15	T50.A16
MMR	T50.B91	T50.B92	T50.B93	T50.B94	T50.B95	T50.B96
Triprolidine	T45.0X1	T45.0X2	T45.0X3	T45.0X4	T45.0X5	T45.0X6
Trisodium hydrogen edetate	T50.6X1	T50.6X2	T50.6X3	T50.6X4	T50.6X5	T50.6X6
Trisoralen	T49.3X1	T49.3X2	T49.3X3	T49.3X4	T49.3X5	T49.3X6
Trisulfapyrimidines	T37.0X1	T37.0X2	T37.0X3	T37.0X4	T37.0X5	T37.0X6
Trithiozine	T44.3X1	T44.3X2	T44.3X3	T44.3X4	T44.3X5	T44.3X6
Tritiozine	T44.3X1	T44.3X2	T44.3X3	T44.3X4	T44.3X5	T44.3X6
Tritoqualine	T45.0X1	T45.0X2	T45.0X3	T45.0X4	T45.0X5	T45.0X6
Trofosfamide	T45.1X1	T45.1X2	T45.1X3	T45.1X4	T45.1X5	T45.1X6
Troleandomycin	T36.3X1	T36.3X2	T36.3X3	T36.3X4	T36.3X5	T36.3X6
Trolnitrate (phosphate)	T46.3X1	T46.3X2	T46.3X3	T46.3X4	T46.3X5	T46.3X6
Tromantadine	T37.5X1	T37.5X2	T37.5X3	T37.5X4	T37.5X5	T37.5X6
Trometamol	T50.2X1	T50.2X2	T50.2X3	T50.2X4	T50.2X5	T50.2X6
Tromethamine	T50.2X1	T50.2X2	T50.2X3	T50.2X4	T50.2X5	T50.2X6
Tronothane	T41.3X1	T41.3X2	T41.3X3	T41.3X4	T41.3X5	T41.3X6
Tropacine	T44.3X1	T44.3X2	T44.3X3	T44.3X4	T44.3X5	T44.3X6
Tropatepine	T44.3X1	T44.3X2	T44.3X3	T44.3X4	T44.3X5	T44.3X6
Tropicamide	T44.3X1	T44.3X2	T44.3X3	T44.3X4	T44.3X5	T44.3X6
Trospium chloride	T44.3X1	T44.3X2	T44.3X3	T44.3X4	T44.3X5	T44.3X6
Troxerutin	T46.991	T46.992	T46.993	T46.994	T46.995	T46.996
Troxidone	T42.2X1	T42.2X2	T42.2X3	T42.2X4	T42.2X5	T42.2X6
Tryparsamide	T37.3X1	T37.3X2	T37.3X3	T37.3X4	T37.3X5	T37.3X6
Trypsin	T45.3X1	T45.3X2	T45.3X3	T45.3X4	T45.3X5	T45.3X6
Tryptizol	T43.011	T43.012	T43.013	T43.014	T43.015	T43.016
TSH	T38.811	T38.812	T38.813	T38.814	T38.815	T38.816
Tuaminoheptane	T48.5X1	T48.5X2	T48.5X3	T48.5X4	T48.5X5	T48.5X6
Tuberculin, purified protein derivative (PPD)	T50.8X1	T50.8X2	T50.8X3	T50.8X4	T50.8X5	T50.8X6
Tubocurare	T48.1X1	T48.1X2	T48.1X3	T48.1X4	T48.1X5	T48.1X6
Tubocurarine (chloride)	T48.1X1	T48.1X2	T48.1X3	T48.1X4	T48.1X5	T48.1X6
Tulobuterol	T48.6X1	T48.6X2	T48.6X3	T48.6X4	T48.6X5	T48.6X6
Turpentine (spirits of)	T52.8X1	T52.8X2	T52.8X3	T52.8X4	—	—
vapor	T52.8X1	T52.8X2	T52.8X3	T52.8X4	—	—
Tybamate	T43.591	T43.592	T43.593	T43.594	T43.595	T43.596
Tyloxapol	T48.4X1	T48.4X2	T48.4X3	T48.4X4	T48.4X5	T48.4X6
Tymazoline	T48.5X1	T48.5X2	T48.5X3	T48.5X4	T48.5X5	T48.5X6
Typhoid-paratyphoid vaccine	T50.A91	T50.A92	T50.A93	T50.A94	T50.A95	T50.A96
Typhus vaccine	T50.A91	T50.A92	T50.A93	T50.A94	T50.A95	T50.A96
Tyropanoate	T50.8X1	T50.8X2	T50.8X3	T50.8X4	T50.8X5	T50.8X6
Tyrothricin	T49.6X1	T49.6X2	T49.6X3	T49.6X4	T49.6X5	T49.6X6
ENT agent	T49.6X1	T49.6X2	T49.6X3	T49.6X4	T49.6X5	T49.6X6
ophthalmic preparation	T49.5X1	T49.5X2	T49.5X3	T49.5X4	T49.5X5	T49.5X6
Ufenamate	T39.391	T39.392	T39.393	T39.394	T39.395	T39.396
Ultraviolet light protectant	T49.3X1	T49.3X2	T49.3X3	T49.3X4	T49.3X5	T49.3X6
Undecenoic acid	T49.0X1	T49.0X2	T49.0X3	T49.0X4	T49.0X5	T49.0X6
Undecoylium	T49.0X1	T49.0X2	T49.0X3	T49.0X4	T49.0X5	T49.0X6
Undecylenic acid (derivatives)	T49.0X1	T49.0X2	T49.0X3	T49.0X4	T49.0X5	T49.0X6
Unna's boot	T49.3X1	T49.3X2	T49.3X3	T49.3X4	T49.3X5	T49.3X6
Unsaturated fatty acid	T46.6X1	T46.6X2	T46.6X3	T46.6X4	T46.6X5	T46.6X6
Uracil mustard	T45.1X1	T45.1X2	T45.1X3	T45.1X4	T45.1X5	T45.1X6
Uramustine	T45.1X1	T45.1X2	T45.1X3	T45.1X4	T45.1X5	T45.1X6
Urapidil	T46.5X1	T46.5X2	T46.5X3	T46.5X4	T46.5X5	T46.5X6
Urari	T48.1X1	T48.1X2	T48.1X3	T48.1X4	T48.1X5	T48.1X6
Urate oxidase	T50.4X1	T50.4X2	T50.4X3	T50.4X4	T50.4X5	T50.4X6
Urea	T47.3X1	T47.3X2	T47.3X3	T47.3X4	T47.3X5	T47.3X6
peroxide	T49.0X1	T49.0X2	T49.0X3	T49.0X4	T49.0X5	T49.0X6
stibamine	T37.4X1	T37.4X2	T37.4X3	T37.4X4	T37.4X5	T37.4X6
topical	T49.8X1	T49.8X2	T49.8X3	T49.8X4	T49.8X5	T49.8X6
Urethane	T45.1X1	T45.1X2	T45.1X3	T45.1X4	T45.1X5	T45.1X6
Urginea (maritima) (scilla) — see Squill						
Uric acid metabolism drug NEC	T50.4X1	T50.4X2	T50.4X3	T50.4X4	T50.4X5	T50.4X6
Uricosuric agent	T50.4X1	T50.4X2	T50.4X3	T50.4X4	T50.4X5	T50.4X6
Urinary anti-infective	T37.8X1	T37.8X2	T37.8X3	T37.8X4	T37.8X5	T37.8X6
Urofollitropin	T38.811	T38.812	T38.813	T38.814	T38.815	T38.816
Urokinase	T45.611	T45.612	T45.613	T45.614	T45.615	T45.616
Urokon	T50.8X1	T50.8X2	T50.8X3	T50.8X4	T50.8X5	T50.8X6
Ursodeoxycholic acid	T50.991	T50.992	T50.993	T50.994	T50.995	T50.996
Ursodiol	T50.991	T50.992	T50.993	T50.994	T50.995	T50.996
Urtica	T62.2X1	T62.2X2	T62.2X3	T62.2X4	—	—
Utility gas — see Gas, utility						

▽ Subterms under main terms may continue to next column or page

Table of Drugs and Chemicals

Tribenoside — Utility gas

Table of Drugs and Chemicals

Substance	Poisoning, Accidental (unintentional)	Poisoning, Intentional Self-harm	Poisoning, Assault	Poisoning, Undetermined	Adverse Effect	Under-dosing
Vaccine NEC	T50.Z91	T50.Z92	T50.Z93	T50.Z94	T50.Z95	T50.Z96
antineoplastic	T50.Z91	T50.Z92	T50.Z93	T50.Z94	T50.Z95	T50.Z96
bacterial NEC	T50.A91	T50.A92	T50.A93	T50.A94	T50.A95	T50.A96
with						
other bacterial component	T50.A21	T50.A22	T50.A23	T50.A24	T50.A25	T50.A26
pertussis component	T50.A11	T50.A12	T50.A13	T50.A14	T50.A15	T50.A16
viral-rickettsial component	T50.A21	T50.A22	T50.A23	T50.A24	T50.A25	T50.A26
mixed NEC	T50.A21	T50.A22	T50.A23	T50.A24	T50.A25	T50.A26
BCG	T50.A91	T50.A92	T50.A93	T50.A94	T50.A95	T50.A96
cholera	T50.A91	T50.A92	T50.A93	T50.A94	T50.A95	T50.A96
diphtheria	T50.A91	T50.A92	T50.A93	T50.A94	T50.A95	T50.A96
with tetanus	T50.A21	T50.A22	T50.A23	T50.A24	T50.A25	T50.A26
and pertussis	T50.A11	T50.A12	T50.A13	T50.A14	T50.A15	T50.A16
influenza	T50.B91	T50.B92	T50.B93	T50.B94	T50.B95	T50.B96
measles	T50.B91	T50.B92	T50.B93	T50.B94	T50.B95	T50.B96
with mumps and rubella	T50.B91	T50.B92	T50.B93	T50.B94	T50.B95	T50.B96
meningococcal	T50.A91	T50.A92	T50.A93	T50.A94	T50.A95	T50.A96
mumps	T50.B91	T50.B92	T50.B93	T50.B94	T50.B95	T50.B96
paratyphoid	T50.A91	T50.A92	T50.A93	T50.A94	T50.A95	T50.A96
pertussis	T50.A11	T50.A12	T50.A13	T50.A14	T50.A15	T50.A16
with diphtheria	T50.A11	T50.A12	T50.A13	T50.A14	T50.A15	T50.A16
and tetanus	T50.A11	T50.A12	T50.A13	T50.A14	T50.A15	T50.A16
with other component	T50.A11	T50.A12	T50.A13	T50.A14	T50.A15	T50.A16
plague	T50.A91	T50.A92	T50.A93	T50.A94	T50.A95	T50.A96
poliomyelitis	T50.B91	T50.B92	T50.B93	T50.B94	T50.B95	T50.B96
poliovirus	T50.B91	T50.B92	T50.B93	T50.B94	T50.B95	T50.B96
rabies	T50.B91	T50.B92	T50.B93	T50.B94	T50.B95	T50.B96
respiratory syncytial virus	T50.B91	T50.B92	T50.B93	T50.B94	T50.B95	T50.B96
rickettsial NEC	T50.A91	T50.A92	T50.A93	T50.A94	T50.A95	T50.A96
with bacterial component	T50.A21	T50.A22	T50.A23	T50.A24	T50.A25	T50.A26
Rocky Mountain spotted fever	T50.A91	T50.A92	T50.A93	T50.A94	T50.A95	T50.A96
rubella	T50.B91	T50.B92	T50.B93	T50.B94	T50.B95	T50.B96
sabin oral	T50.B91	T50.B92	T50.B93	T50.B94	T50.B95	T50.B96
smallpox	T50.B11	T50.B12	T50.B13	T50.B14	T50.B15	T50.B16
TAB	T50.A91	T50.A92	T50.A93	T50.A94	T50.A95	T50.A96
tetanus	T50.A91	T50.A92	T50.A93	T50.A94	T50.A95	T50.A96
typhoid	T50.A91	T50.A92	T50.A93	T50.A94	T50.A95	T50.A96
typhus	T50.A91	T50.A92	T50.A93	T50.A94	T50.A95	T50.A96
viral NEC	T50.B91	T50.B92	T50.B93	T50.B94	T50.B95	T50.B96
yellow fever	T50.B91	T50.B92	T50.B93	T50.B94	T50.B95	T50.B96
Vaccinia immune globulin	T50.Z11	T50.Z12	T50.Z13	T50.Z14	T50.Z15	T50.Z16
Vaginal contraceptives	T49.8X1	T49.8X2	T49.8X3	T49.8X4	T49.8X5	T49.8X6
Valerian						
root	T42.6X1	T42.6X2	T42.6X3	T42.6X4	T42.6X5	T42.6X6
tincture	T42.6X1	T42.6X2	T42.6X3	T42.6X4	T42.6X5	T42.6X6
Valethamate bromide	T44.3X1	T44.3X2	T44.3X3	T44.3X4	T44.3X5	T44.3X6
Valisone	T49.0X1	T49.0X2	T49.0X3	T49.0X4	T49.0X5	T49.0X6
Valium	T42.4X1	T42.4X2	T42.4X3	T42.4X4	T42.4X5	T42.4X6
Valmid	T42.6X1	T42.6X2	T42.6X3	T42.6X4	T42.6X5	T42.6X6
Valnoctamide	T42.6X1	T42.6X2	T42.6X3	T42.6X4	T42.6X5	T42.6X6
Valproate (sodium)	T42.6X1	T42.6X2	T42.6X3	T42.6X4	T42.6X5	T42.6X6
Valproic acid	T42.6X1	T42.6X2	T42.6X3	T42.6X4	T42.6X5	T42.6X6
Valpromide	T42.6X1	T42.6X2	T42.6X3	T42.6X4	T42.6X5	T42.6X6
Vanadium	T56.891	T56.892	T56.893	T56.894	—	—
Vancomycin	T36.8X1	T36.8X2	T36.8X3	T36.8X4	T36.8X5	T36.8X6
Vapor — see also Gas	T59.91	T59.92	T59.93	T59.94		
kiln (carbon monoxide)	T58.8X1	T58.8X2	T58.8X3	T58.8X4	—	—
lead — see lead						
specified source NEC	T59.891	T59.892	T59.893	T59.894	—	—
Vardenafil	T46.7X1	T46.7X2	T46.7X3	T46.7X4	T46.7X5	T46.7X6
Varicose reduction drug	T46.8X1	T46.8X2	T46.8X3	T46.8X4	T46.8X5	T46.8X6
Varnish	T65.4X1	T65.4X2	T65.4X3	T65.4X4	—	—
cleaner	T52.91	T52.92	T52.93	T52.94	—	—
Vaseline	T49.3X1	T49.3X2	T49.3X3	T49.3X4	T49.3X5	T49.3X6
Vasodilan	T46.7X1	T46.7X2	T46.7X3	T46.7X4	T46.7X5	T46.7X6
Vasodilator						
coronary NEC	T46.3X1	T46.3X2	T46.3X3	T46.3X4	T46.3X5	T46.3X6
peripheral NEC	T46.7X1	T46.7X2	T46.7X3	T46.7X4	T46.7X5	T46.7X6
Vasopressin	T38.891	T38.892	T38.893	T38.894	T38.895	T38.896
Vasopressor drugs	T38.891	T38.892	T38.893	T38.894	T38.895	T38.896
Vecuronium bromide	T48.1X1	T48.1X2	T48.1X3	T48.1X4	T48.1X5	T48.1X6
Vegetable extract, astringent	T49.2X1	T49.2X2	T49.2X3	T49.2X4	T49.2X5	T49.2X6
Venlafaxine	T43.211	T43.212	T43.213	T43.214	T43.215	T43.216
Venom, venomous (bite) (sting)	T63.91	T63.92	T63.93	T63.94	—	—
amphibian NEC	T63.831	T63.832	T63.833	T63.834	—	—
animal NEC	T63.891	T63.892	T63.893	T63.894	—	—
ant	T63.421	T63.422	T63.423	T63.424	—	—
Venom, venomous — continued						
arthropod NEC	T63.481	T63.482	T63.483	T63.484	—	—
bee	T63.441	T63.442	T63.443	T63.444	—	—
centipede	T63.411	T63.412	T63.413	T63.414	—	—
fish	T63.591	T63.592	T63.593	T63.594	—	—
frog	T63.811	T63.812	T63.813	T63.814	—	—
hornet	T63.451	T63.452	T63.453	T63.454	—	—
insect NEC	T63.481	T63.482	T63.483	T63.484	—	—
lizard	T63.121	T63.122	T63.123	T63.124	—	—
marine						
animals	T63.691	T63.692	T63.693	T63.694	—	—
bluebottle	T63.611	T63.612	T63.613	T63.614	—	—
jellyfish NEC	T63.621	T63.622	T63.623	T63.624	—	—
Portugese Man-o-war	T63.611	T63.612	T63.613	T63.614	—	—
sea anemone	T63.631	T63.632	T63.633	T63.634	—	—
specified NEC	T63.691	T63.692	T63.693	T63.694	—	—
fish	T63.591	T63.592	T63.593	T63.594	—	—
plants	T63.711	T63.712	T63.713	T63.714	—	—
sting ray	T63.511	T63.512	T63.513	T63.514	—	—
millipede (tropical)	T63.411	T63.412	T63.413	T63.414	—	—
plant NEC	T63.791	T63.792	T63.793	T63.794	—	—
marine	T63.711	T63.712	T63.713	T63.714	—	—
reptile	T63.191	T63.192	T63.193	T63.194	—	—
gila monster	T63.111	T63.112	T63.113	T63.114	—	—
lizard NEC	T63.121	T63.122	T63.123	T63.124	—	—
scorpion	T63.2X1	T63.2X2	T63.2X3	T63.2X4	—	—
snake	T63.001	T63.002	T63.003	T63.004	—	—
African NEC	T63.081	T63.082	T63.083	T63.084	—	—
American (North) (South) NEC	T63.061	T63.062	T63.063	T63.064	—	—
Asian	T63.081	T63.082	T63.083	T63.084	—	—
Australian	T63.071	T63.072	T63.073	T63.074	—	—
cobra	T63.041	T63.042	T63.043	T63.044	—	—
coral snake	T63.021	T63.022	T63.023	T63.024	—	—
rattlesnake	T63.011	T63.012	T63.013	T63.014	—	—
specified NEC	T63.091	T63.092	T63.093	T63.094	—	—
taipan	T63.031	T63.032	T63.033	T63.034	—	—
specified NEC	T63.891	T63.892	T63.893	T63.894	—	—
spider	T63.301	T63.302	T63.303	T63.304	—	—
black widow	T63.311	T63.312	T63.313	T63.314	—	—
brown recluse	T63.331	T63.332	T63.333	T63.334	—	—
specified NEC	T63.391	T63.392	T63.393	T63.394	—	—
tarantula	T63.321	T63.322	T63.323	T63.324	—	—
sting ray	T63.511	T63.512	T63.513	T63.514	—	—
toad	T63.821	T63.822	T63.823	T63.824	—	—
wasp	T63.461	T63.462	T63.463	T63.464	—	—
Venous sclerosing drug NEC	T46.8X1	T46.8X2	T46.8X3	T46.8X4	T46.8X5	T46.8X6
Ventolin — see Albuterol						
Veramon	T42.3X1	T42.3X2	T42.3X3	T42.3X4	T42.3X5	T42.3X6
Verapamil	T46.1X1	T46.1X2	T46.1X3	T46.1X4	T46.1X5	T46.1X6
Veratrine	T46.5X1	T46.5X2	T46.5X3	T46.5X4	T46.5X5	T46.5X6
Veratrum						
album	T62.2X1	T62.2X2	T62.2X3	T62.2X4	—	—
alkaloids	T46.5X1	T46.5X2	T46.5X3	T46.5X4	T46.5X5	T46.5X6
viride	T62.2X1	T62.2X2	T62.2X3	T62.2X4	—	—
Verdigris	T60.3X1	T60.3X2	T60.3X3	T60.3X4	—	—
Veronal	T42.3X1	T42.3X2	T42.3X3	T42.3X4	T42.3X5	T42.3X6
Veroxil	T37.4X1	T37.4X2	T37.4X3	T37.4X4	T37.4X5	T37.4X6
Versenate	T50.6X1	T50.6X2	T50.6X3	T50.6X4	T50.6X5	T50.6X6
Versidyne	T39.8X1	T39.8X2	T39.8X3	T39.8X4	T39.8X5	T39.8X6
Vetrabutine	T48.0X1	T48.0X2	T48.0X3	T48.0X4	T48.0X5	T48.0X6
Vidarabine	T37.5X1	T37.5X2	T37.5X3	T37.5X4	T37.5X5	T37.5X6
Vienna						
green	T57.0X1	T57.0X2	T57.0X3	T57.0X4	—	—
insecticide	T60.2X1	T60.2X2	T60.2X3	T60.2X4	—	—
red	T57.0X1	T57.0X2	T57.0X3	T57.0X4	—	—
pharmaceutical dye	T50.991	T50.992	T50.993	T50.994	T50.995	T50.996
Vigabatrin	T42.6X1	T42.6X2	T42.6X3	T42.6X4	T42.6X5	T42.6X6
Viloxazine	T43.291	T43.292	T43.293	T43.294	T43.295	T43.296
Viminol	T39.8X1	T39.8X2	T39.8X3	T39.8X4	T39.8X5	T39.8X6
Vinbarbital, vinbarbitone	T42.3X1	T42.3X2	T42.3X3	T42.3X4	T42.3X5	T42.3X6
Vinblastine	T45.1X1	T45.1X2	T45.1X3	T45.1X4	T45.1X5	T45.1X6
Vinburnine	T46.7X1	T46.7X2	T46.7X3	T46.7X4	T46.7X5	T46.7X6
Vincamine	T45.1X1	T45.1X2	T45.1X3	T45.1X4	T45.1X5	T45.1X6
Vincristine	T45.1X1	T45.1X2	T45.1X3	T45.1X4	T45.1X5	T45.1X6
Vindesine	T45.1X1	T45.1X2	T45.1X3	T45.1X4	T45.1X5	T45.1X6
Vinesthene, vinethene	T41.0X1	T41.0X2	T41.0X3	T41.0X4	T41.0X5	T41.0X6
Vinorelbine tartrate	T45.1X1	T45.1X2	T45.1X3	T45.1X4	T45.1X5	T45.1X6
Vinpocetine	T46.7X1	T46.7X2	T46.7X3	T46.7X4	T46.7X5	T46.7X6
Vinyl						
acetate	T65.891	T65.892	T65.893	T65.894	—	—
bital	T42.3X1	T42.3X2	T42.3X3	T42.3X4	T42.3X5	T42.3X6

Vaccine NEC — Vinyl

Substance	Poisoning, Accidental (unintentional)	Poisoning, Intentional Self-harm	Poisoning, Assault	Poisoning, Undetermined	Adverse Effect	Under-dosing
Vinyl — continued						
bromide	T65.891	T65.892	T65.893	T65.894	—	—
chloride	T59.891	T59.892	T59.893	T59.894	—	—
ether	T41.0X1	T41.0X2	T41.0X3	T41.0X4	T41.0X5	T41.0X6
Vinylbital	T42.3X1	T42.3X2	T42.3X3	T42.3X4	T42.3X5	T42.3X6
Vinylidene chloride	T65.891	T65.892	T65.893	T65.894	—	—
Vioform	T37.8X1	T37.8X2	T37.8X3	T37.8X4	T37.8X5	T37.8X6
topical	T49.0X1	T49.0X2	T49.0X3	T49.0X4	T49.0X5	T49.0X6
Viomycin	T36.8X1	T36.8X2	T36.8X3	T36.8X4	T36.8X5	T36.8X6
Viosterol	T45.2X1	T45.2X2	T45.2X3	T45.2X4	T45.2X5	T45.2X6
Viper (venom)	T63.091	T63.092	T63.093	T63.094	—	—
Viprynium	T37.4X1	T37.4X2	T37.4X3	T37.4X4	T37.4X5	T37.4X6
Viquidil	T46.7X1	T46.7X2	T46.7X3	T46.7X4	T46.7X5	T46.7X6
Viral vaccine NEC	T50.B91	T50.B92	T50.B93	T50.B94	T50.B95	T50.B96
Virginiamycin	T36.8X1	T36.8X2	T36.8X3	T36.8X4	T36.8X5	T36.8X6
Virugon	T37.5X1	T37.5X2	T37.5X3	T37.5X4	T37.5X5	T37.5X6
Viscous agent	T50.901	T50.902	T50.903	T50.904	T50.905	T50.906
Visine	T49.5X1	T49.5X2	T49.5X3	T49.5X4	T49.5X5	T49.5X6
Visnadine	T46.3X1	T46.3X2	T46.3X3	T46.3X4	T46.3X5	T46.3X6
Vitamin NEC	T45.2X1	T45.2X2	T45.2X3	T45.2X4	T45.2X5	T45.2X6
A	T45.2X1	T45.2X2	T45.2X3	T45.2X4	T45.2X5	T45.2X6
B1	T45.2X1	T45.2X2	T45.2X3	T45.2X4	T45.2X5	T45.2X6
B2	T45.2X1	T45.2X2	T45.2X3	T45.2X4	T45.2X5	T45.2X6
B6	T45.2X1	T45.2X2	T45.2X3	T45.2X4	T45.2X5	T45.2X6
B12	T45.2X1	T45.2X2	T45.2X3	T45.2X4	T45.2X5	T45.2X6
B15	T45.2X1	T45.2X2	T45.2X3	T45.2X4	T45.2X5	T45.2X6
B NEC	T45.2X1	T45.2X2	T45.2X3	T45.2X4	T45.2X5	T45.2X6
nicotinic acid	T46.7X1	T46.7X2	T46.7X3	T46.7X4	T46.7X5	T46.7X6
C	T45.2X1	T45.2X2	T45.2X3	T45.2X4	T45.2X5	T45.2X6
D	T45.2X1	T45.2X2	T45.2X3	T45.2X4	T45.2X5	T45.2X6
D2	T45.2X1	T45.2X2	T45.2X3	T45.2X4	T45.2X5	T45.2X6
D3	T45.2X1	T45.2X2	T45.2X3	T45.2X4	T45.2X5	T45.2X6
E	T45.2X1	T45.2X2	T45.2X3	T45.2X4	T45.2X5	T45.2X6
E acetate	T45.2X1	T45.2X2	T45.2X3	T45.2X4	T45.2X5	T45.2X6
hematopoietic	T45.8X1	T45.8X2	T45.8X3	T45.8X4	T45.8X5	T45.8X6
K1	T45.7X1	T45.7X2	T45.7X3	T45.7X4	T45.7X5	T45.7X6
K2	T45.7X1	T45.7X2	T45.7X3	T45.7X4	T45.7X5	T45.7X6
K NEC	T45.7X1	T45.7X2	T45.7X3	T45.7X4	T45.7X5	T45.7X6
PP	T45.2X1	T45.2X2	T45.2X3	T45.2X4	T45.2X5	T45.2X6
ulceroprotectant	T47.1X1	T47.1X2	T47.1X3	T47.1X4	T47.1X5	T47.1X6
Vleminckx's solution	T49.4X1	T49.4X2	T49.4X3	T49.4X4	T49.4X5	T49.4X6
Voltaren — see Diclofenac sodium						
Warfarin	T45.511	T45.512	T45.513	T45.514	T45.515	T45.516
rodenticide	T60.4X1	T60.4X2	T60.4X3	T60.4X4	—	—
sodium	T60.4X1	T60.4X2	T60.4X3	T60.4X4	—	—
Wasp (sting)	T63.461	T63.462	T63.463	T63.464	—	—
Water						
balance drug	T50.3X1	T50.3X2	T50.3X3	T50.3X4	T50.3X5	T50.3X6
distilled	T50.3X1	T50.3X2	T50.3X3	T50.3X4	T50.3X5	T50.3X6
gas — see Gas, water						
incomplete combustion of — see Carbon, monoxide, fuel, utility						
hemlock	T62.2X1	T62.2X2	T62.2X3	T62.2X4	—	—
moccasin (venom)	T63.061	T63.062	T63.063	T63.064	—	—
purified	T50.3X1	T50.3X2	T50.3X3	T50.3X4	T50.3X5	T50.3X6
Wax (paraffin) (petroleum)	T52.0X1	T52.0X2	T52.0X3	T52.0X4	—	—
automobile	T65.891	T65.892	T65.893	T65.894	—	—
floor	T52.0X1	T52.0X2	T52.0X3	T52.0X4	—	—
Weed killers NEC	T60.3X1	T60.3X2	T60.3X3	T60.3X4	—	—
Welldorm	T42.6X1	T42.6X2	T42.6X3	T42.6X4	T42.6X5	T42.6X6
White						
arsenic	T57.0X1	T57.0X2	T57.0X3	T57.0X4	—	—
hellebore	T62.2X1	T62.2X2	T62.2X3	T62.2X4	—	—
lotion (keratolytic)	T49.4X1	T49.4X2	T49.4X3	T49.4X4	T49.4X5	T49.4X6
spirit	T52.0X1	T52.0X2	T52.0X3	T52.0X4	—	—
Whitewash	T65.891	T65.892	T65.893	T65.894	—	—
Whole blood (human)	T45.8X1	T45.8X2	T45.8X3	T45.8X4	T45.8X5	T45.8X6
Wild						
black cherry	T62.2X1	T62.2X2	T62.2X3	T62.2X4	—	—
poisonous plants NEC	T62.2X1	T62.2X2	T62.2X3	T62.2X4	—	—
Window cleaning fluid	T65.891	T65.892	T65.893	T65.894	—	—
Wintergreen (oil)	T49.3X1	T49.3X2	T49.3X3	T49.3X4	T49.3X5	T49.3X6
Wisterine	T62.2X1	T62.2X2	T62.2X3	T62.2X4	—	—
Witch hazel	T49.2X1	T49.2X2	T49.2X3	T49.2X4	T49.2X5	T49.2X6
Wood alcohol or spirit	T51.1X1	T51.1X2	T51.1X3	T51.1X4	—	—
Wool fat (hydrous)	T49.3X1	T49.3X2	T49.3X3	T49.3X4	T49.3X5	T49.3X6
Woorali	T48.1X1	T48.1X2	T48.1X3	T48.1X4	T48.1X5	T48.1X6
Wormseed, American	T37.4X1	T37.4X2	T37.4X3	T37.4X4	T37.4X5	T37.4X6
Xamoterol	T44.5X1	T44.5X2	T44.5X3	T44.5X4	T44.5X5	T44.5X6
Xanthine diuretics	T50.2X1	T50.2X2	T50.2X3	T50.2X4	T50.2X5	T50.2X6
Xanthinol nicotinate	T46.7X1	T46.7X2	T46.7X3	T46.7X4	T46.7X5	T46.7X6

Substance	Poisoning, Accidental (unintentional)	Poisoning, Intentional Self-harm	Poisoning, Assault	Poisoning, Undetermined	Adverse Effect	Under-dosing
Xanthotoxin	T49.3X1	T49.3X2	T49.3X3	T49.3X4	T49.3X5	T49.3X6
Xantinol nicotinate	T46.7X1	T46.7X2	T46.7X3	T46.7X4	T46.7X5	T46.7X6
Xantocillin	T36.0X1	T36.0X2	T36.0X3	T36.0X4	T36.0X5	T36.0X6
Xenon (127Xe) (133Xe)	T50.8X1	T50.8X2	T50.8X3	T50.8X4	T50.8X5	T50.8X6
Xenysalate	T49.4X1	T49.4X2	T49.4X3	T49.4X4	T49.4X5	T49.4X6
Xibornol	T37.8X1	T37.8X2	T37.8X3	T37.8X4	T37.8X5	T37.8X6
Xigris	T45.511	T45.512	T45.513	T45.514	T45.515	T45.516
Xipamide	T50.2X1	T50.2X2	T50.2X3	T50.2X4	T50.2X5	T50.2X6
Xylene (vapor)	T52.2X1	T52.2X2	T52.2X3	T52.2X4	—	—
Xylocaine (infiltration) (topical)	T41.3X1	T41.3X2	T41.3X3	T41.3X4	T41.3X5	T41.3X6
nerve block (peripheral) (plexus)	T41.3X1	T41.3X2	T41.3X3	T41.3X4	T41.3X5	T41.3X6
spinal	T41.3X1	T41.3X2	T41.3X3	T41.3X4	T41.3X5	T41.3X6
Xylol (vapor)	T52.2X1	T52.2X2	T52.2X3	T52.2X4	—	—
Xylometazoline	T48.5X1	T48.5X2	T48.5X3	T48.5X4	T48.5X5	T48.5X6
Yeast	T45.2X1	T45.2X2	T45.2X3	T45.2X4	T45.2X5	T45.2X6
dried	T45.2X1	T45.2X2	T45.2X3	T45.2X4	T45.2X5	T45.2X6
Yellow						
fever vaccine	T50.B91	T50.B92	T50.B93	T50.B94	T50.B95	T50.B96
jasmine	T62.2X1	T62.2X2	T62.2X3	T62.2X4	—	—
phenolphthalein	T47.2X1	T47.2X2	T47.2X3	T47.2X4	T47.2X5	T47.2X6
Yew	T62.2X1	T62.2X2	T62.2X3	T62.2X4	—	—
Yohimbic acid	T40.991	T40.992	T40.993	T40.994	T40.995	T40.996
Zactane	T39.8X1	T39.8X2	T39.8X3	T39.8X4	T39.8X5	T39.8X6
Zalcitabine	T37.5X1	T37.5X2	T37.5X3	T37.5X4	T37.5X5	T37.5X6
Zaroxolyn	T50.2X1	T50.2X2	T50.2X3	T50.2X4	T50.2X5	T50.2X6
Zephiran (topical)	T49.0X1	T49.0X2	T49.0X3	T49.0X4	T49.0X5	T49.0X6
ophthalmic preparation	T49.5X1	T49.5X2	T49.5X3	T49.5X4	T49.5X5	T49.5X6
Zeranol	T38.7X1	T38.7X2	T38.7X3	T38.7X4	T38.7X5	T38.7X6
Zerone	T51.1X1	T51.1X2	T51.1X3	T51.1X4	—	—
Zidovudine	T37.5X1	T37.5X2	T37.5X3	T37.5X4	T37.5X5	T37.5X6
Zimeldine	T43.221	T43.222	T43.223	T43.224	T43.225	T43.226
Zinc (compounds) (fumes) (vapor)	T56.5X1	T56.5X2	T56.5X3	T56.5X4	—	—
NEC						
anti-infectives	T49.0X1	T49.0X2	T49.0X3	T49.0X4	T49.0X5	T49.0X6
antivaricose	T46.8X1	T46.8X2	T46.8X3	T46.8X4	T46.8X5	T46.8X6
bacitracin	T49.0X1	T49.0X2	T49.0X3	T49.0X4	T49.0X5	T49.0X6
chloride (mouthwash)	T49.6X1	T49.6X2	T49.6X3	T49.6X4	T49.6X5	T49.6X6
chromate	T56.5X1	T56.5X2	T56.5X3	T56.5X4	—	—
gelatin	T49.3X1	T49.3X2	T49.3X3	T49.3X4	T49.3X5	T49.3X6
oxide	T49.3X1	T49.3X2	T49.3X3	T49.3X4	T49.3X5	T49.3X6
plaster	T49.3X1	T49.3X2	T49.3X3	T49.3X4	T49.3X5	T49.3X6
peroxide	T49.0X1	T49.0X2	T49.0X3	T49.0X4	T49.0X5	T49.0X6
pesticides	T56.5X1	T56.5X2	T56.5X3	T56.5X4	—	—
phosphide	T60.4X1	T60.4X2	T60.4X3	T60.4X4	—	—
pyrithionate	T49.4X1	T49.4X2	T49.4X3	T49.4X4	T49.4X5	T49.4X6
stearate	T49.3X1	T49.3X2	T49.3X3	T49.3X4	T49.3X5	T49.3X6
sulfate	T49.5X1	T49.5X2	T49.5X3	T49.5X4	T49.5X5	T49.5X6
ENT agent	T49.6X1	T49.6X2	T49.6X3	T49.6X4	T49.6X5	T49.6X6
ophthalmic solution	T49.5X1	T49.5X2	T49.5X3	T49.5X4	T49.5X5	T49.5X6
topical NEC	T49.0X1	T49.0X2	T49.0X3	T49.0X4	T49.0X5	T49.0X6
undecylenate	T49.0X1	T49.0X2	T49.0X3	T49.0X4	T49.0X5	T49.0X6
Zineb	T60.0X1	T60.0X2	T60.0X3	T60.0X4	—	—
Zinostatin	T45.1X1	T45.1X2	T45.1X3	T45.1X4	T45.1X5	T45.1X6
Zipeprol	T48.3X1	T48.3X2	T48.3X3	T48.3X4	T48.3X5	T48.3X6
Zofenopril	T46.4X1	T46.4X2	T46.4X3	T46.4X4	T46.4X5	T46.4X6
Zolpidem	T42.6X1	T42.6X2	T42.6X3	T42.6X4	T42.6X5	T42.6X6
Zomepirac	T39.391	T39.392	T39.393	T39.394	T39.395	T39.396
Zopiclone	T42.6X1	T42.6X2	T42.6X3	T42.6X4	T42.6X5	T42.6X6
Zorubicin	T45.1X1	T45.1X2	T45.1X3	T45.1X4	T45.1X5	T45.1X6
Zotepine	T43.591	T43.592	T43.593	T43.594	T43.595	T43.596
Zovant	T45.511	T45.512	T45.513	T45.514	T45.515	T45.516
Zoxazolamine	T42.8X1	T42.8X2	T42.8X3	T42.8X4	T42.8X5	T42.8X6
Zuclopenthixol	T43.4X1	T43.4X2	T43.4X3	T43.4X4	T43.4X5	T43.4X6
Zygadenus (venenosus)	T62.2X1	T62.2X2	T62.2X3	T62.2X4	—	—
Zyprexa	T43.591	T43.592	T43.593	T43.594	T43.595	T43.596

ICD-10-CM Index to External Causes

A

Abandonment (causing exposure to weather conditions) (with intent to injure or kill) NEC X58 ☑

Abuse (adult) (child) (mental) (physical) (sexual) X58 ☑

Accident (to) X58 ☑
  aircraft (in transit) (powered) (*see also* Accident, transport, aircraft)
    due to, caused by cataclysm — *see* Forces of nature, by type
  animal-drawn vehicle — *see* Accident, transport, animal-drawn vehicle occupant
  animal-rider — *see* Accident, transport, animal-rider
  automobile — *see* Accident, transport, car occupant
  bare foot water skier V94.4 ☑
  boat, boating (*see also* Accident, watercraft)
    striking swimmer
      powered V94.11 ☑
      unpowered V94.12 ☑
  bus — *see* Accident, transport, bus occupant
  cable car, not on rails V98.0 ☑
    on rails — *see* Accident, transport, streetcar occupant
  car — *see* Accident, transport, car occupant
  caused by, due to
    animal NEC W64 ☑
    chain hoist W24.0 ☑
    cold (excessive) — *see* Exposure, cold
    corrosive liquid, substance — *see* Table of Drugs and Chemicals
    cutting or piercing instrument — *see* Contact, with, by type of instrument
    drive belt W24.0 ☑
    electric
      current — *see* Exposure, electric current
      motor (*see also* Contact, with, by type of machine) W31.3 ☑
        current (of) W86.8 ☑
    environmental factor NEC X58 ☑
    explosive material — *see* Explosion
    fire, flames — *see* Exposure, fire
    firearm missile — *see* Discharge, firearm by type
    heat (excessive) — *see* Heat
    hot — *see* Contact, with, hot
    ignition — *see* Ignition
    lifting device W24.0 ☑
    lightning — *see* subcategory T75.0 ☑
      causing fire — *see* Exposure, fire
    machine, machinery — *see* Contact, with, by type of machine
    natural factor NEC X58 ☑
    pulley (block) W24.0 ☑
    radiation — *see* Radiation
    steam X13.1 ☑
      inhalation X13.0 ☑
      pipe X16 ☑
    thunderbolt — *see* subcategory T75.0 ☑
      causing fire — *see* Exposure, fire
    transmission device W24.1 ☑
  coach — *see* Accident, transport, bus occupant
  coal car — *see* Accident, transport, industrial vehicle occupant
  diving (*see also* Fall, into, water)
    with
      drowning or submersion — *see* Drowning
  forklift — *see* Accident, transport, industrial vehicle occupant
  heavy transport vehicle NOS — *see* Accident, transport, truck occupant
  ice yacht V98.2 ☑
  in
    medical, surgical procedure
      as, or due to misadventure — *see* Misadventure
      causing an abnormal reaction or later complication without mention of misadventure (*see also* Complication of or following, by type of procedure) Y84.9
  land yacht V98.1 ☑
  late effect of — *see* W00-X58 with 7th character S

Accident — *continued*
  logging car — *see* Accident, transport, industrial vehicle occupant
  machine, machinery (*see also* Contact, with, by type of machine)
    on board watercraft V93.69 ☑
      explosion — *see* Explosion, in, watercraft
      fire — *see* Burn, on board watercraft
      powered craft V93.63 ☑
        ferry boat V93.61 ☑
        fishing boat V93.62 ☑
        jetskis V93.63 ☑
        liner V93.61 ☑
        merchant ship V93.60 ☑
        passenger ship V93.61 ☑
        sailboat V93.64 ☑
  mine tram — *see* Accident, transport, industrial vehicle occupant
  mobility scooter (motorized) — *see* Accident, transport, pedestrian, conveyance, specified type NEC
  motor scooter — *see* Accident, transport, motorcyclist
  motor vehicle NOS (traffic) (*see also* Accident, transport) V89.2 ☑
    nontraffic V89.0 ☑
    three-wheeled NOS — *see* Accident, transport, three-wheeled motor vehicle occupant
  motorcycle NOS — *see* Accident, transport, motorcyclist
  nonmotor vehicle NOS (nontraffic) (*see also* Accident, transport) V89.1 ☑
    traffic NOS V89.3 ☑
  nontraffic (victim's mode of transport NOS) V88.9 ☑
    collision (between) V88.7 ☑
      bus and truck V88.5 ☑
      car and:
        bus V88.3 ☑
        pickup V88.2 ☑
        three-wheeled motor vehicle V88.0 ☑
        train V88.6 ☑
        truck V88.4 ☑
        two-wheeled motor vehicle V88.0 ☑
        van V88.2 ☑
      specified vehicle NEC and:
        three-wheeled motor vehicle V88.1 ☑
        two-wheeled motor vehicle V88.1 ☑
    known mode of transport — *see* Accident, transport, by type of vehicle
    noncollision V88.8 ☑
  on board watercraft V93.89 ☑
    powered craft V93.83 ☑
      ferry boat V93.81 ☑
      fishing boat V93.82 ☑
      jetskis V93.83 ☑
      liner V93.81 ☑
      merchant ship V93.80 ☑
      passenger ship V93.81 ☑
    unpowered craft V93.88 ☑
      canoe V93.85 ☑
      inflatable V93.86 ☑
        in tow
          recreational V94.31 ☑
          specified NEC V94.32 ☑
      kayak V93.85 ☑
      sailboat V93.84 ☑
      surf-board V93.88 ☑
      water skis V93.87 ☑
      windsurfer V93.88 ☑
  parachutist V97.29 ☑
    entangled in object V97.21 ☑
    injured on landing V97.22 ☑
  pedal cycle — *see* Accident, transport, pedal cyclist
  pedestrian (on foot)
    with
      another pedestrian W51 ☑
        with fall W03 ☑
          due to ice or snow W00.0 ☑
      on pedestrian conveyance NEC V00.09 ☑
      roller skater (in-line) V00.01 ☑
      skate boarder V00.02 ☑
    transport vehicle — *see* Accident, transport

Accident — *continued*
  pedestrian — *continued*
    on pedestrian conveyance — *see* Accident, transport, pedestrian, conveyance
  pick-up truck or van — *see* Accident, transport, pickup truck occupant
  quarry truck — *see* Accident, transport, industrial vehicle occupant
  railway vehicle (any) (in motion) — *see* Accident, transport, railway vehicle occupant
    due to cataclysm — *see* Forces of nature, by type
  scooter (non-motorized) — *see* Accident, transport, pedestrian, conveyance, scooter
  sequelae of — *see* categories W00-X58 with 7th character S
  skateboard — *see* Accident, transport, pedestrian, conveyance, skateboard
  ski(ing) — *see* Accident, transport, pedestrian, conveyance
    lift V98.3 ☑
  specified cause NEC X58 ☑
  streetcar — *see* Accident, transport, streetcar occupant
  traffic (victim's mode of transport NOS) V87.9 ☑
    collision (between) V87.7 ☑
      bus and truck V87.5 ☑
      car and:
        bus V87.3 ☑
        pickup V87.2 ☑
        three-wheeled motor vehicle V87.0 ☑
        train V87.6 ☑
        truck V87.4 ☑
        two-wheeled motor vehicle V87.0 ☑
        van V87.2 ☑
      specified vehicle NEC and:
        three-wheeled motor vehicle V87.1 ☑
        two-wheeled motor vehicle V87.1 ☑
    known mode of transport — *see* Accident, transport, by type of vehicle
    noncollision V87.8 ☑
  transport (involving injury to) V99 ☑
    18 wheeler — *see* Accident, transport, truck occupant
    agricultural vehicle occupant (nontraffic) V84.9 ☑
      driver V84.5 ☑
      hanger-on V84.7 ☑
      passenger V84.6 ☑
      traffic V84.3 ☑
        driver V84.0 ☑
        hanger-on V84.2 ☑
        passenger V84.1 ☑
      while boarding or alighting V84.4 ☑
    aircraft NEC V97.89 ☑
      military NEC V97.818 ☑
        with civilian aircraft V97.810 ☑
        civilian injured by V97.811 ☑
      occupant injured (in)
        nonpowered craft accident V96.9 ☑
          balloon V96.00 ☑
            collision V96.03 ☑
            crash V96.01 ☑
            explosion V96.05 ☑
            fire V96.04 ☑
            forced landing V96.02 ☑
            specified type NEC V96.09 ☑
          glider V96.20 ☑
            collision V96.23 ☑
            crash V96.21 ☑
            explosion V96.25 ☑
            fire V96.24 ☑
            forced landing V96.22 ☑
            specified type NEC V96.29 ☑
          hang glider V96.10 ☑
            collision V96.13 ☑
            crash V96.11 ☑
            explosion V96.15 ☑
            fire V96.14 ☑
            forced landing V96.12 ☑
            specified type NEC V96.19 ☑
          specified craft NEC V96.8 ☑
        powered craft accident V95.9 ☑
          fixed wing NEC

Accident — continued
  transport — continued
    aircraft — continued
      occupant injured — continued
        powered craft accident — continued
          fixed wing — continued
            commercial V95.30 ☑
              collision V95.33 ☑
              crash V95.31 ☑
              explosion V95.35 ☑
              fire V95.34 ☑
              forced landing V95.32 ☑
              specified type NEC V95.39 ☑
            private V95.20 ☑
              collision V95.23 ☑
              crash V95.21 ☑
              explosion V95.25 ☑
              fire V95.24 ☑
              forced landing V95.22 ☑
              specified type NEC V95.29 ☑
          glider V95.10 ☑
            collision V95.13 ☑
            crash V95.11 ☑
            explosion V95.15 ☑
            fire V95.14 ☑
            forced landing V95.12 ☑
            specified type NEC V95.19 ☑
          helicopter V95.00 ☑
            collision V95.03 ☑
            crash V95.01 ☑
            explosion V95.05 ☑
            fire V95.04 ☑
            forced landing V95.02 ☑
            specified type NEC V95.09 ☑
          spacecraft V95.40 ☑
            collision V95.43 ☑
            crash V95.41 ☑
            explosion V95.45 ☑
            fire V95.44 ☑
            forced landing V95.42 ☑
            specified type NEC V95.49 ☑
          specified craft NEC V95.8 ☑
          ultralight V95.10 ☑
            collision V95.13 ☑
            crash V95.11 ☑
            explosion V95.15 ☑
            fire V95.14 ☑
            forced landing V95.12 ☑
            specified type NEC V95.19 ☑
        specified accident NEC V97.0 ☑
        while boarding or alighting V97.1 ☑
      person (injured by)
        falling from, in or on aircraft V97.0 ☑
        machinery on aircraft V97.89 ☑
        on ground with aircraft involvement V97.39 ☑
        rotating propeller V97.32 ☑
        struck by object falling from aircraft V97.31 ☑
        sucked into aircraft jet V97.33 ☑
        while boarding or alighting aircraft V97.1 ☑
    airport (battery-powered) passenger vehicle — see Accident, transport, industrial vehicle occupant
    all-terrain vehicle occupant (nontraffic) V86.99 ☑
      driver V86.59 ☑
      dune buggy — see Accident, transport, dune buggy occupant
      hanger-on V86.79 ☑
      passenger V86.69 ☑
      snowmobile — see Accident, transport, snowmobile occupant
      traffic V86.39 ☑
        driver V86.09 ☑
        hanger-on V86.29 ☑
        passenger V86.19 ☑
      while boarding or alighting V86.49 ☑
    ambulance occupant (traffic) V86.31 ☑
      driver V86.01 ☑
      hanger-on V86.21 ☑
      nontraffic V86.91 ☑
        driver V86.51 ☑
        hanger-on V86.71 ☑
        passenger V86.61 ☑
      passenger V86.11 ☑
      while boarding or alighting V86.41 ☑

Accident — continued
  transport — continued
    animal-drawn vehicle occupant (in) V80.929 ☑
      collision (with)
        animal V80.12 ☑
          being ridden V80.711 ☑
        animal-drawn vehicle V80.721 ☑
        bus V80.42 ☑
        car V80.42 ☑
        fixed or stationary object V80.82 ☑
        military vehicle V80.920 ☑
        nonmotor vehicle V80.791 ☑
        pedal cycle V80.22 ☑
        pedestrian V80.12 ☑
        pickup V80.42 ☑
        railway train or vehicle V80.62 ☑
        specified motor vehicle NEC V80.52 ☑
        streetcar V80.731 ☑
        truck V80.42 ☑
        two- or three-wheeled motor vehicle V80.32 ☑
        van V80.42 ☑
      noncollision V80.02 ☑
      specified circumstance NEC V80.928 ☑
    animal-rider V80.919 ☑
      collision (with)
        animal V80.11 ☑
          being ridden V80.710 ☑
        animal-drawn vehicle V80.720 ☑
        bus V80.41 ☑
        car V80.41 ☑
        fixed or stationary object V80.81 ☑
        military vehicle V80.910 ☑
        nonmotor vehicle V80.790 ☑
        pedal cycle V80.21 ☑
        pedestrian V80.11 ☑
        pickup V80.41 ☑
        railway train or vehicle V80.61 ☑
        specified motor vehicle NEC V80.51 ☑
        streetcar V80.730 ☑
        truck V80.41 ☑
        two- or three-wheeled motor vehicle V80.31 ☑
        van V80.41 ☑
      noncollision V80.018 ☑
        specified as horse rider V80.010 ☑
      specified circumstance NEC V80.918 ☑
    armored car — see Accident, transport, truck occupant
    battery-powered truck (baggage) (mail) — see Accident, transport, industrial vehicle occupant
    bus occupant V79.9 ☑
      collision (with)
        animal (traffic) V70.9 ☑
          being ridden (traffic) V76.9 ☑
            nontraffic V76.3 ☑
            while boarding or alighting V76.4 ☑
          nontraffic V70.3 ☑
          while boarding or alighting V70.4 ☑
        animal-drawn vehicle (traffic) V76.9 ☑
          nontraffic V76.3 ☑
          while boarding or alighting V76.4 ☑
        bus (traffic) V74.9 ☑
          nontraffic V74.3 ☑
          while boarding or alighting V74.4 ☑
        car (traffic) V73.9 ☑
          nontraffic V73.3 ☑
          while boarding or alighting V73.4 ☑
        motor vehicle NOS (traffic) V79.60 ☑
          nontraffic V79.20 ☑
          specified type NEC (traffic) V79.69 ☑
            nontraffic V79.29 ☑
        pedal cycle (traffic) V71.9 ☑
          nontraffic V71.3 ☑
          while boarding or alighting V71.4 ☑
        pickup truck (traffic) V73.9 ☑
          nontraffic V73.3 ☑
          while boarding or alighting V73.4 ☑
        railway vehicle (traffic) V75.9 ☑
          nontraffic V75.3 ☑
          while boarding or alighting V75.4 ☑
        specified vehicle NEC (traffic) V76.9 ☑
          nontraffic V76.3 ☑
          while boarding or alighting V76.4 ☑
        stationary object (traffic) V77.9 ☑

Accident — continued
  transport — continued
    bus occupant — continued
      collision — continued
        stationary object — continued
          nontraffic V77.3 ☑
          while boarding or alighting V77.4 ☑
        streetcar (traffic) V76.9 ☑
          nontraffic V76.3 ☑
          while boarding or alighting V76.4 ☑
        three wheeled motor vehicle (traffic) V72.9 ☑
          nontraffic V72.3 ☑
          while boarding or alighting V72.4 ☑
        truck (traffic) V74.9 ☑
          nontraffic V74.3 ☑
          while boarding or alighting V74.4 ☑
        two wheeled motor vehicle (traffic) V72.9 ☑
          nontraffic V72.3 ☑
          while boarding or alighting V72.4 ☑
        van (traffic) V73.9 ☑
          nontraffic V73.3 ☑
          while boarding or alighting V73.4 ☑
      driver
        collision (with)
          animal (traffic) V70.5 ☑
            being ridden (traffic) V76.5 ☑
              nontraffic V76.0 ☑
            nontraffic V70.0 ☑
          animal-drawn vehicle (traffic) V76.5 ☑
            nontraffic V76.0 ☑
          bus (traffic) V74.5 ☑
            nontraffic V74.0 ☑
          car (traffic) V73.5 ☑
            nontraffic V73.0 ☑
          motor vehicle NOS (traffic) V79.40 ☑
            nontraffic V79.00 ☑
            specified type NEC (traffic) V79.49 ☑
              nontraffic V79.09 ☑
          pedal cycle (traffic) V71.5 ☑
            nontraffic V71.0 ☑
          pickup truck (traffic) V73.5 ☑
            nontraffic V73.0 ☑
          railway vehicle (traffic) V75.5 ☑
            nontraffic V75.0 ☑
          specified vehicle NEC (traffic) V76.5 ☑
            nontraffic V76.0 ☑
          stationary object (traffic) V77.5 ☑
            nontraffic V77.0 ☑
          streetcar (traffic) V76.5 ☑
            nontraffic V76.0 ☑
          three wheeled motor vehicle (traffic) V72.5 ☑
            nontraffic V72.0 ☑
          truck (traffic) V74.5 ☑
            nontraffic V74.0 ☑
          two wheeled motor vehicle (traffic) V72.5 ☑
            nontraffic V72.0 ☑
          van (traffic) V73.5 ☑
            nontraffic V73.0 ☑
        noncollision accident (traffic) V78.5 ☑
          nontraffic V78.0 ☑
      hanger-on
        collision (with)
          animal (traffic) V70.7 ☑
            being ridden (traffic) V76.7 ☑
              nontraffic V76.2 ☑
            nontraffic V70.2 ☑
          animal-drawn vehicle (traffic) V76.7 ☑
            nontraffic V76.2 ☑
          bus (traffic) V74.7 ☑
            nontraffic V74.2 ☑
          car (traffic) V73.7 ☑
            nontraffic V73.2 ☑
          pedal cycle (traffic) V71.7 ☑
            nontraffic V71.2 ☑
          pickup truck (traffic) V73.7 ☑
            nontraffic V73.2 ☑
          railway vehicle (traffic) V75.7 ☑
            nontraffic V75.2 ☑
          specified vehicle NEC (traffic) V76.7 ☑
            nontraffic V76.2 ☑
          stationary object (traffic) V77.7 ☑
            nontraffic V77.2 ☑
          streetcar (traffic) V76.7 ☑

☑ **Additional Character Required** — Refer to the Tabular List for Character Selection   ▽ **Subterms under main terms may continue to next column or page**

Accident — *continued*
  transport — *continued*
    bus occupant — *continued*
      hanger-on — *continued*
        collision — *continued*
          streetcar — *continued*
            nontraffic V76.2 ☑
            three wheeled motor vehicle (traffic) V72.7 ☑
              nontraffic V72.2 ☑
            truck (traffic) V74.7 ☑
              nontraffic V74.2 ☑
            two wheeled motor vehicle (traffic) V72.7 ☑
              nontraffic V72.2 ☑
            van (traffic) V73.7 ☑
              nontraffic V73.2 ☑
        noncollision accident (traffic) V78.7 ☑
          nontraffic V78.2 ☑
      noncollision accident (traffic) V78.9 ☑
        nontraffic V78.3 ☑
        while boarding or alighting V78.4 ☑
      nontraffic V79.3 ☑
      passenger
        collision (with)
          animal (traffic) V70.6 ☑
            being ridden (traffic) V76.6 ☑
              nontraffic V76.1 ☑
            nontraffic V70.1 ☑
          animal-drawn vehicle (traffic) V76.6 ☑
            nontraffic V76.1 ☑
          bus (traffic) V74.6 ☑
            nontraffic V74.1 ☑
          car (traffic) V73.6 ☑
            nontraffic V73.1 ☑
          motor vehicle NOS (traffic) V79.50 ☑
            nontraffic V79.10 ☑
            specified type NEC (traffic) V79.59 ☑
              nontraffic V79.19 ☑
          pedal cycle (traffic) V71.6 ☑
            nontraffic V71.1 ☑
          pickup truck (traffic) V73.6 ☑
            nontraffic V73.1 ☑
          railway vehicle (traffic) V75.6 ☑
            nontraffic V75.1 ☑
          specified vehicle NEC (traffic) V76.6 ☑
            nontraffic V76.1 ☑
          stationary object (traffic) V77.6 ☑
            nontraffic V77.1 ☑
          streetcar (traffic) V76.6 ☑
            nontraffic V76.1 ☑
          three wheeled motor vehicle (traffic) V72.6 ☑
            nontraffic V72.1 ☑
          truck (traffic) V74.6 ☑
            nontraffic V74.1 ☑
          two wheeled motor vehicle (traffic) V72.6 ☑
            nontraffic V72.1 ☑
          van (traffic) V73.6 ☑
            nontraffic V73.1 ☑
        noncollision accident (traffic) V78.6 ☑
          nontraffic V78.1 ☑
      specified type NEC V79.88 ☑
      military vehicle V79.81 ☑
    cable car, not on rails V98.0 ☑
      on rails — *see* Accident, transport, streetcar occupant
    car occupant V49.9 ☑
      ambulance occupant — *see* Accident, transport, ambulance occupant
      collision (with)
        animal (traffic) V40.9 ☑
          being ridden (traffic) V46.9 ☑
            nontraffic V46.3 ☑
            while boarding or alighting V46.4 ☑
          nontraffic V40.3 ☑
          while boarding or alighting V40.4 ☑
        animal-drawn vehicle (traffic) V46.9 ☑
          nontraffic V46.3 ☑
          while boarding or alighting V46.4 ☑
        bus (traffic) V44.9 ☑
          nontraffic V44.3 ☑
          while boarding or alighting V44.4 ☑
        car (traffic) V43.92 ☑
          nontraffic V43.32 ☑

Accident — *continued*
  transport — *continued*
    car occupant — *continued*
      collision — *continued*
        car — *continued*
          while boarding or alighting V43.42 ☑
        motor vehicle NOS (traffic) V49.60 ☑
          nontraffic V49.20 ☑
          specified type NEC (traffic) V49.69 ☑
            nontraffic V49.29 ☑
        pedal cycle (traffic) V41.9 ☑
          nontraffic V41.3 ☑
          while boarding or alighting V41.4 ☑
        pickup truck (traffic) V43.93 ☑
          nontraffic V43.33 ☑
          while boarding or alighting V43.43 ☑
        railway vehicle (traffic) V45.9 ☑
          nontraffic V45.3 ☑
          while boarding or alighting V45.4 ☑
        specified vehicle NEC (traffic) V46.9 ☑
          nontraffic V46.3 ☑
          while boarding or alighting V46.4 ☑
        sport utility vehicle (traffic) V43.91 ☑
          nontraffic V43.31 ☑
          while boarding or alighting V43.41 ☑
        stationary object (traffic) V47.92 ☑
          nontraffic V47.32 ☑
          while boarding or alighting V47.4 ☑
        streetcar (traffic) V46.9 ☑
          nontraffic V46.3 ☑
          while boarding or alighting V46.4 ☑
        three wheeled motor vehicle (traffic) V42.9 ☑
          nontraffic V42.3 ☑
          while boarding or alighting V42.4 ☑
        truck (traffic) V44.9 ☑
          nontraffic V44.3 ☑
          while boarding or alighting V44.4 ☑
        two wheeled motor vehicle (traffic) V42.9 ☑
          nontraffic V42.3 ☑
          while boarding or alighting V42.4 ☑
        van (traffic) V43.94 ☑
          nontraffic V43.34 ☑
          while boarding or alighting V43.44 ☑
      driver
        collision (with)
          animal (traffic) V40.5 ☑
            being ridden (traffic) V46.5 ☑
              nontraffic V46.0 ☑
            nontraffic V40.0 ☑
          animal-drawn vehicle (traffic) V46.5 ☑
            nontraffic V46.0 ☑
          bus (traffic) V44.5 ☑
            nontraffic V44.0 ☑
          car (traffic) V43.52 ☑
            nontraffic V43.02 ☑
          motor vehicle NOS (traffic) V49.40 ☑
            nontraffic V49.00 ☑
            specified type NEC (traffic) V49.49 ☑
              nontraffic V49.09 ☑
          pedal cycle (traffic) V41.5 ☑
            nontraffic V41.0 ☑
          pickup truck (traffic) V43.53 ☑
            nontraffic V43.03 ☑
          railway vehicle (traffic) V45.5 ☑
            nontraffic V45.0 ☑
          specified vehicle NEC (traffic) V46.5 ☑
            nontraffic V46.0 ☑
          sport utility vehicle (traffic) V43.51 ☑
            nontraffic V43.01 ☑
          stationary object (traffic) V47.52 ☑
            nontraffic V47.02 ☑
          streetcar (traffic) V46.5 ☑
            nontraffic V46.0 ☑
          three wheeled motor vehicle (traffic) V42.5 ☑
            nontraffic V42.0 ☑
          truck (traffic) V44.5 ☑
            nontraffic V44.0 ☑
          two wheeled motor vehicle (traffic) V42.5 ☑
            nontraffic V42.0 ☑
          van (traffic) V43.54 ☑
            nontraffic V43.04 ☑
        noncollision accident (traffic) V48.5 ☑
          nontraffic V48.0 ☑

Accident — *continued*
  transport — *continued*
    car occupant — *continued*
      hanger-on
        collision (with)
          animal (traffic) V40.7 ☑
            being ridden (traffic) V46.7 ☑
              nontraffic V46.2 ☑
            nontraffic V40.2 ☑
          animal-drawn vehicle (traffic) V46.7 ☑
            nontraffic V46.2 ☑
          bus (traffic) V44.7 ☑
            nontraffic V44.2 ☑
          car (traffic) V43.72 ☑
            nontraffic V43.22 ☑
          pedal cycle (traffic) V41.7 ☑
            nontraffic V41.2 ☑
          pickup truck (traffic) V43.73 ☑
            nontraffic V43.23 ☑
          railway vehicle (traffic) V45.7 ☑
            nontraffic V45.2 ☑
          specified vehicle NEC (traffic) V46.7 ☑
            nontraffic V46.2 ☑
          sport utility vehicle (traffic) V43.71 ☑
            nontraffic V43.21 ☑
          stationary object (traffic) V47.7 ☑
            nontraffic V47.2 ☑
          streetcar (traffic) V46.7 ☑
            nontraffic V46.2 ☑
          three wheeled motor vehicle (traffic) V42.7 ☑
            nontraffic V42.2 ☑
          truck (traffic) V44.7 ☑
            nontraffic V44.2 ☑
          two wheeled motor vehicle (traffic) V42.7 ☑
            nontraffic V42.2 ☑
          van (traffic) V43.74 ☑
            nontraffic V43.24 ☑
        noncollision accident (traffic) V48.7 ☑
          nontraffic V48.2 ☑
      noncollision accident (traffic) V48.9 ☑
        nontraffic V48.3 ☑
        while boarding or alighting V48.4 ☑
      nontraffic V49.3 ☑
      passenger
        collision (with)
          animal (traffic) V40.6 ☑
            being ridden (traffic) V46.6 ☑
              nontraffic V46.1 ☑
            nontraffic V40.1 ☑
          animal-drawn vehicle (traffic) V46.6 ☑
            nontraffic V46.1 ☑
          bus (traffic) V44.6 ☑
            nontraffic V44.1 ☑
          car (traffic) V43.62 ☑
            nontraffic V43.12 ☑
          motor vehicle NOS (traffic) V49.50 ☑
            nontraffic V49.10 ☑
            specified type NEC (traffic) V49.59 ☑
              nontraffic V49.19 ☑
          pedal cycle (traffic) V41.6 ☑
            nontraffic V41.1 ☑
          pickup truck (traffic) V43.63 ☑
            nontraffic V43.13 ☑
          railway vehicle (traffic) V45.6 ☑
            nontraffic V45.1 ☑
          specified vehicle NEC (traffic) V46.6 ☑
            nontraffic V46.1 ☑
          sport utility vehicle (traffic) V43.61 ☑
            nontraffic V43.11 ☑
          stationary object (traffic) V47.62 ☑
            nontraffic V47.12 ☑
          streetcar (traffic) V46.6 ☑
            nontraffic V46.1 ☑
          three wheeled motor vehicle (traffic) V42.6 ☑
            nontraffic V42.1 ☑
          truck (traffic) V44.6 ☑
            nontraffic V44.1 ☑
          two wheeled motor vehicle (traffic) V42.6 ☑
            nontraffic V42.1 ☑
          van (traffic) V43.64 ☑
            nontraffic V43.14 ☑
        noncollision accident (traffic) V48.6 ☑

Accident — *continued*
 transport — *continued*
  car occupant — *continued*
   passenger — *continued*
    noncollision accident — *continued*
     nontraffic V48.1 ☑
    specified type NEC V49.88 ☑
    military vehicle V49.81 ☑
  coal car — *see* Accident, transport, industrial vehicle occupant
  construction vehicle occupant (nontraffic) V85.9 ☑
   driver V85.5 ☑
   hanger-on V85.7 ☑
   passenger V85.6 ☑
   traffic V85.3 ☑
    driver V85.0 ☑
    hanger-on V85.2 ☑
    passenger V85.1 ☑
   while boarding or alighting V85.4 ☑
  dirt bike rider — *see* Accident, transport, all-terrain vehicle occupant
  due to cataclysm — *see* Forces of nature, by type
  dune buggy occupant (nontraffic) V86.93 ☑
   driver V86.53 ☑
   hanger-on V86.73 ☑
   passenger V86.63 ☑
   traffic V86.33 ☑
    driver V86.03 ☑
    hanger-on V86.23 ☑
    passenger V86.13 ☑
   while boarding or alighting V86.43 ☑
  forklift — *see* Accident, transport, industrial vehicle occupant
  go cart — *see* Accident, transport, all-terrain vehicle occupant
  golf cart — *see* Accident, transport, all-terrain vehicle occupant
  heavy transport vehicle occupant — *see* Accident, transport, truck occupant
  ice yacht V98.2 ☑
  industrial vehicle occupant (nontraffic) V83.9 ☑
   driver V83.5 ☑
   hanger-on V83.7 ☑
   passenger V83.6 ☑
   traffic V83.3 ☑
    driver V83.0 ☑
    hanger-on V83.2 ☑
    passenger V83.1 ☑
   while boarding or alighting V83.4 ☑
  interurban electric car — *see* Accident, transport, streetcar
  land yacht V98.1 ☑
  logging car — *see* Accident, transport, industrial vehicle occupant
  military vehicle occupant (traffic) V86.34 ☑
   driver V86.04 ☑
   hanger-on V86.24 ☑
   nontraffic V86.94 ☑
    driver V86.54 ☑
    hanger-on V86.74 ☑
    passenger V86.64 ☑
   passenger V86.14 ☑
   while boarding or alighting V86.44 ☑
  mine tram — *see* Accident, transport, industrial vehicle occupant
  motor vehicle NEC occupant (traffic) V86.39 ☑
   driver V86.09 ☑
   hanger-on V86.29 ☑
   nontraffic V86.99 ☑
    driver V86.59 ☑
    hanger-on V86.79 ☑
    passenger V86.69 ☑
   passenger V86.19 ☑
   while boarding or alighting V86.49 ☑
  motorcoach — *see* Accident, transport, bus occupant
  motorcyclist V29.9 ☑
   collision (with)
    animal (traffic) V20.9 ☑
     being ridden (traffic) V26.9 ☑
      nontraffic V26.2 ☑
      while boarding or alighting V26.3 ☑
     nontraffic V20.2 ☑
     while boarding or alighting V20.3 ☑
    animal-drawn vehicle (traffic) V26.9 ☑
     nontraffic V26.2 ☑

Accident — *continued*
 transport — *continued*
  motorcyclist — *continued*
   collision — *continued*
    animal-drawn vehicle — *continued*
     while boarding or alighting V26.3 ☑
    bus (traffic) V24.9 ☑
     nontraffic V24.2 ☑
     while boarding or alighting V24.3 ☑
    car (traffic) V23.9 ☑
     nontraffic V23.2 ☑
     while boarding or alighting V23.3 ☑
    motor vehicle NOS (traffic) V29.60 ☑
     nontraffic V29.20 ☑
     specified type NEC (traffic) V29.69 ☑
      nontraffic V29.29 ☑
    pedal cycle (traffic) V21.9 ☑
     nontraffic V21.2 ☑
     while boarding or alighting V21.3 ☑
    pickup truck (traffic) V23.9 ☑
     nontraffic V23.2 ☑
     while boarding or alighting V23.3 ☑
    railway vehicle (traffic) V25.9 ☑
     nontraffic V25.2 ☑
     while boarding or alighting V25.3 ☑
    specified vehicle NEC (traffic) V26.9 ☑
     nontraffic V26.2 ☑
     while boarding or alighting V26.3 ☑
    stationary object (traffic) V27.9 ☑
     nontraffic V27.2 ☑
     while boarding or alighting V27.3 ☑
    streetcar (traffic) V26.9 ☑
     nontraffic V26.2 ☑
     while boarding or alighting V26.3 ☑
    three wheeled motor vehicle (traffic) V22.9 ☑
     nontraffic V22.2 ☑
     while boarding or alighting V22.3 ☑
    truck (traffic) V24.9 ☑
     nontraffic V24.2 ☑
     while boarding or alighting V24.3 ☑
    two wheeled motor vehicle (traffic) V22.9 ☑
     nontraffic V22.2 ☑
     while boarding or alighting V22.3 ☑
    van (traffic) V23.9 ☑
     nontraffic V23.2 ☑
     while boarding or alighting V23.3 ☑
   driver
    collision (with)
     animal (traffic) V20.4 ☑
      being ridden (traffic) V26.4 ☑
       nontraffic V26.0 ☑
      nontraffic V20.0 ☑
     animal-drawn vehicle (traffic) V26.4 ☑
      nontraffic V26.0 ☑
     bus (traffic) V24.4 ☑
      nontraffic V24.0 ☑
     car (traffic) V23.4 ☑
      nontraffic V23.0 ☑
     motor vehicle NOS (traffic) V29.40 ☑
      nontraffic V29.00 ☑
      specified type NEC (traffic) V29.49 ☑
       nontraffic V29.09 ☑
     pedal cycle (traffic) V21.4 ☑
      nontraffic V21.0 ☑
     pickup truck (traffic) V23.4 ☑
      nontraffic V23.0 ☑
     railway vehicle (traffic) V25.4 ☑
      nontraffic V25.0 ☑
     specified vehicle NEC (traffic) V26.4 ☑
      nontraffic V26.0 ☑
     stationary object (traffic) V27.4 ☑
      nontraffic V27.0 ☑
     streetcar (traffic) V26.4 ☑
      nontraffic V26.0 ☑
     three wheeled motor vehicle (traffic) V22.4 ☑
      nontraffic V22.0 ☑
     truck (traffic) V24.4 ☑
      nontraffic V24.0 ☑
     two wheeled motor vehicle (traffic) V22.4 ☑
      nontraffic V22.0 ☑
     van (traffic) V23.4 ☑
      nontraffic V23.0 ☑
    noncollision accident (traffic) V28.4 ☑

Accident — *continued*
 transport — *continued*
  motorcyclist — *continued*
   driver — *continued*
    noncollision accident — *continued*
     nontraffic V28.0 ☑
    noncollision accident (traffic) V28.9 ☑
     nontraffic V28.2 ☑
     while boarding or alighting V28.3 ☑
   nontraffic V29.3 ☑
   passenger
    collision (with)
     animal (traffic) V20.5 ☑
      being ridden (traffic) V26.5 ☑
       nontraffic V26.1 ☑
      nontraffic V20.1 ☑
     animal-drawn vehicle (traffic) V26.5 ☑
      nontraffic V26.1 ☑
     bus (traffic) V24.5 ☑
      nontraffic V24.1 ☑
     car (traffic) V23.5 ☑
      nontraffic V23.1 ☑
     motor vehicle NOS (traffic) V29.50 ☑
      nontraffic V29.10 ☑
      specified type NEC (traffic) V29.59 ☑
       nontraffic V29.19 ☑
     pedal cycle (traffic) V21.5 ☑
      nontraffic V21.1 ☑
     pickup truck (traffic) V23.5 ☑
      nontraffic V23.1 ☑
     railway vehicle (traffic) V25.5 ☑
      nontraffic V25.1 ☑
     specified vehicle NEC (traffic) V26.5 ☑
      nontraffic V26.1 ☑
     stationary object (traffic) V27.5 ☑
      nontraffic V27.1 ☑
     streetcar (traffic) V26.5 ☑
      nontraffic V26.1 ☑
     three wheeled motor vehicle (traffic) V22.5 ☑
      nontraffic V22.1 ☑
     truck (traffic) V24.5 ☑
      nontraffic V24.1 ☑
     two wheeled motor vehicle (traffic) V22.5 ☑
      nontraffic V22.1 ☑
     van (traffic) V23.5 ☑
      nontraffic V23.1 ☑
    noncollision accident (traffic) V28.5 ☑
     nontraffic V28.1 ☑
   specified type NEC V29.88 ☑
   military vehicle V29.81 ☑
  occupant (of)
   aircraft (powered) V95.9 ☑
    fixed wing
     commercial — *see* Accident, transport, aircraft, occupant, powered, fixed wing, commercial
     private — *see* Accident, transport, aircraft, occupant, powered, fixed wing, private
    nonpowered V96.9 ☑
    specified NEC V95.8 ☑
   airport battery-powered vehicle — *see* Accident, transport, industrial vehicle occupant
   all-terrain vehicle (ATV) — *see* Accident, transport, all-terrain vehicle occupant
   animal-drawn vehicle — *see* Accident, transport, animal-drawn vehicle occupant
   automobile — *see* Accident, transport, car occupant
   balloon V96.00 ☑
   battery-powered vehicle — *see* Accident, transport, industrial vehicle occupant
   bicycle — *see* Accident, transport, pedal cyclist
    motorized — *see* Accident, transport, motorcycle rider
   boat NEC — *see* Accident, watercraft
   bulldozer — *see* Accident, transport, construction vehicle occupant
   bus — *see* Accident, transport, bus occupant
   cable car (on rails) (*see also* Accident, transport, streetcar occupant)
    not on rails V98.0 ☑
   car (*see also* Accident, transport, car occupant)

Accident — continued
  transport — continued
    occupant — continued
      car (see also Accident, transport, car occupant)
        — continued
        cable (on rails) (see also Accident, transport,
          streetcar occupant)
          not on rails V98.0 ☑
      coach — see Accident, transport, bus occupant
      coal-car — see Accident, transport, industrial
        vehicle occupant
      digger — see Accident, transport, construction
        vehicle occupant
      dump truck — see Accident, transport, construc-
        tion vehicle occupant
      earth-leveler — see Accident, transport, con-
        struction vehicle occupant
      farm machinery (self-propelled) — see Acci-
        dent, transport, agricultural vehicle occu-
        pant
      forklift — see Accident, transport, industrial
        vehicle occupant
      glider (unpowered) V96.20 ☑
        hang V96.10 ☑
        powered (microlight) (ultralight) — see Ac-
          cident, transport, aircraft, occupant,
          powered, glider
      glider (unpowered) NEC V96.20 ☑
      hang-glider V96.10 ☑
      harvester — see Accident, transport, agricultur-
        al vehicle occupant
      heavy (transport) vehicle — see Accident,
        transport, truck occupant
      helicopter — see Accident, transport, aircraft,
        occupant, helicopter
      ice-yacht V98.2 ☑
      kite (carrying person) V96.8 ☑
      land-yacht V98.1 ☑
      logging car — see Accident, transport, industri-
        al vehicle occupant
      mechanical shovel — see Accident, transport,
        construction vehicle occupant
      microlight — see Accident, transport, aircraft,
        occupant, powered, glider
      minibus — see Accident, transport, car occu-
        pant
      minivan — see Accident, transport, car occu-
        pant
      moped — see Accident, transport, motorcycle
      motor scooter — see Accident, transport, mo-
        torcycle
      motorcycle (with sidecar) — see Accident,
        transport, motorcycle
      pedal cycle (see also Accident, transport, pedal
        cyclist)
      pick-up (truck) — see Accident, transport,
        pickup truck occupant
      railway (train) (vehicle) (subterranean) (elevat-
        ed) — see Accident, transport, railway
        vehicle occupant
      rickshaw — see Accident, transport, pedal cycle
        motorized — see Accident, transport, three-
          wheeled motor vehicle
        pedal driven — see Accident, transport,
          pedal cyclist
      road-roller — see Accident, transport, construc-
        tion vehicle occupant
      ship NOS V94.9 ☑
      ski-lift (chair) (gondola) V98.3 ☑
      snowmobile — see Accident, transport, snow-
        mobile occupant
      spacecraft, spaceship — see Accident, trans-
        port, aircraft, occupant, spacecraft
      sport utility vehicle — see Accident, transport,
        car occupant
      streetcar (interurban) (operating on public
        street or highway) — see Accident,
        transport, streetcar occupant
      SUV — see Accident, transport, car occupant
      téléférique V98.0 ☑
      three-wheeled vehicle (motorized) (see also
        Accident, transport, three-wheeled motor
        vehicle occupant)
        nonmotorized — see Accident, transport,
          pedal cycle
      tractor (farm) (and trailer) — see Accident,
        transport, agricultural vehicle occupant

Accident — continued
  transport — continued
    occupant — continued
      train — see Accident, transport, railway vehicle
        occupant
      tram — see Accident, transport, streetcar occu-
        pant
        in mine or quarry — see Accident, transport,
          industrial vehicle occupant
      tricycle — see Accident, transport, pedal cycle
        motorized — see Accident, transport, three-
          wheeled motor vehicle
      trolley — see Accident, transport, streetcar oc-
        cupant
        in mine or quarry — see Accident, transport,
          industrial vehicle occupant
      tub, in mine or quarry — see Accident, trans-
        port, industrial vehicle occupant
      ultralight — see Accident, transport, aircraft,
        occupant, powered, glider
      van — see Accident, transport, van occupant
      vehicle NEC V89.9 ☑
        heavy transport — see Accident, transport,
          truck occupant
        motor (traffic) NEC V89.2 ☑
        nontraffic NEC V89.0 ☑
      watercraft NOS V94.9 ☑
        causing drowning B — see Drowning, result-
          ing from accident to boat
  parachutist V97.29 ☑
    after accident to aircraft — see Accident,
      transport, aircraft
    entangled in object V97.21 ☑
    injured on landing V97.22 ☑
  pedal cyclist V19.9 ☑
    collision (with)
      animal (traffic) V10.9 ☑
        being ridden (traffic) V16.9 ☑
          nontraffic V16.2 ☑
          while boarding or alighting V16.3 ☑
        nontraffic V10.2 ☑
        while boarding or alighting V10.3 ☑
      animal-drawn vehicle (traffic) V16.9 ☑
        nontraffic V16.2 ☑
        while boarding or alighting V16.3 ☑
      bus (traffic) V14.9 ☑
        nontraffic V14.2 ☑
        while boarding or alighting V14.3 ☑
      car (traffic) V13.9 ☑
        nontraffic V13.2 ☑
        while boarding or alighting V13.3 ☑
      motor vehicle NOS (traffic) V19.60 ☑
        nontraffic V19.20 ☑
        specified type NEC (traffic) V19.69 ☑
          nontraffic V19.29 ☑
      pedal cycle (traffic) V11.9 ☑
        nontraffic V11.2 ☑
        while boarding or alighting V11.3 ☑
      pickup truck (traffic) V13.9 ☑
        nontraffic V13.2 ☑
        while boarding or alighting V13.3 ☑
      railway vehicle (traffic) V15.9 ☑
        nontraffic V15.2 ☑
        while boarding or alighting V15.3 ☑
      specified vehicle NEC (traffic) V16.9 ☑
        nontraffic V16.2 ☑
        while boarding or alighting V16.3 ☑
      stationary object (traffic) V17.9 ☑
        nontraffic V17.2 ☑
        while boarding or alighting V17.3 ☑
      streetcar (traffic) V16.9 ☑
        nontraffic V16.2 ☑
        while boarding or alighting V16.3 ☑
      three wheeled motor vehicle (traffic)
        V12.9 ☑
        nontraffic V12.2 ☑
        while boarding or alighting V12.3 ☑
      truck (traffic) V14.9 ☑
        nontraffic V14.2 ☑
        while boarding or alighting V14.3 ☑
      two wheeled motor vehicle (traffic) V12.9 ☑
        nontraffic V12.2 ☑
        while boarding or alighting V12.3 ☑
      van (traffic) V13.9 ☑
        nontraffic V13.2 ☑
        while boarding or alighting V13.3 ☑

Accident — continued
  transport — continued
    pedal cyclist — continued
      driver
        collision (with)
          animal (traffic) V10.4 ☑
            being ridden (traffic) V16.4 ☑
              nontraffic V16.0 ☑
            nontraffic V10.0 ☑
          animal-drawn vehicle (traffic) V16.4 ☑
            nontraffic V16.0 ☑
          bus (traffic) V14.4 ☑
            nontraffic V14.0 ☑
          car (traffic) V13.4 ☑
            nontraffic V13.0 ☑
          motor vehicle NOS (traffic) V19.40 ☑
            nontraffic V19.00 ☑
            specified type NEC (traffic) V19.49 ☑
              nontraffic V19.09 ☑
          pedal cycle (traffic) V11.4 ☑
            nontraffic V11.0 ☑
          pickup truck (traffic) V13.4 ☑
            nontraffic V13.0 ☑
          railway vehicle (traffic) V15.4 ☑
            nontraffic V15.0 ☑
          specified vehicle NEC (traffic) V16.4 ☑
            nontraffic V16.0 ☑
          stationary object (traffic) V17.4 ☑
            nontraffic V17.0 ☑
          streetcar (traffic) V16.4 ☑
            nontraffic V16.0 ☑
          three wheeled motor vehicle (traffic)
            V12.4 ☑
            nontraffic V12.0 ☑
          truck (traffic) V14.4 ☑
            nontraffic V14.0 ☑
          two wheeled motor vehicle (traffic)
            V12.4 ☑
            nontraffic V12.0 ☑
          van (traffic) V13.4 ☑
            nontraffic V13.0 ☑
        noncollision accident (traffic) V18.4 ☑
          nontraffic V18.0 ☑
      noncollision accident (traffic) V18.9 ☑
        nontraffic V18.2 ☑
        while boarding or alighting V18.3 ☑
      nontraffic V19.3 ☑
      passenger
        collision (with)
          animal (traffic) V10.5 ☑
            being ridden (traffic) V16.5 ☑
              nontraffic V16.1 ☑
            nontraffic V10.1 ☑
          animal-drawn vehicle (traffic) V16.5 ☑
            nontraffic V16.1 ☑
          bus (traffic) V14.5 ☑
            nontraffic V14.1 ☑
          car (traffic) V13.5 ☑
            nontraffic V13.1 ☑
          motor vehicle NOS (traffic) V19.50 ☑
            nontraffic V19.10 ☑
            specified type NEC (traffic) V19.59 ☑
              nontraffic V19.19 ☑
          pedal cycle (traffic) V11.5 ☑
            nontraffic V11.1 ☑
          pickup truck (traffic) V13.5 ☑
            nontraffic V13.1 ☑
          railway vehicle (traffic) V15.5 ☑
            nontraffic V15.1 ☑
          specified vehicle NEC (traffic) V16.5 ☑
            nontraffic V16.1 ☑
          stationary object (traffic) V17.5 ☑
            nontraffic V17.1 ☑
          streetcar (traffic) V16.5 ☑
            nontraffic V16.1 ☑
          three wheeled motor vehicle (traffic)
            V12.5 ☑
            nontraffic V12.1 ☑
          truck (traffic) V14.5 ☑
            nontraffic V14.1 ☑
          two wheeled motor vehicle (traffic)
            V12.5 ☑
            nontraffic V12.1 ☑
          van (traffic) V13.5 ☑
            nontraffic V13.1 ☑
        noncollision accident (traffic) V18.5 ☑

Accident — *continued*
  transport — *continued*
    pedal cyclist — *continued*
      passenger — *continued*
        noncollision accident — *continued*
          nontraffic V18.1 ☑
        specified type NEC V19.88 ☑
        military vehicle V19.81 ☑
    pedestrian
      conveyance (occupant) V09.9 ☑
        babystroller V00.828 ☑
          collision (with) V09.9 ☑
            animal being ridden or animal drawn vehicle V06.99 ☑
              nontraffic V06.09 ☑
              traffic V06.19 ☑
            bus or heavy transport V04.99 ☑
              nontraffic V04.09 ☑
              traffic V04.19 ☑
            car V03.99 ☑
              nontraffic V03.09 ☑
              traffic V03.19 ☑
            pedal cycle V01.99 ☑
              nontraffic V01.09 ☑
              traffic V01.19 ☑
            pick-up truck or van V03.99 ☑
              nontraffic V03.09 ☑
              traffic V03.19 ☑
            railway (train) (vehicle) V05.99 ☑
              nontraffic V05.09 ☑
              traffic V05.19 ☑
            stationary object V00.822 ☑
            streetcar V06.99 ☑
              nontraffic V06.09 ☑
              traffic V06.19 ☑
            two- or three-wheeled motor vehicle V02.99 ☑
              nontraffic V02.09 ☑
              traffic V02.19 ☑
            vehicle V09.9 ☑
              animal-drawn V06.99 ☑
                nontraffic V06.09 ☑
                traffic V06.19 ☑
              motor
                nontraffic V09.00 ☑
                traffic V09.20 ☑
         fall V00.821 ☑
        nontraffic V09.1 ☑
          involving motor vehicle NEC V09.00 ☑
        traffic V09.3 ☑
          involving motor vehicle NEC V09.20 ☑
        flat-bottomed NEC V00.388 ☑
          collision (with) V09.9 ☑
            animal being ridden or animal drawn vehicle V06.99 ☑
              nontraffic V06.09 ☑
              traffic V06.19 ☑
            bus or heavy transport V04.99 ☑
              nontraffic V04.09 ☑
              traffic V04.19 ☑
            car V03.99 ☑
              nontraffic V03.09 ☑
              traffic V03.19 ☑
            pedal cycle V01.99 ☑
              nontraffic V01.09 ☑
              traffic V01.19 ☑
            pick-up truck or van V03.99 ☑
              nontraffic V03.09 ☑
              traffic V03.19 ☑
            railway (train) (vehicle) V05.99 ☑
              nontraffic V05.09 ☑
              traffic V05.19 ☑
            stationary object V00.382 ☑
            streetcar V06.99 ☑
              nontraffic V06.09 ☑
              traffic V06.19 ☑
            two- or three-wheeled motor vehicle V02.99 ☑
              nontraffic V02.09 ☑
              traffic V02.19 ☑
            vehicle V09.9 ☑
              animal-drawn V06.99 ☑
                nontraffic V06.09 ☑
                traffic V06.19 ☑

pedestrian — *continued*
  conveyance — *continued*
    flat-bottomed — *continued*
      collision — *continued*
        vehicle — *continued*
          motor
            nontraffic V09.00 ☑
            traffic V09.20 ☑
      fall V00.381 ☑
      nontraffic V09.1 ☑
        involving motor vehicle NEC V09.00 ☑
    snow
      board — *see* Accident, transport, pedestrian, conveyance, snow board
      ski — *see* Accident, transport, pedestrian, conveyance, skis (snow)
    traffic V09.3 ☑
      involving motor vehicle NEC V09.20 ☑
    gliding type NEC V00.288 ☑
      collision (with) V09.9 ☑
        animal being ridden or animal drawn vehicle V06.99 ☑
          nontraffic V06.09 ☑
          traffic V06.19 ☑
        bus or heavy transport V04.99 ☑
          nontraffic V04.09 ☑
          traffic V04.19 ☑
        car V03.99 ☑
          nontraffic V03.09 ☑
          traffic V03.19 ☑
        pedal cycle V01.99 ☑
          nontraffic V01.09 ☑
          traffic V01.19 ☑
        pick-up truck or van V03.99 ☑
          nontraffic V03.09 ☑
          traffic V03.19 ☑
        railway (train) (vehicle) V05.99 ☑
          nontraffic V05.09 ☑
          traffic V05.19 ☑
        stationary object V00.282 ☑
        streetcar V06.99 ☑
          nontraffic V06.09 ☑
          traffic V02.19 ☑
        two- or three-wheeled motor vehicle V02.99 ☑
          nontraffic V02.09 ☑
          traffic V02.19 ☑
        vehicle V09.9 ☑
          animal-drawn V06.99 ☑
            nontraffic V06.09 ☑
            traffic V06.19 ☑
          motor
            nontraffic V09.00 ☑
            traffic V09.20 ☑
    fall V00.281 ☑
    heelies — *see* Accident, transport, pedestrian, conveyance, heelies
    ice skate — *see* Accident, transport, pedestrian, conveyance, ice skate
    nontraffic V09.1 ☑
      involving motor vehicle NEC V09.00 ☑
    sled — *see* Accident, transport, pedestrian, conveyance, sled
    traffic V09.3 ☑
      involving motor vehicle NEC V09.20 ☑
      wheelies — *see* Accident, transport, pedestrian, conveyance, heelies
    heelies V00.158 ☑
      colliding with stationary object V00.152 ☑
      fall V00.151 ☑
    ice skates V00.218 ☑
      collision (with) V09.9 ☑
        animal being ridden or animal drawn vehicle V06.99 ☑
          nontraffic V06.09 ☑
          traffic V06.19 ☑

pedestrian — *continued*
  conveyance — *continued*
    ice skates — *continued*
      collision — *continued*
        bus or heavy transport V04.99 ☑
          nontraffic V04.09 ☑
          traffic V04.19 ☑
        car V03.99 ☑
          nontraffic V03.09 ☑
          traffic V03.19 ☑
        pedal cycle V01.99 ☑
          nontraffic V01.09 ☑
          traffic V01.19 ☑
        pick-up truck or van V03.99 ☑
          nontraffic V03.09 ☑
          traffic V03.19 ☑
        railway (train) (vehicle) V05.99 ☑
          nontraffic V05.09 ☑
          traffic V05.19 ☑
        stationary object V00.212 ☑
        streetcar V06.99 ☑
          nontraffic V06.09 ☑
          traffic V06.19 ☑
        two- or three-wheeled motor vehicle V02.99 ☑
          nontraffic V02.09 ☑
          traffic V02.19 ☑
        vehicle V09.9 ☑
          animal-drawn V06.99 ☑
            nontraffic V06.09 ☑
            traffic V06.19 ☑
          motor
            nontraffic V09.00 ☑
            traffic V09.20 ☑
      fall V00.211 ☑
      nontraffic V09.1 ☑
        involving motor vehicle NEC V09.00 ☑
      traffic V09.3 ☑
        involving motor vehicle NEC V09.20 ☑
    motorized mobility scooter V00.838 ☑
      collision with stationary object V00.832 ☑
      fall from V00.831 ☑
    nontraffic V09.1 ☑
      involving motor vehicle V09.00 ☑
        military V09.01 ☑
        specified type NEC V09.09 ☑
    roller skates (non in-line) V00.128 ☑
      collision (with) V09.9 ☑
        animal being ridden or animal drawn vehicle V06.91 ☑
          nontraffic V06.01 ☑
          traffic V06.11 ☑
        bus or heavy transport V04.91 ☑
          nontraffic V04.01 ☑
          traffic V04.11 ☑
        car V03.91 ☑
          nontraffic V03.01 ☑
          traffic V03.11 ☑
        pedal cycle V01.91 ☑
          nontraffic V01.01 ☑
          traffic V01.11 ☑
        pick-up truck or van V03.91 ☑
          nontraffic V03.01 ☑
          traffic V03.11 ☑
        railway (train) (vehicle) V05.91 ☑
          nontraffic V05.01 ☑
          traffic V05.11 ☑
        stationary object V00.122 ☑
        streetcar V06.91 ☑
          nontraffic V06.01 ☑
          traffic V06.11 ☑
        two- or three-wheeled motor vehicle V02.91 ☑
          nontraffic V02.01 ☑
          traffic V02.11 ☑
        vehicle V09.9 ☑
          animal-drawn V06.91 ☑
            nontraffic V06.01 ☑
            traffic V06.11 ☑
          motor
            nontraffic V09.00 ☑

☑ **Additional Character Required** — Refer to the Tabular List for Character Selection   ▽ **Subterms under main terms may continue to next column or page**

Accident — *continued*
  transport — *continued*
    pedestrian — *continued*
      conveyance — *continued*
        roller skates — *continued*
          collision — *continued*
            vehicle — *continued*
              motor — *continued*
                traffic V09.20 ☑
          fall V00.121 ☑
          in-line V00.118 ☑
            collision — *see also* Accident, transport, pedestrian, conveyance occupant, roller skates, collision
              with stationary object V00.112 ☑
            fall V00.111 ☑
            nontraffic V09.1 ☑
              involving motor vehicle NEC V09.00 ☑
            traffic V09.3 ☑
              involving motor vehicle NEC V09.20 ☑
        rolling shoes V00.158 ☑
          colliding with stationary object V00.152 ☑
          fall V00.151 ☑
        rolling type NEC V00.188 ☑
          collision (with) V09.9 ☑
            animal being ridden or animal drawn vehicle V06.99 ☑
              nontraffic V06.09 ☑
              traffic V06.19 ☑
            bus or heavy transport V04.99 ☑
              nontraffic V04.09 ☑
              traffic V04.19 ☑
            car V03.99 ☑
              nontraffic V03.09 ☑
              traffic V03.19 ☑
            pedal cycle V01.99 ☑
              nontraffic V01.09 ☑
              traffic V01.19 ☑
            pick-up truck or van V03.99 ☑
              nontraffic V03.09 ☑
              traffic V03.19 ☑
            railway (train) (vehicle) V05.99 ☑
              nontraffic V05.09 ☑
              traffic V05.19 ☑
            stationary object V00.182 ☑
            streetcar V06.99 ☑
              nontraffic V06.09 ☑
              traffic V06.19 ☑
            two- or three-wheeled motor vehicle V02.99 ☑
              nontraffic V02.09 ☑
              traffic V02.19 ☑
            vehicle V09.9 ☑
              animal-drawn V06.99 ☑
                nontraffic V06.09 ☑
                traffic V06.19 ☑
              motor
                nontraffic V09.00 ☑
                traffic V09.20 ☑
          fall V00.181 ☑
          in-line roller skate — *see* Accident, transport, pedestrian, conveyance, roller skate, in-line
          nontraffic V09.1 ☑
            involving motor vehicle NEC V09.00 ☑
          roller skate — *see* Accident, transport, pedestrian, conveyance, roller skate
          scooter (non-motorized) — *see* Accident, transport, pedestrian, conveyance, scooter
          skateboard — *see* Accident, transport, pedestrian, conveyance, skate-board
          traffic V09.3 ☑
            involving motor vehicle NEC V09.20 ☑
        scooter (non-motorized) V00.148 ☑
          collision (with) V09.9 ☑
            animal being ridden or animal drawn vehicle V06.99 ☑

Accident — *continued*
  transport — *continued*
    pedestrian — *continued*
      conveyance — *continued*
        scooter — *continued*
          collision — *continued*
            animal being ridden or animal drawn vehicle — *continued*
              nontraffic V06.09 ☑
              traffic V06.19 ☑
            bus or heavy transport V04.99 ☑
              nontraffic V04.09 ☑
              traffic V04.19 ☑
            car V03.99 ☑
              nontraffic V03.09 ☑
              traffic V03.19 ☑
            pedal cycle V01.99 ☑
              nontraffic V01.09 ☑
              traffic V01.19 ☑
            pick-up truck or van V03.99 ☑
              nontraffic V03.09 ☑
              traffic V03.19 ☑
            railway (train) (vehicle) V05.99 ☑
              nontraffic V05.09 ☑
              traffic V05.19 ☑
            stationary object V00.142 ☑
            streetcar V06.99 ☑
              nontraffic V06.09 ☑
              traffic V06.19 ☑
            two- or three-wheeled motor vehicle V02.99 ☑
              nontraffic V02.09 ☑
              traffic V02.19 ☑
            vehicle V09.9 ☑
              animal-drawn V06.99 ☑
                nontraffic V06.09 ☑
                traffic V06.19 ☑
              motor
                nontraffic V09.00 ☑
                traffic V09.20 ☑
         fall V00.141 ☑
        nontraffic V09.1 ☑
          involving motor vehicle NEC V09.00 ☑
        traffic V09.3 ☑
          involving motor vehicle NEC V09.20 ☑
        skate board V00.138 ☑
          collision (with) V09.9 ☑
            animal being ridden or animal drawn vehicle V06.92 ☑
              nontraffic V06.02 ☑
              traffic V06.12 ☑
            bus or heavy transport V04.92 ☑
              nontraffic V04.02 ☑
              traffic V04.12 ☑
            car V03.92 ☑
              nontraffic V03.02 ☑
              traffic V03.12 ☑
            pedal cycle V01.92 ☑
              nontraffic V01.02 ☑
              traffic V01.12 ☑
            pick-up truck or van V03.92 ☑
              nontraffic V03.02 ☑
              traffic V03.12 ☑
            railway (train) (vehicle) V05.92 ☑
              nontraffic V05.02 ☑
              traffic V05.12 ☑
            stationary object V00.132 ☑
            streetcar V06.92 ☑
              nontraffic V06.02 ☑
              traffic V06.12 ☑
            two- or three-wheeled motor vehicle V02.92 ☑
              nontraffic V02.02 ☑
              traffic V02.12 ☑
            vehicle V09.9 ☑
              animal-drawn V06.92 ☑
                nontraffic V06.02 ☑
                traffic V06.12 ☑
              motor
                nontraffic V09.00 ☑
                traffic V09.20 ☑
         fall V00.131 ☑
        nontraffic V09.1 ☑

Accident — *continued*
  transport — *continued*
    pedestrian — *continued*
      conveyance — *continued*
        skate board — *continued*
          nontraffic — *continued*
            involving motor vehicle NEC V09.00 ☑
          traffic V09.3 ☑
            involving motor vehicle NEC V09.20 ☑
        skis (snow) V00.328 ☑
          collision (with) V09.9 ☑
            animal being ridden or animal drawn vehicle V06.99 ☑
              nontraffic V06.09 ☑
              traffic V06.19 ☑
            bus or heavy transport V04.99 ☑
              nontraffic V04.09 ☑
              traffic V04.19 ☑
            car V03.99 ☑
              nontraffic V03.09 ☑
              traffic V03.19 ☑
            pedal cycle V01.99 ☑
              nontraffic V01.09 ☑
              traffic V01.19 ☑
            pick-up truck or van V03.99 ☑
              nontraffic V03.09 ☑
              traffic V03.19 ☑
            railway (train) (vehicle) V05.99 ☑
              nontraffic V05.09 ☑
              traffic V05.19 ☑
            stationary object V00.322 ☑
            streetcar V06.99 ☑
              nontraffic V06.09 ☑
              traffic V06.19 ☑
            two- or three-wheeled motor vehicle V02.99 ☑
              nontraffic V02.09 ☑
              traffic V02.19 ☑
            vehicle V09.9 ☑
              animal-drawn V06.99 ☑
                nontraffic V06.09 ☑
                traffic V06.19 ☑
              motor
                nontraffic V09.00 ☑
                traffic V09.20 ☑
         fall V00.321 ☑
        nontraffic V09.1 ☑
          involving motor vehicle NEC V09.00 ☑
        traffic V09.3 ☑
          involving motor vehicle NEC V09.20 ☑
        sled V00.228 ☑
          collision (with) V09.9 ☑
            animal being ridden or animal drawn vehicle V06.99 ☑
              nontraffic V06.09 ☑
              traffic V06.19 ☑
            bus or heavy transport V04.99 ☑
              nontraffic V04.09 ☑
              traffic V04.19 ☑
            car V03.99 ☑
              nontraffic V03.09 ☑
              traffic V03.19 ☑
            pedal cycle V01.99 ☑
              nontraffic V01.09 ☑
              traffic V01.19 ☑
            pick-up truck or van V03.99 ☑
              nontraffic V03.09 ☑
              traffic V03.19 ☑
            railway (train) (vehicle) V05.99 ☑
              nontraffic V05.09 ☑
              traffic V05.19 ☑
            stationary object V00.222 ☑
            streetcar V06.99 ☑
              nontraffic V06.09 ☑
              traffic V06.19 ☑
            two- or three-wheeled motor vehicle V02.99 ☑
              nontraffic V02.09 ☑
              traffic V02.19 ☑
            vehicle V09.9 ☑
              animal-drawn V06.99 ☑
                nontraffic V06.09 ☑

Accident — *continued*
  transport — *continued*
    pedestrian — *continued*
      conveyance — *continued*
        sled — *continued*
          collision — *continued*
            vehicle — *continued*
              animal-drawn — *continued*
                traffic V06.19 ☑
              motor
                nontraffic V09.00 ☑
                traffic V09.20 ☑
          fall V00.221 ☑
          nontraffic V09.1 ☑
            involving motor vehicle NEC
              V09.00 ☑
          traffic V09.3 ☑
            involving motor vehicle NEC
              V09.20 ☑
        snow board V00.318 ☑
          collision (with) V09.9 ☑
            animal being ridden or animal drawn
              vehicle V06.99 ☑
              nontraffic V06.09 ☑
              traffic V06.19 ☑
            bus or heavy transport V04.99 ☑
              nontraffic V04.09 ☑
              traffic V04.19 ☑
            car V03.99 ☑
              nontraffic V03.09 ☑
              traffic V03.19 ☑
            pedal cycle V01.99 ☑
              nontraffic V01.09 ☑
              traffic V01.19 ☑
            pick-up truck or van V03.99 ☑
              nontraffic V03.09 ☑
              traffic V03.19 ☑
            railway (train) (vehicle) V05.99 ☑
              nontraffic V05.09 ☑
              traffic V05.19 ☑
            stationary object V00.312 ☑
            streetcar V06.99 ☑
              nontraffic V06.09 ☑
              traffic V06.19 ☑
            two- or three-wheeled motor vehicle
              V02.99 ☑
              nontraffic V02.09 ☑
              traffic V02.19 ☑
            vehicle V09.9 ☑
              animal-drawn V06.99 ☑
                nontraffic V06.09 ☑
                traffic V06.19 ☑
              motor
                nontraffic V09.00 ☑
                traffic V09.20 ☑
         fall V00.311 ☑
        nontraffic V09.1 ☑
          involving motor vehicle NEC
            V09.00 ☑
        traffic V09.3 ☑
          involving motor vehicle NEC
            V09.20 ☑
      specified type NEC V00.898 ☑
        collision (with) V09.9 ☑
          animal being ridden or animal drawn
            vehicle V06.99 ☑
            nontraffic V06.09 ☑
            traffic V06.19 ☑
          bus or heavy transport V04.99 ☑
            nontraffic V04.09 ☑
            traffic V04.19 ☑
          car V03.99 ☑
            nontraffic V03.09 ☑
            traffic V03.19 ☑
          pedal cycle V01.99 ☑
            nontraffic V01.09 ☑
            traffic V01.19 ☑
          pick-up truck or van V03.99 ☑
            nontraffic V03.09 ☑
            traffic V03.19 ☑
          railway (train) (vehicle) V05.99 ☑
            nontraffic V05.09 ☑
            traffic V05.19 ☑
          stationary object V00.892 ☑
          streetcar V06.99 ☑
            nontraffic V06.09 ☑

Accident — *continued*
  transport — *continued*
    pedestrian — *continued*
      conveyance — *continued*
        specified type — *continued*
          collision — *continued*
            streetcar — *continued*
              traffic V06.19 ☑
            two- or three-wheeled motor vehicle
              V02.99 ☑
              nontraffic V02.09 ☑
              traffic V02.19 ☑
            vehicle V09.9 ☑
              animal-drawn V06.99 ☑
                nontraffic V06.09 ☑
                traffic V06.19 ☑
              motor
                nontraffic V09.00 ☑
                traffic V09.20 ☑
          fall V00.891 ☑
        nontraffic V09.1 ☑
          involving motor vehicle NEC
            V09.00 ☑
        traffic V09.3 ☑
          involving motor vehicle NEC
            V09.20 ☑
      traffic V09.3 ☑
        involving motor vehicle V09.20 ☑
          military V09.21 ☑
          specified type NEC V09.29 ☑
      wheelchair (powered) V00.818 ☑
        collision (with) V09.9 ☑
          animal being ridden or animal drawn
            vehicle V06.99 ☑
            nontraffic V06.09 ☑
            traffic V06.19 ☑
          bus or heavy transport V04.99 ☑
            nontraffic V04.09 ☑
            traffic V04.19 ☑
          car V03.99 ☑
            nontraffic V03.09 ☑
            traffic V03.19 ☑
          pedal cycle V01.99 ☑
            nontraffic V01.09 ☑
            traffic V01.19 ☑
          pick-up truck or van V03.99 ☑
            nontraffic V03.09 ☑
            traffic V03.19 ☑
          railway (train) (vehicle) V05.99 ☑
            nontraffic V05.09 ☑
            traffic V05.19 ☑
          stationary object V00.812 ☑
          streetcar V06.99 ☑
            nontraffic V06.09 ☑
            traffic V06.19 ☑
          two- or three-wheeled motor vehicle
            V02.99 ☑
            nontraffic V02.09 ☑
            traffic V02.19 ☑
          vehicle V09.9 ☑
            animal-drawn V06.99 ☑
              nontraffic V06.09 ☑
              traffic V06.19 ☑
            motor
              nontraffic V09.00 ☑
              traffic V09.20 ☑
        fall V00.811 ☑
       nontraffic V09.1 ☑
         involving motor vehicle NEC
           V09.00 ☑
       traffic V09.3 ☑
         involving motor vehicle NEC
           V09.20 ☑
      wheeled shoe V00.158 ☑
        colliding with stationary object
          V00.152 ☑
        fall V00.151 ☑
      on foot (*see also* Accident, pedestrian)
        collision (with)
          animal being ridden or animal drawn
            vehicle V06.90 ☑
            nontraffic V06.00 ☑
            traffic V06.10 ☑
          bus or heavy transport V04.90 ☑
            nontraffic V04.00 ☑
            traffic V04.10 ☑

Accident — *continued*
  transport — *continued*
    pedestrian — *continued*
      on foot (*see also* Accident, pedestrian) — con-
        tinued
        collision — *continued*
          car V03.90 ☑
            nontraffic V03.00 ☑
            traffic V03.10 ☑
          pedal cycle V01.90 ☑
            nontraffic V01.00 ☑
            traffic V01.10 ☑
          pick-up truck or van V03.90 ☑
            nontraffic V03.00 ☑
            traffic V03.10 ☑
          railway (train) (vehicle) V05.90 ☑
            nontraffic V05.00 ☑
            traffic V05.10 ☑
          streetcar V06.90 ☑
            nontraffic V06.00 ☑
            traffic V06.10 ☑
          two- or three-wheeled motor vehicle
            V02.90 ☑
            nontraffic V02.00 ☑
            traffic V02.10 ☑
          vehicle V09.9 ☑
            animal-drawn V06.90 ☑
              nontraffic V06.00 ☑
              traffic V06.10 ☑
            motor
        nontraffic V09.1 ☑
          involving motor vehicle V09.00 ☑
           military V09.01 ☑
           specified type NEC V09.09 ☑
        traffic V09.3 ☑
          involving motor vehicle V09.20 ☑
           military V09.21 ☑
           specified type NEC V09.29 ☑
    person NEC (unknown way or transportation)
      V99 ☑
      collision (between)
        bus (with)
          heavy transport vehicle (traffic) V87.5 ☑
          nontraffic V88.5 ☑
        car (with)
          bus (traffic) V87.3 ☑
          nontraffic V88.3 ☑
          heavy transport vehicle (traffic) V87.4 ☑
          nontraffic V88.4 ☑
          nontraffic V88.5 ☑
          pick-up truck or van (traffic) V87.2 ☑
          nontraffic V88.2 ☑
          train or railway vehicle (traffic) V87.6 ☑
          nontraffic V88.6 ☑
          two-or three-wheeled motor vehicle
           (traffic) V87.0 ☑
          nontraffic V88.0 ☑
        motor vehicle (traffic) NEC V87.7 ☑
          nontraffic V88.7 ☑
        two-or three-wheeled vehicle (with) (traffic)
          motor vehicle NEC V87.1 ☑
          nontraffic V88.1 ☑
        nonmotor vehicle (collision) (noncollision)
          (traffic) V87.9 ☑
          nontraffic V88.9 ☑
    pickup truck occupant V59.9 ☑
      collision (with)
        animal (traffic) V50.9 ☑
          being ridden (traffic) V56.9 ☑
           nontraffic V56.3 ☑
           while boarding or alighting V56.4 ☑
          nontraffic V50.3 ☑
          while boarding or alighting V50.4 ☑
        animal-drawn vehicle (traffic) V56.9 ☑
          nontraffic V56.3 ☑
          while boarding or alighting V56.4 ☑
        bus (traffic) V54.9 ☑
          nontraffic V54.3 ☑
          while boarding or alighting V54.4 ☑
        car (traffic) V53.9 ☑
          nontraffic V53.3 ☑
          while boarding or alighting V53.4 ☑
        motor vehicle NOS (traffic) V59.60 ☑
          nontraffic V59.20 ☑
          specified type NEC (traffic) V59.69 ☑
           nontraffic V59.29 ☑

Accident — *continued*
  transport — *continued*
    pickup truck occupant — *continued*
      collision — *continued*
        pedal cycle (traffic) V51.9 ☑
          nontraffic V51.3 ☑
          while boarding or alighting V51.4 ☑
        pickup truck (traffic) V53.9 ☑
          nontraffic V53.3 ☑
          while boarding or alighting V53.4 ☑
        railway vehicle (traffic) V55.9 ☑
          nontraffic V55.3 ☑
          while boarding or alighting V55.4 ☑
        specified vehicle NEC (traffic) V56.9 ☑
          nontraffic V56.3 ☑
          while boarding or alighting V56.4 ☑
        stationary object (traffic) V57.9 ☑
          nontraffic V57.3 ☑
          while boarding or alighting V57.4 ☑
        streetcar (traffic) V56.9 ☑
          nontraffic V56.3 ☑
          while boarding or alighting V56.4 ☑
        three wheeled motor vehicle (traffic)
          V52.9 ☑
          nontraffic V52.3 ☑
          while boarding or alighting V52.4 ☑
        truck (traffic) V54.9 ☑
          nontraffic V54.3 ☑
          while boarding or alighting V54.4 ☑
        two wheeled motor vehicle (traffic) V52.9 ☑
          nontraffic V52.3 ☑
          while boarding or alighting V52.4 ☑
        van (traffic) V53.9 ☑
          nontraffic V53.3 ☑
          while boarding or alighting V53.4 ☑
      driver
        collision (with)
          animal (traffic) V50.5 ☑
            being ridden (traffic) V56.5 ☑
              nontraffic V56.0 ☑
            nontraffic V50.0 ☑
          animal-drawn vehicle (traffic) V56.5 ☑
            nontraffic V56.0 ☑
          bus (traffic) V54.5 ☑
            nontraffic V54.0 ☑
          car (traffic) V53.5 ☑
            nontraffic V53.0 ☑
          motor vehicle NOS (traffic) V59.40 ☑
            nontraffic V59.00 ☑
            specified type NEC (traffic) V59.49 ☑
              nontraffic V59.09 ☑
          pedal cycle (traffic) V51.5 ☑
            nontraffic V51.0 ☑
          pickup truck (traffic) V53.5 ☑
            nontraffic V53.0 ☑
          railway vehicle (traffic) V55.5 ☑
            nontraffic V55.0 ☑
          specified vehicle NEC (traffic) V56.5 ☑
            nontraffic V56.0 ☑
          stationary object (traffic) V57.5 ☑
            nontraffic V57.0 ☑
          streetcar (traffic) V56.5 ☑
            nontraffic V56.0 ☑
          three wheeled motor vehicle (traffic)
            V52.5 ☑
            nontraffic V52.0 ☑
          truck (traffic) V54.5 ☑
            nontraffic V54.0 ☑
          two wheeled motor vehicle (traffic)
            V52.5 ☑
            nontraffic V52.0 ☑
          van (traffic) V53.5 ☑
            nontraffic V53.0 ☑
        noncollision accident (traffic) V58.5 ☑
          nontraffic V58.0 ☑
      hanger-on
        collision (with)
          animal (traffic) V50.7 ☑
            being ridden (traffic) V56.7 ☑
              nontraffic V56.2 ☑
            nontraffic V50.2 ☑
          animal-drawn vehicle (traffic) V56.7 ☑
            nontraffic V56.2 ☑
          bus (traffic) V54.7 ☑
            nontraffic V54.2 ☑
          car (traffic) V53.7 ☑

Accident — *continued*
  transport — *continued*
    pickup truck occupant — *continued*
      hanger-on — *continued*
        collision — *continued*
          car — *continued*
            nontraffic V53.2 ☑
          pedal cycle (traffic) V51.7 ☑
            nontraffic V51.2 ☑
          pickup truck (traffic) V53.7 ☑
            nontraffic V53.2 ☑
          railway vehicle (traffic) V55.7 ☑
            nontraffic V55.2 ☑
          specified vehicle NEC (traffic) V56.7 ☑
            nontraffic V56.2 ☑
          stationary object (traffic) V57.7 ☑
            nontraffic V57.2 ☑
          streetcar (traffic) V56.7 ☑
            nontraffic V56.2 ☑
          three wheeled motor vehicle (traffic)
            V52.7 ☑
            nontraffic V52.2 ☑
          truck (traffic) V54.7 ☑
            nontraffic V54.2 ☑
          two wheeled motor vehicle (traffic)
            V52.7 ☑
            nontraffic V52.2 ☑
          van (traffic) V53.7 ☑
            nontraffic V53.2 ☑
        noncollision accident (traffic) V58.7 ☑
          nontraffic V58.2 ☑
      noncollision accident (traffic) V58.9 ☑
        nontraffic V58.3 ☑
        while boarding or alighting V58.4 ☑
      nontraffic V59.3 ☑
      passenger
        collision (with)
          animal (traffic) V50.6 ☑
            being ridden (traffic) V56.6 ☑
              nontraffic V56.1 ☑
            nontraffic V50.1 ☑
          animal-drawn vehicle (traffic) V56.6 ☑
            nontraffic V56.1 ☑
          bus (traffic) V54.6 ☑
            nontraffic V54.1 ☑
          car (traffic) V53.6 ☑
            nontraffic V53.1 ☑
          motor vehicle NOS (traffic) V59.50 ☑
            nontraffic V59.10 ☑
            specified type NEC (traffic) V59.59 ☑
              nontraffic V59.19 ☑
          pedal cycle (traffic) V51.6 ☑
            nontraffic V51.1 ☑
          pickup truck (traffic) V53.6 ☑
            nontraffic V53.1 ☑
          railway vehicle (traffic) V55.6 ☑
            nontraffic V55.1 ☑
          specified vehicle NEC (traffic) V56.6 ☑
            nontraffic V56.1 ☑
          stationary object (traffic) V57.6 ☑
            nontraffic V57.1 ☑
          streetcar (traffic) V56.6 ☑
            nontraffic V56.1 ☑
          three wheeled motor vehicle (traffic)
            V52.6 ☑
            nontraffic V52.1 ☑
          truck (traffic) V54.6 ☑
            nontraffic V54.1 ☑
          two wheeled motor vehicle (traffic)
            V52.6 ☑
            nontraffic V52.1 ☑
          van (traffic) V53.6 ☑
            nontraffic V53.1 ☑
        noncollision accident (traffic) V58.6 ☑
          nontraffic V58.1 ☑
      specified type NEC V59.88 ☑
      military vehicle V59.81 ☑
    quarry truck — *see* Accident, transport, industrial
      vehicle occupant
    race car — *see* Accident, transport, motor vehicle
      NEC occupant
    railway vehicle occupant V81.9 ☑
      collision (with) V81.3 ☑
        motor vehicle (non-military) (traffic)
          V81.1 ☑
          military V81.83 ☑

Accident — *continued*
  transport — *continued*
    railway vehicle occupant — *continued*
      collision — *continued*
        motor vehicle — *continued*
          nontraffic V81.0 ☑
          rolling stock V81.2 ☑
          specified object NEC V81.3 ☑
      during derailment V81.7 ☑
        with antecedent collision B — *see* Accident,
          transport, railway vehicle occupant,
          collision
      explosion V81.81 ☑
      fall (in railway vehicle) V81.5 ☑
        during derailment V81.7 ☑
          with antecedent collision B — *see* Acci-
            dent, transport, railway vehicle
            occupant, collision
        from railway vehicle V81.6 ☑
          during derailment V81.7 ☑
            with antecedent collision B — *see*
              Accident, transport, railway
              vehicle occupant, collision
        while boarding or alighting V81.4 ☑
      fire V81.81 ☑
      object falling onto train V81.82 ☑
      specified type NEC V81.89 ☑
      while boarding or alighting V81.4 ☑
    ski lift V98.3 ☑
    snowmobile occupant (nontraffic) V86.92 ☑
      driver V86.52 ☑
      hanger-on V86.72 ☑
      passenger V86.62 ☑
      traffic V86.32 ☑
        driver V86.02 ☑
        hanger-on V86.22 ☑
        passenger V86.12 ☑
      while boarding or alighting V86.42 ☑
    specified NEC V98.8 ☑
    sport utility vehicle occupant (*see also* Accident,
      transport, car occupant)
      collision (with)
        stationary object (traffic) V47.91 ☑
          nontraffic V47.31 ☑
      driver
        collision (with)
          stationary object (traffic) V47.51 ☑
            nontraffic V47.01 ☑
      passenger
        collision (with)
          stationary object (traffic) V47.61 ☑
            nontraffic V47.11 ☑
    streetcar occupant V82.9 ☑
      collision (with) V82.3 ☑
        motor vehicle (traffic) V82.1 ☑
          nontraffic V82.0 ☑
        rolling stock V82.2 ☑
      during derailment V82.7 ☑
        with antecedent collision B — *see* Accident,
          transport, streetcar occupant, collision
      fall (in streetcar) V82.5 ☑
        during derailment V82.7 ☑
          with antecedent collision B — *see* Acci-
            dent, transport, streetcar occu-
            pant, collision
        from streetcar V82.6 ☑
          during derailment V82.7 ☑
            with antecedent collision B — *see*
              Accident, transport, streetcar
              occupant, collision
        while boarding or alighting V82.4 ☑
      while boarding or alighting V82.4 ☑
      specified type NEC V82.8 ☑
      while boarding or alighting V82.4 ☑
    three-wheeled motor vehicle occupant V39.9 ☑
      collision (with)
        animal (traffic) V30.9 ☑
          being ridden (traffic) V36.9 ☑
            nontraffic V36.3 ☑
            while boarding or alighting V36.4 ☑
          nontraffic V30.3 ☑
          while boarding or alighting V30.4 ☑
        animal-drawn vehicle (traffic) V36.9 ☑
          nontraffic V36.3 ☑
          while boarding or alighting V36.4 ☑
        bus (traffic) V34.9 ☑

Accident — *continued*
  transport — *continued*
    three-wheeled motor vehicle occupant — *continued*
      collision — *continued*
        bus — *continued*
          nontraffic V34.3 ☑
          while boarding or alighting V34.4 ☑
        car (traffic) V33.9 ☑
          nontraffic V33.3 ☑
          while boarding or alighting V33.4 ☑
        motor vehicle NOS (traffic) V39.60 ☑
          nontraffic V39.20 ☑
          specified type NEC (traffic) V39.69 ☑
            nontraffic V39.29 ☑
        pedal cycle (traffic) V31.9 ☑
          nontraffic V31.3 ☑
          while boarding or alighting V31.4 ☑
        pickup truck (traffic) V33.9 ☑
          nontraffic V33.3 ☑
          while boarding or alighting V33.4 ☑
        railway vehicle (traffic) V35.9 ☑
          nontraffic V35.3 ☑
          while boarding or alighting V35.4 ☑
        specified vehicle NEC (traffic) V36.9 ☑
          nontraffic V36.3 ☑
          while boarding or alighting V36.4 ☑
        stationary object (traffic) V37.9 ☑
          nontraffic V37.3 ☑
          while boarding or alighting V37.4 ☑
        streetcar (traffic) V36.9 ☑
          nontraffic V36.3 ☑
          while boarding or alighting V36.4 ☑
        three wheeled motor vehicle (traffic) V32.9 ☑
          nontraffic V32.3 ☑
          while boarding or alighting V32.4 ☑
        truck (traffic) V34.9 ☑
          nontraffic V34.3 ☑
          while boarding or alighting V34.4 ☑
        two wheeled motor vehicle (traffic) V32.9 ☑
          nontraffic V32.3 ☑
          while boarding or alighting V32.4 ☑
        van (traffic) V33.9 ☑
          nontraffic V33.3 ☑
          while boarding or alighting V33.4 ☑
      driver
        collision (with)
          animal (traffic) V30.5 ☑
            being ridden (traffic) V36.5 ☑
              nontraffic V36.0 ☑
            nontraffic V30.0 ☑
          animal-drawn vehicle (traffic) V36.5 ☑
            nontraffic V36.0 ☑
          bus (traffic) V34.5 ☑
            nontraffic V34.0 ☑
          car (traffic) V33.5 ☑
            nontraffic V33.0 ☑
          motor vehicle NOS (traffic) V39.40 ☑
            nontraffic V39.00 ☑
            specified type NEC (traffic) V39.49 ☑
              nontraffic V39.09 ☑
          pedal cycle (traffic) V31.5 ☑
            nontraffic V31.0 ☑
          pickup truck (traffic) V33.5 ☑
            nontraffic V33.0 ☑
          railway vehicle (traffic) V35.5 ☑
            nontraffic V35.0 ☑
          specified vehicle NEC (traffic) V36.5 ☑
            nontraffic V36.0 ☑
          stationary object (traffic) V37.5 ☑
            nontraffic V37.0 ☑
          streetcar (traffic) V36.5 ☑
            nontraffic V36.0 ☑
          three wheeled motor vehicle (traffic) V32.5 ☑
            nontraffic V32.0 ☑
          truck (traffic) V34.5 ☑
            nontraffic V34.0 ☑
          two wheeled motor vehicle (traffic) V32.5 ☑
            nontraffic V32.0 ☑
          van (traffic) V33.5 ☑
            nontraffic V33.0 ☑
        noncollision accident (traffic) V38.5 ☑
          nontraffic V38.0 ☑

Accident — *continued*
  transport — *continued*
    three-wheeled motor vehicle occupant — *continued*
      hanger-on
        collision (with)
          animal (traffic) V30.7 ☑
            being ridden (traffic) V36.7 ☑
              nontraffic V36.2 ☑
            nontraffic V30.2 ☑
          animal-drawn vehicle (traffic) V36.7 ☑
            nontraffic V36.2 ☑
          bus (traffic) V34.7 ☑
            nontraffic V34.2 ☑
          car (traffic) V33.7 ☑
            nontraffic V33.2 ☑
          pedal cycle (traffic) V31.7 ☑
            nontraffic V31.2 ☑
          pickup truck (traffic) V33.7 ☑
            nontraffic V33.2 ☑
          railway vehicle (traffic) V35.7 ☑
            nontraffic V35.2 ☑
          specified vehicle NEC (traffic) V36.7 ☑
            nontraffic V36.2 ☑
          stationary object (traffic) V37.7 ☑
            nontraffic V37.2 ☑
          streetcar (traffic) V36.7 ☑
            nontraffic V36.2 ☑
          three wheeled motor vehicle (traffic) V32.7 ☑
            nontraffic V32.2 ☑
          truck (traffic) V34.7 ☑
            nontraffic V34.2 ☑
          two wheeled motor vehicle (traffic) V32.7 ☑
            nontraffic V32.2 ☑
          van (traffic) V33.7 ☑
            nontraffic V33.2 ☑
        noncollision accident (traffic) V38.7 ☑
          nontraffic V38.2 ☑
      noncollision accident (traffic) V38.9 ☑
        nontraffic V38.3 ☑
        while boarding or alighting V38.4 ☑
      nontraffic V39.3 ☑
      passenger
        collision (with)
          animal (traffic) V30.6 ☑
            being ridden (traffic) V36.6 ☑
              nontraffic V36.1 ☑
            nontraffic V30.1 ☑
          animal-drawn vehicle (traffic) V36.6 ☑
            nontraffic V36.1 ☑
          bus (traffic) V34.6 ☑
            nontraffic V34.1 ☑
          car (traffic) V33.6 ☑
            nontraffic V33.1 ☑
          motor vehicle NOS (traffic) V39.50 ☑
            nontraffic V39.10 ☑
            specified type NEC (traffic) V39.59 ☑
              nontraffic V39.19 ☑
          pedal cycle (traffic) V31.6 ☑
            nontraffic V31.1 ☑
          pickup truck (traffic) V33.6 ☑
            nontraffic V33.1 ☑
          railway vehicle (traffic) V35.6 ☑
            nontraffic V35.1 ☑
          specified vehicle NEC (traffic) V36.6 ☑
            nontraffic V36.1 ☑
          stationary object (traffic) V37.6 ☑
            nontraffic V37.1 ☑
          streetcar (traffic) V36.6 ☑
            nontraffic V36.1 ☑
          three wheeled motor vehicle (traffic) V32.6 ☑
            nontraffic V32.1 ☑
          truck (traffic) V34.6 ☑
            nontraffic V34.1 ☑
          two wheeled motor vehicle (traffic) V32.6 ☑
            nontraffic V32.1 ☑
          van (traffic) V33.6 ☑
            nontraffic V33.1 ☑
        noncollision accident (traffic) V38.6 ☑
          nontraffic V38.1 ☑
      specified type NEC V39.89 ☑
        military vehicle V39.81 ☑

Accident — *continued*
  transport — *continued*
    tractor (farm) (and trailer) — *see* Accident, transport, agricultural vehicle occupant
    tram — *see* Accident, transport, streetcar
      in mine or quarry — *see* Accident, transport, industrial vehicle occupant
    trolley — *see* Accident, transport, streetcar
      in mine or quarry — *see* Accident, transport, industrial vehicle occupant
    truck (heavy) occupant V69.9 ☑
      collision (with)
        animal (traffic) V60.9 ☑
          being ridden (traffic) V66.9 ☑
            nontraffic V66.3 ☑
            while boarding or alighting V66.4 ☑
          nontraffic V60.3 ☑
          while boarding or alighting V60.4 ☑
        animal-drawn vehicle (traffic) V66.9 ☑
          nontraffic V66.3 ☑
          while boarding or alighting V66.4 ☑
        bus (traffic) V64.9 ☑
          nontraffic V64.3 ☑
          while boarding or alighting V64.4 ☑
        car (traffic) V63.9 ☑
          nontraffic V63.3 ☑
          while boarding or alighting V63.4 ☑
        motor vehicle NOS (traffic) V69.60 ☑
          nontraffic V69.20 ☑
          specified type NEC (traffic) V69.69 ☑
            nontraffic V69.29 ☑
        pedal cycle (traffic) V61.9 ☑
          nontraffic V61.3 ☑
          while boarding or alighting V61.4 ☑
        pickup truck (traffic) V63.9 ☑
          nontraffic V63.3 ☑
          while boarding or alighting V63.4 ☑
        railway vehicle (traffic) V65.9 ☑
          nontraffic V65.3 ☑
          while boarding or alighting V65.4 ☑
        specified vehicle NEC (traffic) V66.9 ☑
          nontraffic V66.3 ☑
          while boarding or alighting V66.4 ☑
        stationary object (traffic) V67.9 ☑
          nontraffic V67.3 ☑
          while boarding or alighting V67.4 ☑
        streetcar (traffic) V66.9 ☑
          nontraffic V66.3 ☑
          while boarding or alighting V66.4 ☑
        three wheeled motor vehicle (traffic) V62.9 ☑
          nontraffic V62.3 ☑
          while boarding or alighting V62.4 ☑
        truck (traffic) V64.9 ☑
          nontraffic V64.3 ☑
          while boarding or alighting V64.4 ☑
        two wheeled motor vehicle (traffic) V62.9 ☑
          nontraffic V62.3 ☑
          while boarding or alighting V62.4 ☑
        van (traffic) V63.9 ☑
          nontraffic V63.3 ☑
          while boarding or alighting V63.4 ☑
      driver
        collision (with)
          animal (traffic) V60.5 ☑
            being ridden (traffic) V66.5 ☑
              nontraffic V66.0 ☑
            nontraffic V60.0 ☑
          animal-drawn vehicle (traffic) V66.5 ☑
            nontraffic V66.0 ☑
          bus (traffic) V64.5 ☑
            nontraffic V64.0 ☑
          car (traffic) V63.5 ☑
            nontraffic V63.0 ☑
          motor vehicle NOS (traffic) V69.40 ☑
            nontraffic V69.00 ☑
            specified type NEC (traffic) V69.49 ☑
              nontraffic V69.09 ☑
          pedal cycle (traffic) V61.5 ☑
            nontraffic V61.0 ☑
          pickup truck (traffic) V63.5 ☑
            nontraffic V63.0 ☑
          railway vehicle (traffic) V65.5 ☑
            nontraffic V65.0 ☑
          specified vehicle NEC (traffic) V66.5 ☑
            nontraffic V66.0 ☑

Accident — *continued*
- transport — *continued*
  - truck occupant — *continued*
    - driver — *continued*
      - collision — *continued*
        - stationary object (traffic) V67.5 ☑
          - nontraffic V67.0 ☑
        - streetcar (traffic) V66.5 ☑
          - nontraffic V66.0 ☑
        - three wheeled motor vehicle (traffic) V62.5 ☑
          - nontraffic V62.0 ☑
        - truck (traffic) V64.5 ☑
          - nontraffic V64.0 ☑
        - two wheeled motor vehicle (traffic) V62.5 ☑
          - nontraffic V62.0 ☑
        - van (traffic) V63.5 ☑
          - nontraffic V63.0 ☑
      - noncollision accident (traffic) V68.5 ☑
        - nontraffic V68.0 ☑
    - dump — *see* Accident, transport, construction vehicle occupant
    - hanger-on
      - collision (with)
        - animal (traffic) V60.7 ☑
          - being ridden (traffic) V66.7 ☑
            - nontraffic V66.2 ☑
          - nontraffic V60.2 ☑
        - animal-drawn vehicle (traffic) V66.7 ☑
          - nontraffic V66.2 ☑
        - bus (traffic) V64.7 ☑
          - nontraffic V64.2 ☑
        - car (traffic) V63.7 ☑
          - nontraffic V63.2 ☑
        - pedal cycle (traffic) V61.7 ☑
          - nontraffic V61.2 ☑
        - pickup truck (traffic) V63.7 ☑
          - nontraffic V63.2 ☑
        - railway vehicle (traffic) V65.7 ☑
          - nontraffic V65.2 ☑
        - specified vehicle NEC (traffic) V66.7 ☑
          - nontraffic V66.2 ☑
        - stationary object (traffic) V67.7 ☑
          - nontraffic V67.2 ☑
        - streetcar (traffic) V66.7 ☑
          - nontraffic V66.2 ☑
        - three wheeled motor vehicle (traffic) V62.7 ☑
          - nontraffic V62.2 ☑
        - truck (traffic) V64.7 ☑
          - nontraffic V64.2 ☑
        - two wheeled motor vehicle (traffic) V62.7 ☑
          - nontraffic V62.2 ☑
        - van (traffic) V63.7 ☑
          - nontraffic V63.2 ☑
      - noncollision accident (traffic) V68.7 ☑
        - nontraffic V68.2 ☑
    - noncollision accident (traffic) V68.9 ☑
      - nontraffic V68.3 ☑
      - while boarding or alighting V68.4 ☑
    - nontraffic V69.3 ☑
    - passenger
      - collision (with)
        - animal (traffic) V60.6 ☑
          - being ridden (traffic) V66.6 ☑
            - nontraffic V66.1- ☑
          - nontraffic V60.1 ☑
        - animal-drawn vehicle (traffic) V66.6 ☑
          - nontraffic V66.1 ☑
        - bus (traffic) V64.6 ☑
          - nontraffic V64.1 ☑
        - car (traffic) V63.6 ☑
          - nontraffic V63.1 ☑
        - motor vehicle NOS (traffic) V69.50 ☑
          - nontraffic V69.10 ☑
          - specified type NEC (traffic) V69.59 ☑
            - nontraffic V69.19 ☑
        - pedal cycle (traffic) V61.6 ☑
          - nontraffic V61.1 ☑
        - pickup truck (traffic) V63.6 ☑
          - nontraffic V63.1 ☑
        - railway vehicle (traffic) V65.6 ☑
          - nontraffic V65.1 ☑
        - specified vehicle NEC (traffic) V66.6 ☑

Accident — *continued*
- transport — *continued*
  - truck occupant — *continued*
    - passenger — *continued*
      - collision — *continued*
        - specified vehicle — *continued*
          - nontraffic V66.1 ☑
        - stationary object (traffic) V67.6 ☑
          - nontraffic V67.1 ☑
        - streetcar (traffic) V66.6 ☑
          - nontraffic V66.1 ☑
        - three wheeled motor vehicle (traffic) V62.6 ☑
          - nontraffic V62.1 ☑
        - truck (traffic) V64.6 ☑
          - nontraffic V64.1 ☑
        - two wheeled motor vehicle (traffic) V62.6 ☑
          - nontraffic V62.1 ☑
        - van (traffic) V63.6 ☑
          - nontraffic V63.1 ☑
      - noncollision accident (traffic) V68.6 ☑
        - nontraffic V68.1 ☑
    - pickup — *see* Accident, transport, pickup truck occupant
    - specified type NEC V69.88 ☑
    - military vehicle V69.81 ☑
  - van occupant V59.9 ☑
    - collision (with)
      - animal (traffic) V50.9 ☑
        - being ridden (traffic) V56.9 ☑
          - nontraffic V56.3 ☑
          - while boarding or alighting V56.4 ☑
        - nontraffic V50.3 ☑
        - while boarding or alighting V50.4 ☑
      - animal-drawn vehicle (traffic) V56.9 ☑
        - nontraffic V56.3 ☑
        - while boarding or alighting V56.4 ☑
      - bus (traffic) V54.9 ☑
        - nontraffic V54.3 ☑
        - while boarding or alighting V54.4 ☑
      - car (traffic) V53.9 ☑
        - nontraffic V53.3 ☑
        - while boarding or alighting V53.4 ☑
      - motor vehicle NOS (traffic) V59.60 ☑
        - nontraffic V59.20 ☑
        - specified type NEC (traffic) V59.69 ☑
          - nontraffic V59.29 ☑
      - pedal cycle (traffic) V51.9 ☑
        - nontraffic V51.3 ☑
        - while boarding or alighting V51.4 ☑
      - pickup truck (traffic) V53.9 ☑
        - nontraffic V53.3 ☑
        - while boarding or alighting V53.4 ☑
      - railway vehicle (traffic) V55.9 ☑
        - nontraffic V55.3 ☑
        - while boarding or alighting V55.4 ☑
      - specified vehicle NEC (traffic) V56.9 ☑
        - nontraffic V56.3 ☑
        - while boarding or alighting V56.4 ☑
      - stationary object (traffic) V57.9 ☑
        - nontraffic V57.3 ☑
        - while boarding or alighting V57.4 ☑
      - streetcar (traffic) V56.9 ☑
        - nontraffic V56.3 ☑
        - while boarding or alighting V56.4 ☑
      - three wheeled motor vehicle (traffic) V52.9 ☑
        - nontraffic V52.3 ☑
        - while boarding or alighting V52.4 ☑
      - truck (traffic) V54.9 ☑
        - nontraffic V54.3 ☑
        - while boarding or alighting V54.4 ☑
      - two wheeled motor vehicle (traffic) V52.9 ☑
        - nontraffic V52.3 ☑
        - while boarding or alighting V52.4 ☑
      - van (traffic) V53.9 ☑
        - nontraffic V53.3 ☑
        - while boarding or alighting V53.4 ☑
    - driver
      - collision (with)
        - animal (traffic) V50.5 ☑
          - being ridden (traffic) V56.5 ☑
            - nontraffic V56.0 ☑
          - nontraffic V50.0 ☑
        - animal-drawn vehicle (traffic) V56.5 ☑

Accident — *continued*
- transport — *continued*
  - van occupant — *continued*
    - driver — *continued*
      - collision — *continued*
        - animal-drawn vehicle — *continued*
          - nontraffic V56.0 ☑
        - bus (traffic) V54.5 ☑
          - nontraffic V54.0 ☑
        - car (traffic) V53.5 ☑
          - nontraffic V53.0 ☑
        - motor vehicle NOS (traffic) V59.40 ☑
          - nontraffic V59.00 ☑
          - specified type NEC (traffic) V59.49 ☑
            - nontraffic V59.09 ☑
        - pedal cycle (traffic) V51.5 ☑
          - nontraffic V51.0 ☑
        - pickup truck (traffic) V53.5 ☑
          - nontraffic V53.0 ☑
        - railway vehicle (traffic) V55.5 ☑
          - nontraffic V55.0 ☑
        - specified vehicle NEC (traffic) V56.5 ☑
          - nontraffic V56.0 ☑
        - stationary object (traffic) V57.5 ☑
          - nontraffic V57.0 ☑
        - streetcar (traffic) V56.5 ☑
          - nontraffic V56.0 ☑
        - three wheeled motor vehicle (traffic) V52.5 ☑
          - nontraffic V52.0 ☑
        - truck (traffic) V54.5 ☑
          - nontraffic V54.0 ☑
        - two wheeled motor vehicle (traffic) V52.5 ☑
          - nontraffic V52.0 ☑
        - van (traffic) V53.5 ☑
          - nontraffic V53.0 ☑
      - noncollision accident (traffic) V58.5 ☑
        - nontraffic V58.0 ☑
    - hanger-on
      - collision (with)
        - animal (traffic) V50.7 ☑
          - being ridden (traffic) V56.7 ☑
            - nontraffic V56.2 ☑
          - nontraffic V50.2 ☑
        - animal-drawn vehicle (traffic) V56.7 ☑
          - nontraffic V56.2 ☑
        - bus (traffic) V54.7 ☑
          - nontraffic V54.2 ☑
        - car (traffic) V53.7 ☑
          - nontraffic V53.2 ☑
        - pedal cycle (traffic) V51.7 ☑
          - nontraffic V51.2 ☑
        - pickup truck (traffic) V53.7 ☑
          - nontraffic V53.2 ☑
        - railway vehicle (traffic) V55.7 ☑
          - nontraffic V55.2 ☑
        - specified vehicle NEC (traffic) V56.7 ☑
          - nontraffic V56.2 ☑
        - stationary object (traffic) V57.7 ☑
          - nontraffic V57.2 ☑
        - streetcar (traffic) V56.7 ☑
          - nontraffic V56.2 ☑
        - three wheeled motor vehicle (traffic) V52.7 ☑
          - nontraffic V52.2 ☑
        - truck (traffic) V54.7 ☑
          - nontraffic V54.2 ☑
        - two wheeled motor vehicle (traffic) V52.7 ☑
          - nontraffic V52.2 ☑
        - van (traffic) V53.7 ☑
          - nontraffic V53.2 ☑
      - noncollision accident (traffic) V58.7 ☑
        - nontraffic V58.2 ☑
    - noncollision accident (traffic) V58.9 ☑
      - nontraffic V58.3 ☑
      - while boarding or alighting V58.4 ☑
    - nontraffic V59.3 ☑
    - passenger
      - collision (with)
        - animal (traffic) V50.6 ☑
          - being ridden (traffic) V56.6 ☑
            - nontraffic V56.1 ☑
          - nontraffic V50.1 ☑
        - animal-drawn vehicle (traffic) V56.6 ☑

Accident — *continued*
 transport — *continued*
  van occupant — *continued*
   passenger — *continued*
    collision — *continued*
     animal-drawn vehicle — *continued*
      nontraffic V56.1 ☑
     bus (traffic) V54.6 ☑
      nontraffic V54.1 ☑
     car (traffic) V53.6 ☑
      nontraffic V53.1 ☑
     motor vehicle NOS (traffic) V59.50 ☑
      nontraffic V59.10 ☑
      specified type NEC (traffic) V59.59 ☑
       nontraffic V59.19 ☑
     pedal cycle (traffic) V51.6 ☑
      nontraffic V51.1 ☑
     pickup truck (traffic) V53.6 ☑
      nontraffic V53.1 ☑
     railway vehicle (traffic) V55.6 ☑
      nontraffic V55.1 ☑
     specified vehicle NEC (traffic) V56.6 ☑
      nontraffic V56.1 ☑
     stationary object (traffic) V57.6 ☑
      nontraffic V57.1 ☑
     streetcar (traffic) V56.6 ☑
      nontraffic V56.1 ☑
     three wheeled motor vehicle (traffic) V52.6 ☑
      nontraffic V52.1 ☑
     truck (traffic) V54.6 ☑
      nontraffic V54.1 ☑
     two wheeled motor vehicle (traffic) V52.6 ☑
      nontraffic V52.1 ☑
     van (traffic) V53.6 ☑
      nontraffic V53.1 ☑
    noncollision accident (traffic) V58.6 ☑
     nontraffic V58.1 ☑
    specified type NEC V59.88 ☑
     military vehicle V59.81 ☑
  watercraft occupant — *see* Accident, watercraft
 vehicle NEC V89.9 ☑
  animal-drawn NEC — *see* Accident, transport, animal-drawn vehicle occupant
  special
   agricultural — *see* Accident, transport, agricultural vehicle occupant
   construction — *see* Accident, transport, construction vehicle occupant
   industrial — *see* Accident, transport, industrial vehicle occupant
   three-wheeled NEC (motorized) — *see* Accident, transport, three-wheeled motor vehicle occupant
 watercraft V94.9 ☑
  causing
   drowning B — *see* Drowning, due to, accident to, watercraft
   injury NEC V91.89 ☑
    crushed between craft and object V91.19 ☑
     powered craft V91.13 ☑
      ferry boat V91.11 ☑
      fishing boat V91.12 ☑
      jetskis V91.13 ☑
      liner V91.11 ☑
      merchant ship V91.10 ☑
      passenger ship V91.11 ☑
     unpowered craft V91.18 ☑
      canoe V91.15 ☑
      inflatable V91.16 ☑
      kayak V91.15 ☑
      sailboat V91.14 ☑
      surf-board V91.18 ☑
      windsurfer V91.18 ☑
    fall on board V91.29 ☑
     powered craft V91.23 ☑
      ferry boat V91.21 ☑
      fishing boat V91.22 ☑
      jetskis V91.23 ☑
      liner V91.21 ☑
      merchant ship V91.20 ☑
      passenger ship V91.21 ☑
     unpowered craft
      canoe V91.25 ☑
      inflatable V91.26 ☑

Accident — *continued*
 watercraft — *continued*
  causing — *continued*
   injury — *continued*
    fall on board — *continued*
     unpowered craft — *continued*
      kayak V91.25 ☑
      sailboat V91.24 ☑
    fire on board causing burn V91.09 ☑
     powered craft V91.03 ☑
      ferry boat V91.01 ☑
      fishing boat V91.02 ☑
      jetskis V91.03 ☑
      liner V91.01 ☑
      merchant ship V91.00 ☑
      passenger ship V91.01 ☑
     unpowered craft V91.08 ☑
      canoe V91.05 ☑
      inflatable V91.06 ☑
      kayak V91.05 ☑
      sailboat V91.04 ☑
      surf-board V91.08 ☑
      water skis V91.07 ☑
      windsurfer V91.08 ☑
    hit by falling object V91.39 ☑
     powered craft V91.33 ☑
      ferry boat V91.31 ☑
      fishing boat V91.32 ☑
      jetskis V91.33 ☑
      liner V91.31 ☑
      merchant ship V91.30 ☑
      passenger ship V91.31 ☑
     unpowered craft V91.38 ☑
      canoe V91.35 ☑
      inflatable V91.36 ☑
      kayak V91.35 ☑
      sailboat V91.34 ☑
      surf-board V91.38 ☑
      water skis V91.37 ☑
      windsurfer V91.38 ☑
    specified type NEC V91.89 ☑
     powered craft V91.83 ☑
      ferry boat V91.81 ☑
      fishing boat V91.82 ☑
      jetskis V91.83 ☑
      liner V91.81 ☑
      merchant ship V91.80 ☑
      passenger ship V91.81 ☑
     unpowered craft V91.88 ☑
      canoe V91.85 ☑
      inflatable V91.86 ☑
      kayak V91.85 ☑
      sailboat V91.84 ☑
      surf-board V91.88 ☑
      water skis V91.87 ☑
      windsurfer V91.88 ☑
   due to, caused by cataclysm — *see* Forces of nature, by type
   military NEC V94.818 ☑
    with civilian watercraft V94.810 ☑
    civilian in water injured by V94.811 ☑
   nonpowered, struck by
    nonpowered vessel V94.22 ☑
    powered vessel V94.21 ☑
   specified type NEC V94.89 ☑
   striking swimmer
    powered V94.11 ☑
    unpowered V94.12 ☑

Acid throwing (assault) Y08.89 ☑

Activity (involving) (of victim at time of event) Y93.9
 aerobic and step exercise (class) Y93.A3 (*following* Y93.7)
 alpine skiing Y93.23
 animal care NEC Y93.K9 (*following* Y93.7)
 arts and handcrafts NEC Y93.D9 (*following* Y93.7)
 athletics played as a team or group NEC Y93.69
 athletics played individually NEC Y93.59
 athletics NEC Y93.79
 baking Y93.G3 (*following* Y93.7)
 ballet Y93.41
 barbells Y93.B3 (*following* Y93.7)
 BASE (Building, Antenna, Span, Earth) jumping Y93.33
 baseball Y93.64
 basketball Y93.67
 bathing (personal) Y93.E1 (*following* Y93.7)
 beach volleyball Y93.68

Activity — *continued*
 bike riding Y93.55
 boogie boarding Y93.18
 bowling Y93.54
 boxing Y93.71
 brass instrument playing Y93.J4 (*following* Y93.7)
 building construction Y93.H3 (*following* Y93.7)
 bungee jumping Y93.34
 calisthenics Y93.A2 (*following* Y93.7)
 canoeing (in calm and turbulent water) Y93.16
 capture the flag Y93.6A
 cardiorespiratory exercise NEC Y93.A9 (*following* Y93.7)
 caregiving (providing) NEC Y93.F9 (*following* Y93.7)
  bathing Y93.F1 (*following* Y93.7)
  lifting Y93.F2 (*following* Y93.7)
 cellular
  communication device Y93.C2 (*following* Y93.7)
  telephone Y93.C2 (*following* Y93.7)
 challenge course Y93.A5 (*following* Y93.7)
 cheerleading Y93.45
 circuit training Y93.A4 (*following* Y93.7)
 cleaning
  floor Y93.E5 (*following* Y93.7)
 climbing NEC Y93.39
  mountain Y93.31
  rock Y93.31
  wall Y93.31
 clothing care and maintenance NEC Y93.E9 (*following* Y93.7)
 combatives Y93.75
 computer
  keyboarding Y93.C1 (*following* Y93.7)
  technology NEC Y93.C9 (*following* Y93.7)
 confidence course Y93.A5 (*following* Y93.7)
 construction (building) Y93.H3 (*following* Y93.7)
 cooking and baking Y93.G3 (*following* Y93.7)
 cool down exercises Y93.A2 (*following* Y93.7)
 cricket Y93.69
 crocheting Y93.D1 (*following* Y93.7)
 cross country skiing Y93.24
 dancing (all types) Y93.41
 digging
  dirt Y93.H1 (*following* Y93.7)
 dirt digging Y93.H1 (*following* Y93.7)
 dishwashing Y93.G1 (*following* Y93.7)
 diving (platform) (springboard) Y93.12
  underwater Y93.15
 dodge ball Y93.6A
 downhill skiing Y93.23
 drum playing Y93.J2 (*following* Y93.7)
 dumbbells Y93.B3 (*following* Y93.7)
 electronic
  devices NEC Y93.C9 (*following* Y93.7)
   hand held interactive Y93.C2 (*following* Y93.7)
  game playing (using) (with)
   interactive device Y93.C2 (*following* Y93.7)
   keyboard or other stationary device Y93.C1 (*following* Y93.7)
 elliptical machine Y93.A1 (*following* Y93.7)
 exercise(s)
  machines ((primarily) for)
   cardiorespiratory conditioning Y93.A1 (*following* Y93.7)
   muscle strengthening Y93.B1 (*following* Y93.7)
  muscle strengthening (non-machine) NEC Y93.B9 (*following* Y93.7)
 external motion NEC Y93.I9 (*following* Y93.7)
  rollercoaster Y93.I1 (*following* Y93.7)
 field hockey Y93.65
 figure skating (pairs) (singles) Y93.21
 flag football Y93.62
 floor mopping and cleaning Y93.E5 (*following* Y93.7)
 food preparation and clean up Y93.G1 (*following* Y93.7)
 football (American) NOS Y93.61
  flag Y93.62
  tackle Y93.61
  touch Y93.62
 four square Y93.6A
 free weights Y93.B3 (*following* Y93.7)
 frisbee (ultimate) Y93.74
 furniture
  building Y93.D3 (*following* Y93.7)
  finishing Y93.D3 (*following* Y93.7)
  repair Y93.D3 (*following* Y93.7)
 game playing (electronic)
  using interactive device Y93.C2 (*following* Y93.7)
  using keyboard or other stationary device Y93.C1 (*following* Y93.7)

Activity — *continued*
  gardening Y93.H2 (*following* Y93.7)
  golf Y93.53
  grass drills Y93.A6 (*following* Y93.7)
  grilling and smoking food Y93.G2 (*following* Y93.7)
  grooming and shearing an animal Y93.K3 (*following* Y93.7)
  guerilla drills Y93.A6 (*following* Y93.7)
  gymnastics (rhythmic) Y93.43
  hand held interactive electronic device Y93.C2 (*following* Y93.7)
  handball Y93.73
  handcrafts NEC Y93.D9 (*following* Y93.7)
  hang gliding Y93.35
  hiking (on level or elevated terrain) Y93.Ø1
  hockey (ice) Y93.22
    field Y93.65
  horseback riding Y93.52
  household (interior) maintenance NEC Y93.E9 (*following* Y93.7)
  ice NEC Y93.29
    dancing Y93.21
    hockey Y93.22
    skating Y93.21
  inline roller skating Y93.51
  ironing Y93.E4 (*following* Y93.7)
  judo Y93.75
  jumping jacks Y93.A2 (*following* Y93.7)
  jumping rope Y93.56
  jumping (off) NEC Y93.39
    BASE (Building, Antenna, Span, Earth) Y93.33
    bungee Y93.34
    jacks Y93.A2 (*following* Y93.7)
    rope Y93.56
  karate Y93.75
  kayaking (in calm and turbulent water) Y93.16
  keyboarding (computer) Y93.C1 (*following* Y93.7)
  kickball Y93.6A
  knitting Y93.D1 (*following* Y93.7)
  lacrosse Y93.65
  land maintenance NEC Y93.H9 (*following* Y93.7)
  landscaping Y93.H2 (*following* Y93.7)
  laundry Y93.E2 (*following* Y93.7)
  machines (exercise)
    primarily for cardiorespiratory conditioning Y93.A1 (*following* Y93.7)
    primarily for muscle strengthening Y93.B1 (*following* Y93.7)
  maintenance
    exterior building NEC Y93.H9 (*following* Y93.7)
    household (interior) NEC Y93.E9 (*following* Y93.7)
    land Y93.H9 (*following* Y93.7)
    property Y93.H9 (*following* Y93.7)
  marching (on level or elevated terrain) Y93.Ø1
  martial arts Y93.75
  microwave oven Y93.G3 (*following* Y93.7)
  milking an animal Y93.K2 (*following* Y93.7)
  mopping (floor) Y93.E5 (*following* Y93.7)
  mountain climbing Y93.31
  muscle strengthening
    exercises (non-machine) NEC Y93.B9 (*following* Y93.7)
    machines Y93.B1 (*following* Y93.7)
  musical keyboard (electronic) playing Y93.J1 (*following* Y93.7)
  nordic skiing Y93.24
  obstacle course Y93.A5 (*following* Y93.7)
  oven (microwave) Y93.G3 (*following* Y93.7)
  packing up and unpacking in moving to a new residence Y93.E6 (*following* Y93.7)
  parasailing Y93.19
  percussion instrument playing NEC Y93.J2 (*following* Y93.7)
  personal
    bathing and showering Y93.E1 (*following* Y93.7)
    hygiene NEC Y93.E8 (*following* Y93.7)
    showering Y93.E1 (*following* Y93.7)
  physical games generally associated with school recess, summer camp and children Y93.6A
  physical training NEC Y93.A9 (*following* Y93.7)
  piano playing Y93.J1 (*following* Y93.7)
  pilates Y93.B4 (*following* Y93.7)
  platform diving Y93.12
  playing musical instrument
    brass instrument Y93.J4 (*following* Y93.7)
    drum Y93.J2 (*following* Y93.7)
    musical keyboard (electronic) Y93.J1 (*following* Y93.7)

Activity — *continued*
  playing musical instrument — *continued*
    percussion instrument NEC Y93.J2 (*following* Y93.7)
    piano Y93.J1 (*following* Y93.7)
    string instrument Y93.J3 (*following* Y93.7)
    winds instrument Y93.J4 (*following* Y93.7)
  property maintenance
    exterior NEC Y93.H9 (*following* Y93.7)
    interior NEC Y93.E9 (*following* Y93.7)
  pruning (garden and lawn) Y93.H2 (*following* Y93.7)
  pull-ups Y93.B2 (*following* Y93.7)
  push-ups Y93.B2 (*following* Y93.7)
  racquetball Y93.73
  rafting (in calm and turbulent water) Y93.16
  raking (leaves) Y93.H1 (*following* Y93.7)
  rappelling Y93.32
  refereeing a sports activity Y93.81
  residential relocation Y93.E6 (*following* Y93.7)
  rhythmic gymnastics Y93.43
  rhythmic movement NEC Y93.49
  riding
    horseback Y93.52
    rollercoaster Y93.I1 (*following* Y93.7)
  rock climbing Y93.31
  roller skating (inline) Y93.51
  rollercoaster riding Y93.I1 (*following* Y93.7)
  rough housing and horseplay Y93.83
  rowing (in calm and turbulent water) Y93.16
  rugby Y93.63
  running Y93.02
  SCUBA diving Y93.15
  sewing Y93.D2 (*following* Y93.7)
  shoveling Y93.H1 (*following* Y93.7)
    dirt Y93.H1 (*following* Y93.7)
    snow Y93.H1 (*following* Y93.7)
  showering (personal) Y93.E1 (*following* Y93.7)
  sit-ups Y93.B2 (*following* Y93.7)
  skateboarding Y93.51
  skating (ice) Y93.21
    roller Y93.51
  skiing (alpine) (downhill) Y93.23
    cross country Y93.24
    nordic Y93.24
    water Y93.17
  sledding (snow) Y93.23
  sleeping (sleep) Y93.84
  smoking and grilling food Y93.G2 (*following* Y93.7)
  snorkeling Y93.15
  snow NEC Y93.29
    boarding Y93.23
    shoveling Y93.H1 (*following* Y93.7)
    sledding Y93.23
    tubing Y93.23
  soccer Y93.66
  softball Y93.64
  specified NEC Y93.89
  spectator at an event Y93.82
  sports NEC Y93.79
    sports played as a team or group NEC Y93.69
    sports played individually NEC Y93.59
  springboard diving Y93.12
  squash Y93.73
  stationary bike Y93.A1 (*following* Y93.7)
  step (stepping) exercise (class) Y93.A3 (*following* Y93.7)
  stepper machine Y93.A1 (*following* Y93.7)
  stove Y93.G3 (*following* Y93.7)
  string instrument playing Y93.J3 (*following* Y93.7)
  surfing Y93.18
    wind Y93.18
  swimming Y93.11
  tackle football Y93.61
  tap dancing Y93.41
  tennis Y93.73
  tobogganing Y93.23
  touch football Y93.62
  track and field events (non-running) Y93.57
    running Y93.02
  trampoline Y93.44
  treadmill Y93.A1 (*following* Y93.7)
  trimming shrubs Y93.H2 (*following* Y93.7)
  tubing (in calm and turbulent water) Y93.16
    snow Y93.23
  ultimate frisbee Y93.74
  underwater diving Y93.15
  unpacking in moving to a new residence Y93.E6 (*following* Y93.7)
  use of stove, oven and microwave oven Y93.G3 (*following* Y93.7)

Activity — *continued*
  vacuuming Y93.E3 (*following* Y93.7)
  volleyball (beach) (court) Y93.68
  wake boarding Y93.17
  walking (on level or elevated terrain) Y93.Ø1
    an animal Y93.K1 (*following* Y93.7)
  walking an animal Y93.K1 (*following* Y93.7)
  wall climbing Y93.31
  warm up and cool down exercises Y93.A2 (*following* Y93.7)
  water NEC Y93.19
    aerobics Y93.14
    craft NEC Y93.19
    exercise Y93.14
    polo Y93.13
    skiing Y93.17
    sliding Y93.18
    survival training and testing Y93.19
  weeding (garden and lawn) Y93.H2 (*following* Y93.7)
  wind instrument playing Y93.J4 (*following* Y93.7)
  windsurfing Y93.18
  wrestling Y93.72
  yoga Y93.42
Adverse effect of drugs — *see* Table of Drugs and Chemicals
Aerosinusitis — *see* Air, pressure
After-effect, late — *see* Sequelae
Air
  blast in war operations — *see* War operations, air blast
  pressure
    change, rapid
      during
        ascent W94.29 ☑
          while (in) (surfacing from)
            aircraft W94.23 ☑
            deep water diving W94.21 ☑
            underground W94.22 ☑
        descent W94.39 ☑
          in
            aircraft W94.31 ☑
            water W94.32 ☑
    high, prolonged W94.Ø ☑
    low, prolonged W94.12 ☑
      due to residence or long visit at high altitude W94.11 ☑
Alpine sickness W94.11 ☑
Altitude sickness W94.11 ☑
Anaphylactic shock, anaphylaxis — *see* Table of Drugs and Chemicals
Andes disease W94.11 ☑
Arachnidism, arachnoidism X58 ☑
Arson (with intent to injure or kill) X97 ☑
Asphyxia, asphyxiation
  by
    food (bone) (seed) — *see* categories T17 and T18 ☑
    gas (*see also* Table of Drugs and Chemicals)
      legal
        execution — *see* Legal, intervention, gas
        intervention — *see* Legal, intervention, gas
  from
    fire (*see also* Exposure, fire)
      in war operations — *see* War operations, fire
      ignition — *see* Ignition
    vomitus T17.81 ☑
  in war operations — *see* War operations, restriction of airway
Aspiration
  food (any type) (into respiratory tract) (with asphyxia, obstruction respiratory tract, suffocation) — *see* categories T17 and T18 ☑
  foreign body — *see* Foreign body, aspiration
  vomitus (with asphyxia, obstruction respiratory tract, suffocation) T17.81 ☑
Assassination (attempt) — *see* Assault
Assault (homicidal) (by) (in) YØ9
  arson X97 ☑
  bite (of human being) YØ4.1 ☑
  bodily force YØ4.8 ☑
    bite YØ4.1 ☑
    bumping into YØ4.2 ☑
    sexual — *see* subcategories T74.Ø, T76.Ø ☑
    unarmed fight YØ4.Ø ☑
  bomb X96.9 ☑
    antipersonnel X96.Ø ☑
    fertilizer X96.3 ☑
    gasoline X96.1 ☑

Assault — continued
  bomb — continued
    letter X96.2 ☑
    petrol X96.1 ☑
    pipe X96.3 ☑
    specified NEC X96.8 ☑
  brawl (hand) (fists) (foot) (unarmed) Y04.0 ☑
  burning, burns (by fire) NEC X97 ☑
    acid Y08.89 ☑
    caustic, corrosive substance Y08.89 ☑
    chemical from swallowing caustic, corrosive sub-
        stance — see Table of Drugs and Chemicals
    cigarette(s) X97 ☑
    hot object X98.9 ☑
      fluid NEC X98.2 ☑
      household appliance X98.3 ☑
      specified NEC X98.8 ☑
      steam X98.0 ☑
      tap water X98.1 ☑
      vapors X98.0 ☑
    scalding — see Assault, burning
    steam X98.0 ☑
    vitriol Y08.89 ☑
  caustic, corrosive substance (gas) Y08.89 ☑
  crashing of
    aircraft Y08.81 ☑
    motor vehicle Y03.8 ☑
      pushed in front of Y02.0 ☑
      run over Y03.0 ☑
      specified NEC Y03.8 ☑
  cutting or piercing instrument X99.9 ☑
    dagger X99.2 ☑
    glass X99.0 ☑
    knife X99.1 ☑
    specified NEC X99.8 ☑
    sword X99.2 ☑
  dagger X99.2 ☑
  drowning (in) X92.9 ☑
    bathtub X92.0 ☑
    natural water X92.3 ☑
    specified NEC X92.8 ☑
    swimming pool X92.1 ☑
      following fall X92.2 ☑
  dynamite X96.8 ☑
  explosive(s) (material) X96.9 ☑
  fight (hand) (fists) (foot) (unarmed) Y04.0 ☑
    with weapon — see Assault, by type of weapon
  fire X97 ☑
  firearm X95.9 ☑
    airgun X95.01 ☑
    handgun X93 ☑
    hunting rifle X94.1 ☑
    larger X94.9 ☑
      specified NEC X94.8 ☑
    machine gun X94.2 ☑
    shotgun X94.0 ☑
    specified NEC X95.8 ☑
  from high place Y01 ☑
  gunshot (wound) NEC — see Assault, firearm, by type
  incendiary device X97 ☑
  injury Y09
    to child due to criminal abortion attempt NEC
        Y08.89 ☑
  knife X99.1 ☑
  late effect of — see categories X92-Y08 with 7th
      character S
  placing before moving object NEC Y02.8 ☑
    motor vehicle Y02.0 ☑
  poisoning — see categories T36-T65 with 7th character
      S
  puncture, any part of body — see Assault, cutting or
      piercing instrument
  pushing
    before moving object NEC Y02.8 ☑
      motor vehicle Y02.0 ☑
      subway train Y02.1 ☑
      train Y02.1 ☑
    from high place Y01 ☑
  rape T74.2- ☑
  scalding — see Assault, burning
  sequelae of — see categories X92-Y08 with 7th char-
      acter S
  sexual (by bodily force) T74.2- ☑
  shooting — see Assault, firearm
  specified means NEC Y08.89 ☑

Assault — continued
  stab, any part of body — see Assault, cutting or pierc-
      ing instrument
  steam X98.0 ☑
  striking against
    other person Y04.2 ☑
    sports equipment Y08.09 ☑
      baseball bat Y08.02 ☑
      hockey stick Y08.01 ☑
  struck by
    sports equipment Y08.09 ☑
      baseball bat Y08.02 ☑
      hockey stick Y08.01 ☑
  submersion — see Assault, drowning
  violence Y09
  weapon Y09
    blunt Y00 ☑
    cutting or piercing — see Assault, cutting or
        piercing instrument
    firearm — see Assault, firearm
  wound Y09
    cutting — see Assault, cutting or piercing instru-
        ment
    gunshot — see Assault, firearm
    knife X99.1 ☑
    piercing — see Assault, cutting or piercing instru-
        ment
    puncture — see Assault, cutting or piercing instru-
        ment
    stab — see Assault, cutting or piercing instrument
Attack by mammals NEC W55.89 ☑
Avalanche — see Landslide
Aviator's disease — see Air, pressure

B

Barotitis, barodontalgia, barosinusitis, barotrauma
    (otitic) (sinus) — see Air, pressure
Battered (baby) (child) (person) (syndrome) X58 ☑
Bayonet wound W26.1 ☑
    in
      legal intervention — see Legal, intervention, sharp
          object, bayonet
      war operations — see War operations, combat
    stated as undetermined whether accidental or inten-
        tional Y28.8 ☑
    suicide (attempt) X78.2 ☑
Bean in nose — see categories T17 and T18
Bed set on fire NEC — see Exposure, fire, uncontrolled,
    building, bed
Beheading (by guillotine)
    homicide X99.9 ☑
    legal execution — see Legal, intervention
Bending, injury in — see Overexertion
Bends — see Air, pressure, change
Bite, bitten by
    alligator W58.01 ☑
    arthropod (nonvenomous) NEC W57 ☑
    bull W55.21 ☑
    cat W55.01 ☑
    cow W55.21 ☑
    crocodile W58.11 ☑
    dog W54.0 ☑
    goat W55.31 ☑
    hoof stock NEC W55.31 ☑
    horse W55.11 ☑
    human being (accidentally) W50.3 ☑
      with intent to injure or kill Y04.1 ☑
      as, or caused by, a crowd or human stampede (with
          fall) W52 ☑
      assault Y04.1 ☑
      homicide (attempt) Y04.1 ☑
      in
        fight Y04.1 ☑
    insect (nonvenomous) W57 ☑
    lizard (nonvenomous) W59.01 ☑
    mammal NEC W55.81 ☑
    mammal NEC W55.81 ☑
      marine W56.31 ☑
    marine animal (nonvenomous) W56.81 ☑
    millipede W57 ☑
    moray eel W56.51 ☑
    mouse W53.01 ☑
    person(s) (accidentally) W50.3 ☑
      with intent to injure or kill Y04.1 ☑

Bite, bitten by — continued
    person(s) — continued
      as, or caused by, a crowd or human stampede (with
          fall) W52 ☑
      assault Y04.1 ☑
      homicide (attempt) Y04.1 ☑
      in
        fight Y04.1 ☑
    pig W55.41 ☑
    raccoon W55.51 ☑
    rat W53.11 ☑
    reptile W59.81 ☑
      lizard W59.01 ☑
      snake W59.11 ☑
      turtle W59.21 ☑
        terrestrial W59.81 ☑
    rodent W53.81 ☑
      mouse W53.01 ☑
      rat W53.11 ☑
      specified NEC W53.81 ☑
      squirrel W53.21 ☑
    shark W56.41 ☑
    sheep W55.31 ☑
    snake (nonvenomous) W59.11 ☑
    spider (nonvenomous) W57 ☑
    squirrel W53.21 ☑
Blast (air) in war operations — see War operations, blast
Blizzard X37.2 ☑
Blood alcohol level Y90.9
    less than 20mg/100ml Y90.0
    20-39mg/100ml Y90.1
    40-59mg/100ml Y90.2
    60-79mg/100ml Y90.3
    80-99mg/100ml Y90.4
    100-119mg/100ml Y90.5
    120-199mg/100ml Y90.6
    200-239mg/100ml Y90.7
    presence in blood, level not specified Y90.9
Blow X58 ☑
    by law-enforcing agent, police (on duty) — see Legal,
        intervention, manhandling
    blunt object — see Legal, intervention, blunt object
Blowing up — see Explosion
Brawl (hand) (fists) (foot) Y04.0 ☑
Breakage (accidental) (part of)
    ladder (causing fall) W11 ☑
    scaffolding (causing fall) W12 ☑
Broken
    glass, contact with — see Contact, with, glass
    power line (causing electric shock) W85 ☑
Bumping against, into (accidentally)
    object NEC W22.8 ☑
      with fall — see Fall, due to, bumping against, ob-
          ject
      caused by crowd or human stampede (with fall)
          W52 ☑
      sports equipment W21.9 ☑
    person(s) W51 ☑
      with fall W03 ☑
        due to ice or snow W00.0 ☑
      assault Y04.2 ☑
      caused by, a crowd or human stampede (with fall)
          W52 ☑
      homicide (attempt) Y04.2 ☑
    sports equipment W21.9 ☑
Burn, burned, burning (accidental) (by) (from) (on)
    acid NEC — see Table of Drugs and Chemicals
    bed linen — see Exposure, fire, uncontrolled, in
        building, bed
    blowtorch X08.8 ☑
      with ignition of clothing NEC X06.2 ☑
        nightwear X05 ☑
    bonfire, campfire (controlled) (see also Exposure, fire,
        controlled, not in building)
      uncontrolled — see Exposure, fire, uncontrolled,
          not in building
    candle X08.8 ☑
      with ignition of clothing NEC X06.2 ☑
        nightwear X05 ☑
    caustic liquid, substance (external) (internal) NEC —
        see Table of Drugs and Chemicals
    chemical (external) (internal) (see also Table of Drugs
        and Chemicals)
      in war operations — see War operations. fire
    cigar(s) or cigarette(s) X08.8 ☑

☑ Additional Character Required — Refer to the Tabular List for Character Selection ▽ Subterms under main terms may continue to next column or page

Burn, burned, burning — *continued*
  cigar(s) or cigarette(s) — *continued*
    with ignition of clothing NEC X06.2 ☑
      nightwear X05 ☑
  clothes, clothing NEC (from controlled fire) X06.2 ☑
    with conflagration — *see* Exposure, fire, uncontrolled, building
      not in building or structure — *see* Exposure, fire, uncontrolled, not in building
  cooker (hot) X15.8 ☑
    stated as undetermined whether accidental or intentional Y27.3 ☑
    suicide (attempt) X77.3 ☑
  electric blanket X16 ☑
  engine (hot) X17 ☑
  fire, flames — *see* Exposure, fire
  flare, Very pistol — *see* Discharge, firearm NEC
  heat
    from appliance (electrical) (household) X15.8 ☑
      cooker X15.8 ☑
      hotplate X15.2 ☑
      kettle X15.8 ☑
      light bulb X15.8 ☑
      saucepan X15.3 ☑
      skillet X15.3 ☑
      stated as undetermined whether accidental or intentional Y27.3 ☑
      stove X15.0 ☑
      suicide (attempt) X77.3 ☑
      toaster X15.1 ☑
    in local application or packing during medical or surgical procedure Y63.5
  heating
    appliance, radiator or pipe X16 ☑
  homicide (attempt) — *see* Assault, burning
  hot
    air X14.1 ☑
    cooker X15.8 ☑
    drink X10.0 ☑
    engine X17 ☑
    fat X10.2 ☑
    fluid NEC X12 ☑
    food X10.1 ☑
    gases X14.1 ☑
    heating appliance X16 ☑
    household appliance NEC X15.8 ☑
    kettle X15.8 ☑
    liquid NEC X12 ☑
    machinery X17 ☑
    metal (molten) (liquid) NEC X18 ☑
    object (not producing fire or flames) NEC X19 ☑
    oil (cooking) X10.2 ☑
    pipe(s) X16 ☑
    radiator X16 ☑
    saucepan (glass) (metal) X15.3 ☑
    stove (kitchen) X15.0 ☑
    substance NEC X19 ☑
      caustic or corrosive NEC — *see* Table of Drugs and Chemicals
    toaster X15.1 ☑
    tool X17 ☑
    vapor X13.1 ☑
    water (tap) — *see* Contact, with, hot, tap water
  hotplate X15.2 ☑
    suicide (attempt) X77.3 ☑
  ignition — *see* Ignition
  in war operations — *see* War operations, fire
  inflicted by other person X97 ☑
    by hot objects, hot vapor, and steam — *see* Assault, burning, hot object
  internal, from swallowed caustic, corrosive liquid, substance — *see* Table of Drugs and Chemicals
  iron (hot) X15.8 ☑
    stated as undetermined whether accidental or intentional Y27.3 ☑
    suicide (attempt) X77.3 ☑
  kettle (hot) X15.8 ☑
    stated as undetermined whether accidental or intentional Y27.3 ☑
    suicide (attempt) X77.3 ☑
  lamp (flame) X08.8 ☑
    with ignition of clothing NEC X06.2 ☑
      nightwear X05 ☑
  lighter (cigar) (cigarette) X08.8 ☑
    with ignition of clothing NEC X06.2 ☑
      nightwear X05 ☑

Burn, burned, burning — *continued*
  lightning — *see* subcategory T75.0 ☑
    causing fire — *see* Exposure, fire
  liquid (boiling) (hot) NEC X12 ☑
    stated as undetermined whether accidental or intentional Y27.2 ☑
    suicide (attempt) X77.2 ☑
  local application of externally applied substance in medical or surgical care Y63.5
  machinery (hot) X17 ☑
  matches X08.8 ☑
    with ignition of clothing NEC X06.2 ☑
      nightwear X05 ☑
  mattress — *see* Exposure, fire, uncontrolled, building, bed
  medicament, externally applied Y63.5
  metal (hot) (liquid) (molten) NEC X18 ☑
  nightwear (nightclothes, nightdress, gown, pajamas, robe) X05 ☑
  object (hot) NEC X19 ☑
  on board watercraft
    due to
      accident to watercraft V91.09 ☑
        powered craft V91.03 ☑
          ferry boat V91.01 ☑
          fishing boat V91.02 ☑
          jetskis V91.03 ☑
          liner V91.01 ☑
          merchant ship V91.00 ☑
          passenger ship V91.01 ☑
        unpowered craft V91.08 ☑
          canoe V91.05 ☑
          inflatable V91.06 ☑
          kayak V91.05 ☑
          sailboat V91.04 ☑
          surf-board V91.08 ☑
          water skis V91.07 ☑
          windsurfer V91.08 ☑
      fire on board V93.09 ☑
        ferry boat V93.01 ☑
        fishing boat V93.02 ☑
        jetskis V93.03 ☑
        liner V93.01 ☑
        merchant ship V93.00 ☑
        passenger ship V93.01 ☑
        powered craft NEC V93.03 ☑
        sailboat V93.04 ☑
      specified heat source NEC on board V93.19 ☑
        ferry boat V93.11 ☑
        fishing boat V93.12 ☑
        jetskis V93.13 ☑
        liner V93.11 ☑
        merchant ship V93.10 ☑
        passenger ship V93.11 ☑
        powered craft NEC V93.13 ☑
        sailboat V93.14 ☑
  pipe (hot) X16 ☑
  smoking X08.8 ☑
    with ignition of clothing NEC X06.2 ☑
      nightwear X05 ☑
  powder — *see* Powder burn
  radiator (hot) X16 ☑
  saucepan (hot) (glass) (metal) X15.3 ☑
    stated as undetermined whether accidental or intentional Y27.3 ☑
    suicide (attempt) X77.3 ☑
  self-inflicted X76 ☑
    stated as undetermined whether accidental or intentional Y26 ☑
  stated as undetermined whether accidental or intentional Y27.0 ☑
  steam X13.1 ☑
    pipe X16 ☑
      stated as undetermined whether accidental or intentional Y27.8 ☑
    stated as undetermined whether accidental or intentional Y27.0 ☑
    suicide (attempt) X77.0 ☑
  stove (hot) (kitchen) X15.0 ☑
    stated as undetermined whether accidental or intentional Y27.3 ☑
    suicide (attempt) X77.3 ☑
  substance (hot) NEC X19 ☑
    boiling X12 ☑
      stated as undetermined whether accidental or intentional Y27.2 ☑

Burn, burned, burning — *continued*
  substance — *continued*
    boiling — *continued*
      suicide (attempt) X77.2 ☑
    molten (metal) X18 ☑
    suicide (attempt) NEC X76 ☑
    hot
      household appliance X77.3 ☑
      object X77.9 ☑
    therapeutic misadventure
      heat in local application or packing during medical or surgical procedure Y63.5
      overdose of radiation Y63.2
  toaster (hot) X15.1 ☑
    stated as undetermined whether accidental or intentional Y27.3 ☑
    suicide (attempt) X77.3 ☑
  tool (hot) X17 ☑
  torch, welding X08.8 ☑
    with ignition of clothing NEC X06.2 ☑
      nightwear X05 ☑
  trash fire (controlled) — *see* Exposure, fire, controlled, not in building
    uncontrolled — *see* Exposure, fire, uncontrolled, not in building
  vapor (hot) X13.1 ☑
    stated as undetermined whether accidental or intentional Y27.0 ☑
    suicide (attempt) X77.0 ☑
  Very pistol — *see* Discharge, firearm NEC
Butted by animal W55.82 ☑
  bull W55.22 ☑
  cow W55.22 ☑
  goat W55.32 ☑
  horse W55.12 ☑
  pig W55.42 ☑
  sheep W55.32 ☑

C

Caisson disease — *see* Air, pressure, change
Campfire (exposure to) (controlled) (*see also* Exposure, fire, controlled, not in building)
  uncontrolled — *see* Exposure, fire, uncontrolled, not in building
Capital punishment (any means) — *see* Legal, intervention
Car sickness T75.3 ☑
Casualty (not due to war) NEC X58 ☑
  war — *see* War operations
Cat
  bite W55.01 ☑
  scratch W55.03 ☑
Cataclysm, cataclysmic (any injury) NEC — *see* Forces of nature
Catching fire — *see* Exposure, fire
Caught
  between
    folding object W23.0 ☑
    objects (moving) (stationary and moving) W23.0 ☑
      and machinery — *see* Contact, with, by type of machine
      stationary W23.1 ☑
    sliding door and door frame W23.0 ☑
  by, in
    machinery (moving parts of) — *see* Contact, with, by type of machine
    washing-machine wringer W23.0 ☑
  under packing crate (due to losing grip) W23.1 ☑
Cave-in caused by cataclysmic earth surface movement or eruption — *see* Landslide
Change(s) in air pressure — *see* Air, pressure, change
Choked, choking (on) (any object except food or vomitus)
  food (bone) (seed) — *see* categories T17 and T18 ☑
  vomitus T17.81- ☑
Civil insurrection — *see* War operations
Cloudburst (any injury) X37.8 ☑
Cold, exposure to (accidental) (excessive) (extreme) (natural) (place) NEC — *see* Exposure, cold
Collapse
  building W20.1 ☑
    burning (uncontrolled fire) X00.2 ☑
  dam or man-made structure (causing earth movement) X36.0 ☑
  machinery — *see* Contact, with, by type of machine

Collapse — continued
structure W20.1 ☑
burning (uncontrolled fire) X00.2 ☑
Collision (accidental) NEC (see also Accident, transport)
V89.9 ☑
pedestrian W51 ☑
with fall W03 ☑
due to ice or snow W00.0 ☑
involving pedestrian conveyance — see Accident, transport, pedestrian, conveyance
and
crowd or human stampede (with fall) W52 ☑
object W22.8 ☑
with fall — see Fall, due to, bumping against, object
person(s) — see Collision, pedestrian
transport vehicle NEC V89.9 ☑
and
avalanche, fallen or not moving — see Accident, transport
falling or moving — see Landslide
landslide, fallen or not moving — see Accident, transport
falling or moving — see Landslide
due to cataclysm — see Forces of nature, by type
intentional, purposeful suicide (attempt) — see Suicide, collision
Combustion, spontaneous — see Ignition
Complication (delayed) **of or following** (medical or surgical procedure) Y84.9
with misadventure — see Misadventure
amputation of limb(s) Y83.5
anastomosis (arteriovenous) (blood vessel) (gastrojejunal) (tendon) (natural or artificial material) Y83.2
aspiration (of fluid) Y84.4
tissue Y84.8
biopsy Y84.8
blood
sampling Y84.7
transfusion
procedure Y84.8
bypass Y83.2
catheterization (urinary) Y84.6
cardiac Y84.0
colostomy Y83.3
cystostomy Y83.3
dialysis (kidney) Y84.1
drug — see Table of Drugs and Chemicals
due to misadventure — see Misadventure
duodenostomy Y83.3
electroshock therapy Y84.3
external stoma, creation of Y83.3
formation of external stoma Y83.3
gastrostomy Y83.3
graft Y83.2
hypothermia (medically-induced) Y84.8
implant, implantation (of)
artificial
internal device (cardiac pacemaker) (electrodes in brain) (heart valve prosthesis) (orthopedic) Y83.1
material or tissue (for anastomosis or bypass) Y83.2
with creation of external stoma Y83.3
natural tissues (for anastomosis or bypass) Y83.2
with creation of external stoma Y83.3
infusion
procedure Y84.8
injection — see Table of Drugs and Chemicals
procedure Y84.8
insertion of gastric or duodenal sound Y84.5
insulin-shock therapy Y84.3
paracentesis (abdominal) (thoracic) (aspirative) Y84.4
procedures other than surgical operation — see Complication of or following, by type of procedure
radiological procedure or therapy Y84.2
removal of organ (partial) (total) NEC Y83.6
sampling
blood Y84.7
fluid NEC Y84.4
tissue Y84.8
shock therapy Y84.3
surgical operation NEC (see also Complication of or following, by type of operation) Y83.9
reconstructive NEC Y83.4
with

Complication (delayed) **of or following** — continued
surgical operation (see also Complication of or following, by type of operation) — continued
reconstructive — continued
with — continued
anastomosis, bypass or graft Y83.2
formation of external stoma Y83.3
specified NEC Y83.8
transfusion (see also Table of Drugs and Chemicals)
procedure Y84.8
transplant, transplantation (heart) (kidney) (liver) (whole organ, any) Y83.0
partial organ Y83.4
ureterostomy Y83.3
vaccination (see also Table of Drugs and Chemicals)
procedure Y84.8
Compression
divers' squeeze — see Air, pressure, change
trachea by
food (lodged in esophagus) — see categories T17 and T18 ☑
vomitus (lodged in esophagus) T17.81- ☑
Conflagration — see Exposure, fire, uncontrolled
Constriction (external)
hair W49.01 ☑
jewelry W49.04 ☑
ring W49.04 ☑
rubber band W49.03 ☑
specified item NEC W49.09 ☑
string W49.02 ☑
thread W49.02 ☑
Contact (accidental)
with
abrasive wheel (metalworking) W31.1 ☑
alligator W58.09 ☑
bite W58.01 ☑
crushing W58.03 ☑
strike W58.02 ☑
amphibian W62.9 ☑
frog W62.0 ☑
toad W62.1 ☑
animal (nonvenomous) NEC W64 ☑
marine W56.89 ☑
bite W56.81 ☑
dolphin — see Contact, with, dolphin
fish NEC — see Contact, with, fish
mammal — see Contact, with, mammal, marine
orca — see Contact, with, orca
sea lion — see Contact, with, sea lion
shark — see Contact, with, shark
strike W56.82 ☑
animate mechanical force NEC W64 ☑
arrow W21.89 ☑
not thrown, projected or falling W45.8 ☑
arthropods (nonvenomous) W57 ☑
axe W27.0 ☑
band-saw (industrial) W31.2 ☑
bayonet — see Bayonet wound
bee(s) X58 ☑
bench-saw (industrial) W31.2 ☑
bird W61.99 ☑
bite W61.91 ☑
chicken — see Contact, with, chicken
duck — see Contact, with, duck
goose — see Contact, with, goose
macaw — see Contact, with, macaw
parrot — see Contact, with, parrot
psittacine — see Contact, with, psittacine
strike W61.92 ☑
turkey — see Contact, with, turkey
blender W29.0 ☑
boiling water X12 ☑
stated as undetermined whether accidental or intentional Y27.2 ☑
suicide (attempt) X77.2 ☑
bore, earth-drilling or mining (land) (seabed) W31.0 ☑
buffalo — see Contact, with, hoof stock NEC
bull W55.29 ☑
bite W55.21 ☑
gored W55.22 ☑
strike W55.22 ☑
bumper cars W31.81 ☑
camel — see Contact, with, hoof stock NEC

Contact — continued
with — continued
can
lid W45.2 ☑
opener W27.4 ☑
powered W29.0 ☑
cat W55.09 ☑
bite W55.01 ☑
scratch W55.03 ☑
caterpillar (venomous) X58 ☑
centipede (venomous) X58 ☑
chain
hoist W24.0 ☑
agricultural operations W30.89 ☑
saw W29.3 ☑
chicken W61.39 ☑
peck W61.33 ☑
strike W61.32 ☑
chisel W27.0 ☑
circular saw W31.2 ☑
cobra X58 ☑
combine (harvester) W30.0 ☑
conveyer belt W24.1 ☑
cooker (hot) X15.8 ☑
stated as undetermined whether accidental or intentional Y27.3 ☑
suicide (attempt) X77.3 ☑
coral X58 ☑
cotton gin W31.82 ☑
cow W55.29 ☑
bite W55.21 ☑
strike W55.22 ☑
crane W24.0 ☑
agricultural operations W30.89 ☑
crocodile W58.19 ☑
bite W58.11 ☑
crushing W58.13 ☑
strike W58.12 ☑
dagger W26.1 ☑
stated as undetermined whether accidental or intentional Y28.2 ☑
suicide (attempt) X78.2 ☑
dairy equipment W31.82 ☑
dart W21.89 ☑
not thrown, projected or falling W45.8 ☑
deer — see Contact, with, hoof stock NEC
derrick W24.0 ☑
agricultural operations W30.89 ☑
hay W30.2 ☑
dog W54.8 ☑
bite W54.0 ☑
strike W54.1 ☑
dolphin W56.09 ☑
bite W56.01 ☑
strike W56.02 ☑
donkey — see Contact, with, hoof stock NEC
drill (powered) W29.8 ☑
earth (land) (seabed) W31.0 ☑
nonpowered W27.8 ☑
drive belt W24.0 ☑
agricultural operations W30.89 ☑
dry ice — see Exposure, cold, man-made
dryer (clothes) (powered) (spin) W29.2 ☑
duck W61.69 ☑
bite W61.61 ☑
strike W61.62 ☑
earth (-)
drilling machine (industrial) W31.0 ☑
scraping machine in stationary use W31.83 ☑
edge of stiff paper W45.1 ☑
electric
beater W29.0 ☑
blanket X16 ☑
fan W29.2 ☑
commercial W31.82 ☑
knife W29.1 ☑
mixer W29.0 ☑
elevator (building) W24.0 ☑
agricultural operations W30.89 ☑
grain W30.3 ☑
engine(s), hot NEC X17 ☑
excavating machine W31.0 ☑
farm machine W30.9 ☑
feces — see Contact, with, by type of animal
fer de lance X58 ☑

☑ Additional Character Required — Refer to the Tabular List for Character Selection

Subterms under main terms may continue to next column or page

Contact — *continued*
  with — *continued*
    fish W56.59 ☑
      bite W56.51 ☑
      shark — *see* Contact, with, shark
      strike W56.52 ☑
    flying horses W31.81 ☑
    forging (metalworking) machine W31.1 ☑
    fork W27.4 ☑
    forklift (truck) W24.0 ☑
      agricultural operations W30.89 ☑
    frog W62.0 ☑
    garden
      cultivator (powered) W29.3 ☑
        riding W30.89 ☑
      fork W27.1 ☑
    gas turbine W31.3 ☑
    Gila monster X58 ☑
    giraffe — *see* Contact, with, hoof stock NEC
    glass (sharp) (broken) W25 ☑
      with subsequent fall W18.02 ☑
      assault X99.0 ☑
      due to fall — *see* Fall, by type
      stated as undetermined whether accidental or
        intentional Y28.0 ☑
      suicide (attempt) X78.0 ☑
    goat W55.39 ☑
      bite W55.31 ☑
      strike W55.32 ☑
    goose W61.59 ☑
      bite W61.51 ☑
      strike W61.52 ☑
    hand
      saw W27.0 ☑
      tool (not powered) NEC W27.8 ☑
        powered W29.8 ☑
    harvester W30.0 ☑
    hay-derrick W30.2 ☑
    heating
      appliance (hot) X16 ☑
      pad (electric) X16 ☑
    heat NEC X19 ☑
      from appliance (electrical) (household) — *see*
        Contact, with, hot, household appliance
      heating appliance X16 ☑
    hedge-trimmer (powered) W29.3 ☑
    hoe W27.1 ☑
    hoist (chain) (shaft) NEC W24.0 ☑
      agricultural W30.89 ☑
    hoof stock NEC W55.39 ☑
      bite W55.31 ☑
      strike W55.32 ☑
    hornet(s) X58 ☑
    horse W55.19 ☑
      bite W55.11 ☑
      strike W55.12 ☑
    hot
      air X14.1 ☑
        inhalation X14.0 ☑
      cooker X15.8 ☑
      drinks X10.0 ☑
      engine X17 ☑
      fats X10.2 ☑
      fluids NEC X12 ☑
        assault X98.2 ☑
        suicide (attempt) X77.2 ☑
        undetermined whether accidental or inten-
          tional Y27.2 ☑
      food X10.1 ☑
      gases X14.1 ☑
        inhalation X14.0 ☑
      heating appliance X16 ☑
      household appliance X15.8 ☑
        assault X98.3 ☑
        cooker X15.8 ☑
        hotplate X15.2 ☑
        kettle X15.8 ☑
        light bulb X15.8 ☑
        object NEC X19 ☑
          assault X98.8 ☑
          stated as undetermined whether acciden-
            tal or intentional Y27.9 ☑
          suicide (attempt) X77.8 ☑
        saucepan X15.3 ☑
        skillet X15.3 ☑

Contact — *continued*
  with — *continued*
    hot — *continued*
      household appliance — *continued*
        stated as undetermined whether accidental
          or intentional Y27.3 ☑
        stove X15.0 ☑
        suicide (attempt) X77.3 ☑
        toaster X15.1 ☑
      kettle X15.8 ☑
      light bulb X15.8 ☑
      liquid NEC (*see also* Burn) X12 ☑
        drinks X10.0 ☑
        stated as undetermined whether accidental
          or intentional Y27.2 ☑
        suicide (attempt) X77.2 ☑
        tap water X11.8 ☑
          stated as undetermined whether acciden-
            tal or intentional Y27.1 ☑
          suicide (attempt) X77.1 ☑
      machinery X17 ☑
      metal (molten) (liquid) NEC X18 ☑
      object (not producing fire or flames) NEC X19 ☑
      oil (cooking) X10.2 ☑
      pipe X16 ☑
      plate X15.2 ☑
      radiator X16 ☑
      saucepan (glass) (metal) X15.3 ☑
      skillet X15.3 ☑
      stove (kitchen) X15.0 ☑
      substance NEC X19 ☑
      tap-water X11.8 ☑
        assault X98.1 ☑
        heated on stove X12 ☑
          stated as undetermined whether acciden-
            tal or intentional Y27.2 ☑
          suicide (attempt) X77.2 ☑
        in bathtub X11.0 ☑
        running X11.1 ☑
        stated as undetermined whether accidental
          or intentional Y27.1 ☑
        suicide (attempt) X77.1 ☑
      toaster X15.1 ☑
      tool X17 ☑
      vapors X13.1 ☑
        inhalation X13.0 ☑
      water (tap) X11.8 ☑
        boiling X12 ☑
          stated as undetermined whether acciden-
            tal or intentional Y27.2 ☑
          suicide (attempt) X77.2 ☑
        heated on stove X12 ☑
          stated as undetermined whether acciden-
            tal or intentional Y27.2 ☑
          suicide (attempt) X77.2 ☑
        in bathtub X11.0 ☑
        running X11.1 ☑
        stated as undetermined whether accidental
          or intentional Y27.1 ☑
        suicide (attempt) X77.1 ☑
    hotplate X15.2 ☑
    ice-pick W27.4 ☑
    insect (nonvenomous) NEC W57 ☑
    kettle (hot) X15.8 ☑
    knife W26.0 ☑
      assault X99.1 ☑
      electric W29.1 ☑
      stated as undetermined whether accidental or
        intentional Y28.1 ☑
      suicide (attempt) X78.1 ☑
    lathe (metalworking) W31.1 ☑
      turnings W45.8 ☑
      woodworking W31.2 ☑
    lawnmower (powered) (ridden) W28 ☑
      causing electrocution W86.8 ☑
        suicide (attempt) X83.1 ☑
      unpowered W27.1 ☑
    lift, lifting (devices) W24.0 ☑
      agricultural operations W30.89 ☑
      shaft W24.0 ☑
    liquefied gas — *see* Exposure, cold, man-made
    liquid air, hydrogen, nitrogen — *see* Exposure, cold,
      man-made
    lizard (nonvenomous) W59.09 ☑
      bite W59.01 ☑
      strike W59.02 ☑

Contact — *continued*
  with — *continued*
    llama — *see* Contact, with, hoof stock NEC
    macaw W61.19 ☑
      bite W61.11 ☑
      strike W61.12 ☑
    machine, machinery W31.9 ☑
      abrasive wheel W31.1 ☑
      agricultural including animal-powered
        W30.9 ☑
        combine harvester W30.0 ☑
        grain storage elevator W30.3 ☑
        hay derrick W30.2 ☑
        power take-off device W30.1 ☑
        reaper W30.0 ☑
        specified NEC W30.89 ☑
        thresher W30.0 ☑
        transport vehicle, stationary W30.81 ☑
      band saw W31.2 ☑
      bench saw W31.2 ☑
      circular saw W31.2 ☑
      commercial NEC W31.82 ☑
      drilling, metal (industrial) W31.1 ☑
      earth-drilling W31.0 ☑
      earthmoving or scraping W31.89 ☑
      excavating W31.89 ☑
      forging machine W31.1 ☑
      gas turbine W31.3 ☑
      hot X17 ☑
      internal combustion engine W31.3 ☑
      land drill W31.0 ☑
      lathe W31.1 ☑
      lifting (devices) W24.0 ☑
      metal drill W31.1 ☑
      metalworking (industrial) W31.1 ☑
      milling, metal W31.1 ☑
      mining W31.0 ☑
      molding W31.2 ☑
      overhead plane W31.2 ☑
      power press, metal W31.1 ☑
      prime mover W31.3 ☑
      printing W31.89 ☑
      radial saw W31.2 ☑
      recreational W31.81 ☑
      roller-coaster W31.81 ☑
      rolling mill, metal W31.1 ☑
      sander W31.2 ☑
      seabed drill W31.0 ☑
      shaft
        hoist W31.0 ☑
        lift W31.0 ☑
      specified NEC W31.89 ☑
      spinning W31.89 ☑
      steam engine W31.3 ☑
      transmission W24.1 ☑
      undercutter W31.0 ☑
      water driven turbine W31.3 ☑
      weaving W31.89 ☑
      woodworking or forming (industrial) W31.2 ☑
    mammal (feces) (urine) W55.89 ☑
      bull — *see* Contact, with, bull
      cat — *see* Contact, with, cat
      cow — *see* Contact, with, cow
      goat — *see* Contact, with, goat
      hoof stock — *see* Contact, with, hoof stock
      horse — *see* Contact, with, horse
      marine W56.39 ☑
        dolphin — *see* Contact, with, dolphin
        orca — *see* Contact, with, orca
        sea lion — *see* Contact, with, sea lion
        specified NEC W56.39 ☑
          bite W56.31 ☑
          strike W56.32 ☑
      pig — *see* Contact, with, pig
      raccoon — *see* Contact, with, raccoon
      rodent — *see* Contact, with, rodent
      sheep — *see* Contact, with, sheep
      specified NEC W55.89 ☑
        bite W55.81 ☑
        strike W55.82 ☑
    marine
      animal W56.89 ☑
        bite W56.81 ☑
        dolphin — *see* Contact, with, dolphin
        fish NEC — *see* Contact, with, fish

Contact — *continued*
  with — *continued*
    marine — *continued*
      animal — *continued*
        mammal — *see* Contact, with, mammal, marine
        orca — *see* Contact, with, orca
        sea lion — *see* Contact, with, sea lion
        shark — *see* Contact, with, shark
        strike W56.82 ☑
    meat
      grinder (domestic) W29.0 ☑
        industrial W31.82 ☑
        nonpowered W27.4 ☑
      slicer (domestic) W29.0 ☑
        industrial W31.82 ☑
    merry go round W31.81 ☑
    metal, hot (liquid) (molten) NEC X18 ☑
    millipede W57 ☑
    nail W45.0 ☑
      gun W29.4 ☑
    needle (sewing) W27.3 ☑
      hypodermic W46.0 ☑
        contaminated W46.1 ☑
    object (blunt) NEC
      hot NEC X19
      legal intervention — *see* Legal, intervention, blunt object
      sharp NEC W45.8 ☑
        inflicted by other person NEC W45.8 ☑
          stated as
            intentional homicide (attempt) — *see* Assault, cutting or piercing instrument
        legal intervention — *see* Legal, intervention, sharp object
        self-inflicted X78.9 ☑
    orca W56.29 ☑
      bite W56.21 ☑
      strike W56.22 ☑
    overhead plane W31.2 ☑
    paper (as sharp object) W45.1 ☑
    paper-cutter W27.5 ☑
    parrot W61.09 ☑
      bite W61.01 ☑
      strike W61.02 ☑
    pig W55.49 ☑
      bite W55.41 ☑
      strike W55.42 ☑
    pipe, hot X16 ☑
    pitchfork W27.1 ☑
    plane (metal) (wood) W27.0 ☑
      overhead W31.2 ☑
    plant thorns, spines, sharp leaves or other mechanisms W60 ☑
    powered
      garden cultivator W29.3 ☑
      household appliance, implement, or machine W29.8 ☑
      saw (industrial) W31.2 ☑
        hand W29.8 ☑
    printing machine W31.89 ☑
    psittacine bird W61.29 ☑
      bite W61.21 ☑
      macaw — *see* Contact, with, macaw
      parrot — *see* Contact, with, parrot
      strike W61.22 ☑
    pulley (block) (transmission) W24.0 ☑
      agricultural operations W30.89 ☑
    raccoon W55.59 ☑
      bite W55.51 ☑
      strike W55.52 ☑
    radial-saw (industrial) W31.2 ☑
    radiator (hot) X16 ☑
    rake W27.1 ☑
    rattlesnake X58 ☑
    reaper W30.0 ☑
    reptile W59.89 ☑
      lizard — *see* Contact, with, lizard
      snake — *see* Contact, with, snake
      specified NEC W59.89 ☑
        bite W59.81 ☑
        crushing W59.83 ☑
        strike W59.82 ☑
      turtle — *see* Contact, with, turtle
    rivet gun (powered) W29.4 ☑

Contact — *continued*
  with — *continued*
    road scraper — *see* Accident, transport, construction vehicle
    rodent (feces) (urine) W53.89 ☑
      bite W53.81 ☑
      mouse W53.09 ☑
        bite W53.01 ☑
      rat W53.19 ☑
        bite W53.11 ☑
      specified NEC W53.89 ☑
        bite W53.81 ☑
      squirrel W53.29 ☑
        bite W53.21 ☑
    roller coaster W31.81 ☑
    rope NEC W24.0 ☑
      agricultural operations W30.89 ☑
    saliva — *see* Contact, with, by type of animal
    sander W29.8 ☑
      industrial W31.2 ☑
    saucepan (hot) (glass) (metal) X15.3 ☑
    saw W27.0 ☑
      band (industrial) W31.2 ☑
      bench (industrial) W31.2 ☑
      chain W29.3 ☑
      hand W27.0 ☑
    sawing machine, metal W31.1 ☑
    scissors W27.2 ☑
    scorpion X58 ☑
    screwdriver W27.0 ☑
      powered W29.8 ☑
    sea
      anemone, cucumber or urchin (spine) X58 ☑
      lion W56.19 ☑
        bite W56.11 ☑
        strike W56.12 ☑
    serpent — *see* Contact, with, snake, by type
    sewing-machine (electric) (powered) W29.2 ☑
      not powered W27.8 ☑
    shaft (hoist) (lift) (transmission) NEC W24.0 ☑
      agricultural W30.89 ☑
    shark W56.49 ☑
      bite W56.41 ☑
      strike W56.42 ☑
    shears (hand) W27.2 ☑
      powered (industrial) W31.1 ☑
        domestic W29.2 ☑
    sheep W55.39 ☑
      bite W55.31 ☑
      strike W55.32 ☑
    shovel W27.8 ☑
      steam — *see* Accident, transport, construction vehicle
    snake (nonvenomous) W59.19 ☑
      bite W59.11 ☑
      crushing W59.13 ☑
      strike W59.12 ☑
    spade W27.1 ☑
    spider (venomous) X58 ☑
    spin-drier W29.2 ☑
    spinning machine W31.89 ☑
    splinter W45.8 ☑
    sports equipment W21.9 ☑
    staple gun (powered) W29.8 ☑
    steam X13.1 ☑
      engine W31.3 ☑
      inhalation X13.0 ☑
      pipe X16 ☑
      shovel W31.89 ☑
    stove (hot) (kitchen) X15.0 ☑
    substance, hot NEC X19 ☑
      molten (metal) X18 ☑
    sword W26.1 ☑
      assault X99.2 ☑
      stated as undetermined whether accidental or intentional Y28.2 ☑
      suicide (attempt) X78.2 ☑
    tarantula X58 ☑
    thresher W30.0 ☑
    tin can lid W45.2 ☑
    toad W62.1 ☑
    toaster (hot) X15.1 ☑
    tool W27.8 ☑
      hand (not powered) W27.8 ☑
        auger W27.0 ☑

Contact — *continued*
  with — *continued*
    tool — *continued*
      hand — *continued*
        axe W27.0 ☑
        can opener W27.4 ☑
        chisel W27.0 ☑
        fork W27.4 ☑
        garden W27.1 ☑
        handsaw W27.0 ☑
        hoe W27.1 ☑
        ice-pick W27.4 ☑
        kitchen utensil W27.4 ☑
        manual
          lawn mower W27.1 ☑
          sewing machine W27.8 ☑
        meat grinder W27.4 ☑
        needle (sewing) W27.3 ☑
          hypodermic W46.0 ☑
            contaminated W46.1 ☑
        paper cutter W27.5 ☑
        pitchfork W27.1 ☑
        rake W27.1 ☑
        scissors W27.2 ☑
        screwdriver W27.0 ☑
        specified NEC W27.8 ☑
        workbench W27.0 ☑
      hot X17
      powered W29.8 ☑
        blender W29.0 ☑
          commercial W31.82 ☑
        can opener W29.0 ☑
          commercial W31.82 ☑
        chainsaw W29.3 ☑
        clothes dryer W29.2 ☑
          commercial W31.82 ☑
        dishwasher W29.2 ☑
          commercial W31.82 ☑
        edger W29.3 ☑
        electric fan W29.2 ☑
          commercial W31.82 ☑
        electric knife W29.1 ☑
        food processor W29.0 ☑
          commercial W31.82 ☑
        garbage disposal W29.0 ☑
          commercial W31.82 ☑
        garden tool W29.3 ☑
        hedge trimmer W29.3 ☑
        ice maker W29.0 ☑
          commercial W31.82 ☑
        kitchen appliance W29.0 ☑
          commercial W31.82 ☑
        lawn mower W28 ☑
        meat grinder W29.0 ☑
          commercial W31.82 ☑
        mixer W29.0 ☑
          commercial W31.82 ☑
        rototiller W29.3 ☑
        sewing machine W29.2 ☑
          commercial W31.82 ☑
        washing machine W29.2 ☑
          commercial W31.82 ☑
    transmission device (belt, cable, chain, gear, pinion, shaft) W24.1 ☑
      agricultural operations W30.89 ☑
    turbine (gas) (water-driven) W31.3 ☑
    turkey W61.49 ☑
      peck W61.43 ☑
      strike W61.42 ☑
    turtle (nonvenomous) W59.29 ☑
      bite W59.21 ☑
      strike W59.22 ☑
      terrestrial W59.89 ☑
        bite W59.81 ☑
        crushing W59.83 ☑
        strike W59.82 ☑
    under-cutter W31.0 ☑
    urine — *see* Contact, with, by type of animal
    vehicle
      agricultural use (transport) — *see* Accident, transport, agricultural vehicle
        not on public highway W30.81 ☑
      industrial use (transport) — *see* Accident, transport, industrial vehicle
        not on public highway W31.83 ☑

☑ **Additional Character Required — Refer to the Tabular List for Character Selection**
🔻 **Subterms under main terms may continue to next column or page**

Contact — *continued*
with — *continued*
vehicle — *continued*
off-road use (transport) — *see* Accident, transport, all-terrain or off-road vehicle
not on public highway W31.83 ☑
special construction use (transport) — *see* Accident, transport, construction vehicle
not on public highway W31.83 ☑
venomous
animal X58 ☑
arthropods X58 ☑
lizard X58 ☑
marine animal NEC X58 ☑
marine plant NEC X58 ☑
millipedes (tropical) X58 ☑
plant(s) X58 ☑
snake X58 ☑
spider X58 ☑
viper X58 ☑
washing-machine (powered) W29.2 ☑
wasp X58 ☑
weaving-machine W31.89 ☑
winch W24.0 ☑
agricultural operations W30.89 ☑
wire NEC W24.0 ☑
agricultural operations W30.89 ☑
wood slivers W45.8 ☑
yellow jacket X58 ☑
zebra — *see* Contact, with, hoof stock NEC
Coup de soleil X32 ☑
Crash
aircraft (in transit) (powered) V95.9 ☑
balloon V96.01 ☑
fixed wing NEC (private) V95.21 ☑
commercial V95.31 ☑
glider V96.21 ☑
hang V96.11 ☑
powered V95.11 ☑
helicopter V95.01 ☑
in war operations — *see* War operations, destruction of aircraft
microlight V95.11 ☑
nonpowered V96.9 ☑
specified NEC V96.8 ☑
powered NEC V95.8 ☑
stated as
homicide (attempt) Y08.81 ☑
suicide (attempt) X83.0 ☑
ultralight V95.11 ☑
spacecraft V95.41 ☑
transport vehicle NEC (*see also* Accident, transport) V89.9 ☑
homicide (attempt) Y03.8 ☑
motor NEC (traffic) V89.2 ☑
homicide (attempt) Y03.8 ☑
suicide (attempt) — *see* Suicide, collision
Cruelty (mental) (physical) (sexual) X58 ☑
Crushed (accidentally) X58 ☑
between objects (moving) (stationary and moving) W23.0 ☑
stationary W23.1 ☑
by
alligator W58.03 ☑
avalanche NEC — *see* Landslide
cave-in W20.0 ☑
caused by cataclysmic earth surface movement — *see* Landslide
crocodile W58.13 ☑
crowd or human stampede W52 ☑
falling
aircraft V97.39 ☑
in war operations — *see* War operations, destruction of aircraft
earth, material W20.0 ☑
caused by cataclysmic earth surface movement — *see* Landslide
object NEC W20.8 ☑
landslide NEC — *see* Landslide
lizard (nonvenomous) W59.09 ☑
machinery — *see* Contact, with, by type of machine
reptile NEC W59.89 ☑
snake (nonvenomous) W59.13 ☑
in
machinery — *see* Contact, with, by type of machine

Cut, cutting (any part of body) (accidental) (*see also* Contact, with, by object or machine)
during medical or surgical treatment as misadventure — *see* Index to Diseases and Injuries, Complications
homicide (attempt) — *see* Assault, cutting or piercing instrument
inflicted by other person — *see* Assault, cutting or piercing instrument
legal
execution — *see* Legal, intervention
intervention — *see* Legal, intervention, sharp object
machine NEC (*see also* Contact, with, by type of machine) W31.9 ☑
self-inflicted — *see* Suicide, cutting or piercing instrument
suicide (attempt) — *see* Suicide, cutting or piercing instrument
Cyclone (any injury) X37.1 ☑

D

Decapitation (accidental circumstances) NEC X58 ☑
homicide X99.9 ☑
legal execution — *see* Legal, intervention
Dehydration from lack of water X58 ☑
Deprivation X58 ☑
Derailment (accidental)
railway (rolling stock) (train) (vehicle) (without antecedent collision) V81.7 ☑
with antecedent collision — *see* Accident, transport, railway vehicle occupant
streetcar (without antecedent collision) V82.7 ☑
with antecedent collision — *see* Accident, transport, streetcar occupant
Descent
parachute (voluntary) (without accident to aircraft) V97.29 ☑
due to accident to aircraft — *see* Accident, transport, aircraft
Desertion X58 ☑
Destitution X58 ☑
Disability, late effect or sequela of injury — *see* Sequelae
Discharge (accidental)
airgun W34.010 ☑
assault X95.01 ☑
homicide (attempt) X95.01 ☑
stated as undetermined whether accidental or intentional Y24.0 ☑
suicide (attempt) X74.01 ☑
BB gun — *see* Discharge, airgun
firearm (accidental) W34.00 ☑
assault X95.9 ☑
handgun (pistol) (revolver) W32.0 ☑
assault X93 ☑
homicide (attempt) X93 ☑
legal intervention — *see* Legal, intervention, firearm, handgun
stated as undetermined whether accidental or intentional Y22 ☑
suicide (attempt) X72 ☑
homicide (attempt) X95.9 ☑
hunting rifle W33.02 ☑
assault X94.1 ☑
homicide (attempt) X94.1 ☑
legal intervention
injuring
bystander Y35.032 ☑
law enforcement personnel Y35.031 ☑
suspect Y35.033 ☑
stated as undetermined whether accidental or intentional Y23.1 ☑
suicide (attempt) X73.1 ☑
larger W33.00 ☑
assault X94.9 ☑
homicide (attempt) X94.9 ☑
hunting rifle — *see* Discharge, firearm, hunting rifle
legal intervention — *see* Legal, intervention, firearm by type of firearm
machine gun — *see* Discharge, firearm, machine gun
shotgun — *see* Discharge, firearm, shotgun
specified NEC W33.09 ☑

Discharge — *continued*
firearm — *continued*
larger — *continued*
specified — *continued*
assault X94.8 ☑
homicide (attempt) X94.8 ☑
legal intervention
injuring
bystander Y35.092 ☑
law enforcement personnel Y35.091 ☑
suspect Y35.093 ☑
stated as undetermined whether accidental or intentional Y23.8 ☑
suicide (attempt) X73.8 ☑
stated as undetermined whether accidental or intentional Y23.9 ☑
suicide (attempt) X73.9 ☑
legal intervention
injuring
bystander Y35.002 ☑
law enforcement personnel Y35.001 ☑
suspect Y35.03 ☑
using rubber bullet
injuring
bystander Y35.042 ☑
law enforcement personnel Y35.041 ☑
suspect Y35.043 ☑
machine gun W33.03 ☑
assault X94.2 ☑
homicide (attempt) X94.2 ☑
legal intervention — *see* Legal, intervention, firearm, machine gun
stated as undetermined whether accidental or intentional Y23.3 ☑
suicide (attempt) X73.2 ☑
pellet gun — *see* Discharge, airgun
shotgun W33.01 ☑
assault X94.0 ☑
homicide (attempt) X94.0 ☑
legal intervention — *see* Legal, intervention, firearm, specified NEC
stated as undetermined whether accidental or intentional Y23.0 ☑
suicide (attempt) X73.0 ☑
specified NEC W34.09 ☑
assault X95.8 ☑
homicide (attempt) X95.8 ☑
legal intervention — *see* Legal, intervention, firearm, specified NEC
stated as undetermined whether accidental or intentional Y24.8 ☑
suicide (attempt) X74.8 ☑
stated as undetermined whether accidental or intentional Y24.9 ☑
suicide (attempt) X74.9 ☑
Very pistol W34.09 ☑
assault X95.8 ☑
homicide (attempt) X95.8 ☑
stated as undetermined whether accidental or intentional Y24.8 ☑
suicide (attempt) X74.8 ☑
firework(s) W39 ☑
stated as undetermined whether accidental or intentional Y25 ☑
gas-operated gun NEC W34.018 ☑
airgun — *see* Discharge, airgun
assault X95.09 ☑
homicide (attempt) X95.09 ☑
paintball gun — *see* Discharge, paintball gun
stated as undetermined whether accidental or intentional Y24.8 ☑
suicide (attempt) X74.09 ☑
gun NEC (*see also* Discharge, firearm NEC)
air — *see* Discharge, airgun
BB — *see* Discharge, airgun
for single hand use — *see* Discharge, firearm, handgun
hand — *see* Discharge, firearm, handgun
machine — *see* Discharge, firearm, machine gun
other specified — *see* Discharge, firearm NEC
paintball — *see* Discharge, paintball gun
pellet — *see* Discharge, airgun
handgun — *see* Discharge, firearm, handgun
machine gun — *see* Discharge, firearm, machine gun

Discharge — *continued*
paintball gun W34.011 ☑
assault X95.02 ☑
homicide (attempt) X95.02 ☑
stated as undetermined whether accidental or intentional Y24.8 ☑
suicide (attempt) X74.02 ☑
pistol — *see* Discharge, firearm, handgun
flare — *see* Discharge, firearm, Very pistol
pellet — *see* Discharge, airgun
Very — *see* Discharge, firearm, Very pistol
revolver — *see* Discharge, firearm, handgun
rifle (hunting) — *see* Discharge, firearm, hunting rifle
shotgun — *see* Discharge, firearm, shotgun
spring-operated gun NEC W34.018 ☑
assault X95.09 ☑
homicide (attempt) X95.09 ☑
stated as undetermined whether accidental or intentional Y24.8 ☑
suicide (attempt) X74.09 ☑
Disease
Andes W94.11 ☑
aviator's — *see* Air, pressure
range W94.11 ☑
Diver's disease, palsy, paralysis, squeeze — *see* Air, pressure
Diving (into water) — *see* Accident, diving
Dog bite W54.0 ☑
Dragged by transport vehicle NEC (*see also* Accident, transport) V09.9 ☑
Drinking poison (accidental) — *see* Table of Drugs and Chemicals
Dropped (accidentally) **while being carried or supported by other person** W04 ☑
Drowning (accidental) W74 ☑
assault X92.9 ☑
due to
accident (to)
machinery — *see* Contact, with, by type of machine
watercraft V90.89 ☑
burning V90.29 ☑
powered V90.23 ☑
fishing boat V90.22 ☑
jetskis V90.23 ☑
merchant ship V90.20 ☑
passenger ship V90.21 ☑
unpowered V90.28 ☑
canoe V90.25 ☑
inflatable V90.26 ☑
kayak V90.25 ☑
sailboat V90.24 ☑
water skis V90.27 ☑
crushed V90.39 ☑
powered V90.33 ☑
fishing boat V90.32 ☑
jetskis V90.33 ☑
merchant ship V90.30 ☑
passenger ship V90.31 ☑
unpowered V90.38 ☑
canoe V90.35 ☑
inflatable V90.36 ☑
kayak V90.35 ☑
sailboat V90.34 ☑
water skis V90.37 ☑
overturning V90.09 ☑
powered V90.03 ☑
fishing boat V90.02 ☑
jetskis V90.03 ☑
merchant ship V90.00 ☑
passenger ship V90.01 ☑
unpowered V90.08 ☑
canoe V90.05 ☑
inflatable V90.06 ☑
kayak V90.05 ☑
sailboat V90.04 ☑
sinking V90.19 ☑
powered V90.13 ☑
fishing boat V90.12 ☑
jetskis V90.13 ☑
merchant ship V90.10 ☑
passenger ship V90.11 ☑
unpowered V90.18 ☑
canoe V90.15 ☑
inflatable V90.16 ☑
kayak V90.15 ☑

Drowning — *continued*
due to — *continued*
accident — *continued*
watercraft — *continued*
sinking — *continued*
unpowered — *continued*
sailboat V90.14 ☑
specified type NEC V90.89 ☑
powered V90.83 ☑
fishing boat V90.82 ☑
jetskis V90.83 ☑
merchant ship V90.80 ☑
passenger ship V90.81 ☑
unpowered V90.88 ☑
canoe V90.85 ☑
inflatable V90.86 ☑
kayak V90.85 ☑
sailboat V90.84 ☑
water skis V90.87 ☑
avalanche — *see* Landslide
cataclysmic
earth surface movement NEC — *see* Forces of nature, earth movement
storm — *see* Forces of nature, cataclysmic storm
cloudburst X37.8 ☑
cyclone X37.1 ☑
fall overboard (from) V92.09 ☑
powered craft V92.03 ☑
ferry boat V92.01 ☑
fishing boat V92.02 ☑
jetskis V92.03 ☑
liner V92.01 ☑
merchant ship V92.00 ☑
passenger ship V92.01 ☑
resulting from
accident to watercraft — *see* Drowning, due to, accident to, watercraft
being washed overboard (from) V92.29 ☑
powered craft V92.23 ☑
ferry boat V92.21 ☑
fishing boat V92.22 ☑
jetskis V92.23 ☑
liner V92.21 ☑
merchant ship V92.20 ☑
passenger ship V92.21 ☑
unpowered craft V92.28 ☑
canoe V92.25 ☑
inflatable V92.26 ☑
kayak V92.25 ☑
sailboat V92.24 ☑
surf-board V92.28 ☑
water skis V92.27 ☑
windsurfer V92.28 ☑
motion of watercraft V92.19 ☑
powered craft V92.13 ☑
ferry boat V92.11 ☑
fishing boat V92.12 ☑
jetskis V92.13 ☑
liner V92.11 ☑
merchant ship V92.10 ☑
passenger ship V92.11 ☑
unpowered craft
canoe V92.15 ☑
inflatable V92.16 ☑
kayak V92.15 ☑
sailboat V92.14 ☑
unpowered craft V92.08 ☑
canoe V92.05 ☑
inflatable V92.06 ☑
kayak V92.05 ☑
sailboat V92.04 ☑
surf-board V92.08 ☑
water skis V92.07 ☑
windsurfer V92.08 ☑
hurricane X37.0 ☑
jumping into water from watercraft (involved in accident) (*see also* Drowning, due to, accident to, watercraft)
without accident to or on watercraft W16.711 ☑
tidal wave NEC — *see* Forces of nature, tidal wave
torrential rain X37.8 ☑

Drowning — *continued*
following
fall
into
bathtub W16.211 ☑
bucket W16.221 ☑
fountain — *see* Drowning, following, fall, into, water, specified NEC
quarry — *see* Drowning, following, fall, into, water, specified NEC
reservoir — *see* Drowning, following, fall, into, water, specified NEC
swimming-pool W16.011 ☑
stated as undetermined whether accidental or intentional Y21.3 ☑
striking
bottom W16.021 ☑
wall W16.031 ☑
suicide (attempt) X71.2 ☑
water NOS W16.41 ☑
natural (lake) (open sea) (river) (stream) (pond) W16.111 ☑
striking
bottom W16.121 ☑
side W16.131 ☑
specified NEC W16.311 ☑
striking
bottom W16.321 ☑
wall W16.331 ☑
overboard NEC — *see* Drowning, due to, fall overboard
jump or dive
from boat W16.711 ☑
striking bottom W16.721 ☑
into
fountain — *see* Drowning, following, jump or dive, into, water, specified NEC
quarry — *see* Drowning, following, jump or dive, into, water, specified NEC
reservoir — *see* Drowning, following, jump or dive, into, water, specified NEC
swimming-pool W16.511 ☑
striking
bottom W16.521 ☑
wall W16.531 ☑
suicide (attempt) X71.2 ☑
water NOS W16.91 ☑
natural (lake) (open sea) (river) (stream) (pond) W16.611 ☑
specified NEC W16.811 ☑
bottom W16.821 ☑
striking
bottom W16.821 ☑
wall W16.831 ☑
striking
bottom W16.821 ☑
wall W16.831 ☑
striking bottom W16.621 ☑
homicide (attempt) X92.9 ☑
in
bathtub (accidental) W65 ☑
assault X92.0 ☑
following fall W16.211 ☑
stated as undetermined whether accidental or intentional Y21.1 ☑
stated as undetermined whether accidental or intentional Y21.0 ☑
suicide (attempt) X71.0 ☑
lake — *see* Drowning, in, natural water
natural water (lake) (open sea) (river) (stream) (pond) W69 ☑
assault X92.3 ☑
following
dive or jump W16.611 ☑
striking bottom W16.621 ☑
fall W16.111 ☑
striking
bottom W16.121 ☑
side W16.131 ☑
stated as undetermined whether accidental or intentional Y21.4 ☑
suicide (attempt) X71.3 ☑
quarry — *see* Drowning, in, specified place NEC
quenching tank — *see* Drowning, in, specified place NEC
reservoir — *see* Drowning, in, specified place NEC

☑ **Additional Character Required — Refer to the Tabular List for Character Selection**   ▽ **Subterms under main terms may continue to next column or page**

Drowning — *continued*
- in — *continued*
  - river — *see* Drowning, in, natural water
  - sea — *see* Drowning, in, natural water
  - specified place NEC W73 ☑
    - assault X92.8 ☑
    - following
      - dive or jump W16.811 ☑
        - striking
          - bottom W16.821 ☑
          - wall W16.831 ☑
      - fall W16.311 ☑
        - striking
          - bottom W16.321 ☑
          - wall W16.331 ☑
    - stated as undetermined whether accidental or intentional Y21.8 ☑
    - suicide (attempt) X71.8 ☑
  - stream — *see* Drowning, in, natural water
  - swimming-pool W67 ☑
    - assault X92.1 ☑
      - following fall X92.2 ☑
    - following
      - dive or jump W16.511 ☑
        - striking
          - bottom W16.521 ☑
          - wall W16.531 ☑
      - fall W16.011 ☑
        - striking
          - bottom W16.021 ☑
          - wall W16.031 ☑
    - stated as undetermined whether accidental or intentional Y21.2 ☑
      - following fall Y21.3 ☑
    - suicide (attempt) X71.1 ☑
      - following fall X71.2 ☑
  - war operations — *see* War operations, restriction of airway
- resulting from accident to watercraft — *see* Drowning, due to, accident, watercraft
- self-inflicted X71.9 ☑
- stated as undetermined whether accidental or intentional Y21.9 ☑
- suicide (attempt) X71.9 ☑

E

Earth falling (on) W20.0 ☑
- caused by cataclysmic earth surface movement or eruption — *see* Landslide

Earth (surface) movement NEC — *see* Forces of nature, earth movement

Earthquake (any injury) X34 ☑

Effect(s) (adverse) **of**
- air pressure (any) — *see* Air, pressure
- cold, excessive (exposure to) — *see* Exposure, cold
- heat (excessive) — *see* Heat
- hot place (weather) B — *see* Heat
- insolation X30 ☑
- late — *see* Sequelae
- motion — *see* Motion
- nuclear explosion or weapon in war operations — *see* War operations, nuclear weapon
- radiation — *see* Radiation
- travel — *see* Travel

Electric shock (accidental) (by) (in) — *see* Exposure, electric current

Electrocution (accidental) — *see* Exposure, electric current

Endotracheal tube wrongly placed during anesthetic procedure

Entanglement
- in
  - bed linen, causing suffocation T71 ☑
  - wheel of pedal cycle V19.88 ☑

Entry of foreign body or material — *see* Foreign body

Environmental pollution related condition — *see* category Z57

Execution, legal (any method) — *see* Legal, intervention

Exhaustion
- cold — *see* Exposure, cold
- due to excessive exertion — *see* Overexertion
- heat — *see* Heat

Explosion (accidental) (of) (with secondary fire) W40.9 ☑
- acetylene W40.1 ☑
- aerosol can W36.1 ☑

Explosion — *continued*
- air tank (compressed) (in machinery) W36.2 ☑
- aircraft (in transit) (powered) NEC V95.9 ☑
  - balloon V96.05 ☑
  - fixed wing NEC (private) V95.25 ☑
    - commercial V95.35 ☑
  - glider V96.25 ☑
    - hang V96.15 ☑
    - powered V95.15 ☑
  - helicopter V95.05 ☑
  - in war operations — *see* War operations, destruction of aircraft
  - microlight V95.15 ☑
  - nonpowered V96.9 ☑
    - specified NEC V96.8 ☑
  - powered NEC V95.8 ☑
  - stated as
    - homicide (attempt) Y03.8 ☑
    - suicide (attempt) X83.0 ☑
  - ultralight V95.15 ☑
- anesthetic gas in operating room W40.1 ☑
- antipersonnel bomb W40.8 ☑
  - assault X96.0 ☑
  - homicide (attempt) X96.0 ☑
  - suicide (attempt) X75 ☑
- assault X96.9 ☑
- bicycle tire W37.0 ☑
- blasting (cap) (materials) W40.0 ☑
- boiler (machinery), not on transport vehicle W35 ☑
  - on watercraft — *see* Explosion, in, watercraft
- butane W40.1 ☑
- caused by other person X96.9 ☑
- coal gas W40.1 ☑
- detonator W40.0 ☑
- dump (munitions) W40.8 ☑
- dynamite W40.0 ☑
  - in
    - assault X96.8 ☑
    - homicide (attempt) X96.8 ☑
    - legal intervention
      - injuring
        - bystander Y35.112 ☑
        - law enforcement personnel Y35.111 ☑
        - suspect Y35.113 ☑
    - suicide (attempt) X75 ☑
- explosive (material) W40.9 ☑
  - gas W40.1 ☑
  - in blasting operation W40.0 ☑
  - specified NEC W40.8 ☑
    - in
      - assault X96.8 ☑
      - homicide (attempt) X96.8 ☑
      - legal intervention
        - injuring
          - bystander Y35.192 ☑
          - law enforcement personnel Y35.191 ☑
          - suspect Y35.193 ☑
      - suicide (attempt) X75 ☑
- factory (munitions) W40.8 ☑
- fertilizer bomb W40.8 ☑
  - assault X96.3 ☑
  - homicide (attempt) X96.3 ☑
  - suicide (attempt) X75 ☑
- firearm (parts) NEC W34.19 ☑
  - airgun W34.110 ☑
  - BB gun W34.110 ☑
  - gas, air or spring-operated gun NEC W34.118 ☑
  - hangun W32.1 ☑
  - hunting rifle W33.12 ☑
  - larger firearm W33.10 ☑
    - specified NEC W33.19 ☑
  - machine gun W33.13 ☑
  - paintball gun W34.111 ☑
  - pellet gun W34.110 ☑
  - shotgun W33.11 ☑
  - Very pistol [flare] W34.19 ☑
- fire-damp W40.1 ☑
- fireworks W39 ☑
- gas (coal) (explosive) W40.1 ☑
  - cylinder W36.9 ☑
    - aerosol can W36.1 ☑
    - air tank W36.2 ☑
    - pressurized W36.3 ☑
    - specified NEC W36.8 ☑

Explosion — *continued*
- gasoline (fumes) (tank) not in moving motor vehicle W40.1 ☑
  - bomb W40.8 ☑
    - assault X96.1 ☑
    - homicide (attempt) X96.1 ☑
    - suicide (attempt) X75 ☑
  - in motor vehicle — *see* Accident, transport, by type of vehicle
- grain store W40.8 ☑
- grenade W40.8 ☑
  - in
    - assault X96.8 ☑
    - homicide (attempt) X96.8 ☑
    - legal intervention
      - injuring
        - bystander Y35.192 ☑
        - law enforcement personnel Y35.191 ☑
        - suspect Y35.193 ☑
    - suicide (attempt) X75 ☑
- handgun (parts) — *see* Explosion, firearm, hangun (parts)
- homicide (attempt) X96.9 ☑
  - antipersonnel bomb — *see* Explosion, antipersonnel bomb
  - fertilizer bomb — *see* Explosion, fertilizer bomb
  - gasoline bomb — *see* Explosion, gasoline bomb
  - letter bomb — *see* Explosion, letter bomb
  - pipe bomb — *see* Explosion, pipe bomb
  - specified NEC X96.8 ☑
- hose, pressurized W37.8 ☑
- hot water heater, tank (in machinery) W35 ☑
  - on watercraft — *see* Explosion, in, watercraft
- in, on
  - dump W40.8 ☑
  - factory W40.8 ☑
  - mine (of explosive gases) NEC W40.1 ☑
  - watercraft V93.59 ☑
    - powered craft V93.53 ☑
      - ferry boat V93.51 ☑
      - fishing boat V93.52 ☑
      - jetskis V93.53 ☑
      - liner V93.51 ☑
      - merchant ship V93.50 ☑
      - passenger ship V93.51 ☑
      - sailboat V93.54 ☑
- letter bomb W40.8 ☑
  - assault X96.2 ☑
  - homicide (attempt) X96.2 ☑
  - suicide (attempt) X75 ☑
- machinery (*see also* Contact, with, by type of machine)
  - on board watercraft — *see* Explosion, in, watercraft
  - pressure vessel — *see* Explosion, by type of vessel
- methane W40.1 ☑
- mine W40.1 ☑
- missile NEC W40.8 ☑
- mortar bomb W40.8 ☑
  - in
    - assault X96.8 ☑
    - homicide (attempt) X96.8 ☑
    - legal intervention
      - injuring
        - bystander Y35.192 ☑
        - law enforcement personnel Y35.191 ☑
        - suspect Y35.193 ☑
    - suicide (attempt) X75 ☑
- munitions (dump) (factory) W40.8 ☑
- pipe, pressurized W37.8 ☑
  - bomb W40.8 ☑
    - assault X96.4 ☑
    - homicide (attempt) X96.4 ☑
    - suicide (attempt) X75 ☑
- pressure, pressurized
  - cooker W38 ☑
  - gas tank (in machinery) W36.3 ☑
  - hose W37.8 ☑
  - pipe W37.8 ☑
  - specified device NEC W38 ☑
  - tire W37.8 ☑
    - bicycle W37.0 ☑
  - vessel (in machinery) W38 ☑
- propane W40.1 ☑
- self-inflicted X75 ☑
- shell (artillery) NEC W40.8 ☑
  - during war operations — *see* War operations, explosion

Explosion — continued
  shell — continued
    in
      legal intervention
        injuring
          bystander Y35.122 ☑
          law enforcement personnel Y35.121 ☑
          suspect Y35.123 ☑
      war — see War operations, explosion
  spacecraft V95.45 ☑
  stated as undetermined whether accidental or intentional Y25 ☑
  steam or water lines (in machinery) W37.8 ☑
  stove W40.9 ☑
  suicide (attempt) X75 ☑
  tire, pressurized W37.8 ☑
    bicycle W37.0 ☑
  undetermined whether accidental or intentional Y25 ☑
  vehicle tire NEC W37.8 ☑
    bicycle W37.0 ☑
  war operations — see War operations, explosion
Exposure (to) X58 ☑
  air pressure change — see Air, pressure
  cold (accidental) (excessive) (extreme) (natural) (place) X31 ☑
    assault Y08.89 ☑
    due to
      man-made conditions W93.8 ☑
        dry ice (contact) W93.01 ☑
          inhalation W93.02 ☑
        liquid air (contact) (hydrogen) (nitrogen) W93.11 ☑
          inhalation W93.12 ☑
        refrigeration unit (deep freeze) W93.2 ☑
      suicide (attempt) X83.2 ☑
      weather (conditions) X31 ☑
    homicide (attempt) Y08.89 ☑
    self-inflicted X83.2 ☑
  due to abandonment or neglect X58 ☑
  electric current W86.8 ☑
    appliance (faulty) W86.8 ☑
      domestic W86.0 ☑
    caused by other person Y08.89 ☑
    conductor (faulty) W86.1 ☑
    control apparatus (faulty) W86.1 ☑
    electric power generating plant, distribution station W86.1 ☑
    electroshock gun — see Exposure, electric current, taser
    high-voltage cable W85 ☑
    homicide (attempt) Y08.89 ☑
    legal execution — see Legal, intervention, specified means NEC
    lightning — see subcategory T75.0 ☑
    live rail W86.8 ☑
    misadventure in medical or surgical procedure in electroshock therapy Y63.4
    motor (electric) (faulty) W86.8 ☑
      domestic W86.0 ☑
    self-inflicted X83.1 ☑
    specified NEC W86.8 ☑
      domestic W86.0 ☑
    stun gun — see Exposure, electric current, taser
    suicide (attempt) X83.1 ☑
    taser W86.8 ☑
      assault Y08.89 ☑
      legal intervention — see category Y35 ☑
      self-harm (intentional) X83.8 ☑
      undetermined intent Y33 ☑
    third rail W86.8 ☑
    transformer (faulty) W86.1 ☑
    transmission lines W85 ☑
  environmental tobacco smoke X58 ☑
  excessive
    cold — see Exposure, cold
    heat (natural) NEC X30 ☑
      man-made W92 ☑
  factor(s) NOS X58 ☑
    environmental NEC X58 ☑
    man-made NEC W99 ☑
    natural NEC — see Forces of nature
    specified NEC X58 ☑
  fire, flames (accidental) X08.8 ☑
    assault X97 ☑

Exposure — continued
  fire, flames — continued
    campfire — see Exposure, fire, controlled, not in building
    controlled (in)
      with ignition (of) clothing (see also Ignition, clothes) X06.2 ☑
        nightwear X05 ☑
      bonfire — see Exposure, fire, controlled, not in building
      brazier (in building or structure) (see also Exposure, fire, controlled, building)
        not in building or structure — see Exposure, fire, controlled, not in building
      building or structure X02.0 ☑
        with
          fall from building X02.3 ☑
          from building X02.5 ☑
          injury due to building collapse X02.2 ☑
          smoke inhalation X02.1 ☑
          hit by object from building X02.4 ☑
          specified mode of injury NEC X02.8 ☑
      fireplace, furnace or stove — see Exposure, fire, controlled, building
      not in building or structure X03.0 ☑
        with
          fall X03.3 ☑
          smoke inhalation X03.1 ☑
          hit by object X03.4 ☑
          specified mode of injury NEC X03.8 ☑
      trash — see Exposure, fire, controlled, not in building
    fireplace — see Exposure, fire, controlled, building
    fittings or furniture (in building or structure) (uncontrolled) — see Exposure, fire, uncontrolled, building
    forest (uncontrolled) — see Exposure, fire, uncontrolled, not in building
    grass (uncontrolled) — see Exposure, fire, uncontrolled, not in building
    hay (uncontrolled) — see Exposure, fire, uncontrolled, not in building
    homicide (attempt) X97 ☑
    ignition of highly flammable material X04 ☑
    in, of, on, starting in
      machinery — see Contact, with, by type of machine
      motor vehicle (in motion) (see also Accident, transport, occupant by type of vehicle) V87.8 ☑
        with collision — see Collision
      railway rolling stock, train, vehicle V81.81 ☑
        with collision — see Accident, transport, railway vehicle occupant
      street car (in motion) V82.8 ☑
        with collision — see Accident, transport, streetcar occupant
      transport vehicle NEC (see also Accident, transport)
        with collision — see Collision
      war operations (see also War operations, fire)
        from nuclear explosion — see War operations, nuclear weapons
      watercraft (in transit) (not in transit) V91.09 ☑
        localized — see Burn, on board watercraft, due to, fire on board
        powered craft V91.03 ☑
          ferry boat V91.01 ☑
          fishing boat V91.02 ☑
          jet skis V91.03 ☑
          liner V91.01 ☑
          merchant ship V91.00 ☑
          passenger ship V91.01 ☑
        unpowered craft V91.08 ☑
          canoe V91.05 ☑
          inflatable V91.06 ☑
          kayak V91.05 ☑
          sailboat V91.04 ☑
          surf-board V91.08 ☑
          waterskis V91.07 ☑
          windsurfer V91.08 ☑
    lumber (uncontrolled) — see Exposure, fire, uncontrolled, not in building
    mine (uncontrolled) — see Exposure, fire, uncontrolled, not in building

Exposure — continued
  fire, flames — continued
    prairie (uncontrolled) — see Exposure, fire, uncontrolled, not in building
    resulting from
      explosion — see Explosion
      lightning X08.8 ☑
    self-inflicted X76 ☑
    specified NEC X08.8 ☑
    started by other person X97 ☑
    stated as undetermined whether accidental or intentional Y26 ☑
    stove — see Exposure, fire, controlled, building
    suicide (attempt) X76 ☑
    tunnel (uncontrolled) — see Exposure, fire, uncontrolled, not in building
    uncontrolled
      in building or structure X00.0 ☑
        with
          fall from building X00.3 ☑
          injury due to building collapse X00.2 ☑
          jump from building X00.5 ☑
          smoke inhalation X00.1 ☑
        bed X08.00 ☑
          due to
            cigarette X08.01 ☑
            specified material NEC X08.09 ☑
        furniture NEC X08.20 ☑
          due to
            cigarette X08.21 ☑
            specified material NEC X08.29 ☑
        hit by object from building X00.4 ☑
        sofa X08.10 ☑
          due to
            cigarette X08.11 ☑
            specified material NEC X08.19 ☑
        specified mode of injury NEC X00.8 ☑
      not in building or structure (any) X01.0 ☑
        with
          fall X01.3 ☑
          smoke inhalation X01.1 ☑
          hit by object X01.4 ☑
          specified mode of injury NEC X01.8 ☑
    undetermined whether accidental or intentional Y26 ☑
  forces of nature NEC — see Forces of nature
  G-forces (abnormal) W49.9 ☑
  gravitational forces (abnormal) W49.9 ☑
  heat (natural) NEC — see Heat
  high-pressure jet (hydraulic) (pneumatic) W49.9 ☑
  hydraulic jet W49.9 ☑
  inanimate mechanical force W49.9 ☑
  jet, high-pressure (hydraulic) (pneumatic) W49.9 ☑
  lightning — see subcategory T75.0 ☑
    causing fire — see Exposure, fire
  mechanical forces NEC W49.9 ☑
    animate NEC W64 ☑
    inanimate NEC W49.9 ☑
  noise W42.9 ☑
    supersonic W42.0 ☑
  noxious substance — see Table of Drugs and Chemicals
  pneumatic jet W49.9 ☑
  prolonged in deep-freeze unit or refrigerator W93.2 ☑
  radiation — see Radiation
  smoke (see also Exposure, fire)
    tobacco, second hand Z77.22
  specified factors NEC X58 ☑
  sunlight X32 ☑
    man-made (sun lamp) W89.8 ☑
      tanning bed W89.1 ☑
  supersonic waves W42.0 ☑
  transmission line(s), electric W85 ☑
  vibration W49.9 ☑
  waves
    infrasound W49.9 ☑
    sound W42.9 ☑
    supersonic W42.0 ☑
  weather NEC — see Forces of nature
External cause status Y99.9
  child assisting in compensated work for family Y99.8
  civilian activity done for financial or other compensation Y99.0
  civilian activity done for income or pay Y99.0
  family member assisting in compensated work for other family member Y99.8

External cause status — *continued*
 hobby not done for income Y99.8
 leisure activity Y99.8
 military activity Y99.1
 off-duty activity of military personnel Y99.8
 recreation or sport not for income or while a student
   Y99.8
 specified NEC Y99.8
 student activity Y99.8
 volunteer activity Y99.2

F

Factors, supplemental
 alcohol
  blood level
   less than 20mg/100ml Y90.0
   20-39mg/100ml Y90.1
   40-59mg/100ml Y90.2
   60-79mg/100ml Y90.3
   80-99mg/100ml Y90.4
   100-119mg/100ml Y90.5
   120-199mg/100ml Y90.6
   200-239mg/100ml Y90.7
   240mg/100ml or more Y90.8
  presence in blood, level not specified Y90.9
  presence in blood, but level not specified Y90.9
 environmental-pollution-related condition- see Z57 ☑
 nosocomial condition Y95
 work-related condition Y99.0
Failure
 in suture or ligature during surgical procedure Y65.2
 mechanical, of instrument or apparatus (any) (during
   any medical or surgical procedure) Y65.8
 sterile precautions (during medical and surgical care)
   — *see* Misadventure, failure, sterile precautions,
   by type of procedure
 to
  introduce tube or instrument Y65.4
   endotracheal tube during anesthesia Y65.3
  make curve (transport vehicle) NEC — *see* Accident,
    transport
  remove tube or instrument Y65.4
Fall, falling (accidental) W19 ☑
 building W20.1 ☑
  burning (uncontrolled fire) X00.3 ☑
 down
  embankment W17.81 ☑
  escalator W10.0 ☑
  hill W17.81 ☑
  ladder W11 ☑
  ramp W10.2 ☑
  stairs, steps W10.9 ☑
 due to
  bumping against
   object W18.00 ☑
    sharp glass W18.02 ☑
    specified NEC W18.09 ☑
    sports equipment W18.01 ☑
   person W03 ☑
    due to ice or snow W00.0 ☑
    on pedestrian conveyance — *see* Accident,
      transport, pedestrian, conveyance
  collision with another person W03 ☑
   due to ice or snow W00.0 ☑
   involving pedestrian conveyance — *see* Acci-
     dent, transport, pedestrian, conveyance
  grocery cart tipping over W17.82 ☑
  ice or snow W00.9 ☑
   from one level to another W00.2 ☑
   on stairs or steps W00.1 ☑
  involving pedestrian conveyance — *see* Acci-
    dent, transport, pedestrian, conveyance
  on same level W00.0 ☑
  slipping (on moving sidewalk) W01.0 ☑
   with subsequent striking against object
     W01.10 ☑
    furniture W01.190 ☑
    sharp object W01.119 ☑
     glass W01.110 ☑
     power tool or machine W01.111 ☑
     specified NEC W01.118 ☑
    specified NEC W01.198 ☑
  striking against
   object W18.00 ☑
    sharp glass W18.02 ☑
    specified NEC W18.09 ☑

Fall, falling — *continued*
 due to — *continued*
  striking against — *continued*
   object — *continued*
    sports equipment W18.01 ☑
   person W03 ☑
    due to ice or snow W00.0 ☑
    on pedestrian conveyance — *see* Accident,
      transport, pedestrian, conveyance
 earth (with asphyxia or suffocation (by pressure)) —
   see Earth, falling
 from, off, out of
  aircraft NEC (with accident to aircraft NEC) V97.0 ☑
   while boarding or alighting V97.1 ☑
  balcony W13.0 ☑
  bed W06 ☑
  boat, ship, watercraft NEC (with drowning or sub-
    mersion) — *see* Drowning, due to, fall over-
    board
   with hitting bottom or object V94.0 ☑
  bridge W13.1 ☑
  building W13.9 ☑
   burning (uncontrolled fire) X00.3 ☑
  cavity W17.2 ☑
  chair W07 ☑
  cherry picker W17.89 ☑
  cliff W15 ☑
  dock W17.4 ☑
  embankment W17.81 ☑
  escalator W10.0 ☑
  flagpole W13.8 ☑
  furniture NEC W08 ☑
  grocery cart W17.82 ☑
  haystack W17.89 ☑
  high place NEC W17.89 ☑
   stated as undetermined whether accidental or
     intentional Y30 ☑
  hole W17.2 ☑
  incline W10.2 ☑
  ladder W11 ☑
  lifting device W17.89 ☑
  machine, machinery (*see also* Contact, with, by
    type of machine)
   not in operation W17.89 ☑
  manhole W17.1 ☑
  mobile elevated work platform [MEWP] W17.89 ☑
  motorized mobility scooter W05.2 ☑
  one level to another NEC W17.89 ☑
   intentional, purposeful, suicide (attempt)
     X80 ☑
   stated as undetermined whether accidental or
     intentional Y30 ☑
  pit W17.2 ☑
  playground equipment W09.8 ☑
   jungle gym W09.2 ☑
   slide W09.0 ☑
   swing W09.1 ☑
  quarry W17.89 ☑
  railing W13.9 ☑
  ramp W10.2 ☑
  roof W13.2 ☑
  scaffolding W12 ☑
  scooter (nonmotorized) W05.1 ☑
   motorized mobility W05.2 ☑
  sky lift W17.89 ☑
  stairs, steps W10.9 ☑
   curb W10.1 ☑
   due to ice or snow W00.1 ☑
   escalator W10.0 ☑
   incline W10.2 ☑
   ramp W10.2 ☑
   sidewalk curb W10.1 ☑
   specified NEC W10.8 ☑
  stepladder W11 ☑
  storm drain W17.1 ☑
  streetcar NEC V82.6 ☑
   with antecedent collision — *see* Accident,
     transport, streetcar occupant
   while boarding or alighting V82.4 ☑
  structure NEC W13.8 ☑
   burning (uncontrolled fire) X00.3 ☑
  table W08 ☑
  toilet W18.11 ☑
   with subsequent striking against object
     W18.12 ☑

Fall, falling — *continued*
 from, off, out of — *continued*
  train NEC V81.6 ☑
   during derailment (without antecedent colli-
     sion) V81.7 ☑
    with antecedent collision — *see* Accident,
      transport, railway vehicle occupant
   while boarding or alighting V81.4 ☑
  transport vehicle after collision — *see* Accident,
    transport, by type of vehicle, collision
  tree W14 ☑
  vehicle (in motion) NEC (*see also* Accident, trans-
    port) V89.9 ☑
   motor NEC (*see also* Accident, transport, occu-
     pant, by type of vehicle) V87.8 ☑
   stationary W17.89 ☑
    while boarding or alighting B — *see* Acci-
      dent, transport, by type of vehicle,
      while boarding or alighting
  viaduct W13.8 ☑
  wall W13.8 ☑
  watercraft (*see also* Drowning, due to, fall over-
    board)
   with hitting bottom or object V94.0 ☑
  well W17.0 ☑
  wheelchair, non-moving W05.0 ☑
   powered — *see* Accident, transport, pedestrian,
     conveyance occupant, specified type NEC
  window W13.4 ☑
 in, on
  aircraft NEC V97.0 ☑
   with accident to aircraft V97.0 ☑
   while boarding or alighting V97.1 ☑
  bathtub (empty) W18.2 ☑
   filled W16.212 ☑
    causing drowning W16.211 ☑
  escalator W10.0 ☑
  incline W10.2 ☑
  ladder W11 ☑
  machine, machinery — *see* Contact, with, by type
    of machine
  object, edged, pointed or sharp (with cut) — *see*
    Fall, by type
  playground equipment W09.8 ☑
   jungle gym W09.2 ☑
   slide W09.0 ☑
   swing W09.1 ☑
  ramp W10.2 ☑
  scaffolding W12 ☑
  shower W18.2 ☑
   causing drowning W16.211 ☑
  staircase, stairs, steps W10.9 ☑
   curb W10.1 ☑
   due to ice or snow W00.1 ☑
   escalator W10.0 ☑
   incline W10.2 ☑
   specified NEC W10.8 ☑
  streetcar (without antecedent collision) V82.5 ☑
   with antecedent collision — *see* Accident,
     transport, streetcar occupant
   while boarding or alighting V82.4 ☑
  train (without antecedent collision) V81.5 ☑
   with antecedent collision — *see* Accident,
     transport, railway vehicle occupant
   during derailment (without antecedent colli-
     sion) V81.7 ☑
    with antecedent collision — *see* Accident,
      transport, railway vehicle occupant
   while boarding or alighting V81.4 ☑
  transport vehicle after collision — *see* Accident,
    transport, by type of vehicle, collision
  watercraft V93.39 ☑
   due to
    accident to craft V91.29 ☑
     powered craft V91.23 ☑
      ferry boat V91.21 ☑
      fishing boat V91.22 ☑
      jetskis V91.23 ☑
      liner V91.21 ☑
      merchant ship V91.20 ☑
      passenger ship V91.21 ☑
     unpowered craft
      canoe V91.25 ☑
      inflatable V91.26 ☑
      kayak V91.25 ☑
      sailboat V91.24 ☑

Fall, falling — *continued*
in, on — *continued*
  watercraft — *continued*
    powered craft V93.33 ☑
      ferry boat V93.31 ☑
      fishing boat V93.32 ☑
      jetskis V93.33 ☑
      liner V93.31 ☑
      merchant ship V93.30 ☑
      passenger ship V93.31 ☑
    unpowered craft V93.38 ☑
      canoe V93.35 ☑
      inflatable V93.36 ☑
      kayak V93.35 ☑
      sailboat V93.34 ☑
      surf-board V93.38 ☑
      windsurfer V93.38 ☑
into
  cavity W17.2 ☑
  dock W17.4 ☑
  fire — *see* Exposure, fire, by type
  haystack W17.89 ☑
  hole W17.2 ☑
  lake — *see* Fall, into, water
  lake — *see* Fall, into, water
  manhole W17.1 ☑
  moving part of machinery — *see* Contact, with, by type of machine
  ocean — *see* Fall, into, water
  opening in surface NEC W17.89 ☑
  pit W17.2 ☑
  pond — *see* Fall, into, water
  quarry W17.89 ☑
  river — *see* Fall, into, water
  shaft W17.89 ☑
  storm drain W17.1 ☑
  stream — *see* Fall, into, water
  swimming pool (*see also* Fall, into, water, in, swimming pool)
    empty W17.3 ☑
  tank W17.89 ☑
  water W16.42 ☑
    causing drowning W16.41 ☑
    from watercraft — *see* Drowning, due to, fall overboard
    hitting diving board W21.4 ☑
    in
      bathtub W16.212 ☑
        causing drowning W16.211 ☑
      bucket W16.222 ☑
        causing drowning W16.221 ☑
      natural body of water W16.112 ☑
        causing drowning W16.111 ☑
        striking
          bottom W16.122 ☑
            causing drowning W16.121 ☑
          side W16.132 ☑
            causing drowning W16.131 ☑
      specified water NEC W16.312 ☑
        causing drowning W16.311 ☑
        striking
          bottom W16.322 ☑
            causing drowning W16.321 ☑
          wall W16.332 ☑
            causing drowning W16.331 ☑
      swimming pool W16.012 ☑
        causing drowning W16.011 ☑
        striking
          bottom W16.022 ☑
            causing drowning W16.031 ☑
          wall W16.032 ☑
            causing drowning W16.021 ☑
      utility bucket W16.222 ☑
        causing drowning W16.221 ☑
  well W17.0 ☑
involving
  bed W06 ☑
  chair W07 ☑
  furniture NEC W08 ☑
  glass — *see* Fall, by type
  playground equipment W09.8 ☑
    jungle gym W09.2 ☑
    slide W09.0 ☑
    swing W09.1 ☑
  roller blades — *see* Accident, transport, pedestrian, conveyance

Fall, falling — *continued*
involving — *continued*
  skateboard(s) — *see* Accident, transport, pedestrian, conveyance
  skates (ice) (in line) (roller) — *see* Accident, transport, pedestrian, conveyance
  skis — *see* Accident, transport, pedestrian, conveyance
  table W08 ☑
  wheelchair, non-moving W05.0 ☑
    powered — *see* Accident, transport, pedestrian, conveyance, specified type NEC
object — *see* Struck by, object, falling
off
  toilet W18.11 ☑
    with subsequent striking against object W18.12 ☑
  on same level W18.30 ☑
    due to
      specified NEC W18.39 ☑
      stepping on an object W18.31 ☑
out of
  bed W06 ☑
  building NEC W13.8 ☑
  chair W07 ☑
  furniture NEC W08 ☑
  wheelchair, non-moving W05.0 ☑
    powered — *see* Accident, transport, pedestrian, conveyance, specified type NEC
  window W13.4 ☑
over
  animal W01.0 ☑
  cliff W15 ☑
  embankment W17.81 ☑
  small object W01.0 ☑
rock W20.8 ☑
same level W18.30 ☑
  from
    being crushed, pushed, or stepped on by a crowd or human stampede W52 ☑
    collision, pushing, shoving, by or with other person W03 ☑
    slipping, stumbling, tripping W01.0 ☑
      involving ice or snow W00.0 ☑
      involving skates (ice) (roller), skateboard, skis — *see* Accident, transport, pedestrian, conveyance
snowslide (avalanche) — *see* Landslide
stone W20.8 ☑
structure W20.1 ☑
  burning (uncontrolled fire) X00.3 ☑
through
  bridge W13.1 ☑
  floor W13.3 ☑
  roof W13.2 ☑
  wall W13.8 ☑
  window W13.4 ☑
timber W20.8 ☑
tree (caused by lightning) W20.8 ☑
while being carried or supported by other person(s) W04 ☑
Fallen on by
  animal (not being ridden) NEC W55.89 ☑
Felo-de-se — *see* Suicide
Fight (hand) (fists) (foot) — *see* Assault, fight
Fire (accidental) — *see* Exposure, fire
Firearm discharge — *see* Discharge, firearm
Fireball effects from nuclear explosion in war operations — *see* War operations, nuclear weapons
Fireworks (explosion) W39 ☑
Flash burns from explosion — *see* Explosion
Flood (any injury) (caused by) X38 ☑
  collapse of man-made structure causing earth movement X36.0 ☑
  tidal wave — *see* Forces of nature, tidal wave
Food (any type) **in**
  air passages (with asphyxia, obstruction, or suffocation) — *see* categories T17 and T18
  alimentary tract causing asphyxia (due to compression of trachea) — *see* categories T17 and T18
Forces of nature X39.8 ☑
  avalanche X36.1 ☑
    causing transport accident — *see* Accident, transport, by type of vehicle
  blizzard X37.2 ☑

Forces of nature — *continued*
  cataclysmic storm X37.9 ☑
    with flood X38 ☑
    blizzard X37.2 ☑
    cloudburst X37.8 ☑
    cyclone X37.1 ☑
    dust storm X37.3 ☑
    hurricane X37.0 ☑
    specified storm NEC X37.8 ☑
    storm surge X37.0 ☑
    tornado X37.1 ☑
    twister X37.1 ☑
    typhoon X37.0 ☑
  cloudburst X37.8 ☑
  cold (natural) X31 ☑
  cyclone X37.1 ☑
  dam collapse causing earth movement X36.0 ☑
  dust storm X37.3 ☑
  earth movement X36.1 ☑
    caused by dam or structure collapse X36.0 ☑
    earthquake X34 ☑
  earthquake X34 ☑
  flood (caused by) X38 ☑
    dam collapse X36.0 ☑
    tidal wave B — *see* Forces of nature, tidal wave
  heat (natural) X30 ☑
  hurricane X37.0 ☑
  landslide X36.1 ☑
    causing transport accident — *see* Accident, transport, by type of vehicle
  lightning — *see* subcategory T75.0 ☑
    causing fire — *see* Exposure, fire
  mudslide X36.1 ☑
    causing transport accident — *see* Accident, transport, by type of vehicle
  radiation (natural) X39.08 ☑
    radon X39.01 ☑
  radon X39.01 ☑
  specified force NEC X39.8 ☑
  storm surge X37.0 ☑
  structure collapse causing earth movement X36.0 ☑
  sunlight X32 ☑
  tidal wave X37.41 ☑
    due to
      earthquake X37.41 ☑
      landslide X37.43 ☑
      storm X37.42 ☑
      volcanic eruption X37.41 ☑
  tornado X37.1 ☑
  tsunami X37.41 ☑
  twister X37.1 ☑
  typhoon X37.0 ☑
  volcanic eruption X35 ☑
Foreign body
  aspiration — *see* Index to Diseases and Injuries, Foreign body, respiratory tract
  entering through skin W45.8 ☑
    can lid W45.2 ☑
    nail W45.0 ☑
    paper W45.1 ☑
    specified NEC W45.8 ☑
    splinter W45.8 ☑
Forest fire (exposure to) — *see* Exposure, fire, uncontrolled, not in building
Found injured X58 ☑
  from exposure (to) — *see* Exposure
  on
    highway, road(way), street V89.9 ☑
    railway right of way V81.9 ☑
Fracture (circumstances unknown or unspecified) X58 ☑
  due to specified cause NEC X58 ☑
Freezing — *see* Exposure, cold
Frostbite X31 ☑
  due to man-made conditions — *see* Exposure, cold, man-made
Frozen — *see* Exposure, cold

G

Gored by bull W55.22 ☑
Gunshot wound W34.00 ☑

H

Hailstones, injured by X39.8 ☑

☑ Additional Character Required — Refer to the Tabular List for Character Selection   ▽ Subterms under main terms may continue to next column or page

Hanged herself or himself — *see* Hanging, self-inflicted
Hanging (accidental) (*see also* category) T71 ☑
  legal execution — *see* Legal, intervention, specified
      means NEC
Heat (effects of) (excessive) X30 ☑
  due to
    man-made conditions W92 ☑
      on board watercraft V93.29 ☑
        fishing boat V93.22 ☑
        merchant ship V93.20 ☑
        passenger ship V93.21 ☑
        sailboat V93.24 ☑
        specified powered craft NEC V93.23 ☑
    weather (conditions) X30 ☑
  from
    electric heating apparatus causing burning X16 ☑
    nuclear explosion in war operations — *see* War
      operations, nuclear weapons
  inappropriate in local application or packing in medical
    or surgical procedure Y63.5
Hemorrhage
  delayed following medical or surgical treatment
    without mention of misadventure — *see* Index
      to Diseases and Injuries, Complication(s)
  during medical or surgical treatment as misadventure
    — *see* Index to Diseases and Injuries, Complica-
    tion(s)
High
  altitude (effects) — *see* Air, pressure, low
  level of radioactivity, effects — *see* Radiation
  pressure (effects) — *see* Air, pressure, high
  temperature, effects — *see* Heat
Hit, hitting (accidental) by — *see* Struck by
Hitting against — *see* Striking against
Homicide (attempt) (justifiable) — *see* Assault
Hot
  place, effects (*see also* Heat)
  weather, effects X30 ☑
House fire (uncontrolled) — *see* Exposure, fire, uncon-
  trolled, building
Humidity, causing problem X39.8 ☑
Hunger X58 ☑
Hurricane (any injury) X37.0 ☑
Hypobarism, hypobaropathy — *see* Air, pressure, low

I

Ictus
  caloris (*see also* Heat)
  solaris X30 ☑
Ignition (accidental) (*see also* Exposure, fire) X08.8 ☑
  anesthetic gas in operating room W40.1 ☑
  apparel X06.2 ☑
    from highly flammable material X04 ☑
    nightwear X05 ☑
  bed linen (sheets) (spreads) (pillows) (mattress) — *see*
    Exposure, fire, uncontrolled, building, bed
  benzine X04 ☑
  clothes, clothing NEC (from controlled fire) X06.2 ☑
    from
      highly flammable material X04 ☑
  ether X04 ☑
    in operating room W40.1 ☑
  explosive material — *see* Explosion
  gasoline X04 ☑
  jewelry (plastic) (any) X06.0 ☑
  kerosene X04 ☑
  material
    explosive — *see* Explosion
    highly flammable with secondary explosion X04 ☑
  nightwear X05 ☑
  paraffin X04 ☑
  petrol X04 ☑
Immersion (accidental) (*see also* Drowning)
  hand or foot due to cold (excessive) X31 ☑
Implantation of quills of porcupine W55.89 ☑
Inanition (from) (hunger) X58 ☑
  thirst X58 ☑
Inappropriate operation performed
  correct operation on wrong side or body part (wrong
    side) (wrong site) Y65.53
  operation intended for another patient done on wrong
    patient Y65.52
  wrong operation performed on correct patient Y65.51
Inattention after, at birth (homicidal intent) (infantici-
  dal intent) X58 ☑

Incident, adverse
  device
    anesthesiology Y70.8
      accessory Y70.2
      diagnostic Y70.0
      miscellaneous Y70.8
      monitoring Y70.0
      prosthetic Y70.2
      rehabilitative Y70.1
      surgical Y70.3
      therapeutic Y70.1
    cardiovascular Y71.8
      accessory Y71.2
      diagnostic Y71.0
      miscellaneous Y71.8
      monitoring Y71.0
      prosthetic Y71.2
      rehabilitative Y71.1
      surgical Y71.3
      therapeutic Y71.1
    gastroenterology Y73.8
      accessory Y73.2
      diagnostic Y73.0
      miscellaneous Y73.8
      monitoring Y73.0
      prosthetic Y73.2
      rehabilitative Y73.1
      surgical Y73.3
      therapeutic Y73.1
    general
      hospital Y74.8
        accessory Y74.2
        diagnostic Y74.0
        miscellaneous Y74.8
        monitoring Y74.0
        prosthetic Y74.2
        rehabilitative Y74.1
        surgical Y74.3
        therapeutic Y74.1
      surgical Y81.8
        accessory Y81.2
        diagnostic Y81.0
        miscellaneous Y81.8
        monitoring Y81.0
        prosthetic Y81.2
        rehabilitative Y81.1
        surgical Y81.3
        therapeutic Y81.1
    gynecological Y76.8
      accessory Y76.2
      diagnostic Y76.0
      miscellaneous Y76.8
      monitoring Y76.0
      prosthetic Y76.2
      rehabilitative Y76.1
      surgical Y76.3
      therapeutic Y76.1
    medical Y82.9
      specified type NEC Y82.8
    neurological Y75.8
      accessory Y75.2
      diagnostic Y75.0
      miscellaneous Y75.8
      monitoring Y75.0
      prosthetic Y75.2
      rehabilitative Y75.1
      surgical Y75.3
      therapeutic Y75.1
    obstetrical Y76.8
      accessory Y76.2
      diagnostic Y76.0
      miscellaneous Y76.8
      monitoring Y76.0
      prosthetic Y76.2
      rehabilitative Y76.1
      surgical Y76.3
      therapeutic Y76.1
    ophthalmic Y77.8
      accessory Y77.2
      diagnostic Y77.0
      miscellaneous Y77.8
      monitoring Y77.0
      prosthetic Y77.2
      rehabilitative Y77.1
      surgical Y77.3
      therapeutic Y77.1
    orthopedic Y79.8
      accessory Y79.2

Incident, adverse — *continued*
  device — *continued*
    orthopedic — *continued*
      diagnostic Y79.0
      miscellaneous Y79.8
      monitoring Y79.0
      prosthetic Y79.2
      rehabilitative Y79.1
      surgical Y79.3
      therapeutic Y79.1
    otorhinolaryngological Y72.8
      accessory Y72.2
      diagnostic Y72.0
      miscellaneous Y72.8
      monitoring Y72.0
      prosthetic Y72.2
      rehabilitative Y72.1
      surgical Y72.3
      therapeutic Y72.1
    personal use Y74.8
      accessory Y74.2
      diagnostic Y74.0
      miscellaneous Y74.8
      monitoring Y74.0
      prosthetic Y74.2
      rehabilitative Y74.1
      surgical Y74.3
      therapeutic Y74.1
    physical medicine Y80.8
      accessory Y80.2
      diagnostic Y80.0
      miscellaneous Y80.8
      monitoring Y80.0
      prosthetic Y80.2
      rehabilitative Y80.1
      surgical Y80.3
      therapeutic Y80.1
    plastic surgical Y81.8
      accessory Y81.2
      diagnostic Y81.0
      miscellaneous Y81.8
      monitoring Y81.0
      prosthetic Y81.2
      rehabilitative Y81.1
      surgical Y81.3
      therapeutic Y81.1
    radiological Y78.8
      accessory Y78.2
      diagnostic Y78.0
      miscellaneous Y78.8
      monitoring Y78.0
      prosthetic Y78.2
      rehabilitative Y78.1
      surgical Y78.3
      therapeutic Y78.1
    urology Y73.8
      accessory Y73.2
      diagnostic Y73.0
      miscellaneous Y73.8
      monitoring Y73.0
      prosthetic Y73.2
      rehabilitative Y73.1
      surgical Y73.3
      therapeutic Y73.1
Incineration (accidental) — *see* Exposure, fire
Infanticide — *see* Assault
Infrasound waves (causing injury) W49.9 ☑
Ingestion
  foreign body (causing injury) (with obstruction) — *see*
    Foreign body, alimentary canal
  poisonous
    plant(s) X58 ☑
    substance NEC — *see* Table of Drugs and Chemicals
Inhalation
  excessively cold substance, man-made — *see* Expo-
    sure, cold, man-made
  food (any type) (into respiratory tract) (with asphyxia,
    obstruction respiratory tract, suffocation) — *see*
    categories T17 and T18 ☑
  foreign body — *see* Foreign body, aspiration
  gastric contents (with asphyxia, obstruction respiratory
    passage, suffocation) T17.81- ☑
  hot air or gases X14.0 ☑
  liquid air, hydrogen, nitrogen W93.12 ☑
    suicide (attempt) X83.2 ☑
  steam X13.0 ☑
    assault X98.0 ☑

Inhalation — *continued*
steam — *continued*
stated as undetermined whether accidental or intentional Y27.0 ☑
suicide (attempt) X77.0 ☑
toxic gas — *see* Table of Drugs and Chemicals
vomitus (with asphyxia, obstruction respiratory passage, suffocation) T17.81- ☑
Injury, injured (accidental(ly)) NOS X58 ☑
by, caused by, from
assault — *see* Assault
law-enforcing agent, police, in course of legal intervention — *see* Legal intervention
suicide (attempt) X83.8 ☑
due to, in
civil insurrection — *see* War operations
fight (*see also* Assault, fight) Y04.0 ☑
war operations — *see* War operations
homicide (*see also* Assault) Y09
inflicted (by)
in course of arrest (attempted), suppression of disturbance, maintenance of order, by law-enforcing agents — *see* Legal intervention
other person
stated as
accidental X58 ☑
intentional, homicide (attempt) — *see* Assault
undetermined whether accidental or intentional Y33 ☑
purposely (inflicted) by other person(s) — *see* Assault
self-inflicted X83.8 ☑
stated as accidental X58 ☑
specified cause NEC X58 ☑
undetermined whether accidental or intentional Y33 ☑
Insolation, effects X30 ☑
Insufficient nourishment X58 ☑
Interruption of respiration (by)
food (lodged in esophagus) — *see* categories T17 and T18 ☑
vomitus (lodged in esophagus) T17.81- ☑
Intervention, legal — *see* Legal intervention
Intoxication
drug — *see* Table of Drugs and Chemicals
poison — *see* Table of Drugs and Chemicals

J

Jammed (accidentally)
between objects (moving) (stationary and moving) W23.0 ☑
stationary W23.1 ☑
Jumped, jumping
before moving object NEC X81.8 ☑
motor vehicle X81.0 ☑
subway train X81.1 ☑
train X81.1 ☑
undetermined whether accidental or intentional Y31 ☑
from
boat (into water) voluntarily, without accident (to or on boat) W16.712 ☑
with
accident to or on boat — *see* Accident, watercraft
drowning or submersion W16.711 ☑
suicide (attempt) X71.3 ☑
striking bottom W16.722 ☑
causing drowning W16.721 ☑
building (*see also* Jumped, from, high place) W13.9 ☑
burning (uncontrolled fire) X00.5 ☑
high place NEC W17.89 ☑
suicide (attempt) X80 ☑
undetermined whether accidental or intentional Y30 ☑
structure (*see also* Jumped, from, high place) W13.9 ☑
burning (uncontrolled fire) X00.5 ☑
into water W16.92 ☑
causing drowning W16.91 ☑
from, off watercraft — *see* Jumped, from, boat
in
natural body W16.612 ☑
causing drowning W16.611 ☑

Jumped, jumping — *continued*
into water — *continued*
in — *continued*
natural body — *continued*
striking bottom W16.622 ☑
causing drowning W16.621 ☑
specified place NEC W16.812 ☑
causing drowning W16.811 ☑
striking
bottom W16.822 ☑
causing drowning W16.821 ☑
wall W16.832 ☑
causing drowning W16.831 ☑
swimming pool W16.512 ☑
causing drowning W16.511 ☑
striking
bottom W16.522 ☑
causing drowning W16.521 ☑
wall W16.532 ☑
causing drowning W16.531 ☑
suicide (attempt) X71.3 ☑

K

Kicked by
animal NEC W55.82 ☑
person(s) (accidentally) W50.1 ☑
with intent to injure or kill Y04.0 ☑
as, or caused by, a crowd or human stampede (with fall) W52 ☑
assault Y04.0 ☑
homicide (attempt) Y04.0 ☑
in
fight Y04.0 ☑
legal intervention
injuring
bystander Y35.812 ☑
law enforcement personnel Y35.811 ☑
suspect Y35.813 ☑
Kicking against
object W22.8 ☑
sports equipment W21.9 ☑
stationary wW22.09 ☑
sports equipment W21.89 ☑
person — *see* Striking against, person
sports equipment W21.9 ☑
Killed, killing (accidentally) NOS (*see also* Injury) X58 ☑
in
action — *see* War operations
brawl, fight (hand) (fists) (foot) Y04.0 ☑
by weapon (*see also* Assault)
cutting, piercing — *see* Assault, cutting or piercing instrument
firearm — *see* Discharge, firearm, by type, homicide
self
stated as
accident NOS X58 ☑
suicide — *see* Suicide
undetermined whether accidental or intentional Y33 ☑
Knocked down (accidentally) (by) NOS X58 ☑
animal (not being ridden) NEC (*see also* Struck by, by type of animal)
crowd or human stampede W52 ☑
person W51 ☑
in brawl, fight Y04.0 ☑
transport vehicle NEC (*see also* Accident, transport) V09.9 ☑

L

Laceration NEC — *see* Injury
Lack of
care (helpless person) (infant) (newborn) X58 ☑
food except as result of abandonment or neglect X58 ☑
due to abandonment or neglect X58 ☑
water except as result of transport accident X58 ☑
due to transport accident B — *see* Accident, transport, by type
helpless person, infant, newborn X58 ☑
Landslide (falling on transport vehicle) X36.1 ☑
caused by collapse of man-made structure X36.0 ☑
Late effect — *see* Sequelae

Legal
execution (any method) — *see* Legal, intervention
intervention (by)
baton — *see* Legal, intervention, blunt object, baton
bayonet — *see* Legal, intervention, sharp object, bayonet
blow — *see* Legal, intervention, manhandling
blunt object
baton
injuring
bystander Y35.312 ☑
law enforcement personnel Y35.311 ☑
suspect Y35.313 ☑
injuring
bystander Y35.302 ☑
law enforcement personnel Y35.301 ☑
suspect Y35.303 ☑
specified NEC
injuring
bystander Y35.392 ☑
law enforcement personnel Y35.391 ☑
suspect Y35.393 ☑
stave
injuring
bystander Y35.392 ☑
law enforcement personnel Y35.391 ☑
suspect Y35.393 ☑
bomb — *see* Legal, intervention, explosive
cutting or piercing instrument — *see* Legal, intervention, sharp object
dynamite — *see* Legal, intervention, explosive, dynamite
explosive(s)
dynamite
injuring
bystander Y35.112 ☑
law enforcement personnel Y35.111 ☑
suspect Y35.113 ☑
grenade
injuring
bystander Y35.192 ☑
law enforcement personnel Y35.191 ☑
suspect Y35.193 ☑
injuring
bystander Y35.102 ☑
law enforcement personnel Y35.101 ☑
suspect Y35.103 ☑
mortar bomb
injuring
bystander Y35.192 ☑
law enforcement personnel Y35.191 ☑
suspect Y35.193 ☑
shell
injuring
bystander Y35.122 ☑
law enforcement personnel Y35.121 ☑
suspect Y35.123 ☑
specified NEC
injuring
bystander Y35.192 ☑
law enforcement personnel Y35.191 ☑
suspect Y35.193 ☑
firearm(s) (discharge)
handgun
injuring
bystander Y35.022 ☑
law enforcement personnel Y35.021 ☑
suspect Y35.023 ☑
injuring
bystander Y35.002 ☑
law enforcement personnel Y35.001 ☑
suspect Y35.003 ☑
machine gun
injuring
bystander Y35.012 ☑
law enforcement personnel Y35.011 ☑
suspect Y35.013 ☑
rifle pellet
injuring
bystander Y35.032 ☑
law enforcement personnel Y35.031 ☑
suspect Y35.033 ☑
rubber bullet
injuring
bystander Y35.042 ☑
law enforcement personnel Y35.041 ☑

Legal — *continued*
  intervention — *continued*
    firearm(s) — *continued*
      rubber bullet — *continued*
        injuring — *continued*
          suspect Y35.043 ☑
      shotgun — *see* Legal, intervention, firearm,
        specified NEC
      specified NEC
        injuring
          bystander Y35.092 ☑
          law enforcement personnel Y35.091 ☑
          suspect Y35.093 ☑
    gas (asphyxiation) (poisoning)
      injuring
        bystander Y35.202 ☑
        law enforcement personnel Y35.201 ☑
        suspect Y35.203 ☑
      specified NEC
        injuring
          bystander Y35.292 ☑
          law enforcement personnel Y35.291 ☑
          suspect Y35.293 ☑
      tear gas
        injuring
          bystander Y35.212 ☑
          law enforcement personnel Y35.211 ☑
          suspect Y35.213 ☑
    grenade — *see* Legal, intervention, explosive,
      grenade
    injuring
      bystander Y35.92 ☑
      law enforcement personnel Y35.91 ☑
      suspect Y35.93 ☑
    late effect (of) — *see* with 7th character S Y35 ☑
    manhandling
      injuring
        bystander Y35.812 ☑
        law enforcement personnel Y35.811 ☑
        suspect Y35.813 ☑
    sequelae (of) — *see* with 7th character S Y35 ☑
    sharp objects
      bayonet
        injuring
          bystander Y35.412 ☑
          law enforcement personnel Y35.411 ☑
          suspect Y35.413 ☑
      injuring
        bystander Y35.402 ☑
        law enforcement personnel Y35.401 ☑
        suspect Y35.403 ☑
      specified NEC
        injuring
          bystander Y35.492 ☑
          law enforcement personnel Y35.491 ☑
          suspect Y35.493 ☑
    specified means NEC
      injuring
        bystander Y35.892 ☑
        law enforcement personnel Y35.891 ☑
        suspect Y35.893 ☑
    stabbing — *see* Legal, intervention, sharp object
    stave — *see* Legal, intervention, blunt object, stave
    tear gas — *see* Legal, intervention, gas, tear gas
    truncheon — *see* Legal, intervention, blunt object,
      stave
Lightning (shock) (stroke) (struck by) — *see* subcategory
  T75.0 ☑
  causing fire — *see* Exposure, fire
Loss of control (transport vehicle) NEC — *see* Accident,
  transport
Lost at sea NOS — *see* Drowning, due to, fall overboard
Low
  pressure (effects) — *see* Air, pressure, low
  temperature (effects) — *see* Exposure, cold
Lying before train, vehicle or other moving object
  X81.8 ☑
  subway train X81.1 ☑
  train X81.1 ☑
  undetermined whether accidental or intentional
    Y31 ☑
Lynching — *see* Assault

M

Malfunction (mechanism or component) (of)
  firearm W34.10 ☑
    airgun W34.110 ☑
    BB gun W34.110 ☑
    gas, air or spring-operated gun NEC W34.118 ☑
    handgun W32.1 ☑
    hunting rifle W33.12 ☑
    larger firearm W33.10 ☑
      specified NEC W33.19 ☑
    machine gun W33.13 ☑
    paintball gun W34.111 ☑
    pellet gun W34.110 ☑
    shotgun W33.11 ☑
    specified NEC W34.19 ☑
    Very pistol [flare] W34.19 ☑
  handgun — *see* Malfunction, firearm, handgun
Maltreatment — *see* Perpetrator
Mangled (accidentally) NOS X58 ☑
Manhandling (in brawl, fight) Y04.0 ☑
  legal intervention — *see* Legal, intervention, manhan-
    dling
Manslaughter (nonaccidental) — *see* Assault
Mauled by animal NEC W55.89 ☑
Medical procedure, complication of (delayed or as an
    abnormal reaction without mention of misadven-
    ture) — *see* Complication of or following, by speci-
    fied type of procedure
  due to or as a result of misadventure — *see* Misadven-
    ture
Melting (due to fire) (*see also* Exposure, fire)
  apparel NEC X06.3 ☑
  clothes, clothing NEC X06.3 ☑
    nightwear X05 ☑
  fittings or furniture (burning building) (uncontrolled
    fire) X00.8 ☑
  nightwear X05 ☑
  plastic jewelry X06.1 ☑
Mental cruelty X58 ☑
Military operations (injuries to military and civilians
    occuring during peacetime on military property
    and during routine military exercises and opera-
    tions) (by) (from) (involving) Y37.90- ☑
  air blast Y37.20- ☑
  aircraft
    destruction — *see* Military operations, destruction
      of aircraft
  airway restriction — *see* Military operations, restriction
    of airways
  asphyxiation — *see* Military operations, restriction of
    airways
  biological weapons Y37.6X- ☑
  blast Y37.20- ☑
  blast fragments Y37.20- ☑
  blast wave Y37.20- ☑
  blast wind Y37.20- ☑
  bomb Y37.20- ☑
    dirty Y37.50- ☑
    gasoline Y37.31- ☑
    incendiary Y37.31- ☑
    petrol Y37.31- ☑
  bullet Y37.43- ☑
    incendiary Y37.32- ☑
    rubber Y37.41- ☑
  chemical weapons Y37.7X- ☑
  combat
    hand to hand (unarmed) combat Y37.44- ☑
    using blunt or piercing object Y37.45- ☑
  conflagration — *see* Military operations, fire
  conventional warfare NEC Y37.49- ☑
  depth-charge Y37.01- ☑
  destruction of aircraft Y37.10- ☑
    due to
      air to air missile Y37.11- ☑
      collision with other aircraft Y37.12- ☑
      detonation (accidental) of onboard munitions
        and explosives Y37.14- ☑
      enemy fire or explosives Y37.11- ☑
      explosive placed on aircraft Y37.11- ☑
      onboard fire Y37.13- ☑
      rocket propelled grenade [RPG] Y37.11- ☑
      small arms fire Y37.11- ☑
      surface to air missile Y37.11- ☑
    specified NEC Y37.19- ☑

Military operations — *continued*
  detonation (accidental) of
    onboard marine weapons Y37.05- ☑
    own munitions or munitions launch device Y37.24- ☑
  dirty bomb Y37.50- ☑
  explosion (of) Y37.20- ☑
    aerial bomb Y37.21- ☑
    bomb NOS (*see also* Military operations, bomb(s))
      Y37.20- ☑
    fragments Y37.20- ☑
    grenade Y37.29- ☑
    guided missile Y37.22- ☑
    improvised explosive device [IED] (person-borne)
      (roadside) (vehicle-borne) Y37.23- ☑
    land mine Y37.29- ☑
    marine mine (at sea) (in harbor) Y37.02- ☑
    marine weapon Y37.00- ☑
      specified NEC Y37.09- ☑
    own munitions or munitions launch device (acci-
      dental) Y37.24- ☑
    sea-based artillery shell Y37.03- ☑
    specified NEC Y37.29- ☑
    torpedo Y37.04- ☑
  fire Y37.30- ☑
    specified NEC Y37.39- ☑
  firearms
    discharge Y37.43- ☑
    pellets Y37.42- ☑
  flamethrower Y37.33- ☑
  fragments (from) (of)
    improvised explosive device [IED] (person-borne)
      (roadside) (vehicle-borne) Y37.26- ☑
    munitions Y37.25- ☑
    specified NEC Y37.29- ☑
    weapons Y37.27- ☑
  friendly fire Y37.92- ☑
  hand to hand (unarmed) combat Y37.44- ☑
  hot substances — *see* Military operations, fire
  incendiary bullet Y37.32- ☑
  nuclear weapon (effects of) Y37.50- ☑
    acute radiation exposure Y37.54- ☑
    blast pressure Y37.51- ☑
    direct blast Y37.51- ☑
    direct heat Y37.53- ☑
    fallout exposure Y37.54- ☑
    fireball Y37.53- ☑
    indirect blast (struck or crushed by blast debris)
      (being thrown by blast) Y37.52- ☑
    ionizing radiation (immediate exposure) Y37.54- ☑
    nuclear radiation Y37.54- ☑
    radiation
      ionizing (immediate exposure) Y37.54- ☑
      nuclear Y37.54- ☑
      thermal Y37.53- ☑
    secondary effects Y37.54- ☑
    specified NEC Y37.59- ☑
    thermal radiation Y37.53- ☑
  restriction of air (airway)
    intentional Y37.46- ☑
    unintentional Y37.47- ☑
  rubber bullets Y37.41- ☑
  shrapnel NOS Y37.29- ☑
  suffocation — *see* Military operations, restriction of
    airways
  unconventional warfare NEC Y37.7X- ☑
  underwater blast NOS Y37.00- ☑
  warfare
    conventional NEC Y37.49- ☑
    unconventional NEC Y37.7X- ☑
  weapon of mass destruction [WMD] Y37.91- ☑
  weapons
    biological weapons Y37.6X- ☑
    chemical Y37.7X- ☑
    nuclear (effects of) Y37.50- ☑
      acute radiation exposure Y37.54- ☑
      blast pressure Y37.51- ☑
      direct blast Y37.51- ☑
      direct heat Y37.53- ☑
      fallout exposure Y37.54- ☑
      fireball Y37.53- ☑
      indirect blast (struck or crushed by blast debris)
        (being thrown by blast) Y37.52- ☑
      radiation
        ionizing (immediate exposure) Y37.54- ☑
        nuclear Y37.54- ☑
        thermal Y37.53- ☑

Military operations — continued
  weapons — continued
    nuclear — continued
      secondary effects Y37.54- ☑
      specified NEC Y37.59- ☑
    of mass destruction [WMD] Y37.91- ☑
Misadventure(s) to patient(s) during surgical or medical care Y69
  contaminated medical or biological substance (blood, drug, fluid) Y64.9
    administered (by) NEC Y64.9
      immunization Y64.1
      infusion Y64.0
      injection Y64.1
      specified means NEC Y64.8
      transfusion Y64.0
      vaccination Y64.1
  excessive amount of blood or other fluid during transfusion or infusion Y63.0
  failure
    in dosage Y63.9
      electroshock therapy Y63.4
      inappropriate temperature (too hot or too cold) in local application and packing Y63.5
      infusion
        excessive amount of fluid Y63.0
        incorrect dilution of fluid Y63.1
      insulin-shock therapy Y63.4
      nonadministration of necessary drug or biological substance Y63.6
      overdose — see Table of Drugs and Chemicals radiation, in therapy Y63.2
      radiation
        overdose Y63.2
      specified procedure NEC Y63.8
      transfusion
        excessive amount of blood Y63.0
    mechanical, of instrument or apparatus (any) (during any procedure) Y65.8
    sterile precautions (during procedure) Y62.9
      aspiration of fluid or tissue (by puncture or catheterization, except heart) Y62.6
      biopsy (except needle aspiration) Y62.8
        needle (aspirating) Y62.6
      blood sampling Y62.6
      catheterization Y62.6
        heart Y62.5
      dialysis (kidney) Y62.2
      endoscopic examination Y62.4
      enema Y62.8
      immunization Y62.3
      infusion Y62.1
      injection Y62.3
      needle biopsy Y62.6
      paracentesis (abdominal) (thoracic) Y62.6
      perfusion Y62.2
      puncture (lumbar) Y62.6
      removal of catheter or packing Y62.8
      specified procedure NEC Y62.8
      surgical operation Y62.0
      transfusion Y62.1
      vaccination Y62.3
    suture or ligature during surgical procedure Y65.2
    to introduce or to remove tube or instrument B — see Failure, to
  hemorrhage — see Index to Diseases and Injuries, Complication(s)
  inadvertent exposure of patient to radiation Y63.3
  inappropriate
    operation performed — see Inappropriate operation performed
    temperature (too hot or too cold) in local application or packing Y63.5
  infusion (see also Misadventure, by type, infusion) Y69
    excessive amount of fluid Y63.0
    incorrect dilution of fluid Y63.1
    wrong fluid Y65.1
  mismatched blood in transfusion Y65.0
  nonadministration of necessary drug or biological substance
  overdose — see Table of Drugs and Chemicals radiation (in therapy) Y63.2
  perforation — see Index to Diseases and Injuries, Complication(s)
  performance of inappropriate operation — see Inappropriate operation performed
  puncture — see Index to Diseases and Injuries, Complication(s)

Misadventure(s) to patient(s) during surgical or medical care — continued
  specified type NEC Y65.8
    failure
      suture or ligature during surgical operation Y65.2
      to introduce or to remove tube or instrument B — see Failure, to
    infusion of wrong fluid Y65.1
    performance of inappropriate operation — see Inappropriate operation performed
    transfusion of mismatched blood Y65.0
    wrong
      fluid in infusion Y65.1
      placement of endotracheal tube during anesthetic procedure Y65.3
  transfusion — see Misadventure, by type, transfusion
    excessive amount of blood Y63.0
    mismatched blood Y65.0
  wrong
    drug given in error — see Table of Drugs and Chemicals
    fluid in infusion Y65.1
    placement of endotracheal tube during anesthetic procedure Y65.3
Mismatched blood in transfusion Y65.0
Motion sickness T75.3 ☑
Mountain sickness W94.11 ☑
Mudslide (of cataclysmic nature) — see Landslide
Murder (attempt) — see Assault

N

Nail, contact with W45.0 ☑
  gun W29.4 ☑
Neglect (criminal) (homicidal intent) X58 ☑
Noise (causing injury) (pollution) W42.9 ☑
  supersonic W42.0 ☑
Nonadministration (of)
  drug or biological substance (necessary) Y63.6
  surgical and medical care Y66
Nosocomial condition Y95

O

Object
  falling
    from, in, on, hitting
      machinery — see Contact, with, by type of machine
    set in motion by
      accidental explosion or rupture of pressure vessel W38 ☑
      firearm — see Discharge, firearm, by type
      machine(ry) — see Contact, with, by type of machine
Overdose (drug) — see Table of Drugs and Chemicals radiation Y63.2
Overexertion — see category Y93 ☑
Overexposure (accidental) (to)
  cold (see also Exposure, cold) X31 ☑
    due to man-made conditions — see Exposure, cold, man-made
  heat (see also Heat) X30 ☑
  radiation — see Radiation
  radioactivity W88.0 ☑
  sun (sunburn) X32 ☑
  weather NEC — see Forces of nature
  wind NEC — see Forces of nature
Overheated — see Heat
Overturning (accidental)
  machinery — see Contact, with, by type of machine
  transport vehicle NEC (see also Accident, transport) V89.9 ☑
  watercraft (causing drowning, submersion) (see also Drowning, due to, accident to, watercraft, overturning)
    causing injury except drowning or submersion B — see Accident, watercraft, causing, injury NEC

P

Parachute descent (voluntary) (without accident to aircraft) V97.29 ☑
Pecked by bird W61.99 ☑

Perforation during medical or surgical treatment as misadventure — see Index to Diseases and Injuries, Complication(s)

Perpetrator, perpetration, of assault, maltreatment and neglect (by) Y07.9
  boyfriend Y07.03
  brother Y07.410
    stepbrother Y07.435
  coach Y07.53
  cousin
    female Y07.491
    male Y07.490
  daycare provider Y07.519
    at-home
      adult care Y07.512
      childcare Y07.510
    care center
      adult care Y07.513
      childcare Y07.511
  family member NEC Y07.499
  father Y07.11
    adoptive Y07.13
    foster Y07.420
    stepfather Y07.430
  foster father Y07.420
  foster mother Y07.421
  girl friend Y07.04
  healthcare provider Y07.529
    mental health Y07.521
    specified NEC Y07.528
  husband Y07.01
  instructor Y07.53
  mother Y07.12
    adoptive Y07.14
    foster Y07.421
    stepmother Y07.433
  nonfamily member Y07.50
    specified NEC Y07.59
  nurse Y07.528
  occupational therapist Y07.528
  partner of parent
    female Y07.434
    male Y07.432
  physical therapist Y07.528
  sister Y07.411
  speech therapist Y07.528
  stepbrother Y07.435
  stepfather Y07.430
  stepmother Y07.433
  stepsister Y07.436
  teacher Y07.53
  wife Y07.02

Piercing — see Contact, with, by type of object or machine

Pinched
  between objects (moving) (stationary and moving) W23.0 ☑
  stationary W23.1 ☑

Pinned under machine(ry) — see Contact, with, by type of machine

Place of occurrence Y92.9
  abandoned house Y92.89
  airplane Y92.813
  airport Y92.520
  ambulatory health services establishment NEC Y92.538
  ambulatory surgery center Y92.530
  amusement park Y92.831
  apartment (co-op) — see Place of occurrence, residence, apartment
  assembly hall Y92.29
  bank Y92.510
  barn Y92.71
  baseball field Y92.320
  basketball court Y92.310
  beach Y92.832
  boarding house — see Place of occurrence, residence, boarding house
  boat Y92.814
  bowling alley Y92.39
  bridge Y92.89
  building under construction Y92.61
  bus Y92.811
    station Y92.521
  cafe Y92.511

Place of occurrence — *continued*
  campsite Y92.833
  campus — *see* Place of occurrence, school
  canal Y92.89
  car Y92.810
  casino Y92.59
  children's home — *see* Place of occurrence, residence, institutional, orphanage
  church Y92.22
  cinema Y92.26
  clubhouse Y92.29
  coal pit Y92.64
  college (community) Y92.214
  condominium — *see* Place of occurrence, residence, apartment
  construction area — *see* Place of occurrence, industrial and construction area
  convalescent home — *see* Place of occurrence, residence, institutional, nursing home
  court-house Y92.240
  cricket ground Y92.328
  cultural building Y92.258
    art gallery Y92.250
    museum Y92.251
    music hall Y92.252
    opera house Y92.253
    specified NEC Y92.258
    theater Y92.254
  dancehall Y92.252
  day nursery Y92.210
  dentist office Y92.531
  derelict house Y92.89
  desert Y92.820
  dockyard Y92.62
  dock NOS Y92.89
  doctor's office Y92.531
  dormitory — *see* Place of occurrence, residence, institutional, school dormitory
  dry dock Y92.62
  factory (building) (premises) Y92.63
  farm (land under cultivation) (outbuildings) Y92.79
    barn Y92.71
    chicken coop Y92.72
    field Y92.73
    hen house Y92.72
    house — *see* Place of occurrence, residence, house
    orchard Y92.74
    specified NEC Y92.79
  football field Y92.321
  forest Y92.821
  freeway Y92.411
  gallery Y92.250
  garage (commercial) Y92.59
    boarding house Y92.044
    military base Y92.135
    mobile home Y92.025
    nursing home Y92.124
    orphanage Y92.114
    private house Y92.015
    reform school Y92.155
  gas station Y92.524
  gasworks Y92.69
  golf course Y92.39
  gravel pit Y92.64
  grocery Y92.512
  gymnasium Y92.39
  handball court Y92.318
  harbor Y92.89
  harness racing course Y92.39
  healthcare provider office Y92.531
  highway (interstate) Y92.411
  hill Y92.828
  hockey rink Y92.330
  home — *see* Place of occurrence, residence
  hospice — *see* Place of occurrence, residence, institutional, nursing home
  hospital Y92.239
    cafeteria Y92.233
    corridor Y92.232
    operating room Y92.234
    patient
      bathroom Y92.231
      room Y92.230
    specified NEC Y92.238
  hotel Y92.59
  house (*see also* Place of occurrence, residence)
    abandoned Y92.89
    under construction Y92.61

Place of occurrence — *continued*
  industrial and construction area (yard) Y92.69
    building under construction Y92.61
    dock Y92.62
    dry dock Y92.62
    factory Y92.63
    gasworks Y92.69
    mine Y92.64
    oil rig Y92.65
    pit Y92.64
    power station Y92.69
    shipyard Y92.62
    specified NEC Y92.69
    tunnel under construction Y92.69
    workshop Y92.69
  kindergarten Y92.211
  lacrosse field Y92.328
  lake Y92.828
  library Y92.241
  mall Y92.59
  market Y92.512
  marsh Y92.828
  military
    base — *see* Place of occurrence, residence, institutional, military base
    training ground Y92.84
  mine Y92.64
  mosque Y92.22
  motel Y92.59
  motorway (interstate) Y92.411
  mountain Y92.828
  movie-house Y92.26
  museum Y92.251
  music-hall Y92.252
  not applicable Y92.9
  nuclear power station Y92.69
  nursing home — *see* Place of occurrence, residence, institutional, nursing home
  office building Y92.59
  offshore installation Y92.65
  oil rig Y92.65
  old people's home — *see* Place of occurrence, residence, institutional, specified NEC
  opera-house Y92.253
  orphanage — *see* Place of occurrence, residence, institutional, orphanage
  outpatient surgery center Y92.530
  park (public) Y92.830
    amusement Y92.831
  parking garage Y92.89
    lot Y92.481
  pavement Y92.480
  physician office Y92.531
  polo field Y92.328
  pond Y92.828
  post office Y92.242
  power station Y92.69
  prairie Y92.828
  prison — *see* Place of occurrence, residence, institutional, prison
  public
    administration building Y92.248
      city hall Y92.243
      courthouse Y92.240
      library Y92.241
      post office Y92.242
      specified NEC Y92.248
    building NEC Y92.29
    hall Y92.29
    place NOS Y92.89
  race course Y92.39
  radio station Y92.59
  railway line (bridge) Y92.85
  recreation area Y92.838
    amusement park Y92.831
    beach Y92.832
    campsite Y92.833
    park (public) Y92.830
    seashore Y92.832
    specified NEC Y92.838
  reform school - — *see* Place of occurrence, residence, institutional, reform school
  religious institution Y92.22
  residence (non-institutional) (private) Y92.009
    apartment Y92.039
      bathroom Y92.031
      bedroom Y92.032

Place of occurrence — *continued*
  residence — *continued*
    apartment — *continued*
      kitchen Y92.030
      specified NEC Y92.038
    bathroom Y92.002
    bedroom Y92.003
    boarding house Y92.049
      bathroom Y92.041
      bedroom Y92.042
      driveway Y92.043
      garage Y92.044
      garden Y92.046
      kitchen Y92.040
      specified NEC Y92.048
      swimming pool Y92.045
      yard Y92.046
    dining room Y92.001
    garden Y92.007
    home Y92.009
    house, single family Y92.019
      bathroom Y92.012
      bedroom Y92.013
      dining room Y92.011
      driveway Y92.014
      garage Y92.015
      garden Y92.017
      kitchen Y92.010
      specified NEC Y92.018
      swimming pool Y92.016
      yard Y92.017
    institutional Y92.10
      children's home — *see* Place of occurrence, residence, institutional, orphanage
      hospice — *see* Place of occurrence, residence, institutional, nursing home
      military base Y92.139
        barracks Y92.133
        garage Y92.135
        garden Y92.137
        kitchen Y92.130
        mess hall Y92.131
        specified NEC Y92.138
        swimming pool Y92.136
        yard Y92.137
      nursing home Y92.129
        bathroom Y92.121
        bedroom Y92.122
        driveway Y92.123
        garage Y92.124
        garden Y92.126
        kitchen Y92.120
        specified NEC Y92.128
        swimming pool Y92.125
        yard Y92.126
      orphanage Y92.119
        bathroom Y92.111
        bedroom Y92.112
        driveway Y92.113
        garage Y92.114
        garden Y92.116
        kitchen Y92.110
        specified NEC Y92.118
        swimming pool Y92.115
        yard Y92.116
      prison Y92.149
        bathroom Y92.142
        cell Y92.143
        courtyard Y92.147
        dining room Y92.141
        kitchen Y92.140
        specified NEC Y92.148
        swimming pool Y92.146
      reform school Y92.159
        bathroom Y92.152
        bedroom Y92.153
        dining room Y92.151
        driveway Y92.154
        garage Y92.155
        garden Y92.157
        kitchen Y92.150
        specified NEC Y92.158
        swimming pool Y92.156
        yard Y92.157
      school dormitory Y92.169
        bathroom Y92.162
        bedroom Y92.163
        dining room Y92.161

Place of occurrence — *continued*
  residence — *continued*
    institutional — *continued*
      school dormitory — *continued*
        kitchen Y92.160
        specified NEC Y92.168
      specified NEC Y92.199
        bathroom Y92.192
        bedroom Y92.193
        dining room Y92.191
        driveway Y92.194
        garage Y92.195
        garden Y92.197
        kitchen Y92.190
        specified NEC Y92.198
        swimming pool Y92.196
        yard Y92.197
    kitchen Y92.000
    mobile home Y92.029
      bathroom Y92.022
      bedroom Y92.023
      dining room Y92.021
      driveway Y92.024
      garage Y92.025
      garden Y92.027
      kitchen Y92.020
      specified NEC Y92.028
      swimming pool Y92.026
      yard Y92.027
    specified place in residence NEC Y92.009
    specified residence type NEC Y92.099
      bathroom Y92.091
      bedroom Y92.092
      driveway Y92.093
      garage Y92.094
      garden Y92.096
      kitchen Y92.090
      specified NEC Y92.098
      swimming pool Y92.095
      yard Y92.096
  restaurant Y92.511
  riding school Y92.39
  river Y92.828
  road Y92.488
  rodeo ring Y92.39
  rugby field Y92.328
  same day surgery center Y92.530
  sand pit Y92.64
  school (private) (public) (state) Y92.219
    college Y92.214
    daycare center Y92.210
    elementary school Y92.211
    high school Y92.213
    kindergarten Y92.211
    middle school Y92.212
    specified NEC Y92.218
    trace school Y92.215
    university Y92.214
    vocational school Y92.215
  sea (shore) Y92.832
  senior citizen center Y92.29
  service area
    airport Y92.520
    bus station Y92.521
    gas station Y92.524
    highway rest stop Y92.523
    railway station Y92.522
  shipyard Y92.62
  shop (commercial) Y92.513
  sidewalk Y92.480
  silo Y92.79
  skating rink (roller) Y92.331
    ice Y92.330
  slaughter house Y92.86
  soccer field Y92.322
  specified place NEC Y92.89
  sports area Y92.39
    athletic
      court Y92.318
        basketball Y92.310
        specified NEC Y92.318
        squash Y92.311
        tennis Y92.312
      field Y92.328
        baseball Y92.320
        cricket ground Y92.328
        football Y92.321
        hockey Y92.328

Place of occurrence — *continued*
  sports area — *continued*
    athletic — *continued*
      field — *continued*
        soccer Y92.322
        specified NEC Y92.328
    golf course Y92.39
    gymnasium Y92.39
    riding school Y92.39
    skating rink (roller) Y92.331
      ice Y92.330
    stadium Y92.39
    swimming pool Y92.34
  squash court Y92.311
  stadium Y92.39
  steeplechasing course Y92.39
  store Y92.512
  stream Y92.828
  street and highway Y92.410
    bike path Y92.482
    freeway Y92.411
    highway ramp Y92.415
    interstate highway Y92.411
    local residential or business street Y92.414
    motorway Y92.411
    parking lot Y92.481
    parkway Y92.412
    sidewalk Y92.480
    specified NEC Y92.488
    state road Y92.413
  subway car Y92.816
  supermarket Y92.512
  swamp Y92.828
  swimming pool (public) Y92.34
    private (at) Y92.095
      boarding house Y92.045
      military base Y92.136
      mobile home Y92.026
      nursing home Y92.125
      orphanage Y92.115
      prison Y92.146
      reform school Y92.156
      single family residence Y92.016
  synagogue Y92.22
  television station Y92.59
  tennis court Y92.312
  theater Y92.254
  trade area Y92.59
    bank Y92.510
    cafe Y92.511
    casino Y92.59
    garage Y92.59
    hotel Y92.59
    market Y92.512
    office building Y92.59
    radio station Y92.59
    restaurant Y92.511
    shop Y92.513
    shopping mall Y92.59
    store Y92.512
    supermarket Y92.512
    television station Y92.59
    warehouse Y92.59
  trailer park, residential — *see* Place of occurrence,
    residence, mobile home
  trailer site NOS Y92.89
  train Y92.815
    station Y92.522
  truck Y92.812
  tunnel under construction Y92.69
  university Y92.214
  urgent (health) care center Y92.532
  vehicle (transport) Y92.818
    airplane Y92.813
    boat Y92.814
    bus Y92.811
    car Y92.810
    specified NEC Y92.818
    subway car Y92.816
    train Y92.815
    truck Y92.812
  warehouse Y92.59
  water reservoir Y92.89
  wilderness area Y92.828
    desert Y92.820
    forest Y92.821
    marsh Y92.828
    mountain Y92.828

Place of occurrence — *continued*
  wilderness area — *continued*
    prairie Y92.828
    specified NEC Y92.828
    swamp Y92.828
  workshop Y92.69
  yard, private Y92.096
    boarding house Y92.046
    mobile home Y92.027
    single family house Y92.017
  youth center Y92.29
  zoo (zoological garden) Y92.834
Plumbism — *see* Table of Drugs and Chemicals, lead
Poisoning (accidental) (by) (*see also* Table of Drugs and
  Chemicals)
  by plant, thorns, spines, sharp leaves or other mecha-
    nisms NEC X58 ☑
  carbon monoxide
    generated by
      motor vehicle — *see* Accident, transport
      watercraft (in transit) (not in transit) V93.89 ☑
        ferry boat V93.81 ☑
        fishing boat V93.82 ☑
        jet skis V93.83 ☑
        liner V93.81 ☑
        merchant ship V93.80 ☑
        passenger ship V93.81 ☑
        powered craft NEC V93.83 ☑
  caused by injection of poisons into skin by plant
    thorns, spines, sharp leaves X58 ☑
    marine or sea plants (venomous) X58 ☑
  execution — *see* Legal, intervention, gas
  intervention
    by gas — *see* Legal, intervention, gas
    other specified means — *see* Legal, interven-
      tion, specified means NEC
  exhaust gas
    generated by
      motor vehicle — *see* Accident, transport
      watercraft (in transit) (not in transit) V93.89 ☑
        ferry boat V93.81 ☑
        fishing boat V93.82 ☑
        jet skis V93.83 ☑
        liner V93.81 ☑
        merchant ship V93.80 ☑
        passenger ship V93.81 ☑
        powered craft NEC V93.83 ☑
  fumes or smoke due to
    explosion (*see also* Explosion) W40.9 ☑
    fire — *see* Exposure, fire
    ignition — *see* Ignition
  gas
    in legal intervention — *see* Legal, intervention, gas
    legal execution — *see* Legal, intervention, gas
  in war operations — *see* War operations
  legal
Powder burn (by) (from)
  airgun W34.110 ☑
  BB gun W34.110 ☑
  firearm NEC W34.19 ☑
  gas, air or spring-operated gun NEC W34.118 ☑
  handgun W32.1 ☑
  hunting rifle W33.12 ☑
  larger firearm W33.10 ☑
    specified NEC W33.19 ☑
  machine gun W33.13 ☑
  paintball gun W34.111 ☑
  pellet gun W34.110 ☑
  shotgun W33.11 ☑
  Very pistol [flare] W34.19 ☑
Premature cessation (of) **surgical and medical care**
  Y66
Privation (food) (water) X58 ☑
Procedure (operation)
  correct, on wrong side or body part (wrong side)
    (wrong site) Y65.53
  intended for another patient done on wrong patient
    Y65.52
  performed on patient not scheduled for surgery Y65.52
  performed on wrong patient Y65.52
  wrong, performed on correct patient Y65.51
Prolonged
  sitting in transport vehicle — *see* Travel, by type of
    vehicle
  stay in
    high altitude as cause of anoxia, barodontalgia,
      barotitis or hypoxia W94.11 ☑

Prolonged — *continued*
  stay in — *continued*
    weightless environment X52 ☑
Pulling, excessive — *see* Overexertion
Puncture, puncturing (*see also* Contact, with, by type of object or machine)
  by
    plant thorns, spines, sharp leaves or other mechanisms NEC W60 ☑
  during medical or surgical treatment as misadventure — *see* Index to Diseases and Injuries, Complication(s)
Pushed, pushing (accidental) (injury in) (overexertion) (*see also* Overexertion)
  by other person(s) (accidental) W51 ☑
    with fall W03 ☑
      due to ice or snow W00.0 ☑
    as, or caused by, a crowd or human stampede (with fall) W52 ☑
    before moving object NEC Y02.8 ☑
      motor vehicle Y02.0 ☑
      subway train Y02.1 ☑
      train Y02.1 ☑
    from
      high place NEC
        in accidental circumstances W17.89 ☑
        stated as
          intentional, homicide (attempt) Y01 ☑
          undetermined whether accidental or intentional Y30 ☑
      transport vehicle NEC (*see also* Accident, transport) V89.9 ☑
        stated as
          intentional, homicide (attempt) Y08.89 ☑

R

Radiation (exposure to)
  arc lamps W89.0 ☑
  atomic power plant (malfunction) NEC W88.1 ☑
  complication of or abnormal reaction to medical radiotherapy Y84.2
  electromagnetic, ionizing W88.0 ☑
  gamma rays W88.1 ☑
  in
    war operations (from or following nuclear explosion) — *see* War operations
  inadvertent exposure of patient (receiving test or therapy) Y63.3
  infrared (heaters and lamps) W90.1 ☑
    excessive heat from W92 ☑
  ionized, ionizing (particles, artificially accelerated)
    radioisotopes W88.1 ☑
    specified NEC W88.8 ☑
    x-rays W88.0 ☑
  isotopes, radioactive — *see* Radiation, radioactive isotopes
  laser(s) W90.2 ☑
    in war operations — *see* War operations
    misadventure in medical care Y63.2
  light sources (man-made visible and ultraviolet) W89.9 ☑
    natural X32 ☑
    specified NEC W89.8 ☑
    tanning bed W89.1 ☑
    welding light W89.0 ☑
  man-made visible light W89.9 ☑
    specified NEC W89.8 ☑
    tanning bed W89.1 ☑
    welding light W89.0 ☑
  microwave W90.8 ☑
  misadventure in medical or surgical procedure Y63.2
  natural NEC X39.08 ☑
  radon X39.01 ☑
  overdose (in medical or surgical procedure) Y63.2
  radar W90.0 ☑
  radioactive isotopes (any) W88.1 ☑
    atomic power plant malfunction W88.1 ☑
    misadventure in medical or surgical treatment Y63.2
  radiofrequency W90.0 ☑
  radium NEC W88.1 ☑
  sun X32 ☑
  ultraviolet (light) (man-made) W89.9 ☑
    natural X32 ☑

Radiation — *continued*
  ultraviolet — *continued*
    specified NEC W89.8 ☑
    tanning bed W89.1 ☑
    welding light W89.0 ☑
  welding arc, torch, or light W89.0 ☑
    excessive heat from W92 ☑
  x-rays (hard) (soft) W88.0 ☑
Range disease W94.11 ☑
Rape (attempted) T74.2-
Rat bite W53.11 ☑
Reaction, abnormal to medical procedure (*see also* Complication of or following, by type of procedure) Y84.9
  with misadventure — *see* Misadventure
  biologicals — *see* Table of Drugs and Chemicals
  drugs — *see* Table of Drugs and Chemicals
  vaccine — *see* Table of Drugs and Chemicals
Recoil
  airgun W34.110 ☑
  BB gun W34.110 ☑
  firearm NEC W34.19 ☑
  gas, air or spring-operated gun NEC W34.118 ☑
  handgun W32.1 ☑
  hunting rifle W33.12 ☑
  larger firearm W33.10 ☑
    specified NEC W33.19 ☑
  machine gun W33.13 ☑
  paintball gun W34.111 ☑
  pellet W34.110 ☑
  shotgun W33.11 ☑
  Very pistol [flare] W34.19 ☑
Reduction in
  atmospheric pressure — *see* Air, pressure, change
Rock falling on or hitting (accidentally) (person) W20.8 ☑
  in cave-in W20.0 ☑
Run over (accidentally) (by)
  animal (not being ridden) NEC W55.89 ☑
  machinery — *see* Contact, with, by specified type of machine
  transport vehicle NEC (*see also* Accident, transport) V09.9 ☑
    intentional homicide (attempt) Y03.0 ☑
    motor NEC V09.20 ☑
      intentional homicide (attempt) Y03.0 ☑
Running
  before moving object X81.8 ☑
    motor vehicle X81.0 ☑
Running off, away
  animal (being ridden) (*see also* Accident, transport) V80.918 ☑
    not being ridden W55.89 ☑
  animal-drawn vehicle NEC (*see also* Accident, transport) V80.928 ☑
  highway, road(way), street
    transport vehicle NEC (*see also* Accident, transport) V89.9 ☑
Rupture pressurized devices — *see* Explosion, by type of device

S

Saturnism — *see* Table of Drugs and Chemicals, lead
Scald, scalding (accidental) (by) (from) (in) X19 ☑
  air (hot) X14.1 ☑
  gases (hot) X14.1 ☑
  homicide (attempt) — *see* Assault, burning, hot object
  inflicted by other person
    stated as intentional, homicide (attempt) — *see* Assault, burning, hot object
  liquid (boiling) (hot) NEC X12 ☑
    stated as undetermined whether accidental or intentional Y27.2 ☑
    suicide (attempt) X77.2 ☑
  local application of externally applied substance in medical or surgical care Y63.5
  metal (molten) (liquid) (hot) NEC X18 ☑
  self-inflicted X77.9 ☑
  stated as undetermined whether accidental or intentional Y27.8 ☑
  steam X13.1 ☑
    assault X98.0 ☑
    stated as undetermined whether accidental or intentional Y27.0 ☑
    suicide (attempt) X77.0 ☑

Scald, scalding — *continued*
  suicide (attempt) X77.9 ☑
  vapor (hot) X13.1 ☑
    assault X98.0 ☑
    stated as undetermined whether accidental or intentional Y27.0 ☑
    suicide (attempt) X77.0 ☑
Scratched by
  cat W55.03 ☑
  person(s) (accidentally) W50.4 ☑
    with intent to injure or kill Y04.0 ☑
    as, or caused by, a crowd or human stampede (with fall) W52 ☑
    assault Y04.0 ☑
    homicide (attempt) Y04.0 ☑
    in
      fight Y04.0 ☑
      legal intervention
        injuring
          bystander Y35.892 ☑
          law enforcement personnel Y35.891 ☑
          suspect Y35.893 ☑
Seasickness T75.3 ☑
Self-harm NEC (*see also* External cause by type, undetermined whether accidental or intentional)
  intentional — *see* Suicide
  poisoning NEC — *see* Table of Drugs and Chemicals, poisoning, accidental
Self-inflicted (injury) **NEC** (*see also* External cause by type, undetermined whether accidental or intentional)
  intentional — *see* Suicide
  poisoning NEC — *see* Table of Drugs and Chemicals, poisoning, accidental
Sequelae (of)
  accident NEC — *see* W00-X58 with 7th character S
  assault (homicidal) (any means) — *see* X92-Y08 with 7th character S
  homicide, attempt (any means) — *see* X92-Y08 with 7th character S
  injury undetermined whether accidentally or purposely inflicted — *see* Y21-Y33 with 7th character S
  intentional self-harm (classifiable to X71-X83) — *see* X71-X83 with 7th character S
  legal intervention — *see* with 7th character S Y35 ☑
  motor vehicle accident — *see* V00-V99 with 7th character S
  suicide, attempt (any means) — *see* X71-X83 with 7th character S
  transport accident — *see* V00-V99 with 7th character S
  war operations — *see* War operations
Shock
  electric — *see* Exposure, electric current
  from electric appliance (any) (faulty) W86.8 ☑
    domestic W86.0 ☑
    suicide (attempt) X83.1 ☑
Shooting, shot (accidental(ly)) (*see also* Discharge, firearm, by type)
  herself or himself — *see* Discharge, firearm by type, self-inflicted
  homicide (attempt) — *see* Discharge, firearm by type, homicide
  in war operations — *see* War operations
  inflicted by other person — *see* Discharge, firearm by type, homicide
    accidental — *see* Discharge, firearm, by type of firearm
  legal
    execution — *see* Legal, intervention, firearm
    intervention — *see* Legal, intervention, firearm
  self-inflicted — *see* Discharge, firearm by type, suicide
    accidental — *see* Discharge, firearm, by type of firearm
  suicide (attempt) — *see* Discharge, firearm by type, suicide
Shoving (accidentally) **by other person** — *see* Pushed, by other person
Sickness
  alpine W94.11 ☑
  motion — *see* Motion
  mountain W94.11 ☑

Sinking (accidental)
 watercraft (causing drowning, submersion) (see also
  Drowning, due to, accident to, watercraft, sinking)
  causing injury except drowning or submersion B
   — see Accident, watercraft, causing, injury
   NEC
Siriasis X32 ☑
Slashed wrists — see Cut, self-inflicted
Slipping (accidental) (on same level) (with fall) W01.0 ☑
 without fall W18.40 ☑
  due to
   specified NEC W18.49 ☑
   stepping from one level to another W18.43 ☑
   stepping into hole or opening W18.42 ☑
   stepping on object W18.41 ☑
  on
   ice W00.0 ☑
    with skates — see Accident, transport, pedestri-
     an, conveyance
   mud W01.0 ☑
   oil W01.0 ☑
   snow W00.0 ☑
    with skis — see Accident, transport, pedestrian,
     conveyance
   surface (slippery) (wet) NEC W01.0 ☑
Sliver, wood, contact with W45.8 ☑
Smoldering (due to fire) — see Exposure, fire
Sodomy (attempted) **by force** T74.2 ☑
Sound waves (causing injury) W42.9 ☑
 supersonic W42.0 ☑
Splinter, contact with W45.8 ☑
Stab, stabbing B — see Cut
Starvation X58 ☑
Status of external cause Y99.9
 child assisting in compensated work for family Y99.8
 civilian activity done for financial or other compensation Y99.0
 civilian activity done for income or pay Y99.0
 family member assisting in compensated work for
  other family member Y99.8
 hobby not done for income Y99.8
 leisure activity Y99.8
 military activity Y99.1
 off-duty activity of military personnel Y99.8
 recreation or sport not for income or while a student
  Y99.8
 specified NEC Y99.8
 student activity Y99.8
 volunteer activity Y99.2
Stepped on
 by
  animal (not being ridden) NEC W55.89 ☑
  crowd or human stampede W52 ☑
  person W50.0 ☑
Stepping on
 object W22.8 ☑
  with fall W18.31 ☑
  sports equipment W21.9 ☑
  stationary W22.09 ☑
   sports equipment W21.89 ☑
 person W51 ☑
  by crowd or human stampede W52 ☑
 sports equipment W21.9 ☑
Sting
 arthropod, nonvenomous W57 ☑
 insect, nonvenomous W57 ☑
Storm (cataclysmic) B — see Forces of nature, cataclysmic
  storm
Straining, excessive — see Overexertion
Strangling — see Strangulation
Strangulation (accidental) T71 ☑
Strenuous movements — see category Y93
Striking against
 airbag (automobile) W22.10 ☑
  driver side W22.11 ☑
  front passenger side W22.12 ☑
  specified NEC W22.19 ☑
 bottom when
  diving or jumping into water (in) W16.822 ☑
   causing drowning W16.821 ☑
   from boat W16.722 ☑
    causing drowning W16.721 ☑
   natural body W16.622 ☑
    causing drowning W16.821 ☑
   swimming pool W16.522 ☑
    causing drowning W16.521 ☑

Striking against — continued
 bottom when — continued
  falling into water (in) W16.322 ☑
   causing drowning W16.321 ☑
   fountain — see Striking against, bottom when,
    falling into water, specified NEC
   natural body W16.122 ☑
    causing drowning W16.121 ☑
   reservoir — see Striking against, bottom when,
    falling into water, specified NEC
   specified NEC W16.322 ☑
    causing drowning W16.321 ☑
   swimming pool W16.022 ☑
    causing drowning W16.021 ☑
 diving board (swimming-pool) W21.4 ☑
 object W22.8 ☑
  with
   drowning or submersion — see Drowning
   fall — see Fall, due to, bumping against, object
   caused by crowd or human stampede (with fall)
    W52 ☑
  furniture W22.03 ☑
  lamppost W22.02 ☑
  sports equipment W21.9 ☑
  stationary W22.09 ☑
   sports equipment W21.89 ☑
  wall W22.01 ☑
 person(s) W51 ☑
  with fall W03 ☑
   due to ice or snow W00.0 ☑
  as, or caused by, a crowd or human stampede (with
   fall) W52 ☑
  assault Y04.2 ☑
  homicide (attempt) Y04.2 ☑
 sports equipment W21.9 ☑
 wall (when) W22.01 ☑
  diving or jumping into water (in) W16.832 ☑
   causing drowning W16.831 ☑
   swimming pool W16.532 ☑
    causing drowning W16.531 ☑
  falling into water (in) W16.332 ☑
   causing drowning W16.331 ☑
   fountain — see Striking against, wall when,
    falling into water, specified NEC
   natural body W16.132 ☑
    causing drowning W16.131 ☑
   reservoir — see Striking against, wall when,
    falling into water, specified NEC
   specified NEC W16.332 ☑
    causing drowning W16.331 ☑
   swimming pool W16.032 ☑
    causing drowning W16.031 ☑
  swimming pool (when) W22.042 ☑
   causing drowning W22.041 ☑
   diving or jumping into water W16.532 ☑
    causing drowning W16.531 ☑
   falling into water W16.032 ☑
    causing drowning W16.031 ☑
Struck (accidentally) **by**
 airbag (automobile) W22.10 ☑
  driver side W22.11 ☑
  front passenger side W22.12 ☑
  specified NEC W22.19 ☑
 alligator W58.02 ☑
 animal (not being ridden) NEC W55.89 ☑
 avalanche — see Landslide
 ball (hit) (thrown) W21.00 ☑
  assault Y08.09 ☑
  baseball W21.03 ☑
  basketball W21.05 ☑
  football W21.01 ☑
  golf ball W21.04 ☑
  soccer W21.02 ☑
  softball W21.07 ☑
  specified NEC W21.09 ☑
  volleyball W21.06 ☑
 bat or racquet
  baseball bat W21.11 ☑
   assault Y08.02 ☑
  golf club W21.13 ☑
   assault Y08.09 ☑
  specified NEC W21.19 ☑
   assault Y08.09 ☑
  tennis racquet W21.12 ☑
   assault Y08.09 ☑

Struck (accidentally) **by** — continued
 bullet (see also Discharge, firearm by type)
  in war operations — see War operations
 crocodile W58.12 ☑
 dog W54.1 ☑
 flare, Very pistol — see Discharge, firearm
  NEC
 hailstones X39.8 ☑
 hockey (ice)
  field
   puck W21.221 ☑
   stick W21.211 ☑
  puck W21.220 ☑
  stick W21.210 ☑
   assault Y08.01 ☑
 landslide — see Landslide
 law-enforcement agent (on duty) — see Legal, intervention, manhandling
  with blunt object — see Legal, intervention, blunt
   object
 lightning T75.0 ☑
  causing fire — see Exposure, fire
 machine — see Contact, with, by type of machine
 mammal NEC W55.89 ☑
  marine W56.32 ☑
 marine animal W56.82 ☑
 missile
  firearm — see Discharge, firearm by type
  in war operations — see War operations, missile
 object W22.8 ☑
  blunt W22.8 ☑
   assault Y00 ☑
   suicide (attempt) X79 ☑
   undetermined whether accidental or intention-
    al Y29 ☑
  falling W20.8 ☑
   from, in, on
    building W20.1 ☑
     burning (uncontrolled fire) X00.4 ☑
    cataclysmic
     earth surface movement NEC — see
      Landslide
     storm — see Forces of nature, cata-
      clysmic storm
    cave-in W20.0 ☑
    earthquake X34 ☑
    machine (in operation) — see Contact, with,
     by type of machine
    structure W20.1 ☑
     burning X00.4 ☑
    transport vehicle (in motion) — see Acci-
     dent, transport, by type of vehicle
    watercraft V93.49 ☑
     due to
      accident to craft V91.39 ☑
       powered craft V91.33 ☑
        ferry boat V91.31 ☑
        fishing boat V91.32 ☑
        jetskis V91.33 ☑
        liner V91.31 ☑
        merchant ship V91.30 ☑
        passenger ship V91.31 ☑
       unpowered craft V91.38 ☑
        canoe V91.35 ☑
        inflatable V91.36 ☑
        kayak V91.35 ☑
        sailboat V91.34 ☑
        surf-board V91.38 ☑
        windsurfer V91.38 ☑
      powered craft V93.43 ☑
       ferry boat V93.41 ☑
       fishing boat V93.42 ☑
       jetskis V93.43 ☑
       liner V93.41 ☑
       merchant ship V93.40 ☑
       passenger ship V93.41 ☑
      unpowered craft V93.48 ☑
       sailboat V93.44 ☑
       surf-board V93.48 ☑
       windsurfer V93.48 ☑
  moving NEC W20.8 ☑
  projected W20.8 ☑
   assault Y00 ☑
   in sports W21.9 ☑
    assault Y08.09 ☑
    ball W21.00 ☑

☑ Additional Character Required — Refer to the Tabular List for Character Selection   ▽ Subterms under main terms may continue to next column or page

Struck (accidentally) **by** — *continued*
  object — *continued*
    projected — *continued*
      in sports — *continued*
        ball — *continued*
          baseball W21.03 ☑
          basketball W21.05 ☑
          football W21.01 ☑
          golf ball W21.04 ☑
          soccer W21.02 ☑
          softball W21.07 ☑
          specified NEC W21.09 ☑
          volleyball W21.06 ☑
        bat or racquet
          baseball bat W21.11 ☑
            assault Y08.02 ☑
          golf club W21.13 ☑
            assault Y08.09 ☑
          specified NEC W21.19 ☑
            assault Y08.09 ☑
          tennis racquet W21.12 ☑
            assault Y08.09 ☑
        hockey (ice)
          field
            puck W21.221 ☑
            stick W21.211 ☑
          puck W21.220 ☑
          stick W21.210 ☑
            assault Y08.01 ☑
        specified NEC W21.89 ☑
      set in motion by explosion — *see* Explosion
    thrown W20.8 ☑
      assault Y00 ☑
      in sports W21.9 ☑
        assault Y08.09 ☑
        ball W21.00 ☑
          baseball W21.03 ☑
          basketball W21.05 ☑
          football W21.01 ☑
          golf ball W21.04 ☑
          soccer W21.02 ☑
          soft ball W21.07 ☑
          specified NEC W21.09 ☑
          volleyball W21.06 ☑
        bat or racquet
          baseball bat W21.11 ☑
            assault Y08.02 ☑
          golf club W21.13 ☑
            assault Y08.09 ☑
          specified NEC W21.19 ☑
            assault Y08.09 ☑
          tennis racquet W21.12 ☑
            assault Y08.09 ☑
        hockey (ice)
          field
            puck W21.221 ☑
            stick W21.211 ☑
          puck W21.220 ☑
          stick W21.210 ☑
            assault Y08.01 ☑
        specified NEC W21.89 ☑
    other person(s) W50.0 ☑
      with
        blunt object W22.8 ☑
          intentional, homicide (attempt) Y00 ☑
          sports equipment W21.9 ☑
          undetermined whether accidental or intentional Y29 ☑
        fall W03 ☑
          due to ice or snow W00.0 ☑
      as, or caused by, a crowd or human stampede (with fall) W52 ☑
      assault Y04.2 ☑
      homicide (attempt) Y04.2 ☑
      in legal intervention
        injuring
          bystander Y35.812 ☑
          law enforcement personnel Y35.811 ☑
          suspect Y35.813 ☑
        sports equipment W21.9 ☑
      police (on duty) — *see* Legal, intervention, manhandling
        with blunt object — *see* Legal, intervention, blunt object
    sports equipment W21.9 ☑
      assault Y08.09 ☑

Struck (accidentally) **by** — *continued*
  sports equipment — *continued*
    ball W21.00 ☑
      baseball W21.03 ☑
      basketball W21.05 ☑
      football W21.01 ☑
      golf ball W21.04 ☑
      soccer W21.02 ☑
      soft ball W21.07 ☑
      specified NEC W21.09 ☑
      volleyball W21.06 ☑
    bat or racquet
      baseball bat W21.11 ☑
        assault Y08.02 ☑
      golf club W21.13 ☑
        assault Y08.09 ☑
      specified NEC W21.19 ☑
      tennis racquet W21.12 ☑
        assault Y08.09 ☑
    cleats (shoe) W21.31 ☑
    foot wear NEC W21.39 ☑
    football helmet W21.81 ☑
    hockey (ice)
      field
        puck W21.221 ☑
        stick W21.211 ☑
      puck W21.220 ☑
      stick W21.210 ☑
        assault Y08.01 ☑
    skate blades W21.32 ☑
    specified NEC W21.89 ☑
      assault Y08.09 ☑
  thunderbolt — *see* subcategory T75.0 ☑
    causing fire — *see* Exposure, fire
  transport vehicle NEC (*see also* Accident, transport) V09.9 ☑
    intentional, homicide (attempt) Y03.0 ☑
    motor NEC (*see also* Accident, transport) V09.20 ☑
      homicide Y03.0 ☑
  vehicle (transport) NEC — *see* Accident, transport, by type of vehicle
    stationary (falling from jack, hydraulic lift, ramp) W20.8 ☑
Stumbling
  without fall W18.40 ☑
    due to
      specified NEC W18.49 ☑
      stepping from one level to another W18.43 ☑
      stepping into hole or opening W18.42 ☑
      stepping on object W18.41 ☑
    over
      animal NEC W01.0 ☑
        with fall W18.09 ☑
      carpet, rug or (small) object W22.8 ☑
        with fall W18.09 ☑
      person W51 ☑
        with fall W03 ☑
          due to ice or snow W00.0 ☑
Submersion (accidental) — *see* Drowning
Suffocation (accidental) (by external means) (by pressure) (mechanical) (*see also* category) T71 ☑
  due to, by
    avalanche — *see* Landslide
    explosion — *see* Explosion
    fire — *see* Exposure, fire
    food, any type (aspiration) (ingestion) (inhalation) — *see* categories T17 and T18 ☑
    ignition — *see* Ignition
    landslide — *see* Landslide
    machine(ry) — *see* Contact, with, by type of machine
    vomitus (aspiration) (inhalation) T17.81- ☑
  in
    burning building X00.8 ☑
Suicide, suicidal (attempted) (by) X83.8 ☑
  blunt object X79 ☑
  burning, burns X76 ☑
    hot object X77.9 ☑
      fluid NEC X77.2 ☑
      household appliance X77.3 ☑
      specified NEC X77.8 ☑
      steam X77.0 ☑
      tap water X77.1 ☑
      vapors X77.0 ☑
  caustic substance — *see* Table of Drugs and Chemicals
  cold, extreme X83.2 ☑

Suicide, suicidal — *continued*
  collision of motor vehicle with
    motor vehicle X82.0 ☑
    specified NEC X82.8 ☑
    train X82.1 ☑
    tree X82.2 ☑
  crashing of aircraft X83.0 ☑
  cut (any part of body) X78.9 ☑
  cutting or piercing instrument X78.9 ☑
    dagger X78.2 ☑
    glass X78.0 ☑
    knife X78.1 ☑
    specified NEC X78.8 ☑
    sword X78.2 ☑
  drowning (in) X71.9 ☑
    bathtub X71.0 ☑
    natural water X71.3 ☑
    specified NEC X71.8 ☑
    swimming pool X71.1 ☑
      following fall X71.2 ☑
  electrocution X83.1 ☑
  explosive(s) (material) X75 ☑
  fire, flames X76 ☑
  firearm X74.9 ☑
    airgun X74.01 ☑
    handgun X72 ☑
    hunting rifle X73.1 ☑
    larger X73.9 ☑
      specified NEC X73.8 ☑
    machine gun X73.2 ☑
    shotgun X73.0 ☑
    specified NEC X74.8 ☑
  hanging X83.8 ☑
  hot object — *see* Suicide, burning, hot object
  jumping
    before moving object X81.8 ☑
      motor vehicle X81.0 ☑
      subway train X81.1 ☑
      train X81.1 ☑
    from high place X80 ☑
  late effect of attempt — *see* X71-X83 with 7th character S
  lying before moving object, train, vehicle X81.8 ☑
  poisoning — *see* Table of Drugs and Chemicals
  puncture (any part of body) — *see* Suicide, cutting or piercing instrument
  scald — *see* Suicide, burning, hot object
  sequelae of attempt — *see* X71-X83 with 7th character S
  sharp object (any) — *see* Suicide, cutting or piercing instrument
  shooting — *see* Suicide, firearm
  specified means NEC X83.8 ☑
  stab (any part of body) — *see* Suicide, cutting or piercing instrument
  steam, hot vapors X77.0 ☑
  strangulation X83.8 ☑
  submersion — *see* Suicide, drowning
  suffocation X83.8 ☑
  wound NEC X83.8 ☑
Sunstroke X32 ☑
Supersonic waves (causing injury) W42.0 ☑
Surgical procedure, complication of (delayed or as an abnormal reaction without mention of misadventure) (*see also* Complication of or following, by type of procedure)
  due to or as a result of misadventure — *see* Misadventure
Swallowed, swallowing
  foreign body — *see* Foreign body, alimentary canal
  poison — *see* Table of Drugs and Chemicals
  substance
    caustic or corrosive — *see* Table of Drugs and Chemicals
    poisonous — *see* Table of Drugs and Chemicals

T

Tackle in sport W03 ☑
Terrorism (involving) Y38.80 ☑
  biological weapons Y38.6X- ☑
  chemical weapons Y38.7X- ☑
  conflagration Y38.3X- ☑
  explosion Y38.2X- ☑
    destruction of aircraft Y38.1X- ☑
    marine weapons Y38.0X- ☑

Terrorism — *continued*
    fire Y38.3X- ☑
    firearms Y38.4X- ☑
    hot substances Y38.5X- ☑
    nuclear weapons Y38.5X- ☑
    specified method NEC Y38.89- ☑
Thirst X58 ☑
Threat to breathing
    aspiration — *see* Aspiration
    due to cave-in, falling earth or substance NEC T71 ☑
Thrown (accidentally)
    against part (any) of or object in transport vehicle (in motion) NEC (*see also* Accident, transport)
    from
        high place, homicide (attempt) Y01 ☑
        machinery — *see* Contact, with, by type of machine
        transport vehicle NEC (*see also* Accident, transport) V89.9 ☑
    off — *see* Thrown, from
Thunderbolt — *see* subcategory T75.0 ☑
    causing fire — *see* Exposure, fire
Tidal wave (any injury) NEC — *see* Forces of nature, tidal wave
Took
    overdose (drug) — *see* Table of Drugs and Chemicals
    poison — *see* Table of Drugs and Chemicals
Tornado (any injury) X37.1 ☑
Torrential rain (any injury) X37.8 ☑
Torture X58 ☑
Trampled by animal NEC W55.89 ☑
Trapped (accidentally)
    between objects (moving) (stationary and moving) — *see* Caught
    by part (any) of
        motorcycle V29.88 ☑
        pedal cycle V19.88 ☑
        transport vehicle NEC (*see also* Accident, transport) V89.9 ☑
Travel (effects) (sickness) T75.3 ☑
Tree falling on or hitting (accidentally) (person) W20.8 ☑
Tripping
    without fall W18.40 ☑
    due to
        specified NEC W18.49 ☑
        stepping from one level to another W18.43 ☑
        stepping into hole or opening W18.42 ☑
        stepping on object W18.41 ☑
    over
        animal W01.0 ☑
            with fall W01.0 ☑
        carpet, rug or (small) object W22.8 ☑
            with fall W18.09 ☑
        person W51 ☑
            with fall W03 ☑
                due to ice or snow W00.0 ☑
Twisted by person(s) (accidentally) W50.2 ☑
    with intent to injure or kill Y04.0 ☑
    as, or caused by, a crowd or human stampede (with fall) W52 ☑
    assault Y04.0 ☑
    homicide (attempt) Y04.0 ☑
    in
        fight Y04.0 ☑
        legal intervention — *see* Legal, intervention, manhandling
Twisting, excessive — *see* Overexertion

U

Underdosing of necessary drugs, medicaments or biological substances Y63.6
Undetermined intent (contact) (exposure)
    automobile collision Y32 ☑
    blunt object Y29 ☑
    drowning (submersion) (in) Y21.9 ☑
        bathtub Y21.0 ☑
            after fall Y21.1 ☑
        natural water (lake) (ocean) (pond) (river) (stream) Y21.4 ☑
        specified place NEC Y21.8 ☑
        swimming pool Y21.2 ☑
            after fall Y21.3 ☑
    explosive material Y25 ☑
    fall, jump or push from high place Y30 ☑
    falling, lying or running before moving object Y31 ☑

Undetermined intent — *continued*
    fire Y26 ☑
    firearm discharge Y24.9 ☑
        airgun (BB) (pellet) Y24.0 ☑
        handgun (pistol) (revolver) Y22 ☑
        hunting rifle Y23.1 ☑
        larger Y23.9 ☑
            hunting rifle Y23.1 ☑
            machine gun Y23.3 ☑
            military Y23.2 ☑
            shotgun Y23.0 ☑
            specified type NEC Y23.8 ☑
        machine gun Y23.3 ☑
        military Y23.2 ☑
        shotgun Y23.0 ☑
        specified type NEC Y24.8 ☑
        Very pistol Y24.8 ☑
    hot object Y27.9 ☑
        fluid NEC Y27.2 ☑
        household appliance Y27.3 ☑
        specified object NEC Y27.8 ☑
        steam Y27.0 ☑
        tap water Y27.1 ☑
        vapor Y27.0 ☑
    jump, fall or push from high place Y30 ☑
    lying, falling or running before moving object Y31 ☑
    motor vehicle crash Y32 ☑
    push, fall or jump from high place Y30 ☑
    running, falling or lying before moving object Y31 ☑
    sharp object Y28.9 ☑
        dagger Y28.2 ☑
        glass Y28.0 ☑
        knife Y28.1 ☑
        specified object NEC Y28.8 ☑
        sword Y28.2 ☑
    smoke Y26 ☑
    specified event NEC Y33 ☑

V

Vibration (causing injury) W49.9 ☑
Victim (of)
    avalanche — *see* Landslide
    earth movements NEC — *see* Forces of nature, earth movement
    earthquake X34 ☑
    flood — *see* Flood
    landslide — *see* Landslide
    lightning — *see* subcategory T75.0 ☑
        causing fire — *see* Exposure, fire
    storm (cataclysmic) NEC — *see* Forces of nature, cataclysmic storm
    volcanic eruption X35 ☑
Volcanic eruption (any injury) X35 ☑
Vomitus, gastric contents in air passages (with asphyxia, obstruction or suffocation) T17.81- ☑

W

Walked into stationary object (any) W22.09 ☑
    furniture W22.03 ☑
    lamppost W22.02 ☑
    wall W22.01 ☑
War operations (injuries to military personnel and civilians during war, civil insurrection and peacekeeping missions) (by) (from) (involving) Y36.90 ☑
    after cessation of hostilities Y36.89- ☑
        explosion (of)
            bomb placed during war operations Y36.82- ☑
            mine placed during war operations Y36.81- ☑
        specified NEC Y36.88- ☑
    air blast Y36.20- ☑
    aircraft
        destruction — *see* War operations, destruction of aircraft
        airway restriction — *see* War operations, restriction of airways
    asphyxiation — *see* War operations, restriction of airways
    biological weapons Y36.6X- ☑
    blast Y36.20- ☑
    blast fragments Y36.20- ☑
    blast wave Y36.20- ☑
    blast wind Y36.20- ☑

War operations — *continued*
    bomb Y36.20- ☑
        dirty Y36.50- ☑
        gasoline Y36.31- ☑
        incendiary Y36.31- ☑
        petrol Y36.31- ☑
    bullet Y36.43- ☑
        incendiary Y36.32- ☑
        rubber Y36.41- ☑
    chemical weapons Y36.7X- ☑
    combat
        hand to hand (unarmed) combat Y36.44- ☑
        using blunt or piercing object Y36.45- ☑
    conflagration — *see* War operations, fire
    conventional warfare NEC Y36.49- ☑
    depth-charge Y36.01- ☑
    destruction of aircraft Y36.10- ☑
        due to
            air to air missile Y36.11- ☑
            collision with other aircraft Y36.12- ☑
            detonation (accidental) of onboard munitions and explosives Y36.14- ☑
            enemy fire or explosives Y36.11- ☑
            explosive placed on aircraft Y36.11- ☑
            onboard fire Y36.13- ☑
            rocket propelled grenade [RPG] Y36.11- ☑
            small arms fire Y36.11- ☑
            surface to air missile Y36.11- ☑
        specified NEC Y36.19- ☑
    detonation (accidental) of
        onboard marine weapons Y36.05- ☑
        own munitions or munitions launch device Y36.24- ☑
    dirty bomb Y36.50- ☑
    explosion (of) Y36.20- ☑
        aerial bomb Y36.21- ☑
        after cessation of hostilities
            bomb placed during war operations Y36.82- ☑
            mine placed during war operations Y36.81- ☑
        bomb NOS (*see also* War operations, bomb(s)) Y36.20- ☑
        fragments Y36.20- ☑
        grenade Y36.29- ☑
        guided missile Y36.22- ☑
        improvised explosive device [IED] (person-borne) (roadside) (vehicle-borne) Y36.23- ☑
        land mine Y36.29- ☑
        marine mine (at sea) (in harbor) Y36.02- ☑
        marine weapon Y36.00- ☑
            specified NEC Y36.09- ☑
        own munitions or munitions launch device (accidental) Y36.24- ☑
        sea-based artillery shell Y36.03- ☑
        specified NEC Y36.29- ☑
        torpedo Y36.04- ☑
    fire Y36.30- ☑
        specified NEC Y36.39- ☑
    firearms
        discharge Y36.43- ☑
        pellets Y36.42- ☑
    flamethrower Y36.33- ☑
    fragments (from) (of)
        improvised explosive device [IED] (person-borne) (roadside) (vehicle-borne) Y36.26- ☑
        munitions Y36.25- ☑
        specified NEC Y36.29- ☑
        weapons Y36.27- ☑
    friendly fire Y36.92 ☑
    hand to hand (unarmed) combat Y36.44- ☑
    hot substances — *see* War operations, fire
    incendiary bullet Y36.32- ☑
    nuclear weapon (effects of) Y36.50- ☑
        acute radiation exposure Y36.54- ☑
        blast pressure Y36.51- ☑
        direct blast Y36.51- ☑
        direct heat Y36.53- ☑
        fallout exposure Y36.54- ☑
        fireball Y36.53- ☑
        indirect blast (struck or crushed by blast debris) (being thrown by blast) Y36.52- ☑
        ionizing radiation (immediate exposure) Y36.54- ☑
        nuclear radiation Y36.54- ☑
        radiation
            ionizing (immediate exposure) Y36.54- ☑
            nuclear Y36.54- ☑
            thermal Y36.53- ☑

☑ **Additional Character Required — Refer to the Tabular List for Character Selection**   **Subterms under main terms may continue to next column or page**

War operations — *continued*
  nuclear weapon — *continued*
    secondary effects Y36.54- ☑
    specified NEC Y36.59- ☑
    thermal radiation Y36.53- ☑
  restriction of air (airway)
    intentional Y36.46- ☑
    unintentional Y36.47- ☑
  rubber bullets Y36.41- ☑
  shrapnel NOS Y36.29- ☑
  suffocation — *see* War operations, restriction of airways
  unconventional warfare NEC Y36.7X- ☑
  underwater blast NOS Y36.00- ☑
  warfare
    conventional NEC Y36.49- ☑
    unconventional NEC Y36.7X- ☑
  weapon of mass destruction [WMD] Y36.91 ☑
  weapons
    biological weapons Y36.6X- ☑

War operations — *continued*
  weapons — *continued*
    chemical Y36.7X- ☑
    nuclear (effects of) Y36.50- ☑
      acute radiation exposure Y36.54- ☑
      blast pressure Y36.51- ☑
      direct blast Y36.51- ☑
      direct heat Y36.53- ☑
      fallout exposure Y36.54- ☑
      fireball Y36.53- ☑
      indirect blast (struck or crushed by blast debris) (being thrown by blast) Y36.52- ☑
      radiation
        ionizing (immediate exposure) Y36.54- ☑
        nuclear Y36.54- ☑
        thermal Y36.53- ☑
      secondary effects Y36.54- ☑
      specified NEC Y36.59- ☑
    of mass destruction [WMD] Y36.91 ☑

Washed
  away by flood — *see* Flood
  off road by storm (transport vehicle) — *see* Forces of nature, cataclysmic storm
Weather exposure NEC — *see* Forces of nature
Weightlessness (causing injury) (effects of) (in spacecraft, real or simulated) X52 ☑
Work related condition Y99.0
Wound (accidental) NEC (*see also* Injury) X58 ☑
  battle (*see also* War operations) Y36.90 ☑
  gunshot — *see* Discharge, firearm by type
Wreck transport vehicle NEC (*see also* Accident, transport) V89.9 ☑
Wrong
  device implanted into correct surgical site Y65.51
  fluid in infusion Y65.1
  patient, procedure performed on Y65.52
  procedure (operation) on correct patient Y65.51

ICD-10-CM Tabular List of Diseases and Injuries

Chapter 1. Certain Infectious and Parasitic Diseases (A00–B99)

Chapter Specific Guidelines with Coding Examples

The chapter specific guidelines from the ICD-10-CM Official Guidelines for Coding and Reporting have been provided below. Along with these guidelines are coding examples, contained in the shaded boxes, that have been developed to help illustrate the coding and/or sequencing guidance found in these guidelines.

a. Human immunodeficiency virus (HIV) infections

1) Code only confirmed cases

Code only confirmed cases of HIV infection/illness. This is an exception to the hospital inpatient guideline Section II, H.

In this context, "confirmation" does not require documentation of positive serology or culture for HIV; the provider's diagnostic statement that the patient is HIV positive, or has an HIV-related illness is sufficient.

> *Patient admitted with anemia with possible HIV infection*
>
> **D64.9   Anemia, unspecified**
>
> *Explanation: Only the anemia is coded in this scenario because it has not been confirmed that an HIV infection is present. This is an exception to the guideline Section II, H for hospital inpatient coding.*

2) Selection and sequencing of HIV codes

(a) Patient admitted for HIV-related condition

If a patient is admitted for an HIV-related condition, the principal diagnosis should be B20, Human immunodeficiency virus [HIV] disease followed by additional diagnosis codes for all reported HIV-related conditions.

> *HIV with PCP*
>
> **B20   Human immunodeficiency virus [HIV] disease**
>
> **B59   Pneumocystosis**
>
> *Explanation: Pneumonia due to Pneumocystis carinii is an HIV related condition, so the HIV diagnosis code is reported first, followed by the code for the pneumonia.*

(b) Patient with HIV disease admitted for unrelated condition

If a patient with HIV disease is admitted for an unrelated condition (such as a traumatic injury), the code for the unrelated condition (e.g., the nature of injury code) should be the principal diagnosis. Other diagnoses would be B20 followed by additional diagnosis codes for all reported HIV-related conditions.

> *Unstable angina, native coronary artery atherosclerosis, HIV*
>
> **I25.110   Atherosclerotic heart disease of native coronary artery with unstable angina pectoris**
>
> **B20   Human immunodeficiency virus [HIV] disease**
>
> *Explanation: The arteriosclerotic coronary artery disease and the unstable angina are not related to HIV, so those conditions are reported first using a combination code, and HIV is reported secondarily.*

(c) Whether the patient is newly diagnosed

Whether the patient is newly diagnosed or has had previous admissions/encounters for HIV conditions is irrelevant to the sequencing decision.

> *Newly diagnosed multiple cutaneous Kaposi's sarcoma lesions in previously diagnosed HIV disease*
>
> **B20   Human immunodeficiency virus [HIV] disease**
>
> **C46.0   Kaposi's sarcoma of skin**
>
> *Explanation: Even though the HIV was diagnosed on a previous encounter, it is still sequenced first when coded with an HIV related condition. Kaposi's sarcoma is an HIV-related condition.*

(d) Asymptomatic human immunodeficiency virus

Z21, Asymptomatic human immunodeficiency virus [HIV] infection status, is to be applied when the patient without any documentation of symptoms is listed as being "HIV positive," "known HIV," "HIV test positive," or similar terminology. Do not use this code if the term "AIDS" is used or if the patient is treated for any HIV-related illness or is described as having any condition(s) resulting from his/her HIV positive status; use B20 in these cases.

> *Patient admitted with acute appendicitis. Status positive HIV test on Atripla, with no prior symptoms*
>
> **K35.80   Unspecified acute appendicitis**
>
> **Z21   Asymptomatic human immunodeficiency virus [HIV] infection status**
>
> *Explanation: Code Z21 is sequenced second since documentation indicates that the patient has had a positive HIV test but has been asymptomatic. Being on medication for HIV is not an indication that code B20 is used instead of Z21. Unless there has been documentation that the patient has had current or prior symptoms or HIV-related complications, code B20 is not used. The appendicitis is not an AIDS-related complication and is sequenced first.*

(e) Patients with inconclusive HIV serology

Patients with inconclusive HIV serology, but no definitive diagnosis or manifestations of the illness, may be assigned code R75, Inconclusive laboratory evidence of human immunodeficiency virus [HIV].

(f) Previously diagnosed HIV-related illness

Patients with any known prior diagnosis of an HIV-related illness should be coded to B20. Once a patient has developed an HIV-related illness, the patient should always be assigned code B20 on every subsequent admission/encounter. Patients previously diagnosed with any HIV illness (B20) should never be assigned to R75 or Z21, Asymptomatic human immunodeficiency virus [HIV] infection status

(g) HIV infection in pregnancy, childbirth and the puerperium

During pregnancy, childbirth or the puerperium, a patient admitted (or presenting for a health care encounter) because of an HIV-related illness should receive a principal diagnosis code of O98.7-, Human immunodeficiency [HIV] disease complicating pregnancy, childbirth and the puerperium, followed by B20 and the code(s) for the HIV-related illness(es). Codes from Chapter 15 always take sequencing priority.

Patients with asymptomatic HIV infection status admitted (or presenting for a health care encounter) during pregnancy, childbirth, or the puerperium should receive codes of O98.7- and Z21.

(h) Encounters for testing for HIV

If a patient is being seen to determine his/her HIV status, use code Z11.4, Encounter for screening for human immunodeficiency virus [HIV]. Use additional codes for any associated high risk behavior.

If a patient with signs or symptoms is being seen for HIV testing, code the signs and symptoms. An additional counseling code Z71.7, Human immunodeficiency virus [HIV] counseling, may be used if counseling is provided during the encounter for the test.

When a patient returns to be informed of his/her HIV test results and the test result is negative, use code Z71.7, Human immunodeficiency virus [HIV] counseling.

If the results are positive, see previous guidelines and assign codes as appropriate.

b. Infectious agents as the cause of diseases classified to other chapters

Certain infections are classified in chapters other than Chapter 1 and no organism is identified as part of the infection code. In these instances, it is necessary to use an additional code from Chapter 1 to identify the organism. A code from category B95, Streptococcus, Staphylococcus, and Enterococcus as the cause of diseases classified to other chapters, B96, Other bacterial agents as the cause of diseases classified to other chapters, or B97, Viral agents as the cause of diseases classified to other chapters, is to be used as an additional code to identify the organism. An instructional note will be found at the infection code advising that an additional organism code is required.

E. coli UTI

N39.0	Urinary tract infection, site not specified
B96.20	Unspecified Escherichia coli [E.coli] as the cause of diseases classified elsewhere

Explanation: An instructional note under the code for the urinary tract infection indicates to code also the specific organism.

c. Infections resistant to antibiotics

Many bacterial infections are resistant to current antibiotics. It is necessary to identify all infections documented as antibiotic resistant. Assign a code from category Z16, Resistance to antimicrobial drugs, following the infection code only if the infection code does not identify drug resistance.

Antimycobacterial-resistant primary pulmonary tuberculosis

A15.0	Tuberculosis of lung
Z16.341	Resistance to single antimycobacterial drug

Explanation: Code Z16.341 is assigned as a secondary code to represent the antimycobacterial resistance. This code includes resistance to antimycobacterial drug "NOS"; if multiple drug resistance is not specified, classification defaults to the single drug resistance code.

d. Sepsis, severe sepsis, and septic shock

1) Coding of Sepsis and Severe Sepsis

(a) Sepsis

For a diagnosis of sepsis, assign the appropriate code for the underlying systemic infection. If the type of infection or causal organism is not further specified, assign code A41.9, Sepsis, unspecified organism.

A code from subcategory R65.2, Severe sepsis, should not be assigned unless severe sepsis or an associated acute organ dysfunction is documented.

Gram-negative sepsis

A41.50	Gram-negative sepsis, unspecified

Staphylococcal sepsis

A41.2	Sepsis due to unspecified staphylococcus

Explanation: In both examples above the organism causing the sepsis is identified, therefore A41.9 Sepsis, unspecified organism, would not be appropriate as this code would not capture the highest degree of specificity found in the documentation. Do not use the additional code for severe sepsis unless documented as severe sepsis with acute organ dysfunction.

(i) Negative or inconclusive blood cultures and sepsis

Negative or inconclusive blood cultures do not preclude a diagnosis of sepsis in patients with clinical evidence of the condition; however, the provider should be queried.

(ii) Urosepsis

The term urosepsis is a nonspecific term. It is not to be considered synonymous with sepsis. It has no default code in the Alphabetic Index. Should a provider use this term, he/she must be queried for clarification.

(iii) Sepsis with organ dysfunction

If a patient has sepsis and associated acute organ dysfunction or multiple organ dysfunction (MOD), follow the instructions for coding severe sepsis.

(iv) Acute organ dysfunction that is not clearly associated with the sepsis

If a patient has sepsis and an acute organ dysfunction, but the medical record documentation indicates that the acute organ dysfunction is related to a medical condition other than the sepsis, do not assign a code from subcategory R65.2, Severe sepsis. An acute organ dysfunction must be associated with the sepsis in order to assign the severe sepsis code. If the documentation is not clear as to whether an acute organ dysfunction is related to the sepsis or another medical condition, query the provider.

Sepsis and acute respiratory failure due to COPD exacerbation

A41.9	Sepsis, unspecified organism
J44.1	Chronic obstructive pulmonary disease with (acute) exacerbation
J96.00	Acute respiratory failure, unspecified whether with hypoxia or hypercapnia

Explanation: Although acute organ dysfunction is present in the form of acute respiratory failure, severe sepsis (R65.2) is not coded in this example, as the acute respiratory failure is attributed to the COPD exacerbation rather than the sepsis. Sequencing of these codes would be determined by the circumstances of the admission.

(b) Severe sepsis

The coding of severe sepsis requires a minimum of 2 codes: first a code for the underlying systemic infection, followed by a code from subcategory R65.2, Severe sepsis. If the causal organism is not documented, assign code A41.9, Sepsis, unspecified organism, for the infection. Additional code(s) for the associated acute organ dysfunction are also required.

Due to the complex nature of severe sepsis, some cases may require querying the provider prior to assignment of the codes.

2) Septic shock

(a) Septic shock generally refers to circulatory failure associated with severe sepsis, and therefore, it represents a type of acute organ dysfunction.

For cases of septic shock, the code for the systemic infection should be sequenced first, followed by code R65.21, Severe sepsis with septic shock or code T81.12, Postprocedural septic shock. Any additional codes for the other acute organ dysfunctions should also be assigned. As noted in the sequencing instructions in the Tabular List, the code for septic shock cannot be assigned as a principal diagnosis.

Sepsis with septic shock

A41.9	Sepsis, unspecified organism
R65.21	Severe sepsis with septic shock

Explanation: Documentation of septic shock automatically implies severe sepsis as it is a form of acute organ dysfunction. Septic shock is not coded as the principal diagnosis; it is always preceded by the code for the systemic infection.

3) Sequencing of severe sepsis

If severe sepsis is present on admission, and meets the definition of principal diagnosis, the underlying systemic infection should be assigned as principal diagnosis followed by the appropriate code from subcategory R65.2 as required by the sequencing rules in the Tabular List. A code from subcategory R65.2 can never be assigned as a principal diagnosis.

When severe sepsis develops during an encounter (it was not present on admission), the underlying systemic infection and the appropriate code from subcategory R65.2 should be assigned as secondary diagnoses.

Severe sepsis may be present on admission, but the diagnosis may not be confirmed until sometime after admission. If the documentation is not clear whether severe sepsis was present on admission, the provider should be queried.

4) Sepsis and severe sepsis with a localized infection

If the reason for admission is both sepsis or severe sepsis and a localized infection, such as pneumonia or cellulitis, a code(s) for the underlying systemic infection should be assigned first and the code for the localized infection should be assigned as a secondary diagnosis. If the patient has severe sepsis, a code from subcategory R65.2 should also be assigned as a secondary diagnosis. If the patient is admitted with a localized infection, such as pneumonia, and sepsis/severe sepsis doesn't develop until after admission, the localized infection should be assigned first, followed by the appropriate sepsis/severe sepsis codes.

> *Patient presents with acute renal failure due to severe sepsis from Pseudomonas pneumonia*
>
> **A41.9**   **Sepsis, unspecified organism**
>
> **J15.1**   **Pneumonia due to Pseudomonas**
>
> **R65.20**   **Severe sepsis without septic shock**
>
> **N17.9**   **Acute kidney failure, unspecified**
>
> *Explanation: If all conditions are present on admission, the systemic infection (sepsis) is sequenced first followed by the codes for the localized infection (pneumonia), severe sepsis and any organ dysfunction. If only the pneumonia was present on admission with the sepsis and resulting renal failure developing later in the admission, then the pneumonia would be sequenced first.*

5) Sepsis due to a postprocedural infection

(a) Documentation of causal relationship

As with all postprocedural complications, code assignment is based on the provider's documentation of the relationship between the infection and the procedure.

(b) Sepsis due to a postprocedural infection

For such cases, the postprocedural infection code, such as T80.2, Infections following infusion, transfusion, and therapeutic injection, T81.4, Infection following a procedure, T88.0, Infection following immunization, or O86.0, Infection of obstetric surgical wound, should be coded first, followed by the code for the specific infection. If the patient has severe sepsis, the appropriate code from subcategory R65.2 should also be assigned with the additional code(s) for any acute organ dysfunction.

(c) Postprocedural infection and postprocedural septic shock

In cases where a postprocedural infection has occurred and has resulted in severe sepsis the code for the precipitating complication such as code T81.4, Infection following a procedure, or O86.0, Infection of obstetrical surgical wound should be coded first followed by code R65.20, Severe sepsis without septic shock. A code for the systemic infection should also be assigned.

If a postprocedural infection has resulted in postprocedural septic shock, the code for the precipitating complication such as code T81.4, Infection following a procedure, or O86.0, Infection of obstetrical surgical wound should be coded first followed by code T81.12-, Postprocedural septic shock. A code for the systemic infection should also be assigned.

6) Sepsis and severe sepsis associated with a noninfectious process (condition)

In some cases a noninfectious process (condition), such as trauma, may lead to an infection which can result in sepsis or severe sepsis. If sepsis or severe sepsis is documented as associated with a noninfectious condition, such as a burn or serious injury, and this condition meets the definition for principal diagnosis, the code for the noninfectious condition should be sequenced first, followed by the code for the resulting infection. If severe sepsis is present, a code from subcategory R65.2 should also be assigned with any associated organ dysfunction(s) codes. It is not necessary to assign a code from subcategory R65.1, Systemic inflammatory response syndrome (SIRS) of non-infectious origin, for these cases.

If the infection meets the definition of principal diagnosis, it should be sequenced before the non-infectious condition. When both the associated non-infectious condition and the infection meet the definition of principal diagnosis, either may be assigned as principal diagnosis.

Only one code from category R65, Symptoms and signs specifically associated with systemic inflammation and infection, should be assigned. Therefore, when a non-infectious condition leads to an infection resulting in severe sepsis, assign the appropriate code from subcategory R65.2, Severe sepsis. Do not additionally assign a code from subcategory R65.1, Systemic inflammatory response syndrome (SIRS) of non-infectious origin.

See Section I.C.18. SIRS due to non-infectious process

> *Patient admitted with multiple third-degree burns of upper arm develops severe MSSA sepsis with septic shock, three days into admission*
>
> **T22.391A**   **Burn of third degree of multiple sites of right shoulder and upper arm limb, except wrist and hand, initial encounter**
>
> **A41.01**   **Sepsis due to methicillin susceptible Staphylococcus aureus**
>
> **R65.21**   **Severe sepsis with septic shock**
>
> *Explanation: Severe sepsis is coded rather than SIRS from R65 because it is documented as a severe systemic infectious response with septic shock to a noninfectious condition. The code for the systemic infection is not used as the principal diagnosis because it was not present on admission. The patient was admitted for the burn injury.*

7) Sepsis and septic shock complicating abortion, pregnancy, childbirth, and the puerperium

See Section I.C.15. Sepsis and septic shock complicating abortion, pregnancy, childbirth and the puerperium

8) Newborn sepsis

See Section I.C.16. f. Bacterial sepsis of Newborn

e. Methicillin resistant *Staphylococcus aureus* (MRSA) conditions

1) Selection and sequencing of MRSA codes

(a) Combination codes for MRSA infection

When a patient is diagnosed with an infection that is due to methicillin resistant *Staphylococcus aureus* (MRSA), and that infection has a combination code that includes the causal organism (e.g., sepsis, pneumonia) assign the appropriate combination code for the condition (e.g., code A41.02, Sepsis due to Methicillin resistant Staphylococcus aureus or code J15.212, Pneumonia due to Methicillin resistant Staphylococcus aureus). Do not assign code B95.62, Methicillin resistant Staphylococcus aureus infection as the cause of diseases classified elsewhere, as an additional code, because the combination code includes the type of infection and the MRSA organism. Do not assign a code from subcategory Z16.11, Resistance to penicillins, as an additional diagnosis.

See Section C.1. for instructions on coding and sequencing of sepsis and severe sepsis.

(b) Other codes for MRSA infection

When there is documentation of a current infection (e.g., wound infection, stitch abscess, urinary tract infection) due to MRSA, and that infection does not have a combination code that includes the causal organism, assign the appropriate code to identify the condition along with code B95.62, Methicillin resistant Staphylococcus aureus infection as the cause of diseases classified elsewhere for the MRSA infection. Do not assign a code from subcategory Z16.11, Resistance to penicillins.

(c) Methicillin susceptible Staphylococcus aureus (MSSA) and MRSA colonization

The condition or state of being colonized or carrying MSSA or MRSA is called colonization or carriage, while an individual person is described as being colonized or being a carrier. Colonization means that MSSA or MSRA is present on or in the body without necessarily causing illness. A positive MRSA colonization test might be documented by the provider as "MRSA screen positive" or "MRSA nasal swab positive".

Assign code Z22.322, Carrier or suspected carrier of Methicillin resistant Staphylococcus aureus, for patients documented as having MRSA colonization. Assign code Z22.321, Carrier or suspected carrier of Methicillin susceptible Staphylococcus aureus, for patient documented as having MSSA colonization. Colonization is not necessarily indicative of a disease process or as the cause of a specific condition the patient may have unless documented as such by the provider.

(d) MRSA colonization and infection

If a patient is documented as having both MRSA colonization and infection during a hospital admission, code Z22.322, Carrier or suspected carrier of Methicillin resistant Staphylococcus aureus, and a code for the MRSA infection may both be assigned.

Chapter 1. Certain Infectious and Parasitic Diseases (A00-B99)

INCLUDES diseases generally recognized as communicable or transmissible
Use additional code to identify resistance to antimicrobial drugs (Z16.-)
EXCLUDES 1 certain localized infections—see body system-related chapters
EXCLUDES 2 carrier or suspected carrier of infectious disease (Z22.-)
infectious and parasitic diseases complicating pregnancy, childbirth and the puerperium (O98.-)
infectious and parasitic diseases specific to the perinatal period (P35-P39)
influenza and other acute respiratory infections (J00-J22)

This chapter contains the following blocks:

A00-A09 Intestinal infectious diseases
A15-A19 Tuberculosis
A20-A28 Certain zoonotic bacterial diseases
A30-A49 Other bacterial diseases
A50-A64 Infections with a predominantly sexual mode of transmission
A65-A69 Other spirochetal diseases
A70-A74 Other diseases caused by chlamydiae
A75-A79 Rickettsioses
A80-A89 Viral infections of the central nervous system
A90-A99 Arthropod-borne viral fevers and viral hemorrhagic fevers
B00-B09 Viral infections characterized by skin and mucous membrane lesions
B10 Other human herpesviruses
B15-B19 Viral hepatitis
B20 Human immunodeficiency virus [HIV] disease
B25-B34 Other viral diseases
B35-B49 Mycoses
B50-B64 Protozoal diseases
B65-B83 Helminthiases
B85-B89 Pediculosis, acariasis and other infestations
B90-B94 Sequelae of infectious and parasitic diseases
B95-B97 Bacterial and viral infectious agents
B99 Other infectious diseases

Intestinal Infectious Diseases (A00-A09)

A00 Cholera

CC Excl: For CC codes in category A00, unless otherwise noted: A00.0-A00.9

A00.0 Cholera due to Vibrio cholerae 01, biovar cholerae CC
Classical cholera

A00.1 Cholera due to Vibrio cholerae 01, biovar eltor CC
Cholera eltor

A00.9 Cholera, unspecified CC

A01 Typhoid and paratyphoid fevers

CC Excl: For CC codes in category A01, unless otherwise noted: A01.00-A01.4

A01.0 Typhoid fever
Infection due to Salmonella typhi
A01.00 Typhoid fever, unspecified CC
A01.01 Typhoid meningitis CC
A01.02 Typhoid fever with heart involvement CC
Typhoid endocarditis   Typhoid myocarditis
A01.03 Typhoid pneumonia CC
A01.04 Typhoid arthritis CC
A01.05 Typhoid osteomyelitis CC
A01.09 Typhoid fever with other complications CC
A01.1 Paratyphoid fever A CC
A01.2 Paratyphoid fever B CC
A01.3 Paratyphoid fever C CC
A01.4 Paratyphoid fever, unspecified CC
Infection due to Salmonella paratyphi NOS

A02 Other salmonella infections
INCLUDES infection or foodborne intoxication due to any Salmonella species other than S. typhi and S. paratyphi

A02.0 Salmonella enteritis CC
Salmonellosis
CC Excl: A01.00-A01.09, A01.4-A02.0, A03.9-A05.2, A07.4, A08.0-A09, A48.51-A48.52, K30, K52.1-K52.2, K52.82-K52.9, K58.0-K58.9, K65.0, K65.2, K65.8, K68.12-K68.9, P76.8-P77.9, P78.1, P78.3-P78.89

A02.1 Salmonella sepsis HIV MCC
CC Excl: A02.1, A20.7, A22.7, A26.7, A32.7, A39.2-A39.4, A40.0-A40.1, A40.8-A41.9, A42.7, A48.2-A48.4, A48.8-A49.9, A54.86, B00.7, B37.7, B92, B94.2-B96.89, P36.0-P36.9, P39.2, P39.4-P39.9, R65.10-R65.20, Z16.10-Z16.39

A02.2 Localized salmonella infections
A02.20 Localized salmonella infection, unspecified HIV
A02.21 Salmonella meningitis HIV MCC
CC Excl: A02.21, A17.0-A17.1, A27.81, A39.0, A50.41, A51.41, A52.13, A54.82, A54.84, A54.89-A54.9, A74.81-A74.9, A87.0-A87.9, A96.2, A98.3-A98.4, B26.1, B33.24, B33.4-B33.8, B34.1-B34.2, B34.4-B34.8, B37.5, B38.4, B45.1, B58.2, B92, B94.2-B94.9, B97.10, B97.19, B97.29, B97.5-B97.6, B97.81-B97.89, G00.0-G03.9, G04.2, G32.89, G96.8-G96.9, G98.0-G98.8, G99.8
A02.22 Salmonella pneumonia HIV MCC
CC Excl: A02.22, A15.0-A15.6, A15.8-A15.9, A17.9, A18.82, A18.84, A18.89, A20.2, A21.1, A22.1, A31.0, A37.01, A37.11, A37.81, A37.91, A42.0, A43.0, A48.1, B25.0, B39.0-B39.2, B44.0, B58.3, B59, B67.1, J09.X1-J09.X2, J10.00-J10.1, J11.00-J11.1, J12.0-J12.3, J12.89-J18.1, J18.8-J18.9, J22, J60, J62.0-J67.7, J68.0-J70.4, J70.8-J70.9, J98.4, J98.8-J99, R91.1
A02.23 Salmonella arthritis HIV CC
CC Excl: A02.23, A18.02, A18.09, A39.83-A39.84, A54.40, A54.42-A54.43, A54.82, A54.84, A54.89-A54.9, B06.82, M00.00-M02.30, M02.319, M02.329, M02.339, M02.349, M02.359, M02.369, M02.379-M02.9, M05.40-M05.59, M05.70-M06.09, M06.20-M06.39, M06.80-M07.69, M11.00-M11.9, M12.10-M15.0, M15.3-M15.9, M16.2-M16.9, M17.2-M17.9, M18.2-M18.9, M19.111-M19.93, M24.10-M24.176, M25.00, M25.08-M25.18, M25.40-M25.676, M25.80-M25.9, M35.2, M36.1-M36.4, R29.4
A02.24 Salmonella osteomyelitis HIV CC
CC Excl: A02.24, A18.03-A18.09, M46.20-M46.39, M86.00-M86.9
A02.25 Salmonella pyelonephritis HIV CC
Salmonella tubulo-interstitial nephropathy
CC Excl: A02.25-A02.29
A02.29 Salmonella with other localized infection HIV CC
CC Excl: See code: A02.25
A02.8 Other specified salmonella infections HIV CC
CC Excl:A02.8
A02.9 Salmonella infection, unspecified HIV CC
CC Excl: A02.9

A03 Shigellosis
A03.0 Shigellosis due to Shigella dysenteriae CC
Group A shigellosis [Shiga-Kruse dysentery]
CC Excl: A00.1, A01.00-A01.09, A01.4-A02.0, A03.0, A03.9, A04.9-A05.2, A06.0-A06.2, A06.9, A07.1-A07.9, A08.4-A09, A18.32-A18.39, A18.83, A48.51-A48.52, B37.82, B82.9, J09.X3-J09.X9, J10.2-J10.89, J11.2-J11.89, K30, K31.84, K50.00-K51.919, K52.1-K52.2, K52.82-K55.1, K55.8-K55.9, K58.0-K58.9, P70.0-P70.4, P70.9-P71.9, P72.1, P72.9-P74.4, P74.9, P76.8-P77.9, P78.1, P78.3-P78.89, P94.0
A03.1 Shigellosis due to Shigella flexneri
Group B shigellosis
A03.2 Shigellosis due to Shigella boydii
Group C shigellosis
A03.3 Shigellosis due to Shigella sonnei
Group D shigellosis
A03.8 Other shigellosis
A03.9 Shigellosis, unspecified
Bacillary dysentery NOS

A04 Other bacterial intestinal infections
EXCLUDES 1 bacterial foodborne intoxications, NEC (A05.-)
tuberculous enteritis (A18.32)

CC Excl: For CC codes in category A04, unless otherwise noted: For codes A04.0-A04.4: A02.0, A03.9-A05.0, A05.2, A07.4, A08.0-A09, J09.X3-J09.X9, J10.2-J10.89, J11.2-J11.89, K30, K31.84, K52.1-K52.2, K52.82-K52.9, K58.0-K58.9, K65.0, K65.2, K65.8, K68.12-K68.9, P76.8-P77.9, P78.1, P78.3-P78.89 For codes A04.5-A04.8: A00.1, A01.00-A01.09, A01.4-A02.0, A03.9-A05.2, A06.0-A06.2, A06.9, A07.1-A09, A18.32-A18.39, A18.83, A48.51-A48.52, B37.82, B82.9, J09.X3-J09.X9, J10.2-J10.89, J11.2-J11.89, K30, K31.84, K50.00-K51.919, K52.1-K52.2, K52.82-K55.1, K55.8-K55.9, K58.0-K58.9, P70.0-P70.4, P70.9-P71.9, P72.1, P72.9-P74.4, P74.9, P76.8-P77.9, P78.1, P78.3-P78.89, P94.0

A04.0 Enteropathogenic Escherichia coli infection CC
A04.1 Enterotoxigenic Escherichia coli infection CC
A04.2 Enteroinvasive Escherichia coli infection CC

A04.3 Enterohemorrhagic Escherichia coli infection `CC`

A04.4 Other intestinal Escherichia coli infections `CC`
Escherichia coli enteritis NOS

A04.5 Campylobacter enteritis `CC`

A04.6 Enteritis due to Yersinia enterocolitica `CC`
EXCLUDES 1 extraintestinal yersiniosis (A28.2)

A04.7 Enterocolitis due to Clostridium difficile `CC`
Foodborne intoxication by Clostridium difficile
Pseudomembraneous colitis

A04.8 Other specified bacterial intestinal infections `CC`

A04.9 Bacterial intestinal infection, unspecified `CC`
Bacterial enteritis NOS
CC Excl: A00.1, A01.00-A01.09, A01.4-A02.0, A03.9-A05.0, A05.2, A06.0-A06.2, A06.9, A07.1-A09, A18.32-A18.39, A18.83, B37.82, B82.9, J09.X3-J09.X9, J10.2-J10.89, J11.2-J11.89, K30, K31.84, K52.1-K52.2, K52.82-K52.9, K58.0-K58.9, K65.0, K65.2, K65.8, K68.12-K68.9, P76.8-P77.9, P78.1, P78.3-P78.89

✓4th **A05 Other bacterial foodborne intoxications, not elsewhere classified**
EXCLUDES 1 Clostridium difficile foodborne intoxication and infection (A04.7)
Escherichia coli infection (A04.0-A04.4)
listeriosis (A32.-)
salmonella foodborne intoxication and infection (A02.-)
toxic effect of noxious foodstuffs (T61-T62)

A05.0 Foodborne staphylococcal intoxication `CC`
CC Excl: A00.0-A09, A48.51-A48.52

A05.1 Botulism food poisoning `CC`
Botulism NOS
Classical foodborne intoxication due to Clostridium botulinum
EXCLUDES 1 infant botulism (A48.51)
wound botulism (A48.52)
CC Excl: A04.7-A05.2, A48.51-A48.52

A05.2 Foodborne Clostridium perfringens [Clostridium welchii] intoxication `CC`
Enteritis necroticans
Pig-bel
CC Excl: A02.0, A03.9-A05.2, A07.4, A08.0-A09, A48.51-A48.52, J09.X3-J09.X9, J10.2-J10.89, J11.2-J11.89, K30, K31.84, K52.1-K52.2, K52.82-K52.9, K58.0-K58.9, K65.0, K65.2, K65.8, K68.12-K68.9, P76.8-P77.9, P78.1, P78.3-P78.89

A05.3 Foodborne Vibrio parahaemolyticus intoxication `CC`
CC Excl: See code: A05.0

A05.4 Foodborne Bacillus cereus intoxication `CC`
CC Excl: See code: A05.0

A05.5 Foodborne Vibrio vulnificus intoxication `CC`
CC Excl: See code: A05.0

A05.8 Other specified bacterial foodborne intoxications `CC`
CC Excl: See code: A05.0

A05.9 Bacterial foodborne intoxication, unspecified

✓4th **A06 Amebiasis**
INCLUDES infection due to Entamoeba histolytica
EXCLUDES 1 other protozoal intestinal diseases (A07.-)
EXCLUDES 2 acanthamebiasis (B60.1-)
Naegleriasis (B60.2)

A06.0 Acute amebic dysentery `CC`
Acute amebiasis
Intestinal amebiasis NOS
CC Excl: A06.0-A06.1, A07.4

A06.1 Chronic intestinal amebiasis `CC`
CC Excl: See code: A06.0

A06.2 Amebic nondysenteric colitis `CC`
CC Excl: A02.0, A03.9-A05.0, A05.2, A06.0-A06.2, A06.9, A07.1-A09, B82.9, J09.X3-J09.X9, J10.2-J10.89, J11.2-J11.89, K30, K31.84, K50.00-K51.919, K52.1-K52.2, K52.82-K55.1, K55.8-K55.9, K58.0-K58.9, P76.8-P77.9, P78.1, P78.3-P78.89

A06.3 Ameboma of intestine `CC`
Ameboma NOS
CC Excl: A06.0-A06.6, A06.81-A06.89

A06.4 Amebic liver abscess `MCC`
Hepatic amebiasis
CC Excl: A06.4, K75.0

A06.5 Amebic lung abscess `MCC`
Amebic abscess of lung (and liver)
CC Excl: A06.5, J85.0-J85.2

A06.6 Amebic brain abscess `MCC`
Amebic abscess of brain (and liver) (and lung)
CC Excl: A06.6, G06.0

A06.7 Cutaneous amebiasis

✓5th **A06.8 Amebic infection of other sites**
A06.81 Amebic cystitis `CC`
CC Excl: A06.0-A06.6, A06.81-A06.89

A06.82 Other amebic genitourinary infections `CC`
Amebic balanitis   Amebic vulvovaginitis
Amebic vesiculitis
CC Excl: See code: A06.3

A06.89 Other amebic infections `CC`
Amebic appendicitis   Amebic splenic abscess
CC Excl: See code: A06.3

A06.9 Amebiasis, unspecified

✓4th **A07 Other protozoal intestinal diseases**
CC Excl: For CC codes in category A07, unless otherwise noted: A02.0, A03.9-A05.0, A05.2, A06.0-A06.2, A06.9, A07.1-A09, B82.9, J09.X3-J09.X9, J10.2-J10.89, J11.2-J11.89, K30, K31.84, K52.1-K52.2, K52.82-K52.9, K58.0-K58.9

A07.0 Balantidiasis
Balantidial dysentery

A07.1 Giardiasis [lambliasis] `CC`

A07.2 Cryptosporidiosis `CC`

A07.3 Isosporiasis `HIV` `CC`
Infection due to Isospora belli and Isospora hominis
Intestinal coccidiosis
Isosporosis

A07.4 Cyclosporiasis `CC`
CC Excl: A02.0, A03.9-A05.0, A05.2, A06.0-A06.2, A06.9, A07.1-A09, B82.9, J09.X3-J09.X9, J10.2-J10.89, J11.2-J11.89, K30, K31.84, K52.1-K52.2, K52.82-K52.9, K58.0-K58.9, K65.0, K65.2, K65.8, K68.12-K68.9

A07.8 Other specified protozoal intestinal diseases `CC`
Intestinal microsporidiosis   Sarcocystosis
Intestinal trichomoniasis   Sarcosporidiosis

A07.9 Protozoal intestinal disease, unspecified `CC`
Flagellate diarrhea   Protozoal diarrhea
Protozoal colitis   Protozoal dysentery

✓4th **A08 Viral and other specified intestinal infections**
EXCLUDES 1 influenza with involvement of gastrointestinal tract (J09.X3, J10.2, J11.2)

CC Excl: For CC codes in category A08, unless otherwise noted: A02.0, A03.9-A05.0, A05.2, A06.0-A06.2, A06.9, A07.1-A09, A18.32-A18.39, A18.83, B37.82, B82.9, J09.X3-J09.X9, J10.2-J10.89, J11.2-J11.89, K30, K31.84, K52.1-K52.2, K52.82-K52.9, K58.0-K58.9, K65.0, K65.2, K65.8, K68.12-K68.9, P76.8-P77.9, P78.1, P78.3-P78.89

A08.0 Rotaviral enteritis `CC`

✓5th **A08.1 Acute gastroenteropathy due to Norwalk agent and other small round viruses**
A08.11 Acute gastroenteropathy due to Norwalk agent `CC`
Acute gastroenteropathy due to Norovirus
Acute gastroenteropathy due to Norwalk-like agent

A08.19 Acute gastroenteropathy due to other small round viruses `CC`
Acute gastroenteropathy due to small round virus [SRV] NOS

A08.2 Adenoviral enteritis `CC`

✓5th **A08.3 Other viral enteritis**
A08.31 Calicivirus enteritis `CC`
A08.32 Astrovirus enteritis `CC`
A08.39 Other viral enteritis `CC`
Coxsackie virus enteritis   Enterovirus enteritis NEC
Echovirus enteritis   Torovirus enteritis

A08.4 Viral intestinal infection, unspecified
Viral enteritis NOS   Viral gastroenteropathy NOS
Viral gastroenteritis NOS

A08.8 Other specified intestinal infections

A09 Infectious gastroenteritis and colitis, unspecified `CC`
Infectious colitis NOS
Infectious enteritis NOS
Infectious gastroenteritis NOS
EXCLUDES 1 colitis NOS (K52.9)
diarrhea NOS (R19.7)
enteritis NOS (K52.9)
gastroenteritis NOS (K52.9)
noninfective gastroenteritis and colitis, unspecified (K52.9)
CC Excl: A00.0-A09, A48.51-A48.52

Chapter 1. Certain Infectious and Parasitic Diseases

A15–A18.39

Tuberculosis (A15-A19)

INCLUDES infections due to Mycobacterium tuberculosis and Mycobacterium bovis

EXCLUDES 1 *congenital tuberculosis (P37.0)*
nonspecific reaction to test for tuberculosis without active tuberculosis (R76.1-)
pneumoconiosis associated with tuberculosis, any type in A15 (J65)
positive PPD (R76.11)
positive tuberculin skin test without active tuberculosis (R76.11)
sequelae of tuberculosis (B90.-)
silicotuberculosis (J65)

✓4ᵗʰ A15 Respiratory tuberculosis

A15.0 Tuberculosis of lung   HIV CC
Tuberculous bronchiectasis
Tuberculous fibrosis of lung
Tuberculous pneumonia
Tuberculous pneumothorax
CC Excl: A15.0-A15.6, A15.8-A15.9, A17.9, A18.82, A18.84, A18.89-A19.9, A22.1, A31.0, A31.2-A31.9, A37.01, A37.11, A37.81, A37.91, A48.1, A49.3-A49.9, B25.0, B44.0, B90.9, B92, B94.2-B94.9, B96.0, B96.6-B96.89, J09.X1-J09.X2, J10.00-J10.1, J11.00-J11.1, J12.0-J12.3, J12.89-J18.1, J18.8-J18.9, J44.9, J47.0-J70.4, J70.8-J70.9, J98.4, R91.1

A15.4 Tuberculosis of intrathoracic lymph nodes   HIV CC
Tuberculosis of hilar lymph nodes
Tuberculosis of mediastinal lymph nodes
Tuberculosis of tracheobronchial lymph nodes
EXCLUDES 1 *tuberculosis specified as primary (A15.7)*
CC Excl: See code: A15.0

A15.5 Tuberculosis of larynx, trachea and bronchus   HIV CC
Tuberculosis of bronchus
Tuberculosis of glottis
Tuberculosis of larynx
Tuberculosis of trachea
CC Excl: See code: A15.0

A15.6 Tuberculous pleurisy   HIV CC
Tuberculosis of pleura Tuberculous empyema
EXCLUDES 1 *primary respiratory tuberculosis (A15.7)*
CC Excl: See code: A15.0

A15.7 Primary respiratory tuberculosis   HIV CC
CC Excl: A15.0-A17.82, A17.89-A19.9

A15.8 Other respiratory tuberculosis   HIV CC
Mediastinal tuberculosis
Nasopharyngeal tuberculosis
Tuberculosis of nose
Tuberculosis of sinus [any nasal]
CC Excl: A15.0-A17.82, A17.89, A18.31-A18.39, A18.83, A19.0-A19.9

A15.9 Respiratory tuberculosis unspecified   HIV CC
CC Excl: See code: A15.8

✓4ᵗʰ A17 Tuberculosis of nervous system

A17.0 Tuberculous meningitis   HIV MCC
Tuberculosis of meninges (cerebral)(spinal)
Tuberculous leptomeningitis
EXCLUDES 1 *tuberculous meningoencephalitis (A17.82)*
CC Excl: A02.21, A17.0-A17.1, A17.89-A17.9, A18.82, A18.84, A18.89, A27.81, A31.2-A31.9, A39.0, A49.3-A49.9, A50.41, A51.41, A52.13, A54.82, A54.84, A54.89-A54.9, A87.0-A87.9, B00.3, B02.1, B26.1, B37.5, B38.4, B45.1, B58.2, B90.0, B92, B94.2-B94.9, B96.0, B96.6-B96.89, G00.0-G03.9, G04.2, G32.89, G61.0, G96.8-G96.9, G98.0-G98.8, G99.8

A17.1 Meningeal tuberculoma   HIV MCC
Tuberculoma of meninges (cerebral) (spinal)
EXCLUDES 2 *tuberculoma of brain and spinal cord (A17.81)*
CC Excl: See code: A17.0

✓5ᵗʰ A17.8 Other tuberculosis of nervous system

A17.81 Tuberculoma of brain and spinal cord   HIV MCC
Tuberculous abscess of brain and spinal cord
CC Excl: A17.81-A17.82, A17.89-A17.9, A18.82, A18.84, A18.89, A31.2-A31.9, A49.3-A49.9, B90.0, B92, B94.2-B94.9, B96.0, B96.6-B96.89

A17.82 Tuberculous meningoencephalitis   HIV MCC
Tuberculous myelitis
CC Excl: See code: A17.81

A17.83 Tuberculous neuritis   HIV MCC
Tuberculous mononeuropathy
CC Excl: No Excl

A17.89 Other tuberculosis of nervous system   HIV MCC
Tuberculous polyneuropathy
CC Excl: A17.89-A17.9, A18.82, A18.84, A18.89, A31.2-A31.9, A49.3-A49.9, B90.0, B92, B94.2-B94.9, B96.0, B96.6-B96.89

A17.9 Tuberculosis of nervous system, unspecified   HIV CC
CC Excl: A17.9, A18.82, A18.84, A18.89, A31.2-A31.9, A49.3-A49.9, B92, B94.2-B94.9, B96.0, B96.6-B96.89

✓4ᵗʰ A18 Tuberculosis of other organs

✓5ᵗʰ A18.0 Tuberculosis of bones and joints

A18.01 Tuberculosis of spine   HIV CC
Pott's disease or curvature of spine
Tuberculous arthritis
Tuberculous osteomyelitis of spine
Tuberculous spondylitis
CC Excl: A18.01

A18.02 Tuberculous arthritis of other joints   HIV CC
Tuberculosis of hip (joint)
Tuberculosis of knee (joint)
CC Excl: A18.02

A18.03 Tuberculosis of other bones   HIV CC
Tuberculous mastoiditis
Tuberculous osteomyelitis
CC Excl: A18.01-A18.03

A18.09 Other musculoskeletal tuberculosis   HIV CC
Tuberculous myositis
Tuberculous synovitis
Tuberculous tenosynovitis
CC Excl: A18.01-A18.02, A18.09

✓5ᵗʰ A18.1 Tuberculosis of genitourinary system

A18.10 Tuberculosis of genitourinary system, unspecified   HIV CC
CC Excl: A17.9, A18.10, A18.82, A18.84, A18.89, A31.2-A31.9, A49.3-A49.9, B90.1, B92, B94.2-B94.9, B96.0, B96.6-B96.89

A18.11 Tuberculosis of kidney and ureter   HIV CC
CC Excl: A17.9-A18.13, A18.82, A18.84, A18.89, A31.2-A31.9, A49.3-A49.9, B90.1, B92, B94.2-B94.9, B96.0, B96.6-B96.89

A18.12 Tuberculosis of bladder   HIV CC
CC Excl: See code: A18.11

A18.13 Tuberculosis of other urinary organs   HIV CC
Tuberculous urethritis
CC Excl: See code: A18.11

A18.14 Tuberculosis of prostate   HIV CC A ♂
CC Excl: A17.9, A18.10, A18.14-A18.15, A18.82, A18.84, A18.89, A31.2-A31.9, A49.3-A49.9, B90.1, B92, B94.2-B94.9, B96.0, B96.6-B96.89

A18.15 Tuberculosis of other male genital organs   HIV CC ♂
CC Excl: See code: A18.14

A18.16 Tuberculosis of cervix   HIV CC ♀
CC Excl: A17.9, A18.10, A18.16-A18.18, A18.82, A18.84, A18.89, A31.2-A31.9, A49.3-A49.9, B90.1, B92, B94.2-B94.9, B96.0, B96.6-B96.89

A18.17 Tuberculous female pelvic inflammatory disease   HIV CC ♀
Tuberculous endometritis
Tuberculous oophoritis and salpingitis
CC Excl: See code: A18.16

A18.18 Tuberculosis of other female genital organs   HIV CC ♀
Tuberculous ulceration of vulva
CC Excl: See code: A18.16

A18.2 Tuberculous peripheral lymphadenopathy   HIV CC
Tuberculous adenitis
EXCLUDES 2 *tuberculosis of bronchial and mediastinal lymph nodes (A15.4)*
tuberculosis of mesenteric and retroperitoneal lymph nodes (A18.39)
tuberculous tracheobronchial adenopathy (A15.4)
CC Excl: A17.9, A18.2, A18.82, A18.84, A18.89, A31.2-A31.9, A49.3-A49.9, B92, B94.2-B94.9, B96.0, B96.6-B96.89

✓5ᵗʰ A18.3 Tuberculosis of intestines, peritoneum and mesenteric glands

CC Excl: For CC/MCC codes in subcategory A18.3, unless otherwise noted: A17.9, A18.31-A18.39, A18.82-A18.84, A18.89, A31.2-A31.9, A49.3-A49.9, B92, B94.2-B94.9, B96.0, B96.6-B96.89

A18.31 Tuberculous peritonitis   HIV MCC
Tuberculous ascites

A18.32 Tuberculous enteritis   HIV CC
Tuberculosis of anus and rectum
Tuberculosis of intestine (large) (small)

A18.39 Retroperitoneal tuberculosis   HIV CC
Tuberculosis of mesenteric glands
Tuberculosis of retroperitoneal (lymph glands)

N Newborn: 0   P Pediatric: 0-17   M Maternity: 12-55   A Adult: 15-124   MCC Major CC Condition   PDxMCC PDx acts as own MCC   CC CC Condition   PDxCC PDx acts as own CC

428   ICD-10-CM 2016

A18.4 Tuberculosis of skin and subcutaneous tissue `HIV` `CC`
Erythema induratum, tuberculous
Lupus excedens
Lupus vulgaris NOS
Lupus vulgaris of eyelid
Scrofuloderma
Tuberculosis of external ear
EXCLUDES 2   *lupus erythematosus (L93.-)*
    lupus NOS (M32.9)
    systemic (M32.-)
CC Excl: A15.0-A17.82, A17.89-A19.9

✓5ᵗʰ **A18.5 Tuberculosis of eye**
EXCLUDES 2   *lupus vulgaris of eyelid (A18.4)*

CC Excl: For CC codes in subcategory A18.5, unless otherwise noted: A17.9, A18.50-A18.59, A18.82, A18.84, A18.89, A31.2-A31.9, A49.3-A49.9, B92, B94.2-B94.9, B96.0, B96.6-B96.89

  A18.50 Tuberculosis of eye, unspecified `HIV` `CC`
  A18.51 Tuberculous episcleritis `HIV` `CC`
  A18.52 Tuberculous keratitis `HIV` `CC`
    Tuberculous interstitial keratitis
    Tuberculous keratoconjunctivitis (interstitial) (phlyctenular)
  A18.53 Tuberculous chorioretinitis `HIV` `CC`
  A18.54 Tuberculous iridocyclitis `HIV` `CC`
  A18.59 Other tuberculosis of eye `HIV` `CC`
    Tuberculous conjunctivitis

A18.6 Tuberculosis of (inner) (middle) ear `HIV` `CC`
Tuberculous otitis media
EXCLUDES 2   *tuberculosis of external ear (A18.4)*
    tuberculous mastoiditis (A18.03)
CC Excl: A17.9, A18.6, A18.82, A18.84, A18.89, A31.2-A31.9, A49.3-A49.9, B92, B94.2-B94.9, B96.0, B96.6-B96.89

A18.7 Tuberculosis of adrenal glands `HIV` `CC`
Tuberculous Addison's disease
CC Excl: A17.9, A18.7, A18.82, A18.84, A18.89, A31.2-A31.9, A49.3-A49.9, B92, B94.2-B94.9, B96.0, B96.6-B96.89

✓5ᵗʰ **A18.8 Tuberculosis of other specified organs**
  A18.81 Tuberculosis of thyroid gland `HIV` `CC`
    CC Excl: A17.9, A18.81-A18.82, A18.84, A18.89, A31.2-A31.9, A49.3-A49.9, B92, B94.2-B94.9, B96.0, B96.6-B96.89
  A18.82 Tuberculosis of other endocrine glands `HIV` `CC`
    Tuberculosis of pituitary gland
    Tuberculosis of thymus gland
    CC Excl: A17.9, A18.82, A18.84, A18.89, A31.2-A31.9, A49.3-A49.9, B92, B94.2-B94.9, B96.0, B96.6-B96.89
  A18.83 Tuberculosis of digestive tract organs, not elsewhere classified `HIV` `CC`
    EXCLUDES 1   *tuberculosis of intestine (A18.32)*
    CC Excl: A17.9, A18.31-A18.39, A18.82-A18.84, A18.89, A31.2-A31.9, A49.3-A49.9, B92, B94.2-B94.9, B96.0, B96.6-B96.89
  A18.84 Tuberculosis of heart `HIV` `CC`
    Tuberculous cardiomyopathy
    Tuberculous endocarditis
    Tuberculous myocarditis
    Tuberculous pericarditis
    CC Excl: See code: A18.82
  A18.85 Tuberculosis of spleen `HIV` `CC`
    CC Excl: A17.9-A18.82, A18.84-A18.89, A31.2-A31.9, A49.3-A49.9, B92, B94.2-B94.9, B96.0, B96.6-B96.89
  A18.89 Tuberculosis of other sites `HIV` `CC`
    Tuberculosis of muscle
    Tuberculous cerebral arteritis
    CC Excl: See code: A18.82

✓4ᵗʰ **A19 Miliary tuberculosis**
INCLUDES   disseminated tuberculosis
    generalized tuberculosis
    tuberculous polyserositis

CC Excl: For MCC codes in category A19, unless otherwise noted: A17.9, A18.82, A18.84, A18.89-A19.9, A31.2-A31.9, A49.3-A49.9, B92, B94.2-B94.9, B96.0, B96.6-B96.89

A19.0 Acute miliary tuberculosis of a single specified site `HIV` `MCC`
A19.1 Acute miliary tuberculosis of multiple sites `HIV` `MCC`
A19.2 Acute miliary tuberculosis, unspecified `HIV` `MCC`
A19.8 Other miliary tuberculosis `HIV` `MCC`
A19.9 Miliary tuberculosis, unspecified `HIV` `MCC`

Certain zoonotic bacterial diseases (A20-A28)

✓4ᵗʰ **A20 Plague**
INCLUDES   infection due to Yersinia pestis

A20.0 Bubonic plague `MCC`
    CC Excl: A20.0-A20.9
A20.1 Cellulocutaneous plague `MCC`
    CC Excl: See code: A20.0
A20.2 Pneumonic plague `MCC`
    CC Excl: A20.2-J12.81
A20.3 Plague meningitis `MCC`
    CC Excl: A20.3-A20.8
A20.7 Septicemic plague `MCC`
    CC Excl: A02.1, A20.0-A20.9, A22.7, A26.7, A32.7, A40.0-A40.1, A40.8-A41.9, A42.7, A54.86, B37.7, P36.0-P36.9, P39.2, P39.4-P39.9, R65.10-R65.20
A20.8 Other forms of plague `MCC`
    Abortive plague
    Asymptomatic plague
    Pestis minor
    CC Excl: See code: A20.3
A20.9 Plague, unspecified `MCC`
    CC Excl: A20.9

✓4ᵗʰ **A21 Tularemia**
INCLUDES   deer-fly fever
    infection due to Francisella tularensis
    rabbit fever

A21.0 Ulceroglandular tularemia `CC`
    CC Excl: A21.0
A21.1 Oculoglandular tularemia `CC`
    Ophthalmic tularemia
    CC Excl: A21.1-J12.81
A21.2 Pulmonary tularemia `CC`
    CC Excl: A22.1-A37.01, A37.11, A37.81, A37.91, A48.1, B25.0, B44.0, J09.X1-J09.X2, J10.00-J10.1, J11.00-J11.1, J15.29, J15.5-J18.0, J18.8-J18.9, J22, J60-J70.4, J70.8-J70.9, J98.4, J98.8-J99, R91.1
A21.3 Gastrointestinal tularemia `CC`
    Abdominal tularemia
    CC Excl: A21.3
A21.7 Generalized tularemia `CC`
    CC Excl: A21.0-A21.9
A21.8 Other forms of tularemia `CC`
    CC Excl: See code: A21.7
A21.9 Tulamirea, unspecified `CC`
    CC Excl: See code: A21.7

✓4ᵗʰ **A22 Anthrax**
INCLUDES   infection due to Bacillus anthracis

A22.0 Cutaneous anthrax `CC`
    Malignant carbuncle   Malignant pustule
    CC Excl: A22.0
A22.1 Pulmonary anthrax `MCC`
    Inhalation anthrax   Woolsorter's disease
    Ragpicker's disease
    CC Excl: A15.0-A15.6, A15.8-A15.9, A17.9, A18.82, A18.84, A18.89, A20.2, A21.1-A21.2, A22.1, A31.0, A37.01, A37.11, A37.81,A37.91, A42.0, A43.0, A48.1, B25.0, B39.0-B39.2, B44.0, B58.3, B59, B67.1, J09.X1-J09.X2, J10.00-J10.1, J11.00-J11.1, J12.0-J18.1, J18.8-J18.9, J22, J44.9, J47.0-J70.4, J70.8-J70.9, J98.4, J98.8-J99, Q33.4, R91.1
A22.2 Gastrointestinal anthrax `CC`
    CC Excl: A22.2
A22.7 Anthrax sepsis `PDxMCC` `MCC`
    CC Excl: A02.1-A20.7, A22.7, A26.7, A32.7, A39.2-A39.4, A40.0-A40.1, A40.8-A41.9, A42.7, A48.2-A48.4, A48.8-A49.9, A54.86, B00.7, B37.7, B92, B94.2-B96.89, M00.011-M00.012, M00.021-M00.022, M00.031- M00.032, M00.041-M00.042, M00.051-M00.052, M00.061-M00.062, M00.071-M00.072, P36.0-P36.9, P39.2, P39.4-P39.9, R65.10-R65.20, Z16.10-Z16.39
A22.8 Other forms of anthrax `CC`
    Anthrax meningitis
    CC Excl: A22.8
A22.9 Anthrax, unspecified `CC`
    CC Excl: A22.0-A22.9

✓4ᵗʰ **A23 Brucellosis**
    Malta fever   Undulant fever
    Mediterranean fever

A23.0 Brucellosis due to Brucella melitensis
A23.1 Brucellosis due to Brucella abortus
A23.2 Brucellosis due to Brucella suis
A23.3 Brucellosis due to Brucella canis

✓ Additional Character Required   ✓x7ᵗʰ Placeholder Alert   Unacceptable PDx   Manifestation   Hospital Acquired Condition   EXCLUDES 1 Not Coded Here   EXCLUDES 2 Not Included Here

ICD-10-CM 2016   429

A23.8 **Other brucellosis** `CC`
CC Excl: A23.0-A23.9

A23.9 **Brucellosis, unspecified** `CC`
CC Excl: See code: A23.8

✓4ᵗʰ A24 **Glanders and melioidosis**

A24.0 **Glanders** `CC`
Infection due to Pseudomonas mallei   Malleus
CC Excl: A24.0

A24.1 **Acute and fulminating melioidosis** `CC`
Melioidosis pneumonia   Melioidosis sepsis
CC Excl: A24.1-A24.9

A24.2 **Subacute and chronic melioidosis** `CC`
CC Excl: See code: A24.1

A24.3 **Other melioidosis** `CC`
CC Excl: See code: A24.1

A24.9 **Melioidosis, unspecified** `CC`
Infection due to Pseudomonas pseudomallei NOS
Whitmore's disease
CC Excl: See code: A24.1

✓4ᵗʰ A25 **Rat-bite fevers**

CC Excl: For CC codes in category A25, unless otherwise noted:
A25.0-A25.9

A25.0 **Spirillosis** `CC`
Sodoku

A25.1 **Streptobacillosis** `CC`
Epidemic arthritic erythema   Streptobacillary rat-bite fever
Haverhill fever

A25.9 **Rat-bite fever, unspecified** `CC`

✓4ᵗʰ A26 **Erysipeloid**

A26.0 **Cutaneous erysipeloid**
Erythema migrans

A26.7 **Erysipelothrix sepsis** `PDxMCC` `MCC`
CC Excl: A02.1, A20.7, A22.7, A26.7, A32.7, A39.2-A39.4, A40.0-
A40.1, A40.8-A41.9, A42.7, A48.2-A48.4, A48.8-A49.9, A54.86,
B00.7, B37.7, B92, B94.2-B96.89, R65.10-R65.20, Z16.10-Z16.39

A26.8 **Other forms of erysipeloid**

A26.9 **Erysipeloid, unspecified**

✓4ᵗʰ A27 **Leptospirosis**

CC Excl: For CC/MCC codes in category A27, unless otherwise
noted: A27.0-A27.9

A27.0 **Leptospirosis icterohemorrhagica** `CC`
Leptospiral or spirochetal jaundice (hemorrhagic)
Weil's disease

✓5ᵗʰ A27.8 **Other forms of leptospirosis**

A27.81 **Aseptic meningitis in leptospirosis** `MCC`
CC Excl: A02.21, A17.0-A17.1, A27.0-A27.9, A39.0,
A50.41, A51.41, A52.13, A54.82, A54.84, A54.89-A54.9,
A74.81-A74.9, A87.0-A87.9, A96.2, A98.3-A98.4, B26.1,
B33.24, B33.4-B33.8, B34.1-B34.2, B34.4-B34.8, B37.5,
B38.4, B45.1, B58.2, B92, B94.2-B94.9, B97.10, B97.19,
B97.29, B97.5-B97.6, B97.81-B97.89, G00.0-G03.9, G04.2,
G32.89, G61.0, G96.8-G96.9, G98.0-G98.8, G99.8

A27.89 **Other forms of leptospirosis** `CC`

A27.9 **Leptospirosis, unspecified** `CC`

✓4ᵗʰ A28 **Other zoonotic bacterial diseases, not elsewhere classified**

CC Excl: For CC codes in category A28, unless otherwise noted:
:A26.0, A26.8-A26.9, A28.0, A28.2-A28.9, A32.0-A32.12, A32.81-A32.9

A28.0 **Pasteurellosis** `CC`

A28.1 **Cat-scratch disease** `CC`
Cat-scratch fever
CC Excl: A28.1-B97.21

A28.2 **Extraintestinal yersiniosis** `CC`
EXCLUDES1   enteritis due to Yersinia enterocolitica (A04.6)
plague (A20.-)

A28.8 **Other specified zoonotic bacterial diseases, not** `CC`
elsewhere classified

A28.9 **Zoonotic bacterial disease, unspecified** `CC`

Other bacterial diseases (A30-A49)

✓4ᵗʰ A30 **Leprosy [Hansen's disease]**
INCLUDES   infection due to Mycobacterium leprae
EXCLUDES1   sequelae of leprosy (B92)

A30.0 **Indeterminate leprosy** `CC`
I leprosy
CC Excl: A30.0

A30.1 **Tuberculoid leprosy** `CC`
TT leprosy
CC Excl: A30.1

A30.2 **Borderline tuberculoid leprosy** `CC`
BT leprosy
CC Excl: A30.2-A30.4

A30.3 **Borderline leprosy** `CC`
BB leprosy
CC Excl: See code: A30.2

A30.4 **Borderline lepromatous leprosy** `CC`
BL leprosy
CC Excl: See code: A30.2

A30.5 **Lepromatous leprosy** `CC`
LL leprosy
CC Excl: A30.5

A30.8 **Other forms of leprosy** `CC`
CC Excl: A30.8

A30.9 **Leprosy, unspecified** `CC`
CC Excl: A30.9

✓4ᵗʰ A31 **Infection due to other mycobacteria**

CC Excl: For CC codes in category A31, unless otherwise noted:
A31.0-A31.9

EXCLUDES2   leprosy (A30.-)
tuberculosis (A15-A19)

A31.0 **Pulmonary mycobacterial infection** `CC`
Infection due to Mycobacterium avium
Infection due to Mycobacterium intracellulare [Battey bacillus]
Infection due to Mycobacterium kansasii
CC Excl: A15.0-A15.6, A15.8-A15.9, A17.9, A18.82, A18.84, A18.89,
A22.1, A31.0, A31.2-A31.9, A37.01, A37.11, A37.81, A37.91, A48.1,
A49.3-A49.9, B25.0, B44.0, B90.9, B92, B94.2-B94.9, B96.0, B96.6-
B96.89, J09.X1-J09.X2, J10.00-J10.1, J11.00-J11.1, J12.0-J12.3,
J12.89-J18.1, J18.8-J18.9, J44.9, J47.0-J70.4, J70.8-J70.9, J98.4,
R91.1

A31.1 **Cutaneous mycobacterial infection** `CC`
Buruli ulcer
Infection due to Mycobacterium marinum
Infection due to Mycobacterium ulcerans

A31.2 **Disseminated mycobacterium avium-intracellulare** `HIV` `CC`
complex (DMAC)
MAC sepsis

A31.8 **Other mycobacterial infections** `HIV` `CC`

A31.9 **Mycobacterial infection, unspecified** `HIV` `CC`
Atypical mycobacterial infection NOS
Mycobacteriosis NOS

✓4ᵗʰ A32 **Listeriosis**
INCLUDES   listerial foodborne infection
EXCLUDES1   neonatal (disseminated) listeriosis (P37.2)

CC Excl: For CC/MCC codes in category A32, unless otherwise
noted: A26.0, A26.8-A26.9, A28.0, A28.2-A28.9, A32.0-A32.12,
A32.81-A32.9

A32.0 **Cutaneous listeriosis** `CC`

✓5ᵗʰ A32.1 **Listerial meningitis and meningoencephalitis**

A32.11 **Listerial meningitis** `CC`

A32.12 **Listerial meningoencephalitis** `CC`

A32.7 **Listerial sepsis** `PDxMCC` `MCC`
CC Excl: A02.1, A20.7, A22.7, A26.7, A32.7, A39.2-A39.4, A40.0-
A40.1, A40.8-A41.9, A42.7, A48.2-A48.4, A48.8-A49.9, A54.86,
B00.7, B37.7, B92, B94.2-B96.89, M00.011-M00.012, M00.021-
M00.022, M00.031- M00.032, M00.041-M00.042, M00.051-
M00.052, M00.061-M00.062, M00.071-M00.072, R65.10-R65.20,
Z16.10-Z16.39

✓5ᵗʰ A32.8 **Other forms of listeriosis**

A32.81 **Oculoglandular listeriosis** `CC`

A32.82 **Listerial endocarditis** `CC`

A32.89 **Other forms of listeriosis** `CC`
Listerial cerebral arteritis

A32.9 **Listeriosis, unspecified** `CC`

A33   Tetanus neonatorum   `MCC` `N`
CC Excl: A33-P29.2, P29.4, P29.89-P29.9, P94.1-P94.9, P96.0, P96.3-P96.5, P96.82-P96.89

A34   Obstetrical tetanus   `CC` `M` ♀
CC Excl: A34, O08.0, O08.2-O08.9, O20.0-O20.9, O25.10-O25.3, O26.10-O26.13, O26.30-O26.43, O26.63-O26.819, O26.841-O26.86, O26.891-O26.93, O29.011-O29.93, O35.7X-O35.7X, O44.00-O44.13, O45.8X1-O45.93, O75.4, O75.81, O75.89-O75.9, O80, O90.89, O99.111-O99.285, O99.330-O99.335, O99.350-O99.355, O99.511-O99.73, O99.820-O99.825, O99.840-O9A.53

A35   Other tetanus   `MCC`
Tetanus NOS
> **EXCLUDES 1**   obstetrical tetanus (A34)
>   tetanus neonatorum (A33)
CC Excl: A35, B92, B94.2-B94.9

✓4th **A36   Diphtheria**

> CC Excl: For CC codes in category A36, unless otherwise noted: A36.0-A36.9

A36.0   Pharyngeal diphtheria   `CC`
Diphtheritic membranous angina
Tonsillar diphtheria

A36.1   Nasopharyngeal diphtheria   `CC`

A36.2   Laryngeal diphtheria   `CC`
Diphtheritic laryngotracheitis

A36.3   Cutaneous diphtheria   `CC`
> **EXCLUDES 2**   erythrasma (L08.1)

✓5th **A36.8   Other diphtheria**

A36.81   Diphtheritic cardiomyopathy   `CC`
Diphtheritic myocarditis
CC Excl: A36.81, A52.06, B33.20-B33.22, I00, I01.2-I01.9, I09.0, I09.9, I23.0-I23.3, I23.6-I23.8, I40.0-I41, I51.0, I51.4, I87.8, I99.8-I99.9

A36.82   Diphtheritic radiculomyelitis   `CC`

A36.83   Diphtheritic polyneuritis   `CC`

A36.84   Diphtheritic tubulo-interstitial nephropathy   `CC`

A36.85   Diphtheritic cystitis   `CC`

A36.86   Diphtheritic conjunctivitis   `CC`

A36.89   Other diphtheritic complications   `CC`
Diphtheritic peritonitis

A36.9   Diphtheria, unspecified   `CC`

✓4th **A37   Whooping cough**

> CC Excl: For CC/MCC codes in category A37, unless otherwise noted: For codes A37.00, A37.10, A37.80 and A37.90: A37.00-A37.91 For codes A37.01, A37.11, A37.81 and A37.91: A15.0-A15.6, A15.8-A15.9, A17.9, A18.82, A18.84, A18.89, A21.2, A22.1, A31.0, A37.00-A37.91, A42.0, A43.0, A48.1, B25.0, B39.0-B39.2, B44.0, B58.3, B59, B67.1, J09.X1-J09.X2, J10.00-J10.1, J11.00-J11.1, J12.0-J12.3, J12.89-J18.1, J18.8-J18.9, J22, J44.9, J47.0-J70.4, J70.8-J70.9, J98.4, J98.8-J99, Q33.4, R91.1

✓5th **A37.0   Whooping cough due to Bordetella pertussis**

A37.00   Whooping cough due to Bordetella pertussis without pneumonia   `CC`

A37.01   Whooping cough due to Bordetella pertussis with pneumonia   `PDxMCC` `MCC`

✓5th **A37.1   Whooping cough due to Bordetella parapertussis**

A37.10   Whooping cough due to Bordetella parapertussis without pneumonia   `CC`

A37.11   Whooping cough due to Bordetella parapertussis with pneumonia   `PDxMCC` `MCC`

✓5th **A37.8   Whooping cough due to other Bordetella species**

A37.80   Whooping cough due to other Bordetella species without pneumonia   `CC`

A37.81   Whooping cough due to other Bordetella species with pneumonia   `PDxMCC` `MCC`

✓5th **A37.9   Whooping cough, unspecified species**

A37.90   Whooping cough, unspecified species without pneumonia   `CC`

A37.91   Whooping cough, unspecified species with pneumonia   `PDxMCC` `MCC`

✓4th **A38   Scarlet fever**
> **INCLUDES**   scarlatina
> **EXCLUDES 2**   streptococcal sore throat (J02.0)

> CC Excl: For MCC codes in category A38, unless otherwise noted: A38.0-A38.9, A46, J02.0, J03.00-J03.01

A38.0   Scarlet fever with otitis media   `CC`

A38.1   Scarlet fever with myocarditis   `CC`

A38.8   Scarlet fever with other complications   `CC`

A38.9   Scarlet fever, uncomplicated   `CC`
Scarlet fever, NOS

✓4th **A39   Meningococcal infection**

A39.0   Meningococcal meningitis   `MCC`
CC Excl: A02.21, A17.0-A17.1, A27.81, A39.0, A39.89-A39.9, A49.3-A49.9, A50.41, A51.41, A52.13, A54.82, A54.84, A54.89-A54.9, A87.0-A87.9, B00.3, B02.1, B26.1, B37.5, B38.4, B45.1, B58.2, B92, B94.2-B94.9, B96.0, B96.6-B96.89, G00.0-G03.9, G04.2, G32.89, G61.0, G96.8-G96.9, G98.0-G98.8, G99.8

A39.1   Waterhouse-Friderichsen syndrome   `MCC`
Meningococcal hemorrhagic adrenalitis
Meningococcic adrenal syndrome
CC Excl: A39.1, A39.89-A39.9, A49.3-A49.9, B92, B94.2-B94.9, B96.0, B96.6-B96.89

A39.2   Acute meningococcemia   `MCC`
CC Excl: A02.1, A20.7, A22.7, A26.7, A32.7, A39.2-A39.4, A39.89-A40.1, A40.8-A41.9, A42.7, A49.3-A49.9, A54.86, B00.7, B37.7, B92, B94.2-B94.9, B96.0, B96.6-B96.89, R65.10-R65.20

A39.3   Chronic meningococcemia   `MCC`
CC Excl: See code: A39.2

A39.4   Meningococcemia, unspecified   `MCC`
CC Excl: See code: A39.2

✓5th **A39.5   Meningococcal heart disease**

A39.50   Meningococcal carditis, unspecified   `MCC`
CC Excl: A39.50, A39.89-A39.9, A49.3-A49.9, B92, B94.2-B94.9, B96.0, B96.6-B96.89

A39.51   Meningococcal endocarditis   `MCC`
CC Excl: A39.51, A39.89-A39.9, A49.3-A49.9, B92, B94.2-B94.9, B96.0, B96.6-B96.89

A39.52   Meningococcal myocarditis   `MCC`
CC Excl: A39.52, A49.3-A49.9, B92, B94.2-B94.9, B96.0, B96.6-B96.89

A39.53   Meningococcal pericarditis   `MCC`
CC Excl: A39.53, A39.89-A39.9, A49.3-A49.9, B92, B94.2-B94.9, B96.0, B96.6-B96.89

✓5th **A39.8   Other meningococcal infections**

A39.81   Meningococcal encephalitis   `MCC`
CC Excl: A39.81, A39.89-A39.9, A49.3-A49.9, B92, B94.2-B94.9, B96.0, B96.6-B96.89

A39.82   Meningococcal retrobulbar neuritis   `CC`
CC Excl: A39.82, A39.89-A39.9, A49.3-A49.9, B92, B94.2-B94.9, B96.0, B96.6-B96.89

A39.83   Meningococcal arthritis   `CC`
CC Excl: A39.83-A39.9, A49.3-A49.9, B92, B94.2-B94.9, B96.0, B96.6-B96.89

A39.84   Postmeningococcal arthritis   `CC`
CC Excl: See code: A39.83

A39.89   Other meningococcal infections   `CC`
Meningococcal conjunctivitis
CC Excl: A39.89-A39.9, A49.3-A49.9, B92, B94.2-B94.9, B96.0, B96.6-B96.89

A39.9   Meningococcal infection, unspecified   `CC`
Meningococcal disease NOS
CC Excl: See code: A39.89

✓4th **A40   Streptococcal sepsis**
Code first: postprocedural streptococcal sepsis (T81.4)
streptococcal sepsis during labor (O75.3)
streptococcal sepsis following abortion or ectopic or molar pregnancy (O03-O07, O08.0)
streptococcal sepsis following immunization (T88.0)
streptococcal sepsis following infusion, transfusion or therapeutic injection (T80.2-)
> **EXCLUDES 1**   neonatal (P36.0-P36.1)
>   puerperal sepsis (O85)
>   sepsis due to Streptococcus, group D (A41.81)

> CC Excl: For MCC codes in category A40, unless otherwise noted: A02.1, A20.7, A22.7, A26.7, A32.7, A39.2-A39.4, A40.0-A40.1, A40.8-A41.9, A42.7, A48.2-A48.4, A48.8-A49.9, A54.86, B00.7, B37.7, B92, B94.2-B96.89, M00.011-M00.012, M00.021-M00.022, M00.031-M00.032, M00.041-M00.042, M00.051-M00.052, M00.061-M00.062, M00.071-M00.072, R65.10-R65.20, Z16.10-Z16.39

A40.0   Sepsis due to streptococcus, group A   `MCC`

A40.1   Sepsis due to streptococcus, group B   `MCC`

A40.3   Sepsis due to Streptococcus pneumoniae   `MCC`
Pneumococcal sepsis
CC Excl: No Excl

A40.8   Other streptococcal sepsis   `MCC`

A40.9   Streptococcal sepsis, unspecified   `HIV` `MCC`

✓ Additional Character Required   ✓x7th Placeholder Alert   Unacceptable PDx   Manifestation   Hospital Acquired Condition   **EXCLUDES 1** Not Coded Here   **EXCLUDES 2** Not Included Here

Chapter 1. Certain Infectious and Parasitic Diseases

A41–A49.01

✓4ᵗʰ A41 Other sepsis

Code first: postprocedural sepsis (T81.4)
sepsis during labor (O75.3)
sepsis following abortion, ectopic or molar pregnancy (O03-O07, O08.0)
sepsis following immunization (T88.0)
sepsis following infusion, transfusion or therapeutic injection (T80.2-)

EXCLUDES 1   bacteremia NOS (R78.81)
neonatal (P36.-)
puerperal sepsis (O85)
sepsis NOS (A41.9)
streptococcal sepsis (A40.-)

EXCLUDES 2   sepsis (due to) (in) actinomycotic (A42.7)
sepsis (due to) (in) anthrax (A22.7)
sepsis (due to) (in) candidal (B37.7)
sepsis (due to) (in) Erysipelothrix (A26.7)
sepsis (due to) (in) extraintestinal yersiniosis (A28.2)
sepsis (due to) (in) gonococcal (A54.86)
sepsis (due to) (in) herpesviral (B00.7)
sepsis (due to) (in) listerial (A32.7)
sepsis (due to) (in) melioidosis (A24.1)
sepsis (due to) (in) meningococcal (A39.2-A39.4)
sepsis (due to) (in) plague (A20.7)
sepsis (due to) (in) tularemia (A21.7)
toxic shock syndrome (A48.3)

AHA: 2014, 2Q, 13

CC Excl: For MCC codes in category A41, unless otherwise noted: A02.1, A20.7, A22.7, A26.7, A32.7, A39.2-A39.4, A40.0-A40.1, A40.8-A41.9, A42.7, A48.2-A48.4, A48.8-A49.9, A54.86, B00.7, B37.7, B92, B94.2-B96.89, M00.011-M00.012, M00.021-M00.022, M00.031-M00.032, M00.041-M00.042, M00.051- M00.052, M00.061-M00.062, M00.071-M00.072, R65.10-R65.20, Z16.10-Z16.39

✓5ᵗʰ A41.0 Sepsis due to Staphylococcus aureus

A41.01 Sepsis due to methicillin susceptible Staphylococcus aureus   HIV MCC
MSSA sepsis
Staphylococcus aureus sepsis NOS

A41.02 Sepsis due to methicillin resistant Staphylococcus aureus   HIV MCC

A41.1 Sepsis due to other specified staphylococcus   HIV MCC
Coagulase negative staphylococcus sepsis

A41.2 Sepsis due to unspecified staphylococcus   HIV MCC

A41.3 Sepsis due to Hemophilus influenzae   HIV MCC

A41.4 Sepsis due to anaerobes   HIV MCC
EXCLUDES 1   gas gangrene (A48.0)

✓5ᵗʰ A41.5 Sepsis due to other Gram-negative organisms

A41.50 Gram-negative sepsis, unspecified   HIV MCC
Gram-negative sepsis NOS

A41.51 Sepsis due to Escherichia coli [E. coli]   HIV MCC

A41.52 Sepsis due to Pseudomonas   HIV MCC
Pseudomonas aeroginosa

A41.53 Sepsis due to Serratia   HIV MCC

A41.59 Other Gram-negative sepsis   HIV MCC

✓5ᵗʰ A41.8 Other specified sepsis

A41.81 Sepsis due to Enterococcus   HIV MCC

A41.89 Other specified sepsis   HIV MCC

A41.9 Sepsis, unspecified organism   HIV MCC
Septicemia NOS

✓4ᵗʰ A42 Actinomycosis

EXCLUDES 1   actinomycetoma (B47.1)

A42.0 Pulmonary actinomycosis   HIV CC
CC Excl: A42.0, A42.81-A43.0, A43.8-A43.9, B47.1, J12.81

A42.1 Abdominal actinomycosis   HIV CC
CC Excl: A42.1, A42.81-A42.9, A43.8-A43.9, B47.1

A42.2 Cervicofacial actinomycosis   HIV CC
CC Excl: A42.2, A42.81-A42.9, A43.8-A43.9, B47.1

A42.7 Actinomycotic sepsis   HIV MCC
CC Excl: A02.1, A20.7, A22.7, A26.7, A32.7, A39.2-A39.4, A40.0-A40.1, A40.8-A41.9, A42.7, A48.2-A48.4, A48.8-A49.9, A54.86, B00.7, B37.7, B92, B94.2-B96.89, M00.011-M00.012, M00.021-M00.022, M00.031- M00.032, M00.041-M00.042, M00.051-M00.052, M00.061-M00.062, M00.071-M00.072, R65.10-R65.20, Z16.10-Z16.39

✓5ᵗʰ A42.8 Other forms of actinomycosis

CC Excl: For CC codes in subcategory A42.8, unless otherwise noted: A42.0-A42.2, A42.81-A43.9, B47.1-B47.9, L08.1

A42.81 Actinomycotic meningitis   HIV CC

A42.82 Actinomycotic encephalitis   HIV CC

A42.89 Other forms of actinomycosis   HIV CC

A42.9 Actinomycosis, unspecified   HIV CC
CC Excl: See code: A42.8

✓4ᵗʰ A43 Nocardiosis

A43.0 Pulmonary nocardiosis   HIV CC
CC Excl: A42.0, A42.81-A43.0, A43.8-A43.9, B47.1, J12.81

A43.1 Cutaneous nocardiosis   HIV CC
CC Excl: A42.81-A42.9, A43.1-A43.9, B47.1, L08.1

A43.8 Other forms of nocardiosis   HIV CC
CC Excl: A42.0-A42.2, A42.81-A43.9, B47.1-B47.9, L08.1

A43.9 Nocardiosis, unspecified   HIV CC
CC Excl: See code: A43.8

✓4ᵗʰ A44 Bartonellosis

CC Excl: For CC codes in category A44, unless otherwise noted: A44.0-A44.9, A68.0-A68.9, A69.20-A69.29, A75.0-A79.9, B55.0-B57.5, B60.0

A44.0 Systemic bartonellosis   CC
Oroya fever

A44.1 Cutaneous and mucocutaneous bartonellosis   CC
Verruga peruana

A44.8 Other forms of bartonellosis   CC

A44.9 Bartonellosis, unspecified   CC

A46 Erysipelas

EXCLUDES 1   postpartum or puerperal erysipelas (O86.89)

✓4ᵗʰ A48 Other bacterial diseases, not elsewhere classified

EXCLUDES 1   actinomycetoma (B47.1)

A48.0 Gas gangrene   MCC
Clostridial cellulitis
Clostridial myonecrosis
CC Excl: A48.0, B92, B94.2-B94.9

A48.1 Legionnaires' disease   HIV MCC
CC Excl: A15.0-A15.6, A15.8-A15.9, A17.9, A18.82, A18.84, A18.89, A21.2, A22.1, A31.0, A37.01, A37.11, A37.81, A37.91, A42.0, A43.0, A48.1, B25.0, B39.0-B39.2, B44.0, B58.3, B59, B67.1, J09.X1-J09.X2, J10.00-J10.1, J11.00-J11.1, J12.0-J12.3, J12.89-J18.1, J18.8-J18.9, J22, J44.9, J47.0-J70.4, J70.8-J70.9, J98.4, J98.8-J99, Q33.4, R91.1

A48.2 Nonpneumonic Legionnaires' disease [Pontiac fever]

A48.3 Toxic shock syndrome   MCC
Use additional code to identify the organism (B95, B96)
EXCLUDES 1   endotoxic shock NOS (R57.8)
sepsis NOS (A41.9)
CC Excl: A48.3, G89.0-G89.4, R09.89, R41.0-R41.3, R41.82, R41.9, R44.8-R44.9, R45.83-R45.84, R46.0-R46.89, R52, R57.0-R57.9, R65.21-R68.19, R68.81-R68.83, R68.89-R69

A48.4 Brazilian purpuric fever
Systemic Hemophilus aegyptius infection

✓5ᵗʰ A48.5 Other specified botulism
Non-foodborne intoxication due to toxins of Clostridium botulinum [C. botulinum]
EXCLUDES 1   food poisoning due to toxins of Clostridium botulinum (A05.1)

CC Excl: For CC codes in subcategory A48.5, unless otherwise noted: A04.7, A05.0-A05.2, A48.51-A48.52

A48.51 Infant botulism   CC P

A48.52 Wound botulism   CC
Non-foodborne botulism NOS
Use additional code for associated wound

A48.8 Other specified bacterial diseases

✓4ᵗʰ A49 Bacterial infection of unspecified site

EXCLUDES 1   bacterial agents as the cause of diseases classified elsewhere (B95-B96)
chlamydial infection NOS (A74.9)
meningococcal infection NOS (A39.9)
rickettsial infection NOS (A79.9)
spirochetal infection NOS (A69.9)

✓5ᵗʰ A49.0 Staphylococcal infection, unspecified site

A49.01 Methicillin susceptible Staphylococcus aureus infection, unspecified site
Methicillin susceptible Staphylococcus aureus (MSSA) infection
Staphylococcus aureus infection NOS

N Newborn: 0   P Pediatric: 0-17   M Maternity: 12-55   A Adult: 15-124   MCC Major CC Condition   PDxMCC PDx acts as own MCC   CC CC Condition   PDxCC PDx acts as own CC

432   ICD-10-CM 2016

A49.02　**Methicillin resistant Staphylococcus aureus infection, unspecified site**
Methicillin resistant Staphylococcus aureus (MRSA) infection

A49.1　**Streptococcal infection, unspecified site**

A49.2　**Hemophilus influenzae infection, unspecified site**

A49.3　**Mycoplasma infection, unspecified site**

A49.8　**Other bacterial infections of unspecified site**

A49.9　**Bacterial infection, unspecified**
EXCLUDES1　bacteremia NOS (R78.81)

Infections with a predominantly sexual mode of transmission (A50-A64)

EXCLUDES1　human immunodeficiency virus [HIV] disease (B20)
nonspecific and nongonococcal urethritis (N34.1)
Reiter's disease (M02.3-)

✓4th **A50**　**Congenital syphilis**

✓5th **A50.0**　**Early congenital syphilis, symptomatic**
Any congenital syphilitic condition specified as early or manifest less than two years after birth.

CC Excl: For CC codes in subcategory A50.0, unless otherwise noted: A50.01-A51.46, A51.5-A53.9

A50.01　**Early congenital syphilitic oculopathy** CC

A50.02　**Early congenital syphilitic osteochondropathy** CC

A50.03　**Early congenital syphilitic pharyngitis** CC
Early congenital syphilitic laryngitis

A50.04　**Early congenital syphilitic pneumonia** CC

A50.05　**Early congenital syphilitic rhinitis** CC

A50.06　**Early cutaneous congenital syphilis** CC

A50.07　**Early mucocutaneous congenital syphilis** CC

A50.08　**Early visceral congenital syphilis** CC

A50.09　**Other early congenital syphilis, symptomatic** CC

A50.1　**Early congenital syphilis, latent**
Congenital syphilis without clinical manifestations, with positive serological reaction and negative spinal fluid test, less than two years after birth.

A50.2　**Early congenital syphilis, unspecified** CC
Congenital syphilis NOS less than two years after birth.
CC Excl: A50.01-A51.46, A51.5-A54.85, A54.89-A58, A63.8-A64, B92, B94.2-B94.9, M02.30-M02.342

✓5th **A50.3**　**Late congenital syphilitic oculopathy**
EXCLUDES1　Hutchinson's triad (A50.53)

CC Excl: For CC/MCC codes in subcategory A50.3, unless otherwise noted: A50.01-A51.46, A51.5-A53.9

A50.30　**Late congenital syphilitic oculopathy, unspecified** CC

A50.31　**Late congenital syphilitic interstitial keratitis** CC

A50.32　**Late congenital syphilitic chorioretinitis** CC

A50.39　**Other late congenital syphilitic oculopathy** CC

✓5th **A50.4**　**Late congenital neurosyphilis [juvenile neurosyphilis]**
Use additional code to identify any associated mental disorder
EXCLUDES1　Hutchinson's triad (A50.53)

A50.40　**Late congenital neurosyphilis, unspecified** CC
Juvenile neurosyphilis NOS
CC Excl: A50.01-A51.46, A51.5-A53.9, A56.00-A56.8, A63.8-A64, B92, B94.2-B94.9, N34.1

A50.41　**Late congenital syphilitic meningitis** MCC
CC Excl: A02.21, A17.0-A17.1, A27.81, A39.0, A50.01-A51.46, A51.5-A53.9, A54.82, A54.84, A54.89-A54.9, A56.00-A56.8, A63.8-A64, A87.0-A87.9, B00.3, B02.1, B26.1, B37.5, B38.4, B45.1, B58.2, B92, B94.2-B94.9, G00.0-G03.9, G04.2, G32.89, G61.0, G96.8-G96.9, G98.0-G98.8, G99.8, N34.1

A50.42　**Late congenital syphilitic encephalitis** MCC
CC Excl: A50.01-A51.46, A51.5-A53.9, A56.00-A56.8, A63.8-A64, B92, B94.2-B94.9, N34.1

A50.43　**Late congenital syphilitic polyneuropathy** CC
CC Excl: See code: A50.42

A50.44　**Late congenital syphilitic optic nerve atrophy** CC
CC Excl: A50.01-A51.46, A51.5-A53.9

A50.45　**Juvenile general paresis** CC
Dementia paralytica juvenilis
Juvenile tabetoparetic neurosyphilis
CC Excl: See code: A50.40

A50.49　**Other late congenital neurosyphilis** CC
Juvenile tabes dorsalis
CC Excl: See code: A50.40

✓5th **A50.5**　**Other late congenital syphilis, symptomatic**
Any congenital syphilitic condition specified as late or manifest two years or more after birth.

CC Excl: For CC codes in subcategory A50.5, unless otherwise noted: A50.01-A51.46, A51.5-A53.9

A50.51　**Clutton's joints** CC

A50.52　**Hutchinson's teeth** CC

A50.53　**Hutchinson's triad** CC

A50.54　**Late congenital cardiovascular syphilis** CC

A50.55　**Late congenital syphilitic arthropathy** CC

A50.56　**Late congenital syphilitic osteochondropathy** CC

A50.57　**Syphilitic saddle nose** CC

A50.59　**Other late congenital syphilis, symptomatic** CC

A50.6　**Late congenital syphilis, latent**
Congenital syphilis without clinical manifestations, with positive serological reaction and negative spinal fluid test, two years or more after birth.

A50.7　**Late congenital syphilis, unspecified**
Congenital syphilis NOS two years or more after birth.

A50.9　**Congenital syphilis, unspecified**

✓4th **A51**　**Early syphilis**

A51.0　**Primary genital syphilis**
Syphilitic chancre NOS

A51.1　**Primary anal syphilis**

A51.2　**Primary syphilis of other sites**

✓5th **A51.3**　**Secondary syphilis of skin and mucous membranes**

A51.31　**Condyloma latum** CC
CC Excl: A50.01-A51.46, A51.5-A53.9

A51.32　**Syphilitic alopecia** CC
CC Excl: A50.01-A51.46, A51.5-A54.85, A54.89-A58, A63.8-A64, M02.30-M02.39, N34.1

A51.39　**Other secondary syphilis of skin** CC
Syphilitic leukoderma　Syphilitic mucous patch
EXCLUDES1　late syphilitic leukoderma (A52.79)
CC Excl: See code: A51.31

✓5th **A51.4**　**Other secondary syphilis**

A51.41　**Secondary syphilitic meningitis** MCC
CC Excl: A02.21, A17.0-A17.1, A27.81, A39.0, A50.01-A51.46, A51.5-A54.85, A54.89-A58, A63.8-A64, A74.81-A74.9, A87.0-A87.9, A96.2, A98.3-A98.4, B26.1, B33.24, B33.4-B33.8, B34.1-B34.2, B34.4-B34.8, B37.5, B38.4, B45.1, B58.2, B92, B94.2-B94.9, B97.10, B97.19, B97.29, B97.5-B97.6, B97.81-B97.89, G00.0-G03.9, G04.2, G32.89, G61.0, G96.8-G96.9, G98.0-G98.8, G99.8, M02.30-M02.39, N34.1

A51.42　**Secondary syphilitic female pelvic disease** CC ♀
CC Excl: A50.01-A51.46, A51.5-A54.85, A54.89-A58, A63.8-A64, B92, B94.2-B94.9, M02.30-M02.39, N34.1

A51.43　**Secondary syphilitic oculopathy** CC
Secondary syphilitic chorioretinitis
Secondary syphilitic iridocyclitis, iritis
Secondary syphilitic uveitis
CC Excl: A50.01-A51.46, A51.5-A53.9

A51.44　**Secondary syphilitic nephritis** CC
CC Excl: A50.01-A51.46, A51.5-A54.85, A54.89-A58, A63.8-A64, B92, B94.2-B94.9, M02.30-M02.39, N34.1

A51.45　**Secondary syphilitic hepatitis** CC
CC Excl: A50.01-A51.46, A51.5-A54.85, A54.89-A58, A63.8-A64, K71.0-K71.9, K73.1-K73.8, K74.0-K74.69, K75.2-K76.0, K76.4-K76.5, K76.89-K76.9, M02.30-M02.39, N34.1

A51.46　**Secondary syphilitic osteopathy** CC
CC Excl: A18.09, A50.01-A51.46, A51.5-A54.85, A54.89-A58, A63.8-A64, A66.6, M02.30-M02.39, M84.80-M84.9, M85.10-M85.19, M85.80-M85.89, M86.30-M86.8X9, M89.20-M89.39, M89.50-M89.59, M89.8X0-M89.8X9, M94.1, M94.351-M94.8X9, N34.1

A51.49　**Other secondary syphilitic conditions** CC
Secondary syphilitic lymphadenopathy
Secondary syphilitic myositis
CC Excl: No Excl

A51.5　**Early syphilis, latent**
Syphilis (acquired) without clinical manifestations, with positive serological reaction and negative spinal fluid test, less than two years after infection.

A51.9　**Early syphilis, unspecified**

✓4ᵗʰ **A52 Late syphilis**

✓5ᵗʰ **A52.0 Cardiovascular and cerebrovascular syphilis**

> **CC Excl:** For CC codes in subcategory A52.0, unless otherwise noted: A50.01–A51.46, A51.5–A53.9, A56.00–A56.8, A63.8–A64, B92, B94.2–B94.9, N34.1

A52.00 Cardiovascular syphilis, unspecified   CC

A52.01 Syphilitic aneurysm of aorta   CC

A52.02 Syphilitic aortitis   CC

A52.03 Syphilitic endocarditis   CC
  Syphilitic aortic valve incompetence or stenosis
  Syphilitic mitral valve stenosis
  Syphilitic pulmonary valve regurgitation

A52.04 Syphilitic cerebral arteritis   CC

A52.05 Other cerebrovascular syphilis   CC
  Syphilitic cerebral aneurysm (ruptured) (non-ruptured)
  Syphilitic cerebral thrombosis

A52.06 Other syphilitic heart involvement   CC
  Syphilitic coronary artery disease
  Syphilitic myocarditis
  Syphilitic pericarditis

A52.09 Other cardiovascular syphilis   CC

✓5ᵗʰ **A52.1 Symptomatic neurosyphilis**

> **CC Excl:** For CC/MCC codes in subcategory A52.1, unless otherwise noted: A50.01–A51.46, A51.5–A53.9, A56.00–A56.8, A63.8–A64, B92, B94.2–B94.9, N34.1

A52.10 Symptomatic neurosyphilis, unspecified   CC

A52.11 Tabes dorsalis   CC
  Locomotor ataxia (progressive)
  Tabetic neurosyphilis

A52.12 Other cerebrospinal syphilis   CC

A52.13 Late syphilitic meningitis   MCC
  CC Excl: A02.21, A17.0–A17.1, A27.81, A39.0, A50.01–A51.46, A51.5–A53.9, A54.82, A54.84, A54.89–A54.9, A56.00–A56.8, A63.8–A64, A87.0–A87.9, B00.3, B02.1, B26.1, B37.5, B38.4, B45.1, B58.2, B92, B94.2–B94.9, G00.0–G03.9, G04.2, G32.89, G61.0, G96.8–G96.9, G98.0–G98.8, G99.8, N34.1

A52.14 Late syphilitic encephalitis   MCC

A52.15 Late syphilitic neuropathy   CC
  Late syphilitic acoustic neuritis
  Late syphilitic optic (nerve) atrophy
  Late syphilitic polyneuropathy
  Late syphilitic retrobulbar neuritis

A52.16 Charcôt's arthropathy (tabetic)   CC

A52.17 General paresis   CC
  Dementia paralytica

A52.19 Other symptomatic neurosyphilis   CC
  Syphilitic parkinsonism

A52.2 Asymptomatic neurosyphilis   CC
  CC Excl: See code: A52.1

A52.3 Neurosyphilis, unspecified   CC
  Gumma (syphilitic)   Syphiloma
  Syphilis (late)
  CC Excl: See code: A52.1

✓5ᵗʰ **A52.7 Other symptomatic late syphilis**

> **CC Excl:** For CC codes in subcategory A52.7, unless otherwise noted: A50.01–A51.46, A51.5–A54.85, A54.89–A58, A63.8–A64, M02.30–M02.39, N34.1

A52.71 Late syphilitic oculopathy   CC
  Late syphilitic chorioretinitis
  Late syphilitic episcleritis
  CC Excl: A18.50–A18.59, A50.01–A51.46, A51.5–A54.85, A54.89–A58, A63.8–A64, H15.001–H15.009, H15.091–H15.129, M02.30–M02.39, N34.1

A52.72 Syphilis of lung and bronchus   CC

A52.73 Symptomatic late syphilis of other respiratory organs   CC

A52.74 Syphilis of liver and other viscera   CC
  Late syphilitic peritonitis

A52.75 Syphilis of kidney and ureter   CC
  Syphilitic glomerular disease

A52.76 Other genitourinary symptomatic late syphilis   CC
  Late syphilitic female pelvic inflammatory disease

A52.77 Syphilis of bone and joint   CC

A52.78 Syphilis of other musculoskeletal tissue   CC
  Late syphilitic bursitis
  Syphilis [stage unspecified] of bursa
  Syphilis [stage unspecified] of muscle
  Syphilis [stage unspecified] of synovium
  Syphilis [stage unspecified] of tendon

A52.79 Other symptomatic late syphilis   CC
  Late syphilitic leukoderma   Syphilis of thyroid gland
  Syphilis of adrenal gland   Syphilitic splenomegaly
  Syphilis of pituitary gland
  EXCLUDES 1 *syphilitic leukoderma (secondary) (A51.39)*

A52.8 Late syphilis, latent
  Syphilis (acquired) without clinical manifestations, with positive serological reaction and negative spinal fluid test, two years or more after infection

A52.9 Late syphilis, unspecified

✓4ᵗʰ **A53 Other and unspecified syphilis**

A53.0 Latent syphilis, unspecified as early or late
  Latent syphilis NOS   Positive serological reaction for syphilis

A53.9 Syphilis, unspecified
  Infection due to Treponema pallidum NOS
  Syphilis (acquired) NOS
  EXCLUDES 1 *syphilis NOS under two years of age (A50.2)*

✓4ᵗʰ **A54 Gonococcal infection**

✓5ᵗʰ **A54.0 Gonococcal infection of lower genitourinary tract without periurethral or accessory gland abscess**

> **CC Excl:** For CC codes in subcategory A54.0, unless otherwise noted: A54.00–A54.29, A54.82, A54.84, A54.89–A54.9, A56.00–A56.8, A63.8–A64, B92, B94.2–B94.9, N34.1
>
> **EXCLUDES 1** *gonococcal infection with genitourinary gland abscess (A54.1)*
> *gonococcal infection with periurethral abscess (A54.1)*

A54.00 Gonococcal infection of lower genitourinary tract, unspecified   CC

A54.01 Gonococcal cystitis and urethritis, unspecified   CC

A54.02 Gonococcal vulvovaginitis, unspecified   CC ♀

A54.03 Gonococcal cervicitis, unspecified   CC ♀

A54.09 Other gonococcal infection of lower genitourinary tract   CC

A54.1 Gonococcal infection of lower genitourinary tract with periurethral and accessory gland abscess   CC
  Gonococcal Bartholin's gland abscess
  CC Excl: See code: A54.0

✓5ᵗʰ **A54.2 Gonococcal pelviperitonitis and other gonococcal genitourinary infection**

> **CC Excl:** For CC codes in subcategory A54.2, unless otherwise noted: A54.00–A54.29, A54.82, A54.84, A54.89–A54.9, A56.00–A56.8, A63.8–A64, B92, B94.2–B94.9, N34.1

A54.21 Gonococcal infection of kidney and ureter   CC

A54.22 Gonococcal prostatitis   CC ♂

A54.23 Gonococcal infection of other male genital organs   CC ♂
  Gonococcal epididymitis   Gonococcal orchitis

A54.24 Gonococcal female pelvic inflammatory disease   CC ♀
  Gonococcal pelviperitonitis
  EXCLUDES 1 *gonococcal peritonitis (A54.85)*

A54.29 Other gonococcal genitourinary infections   CC

✓5ᵗʰ **A54.3 Gonococcal infection of eye**

> **CC Excl:** For CC codes in subcategory A54.3, unless otherwise noted: A50.01–A51.46, A51.5–A54.85, A54.89–A58, A63.8–A64, M02.30–M02.39, N34.1

A54.30 Gonococcal infection of eye, unspecified   CC

A54.31 Gonococcal conjunctivitis   CC
  Ophthalmia neonatorum due to gonococcus

A54.32 Gonococcal iridocyclitis   CC

A54.33 Gonococcal keratitis   CC

A54.39 Other gonococcal eye infection   CC
  Gonococcal endophthalmia

N Newborn: 0   P Pediatric: 0-17   M Maternity: 12-55   A Adult: 15-124   **MCC** Major CC Condition   **PDxMCC** PDx acts as own MCC   **CC** CC Condition   **PDxCC** PDx acts as own CC

434

ICD-10-CM 2016

✓5th **A54.4 Gonococcal infection of musculoskeletal system**

> **CC Excl:** For CC codes in subcategory A54.4, unless otherwise noted: A02.23, A17.9, A18.02, A18.09, A18.82, A18.84, A18.89, A39.83-A39.84, A50.01-A51.46, A51.5-A54.85, A54.89-A58, A63.8-A64, B06.82, M00.00-M02.9, M05.40-M05.59, M05.70-M06.09, M06.20-M06.39, M06.80-M07.69, M11.00-M11.9, M12.10-M15.0, M15.3-M15.9, M16.2-M16.9, M17.2-M17.9, M18.2-M18.9, M19.111-M19.93, M24.10-M24.176, M25.00, M25.08-M25.18, M25.40-M25.676, M25.80-M25.9, M35.2, M36.1-M36.4, N34.1, R29.4

     A54.40 Gonococcal infection of musculoskeletal system, unspecified `CC`

     A54.41 Gonococcal spondylopathy `CC`

     A54.42 Gonococcal arthritis `CC`
         EXCLUDES 2   gonococcal infection of spine (A54.41)

     A54.43 Gonococcal osteomyelitis `CC`
         EXCLUDES 2   gonococcal infection of spine (A54.41)

     A54.49 Gonococcal infection of other musculoskeletal tissue `CC`
         Gonococcal bursitis
         Gonococcal myositis
         Gonococcal synovitis
         Gonococcal tenosynovitis

A54.5 Gonococcal pharyngitis

A54.6 Gonococcal infection of anus and rectum

✓5th **A54.8 Other gonococcal infections**

     A54.81 Gonococcal meningitis `MCC`
         CC Excl: A02.21, A17.0-A17.1, A27.81, A39.0, A50.01-A51.46, A51.5-A54.85, A54.89-A58, A63.8-A64, A74.81-A74.9, A87.0-A87.9, A96.2, A98.3-A98.4, B26.1, B33.24, B33.4-B33.8, B34.1-B34.2, B34.4-B34.8, B37.5, B38.4, B45.1, B58.2, B92, B94.2-B94.9, B97.10, B97.19, B97.29, B97.5-B97.6, B97.81-B97.89, G00.0-G03.9, G04.2, G32.89, G61.0, G96.8-G96.9, G98.0-G98.8, G99.8, M02.30-M02.39, N34.1

     A54.82 Gonococcal brain abscess `CC`
         CC Excl: A50.01-A51.46, A51.5-A54.85, A54.89-A58, A63.8-A64, M02.30-M02.39, N25.81-N25.89, N34.1

     A54.83 Gonococcal heart infection `CC`
         Gonococcal endocarditis
         Gonococcal myocarditis
         Gonococcal pericarditis
         CC Excl: A01.00-A01.09, A39.51, A50.01-A51.46, A51.5-A54.85, A54.89-A58, A63.8-A64, A78, B33.20-B33.22, B37.6, B40.0-B40.9, I00, I01.1-I02.0, I05.0-I07.9, I08.1-I08.3, I08.9-I09.1, I09.89-I09.9, I23.0-I23.3, I23.6-I23.8, I33.0-I41, I42.4, I51.0, I51.4, I87.8, I99.8-I99.9, M00.00, M00.08-M00.10, M00.18-M00.20, M00.28-M00.80, M00.88-M00.9, M02.30-M02.39, N34.1, Q22.2, Q23.8-Q23.9, Q24.8, T82.6XXA

     A54.84 Gonococcal pneumonia `CC`
         CC Excl: See code: A54.82

     A54.85 Gonococcal peritonitis `CC`
         EXCLUDES 1   gonococcal pelviperitonitis (A54.24)
         CC Excl: A18.31-A34, A50.01-A51.46, A51.5-A54.85, A54.89-A58, A63.8-A64, K35.2-K35.3, K63.4, K63.89-K63.9, K65.1, K65.3, K65.9, K67, K86.8, K92.89-K92.9, M02.30-M02.39, N34.1, N73.3-N73.4, N73.6, O08.0, O08.82, O85, O86.12, O86.81-O86.89, P78.0, R11.13, T81.60XA, T81.61XA, T81.69XA

     A54.86 Gonococcal sepsis `PDxMCC` `MCC`
         CC Excl: A02.1, A20.7, A22.7, A26.7, A32.7, A39.2-A39.4, A40.0-A40.1, A40.8-A41.9, A42.7, A48.2-A48.4, A48.8-A49.9, A54.86, B00.7, B37.7, B92, B94.2-B96.89, M00.011-M00.012, M00.021-M00.022, M00.031-M00.032, M00.041-M00.042, M00.051-M00.052, M00.061-M00.062, M00.071-M00.072, R65.10-R65.20, Z16.10-Z16.39

     A54.89 Other gonococcal infections `CC`
         Gonococcal keratoderma
         Gonococcal lymphadenitis
         CC Excl: See code: A54.82

A54.9 Gonococcal infection, unspecified `CC`
     CC Excl: See code: A54.82

A55 Chlamydial lymphogranuloma (venereum)
     Climatic or tropical bubo
     Durand-Nicolas-Favre disease
     Esthiomene
     Lymphogranuloma inguinale

✓4th **A56 Other sexually transmitted chlamydial diseases**
     INCLUDES   sexually transmitted diseases due to Chlamydia trachomatis
     EXCLUDES 1   neonatal chlamydial conjunctivitis (P39.1)
              neonatal chlamydial pneumonia (P23.1)
     EXCLUDES 2   chlamydial lymphogranuloma (A55)
              conditions classified to A74-

✓5th **A56.0 Chlamydial infection of lower genitourinary tract**

     A56.00 Chlamydial infection of lower genitourinary tract, unspecified

     A56.01 Chlamydial cystitis and urethritis

     A56.02 Chlamydial vulvovaginitis ♀

     A56.09 Other chlamydial infection of lower genitourinary tract
         Chlamydial cervicitis

✓5th **A56.1 Chlamydial infection of pelviperitoneum and other genitourinary organs**

     A56.11 Chlamydial female pelvic inflammatory disease ♀

     A56.19 Other chlamydial genitourinary infection
         Chlamydial epididymitis
         Chlamydial orchitis

A56.2 Chlamydial infection of genitourinary tract, unspecified

A56.3 Chlamydial infection of anus and rectum

A56.4 Chlamydial infection of pharynx

A56.8 Sexually transmitted chlamydial infection of other sites

A57 Chancroid
     Ulcus molle

A58 Granuloma inguinale
     Donovanosis

✓4th **A59 Trichomoniasis**
     EXCLUDES 2   intestinal trichomoniasis (A07.8)

✓5th **A59.0 Urogenital trichomoniasis**

     A59.00 Urogenital trichomoniasis, unspecified
         Fluor (vaginalis) due to Trichomonas
         Leukorrhea (vaginalis) due to Trichomonas

     A59.01 Trichomonal vulvovaginitis ♀

     A59.02 Trichomonal prostatitis ♂

     A59.03 Trichomonal cystitis and urethritis

     A59.09 Other urogenital trichomoniasis
         Trichomonas cervicitis

A59.8 Trichomoniasis of other sites

A59.9 Trichomoniasis, unspecified

✓4th **A60 Anogenital herpesviral [herpes simplex] infections**

✓5th **A60.0 Herpesviral infection of genitalia and urogenital tract**

     A60.00 Herpesviral infection of urogenital system, unspecified `HIV`

     A60.01 Herpesviral infection of penis `HIV` ♂

     A60.02 Herpesviral infection of other male genital organs ♂

     A60.03 Herpesviral cervicitis ♀

     A60.04 Herpesviral vulvovaginitis `HIV` ♀
         Herpesviral [herpes simplex] ulceration
         Herpesviral [herpes simplex] vaginitis
         Herpesviral [herpes simplex] vulvitis

     A60.09 Herpesviral infection of other urogenital tract `HIV`

A60.1 Herpesviral infection of perianal skin and rectum `HIV`

A60.9 Anogenital herpesviral infection, unspecified `HIV`

✓4th **A63 Other predominantly sexually transmitted diseases, not elsewhere classified**
     EXCLUDES 2   molluscum contagiosum (B08.1)
              papilloma of cervix (D26.0)

A63.0 Anogenital (venereal) warts
     Anogenital warts due to (human) papillomavirus [HPV]
     Condyloma acuminatum

A63.8 Other specified predominantly sexually transmitted diseases

A64 Unspecified sexually transmitted disease

✔ Additional Character Required   ✔x7th Placeholder Alert   Unacceptable PDx   Manifestation   Hospital Acquired Condition   *EXCLUDES 1* Not Coded Here   *EXCLUDES 2* Not Included Here

Other spirochetal diseases (A65-A69)

EXCLUDES 2   leptospirosis (A27.-)
            syphilis (A50–A53)

A65   Nonvenereal syphilis
    Bejel
    Endemic syphilis
    Njovera

✓4th A66   Yaws
    INCLUDES   bouba
                frambesia (tropica)
                pian

A66.0   Initial lesions of yaws
    Chancre of yaws
    Frambesia, initial or primary
    Initial frambesial ulcer
    Mother yaw

A66.1   Multiple papillomata and wet crab yaws
    Frambesioma
    Pianoma
    Plantar or palmar papilloma of yaws

A66.2   Other early skin lesions of yaws
    Cutaneous yaws, less than five years after infection
    Early yaws (cutaneous) (macular) (maculopapular)
        (micropapular) (papular)
    Frambeside of early yaws

A66.3   Hyperkeratosis of yaws
    Ghoul hand
    Hyperkeratosis, palmar or plantar (early) (late) due to yaws
    Worm-eaten soles

A66.4   Gummata and ulcers of yaws
    Gummatous frambeside
    Nodular late yaws (ulcerated)

A66.5   Gangosa
    Rhinopharyngitis mutilans

A66.6   Bone and joint lesions of yaws
    Yaws ganglion
    Yaws goundou
    Yaws gumma, bone
    Yaws gummatous osteitis or periostitis
    Yaws hydrarthrosis
    Yaws osteitis
    Yaws periostitis (hypertrophic)

A66.7   Other manifestations of yaws
    Juxta-articular nodules of yaws
    Mucosal yaws

A66.8   Latent yaws
    Yaws without clinical manifestations, with positive serology

A66.9   Yaws, unspecified

✓4th A67   Pinta [carate]

A67.0   Primary lesions of pinta
    Chancre (primary) of pinta
    Papule (primary) of pinta

A67.1   Intermediate lesions of pinta
    Erythematous plaques of pinta
    Hyperchromic lesions of pinta
    Hyperkeratosis of pinta
    Pintids

A67.2   Late lesions of pinta
    Achromic skin lesions of pinta
    Cicatricial skin lesions of pinta
    Dyschromic skin lesions of pinta

A67.3   Mixed lesions of pinta
    Achromic with hyperchromic skin lesions of pinta [carate]

A67.9   Pinta, unspecified

✓4th A68   Relapsing fevers
    INCLUDES   recurrent fever
    EXCLUDES 2   Lyme disease (A69.2-)

    CC Excl: For CC codes in category A68, unless otherwise noted:
    A44.0–A44.9, A68.0–A68.9, A69.20–A69.29, A75.0–A79.9, B55.0–B57.5, B60.0

A68.0   Louse-borne relapsing fever   CC
    Relapsing fever due to Borrelia recurrentis

A68.1   Tick-borne relapsing fever   CC
    Relapsing fever due to any Borrelia species other than Borrelia recurrentis

A68.9   Relapsing fever, unspecified   CC

✓4th A69   Other spirochetal infections

A69.0   Necrotizing ulcerative stomatitis
    Cancrum oris   Noma
    Fusospirochetal gangrene   Stomatitis gangrenosa

A69.1   Other Vincent's infections   CC
    Fusospirochetal pharyngitis
    Necrotizing ulcerative (acute) gingivitis
    Necrotizing ulcerative (acute) gingivostomatitis
    Spirochetal stomatitis
    Trench mouth
    Vincent's angina
    Vincent's gingivitis
    CC Excl: A69.1

✓5th A69.2   Lyme disease
    Erythema chronicum migrans due to Borrelia burgdorferi

    CC Excl: For CC codes in subcategory A69.2, unless otherwise noted: A44.0–A44.9, A68.0–A68.9, A69.20–A69.29, A75.0–A79.9, B55.0–B57.5, B60.0

    A69.20   Lyme disease, unspecified   CC

    A69.21   Meningitis due to Lyme disease   CC

    A69.22   Other neurologic disorders in Lyme disease   CC
       Cranial neuritis
       Meningoencephalitis
       Polyneuropathy

    A69.23   Arthritis due to Lyme disease   CC

    A69.29   Other conditions associated with Lyme disease   CC
       Myopericarditis due to Lyme disease

A69.8   Other specified spirochetal infections

A69.9   Spirochetal infection, unspecified

Other diseases caused by chlamydiae (A70-A74)

EXCLUDES 1   sexually transmitted chlamydial diseases (A55-A56)

A70   Chlamydia psittaci infections   CC
    Ornithosis
    Parrot fever
    Psittacosis
    CC Excl: A70

✓4th A71   Trachoma
    EXCLUDES 1   sequelae of trachoma (B94.0)

A71.0   Initial stage of trachoma
    Trachoma dubium

A71.1   Active stage of trachoma
    Granular conjunctivitis (trachomatous)
    Trachomatous follicular conjunctivitis
    Trachomatous pannus

A71.9   Trachoma, unspecified

✓4th A74   Other diseases caused by chlamydiae
    EXCLUDES 1   neonatal chlamydial conjunctivitis (P39.1)
               neonatal chlamydial pneumonia (P23.1)
               Reiter's disease (M02.3-)
               sexually transmitted chlamydial diseases (A55-A56)
    EXCLUDES 2   chlamydial pneumonia (J16.0)

A74.0   Chlamydial conjunctivitis
    Paratrachoma

✓5th A74.8   Other chlamydial diseases

    A74.81   Chlamydial peritonitis

    A74.89   Other chlamydial diseases

A74.9   Chlamydial infection, unspecified
    Chlamydiosis NOS

Rickettsioses (A75-A79)

✓4th A75   Typhus fever
    EXCLUDES 1   rickettsiosis due to Ehrlichia sennetsu (A79.81)

    CC Excl: For CC codes in category A75, unless otherwise noted: A44.0–A44.9, A68.0–A68.9, A69.20–A69.29, A75.0–A79.9, B55.0–B57.5, B60.0

A75.0   Epidemic louse-borne typhus fever due to Rickettsia prowazekii   CC
    Classical typhus (fever)
    Epidemic (louse-borne) typhus

A75.1   Recrudescent typhus [Brill's disease]   CC
    Brill-Zinsser disease

A75.2   Typhus fever due to Rickettsia typhi   CC
    Murine (flea-borne) typhus

N Newborn: 0   P Pediatric: 0-17   M Maternity: 12-55   A Adult: 15-124   MCC Major CC Condition   PDxMCC PDx acts as own MCC   CC CC Condition   PDx CC PDx acts as own CC

436   ICD-10-CM 2016

A75.3 Typhus fever due to Rickettsia tsutsugamushi `CC`
Scrub (mite-borne) typhus
Tsutsugamushi fever

A75.9 Typhus fever, unspecified `CC`
Typhus (fever) NOS
CC Excl: A17.82, A44.0-A44.9, A50.42, A52.14, A68.0-A68.9,
A69.20-A69.29, A75.0-A79.9, A81.1, A81.82-A81.89, A83.0-A85.8,
A87.2, A88.0, A88.8, A92.1-A92.8, A93.0, B00.4, B00.82, B01.11-
B01.12, B04, B06.01, B08.09, B08.20-B08.22, B08.60-B08.79, B09-
B10.09, B26.2, B33.1, B45.0, B45.2-B45.9, B55.0-B57.5, B58.2,
B60.0, B75, B97.10, B97.21, G04.00-G04.01, G04.31, G04.81-G05.4,
G37.0, G37.4-G37.5, J09.X3-J09.X9, J10.2-J10.89, J11.2-J11.89,
L44.4, M1A.10-M1A.19, P35.2-P35.9, P37.0-P37.4, P37.8-P37.9,
T56.0X1-T56.0X4 with 7th character A

✓4ᵗʰ **A77 Spotted fever [tick-borne rickettsioses]**

> **CC Excl: For CC codes in category A77, unless otherwise noted:**
> A44.0-A44.9, A68.0-A68.9, A69.20-A69.29, A75.0-A79.9, B55.0-B57.5,
> B60.0

A77.0 Spotted fever due to Rickettsia rickettsii `CC`
Rocky Mountain spotted fever
Sao Paulo fever

A77.1 Spotted fever due to Rickettsia conorii `CC`
African tick typhus
Boutonneuse fever
India tick typhus
Kenya tick typhus
Marseilles fever
Mediterranean tick fever

A77.2 Spotted fever due to Rickettsia siberica `CC`
North Asian tick fever
Siberian tick typhus

A77.3 Spotted fever due to Rickettsia australis `CC`
Queensland tick typhus

✓5ᵗʰ **A77.4 Ehrlichiosis**
EXCLUDES1 Rickettsiosis due to Ehrlichia sennetsu (A79.81)

A77.40 Ehrlichiosis, unspecified `CC`

A77.41 Ehrlichiosis chafeensis [E. chafeensis] `CC`

A77.49 Other ehrlichiosis `CC`

A77.8 Other spotted fevers `CC`

A77.9 Spotted fever, unspecified `CC`
Tick-borne typhus NOS

A78 Q fever `CC`
Infection due to Coxiella burnetii
Nine Mile fever
Quadrilateral fever
CC Excl: See code: A77

✓4ᵗʰ **A79 Other rickettsioses**

A79.0 Trench fever `CC`
Quintan fever   Wolhynian fever
CC Excl: See code: A77

A79.1 Rickettsialpox due to Rickettsia akari `CC`
Kew Garden fever   Vesicular rickettsiosis
CC Excl: A77.0-A79.9

✓5ᵗʰ **A79.8 Other specified rickettsioses**

A79.81 Rickettsiosis due to Ehrlichia sennetsu `CC`
CC Excl: See code: A79.1

A79.89 Other specified rickettsioses `CC`
CC Excl: See code: A79.1

A79.9 Rickettsiosis, unspecified `CC`
Rickettsial infection NOS
CC Excl: See code: A79.1

Viral and prion infections of the central nervous system (A80-A89)

EXCLUDES1 postpolio syndrome (G14)
sequelae of poliomyelitis (B91)
sequelae of viral encephalitis (B94.1)

✓4ᵗʰ **A80 Acute poliomyelitis**

> **CC Excl: For MCC codes in category A80, unless otherwise noted:**
> A80.0-A80.39

A80.0 Acute paralytic poliomyelitis, vaccine-associated `MCC`

A80.1 Acute paralytic poliomyelitis, wild virus, imported `MCC`

A80.2 Acute paralytic poliomyelitis, wild virus, indigenous `MCC`

✓5ᵗʰ **A80.3 Acute paralytic poliomyelitis, other and unspecified**

A80.30 Acute paralytic poliomyelitis, unspecified `MCC`

A80.39 Other acute paralytic poliomyelitis `MCC`

A80.4 Acute nonparalytic poliomyelitis

A80.9 Acute poliomyelitis, unspecified

✓4ᵗʰ **A81 Atypical virus infections of central nervous system**
INCLUDES diseases of the central nervous system caused by prions
Use additional code to identify:
dementia with behavioral disturbance (F02.81)
dementia without behavioral disturbance (F02.80)

✓5ᵗʰ **A81.0 Creutzfeldt-Jakob disease**

A81.00 Creutzfeldt-Jakob disease, unspecified `CC`
Jakob-Creutzfeldt disease, unspecified
CC Excl: A17.82, A50.42, A52.14, A75.9, A79.9, A81.00-
A81.9, A83.0-A85.8, A87.2, A88.0, A88.8, A92.1-A92.2,
A92.4-A92.8, A93.0, B00.4, B00.82, B01.11-B01.12, B04,
B06.01, B08.09, B08.20-B08.22, B08.60-B08.79, B09-
B10.09, B26.2, B33.1, B45.0, B45.2-B45.9, B58.2, B75,
B97.10, G04.00-G04.01, G04.31, G04.81-G05.4, G37.0,
G37.4-G37.5, I67.3, J09.X3-J09.X9, J10.2-J10.89, J11.2-
J11.89, L44.4, M1A.10-M1A.19, P35.2-P35.9, P37.0-P37.4,
P37.8-P37.9, T56.0X1-T56.0X4A

A81.01 Variant Creutzfeldt-Jakob disease `CC`
vCJD
CC Excl: See code: A81.00

A81.09 Other Creutzfeldt-Jakob disease `CC`
CJD
Familial Creutzfeldt-Jakob disease
Iatrogenic Creutzfeldt-Jakob disease
Sporadic Creutzfeldt-Jakob disease
Subacute spongiform encephalopathy (with
dementia)
CC Excl: See code: A81.00

A81.1 Subacute sclerosing panencephalitis `CC`
Dawson's inclusion body encephalitis
Van Bogaert's sclerosing leukoencephalopathy
CC Excl: A81.1, B92, B94.2-B94.9

A81.2 Progressive multifocal leukoencephalopathy `HIV` `CC`
Multifocal leukoencephalopathy NOS
CC Excl: A17.82, A50.42, A52.14, A75.9, A79.9, A81.00-A81.9,
A83.0-A85.8, A87.2, A88.0, A88.8, A92.1-A92.2, A92.4-A92.8, A93.0,
B00.4, B00.82, B01.11-B01.12, B04, B06.01, B08.09, B08.20-B08.22,
B08.60-B08.79, B09-B10.09, B26.2, B27.00-B27.99, B33.1, B45.0,
B45.2-B45.9, B58.2, B75, G04.00-G04.01, G04.31, G04.81-G05.4,
G37.0, G37.4-G37.5, I67.3, J09.X3-J09.X9, J10.2-J10.89, J11.2-
J11.89, L44.4, M1A.10X0-M1A.19X1, P35.2-P35.9, P37.0-P37.4,
P37.8-P37.9, T56.0X1A, T56.0X2A, T56.0X3A, T56.0X4A

✓5ᵗʰ **A81.8 Other atypical virus infections of central nervous system**

A81.81 Kuru `CC`
CC Excl: A81.00-A81.9, I67.3

A81.82 Gerstmann-Sträussler-Scheinker syndrome `HIV` `CC`
GSS syndrome
CC Excl: A81.00-A81.9, A92.30-A92.39, B97.21, I67.3

A81.83 Fatal familial insomnia `HIV` `CC`
FFI
CC Excl: See code: A81.82

**A81.89 Other atypical virus infections of central
nervous system** `HIV` `CC`
CC Excl: See code: A81.82

**A81.9 Atypical virus infection of central nervous system,
unspecified** `HIV` `CC`
Prion diseases of the central nervous system NOS
CC Excl: See code: A81.81

✓4ᵗʰ **A82 Rabies**

> **CC Excl: For CC codes in category A82, unless otherwise noted:**
> A82.0-A82.9

A82.0 Sylvatic rabies `CC`

A82.1 Urban rabies `CC`

A82.9 Rabies, unspecified `CC`

✓4ᵗʰ **A83 Mosquito-borne viral encephalitis**
INCLUDES mosquito-borne viral meningoencephalitis
EXCLUDES2 Venezuelan equine encephalitis (A92.2)
West Nile fever (A92.3-)
West Nile virus (A92.3-)

> **CC Excl: For MCC codes in category A83, unless otherwise noted:**
> A17.82, A50.42, A52.14, A75.9, A79.9, A81.1, A81.82-A81.89, A83.0-
> A85.8, A87.2, A88.0, A88.8, A92.1-A92.8, A93.0, B00.4, B00.82,
> B01.11-B01.12, B04, B06.01, B08.09, B08.20-B08.22, B08.60-B08.79,
> B09-B10.09, B26.2, B27.00-B27.99, B33.1, B45.0, B45.2-B45.9, B58.2,
> B75, B97.10, B97.21, G04.00-G04.01, G04.31, G04.81-G05.4, G37.0,
> G37.4-G37.5, J09.X3-J09.X9, J10.2-J10.89, J11.2-J11.89, L44.4,
> M1A.10X0-M1A.19X1, P35.2-P35.9, P37.0-P37.4, P37.8-P37.9,
> T56.0X1A, T56.0X2A, T56.0X3A, T56.0X4A

A83.0 Japanese encephalitis `MCC`

A83.1 Western equine encephalitis `MCC`

✓ Additional Character Required   ✓x7ᵗʰ Placeholder Alert   Unacceptable PDx   Manifestation   Hospital Acquired Condition   EXCLUDES1 Not Coded Here   EXCLUDES2 Not Included Here

ICD-10-CM 2016   437

A83.2   **Eastern equine encephalitis** `MCC`

A83.3   **St Louis encephalitis** `MCC`

A83.4   **Australian encephalitis** `MCC`
Kunjin virus disease

A83.5   **California encephalitis** `MCC`
California meningoencephalitis
La Crosse encephalitis

A83.6   **Rocio virus disease** `MCC`

A83.8   **Other mosquito-borne viral encephalitis** `MCC`

A83.9   **Mosquito-borne viral encephalitis,** unspecified `MCC`

✓4ᵗʰ **A84**   **Tick-borne viral encephalitis**
> INCLUDES   tick-borne viral meningoencephalitis

> CC Excl: For MCC codes in category A84, unless otherwise noted: A17.82, A50.42, A52.14, A75.9, A79.9, A81.1, A81.82-A81.89, A83.0-A85.8, A87.2, A88.0, A88.8, A92.1-A92.8, A93.0, B00.4, B00.82, B01.11-B01.12, B04, B06.01, B08.09, B08.20-B08.22, B08.60-B08.79, B09-B10.09, B26.2, B27.00-B27.99, B33.1, B45.0, B45.2-B45.9, B58.2, B75, B97.10, B97.21, G04.00-G04.01, G04.31, G04.81-G05.4, G37.0, G37.4-G37.5, J09.X3-J09.X9, J10.2-J10.89, J11.2-J11.89, L44.4, M1A.10X0-M1A.19X1, P35.2-P35.9, P37.0-P37.4, P37.8-P37.9, T56.0X1A, T56.0X2A, T56.0X3A, T56.0X4A

A84.0   **Far Eastern tick-borne encephalitis [Russian spring-summer encephalitis]** `MCC`

A84.1   **Central European tick-borne encephalitis** `MCC`

A84.8   **Other tick-borne viral encephalitis** `MCC`
Louping ill
Powassan virus disease

A84.9   **Tick-borne viral encephalitis,** unspecified `MCC`

✓4ᵗʰ **A85**   **Other viral encephalitis, not elsewhere classified**
> INCLUDES   specified viral encephalomyelitis NEC
> specified viral meningoencephalitis NEC

> EXCLUDES 1   benign myalgic encephalomyelitis (G93.3)
> encephalitis due to cytomegalovirus (B25.8)
> encephalitis due to herpesvirus NEC (B10.0-)
> encephalitis due to herpesvirus [herpes simplex] (B00.4)
> encephalitis due to measles virus (B05.0)
> encephalitis due to mumps virus (B26.2)
> encephalitis due to poliomyelitis virus (A80.-)
> encephalitis due to zoster (B02.0)
> lymphocytic choriomeningitis (A87.2)

> CC Excl: For CC/MCC codes in category A85, unless otherwise noted: A17.82, A50.42, A52.14, A75.9, A79.9, A81.1, A81.82-A81.89, A83.0-A85.8, A87.2, A88.0, A88.8, A92.1-A92.8, A93.0, B00.4, B00.82, B01.11-B01.12, B04, B06.01, B08.09, B08.20-B08.22, B08.60-B08.79, B09-B10.09, B26.2, B27.00-B27.99, B33.1, B45.0, B45.2-B45.9, B58.2, B75, B97.10, B97.21, G04.00-G04.01, G04.31, G04.81-G05.4, G37.0, G37.4-G37.5, H66.40-H66.43, J09.X3-J09.X9, J10.2-J10.89, J11.2-J11.89, L44.4, M1A.10X0-M1A.19X1, M32.0-M32.9, P35.2-P35.9, P37.0-P37.4, P37.8-P37.9, T56.0X1A, T56.0X2A, T56.0X3A, T56.0X4A

A85.0   **Enteroviral encephalitis** `HIV` `CC`
Enteroviral encephalomyelitis

A85.1   **Adenoviral encephalitis** `HIV` `CC`
Adenoviral meningoencephalitis

A85.2   **Arthropod-borne viral encephalitis,** unspecified `MCC`
> EXCLUDES 1   West nile virus with encephalitis (A92.31)

A85.8   **Other specified viral encephalitis** `HIV` `CC`
Encephalitis lethargica
Von Economo-Cruchet disease

A86   **Unspecified viral encephalitis** `HIV` `CC`
Viral encephalomyelitis NOS
Viral meningoencephalitis NOS
> CC Excl: A17.82, A50.42, A52.14, A75.9, A79.9, A81.1, A81.82-A81.89, A83.0-A86, A87.2, A88.0, A88.8-A89, A92.1-A92.2, A92.4-A92.8, A93.0, B00.4, B00.82, B01.11-B01.12, B04, B06.01, B08.09, B08.20-B08.22, B08.60-B08.79, B09-B10.09, B26.2, B27.00-B27.99, B33.1, B45.0, B45.2-B45.9, B58.2, B75, B97.10, G04.00-G04.01, G04.31, G04.81-G05.4, G37.0, G37.4-G37.5, H66.40-H66.43, J09.X3-J09.X9, J10.2-J10.89, J11.2-J11.89, L44.4, M1A.10X0-M1A.19X1, M32.0-M32.9, P35.2-P35.9, P37.0-P37.4, P37.8-P37.9, T56.0X1A, T56.0X2A, T56.0X3A, T56.0X4A

✓4ᵗʰ **A87**   **Viral meningitis**
> EXCLUDES 1   meningitis due to herpesvirus [herpes simplex] (B00.3)
> meningitis due to measles virus (B05.1)
> meningitis due to mumps virus (B26.1)
> meningitis due to poliomyelitis virus (A80.-)
> meningitis due to zoster (B02.1)

> CC Excl: For CC/MCC codes in category A87, unless otherwise noted: A02.21, A17.0-A17.1, A27.81, A39.0, A50.41, A51.41, A52.13, A54.82, A54.84, A54.89-A54.9, A74.81-A74.9, A87.0-A87.9, A96.2, A98.3-A98.4, B26.1, B33.24, B33.4-B33.8, B34.1-B34.2, B34.4-B34.8, B37.5, B38.4, B45.1, B58.2, B92, B94.2-B94.9, B97.10, B97.19, B97.29, B97.5-B97.6, B97.81-B97.89, G00.0-G03.9, G04.2, G32.89, G61.0, G96.8-G96.9, G98.0-G98.8, G99.8

A87.0   **Enteroviral meningitis** `CC`
Coxsackievirus meningitis
Echovirus meningitis

A87.1   **Adenoviral meningitis** `CC`

A87.2   **Lymphocytic choriomeningitis** `CC`
Lymphocytic meningoencephalitis
> CC Excl: A02.21, A17.0-A17.1, A27.81, A39.0, A50.41, A51.41, A52.13, A54.82, A54.84, A54.89-A54.9, A74.81-A74.9, A87.0-A87.9, A92.30-A92.39, A96.2, A98.3-A98.4, B26.1, B33.24, B33.4-B33.8, B34.1-B34.2, B34.4-B34.8, B37.5, B38.4, B45.1, B58.2, B92, B94.2-B94.9, B97.10, B97.19-B97.29, B97.5-B97.6, B97.81-B97.89, G00.0-G03.9, G04.2, G32.89, G61.0, G96.8-G96.9, G98.0-G98.8, G99.8

A87.8   **Other viral meningitis** `CC`

A87.9   **Viral meningitis,** unspecified `CC`

✓4ᵗʰ **A88**   **Other viral infections of central nervous system, not elsewhere classified**
> EXCLUDES 1   viral encephalitis NOS (A86)
> viral meningitis NOS (A87.9)

A88.0   **Enteroviral exanthematous fever [Boston exanthem]** `CC`
> CC Excl: A17.82, A50.42, A52.14, A75.9, A79.9, A81.1, A81.82-A81.89, A83.0-A85.8, A87.2, A88.0, A88.8, A92.1-A92.8, A93.0, B00.4, B00.82, B01.11-B01.12, B04, B06.01, B08.09, B08.20-B08.22, B08.60-B08.79, B09-B10.09, B26.2, B27.00-B27.99, B33.1, B45.0, B45.2-B45.9, B58.2, B75, B97.10, B97.21, G04.00-G04.01, G04.31, G04.81-G05.4, G37.0, G37.4-G37.5, J09.X3-J09.X9, J10.2-J10.89, J11.2-J11.89, L44.4, M1A.10X0-M1A.19X1, P35.2-P35.9, P37.0-P37.4, P37.8-P37.9, T56.0X1A, T56.0X2A, T56.0X3A, T56.0X4A

A88.1   **Epidemic vertigo**

A88.8   **Other specified viral infections of central nervous system** `HIV` `CC`
> CC Excl: See code: A85

A89   **Unspecified viral infection of central nervous system** `HIV` `CC`
> CC Excl: See code: A86

Arthropod-borne viral fevers and viral hemorrhagic fevers (A90-A99)

A90   **Dengue fever [classical dengue]** `CC`
> EXCLUDES 1   dengue hemorrhagic fever (A91)
> CC Excl: A90

A91   **Dengue hemorrhagic fever** `CC`
> CC Excl: A91-A94, A98.0-A98.2, A98.8-A99, B33.1

✓4ᵗʰ **A92**   **Other mosquito-borne viral fevers**
> EXCLUDES 1   Ross River disease (B33.1)

A92.0   **Chikungunya virus disease** `CC`
Chikungunya (hemorrhagic) fever
> CC Excl: See code: A91

A92.1   **O'nyong-nyong fever** `CC`
> CC Excl: A17.82, A50.42, A52.14, A75.9, A79.9, A81.1, A81.82-A81.89, A83.0-A85.8, A87.2, A88.0, A88.8, A91-A94, A98.0-A98.2, A98.8-A99, B00.4, B00.82, B01.11-B01.12, B04, B06.01, B08.09, B08.20-B08.22, B08.60-B08.79, B09-B10.09, B26.2, B27.00-B27.99, B33.1, B45.0, B45.2-B45.9, B58.2, B75, B97.10, B97.21, G04.00-G04.01, G04.31, G04.81-G05.4, G37.0, G37.4-G37.5, J09.X3-J09.X9, J10.2-J10.89, J11.2-J11.89, L44.4, M1A.10X0-M1A.19X1, P35.2-P35.9, P37.0-P37.4, P37.8-P37.9, T56.0X1A, T56.0X2A, T56.0X3A, T56.0X4A

A92.2   **Venezuelan equine fever** `CC`
Venezuelan equine encephalitis
Venezuelan equine encephalomyelitis virus disease
> CC Excl: See code: A92.1

Ⓝ Newborn: 0   Ⓟ Pediatric: 0-17   Ⓜ Maternity: 12-55   Ⓐ Adult: 15-124   `MCC` Major CC Condition   `PDx MCC` PDx acts as own MCC   `CC` CC Condition   `PDx CC` PDx acts as own CC

438   ICD-10-CM 2016

✓5ᵗʰ **A92.3 West Nile virus infection**
West Nile fever

> **CC Excl: For MCC codes in subcategory A92.3, unless otherwise noted:** A17.82, A50.42, A52.14, A75.9, A79.9, A81.1, A81.82-A81.89, A83.0-A85.8, A87.2, A88.0, A88.8, A91-A92.2, A92.4-A94, A98.0-A98.2, A98.8-A99, B00.4, B00.82, B01.11-B01.12, B04, B06.01, B08.09, B08.20-B08.22, B08.60-B08.79, B09-B10.09, B26.2, B27.00-B27.99, B33.1, B45.0, B45.2-B45.9, B75, B97.10, G04.00-G04.01, G04.31, G04.81-G05.4, G37.0, G37.4-G37.5, J09.X3-J09.X9, J10.2-J10.89, J11.2-J11.89, L44.4, P35.2-P35.9, P37.0-P37.4, P37.8-P37.9

A92.30 West Nile virus infection, unspecified `MCC`
West Nile fever NOS
West Nile fever without complications
West Nile virus NOS

A92.31 West Nile virus infection with encephalitis `MCC`
West Nile encephalitis
West Nile encephalomyelitis

A92.32 West Nile virus infection with other neurologic manifestation `MCC`
Use additional code to specify the neurologic manifestation

A92.39 West Nile virus infection with other complications `MCC`
Use additional code to specify the other conditions

A92.4 Rift Valley fever `CC`
CC Excl: See code: A92.1

A92.8 Other specified mosquito-borne viral fevers `CC`
CC Excl: See code: A92.1

A92.9 Mosquito-borne viral fever, unspecified `CC`
CC Excl: See code: A91

✓4ᵗʰ **A93 Other arthropod-borne viral fevers, not elsewhere classified**

A93.0 Oropouche virus disease `CC`
Oropouche fever
CC Excl: A17.82, A50.42, A52.14, A75.9, A79.9, A81.1, A81.82-A81.89, A83.0-A85.8, A87.2, A88.0, A88.8, A91-A94, A98.0-A98.2, A98.8-A99, B00.4, B00.82, B01.11-B01.12, B04, B06.01, B08.09, B08.20-B08.22, B08.60-B08.79, B09-B10.09, B26.2, B27.00-B27.99, B33.1, B45.0, B45.2-B45.9, B58.2, B75, B97.10, B97.21, G04.00-G04.01, G04.31, G04.81-G05.4, G37.0, G37.4-G37.5, J09.X3-J09.X9, J10.2-J10.89, J11.2-J11.89, L44.4, M1A.10-M1A.19, P35.2-P35.9, P37.0-P37.4, P37.8-P37.9, T56.0X1-T56.0X4 with 7th A

A93.1 Sandfly fever `CC`
Pappataci fever
Phlebotomus fever
CC Excl: A91-A94, A98.0-A98.2, A98.8-A99, B33.1

A93.2 Colorado tick fever `CC`
CC Excl: See code: A93.1

A93.8 Other specified arthropod-borne viral fevers `CC`
Piry virus disease
Vesicular stomatitis virus disease [Indiana fever]
CC Excl: See code: A91

A94 Unspecified arthropod-borne viral fever `CC`
Arboviral fever NOS
Arbovirus infection NOS
CC Excl: A91-A94, A98.0-A98.2, A98.8-A99, B33.1

✓4ᵗʰ **A95 Yellow fever**

> **CC Excl: For CC codes in category A95, unless otherwise noted:** A95.0-A95.9

A95.0 Sylvatic yellow fever `CC`
Jungle yellow fever

A95.1 Urban yellow fever `CC`

A95.9 Yellow fever, unspecified `CC`

✓4ᵗʰ **A96 Arenaviral hemorrhagic feverr**

> **CC Excl: For CC codes in category A96, unless otherwise noted:** A74.81-A74.9, A88.1, A96.0-A96.9, A98.3-A98.5, B25.8-B25.9, B33.24-B34.2, B34.4-B34.8, B97.0-B97.89

A96.0 Junin hemorrhagic fever `CC`
Argentinian hemorrhagic fever

A96.1 Machupo hemorrhagic fever `CC`
Bolivian hemorrhagic fever

A96.2 Lassa fever

A96.8 Other arenaviral hemorrhagic fevers `CC`

A96.9 Arenaviral hemorrhagic fever, unspecified `CC`

✓4ᵗʰ **A98 Other viral hemorrhagic fevers, not elsewhere classified**
> **EXCLUDES 1** chikungunya hemorrhagic fever (A92.0)
> dengue hemorrhagic fever (A91)

> **CC Excl: For CC codes in category A98, unless otherwise noted:** A91-A94, A98.0-A98.2, A98.8-A99, B33.1

A98.0 Crimean-Congo hemorrhagic fever `CC`
Central Asian hemorrhagic fever

A98.1 Omsk hemorrhagic fever `CC`

A98.2 Kyasanur Forest disease

A98.3 Marburg virus disease

A98.4 Ebola virus disease

A98.5 Hemorrhagic fever with renal syndrome `CC`
Epidemic hemorrhagic fever
Korean hemorrhagic fever
Russian hemorrhagic fever
Hantaan virus disease
Hantavirus disease with renal manifestations
Nephropathia epidemica
Songo fever
> **EXCLUDES 1** hantavirus (cardio)-pulmonary syndrome (B33.4)
CC Excl: A17.9, A18.10-A18.11, A18.13, A18.82, A18.84, A18.89, A54.21, A54.29, A54.82, A54.84, A54.89-A54.9, A59.00, A59.8-A59.9, A98.5, B37.41-B37.49, B97.21, E08.21-E08.29, E08.618-E08.638, E08.649-E08.8, E09.21-E09.29, E09.618-E09.638, E09.649-E09.8, E10.21-E10.29, E10.618-E10.638, E10.649, E10.69-E10.8, E11.21-E11.29, E11.618-E11.638, E11.649, E11.69-E11.8, E13.21-E13.29, E13.618-E13.638, E13.649-E13.8, M10.30-M10.39, N00.0-N11.0, N11.8-N13.39, N13.6, N14.0-N17.9, N19, N25.0-N26.1, N26.9-N27.9, N28.1-N29, N36.41-N36.43, N36.8-N36.9, N39.8-N39.9, R31.0-R31.9

A98.8 Other specified viral hemorrhagic fevers `CC`

A99 Unspecified viral hemorrhagic fever `CC`
CC Excl: See code: A98

Viral infections characterized by skin and mucous membrane lesions (B00-B09)

✓4ᵗʰ **B00 Herpesviral [herpes simplex] infections**
> **EXCLUDES 1** congenital herpesviral infections (P35.2)
> **EXCLUDES 2** anogenital herpesviral infection (A60.-)
> gammaherpesviral mononucleosis (B27.0-)
> herpangina (B08.5)

B00.0 Eczema herpeticum `HIV`
Kaposi's varicelliform eruption

B00.1 Herpesviral vesicular dermatitis `HIV`
Herpes simplex facialis   Vesicular dermatitis of ear
Herpes simplex labialis   Vesicular dermatitis of lip
Herpes simplex otitis externa

B00.2 Herpesviral gingivostomatitis and pharyngotonsillitis `HIV` `CC`
Herpesviral pharyngitis
CC Excl: B00.2

B00.3 Herpesviral meningitis `HIV` `MCC`
CC Excl: A02.21, A17.0-A17.1, A27.81, A39.0, A50.41, A51.41, A52.13, A54.82, A54.84, A54.89-A54.9, A87.0-A87.9, B00.3, B00.82-B00.9, B02.1, B10.81-B10.89, B26.1, B37.5, B38.4, B45.1, B58.2, B92, B94.2-B94.9, G00.0-G03.9, G04.2, G32.89, G61.0, G96.8-G96.9, G98.0-G98.8, G99.8

B00.4 Herpesviral encephalitis `HIV` `MCC`
Herpesviral meningoencephalitis
Simian B disease
> **EXCLUDES 1** herpesviral encephalitis due to herpesvirus 6 and 7 (B10.01, B10.09)
> non-simplex herpesviral encephalitis (B10.0-)
CC Excl: B00.4-B00.9, B10.01-B10.89, B92, B94.2-B94.9

✓5ᵗʰ **B00.5 Herpesviral ocular disease**

> **CC Excl: For CC codes in subcategory B00.5, unless otherwise noted:** B00.50-B00.59, B00.89-B00.9, B10.81-B10.89

B00.50 Herpesviral ocular disease, unspecified `HIV` `CC`

B00.51 Herpesviral iridocyclitis `HIV` `CC`
Herpesviral iritis
Herpesviral uveitis, anterior

B00.52 Herpesviral keratitis `HIV` `CC`
Herpesviral keratoconjunctivitis

B00.53 Herpesviral conjunctivitis `HIV` `CC`

B00.59 Other herpesviral disease of eye `HIV` `CC`
Herpesviral dermatitis of eyelid

✔ Additional Character Required   ✓x7ᵗʰ Placeholder Alert   Unacceptable PDx   Manifestation   Hospital Acquired Condition   **EXCLUDES 1** Not Coded Here   **EXCLUDES 2** Not Included Here

Chapter 1. Certain Infectious and Parasitic Diseases

B00.7   **Disseminated herpesviral disease**   `HIV` `MCC`
Herpesviral sepsis
CC Excl: A02.1, A20.7, A22.7, A26.7, A32.7, A39.2-A39.4, A40.0-A40.1, A40.8-A41.9, A42.7, A54.86, B00.7, B00.82-B00.9, B10.81-B10.89, B37.7, B92, B94.2-B94.9, R65.10-R65.20

√5ᵗʰ **B00.8**   **Other forms of herpesviral infections**

   B00.81   **Herpesviral hepatitis**   `HIV` `CC`
CC Excl: B00.3, B00.81-B00.9, B10.81-B10.89, B92, B94.2-B94.9

   B00.82   **Herpes simplex myelitis**   `MCC`
CC Excl: A74.81-A74.9, A96.2, A98.3-A98.4, B00.82-B00.9, B01.12, B02.24, B10.81-B10.89, B33.24, B33.4-B33.8, B34.1-B34.2, B34.4-B34.8, B92, B94.2-B94.9, B97.10, B97.19, B97.29, B97.5-B97.6, B97.81-B97.89, G04.00-G04.01, G04.31, G04.81-G04.89, G05.3-G05.4, G37.3

   B00.89   **Other herpesviral infection**   `HIV` `CC`
Herpesviral whitlow
CC Excl: A74.81-A74.9, A96.2, A98.3-A98.4, B00.82-B00.9, B10.81-B10.89, B33.24, B33.4-B33.8, B34.1-B34.2, B34.4-B34.8, B92, B94.2-B94.9, B97.10, B97.19, B97.29, B97.5-B97.6, B97.81-B97.89

B00.9   **Herpesviral infection, unspecified**   `HIV`
Herpes simplex infection NOS

√4ᵗʰ **B01**   **Varicella [chickenpox]**

B01.0   **Varicella meningitis**   `CC`
CC Excl: A74.81-A74.9, A96.2, A98.3-A98.4, B01.0, B01.12, B01.81-B01.9, B08.04, B33.24, B33.4-B33.8, B34.1-B34.2, B34.4-B34.8, B92, B94.2-B94.9, B97.10, B97.19, B97.29, B97.5-B97.6, B97.81-B97.89

√5ᵗʰ **B01.1**   **Varicella encephalitis, myelitis and encephalomyelitis**
Postchickenpox encephalitis, myelitis and encephalomyelitis

   B01.11   **Varicella encephalitis and encephalomyelitis**   `MCC`
Postchickenpox encephalitis and encephalomyelitis
CC Excl: A74.81-A74.9, A96.2, A98.3-A98.4, B01.0-B01.12, B01.81-B01.9, B08.04, B33.24, B33.4-B33.8, B34.1-B34.2, B34.4-B34.8, B92, B94.2-B94.9, B97.10, B97.19, B97.29, B97.5-B97.6, B97.81-B97.89

   B01.12   **Varicella myelitis**   `MCC`
Postchickenpox myelitis
CC Excl: A74.81-A74.9, A96.2, A98.3-A98.4, B00.82, B01.0, B01.12, B01.81-B01.9, B02.24, B08.04, B33.24, B33.4-B33.8, B34.1-B34.2, B34.4-B34.8, B92, B94.2-B94.9, B97.10, B97.19, B97.29, B97.5-B97.6, B97.81-B97.89, G04.00-G04.01, G04.31, G04.81-G04.89, G05.3-G05.4, G37.3

B01.2   **Varicella pneumonia**   `MCC`
CC Excl: A74.81-A74.9, A96.2, A98.3-A98.4, B01.0, B01.12-B01.9, B08.04, B33.24, B33.4-B33.8, B34.1-B34.2, B34.4-B34.8, B92, B94.2-B94.9, B97.10, B97.19, B97.29, B97.5-B97.6, B97.81-B97.89

√5ᵗʰ **B01.8**   **Varicella with other complications**

   B01.81   **Varicella keratitis**   `CC`
CC Excl: See code: B01.0

   B01.89   **Other varicella complications**   `CC`
CC Excl: See code: B01.0

B01.9   **Varicella without complication**   `CC`
Varicella NOS
CC Excl: See code: B01.0

√4ᵗʰ **B02**   **Zoster [herpes zoster]**
INCLUDES   shingles
          zona

B02.0   **Zoster encephalitis**   `HIV` `CC`
Zoster meningoencephalitis
CC Excl: A74.81-A74.9, A96.2, A98.3-A98.4, B00.3, B00.82-B00.9, B02.0-B02.29, B02.7-B02.9, B10.81-B10.89, B33.24, B33.4-B33.8, B34.1-B34.2, B34.4-B34.8, B92, B94.2-B94.9, B97.10, B97.19, B97.29, B97.5-B97.6, B97.81-B97.89

B02.1   **Zoster meningitis**   `HIV` `MCC`
CC Excl: A02.21, A17.0-A17.1, A27.81, A39.0, A50.41, A51.41, A52.13, A54.82, A54.84, A54.89-A54.9, A74.81-A74.9, A87.0-A87.9, A96.2, A98.3-A98.4, B00.3, B00.82-B00.9, B02.0-B02.29, B02.7-B02.9, B10.81-B10.89, B26.1, B33.24, B33.4-B33.8, B34.1-B34.2, B34.4-B34.8, B37.5, B38.4, B45.1, B58.2, B92, B94.2-B94.9, B97.10, B97.19, B97.29, B97.5-B97.6, B97.81-B97.89, G00.0-G03.9, G04.2, G32.89, G61.0, G96.8-G96.9, G98.8, G99.8

√5ᵗʰ **B02.2**   **Zoster with other nervous system involvement**

CC Excl: For CC/MCC codes in subcategory B02.2, unless otherwise noted: A74.81-A74.9, A96.2, A98.3-A98.4, B00.3, B00.82-B00.9, B02.0-B02.29, B02.7-B02.9, B10.81-B10.89, B33.24, B33.4-B33.8, B34.1-B34.2, B34.4-B34.8, B92, B94.2-B94.9, B97.10, B97.19, B97.29, B97.5-B97.6, B97.81-B97.89

   B02.21   **Postherpetic geniculate ganglionitis**   `HIV` `CC`

   B02.22   **Postherpetic trigeminal neuralgia**   `HIV` `CC`

   B02.23   **Postherpetic polyneuropathy**   `HIV` `CC`

   B02.24   **Postherpetic myelitis**   `MCC`
Herpes zoster myelitis
CC Excl: A74.81-A74.9, A96.2, A98.3-A98.4, B00.3, B00.82-B00.9, B01.12, B02.0-B02.29, B02.7-B02.9, B10.81-B10.89, B33.24, B33.4-B33.8, B34.1-B34.2, B34.4-B34.8, B92, B94.2-B94.9, B97.10, B97.19, B97.29, B97.5-B97.6, B97.81-B97.89, G04.00-G04.01, G04.31, G04.81-G04.89, G05.3-G05.4, G37.3

   B02.29   **Other postherpetic nervous system involvement**   `HIV` `CC`
Postherpetic radiculopathy

√5ᵗʰ **B02.3**   **Zoster ocular disease**

CC Excl: For CC codes in subcategory B02.3, unless otherwise noted: B02.30-B02.39

   B02.30   **Zoster ocular disease, unspecified**   `HIV` `CC`

   B02.31   **Zoster conjunctivitis**   `HIV` `CC`

   B02.32   **Zoster iridocyclitis**   `HIV` `CC`

   B02.33   **Zoster keratitis**   `HIV` `CC`
Herpes zoster keratoconjunctivitis

   B02.34   **Zoster scleritis**   `HIV` `CC`

   B02.39   **Other herpes zoster eye disease**   `HIV` `CC`
Zoster blepharitis

B02.7   **Disseminated zoster**   `HIV` `CC`
CC Excl: A60.00-A60.9, A74.81-A74.9, A96.2, A98.3-A98.4, B00.0-B00.2, B00.4-B00.9, B02.0-B02.9, B10.01-B10.89, B33.24, B33.4-B33.8, B34.1-B34.2, B34.4-B34.8, B92, B94.2-B94.9, B97.10, B97.19, B97.29, B97.5-B97.6, B97.81-B97.89

B02.8   **Zoster with other complications**   `HIV` `CC`
Herpes zoster otitis externa
CC Excl: See code: B02.7

B02.9   **Zoster without complications**   `HIV`
Zoster NOS

B03   **Smallpox**   `CC`
NOTE   In 1980 the 33rd World Health Assembly declared that smallpox had been eradicated.
The classification is maintained for surveillance purposes.
CC Excl: B01.0-B01.9, B03, B08.010-B08.04

B04   **Monkeypox**   `CC`
CC Excl: B04-B08.011, B08.09, B08.3, B08.60-B08.79, B09, L44.4

√4ᵗʰ **B05**   **Measles**
INCLUDES   morbilli
EXCLUDES 1   *subacute sclerosing panencephalitis (A81.1)*

B05.0   **Measles complicated by encephalitis**   `MCC`
Postmeasles encephalitis
CC Excl: A74.81-A74.9, A96.2, A98.3-A98.4, B05.0-B05.1, B05.4, B05.89-B05.9, B33.24, B33.4-B33.8, B34.1-B34.2, B34.4-B34.8, B92, B94.2-B94.9, B97.10, B97.19, B97.29, B97.5-B97.6, B97.81-B97.89

B05.1   **Measles complicated by meningitis**   `CC`
Postmeasles meningitis
CC Excl: A74.81-A74.9, A96.2, A98.3-A98.4, B05.1, B05.4, B05.89-B05.9, B33.24, B33.4-B33.8, B34.1-B34.2, B34.4-B34.8, B92, B94.2-B94.9, B97.10, B97.19, B97.29, B97.5-B97.6, B97.81-B97.89

B05.2   **Measles complicated by pneumonia**   `MCC`
Postmeasles pneumonia
CC Excl: A74.81-A74.9, A96.2, A98.3-A98.4, B05.1-B05.2, B05.4, B05.89-B05.9, B33.24, B33.4-B33.8, B34.1-B34.2, B34.4-B34.8, B92, B94.2-B94.9, B97.10, B97.19, B97.29, B97.5-B97.6, B97.81-B97.89

B05.3   **Measles complicated by otitis media**
Postmeasles otitis media

B05.4   **Measles with intestinal complications**   `CC`
CC Excl: See code: B05.1

√5ᵗʰ **B05.8**   **Measles with other complications**

   B05.81   **Measles keratitis and keratoconjunctivitis**   `CC`
CC Excl: A74.81-A74.9, A96.2, A98.3-A98.4, B05.1, B05.4-B05.9, B33.24, B33.4-B33.8, B34.1-B34.2, B34.4-B34.8, B92, B94.2-B94.9, B97.10, B97.19, B97.29, B97.5-B97.6, B97.81-B97.89

   B05.89   **Other measles complications**   `CC`
CC Excl: See code: B05.1

B05.9   **Measles without complication**
Measles NOS

✓4ᵗʰ **B06** **Rubella [German measles]**
> EXCLUDES 1   *congenital rubella (P35.0)*

✓5ᵗʰ   **B06.0**   **Rubella with neurological complications**

> **CC Excl: For CC/MCC codes in subcategory B06.0, unless otherwise noted:** A74.81-A74.9, A96.2, A98.3-A98.4, B06.00-B06.81, B06.89-B06.9, B33.24, B33.4-B33.8, B34.1-B34.2, B34.4-B34.8, B92, B94.2-B94.9, B97.10, B97.19, B97.29, B97.5-B97.6, B97.81-B97.89

> **B06.00**   **Rubella with neurological complication, unspecified**   `CC`

> **B06.01**   **Rubella encephalitis**   `MCC`
> Rubella meningoencephalitis

> **B06.02**   **Rubella meningitis**   `CC`

> **B06.09**   **Other neurological complications of rubella**   `CC`

✓5ᵗʰ   **B06.8**   **Rubella with other complications**

> **B06.81**   **Rubella pneumonia**   `CC`
> CC Excl: See code: B06.00

> **B06.82**   **Rubella arthritis**   `CC`
> CC Excl: A74.81-A74.9, A96.2, A98.3-A98.4, B06.81-B06.9, B33.24, B33.4-B33.8, B34.1-B34.2, B34.4-B34.8, B92, B94.2-B94.9, B97.10, B97.19, B97.29, B97.5-B97.6, B97.81-B97.89

> **B06.89**   **Other rubella complications**   `CC`
> CC Excl: See code: B06.0

B06.9   **Rubella without complication**
> Rubella NOS

✓4ᵗʰ **B07** **Viral warts**
> INCLUDES   verruca simplex
> verruca vulgaris
> viral warts due to human papillomavirus
> EXCLUDES 2   *anogenital (venereal) warts (A63.0)*
> *papilloma of bladder (D41.4)*
> *papilloma of cervix (D26.0)*
> *papilloma larynx (D14.1)*

B07.0   **Plantar wart**
> Verruca plantaris

B07.8   **Other viral warts**
> Common wart
> Flat wart
> Verruca plana

B07.9   **Viral wart, unspecified**

✓4ᵗʰ **B08** **Other viral infections characterized by skin and mucous membrane lesions, not elsewhere classified**
> EXCLUDES 1   *vesicular stomatitis virus disease (A93.8)*

✓5ᵗʰ   **B08.0**   **Other orthopoxvirus infections**
> EXCLUDES 2   *monkeypox (B04)*

✓6ᵗʰ   **B08.01**   **Cowpox and vaccinia not from vaccine**
> **B08.010**   **Cowpox**
> **B08.011**   **Vaccinia not from vaccine**
> EXCLUDES 1   *vaccinia (from vaccination) (generalized) (T88.1)*

> **B08.02**   **Orf virus disease**
> Contagious pustular dermatitis
> Ecthyma contagiosum

> **B08.03**   **Pseudocowpox [milker's node]**

> **B08.04**   **Paravaccinia, unspecified**

> **B08.09**   **Other orthopoxvirus infections**
> Orthopoxvirus infection NOS

B08.1   **Molluscum contagiosum**

✓5ᵗʰ   **B08.2**   **Exanthema subitum [sixth disease]**
> Roseola infantum

> **B08.20**   **Exanthema subitum [sixth disease], unspecified**   `P`
> Roseola infantum, unspecified

> **B08.21**   **Exanthema subitum [sixth disease] due to human herpesvirus 6**   `P`
> Roseola infantum due to human herpesvirus 6

> **B08.22**   **Exanthema subitum [sixth disease] due to human herpesvirus 7**   `P`
> Roseola infantum due to human herpesvirus 7

B08.3   **Erythema infectiosum [fifth disease]**   `CC`
> CC Excl: B08.3-B34.3

B08.4   **Enteroviral vesicular stomatitis with exanthem**
> Hand, foot and mouth disease

B08.5   **Enteroviral vesicular pharyngitis**
> Herpangina

✓5ᵗʰ   **B08.6**   **Parapoxvirus infections**
> **B08.60**   **Parapoxvirus infection, unspecified**
> **B08.61**   **Bovine stomatitis**
> **B08.62**   **Sealpox**
> **B08.69**   **Other parapoxvirus infections**

✓5ᵗʰ   **B08.7**   **Yatapoxvirus infections**
> **B08.70**   **Yatapoxvirus infection, unspecified**
> **B08.71**   **Tanapox virus disease**   `CC`
> CC Excl: B04, B08.010-B08.011, B08.09, B08.3, B08.60-B08.79, B09, L44.4
> **B08.72**   **Yaba pox virus disease**
> Yaba monkey tumor disease
> **B08.79**   **Other yatapoxvirus infections**

B08.8   **Other specified viral infections characterized by skin and mucous membrane lesions**
> Enteroviral lymphonodular pharyngitis
> Foot-and-mouth disease
> Poxvirus NEC

B09 **Unspecified viral infection characterized by skin and mucous membrane lesions**
> Viral enanthema NOS
> Viral exanthema NOS

Other human herpesviruses (B10)

✓4ᵗʰ **B10** **Other human herpesviruses**
> EXCLUDES 2   *cytomegalovirus (B25.9)*
> *Epstein-Barr virus (B27.0-)*
> *herpes NOS (B00.9)*
> *herpes simplex (B00.-)*
> *herpes zoster (B02.-)*
> *human herpesvirus NOS (B00.-)*
> *human herpesvirus 1 and 2 (B00.-)*
> *human herpesvirus 3 (B01.-, B02.-)*
> *human herpesvirus 4 (B27.0-)*
> *human herpesvirus 5 (B25.-)*
> *varicella (B01.-)*
> *zoster (B02.-)*

✓5ᵗʰ   **B10.0**   **Other human herpesvirus encephalitis**
> EXCLUDES 2   *herpes encephalitis NOS (B00.4)*
> *herpes simplex encephalitis (B00.4)*
> *human herpesvirus encephalitis (B00.4)*
> *simian B herpes virus encephalitis (B00.4)*

> **B10.01**   **Human herpesvirus 6 encephalitis**   `HIV` `MCC`
> CC Excl: B00.4, B00.82-B00.9, B10.01-B10.89, B92, B94.2-B94.9

> **B10.09**   **Other human herpesvirus encephalitis**   `HIV` `MCC`
> Human herpesvirus 7 encephalitis
> CC Excl: See code: B10.01

✓5ᵗʰ   **B10.8**   **Other human herpesvirus infection**
> **B10.81**   **Human herpesvirus 6 infection**
> **B10.82**   **Human herpesvirus 7 infection**
> **B10.89**   **Other human herpesvirus infection**
> Human herpesvirus 8 infection
> Kaposi's sarcoma-associated herpesvirus infection

Viral hepatitis (B15-B19)

> EXCLUDES 1   *sequelae of viral hepatitis (B94.2)*
> EXCLUDES 2   *cytomegaloviral hepatitis (B25.1)*
> *herpesviral [herpes simplex] hepatitis (B00.81)*

✓4ᵗʰ **B15** **Acute hepatitis A**
> **B15.0**   **Hepatitis A with hepatic coma**   `MCC`
> CC Excl: A74.81-A74.9, A96.2, A98.3-A98.4, B15.0-B19.9, B33.24, B33.4-B33.8, B34.1-B34.2, B34.4-B34.8, B92, B94.2-B94.9, B97.10, B97.19, B97.29, B97.5-B97.6, B97.81-B97.89

> **B15.9**   **Hepatitis A without hepatic coma**   `CC`
> Hepatitis A (acute)(viral) NOS
> CC Excl: See code: B15.0

✓4ᵗʰ **B16** **Acute hepatitis B**

> **CC Excl: For CC/MCC codes in category B16, unless otherwise noted:** A74.81-A74.9, A96.2, A98.3-A98.4, B15.0-B19.9, B33.24, B33.4-B33.8, B34.1-B34.2, B34.4-B34.8, B92, B94.2-B94.9, B97.10, B97.19, B97.29, B97.5-B97.6, B97.81-B97.89

> **B16.0**   **Acute hepatitis B with delta-agent with hepatic coma**   `MCC`
> **B16.1**   **Acute hepatitis B with delta-agent without hepatic coma**   `CC`
> **B16.2**   **Acute hepatitis B without delta-agent with hepatic coma**   `MCC`

✔ Additional Character Required   ✓x7ᵗʰ Placeholder Alert   Unacceptable PDx   Manifestation   Hospital Acquired Condition   EXCLUDES 1 Not Coded Here   EXCLUDES 2 Not Included Here

ICD-10-CM 2016   **441**

B16.9   **Acute hepatitis B** without delta-agent and without `CC`
hepatic coma
Hepatitis B (acute) (viral) NOS

✓4ᵗʰ **B17**   **Other acute viral hepatitis**

> **CC Excl: For CC/MCC codes in category B17, unless otherwise
noted:** A74.81-A74.9, A96.2, A98.3-A98.4, B15.0-B19.9, B33.24,
B33.4-B33.8, B34.1-B34.2, B34.4-B34.8, B92, B94.2-B94.9, B97.10,
B97.19, B97.29, B97.5-B97.6, B97.81-B97.89

B17.0   **Acute delta-(super) infection** of hepatitis B carrier `CC`

✓5ᵗʰ **B17.1**   **Acute hepatitis C**

     B17.10   **Acute hepatitis C** without hepatic coma `CC`
         Acute hepatitis C NOS

     B17.11   **Acute hepatitis C** with hepatic coma `MCC`

B17.2   **Acute hepatitis E** `CC`

B17.8   **Other** specified acute viral hepatitis `CC`
Hepatitis non-A non-B (acute) (viral) NEC

B17.9   **Acute viral hepatitis,** unspecified `CC`
Acute hepatitis NOS

✓4ᵗʰ **B18**   **Chronic viral hepatitis**

> **CC Excl: For CC codes in category B18, unless otherwise noted:**
A74.81-A74.9, A96.2, A98.3-A98.4, B15.0-B19.9, B33.24, B33.4-B33.8,
B34.1-B34.2, B34.4-B34.8, B92, B94.2-B94.9, B97.10, B97.19, B97.29,
B97.5-B97.6, B97.81-B97.89

B18.0   **Chronic viral hepatitis B** with delta-agent `CC`

B18.1   **Chronic viral hepatitis B** without delta-agent `CC`
Chronic (viral) hepatitis B

B18.2   **Chronic viral** hepatitis C

B18.8   **Other** chronic viral hepatitis `CC`

B18.9   **Chronic viral hepatitis,** unspecified `CC`

✓4ᵗʰ **B19**   **Unspecified viral hepatitis**

> **CC Excl: For CC/MCC codes in category B19, unless otherwise
noted:** A74.81-A74.9, A96.2, A98.3-A98.4, B15.0-B19.9, B33.24,
B33.4-B33.8, B34.1-B34.2, B34.4-B34.8, B92, B94.2-B94.9, B97.10,
B97.19, B97.29, B97.5-B97.6, B97.81-B97.89

B19.0   **Unspecified viral hepatitis** with hepatic coma `MCC`

✓5ᵗʰ **B19.1**   **Unspecified viral** hepatitis B

     B19.10   **Unspecified viral hepatitis B** without hepatic `CC`
         coma
         Unspecified viral hepatitis B NOS

     B19.11   **Unspecified viral hepatitis B** with hepatic coma `MCC`

✓5ᵗʰ **B19.2**   **Unspecified viral** hepatitis C

     B19.20   **Unspecified viral hepatitis C** without hepatic coma `CC`
         Viral hepatitis C NOS

     B19.21   **Unspecified viral hepatitis C** with hepatic coma `MCC`

B19.9   **Unspecified viral hepatitis** without hepatic coma `CC`
Viral hepatitis NOS

Human immunodeficiency virus [HIV] disease (B20)

B20   **Human immunodeficiency virus [HIV] disease** `MCC`
    `INCLUDES`   acquired immune deficiency syndrome [AIDS]
            AIDS-related complex [ARC]
            HIV infection, symptomatic

*Code first human immunodeficiency virus [HIV] disease complicating
pregnancy, childbirth and the puerperium, if applicable (O98.7-)*
Use additional code(s) to identify all manifestations of HIV infection

    `EXCLUDES 1`   *asymptomatic human immunodeficiency virus [HIV] infection
status (Z21)*
            exposure to HIV virus (Z20.6)
            inconclusive serologic evidence of HIV (R75)

> **CC Excl:** B20, B92, B94.2-B94.9

Other viral diseases (B25-B34)

✓4ᵗʰ **B25**   **Cytomegaloviral disease**
    `EXCLUDES 1`   *congenital cytomegalovirus infection (P35.1)*
            cytomegaloviral mononucleosis (B27.1-)

B25.0   **Cytomegaloviral** pneumonitis `PDx MCC` `MCC`
> **CC Excl:** A15.0-A15.6, A15.8-A15.9, A17.9, A18.82, A18.84, A18.89,
A21.2, A22.1, A31.0, A37.01, A37.11, A37.81, A37.91, A42.0, A43.0,
A48.1, B25.0, B39.0-B39.2, B44.0, B58.3, B59, B67.1, J09.X1-J09.X2,
J10.00-J10.1, J11.00-J11.1, J12.0-J12.3, J12.89-J18.1, J18.8-J18.9,
J22, J44.9, J47.0-J70.4, J70.8-J70.9, J98.4, J98.8-J99, Q33.4, R91.1

B25.1   **Cytomegaloviral** hepatitis `PDx CC` `CC`
> **CC Excl:** No Excl

B25.2   **Cytomegaloviral** pancreatitis `PDx MCC` `MCC`
> **CC Excl:** B25.2, K85.0-K86.1, K86.8-K86.9

B25.8   **Other cytomegaloviral diseases** `HIV` `CC`
Cytomegaloviral encephalitis
> **CC Excl:** A96.0-A96.9, A98.3-A98.5, B25.8-B25.9, B33.24-B34.2,
B34.4-B34.8, B97.0-B97.32, B97.39, B97.5-B97.89

B25.9   **Cytomegaloviral disease,** unspecified `HIV` `CC`
> **CC Excl:** See code: B25.8

✓4ᵗʰ **B26**   **Mumps**
    `INCLUDES`   epidemic parotitis
            infectious parotitis

B26.0   **Mumps orchitis** `CC` ♂
> **CC Excl:** A74.81-A74.9, A96.2, A98.3-A98.4, B26.0, B26.82-B26.83,
B26.85-B26.9, B33.24, B33.4-B33.8, B34.1-B34.2, B34.4-B34.8, B92,
B94.2-B94.9, B97.10, B97.19, B97.29, B97.5-B97.6, B97.81-B97.89

B26.1   **Mumps meningitis** `MCC`
> **CC Excl:** A02.21-A17.1, A27.81, A39.0, A50.41, A51.41, A52.13,
A54.82, A54.84, A54.89-A54.9, A74.81-A74.9, A87.0-A87.9, A96.2,
A98.3-A98.4, B00.3, B02.1, B26.1, B26.82-B26.83, B26.85-B26.9,
B33.24, B33.4-B33.8, B34.1-B34.2, B34.4-B34.8, B37.5, B38.4, B45.1,
B58.2, B92, B94.2-B94.9, B97.10, B97.19, B97.29, B97.5-B97.6,
B97.81-B97.89, G00.0-G03.9, G04.2, G32.89, G61.0, G96.8-G96.9,
G98.0-G98.8, G99.8

B26.2   **Mumps encephalitis** `MCC`
> **CC Excl:** A74.81-A74.9, A96.2, A98.3-A98.4, B26.2, B26.82-B26.83,
B26.85-B26.9, B33.24, B33.4-B33.8, B34.1-B34.2, B34.4-B34.8, B92,
B94.2-B94.9, B97.10, B97.19, B97.29, B97.5-B97.6, B97.81-B97.89

B26.3   **Mumps pancreatitis** `CC`
> **CC Excl:** A74.81-A74.9, A96.2, A98.3-A98.4, B26.3, B26.82-B26.83,
B26.85-B26.9, B33.24, B33.4-B33.8, B34.1-B34.2, B34.4-B34.8, B92,
B94.2-B94.9, B97.10, B97.19, B97.29, B97.5-B97.6, B97.81-B97.89

✓5ᵗʰ **B26.8**   **Mumps with** other complications

     B26.81   **Mumps hepatitis** `CC`
>   **CC Excl:** A74.81-A74.9, A96.2, A98.3-A98.4, B26.81-
B26.83, B26.85-B26.9, B33.24, B33.4-B33.8, B34.1-B34.2,
B34.4-B34.8, B92, B94.2-B94.9, B97.10, B97.19, B97.29,
B97.5-B97.6, B97.81-B97.89

     B26.82   **Mumps myocarditis** `CC`
>   **CC Excl:** A74.81-A74.9, A96.2, A98.3-A98.4, B26.82-
B26.83, B26.85-B26.9, B33.24, B33.4-B33.8, B34.1-B34.2,
B34.4-B34.8, B92, B94.2-B94.9, B97.10, B97.19, B97.29,
B97.5-B97.6, B97.81-B97.89

     B26.83   **Mumps nephritis** `CC`
>   **CC Excl:** See code: B26.82

     B26.84   **Mumps polyneuropathy** `CC`
>   **CC Excl:** A74.81-A74.9, A96.2, A98.3-A98.4, B26.82-
B26.9, B33.24, B33.4-B33.8, B34.1-B34.2, B34.4-B34.8,
B92, B94.2-B94.9, B97.10, B97.19, B97.29, B97.5-B97.6,
B97.81-B97.89

     B26.85   **Mumps arthritis** `CC`
>   **CC Excl:** See code: B26.82

     B26.89   **Other mumps complications** `CC`
>   **CC Excl:** See code: B26.82

B26.9   **Mumps without complication**
Mumps NOS
Mumps parotitis NOS

✓4ᵗʰ **B27**   **Infectious mononucleosis**
    `INCLUDES`   glandular fever
            monocytic angina
            Pfeiffer's disease

✓5ᵗʰ **B27.0**   **Gammaherpesviral mononucleosis**
Mononucleosis due to Epstein-Barr virus

     B27.00   **Gammaherpesviral mononucleosis** without
complication

     B27.01   **Gammaherpesviral mononucleosis** with
polyneuropathy

     B27.02   **Gammaherpesviral mononucleosis** with meningitis

     B27.09   **Gammaherpesviral mononucleosis** with other
complications
Hepatomegaly in gammaherpesviral mononucleosis

✓5ᵗʰ **B27.1**   **Cytomegaloviral mononucleosis**

     B27.10   **Cytomegaloviral mononucleosis** without
complications

     B27.11   **Cytomegaloviral mononucleosis** with
polyneuropathy

     B27.12   **Cytomegaloviral mononucleosis** with meningitis

     B27.19   **Cytomegaloviral mononucleosis** with other
complication
Hepatomegaly in cytomegaloviral mononucleosis

N Newborn: 0   P Pediatric: 0-17   M Maternity: 12-55   A Adult: 15-124   `MCC` Major CC Condition   `PDx MCC` PDx acts as own MCC   `CC` CC Condition   `PDx CC` PDx acts as own CC

442   ICD-10-CM 2016

☑5ᵗʰ **B27.8** **Other infectious mononucleosis**

B27.80 **Other infectious mononucleosis without complication**

B27.81 **Other infectious mononucleosis with polyneuropathy**

B27.82 **Other infectious mononucleosis with meningitis**

B27.89 **Other infectious mononucleosis with other complication**
Hepatomegaly in other infectious mononucleosis

☑5ᵗʰ **B27.9** **Infectious mononucleosis, unspecified**

B27.90 **Infectious mononucleosis, unspecified without complication**

B27.91 **Infectious mononucleosis, unspecified with polyneuropathy**

B27.92 **Infectious mononucleosis, unspecified with meningitis**

B27.99 **Infectious mononucleosis, unspecified with other complication**
Hepatomegaly in unspecified infectious mononucleosis

☑4ᵗʰ **B30** **Viral conjunctivitis**
EXCLUDES1 herpesviral [herpes simplex] ocular disease (B00.5)
ocular zoster (B02.3)

B30.0 **Keratoconjunctivitis due to adenovirus**
Epidemic keratoconjunctivitis
Shipyard eye

B30.1 **Conjunctivitis due to adenovirus**
Acute adenoviral follicular conjunctivitis
Swimming-pool conjunctivitis

B30.2 **Viral pharyngoconjunctivitis**

B30.3 **Acute epidemic hemorrhagic conjunctivitis (enteroviral)**
Conjunctivitis due to coxsackievirus 24
Conjunctivitis due to enterovirus 70
Hemorrhagic conjunctivitis (acute)(epidemic)

B30.8 **Other viral conjunctivitis**
Newcastle conjunctivitis

B30.9 **Viral conjunctivitis, unspecified**

☑4ᵗʰ **B33** **Other viral diseases, not elsewhere classified**

B33.0 **Epidemic myalgia**
Bornholm disease

B33.1 **Ross River disease** CC
Epidemic polyarthritis and exanthema
Ross River fever
CC Excl: A17.82, A50.42, A52.14, A75.9, A79.9, A81.1, A81.82-A81.89, A83.0-A85.8, A87.2, A88.0, A88.8, A91-A94, A98.0-A98.2, A98.8-A99, B00.4, B00.82, B01.11-B01.12, B04, B06.01, B08.09, B08.20-B08.22, B08.60-B08.79, B09-B10.09, B26.2, B27.00-B27.99, B33.1, B45.0, B45.2-B45.9, B58.2, B75, B97.10, B97.21, G04.00-G04.01, G04.31, G04.81-G05.4, G37.0, G37.4-G37.5, J09.X3-J09.X9, J10.2-J10.89, J11.2-J11.89, L44.4, M1A.10X0-M1A.19X1, P35.2-P35.9, P37.0-P37.4, P37.8-P37.9, T56.0X1A, T56.0X2A, T56.0X3A, T56.0X4A

☑5ᵗʰ **B33.2** **Viral carditis**
Coxsackie (virus) carditis

B33.20 **Viral carditis, unspecified** CC
CC Excl: A52.06, B33.20-B33.22, I00, I01.2-I01.9, I09.0, I09.9, I23.0-I23.3, I23.6-I23.8, I40.0-I41, I51.0, I51.4, I87.8, I99.8-I99.9

B33.21 **Viral endocarditis** CC
CC Excl: A01.00-A01.09, A39.51, A52.03, A78, B33.21, B37.6, B40.0-B40.9, I00, I01.1, I01.8-I02.0, I05.0-I07.9, I08.1-I08.3, I08.9, I09.1, I09.89-I09.9, I33.0-I39, I42.4, I87.8-I87.9, I99.8-I99.9, Q22.2, Q23.8-Q23.9, Q24.8, T82.6XXA

B33.22 **Viral myocarditis** CC
CC Excl: See code: B33.20

B33.23 **Viral pericarditis** CC
CC Excl: B33.23, I01.0, I09.2, I30.0-I30.9, I31.3-I32, I87.8-I87.9, I99.8-I99.9

B33.24 **Viral cardiomyopathy**

B33.3 **Retrovirus infections, not elsewhere classified**
Retrovirus infection NOS

B33.4 **Hantavirus (cardio)-pulmonary syndrome [HPS] [HCPS]** CC
Hantavirus disease with pulmonary manifestations
Sin nombre virus disease
Use additional code to identify any associated acute kidney failure (N17.9)
EXCLUDES1 hantavirus disease with renal manifestations (A98.5)
hemorrhagic fever with renal manifestations (A98.5)
CC Excl: A74.81-A74.9, A88.1, A96.0-A96.9, A98.3-A98.5, B19.20-B19.21, B25.8-B25.9, B33.24-B34.2, B34.4-B34.8, B97.0-B97.89

B33.8 **Other specified viral diseases**
EXCLUDES1 anogenital human papillomavirus infection (A63.0)
viral warts due to human papillomavirus infection (B07)

☑4ᵗʰ **B34** **Viral infection of unspecified site**
EXCLUDES1 anogenital human papillomavirus infection (A63.0)
cytomegaloviral disease NOS (B25.9)
herpesvirus [herpes simplex] infection NOS (B00.9)
retrovirus infection NOS (B33.3)
viral agents as the cause of diseases classified elsewhere (B97.-)
viral warts due to human papillomavirus infection (B07)

B34.0 **Adenovirus infection, unspecified**

B34.1 **Enterovirus infection, unspecified**
Coxsackievirus infection NOS
Echovirus infection NOS

B34.2 **Coronavirus infection, unspecified**
EXCLUDES1 pneumonia due to SARS-associated coronavirus (J12.81)

B34.3 **Parvovirus infection, unspecified** CC
CC Excl: B08.3, B34.3

B34.4 **Papovavirus infection, unspecified**

B34.8 **Other viral infections of unspecified site**

B34.9 **Viral infection, unspecified**
Viremia NOS

Mycoses (B35-B49)
EXCLUDES2 hypersensitivity pneumonitis due to organic dust (J67.-)
mycosis fungoides (C84.0-)

☑4ᵗʰ **B35** **Dermatophytosis**
INCLUDES favus
infections due to species of Epidermophyton, Micro-sporum and Trichophyton
tinea, any type except those in B36-

B35.0 **Tinea barbae and tinea capitis**
Beard ringworm
Kerion
Scalp ringworm
Sycosis, mycotic

B35.1 **Tinea unguium**
Dermatophytic onychia
Dermatophytosis of nail
Onychomycosis
Ringworm of nails

B35.2 **Tinea manuum**
Dermatophytosis of hand
Hand ringworm

B35.3 **Tinea pedis**
Athlete's foot
Dermatophytosis of foot
Foot ringworm

B35.4 **Tinea corporis**
Ringworm of the body

B35.5 **Tinea imbricata**
Tokelau

B35.6 **Tinea cruris**
Dhobi itch
Groin ringworm
Jock itch

B35.8 **Other dermatophytoses**
Disseminated dermatophytosis
Granulomatous dermatophytosis

B35.9 **Dermatophytosis, unspecified**
Ringworm NOS

☑4ᵗʰ **B36** **Other superficial mycoses**

B36.0 **Pityriasis versicolor**
Tinea flava
Tinea versicolor

☑ Additional Character Required   ☑x7ᵗʰ Placeholder Alert   Unacceptable PDx   Manifestation   Hospital Acquired Condition   EXCLUDES1 Not Coded Here   EXCLUDES2 Not Included Here

Chapter 1. Certain Infectious and Parasitic Diseases

B36.1 Tinea nigra
Keratomycosis nigricans palmaris
Microsporosis nigra
Pityriasis nigra

B36.2 White piedra
Tinea blanca

B36.3 Black piedra

B36.8 Other specified superficial mycoses

B36.9 Superficial mycosis, unspecified

√4ᵗʰ **B37 Candidiasis**

INCLUDES   candidosis
moniliasis

EXCLUDES 1   neonatal candidiasis (P37.5)

B37.0 Candidal stomatitis   HIV CC
Oral thrush
CC Excl: B37.0-B37.9, B48.3, B49, B92, B94.2-B94.9

B37.1 Pulmonary candidiasis   HIV MCC
Candidal bronchitis
Candidal pneumonia
CC Excl: See code: B37.0

B37.2 Candidiasis of skin and nail   HIV
Candidal onychia
Candidal paronychia
EXCLUDES 2   diaper dermatitis (L22)

B37.3 Candidiasis of vulva and vagina   ♀
Candidal vulvovaginitis
Monilial vulvovaginitis
Vaginal thrush

√5ᵗʰ **B37.4 Candidiasis of other urogenital sites**

1 **B37.41 Candidal cystitis and urethritis**   CC
CC Excl: B37.1, B37.41-B37.82, B37.84-B37.9, N25.81-N25.89

B37.42 Candidal balanitis

1 **B37.49 Other urogenital candidiasis**   CC
Candidal pyelonephritis
CC Excl: See code: B37.41

B37.5 Candidal meningitis   HIV MCC
CC Excl: A02.21, A17.0-A17.1, A27.81, A39.0, A50.41, A51.41, A52.13, A54.82, A54.84, A54.89-A54.9, A87.0-A87.9, B00.3, B02.1, B26.1, B37.0-B37.9, B38.4, B45.1, B48.3, B49, B58.2, B92, B94.2-B94.9, G00.0-G03.9, G04.2, G32.89, G61.0, G96.8-G96.9, G98.0-G98.8, G99.8

B37.6 Candidal endocarditis   HIV MCC
CC Excl: B37.0-B37.9, B48.3, B49, B92, B94.2-B94.9

B37.7 Candidal sepsis   PDx MCC MCC
Disseminated candidiasis
Systemic candidiasis
AHA: 2014, 4Q, 46
CC Excl: A02.1, A20.7, A22.7, A26.7, A32.7, A39.2-A39.4, A40.0-A40.1, A40.8-A41.9, A42.7, A48.2-A48.4, A48.8-A49.9, A54.86, B00.7, B37.0-B37.9, B48.3, B49, B92, B94.2-B96.89, R65.10-R65.20, Z16.10-Z16.39

√5ᵗʰ **B37.8 Candidiasis of other sites**

CC Excl: For CC codes in subcategory B37.8, unless otherwise noted: B37.0-B37.9, B48.3, B49, B92, B94.2-B94.9

B37.81 Candidal esophagitis   HIV CC

B37.82 Candidal enteritis   HIV CC
Candidal proctitis

B37.83 Candidal cheilitis   HIV CC

B37.84 Candidal otitis externa   HIV CC

B37.89 Other sites of candidiasis   HIV CC
Candidal osteomyelitis
CC Excl: B37.1, B37.5-B37.82, B37.84-B37.9

B37.9 Candidiasis, unspecified   HIV
Thrush NOS

√4ᵗʰ **B38 Coccidioidomycosis**

B38.0 Acute pulmonary coccidioidomycosis   HIV CC
CC Excl: B38.0-B38.2, B38.7, B38.89-B38.9, B48.3, B49, B92, B94.2-B94.9

B38.1 Chronic pulmonary coccidioidomycosis   HIV CC
CC Excl: B38.0-B39.9

B38.2 Pulmonary coccidioidomycosis, unspecified   HIV CC
CC Excl: See code: B38.1

B38.3 Cutaneous coccidioidomycosis   HIV CC
CC Excl: B38.0-B38.9

B38.4 Coccidioidomycosis meningitis   HIV MCC
CC Excl: A02.21, A17.0-A17.1, A27.81, A39.0, A50.41, A51.41, A52.13, A54.82, A54.84, A54.89-A54.9, A87.0-A87.9, B00.3, B02.1, B26.1, B37.5, B38.4-B38.7, B38.89-B38.9, B45.1, B48.3, B49, B58.2, B92, B94.2-B94.9, G00.0-G03.9, G04.2, G32.89, G61.0, G96.8-G96.9, G98.0-G98.8, G99

B38.7 Disseminated coccidioidomycosis   HIV CC
Generalized coccidioidomycosis
CC Excl: B38.7, B38.89-B38.9, B48.3, B49, B92, B94.2-B94.9

√5ᵗʰ **B38.8 Other forms of coccidioidomycosis**

B38.81 Prostatic coccidioidomycosis   HIV CC ♂
CC Excl: See code: B38.3

B38.89 Other forms of coccidioidomycosis   HIV CC
CC Excl: See code: B38.7

B38.9 Coccidioidomycosis, unspecified   HIV CC
CC Excl: See code: B38.7

√4ᵗʰ **B39 Histoplasmosis**
Code first associated AIDS (B20)
Use additional code for any associated manifestations, such as:
endocarditis (I39)
meningitis (G02)
pericarditis (I32)
retinitis (H32)

B39.0 Acute pulmonary histoplasmosis capsulati   HIV MCC
CC Excl: A22.1, A37.01, A37.11, A37.81, A37.91, A48.1, B25.0, B39.0-B39.4, B39.9, B44.0, B48.3, B49, B92, B94.2-B94.9, J09.X1-J09.X2, J10.00-J10.1, J11.00-J11.1, J12.0-J12.3, J12.89-J18.1, J18.8-J18.9, J44.9, J47.0-J70.4, J70.8-J70.9, J98.4, R91.1

B39.1 Chronic pulmonary histoplasmosis capsulati   HIV MCC
CC Excl: See code: B39.0

B39.2 Pulmonary histoplasmosis capsulati, unspecified   HIV MCC
CC Excl: See code: B39.0

B39.3 Disseminated histoplasmosis capsulati   HIV CC
Generalized histoplasmosis capsulati
CC Excl: B38.0-B39.4

B39.4 Histoplasmosis capsulati, unspecified   HIV
American histoplasmosis

B39.5 Histoplasmosis duboisii   HIV
African histoplasmosis

B39.9 Histoplasmosis, unspecified   HIV

√4ᵗʰ **B40 Blastomycosis**

EXCLUDES 1   Brazilian blastomycosis (B41.-)
keloidal blastomycosis (B48.0)

CC Excl: For CC codes in category B40, unless otherwise noted: B40.0-B40.9, B48.3, B49, B92, B94.2-B94.9

B40.0 Acute pulmonary blastomycosis   CC

B40.1 Chronic pulmonary blastomycosis   CC

B40.2 Pulmonary blastomycosis, unspecified   CC

B40.3 Cutaneous blastomycosis   CC

B40.7 Disseminated blastomycosis   CC
Generalized blastomycosis

√5ᵗʰ **B40.8 Other forms of blastomycosis**

B40.81 Blastomycotic meningoencephalitis   CC
Meningomyelitis due to blastomycosis

B40.89 Other forms of blastomycosis   CC

B40.9 Blastomycosis, unspecified   CC

√4ᵗʰ **B41 Paracoccidioidomycosis**

INCLUDES   Brazilian blastomycosis
Lutz' disease

CC Excl: For CC codes in category B41, unless otherwise noted: B41.0-B41.9, B48.3, B49, B92, B94.2-B94.9

B41.0 Pulmonary paracoccidioidomycosis   CC

B41.7 Disseminated paracoccidioidomycosis   CC
Generalized paracoccidioidomycosis

B41.8 Other forms of paracoccidioidomycosis   CC

B41.9 Paracoccidioidomycosis, unspecified   CC

√4ᵗʰ **B42 Sporotrichosis**

B42.0 Pulmonary sporotrichosis

B42.1 Lymphocutaneous sporotrichosis

B42.7 Disseminated sporotrichosis
Generalized sporotrichosis

---

1   HAC = as SDx not POA, in combination with SDx code T83.51XA also not POA.

✓5ᵗʰ **B42.8** **Other forms of sporotrichosis**

     B42.81 **Cerebral sporotrichosis**
         Meningitis due to sporotrichosis

     B42.82 **Sporotrichosis arthritis**

     B42.89 **Other forms of sporotrichosis**

B42.9 **Sporotrichosis, unspecified**

✓4ᵗʰ **B43** **Chromomycosis and pheomycotic abscess**

B43.0 **Cutaneous chromomycosis**
     Dermatitis verrucosa

B43.1 **Pheomycotic brain abscess**
     Cerebral chromomycosis

B43.2 **Subcutaneous pheomycotic abscess and cyst**

B43.8 **Other forms of chromomycosis**

B43.9 **Chromomycosis, unspecified**

✓4ᵗʰ **B44** **Aspergillosis**

     INCLUDES   aspergilloma

     CC Excl: For CC/MCC codes in category B44, unless otherwise noted: B44.1-B44.7, B44.89-B44.9, B48.3-B48.4, B49, B92, B94.2-B94.9

B44.0 **Invasive pulmonary aspergillosis**   PDxMCC MCC
     CC Excl: A15.0-A15.6, A15.8-A15.9, A17.9, A18.82, A18.84, A18.89, A21.2, A22.1, A31.0, A37.01, A37.11, A37.81, A37.91, A42.0, A43.0, A48.1, B25.0, B39.0-B39.2, B44.0, B58.3, B59, B67.1, J09.X1-J09.X2, J10.00-J10.1, J11.00-J11.1, J12.0-J12.3, J12.89-J18.1, J18.8-J18.9, J22, J44.9, J47.0-J70.4, J70.8-J70.9, J98.4, J98.8-J99, Q33.4, R91.1

B44.1 **Other pulmonary aspergillosis**   CC

B44.2 **Tonsillar aspergillosis**   CC

B44.7 **Disseminated aspergillosis**   CC
     Generalized aspergillosis

✓5ᵗʰ **B44.8** **Other forms of aspergillosis**

     B44.81 **Allergic bronchopulmonary aspergillosis**   CC
         CC Excl: B44.81, J22, J98.8-J98.9

     B44.89 **Other forms of aspergillosis**   CC

B44.9 **Aspergillosis, unspecified**   CC

✓4ᵗʰ **B45** **Cryptococcosis**

     CC Excl: For CC/MCC codes in category B45, unless otherwise noted: B45.0-B45.9, B48.3, B49, B92, B94.2-B94.9

B45.0 **Pulmonary cryptococcosis**   HIV CC
     CC Excl: B45.0, B45.2-B45.9, B48.3, B49, B92, B94.2-B94.9

B45.1 **Cerebral cryptococcosis**   PDxMCC MCC
     Cryptococcal meningitis
     Cryptococcosis meningocerebralis
     CC Excl: A02.21, A17.0-A17.1, A27.81, A39.0, A50.41, A51.41, A52.13, A54.82, A54.84, A54.89-A54.9, A87.0-A87.9, B00.3, B02.1, B26.1, B37.5, B38.4, B45.1, B58.2, E08.40-E08.49, E08.618-E08.638, E08.649-E08.8, E09.40-E09.49, E09.618-E09.638, E09.649-E09.8, E10.40-E10.49, E10.618-E10.638, E10.649, E10.69-E10.8, E11.40-E11.49, E11.618-E11.638, E11.649, E11.69-E11.8, E13.40-E13.49, E13.618-E13.638, E13.649-E13.8, G00.0-G03.9, G04.2, G32.89, G61.0, G96.8-G96.9, G98.0-G98.8, G99.8

B45.2 **Cutaneous cryptococcosis**   HIV CC

B45.3 **Osseous cryptococcosis**   HIV CC

B45.7 **Disseminated cryptococcosis**   HIV CC
     Generalized cryptococcosis

B45.8 **Other forms of cryptococcosis**   HIV CC

B45.9 **Cryptococcosis, unspecified**   HIV CC

✓4ᵗʰ **B46** **Zygomycosis**

     CC Excl: For MCC codes in category B46, unless otherwise noted: B46.0-B46.9, B48.3, B49, B92, B94.2-B94.9

B46.0 **Pulmonary mucormycosis**   MCC

B46.1 **Rhinocerebral mucormycosis**   MCC

B46.2 **Gastrointestinal mucormycosis**   MCC

B46.3 **Cutaneous mucormycosis**   MCC
     Subcutaneous mucormycosis

B46.4 **Disseminated mucormycosis**   MCC
     Generalized mucormycosis

B46.5 **Mucormycosis, unspecified**   MCC

B46.8 **Other zygomycoses**   MCC
     Entomophthoromycosis

B46.9 **Zygomycosis, unspecified**   MCC
     Phycomycosis NOS

✓4ᵗʰ **B47** **Mycetoma**

B47.0 **Eumycetoma**   CC
     Madura foot, mycotic
     Maduromycosis
     CC Excl: B47.0, B48.3, B49, B92, B94.2-B94.9

B47.1 **Actinomycetoma**   HIV CC
     CC Excl: A42.0-A42.2, A42.81-A43.9, B47.1-B47.9, L08.1

B47.9 **Mycetoma, unspecified**   HIV CC
     Madura foot NOS
     CC Excl: A42.81-A42.9, A43.8-A43.9, B47.1-B47.9

✓4ᵗʰ **B48** **Other mycoses, not elsewhere classified**

B48.0 **Lobomycosis**
     Keloidal blastomycosis
     Lobo's disease

B48.1 **Rhinosporidiosis**

B48.2 **Allescheriasis**   CC
     Infection due to Pseudallescheria boydii
     EXCLUDES 1   eumycetoma (B47.0)
     CC Excl: B48.2-B48.3, B49, B92, B94.2-B94.9

B48.3 **Geotrichosis**   CC
     Geotrichum stomatitis
     CC Excl: B48.3-B49

B48.4 **Penicillosis**   CC
     CC Excl: B44.1-B44.7, B44.89-B44.9, B48.3-B48.4, B49, B92, B94.2-B94.9

B48.8 **Other specified mycoses**   HIV CC
     Adiaspiromycosis
     Infection of tissue and organs by Alternaria
     Infection of tissue and organs by Drechslera
     Infection of tissue and organs by Fusarium
     Infection of tissue and organs by saprophytic fungi NEC
     AHA: 2014, 4Q, 46; 2014, 2Q, 13
     CC Excl: B48.3, B48.8-B49, B92, B94.2-B94.9

B49 **Unspecified mycosis**   CC
     Fungemia NOS
     CC Excl: See code: B48.3

Protozoal diseases (B50-B64)

     EXCLUDES 1   amebiasis (A06.-)
         other protozoal intestinal diseases (A07.-)

✓4ᵗʰ **B50** **Plasmodium falciparum malaria**
     INCLUDES   mixed infections of Plasmodium falciparum with any other Plasmodium species

     CC Excl: For CC/MCC codes in category B50, unless otherwise noted: B50.0-B57.5

B50.0 **Plasmodium falciparum malaria with cerebral complications**   CC
     Cerebral malaria NOS

B50.8 **Other severe and complicated Plasmodium falciparum malaria**   CC
     Severe or complicated Plasmodium falciparum malaria NOS

B50.9 **Plasmodium falciparum malaria, unspecified**   MCC

✓4ᵗʰ **B51** **Plasmodium vivax malaria**
     INCLUDES   mixed infections of Plasmodium vivax with other Plasmodium species, except Plasmodium falciparum
     EXCLUDES 1   plasmodium vivax with Plasmodium falciparum (B50.-)

     CC Excl: For CC codes in category B51, unless otherwise noted: B50.0-B57.5

B51.0 **Plasmodium vivax malaria with rupture of spleen**   CC

B51.8 **Plasmodium vivax malaria with other complications**   CC

B51.9 **Plasmodium vivax malaria without complication**   CC
     Plasmodium vivax malaria NOS
     CC Excl: A44.0-A44.9, A68.0-A68.9, A69.20-A69.29, B50.0-B57.5, B60.0

✓4ᵗʰ **B52** **Plasmodium malariae malaria**
     INCLUDES   mixed infections of Plasmodium malariae with other Plasmodium species, except Plasmodium falciparum and Plasmodium vivax
     EXCLUDES 1   Plasmodium falciparum (B50.-)
         Plasmodium vivax (B51.-)

     CC Excl: For CC codes in category B52, unless otherwise noted: B50.0-B57.5

✓ Additional Character Required   ✓x7ᵗʰ Placeholder Alert   Unacceptable PDx   Manifestation   Hospital Acquired Condition   EXCLUDES 1 Not Coded Here   EXCLUDES 2 Not Included Here

ICD-10-CM 2016   445

B52.0 Plasmodium malariae malaria with nephropathy `PDxCC` `CC`
    CC Excl: A17.9, A18.10-A18.11, A18.13, A18.82, A18.84, A18.89, A54.21, A54.29, A54.82, A54.84, A54.89-A54.9, A59.00, A59.8-A59.9, B37.41-B37.49, B50.0-B57.5, E08.21-E08.29, E08.618-E08.638, E08.649-E08.8, E09.21-E09.29, E09.618-E09.638, E09.649-E09.8, E10.21-E10.29, E10.618-E10.638, E10.649, E10.69-E10.8, E11.21-E11.29, E11.618-E11.638, E11.649, E11.69-E11.8, E13.21-E13.29, E13.618-E13.638, E13.649-E13.8, E88.3, M10.30-M10.39, N00.0-N11.0, N11.8-N13.39, N13.6, N14.0-N19, N25.0-N26.1, N26.9-N27.9, N28.1-N29, N36.41-N36.43, N36.8-N36.9, N39.8-N39.9, R31.0-R31.9

B52.8 Plasmodium malariae malaria with other complications `CC`

B52.9 Plasmodium malariae malaria without complication `CC`
    Plasmodium malariae malaria NOS

✓4th **B53 Other specified malaria**

    CC Excl: For CC codes in subcategory B53, unless otherwise noted: B50.0-B57.5

B53.0 Plasmodium ovale malaria `CC`
    EXCLUDES1 Plasmodium ovale with Plasmodium falciparum (B50.-)
    Plasmodium ovale with Plasmodium malariae (B52.-)
    Plasmodium ovale with Plasmodium vivax (B51.-)

B53.1 Malaria due to simian plasmodia `CC`
    EXCLUDES1 Malaria due to simian plasmodia with Plasmodium falciparum (B50.-)
    Malaria due to simian plasmodia with Plasmodium malariae (B52.-)
    Malaria due to simian plasmodia with Plasmodium ovale (B53.0)
    Malaria due to simian plasmodia with Plasmodium vivax (B51.-)

B53.8 Other malaria, not elsewhere classified `CC`

B54 Unspecified malaria `CC`
    CC Excl: B50.0-B57.5, B97.21

✓4th **B55 Leishmaniasis**

    CC Excl: For CC codes in category B55, unless otherwise noted: A44.0-A44.9, A68.0-A68.9, A69.20-A69.29, A75.0-A79.9, B50.0-B57.5, B60.0

B55.0 Visceral leishmaniasis
    Kala-azar
    Post-kala-azar dermal leishmaniasis

B55.1 Cutaneous leishmaniasis `CC`

B55.2 Mucocutaneous leishmaniasis `CC`

B55.9 Leishmaniasis, unspecified `CC`

✓4th **B56 African trypanosomiasis**

    CC Excl: For CC codes in category B56, unless otherwise noted: A44.0-A44.9, A68.0-A68.9, A69.20-A69.29, A75.0-A79.9, B50.0-B57.5, B60.0

B56.0 Gambiense trypanosomiasis `CC`
    Infection due to Trypanosoma brucei gambiense
    West African sleeping sickness

B56.1 Rhodesiense trypanosomiasis `CC`
    East African sleeping sickness
    Infection due to Trypanosoma brucei rhodesiense

B56.9 African trypanosomiasis, unspecified `CC`
    Sleeping sickness NOS

✓4th **B57 Chagas' disease**
    INCLUDES American trypanosomiasis
    infection due to Trypanosoma cruzi

    CC Excl: For CC codes in category B57, unless otherwise noted: A44.0-A44.9, A68.0-A68.9, A69.20-A69.29, A75.0-A79.9, B50.0-B57.5, B60.0

B57.0 Acute Chagas' disease with heart involvement `CC`
    Acute Chagas' disease with myocarditis
    CC Excl: B57.0-B57.2, B92, B94.2-B94.9

B57.1 Acute Chagas' disease without heart involvement `CC`
    Acute Chagas' disease NOS

B57.2 Chagas' disease (chronic) with heart involvement `CC`
    American trypanosomiasis NOS
    Chagas' disease (chronic) NOS
    Chagas' disease (chronic) with myocarditis
    Trypanosomiasis NOS
    CC Excl: See code: B57.0

✓5th **B57.3 Chagas' disease (chronic) with digestive system involvement**

    B57.30 Chagas' disease with digestive system involvement, unspecified `CC`

    B57.31 Megaesophagus in Chagas' disease `CC`

    B57.32 Megacolon in Chagas' disease `CC`

    B57.39 Other digestive system involvement in Chagas' disease `CC`

✓5th **B57.4 Chagas' disease (chronic) with nervous system involvement**

    B57.40 Chagas' disease with nervous system involvement, unspecified `CC`

    B57.41 Meningitis in Chagas' disease `CC`

    B57.42 Meningoencephalitis in Chagas' disease `CC`

    B57.49 Other nervous system involvement in Chagas' disease `CC`

B57.5 Chagas' disease (chronic) with other organ involvement `CC`

✓4th **B58 Toxoplasmosis**
    INCLUDES infection due to Toxoplasma gondii
    EXCLUDES1 congenital toxoplasmosis (P37.1)

✓5th **B58.0 Toxoplasma oculopathy**

    B58.00 Toxoplasma oculopathy, unspecified `HIV` `CC`
      CC Excl: B58.00-B58.9, B94.2-B94.9

    B58.01 Toxoplasma chorioretinitis `HIV` `CC`
      CC Excl: B58.00-B58.01, B58.82-B58.9, B92, B94.2-B94.9

    B58.09 Other toxoplasma oculopathy `HIV` `CC`
      Toxoplasma uveitis
      CC Excl: B58.00-B58.09, B58.82-B58.9, B92, B94.2-B94.9

B58.1 Toxoplasma hepatitis `HIV` `CC`
    CC Excl: B58.00-B58.1, B58.82-B58.9, B92, B94.2-B94.9

B58.2 Toxoplasma meningoencephalitis `HIV` `MCC`
    CC Excl: B58.00-B58.2, B58.82-B58.9, B92, B94.2-B94.9

B58.3 Pulmonary toxoplasmosis `HIV` `MCC`
    CC Excl: A22.1, A37.01, A37.11, A37.81, A37.91, A48.1, B25.0, B44.0, B58.00, B58.3, B58.82-B58.9, B92, B94.2-B94.9, J09.X1-J09.X2, J10.00-J10.1, J11.00-J11.1, J12.0-J12.3, J12.89-J18.1, J18.8-J18.9, J44.9, J47.0-J70.4, J70.8-J70.9, J98.4, R91.1

✓5th **B58.8 Toxoplasmosis with other organ involvement**

    CC Excl: For CC/MCC codes in subcategory B58.8, unless otherwise noted: B58.00, B58.81-B58.9, B92, B94.2-B94.9

    B58.81 Toxoplasma myocarditis `HIV` `MCC`

    B58.82 Toxoplasma myositis `HIV` `CC`
      CC Excl: B58.00, B58.82-B58.9, B92, B94.2-B94.9

    B58.83 Toxoplasma tubulo-interstitial nephropathy `HIV` `CC`
      Toxoplasma pyelonephritis

    B58.89 Toxoplasmosis with other organ involvement `HIV` `CC`

B58.9 Toxoplasmosis, unspecified `HIV` `CC`
    CC Excl: B58.9

B59 Pneumocystosis `HIV` `MCC`
    Pneumonia due to Pneumocystis carinii
    Pneumonia due to Pneumocystis jiroveci
    CC Excl: A22.1, A37.01, A37.11, A37.81, A37.91, A48.1, B25.0, B44.0, B59, B92, B94.2-B94.9, J09.X1-J09.X2, J10.00-J10.1, J11.00-J11.1, J12.0-J12.3, J12.89-J18.1, J18.8-J18.9, J44.9, J47.0-J70.4, J70.8-J70.9, J98.4, R91.1

✓4th **B60 Other protozoal diseases, not elsewhere classified**
    EXCLUDES1 cryptosporidiosis (A07.2)
    intestinal microsporidiosis (A07.8)
    isosporiasis (A07.3)

B60.0 Babesiosis `CC`
    Piroplasmosis
    CC Excl: A44.0-A44.9, A68.0-A68.9, A69.20-A69.29, A75.0-A79.9, B50.0-B57.5, B60.0

✓5th **B60.1 Acanthamebiasis**

    B60.10 Acanthamebiasis, unspecified `CC`
      CC Excl: B59, B60.11, B60.19-B64, B89, B99.8-B99.9, L94.6, M35.2

    B60.11 Meningoencephalitis due to Acanthamoeba (culbertsoni)

    B60.12 Conjunctivitis due to Acanthamoeba

    B60.13 Keratoconjunctivitis due to Acanthamoeba

    B60.19 Other acanthamebic disease `CC`
      CC Excl: See code: B60.10

B60.2 Naegleriasis `CC`
    Primary amebic meningoencephalitis
    CC Excl: See code: B60.10

B60.8 Other specified protozoal diseases `HIV`
    Microsporidiosis

B64 Unspecified protozoal disease

Helminthiases (B65-B83)

✓4ᵗʰ **B65 Schistosomiasis [bilharziasis]**
     INCLUDES   snail fever

     CC Excl: For CC codes in category B65, unless otherwise noted: B65.0-B65.9

     B65.0 Schistosomiasis due to Schistosoma haematobium [urinary schistosomiasis]   CC

     B65.1 Schistosomiasis due to Schistosoma mansoni [intestinal schistosomiasis]   CC

     B65.2 Schistosomiasis due to Schistosoma japonicum   CC
         Asiatic schistosomiasis

     B65.3 Cercarial dermatitis   CC
         Swimmer's itch

     B65.8 Other schistosomiasis   CC
         Infection due to Schistosoma intercalatum
         Infection due to Schistosoma mattheei
         Infection due to Schistosoma mekongi

     B65.9 Schistosomiasis, unspecified

✓4ᵗʰ **B66 Other fluke infections**

     CC Excl: For CC codes in category B66, unless otherwise noted: B66.0-B66.9

     B66.0 Opisthorchiasis   CC
         Infection due to cat liver fluke
         Infection due to Opisthorchis (felineus)(viverrini)

     B66.1 Clonorchiasis   CC
         Chinese liver fluke disease
         Infection due to Clonorchis sinensis
         Oriental liver fluke disease

     B66.2 Dicroceliasis   CC
         Infection due to Dicrocoelium dendriticum
         Lancet fluke infection

     B66.3 Fascioliasis   CC
         Infection due to Fasciola gigantica
         Infection due to Fasciola hepatica
         Infection due to Fasciola indica
         Sheep liver fluke disease

     B66.4 Paragonimiasis   CC
         Infection due to Paragonimus species
         Lung fluke disease
         Pulmonary distomiasis

     B66.5 Fasciolopsiasis   CC
         Infection due to Fasciolopsis buski
         Intestinal distomiasis

     B66.8 Other specified fluke infections   CC
         Echinostomiasis   Nanophyetiasis
         Heterophyiasis   Watsoniasis
         Metagonimiasis

     B66.9 Fluke infection, unspecified

✓4ᵗʰ **B67 Echinococcosis**
     INCLUDES   hydatidosis

     B67.0 Echinococcus granulosus infection of liver   CC
         CC Excl: B67.0, B67.8-B67.99

     B67.1 Echinococcus granulosus infection of lung   CC
         CC Excl: B67.1, B67.8-B67.99, J12.81

     B67.2 Echinococcus granulosus infection of bone   CC
         CC Excl: B67.2, B67.32-B67.39, B67.8-B67.99

     ✓5ᵗʰ **B67.3 Echinococcus granulosus infection, other and multiple sites**

         B67.31 Echinococcus granulosus infection, thyroid gland   CC
             CC Excl: B67.31, B67.8-B67.99

         B67.32 Echinococcus granulosus infection, multiple sites   CC
             CC Excl: B67.2, B67.32-B67.39, B67.8-B67.99

         B67.39 Echinococcus granulosus infection, other sites   CC
             CC Excl: See code: B67.32

     B67.4 Echinococcus granulosus infection, unspecified   CC
         Dog tapeworm (infection)
         CC Excl: B67.4, B67.8-B67.99

     B67.5 Echinococcus multilocularis infection of liver   CC
         CC Excl: B67.5, B67.8-B67.99

     ✓5ᵗʰ **B67.6 Echinococcus multilocularis infection, other and multiple sites**

         B67.61 Echinococcus multilocularis infection, multiple sites   CC
             CC Excl: B67.61-B67.69, B67.8-B67.99

         B67.69 Echinococcus multilocularis infection, other sites   CC
             CC Excl: See code: B67.61

     B67.7 Echinococcus multilocularis infection, unspecified   CC
         CC Excl: B67.7-B67.99

     B67.8 Echinococcosis, unspecified, of liver   CC
         CC Excl: B67.8-B67.99

     ✓5ᵗʰ **B67.9 Echinococcosis, other and unspecified**

         B67.90 Echinococcosis, unspecified   CC
             Echinococcosis NOS
             CC Excl: See code: B67.8

         B67.99 Other echinococcosis   CC
             CC Excl: See code: B67.8

✓4ᵗʰ **B68 Taeniasis**
     EXCLUDES 1   cysticercosis (B69.-)

     B68.0 Taenia solium taeniasis   CC
         Pork tapeworm (infection)
         CC Excl: A00.1, A01.00-A01.09, A01.4-A02.0, A03.9-A05.2, A06.0-A06.2, A06.9, A07.1-A09, A18.32-A18.39, A18.83, A48.51-A48.52, B37.82, B68.0-B71.9, B82.9, J09.X3-J09.X9, J10.2-J10.89, J11.2-J11.89, K30, K31.84, K52.1-K52.2, K52.82-K52.9, K58.0-K58.9, P76.8-P77.9, P78.1, P78.3-P78.89

     B68.1 Taenia saginata taeniasis   CC
         Beef tapeworm (infection)
         Infection due to adult tapeworm Taenia saginata
         CC Excl: B68.0-B71.9

     B68.9 Taeniasis, unspecified   CC
         CC Excl: See code: B68.1

✓4ᵗʰ **B69 Cysticercosis**
     INCLUDES   cysticerciasis infection due to larval form of Taenia solium

     CC Excl: For CC codes in category B69, unless otherwise noted: B68.0-B71.9

     B69.0 Cysticercosis of central nervous system   CC

     B69.1 Cysticercosis of eye   CC

     ✓5ᵗʰ **B69.8 Cysticercosis of other sites**

         B69.81 Myositis in cysticercosis   CC

         B69.89 Cysticercosis of other sites   CC

     B69.9 Cysticercosis, unspecified   CC

✓4ᵗʰ **B70 Diphyllobothriasis and sparganosis**

     CC Excl: For CC codes in category B70, unless otherwise noted: B68.0-B71.9

     B70.0 Diphyllobothriasis   CC
         Diphyllobothrium (adult) (latum) (pacificum) infection
         Fish tapeworm (infection)
         EXCLUDES 2   larval diphyllobothriasis (B70.1)

     B70.1 Sparganosis   CC
         Infection due to Sparganum (mansoni) (proliferum)
         Infection due to Spirometra larva
         Larval diphyllobothriasis
         Spirometrosis

✓4ᵗʰ **B71 Other cestode infections**

     CC Excl: For CC codes in category B71, unless otherwise noted: B68.0-B71.9

     B71.0 Hymenolepiasis   CC
         Dwarf tapeworm infection
         Rat tapeworm (infection)

     B71.1 Dipylidiasis   CC

     B71.8 Other specified cestode infections
         Coenurosis

     B71.9 Cestode infection, unspecified
         Tapeworm (infection) NOS

B72 Dracunculiasis   CC
     INCLUDES   guinea worm infection
               infection due to Dracunculus medinensis
     CC Excl: B72-B74.9

✓4ᵗʰ **B73 Onchocerciasis**
     INCLUDES   onchocerca volvulus infection
               onchocercosis
               river blindness

     CC Excl: For CC codes in category B73, unless otherwise noted: B72-B74.9

     ✓5ᵗʰ **B73.0 Onchocerciasis with eye disease**

         B73.00 Onchocerciasis with eye involvement, unspecified   CC

✓ Additional Character Required   ✗x7ᵗʰ Placeholder Alert   Unacceptable PDx   Manifestation   Hospital Acquired Condition   EXCLUDES 1 Not Coded Here   EXCLUDES 2 Not Included Here

B73.Ø1   **Onchocerciasis with endophthalmitis**   `CC`

B73.Ø2   **Onchocerciasis with glaucoma**   `CC`

B73.Ø9   **Onchocerciasis with other eye involvement**   `CC`
Infestation of eyelid due to onchocerciasis

B73.1   **Onchocerciasis without eye disease**   `CC`

✓4ᵗʰ **B74   Filariasis**
EXCLUDES 2   *onchocerciasis (B73)*
tropical (pulmonary) eosinophilia NOS (J82)

CC Excl: For CC codes in category B74, unless otherwise noted:
B72-B74.9

B74.Ø   **Filariasis due to Wuchereria bancrofti**   `CC`
Bancroftian elephantiasis
Bancroftian filariasis

B74.1   **Filariasis due to Brugia malayi**   `CC`

B74.2   **Filariasis due to Brugia timori**   `CC`

B74.3   **Loiasis**
Calabar swelling
Eyeworm disease of Africa
Loa loa infection

B74.4   **Mansonelliasis**   `CC`
Infection due to Mansonella ozzardi
Infection due to Mansonella perstans
Infection due to Mansonella streptocerca

B74.8   **Other filariases**   `CC`
Dirofilariasis

B74.9   **Filariasis, unspecified**   `CC`

B75   Trichinellosis   `CC`
INCLUDES   infection due to Trichinella species
trichiniasis
CC Excl: A17.82- A5Ø.42, A52.14, A75.9, A79.9, A81.1, A81.82-A81.89,
A83.Ø-A85.8, A87.2, A88.Ø, A88.8, A92.1-A92.8, A93.Ø, BØØ.4, BØØ.82,
BØ1.11-BØ1.12, BØ4, BØ6.Ø1, BØ8.Ø9, BØ8.2Ø-BØ8.22, BØ8.6Ø-BØ8.79, BØ9-
B1Ø.Ø9, B26.2, B33.1, B45.Ø, B45.2-B45.9, B58.2, B75, B97.1Ø, B97.21,
GØ4.ØØ-GØ4.Ø1, GØ4.31, GØ4.81-GØ5.4, G37.Ø, G37.4-G37.5, JØ9.X3-JØ9.X9,
J1Ø.2-J1Ø.89, J11.2-J11.89, L44.4, M1A.1ØXØ-M1A.19X1, P35.2-P35.9, P37.Ø-
P37.4, P37.8-P37.9, T56.ØX1A, T56.ØX2A, T56.ØX3A, T56.ØX4A

✓4ᵗʰ **B76   Hookworm diseases**
INCLUDES   uncinariasis

CC Excl: For CC codes in category B76, unless otherwise noted:
B76.Ø-B76.9

B76.Ø   **Ancylostomiasis**   `CC`
Infection due to Ancylostoma species

B76.1   **Necatoriasis**   `CC`
Infection due to Necator americanus

B76.8   **Other hookworm diseases**   `CC`

B76.9   **Hookworm disease, unspecified**   `CC`
Cutaneous larva migrans NOS

✓4ᵗʰ **B77   Ascariasis**
INCLUDES   ascaridiasis
roundworm infection

B77.Ø   **Ascariasis with intestinal complications**   `CC`
CC Excl: B77.Ø-B78.Ø, B78.7-B82.Ø

✓5ᵗʰ B77.8   **Ascariasis with other complications**

B77.81   **Ascariasis pneumonia**   `PDxMCC` `MCC`
CC Excl: A15.Ø-A15.6, A15.8-A15.9, A17.9, A18.82,
A18.84, A18.89, A21.2, A22.1, A31.Ø, A37.Ø1, A37.11,
A37.81, A37.91, A42.Ø, A43.Ø, A48.1, B25.Ø, B39.Ø-B39.2,
B44.Ø, B58.3, B59, B67.1, B77.Ø-B78.Ø, B78.7-B82.Ø,
JØ9.X1-JØ9.X2, J1Ø.ØØ-J1Ø.1, J11.ØØ-J11.1, J12.Ø-J12.3,
J12.89-J18.1, J18.8-J18.9, J22, J44.9, J47.Ø-J7Ø.4, J7Ø.8-
J7Ø.9, J98.4, J98.8-J99, Q33.4, R91.1

B77.89   **Ascariasis with other complications**   `CC`
CC Excl: B77.Ø-B78.Ø, B78.7-B82.Ø

B77.9   **Ascariasis, unspecified**   `CC`
CC Excl: See code B77.Ø

✓4ᵗʰ **B78   Strongyloidiasis**
EXCLUDES 1   *trichostrongyliasis (B81.2)*

CC Excl: For CC codes in category B78, unless otherwise noted:
B77.Ø-B78.Ø, B78.7-B82.Ø

B78.Ø   **Intestinal strongyloidiasis**   `HIV` `CC`

B78.1   **Cutaneous strongyloidiasis**

B78.7   **Disseminated strongyloidiasis**   `HIV` `CC`

B78.9   **Strongyloidiasis, unspecified**   `HIV` `CC`

B79   Trichuriasis   `CC`
INCLUDES   trichocephaliasis
whipworm (disease)(infection)
CC Excl: See code: B77.89

B8Ø   Enterobiasis   `CC`
INCLUDES   oxyuriasis
pinworm infection
threadworm infection
CC Excl: See code: B77.89

✓4ᵗʰ **B81   Other intestinal helminthiases, not elsewhere classified**
EXCLUDES 1   *angiostrongyliasis due to Parastrongylus cantonensis (B83.2)*

CC Excl: For CC codes in subcategories B81.Ø-B81.2, unless
otherwise noted: B77.Ø-B78.Ø, B78.7-B82.Ø For CC codes in
subcategories B81.3-B81.8: B77.Ø-B78.Ø, B78.7-B83.3, B83.8-B83.9

B81.Ø   **Anisakiasis**   `CC`
Infection due to Anisakis larva

B81.1   **Intestinal capillariasis**   `CC`
Capillariasis NOS
Infection due to Capillaria philippinensis
EXCLUDES 2   *hepatic capillariasis (B83.8)*

B81.2   **Trichostrongyliasis**   `CC`

B81.3   **Intestinal angiostrongyliasis**   `CC`
Angiostrongyliasis due to Parastrongylus costaricensis

B81.4   **Mixed intestinal helminthiases**   `CC`
Infection due to intestinal helminths classified to more than one
of the categories B65.Ø-B81.3 and B81.8
Mixed helminthiasis NOS

B81.8   **Other specified intestinal helminthiases**   `CC`
Infection due to Oesophagostomum species
[esophagostomiasis]
Infection due to Ternidens diminutus [ternidensiasis]

✓4ᵗʰ **B82   Unspecified intestinal parasitism**

B82.Ø   **Intestinal helminthiasis, unspecified**   `CC`
CC Excl: See code: B81.3

B82.9   **Intestinal parasitism, unspecified**

✓4ᵗʰ **B83   Other helminthiases**
EXCLUDES 1   *capillariasis NOS (B81.1)*
EXCLUDES 2   *intestinal capillariasis (B81.1)*

B83.Ø   **Visceral larva migrans**
Toxocariasis

B83.1   **Gnathostomiasis**
Wandering swelling

B83.2   **Angiostrongyliasis due to Parastrongylus cantonensis**
Eosinophilic meningoencephalitis due to Parastrongylus
cantonensis
EXCLUDES 2   *intestinal angiostrongyliasis (B81.3)*

B83.3   **Syngamiasis**
Syngamosis

B83.4   **Internal hirudiniasis**
EXCLUDES 2   *external hirudiniasis (B88.3)*

B83.8   **Other specified helminthiases**
Acanthocephaliasis   Metastrongyliasis
Gongylonemiasis   Thelaziasis
Hepatic capillariasis

B83.9   **Helminthiasis, unspecified**
Worms NOS
EXCLUDES 1   *intestinal helminthiasis NOS (B82.Ø)*

Pediculosis, acariasis and other infestations (B85-B89)

✓4ᵗʰ **B85   Pediculosis and phthiriasis**

B85.Ø   **Pediculosis due to Pediculus humanus capitis**
Head-louse infestation

B85.1   **Pediculosis due to Pediculus humanus corporis**
Body-louse infestation

B85.2   **Pediculosis, unspecified**

B85.3   **Phthiriasis**
Infestation by crab-louse
Infestation by Phthirus pubis

B85.4   **Mixed pediculosis and phthiriasis**
Infestation classifiable to more than one of the categories B85.Ø-
B85.3

B86   Scabies
Sarcoptic itch

✓4ᵗʰ B87 Myiasis
   INCLUDES infestation by larva of flies
   B87.0 Cutaneous myiasis
     Creeping myiasis
   B87.1 Wound myiasis
     Traumatic myiasis
   B87.2 Ocular myiasis
   B87.3 Nasopharyngeal myiasis
     Laryngeal myiasis
   B87.4 Aural myiasis
   ✓5ᵗʰ B87.8 Myiasis of other sites
     B87.81 Genitourinary myiasis
     B87.82 Intestinal myiasis
     B87.89 Myiasis of other sites
   B87.9 Myiasis, unspecified

✓4ᵗʰ B88 Other infestations
   B88.0 Other acariasis
     Acarine dermatitis
     Dermatitis due to Demodex species
     Dermatitis due to Dermanyssus gallinae
     Dermatitis due to Liponyssoides sanguineus
     Trombiculosis
     EXCLUDES 2 scabies (B86)
   B88.1 Tungiasis [sandflea infestation]
   B88.2 Other arthropod infestations
     Scarabiasis
   B88.3 External hirudiniasis
     Leech infestation NOS
     EXCLUDES 2 internal hirudiniasis (B83.4)
   B88.8 Other specified infestations
     Ichthyoparasitism due to Vandellia cirrhosa
     Linguatulosis
     Porocephaliasis
   B88.9 Infestation, unspecified
     Infestation (skin) NOS   Skin parasites NOS
     Infestation by mites NOS

B89 Unspecified parasitic disease

Sequelae of infectious and parasitic diseases (B90-B94)

NOTE Categories B90-B94 are to be used to indicate conditions in categories A00-B89 as the cause of sequelae, which are themselves classified elsewhere. The "sequelae" include conditions specified as such; they also include residuals of diseases classifiable to the above categories if there is evidence that the disease itself is no longer present. Codes from these categories are not to be used for chronic infections. Code chronic current infections to active infectious disease as appropriate.

Code first condition resulting from (sequela) the infectious or parasitic disease

✓4ᵗʰ B90 Sequelae of tuberculosis
   B90.0 Sequelae of central nervous system tuberculosis
   B90.1 Sequelae of genitourinary tuberculosis
   B90.2 Sequelae of tuberculosis of bones and joints
   B90.8 Sequelae of tuberculosis of other organs
     EXCLUDES 2 sequelae of respiratory tuberculosis (B90.9)
   B90.9 Sequelae of respiratory and unspecified tuberculosis
     Sequelae of tuberculosis NOS

B91 Sequelae of poliomyelitis
   EXCLUDES 1 postpolio syndrome (G14)

B92 Sequelae of leprosy

✓4ᵗʰ B94 Sequelae of other and unspecified infectious and parasitic diseases
   B94.0 Sequelae of trachoma
   B94.1 Sequelae of viral encephalitis
   B94.2 Sequelae of viral hepatitis
   B94.8 Sequelae of other specified infectious and parasitic diseases
   B94.9 Sequelae of unspecified infectious and parasitic disease

Bacterial and viral infectious agents (B95-B97)

NOTE These categories are provided for use as supplementary or additional codes to identify the infectious agent(s) in diseases classified elsewhere.

✓4ᵗʰ B95 Streptococcus, Staphylococcus, and Enterococcus as the cause of diseases classified elsewhere
   B95.0 Streptococcus, group A, as the cause of diseases classified elsewhere
   B95.1 Streptococcus, group B, as the cause of diseases classified elsewhere
   B95.2 Enterococcus as the cause of diseases classified elsewhere
   B95.3 Streptococcus pneumoniae as the cause of diseases classified elsewhere
   B95.4 Other streptococcus as the cause of diseases classified elsewhere
   B95.5 Unspecified streptococcus as the cause of diseases classified elsewhere
   ✓5ᵗʰ B95.6 Staphylococcus aureus as the cause of diseases classified elsewhere
     B95.61 Methicillin susceptible Staphylococcus aureus infection as the cause of diseases classified elsewhere
       Methicillin susceptible Staphylococcus aureus (MSSA) infection as the cause of diseases classified elsewhere
       Staphylococcus aureus infection NOS as the cause of diseases classified elsewhere
     B95.62 Methicillin resistant Staphylococcus aureus infection as the cause of diseases classified elsewhere
       Methicillin resistant Staphylococcus aureus (MRSA) infection as the cause of diseases classified elsewhere
   B95.7 Other staphylococcus as the cause of diseases classified elsewhere
   B95.8 Unspecified staphylococcus as the cause of diseases classified elsewhere

✓4ᵗʰ B96 Other bacterial agents as the cause of diseases classified elsewhere
   B96.0 Mycoplasma pneumoniae [M. pneumoniae] as the cause of diseases classified elsewhere
     Pleuro-pneumonia-like-organism [PPLO]
   B96.1 Klebsiella pneumoniae [K. pneumoniae] as the cause of diseases classified elsewhere
   ✓5ᵗʰ B96.2 Escherichia coli [E. coli] as the cause of diseases classified elsewhere
     B96.20 Unspecified Escherichia coli [E. coli] as the cause of diseases classified elsewhere
       Escherichia coli [E. coli] NOS
     B96.21 Shiga toxin-producing Escherichia coli [E. coli] (STEC) O157 as the cause of diseases classified elsewhere
       E. coli O157:H- (nonmotile) with confirmation of Shiga toxin
       E. coli O157 with confirmation of Shiga toxin when H antigen is unknown, or is not H7
       O157:H7 Escherichia coli [E.coli] with or without confirmation of Shiga toxin-production
       Shiga toxin-producing Escherichia coli [E.coli] O157:H7 with or without confirmation of Shiga toxin-production
       STEC O157:H7 with or without confirmation of Shiga toxin-production
     B96.22 Other specified Shiga toxin-producing Escherichia coli [E. coli] (STEC) as the cause of diseases classified elsewhere
       Non-O157 Shiga toxin-producing Escherichia coli [E.coli]
       Non-O157 Shiga toxin-producing Escherichia coli [E.coli] with known O group
     B96.23 Unspecified Shiga toxin-producing Escherichia coli [E. coli] (STEC) as the cause of diseases classified elsewhere
       Shiga toxin-producing Escherichia coli [E. coli] with unspecified O group
       STEC NOS
     B96.29 Other Escherichia coli [E. coli] as the cause of diseases classified elsewhere
       Non-Shiga toxin-producing E. coli
   B96.3 Hemophilus influenzae [H. influenzae] as the cause of diseases classified elsewhere
   B96.4 Proteus (mirabilis) (morganii) as the cause of diseases classified elsewhere

✓ Additional Character Required   ✓x7ᵗʰ Placeholder Alert   Unacceptable PDx   Manifestation   Hospital Acquired Condition   EXCLUDES 1 Not Coded Here   EXCLUDES 2 Not Included Here

ICD-10-CM 2016   449

Chapter 1. Certain Infectious and Parasitic Diseases

B96.5 **Pseudomonas (aeruginosa) (mallei) (pseudomallei) as the cause of diseases classified elsewhere**
    AHA: 2015, 1Q, 18

B96.6 **Bacteroides fragilis [B. fragilis] as the cause of diseases classified elsewhere**

B96.7 **Clostridium perfringens [C. perfringens] as the cause of diseases classified elsewhere**

✓5ᵗʰ **B96.8** **Other specified bacterial agents as the cause of diseases classified elsewhere**

    B96.81 **Helicobacter pylori [H. pylori] as the cause of diseases classified elsewhere**

    B96.82 **Vibrio vulnificus as the cause of diseases classified elsewhere**

    B96.89 **Other specified bacterial agents as the cause of diseases classified elsewhere**

✓4ᵗʰ **B97** **Viral agents as the cause of diseases classified elsewhere**

B97.0 **Adenovirus as the cause of diseases classified elsewhere**

✓5ᵗʰ **B97.1** **Enterovirus as the cause of diseases classified elsewhere**

    B97.10 **Unspecified enterovirus as the cause of diseases classified elsewhere**

    B97.11 **Coxsackievirus as the cause of diseases classified elsewhere**

    B97.12 **Echovirus as the cause of diseases classified elsewhere**

    B97.19 **Other enterovirus as the cause of diseases classified elsewhere**

✓5ᵗʰ **B97.2** **Coronavirus as the cause of diseases classified elsewhere**

    B97.21 **SARS-associated coronavirus as the cause of diseases classified elsewhere** `CC`
        EXCLUDES 1 *pneumonia due to SARS-associated coronavirus (J12.81)*
        CC Excl: A15.0-A15.6, A15.8-A15.9, A17.9, A18.82, A18.84, A18.89, A21.2, A22.1, A31.0, A37.01, A37.11, A37.81, A37.91, A42.0, A43.0, A48.1, B25.0, B34.1-B34.2, B34.4-B34.8, B39.0-B39.2, B44.0, B58.3, B59, B67.1, B97.19-B97.29, B97.5-B97.6, B97.81-B97.89, J09.X1-J09.X2, J10.00-J10.1, J11.00-J11.1, J12.0-J12.3, J12.89-J18.1, J18.8-J18.9, J22, J44.9, J47.0-J70.4, J70.8-J70.9, J98.4, J98.8-J99, Q33.4, R91.1

    B97.29 **Other coronavirus as the cause of diseases classified elsewhere**

✓5ᵗʰ **B97.3** **Retrovirus as the cause of diseases classified elsewhere**
    EXCLUDES 1 *human immunodeficiency virus [HIV] disease (B20)*

B97.30 **Unspecified retrovirus as the cause of diseases classified elsewhere**

B97.31 **Lentivirus as the cause of diseases classified elsewhere**

B97.32 **Oncovirus as the cause of diseases classified elsewhere**

B97.33 **Human T-cell lymphotrophic virus, type I [HTLV-I] as the cause of diseases classified elsewhere** `CC`
    CC Excl: A74.81, A74.9, B33.3-B33.4, B34.1-B34.2, B34.4-B34.8, B97.10, B97.19-B97.29, B97.31-B97.39, B97.5-B97.6, B97.81-B97.89

B97.34 **Human T-cell lymphotrophic virus, type II [HTLV-II] as the cause of diseases classified elsewhere** `CC`
    CC Excl: A74.81, A74.9, B33.3-B33.4, B34.1-B34.2, B34.4-B34.8, B97.10, B97.19-B97.39, B97.5-B97.6, B97.81-B97.89

B97.35 **Human immunodeficiency virus, type 2 [HIV 2] as the cause of diseases classified elsewhere** `CC`
    CC Excl: A74.81, A74.9, B20, B33.3-B33.4, B34.1-B34.2, B34.4-B34.8, B97.10, B97.19-B97.39, B97.5-B97.6, B97.81-B97.89

B97.39 **Other retrovirus as the cause of diseases classified elsewhere**

B97.4 **Respiratory syncytial virus as the cause of diseases classified elsewhere**

B97.5 **Reovirus as the cause of diseases classified elsewhere**

B97.6 **Parvovirus as the cause of diseases classified elsewhere**

B97.7 **Papillomavirus as the cause of diseases classified elsewhere**

✓5ᵗʰ **B97.8** **Other viral agents as the cause of diseases classified elsewhere**

    B97.81 **Human metapneumovirus as the cause of diseases classified elsewhere**

    B97.89 **Other viral agents as the cause of diseases classified elsewhere**

Other infectious diseases (B99)

✓4ᵗʰ **B99** **Other and unspecified infectious diseases**

B99.8 **Other infectious disease** `HIV`

B99.9 **Unspecified infectious disease**

Ⓝ Newborn: 0   ℙ Pediatric: 0-17   Ⓜ Maternity: 12-55   Ⓐ Adult: 15-124   **MCC** Major CC Condition   **PDxMCC** PDx acts as own MCC   **CC** CC Condition   **PDxCC** PDx acts as own CC

450   ICD-10-CM 2016

Chapter 2. Neoplasms (C00–D49)

Chapter Specific Guidelines with Coding Examples

The chapter specific guidelines from the ICD-10-CM Official Guidelines for Coding and Reporting have been provided below. Along with these guidelines are coding examples, contained in the shaded boxes, that have been developed to help illustrate the coding and/or sequencing guidance found in these guidelines.

General guidelines

Chapter 2 of the ICD-10-CM contains the codes for most benign and all malignant neoplasms. Certain benign neoplasms, such as prostatic adenomas, may be found in the specific body system chapters. To properly code a neoplasm it is necessary to determine from the record if the neoplasm is benign, in-situ, malignant, or of uncertain histologic behavior. If malignant, any secondary (metastatic) sites should also be determined.

Primary malignant neoplasms overlapping site boundaries

A primary malignant neoplasm that overlaps two or more contiguous (next to each other) sites should be classified to the subcategory/code .8 ('overlapping lesion'), unless the combination is specifically indexed elsewhere. For multiple neoplasms of the same site that are not contiguous such as tumors in different quadrants of the same breast, codes for each site should be assigned.

A 73-year-old white female with a large rapidly growing malignant tumor in the left breast extending from the upper outer quadrant into the axillary tail

C50.812   **Malignant neoplasm of overlapping sites of left female breast**

Explanation: Because this is a single large tumor that overlaps two contiguous sites, a single code for overlapping sites is assigned.

A 52-year old white female with two distinct lesions of the right breast, one (0.5 cm) in the upper outer quadrant and a second (1.5 cm) in the lower outer quadrant; path report indicates both lesions are malignant

C50.411   **Malignant neoplasm of upper-outer quadrant of breast, female**

C50.511   **Malignant neoplasm of lower-outer quadrant of breast, female**

Explanation: This patient has two distinct malignant lesions of right breast in adjacent quadrants. Because the lesions are not contiguous, two codes are reported.

Malignant neoplasm of ectopic tissue

Malignant neoplasms of ectopic tissue are to be coded to the site of origin mentioned, e.g., ectopic pancreatic malignant neoplasms involving the stomach are coded to pancreas, unspecified (C25.9).

The neoplasm table in the Alphabetic Index should be referenced first. However, if the histological term is documented, that term should be referenced first, rather than going immediately to the Neoplasm Table, in order to determine which column in the Neoplasm Table is appropriate. For example, if the documentation indicates "adenoma," refer to the term in the Alphabetic Index to review the entries under this term and the instructional note to "see also neoplasm, by site, benign." The table provides the proper code based on the type of neoplasm and the site. It is important to select the proper column in the table that corresponds to the type of neoplasm. The Tabular List should then be referenced to verify that the correct code has been selected from the table and that a more specific site code does not exist.

See Section I.C.21. Factors influencing health status and contact with health services, Status, for information regarding Z15.0, codes for genetic susceptibility to cancer.

a. Treatment directed at the malignancy

If the treatment is directed at the malignancy, designate the malignancy as the principal diagnosis.

The only exception to this guideline is if a patient admission/encounter is solely for the administration of chemotherapy, immunotherapy or radiation therapy, assign the appropriate Z51.-- code as the first-listed or principal diagnosis, and the diagnosis or problem for which the service is being performed as a secondary diagnosis.

b. Treatment of secondary site

When a patient is admitted because of a primary neoplasm with metastasis and treatment is directed toward the secondary site only, the secondary neoplasm is designated as the principal diagnosis even though the primary malignancy is still present.

Patient with primary prostate cancer with metastasis to lungs admitted for wedge resection of mass in right lung

C78.01   **Secondary malignant neoplasm of right lung**

C61   **Malignant neoplasm of prostate**

Explanation: Since the admission is for treatment of the lung metastasis, the secondary lung metastasis is sequenced before the primary prostate cancer.

---

c. Coding and sequencing of complications

Coding and sequencing of complications associated with the malignancies or with the therapy thereof are subject to the following guidelines:

1) Anemia associated with malignancy

When admission/encounter is for management of an anemia associated with the malignancy, and the treatment is only for anemia, the appropriate code for the malignancy is sequenced as the principal or first-listed diagnosis followed by the appropriate code for the anemia (such as code D63.0, Anemia in neoplastic disease).

Patient is admitted for treatment of anemia in advanced colon cancer

C18.9   **Malignant neoplasm of colon, unspecified**

D63.0   **Anemia in neoplastic disease**

Explanation: Even though the admission was solely to treat the anemia, this guideline indicates that the code for the malignancy is sequenced first.

---

2) Anemia associated with chemotherapy, immunotherapy and radiation therapy

When the admission/encounter is for management of an anemia associated with an adverse effect of the administration of chemotherapy or immunotherapy and the only treatment is for the anemia, the anemia code is sequenced first followed by the appropriate codes for the neoplasm and the adverse effect (T45.1X5, Adverse effect of antineoplastic and immunosuppressive drugs).

A 56-year-old Hispanic male with grade II follicular lymphoma involving multiple lymph node sites referred for blood transfusion to treat anemia due to chemotherapy

D64.81   **Anemia due to antineoplastic chemotherapy**

C82.18   **Follicular lymphoma grade II, lymph nodes of multiple sites**

T45.1X5A   **Adverse effect of antineoplastic and immunosuppressive drugs, initial encounter**

Explanation: The code for the anemia is sequenced first followed by the code for the malignant neoplasm and lastly the code for the adverse effect.

Chapter 2. Neoplasms

When the admission/encounter is for management of an anemia associated with an adverse effect of radiotherapy, the anemia code should be sequenced first, followed by the appropriate neoplasm code and code Y84.2, Radiological procedure and radiotherapy as the cause of abnormal reaction of the patient, or of later complication, without mention of misadventure at the time of the procedure.

A 55-year-old male with a large malignant rectal tumor has been receiving external radiation therapy to shrink the tumor prior to planned surgery. He is admitted today for a blood transfusion to treat anemia related to radiation therapy.

D64.89   **Other specified anemia**

C20   **Malignant neoplasm of rectum**

Y84.2   **Radiological procedure and radiotherapy as the cause of abnormal reaction of the patient, or of later complication, without mention of misadventure at the time of the procedure**

Explanation: The code for the anemia is sequenced first, followed by the code for the malignancy, and lastly the code for the abnormal reaction due to radiotherapy.

3) Management of dehydration due to the malignancy

When the admission/encounter is for management of dehydration due to the malignancy and only the dehydration is being treated (intravenous rehydration), the dehydration is sequenced first, followed by the code(s) for the malignancy.

4) Treatment of a complication resulting from a surgical procedure

When the admission/encounter is for treatment of a complication resulting from a surgical procedure, designate the complication as the principal or first-listed diagnosis if treatment is directed at resolving the complication.

d. Primary malignancy previously excised

When a primary malignancy has been previously excised or eradicated from its site and there is no further treatment directed to that site and there is no evidence of any existing primary malignancy, a code from category Z85, Personal history of malignant neoplasm, should be used to indicate the former site of the malignancy. Any mention of extension, invasion, or metastasis to another site is coded as a secondary malignant neoplasm to that site. The secondary site may be the principal or first-listed with the Z85 code used as a secondary code.

History of breast cancer, left radical mastectomy 18 months ago with no current treatment; bronchoscopy with lung biopsy shows metastatic disease in the right lung

C78.01   **Secondary malignant neoplasm of right lung**

Z85.3   **Personal history of malignant neoplasm of breast**

Explanation: The patient has undergone a diagnostic procedure that revealed metastatic breast cancer in the right lung. The code for the secondary (metastatic) site is sequenced first followed by a personal history code to identify the former site of the primary malignancy.

e. Admissions/Encounters involving chemotherapy, immunotherapy and radiation therapy

1) Episode of care involves surgical removal of neoplasm

When an episode of care involves the surgical removal of a neoplasm, primary or secondary site, followed by adjunct chemotherapy or radiation treatment during the same episode of care, the code for the neoplasm should be assigned as principal or first-listed diagnosis.

2) Patient admission/encounter solely for administration of chemotherapy, immunotherapy and radiation therapy

If a patient admission/encounter is solely for the administration of chemotherapy, immunotherapy or radiation therapy assign code Z51.0, Encounter for antineoplastic radiation therapy, or Z51.11, Encounter for antineoplastic chemotherapy, or Z51.12, Encounter for antineoplastic immunotherapy as the first-listed or principal diagnosis. If a patient receives more than one of these therapies during the same admission more than one of these codes may be assigned, in any sequence.

The malignancy for which the therapy is being administered should be assigned as a secondary diagnosis.

Patient is admitted for second round of rituximab and fludarabine for his chronic B cell lymphocytic leukemia

Z51.11   **Encounter for antineoplastic chemotherapy**

Z51.12   **Encounter for antineoplastic immunotherapy**

C91.10   **Chronic lymphocytic leukemia of B-cell type not having achieved remission**

Explanation: Rituximab is an antineoplastic immunotherapy while fludarabine is an antineoplastic chemotherapy. The two treatments are often used together. The admission was solely for the purpose of administering this treatment and either can be sequenced first, before the neoplastic condition.

3) Patient admitted for radiation therapy, chemotherapy or immunotherapy and develops complications

When a patient is admitted for the purpose of radiotherapy, immunotherapy or chemotherapy and develops complications such as uncontrolled nausea and vomiting or dehydration, the principal or first-listed diagnosis is Z51.0, Encounter for antineoplastic radiation therapy, or Z51.11, Encounter for antineoplastic chemotherapy, or Z51.12, Encounter for antineoplastic immunotherapy followed by any codes for the complications.

f. Admission/encounter to determine extent of malignancy

When the reason for admission/encounter is to determine the extent of the malignancy, or for a procedure such as paracentesis or thoracentesis, the primary malignancy or appropriate metastatic site is designated as the principal or first-listed diagnosis, even though chemotherapy or radiotherapy is administered.

Patient with left lung cancer with malignant pleural effusion admitted for paracentesis and initiation/administration of chemotherapy

C34.92   **Malignant neoplasm of unspecified part of left bronchus or lung**

J91.0   **Malignant pleural effusion**

Z51.11   **Encounter for antineoplastic chemotherapy**

Explanation: The lung cancer is sequenced before the chemotherapy in this instance because the paracentesis for the malignant effusion is also being performed. An instructional note under the malignant effusion instructs that the lung cancer be sequenced first.

g. Symptoms, signs, and abnormal findings listed in Chapter 18 associated with neoplasms

Symptoms, signs, and ill-defined conditions listed in Chapter 18 characteristic of, or associated with, an existing primary or secondary site malignancy cannot be used to replace the malignancy as principal or first-listed diagnosis, regardless of the number of admissions or encounters for treatment and care of the neoplasm.

See Section I.C.21. Factors influencing health status and contact with health services, Encounter for prophylactic organ removal.

h. Admission/encounter for pain control/management

See Section I.C.6. for information on coding admission/encounter for pain control/management.

i. Malignancy in two or more noncontiguous sites

A patient may have more than one malignant tumor in the same organ. These tumors may represent different primaries or metastatic disease, depending on the site. Should the documentation be unclear, the provider should be queried as to the status of each tumor so that the correct codes can be assigned.

j. Disseminated malignant neoplasm, unspecified

Code C80.0, Disseminated malignant neoplasm, unspecified, is for use only in those cases where the patient has advanced metastatic disease and no known primary or secondary sites are specified. It should not be used in place of assigning codes for the primary site and all known secondary sites.

Patient who has had no medical care for many years is seen today and diagnosed with carcinomatosis

C80.0   **Disseminated malignant neoplasm, unspecified**

Explanation: Carcinomatosis NOS is an "includes" note under this code. Should seldom be used but is available for use in cases such as this.

Chapter 2. Neoplasms

k. Malignant neoplasm without specification of site

Code C80.1, Malignant (primary) neoplasm, unspecified, equates to Cancer, unspecified. This code should only be used when no determination can be made as to the primary site of a malignancy. This code should rarely be used in the inpatient setting.

> *Evaluation of painful hip leads to diagnosis of a metastatic bone lesion from an unknown primary neoplasm source*
>
> **C79.51**   **Secondary malignant neoplasm of bone**
>
> **C80.1**   **Malignant (primary) neoplasm, unspecified**
>
> *Explanation: If only the secondary site is known, use code C80.1 for the unknown primary site.*

l. Sequencing of neoplasm codes

1) Encounter for treatment of primary malignancy

If the reason for the encounter is for treatment of a primary malignancy, assign the malignancy as the principal/first-listed diagnosis. The primary site is to be sequenced first, followed by any metastatic sites.

2) Encounter for treatment of secondary malignancy

When an encounter is for a primary malignancy with metastasis and treatment is directed toward the metastatic (secondary) site(s) only, the metastatic site(s) is designated as the principal/first-listed diagnosis. The primary malignancy is coded as an additional code.

> *Patient has primary colon cancer with metastasis to rib and is evaluated for possible excision of portion of rib bone*
>
> **C79.51**   **Secondary malignant neoplasm of bone**
>
> **C18.9**   **Malignant neoplasm of colon, unspecified**
>
> *Explanation: The treatment for this encounter is focused on the metastasis to the rib bone rather than the primary colon cancer, thus indicating that the bone metastasis is sequenced as the first-listed code.*

3) Malignant neoplasm in a pregnant patient

When a pregnant woman has a malignant neoplasm, a code from subcategory O9A.1-, Malignant neoplasm complicating pregnancy, childbirth, and the puerperium, should be sequenced first, followed by the appropriate code from Chapter 2 to indicate the type of neoplasm.

> *A 30-year-old pregnant female in second trimester evaluated for thyroid malignancy*
>
> **O9A.112**   **Malignant neoplasm complicating pregnancy, second trimester**
>
> **C73**   **Malignant neoplasm of thyroid gland**
>
> *Explanation: Codes from chapter 15 describing complications of pregnancy are sequenced as first-listed codes, further specified by codes from other chapters such as neoplastic, unless the pregnancy is documented as incidental to the condition. See also guideline 1.C.15.a.1.*

4) Encounter for complication associated with a neoplasm

When an encounter is for management of a complication associated with a neoplasm, such as dehydration, and the treatment is only for the complication, the complication is coded first, followed by the appropriate code(s) for the neoplasm.

The exception to this guideline is anemia. When the admission/encounter is for management of an anemia associated with the malignancy, and the treatment is only for anemia, the appropriate code for the malignancy is sequenced as the principal or first-listed diagnosis followed by code D63.0, Anemia in neoplastic disease.

> *Patient with pancreatic cancer is seen for initiation of TPN for cancer-related moderate protein-calorie malnutrition*
>
> **E44.0**   **Moderate protein-calorie malnutrition**
>
> **C25.9**   **Malignant neoplasm of pancreas, unspecified**
>
> *Explanation: The encounter is to initiate treatment for malnutrition, a common complication of many types of neoplasms, and is sequenced first.*

5) Complication from surgical procedure for treatment of a neoplasm

When an encounter is for treatment of a complication resulting from a surgical procedure performed for the treatment of the neoplasm, designate the complication as the principal/first-listed diagnosis. See guideline regarding the coding of a current malignancy versus personal history to determine if the code for the neoplasm should also be assigned.

6) Pathologic fracture due to a neoplasm

When an encounter is for a pathological fracture due to a neoplasm, and the focus of treatment is the fracture, a code from subcategory M84.5, Pathological fracture in neoplastic disease, should be sequenced first, followed by the code for the neoplasm.

If the focus of treatment is the neoplasm with an associated pathological fracture, the neoplasm code should be sequenced first, followed by a code from M84.5 for the pathological fracture.

m. Current malignancy versus personal history of malignancy

When a primary malignancy has been excised but further treatment, such as an additional surgery for the malignancy, radiation therapy or chemotherapy is directed to that site, the primary malignancy code should be used until treatment is completed.

When a primary malignancy has been previously excised or eradicated from its site, there is no further treatment (of the malignancy) directed to that site, and there is no evidence of any existing primary malignancy, a code from category Z85, Personal history of malignant neoplasm, should be used to indicate the former site of the malignancy.

See Section I.C.21. Factors influencing health status and contact with health services, History (of)

> *Female patient with ongoing chemotherapy after right mastectomy for breast cancer*
>
> **C50.911**   **Malignant neoplasm of unspecified site of right female breast**
>
> *Explanation: Even though the breast has been removed, the breast cancer is still being treated with chemotherapy and therefore is still coded as a current condition rather than personal history.*

n. Leukemia, multiple myeloma, and malignant plasma cell neoplasms in remission versus personal history

The categories for leukemia, and category C90, Multiple myeloma and malignant plasma cell neoplasms, have codes indicating whether or not the leukemia has achieved remission. There are also codes Z85.6, Personal history of leukemia, and Z85.79, Personal history of other malignant neoplasms of lymphoid, hematopoietic and related tissues. If the documentation is unclear as to whether the leukemia has achieved remission, the provider should be queried.

See Section I.C.21. Factors influencing health status and contact with health services, History (of)

o. Aftercare following surgery for neoplasm

See Section I.C.21. Factors influencing health status and contact with health services, Aftercare

p. Follow-up care for completed treatment of a malignancy

See Section I.C.21. Factors influencing health status and contact with health services, Follow-up

q. Prophylactic organ removal for prevention of malignancy

See Section I.C. 21, Factors influencing health status and contact with health services, Prophylactic organ removal

r. Malignant neoplasm associated with transplanted organ

A malignant neoplasm of a transplanted organ should be coded as a transplant complication. Assign first the appropriate code from category T86.-, Complications of transplanted organs and tissue, followed by code C80.2, Malignant neoplasm associated with transplanted organ. Use an additional code for the specific malignancy.

Chapter 2. Neoplasms

Chapter 2. Neoplasms (C00-D49)

NOTE

Functional activity

All neoplasms are classified in this chapter, whether they are functionally active or not. An additional code from Chapter 4 may be used, to identify functional activity associated with any neoplasm.

Morphology [Histology]

Chapter 2 classifies neoplasms primarily by site (topography), with broad groupings for behavior, malignant, in situ, benign, etc. The Table of Neoplasms should be used to identify the correct topography code. In a few cases, such as for malignant melanoma and certain neuroendocrine tumors, the morphology (histologic type) is included in the category and codes.

Primary malignant neoplasms overlapping site boundaries

A primary malignant neoplasm that overlaps two or more contiguous (next to each other) sites should be classified to the subcategory/code 8 ("overlapping lesion"), unless the combination is specifically indexed elsewhere. For multiple neoplasms of the same site that are not contiguous, such as tumors in different quadrants of the same breast, codes for each site should be assigned.

Malignant neoplasm of ectopic tissue

Malignant neoplasms of ectopic tissue are to be coded to the site mentioned, e.g., ectopic pancreatic malignant neoplasms are coded to pancreas, unspecified (C25.9).

This chapter contains the following blocks:

C00-C14	Malignant neoplasms of lip, oral cavity and pharynx
C15-C26	Malignant neoplasms of digestive organs
C30-C39	Malignant neoplasms of respiratory and intrathoracic organs
C40-C41	Malignant neoplasms of bone and articular cartilage
C43-C44	Melanoma and other malignant neoplasms of skin
C45-C49	Malignant neoplasms of mesothelial and soft tissue
C50	Malignant neoplasms of breast
C51-C58	Malignant neoplasms of female genital organs
C60-C63	Malignant neoplasms of male genital organs
C64-C68	Malignant neoplasms of urinary tract
C69-C72	Malignant neoplasms of eye, brain and other parts of central nervous system
C73-C75	Malignant neoplasms of thyroid and other endocrine glands
C7A	Malignant neuroendocrine tumors
C7B	Secondary neuroendocrine tumors
C76-C80	Malignant neoplasms of ill-defined, other secondary and unspecified sites
C81-C96	Malignant neoplasms of lymphoid, hematopoietic and related tissue
D00-D09	In situ neoplasms
D10-D36	Benign neoplasms, except benign neuroendocrine tumors
D3A	Benign neuroendocrine tumors
D37-D48	Neoplasms of uncertain behavior, polycythemia vera and myelodysplastic syndromes
D49	Neoplasms of unspecified behavior

MALIGNANT NEOPLASMS (C00-C96)

Malignant neoplasms, stated or presumed to be primary (of specified sites), and certain specified histologies, except neuroendocrine, and of lymphoid, hematopoietic and related tissue (C00-C75)

Malignant neoplasms of lip, oral cavity and pharynx (C00-C14)

✓4ᵗʰ **C00** **Malignant neoplasm of lip**
    Use additional code to identify:
      alcohol abuse and dependence (F10.-)
      history of tobacco use (Z87.891)
      tobacco dependence (F17.-)
      tobacco use (Z72.0)
    EXCLUDES 1   malignant melanoma of lip (C43.0)
          Merkel cell carcinoma of lip (C4A.0)
          other and unspecified malignant neoplasm of skin of lip (C44.0-)

    C00.0 **Malignant neoplasm of external upper lip**
      Malignant neoplasm of lipstick area of upper lip
      Malignant neoplasm of upper lip NOS
      Malignant neoplasm of vermilion border of upper lip

    C00.1 **Malignant neoplasm of external lower lip**
      Malignant neoplasm of lower lip NOS
      Malignant neoplasm of lipstick area of lower lip
      Malignant neoplasm of vermilion border of lower lip

    C00.2 **Malignant neoplasm of external lip, unspecified**
      Malignant neoplasm of vermilion border of lip NOS

    C00.3 **Malignant neoplasm of upper lip, inner aspect**
      Malignant neoplasm of buccal aspect of upper lip
      Malignant neoplasm of frenulum of upper lip
      Malignant neoplasm of mucosa of upper lip
      Malignant neoplasm of oral aspect of upper lip

    C00.4 **Malignant neoplasm of lower lip, inner aspect**
      Malignant neoplasm of buccal aspect of lower lip
      Malignant neoplasm of frenulum of lower lip
      Malignant neoplasm of mucosa of lower lip
      Malignant neoplasm of oral aspect of lower lip

    C00.5 **Malignant neoplasm of lip, unspecified, inner aspect**
      Malignant neoplasm of buccal aspect of lip, unspecified
      Malignant neoplasm of frenulum of lip, unspecified
      Malignant neoplasm of mucosa of lip, unspecified
      Malignant neoplasm of oral aspect of lip, unspecified

    C00.6 **Malignant neoplasm of commissure of lip, unspecified**

    C00.8 **Malignant neoplasm of overlapping sites of lip**

    C00.9 **Malignant neoplasm of lip, unspecified**

C01 **Malignant neoplasm of base of tongue**
    Malignant neoplasm of dorsal surface of base of tongue
    Malignant neoplasm of fixed part of tongue NOS
    Malignant neoplasm of posterior third of tongue
    Use additional code to identify:
      alcohol abuse and dependence (F10.-)
      history of tobacco use (Z87.891)
      tobacco dependence (F17.-)
      tobacco use (Z72.0)

✓4ᵗʰ **C02** **Malignant neoplasm of other and unspecified parts of tongue**
    Use additional code to identify:
      alcohol abuse and dependence (F10.-)
      history of tobacco use (Z87.891)
      tobacco dependence (F17.-)
      tobacco use (Z72.0)

    C02.0 **Malignant neoplasm of dorsal surface of tongue**
      Malignant neoplasm of anterior two-thirds of tongue, dorsal surface
      EXCLUDES 2   malignant neoplasm of dorsal surface of base of tongue (C01)

    C02.1 **Malignant neoplasm of border of tongue**
      Malignant neoplasm of tip of tongue

    C02.2 **Malignant neoplasm of ventral surface of tongue**
      Malignant neoplasm of anterior two-thirds of tongue, ventral surface
      Malignant neoplasm of frenulum linguae

    C02.3 **Malignant neoplasm of anterior two-thirds of tongue, part unspecified**
      Malignant neoplasm of middle third of tongue NOS
      Malignant neoplasm of mobile part of tongue NOS

    C02.4 **Malignant neoplasm of lingual tonsil**
      EXCLUDES 2   malignant neoplasm of tonsil NOS (C09.9)

    C02.8 **Malignant neoplasm of overlapping sites of tongue**
      Malignant neoplasm of two or more contiguous sites of tongue

    C02.9 **Malignant neoplasm of tongue, unspecified**

✓4ᵗʰ **C03** **Malignant neoplasm of gum**
    INCLUDES   malignant neoplasm of alveolar (ridge) mucosa
          malignant neoplasm of gingiva
    Use additional code to identify:
      alcohol abuse and dependence (F10.-)
      history of tobacco use (Z87.891)
      tobacco dependence (F17.-)
      tobacco use (Z72.0)
    EXCLUDES 2   malignant odontogenic neoplasms (C41.0-C41.1)

    C03.0 **Malignant neoplasm of upper gum**

    C03.1 **Malignant neoplasm of lower gum**

    C03.9 **Malignant neoplasm of gum, unspecified**

✓4ᵗʰ **C04** **Malignant neoplasm of floor of mouth**
    Use additional code to identify:
      alcohol abuse and dependence (F10.-)
      history of tobacco use (Z87.891)
      tobacco dependence (F17.-)
      tobacco use (Z72.0)

    C04.0 **Malignant neoplasm of anterior floor of mouth**
      Malignant neoplasm of anterior to the premolar-canine junction

    C04.1 **Malignant neoplasm of lateral floor of mouth**

    C04.8 **Malignant neoplasm of overlapping sites of floor of mouth**

    C04.9 **Malignant neoplasm of floor of mouth, unspecified**

Ⓝ Newborn: 0   Ⓟ Pediatric: 0-17   Ⓜ Maternity: 12-55   Ⓐ Adult: 15-124   MCC Major CC Condition   PDxMCC PDx acts as own MCC   CC CC Condition   PDxCC PDx acts as own CC

454   ICD-10-CM 2016

✓4ᵗʰ C05   Malignant neoplasm of palate
Use additional code to identify:
    alcohol abuse and dependence (F10.-)
    history of tobacco use (Z87.891)
    tobacco dependence (F17.-)
    tobacco use (Z72.0)
    EXCLUDES 1   Kaposi's sarcoma of palate (C46.2)

C05.0   Malignant neoplasm of hard palate

C05.1   Malignant neoplasm of soft palate
      EXCLUDES 2   malignant neoplasm of nasopharyngeal surface of soft palate (C11.3)

C05.2   Malignant neoplasm of uvula

C05.8   Malignant neoplasm of overlapping sites of palate

C05.9   Malignant neoplasm of palate, unspecified
      Malignant neoplasm of roof of mouth

✓4ᵗʰ C06   Malignant neoplasm of other and unspecified parts of mouth
Use additional code to identify:
    alcohol abuse and dependence (F10.-)
    history of tobacco use (Z87.891)
    tobacco dependence (F17.-)
    tobacco use (Z72.0)

C06.0   Malignant neoplasm of cheek mucosa
      Malignant neoplasm of buccal mucosa NOS
      Malignant neoplasm of internal cheek

C06.1   Malignant neoplasm of vestibule of mouth
      Malignant neoplasm of buccal sulcus (upper) (lower)
      Malignant neoplasm of labial sulcus (upper) (lower)

C06.2   Malignant neoplasm of retromolar area

✓5ᵗʰ C06.8   Malignant neoplasm of overlapping sites of other and unspecified parts of mouth

      C06.80   Malignant neoplasm of overlapping sites of unspecified parts of mouth

      C06.89   Malignant neoplasm of overlapping sites of other parts of mouth
         "book leaf" neoplasm [ventral surface of tongue and floor of mouth]

C06.9   Malignant neoplasm of mouth, unspecified
      Malignant neoplasm of minor salivary gland, unspecified site
      Malignant neoplasm of oral cavity NOS

C07   Malignant neoplasm of parotid gland
Use additional code to identify:
    alcohol abuse and dependence (F10.-)
    exposure to environmental tobacco smoke (Z77.22)
    exposure to tobacco smoke in the perinatal period (P96.81)
    history of tobacco use (Z87.891)
    occupational exposure to environmental tobacco smoke (Z57.31)
    tobacco dependence (F17.-)
    tobacco use (Z72.0)

✓4ᵗʰ C08   Malignant neoplasm of other and unspecified major salivary glands
      INCLUDES   malignant neoplasm of salivary ducts
Use additional code to identify:
    alcohol abuse and dependence (F10.-)
    exposure to environmental tobacco smoke (Z77.22)
    exposure to tobacco smoke in the perinatal period (P96.81)
    history of tobacco use (Z87.891)
    occupational exposure to environmental tobacco smoke (Z57.31)
    tobacco dependence (F17.-)
    tobacco use (Z72.0)
    EXCLUDES 1   malignant neoplasms of specified minor salivary glands which are classified according to their anatomical location
    EXCLUDES 2   malignant neoplasms of minor salivary glands NOS (C06.9)
                  malignant neoplasm of parotid gland (C07)

C08.0   Malignant neoplasm of submandibular gland
      Malignant neoplasm of submaxillary gland

C08.1   Malignant neoplasm of sublingual gland

C08.9   Malignant neoplasm of major salivary gland, unspecified
      Malignant neoplasm of salivary gland (major) NOS

✓4ᵗʰ C09   Malignant neoplasm of tonsil
Use additional code to identify:
    alcohol abuse and dependence (F10.-)
    exposure to environmental tobacco smoke (Z77.22)
    exposure to tobacco smoke in the perinatal period (P96.81)
    history of tobacco use (Z87.891)
    occupational exposure to environmental tobacco smoke (Z57.31)
    tobacco dependence (F17.-)
    tobacco use (Z72.0)
    EXCLUDES 2   malignant neoplasm of lingual tonsil (C02.4)
                  malignant neoplasm of pharyngeal tonsil (C11.1)

C09.0   Malignant neoplasm of tonsillar fossa

C09.1   Malignant neoplasm of tonsillar pillar (anterior) (posterior)

C09.8   Malignant neoplasm of overlapping sites of tonsil

C09.9   Malignant neoplasm of tonsil, unspecified
      Malignant neoplasm of tonsil NOS
      Malignant neoplasm of faucial tonsils
      Malignant neoplasm of palatine tonsils

✓4ᵗʰ C10   Malignant neoplasm of oropharynx
Use additional code to identify:
    alcohol abuse and dependence (F10.-)
    exposure to environmental tobacco smoke (Z77.22)
    exposure to tobacco smoke in the perinatal period (P96.81)
    history of tobacco use (Z87.891)
    occupational exposure to environmental tobacco smoke (Z57.31)
    tobacco dependence (F17.-)
    tobacco use (Z72.0)
    EXCLUDES 2   malignant neoplasm of tonsil (C09.-)

C10.0   Malignant neoplasm of vallecula

C10.1   Malignant neoplasm of anterior surface of epiglottis
      Malignant neoplasm of epiglottis, free border [margin]
      Malignant neoplasm of glossoepiglottic fold(s)
      EXCLUDES 2   malignant neoplasm of epiglottis (suprahyoid portion) NOS (C32.1)

C10.2   Malignant neoplasm of lateral wall of oropharynx

C10.3   Malignant neoplasm of posterior wall of oropharynx

C10.4   Malignant neoplasm of branchial cleft
      Malignant neoplasm of branchial cyst [site of neoplasm]

C10.8   Malignant neoplasm of overlapping sites of oropharynx
      Malignant neoplasm of junctional region of oropharynx

C10.9   Malignant neoplasm of oropharynx, unspecified

✓4ᵗʰ C11   Malignant neoplasm of nasopharynx
Use additional code to identify:
    exposure to environmental tobacco smoke (Z77.22)
    exposure to tobacco smoke in the perinatal period (P96.81)
    history of tobacco use (Z87.891)
    occupational exposure to environmental tobacco smoke (Z57.31)
    tobacco dependence (F17.-)
    tobacco use (Z72.0)

C11.0   Malignant neoplasm of superior wall of nasopharynx
      Malignant neoplasm of roof of nasopharynx

C11.1   Malignant neoplasm of posterior wall of nasopharynx
      Malignant neoplasm of adenoid
      Malignant neoplasm of pharyngeal tonsil

C11.2   Malignant neoplasm of lateral wall of nasopharynx
      Malignant neoplasm of fossa of Rosenmüller
      Malignant neoplasm of opening of auditory tube
      Malignant neoplasm of pharyngeal recess

C11.3   Malignant neoplasm of anterior wall of nasopharynx
      Malignant neoplasm of floor of nasopharynx
      Malignant neoplasm of nasopharyngeal (anterior) (posterior) surface of soft palate
      Malignant neoplasm of posterior margin of nasal choana
      Malignant neoplasm of posterior margin of nasal septum

C11.8   Malignant neoplasm of overlapping sites of nasopharynx

C11.9   Malignant neoplasm of nasopharynx, unspecified
      Malignant neoplasm of nasopharyngeal wall NOS

C12   Malignant neoplasm of pyriform sinus
      Malignant neoplasm of pyriform fossa
Use additional code to identify:
    exposure to environmental tobacco smoke (Z77.22)
    exposure to tobacco smoke in the perinatal period (P96.81)
    history of tobacco use (Z87.891)
    occupational exposure to environmental tobacco smoke (Z57.31)
    tobacco dependence (F17.-)
    tobacco use (Z72.0)

✓ Additional Character Required   ✓x7ᵗʰ Placeholder Alert   Unacceptable PDx   Manifestation   Hospital Acquired Condition   *EXCLUDES 1* Not Coded Here   *EXCLUDES 2* Not Included Here

Chapter 2. Neoplasms

☑4ᵗʰ C13 Malignant neoplasm of hypopharynx
Use additional code to identify:
exposure to environmental tobacco smoke (Z77.22)
exposure to tobacco smoke in the perinatal period (P96.81)
history of tobacco use (Z87.891)
occupational exposure to environmental tobacco smoke (Z57.31)
tobacco dependence (F17.-)
tobacco use (Z72.0)
EXCLUDES 2 malignant neoplasm of pyriform sinus (C12)

C13.0 Malignant neoplasm of postcricoid region

C13.1 Malignant neoplasm of aryepiglottic fold, hypopharyngeal aspect
Malignant neoplasm of aryepiglottic fold, marginal zone
Malignant neoplasm of aryepiglottic fold NOS
Malignant neoplasm of interarytenoid fold, marginal zone
Malignant neoplasm of interarytenoid fold NOS
EXCLUDES 2 malignant neoplasm of aryepiglottic fold or interarytenoid fold, laryngeal aspect (C32.1)

C13.2 Malignant neoplasm of posterior wall of hypopharynx

C13.8 Malignant neoplasm of overlapping sites of hypopharynx

C13.9 Malignant neoplasm of hypopharynx, unspecified
Malignant neoplasm of hypopharyngeal wall NOS

☑4ᵗʰ C14 Malignant neoplasm of other and ill-defined sites in the lip, oral cavity and pharynx
Use additional code to identify:
alcohol abuse and dependence (F10.-)
exposure to environmental tobacco smoke (Z77.22)
exposure to tobacco smoke in the perinatal period (P96.81)
history of tobacco use (Z87.891)
occupational exposure to environmental tobacco smoke (Z57.31)
tobacco dependence (F17.-)
tobacco use (Z72.0)
EXCLUDES 1 malignant neoplasm of oral cavity NOS (C06.9)

C14.0 Malignant neoplasm of pharynx, unspecified

C14.2 Malignant neoplasm of Waldeyer's ring

C14.8 Malignant neoplasm of overlapping sites of lip, oral cavity and pharynx
Primary malignant neoplasm of two or more contiguous sites of lip, oral cavity and pharynx
EXCLUDES 1 "book leaf" neoplasm [ventral surface of tongue and floor of mouth] (C06.89)

Malignant neoplasms of digestive organs (C15-C26)
EXCLUDES 1 Kaposi's sarcoma of gastrointestinal sites (C46.4)

☑4ᵗʰ C15 Malignant neoplasm of esophagus
Use additional code to identify:
alcohol abuse and dependence (F10.-)

CC Excl: For CC codes in category C15, unless otherwise noted:
C15.3-C15.9, C26.0, C26.9, C45.7-C45.9, C46.4, C76.8, C7A.00, C7A.098-C7B.00, C7B.1, C80.0-C80.2, D49.0, D49.81-D49.9

C15.3 Malignant neoplasm of upper third of esophagus `cc`

C15.4 Malignant neoplasm of middle third of esophagus `cc`

C15.5 Malignant neoplasm of lower third of esophagus `cc`
EXCLUDES 1 malignant neoplasm of cardio-esophageal junction (C16.0)

C15.8 Malignant neoplasm of overlapping sites of esophagus `cc`

C15.9 Malignant neoplasm of esophagus, unspecified `cc`

☑4ᵗʰ C16 Malignant neoplasm of stomach
Use additional code to identify:
alcohol abuse and dependence (F10.-)
EXCLUDES 2 malignant carcinoid tumor of the stomach (C7A.092)

CC Excl: For CC codes in category C16, unless otherwise noted:
C16.0-C16.9, C26.0, C26.9, C45.7-C45.9, C46.4, C76.8, C7A.00, C7A.092, C7A.094-C7B.00, C7B.1, C80.0-C80.2, D49.0, D49.81-D49.9

C16.0 Malignant neoplasm of cardia `cc`
Malignant neoplasm of cardiac orifice
Malignant neoplasm of cardio-esophageal junction
Malignant neoplasm of esophagus and stomach
Malignant neoplasm of gastro-esophageal junction

C16.1 Malignant neoplasm of fundus of stomach `cc`

C16.2 Malignant neoplasm of body of stomach `cc`

C16.3 Malignant neoplasm of pyloric antrum `cc`
Malignant neoplasm of gastric antrum

C16.4 Malignant neoplasm of pylorus `cc`
Malignant neoplasm of prepylorus
Malignant neoplasm of pyloric canal

C16.5 Malignant neoplasm of lesser curvature of stomach, unspecified `cc`
Malignant neoplasm of lesser curvature of stomach, not classifiable to C16.1-C16.4

C16.6 Malignant neoplasm of greater curvature of stomach, unspecified `cc`
Malignant neoplasm of greater curvature of stomach, not classifiable to C16.0-C16.4

C16.8 Malignant neoplasm of overlapping sites of stomach `cc`

C16.9 Malignant neoplasm of stomach, unspecified `cc`
Gastric cancer NOS

☑4ᵗʰ C17 Malignant neoplasm of small intestine
EXCLUDES 1 malignant carcinoid tumors of the small intestine (C7A.01)

C17.0 Malignant neoplasm of duodenum `cc`
CC Excl: C17.0, C17.8-C17.9, C26.0, C26.9, C45.7-C45.9, C46.4, C7A.00-C7A.010, C7A.019, C7A.098-C7B.00, C7B.1, C76.8, C80.0-C80.2, D49.0, D49.81-D49.9

C17.1 Malignant neoplasm of jejunum `cc`
CC Excl: C17.0, C17.8-C17.9, C26.0, C26.9, C45.7-C45.9, C46.4, C7A.00-C7A.010, C7A.019, C7A.098-C7B.00, C7B.1, C76.8, C80.0-C80.2, D49.0, D49.81-D49.9

C17.2 Malignant neoplasm of ileum `cc`
EXCLUDES 1 malignant neoplasm of ileocecal valve (C18.0)
CC Excl: C17.0, C17.8-C17.9, C26.0, C26.9, C45.7-C45.9, C46.4, C7A.00-C7A.010, C7A.019, C7A.098-C7B.00, C7B.1, C76.8, C80.0-C80.2, D49.0, D49.81-D49.9

C17.3 Meckel's diverticulum, malignant `cc`
EXCLUDES 1 Meckel's diverticulum, congenital (Q43.0)
CC Excl: C17.0, C17.8-C17.9, C26.0, C26.9, C45.7-C45.9, C46.4, C7A.00-C7A.010, C7A.019, C7A.098-C7B.00, C7B.1, C76.8, C80.0-C80.2, D49.0, D49.81-D49.9

C17.8 Malignant neoplasm of overlapping sites of small intestine `cc`
CC Excl: C17.0, C17.8-C17.9, C26.0, C26.9, C45.7-C45.9, C46.4, C7A.00-C7A.010, C7A.019, C7A.098-C7B.00, C7B.1, C76.8, C80.0-C80.2, D49.0, D49.81-D49.9

C17.9 Malignant neoplasm of small intestine, unspecified `cc`
CC Excl: See code: C17.8

☑4ᵗʰ C18 Malignant neoplasm of colon
EXCLUDES 1 malignant carcinoid tumors of the colon (C7A.02-)

C18.0 Malignant neoplasm of cecum `cc`
Malignant neoplasm of ileocecal valve
CC Excl: C18.0, C18.8-C18.9, C26.0, C26.9, C45.7-C45.9, C46.4, C7A.00, C7A.021, C7A.029, C7A.098-C7B.00, C7B.1, C76.8, C80.0-C80.2, D49.0, D49.81-D49.9

C18.1 Malignant neoplasm of appendix `cc`
CC Excl: C18.0, C18.8-C18.9, C26.0, C26.9, C45.7-C45.9, C46.4, C7A.00, C7A.021, C7A.029, C7A.098-C7B.00, C7B.1, C76.8, C80.0-C80.2, D49.0, D49.81-D49.9

C18.2 Malignant neoplasm of ascending colon `cc`
CC Excl: C18.0, C18.8-C18.9, C26.0, C26.9, C45.7-C45.9, C46.4, C7A.00, C7A.021, C7A.029, C7A.098-C7B.00, C7B.1, C76.8, C80.0-C80.2, D49.0, D49.81-D49.9

C18.3 Malignant neoplasm of hepatic flexure `cc`
CC Excl: C18.3, C18.8-C18.9, C26.0, C26.9, C45.7-C45.9, C46.4, C7A.00, C7A.029, C7A.098-C7B.00, C7B.1, C76.8, C80.0-C80.2, D49.0, D49.81-D49.9

C18.4 Malignant neoplasm of transverse colon `cc`
CC Excl: C18.4, C18.8-C18.9, C26.0, C26.9, C45.7-C45.9, C46.4, C7A.00, C7A.023, C7A.029, C7A.098-C7B.00, C7B.1, C76.8, C80.0-C80.2, D49.0, D49.81-D49.9

C18.5 Malignant neoplasm of splenic flexure `cc`
CC Excl: C18.5, C18.8-C18.9, C26.0, C26.9, C45.7-C45.9, C46.4, C7A.00, C7A.029, C7A.098-C7B.00, C7B.1, C76.8, C80.0-C80.2, D49.0, D49.81-D49.9

C18.6 Malignant neoplasm of descending colon `cc`
CC Excl: C18.6, C18.8-C18.9, C26.0, C26.9, C45.7-C45.9, C46.4, C7A.00, C7A.024, C7A.029, C7A.098-C7B.00, C7B.1, C76.8, C80.0-C80.2, D49.0, D49.81-D49.9

C18.7 Malignant neoplasm of sigmoid colon `cc`
Malignant neoplasm of sigmoid (flexure)
EXCLUDES 1 malignant neoplasm of rectosigmoid junction (C19)
CC Excl: C18.7-C18.9, C26.0, C26.9, C45.7-C45.9, C46.4, C7A.00, C7A.025, C7A.029, C7A.098-C7B.00, C7B.1, C76.8, C80.0-C80.2, D49.0, D49.81-D49.9

C18.8 Malignant neoplasm of overlapping sites of colon `cc`
CC Excl: C18.8-C18.9, C26.0, C26.9, C45.7-C45.9, C46.4, C7A.00, C7A.029, C7A.098-C7B.00, C7B.1, C76.8, C80.0-C80.2, D49.0, D49.81-D49.9

C18.9 Malignant neoplasm of colon, unspecified `cc`
Malignant neoplasm of large intestine NOS
CC Excl: See code: C18.8

Ⓝ Newborn: 0 Ⓟ Pediatric: 0-17 Ⓜ Maternity: 12-55 Ⓐ Adult: 15-124 **MCC** Major CC Condition **PDxMCC** PDx acts as own MCC `CC` CC Condition **PDxCC** PDx acts as own CC

456 ICD-10-CM 2016

C19 **Malignant neoplasm of rectosigmoid junction** `CC`
   Malignant neoplasm of colon with rectum
   Malignant neoplasm of rectosigmoid (colon)
   EXCLUDES 1 *malignant carcinoid tumors of the colon (C7A.02-)*
   CC Excl: C19, C21.2-C21.8, C26.0, C26.9, C45.7-C45.9, C46.4, C7A.00, C7A.098-C7B.00, C7B.1, C76.8, C80.0-C80.2, D49.0, D49.81-D49.9

C20 **Malignant neoplasm of rectum** `CC`
   Malignant neoplasm of rectal ampulla
   EXCLUDES 1 *malignant carcinoid tumor of the rectum (C7A.026)*
   CC Excl: C20, C21.2-C21.8, C26.0, C26.9, C45.7-C45.9, C46.4, C7A.00, C7A.026, C7A.098-C7B.00, C7B.1, C76.8, C80.0-C80.2, D49.0, D49.81-D49.9

✓4ᵗʰ C21 **Malignant neoplasm of anus and anal canal**
   EXCLUDES 2 *malignant carcinoid tumors of the colon (C7A.02-)*
      malignant melanoma of anal margin (C43.51)
      malignant melanoma of anal skin (C43.51)
      malignant melanoma of perianal skin (C43.51)
      other and unspecified malignant neoplasm of anal margin (C44.500, C44.510, C44.520, C44.590)
      other and unspecified malignant neoplasm of anal skin (C44.500, C44.510, C44.520, C44.590)
      other and unspecified malignant neoplasm of perianal skin (C44.500, C44.510, C44.520, C44.590)

   C21.0 **Malignant neoplasm of anus, unspecified** `CC`
      CC Excl: C21.0-C21.8, C26.0, C26.9, C45.7-C45.9, C46.4, C76.8, C7A.00, C7A.098-C7B.00, C7B.1, C80.0-C80.2, D49.0, D49.81-D49.9

   C21.1 **Malignant neoplasm of anal canal** `CC`
      Malignant neoplasm of anal sphincter
      CC Excl: See code: C21.0

   C21.2 **Malignant neoplasm of cloacogenic zone** `CC`
      CC Excl: C21.2-C21.8, C26.0, C26.9, C45.7-C45.9, C46.4, C76.8, C7A.00, C7A.098-C7B.00, C7B.1, C80.0-C80.2, D49.0, D49.81-D49.9

   C21.8 **Malignant neoplasm of overlapping sites of rectum, anus and anal canal** `CC`
      Malignant neoplasm of anorectal junction
      Malignant neoplasm of anorectum
      Primary malignant neoplasm of two or more contiguous sites of rectum, anus and anal canal
      CC Excl: See code: C21.2

✓4ᵗʰ C22 **Malignant neoplasm of liver and intrahepatic bile ducts**
   Use additional code to identify:
      alcohol abuse and dependence (F10.-)
      hepatitis B (B16.-, B18.0-B18.1)
      hepatitis C (B17.1-, B18.2)
   EXCLUDES 1 *malignant neoplasm of biliary tract NOS (C24.9)*
      secondary malignant neoplasm of liver and intrahepatic bile duct (C78.7)

   CC Excl: For CC codes in category C22, unless otherwise noted:
   C22.0-C22.9, C26.0, C26.9, C45.7-C45.9, C46.4, C76.8, C7A.00, C7A.098-C7B.00, C7B.1, C80.0-C80.2, D49.0, D49.81-D49.9

   C22.0 **Liver cell carcinoma** `CC`
      Hepatocellular carcinoma
      Hepatoma

   C22.1 **Intrahepatic bile duct carcinoma** `CC`
      Cholangiocarcinoma
      EXCLUDES 1 *malignant neoplasm of hepatic duct (C24.0)*

   C22.2 **Hepatoblastoma** `CC`

   C22.3 **Angiosarcoma of liver** `CC`
      Kupffer cell sarcoma

   C22.4 **Other sarcomas of liver** `CC`

   C22.7 **Other specified carcinomas of liver** `CC`

   C22.8 **Malignant neoplasm of liver, primary, unspecified as to type** `CC`

   C22.9 **Malignant neoplasm of liver, not specified as primary or secondary** `CC`

C23 **Malignant neoplasm of gallbladder** `CC`
   CC Excl: C23, C24.8-C24.9, C26.0, C26.9, C45.7-C45.9, C46.4, C7A.00, C7A.098-C7B.00, C7B.1, C76.8, C80.0-C80.2, D49.0, D49.81-D49.9

✓4ᵗʰ C24 **Malignant neoplasm of other and unspecified parts of biliary tract**
   EXCLUDES 1 *malignant neoplasm of intrahepatic bile duct (C22.1)*

   C24.0 **Malignant neoplasm of extrahepatic bile duct** `CC`
      Malignant neoplasm of biliary duct or passage NOS
      Malignant neoplasm of common bile duct
      Malignant neoplasm of cystic duct
      Malignant neoplasm of hepatic duct
      CC Excl: C24.0, C24.8-C24.9, C26.0, C26.9, C45.7-C45.9, C46.4, C7A.00, C7A.098-C7B.00, C7B.1, C76.8, C80.0-C80.2, D49.0, D49.81-D49.9

   C24.1 **Malignant neoplasm of ampulla of Vater** `CC`
      CC Excl: C24.1-C24.9, C26.0, C26.9, C45.7-C45.9, C46.4, C76.8, C7A.00, C7A.098-C7B.00, C7B.1, C80.0-C80.2, D49.0, D49.81-D49.9

   C24.8 **Malignant neoplasm of overlapping sites of biliary tract** `CC`
      Malignant neoplasm involving both intrahepatic and extrahepatic bile ducts
      Primary malignant neoplasm of two or more contiguous sites of biliary tract
      CC Excl: C24.8-C24.9, C26.0, C26.9, C45.7-C45.9, C46.4, C76.8, C7A.00, C7A.098-C7B.00, C7B.1, C80.0-C80.2, D49.0, D49.81-D49.9

   C24.9 **Malignant neoplasm of biliary tract, unspecified** `CC`
      CC Excl: See code: C24.8

✓4ᵗʰ C25 **Malignant neoplasm of pancreas**
   Use additional code to identify:
      alcohol abuse and dependence (F10.-)

   CC Excl: For CC codes in category C25, unless otherwise noted:
   C25.0-C26.0, C26.9, C45.7-C45.9, C46.4, C76.8, C7A.00, C7A.098-C7B.00, C7B.1, C80.0-C80.2, D49.0, D49.81-D49.9

   C25.0 **Malignant neoplasm of head of pancreas** `CC`
   C25.1 **Malignant neoplasm of body of pancreas** `CC`
   C25.2 **Malignant neoplasm of tail of pancreas** `CC`
   C25.3 **Malignant neoplasm of pancreatic duct** `CC`
   C25.4 **Malignant neoplasm of endocrine pancreas** `CC`
      Malignant neoplasm of islets of Langerhans
      Use additional code to identify any functional activity

   C25.7 **Malignant neoplasm of other parts of pancreas** `CC`
      Malignant neoplasm of neck of pancreas

   C25.8 **Malignant neoplasm of overlapping sites of pancreas** `CC`
   C25.9 **Malignant neoplasm of pancreas, unspecified** `CC`

✓4ᵗʰ C26 **Malignant neoplasm of other and ill-defined digestive organs**
   EXCLUDES 1 *malignant neoplasm of peritoneum and retroperitoneum (C48.-)*

   C26.0 **Malignant neoplasm of intestinal tract, part unspecified**
      Malignant neoplasm of intestine NOS

   C26.1 **Malignant neoplasm of spleen**
      EXCLUDES 1 *Hodgkin lymphoma (C81.-)*
         non-Hodgkin lymphoma (C82-C85)

   C26.9 **Malignant neoplasm of ill-defined sites within the digestive system**
      Malignant neoplasm of alimentary canal or tract NOS
      Malignant neoplasm of gastrointestinal tract NOS
      EXCLUDES 1 *malignant neoplasm of abdominal NOS (C76.2)*
         malignant neoplasm of intra-abdominal NOS (C76.2)

Malignant neoplasms of respiratory and intrathoracic organs (C30-C39)

   INCLUDES malignant neoplasm of middle ear
   EXCLUDES 1 *mesothelioma (C45.-)*

✓4ᵗʰ C30 **Malignant neoplasm of nasal cavity and middle ear**
   C30.0 **Malignant neoplasm of nasal cavity**
      Malignant neoplasm of cartilage of nose
      Malignant neoplasm of nasal concha
      Malignant neoplasm of internal nose
      Malignant neoplasm of septum of nose
      Malignant neoplasm of vestibule of nose
      EXCLUDES 1 *malignant melanoma of skin of nose (C43.31)*
         malignant neoplasm of nasal bone (C41.0)
         malignant neoplasm of nose NOS (C76.0)
         malignant neoplasm of olfactory bulb (C72.2-)
         malignant neoplasm of posterior margin of nasal septum and choana (C11.3)
         malignant neoplasm of turbinates (C41.0)
         other and unspecified malignant neoplasm of skin of nose (C44.301, C44.311, C44.321, C44.391)

   C30.1 **Malignant neoplasm of middle ear**
      Malignant neoplasm of antrum tympanicum
      Malignant neoplasm of auditory tube
      Malignant neoplasm of eustachian tube
      Malignant neoplasm of inner ear
      Malignant neoplasm of mastoid air cells
      Malignant neoplasm of tympanic cavity
      EXCLUDES 1 *malignant melanoma of skin of (external) ear (C43.2-)*
         malignant neoplasm of auricular canal (external) (C43.2-,C44.2-)
         malignant neoplasm of bone of ear (meatus) (C41.0)
         malignant neoplasm of cartilage of ear (C49.0)
         other and unspecified malignant neoplasm of skin of (external) ear (C44.2-)

✓4ᵗʰ C31 Malignant neoplasm of accessory sinuses

    C31.0 Malignant neoplasm of maxillary sinus
        Malignant neoplasm of antrum (Highmore) (maxillary)

    C31.1 Malignant neoplasm of ethmoidal sinus

    C31.2 Malignant neoplasm of frontal sinus

    C31.3 Malignant neoplasm of sphenoid sinus

    C31.8 Malignant neoplasm of overlapping sites of accessory sinuses

    C31.9 Malignant neoplasm of accessory sinus, unspecified

✓4ᵗʰ C32 Malignant neoplasm of larynx
    Use additional code to identify:
        alcohol abuse and dependence (F10.-)
        exposure to environmental tobacco smoke (Z77.22)
        exposure to tobacco smoke in the perinatal period (P96.81)
        history of tobacco use (Z87.891)
        occupational exposure to environmental tobacco smoke (Z57.31)
        tobacco dependence (F17.-)
        tobacco use (Z72.0)

    C32.0 Malignant neoplasm of glottis
        Malignant neoplasm of intrinsic larynx
        Malignant neoplasm of laryngeal commissure
          (anterior)(posterior)
        Malignant neoplasm of vocal cord (true) NOS

    C32.1 Malignant neoplasm of supraglottis
        Malignant neoplasm of aryepiglottic fold or interarytenoid fold,
          laryngeal aspect
        Malignant neoplasm of epiglottis (suprahyoid portion) NOS
        Malignant neoplasm of extrinsic larynx
        Malignant neoplasm of false vocal cord
        Malignant neoplasm of posterior (laryngeal) surface of epiglottis
        Malignant neoplasm of ventricular bands
        EXCLUDES 2   *malignant neoplasm of anterior surface of epiglottis*
             (C10.1)
            malignant neoplasm of aryepiglottic fold or
             interarytenoid fold, hypopharyngeal aspect
             (C13.1)
            malignant neoplasm of aryepiglottic fold or
             interarytenoid fold, marginal zone (C13.1)
            malignant neoplasm of aryepiglottic fold or
             interarytenoid fold NOS (C13.1)

    C32.2 Malignant neoplasm of subglottis

    C32.3 Malignant neoplasm of laryngeal cartilage

    C32.8 Malignant neoplasm of overlapping sites of larynx

    C32.9 Malignant neoplasm of larynx, unspecified

C33 Malignant neoplasm of trachea   `CC`
    Use additional code to identify:
        exposure to environmental tobacco smoke (Z77.22)
        exposure to tobacco smoke in the perinatal period (P96.81)
        history of tobacco use (Z87.891)
        occupational exposure to environmental tobacco smoke (Z57.31)
        tobacco dependence (F17.-)
        tobacco use (Z72.0)
    CC Excl: C33-C34.92, C39.9, C45.7-C45.9, C46.50-C46.52, C76.1, C76.8,
    C78.00-C78.1, C78.30-C78.39, C7A.00, C7A.090, C7A.098-C7B.00, C7B.1,
    C80.0-C80.2, D49.1, D49.81-D49.9

✓4ᵗʰ C34 Malignant neoplasm of bronchus and lung
    Use additional code to identify:
        exposure to environmental tobacco smoke (Z77.22)
        exposure to tobacco smoke in the perinatal period (P96.81)
        history of tobacco use (Z87.891)
        occupational exposure to environmental tobacco smoke (Z57.31)
        tobacco dependence (F17.-)
        tobacco use (Z72.0)
    EXCLUDES 1   *Kaposi's sarcoma of lung (C46.5-)*
           malignant carcinoid tumor of the bronchus and lung (C7A.090)

    ✓5ᵗʰ C34.0 Malignant neoplasm of main bronchus
        Malignant neoplasm of carina
        Malignant neoplasm of hilus (of lung)

        CC Excl: For CC codes in subcategory C34.0, unless
        otherwise noted: C34.00-C34.02, C34.80-C34.92, C39.9,
        C45.7-C45.9, C46.50-C46.52, C76.8, C7A.00, C7A.090,
        C7A.098-C7B.00, C7B.1, C80.0-C80.2, D49.1, D49.81-D49.9

        C34.00 Malignant neoplasm of unspecified main   `CC`
            bronchus

        C34.01 Malignant neoplasm of right main bronchus   `CC`

        C34.02 Malignant neoplasm of left main bronchus   `CC`

    ✓5ᵗʰ C34.1 Malignant neoplasm of upper lobe, bronchus or lung

        CC Excl: For CC codes in subcategory C34.1, unless
        otherwise noted: C34.10-C34.12, C34.80-C34.92, C39.9,
        C45.7-C45.9, C46.50-C46.52, C76.8, C7A.00, C7A.090,
        C7A.098-C7B.00, C7B.1, C80.0-C80.2, D49.1, D49.81-D49.9

        C34.10 Malignant neoplasm of upper lobe, unspecified   `CC`
            bronchus or lung

        C34.11 Malignant neoplasm of upper lobe, right   `CC`
            bronchus or lung

        C34.12 Malignant neoplasm of upper lobe, left   `CC`
            bronchus or lung

    C34.2 Malignant neoplasm of middle lobe, bronchus or lung   `CC`
        CC Excl: C34.2, C34.80-C34.92, C39.9, C45.7-C45.9, C46.50-C46.52,
        C7A.00, C7A.090, C7A.098-C7B.00, C7B.1, C76.8, C80.0-C80.2,
        D49.1, D49.81-D49.9

    ✓5ᵗʰ C34.3 Malignant neoplasm of lower lobe, bronchus or lung

        CC Excl: For CC codes in subcategory C34.3, unless
        otherwise noted: C34.30-C34.92, C39.9, C45.7-C45.9,
        C46.50-C46.52, C76.8, C7A.00, C7A.090, C7A.098-C7B.00,
        C7B.1, C80.0-C80.2, D49.1, D49.81-D49.9

        C34.30 Malignant neoplasm of lower lobe, unspecified   `CC`
            bronchus or lung

        C34.31 Malignant neoplasm of lower lobe, right   `CC`
            bronchus or lung

        C34.32 Malignant neoplasm of lower lobe, left   `CC`
            bronchus or lung

    ✓5ᵗʰ C34.8 Malignant neoplasm of overlapping sites of bronchus and
        lung

        CC Excl: For CC codes in subcategory C34.8, unless
        otherwise noted: C34.80-C34.92, C39.9, C45.7-C45.9,
        C46.50-C46.52, C76.8, C7A.00, C7A.090, C7A.098-C7B.00,
        C7B.1, C80.0-C80.2, D49.1, D49.81-D49.9

        C34.80 Malignant neoplasm of overlapping sites of   `CC`
            unspecified bronchus and lung

        C34.81 Malignant neoplasm of overlapping sites of   `CC`
            right bronchus and lung

        C34.82 Malignant neoplasm of overlapping sites of   `CC`
            left bronchus and lung

    ✓5ᵗʰ C34.9 Malignant neoplasm of unspecified part of bronchus or lung

        CC Excl: For CC codes in subcategory C34.9, unless
        otherwise noted: C34.80-C34.92, C39.9, C45.7-C45.9,
        C46.50-C46.52, C76.8, C7A.00, C7A.090, C7A.098-C7B.00,
        C7B.1, C80.0-C80.2, D49.1, D49.81-D49.9

        C34.90 Malignant neoplasm of unspecified part of   `CC`
            unspecified bronchus or lung
            Lung cancer NOS

        C34.91 Malignant neoplasm of unspecified part of right   `CC`
            bronchus or lung

        C34.92 Malignant neoplasm of unspecified part of left   `CC`
            bronchus or lung

C37 Malignant neoplasm of thymus   `CC`
    EXCLUDES 1   *malignant carcinoid tumor of the thymus (C7A.091)*
    CC Excl: C37, C7A.091

✓4ᵗʰ C38 Malignant neoplasm of heart, mediastinum and pleura
    EXCLUDES 1   *mesothelioma (C45.-)*

    C38.0 Malignant neoplasm of heart   `CC`
        Malignant neoplasm of pericardium
        EXCLUDES 1   *malignant neoplasm of great vessels (C49.3)*
        CC Excl: C38.0, C45.2

    C38.1 Malignant neoplasm of anterior mediastinum   `CC`
        CC Excl: C38.1-C38.3, C38.8, C39.9, C45.7-C45.9, C76.8, C7A.00,
        C7A.098-C7B.00, C7B.1, C80.0-C80.2, D49.1, D49.81-D49.9

    C38.2 Malignant neoplasm of posterior mediastinum   `CC`
        CC Excl: See code: C38.1

    C38.3 Malignant neoplasm of mediastinum, part unspecified   `CC`
        CC Excl: See code: C38.1

    C38.4 Malignant neoplasm of pleura   `CC`
        CC Excl: C38.4-C39.9, C45.0, C45.7-C45.9, C76.8, C7A.00,
        C7A.098-C7B.00, C7B.1, C80.0-C80.2, D49.1, D49.81-D49.9

    C38.8 Malignant neoplasm of overlapping sites of heart,   `CC`
        mediastinum and pleura
        CC Excl: See code: C38.1

▣ Newborn: 0   ▣ Pediatric: 0-17   ▣ Maternity: 12-55   ▣ Adult: 15-124   `MCC` Major CC Condition   `PDxMCC` PDx acts as own MCC   `CC` CC Condition   `PDxCC` PDx acts as own CC

458   ICD-10-CM 2016

✓4ᵗʰ C39　Malignant neoplasm of other and ill-defined sites in the respiratory system and intrathoracic organs
　　　Use additional code to identify:
　　　　exposure to environmental tobacco smoke (Z77.22)
　　　　exposure to tobacco smoke in the perinatal period (P96.81)
　　　　history of tobacco use (Z87.891)
　　　　occupational exposure to environmental tobacco smoke (Z57.31)
　　　　tobacco dependence (F17.-)
　　　　tobacco use (Z72.0)
　　　　EXCLUDES 1　intrathoracic malignant neoplasm NOS (C76.1)
　　　　　　　　thoracic malignant neoplasm NOS (C76.1)

　　C39.0　Malignant neoplasm of upper respiratory tract, part unspecified

　　C39.9　Malignant neoplasm of lower respiratory tract, part unspecified
　　　　Malignant neoplasm of respiratory tract NOS

Malignant neoplasms of bone and articular cartilage (C40-C41)
　　INCLUDES　malignant neoplasm of cartilage (articular) (joint)
　　　　　　malignant neoplasm of periosteum
　　EXCLUDES 1　malignant neoplasm of bone marrow NOS (C96.9)
　　　　　　malignant neoplasm of synovia (C49.-)

✓4ᵗʰ C40　Malignant neoplasm of bone and articular cartilage of limbs
　　　Use additional code to identify major osseous defect, if applicable (M89.7-)

　　✓5ᵗʰ C40.0　Malignant neoplasm of scapula and long bones of upper limb

　　　　CC Excl: For CC codes in subcategory C40.0, unless otherwise noted: C40.00-C40.02, C40.80, C40.92, C41.9, Z51.0

　　　　C40.00　Malignant neoplasm of scapula and long bones of unspecified upper limb　`CC`
　　　　C40.01　Malignant neoplasm of scapula and long bones of right upper limb　`CC`
　　　　C40.02　Malignant neoplasm of scapula and long bones of left upper limb　`CC`

　　✓5ᵗʰ C40.1　Malignant neoplasm of short bones of upper limb

　　　　CC Excl: For CC codes in subcategory C40.1, unless otherwise noted: C40.10-C40.12, C40.80-C40.92, C41.9, Z51.0

　　　　C40.10　Malignant neoplasm of short bones of unspecified upper limb　`CC`
　　　　C40.11　Malignant neoplasm of short bones of right upper limb　`CC`
　　　　C40.12　Malignant neoplasm of short bones of left upper limb　`CC`

　　✓5ᵗʰ C40.2　Malignant neoplasm of long bones of lower limb

　　　　CC Excl: For CC codes in subcategory C40.2, unless otherwise noted: C40.20-C40.22, C40.80-C40.92, C41.9, Z51.0

　　　　C40.20　Malignant neoplasm of long bones of unspecified lower limb　`CC`
　　　　C40.21　Malignant neoplasm of long bones of right lower limb　`CC`
　　　　C40.22　Malignant neoplasm of long bones of left lower limb　`CC`

　　✓5ᵗʰ C40.3　Malignant neoplasm of short bones of lower limb

　　　　CC Excl: For CC codes in subcategory C40.3, unless otherwise noted: C40.30-C40.92, C41.9, Z51.0

　　　　C40.30　Malignant neoplasm of short bones of unspecified lower limb　`CC`
　　　　C40.31　Malignant neoplasm of short bones of right lower limb　`CC`
　　　　C40.32　Malignant neoplasm of short bones of left lower limb　`CC`

　　✓5ᵗʰ C40.8　Malignant neoplasm of overlapping sites of bone and articular cartilage of limb

　　　　CC Excl: For CC codes in subcategory C40.8, unless otherwise noted: C40.00-C41.9, Z51.0

　　　　C40.80　Malignant neoplasm of overlapping sites of bone and articular cartilage of unspecified limb　`CC`
　　　　C40.81　Malignant neoplasm of overlapping sites of bone and articular cartilage of right limb　`CC`
　　　　C40.82　Malignant neoplasm of overlapping sites of bone and articular cartilage of left limb　`CC`

　　✓5ᵗʰ C40.9　Malignant neoplasm of unspecified bones and articular cartilage of limb

　　　　CC Excl: For CC codes in subcategory C40.9, uless otherwise noted: C40.00-C41.9, Z51.0

　　　　C40.90　Malignant neoplasm of unspecified bones and articular cartilage of unspecified limb　`CC`
　　　　C40.91　Malignant neoplasm of unspecified bones and articular cartilage of right limb　`CC`
　　　　C40.92　Malignant neoplasm of unspecified bones and articular cartilage of left limb　`CC`

✓4ᵗʰ C41　Malignant neoplasm of bone and articular cartilage of other and unspecified sites
　　EXCLUDES 1　malignant neoplasm of bones of limbs (C40.-)
　　　　　　malignant neoplasm of cartilage of ear (C49.0)
　　　　　　malignant neoplasm of cartilage of eyelid (C49.0)
　　　　　　malignant neoplasm of cartilage of larynx (C32.3)
　　　　　　malignant neoplasm of cartilage of limbs (C40.-)
　　　　　　malignant neoplasm of cartilage of nose (C30.0)

　　C41.0　Malignant neoplasm of bones of skull and face　`CC`
　　　　Malignant neoplasm of maxilla (superior)
　　　　Malignant neoplasm of orbital bone
　　　　EXCLUDES 2　carcinoma, any type except intraosseous or odontogenic of:
　　　　　　maxillary sinus (C31.0)
　　　　　　upper jaw (C03.0)
　　　　　　malignant neoplasm of jaw bone (lower) (C41.1)
　　　　CC Excl: C40.80-C41.0, C41.9, Z51.0

　　C41.1　Malignant neoplasm of mandible　`CC`
　　　　Malignant neoplasm of inferior maxilla
　　　　Malignant neoplasm of lower jaw bone
　　　　EXCLUDES 2　carcinoma, any type except intraosseous or odontogenic of:
　　　　　　jaw NOS (C03.9)
　　　　　　lower (C03.1)
　　　　　　malignant neoplasm of upper jaw bone (C41.0)
　　　　CC Excl: C40.80-C40.92, C41.1, C41.9, Z51.0

　　C41.2　Malignant neoplasm of vertebral column　`CC`
　　　　EXCLUDES 1　malignant neoplasm of sacrum and coccyx (C41.4)
　　　　CC Excl: C40.80-C40.92, C41.2, C41.9, Z51.0

　　C41.3　Malignant neoplasm of ribs, sternum and clavicle　`CC`
　　　　CC Excl: C40.80-C40.92, C41.3, C41.9, Z51.0

　　C41.4　Malignant neoplasm of pelvic bones, sacrum and coccyx　`CC`
　　　　CC Excl: C40.80-C40.92, C41.4-C41.9, Z51.0

　　C41.9　Malignant neoplasm of bone and articular cartilage, unspecified　`CC`
　　　　CC Excl: C40.00-C41.9, Z51.0

Melanoma and other malignant neoplasms of skin (C43-C44)

✓4ᵗʰ C43　Malignant melanoma of skin
　　EXCLUDES 1　melanoma in situ (D03.-)
　　EXCLUDES 2　malignant melanoma of skin of genital organs (C51-C52, C60.-, C63.-)
　　　　　　Merkel cell carcinoma (C4A.-)
　　　　　　sites other than skin—code to malignant neoplasm of the site

　　C43.0　Malignant melanoma of lip
　　　　EXCLUDES 1　malignant neoplasm of vermilion border of lip (C00.0-C00.2)

　　✓5ᵗʰ C43.1　Malignant melanoma of eyelid, including canthus
　　　　C43.10　Malignant melanoma of unspecified eyelid, including canthus
　　　　C43.11　Malignant melanoma of right eyelid, including canthus
　　　　C43.12　Malignant melanoma of left eyelid, including canthus

　　✓5ᵗʰ C43.2　Malignant melanoma of ear and external auricular canal
　　　　C43.20　Malignant melanoma of unspecified ear and external auricular canal
　　　　C43.21　Malignant melanoma of right ear and external auricular canal
　　　　C43.22　Malignant melanoma of left ear and external auricular canal

　　✓5ᵗʰ C43.3　Malignant melanoma of other and unspecified parts of face
　　　　C43.30　Malignant melanoma of unspecified part of face
　　　　C43.31　Malignant melanoma of nose
　　　　C43.39　Malignant melanoma of other parts of face

　　C43.4　Malignant melanoma of scalp and neck

✓ Additional Character Required　✓x7ᵗʰ Placeholder Alert　Unacceptable PDx　Manifestation　　Hospital Acquired Condition　*EXCLUDES 1* Not Coded Here　*EXCLUDES 2* Not Included Here

ICD-10-CM 2016　　　　　　　　　　　　　　　　　　　　　　　　　　　　　　　　　　　　459

√5ᵗʰ C43.5 Malignant melanoma of trunk
EXCLUDES 2   malignant neoplasm of anus NOS (C21.0)
malignant neoplasm of scrotum (C63.2)

    C43.51 **Malignant melanoma of anal skin**
Malignant melanoma of anal margin
Malignant melanoma of perianal skin

    C43.52 **Malignant melanoma of skin of breast**

    C43.59 **Malignant melanoma of other part of trunk**

√5ᵗʰ C43.6 Malignant melanoma of upper limb, including shoulder

    C43.60 **Malignant melanoma of unspecified upper limb, including shoulder**

    C43.61 **Malignant melanoma of right upper limb, including shoulder**

    C43.62 **Malignant melanoma of left upper limb, including shoulder**

√5ᵗʰ C43.7 Malignant melanoma of lower limb, including hip

    C43.70 **Malignant melanoma of unspecified lower limb, including hip**

    C43.71 **Malignant melanoma of right lower limb, including hip**

    C43.72 **Malignant melanoma of left lower limb, including hip**

    C43.8 **Malignant melanoma of overlapping sites of skin**

    C43.9 **Malignant melanoma of skin, unspecified**
Malignant melanoma of unspecified site of skin

√4ᵗʰ C4A Merkel cell carcinoma

    C4A.0 **Merkel cell carcinoma of lip**
EXCLUDES 1   malignant neoplasm of vermilion border of lip (C00.0-C00.2)

√5ᵗʰ C4A.1 Merkel cell carcinoma of eyelid, including canthus

    C4A.10 **Merkel cell carcinoma of unspecified eyelid, including canthus**

    C4A.11 **Merkel cell carcinoma of right eyelid, including canthus**

    C4A.12 **Merkel cell carcinoma of left eyelid, including canthus**

√5ᵗʰ C4A.2 Merkel cell carcinoma of ear and external auricular canal

    C4A.20 **Merkel cell carcinoma of unspecified ear and external auricular canal**

    C4A.21 **Merkel cell carcinoma of right ear and external auricular canal**

    C4A.22 **Merkel cell carcinoma of left ear and external auricular canal**

√5ᵗʰ C4A.3 Merkel cell carcinoma of other and unspecified parts of face

    C4A.30 **Merkel cell carcinoma of unspecified part of face**

    C4A.31 **Merkel cell carcinoma of nose**

    C4A.39 **Merkel cell carcinoma of other parts of face**

    C4A.4 **Merkel cell carcinoma of scalp and neck**

√5ᵗʰ C4A.5 Merkel cell carcinoma of trunk
EXCLUDES 2   malignant neoplasm of anus NOS (C21.0)
malignant neoplasm of scrotum (C63.2)

    C4A.51 **Merkel cell carcinoma of anal skin**
Merkel cell carcinoma of anal margin
Merkel cell carcinoma of perianal skin

    C4A.52 **Merkel cell carcinoma of skin of breast**

    C4A.59 **Merkel cell carcinoma of other part of trunk**

√5ᵗʰ C4A.6 Merkel cell carcinoma of upper limb, including shoulder

    C4A.60 **Merkel cell carcinoma of unspecified upper limb, including shoulder**

    C4A.61 **Merkel cell carcinoma of right upper limb, including shoulder**

    C4A.62 **Merkel cell carcinoma of left upper limb, including shoulder**

√5ᵗʰ C4A.7 Merkel cell carcinoma of lower limb, including hip

    C4A.70 **Merkel cell carcinoma of unspecified lower limb, including hip**

    C4A.71 **Merkel cell carcinoma of right lower limb, including hip**

    C4A.72 **Merkel cell carcinoma of left lower limb, including hip**

    C4A.8 **Merkel cell carcinoma of overlapping sites**

    C4A.9 **Merkel cell carcinoma, unspecified**
Merkel cell carcinoma of unspecified site

√4ᵗʰ C44 Other and unspecified malignant neoplasm of skin
INCLUDES   malignant neoplasm of sebaceous glands
malignant neoplasm of sweat glands
EXCLUDES 1   Kaposi's sarcoma of skin (C46.0)
malignant melanoma of skin (C43.-)
malignant neoplasm of skin of genital organs (C51-C52, C60-, C63.2)
Merkel cell carcinoma (C4A.-)

√5ᵗʰ C44.0 Other and unspecified malignant neoplasm of skin of lip
EXCLUDES 1   malignant neoplasm of lip (C00.-)

    C44.00 **Unspecified malignant neoplasm of skin of lip**

    C44.01 **Basal cell carcinoma of skin of lip**

    C44.02 **Squamous cell carcinoma of skin of lip**

    C44.09 **Other specified malignant neoplasm of skin of lip**

√5ᵗʰ C44.1 Other and unspecified malignant neoplasm of skin of eyelid, including canthus
EXCLUDES 1   connective tissue of eyelid (C49.0)

    √6ᵗʰ C44.10 Unspecified malignant neoplasm of skin of eyelid, including canthus

      C44.101 **Unspecified malignant neoplasm of skin of unspecified eyelid, including canthus**

      C44.102 **Unspecified malignant neoplasm of skin of right eyelid, including canthus**

      C44.109 **Unspecified malignant neoplasm of skin of left eyelid, including canthus**

    √6ᵗʰ C44.11 Basal cell carcinoma of skin of eyelid, including canthus

      C44.111 **Basal cell carcinoma of skin of unspecified eyelid, including canthus**

      C44.112 **Basal cell carcinoma of skin of right eyelid, including canthus**

      C44.119 **Basal cell carcinoma of skin of left eyelid, including canthus**

    √6ᵗʰ C44.12 Squamous cell carcinoma of skin of eyelid, including canthus

      C44.121 **Squamous cell carcinoma of skin of unspecified eyelid, including canthus**

      C44.122 **Squamous cell carcinoma of skin of right eyelid, including canthus**

      C44.129 **Squamous cell carcinoma of skin of left eyelid, including canthus**

    √6ᵗʰ C44.19 Other specified malignant neoplasm of skin of eyelid, including canthus

      C44.191 **Other specified malignant neoplasm of skin of unspecified eyelid, including canthus**

      C44.192 **Other specified malignant neoplasm of skin of right eyelid, including canthus**

      C44.199 **Other specified malignant neoplasm of skin of left eyelid, including canthus**

√5ᵗʰ C44.2 Other and unspecified malignant neoplasm of skin of ear and external auricular canal
EXCLUDES 1   connective tissue of ear (C49.0)

    √6ᵗʰ C44.20 Unspecified malignant neoplasm of skin of ear and external auricular canal

      C44.201 **Unspecified malignant neoplasm of skin of unspecified ear and external auricular canal**

      C44.202 **Unspecified malignant neoplasm of skin of right ear and external auricular canal**

      C44.209 **Unspecified malignant neoplasm of skin of left ear and external auricular canal**

    √6ᵗʰ C44.21 Basal cell carcinoma of skin of ear and external auricular canal

      C44.211 **Basal cell carcinoma of skin of unspecified ear and external auricular canal**

      C44.212 **Basal cell carcinoma of skin of right ear and external auricular canal**

      C44.219 **Basal cell carcinoma of skin of left ear and external auricular canal**

    √6ᵗʰ C44.22 Squamous cell carcinoma of skin of ear and external auricular canal

      C44.221 **Squamous cell carcinoma of skin of unspecified ear and external auricular canal**

      C44.222 **Squamous cell carcinoma of skin of right ear and external auricular canal**

C44.229   Squamous cell carcinoma of skin of left ear and external auricular canal

☑6th **C44.29**   Other specified malignant neoplasm of skin of ear and external auricular canal

    C44.291   Other specified malignant neoplasm of skin of unspecified ear and external auricular canal

    C44.292   Other specified malignant neoplasm of skin of right ear and external auricular canal

    C44.299   Other specified malignant neoplasm of skin of left ear and external auricular canal

☑5th **C44.3**   Other and unspecified malignant neoplasm of skin of other and unspecified parts of face

   ☑6th **C44.30**   Unspecified malignant neoplasm of skin of other and unspecified parts of face

    C44.300   Unspecified malignant neoplasm of skin of unspecified part of face

    C44.301   Unspecified malignant neoplasm of skin of nose

    C44.309   Unspecified malignant neoplasm of skin of other parts of face

   ☑6th **C44.31**   Basal cell carcinoma of skin of other and unspecified parts of face

    C44.310   Basal cell carcinoma of skin of unspecified parts of face

    C44.311   Basal cell carcinoma of skin of nose

    C44.319   Basal cell carcinoma of skin of other parts of face

   ☑6th **C44.32**   Squamous cell carcinoma of skin of other and unspecified parts of face

    C44.320   Squamous cell carcinoma of skin of unspecified parts of face

    C44.321   Squamous cell carcinoma of skin of nose

    C44.329   Squamous cell carcinoma of skin of other parts of face

   ☑6th **C44.39**   Other specified malignant neoplasm of skin of other and unspecified parts of face

    C44.390   Other specified malignant neoplasm of skin of unspecified parts of face

    C44.391   Other specified malignant neoplasm of skin of nose

    C44.399   Other specified malignant neoplasm of skin of other parts of face

☑5th **C44.4**   Other and unspecified malignant neoplasm of skin of scalp and neck

   C44.40   Unspecified malignant neoplasm of skin of scalp and neck

   C44.41   Basal cell carcinoma of skin of scalp and neck

   C44.42   Squamous cell carcinoma of skin of scalp and neck

   C44.49   Other specified malignant neoplasm of skin of scalp and neck

☑5th **C44.5**   Other and unspecified malignant neoplasm of skin of trunk

    EXCLUDES 1   anus NOS (C21.0)
             scrotum (C63.2)

   ☑6th **C44.50**   Unspecified malignant neoplasm of skin of trunk

    C44.500   Unspecified malignant neoplasm of anal skin
            Unspecified malignant neoplasm of anal margin
            Unspecified malignant neoplasm of perianal skin

    C44.501   Unspecified malignant neoplasm of skin of breast

    C44.509   Unspecified malignant neoplasm of skin of other part of trunk

   ☑6th **C44.51**   Basal cell carcinoma of skin of trunk

    C44.510   Basal cell carcinoma of anal skin
            Basal cell carcinoma of anal margin
            Basal cell carcinoma of perianal skin

    C44.511   Basal cell carcinoma of skin of breast

    C44.519   Basal cell carcinoma of skin of other part of trunk

   ☑6th **C44.52**   Squamous cell carcinoma of skin of trunk

    C44.520   Squamous cell carcinoma of anal skin
            Squamous cell carcinoma of anal margin
            Squamous cell carcinoma of perianal skin

C44.521   Squamous cell carcinoma of skin of breast

C44.529   Squamous cell carcinoma of skin of other part of trunk

☑6th **C44.59**   Other specified malignant neoplasm of skin of trunk

    C44.590   Other specified malignant neoplasm of anal skin
            Other specified malignant neoplasm of anal margin
            Other specified malignant neoplasm of perianal skin

    C44.591   Other specified malignant neoplasm of skin of breast

    C44.599   Other specified malignant neoplasm of skin of other part of trunk

☑5th **C44.6**   Other and unspecified malignant neoplasm of skin of upper limb, including shoulder

   ☑6th **C44.60**   Unspecified malignant neoplasm of skin of upper limb, including shoulder

    C44.601   Unspecified malignant neoplasm of skin of unspecified upper limb, including shoulder

    C44.602   Unspecified malignant neoplasm of skin of right upper limb, including shoulder

    C44.609   Unspecified malignant neoplasm of skin of left upper limb, including shoulder

   ☑6th **C44.61**   Basal cell carcinoma of skin of upper limb, including shoulder

    C44.611   Basal cell carcinoma of skin of unspecified upper limb, including shoulder

    C44.612   Basal cell carcinoma of skin of right upper limb, including shoulder

    C44.619   Basal cell carcinoma of skin of left upper limb, including shoulder

   ☑6th **C44.62**   Squamous cell carcinoma of skin of upper limb, including shoulder

    C44.621   Squamous cell carcinoma of skin of unspecified upper limb, including shoulder

    C44.622   Squamous cell carcinoma of skin of right upper limb, including shoulder

    C44.629   Squamous cell carcinoma of skin of left upper limb, including shoulder

   ☑6th **C44.69**   Other specified malignant neoplasm of skin of upper limb, including shoulder

    C44.691   Other specified malignant neoplasm of skin of unspecified upper limb, including shoulder

    C44.692   Other specified malignant neoplasm of skin of right upper limb, including shoulder

    C44.699   Other specified malignant neoplasm of skin of left upper limb, including shoulder

☑5th **C44.7**   Other and unspecified malignant neoplasm of skin of lower limb, including hip

   ☑6th **C44.70**   Unspecified malignant neoplasm of skin of lower limb, including hip

    C44.701   Unspecified malignant neoplasm of skin of unspecified lower limb, including hip

    C44.702   Unspecified malignant neoplasm of skin of right lower limb, including hip

    C44.709   Unspecified malignant neoplasm of skin of left lower limb, including hip

   ☑6th **C44.71**   Basal cell carcinoma of skin of lower limb, including hip

    C44.711   Basal cell carcinoma of skin of unspecified lower limb, including hip

    C44.712   Basal cell carcinoma of skin of right lower limb, including hip

    C44.719   Basal cell carcinoma of skin of left lower limb, including hip

   ☑6th **C44.72**   Squamous cell carcinoma of skin of lower limb, including hip

    C44.721   Squamous cell carcinoma of skin of unspecified lower limb, including hip

    C44.722   Squamous cell carcinoma of skin of right lower limb, including hip

    C44.729   Squamous cell carcinoma of skin of left lower limb, including hip

---

☑ Additional Character Required   ☑x7th Placeholder Alert   Unacceptable PDx   Manifestation   Hospital Acquired Condition   EXCLUDES 1 Not Coded Here   EXCLUDES 2 Not Included Here

✓6th **C44.79** Other specified malignant neoplasm of skin of lower limb, including hip

    C44.791 Other specified malignant neoplasm of skin of unspecified lower limb, including hip

    C44.792 Other specified malignant neoplasm of skin of right lower limb, including hip

    C44.799 Other specified malignant neoplasm of skin of left lower limb, including hip

✓5th **C44.8** Other and unspecified malignant neoplasm of overlapping sites of skin

    C44.80 Unspecified malignant neoplasm of overlapping sites of skin

    C44.81 Basal cell carcinoma of overlapping sites of skin

    C44.82 Squamous cell carcinoma of overlapping sites of skin

    C44.89 Other specified malignant neoplasm of overlapping sites of skin

✓5th **C44.9** Other and unspecified malignant neoplasm of skin, unspecified

    C44.90 Unspecified malignant neoplasm of skin, unspecified

      Malignant neoplasm of unspecified site of skin

    C44.91 Basal cell carcinoma of skin, unspecified

    C44.92 Squamous cell carcinoma of skin, unspecified

    C44.99 Other specified malignant neoplasm of skin, unspecified

Malignant neoplasms of mesothelial and soft tissue (C45-C49)

✓4th **C45** **Mesothelioma**

    C45.0 Mesothelioma of pleura   CC

      EXCLUDES 1 other malignant neoplasm of pleura (C38.4)

      CC Excl: C38.4, C39.9, C45.0, C45.7-C45.9, C76.8, C7A.00, C7A.098-C7B.00, C7B.1, C80.0-C80.2, D49.1, D49.81-D49.9

    C45.1 Mesothelioma of peritoneum   CC

      Mesothelioma of cul-de-sac

      Mesothelioma of mesentery

      Mesothelioma of mesocolon

      Mesothelioma of omentum

      Mesothelioma of peritoneum (parietal) (pelvic)

      EXCLUDES 1 other malignant neoplasm of soft tissue of peritoneum (C48.-)

      CC Excl: C45.1, C48.0-C48.8, Z51.0

    C45.2 Mesothelioma of pericardium   CC

      EXCLUDES 1 other malignant neoplasm of pericardium (C38.0)

      CC Excl: C38.0, C45.2

    C45.7 Mesothelioma of other sites

    C45.9 Mesothelioma, unspecified

✓4th **C46** **Kaposi's sarcoma**

    Code first any human immunodeficiency virus [HIV] disease (B20)

    C46.0 Kaposi's sarcoma of skin   HIV CC

      CC Excl: C46.0, C46.7-C46.9, Z51.0

    C46.1 Kaposi's sarcoma of soft tissue   HIV CC

      Kaposi's sarcoma of blood vessel

      Kaposi's sarcoma of connective tissue

      Kaposi's sarcoma of fascia

      Kaposi's sarcoma of ligament

      Kaposi's sarcoma of lymphatic(s) NEC

      Kaposi's sarcoma of muscle

      EXCLUDES 2 Kaposi's sarcoma of lymph glands and nodes (C46.3)

      CC Excl: C46.1, C46.7-C46.9, Z51.0

    C46.2 Kaposi's sarcoma of palate   HIV CC

      CC Excl: C46.2, C46.7-C46.9, Z51.0

    C46.3 Kaposi's sarcoma of lymph nodes   HIV CC

      CC Excl: C45.7-C45.9, C46.3, C76.8-C77.9, C7A.00, C7A.098-C7B.01, C7B.1, C80.0-C80.2, D49.81-D49.9

    C46.4 Kaposi's sarcoma of gastrointestinal sites   HIV CC

      CC Excl: C46.4, C46.7-C46.9, Z51.0

✓5th   **C46.5** Kaposi's sarcoma of lung

      CC Excl: For CC codes in subcategory C46.5, unless otherwise noted: C34.80-C34.92, C39.9, C45.7-C45.9, C46.50-C46.52, C76.8, C7A.00, C7A.090, C7A.098-C7B.00, C7B.1, C80.0-C80.2, D49.1, D49.81-D49.9

    C46.50 Kaposi's sarcoma of unspecified lung   HIV CC

    C46.51 Kaposi's sarcoma of right lung   HIV CC

    C46.52 Kaposi's sarcoma of left lung   HIV CC

    C46.7 Kaposi's sarcoma of other sites   HIV CC

      CC Excl: See code: C46.0

    C46.9 Kaposi's sarcoma, unspecified   HIV CC

      Kaposi's sarcoma of unspecified site

      CC Excl: C45.7-C46.9, C51.0-C55, C56.1-C63.9, C64.1-C64.9, C65.1-C65.9, C66.1-C72.9, C76.0-C76.52, C76.8-C7A.00, C7A.093, C7A.098-C80.2, D00.00-D02.4, D04.0-D05.02, D05.10-D05.12, D05.80-D05.92, D06.0-D09.3, D09.8-D09.9, D37.01-D37.6, D37.8-D39.2, D39.8-D39.9, D40.0-D40.12, D40.8-D41.4, D41.8-D43.4, D43.8-D44.7, D44.9, D48.0-D48.62, D48.7-D49.9, Z51.0

✓4th **C47** **Malignant neoplasm of peripheral nerves and autonomic nervous system**

    INCLUDES malignant neoplasm of sympathetic and parasympathetic nerves and ganglia

    EXCLUDES 1 Kaposi's sarcoma of soft tissue (C46.1)

    CC Excl: For CC codes in category C47, unless otherwise noted: Z51.0

    C47.0 Malignant neoplasm of peripheral nerves of head, face and neck   CC

      EXCLUDES 1 malignant neoplasm of peripheral nerves of orbit (C69.6-)

✓5th   **C47.1** Malignant neoplasm of peripheral nerves of upper limb, including shoulder

    C47.10 Malignant neoplasm of peripheral nerves of unspecified upper limb, including shoulder   CC

    C47.11 Malignant neoplasm of peripheral nerves of right upper limb, including shoulder   CC

    C47.12 Malignant neoplasm of peripheral nerves of left upper limb, including shoulder   CC

✓5th   **C47.2** Malignant neoplasm of peripheral nerves of lower limb, including hip

    C47.20 Malignant neoplasm of peripheral nerves of unspecified lower limb, including hip   CC

    C47.21 Malignant neoplasm of peripheral nerves of right lower limb, including hip   CC

    C47.22 Malignant neoplasm of peripheral nerves of left lower limb, including hip   CC

    C47.3 Malignant neoplasm of peripheral nerves of thorax   CC

    C47.4 Malignant neoplasm of peripheral nerves of abdomen   CC

    C47.5 Malignant neoplasm of peripheral nerves of pelvis   CC

    C47.6 Malignant neoplasm of peripheral nerves of trunk, unspecified   CC

      Malignant neoplasm of peripheral nerves of unspecified part of trunk

    C47.8 Malignant neoplasm of overlapping sites of peripheral nerves and autonomic nervous system   CC

    C47.9 Malignant neoplasm of peripheral nerves and autonomic nervous system, unspecified   CC

      Malignant neoplasm of unspecified site of peripheral nerves and autonomic nervous system

✓4th **C48** **Malignant neoplasm of retroperitoneum and peritoneum**

    EXCLUDES 1 Kaposi's sarcoma of connective tissue (C46.1) mesothelioma (C45.-)

    C48.0 Malignant neoplasm of retroperitoneum   CC

      CC Excl: C48.0-Z51.0

    C48.1 Malignant neoplasm of specified parts of peritoneum   CC

      Malignant neoplasm of cul-de-sac

      Malignant neoplasm of mesentery

      Malignant neoplasm of mesocolon

      Malignant neoplasm of omentum

      Malignant neoplasm of parietal peritoneum

      Malignant neoplasm of pelvic peritoneum

      CC Excl: C45.1, C48.0-C48.8, Z51.0

    C48.2 Malignant neoplasm of peritoneum, unspecified   CC

      CC Excl: See code: C48.1

    C48.8 Malignant neoplasm of overlapping sites of retroperitoneum and peritoneum   CC

      CC Excl: See code: C48.1

N Newborn: 0   P Pediatric: 0-17   M Maternity: 12-55   A Adult: 15-124   MCC Major CC Condition   PDxMCC PDx acts as own MCC   CC CC Condition   PDxCC PDx acts as own CC

462   ICD-10-CM 2016

✓4ᵗʰ C49　Malignant neoplasm of other connective and soft tissue
　　　INCLUDES　malignant neoplasm of blood vessel
　　　　　malignant neoplasm of bursa
　　　　　malignant neoplasm of cartilage
　　　　　malignant neoplasm of fascia
　　　　　malignant neoplasm of fat
　　　　　malignant neoplasm of ligament, except uterine
　　　　　malignant neoplasm of lymphatic vessel
　　　　　malignant neoplasm of muscle
　　　　　malignant neoplasm of synovia
　　　　　malignant neoplasm of tendon (sheath)
　　　EXCLUDES 1　*malignant neoplasm of cartilage (of):*
　　　　　　articular (C40-C41)
　　　　　　larynx (C32.3)
　　　　　　nose (C30.0)
　　　　　malignant neoplasm of connective tissue of breast (C50.-)
　　　EXCLUDES 2　*Kaposi's sarcoma of soft tissue (C46.1)*
　　　　　malignant neoplasm of heart (C38.0)
　　　　　malignant neoplasm of peripheral nerves and autonomic
　　　　　　nervous system (C47.-)
　　　　　malignant neoplasm of peritoneum (C48.2)
　　　　　malignant neoplasm of retroperitoneum (C48.0)
　　　　　malignant neoplasm of uterine ligament (C57.3)
　　　　　mesothelioma (C45.-)

> **CC Excl: For CC codes in category C49, unless otherwise noted:**
> Z51.0

　C49.0　**Malignant neoplasm of connective and soft tissue**　CC
　　　of head, face and neck
　　　　Malignant neoplasm of connective tissue of ear
　　　　Malignant neoplasm of connective tissue of eyelid
　　　　EXCLUDES 1　*connective tissue of orbit (C69.6-)*

　✓5ᵗʰ C49.1　**Malignant neoplasm of connective and soft tissue of upper limb, including shoulder**
　　　C49.10　**Malignant neoplasm of connective and soft**　CC
　　　　　tissue of unspecified upper limb, including shoulder
　　　C49.11　**Malignant neoplasm of connective and soft**　CC
　　　　　tissue of right upper limb, including shoulder
　　　C49.12　**Malignant neoplasm of connective and soft**　CC
　　　　　tissue of left upper limb, including shoulder

　✓5ᵗʰ C49.2　**Malignant neoplasm of connective and soft tissue of lower limb, including hip**
　　　C49.20　**Malignant neoplasm of connective and soft**　CC
　　　　　tissue of unspecified lower limb, including hip
　　　C49.21　**Malignant neoplasm of connective and soft**　CC
　　　　　tissue of right lower limb, including hip
　　　C49.22　**Malignant neoplasm of connective and soft**　CC
　　　　　tissue of left lower limb, including hip

　C49.3　**Malignant neoplasm of connective and soft tissue of**　CC
　　　thorax
　　　　Malignant neoplasm of axilla
　　　　Malignant neoplasm of diaphragm
　　　　Malignant neoplasm of great vessels
　　　　EXCLUDES 1　*malignant neoplasm of breast (C50.-)*
　　　　　malignant neoplasm of heart (C38.0)
　　　　　malignant neoplasm of mediastinum (C38.1-C38.3)
　　　　　malignant neoplasm of thymus (C37)

　C49.4　**Malignant neoplasm of connective and soft tissue of**　CC
　　　abdomen
　　　　Malignant neoplasm of abdominal wall
　　　　Malignant neoplasm of hypochondrium

　C49.5　**Malignant neoplasm of connective and soft tissue of**　CC
　　　pelvis
　　　　Malignant neoplasm of buttock
　　　　Malignant neoplasm of groin
　　　　Malignant neoplasm of perineum

　C49.6　**Malignant neoplasm of connective and soft tissue of**　CC
　　　trunk, unspecified
　　　　Malignant neoplasm of back NOS

　C49.8　**Malignant neoplasm of overlapping sites of connective**　CC
　　　and soft tissue
　　　　Primary malignant neoplasm of two or more contiguous sites of
　　　　connective and soft tissue

　C49.9　**Malignant neoplasm of connective and soft tissue,**　CC
　　　unspecified

Malignant neoplasms of breast (C50)

✓4ᵗʰ C50　Malignant neoplasm of breast
　　　INCLUDES　connective tissue of breast
　　　　　Paget's disease of breast
　　　　　Paget's disease of nipple
　　　Use additional code to identify estrogen receptor status (Z17.0, Z17.1)
　　　EXCLUDES 1　*skin of breast (C44.501, C44.511, C44.521, C44.591)*

　✓5ᵗʰ C50.0　**Malignant neoplasm of nipple and areola**
　　　✓6ᵗʰ C50.01　**Malignant neoplasm of nipple and areola, female**
　　　　C50.011　**Malignant neoplasm of nipple and**　♀
　　　　　　areola, right female breast
　　　　C50.012　**Malignant neoplasm of nipple and**　♀
　　　　　　areola, left female breast
　　　　C50.019　**Malignant neoplasm of nipple and**　♀
　　　　　　areola, unspecified female breast
　　　✓6ᵗʰ C50.02　**Malignant neoplasm of nipple and areola, male**
　　　　C50.021　**Malignant neoplasm of nipple and**　♂
　　　　　　areola, right male breast
　　　　C50.022　**Malignant neoplasm of nipple and**　♂
　　　　　　areola, left male breast
　　　　C50.029　**Malignant neoplasm of nipple and**　♂
　　　　　　areola, unspecified male breast

　✓5ᵗʰ C50.1　**Malignant neoplasm of central portion of breast**
　　　✓6ᵗʰ C50.11　**Malignant neoplasm of central portion of breast, female**
　　　　C50.111　**Malignant neoplasm of central portion**　♀
　　　　　　of right female breast
　　　　C50.112　**Malignant neoplasm of central portion**　♀
　　　　　　of left female breast
　　　　C50.119　**Malignant neoplasm of central portion**　♀
　　　　　　of unspecified female breast
　　　✓6ᵗʰ C50.12　**Malignant neoplasm of central portion of breast, male**
　　　　C50.121　**Malignant neoplasm of central portion**　♂
　　　　　　of right male breast
　　　　C50.122　**Malignant neoplasm of central portion**　♂
　　　　　　of left male breast
　　　　C50.129　**Malignant neoplasm of central portion**　♂
　　　　　　of unspecified male breast

　✓5ᵗʰ C50.2　**Malignant neoplasm of upper-inner quadrant of breast**
　　　✓6ᵗʰ C50.21　**Malignant neoplasm of upper-inner quadrant of breast, female**
　　　　C50.211　**Malignant neoplasm of upper-inner**　♀
　　　　　　quadrant of right female breast
　　　　C50.212　**Malignant neoplasm of upper-inner**　♀
　　　　　　quadrant of left female breast
　　　　C50.219　**Malignant neoplasm of upper-inner**　♀
　　　　　　quadrant of unspecified female breast
　　　✓6ᵗʰ C50.22　**Malignant neoplasm of upper-inner quadrant of breast, male**
　　　　C50.221　**Malignant neoplasm of upper-inner**　♂
　　　　　　quadrant of right male breast
　　　　C50.222　**Malignant neoplasm of upper-inner**　♂
　　　　　　quadrant of left male breast
　　　　C50.229　**Malignant neoplasm of upper-inner**　♂
　　　　　　quadrant of unspecified male breast

　✓5ᵗʰ C50.3　**Malignant neoplasm of lower-inner quadrant of breast**
　　　✓6ᵗʰ C50.31　**Malignant neoplasm of lower-inner quadrant of breast, female**
　　　　C50.311　**Malignant neoplasm of lower-inner**　♀
　　　　　　quadrant of right female breast
　　　　C50.312　**Malignant neoplasm of lower-inner**　♀
　　　　　　quadrant of left female breast
　　　　C50.319　**Malignant neoplasm of lower-inner**　♀
　　　　　　quadrant of unspecified female breast
　　　✓6ᵗʰ C50.32　**Malignant neoplasm of lower-inner quadrant of breast, male**
　　　　C50.321　**Malignant neoplasm of lower-inner**　♂
　　　　　　quadrant of right male breast
　　　　C50.322　**Malignant neoplasm of lower-inner**　♂
　　　　　　quadrant of left male breast
　　　　C50.329　**Malignant neoplasm of lower-inner**　♂
　　　　　　quadrant of unspecified male breast

✓ Additional Character Required　✓7ᵗʰ Placeholder Alert　Unacceptable PDx　Manifestation　Hospital Acquired Condition　EXCLUDES 1 Not Coded Here　EXCLUDES 2 Not Included Here

Chapter 2. Neoplasms

✓5th **C50.4 Malignant neoplasm of upper-outer quadrant of breast**

  ✓6th **C50.41 Malignant neoplasm of upper-outer quadrant of breast, female**

    C50.411 Malignant neoplasm of upper-outer quadrant of right female breast ♀

    C50.412 Malignant neoplasm of upper-outer quadrant of left female breast ♀

    C50.419 Malignant neoplasm of upper-outer quadrant of unspecified female breast ♀

  ✓6th **C50.42 Malignant neoplasm of upper-outer quadrant of breast, male**

    C50.421 Malignant neoplasm of upper-outer quadrant of right male breast ♂

    C50.422 Malignant neoplasm of upper-outer quadrant of left male breast ♂

    C50.429 Malignant neoplasm of upper-outer quadrant of unspecified male breast ♂

✓5th **C50.5 Malignant neoplasm of lower-outer quadrant of breast**

  ✓6th **C50.51 Malignant neoplasm of lower-outer quadrant of breast, female**

    C50.511 Malignant neoplasm of lower-outer quadrant of right female breast ♀

    C50.512 Malignant neoplasm of lower-outer quadrant of left female breast ♀

    C50.519 Malignant neoplasm of lower-outer quadrant of unspecified female breast ♀

  ✓6th **C50.52 Malignant neoplasm of lower-outer quadrant of breast, male**

    C50.521 Malignant neoplasm of lower-outer quadrant of right male breast ♂

    C50.522 Malignant neoplasm of lower-outer quadrant of left male breast ♂

    C50.529 Malignant neoplasm of lower-outer quadrant of unspecified male breast ♂

✓5th **C50.6 Malignant neoplasm of axillary tail of breast**

  ✓6th **C50.61 Malignant neoplasm of axillary tail of breast, female**

    C50.611 Malignant neoplasm of axillary tail of right female breast ♀

    C50.612 Malignant neoplasm of axillary tail of left female breast ♀

    C50.619 Malignant neoplasm of axillary tail of unspecified female breast ♀

  ✓6th **C50.62 Malignant neoplasm of axillary tail of breast, male**

    C50.621 Malignant neoplasm of axillary tail of right male breast ♂

    C50.622 Malignant neoplasm of axillary tail of left male breast ♂

    C50.629 Malignant neoplasm of axillary tail of unspecified male breast ♂

✓5th **C50.8 Malignant neoplasm of overlapping sites of breast**

  ✓6th **C50.81 Malignant neoplasm of overlapping sites of breast, female**

    C50.811 Malignant neoplasm of overlapping sites of right female breast ♀

    C50.812 Malignant neoplasm of overlapping sites of left female breast ♀

    C50.819 Malignant neoplasm of overlapping sites of unspecified female breast ♀

  ✓6th **C50.82 Malignant neoplasm of overlapping sites of breast, male**

    C50.821 Malignant neoplasm of overlapping sites of right male breast ♂

    C50.822 Malignant neoplasm of overlapping sites of left male breast ♂

    C50.829 Malignant neoplasm of overlapping sites of unspecified male breast ♂

✓5th **C50.9 Malignant neoplasm of breast of unspecified site**

  ✓6th **C50.91 Malignant neoplasm of breast of unspecified site, female**

    C50.911 Malignant neoplasm of unspecified site of right female breast ♀

    C50.912 Malignant neoplasm of unspecified site of left female breast ♀

    C50.919 Malignant neoplasm of unspecified site of unspecified female breast ♀

  ✓6th **C50.92 Malignant neoplasm of breast of unspecified site, male**

    C50.921 Malignant neoplasm of unspecified site of right male breast ♂

    C50.922 Malignant neoplasm of unspecified site of left male breast ♂

    C50.929 Malignant neoplasm of unspecified site of unspecified male breast ♂

Malignant neoplasms of female genital organs (C51-C58)

INCLUDES   malignant neoplasm of skin of female genital organs

✓4th **C51 Malignant neoplasm of vulva**

  EXCLUDES 1   carcinoma in situ of vulva (D07.1)

  C51.0 Malignant neoplasm of labium majus ♀
    Malignant neoplasm of Bartholin's [greater vestibular] gland

  C51.1 Malignant neoplasm of labium minus ♀

  C51.2 Malignant neoplasm of clitoris ♀

  C51.8 Malignant neoplasm of overlapping sites of vulva ♀

  C51.9 Malignant neoplasm of vulva, unspecified ♀
    Malignant neoplasm of external female genitalia NOS
    Malignant neoplasm of pudendum

C52 Malignant neoplasm of vagina ♀
  EXCLUDES 1   carcinoma in situ of vagina (D07.2)

✓4th **C53 Malignant neoplasm of cervix uteri**
  EXCLUDES 1   carcinoma in situ of cervix uteri (D06.-)

  C53.0 Malignant neoplasm of endocervix ♀

  C53.1 Malignant neoplasm of exocervix ♀

  C53.8 Malignant neoplasm of overlapping sites of cervix uteri ♀

  C53.9 Malignant neoplasm of cervix uteri, unspecified ♀

✓4th **C54 Malignant neoplasm of corpus uteri**

  C54.0 Malignant neoplasm of isthmus uteri ♀
    Malignant neoplasm of lower uterine segment

  C54.1 Malignant neoplasm of endometrium ♀

  C54.2 Malignant neoplasm of myometrium ♀

  C54.3 Malignant neoplasm of fundus uteri ♀

  C54.8 Malignant neoplasm of overlapping sites of corpus uteri ♀

  C54.9 Malignant neoplasm of corpus uteri, unspecified ♀

C55 Malignant neoplasm of uterus, part unspecified ♀

✓4th **C56 Malignant neoplasm of ovary**

  Use additional code to identify any functional activity

  CC Excl: For CC codes in category C56, unless otherwise noted:
  C45.9, C56.1-C57.4, C7A.00, C7A.098-C7B.00, C7B.1, C76.3, C79.60-
  C79.62, C80.0-C80.2

  C56.1 Malignant neoplasm of right ovary CC ♀

  C56.2 Malignant neoplasm of left ovary CC ♀

  C56.9 Malignant neoplasm of unspecified ovary CC ♀

✓4th **C57 Malignant neoplasm of other and unspecified female genital organs**

  ✓5th **C57.0 Malignant neoplasm of fallopian tube**
    Malignant neoplasm of oviduct
    Malignant neoplasm of uterine tube

    C57.00 Malignant neoplasm of unspecified fallopian tube ♀

    C57.01 Malignant neoplasm of right fallopian tube ♀

    C57.02 Malignant neoplasm of left fallopian tube ♀

  ✓5th **C57.1 Malignant neoplasm of broad ligament**

    C57.10 Malignant neoplasm of unspecified broad ligament ♀

    C57.11 Malignant neoplasm of right broad ligament ♀

    C57.12 Malignant neoplasm of left broad ligament ♀

  ✓5th **C57.2 Malignant neoplasm of round ligament**

    C57.20 Malignant neoplasm of unspecified round ligament ♀

    C57.21 Malignant neoplasm of right round ligament ♀

    C57.22 Malignant neoplasm of left round ligament ♀

  C57.3 Malignant neoplasm of parametrium ♀
    Malignant neoplasm of uterine ligament NOS

  C57.4 Malignant neoplasm of uterine adnexa, unspecified ♀

  C57.7 Malignant neoplasm of other specified female genital organs ♀
    Malignant neoplasm of wolffian body or duct

N Newborn: 0   P Pediatric: 0-17   M Maternity: 12-55   A Adult: 15-124   MCC Major CC Condition   PDx MCC PDx acts as own MCC   CC CC Condition   PDx CC PDx acts as own CC

464

ICD-10-CM 2016

C57.8   **Malignant neoplasm of overlapping sites of female genital organs**   ♀
> Primary malignant neoplasm of two or more contiguous sites of the female genital organs whose point of origin cannot be determined
> Primary tubo-ovarian malignant neoplasm whose point of origin cannot be determined
> Primary utero-ovarian malignant neoplasm whose point of origin cannot be determined

C57.9   **Malignant neoplasm of female genital organ, unspecified**   ♀
> Malignant neoplasm of female genitourinary tract NOS

C58   **Malignant neoplasm of placenta**   ♀
> **INCLUDES**   choriocarcinoma NOS
> chorionepithelioma NOS
> **EXCLUDES 1**   chorioadenoma (destruens) (D39.2)
> hydatidiform mole NOS (O01.9)
> invasive hydatidiform mole (D39.2)
> male choriocarcinoma NOS (C62.9-)
> malignant hydatidiform mole (D39.2)

Malignant neoplasms of male genital organs (C60-C63)
> **INCLUDES**   malignant neoplasm of skin of male genital organs

✓4ᵗʰ C60   **Malignant neoplasm of penis**

C60.0   **Malignant neoplasm of prepuce**   ♂
> Malignant neoplasm of foreskin

C60.1   **Malignant neoplasm of glans penis**   ♂

C60.2   **Malignant neoplasm of body of penis**   ♂
> Malignant neoplasm of corpus cavernosum

C60.8   **Malignant neoplasm of overlapping sites of penis**   ♂

C60.9   **Malignant neoplasm of penis, unspecified**   ♂
> Malignant neoplasm of skin of penis NOS

C61   **Malignant neoplasm of prostate**   ♂
> **EXCLUDES 1**   malignant neoplasm of seminal vesicle (C63.7)

✓4ᵗʰ C62   **Malignant neoplasm of testis**
> Use additional code to identify any functional activity

✓5ᵗʰ C62.0   **Malignant neoplasm of undescended testis**
> Malignant neoplasm of ectopic testis
> Malignant neoplasm of retained testis

C62.00   **Malignant neoplasm of unspecified undescended testis**   ♂

C62.01   **Malignant neoplasm of undescended right testis**   ♂

C62.02   **Malignant neoplasm of undescended left testis**   ♂

✓5ᵗʰ C62.1   **Malignant neoplasm of descended testis**
> Malignant neoplasm of scrotal testis

C62.10   **Malignant neoplasm of unspecified descended testis**   ♂

C62.11   **Malignant neoplasm of descended right testis**   ♂

C62.12   **Malignant neoplasm of descended left testis**   ♂

✓5ᵗʰ C62.9   **Malignant neoplasm of testis, unspecified whether descended or undescended**

C62.90   **Malignant neoplasm of unspecified testis, unspecified whether descended or undescended**   ♂
> Malignant neoplasm of testis NOS

C62.91   **Malignant neoplasm of right testis, unspecified whether descended or undescended**   ♂

C62.92   **Malignant neoplasm of left testis, unspecified whether descended or undescended**   ♂

✓4ᵗʰ C63   **Malignant neoplasm of other and unspecified male genital organs**

✓5ᵗʰ C63.0   **Malignant neoplasm of epididymis**

C63.00   **Malignant neoplasm of unspecified epididymis**   ♂

C63.01   **Malignant neoplasm of right epididymis**   ♂

C63.02   **Malignant neoplasm of left epididymis**   ♂

✓5ᵗʰ C63.1   **Malignant neoplasm of spermatic cord**

C63.10   **Malignant neoplasm of unspecified spermatic cord**   ♂

C63.11   **Malignant neoplasm of right spermatic cord**   ♂

C63.12   **Malignant neoplasm of left spermatic cord**   ♂

C63.2   **Malignant neoplasm of scrotum**   ♂
> Malignant neoplasm of skin of scrotum

C63.7   **Malignant neoplasm of other specified male genital organs**   ♂
> Malignant neoplasm of seminal vesicle
> Malignant neoplasm of tunica vaginalis

C63.8   **Malignant neoplasm of overlapping sites of male genital organs**   ♂
> Primary malignant neoplasm of two or more contiguous sites of male genital organs whose point of origin cannot be determined

C63.9   **Malignant neoplasm of male genital organ, unspecified**   ♂
> Malignant neoplasm of male genitourinary tract NOS

Malignant neoplasms of urinary tract (C64-C68)

✓4ᵗʰ C64   **Malignant neoplasm of kidney, except renal pelvis**
> **EXCLUDES 1**   malignant carcinoid tumor of the kidney (C7A.093)
> malignant neoplasm of renal calyces (C65.-)
> malignant neoplasm of renal pelvis (C65.-)

> **CC Excl: For CC codes in category C64, unless otherwise noted:** C45.7-C45.9, C64.1-C64.9, C65.1-C65.9, C68.8-C68.9, C76.8, C7A.00, C7A.093, C7A.098-C7B.00, C7B.1, C80.0-C80.2, D49.5, D49.81-D49.9

C64.1   **Malignant neoplasm of right kidney, except renal pelvis**   CC

C64.2   **Malignant neoplasm of left kidney, except renal pelvis**   CC

C64.9   **Malignant neoplasm of unspecified kidney, except renal pelvis**   CC

✓4ᵗʰ C65   **Malignant neoplasm of renal pelvis**
> **INCLUDES**   malignant neoplasm of pelviureteric junction
> malignant neoplasm of renal calyces

> **CC Excl: For CC codes in category C65, unless otherwise noted:** C45.7-C45.9, C64.1-C64.9, C65.1-C65.9, C68.8-C68.9, C76.8, C7A.00, C7A.093, C7A.098-C7B.00, C7B.1, C80.0-C80.2, D49.5, D49.81-D49.9

C65.1   **Malignant neoplasm of right renal pelvis**   CC

C65.2   **Malignant neoplasm of left renal pelvis**   CC

C65.9   **Malignant neoplasm of unspecified renal pelvis**   CC

✓4ᵗʰ C66   **Malignant neoplasm of ureter**
> **EXCLUDES 1**   malignant neoplasm of ureteric orifice of bladder (C67.6)

> **CC Excl: For CC codes in category C66, unless otherwise noted:** C45.7-C45.9, C66.1-C66.9, C68.8-C68.9, C76.8, C7A.00, C7A.098-C7B.00, C7B.1, C80.0-C80.2, D49.5, D49.81-D49.9

C66.1   **Malignant neoplasm of right ureter**   CC

C66.2   **Malignant neoplasm of left ureter**   CC

C66.9   **Malignant neoplasm of unspecified ureter**   CC

✓4ᵗʰ C67   **Malignant neoplasm of bladder**

C67.0   **Malignant neoplasm of trigone of bladder**

C67.1   **Malignant neoplasm of dome of bladder**

C67.2   **Malignant neoplasm of lateral wall of bladder**

C67.3   **Malignant neoplasm of anterior wall of bladder**

C67.4   **Malignant neoplasm of posterior wall of bladder**

C67.5   **Malignant neoplasm of bladder neck**
> Malignant neoplasm of internal urethral orifice

C67.6   **Malignant neoplasm of ureteric orifice**

C67.7   **Malignant neoplasm of urachus**

C67.8   **Malignant neoplasm of overlapping sites of bladder**

C67.9   **Malignant neoplasm of bladder, unspecified**

✓4ᵗʰ C68   **Malignant neoplasm of other and unspecified urinary organs**
> **EXCLUDES 1**   malignant neoplasm of female genitourinary tract NOS (C57.9)
> malignant neoplasm of male genitourinary tract NOS (C63.9)

C68.0   **Malignant neoplasm of urethra**   CC
> **EXCLUDES 1**   malignant neoplasm of urethral orifice of bladder (C67.5)
> CC Excl: C68.0-C68.9, C79.82

C68.1   **Malignant neoplasm of paraurethral glands**   CC
> CC Excl: See code: C68.0

C68.8   **Malignant neoplasm of overlapping sites of urinary organs**   CC
> Primary malignant neoplasm of two or more contiguous sites of urinary organs whose point of origin cannot be determined
> CC Excl: C64.1-C64.9, C65.1-C65.9, C66.1-C66.9, C68.0-C68.9, C76.3, C79.00-C79.19, C7A.093

C68.9   **Malignant neoplasm of urinary organ, unspecified**   CC
> Malignant neoplasm of urinary system NOS
> CC Excl: See code: C68.8

✓ Additional Character Required   ✓×7ᵗʰ Placeholder Alert   Unacceptable PDx   Manifestation   Hospital Acquired Condition   **EXCLUDES 1** Not Coded Here   **EXCLUDES 2** Not Included Here

Malignant neoplasms of eye, brain and other parts of central nervous system (C69-C72)

✓4ᵗʰ **C69   Malignant neoplasm of eye and adnexa**
> **EXCLUDES 1** *malignant neoplasm of connective tissue of eyelid (C49.Ø)*
> *malignant neoplasm of eyelid (skin) (C43.1-, C44.1-)*
> *malignant neoplasm of optic nerve (C72.3-)*

✓5ᵗʰ **C69.Ø   Malignant neoplasm of conjunctiva**
    C69.ØØ   Malignant neoplasm of unspecified conjunctiva
    C69.Ø1   Malignant neoplasm of right conjunctiva
    C69.Ø2   Malignant neoplasm of left conjunctiva

✓5ᵗʰ **C69.1   Malignant neoplasm of cornea**
    C69.1Ø   Malignant neoplasm of unspecified cornea
    C69.11   Malignant neoplasm of right cornea
    C69.12   Malignant neoplasm of left cornea

✓5ᵗʰ **C69.2   Malignant neoplasm of retina**
> **EXCLUDES 1** *dark area on retina (D49.81)*
> *neoplasm of unspecified behavior of retina and choroid (D49.81)*
> *retinal freckle (D49.81)*

    C69.2Ø   Malignant neoplasm of unspecified retina
    C69.21   Malignant neoplasm of right retina
    C69.22   Malignant neoplasm of left retina

✓5ᵗʰ **C69.3   Malignant neoplasm of choroid**
    C69.3Ø   Malignant neoplasm of unspecified choroid
    C69.31   Malignant neoplasm of right choroid
    C69.32   Malignant neoplasm of left choroid

✓5ᵗʰ **C69.4   Malignant neoplasm of ciliary body**
    C69.4Ø   Malignant neoplasm of unspecified ciliary body
    C69.41   Malignant neoplasm of right ciliary body
    C69.42   Malignant neoplasm of left ciliary body

✓5ᵗʰ **C69.5   Malignant neoplasm of lacrimal gland and duct**
    Malignant neoplasm of lacrimal sac
    Malignant neoplasm of nasolacrimal duct
    C69.5Ø   Malignant neoplasm of unspecified lacrimal gland and duct
    C69.51   Malignant neoplasm of right lacrimal gland and duct
    C69.52   Malignant neoplasm of left lacrimal gland and duct

✓5ᵗʰ **C69.6   Malignant neoplasm of orbit**
    Malignant neoplasm of connective tissue of orbit
    Malignant neoplasm of extraocular muscle
    Malignant neoplasm of peripheral nerves of orbit
    Malignant neoplasm of retrobulbar tissue
    Malignant neoplasm of retro-ocular tissue
> **EXCLUDES 1** *malignant neoplasm of orbital bone (C41.Ø)*

    C69.6Ø   Malignant neoplasm of unspecified orbit
    C69.61   Malignant neoplasm of right orbit
    C69.62   Malignant neoplasm of left orbit

✓5ᵗʰ **C69.8   Malignant neoplasm of overlapping sites of eye and adnexa**
    C69.8Ø   Malignant neoplasm of overlapping sites of unspecified eye and adnexa
    C69.81   Malignant neoplasm of overlapping sites of right eye and adnexa
    C69.82   Malignant neoplasm of overlapping sites of left eye and adnexa

✓5ᵗʰ **C69.9   Malignant neoplasm of unspecified site of eye**
    Malignant neoplasm of eyeball
    C69.9Ø   Malignant neoplasm of unspecified site of unspecified eye
    C69.91   Malignant neoplasm of unspecified site of right eye
    C69.92   Malignant neoplasm of unspecified site of left eye

✓4ᵗʰ **C7Ø   Malignant neoplasm of meninges**
    C7Ø.Ø   Malignant neoplasm of cerebral meninges [CC]
      CC Excl: C45.7-C45.9, C7Ø.Ø, C7Ø.9, C72.9, C76.8, C7A.ØØ, C7A.Ø98-C7B.ØØ, C7B.1, C8Ø.Ø-C8Ø.2, D49.6-D49.9
    C7Ø.1   Malignant neoplasm of spinal meninges [CC]
      CC Excl: C45.7-C45.9, C7Ø.1, C72.9, C76.8, C7A.ØØ, C7A.Ø98-C7B.ØØ, C7B.1, C8Ø.Ø-C8Ø.2, D49.6-D49.9
    C7Ø.9   Malignant neoplasm of meninges, unspecified [CC]
      CC Excl: See code: C7Ø.Ø

✓4ᵗʰ **C71   Malignant neoplasm of brain**
> **EXCLUDES 1** *malignant neoplasm of cranial nerves (C72.2-C72.5)*
> *retrobulbar malignant neoplasm (C69.6-)*

> **CC Excl: For CC codes in category C71, unless otherwise noted:** C45.7-C45.9, C7Ø.Ø, C7Ø.9-C71.9, C72.2Ø-C72.9, C76.8, C7A.ØØ, C7A.Ø98-C7B.ØØ, C7B.1, C8Ø.Ø-C8Ø.2, D49.6-D49.9

    C71.Ø   Malignant neoplasm of cerebrum, except lobes and ventricles [CC]
      Malignant neoplasm of supratentorial NOS
    C71.1   Malignant neoplasm of frontal lobe [CC]
    C71.2   Malignant neoplasm of temporal lobe [CC]
    C71.3   Malignant neoplasm of parietal lobe [CC]
    C71.4   Malignant neoplasm of occipital lobe [CC]
    C71.5   Malignant neoplasm of cerebral ventricle [CC]
> **EXCLUDES 1** *malignant neoplasm of fourth cerebral ventricle (C71.7)*

    C71.6   Malignant neoplasm of cerebellum [CC]
    C71.7   Malignant neoplasm of brain stem [CC]
      Malignant neoplasm of fourth cerebral ventricle
      Infratentorial malignant neoplasm NOS
    C71.8   Malignant neoplasm of overlapping sites of brain [CC]
    C71.9   Malignant neoplasm of brain, unspecified [CC]
      AHA: 2014, 3Q, 3

✓4ᵗʰ **C72   Malignant neoplasm of spinal cord, cranial nerves and other parts of central nervous system**
> **EXCLUDES 1** *malignant neoplasm of meninges (C7Ø.-)*
> *malignant neoplasm of peripheral nerves and autonomic nervous system (C47.-)*

    C72.Ø   Malignant neoplasm of spinal cord [CC]
      CC Excl: C45.7-C45.9, C72.Ø-C72.1, C72.9, C76.8, C7A.ØØ, C7A.Ø98-C7B.ØØ, C7B.1, C8Ø.Ø-C8Ø.2, D49.6-D49.9
    C72.1   Malignant neoplasm of cauda equina [CC]
      CC Excl: See code: C72.Ø

✓5ᵗʰ **C72.2   Malignant neoplasm of olfactory nerve**
    Malignant neoplasm of olfactory bulb
> **CC Excl: For CC codes in subcategory C72.2, unless otherwise noted:** C45.7-C45.9, C72.2Ø-C72.9, C76.8, C7A.ØØ, C7A.Ø98-C7B.ØØ, C7B.1, C8Ø.Ø-C8Ø.2, D49.6-D49.9

    C72.2Ø   Malignant neoplasm of unspecified olfactory nerve [CC]
    C72.21   Malignant neoplasm of right olfactory nerve [CC]
    C72.22   Malignant neoplasm of left olfactory nerve [CC]

✓5ᵗʰ **C72.3   Malignant neoplasm of optic nerve**
> **CC Excl: For CC codes in subcategory C72.3, unless otherwise noted:** C45.7-C45.9, C72.2Ø-C72.9, C76.8, C7A.ØØ, C7A.Ø98-C7B.ØØ, C7B.1, C8Ø.Ø-C8Ø.2, D49.6-D49.9

    C72.3Ø   Malignant neoplasm of unspecified optic nerve [CC]
    C72.31   Malignant neoplasm of right optic nerve [CC]
    C72.32   Malignant neoplasm of left optic nerve [CC]

✓5ᵗʰ **C72.4   Malignant neoplasm of acoustic nerve**
> **CC Excl: For CC codes in subcategory C72.4, unless otherwise noted:** C45.7-C45.9, C72.2Ø-C72.9, C76.8, C7A.ØØ, C7A.Ø98-C7B.ØØ, C7B.1, C8Ø.Ø-C8Ø.2, D49.6-D49.9

    C72.4Ø   Malignant neoplasm of unspecified acoustic nerve [CC]
    C72.41   Malignant neoplasm of right acoustic nerve [CC]
    C72.42   Malignant neoplasm of left acoustic nerve [CC]

✓5ᵗʰ **C72.5   Malignant neoplasm of other and unspecified cranial nerves**
> **CC Excl: For CC codes in subcategory C72.5, unless otherwise noted:** C45.7-C45.9, C72.2Ø-C72.9, C76.8, C7A.ØØ, C7A.Ø98-C7B.ØØ, C7B.1, C8Ø.Ø-C8Ø.2, D49.6-D49.9

    C72.5Ø   Malignant neoplasm of unspecified cranial nerve [CC]
      Malignant neoplasm of cranial nerve NOS
    C72.59   Malignant neoplasm of other cranial nerves [CC]

    C72.9   Malignant neoplasm of central nervous system, unspecified [CC]
      Malignant neoplasm of unspecified site of central nervous system
      Malignant neoplasm of nervous system NOS
      CC Excl: C45.7-C45.9, C7Ø.Ø-C72.9, C7A.ØØ, C7A.Ø98-C7B.ØØ, C7B.1, C76.8, C79.31-C79.49, C8Ø.Ø-C8Ø.2, D49.6-D49.9

Ⓝ Newborn: 0 Ⓟ Pediatric: 0-17 Ⓜ Maternity: 12-55 Ⓐ Adult: 15-124 **MCC** Major CC Condition **PDx MCC** PDx acts as own MCC **CC** CC Condition **PDx CC** PDx acts as own CC

466

ICD-10-CM 2016

Malignant neoplasms of thyroid and other endocrine glands (C73-C75)

C73 Malignant neoplasm of thyroid gland
Use additional code to identify any functional activity

☑4ᵗʰ **C74 Malignant neoplasm of adrenal gland**

> **CC Excl: For CC codes in category C74, unless otherwise noted:** C45.7-C45.9, C74.00-C74.92, C75.9-C7A.00, C7A.098-C7B.00, C7B.1, C76.2, C76.8, C79.70-C79.72, C80.0-C80.2

☑5ᵗʰ **C74.0 Malignant neoplasm of cortex of adrenal gland**
  C74.00 Malignant neoplasm of cortex of unspecified adrenal gland [CC]
  C74.01 Malignant neoplasm of cortex of right adrenal gland [CC]
  C74.02 Malignant neoplasm of cortex of left adrenal gland [CC]

☑5ᵗʰ **C74.1 Malignant neoplasm of medulla of adrenal gland**
  C74.10 Malignant neoplasm of medulla of unspecified adrenal gland [CC]
  C74.11 Malignant neoplasm of medulla of right adrenal gland [CC]
  C74.12 Malignant neoplasm of medulla of left adrenal gland [CC]

☑5ᵗʰ **C74.9 Malignant neoplasm of unspecified part of adrenal gland**
  C74.90 Malignant neoplasm of unspecified part of unspecified adrenal gland [CC]
  C74.91 Malignant neoplasm of unspecified part of right adrenal gland [CC]
  C74.92 Malignant neoplasm of unspecified part of left adrenal gland [CC]

☑4ᵗʰ **C75 Malignant neoplasm of other endocrine glands and related structures**
  EXCLUDES 1 malignant carcinoid tumors (C7A.0-)
  malignant neoplasm of adrenal gland (C74.-)
  malignant neoplasm of endocrine pancreas (C25.4)
  malignant neoplasm of islets of Langerhans (C25.4)
  malignant neoplasm of ovary (C56.-)
  malignant neoplasm of testis (C62.-)
  malignant neoplasm of thymus (C37)
  malignant neoplasm of thyroid gland (C73)
  malignant neuroendocrine tumors (C7A.-)

  C75.0 Malignant neoplasm of parathyroid gland [CC]
    CC Excl: C75.0-C75.9
  C75.1 Malignant neoplasm of pituitary gland [CC]
    CC Excl: C75.1-C75.2, Z51.0
  C75.2 Malignant neoplasm of craniopharyngeal duct [CC]
    CC Excl: See code: C75.1
  C75.3 Malignant neoplasm of pineal gland [CC]
    CC Excl: C75.3-Z51.0
  C75.4 Malignant neoplasm of carotid body [CC]
    CC Excl: C75.4-C75.9
  C75.5 Malignant neoplasm of aortic body and other paraganglia [CC]
    CC Excl: See code: C75.4
  C75.8 Malignant neoplasm with pluriglandular involvement, unspecified [CC]
    CC Excl: C74.00-C75.9
  C75.9 Malignant neoplasm of endocrine gland, unspecified [CC]
    CC Excl: See code: C75.8

Malignant neuroendocrine tumors (C7A)

☑4ᵗʰ **C7A Malignant neuroendocrine tumors**
  Code also any associated multiple endocrine neoplasia [MEN] syndromes (E31.2-)
  Use additional code to identify any associated endocrine syndrome, such as:
  carcinoid syndrome (E34.0)
  EXCLUDES 2 malignant pancreatic islet cell tumors (C25.4)
  Merkel cell carcinoma (C4A.-)

☑5ᵗʰ **C7A.0 Malignant carcinoid tumors**
  C7A.00 Malignant carcinoid tumor of unspecified site [CC]
    CC Excl: C45.7-C45.9, C76.8, C79.89-C7B.00, C7B.09-C80.2, D49.81-D49.9

☑6ᵗʰ **C7A.01 Malignant carcinoid tumors of the small intestine**
  C7A.010 Malignant carcinoid tumor of the duodenum [CC]
    CC Excl: C17.0-C17.9, C26.0, C26.9, C45.7-C45.9, C46.4, C76.8, C7A.00-C7B.00, C7B.1, C80.0-C80.2, D49.0, D49.81-D49.9
  C7A.011 Malignant carcinoid tumor of the jejunum [CC]
    CC Excl: C17.1-C17.9, C26.0, C26.9, C45.7-C45.9, C46.4, C76.8, C7A.00-C7B.00, C7B.1, C80.0-C80.2, D49.0, D49.81-D49.9
  C7A.012 Malignant carcinoid tumor of the ileum [CC]
    CC Excl: C17.2-C17.9, C26.0, C26.9, C45.7-C45.9, C46.4, C76.8, C7A.00-C7B.00, C7B.1, C80.0-C80.2, D49.0, D49.81-D49.9
  C7A.019 Malignant carcinoid tumor of the small intestine, unspecified portion [CC]
    CC Excl: C17.8-C17.9, C26.0, C26.9, C45.7-C45.9, C46.4, C76.8, C7A.00-C7B.00, C7B.1, C80.0-C80.2, D49.0, D49.81-D49.9

☑6ᵗʰ **C7A.02 Malignant carcinoid tumors of the appendix, large intestine, and rectum**
  C7A.020 Malignant carcinoid tumor of the appendix [CC]
    CC Excl: C18.1-C18.9, C26.0, C26.9, C45.7-C45.9, C46.4, C76.8, C7A.00-C7B.00, C7B.1, C80.0-C80.2, D49.0, D49.81-D49.9
  C7A.021 Malignant carcinoid tumor of the cecum [CC]
    CC Excl: C18.0-C18.9, C26.0, C26.9, C45.7-C45.9, C46.4, C76.8, C7A.00-C7B.00, C7B.1, C80.0-C80.2, D49.0, D49.81-D49.9
  C7A.022 Malignant carcinoid tumor of the ascending colon [CC]
    CC Excl: C18.2-C18.9, C26.0, C26.9, C45.7-C45.9, C46.4, C76.8, C7A.00-C7B.00, C7B.1, C80.0-C80.2, D49.0, D49.81-D49.9
  C7A.023 Malignant carcinoid tumor of the transverse colon [CC]
    CC Excl: C18.4-C18.9, C26.0, C26.9, C45.7-C45.9, C46.4, C76.8, C7A.00-C7B.00, C7B.1, C80.0-C80.2, D49.0, D49.81-D49.9
  C7A.024 Malignant carcinoid tumor of the descending colon [CC]
    CC Excl: C18.6-C18.9, C26.0, C26.9, C45.7-C45.9, C46.4, C76.8, C7A.00-C7B.00, C7B.1, C80.0-C80.2, D49.0, D49.81-D49.9
  C7A.025 Malignant carcinoid tumor of the sigmoid colon [CC]
    CC Excl: C18.7-C18.9, C26.0, C26.9, C45.7-C45.9, C46.4, C76.8, C7A.00-C7B.00, C7B.1, C80.0-C80.2, D49.0, D49.81-D49.9
  C7A.026 Malignant carcinoid tumor of the rectum [CC]
    CC Excl: C20-C21.8, C26.0, C26.9, C45.7-C45.9, C46.4, C76.8, C7A.00-C7B.00, C7B.1, C80.0-C80.2, D49.0, D49.81-D49.9
  C7A.029 Malignant carcinoid tumor of the large intestine, unspecified portion [CC]
    Malignant carcinoid tumor of the colon NOS
    CC Excl: C18.8-C18.9, C26.0, C26.9, C45.7-C45.9, C46.4, C76.8, C7A.00-C7B.00, C7B.1, C80.0-C80.2, D49.0, D49.81-D49.9

☑6ᵗʰ **C7A.09 Malignant carcinoid tumors of other sites**
  C7A.090 Malignant carcinoid tumor of the bronchus and lung [CC]
    CC Excl: C34.80-C34.92, C39.9, C45.7-C45.9, C46.50-C46.52, C76.8, C7A.00-C7B.00, C7B.1, C80.0-C80.2, D49.1, D49.81-D49.9
  C7A.091 Malignant carcinoid tumor of the thymus [CC]
    CC Excl: C37-C7A.8
  C7A.092 Malignant carcinoid tumor of the stomach [CC]
    CC Excl: C16.0-C16.9, C26.0, C26.9, C45.7-C45.9, C46.4, C76.8, C7A.00-C7B.00, C7B.1, C80.0-C80.2, D49.0, D49.81-D49.9
  C7A.093 Malignant carcinoid tumor of the kidney [CC]
    CC Excl: C45.7-C45.9, C64.1-C64.9, C65.1-C65.9, C68.8-C68.9, C76.8, C7A.00-C7B.00, C7B.1, C80.0-C80.2, D49.5, D49.81-D49.9

☑ Additional Character Required ☑x7ᵗʰ Placeholder Alert   Unacceptable PDx   Manifestation   Hospital Acquired Condition   **EXCLUDES 1** Not Coded Here   **EXCLUDES 2** Not Included Here

ICD-10-CM 2016   **467**

Chapter 2. Neoplasms

C7A.094–C78.7

C7A.094 Malignant carcinoid tumor of the foregut NOS `cc`
    CC Excl: See code: C7A.092

C7A.095 Malignant carcinoid tumor of the midgut NOS `cc`
    CC Excl: See code: C7A.092

C7A.096 Malignant carcinoid tumor of the hindgut NOS `cc`
    CC Excl: See code: C7A.092

C7A.098 Malignant carcinoid tumors of other sites `cc`
    CC Excl: See code: C7A.00

C7A.1 Malignant poorly differentiated neuroendocrine tumors `cc`
High grade neuroendocrine carcinoma, any site
Malignant poorly differentiated neuroendocrine tumor NOS
Malignant poorly differentiated neuroendocrine carcinoma, any site
    CC Excl: See code: C7A.00

C7A.8 Other malignant neuroendocrine tumors `cc`
    CC Excl: See code: C7A.00

Secondary neuroendocrine tumors (C7B)

✓4ᵗʰ **C7B Secondary neuroendocrine tumors**
Use additional code to identify any functional activity

✓5ᵗʰ **C7B.0 Secondary carcinoid tumors**

C7B.00 Secondary carcinoid tumors, unspecified site

C7B.01 Secondary carcinoid tumors of distant lymph nodes `cc`
    CC Excl: C45.7-C45.9, C46.3, C76.8-C77.9, C7A.00, C7A.098-C80.2, D49.81-D49.9

C7B.02 Secondary carcinoid tumors of liver `cc`
    CC Excl: C45.7-C45.9, C76.8, C78.7-C78.89, C79.89-C7A.00, C7A.098-C80.2, D49.81-D49.9

C7B.03 Secondary carcinoid tumors of bone `cc`
    CC Excl: C45.7-C45.9, C76.8, C79.51-C79.52, C79.89-C7A.00, C7A.098-C80.2, D49.81-D49.9

C7B.04 Secondary carcinoid tumors of peritoneum `cc`
Mesentery metastasis of carcinoid tumor
    CC Excl: C45.7-C45.9, C76.8, C78.6, C78.80-C78.89, C79.89-C7A.00, C7A.098-C80.2, D49.81-D49.9

C7B.09 Secondary carcinoid tumors of other sites `cc`
    CC Excl: C45.7-C45.9, C76.8, C79.89-C7A.00, C7A.098-C80.2, D49.81-D49.9

C7B.1 Secondary Merkel cell carcinoma
Merkel cell carcinoma nodal presentation
Merkel cell carcinoma visceral metastatic presentation

C7B.8 Other secondary neuroendocrine tumors `cc`
    CC Excl: See code: C7B.09

Malignant neoplasms of ill-defined, other secondary and unspecified sites (C76-C80)

✓4ᵗʰ **C76 Malignant neoplasm of other and ill-defined sites**
    EXCLUDES 1   malignant neoplasm of female genitourinary tract NOS (C57.9)
malignant neoplasm of male genitourinary tract NOS (C63.9)
malignant neoplasm of lymphoid, hematopoietic and related tissue (C81-C96)
malignant neoplasm of skin (C44.-)
malignant neoplasm of unspecified site NOS (C80.1)

C76.0 Malignant neoplasm of head, face and neck
Malignant neoplasm of cheek NOS
Malignant neoplasm of nose NOS

C76.1 Malignant neoplasm of thorax
Intrathoracic malignant neoplasm NOS
Malignant neoplasm of axilla NOS
Thoracic malignant neoplasm NOS

C76.2 Malignant neoplasm of abdomen

C76.3 Malignant neoplasm of pelvis
Malignant neoplasm of groin NOS
Malignant neoplasm of sites overlapping systems within the pelvis
Rectovaginal (septum) malignant neoplasm
Rectovesical (septum) malignant neoplasm

✓5ᵗʰ **C76.4 Malignant neoplasm of upper limb**

C76.40 Malignant neoplasm of unspecified upper limb

C76.41 Malignant neoplasm of right upper limb

C76.42 Malignant neoplasm of left upper limb

✓5ᵗʰ **C76.5 Malignant neoplasm of lower limb**

C76.50 Malignant neoplasm of unspecified lower limb

C76.51 Malignant neoplasm of right lower limb

C76.52 Malignant neoplasm of left lower limb

C76.8 Malignant neoplasm of other specified ill-defined sites
Malignant neoplasm of overlapping ill-defined sites

✓4ᵗʰ **C77 Secondary and unspecified malignant neoplasm of lymph nodes**
    EXCLUDES 1   malignant neoplasm of lymph nodes, specified as primary (C81-C86, C88, C96.-)
mesentery metastasis of carcinoid tumor (C7B.04)
secondary carcinoid tumors of distant lymph nodes (C7B.01)

> **CC Excl:** For CC codes in category C77, unless otherwise noted: C45.7-C45.9, C46.3, C76.8-C77.9, C7A.00, C7A.098-C7B.01, C7B.1, C80.0-C80.2, D49.81-D49.9

C77.0 Secondary and unspecified malignant neoplasm of lymph nodes of head, face and neck `cc`
Secondary and unspecified malignant neoplasm of supraclavicular lymph nodes

C77.1 Secondary and unspecified malignant neoplasm of intrathoracic lymph nodes `cc`

C77.2 Secondary and unspecified malignant neoplasm of intra-abdominal lymph nodes `cc`

C77.3 Secondary and unspecified malignant neoplasm of axilla and upper limb lymph nodes `cc`
Secondary and unspecified malignant neoplasm of pectoral lymph nodes

C77.4 Secondary and unspecified malignant neoplasm of inguinal and lower limb lymph nodes `cc`

C77.5 Secondary and unspecified malignant neoplasm of intrapelvic lymph nodes `cc`

C77.8 Secondary and unspecified malignant neoplasm of lymph nodes of multiple regions `cc`

C77.9 Secondary and unspecified malignant neoplasm of lymph node, unspecified `cc`

✓4ᵗʰ **C78 Secondary malignant neoplasm of respiratory and digestive organs**
    EXCLUDES 1   lymph node metastases (C77.0)
secondary carcinoid tumors of liver (C7B.02)
secondary carcinoid tumors of peritoneum (C7B.04)

✓5ᵗʰ **C78.0 Secondary malignant neoplasm of lung**

C78.00 Secondary malignant neoplasm of unspecified lung `cc`
    CC Excl: C45.7-C45.9, C76.8, C78.00-C78.02, C78.30-C78.39, C79.89-C7A.00, C7A.098-C7B.00, C7B.09-C80.2, D49.81-D49.9

C78.01 Secondary malignant neoplasm of right lung `cc`
    CC Excl: See code: C78.00

C78.02 Secondary malignant neoplasm of left lung `cc`
    CC Excl: See code: C78.00

C78.1 Secondary malignant neoplasm of mediastinum `cc`
    CC Excl: C45.7-C45.9, C76.8, C78.1, C78.30-C78.39, C79.89-C7A.00, C7A.098-C7B.00, C7B.09-C80.2, D49.81-D49.9

C78.2 Secondary malignant neoplasm of pleura `cc`
    CC Excl: C45.7-C45.9, C76.8, C78.2-C78.39, C79.89-C7A.00, C7A.098-C7B.00, C7B.09-C80.2, D49.81-D49.9, J91.0

✓5ᵗʰ **C78.3 Secondary malignant neoplasm of other and unspecified respiratory organs**

C78.30 Secondary malignant neoplasm of unspecified respiratory organ `cc`
    CC Excl: C45.7-C45.9, C76.8, C78.00-C78.39, C79.89-C7A.00, C7A.098-C7B.00, C7B.09-C80.2, D49.81-D49.9

C78.39 Secondary malignant neoplasm of other respiratory organs `cc`
    CC Excl: See code: C78.30

C78.4 Secondary malignant neoplasm of small intestine `cc`
    CC Excl: C45.7-C45.9, C76.8, C78.4, C78.80-C78.89, C79.89-C7A.00, C7A.098-C7B.00, C7B.09-C80.2, D49.81-D49.9

C78.5 Secondary malignant neoplasm of large intestine and rectum `cc`
    CC Excl: C45.7-C45.9, C76.8, C78.5, C78.80-C78.89, C79.89-C7A.00, C7A.098-C7B.00, C7B.09-C80.2, D49.81-D49.9

C78.6 Secondary malignant neoplasm of retroperitoneum and peritoneum `cc`
    CC Excl: C45.7-C45.9, C76.8, C78.6, C78.80-C78.89, C79.89-C7A.00, C7A.098-C7B.00, C7B.04-C80.2, D49.81-D49.9

C78.7 Secondary malignant neoplasm of liver and intrahepatic bile duct `cc`
    CC Excl: C45.7-C45.9, C76.8, C78.7-C78.89, C79.89-C7A.00, C7A.098-C7B.00, C7B.02, C7B.09-C80.2, D49.81-D49.9

Ⓝ Newborn: 0   Ⓟ Pediatric: 0-17   Ⓜ Maternity: 12-55   Ⓐ Adult: 15-124   MCC Major CC Condition   PDxMCC PDx acts as own MCC   CC CC Condition   PDxCC PDx acts as own CC

468   ICD-10-CM 2016

C78.8 Secondary malignant neoplasm of other and unspecified digestive organs

> **C78.80 Secondary malignant neoplasm of** unspecified digestive organ   `CC`
> **CC Excl:** C45.7-C45.9, C76.8, C78.4-C78.89, C79.89-C7A.00, C7A.098-C7B.00, C7B.02, C7B.04-C80.2, D49.81-D49.9

> **C78.89 Secondary malignant neoplasm of** other digestive organs   `CC`
> **CC Excl:** See code: C78.80

C79 Secondary malignant neoplasm of other and unspecified sites
> *EXCLUDES 1*   lymph node metastases (C77.0)
> secondary carcinoid tumors (C7B.-)
> secondary neuroendocrine tumors (C7B.-)

C79.0 Secondary malignant neoplasm of kidney and renal pelvis

> **CC Excl: For CC codes in subcategory C79.0, unless otherwise noted:** C45.7-C45.9, C76.8, C79.00-C79.19, C79.89-C7A.00, C7A.098-C7B.00, C7B.09-C80.2, D49.81-D49.9

> **C79.00 Secondary malignant neoplasm of** unspecified kidney and renal pelvis   `CC`

> **C79.01 Secondary malignant neoplasm of** right kidney and renal pelvis   `CC`

> **C79.02 Secondary malignant neoplasm of** left kidney and renal pelvis   `CC`

C79.1 Secondary malignant neoplasm of bladder and other and unspecified urinary organs

> **CC Excl: For CC codes in subcategory C79.1, unless otherwise noted:** C45.7-C45.9, C76.8, C79.00-C79.19, C79.89-C7A.00, C7A.098-C7B.00, C7B.09-C80.2, D49.81-D49.9

> **C79.10 Secondary malignant neoplasm of** unspecified urinary organs   `CC`

> **C79.11 Secondary malignant neoplasm of** bladder   `CC`

> **C79.19 Secondary malignant neoplasm of** other urinary organs   `CC`

C79.2 Secondary malignant neoplasm of skin   `CC`
> *EXCLUDES 1*   secondary Merkel cell carcinoma (C7B.1)
> **CC Excl:** C45.7-C45.9, C76.8, C79.2, C79.89-C7A.00, C7A.098-C7B.00, C7B.09-C80.2, D49.81-D49.9

C79.3 Secondary malignant neoplasm of brain and cerebral meninges

> **C79.31 Secondary malignant neoplasm of** brain   `CC`
> **CC Excl:** C45.7-C45.9, C76.8, C79.31, C79.89-C7A.00, C7A.098-C7B.00, C7B.09-C80.2, D49.81-D49.9

> **C79.32 Secondary malignant neoplasm of** cerebral meninges   `CC`
> **CC Excl:** C45.7-C45.9, C76.8, C79.32-C79.49, C79.89-C7A.00, C7A.098-C7B.00, C7B.09-C80.2, D49.81-D49.9

C79.4 Secondary malignant neoplasm of other and unspecified parts of nervous system

> **C79.40 Secondary malignant neoplasm of** unspecified part of nervous system   `CC`
> **CC Excl:** See code: C79.32

> **C79.49 Secondary malignant neoplasm of** other parts of nervous system   `CC`
> **CC Excl:** See code: C79.32

C79.5 Secondary malignant neoplasm of bone and bone marrow
> *EXCLUDES 1*   secondary carcinoid tumors of bone (C7B.03)

> **C79.51 Secondary malignant neoplasm of** bone   `CC`
> **CC Excl:** C45.7-C45.9, C76.8, C79.51-C79.52, C79.89-C7A.00, C7A.098-C7B.00, C7B.03, C7B.09-C80.2, D49.81-D49.9

> **C79.52 Secondary malignant neoplasm of** bone marrow   `CC`
> **CC Excl:** See code: C79.51

C79.6 Secondary malignant neoplasm of ovary

> **CC Excl: For CC codes in subcategory C79.6, unless otherwise noted:** C45.7-C45.9, C76.8, C79.60-C79.62, C79.89-C7A.00, C7A.098-C7B.00, C7B.09-C80.2, D49.81-D49.9

> **C79.60 Secondary malignant neoplasm of** unspecified ovary   `CC`♀

> **C79.61 Secondary malignant neoplasm of** right ovary   `CC`♀

> **C79.62 Secondary malignant neoplasm of** left ovary   `CC`♀

C79.7 Secondary malignant neoplasm of adrenal gland

> **CC Excl: For CC codes in subcategory C79.7, unless otherwise noted:** C45.7-C45.9, C76.8, C79.70-C79.72, C79.89-C7A.00, C7A.098-C7B.00, C7B.09-C80.2, D49.81-D49.9

> **C79.70 Secondary malignant neoplasm of** unspecified adrenal gland   `CC`

> **C79.71 Secondary malignant neoplasm of** right adrenal gland   `CC`

> **C79.72 Secondary malignant neoplasm of** left adrenal gland   `CC`

C79.8 Secondary malignant neoplasm of other specified sites

> **C79.81 Secondary malignant neoplasm of** breast   `CC`
> **CC Excl:** C45.7-C45.9, C76.8, C79.81, C79.89-C7A.00, C7A.098-C7B.00, C7B.09-C80.2, D49.81-D49.9

> **C79.82 Secondary malignant neoplasm of** genital organs   `CC`
> **CC Excl:** C45.7-C45.9, C76.8, C79.82-C7A.00, C7A.098-C7B.00, C7B.09-C80.2, D49.81-D49.9

> **C79.89 Secondary malignant neoplasm of** other specified sites   `CC`
> **CC Excl:** C45.7-C45.9, C76.8, C79.89-C7A.00, C7A.098-C7B.00, C7B.09-C80.2, D49.81-D49.9

C79.9 Secondary malignant neoplasm of unspecified site   `CC`
> Metastatic cancer NOS
> Metastatic disease NOS
> *EXCLUDES 1*   carcinomatosis NOS (C80.0)
> generalized cancer NOS (C80.0)
> malignant (primary) neoplasm of unspecified site (C80.1)
> **CC Excl:** See code: C79.89

C80 Malignant neoplasm without specification of site
> *EXCLUDES 1*   malignant carcinoid tumor of unspecified site (C7A.00)
> malignant neoplasm of specified multiple sites—code to each site

C80.0 Disseminated malignant neoplasm, unspecified   `CC`
> Carcinomatosis NOS
> Generalized cancer, unspecified site (primary) (secondary)
> Generalized malignancy, unspecified site (primary) (secondary)
> **CC Excl:** See code: C79.89

C80.1 Malignant (primary) neoplasm, unspecified
> Cancer NOS
> Cancer unspecified site (primary)
> Carcinoma unspecified site (primary)
> Malignancy unspecified site (primary)
> *EXCLUDES 1*   secondary malignant neoplasm of unspecified site (C79.9)

C80.2 Malignant neoplasm associated with transplanted organ   `CC`
> Code first complication of transplanted organ (T86.-)
> Use additional code to identify the specific malignancy
> **CC Excl:** See code: C79.89

Malignant neoplasms of lymphoid, hematopoietic and related tissue (C81-C96)

> *EXCLUDES 2*   Kaposi's sarcoma of lymph nodes (C46.3)
> secondary and unspecified neoplasm of lymph nodes (C77.-)
> secondary neoplasm of bone marrow (C79.52)
> secondary neoplasm of spleen (C78.89)

C81 Hodgkin lymphoma
> *EXCLUDES 1*   personal history of Hodgkin lymphoma (Z85.71)

C81.0 Nodular lymphocyte predominant Hodgkin lymphoma

> **C81.00 Nodular lymphocyte predominant Hodgkin lymphoma,** unspecified site   `CC`
> **CC Excl:** C81.00-C81.09, C81.40-C81.49, C81.90, C81.98, D49.81-D49.9

> **C81.01 Nodular lymphocyte predominant Hodgkin lymphoma,** lymph nodes of head, face, and neck   `CC`
> **CC Excl:** C81.00-C81.01, C81.08-C81.09, C81.40-C81.41, C81.48-C81.49, C81.90-C81.91, C81.98, D49.81-D49.9

> **C81.02 Nodular lymphocyte predominant Hodgkin lymphoma,** intrathoracic lymph nodes   `CC`
> **CC Excl:** C81.00-C81.02, C81.08-C81.09, C81.40, C81.42, C81.48-C81.49, C81.90, C81.92, C81.98, D49.81-D49.9

> **C81.03 Nodular lymphocyte predominant Hodgkin lymphoma,** intra-abdominal lymph nodes   `CC`
> **CC Excl:** C81.00, C81.03, C81.08-C81.09, C81.40, C81.43, C81.48-C81.49, C81.90, C81.93, C81.98, D49.81-D49.9

> **C81.04 Nodular lymphocyte predominant Hodgkin lymphoma,** lymph nodes of axilla and upper limb   `CC`
> **CC Excl:** C81.00, C81.04, C81.08-C81.09, C81.40, C81.44, C81.48-C81.49, C81.90, C81.94, C81.98, D49.81-D49.9

✔ Additional Character Required   ✔x7ᵗʰ Placeholder Alert   Unacceptable PDx   Manifestation   Hospital Acquired Condition   *EXCLUDES 1* Not Coded Here   *EXCLUDES 2* Not Included Here

ICD-10-CM 2016   469

Chapter 2. Neoplasms

C81.05   **Nodular lymphocyte predominant Hodgkin lymphoma, lymph nodes of inguinal region and lower limb** `CC`
CC Excl: C81.00, C81.05, C81.08-C81.09, C81.40, C81.45, C81.48-C81.49, C81.90, C81.95, C81.98, D49.81-D49.9

C81.06   **Nodular lymphocyte predominant Hodgkin lymphoma, intrapelvic lymph nodes** `CC`
CC Excl: C81.00, C81.06, C81.08-C81.09, C81.40, C81.46, C81.48-C81.49, C81.90, C81.96, C81.98, D49.81-D49.9

C81.07   **Nodular lymphocyte predominant Hodgkin lymphoma, spleen** `CC`
CC Excl: C81.00, C81.07-C81.09, C81.40, C81.47-C81.49, C81.90, C81.97-C81.98, D49.81-D49.99

C81.08   **Nodular lymphocyte predominant Hodgkin lymphoma, lymph nodes of multiple sites** `CC`
CC Excl: C81.00-C81.09, C81.40-C81.49, C81.90, C81.98, D49.81-D49.9

C81.09   **Nodular lymphocyte predominant Hodgkin lymphoma, extranodal and solid organ sites** `CC`
CC Excl: See code: C81.08

✓5ᵗʰ **C81.1**   **Nodular sclerosis classical Hodgkin lymphoma**

C81.10   **Nodular sclerosis classical Hodgkin lymphoma, unspecified site** `CC`
CC Excl: C81.10-C81.19, C81.90, C81.98, D49.81-D49.9

C81.11   **Nodular sclerosis classical Hodgkin lymphoma, lymph nodes of head, face, and neck** `CC`
CC Excl: C81.10-C81.11, C81.18-C81.19, C81.90-C81.91, C81.98, D49.81-D49.9

C81.12   **Nodular sclerosis classical Hodgkin lymphoma, intrathoracic lymph nodes** `CC`
CC Excl: C81.10, C81.12, C81.18-C81.19, C81.90, C81.92, C81.98, D49.81-D49.9

C81.13   **Nodular sclerosis classical Hodgkin lymphoma, intra-abdominal lymph nodes** `CC`
CC Excl: C81.10, C81.13, C81.18-C81.19, C81.90, C81.93, C81.98, D49.81-D49.9

C81.14   **Nodular sclerosis classical Hodgkin lymphoma, lymph nodes of axilla and upper limb** `CC`
CC Excl: C81.10, C81.14, C81.18-C81.19, C81.90, C81.94, C81.98, D49.81-D49.9

C81.15   **Nodular sclerosis classical Hodgkin lymphoma, lymph nodes of inguinal region and lower limb** `CC`
CC Excl: C81.10, C81.15, C81.18-C81.19, C81.90, C81.95. C81.98, D49.81-D49.9

C81.16   **Nodular sclerosis classical Hodgkin lymphoma, intrapelvic lymph nodes** `CC`
CC Excl: C81.10, C81.16, C81.18-C81.19, C81.90, C81.96, C81.98, D49.81-D49.9

C81.17   **Nodular sclerosis classical Hodgkin lymphoma, spleen** `CC`
CC Excl: C81.10, C81.17-C81.19, C81.90, C81.97-C81.98, D49.81-D49.9

C81.18   **Nodular sclerosis classical Hodgkin lymphoma, lymph nodes of multiple sites** `CC`
CC Excl: C81.10-C81.19, C81.90, C81.98, D49.81-D49.9

C81.19   **Nodular sclerosis classical Hodgkin lymphoma, extranodal and solid organ sites** `CC`
CC Excl: See code: C81.18

✓5ᵗʰ **C81.2**   **Mixed cellularity classical Hodgkin lymphoma**

C81.20   **Mixed cellularity classical Hodgkin lymphoma, unspecified site** `CC`
CC Excl: C81.20-C81.29, C81.90, C81.98, D49.81-D49.9

C81.21   **Mixed cellularity classical Hodgkin lymphoma, lymph nodes of head, face, and neck** `CC`
CC Excl: C81.20-C81.21, C81.28-C81.29, C81.90-C81.91, C81.98, D49.81-D49.9

C81.22   **Mixed cellularity classical Hodgkin lymphoma, intrathoracic lymph nodes** `CC`
CC Excl: C81.20, C81.22, C81.28-C81.29, C81.90, C81.92, C81.98, D49.81-D49.9

C81.23   **Mixed cellularity classical Hodgkin lymphoma, intra-abdominal lymph nodes** `CC`
CC Excl: C81.20, C81.23, C81.28-C81.29, C81.90, C81.93, C81.98, D49.81-D49.9

C81.24   **Mixed cellularity classical Hodgkin lymphoma, lymph nodes of axilla and upper limb** `CC`
CC Excl: C81.20, C81.24, C81.28-C81.29, C81.90, C81.94, C81.98, D49.81-D49.9

C81.25   **Mixed cellularity classical Hodgkin lymphoma, lymph nodes of inguinal region and lower limb** `CC`
CC Excl: C81.20, C81.25, C81.28-C81.29, C81.90, C81.95, C81.98, D49.81-D49.9

C81.26   **Mixed cellularity classical Hodgkin lymphoma, intrapelvic lymph nodes** `CC`
CC Excl: C81.20, C81.26, C81.28-C81.29, C81.90, C81.96, C81.98, D49.81-D49.9

C81.27   **Mixed cellularity classical Hodgkin lymphoma, spleen** `CC`
CC Excl: C81.20, C81.27-C81.29, C81.90, C81.97-C81.98, D49.81-D49.9

C81.28   **Mixed cellularity classical Hodgkin lymphoma, lymph nodes of multiple sites** `CC`
CC Excl: See code: C81.20

C81.29   **Mixed cellularity classical Hodgkin lymphoma, extranodal and solid organ sites** `CC`
CC Excl: See code: C81.20

✓5ᵗʰ **C81.3**   **Lymphocyte-depleted classical Hodgkin lymphoma**

C81.30   **Lymphocyte-depleted classical Hodgkin lymphoma, unspecified site** `CC`
CC Excl: C81.30-C81.39, C81.90, C81.98, D49.81-D49.9

C81.31   **Lymphocyte-depleted classical Hodgkin lymphoma, lymph nodes of head, face, and neck** `CC`
CC Excl: C81.30-C81.31, C81.38-C81.39, C81.91, C81.98, D49.81-D49.9

C81.32   **Lymphocyte-depleted classical Hodgkin lymphoma, intrathoracic lymph nodes** `CC`
CC Excl: C81.30, C81.32, C81.38-C81.39, C81.92, C81.98, D49.81-D49.9

C81.33   **Lymphocyte-depleted classical Hodgkin lymphoma, intra-abdominal lymph nodes** `CC`
CC Excl: C81.30, C81.33, C81.38-C81.39, C81.93, C81.98, D49.81-D49.9

C81.34   **Lymphocyte-depleted classical Hodgkin lymphoma, lymph nodes of axilla and upper limb** `CC`
CC Excl: C81.30, C81.34, C81.38-C81.39, C81.94, C81.98, D49.81-D49.9

C81.35   **Lymphocyte-depleted classical Hodgkin lymphoma, lymph nodes of inguinal region and lower limb** `CC`
CC Excl: C81.30, C81.35, C81.38-C81.39, C81.95, C81.98, D49.81-D49.9

C81.36   **Lymphocyte-depleted classical Hodgkin lymphoma, intrapelvic lymph nodes** `CC`
CC Excl: C81.30, C81.36, C81.38-C81.39, C81.96, C81.98, D49.81-D49.9

C81.37   **Lymphocyte-depleted classical Hodgkin lymphoma, spleen** `CC`
CC Excl: C81.30, C81.37-C81.39, C81.97-C81.98, D49.81-D49.9

C81.38   **Lymphocyte-depleted classical Hodgkin lymphoma, lymph nodes of multiple sites** `CC`
CC Excl: C81.30-C81.39, C81.98, D49.81-D49.9

C81.39   **Lymphocyte-depleted classical Hodgkin lymphoma, extranodal and solid organ sites** `CC`
CC Excl: See code: C81.38

✓5ᵗʰ **C81.4**   **Lymphocyte-rich classical Hodgkin lymphoma**
EXCLUDES 1   nodular lymphocyte predominant Hodgkin lymphoma (C81.0-)

C81.40   **Lymphocyte-rich classical Hodgkin lymphoma, unspecified site** `CC`
CC Excl: C81.00-C81.09, C81.40-C81.49, C81.90, C81.98, D49.81-D49.9

C81.41   **Lymphocyte-rich classical Hodgkin lymphoma, lymph nodes of head, face, and neck** `CC`
CC Excl: C81.00-C81.01, C81.08-C81.09, C81.40-C81.41, C81.48-C81.49, C81.90-C81.91, C81.98, D49.81-D49.9

C81.42   **Lymphocyte-rich classical Hodgkin lymphoma, intrathoracic lymph nodes** `CC`
CC Excl: C81.00, C81.02, C81.08-C81.09, C81.40, C81.42, C81.48-C81.49, C81.90, C81.92, C81.98, D49.81-D49.9

C81.43   **Lymphocyte-rich classical Hodgkin lymphoma, intra-abdominal lymph nodes** `CC`
CC Excl: C81.00, C81.03, C81.08-C81.09, C81.40, C81.43, C81.48-C81.49, C81.90, C81.93, C81.98, D49.81-D49.9

C81.44   **Lymphocyte-rich classical Hodgkin lymphoma, lymph nodes of axilla and upper limb** `CC`
CC Excl: C81.00, C81.04, C81.08-C81.09, C81.40, C81.44, C81.48-C81.49, C81.90, C81.94, C81.98, D49.81-D49.9

C81.45   **Lymphocyte-rich classical Hodgkin lymphoma, lymph nodes of inguinal region and lower limb** `CC`
CC Excl: C81.00, C81.05, C81.08-C81.09, C81.40, C81.48-C81.49, C81.90, C81.95, C81.98, D49.81-D49.9

N Newborn: 0   P Pediatric: 0-17   M Maternity: 12-55   A Adult: 15-124   MCC Major CC Condition   PDx MCC PDx acts as own MCC   CC CC Condition   PDx CC PDx acts as own CC

470

ICD-10-CM 2016

C81.46   **Lymphocyte-rich classical Hodgkin lymphoma, intrapelvic lymph nodes**   CC
    CC Excl: C81.00, C81.06, C81.08-C81.09, C81.40, C81.46, C81.48-C81.49, C81.90, C81.96, C81.98, D49.81-D49.9

C81.47   **Lymphocyte-rich classical Hodgkin lymphoma, spleen**   CC
    CC Excl: C81.00, C81.07-C81.09, C81.40, C81.47-C81.49, C81.90, C81.97-C81.98, D49.81-D49.9

C81.48   **Lymphocyte-rich classical Hodgkin lymphoma, lymph nodes of multiple sites**   CC
    CC Excl: See code: C81.40

C81.49   **Lymphocyte-rich classical Hodgkin lymphoma, extranodal and solid organ sites**   CC
    CC Excl: See code: C81.40

✓5th **C81.7**   **Other classical Hodgkin lymphoma**
    Classical Hodgkin lymphoma NOS

C81.70   **Other classical Hodgkin lymphoma, unspecified site**   CC
    CC Excl: C81.70-C81.90, C81.98, D49.81-D49.9

C81.71   **Other classical Hodgkin lymphoma, lymph nodes of head, face, and neck**   CC
    CC Excl: C81.70-C81.71, C81.78-C81.91, C81.98, D49.81-D49.9

C81.72   **Other classical Hodgkin lymphoma, intrathoracic lymph nodes**   CC
    CC Excl: C81.70, C81.72, C81.78-C81.90, C81.92, C81.98, D49.81-D49.9

C81.73   **Other classical Hodgkin lymphoma, intra-abdominal lymph nodes**   CC
    CC Excl: C81.70, C81.73, C81.78-C81.90, C81.93, C81.98, D49.81-D49.9

C81.74   **Other classical Hodgkin lymphoma, lymph nodes of axilla and upper limb**   CC
    CC Excl: C81.70, C81.74, C81.78-C81.90, C81.94, C81.98, D49.81-D49.9

C81.75   **Other classical Hodgkin lymphoma, lymph nodes of inguinal region and lower limb**   CC
    CC Excl: C81.70, C81.75, C81.78-C81.90, C81.95, C81.98, D49.81-D49.9

C81.76   **Other classical Hodgkin lymphoma, intrapelvic lymph nodes**   CC
    CC Excl: C81.70, C81.76, C81.78-C81.90, C81.96, C81.98, D49.81-D49.9

C81.77   **Other classical Hodgkin lymphoma, spleen**   CC
    CC Excl: C81.70, C81.77-C81.90, C81.97-C81.98, D49.81-D49.

C81.78   **Other classical Hodgkin lymphoma, lymph nodes of multiple sites**   CC
    CC Excl: See code: C81.70

C81.79   **Other classical Hodgkin lymphoma, extranodal and solid organ sites**   CC
    CC Excl: See code: C81.70

✓5th **C81.9**   **Hodgkin lymphoma, unspecified**

C81.90   **Hodgkin lymphoma, unspecified, unspecified site**   CC
    CC Excl: C81.90-C81.98, D49.81-D49.9

C81.91   **Hodgkin lymphoma, unspecified, lymph nodes of head, face, and neck**   CC
    CC Excl: C81.90-C81.91, C81.98, D49.81-D49.9

C81.92   **Hodgkin lymphoma, unspecified, intrathoracic lymph nodes**   CC
    CC Excl: C81.9, C81.92, C81.98, D49.81-D49.9

C81.93   **Hodgkin lymphoma, unspecified, intra-abdominal lymph nodes**   CC
    CC Excl: C81.90, C81.93, C81.98, D49.81-D49.9

C81.94   **Hodgkin lymphoma, unspecified, lymph nodes of axilla and upper limb**   CC
    CC Excl: C81.90, C81.94, C81.98, D49.81-D49.9

C81.95   **Hodgkin lymphoma, unspecified, lymph nodes of inguinal region and lower limb**   CC
    CC Excl: C81.90, C81.95, C81.98, D49.81-D49.9

C81.96   **Hodgkin lymphoma, unspecified, intrapelvic lymph nodes**   CC
    CC Excl: C81.90, C81.96, C81.98, D49.81-D49.9

C81.97   **Hodgkin lymphoma, unspecified, spleen**   CC
    CC Excl: C81.90, C81.97-C81.98, D49.81-D49.9

C81.98   **Hodgkin lymphoma, unspecified, lymph nodes of multiple sites**   CC
    CC Excl: See code: C81.90

C81.99   **Hodgkin lymphoma, unspecified, extranodal and solid organ sites**   CC
    CC Excl: No Excl

✓4th **C82**   **Follicular lymphoma**
    INCLUDES   follicular lymphoma with or without diffuse areas
    EXCLUDES 1   mature T/NK-cell lymphomas (C84.-)
                 personal history of non-Hodgkin lymphoma (Z85.72)

✓5th **C82.0**   **Follicular lymphoma grade I**

C82.00   **Follicular lymphoma grade I, unspecified site**   CC
    CC Excl: C82.00-C82.50, C82.59-C82.69, C82.80-C82.99, C83.10, C83.19, C84.40, C84.49, C84.60, C84.69-C84.70, C84.79-C84.90, C84.99-C84.A0, C84.A9-C84.Z0, C84.Z9, C85.10, C85.19-C85.20, C85.29, C85.80, C85.89-C85.90, C85.99, C86.4, C88.4, C96.4, C96.9, C96.Z, D49.81-D49.9

C82.01   **Follicular lymphoma grade I, lymph nodes of head, face, and neck**   CC
    CC Excl: C82.00-C82.01, C82.08-C82.11, C82.18-C82.21, C82.28-C82.31, C82.38-C82.41, C82.48-C82.49, C82.51, C82.60-C82.61, C82.68-C82.69, C82.80-C82.81, C82.88-C82.91, C82.98-C82.99, C83.11, C84.41, C84.61, C84.71, C84.91, C84.A1, C84.Z1, C85.11, C85.21, C85.81, C85.91, C86.0, D49.81-D49.9

C82.02   **Follicular lymphoma grade I, intrathoracic lymph nodes**   CC
    CC Excl: C82.00, C82.02, C82.08-C82.10, C82.12, C82.18-C82.20, C82.22, C82.28-C82.30, C82.32, C82.38-C82.40, C82.42 C82.48-C82.49, C82.52, C82.60, C82.62, C82.68-C82.69, C82.80, C82.82, C82.88-C82.90, C82.92, C82.98-C82.99, C83.12, C84.42, C84.62, C84.72 C84.92, C84.A2, C84.Z2, C85.12, C85.22, C85.82, C85.92, D49.81-D49.9

C82.03   **Follicular lymphoma grade I, intra-abdominal lymph nodes**   CC
    CC Excl: C82.00, C82.03, C82.08-C82.10, C82.13, C82.18-C82.20, C82.23, C82.28-C82.30, C82.33, C82.38-C82.40, C82.43 C82.48-C82.49, C82.53, C82.60, C82.63, C82.68-C82.69, C82.80, C82.83, C82.88-C82.90, C82.93, C82.98-C82.99, C83.13, C84.43, C84.63, C84.73 C84.93, C84.A3, C84.Z3, C85.13, C85.23, C85.83, C85.93, C86.2-C86.3, D49.81-D49.9

C82.04   **Follicular lymphoma grade I, lymph nodes of axilla and upper limb**   CC
    CC Excl: C82.00, C82.04, C82.08-C82.10, C82.14, C82.18-C82.20, C82.24, C82.28-C82.30, C82.34, C82.38-C82.40, C82.44 C82.48-C82.49, C82.54, C82.60, C82.64, C82.68-C82.69, C82.80, C82.84, C82.88-C82.90, C82.94, C82.98-C82.99, C83.14, C84.44, C84.64, C84.74 C84.94, C84.A4, C84.Z4, C85.14, C85.24, C85.84, C85.94, D49.81-D49.9

C82.05   **Follicular lymphoma grade I, lymph nodes of inguinal region and lower limb**   CC
    CC Excl: C82.00, C82.05, C82.08-C82.10, C82.15, C82.18-C82.20, C82.25, C82.28-C82.30, C82.35, C82.38-C82.40, C82.45 C82.48-C82.49, C82.55, C82.60, C82.65, C82.68-C82.69, C82.80, C82.85, C82.88-C82.90, C82.95, C82.98-C82.99, C83.15, C84.45, C84.65, C84.75 C84.95, C84.A5, C84.Z5, C85.15, C85.25, C85.85, C85.95, D49.81-D49.9

C82.06   **Follicular lymphoma grade I, intrapelvic lymph nodes**   CC
    CC Excl: C82.00, C82.06, C82.08-C82.10, C82.16, C82.18-C82.20, C82.26, C82.28-C82.30, C82.36, C82.38-C82.40, C82.46 C82.48-C82.49, C82.56, C82.60, C82.66, C82.68-C82.69, C82.80, C82.86, C82.88-C82.90, C82.96, C82.98-C82.99, C83.16, C84.46, C84.66, C84.76 C84.96, C84.A6, C84.Z6, C85.16, C85.26, C85.86, C85.96, D49.81-D49.9

C82.07   **Follicular lymphoma grade I, spleen**   CC
    CC Excl: C82.00, C82.07-C82.10, C82.17-C82.20, C82.27-C82.30, C82.37-C82.40, C82.47-C82.49, C82.57, C82.60, C82.67-C82.80, C82.87-C82.90, C82.97-C82.99, C83.17, C84.47, C84.67, C84.77, C84.A7, C84.Z7, C84.97, C85.17, C85.27, C85.87, C85.97, C86.1, D49.81-D49.9

C82.08   **Follicular lymphoma grade I, lymph nodes of multiple sites**   CC
    CC Excl: C82.00-C82.49, C82.58, C82.60-C82.69, C82.80-C82.99, C83.18, C84.48, C84.68, C84.78, C84.98, C84.A8, C84.Z8, C85.18 C85.28, C85.88, C85.98, D49.81-D49.9

C82.09   **Follicular lymphoma grade I, extranodal and solid organ sites**   CC
    CC Excl: C82.00-C82.50, C82.59-C82.99, C83.10, C83.19, C84.40, C84.49-C84.60, C84.69-C84.70, C84.79-C84.A0, C84.A9-C84.Z0, C84.Z9-C84.90, C84.99-C85.10, C85.19-C85.20, C85.29-C85.80, C85.89-C85.90, C85.99, C86.4, C88.4, C96.4, C96.Z-C96.9, D49.81-D49.9

✓5th **C82.1**   **Follicular lymphoma grade II**

C82.10   **Follicular lymphoma grade II, unspecified site**   CC
    CC Excl: See code: C82.00

C82.11   **Follicular lymphoma grade II, lymph nodes of head, face, and neck**   CC
    CC Excl: See code: C82.01

C82.12   **Follicular lymphoma grade II,** intrathoracic **lymph nodes**   `CC`
     CC Excl: See code: C82.02

C82.13   **Follicular lymphoma grade II,** intra-abdominal **lymph nodes**   `CC`
     CC Excl: See code: C82.03

C82.14   **Follicular lymphoma grade II, lymph nodes of axilla and upper limb**   `CC`
     CC Excl: See code: C82.04

C82.15   **Follicular lymphoma grade II, lymph nodes of inguinal region and lower limb**   `CC`
     CC Excl: See code: C82.05

C82.16   **Follicular lymphoma grade II,** intrapelvic **lymph nodes**   `CC`
     CC Excl: See code: C82.06

C82.17   **Follicular lymphoma grade II,** spleen   `CC`
     CC Excl: See code: C82.07

C82.18   **Follicular lymphoma grade II, lymph nodes of multiple sites**   `CC`
     CC Excl: See code: C82.08

C82.19   **Follicular lymphoma grade II,** extranodal and solid organ sites   `CC`
     CC Excl: See code: C82.00

✓5ᵗʰ **C82.2**   **Follicular lymphoma** grade III, unspecified

C82.20   **Follicular lymphoma grade III, unspecified, unspecified site**   `CC`
     CC Excl: See code: C82.00

C82.21   **Follicular lymphoma grade III, unspecified, lymph nodes of** head, face, and neck   `CC`
     CC Excl: See code: C82.01

C82.22   **Follicular lymphoma grade III, unspecified, intrathoracic lymph nodes**   `CC`
     CC Excl: See code: C82.02

C82.23   **Follicular lymphoma grade III, unspecified, intra-abdominal lymph nodes**   `CC`
     CC Excl: See code: C82.03

C82.24   **Follicular lymphoma grade III, unspecified, lymph nodes of** axilla and upper limb   `CC`
     CC Excl: See code: C82.04

C82.25   **Follicular lymphoma grade III, unspecified, lymph nodes of** inguinal region and lower limb   `CC`
     CC Excl: See code: C82.05

C82.26   **Follicular lymphoma grade III, unspecified,** intrapelvic **lymph nodes**   `CC`
     CC Excl: See code: C82.06

C82.27   **Follicular lymphoma grade III, unspecified,** spleen   `CC`
     CC Excl: See code: C82.07

C82.28   **Follicular lymphoma grade III, unspecified, lymph nodes of** multiple sites   `CC`
     CC Excl: See code: C82.08

C82.29   **Follicular lymphoma grade III, unspecified, extranodal and solid organ sites**   `CC`
     CC Excl: See code: C82.00

✓5ᵗʰ **C82.3**   **Follicular lymphoma** grade IIIa

C82.30   **Follicular lymphoma grade IIIa,** unspecified sitesspleen   `CC`
     CC Excl: See code: C82.00

C82.31   **Follicular lymphoma grade IIIa, lymph nodes of** head, face, and neck   `CC`
     CC Excl: See code: C82.01

C82.32   **Follicular lymphoma grade IIIa,** intrathoracic **lymph nodes**   `CC`
     CC Excl: See code: C82.02

C82.33   **Follicular lymphoma grade IIIa,** intra-abdominal **lymph nodes**   `CC`
     CC Excl: See code: C82.03

C82.34   **Follicular lymphoma grade IIIa, lymph nodes of** axilla and upper limb   `CC`
     CC Excl: See code: C82.04

C82.35   **Follicular lymphoma grade IIIa, lymph nodes of** inguinal region and lower limb   `CC`
     CC Excl: See code: C82.05

C82.36   **Follicular lymphoma grade IIIa,** intrapelvic **lymph nodes**   `CC`
     CC Excl: See code: C82.06

C82.37   **Follicular lymphoma grade IIIa,** spleen   `CC`
     CC Excl: See code: C82.07

C82.38   **Follicular lymphoma grade IIIa, lymph nodes of** multiple sites   `CC`
     CC Excl: See code: C82.08

C82.39   **Follicular lymphoma grade IIIa,** extranodal and solid organ sites   `CC`
     CC Excl: See code: C82.00

✓5ᵗʰ **C82.4**   **Follicular lymphoma** grade IIIb

C82.40   **Follicular lymphoma grade IIIb, unspecified site**   `CC`
     CC Excl: See code: C82.00

C82.41   **Follicular lymphoma grade IIIb, lymph nodes of head, face, and neck**   `CC`
     CC Excl: See code: C82.01

C82.42   **Follicular lymphoma grade IIIb,** intrathoracic **lymph nodes**   `CC`
     CC Excl: See code: C82.02

C82.43   **Follicular lymphoma grade IIIb,** intra-abdominal **lymph nodes**   `CC`
     CC Excl: See code: C82.03

C82.44   **Follicular lymphoma grade IIIb, lymph nodes of axilla and upper limb**   `CC`
     CC Excl: See code: C82.04

C82.45   **Follicular lymphoma grade IIIb, lymph nodes of inguinal region and lower limb**   `CC`
     CC Excl: See code: C82.05

C82.46   **Follicular lymphoma grade IIIb,** intrapelvic **lymph nodes**   `CC`
     CC Excl: See code: C82.06

C82.47   **Follicular lymphoma grade IIIb,** spleen   `CC`
     CC Excl: See code: C82.07

C82.48   **Follicular lymphoma grade IIIb, lymph nodes of multiple sites**   `CC`
     CC Excl: See code: C82.08

C82.49   **Follicular lymphoma grade IIIb,** extranodal and solid organ sites   `CC`
     CC Excl: See code: C82.00

✓5ᵗʰ **C82.5**   **Diffuse follicle center lymphoma**

C82.50   **Diffuse follicle center lymphoma, unspecified site**   `HIV` `CC`
     CC Excl: C82.50-C82.59, C83.10-C83.19, C84.40-C84.49, C84.60-C84.Z9, C85.10-C85.29, C85.80-C86.4, C88.4, C96.4, C96.9, C96.Z, D49.81-D49.9

C82.51   **Diffuse follicle center lymphoma, lymph nodes of head, face, and neck**   `HIV` `CC`
     CC Excl: C82.50-C82.51, C82.58-C82.59, C83.10-C83.11, C83.18-C83.19, C84.40-C84.41, C84.48-C84.49, C84.60-C84.61, C84.68-C84.71, C84.78-C84.91, C84.98-C84.A1, C84.A8-C84.Z1, C84.Z8-C84.Z9, C85.10-C85.11, C85.18-C85.21, C85.28-C85.29, C85.80-C85.81 C85.88-C85.91, C85.98-C86.0, C86.4, C88.4, D49.81-D49.9

C82.52   **Diffuse follicle center lymphoma, intrathoracic lymph nodes**   `HIV` `CC`
     CC Excl: C82.50-C82.52, C82.58-C82.59, C83.10, C83.12, C83.18-C83.19, C84.40, C84.42, C84.48-C84.49, C84.60, C84.62, C84.68-C84.70, C84.72, C84.78-C84.90, C84.92, C84.98-C84.A0, C84.A2, C84.A8-C84.Z0, C84.Z2, C84.Z8-C84.Z9, C85.10, C85.12, C85.18-C85.20, C85.22 C85.28-C85.29, C85.80, C85.82, C85.88-C85.90, C85.92, C85.98-C85.99, C86.4, C88.4, D49.81-D49.9

C82.53   **Diffuse follicle center lymphoma, intra-abdominal lymph nodes**   `HIV` `CC`
     CC Excl: C82.50-C82.53, C82.58-C82.59, C83.10, C83.13, C83.18-C83.19, C84.40, C84.43, C84.48-C84.49, C84.60, C84.63, C84.68-C84.70, C84.73, C84.78-C84.90, C84.93, C84.98-C84.A0, C84.A3, C84.A8-C84.Z0, C84.Z3, C84.Z8-C84.Z9, C85.10, C85.13, C85.18-C85.20, C85.23 C85.28-C85.29, C85.80, C85.83, C85.88-C85.90, C85.93, C85.98-C85.99, C86.2-C86.4, C88.4, D49.81-D49.9

C82.54   **Diffuse follicle center lymphoma, lymph nodes of axilla and upper limb**   `HIV` `CC`
     CC Excl: C82.50-C82.54, C82.58-C82.59, C83.10, C83.14, C83.18-C83.19, C84.40, C84.44, C84.48-C84.49, C84.60, C84.64, C84.68-C84.70, C84.74, C84.78-C84.90, C84.94, C84.98-C84.A0, C84.A4, C84.A8-C84.Z0, C84.Z4, C84.Z8-C84.Z9, C85.10, C85.14, C85.18-C85.20, C85.24 C85.28-C85.29, C85.80, C85.84, C85.88-C85.90, C85.94, C85.98-C85.99, C86.4, C88.4, D49.81-D49.9

C82.55   **Diffuse follicle center lymphoma, lymph nodes of inguinal region and lower limb**   `HIV` `CC`
     CC Excl: C82.50-C82.55, C82.58-C82.59, C83.10, C83.15, C83.18-C83.19, C84.40, C84.45, C84.48-C84.49, C84.60, C84.65, C84.68-C84.70, C84.75, C84.78-C84.90, C84.95, C84.98-C84.A0, C84.A5, C84.A8-C84.Z0, C84.Z5, C84.Z8-C84.Z9, C85.10, C85.15, C85.18-C85.20, C85.25 C85.28-C85.29, C85.80, C85.85, C85.88-C85.90, C85.95, C85.98-C85.99, C86.4, C88.4, D49.81-D49.9

N Newborn: 0   P Pediatric: 0-17   M Maternity: 12-55   A Adult: 15-124   MCC Major CC Condition   PDxMCC PDx acts as own MCC   CC CC Condition   PDxCC PDx acts as own CC

472   ICD-10-CM 2016

C82.56 **Diffuse follicle center lymphoma, intrapelvic** `HIV` `CC`
lymph nodes
   CC Excl: C82.50-C82.56, C82.58-C82.59, C83.10, C83.16,
   C83.18-C83.19, C84.40, C84.46, C84.48-C84.49, C84.60,
   C84.66, C84.68-C84.70, C84.76, C84.78-C84.90, C84.96,
   C84.98-C84.A0, C84.A6, C84.A8-C84.Z0, C84.Z6, C84.Z8-
   C84.Z9, C85.10, C85.16, C85.18-C85.20, C85.26 C85.28-
   C85.29, C85.80, C85.86, C85.88-C85.90, C85.96, C85.98-
   C85.99, C86.4, C88.4, D49.81-D49.9

C82.57 **Diffuse follicle center lymphoma, spleen** `HIV` `CC`
   CC Excl: C82.50, C82.57-C82.59, C83.10, C83.17-C83.19,
   C84.40, C84.47-C84.60, C84.67-C84.70, C84.77-C84.A0,
   C84.A7-C84.Z0, C84.Z7-C84.90, C84.97-C85.10, C85.17-
   C85.20, C85.27-C85.80, C85.87-C85.90, C85.97-C85.99,
   C86.1, C86.4, C88.4, D49.81-D49.9

C82.58 **Diffuse follicle center lymphoma, lymph** `HIV` `CC`
nodes of multiple sites
   CC Excl: C82.50-C82.59, C83.10-C83.19, C84.40-C84.49,
   C84.60-C84.Z9, C85.10-C85.29, C85.80-C86.4, C88.4,
   D49.81-D49.9

C82.59 **Diffuse follicle center lymphoma, extranodal** `HIV` `CC`
and solid organ sites
   CC Excl: See code: C82.50

✓5ᵗʰ **C82.6** **Cutaneous follicle center lymphoma**

C82.60 **Cutaneous follicle center lymphoma,** `CC`
unspecified site
   CC Excl: See code: C82.00

C82.61 **Cutaneous follicle center lymphoma, lymph** `CC`
nodes of head, face, and neck
   CC Excl: See code: C82.01

C82.62 **Cutaneous follicle center lymphoma,** `CC`
intrathoracic lymph nodes
   CC Excl: See code: C82.02

C82.63 **Cutaneous follicle center lymphoma,** `CC`
intra-abdominal lymph nodes
   CC Excl: See code: C82.03

C82.64 **Cutaneous follicle center lymphoma, lymph** `CC`
nodes of axilla and upper limb
   CC Excl: See code: C82.04

C82.65 **Cutaneous follicle center lymphoma, lymph** `CC`
nodes of inguinal region and lower limb
   CC Excl: See code: C82.05

C82.66 **Cutaneous follicle center lymphoma, intrapelvic** `CC`
lymph nodes
   CC Excl: See code: C82.06

C82.67 **Cutaneous follicle center lymphoma, spleen** `CC`
   CC Excl: See code: C82.07

C82.68 **Cutaneous follicle center lymphoma, lymph** `CC`
nodes of multiple sites
   CC Excl: See code: C82.08

C82.69 **Cutaneous follicle center lymphoma, extranodal** `CC`
and solid organ sites
   CC Excl: See code: C82.00

✓5ᵗʰ **C82.8** **Other types of follicular lymphoma**

C82.80 **Other types of follicular lymphoma, unspecified** `CC`
site
   CC Excl: See code: C82.00

C82.81 **Other types of follicular lymphoma, lymph** `CC`
nodes of head, face, and neck
   CC Excl: See code: C82.01

C82.82 **Other types of follicular lymphoma, intrathoracic** `CC`
lymph nodes
   CC Excl: See code: C82.02

C82.83 **Other types of follicular lymphoma, intra-** `CC`
abdominal lymph nodes
   CC Excl: See code: C82.03

C82.84 **Other types of follicular lymphoma, lymph** `CC`
nodes of axilla and upper limb
   CC Excl: See code: C82.04

C82.85 **Other types of follicular lymphoma, lymph** `CC`
nodes of inguinal region and lower limb
   CC Excl: See code: C82.05

C82.86 **Other types of follicular lymphoma, intrapelvic** `CC`
lymph nodes
   CC Excl: See code: C82.06

C82.87 **Other types of follicular lymphoma, spleen** `CC`
   CC Excl: See code: C82.07

C82.88 **Other types of follicular lymphoma, lymph** `CC`
nodes of multiple sites
   CC Excl: See code: C82.08

C82.89 **Other types of follicular lymphoma, extranodal** `CC`
and solid organ sites
   CC Excl: See code: C82.00

✓5ᵗʰ **C82.9** **Follicular lymphoma, unspecified**

C82.90 **Follicular lymphoma, unspecified, unspecified** `CC`
site
   CC Excl: See code: C82.00

C82.91 **Follicular lymphoma, unspecified, lymph nodes** `CC`
of head, face, and neck
   CC Excl: See code: C82.01

C82.92 **Follicular lymphoma, unspecified, intrathoracic** `CC`
lymph nodes
   CC Excl: See code: C82.02

C82.93 **Follicular lymphoma, unspecified, intra-** `CC`
abdominal lymph nodes
   CC Excl: See code: C82.03

C82.94 **Follicular lymphoma, unspecified, lymph nodes** `CC`
of axilla and upper limb
   CC Excl: See code: C82.04

C82.95 **Follicular lymphoma, unspecified, lymph nodes** `CC`
of inguinal region and lower limb
   CC Excl: See code: C82.05

C82.96 **Follicular lymphoma, unspecified, intrapelvic** `CC`
lymph nodes
   CC Excl: See code: C82.06

C82.97 **Follicular lymphoma, unspecified, spleen** `CC`
   CC Excl: See code: C82.07

C82.98 **Follicular lymphoma, unspecified, lymph nodes** `CC`
of multiple sites
   CC Excl: See code: C82.08

C82.99 **Follicular lymphoma, unspecified, extranodal** `CC`
and solid organ sites
   CC Excl: See code: C82.00

✓4ᵗʰ **C83** **Non-follicular lymphoma**
   EXCLUDES 1 *personal history of non-Hodgkin lymphoma (Z85.72)*

✓5ᵗʰ **C83.0** **Small cell B-cell lymphoma**
   Lymphoplasmacytic lymphoma
   Nodal marginal zone lymphoma
   Non-leukemic variant of B-CLL
   Splenic marginal zone lymphoma
   EXCLUDES 1 *chronic lymphocytic leukemia (C91.1)*
      mature T/NK-cell lymphomas (C84.-)
      Waldenström macroglobulinemia (C88.0)

C83.00 **Small cell B-cell lymphoma, unspecified site** `HIV` `CC`
   CC Excl: C83.00-C83.09, C83.80-C83.99, C86.5-C86.6,
   D49.81-D49.9

C83.01 **Small cell B-cell lymphoma, lymph nodes of** `HIV` `CC`
head, face, and neck
   CC Excl: C83.00-C83.01, C83.08-C83.09, C83.80-C83.81,
   C83.88-C83.91, C83.98-C83.99, C86.5-C86.6, D49.81-
   D49.9

C83.02 **Small cell B-cell lymphoma, intrathoracic** `HIV` `CC`
lymph nodes
   CC Excl: C83.00-C83.02, C83.08-C83.09, C83.80, C83.82,
   C83.88-C83.90, C83.92, C83.98-C83.99, C86.5-C86.6,
   D49.81-D49.9

C83.03 **Small cell B-cell lymphoma, intra-abdominal** `HIV` `CC`
lymph nodes
   CC Excl: C83.00-C83.03, C83.08-C83.09, C83.80, C83.83,
   C83.88-C83.90, C83.93, C83.98-C83.99, C86.5-C86.6,
   D49.81-D49.9

C83.04 **Small cell B-cell lymphoma, lymph nodes of** `HIV` `CC`
axilla and upper limb
   CC Excl: C83.00-C83.04, C83.08-C83.09, C83.80, C83.84,
   C83.88-C83.90, C83.94, C83.98-C83.99, C86.5-C86.6,
   D49.81-D49.9

C83.05 **Small cell B-cell lymphoma, lymph nodes of** `HIV` `CC`
inguinal region and lower limb
   CC Excl: C83.00-C83.05, C83.08-C83.09, C83.80, C83.85,
   C83.88-C83.90, C83.95, C83.98-C83.99, C86.5-C86.6,
   D49.81-D49.9

C83.06 **Small cell B-cell lymphoma, intrapelvic lymph** `HIV` `CC`
nodes
   CC Excl: C83.00-C83.06, C83.08-C83.09, C83.80, C83.86,
   C83.88-C83.90, C83.96, C83.98-C83.99, C86.5-C86.6,
   D49.81-D49.9

C83.07 **Small cell B-cell lymphoma, spleen** `HIV` `CC`
   CC Excl: C83.00, C83.07-C83.09, C83.80, C83.87-C83.90,
   C83.97-C83.99, C86.5-C86.6, D49.81-D49.9

C83.08 **Small cell B-cell lymphoma, lymph nodes of** `HIV` `CC`
multiple sites
   CC Excl: C83.00-C83.09, C83.80-C83.99, C86.5-C86.6,
   D49.81-D49.9

C83.09 **Small cell B-cell lymphoma, extranodal and** `HIV` `CC`
solid organ sites
   CC Excl: See code: C83.00

☑ Additional Character Required ✓x7ᵗʰ Placeholder Alert Unacceptable PDx Manifestation Hospital Acquired Condition **EXCLUDES 1** Not Coded Here **EXCLUDES 2** Not Included Here

ICD-10-CM 2016   473

✓5ᵗʰ C83.1 Mantle cell lymphoma
Centrocytic lymphoma
Malignant lymphomatous polyposis

C83.10 Mantle cell lymphoma, unspecified site `HIV` `CC`
CC Excl: See code: C82.50

C83.11 Mantle cell lymphoma, lymph nodes of head, `HIV` `CC`
face, and neck
CC Excl: See code: C82.51

C83.12 Mantle cell lymphoma, intrathoracic lymph `HIV` `CC`
nodes
CC Excl: See code: C82.52

C83.13 Mantle cell lymphoma, intra-abdominal `HIV` `CC`
lymph nodes
CC Excl: See code: C82.53

C83.14 Mantle cell lymphoma, lymph nodes of axilla `HIV` `CC`
and upper limb
CC Excl: See code: C82.54

C83.15 Mantle cell lymphoma, lymph nodes of `HIV` `CC`
inguinal region and lower limb
CC Excl: See code: C82.55

C83.16 Mantle cell lymphoma, intrapelvic lymph `HIV` `CC`
nodes
CC Excl: See code: C82.56

C83.17 Mantle cell lymphoma, spleen `HIV` `CC`
CC Excl: See code: C82.57

C83.18 Mantle cell lymphoma, lymph nodes of `HIV` `CC`
multiple sites
CC Excl: See code: C82.58

C83.19 Mantle cell lymphoma, extranodal and solid `HIV` `CC`
organ sites
CC Excl: See code: C82.50

✓5ᵗʰ C83.3 Diffuse large B-cell lymphoma
Anaplastic diffuse large B-cell lymphoma
CD30-positive diffuse large B-cell lymphoma
Centroblastic diffuse large B-cell lymphoma
Diffuse large B-cell lymphoma, subtype not specified
Immunoblastic diffuse large B-cell lymphoma
Plasmablastic diffuse large B-cell lymphoma
T-cell rich diffuse large B-cell lymphoma
EXCLUDES 1   *mature T/NK-cell lymphomas (C84.-)*
mediastinal (thymic) large B-cell lymphoma (C85.2-)

C83.30 Diffuse large B-cell lymphoma, unspecified `HIV` `CC`
site
CC Excl: C83.30-C83.39, D49.81-D49.9

C83.31 Diffuse large B-cell lymphoma, lymph nodes `HIV` `CC`
of head, face, and neck
CC Excl: C83.30-C83.31, C83.38-C83.39, D49.81-D49.9

C83.32 Diffuse large B-cell lymphoma, intrathoracic `HIV` `CC`
lymph nodes
CC Excl: C83.30-C83.32, C83.38-C83.39, D49.81-D49.9

C83.33 Diffuse large B-cell lymphoma, intra- `HIV` `CC`
abdominal lymph nodes
CC Excl: C83.30-C83.33, C83.38-C83.39, D49.81-D49.9

C83.34 Diffuse large B-cell lymphoma, lymph nodes `HIV` `CC`
of axilla and upper limb
CC Excl: C83.30-C83.34, C83.38-C83.39, D49.81-D49.9

C83.35 Diffuse large B-cell lymphoma, lymph nodes `HIV` `CC`
of inguinal region and lower limb
CC Excl: C83.30-C83.35, C83.38-C83.39, D49.81-D49.9

C83.36 Diffuse large B-cell lymphoma, intrapelvic `HIV` `CC`
lymph nodes
CC Excl: C83.30-C83.36, C83.38-C83.39, D49.81-D49.9

C83.37 Diffuse large B-cell lymphoma, spleen `HIV` `CC`
CC Excl: C83.30, C83.37-C83.39, D49.81-D49.9

C83.38 Diffuse large B-cell lymphoma, lymph nodes `HIV` `CC`
of multiple sites
CC Excl: C83.30-C83.39, D49.81-D49.9

C83.39 Diffuse large B-cell lymphoma, extranodal `HIV` `CC`
and solid organ sites
CC Excl: See code: C83.38

✓5ᵗʰ C83.5 Lymphoblastic (diffuse) lymphoma
B-precursor lymphoma
Lymphoblastic B-cell lymphoma
Lymphoblastic lymphoma NOS
Lymphoblastic T-cell lymphoma
T-precursor lymphoma

C83.50 Lymphoblastic (diffuse) lymphoma, `CC`
unspecified site
CC Excl: C83.50-C83.59, D49.81-D49.9

C83.51 Lymphoblastic (diffuse) lymphoma, lymph `CC`
nodes of head, face, and neck
CC Excl: C83.50-C83.51, C83.58-C83.59, D49.81-D49.9

C83.52 Lymphoblastic (diffuse) lymphoma, `CC`
intrathoracic lymph nodes
CC Excl: C83.50, C83.52, C83.58-C83.59, D49.81-D49.9

C83.53 Lymphoblastic (diffuse) lymphoma, intra- `CC`
abdominal lymph nodes
CC Excl: C83.50, C83.53, C83.58-C83.59, D49.81-D49.9

C83.54 Lymphoblastic (diffuse) lymphoma, lymph `CC`
nodes of axilla and upper limb
CC Excl: C83.50, C83.54, C83.58-C83.59, D49.81-D49.9

C83.55 Lymphoblastic (diffuse) lymphoma, lymph `CC`
nodes of inguinal region and lower limb
CC Excl: C83.50, C83.55, C83.58-C83.59, D49.81-D49.9

C83.56 Lymphoblastic (diffuse) lymphoma, intrapelvic `CC`
lymph nodes
CC Excl: C83.50, C83.56, C83.58-C83.59, D49.81-D49.9

C83.57 Lymphoblastic (diffuse) lymphoma, spleen `CC`
CC Excl: C83.50, C83.57-C83.59, D49.81-D49.9

C83.58 Lymphoblastic (diffuse) lymphoma, lymph `CC`
nodes of multiple sites
CC Excl: See code: C83.50

C83.59 Lymphoblastic (diffuse) lymphoma, extranodal `CC`
and solid organ sites
CC Excl: See code: C83.50

✓5ᵗʰ C83.7 Burkitt lymphoma
Atypical Burkitt lymphoma
Burkitt-like lymphoma
EXCLUDES 1   *mature B-cell leukemia Burkitt type (C91.A-)*

C83.70 Burkitt lymphoma, unspecified site `HIV` `CC`
CC Excl: C83.70-C83.79, D49.81-D49.9

C83.71 Burkitt lymphoma, lymph nodes of head, face, `HIV` `CC`
and neck
CC Excl: C83.70-C83.71, C83.78-C83.79, D49.81-D49.9

C83.72 Burkitt lymphoma, intrathoracic lymph nodes `HIV` `CC`
CC Excl: C83.70, C83.72, C83.78-C83.79, D49.81-D49.9

C83.73 Burkitt lymphoma, intra-abdominal lymph `HIV` `CC`
nodes
CC Excl: C83.70, C83.73, C83.78-C83.79, D49.81-D49.9

C83.74 Burkitt lymphoma, lymph nodes of axilla and `HIV` `CC`
upper limb
CC Excl: C83.70, C83.74, C83.78-C83.79, D49.81-D49.9

C83.75 Burkitt lymphoma, lymph nodes of inguinal `HIV` `CC`
region and lower limb
CC Excl: C83.70, C83.75, C83.78-C83.79, D49.81-D49.9

C83.76 Burkitt lymphoma, intrapelvic lymph nodes `HIV` `CC`
CC Excl: C83.70, C83.76, C83.78-C83.79, D49.81-D49.9

C83.77 Burkitt lymphoma, spleen `HIV` `CC`
CC Excl: C83.70, C83.77-C83.79, D49.81-D49.9

C83.78 Burkitt lymphoma, lymph nodes of multiple `HIV` `CC`
sites
CC Excl: See code: C83.70

C83.79 Burkitt lymphoma, extranodal and solid organ `HIV` `CC`
sites
CC Excl: See code: C83.70

✓5ᵗʰ C83.8 Other non-follicular lymphoma
Intravascular large B-cell lymphoma
Lymphoid granulomatosis
Primary effusion B-cell lymphoma
EXCLUDES 1   *mediastinal (thymic) large B-cell lymphoma (C85.2-)*
T-cell rich B-cell lymphoma (C83.3-)

C83.80 Other non-follicular lymphoma, unspecified `HIV` `CC`
site
CC Excl: See code: C83.00

C83.81 Other non-follicular lymphoma, lymph nodes `HIV` `CC`
of head, face, and neck
CC Excl: See code: C83.01

C83.82 Other non-follicular lymphoma, intrathoracic `HIV` `CC`
lymph nodes
CC Excl: See code: C83.02

C83.83 Other non-follicular lymphoma, `HIV` `CC`
intra-abdominal lymph nodes
CC Excl: See code: C83.03

C83.84 Other non-follicular lymphoma, lymph nodes `HIV` `CC`
of axilla and upper limb
CC Excl: See code: C83.04

C83.85 Other non-follicular lymphoma, lymph nodes `HIV` `CC`
of inguinal region and lower limb
CC Excl: See code: C83.05

C83.86   **Other non-follicular lymphoma, intrapelvic** `HIV` `CC`
lymph nodes
CC Excl: See code: C83.06

C83.87   **Other non-follicular lymphoma, spleen** `HIV` `CC`
CC Excl: See code: C83.07

C83.88   **Other non-follicular lymphoma, lymph nodes** `HIV` `CC`
of multiple sites
CC Excl: See code: C83.00

C83.89   **Other non-follicular lymphoma, extranodal** `HIV` `CC`
and solid organ sites
CC Excl: See code: C83.00

✓5ᵗʰ **C83.9**   Non-follicular (diffuse) lymphoma, unspecified

C83.90   **Non-follicular (diffuse) lymphoma,** `HIV` `CC`
unspecified, unspecified site
CC Excl: See code: C83.00

C83.91   **Non-follicular (diffuse) lymphoma,** `HIV` `CC`
unspecified, lymph nodes of head, face, and neck
CC Excl: See code: C83.01

C83.92   **Non-follicular (diffuse) lymphoma,** `HIV` `CC`
unspecified, intrathoracic lymph nodes
CC Excl: See code: C83.02

C83.93   **Non-follicular (diffuse) lymphoma,** `HIV` `CC`
unspecified, intra-abdominal lymph nodes
CC Excl: See code: C83.03

C83.94   **Non-follicular (diffuse) lymphoma,** `HIV` `CC`
unspecified, lymph nodes of axilla and upper limb
CC Excl: See code: C83.04

C83.95   **Non-follicular (diffuse) lymphoma,** `HIV` `CC`
**unspecified, lymph nodes of inguinal region
and lower limb**
CC Excl: See code: C83.05

C83.96   **Non-follicular (diffuse) lymphoma,** `HIV` `CC`
unspecified, intrapelvic lymph nodes
CC Excl: See code: C83.06

C83.97   **Non-follicular (diffuse) lymphoma,** `HIV` `CC`
unspecified, spleen
CC Excl: See code: C83.07

C83.98   **Non-follicular (diffuse) lymphoma,** `HIV` `CC`
unspecified, lymph nodes of multiple sites
CC Excl: See code: C83.00

C83.99   **Non-follicular (diffuse) lymphoma,** `HIV` `CC`
unspecified, extranodal and solid organ sites
CC Excl: See code: C83.00

✓4ᵗʰ **C84**   **Mature T/NK-cell lymphomas**
EXCLUDES 1   personal history of non-Hodgkin lymphoma (Z85.72)

✓5ᵗʰ **C84.0**   **Mycosis fungoides**
EXCLUDES 1   peripheral T-cell lymphoma, not classified (C84.4-)

C84.00   **Mycosis fungoides, unspecified site** `CC`
CC Excl: C82.50, C82.59, C83.10, C83.19, C84.00-C84.09,
C84.40, C84.49, C84.60, C84.69-C84.70, C84.79-C84.90,
C84.99-C84.A0, C84.A9-C84.Z0, C84.Z9, C85.10, C85.19-
C85.20, C85.29, C85.80, C85.89-C85.90, C85.99, C86.4,
C88.4, C96.4, C96.9, C96.Z, D49.81-D49.9

C84.01   **Mycosis fungoides, lymph nodes of head, face,** `CC`
and neck
CC Excl: C82.51, C83.11, C84.00-C84.01, C84.08-C84.09,
C84.41, C84.61, C84.71, C84.91, C84.A1, C84.Z1, C85.11,
C85.21, C85.81, C85.91, C86.0, D49.81-D49.9

C84.02   **Mycosis fungoides, intrathoracic lymph nodes** `CC`
CC Excl: C82.52, C83.12, C84.00, C84.02, C84.08-C84.09,
C84.42, C84.62, C84.72, C84.92, C84.A2, C84.Z2, C85.12,
C85.22, C85.82, C85.92, D49.81-D49.9

C84.03   **Mycosis fungoides, intra-abdominal lymph** `CC`
nodes
CC Excl: C82.53, C83.13, C84.00, C84.03, C84.08-C84.09,
C84.43, C84.63, C84.73, C84.93, C84.A3, C84.Z3, C85.13,
C85.23, C85.83, C85.93, C86.2-C86.3, D49.81-D49.9

C84.04   **Mycosis fungoides, lymph nodes of axilla and** `CC`
upper limb
CC Excl: C82.54, C83.14, C84.00, C84.04, C84.08-C84.09,
C84.44, C84.64, C84.74, C84.94, C84.A4, C84.Z4, C85.14,
C85.24, C85.84, C85.94, D49.81-D49.9

C84.05   **Mycosis fungoides, lymph nodes of inguinal** `CC`
region and lower limb
CC Excl: C82.55, C83.15, C84.00, C84.05, C84.08-C84.09,
C84.45, C84.65, C84.75, C84.95, C84.A5, C84.Z5, C85.15,
C85.25, C85.85, C85.95, D49.81-D49.9

C84.06   **Mycosis fungoides, intrapelvic lymph nodes** `CC`
CC Excl: C82.56, C83.16, C84.00, C84.06, C84.08-C84.09,
C84.46, C84.66, C84.76, C84.96, C84.A6, C84.Z6, C85.16,
C85.26, C85.86, C85.96, D49.81-D49.9

C84.07   **Mycosis fungoides, spleen**
CC Excl: C82.57, C83.17, C84.00, C84.07-C84.09, C84.47,
C84.67, C84.77, C84.97, C84.A7, C84.Z7, C85.17, C85.27,
C85.87, C85.97, C86.1, D49.81-D49.9

C84.08   **Mycosis fungoides, lymph nodes of multiple** `CC`
sites
CC Excl: C82.58, C83.18, C84.00-C84.09, C84.48, C84.68,
C84.78, C84.98, C84.A8, C84.Z8, C85.18, C85.28, C85.88,
C85.98, D49.81-D49.9

C84.09   **Mycosis fungoides, extranodal and solid organ** `CC`
sites
CC Excl: See code: C84.00

✓5ᵗʰ **C84.1**   **Sézary disease**

C84.10   **Sézary disease, unspecified site** `CC`
CC Excl: C82.50, C82.59, C83.10, C83.19, C84.10-C84.19,
C84.40, C84.49, C84.60, C84.69-C84.70, C84.79-C84.90,
C84.99-C84.A0, C84.A9-C84.Z0, C84.Z9, C85.10, C85.19-
C85.20, C85.29, C85.80, C85.89-C85.90, C85.99, C86.4,
C88.4, C96.4, C96.9, C96.Z, D49.81-D49.9

C84.11   **Sézary disease, lymph nodes of head, face, and** `CC`
neck
CC Excl: C82.51, C83.11, C84.10-C84.11, C84.18-C84.19,
C84.41, C84.61, C84.71, C84.91, C84.A1, C84.Z1, C85.11,
C85.21, C85.81, C85.91, C86.0, D49.81-D49.9

C84.12   **Sézary disease, intrathoracic lymph nodes** `CC`
CC Excl: C82.52, C83.12, C84.10, C84.12, C84.18-C84.19,
C84.42, C84.62, C84.72, C84.92, C84.A2, C84.Z2, C85.12,
C85.22, C85.82, C85.92, D49.81-D49.9

C84.13   **Sézary disease, intra-abdominal lymph nodes** `CC`
CC Excl: C82.53, C83.13, C84.10, C84.13, C84.18-C84.19,
C84.43, C84.63, C84.73, C84.93, C84.A3, C84.Z3, C85.13,
C85.23, C85.83, C85.93, C86.2-C86.3, D49.81-D49.9

C84.14   **Sézary disease, lymph nodes of axilla and upper** `CC`
limb
CC Excl: C82.54, C83.14, C84.10, C84.14, C84.18-C84.19,
C84.44, C84.64, C84.74, C84.94, C84.A4, C84.Z4, C85.14,
C85.24, C85.84, C85.94, D49.81-D49.9

C84.15   **Sézary disease, lymph nodes of inguinal region** `CC`
and lower limb
CC Excl: C82.55, C83.15, C84.10, C84.15, C84.18-C84.19,
C84.45, C84.65, C84.75, C84.95, C84.A5, C84.Z5, C85.15,
C85.25, C85.85, C85.95, D49.81-D49.9

C84.16   **Sézary disease, intrapelvic lymph nodes** `CC`
CC Excl: C82.56, C83.16, C84.10, C84.16, C84.18-C84.19,
C84.46, C84.66, C84.76, C84.96, C84.A6, C84.Z6, C85.16,
C85.26, C85.86, C85.96, D49.81-D49.9

C84.17   **Sézary disease, spleen** `CC`
CC Excl: C82.57, C83.17, C84.10, C84.17-C84.19, C84.47,
C84.67, C84.77, C84.97, C84.A7, C84.Z7, C85.17, C85.27,
C85.87, C85.97, C86.1, D49.81-D49.9

C84.18   **Sézary disease, lymph nodes of multiple sites** `CC`
CC Excl: C82.58, C83.18, C84.10-C84.19, C84.48, C84.68,
C84.78, C84.98, C84.A8, C84.Z8, C85.18, C85.28, C85.88,
C85.98, D49.81-D49.9

C84.19   **Sézary disease, extranodal and solid organ sites** `CC`
CC Excl: See code: C84.10

✓5ᵗʰ **C84.4**   **Peripheral T-cell lymphoma, not classified**
Lennert's lymphoma
Lymphoepithelioid lymphoma
Mature T-cell lymphoma, not elsewhere classified

C84.40   **Peripheral T-cell lymphoma, not classified,** `HIV` `CC`
unspecified site
CC Excl: See code: C82.50

C84.41   **Peripheral T-cell lymphoma, not classified,** `HIV` `CC`
lymph nodes of head, face, and neck
CC Excl: See code: C82.51

C84.42   **Peripheral T-cell lymphoma, not classified,** `HIV` `CC`
intrathoracic lymph nodes
CC Excl: See code: C82.52

C84.43   **Peripheral T-cell lymphoma, not classified,** `HIV` `CC`
intra-abdominal lymph nodes
CC Excl: See code: C82.53

C84.44   **Peripheral T-cell lymphoma, not classified,** `HIV` `CC`
lymph nodes of axilla and upper limb
CC Excl: See code: C82.54

C84.45   **Peripheral T-cell lymphoma, not classified,** `HIV` `CC`
lymph nodes of inguinal region and lower limb
CC Excl: See code: C82.55

C84.46   **Peripheral T-cell lymphoma, not classified,** `HIV` `CC`
intrapelvic lymph nodes
CC Excl: See code: C82.56

C84.47   **Peripheral T-cell lymphoma, not classified,** `HIV` `CC`
spleen
CC Excl: See code: C82.57

✓ Additional Character Required   ✓x7ᵗʰ Placeholder Alert   Unacceptable PDx   Manifestation   Hospital Acquired Condition   *EXCLUDES 1* Not Coded Here   *EXCLUDES 2* Not Included Here

C84.48   **Peripheral T-cell lymphoma, not classified, lymph nodes of multiple sites** `HIV` `CC`
CC Excl: See code: C82.58

C84.49   **Peripheral T-cell lymphoma, not classified, extranodal and solid organ sites** `HIV` `CC`
CC Excl: See code: C82.50

√5th **C84.6**   **Anaplastic large cell lymphoma, ALK-positive**
Anaplastic large cell lymphoma, CD30-positive

C84.60   **Anaplastic large cell lymphoma, ALK-positive, unspecified site** `HIV` `CC`
CC Excl: See code: C82.50

C84.61   **Anaplastic large cell lymphoma, ALK-positive, lymph nodes of head, face, and neck** `HIV` `CC`
CC Excl: See code: C82.51

C84.62   **Anaplastic large cell lymphoma, ALK-positive, intrathoracic lymph nodes** `HIV` `CC`
CC Excl: See code: C82.52

C84.63   **Anaplastic large cell lymphoma, ALK-positive, intra-abdominal lymph nodes** `HIV` `CC`
CC Excl: See code: C82.53

C84.64   **Anaplastic large cell lymphoma, ALK-positive, lymph nodes of axilla and upper limb** `HIV` `CC`
CC Excl: See code: C82.54

C84.65   **Anaplastic large cell lymphoma, ALK-positive, lymph nodes of inguinal region and lower limb** `HIV` `CC`
CC Excl: See code: C82.55

C84.66   **Anaplastic large cell lymphoma, ALK-positive, intrapelvic lymph nodes** `HIV` `CC`
CC Excl: See code: C82.56

C84.67   **Anaplastic large cell lymphoma, ALK-positive, spleen** `HIV` `CC`
CC Excl: See code: C82.57

C84.68   **Anaplastic large cell lymphoma, ALK-positive, lymph nodes of multiple sites** `HIV` `CC`
CC Excl: See code: C82.58

C84.69   **Anaplastic large cell lymphoma, ALK-positive, extranodal and solid organ sites** `HIV` `CC`
CC Excl: See code: C82.50

√5th **C84.7**   **Anaplastic large cell lymphoma, ALK-negative**
EXCLUDES 1   *primary cutaneous CD30-positive T-cell proliferations (C86.6-)*

C84.70   **Anaplastic large cell lymphoma, ALK-negative, unspecified site** `HIV` `CC`
CC Excl: See code: C82.50

C84.71   **Anaplastic large cell lymphoma, ALK-negative, lymph nodes of head, face, and neck** `HIV` `CC`
CC Excl: See code: C82.51

C84.72   **Anaplastic large cell lymphoma, ALK-negative, intrathoracic lymph nodes** `HIV` `CC`
CC Excl: See code: C82.52

C84.73   **Anaplastic large cell lymphoma, ALK-negative, intra-abdominal lymph nodes** `HIV` `CC`
CC Excl: See code: C82.53

C84.74   **Anaplastic large cell lymphoma, ALK-negative, lymph nodes of axilla and upper limb** `HIV` `CC`
CC Excl: See code: C82.54

C84.75   **Anaplastic large cell lymphoma, ALK-negative, lymph nodes of inguinal region and lower limb** `HIV` `CC`
CC Excl: See code: C82.55

C84.76   **Anaplastic large cell lymphoma, ALK-negative, intrapelvic lymph nodes** `HIV` `CC`
CC Excl: See code: C82.56

C84.77   **Anaplastic large cell lymphoma, ALK-negative, spleen** `HIV` `CC`
CC Excl: See code: C82.57

C84.78   **Anaplastic large cell lymphoma, ALK-negative, lymph nodes of multiple sites** `HIV` `CC`
CC Excl: See code: C82.58

C84.79   **Anaplastic large cell lymphoma, ALK-negative, extranodal and solid organ sites** `HIV` `CC`
CC Excl: See code: C82.50

√5th **C84.A**   **Cutaneous T-cell lymphoma, unspecified**

C84.A0   **Cutaneous T-cell lymphoma, unspecified, unspecified site** `HIV` `CC`
CC Excl: See code: C82.50

C84.A1   **Cutaneous T-cell lymphoma, unspecified, lymph nodes of head, face, and neck** `HIV` `CC`
CC Excl: See code: C82.51

C84.A2   **Cutaneous T-cell lymphoma, unspecified, intrathoracic lymph nodes** `HIV` `CC`
CC Excl: See code: C82.52

C84.A3   **Cutaneous T-cell lymphoma, unspecified, intra-abdominal lymph nodes** `HIV` `CC`
CC Excl: See code: C82.53

C84.A4   **Cutaneous T-cell lymphoma, unspecified, lymph nodes of axilla and upper limb** `HIV` `CC`
CC Excl: See code: C82.54

C84.A5   **Cutaneous T-cell lymphoma, unspecified, lymph nodes of inguinal region and lower limb** `HIV` `CC`
CC Excl: See code: C82.55

C84.A6   **Cutaneous T-cell lymphoma, unspecified, intrapelvic lymph nodes** `HIV` `CC`
CC Excl: See code: C82.56

C84.A7   **Cutaneous T-cell lymphoma, unspecified, spleen** `HIV` `CC`
CC Excl: See code: C82.57

C84.A8   **Cutaneous T-cell lymphoma, unspecified, lymph nodes of multiple sites** `HIV` `CC`
CC Excl: See code: C82.58

C84.A9   **Cutaneous T-cell lymphoma, unspecified, extranodal and solid organ sites** `HIV` `CC`
CC Excl: See code: C82.50

√5th **C84.Z**   **Other mature T/NK-cell lymphomas**
NOTE   If T-cell lineage or involvement is mentioned in conjunction with a specific lymphoma, code to the more specific description.
EXCLUDES 1   *angioimmunoblastic T-cell lymphoma (C86.5)*
blastic NK-cell lymphoma (C86.4)
enteropathy-type T-cell lymphoma (C86.2)
extranodal NK-cell lymphoma, nasal type (C86.0)
hepatosplenic T-cell lymphoma (C86.1)
primary cutaneous CD30-positive T-cell proliferations (C86.6)
subcutaneous panniculitis-like T-cell lymphoma (C86.3)
T-cell leukemia (C91.1-)

C84.Z0   **Other mature T/NK-cell lymphomas, unspecified site** `HIV` `CC`
CC Excl: See code: C82.50

C84.Z1   **Other mature T/NK-cell lymphomas, lymph nodes of head, face, and neck** `HIV` `CC`
CC Excl: See code: C82.51

C84.Z2   **Other mature T/NK-cell lymphomas, intrathoracic lymph nodes** `HIV` `CC`
CC Excl: See code: C82.52

C84.Z3   **Other mature T/NK-cell lymphomas, intra-abdominal lymph nodes** `HIV` `CC`
CC Excl: See code: C82.53

C84.Z4   **Other mature T/NK-cell lymphomas, lymph nodes of axilla and upper limb** `HIV` `CC`
CC Excl: See code: C82.54

C84.Z5   **Other mature T/NK-cell lymphomas, lymph nodes of inguinal region and lower limb** `HIV` `CC`
CC Excl: See code: C82.55

C84.Z6   **Other mature T/NK-cell lymphomas, intrapelvic lymph nodes** `HIV` `CC`
CC Excl: See code: C82.56

C84.Z7   **Other mature T/NK-cell lymphomas, spleen** `HIV` `CC`
CC Excl: See code: C82.57

C84.Z8   **Other mature T/NK-cell lymphomas, lymph ndoes of multiple sites** `HIV` `CC`
CC Excl: See code: C82.58

C84.Z9   **Other mature T/NK-cell lymphomas, extranodal and solid organ sites** `HIV` `CC`
CC Excl: See code: C82.50

√5th **C84.9**   **Mature T/NK-cell lymphomas, unspecified**
NK/T cell lymphoma NOS
EXCLUDES 1   *mature T-cell lymphoma, not elsewhere classified (C84.4-)*

C84.90   **Mature T/NK-cell lymphomas, unspecified, unspecified site** `HIV` `CC`
CC Excl: See code: C82.50

C84.91   **Mature T/NK-cell lymphomas, unspecified, lymph nodes of head, face, and neck** `HIV` `CC`
CC Excl: See code: C82.51

C84.92   **Mature T/NK-cell lymphomas, unspecified, intrathoracic lymph nodes** `HIV` `CC`
CC Excl: See code: C82.52

C84.93   **Mature T/NK-cell lymphomas, unspecified, intra-abdominal lymph nodes** `HIV` `CC`
CC Excl: See code: C82.53

C84.94 Mature T/NK-cell lymphomas, unspecified, lymph nodes of axilla and upper limb `HIV` `CC`
CC Excl: See code: C82.54

C84.95 Mature T/NK-cell lymphomas, unspecified, lymph nodes of inguinal region and lower limb `HIV` `CC`
CC Excl: See code: C82.55

C84.96 Mature T/NK-cell lymphomas, unspecified, intrapelvic lymph nodes `HIV` `CC`
CC Excl: See code: C82.56

C84.97 Mature T/NK-cell lymphomas, unspecified, spleen `HIV` `CC`
CC Excl: See code: C82.57

C84.98 Mature T/NK-cell lymphomas, unspecified, lymph nodes of multiple sites `HIV` `CC`
CC Excl: See code: C82.58

C84.99 Mature T/NK-cell lymphomas, unspecified, extranodal and solid organ sites `HIV` `CC`
CC Excl: See code: C82.50

√4th **C85** Other specified and unspecified types of non-Hodgkin lymphoma
EXCLUDES 1 other specified types of T/NK-cell lymphoma (C86.-)
personal history of non-Hodgkin lymphoma (Z85.72)

√5th **C85.1** Unspecified B-cell lymphoma
NOTE If B-cell lineage or involvement is mentioned in conjunction with a specific lymphoma, code to the more specific description.

C85.10 Unspecified B-cell lymphoma, unspecified site `HIV` `CC`
CC Excl: See code: C82.50

C85.11 Unspecified B-cell lymphoma, lymph nodes of head, face, and neck `HIV` `CC`
CC Excl: See code: C82.51

C85.12 Unspecified B-cell lymphoma, intrathoracic lymph nodes `HIV` `CC`
CC Excl: See code: C82.52

C85.13 Unspecified B-cell lymphoma, intra-abdominal lymph nodes `HIV` `CC`
CC Excl: See code: C82.53

C85.14 Unspecified B-cell lymphoma, lymph nodes of axilla and upper limb `HIV` `CC`
CC Excl: See code: C82.54

C85.15 Unspecified B-cell lymphoma, lymph nodes of inguinal region and lower limb `HIV` `CC`
CC Excl: See code: C82.55

C85.16 Unspecified B-cell lymphoma, intrapelvic lymph nodes `HIV` `CC`
CC Excl: See code: C82.56

C85.17 Unspecified B-cell lymphoma, spleen `HIV` `CC`
CC Excl: See code: C82.57

C85.18 Unspecified B-cell lymphoma, lymph nodes of multiple sites `HIV` `CC`
CC Excl: See code: C82.58

C85.19 Unspecified B-cell lymphoma, extranodal and solid organ sites `HIV` `CC`
CC Excl: See code: C82.50

√5th **C85.2** Mediastinal (thymic) large B-cell lymphoma

C85.20 Mediastinal (thymic) large B-cell lymphoma, unspecified site `HIV` `CC`
CC Excl: See code: C82.50

C85.21 Mediastinal (thymic) large B-cell lymphoma, lymph nodes of head, face, and neck `HIV` `CC`
CC Excl: See code: C82.51

C85.22 Mediastinal (thymic) large B-cell lymphoma, intrathoracic lymph nodes `HIV` `CC`
CC Excl: See code: C82.52

C85.23 Mediastinal (thymic) large B-cell lymphoma, intra-abdominal lymph nodes `HIV` `CC`
CC Excl: See code: C82.53

C85.24 Mediastinal (thymic) large B-cell lymphoma, lymph nodes of axilla and upper limb `HIV` `CC`
CC Excl: See code: C82.54

C85.25 Mediastinal (thymic) large B-cell lymphoma, lymph nodes of inguinal region and lower limb `HIV` `CC`
CC Excl: See code: C82.55

C85.26 Mediastinal (thymic) large B-cell lymphoma, intrapelvic lymph nodes `HIV` `CC`
CC Excl: See code: C82.56

C85.27 Mediastinal (thymic) large B-cell lymphoma, spleen `HIV` `CC`
CC Excl: See code: C82.57

C85.28 Mediastinal (thymic) large B-cell lymphoma, lymph nodes of multiple sites `HIV` `CC`
CC Excl: See code: C82.58

C85.29 Mediastinal (thymic) large B-cell lymphoma, extranodal and solid organ sites `HIV` `CC`
CC Excl: See code: C82.50

√5th **C85.8** Other specified types of non-Hodgkin lymphoma

C85.80 Other specified types of non-Hodgkin lymphoma, unspecified site `HIV` `CC`
CC Excl: See code: C82.50

C85.81 Other specified types of non-Hodgkin lymphoma, lymph nodes of head, face, and neck `HIV` `CC`
CC Excl: See code: C82.51

C85.82 Other specified types of non-Hodgkin lymphoma, intrathoracic lymph nodes `HIV` `CC`
CC Excl: See code: C82.52

C85.83 Other specified types of non-Hodgkin lymphoma, intra-abdominal lymph nodes `HIV` `CC`
CC Excl: See code: C82.53

C85.84 Other specified types of non-Hodgkin lymphoma, lymph nodes of axilla and upper limb `HIV` `CC`
CC Excl: See code: C82.54

C85.85 Other specified types of non-Hodgkin lymphoma, lymph nodes of inguinal region and lower limb `HIV` `CC`
CC Excl: See code: C82.55

C85.86 Other specified types of non-Hodgkin lymphoma, intrapelvic lymph nodes `HIV` `CC`
CC Excl: See code: C82.56

C85.87 Other specified types of non-Hodgkin lymphoma, spleen `HIV` `CC`
CC Excl: See code: C82.57

C85.88 Other specified types of non-Hodgkin lymphoma, lymph nodes of multiple sites `HIV` `CC`
CC Excl: See code: C82.58

C85.89 Other specified types of non-Hodgkin lymphoma, extranodal and solid organ sites `HIV` `CC`
CC Excl: See code: C82.50

√5th **C85.9** Non-Hodgkin lymphoma, unspecified
Lymphoma NOS
Malignant lymphoma NOS
Non-Hodgkin lymphoma NOS

C85.90 Non-Hodgkin lymphoma, unspecified, unspecified site `HIV` `CC`
CC Excl: See code: C82.50

C85.91 Non-Hodgkin lymphoma, unspecified, lymph nodes of head, face, and neck `HIV` `CC`
CC Excl: See code: C82.51

C85.92 Non-Hodgkin lymphoma, unspecified, intrathoracic lymph nodes `HIV` `CC`
CC Excl: See code: C82.52

C85.93 Non-Hodgkin lymphoma, unspecified, intra-abdominal lymph nodes `HIV` `CC`
CC Excl: See code: C82.53

C85.94 Non-Hodgkin lymphoma, unspecified, lymph nodes of axilla and upper limb `HIV` `CC`
CC Excl: See code: C82.54

C85.95 Non-Hodgkin lymphoma, unspecified, lymph nodes of inguinal region and lower limb `HIV` `CC`
CC Excl: See code: C82.55

C85.96 Non-Hodgkin lymphoma, unspecified, intrapelvic lymph nodes `HIV` `CC`
CC Excl: See code: C82.56

C85.97 Non-Hodgkin lymphoma, unspecified, spleen `HIV` `CC`
CC Excl: See code: C82.57

C85.98 Non-Hodgkin lymphoma, unspecified, lymph nodes of multiple sites `HIV` `CC`
CC Excl: See code: C82.58

C85.99 Non-Hodgkin lymphoma, unspecified, extranodal and solid organ sites `HIV` `CC`
CC Excl: See code: C82.50

√4th **C86** Other specified types of T/NK-cell lymphoma
EXCLUDES 1 anaplastic large cell lymphoma, ALK negative (C84.7-)
anaplastic large cell lymphoma, ALK positive (C84.6-)
mature T/NK-cell lymphomas (C84.-)
other specified types of non-Hodgkin lymphoma (C85.8-)

C86.0 Extranodal NK/T-cell lymphoma, nasal type `HIV` `CC`
CC Excl: See code: C82.51

C86.1 Hepatosplenic T-cell lymphoma `HIV` `CC`
Alpha-beta and gamma delta types
CC Excl: See code: C82.57

Chapter 2. Neoplasms

C86.2   **Enteropathy-type (intestinal) T-cell lymphoma**   HIV CC
Enteropathy associated T-cell lymphoma
CC Excl: See code: C82.53

C86.3   **Subcutaneous panniculitis-like T-cell lymphoma**   HIV CC
CC Excl: See code: C82.53

C86.4   **Blastic NK-cell lymphoma**   HIV CC
CC Excl: See code: C82.50

C86.5   **Angioimmunoblastic T-cell lymphoma**   HIV CC
Angioimmunoblastic lymphadenopathy with dysproteinemia [AILD]
CC Excl: See code: C83.00

C86.6   **Primary cutaneous CD30-positive T-cell proliferations**   HIV CC
Lymphomatoid papulosis
Primary cutaneous anaplastic large cell lymphoma
Primary cutaneous CD30-positive large T-cell lymphoma
CC Excl: See code: C83.00

✓4th **C88**   **Malignant immunoproliferative diseases and certain other B-cell lymphomas**
EXCLUDES 1   B-cell lymphoma, unspecified (C85.1-)
personal history of other malignant neoplasms of lymphoid, hematopoietic and related tissues (Z85.79)

C88.0   **Waldenström macroglobulinemia**
Lymphoplasmacytic lymphoma with IgM-production
Macroglobulinemia (idiopathic) (primary)
EXCLUDES 1   small cell B-cell lymphoma (C83.0)

C88.2   **Heavy chain disease**   CC
Franklin disease
Gamma heavy chain disease
Mu heavy chain disease
CC Excl: C88.2-C88.3, C88.8-C91.32, C91.50-C94.32, C94.80-C95.92, D49.81-D49.9

C88.3   **Immunoproliferative small intestinal disease**   CC
Alpha heavy chain disease
Mediterranean lymphoma
CC Excl: See code: C88.2

C88.4   **Extranodal marginal zone B-cell lymphoma of mucosa-associated lymphoid tissue [MALT-lymphoma]**   HIV CC
Lymphoma of skin-associated lymphoid tissue [SALT-lymphoma]
Lymphoma of bronchial-associated lymphoid tissue [BALT-lymphoma]
EXCLUDES 1   high malignant (diffuse large B-cell) lymphoma (C83.3-)
CC Excl: C82.50-C82.59, C83.10-C83.19, C84.40-C86.4, C88.4, C96.4, C96.Z-C96.9, D49.81-D49.9

C88.8   **Other malignant immunoproliferative diseases**   CC
CC Excl: C88.2-C88.3, C88.8-C95.92, D45-D47.1, D47.3, D47.Z9-D47.9, D48.7-D48.9, D49.81-D49.9

C88.9   **Malignant immunoproliferative disease, unspecified**   CC
Immunoproliferative disease NOS
CC Excl: See code: C88.2

✓4th **C90**   **Multiple myeloma and malignant plasma cell neoplasms**
EXCLUDES 1   personal history of other malignant neoplasms of lymphoid, hematopoietic and related tissues (Z85.79)

CC Excl: For CC codes in category C90, unless otherwise noted:
C88.2-C88.3, C88.8-C95.92, D45-D47.1, D47.3, D47.Z9-D47.9, D48.7-D48.9, D49.81-D49.9

✓5th **C90.0**   **Multiple myeloma**
Kahler's disease   Myelomatosis
Medullary plasmacytoma   Plasma cell myeloma
EXCLUDES 1   solitary myeloma (C90.3-)
solitary plasmactyoma (C90.3-)

C90.00   **Multiple myeloma** not having achieved remission   CC
Multiple myeloma with failed remission
Multiple myeloma NOS

C90.01   **Multiple myeloma** in remission   CC

C90.02   **Multiple myeloma** in relapse   CC

✓5th **C90.1**   **Plasma cell leukemia**
Plasmacytic leukemia

C90.10   **Plasma cell leukemia** not having achieved remission   CC
Plasma cell leukemia with failed remission
Plasma cell leukemia NOS

C90.11   **Plasma cell leukemia** in remission   CC

C90.12   **Plasma cell leukemia** in relapse   CC

✓5th **C90.2**   **Extramedullary plasmacytoma**

C90.20   **Extramedullary plasmacytoma** not having achieved remission   CC
Extramedullary plasmacytoma with failed remission
Extramedullary plasmacytoma NOS

C90.21   **Extramedullary plasmacytoma** in remission   CC

C90.22   **Extramedullary plasmacytoma** in relapse   CC

✓5th **C90.3**   **Solitary plasmacytoma**
Localized malignant plasma cell tumor NOS
Plasmacytoma NOS
Solitary myeloma

C90.30   **Solitary plasmacytoma** not having achieved remission   CC
Solitary plasmacytoma with failed remission
Solitary plasmacytoma NOS

C90.31   **Solitary plasmacytoma** in remission   CC

C90.32   **Solitary plasmacytoma** in relapse   CC

✓4th **C91**   **Lymphoid leukemia**
EXCLUDES 1   personal history of leukemia (Z85.6)

CC Excl: For CC codes in category C91, unless otherwise noted:
C88.2-C88.3, C88.8-C95.92, D45-D47.1, D47.3, D47.Z9-D47.9, D48.7-D48.9, D49.81-D49.9

✓5th **C91.0**   **Acute lymphoblastic leukemia [ALL]**
NOTE   Code C91.0 should only be used for T-cell and B-cell precursor leukemia

C91.00   **Acute lymphoblastic leukemia** not having achieved remission   CC
Acute lymphoblastic leukemia with failed remission
Acute lymphoblastic leukemia NOS

C91.01   **Acute lymphoblastic leukemia,** in remission   CC

C91.02   **Acute lymphoblastic leukemia,** in relapse   CC

✓5th **C91.1**   **Chronic lymphocytic leukemia** of B-cell type
Lymphoplasmacytic leukemia
Richter syndrome
EXCLUDES 1   lymphoplasmacytic lymphoma (C83.0-)

C91.10   **Chronic lymphocytic leukemia of B-cell type** not having achieved remission   CC
Chronic lymphocytic leukemia of B-cell type with failed remission
Chronic lymphocytic leukemia of B-cell type NOS

C91.11   **Chronic lymphocytic leukemia of B-cell type** in remission   CC

C91.12   **Chronic lymphocytic leukemia of B-cell type** in relapse   CC

✓5th **C91.3**   **Prolymphocytic leukemia** of B-cell type

C91.30   **Prolymphocytic leukemia of B-cell type** not having achieved remission   CC
Prolymphocytic leukemia of B-cell type with failed remission
Prolymphocytic leukemia of B-cell type NOS

C91.31   **Prolymphocytic leukemia of B-cell type,** in remission   CC

C91.32   **Prolymphocytic leukemia of B-cell type,** in relapse   CC

✓5th **C91.4**   **Hairy cell leukemia**
Leukemic reticuloendotheliosis

C91.40   **Hairy cell leukemia** not having achieved remission   CC
Hairy cell leukemia with failed remission
Hairy cell leukemia NOS
CC Excl: C82.50, C82.59, C83.10, C83.19, C84.40, C84.49, C84.60, C84.69-C84.70, C84.79-C84.90, C84.99-C84.A0, C84.A9-C84.Z0, C84.Z9, C85.10, C85.19-C85.20, C85.29, C85.80, C85.89-C85.90, C85.99, C86.4, C88.4, C91.40-C91.42, C96.4, C96.9, C96.Z, D49.81-D49.9

C91.41   **Hairy cell leukemia,** in remission   CC
CC Excl: See code: C91.40

C91.42   **Hairy cell leukemia,** in relapse   CC
CC Excl: See code: C91.40

N Newborn: 0   P Pediatric: 0-17   M Maternity: 12-55   A Adult: 15-124   MCC Major CC Condition   PDxMCC PDx acts as own MCC   CC CC Condition   PDxCC PDx acts as own CC

✓5ᵗʰ **C91.5** Adult T-cell **lymphoma/leukemia (HTLV-1-associated)**
Acute variant of adult T-cell lymphoma/leukemia (HTLV-1-associated)
Chronic variant of adult T-cell lymphoma/leukemia (HTLV-1-associated)
Lymphomatoid variant of adult T-cell lymphoma/leukemia (HTLV-1-associated)
Smouldering variant of adult T-cell lymphoma/leukemia (HTLV-1-associated)

     C91.5Ø **Adult T-cell lymphoma/leukemia (HTLV-1-associated)** not having achieved remission   CC A
Adult T-cell lymphoma/leukemia (HTLV-1-associated) with failed remission
Adult T-cell lymphoma/leukemia (HTLV-1-associated) NOS
CC Excl: C88.2-C88.3, C88.8-C91.32, C91.5Ø-C94.32, C94.8Ø-C95.92, D49.81-D49.9

     C91.51 **Adult T-cell lymphoma/leukemia (HTLV-1-associated), in remission**   CC A
CC Excl: See code: C91.5Ø

     C91.52 **Adult T-cell lymphoma/leukemia (HTLV-1-associated), in relapse**   CC A
CC Excl: See code: C91.5Ø

✓5ᵗʰ **C91.6** Prolymphocytic **leukemia of** T-cell type

     C91.6Ø **Prolymphocytic leukemia of T-cell type** not having achieved remission   CC
Prolymphocytic leukemia of T-cell type with failed remission
Prolymphocytic leukemia of T-cell type NOS
CC Excl: See code: C91.5Ø

     C91.61 **Prolymphocytic leukemia of T-cell type, in remission**   CC
CC Excl: See code: C91.5Ø

     C91.62 **Prolymphocytic leukemia of T-cell type, in relapse**   CC
CC Excl: See code: C91.5Ø

✓5ᵗʰ **C91.A** Mature B-cell **leukemia** Burkitt-type
EXCLUDES 1 Burkitt lymphoma (C83.7-)

     C91.AØ **Mature B-cell leukemia Burkitt-type** not having achieved remission   CC
Mature B-cell leukemia Burkitt-type with failed remission
Mature B-cell leukemia Burkitt-type NOS
CC Excl: See code: C91.5Ø

     C91.A1 **Mature B-cell leukemia Burkitt-type, in remission**   CC
CC Excl: See code: C91.5Ø

     C91.A2 **Mature B-cell leukemia Burkitt-type, in relapse**   CC
CC Excl: See code: C91.5Ø

✓5ᵗʰ **C91.Z** Other **lymphoid leukemia**
T-cell large granular lymphocytic leukemia (associated with rheumatoid arthritis)

     C91.ZØ **Other lymphoid leukemia** not having achieved remission   CC
Other lymphoid leukemia with failed remission
Other lymphoid leukemia NOS
CC Excl: See code: C91.5Ø

     C91.Z1 **Other lymphoid leukemia, in remission**   CC
CC Excl: See code: C91.5Ø

     C91.Z2 **Other lymphoid leukemia, in relapse**   CC
CC Excl: See code: C91.5Ø

✓5ᵗʰ **C91.9** Lymphoid leukemia, **unspecified**

     C91.9Ø **Lymphoid leukemia, unspecified** not having achieved remission   CC
Lymphoid leukemia with failed remission
Lymphoid leukemia NOS
CC Excl: See code: C91.5Ø

     C91.91 **Lymphoid leukemia, unspecified, in remission**   CC
CC Excl: See code: C91.5Ø

     C91.92 **Lymphoid leukemia, unspecified, in relapse**   CC
CC Excl: See code: C91.5Ø

✓4ᵗʰ **C92** **Myeloid leukemia**
INCLUDES granulocytic leukemia
myelogenous leukemia
EXCLUDES 1 personal history of leukemia (Z85.6)

CC Excl: For CC codes in category C92, unless otherwise noted: C88.2-C88.3, C88.8-C91.32, C91.5Ø-C94.32, C94.8Ø-C95.92, D49.81-D49.9

✓5ᵗʰ **C92.Ø** Acute myeloblastic **leukemia**
Acute myeloblastic leukemia, minimal differentiation
Acute myeloblastic leukemia (with maturation)
Acute myeloblastic leukemia 1/ETO
Acute myeloblastic leukemia MØ
Acute myeloblastic leukemia M1
Acute myeloblastic leukemia M2
Acute myeloblastic leukemia with t(8;21)
Acute myeloblastic leukemia (without a FAB classification) NOS
Refractory anemia with excess blasts in transformation [RAEB T]
EXCLUDES 1 acute exacerbation of chronic myeloid leukemia (C92.1Ø)
refractory anemia with excess of blasts not in transformation (D46.2-)

     C92.ØØ **Acute myeloblastic leukemia, not having achieved remission**   CC
Acute myeloblastic leukemia with failed remission
Acute myeloblastic leukemia NOS

     C92.Ø1 **Acute myeloblastic leukemia, in remission**   CC

     C92.Ø2 **Acute myeloblastic leukemia, in relapse**   CC

✓5ᵗʰ **C92.1** Chronic **myeloid leukemia, BCR/ABL-positive**
Chronic myelogenous leukemia, Philadelphia chromosome (Ph1) positive
Chronic myelogenous leukemia, t(9;22) (q34;q11)
Chronic myelogenous leukemia with crisis of blast cells
EXCLUDES 1 atypical chronic myeloid leukemia BCR/ABL-negative (C92.2-)
chronic myelomonocytic leukemia (C93.1-)
chronic myeloproliferative disease (D47.1)

     C92.1Ø **Chronic myeloid leukemia, BCR/ABL-positive, not having achieved remission**   CC
Chronic myeloid leukemia, BCR/ABL-positive with failed remission
Chronic myeloid leukemia, BCR/ABL-positive NOS

     C92.11 **Chronic myeloid leukemia, BCR/ABL-positive, in remission**   CC

     C92.12 **Chronic myeloid leukemia, BCR/ABL-positive, in relapse**   CC

✓5ᵗʰ **C92.2** Atypical chronic **myeloid leukemia, BCR/ABL-negative**

     C92.2Ø **Atypical chronic myeloid leukemia, BCR/ABL-negative, not having achieved remission**   CC
Atypical chronic myeloid leukemia, BCR/ABL-negative with failed remission
Atypical chronic myeloid leukemia, BCR/ABL-negative NOS

     C92.21 **Atypical chronic myeloid leukemia, BCR/ABL-negative, in remission**   CC

     C92.22 **Atypical chronic myeloid leukemia, BCR/ABL-negative, in relapse**   CC

✓5ᵗʰ **C92.3** Myeloid **sarcoma**
A malignant tumor of immature myeloid cells
Chloroma
Granulocytic sarcoma

     C92.3Ø **Myeloid sarcoma,** not having achieved remission   CC
Myeloid sarcoma with failed remission
Myeloid sarcoma NOS

     C92.31 **Myeloid sarcoma,** in remission   CC

     C92.32 **Myeloid sarcoma,** in relapse   CC

✓5ᵗʰ **C92.4** Acute promyelocytic **leukemia**
AML M3
AML Me with t(15;17) and variants

     C92.4Ø **Acute promyelocytic leukemia,** not having achieved remission   CC
Acute promyelocytic leukemia with failed remission
Acute promyelocytic leukemia NOS

     C92.41 **Acute promyelocytic leukemia, in remission**   CC

     C92.42 **Acute promyelocytic leukemia, in relapse**   CC

✓ Additional Character Required   ✓x7ᵗʰ Placeholder Alert   Unacceptable PDx   Manifestation   Hospital Acquired Condition   **EXCLUDES 1** Not Coded Here   **EXCLUDES 2** Not Included Here

✓5ᵗʰ C92.5   **Acute myelomonocytic leukemia**
AML M4
AML M4 Eo with inv(16) or t(16;16)

     C92.5Ø   **Acute myelomonocytic leukemia, not having achieved remission**   CC
         Acute myelomonocytic leukemia with failed remission
         Acute myelomonocytic leukemia NOS

     C92.51   **Acute myelomonocytic leukemia, in remission**   CC

     C92.52   **Acute myelomonocytic leukemia, in relapse**   CC

✓5ᵗʰ C92.6   **Acute myeloid leukemia with 11q23-abnormality**
Acute myeloid leukemia with variation of MLL-gene

     C92.6Ø   **Acute myeloid leukemia with 11q23-abnormality** CC **not having achieved remission**
         Acute myeloid leukemia with 11q23-abnormality with failed remission
         Acute myeloid leukemia with 11q23-abnormality NOS

     C92.61   **Acute myeloid leukemia with 11q23-abnormality** CC **in remission**

     C92.62   **Acute myeloid leukemia with 11q23-abnormality** CC **in relapse**

✓5ᵗʰ C92.A   **Acute myeloid leukemia with multilineage dysplasia**
Acute myeloid leukemia with dysplasia of remaining hematopoesis and/or myelodysplastic disease in its history

     C92.AØ   **Acute myeloid leukemia with multilineage** CC **dysplasia, not having achieved remission**
         Acute myeloid leukemia with multilineage dysplasia with failed remission
         Acute myeloid leukemia with multilineage dysplasia NOS

     C92.A1   **Acute myeloid leukemia with multilineage** CC **dysplasia, in remission**

     C92.A2   **Acute myeloid leukemia with multilineage** CC **dysplasia, in relapse**

✓5ᵗʰ C92.Z   **Other myeloid leukemia**

     C92.ZØ   **Other myeloid leukemia not having achieved** CC **remission**
         Myeloid leukemia NEC with failed remission
         Myeloid leukemia NEC

     C92.Z1   **Other myeloid leukemia, in remission**   CC

     C92.Z2   **Other myeloid leukemia, in relapse**   CC

✓5ᵗʰ C92.9   **Myeloid leukemia, unspecified**

     C92.9Ø   **Myeloid leukemia, unspecified, not having** CC **achieved remission**
         Myeloid leukemia, unspecified with failed remission
         Myeloid leukemia, unspecified NOS

     C92.91   **Myeloid leukemia, unspecified in remission**   CC

     C92.92   **Myeloid leukemia, unspecified in relapse**   CC

✓4ᵗʰ C93   **Monocytic leukemia**
     INCLUDES   monocytoid leukemia
     EXCLUDES 1   *personal history of leukemia (Z85.6)*

     CC Excl: For CC codes in category C93, unless otherwise noted:
     C88.2-C88.3, C88.8-C91.32, C91.5Ø-C94.32, C94.8Ø-C95.92, D49.81-D49.9

✓5ᵗʰ C93.Ø   **Acute monoblastic/monocytic leukemia**
AML M5   AML M5b
AML M5a

     C93.ØØ   **Acute monoblastic/monocytic leukemia, not** CC **having achieved remission**
         Acute monoblastic/monocytic leukemia with failed remission
         Acute monoblastic/monocytic leukemia NOS

     C93.Ø1   **Acute monoblastic/monocytic leukemia, in** CC **remission**

     C93.Ø2   **Acute monoblastic/monocytic leukemia, in** CC **relapse**

✓5ᵗʰ C93.1   **Chronic myelomonocytic leukemia**
Chronic monocytic leukemia
CMML-1
CMML-2
CMML with eosinophilia

     C93.1Ø   **Chronic myelomonocytic leukemia not having** CC **achieved remission**
         Chronic myelomonocytic leukemia with failed remission
         Chronic myelomonocytic leukemia NOS

     C93.11   **Chronic myelomonocytic leukemia, in remission**   CC

     C93.12   **Chronic myelomonocytic leukemia, in relapse**   CC

✓5ᵗʰ C93.3   **Juvenile myelomonocytic leukemia**

     C93.3Ø   **Juvenile myelomonocytic leukemia, not** CC P **having achieved remission**
         Juvenile myelomonocytic leukemia with failed remission
         Juvenile myelomonocytic leukemia NOS

     C93.31   **Juvenile myelomonocytic leukemia, in** CC P **remission**

     C93.32   **Juvenile myelomonocytic leukemia, in relapse** CC P

✓5ᵗʰ C93.Z   **Other monocytic leukemia**

     C93.ZØ   **Other monocytic leukemia, not having achieved** CC **remission**
         Other monocytic leukemia NOS

     C93.Z1   **Other monocytic leukemia, in remission**   CC

     C93.Z2   **Other monocytic leukemia, in relapse**   CC

✓5ᵗʰ C93.9   **Monocytic leukemia, unspecified**

     C93.9Ø   **Monocytic leukemia, unspecified, not having** CC **achieved remission**
         Monocytic leukemia, unspecified with failed remission
         Monocytic leukemia, unspecified NOS

     C93.91   **Monocytic leukemia, unspecified in remission**   CC

     C93.92   **Monocytic leukemia, unspecified in relapse**   CC

✓4ᵗʰ C94   **Other leukemias of specified cell type**
     EXCLUDES 1   *leukemic reticuloendotheliosis (C91.4-)*
         myelodysplastic syndromes (D46.-)
         personal history of leukemia (Z85.6)
         plasma cell leukemia (C90.1-)

     CC Excl: For CC codes in category C94, unless otherwise noted:
     C88.2-C88.3, C88.8-C91.32, C91.5Ø-C94.32, C94.8Ø-C95.92, D49.81-D49.9

✓5ᵗʰ C94.Ø   **Acute erythroid leukemia**
Acute myeloid leukemia M6(a)(b)
Erythroleukemia

     C94.ØØ   **Acute erythroid leukemia, not having achieved** CC **remission**
         Acute erythroid leukemia with failed remission
         Acute erythroid leukemia NOS

     C94.Ø1   **Acute erythroid leukemia, in remission**   CC

     C94.Ø2   **Acute erythroid leukemia, in relapse**   CC

✓5ᵗʰ C94.2   **Acute megakaryoblastic leukemia**
Acute myeloid leukemia M7
Acute megakaryocytic leukemia

     C94.2Ø   **Acute megakaryoblastic leukemia not having** CC **achieved remission**
         Acute megakaryoblastic leukemia with failied remission
         Acute megakaryoblastic leukemia NOS

     C94.21   **Acute megakaryoblastic leukemia, in remission**   CC

     C94.22   **Acute megakaryoblastic leukemia, in relapse**   CC

✓5ᵗʰ C94.3   **Mast cell leukemia**

     C94.3Ø   **Mast cell leukemia not having achieved** CC **remission**
         Mast cell leukemia with failed remission
         Mast cell leukemia NOS

     C94.31   **Mast cell leukemia, in remission**   CC

     C94.32   **Mast cell leukemia, in relapse**   CC

✓5ᵗʰ C94.4   **Acute panmyelosis with myelofibrosis**
Acute myelofibrosis
     EXCLUDES 1   *myelofibrosis NOS (D75.81)*
         secondary myelofibrosis NOS (D75.81)

     C94.4Ø   **Acute panmyelosis with myelofibrosis not** CC **having achieved remission**
         Acute myelofibrosis NOS
         Acute panmyelosis with myelofibrosis with failed remission
         Acute panmyelosis NOS
         CC Excl: C88.2-C88.3, C88.8-C88.9, C90.1Ø-C90.11, C90.2Ø-C90.21, C90.3Ø-C90.31, C91.ØØ-C95.92, D45-D47.1, D47.3, D47.Z9-D47.9, D48.7-D48.9

     C94.41   **Acute panmyelosis with myelofibrosis, in** CC **remission**
         CC Excl: See code: C94.4Ø

     C94.42   **Acute panmyelosis with myelofibrosis, in** CC **relapse**
         CC Excl: See code: C94.4Ø

     C94.6   **Myelodysplastic disease, not classified**   CC
         Myeloproliferative disease, not classified
         CC Excl: See code: C94.4Ø

N Newborn: 0   P Pediatric: 0-17   M Maternity: 12-55   A Adult: 15-124   **MCC** Major CC Condition   **PDxMCC** PDx acts as own MCC   **CC** CC Condition   **PDxCC** PDx acts as own CC

480
ICD-10-CM 2016

Chapter 2. Neoplasms

✓5ᵗʰ **C94.8 Other specified leukemias**
Aggressive NK-cell leukemia
Acute basophilic leukemia

     C94.80 Other specified leukemias not having achieved `CC`
remission
Other specified leukemia with failed remission
Other specified leukemias NOS

     C94.81 Other specified leukemias, in remission `CC`

     C94.82 Other specified leukemias, in relapse `CC`

✓4ᵗʰ **C95 Leukemia of unspecified cell type**
EXCLUDES1 personal history of leukemia (Z85.6)

> **CC Excl: For CC codes in category C95, unless otherwise noted:**
> C88.2-C88.3, C88.8-C91.32, C91.50-C94.32, C94.80-C95.92, D49.81-
> D49.9

✓5ᵗʰ **C95.0 Acute leukemia of unspecified cell type**
Acute bilineal leukemia
Acute mixed lineage leukemia
Biphenotypic acute leukemia
Stem cell leukemia of unclear lineage
EXCLUDES1 acute exacerbation of unspecified chronic leukemia
(C95.10)

     C95.00 Acute leukemia of unspecified cell type not `CC`
having achieved remission
Acute leukemia of unspecified cell type with failed
remission
Acute leukemia NOS

     C95.01 Acute leukemia of unspecified cell type, in `CC`
remission

     C95.02 Acute leukemia of unspecified cell type, in `CC`
relapse

✓5ᵗʰ **C95.1 Chronic leukemia of unspecified cell type**

     C95.10 Chronic leukemia of unspecified cell type not `CC`
having achieved remission
Chronic leukemia of unspecified cell type with failed
remission
Chronic leukemia NOS

     C95.11 Chronic leukemia of unspecified cell type, in `CC`
remission

     C95.12 Chronic leukemia of unspecified cell type, in `CC`
relapse

✓5ᵗʰ **C95.9 Leukemia, unspecified**

     C95.90 Leukemia, unspecified not having achieved `CC`
remission
Leukemia, unspecified with failed remission
Leukemia NOS

     C95.91 Leukemia, unspecified, in remission `CC`

     C95.92 Leukemia, unspecified, in relapse `CC`

✓4ᵗʰ **C96 Other and unspecified malignant neoplasms of lymphoid,**
hematopoietic and related tissue
EXCLUDES1 personal history of other malignant neoplasms of lymphoid,
hematopoietic and related tissues (Z85.79)

C96.0 Multifocal and multisystemic (disseminated) `CC`
Langerhans-cell histiocytosis
Histiocytosis X, multisystemic
Letterer-Siwe disease
EXCLUDES1 adult pulmonary Langerhans cell histiocytosis (J84.82)
multifocal and unisystemic Langerhans-cell
histiocytosis (C96.5)
unifocal Langerhans-cell histiocytosis (C96.6)
CC Excl: C82.50, C82.59, C83.10, C83.19, C84.40, C84.49, C84.60,
C84.69-C84.70, C84.79-C84.90, C84.99-C84.A0, C84.A9-C84.Z0,
C84.Z9, C85.10, C85.19-C85.20, C85.29, C85.80, C85.89-C85.90,
C85.99, C86.4, C88.4, C96.0, C96.4, C96.9, C96.Z, D49.81-D49.9

C96.2 Malignant mast cell tumor `CC`
Aggressive systemic mastocytosis
Mast cell sarcoma
EXCLUDES1 indolent mastocytosis (D47.0)
mast cell leukemia (C94.30)
mastocytosis (congenital) (cutaneous) (Q82.2)
CC Excl: C82.50, C82.59, C83.10, C83.19, C84.40, C84.49, C84.60,
C84.69-C84.70, C84.79-C84.90, C84.99-C84.A0, C84.A9-C84.Z0,
C84.Z9, C85.10, C85.19-C85.20, C85.29, C85.80, C85.89-C85.90,
C85.99, C86.4, C88.4, C96.2, C96.4, C96.9, C96.Z, D49.81-D49.9

C96.4 Sarcoma of dendritic cells (accessory cells) `CC`
Follicular dendritic cell sarcoma
Interdigitating dendritic cell sarcoma
Langerhans cell sarcoma
CC Excl: C96.4, C96.9, C96.Z, D49.81-D49.9

C96.5 Multifocal and unisystemic Langerhans-cell histiocytosis `CC`
Hand-Schüller-Christian disease
Histiocytosis X, multifocal
EXCLUDES1 multifocal and multisystemic (disseminated)
Langerhans-cell histiocytosis (C96.0)
unifocal Langerhans-cell histiocytosis (C96.6)
CC Excl: E71.310-E71.32, E71.40-E71.548, E80.4-E80.7, E88.40-
E88.49, H49.811-H49.819

C96.6 Unifocal Langerhans-cell histiocytosis `CC`
Eosinophilic granuloma`CC`
Histiocytosis X, unifocal
Histiocytosis X NOS
Langerhans-cell histiocytosis NOS
EXCLUDES1 multifocal and multisystemic (disseminated)
Langerhans-cell histiocytosis (C96.0)
multifocal and unisystemic Langerhans-cell
histiocytosis (C96.5)
CC Excl: See code: C96.5

C96.A Histiocytic sarcoma `CC`
Malignant histiocytosis
CC Excl: C82.50, C82.59, C83.10, C83.19, C84.40, C84.49, C84.60,
C84.69-C84.70, C84.79-C84.90, C84.99-C84.A0, C84.A9-C84.Z0,
C84.Z9, C85.10, C85.19-C85.20, C85.29, C85.80, C85.89-C85.90,
C85.99, C86.4, C88.4, C96.4, C96.9-C96.Z, D49.81-D49.9

C96.Z Other specified malignant neoplasms of lymphoid, `CC`
hematopoietic and related tissue
CC Excl: See code: C96.4

C96.9 Malignant neoplasm of lymphoid, hematopoietic and `CC`
related tissue, unspecified
CC Excl: See code: C96.4

In situ neoplasms (D00-D09)

`INCLUDES` Bowen's disease
erythroplasia
grade III intraepithelial neoplasia
Queyrat's erythroplasia

✓4ᵗʰ **D00 Carcinoma in situ of oral cavity, esophagus and stomach**
EXCLUDES1 melanoma in situ (D03.-)

✓5ᵗʰ **D00.0 Carcinoma in situ of lip, oral cavity and pharynx**
Use additional code to identify:
exposure to environmental tobacco smoke (Z77.22)
exposure to tobacco smoke in the perinatal period (P96.81)
history of tobacco use (Z87.891)
occupational exposure to environmental tobacco smoke
(Z57.31)
tobacco dependence (F17.-)
tobacco use (Z72.0)
EXCLUDES1 carcinoma in situ of aryepiglottic fold or interarytenoid
fold, laryngeal aspect (D02.0)
carcinoma in situ of epiglottis NOS (D02.0)
carcinoma in situ of epiglottis suprahyoid portion
(D02.0)
carcinoma in situ of skin of lip (D03.0, D04.0)

     D00.00 Carcinoma in situ of oral cavity, unspecified site

     D00.01 Carcinoma in situ of labial mucosa and vermilion
border

     D00.02 Carcinoma in situ of buccal mucosa

     D00.03 Carcinoma in situ of gingiva and edentulous alveolar
ridge

     D00.04 Carcinoma in situ of soft palate

     D00.05 Carcinoma in situ of hard palate

     D00.06 Carcinoma in situ of floor of mouth

     D00.07 Carcinoma in situ of tongue

     D00.08 Carcinoma in situ of pharynx
Carcinoma in situ of aryepiglottic fold NOS
Carcinoma in situ of hypopharyngeal aspect of
aryepiglottic fold
Carcinoma in situ of marginal zone of aryepiglottic
fold

D00.1 Carcinoma in situ of esophagus

D00.2 Carcinoma in situ of stomach

✓4ᵗʰ **D01 Carcinoma in situ of other and unspecified digestive organs**
EXCLUDES1 melanoma in situ (D03.-)

D01.0 Carcinoma in situ of colon
EXCLUDES1 carcinoma in situ of rectosigmoid junction (D01.1)

D01.1 Carcinoma in situ of rectosigmoid junction

D01.2 Carcinoma in situ of rectum

☑ Additional Character Required   ☑x7ᵗʰ Placeholder Alert   Unacceptable PDx   Manifestation   Hospital Acquired Condition   *EXCLUDES1* Not Coded Here   *EXCLUDES2* Not Included Here

D01.3 Carcinoma in situ of **anus and anal canal**
    EXCLUDES 1 *carcinoma in situ of anal margin (D04.5)*
    carcinoma in situ of anal skin (D04.5)
    carcinoma in situ of perianal skin (D04.5)

✓5ᵗʰ **D01.4** Carcinoma in situ of **other and unspecified parts of intestine**
    EXCLUDES 1 *carcinoma in situ of ampulla of Vater (D01.5)*

    D01.40 Carcinoma in situ of **unspecified** part of intestine

    D01.49 Carcinoma in situ of **other** parts of intestine

D01.5 Carcinoma in situ of **liver, gallbladder and bile ducts**
    Carcinoma in situ of ampulla of Vater

D01.7 Carcinoma in situ of **other** specified digestive organs
    Carcinoma in situ of pancreas

D01.9 Carcinoma in situ of digestive organ, **unspecified**

✓4ᵗʰ **D02** **Carcinoma in situ of middle ear and respiratory system**
    Use additional code to identify:
    exposure to environmental tobacco smoke (Z77.22)
    exposure to tobacco smoke in the perinatal period (P96.81)
    history of tobacco use (Z87.891)
    occupational exposure to environmental tobacco smoke (Z57.31)
    tobacco dependence (F17.-)
    tobacco use (Z72.0)
    EXCLUDES 1 *melanoma in situ (D03.-)*

    D02.0 Carcinoma in situ of **larynx**
        Carcinoma in situ of aryepiglottic fold or interarytenoid fold, laryngeal aspect
        Carcinoma in situ of epiglottis (suprahyoid portion)
        EXCLUDES 1 *carcinoma in situ of aryepiglottic fold or interarytenoid fold NOS (D00.08)*
        carcinoma in situ of hypopharyngeal aspect (D00.08)
        carcinoma in situ of marginal zone (D00.08)

    D02.1 Carcinoma in situ of **trachea**

✓5ᵗʰ   **D02.2** Carcinoma in situ of **bronchus and lung**

        D02.20 Carcinoma in situ of **unspecified** bronchus and lung

        D02.21 Carcinoma in situ of **right** bronchus and lung

        D02.22 Carcinoma in situ of **left** bronchus and lung

    D02.3 Carcinoma in situ of **other** parts of respiratory system
        Carcinoma in situ of accessory sinuses
        Carcinoma in situ of middle ear
        Carcinoma in situ of nasal cavities
        EXCLUDES 1 *carcinoma in situ of ear (external) (skin) (D04.2-)*
        carcinoma in situ of nose NOS (D09.8)
        carcinoma in situ of skin of nose (D04.3)

    D02.4 Carcinoma in situ of respiratory system, **unspecified**

✓4ᵗʰ **D03** **Melanoma in situ**

    D03.0 Melanoma in situ of **lip**

✓5ᵗʰ   **D03.1** Melanoma in situ of **eyelid, including canthus**

        D03.10 Melanoma in situ of **unspecified** eyelid, including canthus

        D03.11 Melanoma in situ of **right** eyelid, including canthus

        D03.12 Melanoma in situ of **left** eyelid, including canthus

✓5ᵗʰ   **D03.2** Melanoma in situ of **ear and external auricular canal**

        D03.20 Melanoma in situ of **unspecified** ear and external auricular canal

        D03.21 Melanoma in situ of **right** ear and external auricular canal

        D03.22 Melanoma in situ of **left** ear and external auricular canal

✓5ᵗʰ   **D03.3** Melanoma in situ of **other and unspecified parts of face**

        D03.30 Melanoma in situ of **unspecified** part of face

        D03.39 Melanoma in situ of **other** parts of face

    D03.4 Melanoma in situ of **scalp and neck**

✓5ᵗʰ   **D03.5** Melanoma in situ of **trunk**

        D03.51 Melanoma in situ of **anal skin**
            Melanoma in situ of anal margin
            Melanoma in situ of perianal skin

        D03.52 Melanoma in situ of **breast (skin) (soft tissue)**

        D03.59 Melanoma in situ of **other** part of trunk

✓5ᵗʰ   **D03.6** Melanoma in situ of **upper limb, including shoulder**

        D03.60 Melanoma in situ of **unspecified** upper limb, including shoulder

        D03.61 Melanoma in situ of **right** upper limb, including shoulder

        D03.62 Melanoma in situ of **left** upper limb, including shoulder

✓5ᵗʰ **D03.7** Melanoma in situ of **lower limb, including hip**

    D03.70 Melanoma in situ of **unspecified** lower limb, including hip

    D03.71 Melanoma in situ of **right** lower limb, including hip

    D03.72 Melanoma in situ of **left** lower limb, including hip

D03.8 Melanoma in situ of **other sites**
    Melanoma in situ of scrotum
    EXCLUDES 1 *carcinoma in situ of scrotum (D07.61)*

D03.9 Melanoma in situ, **unspecified**

✓4ᵗʰ **D04** **Carcinoma in situ of skin**
    EXCLUDES 1 *erythroplasia of Queyrat (penis) NOS (D07.4)*
    melanoma in situ (D03.-)

    D04.0 Carcinoma in situ of skin of **lip**
        EXCLUDES 1 *carcinoma in situ of vermilion border of lip (D00.01)*

✓5ᵗʰ   **D04.1** Carcinoma in situ of skin of **eyelid, including canthus**

        D04.10 Carcinoma in situ of skin of **unspecified** eyelid, including canthus

        D04.11 Carcinoma in situ of skin of **right** eyelid, including canthus

        D04.12 Carcinoma in situ of skin of **left** eyelid, including canthus

✓5ᵗʰ   **D04.2** Carcinoma in situ of skin of **ear and external auricular canal**

        D04.20 Carcinoma in situ of skin of **unspecified** ear and external auricular canal

        D04.21 Carcinoma in situ of skin of **right** ear and external auricular canal

        D04.22 Carcinoma in situ of skin of **left** ear and external auricular canal

✓5ᵗʰ   **D04.3** Carcinoma in situ of skin of **other and unspecified parts of face**

        D04.30 Carcinoma in situ of skin of **unspecified** part of face

        D04.39 Carcinoma in situ of skin of **other** parts of face

    D04.4 Carcinoma in situ of skin of **scalp and neck**

    D04.5 Carcinoma in situ of skin of **trunk**
        Carcinoma in situ of anal margin
        Carcinoma in situ of anal skin
        Carcinoma in situ of perianal skin
        Carcinoma in situ of skin of breast
        EXCLUDES 1 *carcinoma in situ of anus NOS (D01.3)*
        carcinoma in situ of scrotum (D07.61)
        carcinoma in situ of skin of genital organs (D07.-)

✓5ᵗʰ   **D04.6** Carcinoma in situ of skin of **upper limb, including shoulder**

        D04.60 Carcinoma in situ of skin of **unspecified** upper limb, including shoulder

        D04.61 Carcinoma in situ of skin of **right** upper limb, including shoulder

        D04.62 Carcinoma in situ of skin of **left** upper limb, including shoulder

✓5ᵗʰ   **D04.7** Carcinoma in situ of skin of **lower limb, including hip**

        D04.70 Carcinoma in situ of skin of **unspecified** lower limb, including hip

        D04.71 Carcinoma in situ of skin of **right** lower limb, including hip

        D04.72 Carcinoma in situ of skin of **left** lower limb, including hip

    D04.8 Carcinoma in situ of skin of **other** sites

    D04.9 Carcinoma in situ of skin, **unspecified**

✓4ᵗʰ **D05** **Carcinoma in situ of breast**
    EXCLUDES 1 *carcinoma in situ of skin of breast (D04.5)*
    melanoma in situ of breast (skin) (D03.5)
    Paget's disease of breast or nipple (C50.-)

✓5ᵗʰ   **D05.0** **Lobular** carcinoma in situ of breast

        D05.00 Lobular carcinoma in situ of **unspecified** breast

        D05.01 Lobular carcinoma in situ of **right** breast

        D05.02 Lobular carcinoma in situ of **left** breast

✓5ᵗʰ   **D05.1** **Intraductal** carcinoma in situ of breast

        D05.10 Intraductal carcinoma in situ of **unspecified** breast

        D05.11 Intraductal carcinoma in situ of **right** breast

        D05.12 Intraductal carcinoma in situ of **left** breast

✓5ᵗʰ   **D05.8** **Other** specified type of carcinoma in situ of breast

        D05.80 Other specified type of carcinoma in situ of **unspecified** breast

        D05.81 Other specified type of carcinoma in situ of **right** breast

---

Ⓝ Newborn: 0   Ⓟ Pediatric: 0-17   Ⓜ Maternity: 12-55   Ⓐ Adult: 15-124   **MCC** Major CC Condition   **PDxMCC** PDx acts as own MCC   **CC** CC Condition   **PDxCC** PDx acts as own CC

D05.82   Other specified type of carcinoma in situ of left breast

☑5ᵗʰ **D05.9   Unspecified type of carcinoma in situ of breast**

D05.90   Unspecified type of carcinoma in situ of unspecified breast

D05.91   Unspecified type of carcinoma in situ of right breast

D05.92   Unspecified type of carcinoma in situ of left breast

☑4ᵗʰ **D06   Carcinoma in situ of cervix uteri**

     INCLUDES   cervical adenocarcinoma in situ
                  cervical intraepithelial glandular neoplasia
                  cervical intraepithelial neoplasia III [CIN III]
                  severe dysplasia of cervix uteri

     EXCLUDES 1   *cervical intraepithelial neoplasia II [CIN II] (N87.1)*
                   cytologic evidence of malignancy of cervix without histologic confirmation (R87.614)
                   high grade squamous intraepithelial lesion (HGSIL) of cervix (R87.613)
                   melanoma in situ of cervix (D03.5)
                   moderate cervical dysplasia (N87.1)

D06.0   Carcinoma in situ of endocervix   ♀

D06.1   Carcinoma in situ of exocervix   ♀

D06.7   Carcinoma in situ of other parts of cervix   ♀

D06.9   Carcinoma in situ of cervix, unspecified   ♀

☑4ᵗʰ **D07   Carcinoma in situ of other and unspecified genital organs**

     EXCLUDES 1   *melanoma in situ of trunk (D03.5)*

D07.0   Carcinoma in situ of endometrium   ♀

D07.1   Carcinoma in situ of vulva   ♀
       Severe dysplasia of vulva
       Vulvar intraepithelial neoplasia III [VIN III]
       EXCLUDES 1   *moderate dysplasia of vulva (N90.1)*
                   vulvar intraepithelial neoplasia II [VIN II] (N90.1)

D07.2   Carcinoma in situ of vagina   ♀
       Severe dysplasia of vagina
       Vaginal intraepithelial neoplasia III [VAIN III]
       EXCLUDES 1   *moderate dysplasia of vagina (N89.1)*
                   vaginal intraepithelial neoplasia II [VIN II] (N89.1)

☑5ᵗʰ **D07.3   Carcinoma in situ of other and unspecified female genital organs**

D07.30   Carcinoma in situ of unspecified female genital organs   ♀

D07.39   Carcinoma in situ of other female genital organs   ♀

D07.4   Carcinoma in situ of penis   ♂
       Erythroplasia of Queyrat NOS

D07.5   Carcinoma in situ of prostate   ♂
       Prostatic intraepithelial neoplasia III (PIN III)
       Severe dysplasia of prostate
       EXCLUDES 1   *dysplasia (mild) (moderate) of prostate (N42.3)*

☑5ᵗʰ **D07.6   Carcinoma in situ of other and unspecified male genital organs**

D07.60   Carcinoma in situ of unspecified male genital organs   ♂

D07.61   Carcinoma in situ of scrotum   ♂

D07.69   Carcinoma in situ of other male genital organs   ♂

☑4ᵗʰ **D09   Carcinoma in situ of other and unspecified sites**

     EXCLUDES 1   *melanoma in situ (D03.-)*

D09.0   Carcinoma in situ of bladder

☑5ᵗʰ **D09.1   Carcinoma in situ of other and unspecified urinary organs**

D09.10   Carcinoma in situ of unspecified urinary organ

D09.19   Carcinoma in situ of other urinary organs

☑5ᵗʰ **D09.2   Carcinoma in situ of eye**

       EXCLUDES 1   *carcinoma in situ of skin of eyelid (D04.1-)*

D09.20   Carcinoma in situ of unspecified eye

D09.21   Carcinoma in situ of right eye

D09.22   Carcinoma in situ of left eye

D09.3   Carcinoma in situ of thyroid and other endocrine glands
       EXCLUDES 1   *carcinoma in situ of endocrine pancreas (D01.7)*
                   carcinoma in situ of ovary (D07.39)
                   carcinoma in situ of testis (D07.69)

D09.8   Carcinoma in situ of other specified sites

D09.9   Carcinoma in situ, unspecified

Benign neoplasms, except benign neuroendocrine tumors (D10-D36)

☑4ᵗʰ **D10   Benign neoplasm of mouth and pharynx**

D10.0   Benign neoplasm of lip
       Benign neoplasm of lip (frenulum) (inner aspect) (mucosa) (vermilion border)
       EXCLUDES 1   *benign neoplasm of skin of lip (D22.0, D23.0)*

D10.1   Benign neoplasm of tongue
       Benign neoplasm of lingual tonsil

D10.2   Benign neoplasm of floor of mouth

☑5ᵗʰ **D10.3   Other and unspecified parts of mouth**

D10.30   Benign neoplasm of unspecified part of mouth

D10.39   Benign neoplasm of other parts of mouth
       Benign neoplasm of minor salivary gland NOS
       EXCLUDES 1   *benign odontogenic neoplasms (D16.4-D16.5)*
                   benign neoplasm of mucosa of lip (D10.0)
                   benign neoplasm of nasopharyngeal surface of soft palate (D10.6)

D10.4   Benign neoplasm of tonsil
       Benign neoplasm of tonsil (faucial) (palatine)
       EXCLUDES 1   *benign neoplasm of lingual tonsil (D10.1)*
                   benign neoplasm of pharyngeal tonsil (D10.6)
                   benign neoplasm of tonsillar fossa (D10.5)
                   benign neoplasm of tonsillar pillars (D10.5)

D10.5   Benign neoplasm of other parts of oropharynx
       Benign neoplasm of epiglottis, anterior aspect
       Benign neoplasm of tonsillar fossa
       Benign neoplasm of tonsillar pillars
       Benign neoplasm of vallecula
       EXCLUDES 1   *benign neoplasm of epiglottis NOS (D14.1)*
                   benign neoplasm of epiglottis, suprahyoid portion (D14.1)

D10.6   Benign neoplasm of nasopharynx
       Benign neoplasm of pharyngeal tonsil
       Benign neoplasm of posterior margin of septum and choanae

D10.7   Benign neoplasm of hypopharynx

D10.9   Benign neoplasm of pharynx, unspecified

☑4ᵗʰ **D11   Benign neoplasm of major salivary glands**

     EXCLUDES 1   *benign neoplasms of specified minor salivary glands which are classified according to their anatomical location*
                   benign neoplasms of minor salivary glands NOS (D10.39)

D11.0   Benign neoplasm of parotid gland

D11.7   Benign neoplasm of other major salivary glands
       Benign neoplasm of sublingual salivary gland
       Benign neoplasm of submandibular salivary gland

D11.9   Benign neoplasm of major salivary gland, unspecified

☑4ᵗʰ **D12   Benign neoplasm of colon, rectum, anus and anal canal**

     EXCLUDES 1   *benign carcinoid tumors of the large intestine, and rectum (D3A.02-)*

D12.0   Benign neoplasm of cecum
       Benign neoplasm of ileocecal valve

D12.1   Benign neoplasm of appendix
       EXCLUDES 1   *benign carcinoid tumor of the appendix (D3A.020)*

D12.2   Benign neoplasm of ascending colon

D12.3   Benign neoplasm of transverse colon
       Benign neoplasm of hepatic flexure
       Benign neoplasm of splenic flexure

D12.4   Benign neoplasm of descending colon

D12.5   Benign neoplasm of sigmoid colon

D12.6   Benign neoplasm of colon, unspecified
       Adenomatosis of colon
       Benign neoplasm of large intestine NOS
       Polyposis (hereditary) of colon
       EXCLUDES 1   *inflammatory polyp of colon (K51.4-)*
                   polyp of colon NOS (K63.5)

D12.7   Benign neoplasm of rectosigmoid junction

D12.8   Benign neoplasm of rectum
       EXCLUDES 1   *benign carcinoid tumor of the rectum (D3A.026)*

D12.9   Benign neoplasm of anus and anal canal
       Benign neoplasm of anus NOS
       EXCLUDES 1   *benign neoplasm of anal margin (D22.5, D23.5)*
                   benign neoplasm of anal skin (D22.5, D23.5)
                   benign neoplasm of perianal skin (D22.5, D23.5)

☑ Additional Character Required   ☑x7ᵗʰ Placeholder Alert   Unacceptable PDx   Manifestation   Hospital Acquired Condition   EXCLUDES 1 Not Coded Here   EXCLUDES 2 Not Included Here

ICD-10-CM 2016   483

Chapter 2. Neoplasms

✓4ᵗʰ **D13 Benign neoplasm of** other and ill-defined parts of digestive system
     EXCLUDES 1   *benign stromal tumors of digestive system (D21.4)*

D13.Ø Benign neoplasm of esophagus

D13.1 Benign neoplasm of stomach
     EXCLUDES 1   *benign carcinoid tumor of the stomach (D3A.Ø92)*

D13.2 Benign neoplasm of duodenum
     EXCLUDES 1   *benign carcinoid tumor of the duodenum (D3A.Ø1Ø)*

✓5ᵗʰ **D13.3 Benign neoplasm of other and unspecified parts of** small intestine
     EXCLUDES 1   *benign carcinoid tumors of the small intestine (D3A.Ø1)*
            benign neoplasm of ileocecal valve (D12.Ø)

     D13.3Ø Benign neoplasm of unspecified part **of small intestine**

     D13.39 Benign neoplasm of other parts **of small intestine**

D13.4 Benign neoplasm of liver
Benign neoplasm of intrahepatic bile ducts

D13.5 Benign neoplasm of extrahepatic bile ducts

D13.6 Benign neoplasm of pancreas
     EXCLUDES 1   *benign neoplasm of endocrine pancreas (D13.7)*

D13.7 Benign neoplasm of endocrine pancreas
Islet cell tumor
Benign neoplasm of islets of Langerhans
Use additional code to identify any functional activity

D13.9 Benign neoplasm of ill-defined sites **within the digestive system**
Benign neoplasm of digestive system NOS
Benign neoplasm of intestine NOS
Benign neoplasm of spleen

✓4ᵗʰ **D14 Benign neoplasm of** middle ear and respiratory system

D14.Ø Benign neoplasm of middle ear, nasal cavity and accessory sinuses
Benign neoplasm of cartilage of nose
     EXCLUDES 1   *benign neoplasm of auricular canal (external) (D22.2-, D23.2-)*
            benign neoplasm of bone of ear (D16.4)
            benign neoplasm of bone of nose (D16.4)
            benign neoplasm of cartilage of ear (D21.Ø)
            benign neoplasm of ear (external)(skin) (D22.2-, D23.2-)
            benign neoplasm of nose NOS (D36.7)
            benign neoplasm of skin of nose (D22.39, D23.39)
            benign neoplasm of olfactory bulb (D33.3)
            benign neoplasm of posterior margin of septum and choanae (D1Ø.6)
            polyp of accessory sinus (J33.8)
            polyp of ear (middle) (H74.4)
            polyp of nasal (cavity) (J33.-)

D14.1 Benign neoplasm of larynx
Adenomatous polyp of larynx
Benign neoplasm of epiglottis (suprahyoid portion)
     EXCLUDES 1   *benign neoplasm of epiglottis, anterior aspect (D1Ø.5)*
            polyp (nonadenomatous) of vocal cord or larynx (J38.1)

D14.2 Benign neoplasm of trachea

✓5ᵗʰ **D14.3 Benign neoplasm of** bronchus and lung
     EXCLUDES 1   *benign carcinoid tumor of the bronchus and lung (D3A.Ø9Ø)*

     D14.3Ø Benign neoplasm of unspecified **bronchus and lung**

     D14.31 Benign neoplasm of right **bronchus and lung**

     D14.32 Benign neoplasm of left **bronchus and lung**

D14.4 Benign neoplasm of respiratory system, unspecified

✓4ᵗʰ **D15 Benign neoplasm of** other and unspecified intrathoracic organs
     EXCLUDES 1   *benign neoplasm of mesothelial tissue (D19.-)*

D15.Ø Benign neoplasm of thymus
     EXCLUDES 1   *benign carcinoid tumor of the thymus (D3A.Ø91)*

D15.1 Benign neoplasm of heart
     EXCLUDES 1   *benign neoplasm of great vessels (D21.3)*

D15.2 Benign neoplasm of mediastinum

D15.7 Benign neoplasm of other specified **intrathoracic organs**

D15.9 Benign neoplasm of intrathoracic organ, unspecified

✓4ᵗʰ **D16 Benign neoplasm of** bone and articular cartilage
     EXCLUDES 1   *benign neoplasm of connective tissue of ear (D21.Ø)*
            benign neoplasm of connective tissue of eyelid (D21.Ø)
            benign neoplasm of connective tissue of larynx (D14.1)
            benign neoplasm of connective tissue of nose (D14.Ø)
            benign neoplasm of synovia (D21.-)

✓5ᵗʰ **D16.Ø Benign neoplasm of** scapula and long bones of upper limb

     D16.ØØ Benign neoplasm of scapula and long bones of unspecified **upper limb**

     D16.Ø1 Benign neoplasm of scapula and long bones of right **upper limb**

     D16.Ø2 Benign neoplasm of scapula and long bones of left **upper limb**

✓5ᵗʰ **D16.1 Benign neoplasm of** short bones of upper limb

     D16.1Ø Benign neoplasm of short bones of unspecified **upper limb**

     D16.11 Benign neoplasm of short bones of right **upper limb**

     D16.12 Benign neoplasm of short bones of left **upper limb**

✓5ᵗʰ **D16.2 Benign neoplasm of** long bones of lower limb

     D16.2Ø Benign neoplasm of long bones of unspecified **lower limb**

     D16.21 Benign neoplasm of long bones of right **lower limb**

     D16.22 Benign neoplasm of long bones of left **lower limb**

✓5ᵗʰ **D16.3 Benign neoplasm of** short bones of lower limb

     D16.3Ø Benign neoplasm of short bones of unspecified **lower limb**

     D16.31 Benign neoplasm of short bones of right **lower limb**

     D16.32 Benign neoplasm of short bones of left **lower limb**

D16.4 Benign neoplasm of bones of skull and face
Benign neoplasm of maxilla (superior)
Benign neoplasm of orbital bone
Keratocyst of maxilla
Keratocystic odontogenic tumor of maxilla
     EXCLUDES 1   *benign neoplasm of lower jaw bone (D16.5)*

D16.5 Benign neoplasm of lower jaw bone
Keratocyst of mandible
Keratocystic odontogenic tumor of mandible

D16.6 Benign neoplasm of vertebral column
     EXCLUDES 1   *benign neoplasm of sacrum and coccyx (D16.8)*

D16.7 Benign neoplasm of ribs, sternum and clavicle

D16.8 Benign neoplasm of pelvic bones, sacrum and coccyx

D16.9 Benign neoplasm of bone and articular cartilage, unspecified

✓4ᵗʰ **D17 Benign** lipomatous **neoplasm**

D17.Ø Benign lipomatous neoplasm of skin and subcutaneous tissue of head, face and neck

D17.1 Benign lipomatous neoplasm of skin and subcutaneous tissue of trunk

✓5ᵗʰ **D17.2 Benign lipomatous neoplasm of** skin and subcutaneous tissue of limb

     D17.2Ø Benign lipomatous neoplasm of skin and subcutaneous tissue of unspecified limb

     D17.21 Benign lipomatous neoplasm of skin and subcutaneous tissue of right arm

     D17.22 Benign lipomatous neoplasm of skin and subcutaneous tissue of left arm

     D17.23 Benign lipomatous neoplasm of skin and subcutaneous tissue of right leg

     D17.24 Benign lipomatous neoplasm of skin and subcutaneous tissue of left leg

✓5ᵗʰ **D17.3 Benign lipomatous neoplasm of** skin and subcutaneous tissue of other and unspecified sites

     D17.3Ø Benign lipomatous neoplasm of skin and subcutaneous tissue of unspecified sites

     D17.39 Benign lipomatous neoplasm of skin and subcutaneous tissue of other sites

D17.4 Benign lipomatous neoplasm of intrathoracic organs

D17.5 Benign lipomatous neoplasm of intra-abdominal organs
     EXCLUDES 1   *benign lipomatous neoplasm of peritoneum and retroperitoneum (D17.79)*

D17.6 Benign lipomatous neoplasm of spermatic cord   ♂

✓5ᵗʰ **D17.7 Benign lipomatous neoplasm of** other sites

     D17.71 Benign lipomatous neoplasm of kidney

     D17.72 Benign lipomatous neoplasm of other genitourinary organ

---

Ⓝ Newborn: 0   Ⓟ Pediatric: 0-17   Ⓜ Maternity: 12-55   Ⓐ Adult: 15-124   **MCC** Major CC Condition   **PDxMCC** PDx acts as own MCC   **CC** CC Condition   **PDxCC** PDx acts as own CC

D17.79   **Benign lipomatous neoplasm of** other sites
Benign lipomatous neoplasm of peritoneum
Benign lipomatous neoplasm of retroperitoneum

D17.9   **Benign lipomatous neoplasm,** unspecified
Lipoma NOS

☑4ᵗʰ **D18**   **Hemangioma and lymphangioma, any site**
EXCLUDES 1   benign neoplasm of glomus jugulare (D35.6)
blue or pigmented nevus (D22.-)
nevus NOS (D22.-)
vascular nevus (Q82.5)

☑5ᵗʰ **D18.0**   **Hemangioma**
Angioma NOS
Cavernous nevus

   D18.00   **Hemangioma** unspecified site

   D18.01   **Hemangioma of** skin and subcutaneous tissue

   D18.02   **Hemangioma of** intracranial structures

   D18.03   **Hemangioma of** intra-abdominal structures

   D18.09   **Hemangioma of** other sites

  D18.1   **Lymphangioma, any site**

☑4ᵗʰ **D19**   **Benign neoplasm of** mesothelial tissue

  D19.0   **Benign neoplasm of mesothelial tissue of** pleura

  D19.1   **Benign neoplasm of mesothelial tissue of** peritoneum

  D19.7   **Benign neoplasm of mesothelial tissue of** other sites

  D19.9   **Benign neoplasm of mesothelial tissue,** unspecified
Benign mesothelioma NOS

☑4ᵗʰ **D20**   **Benign neoplasm of soft tissue of** retroperitoneum and peritoneum
EXCLUDES 1   benign lipomatous neoplasm of peritoneum and retroperitoneum (D17.79)
benign neoplasm of mesothelial tissue (D19.-)

  D20.0   **Benign neoplasm of soft tissue of** retroperitoneum

  D20.1   **Benign neoplasm of soft tissue of** peritoneum

☑4ᵗʰ **D21**   **Other benign neoplasms of** connective and other soft tissue
INCLUDES   benign neoplasm of blood vessel
benign neoplasm of bursa
benign neoplasm of cartilage
benign neoplasm of fascia
benign neoplasm of fat
benign neoplasm of ligament, except uterine
benign neoplasm of lymphatic channel
benign neoplasm of muscle
benign neoplasm of synovia
benign neoplasm of tendon (sheath)
benign stromal tumors
EXCLUDES 1   benign neoplasm of articular cartilage (D16.-)
benign neoplasm of cartilage of larynx (D14.1)
benign neoplasm of cartilage of nose (D14.0)
benign neoplasm of connective tissue of breast (D24.-)
benign neoplasm of peripheral nerves and autonomic nervous system (D36.1-)
benign neoplasm of peritoneum (D20.1)
benign neoplasm of retroperitoneum (D20.0)
benign neoplasm of uterine ligament, any (D28.2)
benign neoplasm of vascular tissue (D18.-)
hemangioma (D18.0-)
lipomatous neoplasm (D17.-)
lymphangioma (D18.1)
uterine leiomyoma (D25.-)

  D21.0   **Benign neoplasm of connective and other soft tissue of** head, face and neck
Benign neoplasm of connective tissue of ear
Benign neoplasm of connective tissue of eyelid
EXCLUDES 1   benign neoplasm of connective tissue of orbit (D31.6-)

☑5ᵗʰ **D21.1**   **Benign neoplasm of connective and other soft tissue of** upper limb, including shoulder

   D21.10   **Benign neoplasm of connective and other soft tissue of** unspecified **upper limb, including shoulder**

   D21.11   **Benign neoplasm of connective and other soft tissue of** right **upper limb, including shoulder**

   D21.12   **Benign neoplasm of connective and other soft tissue of** left **upper limb, including shoulder**

☑5ᵗʰ **D21.2**   **Benign neoplasm of connective and other soft tissue of** lower limb, including hip

   D21.20   **Benign neoplasm of connective and other soft tissue of** unspecified **lower limb, including hip**

   D21.21   **Benign neoplasm of connective and other soft tissue of** right **lower limb, including hip**

   D21.22   **Benign neoplasm of connective and other soft tissue of** left **lower limb, including hip**

  D21.3   **Benign neoplasm of connective and other soft tissue of** thorax
Benign neoplasm of axilla
Benign neoplasm of diaphragm
Benign neoplasm of great vessels
EXCLUDES 1   benign neoplasm of heart (D15.1)
benign neoplasm of mediastinum (D15.2)
benign neoplasm of thymus (D15.0)

  D21.4   **Benign neoplasm of connective and other soft tissue of** abdomen
Benign stromal tumors of abdomen

  D21.5   **Benign neoplasm of connective and other soft tissue of** pelvis
EXCLUDES 1   benign neoplasm of any uterine ligament (D28.2)
uterine leiomyoma (D25.-)

  D21.6   **Benign neoplasm of connective and other soft tissue of** trunk, unspecified
Benign neoplasm of back NOS

  D21.9   **Benign neoplasm of connective and other soft tissue,** unspecified

☑4ᵗʰ **D22**   **Melanocytic nevi**
INCLUDES   atypical nevus
blue hairy pigmented nevus
nevus NOS

  D22.0   **Melanocytic nevi of** lip

☑5ᵗʰ **D22.1**   **Melanocytic nevi of** eyelid, including canthus

   D22.10   **Melanocytic nevi of** unspecified **eyelid, including canthus**

   D22.11   **Melanocytic nevi of** right **eyelid, including canthus**

   D22.12   **Melanocytic nevi of** left **eyelid, including canthus**

☑5ᵗʰ **D22.2**   **Melanocytic nevi of** ear and external auricular canal

   D22.20   **Melanocytic nevi of** unspecified **ear and external auricular canal**

   D22.21   **Melanocytic nevi of** right **ear and external auricular canal**

   D22.22   **Melanocytic nevi of** left **ear and external auricular canal**

☑5ᵗʰ **D22.3**   **Melanocytic nevi of** other and unspecified parts of face

   D22.30   **Melanocytic nevi of** unspecified **part of face**

   D22.39   **Melanocytic nevi of** other **parts of face**

  D22.4   **Melanocytic nevi of** scalp and neck

  D22.5   **Melanocytic nevi of** trunk
Melanocytic nevi of anal margin
Melanocytic nevi of anal skin
Melanocytic nevi of perianal skin
Melanocytic nevi of skin of breast

☑5ᵗʰ **D22.6**   **Melanocytic nevi of** upper limb, including shoulder

   D22.60   **Melanocytic nevi of** unspecified **upper limb, including shoulder**

   D22.61   **Melanocytic nevi of** right **upper limb, including shoulder**

   D22.62   **Melanocytic nevi of** left **upper limb, including shoulder**

☑5ᵗʰ **D22.7**   **Melanocytic nevi of** lower limb, including hip

   D22.70   **Melanocytic nevi of** unspecified **lower limb, including hip**

   D22.71   **Melanocytic nevi of** right **lower limb, including hip**

   D22.72   **Melanocytic nevi of** left **lower limb, including hip**

  D22.9   **Melanocytic nevi,** unspecified

☑4ᵗʰ **D23**   **Other benign neoplasms of** skin
INCLUDES   benign neoplasm of hair follicles
benign neoplasm of sebaceous glands
benign neoplasm of sweat glands
EXCLUDES 1   benign lipomatous neoplasms of skin (D17.0-D17.3)
melanocytic nevi (D22.-)

  D23.0   **Other benign neoplasm of skin of** lip
EXCLUDES 1   benign neoplasm of vermilion border of lip (D10.0)

☑5ᵗʰ **D23.1**   **Other benign neoplasm of skin of** eyelid, including canthus

   D23.10   **Other benign neoplasm of skin of** unspecified **eyelid, including canthus**

   D23.11   **Other benign neoplasm of skin of** right **eyelid, including canthus**

   D23.12   **Other benign neoplasm of skin of** left **eyelid, including canthus**

√5ᵗʰ D23.2 Other benign neoplasm of skin of ear and external auricular canal
- **D23.2Ø** Other benign neoplasm of skin of unspecified ear and external auricular canal
- **D23.21** Other benign neoplasm of skin of right ear and external auricular canal
- **D23.22** Other benign neoplasm of skin of left ear and external auricular canal

√5ᵗʰ D23.3 Other benign neoplasm of skin of other and unspecified parts of face
- **D23.3Ø** Other benign neoplasm of skin of unspecified part of face
- **D23.39** Other benign neoplasm of skin of other parts of face

D23.4 Other benign neoplasm of skin of scalp and neck

D23.5 Other benign neoplasm of skin of trunk
Other benign neoplasm of anal margin
Other benign neoplasm of anal skin
Other benign neoplasm of perianal skin
Other benign neoplasm of skin of breast
EXCLUDES 1 benign neoplasm of anus NOS (D12.9)

√5ᵗʰ D23.6 Other benign neoplasm of skin of upper limb, including shoulder
- **D23.6Ø** Other benign neoplasm of skin of unspecified upper limb, including shoulder
- **D23.61** Other benign neoplasm of skin of right upper limb, including shoulder
- **D23.62** Other benign neoplasm of skin of left upper limb, including shoulder

√5ᵗʰ D23.7 Other benign neoplasm of skin of lower limb, including hip
- **D23.7Ø** Other benign neoplasm of skin of unspecified lower limb, including hip
- **D23.71** Other benign neoplasm of skin of right lower limb, including hip
- **D23.72** Other benign neoplasm of skin of left lower limb, including hip

D23.9 Other benign neoplasm of skin, unspecified

√4ᵗʰ D24 Benign neoplasm of breast
INCLUDES benign neoplasm of connective tissue of breast
benign neoplasm of soft parts of breast
fibroadenoma of breast
EXCLUDES 2 adenofibrosis of breast (N60.2)
benign cyst of breast (N60.-)
benign mammary dysplasia (N60.-)
benign neoplasm of skin of breast (D22.5, D23.5)
fibrocystic disease of breast (N60.-)
- **D24.1** Benign neoplasm of right breast
- **D24.2** Benign neoplasm of left breast
- **D24.9** Benign neoplasm of unspecified breast

√4ᵗʰ D25 Leiomyoma of uterus
INCLUDES uterine fibroid
uterine fibromyoma
uterine myoma
- **D25.Ø** Submucous leiomyoma of uterus ♀
- **D25.1** Intramural leiomyoma of uterus ♀
  Interstitial leiomyoma of uterus
- **D25.2** Subserosal leiomyoma of uterus ♀
  Subperitoneal leiomyoma of uterus
- **D25.9** Leiomyoma of uterus, unspecified ♀

√4ᵗʰ D26 Other benign neoplasms of uterus
- **D26.Ø** Other benign neoplasm of cervix uteri ♀
- **D26.1** Other benign neoplasm of corpus uteri ♀
- **D26.7** Other benign neoplasm of other parts of uterus ♀
- **D26.9** Other benign neoplasm of uterus, unspecified ♀

√4ᵗʰ D27 Benign neoplasm of ovary
Use additional code to identify any functional activity
EXCLUDES 2 corpus albicans cyst (N83.2)
corpus luteum cyst (N83.1)
endometrial cyst (N80.1)
follicular (atretic) cyst (N83.0)
graafian follicle cyst (N83.0)
ovarian cyst NEC (N83.2)
ovarian retention cyst (N83.2)
- **D27.Ø** Benign neoplasm of right ovary ♀
- **D27.1** Benign neoplasm of left ovary ♀
- **D27.9** Benign neoplasm of unspecified ovary ♀

√4ᵗʰ D28 Benign neoplasm of other and unspecified female genital organs
INCLUDES adenomatous polyp
benign neoplasm of skin of female genital organs
benign teratoma
EXCLUDES 1 epoophoron cyst (Q50.5)
fimbrial cyst (Q50.4)
Gartner's duct cyst (Q52.4)
parovarian cyst (Q50.5)
- **D28.Ø** Benign neoplasm of vulva ♀
- **D28.1** Benign neoplasm of vagina ♀
- **D28.2** Benign neoplasm of uterine tubes and ligaments ♀
  Benign neoplasm of fallopian tube
  Benign neoplasm of uterine ligament (broad) (round)
- **D28.7** Benign neoplasm of other specified female genital organs ♀
- **D28.9** Benign neoplasm of female genital organ, unspecified ♀

√4ᵗʰ D29 Benign neoplasm of male genital organs
INCLUDES benign neoplasm of skin of male genital organs
- **D29.Ø** Benign neoplasm of penis ♂
- **D29.1** Benign neoplasm of prostate ♂
  EXCLUDES 1 enlarged prostate (N40.-)
- **√5ᵗʰ D29.2** Benign neoplasm of testis
  Use additional code to identify any functional activity
  - **D29.2Ø** Benign neoplasm of unspecified testis ♂
  - **D29.21** Benign neoplasm of right testis ♂
  - **D29.22** Benign neoplasm of left testis ♂
- **√5ᵗʰ D29.3** Benign neoplasm of epididymis
  - **D29.3Ø** Benign neoplasm of unspecified epididymis ♂
  - **D29.31** Benign neoplasm of right epididymis ♂
  - **D29.32** Benign neoplasm of left epididymis ♂
- **D29.4** Benign neoplasm of scrotum
  Benign neoplasm of skin of scrotum
- **D29.8** Benign neoplasm of other specified male genital organs ♂
  Benign neoplasm of seminal vesicle
  Benign neoplasm of spermatic cord
  Benign neoplasm of tunica vaginalis
- **D29.9** Benign neoplasm of male genital organ, unspecified ♂

√4ᵗʰ D30 Benign neoplasm of urinary organs
- **√5ᵗʰ D30.Ø** Benign neoplasm of kidney
  EXCLUDES 1 benign carcinoid tumor of the kidney (D3A.Ø93)
  benign neoplasm of renal calyces (D30.1-)
  benign neoplasm of renal pelvis (D30.1-)
  - **D30.00** Benign neoplasm of unspecified kidney
  - **D30.01** Benign neoplasm of right kidney
  - **D30.02** Benign neoplasm of left kidney
- **√5ᵗʰ D30.1** Benign neoplasm of renal pelvis
  - **D30.10** Benign neoplasm of unspecified renal pelvis
  - **D30.11** Benign neoplasm of right renal pelvis
  - **D30.12** Benign neoplasm of left renal pelvis
- **√5ᵗʰ D30.2** Benign neoplasm of ureter
  EXCLUDES 1 benign neoplasm of ureteric orifice of bladder (D30.3)
  - **D30.20** Benign neoplasm of unspecified ureter
  - **D30.21** Benign neoplasm of right ureter
  - **D30.22** Benign neoplasm of left ureter
- **D30.3** Benign neoplasm of bladder
  Benign neoplasm of ureteric orifice of bladder
  Benign neoplasm of urethral orifice of bladder
- **D30.4** Benign neoplasm of urethra
  EXCLUDES 1 benign neoplasm of urethral orifice of bladder (D30.3)
- **D30.8** Benign neoplasm of other specified urinary organs
  Benign neoplasm of paraurethral glands
- **D30.9** Benign neoplasm of urinary organ, unspecified
  Benign neoplasm of urinary system NOS

√4ᵗʰ D31 Benign neoplasm of eye and adnexa
EXCLUDES 1 benign neoplasm of connective tissue of eyelid (D21.0)
benign neoplasm of optic nerve (D33.3)
benign neoplasm of skin of eyelid (D22.1-, D23.1-)
- **√5ᵗʰ D31.Ø** Benign neoplasm of conjunctiva
  - **D31.00** Benign neoplasm of unspecified conjunctiva
  - **D31.01** Benign neoplasm of right conjunctiva
  - **D31.02** Benign neoplasm of left conjunctiva
- **√5ᵗʰ D31.1** Benign neoplasm of cornea
  - **D31.10** Benign neoplasm of unspecified cornea

D31.11   **Benign neoplasm of** right cornea

D31.12   **Benign neoplasm of** left cornea

✓5ᵗʰ   **D31.2**   **Benign neoplasm of** retina

> **EXCLUDES 1**   *dark area on retina (D49.81)*
> *hemangioma of retina (D49.81)*
> *neoplasm of unspecified behavior of retina and choroid*
> *(D49.81)*
> *retinal freckle (D49.81)*

D31.20   **Benign neoplasm of** unspecified retina

D31.21   **Benign neoplasm of** right retina

D31.22   **Benign neoplasm of** left retina

✓5ᵗʰ   **D31.3**   **Benign neoplasm of** choroid

D31.30   **Benign neoplasm of** unspecified choroid

D31.31   **Benign neoplasm of** right choroid

D31.32   **Benign neoplasm of** left choroid

✓5ᵗʰ   **D31.4**   **Benign neoplasm of** ciliary body

D31.40   **Benign neoplasm of** unspecified ciliary body

D31.41   **Benign neoplasm of** right ciliary body

D31.42   **Benign neoplasm of** left ciliary body

✓5ᵗʰ   **D31.5**   **Benign neoplasm of** lacrimal gland and duct

> Benign neoplasm of lacrimal sac
> Benign neoplasm of nasolacrimal duct

D31.50   **Benign neoplasm of** unspecified lacrimal gland and duct

D31.51   **Benign neoplasm of** right lacrimal gland and duct

D31.52   **Benign neoplasm of** left lacrimal gland and duct

✓5ᵗʰ   **D31.6**   **Benign neoplasm of** unspecified site of orbit

> Benign neoplasm of connective tissue of orbit
> Benign neoplasm of extraocular muscle
> Benign neoplasm of peripheral nerves of orbit
> Benign neoplasm of retrobulbar tissue
> Benign neoplasm of retro-ocular tissue
> **EXCLUDES 1**   *benign neoplasm of orbital bone (D16.4)*

D31.60   **Benign neoplasm of** unspecified site of unspecified orbit

D31.61   **Benign neoplasm of** unspecified site of right orbit

D31.62   **Benign neoplasm of** unspecified site of left orbit

✓5ᵗʰ   **D31.9**   **Benign neoplasm of** unspecified part of eye

> Benign neoplasm of eyeball

D31.90   **Benign neoplasm of** unspecified part of unspecified eye

D31.91   **Benign neoplasm of** unspecified part of right eye

D31.92   **Benign neoplasm of** unspecified part of left eye

✓4ᵗʰ   **D32**   **Benign neoplasm of** meninges

D32.0   **Benign neoplasm of** cerebral meninges

D32.1   **Benign neoplasm of** spinal meninges

D32.9   **Benign neoplasm of** meninges, unspecified

> Meningioma NOS

✓4ᵗʰ   **D33**   **Benign neoplasm of** brain and other parts of central nervous system

> **EXCLUDES 1**   *angioma (D18.0-)*
> *benign neoplasm of meninges (D32.-)*
> *benign neoplasm of peripheral nerves and autonomic nervous*
> *system (D36.1-)*
> *hemangioma (D18.0-)*
> *neurofibromatosis (Q85.0-)*
> *retro-ocular benign neoplasm (D31.6-)*

D33.0   **Benign neoplasm of** brain, supratentorial

> Benign neoplasm of cerebral ventricle
> Benign neoplasm of cerebrum
> Benign neoplasm of frontal lobe
> Benign neoplasm of occipital lobe
> Benign neoplasm of parietal lobe
> Benign neoplasm of temporal lobe
> **EXCLUDES 1**   *benign neoplasm of fourth ventricle (D33.1)*

D33.1   **Benign neoplasm of** brain, infratentorial

> Benign neoplasm of brain stem
> Benign neoplasm of cerebellum
> Benign neoplasm of fourth ventricle

D33.2   **Benign neoplasm of** brain, unspecified

D33.3   **Benign neoplasm of** cranial nerves

> Benign neoplasm of olfactory bulb

D33.4   **Benign neoplasm of** spinal cord

D33.7   **Benign neoplasm of** other specified parts of central nervous system

D33.9   **Benign neoplasm of** central nervous system, unspecified

> Benign neoplasm of nervous system (central) NOS

D34   **Benign neoplasm of** thyroid gland

> Use additional code to identify any functional activity

✓4ᵗʰ   **D35**   **Benign neoplasm of** other and unspecified endocrine glands

> Use additional code to identify any functional activity
> **EXCLUDES 1**   *benign neoplasm of endocrine pancreas (D13.7)*
> *benign neoplasm of ovary (D27.-)*
> *benign neoplasm of testis (D29.2-)*
> *benign neoplasm of thymus (D15.0)*

✓5ᵗʰ   **D35.0**   **Benign neoplasm of** adrenal gland

D35.00   **Benign neoplasm of** unspecified adrenal gland

D35.01   **Benign neoplasm of** right adrenal gland

D35.02   **Benign neoplasm of** left adrenal gland

D35.1   **Benign neoplasm of** parathyroid gland

D35.2   **Benign neoplasm of** pituitary gland

> **AHA:** 2014, 3Q, 22

D35.3   **Benign neoplasm of** craniopharyngeal duct

D35.4   **Benign neoplasm of** pineal gland

D35.5   **Benign neoplasm of** carotid body

D35.6   **Benign neoplasm of** aortic body and other paraganglia

> Benign tumor of glomus jugulare

D35.7   **Benign neoplasm of** other specified endocrine glands

D35.9   **Benign neoplasm of** endocrine gland, unspecified

> Benign neoplasm of unspecified endocrine gland

✓4ᵗʰ   **D36**   **Benign neoplasm of** other and unspecified sites

D36.0   **Benign neoplasm of** lymph nodes

> **EXCLUDES 1**   *lymphangioma (D18.1)*

✓5ᵗʰ   **D36.1**   **Benign neoplasm of** peripheral nerves and autonomic nervous system

> **EXCLUDES 1**   *benign neoplasm of peripheral nerves of orbit (D31.6-)*
> *neurofibromatosis (Q85.0-)*

D36.10   **Benign neoplasm of peripheral nerves and autonomic nervous system,** unspecified

D36.11   **Benign neoplasm of peripheral nerves and autonomic nervous system of** face, head, and neck

D36.12   **Benign neoplasm of peripheral nerves and autonomic nervous system,** upper limb, including shoulder

D36.13   **Benign neoplasm of peripheral nerves and autonomic nervous system of** lower limb, including hip

D36.14   **Benign neoplasm of peripheral nerves and autonomic nervous system of** thorax

D36.15   **Benign neoplasm of peripheral nerves and autonomic nervous system of** abdomen

D36.16   **Benign neoplasm of peripheral nerves and autonomic nervous system of** pelvis

D36.17   **Benign neoplasm of peripheral nerves and autonomic nervous system of** trunk, unspecified

D36.7   **Benign neoplasm of** other specified sites

> Benign neoplasm of nose NOS

D36.9   **Benign neoplasm,** unspecified site

Benign neuroendocrine tumors (D3A)

✓4ᵗʰ   **D3A**   **Benign neuroendocrine tumors**

> Code also any associated multiple endocrine neoplasia [MEN] syndromes (E31.2-)
> Use additional code to identify any associated endocrine syndrome, such as:
> carcinoid syndrome (E34.0)
> **EXCLUDES 2**   *benign pancreatic islet cell tumors (D13.7)*

✓5ᵗʰ   **D3A.0**   **Benign** carcinoid tumors

D3A.00   **Benign carcinoid tumor of** unspecified site

> Carcinoid tumor NOS

✓6ᵗʰ   D3A.01   **Benign carcinoid tumors of the** small intestine

D3A.010   **Benign carcinoid tumor of the** duodenum

D3A.011   **Benign carcinoid tumor of the** jejunum

D3A.012   **Benign carcinoid tumor of the** ileum

D3A.019   **Benign carcinoid tumor of the small intestine,** unspecified portion

✓6ᵗʰ   D3A.02   **Benign carcinoid tumors of the** appendix, large intestine, and rectum

D3A.020   **Benign carcinoid tumor of the** appendix

☑ Additional Character Required   ✗ʎ7ᵗʰ Placeholder Alert   Unacceptable PDx   Manifestation   Hospital Acquired Condition   **EXCLUDES 1** Not Coded Here   **EXCLUDES 2** Not Included Here

ICD-10-CM 2016   487

Chapter 2. Neoplasms

D3A.021   **Benign carcinoid tumor of the** cecum

D3A.022   **Benign carcinoid tumor of the** ascending colon

D3A.023   **Benign carcinoid tumor of the** transverse colon

D3A.024   **Benign carcinoid tumor of the** descending colon

D3A.025   **Benign carcinoid tumor of the** sigmoid colon

D3A.026   **Benign carcinoid tumor of the** rectum

D3A.029   **Benign carcinoid tumor of the** large intestine, unspecified portion
     Benign carcinoid tumor of the colon NOS

✓6ᵗʰ   **D3A.09   Benign carcinoid tumors of** other sites

D3A.090   **Benign carcinoid tumor of the** bronchus and lung

D3A.091   **Benign carcinoid tumor of the** thymus

D3A.092   **Benign carcinoid tumor of the** stomach

D3A.093   **Benign carcinoid tumor of the** kidney

D3A.094   **Benign carcinoid tumor of the** foregut NOS

D3A.095   **Benign carcinoid tumor of the** midgut NOS

D3A.096   **Benign carcinoid tumor of the** hindgut NOS

D3A.098   **Benign carcinoid tumors of** other sites

D3A.8   Other benign neuroendocrine tumors
     Neuroendocrine tumor NOS

Neoplasms of uncertain behavior, polycythemia vera and myelodysplastic syndromes (D37-D48)

NOTE   Categories D37-D44, and D48 classify by site neoplasms of uncertain behavior, i.e., histologic confirmation whether the neoplasm is malignant or benign cannot be made.

EXCLUDES 1   *neoplasms of unspecified behavior (D49.-)*

✓4ᵗʰ   **D37   Neoplasm of uncertain behavior of** oral cavity and digestive organs

EXCLUDES 1   *stromal tumors of uncertain behavior of digestive system (D48.1)*

✓5ᵗʰ   **D37.0   Neoplasm of uncertain behavior of** lip, oral cavity and pharynx

EXCLUDES 1   *neoplasm of uncertain behavior of aryepiglottic fold or interarytenoid fold, laryngeal aspect (D38.0)*
neoplasm of uncertain behavior of epiglottis NOS (D38.0)
neoplasm of uncertain behavior of skin of lip (D48.5)
neoplasm of uncertain behavior of suprahyoid portion of epiglottis (D38.0)

D37.01   **Neoplasm of uncertain behavior of** lip
     Neoplasm of uncertain behavior of vermilion border of lip

D37.02   **Neoplasm of uncertain behavior of** tongue

✓6ᵗʰ   **D37.03   Neoplasm of uncertain behavior of the** major salivary glands

D37.030   **Neoplasm of uncertain behavior of the** parotid salivary glands

D37.031   **Neoplasm of uncertain behavior of the** sublingual salivary glands

D37.032   **Neoplasm of uncertain behavior of the** submandibular salivary glands

D37.039   **Neoplasm of uncertain behavior of the** major salivary glands, unspecified

D37.04   **Neoplasm of uncertain behavior of the** minor salivary glands
     Neoplasm of uncertain behavior of submucosal salivary glands of lip
     Neoplasm of uncertain behavior of submucosal salivary glands of cheek
     Neoplasm of uncertain behavior of submucosal salivary glands of hard palate
     Neoplasm of uncertain behavior of submucosal salivary glands of soft palate

D37.05   **Neoplasm of uncertain behavior of** pharynx
     Neoplasm of uncertain behavior of aryepiglottic fold of pharynx NOS
     Neoplasm of uncertain behavior of hypopharyngeal aspect of aryepiglottic fold of pharynx
     Neoplasm of uncertain behavior of marginal zone of aryepiglottic fold of pharynx

D37.09   **Neoplasm of uncertain behavior of** other specified sites of the oral cavity

D37.1   **Neoplasm of uncertain behavior of** stomach

D37.2   **Neoplasm of uncertain behavior of** small intestine

D37.3   **Neoplasm of uncertain behavior of** appendix

D37.4   **Neoplasm of uncertain behavior of** colon

D37.5   **Neoplasm of uncertain behavior of** rectum
     Neoplasm of uncertain behavior of rectosigmoid junction

D37.6   **Neoplasm of uncertain behavior of** liver, gallbladder and bile ducts
     Neoplasm of uncertain behavior of ampulla of Vater

D37.8   **Neoplasm of uncertain behavior of** other specified digestive organs
     Neoplasm of uncertain behavior of anal canal
     Neoplasm of uncertain behavior of anal sphincter
     Neoplasm of uncertain behavior of anus NOS
     Neoplasm of uncertain behavior of esophagus
     Neoplasm of uncertain behavior of intestine NOS
     Neoplasm of uncertain behavior of pancreas

EXCLUDES 1   *neoplasm of uncertain behavior of anal margin (D48.5)*
neoplasm of uncertain behavior of anal skin (D48.5)
neoplasm of uncertain behavior of perianal skin (D48.5)

D37.9   **Neoplasm of uncertain behavior of** digestive organ, unspecified

✓4ᵗʰ   **D38   Neoplasm of uncertain behavior of** middle ear and respiratory and intrathoracic organs

EXCLUDES 1   *neoplasm of uncertain behavior of heart (D48.7)*

D38.0   **Neoplasm of uncertain behavior of** larynx
     Neoplasm of uncertain behavior of aryepiglottic fold or interarytenoid fold, laryngeal aspect
     Neoplasm of uncertain behavior of epiglottis (suprahyoid portion)

EXCLUDES 1   *neoplasm of uncertain behavior of aryepiglottic fold or interarytenoid fold NOS (D37.05)*
neoplasm of uncertain behavior of hypopharyngeal aspect of aryepiglottic fold (D37.05)
neoplasm of uncertain behavior of marginal zone of aryepiglottic fold (D37.05)

D38.1   **Neoplasm of uncertain behavior of** trachea, bronchus and lung

D38.2   **Neoplasm of uncertain behavior of** pleura

D38.3   **Neoplasm of uncertain behavior of** mediastinum

D38.4   **Neoplasm of uncertain behavior of** thymus

D38.5   **Neoplasm of uncertain behavior of** other respiratory organs
     Neoplasm of uncertain behavior of accessory sinuses
     Neoplasm of uncertain behavior of cartilage of nose
     Neoplasm of uncertain behavior of middle ear
     Neoplasm of uncertain behavior of nasal cavities

EXCLUDES 1   *neoplasm of uncertain behavior of ear (external) (skin) (D48.5)*
neoplasm of uncertain behavior of nose NOS (D48.7)
neoplasm of uncertain behavior of skin of nose (D48.5)

D38.6   **Neoplasm of uncertain behavior of** respiratory organ, unspecified

✓4ᵗʰ   **D39   Neoplasm of uncertain behavior of** female genital organs

D39.0   **Neoplasm of uncertain behavior of** uterus   ♀

✓5ᵗʰ   **D39.1   Neoplasm of uncertain behavior of** ovary
     Use additional code to identify any functional activity

D39.10   **Neoplasm of uncertain behavior of** unspecified ovary   ♀

D39.11   **Neoplasm of uncertain behavior of** right ovary   ♀

D39.12   **Neoplasm of uncertain behavior of** left ovary   ♀

D39.2   **Neoplasm of uncertain behavior of** placenta   ♀
     Chorioadenoma destruens
     Invasive hydatidiform mole
     Malignant hydatidiform mole

EXCLUDES 1   *hydatidiform mole NOS (O01.9)*

D39.8   **Neoplasm of uncertain behavior of** other specified female genital organs   ♀
     Neoplasm of uncertain behavior of skin of female genital organs

D39.9   **Neoplasm of uncertain behavior of** female genital organ, unspecified   ♀

✓4ᵗʰ   **D40   Neoplasm of uncertain behavior of** male genital organs

D40.0   **Neoplasm of uncertain behavior of** prostate   ♂

✓5ᵗʰ   **D40.1   Neoplasm of uncertain behavior of** testis

D40.10   **Neoplasm of uncertain behavior of** unspecified testis   ♂

D40.11   **Neoplasm of uncertain behavior of** right testis   ♂

D40.12   **Neoplasm of uncertain behavior of** left testis   ♂

Ⓝ Newborn: 0   Ⓟ Pediatric: 0-17   Ⓜ Maternity: 12-55   Ⓐ Adult: 15-124   **MCC** Major CC Condition   **PDxMCC** PDx acts as own MCC   **CC** CC Condition   **PDxCC** PDx acts as own CC

488   ICD-10-CM 2016

D40.8   **Neoplasm of uncertain behavior of other specified male genital organs**   ♂
Neoplasm of uncertain behavior of skin of male genital organs

D40.9   **Neoplasm of uncertain behavior of male genital organ, unspecified**   ♂

☑4ᵗʰ **D41**   **Neoplasm of uncertain behavior of urinary organs**

   ☑5ᵗʰ **D41.0**   **Neoplasm of uncertain behavior of kidney**
     EXCLUDES 1   *neoplasm of uncertain behavior of renal pelvis (D41.1-)*

     D41.00   **Neoplasm of uncertain behavior of unspecified kidney**

     D41.01   **Neoplasm of uncertain behavior of right kidney**

     D41.02   **Neoplasm of uncertain behavior of left kidney**

   ☑5ᵗʰ **D41.1**   **Neoplasm of uncertain behavior of renal pelvis**

     D41.10   **Neoplasm of uncertain behavior of unspecified renal pelvis**

     D41.11   **Neoplasm of uncertain behavior of right renal pelvis**

     D41.12   **Neoplasm of uncertain behavior of left renal pelvis**

   ☑5ᵗʰ **D41.2**   **Neoplasm of uncertain behavior of ureter**

     D41.20   **Neoplasm of uncertain behavior of unspecified ureter**

     D41.21   **Neoplasm of uncertain behavior of right ureter**

     D41.22   **Neoplasm of uncertain behavior of left ureter**

   D41.3   **Neoplasm of uncertain behavior of urethra**

   D41.4   **Neoplasm of uncertain behavior of bladder**

   D41.8   **Neoplasm of uncertain behavior of other specified urinary organs**

   D41.9   **Neoplasm of uncertain behavior of unspecified urinary organ**

☑4ᵗʰ **D42**   **Neoplasm of uncertain behavior of meninges**

   D42.0   **Neoplasm of uncertain behavior of cerebral meninges**

   D42.1   **Neoplasm of uncertain behavior of spinal meninges**

   D42.9   **Neoplasm of uncertain behavior of meninges, unspecified**

☑4ᵗʰ **D43**   **Neoplasm of uncertain behavior of brain and central nervous system**
     EXCLUDES 1   *neoplasm of uncertain behavior of peripheral nerves and autonomic nervous system (D48.2)*

   D43.0   **Neoplasm of uncertain behavior of brain, supratentorial**
Neoplasm of uncertain behavior of cerebral ventricle
Neoplasm of uncertain behavior of cerebrum
Neoplasm of uncertain behavior of frontal lobe
Neoplasm of uncertain behavior of occipital lobe
Neoplasm of uncertain behavior of parietal lobe
Neoplasm of uncertain behavior of temporal lobe
     EXCLUDES 1   *neoplasm of uncertain behavior of fourth ventricle (D43.1)*

   D43.1   **Neoplasm of uncertain behavior of brain, infratentorial**
Neoplasm of uncertain behavior of brain stem
Neoplasm of uncertain behavior of cerebellum
Neoplasm of uncertain behavior of fourth ventricle

   D43.2   **Neoplasm of uncertain behavior of brain, unspecified**

   D43.3   **Neoplasm of uncertain behavior of cranial nerves**

   D43.4   **Neoplasm of uncertain behavior of spinal cord**

   D43.8   **Neoplasm of uncertain behavior of other specified parts of central nervous system**

   D43.9   **Neoplasm of uncertain behavior of central nervous system, unspecified**
Neoplasm of uncertain behavior of nervous system (central) NOS

☑4ᵗʰ **D44**   **Neoplasm of uncertain behavior of endocrine glands**
     EXCLUDES 1   *multiple endocrine adenomatosis (E31.2-)*
             multiple endocrine neoplasia (E31.2-)
             neoplasm of uncertain behavior of endocrine pancreas (D37.8)
             neoplasm of uncertain behavior of ovary (D39.1-)
             neoplasm of uncertain behavior of testis (D40.1-)
             neoplasm of uncertain behavior of thymus (D38.4)

   D44.0   **Neoplasm of uncertain behavior of thyroid gland**

   ☑5ᵗʰ **D44.1**   **Neoplasm of uncertain behavior of adrenal gland**
Use additional code to identify any functional activity

     D44.10   **Neoplasm of uncertain behavior of unspecified adrenal gland**

     D44.11   **Neoplasm of uncertain behavior of right adrenal gland**

     D44.12   **Neoplasm of uncertain behavior of left adrenal gland**

   D44.2   **Neoplasm of uncertain behavior of parathyroid gland**

   D44.3   **Neoplasm of uncertain behavior of pituitary gland**
Use additional code to identify any functional activity

   D44.4   **Neoplasm of uncertain behavior of craniopharyngeal duct**

   D44.5   **Neoplasm of uncertain behavior of pineal gland**

   D44.6   **Neoplasm of uncertain behavior of carotid body**

   D44.7   **Neoplasm of uncertain behavior of aortic body and other paraganglia**

   D44.9   **Neoplasm of uncertain behavior of unspecified endocrine gland**

D45   **Polycythemia vera**
     EXCLUDES 1   *familial polycythemia (D75.0)*
             secondary polycythemia (D75.1)

☑4ᵗʰ **D46**   **Myelodysplastic syndromes**
Use additional code for adverse effect, if applicable, to identify drug (T36-T50 with fifth or sixth character 5)
     EXCLUDES 2   *drug-induced aplastic anemia (D61.1)*

   D46.0   **Refractory anemia without ring sideroblasts, so stated**
Refractory anemia without sideroblasts, without excess of blasts

   D46.1   **Refractory anemia with ring sideroblasts**
RARS

   ☑5ᵗʰ **D46.2**   **Refractory anemia with excess of blasts**

     D46.20   **Refractory anemia with excess of blasts, unspecified**
RAEB NOS

     D46.21   **Refractory anemia with excess of blasts 1**
RAEB 1

     D46.22   **Refractory anemia with excess of blasts 2**   CC
RAEB 2
CC Excl: C88.2-C88.3, C88.8-C88.9, C90.10-C90.11, C90.20-C90.21, C90.30-C90.31, C91.00-C95.92, D45-D47.1, D47.3, D47.Z9-D47.9, D48.7-D48.9

   D46.A   **Refractory cytopenia with multilineage dysplasia**

   D46.B   **Refractory cytopenia with multilineage dysplasia and ring sideroblasts**
RCMD RS

   D46.C   **Myelodysplastic syndrome with isolated del(5q) chromosomal abnormality**   CC
Myelodysplastic syndrome with 5q deletion
5q minus syndrome NOS
CC Excl: See code: D46.22

   D46.4   **Refractory anemia, unspecified**

   D46.Z   **Other myelodysplastic syndromes**
     EXCLUDES 1   *chronic myelomonocytic leukemia (C93.1-)*

   D46.9   **Myelodysplastic syndrome, unspecified**
Myelodysplasia NOS

☑4ᵗʰ **D47**   **Other neoplasms of uncertain behavior of lymphoid, hematopoietic and related tissue**

   D47.0   **Histiocytic and mast cell tumors of uncertain behavior**   CC
Indolent systemic mastocytosis
Mast cell tumor NOS
Mastocytoma NOS
     EXCLUDES 1   *malignant mast cell tumor (C96.2)*
             mastocytosis (congenital) (cutaneous) (Q82.2)
CC Excl: C88.8, C94.40-C94.6, D45-D47.1, D47.3, D47.Z9-D47.9, D75.81, Z51.0

   D47.1   **Chronic myeloproliferative disease**   CC
Chronic neutrophilic leukemia
Myeloproliferative disease, unspecified
     EXCLUDES 1   *atypical chronic myeloid leukemia BCR/ABL-negative (C92.2-)*
             chronic myeloid leukemia BCR/ABL-positive (C92.1-)
             myelofibrosis NOS (D75.81)
             myelophthisic anemia (D61.82)
             myelophthisis (D61.82)
             secondary myelofibrosis NOS (D75.81)
CC Excl: See code: D46.22

   D47.2   **Monoclonal gammopathy**
Monoclonal gammopathy of undetermined significance [MGUS]

   D47.3   **Essential (hemorrhagic) thrombocythemia**
Essential thrombocytosis
Idiopathic hemorrhagic thrombocythemia

   D47.4   **Osteomyelofibrosis**
Chronic idiopathic myelofibrosis
Myelofibrosis (idiopathic) (with myeloid metaplasia)
Myelosclerosis (megakaryocytic) with myeloid metaplasia
Secondary myelofibrosis in myeloproliferative disease
     EXCLUDES 1   *acute myelofibrosis (C94.4-)*

☑ Additional Character Required   ☑x7ᵗʰ Placeholder Alert   Unacceptable PDx   Manifestation   Hospital Acquired Condition   EXCLUDES 1 Not Coded Here   EXCLUDES 2 Not Included Here

ICD-10-CM 2016   489

Chapter 2. Neoplasms

D47.Z–D49.9

√5ᵗʰ **D47.Z** **Other** specified neoplasms of uncertain behavior of lymphoid, hematopoietic and related tissue

  D47.Z1 **Post-transplant lymphoproliferative disorder (PTLD)** CC
    Code first complications of transplanted organs and tissue (T86.-)
    CC Excl: D47.Z1, D78.81-D78.89, E89.810-E89.89, H59.011-H59.019, H59.031-H59.099, H59.811-H59.89, H95.811-H95.89, I97.3, M96.89, N98.1-N98.9, T86.850-T86.859, T86.90-T86.99

  D47.Z9 **Other specified neoplasms of uncertain behavior of lymphoid, hematopoietic and related tissue** CC
    Histiocytic tumors of uncertain behavior
    CC Excl: C88.2-C88.3, C88.8-C88.9, C90.10-C90.11, C90.20-C90.21, C90.30-C90.31, C91.00-C95.92, D45-D47.1, D47.3, D47.Z9-D47.9, D48.7-D48.9

D47.9 **Neoplasm of uncertain behavior of lymphoid, hematopoietic and related tissue, unspecified** CC
  Lymphoproliferative disease NOS
  CC Excl: See code: D47.Z9

√4ᵗʰ **D48** **Neoplasm of uncertain behavior of other and unspecified sites**
  EXCLUDES 1   neurofibromatosis (nonmalignant) (Q85.0-)

D48.0 **Neoplasm of uncertain behavior of bone and articular cartilage**
  EXCLUDES 1   neoplasm of uncertain behavior of cartilage of ear (D48.1)
    neoplasm of uncertain behavior of cartilage of larynx (D38.0)
    neoplasm of uncertain behavior of cartilage of nose (D38.5)
    neoplasm of uncertain behavior of connective tissue of eyelid (D48.1)
    neoplasm of uncertain behavior of synovia (D48.1)

D48.1 **Neoplasm of uncertain behavior of connective and other soft tissue**
  Neoplasm of uncertain behavior of connective tissue of ear
  Neoplasm of uncertain behavior of connective tissue of eyelid
  Stromal tumors of uncertain behavior of digestive system
  EXCLUDES 1   neoplasm of uncertain behavior of articular cartilage (D48.0)
    neoplasm of uncertain behavior of cartilage of larynx (D38.0)
    neoplasm of uncertain behavior of cartilage of nose (D38.5)
    neoplasm of uncertain behavior of connective tissue of breast (D48.6-)

D48.2 **Neoplasm of uncertain behavior of peripheral nerves and autonomic nervous system**
  EXCLUDES 1   neoplasm of uncertain behavior of peripheral nerves of orbit (D48.7)

D48.3 **Neoplasm of uncertain behavior of retroperitoneum**

D48.4 **Neoplasm of uncertain behavior of peritoneum**

D48.5 **Neoplasm of uncertain behavior of skin**
  Neoplasm of uncertain behavior of anal margin
  Neoplasm of uncertain behavior of anal skin
  Neoplasm of uncertain behavior of perianal skin
  Neoplasm of uncertain behavior of skin of breast
  EXCLUDES 1   neoplasm of uncertain behavior of anus NOS (D37.8)
    neoplasm of uncertain behavior of skin of genital organs (D39.8, D40.8)
    neoplasm of uncertain behavior of vermilion border of lip (D37.0)

√5ᵗʰ **D48.6** **Neoplasm of uncertain behavior of breast**
  Neoplasm of uncertain behavior of connective tissue of breast
  Cystosarcoma phyllodes
  EXCLUDES 1   neoplasm of uncertain behavior of skin of breast (D48.5)

  D48.60 **Neoplasm of uncertain behavior of unspecified breast**

  D48.61 **Neoplasm of uncertain behavior of right breast**

  D48.62 **Neoplasm of uncertain behavior of left breast**

D48.7 **Neoplasm of uncertain behavior of other specified sites**
  Neoplasm of uncertain behavior of eye
  Neoplasm of uncertain behavior of heart
  Neoplasm of uncertain behavior of peripheral nerves of orbit
  EXCLUDES 1   neoplasm of uncertain behavior of connective tissue (D48.1)
    neoplasm of uncertain behavior of skin of eyelid (D48.5)

D48.9 **Neoplasm of uncertain behavior, unspecified**

Neoplasms of unspecified behavior (D49)

√4ᵗʰ **D49** **Neoplasms of unspecified behavior**
  NOTE   Category D49 classifies by site neoplasms of unspecified morphology and behavior. The term "mass", unless otherwise stated, is not to be regarded as a neoplastic growth.
  INCLUDES   "growth" NOS
    neoplasm NOS
    new growth NOS
    tumor NOS
  EXCLUDES 1   neoplasms of uncertain behavior (D37-D44, D48)

D49.0 **Neoplasm of unspecified behavior of digestive system**
  EXCLUDES 1   neoplasm of unspecified behavior of margin of anus (D49.2)
    neoplasm of unspecified behavior of perianal skin (D49.2)
    neoplasm of unspecified behavior of skin of anus (D49.2)

D49.1 **Neoplasm of unspecified behavior of respiratory system**

D49.2 **Neoplasm of unspecified behavior of bone, soft tissue, and skin**
  EXCLUDES 1   neoplasm of unspecified behavior of anal canal (D49.0)
    neoplasm of unspecified behavior of anus NOS (D49.0)
    neoplasm of unspecified behavior of bone marrow (D49.89)
    neoplasm of unspecified behavior of cartilage of larynx (D49.1)
    neoplasm of unspecified behavior of cartilage of nose (D49.1)
    neoplasm of unspecified behavior of connective tissue of breast (D49.3)
    neoplasm of unspecified behavior of skin of genital organs (D49.5)
    neoplasm of unspecified behavior of vermilion border of lip (D49.0)

D49.3 **Neoplasm of unspecified behavior of breast**
  EXCLUDES 1   neoplasm of unspecified behavior of skin of breast (D49.2)

D49.4 **Neoplasm of unspecified behavior of bladder**

D49.5 **Neoplasm of unspecified behavior of other genitourinary organs**

D49.6 **Neoplasm of unspecified behavior of brain**
  EXCLUDES 1   neoplasm of unspecified behavior of cerebral meninges (D49.7)
    neoplasm of unspecified behavior of cranial nerves (D49.7)

D49.7 **Neoplasm of unspecified behavior of endocrine glands and other parts of nervous system**
  EXCLUDES 1   neoplasm of unspecified behavior of peripheral, sympathetic, and parasympathetic nerves and ganglia (D49.2)

√5ᵗʰ **D49.8** **Neoplasm of unspecified behavior of other specified sites**
  EXCLUDES 1   neoplasm of unspecified behavior of eyelid (skin) (D49.2)
    neoplasm of unspecified behavior of eyelid cartilage (D49.2)
    neoplasm of unspecified behavior of great vessels (D49.2)
    neoplasm of unspecified behavior of optic nerve (D49.7)

  D49.81 **Neoplasm of unspecified behavior of retina and choroid**
    Dark area on retina
    Retinal freckle

  D49.89 **Neoplasm of unspecified behavior of other specified sites**

D49.9 **Neoplasm of unspecified behavior of unspecified site**

N Newborn: 0   P Pediatric: 0-17   M Maternity: 12-55   A Adult: 15-124   **MCC** Major CC Condition   **PDx MCC** PDx acts as own MCC   CC CC Condition   **PDx CC** PDx acts as own CC

490

ICD-10-CM 2016

Chapter 3. Disease of the Blood and Blood-Forming Organs and Certain Disorders Involving the Immune Mechanism (D5Ø–D89)

Chapter Specific Coding Guidelines and Examples
Reserved for future guideline expansion

Chapter 3. Diseases of the Blood and Blood-forming Organs and Certain Disorders Involving the Immune Mechanism (D50-D89)

EXCLUDES 2   autoimmune disease (systemic) NOS (M35.9)
certain conditions originating in the perinatal period (P00-P96)
complications of pregnancy, childbirth and the puerperium (O00-O9A)
congenital malformations, deformations and chromosomal abnormalities (Q00-Q99)
endocrine, nutritional and metabolic diseases (E00-E88)
human immunodeficiency virus [HIV] disease (B20)
injury, poisoning and certain other consequences of external causes (S00-T88)
neoplasms (C00-D49)
symptoms, signs and abnormal clinical and laboratory findings, not elsewhere classified (R00-R94)

This chapter contains the following blocks:

D50-D53	Nutritional anemias
D55-D59	Hemolytic anemias
D60-D64	Aplastic and other anemias and other bone marrow failure syndromes
D65-D69	Coagulation defects, purpura and other hemorrhagic conditions
D70-D77	Other disorders of blood and blood-forming organs
D78	Intraoperative and postprocedural complications of the spleen
D80-D89	Certain disorders involving the immune mechanism

Nutritional anemias (D50-D53)

✓4ᵗʰ **D50   Iron deficiency anemia**
INCLUDES   asiderotic anemia
hypochromic anemia

D50.0   Iron deficiency anemia secondary to blood loss (chronic)
Posthemorrhagic anemia (chronic)
EXCLUDES 1   acute posthemorrhagic anemia (D62)
congenital anemia from fetal blood loss (P61.3)

D50.1   Sideropenic dysphagia
Kelly-Paterson syndrome
Plummer-Vinson syndrome

D50.8   Other iron deficiency anemias
Iron deficiency anemia due to inadequate dietary iron intake

D50.9   Iron deficiency anemia, unspecified

✓4ᵗʰ **D51   Vitamin B12 deficiency anemia**
EXCLUDES 1   vitamin B12 deficiency (E53.8)

D51.0   Vitamin B12 deficiency anemia due to intrinsic factor deficiency
Addison anemia
Biermer anemia
Pernicious (congenital) anemia
Congenital intrinsic factor deficiency

D51.1   Vitamin B12 deficiency anemia due to selective vitamin B12 malabsorption with proteinuria
Imerslund (Gräsbeck) syndrome
Megaloblastic hereditary anemia

D51.2   Transcobalamin II deficiency

D51.3   Other dietary vitamin B12 deficiency anemia
Vegan anemia

D51.8   Other vitamin B12 deficiency anemias

D51.9   Vitamin B12 deficiency anemia, unspecified

✓4ᵗʰ **D52   Folate deficiency anemia**
EXCLUDES 1   folate deficiency without anemia (E53.8)

D52.0   Dietary folate deficiency anemia
Nutritional megaloblastic anemia

D52.1   Drug-induced folate deficiency anemia
Use additional code for adverse effect, if applicable, to identify drug (T36-T50 with fifth or sixth character 5)

D52.8   Other folate deficiency anemias

D52.9   Folate deficiency anemia, unspecified
Folic acid deficiency anemia NOS

✓4ᵗʰ **D53   Other nutritional anemias**
INCLUDES   megaloblastic anemia unresponsive to vitamin B12 or folate therapy

D53.0   Protein deficiency anemia
Amino-acid deficiency anemia
Orotaciduric anemia
EXCLUDES 1   Lesch-Nyhan syndrome (E79.1)

D53.1   Other megaloblastic anemias, not elsewhere classified
Megaloblastic anemia NOS
EXCLUDES 1   Di Guglielmo's disease (C94.0)

D53.2   Scorbutic anemia
EXCLUDES 1   scurvy (E54)

D53.8   Other specified nutritional anemias
Anemia associated with deficiency of copper
Anemia associated with deficiency of molybdenum
Anemia associated with deficiency of zinc
EXCLUDES 1   nutritional deficiencies without anemia, such as:
copper deficiency NOS (E61.0)
molybdenum deficiency NOS (E61.5)
zinc deficiency NOS (E60)

D53.9   Nutritional anemia, unspecified
Simple chronic anemia
EXCLUDES 1   anemia NOS (D64.9)

Hemolytic anemias (D55-D59)

✓4ᵗʰ **D55   Anemia due to enzyme disorders**
EXCLUDES 1   drug-induced enzyme deficiency anemia (D59.2)

D55.0   Anemia due to glucose-6-phosphate dehydrogenase [G6PD] deficiency
Favism
G6PD deficiency anemia

D55.1   Anemia due to other disorders of glutathione metabolism
Anemia (due to) enzyme deficiencies, except G6PD, related to the hexose monophosphate [HMP] shunt pathway
Anemia (due to) hemolytic nonspherocytic (hereditary), type I

D55.2   Anemia due to disorders of glycolytic enzymes
Hemolytic nonspherocytic (hereditary) anemia, type II
Hexokinase deficiency anemia
Pyruvate kinase [PK] deficiency anemia
Triose-phosphate isomerase deficiency anemia
EXCLUDES 1   disorders of glycolysis not associated with anemia (E74.8)

D55.3   Anemia due to disorders of nucleotide metabolism

D55.8   Other anemias due to enzyme disorders

D55.9   Anemia due to enzyme disorder, unspecified

✓4ᵗʰ **D56   Thalassemia**
EXCLUDES 1   sickle-cell thalassemia (D57.4-)

D56.0   Alpha thalassemia
Alpha thalassemia major
Hemoglobin H Constant Spring
Hemoglobin H disease
Hydrops fetalis due to alpha thalassemia
Severe alpha thalassemia
Triple gene defect alpha thalassemia
Use additional code, if applicable, for hydrops fetalis due to alpha thalassemia (P56.99)
EXCLUDES 1   alpha thalassemia trait or minor (D56.3)
asymptomatic alpha thalassemia (D56.3)
hydrops fetalis due to isoimmunization (P56.0)
hydrops fetalis not due to immune hemolysis (P83.2)

D56.1   Beta thalassemia
Beta thalassemia major
Cooley's anemia
Homozygous beta thalassemia
Severe beta thalassemia
Thalassemia intermedia
Thalassemia major
EXCLUDES 1   beta thalassemia minor (D56.3)
beta thalassemia trait (D56.3)
delta-beta thalassemia (D56.2)
hemoglobin E-beta thalassemia (D56.5)
sickle-cell beta thalassemia (D57.4-)

D56.2   Delta-beta thalassemia
Homozygous delta-beta thalassemia
EXCLUDES 1   delta-beta thalassemia minor (D56.3)
delta-beta thalassemia trait (D56.3)

D56.3   Thalassemia minor
Alpha thalassemia minor
Alpha thalassemia silent carrier
Alpha thalassemia trait
Beta thalassemia minor
Beta thalassemia trait
Delta-beta thalassemia minor
Delta-beta thalassemia trait
Thalassemia trait NOS
EXCLUDES 1   alpha thalassemia (D56.0)
beta thalassemia (D56.1)
delta-beta thalassemia (D56.2)
hemoglobin E-beta thalassemia (D56.5)
sickle-cell trait (D57.3)

D56.4 Hereditary persistence of fetal hemoglobin [HPFH]

D56.5 Hemoglobin E-beta **thalassemia**
> EXCLUDES 1   *beta thalassemia (D56.1)*
> *beta thalassemia minor (D56.3)*
> *beta thalassemia trait (D56.3)*
> *delta-beta thalassemia (D56.2)*
> *delta-beta thalassemia trait (D56.3)*
> *hemoglobin E disease (D58.2)*
> *other hemoglobinopathies (D58.2)*
> *sickle-cell beta thalassemia (D57.4-)*

D56.8 Other **thalassemias**
Dominant thalassemia
Hemoglobin C thalassemia
Mixed thalassemia
Thalassemia with other hemoglobinopathy
> EXCLUDES 1   *hemoglobin C disease (D58.2)*
> *hemoglobin E disease (D58.2)*
> *other hemoglobinopathies (D58.2)*
> *sickle-cell anemia (D57.-)*
> *sickle-cell thalassemia (D57.4)*

D56.9 Thalassemia, **unspecified**
Mediterranean anemia (with other hemoglobinopathy)

☑4ᵗʰ **D57** Sickle-cell **disorders**
Use additional code for any associated fever (R50.81)
> EXCLUDES 1   *other hemoglobinopathies (D58.-)*

> CC Excl: For MCC codes in category D57, unless otherwise noted:
> D47.4, D50.0-D64.9, D68.312, D68.51-D68.69, D75.81, D75.89-D75.9, D77, D89.2

☑6ᵗʰ **D57.0** **Hb-SS disease** with crisis
Sickle-cell disease NOS with crisis
Hb-SS disease with vasoocclusive pain

> **D57.00** **Hb-SS disease** with crisis, unspecified   `MCC`
> **D57.01** **Hb-SS disease** with acute chest syndrome   `MCC`
> **D57.02** **Hb-SS disease** with splenic sequestration   `MCC`

D57.1 Sickle-cell **disease** without crisis
Hb-SS disease without crisis
Sickle-cell anemia NOS
Sickle-cell disease NOS
Sickle-cell disorder NOS

☑5ᵗʰ **D57.2** Sickle-cell/**Hb-C disease**
Hb-SC disease
Hb-S/Hb-C disease

> **D57.20** **Sickle-cell/Hb-C disease** without crisis
> ☑6ᵗʰ **D57.21** **Sickle-cell/Hb-C disease** with crisis
> > **D57.211** **Sickle-cell/Hb-C disease** with acute chest syndrome   `PDxCC` `MCC`
> > **D57.212** **Sickle-cell/Hb-C disease** with splenic sequestration   `MCC`
> > **D57.219** **Sickle-cell/Hb-C disease** with crisis, unspecified   `MCC`
> > Sickle-cell/Hb-C disease with crisis NOS

D57.3 Sickle-cell **trait**
Hb-S trait
Heterozygous hemoglobin S

☑5ᵗʰ **D57.4** Sickle-cell **thalassemia**
Sickle-cell beta thalassemia
Thalassemia Hb-S disease

> **D57.40** **Sickle-cell thalassemia** without crisis
> Microdrepanocytosis
> Sickle-cell thalassemia NOS
> ☑6ᵗʰ **D57.41** **Sickle-cell thalassemia** with crisis
> Sickle-cell thalassemia with vasoocclusive pain
> > **D57.411** **Sickle-cell thalassemia** with acute chest syndrome   `PDxCC` `MCC`
> > **D57.412** **Sickle-cell thalassemia** with splenic sequestration   `MCC`
> > **D57.419** **Sickle-cell thalassemia** with crisis, unspecified   `MCC`
> > Sickle-cell thalassemia with crisis NOS

☑5ᵗʰ **D57.8** Other **sickle-cell disorders**
Hb-SD disease
Hb-SE disease

> **D57.80** **Other sickle-cell disorders** without crisis
> ☑6ᵗʰ **D57.81** **Other sickle-cell disorders** with crisis
> > **D57.811** **Other sickle-cell disorders** with acute chest syndrome   `MCC`
> > **D57.812** **Other sickle-cell disorders** with splenic sequestration   `MCC`

D57.819 **Other sickle-cell disorders** with crisis, unspecified   `MCC`
Other sickle-cell disorders with crisis NOS

☑4ᵗʰ **D58** Other hereditary **hemolytic anemias**
> EXCLUDES 1   *hemolytic anemia of the newborn (P55.-)*

D58.0 Hereditary **spherocytosis**
Acholuric (familial) jaundice
Congenital (spherocytic) hemolytic icterus
Minkowski-Chauffard syndrome

D58.1 Hereditary **elliptocytosis**
Elliptocytosis (congenital)
Ovalocytosis (congenital) (hereditary)

D58.2 Other **hemoglobinopathies**
Abnormal hemoglobin NOS
Congenital Heinz body anemia
Hb-C disease
Hb-D disease
Hb-E disease
Hemoglobinopathy NOS
Unstable hemoglobin hemolytic disease
> EXCLUDES 1   *familial polycythemia (D75.0)*
> *Hb-M disease (D74.0)*
> *hemoglobin E-beta thalassemia (D56.5)*
> *hereditary persistence of fetal hemoglobin [HPFH] (D56.4)*
> *high-altitude polycythemia (D75.1)*
> *methemoglobinemia (D74.-)*
> *other hemoglobinopathies with thalassemia (D56.8)*

D58.8 Other specified hereditary **hemolytic anemias**   `CC`
Stomatocytosis
CC Excl: D50.0-D64.9, D75.9, P61.2-P61.4

D58.9 Hereditary **hemolytic anemia, unspecified**   `CC`
CC Excl: See code: D58.8

☑4ᵗʰ **D59** Acquired **hemolytic anemia**

> CC Excl: For CC/MCC codes in category D59, unless otherwise noted: D47.4, D50.0-D64.9, D68.312, D68.51-D68.69, D75.81, D75.89-D75.9, D77, D89.2

D59.0 Drug-induced autoimmune **hemolytic anemia**   `CC`
Use additional code for adverse effect, if applicable, to identify drug (T36-T50 with fifth or sixth character 5)

D59.1 Other autoimmune **hemolytic anemias**   `CC`
Autoimmune hemolytic disease (cold type) (warm type)
Chronic cold hemagglutinin disease
Cold agglutinin disease
Cold agglutinin hemoglobinuria
Cold type (secondary) (symptomatic) hemolytic anemia
Warm type (secondary) (symptomatic) hemolytic anemia
> EXCLUDES 1   *Evans syndrome (D69.41)*
> *hemolytic disease of newborn (P55.-)*
> *paroxysmal cold hemoglobinuria (D59.6)*

D59.2 Drug-induced nonautoimmune **hemolytic anemia**   `CC`
Drug-induced enzyme deficiency anemia
Use additional code for adverse effect, if applicable, to identify drug (T36-T50 with fifth or sixth character 5)

D59.3 Hemolytic-uremic **syndrome**   `MCC`
Use additional code to identify associated:
E. coli infection (B96.2-)
Pneumococcal pneumonia (J13)
Shigella dysenteriae (A03.9)

D59.4 Other nonautoimmune **hemolytic anemias**   `CC`
Mechanical hemolytic anemia
Microangiopathic hemolytic anemia
Toxic hemolytic anemia

D59.5 Paroxysmal nocturnal hemoglobinuria [Marchiafava-Micheli]
> EXCLUDES 1   *hemoglobinuria NOS (R82.3)*

D59.6 Hemoglobinuria **due to hemolysis from other external causes**
Hemoglobinuria from exertion
March hemoglobinuria
Paroxysmal cold hemoglobinuria
Use additional code (Chapter 20) to identify external cause
> EXCLUDES 1   *hemoglobinuria NOS (R82.3)*

D59.8 Other acquired **hemolytic anemias**

D59.9 Acquired hemolytic anemia, **unspecified**   `CC`
Idiopathic hemolytic anemia, chronic

☑ Additional Character Required   ☑7ᵗʰ Placeholder Alert   Unacceptable PDx   Manifestation   Hospital Acquired Condition   EXCLUDES 1 Not Coded Here   EXCLUDES 2 Not Included Here

Chapter 3. Disease of the Blood and Blood-Forming Organs

Aplastic and other anemias and other bone marrow failure syndromes (D60-D64)

✓4th D60 Acquired pure red cell aplasia [erythroblastopenia]
- INCLUDES red cell aplasia (acquired) (adult) (with thymoma)
- EXCLUDES1 congenital red cell aplasia (D61.01)

> CC Excl: For CC/MCC codes in category D60, unless otherwise noted: D47.4, D50.0-D64.9, D68.312, D68.51-D68.69, D75.81, D75.89-D75.9, D77, D89.2

- **D60.0** Chronic acquired pure red cell aplasia   MCC
- **D60.1** Transient acquired pure red cell aplasia   MCC
- **D60.8** Other acquired pure red cell aplasias   MCC
- **D60.9** Acquired pure red cell aplasia, unspecified   MCC

✓4th D61 Other aplastic anemias and other bone marrow failure syndromes
- EXCLUDES1 neutropenia (D70.-)
- AHA: 2014, 4Q, 22

- **✓5th D61.0 Constitutional aplastic anemia**

  - **D61.01 Constitutional (pure) red blood cell aplasia**   CC
    - Blackfan-Diamond syndrome
    - Congenital (pure) red cell aplasia
    - Familial hypoplastic anemia
    - Primary (pure) red cell aplasia
    - Red cell (pure) aplasia of infants
    - EXCLUDES1 acquired red cell aplasia (D60.9)
    - CC Excl: D50.0-D61.3, D61.89-D64.9, D75.9, P61.2-P61.4

  - **D61.09 Other constitutional aplastic anemia**   CC
    - Fanconi's anemia
    - Pancytopenia with malformations
    - CC Excl: D50.0-D61.3, D61.89-D64.9, D69.3-D69.49, D75.9, P61.2-P61.4

- **D61.1 Drug-induced aplastic anemia**   MCC
  - Use additional code for adverse effect, if applicable, to identify drug (T36-T50 with fifth or sixth character 5)
  - CC Excl: D47.4, D50.0-D64.9, D68.312, D68.51-D68.69, D75.81, D75.89-D75.9, D77, D89.2

- **D61.2 Aplastic anemia due to other external agents**   MCC
  - Code first, if applicable, toxic effects of substances chiefly nonmedicinal as to source (T51-T65)
  - CC Excl: See code: D61.1

- **D61.3 Idiopathic aplastic anemia**   MCC
  - CC Excl: See code: D61.1

- **✓5th D61.8 Other specified aplastic anemias and other bone marrow failure syndromes**

  > CC Excl: For CC/MCC codes in subcategory D61.8, unless otherwise noted: D60.0-D60.9, D61.1-D64.9, D70.0-D70.9, D72.810-D72.820, D72.823, D72.825-D72.829, D75.9, D76.1-D76.3, P61.2

  - **✓6th D61.81 Pancytopenia**
    - EXCLUDES1 pancytopenia (due to) (with) aplastic anemia (D61.9)
      pancytopenia (due to) (with) bone marrow infiltration (D61.82)
      pancytopenia (due to) (with) congenital (pure) red cell aplasia (D61.01)
      pancytopenia (due to) (with) hairy cell leukemia (C91.4-)
      pancytopenia (due to) (with) human immunodeficiency virus disease (B20)
      pancytopenia (due to) (with) leukoerythroblastic anemia (D61.82)
      pancytopenia (due to) (with) myelodysplastic syndromes (D46.-)
      pancytopenia (due to) (with) myeloproliferative disease (D47.1)

    - **D61.810 Antineoplastic chemotherapy induced pancytopenia**   MCC
      - EXCLUDES2 aplastic anemia due to antineoplastic chemotherapy (D61.1)

    - **D61.811 Other drug-induced pancytopenia**   MCC
      - EXCLUDES2 aplastic anemia due to drugs (D61.1)

    - **D61.818 Other pancytopenia**   CC

- **D61.82 Myelophthisis**   CC
  - Leukoerythroblastic anemia
  - Myelophthisic anemia
  - Panmyelophthisis
  - Code also the underlying disorder, such as:
    malignant neoplasm of breast (C50.-)
    tuberculosis (A15.-)
  - EXCLUDES1 idiopathic myelofibrosis (D47.1)
    myelofibrosis NOS (D75.81)
    myelofibrosis with myeloid metaplasia (D47.4)
    primary myelofibrosis (D47.1)
    secondary myelofibrosis (D75.81)

- **D61.89 Other specified aplastic anemias and other bone marrow failure syndromes**   MCC
  - CC Excl: See code: D61.1

- **D61.9 Aplastic anemia, unspecified**   CC
  - Hypoplastic anemia NOS
  - Medullary hypoplasia
  - CC Excl: See code: D61.1

D62 Acute posthemorrhagic anemia   CC
- EXCLUDES1 anemia due to chronic blood loss (D50.0)
  blood loss anemia NOS (D50.0)
  congenital anemia from fetal blood loss (P61.3)
- CC Excl: D47.4, D50.0-D64.9, D68.312, D68.51-D68.69, D75.81, D75.89-D75.9, D77, D89.2, T79.2XXA

✓4th D63 Anemia in chronic diseases classified elsewhere

- **D63.0 Anemia in neoplastic disease**
  - Code first neoplasm (C00-D49)
  - EXCLUDES1 anemia due to antineoplastic chemotherapy (D64.81)
    aplastic anemia due to antineoplastic chemotherapy (D61.1)

- **D63.1 Anemia in chronic kidney disease**
  - Erythropoietin resistant anemia (EPO resistant anemia)
  - Code first underlying chronic kidney disease (CKD) (N18.-)

- **D63.8 Anemia in other chronic diseases classified elsewhere**
  - Code first underlying disease, such as:
    diphyllobothriasis (B70.0)
    hookworm disease (B76.0-B76.9)
    hypothyroidism (E00.0-E03.9)
    malaria (B50.0-B54)
    symptomatic late syphilis (A52.79)
    tuberculosis (A18.89)

✓4th D64 Other anemias
- EXCLUDES1 refractory anemia (D46.-)
  refractory anemia with excess blasts in transformation [RAEB T] (C92.0-)

- **D64.0 Hereditary sideroblastic anemia**
  - Sex-linked hypochromic sideroblastic anemia

- **D64.1 Secondary sideroblastic anemia due to disease**
  - Code first underlying disease

- **D64.2 Secondary sideroblastic anemia due to drugs and toxins**
  - Code first poisoning due to drug or toxin, if applicable (T36-T65 with fifth or sixth character 1-4 or 6)
  - Use additional code for adverse effect, if applicable, to identify drug (T36-T50 with fifth or sixth character 5)

- **D64.3 Other sideroblastic anemias**
  - Sideroblastic anemia NOS
  - Pyridoxine-responsive sideroblastic anemia NEC

- **D64.4 Congenital dyserythropoietic anemia**
  - Dyshematopoietic anemia (congenital)
  - EXCLUDES1 Blackfan-Diamond syndrome (D61.01)
    Di Guglielmo's disease (C94.0)

- **✓5th D64.8 Other specified anemias**

  - **D64.81 Anemia due to antineoplastic chemotherapy**
    - Antineoplastic chemotherapy induced anemia
    - EXCLUDES1 anemia in neoplastic disease (D63.0)
      aplastic anemia due to antineoplastic chemotherapy (D61.1)
    - AHA: 2014, 4Q, 22

  - **D64.89 Other specified anemias**
    - Infantile pseudoleukemia

- **D64.9 Anemia, unspecified**

N Newborn: 0   P Pediatric: 0-17   M Maternity: 12-55   A Adult: 15-124   MCC Major CC Condition   PDxMCC PDx acts as own MCC   CC CC Condition   PDxCC PDx acts as own CC

494   ICD-10-CM 2016

Coagulation defects, purpura and other hemorrhagic conditions (D65-D69)

D65 Disseminated intravascular coagulation [defibrination syndrome] `MCC`
  Afibrinogenemia, acquired
  Consumption coagulopathy
  Diffuse or disseminated intravascular coagulation [DIC]
  Fibrinolytic hemorrhage, acquired
  Fibrinolytic purpura
  Purpura fulminans
  EXCLUDES 1 *disseminated intravascular coagulation (complicating):*
        abortion or ectopic or molar pregnancy (O00-O07, O08.1)
        in newborn (P60)
        pregnancy, childbirth and the puerperium (O45.0, O46.0, O67.0, O72.3)
  CC Excl: D47.4, D65-D69.9, D75.81-D75.9, D77, D89.2

D66 Hereditary factor VIII deficiency `MCC`
  Classical hemophilia
  Deficiency factor VIII (with functional defect)
  Hemophilia A
  Hemophilia NOS
  EXCLUDES 1 *factor VIII deficiency with vascular defect (D68.0)*
  CC Excl: See code: D65

D67 Hereditary factor IX deficiency `MCC`
  Christmas disease
  Factor IX deficiency (with functional defect)
  Hemophilia B
  Plasma thromboplastin component [PTC] deficiency
  CC Excl: See code: D65

✓4ᵗʰ **D68 Other coagulation defects**
  EXCLUDES 1 *abnormal coagulation profile (R79.1)*
        coagulation defects complicating abortion or ectopic or molar pregnancy (O00-O07, O08.1)
        coagulation defects complicating pregnancy, childbirth and the puerperium (O45.0, O46.0, O67.0, O72.3)

  D68.0 Von Willebrand's disease `CC`
    Angiohemophilia
    Factor VIII deficiency with vascular defect
    Vascular hemophilia
    EXCLUDES 1 *capillary fragility (hereditary) (D69.8)*
          factor VIII deficiency NOS (D66)
          factor VIII deficiency with functional defect (D66)
    CC Excl: See code: D65

  D68.1 Hereditary factor XI deficiency `CC`
    Hemophilia C
    Plasma thromboplastin antecedent [PTA] deficiency
    Rosenthal's disease
    CC Excl: See code: D65

  D68.2 Hereditary deficiency of other clotting factors `CC`
    AC globulin deficiency
    Congenital afibrinogenemia
    Deficiency of factor I [fibrinogen]
    Deficiency of factor II [prothrombin]
    Deficiency of factor V [labile]
    Deficiency of factor VII [stable]
    Deficiency of factor X [Stuart-Prower]
    Deficiency of factor XII [Hageman]
    Deficiency of factor XIII [fibrin stabilizing]
    Dysfibrinogenemia (congenital)
    Hypoproconvertinemia
    Owren's disease
    Proaccelerin deficiency
    CC Excl: See code: D65

✓5ᵗʰ **D68.3 Hemorrhagic disorder due to circulating anticoagulants**

    ✓6ᵗʰ **D68.31 Hemorrhagic disorder due to intrinsic circulating anticoagulants, antibodies, or inhibitors**

          D68.311 Acquired hemophilia `CC`
              Autoimmune hemophilia
              Autoimmune inhibitors to clotting factors
              Secondary hemophilia
              CC Excl: D47.4, D65-D69.9, D75.82-D75.9, D77, D89.2

          D68.312 Antiphospholipid antibody with hemorrhagic disorder `CC`
              Lupus anticoagulant (LAC) with hemorrhagic disorder
              Systemic lupus erythematosus [SLE] inhibitor with hemorrhagic disorder
              EXCLUDES 1 *antiphospholipid antibody, finding without diagnosis (R76.0)*
                    antiphospholipid antibody syndrome (D68.61)
                    antiphospholipid antibody with hypercoagulable state (D68.61)
                    lupus anticoagulant (LAC) finding without diagnosis (R76.0)
                    lupus anticoagulant (LAC) with hypercoagulable state (D68.62)
                    systemic lupus erythematosus [SLE] inhibitor finding without diagnosis (R76.0)
                    systemic lupus erythematosus [SLE] inhibitor with hypercoagulable state (D68.62)
              CC Excl: D47.4, D68.311-D68.318, D68.51-D68.69, D70.0-D72.9, D73.81, D75.81, D75.89-D77, D89.2

          D68.318 Other hemorrhagic disorder due to intrinsic circulating anticoagulants, antibodies, or inhibitors `CC`
              Antithromboplastinemia
              Antithromboplastinogenemia
              Hemorrhagic disorder due to intrinsic increase in antithrombin
              Hemorrhagic disorder due to intrinsic increase in anti-VIIIa
              Hemorrhagic disorder due to intrinsic increase in anti-IXa
              Hemorrhagic disorder due to intrinsic increase in anti-XIa
              CC Excl: See code: D68.311

    D68.32 Hemorrhagic disorder due to extrinsic circulating anticoagulants `CC`
        Drug-induced hemorrhagic disorder
        Hemorrhagic disorder due to increase in anti-IIa
        Hemorrhagic disorder due to increase in anti-Xa
        Hyperheparinemia
        Use additional code for adverse effect, if applicable, to identify drug (T45.515, T45.525)
        CC Excl: D47.4, D65-D69.9, D75.81-D75.9, D77, D89.2

  D68.4 Acquired coagulation factor deficiency `CC`
    Deficiency of coagulation factor due to liver disease
    Deficiency of coagulation factor due to vitamin K deficiency
    EXCLUDES 1 *vitamin K deficiency of newborn (P53)*
    CC Excl: See code: D68.32

✓5ᵗʰ **D68.5 Primary thrombophilia**
    Primary hypercoagulable states
    EXCLUDES 1 *antiphospholipid syndrome (D68.61)*
          lupus anticoagulant (D68.62)
          secondary activated protein C resistance (D68.69)
          secondary antiphospholipid antibody syndrome (D68.69)
          secondary lupus anticoagulant with hypercoagulable state (D68.69)
          secondary systemic lupus erythematosus [SLE] inhibitor with hypercoagulable state (D68.69)
          systemic lupus erythematosus [SLE] inhibitor finding without diagnosis (R76.0)
          systemic lupus erythematosus [SLE] inhibitor with hemorrhagic disorder (D68.312)
          thrombotic thrombocytopenic purpura (M31.1)

    CC Excl: For CC codes in subcategory D68.5, unless otherwise noted: D47.4, D68.312, D68.51-D68.69, D70.0-D72.9, D73.81, D75.81, D75.89-D75.9, D76.1-D77, D89.2

    D68.51 Activated protein C resistance `CC`
        Factor V Leiden mutation

    D68.52 Prothrombin gene mutation `CC`

✓ Additional Character Required   ✓x7ᵗʰ Placeholder Alert   Unacceptable PDx   Manifestation   Hospital Acquired Condition   *EXCLUDES 1* Not Coded Here   *EXCLUDES 2* Not Included Here

ICD-10-CM 2016   495

Chapter 3. Disease of the Blood and Blood-Forming Organs

D68.59   **Other primary thrombophilia**   `CC`
Antithrombin III deficiency
Hypercoagulable state NOS
Primary hypercoagulable state NEC
Primary thrombophilia NEC
Protein C deficiency
Protein S deficiency
Thrombophilia NOS

√5ᵗʰ **D68.6**   **Other thrombophilia**
Other hypercoagulable states
EXCLUDES 1   *diffuse or disseminated intravascular coagulation [DIC] (D65)*
heparin induced thrombocytopenia (HIT) (D75.82)
hyperhomocysteinemia (E72.11)

CC Excl: For CC codes in subcategory D68.6, unless otherwise noted: D47.4, D68.312, D68.51-D68.69, D70.0-D72.9, D73.81, D75.81, D75.89-D75.9, D76.1-D77, D89.2

D68.61   **Antiphospholipid syndrome**   `CC`
Anticardiolipin syndrome
Antiphospholipid antibody syndrome
EXCLUDES 1   *antiphospholipid antibody, finding without diagnosis (R76.0)*
antiphospholipid antibody with hemorrhagic disorder (D68.312)
lupus anticoagulant syndrome (D68.62)

D68.62   **Lupus anticoagulant syndrome**   `CC`
Lupus anticoagulant
Presence of systemic lupus erythematosus [SLE] inhibitor
EXCLUDES 1   *anticardiolipin syndrome (D68.61)*
antiphospholipid syndrome (D68.61)
lupus anticoagulant (LAC) finding without diagnosis (R79.0)
lupus anticoagulant (LAC) with hemorrhagic disorder (D68.312)

D68.69   **Other thrombophilia**   `CC`
Hypercoagulable states NEC
Secondary hypercoagulable state NOS

D68.8   **Other specified coagulation defects**   `CC`
EXCLUDES 1   *hemorrhagic disease of newborn (P53)*
CC Excl: See code: D68.32

D68.9   **Coagulation defect, unspecified**   `CC`
CC Excl: See code: D68.32

√4ᵗʰ **D69**   **Purpura and other hemorrhagic conditions**
EXCLUDES 1   *benign hypergammaglobulinemic purpura (D89.0)*
cryoglobulinemic purpura (D89.1)
essential (hemorrhagic) thrombocythemia (D47.3)
hemorrhagic thrombocythemia (D47.3)
purpura fulminans (D65)
thrombotic thrombocytopenic purpura (M31.1)
Waldenström hypergammaglobulinemic purpura (D89.0)

CC Excl: For CC codes in category D69, unless otherwise noted: D47.4, D65-D69.9, D75.81-D75.9, D77, D89.2

D69.0   **Allergic purpura**   `CC`
Allergic vasculitis
Nonthrombocytopenic hemorrhagic purpura
Nonthrombocytopenic idiopathic purpura
Purpura anaphylactoid
Purpura Henoch(-Schönlein)
Purpura rheumatica
Vascular purpura
EXCLUDES 1   *thrombocytopenic hemorrhagic purpura (D69.3)*

D69.1   **Qualitative platelet defects**
Bernard-Soulier [giant platelet] syndrome
Glanzmann's disease
Grey platelet syndrome
Thromboasthenia (hemorrhagic) (hereditary)
Thrombocytopathy
EXCLUDES 1   *von Willebrand's disease (D68.0)*

D69.2   **Other nonthrombocytopenic purpura**
Purpura NOS
Purpura simplex
Senile purpura

D69.3   **Immune thrombocytopenic purpura**   `CC`
Hemorrhagic (thrombocytopenic) purpura
Idiopathic thrombocytopenic purpura
Tidal platelet dysgenesis

√5ᵗʰ **D69.4**   **Other primary thrombocytopenia**
EXCLUDES 1   *transient neonatal thrombocytopenia (P61.0)*
Wiskott-Aldrich syndrome (D82.0)

D69.41   **Evans syndrome**   `CC`

D69.42   **Congenital and hereditary thrombocytopenia purpura**   `CC`
Congenital thrombocytopenia
Hereditary thrombocytopenia
Code first congenital or hereditary disorder, such as:
thrombocytopenia with absent radius (TAR syndrome) (Q87.2)

D69.49   **Other primary thrombocytopenia**
Megakaryocytic hypoplasia
Primary thrombocytopenia NOS

√5ᵗʰ **D69.5**   **Secondary thrombocytopenia**
EXCLUDES 1   *heparin induced thrombocytopenia (HIT) (D75.82)*
transient thrombocytopenia of newborn (P61.0)

D69.51   **Posttransfusion purpura**
Posttransfusion purpura from whole blood (fresh) or blood products
PTP

D69.59   **Other secondary thrombocytopenia**
AHA: 2014, 4Q, 22

D69.6   **Thrombocytopenia, unspecified**

D69.8   **Other specified hemorrhagic conditions**
Capillary fragility (hereditary)
Vascular pseudohemophilia

D69.9   **Hemorrhagic condition, unspecified**

Other disorders of blood and blood-forming organs (D70-D77)

√4ᵗʰ **D70**   **Neutropenia**
INCLUDES   agranulocytosis
decreased absolute neurophile count (ANC)
Use additional code for any associated:
fever (R50.81)
mucositis (J34.81, K12.3-, K92.81, N76.81)
EXCLUDES 1   *neutropenic splenomegaly (D73.81)*
transient neonatal neutropenia (P61.5)

D70.0   **Congenital agranulocytosis**
Congenital neutropenia
Infantile genetic agranulocytosis
Kostmann's disease

D70.1   **Agranulocytosis secondary to cancer chemotherapy**
Code also underlying neoplasm
Use additional code for adverse effect, if applicable, to identify drug (T45.1X5)
AHA: 2014, 4Q, 22

D70.2   **Other drug-induced agranulocytosis**
Use additional code for adverse effect, if applicable, to identify drug (T36-T50 with fifth or sixth character 5)

D70.3   **Neutropenia due to infection**

D70.4   **Cyclic neutropenia**
Cyclic hematopoiesis
Periodic neutropenia

D70.8   **Other neutropenia**

D70.9   **Neutropenia, unspecified**

D71   **Functional disorders of polymorphonuclear neutrophils**
Cell membrane receptor complex [CR3] defect
Chronic (childhood) granulomatous disease
Congenital dysphagocytosis
Progressive septic granulomatosis

√4ᵗʰ **D72**   **Other disorders of white blood cells**
EXCLUDES 1   *basophilia (D72.824)*
immunity disorders (D80-D89)
neutropenia (D70)
preleukemia (syndrome) (D46.9)

D72.0   **Genetic anomalies of leukocytes**
Alder (granulation) (granulocyte) anomaly
Alder syndrome
Hereditary leukocytic hypersegmentation
Hereditary leukocytic hyposegmentation
Hereditary leukomelanopathy
May-Hegglin (granulation) (granulocyte) anomaly
May-Hegglin syndrome
Pelger-Huët (granulation) (granulocyte) anomaly
Pelger-Huët syndrome
EXCLUDES 1   *Chédiak (-Steinbrinck)-Higashi syndrome (E70.330)*

N Newborn: 0   P Pediatric: 0-17   M Maternity: 12-55   A Adult: 15-124   MCC Major CC Condition   PDxMCC PDx acts as own MCC   CC CC Condition   PDxCC PDx acts as own CC

496

ICD-10-CM 2016

D72.1 Eosinophilia
Allergic eosinophilia
Hereditary eosinophilia
> EXCLUDES 1   *Löffler's syndrome (J82)*
> *pulmonary eosinophilia (J82)*

✓5ᵗʰ D72.8 Other specified disorders of white blood cells
> EXCLUDES 1   *leukemia (C91-C95)*

✓6ᵗʰ D72.81 Decreased white blood cell count
> EXCLUDES 1   *neutropenia (D70.-)*

D72.810 Lymphocytopenia
Decreased lymphocytes

D72.818 Other decreased white blood cell count
Basophilic leukopenia
Eosinophilic leukopenia
Monocytopenia
Other decreased leukocytes
Plasmacytopenia

D72.819 Decreased white blood cell count, unspecified
Decreased leukocytes, unspecified
Leukocytopenia, unspecified
Leukopenia
> EXCLUDES 1   *malignant leukopenia (D70.9)*

✓6ᵗʰ D72.82 Elevated white blood cell count
> EXCLUDES 1   *eosinophilia (D72.1)*

D72.820 Lymphocytosis (symptomatic)
Elevated lymphocytes

D72.821 Monocytosis (symptomatic)
> EXCLUDES 1   *infectious mononucleosis (B27.-)*

D72.822 Plasmacytosis

D72.823 Leukemoid reaction
Basophilic leukemoid reaction
Leukemoid reaction NOS
Lymphocytic leukemoid reaction
Monocytic leukemoid reaction
Myelocytic leukemoid reaction
Neutrophilic leukemoid reaction

D72.824 Basophilia

D72.825 Bandemia
Bandemia without diagnosis of specific infection
> EXCLUDES 1   *confirmed infection—code to infection*
> *leukemia (C91.-, C92.-, C93.-, C94.-, C95.-)*

D72.828 Other elevated white blood cell count

D72.829 Elevated white blood cell count, unspecified
Elevated leukocytes, unspecified
Leukocytosis, unspecified

D72.89 Other specified disorders of white blood cells
Abnormality of white blood cells NEC

D72.9 Disorder of white blood cells, unspecified
Abnormal leukocyte differential NOS

✓4ᵗʰ D73 Diseases of spleen

D73.0 Hyposplenism
Atrophy of spleen
> EXCLUDES 1   *asplenia (congenital) (Q89.01)*
> *postsurgical absence of spleen (Z90.81)*

D73.1 Hypersplenism
> EXCLUDES 1   *neutropenic splenomegaly (D73.81)*
> *primary splenic neutropenia (D73.81)*
> *splenitis, splenomegaly in late syphilis (A52.79)*
> *splenitis, splenomegaly in tuberculosis (A18.85)*
> *splenomegaly NOS (R16.1)*
> *splenomegaly congenital (Q89.0)*

D73.2 Chronic congestive splenomegaly

D73.3 Abscess of spleen

D73.4 Cyst of spleen

D73.5 Infarction of spleen
Splenic rupture, nontraumatic
Torsion of spleen
> EXCLUDES 1   *rupture of spleen due to Plasmodium vivax malaria (B51.0)*
> *traumatic rupture of spleen (S36.03-)*

✓5ᵗʰ D73.8 Other diseases of spleen

D73.81 Neutropenic splenomegaly
Werner-Schultz disease

D73.89 Other diseases of spleen
Fibrosis of spleen NOS
Perisplenitis
Splenitis NOS

D73.9 Disease of spleen, unspecified

✓4ᵗʰ D74 Methemoglobinemia

> **CC Excl: For CC codes in category D74, unless otherwise noted:**
> D56.4, D58.2-D59.2, D59.4-D59.9, D64.4-D64.9, D74.0-D74.9, D75.9

D74.0 Congenital methemoglobinemia   CC
Congenital NADH-methemoglobin reductase deficiency
Hemoglobin-M [Hb-M] disease
Methemoglobinemia, hereditary

D74.8 Other methemoglobinemias   CC
Acquired methemoglobinemia (with sulfhemoglobinemia)
Toxic methemoglobinemia

D74.9 Methemoglobinemia, unspecified   CC

✓4ᵗʰ D75 Other and unspecified diseases of blood and blood-forming organs
> EXCLUDES 2   *acute lymphadenitis (L04.-)*
> *chronic lymphadenitis (I88.1)*
> *enlarged lymph nodes (R59.-)*
> *hypergammaglobulinemia NOS (D89.2)*
> *lymphadenitis NOS (I88.9)*
> *mesenteric lymphadenitis (acute) (chronic) (I88.0)*

D75.0 Familial erythrocytosis
Benign polycythemia
Familial polycythemia
> EXCLUDES 1   *hereditary ovalocytosis (D58.1)*

D75.1 Secondary polycythemia
Acquired polycythemia
Emotional polycythemia
Erythrocytosis NOS
Hypoxemic polycythemia
Nephrogenous polycythemia
Polycythemia due to erythropoietin
Polycythemia due to fall in plasma volume
Polycythemia due to high altitude
Polycythemia due to stress
Polycythemia NOS
Relative polycythemia
> EXCLUDES 1   *polycythemia neonatorum (P61.1)*
> *polycythemia vera (D45)*

✓5ᵗʰ D75.8 Other specified diseases of blood and blood-forming organs

D75.81 *Myelofibrosis*   CC
Myelofibrosis NOS
Secondary myelofibrosis NOS
Code first the underlying disorder, such as:
   malignant neoplasm of breast (C50.-)
Use additional code, if applicable, for associated therapy-related myelodysplastic syndrome (D46.-)
Use additional code for adverse effect, if applicable, to identify drug (T45.1X5)
> EXCLUDES 1   *acute myelofibrosis (C94.4-)*
> *idiopathic myelofibrosis (D47.1)*
> *leukoerythroblastic anemia (D61.82)*
> *myelofibrosis with myeloid metaplasia (D47.4)*
> *myelophthisic anemia (D61.82)*
> *myelophthisis (D61.82)*
> *primary myelofibrosis (D47.1)*

> **CC Excl:** C88.2-C88.3, C88.8-C88.9, C90.10-C90.11, C90.20-C90.21, C90.30-C90.31, C91.00-C95.92, D45-D47.1, D47.3, D47.Z9-D47.9, D48.7-D48.9

D75.82 Heparin induced thrombocytopenia (HIT)

D75.89 Other specified diseases of blood and blood-forming organs

D75.9 Disease of blood and blood-forming organs, unspecified

✓ Additional Character Required   ✓x7ᵗʰ Placeholder Alert   Unacceptable PDx   Manifestation   Hospital Acquired Condition   EXCLUDES 1 Not Coded Here   EXCLUDES 2 Not Included Here

✓4th D76 Other specified diseases with participation of lymphoreticular and reticulohistiocytic tissue

    EXCLUDES 1   (Abt-) Letterer-Siwe disease (C96.0)
         eosinophilic granuloma (C96.6)
         Hand-Schüller-Christian disease (C96.5)
         histiocytic sarcoma (C96.A)
         histiocytosis X, multifocal (C96.5)
         histiocytosis X, unifocal (C96.6)
         Langerhans-cell histiocytosis, multifocal (C96.5)
         Langerhans-cell histiocytosis NOS (C96.6)
         Langerhans-cell histiocytosis, unifocal (C96.6)
         leukemic reticuloendotheliosis or reticulosis (C91.4-)
         lipomelanotic reticuloendotheliosis or reticulosis (I89.8)
         malignant histiocytosis (C96.A)

D76.1 Hemophagocytic lymphohistiocytosis CC
    Familial hemophagocytic reticulosis
    Histiocytoses of mononuclear phagocytes
    CC Excl: D60.0-D60.9, D61.1-D61.9, D65, D69.3-D70.9, D72.818-D72.819, D75.82, D75.9

D76.2 Hemophagocytic syndrome, infection-associated CC
    Use additional code to identify infectious agent or disease
    CC Excl: See code: D76.1

D76.3 Other histiocytosis syndromes CC
    Reticulohistiocytoma (giant-cell)
    Sinus histiocytosis with massive lymphadenopathy
    Xanthogranuloma
    CC Excl: See code: D76.1

D77 Other disorders of blood and blood-forming organs in diseases classified elsewhere

    Code first underlying disease, such as:
         amyloidosis (E85.-)
         congenital early syphilis (A50.0)
         echinococcosis (B67.0-B67.9)
         malaria (B50.0-B54)
         schistosomiasis [bilharziasis] (B65.0-B65.9)
         vitamin C deficiency (E54)
    EXCLUDES 1   rupture of spleen due to Plasmodium vivax malaria (B51.0)
         splenitis, splenomegaly in late syphilis (A52.79)
         splenitis, splenomegaly in tuberculosis (A18.85)

Intraoperative and postprocedural complications of the spleen (D78)

✓4th D78 Intraoperative and postprocedural complications of the spleen

✓5th D78.0 Intraoperative hemorrhage and hematoma of the spleen complicating a procedure
    EXCLUDES 1   intraoperative hemorrhage and hematoma of the spleen due to accidental puncture or laceration during a procedure (D78.1-)

    D78.01 Intraoperative hemorrhage and hematoma CC **of the spleen complicating a procedure on the spleen**
        CC Excl: D78.01-D78.02, D78.21-D78.89, H95.811-H95.89, I85.01, I85.11, I97.3, K21.9, K22.8, K23-K25.0, K25.2, K25.4, K25.6, K26.0, K26.2, K26.4, K26.6, K27.0, K27.2, K27.4, K27.6, K28.0, K28.2, K28.4, K28.6, K29.01, K29.21, K29.31, K29.41, K29.51, K29.61, K29.71, K29.81, K29.91, K31.811, K55.21, K57.01, K57.11, K57.13, K57.21, K57.31, K57.33, K57.41, K57.51, K57.53, K57.81, K57.91, K57.93, K62.5, K92.0-K92.2, M96.89, N98.1-N98.9, P54.1-P54.3, T81.10XA, T81.11XA, T81.12XA, T81.19XA, T81.82XA, T81.89XA, T81.9XXA

    D78.02 Intraoperative hemorrhage and hematoma CC **of the spleen complicating other procedure**
        CC Excl: See code: D78.01

✓5th D78.1 Accidental puncture and laceration of the spleen during a procedure

    D78.11 Accidental puncture and laceration of the CC **spleen during a procedure on the spleen**
        CC Excl: D78.11-D78.12, D78.81-D78.89, E36.11-E36.8, E89.810-E89.89, G96.11, G97.41-G97.49, H59.011-H59.019, H59.031-H59.099, H59.211-H59.229, H59.811-H59.89, H95.31-H95.32, H95.811-H95.89, I97.3, I97.51-I97.52, J95.71-J95.72, K91.71-K91.72, L76.11-L76.12, L76.81-L76.82, M96.820-M96.821, M96.89, N98.1-N98.9, N99.71-N99.72, T81.82XXA, T81.89XX1, T81.9XXA

    D78.12 Accidental puncture and laceration of the CC **spleen during other procedure**
        CC Excl: See code: D78.11

✓5th D78.2 Postprocedural hemorrhage and hematoma of the spleen following a procedure

    D78.21 Postprocedural hemorrhage and hematoma of CC **the spleen following a procedure on the spleen**
        CC Excl: See code: D78.01

    D78.22 Postprocedural hemorrhage and hematoma of CC **the spleen following other procedure**
        CC Excl: See code: D78.01

✓5th D78.8 Other intraoperative and postprocedural complications of the spleen
    Use additional code, if applicable, to further specify disorder

    D78.81 Other intraoperative complications CC **of the spleen**
        CC Excl: D78.81-D78.89, H95.811-H95.89, I97.3, M96.89, N98.1-N98.9, T81.82XA, T81.89XA, T81.9XXA

    D78.89 Other postprocedural complications CC **of the spleen**
        CC Excl: See code: D78.81

Certain disorders involving the immune mechanism (D80-D89)

    INCLUDES   defects in the complement system
         immunodeficiency disorders, except human immunodeficiency virus [HIV] disease
         sarcoidosis
    EXCLUDES 1   autoimmune disease (systemic) NOS (M35.9)
         functional disorders of polymorphonuclear neutrophils (D71)
         human immunodeficiency virus [HIV] disease (B20)

✓4th D80 Immunodeficiency with predominantly antibody defects

    CC Excl: For CC codes in category D80, unless otherwise noted: D80.0, D80.3-D81.2, D81.4, D81.6-D81.7, D81.89-D84.0, D84.8-D84.9, D89.3, D89.82-D89.9

    D80.0 Hereditary hypogammaglobulinemia CC
        Autosomal recessive agammaglobulinemia (Swiss type)
        X-linked agammaglobulinemia [Bruton] (with growth hormone deficiency)

    D80.1 Nonfamilial hypogammaglobulinemia CC
        Agammaglobulinemia with immunoglobulin-bearing B-lymphocytes
        Common variable agammaglobulinemia [CVAgamma]
        Hypogammaglobulinemia NOS
        CC Excl: D80.0-D81.2, D81.4, D81.6-D81.7, D81.89-D84.0, D84.8-D84.9, D89.3, D89.82-D89.9

    D80.2 Selective deficiency of immunoglobulin A [IgA] CC

    D80.3 Selective deficiency of immunoglobulin G [IgG] subclasses CC

    D80.4 Selective deficiency of immunoglobulin M [IgM] CC

    D80.5 Immunodeficiency with increased immunoglobulin M [IgM] CC

    D80.6 Antibody deficiency with near-normal immunoglobulins CC **or with hyperimmunoglobulinemia**

    D80.7 Transient hypogammaglobulinemia of infancy CC N

    D80.8 Other immunodeficiencies with predominantly CC **antibody defects**
        Kappa light chain deficiency

    D80.9 Immunodeficiency with predominantly antibody CC **defects, unspecified**

✓4th D81 Combined immunodeficiencies
    EXCLUDES 1   autosomal recessive agammaglobulinemia (Swiss type) (D80.0)

    CC Excl: For CC codes in category D81, unless otherwise noted: D80.0, D80.3-D81.2, D81.4, D81.6-D81.7, D81.89-D84.0, D84.8-D84.9, D89.3, D89.82-D89.9

    D81.0 Severe combined immunodeficiency [SCID] with reticular CC **dysgenesis**

    D81.1 Severe combined immunodeficiency [SCID] with low CC **T- and B-cell numbers**

    D81.2 Severe combined immunodeficiency [SCID] with low CC **or normal B-cell numbers**

    D81.3 Adenosine deaminase [ADA] deficiency CC
        CC Excl: D81.3, D81.5, D81.810, D84.1, E76.01-E76.9, E79.1-E80.29, E80.4-E80.7, E88.81

    D81.4 Nezelof's syndrome CC

    D81.5 Purine nucleoside phosphorylase [PNP] deficiency CC
        CC Excl: See code: D81.3

    D81.6 Major histocompatibility complex class I deficiency CC
        Bare lymphocyte syndrome

    D81.7 Major histocompatibility complex class II deficiency CC

☑5ᵗʰ **D81.8 Other combined immunodeficiencies**

☑6ᵗʰ **D81.81 Biotin-dependent carboxylase deficiency**
Multiple carboxylase deficiency
EXCLUDES1 *biotin-dependent carboxylase deficiency due to dietary deficiency of biotin (E53.8)*

D81.810 Biotinidase deficiency

D81.818 Other biotin-dependent carboxylase deficiency
Holocarboxylase synthetase deficiency
Other multiple carboxylase deficiency

D81.819 Biotin-dependent carboxylase deficiency, unspecified
Multiple carboxylase deficiency, unspecified

D81.89 Other combined immunodeficiencies CC

D81.9 Combined immunodeficiency, unspecified CC
Severe combined immunodeficiency disorder [SCID] NOS

☑4ᵗʰ **D82 Immunodeficiency associated with other major defects**
EXCLUDES1 *ataxia telangiectasia [Louis-Bar] (G11.3)*

D82.0 Wiskott-Aldrich syndrome CC
Immunodeficiency with thrombocytopenia and eczema
CC Excl: See code: D80

D82.1 Di George's syndrome CC
Pharyngeal pouch syndrome
Thymic alymphoplasia
Thymic aplasia or hypoplasia with immunodeficiency
CC Excl: See code: D80

D82.2 Immunodeficiency with short-limbed stature

D82.3 Immunodeficiency following hereditary defective response to Epstein-Barr virus
X-linked lymphoproliferative disease

D82.4 Hyperimmunoglobulin E [IgE] syndrome

D82.8 Immunodeficiency associated with other specified major defects

D82.9 Immunodeficiency associated with major defect, unspecified

☑4ᵗʰ **D83 Common variable immunodeficiency**

CC Excl: For CC codes in category D83, unless otherwise noted:
D80.0, D80.3-D81.2, D81.4, D81.6-D81.7, D81.89-D84.0, D84.8-D84.9, D89.3, D89.82-D89.9

D83.0 Common variable immunodeficiency with predominant abnormalities of B-cell numbers and function CC

D83.1 Common variable immunodeficiency with predominant immunoregulatory T-cell disorders CC

D83.2 Common variable immunodeficiency with autoantibodies to B- or T-cells CC

D83.8 Other common variable immunodeficiencies CC

D83.9 Common variable immunodeficiency, unspecified CC

☑4ᵗʰ **D84 Other immunodeficiencies**

D84.0 Lymphocyte function antigen-1 [LFA-1] defect

D84.1 Defects in the complement system
C1 esterase inhibitor [C1-INH] deficiency

D84.8 Other specified immunodeficiencies CC
CC Excl: See code: D83

D84.9 Immunodeficiency, unspecified CC
CC Excl: See code: D83

☑4ᵗʰ **D86 Sarcoidosis**

D86.0 Sarcoidosis of lung

D86.1 Sarcoidosis of lymph nodes

D86.2 Sarcoidosis of lung with sarcoidosis of lymph nodes

D86.3 Sarcoidosis of skin

☑5ᵗʰ **D86.8 Sarcoidosis of other sites**

D86.81 Sarcoid meningitis

D86.82 Multiple cranial nerve palsies in sarcoidosis

D86.83 Sarcoid iridocyclitis

D86.84 Sarcoid pyelonephritis
Tubulo-interstitial nephropathy in sarcoidosis

D86.85 Sarcoid myocarditis

D86.86 Sarcoid arthropathy
Polyarthritis in sarcoidosis

D86.87 Sarcoid myositis

D86.89 Sarcoidosis of other sites
Hepatic granuloma
Uveoparotid fever [Heerfordt]

D86.9 Sarcoidosis, unspecified

☑4ᵗʰ **D89 Other disorders involving the immune mechanism, not elsewhere classified**
EXCLUDES1 *hyperglobulinemia NOS (R77.1)*
monoclonal gammopathy (of undetermined significance) (D47.2)
EXCLUDES2 *transplant failure and rejection (T86.-)*

D89.0 Polyclonal hypergammaglobulinemia
Benign hypergammaglobulinemic purpura
Polyclonal gammopathy NOS

D89.1 Cryoglobulinemia
Cryoglobulinemic purpura
Cryoglobulinemic vasculitis
Essential cryoglobulinemia
Idiopathic cryoglobulinemia
Mixed cryoglobulinemia
Primary cryoglobulinemia
Secondary cryoglobulinemia

D89.2 Hypergammaglobulinemia, unspecified

D89.3 Immune reconstitution syndrome
Immune reconstitution inflammatory syndrome [IRIS]
Use additional code for adverse effect, if applicable, to identify drug (T36-T50 with fifth or sixth character 5)

☑5ᵗʰ **D89.8 Other specified disorders involving the immune mechanism, not elsewhere classified**

☑6ᵗʰ **D89.81 Graft-versus-host disease**
Code first underlying cause, such as:
complications of transplanted organs and tissue (T86.-)
complications of blood transfusion (T80.89)
Use additional code to identify associated manifestations, such as:
desquamative dermatitis (L30.8)
diarrhea (R19.7)
elevated bilirubin (R17)
hair loss (L65.9)

CC Excl: For CC codes in subcategory D89.81, unless otherwise noted: D78.81-D78.89, D89.810-D89.813, E89.810-E89.89, H59.011-H59.019, H59.031-H59.099, H59.811-H59.89, H95.811-H95.89, I97.3, M96.89, N98.1-N98.9, T86.00-T86.09

D89.810 Acute graft-versus-host disease CC

D89.811 Chronic graft-versus-host disease CC

D89.812 Acute on chronic graft-versus-host disease CC

D89.813 Graft-versus-host disease, unspecified CC

D89.82 Autoimmune lymphoproliferative syndrome [ALPS]

D89.89 Other specified disorders involving the immune mechanism, not elsewhere classified
EXCLUDES1 *human immunodeficiency virus disease (B20)*

D89.9 Disorder involving the immune mechanism, unspecified
Immune disease NOS

☑ Additional Character Required   ☑x7ᵗʰ Placeholder Alert   Unacceptable PDx   Manifestation   Hospital Acquired Condition   EXCLUDES1 Not Coded Here   EXCLUDES2 Not Included Here

Chapter 4. Endocrine, Nutritional, and Metabolic Diseases (EØØ–E89)

Chapter Specific Guidelines with Coding Examples

The chapter specific guidelines from the ICD-10-CM Official Guidelines for Coding and Reporting have been provided below. Along with these guidelines are coding examples, contained in the shaded boxes, that have been developed to help illustrate the coding and/or sequencing guidance found in these guidelines.

a. Diabetes mellitus

The diabetes mellitus codes are combination codes that include the type of diabetes mellitus, the body system affected, and the complications affecting that body system. As many codes within a particular category as are necessary to describe all of the complications of the disease may be used. They should be sequenced based on the reason for a particular encounter. Assign as many codes from categories E08–E13 as needed to identify all of the associated conditions that the patient has.

> Patient is seen for uncontrolled diabetes, type 2, with diabetic polyneuropathy and diabetic retinopathy with macular edema
>
> **E11.65**   **Type 2 diabetes mellitus with hyperglycemia**
>
> **E11.311**   **Type 2 diabetes mellitus with unspecified diabetic retinopathy with macular edema**
>
> **E11.42**   **Type 2 diabetes mellitus with diabetic polyneuropathy**
>
> *Explanation*: Use as many codes to describe the diabetic complications as needed. Many are combination codes that describe more than one condition. Code first the reason for the encounter. "Uncontrolled" is described as "with hyperglycemia."

1) Type of diabetes

The age of a patient is not the sole determining factor, though most type 1 diabetics develop the condition before reaching puberty. For this reason type 1 diabetes mellitus is also referred to as juvenile diabetes.

> A 45-year-old patient is diagnosed with Type 1 diabetes
>
> **E10.9**   **Type 1 diabetes mellitus without complications**
>
> *Explanation*: Although most type 1 diabetics are diagnosed in childhood or adolescence, it can also begin in adults.

2) Type of diabetes mellitus not documented

If the type of diabetes mellitus is not documented in the medical record the default is E11.-, Type 2 diabetes mellitus.

> Office visit lists diabetes and hypertension on patient problem list
>
> **E11.9**   **Type 2 diabetes mellitus without complications**
>
> **I10**   **Essential (primary) hypertension**
>
> *Explanation*: Since the type of diabetes was not documented and no complications were noted, the default code is E11.9.

3) Diabetes mellitus and the use of insulin

If the documentation in a medical record does not indicate the type of diabetes but does indicate that the patient uses insulin, code E11, Type 2 diabetes mellitus, should be assigned. Code Z79.4, Long-term (current) use of insulin, should also be assigned to indicate that the patient uses insulin. Code Z79.4 should not be assigned if insulin is given temporarily to bring a type 2 patient's blood sugar under control during an encounter.

> Office visit lists chronic diabetes with daily insulin use on patient problem list
>
> **E11.9**   **Type 2 diabetes mellitus without complications**
>
> **Z79.4**   **Long-term (current) use of insulin**
>
> *Explanation*: Do not assume that a patient on insulin must have type 1 diabetes. The default for diabetes without further specification defaults to type 2. Add the code for long-term use of insulin.

4) Diabetes mellitus in pregnancy and gestational diabetes

See Section I.C.15. Diabetes mellitus in pregnancy.

See Section I.C.15. Gestational (pregnancy induced) diabetes

5) Complications due to insulin pump malfunction

(a) Underdose of insulin due to insulin pump failure

An underdose of insulin due to an insulin pump failure should be assigned to a code from subcategory T85.6, Mechanical complication of other specified internal and external prosthetic devices, implants and grafts, that specifies the type of pump malfunction, as the principal or first-listed code, followed by code T38.3X6-, Underdosing of insulin and oral hypoglycemic [antidiabetic] drugs. Additional codes for the type of diabetes mellitus and any associated complications due to the underdosing should also be assigned.

> A 24-year-old type 1 diabetic male treated in ED for hyperglycemia; insulin pump found to be malfunctioning and underdosing
>
> **T85.614A**   **Breakdown (mechanical) of insulin pump, initial encounter**
>
> **T38.3X6A**   **Underdosing of insulin and oral hypoglycemic [antidiabetic] drugs, initial encounter**
>
> **E10.65**   **Type 1 diabetes mellitus with hyperglycemia**
>
> *Explanation*: The complication code for the mechanical breakdown of the pump is sequenced first, followed by the underdosing code and type of diabetes with complication. Code all other diabetic complication codes necessary to describe the patient's condition.

(b) Overdose of insulin due to insulin pump failure

The principal or first-listed code for an encounter due to an insulin pump malfunction resulting in an overdose of insulin, should also be T85.6-, Mechanical complication of other specified internal and external prosthetic devices, implants and grafts, followed by code T38.3X1-, Poisoning by insulin and oral hypoglycemic [antidiabetic] drugs, accidental (unintentional).

> A 24-year-old type 1 diabetic male found down with diabetic coma, brought into ED and treated for hypoglycemia; insulin pump found to be malfunctioning and overdosing
>
> **T85.614A**   **Breakdown (mechanical) of insulin pump, initial encounter**
>
> **T38.3X1A**   **Poisoning by insulin and oral hypoglycemic [antidiabetic] drugs, accidental (unintentional), initial encounter**
>
> **E10.641**   **Type 1 diabetes mellitus with hypoglycemia with coma**
>
> *Explanation*: The complication code for the mechanical breakdown of the pump is sequenced first, followed by the poisoning code and type of diabetes with complication. All the characters in the combination code must be used to form a valid code and to fully describe the type of diabetes, the hypoglycemia, and the coma.

6) Secondary diabetes mellitus

Codes under categories E08, Diabetes mellitus due to underlying condition, E09, Drug or chemical induced diabetes mellitus, and E13, Other specified diabetes mellitus, identify complications/manifestations associated with secondary diabetes mellitus. Secondary diabetes is always caused by another condition or event (e.g., cystic fibrosis, malignant neoplasm of pancreas, pancreatectomy, adverse effect of drug, or poisoning).

(a) Secondary diabetes mellitus and the use of insulin

For patients who routinely use insulin, code Z79.4, Long-term (current) use of insulin, should also be assigned. Code Z79.4 should not be assigned if insulin is given temporarily to bring a patient's blood sugar under control during an encounter.

Type 2 diabetic with no complications, normally only on oral metformin, is given insulin for three days to maintain glucose control while in the hospital recovering from surgery

E11.9　　Type 2 diabetes mellitus without complications

No code is used for insulin use

Explanation: Do not code the long term (current) use of insulin when only provided temporarily.

Type 2 diabetic with diabetic polyneuropathy on insulin

E11.42　　Type 2 diabetes mellitus with diabetic polyneuropathy

Z79.4　　Long-term (current) use of insulin

Explanation: Add the Z code for the long-term use of insulin because the insulin is taken chronically.

(b) Assigning and sequencing secondary diabetes codes and its causes

The sequencing of the secondary diabetes codes in relationship to codes for the cause of the diabetes is based on the Tabular List instructions for categories E08, E09 and E13.

(i) Secondary diabetes mellitus due to pancreatectomy

For postpancreatectomy diabetes mellitus (lack of insulin due to the surgical removal of all or part of the pancreas), assign code E89.1, Postprocedural hypoinsulinemia. Assign a code from category E13 and a code from subcategory Z90.41-, Acquired absence of pancreas, as additional codes.

Patient with newly diagnosed diabetes after surgical removal of part of pancreas

E89.1　　Postprocedural hypoinsulinemia

E13.9　　Other specified diabetes mellitus without complications

Z90.411　　Acquired partial absence of pancreas

Explanation: Sequence the postprocedural complication of the hypoinsulinemia due to the partial removal of the pancreas as the first-listed code, followed by the other specified diabetes (NEC) with or without complications and the partial or total acquired absence of the pancreas.

(ii) Secondary diabetes due to drugs

Secondary diabetes may be caused by an adverse effect of correctly administered medications, poisoning or sequela of poisoning.

See section I.C.19.e for coding of adverse effects and poisoning, and section I.C.20 for external cause code reporting.

Initial encounter for corticosteroid-induced diabetes mellitus

E09.9　　Drug or chemical induced diabetes mellitus without complications

T38.0X5A　　Adverse effect of glucocorticoids and synthetic analogues, initial encounter

Explanation: If the diabetes is caused by an adverse effect of a drug, the diabetic condition is coded first. If it occurs from a poisoning or overdose, the poisoning code causing the diabetes is sequenced first.

Chapter 4. Endocrine, Nutritional and Metabolic Diseases (E00-E89)

NOTE All neoplasms, whether functionally active or not, are classified in Chapter 2. Appropriate codes in this chapter (i.e. E05.8, E07.0, E16-E31, E34-) may be used as additional codes to indicate either functional activity by neoplasms and ectopic endocrine tissue or hyperfunction and hypofunction of endocrine glands associated with neoplasms and other conditions classified elsewhere.

EXCLUDES 1 transitory endocrine and metabolic disorders specific to newborn (P70-P74)

This chapter contains the following blocks:
E00-E07	Disorders of thyroid gland
E08-E13	Diabetes mellitus
E15-E16	Other disorders of glucose regulation and pancreatic internal secretion
E20-E35	Disorders of other endocrine glands
E36	Intraoperative complications of endocrine system
E40-E46	Malnutrition
E50-E64	Other nutritional deficiencies
E65-E68	Overweight, obesity and other hyperalimentation
E70-E88	Metabolic disorders
E89	Postprocedural endocrine and metabolic complications and disorders, not elsewhere classified

Disorders of thyroid gland (E00-E07)

✓4ᵗʰ E00 Congenital iodine-deficiency syndrome
Use additional code (F70-F79) to identify associated intellectual disabilities
EXCLUDES 1 subclinical iodine-deficiency hypothyroidism (E02)

E00.0 Congenital iodine-deficiency syndrome, neurological type
Endemic cretinism, neurological type

E00.1 Congenital iodine-deficiency syndrome, myxedematous type
Endemic hypothyroid cretinism
Endemic cretinism, myxedematous type

E00.2 Congenital iodine-deficiency syndrome, mixed type
Endemic cretinism, mixed type

E00.9 Congenital iodine-deficiency syndrome, unspecified
Congenital iodine-deficiency hypothyroidism NOS
Endemic cretinism NOS

✓4ᵗʰ E01 Iodine-deficiency related thyroid disorders and allied conditions
EXCLUDES 1 congenital iodine-deficiency syndrome (E00.-)
subclinical iodine-deficiency hypothyroidism (E02)

E01.0 Iodine-deficiency related diffuse (endemic) goiter

E01.1 Iodine-deficiency related multinodular (endemic) goiter
Iodine-deficiency related nodular goiter

E01.2 Iodine-deficiency related (endemic) goiter, unspecified
Endemic goiter NOS

E01.8 Other iodine-deficiency related thyroid disorders and allied conditions
Acquired iodine-deficiency hypothyroidism NOS

E02 Subclinical iodine-deficiency hypothyroidism

✓4ᵗʰ E03 Other hypothyroidism
EXCLUDES 1 iodine-deficiency related hypothyroidism (E00-E02)
postprocedural hypothyroidism (E89.0)

E03.0 Congenital hypothyroidism with diffuse goiter
Congenital parenchymatous goiter (nontoxic)
Congenital goiter (nontoxic) NOS
EXCLUDES 1 transitory congenital goiter with normal function (P72.0)

E03.1 Congenital hypothyroidism without goiter
Aplasia of thyroid (with myxedema)
Congenital atrophy of thyroid
Congenital hypothyroidism NOS

E03.2 Hypothyroidism due to medicaments and other exogenous substances
Code first poisoning due to drug or toxin, if applicable (T36-T65 with fifth or sixth character 1-4 or 6)
Use additional code for adverse effect, if applicable, to identify drug (T36-T50 with fifth or sixth character 5)

E03.3 Postinfectious hypothyroidism

E03.4 Atrophy of thyroid (acquired)
EXCLUDES 1 congenital atrophy of thyroid (E03.1)

E03.5 Myxedema coma MCC
CC Excl: B15.0-B19.9, E03.5, E08.00-E08.59, E08.618-E08.638, E08.641-E09.59, E09.618-E09.638, E09.641-E10.59, E10.618-E10.638, E10.641-E10.649, E10.69-E11.59, E11.618-E11.638, E11.641-E11.649, E11.69-E13.59, E13.618-E13.638, E13.641-E16.2, E89.1, G32.89, G89.0-G89.4, G93.81-G93.9, G96.8-G96.9, G98.0-G98.8, G99.8, I60.00-I62.9, K72.91, R40.0-R40.2124, R40.2210-R40.2224, R40.2310-R40.2324, R40.2340-R40.2344, R40.3-R41.3, R41.82, R41.9-R42, R44.8-R44.9, R45.83-R45.84, R46.0-R46.89, R52, R55, R68.0-R68.19, R68.81-R68.83, R68.89-R69; S02.0XX-S06.9X9 with 7th character A

E03.8 Other specified hypothyroidism

E03.9 Hypothyroidism, unspecified
Myxedema NOS

✓4ᵗʰ E04 Other nontoxic goiter
EXCLUDES 1 congenital goiter (NOS) (diffuse) (parenchymatous) (E03.0)
iodine-deficiency related goiter (E00-E02)

E04.0 Nontoxic diffuse goiter
Diffuse (colloid) nontoxic goiter
Simple nontoxic goiter

E04.1 Nontoxic single thyroid nodule
Colloid nodule (cystic) (thyroid)   Thyroid (cystic) nodule NOS
Nontoxic uninodular goiter

E04.2 Nontoxic multinodular goiter
Cystic goiter NOS
Multinodular (cystic) goiter NOS

E04.8 Other specified nontoxic goiter

E04.9 Nontoxic goiter, unspecified
Goiter NOS
Nodular goiter (nontoxic) NOS

✓4ᵗʰ E05 Thyrotoxicosis [hyperthyroidism]
EXCLUDES 1 chronic thyroiditis with transient thyrotoxicosis (E06.2)
neonatal thyrotoxicosis (P72.1)

CC Excl: For MCC codes in category E05, unless otherwise noted: A17.9-A18.82, A18.84, A18.89, E00.0-E03.4, E03.8-E07.1, E07.89-E07.9, E30.9, E34.1, E34.50-E35, E89.0

✓5ᵗʰ E05.0 Thyrotoxicosis with diffuse goiter
Exophthalmic or toxic goiter NOS
Graves' disease
Toxic diffuse goiter

E05.00 Thyrotoxicosis with diffuse goiter without thyrotoxic crisis or storm

E05.01 Thyrotoxicosis with diffuse goiter with thyrotoxic crisis or storm MCC

✓5ᵗʰ E05.1 Thyrotoxicosis with toxic single thyroid nodule
Thyrotoxicosis with toxic uninodular goiter

E05.10 Thyrotoxicosis with toxic single thyroid nodule without thyrotoxic crisis or storm

E05.11 Thyrotoxicosis with toxic single thyroid nodule with thyrotoxic crisis or storm MCC

✓5ᵗʰ E05.2 Thyrotoxicosis with toxic multinodular goiter
Toxic nodular goiter NOS

E05.20 Thyrotoxicosis with toxic multinodular goiter without thyrotoxic crisis or storm

E05.21 Thyrotoxicosis with toxic multinodular goiter with thyrotoxic crisis or storm MCC

✓5ᵗʰ E05.3 Thyrotoxicosis from ectopic thyroid tissue

E05.30 Thyrotoxicosis from ectopic thyroid tissue without thyrotoxic crisis or storm

E05.31 Thyrotoxicosis from ectopic thyroid tissue with thyrotoxic crisis or storm MCC

✓5ᵗʰ E05.4 Thyrotoxicosis factitia

E05.40 Thyrotoxicosis factitia without thyrotoxic crisis or storm

E05.41 Thyrotoxicosis factitia with thyrotoxic crisis or storm MCC

✓5ᵗʰ E05.8 Other thyrotoxicosis
Overproduction of thyroid-stimulating hormone

E05.80 Other thyrotoxicosis without thyrotoxic crisis or storm

E05.81 Other thyrotoxicosis with thyrotoxic crisis or storm MCC

✓5ᵗʰ E05.9 Thyrotoxicosis, unspecified
Hyperthyroidism NOS

E05.90 Thyrotoxicosis, unspecified without thyrotoxic crisis or storm

N Newborn: 0   P Pediatric: 0-17   M Maternity: 12-55   A Adult: 15-124   MCC Major CC Condition   PDxMCC PDx acts as own MCC   CC CC Condition   PDxCC PDx acts as own CC

502

ICD-10-CM 2016

E05.91   **Thyrotoxicosis, unspecified with thyrotoxic crisis or storm** `MCC`

☑️**4th** **E06**   **Thyroiditis**
     EXCLUDES 1   *postpartum thyroiditis (O90.5)*

   E06.0   **Acute thyroiditis** `CC`
       Abscess of thyroid
       Pyogenic thyroiditis
       Suppurative thyroiditis
       Use additional code (B95-B97) to identify infectious agent
       CC Excl: E06.0-E06.9

   E06.1   **Subacute thyroiditis**
       de Quervain thyroiditis   Nonsuppurative thyroiditis
       Giant-cell thyroiditis   Viral thyroiditis
       Granulomatous thyroiditis
       EXCLUDES 1   *autoimmune thyroiditis (E06.3)*

   E06.2   **Chronic thyroiditis with transient thyrotoxicosis**
       EXCLUDES 1   *autoimmune thyroiditis (E06.3)*

   E06.3   **Autoimmune thyroiditis**
       Hashimoto's thyroiditis
       Hashitoxicosis (transient)
       Lymphadenoid goiter
       Lymphocytic thyroiditis
       Struma lymphomatosa

   E06.4   **Drug-induced thyroiditis**
       Use additional code for adverse effect, if applicable, to identify drug (T36-T50 with fifth or sixth character 5)

   E06.5   **Other chronic thyroiditis**
       Chronic fibrous thyroiditis
       Chronic thyroiditis NOS
       Ligneous thyroiditis
       Riedel thyroiditis

   E06.9   **Thyroiditis, unspecified**

☑️**4th** **E07**   **Other disorders of thyroid**

   E07.0   **Hypersecretion of calcitonin**
       C-cell hyperplasia of thyroid
       Hypersecretion of thyrocalcitonin

   E07.1   **Dyshormogenetic goiter**
       Familial dyshormogenetic goiter
       Pendred's syndrome
       EXCLUDES 1   *transitory congenital goiter with normal function (P72.0)*

☑️**5th**   **E07.8**   **Other specified disorders of thyroid**
     E07.81   **Sick-euthyroid syndrome**
         Euthyroid sick-syndrome
     E07.89   **Other specified disorders of thyroid**
         Abnormality of thyroid-binding globulin
         Hemorrhage of thyroid
         Infarction of thyroid

   E07.9   **Disorder of thyroid, unspecified**

Diabetes mellitus (E08-E13)

☑️**4th** **E08**   **Diabetes mellitus due to underlying condition**
     Code first the underlying condition, such as:
       congenital rubella (P35.0)
       cushing's syndrome (E24.-)
       cystic fibrosis (E84.-)
       malignant neoplasm (C00-C96)
       malnutrition (E40-E46)
       pancreatitis and other diseases of the pancreas (K85.-, K86.-)
     Use additional code to identify any insulin use (Z79.4)
     EXCLUDES 1   *drug or chemical induced diabetes mellitus (E09.-)*
         gestational diabetes (O24.4-)
         neonatal diabetes mellitus (P70.2)
         postpancreatectomy diabetes mellitus (E13.-)
         postprocedural diabetes mellitus (E13.-)
         secondary diabetes mellitus NEC (E13.-)
         type 1 diabetes mellitus (E10.-)
         type 2 diabetes mellitus (E11.-)
     AHA: 2013, 4Q, 114; 2013, 3Q, 20

     CC Excl: For MCC codes in category E08, unless otherwise noted:
     E08.00-E08.59, E08.618-E08.638, E08.641-E09.59, E09.618-E09.638,
     E09.641-E10.59, E10.618-E10.638, E10.641-E10.649, E10.69-E11.59,
     E11.618-E11.638, E11.641-E11.649, E11.69-E13.59, E13.618-E13.638,
     E13.641-E16.2, E30.9, E34.1, E34.8-E35, E89.1

☑️**5th**   **E08.0**   **Diabetes mellitus due to underlying condition with hyperosmolarity**
     E08.00   *Diabetes mellitus due to underlying condition with hyperosmolarity without nonketotic hyperglycemic-hyperosmolar coma (NKHHC)* `MCC`
     E08.01   *Diabetes mellitus due to underlying condition with hyperosmolarity with coma* `MCC`

☑️**5th**   **E08.1**   **Diabetes mellitus due to underlying condition with ketoacidosis**
     E08.10   *Diabetes mellitus due to underlying condition with ketoacidosis without coma* `MCC`
     E08.11   *Diabetes mellitus due to underlying condition with ketoacidosis with coma* `MCC`

☑️**5th**   **E08.2**   **Diabetes mellitus due to underlying condition with kidney complications**
     E08.21   *Diabetes mellitus due to underlying condition with diabetic nephropathy*
       Diabetes mellitus due to underlying condition with intercapillary glomerulosclerosis
       Diabetes mellitus due to underlying condition with intracapillary glomerulonephrosis
       Diabetes mellitus due to underlying condition with Kimmelstiel-Wilson disease
     E08.22   *Diabetes mellitus due to underlying condition with diabetic chronic kidney disease*
       Use additional code to identify stage of chronic kidney disease (N18.1-N18.6)
     E08.29   *Diabetes mellitus due to underlying condition with other diabetic kidney complication*
       Renal tubular degeneration in diabetes mellitus due to underlying condition

☑️**5th**   **E08.3**   **Diabetes mellitus due to underlying condition with ophthalmic complications**
   ☑️**6th**   **E08.31**   **Diabetes mellitus due to underlying condition with unspecified diabetic retinopathy**
       E08.311   *Diabetes mellitus due to underlying condition with unspecified diabetic retinopathy with macular edema*
       E08.319   *Diabetes mellitus due to underlying condition with unspecified diabetic retinopathy without macular edema*
   ☑️**6th**   **E08.32**   **Diabetes mellitus due to underlying condition with mild nonproliferative diabetic retinopathy**
       Diabetes mellitus due to underlying condition with nonproliferative diabetic retinopathy NOS
       E08.321   *Diabetes mellitus due to underlying condition with mild nonproliferative diabetic retinopathy with macular edema*
       E08.329   *Diabetes mellitus due to underlying condition with mild nonproliferative diabetic retinopathy without macular edema*
   ☑️**6th**   **E08.33**   **Diabetes mellitus due to underlying condition with moderate nonproliferative diabetic retinopathy**
       E08.331   *Diabetes mellitus due to underlying condition with moderate nonproliferative diabetic retinopathy with macular edema*
       E08.339   *Diabetes mellitus due to underlying condition with moderate nonproliferative diabetic retinopathy without macular edema*
   ☑️**6th**   **E08.34**   **Diabetes mellitus due to underlying condition with severe nonproliferative diabetic retinopathy**
       E08.341   *Diabetes mellitus due to underlying condition with severe nonproliferative diabetic retinopathy with macular edema*
       E08.349   *Diabetes mellitus due to underlying condition with severe nonproliferative diabetic retinopathy without macular edema*
   ☑️**6th**   **E08.35**   **Diabetes mellitus due to underlying condition with proliferative diabetic retinopathy**
       E08.351   *Diabetes mellitus due to underlying condition with proliferative diabetic retinopathy with macular edema*
       E08.359   *Diabetes mellitus due to underlying condition with proliferative diabetic retinopathy without macular edema*
     E08.36   *Diabetes mellitus due to underlying condition with diabetic cataract*

☑️ Additional Character Required   ☑️x7th Placeholder Alert   Unacceptable PDx   Manifestation   Hospital Acquired Condition   **EXCLUDES 1** Not Coded Here   **EXCLUDES 2** Not Included Here

ICD-10-CM 2016   503

E08.39   *Diabetes mellitus due to underlying condition with other diabetic ophthalmic complication*
Use additional code to identify manifestation, such as: diabetic glaucoma (H40-H42)

✓5ᵗʰ **E08.4**   **Diabetes mellitus due to underlying condition with neurological complications**

E08.40   *Diabetes mellitus due to underlying condition with diabetic neuropathy, unspecified*

E08.41   *Diabetes mellitus due to underlying condition with diabetic mononeuropathy*

E08.42   *Diabetes mellitus due to underlying condition with diabetic polyneuropathy*
Diabetes mellitus due to underlying condition with diabetic neuralgia

E08.43   *Diabetes mellitus due to underlying condition with diabetic autonomic (poly)neuropathy*
Diabetes mellitus due to underlying condition with diabetic gastroparesis
AHA: 2013, 4Q, 114

E08.44   *Diabetes mellitus due to underlying condition with diabetic amyotrophy*

E08.49   *Diabetes mellitus due to underlying condition with other diabetic neurological complication*

✓5ᵗʰ **E08.5**   **Diabetes mellitus due to underlying condition with circulatory complications**

E08.51   *Diabetes mellitus due to underlying condition with diabetic peripheral angiopathy without gangrene*

E08.52   *Diabetes mellitus due to underlying condition with diabetic peripheral angiopathy with gangrene* **PDxCC CC**
Diabetes mellitus due to underlying condition with diabetic gangrene
CC Excl: G89.0-G89.4, I70.261-I70.269, I96, R41.0-R41.3, R41.82, R41.9, R44.8-R44.9, R45.83-R45.84, R46.0-R46.89, R52, R68.0-R68.19, R68.81-R68.83, R68.89-R69

E08.59   *Diabetes mellitus due to underlying condition with other circulatory complications*

✓5ᵗʰ **E08.6**   **Diabetes mellitus due to underlying condition with other specified complications**

✓6ᵗʰ **E08.61**   **Diabetes mellitus due to underlying condition with diabetic arthropathy**

E08.610   *Diabetes mellitus due to underlying condition with diabetic neuropathic arthropathy*
Diabetes mellitus due to underlying condition with Charcôt's joints

E08.618   *Diabetes mellitus due to underlying condition with other diabetic arthropathy*

✓6ᵗʰ **E08.62**   **Diabetes mellitus due to underlying condition with skin complications**

E08.620   *Diabetes mellitus due to underlying condition with diabetic dermatitis*
Diabetes mellitus due to underlying condition with diabetic necrobiosis lipoidica

E08.621   *Diabetes mellitus due to underlying condition with foot ulcer*
Use additional code to identify site of ulcer (L97.4-, L97.5-)

E08.622   *Diabetes mellitus due to underlying condition with other skin ulcer*
Use additional code to identify site of ulcer (L97.1-L97.9, L98.41-L98.49)

E08.628   *Diabetes mellitus due to underlying condition with other skin complications*

✓6ᵗʰ **E08.63**   **Diabetes mellitus due to underlying condition with oral complications**

E08.630   *Diabetes mellitus due to underlying condition with periodontal disease*

E08.638   *Diabetes mellitus due to underlying condition with other oral complications*

✓6ᵗʰ **E08.64**   **Diabetes mellitus due to underlying condition with hypoglycemia**

E08.641   *Diabetes mellitus due to underlying condition with hypoglycemia with coma* **MCC**

E08.649   *Diabetes mellitus due to underlying condition with hypoglycemia without coma*

E08.65   *Diabetes mellitus due to underlying condition with hyperglycemia*

E08.69   *Diabetes mellitus due to underlying condition with other specified complication*
Use additional code to identify complication

E08.8   **Diabetes mellitus due to underlying condition with unspecified complications**

E08.9   **Diabetes mellitus due to underlying condition without complications**

✓4ᵗʰ **E09**   **Drug or chemical induced diabetes mellitus**
Code first poisoning due to drug or toxin, if applicable (T36-T65 with fifth or sixth character 1-4 or 6)
Use additional code for adverse effect, if applicable, to identify drug (T36-T50 with fifth or sixth character 5)
Use additional code to identify any insulin use (Z79.4)
EXCLUDES 1   diabetes mellitus due to underlying condition (E08.-)
gestational diabetes (O24.4-)
neonatal diabetes mellitus (P70.2)
postpancreatectomy diabetes mellitus (E13.-)
postprocedural diabetes mellitus (E13.-)
secondary diabetes mellitus NEC (E13.-)
type 1 diabetes mellitus (E10.-)
type 2 diabetes mellitus (E11.-)
AHA: 2013, 4Q, 114; 2013, 3Q, 20

CC Excl: For MCC codes in category E09, unless otherwise noted:
E08.00-E08.59, E08.618-E08.638, E08.641-E09.59, E09.618-E09.638, E09.641-E10.59, E10.618-E10.638, E10.641-E10.649, E10.69-E11.59, E11.618-E11.638, E11.641-E11.649, E11.69-E13.59, E13.618-E13.638, E13.641-E16.2, E30.9, E34.1, E34.8-E35, E89.1

✓5ᵗʰ **E09.0**   **Drug or chemical induced diabetes mellitus with hyperosmolarity**

E09.00   **Drug or chemical induced diabetes mellitus with hyperosmolarity without nonketotic hyperglycemic-hyperosmolar coma (NKHHC)** **MCC**

E09.01   **Drug or chemical induced diabetes mellitus with hyperosmolarity with coma** **MCC**

✓5ᵗʰ **E09.1**   **Drug or chemical induced diabetes mellitus with ketoacidosis**

E09.10   **Drug or chemical induced diabetes mellitus with ketoacidosis without coma** **MCC**

E09.11   **Drug or chemical induced diabetes mellitus with ketoacidosis with coma** **MCC**

✓5ᵗʰ **E09.2**   **Drug or chemical induced diabetes mellitus with kidney complications**

E09.21   **Drug or chemical induced diabetes mellitus with diabetic nephropathy**
Drug or chemical induced diabetes mellitus with intercapillary glomerulosclerosis
Drug or chemical induced diabetes mellitus with intracapillary glomerulonephrosis
Drug or chemical induced diabetes mellitus with Kimmelstiel-Wilson disease

E09.22   **Drug or chemical induced diabetes mellitus with diabetic chronic kidney disease**
Use additional code to identify stage of chronic kidney disease (N18.1-N18.6)

E09.29   **Drug or chemical induced diabetes mellitus with other diabetic kidney complication**
Drug or chemical induced diabetes mellitus with renal tubular degeneration

✓5ᵗʰ **E09.3**   **Drug or chemical induced diabetes mellitus with ophthalmic complications**

✓6ᵗʰ **E09.31**   **Drug or chemical induced diabetes mellitus with unspecified diabetic retinopathy**

E09.311   **Drug or chemical induced diabetes mellitus with unspecified diabetic retinopathy with macular edema**

E09.319   **Drug or chemical induced diabetes mellitus with unspecified diabetic retinopathy without macular edema**

✓6ᵗʰ **E09.32**   **Drug or chemical induced diabetes mellitus with mild nonproliferative diabetic retinopathy**
Drug or chemical induced diabetes mellitus with nonproliferative diabetic retinopathy NOS

E09.321   **Drug or chemical induced diabetes mellitus with mild nonproliferative diabetic retinopathy with macular edema**

E09.329   **Drug or chemical induced diabetes mellitus with mild nonproliferative diabetic retinopathy without macular edema**

✓6th **E09.33** **Drug or chemical induced diabetes mellitus with moderate nonproliferative diabetic retinopathy**

   E09.331 **Drug or chemical induced diabetes mellitus with moderate nonproliferative diabetic retinopathy with macular edema**

   E09.339 **Drug or chemical induced diabetes mellitus with moderate nonproliferative diabetic retinopathy without macular edema**

✓6th **E09.34** **Drug or chemical induced diabetes mellitus with severe nonproliferative diabetic retinopathy**

   E09.341 **Drug or chemical induced diabetes mellitus with severe nonproliferative diabetic retinopathy with macular edema**

   E09.349 **Drug or chemical induced diabetes mellitus with severe nonproliferative diabetic retinopathy without macular edema**

✓6th **E09.35** **Drug or chemical induced diabetes mellitus with proliferative diabetic retinopathy**

   E09.351 **Drug or chemical induced diabetes mellitus with proliferative diabetic retinopathy with macular edema**

   E09.359 **Drug or chemical induced diabetes mellitus with proliferative diabetic retinopathy without macular edema**

   E09.36 **Drug or chemical induced diabetes mellitus with diabetic cataract**

   E09.39 **Drug or chemical induced diabetes mellitus with other diabetic ophthalmic complication**
Use additional code to identify manifestation, such as: diabetic glaucoma (H40-H42)

✓5th **E09.4** **Drug or chemical induced diabetes mellitus with neurological complications**

   E09.40 **Drug or chemical induced diabetes mellitus with neurological complications with diabetic neuropathy, unspecified**

   E09.41 **Drug or chemical induced diabetes mellitus with neurological complications with diabetic mononeuropathy**

   E09.42 **Drug or chemical induced diabetes mellitus with neurological complications with diabetic polyneuropathy**
Drug or chemical induced diabetes mellitus with diabetic neuralgia

   E09.43 **Drug or chemical induced diabetes mellitus with neurological complications with diabetic autonomic (poly)neuropathy**
Drug or chemical induced diabetes mellitus with diabetic gastroparesis
AHA: 2013, 4Q, 114

   E09.44 **Drug or chemical induced diabetes mellitus with neurological complications with diabetic amyotrophy**

   E09.49 **Drug or chemical induced diabetes mellitus with neurological complications with other diabetic neurological complication**

✓5th **E09.5** **Drug or chemical induced diabetes mellitus with circulatory complications**

   E09.51 **Drug or chemical induced diabetes mellitus with diabetic peripheral angiopathy without gangrene**

   E09.52 **Drug or chemical induced diabetes mellitus with diabetic peripheral angiopathy with gangrene** PDxCC CC
Drug or chemical induced diabetes mellitus with diabetic gangrene
CC Excl: G89.0-G89.4, I70.261-I70.269, I96, R41.0-R41.3, R41.82, R41.9, R44.8-R44.9, R45.83-R45.84, R46.0-R46.89, R52, R68.0-R68.19, R68.81-R68.83, R68.89-R69

   E09.59 **Drug or chemical induced diabetes mellitus with other circulatory complications**

✓5th **E09.6** **Drug or chemical induced diabetes mellitus with other specified complications**

✓6th **E09.61** **Drug or chemical induced diabetes mellitus with diabetic arthropathy**

   E09.610 **Drug or chemical induced diabetes mellitus with diabetic neuropathic arthropathy**
Drug or chemical induced diabetes mellitus with Charcôt's joints

   E09.618 **Drug or chemical induced diabetes mellitus with other diabetic arthropathy**

✓6th **E09.62** **Drug or chemical induced diabetes mellitus with skin complications**

   E09.620 **Drug or chemical induced diabetes mellitus with diabetic dermatitis**
Drug or chemical induced diabetes mellitus with diabetic necrobiosis lipoidica

   E09.621 **Drug or chemical induced diabetes mellitus with foot ulcer**
Use additional code to identify site of ulcer (L97.4-, L97.5-)

   E09.622 **Drug or chemical induced diabetes mellitus with other skin ulcer**
Use additional code to identify site of ulcer (L97.1-L97.9, L98.41-L98.49)

   E09.628 **Drug or chemical induced diabetes mellitus with other skin complications**

✓6th **E09.63** **Drug or chemical induced diabetes mellitus with oral complications**

   E09.630 **Drug or chemical induced diabetes mellitus with periodontal disease**

   E09.638 **Drug or chemical induced diabetes mellitus with other oral complications**

✓6th **E09.64** **Drug or chemical induced diabetes mellitus with hypoglycemia**

   E09.641 **Drug or chemical induced diabetes mellitus with hypoglycemia with coma** MCC

   E09.649 **Drug or chemical induced diabetes mellitus with hypoglycemia without coma**

   E09.65 **Drug or chemical induced diabetes mellitus with hyperglycemia**

   E09.69 **Drug or chemical induced diabetes mellitus with other specified complication**
Use additional code to identify complication

   E09.8 **Drug or chemical induced diabetes mellitus with unspecified complications**

   E09.9 **Drug or chemical induced diabetes mellitus without complications**

✓4th **E10** **Type 1 diabetes mellitus**
INCLUDES   brittle diabetes (mellitus)
diabetes (mellitus) due to autoimmune process
diabetes (mellitus) due to immune mediated pancreatic islet beta-cell destruction
idiopathic diabetes (mellitus)
juvenile onset diabetes (mellitus)
ketosis-prone diabetes (mellitus)
EXCLUDES 1   *diabetes mellitus due to underlying condition (E08.-)*
drug or chemical induced diabetes mellitus (E09.-)
gestational diabetes (O24.4-)
hyperglycemia NOS (R73.9)
neonatal diabetes mellitus (P70.2)
postpancreatectomy diabetes mellitus (E13.-)
postprocedural diabetes mellitus (E13.-)
secondary diabetes mellitus NEC (E13.-)
type 2 diabetes mellitus (E11.-)
AHA: 2013, 4Q, 114; 2013, 3Q, 20

CC Excl: For MCC codes in category E10, unless otherwise noted:
E08.00-E08.59, E08.618-E08.638, E08.641-E09.59, E09.618-E09.638, E09.641-E10.59, E10.618-E10.638, E10.641-E10.649, E10.69-E11.59, E11.618-E11.638, E11.641-E11.649, E11.69-E13.59, E13.618-E13.638, E13.641-E16.2, E30.9, E34.1, E34.50-E35, E89.1

✓5th **E10.1** **Type 1 diabetes mellitus with ketoacidosis**
AHA: 2013, 3Q, 20

   E10.10 **Type 1 diabetes mellitus with ketoacidosis without coma** MCC

   E10.11 **Type 1 diabetes mellitus with ketoacidosis with coma** MCC

✓5th **E10.2** **Type 1 diabetes mellitus with kidney complications**

   E10.21 **Type 1 diabetes mellitus with diabetic nephropathy**
Type 1 diabetes mellitus with intercapillary glomerulosclerosis
Type 1 diabetes mellitus with intracapillary glomerulonephrosis
Type 1 diabetes mellitus with Kimmelstiel-Wilson disease

   E10.22 **Type 1 diabetes mellitus with diabetic chronic kidney disease**
Use additional code to identify stage of chronic kidney disease (N18.1-N18.6)

✔ Additional Character Required   ✔x7th Placeholder Alert   Unacceptable PDx   Manifestation   Hospital Acquired Condition   EXCLUDES1 Not Coded Here   EXCLUDES2 Not Included Here

ICD-10-CM 2016   505

E10.29 Type 1 diabetes mellitus with **other diabetic kidney complication**
  Type 1 diabetes mellitus with renal tubular degeneration

✓5th **E10.3** Type 1 diabetes mellitus with **ophthalmic complications**

✓6th **E10.31** Type 1 diabetes mellitus with **unspecified diabetic retinopathy**

E10.311 Type 1 diabetes mellitus with **unspecified diabetic retinopathy with macular edema**

E10.319 Type 1 diabetes mellitus with **unspecified diabetic retinopathy** without macular edema

✓6th **E10.32** Type 1 diabetes mellitus with **mild nonproliferative diabetic retinopathy**
  Type 1 diabetes mellitus with nonproliferative diabetic retinopathy NOS

E10.321 Type 1 diabetes mellitus with **mild nonproliferative diabetic retinopathy with macular edema**

E10.329 Type 1 diabetes mellitus with **mild nonproliferative diabetic retinopathy without macular edema**

✓6th **E10.33** Type 1 diabetes mellitus with **moderate nonproliferative diabetic retinopathy**

E10.331 Type 1 diabetes mellitus with **moderate nonproliferative diabetic retinopathy with macular edema**

E10.339 Type 1 diabetes mellitus with **moderate nonproliferative diabetic retinopathy without macular edema**

✓6th **E10.34** Type 1 diabetes mellitus with **severe nonproliferative diabetic retinopathy**

E10.341 Type 1 diabetes mellitus with **severe nonproliferative diabetic retinopathy with macular edema**

E10.349 Type 1 diabetes mellitus with **severe nonproliferative diabetic retinopathy without macular edema**

✓6th **E10.35** Type 1 diabetes mellitus with **proliferative diabetic retinopathy**

E10.351 Type 1 diabetes mellitus with **proliferative diabetic retinopathy with macular edema**

E10.359 Type 1 diabetes mellitus with **proliferative diabetic retinopathy without macular edema**

E10.36 Type 1 diabetes mellitus with diabetic **cataract**

E10.39 Type 1 diabetes mellitus with **other diabetic ophthalmic complication**
  Use additional code to identify manifestation, such as: diabetic glaucoma (H40-H42)

✓5th **E10.4** Type 1 diabetes mellitus with **neurological complications**

E10.40 Type 1 diabetes mellitus with diabetic **neuropathy, unspecified**

E10.41 Type 1 diabetes mellitus with diabetic **mononeuropathy**

E10.42 Type 1 diabetes mellitus with diabetic **polyneuropathy**
  Type 1 diabetes mellitus with diabetic neuralgia

E10.43 Type 1 diabetes mellitus with diabetic **autonomic (poly)neuropathy**
  Type 1 diabetes mellitus with diabetic gastroparesis
  AHA: 2013, 4Q, 114

E10.44 Type 1 diabetes mellitus with diabetic **amyotrophy**

E10.49 Type 1 diabetes mellitus with **other diabetic neurological complication**

✓5th **E10.5** Type 1 diabetes mellitus with **circulatory complications**

E10.51 Type 1 diabetes mellitus with diabetic **peripheral angiopathy without gangrene**

E10.52 Type 1 diabetes mellitus with diabetic **peripheral angiopathy with gangrene** `PDxCC` `CC`
  Type 1 diabetes mellitus with diabetic gangrene
  CC Excl: G89.0-G89.4, I70.261-I70.269, I96, R41.0-R41.3, R41.82, R41.9, R44.8-R44.9, R45.83-R45.84, R46.0-R46.89, R52, R68.0-R68.19, R68.81-R68.83, R68.89-R69

E10.59 Type 1 diabetes mellitus with **other circulatory complications**

✓5th **E10.6** Type 1 diabetes mellitus with **other specified complications**

✓6th **E10.61** Type 1 diabetes mellitus with **diabetic arthropathy**

E10.610 Type 1 diabetes mellitus with **diabetic neuropathic arthropathy**
  Type 1 diabetes mellitus with Charcôt's joints

E10.618 Type 1 diabetes mellitus with **other diabetic arthropathy**

✓6th **E10.62** Type 1 diabetes mellitus with **skin complications**

E10.620 Type 1 diabetes mellitus with **diabetic dermatitis**
  Type 1 diabetes mellitus with diabetic necrobiosis lipoidica

E10.621 Type 1 diabetes mellitus with **foot ulcer**
  Use additional code to identify site of ulcer (L97.4-, L97.5-)

E10.622 Type 1 diabetes mellitus with **other skin ulcer**
  Use additional code to identify site of ulcer (L97.1-L97.9, L98.41-L98.49)

E10.628 Type 1 diabetes mellitus with **other skin complications**

✓6th **E10.63** Type 1 diabetes mellitus with **oral complications**

E10.630 Type 1 diabetes mellitus with **periodontal disease**

E10.638 Type 1 diabetes mellitus with **other oral complications**

✓6th **E10.64** Type 1 diabetes mellitus with **hypoglycemia**

E10.641 Type 1 diabetes mellitus with **hypoglycemia with coma** `MCC`

E10.649 Type 1 diabetes mellitus with **hypoglycemia without coma**

E10.65 Type 1 diabetes mellitus with **hyperglycemia**
  AHA: 2013, 3Q, 20

E10.69 Type 1 diabetes mellitus with **other specified complication**
  Use additional code to identify complication

E10.8 Type 1 diabetes mellitus with **unspecified complications**

E10.9 Type 1 diabetes mellitus **without complications**

✓4th **E11** **Type 2 diabetes mellitus**
  `INCLUDES` diabetes (mellitus) due to insulin secretory defect
  diabetes NOS
  insulin resistant diabetes (mellitus)
  Use additional code to identify any insulin use (Z79.4)
  `EXCLUDES 1` diabetes mellitus due to underlying condition (E08.-)
  drug or chemical induced diabetes mellitus (E09.-)
  gestational diabetes (O24.4-)
  neonatal diabetes mellitus (P70.2)
  postpancreatectomy diabetes mellitus (E13.-)
  postprocedural diabetes mellitus (E13.-)
  secondary diabetes mellitus NEC (E13.-)
  type 1 diabetes mellitus (E10.-)
  AHA: 2013, 4Q, 114; 2013, 3Q, 20; 2013, 1Q, 26

  CC Excl: For MCC codes in category E11, unless otherwise noted:
  E08.00-E08.59, E08.618-E08.638, E08.641-E09.59, E09.618-E09.638, E09.641-E10.59, E10.618-E10.638, E10.641-E10.649, E10.69-E11.59, E11.618-E11.638, E11.641-E11.649, E11.69-E13.59, E13.618-E13.638, E13.641-E16.2, E30.9, E34.1, E34.8-E35, E89.1

✓5th **E11.0** Type 2 diabetes mellitus with **hyperosmolarity**

E11.00 **Type 2 diabetes mellitus with hyperosmolarity without nonketotic hyperglycemic-hyperosmolar coma (NKHHC)** `MCC`

E11.01 **Type 2 diabetes mellitus with hyperosmolarity with coma** `MCC`

✓5th **E11.2** Type 2 diabetes mellitus with **kidney complications**

E11.21 Type 2 diabetes mellitus with diabetic **nephropathy**
  Type 2 diabetes mellitus with intercapillary glomerulosclerosis
  Type 2 diabetes mellitus with intracapillary glomerulonephrosis
  Type 2 diabetes mellitus with Kimmelstiel-Wilson disease

E11.22 Type 2 diabetes mellitus with diabetic **chronic kidney disease**
  Use additional code to identify stage of chronic kidney disease (N18.1-N18.6)

N Newborn: 0   P Pediatric: 0-17   M Maternity: 12-55   A Adult: 15-124   MCC Major CC Condition   PDxMCC PDx acts as own MCC   CC CC Condition   PDxCC PDx acts as own CC

506

ICD-10-CM 2016

E11.29 Type 2 diabetes mellitus with **other** diabetic kidney complication
> Type 2 diabetes mellitus with renal tubular degeneration

✓5th **E11.3** Type 2 diabetes mellitus with **ophthalmic complications**

  ✓6th **E11.31** Type 2 diabetes mellitus with **unspecified diabetic retinopathy**

    E11.311 Type 2 diabetes mellitus with unspecified diabetic retinopathy **with macular edema**

    E11.319 Type 2 diabetes mellitus with unspecified diabetic retinopathy **without macular edema**

  ✓6th **E11.32** Type 2 diabetes mellitus with **mild nonproliferative diabetic retinopathy**
> Type 2 diabetes mellitus with nonproliferative diabetic retinopathy NOS

    E11.321 Type 2 diabetes mellitus with mild nonproliferative diabetic retinopathy **with macular edema**

    E11.329 Type 2 diabetes mellitus with mild nonproliferative diabetic retinopathy **without macular edema**

  ✓6th **E11.33** Type 2 diabetes mellitus with **moderate nonproliferative diabetic retinopathy**

    E11.331 Type 2 diabetes mellitus with moderate nonproliferative diabetic retinopathy **with macular edema**

    E11.339 Type 2 diabetes mellitus with moderate nonproliferative diabetic retinopathy **without macular edema**

  ✓6th **E11.34** Type 2 diabetes mellitus with **severe nonproliferative diabetic retinopathy**

    E11.341 Type 2 diabetes mellitus with severe nonproliferative diabetic retinopathy **with macular edema**

    E11.349 Type 2 diabetes mellitus with severe nonproliferative diabetic retinopathy **without macular edema**

  ✓6th **E11.35** Type 2 diabetes mellitus with **proliferative diabetic retinopathy**

    E11.351 Type 2 diabetes mellitus with proliferative diabetic retinopathy **with macular edema**

    E11.359 Type 2 diabetes mellitus with proliferative diabetic retinopathy **without macular edema**

  E11.36 Type 2 diabetes mellitus with diabetic **cataract**

  E11.39 Type 2 diabetes mellitus with **other** diabetic ophthalmic complication
> Use additional code to identify manifestation, such as: diabetic glaucoma (H40-H42)

✓5th **E11.4** Type 2 diabetes mellitus with **neurological complications**

  E11.40 Type 2 diabetes mellitus with diabetic **neuropathy, unspecified**
> **AHA:** 2013, 4Q, 129

  E11.41 Type 2 diabetes mellitus with diabetic **mononeuropathy**

  E11.42 Type 2 diabetes mellitus with diabetic **polyneuropathy**
> Type 2 diabetes mellitus with diabetic neuralgia

  E11.43 Type 2 diabetes mellitus with diabetic **autonomic (poly)neuropathy**
> Type 2 diabetes mellitus with diabetic gastroparesis
> **AHA:** 2013, 4Q, 114

  E11.44 Type 2 diabetes mellitus with diabetic **amyotrophy**

  E11.49 Type 2 diabetes mellitus with **other** diabetic neurological complication

✓5th **E11.5** Type 2 diabetes mellitus with **circulatory complications**

  E11.51 Type 2 diabetes mellitus with diabetic **peripheral angiopathy without gangrene**

  E11.52 Type 2 diabetes mellitus with diabetic **peripheral angiopathy with gangrene**   `PDx CC` `CC`
> Type 2 diabetes mellitus with diabetic gangrene
> **CC Excl:** G89.0-G89.4, I70.261-I70.269, I96, R41.0-R41.3, R41.82, R41.9, R44.8-R44.9, R45.83-R45.84, R46.0-R46.89, R52, R68.0-R68.19, R68.81-R68.83, R68.89-R69

  E11.59 Type 2 diabetes mellitus with **other** circulatory complications

✓5th **E11.6** Type 2 diabetes mellitus with **other specified complications**

  ✓6th **E11.61** Type 2 diabetes mellitus with **diabetic arthropathy**

    E11.610 Type 2 diabetes mellitus with **diabetic neuropathic arthropathy**
> Type 2 diabetes mellitus with Charcôt's joints

    E11.618 Type 2 diabetes mellitus with **other diabetic arthropathy**

  ✓6th **E11.62** Type 2 diabetes mellitus with **skin complications**

    E11.620 Type 2 diabetes mellitus with **diabetic dermatitis**
> Type 2 diabetes mellitus with diabetic necrobiosis lipoidica

    E11.621 Type 2 diabetes mellitus with **foot ulcer**
> Use additional code to identify site of ulcer (L97.4-, L97.5-)

    E11.622 Type 2 diabetes mellitus with **other skin ulcer**
> Use additional code to identify site of ulcer (L97.1-L97.9, L98.41-L98.49)

    E11.628 Type 2 diabetes mellitus with **other skin complications**

  ✓6th **E11.63** Type 2 diabetes mellitus with **oral complications**

    E11.630 Type 2 diabetes mellitus with **periodontal disease**

    E11.638 Type 2 diabetes mellitus with **other oral complications**

  ✓6th **E11.64** Type 2 diabetes mellitus with **hypoglycemia**

    E11.641 Type 2 diabetes mellitus with **hypoglycemia with coma**   `MCC`

    E11.649 Type 2 diabetes mellitus with **hypoglycemia without coma**

  E11.65 Type 2 diabetes mellitus with **hyperglycemia**
> **AHA:** 2013, 3Q, 20

  E11.69 Type 2 diabetes mellitus with **other specified complication**
> Use additional code to identify complication

E11.8 Type 2 diabetes mellitus with **unspecified complications**

13 **E11.9** Type 2 diabetes mellitus **without complications**

✓4th **E13** Other specified **diabetes mellitus**
> Diabetes mellitus due to genetic defects of beta-cell function
> Diabetes mellitus due to genetic defects in insulin action
> Postpancreatectomy diabetes mellitus
> Postprocedural diabetes mellitus
> Secondary diabetes mellitus NEC
> Use additional code to identify any insulin use (Z79.4)
>
> **EXCLUDES 1**   diabetes (mellitus) due to autoimmune process (E10.-)
> diabetes (mellitus) due to immune mediated pancreatic islet beta-cell destruction (E10.-)
> diabetes mellitus due to underlying condition (E08.-)
> drug or chemical induced diabetes mellitus (E09.-)
> gestational diabetes (O24.4-)
> neonatal diabetes mellitus (P70.2)
> type 2 diabetes mellitus (E11.-)
>
> **AHA:** 2013, 4Q, 114; 2013, 3Q, 20

> **CC Excl: For MCC codes in category E13, unless otherwise noted:**
> E08.00-E08.59, E08.618-E08.638, E08.641-E09.59, E09.618-E09.638,
> E09.641-E10.59, E10.618-E10.638, E10.641-E10.649, E10.69-E11.59,
> E11.618-E11.638, E11.641-E11.649, E11.69-E13.59, E13.618-E13.638,
> E13.641-E16.2, E30.9, E34.1, E34.8-E35, E89.1

  ✓6th **E13.0** Other specified diabetes mellitus with **hyperosmolarity**

    E13.00 Other specified diabetes mellitus with **hyperosmolarity without nonketotic hyperglycemic-hyperosmolar coma (NKHHC)**   `MCC`

    E13.01 Other specified diabetes mellitus with **hyperosmolarity with coma**   `MCC`

  ✓5th **E13.1** Other specified diabetes mellitus with **ketoacidosis**
> **AHA:** 2013, 1Q, 26

    E13.10 Other specified diabetes mellitus with **ketoacidosis without coma**   `MCC`

    E13.11 Other specified diabetes mellitus with **ketoacidosis with coma**   `MCC`

---

13 Questionable admission when used as PDx.

✓ Additional Character Required   ✓x7th Placeholder Alert   Unacceptable PDx   Manifestation   Hospital Acquired Condition   **EXCLUDES 1** Not Coded Here   **EXCLUDES 2** Not Included Here

Chapter 4. Endocrine, Nutritional, and Metabolic Diseases

✓5th **E13.2** **Other specified diabetes mellitus with kidney complications**

     E13.21 **Other specified diabetes mellitus with diabetic nephropathy**
         Other specified diabetes mellitus with intercapillary glomerulosclerosis
         Other specified diabetes mellitus with intracapillary glomerulonephrosis
         Other specified diabetes mellitus with Kimmelstiel-Wilson disease

     E13.22 **Other specified diabetes mellitus with diabetic chronic kidney disease**
         Use additional code to identify stage of chronic kidney disease (N18.1-N18.6)

     E13.29 **Other specified diabetes mellitus with other diabetic kidney complication**
         Other specified diabetes mellitus with renal tubular degeneration

✓5th **E13.3** **Other specified diabetes mellitus with ophthalmic complications**

     ✓6th **E13.31** **Other specified diabetes mellitus with unspecified diabetic retinopathy**

         E13.311 **Other specified diabetes mellitus with unspecified diabetic retinopathy with macular edema**

         E13.319 **Other specified diabetes mellitus with unspecified diabetic retinopathy without macular edema**

     ✓6th **E13.32** **Other specified diabetes mellitus with mild nonproliferative diabetic retinopathy**
         Other specified diabetes mellitus with nonproliferative diabetic retinopathy NOS

         E13.321 **Other specified diabetes mellitus with mild nonproliferative diabetic retinopathy with macular edema**

         E13.329 **Other specified diabetes mellitus with mild nonproliferative diabetic retinopathy without macular edema**

     ✓6th **E13.33** **Other specified diabetes mellitus with moderate nonproliferative diabetic retinopathy**

         E13.331 **Other specified diabetes mellitus with moderate nonproliferative diabetic retinopathy with macular edema**

         E13.339 **Other specified diabetes mellitus with moderate nonproliferative diabetic retinopathy without macular edema**

     ✓6th **E13.34** **Other specified diabetes mellitus with severe nonproliferative diabetic retinopathy**

         E13.341 **Other specified diabetes mellitus with severe nonproliferative diabetic retinopathy with macular edema**

         E13.349 **Other specified diabetes mellitus with severe nonproliferative diabetic retinopathy without macular edema**

     ✓6th **E13.35** **Other specified diabetes mellitus with proliferative diabetic retinopathy**

         E13.351 **Other specified diabetes mellitus with proliferative diabetic retinopathy with macular edema**

         E13.359 **Other specified diabetes mellitus with proliferative diabetic retinopathy without macular edema**

     E13.36 **Other specified diabetes mellitus with diabetic cataract**

     E13.39 **Other specified diabetes mellitus with other diabetic ophthalmic complication**
         Use additional code to identify manifestation, such as: diabetic glaucoma (H40-H42)

✓5th **E13.4** **Other specified diabetes mellitus with neurological complications**

     E13.40 **Other specified diabetes mellitus with diabetic neuropathy, unspecified**

     E13.41 **Other specified diabetes mellitus with diabetic mononeuropathy**

     E13.42 **Other specified diabetes mellitus with diabetic polyneuropathy**
         Other specified diabetes mellitus with diabetic neuralgia

     E13.43 **Other specified diabetes mellitus with diabetic autonomic (poly)neuropathy**
         Other specified diabetes mellitus with diabetic gastroparesis
         AHA: 2013, 4Q, 114

     E13.44 **Other specified diabetes mellitus with diabetic amyotrophy**

     E13.49 **Other specified diabetes mellitus with other diabetic neurological complication**

✓5th **E13.5** **Other specified diabetes mellitus with circulatory complications**

     E13.51 **Other specified diabetes mellitus with diabetic peripheral angiopathy without gangrene**

     E13.52 **Other specified diabetes mellitus with diabetic peripheral angiopathy with gangrene**   PDxCC CC
         Other specified diabetes mellitus with diabetic gangrene
         CC Excl: G89.0-G89.4, I70.261-I70.269, I96, R41.0-R41.3, R41.82, R41.9, R44.8-R44.9, R45.83-R45.84, R46.0-R46.89, R52, R68.0-R68.19, R68.81-R68.83, R68.89-R69

     E13.59 **Other specified diabetes mellitus with other circulatory complications**

✓5th **E13.6** **Other specified diabetes mellitus with other specified complications**

     ✓6th **E13.61** **Other specified diabetes mellitus with diabetic arthropathy**

         E13.610 **Other specified diabetes mellitus with diabetic neuropathic arthropathy**
         Other specified diabetes mellitus with Charcôt's joints

         E13.618 **Other specified diabetes mellitus with other diabetic arthropathy**

     ✓6th **E13.62** **Other specified diabetes mellitus with skin complications**

         E13.620 **Other specified diabetes mellitus with diabetic dermatitis**
         Other specified diabetes mellitus with diabetic necrobiosis lipoidica

         E13.621 **Other specified diabetes mellitus with foot ulcer**
         Use additional code to identify site of ulcer (L97.4-, L97.5-)

         E13.622 **Other specified diabetes mellitus with other skin ulcer**
         Use additional code to identify site of ulcer (L97.1-L97.9, L98.41-L98.49)

         E13.628 **Other specified diabetes mellitus with other skin complications**

     ✓6th **E13.63** **Other specified diabetes mellitus with oral complications**

         E13.630 **Other specified diabetes mellitus with periodontal disease**

         E13.638 **Other specified diabetes mellitus with other oral complications**

     ✓6th **E13.64** **Other specified diabetes mellitus with hypoglycemia**

         E13.641 **Other specified diabetes mellitus with hypoglycemia with coma**   MCC

         E13.649 **Other specified diabetes mellitus with hypoglycemia without coma**

     E13.65 **Other specified diabetes mellitus with hyperglycemia**

     E13.69 **Other specified diabetes mellitus with other specified complication**
         Use additional code to identify complication

E13.8 **Other specified diabetes mellitus with unspecified complications**

[13] **E13.9** **Other specified diabetes mellitus without complications**

___

[13] Questionable admission when used as PDx.

N Newborn: 0   P Pediatric: 0-17   M Maternity: 12-55   A Adult: 15-124   MCC Major CC Condition   PDxMCC PDx acts as own MCC   CC CC Condition   PDxCC PDx acts as own CC

508   ICD-10-CM 2016

Other disorders of glucose regulation and pancreatic internal secretion (E15-E16)

E15   Nondiabetic hypoglycemic coma   `CC`
INCLUDES   drug-induced insulin coma in nondiabetic
hyperinsulinism with hypoglycemic coma
hypoglycemic coma NOS

CC Excl: E08.00-E08.59, E08.618-E08.638, E08.641-E09.59, E09.618-
E09.638, E09.641-E10.59, E10.618-E10.638, E10.641-E10.649, E10.69-
E11.59, E11.618-E11.638, E11.641-E11.649, E11.69-E13.59, E13.618-
E13.638, E13.641-E16.2, E30.9, E34.1, E34.50-E35, E89.1

✓4th E16   Other disorders of pancreatic internal secretion

E16.0   Drug-induced hypoglycemia without coma
Use additional code for adverse effect, if applicable, to identify
drug (T36-T50 with fifth or sixth character 5)

E16.1   Other hypoglycemia
Functional hyperinsulinism
Functional nonhyperinsulinemic hypoglycemia
Hyperinsulinism NOS
Hyperplasia of pancreatic islet beta cells NOS
EXCLUDES 1   hypoglycemia in infant of diabetic mother (P70.1)
neonatal hypoglycemia (P70.4)

E16.2   Hypoglycemia, unspecified

E16.3   Increased secretion of glucagon
Hyperplasia of pancreatic endocrine cells with glucagon excess

E16.4   Increased secretion of gastrin
Hypergastrinemia
Hyperplasia of pancreatic endocrine cells with gastrin excess
Zollinger-Ellison syndrome

E16.8   Other specified disorders of pancreatic internal secretion
Increased secretion from endocrine pancreas of growth
hormone-releasing hormone
Increased secretion from endocrine pancreas of pancreatic
polypeptide
Increased secretion from endocrine pancreas of somatostatin
Increased secretion from endocrine pancreas of vasoactive-
intestinal polypeptide

E16.9   Disorder of pancreatic internal secretion, unspecified
Islet-cell hyperplasia NOS
Pancreatic endocrine cell hyperplasia NOS

Disorders of other endocrine glands (E20-E35)

EXCLUDES 1   galactorrhea (N64.3)
gynecomastia (N62)

✓4th E20   Hypoparathyroidism
EXCLUDES 1   Di George's syndrome (D82.1)
postprocedural hypoparathyroidism (E89.2)
tetany NOS (R29.0)
transitory neonatal hypoparathyroidism (P71.4)

E20.0   Idiopathic hypoparathyroidism

E20.1   Pseudohypoparathyroidism

E20.8   Other hypoparathyroidism

E20.9   Hypoparathyroidism, unspecified
Parathyroid tetany

✓4th E21   Hyperparathyroidism and other disorders of parathyroid gland
EXCLUDES 1   adult osteomalacia (M83.-)
ectopic hyperparathyroidism (E34.2)
familial hypocalciuric hypercalcemia (E83.52)
hungry bone syndrome (E83.81)
infantile and juvenile osteomalacia (E55.0)

E21.0   Primary hyperparathyroidism
Hyperplasia of parathyroid
Osteitis fibrosa cystica generalisata [von Recklinghausen's
disease of bone]

E21.1   Secondary hyperparathyroidism, not elsewhere classified
EXCLUDES 1   secondary hyperparathyroidism of renal origin (N25.81)

E21.2   Other hyperparathyroidism
Tertiary hyperparathyroidism
EXCLUDES 1   familial hypocalciuric hypercalcemia (E83.52)

E21.3   Hyperparathyroidism, unspecified

E21.4   Other specified disorders of parathyroid gland

E21.5   Disorder of parathyroid gland, unspecified

✓4th E22   Hyperfunction of pituitary gland
EXCLUDES 1   Cushing's syndrome (E24.-)
Nelson's syndrome (E24.1)
overproduction of ACTH not associated with Cushing's disease
(E27.0)
overproduction of pituitary ACTH (E24.0)
overproduction of thyroid-stimulating hormone (E05.8-)

E22.0   Acromegaly and pituitary gigantism
Overproduction of growth hormone
EXCLUDES 1   constitutional gigantism (E34.4)
constitutional tall stature (E34.4)
increased secretion from endocrine pancreas of growth
hormone-releasing hormone (E16.8)

E22.1   Hyperprolactinemia   `CC`
Use additional code for adverse effect, if applicable, to identify
drug (T36-T50 with fifth or sixth character 5)
CC Excl: E22.1-E22.9

E22.2   Syndrome of inappropriate secretion of antidiuretic hormone   `CC`
CC Excl: E22.0-E23.7, E24.1, E30.9, E34.1, E34.4, E34.8-E35, E89.3

E22.8   Other hyperfunction of pituitary gland   `CC`
Central precocious puberty
CC Excl: See code: E22.1

E22.9   Hyperfunction of pituitary gland, unspecified   `CC`
CC Excl: See code: E22.1

✓4th E23   Hypofunction and other disorders of the pituitary gland
INCLUDES   the listed conditions whether the disorder is in the pituitary
or the hypothalamus
EXCLUDES 1   postprocedural hypopituitarism (E89.3)

E23.0   Hypopituitarism   `CC`
Fertile eunuch syndrome
Hypogonadotropic hypogonadism
Idiopathic growth hormone deficiency
Isolated deficiency of gonadotropin
Isolated deficiency of growth hormone
Isolated deficiency of pituitary hormone
Kallmann's syndrome
Lorain-Levi short stature
Necrosis of pituitary gland (postpartum)
Panhypopituitarism
Pituitary cachexia
Pituitary insufficiency NOS
Pituitary short stature
Sheehan's syndrome
Simmonds' disease
CC Excl: E22.0-E23.7, E24.1, E30.9, E34.1, E34.4-E35, E89.3

E23.1   Drug-induced hypopituitarism
Use additional code for adverse effect, if applicable, to identify
drug (T36-T50 with fifth or sixth character 5)

E23.2   Diabetes insipidus   `CC`
EXCLUDES 1   nephrogenic diabetes insipidus (N25.1)
CC Excl: E22.1-E23.7, E24.1, E30.9, E34.1, E34.50-E35, E89.3

E23.3   Hypothalamic dysfunction, not elsewhere classified
EXCLUDES 1   Prader-Willi syndrome (Q87.1)
Russell-Silver syndrome (Q87.1)

E23.6   Other disorders of pituitary gland
Abscess of pituitary
Adiposogenital dystrophy

E23.7   Disorder of pituitary gland, unspecified

✓4th E24   Cushing's syndrome
EXCLUDES 1   congenital adrenal hyperplasia (E25.0)

CC Excl: For CC codes in category E24, unless otherwise noted:
E24.0, E24.2-E26.9, E30.9, E34.1, E34.50-E35

E24.0   Pituitary-dependent Cushing's disease   `CC`
Overproduction of pituitary ACTH
Pituitary-dependent hypercorticalism

E24.1   Nelson's syndrome

E24.2   Drug-induced Cushing's syndrome   `CC`
Use additional code for adverse effect, if applicable, to identify
drug (T36-T50 with fifth or sixth character 5)

E24.3   Ectopic ACTH syndrome   `CC`

E24.4   Alcohol-induced pseudo-Cushing's syndrome   `CC`

E24.8   Other Cushing's syndrome   `CC`

E24.9   Cushing's syndrome, unspecified   `CC`

✓ Additional Character Required   ✓x7th Placeholder Alert   Unacceptable PDx   Manifestation   Hospital Acquired Condition   EXCLUDES 1 Not Coded Here   EXCLUDES 2 Not Included Here

Chapter 4. Endocrine, Nutritional, and Metabolic Diseases

✓4th E25 Adrenogenital disorders

INCLUDES adrenogenital syndromes, virilizing or feminizing, whether acquired or due to adrenal hyperplasia consequent on inborn enzyme defects in hormone synthesis
female adrenal pseudohermaphroditism
female heterosexual precocious pseudopuberty
male isosexual precocious pseudopuberty
male macrogenitosomia praecox
male sexual precocity with adrenal hyperplasia
male virilization (female)

EXCLUDES 1 indeterminate sex and pseudohermaphroditism (Q56)
chromosomal abnormalities (Q90-Q99)

E25.0 Congenital adrenogenital disorders associated with enzyme deficiency
Congenital adrenal hyperplasia
21-Hydroxylase deficiency
Salt-losing congenital adrenal hyperplasia

E25.8 Other adrenogenital disorders
Idiopathic adrenogenital disorder
Use additional code for adverse effect, if applicable, to identify drug (T36-T50 with fifth or sixth character 5)

E25.9 Adrenogenital disorder, unspecified
Adrenogenital syndrome NOS

✓4th E26 Hyperaldosteronism

✓5th E26.0 Primary hyperaldosteronism

E26.01 Conn's syndrome
Code also adrenal adenoma (D35.0-)

E26.02 Glucocorticoid-remediable aldosteronism
Familial aldosteronism type I

E26.09 Other primary hyperaldosteronism
Primary aldosteronism due to adrenal hyperplasia (bilateral)

E26.1 Secondary hyperaldosteronism

✓5th E26.8 Other hyperaldosteronism

E26.81 Bartter's syndrome

E26.89 Other hyperaldosteronism

E26.9 Hyperaldosteronism, unspecified
Aldosteronism NOS
Hyperaldosteronism NOS

✓4th E27 Other disorders of adrenal gland

CC Excl: For CC codes in category E27, unless otherwise noted:
A17.9, A18.7, A18.82, A18.84, A18.89, E27.0-E27.9, E30.9, E34.1, E34.50-E35, E89.6

E27.0 Other adrenocortical overactivity   CC
Overproduction of ACTH, not associated with Cushing's disease
Premature adrenarche
EXCLUDES 1 Cushing's syndrome (E24.-)

E27.1 Primary adrenocortical insufficiency   CC
Addison's disease
Autoimmune adrenalitis
EXCLUDES 1 Addison only phenotype adrenoleukodystrophy (E71.528)
amyloidosis (E85.-)
tuberculous Addison's disease (A18.7)
Waterhouse-Friderichsen syndrome (A39.1)

E27.2 Addisonian crisis   CC
Adrenal crisis
Adrenocortical crisis

E27.3 Drug-induced adrenocortical insufficiency   CC
Use additional code for adverse effect, if applicable, to identify drug (T36-T50 with fifth or sixth character 5)

✓5th E27.4 Other and unspecified adrenocortical insufficiency
EXCLUDES 1 adrenoleukodystrophy [Addison-Schilder] (E71.528)
Waterhouse-Friderichsen syndrome (A39.1)

E27.40 Unspecified adrenocortical insufficiency   CC
Adrenocortical insufficiency NOS
Hypoaldosteronism

E27.49 Other adrenocortical insufficiency   CC
Adrenal hemorrhage
Adrenal infarction

E27.5 Adrenomedullary hyperfunction   CC
Adrenomedullary hyperplasia
Catecholamine hypersecretion

E27.8 Other specified disorders of adrenal gland
Abnormality of cortisol-binding globulin

E27.9 Disorder of adrenal gland, unspecified

✓4th E28 Ovarian dysfunction
EXCLUDES 1 isolated gonadotropin deficiency (E23.0)
postprocedural ovarian failure (E89.4-)

E28.0 Estrogen excess   ♀
Use additional code for adverse effect, if applicable, to identify drug (T36-T50 with fifth or sixth character 5)

E28.1 Androgen excess   ♀
Hypersecretion of ovarian androgens
Use additional code for adverse effect, if applicable, to identify drug (T36-T50 with fifth or sixth character 5)

E28.2 Polycystic ovarian syndrome   ♀
Sclerocystic ovary syndrome
Stein-Leventhal syndrome

✓5th E28.3 Primary ovarian failure
EXCLUDES 1 pure gonadal dysgenesis (Q99.1)
Turner's syndrome (Q96.-)

✓6th E28.31 Premature menopause

E28.310 Symptomatic premature menopause   A♀
Symptoms such as flushing, sleeplessness, headache, lack of concentration, associated with premature menopause

E28.319 Asymptomatic premature menopause   A♀
Premature menopause NOS

E28.39 Other primary ovarian failure   ♀
Decreased estrogen
Resistant ovary syndrome

E28.8 Other ovarian dysfunction   ♀
Ovarian hyperfunction NOS
EXCLUDES 1 postprocedural ovarian failure (E89.4-)

E28.9 Ovarian dysfunction, unspecified   ♀

✓4th E29 Testicular dysfunction
EXCLUDES 1 androgen insensitivity syndrome (E34.5-)
azoospermia or oligospermia NOS (N46.0-N46.1)
isolated gonadotropin deficiency (E23.0)
Klinefelter's syndrome (Q98.0-Q98.2, Q98.4)

E29.0 Testicular hyperfunction   ♂
Hypersecretion of testicular hormones

E29.1 Testicular hypofunction   ♂
Defective biosynthesis of testicular androgen NOS
5-delta-Reductase deficiency (with male pseudohermaphroditism)
Testicular hypogonadism NOS
Use additional code for adverse effect, if applicable, to identify drug (T36-T50 with fifth or sixth character 5)
EXCLUDES 1 postprocedural testicular hypofunction (E89.5)

E29.8 Other testicular dysfunction   ♂

E29.9 Testicular dysfunction, unspecified   ♂

✓4th E30 Disorders of puberty, not elsewhere classified

E30.0 Delayed puberty
Constitutional delay of puberty
Delayed sexual development

E30.1 Precocious puberty   P
Precocious menstruation
EXCLUDES 1 Albright (-McCune) (-Sternberg) syndrome (Q78.1)
central precocious puberty (E22.8)
congenital adrenal hyperplasia (E25.0)
female heterosexual precocious pseudopuberty (E25.-)
male isosexual precocious pseudopuberty (E25.-)

E30.8 Other disorders of puberty   P
Premature thelarche

E30.9 Disorder of puberty, unspecified

✓4th E31 Polyglandular dysfunction
EXCLUDES 1 ataxia telangiectasia [Louis-Bar] (G11.3)
dystrophia myotonica [Steinert] (G71.11)
pseudohypoparathyroidism (E20.1)

E31.0 Autoimmune polyglandular failure
Schmidt's syndrome

E31.1 Polyglandular hyperfunction
EXCLUDES 1 multiple endocrine adenomatosis (E31.2-)
multiple endocrine neoplasia (E31.2-)

N Newborn: 0   P Pediatric: 0-17   M Maternity: 12-55   A Adult: 15-124   MCC Major CC Condition   PDxMCC PDx acts as own MCC   CC CC Condition   PDxCC PDx acts as own CC

510   ICD-10-CM 2016

☑5ᵗʰ **E31.2 Multiple endocrine neoplasia [MEN] syndromes**
Multiple endocrine adenomatosis
Code also any associated malignancies and other conditions
associated with the syndromes

     E31.20 Multiple endocrine neoplasia [MEN] syndrome,
unspecified
Multiple endocrine adenomatosis NOS
Multiple endocrine neoplasia [MEN] syndrome NOS

     E31.21 Multiple endocrine neoplasia [MEN] type I
Wermer's syndrome

     E31.22 Multiple endocrine neoplasia [MEN] type IIA
Sipple's syndrome

     E31.23 Multiple endocrine neoplasia [MEN] type IIB

E31.8 Other polyglandular dysfunction

E31.9 Polyglandular dysfunction, unspecified

☑4ᵗʰ **E32 Diseases of thymus**
EXCLUDES 1   *aplasia or hypoplasia of thymus with immunodeficiency (D82.1)*
myasthenia gravis (G70.0)

E32.0 Persistent hyperplasia of thymus
Hypertrophy of thymus

E32.1 Abscess of thymus   CC
CC Excl: E30.9, E32.0-E32.9, E34.1, E34.50-E35

E32.8 Other diseases of thymus
EXCLUDES 1   *aplasia or hypoplasia with immunodeficiency (D82.1)*
thymoma (D15.0)

E32.9 Disease of thymus, unspecified

☑4ᵗʰ **E34 Other endocrine disorders**
EXCLUDES 1   *pseudohypoparathyroidism (E20.1)*

E34.0 Carcinoid syndrome   CC
    NOTE   May be used as an additional code to identify
functional activity associated with a carcinoid tumor.
CC Excl: E30.9, E34.0-E34.2, E34.50-E35

E34.1 Other hypersecretion of intestinal hormones

E34.2 Ectopic hormone secretion, not elsewhere classified
EXCLUDES 1   *ectopic ACTH syndrome (E24.3)*

E34.3 Short stature due to endocrine disorder
Constitutional short stature
Laron-type short stature
EXCLUDES 1   *achondroplastic short stature (Q77.4)*
hypochondroplastic short stature (Q77.4)
nutritional short stature (E45)
pituitary short stature (E23.0)
progeria (E34.8)
renal short stature (N25.0)
Russell-Silver syndrome (Q87.1)
short-limbed stature with immunodeficiency (D82.2)
short stature in specific dysmorphic syndromes— code
to syndrome—see Alphabetical Index
short stature NOS (R62.52)

E34.4 Constitutional tall stature
Constitutional gigantism

☑5ᵗʰ **E34.5 Androgen insensitivity syndrome**

     E34.50 Androgen insensitivity syndrome, unspecified
Androgen insensitivity NOS

     E34.51 Complete androgen insensitivity syndrome
Complete androgen insensitivity
de Quervain syndrome
Goldberg-Maxwell syndrome

     E34.52 Partial androgen insensitivity syndrome
Partial androgen insensitivity
Reifenstein syndrome

E34.8 Other specified endocrine disorders
Pineal gland dysfunction   Progeria
EXCLUDES 2   *pseudohypoparathyroidism (E20.1)*

E34.9 Endocrine disorder, unspecified
Endocrine disturbance NOS
Hormone disturbance NOS

E35 **Disorders of endocrine glands in diseases classified elsewhere**
Code first underlying disease, such as:
late congenital syphilis of thymus gland [Dubois disease] (A50.5)
Use additional code, if applicable, to identify:
sequelae of tuberculosis of other organs (B90.8)
EXCLUDES 1   *Echinococcus granulosus infection of thyroid gland (B67.3)*
meningococcal hemorrhagic adrenalitis (A39.1)
syphilis of endocrine gland (A52.79)
tuberculosis of adrenal gland, except calcification (A18.7)
tuberculosis of endocrine gland NEC (A18.82)
tuberculosis of thyroid gland (A18.81)
Waterhouse-Friderichsen syndrome (A39.1)

☑4ᵗʰ **E36 Intraoperative complications of endocrine system**
EXCLUDES 2   *postprocedural endocrine and metabolic complications and*
disorders, not elsewhere classified (E89.-)

☑5ᵗʰ **E36.0 Intraoperative hemorrhage and hematoma of an endocrine**
system organ or structure complicating a procedure
EXCLUDES 1   *intraoperative hemorrhage and hematoma of an*
endocrine system organ or structure due to
accidental puncture or laceration during a
procedure (E36.1-)

     E36.01 Intraoperative hemorrhage and hematoma of   CC
an endocrine system organ or structure
complicating an endocrine system procedure
CC Excl: E36.01-E36.02, E36.8, E89.810-E89.89, H95.811-
H95.89, I85.01, I85.11, I97.3, K21.9, K22.8, K23-K25.0,
K25.2, K25.4, K25.6, K26.0, K26.2, K26.4, K26.6, K27.0,
K27.2, K27.4, K27.6, K28.0, K28.2, K28.4, K28.6, K29.01,
K29.21, K29.31, K29.41, K29.51, K29.61, K29.71, K29.81,
K29.91, K31.811, K55.21, K57.01, K57.11, K57.13, K57.21,
K57.31, K57.33, K57.41, K57.51, K57.53, K57.81, K57.91,
K57.93, K62.5, K92.0-K92.2, M96.89, N98.1-N98.9, P54.1-
P54.3, T81.10XA, T81.11XA, T81.12XA, T81.19XA,
T81.82XA, T81.89XA, T81.9XXA

     E36.02 Intraoperative hemorrhage and hematoma of   CC
an endocrine system organ or structure
complicating other procedure
CC Excl: See code: E36.01

☑5ᵗʰ **E36.1 Accidental puncture and laceration of an endocrine system**
organ or structure during a procedure

     E36.11 Accidental puncture and laceration of an   CC
endocrine system organ or structure during an
endocrine system procedure
CC Excl: D78.11-D78.12, D78.81-D78.89, E36.11-E36.8,
E89.810-E89.89, G96.11, G97.41, G97.48-G97.49,
H59.011-H59.019, H59.031-H59.099, H59.211-H59.229,
H59.811-H59.89, H95.31-H95.32, H95.811-H95.89, I97.3,
I97.51-I97.52, J95.71-J95.72, K91.71-K91.72, L76.11-
L76.12, L76.81-L76.82, M96.820-M96.821, M96.89,
N98.1-N98.9, N99.71-N99.72, T81.82XA, T81.89XA,
T81.9XXA

     E36.12 Accidental puncture and laceration of an   CC
endocrine system organ or structure during
other procedure
CC Excl: See code: E36.11

E36.8 Other intraoperative complications of endocrine system
Use additional code, if applicable, to further specify disorder

Malnutrition (E40-E46)

EXCLUDES 1   *intestinal malabsorption (K90.-)*
sequelae of protein-calorie malnutrition (E64.0)
EXCLUDES 2   *nutritional anemias (D50-D53)*
starvation (T73.0)

E40 Kwashiorkor   MCC
Severe malnutrition with nutritional edema with dyspigmentation
of skin and hair
EXCLUDES 1   *marasmic kwashiorkor (E42)*
CC Excl: E40-E46, E64.0

E41 Nutritional marasmus   MCC
Severe malnutrition with marasmus
EXCLUDES 1   *marasmic kwashiorkor (E42)*
CC Excl: See code: E40

E42 Marasmic kwashiorkor   MCC
Intermediate form severe protein-calorie malnutrition
Severe protein-calorie malnutrition with signs of both kwashiorkor
and marasmus
CC Excl: See code: E40

E43 Unspecified severe protein-calorie malnutrition   MCC
Starvation edema
CC Excl: See code: E40

☑ Additional Character Required   ☑x7ᵗʰ Placeholder Alert   Unacceptable PDx   Manifestation   Hospital Acquired Condition   *EXCLUDES 1* Not Coded Here   *EXCLUDES 2* Not Included Here

ICD-10-CM 2016   511

Chapter 4. Endocrine, Nutritional, and Metabolic Diseases

E44–E63.9

✓4ᵗʰ **E44   Protein-calorie malnutrition of moderate and mild degree**

E44.0   **Moderate** protein-calorie malnutrition   CC

E44.1   **Mild** protein-calorie malnutrition   CC

E45   Retarded development following protein-calorie   CC
malnutrition
Nutritional short stature
Nutritional stunting
Physical retardation due to malnutrition
CC Excl: See code: E40

E46   Unspecified protein-calorie malnutrition   CC
Malnutrition NOS
Protein-calorie imbalance NOS
EXCLUDES 1   *nutritional deficiency NOS (E63.9)*
CC Excl: See code: E40

Other nutritional deficiencies (E50-E64)

EXCLUDES 2   *nutritional anemias (D50-D53)*

✓4ᵗʰ **E50   Vitamin A deficiency**
EXCLUDES 1   *sequelae of vitamin A deficiency (E64.1)*

E50.0   **Vitamin A deficiency with** conjunctival xerosis

E50.1   **Vitamin A deficiency with** Bitot's spot and conjunctival
xerosis
Bitot's spot in the young child

E50.2   **Vitamin A deficiency with** corneal xerosis

E50.3   **Vitamin A deficiency with** corneal ulceration and xerosis

E50.4   **Vitamin A deficiency with** keratomalacia

E50.5   **Vitamin A deficiency with** night blindness

E50.6   **Vitamin A deficiency with** xerophthalmic scars of cornea

E50.7   **Other ocular manifestations** of vitamin A deficiency
Xerophthalmia NOS

E50.8   **Other manifestations** of vitamin A deficiency
Follicular keratosis
Xeroderma

E50.9   **Vitamin A deficiency,** unspecified
Hypovitaminosis A NOS

✓4ᵗʰ **E51   Thiamine deficiency**
EXCLUDES 1   *sequelae of thiamine deficiency (E64.8)*

CC Excl: For CC codes in category E51, unless otherwise noted:
D81.818-D81.819, E51.11-E53.9, E56.0, E56.8-E63.9, E64.8-E64.9

✓5ᵗʰ   E51.1   Beriberi

E51.11   **Dry beriberi**   CC
Beriberi NOS
Beriberi with polyneuropathy

E51.12   **Wet beriberi**   CC
Beriberi with cardiovascular manifestations
Cardiovascular beriberi
Shoshin disease

E51.2   **Wernicke's encephalopathy**   CC

E51.8   **Other manifestations** of thiamine deficiency   CC

E51.9   **Thiamine deficiency,** unspecified   CC

E52   Niacin deficiency [pellagra]
Niacin (-tryptophan) deficiency
Nicotinamide deficiency
Pellagra (alcoholic)
EXCLUDES 1   *sequelae of niacin deficiency (E64.8)*

✓4ᵗʰ **E53   Deficiency of** other B group vitamins
EXCLUDES 1   *sequelae of vitamin B deficiency (E64.8)*

E53.0   **Riboflavin deficiency**   CC
Ariboflavinosis
Vitamin B2 deficiency
CC Excl: See code: E51

E53.1   **Pyridoxine deficiency**
Vitamin B6 deficiency
EXCLUDES 1   *pyridoxine-responsive sideroblastic anemia (D64.3)*

E53.8   **Deficiency of** other specified B group vitamins
Biotin deficiency
Cyanocobalamin deficiency
Folate deficiency
Folic acid deficiency
Pantothenic acid deficiency
Vitamin B12 deficiency
EXCLUDES 1   *folate deficiency anemia (D52.-)*
vitamin B12 deficiency anemia (D51.-)

E53.9   **Vitamin B deficiency,** unspecified

E54   Ascorbic acid deficiency
Deficiency of vitamin C
Scurvy
EXCLUDES 1   *scorbutic anemia (D53.2)*
sequelae of vitamin C deficiency (E64.2)

✓4ᵗʰ **E55   Vitamin D deficiency**
EXCLUDES 1   *adult osteomalacia (M83.-)*
osteoporosis (M80.-)
sequelae of rickets (E64.3)

E55.0   **Rickets, active**   CC
Infantile osteomalacia
Juvenile osteomalacia
EXCLUDES 1   *celiac rickets (K90.0)*
Crohn's rickets (K50.-)
hereditary vitamin D-dependent rickets (E83.32)
inactive rickets (E64.3)
renal rickets (N25.0)
sequelae of rickets (E64.3)
vitamin D-resistant rickets (E83.31)
CC Excl: E55.0-E63.9, E64.3-E64.9, M83.0-M83.9

E55.9   **Vitamin D deficiency,** unspecified
Avitaminosis D

✓4ᵗʰ **E56   Other vitamin deficiencies**
EXCLUDES 1   *sequelae of other vitamin deficiencies (E64.8)*

E56.0   **Deficiency of** vitamin E

E56.1   **Deficiency of** vitamin K
EXCLUDES 1   *deficiency of coagulation factor due to vitamin K*
deficiency (D68.4)
vitamin K deficiency of newborn (P53)

E56.8   **Deficiency of** other vitamins

E56.9   **Vitamin deficiency,** unspecified

E58   Dietary calcium deficiency
EXCLUDES 1   *disorders of calcium metabolism (E83.5-)*
sequelae of calcium deficiency (E64.8)

E59   Dietary selenium deficiency
Keshan disease
EXCLUDES 1   *sequelae of selenium deficiency (E64.8)*

E60   Dietary zinc deficiency

✓4ᵗʰ **E61   Deficiency of other nutrient elements**
Use additional code for adverse effect, if applicable, to identify drug
(T36-T50 with fifth or sixth character 5)
EXCLUDES 1   *disorders of mineral metabolism (E83.-)*
iodine deficiency related thyroid disorders (E00-E02)
sequelae of malnutrition and other nutritional deficiencies
(E64.-)

E61.0   **Copper deficiency**

E61.1   **Iron deficiency**
EXCLUDES 1   *iron deficiency anemia (D50.-)*

E61.2   **Magnesium deficiency**

E61.3   **Manganese deficiency**

E61.4   **Chromium deficiency**

E61.5   **Molybdenum deficiency**

E61.6   **Vanadium deficiency**

E61.7   **Deficiency of** multiple nutrient elements

E61.8   **Deficiency of** other specified nutrient elements

E61.9   **Deficiency of nutrient element,** unspecified

✓4ᵗʰ **E63   Other nutritional deficiencies**
EXCLUDES 1   *dehydration (E86.0)*
failure to thrive, adult (R62.7)
failure to thrive, child (R62.51)
feeding problems in newborn (P92.-)
sequelae of malnutrition and other nutritional deficiencies
(E64.-)

E63.0   **Essential fatty acid [EFA] deficiency**

E63.1   **Imbalance of constituents of food intake**

E63.8   **Other specified nutritional deficiencies**

E63.9   **Nutritional deficiency,** unspecified

N Newborn: 0   P Pediatric: 0-17   M Maternity: 12-55   A Adult: 15-124   MCC Major CC Condition   PDxMCC PDx acts as own MCC   CC CC Condition   PDxCC PDx acts as own CC

✓4ᵗʰ **E64   Sequelae of malnutrition and other nutritional deficiencies**
> **NOTE**   This category is to be used to indicate conditions in categories E43, E44, E46, E50-E63 as the cause of sequelae, which are themselves classified elsewhere. The 'sequelae' include conditions specified as such; they also include the late effects of diseases classifiable to the above categories if the disease itself is no longer present
>
> Code first condition resulting from (sequela) of malnutrition and other nutritional deficiencies

E64.0   Sequelae of protein-calorie malnutrition   CC
> **EXCLUDES 2**   retarded development following protein-calorie malnutrition (E45)
>
> **CC Excl:** E40-E46, E64.0

E64.1   Sequelae of vitamin A deficiency

E64.2   Sequelae of vitamin C deficiency

E64.3   Sequelae of rickets

E64.8   Sequelae of other nutritional deficiencies

E64.9   Sequelae of unspecified nutritional deficiency

Overweight, obesity and other hyperalimentation (E65-E68)

E65   Localized adiposity
> Fat pad

✓4ᵗʰ **E66   Overweight and obesity**
> Code first obesity complicating pregnancy, childbirth and the puerperium, if applicable (O99.21-)
> Use additional code to identify body mass index (BMI), if known (Z68.-)
> **EXCLUDES 1**   adiposogenital dystrophy (E23.6)
> lipomatosis NOS (E88.2)
> lipomatosis dolorosa [Dercum] (E88.2)
> Prader-Willi syndrome (Q87.1)

✓5ᵗʰ **E66.0   Obesity due to excess calories**
> 2   **E66.01   Morbid (severe) obesity due to excess calories**
> > **EXCLUDES 1**   morbid (severe) obesity with alveolar hypoventilation (E66.2)
>
> 13 **E66.09   Other obesity due to excess calories**

13 **E66.1   Drug-induced obesity**
> Use additional code for adverse effect, if applicable, to identify drug (T36-T50 with fifth or sixth character 5)

E66.2   Morbid (severe) obesity with alveolar hypoventilation   CC
> Pickwickian syndrome
> **CC Excl:** E66.2-I27.81, I27.89-I27.9

E66.3   Overweight

13 **E66.8   Other obesity**

13 **E66.9   Obesity, unspecified**
> Obesity NOS

✓4ᵗʰ **E67   Other hyperalimentation**
> **EXCLUDES 1**   hyperalimentation NOS (R63.2)
> sequelae of hyperalimentation (E68)

E67.0   Hypervitaminosis A

E67.1   Hypercarotinemia

E67.2   Megavitamin-B6 syndrome

E67.3   Hypervitaminosis D

E67.8   Other specified hyperalimentation

E68   Sequelae of hyperalimentation
> Code first condition resulting from (sequela) of hyperalimentation

Metabolic disorders (E70-E88)

> **EXCLUDES 1**   androgen insensitivity syndrome (E34.5-)
> congenital adrenal hyperplasia (E25.0)
> Ehlers-Danlos syndrome (Q79.6)
> hemolytic anemias attributable to enzyme disorders (D55.-)
> Marfan's syndrome (Q87.4)
> 5-alpha-reductase deficiency (E29.1)

✓4ᵗʰ **E70   Disorders of aromatic amino-acid metabolism**

> **CC Excl: For CC codes in category E70, unless otherwise noted:** C88.0, D47.2, D89.0-D89.1, E70.0-E71.30, E72.00-E72.02, E72.04-E74.9, E75.21-E75.22, E75.240-E75.249, E75.3, E75.5-E75.6, E77.0-E78.70, E78.79-E78.9, E88.09-E88.2, E88.89

E70.0   Classical phenylketonuria   CC

E70.1   Other hyperphenylalaninemias   CC

✓5ᵗʰ **E70.2   Disorders of tyrosine metabolism**
> **EXCLUDES 1**   transitory tyrosinemia of newborn (P74.5)

E70.20   Disorder of tyrosine metabolism, unspecified   CC

E70.21   Tyrosinemia   CC
> Hypertyrosinemia

E70.29   Other disorders of tyrosine metabolism   CC
> Alkaptonuria
> Ochronosis

✓5ᵗʰ **E70.3   Albinism**

E70.30   Albinism, unspecified   CC

✓6ᵗʰ **E70.31   Ocular albinism**
> **E70.310   X-linked ocular albinism**   CC
> **E70.311   Autosomal recessive ocular albinism**   CC
> **E70.318   Other ocular albinism**   CC
> **E70.319   Ocular albinism, unspecified**   CC

✓6ᵗʰ **E70.32   Oculocutaneous albinism**
> **EXCLUDES 1**   Chediak-Higashi syndrome (E70.330)
> Hermansky-Pudlak syndrome (E70.331)

> **E70.320   Tyrosinase negative oculocutaneous albinism**   CC
> > Albinism I
> > Oculocutaneous albinism ty-neg

> **E70.321   Tyrosinase positive oculocutaneous albinism**   CC
> > Albinism II
> > Oculocutaneous albinism ty-pos

> **E70.328   Other oculocutaneous albinism**   CC
> > Cross syndrome

> **E70.329   Oculocutaneous albinism, unspecified**   CC

✓6ᵗʰ **E70.33   Albinism with hematologic abnormality**
> **E70.330   Chediak-Higashi syndrome**   CC
> **E70.331   Hermansky-Pudlak syndrome**   CC
> **E70.338   Other albinism with hematologic abnormality**   CC
> **E70.339   Albinism with hematologic abnormality, unspecified**   CC

E70.39   Other specified albinism   CC
> Piebaldism

✓5ᵗʰ **E70.4   Disorders of histidine metabolism**
> **E70.40   Disorders of histidine metabolism, unspecified**   CC
> **E70.41   Histidinemia**   CC
> **E70.49   Other disorders of histidine metabolism**   CC

E70.5   Disorders of tryptophan metabolism   CC

E70.8   Other disorders of aromatic amino-acid metabolism   CC

E70.9   Disorder of aromatic amino-acid metabolism, unspecified   CC

✓4ᵗʰ **E71   Disorders of branched-chain amino-acid metabolism and fatty-acid metabolism**

E71.0   Maple-syrup-urine disease   CC
> **CC Excl:** See code: E70

✓5ᵗʰ **E71.1   Other disorders of branched-chain amino-acid metabolism**

> **CC Excl: For CC codes in subcategory E71.1, unless otherwise noted:** C88.0, D47.2, D89.0-D89.1, E70.0-E71.30, E72.00-E72.02, E72.04-E74.9, E75.21-E75.22, E75.240-E75.249, E75.3, E75.5-E75.6, E77.0-E78.70, E78.79-E78.9, E88.09-E88.2, E88.89

✓6ᵗʰ **E71.11   Branched-chain organic acidurias**
> **E71.110   Isovaleric acidemia**   CC
> **E71.111   3-methylglutaconic aciduria**   CC
> **E71.118   Other branched-chain organic acidurias**   CC

✓6ᵗʰ **E71.12   Disorders of propionate metabolism**
> **E71.120   Methylmalonic acidemia**   CC
> **E71.121   Propionic acidemia**   CC
> **E71.128   Other disorders of propionate metabolism**   CC

E71.19   Other disorders of branched-chain amino-acid metabolism   CC
> Hyperleucine-isoleucinemia
> Hypervalinemia

E71.2   Disorder of branched-chain amino-acid metabolism, unspecified   CC
> **CC Excl:** See code: E70

---

2   HAC = as PDx in combination with one of the following procedure codes: 0D16[0,4,8][7,J,K,Z][9,A,B,L] or 0DV64CZ **AND** in combination with SDx, not POA, of K68.11, K95.01, K95.81 or T81.4XXA.

13 Questionable admission when used as PDx.

☑ Additional Character Required   ✓x7ᵗʰ Placeholder Alert   Unacceptable PDx   Manifestation   Hospital Acquired Condition   **EXCLUDES 1** Not Coded Here   **EXCLUDES 2** Not Included Here

E71.3 Disorders of fatty-acid metabolism
>*EXCLUDES 1* peroxisomal disorders (E71.5)
>Refsum's disease (G60.1)
>Schilder's disease (G37.0)
>*EXCLUDES 2* carnitine deficiency due to inborn error of metabolism (E71.42)

>**CC Excl:** For CC codes in subcategory E71.3, unless otherwise noted: C96.5-C96.6, E71.39-E71.548, E80.3, E88.40-E88.49, E88.89, H49.811-H49.819

E71.30 Disorder of fatty-acid metabolism, unspecified

E71.31 Disorders of fatty-acid oxidation
E71.310 Long chain/very long chain acyl CoA dehydrogenase deficiency
LCAD
VLCAD
E71.311 Medium chain acyl CoA dehydrogenase deficiency
MCAD
E71.312 Short chain acyl CoA dehydrogenase deficiency
SCAD
E71.313 Glutaric aciduria type II
Glutaric aciduria type II A
Glutaric aciduria type II B
Glutaric aciduria type II C
>*EXCLUDES 1* glutaric aciduria (type 1) NOS (E72.3)
E71.314 Muscle carnitine palmitoyltransferase deficiency
E71.318 Other disorders of fatty-acid oxidation
E71.32 Disorders of ketone metabolism
E71.39 Other disorders of fatty-acid metabolism
>**CC Excl:** E71.310-E71.32, E71.40-E71.548, E80.4-E80.7, E88.40-E88.49, H49.811-H49.819

E71.4 Disorders of carnitine metabolism
>*EXCLUDES 1* muscle carnitine palmitoyltransferase deficiency (E71.314)

E71.40 Disorder of carnitine metabolism, unspecified
E71.41 Primary carnitine deficiency
E71.42 Carnitine deficiency due to inborn errors of metabolism
Code also associated inborn error or metabolism
E71.43 Iatrogenic carnitine deficiency
Carnitine deficiency due to hemodialysis
Carnitine deficiency due to Valproic acid therapy
E71.44 Other secondary carnitine deficiency
E71.440 Ruvalcaba-Myhre-Smith syndrome
E71.448 Other secondary carnitine deficiency

E71.5 Peroxisomal disorders
>*EXCLUDES 1* Schilder's disease (G37.0)

>**CC Excl:** For CC codes in subcategory E71.5, unless otherwise noted: C96.5-C96.6, E71.310-E71.448, E80.3-E80.7, E88.40-E88.49, E88.89, H49.811-H49.819

E71.50 Peroxisomal disorder, unspecified
E71.51 Disorders of peroxisome biogenesis
Group 1 peroxisomal disorders
>*EXCLUDES 1* Refsum's disease (G60.1)
E71.510 Zellweger syndrome
E71.511 Neonatal adrenoleukodystrophy
>*EXCLUDES 1* X-linked adrenoleukodystrophy (E71.52-)
E71.518 Other disorders of peroxisome biogenesis
E71.52 X-linked adrenoleukodystrophy
E71.520 Childhood cerebral X-linked adrenoleukodystrophy
E71.521 Adolescent X-linked adrenoleukodystrophy
E71.522 Adrenomyeloneuropathy
E71.528 Other X-linked adrenoleukodystrophy
Addison only phenotype adrenoleukodystrophy
Addison-Schilder adrenoleukodystrophy
E71.529 X-linked adrenoleukodystrophy, unspecified type
E71.53 Other group 2 peroxisomal disorders

E71.54 Other peroxisomal disorders
E71.540 Rhizomelic chondrodysplasia punctata
>*EXCLUDES 1* chondrodysplasia punctata NOS (Q77.3)
E71.541 Zellweger-like syndrome
E71.542 Other group 3 peroxisomal disorders
E71.548 Other peroxisomal disorders

E72 Other disorders of amino-acid metabolism
>*EXCLUDES 1* disorders of:
>aromatic amino-acid metabolism (E70.-)
>branched-chain amino-acid metabolism (E71.0-E71.2)
>fatty-acid metabolism (E71.3)
>purine and pyrimidine metabolism (E79.-)
>gout (M1A.-, M10.-)

>**CC Excl:** For CC codes in category E72, unless otherwise noted: C88.0, D47.2, D89.0-D89.1, E70.0-E71.30, E72.00-E72.02, E72.04-E74.9, E75.21-E75.22, E75.240-E75.249, E75.3, E75.5-E75.6, E77.0-E78.70, E78.79-E78.9, E88.09-E88.2, E88.89

E72.0 Disorders of amino-acid transport
>*EXCLUDES 1* disorders of tryptophan metabolism (E70.5)

E72.00 Disorders of amino-acid transport, unspecified
E72.01 Cystinuria
E72.02 Hartnup's disease
E72.03 Lowe's syndrome
Use additional code for associated glaucoma (H42)
>**CC Excl:** No Excl
E72.04 Cystinosis
Fanconi (-de Toni) (-Debré) syndrome with cystinosis
>*EXCLUDES 1* Fanconi (-de Toni) (-Debré) syndrome without cystinosis (E72.09)
E72.09 Other disorders of amino-acid transport
Fanconi (-de Toni) (-Debré) syndrome, unspecified

E72.1 Disorders of sulfur-bearing amino-acid metabolism
>*EXCLUDES 1* cystinosis (E72.04)
>cystinuria (E72.01)
>transcobalamin II deficiency (D51.2)

E72.10 Disorders of sulfur-bearing amino-acid metabolism, unspecified
E72.11 Homocystinuria
Cystathionine synthase deficiency
E72.12 Methylenetetrahydrofolate reductase deficiency
E72.19 Other disorders of sulfur-bearing amino-acid metabolism
Cystathioninuria
Methioninemia
Sulfite oxidase deficiency

E72.2 Disorders of urea cycle metabolism
>*EXCLUDES 1* disorders of ornithine metabolism (E72.4)

E72.20 Disorder of urea cycle metabolism, unspecified
Hyperammonemia
>*EXCLUDES 1* hyperammonemia- hyperornithinemia-homocitrullinemia syndrome (E72.4)
>transient hyperammonemia of newborn (P74.6)
E72.21 Argininemia
E72.22 Arginosuccinic aciduria
E72.23 Citrullinemia
E72.29 Other disorders of urea cycle metabolism

E72.3 Disorders of lysine and hydroxylysine metabolism
Glutaric aciduria NOS
Glutaric aciduria (type I)
Hydroxylysinemia
Hyperlysinemia
>*EXCLUDES 1* glutaric aciduria type II (E71.313)
>Refsum's disease (G60.1)
>Zellweger syndrome (E71.510)

E72.4 Disorders of ornithine metabolism
Hyperammonemia-hyperornithinemia-homocitrullinemia syndrome
Ornithinemia (types I, II)
Ornithine transcarbamylase deficiency
>*EXCLUDES 1* hereditary choroidal dystrophy (H31.2-)

E72.5 Disorders of glycine metabolism
E72.50 Disorder of glycine metabolism, unspecified
E72.51 Non-ketotic hyperglycinemia
E72.52 Trimethylaminuria

E72.53   **Hyperoxaluria**   `CC`
Oxalosis
Oxaluria

E72.59   **Other disorders of glycine metabolism**   `CC`
D-glycericacidemia
Hyperhydroxyprolinemia
Hyperprolinemia (types I, II)
Sarcosinemia

E72.8   **Other specified disorders of amino-acid metabolism**   `CC`
Disorders of beta-amino-acid metabolism
Disorders of gamma-glutamyl cycle

E72.9   **Disorder of amino-acid metabolism, unspecified**   `CC`

✓4th **E73**   **Lactose intolerance**

E73.0   **Congenital lactase deficiency**

E73.1   **Secondary lactase deficiency**

E73.8   **Other lactose intolerance**

E73.9   **Lactose intolerance, unspecified**

✓4th **E74**   **Other disorders of carbohydrate metabolism**
> EXCLUDES 1   *diabetes mellitus (E08-E13)*
> *hypoglycemia NOS (E16.2)*
> *increased secretion of glucagon (E16.3)*
> *mucopolysaccharidosis (E76.0-E76.3)*

> **CC Excl: For CC codes in category E74, unless otherwise noted:**
> C88.0, D47.2, D89.0-D89.1, E70.0-E71.30, E72.00-E72.02, E72.04-E74.9, E75.21-E75.22, E75.240-E75.249, E75.3, E75.5-E75.6, E77.0-E78.70, E78.79-E78.9, E88.09-E88.2, E88.89

✓5th **E74.0**   **Glycogen storage disease**

E74.00   **Glycogen storage disease, unspecified**   `CC`

E74.01   **von Gierke disease**   `CC`
Type I glycogen storage disease

E74.02   **Pompe disease**   `CC`
Cardiac glycogenosis
Type II glycogen storage disease

E74.03   **Cori disease**   `CC`
Forbes disease
Type III glycogen storage disease

E74.04   **McArdle disease**   `CC`
Type V glycogen storage disease

E74.09   **Other glycogen storage disease**   `CC`
Andersen disease
Hers disease
Tauri disease
Glycogen storage disease, types 0, IV, VI-XI
Liver phosphorylase deficiency
Muscle phosphofructokinase deficiency

✓5th **E74.1**   **Disorders of fructose metabolism**
> EXCLUDES 1   *muscle phosphofructokinase deficiency (E74.09)*

E74.10   **Disorder of fructose metabolism, unspecified**

E74.11   **Essential fructosuria**
Fructokinase deficiency

E74.12   **Hereditary fructose intolerance**
Fructosemia

E74.19   **Other disorders of fructose metabolism**
Fructose-1, 6-diphosphatase deficiency

✓5th **E74.2**   **Disorders of galactose metabolism**

E74.20   **Disorders of galactose metabolism, unspecified**   `CC`

E74.21   **Galactosemia**   `CC`

E74.29   **Other disorders of galactose metabolism**   `CC`
Galactokinase deficiency

✓5th **E74.3**   **Other disorders of intestinal carbohydrate absorption**
> EXCLUDES 2   *lactose intolerance (E73.-)*

E74.31   **Sucrase-isomaltase deficiency**

E74.39   **Other disorders of intestinal carbohydrate absorption**
Disorder of intestinal carbohydrate absorption NOS
Glucose-galactose malabsorption
Sucrase deficiency

E74.4   **Disorders of pyruvate metabolism and gluconeogenesis**   `CC`
Deficiency of phosphoenolpyruvate carboxykinase
Deficiency of pyruvate carboxylase
Deficiency of pyruvate dehydrogenase
> EXCLUDES 1   *disorders of pyruvate metabolism and gluconeogenesis with anemia (D55.-)*
> *Leigh's syndrome (G31.82)*

E74.8   **Other specified disorders of carbohydrate metabolism**   `CC`
Essential pentosuria
Renal glycosuria

E74.9   **Disorder of carbohydrate metabolism, unspecified**

✓4th **E75**   **Disorders of sphingolipid metabolism and other lipid storage disorders**
> EXCLUDES 1   *mucolipidosis, types I-III (E77.0-E77.1)*
> *Refsum's disease (G60.1)*

✓5th **E75.0**   **GM2 gangliosidosis**

> **CC Excl: For CC codes in subcategory E75.0, unless otherwise noted:** E75.00-E75.19, E75.4, F84.2, G13.2-G13.8, G30.0-G31.82, G31.84-G31.9, G91.4, G94

E75.00   **GM2 gangliosidosis, unspecified**   `CC`

E75.01   **Sandhoff disease**   `CC`

E75.02   **Tay-Sachs disease**   `CC`

E75.09   **Other GM2 gangliosidosis**   `CC`
Adult GM2 gangliosidosis
Juvenile GM2 gangliosidosis

✓5th **E75.1**   **Other and unspecified gangliosidosis**

> **CC Excl: For CC codes in subcategory E75.1, unless otherwise noted:** E75.00-E75.19, E75.4, F84.2, G13.2-G13.8, G30.0-G31.82, G31.84-G31.9, G91.4, G94

E75.10   **Unspecified gangliosidosis**   `CC`
Gangliosidosis NOS

E75.11   **Mucolipidosis IV**   `CC`

E75.19   **Other gangliosidosis**
GM1 gangliosidosis
GM3 gangliosidosis

✓5th **E75.2**   **Other sphingolipidosis**
> EXCLUDES 1   *adrenoleukodystrophy [Addison-Schilder] (E71.528)*

> **CC Excl: For CC codes in subcategory E75.2, unless otherwise noted:** E75.00-E75.19, E75.23, E75.25-E75.29, E75.4, F84.2, G13.2-G13.8, G31.2-G31.82, G32.89, G91.4, G93.81, G93.89-G94, G96.8-G96.9, G98.0-G98.8, G99.8

E75.21   **Fabry (-Anderson) disease**

E75.22   **Gaucher disease**

E75.23   **Krabbe disease**   `CC`

✓6th **E75.24**   **Niemann-Pick disease**

E75.240   **Niemann-Pick disease type A**

E75.241   **Niemann-Pick disease type B**

E75.242   **Niemann-Pick disease type C**

E75.243   **Niemann-Pick disease type D**

E75.248   **Other Niemann-Pick disease**

E75.249   **Niemann-Pick disease, unspecified**

E75.25   **Metachromatic leukodystrophy**   `CC`

E75.29   **Other sphingolipidosis**   `CC`
Farber's syndrome
Sulfatase deficiency
Sulfatide lipidosis

E75.3   **Sphingolipidosis, unspecified**

E75.4   **Neuronal ceroid lipofuscinosis**   `CC`
Batten disease
Bielschowsky-Jansky disease
Kufs disease
Spielmeyer-Vogt disease
CC Excl: See code: E75.0

E75.5   **Other lipid storage disorders**
Cerebrotendinous cholesterosis [van Bogaert-Scherer-Epstein]
Wolman's disease

E75.6   **Lipid storage disorder, unspecified**

✓4th **E76**   **Disorders of glycosaminoglycan metabolism**

> **CC Excl: For CC codes in category E76, unless otherwise noted:** D81.3, D81.5, D81.810, D84.1, E76.01-E76.9, E79.1-E80.29, E80.4-E80.7, E85.0, E85.9, E88.81

✓5th **E76.0**   **Mucopolysaccharidosis, type I**

E76.01   **Hurler's syndrome**   `CC`

E76.02   **Hurler-Scheie syndrome**   `CC`

E76.03   **Scheie's syndrome**   `CC`

E76.1   **Mucopolysaccharidosis, type II**   `CC`
Hunter's syndrome

✓5th **E76.2**   **Other mucopolysaccharidoses**

✓6th **E76.21**   **Morquio mucopolysaccharidoses**

E76.210   **Morquio A mucopolysaccharidoses**   `CC`
Classic Morquio syndrome
Morquio syndrome A
Mucopolysaccharidosis, type IVA

✓ Additional Character Required   ✓x7th Placeholder Alert   Unacceptable PDx   Manifestation   4 Hospital Acquired Condition   EXCLUDES 1 Not Coded Here   EXCLUDES 2 Not Included Here

E76.211   **Morquio B mucopolysaccharidoses** CC
Morquio-like mucopolysaccharidoses
Morquio-like syndrome
Morquio syndrome B
Mucopolysaccharidosis, type IVB

E76.219   **Morquio mucopolysaccharidoses, unspecified** CC
Morquio syndrome
Mucopolysaccharidosis, type IV

E76.22   **Sanfilippo mucopolysaccharidoses** CC
Mucopolysaccharidosis, type III (A) (B) (C) (D)
Sanfilippo A syndrome
Sanfilippo B syndrome
Sanfilippo C syndrome
Sanfilippo D syndrome

E76.29   **Other mucopolysaccharidoses** CC
beta-Glucuronidase deficiency
Maroteaux-Lamy (mild) (severe) syndrome
Mucopolysaccharidosis, types VI, VII

E76.3   **Mucopolysaccharidosis, unspecified** CC

E76.8   **Other disorders of glucosaminoglycan metabolism** CC

E76.9   **Glucosaminoglycan metabolism disorder, unspecified** CC

✓4th **E77**   **Disorders of glycoprotein metabolism**

E77.0   **Defects in post-translational modification of lysosomal enzymes**
Mucolipidosis II [I-cell disease]
Mucolipidosis III [pseudo-Hurler polydystrophy]

E77.1   **Defects in glycoprotein degradation**
Aspartylglucosaminuria
Fucosidosis
Mannosidosis
Sialidosis [mucolipidosis I]
CC Excl: See code: E76

E77.8   **Other disorders of glycoprotein metabolism**

E77.9   **Disorder of glycoprotein metabolism, unspecified**

✓4th **E78**   **Disorders of lipoprotein metabolism and other lipidemias**
EXCLUDES 1   sphingolipidosis (E75.0-E75.3)

E78.0   **Pure hypercholesterolemia**
Familial hypercholesterolemia
Fredrickson's hyperlipoproteinemia, type IIa
Hyperbetalipoproteinemia
Hyperlipidemia, Group A
Low-density-lipoprotein-type [LDL] hyperlipoproteinemia

E78.1   **Pure hyperglyceridemia**
Elevated fasting triglycerides
Endogenous hyperglyceridemia
Fredrickson's hyperlipoproteinemia, type IV
Hyperlipidemia, group B
Hyperprebetalipoproteinemia
Very-low-density-lipoprotein-type [VLDL] hyperlipoproteinemia

E78.2   **Mixed hyperlipidemia**
Broad- or floating-betalipoproteinemia
Combined hyperlipidemia NOS
Elevated cholesterol with elevated triglycerides NEC
Fredrickson's hyperlipoproteinemia, type IIb or III
Hyperbetalipoproteinemia with prebetalipoproteinemia
Hypercholesteremia with endogenous hyperglyceridemia
Hyperlipidemia, group C
Tubo-eruptive xanthoma
Xanthoma tuberosum
EXCLUDES 1   cerebrotendinous cholesterosis [van Bogaert-Scherer-Epstein] (E75.5)
familial combined hyperlipidemia (E78.4)

E78.3   **Hyperchylomicronemia**
Chylomicron retention disease
Fredrickson's hyperlipoproteinemia, type I or V
Hyperlipidemia, group D
Mixed hyperglyceridemia

E78.4   **Other hyperlipidemia**
Familial combined hyperlipidemia

E78.5   **Hyperlipidemia, unspecified**

E78.6   **Lipoprotein deficiency**
Abetalipoproteinemia
Depressed HDL cholesterol
High-density lipoprotein deficiency
Hypoalphalipoproteinemia
Hypobetalipoproteinemia (familial)
Lecithin cholesterol acyltransferase deficiency
Tangier disease

✓5th **E78.7**   **Disorders of bile acid and cholesterol metabolism**
EXCLUDES 1   Niemann-Pick disease type C (E75.242)

E78.70   **Disorder of bile acid and cholesterol metabolism, unspecified**

E78.71   **Barth syndrome** CC
CC Excl: E78.71-E78.72, Q87.1-Q87.89, Q89.8, Q99.2

E78.72   **Smith-Lemli-Opitz syndrome** CC
CC Excl: See code: E78.71

E78.79   **Other disorders of bile acid and cholesterol metabolism**

✓5th **E78.8**   **Other disorders of lipoprotein metabolism**

E78.81   **Lipoid dermatoarthritis**

E78.89   **Other lipoprotein metabolism disorders**

E78.9   **Disorder of lipoprotein metabolism, unspecified**

✓4th **E79**   **Disorders of purine and pyrimidine metabolism**
EXCLUDES 1   Ataxia-telangiectasia (Q87.1)
Bloom's syndrome (Q82.8)
Cockayne's syndrome (Q87.1)
calculus of kidney (N20.0)
combined immunodeficiency disorders (D81.-)
Fanconi's anemia (D61.09)
gout (M1A.-, M10.-)
orotaciduric anemia (D53.0)
progeria (E34.8)
Werner's syndrome (E34.8)
xeroderma pigmentosum (Q82.1)

CC Excl: For CC codes in category E79, unless otherwise noted:
D81.3, D81.5, D81.810, D84.1, E76.01-E76.9, E79.1-E80.29, E80.4-E80.7, E88.81

E79.0   **Hyperuricemia without signs of inflammatory arthritis and tophaceous disease**
Asymptomatic hyperuricemia

E79.1   **Lesch-Nyhan syndrome** CC
HGPRT deficiency

E79.2   **Myoadenylate deaminase deficiency** CC

E79.8   **Other disorders of purine and pyrimidine metabolism** CC
Hereditary xanthinuria

E79.9   **Disorder of purine and pyrimidine metabolism, unspecified** CC

✓4th **E80**   **Disorders of porphyrin and bilirubin metabolism**
INCLUDES   defects of catalase and peroxidase

CC Excl: For CC codes in category E80, unless otherwise noted:
D81.3, D81.5, D81.810, D84.1, E76.01-E76.9, E79.1-E80.29, E80.4-E80.7, E88.81

E80.0   **Hereditary erythropoietic porphyria** CC
Congenital erythropoietic porphyria
Erythropoietic protoporphyria

E80.1   **Porphyria cutanea tarda** CC

✓5th **E80.2**   **Other and unspecified porphyria**

E80.20   **Unspecified porphyria** CC
Porphyria NOS

E80.21   **Acute intermittent (hepatic) porphyria** CC

E80.29   **Other porphyria** CC
Hereditary coproporphyria

E80.3   **Defects of catalase and peroxidase** CC
Acatalasia [Takahara]
CC Excl: E71.310-E71.32, E71.40-E71.548, E80.4-E80.7, E88.40-E88.49, H49.811-H49.819

E80.4   **Gilbert syndrome**

E80.5   **Crigler-Najjar syndrome**

E80.6   **Other disorders of bilirubin metabolism**
Dubin-Johnson syndrome
Rotor's syndrome

E80.7   **Disorder of bilirubin metabolism, unspecified**

✓4th **E83**   **Disorders of mineral metabolism**
EXCLUDES 1   dietary mineral deficiency (E58-E61)
parathyroid disorders (E20-E21)
vitamin D deficiency (E55.-)

✓5th **E83.0**   **Disorders of copper metabolism**

E83.00   **Disorder of copper metabolism, unspecified**

E83.01   **Wilson's disease**
Code also associated Kayser Fleischer ring (H18.04-)

E83.09   **Other disorders of copper metabolism**
Menkes' (kinky hair) (steely hair) disease

✓5th **E83.1 Disorders of iron metabolism**
> *EXCLUDES 1*   iron deficiency anemia (D50.-)
> sideroblastic anemia (D64.0-D64.3)

E83.10 Disorder of iron metabolism, unspecified

✓6th **E83.11 Hemochromatosis**

E83.110 Hereditary hemochromatosis
Bronzed diabetes
Pigmentary cirrhosis (of liver)
Primary (hereditary) hemochromatosis

E83.111 Hemochromatosis due to repeated red blood cell transfusions
Iron overload due to repeated red blood cell transfusions
Transfusion (red blood cell) associated hemochromatosis

E83.118 Other hemochromatosis

E83.119 Hemochromatosis, unspecified

E83.19 Other disorders of iron metabolism
Use additional code, if applicable, for idiopathic pulmonary hemosiderosis (J84.03)

E83.2 Disorders of zinc metabolism
Acrodermatitis enteropathica

✓5th **E83.3 Disorders of phosphorus metabolism and phosphatases**
> *EXCLUDES 1*   adult osteomalacia (M83.-)
> osteoporosis (M80.-)

E83.30 Disorder of phosphorus metabolism, unspecified

E83.31 Familial hypophosphatemia
Vitamin D-resistant osteomalacia
Vitamin D-resistant rickets
> *EXCLUDES 1*   vitamin D-deficiency rickets (E55.0)

E83.32 Hereditary vitamin D-dependent rickets (type 1) (type 2)
25-hydroxyvitamin D 1-alpha-hydroxylase deficiency
Pseudovitamin D deficiency
Vitamin D receptor defect

E83.39 Other disorders of phosphorus metabolism
Acid phosphatase deficiency
Hypophosphatasia

✓5th **E83.4 Disorders of magnesium metabolism**

E83.40 Disorders of magnesium metabolism, unspecified

E83.41 Hypermagnesemia

E83.42 Hypomagnesemia

E83.49 Other disorders of magnesium metabolism

✓5th **E83.5 Disorders of calcium metabolism**
> *EXCLUDES 1*   chondrocalcinosis (M11.1-M11.2)
> hungry bone syndrome (E83.81)
> hyperparathyroidism (E21.0-E21.3)

E83.50 Unspecified disorder of calcium metabolism

E83.51 Hypocalcemia

E83.52 Hypercalcemia
Familial hypocalciuric hypercalcemia

E83.59 Other disorders of calcium metabolism
Idiopathic hypercalciuria

✓5th **E83.8 Other disorders of mineral metabolism**

E83.81 Hungry bone syndrome

E83.89 Other disorders of mineral metabolism

E83.9 Disorder of mineral metabolism, unspecified

✓4th **E84 Cystic fibrosis**
> *INCLUDES*   mucoviscidosis

> **CC Excl: For CC/MCC codes in category E84, unless otherwise noted:** E84.0-E84.9

E84.0 Cystic fibrosis with pulmonary manifestations   MCC
Use additional code to identify any infectious organism present, such as:
Pseudomonas (B96.5)

✓5th **E84.1 Cystic fibrosis with intestinal manifestations**

E84.11 Meconium ileus in cystic fibrosis   MCC N
> *EXCLUDES 1*   meconium ileus not due to cystic fibrosis (P76.0)

E84.19 Cystic fibrosis with other intestinal manifestations   CC
Distal intestinal obstruction syndrome

E84.8 Cystic fibrosis with other manifestations   CC

E84.9 Cystic fibrosis, unspecified   CC

✓4th **E85 Amyloidosis**
> *EXCLUDES 1*   Alzheimer's disease (G30.0-)

> **CC Excl: For CC codes in category E85, unless otherwise noted:** E85.0-E85.9, E88.81

E85.0 Non-neuropathic heredofamilial amyloidosis   CC
Familial Mediterranean fever
Hereditary amyloid nephropathy
AHA: 2012, 4Q, 99

E85.1 Neuropathic heredofamilial amyloidosis   CC
Amyloid polyneuropathy (Portuguese)

E85.2 Heredofamilial amyloidosis, unspecified   CC

E85.3 Secondary systemic amyloidosis   CC
Hemodialysis-associated amyloidosis

E85.4 Organ-limited amyloidosis   CC
Localized amyloidosis

E85.8 Other amyloidosis   CC

E85.9 Amyloidosis, unspecified   CC

✓4th **E86 Volume depletion**
> *EXCLUDES 1*   dehydration of newborn (P74.1)
> hypovolemic shock NOS (R57.1)
> postprocedural hypovolemic shock (T81.19)
> traumatic hypovolemic shock (T79.4)

E86.0 Dehydration
AHA: 2014, 1Q, 7

E86.1 Hypovolemia
Depletion of volume of plasma

E86.9 Volume depletion, unspecified

✓4th **E87 Other disorders of fluid, electrolyte and acid-base balance**
> *EXCLUDES 1*   diabetes insipidus (E23.2)
> electrolyte imbalance associated with hyperemesis gravidarum (O21.1)
> electrolyte imbalance following ectopic or molar pregnancy (O08.5)
> familial periodic paralysis (G72.3)

> **CC Excl: For CC codes in category E87, unless otherwise noted:** E86.0-E87.8

E87.0 Hyperosmolality and hypernatremia   CC
Sodium [Na] excess
Sodium [Na] overload
AHA: 2014, 1Q, 7

E87.1 Hypo-osmolality and hyponatremia   CC
Sodium [Na] deficiency
> *EXCLUDES 1*   syndrome of inappropriate secretion of antidiuretic hormone (E22.2)
AHA: 2014, 1Q, 7

E87.2 Acidosis   CC
Acidosis NOS
Lactic acidosis
Metabolic acidosis
Respiratory acidosis
> *EXCLUDES 1*   diabetic acidosis—see categories E08-E10, E13 with ketoacidosis

E87.3 Alkalosis   CC
Alkalosis NOS
Metabolic alkalosis
Respiratory alkalosis

E87.4 Mixed disorder of acid-base balance   CC

E87.5 Hyperkalemia
Potassium [K] excess
Potassium [K] overload

E87.6 Hypokalemia
Potassium [K] deficiency

✓5th **E87.7 Fluid overload**
> *EXCLUDES 1*   edema NOS (R60.9)
> fluid retention (R60.9)

E87.70 Fluid overload, unspecified

E87.71 Transfusion associated circulatory overload
Fluid overload due to transfusion (blood) (blood components)
TACO

E87.79 Other fluid overload

E87.8 Other disorders of electrolyte and fluid balance, not elsewhere classified
Electrolyte imbalance NOS
Hyperchloremia
Hypochloremia

✓ Additional Character Required   ✓x7th Placeholder Alert   Unacceptable PDx   Manifestation   Hospital Acquired Condition   *EXCLUDES 1* Not Coded Here   *EXCLUDES 2* Not Included Here

ICD-10-CM 2016   517

Chapter 4. Endocrine, Nutritional, and Metabolic Diseases

✓4ᵗʰ **E88 Other and unspecified metabolic disorders**
Use additional codes for associated conditions
     EXCLUDES 1   *histiocytosis X (chronic) (C96.6)*

✓5ᵗʰ **E88.0 Disorders of plasma-protein metabolism, not elsewhere classified**
     EXCLUDES 1   *disorder of lipoprotein metabolism (E78.-)*
         monoclonal gammopathy (of undetermined significance) (D47.2)
         polyclonal hypergammaglobulinemia (D89.0)
         Waldenström's macroglobulinemia (C88.0)

     E88.01 Alpha-1-antitrypsin deficiency
         AAT deficiency

     E88.09 Other disorders of plasma-protein metabolism, not elsewhere classified
         Bisalbuminemia

   E88.1 Lipodystrophy, not elsewhere classified
     Lipodystrophy NOS
     EXCLUDES 1   *Whipple's disease (K90.81)*

   E88.2 Lipomatosis, not elsewhere classified
     Lipomatosis NOS
     Lipomatosis (Check) dolorosa [Dercum]

   E88.3 Tumor lysis syndrome   MCC
     Tumor lysis syndrome (spontaneous)
     Tumor lysis syndrome following antineoplastic drug chemotherapy
     Use additional code for adverse effect, if applicable, to identify drug (T45.1X5)
     CC Excl: E08.21-E08.29, E09.21-E09.29, E88.3, N00.0-N01.9, N02.8-N02.9, N04.7-N05.1, N05.6-N06.1, N06.6-N07.1, N07.6-N08, N14.0-N15.0, N15.8-N17.9

✓5ᵗʰ **E88.4 Mitochondrial metabolism disorders**
     EXCLUDES 1   *disorders of pyruvate metabolism (E74.4)*
         Kearns-Sayre syndrome (H49.81)
         Leber's disease (H47.22)
         Leigh's encephalopathy (G31.82)
         Mitochondrial myopathy, NEC (G71.3)
         Reye's syndrome (G93.7)

     CC Excl: For CC codes in subcategory E88.4, unless otherwise noted: C96.5-C96.6, E71.310-E71.548, E80.3-E80.7, E88.89

     E88.40 Mitochondrial metabolism disorder, unspecified   CC

     E88.41 MELAS syndrome   CC
         Mitochondrial myopathy, encephalopathy, lactic acidosis and stroke-like episodes

     E88.42 MERRF syndrome   CC
         Myoclonic epilepsy associated with ragged-red fibers
         Code also myoclonic epilepsy (G40.3-)

     E88.49 Other mitochondrial metabolism disorders   CC

✓5ᵗʰ **E88.8 Other specified metabolic disorders**
     E88.81 Metabolic syndrome
         Dysmetabolic syndrome X
         Use additional codes for associated manifestations, such as:
            obesity (E66.-)

     E88.89 Other specified metabolic disorders
         Launois-Bensaude adenolipomatosis
         EXCLUDES 1   *adult pulmonary Langerhans cell histiocytosis (J84.82)*
         CC Excl: E71.310-E71.32, E71.40-E71.548, E80.4-E80.7, E88.40-E88.49, H49.811-H49.819

   E88.9 Metabolic disorder, unspecified

✓4ᵗʰ **E89 Postprocedural endocrine and metabolic complications and disorders, not elsewhere classified**
     EXCLUDES 2   *intraoperative complications of endocrine system organ or structure (E36.0-, E36.1-, E36.8)*

   E89.0 Postprocedural hypothyroidism
     Postirradiation hypothyroidism
     Postsurgical hypothyroidism

   E89.1 Postprocedural hypoinsulinemia   CC
     Postpancreatectomy hyperglycemia
     Postsurgical hypoinsulinemia
     Use additional code, if applicable, to identify:
         acquired absence of pancreas (Z90.41-)
         diabetes mellitus (postpancreatectomy) (postprocedural) (E13.-)
         insulin use (Z79.4)
     EXCLUDES 1   *transient postprocedural hyperglycemia (R73.9)*
         transient postprocedural hypoglycemia (E16.2)
     CC Excl: E08.00-E08.59, E08.618-E08.638, E08.641-E09.59, E09.618-E09.638, E09.641-E10.59, E10.618-E10.638, E10.641-E10.649, E10.69-E11.59, E11.618-E11.638, E11.641-E11.649, E11.69-E13.59, E13.618-E13.638, E13.641-E16.2, E30.9, E34.1, E34.50-E35, E89.1

   E89.2 Postprocedural hypoparathyroidism
     Parathyroprival tetany

   E89.3 Postprocedural hypopituitarism
     Postirradiation hypopituitarism

✓5ᵗʰ **E89.4 Postprocedural ovarian failure**
     E89.40 Asymptomatic postprocedural ovarian failure   ♀
         Postprocedural ovarian failure NOS

     E89.41 Symptomatic postprocedural ovarian failure   ♀
         Symptoms such as flushing, sleeplessness, headache, lack of concentration, associated with postprocedural menopause

   E89.5 Postprocedural testicular hypofunction   ♂

   E89.6 Postprocedural adrenocortical (-medullary) hypofunction   CC
     CC Excl: A17.9, A18.7, A18.82, A18.84, A18.89, E27.0-E27.9, E30.9, E34.1, E34.50-E35, E89.6

✓5ᵗʰ **E89.8 Other postprocedural endocrine and metabolic complications and disorders**
   ✓6ᵗʰ **E89.81 Postprocedural hemorrhage and hematoma of an endocrine system organ or structure following a procedure**
     E89.810 Postprocedural hemorrhage and hematoma of an endocrine system organ or structure following an endocrine system procedure   CC
         CC Excl: E36.8, E89.810-E89.89, H95.811-H95.89, I97.3, M96.89, N98.1-N98.9, T81.82 with 7th character A, T81.89X-T81.9XX with 7th A

     E89.811 Postprocedural hemorrhage and hematoma of an endocrine system organ or structure following other procedure   CC
         CC Excl: See code E89.810

     E89.89 Other postprocedural endocrine and metabolic complications and disorders   CC
         Use additional code, if applicable, to further specify disorder
     CC Excl: See code E89.810

N Newborn: 0   P Pediatric: 0-17   M Maternity: 12-55   A Adult: 15-124   MCC Major CC Condition   PDxMCC PDx acts as own MCC   CC CC Condition   PDxCC PDx acts as own CC

Chapter 5. Mental, Behavioral and Neurodevelopmental Disorders (F01–F99)

Chapter Specific Guidelines with Coding Examples

The chapter specific guidelines from the ICD-10-CM Official Guidelines for Coding and Reporting have been provided below. Along with these guidelines are coding examples, contained in the shaded boxes, that have been developed to help illustrate the coding and/or sequencing guidance found in these guidelines.

a. Pain disorders related to psychological factors

Assign code F45.41, for pain that is exclusively related to psychological disorders. As indicated by the Excludes 1 note under category G89, a code from category G89 should not be assigned with code F45.41.

> Perceived abdominal pain determined to be persistent somatoform pain disorder
>
> **F45.41   Pain disorder exclusively related to psychological factors**
>
> *Explanation*: This pain was diagnosed as being exclusively psychological; therefore, no code from category G89 is added.

Code F45.42, Pain disorders with related psychological factors, should be used with a code from category G89, Pain, not elsewhere classified, if there is documentation of a psychological component for a patient with acute or chronic pain.

See Section I.C.6. Pain

b. Mental and behavioral disorders due to psychoactive substance use

1) In remission

Selection of codes for "in remission" for categories F10-F19, Mental and behavioral disorders due to psychoactive substance use (categories F10-F19 with -.21) requires the provider's clinical judgment. The appropriate codes for "in remission" are assigned only on the basis of provider documentation (as defined in the Official Guidelines for Coding and Reporting).

> Medical history: Opioid dependence in remission
>
> **F11.21   Opioid dependence, in remission**
>
> *Explanation*: The "in remission" codes are assigned when the provider documents the remission.

2) Psychoactive substance use, abuse and dependence

When the provider documentation refers to use, abuse and dependence of the same substance (e.g. alcohol, opioid, cannabis, etc.), only one code should be assigned to identify the pattern of use based on the following hierarchy:

- If both use and abuse are documented, assign only the code for abuse
- If both abuse and dependence are documented, assign only the code for dependence
- If use, abuse and dependence are all documented, assign only the code for dependence
- If both use and dependence are documented, assign only the code for dependence.

> History and physical notes cannabis dependence; progress note says cannabis abuse
>
> **F12.20   Cannabis dependence, uncomplicated**
>
> *Explanation*: In the hierarchy, the dependence code is used if both abuse and dependence are documented.

> Discharge summary says cocaine abuse; progress notes list cocaine use
>
> **F14.10   Cocaine abuse, uncomplicated**
>
> *Explanation*: In the hierarchy, the abuse code is used if both abuse and use are documented.

3) Psychoactive Substance Use

As with all other diagnoses, the codes for psychoactive substance use (F10.9-, F11.9-, F12.9-, F13.9-, F14.9-, F15.9-, F16.9-) should only be assigned based on provider documentation and when they meet the definition of a reportable diagnosis (see Section III, Reporting Additional Diagnoses). The codes are to be used only when the psychoactive substance use is associated with a mental or behavioral disorder, and such a relationship is documented by the provider.

> ED reports that a 27-year-old female tripped and broke her right ankle. Her friends reported that they were drinking and dancing at a nightclub.
>
> **S82.891A   Other fracture of right lower leg, initial encounter for closed fracture**
>
> **W01.0XXA   Fall on same level from slipping, tripping and stumbling, initial encounter**
>
> **Y92.252   Music hall as the place of occurrence of the external cause**
>
> **Y93.41   Activity, dancing**
>
> *Explanation*: Note that no code was added for alcohol use or abuse. Unless it is specifically associated with a diagnosis by provider documentation and meets the definition of a reportable diagnosis, it is not assigned. However, if the documentation from the provider stated: "The patient tripped, fell and fractured her right ankle while dancing due to her elevated blood alcohol, consistent with her ongoing alcohol abuse," the following code would be added:
>
> **F10.10   Alcohol abuse, uncomplicated**

Chapter 5. Mental, Behavioral, and Neurodevelopmental Disorders (F01-F99)

INCLUDES disorders of psychological development

EXCLUDES 2 symptoms, signs and abnormal clinical laboratory findings, not elsewhere classified (R00-R99)

This chapter contains the following blocks:

F01-F09 Mental disorders due to known physiological conditions
F10-F19 Mental and behavioral disorders due to psychoactive substance use
F20-F29 Schizophrenia, schizotypal, delusional, and other non-mood psychotic disorders
F30-F39 Mood [affective] disorders
F40-F48 Anxiety, dissociative, stress-related, somatoform and other nonpsychotic mental disorders
F50-F59 Behavioral syndromes associated with physiological disturbances and physical factors
F60-F69 Disorders of adult personality and behavior
F70-F79 Intellectual disabilities
F80-F89 Pervasive and specific developmental disorders
F90-F98 Behavioral and emotional disorders with onset usually occurring in childhood and adolescence
F99 Unspecified mental disorder

Mental disorders due to known physiological conditions (F01-F09)

NOTE This block comprises a range of mental disorders grouped together on the basis of their having in common a demonstrable etiology in cerebral disease, brain injury, or other insult leading to cerebral dysfunction. The dysfunction may be primary, as in diseases, injuries, and insults that affect the brain directly and selectively; or secondary, as in systemic diseases and disorders that attack the brain only as one of the multiple organs or systems of the body that are involved.

✓4th F01 Vascular dementia

Vascular dementia as a result of infarction of the brain due to vascular disease, including hypertensive cerebrovascular disease.

INCLUDES arteriosclerotic dementia

Code first the underlying physiological condition or sequelae of cerebrovascular disease.

✓5th F01.5 Vascular dementia

F01.50 Vascular dementia without behavioral disturbance   A

F01.51 Vascular dementia with behavioral disturbance   CC A

Vascular dementia with aggressive behavior
Vascular dementia with combative behavior
Vascular dementia with violent behavior
Use additional code, if applicable, to identify wandering in vascular dementia (Z91.83)
CC Excl: F01.51

✓4th F02 Dementia in other diseases classified elsewhere

Code first the underlying physiological condition, such as:
Alzheimer's (G30.-)
cerebral lipidosis (E75.4)
Creutzfeldt-Jakob disease (A81.0-)
dementia with Lewy bodies (G31.83)
epilepsy and recurrent seizures (G40.-)
frontotemporal dementia (G31.09)
hepatolenticular degeneration (E83.0)
human immunodeficiency virus [HIV] disease (B20)
hypercalcemia (E83.52)
hypothyroidism, acquired (E00-E03.-)
intoxications (T36-T65)
Jakob-Creutzfeldt disease (A81.0-)
multiple sclerosis (G35)
neurosyphilis (A52.17)
niacin deficiency [pellagra] (E52)
Parkinson's disease (G20)
Pick's disease (G31.01)
polyarteritis nodosa (M30.0)
systemic lupus erythematosus (M32.-)
trypanosomiasis (B56.-, B57.-)
vitamin B deficiency (E53.8)

EXCLUDES 1 dementia with Parkinsonism (G31.83)
EXCLUDES 2 dementia in alcohol and psychoactive substance disorders (F10-F19, with .17, .27, .97)
vascular dementia (F01.5-)

✓5th F02.8 Dementia in other diseases classified elsewhere

F02.80 *Dementia in other diseases classified elsewhere without behavioral disturbance*
Dementia in other diseases classified elsewhere NOS

F02.81 *Dementia in other diseases classified elsewhere with behavioral disturbance*   CC
Dementia in other diseases classified elsewhere with aggressive behavior
Dementia in other diseases classified elsewhere with combative behavior
Dementia in other diseases classified elsewhere with violent behavior
Use additional code, if applicable, to identify wandering in dementia in conditions classified elsewhere (Z91.83)
CC Excl: F02.81, F03.91

✓4th F03 Unspecified dementia

Presenile dementia NOS   Senile dementia NOS
Presenile psychosis NOS   Senile dementia depressed
Primary degenerative dementia NOS   or paranoid type
Senile dementia NOS   Senile psychosis NOS

EXCLUDES 1 senility NOS (R41.81)
EXCLUDES 2 mild memory disturbance due to known physiological condition (F06.8)
senile dementia with delirium or acute confusional state (F05)

✓5th F03.9 Unspecified dementia

F03.90 Unspecified dementia without behavioral   HIV A
disturbance
Dementia NOS
AHA: 2012, 4Q, 92

F03.91 Unspecified dementia with behavioral   CC A
disturbance
Unspecified dementia with aggressive behavior
Unspecified dementia with combative behavior
Unspecified dementia with violent behavior
Use additional code, if applicable, to identify wandering in unspecified dementia (Z91.83)
CC Excl: See code: F02.81

F04 Amnestic disorder due to known physiological condition

Korsakov's psychosis or syndrome, nonalcoholic
Code first the underlying physiological condition
EXCLUDES 1 amnesia NOS (R41.3)
anterograde amnesia (R41.1)
dissociative amnesia (F44.0)
retrograde amnesia (R41.2)
EXCLUDES 2 alcohol-induced or unspecified Korsakov's syndrome (F10.26, F10.96)
Korsakov's syndrome induced by other psychoactive substances (F13.26, F13.96, F19.16, F19.26, F19.96)

F05 Delirium due to known physiological condition   CC

Acute or subacute brain syndrome
Acute or subacute confusional state (nonalcoholic)
Acute or subacute infective psychosis
Acute or subacute organic reaction
Acute or subacute psycho-organic syndrome
Delirium of mixed etiology
Delirium superimposed on dementia
Sundowning
Code first the underlying physiological condition
EXCLUDES 1 delirium NOS (R41.0)
EXCLUDES 2 delirium tremens alcohol-induced or unspecified (F10.231, F10.921)
CC Excl: F05, R45.851

✓4th F06 Other mental disorders due to known physiological condition

INCLUDES mental disorders due to endocrine disorder
mental disorders due to exogenous hormone
mental disorders due to exogenous toxic substance
mental disorders due to primary cerebral disease
mental disorders due to somatic illness
mental disorders due to systemic disease affecting the brain
Code first the underlying physiological condition
EXCLUDES 1 unspecified dementia (F03)
EXCLUDES 2 delirium due to known physiological condition (F05)
dementia as classified in F01-F02
other mental disorders associated with alcohol and other psychoactive substances (F10-F19)

N Newborn: 0   P Pediatric: 0-17   M Maternity: 12-55   A Adult: 15-124   MCC Major CC Condition   PDxMCC PDx acts as own MCC   CC CC Condition   PDxCC PDx acts as own CC

520   ICD-10-CM 2016

F06.0 **Psychotic disorder with hallucinations** due to known physiological condition   `CC`
Organic hallucinatory state (nonalcoholic)
EXCLUDES 2   *hallucinations and perceptual disturbance induced by alcohol and other psychoactive substances (F10-F19 with .151, .251, .951)*
schizophrenia (F20.-)
CC Excl: F02.80-F02.81, F04-F06.8, F10.10-F11.19, F11.21-F13.19, F13.21-F14.19, F14.21-F15.19, F15.21-F16.19, F16.21-F16.99, F17.203-F17.209, F17.213-F17.219, F17.223-F17.229, F17.293-F18.19, F18.21-F19.19, F19.21-F19.99, F53, F55.0-F55.8, R78.0

F06.1 **Catatonic disorder** due to known physiological condition
EXCLUDES 1   *catatonic stupor (R40.1)*
stupor NOS (R40.1)
EXCLUDES 2   *catatonic schizophrenia (F20.2)*
dissociative stupor (F44.2)

F06.2 **Psychotic disorder with delusions** due to known physiological condition   `CC`
Paranoid and paranoid-hallucinatory organic states
Schizophrenia-like psychosis in epilepsy
EXCLUDES 2   *alcohol and drug-induced psychotic disorder (F10-F19 with .150, .250, .950)*
brief psychotic disorder (F23)
delusional disorder (F22)
schizophrenia (F20.-)
CC Excl: See code: F06.0

☑5ᵗʰ **F06.3** **Mood disorder** due to known physiological condition
EXCLUDES 2   *mood disorders due to alcohol and other psychoactive substances (F10-F19 with .14, .24, .94)*
mood disorders, not due to known physiological condition or unspecified (F30-F39)

     F06.30 **Mood disorder** due to known physiological condition, **unspecified**

     F06.31 **Mood disorder** due to known physiological condition with **depressive features**

     F06.32 **Mood disorder** due to known physiological condition with **major depressive-like episode**

     F06.33 **Mood disorder** due to known physiological condition with **manic features**

     F06.34 **Mood disorder** due to known physiological condition with **mixed features**

F06.4 **Anxiety disorder** due to known physiological condition
EXCLUDES 2   *anxiety disorders due to alcohol and other psychoactive substances (F10-F19 with .180, .280, .980)*
anxiety disorders, not due to known physiological condition or unspecified (F40.-, F41.-)

F06.8 **Other specified mental disorders** due to known physiological condition   `HIV`
Epileptic psychosis NOS
Organic dissociative disorder
Organic emotionally labile [asthenic] disorder

☑4ᵗʰ **F07** **Personality and behavioral disorders due to known physiological condition**
Code first the underlying physiological condition

F07.0 **Personality change** due to known physiological condition
Frontal lobe syndrome
Limbic epilepsy personality syndrome
Lobotomy syndrome
Organic personality disorder
Organic pseudopsychopathic personality
Organic pseudoretarded personality
Postleucotomy syndrome
Code first underlying physiological condition
EXCLUDES 1   *mild cognitive impairment (G31.84)*
postconcussional syndrome (F07.81)
postencephalitic syndrome (F07.89)
signs and symptoms involving emotional state (R45.-)
EXCLUDES 2   *specific personality disorder (F60.-)*

☑5ᵗʰ **F07.8** **Other personality and behavioral disorders** due to known physiological condition

     F07.81 **Postconcussional syndrome**
Postcontusional syndrome (encephalopathy)
Post-traumatic brain syndrome, nonpsychotic
Use additional code to identify associated post-traumatic headache, if applicable (G44.3-)
EXCLUDES 1   *current concussion (brain) (S06.0-)*
postencephalitic syndrome (F07.89)

     F07.89 **Other personality and behavioral disorders** due to known physiological condition
Postencephalitic syndrome
Right hemispheric organic affective disorder

F07.9 **Unspecified personality and behavioral disorder** due to known physiological condition   `HIV`
Organic psychosyndrome

F09 **Unspecified mental disorder due to known physiological condition**   `HIV`
Mental disorder NOS due to known physiological condition
Organic brain syndrome NOS
Organic mental disorder NOS
Organic psychosis NOS
Symptomatic psychosis NOS
Code first the underlying physiological condition
EXCLUDES 1   *psychosis NOS (F29)*

Mental and behavioral disorders due to psychoactive substance use (F10-F19)

☑4ᵗʰ **F10** **Alcohol related disorders**
Use additional code for blood alcohol level, if applicable (Y90.-)

> **CC Excl: For CC codes in category F10, unless otherwise noted:** F02.80-F02.81, F04-F06.8, F10.10-F11.19, F11.21-F13.19, F13.21-F14.19, F14.21-F15.19, F15.21-F16.19, F16.21-F16.99, F17.203-F17.209, F17.213-F17.219, F17.223-F17.229, F17.293-F18.19, F18.21-F19.19, F19.21-F19.99, F53, F55.0-F55.8, R78.0

☑5ᵗʰ **F10.1** **Alcohol abuse**
EXCLUDES 1   *alcohol dependence (F10.2-)*
alcohol use, unspecified (F10.9-)

     F10.10 **Alcohol abuse, uncomplicated**

☑6ᵗʰ **F10.12** **Alcohol abuse with intoxication**
     F10.120 **Alcohol abuse with intoxication, uncomplicated**
     F10.121 **Alcohol abuse with intoxication delirium**   `CC`
     F10.129 **Alcohol abuse with intoxication, unspecified**

     F10.14 **Alcohol abuse with alcohol-induced mood disorder**   `CC`

☑6ᵗʰ **F10.15** **Alcohol abuse with alcohol-induced psychotic disorder**
     F10.150 **Alcohol abuse with alcohol-induced psychotic disorder with delusions**
     F10.151 **Alcohol abuse with alcohol-induced psychotic disorder with hallucinations**   `CC`
     F10.159 **Alcohol abuse with alcohol-induced psychotic disorder, unspecified**   `CC`

☑6ᵗʰ **F10.18** **Alcohol abuse with other alcohol-induced disorders**
     F10.180 **Alcohol abuse with alcohol-induced anxiety disorder**   `CC`
     F10.181 **Alcohol abuse with alcohol-induced sexual dysfunction**
     F10.182 **Alcohol abuse with alcohol-induced sleep disorder**
     F10.188 **Alcohol abuse with other alcohol-induced disorder**   `CC`

     F10.19 **Alcohol abuse with unspecified alcohol-induced disorder**   `CC`

☑5ᵗʰ **F10.2** **Alcohol dependence**
EXCLUDES 1   *alcohol abuse (F10.1-)*
alcohol use, unspecified (F10.9-)
EXCLUDES 2   *toxic effect of alcohol (T51.0-)*

     F10.20 **Alcohol dependence, uncomplicated**

     F10.21 **Alcohol dependence, in remission**

☑6ᵗʰ **F10.22** **Alcohol dependence with intoxication**
Acute drunkenness (in alcoholism)
EXCLUDES 1   *alcohol dependence with withdrawal (F10.23-)*
     F10.220 **Alcohol dependence with intoxication, uncomplicated**
     F10.221 **Alcohol dependence with intoxication delirium**   `CC`
     F10.229 **Alcohol dependence with intoxication, unspecified**

☑6ᵗʰ **F10.23** **Alcohol dependence with withdrawal**
EXCLUDES 1   *Alcohol dependence with intoxication (F10.22-)*
     F10.230 **Alcohol dependence with withdrawal, uncomplicated**   `CC`
     F10.231 **Alcohol dependence with withdrawal delirium**   `CC`

☑ Additional Character Required   ☑x7ᵗʰ Placeholder Alert   Unacceptable PDx   ■ Manifestation   Hospital Acquired Condition   *EXCLUDES 1* Not Coded Here   *EXCLUDES 2* Not Included Here

F10.232 **Alcohol dependence with withdrawal with perceptual disturbance** [CC]

F10.239 **Alcohol dependence with withdrawal, unspecified** [CC]

F10.24 **Alcohol dependence with alcohol-induced mood disorder** [CC]

✓6ᵗʰ **F10.25** **Alcohol dependence with alcohol-induced psychotic disorder**

F10.250 **Alcohol dependence with alcohol-induced psychotic disorder with delusions**

F10.251 **Alcohol dependence with alcohol-induced psychotic disorder with hallucinations** [CC]

F10.259 **Alcohol dependence with alcohol-induced psychotic disorder, unspecified** [CC]

F10.26 **Alcohol dependence with alcohol-induced persisting amnestic disorder**

F10.27 **Alcohol dependence with alcohol-induced persisting dementia** [CC]

✓6ᵗʰ **F10.28** **Alcohol dependence with other alcohol-induced disorders**

F10.280 **Alcohol dependence with alcohol-induced anxiety disorder** [CC]

F10.281 **Alcohol dependence with alcohol-induced sexual dysfunction** [CC]

F10.282 **Alcohol dependence with alcohol-induced sleep disorder**

F10.288 **Alcohol dependence with other alcohol-induced disorder** [CC]

F10.29 **Alcohol dependence with unspecified alcohol-induced disorder** [CC]

✓5ᵗʰ **F10.9** **Alcohol use, unspecified**

　EXCLUDES 1　*alcohol abuse (F10.1-)*
　　　　　　alcohol dependence (F10.2-)

✓6ᵗʰ **F10.92** **Alcohol use, unspecified with intoxication**

F10.920 **Alcohol use, unspecified with intoxication, uncomplicated**

F10.921 **Alcohol use, unspecified with intoxication delirium** [CC]

F10.929 **Alcohol use, unspecified with intoxication, unspecified**

F10.94 **Alcohol use, unspecified with alcohol-induced mood disorder** [CC]

✓6ᵗʰ **F10.95** **Alcohol use, unspecified with alcohol-induced psychotic disorder**

F10.950 **Alcohol use, unspecified with alcohol-induced psychotic disorder with delusions**

F10.951 **Alcohol use, unspecified with alcohol-induced psychotic disorder with hallucinations** [CC]

F10.959 **Alcohol use, unspecified with alcohol-induced psychotic disorder, unspecified** [CC]

F10.96 **Alcohol use, unspecified with alcohol-induced persisting amnestic disorder**

F10.97 **Alcohol use, unspecified with alcohol-induced persisting dementia**

✓6ᵗʰ **F10.98** **Alcohol use, unspecified with other alcohol-induced disorders**

F10.980 **Alcohol use, unspecified with alcohol-induced anxiety disorder** [CC]

F10.981 **Alcohol use, unspecified with alcohol-induced sexual dysfunction** [CC]

F10.982 **Alcohol use, unspecified with alcohol-induced sleep disorder**

F10.988 **Alcohol use, unspecified with other alcohol-induced disorder** [CC]

F10.99 **Alcohol use, unspecified with unspecified alcohol-induced disorder** [CC]

✓4ᵗʰ **F11** **Opioid related disorders**

> **CC Excl: For CC codes in category F11, unless otherwise noted:**
> F02.80-F02.81, F04-F06.8, F10.10-F11.19, F11.21-F13.19, F13.21-F14.19, F14.21-F15.19, F15.21-F16.19, F16.21-F16.99, F17.203-F17.209, F17.213-F17.219, F17.223-F17.229, F17.293-F18.19, F18.21-F19.19, F19.21-F19.99, F53, F55.0-F55.8, R78.0

✓5ᵗʰ **F11.1** **Opioid abuse**

　EXCLUDES 1　*opioid dependence (F11.2-)*
　　　　　　opioid use, unspecified (F11.9-)

F11.10 **Opioid abuse, uncomplicated**

✓6ᵗʰ **F11.12** **Opioid abuse with intoxication**

F11.120 **Opioid abuse with intoxication, uncomplicated**

F11.121 **Opioid abuse with intoxication delirium** [CC]

F11.122 **Opioid abuse with intoxication with perceptual disturbance**

F11.129 **Opioid abuse with intoxication, unspecified**

F11.14 **Opioid abuse with opioid-induced mood disorder**

✓6ᵗʰ **F11.15** **Opioid abuse with opioid-induced psychotic disorder**

F11.150 **Opioid abuse with opioid-induced psychotic disorder with delusions** [CC]

F11.151 **Opioid abuse with opioid-induced psychotic disorder with hallucinations** [CC]

F11.159 **Opioid abuse with opioid-induced psychotic disorder, unspecified**

✓6ᵗʰ **F11.18** **Opioid abuse with other opioid-induced disorder**

F11.181 **Opioid abuse with opioid-induced sexual dysfunction**

F11.182 **Opioid abuse with opioid-induced sleep disorder**

F11.188 **Opioid abuse with other opioid-induced disorder**

F11.19 **Opioid abuse with unspecified opioid-induced disorder**

✓5ᵗʰ **F11.2** **Opioid dependence**

　EXCLUDES 1　*opioid abuse (F11.1-)*
　　　　　　opioid use, unspecified (F11.9-)
　EXCLUDES 2　*opioid poisoning (T40.0-T40.2-)*

F11.20 **Opioid dependence, uncomplicated** [CC]
　　　CC Excl: No excl

F11.21 **Opioid dependence, in remission**

✓6ᵗʰ **F11.22** **Opioid dependence with intoxication**
　　　EXCLUDES 1　*opioid dependence with withdrawal (F11.23)*

F11.220 **Opioid dependence with intoxication, uncomplicated**
　　　CC Excl: No excl

F11.221 **Opioid dependence with intoxication delirium** [CC]
　　　CC Excl: F02.80-F02.81, F04- F06.8, F10.10-F11.19, F11.21-F13.19, F13.21- F14.19, F14.21-F15.19, F15.21-F16.19, F16.21-F16.99, F17.203-F17.209, F17.213- F17.219, F17.223-F17.229, F17.293-F18.19, F18.21-F19.19, F19.21-F19.99, F53, F55.0-F55.8, R78.0

F11.222 **Opioid dependence with intoxication with perceptual disturbance** [CC]
　　　CC Excl: No excl

F11.229 **Opioid dependence with intoxication, unspecified**

F11.23 **Opioid dependence with withdrawal** [CC]
　　　EXCLUDES 1　*opioid dependence with intoxication (F11.22-)*
　　　CC Excl: See code: F11.221

F11.24 **Opioid dependence with opioid-induced mood disorder**

✓6ᵗʰ **F11.25** **Opioid dependence with opioid-induced psychotic disorder**

F11.250 **Opioid dependence with opioid-induced psychotic disorder with delusions** [CC]
　　　CC Excl: See code: F11.221

F11.251 **Opioid dependence with opioid-induced psychotic disorder with hallucinations** [CC]
　　　CC Excl: See code: F11.221

F11.259   Opioid dependence with opioid-induced psychotic disorder, unspecified   CC
     CC Excl: No excl

✓6th   **F11.28**   Opioid dependence with other opioid-induced disorder

F11.281   Opioid dependence with opioid-induced sexual dysfunction   CC
     CC Excl: No excl

F11.282   Opioid dependence with opioid-induced sleep disorder   CC
     CC Excl: No excl

F11.288   Opioid dependence with other opioid-induced disorder   CC
     CC Excl: No excl

F11.29   Opioid dependence with unspecified opioid-induced disorder

✓5th   **F11.9**   Opioid use, unspecified
     EXCLUDES 1   opioid abuse (F11.1-)
                   opioid dependence (F11.2-)

F11.90   Opioid use, unspecified, uncomplicated

✓6th   **F11.92**   Opioid use, unspecified with intoxication
     EXCLUDES 1   opioid use, unspecified with withdrawal (F11.93)

F11.920   Opioid use, unspecified with intoxication, uncomplicated

F11.921   Opioid use, unspecified with intoxication delirium   CC
     CC Excl: See code: F11.221

F11.922   Opioid use, unspecified with intoxication with perceptual disturbance

F11.929   Opioid use, unspecified with intoxication, unspecified

F11.93   Opioid use, unspecified with withdrawal   CC
     EXCLUDES 1   opioid use, unspecified with intoxication (F11.92-)
     CC Excl: See code: F11.221

F11.94   Opioid use, unspecified with opioid-induced mood disorder

✓6th   **F11.95**   Opioid use, unspecified with opioid-induced psychotic disorder

F11.950   Opioid use, unspecified with opioid-induced psychotic disorder with delusions   CC
     CC Excl: See code: F11.221

F11.951   Opioid use, unspecified with opioid-induced psychotic disorder with hallucinations   CC
     CC Excl: See code: F11.221

F11.959   Opioid use, unspecified with opioid-induced psychotic disorder, unspecified

✓6th   **F11.98**   Opioid use, unspecified with other specified opioid-induced disorder

F11.981   Opioid use, unspecified with opioid-induced sexual dysfunction

F11.982   Opioid use, unspecified with opioid-induced sleep disorder

F11.988   Opioid use, unspecified with other opioid-induced disorder

F11.99   Opioid use, unspecified with unspecified opioid-induced disorder

✓4th   **F12**   **Cannabis related disorders**
     INCLUDES   marijuana

CC Excl: For CC codes in category F12, unless otherwise noted:
F02.80-F02.81, F04-F06.8, F10.10-F11.19, F11.21-F13.19, F13.21-F14.19, F14.21-F15.19, F15.21-F16.19, F16.21-F16.99, F17.203-F17.209, F17.213-F17.219, F17.223-F17.229, F17.293-F18.19, F18.21-F19.19, F19.21-F19.99, F53, F55.0-F55.8, R78.0

✓5th   **F12.1**   Cannabis abuse
     EXCLUDES 1   cannabis dependence (F12.2-)
                   cannabis use, unspecified (F12.9-)

F12.10   Cannabis abuse, uncomplicated

✓6th   **F12.12**   Cannabis abuse with intoxication

F12.120   Cannabis abuse with intoxication, uncomplicated

F12.121   Cannabis abuse with intoxication delirium   CC

F12.122   Cannabis abuse with intoxication with perceptual disturbance

F12.129   Cannabis abuse with intoxication, unspecified

✓6th   **F12.15**   Cannabis abuse with psychotic disorder

F12.150   Cannabis abuse with psychotic disorder with delusions   CC

F12.151   Cannabis abuse with psychotic disorder with hallucinations   CC

F12.159   Cannabis abuse with psychotic disorder, unspecified

✓6th   **F12.18**   Cannabis abuse with other cannabis-induced disorder

F12.180   Cannabis abuse with cannabis-induced anxiety disorder

F12.188   Cannabis abuse with other cannabis-induced disorder

F12.19   Cannabis abuse with unspecified cannabis-induced disorder

✓5th   **F12.2**   Cannabis dependence
     EXCLUDES 1   cannabis abuse (F12.1-)
                   cannabis use, unspecified (F12.9-)
     EXCLUDES 2   cannabis poisoning (T40.7-)

F12.20   Cannabis dependence, uncomplicated

F12.21   Cannabis dependence, in remission

✓6th   **F12.22**   Cannabis dependence with intoxication

F12.220   Cannabis dependence with intoxication, uncomplicated

F12.221   Cannabis dependence with intoxication delirium   CC

F12.222   Cannabis dependence with intoxication with perceptual disturbance

F12.229   Cannabis dependence with intoxication, unspecified

✓6th   **F12.25**   Cannabis dependence with psychotic disorder

F12.250   Cannabis dependence with psychotic disorder with delusions   CC

F12.251   Cannabis dependence with psychotic disorder with hallucinations   CC

F12.259   Cannabis dependence with psychotic disorder, unspecified

✓6th   **F12.28**   Cannabis dependence with other cannabis-induced disorder

F12.280   Cannabis dependence with cannabis-induced anxiety disorder

F12.288   Cannabis dependence with other cannabis-induced disorder

F12.29   Cannabis dependence with unspecified cannabis-induced disorder

✓5th   **F12.9**   Cannabis use, unspecified
     EXCLUDES 1   cannabis abuse (F12.1-)
                   cannabis dependence (F12.2-)

F12.90   Cannabis use, unspecified, uncomplicated

✓6th   **F12.92**   Cannabis use, unspecified with intoxication

F12.920   Cannabis use, unspecified with intoxication, uncomplicated

F12.921   Cannabis use, unspecified with intoxication delirium   CC

F12.922   Cannabis use, unspecified with intoxication with perceptual disturbance

F12.929   Cannabis use, unspecified with intoxication, unspecified

✓6th   **F12.95**   Cannabis use, unspecified with psychotic disorder

F12.950   Cannabis use, unspecified with psychotic disorder with delusions   CC

F12.951   Cannabis use, unspecified with psychotic disorder with hallucinations   CC

F12.959   Cannabis use, unspecified with psychotic disorder, unspecified

✓6th   **F12.98**   Cannabis use, unspecified with other cannabis-induced disorder

F12.980   Cannabis use, unspecified with anxiety disorder

F12.988   Cannabis use, unspecified with other cannabis-induced disorder

F12.99   Cannabis use, unspecified with unspecified cannabis-induced disorder

---

✓ Additional Character Required   ✓x7th Placeholder Alert   Unacceptable PDx   Manifestation   Hospital Acquired Condition   **EXCLUDES 1** Not Coded Here   **EXCLUDES 2** Not Included Here

✓4th **F13** **Sedative, hypnotic, or anxiolytic related disorders**

> **CC Excl: For CC codes in category F13, unless otherwise noted:**
> F02.80-F02.81, F04-F06.8, F10.10-F11.19, F11.21-F13.19, F13.21-
> F14.19, F14.21-F15.19, F15.21-F16.19, F16.21-F16.99, F17.203-
> F17.209, F17.213-F17.219, F17.223-F17.229, F17.293- F18.19, F18.21-
> F19.19, F19.21-F19.99, F53, F55.0-F55.8, R78.0

✓5th **F13.1** **Sedative, hypnotic or anxiolytic-related abuse**

> *EXCLUDES 1*   *sedative, hypnotic or anxiolytic-related dependence (F13.2-)*
> *sedative, hypnotic, or anxiolytic use, unspecified (F13.9-)*

F13.10 **Sedative, hypnotic or anxiolytic abuse, uncomplicated**

✓6th **F13.12** **Sedative, hypnotic or anxiolytic abuse with intoxication**

     F13.120 **Sedative, hypnotic or anxiolytic abuse with intoxication, uncomplicated**

     F13.121 **Sedative, hypnotic or anxiolytic abuse with intoxication delirium**   CC

     F13.129 **Sedative, hypnotic or anxiolytic abuse with intoxication, unspecified**

F13.14 **Sedative, hypnotic or anxiolytic abuse with sedative, hypnotic or anxiolytic-induced mood disorder**

✓6th **F13.15** **Sedative, hypnotic or anxiolytic abuse with sedative, hypnotic or anxiolytic-induced psychotic disorder**

     F13.150 **Sedative, hypnotic or anxiolytic abuse with sedative, hypnotic or anxiolytic-induced psychotic disorder with delusions**   CC

     F13.151 **Sedative, hypnotic or anxiolytic abuse with sedative, hypnotic or anxiolytic-induced psychotic disorder with hallucinations**   CC

     F13.159 **Sedative, hypnotic or anxiolytic abuse with sedative, hypnotic or anxiolytic-induced psychotic disorder, unspecified**

✓6th **F13.18** **Sedative, hypnotic or anxiolytic abuse with other sedative, hypnotic or anxiolytic-induced disorders**

     F13.180 **Sedative, hypnotic or anxiolytic abuse with sedative, hypnotic or anxiolytic-induced anxiety disorder**

     F13.181 **Sedative, hypnotic or anxiolytic abuse with sedative, hypnotic or anxiolytic-induced sexual dysfunction**

     F13.182 **Sedative, hypnotic or anxiolytic abuse with sedative, hypnotic or anxiolytic-induced sleep disorder**

     F13.188 **Sedative, hypnotic or anxiolytic abuse with other sedative, hypnotic or anxiolytic-induced disorder**

F13.19 **Sedative, hypnotic or anxiolytic abuse with unspecified sedative, hypnotic or anxiolytic-induced disorder**

✓5th **F13.2** **Sedative, hypnotic or anxiolytic-related dependence**

> *EXCLUDES 1*   *sedative, hypnotic or anxiolytic-related abuse (F13.1-)*
> *sedative, hypnotic, or anxiolytic use, unspecified (F13.9-)*
> *EXCLUDES 2*   *sedative, hypnotic, or anxiolytic poisoning (T42.-)*

F13.20 **Sedative, hypnotic or anxiolytic dependence, uncomplicated**   CC
     CC Excl: No excl

F13.21 **Sedative, hypnotic or anxiolytic dependence, in remission**

✓6th **F13.22** **Sedative, hypnotic or anxiolytic dependence with intoxication**

> *EXCLUDES 1*   *sedative, hypnotic or anxiolytic dependence with withdrawal (F13.23-)*

     F13.220 **Sedative, hypnotic or anxiolytic dependence with intoxication, uncomplicated**

     F13.221 **Sedative, hypnotic or anxiolytic dependence with intoxication delirium**   CC
         CC Excl: See code: F13

     F13.229 **Sedative, hypnotic or anxiolytic dependence with intoxication, unspecified**

✓6th **F13.23** **Sedative, hypnotic or anxiolytic dependence with withdrawal**

> *EXCLUDES 1*   *sedative, hypnotic or anxiolytic dependence with intoxication (F13.22-)*

     F13.230 **Sedative, hypnotic or anxiolytic dependence with withdrawal, uncomplicated**   CC
         CC Excl: See code: F13

     F13.231 **Sedative, hypnotic or anxiolytic dependence with withdrawal delirium**   CC
         CC Excl: See code: F13

     F13.232 **Sedative, hypnotic or anxiolytic dependence with withdrawal with perceptual disturbance**   CC
         CC Excl: See code: F13

     F13.239 **Sedative, hypnotic or anxiolytic dependence with withdrawal, unspecified**   CC
         CC Excl: See code: F13

F13.24 **Sedative, hypnotic or anxiolytic dependence with sedative, hypnotic or anxiolytic-induced mood disorder**

✓6th **F13.25** **Sedative, hypnotic or anxiolytic dependence with sedative, hypnotic or anxiolytic-induced psychotic disorder**

     F13.250 **Sedative, hypnotic or anxiolytic dependence with sedative, hypnotic or anxiolytic-induced psychotic disorder with delusions**   CC
         CC Excl: See code: F13

     F13.251 **Sedative, hypnotic or anxiolytic dependence with sedative, hypnotic or anxiolytic-induced psychotic disorder with hallucinations**   CC
         CC Excl: See code: F13

     F13.259 **Sedative, hypnotic or anxiolytic dependence with sedative, hypnotic or anxiolytic-induced psychotic disorder, unspecified**   CC
         CC Excl: No Excl

F13.26 **Sedative, hypnotic or anxiolytic dependence with sedative, hypnotic or anxiolytic-induced persisting amnestic disorder**   CC
     CC Excl: No Excl

F13.27 **Sedative, hypnotic or anxiolytic dependence with sedative, hypnotic or anxiolytic-induced persisting dementia**   CC
     CC Excl: See code: F13

✓6th **F13.28** **Sedative, hypnotic or anxiolytic dependence with other sedative, hypnotic or anxiolytic-induced disorders**

     F13.280 **Sedative, hypnotic or anxiolytic dependence with sedative, hypnotic or anxiolytic-induced anxiety disorder**   CC
         CC Excl: No Excl

     F13.281 **Sedative, hypnotic or anxiolytic dependence with sedative, hypnotic or anxiolytic-induced sexual dysfunction**   CC
         CC Excl: No Excl

     F13.282 **Sedative, hypnotic or anxiolytic dependence with sedative, hypnotic or anxiolytic-induced sleep disorder**   CC
         CC Excl: No Excl

     F13.288 **Sedative, hypnotic or anxiolytic dependence with other sedative, hypnotic or anxiolytic-induced disorder**   CC
         CC Excl: No Excl

F13.29 **Sedative, hypnotic or anxiolytic dependence with unspecified sedative, hypnotic or anxiolytic-induced disorder**

✓5th **F13.9** **Sedative, hypnotic or anxiolytic-related use, unspecified**

> *EXCLUDES 1*   *sedative, hypnotic or anxiolytic-related abuse (F13.1-)*
> *sedative, hypnotic or anxiolytic-related dependence (F13.2-)*

F13.90 **Sedative, hypnotic, or anxiolytic use, unspecified, uncomplicated**

✓6th **F13.92** **Sedative, hypnotic or anxiolytic use, unspecified with intoxication**

> *EXCLUDES 1*   *sedative, hypnotic or anxiolytic use, unspecified with withdrawal (F13.93-)*

N Newborn: 0   P Pediatric: 0-17   M Maternity: 12-55   A Adult: 15-124   MCC Major CC Condition   PDxMCC PDx acts as own MCC   CC CC Condition   PDxCC PDx acts as own CC

F13.920   Sedative, hypnotic or anxiolytic use, unspecified with intoxication, uncomplicated

F13.921   Sedative, hypnotic or anxiolytic use, unspecified with intoxication delirium   `CC`

F13.929   Sedative, hypnotic or anxiolytic use, unspecified with intoxication, unspecified

✓6th **F13.93**   Sedative, hypnotic or anxiolytic use, unspecified with withdrawal

> EXCLUDES 1   *sedative, hypnotic or anxiolytic use, unspecified with intoxication (F13.92-)*

F13.930   Sedative, hypnotic or anxiolytic use, unspecified with withdrawal, uncomplicated   `CC`

F13.931   Sedative, hypnotic or anxiolytic use, unspecified with withdrawal delirium   `CC`

F13.932   Sedative, hypnotic or anxiolytic use, unspecified with withdrawal with perceptual disturbances   `CC`

F13.939   Sedative, hypnotic or anxiolytic use, unspecified with withdrawal, unspecified   `CC`

F13.94   Sedative, hypnotic or anxiolytic use, unspecified with sedative, hypnotic or anxiolytic-induced mood disorder

✓6th **F13.95**   Sedative, hypnotic or anxiolytic use, unspecified with sedative, hypnotic or anxiolytic-induced psychotic disorder

F13.950   Sedative, hypnotic or anxiolytic use, unspecified with sedative, hypnotic or anxiolytic-induced psychotic disorder with delusions   `CC`

F13.951   Sedative, hypnotic or anxiolytic use, unspecified with sedative, hypnotic or anxiolytic-induced psychotic disorder with hallucinations   `CC`

F13.959   Sedative, hypnotic or anxiolytic use, unspecified with sedative, hypnotic or anxiolytic-induced psychotic disorder, unspecified

F13.96   Sedative, hypnotic or anxiolytic use, unspecified with sedative, hypnotic or anxiolytic-induced persisting amnestic disorder

F13.97   Sedative, hypnotic or anxiolytic use, unspecified with sedative, hypnotic or anxiolytic-induced persisting dementia   `CC`

✓6th **F13.98**   Sedative, hypnotic or anxiolytic use, unspecified with other sedative, hypnotic or anxiolytic-induced disorders

F13.980   Sedative, hypnotic or anxiolytic use, unspecified with sedative, hypnotic or anxiolytic-induced anxiety disorder

F13.981   Sedative, hypnotic or anxiolytic use, unspecified with sedative, hypnotic or anxiolytic-induced sexual dysfunction

F13.982   Sedative, hypnotic or anxiolytic use, unspecified with sedative, hypnotic or anxiolytic-induced sleep disorder

F13.988   Sedative, hypnotic or anxiolytic use, unspecified with other sedative, hypnotic or anxiolytic-induced disorder

F13.99   Sedative, hypnotic or anxiolytic use, unspecified with unspecified sedative, hypnotic or anxiolytic-induced disorder

✓4th **F14**   **Cocaine related disorders**

> EXCLUDES 2   *other stimulant-related disorders (F15.-)*

CC Excl: For CC codes in category F14, unless otherwise noted:
F02.80-F02.81, F04-F06.8, F10.10-F11.19, F11.21-F13.19, F13.21-F14.19, F14.21-F15.19, F15.21-F16.19, F16.21-F16.99, F17.203-F17.209, F17.213-F17.219, F17.223-F17.229, F17.293-F18.19, F18.21-F19.19, F19.21-F19.99, F53, F55.0-F55.8, R78.0

✓5th **F14.1**   Cocaine abuse

> EXCLUDES 1   *cocaine dependence (F14.2-)*
> *cocaine use, unspecified (F14.9-)*

F14.10   Cocaine abuse, uncomplicated

✓6th **F14.12**   Cocaine abuse with intoxication

F14.120   Cocaine abuse with intoxication, uncomplicated

F14.121   Cocaine abuse with intoxication with delirium   `CC`

F14.122   Cocaine abuse with intoxication with perceptual disturbance

F14.129   Cocaine abuse with intoxication, unspecified

F14.14   Cocaine abuse with cocaine-induced mood disorder

✓6th **F14.15**   Cocaine abuse with cocaine-induced psychotic disorder

F14.150   Cocaine abuse with cocaine-induced psychotic disorder with delusions   `CC`

F14.151   Cocaine abuse with cocaine-induced psychotic disorder with hallucinations   `CC`

F14.159   Cocaine abuse with cocaine-induced psychotic disorder, unspecified

✓6th **F14.18**   Cocaine abuse with other cocaine-induced disorder

F14.180   Cocaine abuse with cocaine-induced anxiety disorder

F14.181   Cocaine abuse with cocaine-induced sexual dysfunction

F14.182   Cocaine abuse with cocaine-induced sleep disorder

F14.188   Cocaine abuse with other cocaine-induced disorder

F14.19   Cocaine abuse with unspecified cocaine-induced disorder

✓5th **F14.2**   Cocaine dependence

> EXCLUDES 1   *cocaine abuse (F14.1-)*
> *cocaine use, unspecified (F14.9-)*
> EXCLUDES 2   *cocaine poisoning (T40.5-)*

F14.20   Cocaine dependence, uncomplicated   `CC`
     CC Excl: No Excl

F14.21   Cocaine dependence, in remission

✓6th **F14.22**   Cocaine dependence with intoxication

> EXCLUDES 1   *cocaine dependence with withdrawal (F14.23)*

F14.220   Cocaine dependence with intoxication, uncomplicated

F14.221   Cocaine dependence with intoxication delirium   `CC`

F14.222   Cocaine dependence with intoxication with perceptual disturbance   `CC`
     CC Excl: No Excl

F14.229   Cocaine dependence with intoxication, unspecified   `CC`
     CC Excl: No Excl

F14.23   Cocaine dependence with withdrawal   `CC`

> EXCLUDES 1   *cocaine dependence with intoxication (F14.22-)*

F14.24   Cocaine dependence with cocaine-induced mood disorder

✓6th **F14.25**   Cocaine dependence with cocaine-induced psychotic disorder

F14.250   Cocaine dependence with cocaine-induced psychotic disorder with delusions   `CC`

F14.251   Cocaine dependence with cocaine-induced psychotic disorder with hallucinations   `CC`

F14.259   Cocaine dependence with cocaine-induced psychotic disorder, unspecified   `CC`
     CC Excl: No Excl

✓6th **F14.28**   Cocaine dependence with other cocaine-induced disorder

F14.280   Cocaine dependence with cocaine-induced anxiety disorder   `CC`
     CC Excl: No Excl

F14.281   Cocaine dependence with cocaine-induced sexual dysfunction   `CC`
     CC Excl: No Excl

F14.282   Cocaine dependence with cocaine-induced sleep disorder   `CC`
     CC Excl: No Excl

F14.288   Cocaine dependence with other cocaine-induced disorder   `CC`
     CC Excl: No Excl

F14.29   Cocaine dependence with unspecified cocaine-induced disorder

✓5th **F14.9**   Cocaine use, unspecified
> EXCLUDES 1   cocaine abuse (F14.1-)
>   cocaine dependence (F14.2-)

     F14.90   Cocaine use, unspecified, uncomplicated

✓6th   **F14.92**   Cocaine use, unspecified with intoxication
         F14.920   Cocaine use, unspecified with intoxication, uncomplicated
         F14.921   Cocaine use, unspecified with intoxication delirium   CC
         F14.922   Cocaine use, unspecified with intoxication with perceptual disturbance
         F14.929   Cocaine use, unspecified with intoxication, unspecified

     F14.94   Cocaine use, unspecified with cocaine-induced mood disorder

✓6th   **F14.95**   Cocaine use, unspecified with cocaine-induced psychotic disorder
         F14.950   Cocaine use, unspecified with cocaine-induced psychotic disorder with delusions   CC
         F14.951   Cocaine use, unspecified with cocaine-induced psychotic disorder with hallucinations   CC
         F14.959   Cocaine use, unspecified with cocaine-induced psychotic disorder, unspecified

✓6th   **F14.98**   Cocaine use, unspecified with other specified cocaine-induced disorder
         F14.980   Cocaine use, unspecified with cocaine-induced anxiety disorder
         F14.981   Cocaine use, unspecified with cocaine-induced sexual dysfunction
         F14.982   Cocaine use, unspecified with cocaine-induced sleep disorder
         F14.988   Cocaine use, unspecified with other cocaine-induced disorder

     F14.99   Cocaine use, unspecified with unspecified cocaine-induced disorder

✓4th **F15**   **Other stimulant related disorders**
> INCLUDES   amphetamine-related disorders
>   caffeine
> EXCLUDES 2   cocaine-related disorders (F14.-)

> **CC Excl: For CC codes in category F15, unless otherwise noted:**
> F02.80-F02.81, F04-F06.8, F10.10-F11.19, F11.21-F13.19, F13.21-
> F14.19, F14.21-F15.19, F15.21-F16.19, F16.21-F16.99, F17.203-
> F17.209, F17.213-F17.219, F17.223-F17.229, F17.293-F18.19, F18.21-
> F19.19, F19.21-F19.99, F53, F55.0-F55.8, R78.0

✓5th **F15.1**   Other stimulant abuse
> EXCLUDES 1   other stimulant dependence (F15.2-)
>   other stimulant use, unspecified (F15.9-)

     F15.10   Other stimulant abuse, uncomplicated

✓6th   **F15.12**   Other stimulant abuse with intoxication
         F15.120   Other stimulant abuse with intoxication, uncomplicated
         F15.121   Other stimulant abuse with intoxication delirium   CC
         F15.122   Other stimulant abuse with intoxication with perceptual disturbance
         F15.129   Other stimulant abuse with intoxication, unspecified

     F15.14   Other stimulant abuse with stimulant-induced mood disorder

✓6th   **F15.15**   Other stimulant abuse with stimulant-induced psychotic disorder
         F15.150   Other stimulant abuse with stimulant-induced psychotic disorder with delusions   CC
         F15.151   Other stimulant abuse with stimulant-induced psychotic disorder with hallucinations   CC
         F15.159   Other stimulant abuse with stimulant-induced psychotic disorder, unspecified

✓6th   **F15.18**   Other stimulant abuse with other stimulant-induced disorder
         F15.180   Other stimulant abuse with stimulant-induced anxiety disorder

         F15.181   Other stimulant abuse with stimulant-induced sexual dysfunction
         F15.182   Other stimulant abuse with stimulant-induced sleep disorder
         F15.188   Other stimulant abuse with other stimulant-induced disorder

     F15.19   Other stimulant abuse with unspecified stimulant-induced disorder

✓5th **F15.2**   Other stimulant dependence
> EXCLUDES 1   other stimulant abuse (F15.1-)
>   other stimulant use, unspecified (F15.9-)

     F15.20   Other stimulant dependence, uncomplicated   CC
         CC Excl: No Excl

     F15.21   Other stimulant dependence, in remission

✓6th   **F15.22**   Other stimulant dependence with intoxication
> EXCLUDES 1   other stimulant dependence with withdrawal (F15.23)

         F15.220   Other stimulant dependence with intoxication, uncomplicated
         F15.221   Other stimulant dependence with intoxication delirium   CC
         F15.222   Other stimulant dependence with intoxication with perceptual disturbance   CC
           CC Excl: No Excl
         F15.229   Other stimulant dependence with intoxication, unspecified

     F15.23   Other stimulant dependence with withdrawal   CC
> EXCLUDES 1   other stimulant dependence with intoxication (F15.22-)

     F15.24   Other stimulant dependence with stimulant-induced mood disorder

✓6th   **F15.25**   Other stimulant dependence with stimulant-induced psychotic disorder
         F15.250   Other stimulant dependence with stimulant-induced psychotic disorder with delusions   CC
         F15.251   Other stimulant dependence with stimulant-induced psychotic disorder with hallucinations   CC
         F15.259   Other stimulant dependence with stimulant-induced psychotic disorder, unspecified   CC
           CC Excl: No Excl

✓6th   **F15.28**   Other stimulant dependence with other stimulant-induced disorder
         F15.280   Other stimulant dependence with stimulant-induced anxiety disorder   CC
           CC Excl: No Excl
         F15.281   Other stimulant dependence with stimulant-induced sexual dysfunction   CC
           CC Excl: No Excl
         F15.282   Other stimulant dependence with stimulant-induced sleep disorder   CC
           CC Excl: No Excl
         F15.288   Other stimulant dependence with other stimulant-induced disorder   CC
           CC Excl: No Excl

     F15.29   Other stimulant dependence with unspecified stimulant-induced disorder

✓5th **F15.9**   Other stimulant use, unspecified
> EXCLUDES 1   other stimulant abuse (F15.1-)
>   other stimulant dependence (F15.2-)

     F15.90   Other stimulant use, unspecified, uncomplicated

✓6th   **F15.92**   Other stimulant use, unspecified with intoxication
> EXCLUDES 1   other stimulant use, unspecified with withdrawal (F15.93)

         F15.920   Other stimulant use, unspecified with intoxication, uncomplicated
         F15.921   Other stimulant use, unspecified with intoxication delirium   CC
         F15.922   Other stimulant use, unspecified with intoxication with perceptual disturbance
         F15.929   Other stimulant use, unspecified with intoxication, unspecified

     F15.93   Other stimulant use, unspecified with withdrawal   CC
> EXCLUDES 1   other stimulant use, unspecified with intoxication (F15.92-)

N Newborn: 0   P Pediatric: 0-17   M Maternity: 12-55   A Adult: 15-124   MCC Major CC Condition   PDxMCC PDx acts as own MCC   CC CC Condition   PDxCC PDx acts as own CC

F15.94   **Other stimulant use, unspecified with stimulant-induced** mood disorder

✓6ᵗʰ F15.95   **Other stimulant use, unspecified with stimulant-induced** psychotic disorder

F15.950   **Other stimulant use, unspecified with stimulant-induced psychotic disorder with** delusions [cc]

F15.951   **Other stimulant use, unspecified with stimulant-induced psychotic disorder with** hallucinations [cc]

F15.959   **Other stimulant use, unspecified with stimulant-induced psychotic disorder,** unspecified

✓6ᵗʰ F15.98   **Other stimulant use, unspecified with** other **stimulant-induced disorder**

F15.980   **Other stimulant use, unspecified with stimulant-induced** anxiety disorder

F15.981   **Other stimulant use, unspecified with stimulant-induced** sexual dysfunction

F15.982   **Other stimulant use, unspecified with stimulant-induced** sleep disorder

F15.988   **Other stimulant use, unspecified with** other **stimulant-induced disorder**

F15.99   **Other stimulant use, unspecified with** unspecified **stimulant-induced disorder**

✓4ᵗʰ **F16   Hallucinogen related disorders**
INCLUDES	ecstasy
	PCP
	phencyclidine

CC Excl: For CC codes in category F16, unless otherwise noted:
F02.80-F02.81, F04-F06.8, F10.10-F11.19, F11.21-F13.19, F13.21-F14.19, F14.21-F15.19, F15.21-F16.19, F16.21-F16.99, F17.203-F17.209, F17.213-F17.219, F17.223-F17.229, F17.293-F18.19, F18.21-F19.19, F19.21-F19.99, F53, F55.0-F55.8, R78.0

✓5ᵗʰ F16.1   **Hallucinogen** abuse
| EXCLUDES 1 | *hallucinogen dependence (F16.2-)* |
| | *hallucinogen use, unspecified (F16.9-)* |

F16.10   **Hallucinogen abuse,** uncomplicated

✓6ᵗʰ F16.12   **Hallucinogen abuse with** intoxication

F16.120   **Hallucinogen abuse with intoxication,** uncomplicated

F16.121   **Hallucinogen abuse with intoxication with** delirium [cc]

F16.122   **Hallucinogen abuse with intoxication with** perceptual disturbance

F16.129   **Hallucinogen abuse with intoxication,** unspecified

F16.14   **Hallucinogen abuse with hallucinogen-induced** mood disorder

✓6ᵗʰ F16.15   **Hallucinogen abuse with hallucinogen-induced** psychotic disorder

F16.150   **Hallucinogen abuse with hallucinogen-induced psychotic disorder with** delusions [cc]

F16.151   **Hallucinogen abuse with hallucinogen-induced psychotic disorder with** hallucinations [cc]

F16.159   **Hallucinogen abuse with hallucinogen-induced psychotic disorder,** unspecified

✓6ᵗʰ F16.18   **Hallucinogen abuse with** other **hallucinogen-induced disorder**

F16.180   **Hallucinogen abuse with hallucinogen-induced** anxiety disorder

F16.183   **Hallucinogen abuse with hallucinogen-induced** persisting perception disorder (flashbacks)

F16.188   **Hallucinogen abuse with** other **hallucinogen-induced disorder**

F16.19   **Hallucinogen abuse with** unspecified **hallucinogen-induced disorder**

✓5ᵗʰ F16.2   **Hallucinogen** dependence
| EXCLUDES 1 | *hallucinogen abuse (F16.1-)* |
| | *hallucinoge n use, unspecified (F16.9-)* |

F16.20   **Hallucinogen dependence,** uncomplicated [cc]
         CC Excl: No Excl

F16.21   **Hallucinogen dependence,** in remission

✓6ᵗʰ F16.22   **Hallucinogen dependence with** intoxication

F16.220   **Hallucinogen dependence with intoxication,** uncomplicated

F16.221   **Hallucinogen dependence with intoxication with** delirium [cc]

F16.229   **Hallucinogen dependence with intoxication,** unspecified

F16.24   **Hallucinogen dependence with hallucinogen-induced** mood disorder

✓6ᵗʰ F16.25   **Hallucinogen dependence with hallucinogen-induced** psychotic disorder

F16.250   **Hallucinogen dependence with hallucinogen-induced psychotic disorder with** delusions [cc]

F16.251   **Hallucinogen dependence with hallucinogen-induced psychotic disorder with** hallucinations [cc]

F16.259   **Hallucinogen dependence with hallucinogen-induced psychotic disorder,** unspecified [cc]
         CC Excl: No Excl

✓6ᵗʰ F16.28   **Hallucinogen dependence with** other **hallucinogen-induced disorder**

F16.280   **Hallucinogen dependence with hallucinogen-induced** anxiety disorder [cc]
         CC Excl: No Excl

F16.283   **Hallucinogen dependence with hallucinogen** persisting perception disorder (flashbacks) [cc]
         CC Excl: No Excl

F16.288   **Hallucinogen dependence with** other **hallucinogen-induced disorder** [cc]
         CC Excl: No Excl

F16.29   **Hallucinogen dependence with** unspecified **hallucinogen-induced disorder**

✓5ᵗʰ F16.9   **Hallucinogen use,** unspecified
| EXCLUDES 1 | *hallucinogen abuse (F16.1-)* |
| | *hallucinogen dependence (F16.2-)* |

F16.90   **Hallucinogen use, unspecified,** uncomplicated

✓6ᵗʰ F16.92   **Hallucinogen use, unspecified with** intoxication

F16.920   **Hallucinogen use, unspecified with intoxication,** uncomplicated

F16.921   **Hallucinogen use, unspecified with intoxication with** delirium [cc]

F16.929   **Hallucinogen use, unspecified with intoxication,** unspecified

F16.94   **Hallucinogen use, unspecified with hallucinogen-induced** mood disorder

✓6ᵗʰ F16.95   **Hallucinogen use, unspecified with hallucinogen-induced** psychotic disorder

F16.950   **Hallucinogen use, unspecified with hallucinogen-induced psychotic disorder with** delusions [cc]

F16.951   **Hallucinogen use, unspecified with hallucinogen-induced psychotic disorder with** hallucinations [cc]

F16.959   **Hallucinogen use, unspecified with hallucinogen-induced psychotic disorder,** unspecified

✓6ᵗʰ F16.98   **Hallucinogen use, unspecified with** other **specified hallucinogen-induced disorder**

F16.980   **Hallucinogen use, unspecified with hallucinogen-induced** anxiety disorder

F16.983   **Hallucinogen use, unspecified with hallucinogen** persisting perception disorder (flashbacks)

F16.988   **Hallucinogen use, unspecified with** other **hallucinogen-induced disorder**

F16.99   **Hallucinogen use, unspecified with** unspecified **hallucinogen-induced disorder**

✓4ᵗʰ F17   Nicotine dependence

    EXCLUDES 1   history of tobacco dependence (Z87.891)
         tobacco use NOS (Z72.0)
    EXCLUDES 2   tobacco use (smoking) during pregnancy, childbirth and the puerperium (O99.33-)
         toxic effect of nicotine (T65.2-)
    AHA: 2013, 4Q, 108-109

> **CC Excl: For CC codes in category F17, unless otherwise noted:**
> F02.80-F02.81, F04-F06.8, F10.10-F11.19, F11.21-F13.19, F13.21-
> F14.19, F14.21-F15.19, F15.21-F16.19, F16.21-F16.99, F17.203-
> F17.209, F17.213-F17.219, F17.223-F17.229, F17.293-F18.19, F18.21-
> F19.19, F19.21-F19.99, F53, F55.0-F55.8, R78.0

✓5ᵗʰ F17.2   Nicotine dependence

   ✓6ᵗʰ F17.20   Nicotine dependence, unspecified
      F17.200   Nicotine dependence, unspecified, uncomplicated
      F17.201   Nicotine dependence, unspecified, in remission
      F17.203   Nicotine dependence unspecified, withdrawal   CC
      F17.208   Nicotine dependence, unspecified, with other nicotine-induced disorders
      F17.209   Nicotine dependence, unspecified, with unspecified nicotine-induced disorders

   ✓6ᵗʰ F17.21   Nicotine dependence, cigarettes
      F17.210   Nicotine dependence, cigarettes, uncomplicated
      F17.211   Nicotine dependence, cigarettes, in remission
      F17.213   Nicotine dependence, cigarettes, with withdrawal   CC
      F17.218   Nicotine dependence, cigarettes, with other nicotine-induced disorders
      F17.219   Nicotine dependence, cigarettes, with unspecified nicotine-induced disorders

   ✓6ᵗʰ F17.22   Nicotine dependence, chewing tobacco
      F17.220   Nicotine dependence, chewing tobacco, uncomplicated
      F17.221   Nicotine dependence, chewing tobacco, in remission
      F17.223   Nicotine dependence, chewing tobacco, with withdrawal   CC
      F17.228   Nicotine dependence, chewing tobacco, with other nicotine-induced disorders
      F17.229   Nicotine dependence, chewing tobacco, with unspecified nicotine-induced disorders

   ✓6ᵗʰ F17.29   Nicotine dependence, other tobacco product
      F17.290   Nicotine dependence, other tobacco product, uncomplicated
      F17.291   Nicotine dependence, other tobacco product, in remission
      F17.293   Nicotine dependence, other tobacco product, with withdrawal   CC
      F17.298   Nicotine dependence, other tobacco product, with other nicotine-induced disorders
      F17.299   Nicotine dependence, other tobacco product, with unspecified nicotine-induced disorders

✓4ᵗʰ F18   Inhalant related disorders
    INCLUDES   volatile solvents

> **CC Excl: For CC codes in category F18, unless otherwise noted:**
> F02.80-F02.81, F04-F06.8, F10.10-F11.19, F11.21-F13.19, F13.21-
> F14.19, F14.21-F15.19, F15.21-F16.19, F16.21-F16.99, F17.203-
> F17.209, F17.213-F17.219, F17.223-F17.229, F17.293-F18.19, F18.21-
> F19.19, F19.21-F19.99, F53, F55.0-F55.8, R78.0

✓5ᵗʰ F18.1   Inhalant abuse
    EXCLUDES 1   inhalant dependence (F18.2-)
         inhalant use, unspecified (F18.9-)

     F18.10   Inhalant abuse, uncomplicated
   ✓6ᵗʰ F18.12   Inhalant abuse with intoxication
      F18.120   Inhalant abuse with intoxication, uncomplicated
      F18.121   Inhalant abuse with intoxication delirium   CC

      F18.129   Inhalant abuse with intoxication, unspecified
     F18.14   Inhalant abuse with inhalant-induced mood disorder
   ✓6ᵗʰ F18.15   Inhalant abuse with inhalant-induced psychotic disorder
      F18.150   Inhalant abuse with inhalant-induced psychotic disorder with delusions   CC
      F18.151   Inhalant abuse with inhalant-induced psychotic disorder with hallucinations   CC
      F18.159   Inhalant abuse with inhalant-induced psychotic disorder, unspecified
     F18.17   Inhalant abuse with inhalant-induced dementia   CC
   ✓6ᵗʰ F18.18   Inhalant abuse with other inhalant-induced disorders
      F18.180   Inhalant abuse with inhalant-induced anxiety disorder
      F18.188   Inhalant abuse with other inhalant-induced disorder
     F18.19   Inhalant abuse with unspecified inhalant-induced disorder

✓5ᵗʰ F18.2   Inhalant dependence
    EXCLUDES 1   inhalant abuse (F18.1-)
         inhalant use, unspecified (F18.9-)

     F18.20   Inhalant dependence, uncomplicated   CC
      CC Excl: No Excl
     F18.21   Inhalant dependence, in remission
   ✓6ᵗʰ F18.22   Inhalant dependence with intoxication
      F18.220   Inhalant dependence with intoxication, uncomplicated
      F18.221   Inhalant dependence with intoxication delirium   CC
      F18.229   Inhalant dependence with intoxication, unspecified
     F18.24   Inhalant dependence with inhalant-induced mood disorder
   ✓6ᵗʰ F18.25   Inhalant dependence with inhalant-induced psychotic disorder
      F18.250   Inhalant dependence with inhalant-induced psychotic disorder with delusions   CC
      F18.251   Inhalant dependence with inhalant-induced psychotic disorder with hallucinations   CC
      F18.259   Inhalant dependence with inhalant-induced psychotic disorder, unspecified   CC
       CC Excl: No Excl
     F18.27   Inhalant dependence with inhalant-induced dementia   CC
   ✓6ᵗʰ F18.28   Inhalant dependence with other inhalant-induced disorders
      F18.280   Inhalant dependence with inhalant-induced anxiety disorder   CC
       CC Excl: No Excl
      F18.288   Inhalant dependence with other inhalant-induced disorder   CC
       CC Excl: No Excl
     F18.29   Inhalant dependence with unspecified inhalant-induced disorder

✓5ᵗʰ F18.9   Inhalant use, unspecified
    EXCLUDES 1   inhalant abuse (F18.1-)
         inhalant dependence (F18.2-)

     F18.90   Inhalant use, unspecified, uncomplicated
   ✓6ᵗʰ F18.92   Inhalant use, unspecified with intoxication
      F18.920   Inhalant use, unspecified with intoxication, uncomplicated
      F18.921   Inhalant use, unspecified with intoxication with delirium   CC
      F18.929   Inhalant use, unspecified with intoxication, unspecified
     F18.94   Inhalant use, unspecified with inhalant-induced mood disorder
   ✓6ᵗʰ F18.95   Inhalant use, unspecified with inhalant-induced psychotic disorder
      F18.950   Inhalant use, unspecified with inhalant-induced psychotic disorder with delusions   CC

F18.951   Inhalant use, unspecified with inhalant-induced psychotic disorder with **hallucinations**   CC

F18.959   Inhalant use, unspecified with inhalant-induced psychotic disorder, **unspecified**

F18.97   Inhalant use, unspecified with inhalant-induced **persisting dementia**   CC

✓6ᵗʰ   F18.98   Inhalant use, unspecified with other inhalant-induced disorders

F18.980   Inhalant use, unspecified with inhalant-induced **anxiety disorder**

F18.988   Inhalant use, unspecified with other inhalant-induced disorder

F18.99   Inhalant use, unspecified with **unspecified** inhalant-induced disorder

✓4ᵗʰ   **F19**   **Other psychoactive substance related disorders**

INCLUDES   polysubstance drug use (indiscriminate drug use)

CC Excl: For CC codes in category F19, unless otherwise noted:
F02.80–F02.81, F04–F06.8, F10.10–F11.19, F11.21–F13.19, F13.21–F14.19, F14.21–F15.19, F15.21–F16.19, F16.21–F16.99, F17.203–F17.209, F17.213–F17.219, F17.223–F17.229, F17.293–F18.19, F18.21–F19.19, F19.21–F19.99, F53, F55.0–F55.8, R78.0

✓5ᵗʰ   **F19.1**   **Other psychoactive substance abuse**

EXCLUDES 1   other psychoactive substance dependence (F19.2-)
other psychoactive substance use, unspecified (F19.9-)

F19.10   **Other psychoactive substance abuse, uncomplicated**

✓6ᵗʰ   F19.12   **Other psychoactive substance abuse with intoxication**

F19.120   **Other psychoactive substance abuse with intoxication, uncomplicated**

F19.121   **Other psychoactive substance abuse with intoxication delirium**   CC

F19.122   **Other psychoactive substance abuse with intoxication with perceptual disturbances**

F19.129   **Other psychoactive substance abuse with intoxication, unspecified**

F19.14   **Other psychoactive substance abuse with psychoactive substance-induced mood disorder**

✓6ᵗʰ   F19.15   **Other psychoactive substance abuse with psychoactive substance-induced psychotic disorder**

F19.150   **Other psychoactive substance abuse with psychoactive substance-induced psychotic disorder with delusions**   CC

F19.151   **Other psychoactive substance abuse with psychoactive substance-induced psychotic disorder with hallucinations**   CC

F19.159   **Other psychoactive substance abuse with psychoactive substance-induced psychotic disorder, unspecified**

F19.16   **Other psychoactive substance abuse with psychoactive substance-induced persisting amnestic disorder**

F19.17   **Other psychoactive substance abuse with psychoactive substance-induced persisting dementia**   CC

✓6ᵗʰ   F19.18   **Other psychoactive substance abuse with other psychoactive substance-induced disorders**

F19.180   **Other psychoactive substance abuse with psychoactive substance-induced anxiety disorder**

F19.181   **Other psychoactive substance abuse with psychoactive substance-induced sexual dysfunction**

F19.182   **Other psychoactive substance abuse with psychoactive substance-induced sleep disorder**

F19.188   **Other psychoactive substance abuse with other psychoactive substance-induced disorder**

F19.19   **Other psychoactive substance abuse with unspecified psychoactive substance-induced disorder**

✓5ᵗʰ   **F19.2**   **Other psychoactive substance dependence**

EXCLUDES 1   other psychoactive substance abuse (F19.1-)
other psychoactive substance use, unspecified (F19.9-)

F19.20   **Other psychoactive substance dependence, uncomplicated**   CC
CC Excl: No Excl

F19.21   **Other psychoactive substance dependence, in remission**

✓6ᵗʰ   F19.22   **Other psychoactive substance dependence with intoxication**

EXCLUDES 1   other psychoactive substance dependence with withdrawal (F19.23-)

F19.220   **Other psychoactive substance dependence with intoxication, uncomplicated**

F19.221   **Other psychoactive substance dependence with intoxication delirium**   CC

F19.222   **Other psychoactive substance dependence with intoxication with perceptual disturbance**   CC
CC Excl: No Excl

F19.229   **Other psychoactive substance dependence with intoxication, unspecified**

✓6ᵗʰ   F19.23   **Other psychoactive substance dependence with withdrawal**

EXCLUDES 1   other psychoactive substance dependence with intoxication (F19.22-)

F19.230   **Other psychoactive substance dependence with withdrawal, uncomplicated**   CC

F19.231   **Other psychoactive substance dependence with withdrawal delirium**   CC

F19.232   **Other psychoactive substance dependence with withdrawal with perceptual disturbance**   CC

F19.239   **Other psychoactive substance dependence with withdrawal, unspecified**   CC

F19.24   **Other psychoactive substance dependence with psychoactive substance-induced mood disorder**

✓6ᵗʰ   F19.25   **Other psychoactive substance dependence with psychoactive substance-induced psychotic disorder**

F19.250   **Other psychoactive substance dependence with psychoactive substance-induced psychotic disorder with delusions**   CC

F19.251   **Other psychoactive substance dependence with psychoactive substance-induced psychotic disorder with hallucinations**   CC

F19.259   **Other psychoactive substance dependence with psychoactive substance-induced psychotic disorder, unspecified**   CC
CC Excl: No Excl

F19.26   **Other psychoactive substance dependence with psychoactive substance-induced persisting amnestic disorder**   CC
CC Excl: No Excl

F19.27   **Other psychoactive substance dependence with psychoactive substance-induced persisting dementia**   CC

✓6ᵗʰ   F19.28   **Other psychoactive substance dependence with other psychoactive substance-induced disorders**

F19.280   **Other psychoactive substance dependence with psychoactive substance-induced anxiety disorder**   CC
CC Excl: No Excl

F19.281   **Other psychoactive substance dependence with psychoactive substance-induced sexual dysfunction**   CC
CC Excl: No Excl

F19.282   **Other psychoactive substance dependence with psychoactive substance-induced sleep disorder**   CC
CC Excl: No Excl

F19.288   **Other psychoactive substance dependence with other psychoactive substance-induced disorder**   CC
CC Excl: No Excl

F19.29   **Other psychoactive substance dependence with unspecified psychoactive substance-induced disorder**

✓ Additional Character Required   ✓x7ᵗʰ Placeholder Alert   Unacceptable PDx   Manifestation   Hospital Acquired Condition   EXCLUDES 1 Not Coded Here   EXCLUDES 2 Not Included Here

ICD-10-CM 2016   529

Chapter 5. Mental, Behavioral and Neurodevelopmental Disorders

F18.951–F19.29

√5th F19.9 Other psychoactive substance use, unspecified
> **EXCLUDES 1**   *other psychoactive substance abuse (F19.1-)*
> *other psychoactive substance dependence (F19.2-)*

F19.90 Other psychoactive substance use, unspecified, uncomplicated

√6th F19.92 Other psychoactive substance use, unspecified with intoxication
> **EXCLUDES 1**   *other psychoactive substance use, unspecified with withdrawal (F19.93)*

> **F19.920 Other psychoactive substance use, unspecified with intoxication, uncomplicated**

> **F19.921 Other psychoactive substance use, unspecified with intoxication with delirium**   CC

> **F19.922 Other psychoactive substance use, unspecified with intoxication with perceptual disturbance**

> **F19.929 Other psychoactive substance use, unspecified with intoxication, unspecified**

√6th F19.93 Other psychoactive substance use, unspecified with withdrawal
> **EXCLUDES 1**   *other psychoactive substance use, unspecified with intoxication (F19.92-)*

> **F19.930 Other psychoactive substance use, unspecified with withdrawal, uncomplicated**   CC

> **F19.931 Other psychoactive substance use, unspecified with withdrawal delirium**   CC

> **F19.932 Other psychoactive substance use, unspecified with withdrawal with perceptual disturbance**   CC

> **F19.939 Other psychoactive substance use, unspecified with withdrawal, unspecified**   CC

F19.94 Other psychoactive substance use, unspecified with psychoactive substance-induced mood disorder

√6th F19.95 Other psychoactive substance use, unspecified with psychoactive substance-induced psychotic disorder

> **F19.950 Other psychoactive substance use, unspecified with psychoactive substance-induced psychotic disorder with delusions**   CC

> **F19.951 Other psychoactive substance use, unspecified with psychoactive substance-induced psychotic disorder with hallucinations**

> **F19.959 Other psychoactive substance use, unspecified with psychoactive substance-induced psychotic disorder, unspecified**

F19.96 Other psychoactive substance use, unspecified with psychoactive substance-induced persisting amnestic disorder

F19.97 Other psychoactive substance use, unspecified with psychoactive substance-induced persisting dementia   CC

√6th F19.98 Other psychoactive substance use, unspecified with other psychoactive substance-induced disorders

> **F19.980 Other psychoactive substance use, unspecified with psychoactive substance-induced anxiety disorder**

> **F19.981 Other psychoactive substance use, unspecified with psychoactive substance-induced sexual dysfunction**

> **F19.982 Other psychoactive substance use, unspecified with psychoactive substance-induced sleep disorder**

> **F19.988 Other psychoactive substance use, unspecified with other psychoactive substance-induced disorder**

F19.99 Other psychoactive substance use, unspecified with unspecified psychoactive substance-induced disorder

Schizophrenia, schizotypal, delusional, and other non-mood psychotic disorders (F20-F29)

√4th F20 Schizophrenia
> **EXCLUDES 1**   *brief psychotic disorder (F23)*
> *cyclic schizophrenia (F25.0)*
> *mood [affective] disorders with psychotic symptoms (F30.2, F31.2, F31.5, F31.64, F32.3, F33.3)*
> *schizoaffective disorder (F25.-)*
> *schizophrenic reaction NOS (F23)*
> **EXCLUDES 2**   *schizophrenic reaction in:*
> *alcoholism (F10.15-, F10.25-, F10.95-)*
> *brain disease (F06.2)*
> *epilepsy (F06.2)*
> *psychoactive drug use (F11-F19 with .15, .25, .95)*
> *schizotypal disorder (F21)*

> **CC Excl:** For CC codes in category F20, unless otherwise noted:
> F07.0-F07.81, F07.9-F09, F20.0-F48.1, F48.8-F51.03, F51.12, F51.19, F51.3-F51.9, F52.5, F54, F59-F63.2, F63.81-F63.9, F68.10-F80.2, F80.4, F80.89-F84.0, F84.3-F99, G44.201-G44.229, H93.25, R45.1-R45.2, R45.5-R45.82, R45.86-R45.87

> **F20.0 Paranoid schizophrenia**   CC
> Paraphrenic schizophrenia
> **EXCLUDES 1**   *involutional paranoid state (F22)*
> *paranoia (F22)*

> **F20.1 Disorganized schizophrenia**   CC
> Hebephrenic schizophrenia
> Hebephrenia

> **F20.2 Catatonic schizophrenia**   CC
> Schizophrenic catalepsy
> Schizophrenic catatonia
> Schizophrenic flexibilitas cerea
> **EXCLUDES 1**   *catatonic stupor (R40.1)*

> **F20.3 Undifferentiated schizophrenia**
> Atypical schizophrenia
> **EXCLUDES 1**   *acute schizophrenia-like psychotic disorder (F23)*
> **EXCLUDES 2**   *post-schizophrenic depression (F32.8)*

> **F20.5 Residual schizophrenia**   CC
> Restzustand (schizophrenic)
> Schizophrenic residual state

> **√5th F20.8 Other schizophrenia**

> > **F20.81 Schizophreniform disorder**   CC
> > Schizophreniform psychosis NOS

> > **F20.89 Other schizophrenia**   CC
> > Cenesthopathic schizophrenia
> > Simple schizophrenia

> **F20.9 Schizophrenia, unspecified**

F21 Schizotypal disorder
> Borderline schizophrenia
> Latent schizophrenia
> Latent schizophrenic reaction
> Prepsychotic schizophrenia
> Prodromal schizophrenia
> Pseudoneurotic schizophrenia
> Pseudopsychopathic schizophrenia
> Schizotypal personality disorder
> **EXCLUDES 2**   *Asperger's syndrome (F84.5)*
> *schizoid personality disorder (F60.1)*

F22 Delusional disorders
> Delusional dysmorphophobia
> Involutional paranoid state
> Paranoia
> Paranoia querulans
> Paranoid psychosis
> Paranoid state
> Paraphrenia (late)
> Sensitiver Beziehungswahn
> **EXCLUDES 1**   *mood [affective] disorders with psychotic symptoms (F30.2, F31.2, F31.5, F31.64, F32.3, F33.3)*
> *paranoid schizophrenia (F20.0)*
> **EXCLUDES 2**   *paranoid personality disorder (F60.0)*
> *paranoid psychosis, psychogenic (F23)*
> *paranoid reaction (F23)*

F23 Brief psychotic disorder   CC
> Paranoid reaction
> Psychogenic paranoid psychosis
> **EXCLUDES 2**   *mood [affective] disorders with psychotic symptoms (F30.2, F31.2, F31.64, F32.3, F33.3)*
> **CC Excl:** No Excl

N Newborn: 0   P Pediatric: 0-17   M Maternity: 12-55   A Adult: 15-124   MCC Major CC Condition   PDx MCC PDx acts as own MCC   CC CC Condition   PDx CC PDx acts as own CC

530   ICD-10-CM 2016

F24   **Shared psychotic disorder**
Folie à deux
Induced paranoid disorder
Induced psychotic disorder

☑4ᵗʰ **F25**   **Schizoaffective disorders**
EXCLUDES1   *mood [affective] disorders with psychotic symptoms (F30.2, F31.2, F31.5, F31.64, F32.3, F33.3)*
schizophrenia (F20.-)

    F25.0   **Schizoaffective disorder, bipolar type**
Cyclic schizophrenia
Schizoaffective disorder, manic type
Schizoaffective disorder, mixed type
Schizoaffective psychosis, bipolar type
Schizophreniform psychosis, manic type

    F25.1   **Schizoaffective disorder, depressive type**
Schizoaffective psychosis, depressive type
Schizophreniform psychosis, depressive type

    F25.8   **Other schizoaffective disorders**

    F25.9   **Schizoaffective disorder, unspecified**
Schizoaffective psychosis NOS

F28   **Other psychotic disorder not due to a substance or known**   `HIV`
physiological condition
Chronic hallucinatory psychosis

F29   **Unspecified psychosis not due to a substance or known**   `HIV`
physiological condition
Psychosis NOS
EXCLUDES1   *mental disorder NOS (F99)*
unspecified mental disorder due to known physiological condition (F09)

Mood [affective] disorders (F30-F39)

☑4ᵗʰ **F30**   **Manic episode**
INCLUDES   bipolar disorder, single manic episode
mixed affective episode
EXCLUDES1   *bipolar disorder (F31.-)*
major depressive disorder, recurrent (F33.-)
major depressive disorder, single episode (F32.-)

> **CC Excl: For CC codes in category F30, unless otherwise noted:**
> F07.0-F07.81, F07.9-F09, F20.0-F48.1, F48.8-F51.03, F51.12, F51.19,
> F51.3-F51.9, F52.5, F54, F59-F63.2, F63.81-F63.9, F68.10-F80.2, F80.4,
> F80.89-F84.0, F84.3-F99, G44.201-G44.229, H93.25, R45.1-R45.2,
> R45.5-R45.82, R45.86-R45.87

    ☑5ᵗʰ **F30.1**   **Manic episode without psychotic symptoms**
       F30.10   **Manic episode without psychotic symptoms, unspecified**   `CC`
       F30.11   **Manic episode without psychotic symptoms, mild**   `CC`
       F30.12   **Manic episode without psychotic symptoms, moderate**   `CC`
       F30.13   **Manic episode, severe, without psychotic symptoms**   `CC`
          CC Excl: F30.13-F30.2, F31.13-F31.2, F31.4-F31.5, F31.63-F31.64

    F30.2   **Manic episode, severe with psychotic symptoms**   `CC`
Manic stupor
Mania with mood-congruent psychotic symptoms
Mania with mood-incongruent psychotic symptoms

    F30.3   **Manic episode in partial remission**

    F30.4   **Manic episode in full remission**

    F30.8   **Other manic episodes**
Hypomania

    F30.9   **Manic episode, unspecified**   `CC`
Mania NOS

☑4ᵗʰ **F31**   **Bipolar disorder**
INCLUDES   manic-depressive illness
manic-depressive psychosis
manic-depressive reaction
EXCLUDES1   *bipolar disorder, single manic episode (F30.-)*
major depressive disorder, single episode (F32.-)
major depressive disorder, recurrent (F33.-)
EXCLUDES2   *cyclothymia (F34.0)*

> **CC Excl: For CC codes in category F31, unless otherwise noted:**
> F07.0-F07.81, F07.9-F09, F20.0-F48.1, F48.8-F51.03, F51.12, F51.19,
> F51.3-F51.9, F52.5, F54, F59-F63.2, F63.81-F63.9, F68.10-F80.2, F80.4,
> F80.89-F84.0, F84.3-F99, G44.201-G44.229, H93.25, R45.1-R45.2,
> R45.5-R45.82, R45.86-R45.87

    F31.0   **Bipolar disorder, current episode hypomanic**   `CC`

    ☑5ᵗʰ **F31.1**   **Bipolar disorder, current episode manic without psychotic features**
       F31.10   **Bipolar disorder, current episode manic without psychotic features, unspecified**   `CC`
       F31.11   **Bipolar disorder, current episode manic without psychotic features, mild**   `CC`
       F31.12   **Bipolar disorder, current episode manic without psychotic features, moderate**   `CC`
       F31.13   **Bipolar disorder, current episode manic without psychotic features, severe**   `CC`
          CC Excl: F31.13-F31.2, F31.63-F31.64

    F31.2   **Bipolar disorder, current episode manic severe with psychotic features**   `CC`
Bipolar disorder, current episode manic with mood-congruent psychotic symptoms
Bipolar disorder, current episode manic with mood-incongruent psychotic symptoms

    ☑5ᵗʰ **F31.3**   **Bipolar disorder, current episode depressed, mild or moderate severity**
       F31.30   **Bipolar disorder, current episode depressed, mild or moderate severity, unspecified**   `CC`
       F31.31   **Bipolar disorder, current episode depressed, mild**   `CC`
       F31.32   **Bipolar disorder, current episode depressed, moderate**   `CC`

    F31.4   **Bipolar disorder, current episode depressed, severe, without psychotic features**   `CC`
          CC Excl: F31.13-F31.2, F31.4-F31.5, F31.63-F31.64

    F31.5   **Bipolar disorder, current episode depressed, severe, with psychotic features**   `CC`
Bipolar disorder, current episode depressed with mood-incongruent psychotic symptoms
Bipolar disorder, current episode depressed with mood-congruent psychotic symptoms

    ☑5ᵗʰ **F31.6**   **Bipolar disorder, current episode mixed**
       F31.60   **Bipolar disorder, current episode mixed, unspecified**   `CC`
       F31.61   **Bipolar disorder, current episode mixed, mild**   `CC`
       F31.62   **Bipolar disorder, current episode mixed, moderate**   `CC`
       F31.63   **Bipolar disorder, current episode mixed, severe, without psychotic features**   `CC`
          CC Excl: See code: F31.4
       F31.64   **Bipolar disorder, current episode mixed, severe, with psychotic features**   `CC`
Bipolar disorder, current episode mixed with mood-congruent psychotic symptoms
Bipolar disorder, current episode mixed with mood-incongruent psychotic symptoms

    ☑5ᵗʰ **F31.7**   **Bipolar disorder, currently in remission**
       F31.70   **Bipolar disorder, currently in remission, most recent episode unspecified**
       F31.71   **Bipolar disorder, in partial remission, most recent episode hypomanic**
       F31.72   **Bipolar disorder, in full remission, most recent episode hypomanic**
       F31.73   **Bipolar disorder, in partial remission, most recent episode manic**
       F31.74   **Bipolar disorder, in full remission, most recent episode manic**
       F31.75   **Bipolar disorder, in partial remission, most recent episode depressed**
       F31.76   **Bipolar disorder, in full remission, most recent episode depressed**
       F31.77   **Bipolar disorder, in partial remission, most recent episode mixed**
       F31.78   **Bipolar disorder, in full remission, most recent episode mixed**

    ☑5ᵗʰ **F31.8**   **Other bipolar disorders**
       F31.81   **Bipolar II disorder**   `CC`
       F31.89   **Other bipolar disorder**   `CC`
Recurrent manic episodes NOS

    F31.9   **Bipolar disorder, unspecified**

√4ᵗʰ **F32 Major depressive disorder, single episode**
INCLUDES single episode of agitated depression
single episode of depressive reaction
single episode of major depression
single episode of psychogenic depression
single episode of reactive depression
single episode of vital depression
EXCLUDES 1 bipolar disorder (F31.-)
manic episode (F30.-)
recurrent depressive disorder (F33.-)
EXCLUDES 2 adjustment disorder (F43.2)

CC Excl: For CC codes in category F32, unless otherwise noted:
F32.0-F32.3, F33.0-F33.40, F33.9

F32.0 Major depressive disorder, single episode, mild CC
F32.1 Major depressive disorder, single episode, moderate CC
F32.2 Major depressive disorder, single episode, severe without psychotic features CC
F32.3 Major depressive disorder, single episode, severe with psychotic features CC
Single episode of major depression with mood-congruent psychotic symptoms
Single episode of major depression with mood-incongruent psychotic symptoms
Single episode of major depression with psychotic symptoms
Single episode of psychogenic depressive psychosis
Single episode of psychotic depression
Single episode of reactive depressive psychosis
F32.4 Major depressive disorder, single episode, in partial remission
F32.5 Major depressive disorder, single episode, in full remission
F32.8 Other depressive episodes
Atypical depression
Post-schizophrenic depression
Single episode of 'masked' depression NOS
F32.9 Major depressive disorder, single episode, unspecified
Depression NOS
Depressive disorder NOS
Major depression NOS
AHA: 2013, 4Q, 107

√4ᵗʰ **F33 Major depressive disorder, recurrent**
Recurrent episodes of depressive reaction
Recurrent episodes of endogenous depression
Recurrent episodes of major depression
Recurrent episodes of psychogenic depression
Recurrent episodes of reactive depression
Recurrent episodes of seasonal depressive disorder
Recurrent episodes of vital depression
EXCLUDES 1 bipolar disorder (F31.-)
manic episode (F30.-)

F33.0 Major depressive disorder, recurrent, mild CC
CC Excl: See code: F32
F33.1 Major depressive disorder, recurrent, moderate CC
CC Excl: See code: F32
F33.2 Major depressive disorder, recurrent, severe without psychotic features CC
CC Excl: See code: F32
F33.3 Major depressive disorder, recurrent, severe with psychotic symptoms CC
Endogenous depression with psychotic symptoms
Recurrent severe episodes of major depression with mood-congruent psychotic symptoms
Recurrent severe episodes of major depression with mood-incongruent psychotic symptoms
Recurrent severe episodes of major depression with psychotic symptoms
Recurrent severe episodes of psychogenic depressive psychosis
Recurrent severe episodes of psychotic depression
Recurrent severe episodes of reactive depressive psychosis
CC Excl: F07.0-F07.81, F07.9-F09, F20.0-F48.1, F48.8-F51.03, F51.12, F51.19, F51.3-F51.9, F52.5, F54, F59-F63.2, F63.81-F63.9, F68.10-F80.4, F80.89-F84.0, F84.3-F99, G44.201-G44.229, H93.25, R45.1-R45.2, R45.5-R45.82, R45.86-R45.87

√5ᵗʰ **F33.4 Major depressive disorder, recurrent, in remission**
F33.40 Major depressive disorder, recurrent, in remission, unspecified CC
CC Excl: See code: F32
F33.41 Major depressive disorder, recurrent, in partial remission
F33.42 Major depressive disorder, recurrent, in full remission

F33.8 Other recurrent depressive disorders CC
Recurrent brief depressive episodes
CC Excl: See code: F33.3
F33.9 Major depressive disorder, recurrent, unspecified CC
Monopolar depression NOS
CC Excl: See code: F32

√4ᵗʰ **F34 Persistent mood [affective] disorders**
F34.0 Cyclothymic disorder
Affective personality disorder
Cycloid personality
Cyclothymia
Cyclothymic personality
F34.1 Dysthymic disorder
Depressive neurosis
Depressive personality disorder
Dysthymia
Neurotic depression
Persistent anxiety depression
EXCLUDES 2 anxiety depression (mild or not persistent) (F41.8)
F34.8 Other persistent mood [affective] disorders CC
CC Excl: See code: F33.3
F34.9 Persistent mood [affective] disorder, unspecified CC
CC Excl: See code: F33.3
F39 Unspecified mood [affective] disorder
Affective psychosis NOS

Anxiety, dissociative, stress-related, somatoform and other nonpsychotic mental disorders (F40-F48)

√4ᵗʰ **F40 Phobic anxiety disorders**
√5ᵗʰ **F40.0 Agoraphobia**
F40.00 Agoraphobia, unspecified
F40.01 Agoraphobia with panic disorder
Panic disorder with agoraphobia
EXCLUDES 1 panic disorder without agoraphobia (F41.0)
F40.02 Agoraphobia without panic disorder
√5ᵗʰ **F40.1 Social phobias**
Anthropophobia
Social anxiety disorder of childhood
Social neurosis
F40.10 Social phobia, unspecified
F40.11 Social phobia, generalized
√5ᵗʰ **F40.2 Specific (isolated) phobias**
EXCLUDES 2 dysmorphophobia (nondelusional) (F45.22)
nosophobia (F45.22)
√6ᵗʰ **F40.21 Animal type phobia**
F40.210 Arachnophobia
Fear of spiders
F40.218 Other animal type phobia
√6ᵗʰ **F40.22 Natural environment type phobia**
F40.220 Fear of thunderstorms
F40.228 Other natural environment type phobia
√6ᵗʰ **F40.23 Blood, injection, injury type phobia**
F40.230 Fear of blood
F40.231 Fear of injections and transfusions
F40.232 Fear of other medical care
F40.233 Fear of injury
√6ᵗʰ **F40.24 Situational type phobia**
F40.240 Claustrophobia
F40.241 Acrophobia
F40.242 Fear of bridges
F40.243 Fear of flying
F40.248 Other situational type phobia
√6ᵗʰ **F40.29 Other specified phobia**
F40.290 Androphobia
Fear of men
F40.291 Gynephobia
Fear of women
F40.298 Other specified phobia
F40.8 Other phobic anxiety disorders
Phobic anxiety disorder of childhood
F40.9 Phobic anxiety disorder, unspecified
Phobia NOS
Phobic state NOS

✓4th F41 Other anxiety disorders
EXCLUDES 2   anxiety in:
- acute stress reaction (F43.0)
- transient adjustment reaction (F43.2)
- neurasthenia (F48.8)
- psychophysiologic disorders (F45.-)
- separation anxiety (F93.0)

F41.0 Panic disorder [episodic paroxysmal anxiety] without agoraphobia
- Panic attack
- Panic state
- EXCLUDES 1   panic disorder with agoraphobia (F40.01)

F41.1 Generalized anxiety disorder
- Anxiety neurosis
- Anxiety reaction
- Anxiety state
- Overanxious disorder
- EXCLUDES 2   neurasthenia (F48.8)

F41.3 Other mixed anxiety disorders

F41.8 Other specified anxiety disorders
- Anxiety depression (mild or not persistent)
- Anxiety hysteria
- Mixed anxiety and depressive disorder

F41.9 Anxiety disorder, unspecified
- Anxiety NOS

F42 Obsessive-compulsive disorder
- Anancastic neurosis
- Obsessive-compulsive neurosis
- EXCLUDES 2   obsessive-compulsive personality (disorder) (F60.5)
  obsessive-compulsive symptoms occurring in depression (F32-F33)
  obsessive-compulsive symptoms occurring in schizophrenia (F20.-)

✓4th F43 Reaction to severe stress, and adjustment disorders

F43.0 Acute stress reaction
- Acute crisis reaction
- Acute reaction to stress
- Combat and operational stress reaction
- Combat fatigue
- Crisis state
- Psychic shock

✓5th F43.1 Post-traumatic stress disorder (PTSD)
- Traumatic neurosis

   F43.10 Post-traumatic stress disorder, unspecified

   F43.11 Post-traumatic stress disorder, acute

   F43.12 Post-traumatic stress disorder, chronic

✓5th F43.2 Adjustment disorders
- Culture shock
- Grief reaction
- Hospitalism in children
- EXCLUDES 2   separation anxiety disorder of childhood (F93.0)

   F43.20 Adjustment disorder, unspecified

   F43.21 Adjustment disorder with depressed mood
     AHA: 2014, 1Q, 25

   F43.22 Adjustment disorder with anxiety

   F43.23 Adjustment disorder with mixed anxiety and depressed mood

   F43.24 Adjustment disorder with disturbance of conduct

   F43.25 Adjustment disorder with mixed disturbance of emotions and conduct

   F43.29 Adjustment disorder with other symptoms

F43.8 Other reactions to severe stress

F43.9 Reaction to severe stress, unspecified

✓4th F44 Dissociative and conversion disorders
INCLUDES   conversion hysteria
- conversion reaction
- hysteria
- hysterical psychosis
- EXCLUDES 2   malingering [conscious simulation] (Z76.5)

F44.0 Dissociative amnesia
- EXCLUDES 1   amnesia NOS (R41.3)
  anterograde amnesia (R41.1)
  retrograde amnesia (R41.2)
- EXCLUDES 2   alcohol-or other psychoactive substance-induced amnestic disorder (F10, F13, F19 with .26, .96)
  amnestic disorder due to known physiological condition (F04)
  postictal amnesia in epilepsy (G40.-)

F44.1 Dissociative fugue
- EXCLUDES 2   postictal fugue in epilepsy (G40.-)

F44.2 Dissociative stupor
- EXCLUDES 1   catatonic stupor (R40.1)
  stupor NOS (R40.1)
- EXCLUDES 2   catatonic disorder due to known physiological condition (F06.1)
  depressive stupor (F32, F33)
  manic stupor (F30, F31)

F44.4 Conversion disorder with motor symptom or deficit
- Dissociative motor disorders
- Psychogenic aphonia
- Psychogenic dysphonia

F44.5 Conversion disorder with seizures or convulsions
- Dissociative convulsions

F44.6 Conversion disorder with sensory symptom or deficit
- Dissociative anesthesia and sensory loss
- Psychogenic deafness

F44.7 Conversion disorder with mixed symptom presentation

✓5th F44.8 Other dissociative and conversion disorders

   F44.81 Dissociative identity disorder
- Multiple personality disorder

   F44.89 Other dissociative and conversion disorders
- Ganser's syndrome
- Psychogenic confusion
- Psychogenic twilight state
- Trance and possession disorders

F44.9 Dissociative and conversion disorder, unspecified
- Dissociative disorder NOS

✓4th F45 Somatoform disorders
EXCLUDES 2   dissociative and conversion disorders (F44.-)
- factitious disorders (F68.1-)
- hair-plucking (F63.3)
- lalling (F80.0)
- lisping (F80.0)
- malingering [conscious simulation] (Z76.5)
- nail-biting (F98.8)
- psychological or behavioral factors associated with disorders or diseases classified elsewhere (F54)
- sexual dysfunction, not due to a substance or known physiological condition (F52.-)
- thumb-sucking (F98.8)
- tic disorders (in childhood and adolescence) (F95.-)
- Tourette's syndrome (F95.2)
- trichotillomania (F63.3)

F45.0 Somatization disorder
- Briquet's disorder
- Multiple psychosomatic disorder

F45.1 Undifferentiated somatoform disorder
- Undifferentiated psychosomatic disorder

✓5th F45.2 Hypochondriacal disorders
- EXCLUDES 2   delusional dysmorphophobia (F22)
  fixed delusions about bodily functions or shape (F22)

   F45.20 Hypochondriacal disorder, unspecified

   F45.21 Hypochondriasis
- Hypochondriacal neurosis

   F45.22 Body dysmorphic disorder
- Dysmorphophobia (nondelusional)
- Nosophobia

   F45.29 Other hypochondriacal disorders

✓5th F45.4 Pain disorders related to psychological factors
- EXCLUDES 1   pain NOS (R52)

   F45.41 Pain disorder exclusively related to psychological factors
- Somatoform pain disorder (persistent)

   F45.42 Pain disorder with related psychological factors
- Code also associated acute or chronic pain (G89.-)

F45.8 Other somatoform disorders
- Psychogenic dysmenorrhea
- Psychogenic dysphagia, including "globus hystericus"
- Psychogenic pruritus
- Psychogenic torticollis
- Somatoform autonomic dysfunction
- Teeth grinding
- EXCLUDES 1   sleep related teeth grinding (G47.63)

F45.9 Somatoform disorder, unspecified
- Psychosomatic disorder NOS

✓ Additional Character Required   ✓x7th Placeholder Alert   Unacceptable PDx   Manifestation   Hospital Acquired Condition   EXCLUDES 1 Not Coded Here   EXCLUDES 2 Not Included Here

ICD-10-CM 2016   533

F41–F45.9

Chapter 5. Mental, Behavioral and Neurodevelopmental Disorders

√4th **F48   Other nonpsychotic mental disorders**

F48.1   Depersonalization-derealization syndrome

F48.2   Pseudobulbar affect

Involuntary emotional expression disorder

Code first underlying cause, if known, such as:

amyotrophic lateral sclerosis (G12.21)

multiple sclerosis (G35)

sequelae of cerebrovascular disease (I69.-)

sequelae of traumatic intracranial injury (S06.-)

F48.8   Other specified nonpsychotic mental disorders

Dhat syndrome

Neurasthenia

Occupational neurosis, including writer's cramp

Psychasthenia

Psychasthenic neurosis

Psychogenic syncope

F48.9   Nonpsychotic mental disorder, unspecified

Neurosis NOS

Behavioral syndromes associated with physiological disturbances and physical factors (F50-F59)

√4th **F50   Eating disorders**

EXCLUDES 1   anorexia NOS (R63.0)

feeding difficulties (R63.3)

polyphagia (R63.2)

EXCLUDES 2   feeding disorder in infancy or childhood (F98.2-)

> CC Excl: For CC codes in category F50, unless otherwise noted:
> F45.9, F50.00-F50.9, F59, F98.21-F98.3

√5th **F50.0   Anorexia nervosa**

EXCLUDES 1   loss of appetite (R63.0)

psychogenic loss of appetite (F50.8)

F50.00   Anorexia nervosa, unspecified   CC

F50.01   Anorexia nervosa, restricting type   CC

F50.02   Anorexia nervosa, binge eating/purging type   CC

EXCLUDES 1   bulimia nervosa (F50.2)

F50.2   Bulimia nervosa   CC

Bulimia NOS

Hyperorexia nervosa

EXCLUDES 1   anorexia nervosa, binge eating/purging type (F50.02)

CC Excl: F50.00-F50.9, F98.21-F98.29

F50.8   Other eating disorders

Pica in adults

Psychogenic loss of appetite

EXCLUDES 2   pica of infancy and childhood (F98.3)

F50.9   Eating disorder, unspecified

Atypical anorexia nervosa

Atypical bulimia nervosa

√4th **F51   Sleep disorders not due to a substance or known physiological condition**

EXCLUDES 2   organic sleep disorders (G47.-)

√5th **F51.0   Insomnia not due to a substance or known physiological condition**

EXCLUDES 2   alcohol related insomnia (F10.182, F10.282, F10.982)

drug-related insomnia (F11.182, F11.282, F11.982, F13.182, F13.282, F13.982, F14.182, F14.282, F14.982, F15.182, F15.282, F15.982, F19.182, F19.282, F19.982)

insomnia NOS (G47.0-)

insomnia due to known physiological condition (G47.0-)

organic insomnia (G47.0-)

sleep deprivation (Z72.820)

F51.01   Primary insomnia

Idiopathic insomnia

F51.02   Adjustment insomnia

F51.03   Paradoxical insomnia

F51.04   Psychophysiologic insomnia

F51.05   Insomnia due to other mental disorder

Code also associated mental disorder

F51.09   Other insomnia not due to a substance or known physiological condition

√5th **F51.1   Hypersomnia not due to a substance or known physiological condition**

EXCLUDES 2   alcohol related hypersomnia (F10.182, F10.282, F10.982)

drug-related hypersomnia (F11.182, F11.282, F11.982, F13.182, F13.282, F13.982, F14.182, F14.282, F14.982, F15.182, F15.282, F15.982, F19.182, F19.282, F19.982)

hypersomnia NOS (G47.10)

hypersomnia due to known physiological condition (G47.10)

idiopathic hypersomnia (G47.11, G47.12)

narcolepsy (G47.4-)

F51.11   Primary hypersomnia

F51.12   Insufficient sleep syndrome

EXCLUDES 1   sleep deprivation (Z72.820)

F51.13   Hypersomnia due to other mental disorder

Code also associated mental disorder

F51.19   Other hypersomnia not due to a substance or known physiological condition

F51.3   Sleepwalking [somnambulism]

F51.4   Sleep terrors [night terrors]

F51.5   Nightmare disorder

Dream anxiety disorder

F51.8   Other sleep disorders not due to a substance or known physiological condition

F51.9   Sleep disorder not due to a substance or known physiological condition, unspecified

Emotional sleep disorder NOS

√4th **F52   Sexual dysfunction not due to a substance or known physiological condition**

EXCLUDES 2   Dhat syndrome (F48.8)

F52.0   Hypoactive sexual desire disorder

Anhedonia (sexual)

Lack or loss of sexual desire

EXCLUDES 1   decreased libido (R68.82)

F52.1   Sexual aversion disorder

Sexual aversion and lack of sexual enjoyment

√5th **F52.2   Sexual arousal disorders**

Failure of genital response

F52.21   Male erectile disorder   ♂

Psychogenic impotence

EXCLUDES 1   impotence of organic origin (N52.-)

impotence NOS (N52.-)

F52.22   Female sexual arousal disorder   ♀

Frigidity

√5th **F52.3   Orgasmic disorder**

Inhibited orgasm

Psychogenic anorgasmy

F52.31   Female orgasmic disorder   ♀

F52.32   Male orgasmic disorder   ♂

F52.4   Premature ejaculation   ♂

F52.5   Vaginismus not due to a substance or known physiological condition   ♀

Psychogenic vaginismus

EXCLUDES 2   vaginismus (due to a known physiological condition) (N94.2)

F52.6   Dyspareunia not due to a substance or known physiological condition   ♀

Psychogenic dyspareunia

EXCLUDES 2   dyspareunia (due to a known physiological condition) (N94.1)

F52.8   Other sexual dysfunction not due to a substance or known physiological condition

Excessive sexual drive

Nymphomania

Satyriasis

F52.9   Unspecified sexual dysfunction not due to a substance or known physiological condition

Sexual dysfunction NOS

F53   Puerperal psychosis   ♀

Postpartum depression

EXCLUDES 1   mood disorders with psychotic features (F30.2, F31.2, F31.5, F31.64, F32.3, F33.3)

postpartum dysphoria (O90.6)

psychosis in schizophrenia, schizotypal, delusional, and other psychotic disorders (F20-F29)

N Newborn: 0   P Pediatric: 0-17   M Maternity: 12-55   A Adult: 15-124   MCC Major CC Condition   PDxMCC PDx acts as own MCC   CC CC Condition   PDxCC PDx acts as own CC

534   ICD-10-CM 2016

F54 Psychological and behavioral factors associated with disorders or diseases classified elsewhere

Psychological factors affecting physical conditions

Code first the associated physical disorder, such as:
asthma (J45.-)
dermatitis (L23-L25)
gastric ulcer (K25.-)
mucous colitis (K58.-)
ulcerative colitis (K51.-)
urticaria (L50.-)
EXCLUDES 2 *tension-type headache (G44.2)*

✓4ᵗʰ F55 Abuse of non-psychoactive substances

EXCLUDES 2 *abuse of psychoactive substances (F10-F19)*

F55.0 Abuse of antacids

F55.1 Abuse of herbal or folk remedies

F55.2 Abuse of laxatives

F55.3 Abuse of steroids or hormones

F55.4 Abuse of vitamins

F55.8 Abuse of other non-psychoactive substances

F59 Unspecified behavioral syndromes associated with physiological disturbances and physical factors

Psychogenic physiological dysfunction NOS

Disorders of adult personality and behavior (F60-F69)

✓4ᵗʰ F60 Specific personality disorders

F60.0 Paranoid personality disorder
Expansive paranoid personality (disorder)
Fanatic personality (disorder)
Paranoid personality (disorder)
Querulant personality (disorder)
Sensitive paranoid personality (disorder)
EXCLUDES 2 *paranoia (F22)*
paranoia querulans (F22)
paranoid psychosis (F22)
paranoid schizophrenia (F20.0)
paranoid state (F22)

F60.1 Schizoid personality disorder
EXCLUDES 2 *Asperger's syndrome (F84.5)*
delusional disorder (F22)
schizoid disorder of childhood (F84.5)
schizophrenia (F20.-)
schizotypal disorder (F21)

F60.2 Antisocial personality disorder
Amoral personality (disorder)
Asocial personality (disorder)
Dissocial personality disorder
Psychopathic personality (disorder)
Sociopathic personality (disorder)
EXCLUDES 1 *conduct disorders (F91.-)*
EXCLUDES 2 *borderline personality disorder (F60.3)*

F60.3 Borderline personality disorder
Aggressive personality (disorder)
Emotionally unstable personality disorder
Explosive personality (disorder)
EXCLUDES 2 *antisocial personality disorder (F60.2)*

F60.4 Histrionic personality disorder
Hysterical personality (disorder)
Psychoinfantile personality (disorder)

F60.5 Obsessive-compulsive personality disorder
Anankastic personality (disorder)
Compulsive personality (disorder)
Obsessional personality (disorder)
EXCLUDES 2 *obsessive-compulsive disorder (F42)*

F60.6 Avoidant personality disorder
Anxious personality disorder

F60.7 Dependent personality disorder
Asthenic personality (disorder)
Inadequate personality (disorder)
Passive personality (disorder)

✓5ᵗʰ F60.8 Other specific personality disorders

F60.81 Narcissistic personality disorder

F60.89 Other specific personality disorders
Eccentric personality disorder
"Haltlose" type personality disorder
Immature personality disorder
Passive-aggressive personality disorder
Psychoneurotic personality disorder
Self-defeating personality disorder

F60.9 Personality disorder, unspecified
Character disorder NOS
Character neurosis NOS
Pathological personality NOS

✓4ᵗʰ F63 Impulse disorders

EXCLUDES 2 *habitual excessive use of alcohol or psychoactive substances (F10-F19)*
impulse disorders involving sexual behavior (F65.-)

F63.0 Pathological gambling
Compulsive gambling
EXCLUDES 1 *gambling and betting NOS (Z72.6)*
EXCLUDES 2 *excessive gambling by manic patients (F30, F31)*
gambling in antisocial personality disorder (F60.2)

F63.1 Pyromania
Pathological fire-setting
EXCLUDES 2 *fire-setting (by) (in):*
adult with antisocial personality disorder (F60.2)
alcohol or psychoactive substance intoxication (F10-F19)
conduct disorders (F91.-)
mental disorders due to known physiological condition (F01-F09)
schizophrenia (F20.-)

F63.2 Kleptomania
Pathological stealing
EXCLUDES 1 *shoplifting as the reason for observation for suspected mental disorder (Z03.8)*
EXCLUDES 2 *depressive disorder with stealing (F31-F33)*
stealing due to underlying mental condition—code to mental condition
stealing in mental disorders due to known physiological condition (F01-F09)

F63.3 Trichotillomania
Hair plucking
EXCLUDES 2 *other stereotyped movement disorder (F98.4)*

✓5ᵗʰ F63.8 Other impulse disorders

F63.81 Intermittent explosive disorder

F63.89 Other impulse disorders

F63.9 Impulse disorder, unspecified
Impulse control disorder NOS

✓4ᵗʰ F64 Gender identity disorders

F64.1 Gender identity disorder in adolescence and adulthood
Dual role transvestism
Transsexualism
Use additional code to identify sex reassignment status (Z87.890)
EXCLUDES 1 *gender identity disorder in childhood (F64.2)*
EXCLUDES 2 *fetishistic transvestism (F65.1)*

F64.2 Gender identity disorder of childhood   P
EXCLUDES 1 *gender identity disorder in adolescence and adulthood (F64.1)*
EXCLUDES 2 *sexual maturation disorder (F66)*

F64.8 Other gender identity disorders

F64.9 Gender identity disorder, unspecified
Gender-role disorder NOS

✓4ᵗʰ F65 Paraphilias

F65.0 Fetishism

F65.1 Transvestic fetishism
Fetishistic transvestism

F65.2 Exhibitionism

F65.3 Voyeurism

F65.4 Pedophilia

✓5ᵗʰ F65.5 Sadomasochism

F65.50 Sadomasochism, unspecified

F65.51 Sexual masochism

F65.52 Sexual sadism

✓5ᵗʰ F65.8 Other paraphilias

F65.81 Frotteurism

F65.89 Other paraphilias
Necrophilia

F65.9 Paraphilia, unspecified
Sexual deviation NOS

F66 Other sexual disorders
Sexual maturation disorder
Sexual relationship disorder

✓ Additional Character Required   ✓x7ᵗʰ Placeholder Alert   Unacceptable PDx   Manifestation   Hospital Acquired Condition   EXCLUDES 1 Not Coded Here   EXCLUDES 2 Not Included Here

Chapter 5. Mental, Behavioral and Neurodevelopmental Disorders

F68–F84.0

✓4ᵗʰ **F68 Other disorders of adult personality and behavior**

✓5ᵗʰ **F68.1 Factitious disorder**
Compensation neurosis
Elaboration of physical symptoms for psychological reasons
Hospital hopper syndrome
Münchhausen's syndrome
Peregrinating patient
EXCLUDES 2   *factitial dermatitis (L98.1)*
person feigning illness (with obvious motivation) (Z76.5)

     F68.10 Factitious disorder, unspecified   CC
         CC Excl: F07.0-F07.81, F07.9-F09, F20.0-F48.1, F48.8-F51.03, F51.12, F51.19, F51.3-F51.9, F52.5, F54, F59-F63.2, F63.81-F63.9, F68.10-F80.2, F80.4, F80.89-F84.0, F84.3-F99, G44.201-G44.229, H93.25, R45.1-R45.2, R45.5-R45.82, R45.86-R45.87

     F68.11 Factitious disorder with predominantly psychological signs and symptoms

     F68.12 Factitious disorder with predominantly physical   CC
signs and symptoms
         CC Excl: See code: F68.10

     F68.13 Factitious disorder with combined psychological and physical signs and symptoms

   F68.8 Other specified disorders of adult personality and behavior

F69 Unspecified disorder of adult personality and behavior   A

Intellectual Disabilities (F70–F79)

Code first any associated physical or developmental disorders
EXCLUDES 1   *borderline intellectual functioning, IQ above 70 to 84 (R41.83)*

F70 Mild intellectual disabilities
IQ level 50-55 to approximately 70
Mild mental subnormality

F71 Moderate intellectual disabilities
IQ level 35-40 to 50-55
Moderate mental subnormality

F72 Severe intellectual disabilities   CC
IQ 20-25 to 35-40
Severe mental subnormality
CC Excl: F72-F73

F73 Profound intellectual disabilities   CC
IQ level below 20-25
Profound mental subnormality
CC Excl: See code: F72

F78 Other intellectual disabilities

F79 Unspecified intellectual disabilities
Mental deficiency NOS
Mental subnormality NOS

Pervasive and specific developmental disorders (F80-F89)

✓4ᵗʰ **F80 Specific developmental disorders of speech and language**

   F80.0 Phonological disorder
Dyslalia
Functional speech articulation disorder
Lalling
Lisping
Phonological developmental disorder
Speech articulation developmental disorder
EXCLUDES 1   *speech articulation impairment due to aphasia NOS (R47.01)*
speech articulation impairment due to apraxia (R48.2)
EXCLUDES 2   *speech articulation impairment due to hearing loss (F80.4)*
speech articulation impairment due to intellectual disabilities (F70-F79)
speech articulation impairment with expressive language developmental disorder (F80.1)
speech articulation impairment with mixed receptive expressive language developmental disorder (F80.2)

   F80.1 Expressive language disorder
Developmental dysphasia or aphasia, expressive type
EXCLUDES 1   *dysphasia and aphasia NOS (R47.-)*
mixed receptive-expressive language disorder (F80.2)
EXCLUDES 2   *acquired aphasia with epilepsy [Landau-Kleffner] (G40.80-)*
intellectual disabilities (F70-F79)
pervasive developmental disorders (F84.-)
selective mutism (F94.0)

   F80.2 Mixed receptive-expressive language disorder
Developmental dysphasia or aphasia, receptive type
Developmental Wernicke's aphasia
EXCLUDES 1   *central auditory processing disorder (H93.25)*
dysphasia or aphasia NOS (R47.-)
expressive language disorder (F80.1)
expressive type dysphasia or aphasia (F80.1)
word deafness (H93.25)
EXCLUDES 2   *acquired aphasia with epilepsy [Landau-Kleffner] (G40.80-)*
intellectual disabilities (F70-F79)
pervasive developmental disorders (F84.-)
selective mutism (F94.0)

   F80.4 Speech and language development delay due to hearing loss
Code also type of hearing loss (H90.-, H91.-)

✓5ᵗʰ **F80.8 Other developmental disorders of speech and language**

     F80.81 Childhood onset fluency disorder
Cluttering NOS
Stuttering NOS
EXCLUDES 1   *adult onset fluency disorder (F98.5)*
fluency disorder in conditions classified elsewhere (R47.82)
fluency disorder (stuttering) following cerebrovascular disease (I69. with final characters-23)

     F80.89 Other developmental disorders of speech and language

   F80.9 Developmental disorder of speech and language, unspecified
Communication disorder NOS
Language disorder NOS

✓4ᵗʰ **F81 Specific developmental disorders of scholastic skills**

   F81.0 Specific reading disorder
"Backward reading"
Developmental dyslexia
Specific reading retardation
EXCLUDES 1   *alexia NOS (R48.0)*
dyslexia NOS (R48.0)

   F81.2 Mathematics disorder
Developmental acalculia
Developmental arithmetical disorder
Developmental Gerstmann's syndrome
EXCLUDES 1   *acalculia NOS (R48.8)*
EXCLUDES 2   *arithmetical difficulties associated with a reading disorder (F81.0)*
arithmetical difficulties associated with a spelling disorder (F81.81)
arithmetical difficulties due to inadequate teaching (Z55.8)

✓5ᵗʰ **F81.8 Other developmental disorders of scholastic skills**

     F81.81 Disorder of written expression
Specific spelling disorder

     F81.89 Other developmental disorders of scholastic skills

   F81.9 Developmental disorder of scholastic skills, unspecified
Knowledge acquisition disability NOS
Learning disability NOS
Learning disorder NOS

F82 Specific developmental disorder of motor function
Clumsy child syndrome
Developmental coordination disorder
Developmental dyspraxia
EXCLUDES 1   *abnormalities of gait and mobility (R26.-)*
lack of coordination (R27.-)
EXCLUDES 2   *lack of coordination secondary to intellectual disabilities (F70-F79)*

✓4ᵗʰ **F84 Pervasive developmental disorders**
Use additional code to identify any associated medical condition and intellectual disabilities

CC Excl: For CC codes in category F84, unless otherwise noted:
F07.0-F07.81, F07.9-F09, F20.0-F48.1, F48.8-F51.03, F51.12, F51.19, F51.3-F51.9, F52.5, F54, F59-F63.2, F63.81-F63.9, F68.10-F80.2, F80.4, F80.89-F84.0, F84.3-F99, G44.201-G44.229, H93.25, R45.1-R45.2, R45.5-R45.82, R45.86-R45.87

   F84.0 Autistic disorder   CC
Infantile autism
Infantile psychosis
Kanner's syndrome
EXCLUDES 1   *Asperger's syndrome (F84.5)*

N Newborn: 0   P Pediatric: 0-17   M Maternity: 12-55   A Adult: 15-124   MCC Major CC Condition   PDxMCC PDx acts as own MCC   CC CC Condition   PDxCC PDx acts as own CC

536

ICD-10-CM 2016

F84.2 Rett's syndrome `CC`
> EXCLUDES 1   *Asperger's syndrome (F84.5)*
> *Autistic disorder (F84.0)*
> *Other childhood disintegrative disorder (F84.3)*
> **CC Excl:** E75.00-E75.19, E75.4, F84.2, G13.2-G13.8, G30.0-G31.82,
> G31.84-G31.9, G91.4, G94

F84.3 Other childhood disintegrative disorder `CC` `P`
> Dementia infantilis
> Disintegrative psychosis
> Heller's syndrome
> Symbiotic psychosis
> Use additional code to identify any associated neurological
>   condition
> > EXCLUDES 1   *Asperger's syndrome (F84.5)*
> > *Autistic disorder (F84.0)*
> > *Rett's syndrome (F84.2)*

F84.5 Asperger's syndrome `CC`
> Asperger's disorder
> Autistic psychopathy
> Schizoid disorder of childhood

F84.8 Other pervasive developmental disorders `CC`
> Overactive disorder associated with intellectual disabilities
>   and stereotyped movements

F84.9 Pervasive developmental disorder, unspecified `CC`
> Atypical autism

F88 Other disorders of psychological development
> Developmental agnosia

F89 Unspecified disorder of psychological development
> Developmental disorder NOS

Behavioral and emotional disorders with onset usually occurring in childhood and adolescence (F90-F98)

> NOTE   Codes within categories F90-F98 may be used regardless of the age
> of a patient. These disorders generally have onset within the
> childhood or adolescent years, but may continue throughout life or
> not be diagnosed until adulthood

☑4ᵗʰ **F90 Attention-deficit hyperactivity disorders**
> INCLUDES   attention deficit disorder with hyperactivity
> attention deficit syndrome with hyperactivity
> > EXCLUDES 2   *anxiety disorders (F40.-, F41.-)*
> > *mood [affective] disorders (F30-F39)*
> > *pervasive developmental disorders (F84.-)*
> > *schizophrenia (F20.-)*

F90.0 Attention-deficit hyperactivity disorder, predominantly inattentive type

F90.1 Attention-deficit hyperactivity disorder, predominantly hyperactive type

F90.2 Attention-deficit hyperactivity disorder, combined type

F90.8 Attention-deficit hyperactivity disorder, other type

F90.9 Attention-deficit hyperactivity disorder, unspecified type
> Attention-deficit hyperactivity disorder of childhood or
>   adolescence NOS
> Attention-deficit hyperactivity disorder NOS

☑4ᵗʰ **F91 Conduct disorders**
> EXCLUDES 1   *antisocial behavior (Z72.81-)*
> *antisocial personality disorder (F60.2)*
> EXCLUDES 2   *conduct problems associated with attention-deficit*
> *hyperactivity disorder (F90.-)*
> *mood [affective] disorders (F30-F39)*
> *pervasive developmental disorders (F84.-)*
> *schizophrenia (F20.-)*

F91.0 Conduct disorder confined to family context

F91.1 Conduct disorder, childhood-onset type
> Unsocialized conduct disorder
> Conduct disorder, solitary aggressive type
> Unsocialized aggressive disorder

F91.2 Conduct disorder, adolescent-onset type
> Socialized conduct disorder
> Conduct disorder, group type

F91.3 Oppositional defiant disorder

F91.8 Other conduct disorders

F91.9 Conduct disorder, unspecified
> Behavioral disorder NOS
> Conduct disorder NOS
> Disruptive behavior disorder NOS

☑4ᵗʰ **F93 Emotional disorders with onset specific to childhood**
F93.0 Separation anxiety disorder of childhood `P`
> > EXCLUDES 2   *mood [affective] disorders (F30-F39)*
> > *nonpsychotic mental disorders (F40-F48)*
> > *phobic anxiety disorder of childhood (F40.8)*
> > *social phobia (F40.1)*

F93.8 Other childhood emotional disorders `P`
> Identity disorder
> > EXCLUDES 2   *gender identity disorder of childhood (F64.2)*

F93.9 Childhood emotional disorder, unspecified `P`

☑4ᵗʰ **F94 Disorders of social functioning with onset specific to childhood and adolescence**
F94.0 Selective mutism
> Elective mutism
> > EXCLUDES 2   *pervasive developmental disorders (F84.-)*
> > *schizophrenia (F20.-)*
> > *specific developmental disorders of speech and*
> > *language (F80.-)*
> > *transient mutism as part of separation anxiety in young*
> > *children (F93.0)*

F94.1 Reactive attachment disorder of childhood `P`
> Use additional code to identify any associated failure to thrive or
>   growth retardation
> > EXCLUDES 1   *disinhibited attachment disorder of childhood (F94.1)*
> > *normal variation in pattern of selective attachment*
> > EXCLUDES 2   *Asperger's syndrome (F84.5)*
> > *maltreatment syndromes (T74.-)*
> > *sexual or physical abuse in childhood, resulting in*
> > *psychosocial problems (Z62.81-)*

F94.2 Disinhibited attachment disorder of childhood `P`
> Affectionless psychopathy
> Institutional syndrome
> > EXCLUDES 1   *reactive attachment disorder of childhood (F94.1)*
> > EXCLUDES 2   *Asperger's syndrome (F84.5)*
> > *attention-deficit hyperactivity disorders (F90.-)*
> > *hospitalism in children (F43.2-)*

F94.8 Other childhood disorders of social functioning `P`
F94.9 Childhood disorder of social functioning, unspecified `P`

☑4ᵗʰ **F95 Tic disorder**
F95.0 Transient tic disorder
F95.1 Chronic motor or vocal tic disorder
F95.2 Tourette's disorder
> Combined vocal and multiple motor tic disorder [de la Tourette]
> Tourette's syndrome

F95.8 Other tic disorders
F95.9 Tic disorder, unspecified
> Tic NOS

☑4ᵗʰ **F98 Other behavioral and emotional disorders with onset usually occurring in childhood and adolescence**
> EXCLUDES 2   *breath-holding spells (R06.89)*
> *gender identity disorder of childhood (F64.2)*
> *Kleine-Levin syndrome (G47.13)*
> *obsessive-compulsive disorder (F42)*
> *sleep disorders not due to a substance or known physiological*
> *condition (F51.-)*

F98.0 Enuresis not due to a substance or known physiological condition
> Enuresis (primary) (secondary) of nonorganic origin
> Functional enuresis
> Psychogenic enuresis
> Urinary incontinence of nonorganic origin
> > EXCLUDES 1   *enuresis NOS (R32)*

F98.1 Encopresis not due to a substance or known physiological condition
> Functional encopresis
> Incontinence of feces of nonorganic origin
> Psychogenic encopresis
> Use additional code to identify the cause of any coexisting
>   constipation
> > EXCLUDES 1   *encopresis NOS (R15.-)*

☑5ᵗʰ **F98.2 Other feeding disorders of infancy and childhood**
> > EXCLUDES 1   *feeding difficulties (R63.3)*
> > EXCLUDES 2   *anorexia nervosa and other eating disorders (F50.-)*
> > *feeding problems of newborn (P92.-)*
> > *pica of infancy or childhood (F98.3)*

F98.21 Rumination disorder of infancy `P`
F98.29 Other feeding disorders of infancy and early childhood `P`

☑ Additional Character Required   ✓x7ᵗʰ Placeholder Alert   Unacceptable PDx   Manifestation   Hospital Acquired Condition   EXCLUDES 1 Not Coded Here   EXCLUDES 2 Not Included Here

F98.3 Pica of infancy and childhood   P

F98.4 Stereotyped movement disorders
Stereotype/habit disorder
EXCLUDES 1 *abnormal involuntary movements (R25.-)*
EXCLUDES 2 *compulsions in obsessive-compulsive disorder (F42)*
hair plucking (F63.3)
movement disorders of organic origin (G20-G25)
nail-biting (F98.8)
nose-picking (F98.8)
stereotypies that are part of a broader psychiatric condition (F01-F95)
thumb-sucking (F98.8)
tic disorders (F95.-)
trichotillomania (F63.3)

F98.5 Adult onset fluency disorder
EXCLUDES 1 *childhood onset fluency disorder (F80.81)*
dysphasia (R47.02)
fluency disorder in conditions classified elsewhere (R47.82)
fluency disorder (stuttering) following cerebrovascular disease (I69. with final characters -23)
tic disorders (F95.-)

F98.8 Other specified behavioral and emotional disorders with   P
onset usually occurring in childhood and adolescence
Excessive masturbation
Nail-biting
Nose-picking
Thumb-sucking

F98.9 Unspecified behavioral and emotional disorders with   P
onset usually occurring in childhood and adolescence

Unspecified mental disorder (F99)

F99 Mental disorder, not otherwise specified
Mental illness NOS
EXCLUDES 1 *unspecified mental disorder due to known physiological condition (F09)*

Chapter 6. Diseases of the Nervous System (G00-G99)

Chapter Specific Guidelines with Coding Examples

The chapter specific guidelines from the ICD-10-CM Official Guidelines for Coding and Reporting have been provided below. Along with these guidelines are coding examples, contained in the shaded boxes, that have been developed to help illustrate the coding and/or sequencing guidance found in these guidelines.

a. Dominant/nondominant side

Codes from category G81, Hemiplegia and hemiparesis, and subcategories G83.1, Monoplegia of lower limb, G83.2, Monoplegia of upper limb, and G83.3, Monoplegia, unspecified, identify whether the dominant or nondominant side is affected. Should the affected side be documented, but not specified as dominant or nondominant, and the classification system does not indicate a default, code selection is as follows:

- For ambidextrous patients, the default should be dominant.
- If the left side is affected, the default is non-dominant.
- If the right side is affected, the default is dominant.

> Hemiplegia affecting left side of ambidextrous patient
>
> **G81.92   Hemiplegia, unspecified affecting left dominant side**
>
> *Explanation:* Documentation states that the left side is affected and dominant is used for ambidextrous persons.

> Right spastic hemiplegia, unknown whether patient is right- or left-handed
>
> **G81.11   Spastic hemiplegia affecting right dominant side**
>
> *Explanation:* Since it is unknown whether the patient is right- or left-handed, if the right side is affected, the default is dominant.

b. Pain—Category G89

1) General coding information

Codes in category G89, Pain, not elsewhere classified, may be used in conjunction with codes from other categories and chapters to provide more detail about acute or chronic pain and neoplasm-related pain, unless otherwise indicated below.

If the pain is not specified as acute or chronic, post-thoracotomy, postprocedural, or neoplasm-related, do not assign codes from category G89.

A code from category G89 should not be assigned if the underlying (definitive) diagnosis is known, unless the reason for the encounter is pain control/ management and not management of the underlying condition.

When an admission or encounter is for a procedure aimed at treating the underlying condition (e.g., spinal fusion, kyphoplasty), a code for the underlying condition (e.g., vertebral fracture, spinal stenosis) should be assigned as the principal diagnosis. No code from category G89 should be assigned.

> Elderly patient with back pain is admitted for outpatient kyphoplasty for age-related osteopathic compression fracture at vertebra T3
>
> **M80.08XA   Age-related osteoporosis with current pathological fracture, vertebra(e), initial encounter**
>
> *Explanation:* No code is assigned for the pain as it is inherent in the underlying condition being treated.

(a) Category G89 codes as principal or first-listed diagnosis

Category G89 codes are acceptable as principal diagnosis or the first-listed code:

- When pain control or pain management is the reason for the admission/encounter (e.g., a patient with displaced intervertebral disc, nerve impingement and severe back pain presents for injection of steroid into the spinal canal). The underlying cause of the pain should be reported as an additional diagnosis, if known.

> Patient presents for a steroid injection for control of pain of chronic right knee due to primary degenerative joint disease
>
> **G89.29   Other chronic pain**
>
> **M17.11   Unilateral primary osteoarthritis, right knee**
>
> *Explanation:* Since the encounter is for control of pain, not treating the underlying condition, the pain code is sequenced first followed by the underlying condition. The M25 pain code is not necessary as the underlying condition code represents the specific site.

- When a patient is admitted for the insertion of a neurostimulator for pain control, assign the appropriate pain code as the principal or first-listed diagnosis. When an admission or encounter is for a procedure aimed at treating the underlying condition and a neurostimulator is inserted for pain control during the same admission/encounter, a code for the underlying condition should be assigned as the principal diagnosis and the appropriate pain code should be assigned as a secondary diagnosis.

(b) Use of category G89 codes in conjunction with site specific pain codes

(i) Assigning category G89 and site-specific pain codes

Codes from category G89 may be used in conjunction with codes that identify the site of pain (including codes from chapter 18) if the category G89 code provides additional information. For example, if the code describes the site of the pain, but does not fully describe whether the pain is acute or chronic, then both codes should be assigned.

> Patient is seen to evaluate chronic left shoulder pain
>
> **M25.512   Pain in left shoulder**
>
> **G89.29   Other chronic pain**
>
> *Explanation:* No underlying condition has been determined yet so the pain would be the reason for the visit. The M25 pain code in this instance does not fully describe the condition as it does not represent that the pain is chronic. The G89 chronic pain code is assigned to provide specificity.

(ii) Sequencing of category G89 codes with site-specific pain codes

The sequencing of category G89 codes with site-specific pain codes (including chapter 18 codes), is dependent on the circumstances of the encounter/admission as follows:

- If the encounter is for pain control or pain management, assign the code from category G89 followed by the code identifying the specific site of pain (e.g., encounter for pain management for acute neck pain from trauma is assigned code G89.11, Acute pain due to trauma, followed by code M54.2, Cervicalgia, to identify the site of pain).

> Management of acute, traumatic right knee pain
>
> **G89.11   Acute pain due to trauma**
>
> **M25.561   Pain in right knee**
>
> *Explanation:* The reason for the encounter is to manage or control the pain, not to treat or evaluate an underlying condition. The G89 pain code is assigned as the principal diagnosis but in this instance does not fully describe the condition as it does not include the site and laterality. The M25 pain code is added to provide this information.

- If the encounter is for any other reason except pain control or pain management, and a related definitive diagnosis has not been established (confirmed) by the provider, assign the code for the specific site of pain first, followed by the appropriate code from category G89.

> Tests are performed to investigate the source of the patient's chronic epigastric abdominal pain
>
> **R10.13**   **Epigastric pain**
>
> **G89.29**   **Other chronic pain**
>
> *Explanation*: In this instance the patient's epigastric pain is not being treated; rather the source of the pain is being investigated. A code from chapter 18 for epigastric pain is sequenced before the additional specificity of the G89 code for the chronic pain.

2) Pain due to devices, implants and grafts

See Section I.C.19. Pain due to medical devices

3) Postoperative Pain

The provider's documentation should be used to guide the coding of postoperative pain, as well as *Section III. Reporting Additional Diagnoses* and *Section IV. Diagnostic Coding and Reporting in the Outpatient Setting*.

The default for post-thoracotomy and other postoperative pain not specified as acute or chronic is the code for the acute form.

Routine or expected postoperative pain immediately after surgery should not be coded.

> Pain pump dose is increased for the patient's unexpected, extreme pain post-thoracotomy
>
> **G89.12**   **Acute post-thoracotomy pain**
>
> *Explanation*: When acute or chronic is not documented, default to acute. The use of "unexpected, extreme" and the increase of medication dosage indicate that the pain was more than routine or expected.

(a) Postoperative pain not associated with specific postoperative complication

Postoperative pain not associated with a specific postoperative complication is assigned to the appropriate postoperative pain code in category G89.

(b) Postoperative pain associated with specific postoperative complication

Postoperative pain associated with a specific postoperative complication (such as painful wire sutures) is assigned to the appropriate code(s) found in Chapter 19, Injury, poisoning, and certain other consequences of external causes. If appropriate, use additional code(s) from category G89 to identify acute or chronic pain (G89.18 or G89.28).

4) Chronic pain

Chronic pain is classified to subcategory G89.2. There is no time frame defining when pain becomes chronic pain. The provider's documentation should be used to guide use of these codes.

5) Neoplasm related pain

Code G89.3 is assigned to pain documented as being related, associated or due to cancer, primary or secondary malignancy, or tumor. This code is assigned regardless of whether the pain is acute or chronic.

This code may be assigned as the principal or first-listed code when the stated reason for the admission/encounter is documented as pain control/pain management. The underlying neoplasm should be reported as an additional diagnosis.

> Pain medication adjustment for chronic pain from bone metastasis
>
> **G89.3**   **Neoplasm related pain (acute)(chronic)**
>
> **C79.51**   **Secondary malignant neoplasm of bone**
>
> *Explanation*: Since the encounter was for pain medication management, the pain, rather than the neoplasm, was the reason for the encounter and is sequenced first. This "neoplasm-related pain" code includes both acute and chronic pain.

When the reason for the admission/encounter is management of the neoplasm and the pain associated with the neoplasm is also documented, code G89.3 may be assigned as an additional diagnosis. It is not necessary to assign an additional code for the site of the pain.

See Section I.C.2 for instructions on the sequencing of neoplasms for all other stated reasons for the admission/encounter (except for pain control/pain management).

> Patient with lung cancer presents with acute hip pain and is evaluated and found to have iliac bone metastasis
>
> **C79.51**   **Secondary malignant neoplasm of bone**
>
> **C34.90**   **Malignant neoplasm of unspecified part of unspecified bronchus or lung**
>
> **G89.3**   **Neoplasm related pain (acute)(chronic)**
>
> *Explanation*: The reason for the encounter was the evaluation and diagnosis of the bone metastasis, whose code would be assigned as first-listed, followed by codes for the primary neoplasm and the pain due to the iliac bone metastasis.

6) Chronic pain syndrome

Central pain syndrome (G89.0) and chronic pain syndrome (G89.4) are different than the term "chronic pain," and therefore codes should only be used when the provider has specifically documented this condition.

See Section I.C.5. Pain disorders related to psychological factors

Chapter 6. Diseases of the Nervous System (G00-G99)

EXCLUDES 2   *certain conditions originating in the perinatal period (P04-P96)*
certain infectious and parasitic diseases (A00-B99)
complications of pregnancy, childbirth and the puerperium (O00-O9A)
congenital malformations, deformations, and chromosomal abnormalities (Q00-Q99)
endocrine, nutritional and metabolic diseases (E00-E88)
injury, poisoning and certain other consequences of external causes (S00-T88)
neoplasms (C00-D49)
symptoms, signs and abnormal clinical and laboratory findings, not elsewhere classified (R00-R94)

This chapter contains the following blocks:

G00-G09   Inflammatory diseases of the central nervous system
G10-G14   Systemic atrophies primarily affecting the central nervous system
G20-G26   Extrapyramidal and movement disorders
G30-G32   Other degenerative diseases of the nervous system
G35-G37   Demyelinating diseases of the central nervous system
G40-G47   Episodic and paroxysmal disorders
G50-G59   Nerve, nerve root and plexus disorders
G60-G65   Polyneuropathies and other disorders of the peripheral nervous system
G70-G73   Diseases of myoneural junction and muscle
G80-G83   Cerebral palsy and other paralytic syndromes
G89-G99   Other disorders of the nervous system

Inflammatory diseases of the central nervous system (G00-G09)

✓4ᵗʰ **G00   Bacterial meningitis, not elsewhere classified**
INCLUDES   bacterial arachnoiditis
bacterial leptomeningitis
bacterial meningitis
bacterial pachymeningitis
EXCLUDES 1   *bacterial:*
meningoencephalitis (G04.2)
meningomyelitis (G04.2)

CC Excl: For MCC codes in category G00, unless otherwise noted:
A02.21, A17.0-A17.1, A27.81, A39.0, A50.41, A51.41, A52.13, A54.82, A54.84, A54.89-A54.9, A87.0-A87.9, B00.3, B02.1, B26.1, B37.5, B38.4, B45.1, B58.2, E08.40-E08.49, E08.618-E08.638, E08.649-E08.8, E09.40-E09.49, E09.618-E09.638, E09.649-E09.8, E10.40-E10.49, E10.618-E10.638, E10.649, E10.69-E10.8, E11.40-E11.49, E11.618-E11.638, E11.649, E11.69-E11.8, E13.40-E13.49, E13.618-E13.638, E13.649-E13.8, G00.0-G03.9, G04.2, G32.89, G61.0, G96.8-G96.9, G98.0-G98.8, G99.8

G00.0   Hemophilus meningitis   MCC
Meningitis due to Hemophilus influenzae

G00.1   Pneumococcal meningitis   MCC

G00.2   Streptococcal meningitis   MCC
Use additional code to further identify organism (B95.0-B95.5)

G00.3   Staphylococcal meningitis   MCC
Use additional code to further identify organism (B95.61-B95.8)

G00.8   Other bacterial meningitis   MCC
Meningitis due to Escherichia coli
Meningitis due to Friedländer's bacillus
Meningitis due to Klebsiella
Use additional code to further identify organism (B96.-)

G00.9   Bacterial meningitis, unspecified   MCC
Meningitis due to gram-negative bacteria, unspecified
Purulent meningitis NOS
Pyogenic meningitis NOS
Suppurative meningitis NOS

G01   Meningitis in bacterial diseases classified elsewhere   MCC
Code first underlying disease
EXCLUDES 1   *meningitis (in):*
gonococcal (A54.81)
leptospirosis (A27.81)
listeriosis (A32.11)
Lyme disease (A69.21)
meningococcal (A39.0)
neurosyphilis (A52.13)
tuberculosis (A17.0)
meningoencephalitis and meningomyelitis in bacterial diseases classified elsewhere (G05)
CC Excl: See code: G00

G02   Meningitis in other infectious and parasitic diseases classified elsewhere   MCC
Code first underlying disease, such as:
African trypanosomiasis (B56.-)
poliovirus infection (A80.-)
EXCLUDES 1   *candidal meningitis (B37.5)*
coccidioidomycosis meningitis (B38.4)
cryptococcal meningitis (B45.1)
herpesviral [herpes simplex] meningitis (B00.3)
infectious mononucleosis complicated by meningitis (B27.- with fourth character 2)
measles complicated by meningitis (B05.1)
meningoencephalitis and meningomyelitis in other infectious and parasitic diseases classified elsewhere (G05)
mumps meningitis (B26.1)
rubella meningitis (B06.02)
varicella [chickenpox] meningitis (B01.0)
zoster meningitis (B02.1)
CC Excl: A02.21, A17.0-A17.1, A27.81, A39.0, A50.41, A51.41, A52.13, A54.82, A54.84, A54.89-A54.9, A87.0-A87.9, B00.3, B02.1, B26.1, B37.5, B38.4, B45.1, B58.2, G00.0-G03.9, G04.2, G32.89, G61.0, G96.8-G96.9, G98.0-G98.8, G99.8

✓4ᵗʰ **G03   Meningitis due to other and unspecified causes**
INCLUDES   arachnoiditis NOS
leptomeningitis NOS
meningitis NOS
pachymeningitis NOS
EXCLUDES 1   *meningoencephalitis (G04.-)*
meningomyelitis (G04.-)

G03.0   Nonpyogenic meningitis   MCC
Aseptic meningitis
Nonbacterial meningitis
CC Excl: See code: G00

G03.1   Chronic meningitis   CC
CC Excl: See code: G00

G03.2   Benign recurrent meningitis [Mollaret]   CC
CC Excl: A02.21, A17.0-A17.1, A27.81, A39.0, A50.41, A51.41, A52.13, A54.82, A54.84, A54.89-A54.9, A74.81-A74.9, A87.0-A87.9, A96.2, A98.3-A98.4, B26.1, B33.24, B33.4-B33.8, B34.1-B34.2, B34.4-B34.8, B37.5, B38.4, B45.1, B58.2, B92, B94.2-B94.9, B97.10, B97.19, B97.29, B97.5-B97.6, B97.81-B97.89, G00.0-G03.9, G04.2, G32.89, G61.0, G96.8-G96.9, G98.0-G98.8, G99.8

G03.8   Meningitis due to other specified causes   MCC
CC Excl: See code: G00

G03.9   Meningitis, unspecified   MCC
Arachnoiditis (spinal) NOS
CC Excl: See code: G00

✓4ᵗʰ **G04   Encephalitis, myelitis and encephalomyelitis**
INCLUDES   acute ascending myelitis
meningoencephalitis
meningomyelitis
EXCLUDES 1   *encephalopathy NOS (G93.40)*
EXCLUDES 2   *acute transverse myelitis (G37.3-)*
alcoholic encephalopathy (G31.2)
benign myalgic encephalomyelitis (G93.3)
multiple sclerosis (G35)
subacute necrotizing myelitis (G37.4)
toxic encephalitis (G92)
toxic encephalopathy (G92)

✓5ᵗʰ **G04.0   Acute disseminated encephalitis and encephalomyelitis (ADEM)**
EXCLUDES 1   *acute necrotizing hemorrhagic encephalopathy (G04.3-)*
other noninfectious acute disseminated encephalomyelitis (noninfectious ADEM) (G04.81)

G04.00   Acute disseminated encephalitis and encephalomyelitis, unspecified   MCC
CC Excl: A02.21, A17.0-A17.1, A17.82, A27.81, A39.0, A50.41-A50.42, A51.41, A52.13-A52.14, A54.82, A54.84, A54.89-A54.9, A81.1, A81.82-A81.89, A83.0-A85.8, A87.0-A88.0, A88.8, A92.1-A92.8, A93.0, A96.2, A98.3-A98.4, B00.3-B00.4, B00.89-B01.11, B01.81-B02.23, B02.29, B02.7-B02.9, B04, B06.01, B08.04-B08.09, B08.20-B08.22, B08.60-B08.79, B09-B10.89, B26.1-B26.2, B27.00-B27.99, B33.1, B33.24, B33.4-B33.8, B34.1-B34.2, B34.4-B34.8, B37.5, B38.4, B45.1, B58.2, B92, B94.2-B94.9, B97.10, B97.19-B97.29, B97.5-B97.6, B97.81-B97.89, G00.0-G04.01, G04.2, G04.31, G04.81-G05.4, G32.89, G37.0, G37.4-G37.5, G61.0, G96.8-G96.9, G98.0-G98.8, G99.8, J09.X3-J09.X9, J10.2-J10.89, J11.2-J11.89, L44.4, P35.2-P35.9, P37.0-P37.4, P37.8-P37.9

✓ Additional Character Required   ✓x7ᵗʰ Placeholder Alert   Unacceptable PDx   Manifestation   Hospital Acquired Condition   EXCLUDES 1 Not Coded Here   EXCLUDES 2 Not Included Here

Chapter 6. Diseases of the Nervous System

G04.01   Postinfectious acute disseminated encephalitis and encephalomyelitis (postinfectious ADEM)   `MCC`

EXCLUDES 1   post chickenpox encephalitis (B01.1)
post measles encephalitis (B05.0)
post measles myelitis (B05.1)

CC Excl: See code: G04.00

G04.02   Postimmunization acute disseminated encephalitis, myelitis and encephalomyelitis   `MCC`

Encephalitis, postimmunization
Encephalomyelitis, postimmunization

Use additional code to identify the vaccine (T50.A-, T50.B-, T50Z-)

CC Excl: No Excl

G04.1   **Tropical spastic paraplegia**   `CC`

CC Excl: G04.1, G11.0-G12.9, G32.0-G37.3, G37.5-G37.9, G80.0-G80.2, G80.4-G83.9, G90.01-G90.09, G90.2, G90.4-G90.9, G92, G93.40-G93.49, G93.81, G93.89-G93.9, G95.0-G95.9, G96.8-G96.9, G98.0-G99.8, I67.83, R53.2

G04.2   **Bacterial meningoencephalitis and meningomyelitis, not elsewhere classified**   `MCC`

CC Excl: See code: G00

✓5ᵗʰ   **G04.3**   **Acute necrotizing hemorrhagic encephalopathy**

EXCLUDES 1   acute disseminated encephalitis and encephalomyelitis (G04.0-)

G04.30   Acute necrotizing hemorrhagic encephalopathy, unspecified   `MCC`

CC Excl: No Excl

G04.31   Postinfectious acute necrotizing hemorrhagic encephalopathy   `MCC`

CC Excl: See code: G04.00

G04.32   Postimmunization acute necrotizing hemorrhagic encephalopathy   `MCC`

Use additional code to identify the vaccine (T50.A-, T50.B-, T50Z-)

CC Excl: No Excl

G04.39   Other acute necrotizing hemorrhagic encephalopathy   `MCC`

Code also underlying etiology, if applicable

CC Excl: No Excl

✓5ᵗʰ   **G04.8**   **Other encephalitis, myelitis and encephalomyelitis**

Code also any associated seizure (G40.-, R56.9)

G04.81   Other encephalitis and encephalomyelitis   `HIV` `MCC`

Noninfectious acute disseminated encephalomyelitis (noninfectious ADEM)

CC Excl: See code: G04.00

G04.89   Other myelitis   `HIV` `MCC`

CC Excl: See code: G04.00

✓5ᵗʰ   **G04.9**   **Encephalitis, myelitis and encephalomyelitis, unspecified**

G04.90   Encephalitis and encephalomyelitis, unspecified   `HIV` `MCC`

Ventriculitis (cerebral) NOS

CC Excl: A17.82, A28.1, A50.42, A52.14, A75.9, A79.9, A81.1, A81.82-A81.89, A83.0-A85.8, A87.2, A88.0, A88.8, A92.1-A92.8, A93.0, B00.4, B00.82, B01.11-B01.12, B04, B06.01, B08.09, B08.20-B08.22, B08.60-B08.79, B09-B10.09, B26.2, B27.00-B27.99, B33.1, B45.0, B45.2-B45.9, B54, B58.2, B75, B97.10, B97.21, G04.00-G04.01, G04.31, G04.81-G05.4, G37.0, G37.4-G37.5, H66.40-H66.43, J09.X3-J09.X9, J10.2-J10.89, J11.2-J11.89, L44.4, M1A.10X0-M1A.19X1, M32.0-M32.9, P35.2-P35.9, P37.0-P37.4, P37.8-P37.9, T56.0X1A, T56.0X2A, T56.0X3A, T56.0X4A

G04.91   Myelitis, unspecified   `HIV` `MCC`

CC Excl: See code: G04.90

✓4ᵗʰ   **G05**   **Encephalitis, myelitis and encephalomyelitis in diseases classified elsewhere**

Code first underlying disease, such as:
human immunodeficiency virus [HIV] disease (B20)
poliovirus (A80.-)
suppurative otitis media (H66.01-H66.4)
trichinellosis (B75)

EXCLUDES 1   adenoviral encephalitis, myelitis and encephalomyelitis (A85.1)
congenital toxoplasmosis encephalitis, myelitis and encephalomyelitis (P37.1)
cytomegaloviral encephalitis, myelitis and encephalomyelitis (B25.8)
encephalitis, myelitis and encephalomyelitis (in) measles (B05.0)
encephalitis, myelitis and encephalomyelitis (in) systemic lupus erythematosus (M32.19)
enteroviral encephalitis, myelitis and encephalomyelitis (A85.0)
eosinophilic meningoencephalitis (B83.2)
herpesviral [herpes simplex] encephalitis, myelitis and encephalomyelitis (B00.4)
listerial encephalitis, myelitis and encephalomyelitis (A32.12)
meningococcal encephalitis, myelitis and encephalomyelitis (A39.81)
mumps encephalitis, myelitis and encephalomyelitis (B26.2)
postchickenpox encephalitis, myelitis and encephalomyelitis (B01.1-)
rubella encephalitis, myelitis and encephalomyelitis (B06.01)
toxoplasmosis encephalitis, myelitis and encephalomyelitis (B58.2)
zoster encephalitis, myelitis and encephalomyelitis (B02.0)

G05.3   *Encephalitis and encephalomyelitis in diseases classified elsewhere*   `MCC`

Meningoencephalitis in diseases classified elsewhere

CC Excl: See code: G04.00

G05.4   *Myelitis in diseases classified elsewhere*   `MCC`

Meningomyelitis in diseases classified elsewhere

CC Excl: See code: G04.00

✓4ᵗʰ   **G06**   **Intracranial and intraspinal abscess and granuloma**

Use additional code (B95-B97) to identify infectious agent

G06.0   Intracranial abscess and granuloma   `MCC`

Brain [any part] abscess (embolic)
Cerebellar abscess (embolic)
Cerebral abscess (embolic)
Intracranial epidural abscess or granuloma
Intracranial extradural abscess or granuloma
Intracranial subdural abscess or granuloma
Otogenic abscess (embolic)

EXCLUDES 1   tuberculous intracranial abscess and granuloma (A17.81)

CC Excl: A06.6, A17.81, E08.40-E08.49, E08.618-E08.638, E08.649-E08.8, E09.40-E09.49, E09.618-E09.638, E09.649-E09.8, E10.40-E10.49, E10.618-E10.638, E10.649, E10.69-E10.8, E11.40-E11.49, E11.618-E11.638, E11.649, E11.69-E11.8, E13.40-E13.49, E13.618-E13.638, E13.649-E13.8, G06.0-G08, G93.81, G93.89-G93.9

G06.1   Intraspinal abscess and granuloma   `MCC`

Abscess (embolic) of spinal cord [any part]
Intraspinal epidural abscess or granuloma
Intraspinal extradural abscess or granuloma
Intraspinal subdural abscess or granuloma

EXCLUDES 1   tuberculous intraspinal abscess and granuloma (A17.81)

CC Excl: A06.6, A17.81, E08.40-E08.49, E08.618-E08.638, E08.649-E08.8, E09.40-E09.49, E09.618-E09.638, E09.649-E09.8, E10.40-E10.49, E10.618-E10.638, E10.649, E10.69-E10.8, E11.40-E11.49, E11.618-E11.638, E11.649, E11.69-E11.8, E13.40-E13.49, E13.618-E13.638, E13.649-E13.8, G06.1

G06.2   Extradural and subdural abscess, unspecified   `MCC`

CC Excl: A06.6, A17.81, E08.40-E08.49, E08.618-E08.638, E08.649-E08.8, E09.40-E09.49, E09.618-E09.638, E09.649-E09.8, E10.40-E10.49, E10.618-E10.638, E10.649, E10.69-E10.8, E11.40-E11.49, E11.618-E11.638, E11.649, E11.69-E11.8, E13.40-E13.49, E13.618-E13.638, E13.649-E13.8, G06.0-G08

G07   *Intracranial and intraspinal abscess and granuloma in diseases classified elsewhere*   `MCC`

Code first underlying disease, such as:
schistosomiasis granuloma of brain (B65.-)

EXCLUDES 1   abscess of brain:
amebic (A06.6)
chromomycotic (B43.1)
gonococcal (A54.82)
tuberculous (A17.81)
tuberculoma of meninges (A17.1)

CC Excl: See code: G06.2

N Newborn: 0   P Pediatric: 0-17   M Maternity: 12-55   A Adult: 15-124   `MCC` Major CC Condition   `PDxMCC` PDx acts as own MCC   `CC` CC Condition   `PDxCC` PDx acts as own CC

542   ICD-10-CM 2016

G08   **Intracranial and intraspinal phlebitis and thrombophlebitis** `MCC`

Septic embolism of intracranial or intraspinal venous sinuses and veins

Septic endophlebitis of intracranial or intraspinal venous sinuses and veins

Septic phlebitis of intracranial or intraspinal venous sinuses and veins

Septic thrombophlebitis of intracranial or intraspinal venous sinuses and veins

Septic thrombosis of intracranial or intraspinal venous sinuses and veins

   EXCLUDES 1   *intracranial phlebitis and thrombophlebitis complicating: abortion, ectopic or molar pregnancy (O00-O07, O08.7)*
pregnancy, childbirth and the puerperium (O22.5, O87.3)
nonpyogenic intracranial phlebitis and thrombophlebitis (I67.6)

   EXCLUDES 2   *intracranial phlebitis and thrombophlebitis complicating nonpyogenic intraspinal phlebitis and thrombophlebitis (G95.1)*

   CC Excl: See code: G06.2

G09   **Sequelae of inflammatory diseases of central nervous system**

   `NOTE`   Category G09 is to be used to indicate conditions whose primary classification is to G00-G08 as the cause of sequelae, themselves classifiable elsewhere. The "sequelae" include conditions specified as residuals.

   Code first condition resulting from (sequela) of inflammatory diseases of central nervous system

Systemic atrophies primarily affecting the central nervous system (G10-G14)

G10   **Huntington's disease** `CC`

Huntington's chorea

Huntington's dementia

   CC Excl: G04.1, G20, G21.11-G21.9, G32.89-G37.2, G37.5-G37.9, G80.0-G80.2, G80.4-G80.9, G82.20-G83.0, G92, G93.1, G93.40-G93.6, G93.81, G93.89-G93.9, G96.8-G96.9, G98.0-G98.8, G99.8, I67.83, R53.2

`√4ᵗʰ` **G11**   **Hereditary ataxia**

   EXCLUDES 2   *cerebral palsy (G80.-)*
hereditary and idiopathic neuropathy (G60.-)
metabolic disorders (E70-E88)

   CC Excl: For CC codes in category G11, unless otherwise noted:
G04.1, G10-G12.9, G21.0, G23.0-G25.79, G25.82-G26, G32.0-G37.3, G37.5-G37.9, G80.0-G83.9, G90.01-G90.09, G90.2-G90.9, G92-G93.1, G93.40-G93.49, G93.81, G93.89-G93.9, G95.0-G95.9, G96.8-G96.9, G98.0-G99.8, I67.83, R53.2

G11.0   **Congenital nonprogressive ataxia** `CC`

G11.1   **Early-onset cerebellar ataxia** `CC`

Early-onset cerebellar ataxia with essential tremor

Early-onset cerebellar ataxia with myoclonus [Hunt's ataxia]

Early-onset cerebellar ataxia with retained tendon reflexes

Friedreich's ataxia (autosomal recessive)

X-linked recessive spinocerebellar ataxia

G11.2   **Late-onset cerebellar ataxia** `CC` `A`

G11.3   **Cerebellar ataxia with defective DNA repair** `CC`

Ataxia telangiectasia [Louis-Bar]

   EXCLUDES 2   *Cockayne's syndrome (Q87.1)*
other disorders of purine and pyrimidine metabolism (E79.-)
xeroderma pigmentosum (Q82.1)

G11.4   **Hereditary spastic paraplegia** `CC`

   CC Excl: G04.1, G10-G12.9, G21.0, G23.0-G25.79, G25.82-G26, G32.0-G37.3, G37.5-G37.9, G80.0-G83.9, G90.01-G90.09, G90.2-G90.9, G92, G93.1, G93.40-G93.49, G93.81, G93.89-G93.9, G95.0-G95.9, G96.12-G96.9, G97.1, G98.0-G99.8, I67.83, R53.2

G11.8   **Other hereditary ataxias** `CC`

G11.9   **Hereditary ataxia, unspecified** `CC`

Hereditary cerebellar ataxia NOS

Hereditary cerebellar degeneration

Hereditary cerebellar disease

Hereditary cerebellar syndrome

   CC Excl: G11.0-G11.9, G32.81

`√4ᵗʰ` **G12**   **Spinal muscular atrophy and related syndromes**

   CC Excl: For CC codes in category G12, unless otherwise noted:
E08.40-E08.49, E08.618-E08.638, E08.649-E08.8, E09.40-E09.49, E09.618-E09.638, E09.649-E09.8, E10.40-E10.49, E10.618-E10.638, E10.649, E10.69-E10.8, E11.40-E11.49, E11.618-E11.638, E11.649, E11.69-E11.8, E13.40-E13.49, E13.618-E13.638, E13.649-E13.8, G11.3, G11.8-G12.9, G32.0, G32.89, G90.01-G90.09, G90.2, G90.4-G90.9, G95.0-G95.9, G96.8-G96.9, G98.0-G99.8

G12.0   **Infantile spinal muscular atrophy, type I [Werdnig-Hoffman]** `CC`

G12.1   **Other inherited spinal muscular atrophy** `CC`

Adult form spinal muscular atrophy

Childhood form, type II spinal muscular atrophy

Distal spinal muscular atrophy

Juvenile form, type III spinal muscular atrophy [Kugelberg-Welander]

Progressive bulbar palsy of childhood [Fazio-Londe]

Scapuloperoneal form spinal muscular atrophy

`√5ᵗʰ` **G12.2**   **Motor neuron disease**

G12.20   **Motor neuron disease, unspecified** `CC`

G12.21   **Amyotrophic lateral sclerosis** `CC` `A`

Progressive spinal muscle atrophy

G12.22   **Progressive bulbar palsy** `CC`

G12.29   **Other motor neuron disease** `CC`

Familial motor neuron disease

Primary lateral sclerosis

G12.8   **Other spinal muscular atrophies and related syndromes** `CC`

G12.9   **Spinal muscular atrophy, unspecified** `CC`

`√4ᵗʰ` **G13**   **Systemic atrophies primarily affecting central nervous system in diseases classified elsewhere**

G13.0   *Paraneoplastic neuromyopathy and neuropathy*

Carcinomatous neuromyopathy

Sensorial paraneoplastic neuropathy [Denny Brown]

   Code first underlying neoplasm (C00-D49)

G13.1   *Other systemic atrophy primarily affecting central nervous system in neoplastic disease*

Paraneoplastic limbic encephalopathy

   Code first underlying neoplasm (C00-D49)

G13.2   *Systemic atrophy primarily affecting the central nervous system in myxedema*

   Code first underlying disease, such as:
hypothyroidism (E03.-)
myxedematous congenital iodine deficiency (E00.1)

G13.8   *Systemic atrophy primarily affecting central nervous system in other diseases classified elsewhere*

   Code first underlying disease

G14   **Postpolio syndrome**

Postpolio myelitic syndrome

   EXCLUDES 1   *sequelae of poliomyelitis (B91)*

Extrapyramidal and movement disorders (G20-G26)

G20   **Parkinson's disease**

Hemiparkinsonism

Idiopathic Parkinsonism or Parkinson's disease

Paralysis agitans

Parkinsonism or Parkinson's disease NOS

Primary Parkinsonism or Parkinson's disease

   EXCLUDES 1   *dementia with Parkinsonism (G31.83)*

`√4ᵗʰ` **G21**   **Secondary parkinsonism**

   EXCLUDES 1   *dementia with Parkinsonism (G31.83)*
Huntington's disease (G10)
Shy-Drager syndrome (G90.3)
syphilitic Parkinsonism (A52.19)

G21.0   **Malignant neuroleptic syndrome** `MCC`

Use additional code for adverse effect, if applicable, to identify drug (T43.3X5, T43.4X5, T43.505, T43.595)

   EXCLUDES 1   *neuroleptic induced parkinsonism (G21.11)*

   CC Excl: G10, G21.0, G23.0-G25.79, G25.82-G26, G80.3, G81.00-G81.94, G90.3, G93.2, G93.40-G93.49, I67.83

`√5ᵗʰ` **G21.1**   **Other drug-induced secondary parkinsonism**

G21.11   **Neuroleptic induced parkinsonism** `CC`

Use additional code for adverse effect, if applicable, to identify drug (T43.3X5, T43.4X5, T43.505, T43.595)

   EXCLUDES 1   *malignant neuroleptic syndrome (G21.0)*

   CC Excl: G20-G21.9

G21.19   **Other drug induced secondary parkinsonism** `CC`

Use additional code for adverse effect, if applicable, to identify drug (T36-T50 with fifth or sixth character 5)

   CC Excl: See code: G21.11

G21.2   **Secondary parkinsonism due to other external agents** `CC`

Code first (T51-T65) to identify external agent

   CC Excl: See code: G21.11

G21.3   **Postencephalitic parkinsonism** `CC`

   CC Excl: See code: G21.11

G21.4   **Vascular parkinsonism**

`✓` Additional Character Required   `√xᵗʰ` Placeholder Alert   Unacceptable PDx   Manifestation   Hospital Acquired Condition   *EXCLUDES 1* Not Coded Here   *EXCLUDES 2* Not Included Here

Chapter 6. Diseases of the Nervous System

G21.8 Other secondary parkinsonism ᶜᶜ
CC Excl: See code: G21.11

G21.9 Secondary parkinsonism, unspecified ᶜᶜ
CC Excl: See code: G21.11

✓4ᵗʰ **G23** Other degenerative diseases of basal ganglia
EXCLUDES 2 *multi-system degeneration of the autonomic nervous system (G90.3)*

CC Excl: For CC codes in category G23, unless otherwise noted:
G20, G21.11-G21.9, G90.01-G90.09, G93.40-G93.49, I67.83

G23.0 Hallervorden-Spatz disease ᶜᶜ
Pigmentary pallidal degeneration

G23.1 Progressive supranuclear ophthalmoplegia ᶜᶜ
[Steele-Richardson-Olszewski]
Progressive supranuclear palsy

G23.2 Striatonigral degeneration ᶜᶜ

G23.8 Other specified degenerative diseases of basal ganglia ᶜᶜ
Calcification of basal ganglia

G23.9 Degenerative disease of basal ganglia, unspecified ᶜᶜ

✓4ᵗʰ **G24** Dystonia
INCLUDES dyskinesia
EXCLUDES 2 *athetoid cerebral palsy (G80.3)*

CC Excl: For CC codes in category G24, unless otherwise noted:
G20, G21.11-G21.9, G25.70-G25.79, G25.89-G26, G80.3, G93.40-G93.49, I67.8

✓5ᵗʰ **G24.0** Drug induced dystonia
Use additional code for adverse effect, if applicable, to identify drug (T36-T50 with fifth or sixth character5)

G24.01 Drug induced subacute dyskinesia
Drug induced blepharospasm
Drug induced orofacial dyskinesia
Neuroleptic induced tardive dyskinesia
Tardive dyskinesia

G24.02 Drug induced acute dystonia ᶜᶜ
Acute dystonic reaction to drugs
Neuroleptic induced acute dystonia

G24.09 Other drug induced dystonia ᶜᶜ

G24.1 Genetic torsion dystonia
Dystonia deformans progressiva
Dystonia musculorum deformans
Familial torsion dystonia
Idiopathic familial dystonia
Idiopathic (torsion) dystonia NOS
(Schwalbe-) Ziehen-Oppenheim disease

G24.2 Idiopathic nonfamilial dystonia ᶜᶜ

G24.3 Spasmodic torticollis
EXCLUDES 1 *congenital torticollis (Q68.0)*
hysterical torticollis (F44.4)
ocular torticollis (R29.891)
psychogenic torticollis (F45.8)
torticollis NOS (M43.6)
traumatic recurrent torticollis (S13.4)

G24.4 Idiopathic orofacial dystonia
Orofacial dyskinesia
EXCLUDES 1 *drug induced orofacial dyskinesia (G24.01)*

G24.5 Blepharospasm
EXCLUDES 1 *drug induced blepharospasm (G24.01)*

G24.8 Other dystonia ᶜᶜ
Acquired torsion dystonia NOS

G24.9 Dystonia, unspecified
Dyskinesia NOS

✓4ᵗʰ **G25** Other extrapyramidal and movement disorders
EXCLUDES 2 *sleep related movement disorders (G47.6-)*

G25.0 Essential tremor
Familial tremor
EXCLUDES 1 *tremor NOS (R25.1)*

G25.1 Drug-induced tremor
Use additional code for adverse effect, if applicable, to identify drug (T36-T50 with fifth or sixth character 5)

G25.2 Other specified forms of tremor
Intention tremor

G25.3 Myoclonus
Drug-induced myoclonus
Palatal myoclonus
Use additional code for adverse effect, if applicable, to identify drug (T36-T50 with fifth or sixth character 5)
EXCLUDES 1 *facial myokymia (G51.4)*
myoclonic epilepsy (G40.-)

G25.4 Drug-induced chorea
Use additional code for adverse effect, if applicable, to identify drug (T36-T50 with fifth or sixth character 5)

G25.5 Other chorea
Chorea NOS
EXCLUDES 1 *chorea NOS with heart involvement (I02.0)*
Huntington's chorea (G10)
rheumatic chorea (I02.-)
Sydenham's chorea (I02.-)

✓5ᵗʰ **G25.6** Drug induced tics and other tics of organic origin

G25.61 Drug induced tics
Use additional code for adverse effect, if applicable, to identify drug (T36-T50 with fifth or sixth character 5)

G25.69 Other tics of organic origin
EXCLUDES 1 *habit spasm (F95.9)*
tic NOS (F95.9)
Tourette's syndrome (F95.2)

✓5ᵗʰ **G25.7** Other and unspecified drug induced movement disorders
Use additional code for adverse effect, if applicable, to identify drug (T36-T50 with fifth or sixth character 5)

G25.70 Drug induced movement disorder, unspecified

G25.71 Drug induced akathisia
Drug induced acathisia
Neuroleptic induced acute akathisia

G25.79 Other drug induced movement disorders

✓5ᵗʰ **G25.8** Other specified extrapyramidal and movement disorders

G25.81 Restless legs syndrome

G25.82 Stiff-man syndrome ᶜᶜ
CC Excl: G04.1, G10, G12.22, G20-G21.9, G24.01-G25.79, G25.82-G26, G32.89-G37.2, G37.5-G37.9, G80.0-G80.9, G82.20-G83.0, G92, G93.1, G93.40-G93.6, G93.81, G93.89-G93.9, G96.8-G96.9

G25.83 Benign shuddering attacks

G25.89 Other specified extrapyramidal and movement disorders

G25.9 Extrapyramidal and movement disorder, unspecified ᶜᶜ
CC Excl: See code: G25.82

G26 *Extrapyramidal and movement disorders in diseases classified elsewhere*
Code first underlying disease

Other degenerative diseases of the nervous system (G30-G32)

✓4ᵗʰ **G30** Alzheimer's disease
INCLUDES Alzheimer's dementia senile and presenile forms
Use additional code to identify:
delirium, if applicable (F05)
dementia with behavioral disturbance (F02.81)
dementia without behavioral disturbance (F02.80)
EXCLUDES 1 *senile degeneration of brain NEC (G31.1)*
senile dementia NOS (F03)
senility NOS (R41.81)

G30.0 Alzheimer's disease with early onset

G30.1 Alzheimer's disease with late onset ᴀ

G30.8 Other Alzheimer's disease

G30.9 Alzheimer's disease, unspecified
AHA: 2012, 4Q, 95

✓4ᵗʰ **G31** Other degenerative diseases of nervous system, not elsewhere classified
Use additional code to identify:
dementia with behavioral disturbance (F02.81)
dementia without behavioral disturbance (F02.80)
EXCLUDES 2 *Reye's syndrome (G93.7)*

✓5ᵗʰ **G31.0** Frontotemporal dementia

G31.01 Pick's disease
Primary progressive aphasia
Progressive isolated aphasia

G31.09 Other frontotemporal dementia
Frontal dementia

G31.1 Senile degeneration of brain, not elsewhere classified
EXCLUDES 1 *Alzheimer's disease (G30.-)*
senility NOS (R41.81)

ℕ Newborn: 0   ℙ Pediatric: 0-17   �Ⅿ Maternity: 12-55   Ⓐ Adult: 15-124   **MCC** Major CC Condition   **PDxMCC** PDx acts as own MCC   ᶜᶜ CC Condition   **PDxCC** PDx acts as own CC

G31.2 Degeneration of nervous system due to alcohol
Alcoholic cerebellar ataxia
Alcoholic cerebellar degeneration
Alcoholic cerebral degeneration
Alcoholic encephalopathy
Dysfunction of the autonomic nervous system due to alcohol
Code also associated alcoholism (F10.-)

√5th **G31.8 Other specified degenerative diseases of nervous system**

> CC Excl: For CC codes in subcategory G31.8, unless otherwise noted: E75.00-E75.19, E75.4, F84.2, G13.2-G13.8, G30.0-G31.82, G31.84-G31.9, G91.4, G94

G31.81 Alpers disease   `CC`
Grey-matter degeneration

G31.82 Leigh's disease   `CC`
Subacute necrotizing encephalopathy

G31.83 Dementia with Lewy bodies
Dementia with Parkinsonism   Lewy body disease
Lewy body dementia

G31.84 Mild cognitive impairment, so stated
> EXCLUDES 1   age related cognitive decline (R41.81)
> altered mental status (R41.82)
> cerebral degeneration (G31.9)
> change in mental status (R41.82)
> cognitive deficits following (sequelae of)
> cerebral hemorrhage or infarction
> (I69.01, I69.11, I69.21, I69.31, I69.81,
> I69.91)
> cognitive impairment due to intracranial or
> head injury (S06.-)
> dementia (F01.-, F02.-, F03)
> mild memory disturbance (F06.8)
> neurologic neglect syndrome (R41.4)
> personality change, nonpsychotic (F68.8)

G31.85 Corticobasal degeneration

G31.89 Other specified degenerative diseases of nervous system

G31.9 Degenerative disease of nervous system, unspecified

√4th **G32 Other degenerative disorders of nervous system in diseases classified elsewhere**

G32.0 Subacute combined degeneration of spinal cord in diseases classified elsewhere   `CC`
Dana-Putnam syndrome
Sclerosis of spinal cord (combined) (dorsolateral) (posterolateral)
Code first underlying disease, such as:
vitamin B12 deficiency (E53.8)
vitamin B12 deficiency:
anemia (D51.9)
dietary (D51.3)
pernicious (D51.0)
> EXCLUDES 1   syphilitic combined degeneration of spinal cord
> (A52.11)
CC Excl: G04.1, G11.3, G11.8-G12.9, G32.0, G32.89-G37.3, G37.5-G37.9, G80.0-G80.2, G80.4-G83.9, G90.01-G90.09, G90.2, G90.4-G90.9, G93.1, G93.40-G93.49, G95.0-G95.9, G96.12-G96.9, G97.1, G98.0-G99.8, I67.83, R53.2

√5th **G32.8 Other specified degenerative disorders of nervous system in diseases classified elsewhere**
Code first underlying disease, such as:
amyloidosis cerebral degeneration (E85.-)
cerebral degeneration (due to) hypothyroidism (E00.0-E03.9)
cerebral degeneration (due to) neoplasm (C00-D49)
cerebral degeneration (due to) vitamin B deficiency, except thiamine (E52-E53.-)
> EXCLUDES 1   superior hemorrhagic polioencephalitis [Wernicke's
> encephalopathy] (E51.2)

G32.81 Cerebellar ataxia in diseases classified elsewhere   `CC`
Code first underlying disease, such as:
celiac disease (with gluten ataxia) (K90.0)
cerebellar ataxia (in) neoplastic disease (paraneoplastic cerebellar degeneration) (C00-D49)
non-celiac gluten ataxia (M35.9)
> EXCLUDES 1   systemic atrophy primarily affecting the
> central nervous system in alcoholic
> cerebellar ataxia (G31.2)
> systemic atrophy primarily affecting the
> central nervous system in myxedema
> (G13.2)
CC Excl: G04.1, G10-G12.9, G21.0, G23.0-G25.79, G25.82-G26, G32.0-G37.3, G37.5-G37.9, G80.0-G83.9, G90.01-G90.09, G90.2-G90.9, G92-G93.1, G93.40-G93.49, G93.81, G93.89-G93.9, G95.0-G95.9, G96.8-G96.9, G98.0-G99.8, I67.83, R53.2

G32.89 Other specified degenerative disorders of nervous system in diseases classified elsewhere
Degenerative encephalopathy in diseases classified elsewhere

Demyelinating diseases of the central nervous system (G35-G37)

G35 Multiple sclerosis
Disseminated multiple sclerosis
Generalized multiple sclerosis
Multiple sclerosis NOS
Multiple sclerosis of brain stem
Multiple sclerosis of cord

√4th **G36 Other acute disseminated demyelination**
> EXCLUDES 1   postinfectious encephalitis and encephalomyelitis NOS (G04.01)

G36.0 Neuromyelitis optica [Devic]   `CC`
Demyelination in optic neuritis
> EXCLUDES 1   optic neuritis NOS (H46)
CC Excl: G36.0, G93.40-G93.49, I67.83

G36.1 Acute and subacute hemorrhagic leukoencephalitis [Hurst]   `CC`
CC Excl: G04.1, G10-G12.9, G21.0, G24.01-G25.79, G25.82-G26, G32.0-G37.3, G37.5-G37.9, G80.0-G83.9, G90.01-G90.09, G90.2, G90.4-G90.9, G92, G93.40-G93.49, G93.81, G93.89-G93.9, G95.0-G95.9, G96.8-G96.9, G98.0-G99.8, I67.83, R53.2

G36.8 Other specified acute disseminated demyelination   `CC`
CC Excl: See code: G36.1

G36.9 Acute disseminated demyelination, unspecified   `HIV` `CC`
CC Excl: See code: G36.1

√4th **G37 Other demyelinating diseases of central nervous system**

G37.0 Diffuse sclerosis of central nervous system   `CC`
Periaxial encephalitis
Schilder's disease
> EXCLUDES 1   X linked adrenoleukodystrophy (E71.52-)
CC Excl: A92.30-A92.39, B97.21, G93.40-G93.49, I67.83

G37.1 Central demyelination of corpus callosum   `CC`
CC Excl: See code: G36.1

G37.2 Central pontine myelinolysis   `CC`
CC Excl: See code: G36.1

G37.3 Acute transverse myelitis in demyelinating disease of central nervous system   `CC`
Acute transverse myelitis NOS
Acute transverse myelopathy
> EXCLUDES 1   multiple sclerosis (G35)
> neuromyelitis optica [Devic] (G36.0)
CC Excl: A02.21, A17.0-A17.1, A27.81, A39.0, A50.41, A51.41, A52.13, A54.82, A54.84, A54.89-A54.9, A87.0-A87.9, A96.2, A98.3-A98.4, B00.3, B00.89-B00.9, B02.0-B02.23, B02.29, B02.7-B02.9, B10.81-B10.89, B26.1, B33.24, B33.4-B33.8, B34.1-B34.2, B34.4-B34.8, B37.5, B38.4, B45.1, B58.2, B92, B94.2-B94.9, B97.10, B97.19, B97.29, B97.5-B97.6, B97.81-B97.89, E08.40-E08.49, E09.40-E09.49, E10.40-E10.49, E11.40-E11.49, E13.40-E13.49, G00.0-G03.9, G04.1-G04.2, G11.3, G11.8-G12.9, G32.0, G32.89-G37.2, G37.5-G37.9, G61.0, G80.0-G80.2, G80.4-G83.9, G90.01-G90.09, G90.2, G90.4-G90.9, G93.1, G93.40-G93.49, G95.0-G95.9, G96.12-G96.9, G97.1, G98.0-G99.8, I67.83, R53.2

G37.4 Subacute necrotizing myelitis of central nervous system   `HIV` `MCC`
CC Excl: A17.82, A28.1, A50.42, A52.14, A75.9, A79.9, A81.1, A81.82-A81.89, A83.0-A85.8, A87.2, A88.0, A88.8, A92.1-A92.8, A93.0, B00.4, B00.82, B01.11-B01.12, B04, B06.01, B08.09, B08.20-B08.22, B08.60-B08.79, B09-B10.09, B26.2, B27.00-B27.99, B33.1, B45.0, B45.2-B45.9, B54, B58.2, B75, B97.10, B97.21, G04.00-G04.01, G04.31, G04.81-G05.4, G37.0, G37.4-G37.5, H66.40-H66.43, J09.X3-J09.X9, J10.2-J10.89, J11.2-J11.89, L44.4, M1A.10X0-M1A.19X1, M32.0-M32.9, P35.2-P35.9, P37.0-P37.4, P37.8-P37.9, T56.0X1A, T56.0X2A, T56.0X3A, T56.0X4A

G37.5 Concentric sclerosis [Balo] of central nervous system   `CC`
CC Excl: See code: G37.0

G37.8 Other specified demyelinating diseases of central nervous system   `CC`
CC Excl: See code: G36.1

G37.9 Demyelinating disease of central nervous system, unspecified   `HIV` `CC`
CC Excl: See code: G36.1

Chapter 6. Diseases of the Nervous System

G40–G40.3

Episodic and paroxysmal disorders (G40-G47)

√4th G40 Epilepsy and recurrent seizures

NOTE The following terms are to be considered equivalent to intractable: pharmacoresistant (pharmacologically resistant), treatment resistant, refractory (medically) and poorly controlled

EXCLUDES 1 conversion disorder with seizures (F44.5)
convulsions NOS (R56.9)
hippocampal sclerosis (G93.81)
mesial temporal sclerosis (G93.81)
post traumatic seizures (R56.1)
seizure (convulsive) NOS (R56.9)
seizure of newborn (P90)
temporal sclerosis (G93.81)
Todd's paralysis (G83.8)

√5th G40.0 Localization-related (focal) (partial) idiopathic epilepsy and epileptic syndromes with seizures of localized onset
Benign childhood epilepsy with centrotemporal EEG spikes
Childhood epilepsy with occipital EEG paroxysms
EXCLUDES 1 adult onset localization-related epilepsy (G40.1-, G40.2-)

√6th G40.00 Localization-related (focal) (partial) idiopathic epilepsy and epileptic syndromes with seizures of localized onset, not intractable
Localization-related (focal) (partial) idiopathic epilepsy and epileptic syndromes with seizures of localized onset without intractability

G40.001 Localization-related (focal) (partial) idiopathic epilepsy and epileptic syndromes with seizures of localized onset, not intractable, with status epilepticus CC
CC Excl: G32.89, G40.001-G40.919, G93.40-G93.49, G93.9, G96.8-G96.9, G98.0-G98.8, G99.8, I67.83, R56.1

G40.009 Localization-related (focal) (partial) idiopathic epilepsy and epileptic syndromes with seizures of localized onset, not intractable, without status epilepticus CC
Localization-related (focal) (partial) idiopathic epilepsy and epileptic syndromes with seizures of localized onset NOS
CC Excl: See code: G40.001

√6th G40.01 Localization-related (focal) (partial) idiopathic epilepsy and epileptic syndromes with seizures of localized onset, intractable

CC Excl: For CC codes in subcategory G40.01, unless otherwise noted: E08.40-E08.49, E09.40-E09.49, E10.40-E10.49, E11.40-E11.49, E13.40-E13.49, G32.89, G40.001-G40.919, G93.81, G93.89-G93.9, G96.8-G96.9, G98.0-G98.8, G99.8, R56.1

G40.011 Localization-related (focal) (partial) idiopathic epilepsy and epileptic syndromes with seizures of localized onset, intractable, with status epilepticus CC

G40.019 Localization-related (focal) (partial) idiopathic epilepsy and epileptic syndromes with seizures of localized onset, intractable, without status epilepticus CC

√5th G40.1 Localization-related (focal) (partial) symptomatic epilepsy and epileptic syndromes with simple partial seizures
Attacks without alteration of consciousness
Epilepsia partialis continua [Kozhevnikof]
Simple partial seizures developing into secondarily generalized seizures

√6th G40.10 Localization-related (focal) (partial) symptomatic epilepsy and epileptic syndromes with simple partial seizures, not intractable
Localization-related (focal) (partial) symptomatic epilepsy and epileptic syndromes with simple partial seizures without intractability

CC Excl: For CC codes in subcategory G40.10, unless otherwise noted: G32.89, G40.001-G40.919, G93.40-G93.49, G93.9, G96.8-G96.9, G98.0-G98.8, G99.8, I67.83, R56.1

G40.101 Localization-related (focal) (partial) symptomatic epilepsy and epileptic syndromes with simple partial seizures, not intractable, with status epilepticus CC

G40.109 Localization-related (focal) (partial) symptomatic epilepsy and epileptic syndromes with simple partial seizures, not intractable, without status epilepticus CC
Localization-related (focal) (partial) symptomatic epilepsy and epileptic syndromes with simple partial seizures NOS

√6th G40.11 Localization-related (focal) (partial) symptomatic epilepsy and epileptic syndromes with simple partial seizures, intractable

CC Excl: For CC codes in subcategory G40.11, unless otherwise noted: E08.40-E08.49, E09.40-E09.49, E10.40-E10.49, E11.40-E11.49, E13.40-E13.49, G32.89, G40.001-G40.919, G93.81, G93.89-G93.9, G96.8-G96.9, G98.0-G98.8, G99.8, R56.1

G40.111 Localization-related (focal) (partial) symptomatic epilepsy and epileptic syndromes with simple partial seizures, intractable, with status epilepticus CC

G40.119 Localization-related (focal) (partial) symptomatic epilepsy and epileptic syndromes with simple partial seizures, intractable, without status epilepticus CC

√5th G40.2 Localization-related (focal) (partial) symptomatic epilepsy and epileptic syndromes with complex partial seizures
Attacks with alteration of consciousness, often with automatisms
Complex partial seizures developing into secondarily generalized seizures

√6th G40.20 Localization-related (focal) (partial) symptomatic epilepsy and epileptic syndromes with complex partial seizures, not intractable
Localization-related (focal) (partial) symptomatic epilepsy and epileptic syndromes with complex partial seizures without intractability

CC Excl: For CC codes in subcategory G40.20, unless otherwise noted: G32.89, G40.001-G40.919, G93.40-G93.49, G93.9, G96.8-G96.9, G98.0-G98.8, G99.8, I67.83, R56.1

G40.201 Localization-related (focal) (partial) symptomatic epilepsy and epileptic syndromes with complex partial seizures, not intractable, with status epilepticus CC

G40.209 Localization-related (focal) (partial) symptomatic epilepsy and epileptic syndromes with complex partial seizures, not intractable, without status epilepticus CC
Localization-related (focal) (partial) symptomatic epilepsy and epileptic syndromes with complex partial seizures NOS

√6th G40.21 Localization-related (focal) (partial) symptomatic epilepsy and epileptic syndromes with complex partial seizures, intractable

CC Excl: For CC codes in subcategory G40.21, unless otherwise noted: E08.40-E08.49, E09.40-E09.49, E10.40-E10.49, E11.40-E11.49, E13.40-E13.49, G32.89, G40.001-G40.919, G93.81, G93.89-G93.9, G96.8-G96.9, G98.0-G98.8, G99.8, R56.1

G40.211 Localization-related (focal) (partial) symptomatic epilepsy and epileptic syndromes with complex partial seizures, intractable, with status epilepticus CC

G40.219 Localization-related (focal) (partial) symptomatic epilepsy and epileptic syndromes with complex partial seizures, intractable, without status epilepticus CC

√5th G40.3 Generalized idiopathic epilepsy and epileptic syndromes
Code also MERRF syndrome, if applicable (E88.42)

CC Excl: For MCC codes in subcategory G40.3, unless otherwise noted: E08.40-E08.49, E08.618-E08.638, E08.649-E08.8, E09.40-E09.49, E09.618-E09.638, E09.649-E09.8, E10.40-E10.49, E10.618-E10.638, E10.649, E10.69-E10.8, E11.40-E11.49, E11.618-E11.638, E11.649, E11.69-E11.8, E13.40-E13.49, E13.618-E13.638, E13.649-E13.8, G32.89, G40.001-G40.919, G93.81, G93.89-G93.9, G96.8-G96.9, G98.0-G98.8, G99.8, R56.1

√6ᵗʰ **G40.30 Generalized idiopathic epilepsy and epileptic syndromes, not intractable**
  Generalized idiopathic epilepsy and epileptic syndromes without intractability

  G40.301 Generalized idiopathic epilepsy and epileptic syndromes, not intractable, with status epilepticus MCC

  G40.309 Generalized idiopathic epilepsy and epileptic syndromes, not intractable, without status epilepticus
    Generalized idiopathic epilepsy and epileptic syndromes NOS

√6ᵗʰ **G40.31 Generalized idiopathic epilepsy and epileptic syndromes, intractable**

  G40.311 Generalized idiopathic epilepsy and epileptic syndromes, intractable, with status epilepticus MCC

  G40.319 Generalized idiopathic epilepsy and epileptic syndromes, intractable, without status epilepticus MCC

√5ᵗʰ **G40.A Absence epileptic syndrome**
  Childhood absence epilepsy [pyknolepsy]
  Juvenile absence epilepsy
  Absence epileptic syndrome, NOS

  CC Excl: For CC codes in subcategory G40.A, unless otherwise noted: E08.40-E08.49, E09.40-E09.49, E10.40-E10.49, E11.40-E11.49, E13.40-E13.49, G32.89, G40.001-G40.919, G93.81, G93.89-G93.9, G96.8-G96.9, G98.0-G98.8, G99.8, R56.1

  √6ᵗʰ **G40.A0 Absence epileptic syndrome, not intractable**
    G40.A01 Absence epileptic syndrome, not intractable, with status epilepticus
    G40.A09 Absence epileptic syndrome, not intractable, without status epilepticus

  √6ᵗʰ **G40.A1 Absence epileptic syndrome, intractable**
    G40.A11 Absence epileptic syndrome, intractable, with status epilepticus CC
    G40.A19 Absence epileptic syndrome, intractable, without status epilepticus CC

√5ᵗʰ **G40.B Juvenile myoclonic epilepsy [impulsive petit mal]**

  CC Excl: For CC codes in subcategory G40.B, unless otherwise noted: E08.40-E08.49, E09.40-E09.49, E10.40-E10.49, E11.40-E11.49, E13.40-E13.49, G32.89, G40.001-G40.919, G93.81, G93.89-G93.9, G96.8-G96.9, G98.0-G98.8, G99.8, R56.1

  √6ᵗʰ **G40.B0 Juvenile myoclonic epilepsy, not intractable**
    G40.B01 Juvenile myoclonic epilepsy, not intractable, with status epilepticus CC
    G40.B09 Juvenile myoclonic epilepsy, not intractable, without status epilepticus CC

  √6ᵗʰ **G40.B1 Juvenile myoclonic epilepsy, intractable**
    G40.B11 Juvenile myoclonic epilepsy, intractable, with status epilepticus CC
    G40.B19 Juvenile myoclonic epilepsy, intractable, without status epilepticus CC

√5ᵗʰ **G40.4 Other generalized epilepsy and epileptic syndromes**
  Epilepsy with grand mal seizures on awakening
  Epilepsy with myoclonic absences
  Epilepsy with myoclonic-astatic seizures
  Grand mal seizure NOS
  Nonspecific atonic epileptic seizures
  Nonspecific clonic epileptic seizures
  Nonspecific myoclonic epileptic seizures
  Nonspecific tonic epileptic seizures
  Nonspecific tonic-clonic epileptic seizures
  Symptomatic early myoclonic encephalopathy

  √6ᵗʰ **G40.40 Other generalized epilepsy and epileptic syndromes, not intractable**
    Other generalized epilepsy and epileptic syndromes without intractability
    Other generalized epilepsy and epileptic syndromes NOS
    G40.401 Other generalized epilepsy and epileptic syndromes, not intractable, with status epilepticus
    G40.409 Other generalized epilepsy and epileptic syndromes, not intractable, without status epilepticus

√6ᵗʰ **G40.41 Other generalized epilepsy and epileptic syndromes, intractable**

  CC Excl: For CC codes in subcategory G40.41, unless otherwise noted: E08.40-E08.49, E09.40-E09.49, E10.40-E10.49, E11.40-E11.49, E13.40-E13.49, G32.89, G40.001-G40.919, G93.81, G93.89-G93.9, G96.8-G96.9, G98.0-G98.8, G99.8, R56.1

  G40.411 Other generalized epilepsy and epileptic syndromes, intractable, with status epilepticus CC

  G40.419 Other generalized epilepsy and epileptic syndromes, intractable, without status epilepticus CC

√5ᵗʰ **G40.5 Epileptic seizures related to external causes**
  Epileptic seizures related to alcohol
  Epileptic seizures related to drugs
  Epileptic seizures related to hormonal changes
  Epileptic seizures related to sleep deprivation
  Epileptic seizures related to stress
  Use additional code for adverse effect, if applicable, to identify drug (T36-T50 with fifth or sixth character 5)
  Code also, if applicable, associated epilepsy and recurrent seizures (G40.-)

  CC Excl: For CC codes in subcategory G40.5, unless otherwise noted: E08.40-E08.49, E09.40-E09.49, E10.40-E10.49, E11.40-E11.49, E13.40-E13.49, G32.89, G40.001-G40.919, G93.81, G93.89-G93.9, G96.8-G96.9, G98.0-G98.8, G99.8, R56.1

  √6ᵗʰ **G40.50 Epileptic seizures related to external causes, not intractable**
    G40.501 Epileptic seizures related to external causes, not intractable, with status epilepticus CC
    G40.509 Epileptic seizures related to external causes, not intractable, without status epilepticus CC
      Epileptic seizures related to external causes, NOS

√5ᵗʰ **G40.8 Other epilepsy and recurrent seizures**
  Epilepsies and epileptic syndromes undetermined as to whether they are focal or generalized
  Landau-Kleffner syndrome

  CC Excl: For CC codes in subcategory G40.8, unless otherwise noted: E08.40-E08.49, E09.40-E09.49, E10.40-E10.49, E11.40-E11.49, E13.40-E13.49, G32.89, G40.001-G40.919, G93.81, G93.89-G93.9, G96.8-G96.9, G98.0-G98.8, G99.8, R56.1

  √6ᵗʰ **G40.80 Other epilepsy**
    G40.801 Other epilepsy, not intractable, with status epilepticus CC
      Other epilepsy without intractability with status epilepticus
    G40.802 Other epilepsy, not intractable, without status epilepticus CC
      Other epilepsy without intractability without status epilepticus
    G40.803 Other epilepsy, intractable, with status epilepticus CC
    G40.804 Other epilepsy, intractable, without status epilepticus CC

  √6ᵗʰ **G40.81 Lennox-Gastaut syndrome**
    G40.811 Lennox-Gastaut syndrome, not intractable, with status epilepticus CC
    G40.812 Lennox-Gastaut syndrome, not intractable, without status epilepticus CC
    G40.813 Lennox-Gastaut syndrome, intractable, with status epilepticus CC
    G40.814 Lennox-Gastaut syndrome, intractable, without status epilepticus CC

  √6ᵗʰ **G40.82 Epileptic spasms**
    Infantile spasms
    Salaam attacks
    West's syndrome
    G40.821 Epileptic spasms, not intractable, with status epilepticus CC
      CC Excl: G32.89, G40.001-G40.919, G93.40-G93.49, G93.9, G96.8-G96.9, G98.0-G98.8, G99.8, I67.83, R56.1

☑ Additional Character Required √x7ᵗʰ Placeholder Alert Unacceptable PDx Manifestation Hospital Acquired Condition **EXCLUDES 1** Not Coded Here **EXCLUDES 2** Not Included Here

G40.822   **Epileptic spasms, not intractable, without status epilepticus**   CC
     CC Excl: See code: G40.821

G40.823   **Epileptic spasms, intractable, with status epilepticus**   CC

G40.824   **Epileptic spasms, intractable, without status epilepticus**   CC

G40.89   **Other seizures**   CC
     EXCLUDES 1   *post traumatic seizures (R56.1)*
        recurrent seizures NOS (G40.909)
        seizure NOS (R56.9)

✓5th **G40.9**   **Epilepsy, unspecified**

> **CC Excl:** For CC codes in subcategory G40.9, unless otherwise noted: E08.40-E08.49, E09.40-E09.49, E10.40-E10.49, E11.40-E11.49, E13.40-E13.49, G32.89, G40.001-G40.919, G93.81, G93.89-G93.9, G96.8-G96.9, G98.0-G98.8, G99.8, R56.1

✓6th **G40.90**   **Epilepsy, unspecified, not intractable**
     Epilepsy, unspecified, without intractability

G40.901   **Epilepsy, unspecified, not intractable, with status epilepticus**

G40.909   **Epilepsy, unspecified, not intractable, without status epilepticus**
     Epilepsy NOS
     Epileptic convulsions NOS
     Epileptic fits NOS
     Epileptic seizures NOS
     Recurrent seizures NOS
     Seizure disorder NOS

✓6th **G40.91**   **Epilepsy, unspecified, intractable**
     Intractable seizure disorder NOS

G40.911   **Epilepsy, unspecified, intractable, with status epilepticus**   CC

G40.919   **Epilepsy, unspecified, intractable, without status epilepticus**   CC

✓4th **G43**   **Migraine**
     NOTE   The following terms are to be considered equivalent to intractable: pharmacoresistant (pharmacologically resistant), treatment resistant, refractory (medically) and poorly controlled
     Use additional code for adverse effect, if applicable, to identify drug (T36-T50 with fifth or sixth character 5)
     EXCLUDES 1   *headache NOS (R51)*
        lower half migraine (G44.00)
     EXCLUDES 2   *headache syndromes (G44.-)*

✓5th **G43.0**   **Migraine without aura**
     Common migraine
     EXCLUDES 1   *chronic migraine without aura (G43.7-)*

✓6th **G43.00**   **Migraine without aura, not intractable**
     Migraine without aura without mention of refractory migraine

G43.001   **Migraine without aura, not intractable, with status migrainosus**

G43.009   **Migraine without aura, not intractable, without status migrainosus**
     Migraine without aura NOS

✓6th **G43.01**   **Migraine without aura, intractable**
     Migraine without aura with refractory migraine

G43.011   **Migraine without aura, intractable, with status migrainosus**

G43.019   **Migraine without aura, intractable, without status migrainosus**

✓5th **G43.1**   **Migraine with aura**
     Basilar migraine
     Classical migraine
     Migraine equivalents
     Migraine preceded or accompanied by transient focal neurological phenomena
     Migraine triggered seizures
     Migraine with acute-onset aura
     Migraine with aura without headache (migraine equivalents)
     Migraine with prolonged aura
     Migraine with typical aura
     Retinal migraine
     Code also any associated seizure (G40.-, R56.9)
     EXCLUDES 1   *persistent migraine aura (G43.5-, G43.6-)*

✓6th **G43.10**   **Migraine with aura, not intractable**
     Migraine with aura without mention of refractory migraine

G43.101   **Migraine with aura, not intractable, with status migrainosus**

G43.109   **Migraine with aura, not intractable, without status migrainosus**
     Migraine with aura NOS

✓6th **G43.11**   **Migraine with aura, intractable**
     Migraine with aura with refractory migraine

G43.111   **Migraine with aura, intractable, with status migrainosus**

G43.119   **Migraine with aura, intractable, without status migrainosus**

✓5th **G43.4**   **Hemiplegic migraine**
     Familial migraine
     Sporadic migraine

✓6th **G43.40**   **Hemiplegic migraine, not intractable**
     Hemiplegic migraine without refractory migraine

G43.401   **Hemiplegic migraine, not intractable, with status migrainosus**

G43.409   **Hemiplegic migraine, not intractable, without status migrainosus**
     Hemiplegic migraine NOS

✓6th **G43.41**   **Hemiplegic migraine, intractable**
     Hemiplegic migraine with refractory migraine

G43.411   **Hemiplegic migraine, intractable, with status migrainosus**

G43.419   **Hemiplegic migraine, intractable, without status migrainosus**

✓5th **G43.5**   **Persistent migraine aura without cerebral infarction**

✓6th **G43.50**   **Persistent migraine aura without cerebral infarction, not intractable**
     Persistent migraine aura without cerebral infarction, without refractory migraine

G43.501   **Persistent migraine aura without cerebral infarction, not intractable, with status migrainosus**

G43.509   **Persistent migraine aura without cerebral infarction, not intractable, without status migrainosus**
     Persistent migraine aura NOS

✓6th **G43.51**   **Persistent migraine aura without cerebral infarction, intractable**
     Persistent migraine aura without cerebral infarction, with refractory migraine

G43.511   **Persistent migraine aura without cerebral infarction, intractable, with status migrainosus**

G43.519   **Persistent migraine aura without cerebral infarction, intractable, without status migrainosus**

✓5th **G43.6**   **Persistent migraine aura with cerebral infarction**
     Code also the type of cerebral infarction (I63.-)

> **CC Excl:** For CC codes in subcategory G43.6, unless otherwise noted: G43.601-G43.619, I63.00-I66.9

✓6th **G43.60**   **Persistent migraine aura with cerebral infarction, not intractable**
     Persistent migraine aura with cerebral infarction, without refractory migraine

G43.601   **Persistent migraine aura with cerebral infarction, not intractable, with status migrainosus**   CC

G43.609   **Persistent migraine aura with cerebral infarction, not intractable, without status migrainosus**   CC

✓6th **G43.61**   **Persistent migraine aura with cerebral infarction, intractable**
     Persistent migraine aura with cerebral infarction, with refractory migraine

G43.611   **Persistent migraine aura with cerebral infarction, intractable, with status migrainosus**   CC

G43.619   **Persistent migraine aura with cerebral infarction, intractable, without status migrainosus**   CC

✓5th **G43.7**   **Chronic migraine without aura**
     Transformed migraine
     EXCLUDES 1   *migraine without aura (G43.0-)*

✓6th **G43.70**   **Chronic migraine without aura, not intractable**
     Chronic migraine without aura, without refractory migraine

G43.701 **Chronic migraine without aura, not intractable,** with status migrainosus

G43.709 **Chronic migraine without aura, not intractable,** without status migrainosus
Chronic migraine without aura NOS

✓6th **G43.71** **Chronic migraine without aura, intractable**
Chronic migraine without aura, with refractory migraine

G43.711 **Chronic migraine without aura, intractable,** with status migrainosus

G43.719 **Chronic migraine without aura, intractable,** without status migrainosus

✓5th **G43.A** **Cyclical vomiting**

G43.A0 **Cyclical vomiting,** not intractable
Cyclical vomiting, without refractory migraine

G43.A1 **Cyclical vomiting,** intractable
Cyclical vomiting, with refractory migraine

✓5th **G43.B** **Ophthalmoplegic migraine**

G43.B0 **Ophthalmoplegic migraine,** not intractable
Ophthalmoplegic migraine, without refractory migraine

G43.B1 **Ophthalmoplegic migraine,** intractable
Ophthalmoplegic migraine, with refractory migraine

✓5th **G43.C** **Periodic headache syndromes in child or adult**

G43.C0 **Periodic headache syndromes in child or adult,** not intractable
Periodic headache syndromes in child or adult, without refractory migraine

G43.C1 **Periodic headache syndromes in child or adult, intractable**
Periodic headache syndromes in child or adult, with refractory migraine

✓5th **G43.D** **Abdominal migraine**

G43.D0 **Abdominal migraine,** not intractable
Abdominal migraine, without refractory migraine

G43.D1 **Abdominal migraine,** intractable
Abdominal migraine, with refractory migraine

✓5th **G43.8** **Other migraine**

✓6th **G43.80** **Other migraine,** not intractable
Other migraine, without refractory migraine

G43.801 **Other migraine, not intractable,** with status migrainosus

G43.809 **Other migraine, not intractable,** without status migrainosus

✓6th **G43.81** **Other migraine,** intractable
Other migraine, with refractory migraine

G43.811 **Other migraine, intractable,** with status migrainosus

G43.819 **Other migraine, intractable,** without status migrainosus

✓6th **G43.82** **Menstrual migraine,** not intractable
Menstrual headache, not intractable
Menstrual migraine, without refractory migraine
Menstrually related migraine, not intractable
Pre-menstrual headache, not intractable
Pre-menstrual migraine, not intractable
Pure menstrual migraine, not intractable
Code also associated premenstrual tension syndrome (N94.3)

G43.821 **Menstrual migraine, not intractable, with status migrainosus** ♀

G43.829 **Menstrual migraine, not intractable, without status migrainosus** ♀
Menstrual migraine NOS

✓6th **G43.83** **Menstrual migraine,** intractable
Menstrual headache, intractable
Menstrual migraine, with refractory migraine
Menstrually related migraine, intractable
Pre-menstrual headache, intractable
Pre-menstrual migraine, intractable
Pure menstrual migraine, intractable
Code also associated premenstrual tension syndrome (N94.3)

G43.831 **Menstrual migraine, intractable, with status migrainosus** ♀

G43.839 **Menstrual migraine, intractable, without status migrainosus** ♀

✓5th **G43.9** **Migraine, unspecified**

✓6th **G43.90** **Migraine, unspecified,** not intractable
Migraine, unspecified, without refractory migraine

G43.901 **Migraine, unspecified, not intractable, with status migrainosus**
Status migrainosus NOS

G43.909 **Migraine, unspecified, not intractable, without status migrainosus**
Migraine NOS

✓6th **G43.91** **Migraine, unspecified,** intractable
Migraine, unspecified, with refractory migraine

G43.911 **Migraine, unspecified, intractable, with status migrainosus**

G43.919 **Migraine, unspecified, intractable, without status migrainosus**

✓4th **G44** **Other headache syndromes**
EXCLUDES 1   headache NOS (R51)
EXCLUDES 2   atypical facial pain (G50.1)
headache due to lumbar puncture (G97.1)
migraines (G43.-)
trigeminal neuralgia (G50.0)

✓5th **G44.0** **Cluster headaches and other trigeminal autonomic cephalgias (TAC)**

✓6th **G44.00** **Cluster headache syndrome,** unspecified
Ciliary neuralgia   Lower half migraine
Cluster headache NOS   Migrainous neuralgia
Histamine cephalgia

G44.001 **Cluster headache syndrome, unspecified, intractable**

G44.009 **Cluster headache syndrome, unspecified, not intractable**
Cluster headache syndrome NOS

✓6th **G44.01** **Episodic cluster headache**

G44.011 **Episodic cluster headache, intractable**

G44.019 **Episodic cluster headache, not intractable**
Episodic cluster headache NOS

✓6th **G44.02** **Chronic cluster headache**

G44.021 **Chronic cluster headache, intractable**

G44.029 **Chronic cluster headache, not intractable**
Chronic cluster headache NOS

✓6th **G44.03** **Episodic paroxysmal hemicrania**
Paroxysmal hemicrania NOS

G44.031 **Episodic paroxysmal hemicrania, intractable**

G44.039 **Episodic paroxysmal hemicrania, not intractable**
Episodic paroxysmal hemicrania NOS

✓6th **G44.04** **Chronic paroxysmal hemicrania**

G44.041 **Chronic paroxysmal hemicrania, intractable**

G44.049 **Chronic paroxysmal hemicrania, not intractable**
Chronic paroxysmal hemicrania NOS

✓6th **G44.05** **Short lasting unilateral neuralgiform headache with conjunctival injection and tearing (SUNCT)**

G44.051 **Short lasting unilateral neuralgiform headache with conjunctival injection and tearing (SUNCT), intractable**

G44.059 **Short lasting unilateral neuralgiform headache with conjunctival injection and tearing (SUNCT), not intractable**
Short lasting unilateral neuralgiform headache with conjunctival injection and tearing (SUNCT) NOS

✓6th **G44.09** **Other trigeminal autonomic cephalgias (TAC)**

G44.091 **Other trigeminal autonomic cephalgias (TAC), intractable**

G44.099 **Other trigeminal autonomic cephalgias syndrome (TAC), not intractable**

G44.1 **Vascular headache, not elsewhere classified**
EXCLUDES 2   cluster headache (G44.0)
complicated headache syndromes (G44.5-)
drug-induced headache (G44.4-)
migraine (G43.-)
other specified headache syndromes (G44.8-)
post-traumatic headache (G44.3-)
tension-type headache (G44.2-)

✓ Additional Character Required   ✓x7th Placeholder Alert   Unacceptable PDx   Manifestation   Hospital Acquired Condition   EXCLUDES 1 Not Coded Here   EXCLUDES 2 Not Included Here

✓5ᵗʰ **G44.2 Tension-type headache**

  ✓6ᵗʰ **G44.20 Tension-type headache,** unspecified

    G44.201 Tension-type headache, unspecified, intractable

    G44.209 Tension-type headache, unspecified, not intractable

      Tension headache NOS

  ✓6ᵗʰ **G44.21 Episodic tension-type headache**

    G44.211 Episodic tension-type headache, intractable

    G44.219 Episodic tension-type headache, not intractable

      Episodic tension-type headache NOS

  ✓6ᵗʰ **G44.22 Chronic tension-type headache**

    G44.221 Chronic tension-type headache, intractable

    G44.229 Chronic tension-type headache, not intractable

      Chronic tension-type headache NOS

✓5ᵗʰ **G44.3 Post-traumatic headache**

  ✓6ᵗʰ **G44.30 Post-traumatic headache,** unspecified

    G44.301 Post-traumatic headache, unspecified, intractable

    G44.309 Post-traumatic headache, unspecified, not intractable

      Post-traumatic headache NOS

  ✓6ᵗʰ **G44.31 Acute post-traumatic headache**

    G44.311 Acute post-traumatic headache, intractable

    G44.319 Acute post-traumatic headache, not intractable

      Acute post-traumatic headache NOS

  ✓6ᵗʰ **G44.32 Chronic post-traumatic headache**

    G44.321 Chronic post-traumatic headache, intractable

    G44.329 Chronic post-traumatic headache, not intractable

      Chronic post-traumatic headache NOS

✓5ᵗʰ **G44.4 Drug-induced headache, not elsewhere classified**

  Medication overuse headache

  Use additional code for adverse effect, if applicable, to identify drug (T36-T50 with fifth or sixth character 5)

  G44.40 Drug-induced headache, not elsewhere classified, not intractable

  G44.41 Drug-induced headache, not elsewhere classified, intractable

✓5ᵗʰ **G44.5 Complicated headache syndromes**

  G44.51 Hemicrania continua

  G44.52 New daily persistent headache (NDPH)

  G44.53 Primary thunderclap headache

  G44.59 Other complicated headache syndrome

✓5ᵗʰ **G44.8 Other specified headache syndromes**

  G44.81 Hypnic headache

  G44.82 Headache associated with sexual activity

    Orgasmic headache

    Preorgasmic headache

  G44.83 Primary cough headache

  G44.84 Primary exertional headache

  G44.85 Primary stabbing headache

  G44.89 Other headache syndrome

✓4ᵗʰ **G45 Transient cerebral ischemic attacks and related syndromes**

  EXCLUDES 1   neonatal cerebral ischemia (P91.0)

                 transient retinal artery occlusion (H34.0-)

> **CC Excl: For CC codes in category G45, unless otherwise noted:**
> E08.51-E08.59, E08.618-E08.638, E08.649-E08.8, E09.51-E09.59,
> E09.618-E09.638, E09.649-E09.8, E10.51-E10.59, E10.618-E10.638,
> E10.649, E10.69-E10.8, E11.51-E11.59, E11.618-E11.638, E11.649,
> E11.69-E11.8, E13.51-E13.59, E13.618-E13.638, E13.649-E13.8, G45.0-
> G45.2, G45.8-G46.2, I63.00-I63.29, I65.01-I65.9, I67.841-I67.848,
> I87.8-I87.9, I99.8-I99.9

G45.0 Vertebro-basilar artery syndrome   CC

G45.1 Carotid artery syndrome (hemispheric)   CC

G45.2 Multiple and bilateral precerebral artery syndromes   CC

G45.3 Amaurosis fugax   CC

  CC Excl: G45.3-H34.9

G45.4 Transient global amnesia

  EXCLUDES 1   amnesia NOS (R41.3)

G45.8 Other transient cerebral ischemic attacks and related syndromes   CC

G45.9 Transient cerebral ischemic attack, unspecified   CC

  Spasm of cerebral artery

  TIA

  Transient cerebral ischemia NOS

✓4ᵗʰ **G46 Vascular syndromes of brain in cerebrovascular diseases**

  Code first underlying cerebrovascular disease (I60-I69)

> **CC Excl: For CC codes in category G46, unless otherwise noted:**
> E08.51-E08.59, E08.618-E08.638, E08.649-E08.8, E09.51-E09.59,
> E09.618-E09.638, E09.649-E09.8, E10.51-E10.59, E10.618-E10.638,
> E10.649, E10.69-E10.8, E11.51-E11.59, E11.618-E11.638, E11.649,
> E11.69-E11.8, E13.51-E13.59, E13.618-E13.638, E13.649-E13.8, G45.0-
> G45.2, G45.8-G46.2, I63.00-I63.29, I65.01-I65.9, I67.841-I67.848,
> I87.8-I87.9, I99.8-I99.9

G46.0 Middle cerebral artery syndrome   CC

G46.1 Anterior cerebral artery syndrome   CC

G46.2 Posterior cerebral artery syndrome   CC

G46.3 Brain stem stroke syndrome

  Benedikt syndrome   Millard-Gubler syndrome

  Claude syndrome   Wallenberg syndrome

  Foville syndrome   Weber syndrome

G46.4 Cerebellar stroke syndrome

G46.5 Pure motor lacunar syndrome

G46.6 Pure sensory lacunar syndrome

G46.7 Other lacunar syndromes

G46.8 Other vascular syndromes of brain in cerebrovascular diseases

✓4ᵗʰ **G47 Sleep disorders**

  EXCLUDES 2   nightmares (F51.5)

             nonorganic sleep disorders (F51.-)

             sleep terrors (F51.4)

             sleepwalking (F51.3)

  ✓5ᵗʰ **G47.0 Insomnia**

    EXCLUDES 2   alcohol related insomnia (F10.182, F10.282, F10.982)

           drug-related insomnia (F11.182, F11.282, F11.982,
                  F13.182, F13.282, F13.982, F14.182,
                  F14.282, F14.982, F15.182, F15.282, F15.982,
                  F19.182, F19.282, F19.982)

           idiopathic insomnia (F51.01)

           insomnia due to a mental disorder (F51.05)

           insomnia not due to a substance or known
                physiological condition (F51.0-)

           nonorganic insomnia (F51.0-)

           primary insomnia (F51.01)

           sleep apnea (G47.3-)

    G47.00 Insomnia, unspecified

      Insomnia NOS

    G47.01 Insomnia due to medical condition

      Code also associated medical condition

    G47.09 Other insomnia

  ✓5ᵗʰ **G47.1 Hypersomnia**

    EXCLUDES 2   alcohol-related hypersomnia (F10.182, F10.282,
                  F10.982)

           drug-related hypersomnia (F11.182, F11.282, F11.982,
                  F13.182, F13.282, F13.982, F14.182, F14.282,
                  F14.982, F15.182, F15.282, F15.982, F19.182,
                  F19.282, F19.982)

           hypersomnia due to a mental disorder (F51.13)

           hypersomnia not due to a substance or known
                physiological condition (F51.1-)

           primary hypersomnia (F51.11)

           sleep apnea (G47.3-)

    G47.10 Hypersomnia, unspecified

      Hypersomnia NOS

    G47.11 Idiopathic hypersomnia with long sleep time

      Idiopathic hypersomnia NOS

    G47.12 Idiopathic hypersomnia without long sleep time

    G47.13 Recurrent hypersomnia

      Kleine-Levin syndrome

      Menstrual related hypersomnia

    G47.14 Hypersomnia due to medical condition

      Code also associated medical condition

    G47.19 Other hypersomnia

N Newborn: 0   P Pediatric: 0-17   M Maternity: 12-55   A Adult: 15-124   MCC Major CC Condition   PDx MCC PDx acts as own MCC   CC CC Condition   PDx CC PDx acts as own CC

550   ICD-10-CM 2016

☑5ᵗʰ **G47.2 Circadian rhythm sleep disorders**
Disorders of the sleep wake schedule
Inversion of nyctohemeral rhythm
Inversion of sleep rhythm

G47.20 Circadian rhythm sleep disorder, unspecified type
Sleep wake schedule disorder NOS

G47.21 Circadian rhythm sleep disorder, delayed sleep phase type
Delayed sleep phase syndrome

G47.22 Circadian rhythm sleep disorder, advanced sleep phase type

G47.23 Circadian rhythm sleep disorder, irregular sleep wake type
Irregular sleep-wake pattern

G47.24 Circadian rhythm sleep disorder, free running type

G47.25 Circadian rhythm sleep disorder, jet lag type

G47.26 Circadian rhythm sleep disorder, shift work type

G47.27 Circadian rhythm sleep disorder in conditions classified elsewhere
Code first underlying condition

G47.29 Other circadian rhythm sleep disorder

☑5ᵗʰ **G47.3 Sleep apnea**
Code also any associated underlying condition
EXCLUDES1 *apnea NOS (R06.81)*
    Cheyne-Stokes breathing (R06.3)
    pickwickian syndrome (E66.2)
    sleep apnea of newborn (P28.3)

G47.30 Sleep apnea, unspecified
Sleep apnea NOS

G47.31 Primary central sleep apnea

G47.32 High altitude periodic breathing

G47.33 Obstructive sleep apnea (adult) (pediatric)
EXCLUDES1 *obstructive sleep apnea of newborn (P28.3)*

G47.34 Idiopathic sleep related nonobstructive alveolar hypoventilation
Sleep related hypoxia

G47.35 Congenital central alveolar hypoventilation syndrome

G47.36 Sleep related hypoventilation in conditions classified elsewhere
Sleep related hypoxemia in conditions classified elsewhere
Code first underlying condition

G47.37 Central sleep apnea in conditions classified elsewhere
Code first underlying condition

G47.39 Other sleep apnea

☑5ᵗʰ **G47.4 Narcolepsy and cataplexy**

☑6ᵗʰ **G47.41 Narcolepsy**

G47.411 Narcolepsy with cataplexy

G47.419 Narcolepsy without cataplexy
Narcolepsy NOS

☑6ᵗʰ **G47.42 Narcolepsy in conditions classified elsewhere**
Code first underlying condition

G47.421 Narcolepsy in conditions classified elsewhere with cataplexy

G47.429 Narcolepsy in conditions classified elsewhere without cataplexy

☑5ᵗʰ **G47.5 Parasomnia**
EXCLUDES1 *alcohol induced parasomnia (F10.182, F10.282, F10.982)*
    drug induced parasomnia (F11.182, F11.282, F11.982, F13.182, F13.282, F13.982, F14.182, F14.282, F14.982, F15.182, F15.282, F15.982, F19.182, F19.282, F19.982)
    parasomnia not due to a substance or known physiological condition (F51.8)

G47.50 Parasomnia, unspecified
Parasomnia NOS

G47.51 Confusional arousals

G47.52 REM sleep behavior disorder

G47.53 Recurrent isolated sleep paralysis

G47.54 Parasomnia in conditions classified elsewhere
Code first underlying condition

G47.59 Other parasomnia

☑5ᵗʰ **G47.6 Sleep related movement disorders**
EXCLUDES2 *restless legs syndrome (G25.81)*

G47.61 Periodic limb movement disorder

G47.62 Sleep related leg cramps

G47.63 Sleep related bruxism
EXCLUDES1 *psychogenic bruxism (F45.8)*

G47.69 Other sleep related movement disorders

G47.8 Other sleep disorders

G47.9 Sleep disorder, unspecified
Sleep disorder NOS

Nerve, nerve root and plexus disorders (G50-G59)

EXCLUDES1 *current traumatic nerve, nerve root and plexus disorders—see Injury, nerve by body region*
    neuralgia NOS (M79.2)
    neuritis NOS (M79.2)
    peripheral neuritis in pregnancy (O26.82-)
    radiculitis NOS (M54.1-)

☑4ᵗʰ **G50 Disorders of trigeminal nerve**
INCLUDES disorders of 5th cranial nerve

G50.0 Trigeminal neuralgia
Syndrome of paroxysmal facial pain
Tic douloureux

G50.1 Atypical facial pain

G50.8 Other disorders of trigeminal nerve

G50.9 Disorder of trigeminal nerve, unspecified

☑4ᵗʰ **G51 Facial nerve disorders**
INCLUDES disorders of 7th cranial nerve

G51.0 Bell's palsy
Facial palsy

G51.1 Geniculate ganglionitis
EXCLUDES1 *postherpetic geniculate ganglionitis (B02.21)*

G51.2 Melkersson's syndrome
Melkersson-Rosenthal syndrome

G51.3 Clonic hemifacial spasm

G51.4 Facial myokymia

G51.8 Other disorders of facial nerve

G51.9 Disorder of facial nerve, unspecified

☑4ᵗʰ **G52 Disorders of other cranial nerves**
EXCLUDES2 *disorders of acoustic [8th] nerve (H93.3)*
    disorders of optic [2nd] nerve (H46, H47.0)
    paralytic strabismus due to nerve palsy (H49.0-H49.2)

G52.0 Disorders of olfactory nerve
Disorders of 1st cranial nerve

G52.1 Disorders of glossopharyngeal nerve
Disorder of 9th cranial nerve
Glossopharyngeal neuralgia

G52.2 Disorders of vagus nerve
Disorders of pneumogastric [10th] nerve

G52.3 Disorders of hypoglossal nerve
Disorders of 12th cranial nerve

G52.7 Disorders of multiple cranial nerves
Polyneuritis cranialis

G52.8 Disorders of other specified cranial nerves

G52.9 Cranial nerve disorder, unspecified

G53 Cranial nerve disorders in diseases classified elsewhere
Code first underlying disease, such as:
   neoplasm (C00-D49)
EXCLUDES1 *multiple cranial nerve palsy in sarcoidosis (D86.82)*
    multiple cranial nerve palsy in syphilis (A52.15)
    postherpetic geniculate ganglionitis (B02.21)
    postherpetic trigeminal neuralgia (B02.22)

☑4ᵗʰ **G54 Nerve root and plexus disorders**
EXCLUDES1 *current traumatic nerve root and plexus disorders—see nerve injury by body region*
    intervertebral disc disorders (M50-M51)
    neuritis or radiculitis brachial NOS (M54.13)
    neuritis or radiculitis lumbar NOS (M54.16)
    neuritis or radiculitis lumbosacral NOS (M54.17)
    neuritis or radiculitis thoracic NOS (M54.14)
    radiculitis NOS (M54.10)
    radiculopathy NOS (M54.10)
    spondylosis (M47.-)

G54.0 Brachial plexus disorders
Thoracic outlet syndrome

G54.1 Lumbosacral plexus disorders

G54.2 Cervical root disorders, not elsewhere classified

G54.3 Thoracic root disorders, not elsewhere classified

G54.4 Lumbosacral root disorders, not elsewhere classified

G54.5 Neuralgic amyotrophy
Parsonage-Aldren-Turner syndrome
Shoulder-girdle neuritis
> **EXCLUDES 1** neuralgic amyotrophy in diabetes mellitus (E08-E13 with .44)

G54.6 Phantom limb syndrome with pain

G54.7 Phantom limb syndrome without pain
Phantom limb syndrome NOS

G54.8 Other nerve root and plexus disorders

G54.9 Nerve root and plexus disorder, unspecified

G55 *Nerve root and plexus compressions in diseases classified elsewhere*
Code first underlying disease, such as:
neoplasm (C00-D49)
> **EXCLUDES 1** nerve root compression (due to) (in) ankylosing spondylitis (M45.-)
> nerve root compression (due to) (in) dorsopathies (M53.-, M54.-)
> nerve root compression (due to) (in) intervertebral disc disorders (M50.1-, M51.1-)
> nerve root compression (due to) (in) spondylopathies (M46.-, M48.-)

☑4ᵗʰ G56 Mononeuropathies of upper limb
> **EXCLUDES 1** current traumatic nerve disorder—see nerve injury by body region

☑5ᵗʰ G56.0 Carpal tunnel syndrome
    G56.00 Carpal tunnel syndrome, unspecified upper limb
    G56.01 Carpal tunnel syndrome, right upper limb
    G56.02 Carpal tunnel syndrome, left upper limb

☑5ᵗʰ G56.1 Other lesions of median nerve
    G56.10 Other lesions of median nerve, unspecified upper limb
    G56.11 Other lesions of median nerve, right upper limb
    G56.12 Other lesions of median nerve, left upper limb

☑5ᵗʰ G56.2 Lesion of ulnar nerve
Tardy ulnar nerve palsy
    G56.20 Lesion of ulnar nerve, unspecified upper limb
    G56.21 Lesion of ulnar nerve, right upper limb
    G56.22 Lesion of ulnar nerve, left upper limb

☑5ᵗʰ G56.3 Lesion of radial nerve
    G56.30 Lesion of radial nerve, unspecified upper limb
    G56.31 Lesion of radial nerve, right upper limb
    G56.32 Lesion of radial nerve, left upper limb

☑5ᵗʰ G56.4 Causalgia of upper limb
Complex regional pain syndrome II of upper limb
> **EXCLUDES 1** complex regional pain syndrome I of lower limb (G90.52-)
> complex regional pain syndrome I of upper limb (G90.51-)
> complex regional pain syndrome II of lower limb (G57.7-)
> reflex sympathetic dystrophy of lower limb (G90.52-)
> reflex sympathetic dystrophy of upper limb (G90.51-)

    G56.40 Causalgia of unspecified upper limb
    G56.41 Causalgia of right upper limb
    G56.42 Causalgia of left upper limb

☑5ᵗʰ G56.8 Other specified mononeuropathies of upper limb
Interdigital neuroma of upper limb
    G56.80 Other specified mononeuropathies of unspecified upper limb
    G56.81 Other specified mononeuropathies of right upper limb
    G56.82 Other specified mononeuropathies of left upper limb

☑5ᵗʰ G56.9 Unspecified mononeuropathy of upper limb
    G56.90 Unspecified mononeuropathy of unspecified upper limb
    G56.91 Unspecified mononeuropathy of right upper limb
    G56.92 Unspecified mononeuropathy of left upper limb

☑4ᵗʰ G57 Mononeuropathies of lower limb
> **EXCLUDES 1** current traumatic nerve disorder—see nerve injury by body region

☑5ᵗʰ G57.0 Lesion of sciatic nerve
> **EXCLUDES 1** sciatica NOS (M54.3-)
> **EXCLUDES 2** sciatica attributed to intervertebral disc disorder (M51.1-)

    G57.00 Lesion of sciatic nerve, unspecified lower limb
    G57.01 Lesion of sciatic nerve, right lower limb
    G57.02 Lesion of sciatic nerve, left lower limb

☑5ᵗʰ G57.1 Meralgia paresthetica
Lateral cutaneous nerve of thigh syndrome
    G57.10 Meralgia paresthetica, unspecified lower limb
    G57.11 Meralgia paresthetica, right lower limb
    G57.12 Meralgia paresthetica, left lower limb

☑5ᵗʰ G57.2 Lesion of femoral nerve
    G57.20 Lesion of femoral nerve, unspecified lower limb
    G57.21 Lesion of femoral nerve, right lower limb
    G57.22 Lesion of femoral nerve, left lower limb

☑5ᵗʰ G57.3 Lesion of lateral popliteal nerve
Peroneal nerve palsy
    G57.30 Lesion of lateral popliteal nerve, unspecified lower limb
    G57.31 Lesion of lateral popliteal nerve, right lower limb
    G57.32 Lesion of lateral popliteal nerve, left lower limb

☑5ᵗʰ G57.4 Lesion of medial popliteal nerve
    G57.40 Lesion of medial popliteal nerve, unspecified lower limb
    G57.41 Lesion of medial popliteal nerve, right lower limb
    G57.42 Lesion of medial popliteal nerve, left lower limb

☑5ᵗʰ G57.5 Tarsal tunnel syndrome
    G57.50 Tarsal tunnel syndrome, unspecified lower limb
    G57.51 Tarsal tunnel syndrome, right lower limb
    G57.52 Tarsal tunnel syndrome, left lower limb

☑5ᵗʰ G57.6 Lesion of plantar nerve
Morton's metatarsalgia
    G57.60 Lesion of plantar nerve, unspecified lower limb
    G57.61 Lesion of plantar nerve, right lower limb
    G57.62 Lesion of plantar nerve, left lower limb

☑5ᵗʰ G57.7 Causalgia of lower limb
Complex regional pain syndrome II of lower limb
> **EXCLUDES 1** complex regional pain syndrome I of lower limb (G90.52-)
> complex regional pain syndrome I of upper limb (G90.51-)
> complex regional pain syndrome II of upper limb (G56.4-)
> reflex sympathetic dystrophy of lower limb (G90.52-)
> reflex sympathetic dystrophy of upper limb (G90.51-)

    G57.70 Causalgia of unspecified lower limb
    G57.71 Causalgia of right lower limb
    G57.72 Causalgia of left lower limb

☑5ᵗʰ G57.8 Other specified mononeuropathies of lower limb
Interdigital neuroma of lower limb
    G57.80 Other specified mononeuropathies of unspecified lower limb
    G57.81 Other specified mononeuropathies of right lower limb
    G57.82 Other specified mononeuropathies of left lower limb

☑5ᵗʰ G57.9 Unspecified mononeuropathy of lower limb
    G57.90 Unspecified mononeuropathy of unspecified lower limb
    G57.91 Unspecified mononeuropathy of right lower limb
    G57.92 Unspecified mononeuropathy of left lower limb

☑4ᵗʰ G58 Other mononeuropathies
    G58.0 Intercostal neuropathy
    G58.7 Mononeuritis multiplex
    G58.8 Other specified mononeuropathies
    G58.9 Mononeuropathy, unspecified

G59   *Mononeuropathy in diseases classified elsewhere*
     Code first underlying disease
       EXCLUDES 1   *diabetic mononeuropathy (E08-E13 with .41)*
              syphilitic nerve paralysis (A52.19)
              syphilitic neuritis (A52.15)
              tuberculous mononeuropathy (A17.83)

Polyneuropathies and other disorders of the peripheral nervous system (G60-G65)

     EXCLUDES 1   *neuralgia NOS (M79.2)*
              neuritis NOS (M79.2)
              peripheral neuritis in pregnancy (O26.82-)
              radiculitis NOS (M54.10)

✓4ᵗʰ G60   Hereditary and idiopathic neuropathy
     G60.0   Hereditary motor and sensory neuropathy
         Charcôt-Marie-Tooth disease
         Déjérine-Sottas disease
         Hereditary motor and sensory neuropathy, types I-IV
         Hypertrophic neuropathy of infancy
         Peroneal muscular atrophy (axonal type) (hypertrophic type)
         Roussy-Levy syndrome

     G60.1   Refsum's disease   `CC`
         Infantile Refsum disease
         AHA: 2014, 2Q, 4
         CC Excl: E11.42, G13.0-G13.1, G50.0-G65.2, M34.83

     G60.2   Neuropathy in association with hereditary ataxia

     G60.3   Idiopathic progressive neuropathy

     G60.8   Other hereditary and idiopathic neuropathies
         Dominantly inherited sensory neuropathy
         Morvan's disease
         Nelaton's syndrome
         Recessively inherited sensory neuropathy

     G60.9   Hereditary and idiopathic neuropathy, unspecified

✓4ᵗʰ G61   Inflammatory polyneuropathy
     G61.0   Guillain-Barre syndrome   `CC`
         Acute (post-)infective polyneuritis
         Miller Fisher syndrome
         AHA: 2014, 2Q, 4
         CC Excl: A02.21, A17.0-A17.1, A27.81, A39.0, A39.89-A39.9, A49.3-A49.9, A50.41, A51.41, A52.13, A54.82, A54.84, A54.89-A54.9, A87.0-A87.9, B00.3, B02.1, B26.1, B37.5, B38.4, B45.1, B58.2, B92, B94.2-B94.9, B96.0, B96.6-B96.89, G00.0-G03.9, G04.2, G32.89, G61.0, G96.8-G96.9, G98.0-G98.8, G99.8

     G61.1   Serum neuropathy
         Use additional code for adverse effect, if applicable, to identify serum (T50.-)

     ✓5ᵗʰ G61.8   Other inflammatory polyneuropathies
         G61.81   Chronic inflammatory demyelinating   `CC`
               polyneuritis
               CC Excl: G51.0-G54.5, G54.8-G60.9, G61.81-G61.89, G62.81, G62.89, G64

         G61.89   Other inflammatory polyneuropathies

     G61.9   Inflammatory polyneuropathy, unspecified

✓4ᵗʰ G62   Other and unspecified polyneuropathies
     G62.0   Drug-induced polyneuropathy
         Use additional code for adverse effect, if applicable, to identify drug (T36-T50 with fifth or sixth character 5)

     G62.1   Alcoholic polyneuropathy

     G62.2   Polyneuropathy due to other toxic agents
         Code first (T51-T65) to identify toxic agent

     ✓5ᵗʰ G62.8   Other specified polyneuropathies
         G62.81   Critical illness polyneuropathy   `CC`
               Acute motor neuropathy
               CC Excl: G51.0-G54.5, G54.8-G60.9, G61.81-G61.9, G62.81, G62.89-G62.9, G64

         G62.82   Radiation-induced polyneuropathy
               Use additional external cause code (W88-W90, X39.0-) to identify cause

         G62.89   Other specified polyneuropathies

     G62.9   Polyneuropathy, unspecified
         Neuropathy NOS

G63   *Polyneuropathy in diseases classified elsewhere*
     Code first underlying disease, such as:
         amyloidosis (E85.-)
         endocrine disease, except diabetes (E00-E07, E15-E16, E20-E34)
         metabolic diseases (E70-E88)
         neoplasm (C00-D49)
         nutritional deficiency (E40-E64)
     EXCLUDES 1   *polyneuropathy (in):*
              diabetes mellitus (E08-E13 with .42)
              diphtheria (A36.83)
              infectious mononucleosis (B27.0-B27.9 with 1)
              Lyme disease (A69.22)
              mumps (B26.84)
              postherpetic (B02.23)
              rheumatoid arthritis (M05.33)
              scleroderma (M34.83)
              systemic lupus erythematosus (M32.19)
     AHA: 2012, 4Q, 99

G64   Other disorders of peripheral nervous system
     Disorder of peripheral nervous system NOS

✓4ᵗʰ G65   Sequelae of inflammatory and toxic polyneuropathies
     Code first condition resulting from (sequela) of inflammatory and toxic polyneuropathies
     G65.0   Sequelae of Guillain-Barré syndrome
     G65.1   Sequelae of other inflammatory polyneuropathy
     G65.2   Sequelae of toxic polyneuropathy

Diseases of myoneural junction and muscle (G70-G73)

✓4ᵗʰ G70   Myasthenia gravis and other myoneural disorders
     EXCLUDES 1   *botulism (A05.1, A48.51-A48.52)*
              transient neonatal myasthenia gravis (P94.0)

     CC Excl: For CC/MCC codes in category G70, unless otherwise noted: E08.40-E08.49, E08.618-E08.638, E08.649-E08.8, E09.40-E09.49, E09.618-E09.638, E09.649-E09.8, E10.40-E10.49, E10.618-E10.638, E10.649, E10.69-E10.8, E11.40-E11.49, E11.618-E11.638, E11.649, E11.69-E11.8, E13.40-E13.49, E13.618-E13.638, E13.649-E13.8, G32.89, G70.00-G70.01, G70.80-G70.81, G73.1-G73.3, G96.8-G96.9, G98.0-G98.8, G99.8

     ✓5ᵗʰ G70.0   Myasthenia gravis
         G70.00   Myasthenia gravis without (acute) exacerbation
               Myasthenia gravis NOS
         G70.01   Myasthenia gravis with (acute) exacerbation   `MCC`
               Myasthenia gravis in crisis

     G70.1   Toxic myoneural disorders
         Code first (T51-T65) to identify toxic agent

     G70.2   Congenital and developmental myasthenia

     ✓5ᵗʰ G70.8   Other specified myoneural disorders
         G70.80   Lambert-Eaton syndrome, unspecified   `CC`
               Lambert-Eaton syndrome NOS
         G70.81   *Lambert-Eaton syndrome in disease classified*   `CC`
               elsewhere
               Code first underlying disease
               EXCLUDES 1   *Lambert-Eaton syndrome in neoplastic disease (G73.1)*
         G70.89   Other specified myoneural disorders

     G70.9   Myoneural disorder, unspecified

✓ Additional Character Required   **✓x7ᵗʰ** Placeholder Alert   Unacceptable PDx   Manifestation   Hospital Acquired Condition   **EXCLUDES 1** Not Coded Here   **EXCLUDES 2** Not Included Here

ICD-10-CM 2016   553

Chapter 6. Diseases of the Nervous System

G71–G80.4

✓4ᵗʰ **G71 Primary disorders of muscles**

EXCLUDES 2   arthrogryposis multiplex congenita (Q74.3)
     metabolic disorders (E70-E88)
     myositis (M60.-)

G71.0 Muscular dystrophy   CC

Autosomal recessive, childhood type, muscular dystrophy resembling Duchenne or Becker muscular dystrophy
Benign [Becker] muscular dystrophy
Benign scapuloperoneal muscular dystrophy with early contractures [Emery-Dreifuss]
Congenital muscular dystrophy NOS
Congenital muscular dystrophy with specific morphological abnormalities of the muscle fiber
Distal muscular dystrophy
Facioscapulohumeral muscular dystrophy
Limb-girdle muscular dystrophy
Ocular muscular dystrophy
Oculopharyngeal muscular dystrophy
Scapuloperoneal muscular dystrophy
Severe [Duchenne] muscular dystrophy
CC Excl: E08.40-E08.49, E08.618-E08.638, E08.649-E08.8, E09.40-E09.49, E09.618-E09.638, E09.649-E09.8, E10.40-E10.49, E10.618-E10.638, E10.649, E10.69-E10.8, E11.40-E11.49, E11.618-E11.638, E11.649, E11.69-E11.8, E13.40-E13.49, E13.618-E13.638, E13.649-E13.8, G32.89, G71.0, G71.2, G96.8-G96.9, G98.0-G98.8, G99.8

✓5ᵗʰ **G71.1 Myotonic disorders**

G71.11 Myotonic muscular dystrophy
Dystrophia myotonica [Steinert]
Myotonia atrophica
Myotonic dystrophy
Proximal myotonic myopathy (PROMM)
Steinert disease

G71.12 Myotonia congenita
Acetazolamide responsive myotonia congenita
Dominant myotonia congenita [Thomsen disease]
Myotonia levior
Recessive myotonia congenita [Becker disease]

G71.13 Myotonic chondrodystrophy
Chondrodystrophic myotonia
Congenital myotonic chondrodystrophy
Schwartz-Jampel disease

G71.14 Drug induced myotonia
Use additional code for adverse effect, if applicable, to identify drug (T36-T50 with fifth or sixth character 5)

G71.19 Other specified myotonic disorders
Myotonia fluctuans
Myotonia permanens
Neuromyotonia [Isaacs]
Paramyotonia congenita (of von Eulenburg)
Pseudomyotonia
Symptomatic myotonia

G71.2 Congenital myopathies   CC
Central core disease   Myotubular (centronuclear)
Fiber-type disproportion   myopathy
Minicore disease   Nemaline myopathy
Multicore disease
EXCLUDES 1   arthrogryposis multiplex congenita (Q74.3)
CC Excl: See code: G71.0

G71.3 Mitochondrial myopathy, not elsewhere classified
EXCLUDES 1   Kearns-Sayre syndrome (H49.81)
     Leber's disease (H47.21)
     Leigh's encephalopathy (G31.82)
     mitochondrial metabolism disorders (E88.4-)
     Reye's syndrome (G93.7)

G71.8 Other primary disorders of muscles

G71.9 Primary disorder of muscle, unspecified
Hereditary myopathy NOS

✓4ᵗʰ **G72 Other and unspecified myopathies**
EXCLUDES 1   arthrogryposis multiplex congenita (Q74.3)
     dermatopolymyositis (M33.-)
     ischemic infarction of muscle (M62.2-)
     myositis (M60.-)
     polymyositis (M33.2-)

G72.0 Drug-induced myopathy   CC
Use additional code for adverse effect, if applicable, to identify drug (T36-T50 with fifth or sixth character 5)
CC Excl: G32.89, G70.00-G72.3, G72.81-G73.7, G96.8-G96.9, G98.0-G98.8, G99.8

G72.1 Alcoholic myopathy   CC
Use additional code to identify alcoholism (F10.-)
CC Excl: See code: G72.0

G72.2 Myopathy due to other toxic agents   CC
Code first (T51-T65) to identify toxic agent
CC Excl: See code: G72.0

G72.3 Periodic paralysis
Familial periodic paralysis
Hyperkalemic periodic paralysis (familial)
Hypokalemic periodic paralysis (familial)
Myotonic periodic paralysis (familial)
Normokalemic paralysis (familial)
Potassium sensitive periodic paralysis
EXCLUDES 1   paramyotonia congenita (of von Eulenburg) (G71.19)

✓5ᵗʰ **G72.4 Inflammatory and immune myopathies, not elsewhere classified**

G72.41 Inclusion body myositis [IBM]

G72.49 Other inflammatory and immune myopathies, not elsewhere classified
Inflammatory myopathy NOS

✓5ᵗʰ **G72.8 Other specified myopathies**

G72.81 Critical illness myopathy   CC
Acute necrotizing myopathy
Acute quadriplegic myopathy
Intensive care (ICU) myopathy
Myopathy of critical illness
CC Excl: G70.1-G72.3, G72.81-G73.7

G72.89 Other specified myopathies

G72.9 Myopathy, unspecified

✓4ᵗʰ **G73 Disorders of myoneural junction and muscle in diseases classified elsewhere**

G73.1 Lambert-Eaton syndrome in neoplastic disease   CC
Code first underlying neoplasm (C00-D49)
EXCLUDES 1   Lambert-Eaton syndrome not associated with neoplasm (G70.80-G70.81)
CC Excl: E08.40-E08.49, E08.618-E08.638, E08.649-E08.8, E09.40-E09.49, E09.618-E09.638, E09.649-E09.8, E10.40-E10.49, E10.618-E10.638, E10.649, E10.69-E10.8, E11.40-E11.49, E11.618-E11.638, E11.649, E11.69-E11.8, E13.40-E13.49, E13.618-E13.638, E13.649-E13.8, G32.89, G70.00-G70.01, G70.80-G70.81, G73.1-G73.3, G96.8-G96.9, G98.0-G98.8, G99.8

G73.3 Myasthenic syndromes in other diseases classified elsewhere   CC
Code first underlying disease, such as:
     neoplasm (C00-D49)
     thyrotoxicosis (E05.-)
CC Excl: See code: G73.1

G73.7 Myopathy in diseases classified elsewhere
Code first underlying disease, such as:
     hyperparathyroidism (E21.0, E21.3)
     hypoparathyroidism (E20.-)
     glycogen storage disease (E74.0)
     lipid storage disorders (E75.-)
EXCLUDES 1   myopathy in:
     rheumatoid arthritis (M05.4-)
     sarcoidosis (D86.87)
     scleroderma (M34.82)
     sicca syndrome [Sjögren] (M35.03)
     systemic lupus erythematosus (M32.19)

Cerebral palsy and other paralytic syndromes (G80-G83)

✓4ᵗʰ **G80 Cerebral palsy**
EXCLUDES 1   hereditary spastic paraplegia (G11.4)

G80.0 Spastic quadriplegic cerebral palsy   MCC
Congenital spastic paralysis (cerebral)
CC Excl: E08.40-E08.49, E08.618-E08.638, E08.649-E08.8, E09.40-E09.49, E09.618-E09.638, E09.649-E09.8, E10.40-E10.49, E10.618-E10.638, E10.649, E10.69-E10.8, E11.40-E11.49, E11.618-E11.638, E11.649, E11.69-E11.8, E13.40-E13.49, E13.618-E13.638, E13.649-E13.8, G04.1, G32.89, G80.0-G80.2, G80.4-G83.9, G90.1, G93.81, G93.89-G93.9, G96.8-G96.9, G98.0-G98.8, G99.8, Q06.0-Q06.1, Q06.3, Q06.8-Q06.9, Q07.8-Q07.9, R53.2

G80.1 Spastic diplegic cerebral palsy   CC
Spastic cerebral palsy NOS
CC Excl: G80.1, G93.40-G93.49, I67.83

G80.2 Spastic hemiplegic cerebral palsy   CC
CC Excl: G80.2, G93.40-G93.49, I67.83

G80.3 Athetoid cerebral palsy   CC
Double athetosis (syndrome)   Dystonic cerebral palsy
Dyskinetic cerebral palsy   Vogt disease
CC Excl: G20, G21.11-G21.9, G25.70-G25.79, G25.89-G26, G80.0-G80.9, G93.40-G93.49, I67.83

G80.4 Ataxic cerebral palsy

N Newborn: 0   P Pediatric: 0-17   M Maternity: 12-55   A Adult: 15-124   MCC Major CC Condition   PDxMCC PDx acts as own MCC   CC CC Condition   PDxCC PDx acts as own CC

554   ICD-10-CM 2016

Chapter 6. Diseases of the Nervous System

G80.8   Other **cerebral palsy**
     Mixed cerebral palsy syndromes

G80.9   **Cerebral palsy, unspecified**
     Cerebral palsy NOS

✓4ᵗʰ **G81**   **Hemiplegia and hemiparesis**
     NOTE   This category is to be used only when hemiplegia (complete)(incomplete) is reported without further specification, or is stated to be old or longstanding but of unspecified cause. The category is also for use in multiple coding to identify these types of hemiplegia resulting from any cause.
     EXCLUDES1   *congenital cerebral palsy (G80.-)*
         hemiplegia and hemiparesis due to sequela of cerebrovascular disease (I69.05-, I69.15-, I69.25-, I69.35-, I69.85-, I69.95-)
     AHA: 2015, 1Q, 25

> **CC Excl: For CC codes in category G81, unless otherwise noted:** G04.1, G11.0-G12.9, G32.0-G37.3, G37.5-G37.9, G80.0-G80.2, G80.4-G83.9, G90.01-G90.09, G90.2, G90.4-G90.9, G92, G93.40-G93.49, G93.81, G93.89-G93.9, G95.0-G95.9, G96.8-G96.9, G98.0-G99.8, I67.83, R53.2

✓5ᵗʰ   **G81.0**   **Flaccid** hemiplegia
     G81.00   Flaccid hemiplegia affecting **unspecified** side   CC
     G81.01   Flaccid hemiplegia affecting **right dominant side**   CC
     G81.02   Flaccid hemiplegia affecting **left dominant side**   CC
     G81.03   Flaccid hemiplegia affecting **right nondominant side**   CC
     G81.04   Flaccid hemiplegia affecting **left nondominant side**

✓5ᵗʰ   **G81.1**   **Spastic** hemiplegia
     G81.10   Spastic hemiplegia affecting **unspecified** side   CC
     G81.11   Spastic hemiplegia affecting **right dominant side**   CC
     G81.12   Spastic hemiplegia affecting **left dominant side**   CC
     G81.13   Spastic hemiplegia affecting **right nondominant side**   CC
     G81.14   Spastic hemiplegia affecting **left nondominant side**

✓5ᵗʰ   **G81.9**   **Hemiplegia, unspecified**
     AHA: 2014, 1Q, 23
     G81.90   Hemiplegia, unspecified affecting **unspecified** side   CC
     G81.91   Hemiplegia, unspecified affecting **right dominant side**   CC
     G81.92   Hemiplegia, unspecified affecting **left dominant side**   CC
     G81.93   Hemiplegia, unspecified affecting **right nondominant side**   CC
     G81.94   Hemiplegia, unspecified affecting **left nondominant side**   CC

✓4ᵗʰ **G82**   **Paraplegia (paraparesis) and quadriplegia (quadriparesis)**
     NOTE   This category is to be used only when the listed conditions are reported without further specification, or are stated to be old or longstanding but of unspecified cause. The category is also for use in multiple coding to identify these conditions resulting from any cause
     EXCLUDES1   *congenital cerebral palsy (G80.-)*
         functional quadriplegia (R53.2)
         hysterical paralysis (F44.4)

✓5ᵗʰ   **G82.2**   **Paraplegia**
     Paralysis of both lower limbs NOS
     Paraparesis (lower) NOS
     Paraplegia (lower) NOS

> **CC Excl: For CC codes in subcategory G82.2, unless otherwise noted:** See code: G81

     G82.20   **Paraplegia, unspecified**   CC
     G82.21   **Paraplegia, complete**   CC
     G82.22   **Paraplegia, incomplete**   CC

✓5ᵗʰ   **G82.5**   **Quadriplegia**

> **CC Excl: For MCC codes in subcategory G82.5, unless otherwise noted:** See code: G80.0

     G82.50   **Quadriplegia, unspecified**   MCC
     G82.51   **Quadriplegia, C1-C4 complete**   MCC
     G82.52   **Quadriplegia, C1-C4 incomplete**   MCC
     G82.53   **Quadriplegia, C5-C7 complete**   MCC
     G82.54   **Quadriplegia, C5-C7 incomplete**   MCC

✓4ᵗʰ **G83**   **Other paralytic syndromes**
     NOTE   This category is to be used only when the listed conditions are reported without further specification, or are stated to be old or longstanding but of unspecified cause. The category is also for use in multiple coding to identify these conditions resulting from any cause.
     INCLUDES   paralysis (complete) (incomplete), except as in G80-G82

     G83.0   **Diplegia of upper limbs**   CC
         Diplegia (upper)   Paralysis of both upper limbs
         CC Excl: G32.89, G82.50-G83.0, G83.5-G83.9, G96.8-G96.9, G98.0-G98.8, G99.8, R53.2

✓5ᵗʰ   **G83.1**   **Monoplegia of lower limb**
     Paralysis of lower limb
     EXCLUDES1   *monoplegia of lower limbs due to sequela of cerebrovascular disease (I69.04-, I69.14-, I69.24-, I69.34-, I69.84-, I69.94-)*
     G83.10   Monoplegia of lower limb affecting **unspecified** side
     G83.11   Monoplegia of lower limb affecting **right dominant side**
     G83.12   Monoplegia of lower limb affecting **left dominant side**
     G83.13   Monoplegia of lower limb affecting **right nondominant side**
     G83.14   Monoplegia of lower limb affecting **left nondominant side**

✓5ᵗʰ   **G83.2**   **Monoplegia of upper limb**
     Paralysis of upper limb
     EXCLUDES1   *monoplegia of upper limbs due to sequela of cerebrovascular disease (I69.03-, I69.13-, I69.23-, I69.33-, I69.83-, I69.93-)*
     G83.20   Monoplegia of upper limb affecting **unspecified** side
     G83.21   Monoplegia of upper limb affecting **right dominant side**
     G83.22   Monoplegia of upper limb affecting **left dominant side**
     G83.23   Monoplegia of upper limb affecting **right nondominant side**
     G83.24   Monoplegia of upper limb affecting **left nondominant side**

✓5ᵗʰ   **G83.3**   **Monoplegia, unspecified**
     G83.30   Monoplegia, unspecified affecting **unspecified** side
     G83.31   Monoplegia, unspecified affecting **right dominant side**
     G83.32   Monoplegia, unspecified affecting **left dominant side**
     G83.33   Monoplegia, unspecified affecting **right nondominant side**
     G83.34   Monoplegia, unspecified affecting **left nondominant side**

     G83.4   **Cauda equina syndrome**   CC
         Neurogenic bladder due to cauda equina syndrome
         EXCLUDES1   *cord bladder NOS (G95.89)*
             neurogenic bladder NOS (N31.9)
         CC Excl: G04.1, G32.89, G82.20-G82.54, G83.10-G83.14, G83.4-G83.9, G96.8-G96.9, G98.0-G98.8, G99.8, R53.2

     G83.5   **Locked-in state**   MCC
         CC Excl: G04.1, G32.89, G80.0-G80.2, G80.4-G83.9, G92, G93.40-G93.49, G93.81, G93.89-G93.9, G96.8-G96.9, G98.0-G98.8, G99.8, I67.83, R53.2

✓5ᵗʰ   **G83.8**   **Other specified paralytic syndromes**
     EXCLUDES1   *paralytic syndromes due to current spinal cord injury—code to spinal cord injury (S14, S24, S34)*
     G83.81   **Brown-Séquard syndrome**
     G83.82   **Anterior cord syndrome**
     G83.83   **Posterior cord syndrome**
     G83.84   **Todd's paralysis (postepileptic)**
     G83.89   **Other specified paralytic syndromes**

     G83.9   **Paralytic syndrome, unspecified**

✓ Additional Character Required   ✓ₓ7ᵗʰ Placeholder Alert   Unacceptable PDx   Manifestation   Hospital Acquired Condition   **EXCLUDES1** Not Coded Here   **EXCLUDES2** Not Included Here

ICD-10-CM 2016   555

(left margin) **Chapter 6. Diseases of the Nervous System**

Other disorders of the nervous system (G89-G99)

✓4ᵗʰ G89 Pain, not elsewhere classified

Code also related psychological factors associated with pain (F45.42)

EXCLUDES 1 *generalized pain NOS (R52)*
pain disorders exclusively related to psychological factors (F45.41)
pain NOS (R52)

EXCLUDES 2 *atypical face pain (G50.1)*
headache syndromes (G44.-)
localized pain, unspecified type—code to pain by site, such as:
   abdomen pain (R10.-)
   back pain (M54.9)
   breast pain (N64.4)
   chest pain (R07.1-R07.9)
   ear pain (H92.0-)
   eye pain (H57.1)
   headache (R51)
   joint pain (M25.5-)
   limb pain (M79.6-)
   lumbar region pain (M54.5)
   painful urination (R30.9)
   pelvic and perineal pain (R10.2)
   renal colic (N23)
   shoulder pain (M25.51-)
   spine pain (M54.-)
   throat pain (R07.0)
   tongue pain (K14.6)
   tooth pain (K08.8)
migraines (G43.-)
myalgia (M79.1)
pain from prosthetic devices, implants, and grafts (T82.84, T83.84, T84.84, T85.84)
phantom limb syndrome with pain (G54.6)
vulvar vestibulitis (N94.810)
vulvodynia (N94.81-)

G89.0 Central pain syndrome
Déjérine-Roussy syndrome
Myelopathic pain syndrome
Thalamic pain syndrome (hyperesthetic)

✓5ᵗʰ G89.1 Acute pain, not elsewhere classified

G89.11 Acute pain due to trauma

G89.12 Acute post-thoracotomy pain
Post-thoracotomy pain NOS

G89.18 Other acute postprocedural pain
Postoperative pain NOS
Postprocedural pain NOS

✓5ᵗʰ G89.2 Chronic pain, not elsewhere classified

EXCLUDES 1 *causalgia, lower limb (G57.7-)*
causalgia, upper limb (G56.4-)
central pain syndrome (G89.0)
chronic pain syndrome (G89.4)
complex regional pain syndrome II, lower limb (G57.7-)
complex regional pain syndrome II, upper limb (G56.4-)
neoplasm related chronic pain (G89.3)
reflex sympathetic dystrophy (G90.5-)

G89.21 Chronic pain due to trauma

G89.22 Chronic post-thoracotomy pain

G89.28 Other chronic postprocedural pain
Other chronic postoperative pain

G89.29 Other chronic pain

G89.3 Neoplasm related pain (acute) (chronic)
Cancer associated pain
Pain due to malignancy (primary) (secondary)
Tumor associated pain

G89.4 Chronic pain syndrome
Chronic pain associated with significant psychosocial dysfunction

✓4ᵗʰ G90 Disorders of autonomic nervous system

EXCLUDES 1 *dysfunction of the autonomic nervous system due to alcohol (G31.2)*

✓5ᵗʰ G90.0 Idiopathic peripheral autonomic neuropathy

G90.01 Carotid sinus syncope
Carotid sinus syndrome

G90.09 Other idiopathic peripheral autonomic neuropathy
Idiopathic peripheral autonomic neuropathy NOS

G90.1 Familial dysautonomia [Riley-Day]

G90.2 Horner's syndrome
Bernard(-Horner) syndrome
Cervical sympathetic dystrophy or paralysis

G90.3 Multi-system degeneration of the autonomic nervous system   CC
Neurogenic orthostatic hypotension [Shy-Drager]
EXCLUDES 1 *orthostatic hypotension NOS (I95.1)*
CC Excl: G20-G21.9, G90.01-G90.09, G93.40-G93.49, I67.83

G90.4 Autonomic dysreflexia
Use additional code to identify the cause, such as:
  fecal impaction (K56.41)
  pressure ulcer (pressure area) (L89.-)
  urinary tract infection (N39.0)

✓5ᵗʰ G90.5 Complex regional pain syndrome I (CRPS I)
Reflex sympathetic dystrophy
EXCLUDES 1 *causalgia of lower limb (G57.7-)*
causalgia of upper limb (G56.4-)
complex regional pain syndrome II of lower limb (G57.7-)
complex regional pain syndrome II of upper limb (G56.4-)

G90.50 Complex regional pain syndrome I, unspecified   CC
CC Excl: G90.50-G90.59

✓6ᵗʰ G90.51 Complex regional pain syndrome I of upper limb

> **CC Excl: For CC codes in subcategory G90.51, unless otherwise noted:** E08.40-E08.49, E09.40-E09.49, E10.40-E10.49, E11.40-E11.49, E13.40-E13.49, G04.1, G11.3, G11.8-G12.9, G32.0, G32.89-G37.3, G37.5-G37.9, G80.0-G80.2, G80.4-G83.9, G90.01-G90.09, G90.2, G90.4-G90.9, G93.1, G93.40-G93.49, G95.0-G95.9, G96.12-G96.9, G97.1, G98.0-G99.8, I67.83, R53.2

    G90.511 Complex regional pain syndrome I of right upper limb   CC
    G90.512 Complex regional pain syndrome I of left upper limb   CC
    G90.513 Complex regional pain syndrome I of upper limb, bilateral   CC
    G90.519 Complex regional pain syndrome I of unspecified upper limb   CC

✓6ᵗʰ G90.52 Complex regional pain syndrome I of lower limb

> **CC Excl: For CC codes in subcategory G90.52, unless otherwise noted:** E08.40-E08.49, E09.40-E09.49, E10.40-E10.49, E11.40-E11.49, E13.40-E13.49, G04.1, G11.3, G11.8-G12.9, G32.0, G32.89-G37.3, G37.5-G37.9, G80.0-G80.2, G80.4-G83.9, G90.01-G90.09, G90.2, G90.4-G90.9, G93.1, G93.40-G93.49, G95.0-G95.9, G96.12-G96.9, G97.1, G98.0-G99.8, I67.83, R53.2

    G90.521 Complex regional pain syndrome I of right lower limb   CC
    G90.522 Complex regional pain syndrome I of left lower limb   CC
    G90.523 Complex regional pain syndrome I of lower limb, bilateral   CC
    G90.529 Complex regional pain syndrome I of unspecified lower limb   CC

G90.59 Complex regional pain syndrome I of other specified site   CC
CC Excl: See code: G90.52

G90.8 Other disorders of autonomic nervous system

G90.9 Disorder of the autonomic nervous system, unspecified

✓4ᵗʰ G91 Hydrocephalus

INCLUDES acquired hydrocephalus
EXCLUDES 1 *Arnold-Chiari syndrome with hydrocephalus (Q07.-)*
congenital hydrocephalus (Q03.-)
spina bifida with hydrocephalus (Q05.-)

> **CC Excl: For CC codes in subcategories G91.0 & G91.2, unless otherwise noted:** G91.0-G91.3, G91.8-G91.9
> **For CC codes in subcategories G91.1, G91.3-G91.9, unless otherwise noted:** E08.40-E08.49, E08.618-E08.638, E08.649-E08.8, E09.40-E09.49, E09.618-E09.638, E09.649-E09.8, E10.40-E10.49, E10.618-E10.638, E10.649, E10.69-E10.8, E11.40-E11.49, E11.618-E11.638, E11.649, E11.69-E11.8, E13.40-E13.49, E13.618-E13.638, E13.649-E13.8, G13.2-G13.8, G31.2, G31.83-G31.9, G90.1, G91.0-G91.9, G93.81, G93.89-G94, Q03.0-Q03.9, Q04.4-Q04.8, Q05.0-Q05.4, Q05.9-Q06.1, Q06.3, Q06.8-Q06.9, Q07.02-Q07.9

G91.0 Communicating hydrocephalus   CC
Secondary normal pressure hydrocephalus

G91.1 Obstructive hydrocephalus   CC

G91.2 (Idiopathic) normal pressure hydrocephalus   CC
Normal pressure hydrocephalus NOS

N Newborn: 0   **P** Pediatric: 0-17   **M** Maternity: 12-55   **A** Adult: 15-124   **MCC** Major CC Condition   **PDxMCC** PDx acts as own MCC   **CC** CC Condition   **PDxCC** PDx acts as own CC
556   ICD-10-CM 2016

*(left margin, bottom)* G89-G91.2

G91.3 Post-traumatic **hydrocephalus, unspecified** `CC`

G91.4 *Hydrocephalus in diseases classified elsewhere*

  Code first underlying condition, such as:
    congenital syphilis (A50.4-)
    neoplasm (C00-D49)

  EXCLUDES 1 *hydrocephalus due to congenital toxoplasmosis (P37.1)*
  AHA: 2014, 3Q, 3

G91.8 Other **hydrocephalus** `CC`

G91.9 **Hydrocephalus, unspecified** `CC`

G92 **Toxic encephalopathy** `MCC`

  Toxic encephalitis
  Toxic metabolic encephalopathy
  Code first (T51-T65) to identify toxic agent
  CC Excl: A17.82, A17.9, A18.82, A18.84, A18.89, A39.81, A50.42, A52.14, A83.0-A85.1, A85.8-A86, A88.8-A89, B00.4, B01.11, B10.01-B10.09, B26.2, B58.2, E08.40-E08.49, E08.618-E08.638, E08.649-E08.8, E09.40-E09.49, E09.618-E09.638, E09.649-E09.8, E10.40-E10.49, E10.618-E10.638, E10.649, E10.69-E10.8, E11.40-E11.49, E11.618-E11.638, E11.649, E11.69-E11.8, E13.40-E13.49, E13.618-E13.638, E13.649-E13.8, G04.00-G04.01, G04.31, G04.81-G05.4, G32.89, G37.3-G37.4, G92, G93.40-G93.49, G93.81, G93.89-G93.9, G96.8-G96.9, G98.0-G98.8, G99.8, I67.83

`✔4ᵗʰ` **G93** **Other disorders of brain**

G93.0 **Cerebral cysts**
  Arachnoid cyst
  Porencephalic cyst, acquired
  EXCLUDES 1 *acquired periventricular cysts of newborn (P91.1)*
  congenital cerebral cysts (Q04.6)

G93.1 **Anoxic brain damage, not elsewhere classified** `CC`
  EXCLUDES 1 *cerebral anoxia due to anesthesia during labor and delivery (O74.3)*
  cerebral anoxia due to anesthesia during the puerperium (O89.2)
  neonatal anoxia (P84)
  CC Excl: E08.40-E08.49, E08.618-E08.638, E08.649-E08.8, E09.40-E09.49, E09.618-E09.638, E09.649-E09.8, E10.40-E10.49, E10.618-E10.638, E10.649, E10.69-E10.8, E11.40-E11.49, E11.618-E11.638, E11.649, E11.69-E11.8, E13.40-E13.49, E13.618-E13.638, E13.649-E13.8, G32.89, G93.1-G93.2, G96.8-G96.9, G98.0-G98.8, G99.8

G93.2 **Benign intracranial hypertension**
  EXCLUDES 1 *hypertensive encephalopathy (I67.4)*

G93.3 **Postviral fatigue syndrome**
  Benign myalgic encephalomyelitis
  EXCLUDES 1 *chronic fatigue syndrome NOS (R53.82)*

`✔5ᵗʰ` **G93.4** **Other and unspecified encephalopathy**
  EXCLUDES 1 *alcoholic encephalopathy (G31.2)*
  encephalopathy in diseases classified elsewhere (G94)
  hypertensive encephalopathy (I67.4)
  toxic (metabolic) encephalopathy (G92)

  G93.40 **Encephalopathy, unspecified** `HIV` `MCC`
    CC Excl: G21.0, G83.5, G93.41-G93.49, I67.83

  G93.41 **Metabolic encephalopathy** `HIV` `MCC`
    Septic encephalopathy
    CC Excl: G21.0, G83.5, G93.40, G93.49, I67.83

  G93.49 **Other encephalopathy** `HIV` `MCC`
    Encephalopathy NEC
    CC Excl: G21.0, G83.5, G93.40-G93.41

G93.5 **Compression of brain** `MCC`
  Arnold-Chiari type 1 compression of brain
  Compression of brain (stem)
  Herniation of brain (stem)
  EXCLUDES 1 *diffuse traumatic compression of brain (S06.2-)*
  focal traumatic compression of brain (S06.3-)
  CC Excl: G81.90, G93.82

G93.6 **Cerebral edema** `MCC`
  EXCLUDES 1 *cerebral edema due to birth injury (P11.0)*
  traumatic cerebral edema (S06.1-)
  CC Excl: G93.6, G93.82

G93.7 **Reye's syndrome** `MCC` `P`
  Code first (T39.0-), if salicylates-induced
  CC Excl: G93.7

`✔5ᵗʰ` **G93.8** **Other specified disorders of brain**

  G93.81 **Temporal sclerosis**
    Hippocampal sclerosis
    Mesial temporal sclerosis

G93.82 **Brain death** `MCC`
  CC Excl: B15.0-B19.9, E03.5, E08.00-E08.59, E08.618-E09.59, E09.618-E10.59, E10.618-E10.649, E10.69-E11.59, E11.618-E11.649, E11.69-E13.59, E13.618-E16.2, E89.1, G32.89, G89.0-G89.4, G93.81-G93.9, G96.8-G96.9, G98.0-G98.8, G99.8, I60.00-I62.9, K72.91, R40.0-R40.2124, R40.2210-R40.2224, R40.2310-R40.2324, R40.2340-R40.2344, R40.3-R41.3, R41.82, R41.9-R42, R44.8-R44.9, R45.83-R45.84, R46.0-R46.89, R52, R55, R68.0-R68.19, R68.81-R68.83, R68.89-R69, S02.0XX-S02.19X with 7th [A, B], S02.91X with 7th [A, B], S06.0X0-S06.9X9 with 7th A

G93.89 **Other specified disorders of brain**
  Postradiation encephalopathy

G93.9 **Disorder of brain, unspecified** `HIV`

G94 *Other disorders of brain in diseases classified elsewhere*
  Code first underlying disease
  EXCLUDES 1 *encephalopathy in congenital syphilis (A50.49)*
  encephalopathy in influenza (J09.X9, J10.81, J11.81)
  encephalopathy in syphilis (A52.19)
  hydrocephalus in diseases classified elsewhere (G91.4)

`✔4ᵗʰ` **G95** **Other and unspecified diseases of spinal cord**
  EXCLUDES 2 *myelitis (G04.-)*

G95.0 **Syringomyelia and syringobulbia** `CC`
  CC Excl: G04.1, G11.3, G11.8-G12.9, G32.0, G32.89-G37.3, G37.5-G37.9, G80.0-G80.2, G80.4-G83.9, G90.01-G90.09, G90.2, G90.4-G90.9, G93.40-G93.49, G93.81, G93.89-G93.9, G95.0-G95.9, G96.12-G96.9, G97.1, G98.0-G99.8, I67.83, R53.2

`✔5ᵗʰ` **G95.1** **Vascular myelopathies**
  EXCLUDES 2 *intraspinal phlebitis and thrombophlebitis, except non-pyogenic (G08)*

  G95.11 **Acute infarction of spinal cord (embolic) (nonembolic)** `MCC`
    Anoxia of spinal cord
    Arterial thrombosis of spinal cord
    CC Excl: E08.40-E08.49, E09.40-E09.49, E10.40-E10.49, E11.40-E11.49, E13.40-E13.49, G04.1, G11.3, G11.8-G12.9, G32.0, G32.89-G37.3, G37.5-G37.9, G80.0-G80.2, G80.4-G83.9, G90.01-G90.09, G90.2, G90.4-G90.9, G93.40-G93.49, G95.0-G95.9, G96.12-G96.9, G97.1, G98.0-G99.8, I67.83, R53.2

  G95.19 **Other vascular myelopathies** `MCC`
    Edema of spinal cord
    Hematomyelia
    Nonpyogenic intraspinal phlebitis and thrombophlebitis
    Subacute necrotic myelopathy
    CC Excl: See code: G95.11

`✔5ᵗʰ` **G95.2** **Other and unspecified cord compression**

  G95.20 **Unspecified cord compression** `HIV` `CC`
    CC Excl: E08.40-E08.49, E09.40-E09.49, E10.40-E10.49, E11.40-E11.49, E13.40-E13.49, G04.1, G11.3-G12.9, G32.0, G32.89-G37.3, G37.5-G37.9, G80.0-G80.2, G80.4-G83.9, G90.01-G90.09, G90.2, G90.4-G90.9, G93.1, G93.40-G93.49, G95.0-G95.9, G96.12-G96.9, G97.1, G98.0-G99.8, I67.83, R53.2

  G95.29 **Other cord compression** `HIV` `CC`
    CC Excl: See code: G95.20

`✔5ᵗʰ` **G95.8** **Other specified diseases of spinal cord**
  EXCLUDES 1 *neurogenic bladder NOS (N31.9)*
  neurogenic bladder due to cauda equina syndrome (G83.4)
  neuromuscular dysfunction of bladder without spinal cord lesion (N31.-)

  G95.81 **Conus medullaris syndrome** `CC`
    CC Excl: See code: G90.51

  G95.89 **Other specified diseases of spinal cord** `CC`
    Cord bladder NOS
    Drug-induced myelopathy
    Radiation-induced myelopathy
    EXCLUDES 1 *myelopathy NOS (G95.9)*
    CC Excl: See code: G90.51

G95.9 **Disease of spinal cord, unspecified** `HIV` `CC`
  Myelopathy NOS
  CC Excl: See code: G95.20

`✔4ᵗʰ` **G96** **Other disorders of central nervous system**

G96.0 **Cerebrospinal fluid leak** `CC`
  EXCLUDES 1 *cerebrospinal fluid leak from spinal puncture (G97.0)*
  CC Excl: E08.40-E08.49, E08.618-E08.638, E08.649-E08.8, E09.40-E09.49, E09.618-E09.638, E09.649-E09.8, E10.40-E10.49, E10.618-E10.638, E10.649, E10.69-E10.8, E11.40-E11.49, E11.618-E11.638, E11.649, E11.69-E11.8, E13.40-E13.49, E13.618-E13.638, E13.649-E13.8, G32.89, G96.0, G96.8-G96.9, G98.0-G98.8, G99.8

✔ Additional Character Required ✔x7ᵗʰ Placeholder Alert Unacceptable PDx Manifestation Hospital Acquired Condition **EXCLUDES 1** Not Coded Here **EXCLUDES 2** Not Included Here

ICD-10-CM 2016

557

Chapter 6. Diseases of the Nervous System

G96.1–G99.8

✓5ᵗʰ **G96.1** **Disorders of meninges, not elsewhere classified**

    G96.11 **Dural tear** `CC`

        EXCLUDES 1 *accidental puncture or laceration of dura during a procedure (G97.41)*

        AHA: 2014, 4Q, 24

        CC Excl: D78.11-D78.12, D78.81-D78.89, E36.11-E36.8, E89.810-E89.89, G96.11, G97.41, G97.48-G97.49, H59.011-H59.019, H59.031-H59.099, H59.211-H59.229, H59.811-H59.89, H95.31-H95.32, H95.811-H95.89, I97.3, I97.51-I97.52, J95.71-J95.72, K91.71-K91.72, L76.11-L76.12, L76.81-L76.82, M96.820-M96.821, M96.89, N98.1-N98.9, N99.71-N99.72, T81.82XA, T81.89XA, T81.9XXA

    G96.12 **Meningeal adhesions (cerebral) (spinal)**

    G96.19 **Other disorders of meninges, not elsewhere classified**

  G96.8 **Other specified disorders of central nervous system**

  G96.9 **Disorder of central nervous system, unspecified** `HIV`

✓4ᵗʰ **G97** **Intraoperative and postprocedural complications and disorders of nervous system, not elsewhere classified**

    EXCLUDES 2 *intraoperative and postprocedural cerebrovascular infarction (I97.81-, I97.82-)*

  G97.0 **Cerebrospinal fluid leak from spinal puncture** `CC`

    CC Excl: D78.81-D78.89, E36.8, E89.810-E89.89, G97.0, G97.2-G97.32, G97.81-G97.82, H59.011-H59.019, H59.031-H59.099, H59.811-H59.89, H95.811-H95.89, I97.3, I97.810-I97.821, L76.81-L76.82, M96.89, N98.1-N98.9, T81.82XA, T81.89XA, T81.9XXA

  G97.1 **Other reaction to spinal and lumbar puncture**

    Headache due to lumbar puncture

  G97.2 **Intracranial hypotension following ventricular shunting** `CC`

    CC Excl: See code: G97.0

✓5ᵗʰ **G97.3** **Intraoperative hemorrhage and hematoma of a nervous system organ or structure complicating a procedure**

    EXCLUDES 1 *intraoperative hemorrhage and hematoma of a nervous system organ or structure due to accidental puncture and laceration during a procedure (G97.4-)*

    G97.31 **Intraoperative hemorrhage and hematoma of a nervous system organ or structure complicating a nervous system procedure** `CC`

        CC Excl: G97.4, G97.2-G97.32, G97.81-G97.82, H95.811-H95.89, I97.3, I97.810-I97.821, M96.89, N98.1-N98.9, T81.82XA, T81.89XA, T81.9XXA

    G97.32 **Intraoperative hemorrhage and hematoma of a nervous system organ or structure complicating other procedure** `CC`

        CC Excl: See code: G97.31

✓5ᵗʰ **G97.4** **Accidental puncture and laceration of a nervous system organ or structure during a procedure**

    CC Excl: For CC codes in subcategory G97.4, unless otherwise noted: D78.11-D78.12, D78.81-D78.89, E36.11-E36.8, E89.810-E89.89, G96.11, G97.41, G97.48-G97.49, H59.011-H59.019, H59.031-H59.099, H59.211-H59.229, H59.811-H59.89, H95.31-H95.32, H95.811-H95.89, I97.3, I97.51-I97.52, J95.71-J95.72, K91.71-K91.72, L76.11-L76.12, L76.81-L76.82, M96.820-M96.821, M96.89, N98.1-N98.9, N99.71-N99.72, T81.82XA, T81.89XA, T81.9XXA

    G97.41 **Accidental puncture or laceration of dura during a procedure** `CC`

        Incidental (inadvertent) durotomy

        AHA: 2014, 4Q, 24

    G97.48 **Accidental puncture and laceration of other nervous system organ or structure during a nervous system procedure** `CC`

    G97.49 **Accidental puncture and laceration of other nervous system organ or structure during other procedure** `CC`

✓5ᵗʰ **G97.5** **Postprocedural hemorrhage and hematoma of a nervous system organ or structure following a procedure**

    G97.51 **Postprocedural hemorrhage and hematoma of a nervous system organ or structure following a nervous system procedure** `CC`

        CC Excl: G97.51-G97.52, H95.811-H95.89, I85.01, I85.11, I97.3, K21.9, K22.8, K23-K25.0, K25.2, K25.4, K25.6, K26.0, K26.2, K26.4, K26.6, K27.0, K27.2, K27.4, K27.6, K28.0, K28.2, K28.4, K28.6, K29.01, K29.21, K29.31, K29.41, K29.51, K29.61, K29.71, K29.81, K29.91, K31.811, K55.21, K57.01, K57.11, K57.13, K57.21, K57.31, K57.33, K57.41, K57.51, K57.53, K57.81, K57.91, K57.93, K62.5, K92.0-K92.2, M96.89, N98.1-N98.9, P54.1-P54.3, T81.10XA, T81.11XA, T81.12XA, T81.19XA, T81.82XA, T81.89XA, T81.9XXA

    G97.52 **Postprocedural hemorrhage and hematoma of a nervous system organ or structure following other procedure** `CC`

        CC Excl: See code: G97.51

✓5ᵗʰ **G97.8** **Other intraoperative and postprocedural complications and disorders of nervous system**

    Use additional code to further specify disorder

    G97.81 **Other intraoperative complications of nervous system** `CC`

        CC Excl: See code: G97.0

    G97.82 **Other postprocedural complications and disorders of nervous system** `CC`

        CC Excl: See code: G97.0

✓4ᵗʰ **G98** **Other disorders of nervous system not elsewhere classified**

    INCLUDES nervous system disorder NOS

  G98.0 **Neurogenic arthritis, not elsewhere classified**

    Nonsyphilitic neurogenic arthropathy NEC

    Nonsyphilitic neurogenic spondylopathy NEC

    EXCLUDES 1 *spondylopathy (in):*

        syringomyelia and syringobulbia (G95.0)

        tabes dorsalis (A52.11)

  G98.8 **Other disorders of nervous system** `HIV`

    Nervous system disorder NOS

✓4ᵗʰ **G99** **Other disorders of nervous system in diseases classified elsewhere**

  G99.0 *Autonomic neuropathy in diseases classified elsewhere* `CC`

    Code first underlying disease, such as:

      amyloidosis (E85.-)

      gout (M1A.-, M10.-)

      hyperthyroidism (E05.-)

    EXCLUDES 1 *diabetic autonomic neuropathy (E08-E13 with .43)*

    CC Excl: G90.01-G90.09, G90.2, G90.50-G90.9, G93.40-G93.49, G99.0, I67.83

  G99.2 *Myelopathy in diseases classified elsewhere* `CC`

    Code first underlying disease, such as:

      neoplasm (C00-D49)

    EXCLUDES 1 *myelopathy in:*

      intervertebral disease (M50.0-, M51.0-)

      spondylosis (M47.0-, M47.1-)

    CC Excl: E08.40-E08.49, E09.40-E09.49, E10.40-E10.49, E11.40-E11.49, E13.40-E13.49, G04.1, G11.3, G11.8-G12.9, G32.0, G32.89-G37.3, G37.5-G37.9, G80.0-G80.2, G80.4-G83.9, G90.01-G90.09, G90.2, G90.4-G90.9, G93.1, G93.40-G93.49, G95.0-G95.9, G96.12-G96.9, G97.1, G98.0-G99.8, I67.83, R53.2

  G99.8 *Other specified disorders of nervous system in diseases classified elsewhere*

    Code first underlying disorder, such as:

      amyloidosis (E85.-)

      avitaminosis (E56.9)

    EXCLUDES 1 *nervous system involvement in:*

      cysticercosis (B69.0)

      rubella (B06.0-)

      syphilis (A52.1-)

Ⓝ Newborn: 0   Ⓟ Pediatric: 0-17   Ⓜ Maternity: 12-55   Ⓐ Adult: 15-124   **MCC** Major CC Condition   **PDxMCC** PDx acts as own MCC   **CC** CC Condition   **PDxCC** PDx acts as own CC

558   ICD-10-CM 2016

Chapter 7. Diseases of the Eye and Adnexa (H00–H59)

Chapter Specific Guidelines with Coding Examples

The chapter specific guidelines from the ICD-10-CM Official Guidelines for Coding and Reporting have been provided below. Along with these guidelines are coding examples, contained in the shaded boxes, that have been developed to help illustrate the coding and/or sequencing guidance found in these guidelines.

a. Glaucoma

1) Assigning glaucoma codes

Assign as many codes from category H40, Glaucoma, as needed to identify the type of glaucoma, the affected eye, and the glaucoma stage.

2) Bilateral glaucoma with same type and stage

When a patient has bilateral glaucoma and both eyes are documented as being the same type and stage, and there is a code for bilateral glaucoma, report only the code for the type of glaucoma, bilateral, with the seventh character for the stage.

> Bilateral severe stage pigmentary glaucoma
>
> **H40.1333   Pigmentary glaucoma, bilateral, severe stage**
>
> *Explanation*: In this scenario, the patient has the same type and stage of glaucoma in both eyes. As this type of glaucoma has a code for bilateral, assign only the code for the bilateral glaucoma with the seventh character for the stage.

When a patient has bilateral glaucoma and both eyes are documented as being the same type and stage, and the classification does not provide a code for bilateral glaucoma (i.e. subcategories H40.10, H40.11 and H40.20) report only one code for the type of glaucoma with the appropriate seventh character for the stage.

> Bilateral, mild stage, primary open-angle glaucoma
>
> **H40.11X1   Primary open-angle glaucoma, mild stage**
>
> *Explanation*: In this scenario, the patient has glaucoma of the same type and stage of both eyes, but there is no code specifically for bilateral glaucoma. Only one code is assigned with the appropriate seventh character for the stage.

3) Bilateral glaucoma stage with different types or stages

When a patient has bilateral glaucoma and each eye is documented as having a different type or stage, and the classification distinguishes laterality, assign the appropriate code for each eye rather than the code for bilateral glaucoma.

> Bilateral chronic angle-closure glaucoma; right eye is documented as mild stage and left eye as moderate stage
>
> **H40.2211   Chronic angle-closure glaucoma, right eye, mild stage**
>
> **H40.2222   Chronic angle-closure glaucoma, left eye, moderate stage**
>
> *Explanation*: In this scenario the patient has the same type of glaucoma in both eyes, but each eye is at a different stage. Because the subcategory for this condition identifies laterality, one code is assigned for the right eye and one code is assigned for the left eye, each with the appropriate seventh character for the stage appended.

When a patient has bilateral glaucoma and each eye is documented as having a different type, and the classification does not distinguish laterality (i.e. subcategories H40.10, H40.11 and H40.20), assign one code for each type of glaucoma with the appropriate seventh character for the stage.

> Documentation relates mild, unspecified primary angle-closure glaucoma of the left eye with mild primary open-angle glaucoma of the right eye
>
> **H40.20X1   Unspecified primary angle-closure glaucoma, mild stage**
>
> **H40.11X1   Primary open-angle glaucoma, mild stage**
>
> *Explanation*: In this scenario the patient has a different type of glaucoma in each eye and the classification does not distinguish laterality. A code for each type of glaucoma is assigned, each with the appropriate seventh character for the stage.

When a patient has bilateral glaucoma and each eye is documented as having the same type, but different stage, and the classification does not distinguish laterality (i.e. subcategories H40.10, H40.11 and H40.20), assign a code for the type of glaucoma for each eye with the seventh character for the specific glaucoma stage documented for each eye.

> Bilateral primary open-angle glaucoma; the right eye is documented to be in mild stage and the left eye as being in moderate stage
>
> **H40.11X2   Primary open-angle glaucoma, moderate stage**
>
> **H40.11X1   Primary open-angle glaucoma, mild stage**
>
> *Explanation*: In this scenario the patient has the same type of glaucoma in each eye but each eye is at a different stage, and the classification does not distinguish laterality at this subcategory level. Two codes are assigned; both codes represent the same type of glaucoma but each has a different seventh character identifying the appropriate stage for each eye.

4) Patient admitted with glaucoma and stage evolves during the admission

If a patient is admitted with glaucoma and the stage progresses during the admission, assign the code for highest stage documented.

> Patient admitted with mild low-tension glaucoma of the right eye, which progresses to moderate stage during the patient's stay
>
> **H40.1212   Low-tension glaucoma, right eye, moderate stage**
>
> *Explanation*: When the glaucoma stage progresses during an admission, assign only the code for the highest stage documented.

5) Indeterminate stage glaucoma

Assignment of the seventh character "4" for "indeterminate stage" should be based on the clinical documentation. The seventh character "4" is used for glaucomas whose stage cannot be clinically determined. This seventh character should not be confused with the seventh character "0", unspecified, which should be assigned when there is no documentation regarding the stage of the glaucoma.

Chapter 7. Diseases of the Eye and Adnexa (H00–H59)

NOTE Use an external cause code following the code for the eye condition, if applicable, to identify the cause of the eye condition.

EXCLUDES 2 *certain conditions originating in the perinatal period (P04-P96)*
certain infectious and parasitic diseases (A00-B99)
complications of pregnancy, childbirth and the puerperium (O00-O9A)
congenital malformations, deformations, and chromosomal abnormalities (Q00-Q99)
diabetes mellitus related eye conditions (E09.3-, E10.3-, E11.3-, E13.3-)
endocrine, nutritional and metabolic diseases (E00-E88)
injury (trauma) of eye and orbit (S05.-)
injury, poisoning and certain other consequences of external causes (S00-T88)
neoplasms (C00-D49)
symptoms, signs and abnormal clinical and laboratory findings, not elsewhere classified (R00-R94)
syphilis related eye disorders (A50.01, A50.3-, A51.43, A52.71)

This chapter contains the following blocks:

H00-H05	Disorders of eyelid, lacrimal system and orbit
H10-H11	Disorders of conjunctiva
H15-H22	Disorders of sclera, cornea, iris and ciliary body
H25-H28	Disorders of lens
H30-H36	Disorders of choroid and retina
H40-H42	Glaucoma
H43-H44	Disorders of vitreous body and globe
H46-H47	Disorders of optic nerve and visual pathways
H49-H52	Disorders of ocular muscles, binocular movement, accommodation and refraction
H53-H54	Visual disturbances and blindness
H55-H57	Other disorders of eye and adnexa
H59	Intraoperative and postprocedural complications and disorders of eye and adnexa, not elsewhere classified

Disorders of eyelid, lacrimal system and orbit (H00-H05)

EXCLUDES 2 *open wound of eyelid (S01.1-)*
superficial injury of eyelid (S00.1-, S00.2-)

✓4ᵗʰ **H00 Hordeolum and chalazion**

✓5ᵗʰ **H00.0 Hordeolum (externum) (internum) of eyelid**

✓6ᵗʰ **H00.01 Hordeolum externum**
Hordeolum NOS
Stye

H00.011 Hordeolum externum right upper **eyelid**
H00.012 Hordeolum externum right lower **eyelid**
H00.013 Hordeolum externum right eye, unspecified **eyelid**
H00.014 Hordeolum externum left upper **eyelid**
H00.015 Hordeolum externum left lower **eyelid**
H00.016 Hordeolum externum left eye, unspecified **eyelid**
H00.019 Hordeolum externum unspecified eye, unspecified **eyelid**

✓6ᵗʰ **H00.02 Hordeolum internum**
Infection of meibomian gland

H00.021 Hordeolum internum right upper **eyelid**
H00.022 Hordeolum internum right lower **eyelid**
H00.023 Hordeolum internum right eye, unspecified **eyelid**
H00.024 Hordeolum internum left upper **eyelid**
H00.025 Hordeolum internum left lower **eyelid**
H00.026 Hordeolum internum left eye, unspecified **eyelid**
H00.029 Hordeolum internum unspecified eye, unspecified **eyelid**

✓6ᵗʰ **H00.03 Abscess of eyelid**
Furuncle of eyelid

H00.031 Abscess of right upper **eyelid**
H00.032 Abscess of right lower **eyelid**
H00.033 Abscess of eyelid right eye, unspecified **eyelid**
H00.034 Abscess of left upper **eyelid**
H00.035 Abscess of left lower **eyelid**
H00.036 Abscess of eyelid left eye, unspecified **eyelid**
H00.039 Abscess of eyelid unspecified eye, unspecified **eyelid**

✓5ᵗʰ **H00.1 Chalazion**
Meibomian (gland) cyst
EXCLUDES 2 *infected meibomian gland (H00.02-)*

H00.11 Chalazion right upper **eyelid**
H00.12 Chalazion right lower **eyelid**
H00.13 Chalazion right eye, unspecified **eyelid**
H00.14 Chalazion left upper **eyelid**
H00.15 Chalazion left lower **eyelid**
H00.16 Chalazion left eye, unspecified **eyelid**
H00.19 Chalazion unspecified eye, unspecified **eyelid**

✓4ᵗʰ **H01 Other inflammation of eyelid**

✓5ᵗʰ **H01.0 Blepharitis**
EXCLUDES 1 *blepharoconjunctivitis (H10.5-)*

✓6ᵗʰ **H01.00 Unspecified blepharitis**
H01.001 Unspecified blepharitis right upper **eyelid**
H01.002 Unspecified blepharitis right lower **eyelid**
H01.003 Unspecified blepharitis right eye, unspecified **eyelid**
H01.004 Unspecified blepharitis left upper **eyelid**
H01.005 Unspecified blepharitis left lower **eyelid**
H01.006 Unspecified blepharitis left eye, unspecified **eyelid**
H01.009 Unspecified blepharitis unspecified eye, unspecified **eyelid**

✓6ᵗʰ **H01.01 Ulcerative blepharitis**
H01.011 Ulcerative blepharitis right upper **eyelid**
H01.012 Ulcerative blepharitis right lower **eyelid**
H01.013 Ulcerative blepharitis right eye, unspecified **eyelid**
H01.014 Ulcerative blepharitis left upper **eyelid**
H01.015 Ulcerative blepharitis left lower **eyelid**
H01.016 Ulcerative blepharitis left eye, unspecified **eyelid**
H01.019 Ulcerative blepharitis unspecified eye, unspecified **eyelid**

✓6ᵗʰ **H01.02 Squamous blepharitis**
H01.021 Squamous blepharitis right upper **eyelid**
H01.022 Squamous blepharitis right lower **eyelid**
H01.023 Squamous blepharitis right eye, unspecified **eyelid**
H01.024 Squamous blepharitis left upper **eyelid**
H01.025 Squamous blepharitis left lower **eyelid**
H01.026 Squamous blepharitis left eye, unspecified **eyelid**
H01.029 Squamous blepharitis unspecified eye, unspecified **eyelid**

✓5ᵗʰ **H01.1 Noninfectious dermatoses of eyelid**

✓6ᵗʰ **H01.11 Allergic dermatitis of eyelid**
Contact dermatitis of eyelid

H01.111 Allergic dermatitis of right upper **eyelid**
H01.112 Allergic dermatitis of right lower **eyelid**
H01.113 Allergic dermatitis of right eye, unspecified **eyelid**
H01.114 Allergic dermatitis of left upper **eyelid**
H01.115 Allergic dermatitis of left lower **eyelid**
H01.116 Allergic dermatitis of left eye, unspecified **eyelid**
H01.119 Allergic dermatitis of unspecified eye, unspecified **eyelid**

✓6ᵗʰ **H01.12 Discoid lupus erythematosus of eyelid**
H01.121 Discoid lupus erythematosus of right upper **eyelid**
H01.122 Discoid lupus erythematosus of right lower **eyelid**
H01.123 Discoid lupus erythematosus of right eye, unspecified **eyelid**
H01.124 Discoid lupus erythematosus of left upper **eyelid**
H01.125 Discoid lupus erythematosus of left lower **eyelid**
H01.126 Discoid lupus erythematosus of left eye, unspecified **eyelid**
H01.129 Discoid lupus erythematosus of unspecified eye, unspecified **eyelid**

N Newborn: 0   **P** Pediatric: 0-17   **M** Maternity: 12-55   **A** Adult: 15-124   **MCC** Major CC Condition   **PDxMCC** PDx acts as own MCC   **CC** CC Condition   **PDxCC** PDx acts as own CC

☑6ᵗʰ **H01.13** Eczematous dermatitis of eyelid

     H01.131 Eczematous dermatitis of right upper eyelid

     H01.132 Eczematous dermatitis of right lower eyelid

     H01.133 Eczematous dermatitis of right eye, unspecified eyelid

     H01.134 Eczematous dermatitis of left upper eyelid

     H01.135 Eczematous dermatitis of left lower eyelid

     H01.136 Eczematous dermatitis of left eye, unspecified eyelid

     H01.139 Eczematous dermatitis of unspecified eye, unspecified eyelid

☑6ᵗʰ **H01.14** Xeroderma of eyelid

     H01.141 Xeroderma of right upper eyelid

     H01.142 Xeroderma of right lower eyelid

     H01.143 Xeroderma of right eye, unspecified eyelid

     H01.144 Xeroderma of left upper eyelid

     H01.145 Xeroderma of left lower eyelid

     H01.146 Xeroderma of left eye, unspecified eyelid

     H01.149 Xeroderma of unspecified eye, unspecified eyelid

H01.8 Other specified inflammations of eyelid

H01.9 Unspecified inflammation of eyelid

     Inflammation of eyelid NOS

☑4ᵗʰ **H02** Other disorders of eyelid

     EXCLUDES 1   congenital malformations of eyelid (Q10.0-Q10.3)

☑5ᵗʰ **H02.0** Entropion and trichiasis of eyelid

☑6ᵗʰ **H02.00** Unspecified entropion of eyelid

     H02.001 Unspecified entropion of right upper eyelid

     H02.002 Unspecified entropion of right lower eyelid

     H02.003 Unspecified entropion of right eye, unspecified eyelid

     H02.004 Unspecified entropion of left upper eyelid

     H02.005 Unspecified entropion of left lower eyelid

     H02.006 Unspecified entropion of left eye, unspecified eyelid

     H02.009 Unspecified entropion of unspecified eye, unspecified eyelid

☑6ᵗʰ **H02.01** Cicatricial entropion of eyelid

     H02.011 Cicatricial entropion of right upper eyelid

     H02.012 Cicatricial entropion of right lower eyelid

     H02.013 Cicatricial entropion of right eye, unspecified eyelid

     H02.014 Cicatricial entropion of left upper eyelid

     H02.015 Cicatricial entropion of left lower eyelid

     H02.016 Cicatricial entropion of left eye, unspecified eyelid

     H02.019 Cicatricial entropion of unspecified eye, unspecified eyelid

☑6ᵗʰ **H02.02** Mechanical entropion of eyelid

     H02.021 Mechanical entropion of right upper eyelid

     H02.022 Mechanical entropion of right lower eyelid

     H02.023 Mechanical entropion of right eye, unspecified eyelid

     H02.024 Mechanical entropion of left upper eyelid

     H02.025 Mechanical entropion of left lower eyelid

     H02.026 Mechanical entropion of left eye, unspecified eyelid

     H02.029 Mechanical entropion of unspecified eye, unspecified eyelid

☑6ᵗʰ **H02.03** Senile entropion of eyelid

     H02.031 Senile entropion of right upper eyelid   🅰

     H02.032 Senile entropion of right lower eyelid   🅰

     H02.033 Senile entropion of right eye, unspecified eyelid   🅰

     H02.034 Senile entropion of left upper eyelid   🅰

     H02.035 Senile entropion of left lower eyelid   🅰

     H02.036 Senile entropion of left eye, unspecified eyelid   🅰

     H02.039 Senile entropion of unspecified eye, unspecified eyelid   🅰

☑6ᵗʰ **H02.04** Spastic entropion of eyelid

     H02.041 Spastic entropion of right upper eyelid

     H02.042 Spastic entropion of right lower eyelid

     H02.043 Spastic entropion of right eye, unspecified eyelid

     H02.044 Spastic entropion of left upper eyelid

     H02.045 Spastic entropion of left lower eyelid

     H02.046 Spastic entropion of left eye, unspecified eyelid

     H02.049 Spastic entropion of unspecified eye, unspecified eyelid

☑6ᵗʰ **H02.05** Trichiasis without entropian

     H02.051 Trichiasis without entropian right upper eyelid

     H02.052 Trichiasis without entropian right lower eyelid

     H02.053 Trichiasis without entropian right eye, unspecified eyelid

     H02.054 Trichiasis without entropian left upper eyelid

     H02.055 Trichiasis without entropian left lower eyelid

     H02.056 Trichiasis without entropian left eye, unspecified eyelid

     H02.059 Trichiasis without entropian unspecified eye, unspecified eyelid

☑5ᵗʰ **H02.1** Ectropion of eyelid

☑6ᵗʰ **H02.10** Unspecified ectropion of eyelid

     H02.101 Unspecified ectropion of right upper eyelid

     H02.102 Unspecified ectropion of right lower eyelid

     H02.103 Unspecified ectropion of right eye, unspecified eyelid

     H02.104 Unspecified ectropion of left upper eyelid

     H02.105 Unspecified ectropion of left lower eyelid

     H02.106 Unspecified ectropion of left eye, unspecified eyelid

     H02.109 Unspecified ectropion of unspecified eye, unspecified eyelid

☑6ᵗʰ **H02.11** Cicatricial ectropion of eyelid

     H02.111 Cicatricial ectropion of right upper eyelid

     H02.112 Cicatricial ectropion of right lower eyelid

     H02.113 Cicatricial ectropion of right eye, unspecified eyelid

     H02.114 Cicatricial ectropion of left upper eyelid

     H02.115 Cicatricial ectropion of left lower eyelid

     H02.116 Cicatricial ectropion of left eye, unspecified eyelid

     H02.119 Cicatricial ectropion of unspecified eye, unspecified eyelid

☑6ᵗʰ **H02.12** Mechanical ectropion of eyelid

     H02.121 Mechanical ectropion of right upper eyelid

     H02.122 Mechanical ectropion of right lower eyelid

     H02.123 Mechanical ectropion of right eye, unspecified eyelid

     H02.124 Mechanical ectropion of left upper eyelid

     H02.125 Mechanical ectropion of left lower eyelid

     H02.126 Mechanical ectropion of left eye, unspecified eyelid

     H02.129 Mechanical ectropion of unspecified eye, unspecified eyelid

☑6ᵗʰ **H02.13** Senile ectropion of eyelid

     H02.131 Senile ectropion of right upper eyelid   🅰

     H02.132 Senile ectropion of right lower eyelid   🅰

     H02.133 Senile ectropion of right eye, unspecified eyelid   🅰

     H02.134 Senile ectropion of left upper eyelid   🅰

     H02.135 Senile ectropion of left lower eyelid   🅰

     H02.136 Senile ectropion of left eye, unspecified eyelid   🅰

     H02.139 Senile ectropion of unspecified eye, unspecified eyelid   🅰

☑6ᵗʰ **H02.14** Spastic ectropion of eyelid

     H02.141 Spastic ectropion of right upper eyelid

     H02.142 Spastic ectropion of right lower eyelid

☑ Additional Character Required   ☑x7ᵗʰ Placeholder Alert   Unacceptable PDx   Manifestation   Hospital Acquired Condition   EXCLUDES 1 Not Coded Here   EXCLUDES 2 Not Included Here

H02.143   Spastic ectropion of right eye, unspecified eyelid
H02.144   Spastic ectropion of left upper eyelid
H02.145   Spastic ectropion of left lower eyelid
H02.146   Spastic ectropion of left eye, unspecified eyelid
H02.149   Spastic ectropion of unspecified eye, unspecified eyelid

✓5th H02.2   Lagophthalmos

✓6th H02.20   Unspecified lagophthalmos
H02.201   Unspecified lagophthalmos right upper eyelid
H02.202   Unspecified lagophthalmos right lower eyelid
H02.203   Unspecified lagophthalmos right eye, unspecified eyelid
H02.204   Unspecified lagophthalmos left upper eyelid
H02.205   Unspecified lagophthalmos left lower eyelid
H02.206   Unspecified lagophthalmos left eye, unspecified eyelid
H02.209   Unspecified lagophthalmos unspecified eye, unspecified eyelid

✓6th H02.21   Cicatricial lagophthalmos
H02.211   Cicatricial lagophthalmos right upper eyelid
H02.212   Cicatricial lagophthalmos right lower eyelid
H02.213   Cicatricial lagophthalmos right eye, unspecified eyelid
H02.214   Cicatricial lagophthalmos left upper eyelid
H02.215   Cicatricial lagophthalmos left lower eyelid
H02.216   Cicatricial lagophthalmos left eye, unspecified eyelid
H02.219   Cicatricial lagophthalmos unspecified eye, unspecified eyelid

✓6th H02.22   Mechanical lagophthalmos
H02.221   Mechanical lagophthalmos right upper eyelid
H02.222   Mechanical lagophthalmos right lower eyelid
H02.223   Mechanical lagophthalmos right eye, unspecified eyelid
H02.224   Mechanical lagophthalmos left upper eyelid
H02.225   Mechanical lagophthalmos left lower eyelid
H02.226   Mechanical lagophthalmos left eye, unspecified eyelid
H02.229   Mechanical lagophthalmos unspecified eye, unspecified eyelid

✓6th H02.23   Paralytic lagophthalmos
H02.231   Paralytic lagophthalmos right upper eyelid
H02.232   Paralytic lagophthalmos right lower eyelid
H02.233   Paralytic lagophthalmos right eye, unspecified eyelid
H02.234   Paralytic lagophthalmos left upper eyelid
H02.235   Paralytic lagophthalmos left lower eyelid
H02.236   Paralytic lagophthalmos left eye, unspecified eyelid
H02.239   Paralytic lagophthalmos unspecified eye, unspecified eyelid

✓5th H02.3   Blepharochalasis
Pseudoptosis
H02.30   Blepharochalasis unspecified eye, unspecified eyelid
H02.31   Blepharochalasis right upper eyelid
H02.32   Blepharochalasis right lower eyelid
H02.33   Blepharochalasis right eye, unspecified eyelid
H02.34   Blepharochalasis left upper eyelid
H02.35   Blepharochalasis left lower eyelid
H02.36   Blepharochalasis left eye, unspecified eyelid

✓5th H02.4   Ptosis of eyelid

✓6th H02.40   Unspecified ptosis of eyelid
H02.401   Unspecified ptosis of right eyelid
H02.402   Unspecified ptosis of left eyelid
H02.403   Unspecified ptosis of bilateral eyelids
H02.409   Unspecified ptosis of unspecified eyelid

✓6th H02.41   Mechanical ptosis of eyelid
H02.411   Mechanical ptosis of right eyelid
H02.412   Mechanical ptosis of left eyelid
H02.413   Mechanical ptosis of bilateral eyelids
H02.419   Mechanical ptosis of unspecified eyelid

✓6th H02.42   Myogenic ptosis of eyelid
H02.421   Myogenic ptosis of right eyelid
H02.422   Myogenic ptosis of left eyelid
H02.423   Myogenic ptosis of bilateral eyelids
H02.429   Myogenic ptosis of unspecified eyelid

✓6th H02.43   Paralytic ptosis of eyelid
Neurogenic ptosis of eyelid
H02.431   Paralytic ptosis of right eyelid
H02.432   Paralytic ptosis of left eyelid
H02.433   Paralytic ptosis of bilateral eyelids
H02.439   Paralytic ptosis unspecified eyelid

✓5th H02.5   Other disorders affecting eyelid function
EXCLUDES 2   blepharospasm (G24.5)
organic tic (G25.69)
psychogenic tic (F95.-)

✓6th H02.51   Abnormal innervation syndrome
H02.511   Abnormal innervation syndrome right upper eyelid
H02.512   Abnormal innervation syndrome right lower eyelid
H02.513   Abnormal innervation syndrome right eye, unspecified eyelid
H02.514   Abnormal innervation syndrome left upper eyelid
H02.515   Abnormal innervation syndrome left lower eyelid
H02.516   Abnormal innervation syndrome left eye, unspecified eyelid
H02.519   Abnormal innervation syndrome unspecified eye, unspecified eyelid

✓6th H02.52   Blepharophimosis
Ankyloblepharon
H02.521   Blepharophimosis right upper eyelid
H02.522   Blepharophimosis right lower eyelid
H02.523   Blepharophimosis right eye, unspecified eyelid
H02.524   Blepharophimosis left upper eyelid
H02.525   Blepharophimosis left lower eyelid
H02.526   Blepharophimosis left eye, unspecified eyelid
H02.529   Blepharophimosis unspecified eye, unspecified lid

✓6th H02.53   Eyelid retraction
Eyelid lag
H02.531   Eyelid retraction right upper eyelid
H02.532   Eyelid retraction right lower eyelid
H02.533   Eyelid retraction right eye, unspecified eyelid
H02.534   Eyelid retraction left upper eyelid
H02.535   Eyelid retraction left lower eyelid
H02.536   Eyelid retraction left eye, unspecified eyelid
H02.539   Eyelid retraction unspecified eye, unspecified lid

H02.59   Other disorders affecting eyelid function
Deficient blink reflex
Sensory disorders

✓5th H02.6   Xanthelasma of eyelid
H02.60   Xanthelasma of unspecified eye, unspecified eyelid
H02.61   Xanthelasma of right upper eyelid
H02.62   Xanthelasma of right lower eyelid
H02.63   Xanthelasma of right eye, unspecified eyelid
H02.64   Xanthelasma of left upper eyelid

H02.65   **Xanthelasma of left lower eyelid**

H02.66   **Xanthelasma of left eye, unspecified eyelid**

✓5ᵗʰ   **H02.7**   **Other and unspecified degenerative disorders of eyelid and periocular area**

   H02.70   **Unspecified degenerative disorders of eyelid and periocular area**

   ✓6ᵗʰ   H02.71   **Chloasma of eyelid and periocular area**
     Dyspigmentation of eyelid
     Hyperpigmentation of eyelid

     H02.711   **Chloasma of right upper eyelid and periocular area**

     H02.712   **Chloasma of right lower eyelid and periocular area**

     H02.713   **Chloasma of right eye, unspecified eyelid and periocular area**

     H02.714   **Chloasma of left upper eyelid and periocular area**

     H02.715   **Chloasma of left lower eyelid and periocular area**

     H02.716   **Chloasma of left eye, unspecified eyelid and periocular area**

     H02.719   **Chloasma of unspecified eye, unspecified eyelid and periocular area**

   ✓6ᵗʰ   H02.72   **Madarosis of eyelid and periocular area**
     Hypotrichosis of eyelid

     H02.721   **Madarosis of right upper eyelid and periocular area**

     H02.722   **Madarosis of right lower eyelid and periocular area**

     H02.723   **Madarosis of right eye, unspecified eyelid and periocular area**

     H02.724   **Madarosis of left upper eyelid and periocular area**

     H02.725   **Madarosis of left lower eyelid and periocular area**

     H02.726   **Madarosis of left eye, unspecified eyelid and periocular area**

     H02.729   **Madarosis of unspecified eye, unspecified eyelid and periocular area**

   ✓6ᵗʰ   H02.73   **Vitiligo of eyelid and periocular area**
     Hypopigmentation of eyelid

     H02.731   **Vitiligo of right upper eyelid and periocular area**

     H02.732   **Vitiligo of right lower eyelid and periocular area**

     H02.733   **Vitiligo of right eye, unspecified eyelid and periocular area**

     H02.734   **Vitiligo of left upper eyelid and periocular area**

     H02.735   **Vitiligo of left lower eyelid and periocular area**

     H02.736   **Vitiligo of left eye, unspecified eyelid and periocular area**

     H02.739   **Vitiligo of unspecified eye, unspecified eyelid and periocular area**

   H02.79   **Other degenerative disorders of eyelid and periocular area**

✓5ᵗʰ   **H02.8**   **Other specified disorders of eyelid**

   ✓6ᵗʰ   H02.81   **Retained foreign body in eyelid**
     Use additional code to identify the type of retained foreign body (Z18.-)
     EXCLUDES 1   *laceration of eyelid with foreign body (S01.12-)*
       retained intraocular foreign body (H44.6-, H44.7-)
       superficial foreign body of eyelid and periocular area (S00.25-)

     H02.811   **Retained foreign body in right upper eyelid**

     H02.812   **Retained foreign body in right lower eyelid**

     H02.813   **Retained foreign body in right eye, unspecified eyelid**

     H02.814   **Retained foreign body in left upper eyelid**

     H02.815   **Retained foreign body in left lower eyelid**

     H02.816   **Retained foreign body in left eye, unspecified eyelid**

     H02.819   **Retained foreign body in unspecified eye, unspecified eyelid**

   ✓6ᵗʰ   H02.82   **Cysts of eyelid**
     Sebaceous cyst of eyelid

     H02.821   **Cysts of right upper eyelid**

     H02.822   **Cysts of right lower eyelid**

     H02.823   **Cysts of right eye, unspecified eyelid**

     H02.824   **Cysts of left upper eyelid**

     H02.825   **Cysts of left lower eyelid**

     H02.826   **Cysts of left eye, unspecified eyelid**

     H02.829   **Cysts of unspecified eye, unspecified eyelid**

   ✓6ᵗʰ   H02.83   **Dermatochalasis of eyelid**

     H02.831   **Dermatochalasis of right upper eyelid**

     H02.832   **Dermatochalasis of right lower eyelid**

     H02.833   **Dermatochalasis of right eye, unspecified eyelid**

     H02.834   **Dermatochalasis of left upper eyelid**

     H02.835   **Dermatochalasis of left lower eyelid**

     H02.836   **Dermatochalasis of left eye, unspecified eyelid**

     H02.839   **Dermatochalasis of unspecified eye, unspecified eyelid**

   ✓6ᵗʰ   H02.84   **Edema of eyelid**
     Hyperemia of eyelid

     H02.841   **Edema of right upper eyelid**

     H02.842   **Edema of right lower eyelid**

     H02.843   **Edema of right eye, unspecified eyelid**

     H02.844   **Edema of left upper eyelid**

     H02.845   **Edema of left lower eyelid**

     H02.846   **Edema of left eye, unspecified eyelid**

     H02.849   **Edema of unspecified eye, unspecified eyelid**

   ✓6ᵗʰ   H02.85   **Elephantiasis of eyelid**

     H02.851   **Elephantiasis of right upper eyelid**

     H02.852   **Elephantiasis of right lower eyelid**

     H02.853   **Elephantiasis of right eye, unspecified eyelid**

     H02.854   **Elephantiasis of left upper eyelid**

     H02.855   **Elephantiasis of left lower eyelid**

     H02.856   **Elephantiasis of left eye, unspecified eyelid**

     H02.859   **Elephantiasis of unspecified eye, unspecified eyelid**

   ✓6ᵗʰ   H02.86   **Hypertrichosis of eyelid**

     H02.861   **Hypertrichosis of right upper eyelid**

     H02.862   **Hypertrichosis of right lower eyelid**

     H02.863   **Hypertrichosis of right eye, unspecified eyelid**

     H02.864   **Hypertrichosis of left upper eyelid**

     H02.865   **Hypertrichosis of left lower eyelid**

     H02.866   **Hypertrichosis of left eye, unspecified eyelid**

     H02.869   **Hypertrichosis of unspecified eye, unspecified eyelid**

   ✓6ᵗʰ   H02.87   **Vascular anomalies of eyelid**

     H02.871   **Vascular anomalies of right upper eyelid**

     H02.872   **Vascular anomalies of right lower eyelid**

     H02.873   **Vascular anomalies of right eye, unspecified eyelid**

     H02.874   **Vascular anomalies of left upper eyelid**

     H02.875   **Vascular anomalies of left lower eyelid**

     H02.876   **Vascular anomalies of left eye, unspecified eyelid**

     H02.879   **Vascular anomalies of unspecified eye, unspecified eyelid**

   H02.89   **Other specified disorders of eyelid**
     Hemorrhage of eyelid

  H02.9   **Unspecified disorder of eyelid**
   Disorder of eyelid NOS

✓4ᵗʰ   **H04**   **Disorders of lacrimal system**
   EXCLUDES 1   *congenital malformations of lacrimal system (Q10.4-Q10.6)*

   ✓5ᵗʰ   **H04.0**   **Dacryoadenitis**

     ✓6ᵗʰ   H04.00   **Unspecified dacryoadenitis**

       H04.001   **Unspecified dacryoadenitis, right lacrimal gland**

✓ Additional Character Required   ✓x7ᵗʰ Placeholder Alert   Unacceptable PDx   Manifestation   Hospital Acquired Condition   **EXCLUDES 1** Not Coded Here   **EXCLUDES 2** Not Included Here

ICD-10-CM 2016   563

Chapter 7. Diseases of the Eye and Adnexa

H02.65–H04.001

Chapter 7. Diseases of the Eye and Adnexa

H04.002–H04.412

H04.002   Unspecified dacryoadenitis, left lacrimal gland

H04.003   Unspecified dacryoadenitis, bilateral lacrimal glands

H04.009   Unspecified dacryoadenitis, unspecified lacrimal gland

✓6ᵗʰ **H04.01   Acute dacryoadenitis**

H04.011   Acute dacryoadenitis, right lacrimal gland

H04.012   Acute dacryoadenitis, left lacrimal gland

H04.013   Acute dacryoadenitis, bilateral lacrimal glands

H04.019   Acute dacryoadenitis, unspecified lacrimal gland

✓6ᵗʰ **H04.02   Chronic dacryoadenitis**

H04.021   Chronic dacryoadenitis, right lacrimal gland

H04.022   Chronic dacryoadenitis, left lacrimal gland

H04.023   Chronic dacryoadenitis, bilateral lacrimal glands

H04.029   Chronic dacryoadenitis, unspecified lacrimal gland

✓6ᵗʰ **H04.03   Chronic enlargement of lacrimal gland**

H04.031   Chronic enlargement of right lacrimal gland

H04.032   Chronic enlargement of left lacrimal gland

H04.033   Chronic enlargement of bilateral lacrimal glands

H04.039   Chronic enlargement of unspecified lacrimal gland

✓5ᵗʰ **H04.1   Other disorders of lacrimal gland**

✓6ᵗʰ **H04.11   Dacryops**

H04.111   Dacryops of right lacrimal gland

H04.112   Dacryops of left lacrimal gland

H04.113   Dacryops of bilateral lacrimal glands

H04.119   Dacryops of unspecified lacrimal gland

✓6ᵗʰ **H04.12   Dry eye syndrome**
Tear film insufficiency, NOS

H04.121   Dry eye syndrome of right lacrimal gland

H04.122   Dry eye syndrome of left lacrimal gland

H04.123   Dry eye syndrome of bilateral lacrimal glands

H04.129   Dry eye syndrome of unspecified lacrimal gland

✓6ᵗʰ **H04.13   Lacrimal cyst**
Lacrimal cystic degeneration

H04.131   Lacrimal cyst, right lacrimal gland

H04.132   Lacrimal cyst, left lacrimal gland

H04.133   Lacrimal cyst, bilateral lacrimal glands

H04.139   Lacrimal cyst, unspecified lacrimal gland

✓6ᵗʰ **H04.14   Primary lacrimal gland atrophy**

H04.141   Primary lacrimal gland atrophy, right lacrimal gland

H04.142   Primary lacrimal gland atrophy, left lacrimal gland

H04.143   Primary lacrimal gland atrophy, bilateral lacrimal glands

H04.149   Primary lacrimal gland atrophy, unspecified lacrimal gland

✓6ᵗʰ **H04.15   Secondary lacrimal gland atrophy**

H04.151   Secondary lacrimal gland atrophy, right lacrimal gland

H04.152   Secondary lacrimal gland atrophy, left lacrimal gland

H04.153   Secondary lacrimal gland atrophy, bilateral lacrimal glands

H04.159   Secondary lacrimal gland atrophy, unspecified lacrimal gland

✓6ᵗʰ **H04.16   Lacrimal gland dislocation**

H04.161   Lacrimal gland dislocation, right lacrimal gland

H04.162   Lacrimal gland dislocation, left lacrimal gland

H04.163   Lacrimal gland dislocation, bilateral lacrimal glands

H04.169   Lacrimal gland dislocation, unspecified lacrimal gland

H04.19   Other specified disorders of lacrimal gland

✓5ᵗʰ **H04.2   Epiphora**

✓6ᵗʰ **H04.20   Unspecified epiphora**

H04.201   Unspecified epiphora, right lacrimal gland

H04.202   Unspecified epiphora, left lacrimal gland

H04.203   Unspecified epiphora, bilateral lacrimal glands

H04.209   Unspecified epiphora, unspecified lacrimal gland

✓6ᵗʰ **H04.21   Epiphora due to excess lacrimation**

H04.211   Epiphora due to excess lacrimation, right lacrimal gland

H04.212   Epiphora due to excess lacrimation, left lacrimal gland

H04.213   Epiphora due to excess lacrimation, bilateral lacrimal glands

H04.219   Epiphora due to excess lacrimation, unspecified lacrimal gland

✓6ᵗʰ **H04.22   Epiphora due to insufficient drainage**

H04.221   Epiphora due to insufficient drainage, right lacrimal gland

H04.222   Epiphora due to insufficient drainage, left lacrimal gland

H04.223   Epiphora due to insufficient drainage, bilateral lacrimal glands

H04.229   Epiphora due to insufficient drainage, unspecified lacrimal gland

✓5ᵗʰ **H04.3   Acute and unspecified inflammation of lacrimal passages**
EXCLUDES 1   neonatal dacryocystitis (P39.1)

✓6ᵗʰ **H04.30   Unspecified dacryocystitis**

H04.301   Unspecified dacryocystitis of right lacrimal passage

H04.302   Unspecified dacryocystitis of left lacrimal passage

H04.303   Unspecified dacryocystitis of bilateral lacrimal passages

H04.309   Unspecified dacryocystitis of unspecified lacrimal passage

✓6ᵗʰ **H04.31   Phlegmonous dacryocystitis**

H04.311   Phlegmonous dacryocystitis of right lacrimal passage

H04.312   Phlegmonous dacryocystitis of left lacrimal passage

H04.313   Phlegmonous dacryocystitis of bilateral lacrimal passages

H04.319   Phlegmonous dacryocystitis of unspecified lacrimal passage

✓6ᵗʰ **H04.32   Acute dacryocystitis**
Acute dacryopericystitis

H04.321   Acute dacryocystitis of right lacrimal passage

H04.322   Acute dacryocystitis of left lacrimal passage

H04.323   Acute dacryocystitis of bilateral lacrimal passages

H04.329   Acute dacryocystitis of unspecified lacrimal passage

✓6ᵗʰ **H04.33   Acute lacrimal canaliculitis**

H04.331   Acute lacrimal canaliculitis of right lacrimal passage

H04.332   Acute lacrimal canaliculitis of left lacrimal passage

H04.333   Acute lacrimal canaliculitis of bilateral lacrimal passages

H04.339   Acute lacrimal canaliculitis of unspecified lacrimal passage

✓5ᵗʰ **H04.4   Chronic inflammation of lacrimal passages**

✓6ᵗʰ **H04.41   Chronic dacryocystitis**

H04.411   Chronic dacryocystitis of right lacrimal passage

H04.412   Chronic dacryocystitis of left lacrimal passage

Ⓝ Newborn: 0   Ⓟ Pediatric: 0-17   Ⓜ Maternity: 12-55   Ⓐ Adult: 15-124   **MCC** Major CC Condition   **PDxMCC** PDx acts as own MCC   **CC** CC Condition   **PDxCC** PDx acts as own CC

H04.413   **Chronic dacryocystitis of** bilateral **lacrimal passages**

H04.419   **Chronic dacryocystitis of** unspecified **lacrimal passage**

✓6ᵗʰ   **H04.42**   Chronic **lacrimal** canaliculitis

H04.421   **Chronic lacrimal canaliculitis of** right **lacrimal passage**

H04.422   **Chronic lacrimal canaliculitis of** left **lacrimal passage**

H04.423   **Chronic lacrimal canaliculitis of** bilateral **lacrimal passages**

H04.429   **Chronic lacrimal canaliculitis of** unspecified **lacrimal passage**

✓6ᵗʰ   **H04.43**   Chronic **lacrimal** mucocele

H04.431   **Chronic lacrimal mucocele of** right **lacrimal passage**

H04.432   **Chronic lacrimal mucocele of** left **lacrimal passage**

H04.433   **Chronic lacrimal mucocele of** bilateral **lacrimal passages**

H04.439   **Chronic lacrimal mucocele of** unspecified **lacrimal passage**

✓5ᵗʰ   **H04.5**   Stenosis and insufficiency of lacrimal passages

✓6ᵗʰ   **H04.51**   Dacryolith

H04.511   **Dacryolith of** right **lacrimal passage**

H04.512   **Dacryolith of** left **lacrimal passage**

H04.513   **Dacryolith of** bilateral **lacrimal passages**

H04.519   **Dacryolith of** unspecified **lacrimal passage**

✓6ᵗʰ   **H04.52**   Eversion **of lacrimal** punctum

H04.521   **Eversion of** right **lacrimal punctum**

H04.522   **Eversion of** left **lacrimal punctum**

H04.523   **Eversion of** bilateral **lacrimal punctum**

H04.529   **Eversion of** unspecified **lacrimal punctum**

✓6ᵗʰ   **H04.53**   Neonatal obstruction **of nasolacrimal duct**

EXCLUDES 1   *congenital stenosis and stricture of lacrimal duct (Q10.5)*

H04.531   **Neonatal obstruction of** right **nasolacrimal duct**   N

H04.532   **Neonatal obstruction of** left **nasolacrimal duct**   N

H04.533   **Neonatal obstruction of** bilateral **nasolacrimal duct**   N

H04.539   **Neonatal obstruction of** unspecified **nasolacrimal duct**   N

✓6ᵗʰ   **H04.54**   Stenosis of lacrimal canaliculi

H04.541   **Stenosis of** right **lacrimal canaliculi**

H04.542   **Stenosis of** left **lacrimal canaliculi**

H04.543   **Stenosis of** bilateral **lacrimal canaliculi**

H04.549   **Stenosis of** unspecified **lacrimal canaliculi**

✓6ᵗʰ   **H04.55**   Acquired stenosis of nasolacrimal duct

H04.551   **Acquired stenosis of** right **nasolacrimal duct**

H04.552   **Acquired stenosis of** left **nasolacrimal duct**

H04.553   **Acquired stenosis of** bilateral **nasolacrimal duct**

H04.559   **Acquired stenosis of** unspecified **nasolacrimal duct**

✓6ᵗʰ   **H04.56**   Stenosis of lacrimal punctum

H04.561   **Stenosis of** right **lacrimal punctum**

H04.562   **Stenosis of** left **lacrimal punctum**

H04.563   **Stenosis of** bilateral **lacrimal punctum**

H04.569   **Stenosis of** unspecified **lacrimal punctum**

✓6ᵗʰ   **H04.57**   Stenosis of lacrimal sac

H04.571   **Stenosis of** right **lacrimal sac**

H04.572   **Stenosis of** left **lacrimal sac**

H04.573   **Stenosis of** bilateral **lacrimal sac**

H04.579   **Stenosis of** unspecified **lacrimal sac**

✓5ᵗʰ   **H04.6**   Other changes of lacrimal passages

✓6ᵗʰ   **H04.61**   Lacrimal fistula

H04.611   **Lacrimal fistula** right **lacrimal passage**

H04.612   **Lacrimal fistula** left **lacrimal passage**

H04.613   **Lacrimal fistula** bilateral **lacrimal passages**

H04.619   **Lacrimal fistula** unspecified **lacrimal passage**

H04.69   **Other changes of lacrimal passages**

✓5ᵗʰ   **H04.8**   Other disorders of lacrimal system

✓6ᵗʰ   **H04.81**   Granuloma of lacrimal passages

H04.811   **Granuloma of** right **lacrimal passage**

H04.812   **Granuloma of** left **lacrimal passage**

H04.813   **Granuloma of** bilateral **lacrimal passages**

H04.819   **Granuloma of** unspecified **lacrimal passage**

H04.89   **Other disorders of lacrimal system**

H04.9   **Disorder of lacrimal system, unspecified**

✓4ᵗʰ   **H05**   **Disorders of orbit**

EXCLUDES 1   *congenital malformation of orbit (Q10.7)*

✓5ᵗʰ   **H05.0**   Acute inflammation of orbit

H05.00   **Unspecified acute inflammation of orbit**

✓6ᵗʰ   **H05.01**   Cellulitis **of orbit**

Abscess of orbit

> **CC Excl: For CC codes in subcategory H05.01, unless otherwise noted:** H05.00-H05.049

H05.011   **Cellulitis of** right **orbit**   CC

H05.012   **Cellulitis of** left **orbit**   CC

H05.013   **Cellulitis of** bilateral **orbits**   CC

H05.019   **Cellulitis of** unspecified **orbit**   CC

✓6ᵗʰ   **H05.02**   Osteomyelitis **of orbit**

> **CC Excl: For CC codes in subcategory H05.02, unless otherwise noted:** A02.24, A17.9, A18.03-A18.09, A18.82, A18.84, A18.89, H05.021-H05.029, M46.20-M46.39, M86.00-M86.9

H05.021   **Osteomyelitis of** right **orbit**   CC

H05.022   **Osteomyelitis of** left **orbit**   CC

H05.023   **Osteomyelitis of** bilateral **orbits**   CC

H05.029   **Osteomyelitis of** unspecified **orbit**   CC

✓6ᵗʰ   **H05.03**   Periostitis **of orbit**

> **CC Excl: For CC codes in subcategory H05.03, unless otherwise noted:** A02.24, A17.9, A18.03-A18.09, A18.82, A18.84, A18.89, H05.031-H05.039, M46.20-M46.39, M86.00-M86.9

H05.031   **Periostitis of** right **orbit**   CC

H05.032   **Periostitis of** left **orbit**   CC

H05.033   **Periostitis of** bilateral **orbits**   CC

H05.039   **Periostitis of** unspecified **orbit**   CC

✓6ᵗʰ   **H05.04**   Tenonitis **of orbit**

H05.041   **Tenonitis of** right **orbit**

H05.042   **Tenonitis of** left **orbit**

H05.043   **Tenonitis of** bilateral **orbits**

H05.049   **Tenonitis of** unspecified **orbit**

✓5ᵗʰ   **H05.1**   Chronic inflammatory disorders of orbit

H05.10   **Unspecified chronic inflammatory disorders of orbit**

✓6ᵗʰ   **H05.11**   Granuloma of orbit

Pseudotumor (inflammatory) of orbit

H05.111   **Granuloma of** right **orbit**

H05.112   **Granuloma of** left **orbit**

H05.113   **Granuloma of** bilateral **orbits**

H05.119   **Granuloma of** unspecified **orbit**

✓6ᵗʰ   **H05.12**   Orbital myositis

H05.121   **Orbital myositis,** right **orbit**

H05.122   **Orbital myositis,** left **orbit**

H05.123   **Orbital myositis,** bilateral

H05.129   **Orbital myositis,** unspecified **orbit**

✓5ᵗʰ   **H05.2**   Exophthalmic conditions

H05.20   **Unspecified exophthalmos**

✓6ᵗʰ   **H05.21**   Displacement (lateral) of globe

H05.211   **Displacement (lateral) of globe,** right **eye**

H05.212   **Displacement (lateral) of globe,** left **eye**

H05.213   **Displacement (lateral) of globe,** bilateral

H05.219   **Displacement (lateral) of globe,** unspecified **eye**

✓6ᵗʰ   **H05.22**   Edema of orbit

Orbital congestion

H05.221   **Edema of** right **orbit**

H05.222   **Edema of** left **orbit**

H05.223   **Edema of** bilateral **orbit**

H05.229   **Edema of** unspecified **orbit**

✓ Additional Character Required   ✓x7ᵗʰ Placeholder Alert   Unacceptable PDx   Manifestation   Hospital Acquired Condition   EXCLUDES 1 Not Coded Here   EXCLUDES 2 Not Included Here

✓6ᵗʰ **H05.23 Hemorrhage of orbit**
     H05.231 Hemorrhage of right orbit
     H05.232 Hemorrhage of left orbit
     H05.233 Hemorrhage of bilateral orbit
     H05.239 Hemorrhage of unspecified orbit

✓6ᵗʰ **H05.24 Constant exophthalmos**
     H05.241 Constant exophthalmos, right eye
     H05.242 Constant exophthalmos, left eye
     H05.243 Constant exophthalmos, bilateral
     H05.249 Constant exophthalmos, unspecified eye

✓6ᵗʰ **H05.25 Intermittent exophthalmos**
     H05.251 Intermittent exophthalmos, right eye
     H05.252 Intermittent exophthalmos, left eye
     H05.253 Intermittent exophthalmos, bilateral
     H05.259 Intermittent exophthalmos, unspecified eye

✓6ᵗʰ **H05.26 Pulsating exophthalmos**
     H05.261 Pulsating exophthalmos, right eye
     H05.262 Pulsating exophthalmos, left eye
     H05.263 Pulsating exophthalmos, bilateral
     H05.269 Pulsating exophthalmos, unspecified eye

✓5ᵗʰ **H05.3 Deformity of orbit**
     EXCLUDES 1   congenital deformity of orbit (Q10.7)
                 hypertelorism (Q75.2)

     H05.30 Unspecified deformity of orbit

✓6ᵗʰ **H05.31 Atrophy of orbit**
     H05.311 Atrophy of right orbit
     H05.312 Atrophy of left orbit
     H05.313 Atrophy of bilateral orbit
     H05.319 Atrophy of unspecified orbit

✓6ᵗʰ **H05.32 Deformity of orbit due to bone disease**
     Code also associated bone disease
     H05.321 Deformity of right orbit due to bone disease
     H05.322 Deformity of left orbit due to bone disease
     H05.323 Deformity of bilateral orbits due to bone disease
     H05.329 Deformity of unspecified orbit due to bone disease

✓6ᵗʰ **H05.33 Deformity of orbit due to trauma or surgery**
     H05.331 Deformity of right orbit due to trauma or surgery
     H05.332 Deformity of left orbit due to trauma or surgery
     H05.333 Deformity of bilateral orbits due to trauma or surgery
     H05.339 Deformity of unspecified orbit due to trauma or surgery

✓6ᵗʰ **H05.34 Enlargement of orbit**
     H05.341 Enlargement of right orbit
     H05.342 Enlargement of left orbit
     H05.343 Enlargement of bilateral orbits
     H05.349 Enlargement of unspecified orbit

✓6ᵗʰ **H05.35 Exostosis of orbit**
     H05.351 Exostosis of right orbit
     H05.352 Exostosis of left orbit
     H05.353 Exostosis of bilateral orbits
     H05.359 Exostosis of unspecified orbit

✓5ᵗʰ **H05.4 Enophthalmos**

✓6ᵗʰ **H05.40 Unspecified enophthalmos**
     H05.401 Unspecified enophthalmos, right eye
     H05.402 Unspecified enophthalmos, left eye
     H05.403 Unspecified enophthalmos, bilateral
     H05.409 Unspecified enophthalmos, unspecified eye

✓6ᵗʰ **H05.41 Enophthalmos due to atrophy of orbital tissue**
     H05.411 Enophthalmos due to atrophy of orbital tissue, right eye
     H05.412 Enophthalmos due to atrophy of orbital tissue, left eye
     H05.413 Enophthalmos due to atrophy of orbital tissue, bilateral
     H05.419 Enophthalmos due to atrophy of orbital tissue, unspecified eye

✓6ᵗʰ **H05.42 Enophthalmos due to trauma or surgery**
     H05.421 Enophthalmos due to trauma or surgery, right eye
     H05.422 Enophthalmos due to trauma or surgery, left eye
     H05.423 Enophthalmos due to trauma or surgery, bilateral
     H05.429 Enophthalmos due to trauma or surgery, unspecified eye

✓5ᵗʰ **H05.5 Retained (old) foreign body following penetrating wound of orbit**
     Retrobulbar foreign body
     Use additional code to identify the type of retained foreign body (Z18.-)
     EXCLUDES 1   current penetrating wound of orbit (S05.4-)
     EXCLUDES 2   retained foreign body of eyelid (H02.81-)
                 retained intraocular foreign body (H44.6-, H44.7-)

     H05.50 Retained (old) foreign body following penetrating wound of unspecified orbit
     H05.51 Retained (old) foreign body following penetrating wound of right orbit
     H05.52 Retained (old) foreign body following penetrating wound of left orbit
     H05.53 Retained (old) foreign body following penetrating wound of bilateral orbits

✓5ᵗʰ **H05.8 Other disorders of orbit**

✓6ᵗʰ **H05.81 Cyst of orbit**
     Encephalocele of orbit
     H05.811 Cyst of right orbit
     H05.812 Cyst of left orbit
     H05.813 Cyst of bilateral orbits
     H05.819 Cyst of unspecified orbit

✓6ᵗʰ **H05.82 Myopathy of extraocular muscles**
     H05.821 Myopathy of extraocular muscles, right orbit
     H05.822 Myopathy of extraocular muscles, left orbit
     H05.823 Myopathy of extraocular muscles, bilateral
     H05.829 Myopathy of extraocular muscles, unspecified orbit

     H05.89 Other disorders of orbit
     H05.9 Unspecified disorder of orbit

Disorders of conjunctiva (H10-H11)

✓4ᵗʰ **H10 Conjunctivitis**
     EXCLUDES 1   keratoconjunctivitis (H16.2-)

✓5ᵗʰ **H10.0 Mucopurulent conjunctivitis**

✓6ᵗʰ **H10.01 Acute follicular conjunctivitis**
     H10.011 Acute follicular conjunctivitis, right eye
     H10.012 Acute follicular conjunctivitis, left eye
     H10.013 Acute follicular conjunctivitis, bilateral
     H10.019 Acute follicular conjunctivitis, unspecified eye

✓6ᵗʰ **H10.02 Other mucopurulent conjunctivitis**
     H10.021 Other mucopurulent conjunctivitis, right eye
     H10.022 Other mucopurulent conjunctivitis, left eye
     H10.023 Other mucopurulent conjunctivitis, bilateral
     H10.029 Other mucopurulent conjunctivitis, unspecified eye

✓5ᵗʰ **H10.1 Acute atopic conjunctivitis**
     Acute papillary conjunctivitis
     H10.10 Acute atopic conjunctivitis, unspecified eye
     H10.11 Acute atopic conjunctivitis, right eye
     H10.12 Acute atopic conjunctivitis, left eye
     H10.13 Acute atopic conjunctivitis, bilateral

N Newborn: 0   P Pediatric: 0-17   M Maternity: 12-55   A Adult: 15-124   MCC Major CC Condition   PDxMCC PDx acts as own MCC   CC CC Condition   PDxCC PDx acts as own CC

566   ICD-10-CM 2016

✓5th **H10.2** Other acute **conjunctivitis**

✓6th **H10.21** **Acute** toxic **conjunctivitis**
Acute chemical conjunctivitis
Code first (T51-T65) to identify chemical and intent
EXCLUDES 1 *burn and corrosion of eye and adnexa (T26.-)*

H10.211 **Acute toxic conjunctivitis,** right **eye**
H10.212 **Acute toxic conjunctivitis,** left **eye**
H10.213 **Acute toxic conjunctivitis,** bilateral
H10.219 **Acute toxic conjunctivitis,** unspecified **eye**

✓6th **H10.22** **Pseudomembranous conjunctivitis**
H10.221 **Pseudomembranous conjunctivitis,** right **eye**
H10.222 **Pseudomembranous conjunctivitis,** left **eye**
H10.223 **Pseudomembranous conjunctivitis,** bilateral
H10.229 **Pseudomembranous conjunctivitis,** unspecified **eye**

✓6th **H10.23** **Serous** conjunctivitis, except viral
EXCLUDES 1 *viral conjunctivitis (B30.-)*
H10.231 **Serous conjunctivitis, except viral,** right **eye**
H10.232 **Serous conjunctivitis, except viral,** left **eye**
H10.233 **Serous conjunctivitis, except viral,** bilateral
H10.239 **Serous conjunctivitis, except viral,** unspecified **eye**

✓5th **H10.3** **Unspecified acute conjunctivitis**
EXCLUDES 1 *ophthalmia neonatorum NOS (P39.1)*
H10.30 **Unspecified acute conjunctivitis,** unspecified **eye**
H10.31 **Unspecified acute conjunctivitis,** right **eye**
H10.32 **Unspecified acute conjunctivitis,** left **eye**
H10.33 **Unspecified acute conjunctivitis,** bilateral

✓5th **H10.4** Chronic **conjunctivitis**

✓6th **H10.40** **Unspecified chronic conjunctivitis**
H10.401 **Unspecified chronic conjunctivitis,** right **eye**
H10.402 **Unspecified chronic conjunctivitis,** left **eye**
H10.403 **Unspecified chronic conjunctivitis,** bilateral
H10.409 **Unspecified chronic conjunctivitis,** unspecified **eye**

✓6th **H10.41** **Chronic** giant papillary **conjunctivitis**
H10.411 **Chronic giant papillary conjunctivitis,** right **eye**
H10.412 **Chronic giant papillary conjunctivitis,** left **eye**
H10.413 **Chronic giant papillary conjunctivitis,** bilateral
H10.419 **Chronic giant papillary conjunctivitis,** unspecified **eye**

✓6th **H10.42** **Simple** chronic **conjunctivitis**
H10.421 **Simple chronic conjunctivitis,** right **eye**
H10.422 **Simple chronic conjunctivitis,** left **eye**
H10.423 **Simple chronic conjunctivitis,** bilateral
H10.429 **Simple chronic conjunctivitis,** unspecified **eye**

✓6th **H10.43** **Chronic** follicular **conjunctivitis**
H10.431 **Chronic follicular conjunctivitis,** right **eye**
H10.432 **Chronic follicular conjunctivitis,** left **eye**
H10.433 **Chronic follicular conjunctivitis,** bilateral
H10.439 **Chronic follicular conjunctivitis,** unspecified **eye**

H10.44 **Vernal** conjunctivitis
EXCLUDES 1 *vernal keratoconjunctivitis with limbar and corneal involvement (H16.26-)*

H10.45 **Other chronic** allergic **conjunctivitis**

✓5th **H10.5** **Blepharoconjunctivitis**

✓6th **H10.50** **Unspecified blepharoconjunctivitis**
H10.501 **Unspecified blepharoconjunctivitis,** right **eye**
H10.502 **Unspecified blepharoconjunctivitis,** left **eye**

H10.503 **Unspecified blepharoconjunctivitis,** bilateral
H10.509 **Unspecified blepharoconjunctivitis,** unspecified **eye**

✓6th **H10.51** **Ligneous** conjunctivitis
H10.511 **Ligneous conjunctivitis,** right **eye**
H10.512 **Ligneous conjunctivitis,** left **eye**
H10.513 **Ligneous conjunctivitis,** bilateral
H10.519 **Ligneous conjunctivitis,** unspecified **eye**

✓6th **H10.52** **Angular** blepharoconjunctivitis
H10.521 **Angular blepharoconjunctivitis,** right **eye**
H10.522 **Angular blepharoconjunctivitis,** left **eye**
H10.523 **Angular blepharoconjunctivitis,** bilateral
H10.529 **Angular blepharoconjunctivitis,** unspecified **eye**

✓6th **H10.53** **Contact** blepharoconjunctivitis
H10.531 **Contact blepharoconjunctivitis,** right **eye**
H10.532 **Contact blepharoconjunctivitis,** left **eye**
H10.533 **Contact blepharoconjunctivitis,** bilateral
H10.539 **Contact blepharoconjunctivitis,** unspecified **eye**

✓5th **H10.8** **Other conjunctivitis**

✓6th **H10.81** **Pingueculitis**
EXCLUDES 1 *pinguecula (H11.15-)*
H10.811 **Pingueculitis,** right **eye**
H10.812 **Pingueculitis,** left **eye**
H10.813 **Pingueculitis,** bilateral
H10.819 **Pingueculitis,** unspecified **eye**

H10.89 **Other conjunctivitis**

H10.9 **Unspecified conjunctivitis**

✓4th **H11** **Other disorders of conjunctiva**
EXCLUDES 1 *keratoconjunctivitis (H16.2-)*

✓5th **H11.0** **Pterygium of eye**
EXCLUDES 1 *pseudopterygium (H11.81-)*

✓6th **H11.00** **Unspecified** pterygium of eye
H11.001 **Unspecified pterygium of** right **eye**
H11.002 **Unspecified pterygium of** left **eye**
H11.003 **Unspecified pterygium of eye,** bilateral
H11.009 **Unspecified pterygium of** unspecified **eye**

✓6th **H11.01** **Amyloid** pterygium
H11.011 **Amyloid pterygium of** right **eye**
H11.012 **Amyloid pterygium of** left **eye**
H11.013 **Amyloid pterygium of eye,** bilateral
H11.019 **Amyloid pterygium of** unspecified **eye**

✓6th **H11.02** **Central** pterygium of eye
H11.021 **Central pterygium of** right **eye**
H11.022 **Central pterygium of** left **eye**
H11.023 **Central pterygium of eye,** bilateral
H11.029 **Central pterygium of** unspecified **eye**

✓6th **H11.03** **Double** pterygium of eye
H11.031 **Double pterygium of** right **eye**
H11.032 **Double pterygium of** left **eye**
H11.033 **Double pterygium of eye,** bilateral
H11.039 **Double pterygium of** unspecified **eye**

✓6th **H11.04** **Peripheral** pterygium of eye, stationary
H11.041 **Peripheral pterygium, stationary,** right **eye**
H11.042 **Peripheral pterygium, stationary,** left **eye**
H11.043 **Peripheral pterygium, stationary,** bilateral
H11.049 **Peripheral pterygium, stationary,** unspecified **eye**

✓6th **H11.05** **Peripheral** pterygium of eye, progressive
H11.051 **Peripheral pterygium, progressive,** right **eye**
H11.052 **Peripheral pterygium, progressive,** left **eye**
H11.053 **Peripheral pterygium, progressive,** bilateral
H11.059 **Peripheral pterygium, progressive,** unspecified **eye**

H11.06 Recurrent pterygium of eye
- H11.061 Recurrent pterygium of right eye
- H11.062 Recurrent pterygium of left eye
- H11.063 Recurrent pterygium of eye, bilateral
- H11.069 Recurrent pterygium of unspecified eye

H11.1 Conjunctival degenerations and deposits
EXCLUDES 2 pseudopterygium (H11.81)
- H11.10 Unspecified conjunctival degenerations

H11.11 Conjunctival deposits
- H11.111 Conjunctival deposits, right eye
- H11.112 Conjunctival deposits, left eye
- H11.113 Conjunctival deposits, bilateral
- H11.119 Conjunctival deposits, unspecified eye

H11.12 Conjunctival concretions
- H11.121 Conjunctival concretions, right eye
- H11.122 Conjunctival concretions, left eye
- H11.123 Conjunctival concretions, bilateral
- H11.129 Conjunctival concretions, unspecified eye

H11.13 Conjunctival pigmentations
Conjunctival argyrosis [argyria]
- H11.131 Conjunctival pigmentations, right eye
- H11.132 Conjunctival pigmentations, left eye
- H11.133 Conjunctival pigmentations, bilateral
- H11.139 Conjunctival pigmentations, unspecified eye

H11.14 Conjunctival xerosis, unspecified
EXCLUDES 1 xerosis of conjunctiva due to vitamin A deficiency (E50.0, E50.1)
- H11.141 Conjunctival xerosis, unspecified, right eye
- H11.142 Conjunctival xerosis , unspecified, left eye
- H11.143 Conjunctival xerosis, unspecified, bilateral
- H11.149 Conjunctival xerosis, unspecified, unspecified eye

H11.15 Pinguecula
EXCLUDES 1 pingueculitis (H10.81-)
- H11.151 Pinguecula, right eye
- H11.152 Pinguecula, left eye
- H11.153 Pinguecula, bilateral
- H11.159 Pinguecula, unspecified eye

H11.2 Conjunctival scars
H11.21 Conjunctival adhesions and strands (localized)
- H11.211 Conjunctival adhesions and strands (localized), right eye
- H11.212 Conjunctival adhesions and strands (localized), left eye
- H11.213 Conjunctival adhesions and strands (localized), bilateral
- H11.219 Conjunctival adhesions and strands (localized), unspecified eye

H11.22 Conjunctival granuloma
- H11.221 Conjunctival granuloma, right eye
- H11.222 Conjunctival granuloma, left eye
- H11.223 Conjunctival granuloma, bilateral
- H11.229 Conjunctival granuloma, unspecified

H11.23 Symblepharon
- H11.231 Symblepharon, right eye
- H11.232 Symblepharon, left eye
- H11.233 Symblepharon, bilateral
- H11.239 Symblepharon, unspecified eye

H11.24 Scarring of conjunctiva
- H11.241 Scarring of conjunctiva, right eye
- H11.242 Scarring of conjunctiva, left eye
- H11.243 Scarring of conjunctiva, bilateral
- H11.249 Scarring of conjunctiva, unspecified eye

H11.3 Conjunctival hemorrhage
Subconjunctival hemorrhage
- H11.30 Conjunctival hemorrhage, unspecified eye
- H11.31 Conjunctival hemorrhage, right eye
- H11.32 Conjunctival hemorrhage, left eye
- H11.33 Conjunctival hemorrhage, bilateral

H11.4 Other conjunctival vascular disorders and cysts
H11.41 Vascular abnormalities of conjunctiva
Conjunctival aneurysm
- H11.411 Vascular abnormalities of conjunctiva, right eye
- H11.412 Vascular abnormalities of conjunctiva, left eye
- H11.413 Vascular abnormalities of conjunctiva, bilateral
- H11.419 Vascular abnormalities of conjunctiva, unspecified eye

H11.42 Conjunctival edema
- H11.421 Conjunctival edema, right eye
- H11.422 Conjunctival edema, left eye
- H11.423 Conjunctival edema, bilateral
- H11.429 Conjunctival edema, unspecified eye

H11.43 Conjunctival hyperemia
- H11.431 Conjunctival hyperemia, right eye
- H11.432 Conjunctival hyperemia, left eye
- H11.433 Conjunctival hyperemia, bilateral
- H11.439 Conjunctival hyperemia, unspecified eye

H11.44 Conjunctival cysts
- H11.441 Conjunctival cysts, right eye
- H11.442 Conjunctival cysts, left eye
- H11.443 Conjunctival cysts, bilateral
- H11.449 Conjunctival cysts, unspecified eye

H11.8 Other specified disorders of conjunctiva
H11.81 Pseudopterygium of conjunctiva
- H11.811 Pseudopterygium of conjunctiva, right eye
- H11.812 Pseudopterygium of conjunctiva, left eye
- H11.813 Pseudopterygium of conjunctiva, bilateral
- H11.819 Pseudopterygium of conjunctiva, unspecified eye

H11.82 Conjunctivochalasis
- H11.821 Conjunctivochalasis, right eye
- H11.822 Conjunctivochalasis, left eye
- H11.823 Conjunctivochalasis, bilateral
- H11.829 Conjunctivochalasis, unspecified eye
- H11.89 Other specified disorders of conjunctiva
- H11.9 Unspecified disorder of conjunctiva

Disorders of sclera, cornea, iris and ciliary body (H15-H22)

H15 Disorders of sclera
H15.0 Scleritis
H15.00 Unspecified scleritis
- H15.001 Unspecified scleritis, right eye
- H15.002 Unspecified scleritis, left eye
- H15.003 Unspecified scleritis, bilateral
- H15.009 Unspecified scleritis, unspecified eye

H15.01 Anterior scleritis
- H15.011 Anterior scleritis, right eye
- H15.012 Anterior scleritis, left eye
- H15.013 Anterior scleritis, bilateral
- H15.019 Anterior scleritis, unspecified eye

H15.02 Brawny scleritis
- H15.021 Brawny scleritis, right eye
- H15.022 Brawny scleritis, left eye
- H15.023 Brawny scleritis, bilateral
- H15.029 Brawny scleritis, unspecified eye

H15.03 Posterior scleritis
Sclerotenonitis
- H15.031 Posterior scleritis, right eye
- H15.032 Posterior scleritis, left eye
- H15.033 Posterior scleritis, bilateral
- H15.039 Posterior scleritis, unspecified eye

H15.04 Scleritis with corneal involvement
- H15.041 Scleritis with corneal involvement, right eye
- H15.042 Scleritis with corneal involvement, left eye
- H15.043 Scleritis with corneal involvement, bilateral

H15.049   **Scleritis with corneal involvement, unspecified eye**

✓6ᵗʰ **H15.05**   **Scleromalacia perforans**

H15.051   **Scleromalacia perforans**, right eye

H15.052   **Scleromalacia perforans**, left eye

H15.053   **Scleromalacia perforans**, bilateral

H15.059   **Scleromalacia perforans**, unspecified eye

✓6ᵗʰ **H15.09**   **Other scleritis**
> Scleral abscess

H15.091   **Other scleritis**, right eye

H15.092   **Other scleritis**, left eye

H15.093   **Other scleritis**, bilateral

H15.099   **Other scleritis**, unspecified eye

✓5ᵗʰ **H15.1**   **Episcleritis**

✓6ᵗʰ **H15.10**   **Unspecified episcleritis**

H15.101   **Unspecified episcleritis**, right eye

H15.102   **Unspecified episcleritis**, left eye

H15.103   **Unspecified episcleritis**, bilateral

H15.109   **Unspecified episcleritis**, unspecified eye

✓6ᵗʰ **H15.11**   **Episcleritis periodica fugax**

H15.111   **Episcleritis periodica fugax**, right eye

H15.112   **Episcleritis periodica fugax**, left eye

H15.113   **Episcleritis periodica fugax**, bilateral

H15.119   **Episcleritis periodica fugax**, unspecified eye

✓6ᵗʰ **H15.12**   **Nodular episcleritis**

H15.121   **Nodular episcleritis**, right eye

H15.122   **Nodular episcleritis**, left eye

H15.123   **Nodular episcleritis**, bilateral

H15.129   **Nodular episcleritis**, unspecified eye

✓5ᵗʰ **H15.8**   **Other disorders of sclera**
> EXCLUDES 2   blue sclera (Q13.5)
>   degenerative myopia (H44.2-)

✓6ᵗʰ **H15.81**   **Equatorial staphyloma**

H15.811   **Equatorial staphyloma**, right eye

H15.812   **Equatorial staphyloma**, left eye

H15.813   **Equatorial staphyloma**, bilateral

H15.819   **Equatorial staphyloma**, unspecified eye

✓6ᵗʰ **H15.82**   **Localized anterior staphyloma**

H15.821   **Localized anterior staphyloma**, right eye

H15.822   **Localized anterior staphyloma**, left eye

H15.823   **Localized anterior staphyloma**, bilateral

H15.829   **Localized anterior staphyloma, unspecified eye**

✓6ᵗʰ **H15.83**   **Staphyloma posticum**

H15.831   **Staphyloma posticum**, right eye

H15.832   **Staphyloma posticum**, left eye

H15.833   **Staphyloma posticum**, bilateral

H15.839   **Staphyloma posticum**, unspecified eye

✓6ᵗʰ **H15.84**   **Scleral ectasia**

H15.841   **Scleral ectasia**, right eye

H15.842   **Scleral ectasia**, left eye

H15.843   **Scleral ectasia**, bilateral

H15.849   **Scleral ectasia**, unspecified eye

✓6ᵗʰ **H15.85**   **Ring staphyloma**

H15.851   **Ring staphyloma**, right eye

H15.852   **Ring staphyloma**, left eye

H15.853   **Ring staphyloma**, bilateral

H15.859   **Ring staphyloma**, unspecified eye

H15.89   **Other disorders of sclera**

H15.9   **Unspecified disorder of sclera**

✓4ᵗʰ **H16**   **Keratitis**

✓5ᵗʰ **H16.0**   **Corneal ulcer**

✓6ᵗʰ **H16.00**   **Unspecified corneal ulcer**

H16.001   **Unspecified corneal ulcer**, right eye

H16.002   **Unspecified corneal ulcer**, left eye

H16.003   **Unspecified corneal ulcer**, bilateral

H16.009   **Unspecified corneal ulcer**, unspecified eye

✓6ᵗʰ **H16.01**   **Central corneal ulcer**

H16.011   **Central corneal ulcer**, right eye

H16.012   **Central corneal ulcer**, left eye

H16.013   **Central corneal ulcer**, bilateral

H16.019   **Central corneal ulcer**, unspecified eye

✓6ᵗʰ **H16.02**   **Ring corneal ulcer**

H16.021   **Ring corneal ulcer**, right eye

H16.022   **Ring corneal ulcer**, left eye

H16.023   **Ring corneal ulcer**, bilateral

H16.029   **Ring corneal ulcer**, unspecified eye

✓6ᵗʰ **H16.03**   **Corneal ulcer with hypopyon**

H16.031   **Corneal ulcer with hypopyon**, right eye

H16.032   **Corneal ulcer with hypopyon**, left eye

H16.033   **Corneal ulcer with hypopyon**, bilateral

H16.039   **Corneal ulcer with hypopyon, unspecified eye**

✓6ᵗʰ **H16.04**   **Marginal corneal ulcer**

H16.041   **Marginal corneal ulcer**, right eye

H16.042   **Marginal corneal ulcer**, left eye

H16.043   **Marginal corneal ulcer**, bilateral

H16.049   **Marginal corneal ulcer**, unspecified eye

✓6ᵗʰ **H16.05**   **Mooren's corneal ulcer**

H16.051   **Mooren's corneal ulcer**, right eye

H16.052   **Mooren's corneal ulcer**, left eye

H16.053   **Mooren's corneal ulcer**, bilateral

H16.059   **Mooren's corneal ulcer**, unspecified eye

✓6ᵗʰ **H16.06**   **Mycotic corneal ulcer**

H16.061   **Mycotic corneal ulcer**, right eye

H16.062   **Mycotic corneal ulcer**, left eye

H16.063   **Mycotic corneal ulcer**, bilateral

H16.069   **Mycotic corneal ulcer**, unspecified eye

✓6ᵗʰ **H16.07**   **Perforated corneal ulcer**

H16.071   **Perforated corneal ulcer**, right eye

H16.072   **Perforated corneal ulcer**, left eye

H16.073   **Perforated corneal ulcer**, bilateral

H16.079   **Perforated corneal ulcer**, unspecified eye

✓5ᵗʰ **H16.1**   **Other and unspecified superficial keratitis without conjunctivitis**

✓6ᵗʰ **H16.10**   **Unspecified superficial keratitis**

H16.101   **Unspecified superficial keratitis**, right eye

H16.102   **Unspecified superficial keratitis**, left eye

H16.103   **Unspecified superficial keratitis**, bilateral

H16.109   **Unspecified superficial keratitis, unspecified eye**

✓6ᵗʰ **H16.11**   **Macular keratitis**
> Areolar keratitis
> Nummular keratitis
> Stellate keratitis
> Striate keratitis

H16.111   **Macular keratitis**, right eye

H16.112   **Macular keratitis**, left eye

H16.113   **Macular keratitis**, bilateral

H16.119   **Macular keratitis**, unspecified eye

✓6ᵗʰ **H16.12**   **Filamentary keratitis**

H16.121   **Filamentary keratitis**, right eye

H16.122   **Filamentary keratitis**, left eye

H16.123   **Filamentary keratitis**, bilateral

H16.129   **Filamentary keratitis**, unspecified eye

✓6ᵗʰ **H16.13**   **Photokeratitis**
> Snow blindness
> Welders keratitis

H16.131   **Photokeratitis**, right eye

H16.132   **Photokeratitis**, left eye

H16.133   **Photokeratitis**, bilateral

H16.139   **Photokeratitis**, unspecified eye

✓6ᵗʰ **H16.14**   **Punctate keratitis**

H16.141   **Punctate keratitis**, right eye

H16.142   **Punctate keratitis**, left eye

H16.143   **Punctate keratitis**, bilateral

H16.149   **Punctate keratitis**, unspecified eye

✓5ᵗʰ **H16.2**   **Keratoconjunctivitis**

✓6ᵗʰ **H16.20**   **Unspecified keratoconjunctivitis**
> Superficial keratitis with conjunctivitis NOS

H16.201   **Unspecified keratoconjunctivitis, right eye**

H16.202   **Unspecified keratoconjunctivitis, left eye**

☑ Additional Character Required   ☑x7ᵗʰ Placeholder Alert   Unacceptable PDx   Manifestation   Hospital Acquired Condition   EXCLUDES 1 Not Coded Here   EXCLUDES 2 Not Included Here

Chapter 7. Diseases of the Eye and Adnexa

H16.203–H17.819

H16.203   Unspecified keratoconjunctivitis, bilateral

H16.209   Unspecified keratoconjunctivitis, unspecified eye

√6ᵗʰ **H16.21**   **Exposure keratoconjunctivitis**

H16.211   Exposure keratoconjunctivitis, right eye

H16.212   Exposure keratoconjunctivitis, left eye

H16.213   Exposure keratoconjunctivitis, bilateral

H16.219   Exposure keratoconjunctivitis, unspecified eye

√6ᵗʰ **H16.22**   **Keratoconjunctivitis sicca, not specified as Sjögren's**

    EXCLUDES 1   *Sjögren's syndrome (M35.01)*

H16.221   Keratoconjunctivitis sicca, not specified as Sjögren's, right eye

H16.222   Keratoconjunctivitis sicca, not specified as Sjögren's, left eye

H16.223   Keratoconjunctivitis sicca, not specified as Sjögren's, bilateral

H16.229   Keratoconjunctivitis sicca, not specified as Sjögren's, unspecified eye

√6ᵗʰ **H16.23**   **Neurotrophic keratoconjunctivitis**

H16.231   Neurotrophic keratoconjunctivitis, right eye

H16.232   Neurotrophic keratoconjunctivitis, left eye

H16.233   Neurotrophic keratoconjunctivitis, bilateral

H16.239   Neurotrophic keratoconjunctivitis, unspecified eye

√6ᵗʰ **H16.24**   **Ophthalmia nodosa**

H16.241   Ophthalmia nodosa, right eye

H16.242   Ophthalmia nodosa, left eye

H16.243   Ophthalmia nodosa, bilateral

H16.249   Ophthalmia nodosa, unspecified eye

√6ᵗʰ **H16.25**   **Phlyctenular keratoconjunctivitis**

H16.251   Phlyctenular keratoconjunctivitis, right eye

H16.252   Phlyctenular keratoconjunctivitis, left eye

H16.253   Phlyctenular keratoconjunctivitis, bilateral

H16.259   Phlyctenular keratoconjunctivitis, unspecified eye

√6ᵗʰ **H16.26**   **Vernal keratoconjunctivitis, with limbar and corneal involvement**

    EXCLUDES 1   *vernal conjunctivitis without limbar and corneal involvement (H10.44)*

H16.261   Vernal keratoconjunctivitis, with limbar and corneal involvement, right eye

H16.262   Vernal keratoconjunctivitis, with limbar and corneal involvement, left eye

H16.263   Vernal keratoconjunctivitis, with limbar and corneal involvement, bilateral

H16.269   Vernal keratoconjunctivitis, with limbar and corneal involvement, unspecified eye

√6ᵗʰ **H16.29**   **Other keratoconjunctivitis**

H16.291   Other keratoconjunctivitis, right eye

H16.292   Other keratoconjunctivitis, left eye

H16.293   Other keratoconjunctivitis, bilateral

H16.299   Other keratoconjunctivitis, unspecified eye

√5ᵗʰ **H16.3**   **Interstitial and deep keratitis**

√6ᵗʰ **H16.30**   **Unspecified interstitial keratitis**

H16.301   Unspecified interstitial keratitis, right eye

H16.302   Unspecified interstitial keratitis, left eye

H16.303   Unspecified interstitial keratitis, bilateral

H16.309   Unspecified interstitial keratitis, unspecified eye

√6ᵗʰ **H16.31**   **Corneal abscess**

H16.311   Corneal abscess, right eye

H16.312   Corneal abscess, left eye

H16.313   Corneal abscess, bilateral

H16.319   Corneal abscess, unspecified eye

√6ᵗʰ **H16.32**   **Diffuse interstitial keratitis**

    Cogan's syndrome

H16.321   Diffuse interstitial keratitis, right eye

H16.322   Diffuse interstitial keratitis, left eye

H16.323   Diffuse interstitial keratitis, bilateral

H16.329   Diffuse interstitial keratitis, unspecified eye

√6ᵗʰ **H16.33**   **Sclerosing keratitis**

H16.331   Sclerosing keratitis, right eye

H16.332   Sclerosing keratitis, left eye

H16.333   Sclerosing keratitis, bilateral

H16.339   Sclerosing keratitis, unspecified eye

√6ᵗʰ **H16.39**   **Other interstitial and deep keratitis**

H16.391   Other interstitial and deep keratitis, right eye

H16.392   Other interstitial and deep keratitis, left eye

H16.393   Other interstitial and deep keratitis, bilateral

H16.399   Other interstitial and deep keratitis, unspecified eye

√5ᵗʰ **H16.4**   **Corneal neovascularization**

√6ᵗʰ **H16.40**   **Unspecified corneal neovascularization**

H16.401   Unspecified corneal neovascularization, right eye

H16.402   Unspecified corneal neovascularization, left eye

H16.403   Unspecified corneal neovascularization, bilateral

H16.409   Unspecified corneal neovascularization, unspecified eye

√6ᵗʰ **H16.41**   **Ghost vessels (corneal)**

H16.411   Ghost vessels (corneal), right eye

H16.412   Ghost vessels (corneal), left eye

H16.413   Ghost vessels (corneal), bilateral

H16.419   Ghost vessels (corneal), unspecified eye

√6ᵗʰ **H16.42**   **Pannus (corneal)**

H16.421   Pannus (corneal), right eye

H16.422   Pannus (corneal), left eye

H16.423   Pannus (corneal), bilateral

H16.429   Pannus (corneal), unspecified eye

√6ᵗʰ **H16.43**   **Localized vascularization of cornea**

H16.431   Localized vascularization of cornea, right eye

H16.432   Localized vascularization of cornea, left eye

H16.433   Localized vascularization of cornea, bilateral

H16.439   Localized vascularization of cornea, unspecified eye

√6ᵗʰ **H16.44**   **Deep vascularization of cornea**

H16.441   Deep vascularization of cornea, right eye

H16.442   Deep vascularization of cornea, left eye

H16.443   Deep vascularization of cornea, bilateral

H16.449   Deep vascularization of cornea, unspecified eye

H16.8   **Other keratitis**

H16.9   **Unspecified keratitis**

√4ᵗʰ **H17**   **Corneal scars and opacities**

√5ᵗʰ **H17.0**   **Adherent leukoma**

H17.00   Adherent leukoma, unspecified eye

H17.01   Adherent leukoma, right eye

H17.02   Adherent leukoma, left eye

H17.03   Adherent leukoma, bilateral

√5ᵗʰ **H17.1**   **Central corneal opacity**

H17.10   Central corneal opacity, unspecified eye

H17.11   Central corneal opacity, right eye

H17.12   Central corneal opacity, left eye

H17.13   Central corneal opacity, bilateral

√5ᵗʰ **H17.8**   **Other corneal scars and opacities**

√6ᵗʰ **H17.81**   **Minor opacity of cornea**

    Corneal nebula

H17.811   Minor opacity of cornea, right eye

H17.812   Minor opacity of cornea, left eye

H17.813   Minor opacity of cornea, bilateral

H17.819   Minor opacity of cornea, unspecified eye

Ⓝ Newborn: 0   Ⓟ Pediatric: 0-17   Ⓜ Maternity: 12-55   Ⓐ Adult: 15-124   **MCC** Major CC Condition   **PDx MCC** PDx acts as own MCC   **CC** CC Condition   **PDx CC** PDx acts as own CC

570   ICD-10-CM 2016

✓6ᵗʰ **H17.82** Peripheral opacity of cornea
    H17.821 Peripheral opacity of cornea, right eye
    H17.822 Peripheral opacity of cornea, left eye
    H17.823 Peripheral opacity of cornea, bilateral
    H17.829 Peripheral opacity of cornea, unspecified eye
  H17.89 Other corneal scars and opacities
 H17.9 Unspecified corneal scar and opacity

✓4ᵗʰ **H18** Other disorders of cornea
  ✓5ᵗʰ **H18.0** Corneal pigmentations and deposits
    ✓6ᵗʰ **H18.00** Unspecified corneal deposit
      H18.001 Unspecified corneal deposit, right eye
      H18.002 Unspecified corneal deposit, left eye
      H18.003 Unspecified corneal deposit, bilateral
      H18.009 Unspecified corneal deposit, unspecified eye
    ✓6ᵗʰ **H18.01** Anterior corneal pigmentations
      Staehli's line
      H18.011 Anterior corneal pigmentations, right eye
      H18.012 Anterior corneal pigmentations, left eye
      H18.013 Anterior corneal pigmentations, bilateral
      H18.019 Anterior corneal pigmentations, unspecified eye
    ✓6ᵗʰ **H18.02** Argentous corneal deposits
      H18.021 Argentous corneal deposits, right eye
      H18.022 Argentous corneal deposits, left eye
      H18.023 Argentous corneal deposits, bilateral
      H18.029 Argentous corneal deposits, unspecified eye
    ✓6ᵗʰ **H18.03** Corneal deposits in metabolic disorders
      Code also associated metabolic disorder
      H18.031 Corneal deposits in metabolic disorders, right eye
      H18.032 Corneal deposits in metabolic disorders, left eye
      H18.033 Corneal deposits in metabolic disorders, bilateral
      H18.039 Corneal deposits in metabolic disorders, unspecified eye
    ✓6ᵗʰ **H18.04** Kayser-Fleischer ring
      Code also associated Wilson's disease (E83.01)
      H18.041 Kayser-Fleischer ring, right eye
      H18.042 Kayser-Fleischer ring, left eye
      H18.043 Kayser-Fleischer ring, bilateral
      H18.049 Kayser-Fleischer ring, unspecified eye
    ✓6ᵗʰ **H18.05** Posterior corneal pigmentations
      Krukenberg's spindle
      H18.051 Posterior corneal pigmentations, right eye
      H18.052 Posterior corneal pigmentations, left eye
      H18.053 Posterior corneal pigmentations, bilateral
      H18.059 Posterior corneal pigmentations, unspecified eye
    ✓6ᵗʰ **H18.06** Stromal corneal pigmentations
      Hematocornea
      H18.061 Stromal corneal pigmentations, right eye
      H18.062 Stromal corneal pigmentations, left eye
      H18.063 Stromal corneal pigmentations, bilateral
      H18.069 Stromal corneal pigmentations, unspecified eye
  ✓5ᵗʰ **H18.1** Bullous keratopathy
    H18.10 Bullous keratopathy, unspecified eye
    H18.11 Bullous keratopathy, right eye
    H18.12 Bullous keratopathy, left eye
    H18.13 Bullous keratopathy, bilateral
  ✓5ᵗʰ **H18.2** Other and unspecified corneal edema
    H18.20 Unspecified corneal edema
    ✓6ᵗʰ **H18.21** Corneal edema secondary to contact lens
      EXCLUDES 2 *other corneal disorders due to contact lens (H18.82-)*
      H18.211 Corneal edema secondary to contact lens, right eye
      H18.212 Corneal edema secondary to contact lens, left eye

      H18.213 Corneal edema secondary to contact lens, bilateral
      H18.219 Corneal edema secondary to contact lens, unspecified eye
    ✓6ᵗʰ **H18.22** Idiopathic corneal edema
      H18.221 Idiopathic corneal edema, right eye
      H18.222 Idiopathic corneal edema, left eye
      H18.223 Idiopathic corneal edema, bilateral
      H18.229 Idiopathic corneal edema, unspecified eye
    ✓6ᵗʰ **H18.23** Secondary corneal edema
      H18.231 Secondary corneal edema, right eye
      H18.232 Secondary corneal edema, left eye
      H18.233 Secondary corneal edema, bilateral
      H18.239 Secondary corneal edema, unspecified eye
  ✓5ᵗʰ **H18.3** Changes of corneal membranes
    H18.30 Unspecified corneal membrane change
    ✓6ᵗʰ **H18.31** Folds and rupture in Bowman's membrane
      H18.311 Folds and rupture in Bowman's membrane, right eye
      H18.312 Folds and rupture in Bowman's membrane, left eye
      H18.313 Folds and rupture in Bowman's membrane, bilateral
      H18.319 Folds and rupture in Bowman's membrane, unspecified eye
    ✓6ᵗʰ **H18.32** Folds in Descemet's membrane
      H18.321 Folds in Descemet's membrane, right eye
      H18.322 Folds in Descemet's membrane, left eye
      H18.323 Folds in Descemet's membrane, bilateral
      H18.329 Folds in Descemet's membrane, unspecified eye
    ✓6ᵗʰ **H18.33** Rupture in Descemet's membrane
      H18.331 Rupture in Descemet's membrane, right eye
      H18.332 Rupture in Descemet's membrane, left eye
      H18.333 Rupture in Descemet's membrane, bilateral
      H18.339 Rupture in Descemet's membrane, unspecified eye
  ✓5ᵗʰ **H18.4** Corneal degeneration
    EXCLUDES 1 *Mooren's ulcer (H16.0-)*
      recurrent erosion of cornea (H18.83-)
    H18.40 Unspecified corneal degeneration
    ✓6ᵗʰ **H18.41** Arcus senilis
      Senile corneal changes
      H18.411 Arcus senilis, right eye
      H18.412 Arcus senilis, left eye
      H18.413 Arcus senilis, bilateral
      H18.419 Arcus senilis, unspecified eye
    ✓6ᵗʰ **H18.42** Band keratopathy
      H18.421 Band keratopathy, right eye
      H18.422 Band keratopathy, left eye
      H18.423 Band keratopathy, bilateral
      H18.429 Band keratopathy, unspecified eye
    H18.43 Other calcerous corneal degeneration
    ✓6ᵗʰ **H18.44** Keratomalacia
      EXCLUDES 1 *keratomalacia due to vitamin A deficiency (E50.4)*
      H18.441 Keratomalacia, right eye
      H18.442 Keratomalacia, left eye
      H18.443 Keratomalacia, bilateral
      H18.449 Keratomalacia, unspecified eye
    ✓6ᵗʰ **H18.45** Nodular corneal degeneration
      H18.451 Nodular corneal degeneration, right eye
      H18.452 Nodular corneal degeneration, left eye
      H18.453 Nodular corneal degeneration, bilateral
      H18.459 Nodular corneal degeneration, unspecified eye
    ✓6ᵗʰ **H18.46** Peripheral corneal degeneration
      H18.461 Peripheral corneal degeneration, right eye
      H18.462 Peripheral corneal degeneration, left eye
      H18.463 Peripheral corneal degeneration, bilateral

☑ Additional Character Required   ✓x7ᵗʰ Placeholder Alert   Unacceptable PDx   Manifestation   Hospital Acquired Condition   **EXCLUDES 1** Not Coded Here   *EXCLUDES 2* Not Included Here

Chapter 7. Diseases of the Eye and Adnexa

H18.469   Peripheral corneal degeneration, unspecified eye

H18.49   **Other corneal degeneration**

√5ᵗʰ H18.5   **Hereditary corneal dystrophies**

H18.50   Unspecified hereditary corneal dystrophies

H18.51   Endothelial corneal dystrophy
Fuchs' dystrophy

H18.52   Epithelial (juvenile) corneal dystrophy

H18.53   Granular corneal dystrophy

H18.54   Lattice corneal dystrophy

H18.55   Macular corneal dystrophy

H18.59   Other hereditary corneal dystrophies

√5ᵗʰ H18.6   **Keratoconus**

√6ᵗʰ H18.60   **Keratoconus, unspecified**

H18.601   Keratoconus, unspecified, right eye
H18.602   Keratoconus, unspecified, left eye
H18.603   Keratoconus, unspecified, bilateral
H18.609   Keratoconus, unspecified, unspecified eye

√6ᵗʰ H18.61   **Keratoconus, stable**

H18.611   Keratoconus, stable, right eye
H18.612   Keratoconus, stable, left eye
H18.613   Keratoconus, stable, bilateral
H18.619   Keratoconus, stable, unspecified eye

√6ᵗʰ H18.62   **Keratoconus, unstable**
Acute hydrops

H18.621   Keratoconus, unstable, right eye
H18.622   Keratoconus, unstable, left eye
H18.623   Keratoconus, unstable, bilateral
H18.629   Keratoconus, unstable, unspecified eye

√5ᵗʰ H18.7   **Other and unspecified corneal deformities**
EXCLUDES 1 *congenital malformations of cornea (Q13.3-Q13.4)*

H18.70   Unspecified corneal deformity

√6ᵗʰ H18.71   **Corneal ectasia**

H18.711   Corneal ectasia, right eye
H18.712   Corneal ectasia, left eye
H18.713   Corneal ectasia, bilateral
H18.719   Corneal ectasia, unspecified eye

√6ᵗʰ H18.72   **Corneal staphyloma**

H18.721   Corneal staphyloma, right eye
H18.722   Corneal staphyloma, left eye
H18.723   Corneal staphyloma, bilateral
H18.729   Corneal staphyloma, unspecified eye

√6ᵗʰ H18.73   **Descemetocele**

H18.731   Descemetocele, right eye
H18.732   Descemetocele, left eye
H18.733   Descemetocele, bilateral
H18.739   Descemetocele, unspecified eye

√6ᵗʰ H18.79   **Other corneal deformities**

H18.791   Other corneal deformities, right eye
H18.792   Other corneal deformities, left eye
H18.793   Other corneal deformities, bilateral
H18.799   Other corneal deformities, unspecified eye

√5ᵗʰ H18.8   **Other specified disorders of cornea**

√6ᵗʰ H18.81   **Anesthesia and hypoesthesia of cornea**

H18.811   Anesthesia and hypoesthesia of cornea, right eye
H18.812   Anesthesia and hypoesthesia of cornea, left eye
H18.813   Anesthesia and hypoesthesia of cornea, bilateral
H18.819   Anesthesia and hypoesthesia of cornea, unspecified eye

√6ᵗʰ H18.82   **Corneal disorder due to contact lens**
EXCLUDES 2 *corneal edema due to contact lens (H18.21-)*

H18.821   Corneal disorder due to contact lens, right eye
H18.822   Corneal disorder due to contact lens, left eye
H18.823   Corneal disorder due to contact lens, bilateral
H18.829   Corneal disorder due to contact lens, unspecified eye

√6ᵗʰ H18.83   **Recurrent erosion of cornea**

H18.831   Recurrent erosion of cornea, right eye
H18.832   Recurrent erosion of cornea, left eye
H18.833   Recurrent erosion of cornea, bilateral
H18.839   Recurrent erosion of cornea, unspecified eye

√6ᵗʰ H18.89   **Other specified disorders of cornea**

H18.891   Other specified disorders of cornea, right eye
H18.892   Other specified disorders of cornea, left eye
H18.893   Other specified disorders of cornea, bilateral
H18.899   Other specified disorders of cornea, unspecified eye

H18.9   **Unspecified disorder of cornea**

√4ᵗʰ **H20   Iridocyclitis**

CC Excl: For CC codes in category H20, unless otherwise noted:
A18.54, H20.00-H20.9

√5ᵗʰ H20.0   **Acute and subacute iridocyclitis**
Acute anterior uveitis
Acute cyclitis
Acute iritis
Subacute anterior uveitis
Subacute cyclitis
Subacute iritis
EXCLUDES 1 *iridocyclitis, iritis, uveitis (due to) (in) diabetes mellitus (E08-E13 with .39)*
iridocyclitis, iritis, uveitis (due to) (in) diphtheria (A36.89)
iridocyclitis, iritis, uveitis (due to) (in) gonococcal (A54.32)
iridocyclitis, iritis, uveitis (due to) (in) herpes (simplex) (B00.51)
iridocyclitis, iritis, uveitis (due to) (in) herpes zoster (B02.32)
iridocyclitis, iritis, uveitis (due to) (in) late congenital syphilis (A50.39)
iridocyclitis, iritis, uveitis (due to) (in) late syphilis (A52.71)
iridocyclitis, iritis, uveitis (due to) (in) sarcoidosis (D86.83)
iridocyclitis, iritis, uveitis (due to) (in) syphilis (A51.43)
iridocyclitis, iritis, uveitis (due to) (in) toxoplasmosis (B58.09)
iridocyclitis, iritis, uveitis (due to) (in) tuberculosis (A18.54)

H20.00   **Unspecified acute and subacute iridocyclitis**   CC

√6ᵗʰ H20.01   **Primary iridocyclitis**

H20.011   Primary iridocyclitis, right eye   CC
H20.012   Primary iridocyclitis, left eye   CC
H20.013   Primary iridocyclitis, bilateral   CC
H20.019   Primary iridocyclitis, unspecified eye   CC

√6ᵗʰ H20.02   **Recurrent acute iridocyclitis**

H20.021   Recurrent acute iridocyclitis, right eye   CC
H20.022   Recurrent acute iridocyclitis, left eye   CC
H20.023   Recurrent acute iridocyclitis, bilateral   CC
H20.029   Recurrent acute iridocyclitis, unspecified eye   CC

√6ᵗʰ H20.03   **Secondary infectious iridocyclitis**

H20.031   Secondary infectious iridocyclitis, right eye   CC
H20.032   Secondary infectious iridocyclitis, left eye   CC
H20.033   Secondary infectious iridocyclitis, bilateral   CC
H20.039   Secondary infectious iridocyclitis, unspecified eye   CC

√6ᵗʰ H20.04   **Secondary noninfectious iridocyclitis**

H20.041   Secondary noninfectious iridocyclitis, right eye
H20.042   Secondary noninfectious iridocyclitis, left eye
H20.043   Secondary noninfectious iridocyclitis, bilateral
H20.049   Secondary noninfectious iridocyclitis, unspecified eye

✓6ᵗʰ **H20.05 Hypopyon**
     H20.051 Hypopyon, **right eye**
     H20.052 Hypopyon, **left eye**
     H20.053 Hypopyon, **bilateral**
     H20.059 Hypopyon, **unspecified eye**

✓5ᵗʰ **H20.1 Chronic iridocyclitis**
     Use additional code for any associated cataract (H26.21-)
     EXCLUDES 2   *posterior cyclitis (H30.2-)*
     H20.10 Chronic iridocyclitis, **unspecified eye**
     H20.11 Chronic iridocyclitis, **right eye**
     H20.12 Chronic iridocyclitis, **left eye**
     H20.13 Chronic iridocyclitis, **bilateral**

✓5ᵗʰ **H20.2 Lens-induced iridocyclitis**
     H20.20 Lens-induced iridocyclitis, **unspecified eye**
     H20.21 Lens-induced iridocyclitis, **right eye**
     H20.22 Lens-induced iridocyclitis, **left eye**
     H20.23 Lens-induced iridocyclitis, **bilateral**

✓5ᵗʰ **H20.8 Other iridocyclitis**
     EXCLUDES 2   *glaucomatocyclitis crises (H40.4-)*
                posterior cyclitis (H30.2-)
                sympathetic uveitis (H44.13-)

     ✓6ᵗʰ **H20.81 Fuchs' heterochromic cyclitis**
         H20.811 Fuchs' heterochromic cyclitis, **right eye**
         H20.812 Fuchs' heterochromic cyclitis, **left eye**
         H20.813 Fuchs' heterochromic cyclitis, **bilateral**
         H20.819 Fuchs' heterochromic cyclitis, **unspecified eye**

     ✓6ᵗʰ **H20.82 Vogt-Koyanagi syndrome**
         H20.821 Vogt-Koyanagi syndrome, **right eye**
         H20.822 Vogt-Koyanagi syndrome, **left eye**
         H20.823 Vogt-Koyanagi syndrome, **bilateral**
         H20.829 Vogt-Koyanagi syndrome, **unspecified eye**

H20.9 Unspecified iridocyclitis   `CC`
     Uveitis NOS

✓4ᵗʰ **H21 Other disorders of iris and ciliary body**
     EXCLUDES 2   *sympathetic uveitis (H44.1-)*

✓5ᵗʰ **H21.0 Hyphema**
     EXCLUDES 1   *traumatic hyphema (S05.1-)*
     H21.00 Hyphema, **unspecified eye**
     H21.01 Hyphema, **right eye**
     H21.02 Hyphema, **left eye**
     H21.03 Hyphema, **bilateral**

✓5ᵗʰ **H21.1 Other vascular disorders of iris and ciliary body**
     Neovascularization of iris or ciliary body
     Rubeosis iridis
     Rubeosis of iris

     ✓6ᵗʰ **H21.1X Other vascular disorders of iris and ciliary body**
         H21.1X1 Other vascular disorders of iris and ciliary body, **right eye**
         H21.1X2 Other vascular disorders of iris and ciliary body, **left eye**
         H21.1X3 Other vascular disorders of iris and ciliary body, **bilateral**
         H21.1X9 Other vascular disorders of iris and ciliary body, **unspecified eye**

✓5ᵗʰ **H21.2 Degeneration of iris and ciliary body**

     ✓6ᵗʰ **H21.21 Degeneration of chamber angle**
         H21.211 Degeneration of chamber angle, **right eye**
         H21.212 Degeneration of chamber angle, **left eye**
         H21.213 Degeneration of chamber angle, **bilateral**
         H21.219 Degeneration of chamber angle, **unspecified eye**

     ✓6ᵗʰ **H21.22 Degeneration of ciliary body**
         H21.221 Degeneration of ciliary body, **right eye**
         H21.222 Degeneration of ciliary body, **left eye**
         H21.223 Degeneration of ciliary body, **bilateral**
         H21.229 Degeneration of ciliary body, **unspecified eye**

     ✓6ᵗʰ **H21.23 Degeneration of iris (pigmentary)**
         Translucency of iris
         H21.231 Degeneration of iris (pigmentary), **right eye**

H21.232 Degeneration of iris (pigmentary), **left eye**
H21.233 Degeneration of iris (pigmentary), **bilateral**
H21.239 Degeneration of iris (pigmentary), **unspecified eye**

✓6ᵗʰ **H21.24 Degeneration of pupillary margin**
     H21.241 Degeneration of pupillary margin, **right eye**
     H21.242 Degeneration of pupillary margin, **left eye**
     H21.243 Degeneration of pupillary margin, **bilateral**
     H21.249 Degeneration of pupillary margin, **unspecified eye**

✓6ᵗʰ **H21.25 Iridoschisis**
     H21.251 Iridoschisis, **right eye**
     H21.252 Iridoschisis, **left eye**
     H21.253 Iridoschisis, **bilateral**
     H21.259 Iridoschisis, **unspecified eye**

✓6ᵗʰ **H21.26 Iris atrophy (essential) (progressive)**
     H21.261 Iris atrophy (essential) (progressive), **right eye**
     H21.262 Iris atrophy (essential) (progressive), **left eye**
     H21.263 Iris atrophy (essential) (progressive), **bilateral**
     H21.269 Iris atrophy (essential) (progressive), **unspecified eye**

✓6ᵗʰ **H21.27 Miotic pupillary cyst**
     H21.271 Miotic pupillary cyst, **right eye**
     H21.272 Miotic pupillary cyst, **left eye**
     H21.273 Miotic pupillary cyst, **bilateral**
     H21.279 Miotic pupillary cyst, **unspecified eye**

H21.29 Other iris atrophy

✓5ᵗʰ **H21.3 Cyst of iris, ciliary body and anterior chamber**
     EXCLUDES 2   *miotic pupillary cyst (H21.27-)*

     ✓6ᵗʰ **H21.30 Idiopathic cysts of iris, ciliary body or anterior chamber**
         Cyst of iris, ciliary body or anterior chamber NOS
         H21.301 Idiopathic cysts of iris, ciliary body or anterior chamber, **right eye**
         H21.302 Idiopathic cysts of iris, ciliary body or anterior chamber, **left eye**
         H21.303 Idiopathic cysts of iris, ciliary body or anterior chamber, **bilateral**
         H21.309 Idiopathic cysts of iris, ciliary body or anterior chamber, **unspecified eye**

     ✓6ᵗʰ **H21.31 Exudative cysts of iris or anterior chamber**
         H21.311 Exudative cysts of iris or anterior chamber, **right eye**
         H21.312 Exudative cysts of iris or anterior chamber, **left eye**
         H21.313 Exudative cysts of iris or anterior chamber, **bilateral**
         H21.319 Exudative cysts of iris or anterior chamber, **unspecified eye**

     ✓6ᵗʰ **H21.32 Implantation cysts of iris, ciliary body or anterior chamber**
         H21.321 Implantation cysts of iris, ciliary body or anterior chamber, **right eye**
         H21.322 Implantation cysts of iris, ciliary body or anterior chamber, **left eye**
         H21.323 Implantation cysts of iris, ciliary body or anterior chamber, **bilateral**
         H21.329 Implantation cysts of iris, ciliary body or anterior chamber, **unspecified eye**

     ✓6ᵗʰ **H21.33 Parasitic cyst of iris, ciliary body or anterior chamber**

         CC Excl: For CC codes in subcategory H21.33, unless otherwise noted: H20.051-H20.059, H21.331-H21.339, H33.121-H33.129, H44.001-H44.029, H44.121-H44.129, H44.19

         H21.331 Parasitic cyst of iris, ciliary body or anterior chamber, **right eye**   `CC`
         H21.332 Parasitic cyst of iris, ciliary body or anterior chamber, **left eye**   `CC`

Chapter 7. Diseases of the Eye and Adnexa *(left margin)*

H21.333　Parasitic cyst of iris, ciliary body or anterior chamber, **bilateral**　`CC`

H21.339　Parasitic cyst of iris, ciliary body or anterior chamber, **unspecified eye**　`CC`

✓6th　H21.34　Primary cyst of pars plana

H21.341　Primary cyst of pars plana, **right eye**

H21.342　Primary cyst of pars plana, **left eye**

H21.343　Primary cyst of pars plana, **bilateral**

H21.349　Primary cyst of pars plana, **unspecified eye**

✓6th　H21.35　Exudative cyst of pars plana

H21.351　Exudative cyst of pars plana, **right eye**

H21.352　Exudative cyst of pars plana, **left eye**

H21.353　Exudative cyst of pars plana, **bilateral**

H21.359　Exudative cyst of pars plana, **unspecified eye**

✓5th　**H21.4　Pupillary membranes**
Iris bombé
Pupillary occlusion
Pupillary seclusion
　EXCLUDES 1　*congenital pupillary membranes (Q13.8)*

H21.40　Pupillary membranes, **unspecified eye**

H21.41　Pupillary membranes, **right eye**

H21.42　Pupillary membranes, **left eye**

H21.43　Pupillary membranes, **bilateral**

✓5th　**H21.5　Other and unspecified adhesions and disruptions of iris and ciliary body**
　EXCLUDES 1　*corectopia (Q13.2)*

✓6th　H21.50　Unspecified adhesions of iris
Synechia (iris) NOS

H21.501　Unspecified adhesions of iris, **right eye**

H21.502　Unspecified adhesions of iris, **left eye**

H21.503　Unspecified adhesions of iris, **bilateral**

H21.509　Unspecified adhesions of iris and ciliary body, **unspecified eye**

✓6th　H21.51　Anterior synechiae (iris)

H21.511　Anterior synechiae (iris), **right eye**

H21.512　Anterior synechiae (iris), **left eye**

H21.513　Anterior synechiae (iris), **bilateral**

H21.519　Anterior synechiae (iris), **unspecified eye**

✓6th　H21.52　Goniosynechiae

H21.521　Goniosynechiae, **right eye**

H21.522　Goniosynechiae, **left eye**

H21.523　Goniosynechiae, **bilateral**

H21.529　Goniosynechiae, **unspecified eye**

✓6th　H21.53　Iridodialysis

H21.531　Iridodialysis, **right eye**

H21.532　Iridodialysis, **left eye**

H21.533　Iridodialysis, **bilateral**

H21.539　Iridodialysis, **unspecified eye**

✓6th　H21.54　Posterior synechiae (iris)

H21.541　Posterior synechiae (iris), **right eye**

H21.542　Posterior synechiae (iris), **left eye**

H21.543　Posterior synechiae (iris), **bilateral**

H21.549　Posterior synechiae (iris), **unspecified eye**

✓6th　H21.55　Recession of chamber angle

H21.551　Recession of chamber angle, **right eye**

H21.552　Recession of chamber angle, **left eye**

H21.553　Recession of chamber angle, **bilateral**

H21.559　Recession of chamber angle, **unspecified eye**

✓6th　H21.56　Pupillary abnormalities
Deformed pupil
Ectopic pupil
Rupture of sphincter, pupil
　EXCLUDES 1　*congenital deformity of pupil (Q13.2-)*

H21.561　Pupillary abnormality, **right eye**

H21.562　Pupillary abnormality, **left eye**

H21.563　Pupillary abnormality, **bilateral**

H21.569　Pupillary abnormality, **unspecified eye**

✓5th　**H21.8　Other specified disorders of iris and ciliary body**

H21.81　Floppy iris syndrome
Intraoperative floppy iris syndrome (IFIS)
Use additional code for adverse effect, if applicable, to identify drug (T36-T50 with fifth or sixth character 5)

H21.82　Plateau iris syndrome (post-iridectomy) (postprocedural)

H21.89　Other specified disorders of iris and ciliary body

H21.9　Unspecified disorder of iris and ciliary body

H22　Disorders of iris and ciliary body in diseases classified elsewhere
Code first underlying disease, such as:
gout (M1A.-, M10.-)
leprosy (A30.-)
parasitic disease (B89)

Disorders of lens (H25-H28)

✓4th　**H25　Age-related cataract**
Senile cataract
　EXCLUDES 2　*capsular glaucoma with pseudoexfoliation of lens (H40.1-)*

✓5th　**H25.0　Age-related incipient cataract**

✓6th　H25.01　Cortical age-related cataract

H25.011　Cortical age-related cataract, **right eye**　`A`

H25.012　Cortical age-related cataract, **left eye**　`A`

H25.013　Cortical age-related cataract, **bilateral**　`A`

H25.019　Cortical age-related cataract, **unspecified eye**　`A`

✓6th　H25.03　Anterior subcapsular polar age-related cataract

H25.031　Anterior subcapsular polar age-related cataract, **right eye**　`A`

H25.032　Anterior subcapsular polar age-related cataract, **left eye**　`A`

H25.033　Anterior subcapsular polar age-related cataract, **bilateral**　`A`

H25.039　Anterior subcapsular polar age-related cataract, **unspecified eye**　`A`

✓6th　H25.04　Posterior subcapsular polar age-related cataract

H25.041　Posterior subcapsular polar age-related cataract, **right eye**　`A`

H25.042　Posterior subcapsular polar age-related cataract, **left eye**　`A`

H25.043　Posterior subcapsular polar age-related cataract, **bilateral**　`A`

H25.049　Posterior subcapsular polar age-related cataract, **unspecified eye**　`A`

✓6th　H25.09　Other age-related incipient cataract
Coronary age-related cataract
Punctate age-related cataract
Water clefts

H25.091　Other age-related incipient cataract, **right eye**　`A`

H25.092　Other age-related incipient cataract, **left eye**　`A`

H25.093　Other age-related incipient cataract, **bilateral**　`A`

H25.099　Other age-related incipient cataract, **unspecified eye**　`A`

✓5th　**H25.1　Age-related nuclear cataract**
Cataracta brunescens
Nuclear sclerosis cataract

H25.10　Age-related nuclear cataract, **unspecified eye**　`A`

H25.11　Age-related nuclear cataract, **right eye**　`A`

H25.12　Age-related nuclear cataract, **left eye**　`A`

H25.13　Age-related nuclear cataract, **bilateral**　`A`

✓5th　**H25.2　Age-related cataract, morgagnian type**
Age-related hypermature cataract

H25.20　Age-related cataract, morgagnian type, **unspecified eye**　`A`

H25.21　Age-related cataract, morgagnian type, **right eye**　`A`

H25.22　Age-related cataract, morgagnian type, **left eye**　`A`

H25.23　Age-related cataract, morgagnian type, **bilateral**　`A`

H21.333–H25.23 *(left margin)*

N Newborn: 0　P Pediatric: 0-17　M Maternity: 12-55　A Adult: 15-124　MCC Major CC Condition　PDxMCC PDx acts as own MCC　CC CC Condition　PDxCC PDx acts as own CC

574　　　　ICD-10-CM 2016

√5ᵗʰ **H25.8** Other **age-related cataract**

  √6ᵗʰ **H25.81** **Combined forms** of age-related cataract

   H25.811 **Combined forms of age-related cataract, right eye** Ⓐ

   H25.812 **Combined forms of age-related cataract, left eye** Ⓐ

   H25.813 **Combined forms of age-related cataract, bilateral** Ⓐ

   H25.819 **Combined forms of age-related cataract, unspecified eye** Ⓐ

  H25.89 Other **age-related cataract** Ⓐ

H25.9 Unspecified **age-related cataract** Ⓐ

√4ᵗʰ **H26** **Other cataract**

  EXCLUDES 1 congenital cataract (Q12.0)

  √5ᵗʰ **H26.0** **Infantile and juvenile cataract**

    √6ᵗʰ **H26.00** Unspecified in**fantile and juvenile cataract**

   H26.001 **Unspecified infantile and juvenile cataract, right eye** Ⓟ

   H26.002 **Unspecified infantile and juvenile cataract, left eye** Ⓟ

   H26.003 **Unspecified infantile and juvenile cataract, bilateral** Ⓟ

   H26.009 **Unspecified infantile and juvenile cataract, unspecified eye** Ⓟ

    √6ᵗʰ **H26.01** **Infantile and juvenile cortical, lamellar, or zonular cataract**

   H26.011 **Infantile and juvenile cortical, lamellar, or zonular cataract, right eye** Ⓟ

   H26.012 **Infantile and juvenile cortical, lamellar, or zonular cataract, left eye** Ⓟ

   H26.013 **Infantile and juvenile cortical, lamellar, or zonular cataract, bilateral** Ⓟ

   H26.019 **Infantile and juvenile cortical, lamellar, or zonular cataract, unspecified eye** Ⓟ

    √6ᵗʰ **H26.03** **Infantile and juvenile nuclear cataract**

   H26.031 **Infantile and juvenile nuclear cataract, right eye** Ⓟ

   H26.032 **Infantile and juvenile nuclear cataract, left eye** Ⓟ

   H26.033 **Infantile and juvenile nuclear cataract, bilateral** Ⓟ

   H26.039 **Infantile and juvenile nuclear cataract, unspecified eye** Ⓟ

    √6ᵗʰ **H26.04** **Anterior subcapsular polar infantile and juvenile cataract**

   H26.041 **Anterior subcapsular polar infantile and juvenile cataract, right eye** Ⓟ

   H26.042 **Anterior subcapsular polar infantile and juvenile cataract, left eye** Ⓟ

   H26.043 **Anterior subcapsular polar infantile and juvenile cataract, bilateral** Ⓟ

   H26.049 **Anterior subcapsular polar infantile and juvenile cataract, unspecified eye** Ⓟ

    √6ᵗʰ **H26.05** **Posterior subcapsular polar infantile and juvenile cataract**

   H26.051 **Posterior subcapsular polar infantile and juvenile cataract, right eye** Ⓟ

   H26.052 **Posterior subcapsular polar infantile and juvenile cataract, left eye** Ⓟ

   H26.053 **Posterior subcapsular polar infantile and juvenile cataract, bilateral** Ⓟ

   H26.059 **Posterior subcapsular polar infantile and juvenile cataract, unspecified eye** Ⓟ

    √6ᵗʰ **H26.06** **Combined forms** of infantile and juvenile cataract

   H26.061 **Combined forms of infantile and juvenile cataract, right eye** Ⓟ

   H26.062 **Combined forms of infantile and juvenile cataract, left eye** Ⓟ

   H26.063 **Combined forms of infantile and juvenile cataract, bilateral** Ⓟ

   H26.069 **Combined forms of infantile and juvenile cataract, unspecified eye** Ⓟ

    H26.09 Other **infantile and juvenile cataract** Ⓟ

√5ᵗʰ **H26.1** **Traumatic cataract**

  Use additional code (Chapter 20) to identify external cause

  √6ᵗʰ **H26.10** **Unspecified traumatic cataract**

   H26.101 **Unspecified traumatic cataract, right eye**

   H26.102 **Unspecified traumatic cataract, left eye**

   H26.103 **Unspecified traumatic cataract, bilateral**

   H26.109 **Unspecified traumatic cataract, unspecified eye**

  √6ᵗʰ **H26.11** **Localized traumatic opacities**

   H26.111 **Localized traumatic opacities, right eye**

   H26.112 **Localized traumatic opacities, left eye**

   H26.113 **Localized traumatic opacities, bilateral**

   H26.119 **Localized traumatic opacities, unspecified eye**

  √6ᵗʰ **H26.12** **Partially resolved traumatic cataract**

   H26.121 **Partially resolved traumatic cataract, right eye**

   H26.122 **Partially resolved traumatic cataract, left eye**

   H26.123 **Partially resolved traumatic cataract, bilateral**

   H26.129 **Partially resolved traumatic cataract, unspecified eye**

  √6ᵗʰ **H26.13** **Total traumatic cataract**

   H26.131 **Total traumatic cataract, right eye**

   H26.132 **Total traumatic cataract, left eye**

   H26.133 **Total traumatic cataract, bilateral**

   H26.139 **Total traumatic cataract, unspecified eye**

√5ᵗʰ **H26.2** **Complicated cataract**

  H26.20 **Unspecified complicated cataract**

    Cataracta complicata NOS

  √6ᵗʰ **H26.21** **Cataract with neovascularization**

    Code also associated condition, such as:

      chronic iridocyclitis (H20.1-)

   H26.211 **Cataract with neovascularization, right eye**

   H26.212 **Cataract with neovascularization, left eye**

   H26.213 **Cataract with neovascularization, bilateral**

   H26.219 **Cataract with neovascularization, unspecified eye**

  √6ᵗʰ **H26.22** **Cataract secondary to ocular disorders (degenerative) (inflammatory)**

    Code also associated ocular disorder

   H26.221 **Cataract secondary to ocular disorders (degenerative) (inflammatory), right eye**

   H26.222 **Cataract secondary to ocular disorders (degenerative) (inflammatory), left eye**

   H26.223 **Cataract secondary to ocular disorders (degenerative) (inflammatory), bilateral**

   H26.229 **Cataract secondary to ocular disorders (degenerative) (inflammatory), unspecified eye**

  √6ᵗʰ **H26.23** **Glaucomatous flecks (subcapsular)**

    Code first underlying glaucoma (H40-H42)

   H26.231 **Glaucomatous flecks (subcapsular), right eye**

   H26.232 **Glaucomatous flecks (subcapsular), left eye**

   H26.233 **Glaucomatous flecks (subcapsular), bilateral**

   H26.239 **Glaucomatous flecks (subcapsular), unspecified eye**

√5ᵗʰ **H26.3** **Drug-induced cataract**

  Toxic cataract

  Use additional code for adverse effect, if applicable, to identify drug (T36-T50 with fifth or sixth character 5)

  H26.30 **Drug-induced cataract, unspecified eye**

  H26.31 **Drug-induced cataract, right eye**

  H26.32 **Drug-induced cataract, left eye**

  H26.33 **Drug-induced cataract, bilateral**

√5ᵗʰ **H26.4** **Secondary cataract**

  H26.40 **Unspecified secondary cataract**

  √6ᵗʰ **H26.41** **Soemmering's ring**

   H26.411 **Soemmering's ring, right eye**

   H26.412 **Soemmering's ring, left eye**

Chapter 7. Diseases of the Eye and Adnexa

H26.413   **Soemmering's ring**, bilateral
H26.419   **Soemmering's ring**, unspecified eye

✓6ᵗʰ **H26.49 Other secondary cataract**
H26.491   **Other secondary cataract**, right eye
H26.492   **Other secondary cataract**, left eye
H26.493   **Other secondary cataract**, bilateral
H26.499   **Other secondary cataract**, unspecified eye

H26.8 Other specified cataract
H26.9 Unspecified cataract

✓4ᵗʰ **H27 Other disorders of lens**
    EXCLUDES 1   *congenital lens malformations (Q12.-)*
        mechanical complications of intraocular lens implant (T85.2)
        pseudophakia (Z96.1)

✓5ᵗʰ **H27.0 Aphakia**
    Acquired absence of lens
    Acquired aphakia
    Aphakia due to trauma
      EXCLUDES 1   *cataract extraction status (Z98.4-)*
          congenital absence of lens (Q12.3)
          congenital aphakia (Q12.3)

H27.00   **Aphakia, unspecified eye**
H27.01   **Aphakia, right eye**
H27.02   **Aphakia, left eye**
H27.03   **Aphakia, bilateral**

✓5ᵗʰ **H27.1 Dislocation of lens**
H27.10   **Unspecified dislocation of lens**

    ✓6ᵗʰ **H27.11 Subluxation of lens**
H27.111   **Subluxation of lens**, right eye
H27.112   **Subluxation of lens**, left eye
H27.113   **Subluxation of lens**, bilateral
H27.119   **Subluxation of lens**, unspecified eye

    ✓6ᵗʰ **H27.12 Anterior dislocation of lens**
H27.121   **Anterior dislocation of lens**, right eye
H27.122   **Anterior dislocation of lens**, left eye
H27.123   **Anterior dislocation of lens**, bilateral
H27.129   **Anterior dislocation of lens**, unspecified eye

    ✓6ᵗʰ **H27.13 Posterior dislocation of lens**
H27.131   **Posterior dislocation of lens**, right eye
H27.132   **Posterior dislocation of lens**, left eye
H27.133   **Posterior dislocation of lens**, bilateral
H27.139   **Posterior dislocation of lens**, unspecified eye

H27.8 Other specified disorders of lens
H27.9 Unspecified disorder of lens

H28 Cataract in diseases classified elsewhere
    Code first underlying disease, such as:
      hypoparathyroidism (E20.-)
      myotonia (G71.1-)
      myxedema (E03.-)
      protein-calorie malnutrition (E40-E46)
      EXCLUDES 1   *cataract in diabetes mellitus (E08.36, E09.36, E10.36, E11.36, E13.36)*

Disorders of choroid and retina (H30-H36)

✓4ᵗʰ **H30 Chorioretinal inflammation**

    CC Excl: For CC codes in category H30, unless otherwise noted:
    H30.001-H30.93

✓5ᵗʰ **H30.0 Focal chorioretinal inflammation**
    Focal chorioretinitis
    Focal choroiditis
    Focal retinitis
    Focal retinochoroiditis

    ✓6ᵗʰ **H30.00 Unspecified focal chorioretinal inflammation**
    Focal chorioretinitis NOS
    Focal choroiditis NOS
    Focal retinitis NOS
    Focal retinochoroiditis NOS
H30.001   **Unspecified focal chorioretinal inflammation**, right eye
H30.002   **Unspecified focal chorioretinal inflammation**, left eye
H30.003   **Unspecified focal chorioretinal inflammation**, bilateral

H30.009   **Unspecified focal chorioretinal inflammation**, unspecified eye

✓6ᵗʰ **H30.01 Focal chorioretinal inflammation, juxtapapillary**
H30.011   **Focal chorioretinal inflammation, juxtapapillary**, right eye
H30.012   **Focal chorioretinal inflammation, juxtapapillary**, left eye
H30.013   **Focal chorioretinal inflammation, juxtapapillary**, bilateral
H30.019   **Focal chorioretinal inflammation, juxtapapillary**, unspecified eye

✓6ᵗʰ **H30.02 Focal chorioretinal inflammation of posterior pole**
H30.021   **Focal chorioretinal inflammation of posterior pole**, right eye
H30.022   **Focal chorioretinal inflammation of posterior pole**, left eye
H30.023   **Focal chorioretinal inflammation of posterior pole**, bilateral
H30.029   **Focal chorioretinal inflammation of posterior pole**, unspecified eye

✓6ᵗʰ **H30.03 Focal chorioretinal inflammation, peripheral**
H30.031   **Focal chorioretinal inflammation, peripheral**, right eye
H30.032   **Focal chorioretinal inflammation, peripheral**, left eye
H30.033   **Focal chorioretinal inflammation, peripheral**, bilateral
H30.039   **Focal chorioretinal inflammation, peripheral**, unspecified eye

✓6ᵗʰ **H30.04 Focal chorioretinal inflammation, macular or paramacular**
H30.041   **Focal chorioretinal inflammation, macular or paramacular**, right eye
H30.042   **Focal chorioretinal inflammation, macular or paramacular**, left eye
H30.043   **Focal chorioretinal inflammation, macular or paramacular**, bilateral
H30.049   **Focal chorioretinal inflammation, macular or paramacular**, unspecified eye

✓5ᵗʰ **H30.1 Disseminated chorioretinal inflammation**
    Disseminated chorioretinitis
    Disseminated choroiditis
    Disseminated retinitis
    Disseminated retinochoroiditis
      EXCLUDES 2   *exudative retinopathy (H35.02-)*

    ✓6ᵗʰ **H30.10 Unspecified disseminated chorioretinal inflammation**
    Disseminated chorioretinitis NOS
    Disseminated choroiditis NOS
    Disseminated retinitis NOS
    Disseminated retinochoroiditis NOS
H30.101   **Unspecified disseminated chorioretinal inflammation**, right eye   CC
H30.102   **Unspecified disseminated chorioretinal inflammation**, left eye   CC
H30.103   **Unspecified disseminated chorioretinal inflammation**, bilateral   CC
H30.109   **Unspecified disseminated chorioretinal inflammation**, unspecified eye   CC

    ✓6ᵗʰ **H30.11 Disseminated chorioretinal inflammation of posterior pole**
H30.111   **Disseminated chorioretinal inflammation of posterior pole**, right eye   CC
H30.112   **Disseminated chorioretinal inflammation of posterior pole**, left eye   CC
H30.113   **Disseminated chorioretinal inflammation of posterior pole**, bilateral   CC
H30.119   **Disseminated chorioretinal inflammation of posterior pole**, unspecified eye   CC

    ✓6ᵗʰ **H30.12 Disseminated chorioretinal inflammation, peripheral**
H30.121   **Disseminated chorioretinal inflammation, peripheral** right eye   CC

N Newborn: 0   P Pediatric: 0-17   M Maternity: 12-55   A Adult: 15-124   MCC Major CC Condition   PDxMCC PDx acts as own MCC   CC CC Condition   PDxCC PDx acts as own CC

576   ICD-10-CM 2016

H30.122 **Disseminated chorioretinal inflammation, peripheral, left eye** `CC`

H30.123 **Disseminated chorioretinal inflammation, peripheral, bilateral** `CC`

H30.129 **Disseminated chorioretinal inflammation, peripheral, unspecified eye** `CC`

✓6ᵗʰ **H30.13 Disseminated chorioretinal inflammation, generalized**

H30.131 **Disseminated chorioretinal inflammation, generalized, right eye** `CC`

H30.132 **Disseminated chorioretinal inflammation, generalized, left eye** `CC`

H30.133 **Disseminated chorioretinal inflammation, generalized, bilateral** `CC`

H30.139 **Disseminated chorioretinal inflammation, generalized, unspecified eye** `CC`

✓6ᵗʰ **H30.14 Acute posterior multifocal placoid pigment epitheliopathy**

H30.141 **Acute posterior multifocal placoid pigment epitheliopathy, right eye** `CC`

H30.142 **Acute posterior multifocal placoid pigment epitheliopathy, left eye** `CC`

H30.143 **Acute posterior multifocal placoid pigment epitheliopathy, bilateral** `CC`

H30.149 **Acute posterior multifocal placoid pigment epitheliopathy, unspecified eye** `CC`

✓5ᵗʰ **H30.2 Posterior cyclitis**
Pars planitis

H30.20 **Posterior cyclitis, unspecified eye**

H30.21 **Posterior cyclitis, right eye**

H30.22 **Posterior cyclitis, left eye**

H30.23 **Posterior cyclitis, bilateral**

✓5ᵗʰ **H30.8 Other chorioretinal inflammations**

✓6ᵗʰ **H30.81 Harada's disease**

H30.811 **Harada's disease, right eye**

H30.812 **Harada's disease, left eye**

H30.813 **Harada's disease, bilateral**

H30.819 **Harada's disease, unspecified eye**

✓6ᵗʰ **H30.89 Other chorioretinal inflammations**

H30.891 **Other chorioretinal inflammations, right eye** `CC`

H30.892 **Other chorioretinal inflammations, left eye** `CC`

H30.893 **Other chorioretinal inflammations, bilateral** `CC`

H30.899 **Other chorioretinal inflammations, unspecified eye** `CC`

✓5ᵗʰ **H30.9 Unspecified chorioretinal inflammation**
Chorioretinitis NOS
Choroiditis NOS
Neuroretinitis NOS
Retinitis NOS
Retinochoroiditis NOS

H30.90 **Unspecified chorioretinal inflammation, unspecified eye** `CC`

H30.91 **Unspecified chorioretinal inflammation, right eye** `CC`

H30.92 **Unspecified chorioretinal inflammation, left eye** `CC`

H30.93 **Unspecified chorioretinal inflammation, bilateral** `CC`

✓4ᵗʰ **H31 Other disorders of choroid**

CC Excl: For CC codes in category H31, unless otherwise noted:
H31.301-H32

✓5ᵗʰ **H31.0 Chorioretinal scars**
EXCLUDES 2   *postsurgical chorioretinal scars (H59.81-)*

✓6ᵗʰ **H31.00 Unspecified chorioretinal scars**

H31.001 **Unspecified chorioretinal scars, right eye**

H31.002 **Unspecified chorioretinal scars, left eye**

H31.003 **Unspecified chorioretinal scars, bilateral**

H31.009 **Unspecified chorioretinal scars, unspecified eye**

✓6ᵗʰ **H31.01 Macula scars of posterior pole (postinflammatory) (post-traumatic)**
EXCLUDES 1   *postprocedural chorioretinal scar (H59.81-)*

H31.011 **Macula scars of posterior pole (postinflammatory) (post-traumatic), right eye**

H31.012 **Macula scars of posterior pole (postinflammatory) (post-traumatic), left eye**

H31.013 **Macula scars of posterior pole (postinflammatory) (post-traumatic), bilateral**

H31.019 **Macula scars of posterior pole (postinflammatory) (post-traumatic), unspecified eye**

✓6ᵗʰ **H31.02 Solar retinopathy**

H31.021 **Solar retinopathy, right eye**

H31.022 **Solar retinopathy, left eye**

H31.023 **Solar retinopathy, bilateral**

H31.029 **Solar retinopathy, unspecified eye**

✓6ᵗʰ **H31.09 Other chorioretinal scars**

H31.091 **Other chorioretinal scars, right eye**

H31.092 **Other chorioretinal scars, left eye**

H31.093 **Other chorioretinal scars, bilateral**

H31.099 **Other chorioretinal scars, unspecified eye**

✓5ᵗʰ **H31.1 Choroidal degeneration**
EXCLUDES 2   *angioid streaks of macula (H35.33)*

✓6ᵗʰ **H31.10 Unspecified choroidal degeneration**
Choroidal sclerosis NOS

H31.101 **Choroidal degeneration, unspecified, right eye**

H31.102 **Choroidal degeneration, unspecified, left eye**

H31.103 **Choroidal degeneration, unspecified, bilateral**

H31.109 **Choroidal degeneration, unspecified, unspecified eye**

✓6ᵗʰ **H31.11 Age-related choroidal atrophy**

H31.111 **Age-related choroidal atrophy, right eye** `A`

H31.112 **Age-related choroidal atrophy, left eye** `A`

H31.113 **Age-related choroidal atrophy, bilateral** `A`

H31.119 **Age-related choroidal atrophy, unspecified eye** `A`

✓6ᵗʰ **H31.12 Diffuse secondary atrophy of choroid**

H31.121 **Diffuse secondary atrophy of choroid, right eye**

H31.122 **Diffuse secondary atrophy of choroid, left eye**

H31.123 **Diffuse secondary atrophy of choroid, bilateral**

H31.129 **Diffuse secondary atrophy of choroid, unspecified eye**

✓5ᵗʰ **H31.2 Hereditary choroidal dystrophy**
EXCLUDES 2   *hyperornithinemia (E72.4)*
           ornithinemia (E72.4)

H31.20 **Hereditary choroidal dystrophy, unspecified**

H31.21 **Choroideremia**

H31.22 **Choroidal dystrophy (central areolar) (generalized) (peripapillary)**

H31.23 **Gyrate atrophy, choroid**

H31.29 **Other hereditary choroidal dystrophy**

✓5ᵗʰ **H31.3 Choroidal hemorrhage and rupture**

✓6ᵗʰ **H31.30 Unspecified choroidal hemorrhage**

H31.301 **Unspecified choroidal hemorrhage, right eye**

H31.302 **Unspecified choroidal hemorrhage, left eye**

H31.303 **Unspecified choroidal hemorrhage, bilateral**

H31.309 **Unspecified choroidal hemorrhage, unspecified eye**

✓6ᵗʰ **H31.31 Expulsive choroidal hemorrhage**

H31.311 **Expulsive choroidal hemorrhage, right eye**

H31.312 **Expulsive choroidal hemorrhage, left eye**

✓ Additional Character Required   ✗7ᵗʰ Placeholder Alert   Unacceptable PDx   Manifestation   Hospital Acquired Condition   *EXCLUDES 1* Not Coded Here   *EXCLUDES 2* Not Included Here

Chapter 7. Diseases of the Eye and Adnexa

H31.313   **Expulsive choroidal hemorrhage,** bilateral

H31.319   **Expulsive choroidal hemorrhage,** unspecified eye

✓6ᵗʰ **H31.32**   **Choroidal rupture**

H31.321   **Choroidal rupture,** right eye   `CC`

H31.322   **Choroidal rupture,** left eye   `CC`

H31.323   **Choroidal rupture,** bilateral   `CC`

H31.329   **Choroidal rupture,** unspecified eye   `CC`

✓5ᵗʰ **H31.4**   **Choroidal detachment**

✓6ᵗʰ **H31.40**   **Unspecified choroidal detachment**

H31.401   **Unspecified choroidal detachment,** right eye   `CC`

H31.402   **Unspecified choroidal detachment,** left eye   `CC`

H31.403   **Unspecified choroidal detachment,** bilateral   `CC`

H31.409   **Unspecified choroidal detachment,** unspecified eye   `CC`

✓6ᵗʰ **H31.41**   **Hemorrhagic choroidal detachment**

H31.411   **Hemorrhagic choroidal detachment,** right eye   `CC`

H31.412   **Hemorrhagic choroidal detachment,** left eye   `CC`

H31.413   **Hemorrhagic choroidal detachment,** bilateral   `CC`

H31.419   **Hemorrhagic choroidal detachment,** unspecified eye   `CC`

✓6ᵗʰ **H31.42**   **Serous choroidal detachment**

H31.421   **Serous choroidal detachment,** right eye   `CC`

H31.422   **Serous choroidal detachment,** left eye   `CC`

H31.423   **Serous choroidal detachment,** bilateral   `CC`

H31.429   **Serous choroidal detachment,** unspecified eye   `CC`

H31.8   **Other specified disorders of choroid**

H31.9   **Unspecified disorder of choroid**

H32   ***Chorioretinal disorders in diseases classified elsewhere***

Code first underlying disease, such as:
congenital toxoplasmosis (P37.1)
histoplasmosis (B39.-)
leprosy (A30.-)

EXCLUDES 1   *chorioretinitis (in):*
toxoplasmosis (acquired) (B58.01)
tuberculosis (A18.53)

✓4ᵗʰ **H33**   **Retinal detachments and breaks**

> **CC Excl: For CC codes in category H33, unless otherwise noted:**
> H33.001-H33.119, H33.191-H33.8, H35.70-H35.739

EXCLUDES 1   *detachment of retinal pigment epithelium (H35.72-, H35.73-)*

✓5ᵗʰ **H33.0**   **Retinal detachment with retinal break**

Rhegmatogenous retinal detachment

EXCLUDES 1   *serous retinal detachment (without retinal break) (H33.2-)*

✓6ᵗʰ **H33.00**   **Unspecified retinal detachment with retinal break**

H33.001   **Unspecified retinal detachment with retinal break,** right eye

H33.002   **Unspecified retinal detachment with retinal break,** left eye

H33.003   **Unspecified retinal detachment with retinal break,** bilateral

H33.009   **Unspecified retinal detachment with retinal break,** unspecified eye

✓6ᵗʰ **H33.01**   **Retinal detachment with single break**

H33.011   **Retinal detachment with single break,** right eye

H33.012   **Retinal detachment with single break,** left eye

H33.013   **Retinal detachment with single break,** bilateral

H33.019   **Retinal detachment with single break,** unspecified eye

✓6ᵗʰ **H33.02**   **Retinal detachment with multiple breaks**

H33.021   **Retinal detachment with multiple breaks,** right eye

H33.022   **Retinal detachment with multiple breaks,** left eye

H33.023   **Retinal detachment with multiple breaks,** bilateral

H33.029   **Retinal detachment with multiple breaks,** unspecified eye

✓6ᵗʰ **H33.03**   **Retinal detachment with** giant retinal tear

H33.031   **Retinal detachment with giant retinal tear,** right eye

H33.032   **Retinal detachment with giant retinal tear,** left eye

H33.033   **Retinal detachment with giant retinal tear,** bilateral

H33.039   **Retinal detachment with giant retinal tear,** unspecified eye

✓6ᵗʰ **H33.04**   **Retinal detachment with** retinal dialysis

H33.041   **Retinal detachment with retinal dialysis,** right eye

H33.042   **Retinal detachment with retinal dialysis,** left eye

H33.043   **Retinal detachment with retinal dialysis,** bilateral

H33.049   **Retinal detachment with retinal dialysis,** unspecified eye

✓6ᵗʰ **H33.05**   **Total** retinal detachment

H33.051   **Total retinal detachment,** right eye

H33.052   **Total retinal detachment,** left eye

H33.053   **Total retinal detachment,** bilateral

H33.059   **Total retinal detachment,** unspecified eye

✓5ᵗʰ **H33.1**   **Retinoschisis and retinal cysts**

EXCLUDES 1   *congenital retinoschisis (Q14.1)*
microcystoid degeneration of retina (H35.42-)

✓6ᵗʰ **H33.10**   **Unspecified retinoschisis**

H33.101   **Unspecified retinoschisis,** right eye

H33.102   **Unspecified retinoschisis,** left eye

H33.103   **Unspecified retinoschisis,** bilateral

H33.109   **Unspecified retinoschisis,** unspecified eye

✓6ᵗʰ **H33.11**   **Cyst of ora serrata**

H33.111   **Cyst of ora serrata,** right eye

H33.112   **Cyst of ora serrata,** left eye

H33.113   **Cyst of ora serrata,** bilateral

H33.119   **Cyst of ora serrata,** unspecified eye

✓6ᵗʰ **H33.12**   **Parasitic cyst of retina**

> **CC Excl: For CC codes in subcategory H33.12, unless otherwise noted:** H20.051-H20.059, H21.331-H21.339, H33.121-H33.129, H44.001-H44.029, H44.121-H44.129, H44.19

H33.121   **Parasitic cyst of retina,** right eye   `CC`

H33.122   **Parasitic cyst of retina,** left eye   `CC`

H33.123   **Parasitic cyst of retina,** bilateral   `CC`

H33.129   **Parasitic cyst of retina,** unspecified eye   `CC`

✓6ᵗʰ **H33.19**   **Other retinoschisis and retinal cysts**

Pseudocyst of retina

H33.191   **Other retinoschisis and retinal cysts,** right eye

H33.192   **Other retinoschisis and retinal cysts,** left eye

H33.193   **Other retinoschisis and retinal cysts,** bilateral

H33.199   **Other retinoschisis and retinal cysts,** unspecified eye

✓5ᵗʰ **H33.2**   **Serous retinal detachment**

Retinal detachment NOS

Retinal detachment without retinal break

EXCLUDES 1   *central serous chorioretinopathy (H35.71-)*

H33.20   **Serous retinal detachment,** unspecified eye   `CC`

H33.21   **Serous retinal detachment,** right eye   `CC`

H33.22   **Serous retinal detachment,** left eye   `CC`

H33.23   **Serous retinal detachment,** bilateral   `CC`

Ⓝ Newborn: 0   Ⓟ Pediatric: 0-17   Ⓜ Maternity: 12-55   Ⓐ Adult: 15-124   **MCC** Major CC Condition   **PDxMCC** PDx acts as own MCC   **CC** CC Condition   **PDxCC** PDx acts as own CC

578   ICD-10-CM 2016

Chapter 7. Diseases of the Eye and Adnexa

✓5ᵗʰ **H33.3 Retinal breaks without detachment**
    EXCLUDES 1   chorioretinal scars after surgery for detachment
         (H59.81-)
         peripheral retinal degeneration without break (H35.4-)

    ✓6ᵗʰ **H33.30 Unspecified retinal break**
       H33.301   **Unspecified retinal break, right eye**
       H33.302   **Unspecified retinal break, left eye**
       H33.303   **Unspecified retinal break, bilateral**
       H33.309   **Unspecified retinal break, unspecified eye**

    ✓6ᵗʰ **H33.31 Horseshoe tear of retina without detachment**
       Operculum of retina without detachment
       H33.311   **Horseshoe tear of retina without detachment, right eye**
       H33.312   **Horseshoe tear of retina without detachment, left eye**
       H33.313   **Horseshoe tear of retina without detachment, bilateral**
       H33.319   **Horseshoe tear of retina without detachment, unspecified eye**

    ✓6ᵗʰ **H33.32 Round hole of retina without detachment**
       H33.321   **Round hole, right eye**
       H33.322   **Round hole, left eye**
       H33.323   **Round hole, bilateral**
       H33.329   **Round hole, unspecified eye**

    ✓6ᵗʰ **H33.33 Multiple defects of retina without detachment**
       H33.331   **Multiple defects of retina without detachment, right eye**
       H33.332   **Multiple defects of retina without detachment, left eye**
       H33.333   **Multiple defects of retina without detachment, bilateral**
       H33.339   **Multiple defects of retina without detachment, unspecified eye**

✓5ᵗʰ **H33.4 Traction detachment of retina**
     Proliferative vitreo-retinopathy with retinal detachment
    H33.40   **Traction detachment of retina, unspecified eye** CC
    H33.41   **Traction detachment of retina, right eye** CC
    H33.42   **Traction detachment of retina, left eye** CC
    H33.43   **Traction detachment of retina, bilateral** CC

    H33.8 Other retinal detachments CC

✓4ᵗʰ **H34 Retinal vascular occlusions**

    CC Excl: For CC codes in category H34, unless otherwise noted:
    G45.3, H34.00-H34.9

    EXCLUDES 1   amaurosis fugax (G45.3)

✓5ᵗʰ **H34.0 Transient retinal artery occlusion**
    H34.00   **Transient retinal artery occlusion, unspecified eye** CC
    H34.01   **Transient retinal artery occlusion, right eye** CC
    H34.02   **Transient retinal artery occlusion, left eye** CC
    H34.03   **Transient retinal artery occlusion, bilateral** CC

✓5ᵗʰ **H34.1 Central retinal artery occlusion**
    H34.10   **Central retinal artery occlusion, unspecified eye** CC
    H34.11   **Central retinal artery occlusion, right eye** CC
    H34.12   **Central retinal artery occlusion, left eye** CC
    H34.13   **Central retinal artery occlusion, bilateral** CC

✓5ᵗʰ **H34.2 Other retinal artery occlusions**
    ✓6ᵗʰ **H34.21 Partial retinal artery occlusion**
      Hollenhorst's plaque
      Retinal microembolism
      H34.211   **Partial retinal artery occlusion, right eye** CC
      H34.212   **Partial retinal artery occlusion, left eye** CC
      H34.213   **Partial retinal artery occlusion, bilateral** CC
      H34.219   **Partial retinal artery occlusion, unspecified eye** CC

    ✓6ᵗʰ **H34.23 Retinal artery branch occlusion**
      H34.231   **Retinal artery branch occlusion, right eye** CC
      H34.232   **Retinal artery branch occlusion, left eye** CC
      H34.233   **Retinal artery branch occlusion, bilateral** CC

    H34.239   **Retinal artery branch occlusion, unspecified eye** CC

✓5ᵗʰ **H34.8 Other retinal vascular occlusions**
    ✓6ᵗʰ **H34.81 Central retinal vein occlusion**
      H34.811   **Central retinal vein occlusion, right eye** CC
      H34.812   **Central retinal vein occlusion, left eye** CC
      H34.813   **Central retinal vein occlusion, bilateral** CC
      H34.819   **Central retinal vein occlusion, unspecified eye** CC

    ✓6ᵗʰ **H34.82 Venous engorgement**
      Incipient retinal vein occlusion
      Partial retinal vein occlusion
      H34.821   **Venous engorgement, right eye**
      H34.822   **Venous engorgement, left eye**
      H34.823   **Venous engorgement, bilateral**
      H34.829   **Venous engorgement, unspecified eye**

    ✓6ᵗʰ **H34.83 Tributary (branch) retinal vein occlusion**
      H34.831   **Tributary (branch) retinal vein occlusion, right eye**
      H34.832   **Tributary (branch) retinal vein occlusion, left eye**
      H34.833   **Tributary (branch) retinal vein occlusion, bilateral**
      H34.839   **Tributary (branch) retinal vein occlusion, unspecified eye**

    H34.9 Unspecified retinal vascular occlusion CC

✓4ᵗʰ **H35 Other retinal disorders**
    EXCLUDES 2   diabetic retinal disorders (E08.311- E08.359, E09.311- E09.359, E10.311- E10.359, E11.311- E11.359, E13.311- E13.359)

✓5ᵗʰ **H35.0 Background retinopathy and retinal vascular changes**
    Code also any associated hypertension (I10.-)
    H35.00 Unspecified background retinopathy

    ✓6ᵗʰ **H35.01 Changes in retinal vascular appearance**
      Retinal vascular sheathing
      H35.011   **Changes in retinal vascular appearance, right eye**
      H35.012   **Changes in retinal vascular appearance, left eye**
      H35.013   **Changes in retinal vascular appearance, bilateral**
      H35.019   **Changes in retinal vascular appearance, unspecified eye**

    ✓6ᵗʰ **H35.02 Exudative retinopathy**
      Coats retinopathy
      H35.021   **Exudative retinopathy, right eye**
      H35.022   **Exudative retinopathy, left eye**
      H35.023   **Exudative retinopathy, bilateral**
      H35.029   **Exudative retinopathy, unspecified eye**

    ✓6ᵗʰ **H35.03 Hypertensive retinopathy**
      H35.031   **Hypertensive retinopathy, right eye**
      H35.032   **Hypertensive retinopathy, left eye**
      H35.033   **Hypertensive retinopathy, bilateral**
      H35.039   **Hypertensive retinopathy, unspecified eye**

    ✓6ᵗʰ **H35.04 Retinal micro-aneurysms, unspecified**
      H35.041   **Retinal micro-aneurysms, unspecified, right eye**
      H35.042   **Retinal micro-aneurysms, unspecified, left eye**
      H35.043   **Retinal micro-aneurysms, unspecified, bilateral**
      H35.049   **Retinal micro-aneurysms, unspecified, unspecified eye**

    ✓6ᵗʰ **H35.05 Retinal neovascularization, unspecified**
      H35.051   **Retinal neovascularization, unspecified, right eye**
      H35.052   **Retinal neovascularization, unspecified, left eye**
      H35.053   **Retinal neovascularization, unspecified, bilateral**
      H35.059   **Retinal neovascularization, unspecified, unspecified eye**

✓ Additional Character Required   ✓x7ᵗʰ Placeholder Alert   Unacceptable PDx   Manifestation   Hospital Acquired Condition   *EXCLUDES 1* Not Coded Here   *EXCLUDES 2* Not Included Here

Chapter 7. Diseases of the Eye and Adnexa

✓6ᵗʰ **H35.06** **Retinal vasculitis**
Eales disease
Retinal perivasculitis
H35.061 **Retinal vasculitis, right eye**
H35.062 **Retinal vasculitis, left eye**
H35.063 **Retinal vasculitis, bilateral**
H35.069 **Retinal vasculitis, unspecified eye**

✓6ᵗʰ **H35.07** **Retinal telangiectasis**
H35.071 **Retinal telangiectasis, right eye**
H35.072 **Retinal telangiectasis, left eye**
H35.073 **Retinal telangiectasis, bilateral**
H35.079 **Retinal telangiectasis, unspecified eye**

H35.09 **Other intraretinal microvascular abnormalities**
Retinal varices

✓5ᵗʰ **H35.1** **Retinopathy of prematurity**

✓6ᵗʰ **H35.10** **Retinopathy of prematurity, unspecified**
Retinopathy of prematurity NOS
H35.101 **Retinopathy of prematurity, unspecified, right eye**
H35.102 **Retinopathy of prematurity, unspecified, left eye**
H35.103 **Retinopathy of prematurity, unspecified, bilateral**
H35.109 **Retinopathy of prematurity, unspecified, unspecified eye**

✓6ᵗʰ **H35.11** **Retinopathy of prematurity, stage 0**
H35.111 **Retinopathy of prematurity, stage 0, right eye**
H35.112 **Retinopathy of prematurity, stage 0, left eye**
H35.113 **Retinopathy of prematurity, stage 0, bilateral**
H35.119 **Retinopathy of prematurity, stage 0, unspecified eye**

✓6ᵗʰ **H35.12** **Retinopathy of prematurity, stage 1**
H35.121 **Retinopathy of prematurity, stage 1, right eye**
H35.122 **Retinopathy of prematurity, stage 1, left eye**
H35.123 **Retinopathy of prematurity, stage 1, bilateral**
H35.129 **Retinopathy of prematurity, stage 1, unspecified eye**

✓6ᵗʰ **H35.13** **Retinopathy of prematurity, stage 2**
H35.131 **Retinopathy of prematurity, stage 2, right eye**
H35.132 **Retinopathy of prematurity, stage 2, left eye**
H35.133 **Retinopathy of prematurity, stage 2, bilateral**
H35.139 **Retinopathy of prematurity, stage 2, unspecified eye**

✓6ᵗʰ **H35.14** **Retinopathy of prematurity, stage 3**
H35.141 **Retinopathy of prematurity, stage 3, right eye**
H35.142 **Retinopathy of prematurity, stage 3, left eye**
H35.143 **Retinopathy of prematurity, stage 3, bilateral**
H35.149 **Retinopathy of prematurity, stage 3, unspecified eye**

✓6ᵗʰ **H35.15** **Retinopathy of prematurity, stage 4**
H35.151 **Retinopathy of prematurity, stage 4, right eye**
H35.152 **Retinopathy of prematurity, stage 4, left eye**
H35.153 **Retinopathy of prematurity, stage 4, bilateral**
H35.159 **Retinopathy of prematurity, stage 4, unspecified eye**

✓6ᵗʰ **H35.16** **Retinopathy of prematurity, stage 5**
H35.161 **Retinopathy of prematurity, stage 5, right eye**
H35.162 **Retinopathy of prematurity, stage 5, left eye**
H35.163 **Retinopathy of prematurity, stage 5, bilateral**

H35.169 **Retinopathy of prematurity, stage 5, unspecified eye**

✓6ᵗʰ **H35.17** **Retrolental fibroplasia**
H35.171 **Retrolental fibroplasia, right eye**
H35.172 **Retrolental fibroplasia, left eye**
H35.173 **Retrolental fibroplasia, bilateral**
H35.179 **Retrolental fibroplasia, unspecified eye**

✓5ᵗʰ **H35.2** **Other non-diabetic proliferative retinopathy**
Proliferative vitreo-retinopathy
EXCLUDES 1 *proliferative vitreo-retinopathy with retinal detachment (H33.4-)*
H35.20 **Other non-diabetic proliferative retinopathy, unspecified eye**
H35.21 **Other non-diabetic proliferative retinopathy, right eye**
H35.22 **Other non-diabetic proliferative retinopathy, left eye**
H35.23 **Other non-diabetic proliferative retinopathy, bilateral**

✓5ᵗʰ **H35.3** **Degeneration of macula and posterior pole**
H35.30 **Unspecified macular degeneration** Ⓐ
Age-related macular degeneration
H35.31 **Nonexudative age-related macular degeneration** Ⓐ
Atrophic age-related macular degeneration
H35.32 **Exudative age-related macular degeneration** Ⓐ
H35.33 **Angioid streaks of macula**

✓6ᵗʰ **H35.34** **Macular cyst, hole, or pseudohole**
H35.341 **Macular cyst, hole, or pseudohole, right eye**
H35.342 **Macular cyst, hole, or pseudohole, left eye**
H35.343 **Macular cyst, hole, or pseudohole, bilateral**
H35.349 **Macular cyst, hole, or pseudohole, unspecified eye**

✓6ᵗʰ **H35.35** **Cystoid macular degeneration**
EXCLUDES 1 *cystoid macular edema following cataract surgery (H59.03-)*
H35.351 **Cystoid macular degeneration, right eye**
H35.352 **Cystoid macular degeneration, left eye**
H35.353 **Cystoid macular degeneration, bilateral**
H35.359 **Cystoid macular degeneration, unspecified eye**

✓6ᵗʰ **H35.36** **Drusen (degenerative) of macula**
H35.361 **Drusen (degenerative) of macula, right eye**
H35.362 **Drusen (degenerative) of macula, left eye**
H35.363 **Drusen (degenerative) of macula, bilateral**
H35.369 **Drusen (degenerative) of macula, unspecified eye**

✓6ᵗʰ **H35.37** **Puckering of macula**
H35.371 **Puckering of macula, right eye**
H35.372 **Puckering of macula, left eye**
H35.373 **Puckering of macula, bilateral**
H35.379 **Puckering of macula, unspecified eye**

✓6ᵗʰ **H35.38** **Toxic maculopathy**
Code first poisoning due to drug or toxin, if applicable (T36-T65 with fifth or sixth character 1-4 or 6)
Use additional code for adverse effect, if applicable, to identify drug (T36-T50 with fifth or sixth character 5)
H35.381 **Toxic maculopathy, right eye**
H35.382 **Toxic maculopathy, left eye**
H35.383 **Toxic maculopathy, bilateral**
H35.389 **Toxic maculopathy, unspecified eye**

✓5ᵗʰ **H35.4** **Peripheral retinal degeneration**
EXCLUDES 1 *hereditary retinal degeneration (dystrophy) (H35.5-) peripheral retinal degeneration with retinal break (H33.3-)*
H35.40 **Unspecified peripheral retinal degeneration**

✓6ᵗʰ **H35.41** **Lattice degeneration of retina**
Palisade degeneration of retina
H35.411 **Lattice degeneration of retina, right eye**
H35.412 **Lattice degeneration of retina, left eye**
H35.413 **Lattice degeneration of retina, bilateral**

H35.419   **Lattice degeneration of retina, unspecified eye**

✓6ᵗʰ **H35.42**   **Microcystoid degeneration of retina**

H35.421   **Microcystoid degeneration of retina, right eye**

H35.422   **Microcystoid degeneration of retina, left eye**

H35.423   **Microcystoid degeneration of retina, bilateral**

H35.429   **Microcystoid degeneration of retina, unspecified eye**

✓6ᵗʰ **H35.43**   **Paving stone degeneration of retina**

H35.431   **Paving stone degeneration of retina, right eye**

H35.432   **Paving stone degeneration of retina, left eye**

H35.433   **Paving stone degeneration of retina, bilateral**

H35.439   **Paving stone degeneration of retina, unspecified eye**

✓6ᵗʰ **H35.44**   **Age-related reticular degeneration of retina**

H35.441   **Age-related reticular degeneration of retina, right eye**   A

H35.442   **Age-related reticular degeneration of retina, left eye**   A

H35.443   **Age-related reticular degeneration of retina, bilateral**   A

H35.449   **Age-related reticular degeneration of retina, unspecified eye**   A

✓6ᵗʰ **H35.45**   **Secondary pigmentary degeneration**

H35.451   **Secondary pigmentary degeneration, right eye**

H35.452   **Secondary pigmentary degeneration, left eye**

H35.453   **Secondary pigmentary degeneration, bilateral**

H35.459   **Secondary pigmentary degeneration, unspecified eye**

✓6ᵗʰ **H35.46**   **Secondary vitreoretinal degeneration**

H35.461   **Secondary vitreoretinal degeneration, right eye**

H35.462   **Secondary vitreoretinal degeneration, left eye**

H35.463   **Secondary vitreoretinal degeneration, bilateral**

H35.469   **Secondary vitreoretinal degeneration, unspecified eye**

✓5ᵗʰ **H35.5**   **Hereditary retinal dystrophy**

EXCLUDES 1   *dystrophies primarily involving Bruch's membrane (H31.1-)*

H35.50   **Unspecified hereditary retinal dystrophy**

H35.51   **Vitreoretinal dystrophy**

H35.52   **Pigmentary retinal dystrophy**
Albipunctate retinal dystrophy
Retinitis pigmentosa
Tapetoretinal dystrophy

H35.53   **Other dystrophies primarily involving the sensory retina**
Stargardt's disease

H35.54   **Dystrophies primarily involving the retinal pigment epithelium**
Vitelliform retinal dystrophy

✓5ᵗʰ **H35.6**   **Retinal hemorrhage**

H35.60   **Retinal hemorrhage, unspecified eye**

H35.61   **Retinal hemorrhage, right eye**

H35.62   **Retinal hemorrhage, left eye**

H35.63   **Retinal hemorrhage, bilateral**

✓5ᵗʰ **H35.7**   **Separation of retinal layers**

EXCLUDES 1   *retinal detachment (serous) (H33.2-)
rhegmatogenous retinal detachment (H33.0-)*

CC Excl: For CC codes in subcategory H35.7, unless otherwise noted: H33.001-H33.119, H33.191-H33.8, H35.70-H35.739

H35.70   **Unspecified separation of retinal layers**   CC

✓6ᵗʰ **H35.71**   **Central serous chorioretinopathy**

H35.711   **Central serous chorioretinopathy, right eye**

H35.712   **Central serous chorioretinopathy, left eye**

H35.713   **Central serous chorioretinopathy, bilateral**

H35.719   **Central serous chorioretinopathy, unspecified eye**

✓6ᵗʰ **H35.72**   **Serous detachment of retinal pigment epithelium**

H35.721   **Serous detachment of retinal pigment epithelium, right eye**   CC

H35.722   **Serous detachment of retinal pigment epithelium, left eye**   CC

H35.723   **Serous detachment of retinal pigment epithelium, bilateral**   CC

H35.729   **Serous detachment of retinal pigment epithelium, unspecified eye**   CC

✓6ᵗʰ **H35.73**   **Hemorrhagic detachment of retinal pigment epithelium**

H35.731   **Hemorrhagic detachment of retinal pigment epithelium, right eye**   CC

H35.732   **Hemorrhagic detachment of retinal pigment epithelium, left eye**   CC

H35.733   **Hemorrhagic detachment of retinal pigment epithelium, bilateral**   CC

H35.739   **Hemorrhagic detachment of retinal pigment epithelium, unspecified eye**   CC

✓5ᵗʰ **H35.8**   **Other specified retinal disorders**

EXCLUDES 2   *retinal hemorrhage (H35.6-)*

H35.81   **Retinal edema**
Retinal cotton wool spots

H35.82   **Retinal ischemia**   CC
CC Excl: H35.60-H35.63, H35.81-H35.89

H35.89   **Other specified retinal disorders**

H35.9   **Unspecified retinal disorder**

H36   ***Retinal disorders in diseases classified elsewhere***
*Code first underlying disease, such as:
lipid storage disorders (E75.-)
sickle-cell disorders (D57.-)*

EXCLUDES 1   *arteriosclerotic retinopathy (H35.0-)
diabetic retinopathy (E08.3-, E09.3-, E10.3-, E11.3-, E13.3-)*

Glaucoma (H40-H42)

✓4ᵗʰ **H40**   **Glaucoma**

EXCLUDES 1   *absolute glaucoma (H44.51-)
congenital glaucoma (Q15.0)
traumatic glaucoma due to birth injury (P15.3)*

✓5ᵗʰ **H40.0**   **Glaucoma suspect**

✓6ᵗʰ **H40.00**   **Preglaucoma, unspecified**

H40.001   **Preglaucoma, unspecified, right eye**

H40.002   **Preglaucoma, unspecified, left eye**

H40.003   **Preglaucoma, unspecified, bilateral**

H40.009   **Preglaucoma, unspecified, unspecified eye**

✓6ᵗʰ **H40.01**   **Open angle with borderline findings, low risk**
Open angle, low risk

H40.011   **Open angle with borderline findings, low risk, right eye**

H40.012   **Open angle with borderline findings, low risk, left eye**

H40.013   **Open angle with borderline findings, low risk, bilateral**

H40.019   **Open angle with borderline findings, low risk, unspecified eye**

✓6ᵗʰ **H40.02**   **Open angle with borderline findings, high risk**
Open angle, high risk

H40.021   **Open angle with borderline findings, high risk, right eye**

H40.022   **Open angle with borderline findings, high risk, left eye**

H40.023   **Open angle with borderline findings, high risk, bilateral**

H40.029   **Open angle with borderline findings, high risk, unspecified eye**

✓ Additional Character Required   ✓x7ᵗʰ Placeholder Alert   Unacceptable PDx   Manifestation   Hospital Acquired Condition   EXCLUDES 1 Not Coded Here   EXCLUDES 2 Not Included Here

ICD-10-CM 2016   581

Chapter 7. Diseases of the Eye and Adnexa

√6th **H40.03** Anatomical narrow **angle**
　　　　Primary angle closure suspect
　　　H40.031 Anatomical narrow angle, right **eye**
　　　H40.032 Anatomical narrow angle, left **eye**
　　　H40.033 Anatomical narrow angle, bilateral
　　　H40.039 Anatomical narrow angle, unspecified **eye**

√6th **H40.04** Steroid responder
　　　H40.041 Steroid responder, right **eye**
　　　H40.042 Steroid responder, left **eye**
　　　H40.043 Steroid responder, bilateral
　　　H40.049 Steroid responder, unspecified **eye**

√6th **H40.05** Ocular hypertension
　　　H40.051 Ocular hypertension, right **eye**
　　　H40.052 Ocular hypertension, left **eye**
　　　H40.053 Ocular hypertension, bilateral
　　　H40.059 Ocular hypertension, unspecified **eye**

√6th **H40.06** Primary angle **closure** without glaucoma damage
　　　H40.061 Primary angle closure without glaucoma damage, right **eye**
　　　H40.062 Primary angle closure without glaucoma damage, left **eye**
　　　H40.063 Primary angle closure without glaucoma damage, bilateral
　　　H40.069 Primary angle closure without glaucoma damage, unspecified **eye**

√5th **H40.1** Open-angle glaucoma

> One of the following 7th characters is to be assigned to each code in subcategories H40.10, H40.11, H40.12-, H40.13-, and H40.14- to designate the stage of glaucoma.
> Ø　stage unspecified
> 1　mild stage
> 2　moderate stage
> 3　severe stage
> 4　indeterminate stage

√x7th **H40.10** Unspecified **open-angle glaucoma**

√x7th **H40.11** Primary **open-angle glaucoma**
　　　Chronic simple glaucoma

√6th **H40.12** Low-tension **glaucoma**
　√7th **H40.121** Low-tension glaucoma, right **eye**
　√7th **H40.122** Low-tension glaucoma, left **eye**
　√7th **H40.123** Low-tension glaucoma, bilateral
　√7th **H40.129** Low-tension glaucoma, unspecified **eye**

√6th **H40.13** Pigmentary **glaucoma**
　√7th **H40.131** Pigmentary glaucoma, right **eye**
　√7th **H40.132** Pigmentary glaucoma, left **eye**
　√7th **H40.133** Pigmentary glaucoma, bilateral
　√7th **H40.139** Pigmentary glaucoma, unspecified **eye**

√6th **H40.14** Capsular glaucoma with pseudoexfoliation **of lens**
　√7th **H40.141** Capsular glaucoma with pseudoexfoliation of lens, right **eye**
　√7th **H40.142** Capsular glaucoma with pseudoexfoliation of lens, left **eye**
　√7th **H40.143** Capsular glaucoma with pseudoexfoliation of lens, bilateral
　√7th **H40.149** Capsular glaucoma with pseudoexfoliation of lens, unspecified **eye**

√6th **H40.15** Residual **stage** of open-angle glaucoma
　　　H40.151 Residual stage of open-angle glaucoma, right **eye**
　　　H40.152 Residual stage of open-angle glaucoma, left **eye**
　　　H40.153 Residual stage of open-angle glaucoma, bilateral
　　　H40.159 Residual stage of open-angle glaucoma, unspecified **eye**

√5th **H40.2** Primary angle-closure glaucoma
> EXCLUDES 1　aqueous misdirection (H40.83-)
> 　　　　malignant glaucoma (H40.83-)

> One of the following 7th characters is to be assigned to each code in subcategories H40.20 and H40.22- to designate the stage of glaucoma.
> Ø　stage unspecified
> 1　mild stage
> 2　moderate stage
> 3　severe stage
> 4　indeterminate stage

> **CC Excl: For CC codes in subcategory H40.2, unless otherwise noted:** H40.211-H40.219

√x7th **H40.20** Unspecified **primary angle-closure glaucoma**

√6th **H40.21** Acute **angle-closure glaucoma**
　　　Acute angle-closure glaucoma attack
　　　Acute angle-closure glaucoma crisis
　　　H40.211 Acute angle-closure glaucoma, right **eye**　　CC
　　　H40.212 Acute angle-closure glaucoma, left **eye**　　CC
　　　H40.213 Acute angle-closure glaucoma, bilateral　　CC
　　　H40.219 Acute angle-closure glaucoma, unspecified **eye**　　CC

√6th **H40.22** Chronic **angle-closure glaucoma**
　　　Chronic primary angle-closure glaucoma
　√7th **H40.221** Chronic angle-closure glaucoma, right **eye**
　√7th **H40.222** Chronic angle-closure glaucoma, left **eye**
　√7th **H40.223** Chronic angle-closure glaucoma, bilateral
　√7th **H40.229** Chronic angle-closure glaucoma, unspecified **eye**

√6th **H40.23** Intermittent **angle-closure glaucoma**
　　　H40.231 Intermittent angle-closure glaucoma, right **eye**
　　　H40.232 Intermittent angle-closure glaucoma, left **eye**
　　　H40.233 Intermittent angle-closure glaucoma, bilateral
　　　H40.239 Intermittent angle-closure glaucoma, unspecified **eye**

√6th **H40.24** Residual **stage** of angle-closure glaucoma
　　　H40.241 Residual stage of angle-closure glaucoma, right **eye**
　　　H40.242 Residual stage of angle-closure glaucoma, left **eye**
　　　H40.243 Residual stage of angle-closure glaucoma, bilateral
　　　H40.249 Residual stage of angle-closure glaucoma, unspecified **eye**

√5th **H40.3** Glaucoma secondary **to eye** trauma
　　　Code also underlying condition

> One of the following 7th characters is to be assigned to each code in subcategory H40.3- to designate the stage of glaucoma.
> Ø　stage unspecified
> 1　mild stage
> 2　moderate stage
> 3　severe stage
> 4　indeterminate stage

√x7th **H40.30** Glaucoma secondary to eye trauma, unspecified **eye**
√x7th **H40.31** Glaucoma secondary to eye trauma, right **eye**
√x7th **H40.32** Glaucoma secondary to eye trauma, left **eye**
√x7th **H40.33** Glaucoma secondary to eye trauma, bilateral

N Newborn: 0　P Pediatric: 0-17　M Maternity: 12-55　A Adult: 15-124　MCC Major CC Condition　PDxMCC PDx acts as own MCC　CC CC Condition　PDxCC PDx acts as own CC

582　　　　　ICD-10-CM 2016

✓5ᵗʰ H40.4 Glaucoma secondary to eye inflammation
Code also underlying condition

One of the following 7th characters is to be assigned to each code in subcategory H40.4- to designate the stage of glaucoma.
0 stage unspecified
1 mild stage
2 moderate stage
3 severe stage
4 indeterminate stage

✓x7ᵗʰ H40.40 Glaucoma secondary to eye inflammation, unspecified eye
✓x7ᵗʰ H40.41 Glaucoma secondary to eye inflammation, right eye
✓x7ᵗʰ H40.42 Glaucoma secondary to eye inflammation, left eye
✓x7ᵗʰ H40.43 Glaucoma secondary to eye inflammation, bilateral

✓5ᵗʰ H40.5 Glaucoma secondary to other eye disorders
Code also underlying eye disorder

One of the following 7th characters is to be assigned to each code in subcategory H40.5- to designate the stage of glaucoma.
0 stage unspecified
1 mild stage
2 moderate stage
3 severe stage
4 indeterminate stage

✓x7ᵗʰ H40.50 Glaucoma secondary to other eye disorders, unspecified eye
✓x7ᵗʰ H40.51 Glaucoma secondary to other eye disorders, right eye
✓x7ᵗʰ H40.52 Glaucoma secondary to other eye disorders, left eye
✓x7ᵗʰ H40.53 Glaucoma secondary to other eye disorders, bilateral

✓5ᵗʰ H40.6 Glaucoma secondary to drugs
Use additional code for adverse effect, if applicable, to identify drug (T36-T50 with fifth or sixth character 5)

One of the following 7th characters is to be assigned to each code in subcategory H40.6- to designate the stage of glaucoma.
0 stage unspecified
1 mild stage
2 moderate stage
3 severe stage
4 indeterminate stage

✓x7ᵗʰ H40.60 Glaucoma secondary to drugs, unspecified eye
✓x7ᵗʰ H40.61 Glaucoma secondary to drugs, right eye
✓x7ᵗʰ H40.62 Glaucoma secondary to drugs, left eye
✓x7ᵗʰ H40.63 Glaucoma secondary to drugs, bilateral

✓5ᵗʰ H40.8 Other glaucoma
    ✓6ᵗʰ H40.81 Glaucoma with increased episcleral venous pressure
        H40.811 Glaucoma with increased episcleral venous pressure, right eye
        H40.812 Glaucoma with increased episcleral venous pressure, left eye
        H40.813 Glaucoma with increased episcleral venous pressure, bilateral
        H40.819 Glaucoma with increased episcleral venous pressure, unspecified eye
    ✓6ᵗʰ H40.82 Hypersecretion glaucoma
        H40.821 Hypersecretion glaucoma, right eye
        H40.822 Hypersecretion glaucoma, left eye
        H40.823 Hypersecretion glaucoma, bilateral
        H40.829 Hypersecretion glaucoma, unspecified eye
    ✓6ᵗʰ H40.83 Aqueous misdirection
        Malignant glaucoma
        H40.831 Aqueous misdirection, right eye
        H40.832 Aqueous misdirection, left eye
        H40.833 Aqueous misdirection, bilateral
        H40.839 Aqueous misdirection, unspecified eye
    H40.89 Other specified glaucoma
H40.9 Unspecified glaucoma

H42 *Glaucoma in diseases classified elsewhere*
Code first underlying condition, such as:
  amyloidosis (E85.-)
  aniridia (Q13.1)
  Lowe's syndrome (E72.03)
  Reiger's anomaly (Q13.81)
  specified metabolic disorder (E70-E88)
EXCLUDES1 *glaucoma (in):*
    diabetes mellitus (E08.39, E09.39, E10.39, E11.39, E13.39)
    onchocerciasis (B73.02)
    syphilis (A52.71)
    tuberculous (A18.59)

Disorders of vitreous body and globe (H43-H44)

✓4ᵗʰ H43 Disorders of vitreous body
  ✓5ᵗʰ H43.0 Vitreous prolapse
    EXCLUDES1 *traumatic vitreous prolapse (S05.2-)*
    vitreous syndrome following cataract surgery (H59.0-)
    H43.00 Vitreous prolapse, unspecified eye
    H43.01 Vitreous prolapse, right eye
    H43.02 Vitreous prolapse, left eye
    H43.03 Vitreous prolapse, bilateral
  ✓5ᵗʰ H43.1 Vitreous hemorrhage
    H43.10 Vitreous hemorrhage, unspecified eye
    H43.11 Vitreous hemorrhage, right eye
    H43.12 Vitreous hemorrhage, left eye
    H43.13 Vitreous hemorrhage, bilateral
  ✓5ᵗʰ H43.2 Crystalline deposits in vitreous body
    H43.20 Crystalline deposits in vitreous body, unspecified eye
    H43.21 Crystalline deposits in vitreous body, right eye
    H43.22 Crystalline deposits in vitreous body, left eye
    H43.23 Crystalline deposits in vitreous body, bilateral
  ✓5ᵗʰ H43.3 Other vitreous opacities
    ✓6ᵗʰ H43.31 Vitreous membranes and strands
        H43.311 Vitreous membranes and strands, right eye
        H43.312 Vitreous membranes and strands, left eye
        H43.313 Vitreous membranes and strands, bilateral
        H43.319 Vitreous membranes and strands, unspecified eye
    ✓6ᵗʰ H43.39 Other vitreous opacities
        Vitreous floaters
        H43.391 Other vitreous opacities, right eye
        H43.392 Other vitreous opacities, left eye
        H43.393 Other vitreous opacities, bilateral
        H43.399 Other vitreous opacities, unspecified eye
  ✓5ᵗʰ H43.8 Other disorders of vitreous body
    EXCLUDES1 *proliferative vitreo-retinopathy with retinal detachment (H33.4-)*
    EXCLUDES2 *vitreous abscess (H44.02-)*
    ✓6ᵗʰ H43.81 Vitreous degeneration
        Vitreous detachment
        H43.811 Vitreous degeneration, right eye
        H43.812 Vitreous degeneration, left eye
        H43.813 Vitreous degeneration, bilateral
        H43.819 Vitreous degeneration, unspecified eye
    ✓6ᵗʰ H43.82 Vitreomacular adhesion
        Vitreomacular traction
        H43.821 Vitreomacular adhesion, right eye A
        H43.822 Vitreomacular adhesion, left eye A
        H43.823 Vitreomacular adhesion, bilateral A
        H43.829 Vitreomacular adhesion, unspecified eye A
    H43.89 Other disorders of vitreous body
  H43.9 Unspecified disorder of vitreous body

Chapter 7. Diseases of the Eye and Adnexa

H44   Disorders of globe
INCLUDES   disorders affecting multiple structures of eye

H44.0   Purulent endophthalmitis
Use additional code to identify organism
EXCLUDES 1   bleb associated endophthalmitis (H59.4-)

H44.00   Unspecified purulent endophthalmitis

> CC Excl: For CC codes in subcategory H44.00, unless otherwise noted: H20.051-H20.059, H21.331-H21.339, H33.121-H33.129, H44.001-H44.029, H44.121-H44.129, H44.19

H44.001   Unspecified purulent endophthalmitis, right eye   CC

H44.002   Unspecified purulent endophthalmitis, left eye   CC

H44.003   Unspecified purulent endophthalmitis, bilateral   CC

H44.009   Unspecified purulent endophthalmitis, unspecified eye   CC

H44.01   Panophthalmitis (acute)

> CC Excl: For CC codes in subcategory H44.01, unless otherwise noted: H20.051-H20.059, H21.331-H21.339, H33.121-H33.129, H44.001-H44.029, H44.121-H44.129, H44.19

H44.011   Panophthalmitis (acute), right eye   CC

H44.012   Panophthalmitis (acute), left eye   CC

H44.013   Panophthalmitis (acute), bilateral   CC

H44.019   Panophthalmitis (acute), unspecified eye   CC

H44.02   Vitreous abscess (chronic)

> CC Excl: For CC codes in subcategory H44.02, unless otherwise noted: H16.241-H16.249, H21.331-H21.339, H33.121-H33.129, H44.001-H44.19

H44.021   Vitreous abscess (chronic), right eye   CC

H44.022   Vitreous abscess (chronic), left eye   CC

H44.023   Vitreous abscess (chronic), bilateral   CC

H44.029   Vitreous abscess (chronic), unspecified eye   CC

H44.1   Other endophthalmitis
EXCLUDES 1   bleb associated endophthalmitis (H59.4-)
EXCLUDES 2   ophthalmia nodosa (H16.2-)

H44.11   Panuveitis

> CC Excl: For CC codes in subcategory H44.11, unless otherwise noted: H44.111-H44.119, H44.131-H44.139

H44.111   Panuveitis, right eye   CC

H44.112   Panuveitis, left eye   CC

H44.113   Panuveitis, bilateral   CC

H44.119   Panuveitis, unspecified eye   CC

H44.12   Parasitic endophthalmitis, unspecified

> CC Excl: For CC codes in subcategory H44.12, unless otherwise noted: H20.051-H20.059, H21.331-H21.339, H33.121-H33.129, H44.001-H44.029, H44.121-H44.129, H44.19

H44.121   Parasitic endophthalmitis, unspecified, right eye   CC

H44.122   Parasitic endophthalmitis, unspecified, left eye   CC

H44.123   Parasitic endophthalmitis, unspecified, bilateral   CC

H44.129   Parasitic endophthalmitis, unspecified, unspecified eye   CC

H44.13   Sympathetic uveitis

> CC Excl: For CC codes in subcategory H44.13 unless otherwise noted: H44.111-H44.119, H44.131-H44.139

H44.131   Sympathetic uveitis, right eye   CC

H44.132   Sympathetic uveitis, left eye   CC

H44.133   Sympathetic uveitis, bilateral   CC

H44.139   Sympathetic uveitis, unspecified eye   CC

H44.19   Other endophthalmitis   CC
CC Excl: H20.051-H20.059, H21.331-H21.339, H33.121-H33.129, H44.001-H44.029, H44.121-H44.129, H44.19

H44.2   Degenerative myopia
Malignant myopia

H44.20   Degenerative myopia, unspecified eye

H44.21   Degenerative myopia, right eye

H44.22   Degenerative myopia, left eye

H44.23   Degenerative myopia, bilateral

H44.3   Other and unspecified degenerative disorders of globe

H44.30   Unspecified degenerative disorder of globe

H44.31   Chalcosis

H44.311   Chalcosis, right eye

H44.312   Chalcosis, left eye

H44.313   Chalcosis, bilateral

H44.319   Chalcosis, unspecified eye

H44.32   Siderosis of eye

H44.321   Siderosis of eye, right eye

H44.322   Siderosis of eye, left eye

H44.323   Siderosis of eye, bilateral

H44.329   Siderosis of eye, unspecified eye

H44.39   Other degenerative disorders of globe

H44.391   Other degenerative disorders of globe, right eye

H44.392   Other degenerative disorders of globe, left eye

H44.393   Other degenerative disorders of globe, bilateral

H44.399   Other degenerative disorders of globe, unspecified eye

H44.4   Hypotony of eye

H44.40   Unspecified hypotony of eye

H44.41   Flat anterior chamber hypotony of eye

H44.411   Flat anterior chamber hypotony of right eye

H44.412   Flat anterior chamber hypotony of left eye

H44.413   Flat anterior chamber hypotony of eye, bilateral

H44.419   Flat anterior chamber hypotony of unspecified eye

H44.42   Hypotony of eye due to ocular fistula

H44.421   Hypotony of right eye due to ocular fistula

H44.422   Hypotony of left eye due to ocular fistula

H44.423   Hypotony of eye due to ocular fistula, bilateral

H44.429   Hypotony of unspecified eye due to ocular fistula

H44.43   Hypotony of eye due to other ocular disorders

H44.431   Hypotony of eye due to other ocular disorders, right eye

H44.432   Hypotony of eye due to other ocular disorders, left eye

H44.433   Hypotony of eye due to other ocular disorders, bilateral

H44.439   Hypotony of eye due to other ocular disorders, unspecified eye

H44.44   Primary hypotony of eye

H44.441   Primary hypotony of right eye

H44.442   Primary hypotony of left eye

H44.443   Primary hypotony of eye, bilateral

H44.449   Primary hypotony of unspecified eye

H44.5   Degenerated conditions of globe

H44.50   Unspecified degenerated conditions of globe

H44.51   Absolute glaucoma

H44.511   Absolute glaucoma, right eye

H44.512   Absolute glaucoma, left eye

H44.513   Absolute glaucoma, bilateral

H44.519   Absolute glaucoma, unspecified eye

H44.52   Atrophy of globe
Phthisis bulbi

H44.521   Atrophy of globe, right eye

H44.522   Atrophy of globe, left eye

H44.523   Atrophy of globe, bilateral

H44.529   Atrophy of globe, unspecified eye

H44.53   Leucocoria

H44.531   Leucocoria, right eye

N Newborn: 0   P Pediatric: 0-17   M Maternity: 12-55   A Adult: 15-124   MCC Major CC Condition   PDxMCC PDx acts as own MCC   CC CC Condition   PDxCC PDx acts as own CC

H44.532   Leucocoria, left eye
H44.533   Leucocoria, bilateral
H44.539   Leucocoria, unspecified eye

✓5ᵗʰ **H44.6   Retained (old) intraocular foreign body, magnetic**
Use additional code to identify magnetic foreign body (Z18.11)
EXCLUDES 1   current intraocular foreign body (S05.-)
EXCLUDES 2   retained foreign body in eyelid (H02.81-)
retained (old) foreign body following penetrating wound of orbit (H05.5-)
retained (old) intraocular foreign body, nonmagnetic (H44.7-)

✓6ᵗʰ **H44.60   Unspecified retained (old) intraocular foreign body, magnetic**
H44.601   Unspecified retained (old) intraocular foreign body, magnetic, right eye
H44.602   Unspecified retained (old) intraocular foreign body, magnetic, left eye
H44.603   Unspecified retained (old) intraocular foreign body, magnetic, bilateral
H44.609   Unspecified retained (old) intraocular foreign body, magnetic, unspecified eye

✓6ᵗʰ **H44.61   Retained (old) magnetic foreign body in anterior chamber**
H44.611   Retained (old) magnetic foreign body in anterior chamber, right eye
H44.612   Retained (old) magnetic foreign body in anterior chamber, left eye
H44.613   Retained (old) magnetic foreign body in anterior chamber, bilateral
H44.619   Retained (old) magnetic foreign body in anterior chamber, unspecified eye

✓6ᵗʰ **H44.62   Retained (old) magnetic foreign body in iris or ciliary body**
H44.621   Retained (old) magnetic foreign body in iris or ciliary body, right eye
H44.622   Retained (old) magnetic foreign body in iris or ciliary body, left eye
H44.623   Retained (old) magnetic foreign body in iris or ciliary body, bilateral
H44.629   Retained (old) magnetic foreign body in iris or ciliary body, unspecified eye

✓6ᵗʰ **H44.63   Retained (old) magnetic foreign body in lens**
H44.631   Retained (old) magnetic foreign body in lens, right eye
H44.632   Retained (old) magnetic foreign body in lens, left eye
H44.633   Retained (old) magnetic foreign body in lens, bilateral
H44.639   Retained (old) magnetic foreign body in lens, unspecified eye

✓6ᵗʰ **H44.64   Retained (old) magnetic foreign body in posterior wall of globe**
H44.641   Retained (old) magnetic foreign body in posterior wall of globe, right eye
H44.642   Retained (old) magnetic foreign body in posterior wall of globe, left eye
H44.643   Retained (old) magnetic foreign body in posterior wall of globe, bilateral
H44.649   Retained (old) magnetic foreign body in posterior wall of globe, unspecified eye

✓6ᵗʰ **H44.65   Retained (old) magnetic foreign body in vitreous body**
H44.651   Retained (old) magnetic foreign body in vitreous body, right eye
H44.652   Retained (old) magnetic foreign body in vitreous body, left eye
H44.653   Retained (old) magnetic foreign body in vitreous body, bilateral
H44.659   Retained (old) magnetic foreign body in vitreous body, unspecified eye

✓6ᵗʰ **H44.69   Retained (old) intraocular foreign body, magnetic, in other or multiple sites**
H44.691   Retained (old) intraocular foreign body, magnetic, in other or multiple sites, right eye
H44.692   Retained (old) intraocular foreign body, magnetic, in other or multiple sites, left eye

H44.693   Retained (old) intraocular foreign body, magnetic, in other or multiple sites, bilateral
H44.699   Retained (old) intraocular foreign body, magnetic, in other or multiple sites, unspecified eye

✓5ᵗʰ **H44.7   Retained (old) intraocular foreign body, nonmagnetic**
Use additional code to identify nonmagnetic foreign body (Z18.01-Z18.10, Z18.12, Z18.2-Z18.9)
EXCLUDES 1   current intraocular foreign body (S05.-)
EXCLUDES 2   retained foreign body in eyelid (H02.81-)
retained (old) foreign body following penetrating wound of orbit (H05.5-)
retained (old) intraocular foreign body, magnetic (H44.6-)

✓6ᵗʰ **H44.70   Unspecified retained (old) intraocular foreign body, nonmagnetic**
H44.701   Unspecified retained (old) intraocular foreign body, nonmagnetic, right eye
H44.702   Unspecified retained (old) intraocular foreign body, nonmagnetic, left eye
H44.703   Unspecified retained (old) intraocular foreign body, nonmagnetic, bilateral
H44.709   Unspecified retained (old) intraocular foreign body, nonmagnetic, unspecified eye
Retained (old) intraocular foreign body NOS

✓6ᵗʰ **H44.71   Retained (nonmagnetic) (old) foreign body in anterior chamber**
H44.711   Retained (nonmagnetic) (old) foreign body in anterior chamber, right eye
H44.712   Retained (nonmagnetic) (old) foreign body in anterior chamber, left eye
H44.713   Retained (nonmagnetic) (old) foreign body in anterior chamber, bilateral
H44.719   Retained (nonmagnetic) (old) foreign body in anterior chamber, unspecified eye

✓6ᵗʰ **H44.72   Retained (nonmagnetic) (old) foreign body in iris or ciliary body**
H44.721   Retained (nonmagnetic) (old) foreign body in iris or ciliary body, right eye
H44.722   Retained (nonmagnetic) (old) foreign body in iris or ciliary body, left eye
H44.723   Retained (nonmagnetic) (old) foreign body in iris or ciliary body, bilateral
H44.729   Retained (nonmagnetic) (old) foreign body in iris or ciliary body, unspecified eye

✓6ᵗʰ **H44.73   Retained (nonmagnetic) (old) foreign body in lens**
H44.731   Retained (nonmagnetic) (old) foreign body in lens, right eye
H44.732   Retained (nonmagnetic) (old) foreign body in lens, left eye
H44.733   Retained (nonmagnetic) (old) foreign body in lens, bilateral
H44.739   Retained (nonmagnetic) (old) foreign body in lens, unspecified eye

✓6ᵗʰ **H44.74   Retained (nonmagnetic) (old) foreign body in posterior wall of globe**
H44.741   Retained (nonmagnetic) (old) foreign body in posterior wall of globe, right eye
H44.742   Retained (nonmagnetic) (old) foreign body in posterior wall of globe, left eye
H44.743   Retained (nonmagnetic) (old) foreign body in posterior wall of globe, bilateral
H44.749   Retained (nonmagnetic) (old) foreign body in posterior wall of globe, unspecified eye

✓6ᵗʰ **H44.75   Retained (nonmagnetic) (old) foreign body in vitreous body**
H44.751   Retained (nonmagnetic) (old) foreign body in vitreous body, right eye
H44.752   Retained (nonmagnetic) (old) foreign body in vitreous body, left eye
H44.753   Retained (nonmagnetic) (old) foreign body in vitreous body, bilateral
H44.759   Retained (nonmagnetic) (old) foreign body in vitreous body, unspecified eye

☑ Additional Character Required   ✓x7ᵗʰ Placeholder Alert   Unacceptable PDx   Manifestation   Hospital Acquired Condition   *EXCLUDES 1* Not Coded Here   *EXCLUDES 2* Not Included Here

ICD-10-CM 2016   **585**

Chapter 7. Diseases of the Eye and Adnexa

H44.532–H44.759

√6ᵗʰ **H44.79 Retained (old) intraocular foreign body, nonmagnetic, in other or multiple sites**

    H44.791 Retained (old) intraocular foreign body, nonmagnetic, in other or multiple sites, right eye

    H44.792 Retained (old) intraocular foreign body, nonmagnetic, in other or multiple sites, left eye

    H44.793 Retained (old) intraocular foreign body, nonmagnetic, in other or multiple sites, bilateral

    H44.799 Retained (old) intraocular foreign body, nonmagnetic, in other or multiple sites, unspecified eye

√5ᵗʰ **H44.8 Other disorders of globe**

    √6ᵗʰ **H44.81 Hemophthalmos**

        H44.811 Hemophthalmos, right eye

        H44.812 Hemophthalmos, left eye

        H44.813 Hemophthalmos, bilateral

        H44.819 Hemophthalmos, unspecified eye

    √6ᵗʰ **H44.82 Luxation of globe**

        H44.821 Luxation of globe, right eye

        H44.822 Luxation of globe, left eye

        H44.823 Luxation of globe, bilateral

        H44.829 Luxation of globe, unspecified eye

    H44.89 Other disorders of globe

H44.9 Unspecified disorder of globe

Disorders of optic nerve and visual pathways (H46-H47)

√4ᵗʰ **H46 Optic neuritis**

    EXCLUDES 2 *ischemic optic neuropathy (H47.01-)*

              neuromyelitis optica [Devic] (G36.0)

    CC Excl: For CC codes in category H46, unless otherwise noted: H46.00-H46.9

    √5ᵗʰ **H46.0 Optic papillitis**

        H46.00 Optic papillitis, unspecified eye CC

        H46.01 Optic papillitis, right eye CC

        H46.02 Optic papillitis, left eye CC

        H46.03 Optic papillitis, bilateral CC

    √5ᵗʰ **H46.1 Retrobulbar neuritis**

        Retrobulbar neuritis NOS

        EXCLUDES 1 *syphilitic retrobulbar neuritis (A52.15)*

        H46.10 Retrobulbar neuritis, unspecified eye CC

        H46.11 Retrobulbar neuritis, right eye CC

        H46.12 Retrobulbar neuritis, left eye CC

        H46.13 Retrobulbar neuritis, bilateral CC

    H46.2 Nutritional optic neuropathy

    H46.3 Toxic optic neuropathy

        Code first (T51-T65) to identify cause

    H46.8 Other optic neuritis CC

    H46.9 Unspecified optic neuritis CC

√4ᵗʰ **H47 Other disorders of optic [2nd] nerve and visual pathways**

    √5ᵗʰ **H47.0 Disorders of optic nerve, not elsewhere classified**

        √6ᵗʰ **H47.01 Ischemic optic neuropathy**

            H47.011 Ischemic optic neuropathy, right eye

            H47.012 Ischemic optic neuropathy, left eye

            H47.013 Ischemic optic neuropathy, bilateral

            H47.019 Ischemic optic neuropathy, unspecified eye

        √6ᵗʰ **H47.02 Hemorrhage in optic nerve sheath**

            H47.021 Hemorrhage in optic nerve sheath, right eye

            H47.022 Hemorrhage in optic nerve sheath, left eye

            H47.023 Hemorrhage in optic nerve sheath, bilateral

            H47.029 Hemorrhage in optic nerve sheath, unspecified eye

        √6ᵗʰ **H47.03 Optic nerve hypoplasia**

            H47.031 Optic nerve hypoplasia, right eye

            H47.032 Optic nerve hypoplasia, left eye

            H47.033 Optic nerve hypoplasia, bilateral

            H47.039 Optic nerve hypoplasia, unspecified eye

√6ᵗʰ **H47.09 Other disorders of optic nerve, not elsewhere classified**

    Compression of optic nerve

    H47.091 Other disorders of optic nerve, not elsewhere classified, right eye

    H47.092 Other disorders of optic nerve, not elsewhere classified, left eye

    H47.093 Other disorders of optic nerve, not elsewhere classified, bilateral

    H47.099 Other disorders of optic nerve, not elsewhere classified, unspecified eye

√5ᵗʰ **H47.1 Papilledema**

    H47.10 Unspecified papilledema CC

        CC Excl: A17.9, A18.50-A18.59, A18.82, A18.84, A18.89, A39.82, E08.311-E08.39, E08.618-E08.638, E08.649-E08.8, E09.311-E09.39, E09.618-E09.638, E09.649-E09.8, E10.311-E10.39, E10.618-E10.638, E10.649, E10.69-E10.8, E11.311-E11.39, E11.618-E11.638, E11.649, E11.69-E11.8, E13.311-E13.39, E13.618-E13.638, E13.649-E13.8, H47.10-H47.13, H47.231-H47.239, H47.331-H47.339, H57.8-H57.9, H59.40-H59.43, Q11.3, Q15.8-Q15.9

    H47.11 Papilledema associated with increased intracranial pressure CC

        CC Excl: See code: H47.10

    H47.12 Papilledema associated with decreased ocular pressure

    H47.13 Papilledema associated with retinal disorder

    √6ᵗʰ **H47.14 Foster-Kennedy syndrome**

        H47.141 Foster-Kennedy syndrome, right eye

        H47.142 Foster-Kennedy syndrome, left eye

        H47.143 Foster-Kennedy syndrome, bilateral

        H47.149 Foster-Kennedy syndrome, unspecified eye

√5ᵗʰ **H47.2 Optic atrophy**

    H47.20 Unspecified optic atrophy

    √6ᵗʰ **H47.21 Primary optic atrophy**

        H47.211 Primary optic atrophy, right eye

        H47.212 Primary optic atrophy, left eye

        H47.213 Primary optic atrophy, bilateral

        H47.219 Primary optic atrophy, unspecified eye

    H47.22 Hereditary optic atrophy

        Leber's optic atrophy

    √6ᵗʰ **H47.23 Glaucomatous optic atrophy**

        H47.231 Glaucomatous optic atrophy, right eye

        H47.232 Glaucomatous optic atrophy, left eye

        H47.233 Glaucomatous optic atrophy, bilateral

        H47.239 Glaucomatous optic atrophy, unspecified eye

    √6ᵗʰ **H47.29 Other optic atrophy**

        Temporal pallor of optic disc

        H47.291 Other optic atrophy, right eye

        H47.292 Other optic atrophy, left eye

        H47.293 Other optic atrophy, bilateral

        H47.299 Other optic atrophy, unspecified eye

√5ᵗʰ **H47.3 Other disorders of optic disc**

    √6ᵗʰ **H47.31 Coloboma of optic disc**

        H47.311 Coloboma of optic disc, right eye

        H47.312 Coloboma of optic disc, left eye

        H47.313 Coloboma of optic disc, bilateral

        H47.319 Coloboma of optic disc, unspecified eye

    √6ᵗʰ **H47.32 Drusen of optic disc**

        H47.321 Drusen of optic disc, right eye

        H47.322 Drusen of optic disc, left eye

        H47.323 Drusen of optic disc, bilateral

        H47.329 Drusen of optic disc, unspecified eye

    √6ᵗʰ **H47.33 Pseudopapilledema of optic disc**

        H47.331 Pseudopapilledema of optic disc, right eye

        H47.332 Pseudopapilledema of optic disc, left eye

        H47.333 Pseudopapilledema of optic disc, bilateral

        H47.339 Pseudopapilledema of optic disc, unspecified eye

    √6ᵗʰ **H47.39 Other disorders of optic disc**

        H47.391 Other disorders of optic disc, right eye

        H47.392 Other disorders of optic disc, left eye

N Newborn: 0   P Pediatric: 0-17   M Maternity: 12-55   A Adult: 15-124   **MCC** Major CC Condition   **PDxMCC** PDx acts as own MCC   CC CC Condition   **PDxCC** PDx acts as own CC

586   ICD-10-CM 2016

H47.393 Other disorders of optic disc, bilateral

H47.399 Other disorders of optic disc, unspecified eye

✓5ᵗʰ **H47.4 Disorders of optic chiasm**
Code also underlying condition

CC Excl: For CC codes in subcategory H47.4, unless otherwise noted: H47.41-H47.539

H47.41 Disorders of optic chiasm in (due to) inflammatory disorders   CC

H47.42 Disorders of optic chiasm in (due to) neoplasm   CC

H47.43 Disorders of optic chiasm in (due to) vascular disorders   CC

H47.49 Disorders of optic chiasm in (due to) other disorders   CC

✓5ᵗʰ **H47.5 Disorders of other visual pathways**
Disorders of optic tracts, geniculate nuclei and optic radiations
Code also underlying condition

CC Excl: For CC codes in subcategory H47.5, unless otherwise noted: H47.41-H47.539

✓6ᵗʰ H47.51 Disorders of visual pathways in (due to) inflammatory disorders

H47.511 Disorders of visual pathways in (due to) inflammatory disorders, right side   CC

H47.512 Disorders of visual pathways in (due to) inflammatory disorders, left side   CC

H47.519 Disorders of visual pathways in (due to) inflammatory disorders, unspecified side   CC

✓6ᵗʰ H47.52 Disorders of visual pathways in (due to) neoplasm

H47.521 Disorders of visual pathways in (due to) neoplasm, right side   CC

H47.522 Disorders of visual pathways in (due to) neoplasm, left side   CC

H47.529 Disorders of visual pathways in (due to) neoplasm, unspecified side   CC

✓6ᵗʰ H47.53 Disorders of visual pathways in (due to) vascular disorders

H47.531 Disorders of visual pathways in (due to) vascular disorders, right side   CC

H47.532 Disorders of visual pathways in (due to) vascular disorders, left side   CC

H47.539 Disorders of visual pathways in (due to) vascular disorders, unspecified side   CC

✓5ᵗʰ **H47.6 Disorders of visual cortex**
Code also underlying condition
EXCLUDES 1 injury to visual cortex S04.04

CC Excl: For CC codes in subcategory H47.6, unless otherwise noted: H47.611-H47.9

✓6ᵗʰ H47.61 Cortical blindness

H47.611 Cortical blindness, right side of brain

H47.612 Cortical blindness, left side of brain

H47.619 Cortical blindness, unspecified side of brain

✓6ᵗʰ H47.62 Disorders of visual cortex in (due to) inflammatory disorders

H47.621 Disorders of visual cortex in (due to) inflammatory disorders, right side of brain   CC

H47.622 Disorders of visual cortex in (due to) inflammatory disorders, left side of brain   CC

H47.629 Disorders of visual cortex in (due to) inflammatory disorders, unspecified side of brain   CC

✓6ᵗʰ H47.63 Disorders of visual cortex in (due to) neoplasm

H47.631 Disorders of visual cortex in (due to) neoplasm, right side of brain   CC

H47.632 Disorders of visual cortex in (due to) neoplasm, left side of brain   CC

H47.639 Disorders of visual cortex in (due to) neoplasm, unspecified side of brain   CC

✓6ᵗʰ H47.64 Disorders of visual cortex in (due to) vascular disorders

H47.641 Disorders of visual cortex in (due to) vascular disorders, right side of brain   CC

H47.642 Disorders of visual cortex in (due to) vascular disorders, left side of brain   CC

H47.649 Disorders of visual cortex in (due to) vascular disorders, unspecified side of brain   CC

H47.9 Unspecified disorder of visual pathways

Disorders of ocular muscles, binocular movement, accommodation and refraction (H49-H52)

EXCLUDES 2 nystagmus and other irregular eye movements (H55)

✓4ᵗʰ **H49 Paralytic strabismus**
EXCLUDES 2 internal ophthalmoplegia (H52.51-)
internuclear ophthalmoplegia (H51.2-)
progressive supranuclear ophthalmoplegia (G23.1)

✓5ᵗʰ **H49.0 Third [oculomotor] nerve palsy**

H49.00 Third [oculomotor] nerve palsy, unspecified eye

H49.01 Third [oculomotor] nerve palsy, right eye

H49.02 Third [oculomotor] nerve palsy, left eye

H49.03 Third [oculomotor] nerve palsy, bilateral

✓5ᵗʰ **H49.1 Fourth [trochlear] nerve palsy**

H49.10 Fourth [trochlear] nerve palsy, unspecified eye

H49.11 Fourth [trochlear] nerve palsy, right eye

H49.12 Fourth [trochlear] nerve palsy, left eye

H49.13 Fourth [trochlear] nerve palsy, bilateral

✓5ᵗʰ **H49.2 Sixth [abducent] nerve palsy**

H49.20 Sixth [abducent] nerve palsy, unspecified eye

H49.21 Sixth [abducent] nerve palsy, right eye

H49.22 Sixth [abducent] nerve palsy, left eye

H49.23 Sixth [abducent] nerve palsy, bilateral

✓5ᵗʰ **H49.3 Total (external) ophthalmoplegia**

H49.30 Total (external) ophthalmoplegia, unspecified eye

H49.31 Total (external) ophthalmoplegia, right eye

H49.32 Total (external) ophthalmoplegia, left eye

H49.33 Total (external) ophthalmoplegia, bilateral

✓5ᵗʰ **H49.4 Progressive external ophthalmoplegia**
EXCLUDES 1 Kearns-Sayre syndrome (H49.81-)

H49.40 Progressive external ophthalmoplegia, unspecified eye

H49.41 Progressive external ophthalmoplegia, right eye

H49.42 Progressive external ophthalmoplegia, left eye

H49.43 Progressive external ophthalmoplegia, bilateral

✓5ᵗʰ **H49.8 Other paralytic strabismus**

CC Excl: For CC codes in subcategory H49.8, unless otherwise noted: C96.5-C96.6, E71.310-E71.548, E80.3-E80.7, E88.89

✓6ᵗʰ H49.81 Kearns-Sayre syndrome
Progressive external ophthalmoplegia with pigmentary retinopathy
Use additional code for other manifestation, such as: heart block (I45.9)

H49.811 Kearns-Sayre syndrome, right eye   CC

H49.812 Kearns-Sayre syndrome, left eye   CC

H49.813 Kearns-Sayre syndrome, bilateral   CC

H49.819 Kearns-Sayre syndrome, unspecified eye   CC

✓6ᵗʰ H49.88 Other paralytic strabismus
External ophthalmoplegia NOS

H49.881 Other paralytic strabismus, right eye

H49.882 Other paralytic strabismus, left eye

H49.883 Other paralytic strabismus, bilateral

H49.889 Other paralytic strabismus, unspecified eye

H49.9 Unspecified paralytic strabismus

✓4ᵗʰ **H50 Other strabismus**

✓5ᵗʰ **H50.0 Esotropia**
Convergent concomitant strabismus
EXCLUDES 1 intermittent esotropia (H50.31-, H50.32)

H50.00 Unspecified esotropia

Chapter 7. Diseases of the Eye and Adnexa

H50.01–H52.512

√6ᵗʰ **H50.01 Monocular esotropia**
     H50.011 Monocular esotropia, right eye
     H50.012 Monocular esotropia, left eye

√6ᵗʰ **H50.02 Monocular esotropia with A pattern**
     H50.021 Monocular esotropia with A pattern, right eye
     H50.022 Monocular esotropia with A pattern, left eye

√6ᵗʰ **H50.03 Monocular esotropia with V pattern**
     H50.031 Monocular esotropia with V pattern, right eye
     H50.032 Monocular esotropia with V pattern, left eye

√6ᵗʰ **H50.04 Monocular esotropia with other noncomitancies**
     H50.041 Monocular esotropia with other noncomitancies, right eye
     H50.042 Monocular esotropia with other noncomitancies, left eye

H50.05 Alternating esotropia
H50.06 Alternating esotropia with A pattern
H50.07 Alternating esotropia with V pattern
H50.08 Alternating esotropia with other noncomitancies

√5ᵗʰ **H50.1 Exotropia**
     Divergent concomitant strabismus
     EXCLUDES 1   intermittent exotropia (H50.33-, H50.34)

H50.10 Unspecified exotropia

√6ᵗʰ **H50.11 Monocular exotropia**
     H50.111 Monocular exotropia, right eye
     H50.112 Monocular exotropia, left eye

√6ᵗʰ **H50.12 Monocular exotropia with A pattern**
     H50.121 Monocular exotropia with A pattern, right eye
     H50.122 Monocular exotropia with A pattern, left eye

√6ᵗʰ **H50.13 Monocular exotropia with V pattern**
     H50.131 Monocular exotropia with V pattern, right eye
     H50.132 Monocular exotropia with V pattern, left eye

√6ᵗʰ **H50.14 Monocular exotropia with other noncomitancies**
     H50.141 Monocular exotropia with other noncomitancies, right eye
     H50.142 Monocular exotropia with other noncomitancies, left eye

H50.15 Alternating exotropia
H50.16 Alternating exotropia with A pattern
H50.17 Alternating exotropia with V pattern
H50.18 Alternating exotropia with other noncomitancies

√5ᵗʰ **H50.2 Vertical strabismus**
     Hypertropia
H50.21 Vertical strabismus, right eye
H50.22 Vertical strabismus, left eye

√5ᵗʰ **H50.3 Intermittent heterotropia**
H50.30 Unspecified intermittent heterotropia

√6ᵗʰ **H50.31 Intermittent monocular esotropia**
     H50.311 Intermittent monocular esotropia, right eye
     H50.312 Intermittent monocular esotropia, left eye

H50.32 Intermittent alternating esotropia

√6ᵗʰ **H50.33 Intermittent monocular exotropia**
     H50.331 Intermittent monocular exotropia, right eye
     H50.332 Intermittent monocular exotropia, left eye

H50.34 Intermittent alternating exotropia

√5ᵗʰ **H50.4 Other and unspecified heterotropia**
H50.40 Unspecified heterotropia

√6ᵗʰ **H50.41 Cyclotropia**
     H50.411 Cyclotropia, right eye
     H50.412 Cyclotropia, left eye

H50.42 Monofixation syndrome
H50.43 Accommodative component in esotropia

√5ᵗʰ **H50.5 Heterophoria**
H50.50 Unspecified heterophoria

H50.51 Esophoria
H50.52 Exophoria
H50.53 Vertical heterophoria
H50.54 Cyclophoria
H50.55 Alternating heterophoria

√5ᵗʰ **H50.6 Mechanical strabismus**
H50.60 Mechanical strabismus, unspecified

√6ᵗʰ **H50.61 Brown's sheath syndrome**
     H50.611 Brown's sheath syndrome, right eye
     H50.612 Brown's sheath syndrome, left eye

H50.69 Other mechanical strabismus
     Strabismus due to adhesions
     Traumatic limitation of duction of eye muscle

√5ᵗʰ **H50.8 Other specified strabismus**

√6ᵗʰ **H50.81 Duane's syndrome**
     H50.811 Duane's syndrome, right eye
     H50.812 Duane's syndrome, left eye

H50.89 Other specified strabismus

H50.9 Unspecified strabismus

√4ᵗʰ **H51 Other disorders of binocular movement**
H51.0 Palsy (spasm) of conjugate gaze

√5ᵗʰ **H51.1 Convergence insufficiency and excess**
H51.11 Convergence insufficiency
H51.12 Convergence excess

√5ᵗʰ **H51.2 Internuclear ophthalmoplegia**
H51.20 Internuclear ophthalmoplegia, unspecified eye
H51.21 Internuclear ophthalmoplegia, right eye
H51.22 Internuclear ophthalmoplegia, left eye
H51.23 Internuclear ophthalmoplegia, bilateral

H51.8 Other specified disorders of binocular movement
H51.9 Unspecified disorder of binocular movement

√4ᵗʰ **H52 Disorders of refraction and accommodation**

√5ᵗʰ **H52.0 Hypermetropia**
H52.00 Hypermetropia, unspecified eye
H52.01 Hypermetropia, right eye
H52.02 Hypermetropia, left eye
H52.03 Hypermetropia, bilateral

√5ᵗʰ **H52.1 Myopia**
     EXCLUDES 1   degenerative myopia (H44.2-)
H52.10 Myopia, unspecified eye
H52.11 Myopia, right eye
H52.12 Myopia, left eye
H52.13 Myopia, bilateral

√5ᵗʰ **H52.2 Astigmatism**

√6ᵗʰ **H52.20 Unspecified astigmatism**
     H52.201 Unspecified astigmatism, right eye
     H52.202 Unspecified astigmatism, left eye
     H52.203 Unspecified astigmatism, bilateral
     H52.209 Unspecified astigmatism, unspecified eye

√6ᵗʰ **H52.21 Irregular astigmatism**
     H52.211 Irregular astigmatism, right eye
     H52.212 Irregular astigmatism, left eye
     H52.213 Irregular astigmatism, bilateral
     H52.219 Irregular astigmatism, unspecified eye

√6ᵗʰ **H52.22 Regular astigmatism**
     H52.221 Regular astigmatism, right eye
     H52.222 Regular astigmatism, left eye
     H52.223 Regular astigmatism, bilateral
     H52.229 Regular astigmatism, unspecified eye

√5ᵗʰ **H52.3 Anisometropia and aniseikonia**
H52.31 Anisometropia
H52.32 Aniseikonia

H52.4 Presbyopia

√5ᵗʰ **H52.5 Disorders of accommodation**

√6ᵗʰ **H52.51 Internal ophthalmoplegia (complete) (total)**
     H52.511 Internal ophthalmoplegia (complete) (total), right eye
     H52.512 Internal ophthalmoplegia (complete) (total), left eye

Ⓝ Newborn: 0   Ⓟ Pediatric: 0-17   Ⓜ Maternity: 12-55   Ⓐ Adult: 15-124   **MCC** Major CC Condition   **PDxMCC** PDx acts as own MCC   **CC** CC Condition   **PDxCC** PDx acts as own CC

588   ICD-10-CM 2016

H52.513   Internal ophthalmoplegia (complete) (total), **bilateral**

H52.519   Internal ophthalmoplegia (complete) (total), **unspecified** eye

☑6ᵗʰ **H52.52**   **Paresis** of accommodation

H52.521   **Paresis of accommodation, right** eye

H52.522   **Paresis of accommodation, left** eye

H52.523   **Paresis of accommodation, bilateral**

H52.529   **Paresis of accommodation, unspecified** eye

☑6ᵗʰ **H52.53**   **Spasm** of accommodation

H52.531   **Spasm of accommodation, right** eye

H52.532   **Spasm of accommodation, left** eye

H52.533   **Spasm of accommodation, bilateral**

H52.539   **Spasm of accommodation, unspecified** eye

H52.6   **Other disorders of refraction**

H52.7   **Unspecified disorder of refraction**

Visual disturbances and blindness (H53-H54)

☑4ᵗʰ **H53**   **Visual disturbances**

☑5ᵗʰ **H53.0**   **Amblyopia ex anopsia**

> **EXCLUDES 1**   *amblyopia due to vitamin A deficiency (E50.5)*

☑6ᵗʰ **H53.00**   **Unspecified** amblyopia

H53.001   **Unspecified amblyopia, right** eye

H53.002   **Unspecified amblyopia, left** eye

H53.003   **Unspecified amblyopia, bilateral**

H53.009   **Unspecified amblyopia, unspecified** eye

☑6ᵗʰ **H53.01**   **Deprivation** amblyopia

H53.011   **Deprivation amblyopia, right** eye

H53.012   **Deprivation amblyopia, left** eye

H53.013   **Deprivation amblyopia, bilateral**

H53.019   **Deprivation amblyopia, unspecified** eye

☑6ᵗʰ **H53.02**   **Refractive** amblyopia

H53.021   **Refractive amblyopia, right** eye

H53.022   **Refractive amblyopia, left** eye

H53.023   **Refractive amblyopia, bilateral**

H53.029   **Refractive amblyopia, unspecified** eye

☑6ᵗʰ **H53.03**   **Strabismic** amblyopia

> **EXCLUDES 1**   *strabismus (H50.-)*

H53.031   **Strabismic amblyopia, right** eye

H53.032   **Strabismic amblyopia, left** eye

H53.033   **Strabismic amblyopia, bilateral**

H53.039   **Strabismic amblyopia, unspecified** eye

☑5ᵗʰ **H53.1**   **Subjective visual disturbances**

> **CC Excl: For CC codes in subcategory H53.1, unless otherwise noted:** H53.10–H53.139, H53.16, R44.1, R48.3

> **EXCLUDES 1**   *subjective visual disturbances due to vitamin A deficiency (E50.5)*
> *visual hallucinations (R44.1)*

H53.10   **Unspecified** subjective visual disturbances

H53.11   **Day blindness**
Hemeralopia

☑6ᵗʰ **H53.12**   **Transient** visual loss
Scintillating scotoma

> **EXCLUDES 1**   *amaurosis fugax (G45.3-)*
> *transient retinal artery occlusion (H34.0-)*

H53.121   **Transient visual loss, right** eye

H53.122   **Transient visual loss, left** eye

H53.123   **Transient visual loss, bilateral**

H53.129   **Transient visual loss, unspecified** eye

☑6ᵗʰ **H53.13**   **Sudden** visual loss

H53.131   **Sudden visual loss, right** eye

H53.132   **Sudden visual loss, left** eye

H53.133   **Sudden visual loss, bilateral**

H53.139   **Sudden visual loss, unspecified** eye

☑6ᵗʰ **H53.14**   **Visual discomfort**
Asthenopia
Photophobia

H53.141   **Visual discomfort, right** eye

H53.142   **Visual discomfort, left** eye

H53.143   **Visual discomfort, bilateral**

H53.149   **Visual discomfort, unspecified**

H53.15   **Visual distortions of shape and size**
Metamorphopsia

H53.16   **Psychophysical visual disturbances**

H53.19   **Other subjective visual disturbances**
Visual halos

H53.2   **Diplopia**
Double vision

☑5ᵗʰ **H53.3**   **Other and unspecified disorders of binocular vision**

H53.30   **Unspecified disorder of binocular vision**

H53.31   **Abnormal retinal correspondence**

H53.32   **Fusion with defective stereopsis**

H53.33   **Simultaneous visual perception without fusion**

H53.34   **Suppression of binocular vision**

☑5ᵗʰ **H53.4**   **Visual field defects**

H53.40   **Unspecified** visual field defects

☑6ᵗʰ **H53.41**   **Scotoma involving central area**
Central scotoma

H53.411   **Scotoma involving central area, right** eye

H53.412   **Scotoma involving central area, left** eye

H53.413   **Scotoma involving central area, bilateral**

H53.419   **Scotoma involving central area, unspecified** eye

☑6ᵗʰ **H53.42**   **Scotoma of blind spot area**
Enlarged blind spot

H53.421   **Scotoma of blind spot area, right** eye

H53.422   **Scotoma of blind spot area, left** eye

H53.423   **Scotoma of blind spot area, bilateral**

H53.429   **Scotoma of blind spot area, unspecified** eye

☑6ᵗʰ **H53.43**   **Sector or arcuate defects**
Arcuate scotoma
Bjerrum scotoma

H53.431   **Sector or arcuate defects, right** eye

H53.432   **Sector or arcuate defects, left** eye

H53.433   **Sector or arcuate defects, bilateral**

H53.439   **Sector or arcuate defects, unspecified** eye

☑6ᵗʰ **H53.45**   **Other localized visual field defect**
Peripheral visual field defect
Ring scotoma NOS
Scotoma NOS

H53.451   **Other localized visual field defect, right** eye

H53.452   **Other localized visual field defect, left** eye

H53.453   **Other localized visual field defect, bilateral**

H53.459   **Other localized visual field defect, unspecified** eye

☑6ᵗʰ **H53.46**   **Homonymous bilateral field defects**
Homonymous hemianopia
Homonymous hemianopsia
Quadrant anopia
Quadrant anopsia

H53.461   **Homonymous bilateral field defects, right** side

H53.462   **Homonymous bilateral field defects, left** side

H53.469   **Homonymous bilateral field defects, unspecified** side
Homonymous bilateral field defects NOS

H53.47   **Heteronymous bilateral field defects**
Heteronymous hemianop(s)ia

☑6ᵗʰ **H53.48**   **Generalized contraction of visual field**

H53.481   **Generalized contraction of visual field, right** eye

H53.482   **Generalized contraction of visual field, left** eye

H53.483   **Generalized contraction of visual field, bilateral**

H53.489   **Generalized contraction of visual field, unspecified** eye

☑5ᵗʰ **H53.5**   **Color vision deficiencies**
Color blindness

> **EXCLUDES 2**   *day blindness (H53.11)*

H53.50   **Unspecified color vision deficiencies**
Color blindness NOS

✔ Additional Character Required   ✔x7ᵗʰ Placeholder Alert   Unacceptable PDx   ■ Manifestation   Hospital Acquired Condition   **EXCLUDES 1** Not Coded Here   **EXCLUDES 2** Not Included Here

ICD-10-CM 2016   **589**

H53.51   **Achromatopsia**

H53.52   **Acquired color vision deficiency**

H53.53   **Deuteranomaly**
Deuteranopia

H53.54   **Protanomaly**
Protanopia

H53.55   **Tritanomaly**
Tritanopia

H53.59   **Other color vision deficiencies**

✓5ᵗʰ **H53.6**   **Night blindness**
EXCLUDES 1   night blindness due to vitamin A deficiency (E50.5)

H53.60   **Unspecified night blindness**

H53.61   **Abnormal dark adaptation curve**

H53.62   **Acquired night blindness**

H53.63   **Congenital night blindness**

H53.69   **Other night blindness**

✓5ᵗʰ **H53.7**   **Vision sensitivity deficiencies**

H53.71   **Glare sensitivity**

H53.72   **Impaired contrast sensitivity**

H53.8   **Other visual disturbances**

H53.9   **Unspecified visual disturbance**

✓4ᵗʰ **H54**   **Blindness and low vision**
NOTE   For definition of visual impairment categories see table below
Code first any associated underlying cause of the blindness
EXCLUDES 1   amaurosis fugax (G45.3)

H54.0   **Blindness, both eyes**
Visual impairment categories 3, 4, 5 in both eyes.

✓5ᵗʰ **H54.1**   **Blindness, one eye, low vision other eye**
Visual impairment categories 3, 4, 5 in one eye, with categories 1 or 2 in the other eye.

H54.10   **Blindness, one eye, low vision other eye, unspecified eyes**

H54.11   **Blindness, right eye, low vision left eye**

H54.12   **Blindness, left eye, low vision right eye**

H54.2   **Low vision, both eyes**
Visual impairment categories 1 or 2 in both eyes.

H54.3   **Unqualified visual loss, both eyes**
Visual impairment category 9 in both eyes.

✓5ᵗʰ **H54.4**   **Blindness, one eye**
Visual impairment categories 3, 4, 5 in one eye [normal vision in other eye]

H54.40   **Blindness, one eye, unspecified eye**

H54.41   **Blindness, right eye, normal vision left eye**

H54.42   **Blindness, left eye, normal vision right eye**

✓5ᵗʰ **H54.5**   **Low vision, one eye**
Visual impairment categories 1 or 2 in one eye [normal vision in other eye].

H54.50   **Low vision, one eye, unspecified eye**

H54.51   **Low vision, right eye, normal vision left eye**

H54.52   **Low vision, left eye, normal vision right eye**

✓5ᵗʰ **H54.6**   **Unqualified visual loss, one eye**
Visual impairment category 9 in one eye [normal vision in other eye].

H54.60   **Unqualified visual loss, one eye, unspecified**

H54.61   **Unqualified visual loss, right eye, normal vision left eye**

H54.62   **Unqualified visual loss, left eye, normal vision right eye**

H54.7   **Unspecified visual loss**
Visual impairment category 9 NOS

H54.8   **Legal blindness, as defined in USA**
Blindness NOS according to USA definition
EXCLUDES 1   legal blindness with specification of impairment level (H54.0-H54.7)

NOTE   The following table gives a classification of severity of visual impairment recommended by a WHO Study Group on the Prevention of Blindness, Geneva, 6-10 November l972.

The term "low vision" in category H54 comprises categories 1 and 2 of the table, the term "blindness" categories 3, 4 and 5, and the term "unqualified visual loss" category 9.

If the extent of the visual field is taken into account, patients with a field no greater than 10 but greater than 5 around central fixation should be placed in category 3 and patients with a field nocategory greater than 5 around central fixation should be placed in 4, even if the central acuity is not impaired.

Category of visual impairment	Visual acuity with best possible correction	
	Maximum less than:	Minimum equal to or better than:
1	6/18 3/10 (0.3) 20/70	6/60 1/10 (0.1) 20/200
2	6/60 1/10 (0.1) 20/200	3/60 1/20 (0.5) 20/400
3	3/60 1/20 (0.05) 20/400	1/60 (finger counting at one meter) 1/50 (0.02) 5/300 (20/1200)
4	1/60 (finger counting at one meter) 1/50 (0.02) 5/300	Light perception
5	No light perception	
9	Undetermined or unspecified	

Other disorders of eye and adnexa (H55-H59)

✓4ᵗʰ **H55**   **Nystagmus and other irregular eye movements**

✓5ᵗʰ **H55.0**   **Nystagmus**

H55.00   **Unspecified nystagmus**

H55.01   **Congenital nystagmus**

H55.02   **Latent nystagmus**

H55.03   **Visual deprivation nystagmus**

H55.04   **Dissociated nystagmus**

H55.09   **Other forms of nystagmus**

✓5ᵗʰ **H55.8**   **Other irregular eye movements**

H55.81   **Saccadic eye movements**

H55.89   **Other irregular eye movements**

✓4ᵗʰ **H57**   **Other disorders of eye and adnexa**

✓5ᵗʰ **H57.0**   **Anomalies of pupillary function**

H57.00   **Unspecified anomaly of pupillary function**

H57.01   **Argyll Robertson pupil, atypical**
EXCLUDES 1   syphilitic Argyll Robertson pupil (A52.19)

H57.02   **Anisocoria**

H57.03   **Miosis**

H57.04   **Mydriasis**

✓6ᵗʰ **H57.05**   **Tonic pupil**

H57.051   **Tonic pupil, right eye**

H57.052   **Tonic pupil, left eye**

H57.053   **Tonic pupil, bilateral**

H57.059   **Tonic pupil, unspecified eye**

H57.09   **Other anomalies of pupillary function**

✓5ᵗʰ **H57.1**   **Ocular pain**

H57.10   **Ocular pain, unspecified eye**

H57.11   **Ocular pain, right eye**

H57.12   **Ocular pain, left eye**

H57.13   **Ocular pain, bilateral**

H57.8   **Other specified disorders of eye and adnexa**

H57.9   **Unspecified disorder of eye and adnexa**

Ⓝ Newborn: 0   Ⓟ Pediatric: 0-17   Ⓜ Maternity: 12-55   Ⓐ Adult: 15-124   **MCC** Major CC Condition   **PDxMCC** PDx acts as own MCC   **CC** CC Condition   **PDxCC** PDx acts as own CC

590

ICD-10-CM 2016

H53.51–H57.9

✓4th **H59** **Intraoperative and postprocedural complications and disorders of eye and adnexa, not elsewhere classified**

EXCLUDES 1　mechanical complication of intraocular lens (T85.2)
mechanical complication of other ocular prosthetic devices, implants and grafts (T85.3)
pseudophakia (Z96.1)
secondary cataracts (H26.4-)

✓5th **H59.0** **Disorders of the eye** following cataract surgery

CC Excl: For CC codes in subcategory H59.0, unless otherwise noted: H59.011-H59.019, H59.031-H59.099, H59.811-H59.89, H95.811-H95.89, I97.3, M96.89, N98.1-N98.9, T81.82XA, T81.89XA, T81.9XXA

✓6th **H59.01** **Keratopathy (bullous aphakic)** following cataract surgery
Vitreal corneal syndrome
Vitreous (touch) syndrome

H59.011 Keratopathy (bullous aphakic) following cataract surgery, right eye 　CC

H59.012 Keratopathy (bullous aphakic) following cataract surgery, left eye 　CC

H59.013 Keratopathy (bullous aphakic) following cataract surgery, bilateral 　CC

H59.019 Keratopathy (bullous aphakic) following cataract surgery, unspecified eye 　CC

✓6th **H59.02** **Cataract (lens) fragments** in eye following cataract surgery

H59.021 Cataract (lens) fragments in eye following cataract surgery, right eye

H59.022 Cataract (lens) fragments in eye following cataract surgery, left eye

H59.023 Cataract (lens) fragments in eye following cataract surgery, bilateral

H59.029 Cataract (lens) fragments in eye following cataract surgery, unspecified eye

✓6th **H59.03** **Cystoid macular edema** following cataract surgery

H59.031 Cystoid macular edema following cataract surgery, right eye 　CC

H59.032 Cystoid macular edema following cataract surgery, left eye 　CC

H59.033 Cystoid macular edema following cataract surgery, bilateral 　CC

H59.039 Cystoid macular edema following cataract surgery, unspecified eye 　CC

✓6th **H59.09** **Other disorders** of the eye following cataract surgery

H59.091 Other disorders of the right eye following cataract surgery 　CC

H59.092 Other disorders of the left eye following cataract surgery 　CC

H59.093 Other disorders of the eye following cataract surgery, bilateral 　CC

H59.099 Other disorders of unspecified eye following cataract surgery 　CC

✓5th **H59.1** **Intraoperative hemorrhage and hematoma** of eye and adnexa complicating a procedure

EXCLUDES 1　intraoperative hemorrhage and hematoma of eye and adnexa due to accidental puncture or laceration during a procedure (H59.2-)

CC Excl: For CC codes in subcategory H59.1, unless otherwise noted: H59.011-H59.019, H59.031-H59.129, H59.311-H59.329, H59.811-H59.89, H95.811-H95.89, I85.01, I85.11, I97.3, K21.9, K22.8, K23-K25.0, K25.2, K25.4, K25.6, K26.0, K26.2, K26.4, K26.6, K27.0, K27.2, K27.4, K27.6, K28.0, K28.2, K28.4, K28.6, K29.01, K29.21, K29.31, K29.41, K29.51, K29.61, K29.71, K29.81, K29.91, K31.811, K55.21, K57.01, K57.11, K57.13, K57.21, K57.31, K57.33, K57.41, K57.51, K57.53, K57.81, K57.91, K57.93, K62.5, K92.0-K92.2, M96.89, N98.1-N98.9, P54.1-P54.3, T81.10XA, T81.11XA, T81.12XA, T81.19XA, T81.82XA, T81.89XA, T81.9XXA

✓6th **H59.11** **Intraoperative hemorrhage and hematoma of eye and adnexa** complicating an ophthalmic procedure

H59.111 Intraoperative hemorrhage and hematoma of right eye and adnexa complicating an ophthalmic procedure 　CC

H59.112 Intraoperative hemorrhage and hematoma of left eye and adnexa complicating an ophthalmic procedure 　CC

H59.113 Intraoperative hemorrhage and hematoma of eye and adnexa complicating an ophthalmic procedure, bilateral 　CC

H59.119 Intraoperative hemorrhage and hematoma of unspecified eye and adnexa complicating an ophthalmic procedure 　CC

✓6th **H59.12** **Intraoperative hemorrhage and hematoma of eye and adnexa complicating** other procedure

H59.121 Intraoperative hemorrhage and hematoma of right eye and adnexa complicating other procedure 　CC

H59.122 Intraoperative hemorrhage and hematoma of left eye and adnexa complicating other procedure 　CC

H59.123 Intraoperative hemorrhage and hematoma of eye and adnexa complicating other procedure, bilateral 　CC

H59.129 Intraoperative hemorrhage and hematoma of unspecified eye and adnexa complicating other procedure 　CC

✓5th **H59.2** **Accidental puncture and laceration** of eye and adnexa during a procedure

CC Excl: For CC codes in subcategory H59.2, unless otherwise noted: D78.11-D78.12, D78.81-D78.89, E36.11-E36.8, E89.810-E89.89, G96.11, G97.41, G97.48-G97.49, H59.011-H59.019, H59.031-H59.099, H59.211-H59.229, H59.811-H59.89, H95.31-H95.32, H95.811-H95.89, I97.3, I97.51-I97.52, J95.71-J95.72, K91.71-K91.72, L76.11-L76.12, L76.81-L76.82, M96.820-M96.821, M96.89, N98.1-N98.9, N99.71-N99.72, T81.82XA, T81.89XA, T81.9XXA

✓6th **H59.21** **Accidental puncture and laceration of eye and adnexa during an** ophthalmic procedure

H59.211 Accidental puncture and laceration of right eye and adnexa during an ophthalmic procedure 　CC

H59.212 Accidental puncture and laceration of left eye and adnexa during an ophthalmic procedure 　CC

H59.213 Accidental puncture and laceration of eye and adnexa during an ophthalmic procedure, bilateral 　CC

H59.219 Accidental puncture and laceration of unspecified eye and adnexa during an ophthalmic procedure 　CC

✓6th **H59.22** **Accidental puncture and laceration of eye and adnexa during** other procedure

H59.221 Accidental puncture and laceration of right eye and adnexa during other procedure 　CC

H59.222 Accidental puncture and laceration of left eye and adnexa during other procedure 　CC

H59.223 Accidental puncture and laceration of eye and adnexa during other procedure, bilateral 　CC

H59.229 Accidental puncture and laceration of unspecified eye and adnexa during other procedure 　CC

✓5th **H59.3** **Postprocedural hemorrhage and hematoma** of eye and adnexa following a procedure

CC Excl: For CC codes in subcategory H59.3, unless otherwise noted: See code: H59.1

✓6th **H59.31** **Postprocedural hemorrhage and hematoma of eye and adnexa following an** ophthalmic procedure

H59.311 Postprocedural hemorrhage and hematoma of right eye and adnexa following an ophthalmic procedure 　CC

H59.312 Postprocedural hemorrhage and hematoma of left eye and adnexa following an ophthalmic procedure 　CC

H59.313 Postprocedural hemorrhage and hematoma of eye and adnexa following an ophthalmic procedure, bilateral 　CC

H59.319 Postprocedural hemorrhage and hematoma of unspecified eye and adnexa following an ophthalmic procedure 　CC

✓ Additional Character Required　✓x7th Placeholder Alert　Unacceptable PDx　Manifestation　Hospital Acquired Condition　EXCLUDES 1 Not Coded Here　EXCLUDES 2 Not Included Here

Chapter 7. Diseases of the Eye and Adnexa

☑6ᵗʰ **H59.32 Postprocedural hemorrhage and hematoma of eye and adnexa following** other procedure

    H59.321 Postprocedural hemorrhage and   CC
        hematoma of right **eye and adnexa following other procedure**

    H59.322 Postprocedural hemorrhage and   CC
        hematoma of left **eye and adnexa following other procedure**

    H59.323 Postprocedural hemorrhage and   CC
        hematoma of eye and adnexa following other procedure, bilateral

    H59.329 Postprocedural hemorrhage and   CC
        hematoma of unspecified **eye and adnexa following other procedure**

☑5ᵗʰ **H59.4 Inflammation (infection) of** postprocedural bleb
    Postprocedural blebitis

    EXCLUDES 1   *filtering (vitreous) bleb after glaucoma surgery status (Z98.83)*

    H59.40 Inflammation (infection) of postprocedural bleb, unspecified

    H59.41 Inflammation (infection) of postprocedural bleb, stage 1

    H59.42 Inflammation (infection) of postprocedural bleb, stage 2

    H59.43 Inflammation (infection) of postprocedural bleb, stage 3
        Bleb endophthalmitis

☑5ᵗʰ **H59.8 Other intraoperative and postprocedural complications and disorders of eye and adnexa, not elsewhere classified**

    CC Excl: For CC codes in subcategory H59.8, unless otherwise noted: H59.011-H59.019, H59.031-H59.099, H59.811-H59.89, H95.811-H95.89, I97.3, M96.89, N98.1-N98.9, T81.82XA, T81.89XA, T81.9XXA

☑6ᵗʰ **H59.81 Chorioretinal scars after surgery for detachment**

    H59.811 Chorioretinal scars after surgery for   CC
        detachment, right **eye**

    H59.812 Chorioretinal scars after surgery for   CC
        detachment, left **eye**

    H59.813 Chorioretinal scars after surgery for   CC
        detachment, bilateral

    H59.819 Chorioretinal scars after surgery for
        detachment, unspecified **eye**

    H59.88 Other intraoperative complications of eye and   CC
        adnexa, not elsewhere classified

    H59.89 Other postprocedural complications and   CC
        disorders of eye and adnexa, not elsewhere classified

N Newborn: 0   P Pediatric: 0-17   M Maternity: 12-55   A Adult: 15-124   **MCC** Major CC Condition   **PDx MCC** PDx acts as own MCC   CC CC Condition   **PDx CC** PDx acts as own CC

592   ICD-10-CM 2016

Chapter 8. Diseases of the Ear and Mastoid Process (H60–H95)

Chapter Specific Coding Guidelines and Examples
Reserved for future guideline expansion.

Chapter 8. Diseases of the Ear and Mastoid Process (H60-H95)

NOTE   Use an external cause code following the code for the ear condition, if applicable, to identify the cause of the ear condition.

EXCLUDES 2   certain conditions originating in the perinatal period (P04-P96)
certain infectious and parasitic diseases (A00-B99)
complications of pregnancy, childbirth and the puerperium (O00-O9A)
congenital malformations, deformations and chromosomal abnormalities (Q00-Q99)
endocrine, nutritional and metabolic diseases (E00-E88)
injury, poisoning and certain other consequences of external causes (S00-T88)
neoplasms (C00-D49)
symptoms, signs and abnormal clinical and laboratory findings, not elsewhere classified (R00-R94)

This chapter contains the following blocks:

H60-H62   Diseases of external ear
H65-H75   Diseases of middle ear and mastoid
H80-H83   Diseases of inner ear
H90-H94   Other disorders of ear
H95   Intraoperative and postprocedural complications and disorders of ear and mastoid process, not elsewhere classified

Diseases of external ear (H60-H62)

✓4ᵗʰ H60   Otitis externa

✓5ᵗʰ H60.0   Abscess of external ear
Boil of external ear
Carbuncle of auricle or external auditory canal
Furuncle of external ear

    H60.00   Abscess of external ear, unspecified ear
    H60.01   Abscess of right external ear
    H60.02   Abscess of left external ear
    H60.03   Abscess of external ear, bilateral

✓5ᵗʰ H60.1   Cellulitis of external ear
Cellulitis of auricle
Cellulitis of external auditory canal

    H60.10   Cellulitis of external ear, unspecified ear
    H60.11   Cellulitis of right external ear
    H60.12   Cellulitis of left external ear
    H60.13   Cellulitis of external ear, bilateral

✓5ᵗʰ H60.2   Malignant otitis externa

> **CC Excl: For CC codes in subcategory H60.2, unless otherwise noted:** H60.20-H60.23, H70.001-H70.13

    H60.20   Malignant otitis externa, unspecified ear   CC
    H60.21   Malignant otitis externa, right ear   CC
    H60.22   Malignant otitis externa, left ear   CC
    H60.23   Malignant otitis externa, bilateral   CC

✓5ᵗʰ H60.3   Other infective otitis externa

   ✓6ᵗʰ H60.31   Diffuse otitis externa
    H60.311   Diffuse otitis externa, right ear
    H60.312   Diffuse otitis externa, left ear
    H60.313   Diffuse otitis externa, bilateral
    H60.319   Diffuse otitis externa, unspecified ear

   ✓6ᵗʰ H60.32   Hemorrhagic otitis externa
    H60.321   Hemorrhagic otitis externa, right ear
    H60.322   Hemorrhagic otitis externa, left ear
    H60.323   Hemorrhagic otitis externa, bilateral
    H60.329   Hemorrhagic otitis externa, unspecified ear

   ✓6ᵗʰ H60.33   Swimmer's ear
    H60.331   Swimmer's ear, right ear
    H60.332   Swimmer's ear, left ear
    H60.333   Swimmer's ear, bilateral
    H60.339   Swimmer's ear, unspecified ear

   ✓6ᵗʰ H60.39   Other infective otitis externa
    H60.391   Other infective otitis externa, right ear
    H60.392   Other infective otitis externa, left ear
    H60.393   Other infective otitis externa, bilateral
    H60.399   Other infective otitis externa, unspecified ear

✓5ᵗʰ H60.4   Cholesteatoma of external ear
Keratosis obturans of external ear (canal)

   EXCLUDES 2   cholesteatoma of middle ear (H71.-)
    recurrent cholesteatoma of postmastoidectomy cavity (H95.0-)

    H60.40   Cholesteatoma of external ear, unspecified ear
    H60.41   Cholesteatoma of right external ear
    H60.42   Cholesteatoma of left external ear
    H60.43   Cholesteatoma of external ear, bilateral

✓5ᵗʰ H60.5   Acute noninfective otitis externa

   ✓6ᵗʰ H60.50   Unspecified acute noninfective otitis externa
Acute otitis externa NOS
    H60.501   Unspecified acute noninfective otitis externa, right ear
    H60.502   Unspecified acute noninfective otitis externa, left ear
    H60.503   Unspecified acute noninfective otitis externa, bilateral
    H60.509   Unspecified acute noninfective otitis externa, unspecified ear

   ✓6ᵗʰ H60.51   Acute actinic otitis externa
    H60.511   Acute actinic otitis externa, right ear
    H60.512   Acute actinic otitis externa, left ear
    H60.513   Acute actinic otitis externa, bilateral
    H60.519   Acute actinic otitis externa, unspecified ear

   ✓6ᵗʰ H60.52   Acute chemical otitis externa
    H60.521   Acute chemical otitis externa, right ear
    H60.522   Acute chemical otitis externa, left ear
    H60.523   Acute chemical otitis externa, bilateral
    H60.529   Acute chemical otitis externa, unspecified ear

   ✓6ᵗʰ H60.53   Acute contact otitis externa
    H60.531   Acute contact otitis externa, right ear
    H60.532   Acute contact otitis externa, left ear
    H60.533   Acute contact otitis externa, bilateral
    H60.539   Acute contact otitis externa, unspecified ear

   ✓6ᵗʰ H60.54   Acute eczematoid otitis externa
    H60.541   Acute eczematoid otitis externa, right ear
    H60.542   Acute eczematoid otitis externa, left ear
    H60.543   Acute eczematoid otitis externa, bilateral
    H60.549   Acute eczematoid otitis externa, unspecified ear

   ✓6ᵗʰ H60.55   Acute reactive otitis externa
    H60.551   Acute reactive otitis externa, right ear
    H60.552   Acute reactive otitis externa, left ear
    H60.553   Acute reactive otitis externa, bilateral
    H60.559   Acute reactive otitis externa, unspecified ear

   ✓6ᵗʰ H60.59   Other noninfective acute otitis externa
    H60.591   Other noninfective acute otitis externa, right ear
    H60.592   Other noninfective acute otitis externa, left ear
    H60.593   Other noninfective acute otitis externa, bilateral
    H60.599   Other noninfective acute otitis externa, unspecified ear

✓5ᵗʰ H60.6   Unspecified chronic otitis externa
    H60.60   Unspecified chronic otitis externa, unspecified ear
    H60.61   Unspecified chronic otitis externa, right ear
    H60.62   Unspecified chronic otitis externa, left ear
    H60.63   Unspecified chronic otitis externa, bilateral

✓5ᵗʰ H60.8   Other otitis externa

   ✓6ᵗʰ H60.8X   Other otitis externa
    H60.8X1   Other otitis externa, right ear
    H60.8X2   Other otitis externa, left ear
    H60.8X3   Other otitis externa, bilateral
    H60.8X9   Other otitis externa, unspecified ear

✓5ᵗʰ H60.9   Unspecified otitis externa
    H60.90   Unspecified otitis externa, unspecified ear
    H60.91   Unspecified otitis externa, right ear

N Newborn: 0   P Pediatric: 0-17   M Maternity: 12-55   A Adult: 15-124   MCC Major CC Condition   PDxMCC PDx acts as own MCC   CC CC Condition   PDxCC PDx acts as own CC

594   ICD-10-CM 2016

H60.92   Unspecified otitis externa, left ear

H60.93   Unspecified otitis externa, bilateral

✓4ᵗʰ **H61   Other disorders of external ear**

✓5ᵗʰ   **H61.0   Chondritis and perichondritis of external ear**
Chondrodermatitis nodularis chronica helicis
Perichondritis of auricle
Perichondritis of pinna

✓6ᵗʰ   **H61.00   Unspecified perichondritis of external ear**

H61.001   Unspecified perichondritis of right external ear

H61.002   Unspecified perichondritis of left external ear

H61.003   Unspecified perichondritis of external ear, bilateral

H61.009   Unspecified perichondritis of external ear, unspecified ear

✓6ᵗʰ   **H61.01   Acute perichondritis of external ear**

H61.011   Acute perichondritis of right external ear

H61.012   Acute perichondritis of left external ear

H61.013   Acute perichondritis of external ear, bilateral

H61.019   Acute perichondritis of external ear, unspecified ear

✓6ᵗʰ   **H61.02   Chronic perichondritis of external ear**

H61.021   Chronic perichondritis of right external ear

H61.022   Chronic perichondritis of left external ear

H61.023   Chronic perichondritis of external ear, bilateral

H61.029   Chronic perichondritis of external ear, unspecified ear

✓6ᵗʰ   **H61.03   Chondritis of external ear**
Chondritis of auricle   Chondritis of pinna
AHA: 2015, 1Q, 18

H61.031   Chondritis of right external ear

H61.032   Chondritis of left external ear

H61.033   Chondritis of external ear, bilateral

H61.039   Chondritis of external ear, unspecified ear

✓5ᵗʰ   **H61.1   Noninfective disorders of pinna**
EXCLUDES2   cauliflower ear (M95.1-)
           gouty tophi of ear (M1A.-)

✓6ᵗʰ   **H61.10   Unspecified noninfective disorders of pinna**
Disorder of pinna NOS

H61.101   Unspecified noninfective disorders of pinna, right ear

H61.102   Unspecified noninfective disorders of pinna, left ear

H61.103   Unspecified noninfective disorders of pinna, bilateral

H61.109   Unspecified noninfective disorders of pinna, unspecified ear

✓6ᵗʰ   **H61.11   Acquired deformity of pinna**
Acquired deformity of auricle
EXCLUDES2   cauliflower ear (M95.1-)

H61.111   Acquired deformity of pinna, right ear

H61.112   Acquired deformity of pinna, left ear

H61.113   Acquired deformity of pinna, bilateral

H61.119   Acquired deformity of pinna, unspecified ear

✓6ᵗʰ   **H61.12   Hematoma of pinna**
Hematoma of auricle

H61.121   Hematoma of pinna, right ear

H61.122   Hematoma of pinna, left ear

H61.123   Hematoma of pinna, bilateral

H61.129   Hematoma of pinna, unspecified ear

✓6ᵗʰ   **H61.19   Other noninfective disorders of pinna**

H61.191   Noninfective disorders of pinna, right ear

H61.192   Noninfective disorders of pinna, left ear

H61.193   Noninfective disorders of pinna, bilateral

H61.199   Noninfective disorders of pinna, unspecified ear

✓5ᵗʰ   **H61.2   Impacted cerumen**
Wax in ear

13 H61.20   Impacted cerumen, unspecified ear

13 H61.21   Impacted cerumen, right ear

13 H61.22   Impacted cerumen, left ear

13 H61.23   Impacted cerumen, bilateral

✓5ᵗʰ   **H61.3   Acquired stenosis of external ear canal**
Collapse of external ear canal
EXCLUDES1   postprocedural stenosis of external ear canal (H95.81-)

✓6ᵗʰ   **H61.30   Acquired stenosis of external ear canal, unspecified**

H61.301   Acquired stenosis of right external ear canal, unspecified

H61.302   Acquired stenosis of left external ear canal, unspecified

H61.303   Acquired stenosis of external ear canal, unspecified, bilateral

H61.309   Acquired stenosis of external ear canal, unspecified, unspecified ear

✓6ᵗʰ   **H61.31   Acquired stenosis of external ear canal secondary to trauma**

H61.311   Acquired stenosis of right external ear canal secondary to trauma

H61.312   Acquired stenosis of left external ear canal secondary to trauma

H61.313   Acquired stenosis of external ear canal secondary to trauma, bilateral

H61.319   Acquired stenosis of external ear canal secondary to trauma, unspecified ear

✓6ᵗʰ   **H61.32   Acquired stenosis of external ear canal secondary to inflammation and infection**

H61.321   Acquired stenosis of right external ear canal secondary to inflammation and infection

H61.322   Acquired stenosis of left external ear canal secondary to inflammation and infection

H61.323   Acquired stenosis of external ear canal secondary to inflammation and infection, bilateral

H61.329   Acquired stenosis of external ear canal secondary to inflammation and infection, unspecified ear

✓6ᵗʰ   **H61.39   Other acquired stenosis of external ear canal**

H61.391   Other acquired stenosis of right external ear canal

H61.392   Other acquired stenosis of left external ear canal

H61.393   Other acquired stenosis of external ear canal, bilateral

H61.399   Other acquired stenosis of external ear canal, unspecified ear

✓5ᵗʰ   **H61.8   Other specified disorders of external ear**

✓6ᵗʰ   **H61.81   Exostosis of external canal**

H61.811   Exostosis of right external canal

H61.812   Exostosis of left external canal

H61.813   Exostosis of external canal, bilateral

H61.819   Exostosis of external canal, unspecified ear

✓6ᵗʰ   **H61.89   Other specified disorders of external ear**

H61.891   Other specified disorders of right external ear

H61.892   Other specified disorders of left external ear

H61.893   Other specified disorders of external ear, bilateral

H61.899   Other specified disorders of external ear, unspecified ear

✓5ᵗʰ   **H61.9   Disorder of external ear, unspecified**

H61.90   Disorder of external ear, unspecified, unspecified ear

H61.91   Disorder of right external ear, unspecified

H61.92   Disorder of left external ear, unspecified

H61.93   Disorder of external ear, unspecified, bilateral

---

13 Questionable admission when used as PDx.

✓ Additional Character Required   ✓x7ᵗʰ Placeholder Alert   Unacceptable PDx   Manifestation   Hospital Acquired Condition   EXCLUDES1 Not Coded Here   EXCLUDES2 Not Included Here

Chapter 8. Diseases of the Ear and Mastoid Process

☑4ᵗʰ H62 Disorders of external ear in diseases classified elsewhere

☑5ᵗʰ H62.4 Otitis externa in other diseases classified elsewhere

Code first underlying disease, such as:
erysipelas (A46)
impetigo (L01.0)

EXCLUDES 1   *otitis externa (in):*
candidiasis (B37.84)
herpes viral [herpes simplex] (B00.1)
herpes zoster (B02.8)

H62.40 Otitis externa in other diseases classified elsewhere, unspecified ear

H62.41 Otitis externa in other diseases classified elsewhere, right ear

H62.42 Otitis externa in other diseases classified elsewhere, left ear

H62.43 Otitis externa in other diseases classified elsewhere, bilateral

☑5ᵗʰ H62.8 Other disorders of external ear in diseases classified elsewhere

Code first underlying disease, such as:
gout (M1A.-, M10.-)

☑6ᵗʰ H62.8X Other disorders of external ear in diseases classified elsewhere

H62.8X1 Other disorders of right external ear in diseases classified elsewhere

H62.8X2 Other disorders of left external ear in diseases classified elsewhere

H62.8X3 Other disorders of external ear in diseases classified elsewhere, bilateral

H62.8X9 Other disorders of external ear in diseases classified elsewhere, unspecified ear

Diseases of middle ear and mastoid (H65-H75)

☑4ᵗʰ H65 Nonsuppurative otitis media

INCLUDES   nonsuppurative otitis media with myringitis

Use additional code for any associated perforated tympanic membrane (H72.-)

Use additional code to identify:
exposure to environmental tobacco smoke (Z77.22)
exposure to tobacco smoke in the perinatal period (P96.81)
history of tobacco use (Z87.891)
occupational exposure to environmental tobacco smoke (Z57.31)
tobacco dependence (F17.-)
tobacco use (Z72.0)

☑5ᵗʰ H65.0 Acute serous otitis media

Acute and subacute secretory otitis

H65.00 Acute serous otitis media, unspecified ear

H65.01 Acute serous otitis media, right ear

H65.02 Acute serous otitis media, left ear

H65.03 Acute serous otitis media, bilateral

H65.04 Acute serous otitis media, recurrent, right ear

H65.05 Acute serous otitis media, recurrent, left ear

H65.06 Acute serous otitis media, recurrent, bilateral

H65.07 Acute serous otitis media, recurrent, unspecified ear

☑5ᵗʰ H65.1 Other acute nonsuppurative otitis media

EXCLUDES 1   *otitic barotrauma (T70.0)*
otitis media (acute) NOS (H66.9)

☑6ᵗʰ H65.11 Acute and subacute allergic otitis media (mucoid) (sanguinous) (serous)

H65.111 Acute and subacute allergic otitis media (mucoid) (sanguinous) (serous), right ear

H65.112 Acute and subacute allergic otitis media (mucoid) (sanguinous) (serous), left ear

H65.113 Acute and subacute allergic otitis media (mucoid) (sanguinous) (serous), bilateral

H65.114 Acute and subacute allergic otitis media (mucoid) (sanguinous) (serous), recurrent, right ear

H65.115 Acute and subacute allergic otitis media (mucoid) (sanguinous) (serous), recurrent, left ear

H65.116 Acute and subacute allergic otitis media (mucoid) (sanguinous) (serous), recurrent, bilateral

H65.117 Acute and subacute allergic otitis media (mucoid) (sanguinous) (serous), recurrent, unspecified ear

H65.119 Acute and subacute allergic otitis media (mucoid) (sanguinous) (serous), unspecified ear

☑6ᵗʰ H65.19 Other acute nonsuppurative otitis media

Acute and subacute mucoid otitis media
Acute and subacute nonsuppurative otitis media NOS
Acute and subacute sanguinous otitis media
Acute and subacute seromucinous otitis media

H65.191 Other acute nonsuppurative otitis media, right ear

H65.192 Other acute nonsuppurative otitis media, left ear

H65.193 Other acute nonsuppurative otitis media, bilateral

H65.194 Other acute nonsuppurative otitis media, recurrent, right ear

H65.195 Other acute nonsuppurative otitis media, recurrent, left ear

H65.196 Other acute nonsuppurative otitis media, recurrent, bilateral

H65.197 Other acute nonsuppurative otitis media, recurrent, unspecified ear

H65.199 Other acute nonsuppurative otitis media, unspecified ear

☑5ᵗʰ H65.2 Chronic serous otitis media

Chronic tubotympanal catarrh

H65.20 Chronic serous otitis media, unspecified ear

H65.21 Chronic serous otitis media, right ear

H65.22 Chronic serous otitis media, left ear

H65.23 Chronic serous otitis media, bilateral

☑5ᵗʰ H65.3 Chronic mucoid otitis media

Chronic mucinous otitis media
Chronic secretory otitis media
Chronic transudative otitis media
Glue ear

EXCLUDES 1   *adhesive middle ear disease (H74.1)*

H65.30 Chronic mucoid otitis media, unspecified ear

H65.31 Chronic mucoid otitis media, right ear

H65.32 Chronic mucoid otitis media, left ear

H65.33 Chronic mucoid otitis media, bilateral

☑5ᵗʰ H65.4 Other chronic nonsuppurative otitis media

☑6ᵗʰ H65.41 Chronic allergic otitis media

H65.411 Chronic allergic otitis media, right ear

H65.412 Chronic allergic otitis media, left ear

H65.413 Chronic allergic otitis media, bilateral

H65.419 Chronic allergic otitis media, unspecified ear

☑6ᵗʰ H65.49 Other chronic nonsuppurative otitis media

Chronic exudative otitis media
Chronic nonsuppurative otitis media NOS
Chronic otitis media with effusion (nonpurulent)
Chronic seromucinous otitis media

H65.491 Other chronic nonsuppurative otitis media, right ear

H65.492 Other chronic nonsuppurative otitis media, left ear

H65.493 Other chronic nonsuppurative otitis media, bilateral

H65.499 Other chronic nonsuppurative otitis media, unspecified ear

☑5ᵗʰ H65.9 Unspecified nonsuppurative otitis media

Allergic otitis media NOS
Catarrhal otitis media NOS
Exudative otitis media NOS
Mucoid otitis media NOS
Otitis media with effusion (nonpurulent) NOS
Secretory otitis media NOS
Seromucinous otitis media NOS
Serous otitis media NOS
Transudative otitis media NOS

H65.90 Unspecified nonsuppurative otitis media, unspecified ear

H65.91 Unspecified nonsuppurative otitis media, right ear

H65.92 Unspecified nonsuppurative otitis media, left ear

H65.93 Unspecified nonsuppurative otitis media, bilateral

N Newborn: 0   **P** Pediatric: 0-17   **M** Maternity: 12-55   **A** Adult: 15-124   **MCC** Major CC Condition   **PDxMCC** PDx acts as own MCC   **CC** CC Condition   **PDxCC** PDx acts as own CC

596   ICD-10-CM 2016

☑4ᵗʰ **H66 Suppurative and unspecified otitis media**
INCLUDES suppurative and unspecified otitis media with myringitis
Use additional code to identify:
exposure to environmental tobacco smoke (Z77.22)
exposure to tobacco smoke in the perinatal period (P96.81)
history of tobacco use (Z87.891)
occupational exposure to environmental tobacco smoke (Z57.31)
tobacco dependence (F17.-)
tobacco use (Z72.0)

☑5ᵗʰ **H66.0 Acute suppurative otitis media**

☑6ᵗʰ **H66.00 Acute suppurative otitis media without spontaneous rupture of ear drum**

H66.001 Acute suppurative otitis media without spontaneous rupture of ear drum, right ear

H66.002 Acute suppurative otitis media without spontaneous rupture of ear drum, left ear

H66.003 Acute suppurative otitis media without spontaneous rupture of ear drum, bilateral

H66.004 Acute suppurative otitis media without spontaneous rupture of ear drum, recurrent, right ear

H66.005 Acute suppurative otitis media without spontaneous rupture of ear drum, recurrent, left ear

H66.006 Acute suppurative otitis media without spontaneous rupture of ear drum, recurrent, bilateral

H66.007 Acute suppurative otitis media without spontaneous rupture of ear drum, recurrent, unspecified ear

H66.009 Acute suppurative otitis media without spontaneous rupture of ear drum, unspecified ear

☑6ᵗʰ **H66.01 Acute suppurative otitis media with spontaneous rupture of ear drum**

H66.011 Acute suppurative otitis media with spontaneous rupture of ear drum, right ear

H66.012 Acute suppurative otitis media with spontaneous rupture of ear drum, left ear

H66.013 Acute suppurative otitis media with spontaneous rupture of ear drum, bilateral

H66.014 Acute suppurative otitis media with spontaneous rupture of ear drum, recurrent, right ear

H66.015 Acute suppurative otitis media with spontaneous rupture of ear drum, recurrent, left ear

H66.016 Acute suppurative otitis media with spontaneous rupture of ear drum, recurrent, bilateral

H66.017 Acute suppurative otitis media with spontaneous rupture of ear drum, recurrent, unspecified ear

H66.019 Acute suppurative otitis media with spontaneous rupture of ear drum, unspecified ear

☑5ᵗʰ **H66.1 Chronic tubotympanic suppurative otitis media**
Benign chronic suppurative otitis media
Chronic tubotympanic disease
Use additional code for any associated perforated tympanic membrane (H72.-)

H66.10 Chronic tubotympanic suppurative otitis media, unspecified

H66.11 Chronic tubotympanic suppurative otitis media, right ear

H66.12 Chronic tubotympanic suppurative otitis media, left ear

H66.13 Chronic tubotympanic suppurative otitis media, bilateral

☑5ᵗʰ **H66.2 Chronic atticoantral suppurative otitis media**
Chronic atticoantral disease
Use additional code for any associated perforated tympanic membrane (H72.-)

H66.20 Chronic atticoantral suppurative otitis media, unspecified ear

H66.21 Chronic atticoantral suppurative otitis media, right ear

H66.22 Chronic atticoantral suppurative otitis media, left ear

H66.23 Chronic atticoantral suppurative otitis media, bilateral

☑5ᵗʰ **H66.3 Other chronic suppurative otitis media**
Chronic suppurative otitis media NOS
Use additional code for any associated perforated tympanic membrane (H72.-)
EXCLUDES1 tuberculous otitis media (A18.6)

☑6ᵗʰ **H66.3X Other chronic suppurative otitis media**

H66.3X1 Other chronic suppurative otitis media, right ear

H66.3X2 Other chronic suppurative otitis media, left ear

H66.3X3 Other chronic suppurative otitis media, bilateral

H66.3X9 Other chronic suppurative otitis media, unspecified ear

☑5ᵗʰ **H66.4 Suppurative otitis media, unspecified**
Purulent otitis media NOS
Use additional code for any associated perforated tympanic membrane (H72.-)

H66.40 Suppurative otitis media, unspecified, unspecified ear

H66.41 Suppurative otitis media, unspecified, right ear

H66.42 Suppurative otitis media, unspecified, left ear

H66.43 Suppurative otitis media, unspecified, bilateral

☑5ᵗʰ **H66.9 Otitis media, unspecified**
Otitis media NOS
Acute otitis media NOS
Chronic otitis media NOS
Use additional code for any associated perforated tympanic membrane (H72.-)

H66.90 Otitis media, unspecified, unspecified ear

H66.91 Otitis media, unspecified, right ear

H66.92 Otitis media, unspecified, left ear

H66.93 Otitis media, unspecified, bilateral

☑4ᵗʰ **H67 Otitis media in diseases classified elsewhere**
Code first underlying disease, such as:
viral disease NEC (B00-B34)
Use additional code for any associated perforated tympanic membrane (H72.-)
EXCLUDES1 otitis media in:
influenza (J09.X9, J10.83, J11.83)
measles (B05.3)
scarlet fever (A38.0)
tuberculosis (A18.6)

H67.1 Otitis media in diseases classified elsewhere, right ear

H67.2 Otitis media in diseases classified elsewhere, left ear

H67.3 Otitis media in diseases classified elsewhere, bilateral

H67.9 Otitis media in diseases classified elsewhere, unspecified ear

☑4ᵗʰ **H68 Eustachian salpingitis and obstruction**

☑5ᵗʰ **H68.0 Eustachian salpingitis**

☑6ᵗʰ **H68.00 Unspecified Eustachian salpingitis**

H68.001 Unspecified Eustachian salpingitis, right ear

H68.002 Unspecified Eustachian salpingitis, left ear

H68.003 Unspecified Eustachian salpingitis, bilateral

H68.009 Unspecified Eustachian salpingitis, unspecified ear

☑6ᵗʰ **H68.01 Acute Eustachian salpingitis**

H68.011 Acute Eustachian salpingitis, right ear

H68.012 Acute Eustachian salpingitis, left ear

H68.013 Acute Eustachian salpingitis, bilateral

H68.019 Acute Eustachian salpingitis, unspecified ear

☑6ᵗʰ **H68.02 Chronic Eustachian salpingitis**

H68.021 Chronic Eustachian salpingitis, right ear

H68.022 Chronic Eustachian salpingitis, left ear

H68.023 Chronic Eustachian salpingitis, bilateral

H68.029 Chronic Eustachian salpingitis, unspecified ear

Chapter 8. Diseases of the Ear and Mastoid Process

√5ᵗʰ **H68.1** **Obstruction** of Eustachian tube
Stenosis of Eustachian tube
Stricture of Eustachian tube

  √6ᵗʰ **H68.10** **Unspecified** obstruction of Eustachian tube

    H68.101 Unspecified obstruction of Eustachian tube, **right ear**

    H68.102 Unspecified obstruction of Eustachian tube, **left ear**

    H68.103 Unspecified obstruction of Eustachian tube, **bilateral**

    H68.109 Unspecified obstruction of Eustachian tube, **unspecified** ear

  √6ᵗʰ **H68.11** **Osseous** obstruction of Eustachian tube

    H68.111 Osseous obstruction of Eustachian tube, **right ear**

    H68.112 Osseous obstruction of Eustachian tube, **left ear**

    H68.113 Osseous obstruction of Eustachian tube, **bilateral**

    H68.119 Osseous obstruction of Eustachian tube, **unspecified** ear

  √6ᵗʰ **H68.12** **Intrinsic cartilagenous** obstruction of Eustachian tube

    H68.121 Intrinsic cartilagenous obstruction of Eustachian tube, **right ear**

    H68.122 Intrinsic cartilagenous obstruction of Eustachian tube, **left ear**

    H68.123 Intrinsic cartilagenous obstruction of Eustachian tube, **bilateral**

    H68.129 Intrinsic cartilagenous obstruction of Eustachian tube, **unspecified** ear

  √6ᵗʰ **H68.13** **Extrinsic cartilagenous** obstruction of Eustachian tube
Compression of Eustachian tube

    H68.131 Extrinsic cartilagenous obstruction of Eustachian tube, **right ear**

    H68.132 Extrinsic cartilagenous obstruction of Eustachian tube, **left ear**

    H68.133 Extrinsic cartilagenous obstruction of Eustachian tube, **bilateral**

    H68.139 Extrinsic cartilagenous obstruction of Eustachian tube, **unspecified** ear

√4ᵗʰ **H69** **Other and unspecified disorders of Eustachian tube**

  √5ᵗʰ **H69.0** **Patulous** Eustachian tube

    H69.00 Patulous Eustachian tube, **unspecified** ear

    H69.01 Patulous Eustachian tube, **right ear**

    H69.02 Patulous Eustachian tube, **left ear**

    H69.03 Patulous Eustachian tube, **bilateral**

  √5ᵗʰ **H69.8** **Other specified disorders of Eustachian tube**

    H69.80 Other specified disorders of Eustachian tube, **unspecified** ear

    H69.81 Other specified disorders of Eustachian tube, **right ear**

    H69.82 Other specified disorders of Eustachian tube, **left ear**

    H69.83 Other specified disorders of Eustachian tube, **bilateral**

  √5ᵗʰ **H69.9** **Unspecified Eustachian tube disorder**

    H69.90 Unspecified Eustachian tube disorder, **unspecified** ear

    H69.91 Unspecified Eustachian tube disorder, **right ear**

    H69.92 Unspecified Eustachian tube disorder, **left ear**

    H69.93 Unspecified Eustachian tube disorder, **bilateral**

√4ᵗʰ **H70** **Mastoiditis and related conditions**

  √5ᵗʰ **H70.0** **Acute mastoiditis**
Abscess of mastoid
Empyema of mastoid

> **CC Excl:** For CC codes in subcategory H70.0, unless otherwise noted: A17.9, A18.6, A18.82, A18.84, A18.89, H70.001-H70.93, H75.00-H75.83, H93.8X1-H93.93, H94.80-H95.199, Q16.1, Q16.9, Q17.3-Q17.9

  √6ᵗʰ **H70.00** **Acute mastoiditis** without complications

    H70.001 Acute mastoiditis without complications, **right ear**   CC

    H70.002 Acute mastoiditis without complications, **left ear**   CC

    H70.003 Acute mastoiditis without complications, **bilateral**   CC

    H70.009 Acute mastoiditis without complications, **unspecified eard**   CC

  √6ᵗʰ **H70.01** **Subperiosteal abscess** of mastoid

    H70.011 Subperiosteal abscess of mastoid, **right ear**   CC

    H70.012 Subperiosteal abscess of mastoid, **left ear**   CC

    H70.013 Subperiosteal abscess of mastoid, **bilateral**   CC

    H70.019 Subperiosteal abscess of mastoid, **unspecified** ear   CC

  √6ᵗʰ **H70.09** **Acute mastoiditis** with other complications

    H70.091 Acute mastoiditis with other complications, **right ear**   CC

    H70.092 Acute mastoiditis with other complications, **left ear**   CC

    H70.093 Acute mastoiditis with other complications, **bilateral**   CC

    H70.099 Acute mastoiditis with other complications, **unspecified** ear   CC

  √5ᵗʰ **H70.1** **Chronic** mastoiditis
Caries of mastoid
Fistula of mastoid

    EXCLUDES 1 tuberculous mastoiditis (A18.03)

    H70.10 Chronic mastoiditis, **unspecified** ear

    H70.11 Chronic mastoiditis, **right ear**

    H70.12 Chronic mastoiditis, **left ear**

    H70.13 Chronic mastoiditis, **bilateral**

  √5ᵗʰ **H70.2** **Petrositis**
Inflammation of petrous bone

  √6ᵗʰ **H70.20** **Unspecified** petrositis

    H70.201 Unspecified petrositis, **right ear**

    H70.202 Unspecified petrositis, **left ear**

    H70.203 Unspecified petrositis, **bilateral**

    H70.209 Unspecified petrositis, **unspecified** ear

  √6ᵗʰ **H70.21** **Acute** petrositis

    H70.211 Acute petrositis, **right ear**

    H70.212 Acute petrositis, **left ear**

    H70.213 Acute petrositis, **bilateral**

    H70.219 Acute petrositis, **unspecified** ear

  √6ᵗʰ **H70.22** **Chronic petrositis**

    H70.221 Chronic petrositis, **right ear**

    H70.222 Chronic petrositis, **left ear**

    H70.223 Chronic petrositis, **bilateral**

    H70.229 Chronic petrositis, **unspecified** ear

  √5ᵗʰ **H70.8** **Other mastoiditis and related conditions**

    EXCLUDES 1 preauricular sinus and cyst (Q18.1)
sinus, fistula, and cyst of branchial cleft (Q18.0)

  √6ᵗʰ **H70.81** **Postauricular fistula**

    H70.811 Postauricular fistula, **right ear**

    H70.812 Postauricular fistula, **left ear**

    H70.813 Postauricular fistula, **bilateral**

    H70.819 Postauricular fistula, **unspecified** ear

  √6ᵗʰ **H70.89** **Other** mastoiditis and related conditions

    H70.891 Other mastoiditis and related conditions, **right ear**

    H70.892 Other mastoiditis and related conditions, **left ear**

    H70.893 Other mastoiditis and related conditions, **bilateral**

    H70.899 Other mastoiditis and related conditions, **unspecified** ear

  √5ᵗʰ **H70.9** **Unspecified** mastoiditis

    H70.90 Unspecified mastoiditis, **unspecified** ear

    H70.91 Unspecified mastoiditis, **right ear**

    H70.92 Unspecified mastoiditis, **left ear**

    H70.93 Unspecified mastoiditis, **bilateral**

N Newborn: 0   P Pediatric: 0-17   M Maternity: 12-55   A Adult: 15-124   MCC Major CC Condition   PDxMCC PDx acts as own MCC   CC CC Condition   PDxCC PDx acts as own CC

598

ICD-10-CM 2016

☑4ᵗʰ **H71** **Cholesteatoma of middle ear**
     EXCLUDES 2   *cholesteatoma of external ear (H60.4-)*
            recurrent cholesteatoma of postmastoidectomy cavity (H95.0-)

   ☑5ᵗʰ **H71.0** **Cholesteatoma of** attic
     H71.00   **Cholesteatoma of attic,** unspecified **ear**
     H71.01   **Cholesteatoma of attic,** right **ear**
     H71.02   **Cholesteatoma of attic,** left **ear**
     H71.03   **Cholesteatoma of attic,** bilateral

   ☑5ᵗʰ **H71.1** **Cholesteatoma of** tympanum
     H71.10   **Cholesteatoma of tympanum,** unspecified **ear**
     H71.11   **Cholesteatoma of tympanum,** right **ear**
     H71.12   **Cholesteatoma of tympanum,** left **ear**
     H71.13   **Cholesteatoma of tympanum,** bilateral

   ☑5ᵗʰ **H71.2** **Cholesteatoma of** mastoid
     H71.20   **Cholesteatoma of mastoid,** unspecified **ear**
     H71.21   **Cholesteatoma of mastoid,** right **ear**
     H71.22   **Cholesteatoma of mastoid,** left **ear**
     H71.23   **Cholesteatoma of mastoid,** bilateral

   ☑5ᵗʰ **H71.3** Diffuse cholesteatosis
     H71.30   **Diffuse cholesteatosis,** unspecified **ear**
     H71.31   **Diffuse cholesteatosis,** right **ear**
     H71.32   **Diffuse cholesteatosis,** left **ear**
     H71.33   **Diffuse cholesteatosis,** bilateral

   ☑5ᵗʰ **H71.9** Unspecified cholesteatoma
     H71.90   **Unspecified cholesteatoma,** unspecified **ear**
     H71.91   **Unspecified cholesteatoma,** right **ear**
     H71.92   **Unspecified cholesteatoma,** left **ear**
     H71.93   **Unspecified cholesteatoma,** bilateral

☑4ᵗʰ **H72** **Perforation of tympanic membrane**
     INCLUDES   persistent post-traumatic perforation of ear drum
            postinflammatory perforation of ear drum
     Code first any associated otitis media (H65.-, H66.1-, H66.2-, H66.3-,
         H66.4-, H66.9-, H67.-)
     EXCLUDES 1   *acute suppurative otitis media with rupture of the tympanic*
            membrane (H66.01-)
            traumatic rupture of ear drum (S09.2-)

   ☑5ᵗʰ **H72.0** Central **perforation of tympanic membrane**
     H72.00   **Central perforation of tympanic membrane,**
            unspecified **ear**
     H72.01   **Central perforation of tympanic membrane,** right
            ear
     H72.02   **Central perforation of tympanic membrane,** left **ear**
     H72.03   **Central perforation of tympanic membrane,**
            bilateral

   ☑5ᵗʰ **H72.1** Attic **perforation of tympanic membrane**
     Perforation of pars flaccida
     H72.10   **Attic perforation of tympanic membrane,**
            unspecified **ear**
     H72.11   **Attic perforation of tympanic membrane,** right **ear**
     H72.12   **Attic perforation of tympanic membrane,** left **ear**
     H72.13   **Attic perforation of tympanic membrane,** bilateral

   ☑5ᵗʰ **H72.2** Other marginal perforations of tympanic membrane
     ☑6ᵗʰ **H72.2X**   Other marginal **perforations of tympanic membrane**
         H72.2X1   **Other marginal perforations of tympanic**
              membrane, right **ear**
         H72.2X2   **Other marginal perforations of tympanic**
              membrane, left **ear**
         H72.2X3   **Other marginal perforations of tympanic**
              membrane, bilateral
         H72.2X9   **Other marginal perforations of tympanic**
              membrane, unspecified **ear**

   ☑5ᵗʰ **H72.8** Other **perforations of tympanic membrane**
     ☑6ᵗʰ **H72.81**   Multiple **perforations of tympanic membrane**
         H72.811   **Multiple perforations of tympanic**
              membrane, right **ear**
         H72.812   **Multiple perforations of tympanic**
              membrane, left **ear**
         H72.813   **Multiple perforations of tympanic**
              membrane, bilateral
         H72.819   **Multiple perforations of tympanic**
              membrane, unspecified **ear**

   ☑6ᵗʰ **H72.82**   Total **perforations of tympanic membrane**
     H72.821   **Total perforations of tympanic**
            membrane, right **ear**
     H72.822   **Total perforations of tympanic**
            membrane, left **ear**
     H72.823   **Total perforations of tympanic**
            membrane, bilateral
     H72.829   **Total perforations of tympanic**
            membrane, unspecified **ear**

   ☑5ᵗʰ **H72.9** Unspecified **perforation of tympanic membrane**
     H72.90   **Unspecified perforation of tympanic membrane,**
            unspecified **ear**
     H72.91   **Unspecified perforation of tympanic membrane,**
            right **ear**
     H72.92   **Unspecified perforation of tympanic membrane,** left
            ear
     H72.93   **Unspecified perforation of tympanic membrane,**
            bilateral

☑4ᵗʰ **H73** **Other disorders of tympanic membrane**
   ☑5ᵗʰ **H73.0** Acute **myringitis**
     EXCLUDES 1   *acute myringitis with otitis media (H65, H66)*
     ☑6ᵗʰ **H73.00**   Unspecified **acute myringitis**
         Acute tympanitis NOS
         H73.001   **Acute myringitis,** right **ear**
         H73.002   **Acute myringitis,** left **ear**
         H73.003   **Acute myringitis,** bilateral
         H73.009   **Acute myringitis,** unspecified **ear**
     ☑6ᵗʰ **H73.01**   Bullous **myringitis**
         H73.011   **Bullous myringitis,** right **ear**
         H73.012   **Bullous myringitis,** left **ear**
         H73.013   **Bullous myringitis,** bilateral
         H73.019   **Bullous myringitis,** unspecified **ear**
     ☑6ᵗʰ **H73.09**   Other **acute myringitis**
         H73.091   **Other acute myringitis,** right **ear**
         H73.092   **Other acute myringitis,** left **ear**
         H73.093   **Other acute myringitis,** bilateral
         H73.099   **Other acute myringitis,** unspecified **ear**

   ☑5ᵗʰ **H73.1** Chronic **myringitis**
     Chronic tympanitis
     EXCLUDES 1   *chronic myringitis with otitis media (H65, H66)*
     H73.10   **Chronic myringitis,** unspecified **ear**
     H73.11   **Chronic myringitis,** right **ear**
     H73.12   **Chronic myringitis,** left **ear**
     H73.13   **Chronic myringitis,** bilateral

   ☑5ᵗʰ **H73.2** Unspecified **myringitis**
     H73.20   **Unspecified myringitis,** unspecified **ear**
     H73.21   **Unspecified myringitis,** right **ear**
     H73.22   **Unspecified myringitis,** left **ear**
     H73.23   **Unspecified myringitis,** bilateral

   ☑5ᵗʰ **H73.8** Other specified disorders of tympanic membrane
     ☑6ᵗʰ **H73.81**   Atrophic flaccid **tympanic membrane**
         H73.811   **Atrophic flaccid tympanic membrane,**
              right **ear**
         H73.812   **Atrophic flaccid tympanic membrane,**
              left **ear**
         H73.813   **Atrophic flaccid tympanic membrane,**
              bilateral
         H73.819   **Atrophic flaccid tympanic membrane,**
              unspecified **ear**
     ☑6ᵗʰ **H73.82**   Atrophic nonflaccid **tympanic membrane**
         H73.821   **Atrophic nonflaccid tympanic membrane,**
              right **ear**
         H73.822   **Atrophic nonflaccid tympanic membrane,**
              left **ear**
         H73.823   **Atrophic nonflaccid tympanic membrane,**
              bilateral
         H73.829   **Atrophic nonflaccid tympanic membrane,**
              unspecified **ear**
     ☑6ᵗʰ **H73.89**   Other specified disorders of tympanic membrane
         H73.891   **Other specified disorders of tympanic**
              membrane, right **ear**
         H73.892   **Other specified disorders of tympanic**
              membrane, left **ear**

☑ Additional Character Required   ☑x7ᵗʰ Placeholder Alert   Unacceptable PDx   Manifestation   Hospital Acquired Condition   EXCLUDES 1 Not Coded Here   EXCLUDES 2 Not Included Here

ICD-10-CM 2016   **599**

Chapter 8. Diseases of the Ear and Mastoid Process

H71–H73.892

H73.893 **Other specified disorders of tympanic membrane,** bilateral

H73.899 **Other specified disorders of tympanic membrane,** unspecified ear

✓5ᵗʰ **H73.9** Unspecified **disorder of tympanic membrane**

H73.90 **Unspecified disorder of tympanic membrane,** unspecified ear

H73.91 **Unspecified disorder of tympanic membrane,** right ear

H73.92 **Unspecified disorder of tympanic membrane,** left ear

H73.93 **Unspecified disorder of tympanic membrane,** bilateral

✓4ᵗʰ **H74 Other disorders of middle ear mastoid**
   EXCLUDES 2   *mastoiditis (H70.-)*

✓5ᵗʰ **H74.0 Tympanosclerosis**

H74.01 **Tympanosclerosis,** right ear

H74.02 **Tympanosclerosis,** left ear

H74.03 **Tympanosclerosis,** bilateral

H74.09 **Tympanosclerosis,** unspecified ear

✓5ᵗʰ **H74.1 Adhesive middle ear disease**
   Adhesive otitis
   EXCLUDES 1   *glue ear (H65.3-)*

H74.11 **Adhesive** right **middle ear disease**

H74.12 **Adhesive** left **middle ear disease**

H74.13 **Adhesive middle ear disease,** bilateral

H74.19 **Adhesive middle ear disease,** unspecified ear

✓5ᵗʰ **H74.2 Discontinuity and dislocation of ear ossicles**

H74.20 **Discontinuity and dislocation of ear ossicles,** unspecified ear

H74.21 **Discontinuity and dislocation of** right **ear ossicles**

H74.22 **Discontinuity and dislocation of** left **ear ossicles**

H74.23 **Discontinuity and dislocation of ear ossicles,** bilateral

✓5ᵗʰ **H74.3 Other acquired abnormalities of ear ossicles**

✓6ᵗʰ **H74.31** Ankylosis **of ear ossicles**

H74.311 **Ankylosis of ear ossicles,** right ear

H74.312 **Ankylosis of ear ossicles,** left ear

H74.313 **Ankylosis of ear ossicles,** bilateral

H74.319 **Ankylosis of ear ossicles,** unspecified ear

✓6ᵗʰ **H74.32** Partial loss **of ear ossicles**

H74.321 **Partial loss of ear ossicles,** right ear

H74.322 **Partial loss of ear ossicles,** left ear

H74.323 **Partial loss of ear ossicles,** bilateral

H74.329 **Partial loss of ear ossicles,** unspecified ear

✓6ᵗʰ **H74.39** Other **acquired abnormalities of ear ossicles**

H74.391 **Other acquired abnormalities of** right **ear ossicles**

H74.392 **Other acquired abnormalities of** left **ear ossicles**

H74.393 **Other acquired abnormalities of ear ossicles,** bilateral

H74.399 **Other acquired abnormalities of ear ossicles,** unspecified ear

✓5ᵗʰ **H74.4 Polyp of middle ear**

H74.40 **Polyp of middle ear,** unspecified ear

H74.41 **Polyp of** right **middle ear**

H74.42 **Polyp of** left **middle ear**

H74.43 **Polyp of middle ear,** bilateral

✓5ᵗʰ **H74.8 Other specified disorders of middle ear and mastoid**

✓6ᵗʰ **H74.8X** Other specified disorders of middle ear and mastoid

H74.8X1 **Other specified disorders of** right **middle ear and mastoid**

H74.8X2 **Other specified disorders of** left **middle ear and mastoid**

H74.8X3 **Other specified disorders of middle ear and mastoid,** bilateral

H74.8X9 **Other specified disorders of middle ear and mastoid,** unspecified ear

✓5ᵗʰ **H74.9 Unspecified disorder of middle ear and mastoid**

H74.90 **Unspecified disorder of middle ear and mastoid,** unspecified ear

H74.91 **Unspecified disorder of** right **middle ear and mastoid**

H74.92 **Unspecified disorder of** left **middle ear and mastoid**

H74.93 **Unspecified disorder of middle ear and mastoid,** bilateral

✓4ᵗʰ **H75 Other disorders of middle ear and mastoid in diseases classified elsewhere**
   Code first underlying disease

✓5ᵗʰ **H75.0 Mastoiditis in infectious and parasitic diseases classified elsewhere**
   EXCLUDES 1   *mastoiditis (in):*
      syphilis (A52.77)
      tuberculosis (A18.03)

H75.00 *Mastoiditis in infectious and parasitic diseases classified elsewhere, unspecified ear*

H75.01 *Mastoiditis in infectious and parasitic diseases classified elsewhere, right ear*

H75.02 *Mastoiditis in infectious and parasitic diseases classified elsewhere, left ear*

H75.03 *Mastoiditis in infectious and parasitic diseases classified elsewhere, bilateral*

✓5ᵗʰ **H75.8 Other specified disorders of middle ear and mastoid in diseases classified elsewhere**

H75.80 *Other specified disorders of middle ear and mastoid in diseases classified elsewhere, unspecified ear*

H75.81 *Other specified disorders of right middle ear and mastoid in diseases classified elsewhere*

H75.82 *Other specified disorders of left middle ear and mastoid in diseases classified elsewhere*

H75.83 *Other specified disorders of middle ear and mastoid in diseases classified elsewhere, bilateral*

Diseases of inner ear (H80-H83)

✓4ᵗʰ **H80 Otosclerosis**
   INCLUDES   Otospongiosis

✓5ᵗʰ **H80.0 Otosclerosis involving oval window,** nonobliterative

H80.00 **Otosclerosis involving oval window, nonobliterative,** unspecified ear

H80.01 **Otosclerosis involving oval window, nonobliterative,** right ear

H80.02 **Otosclerosis involving oval window, nonobliterative,** left ear

H80.03 **Otosclerosis involving oval window, nonobliterative,** bilateral

✓5ᵗʰ **H80.1 Otosclerosis involving oval window,** obliterative

H80.10 **Otosclerosis involving oval window, obliterative,** unspecified ear

H80.11 **Otosclerosis involving oval window, obliterative,** right ear

H80.12 **Otosclerosis involving oval window, obliterative,** left ear

H80.13 **Otosclerosis involving oval window, obliterative,** bilateral

✓5ᵗʰ **H80.2** Cochlear **otosclerosis**
   Otosclerosis involving otic capsule
   Otosclerosis involving round window

H80.20 **Cochlear otosclerosis,** unspecified ear

H80.21 **Cochlear otosclerosis,** right ear

H80.22 **Cochlear otosclerosis,** left ear

H80.23 **Cochlear otosclerosis,** bilateral

✓5ᵗʰ **H80.8** Other **otosclerosis**

H80.80 **Other otosclerosis,** unspecified ear

H80.81 **Other otosclerosis,** right ear

H80.82 **Other otosclerosis,** left ear

H80.83 **Other otosclerosis,** bilateral

✓5ᵗʰ **H80.9** Unspecified **otosclerosis**

H80.90 **Unspecified otosclerosis,** unspecified ear

H80.91 **Unspecified otosclerosis,** right ear

H80.92 **Unspecified otosclerosis,** left ear

H80.93 **Unspecified otosclerosis,** bilateral

✓4ᵗʰ H81 Disorders of vestibular function
    EXCLUDES 1 *epidemic vertigo (A88.1)*
           vertigo NOS (R42)

   ✓5ᵗʰ H81.Ø Ménière's disease
     Labyrinthine hydrops
     Ménière's syndrome or vertigo
     H81.Ø1 Ménière's disease, right ear
     H81.Ø2 Ménière's disease, left ear
     H81.Ø3 Ménière's disease, bilateral
     H81.Ø9 Ménière's disease, unspecified ear

   ✓5ᵗʰ H81.1 Benign paroxysmal vertigo
     H81.1Ø Benign paroxysmal vertigo, unspecified ear
     H81.11 Benign paroxysmal vertigo, right ear
     H81.12 Benign paroxysmal vertigo, left ear
     H81.13 Benign paroxysmal vertigo, bilateral

   ✓5ᵗʰ H81.2 Vestibular neuronitis
     H81.2Ø Vestibular neuronitis, unspecified ear
     H81.21 Vestibular neuronitis, right ear
     H81.22 Vestibular neuronitis, left ear
     H81.23 Vestibular neuronitis, bilateral

   ✓5ᵗʰ H81.3 Other peripheral vertigo
    ✓6ᵗʰ H81.31 Aural vertigo
      H81.311 Aural vertigo, right ear
      H81.312 Aural vertigo, left ear
      H81.313 Aural vertigo, bilateral
      H81.319 Aural vertigo, unspecified ear
    ✓6ᵗʰ H81.39 Other peripheral vertigo
      Lermoyez' syndrome
      Otogenic vertigo
      Peripheral vertigo NOS
      H81.391 Other peripheral vertigo, right ear
      H81.392 Other peripheral vertigo, left ear
      H81.393 Other peripheral vertigo, bilateral
      H81.399 Other peripheral vertigo, unspecified ear

   ✓5ᵗʰ H81.4 Vertigo of central origin
     Central positional nystagmus
     H81.41 Vertigo of central origin, right ear
     H81.42 Vertigo of central origin, left ear
     H81.43 Vertigo of central origin, bilateral
     H81.49 Vertigo of central origin, unspecified ear

   ✓5ᵗʰ H81.8 Other disorders of vestibular function
    ✓6ᵗʰ H81.8X Other disorders of vestibular function
      H81.8X1 Other disorders of vestibular function, right ear
      H81.8X2 Other disorders of vestibular function, left ear
      H81.8X3 Other disorders of vestibular function, bilateral
      H81.8X9 Other disorders of vestibular function, unspecified ear

   ✓5ᵗʰ H81.9 Unspecified disorder of vestibular function
     Vertiginous syndrome NOS
     H81.9Ø Unspecified disorder of vestibular function, unspecified ear
     H81.91 Unspecified disorder of vestibular function, right ear
     H81.92 Unspecified disorder of vestibular function, left ear
     H81.93 Unspecified disorder of vestibular function, bilateral

✓4ᵗʰ H82 Vertiginous syndromes in diseases classified elsewhere
    Code first underlying disease
    EXCLUDES 1 *epidemic vertigo (A88.1)*
   H82.1 *Vertiginous syndromes in diseases classified elsewhere, right ear*
   H82.2 *Vertiginous syndromes in diseases classified elsewhere, left ear*
   H82.3 *Vertiginous syndromes in diseases classified elsewhere, bilateral*
   H82.9 *Vertiginous syndromes in diseases classified elsewhere, unspecified ear*

✓4ᵗʰ H83 Other diseases of inner ear
   ✓5ᵗʰ H83.Ø Labyrinthitis
     H83.Ø1 Labyrinthitis, right ear
     H83.Ø2 Labyrinthitis, left ear
     H83.Ø3 Labyrinthitis, bilateral
     H83.Ø9 Labyrinthitis, unspecified ear

   ✓5ᵗʰ H83.1 Labyrinthine fistula
     H83.11 Labyrinthine fistula, right ear
     H83.12 Labyrinthine fistula, left ear
     H83.13 Labyrinthine fistula, bilateral
     H83.19 Labyrinthine fistula, unspecified ear

   ✓5ᵗʰ H83.2 Labyrinthine dysfunction
     Labyrinthine hypersensitivity
     Labyrinthine hypofunction
     Labyrinthine loss of function
    ✓6ᵗʰ H83.2X Labyrinthine dysfunction
      H83.2X1 Labyrinthine dysfunction, right ear
      H83.2X2 Labyrinthine dysfunction, left ear
      H83.2X3 Labyrinthine dysfunction, bilateral
      H83.2X9 Labyrinthine dysfunction, unspecified ear

   ✓5ᵗʰ H83.3 Noise effects on inner ear
     Acoustic trauma of inner ear
     Noise-induced hearing loss of inner ear
    ✓6ᵗʰ H83.3X Noise effects on inner ear
      H83.3X1 Noise effects on right inner ear
      H83.3X2 Noise effects on left inner ear
      H83.3X3 Noise effects on inner ear, bilateral
      H83.3X9 Noise effects on inner ear, unspecified ear

   ✓5ᵗʰ H83.8 Other specified diseases of inner ear
    ✓6ᵗʰ H83.8X Other specified diseases of inner ear
      H83.8X1 Other specified diseases of right inner ear
      H83.8X2 Other specified diseases of left inner ear
      H83.8X3 Other specified diseases of inner ear, bilateral
      H83.8X9 Other specified diseases of inner ear, unspecified ear

   ✓5ᵗʰ H83.9 Unspecified disease of inner ear
     H83.9Ø Unspecified disease of inner ear, unspecified ear
     H83.91 Unspecified disease of right inner ear
     H83.92 Unspecified disease of left inner ear
     H83.93 Unspecified disease of inner ear, bilateral

Other disorders of ear (H9Ø-H94)

✓4ᵗʰ H9Ø Conductive and sensorineural hearing loss
    EXCLUDES 1 *deaf nonspeaking NEC (H91.3)*
           deafness NOS (H91.9-)
           hearing loss NOS (H91.9-)
           noise-induced hearing loss (H83.3-)
           ototoxic hearing loss (H91.Ø-)
           sudden (idiopathic) hearing loss (H91.2-)

   H9Ø.Ø Conductive hearing loss, bilateral

   ✓5ᵗʰ H9Ø.1 Conductive hearing loss, unilateral with unrestricted hearing on the contralateral side
     H9Ø.11 Conductive hearing loss, unilateral, right ear, with unrestricted hearing on the contralateral side
     H9Ø.12 Conductive hearing loss, unilateral, left ear, with unrestricted hearing on the contralateral side

   H9Ø.2 Conductive hearing loss, unspecified
     Conductive deafness NOS

   H9Ø.3 Sensorineural hearing loss, bilateral

   ✓5ᵗʰ H9Ø.4 Sensorineural hearing loss, unilateral with unrestricted hearing on the contralateral side
     H9Ø.41 Sensorineural hearing loss, unilateral, right ear, with unrestricted hearing on the contralateral side
     H9Ø.42 Sensorineural hearing loss, unilateral, left ear, with unrestricted hearing on the contralateral side

   H9Ø.5 Unspecified sensorineural hearing loss

Central hearing loss NOS	Perceptive hearing loss NOS
Congenital deafness NOS	Sensorineural deafness NOS
Neural hearing loss NOS	Sensory hearing loss NOS

     EXCLUDES 1 *abnormal auditory perception (H93.2-)*
            psychogenic deafness (F44.6)

   H9Ø.6 Mixed conductive and sensorineural hearing loss, bilateral

   ✓5ᵗʰ H9Ø.7 Mixed conductive and sensorineural hearing loss, unilateral with unrestricted hearing on the contralateral side
     H9Ø.71 Mixed conductive and sensorineural hearing loss, unilateral, right ear, with unrestricted hearing on the contralateral side

---

✓ Additional Character Required   ✓x7ᵗʰ Placeholder Alert   Unacceptable PDx   Manifestation   Hospital Acquired Condition   **EXCLUDES 1** Not Coded Here   **EXCLUDES 2** Not Included Here

ICD-10-CM 2016   601

Chapter 8. Diseases of the Ear and Mastoid Process

H81–H90.71

Chapter 8. Diseases of the Ear and Mastoid Process

H90.72–H93.8X9

H90.72   **Mixed conductive and sensorineural hearing loss, unilateral, left ear, with unrestricted hearing on the contralateral side**

H90.8   Mixed conductive and sensorineural hearing loss, unspecified

✓4th **H91   Other and unspecified hearing loss**

     EXCLUDES 1   *abnormal auditory perception (H93.2-)*
         hearing loss as classified in H90-
         impacted cerumen (H61.2-)
         noise-induced hearing loss (H83.3-)
         psychogenic deafness (F44.6)
         transient ischemic deafness (H93.01-)

✓5th **H91.0   Ototoxic hearing loss**

     Code first poisoning due to drug or toxin, if applicable (T36-T65 with fifth or sixth character 1-4 or 6)
     Use additional code for adverse effect, if applicable, to identify drug (T36-T50 with fifth or sixth character 5)

     H91.01   Ototoxic hearing loss, right ear
     H91.02   Ototoxic hearing loss, left ear
     H91.03   Ototoxic hearing loss, bilateral
     H91.09   Ototoxic hearing loss, unspecified ear

✓5th **H91.1   Presbycusis**

     Presbyacusia

     H91.10   Presbycusis, unspecified ear
     H91.11   Presbycusis, right ear
     H91.12   Presbycusis, left ear
     H91.13   Presbycusis, bilateral

✓5th **H91.2   Sudden idiopathic hearing loss**

     Sudden hearing loss NOS

     H91.20   Sudden idiopathic hearing loss, unspecified ear
     H91.21   Sudden idiopathic hearing loss, right ear
     H91.22   Sudden idiopathic hearing loss, left ear
     H91.23   Sudden idiopathic hearing loss, bilateral

H91.3   Deaf nonspeaking, not elsewhere classified

✓5th **H91.8   Other specified hearing loss**

     ✓6th **H91.8X   Other specified hearing loss**

         H91.8X1   Other specified hearing loss, right ear
         H91.8X2   Other specified hearing loss, left ear
         H91.8X3   Other specified hearing loss, bilateral
         H91.8X9   Other specified hearing loss, unspecified ear

✓5th **H91.9   Unspecified hearing loss**

     Deafness NOS
     High frequency deafness
     Low frequency deafness

     H91.90   Unspecified hearing loss, unspecified ear
     H91.91   Unspecified hearing loss, right ear
     H91.92   Unspecified hearing loss, left ear
     H91.93   Unspecified hearing loss, bilateral

✓4th **H92   Otalgia and effusion of ear**

✓5th **H92.0   Otalgia**

     H92.01   Otalgia, right ear
     H92.02   Otalgia, left ear
     H92.03   Otalgia, bilateral
     H92.09   Otalgia, unspecified ear

✓5th **H92.1   Otorrhea**

     EXCLUDES 1   *leakage of cerebrospinal fluid through ear (G96.0)*

     H92.10   Otorrhea, unspecified ear
     H92.11   Otorrhea, right ear
     H92.12   Otorrhea, left ear
     H92.13   Otorrhea, bilateral

✓5th **H92.2   Otorrhagia**

     EXCLUDES 1   *traumatic otorrhagia—code to injury*

     H92.20   Otorrhagia, unspecified ear
     H92.21   Otorrhagia, right ear
     H92.22   Otorrhagia, left ear
     H92.23   Otorrhagia, bilateral

✓4th **H93   Other disorders of ear, not elsewhere classified**

✓5th **H93.0   Degenerative and vascular disorders of ear**

     EXCLUDES 1   *presbycusis (H91.1)*

     ✓6th **H93.01   Transient ischemic deafness**

         H93.011   Transient ischemic deafness, right ear
         H93.012   Transient ischemic deafness, left ear
         H93.013   Transient ischemic deafness, bilateral
         H93.019   Transient ischemic deafness, unspecified ear

     ✓6th **H93.09   Unspecified degenerative and vascular disorders of ear**

         H93.091   Unspecified degenerative and vascular disorders of right ear
         H93.092   Unspecified degenerative and vascular disorders of left ear
         H93.093   Unspecified degenerative and vascular disorders of ear, bilateral
         H93.099   Unspecified degenerative and vascular disorders of unspecified ear

✓5th **H93.1   Tinnitus**

     H93.11   Tinnitus, right ear
     H93.12   Tinnitus, left ear
     H93.13   Tinnitus, bilateral
     H93.19   Tinnitus, unspecified ear

✓5th **H93.2   Other abnormal auditory perceptions**

     EXCLUDES 2   *auditory hallucinations (R44.0)*

     ✓6th **H93.21   Auditory recruitment**

         H93.211   Auditory recruitment, right ear
         H93.212   Auditory recruitment, left ear
         H93.213   Auditory recruitment, bilateral
         H93.219   Auditory recruitment, unspecified ear

     ✓6th **H93.22   Diplacusis**

         H93.221   Diplacusis, right ear
         H93.222   Diplacusis, left ear
         H93.223   Diplacusis, bilateral
         H93.229   Diplacusis, unspecified ear

     ✓6th **H93.23   Hyperacusis**

         H93.231   Hyperacusis, right ear
         H93.232   Hyperacusis, left ear
         H93.233   Hyperacusis, bilateral
         H93.239   Hyperacusis, unspecified ear

     ✓6th **H93.24   Temporary auditory threshold shift**

         H93.241   Temporary auditory threshold shift, right ear
         H93.242   Temporary auditory threshold shift, left ear
         H93.243   Temporary auditory threshold shift, bilateral
         H93.249   Temporary auditory threshold shift, unspecified ear

     H93.25   Central auditory processing disorder
         Congenital auditory imperception
         Word deafness
         EXCLUDES 1   *mixed receptive-expressive language disorder (F80.2)*

     ✓6th **H93.29   Other abnormal auditory perceptions**

         H93.291   Other abnormal auditory perceptions, right ear
         H93.292   Other abnormal auditory perceptions, left ear
         H93.293   Other abnormal auditory perceptions, bilateral
         H93.299   Other abnormal auditory perceptions, unspecified ear

✓5th **H93.3   Disorders of acoustic nerve**

     Disorder of 8th cranial nerve
     EXCLUDES 1   *acoustic neuroma (D33.3)*
         syphilitic acoustic neuritis (A52.15)

     ✓6th **H93.3X   Disorders of acoustic nerve**

         H93.3X1   Disorders of right acoustic nerve
         H93.3X2   Disorders of left acoustic nerve
         H93.3X3   Disorders of bilateral acoustic nerves
         H93.3X9   Disorders of unspecified acoustic nerve

✓5th **H93.8   Other specified disorders of ear**

     ✓6th **H93.8X   Other specified disorders of ear**

         H93.8X1   Other specified disorders of right ear
         H93.8X2   Other specified disorders of left ear
         H93.8X3   Other specified disorders of ear, bilateral
         H93.8X9   Other specified disorders of ear, unspecified ear

N Newborn: 0   P Pediatric: 0-17   M Maternity: 12-55   A Adult: 15-124   MCC Major CC Condition   PDxMCC PDx acts as own MCC   CC CC Condition   PDxCC PDx acts as own CC

602

ICD-10-CM 2016

✓5ᵗʰ **H93.9　Unspecified disorder of ear**

　　H93.90　Unspecified disorder of ear, unspecified ear

　　H93.91　Unspecified disorder of right ear

　　H93.92　Unspecified disorder of left ear

　　H93.93　Unspecified disorder of ear, bilateral

✓4ᵗʰ **H94　Other disorders of ear in diseases classified elsewhere**

　✓5ᵗʰ **H94.0　Acoustic neuritis in infectious and parasitic diseases classified elsewhere**

　　　Code first underlying disease, such as:
　　　　parasitic disease (B65-B89)

　　　　EXCLUDES1　*acoustic neuritis (in):*
　　　　　　herpes zoster (B02.29)
　　　　　　syphilis (A52.15)

　　H94.00　***Acoustic neuritis in infectious and parasitic diseases classified elsewhere, unspecified ear***

　　H94.01　***Acoustic neuritis in infectious and parasitic diseases classified elsewhere, right ear***

　　H94.02　***Acoustic neuritis in infectious and parasitic diseases classified elsewhere, left ear***

　　H94.03　***Acoustic neuritis in infectious and parasitic diseases classified elsewhere, bilateral***

　✓5ᵗʰ **H94.8　Other specified disorders of ear in diseases classified elsewhere**

　　　Code first underlying disease, such as:
　　　　congenital syphilis (A50.0)

　　　　EXCLUDES1　*aural myiasis (B87.4)*
　　　　　　syphilitic labyrinthitis (A52.79)

　　H94.80　***Other specified disorders of ear in diseases classified elsewhere, unspecified ear***

　　H94.81　***Other specified disorders of right ear in diseases classified elsewhere***

　　H94.82　***Other specified disorders of left ear in diseases classified elsewhere***

　　H94.83　***Other specified disorders of ear in diseases classified elsewhere, bilateral***

Intraoperative and postprocedural complications and disorders of ear and mastoid process, not elsewhere classified (H95)

✓4ᵗʰ **H95　Intraoperative and postprocedural complications and disorders of ear and mastoid process, not elsewhere classified**

　✓5ᵗʰ **H95.0　Recurrent cholesteatoma of postmastoidectomy cavity**

　　H95.00　Recurrent cholesteatoma of postmastoidectomy cavity, unspecified ear

　　H95.01　Recurrent cholesteatoma of postmastoidectomy cavity, right ear

　　H95.02　Recurrent cholesteatoma of postmastoidectomy cavity, left ear

　　H95.03　Recurrent cholesteatoma of postmastoidectomy cavity, bilateral ears

　✓5ᵗʰ **H95.1　Other disorders of ear and mastoid process following mastoidectomy**

　　✓6ᵗʰ **H95.11　Chronic inflammation of postmastoidectomy cavity**

　　　H95.111　Chronic inflammation of postmastoidectomy cavity, right ear

　　　H95.112　Chronic inflammation of postmastoidectomy cavity, left ear

　　　H95.113　Chronic inflammation of postmastoidectomy cavity, bilateral ears

　　　H95.119　Chronic inflammation of postmastoidectomy cavity, unspecified ear

　　✓6ᵗʰ **H95.12　Granulation of postmastoidectomy cavity**

　　　H95.121　Granulation of postmastoidectomy cavity, right ear

　　　H95.122　Granulation of postmastoidectomy cavity, left ear

　　　H95.123　Granulation of postmastoidectomy cavity, bilateral ears

　　　H95.129　Granulation of postmastoidectomy cavity, unspecified ear

　　✓6ᵗʰ **H95.13　Mucosal cyst of postmastoidectomy cavity**

　　　H95.131　Mucosal cyst of postmastoidectomy cavity, right ear

　　　H95.132　Mucosal cyst of postmastoidectomy cavity, left ear

　　　H95.133　Mucosal cyst of postmastoidectomy cavity, bilateral ears

　　　H95.139　Mucosal cyst of postmastoidectomy cavity, unspecified ear

　　✓6ᵗʰ **H95.19　Other disorders following mastoidectomy**

　　　H95.191　Other disorders following mastoidectomy, right ear

　　　H95.192　Other disorders following mastoidectomy, left ear

　　　H95.193　Other disorders following mastoidectomy, bilateral ears

　　　H95.199　Other disorders following mastoidectomy, unspecified ear

　✓5ᵗʰ **H95.2　Intraoperative hemorrhage and hematoma of ear and mastoid process complicating a procedure**

　　　EXCLUDES1　*intraoperative hemorrhage and hematoma of ear and mastoid process due to accidental puncture or laceration during a procedure (H95.3-)*

　　H95.21　Intraoperative hemorrhage and hematoma of ear and mastoid process complicating a procedure on the ear and mastoid process　　[CC]
　　　CC Excl: H95.21-H95.22, H95.41-H95.89, I85.01, I85.11, I97.3, K21.9, K22.8, K23-K25.0, K25.2, K25.4, K25.6, K26.0, K26.2, K26.4, K26.6, K27.0, K27.2, K27.4, K27.6, K28.0, K28.2, K28.4, K28.6, K29.01, K29.21, K29.31, K29.41, K29.51, K29.61, K29.71, K29.81, K29.91, K31.811, K55.21, K57.01, K57.11, K57.13, K57.21, K57.31, K57.33, K57.41, K57.51, K57.53, K57.81, K57.91, K57.93, K62.5, K92.0-K92.2, M96.89, N98.1-N98.9, P54.1-P54.3, T81.10XA, T81.11XA, T81.12XA, T81.19XA, T81.82XA, T81.89XA, T81.9XXA

　　H95.22　Intraoperative hemorrhage and hematoma of of ear and mastoid process complicating other procedure　　[CC]
　　　CC Excl: See code: H95.21

　✓5ᵗʰ **H95.3　Accidental puncture and laceration of ear and mastoid process during a procedure**

　　　CC Excl: For CC codes in subcategory H95.3, unless otherwise noted: D78.11-D78.12, D78.81-D78.89, E36.11-E36.8, E89.810-E89.89, G96.11, G97.41, G97.48-G97.49, H59.011-H59.019, H59.031-H59.099, H59.211-H59.229, H59.811-H59.89, H95.31-H95.32, H95.811-H95.89, I97.3, I97.51-I97.52, J95.71-J95.72, K91.71-K91.72, L76.11-L76.12, L76.81-L76.82, M96.820-M96.821, M96.89, N98.1-N98.9, N99.71-N99.72, T81.82XA, T81.89XA, T81.9XXA

　　H95.31　Accidental puncture and laceration of the ear and mastoid process during a procedure on the ear and mastoid process　　[CC]

　　H95.32　Accidental puncture and laceration of the ear and mastoid process during other procedure　　[CC]

　✓5ᵗʰ **H95.4　Postprocedural hemorrhage and hematoma of ear and mastoid process following a procedure**

　　H95.41　Postprocedural hemorrhage and hematoma of ear and mastoid process following a procedure on the ear and mastoid process　　[CC]
　　　CC Excl: See code: H95.21

　　H95.42　Postprocedural hemorrhage and hematoma of ear and mastoid process following other procedure　　[CC]
　　　CC Excl: See code: H95.21

　✓5ᵗʰ **H95.8　Other intraoperative and postprocedural complications and disorders of the ear and mastoid process, not elsewhere classified**

　　　EXCLUDES2　*postprocedural complications and disorders following mastoidectomy (H95.0-, H95.1-)*

　　　CC Excl: For CC codes in subcategory H95.8, unless otherwise noted: D78.81-D78.89, E36.8, E89.810-E89.89, H59.011-H59.019, H59.031-H59.099, H59.811-H59.89, H95.811-H95.89, I97.3, L76.81-L76.82, M96.89, N98.1-N98.9, T81.82XA, T81.89XA, T81.9XXA

　　✓6ᵗʰ **H95.81　Postprocedural stenosis of external ear canal**

　　　H95.811　Postprocedural stenosis of right external ear canal　　[CC]

　　　H95.812　Postprocedural stenosis of left external ear canal　　[CC]

　　　H95.813　Postprocedural stenosis of external ear canal, bilateral　　[CC]

　　　H95.819　Postprocedural stenosis of unspecified external ear canal　　[CC]

✓ Additional Character Required　　✓x7ᵗʰ Placeholder Alert　　Unacceptable PDx　　Manifestation　　Hospital Acquired Condition　　**EXCLUDES1** Not Coded Here　　**EXCLUDES2** Not Included Here

ICD-10-CM 2016　　　　　　　　　　　　　　　　　　　　　　　　　　　　　603

Chapter 8. Diseases of the Ear and Mastoid Process

H95.88   **Other intraoperative complications and**   `CC`
          disorders of the ear and mastoid process,
          not elsewhere classified
             Use additional code, if applicable, to further specify
             disorder

H95.89   **Other postprocedural complications and**   `CC`
          disorders of the ear and mastoid process, not
          elsewhere classified
             Use additional code, if applicable, to further specify
             disorder

N Newborn: 0   P Pediatric: 0-17   M Maternity: 12-55   A Adult: 15-124   **MCC** Major CC Condition   **PDxMCC** PDx acts as own MCC   **CC** CC Condition   **PDxCC** PDx acts as own CC

604   ICD-10-CM 2016

Chapter 9. Diseases of the Circulatory System (I00–I99)

Chapter Specific Guidelines with Coding Examples

The chapter specific guidelines from the ICD-10-CM Official Guidelines for Coding and Reporting have been provided below. Along with these guidelines are coding examples, contained in the shaded boxes, that have been developed to help illustrate the coding and/or sequencing guidance found in these guidelines.

a. Hypertension

1) Hypertension with heart disease

Heart conditions classified to I50.- or I51.4-I51.9, are assigned to a code from category I11, Hypertensive heart disease, when a causal relationship is stated (due to hypertension) or implied (hypertensive). Use an additional code from category I50, Heart failure, to identify the type of heart failure in those patients with heart failure.

The same heart conditions (I50.-, I51.4-I51.9) with hypertension, but without a stated causal relationship, are coded separately. Sequence according to the circumstances of the admission/encounter.

Hypertensive heart disease with left heart failure

| I11.0 | Hypertensive heart disease with heart failure |
| I50.1 | Left ventricular failure |

Explanation: A causal relationship between hypertension and heart disease must be stated or implied to report codes from category I11 Hypertensive heart disease. Use an additional code to identify type of heart failure (I50.-).

2) Hypertensive chronic kidney disease

Assign codes from category I12, Hypertensive chronic kidney disease, when both hypertension and a condition classifiable to category N18, Chronic kidney disease (CKD), are present. Unlike hypertension with heart disease, ICD-10-CM presumes a cause-and-effect relationship and classifies chronic kidney disease with hypertension as hypertensive chronic kidney disease.

The appropriate code from category N18 should be used as a secondary code with a code from category I12 to identify the stage of chronic kidney disease.

See Section I.C.14. Chronic kidney disease.

If a patient has hypertensive chronic kidney disease and acute renal failure, an additional code for the acute renal failure is required.

Patient is admitted with stage IV chronic kidney disease (CKD). The physician has also documented hypertension for this patient.

| I12.9 | Hypertensive chronic kidney disease with stage 1 through stage 4 chronic kidney disease, or unspecified chronic kidney disease |
| N18.4 | Chronic kidney disease, stage 4 (severe) |

Explanation: A causal relationship between hypertension and chronic kidney disease (CKD) is **assumed** unless otherwise documented. Use an additional code to identify the stage of chronic kidney disease.

3) Hypertensive heart and chronic kidney disease

Assign codes from combination category I13, Hypertensive heart and chronic kidney disease, when both hypertensive kidney disease and hypertensive heart disease are stated in the diagnosis. Assume a relationship between the hypertension and the chronic kidney disease, whether or not the condition is so designated. If heart failure is present, assign an additional code from category I50 to identify the type of heart failure.

The appropriate code from category N18, Chronic kidney disease, should be used as a secondary code with a code from category I13 to identify the stage of chronic kidney disease.

See Section I.C.14. Chronic kidney disease.

The codes in category I13, Hypertensive heart and chronic kidney disease, are combination codes that include hypertension, heart disease and chronic kidney disease. The Includes note at I13 specifies that the conditions included at I11 and I12 are included together in I13. If a patient has hypertension, heart disease and chronic kidney disease then a code from I13 should be used, not individual codes for hypertension, heart disease and chronic kidney disease, or codes from I11 or I12.

For patients with both acute renal failure and chronic kidney disease an additional code for acute renal failure is required.

Hypertensive heart and kidney disease with congestive heart failure and stage 2 chronic kidney disease

I13.0	Hypertensive heart and chronic kidney disease with heart failure and stage 1 through stage 4 chronic kidney disease, or unspecified chronic kidney disease
I50.9	Heart failure, unspecified
N18.2	Chronic kidney disease, stage 2 (mild)

Explanation: Combination codes in category I13 are used to report conditions classifiable to *both* categories I11 and I12. Do not report conditions classifiable to I11 and I12 separately. Use additional codes to report type of heart failure and stage of CKD.

4) Hypertensive cerebrovascular disease

For hypertensive cerebrovascular disease, first assign the appropriate code from categories I60-I69, followed by the appropriate hypertension code.

Rupture of cerebral aneurysm caused by malignant hypertension

| I60.8 | Other nontraumatic subarachnoid hemorrhage |
| I10 | Essential (primary) hypertension |

Explanation: Hypertensive cerebrovascular disease requires two codes: the appropriate I60-I69 code followed by the appropriate hypertension code.

5) Hypertensive retinopathy

Subcategory H35.0, Background retinopathy and retinal vascular changes, should be used with a code from category I10 – I15, Hypertensive disease to include the systemic hypertension. The sequencing is based on the reason for the encounter.

Hypertensive retinopathy of the right eye

| H35.031 | Hypertensive retinopathy, right eye |
| I10 | Essential (primary) hypertension |

Explanation: Hypertensive retinopathy requires two codes: the appropriate subcategory H35.0 code and a code for the hypertension.

6) Hypertension, secondary

Secondary hypertension is due to an underlying condition. Two codes are required: one to identify the underlying etiology and one from category I15 to identify the hypertension. Sequencing of codes is determined by the reason for admission/encounter.

Renovascular hypertension due to renal artery atherosclerosis

| I15.0 | Renovascular hypertension |
| I70.1 | Atherosclerosis of renal artery |

Explanation: Secondary hypertension requires two codes: a code to identify the etiology and the appropriate I15 code.

7) Hypertension, transient

Assign code R03.0, Elevated blood pressure reading without diagnosis of hypertension, unless patient has an established diagnosis of hypertension. Assign code O13.-, Gestational [pregnancy-induced] hypertension without significant proteinuria, or O14.-, Pre-eclampsia, for transient hypertension of pregnancy.

8) Hypertension, controlled

This diagnostic statement usually refers to an existing state of hypertension under control by therapy. Assign the appropriate code from categories I10-I15, Hypertensive diseases.

9) Hypertension, uncontrolled

Uncontrolled hypertension may refer to untreated hypertension or hypertension not responding to current therapeutic regimen. In either case, assign the appropriate code from categories I10-I15, Hypertensive diseases.

b. Atherosclerotic coronary artery disease and angina

ICD-10-CM has combination codes for atherosclerotic heart disease with angina pectoris. The subcategories for these codes are I25.11, Atherosclerotic heart disease of native coronary artery with angina pectoris and I25.7,

Chapter 9. Diseases of the Circulatory System

Atherosclerosis of coronary artery bypass graft(s) and coronary artery of transplanted heart with angina pectoris.

When using one of these combination codes it is not necessary to use an additional code for angina pectoris. A causal relationship can be assumed in a patient with both atherosclerosis and angina pectoris, unless the documentation indicates the angina is due to something other than the atherosclerosis.

If a patient with coronary artery disease is admitted due to an acute myocardial infarction (AMI), the AMI should be sequenced before the coronary artery disease.

See Section I.C.9. Acute myocardial infarction (AMI)

> Patient is being seen for spastic angina pectoris. She also has a documented history of progressive coronary artery disease of the native vessels.
>
> **I25.111   Atherosclerotic heart disease of native coronary artery with angina pectoris with documented spasm**
>
> *Explanation*: Report the combination code for atherosclerotic heart disease (coronary artery disease) with angina pectoris. A causal relationship is assumed in a patient with both atherosclerosis and angina pectoris, unless the documentation indicates the angina is due to something other than the atherosclerosis. When using one of these combination codes, it is not necessary to use an additional code for angina pectoris.

c. Intraoperative and postprocedural cerebrovascular accident

Medical record documentation should clearly specify the cause- and- effect relationship between the medical intervention and the cerebrovascular accident in order to assign a code for intraoperative or postprocedural cerebrovascular accident.

Proper code assignment depends on whether it was an infarction or hemorrhage and whether it occurred intraoperatively or postoperatively. If it was a cerebral hemorrhage, code assignment depends on the type of procedure performed.

> Embolic cerebral infarction of the right middle cerebral artery that occurred during hip replacement surgery. The surgeon documented as due to the surgery.
>
> **I97.811   Intraoperative cerebrovascular infarction during other surgery**
>
> **I63.411   Cerebral infarction due to embolism of right middle cerebral artery**
>
> *Explanation*: Code assignment for intraoperative or postprocedural cerebrovascular accident is based on the provider's documentation of a cause-and-effect relationship between the condition and the procedure. Proper code assignment also depends on whether the cerebrovascular accident was an infarction or hemorrhage, occurred intraoperatively or postoperatively, and the type of procedure performed.

d. Sequelae of cerebrovascular disease

1) Category I69, Sequelae of cerebrovascular disease

Category I69 is used to indicate conditions classifiable to categories I60-I67 as the causes of sequela (neurologic deficits), themselves classified elsewhere. These "late effects" include neurologic deficits that persist after initial onset of conditions classifiable to categories I60-I67. The neurologic deficits caused by cerebrovascular disease may be present from the onset or may arise at any time after the onset of the condition classifiable to categories I60-I67.

Codes from category I69, Sequelae of cerebrovascular disease, that specify hemiplegia, hemiparesis and monoplegia identify whether the dominant or nondominant side is affected. Should the affected side be documented, but not specified as dominant or nondominant, and the classification system does not indicate a default, code selection is as follows:

- For ambidextrous patients, the default should be dominant.
- If the left side is affected, the default is non-dominant.
- If the right side is affected, the default is dominant.

2) Codes from category I69 with codes from I60–I67

Codes from category I69 may be assigned on a health care record with codes from I60-I67, if the patient has a current cerebrovascular disease and deficits from an old cerebrovascular disease.

3) Codes from category I69 and Personal history of transient ischemic attack (TIA) and cerebral infarction (Z86.73)

Codes from category I69 should not be assigned if the patient does not have neurologic deficits.

See Section I.C.21. 4. History (of) for use of personal history codes

> Flaccid hemiparesis of the right side due to old cerebral infarction
>
> **I69.351   Hemiplegia and hemiparesis following cerebral infarction affecting right dominant side**
>
> *Explanation*: Sequela codes specify the residual effect that remains after the acute phase of a previous illness or injury (I60–I67). The "sequelae" include conditions specified as such or as residuals, which may occur at any time, even months or years, after the onset of the causal condition. There is no time limit restricting the reporting of sequela (late effect) codes. For this scenario, the documentation indicates that the right side is affected but does not note which side is the patient's dominant side, e.g., right or left. The default is to assume the right side is the dominant side.

e. Acute myocardial infarction (AMI)

1) ST elevation myocardial infarction (STEMI) and non ST elevation myocardial infarction (NSTEMI)

The ICD-10-CM codes for acute myocardial infarction (AMI) identify the site, such as anterolateral wall or true posterior wall. Subcategories I21.0-I21.2 and code I21.3 are used for ST elevation myocardial infarction (STEMI). Code I21.4, Non-ST elevation (NSTEMI) myocardial infarction, is used for non ST elevation myocardial infarction (NSTEMI) and nontransmural MIs.

If NSTEMI evolves to STEMI, assign the STEMI code. If STEMI converts to NSTEMI due to thrombolytic therapy, it is still coded as STEMI.

For encounters occurring while the myocardial infarction is equal to, or less than, four weeks old, including transfers to another acute setting or a postacute setting, and the patient requires continued care for the myocardial infarction, codes from category I21 may continue to be reported. For encounters after the 4 week time frame and the patient is still receiving care related to the myocardial infarction, the appropriate aftercare code should be assigned, rather than a code from category I21. For old or healed myocardial infarctions not requiring further care, code I25.2, Old myocardial infarction, may be assigned.

> Acute inferior NSTEMI evolved into STEMI
>
> **I21.19   ST elevation (STEMI) myocardial infarction involving other coronary artery of inferior wall**
>
> *Explanation*: If an NSTEMI converts to a STEMI, report only the STEMI code.

2) Acute myocardial infarction, unspecified

Code I21.3, ST elevation (STEMI) myocardial infarction of unspecified site, is the default for unspecified acute myocardial infarction. If only STEMI or transmural MI without the site is documented, assign code I21.3.

3) AMI documented as nontransmural or subendocardial but site provided

If an AMI is documented as nontransmural or subendocardial, but the site is provided, it is still coded as a subendocardial AMI.

See Section I.C.21.3 for information on coding status post administration of tPA in a different facility within the last 24 hours.

> Acute inferior subendocardial myocardial infarction (NSTEMI)
>
> **I21.4   Non-ST elevation (NSTEMI) myocardial infarction**
>
> *Explanation*: An AMI documented as subendocardial or nontransmural is coded as such (I21.4, I22.2), even if the site of infarction is specified.

4) Subsequent acute myocardial infarction

A code from category I22, Subsequent ST elevation (STEMI) and non ST elevation (NSTEMI) myocardial infarction, is to be used when a patient who has suffered an AMI has a new AMI within the 4 week time frame of the initial AMI. A code from category I22 must be used in conjunction with a code from category I21. The sequencing of the I22 and I21 codes depends on the circumstances of the encounter.

> Acute inferior STEMI status post acute NSTEMI two weeks ago.
>
> **I22.1   Subsequent ST elevation (STEMI) myocardial infarction of inferior wall**
>
> **I21.4   Non-ST elevation (NSTEMI) myocardial infarction**
>
> *Explanation*: A code from I22 must be used in conjunction with a code from I21 when a patient who has suffered an AMI has a new AMI within four weeks of the initial one. Category I22 is never reported alone. The guidelines for assigning the correct I22 code are the same as those for reporting the initial MI (I21). Sequencing is determined by the circumstances of the encounter.

Chapter 9. Diseases of the Circulatory System (I00-I99)

EXCLUDES 2   certain conditions originating in the perinatal period (P04-P96)
certain infectious and parasitic diseases (A00-B99)
complications of pregnancy, childbirth and the puerperium (O00-O9A)
congenital malformations, deformations, and chromosomal abnormalities (Q00-Q99)
endocrine, nutritional and metabolic diseases (E00-E88)
injury, poisoning and certain other consequences of external causes (S00-T88)
neoplasms (C00-D49)
symptoms, signs and abnormal clinical and laboratory findings, not elsewhere classified (R00-R94)
systemic connective tissue disorders (M30-M36)
transient cerebral ischemic attacks and related syndromes (G45.-)

This chapter contains the following blocks:

I00-I02	Acute rheumatic fever
I05-I09	Chronic rheumatic heart diseases
I10-I15	Hypertensive diseases
I20-I25	Ischemic heart diseases
I26-I28	Pulmonary heart disease and diseases of pulmonary circulation
I30-I52	Other forms of heart disease
I60-I69	Cerebrovascular diseases
I70-I79	Diseases of arteries, arterioles and capillaries
I80-I89	Diseases of veins, lymphatic vessels and lymph nodes, not elsewhere classified
I95-I99	Other and unspecified disorders of the circulatory system

Acute rheumatic fever (I00-I02)

I00   **Rheumatic fever without heart involvement**
   INCLUDES   arthritis, rheumatic, acute or subacute
   EXCLUDES 1   rheumatic fever with heart involvement (I01.0-I01.9)

✓4ᵗʰ I01   **Rheumatic fever with heart involvement**
   EXCLUDES 1   chronic diseases of rheumatic origin (I05-I09) unless rheumatic fever is also present or there is evidence of reactivation or activity of the rheumatic process.

I01.0   **Acute rheumatic pericarditis**   `CC`
Any condition in I00 with pericarditis
Rheumatic pericarditis (acute)
   EXCLUDES 1   acute pericarditis not specified as rheumatic (I30.-)
   CC Excl: B33.23, I01.0, I09.2, I30.0-I30.9, I31.3-I32, I87.8-I87.9, I99.8-I99.9

I01.1   **Acute rheumatic endocarditis**   `CC`
Any condition in I00 with endocarditis or valvulitis
Acute rheumatic valvulitis
   CC Excl: A01.00-A01.09, A39.51, A52.03, A78, B33.21, B37.6, I00, I01.1, I01.8-I02.0, I05.0-I07.9, I08.1-I08.3, I08.9, I09.1, I09.89-I09.9, I33.0-I39, I42.4, I87.8-I87.9, I99.8-I99.9, Q22.2, Q23.8-Q23.9, Q24.8, T82.6XXA

I01.2   **Acute rheumatic myocarditis**   `CC`
Any condition in I00 with myocarditis
   CC Excl: A52.06, B33.22, I00, I01.2-I01.9, I09.0, I09.9, I23.0-I23.3, I23.6-I23.8, I40.0-I41, I51.0, I51.4, I87.8-I87.9, I99.8-I99.9

I01.8   **Other acute rheumatic heart disease**   `CC`
Any condition in I00 with other or multiple types of heart involvement
Acute rheumatic pancarditis
   CC Excl: I01.0-I09.9, I50.20-I50.43

I01.9   **Acute rheumatic heart disease, unspecified**   `CC`
Any condition in I00 with unspecified type of heart involvement
Rheumatic carditis, acute
Rheumatic heart disease, active or acute
   CC Excl: I01.0-I09.9

✓4ᵗʰ I02   **Rheumatic chorea**
   INCLUDES   Sydenham's chorea
   EXCLUDES 1   chorea NOS (G25.5)
     Huntington's chorea (G10)

I02.0   **Rheumatic chorea with heart involvement**   `CC`
Chorea NOS with heart involvement
Rheumatic chorea with heart involvement of any type classifiable under I01-
   CC Excl: See code: I01.8

I02.9   **Rheumatic chorea without heart involvement**   `CC`
Rheumatic chorea NOS
   CC Excl: See code: I01.9

Chronic rheumatic heart diseases (I05-I09)

✓4ᵗʰ I05   **Rheumatic mitral valve diseases**
   INCLUDES   conditions classifiable to both I05.0 and I05.2-I05.9, whether specified as rheumatic or not
   EXCLUDES 1   mitral valve disease specified as nonrheumatic (I34.-)
     mitral valve disease with aortic and/or tricuspid valve involvement (I08.-)

I05.0   **Rheumatic mitral stenosis**
Mitral (valve) obstruction (rheumatic)

I05.1   **Rheumatic mitral insufficiency**
Rheumatic mitral incompetence
Rheumatic mitral regurgitation
   EXCLUDES 1   mitral insufficiency not specified as rheumatic (I34.0)

I05.2   **Rheumatic mitral stenosis with insufficiency**
Rheumatic mitral stenosis with incompetence or regurgitation

I05.8   **Other rheumatic mitral valve diseases**
Rheumatic mitral (valve) failure

I05.9   **Rheumatic mitral valve disease, unspecified**
Rheumatic mitral (valve) disorder (chronic) NOS

✓4ᵗʰ I06   **Rheumatic aortic valve diseases**
   EXCLUDES 1   aortic valve disease not specified as rheumatic (I35.-)
     aortic valve disease with mitral and/or tricuspid valve involvement (I08.-)

I06.0   **Rheumatic aortic stenosis**
Rheumatic aortic (valve) obstruction

I06.1   **Rheumatic aortic insufficiency**
Rheumatic aortic incompetence
Rheumatic aortic regurgitation

I06.2   **Rheumatic aortic stenosis with insufficiency**
Rheumatic aortic stenosis with incompetence or regurgitation

I06.8   **Other rheumatic aortic valve diseases**

I06.9   **Rheumatic aortic valve disease, unspecified**
Rheumatic aortic (valve) disease NOS

✓4ᵗʰ I07   **Rheumatic tricuspid valve diseases**
   INCLUDES   rheumatic tricuspid valve diseases specified as rheumatic or unspecified
   EXCLUDES 1   tricuspid valve disease specified as nonrheumatic (I36.-)
     tricuspid valve disease with aortic and/or mitral valve involvement (I08.-)

I07.0   **Rheumatic tricuspid stenosis**
Tricuspid (valve) stenosis (rheumatic)

I07.1   **Rheumatic tricuspid insufficiency**
Tricuspid (valve) insufficiency (rheumatic)

I07.2   **Rheumatic tricuspid stenosis and insufficiency**

I07.8   **Other rheumatic tricuspid valve diseases**

I07.9   **Rheumatic tricuspid valve disease, unspecified**
Rheumatic tricuspid valve disorder NOS

✓4ᵗʰ I08   **Multiple valve diseases**
   INCLUDES   multiple valve diseases specified as rheumatic or unspecified
   EXCLUDES 1   endocarditis, valve unspecified (I38)
     multiple valve disease specified a nonrheumatic (I34.-, I35.-, I36.-, I37.-, I38.-, Q22.-, Q23.-, Q24.8-)
     rheumatic valve disease NOS (I09.1)

I08.0   **Rheumatic disorders of both mitral and aortic valves**
Involvement of both mitral and aortic valves specified as rheumatic or unspecified

I08.1   **Rheumatic disorders of both mitral and tricuspid valves**

I08.2   **Rheumatic disorders of both aortic and tricuspid valves**

I08.3   **Combined rheumatic disorders of mitral, aortic and tricuspid valves**

I08.8   **Other rheumatic multiple valve diseases**

I08.9   **Rheumatic multiple valve disease, unspecified**

✓4ᵗʰ I09   **Other rheumatic heart diseases**

I09.0   **Rheumatic myocarditis**   `CC`
   EXCLUDES 1   myocarditis not specified as rheumatic (I51.4)
   CC Excl: I00, I01.2-I01.9, I09.0, I09.9, I23.0-I23.3, I23.6-I23.8, I40.0-I41, I51.0, I51.4, I87.8-I87.9, I99.8-I99.9

I09.1   **Rheumatic diseases of endocardium, valve unspecified**
Rheumatic endocarditis (chronic)
Rheumatic valvulitis (chronic)
   EXCLUDES 1   endocarditis, valve unspecified (I38)

✔ Additional Character Required   ✔x7ᵗʰ Placeholder Alert   Unacceptable PDx   Manifestation   Hospital Acquired Condition   **EXCLUDES 1** Not Coded Here   **EXCLUDES 2** Not Included Here

Chapter 9. Diseases of the Circulatory System

I09.2 Chronic rheumatic pericarditis CC
Adherent pericardium, rheumatic
Chronic rheumatic mediastinopericarditis
Chronic rheumatic myopericarditis
EXCLUDES 1 chronic pericarditis not specified as rheumatic (I31.-)
CC Excl: B33.23, I01.0, I09.2, I30.0-I30.9, I31.3-I32, I87.8-I87.9, I99.8-I99.9

✓5th **I09.8 Other specified rheumatic heart diseases**
I09.81 Rheumatic heart failure CC
Use additional code to identify type of heart failure (I50.-)
CC Excl: I09.81, I09.9, I11.0, I50.1-I50.9, I87.8-I87.9, I99.8-I99.9

I09.89 Other specified rheumatic heart diseases
Rheumatic disease of pulmonary valve

I09.9 Rheumatic heart disease, unspecified
Rheumatic carditis
EXCLUDES 1 rheumatoid carditis (M05.31)

Hypertensive diseases (I10-I15)

Use additional code to identify:
exposure to environmental tobacco smoke (Z77.22)
history of tobacco use (Z87.891)
occupational exposure to environmental tobacco smoke (Z57.31)
tobacco dependence (F17.-)
tobacco use (Z72.0)
EXCLUDES 1 hypertensive disease complicating pregnancy, childbirth and the puerperium (O10-O11, O13-O16)
neonatal hypertension (P29.2)
primary pulmonary hypertension (I27.0)

13**I10 Essential (primary) hypertension**
INCLUDES high blood pressure
hypertension (arterial) (benign) (essential) (malignant) (primary) (systemic)
EXCLUDES 1 hypertensive disease complicating pregnancy, childbirth and the puerperium (O10-O11, O13-O16)
EXCLUDES 2 essential (primary) hypertension involving vessels of brain (I60-I69)
essential (primary) hypertension involving vessels of eye (H35.0-)

✓4th **I11 Hypertensive heart disease**
INCLUDES any condition in I51.4-I51.9 due to hypertension
I11.0 Hypertensive heart disease with heart failure
Hypertensive heart failure
Use additional code to identify type of heart failure (I50.-)
I11.9 Hypertensive heart disease without heart failure
Hypertensive heart disease NOS

✓4th **I12 Hypertensive chronic kidney disease**
INCLUDES any condition in N18- and N26- due to hypertension
arteriosclerosis of kidney
arteriosclerotic nephritis (chronic) (interstitial)
hypertensive nephropathy
nephrosclerosis
EXCLUDES 1 hypertension due to kidney disease (I15.0, I15.1)
renovascular hypertension (I15.0)
secondary hypertension (I15.-)
EXCLUDES 2 acute kidney failure (N17.-)
I12.0 Hypertensive chronic kidney disease with stage 5 chronic kidney disease or end stage renal disease CC
Use additional code to identify the stage of chronic kidney disease (N18.5, N18.6)
CC Excl: I10-I15.9, I87.8-I87.9, I99.8-I99.9, N18.6, N26.2
I12.9 Hypertensive chronic kidney disease with stage 1 through stage 4 chronic kidney disease, or unspecified chronic kidney disease
Hypertensive chronic kidney disease NOS
Hypertensive renal disease NOS
Use additional code to identify the stage of chronic kidney disease (N18.1-N18.4, N18.9)

✓4th **I13 Hypertensive heart and chronic kidney disease**
INCLUDES any condition in I11- with any condition in I12-
cardiorenal disease
cardiovascular renal disease
CC Excl: For CC codes in category I13, unless otherwise noted: I10-I15.9, I87.8-I87.9, I99.8-I99.9, N26.2

I13.0 Hypertensive heart and chronic kidney disease with heart failure and stage 1 through stage 4 chronic kidney disease, or unspecified chronic kidney disease CC
Use additional code to identify type of heart failure (I50.-)
Use additional code to identify stage of chronic kidney disease (N18.1-N18.4, N18.9)

✓5th **I13.1 Hypertensive heart and chronic kidney disease without heart failure**
I13.10 Hypertensive heart and chronic kidney disease without heart failure, with stage 1 through stage 4 chronic kidney disease, or unspecified chronic kidney disease
Hypertensive heart disease and hypertensive chronic kidney disease NOS
Use additional code to identify the stage of chronic kidney disease (N18.1-N18.4, N18.9)
I13.11 Hypertensive heart and chronic kidney disease without heart failure, with stage 5 chronic kidney disease, or end stage renal disease CC
Use additional code to identify the stage of chronic kidney disease (N18.5, N18.6)
I13.2 Hypertensive heart and chronic kidney disease with heart failure and with stage 5 chronic kidney disease, or end stage renal disease CC
Use additional code to identify type of heart failure (I50.-)
Use additional code to identify the stage of chronic kidney disease (N18.5, N18.6)

✓4th **I15 Secondary hypertension**
Code also underlying condition
EXCLUDES 1 postprocedural hypertension (I97.3)
EXCLUDES 2 secondary hypertension involving vessels of brain (I60-I69)
secondary hypertension involving vessels of eye (H35.0-)
I15.0 Renovascular hypertension
I15.1 Hypertension secondary to other renal disorders
I15.2 Hypertension secondary to endocrine disorders
I15.8 Other secondary hypertension
I15.9 Secondary hypertension, unspecified

Ischemic heart diseases (I20-I25)

Use additional code to identify presence of hypertension (I10-I15)

✓4th **I20 Angina pectoris**
Use additional code to identify:
exposure to environmental tobacco smoke (Z77.22)
history of tobacco use (Z87.891)
occupational exposure to environmental tobacco smoke (Z57.31)
tobacco dependence (F17.-)
tobacco use (Z72.0)
EXCLUDES 1 angina pectoris with atherosclerotic heart disease of native coronary arteries (I25.1-)
atherosclerosis of coronary artery bypass graft(s) and coronary artery of transplanted heart with angina pectoris (I25.7-)
postinfarction angina (I23.7)
I20.0 Unstable angina CC
Accelerated angina
Crescendo angina
De novo effort angina
Intermediate coronary syndrome
Preinfarction syndrome
Worsening effort angina
CC Excl: I09.81, I11.0, I13.0, I13.2, I20.0-I22.9, I24.0, I24.8-I24.9, I25.5-I25.6, I25.82-I25.83, I25.89-I25.9, I50.1, I50.9, I87.8-I87.9, I99.8-I99.9, R57.0, R57.9
I20.1 Angina pectoris with documented spasm CC
Angiospastic angina
Prinzmetal angina
Spasm-induced angina
Variant angina
CC Excl: I20.0-I22.9, I24.0, I24.8-I24.9, I25.5-I25.6, I25.89-I25.9, I87.8-I87.9, I99.8-I99.9
I20.8 Other forms of angina pectoris
Angina equivalent
Angina of effort
Coronary slow flow syndrome
Stenocardia
Use additional code(s) for symptoms associated with angina equivalent

---
13 Questionable admission when used as PDx.

I20.9   **Angina pectoris,** unspecified
     Angina NOS
     Anginal syndrome
     Cardiac angina
     Ischemic chest pain

✓4ᵗʰ I21   **ST elevation (STEMI) and non-ST elevation (NSTEMI) myocardial infarction**
     INCLUDES   cardiac infarction
         coronary (artery) embolism
         coronary (artery) occlusion
         coronary (artery) rupture
         coronary (artery) thrombosis
         infarction of heart, myocardium, or ventricle
         myocardial infarction specified as acute or with a stated
             duration of 4 weeks (28 days) or less from onset
     Use additional code, if applicable, to identify:
       exposure to environmental tobacco smoke (Z77.22)
       history of tobacco use (Z87.891)
       occupational exposure to environmental tobacco smoke (Z57.31)
       status post administration of tPA (rtPA) in a different facility within
          the last 24 hours prior to admission to current facility (Z92.82)
       tobacco dependence (F17.-)
       tobacco use (Z72.0)
     EXCLUDES 2   *old myocardial infarction (I25.2)*
         postmyocardial infarction syndrome (I24.1)
         subsequent myocardial infarction (I22.-)
     AHA: 2013, 1Q, 25; 2012, 4Q, 96, 102-103

> **CC Excl: For MCC codes in category I21, unless otherwise noted:**
> I21.01-I22.9, I87.8-I87.9, I99.8-I99.9

✓5ᵗʰ I21.0   **ST elevation (STEMI) myocardial infarction of** anterior wall

     I21.01   **ST elevation (STEMI) myocardial infarction**   MCC
          involving left main coronary artery

     I21.02   **ST elevation (STEMI) myocardial infarction**   MCC
          involving left anterior descending coronary artery
          ST elevation (STEMI) myocardial infarction involving
            diagonal coronary artery
          AHA: 2013, 1Q, 25

     I21.09   **ST elevation (STEMI) myocardial infarction**   MCC
          involving other coronary artery of anterior wall
          Acute transmural myocardial infarction of anterior wall
          Anteroapical transmural (Q wave) infarction (acute)
          Anterolateral transmural (Q wave) infarction (acute)
          Anteroseptal transmural (Q wave) infarction (acute)
          Transmural (Q wave) infarction (acute) (of) anterior
            (wall) NOS
          AHA: 2012, 4Q, 102-103

✓5ᵗʰ I21.1   **ST elevation (STEMI) myocardial infarction of** inferior wall

     I21.11   **ST elevation (STEMI) myocardial infarction**   MCC
          involving right coronary artery
          Inferoposterior transmural (Q wave) infarction (acute)

     I21.19   **ST elevation (STEMI) myocardial infarction**   MCC
          involving other coronary artery of inferior wall
          Acute transmural myocardial infarction of inferior wall
          Inferolateral transmural (Q wave) infarction (acute)
          Transmural (Q wave) infarction (acute) (of)
            diaphragmatic wall
          Transmural (Q wave) infarction (acute) (of) inferior
            (wall) NOS
          EXCLUDES 2   *ST elevation (STEMI) myocardial infarction*
            involving left circumflex coronary artery
            (I21.21)
          AHA: 2012, 4Q, 96

✓5ᵗʰ I21.2   **ST elevation (STEMI) myocardial infarction of** other sites

     I21.21   **ST elevation (STEMI) myocardial infarction**   MCC
          involving left circumflex coronary artery
          ST elevation (STEMI) myocardial infarction involving
            oblique marginal coronary artery

     I21.29   **ST elevation (STEMI) myocardial infarction**   MCC
          involving other sites
          Acute transmural myocardial infarction of other sites
          Apical-lateral transmural (Q wave) infarction (acute)
          Basal-lateral transmural (Q wave) infarction (acute)
          High lateral transmural (Q wave) infarction (acute)
          Lateral (wall) NOS transmural (Q wave) infarction
            (acute)
          Posterior (true) transmural (Q wave) infarction (acute)
          Posterobasal transmural (Q wave) infarction (acute)
          Posterolateral transmural (Q wave) infarction (acute)
          Posteroseptal transmural (Q wave) infarction (acute)
          Septal transmural (Q wave) infarction (acute) NOS

I21.3   **ST elevation (STEMI) myocardial infarction of**   MCC
     unspecified site
     Acute transmural myocardial infarction of unspecified site
     Myocardial infarction (acute) NOS
     Transmural (Q wave) myocardial infarction NOS

I21.4   **Non-ST elevation (NSTEMI) myocardial infarction**   MCC
     Acute subendocardial myocardial infarction
     Non-Q wave myocardial infarction NOS
     Nontransmural myocardial infarction NOS

✓4ᵗʰ I22   **Subsequent ST elevation (STEMI) and non-ST elevation (NSTEMI) myocardial infarction**
     INCLUDES   acute myocardial infarction occurring within four weeks (28
            days) of a previous acute myocardial infarction,
            regardless of site
         cardiac infarction
         coronary (artery) embolism
         coronary (artery) occlusion
         coronary (artery) rupture
         coronary (artery) thrombosis
         infarction of heart, myocardium, or ventricle
         recurrent myocardial infarction
         reinfarction of myocardium
         rupture of heart, myocardium, or ventricle
     Use additional code, if applicable, to identify:
       exposure to environmental tobacco smoke (Z77.22)
       history of tobacco use (Z87.891)
       occupational exposure to environmental tobacco smoke (Z57.31)
       status post administration of tPA (rtPA) in a different facility within
          the last 24 hours prior to admission to current facility (Z92.82)
       tobacco dependence (F17.-)
       tobacco use (Z72.0))
     AHA: 2013, 1Q, 25; 2012, 4Q, 97, 102-103

> **CC Excl: For MCC codes in category I22, unless otherwise noted:**
> See code: I21

I22.0   **Subsequent ST elevation (STEMI) myocardial infarction**   MCC
     of anterior wall
     Subsequent acute transmural myocardial infarction of anterior
       wall
     Subsequent transmural (Q wave) infarction (acute)(of) anterior
       (wall) NOS
     Subsequent anteroapical transmural (Q wave) infarction (acute)
     Subsequent anterolateral transmural (Q wave) infarction (acute)
     Subsequent anteroseptal transmural (Q wave) infarction (acute)

I22.1   **Subsequent ST elevation (STEMI) myocardial infarction**   MCC
     of inferior wall
     Subsequent acute transmural myocardial infarction of inferior
       wall
     Subsequent transmural (Q wave) infarction (acute)(of)
       diaphragmatic wall
     Subsequent transmural (Q wave) infarction (acute)(of) inferior
       (wall) NOS
     Subsequent inferolateral transmural (Q wave) infarction (acute)
     Subsequent inferoposterior transmural (Q wave) infarction
       (acute)
     AHA: 2012, 4Q, 102

I22.2   **Subsequent non-ST elevation (NSTEMI) myocardial**   MCC
     infarction
     Subsequent acute subendocardial myocardial infarction
     Subsequent non-Q wave myocardial infarction NOS
     Subsequent nontransmural myocardial infarction NOS

I22.8   **Subsequent ST elevation (STEMI) myocardial infarction**   MCC
     of other sites
     Subsequent acute transmural myocardial infarction of other
       sites
     Subsequent apical-lateral transmural (Q wave) myocardial
       infarction (acute)
     Subsequent basal-lateral transmural (Q wave) myocardial
       infarction (acute)
     Subsequent high lateral transmural (Q wave) myocardial
       infarction (acute)
     Subsequent transmural (Q wave) myocardial infarction
       (acute)(of) lateral (wall) NOS
     Subsequent posterior (true)transmural (Q wave) myocardial
       infarction (acute)
     Subsequent posterobasal transmural (Q wave) myocardial
       infarction (acute)
     Subsequent posterolateral transmural (Q wave) myocardial
       infarction (acute)
     Subsequent posteroseptal transmural (Q wave) myocardial
       infarction (acute)
     Subsequent septal NOS transmural (Q wave) myocardial
       infarction (acute)

✅ Additional Character Required   ✓x7ᵗʰ Placeholder Alert   Unacceptable PDx   Manifestation   Hospital Acquired Condition   EXCLUDES 1 Not Coded Here   EXCLUDES 2 Not Included Here

I22.9   **Subsequent ST elevation (STEMI) myocardial infarction of unspecified site** `MCC`
> Subsequent acute myocardial infarction of unspecified site
> Subsequent myocardial infarction (acute) NOS

✓4th I23   **Certain current complications following ST elevation (STEMI) and non-ST elevation (NSTEMI) myocardial infarction (within the 28 day period)**

> **CC Excl: For CC/MCC codes in category I23, unless otherwise noted:** E78.71-E78.72, I23.0-I23.8, I40.0-I41, I51.0-I51.2, I51.4, I87.8-I87.9, I97.0-I97.191, I99.8-I99.9, P29.3, Q20.0-Q21.9, Q23.8-Q23.9, Q24.8-Q24.9, Q27.30, Q27.4, Q28.0-Q28.1, Q28.8-Q28.9, Q87.1-Q87.89, Q89.7-Q89.8, Q99.2

I23.0   **Hemopericardium as current complication following acute myocardial infarction** `CC` `A`
> *EXCLUDES 1*   hemopericardium not specified as current complication following acute myocardial infarction (I31.2)

I23.1   **Atrial septal defect as current complication following acute myocardial infarction** `CC` `A`
> *EXCLUDES 1*   acquired atrial septal defect not specified as current complication following acute myocardial infarction (I51.0)

I23.2   **Ventricular septal defect as current complication following acutemyocardial infarction** `CC` `A`
> *EXCLUDES 1*   acquired ventricular septal defect not specified as current complication following acute myocardial infarction (I51.0)

I23.3   **Rupture of cardiac wall without hemopericardium as current complication following acute myocardial infarction** `CC` `A`

I23.4   **Rupture of chordae tendineae as current complication following acute myocardial infarction** `MCC`
> *EXCLUDES 1*   rupture of chordae tendineae not specified as current complication following acute myocardial infarction (I51.1)
> **CC Excl:** I23.0-I23.4, I23.6-I23.8, I51.0-I51.1, I87.8-I87.9, I99.8-I99.9

I23.5   **Rupture of papillary muscle as current complication following acute myocardial infarction** `MCC`
> *EXCLUDES 1*   rupture of papillary muscle not specified as current complication following acute myocardial infarction (I51.2)
> **CC Excl:** I23.0-I23.3, I23.5-I23.8, I51.0, I51.2, I87.8-I87.9, I99.8-I99.9

I23.6   **Thrombosis of atrium, auricular appendage, and ventricle as current complications following acute myocardial infarction** `CC` `A`
> *EXCLUDES 1*   thrombosis of atrium, auricular appendage, and ventricle not specified as current complication following acute myocardial infarction (I51.3)

I23.7   **Postinfarction angina** `CC` `A`

I23.8   **Other current complications following acute myocardial infarction** `CC` `A`

✓4th I24   **Other acute ischemic heart diseases**
> *EXCLUDES 1*   angina pectoris (I20.-)
> transient myocardial ischemia in newborn (P29.4)

> **CC Excl: For CC codes in category I24, unless otherwise noted:** I20.0-I22.9, I24.0-I24.9, I25.5-I25.6, I25.89-I25.9, I87.8-I87.9, I99.8-I99.9

I24.0   **Acute coronary thrombosis not resulting in myocardial infarction** `CC`
> Acute coronary (artery) (vein) embolism not resulting in myocardial infarction
> Acute coronary (artery) (vein) occlusion not resulting in myocardial infarction
> Acute coronary (artery) (vein) thromboembolism not resulting in myocardial infarction
> *EXCLUDES 1*   atherosclerotic heart disease (I25.1-)
> **AHA:** 2013, 1Q, 24

I24.1   **Dressler's syndrome** `CC`
> Postmyocardial infarction syndrome
> *EXCLUDES 1*   postinfarction angina (I23.7)
> **CC Excl:** I24.0-I24.9, I87.8-I87.9, I99.8-I99.9

I24.8   **Other forms of acute ischemic heart disease** `CC`

I24.9   **Acute ischemic heart disease, unspecified** `CC`
> *EXCLUDES 1*   ischemic heart disease (chronic) NOS (I25.9)

✓4th I25   **Chronic ischemic heart disease**
> Use additional code to identify:
> chronic total occlusion of coronary artery (I25.82)
> exposure to environmental tobacco smoke (Z77.22)
> history of tobacco use (Z87.891)
> occupational exposure to environmental tobacco smoke (Z57.31)
> tobacco dependence (F17.-)
> tobacco use (Z72.0)

I25.1   **Atherosclerotic heart disease of** native **coronary artery**
> Atherosclerotic cardiovascular disease
> Coronary (artery) atheroma
> Coronary (artery) atherosclerosis
> Coronary (artery) disease
> Coronary (artery) sclerosis
> Use additional code, if applicable, to identify:
> coronary atherosclerosis due to calcified coronary lesion (I25.84)
> coronary atherosclerosis due to lipid rich plaque (I25.83)
> *EXCLUDES 2*   atheroembolism (I75.-)
> atherosclerosis of coronary artery bypass graft(s) and transplanted heart (I25.7-)

I25.10   **Atherosclerotic heart disease of native coronary artery** without angina pectoris `A`
> Atherosclerotic heart disease NOS
> **AHA:** 2012, 4Q, 92

✓6th I25.11   **Atherosclerotic heart disease of native coronary artery** with angina pectoris

> **I25.110**   **Atherosclerotic heart disease of native coronary artery with** unstable **angina pectoris** `PDxCC` `CC` `A`
> > *EXCLUDES 1*   unstable angina without atherosclerotic heart disease (I20.0)
> > **CC Excl:** I09.81, I11.0, I13.0, I13.2, I20.0-I22.9, I24.0, I24.8-I24.9, I25.5-I25.6, I25.82-I25.83, I25.89-I25.9, I50.1, I50.9, I87.8-I87.9, I99.8-I99.9, R57.0, R57.9

> **I25.111**   **Atherosclerotic heart disease of native coronary artery with angina pectoris with** documented spasm `A`
> > *EXCLUDES 1*   angina pectoris with documented spasm without atherosclerotic heart disease (I20.1)

> **I25.118**   **Atherosclerotic heart disease of native coronary artery with** other forms of **angina pectoris** `A`
> > *EXCLUDES 1*   other forms of angina pectoris without atherosclerotic heart disease (I20.8)

> **I25.119**   **Atherosclerotic heart disease of native coronary artery with** unspecified **angina pectoris** `A`
> > Atherosclerotic heart disease with angina NOS
> > Atherosclerotic heart disease with ischemic chest pain
> > *EXCLUDES 1*   unspecified angina pectoris without atherosclerotic heart disease (I20.9)

I25.2   **Old myocardial infarction**
> Healed myocardial infarction
> Past myocardial infarction diagnosed by ECG or other investigation, but currently presenting no symptoms

I25.3   **Aneurysm of heart** `CC`
> Mural aneurysm
> Ventricular aneurysm
> **CC Excl:** I25.3-I25.41

✓5th I25.4   **Coronary artery aneurysm and dissection**

> **I25.41**   **Coronary artery aneurysm**
> > Coronary arteriovenous fistula, acquired
> > *EXCLUDES 1*   congenital coronary (artery) aneurysm (Q24.5)

> **I25.42**   **Coronary artery dissection** `MCC`
> > **CC Excl:** I25.42, I77.2-I77.3, I77.5-I77.6, I77.79, I77.89-I77.9, M31.8-M31.9

I25.5   **Ischemic cardiomyopathy**
> *EXCLUDES 2*   coronary atherosclerosis (I25.1-, I25.7-)

I25.6   **Silent myocardial ischemia**

`N` Newborn: 0   `P` Pediatric: 0-17   `M` Maternity: 12-55   `A` Adult: 15-124   `MCC` Major CC Condition   `PDxMCC` PDx acts as own MCC   `CC` CC Condition   `PDxCC` PDx acts as own CC

610   ICD-10-CM 2016

✓5ᵗʰ I25.7   **Atherosclerosis of coronary artery bypass graft(s) and coronary artery of transplanted heart with angina pectoris**
Use additional code, if applicable, to identify:
coronary atherosclerosis due to calcified coronary lesion (I25.84)
coronary atherosclerosis due to lipid rich plaque (I25.83)
EXCLUDES 1   *atherosclerosis of bypass graft(s) of transplanted heart without angina pectoris (I25.812)*
atherosclerosis of coronary artery bypass graft(s) without angina pectoris (I25.810)
atherosclerosis of native coronary artery of transplanted heart without angina pectoris (I25.811)
embolism or thrombus of coronary artery bypass graft(s) (T82.8-)

✓6ᵗʰ I25.70   **Atherosclerosis of coronary artery bypass graft(s), unspecified, with angina pectoris**

    I25.700   **Atherosclerosis of coronary** [PDx CC] [CC] [A] **artery bypass graft(s), unspecified, with unstable angina pectoris**
EXCLUDES 1   *unstable angina pectoris without atherosclerosis of coronary artery bypass graft (I20.0)*
CC Excl: I09.81, I11.0, I13.0, I13.2, I20.0-I22.9, I24.0, I24.8-I24.9, I25.5-I25.6, I25.82-I25.83, I25.89-I25.9, I50.1, I50.9, I87.8-I87.9, I99.8-I99.9, R57.0, R57.9

    I25.701   **Atherosclerosis of coronary artery** [A] **bypass graft(s), unspecified, with angina pectoris with documented spasm**
EXCLUDES 1   *angina pectoris with documented spasm without atherosclerosis of coronary artery bypass graft (I20.1)*

    I25.708   **Atherosclerosis of coronary artery** [A] **bypass graft(s), unspecified, with other forms of angina pectoris**
EXCLUDES 1   *other forms of angina pectoris without atherosclerosis of coronary artery bypass graft (I20.8)*

    I25.709   **Atherosclerosis of coronary artery** [A] **bypass graft(s), unspecified, with unspecified angina pectoris**
EXCLUDES 1   *unspecified angina pectoris without atherosclerosis of coronary artery bypass graft (I20.9)*

✓6ᵗʰ I25.71   **Atherosclerosis of autologous vein coronary artery bypass graft(s) with angina pectoris**

CC Excl: For CC codes in subcategory I25.71, unless otherwise noted: I25.10-I25.119, I25.700-I25.799, I25.811-I25.84

    I25.710   **Atherosclerosis of autologous** [PDx CC] [CC] [A] **vein coronary artery bypass graft(s) with unstable angina pectoris**
EXCLUDES 1   *unstable angina without atherosclerosis of autologous vein coronary artery bypass graft(s) (I20.0)*
CC Excl: I09.81-I11.0, I13.0, I13.2, I20.0-I22.9, I24.0, I24.8-I25.119, I25.5-I25.739, I25.760-I25.799, I25.812-I25.9, I50.1, I50.9, I87.8-I87.9, I99.8-I99.9, R57.0, R57.9

    I25.711   **Atherosclerosis of autologous vein** [CC] [A] **coronary artery bypass graft(s) with angina pectoris with documented spasm**
EXCLUDES 1   *angina pectoris with documented spasm without atherosclerosis of autologous vein coronary artery bypass graft(s) (I20.1)*

    I25.718   **Atherosclerosis of autologous vein** [CC] [A] **coronary artery bypass graft(s) with other forms of angina pectoris**
EXCLUDES 1   *other forms of angina pectoris without atherosclerosis of autologous vein coronary artery bypass graft(s) (I20.8)*

    I25.719   **Atherosclerosis of autologous vein** [CC] [A] **coronary artery bypass graft(s) with unspecified angina pectoris**
EXCLUDES 1   *unspecified angina pectoris without atherosclerosis of autologous vein coronary artery bypass graft(s) (I20.9)*

✓6ᵗʰ I25.72   **Atherosclerosis of autologous artery coronary artery bypass graft(s) with angina pectoris**
Atherosclerosis of internal mammary artery graft with angina pectoris

CC Excl: For CC codes in subcategories I25.72, unless otherwise noted: I25.10-I25.119, I25.700-I25.738

    I25.720   **Atherosclerosis of autologous** [PDx CC] [CC] [A] **artery coronary artery bypass graft(s) with unstable angina pectoris**
EXCLUDES 1   *unstable angina without atherosclerosis of autologous artery coronary artery bypass graft(s) (I20.0)*
CC Excl: See code: I25.710

    I25.721   **Atherosclerosis of autologous artery** [CC] [A] **coronary artery bypass graft(s) with angina pectoris with documented spasm**
EXCLUDES 1   *angina pectoris with documented spasm without atherosclerosis of autologous artery coronary artery bypass graft(s) (I20.1)*

    I25.728   **Atherosclerosis of autologous artery** [CC] [A] **coronary artery bypass graft(s) with other forms of angina pectoris**
EXCLUDES 1   *other forms of angina pectoris without atherosclerosis of autologous artery coronary artery bypass graft(s) (I20.8)*

    I25.729   **Atherosclerosis of autologous artery** [CC] [A] **coronary artery bypass graft(s) with unspecified angina pectoris**
EXCLUDES 1   *unspecified angina pectoris without atherosclerosis of autologous artery coronary artery bypass graft(s) (I20.9)*

✓6ᵗʰ I25.73   **Atherosclerosis of nonautologous biological coronary artery bypass graft(s) with angina pectoris**

CC Excl: For CC codes in subcategories I25.73, unless otherwise noted: I25.10-I25.119, I25.700-I25.738

    I25.730   **Atherosclerosis of** [PDx CC] [CC] [A] **nonautologous biological coronary artery bypass graft(s) with unstable angina pectoris**
EXCLUDES 1   *unstable angina without atherosclerosis of nonautologous biological coronary artery bypass graft(s) (I20.0)*
CC Excl: See code: I25.710

    I25.731   **Atherosclerosis of nonautologous** [CC] [A] **biological coronary artery bypass graft(s) with angina pectoris with documented spasm**
EXCLUDES 1   *angina pectoris with documented spasm without atherosclerosis of nonautologous biological coronary artery bypass graft(s) (I20.1)*

    I25.738   **Atherosclerosis of nonautologous** [CC] [A] **biological coronary artery bypass graft(s) with other forms of angina pectoris**
EXCLUDES 1   *other forms of angina pectoris without atherosclerosis of nonautologous biological coronary artery bypass graft(s) (I20.8)*

✓ Additional Character Required   ✓x7ᵗʰ Placeholder Alert   Unacceptable PDx   Manifestation   Hospital Acquired Condition   **EXCLUDES 1** Not Coded Here   **EXCLUDES 2** Not Included Here

I25.739 Atherosclerosis of nonautologous `CC` `A` biological coronary artery bypass graft(s) with **unspecified** angina pectoris
> *EXCLUDES 1* *unspecified angina pectoris without atherosclerosis of nonautologous biological coronary artery bypass graft(s) (I20.9)*

✓6ᵗʰ **I25.75** Atherosclerosis of **native** coronary artery of **transplanted heart** with angina pectoris
> *EXCLUDES 1* *atherosclerosis of native coronary artery of transplanted heart without angina pectoris (I25.811)*

> **CC Excl: For CC codes in subcategory I25.75, unless otherwise noted:** I25.10-I25.119, I25.700-I25.799, I25.811-I25.84

I25.750 Atherosclerosis of native `PDxCC` `CC` coronary artery of transplanted heart with **unstable** angina
> **CC Excl:** I09.81, I11.0, I13.0, I13.2, I20.0-I22.9, I24.0, I24.8-I25.119, I25.5-I25.799, I25.811-I25.9, I50.1, I50.9, I87.8-I87.9, I99.8-I99.9, R57.0, R57.9

I25.751 Atherosclerosis of native coronary `CC` artery of transplanted heart with angina pectoris with **documented spasm**

I25.758 Atherosclerosis of native coronary `CC` artery of transplanted heart with **other forms** of angina pectoris

I25.759 Atherosclerosis of native coronary `CC` artery of transplanted heart with **unspecified** angina pectoris

✓6ᵗʰ **I25.76** Atherosclerosis of **bypass graft** of coronary artery of **transplanted heart** with angina pectoris
> *EXCLUDES 1* *atherosclerosis of bypass graft of coronary artery of transplanted heart without angina pectoris (I25.812)*

> **CC Excl: For CC codes in subcategory I25.76, unless otherwise noted:** I25.10-I25.119, I25.700-I25.759, I25.790-I25.799, I25.811, I25.82-I25.84

I25.760 Atherosclerosis of bypass `PDxCC` `CC` `A` graft of coronary artery of transplanted heart with **unstable** angina
> **CC Excl:** I09.81-I11.0, I13.0, I13.2, I20.0-I22.9, I24.0, I24.8-I25.119, I25.5-I25.759, I25.790-I25.799, I25.811, I25.82-I25.9, I50.1, I50.9, I87.8-I87.9, I99.8-I99.9, R57.0, R57.9

I25.761 Atherosclerosis of bypass graft of `CC` `A` coronary artery of transplanted heart with angina pectoris with **documented spasm**

I25.768 Atherosclerosis of bypass graft of `CC` `A` coronary artery of transplanted heart with **other forms** of angina pectoris

I25.769 Atherosclerosis of bypass graft of `CC` `A` coronary artery of transplanted heart with **unspecified** angina pectoris

✓6ᵗʰ **I25.79** Atherosclerosis of **other** coronary artery bypass graft(s) with angina pectoris

> **CC Excl: For CC codes in subcategory I25.79, unless otherwise noted:** No exclusion

I25.790 Atherosclerosis of other `PDxCC` `CC` `A` coronary artery bypass graft(s) with **unstable** angina pectoris
> *EXCLUDES 1* *unstable angina without atherosclerosis of other coronary artery bypass graft(s) (I20.0)*
> **CC Excl:** I09.81, I11.0, I13.0, I13.2, I20.0-I22.9, I24.0, I24.8-I24.9, I25.5-I25.6, I25.82-I25.83, I25.89-I25.9, I50.1, I50.9, I87.8-I87.9, I99.8-I99.9, R57.0, R57.9

I25.791 Atherosclerosis of other coronary `CC` `A` artery bypass graft(s) with angina pectoris with **documented spasm**
> *EXCLUDES 1* *angina pectoris with documented spasm without atherosclerosis of other coronary artery bypass graft(s) (I20.1)*
> **CC Excl:** No Excl

I25.798 Atherosclerosis of other coronary `CC` `A` artery bypass graft(s) with **other forms** of angina pectoris
> *EXCLUDES 1* *other forms of angina pectoris without atherosclerosis of other coronary artery bypass graft(s) (I20.8)*
> **CC Excl:** No Excl

I25.799 Atherosclerosis of other coronary `CC` `A` artery bypass graft(s) with **unspecified** angina pectoris
> *EXCLUDES 1* *unspecified angina pectoris without atherosclerosis of other coronary artery bypass graft(s) (I20.9)*
> **CC Excl:** No Excl

✓5ᵗʰ **I25.8** **Other forms of chronic ischemic heart disease**

✓6ᵗʰ **I25.81** Atherosclerosis of **other coronary vessels without** angina pectoris
> Use additional code, if applicable, to identify:
> coronary atherosclerosis due to calcified coronary lesion (I25.84)
> coronary atherosclerosis due to lipid rich plaque (I25.83)
> *EXCLUDES 1* *atherosclerotic heart disease of native coronary artery without angina pectoris (I25.10)*

I25.810 Atherosclerosis of coronary artery `CC` `A` bypass graft(s) without angina pectoris
> Atherosclerosis of coronary artery bypass graft NOS
> *EXCLUDES 1* *atherosclerosis of coronary bypass graft(s) with angina pectoris (I25.70--I25.73-, I25.79-)*
> **CC Excl:** No excl

I25.811 Atherosclerosis of **native coronary** `CC` artery of **transplanted heart without** angina pectoris
> Atherosclerosis of native coronary artery of transplanted heart NOS
> *EXCLUDES 1* *atherosclerosis of native coronary artery of transplanted heart with angina pectoris (I25.75-)*
> **CC Excl:** See code: I25.75

I25.812 Atherosclerosis of **bypass graft** of `CC` `A` coronary artery of **transplanted heart** without angina pectoris
> Atherosclerosis of bypass graft of transplanted heart NOS
> *EXCLUDES 1* *atherosclerosis of bypass graft of transplanted heart with angina pectoris (I25.76)*
> **CC Excl:** See code: I25.76

I25.82 **Chronic total occlusion of coronary artery**
> Complete occlusion of coronary artery
> Total occlusion of coronary artery
> Code first coronary atherosclerosis (I25.1-, I25.7-, I25.81-)
> *EXCLUDES 1* *acute coronary occlusion with myocardial infarction (I21.-, I22.-)*
> *acute coronary occlusion without myocardial infarction (I24.0)*

I25.83 **Coronary atherosclerosis due to lipid rich plaque** `A`
> Code first coronary atherosclerosis (I25.1-, I25.7-, I25.81-)

I25.84 **Coronary atherosclerosis due to calcified coronary lesion**
> Coronary atherosclerosis due to severely calcified coronary lesion
> Code first coronary atherosclerosis (I25.1-, I25.7-, I25.81-)

I25.89 **Other forms of chronic ischemic heart disease**

`N` Newborn: 0　`P` Pediatric: 0-17　`M` Maternity: 12-55　`A` Adult: 15-124　`MCC` Major CC Condition　`PDxMCC` PDx acts as own MCC　`CC` CC Condition　`PDxCC` PDx acts as own CC

   I25.9   **Chronic ischemic heart disease,** unspecified
       Ischemic heart disease (chronic) NOS

Pulmonary heart disease and diseases of pulmonary circulation (I26-I28)

✓4ᵗʰ **I26**   **Pulmonary embolism**
    Pulmonary (acute) (artery)(vein) infarction
    Pulmonary (acute) (artery)(vein) thromboembolism
    Pulmonary (acute) (artery)(vein) thrombosis
    EXCLUDES 2   *chronic pulmonary embolism (I27.82)*
       personal history of pulmonary embolism (Z86.711)
       pulmonary embolism due to trauma (T79.0, T79.1)
       pulmonary embolism due to complications of surgical and medical care (T80.0, T81.7-, T82.8-)
       pulmonary embolism complicating abortion, ectopic or molar pregnancy (O00-O07, O08.2)
       pulmonary embolism complicating pregnancy, childbirth and the puerperium (O88.-)
       septic (non-pulmonary) arterial embolism (I76)

✓5ᵗʰ   **I26.0**   **Pulmonary embolism with acute cor pulmonale**
       I26.01   **Septic pulmonary embolism with acute cor pulmonale**   PDxMCC MCC
          Code first underlying infection
          CC Excl: I26.01-I26.99, I27.2-I27.9, I74.01-I74.10, I74.19, I87.8-I87.9, I99.8-I99.9
      3   **I26.02**   **Saddle embolus of pulmonary artery with acute cor pulmonale**   PDxMCC MCC
          CC Excl: See code: I26.01
      3   **I26.09**   **Other pulmonary embolism with acute cor pulmonale**   PDxMCC MCC
          Acute cor pulmonale NOS
          AHA: 2014, 4Q, 21
          CC Excl: See code: I26.01

✓5ᵗʰ   **I26.9**   **Pulmonary embolism without acute cor pulmonale**
       I26.90   **Septic pulmonary embolism without acute cor pulmonale**   MCC
          Code first underlying infection
          CC Excl: I26.01-I26.99, I27.82, I74.01-I74.10, I74.19, I87.8-I87.9, I99.8-I99.9, T80.0XXA, T81.718A, T81.72XA, T82.817A, T82.818A
      3   **I26.92**   **Saddle embolus of pulmonary artery without acute cor pulmonale**   MCC
          CC Excl: I26.01-I26.99, I27.82, I74.01-I74.10, I74.19, I87.8-I87.9, I99.8-I99.9
      3   **I26.99**   **Other pulmonary embolism without acute cor pulmonale**   MCC
          Acute pulmonary embolism NOS
          Pulmonary embolism NOS
          CC Excl: I26.01-I26.99, I27.82, I74.01-I74.10, I74.19, I87.8-I87.9, I99.8-I99.9, T80.0XXA, T81.718A, T82.72XA, T82.817A, T82.818A

✓4ᵗʰ **I27**   **Other pulmonary heart diseases**
    I27.0   **Primary pulmonary hypertension**   CC
       EXCLUDES 1   *pulmonary hypertension NOS (I27.2)*
           secondary pulmonary hypertension (I27.2)
       CC Excl: E66.2, I27.0, I27.2, I27.81, I27.89-I27.9, I28.8-I28.9, I87.8-I87.9, I99.8-I99.9
    I27.1   **Kyphoscoliotic heart disease**   CC
       CC Excl: E66.2, I27.0-I27.81, I27.89-I27.9
    I27.2   **Other secondary pulmonary hypertension**
       Pulmonary hypertension NOS
       Code also associated underlying condition
       AHA: 2014, 4Q, 21

✓5ᵗʰ   **I27.8**   **Other specified pulmonary heart diseases**
       I27.81   **Cor pulmonale (chronic)**
          Cor pulmonale NOS
          EXCLUDES 1   *acute cor pulmonale (I26.0-)*
          AHA: 2014, 4Q, 21
       I27.82   **Chronic pulmonary embolism**   CC
          Use additional code, if applicable, for associated long-term (current) use of anticoagulants (Z79.01)
          EXCLUDES 1   *personal history of pulmonary embolism (Z86.711)*
          CC Excl: I26.01-I26.99, I27.82, I74.01-I74.10, I74.19, I87.8-I87.9, I99.8-I99.9
       I27.89   **Other specified pulmonary heart diseases**
          Eisenmenger's complex
          Eisenmenger's syndrome
          EXCLUDES 1   *Eisenmenger's defect (Q21.8)*

    I27.9   **Pulmonary heart disease, unspecified**
       Chronic cardiopulmonary disease

✓4ᵗʰ **I28**   **Other diseases of pulmonary vessels**
    I28.0   **Arteriovenous fistula of pulmonary vessels**   CC
       EXCLUDES 1   *congenital arteriovenous fistula (Q25.72)*
       CC Excl: I28.0-I28.9
    I28.1   **Aneurysm of pulmonary artery**   CC
       EXCLUDES 1   *congenital aneurysm (Q25.79)*
           congenital arteriovenous aneurysm (Q25.72)
       CC Excl: See code: I28.0
    I28.8   **Other diseases of pulmonary vessels**
       Pulmonary arteritis
       Pulmonary endarteritis
       Rupture of pulmonary vessels
       Stenosis of pulmonary vessels
       Stricture of pulmonary vessels
    I28.9   **Disease of pulmonary vessels, unspecified**

Other forms of heart disease (I30-I52)

✓4ᵗʰ **I30**   **Acute pericarditis**
    INCLUDES   acute mediastinopericarditis
          acute myopericarditis
          acute pericardial effusion
          acute pleuropericarditis
          acute pneumopericarditis
    EXCLUDES 1   *Dressler's syndrome (I24.1)*
          rheumatic pericarditis (acute) (I01.0)

    CC Excl: For CC codes in category I30, unless otherwise noted: I01.0, I09.2, I30.0-I30.9, I31.3-I32, I87.8-I87.9, I99.8-I99.9

    I30.0   **Acute nonspecific idiopathic pericarditis**   CC
    I30.1   **Infective pericarditis**   CC
       Pneumococcal pericarditis
       Pneumopyopericardium
       Purulent pericarditis
       Pyopericarditis
       Pyopericardium
       Pyopneumopericardium
       Staphylococcal pericarditis
       Streptococcal pericarditis
       Suppurative pericarditis
       Viral pericarditis
       Use additional code (B95-B97) to identify infectious agent
    I30.8   **Other forms of acute pericarditis**   CC
    I30.9   **Acute pericarditis, unspecified**   CC

✓4ᵗʰ **I31**   **Other diseases of pericardium**
    EXCLUDES 1   *diseases of pericardium specified as rheumatic (I09.2)*
          postcardiotomy syndrome (I97.0)
          traumatic injury to pericardium (S26.-)
    I31.0   **Chronic adhesive pericarditis**   CC
       Accretio cordis   Adhesive mediastinopericarditis
       Adherent pericardium
       CC Excl: I31.0-I31.9, I87.8-I87.9, I99.8-I99.9
    I31.1   **Chronic constrictive pericarditis**   CC
       Concretio cordis   Pericardial calcification
       CC Excl: See code: I31.0
    I31.2   **Hemopericardium, not elsewhere classified**   CC
       EXCLUDES 1   *hemopericardium as current complication following acute myocardial infarction (I23.0)*
       CC Excl: See code: I31.0
    I31.3   **Pericardial effusion (noninflammatory)**
       Chylopericardium
       EXCLUDES 1   *acute pericardial effusion (I30.9)*
       CC Excl: B33.23, I01.0, I09.2, I30.0-I30.9, I31.3-I32, I87.8-I87.9, I99.8-I99.9
    I31.4   **Cardiac tamponade**   CC
       Code first underlying cause
       CC Excl: See code: I31.3
    I31.8   **Other specified diseases of pericardium**   CC
       Epicardial plaques   Focal pericardial adhesions
       CC Excl: See code: I31.3
    I31.9   **Disease of pericardium, unspecified**   CC
       Pericarditis (chronic) NOS
       CC Excl: See code: I31.3

---

3   HAC = as SDx not POA, in combination with one of the following procedure codes: Ø5R[9,B]Ø[1,2,3,4,J][9,A,Z]; Ø5R[9,B]Ø[7,K]Z; Ø5R[A,E]Ø[Ø,1,3,J][9,A,Z]; Ø5R[A,E]Ø[7,K]Z; Ø5R[C,D,T,U,V,W]Ø[7,K]Z; Ø5R[C,D,T,U,V,W]ØJ[9,A,Z]; Ø5R[R,S]Ø[1,3,J][9,A,Z]; Ø5R[R,S]Ø[7,K]Z; Ø5U[9,B]ØBZ; Ø5U[A,E,R,S]ØBZ.

✓ Additional Character Required   ✓x7ᵗʰ Placeholder Alert   Unacceptable PDx   Manifestation   Hospital Acquired Condition   EXCLUDES 1 Not Coded Here   EXCLUDES 2 Not Included Here

Chapter 9. Diseases of the Circulatory System

I32   **Pericarditis in diseases classified elsewhere**   `CC`

Code first underlying disease

EXCLUDES 1   pericarditis (in):
     coxsackie (virus) (B33.23)
     gonococcal (A54.83)
     meningococcal (A39.53)
     rheumatoid (arthritis) (M05.31)
     syphilitic (A52.06)
     systemic lupus erythematosus (M32.12)
     tuberculosis (A18.84)

CC Excl: I01.0, I09.2, I30.0-I30.9, I31.3-I32, I87.8-I87.9, I99.8-I99.9

✓4ᵗʰ I33   **Acute and subacute endocarditis**

EXCLUDES 1   acute rheumatic endocarditis (I01.1)
     endocarditis NOS (I38)

I33.0   **Acute and subacute infective endocarditis**   `HIV` `MCC`
Bacterial endocarditis (acute) (subacute)
Infective endocarditis (acute) (subacute) NOS
Endocarditis lenta (acute) (subacute)
Malignant endocarditis (acute) (subacute)
Purulent endocarditis (acute) (subacute)
Septic endocarditis (acute) (subacute)
Ulcerative endocarditis (acute) (subacute)
Vegetative endocarditis (acute) (subacute)
Use additional code (B95-B97) to identify infectious agent
CC Excl: I01.1-I08.3, I09.1, I33.0-I33.9, I38-I39, I87.8-I87.9, I99.8-I99.9

I33.9   **Acute and subacute endocarditis, unspecified**   `HIV` `MCC`
Acute endocarditis NOS
Acute myoendocarditis NOS
Acute periendocarditis NOS
Subacute endocarditis NOS
Subacute myoendocarditis NOS
Subacute periendocarditis NOS
CC Excl: See code: I33.0

✓4ᵗʰ I34   **Nonrheumatic mitral valve disorders**

EXCLUDES 1   mitral valve disease (I05.9)
     mitral valve failure (I05.8)
     mitral valve stenosis (I05.0)
     mitral valve disorder of unspecified cause with diseases of aortic and/or tricuspid valve(s) (I08.-)
     mitral valve disorder of unspecified cause with mitral stenosis or obstruction (I05.0)
     mitral valve disorder specified as congenital (Q23.2, Q23.3)
     mitral valve disorder specified as rheumatic (I05.-)

I34.0   **Nonrheumatic mitral (valve) insufficiency**
Nonrheumatic mitral (valve) incompetence NOS
Nonrheumatic mitral (valve) regurgitation NOS

I34.1   **Nonrheumatic mitral (valve) prolapse**
Floppy nonrheumatic mitral valve syndrome
EXCLUDES 1   Marfan's syndrome (Q87.4-)

I34.2   **Nonrheumatic mitral (valve) stenosis**

I34.8   **Other nonrheumatic mitral valve disorders**

I34.9   **Nonrheumatic mitral valve disorder, unspecified**

✓4ᵗʰ I35   **Nonrheumatic aortic valve disorders**

EXCLUDES 1   aortic valve disorder of unspecified cause but with diseases of mitral and/or tricuspid valve(s) (I08.-)
     aortic valve disorder specified as congenital (Q23.0, Q23.1)
     aortic valve disorder specified as rheumatic (I06.-)
     hypertrophic subaortic stenosis (I42.1)

I35.0   **Nonrheumatic aortic (valve) stenosis**

I35.1   **Nonrheumatic aortic (valve) insufficiency**
Nonrheumatic aortic (valve) incompetence NOS
Nonrheumatic aortic (valve) regurgitation NOS

I35.2   **Nonrheumatic aortic (valve) stenosis with insufficiency**

I35.8   **Other nonrheumatic aortic valve disorders**

I35.9   **Nonrheumatic aortic valve disorder, unspecified**

✓4ᵗʰ I36   **Nonrheumatic tricuspid valve disorders**

EXCLUDES 1   tricuspid valve disorders of unspecified cause (I07.-)
     tricuspid valve disorders specified as congenital (Q22.4, Q22.8, Q22.9)
     tricuspid valve disorders specified as rheumatic (I07.-)
     tricuspid valve disorders with aortic and/or mitral valve involvement (I08.-)

I36.0   **Nonrheumatic tricuspid (valve) stenosis**

I36.1   **Nonrheumatic tricuspid (valve) insufficiency**
Nonrheumatic tricuspid (valve) incompetence
Nonrheumatic tricuspid (valve) regurgitation

I36.2   **Nonrheumatic tricuspid (valve) stenosis with insufficiency**

I36.8   **Other nonrheumatic tricuspid valve disorders**

I36.9   **Nonrheumatic tricuspid valve disorder, unspecified**

✓4ᵗʰ I37   **Nonrheumatic pulmonary valve disorders**

EXCLUDES 1   pulmonary valve disorder specified as congenital (Q22.1, Q22.2, Q22.3)
     pulmonary valve disorder specified as rheumatic (I09.89)

I37.0   **Nonrheumatic pulmonary valve stenosis**

I37.1   **Nonrheumatic pulmonary valve insufficiency**
Nonrheumatic pulmonary valve incompetence
Nonrheumatic pulmonary valve regurgitation

I37.2   **Nonrheumatic pulmonary valve stenosis with insufficiency**

I37.8   **Other nonrheumatic pulmonary valve disorders**

I37.9   **Nonrheumatic pulmonary valve disorder, unspecified**

I38   **Endocarditis, valve unspecified**   `CC`

INCLUDES   endocarditis (chronic) NOS
valvular incompetence NOS
valvular insufficiency NOS
valvular regurgitation NOS
valvular stenosis NOS
valvulitis (chronic) NOS

EXCLUDES 1   congenital insufficiency of cardiac valve NOS (Q24.8)
     congenital stenosis of cardiac valve NOS (Q24.8)
     endocardial fibroelastosis (I42.4)
     endocarditis specified as rheumatic (I09.1)

CC Excl: I38-I39, I87.8-I87.9, I99.8-I99.9

I39   **Endocarditis and heart valve disorders in diseases classified elsewhere**   `CC`

Code first underlying disease, such as:
     Q fever (A78)

EXCLUDES 1   endocardial involvement in:
     candidiasis (B37.6)
     gonococcal infection (A54.83)
     Libman-Sacks disease (M32.11)
     listerosis (A32.82)
     meningococcal infection (A39.51)
     rheumatoid arthritis (M05.31)
     syphilis (A52.03)
     tuberculosis (A18.84)
     typhoid fever (A01.02)

CC Excl: See code: I38

✓4ᵗʰ I40   **Acute myocarditis**

INCLUDES   subacute myocarditis

EXCLUDES 1   acute rheumatic myocarditis (I01.2)

CC Excl: For MCC codes in category I40, unless otherwise noted: I01.2, I09.0, I23.0-I23.3, I23.6-I23.8, I40.0-I41, I51.0, I51.4, I87.8-I87.9, I99.8-I99.9

I40.0   **Infective myocarditis**   `HIV` `MCC`
Septic myocarditis
Use additional code (B95-B97) to identify infectious agent

I40.1   **Isolated myocarditis**   `HIV` `MCC`
Fiedler's myocarditis
Giant cell myocarditis
Idiopathic myocarditis

I40.8   **Other acute myocarditis**   `HIV` `MCC`

I40.9   **Acute myocarditis, unspecified**   `HIV` `MCC`

I41   **Myocarditis in diseases classified elsewhere**   `MCC`

Code first underlying disease, such as:
     typhus (A75.0-A75.9)

EXCLUDES 1   myocarditis (in):
     Chagas' disease (chronic) (B57.2)
       acute (B57.0)
     coxsackie (virus) infection (B33.22)
     diphtheritic (A36.81)
     gonococcal (A54.83)
     influenzal (J09.X9, J10.82, J11.82)
     meningococcal (A39.52)
     mumps (B26.82)
     rheumatoid arthritis (M05.31)
     sarcoid (D86.85)
     syphilis (A52.06)
     toxoplasmosis (B58.81)
     tuberculous (A18.84)

CC Excl: See code: I40

N Newborn: 0   P Pediatric: 0-17   M Maternity: 12-55   A Adult: 15-124   `MCC` Major CC Condition   `PDxMCC` PDx acts as own MCC   `CC` CC Condition   `PDxCC` PDx acts as own CC

✓4th **I42 Cardiomyopathy**

INCLUDES myocardiopathy

Code first pre-existing cardiomyopathy complicating pregnancy and puerperium (O99.4)

EXCLUDES 1 ischemic cardiomyopathy (I25.5)

peripartum cardiomyopathy (O90.3)

EXCLUDES 2 ventricular hypertrophy (I51.7)

CC Excl: For CC codes in category I42, unless otherwise noted: I09.81, I11.0, I13.0, I13.2, I25.10-I25.119, I25.5-I25.799, I25.811-I25.9, I42.0-I44.1, I44.30-I44.39, I45.2-I45.4, I45.81-I45.89, I48.0-I49.1, I49.3-I49.8, I50.1, I50.9, I87.8-I87.9, I99.8-I99.9, Q24.6, R00.0-R00.2, R57.0, R57.9

I42.0 Dilated cardiomyopathy CC

Congestive cardiomyopathy

I42.1 Obstructive hypertrophic cardiomyopathy CC

Hypertrophic subaortic stenosis (idiopathic)

I42.2 Other hypertrophic cardiomyopathy CC

Nonobstructive hypertrophic cardiomyopathy

I42.3 Endomyocardial (eosinophilic) disease CC

Endomyocardial (tropical) fibrosis

Löffler's endocarditis

I42.4 Endocardial fibroelastosis CC

Congenital cardiomyopathy

Elastomyofibrosis

I42.5 Other restrictive cardiomyopathy CC

Constrictive cardiomyopathy NOS

I42.6 Alcoholic cardiomyopathy CC

Code also presence of alcoholism (F10.-)

I42.7 Cardiomyopathy due to drug and external agent CC

Code first poisoning due to drug or toxin, if applicable (T36-T65 with fifth or sixth character 1-4 or 6)

Use additional code for adverse effect, if applicable, to identify drug (T36-T50 with fifth or sixth character 5)

I42.8 Other cardiomyopathies CC

I42.9 Cardiomyopathy, unspecified CC

Cardiomyopathy (primary) (secondary) NOS

I43 Cardiomyopathy in diseases classified elsewhere CC

Code first underlying disease, such as:

amyloidosis (E85.-)

glycogen storage disease (E74.0)

gout (M10.0-)

thyrotoxicosis (E05.0-E05.9-)

EXCLUDES 1 cardiomyopathy (in):

coxsackie (virus) (B33.24)

diphtheria (A36.81)

sarcoidosis (D86.85)

tuberculosis (A18.84)

CC Excl: See code: I42

✓4th **I44 Atrioventricular and left bundle-branch block**

I44.0 Atrioventricular block, first degree

I44.1 Atrioventricular block, second degree

Atrioventricular block, type I and II

Möbitz block, type I and II

Second degree block, type I and II

Wenckebach's block

I44.2 Atrioventricular block, complete CC

Complete heart block NOS

Third degree block

CC Excl: I44.0-I49.02, I49.2, I49.8, I87.8-I87.9, I99.8-I99.9, R00.1

✓5th **I44.3 Other and unspecified atrioventricular block**

Atrioventricular block NOS

I44.30 Unspecified atrioventricular block

I44.39 Other atrioventricular block

13 **I44.4 Left anterior fascicular block**

13 **I44.5 Left posterior fascicular block**

✓5th **I44.6 Other and unspecified fascicular block**

13 **I44.60 Unspecified fascicular block**

Left bundle-branch hemiblock NOS

13 **I44.69 Other fascicular block**

13 **I44.7 Left bundle-branch block, unspecified**

✓4th **I45 Other conduction disorders**

CC Excl: For CC codes in category I45, unless otherwise noted: I44.0-I49.02, I49.2, I49.8, I87.8-I87.9, I99.8-I99.9, R00.1

13 **I45.0 Right fascicular block**

✓5th **I45.1 Other and unspecified right bundle-branch block**

13 **I45.10 Unspecified right bundle-branch block**

Right bundle-branch block NOS

13 **I45.19 Other right bundle-branch block**

I45.2 Bifascicular block CC

I45.3 Trifascicular block CC

I45.4 Nonspecific intraventricular block

Bundle-branch block NOS

I45.5 Other specified heart block

Sinoatrial block   Sinoauricular block

EXCLUDES 1 heart block NOS (I45.9)

I45.6 Pre-excitation syndrome

Accelerated atrioventricular conduction

Accessory atrioventricular conduction

Anomalous atrioventricular excitation

Lown-Ganong-Levine syndrome

Pre-excitation atrioventricular conduction

Wolff-Parkinson-White syndrome

✓5th **I45.8 Other specified conduction disorders**

I45.81 Long QT syndrome

I45.89 Other specified conduction disorders CC

Atrioventricular [AV] dissociation

Interference dissociation

Isorhythmic dissociation

Nonparoxysmal AV nodal tachycardia

AHA: 2013, 2Q, 31

I45.9 Conduction disorder, unspecified

Heart block NOS

Stokes-Adams syndrome

✓4th **I46 Cardiac arrest**

EXCLUDES 1 cardiogenic shock (R57.0)

CC Excl: For MCC codes in category I46, unless otherwise noted: I46.2-I49.02, I49.2, I87.8-I87.9, I99.8-I99.9

10 **I46.2 Cardiac arrest due to underlying cardiac condition** MCC

Code first underlying cardiac condition

10 **I46.8 Cardiac arrest due to other underlying condition** MCC

Code first underlying condition

10 **I46.9 Cardiac arrest, cause unspecified** MCC

✓4th **I47 Paroxysmal tachycardia**

Code first tachycardia complicating:

abortion or ectopic or molar pregnancy (O00-O07, O08.8)

obstetric surgery and procedures (O75.4)

EXCLUDES 1 tachycardia NOS (R00.0)

sinoauricular tachycardia NOS (R00.0)

sinus [sinusal] tachycardia NOS (R00.0)

CC Excl: For CC codes in category I47, unless otherwise noted: See code: I45

I47.0 Re-entry ventricular arrhythmia CC

I47.1 Supraventricular tachycardia CC

Atrial (paroxysmal) tachycardia

Atrioventricular [AV] (paroxysmal) tachycardia

Atrioventricular re-entrant (nodal) tachycardia [AVNRT] [AVRT]

Junctional (paroxysmal) tachycardia

Nodal (paroxysmal) tachycardia

I47.2 Ventricular tachycardia CC

AHA: 2013, 3Q, 23

I47.9 Paroxysmal tachycardia, unspecified

Bouveret (-Hoffman) syndrome

✓4th **I48 Atrial fibrillation and flutter**

CC Excl: For CC codes in category I48, unless otherwise noted: See code: I45

I48.0 Paroxysmal atrial fibrillation

I48.1 Persistent atrial fibrillation CC

I48.2 Chronic atrial fibrillation

Permanent atrial fibrillation

I48.3 Typical atrial flutter CC

Type I atrial flutter

I48.4 Atypical atrial flutter CC

Type II atrial flutter

✓5th **I48.9 Unspecified atrial fibrillation and atrial flutter**

I48.91 Unspecified atrial fibrillation

I48.92 Unspecified atrial flutter CC

---

10 MCC only if patient is discharged alive.

13 Questionable admission when used as PDx.

✓ Additional Character Required ✓x7th Placeholder Alert Unacceptable PDx Manifestation Hospital Acquired Condition EXCLUDES 1 Not Coded Here EXCLUDES 2 Not Included Here

✓4th I49   Other cardiac arrhythmias

CC Excl: For MCC codes in category I49, unless otherwise noted: See code: I45

Code first cardiac arrhythmia complicating:
- abortion or ectopic or molar pregnancy (O00-O07, O08.8)
- obstetric surgery and procedures (O75.4)

> EXCLUDES 1   bradycardia NOS (R00.1)
> neonatal dysrhythmia (P29.1-)
> sinoatrial bradycardia (R00.1)
> sinus bradycardia (R00.1)
> vagal bradycardia (R00.1)

✓5th I49.0   Ventricular fibrillation and flutter

   10   **I49.01   Ventricular fibrillation**   `MCC`

   I49.02   Ventricular flutter   `MCC`

I49.1   Atrial premature depolarization
Atrial premature beats

I49.2   Junctional premature depolarization   `CC`

I49.3   Ventricular premature depolarization

✓5th I49.4   Other and unspecified premature depolarization

   I49.40   Unspecified premature depolarization
Premature beats NOS

   I49.49   Other premature depolarization
Ectopic beats   Extrasystolic arrhythmias
Extrasystoles   Premature contractions

I49.5   Sick sinus syndrome
Tachycardia-bradycardia syndrome

I49.8   Other specified cardiac arrhythmias
Coronary sinus rhythm disorder   Nodal rhythm disorder
Ectopic rhythm disorder

I49.9   Cardiac arrhythmia, unspecified
Arrhythmia (cardiac) NOS

✓4th I50   Heart failure

Code first:
- heart failure complicating abortion or ectopic or molar pregnancy (O00-O07, O08.8)
- heart failure following surgery (I97.13-)
- heart failure due to hypertension (I11.0)
- heart failure due to hypertension with chronic kidney disease (I13.-)
- obstetric surgery and procedures (O75.4)
- rheumatic heart failure (I09.81)

> EXCLUDES 1   cardiac arrest (I46.-)
> neonatal cardiac failure (P29.0)

AHA: 2014, 1Q, 25; 2013, 2Q, 33

CC Excl: For CC/MCC codes in category I50, unless otherwise noted: I09.81, I11.0, I50.1-I50.9, I87.8-I87.9, I99.8-I99.9, J81.0

I50.1   Left ventricular failure   `CC`
Cardiac asthma
Edema of lung with heart disease NOS
Edema of lung with heart failure
Left heart failure
Pulmonary edema with heart disease NOS
Pulmonary edema with heart failure

> EXCLUDES 1   edema of lung without heart disease or heart failure (J81.-)
> pulmonary edema without heart disease or failure (J81.-)

CC Excl: I09.81, I11.0, I50.1-I50.9, I87.8-I87.9, I99.8-I99.9

✓5th I50.2   Systolic (congestive) heart failure

> EXCLUDES 1   combined systolic (congestive) and diastolic (congestive) heart failure (I50.4-)

   I50.20   Unspecified systolic (congestive) heart failure   `CC`

   I50.21   Acute systolic (congestive) heart failure   `MCC`

   I50.22   Chronic systolic (congestive) heart failure   `CC`

   I50.23   Acute on chronic systolic (congestive) heart failure   `MCC`

✓5th I50.3   Diastolic (congestive) heart failure

> EXCLUDES 1   combined systolic (congestive) and diastolic (congestive) heart failure (I50.4-)

   I50.30   Unspecified diastolic (congestive) heart failure   `CC`

   I50.31   Acute diastolic (congestive) heart failure   `MCC`

   I50.32   Chronic diastolic (congestive) heart failure   `CC`

   I50.33   Acute on chronic diastolic (congestive) heart failure   `MCC`

✓5th I50.4   Combined systolic (congestive) and diastolic (congestive) heart failure

   I50.40   Unspecified combined systolic (congestive) and diastolic (congestive) heart failure   `CC`

   I50.41   Acute combined systolic (congestive) and diastolic (congestive) heart failure   `MCC`

   I50.42   Chronic combined systolic (congestive) and diastolic (congestive) heart failure   `CC`

   I50.43   Acute on chronic combined systolic (congestive) and diastolic (congestive) heart failure   `MCC`

I50.9   Heart failure, unspecified
Biventricular (heart) failure NOS
Cardiac, heart or myocardial failure NOS
Congestive heart disease
Congestive heart failure NOS
Right ventricular failure (secondary to left heart failure)

> EXCLUDES 1   fluid overload (E87.70)

AHA: 2014, 4Q, 21; 2012, 4Q, 92

✓4th I51   Complications and ill-defined descriptions of heart disease

> EXCLUDES 1   any condition in I51.4-I51.9 due to hypertension (I11.-)
> any condition in I51.4-I51.9 due to hypertension and chronic kidney disease (I13.-)
> heart disease specified as rheumatic (I00-I09)

I51.0   Cardiac septal defect, acquired   `CC` `A`
Acquired septal atrial defect (old)
Acquired septal auricular defect (old)
Acquired septal ventricular defect (old)

> EXCLUDES 1   cardiac septal defect as current complication following acute myocardial infarction (I23.1, I23.2)

CC Excl: E78.71-E78.72, I23.0-I23.8, I40.0-I41, I51.0-I51.2, I51.4, I87.8-I87.9, I97.0-I97.191, I99.8-I99.9, P29.3, Q20.0-Q21.9, Q23.8-Q23.9, Q24.8-Q24.9, Q27.30, Q27.4, Q28.0-Q28.1, Q28.8-Q28.9, Q87.1-Q87.89, Q89.7-Q89.8, Q99.2

I51.1   Rupture of chordae tendineae, not elsewhere classified   `MCC`

> EXCLUDES 1   rupture of chordae tendineae as current complication following acute myocardial infarction (I23.4)

CC Excl: I23.0-I23.4, I23.6-I23.8, I51.0-I51.1, I87.8-I87.9, I99.8-I99.9

I51.2   Rupture of papillary muscle, not elsewhere classified   `MCC`

> EXCLUDES 1   rupture of papillary muscle as current complication following acute myocardial infarction (I23.5)

CC Excl: I23.0-I23.3, I23.5-I23.8, I51.0, I51.2, I87.8-I87.9, I99.8-I99.9

I51.3   Intracardiac thrombosis, not elsewhere classified
Apical thrombosis (old)   Mural thrombosis (old)
Atrial thrombosis (old)   Ventricular thrombosis (old)
Auricular thrombosis (old)

> EXCLUDES 1   intracardiac thrombosis as current complication following acute myocardial infarction (I23.6)

AHA: 2013, 1Q, 24

I51.4   Myocarditis, unspecified
Chronic (interstitial) myocarditis   Myocarditis NOS
Myocardial fibrosis

> EXCLUDES 1   acute or subacute myocarditis (I40.-)

I51.5   Myocardial degeneration
Fatty degeneration of heart or myocardium
Myocardial disease
Senile degeneration of heart or myocardium

I51.7   Cardiomegaly
Cardiac dilatation   Ventricular dilatation
Cardiac hypertrophy

✓5th I51.8   Other ill-defined heart diseases

   I51.81   Takotsubo syndrome   `CC`
Reversible left ventricular dysfunction following sudden emotional stress
Stress induced cardiomyopathy
Takotsubo cardiomyopathy
Transient left ventricular apical ballooning syndrome

   CC Excl: I09.81, I11.0, I50.1-I50.9, I51.81, I51.9-I52, I87.8-I87.9, I99.8-I99.9

   I51.89   Other ill-defined heart diseases
Carditis (acute)(chronic)
Pancarditis (acute)(chronic)

I51.9   Heart disease, unspecified

---

10 MCC only if patient is discharged alive.

N Newborn: 0   P Pediatric: 0-17   M Maternity: 12-55   A Adult: 15-124   `MCC` Major CC Condition   `PDxMCC` PDx acts as own MCC   `CC` CC Condition   `PDxCC` PDx acts as own CC

I52   *Other heart disorders in diseases classified elsewhere*
> *Code first underlying disease, such as:*
> *congenital syphilis (A50.5)*
> *mucopolysaccharidosis (E76.3)*
> *schistosomiasis (B65.0-B65.9)*
>> **EXCLUDES 1**   *heart disease (in):*
>> *gonococcal infection (A54.83)*
>> *meningococcal infection (A39.50)*
>> *rheumatoid arthritis (M05.31)*
>> *syphilis (A52.06)*

Cerebrovascular diseases (I60-I69)

Use additional code to identify presence of:
alcohol abuse and dependence (F10.-)
exposure to environmental tobacco smoke (Z77.22)
history of tobacco use (Z87.891)
hypertension (I10-I15)
occupational exposure to environmental tobacco smoke (Z57.31)
tobacco dependence (F17.-)
tobacco use (Z72.0)
> **EXCLUDES 1**   *transient cerebral ischemic attacks and related syndromes (G45.-)*
> *traumatic intracranial hemorrhage (S06.-)*

AHA: 2014, 3Q, 5; 2012, 4Q, 91-92

✓4ᵗʰ **I60**   **Nontraumatic subarachnoid hemorrhage**
> **INCLUDES**   ruptured cerebral aneurysm
> **EXCLUDES 1**   *sequelae of subarachnoid hemorrhage (I69.0-)*
> *syphilitic ruptured cerebral aneurysm (A52.05)*

> **CC Excl: For MCC codes in category I60, unless otherwise noted:**
> E03.5, G93.82, I60.00-I62.9, I87.8-I87.9, I99.8-I99.9, R40.0-R40.2124,
> R40.2210-R40.2224, R40.2310-R40.2324, R40.2340-R40.2344, R40.3-
> R40.4, S02.0XX-S02.19X with 7th [A, B], S02.91X with 7th [A, B],
> S06.0X0-S06.9X9 with 7th A

   ✓5ᵗʰ **I60.0**   **Nontraumatic subarachnoid hemorrhage from** carotid siphon and bifurcation

     I60.00   **Nontraumatic subarachnoid hemorrhage from** unspecified **carotid siphon and bifurcation** `MCC`

     I60.01   **Nontraumatic subarachnoid hemorrhage from** right **carotid siphon and bifurcation** `MCC`

     I60.02   **Nontraumatic subarachnoid hemorrhage from** left **carotid siphon and bifurcation** `MCC`

   ✓5ᵗʰ **I60.1**   **Nontraumatic subarachnoid hemorrhage from** middle cerebral artery

     I60.10   **Nontraumatic subarachnoid hemorrhage from** unspecified **middle cerebral artery** `MCC`

     I60.11   **Nontraumatic subarachnoid hemorrhage from** right **middle cerebral artery** `MCC`

     I60.12   **Nontraumatic subarachnoid hemorrhage from** left **middle cerebral artery** `MCC`

   ✓5ᵗʰ **I60.2**   **Nontraumatic subarachnoid hemorrhage from** anterior communicating artery

     I60.20   **Nontraumatic subarachnoid hemorrhage from** unspecified **anterior communicating artery** `MCC`

     I60.21   **Nontraumatic subarachnoid hemorrhage from** right **anterior communicating artery** `MCC`

     I60.22   **Nontraumatic subarachnoid hemorrhage from** left **anterior communicating artery** `MCC`

   ✓5ᵗʰ **I60.3**   **Nontraumatic subarachnoid hemorrhage from** posterior communicating artery

     I60.30   **Nontraumatic subarachnoid hemorrhage from** unspecified **posterior communicating artery** `MCC`

     I60.31   **Nontraumatic subarachnoid hemorrhage from** right **posterior communicating artery** `MCC`

     I60.32   **Nontraumatic subarachnoid hemorrhage from** left **posterior communicating artery** `MCC`

   I60.4   **Nontraumatic subarachnoid hemorrhage from** basilar artery `MCC`

   ✓5ᵗʰ **I60.5**   **Nontraumatic subarachnoid hemorrhage from** vertebral artery

     I60.50   **Nontraumatic subarachnoid hemorrhage from** unspecified **vertebral artery** `MCC`

     I60.51   **Nontraumatic subarachnoid hemorrhage from** right **vertebral artery** `MCC`

     I60.52   **Nontraumatic subarachnoid hemorrhage from** left **vertebral artery** `MCC`

   I60.6   **Nontraumatic subarachnoid hemorrhage from** other **intracranial arteries** `MCC`

   I60.7   **Nontraumatic subarachnoid hemorrhage from** unspecified intracranial artery `MCC`
> Ruptured (congenital) berry aneurysm
> Ruptured (congenital) cerebral aneurysm
> Subarachnoid hemorrhage (nontraumatic) from cerebral artery NOS
> Subarachnoid hemorrhage (nontraumatic) from communicating artery NOS
>> **EXCLUDES 1**   *berry aneurysm, nonruptured (I67.1)*

   I60.8   **Other nontraumatic subarachnoid hemorrhage** `MCC`
> Meningeal hemorrhage
> Rupture of cerebral arteriovenous malformation

   I60.9   **Nontraumatic subarachnoid hemorrhage,** unspecified `MCC`

✓4ᵗʰ **I61**   **Nontraumatic intracerebral hemorrhage**
> **EXCLUDES 1**   *sequelae of intracerebral hemorrhage (I69.1-)*

> **CC Excl: For MCC codes in category I61, unless otherwise noted:**
> See code: I60

   I61.0   **Nontraumatic intracerebral hemorrhage in** hemisphere, subcortical `MCC`
> Deep intracerebral hemorrhage (nontraumatic)

   I61.1   **Nontraumatic intracerebral hemorrhage in** hemisphere, cortical `MCC`
> Cerebral lobe hemorrhage (nontraumatic)
> Superficial intracerebral hemorrhage (nontraumatic)

   I61.2   **Nontraumatic intracerebral hemorrhage in** hemisphere, unspecified `MCC`

   I61.3   **Nontraumatic intracerebral hemorrhage in** brain stem `MCC`

   I61.4   **Nontraumatic intracerebral hemorrhage in** cerebellum `MCC`

   I61.5   **Nontraumatic intracerebral hemorrhage,** intraventricular `MCC`

   I61.6   **Nontraumatic intracerebral hemorrhage,** multiple localized `MCC`

   I61.8   **Other nontraumatic intracerebral hemorrhage** `MCC`

   I61.9   **Nontraumatic intracerebral hemorrhage,** unspecified `MCC`

✓4ᵗʰ **I62**   **Other and unspecified nontraumatic intracranial hemorrhage**
> **EXCLUDES 1**   *sequelae of intracranial hemorrhage (I69.2)*

> **CC Excl: For CC/MCC codes in category I62, unless otherwise noted:** See code: I60

   ✓5ᵗʰ **I62.0**   **Nontraumatic** subdural **hemorrhage**

     I62.00   **Nontraumatic subdural hemorrhage,** unspecified `MCC`

     I62.01   **Nontraumatic** acute **subdural hemorrhage** `MCC`

     I62.02   **Nontraumatic** subacute **subdural hemorrhage** `MCC`

     I62.03   **Nontraumatic** chronic **subdural hemorrhage** `MCC`

   I62.1   **Nontraumatic** extradural **hemorrhage** `MCC`
> Nontraumatic epidural hemorrhage

   I62.9   **Nontraumatic intracranial hemorrhage,** unspecified `CC`

✓4ᵗʰ **I63**   **Cerebral infarction**
> **INCLUDES**   occlusion and stenosis of cerebral and precerebral arteries, resulting in cerebral infarction
> Use additional code, if applicable, to identify status post administration of tPA (rtPA) in a different facility within the last 24 hours prior to admission to current facility (Z92.82)
> **EXCLUDES 1**   *sequelae of cerebral infarction (I69.3-)*

AHA: 2014, 1Q, 23

   ✓5ᵗʰ **I63.0**   **Cerebral infarction due to** thrombosis **of** precerebral **arteries**

> **CC Excl: For MCC codes in subcategory I63.0, unless otherwise noted:** E08.51-E08.59, E08.618-E08.638,
> E08.649-E08.8, E09.51-E09.59, E09.618-E09.638, E09.649-
> E09.8, E10.51-E10.59, E10.618-E10.638, E10.649, E10.69-
> E10.8, E11.51-E11.59, E11.618-E11.638, E11.649, E11.69-
> E11.8, E13.51-E13.59, E13.618-E13.638, E13.649-E13.8,
> G43.601-G43.619, I63.00-I63.29, I65.01-I65.9, I87.8-I87.9,
> I99.8-I99.9

     I63.00   **Cerebral infarction due to thrombosis of** unspecified **precerebral artery** `MCC`

     ✓6ᵗʰ **I63.01**   **Cerebral infarction due to thrombosis of** vertebral artery

       I63.011   **Cerebral infarction due to thrombosis of** right **vertebral artery** `MCC`

       I63.012   **Cerebral infarction due to thrombosis of** left **vertebral artery** `MCC`

       I63.019   **Cerebral infarction due to thrombosis of** unspecified **vertebral artery** `MCC`

     I63.02   **Cerebral infarction due to thrombosis of** basilar artery `MCC`

✓ Additional Character Required   ✓ₓ7ᵗʰ Placeholder Alert   Unacceptable PDx   Manifestation   Hospital Acquired Condition   **EXCLUDES 1** Not Coded Here   **EXCLUDES 2** Not Included Here

ICD-10-CM 2016   617

✓6ᵗʰ I63.03 Cerebral infarction due to thrombosis of carotid artery

    I63.031 Cerebral infarction due to thrombosis **MCC** of right carotid artery

    I63.032 Cerebral infarction due to thrombosis **MCC** of left carotid artery

    I63.039 Cerebral infarction due to thrombosis **MCC** of unspecified carotid artery

  I63.09 Cerebral infarction due to thrombosis of other **MCC** precerebral artery

✓5ᵗʰ I63.1 Cerebral infarction due to embolism of precerebral arteries

> **CC Excl: For MCC codes in subcategory I63.1, unless otherwise noted:** E08.51-E08.59, E08.618-E08.638, E08.649-E08.8, E09.51-E09.59, E09.618-E09.638, E09.649-E09.8, E10.51-E10.59, E10.618-E10.638, E10.649, E10.69-E10.8, E11.51-E11.59, E11.618-E11.638, E11.649, E11.69-E11.8, E13.51-E13.59, E13.618-E13.638, E13.649-E13.8, G43.601-G43.619, I63.00-I63.29, I65.01-I65.9, I87.8-I87.9, I99.8-I99.9

  I63.10 Cerebral infarction due to embolism of **MCC** unspecified precerebral artery

✓6ᵗʰ I63.11 Cerebral infarction due to embolism of vertebral artery

    I63.111 Cerebral infarction due to embolism **MCC** of right vertebral artery

    I63.112 Cerebral infarction due to embolism **MCC** of left vertebral artery

    I63.119 Cerebral infarction due to embolism **MCC** of unspecified vertebral artery

  I63.12 Cerebral infarction due to embolism of basilar **MCC** artery

✓6ᵗʰ I63.13 Cerebral infarction due to embolism of carotid artery

    I63.131 Cerebral infarction due to embolism **MCC** of right carotid artery

    I63.132 Cerebral infarction due to embolism **MCC** of left carotid artery

    I63.139 Cerebral infarction due to embolism **MCC** of unspecified carotid artery

  I63.19 Cerebral infarction due to embolism of other **MCC** precerebral artery

✓5ᵗʰ I63.2 Cerebral infarction due to unspecified occlusion or stenosis of precerebral arteries

> **CC Excl: For MCC codes in subcategory I63.2, unless otherwise noted:** E08.51-E08.59, E08.618-E08.638, E08.649-E08.8, E09.51-E09.59, E09.618-E09.638, E09.649-E09.8, E10.51-E10.59, E10.618-E10.638, E10.649, E10.69-E10.8, E11.51-E11.59, E11.618-E11.638, E11.649, E11.69-E11.8, E13.51-E13.59, E13.618-E13.638, E13.649-E13.8, G43.601-G43.619, I63.00-I63.29, I65.01-I65.9, I87.8-I87.9, I99.8-I99.9

  I63.20 Cerebral infarction due to unspecified occlusion **MCC** or stenosis of unspecified precerebral arteries

✓6ᵗʰ I63.21 Cerebral infarction due to unspecified occlusion or stenosis of vertebral arteries

    I63.211 Cerebral infarction due to unspecified **MCC** occlusion or stenosis of right vertebral arteries

    I63.212 Cerebral infarction due to unspecified **MCC** occlusion or stenosis of left vertebral arteries

    I63.219 Cerebral infarction due to unspecified **MCC** occlusion or stenosis of unspecified vertebral arteries

  I63.22 Cerebral infarction due to unspecified occlusion **MCC** or stenosis of basilar arteries

✓6ᵗʰ I63.23 Cerebral infarction due to unspecified occlusion or stenosis of carotid arteries

    I63.231 Cerebral infarction due to unspecified **MCC** occlusion or stenosis of right carotid arteries

    I63.232 Cerebral infarction due to unspecified **MCC** occlusion or stenosis of left carotid arteries

    I63.239 Cerebral infarction due to unspecified **MCC** occlusion or stenosis of unspecified carotid arteries

  I63.29 Cerebral infarction due to unspecified occlusion **MCC** or stenosis of other precerebral arteries

✓5ᵗʰ I63.3 Cerebral infarction due to thrombosis of cerebral arteries

> **CC Excl: For MCC codes in subcategory I63.3, unless otherwise noted:** E08.51-E08.59, E08.618-E08.638, E08.649-E08.8, E09.51-E09.59, E09.618-E09.638, E09.649-E09.8, E10.51-E10.59, E10.618-E10.638, E10.649, E10.69-E10.8, E11.51-E11.59, E11.618-E11.638, E11.649, E11.69-E11.8, E13.51-E13.59, E13.618-E13.638, E13.649-E13.8, G43.601-G43.619, I63.30-I63.9, I66.01-I66.9, I87.8-I87.9, I99.8-I99.9

  I63.30 Cerebral infarction due to thrombosis of **MCC** unspecified cerebral artery

✓6ᵗʰ I63.31 Cerebral infarction due to thrombosis of middle cerebral artery

    I63.311 Cerebral infarction due to thrombosis **MCC** of right middle cerebral artery

    I63.312 Cerebral infarction due to thrombosis **MCC** of left middle cerebral artery

    I63.319 Cerebral infarction due to thrombosis **MCC** of unspecified middle cerebral artery

✓6ᵗʰ I63.32 Cerebral infarction due to thrombosis of anterior cerebral artery

    I63.321 Cerebral infarction due to thrombosis **MCC** of right anterior cerebral artery

    I63.322 Cerebral infarction due to thrombosis **MCC** of left anterior cerebral artery

    I63.329 Cerebral infarction due to thrombosis **MCC** of unspecified anterior cerebral artery

✓6ᵗʰ I63.33 Cerebral infarction due to thrombosis of posterior cerebral artery

    I63.331 Cerebral infarction due to thrombosis **MCC** of right posterior cerebral artery

    I63.332 Cerebral infarction due to thrombosis **MCC** of left posterior cerebral artery

    I63.339 Cerebral infarction due to thrombosis **MCC** of unspecified posterior cerebral artery

✓6ᵗʰ I63.34 Cerebral infarction due to thrombosis of cerebellar artery

    I63.341 Cerebral infarction due to thrombosis **MCC** of right cerebellar artery

    I63.342 Cerebral infarction due to thrombosis **MCC** of left cerebellar artery

    I63.349 Cerebral infarction due to thrombosis **MCC** of unspecified cerebellar artery

  I63.39 Cerebral infarction due to thrombosis of other **MCC** cerebral artery

✓5ᵗʰ I63.4 Cerebral infarction due to embolism of cerebral arteries

> **CC Excl: For MCC codes in subcategory I63.4, unless otherwise noted:** E08.51-E08.59, E08.618-E08.638, E08.649-E08.8, E09.51-E09.59, E09.618-E09.638, E09.649-E09.8, E10.51-E10.59, E10.618-E10.638, E10.649, E10.69-E10.8, E11.51-E11.59, E11.618-E11.638, E11.649, E11.69-E11.8, E13.51-E13.59, E13.618-E13.638, E13.649-E13.8, G43.601-G43.619, I63.30-I63.9, I66.01-I66.9, I87.8-I87.9, I99.8-I99.9

  I63.40 Cerebral infarction due to embolism of **MCC** unspecified cerebral artery

✓6ᵗʰ I63.41 Cerebral infarction due to embolism of middle cerebral artery

    I63.411 Cerebral infarction due to embolism **MCC** of right middle cerebral artery

    I63.412 Cerebral infarction due to embolism **MCC** of left middle cerebral artery

    I63.419 Cerebral infarction due to embolism **MCC** of unspecified middle cerebral artery

✓6ᵗʰ I63.42 Cerebral infarction due to embolism of anterior cerebral artery

    I63.421 Cerebral infarction due to embolism **MCC** of right anterior cerebral artery

    I63.422 Cerebral infarction due to embolism **MCC** of left anterior cerebral artery

    I63.429 Cerebral infarction due to embolism **MCC** of unspecified anterior cerebral artery

✓6ᵗʰ I63.43 Cerebral infarction due to embolism of posterior cerebral artery

    I63.431 Cerebral infarction due to embolism **MCC** of right posterior cerebral artery

    I63.432 Cerebral infarction due to embolism **MCC** of left posterior cerebral artery

I63.439   Cerebral infarction due to embolism `MCC`
of unspecified posterior cerebral artery

✓6ᵗʰ   **I63.44**   **Cerebral infarction due to embolism of cerebellar artery**

I63.441   Cerebral infarction due to embolism `MCC`
of right cerebellar artery

I63.442   Cerebral infarction due to embolism `MCC`
of left cerebellar artery

I63.449   Cerebral infarction due to embolism `MCC`
of unspecified cerebellar artery

I63.49   Cerebral infarction due to embolism of other `MCC`
cerebral artery

✓5ᵗʰ   **I63.5**   **Cerebral infarction due to unspecified occlusion or stenosis of cerebral arteries**

> **CC Excl: For MCC codes in subcategory I63.5, unless otherwise noted:** E08.51-E08.59, E08.618-E08.638, E08.649-E08.8, E09.51-E09.59, E09.618-E09.638, E09.649-E09.8, E10.51-E10.59, E10.618-E10.638, E10.649, E10.69-E10.8, E11.51-E11.59, E11.618-E11.638, E11.649, E11.69-E11.8, E13.51-E13.59, E13.618-E13.638, E13.649-E13.8, G43.601-G43.619, I63.30-I63.9, I66.01-I66.9, I87.8-I87.9, I99.8-I99.9

I63.50   Cerebral infarction due to unspecified occlusion `MCC`
or stenosis of unspecified cerebral artery

✓6ᵗʰ   **I63.51**   **Cerebral infarction due to unspecified occlusion or stenosis of middle cerebral artery**

I63.511   Cerebral infarction due to unspecified `MCC`
occlusion or stenosis of right middle
cerebral artery

I63.512   Cerebral infarction due to unspecified `MCC`
occlusion or stenosis of left middle
cerebral artery

I63.519   Cerebral infarction due to unspecified `MCC`
occlusion or stenosis of unspecified
middle cerebral artery

✓6ᵗʰ   **I63.52**   **Cerebral infarction due to unspecified occlusion or stenosis of anterior cerebral artery**

I63.521   Cerebral infarction due to unspecified `MCC`
occlusion or stenosis of right anterior
cerebral artery

I63.522   Cerebral infarction due to unspecified `MCC`
occlusion or stenosis of left anterior
cerebral artery

I63.529   Cerebral infarction due to unspecified `MCC`
occlusion or stenosis of unspecified
anterior cerebral artery

✓6ᵗʰ   **I63.53**   **Cerebral infarction due to unspecified occlusion or stenosis of posterior cerebral artery**

I63.531   Cerebral infarction due to unspecified `MCC`
occlusion or stenosis of right posterior
cerebral artery

I63.532   Cerebral infarction due to unspecified `MCC`
occlusion or stenosis of left posterior
cerebral artery

I63.539   Cerebral infarction due to unspecified `MCC`
occlusion or stenosis of unspecified
posterior cerebral artery

✓6ᵗʰ   **I63.54**   **Cerebral infarction due to unspecified occlusion or stenosis of cerebellar artery**

I63.541   Cerebral infarction due to unspecified `MCC`
occlusion or stenosis of right
cerebellar artery

I63.542   Cerebral infarction due to unspecified `MCC`
occlusion or stenosis of left
cerebellar artery

I63.549   Cerebral infarction due to unspecified `MCC`
occlusion or stenosis of unspecified
cerebellar artery

I63.59   Cerebral infarction due to unspecified occlusion `MCC`
or stenosis of other cerebral artery

I63.6   **Cerebral infarction due to cerebral venous thrombosis, nonpyogenic**   `MCC`
CC Excl: See code: I63.5

I63.8   **Other cerebral infarction**   `MCC`
CC Excl:.See code: I63.5

I63.9   **Cerebral infarction, unspecified**   `MCC`
Stroke NOS
AHA: 2015, 1Q, 25
CC Excl: See code: I63.5

✓4ᵗʰ   **I65**   **Occlusion and stenosis of precerebral arteries, not resulting in cerebral infarction**

`INCLUDES`   embolism of precerebral artery
narrowing of precerebral artery
obstruction (complete) (partial) of precerebral artery
thrombosis of precerebral artery

`EXCLUDES 1`   insufficiency, NOS, of precerebral artery (G45.-)
insufficiency of precerebral arteries causing cerebral infarction (I63.0-I63.2)

✓5ᵗʰ   **I65.0**   **Occlusion and stenosis of vertebral artery**

I65.01   Occlusion and stenosis of right vertebral artery

I65.02   Occlusion and stenosis of left vertebral artery

I65.03   Occlusion and stenosis of bilateral vertebral arteries

I65.09   Occlusion and stenosis of unspecified vertebral artery

I65.1   **Occlusion and stenosis of basilar artery**

✓5ᵗʰ   **I65.2**   **Occlusion and stenosis of carotid artery**

I65.21   Occlusion and stenosis of right carotid artery

I65.22   Occlusion and stenosis of left carotid artery

I65.23   Occlusion and stenosis of bilateral carotid arteries

I65.29   Occlusion and stenosis of unspecified carotid artery

I65.8   **Occlusion and stenosis of other precerebral arteries**

I65.9   **Occlusion and stenosis of unspecified precerebral artery**
Occlusion and stenosis of precerebral artery NOS

✓4ᵗʰ   **I66**   **Occlusion and stenosis of cerebral arteries, not resulting in cerebral infarction**

`INCLUDES`   embolism of cerebral artery
narrowing of cerebral artery
obstruction (complete) (partial) of cerebral artery
thrombosis of cerebral artery

`EXCLUDES 1`   occlusion and stenosis of cerebral artery causing cerebral infarction (I63.3-I63.5)

✓5ᵗʰ   **I66.0**   **Occlusion and stenosis of middle cerebral artery**

I66.01   Occlusion and stenosis of right middle cerebral artery

I66.02   Occlusion and stenosis of left middle cerebral artery

I66.03   Occlusion and stenosis of bilateral middle cerebral arteries

I66.09   Occlusion and stenosis of unspecified middle cerebral artery

✓5ᵗʰ   **I66.1**   **Occlusion and stenosis of anterior cerebral artery**

I66.11   Occlusion and stenosis of right anterior cerebral artery

I66.12   Occlusion and stenosis of left anterior cerebral artery

I66.13   Occlusion and stenosis of bilateral anterior cerebral arteries

I66.19   Occlusion and stenosis of unspecified anterior cerebral artery

✓5ᵗʰ   **I66.2**   **Occlusion and stenosis of posterior cerebral artery**

I66.21   Occlusion and stenosis of right posterior cerebral artery

I66.22   Occlusion and stenosis of left posterior cerebral artery

I66.23   Occlusion and stenosis of bilateral posterior cerebral arteries

I66.29   Occlusion and stenosis of unspecified posterior cerebral artery

I66.3   **Occlusion and stenosis of cerebellar arteries**

I66.8   **Occlusion and stenosis of other cerebral arteries**
Occlusion and stenosis of perforating arteries

I66.9   **Occlusion and stenosis of unspecified cerebral artery**

✓4ᵗʰ   **I67**   **Other cerebrovascular diseases**

`EXCLUDES 1`   sequelae of the listed conditions (I69.8)

I67.0   **Dissection of cerebral arteries, nonruptured**   `MCC`
`EXCLUDES 1`   ruptured cerebral arteries (I60.7)
CC Excl: I77.2-I77.3, I77.5-I77.6, I77.89-I77.9, M31.8-M31.9

I67.1   **Cerebral aneurysm, nonruptured**
Cerebral aneurysm NOS
Cerebral arteriovenous fistula, acquired
Internal carotid artery aneurysm, intracranial portion
Internal carotid artery aneurysm, NOS
`EXCLUDES 1`   congenital cerebral aneurysm, nonruptured (Q28.-)
ruptured cerebral aneurysm (I60.7)

I67.2   **Cerebral atherosclerosis**   ◭
Atheroma of cerebral and precerebral arteries

✔ Additional Character Required   ✔x7ᵗʰ Placeholder Alert   Unacceptable PDx   **Manifestation**   Hospital Acquired Condition   `EXCLUDES 1` Not Coded Here   `EXCLUDES 2` Not Included Here

I67.3 Progressive vascular leukoencephalopathy `HIV` `CC`
Binswanger's disease
CC Excl: A17.82, A50.42, A52.14, A75.9, A79.9, A81.00-A81.9, A83.0-A85.8, A87.2, A88.0, A88.8, A92.1-A92.2, A92.4-A92.8, A93.0, B00.4, B00.82, B01.11-B01.12, B04, B06.01, B08.09, B08.20-B08.22, B08.60-B08.79, B09-B10.09, B26.2, B27.00-B27.99, B33.1, B45.0, B45.2-B45.9, B58.2, B75, G04.00-G04.01, G04.31, G04.81-G05.4, G37.0, G37.4-G37.5, I67.3, J09.X3-J09.X9, J10.2-J10.89, J11.2-J11.89, L44.4, M1A.10X0-M1A.19X1, P35.2-P35.9, P37.0-P37.4, P37.8-P37.9, T56.0X1A, T56.0X2A, T56.0X3A, T56.0X4A

I67.4 Hypertensive encephalopathy `CC`
CC Excl: E08.51-E08.59, E08.618-E08.638, E08.649-E08.8, E09.51-E09.59, E09.618-E09.638, E09.649-E09.8, E10.51-E10.59, E10.618-E10.638, E10.649, E10.69-E10.8, E11.51-E11.59, E11.618-E11.638, E11.649, E11.69-E11.8, E13.51-E13.59, E13.618-E13.638, E13.649-E13.8, I67.4, I87.8-I87.9, I99.8-I99.9

I67.5 Moyamoya disease `CC`
CC Excl: E08.51-E08.59, E08.618-E08.638, E08.649-E08.8, E09.51-E09.59, E09.618-E09.638, E09.649-E09.8, E10.51-E10.59, E10.618-E10.638, E10.649, E10.69-E10.8, E11.51-E11.59, E11.618-E11.638, E11.649, E11.69-E11.8, E13.51-E13.59, E13.618-E13.638, E13.649-E13.8, I67.5, I87.8-I87.9, I99.8-I99.9

I67.6 Nonpyogenic thrombosis of intracranial venous system `CC`
Nonpyogenic thrombosis of cerebral vein
Nonpyogenic thrombosis of intracranial venous sinus
EXCLUDES 1 *nonpyogenic thrombosis of intracranial venous system causing infarction (I63.6)*
CC Excl: E08.51-E08.59, E08.618-E08.638, E08.649-E08.8, E09.51-E09.59, E09.618-E09.638, E09.649-E09.8, E10.51-E10.59, E10.618-E10.638, E10.649, E10.69-E10.8, E11.51-E11.59, E11.618-E11.638, E11.649, E11.69-E11.8, E13.51-E13.59, E13.618-E13.638, E13.649-E13.8, I67.6, I87.8-I87.9, I99.8-I99.9

I67.7 Cerebral arteritis, not elsewhere classified `CC`
Granulomatous angiitis of the nervous system
EXCLUDES 1 *allergic granulomatous angiitis (M30.1)*
CC Excl: E08.51-E08.59, E08.618-E08.638, E08.649-E08.8, E09.51-E09.59, E09.618-E09.638, E09.649-E09.8, E10.51-E10.59, E10.618-E10.638, E10.649, E10.69-E10.8, E11.51-E11.59, E11.618-E11.638, E11.649, E11.69-E11.8, E13.51-E13.59, E13.618-E13.638, E13.649-E13.8, I67.7, I68.2, I87.8-I87.9, I99.8-I99.9

√5th I67.8 Other specified cerebrovascular diseases

I67.81 Acute cerebrovascular insufficiency `CC`
Acute cerebrovascular insufficiency unspecified as to location or reversibility
CC Excl: E08.51-E08.59, E08.618-E08.638, E08.649-E08.8, E09.51-E09.59, E09.618-E09.638, E09.649-E09.8, E10.51-E10.59, E10.618-E10.638, E10.649, E10.69-E10.8, E11.51-E11.59, E11.618-E11.638, E11.649, E11.69-E11.8, E13.51-E13.59, E13.618-E13.638, E13.649-E13.8, G45.0-G45.2, G45.8-G46.2, I60.00-I62.9, I63.30-I63.9, I66.01-I66.9, I67.81-I67.82, I67.841-I67.89, I87.8-I87.9 I99.8-I99.9

I67.82 Cerebral ischemia `CC`
Chronic cerebral ischemia
CC Excl: See code: I67.81

I67.83 Posterior reversible encephalopathy syndrome `HIV` `MCC`
PRES
CC Excl: G21.0, G83.5, G93.40-G93.41

√6th I67.84 Cerebral vasospasm and vasoconstriction

I67.841 Reversible cerebrovascular vasoconstriction syndrome `CC`
Call-Fleming syndrome
Code first underlying condition, if applicable, such as eclampsia (O15.00-O15.9)
CC Excl: E08.51-E08.59, E08.618-E08.638, E08.649-E08.8, E09.51-E09.59, E09.618-E09.638, E09.649-E09.8, E10.51-E10.59, E10.618-E10.638, E10.649, E10.69-E10.8, E11.51-E11.59, E11.618-E11.638, E11.649, E11.69-E11.8, E13.51-E13.59, E13.618-E13.638, E13.649-E13.8, G45.0-G45.2, G45.8-G46.2, I63.00-I63.29, I65.01-I65.9, I67.841-I67.848, I87.8-I87.9, I99.8-I99.9

I67.848 Other cerebrovascular vasospasm and vasoconstriction `CC`
CC Excl: See code: I67.841

I67.89 Other cerebrovascular disease `CC`
CC Excl: See code: I67.81

I67.9 Cerebrovascular disease, unspecified

√4th I68 Cerebrovascular disorders in diseases classified elsewhere

I68.0 *Cerebral amyloid angiopathy*
Code first underlying amyloidosis (E85.-)

I68.2 *Cerebral arteritis in other diseases classified elsewhere* `CC`
Code first underlying disease
EXCLUDES 1 *cerebral arteritis (in):*
listerosis (A32.89)
systemic lupus erythematosus (M32.19)
syphilis (A52.04)
tuberculosis (A18.89)
CC Excl: See code: I67.7

I68.8 *Other cerebrovascular disorders in diseases classified elsewhere*
Code first underlying disease
EXCLUDES 1 *syphilitic cerebral aneurysm (A52.05)*

√4th I69 Sequelae of cerebrovascular disease
NOTE Category I69 is to be used to indicate conditions in I60-I67 as the cause of sequelae. The "sequelae" include conditions specified as such or as residuals which may occur at any time after the onset of the causal condition
EXCLUDES 1 *personal history of cerebral infarction without residual deficit (Z86.73)*
personal history of prolonged reversible ischemic neurologic deficit (PRIND) (Z86.73)
personal history of reversible ischemic neurologcial deficit (RIND) (Z86.73)
sequelae of traumatic intracranial injury (S06.-)
transient ischemic attack (TIA) (G45.9)
AHA: 2012, 4Q, 106

√5th I69.0 Sequelae of nontraumatic subarachnoid hemorrhage

I69.00 Unspecified sequelae of nontraumatic subarachnoid hemorrhage

I69.01 Cognitive deficits following nontraumatic subarachnoid hemorrhage

√6th I69.02 Speech and language deficits following nontraumatic subarachnoid hemorrhage

I69.020 Aphasia following nontraumatic subarachnoid hemorrhage

I69.021 Dysphasia following nontraumatic subarachnoid hemorrhage

I69.022 Dysarthria following nontraumatic subarachnoid hemorrhage

I69.023 Fluency disorder following nontraumatic subarachnoid hemorrhage
Stuttering following nontraumatic subarachnoid hemorrhage

I69.028 Other speech and language deficits following nontraumatic subarachnoid hemorrhage

√6th I69.03 Monoplegia of upper limb following nontraumatic subarachnoid hemorrhage

I69.031 Monoplegia of upper limb following nontraumatic subarachnoid hemorrhage affecting right dominant side

I69.032 Monoplegia of upper limb following nontraumatic subarachnoid hemorrhage affecting left dominant side

I69.033 Monoplegia of upper limb following nontraumatic subarachnoid hemorrhage affecting right non-dominant side

I69.034 Monoplegia of upper limb following nontraumatic subarachnoid hemorrhage affecting left non-dominant side

I69.039 Monoplegia of upper limb following nontraumatic subarachnoid hemorrhage affecting unspecified side

√6th I69.04 Monoplegia of lower limb following nontraumatic subarachnoid hemorrhage

I69.041 Monoplegia of lower limb following nontraumatic subarachnoid hemorrhage affecting right dominant side

I69.042 Monoplegia of lower limb following nontraumatic subarachnoid hemorrhage affecting left dominant side

I69.043 Monoplegia of lower limb following nontraumatic subarachnoid hemorrhage affecting right non-dominant side

I69.044 Monoplegia of lower limb following nontraumatic subarachnoid hemorrhage affecting left non-dominant side

I69.049 Monoplegia of lower limb following nontraumatic subarachnoid hemorrhage affecting unspecified side

✓6ᵗʰ **I69.05 Hemiplegia and hemiparesis following nontraumatic subarachnoid hemorrhage**
AHA: 2015, 1Q, 25

     I69.051 Hemiplegia and hemiparesis following cc **nontraumatic subarachnoid hemorrhage affecting right dominant side**
CC Excl: I69.051-I69.052, I69.151-I69.152, I69.251-I69.252, I69.351-I69.352, I69.851-I69.852, I69.951-I69.952

     I69.052 Hemiplegia and hemiparesis following cc **nontraumatic subarachnoid hemorrhage affecting left dominant side**
CC Excl: See code: I69.051

     I69.053 Hemiplegia and hemiparesis following cc **nontraumatic subarachnoid hemorrhage affecting right non-dominant side**
CC Excl: I69.053-I69.054, I69.153-I69.154, I69.253-I69.254, I69.353-I69.354, I69.853-I69.854, I69.953-I69.954

     I69.054 Hemiplegia and hemiparesis following cc **nontraumatic subarachnoid hemorrhage affecting left non-dominant side**
CC Excl: See code: I69.053

     I69.059 Hemiplegia and hemiparesis following cc **nontraumatic subarachnoid hemorrhage affecting unspecified side**
CC Excl: I69.059-I69.159, I69.259, I69.359, I69.859, I69.959

✓6ᵗʰ **I69.06 Other paralytic syndrome following nontraumatic subarachnoid hemorrhage**
Use additional code to identify type of paralytic syndrome, such as:
locked-in state (G83.5)
quadriplegia (G82.5-)

     EXCLUDES 1   hemiplegia/hemiparesis following nontraumatic subarachnoid hemorrhage (I69.05-)
monoplegia of lower limb following nontraumatic subarachnoid hemorrhage (I69.04-)
monoplegia of upper limb following nontraumatic subarachnoid hemorrhage (I69.03-)

     I69.061 Other paralytic syndrome following nontraumatic subarachnoid hemorrhage affecting right dominant side

     I69.062 Other paralytic syndrome following nontraumatic subarachnoid hemorrhage affecting left dominant side

     I69.063 Other paralytic syndrome following nontraumatic subarachnoid hemorrhage affecting right non-dominant side

     I69.064 Other paralytic syndrome following nontraumatic subarachnoid hemorrhage affecting left non-dominant side

     I69.065 Other paralytic syndrome following nontraumatic subarachnoid hemorrhage, bilateral

     I69.069 Other paralytic syndrome following nontraumatic subarachnoid hemorrhage affecting unspecified side

✓6ᵗʰ **I69.09 Other sequelae of nontraumatic subarachnoid hemorrhage**

     I69.090 Apraxia following nontraumatic subarachnoid hemorrhage

     I69.091 Dysphagia following nontraumatic subarachnoid hemorrhage
Use additional code to identify the type of dysphagia, if known (R13.1-)

     I69.092 Facial weakness following nontraumatic subarachnoid hemorrhage
Facial droop following nontraumatic subarachnoid hemorrhage

     I69.093 Ataxia following nontraumatic subarachnoid hemorrhage

     I69.098 Other sequelae following nontraumatic subarachnoid hemorrhage
Alterations of sensation following nontraumatic subarachnoid hemorrhage
Disturbance of vision following nontraumatic subarachnoid hemorrhage
Use additional code to identify the sequelae

✓5ᵗʰ **I69.1 Sequelae of nontraumatic intracerebral hemorrhage**

     I69.10 Unspecified sequelae of nontraumatic intracerebral hemorrhage

     I69.11 Cognitive deficits following nontraumatic intracerebral hemorrhage

✓6ᵗʰ   **I69.12 Speech and language deficits following nontraumatic intracerebral hemorrhage**

         I69.120 Aphasia following nontraumatic intracerebral hemorrhage

         I69.121 Dysphasia following nontraumatic intracerebral hemorrhage

         I69.122 Dysarthria following nontraumatic intracerebral hemorrhage

         I69.123 Fluency disorder following nontraumatic intracerebral hemorrhage
Stuttering following nontraumatic subarachnoid hemorrhage

         I69.128 Other speech and language deficits following nontraumatic intracerebral hemorrhage

✓6ᵗʰ   **I69.13 Monoplegia of upper limb following nontraumatic intracerebral hemorrhage**

         I69.131 Monoplegia of upper limb following nontraumatic intracerebral hemorrhage affecting right dominant side

         I69.132 Monoplegia of upper limb following nontraumatic intracerebral hemorrhage affecting left dominant side

         I69.133 Monoplegia of upper limb following nontraumatic intracerebral hemorrhage affecting right non-dominant side

         I69.134 Monoplegia of upper limb following nontraumatic intracerebral hemorrhage affecting left non-dominant side

         I69.139 Monoplegia of upper limb following nontraumatic intracerebral hemorrhage affecting unspecified side

✓6ᵗʰ   **I69.14 Monoplegia of lower limb following nontraumatic intracerebral hemorrhage**

         I69.141 Monoplegia of lower limb following nontraumatic intracerebral hemorrhage affecting right dominant side

         I69.142 Monoplegia of lower limb following nontraumatic intracerebral hemorrhage affecting left dominant side

         I69.143 Monoplegia of lower limb following nontraumatic intracerebral hemorrhage affecting right non-dominant side

         I69.144 Monoplegia of lower limb following nontraumatic intracerebral hemorrhage affecting left non-dominant side

         I69.149 Monoplegia of lower limb following nontraumatic intracerebral hemorrhage affecting unspecified side

✓6ᵗʰ   **I69.15 Hemiplegia and hemiparesis following nontraumatic intracerebral hemorrhage**
AHA: 2015, 1Q, 25

         I69.151 Hemiplegia and hemiparesis following cc **nontraumatic intracerebral hemorrhage affecting right dominant side**
CC Excl: I69.051-I69.052, I69.151-I69.152, I69.251-I69.252, I69.351-I69.352, I69.851-I69.852, I69.951-I69.952

         I69.152 Hemiplegia and hemiparesis following cc **nontraumatic intracerebral hemorrhage affecting left dominant side**
CC Excl: See code: I69.151

✓ Additional Character Required   ✓x7ᵗʰ Placeholder Alert   Unacceptable PDx   Manifestation   Hospital Acquired Condition   *EXCLUDES 1* Not Coded Here   *EXCLUDES 2* Not Included Here

ICD-10-CM 2016   621

I69.153   **Hemiplegia and hemiparesis following** `CC`
nontraumatic intracerebral hemorrhage
affecting right non-dominant **side**
      CC Excl: I69.Ø53-I69.Ø54, I69.153-I69.154,
      I69.253-I69.254, I69.353-I69.354, I69.853-
      I69.854, I69.953-I69.954

I69.154   **Hemiplegia and hemiparesis following** `CC`
nontraumatic intracerebral hemorrhage
affecting left non-dominant **side**
      CC Excl: See code: I69.153

I69.159   **Hemiplegia and hemiparesis following** `CC`
nontraumatic intracerebral hemorrhage
affecting unspecified **side**
      CC Excl: I69.Ø59, I69.159, I69.259, I69.359,
      I69.859, I69.959

✓6ᵗʰ **I69.16**   **Other paralytic syndrome following nontraumatic**
intracerebral hemorrhage
      Use additional code to identify type of paralytic
            syndrome, such as:
      locked-in state (G83.5)
      quadriplegia (G82.5-)
      EXCLUDES 1   *hemiplegia/hemiparesis following*
                  nontraumatic intracerebral
                  hemorrhage (I69.15-)
                  monoplegia of lower limb following
                  nontraumatic intracerebral hemorrhage
                  (I69.14-)
                  monoplegia of upper limb following
                  nontraumatic intracerebral hemorrhage
                  (I69.13-)

I69.161   **Other paralytic syndrome following**
nontraumatic intracerebral hemorrhage
affecting right dominant **side**

I69.162   **Other paralytic syndrome following**
nontraumatic intracerebral hemorrhage
affecting left dominant **side**

I69.163   **Other paralytic syndrome following**
nontraumatic intracerebral hemorrhage
affecting right non-dominant **side**

I69.164   **Other paralytic syndrome following**
nontraumatic intracerebral hemorrhage
affecting left non-dominant **side**

I69.165   **Other paralytic syndrome following**
nontraumatic intracerebral hemorrhage,
bilateral

I69.169   **Other paralytic syndrome following**
nontraumatic intracerebral hemorrhage
affecting unspecified **side**

✓6ᵗʰ **I69.19**   **Other sequelae of nontraumatic intracerebral**
hemorrhage

I69.19Ø   **Apraxia following nontraumatic**
intracerebral hemorrhage

I69.191   **Dysphagia following nontraumatic**
intracerebral hemorrhage
      Use additional code to identify the type of
            dysphagia, if known (R13.1-)

I69.192   **Facial weakness following nontraumatic**
intracerebral hemorrhage
      Facial droop following nontraumatic
            intracerebral hemorrhage

I69.193   **Ataxia following nontraumatic**
intracerebral hemorrhage

I69.198   **Other sequelae of nontraumatic**
intracerebral hemorrhage
      Alteration of sensations following
            nontraumatic intracerebral
            hemorrhage
      Disturbance of vision following
            nontraumatic intracerebral
            hemorrhage
      Use additional code to identify the
            sequelae

✓5ᵗʰ **I69.2**   **Sequelae of other nontraumatic** intracranial **hemorrhage**

I69.2Ø   **Unspecified** sequelae of other nontraumatic
intracranial hemorrhage

I69.21   **Cognitive deficits following other nontraumatic**
intracranial hemorrhage

✓6ᵗʰ **I69.22**   **Speech and** language deficits **following other**
nontraumatic intracranial hemorrhage

I69.22Ø   **Aphasia following other nontraumatic**
intracranial hemorrhage

I69.221   **Dysphasia following other nontraumatic**
intracranial hemorrhage

I69.222   **Dysarthria following other nontraumatic**
intracranial hemorrhage

I69.223   **Fluency disorder following other**
nontraumatic intracranial hemorrhage
      Stuttering following nontraumatic
            subarachnoid hemorrhage

I69.228   **Other speech and language deficits**
following other nontraumatic intracranial
hemorrhage

✓6ᵗʰ **I69.23**   **Monoplegia of upper limb following other**
nontraumatic intracranial hemorrhage

I69.231   **Monoplegia of upper limb following other**
nontraumatic intracranial hemorrhage
affecting right dominant **side**

I69.232   **Monoplegia of upper limb following other**
nontraumatic intracranial hemorrhage
affecting left dominant **side**

I69.233   **Monoplegia of upper limb following other**
nontraumatic intracranial hemorrhage
affecting right non-dominant **side**

I69.234   **Monoplegia of upper limb following other**
nontraumatic intracranial hemorrhage
affecting left non-dominant **side**

I69.239   **Monoplegia of upper limb following other**
nontraumatic intracranial hemorrhage
affecting unspecified **side**

✓6ᵗʰ **I69.24**   **Monoplegia of** lower limb **following other**
nontraumatic intracranial hemorrhage

I69.241   **Monoplegia of lower limb following other**
nontraumatic intracranial hemorrhage
affecting right dominant **side**

I69.242   **Monoplegia of lower limb following other**
nontraumatic intracranial hemorrhage
affecting left dominant **side**

I69.243   **Monoplegia of lower limb following other**
nontraumatic intracranial hemorrhage
affecting right non-dominant **side**

I69.244   **Monoplegia of lower limb following other**
nontraumatic intracranial hemorrhage
affecting left non-dominant **side**

I69.249   **Monoplegia of lower limb following other**
nontraumatic intracranial hemorrhage
affecting unspecified **side**

✓6ᵗʰ **I69.25**   **Hemiplegia and** hemiparesis **following other**
nontraumatic intracranial hemorrhage
      AHA: 2015, 1Q, 25

I69.251   **Hemiplegia and hemiparesis following** `CC`
other nontraumatic intracranial
hemorrhage affecting right
dominant side
      CC Excl: See code: I69.151

I69.252   **Hemiplegia and hemiparesis following** `CC`
other nontraumatic intracranial
hemorrhage affecting left
dominant side
      CC Excl: See code: I69.151

I69.253   **Hemiplegia and hemiparesis following** `CC`
other nontraumatic intracranial
hemorrhage affecting right
non-dominant side
      CC Excl: See code: I69.153

I69.254   **Hemiplegia and hemiparesis following** `CC`
other nontraumatic intracranial
hemorrhage affecting left
non-dominant side
      CC Excl: See code: I69.153

I69.259   **Hemiplegia and hemiparesis following** `CC`
other nontraumatic intracranial
hemorrhage affecting unspecified **side**
      CC Excl: See code: I69.159

Ⓝ Newborn: 0   Ⓟ Pediatric: 0-17   Ⓜ Maternity: 12-55   Ⓐ Adult: 15-124   `MCC` Major CC Condition   `PDxMCC` PDx acts as own MCC   `CC` CC Condition   `PDxCC` PDx acts as own CC

622   ICD-10-CM 2016

☑6ᵗʰ **I69.26** **Other paralytic syndrome** following other nontraumatic intracranial hemorrhage

Use additional code to identify type of paralytic syndrome, such as:
locked-in state (G83.5)
quadriplegia (G82.5-)

EXCLUDES 1 *hemiplegia/hemiparesis following other nontraumatic intracranial hemorrhage (I69.25-)*
monoplegia of lower limb following other nontraumatic intracranial hemorrhage (I69.24-)
monoplegia of upper limb following other nontraumatic intracranial hemorrhage (I69.23-)

I69.261 **Other paralytic syndrome following other nontraumatic intracranial hemorrhage affecting right dominant side**

I69.262 **Other paralytic syndrome following other nontraumatic intracranial hemorrhage affecting left dominant side**

I69.263 **Other paralytic syndrome following other nontraumatic intracranial hemorrhage affecting right non-dominant side**

I69.264 **Other paralytic syndrome following other nontraumatic intracranial hemorrhage affecting left non-dominant side**

I69.265 **Other paralytic syndrome following other nontraumatic intracranial hemorrhage, bilateral**

I69.269 **Other paralytic syndrome following other nontraumatic intracranial hemorrhage affecting unspecified side**

☑6ᵗʰ **I69.29** **Other sequelae** of other nontraumatic intracranial hemorrhage

I69.290 **Apraxia following other nontraumatic intracranial hemorrhage**

I69.291 **Dysphagia following other nontraumatic intracranial hemorrhage**

Use additional code to identify the type of dysphagia, if known (R13.1-)

I69.292 **Facial weakness following other nontraumatic intracranial hemorrhage**

Facial droop following other nontraumatic intracranial hemorrhage

I69.293 **Ataxia following other nontraumatic intracranial hemorrhage**

I69.298 **Other sequelae of other nontraumatic intracranial hemorrhage**

Alteration of sensation following other nontraumatic intracranial hemorrhage
Disturbance of vision following other nontraumatic intracranial hemorrhage
Use additional code to identify the sequelae

☑5ᵗʰ **I69.3** **Sequelae of** cerebral infarction

Sequelae of stroke NOS
AHA: 2013, 4Q, 127-128; 2012, 4Q, 92, 94

I69.30 **Unspecified sequelae of cerebral infarction**

I69.31 **Cognitive deficits following cerebral infarction**

☑6ᵗʰ **I69.32** **Speech and language deficits following cerebral infarction**

I69.320 **Aphasia following cerebral infarction**

I69.321 **Dysphasia following cerebral infarction**
AHA: 2012, 4Q, 91

I69.322 **Dysarthria following cerebral infarction**

I69.323 **Fluency disorder following cerebral infarction**

Stuttering following nontraumatic subarachnoid hemorrhage

I69.328 **Other speech and language deficits following cerebral infarction**

☑6ᵗʰ **I69.33** **Monoplegia of upper limb following cerebral infarction**

I69.331 **Monoplegia of upper limb following cerebral infarction affecting right dominant side**

I69.332 **Monoplegia of upper limb following cerebral infarction affecting left dominant side**

I69.333 **Monoplegia of upper limb following cerebral infarction affecting right non-dominant side**

I69.334 **Monoplegia of upper limb following cerebral infarction affecting left non-dominant side**

I69.339 **Monoplegia of upper limb following cerebral infarction affecting unspecified side**

☑6ᵗʰ **I69.34** **Monoplegia of lower limb following cerebral infarction**

I69.341 **Monoplegia of lower limb following cerebral infarction affecting right dominant side**

I69.342 **Monoplegia of lower limb following cerebral infarction affecting left dominant side**

I69.343 **Monoplegia of lower limb following cerebral infarction affecting right non-dominant side**

I69.344 **Monoplegia of lower limb following cerebral infarction affecting left non-dominant side**

I69.349 **Monoplegia of lower limb following cerebral infarction affecting unspecified side**

☑6ᵗʰ **I69.35** **Hemiplegia and hemiparesis following cerebral infarction**
AHA: 2015, 1Q, 25

I69.351 **Hemiplegia and hemiparesis following cerebral infarction affecting right dominant side** CC

CC Excl: I69.051-I69.052, I69.151-I69.152, I69.251-I69.252, I69.351-I69.352, I69.851-I69.852, I69.951-I69.952

I69.352 **Hemiplegia and hemiparesis following cerebral infarction affecting left dominant side** CC

CC Excl: See code: I69.351

I69.353 **Hemiplegia and hemiparesis following cerebral infarction affecting right non-dominant side** CC

CC Excl: I69.053-I69.054, I69.153-I69.154, I69.253-I69.254, I69.353-I69.354, I69.853-I69.854, I69.953-I69.954

I69.354 **Hemiplegia and hemiparesis following cerebral infarction affecting left non-dominant side** CC

AHA: 2012, 4Q, 91
CC Excl: See code: I69.353

I69.359 **Hemiplegia and hemiparesis following cerebral infarction affecting unspecified side** CC

CC Excl: I69.059, I69.159, I69.259, I69.359, I69.859, I69.959

☑6ᵗʰ **I69.36** **Other paralytic syndrome following cerebral infarction**

Use additional code to identify type of paralytic syndrome, such as:
locked-in state (G83.5)
quadriplegia (G82.5-)

EXCLUDES 1 *hemiplegia/hemiparesis following cerebral infarction (I69.35-)*
monoplegia of lower limb following cerebral infarction (I69.34-)
monoplegia of upper limb following cerebral infarction (I69.33-)

I69.361 **Other paralytic syndrome following cerebral infarction affecting right dominant side**

I69.362 **Other paralytic syndrome following cerebral infarction affecting left dominant side**

I69.363 **Other paralytic syndrome following cerebral infarction affecting right non-dominant side**

I69.364 **Other paralytic syndrome following cerebral infarction affecting left non-dominant side**

I69.365 **Other paralytic syndrome following cerebral infarction, bilateral**

☑ Additional Character Required   ☑x7ᵗʰ Placeholder Alert   Unacceptable PDx   Manifestation   Hospital Acquired Condition   EXCLUDES 1 Not Coded Here   EXCLUDES 2 Not Included Here

ICD-10-CM 2016   623

I69.369 Other paralytic syndrome following cerebral infarction affecting unspecified side

✓6ᵗʰ **I69.39** Other sequelae of cerebral infarction

I69.390 Apraxia following cerebral infarction

I69.391 Dysphagia following cerebral infarction
　Use additional code to identify the type of dysphagia, if known (R13.1-)

I69.392 Facial weakness following cerebral infarction
　Facial droop following cerebral infarction

I69.393 Ataxia following cerebral infarction

I69.398 Other sequelae of cerebral infarction
　Alteration of sensation following cerebral infarction
　Disturbance of vision following cerebral infarction
　Use additional code to identify the sequelae

✓5ᵗʰ **I69.8** Sequelae of other cerebrovascular diseases
　EXCLUDES 1　sequelae of traumatic intracranial injury (S06.-)

I69.80 Unspecified sequelae of other cerebrovascular disease

I69.81 Cognitive deficits following other cerebrovascular disease

✓6ᵗʰ **I69.82** Speech and language deficits following other cerebrovascular disease

I69.820 Aphasia following other cerebrovascular disease

I69.821 Dysphasia following other cerebrovascular disease

I69.822 Dysarthria following other cerebrovascular disease

I69.823 Fluency disorder following other cerebrovascular disease
　Stuttering following nontraumatic subarachnoid hemorrhage

I69.828 Other speech and language deficits following other cerebrovascular disease

✓6ᵗʰ **I69.83** Monoplegia of upper limb following other cerebrovascular disease

I69.831 Monoplegia of upper limb following other cerebrovascular disease affecting right dominant side

I69.832 Monoplegia of upper limb following other cerebrovascular disease affecting left dominant side

I69.833 Monoplegia of upper limb following other cerebrovascular disease affecting right non-dominant side

I69.834 Monoplegia of upper limb following other cerebrovascular disease affecting left non-dominant side

I69.839 Monoplegia of upper limb following other cerebrovascular disease affecting unspecified side

✓6ᵗʰ **I69.84** Monoplegia of lower limb following other cerebrovascular disease

I69.841 Monoplegia of lower limb following other cerebrovascular disease affecting right dominant side

I69.842 Monoplegia of lower limb following other cerebrovascular disease affecting left dominant side

I69.843 Monoplegia of lower limb following other cerebrovascular disease affecting right non-dominant side

I69.844 Monoplegia of lower limb following other cerebrovascular disease affecting left non-dominant side

I69.849 Monoplegia of lower limb following other cerebrovascular disease affecting unspecified side

✓6ᵗʰ **I69.85** Hemiplegia and hemiparesis following other cerebrovascular disease
　AHA: 2015, 1Q, 25

I69.851 Hemiplegia and hemiparesis following CC other cerebrovascular disease affecting right dominant side
　CC Excl: See code: I69.051

I69.852 Hemiplegia and hemiparesis following CC other cerebrovascular disease affecting left dominant side
　CC Excl: See code: I69.051

I69.853 Hemiplegia and hemiparesis following CC other cerebrovascular disease affecting right non-dominant side
　CC Excl: See code: I69.053

I69.854 Hemiplegia and hemiparesis following CC other cerebrovascular disease affecting left non-dominant side
　CC Excl: See code: I69.053

I69.859 Hemiplegia and hemiparesis following CC other cerebrovascular disease affecting unspecified side
　CC Excl: See code: I69.059

✓6ᵗʰ **I69.86** Other paralytic syndrome following other cerebrovascular disease
　Use additional code to identify type of paralytic syndrome, such as:
　locked-in state (G83.5)
　quadriplegia (G82.5-)
　EXCLUDES 1　hemiplegia/hemiparesis following other cerebrovascular disease (I69.85-)
　monoplegia of lower limb following other cerebrovascular disease (I69.84-)
　monoplegia of upper limb following other cerebrovascular disease (I69.83-)

I69.861 Other paralytic syndrome following other cerebrovascular disease affecting right dominant side

I69.862 Other paralytic syndrome following other cerebrovascular disease affecting left dominant side

I69.863 Other paralytic syndrome following other cerebrovascular disease affecting right non-dominant side

I69.864 Other paralytic syndrome following other cerebrovascular disease affecting left non-dominant side

I69.865 Other paralytic syndrome following other cerebrovascular disease, bilateral

I69.869 Other paralytic syndrome following other cerebrovascular disease affecting unspecified side

✓6ᵗʰ **I69.89** Other sequelae of other cerebrovascular disease

I69.890 Apraxia following other cerebrovascular disease

I69.891 Dysphagia following other cerebrovascular disease
　Use additional code to identify the type of dysphagia, if known (R13.1-)

I69.892 Facial weakness following other cerebrovascular disease
　Facial droop following other cerebrovascular disease

I69.893 Ataxia following other cerebrovascular disease

I69.898 Other sequelae of other cerebrovascular disease
　Alteration of sensation following other cerebrovascular disease
　Disturbance of vision following other cerebrovascular disease
　Use additional code to identify the sequelae

✓5ᵗʰ **I69.9** Sequelae of unspecified cerebrovascular diseases
　EXCLUDES 1　sequelae of stroke (I69.3)
　sequelae of traumatic intracranial injury (S06.-)

I69.90 Unspecified sequelae of unspecified cerebrovascular disease

I69.91 Cognitive deficits following unspecified cerebrovascular disease

✓6ᵗʰ **I69.92** Speech and language deficits following unspecified cerebrovascular disease

I69.920 Aphasia following unspecified cerebrovascular disease

I69.921 Dysphasia following unspecified cerebrovascular disease

I69.922 Dysarthria following unspecified cerebrovascular disease

N Newborn: 0　　P Pediatric: 0-17　　M Maternity: 12-55　　A Adult: 15-124　　MCC Major CC Condition　　PDxMCC PDx acts as own MCC　　CC CC Condition　　PDxCC PDx acts as own CC

624　　ICD-10-CM 2016

I69.923   **Fluency disorder following unspecified cerebrovascular disease**
    Stuttering following nontraumatic subarachnoid hemorrhage

I69.928   **Other speech and language deficits following unspecified cerebrovascular disease**

✓6ᵗʰ   **I69.93   Monoplegia of upper limb following unspecified cerebrovascular disease**

I69.931   **Monoplegia of upper limb following unspecified cerebrovascular disease affecting right dominant side**

I69.932   **Monoplegia of upper limb following unspecified cerebrovascular disease affecting left dominant side**

I69.933   **Monoplegia of upper limb following unspecified cerebrovascular disease affecting right non-dominant side**

I69.934   **Monoplegia of upper limb following unspecified cerebrovascular disease affecting left non-dominant side**

I69.939   **Monoplegia of upper limb following unspecified cerebrovascular disease affecting unspecified side**

✓6ᵗʰ   **I69.94   Monoplegia of lower limb following unspecified cerebrovascular disease**

I69.941   **Monoplegia of lower limb following unspecified cerebrovascular disease affecting right dominant side**

I69.942   **Monoplegia of lower limb following unspecified cerebrovascular disease affecting left dominant side**

I69.943   **Monoplegia of lower limb following unspecified cerebrovascular disease affecting right non-dominant side**

I69.944   **Monoplegia of lower limb following unspecified cerebrovascular disease affecting left non-dominant side**

I69.949   **Monoplegia of lower limb following unspecified cerebrovascular disease affecting unspecified side**

✓6ᵗʰ   **I69.95   Hemiplegia and hemiparesis following unspecified cerebrovascular disease**
    AHA: 2015, 1Q, 25

I69.951   **Hemiplegia and hemiparesis following unspecified cerebrovascular disease affecting right dominant side** `CC`
    CC Excl: I69.051–I69.052, I69.151–I69.152, I69.251–I69.252, I69.351–I69.352, I69.851–I69.852, I69.951–I69.952

I69.952   **Hemiplegia and hemiparesis following unspecified cerebrovascular disease affecting left dominant side** `CC`
    CC Excl: See code: I69.951

I69.953   **Hemiplegia and hemiparesis following unspecified cerebrovascular disease affecting right non-dominant side** `CC`
    CC Excl: I69.053–I69.054, I69.153–I69.154, I69.253–I69.254, I69.353–I69.354, I69.853–I69.854, I69.953–I69.954

I69.954   **Hemiplegia and hemiparesis following unspecified cerebrovascular disease affecting left non-dominant side** `CC`
    CC Excl: See code: I69.953

I69.959   **Hemiplegia and hemiparesis following unspecified cerebrovascular disease affecting unspecified side** `CC`
    CC Excl: I69.059, I69.159, I69.259, I69.359, I69.859, I69.959

✓6ᵗʰ   **I69.96   Other paralytic syndrome following unspecified cerebrovascular disease**
    Use additional code to identify type of paralytic syndrome, such as:
     locked-in state (G83.5)
     quadriplegia (G82.5-)
    EXCLUDES 1   *hemiplegia/hemiparesis following unspecified cerebrovascular disease (I69.95-)*
     monoplegia of lower limb following unspecified cerebrovascular disease (I69.94-)
     monoplegia of upper limb following unspecified cerebrovascular disease (I69.93-)

I69.961   **Other paralytic syndrome following unspecified cerebrovascular disease affecting right dominant side**

I69.962   **Other paralytic syndrome following unspecified cerebrovascular disease affecting left dominant side**

I69.963   **Other paralytic syndrome following unspecified cerebrovascular disease affecting right non-dominant side**

I69.964   **Other paralytic syndrome following unspecified cerebrovascular disease affecting left non-dominant side**

I69.965   **Other paralytic syndrome following unspecified cerebrovascular disease, bilateral**

I69.969   **Other paralytic syndrome following unspecified cerebrovascular disease affecting unspecified side**

✓6ᵗʰ   **I69.99   Other sequelae of unspecified cerebrovascular disease**

I69.990   **Apraxia following unspecified cerebrovascular disease**

I69.991   **Dysphagia following unspecified cerebrovascular disease**
    Use additional code to identify the type of dysphagia, if known (R13.1-)

I69.992   **Facial weakness following unspecified cerebrovascular disease**
    Facial droop following unspecified cerebrovascular disease

I69.993   **Ataxia following unspecified cerebrovascular disease**

I69.998   **Other sequelae following unspecified cerebrovascular disease**
    Alteration in sensation following unspecified cerebrovascular disease
    Disturbance of vision following unspecified cerebrovascular disease
    Use additional code to identify the sequelae

Diseases of arteries, arterioles and capillaries (I70-I79)

✓4ᵗʰ   **I70   Atherosclerosis**
    INCLUDES   arteriolosclerosis
     arterial degeneration
     arteriosclerosis
     arteriosclerotic vascular disease
     arteriovascular degeneration
     atheroma
     endarteritis deformans or obliterans
     senile arteritis
     senile endarteritis
     vascular degeneration
    Use additional code to identify:
     exposure to environmental tobacco smoke (Z77.22)
     history of tobacco use (Z87.891)
     occupational exposure to environmental tobacco smoke (Z57.31)
     tobacco dependence (F17.-)
     tobacco use (Z72.0)
    EXCLUDES 2   *arteriosclerotic cardiovascular disease (I25.1-)*
     arteriosclerotic heart disease (I25.1-)
     atheroembolism (I75.-)
     cerebral atherosclerosis (I67.2)
     coronary atherosclerosis (I25.1-)
     mesenteric atherosclerosis (K55.1)
     precerebral atherosclerosis (I67.2)
     primary pulmonary atherosclerosis (I27.0)

✓ Additional Character Required   ✓x7ᵗʰ Placeholder Alert   Unacceptable PDx   Manifestation   Hospital Acquired Condition   **EXCLUDES 1** Not Coded Here   **EXCLUDES 2** Not Included Here

ICD-10-CM 2016   625

Chapter 9. Diseases of the Circulatory System

I69.923–I70

Chapter 9. Diseases of the Circulatory System

I70.0   **Atherosclerosis of** aorta   [A]

I70.1   **Atherosclerosis of** renal artery   [A]
Goldblatt's kidney
> EXCLUDES 2   atherosclerosis of renal arterioles (I12.-)

✓5ᵗʰ **I70.2**   **Atherosclerosis of** native **arteries of the** extremities
Mönckeberg's (medial) sclerosis
Use additional code, if applicable, to identify chronic total occlusion of artery of extremity (I70.92)
> EXCLUDES 2   atherosclerosis of bypass graft of extremities (I70.30-I70.79)

✓6ᵗʰ   **I70.20**   **Unspecified** atherosclerosis of native arteries of extremities
- **I70.201**   Unspecified atherosclerosis of native arteries of extremities, right leg   [A]
- **I70.202**   Unspecified atherosclerosis of native arteries of extremities, left leg   [A]
- **I70.203**   Unspecified atherosclerosis of native arteries of extremities, bilateral legs   [A]
- **I70.208**   Unspecified atherosclerosis of native arteries of extremities, other extremity   [A]
- **I70.209**   Unspecified atherosclerosis of native arteries of extremities, unspecified extremity   [A]

✓6ᵗʰ   **I70.21**   **Atherosclerosis of native arteries of extremities with** intermittent claudication
- **I70.211**   Atherosclerosis of native arteries of extremities with intermittent claudication, right leg   [A]
- **I70.212**   Atherosclerosis of native arteries of extremities with intermittent claudication, left leg   [A]
- **I70.213**   Atherosclerosis of native arteries of extremities with intermittent claudication, bilateral legs   [A]
- **I70.218**   Atherosclerosis of native arteries of extremities with intermittent claudication, other extremity   [A]
- **I70.219**   Atherosclerosis of native arteries of extremities with intermittent claudication, unspecified extremity   [A]

✓6ᵗʰ   **I70.22**   **Atherosclerosis of native arteries of extremities with** rest pain
> INCLUDES   any condition classifiable to I70.21-
- **I70.221**   Atherosclerosis of native arteries of extremities with rest pain, right leg   [A]
- **I70.222**   Atherosclerosis of native arteries of extremities with rest pain, left leg   [A]
- **I70.223**   Atherosclerosis of native arteries of extremities with rest pain, bilateral legs   [A]
- **I70.228**   Atherosclerosis of native arteries of extremities with rest pain, other extremity   [A]
- **I70.229**   Atherosclerosis of native arteries of extremities with rest pain, unspecified extremity   [A]

✓6ᵗʰ   **I70.23**   **Atherosclerosis of native arteries of** right leg **with** ulceration
> INCLUDES   any condition classifiable to I70.211 and I70.221
Use additional code to identify severity of ulcer (L97.-)
- **I70.231**   Atherosclerosis of native arteries of right leg with ulceration of thigh   [A]
- **I70.232**   Atherosclerosis of native arteries of right leg with ulceration of calf   [A]
- **I70.233**   Atherosclerosis of native arteries of right leg with ulceration of ankle   [A]
- **I70.234**   Atherosclerosis of native arteries of right leg with ulceration of heel and midfoot   [A]
  Atherosclerosis of native arteries of right leg with ulceration of plantar surface of midfoot
- **I70.235**   Atherosclerosis of native arteries of right leg with ulceration of other part of foot   [A]
  Atherosclerosis of native arteries of right leg extremities with ulceration of toe
- **I70.238**   Atherosclerosis of native arteries of right leg with ulceration of other part of lower right leg   [A]

- **I70.239**   Atherosclerosis of native arteries of right leg with ulceration of unspecified site   [A]

✓6ᵗʰ   **I70.24**   **Atherosclerosis of native arteries of** left leg **with** ulceration
> INCLUDES   any condition classifiable to I70.212 and I70.222
Use additional code to identify severity of ulcer (L97.-)
- **I70.241**   Atherosclerosis of native arteries of left leg with ulceration of thigh   [A]
- **I70.242**   Atherosclerosis of native arteries of left leg with ulceration of calf   [A]
- **I70.243**   Atherosclerosis of native arteries of left leg with ulceration of ankle   [A]
- **I70.244**   Atherosclerosis of native arteries of left leg with ulceration of heel and midfoot   [A]
  Atherosclerosis of native arteries of left leg with ulceration of plantar surface of midfoot
- **I70.245**   Atherosclerosis of native arteries of left leg with ulceration of other part of foot   [A]
  Atherosclerosis of native arteries of left leg extremities with ulceration of toe
- **I70.248**   Atherosclerosis of native arteries of left leg with ulceration of other part of lower left leg   [A]
- **I70.249**   Atherosclerosis of native arteries of left leg with ulceration of unspecified site   [A]

I70.25   **Atherosclerosis of native arteries of** other **extremities with** ulceration   [A]
> INCLUDES   any condition classifiable to I70.218 and I70.228
Use additional code to identify the severity of the ulcer (L98.49-)

✓6ᵗʰ   **I70.26**   **Atherosclerosis of native arteries of extremities with** gangrene
> INCLUDES   any condition classifiable to I70.21-, I70.22-, I70.23-, I70.24-, and I70.25-
Use additional code to identify the severity of any ulcer (L97.-, L98.49-), if applicable

> **CC Excl:** For CC codes in subcategory I70.26, unless otherwise noted: G89.0-G89.4, I70.261-I70.269, I96, R41.0-R41.3, R41.82, R41.9, R44.8-R44.9, R45.83-R45.84, R46.0-R46.89, R52, R68.0-R68.19, R68.81-R68.83, R68.89-R69

- **I70.261**   Atherosclerosis of native arteries of extremities with gangrene, right leg   [CC] [A]
- **I70.262**   Atherosclerosis of native arteries of extremities with gangrene, left leg   [CC] [A]
- **I70.263**   Atherosclerosis of native arteries of extremities with gangrene, bilateral legs   [CC] [A]
- **I70.268**   Atherosclerosis of native arteries of extremities with gangrene, other extremity   [CC] [A]
- **I70.269**   Atherosclerosis of native arteries of extremities with gangrene, unspecified extremity   [CC] [A]

✓6ᵗʰ   **I70.29**   **Other** atherosclerosis of native arteries of extremities
- **I70.291**   Other atherosclerosis of native arteries of extremities, right leg   [A]
- **I70.292**   Other atherosclerosis of native arteries of extremities, left leg   [A]
- **I70.293**   Other atherosclerosis of native arteries of extremities, bilateral legs   [A]
- **I70.298**   Other atherosclerosis of native arteries of extremities, other extremity   [A]
- **I70.299**   Other atherosclerosis of native arteries of extremities, unspecified extremity   [A]

✓5ᵗʰ **I70.3**   **Atherosclerosis of** unspecified type of bypass graft(s) **of the** extremities
Use additional code, if applicable, to identify chronic total occlusion of artery of extremity (I70.92)
> EXCLUDES 1   embolism or thrombus of bypass graft(s) of extremities (T82.8-)

✓6ᵗʰ   **I70.30**   **Unspecified** atherosclerosis of unspecified type of bypass graft(s) of the extremities

[N] Newborn: 0   [P] Pediatric: 0-17   [M] Maternity: 12-55   [A] Adult: 15-124   [MCC] Major CC Condition   [PDxMCC] PDx acts as own MCC   [CC] CC Condition   [PDxCC] PDx acts as own CC

626   ICD-10-CM 2016

I70.301 Unspecified atherosclerosis of unspecified type of bypass graft(s) of the extremities, right leg   A

I70.302 Unspecified atherosclerosis of unspecified type of bypass graft(s) of the extremities, left leg   A

I70.303 Unspecified atherosclerosis of unspecified type of bypass graft(s) of the extremities, bilateral legs   A

I70.308 Unspecified atherosclerosis of unspecified type of bypass graft(s) of the extremities, other extremity   A

I70.309 Unspecified atherosclerosis of unspecified type of bypass graft(s) of the extremities, unspecified extremity   A

√6ᵗʰ **I70.31** Atherosclerosis of unspecified type of bypass graft(s) of the extremities with intermittent claudication

I70.311 Atherosclerosis of unspecified type of bypass graft(s) of the extremities with intermittent claudication, right leg   A

I70.312 Atherosclerosis of unspecified type of bypass graft(s) of the extremities with intermittent claudication, left leg   A

I70.313 Atherosclerosis of unspecified type of bypass graft(s) of the extremities with intermittent claudication, bilateral legs   A

I70.318 Atherosclerosis of unspecified type of bypass graft(s) of the extremities with intermittent claudication, other extremity   A

I70.319 Atherosclerosis of unspecified type of bypass graft(s) of the extremities with intermittent claudication, unspecified extremity   A

√6ᵗʰ **I70.32** Atherosclerosis of unspecified type of bypass graft(s) of the extremities with rest pain
INCLUDES any condition classifiable to I70.31-

I70.321 Atherosclerosis of unspecified type of bypass graft(s) of the extremities with rest pain, right leg   A

I70.322 Atherosclerosis of unspecified type of bypass graft(s) of the extremities with rest pain, left leg   A

I70.323 Atherosclerosis of unspecified type of bypass graft(s) of the extremities with rest pain, bilateral legs   A

I70.328 Atherosclerosis of unspecified type of bypass graft(s) of the extremities with rest pain, other extremity   A

I70.329 Atherosclerosis of unspecified type of bypass graft(s) of the extremities with rest pain, unspecified extremity   A

√6ᵗʰ **I70.33** Atherosclerosis of unspecified type of bypass graft(s) of the right leg with ulceration
INCLUDES any condition classifiable to I70.311 and I70.321
Use additional code to identify severity of ulcer (L97.-)

> **CC Excl: For CC codes in subcategory I70.33, unless otherwise noted:** I70.231–I70.25, L44.8-L45, L94.2, L94.4, L97.101-L97.929, L98.411-L98.499, L98.8, L99

I70.331 Atherosclerosis of unspecified type of bypass graft(s) of the right leg with ulceration of thigh   PDxCC CC A

I70.332 Atherosclerosis of unspecified type of bypass graft(s) of the right leg with ulceration of calf   PDxCC CC A

I70.333 Atherosclerosis of unspecified type of bypass graft(s) of the right leg with ulceration of ankle   PDxCC CC A

I70.334 Atherosclerosis of unspecified type of bypass graft(s) of the right leg with ulceration of heel and midfoot   PDxCC CC A
Atherosclerosis of unspecified type of bypass graft(s) of right leg with ulceration of plantar surface of midfoot

I70.335 Atherosclerosis of unspecified type of bypass graft(s) of the right leg with ulceration of other part of foot   A
Atherosclerosis of unspecified type of bypass graft(s) of the right leg with ulceration of toe

I70.338 Atherosclerosis of unspecified type of bypass graft(s) of the right leg with ulceration of other part of lower leg   PDxCC CC A

I70.339 Atherosclerosis of unspecified type of bypass graft(s) of the right leg with ulceration of unspecified site   PDxCC CC A

√6ᵗʰ **I70.34** Atherosclerosis of unspecified type of bypass graft(s) of the left leg with ulceration
INCLUDES any condition classifiable to I70.312 and I70.322
Use additional code to identify severity of ulcer (L97.-)

I70.341 Atherosclerosis of unspecified type of bypass graft(s) of the left leg with ulceration of thigh   PDxCC CC A

I70.342 Atherosclerosis of unspecified type of bypass graft(s) of the left leg with ulceration of calf   PDxCC CC A

I70.343 Atherosclerosis of unspecified type of bypass graft(s) of the left leg with ulceration of ankle   PDxCC CC A

I70.344 Atherosclerosis of unspecified type of bypass graft(s) of the left leg with ulceration of heel and midfoot   PDxCC CC A
Atherosclerosis of unspecified type of bypass graft(s) of left leg with ulceration of plantar surface of midfoot

I70.345 Atherosclerosis of unspecified type of bypass graft(s) of the left leg with ulceration of other part of foot   A
Atherosclerosis of unspecified type of bypass graft(s) of the left leg with ulceration of toe

I70.348 Atherosclerosis of unspecified type of bypass graft(s) of the left leg with ulceration of other part of lower leg   PDxCC CC A

I70.349 Atherosclerosis of unspecified type of bypass graft(s) of the left leg with ulceration of unspecified site   PDxCC CC A

I70.35 Atherosclerosis of unspecified type of bypass graft(s) of other extremity with ulceration   A
INCLUDES any condition classifiable to I70.318 and I70.328
Use additional code to identify severity of ulcer (L98.49-)

√6ᵗʰ **I70.36** Atherosclerosis of unspecified type of bypass graft(s) of the extremities with gangrene
INCLUDES any condition classifiable to I70.31-, I70.32-, I70.33-, I70.34-, I70.35
Use additional code to identify the severity of any ulcer (L97.-, L98.49-), if applicable

I70.361 Atherosclerosis of unspecified type of bypass graft(s) of the extremities with gangrene, right leg   PDxCC CC A
CC Excl: G89.0-G89.4, I70.261-I70.269, I96, R41.0-R41.3, R41.82, R41.9, R44.8-R44.9, R45.83-R45.84, R46.0-R46.89, R52, R68.0-R68.19, R68.81-R68.83, R68.89-R69

I70.362 Atherosclerosis of unspecified type of bypass graft(s) of the extremities with gangrene, left leg   PDxCC CC A
CC Excl: See code: I70.361

I70.363 Atherosclerosis of unspecified type of bypass graft(s) of the extremities with gangrene, bilateral legs   PDxCC CC A
CC Excl: See code: I70.361

I70.368 Atherosclerosis of unspecified type of bypass graft(s) of the extremities with gangrene, other extremity   PDxCC CC A
CC Excl: See code: I70.361

I70.369 Atherosclerosis of unspecified type of bypass graft(s) of the extremities with gangrene, unspecified extremity   PDxCC CC A
CC Excl: See code: I70.361

√ Additional Character Required   √x7ᵗʰ Placeholder Alert   Unacceptable PDx   Manifestation   Hospital Acquired Condition   EXCLUDES 1 Not Coded Here   EXCLUDES 2 Not Included Here

✓6th **I70.39** **Other** atherosclerosis of unspecified type of bypass graft(s) of the extremities

I70.391 Other atherosclerosis of unspecified type of bypass graft(s) of the extremities, **right leg** Ⓐ

I70.392 Other atherosclerosis of unspecified type of bypass graft(s) of the extremities, **left leg** Ⓐ

I70.393 Other atherosclerosis of unspecified type of bypass graft(s) of the extremities, **bilateral legs** Ⓐ

I70.398 Other atherosclerosis of unspecified type of bypass graft(s) of the extremities, **other extremity** Ⓐ

I70.399 Other atherosclerosis of unspecified type of bypass graft(s) of the extremities, **unspecified extremity** Ⓐ

✓5th **I70.4** **Atherosclerosis of** autologous vein bypass graft(s) of the extremities

Use additional code, if applicable, to identify chronic total occlusion of artery of extremity (I70.92)

✓6th **I70.40** **Unspecified** atherosclerosis of autologous vein bypass graft(s) of the extremities

I70.401 Unspecified atherosclerosis of autologous vein bypass graft(s) of the extremities, **right leg** Ⓐ

I70.402 Unspecified atherosclerosis of autologous vein bypass graft(s) of the extremities, **left leg** Ⓐ

I70.403 Unspecified atherosclerosis of autologous vein bypass graft(s) of the extremities, **bilateral legs** Ⓐ

I70.408 Unspecified atherosclerosis of autologous vein bypass graft(s) of the extremities, **other extremity** Ⓐ

I70.409 Unspecified atherosclerosis of autologous vein bypass graft(s) of the extremities, **unspecified extremity** Ⓐ

✓6th **I70.41** **Atherosclerosis of autologous vein bypass graft(s) of the extremities with** intermittent claudication

I70.411 Atherosclerosis of autologous vein bypass graft(s) of the extremities with intermittent claudication, **right leg** Ⓐ

I70.412 Atherosclerosis of autologous vein bypass graft(s) of the extremities with intermittent claudication, **left leg** Ⓐ

I70.413 Atherosclerosis of autologous vein bypass graft(s) of the extremities with intermittent claudication, **bilateral legs** Ⓐ

I70.418 Atherosclerosis of autologous vein bypass graft(s) of the extremities with intermittent claudication, **other extremity** Ⓐ

I70.419 Atherosclerosis of autologous vein bypass graft(s) of the extremities with intermittent claudication, **unspecified extremity** Ⓐ

✓6th **I70.42** **Atherosclerosis of autologous vein bypass graft(s) of the extremities with** rest pain

INCLUDES any condition classifiable to I70.41-

I70.421 Atherosclerosis of autologous vein bypass graft(s) of the extremities with rest pain, **right leg** Ⓐ

I70.422 Atherosclerosis of autologous vein bypass graft(s) of the extremities with rest pain, **left leg** Ⓐ

I70.423 Atherosclerosis of autologous vein bypass graft(s) of the extremities with rest pain, **bilateral legs** Ⓐ

I70.428 Atherosclerosis of autologous vein bypass graft(s) of the extremities with rest pain, **other extremity** Ⓐ

I70.429 Atherosclerosis of autologous vein bypass graft(s) of the extremities with rest pain, **unspecified extremity** Ⓐ

✓6th **I70.43** **Atherosclerosis of autologous vein bypass graft(s) of the** right leg with ulceration

INCLUDES any condition classifiable to I70.411 and I70.421

Use additional code to identify severity of ulcer (L97.-)

CC Excl: For CC codes in subcategory I70.43, unless otherwise noted: I70.231-I70.25, L44.8-L45, L94.2, L94.4, L97.101-L97.929, L98.411-L98.499, L98.8, L99

I70.431 Atherosclerosis of autologous vein bypass graft(s) of the right leg with ulceration of **thigh** PDxCC CC Ⓐ

I70.432 Atherosclerosis of autologous vein bypass graft(s) of the right leg with ulceration of **calf** PDxCC CC Ⓐ

I70.433 Atherosclerosis of autologous vein bypass graft(s) of the right leg with ulceration of **ankle** PDxCC CC Ⓐ

I70.434 Atherosclerosis of autologous vein bypass graft(s) of the right leg with ulceration of **heel and midfoot** PDxCC CC Ⓐ

Atherosclerosis of autologous vein bypass graft(s) of right leg with ulceration of plantar surface of midfoot

I70.435 Atherosclerosis of autologous vein bypass graft(s) of the right leg with ulceration of **other part of foot** Ⓐ

Atherosclerosis of autologous vein bypass graft(s) of right leg with ulceration of toe

I70.438 Atherosclerosis of autologous vein bypass graft(s) of the right leg with ulceration of **other part of lower leg** PDxCC CC Ⓐ

I70.439 Atherosclerosis of autologous vein bypass graft(s) of the right leg with ulceration of **unspecified** site PDxCC CC Ⓐ

✓6th **I70.44** **Atherosclerosis of autologous vein bypass graft(s) of the** left leg with ulceration

INCLUDES any condition classifiable to I70.412 and I70.422

Use additional code to identify severity of ulcer (L97.-)

I70.441 Atherosclerosis of autologous vein bypass graft(s) of the left leg with ulceration of **thigh** PDxCC CC Ⓐ

I70.442 Atherosclerosis of autologous vein bypass graft(s) of the left leg with ulceration of **calf** PDxCC CC Ⓐ

I70.443 Atherosclerosis of autologous vein bypass graft(s) of the left leg with ulceration of **ankle** PDxCC CC Ⓐ

I70.444 Atherosclerosis of autologous vein bypass graft(s) of the left leg with ulceration of **heel and midfoot** PDxCC CC Ⓐ

Atherosclerosis of autologous vein bypass graft(s) of left leg with ulceration of plantar surface of midfoot

I70.445 Atherosclerosis of autologous vein bypass graft(s) of the left leg with ulceration of **other part of foot** Ⓐ

Atherosclerosis of autologous vein bypass graft(s) of left leg with ulceration of toe

I70.448 Atherosclerosis of autologous vein bypass graft(s) of the left leg with ulceration of **other part of lower leg** PDxCC CC Ⓐ

I70.449 Atherosclerosis of autologous vein bypass graft(s) of the left leg with ulceration of **unspecified** site PDxCC CC Ⓐ

I70.45 **Atherosclerosis of autologous vein bypass graft(s) of** other extremity with ulceration Ⓐ

INCLUDES any condition classifiable to I70.418, I70.428, and I70.438

Use additional code to identify severity of ulcer (L98.49)

Ⓝ Newborn: 0   Ⓟ Pediatric: 0-17   Ⓜ Maternity: 12-55   Ⓐ Adult: 15-124   MCC Major CC Condition   PDxMCC PDx acts as own MCC   CC CC Condition   PDxCC PDx acts as own CC

628   ICD-10-CM 2016

✓6ᵗʰ I70.46 Atherosclerosis of autologous vein bypass graft(s) of the extremities with gangrene
> **INCLUDES** any condition classifiable to I70.41-, I70.42-, and I70.43-, I70.44-, I70.45
> Use additional code to identify the severity of any ulcer (L97.-, L98.49-), if applicable

     I70.461 Atherosclerosis of autologous `PDxCC` `CC` `A` **vein bypass graft(s) of the extremities with gangrene, right leg**
> CC Excl: G89.0-G89.4, I70.261-I70.269, I96, R41.0-R41.3, R41.82, R41.9, R44.8-R44.9, R45.83-R45.84, R46.0-R46.89, R52, R68.0-R68.19, R68.81-R68.83, R68.89-R69

     I70.462 Atherosclerosis of autologous `PDxCC` `CC` `A` **vein bypass graft(s) of the extremities with gangrene, left leg**
> CC Excl: See code: I70.461

     I70.463 Atherosclerosis of autologous `PDxCC` `CC` `A` **vein bypass graft(s) of the extremities with gangrene, bilateral legs**
> CC Excl: See code: I70.461

     I70.468 Atherosclerosis of autologous `PDxCC` `CC` `A` **vein bypass graft(s) of the extremities with gangrene, other extremity**
> CC Excl: See code: I70.461

     I70.469 Atherosclerosis of autologous `PDxCC` `CC` `A` **vein bypass graft(s) of the extremities with gangrene, unspecified extremity**
> CC Excl: See code: I70.461

✓6ᵗʰ I70.49 Other atherosclerosis of autologous vein bypass graft(s) of the extremities

     I70.491 Other atherosclerosis of autologous `A` **vein bypass graft(s) of the extremities, right leg**

     I70.492 Other atherosclerosis of autologous `A` **vein bypass graft(s) of the extremities, left leg**

     I70.493 Other atherosclerosis of autologous `A` **vein bypass graft(s) of the extremities, bilateral legs**

     I70.498 Other atherosclerosis of autologous `A` **vein bypass graft(s) of the extremities, other extremity**

     I70.499 Other atherosclerosis of autologous `A` **vein bypass graft(s) of the extremities, unspecified extremity**

✓6ᵗʰ I70.5 Atherosclerosis of nonautologous biological bypass graft(s) of the extremities
> Use additional code, if applicable, to identify chronic total occlusion of artery of extremity (I70.92)

✓6ᵗʰ I70.50 Unspecified atherosclerosis of nonautologous biological bypass graft(s) of the extremities

     I70.501 Unspecified atherosclerosis of `A` **nonautologous biological bypass graft(s) of the extremities, right leg**

     I70.502 Unspecified atherosclerosis of `A` **nonautologous biological bypass graft(s) of the extremities, left leg**

     I70.503 Unspecified atherosclerosis of `A` **nonautologous biological bypass graft(s) of the extremities, bilateral legs**

     I70.508 Unspecified atherosclerosis of `A` **nonautologous biological bypass graft(s) of the extremities, other extremity**

     I70.509 Unspecified atherosclerosis of `A` **nonautologous biological bypass graft(s) of the extremities, unspecified extremity**

✓6ᵗʰ I70.51 Atherosclerosis of nonautologous biological bypass graft(s) of the extremities with intermittent claudication

     I70.511 Atherosclerosis of nonautologous `A` **biological bypass graft(s) of the extremities with intermittent claudication, right leg**

     I70.512 Atherosclerosis of nonautologous `A` **biological bypass graft(s) of the extremities with intermittent claudication, left leg**

     I70.513 Atherosclerosis of nonautologous `A` **biological bypass graft(s) of the extremities with intermittent claudication, bilateral legs**

     I70.518 Atherosclerosis of nonautologous `A` **biological bypass graft(s) of the extremities with intermittent claudication, other extremity**

     I70.519 Atherosclerosis of nonautologous `A` **biological bypass graft(s) of the extremities with intermittent claudication, unspecified extremity**

✓6ᵗʰ I70.52 Atherosclerosis of nonautologous biological bypass graft(s) of the extremities with rest pain
> **INCLUDES** any condition classifiable to I70.51-

     I70.521 Atherosclerosis of nonautologous `A` **biological bypass graft(s) of the extremities with rest pain, right leg**

     I70.522 Atherosclerosis of nonautologous `A` **biological bypass graft(s) of the extremities with rest pain, left leg**

     I70.523 Atherosclerosis of nonautologous `A` **biological bypass graft(s) of the extremities with rest pain, bilateral legs**

     I70.528 Atherosclerosis of nonautologous `A` **biological bypass graft(s) of the extremities with rest pain, other extremity**

     I70.529 Atherosclerosis of nonautologous `A` **biological bypass graft(s) of the extremities with rest pain, unspecified extremity**

✓6ᵗʰ I70.53 Atherosclerosis of nonautologous biological bypass graft(s) of the right leg with ulceration
> **INCLUDES** any condition classifiable to I70.511 and I70.521
> Use additional code to identify severity of ulcer (L97.-)

> CC Excl: For CC codes in subcategory I70.53, unless otherwise noted: I70.231-I70.25, L44.8-L45, L94.2, L94.4, L97.101-L97.929, L98.411-L98.499, L98.8, L99

     I70.531 Atherosclerosis of biological `PDxCC` `CC` `A` **nonautologous bypass graft(s) of the right leg with ulceration of thigh**

     I70.532 Atherosclerosis of biological `PDxCC` `CC` `A` **nonautologous bypass graft(s) of the right leg with ulceration of calf**

     I70.533 Atherosclerosis of `PDxCC` `CC` `A` **nonautologous biological bypass graft(s) of the right leg with ulceration of ankle**

     I70.534 Atherosclerosis of `PDxCC` `CC` `A` **nonautologous biological bypass graft(s) of the right leg with ulceration of heel and midfoot**
> Atherosclerosis of nonautologous biological bypass graft(s) of right leg with ulceration of plantar surface of midfoot

     I70.535 Atherosclerosis of nonautologous `A` **biological bypass graft(s) of the right leg with ulceration of other part of foot**
> Atherosclerosis of nonautologous biological bypass graft(s) of the right leg with ulceration of toe

     I70.538 Atherosclerosis of `PDxCC` `CC` `A` **nonautologous biological bypass graft(s) of the right leg with ulceration of other part of lower leg**

     I70.539 Atherosclerosis of `PDxCC` `CC` `A` **nonautologous biological bypass graft(s) of the right leg with ulceration of unspecified site**

✓6ᵗʰ I70.54 Atherosclerosis of nonautologous biological bypass graft(s) of the left leg with ulceration
> **INCLUDES** any condition classifiable to I70.512 and I70.522
> Use additional code to identify severity of ulcer (L97.-)

     I70.541 Atherosclerosis of `PDxCC` `CC` `A` **nonautologous biological bypass graft(s) of the left leg with ulceration of thigh**

     I70.542 Atherosclerosis of `PDxCC` `CC` `A` **nonautologous biological bypass graft(s) of the left leg with ulceration of calf**

✓ Additional Character Required   ✓x7ᵗʰ Placeholder Alert   Unacceptable PDx   Manifestation   Hospital Acquired Condition   **EXCLUDES 1** Not Coded Here   *EXCLUDES 2* Not Included Here

ICD-10-CM 2016   629

I70.543   **Atherosclerosis of** `PDxCC` `CC` `A`
nonautologous biological bypass graft(s)
of the left leg with ulceration of ankle

I70.544   **Atherosclerosis of** `PDxCC` `CC` `A`
nonautologous biological bypass graft(s)
of the left leg with ulceration of heel and
midfoot
> Atherosclerosis of nonautologous
> biological bypass graft(s) of left leg
> with ulceration of plantar surface of
> midfoot

I70.545   **Atherosclerosis of nonautologous** `A`
biological bypass graft(s) of the left leg
with ulceration of other part of foot
> Atherosclerosis of nonautologous
> biological bypass graft(s) of the left leg
> with ulceration of toe

I70.548   **Atherosclerosis of** `PDxCC` `CC` `A`
nonautologous biological bypass
graft(s) of the left leg with ulceration
of other part of lower leg

I70.549   **Atherosclerosis of** `PDxCC` `CC` `A`
nonautologous biological bypass
graft(s) of the left leg with ulceration
of unspecified site

I70.55   **Atherosclerosis of nonautologous biological** `A`
bypass graft(s) of other extremity with ulceration
`INCLUDES`   any condition classifiable to I70.518,
I70.528, and I70.538
Use additional code to identify severity of ulcer
(L98.49)

✓6ᵗʰ **I70.56**   **Atherosclerosis of nonautologous biological bypass**
graft(s) of the extremities with gangrene
`INCLUDES`   any condition classifiable to I70.51-, I70.52-,
and I70.53-, I70.54-, I70.55
Use additional code to identify the severity of any
ulcer (L97.-, L98.49-), if applicable

I70.561   **Atherosclerosis of** `PDxCC` `CC` `A`
nonautologous biological bypass graft(s)
of the extremities with gangrene, right leg
CC Excl: G89.0-G89.4, I70.261-I70.269, I96,
R41.0-R41.3, R41.82, R41.9, R44.8-R44.9,
R45.83-R45.84, R46.0-R46.89, R52, R68.0-
R68.19, R68.81-R68.83, R68.89-R69

I70.562   **Atherosclerosis of** `PDxCC` `CC` `A`
nonautologous biological bypass graft(s)
of the extremities with gangrene, left leg
CC Excl: See code: I70.561

I70.563   **Atherosclerosis of** `PDxCC` `CC` `A`
nonautologous biological bypass graft(s)
of the extremities with gangrene,
bilateral legs
CC Excl: See code: I70.561

I70.568   **Atherosclerosis of** `PDxCC` `CC` `A`
nonautologous biological bypass graft(s)
of the extremities with gangrene, other
extremity
CC Excl: See code: I70.561

I70.569   **Atherosclerosis of** `PDxCC` `CC` `A`
nonautologous biological bypass graft(s)
of the extremities with gangrene,
unspecified extremity
CC Excl: See code: I70.561

✓6ᵗʰ **I70.59**   **Other atherosclerosis of nonautologous biological**
bypass graft(s) of the extremities

I70.591   **Other atherosclerosis of** `A`
biological nonautologous bypass
graft(s) of the extremities, right leg

I70.592   **Other atherosclerosis of** `A`
nonautologous biological bypass
graft(s) of the extremities, left leg

I70.593   **Other atherosclerosis of** `A`
nonautologous biological bypass
graft(s) of the extremities,
bilateral legs

I70.598   **Other atherosclerosis of** `A`
nonautologous biological bypass
graft(s) of the extremities,
other extremity

I70.599   **Other atherosclerosis of** `A`
nonautologous biological bypass
graft(s) of the extremities,
unspecified extremity

✓5ᵗʰ **I70.6**   **Atherosclerosis of nonbiological bypass graft(s) of the**
extremities
Use additional code, if applicable, to identify chronic total
occlusion of artery of extremity (I70.92)

✓6ᵗʰ **I70.60**   **Unspecified atherosclerosis of nonbiological bypass**
graft(s) of the extremities

I70.601   **Unspecified atherosclerosis of** `A`
nonbiological bypass graft(s) of the
extremities, right leg

I70.602   **Unspecified atherosclerosis of** `A`
nonbiological bypass graft(s) of the
extremities, left leg

I70.603   **Unspecified atherosclerosis of** `A`
nonbiological bypass graft(s) of the
extremities, bilateral legs

I70.608   **Unspecified atherosclerosis of** `A`
nonbiological bypass graft(s) of the
extremities, other extremity

I70.609   **Unspecified atherosclerosis of** `A`
nonbiological bypass graft(s) of the
extremities, unspecified extremity

✓6ᵗʰ **I70.61**   **Atherosclerosis of nonbiological bypass graft(s) of**
the extremities with intermittent claudication

I70.611   **Atherosclerosis of nonbiological** `A`
bypass graft(s) of the extremities with
intermittent claudication, right leg

I70.612   **Atherosclerosis of nonbiological** `A`
bypass graft(s) of the extremities with
intermittent claudication, left leg

I70.613   **Atherosclerosis of nonbiological** `A`
bypass graft(s) of the extremities with
intermittent claudication, bilateral legs

I70.618   **Atherosclerosis of nonbiological** `A`
bypass graft(s) of the extremities with
intermittent claudication,
other extremity

I70.619   **Atherosclerosis of nonbiological** `A`
bypass graft(s) of the extremities with
intermittent claudication, unspecified
extremity

✓6ᵗʰ **I70.62**   **Atherosclerosis of nonbiological bypass graft(s) of**
the extremities with rest pain
`INCLUDES`   any condition classifiable to I70.61-

I70.621   **Atherosclerosis of nonbiological** `A`
bypass graft(s) of the extremities with
rest pain, right leg

I70.622   **Atherosclerosis of nonbiological** `A`
bypass graft(s) of the extremities
with rest pain, left leg

I70.623   **Atherosclerosis of nonbiological** `A`
bypass graft(s) of the extremities with rest
pain, bilateral legs

I70.628   **Atherosclerosis of nonbiological** `A`
bypass graft(s) of the extremities
with rest pain, other extremity

I70.629   **Atherosclerosis of nonbiological** `A`
bypass graft(s) of the extremities
with rest pain, unspecified extremity

✓6ᵗʰ **I70.63**   **Atherosclerosis of nonbiological bypass graft(s) of**
the right leg with ulceration
`INCLUDES`   any condition classifiable to I70.611 and
I70.621
Use additional code to identify severity of ulcer (L97.-)

> CC Excl: For CC codes in subcategory I70.63,
> unless otherwise noted: I70.231-I70.25, L44.8-
> L45, L94.2, L94.4, L97.101-L97.929, L98.411-
> L98.499, L98.8, L99

I70.631   **Atherosclerosis of** `PDxCC` `CC` `A`
nonbiological bypass graft(s) of the
right leg with ulceration of thigh

I70.632   **Atherosclerosis of** `PDxCC` `CC` `A`
nonbiological bypass graft(s) of the
right leg with ulceration of calf

I70.633   **Atherosclerosis of** `PDxCC` `CC` `A`
nonbiological bypass graft(s) of the
right leg with ulceration of ankle

I70.634   **Atherosclerosis of** `PDxCC` `CC` `A`
nonbiological bypass graft(s) of the
right leg with ulceration of heel and
midfoot
Atherosclerosis of nonbiological bypass
graft(s) of right leg with ulceration of
plantar surface of midfoot

I70.635   **Atherosclerosis of nonbiological** `A`
bypass graft(s) of the right leg with
ulceration of other part of foot
Atherosclerosis of nonbiological bypass
graft(s) of the right leg with ulceration
of toe

I70.638   **Atherosclerosis of** `PDxCC` `CC` `A`
nonbiological bypass graft(s) of the
right leg with ulceration of other part
of lower leg

I70.639   **Atherosclerosis of** `PDxCC` `CC` `A`
nonbiological bypass graft(s) of the
right leg with ulceration of unspecified
site

✓6ᵗʰ **I70.64**   **Atherosclerosis of nonbiological bypass graft(s) of**
the left leg with ulceration
`INCLUDES`   any condition classifiable to I70.612 and
I70.622
Use additional code to identify severity of ulcer (L97.-)

I70.641   **Atherosclerosis of** `PDxCC` `CC` `A`
nonbiological bypass graft(s) of the
left leg with ulceration of thigh

I70.642   **Atherosclerosis of** `PDxCC` `CC` `A`
nonbiological bypass graft(s) of the
left leg with ulceration of calf

I70.643   **Atherosclerosis of** `PDxCC` `CC` `A`
nonbiological bypass graft(s) of the
left leg with ulceration of ankle

I70.644   **Atherosclerosis of** `PDxCC` `CC` `A`
nonbiological bypass graft(s) of the
left leg with ulceration of heel and
midfoot
Atherosclerosis of nonbiological bypass
graft(s) of left leg with ulceration of
plantar surface of midfoot

I70.645   **Atherosclerosis of nonbiological** `A`
bypass graft(s) of the left leg with
ulceration of other part of foot
Atherosclerosis of nonbiological bypass
graft(s) of the left leg with ulceration
of toe

I70.648   **Atherosclerosis of** `PDxCC` `CC` `A`
nonbiological bypass graft(s) of the
left leg with ulceration of other part of
lower leg

I70.649   **Atherosclerosis of** `PDxCC` `CC` `A`
nonbiological bypass graft(s) of the
left leg with ulceration of unspecified site

I70.65   **Atherosclerosis of nonbiological bypass graft(s)** `A`
of other extremity with ulceration
`INCLUDES`   any condition classifiable to I70.618 and
I70.628
Use additional code to identify severity of ulcer
(L98.49)

✓6ᵗʰ **I70.66**   **Atherosclerosis of nonbiological bypass graft(s) of**
the extremities with gangrene
`INCLUDES`   any condition classifiable to I70.61-, I70.62-,
I70.63-, I70.64-, I70.65
Use additional code to identify the severity of any
ulcer (L97.-, L98.49-), if applicable

I70.661   **Atherosclerosis of** `PDxCC` `CC` `A`
nonbiological bypass graft(s) of the
extremities with gangrene, right leg
CC Excl: G89.0-G89.4, I70.261-I70.269, I96,
R41.0-R41.3, R41.82, R41.9, R44.8-R44.9,
R45.83-R45.84, R46.0-R46.89, R52, R68.0-
R68.19, R68.81-R68.83, R68.89-R69

I70.662   **Atherosclerosis of** `PDxCC` `CC` `A`
nonbiological bypass graft(s) of the
extremities with gangrene, left leg
CC Excl: See code: I70.661

I70.663   **Atherosclerosis of** `PDxCC` `CC` `A`
nonbiological bypass graft(s) of the
extremities with gangrene, bilateral legs
CC Excl: See code: I70.661

I70.668   **Atherosclerosis of** `PDxCC` `CC` `A`
nonbiological bypass graft(s) of the
extremities with gangrene, other
extremity
CC Excl: See code: I70.661

I70.669   **Atherosclerosis of** `PDxCC` `CC` `A`
nonbiological bypass graft(s) of the
extremities with gangrene, unspecified
extremity
CC Excl: See code: I70.661

✓6ᵗʰ **I70.69**   **Other atherosclerosis of nonbiological bypass**
graft(s) of the extremities

I70.691   **Other atherosclerosis of nonbiological** `A`
bypass graft(s) of the extremities,
right leg

I70.692   **Other atherosclerosis of nonbiological** `A`
bypass graft(s) of the extremities,
left leg

I70.693   **Other atherosclerosis of nonbiological** `A`
bypass graft(s) of the extremities,
bilateral legs

I70.698   **Other atherosclerosis of nonbiological** `A`
bypass graft(s) of the extremities,
other extremity

I70.699   **Other atherosclerosis of nonbiological** `A`
bypass graft(s) of the extremities,
unspecified extremity

✓5ᵗʰ **I70.7**   **Atherosclerosis of other type of bypass graft(s) of the**
extremities
Use additional code, if applicable, to identify chronic total
occlusion of artery of extremity (I70.92)

✓6ᵗʰ **I70.70**   **Unspecified atherosclerosis of other type of bypass**
graft(s) of the extremities

I70.701   **Unspecified atherosclerosis of other** `A`
type of bypass graft(s) of the
extremities, right leg

I70.702   **Unspecified atherosclerosis of other** `A`
type of bypass graft(s) of the
extremities, left leg

I70.703   **Unspecified atherosclerosis of other** `A`
type of bypass graft(s) of the
extremities, bilateral legs

I70.708   **Unspecified atherosclerosis of other** `A`
type of bypass graft(s) of the
extremities, other extremity

I70.709   **Unspecified atherosclerosis of other** `A`
type of bypass graft(s) of the
extremities, unspecified extremity

✓6ᵗʰ **I70.71**   **Atherosclerosis of other type of bypass graft(s) of**
the extremities with intermittent claudication

I70.711   **Atherosclerosis of other type of bypass** `A`
graft(s) of the extremities with
intermittent claudication, right leg

I70.712   **Atherosclerosis of other type of bypass** `A`
graft(s) of the extremities with
intermittent claudication, left leg

I70.713   **Atherosclerosis of other type of bypass** `A`
graft(s) of the extremities with
intermittent claudication, bilateral legs

I70.718   **Atherosclerosis of other type of bypass** `A`
graft(s) of the extremities with
intermittent claudication, other extremity

I70.719   **Atherosclerosis of other type of bypass** `A`
graft(s) of the extremities with
intermittent claudication, unspecified
extremity

✓6ᵗʰ **I70.72**   **Atherosclerosis of other type of bypass graft(s) of**
the extremities with rest pain
`INCLUDES`   any condition classifiable to I70.71-

I70.721   **Atherosclerosis of other type of bypass** `A`
graft(s) of the extremities with rest pain,
right leg

I70.722   **Atherosclerosis of other type of bypass** `A`
graft(s) of the extremities with rest pain,
left leg

I70.723   **Atherosclerosis of other type of bypass** `A`
graft(s) of the extremities with rest pain,
bilateral legs

I70.728   **Atherosclerosis of other type of bypass** `A`
graft(s) of the extremities with rest pain,
other extremity

✅ Additional Character Required   ✓x7ᵗʰ Placeholder Alert   Unacceptable PDx   Manifestation   Hospital Acquired Condition   `EXCLUDES 1` Not Coded Here   `EXCLUDES 2` Not Included Here

ICD-10-CM 2016   631

I70.729   **Atherosclerosis of other type of bypass graft(s) of the extremities with rest pain, unspecified extremity** A

√6th   **I70.73**   **Atherosclerosis of other type of bypass graft(s) of the right leg with ulceration**
INCLUDES   any condition classifiable to I70.711 and I70.721
Use additional code to identify severity of ulcer (L97.-)

> **CC Excl: For CC codes in subcategory I70.73, unless otherwise noted:** I70.231-I70.25, L44.8-L45, L94.2, L94.4, L97.101-L97.929, L98.411-L98.499, L98.8, L99

I70.731   **Atherosclerosis of other type of bypass graft(s) of the right leg with ulceration of thigh** PDxCC CC A

I70.732   **Atherosclerosis of other type of bypass graft(s) of the right leg with ulceration of calf** PDxCC CC A

I70.733   **Atherosclerosis of other type of bypass graft(s) of the right leg with ulceration of ankle** PDxCC CC A

I70.734   **Atherosclerosis of other type of bypass graft(s) of the right leg with ulceration of heel and midfoot** PDxCC CC A
Atherosclerosis of other type of bypass graft(s) of right leg with ulceration of plantar surface of midfoot

I70.735   **Atherosclerosis of other type of bypass graft(s) of the right leg with ulceration of other part of foot** A
Atherosclerosis of other type of bypass graft(s) of right leg with ulceration of toe

I70.738   **Atherosclerosis of other type of bypass graft(s) of the right leg with ulceration of other part of lower leg** PDxCC CC A

I70.739   **Atherosclerosis of other type of bypass graft(s) of the right leg with ulceration of unspecified site** PDxCC CC A

√6th   **I70.74**   **Atherosclerosis of other type of bypass graft(s) of the left leg with ulceration**
INCLUDES   any condition classifiable to I70.712 and I70.722
Use additional code to identify severity of ulcer (L97.-)

I70.741   **Atherosclerosis of other type of bypass graft(s) of the left leg with ulceration of thigh** PDxCC CC A

I70.742   **Atherosclerosis of other type of bypass graft(s) of the left leg with ulceration of calf** PDxCC CC A

I70.743   **Atherosclerosis of other type of bypass graft(s) of the left leg with ulceration of ankle** PDxCC CC A

I70.744   **Atherosclerosis of other type of bypass raft(s) of the left leg with ulceration of heel and midfoot** PDxCC CC A
Atherosclerosis of other type of bypass graft(s) of left leg with ulceration of plantar surface of midfoot

I70.745   **Atherosclerosis of other type of bypass graft(s) of the left leg with ulceration of other part of foot** A
Atherosclerosis of other type of bypass graft(s) of left leg with ulceration of toe

I70.748   **Atherosclerosis of other type of bypass graft(s) of the left leg with ulceration of other part of lower leg** PDxCC CC A

I70.749   **Atherosclerosis of other type of bypass graft(s) of the left leg with ulceration of unspecified site** PDxCC CC A

I70.75   **Atherosclerosis of other type of bypass graft(s) of other extremity with ulceration** A
INCLUDES   any condition classifiable to I70.718 and I70.728
Use additional code to identify severity of ulcer (L98.49)

√6th   **I70.76**   **Atherosclerosis of other type of bypass graft(s) of the extremities with gangrene**
INCLUDES   any condition classifiable to I70.71-, I70.72-, I70.73-, I70.74-, I70.75
Use additional code to identify the severity of any ulcer (L97.-, L98.49-), if applicable

I70.761   **Atherosclerosis of other type of bypass graft(s) of the extremities with gangrene, right leg** PDxCC CC A
CC Excl: G89.0-G89.4, I70.261-I70.269, I96, R41.0-R41.3, R41.82, R41.9, R44.8-R44.9, R45.83-R45.84, R46.0-R46.89, R52, R68.0-R68.19, R68.81-R68.83, R68.89-R69

I70.762   **Atherosclerosis of other type of bypass graft(s) of the extremities with gangrene, left leg** PDxCC CC A
CC Excl: See code: I70.761

I70.763   **Atherosclerosis of other type of bypass graft(s) of the extremities with gangrene, bilateral legs** PDxCC CC A
CC Excl: See code: I70.761

I70.768   **Atherosclerosis of other type of bypass graft(s) of the extremities with gangrene, other extremity** PDxCC CC A
CC Excl: See code: I70.761

I70.769   **Atherosclerosis of other type of bypass graft(s) of the extremities with gangrene, unspecified extremity** PDxCC CC A
CC Excl: See code: I70.761

√6th   **I70.79**   **Other atherosclerosis of other type of bypass graft(s) of the extremities**

I70.791   **Other atherosclerosis of other type of bypass graft(s) of the extremities, right leg** A

I70.792   **Other atherosclerosis of other type of bypass graft(s) of the extremities, left leg** A

I70.793   **Other atherosclerosis of other type of bypass graft(s) of the extremities, bilateral legs** A

I70.798   **Other atherosclerosis of other type of bypass graft(s) of the extremities, other extremity** A

I70.799   **Other atherosclerosis of other type of bypass graft(s) of the extremities, unspecified extremity** A

I70.8   **Atherosclerosis of other arteries** A

√5th   **I70.9**   **Other and unspecified atherosclerosis**

I70.90   **Unspecified atherosclerosis** A

I70.91   **Generalized atherosclerosis** A

I70.92   **Chronic total occlusion of artery of the extremities** CC A
Complete occlusion of artery of the extremities
Total occlusion of artery of the extremities
Code first atherosclerosis of arteries of the extremities (I70.2-, I70.3-, I70.4-, I70.5-, I70.6-, I70.7-)
CC Excl: I70.92, I73.81-I77.2, I77.5-I77.6, I77.810-I77.819, I79.1-I79.8, M31.8-M31.9

√4th   **I71**   **Aortic aneurysm and dissection**
EXCLUDES 1   aortic ectasia (I77.81-)
syphilitic aortic aneurysm (A52.01)
traumatic aortic aneurysm (S25.09, S35.09)

> **CC Excl: For MCC codes in category I71, unless otherwise noted:** E08.51-E08.59, E08.618-E08.638, E08.649-E08.8, E09.51-E09.59, E09.618-E09.638, E09.649-E09.8, E10.51-E10.59, E10.618-E10.638, E10.649, E10.69-E10.8, E11.51-E11.59, E11.618-E11.638, E11.649, E11.69-E11.8, E13.51-E13.59, E13.618-E13.638, E13.649-E13.8, I71.00-I71.9, I77.810-I77.819, I79.0, I87.8-I87.9, I99.8-I99.9

√5th   **I71.0**   **Dissection of aorta**

I71.00   **Dissection of unspecified site of aorta** MCC

I71.01   **Dissection of thoracic aorta** MCC

I71.02   **Dissection of abdominal aorta** MCC

I71.03   **Dissection of thoracoabdominal aorta** MCC

I71.1   **Thoracic aortic aneurysm, ruptured** MCC

I71.2   **Thoracic aortic aneurysm, without rupture**

I71.3   **Abdominal aortic aneurysm, ruptured** MCC

I71.4   **Abdominal aortic aneurysm, without rupture**

I71.5   **Thoracoabdominal aortic aneurysm, ruptured** MCC

I71.6   **Thoracoabdominal aortic aneurysm, without rupture**

N Newborn: 0   P Pediatric: 0-17   M Maternity: 12-55   A Adult: 15-124   MCC Major CC Condition   PDxMCC PDx acts as own MCC   CC CC Condition   PDxCC PDx acts as own CC

632   ICD-10-CM 2016

I71.8 Aortic aneurysm of unspecified site, ruptured   MCC
Rupture of aorta NOS

I71.9 Aortic aneurysm of unspecified site, without rupture
Aneurysm of aorta
Dilatation of aorta
Hyaline necrosis of aorta

√4th **I72 Other aneurysm**
INCLUDES   aneurysm (cirsoid) (false) (ruptured)
EXCLUDES 2   acquired aneurysm (I77.0)
aneurysm (of) aorta (I71.-)
aneurysm (of) arteriovenous NOS (Q27.3-)
carotid artery dissection (I77.71)
cerebral (nonruptured) aneurysm (I67.1)
coronary aneurysm (I25.4)
coronary artery dissection (I25.42)
dissection of artery NEC (I77.79)
heart aneurysm (I25.3)
iliac artery dissection (I77.72)
pulmonary artery aneurysm (I28.1)
renal artery dissection (I77.73)
retinal aneurysm (H35.0)
ruptured cerebral aneurysm (I60.7)
varicose aneurysm (I77.0)
vertebral artery dissection (I77.74)

I72.0 Aneurysm of carotid artery
Aneurysm of common carotid artery
Aneurysm of external carotid artery
Aneurysm of internal carotid artery, extracranial portion
EXCLUDES 1   aneurysm of internal carotid artery, intracranial portion (I67.1)
aneurysm of internal carotid artery NOS (I67.1)

I72.1 Aneurysm of artery of upper extremity

I72.2 Aneurysm of renal artery

I72.3 Aneurysm of iliac artery

I72.4 Aneurysm of artery of lower extremity

I72.8 Aneurysm of other specified arteries

I72.9 Aneurysm of unspecified site

√4th **I73 Other peripheral vascular diseases**
EXCLUDES 2   chilblains (T69.1)
frostbite (T33- T34)
immersion hand or foot (T69.0-)
spasm of cerebral artery (G45.9)

√5th **I73.0 Raynaud's syndrome**
Raynaud's disease
Raynaud's phenomenon (secondary)

I73.00 Raynaud's syndrome without gangrene

I73.01 Raynaud's syndrome with gangrene   PDxCC   CC
CC Excl: G89.0-G89.4, I70.261-I70.269, I96, R41.0-R41.3, R41.82, R41.9, R44.8-R44.9, R45.83-R45.84, R46.0-R46.89, R52, R68.0-R68.19, R68.81-R68.83, R68.89-R69

I73.1 Thromboangiitis obliterans [Buerger's disease]

√5th **I73.8 Other specified peripheral vascular diseases**
EXCLUDES 1   diabetic (peripheral) angiopathy (E08-E13 with .51-.52)

I73.81 Erythromelalgia

I73.89 Other specified peripheral vascular diseases
Acrocyanosis
Erythrocyanosis
Simple acroparesthesia [Schultze's type]
Vasomotor acroparesthesia [Nothnagel's type]

I73.9 Peripheral vascular disease, unspecified
Intermittent claudication
Peripheral angiopathy NOS
Spasm of artery
EXCLUDES 1   atherosclerosis of the extremities (I70.2--I70.7-)

√4th **I74 Arterial embolism and thrombosis**
Embolic infarction
Embolic occlusion
Thrombotic infarction
Thrombotic occlusion
Code first:
embolism and thrombosis complicating abortion or ectopic or molar pregnancy (O00-O07, O08.2)
embolism and thrombosis complicating pregnancy, childbirth and the puerperium (O88.-)
EXCLUDES 2   atheroembolism (I75.-)
basilar embolism and thrombosis (I63.0-I63.2, I65.1)
carotid embolism and thrombosis (I63.0-I63.2, I65.2)
cerebral embolism and thrombosis (I63.3-I63.5, I66-)
coronary embolism and thrombosis (I21-I25)
mesenteric embolism and thrombosis (K55.0)
ophthalmic embolism and thrombosis (H34.-)
precerebral embolism and thrombosis NOS (I63.0-I63.2, I65.9)
pulmonary embolism and thrombosis (I26.-)
renal embolism and thrombosis (N28.0)
retinal embolism and thrombosis (H34.-)
septic embolism and thrombosis (I76)
vertebral embolism and thrombosis (I63.0-I63.2, I65.0)

√5th **I74.0 Embolism and thrombosis of abdominal aorta**

I74.01 Saddle embolus of abdominal aorta   MCC
CC Excl: I26.01-I26.99, I27.82, I74.01-I74.10, I74.19, I87.8-I87.9, I99.8-I99.9

I74.09 Other arterial embolism and thrombosis of abdominal aorta   CC
Aortic bifurcation syndrome   Leriche's syndrome
Aortoiliac obstruction
CC Excl: See code: I74.01

√5th **I74.1 Embolism and thrombosis of other and unspecified parts of aorta**

I74.10 Embolism and thrombosis of unspecified parts of aorta   CC
CC Excl: See code: I74.01

I74.11 Embolism and thrombosis of thoracic aorta   CC
CC Excl: E08.51-E08.59, E08.618-E08.638, E08.649-E08.8, E09.51-E09.59, E09.618-E09.638, E09.649-E09.8, E10.51-E10.59, E10.618-E10.638, E10.649, E10.69-E10.8, E11.51-E11.59, E11.618-E11.638, E11.649, E11.69-E11.8, E13.51-E13.59, E13.618-E13.638, E13.649-E13.8, I74.11, I74.8-I74.9, I76, I87.8-I87.9, I99.8-I99.9

I74.19 Embolism and thrombosis of other parts of aorta   CC
CC Excl: I26.01-I26.99, I27.82, I74.01-I74.10, I74.19, I87.8-I87.9, I99.8-I99.9

I74.2 Embolism and thrombosis of arteries of the upper extremities   CC
CC Excl: E08.51-E08.59, E08.618-E08.638, E08.649-E08.8, E09.51-E09.59, E09.618-E09.638, E09.649-E09.8, E10.51-E10.59, E10.618-E10.638, E10.649, E10.69-E10.8, E11.51-E11.59, E11.618-E11.638, E11.649, E11.69-E11.8, E13.51-E13.59, E13.618-E13.638, E13.649-E13.8, I74.2, I74.8-I74.9, I76, I87.8-I87.9, I99.8-I99.9

I74.3 Embolism and thrombosis of arteries of the lower extremities   CC
CC Excl: E08.51-E08.59, E08.618-E08.638, E08.649-E08.8, E09.51-E09.59, E09.618-E09.638, E09.649-E09.8, E10.51-E10.59, E10.618-E10.638, E10.649, E10.69-E10.8, E11.51-E11.59, E11.618-E11.638, E11.649, E11.69-E11.8, E13.51-E13.59, E13.618-E13.638, E13.649-E13.8, I74.3-I74.4, I74.8-I74.9, I76, I87.8-I87.9, I99.8-I99.9

I74.4 Embolism and thrombosis of arteries of extremities, unspecified   CC
Peripheral arterial embolism NOS
CC Excl: See code: I74.3

I74.5 Embolism and thrombosis of iliac artery   CC
CC Excl: E08.51-E08.59, E08.618-E08.638, E08.649-E08.8, E09.51-E09.59, E09.618-E09.638, E09.649-E09.8, E10.51-E10.59, E10.618-E10.638, E10.649, E10.69-E10.8, E11.51-E11.59, E11.618-E11.638, E11.649, E11.69-E11.8, E13.51-E13.59, E13.618-E13.638, E13.649-E13.8, I74.5-I74.9, I76, I87.8-I87.9, I99.8-I99.9

I74.8 Embolism and thrombosis of other arteries   CC
CC Excl: E08.51-E08.59, E08.618-E08.638, E08.649-E08.8, E09.51-E09.59, E09.618-E09.638, E09.649-E09.8, E10.51-E10.59, E10.618-E10.638, E10.649, E10.69-E10.8, E11.51-E11.59, E11.618-E11.638, E11.649, E11.69-E11.8, E13.51-E13.59, E13.618-E13.638, E13.649-E13.8, I74.8-I74.9, I76, I87.8-I87.9, I99.8-I99.9

I74.9 Embolism and thrombosis of unspecified artery   CC
CC Excl: See code: I74.8

✔ Additional Character Required   ✔x7th Placeholder Alert   Unacceptable PDx   Manifestation   Hospital Acquired Condition   EXCLUDES 1 Not Coded Here   EXCLUDES 2 Not Included Here

ICD-10-CM 2016   633

Chapter 9. Diseases of the Circulatory System

✓4ᵗʰ I75   Atheroembolism
Atherothrombotic microembolism
Cholesterol embolism

✓5ᵗʰ I75.0   Atheroembolism of extremities

✓6ᵗʰ I75.01   Atheroembolism of upper extremity

> **CC Excl:** For CC codes in subcategory I75.01, unless otherwise noted: E08.51-E08.59, E08.618-E08.638, E08.649-E08.8, E09.51-E09.59, E09.618-E09.638, E09.649-E09.8, E10.51-E10.59, E10.618-E10.638, E10.649, E10.69-E10.8, E11.51-E11.59, E11.618-E11.638, E11.649, E11.69-E11.8, E13.51-E13.59, E13.618-E13.638, E13.649-E13.8, I74.8-I75.019, I76, I87.8-I87.9, I99.8-I99.9

     I75.011   Atheroembolism of right upper extremity   CC

     I75.012   Atheroembolism of left upper extremity   CC

     I75.013   Atheroembolism of bilateral upper extremities   CC

     I75.019   Atheroembolism of unspecified upper extremity   CC

✓6ᵗʰ I75.02   Atheroembolism of lower extremity

> **CC Excl:** For CC codes in subcategory I75.02, unless otherwise noted: E08.51-E08.59, E08.618-E08.638, E08.649-E08.8, E09.51-E09.59, E09.618-E09.638, E09.649-E09.8, E10.51-E10.59, E10.618-E10.638, E10.649, E10.69-E10.8, E11.51-E11.59, E11.618-E11.638, E11.649, E11.69-E11.8, E13.51-E13.59, E13.618-E13.638, E13.649-E13.8, I74.8-I74.9, I75.021-I75.029, I76, I87.8-I87.9, I99.8-I99.9

     I75.021   Atheroembolism of right lower extremity   CC

     I75.022   Atheroembolism of left lower extremity   CC

     I75.023   Atheroembolism of bilateral lower extremities   CC

     I75.029   Atheroembolism of unspecified lower extremity   CC

✓5ᵗʰ I75.8   Atheroembolism of other sites

     I75.81   Atheroembolism of kidney   CC
Use additional code for any associated acute kidney failure and chronic kidney disease (N17.-, N18.-)
> **CC Excl:** E08.51-E08.59, E08.618-E08.638, E08.649-E08.8, E09.51-E09.59, E09.618-E09.638, E09.649-E09.8, E10.51-E10.59, E10.618-E10.638, E10.649, E10.69-E10.8, E11.51-E11.59, E11.618-E11.638, E11.649, E11.69-E11.8, E13.51-E13.59, E13.618-E13.638, E13.649-E13.8, I74.8-I74.9, I75.81, I76, I87.8-I87.9, I99.8-I99.9

     I75.89   Atheroembolism of other site   CC
> **CC Excl:** E08.51-E08.59, E08.618-E08.638, E08.649-E08.8, E09.51-E09.59, E09.618-E09.638, E09.649-E09.8, E10.51-E10.59, E10.618-E10.638, E10.649, E10.69-E10.8, E11.51-E11.59, E11.618-E11.638, E11.649, E11.69-E11.8, E13.51-E13.59, E13.618-E13.638, E13.649-E13.8, I74.8-I74.9, I75.89-I76, I87.8-I87.9, I99.8-I99.9

I76   Septic arterial embolism   CC
Code first underlying infection, such as:
   infective endocarditis (I33.0)
   lung abscess (J85.-)
Use additional code to identify the site of the embolism (I74.-)
> *EXCLUDES 2*   septic pulmonary embolism (I26.01, I26.90)
CC Excl: See code: I74.8

✓4ᵗʰ I77   Other disorders of arteries and arterioles
> *EXCLUDES 2*   collagen (vascular) diseases (M30-M36)
>   hypersensitivity angiitis (M31.0)
>   pulmonary artery (I28.-)

I77.0   Arteriovenous fistula, acquired
Aneurysmal varix
Arteriovenous aneurysm, acquired
> *EXCLUDES 1*   arteriovenous aneurysm NOS (Q27.3-)
>   presence of arteriovenous shunt (fistula) for dialysis (Z99.2)
>   traumatic—see injury of blood vessel by body region
> *EXCLUDES 2*   cerebral (I67.1)
>   coronary (I25.4)

I77.1   Stricture of artery
Narrowing of artery

I77.2   Rupture of artery   CC
Erosion of artery
Fistula of artery
Ulcer of artery
> *EXCLUDES 1*   traumatic rupture of artery—see injury of blood vessel by body region
CC Excl: I25.42, I67.0, I77.2, I77.72-I77.79

I77.3   Arterial fibromuscular dysplasia
Fibromuscular hyperplasia (of) carotid artery
Fibromuscular hyperplasia (of) renal artery

I77.4   Celiac artery compression syndrome   CC
CC Excl: I77.4

I77.5   Necrosis of artery   CC
CC Excl: I77.5, M31.8-M31.9

I77.6   Arteritis, unspecified
Aortitis NOS
Endarteritis NOS
> *EXCLUDES 1*   arteritis or endarteritis:
>   aortic arch (M31.4)
>   cerebral NEC (I67.7)
>   coronary (I25.89)
>   deformans (I70.-)
>   giant cell (M31.5., M31.6)
>   obliterans (I70.-)
>   senile (I70.-)

✓5ᵗʰ I77.7   Other arterial dissection
> *EXCLUDES 2*   dissection of aorta (I71.0-)
>   dissection of coronary artery (I25.42)

> **CC Excl:** For MCC codes in subcategory I77.7, unless otherwise noted: I77.2-I77.3, I77.5-I77.6, I77.89-I77.9, M31.8-M31.9

     I77.71   Dissection of carotid artery   MCC

     I77.72   Dissection of iliac artery   MCC

     I77.73   Dissection of renal artery   MCC

     I77.74   Dissection of vertebral artery   MCC

     I77.79   Dissection of other artery   MCC

✓5ᵗʰ I77.8   Other specified disorders of arteries and arterioles

✓6ᵗʰ I77.81   Aortic ectasia
Ectasis aorta
> *EXCLUDES 1*   aortic aneurysm and dissection (I71.0-)

     I77.810   Thoracic aortic ectasia

     I77.811   Abdominal aortic ectasia

     I77.812   Thoracoabdominal aortic ectasia

     I77.819   Aortic ectasia, unspecified site

     I77.89   Other specified disorders of arteries and arterioles

I77.9   Disorder of arteries and arterioles, unspecified

✓4ᵗʰ I78   Diseases of capillaries

I78.0   Hereditary hemorrhagic telangiectasia
Rendu-Osler-Weber disease

I78.1   Nevus, non-neoplastic
Araneus nevus
Senile nevus
Spider nevus
Stellar nevus
> *EXCLUDES 1*   nevus NOS (D22.-)
>   vascular NOS (Q82.5)
> *EXCLUDES 2*   blue nevus (D22.-)
>   flammeus nevus (Q82.5)
>   hairy nevus (D22.-)
>   melanocytic nevus (D22.-)
>   pigmented nevus (D22.-)
>   portwine nevus (Q82.5)
>   sanguineous nevus (Q82.5)
>   strawberry nevus (Q82.5)
>   verrucous nevus (Q82.5)

I78.8   Other diseases of capillaries

I78.9   Disease of capillaries, unspecified

✓4ᵗʰ I79   Disorders of arteries, arterioles and capillaries in diseases classified elsewhere

I79.0   Aneurysm of aorta in diseases classified elsewhere
Code first underlying disease
> *EXCLUDES 1*   syphilitic aneurysm (A52.01)

I79.1   Aortitis in diseases classified elsewhere
Code first underlying disease
> *EXCLUDES 1*   syphilitic aortitis (A52.02)

Ⓝ Newborn: 0   Ⓟ Pediatric: 0-17   Ⓜ Maternity: 12-55   Ⓐ Adult: 15-124   **MCC** Major CC Condition   **PDxMCC** PDx acts as own MCC   **CC** CC Condition   **PDxCC** PDx acts as own CC

I79.8 **Other disorders of arteries, arterioles and capillaries in diseases classified elsewhere**

Code first underlying disease, such as:
amyloidosis (E85.-)

EXCLUDES 1   *diabetic (peripheral) angiopathy (E08-E13 with .51-.52)*
syphilitic endarteritis (A52.09)
tuberculous endarteritis (A18.89)

Diseases of veins, lymphatic vessels and lymph nodes, not elsewhere classified (I80-I89)

✓4th **I80**   **Phlebitis and thrombophlebitis**

INCLUDES   endophlebitis
inflammation, vein
periphlebitis
suppurative phlebitis

Code first:
phlebitis and thrombophlebitis complicating abortion, ectopic or molar pregnancy (O00-O07, O08.7)
phlebitis and thrombophlebitis complicating pregnancy, childbirth and the puerperium (O22.-, O87.-)

EXCLUDES 1   *venous embolism and thrombosis of lower extremities ((I82.4-, I82.5-, I82.81-)*

CC Excl: For CC codes in category I80, unless otherwise noted:
E08.51-E08.59, E08.618-E08.638, E08.649-E08.8, E09.51-E09.59,
E09.618-E09.638, E09.649-E09.8, E10.51-E10.59, E10.618-E10.638,
E10.649, E10.69-E10.8, E11.51-E11.59, E11.618-E11.638, E11.649,
E11.69-E11.8, E13.51-E13.59, E13.618-E13.638, E13.649-E13.8, I80.00-
I80.9, I87.8-I87.9, I99.8-I99.9

✓5th **I80.0**   **Phlebitis and thrombophlebitis of superficial vessels of lower extremities**
Phlebitis and thrombophlebitis of femoropopliteal vein

I80.00   **Phlebitis and thrombophlebitis of superficial vessels of unspecified lower extremity**

I80.01   **Phlebitis and thrombophlebitis of superficial vessels of right lower extremity**

I80.02   **Phlebitis and thrombophlebitis of superficial vessels of left lower extremity**

I80.03   **Phlebitis and thrombophlebitis of superficial vessels of lower extremities, bilateral**

✓5th **I80.1**   **Phlebitis and thrombophlebitis of femoral vein**

I80.10   **Phlebitis and thrombophlebitis of unspecified femoral vein**   CC

I80.11   **Phlebitis and thrombophlebitis of right femoral vein**   CC

I80.12   **Phlebitis and thrombophlebitis of left femoral vein**   CC

I80.13   **Phlebitis and thrombophlebitis of femoral vein, bilateral**   CC

✓5th **I80.2**   **Phlebitis and thrombophlebitis of other and unspecified deep vessels of lower extremities**

✓6th **I80.20**   **Phlebitis and thrombophlebitis of unspecified deep vessels of lower extremities**

I80.201   **Phlebitis and thrombophlebitis of unspecified deep vessels of right lower extremity**   CC

I80.202   **Phlebitis and thrombophlebitis of unspecified deep vessels of left lower extremity**   CC

I80.203   **Phlebitis and thrombophlebitis of unspecified deep vessels of lower extremities, bilateral**   CC

I80.209   **Phlebitis and thrombophlebitis of unspecified deep vessels of unspecified lower extremity**   CC

✓6th **I80.21**   **Phlebitis and thrombophlebitis of iliac vein**

I80.211   **Phlebitis and thrombophlebitis of right iliac vein**   CC

I80.212   **Phlebitis and thrombophlebitis of left iliac vein**   CC

I80.213   **Phlebitis and thrombophlebitis of iliac vein, bilateral**   CC

I80.219   **Phlebitis and thrombophlebitis of unspecified iliac vein**   CC

✓6th **I80.22**   **Phlebitis and thrombophlebitis of popliteal vein**

I80.221   **Phlebitis and thrombophlebitis of right popliteal vein**   CC

I80.222   **Phlebitis and thrombophlebitis of left popliteal vein**   CC

I80.223   **Phlebitis and thrombophlebitis of popliteal vein, bilateral**   CC

I80.229   **Phlebitis and thrombophlebitis of unspecified popliteal vein**   CC

✓6th **I80.23**   **Phlebitis and thrombophlebitis of tibial vein**

I80.231   **Phlebitis and thrombophlebitis of right tibial vein**   CC

I80.232   **Phlebitis and thrombophlebitis of left tibial vein**   CC

I80.233   **Phlebitis and thrombophlebitis of tibial vein, bilateral**   CC

I80.239   **Phlebitis and thrombophlebitis of unspecified tibial vein**   CC

✓6th **I80.29**   **Phlebitis and thrombophlebitis of other deep vessels of lower extremities**

I80.291   **Phlebitis and thrombophlebitis of other deep vessels of right lower extremity**   CC

I80.292   **Phlebitis and thrombophlebitis of other deep vessels of left lower extremity**   CC

I80.293   **Phlebitis and thrombophlebitis of other deep vessels of lower extremity, bilateral**   CC

I80.299   **Phlebitis and thrombophlebitis of other deep vessels of unspecified lower extremity**   CC

I80.3   **Phlebitis and thrombophlebitis of lower extremities, unspecified**

I80.8   **Phlebitis and thrombophlebitis of other sites**

I80.9   **Phlebitis and thrombophlebitis of unspecified site**

I81   **Portal vein thrombosis**   MCC
Portal (vein) obstruction
EXCLUDES 2   *hepatic vein thrombosis (I82.0)*
phlebitis of portal vein (K75.1)
CC Excl: E08.51-E08.59, E08.618-E08.638, E08.649-E08.8, E09.51-E09.59,
E09.618-E09.638, E09.649-E09.8, E10.51-E10.59, E10.618-E10.638, E10.649,
E10.69-E10.8, E11.51-E11.59, E11.618-E11.638, E11.649, E11.69-E11.8,
E13.51-E13.59, E13.618-E13.638, E13.649-E13.8, I81, I82.210-I82.211,
I82.290-I82.291, I82.401-I82.91, I87.8-I87.9, I99.8-I99.9

✓4th **I82**   **Other venous embolism and thrombosis**
Code first venous embolism and thrombosis complicating:
abortion, ectopic or molar pregnancy (O00-O07, O08.7)
pregnancy, childbirth and the puerperium (O22.-, O87.-)
EXCLUDES 2   *venous embolism and thrombosis (of):*
cerebral (I63.6, I67.6)
coronary (I21-I25)
intracranial and intraspinal, septic or NOS (G08)
intracranial, nonpyogenic (I67.6)
intraspinal, nonpyogenic (G95.1)
mesenteric (K55.0)
portal (I81)
pulmonary (I26.-)

I82.0   **Budd-Chiari syndrome**   MCC
Hepatic vein thrombosis
CC Excl: E08.51-E08.59, E08.618-E08.638, E08.649-E08.8, E09.51-
E09.59, E09.618-E09.638, E09.649-E09.8, E10.51-E10.59, E10.618-
E10.638, E10.649, E10.69-E10.8, E11.51-E11.59, E11.618-E11.638,
E11.649, E11.69-E11.8, E13.51-E13.59, E13.618-E13.638, E13.649-
E13.8, I82.0, I82.210-I82.211, I82.290-I82.291, I82.401-I82.91, I87.8-
I87.9, I99.8-I99.9

I82.1   **Thrombophlebitis migrans**   CC
CC Excl: E08.51-E08.59, E08.618-E08.638, E08.649-E08.8, E09.51-
E09.59, E09.618-E09.638, E09.649-E09.8, E10.51-E10.59, E10.618-
E10.638, E10.649, E10.69-E10.8, E11.51-E11.59, E11.618-E11.638,
E11.649, E11.69-E11.8, E13.51-E13.59, E13.618-E13.638, E13.649-
E13.8, I82.1-I82.211, I82.290-I82.291, I82.401-I82.91, I87.8-I87.9,
I99.8-I99.9

✓ Additional Character Required   ✓x7th Placeholder Alert   Unacceptable PDx   Manifestation   Hospital Acquired Condition   EXCLUDES 1 Not Coded Here   EXCLUDES 2 Not Included Here

Chapter 9. Diseases of the Circulatory System

✓5ᵗʰ I82.2 Embolism and thrombosis of vena cava and other thoracic veins

✓6ᵗʰ I82.21 Embolism and thrombosis of superior vena cava

I82.210 Acute embolism and thrombosis of superior vena cava CC

Embolism and thrombosis of superior vena cava NOS

CC Excl: E08.51-E08.59, E08.618-E08.638, E08.649-E08.8, E09.51-E09.59, E09.618-E09.638, E09.649-E09.8, E10.51-E10.59, E10.618-E10.638, E10.649, E10.69-E10.8, E11.51-E11.59, E11.618-E11.638, E11.649, E11.69-E11.8, E13.51-E13.59, E13.618-E13.638, E13.649-E13.8, I82.210-I82.211, I82.290-I82.291, I82.401-I82.91, I87.8-I87.9, I99.8-I99.9

I82.211 Chronic embolism and thrombosis of superior vena cava CC

CC Excl: See code: I82.210

✓6ᵗʰ I82.22 Embolism and thrombosis of inferior vena cava

I82.220 Acute embolism and thrombosis of inferior vena cava MCC

Embolism and thrombosis of inferior vena cava NOS

CC Excl: E08.51-E08.59, E08.618-E08.638, E08.649-E08.8, E09.51-E09.59, E09.618-E09.638, E09.649-E09.8, E10.51-E10.59, E10.618-E10.638, E10.649, E10.69-E10.8, E11.51-E11.59, E11.618-E11.638, E11.649, E11.69-E11.8, E13.51-E13.59, E13.618-E13.638, E13.649-E13.8, I82.210-I82.291, I82.401-I82.91, I87.8-I87.9, I99.8-I99.9

I82.221 Chronic embolism and thrombosis of inferior vena cava MCC

CC Excl: See code: I82.220

✓6ᵗʰ I82.29 Embolism and thrombosis of other thoracic veins

Embolism and thrombosis of brachiocephalic (innominate) vein

I82.290 Acute embolism and thrombosis of other thoracic veins CC

CC Excl: See code: I82.210

I82.291 Chronic embolism and thrombosis of other thoracic veins CC

CC Excl: See code: I82.210

I82.3 Embolism and thrombosis of renal vein CC

CC Excl: E08.51-E08.59, E08.618-E08.638, E08.649-E08.8, E09.51-E09.59, E09.618-E09.638, E09.649-E09.8, E10.51-E10.59, E10.618-E10.638, E10.649, E10.69-E10.8, E11.51-E11.59, E11.618-E11.638, E11.649, E11.69-E11.8, E13.51-E13.59, E13.618-E13.638, E13.649-E13.8, I82.210-I82.211, I82.290-I82.91, I87.8-I87.9, I99.8-I99.9

✓5ᵗʰ I82.4 Acute embolism and thrombosis of deep veins of lower extremity

CC Excl: For CC codes in subcategory I82.4, unless otherwise noted: E08.51-E08.59, E08.618-E08.638, E08.649-E08.8, E09.51-E09.59, E09.618-E09.638, E09.649-E09.8, E10.51-E10.59, E10.618-E10.638, E10.649, E10.69-E10.8, E11.51-E11.59, E11.618-E11.638, E11.649, E11.69-E11.8, E13.51-E13.59, E13.618-E13.638, E13.649-E13.8, I82.210-I82.211, I82.290-I82.291, I82.401-I82.91, I87.8-I87.9, I99.8-I99.9

✓6ᵗʰ I82.40 Acute embolism and thrombosis of unspecified deep veins of lower extremity

Deep vein thrombosis NOS
DVT NOS

EXCLUDES 1   acute embolism and thrombosis of unspecified deep veins of distal lower extremity (I82.4Z-)
acute embolism and thrombosis of unspecified deep veins of proximal lower extremity (I82.4Y-)

[3] I82.401 Acute embolism and thrombosis of unspecified deep veins of right lower extremity CC

[3] I82.402 Acute embolism and thrombosis of unspecified deep veins of left lower extremity CC

[3] I82.403 Acute embolism and thrombosis of unspecified deep veins of lower extremity, bilateral CC

[3] I82.409 Acute embolism and thrombosis of unspecified deep veins of unspecified lower extremity CC

✓6ᵗʰ I82.41 Acute embolism and thrombosis of femoral vein

[3] I82.411 Acute embolism and thrombosis of right femoral vein CC

[3] I82.412 Acute embolism and thrombosis of left femoral vein CC

[3] I82.413 Acute embolism and thrombosis of femoral vein, bilateral CC

[3] I82.419 Acute embolism and thrombosis of unspecified femoral vein CC

✓6ᵗʰ I82.42 Acute embolism and thrombosis of iliac vein

[3] I82.421 Acute embolism and thrombosis of right iliac vein CC

[3] I82.422 Acute embolism and thrombosis of left iliac vein CC

[3] I82.423 Acute embolism and thrombosis of iliac vein, bilateral CC

[3] I82.429 Acute embolism and thrombosis of unspecified iliac vein CC

✓6ᵗʰ I82.43 Acute embolism and thrombosis of popliteal vein

[3] I82.431 Acute embolism and thrombosis of right popliteal vein CC

[3] I82.432 Acute embolism and thrombosis of left popliteal vein CC

[3] I82.433 Acute embolism and thrombosis of popliteal vein, bilateral CC

[3] I82.439 Acute embolism and thrombosis of unspecified popliteal vein CC

✓6ᵗʰ I82.44 Acute embolism and thrombosis of tibial vein

[3] I82.441 Acute embolism and thrombosis of right tibial vein CC

[3] I82.442 Acute embolism and thrombosis of left tibial vein CC

[3] I82.443 Acute embolism and thrombosis of tibial vein, bilateral CC

[3] I82.449 Acute embolism and thrombosis of unspecified tibial vein CC

✓6ᵗʰ I82.49 Acute embolism and thrombosis of other specified deep vein of lower extremity

[3] I82.491 Acute embolism and thrombosis of other specified deep vein of right lower extremity CC

[3] I82.492 Acute embolism and thrombosis of other specified deep vein of left lower extremity CC

[3] I82.493 Acute embolism and thrombosis of other specified deep vein of lower extremity, bilateral CC

[3] I82.499 Acute embolism and thrombosis of other specified deep vein of unspecified lower extremity CC

✓6ᵗʰ I82.4Y Acute embolism and thrombosis of unspecified deep veins of proximal lower extremity

Acute embolism and thrombosis of deep vein of thigh NOS
Acute embolism and thrombosis of deep vein of upper leg NOS

[3] I82.4Y1 Acute embolism and thrombosis of unspecified deep veins of right proximal lower extremity CC

[3] I82.4Y2 Acute embolism and thrombosis of unspecified deep veins of left proximal lower extremity CC

[3] I82.4Y3 Acute embolism and thrombosis of unspecified deep veins of proximal lower extremity, bilateral CC

[3] I82.4Y9 Acute embolism and thrombosis of unspecified deep veins of unspecified proximal lower extremity CC

✓6ᵗʰ I82.4Z Acute embolism and thrombosis of unspecified deep veins of distal lower extremity

Acute embolism and thrombosis of deep vein of calf NOS
Acute embolism and thrombosis of deep vein of lower leg NOS

[3] I82.4Z1 Acute embolism and thrombosis of unspecified deep veins of right distal lower extremity CC

---

[3] HAC = as SDx not POA, in combination with one of the following procedure codes: ØSR[9,B]Ø[1,2,3,4,J][9,A,Z]; ØSR[9,B]Ø[7,K]Z; ØSR[A,E]Ø[Ø,1,3,J][9,A,Z]; ØSR[A,E]Ø[7,K]Z; ØSR[C,D,T,U,V,W]Ø[7,K]Z; ØSR[C,D,T,U,V,W]ØJ[9,A,Z]; ØSR[R,S]Ø[1,3,J][9,A,Z]; ØSR[R,S]Ø[7,K]Z; ØSU[9,B]ØBZ; ØSU[A,E,R,S]ØBZ.

N Newborn: 0   P Pediatric: 0-17   M Maternity: 12-55   A Adult: 15-124   MCC Major CC Condition   PDxMCC PDx acts as own MCC   CC CC Condition   PDxCC PDx acts as own CC

636   ICD-10-CM 2016

3 **I82.4Z2** **Acute embolism and thrombosis of** CC
**unspecified deep veins of left distal
lower extremity**

3 **I82.4Z3** **Acute embolism and thrombosis of** CC
**unspecified deep veins of distal lower
extremity, bilateral**

3 **I82.4Z9** **Acute embolism and thrombosis of** CC
**unspecified deep veins of unspecified
distal lower extremity**

√5th **I82.5** **Chronic embolism and thrombosis of deep veins of lower
extremity**
Use additional code, if applicable, for associated long-term
(current) use of anticoagulants (Z79.01)
EXCLUDES 1 *personal history of venous embolism and thrombosis
(Z86.718)*

**CC Excl: For CC codes in subcategory I82.5, unless
otherwise noted:** See code: I82.4

√6th **I82.50** **Chronic embolism and thrombosis of unspecified
deep veins of lower extremity**
EXCLUDES 1 *chronic embolism and thrombosis of
unspecified deep veins of distal lower
extremity (I82.5Z-)
chronic embolism and thrombosis of
unspecified deep veins of proximal lower
extremity (I82.5Y-)*

I82.501 **Chronic embolism and thrombosis of** CC
**unspecified deep veins of right lower
extremity**

I82.502 **Chronic embolism and thrombosis of** CC
**unspecified deep veins of left lower
extremity**

I82.503 **Chronic embolism and thrombosis of** CC
**unspecified deep veins of lower extremity,
bilateral**

I82.509 **Chronic embolism and thrombosis of** CC
**unspecified deep veins of unspecified
lower extremity**

√6th **I82.51** **Chronic embolism and thrombosis of femoral vein**

I82.511 **Chronic embolism and thrombosis of** CC
right femoral vein

I82.512 **Chronic embolism and thrombosis of** CC
left femoral vein

I82.513 **Chronic embolism and thrombosis of** CC
femoral vein, bilateral

I82.519 **Chronic embolism and thrombosis of** CC
unspecified femoral vein

√6th **I82.52** **Chronic embolism and thrombosis of iliac vein**

I82.521 **Chronic embolism and thrombosis of** CC
right iliac vein

I82.522 **Chronic embolism and thrombosis of** CC
left iliac vein

I82.523 **Chronic embolism and thrombosis of** CC
iliac vein, bilateral

I82.529 **Chronic embolism and thrombosis of** CC
unspecified iliac vein

√6th **I82.53** **Chronic embolism and thrombosis of popliteal vein**

I82.531 **Chronic embolism and thrombosis of** CC
right popliteal vein

I82.532 **Chronic embolism and thrombosis of** CC
left popliteal vein

I82.533 **Chronic embolism and thrombosis of** CC
popliteal vein, bilateral

I82.539 **Chronic embolism and thrombosis of** CC
unspecified popliteal vein

√6th **I82.54** **Chronic embolism and thrombosis of tibial vein**

I82.541 **Chronic embolism and thrombosis of** CC
right tibial vein

I82.542 **Chronic embolism and thrombosis of** CC
left tibial vein

I82.543 **Chronic embolism and thrombosis of** CC
tibial vein, bilateral

I82.549 **Chronic embolism and thrombosis of** CC
unspecified tibial vein

√6th **I82.59** **Chronic embolism and thrombosis of other specified
deep vein of lower extremity**

I82.591 **Chronic embolism and thrombosis of** CC
**other specified deep vein of right lower
extremity**

I82.592 **Chronic embolism and thrombosis of** CC
**other specified deep vein of left lower
extremity**

I82.593 **Chronic embolism and thrombosis of** CC
**other specified deep vein of lower
extremity, bilateral**

I82.599 **Chronic embolism and thrombosis of** CC
**other specified deep vein of unspecified
lower extremity**

√6th **I82.5Y** **Chronic embolism and thrombosis of unspecified
deep veins of proximal lower extremity**
Chronic embolism and thrombosis of deep veins of
thigh NOS
Chronic embolism and thrombosis of deep veins of
upper leg NOS

I82.5Y1 **Chronic embolism and thrombosis of** CC
**unspecified deep veins of right proximal
lower extremity**

I82.5Y2 **Chronic embolism and thrombosis of** CC
**unspecified deep veins of left proximal
lower extremity**

I82.5Y3 **Chronic embolism and thrombosis of** CC
**unspecified deep veins of proximal lower
extremity, bilateral**

I82.5Y9 **Chronic embolism and thrombosis of** CC
**unspecified deep veins of unspecified
proximal lower extremity**

√6th **I82.5Z** **Chronic embolism and thrombosis of unspecified
deep veins of distal lower extremity**
Chronic embolism and thrombosis of deep veins of
calf NOS
Chronic embolism and thrombosis of deep veins of
lower leg NOS

I82.5Z1 **Chronic embolism and thrombosis of** CC
**unspecified deep veins of right distal
lower extremity**

I82.5Z2 **Chronic embolism and thrombosis of** CC
**unspecified deep veins of left distal
lower extremity**

I82.5Z3 **Chronic embolism and thrombosis of** CC
**unspecified deep veins of distal lower
extremity, bilateral**

I82.5Z9 **Chronic embolism and thrombosis of** CC
**unspecified deep veins of unspecified
distal lower extremity**

√5th **I82.6** **Acute embolism and thrombosis of veins of upper extremity**

**CC Excl: For CC codes in subcategory I82.6, unless
otherwise noted:** See code: I82.4

√6th **I82.60** **Acute embolism and thrombosis of unspecified veins
of upper extremity**

I82.601 **Acute embolism and thrombosis of** CC
**unspecified veins of right upper
extremity**

I82.602 **Acute embolism and thrombosis of** CC
**unspecified veins of left upper
extremity**

I82.603 **Acute embolism and thrombosis of** CC
**unspecified veins of upper extremity,
bilateral**

I82.609 **Acute embolism and thrombosis of** CC
**unspecified veins of unspecified upper
extremity**

√6th **I82.61** **Acute embolism and thrombosis of superficial veins
of upper extremity**
Acute embolism and thrombosis of antecubital vein
Acute embolism and thrombosis of basilic vein
Acute embolism and thrombosis of cephalic vein

I82.611 **Acute embolism and thrombosis of** CC
**superficial veins of right upper
extremity**

I82.612 **Acute embolism and thrombosis of** CC
**superficial veins of left upper
extremity**

---

3   HAC = as SDx not POA, in combination with one of the following procedure codes: 0SR[9,B]0[1,2,3,4,J][9,A,Z]; 0SR[9,B]0[7,K]Z; 0SR[A,E]0[0,1,3,J][9,A,Z]; 0SR[A,E]0[7,K]Z;
0SR[C,D,T,U,V,W]0[7,K]Z; 0SR[C,D,T,U,V,W]0J[9,A,Z]; 0SR[R,S]0[1,3,J][9,A,Z]; 0SR[R,S]0[7,K]Z; 0SU[9,B]0BZ; 0SU[A,E,R,S]0BZ.

I82.613   **Acute embolism and thrombosis of superficial veins of upper extremity, bilateral**   CC

I82.619   **Acute embolism and thrombosis of superficial veins of unspecified upper extremity**   CC

√6ᵗʰ I82.62   **Acute embolism and thrombosis of deep veins of upper extremity**
Acute embolism and thrombosis of brachial vein
Acute embolism and thrombosis of radial vein
Acute embolism and thrombosis of ulnar vein

I82.621   **Acute embolism and thrombosis of deep veins of right upper extremity**   CC

I82.622   **Acute embolism and thrombosis of deep veins of left upper extremity**   CC

I82.623   **Acute embolism and thrombosis of deep veins of upper extremity, bilateral**   CC

I82.629   **Acute embolism and thrombosis of deep veins of unspecified upper extremity**   CC

√5ᵗʰ I82.7   **Chronic embolism and thrombosis of veins of upper extremity**
Use additional code, if applicable, for associated long-term (current) use of anticoagulants (Z79.01)
   EXCLUDES 1   *personal history of venous embolism and thrombosis (Z86.718)*

> **CC Excl:** For CC codes in subcategory I82.7, unless otherwise noted: See code: I82.4

√6ᵗʰ I82.70   **Chronic embolism and thrombosis of unspecified veins of upper extremity**

I82.701   **Chronic embolism and thrombosis of unspecified veins of right upper extremity**   CC

I82.702   **Chronic embolism and thrombosis of unspecified veins of left upper extremity**   CC

I82.703   **Chronic embolism and thrombosis of unspecified veins of upper extremity, bilateral**   CC

I82.709   **Chronic embolism and thrombosis of unspecified veins of unspecified upper extremity**   CC

√6ᵗʰ I82.71   **Chronic embolism and thrombosis of superficial veins of upper extremity**
Chronic embolism and thrombosis of antecubital vein
Chronic embolism and thrombosis of basilic vein
Chronic embolism and thrombosis of cephalic vein

I82.711   **Chronic embolism and thrombosis of superficial veins of right upper extremity**   CC

I82.712   **Chronic embolism and thrombosis of superficial veins of left upper extremity**   CC

I82.713   **Chronic embolism and thrombosis of superficial veins of upper extremity, bilateral**   CC

I82.719   **Chronic embolism and thrombosis of superficial veins of unspecified upper extremity**   CC

√6ᵗʰ I82.72   **Chronic embolism and thrombosis of deep veins of upper extremity**
Chronic embolism and thrombosis of brachial vein
Chronic embolism and thrombosis of radial vein
Chronic embolism and thrombosis of ulnar vein

I82.721   **Chronic embolism and thrombosis of deep veins of right upper extremity**   CC

I82.722   **Chronic embolism and thrombosis of deep veins of left upper extremity**   CC

I82.723   **Chronic embolism and thrombosis of deep veins of upper extremity, bilateral**   CC

I82.729   **Chronic embolism and thrombosis of deep veins of unspecified upper extremity**   CC

√5ᵗʰ I82.A   **Embolism and thrombosis of axillary vein**

> **CC Excl:** For CC codes in subcategory I82.A, unless otherwise noted: See code: I82.4

√6ᵗʰ I82.A1   **Acute embolism and thrombosis of axillary vein**

I82.A11   **Acute embolism and thrombosis of right axillary vein**   CC

I82.A12   **Acute embolism and thrombosis of left axillary vein**   CC

I82.A13   **Acute embolism and thrombosis of axillary vein, bilateral**   CC

I82.A19   **Acute embolism and thrombosis of unspecified axillary vein**   CC

√6ᵗʰ I82.A2   **Chronic embolism and thrombosis of axillary vein**

I82.A21   **Chronic embolism and thrombosis of right axillary vein**   CC

I82.A22   **Chronic embolism and thrombosis of left axillary vein**   CC

I82.A23   **Chronic embolism and thrombosis of axillary vein, bilateral**   CC

I82.A29   **Chronic embolism and thrombosis of unspecified axillary vein**   CC

√5ᵗʰ I82.B   **Embolism and thrombosis of subclavian vein**

> **CC Excl:** For CC codes in subcategory I82.B, unless otherwise noted: E08.51-E08.59, E08.618-E08.638, E08.649-E08.8, E09.51-E09.59, E09.618-E09.638, E09.649-E09.8, E10.51-E10.59, E10.618-E10.638, E10.649, E10.69-E10.8, E11.51-E11.59, E11.618-E11.638, E11.649, E11.69-E11.8, E13.51-E13.59, E13.618-E13.638, E13.649-E13.8, I82.210-I82.211, I82.290-I82.291, I82.401-I82.91, I87.8-I87.9, I99.8-I99.9

√6ᵗʰ I82.B1   **Acute embolism and thrombosis of subclavian vein**

I82.B11   **Acute embolism and thrombosis of right subclavian vein**   CC

I82.B12   **Acute embolism and thrombosis of left subclavian vein**   CC

I82.B13   **Acute embolism and thrombosis of subclavian vein, bilateral**   CC

I82.B19   **Acute embolism and thrombosis of unspecified subclavian vein**   CC

√6ᵗʰ I82.B2   **Chronic embolism and thrombosis of subclavian vein**

I82.B21   **Chronic embolism and thrombosis of right subclavian vein**   CC

I82.B22   **Chronic embolism and thrombosis of left subclavian vein**   CC

I82.B23   **Chronic embolism and thrombosis of subclavian vein, bilateral**   CC

I82.B29   **Chronic embolism and thrombosis of unspecified subclavian vein**   CC

√5ᵗʰ I82.C   **Embolism and thrombosis of internal jugular vein**

> **CC Excl:** For CC codes in subcategory I82.C, unless otherwise noted: See code: I82.B

√6ᵗʰ I82.C1   **Acute embolism and thrombosis of internal jugular vein**

I82.C11   **Acute embolism and thrombosis of right internal jugular vein**   CC

I82.C12   **Acute embolism and thrombosis of left internal jugular vein**   CC

I82.C13   **Acute embolism and thrombosis of internal jugular vein, bilateral**   CC

I82.C19   **Acute embolism and thrombosis of unspecified internal jugular vein**   CC

√6ᵗʰ I82.C2   **Chronic embolism and thrombosis of internal jugular vein**

I82.C21   **Chronic embolism and thrombosis of right internal jugular vein**   CC

I82.C22   **Chronic embolism and thrombosis of left internal jugular vein**   CC

I82.C23   **Chronic embolism and thrombosis of internal jugular vein, bilateral**   CC

I82.C29   **Chronic embolism and thrombosis of unspecified internal jugular vein**   CC

√5ᵗʰ I82.8   **Embolism and thrombosis of other specified veins**
Use additional code, if applicable, for associated long-term (current) use of anticoagulants (Z79.01)

> **CC Excl:** For CC codes in subcategory I82.8, unless otherwise noted: See code: I82.B

N Newborn: 0   P Pediatric: 0-17   M Maternity: 12-55   A Adult: 15-124   MCC Major CC Condition   PDxMCC PDx acts as own MCC   CC CC Condition   PDxCC PDx acts as own CC

638   ICD-10-CM 2016

☑6ᵗʰ I82.81 Embolism and thrombosis of superficial veins of lower extremities
    Embolism and thrombosis of saphenous vein (greater) (lesser)

      I82.811 Embolism and thrombosis of superficial veins of right lower extremities `CC`

      I82.812 Embolism and thrombosis of superficial veins of left lower extremities `CC`

      I82.813 Embolism and thrombosis of superficial veins of lower extremities, bilateral `CC`

      I82.819 Embolism and thrombosis of superficial veins of unspecified lower extremities `CC`

☑6ᵗʰ I82.89 Embolism and thrombosis of other specified veins

      I82.890 Acute embolism and thrombosis of other specified veins `CC`

      I82.891 Chronic embolism and thrombosis of other specified veins `CC`

☑5ᵗʰ I82.9 Embolism and thrombosis of unspecified vein

> **CC Excl: For CC codes in subcategory I82.9, unless otherwise noted:** See code: I82.B

      I82.90 Acute embolism and thrombosis of unspecified vein `CC`
         Embolism of vein NOS
         Thrombosis (vein) NOS

      I82.91 Chronic embolism and thrombosis of unspecified vein `CC`

☑4ᵗʰ I83 Varicose veins of lower extremities
    EXCLUDES 1 varicose veins complicating pregnancy (O22.0-)
              varicose veins complicating the puerperium (O87.4)

☑5ᵗʰ I83.0 Varicose veins of lower extremities with ulcer
    Use additional code to identify severity of ulcer (L97.-)

    ☑6ᵗʰ I83.00 Varicose veins of unspecified lower extremity with ulcer

      I83.001 Varicose veins of unspecified lower extremity with ulcer of thigh `A`

      I83.002 Varicose veins of unspecified lower extremity with ulcer of calf `A`

      I83.003 Varicose veins of unspecified lower extremity with ulcer of ankle `A`

      I83.004 Varicose veins of unspecified lower extremity with ulcer of heel and midfoot `A`
         Varicose veins of unspecified lower extremity with ulcer of plantar surface of midfoot

      I83.005 Varicose veins of unspecified lower extremity with ulcer other part of foot `A`
         Varicose veins of unspecified lower extremity with ulcer of toe

      I83.008 Varicose veins of unspecified lower extremity with ulcer other part of lower leg `A`

      I83.009 Varicose veins of unspecified lower extremity with ulcer of unspecified site `A`

    ☑6ᵗʰ I83.01 Varicose veins of right lower extremity with ulcer

      I83.011 Varicose veins of right lower extremity with ulcer of thigh `A`

      I83.012 Varicose veins of right lower extremity with ulcer of calf `A`

      I83.013 Varicose veins of right lower extremity with ulcer of ankle `A`

      I83.014 Varicose veins of right lower extremity with ulcer of heel and midfoot `A`
         Varicose veins of right lower extremity with ulcer of plantar surface of midfoot

      I83.015 Varicose veins of right lower extremity with ulcer other part of foot `A`
         Varicose veins of right lower extremity with ulcer of toe

      I83.018 Varicose veins of right lower extremity with ulcer other part of lower leg `A`

      I83.019 Varicose veins of right lower extremity with ulcer of unspecified site `A`

☑6ᵗʰ I83.02 Varicose veins of left lower extremity with ulcer

      I83.021 Varicose veins of left lower extremity with ulcer of thigh `A`

      I83.022 Varicose veins of left lower extremity with ulcer of calf `A`

      I83.023 Varicose veins of left lower extremity with ulcer of ankle `A`

      I83.024 Varicose veins of left lower extremity with ulcer of heel and midfoot `A`
         Varicose veins of left lower extremity with ulcer of plantar surface of midfoot

      I83.025 Varicose veins of left lower extremity with ulcer other part of foot `A`
         Varicose veins of left lower extremity with ulcer of toe

      I83.028 Varicose veins of left lower extremity with ulcer other part of lower leg `A`

      I83.029 Varicose veins of left lower extremity with ulcer of unspecified site `A`

☑5ᵗʰ I83.1 Varicose veins of lower extremities with inflammation
    Stasis dermatitis

      I83.10 Varicose veins of unspecified lower extremity with inflammation `A`

      I83.11 Varicose veins of right lower extremity with inflammation `A`

      I83.12 Varicose veins of left lower extremity with inflammation `A`

☑5ᵗʰ I83.2 Varicose veins of lower extremities with both ulcer and inflammation

> **CC Excl: For CC codes in subcategory I83.2, unless otherwise noted:** I83.001-I83.229, I83.90-I83.93

    Use additional code to identify severity of ulcer (L97.-)

    ☑6ᵗʰ I83.20 Varicose veins of unspecified lower extremity with both ulcer and inflammation

      I83.201 Varicose veins of unspecified lower extremity with both ulcer of thigh and inflammation `CC` `A`

      I83.202 Varicose veins of unspecified lower extremity with both ulcer of calf and inflammation `CC` `A`

      I83.203 Varicose veins of unspecified lower extremity with both ulcer of ankle and inflammation `CC` `A`

      I83.204 Varicose veins of unspecified lower extremity with both ulcer of heel and midfoot and inflammation `CC` `A`
         Varicose veins of unspecified lower extremity with both ulcer of plantar surface of midfoot and inflammation

      I83.205 Varicose veins of unspecified lower extremity with both ulcer of other part of foot and inflammation `CC` `A`
         Varicose veins of unspecified lower extremity with both ulcer of toe and inflammation

      I83.208 Varicose veins of unspecified lower extremity with both ulcer of other part of lower extremity and inflammation `CC` `A`

      I83.209 Varicose veins of unspecified lower extremity with both ulcer of unspecified site and inflammation `CC` `A`

    ☑6ᵗʰ I83.21 Varicose veins of right lower extremity with both ulcer and inflammation

      I83.211 Varicose veins of right lower extremity with both ulcer of thigh and inflammation `CC` `A`

      I83.212 Varicose veins of right lower extremity with both ulcer of calf and inflammation `CC` `A`

      I83.213 Varicose veins of right lower extremity with both ulcer of ankle and inflammation `CC` `A`

      I83.214 Varicose veins of right lower extremity with both ulcer of heel and midfoot and inflammation `CC` `A`
         Varicose veins of right lower extremity with both ulcer of plantar surface of midfoot and inflammation

---

☑ Additional Character Required   ✓x7ᵗʰ Placeholder Alert   Unacceptable PDx   Manifestation   Hospital Acquired Condition   *EXCLUDES 1* Not Coded Here   *EXCLUDES 2* Not Included Here

ICD-10-CM 2016   **639**

Chapter 9. Diseases of the Circulatory System

I83.215–I87.019

I83.215   **Varicose veins of right lower extremity with both ulcer** other **part of foot and inflammation**   `CC` `A`
> Varicose veins of right lower extremity with both ulcer of toe and inflammation

I83.218   **Varicose veins of right lower extremity with both ulcer of** other **part of lower extremity and inflammation**   `CC` `A`

I83.219   **Varicose veins of right lower extremity with both ulcer of unspecified site and inflammation**   `CC` `A`

✓6ᵗʰ **I83.22**   **Varicose veins of** left **lower extremity with both ulcer and inflammation**

I83.221   **Varicose veins of left lower extremity with both ulcer of** thigh **and inflammation**   `CC` `A`

I83.222   **Varicose veins of left lower extremity with both ulcer of** calf **and inflammation**   `CC` `A`

I83.223   **Varicose veins of left lower extremity with both ulcer of** ankle **and inflammation**   `CC` `A`

I83.224   **Varicose veins of left lower extremity with both ulcer of** heel and midfoot **and inflammation**   `CC` `A`
> Varicose veins of left lower extremity with both ulcer of plantar surface of midfoot and inflammation

I83.225   **Varicose veins of left lower extremity with both ulcer** other **part of foot and inflammation**   `CC` `A`
> Varicose veins of left lower extremity with both ulcer of toe and inflammation

I83.228   **Varicose veins of left lower extremity with both ulcer of** other **part of lower extremity and inflammation**   `CC` `A`

I83.229   **Varicose veins of left lower extremity with both ulcer of unspecified site and inflammation**   `CC` `A`

✓5ᵗʰ **I83.8**   **Varicose veins of lower extremities with** other complications

✓6ᵗʰ **I83.81**   **Varicose veins of lower extremities with** pain

I83.811   **Varicose veins of** right **lower extremities with pain**   `A`

I83.812   **Varicose veins of** left **lower extremities with pain**   `A`

I83.813   **Varicose veins of** bilateral **lower extremities with pain**   `A`

I83.819   **Varicose veins of** unspecified **lower extremities with pain**   `A`

✓6ᵗʰ **I83.89**   **Varicose veins of lower extremities with** other **complications**
> Varicose veins of lower extremities with edema
> Varicose veins of lower extremities with swelling

I83.891   **Varicose veins of** right **lower extremities with other complications**   `A`

I83.892   **Varicose veins of** left **lower extremities with other complications**   `A`

I83.893   **Varicose veins of** bilateral **lower extremities with other complications**   `A`

I83.899   **Varicose veins of** unspecified **lower extremities with other complications**   `A`

✓5ᵗʰ **I83.9**   **Asymptomatic varicose veins of lower extremities**
> Phlebectasia of lower extremities
> Varicose veins of lower extremities
> Varix of lower extremities

I83.90   **Asymptomatic varicose veins of** unspecified **lower extremity**   `A`
> Varicose veins NOS

I83.91   **Asymptomatic varicose veins of** right **lower extremity**   `A`

I83.92   **Asymptomatic varicose veins of** left **lower extremity**   `A`

I83.93   **Asymptomatic varicose veins of** bilateral **lower extremities**   `A`

✓4ᵗʰ **I85**   **Esophageal varices**
Use additional code to identify:
   alcohol abuse and dependence (F10.-)

✓5ᵗʰ **I85.0**   **Esophageal varices**
> Idiopathic esophageal varices
> Primary esophageal varices

I85.00   **Esophageal varices** without bleeding   `CC`
> Esophageal varices NOS
> **CC Excl:** E16.4, I85.00-I85.01, I85.11, I87.8-I87.9, I99.8-I99.9, K22.6, K25.0-K28.9, K29.01, K29.21, K29.31, K29.41, K29.51, K29.61, K29.71, K29.81, K29.91, K31.811, K92.0-K92.2

I85.01   **Esophageal varices** with bleeding   `MCC`
> **CC Excl:** E16.4, I85.01, I85.11, I87.8-I87.9, I99.8-I99.9, K22.10-K22.11, K22.6-K22.719, K25.0-K28.9, K29.01, K29.21, K29.31, K29.41, K29.51, K29.61, K29.71, K29.81, K29.91, K31.811, K55.21, K57.01, K57.11, K57.13, K57.21, K57.31, K57.33, K57.41, K57.51, K57.53, K57.81, K57.91, K57.93, K62.5, K92.0-K92.2

✓5ᵗʰ **I85.1**   **Secondary esophageal varices**
> Esophageal varices secondary to alcoholic liver disease
> Esophageal varices secondary to cirrhosis of liver
> Esophageal varices secondary to schistosomiasis
> Esophageal varices secondary to toxic liver disease
> Code first underlying disease

I85.10   **Secondary esophageal varices** without bleeding   `CC`
> **CC Excl:** E16.4, I85.00-I85.11, I87.8-I87.9, I99.8-I99.9, K22.6, K25.0-K28.9, K29.01, K29.21, K29.31, K29.41, K29.51, K29.61, K29.71, K29.81, K29.91, K31.811, K92.0-K92.2

I85.11   **Secondary esophageal varices** with bleeding   `MCC`
> **CC Excl:** I85.01, I85.11, I87.8-I87.9, I99.8-I99.9

✓4ᵗʰ **I86**   **Varicose veins of other sites**
> `EXCLUDES 1`   varicose veins of unspecified site (I83.9-)
> `EXCLUDES 2`   retinal varices (H35.0-)

I86.0   **Sublingual** varices

I86.1   **Scrotal** varices   ♂
> Varicocele

I86.2   **Pelvic** varices

I86.3   **Vulval** varices   ♀
> `EXCLUDES 1`   vulval varices complicating childbirth and the puerperium (O87.8)
>   vulval varices complicating pregnancy (O22.1-)

I86.4   **Gastric** varices

I86.8   **Varicose veins of** other specified **sites**   `A`
> Varicose ulcer of nasal septum

✓4ᵗʰ **I87**   **Other disorders of veins**

✓5ᵗʰ **I87.0**   **Postthrombotic syndrome**
> Chronic venous hypertension due to deep vein thrombosis
> Postphlebitic syndrome
> `EXCLUDES 1`   chronic venous hypertension without deep vein thrombosis (I87.3-)

> **CC Excl: For CC codes in subcategory I87.0, unless otherwise noted:** I80.00-I80.9

✓6ᵗʰ **I87.00**   **Postthrombotic syndrome** without complications
> Asymptomatic postthrombotic syndrome

I87.001   **Postthrombotic syndrome without complications of** right lower **extremity**

I87.002   **Postthrombotic syndrome without complications of** left lower **extremity**

I87.003   **Postthrombotic syndrome without complications of** bilateral lower **extremity**

I87.009   **Postthrombotic syndrome without complications of** unspecified **extremity**
> Postthrombotic syndrome NOS

✓6ᵗʰ **I87.01**   **Postthrombotic syndrome with** ulcer
> Use additional code to specify site and severity of ulcer (L97.-)

I87.011   **Postthrombotic syndrome with ulcer of** right lower **extremity**   `CC`

I87.012   **Postthrombotic syndrome with ulcer of** left lower **extremity**   `CC`

I87.013   **Postthrombotic syndrome with ulcer of** bilateral lower **extremity**   `CC`

I87.019   **Postthrombotic syndrome with ulcer of** unspecified lower **extremity**   `CC`

`N` Newborn: 0   `P` Pediatric: 0-17   `M` Maternity: 12-55   `A` Adult: 15-124   `MCC` Major CC Condition   `PDxMCC` PDx acts as own MCC   `CC` CC Condition   `PDxCC` PDx acts as own CC

640   ICD-10-CM 2016

✓6ᵗʰ I87.02 Postthrombotic syndrome with inflammation

I87.021   Postthrombotic syndrome with inflammation of right lower extremity

I87.022   Postthrombotic syndrome with inflammation of left lower extremity

I87.023   Postthrombotic syndrome with inflammation of bilateral lower extremity

I87.029   Postthrombotic syndrome with inflammation of unspecified lower extremity

✓6ᵗʰ I87.03 Postthrombotic syndrome with ulcer and inflammation

Use additional code to specify site and severity of ulcer (L97.-)

I87.031   Postthrombotic syndrome with ulcer and inflammation of right lower extremity   CC

I87.032   Postthrombotic syndrome with ulcer and inflammation of left lower extremity   CC

I87.033   Postthrombotic syndrome with ulcer and inflammation of bilateral lower extremity   CC

I87.039   Postthrombotic syndrome with ulcer and inflammation of unspecified lower extremity   CC

✓6ᵗʰ I87.09 Postthrombotic syndrome with other complications

I87.091   Postthrombotic syndrome with other complications of right lower extremity

I87.092   Postthrombotic syndrome with other complications of left lower extremity

I87.093   Postthrombotic syndrome with other complications of bilateral lower extremity

I87.099   Postthrombotic syndrome with other complications of unspecified lower extremity

I87.1 Compression of vein   CC

Stricture of vein

Vena cava syndrome (inferior) (superior)

EXCLUDES 2   compression of pulmonary vein (I28.8)

CC Excl: I87.1

I87.2 Venous insufficiency (chronic) (peripheral)

✓5ᵗʰ I87.3 Chronic venous hypertension (idiopathic)

Stasis edema

EXCLUDES 1   chronic venous hypertension due to deep vein thrombosis (I87.0-)

varicose veins of lower extremities (I83.-)

CC Excl: For CC codes in subcategory I87.3, unless otherwise noted: I83.001-I83.229, I83.90-I83.93, I87.2, I87.8-I87.9, I99.8-I99.9

✓6ᵗʰ I87.30 Chronic venous hypertension (idiopathic) without complications

Asymptomatic chronic venous hypertension (idiopathic)

I87.301   Chronic venous hypertension (idiopathic) without complications of right lower extremity

I87.302   Chronic venous hypertension (idiopathic) without complications of left lower extremity

I87.303   Chronic venous hypertension (idiopathic) without complications of bilateral lower extremity

I87.309   Chronic venous hypertension (idiopathic) without complications of unspecified lower extremity

Chronic venous hypertension NOS

✓6ᵗʰ I87.31 Chronic venous hypertension (idiopathic) with ulcer

Use additional code to specify site and severity of ulcer (L97.-)

I87.311   Chronic venous hypertension (idiopathic) with ulcer of right lower extremity   CC

I87.312   Chronic venous hypertension (idiopathic) with ulcer of left lower extremity   CC

I87.313   Chronic venous hypertension (idiopathic) with ulcer of bilateral lower extremity   CC

I87.319   Chronic venous hypertension (idiopathic) with ulcer of unspecified lower extremity   CC

✓6ᵗʰ I87.32 Chronic venous hypertension (idiopathic) with inflammation

I87.321   Chronic venous hypertension (idiopathic) with inflammation of right lower extremity

I87.322   Chronic venous hypertension (idiopathic) with inflammation of left lower extremity

I87.323   Chronic venous hypertension (idiopathic) with inflammation of bilateral lower extremity

I87.329   Chronic venous hypertension (idiopathic) with inflammation of unspecified lower extremity

✓6ᵗʰ I87.33 Chronic venous hypertension (idiopathic) with ulcer and inflammation

Use additional code to specify site and severity of ulcer (L97.-)

I87.331   Chronic venous hypertension (idiopathic) with ulcer and inflammation of right lower extremity   CC

I87.332   Chronic venous hypertension (idiopathic) with ulcer and inflammation of left lower extremity   CC

I87.333   Chronic venous hypertension (idiopathic) with ulcer and inflammation of bilateral lower extremity   CC

I87.339   Chronic venous hypertension (idiopathic) with ulcer and inflammation of unspecified lower extremity   CC

✓6ᵗʰ I87.39 Chronic venous hypertension (idiopathic) with other complications

I87.391   Chronic venous hypertension (idiopathic) with other complications of right lower extremity

I87.392   Chronic venous hypertension (idiopathic) with other complications of left lower extremity

I87.393   Chronic venous hypertension (idiopathic) with other complications of bilateral lower extremity

I87.399   Chronic venous hypertension (idiopathic) with other complications of unspecified lower extremity

I87.8 Other specified disorders of veins

Phlebosclerosis

Venofibrosis

I87.9 Disorder of vein, unspecified

✓4ᵗʰ I88 Nonspecific lymphadenitis

EXCLUDES 1   acute lymphadenitis, except mesenteric (L04.-)

enlarged lymph nodes NOS (R59.-)

human immunodeficiency virus [HIV] disease resulting in generalized lymphadenopathy (B20)

I88.0 Nonspecific mesenteric lymphadenitis

Mesenteric lymphadenitis (acute)(chronic)

I88.1 Chronic lymphadenitis, except mesenteric

Adenitis

Lymphadenitis

I88.8 Other nonspecific lymphadenitis

I88.9 Nonspecific lymphadenitis, unspecified

Lymphadenitis NOS

✓4ᵗʰ I89 Other noninfective disorders of lymphatic vessels and lymph nodes

EXCLUDES 1   chylocele, tunica vaginalis (nonfilarial) NOS (N50.8)

enlarged lymph nodes NOS (R59.-)

filarial chylocele (B74.-)

hereditary lymphedema (Q82.0)

I89.0 Lymphedema, not elsewhere classified

Elephantiasis (nonfilarial) NOS

Lymphangiectasis

Obliteration, lymphatic vessel

Praecox lymphedema

Secondary lymphedema

EXCLUDES 1   postmastectomy lymphedema (I97.2)

I89.1 Lymphangitis

Chronic lymphangitis

Lymphangitis NOS

Subacute lymphangitis

EXCLUDES 1   acute lymphangitis (L03.-)

✓ Additional Character Required   ✓x7ᵗʰ Placeholder Alert   Unacceptable PDx   Manifestation   Hospital Acquired Condition   EXCLUDES 1 Not Coded Here   EXCLUDES 2 Not Included Here

I89.8   **Other specified noninfective disorders of lymphatic vessels and lymph nodes**
Chylocele (nonfilarial)
Chylous ascites
Chylous cyst
Lipomelanotic reticulosis
Lymph node or vessel fistula
Lymph node or vessel infarction
Lymph node or vessel rupture

I89.9   **Noninfective disorder of lymphatic vessels and lymph nodes, unspecified**
Disease of lymphatic vessels NOS

Other and unspecified disorders of the circulatory system (I95-I99)

✓4ᵗʰ **I95**   **Hypotension**
> **EXCLUDES 1**   *cardiovascular collapse (R57.9)*
> *maternal hypotension syndrome (O26.5-)*
> *nonspecific low blood pressure reading NOS (R03.1)*

     I95.0   **Idiopathic hypotension**

     I95.1   **Orthostatic hypotension**
Hypotension, postural
> **EXCLUDES 1**   *neurogenic orthostatic hypotension [Shy-Drager] (G90.3)*
> *orthostatic hypotension due to drugs (I95.2)*

     I95.2   **Hypotension due to drugs**
Orthostatic hypotension due to drugs
Use additional code for adverse effect, if applicable, to identify drug (T36-T50 with fifth or sixth character 5)

     I95.3   **Hypotension of hemodialysis**
Intra-dialytic hypotension

     ✓5ᵗʰ **I95.8**   **Other hypotension**

         I95.81   **Postprocedural hypotension**

         I95.89   **Other hypotension**
Chronic hypotension

     I95.9   **Hypotension, unspecified**

I96   **Gangrene, not elsewhere classified**   `CC`
Gangrenous cellulitis
> **EXCLUDES 1**   *gangrene in atherosclerosis of native arteries of the extremities (I70.26)*
> *gangrene in diabetes mellitus (E08-E13)*
> *gangrene in hernia (K40.1, K40.4, K41.1, K41.4, K42.1, K43.1-, K44.1, K45.1, K46.1)*
> *gangrene in other peripheral vascular diseases (I73.-)*
> *gangrene of certain specified sites—see Alphabetical Index*
> *gas gangrene (A48.0)*
> *pyoderma gangrenosum (L88)*

AHA: 2013, 2Q, 34
CC Excl: G89.0-G89.4, I70.261-I70.269, I96, R41.0-R41.3, R41.82, R41.9, R44.8-R44.9, R45.83-R45.84, R46.0-R46.89, R52, R68.0-R68.19, R68.81-R68.83, R68.89-R69

✓4ᵗʰ **I97**   **Intraoperative and postprocedural complications and disorders of circulatory system, not elsewhere classified**
> **EXCLUDES 2**   *postprocedural shock (T81.1-)*

     I97.0   **Postcardiotomy syndrome**

     ✓5ᵗʰ **I97.1**   **Other postprocedural cardiac functional disturbances**
> **EXCLUDES 2**   *acute pulmonary insufficiency following thoracic surgery (J95.1)*
> *intraoperative cardiac functional disturbances (I97.7-)*

> **CC Excl: For CC codes in subcategory I97.1, unless otherwise noted:** D78.81-D78.89, E36.8, E89.810-E89.89, H59.011-H59.019, H59.031-H59.099, H59.811-H59.89, H95.811-H95.89, I97.110-I97.191, I97.3, I97.710-I97.791, I97.88-I97.89, L76.81-L76.82, M96.89, N98.1-N98.9, T81.82XA, T81.89XA, T81.9XXA

         ✓6ᵗʰ **I97.11**   **Postprocedural cardiac insufficiency**

             I97.110   **Postprocedural cardiac insufficiency following cardiac surgery**   `CC`

             I97.111   **Postprocedural cardiac insufficiency following other surgery**   `CC`

         ✓6ᵗʰ **I97.12**   **Postprocedural cardiac arrest**

             I97.120   **Postprocedural cardiac arrest following cardiac surgery**   `CC`

             I97.121   **Postprocedural cardiac arrest following other surgery**   `CC`

         ✓6ᵗʰ **I97.13**   **Postprocedural heart failure**
Use additional code to identify the heart failure (I50.-)

             I97.130   **Postprocedural heart failure following cardiac surgery**   `CC`

             I97.131   **Postprocedural heart failure following other surgery**   `CC`

         ✓6ᵗʰ **I97.19**   **Other postprocedural cardiac functional disturbances**
Use additional code, if applicable, to further specify disorder

             I97.190   **Other postprocedural cardiac functional disturbances following cardiac surgery**   `CC`

             I97.191   **Other postprocedural cardiac functional disturbances following other surgery**   `CC`

     I97.2   **Postmastectomy lymphedema syndrome**   `A`
Elephantiasis due to mastectomy
Obliteration of lymphatic vessels

     I97.3   **Postprocedural hypertension**

     ✓5ᵗʰ **I97.4**   **Intraoperative hemorrhage and hematoma of a circulatory system organ or structure complicating a procedure**
> **EXCLUDES 1**   *intraoperative hemorrhage and hematoma of a circulatory system organ or structure due to accidental puncture and laceration during a procedure (I97.5-)*
> **EXCLUDES 2**   *intraoperative cerebrovascular hemorrhage complicating a procedure (G97.3-)*

> **CC Excl: For CC codes in subcategory I97.4, unless otherwise noted:** H95.811-H95.89, I85.01, I85.11, I97.3-I97.42, I97.610-I97.62, K21.9, K22.8, K23-K25.0, K25.2, K25.4, K25.6, K26.0, K26.2, K26.4, K26.6, K27.0, K27.2, K27.4, K27.6, K28.0, K28.2, K28.4, K28.6, K29.01, K29.21, K29.31, K29.41, K29.51, K29.61, K29.71, K29.81, K29.91, K31.811, K55.21, K57.01, K57.11, K57.13, K57.21, K57.31, K57.33, K57.41, K57.51, K57.53, K57.81, K57.91, K57.93, K62.5, K92.0-K92.2, M96.89, N98.1-N98.9, P54.1-P54.3, T81.10XA, T81.11XA,T81.12XA, T81.19XA,T81.82XA, T81.89XA, T81.9XXA

         ✓6ᵗʰ **I97.41**   **Intraoperative hemorrhage and hematoma of a circulatory system organ or structure complicating a circulatory system procedure**

             I97.410   **Intraoperative hemorrhage and hematoma of a circulatory system organ or structure complicating a cardiac catheterization**   `CC`

             I97.411   **Intraoperative hemorrhage and hematoma of a circulatory system organ or structure complicating a cardiac bypass**   `CC`

             I97.418   **Intraoperative hemorrhage and hematoma of a circulatory system organ or structure complicating other circulatory system procedure**   `CC`

         I97.42   **Intraoperative hemorrhage and hematoma of a circulatory system organ or structure complicating other procedure**   `CC`

     ✓5ᵗʰ **I97.5**   **Accidental puncture and laceration of a circulatory system organ or structure during a procedure**
> **EXCLUDES 2**   *accidental puncture and laceration of brain during a procedure (G97.4-)*

         I97.51   **Accidental puncture and laceration of a circulatory system organ or structure during a circulatory system procedure**   `CC`
CC Excl: D78.11-D78.12, D78.81-D78.89, E36.11-E36.8, E89.810-E89.89, G96.11, G97.41-G97.49, H59.011-H59.019, H59.031-H59.099, H59.211-H59.229, H59.811-H59.89, H95.31-H95.32, H95.811-H95.89, I97.3, I97.51-I97.52, J95.71-J95.72, K91.71-K91.72, L76.11-L76.12, L76.81-L76.82, M96.820-M96.821, M96.89, N98.1-N98.9, N99.71-N99.72, T81.10XA, T81.11XA,T81.12XA, T81.19XA,T81.82XA, T81.89XA, T81.9XXA

         I97.52   **Accidental puncture and laceration of a circulatory system organ or structure during other procedure**   `CC`
CC Excl: See code: I97.51

N Newborn: 0   P Pediatric: 0-17   M Maternity: 12-55   A Adult: 15-124   **MCC** Major CC Condition   **PDxMCC** PDx acts as own MCC   CC CC Condition   **PDxCC** PDx acts as own CC

642   ICD-10-CM 2016

I89.8–I97.52

✓5ᵗʰ **I97.6** **Postprocedural hemorrhage and hematoma of a circulatory system organ or structure following a procedure**
         EXCLUDES 2   *postprocedural cerebrovascular hemorrhage complicating a procedure (G97.5-)*

         CC Excl: For CC codes in subcategory I97.6, unless otherwise noted: See code: I97.4

     ✓6ᵗʰ **I97.61** **Postprocedural hemorrhage and hematoma of a circulatory system organ or structure following a circulatory system procedure**

         I97.610 Postprocedural hemorrhage and hematoma of a circulatory system organ or structure following a cardiac catheterization   `CC`

         I97.611 Postprocedural hemorrhage and hematoma of a circulatory system organ or structure following cardiac bypass   `CC`

         I97.618 Postprocedural hemorrhage and hematoma of a circulatory system organ or structure following other circulatory system procedure   `CC`

     I97.62 **Postprocedural hemorrhage and hematoma of a circulatory system organ or structure following other procedure**   `CC`

✓5ᵗʰ **I97.7** **Intraoperative cardiac functional disturbances**
         EXCLUDES 2   *acute pulmonary insufficiency following thoracic surgery (J95.1)*
                  postprocedural cardiac functional disturbances (I97.1-)

         CC Excl: For CC codes in subcategory I97.7, unless otherwise noted: D78.81-D78.89, E36.8, E89.810-E89.89, H59.011-H59.019, H59.031-H59.099, H59.811-H59.89, H95.811-H95.89, I97.110-I97.191, I97.3, I97.710-I97.791, I97.88-I97.89, L76.81-L76.82, M96.89, N98.1-N98.9, T81.82XA,T81.89XA,T81.9XXA

     ✓6ᵗʰ **I97.71** **Intraoperative cardiac arrest**
         I97.710 Intraoperative cardiac arrest during cardiac surgery   `CC`
         I97.711 Intraoperative cardiac arrest during other surgery   `CC`

     ✓6ᵗʰ **I97.79** **Other intraoperative cardiac functional disturbances**
         Use additional code, if applicable, to further specify disorder
         I97.790 Other intraoperative cardiac functional disturbances during cardiac surgery   `CC`
         I97.791 Other intraoperative cardiac functional disturbances during other surgery   `CC`

✓5ᵗʰ **I97.8** **Other intraoperative and postprocedural complications and disorders of the circulatory system, not elsewhere classified**
         Use additional code, if applicable, to further specify disorder

     ✓6ᵗʰ **I97.81** **Intraoperative cerebrovascular infarction**
         I97.810 Intraoperative cerebrovascular infarction during cardiac surgery   `CC`
         CC Excl: D78.81-D78.89, E36.8, E89.810-E89.89, G97.0, G97.2-G97.32, G97.81-G97.82, H59.011-H59.019, H59.031-H59.099, H59.811-H59.89, H95.811-H95.89, I97.3, I97.810-I97.821, L76.81-L76.82, M96.89, N98.1-N98.9, T81.10XA, T81.11XA,T81.12XA, T81.19XA,T81.82XA, T81.89XA, T81.9XXA

         I97.811 Intraoperative cerebrovascular infarction during other surgery   `CC`
         CC Excl: See code: I97.810

     ✓6ᵗʰ **I97.82** **Postprocedural cerebrovascular infarction**
         I97.820 Postprocedural cerebrovascular infarction during cardiac surgery   `CC`
         CC Excl: See code: I97.810

         I97.821 Postprocedural cerebrovascular infarction during other surgery   `CC`
         CC Excl: See code: I97.810

         I97.88 Other intraoperative complications of the circulatory system, not elsewhere classified   `CC`
         CC Excl: See code: I97.1

         I97.89 Other postprocedural complications and disorders of the circulatory system, not elsewhere classified   `CC`
         CC Excl: See code: I97.1

✓4ᵗʰ **I99** **Other and unspecified disorders of circulatory system**
     I99.8 Other disorder of circulatory system
     I99.9 Unspecified disorder of circulatory system

Chapter 10. Diseases of the Respiratory System (J00–J99)

Chapter Specific Guidelines with Coding Examples

The chapter specific guidelines from the ICD-10-CM Official Guidelines for Coding and Reporting have been provided below. Along with these guidelines are coding examples, contained in the shaded boxes, that have been developed to help illustrate the coding and/or sequencing guidance found in these guidelines.

a. Chronic obstructive pulmonary disease [COPD] and asthma

1) Acute exacerbation of chronic obstructive bronchitis and asthma

The codes in categories J44 and J45 distinguish between uncomplicated cases and those in acute exacerbation. An acute exacerbation is a worsening or a decompensation of a chronic condition. An acute exacerbation is not equivalent to an infection superimposed on a chronic condition, though an exacerbation may be triggered by an infection.

Acute streptococcal bronchitis with acute exacerbation of COPD

J20.2   **Acute bronchitis due to streptococcus**

J44.0   **Chronic obstructive pulmonary disease with acute lower respiratory infection**

J44.1   **Chronic obstructive pulmonary disease with (acute) exacerbation**

Explanation: ICD-10-CM uses combination codes to create organism-specific classifications for acute bronchitis. Category J44 codes include combination codes with severity components, which differentiate between COPD with acute lower respiratory infection (acute bronchitis), COPD with acute exacerbation, and COPD without mention of a complication (unspecified).

An acute exacerbation is a worsening or a decompensation of a chronic condition. An acute exacerbation is not equivalent to an infection superimposed on a chronic condition, though an exacerbation may be triggered by an infection, as in this example.

Exacerbation of moderate persistent asthma with status asthmaticus

J45.42   **Moderate persistent asthma with status asthmaticus**

Explanation: Category J45 Asthma includes severity-specific subcategories and fifth-character codes to distinguish between uncomplicated cases, those in acute exacerbation, and those with status asthmaticus.

---

b. Acute respiratory failure

1) Acute respiratory failure as principal diagnosis

A code from subcategory J96.0, Acute respiratory failure, or subcategory J96.2, Acute and chronic respiratory failure, may be assigned as a principal diagnosis when it is the condition established after study to be chiefly responsible for occasioning the admission to the hospital, and the selection is supported by the Alphabetic Index and Tabular List. However, chapter-specific coding guidelines (such as obstetrics, poisoning, HIV, newborn) that provide sequencing direction take precedence.

Acute hypoxic respiratory failure due to COPD exacerbation

J96.01   **Acute respiratory failure with hypoxia**

J44.1   **Chronic obstructive pulmonary disease with (acute) exacerbation**

Explanation: Category J96 classifies respiratory failure with combination codes that designate the severity and the presence of hypoxia and hypercapnia. Code J96.01 is sequenced as the first-listed diagnosis, as the reason for the admission. Respiratory failure may be assigned as a principal diagnosis when it is the condition established after study to be chiefly responsible for occasioning the admission to the hospital and the selection is supported by the Alphabetic Index and Tabular List.

---

2) Acute respiratory failure as secondary diagnosis

Respiratory failure may be listed as a secondary diagnosis if it occurs after admission, or if it is present on admission, but does not meet the definition of principal diagnosis.

Acute respiratory failure due to accidental oxycodone overdose

T40.2X1A   **Poisoning by other opioids, accidental (unintentional), initial encounter**

J96.00   **Acute respiratory failure, unspecified whether with hypoxia or hypercapnia**

Explanation: Respiratory failure may be assigned as a principal diagnosis when it is the condition established after study to be chiefly responsible for occasioning the admission to the hospital, and the selection is supported by the Alphabetic Index and Tabular List. However, chapter-specific coding guidelines, such as poisoning, that provide sequencing direction take precedence. When coding a poisoning or reaction to the improper use of a medication (e.g. overdose, wrong substance given or taken in error, wrong route of administration), first assign the appropriate code from categories T36–T50. Use additional code(s) for all manifestations of the poisoning. In this instance, the respiratory failure is a manifestation of the poisoning and is sequenced as a secondary diagnosis.

Acute pneumococcal pneumonia with subsequent development of acute respiratory failure

J13   **Pneumonia due to Streptococcus pneumoniae**

J96.00   **Acute respiratory failure, unspecified whether with hypoxia or hypercapnia**

Explanation: Acute respiratory failure may be listed as a secondary diagnosis if it occurs after admission, or if it is present on admission but does not meet the definition of principal diagnosis.

---

3) Sequencing of acute respiratory failure and another acute condition

When a patient is admitted with respiratory failure and another acute condition, (e.g., myocardial infarction, cerebrovascular accident, aspiration pneumonia), the principal diagnosis will not be the same in every situation. This applies whether the other acute condition is a respiratory or nonrespiratory condition. Selection of the principal diagnosis will be dependent on the circumstances of admission. If both the respiratory failure and the other acute condition are equally responsible for occasioning the admission to the hospital, and there are no chapter-specific sequencing rules, the guideline regarding two or more diagnoses that equally meet the definition for principal diagnosis (*Section II, C.*) may be applied in these situations.

If the documentation is not clear as to whether acute respiratory failure and another condition are equally responsible for occasioning the admission, query the provider for clarification.

Acute pneumococcal pneumonia and acute respiratory failure, both present on admission

J96.00   **Acute respiratory failure, unspecified whether with hypoxia or hypercapnia**

J13   **Pneumonia due to Streptococcus pneumoniae**

Explanation: When a patient is admitted with respiratory failure and another acute condition, such as a bacterial pneumonia, the principal diagnosis is not the same in every situation. This applies whether the other acute condition is a respiratory or nonrespiratory condition. The principal diagnosis depends on the circumstances of admission.

---

c. Influenza due to certain identified influenza viruses

Code only confirmed cases of influenza due to certain identified influenza viruses (category J09), and due to other identified influenza virus (category J10). This is an exception to the hospital inpatient guideline Section II, H. (Uncertain Diagnosis).

In this context, "confirmation" does not require documentation of positive laboratory testing specific for avian or other novel influenza A or other identified influenza virus. However, coding should be based on the provider's diagnostic statement that the patient has avian influenza, or other novel influenza A, for category J09, or has another particular identified strain of influenza, such as H1N1 or H3N2, but not identified as novel or variant, for category J10.

If the provider records "suspected" or "possible" or "probable" avian influenza, or novel influenza, or other identified influenza, then the appropriate influenza code from category J11, Influenza due to unidentified influenza virus, should be assigned. A code from category J09, Influenza due to certain identified influenza viruses, should not be assigned nor should a code from category J10, Influenza due to other identified influenza virus.

> Influenza due to avian influenza virus with pneumonia
>
> **J09.X1   Influenza due to identified novel influenza A virus with pneumonia**
>
> *Explanation*: Codes in category J09 Influenza due to certain identified influenza viruses should be assigned only for confirmed cases. "Confirmation" does not require positive laboratory testing of a specific influenza virus but does need to be based on the provider's diagnostic statement, which should not include terms such as "possible," "probable," or "suspected."

d. Ventilator associated pneumonia

1) Documentation of ventilator associated pneumonia

As with all procedural or postprocedural complications, code assignment is based on the provider's documentation of the relationship between the condition and the procedure.

Code J95.851, Ventilator associated pneumonia, should be assigned only when the provider has documented ventilator associated pneumonia (VAP). An additional code to identify the organism (e.g., Pseudomonas aeruginosa, code B96.5) should also be assigned. Do not assign an additional code from categories J12-J18 to identify the type of pneumonia.

Code J95.851 should not be assigned for cases where the patient has pneumonia and is on a mechanical ventilator and the provider has not specifically stated that the pneumonia is ventilator-associated pneumonia. If the documentation is unclear as to whether the patient has a pneumonia that is a complication attributable to the mechanical ventilator, query the provider.

2) Ventilator associated pneumonia develops after admission

A patient may be admitted with one type of pneumonia (e.g., code J13, Pneumonia due to Streptococcus pneumonia) and subsequently develop VAP. In this instance, the principal diagnosis would be the appropriate code from categories J12-J18 for the pneumonia diagnosed at the time of admission. Code J95.851, Ventilator associated pneumonia, would be assigned as an additional diagnosis when the provider has also documented the presence of ventilator associated pneumonia.

> Patient with pneumonia due to *Klebsiella pneumoniae* develops superimposed MRSA ventilator-associated pneumonia
>
> **J15.0   Pneumonia due to Klebsiella pneumoniae**
>
> **J95.851   Ventilator associated pneumonia**
>
> **B95.62   Methicillin resistant Staphylococcus aureus infection as the cause of diseases classified elsewhere**
>
> *Explanation*: Code assignment for ventilator-associated pneumonia is based on the provider's documentation of the relationship between the condition and the procedure and is reported only when the provider has documented ventilator-associated pneumonia (VAP).
>
> A patient may be admitted with one type of pneumonia and subsequently develop VAP. In this example, the principal diagnosis code describes the pneumonia diagnosed at the time of admission, with code J95.851 Ventilator associated pneumonia, assigned as secondary.

Chapter 10. Diseases of the Respiratory System

Chapter 10. Diseases of the Respiratory System (J00-J99)

NOTE   When a respiratory condition is described as occurring in more than one site and is not specifically indexed, it should be classified to the lower anatomic site (e.g. tracheobronchitis to bronchitis in J40).

Use additional code, where applicable, to identify:
exposure to environmental tobacco smoke (Z77.22)
exposure to tobacco smoke in the perinatal period (P96.81)
history of tobacco use (Z87.891)
occupational exposure to environmental tobacco smoke (Z57.31)
tobacco dependence (F17.-)
tobacco use (Z72.0)

EXCLUDES 2 *certain conditions originating in the perinatal period (P04-P96)*
certain infectious and parasitic diseases (A00-B99)
complications of pregnancy, childbirth and the puerperium (O00-O9A)
congenital malformations, deformations and chromosomal abnormalities (Q00-Q99)
endocrine, nutritional and metabolic diseases (E00-E88)
injury, poisoning and certain other consequences of external causes (S00-T88)
neoplasms (C00-D49)
smoke inhalation (T59.81-)
symptoms, signs and abnormal clinical and laboratory findings, not elsewhere classified (R00-R94)

This chapter contains the following blocks:

J00-J06	Acute upper respiratory infections
J09-J18	Influenza and pneumonia
J20-J22	Other acute lower respiratory infections
J30-J39	Other diseases of upper respiratory tract
J40-J47	Chronic lower respiratory diseases
J60-J70	Lung diseases due to external agents
J80-J84	Other respiratory diseases principally affecting the interstitium
J85-J86	Suppurative and necrotic conditions of the lower respiratory tract
J90-J94	Other diseases of the pleura
J95	Intraoperative and postprocedural complications and disorders of respiratory system, not elsewhere classified
J96-J99	Other diseases of the respiratory system

Acute upper respiratory infections (J00-J06)

EXCLUDES 1 *chronic obstructive pulmonary disease with acute lower respiratory infection (J44.0)*
influenza virus with other respiratory manifestations (J09.X2, J10.1, J11.1)

J00   Acute nasopharyngitis (common cold)
Acute rhinitis   Infective rhinitis
Coryza (acute)   Nasal catarrh, acute
Infective nasopharyngitis NOS   Nasopharyngitis NOS

EXCLUDES 1 *acute pharyngitis (J02.-)*
acute sore throat NOS (J02.9)
pharyngitis NOS (J02.9)
rhinitis NOS (J31.0)
sore throat NOS (J02.9)

EXCLUDES 2 *allergic rhinitis (J30.1-J30.9)*
chronic pharyngitis (J31.2)
chronic rhinitis (J31.0)
chronic sore throat (J31.2)
nasopharyngitis, chronic (J31.1)
vasomotor rhinitis (J30.0)

✓4ᵗʰ J01   Acute sinusitis
INCLUDES   acute abscess of sinus
acute empyema of sinus
acute infection of sinus
acute inflammation of sinus
acute suppuration of sinus
Use additional code (B95-B97) to identify infectious agent

EXCLUDES 1 *sinusitis NOS (J32.9)*
EXCLUDES 2 *chronic sinusitis (J32.0-J32.8)*

✓5ᵗʰ J01.0   Acute maxillary sinusitis
Acute antritis
     J01.00   Acute maxillary sinusitis, unspecified
     J01.01   Acute recurrent maxillary sinusitis

✓5ᵗʰ J01.1   Acute frontal sinusitis
     J01.10   Acute frontal sinusitis, unspecified
     J01.11   Acute recurrent frontal sinusitis

✓5ᵗʰ J01.2   Acute ethmoidal sinusitis
     J01.20   Acute ethmoidal sinusitis, unspecified
     J01.21   Acute recurrent ethmoidal sinusitis

✓5ᵗʰ J01.3   Acute sphenoidal sinusitis
     J01.30   Acute sphenoidal sinusitis, unspecified
     J01.31   Acute recurrent sphenoidal sinusitis

✓5ᵗʰ J01.4   Acute pansinusitis
     J01.40   Acute pansinusitis, unspecified
     J01.41   Acute recurrent pansinusitis

✓5ᵗʰ J01.8   Other acute sinusitis
     J01.80   Other acute sinusitis
         Acute sinusitis involving more than one sinus but not pansinusitis
     J01.81   Other acute recurrent sinusitis
         Acute recurrent sinusitis involving more than one sinus but not pansinusitis

✓5ᵗʰ J01.9   Acute sinusitis, unspecified
     J01.90   Acute sinusitis, unspecified
     J01.91   Acute recurrent sinusitis, unspecified

✓4ᵗʰ J02   Acute pharyngitis
INCLUDES   acute sore throat
EXCLUDES 1 *acute laryngopharyngitis (J06.0)*
peritonsillar abscess (J36)
pharyngeal abscess (J39.1)
retropharyngeal abscess (J39.0)
EXCLUDES 2 *chronic pharyngitis (J31.2)*

J02.0   Streptococcal pharyngitis
Septic pharyngitis
Streptococcal sore throat
EXCLUDES 2 *scarlet fever (A38.-)*

J02.8   Acute pharyngitis due to other specified organisms
Use additional code (B95-B97) to identify infectious agent
EXCLUDES 1 *acute pharyngitis due to coxsackie virus (B08.5)*
acute pharyngitis due to gonococcus (A54.5)
acute pharyngitis due to herpes [simplex] virus (B00.2)
acute pharyngitis due to infectious mononucleosis (B27.-)
enteroviral vesicular pharyngitis (B08.5)

J02.9   Acute pharyngitis, unspecified
Gangrenous pharyngitis (acute)
Infective pharyngitis (acute) NOS
Pharyngitis (acute) NOS
Sore throat (acute) NOS
Suppurative pharyngitis (acute)
Ulcerative pharyngitis (acute)

✓4ᵗʰ J03   Acute tonsillitis
EXCLUDES 1 *acute sore throat (J02.-)*
hypertrophy of tonsils (J35.1)
peritonsillar abscess (J36)
sore throat NOS (J02.9)
streptococcal sore throat (J02.0)
EXCLUDES 2 *chronic tonsillitis (J35.0)*

✓5ᵗʰ J03.0   Streptococcal tonsillitis
     J03.00   Acute streptococcal tonsillitis, unspecified
     J03.01   Acute recurrent streptococcal tonsillitis

✓5ᵗʰ J03.8   Acute tonsillitis due to other specified organisms
Use additional code (B95-B97) to identify infectious agent
EXCLUDES 1 *diphtheritic tonsillitis (A36.0)*
herpesviral pharyngotonsillitis (B00.2)
streptococcal tonsillitis (J03.0)
tuberculous tonsillitis (A15.8)
Vincent's tonsillitis (A69.1)
     J03.80   Acute tonsillitis due to other specified organisms
     J03.81   Acute recurrent tonsillitis due to other specified organisms

✓5ᵗʰ J03.9   Acute tonsillitis, unspecified
Follicular tonsillitis (acute)   Tonsillitis (acute) NOS
Gangrenous tonsillitis (acute)   Ulcerative tonsillitis (acute)
Infective tonsillitis (acute)
     J03.90   Acute tonsillitis, unspecified
     J03.91   Acute recurrent tonsillitis, unspecified

✓4ᵗʰ J04   Acute laryngitis and tracheitis
Use additional code (B95-B97) to identify infectious agent
EXCLUDES 1 *acute obstructive laryngitis [croup] and epiglottitis (J05.-)*
EXCLUDES 2 *laryngismus (stridulus) (J38.5)*

N Newborn: 0   **P** Pediatric: 0-17   **M** Maternity: 12-55   **A** Adult: 15-124   **MCC** Major CC Condition   **PDxMCC** PDx acts as own MCC   **CC** CC Condition   **PDxCC** PDx acts as own CC

J04.0 **Acute** laryngitis
Edematous laryngitis (acute)   Suppurative laryngitis (acute)
Laryngitis (acute) NOS   Ulcerative laryngitis (acute)
Subglottic laryngitis (acute)
EXCLUDES 1 acute obstructive laryngitis (J05.0)
EXCLUDES 2 chronic laryngitis (J37.0)

☑5ᵗʰ **J04.1** **Acute** tracheitis
Acute viral tracheitis   Tracheitis (acute) NOS
Catarrhal tracheitis (acute)
EXCLUDES 2 chronic tracheitis (J42)

    J04.10 **Acute tracheitis** without obstruction

    J04.11 **Acute tracheitis** with obstruction   `MCC`
CC Excl: A15.8-A15.9, A17.9, A18.82, A18.84, A18.89,
J04.10-J04.2, J05.10-J05.11, J22, J98.8-J98.9

    J04.2 **Acute** laryngotracheitis
Laryngotracheitis NOS
Tracheitis (acute) with laryngitis (acute)
EXCLUDES 1 acute obstructive laryngotracheitis (J05.0)
EXCLUDES 2 chronic laryngotracheitis (J37.1)

☑5ᵗʰ **J04.3** **Supraglottitis, unspecified**

    J04.30 **Supraglottitis, unspecified,** without obstruction

    J04.31 **Supraglottitis, unspecified,** with obstruction   `MCC`
CC Excl: A15.8-A15.9, A17.9, A18.82, A18.84, A18.89,
J04.0-J04.2, J05.10-J05.11, J22, J98.8-J98.9

☑4ᵗʰ **J05** **Acute obstructive laryngitis [croup] and epiglottitis**
Use additional code (B95-B97) to identify infectious agent

    J05.0 **Acute obstructive laryngitis [croup]**
Obstructive laryngitis (acute) NOS
Obstructive laryngotracheitis NOS

☑5ᵗʰ **J05.1** **Acute epiglottitis**
EXCLUDES 2 epiglottitis, chronic (J37.0)

    J05.10 **Acute epiglottitis** without obstruction   `CC`
Epiglottitis NOS
CC Excl: J04.31, J05.10-J05.11

    J05.11 **Acute epiglottitis** with obstruction   `MCC`
CC Excl: See code: J04.31

☑4ᵗʰ **J06** **Acute upper respiratory infections of multiple and unspecified sites**
EXCLUDES 1 acute respiratory infection NOS (J22)
streptococcal pharyngitis (J02.0)3

    J06.0 **Acute laryngopharyngitis**

    J06.9 **Acute upper respiratory infection, unspecified**
Upper respiratory disease, acute
Upper respiratory infection NOS

Influenza and pneumonia (J09-J18)

EXCLUDES 2 allergic or eosinophilic pneumonia (J82)
aspiration pneumonia NOS (J69.0)
congenital pneumonia (P23.9)
lipid pneumonia (J69.1)
meconium pneumonia (P24.01)
neonatal aspiration pneumonia (P24.-)
pneumonia due to solids and liquids (J69.-)
rheumatic pneumonia (I00)
ventilator associated pneumonia (J95.851)

☑4ᵗʰ **J09** **Influenza due to** certain **identified influenza viruses**
EXCLUDES 1 seasonal influenza due to other identified influenza virus (J10.-)
seasonal influenza due to unidentified influenza virus (J11.-)

☑5ᵗʰ **J09.X** **Influenza due to identified** novel **influenza A virus**
Avian influenza
Bird influenza
Influenza A/H5N1
Influenza of other animal origin, not bird or swine
Swine influenza virus (viruses that normally cause infections in pigs)

    J09.X1 **Influenza due to identified novel influenza A** `HIV` `MCC`
virus with pneumonia
Code also, if applicable, associated:
lung abscess (J85.1)
other specified type of pneumonia
CC Excl: A15.0-A15.6, A15.8-A15.9, A17.9, A18.82,
A18.84, A18.89, A21.2, A22.1, A31.0, A37.01, A37.11,
A37.81, A37.91, A42.0, A43.0, A48.1, B25.0, B39.0-B39.2,
B44.0, B58.3, B59, B67.1, J09.X1-J09.X2, J10.00-J10.1,
J11.00-J11.1, J12.0-J12.3, J12.89-J18.1, J18.8-J18.9, J22,
J44.9, J47.0-J70.4, J70.8-J70.9, J98.4, J98.8-J99, Q33.4,
R91.1

J09.X2 **Influenza due to identified novel influenza A virus**
with **other respiratory manifestations**
Influenza due to identified novel influenza A virus NOS
Influenza due to identified novel influenza A virus with laryngitis
Influenza due to identified novel influenza A virus with pharyngitis
Influenza due to identified novel influenza A virus with upper respiratory symptoms
Use additional code, if applicable, for associated:
pleural effusion (J91.8)
sinusitis (J01.-)

J09.X3 **Influenza due to identified novel influenza A virus**
with **gastrointestinal manifestations**
Influenza due to identified novel influenza A virus gastroenteritis
EXCLUDES 1 'intestinal flu' [viral gastroenteritis] (A08.-)

J09.X9 **Influenza due to identified novel influenza A virus**
with **other manifestations**
Influenza due to identified novel influenza A virus with encephalopathy
Influenza due to identified novel influenza A virus with myocarditis
Influenza due to identified novel influenza A virus with otitis media
Use additional code to identify manifestation

☑4ᵗʰ **J10** **Influenza due to** other **identified influenza virus**
EXCLUDES 1 influenza due to avian influenza virus (J09.X-)
influenza due to swine flu (J09.X-)
influenza due to unidentifed influenza virus (J11.-)

☑5ᵗʰ **J10.0** **Influenza due to other identified influenza virus with pneumonia**
Code also associated lung abscess, if applicable (J85.1)

    J10.00 **Influenza due to other identified influenza**   `MCC`
virus with unspecified type **of pneumonia**
CC Excl: See code: J09.X1

    J10.01 **Influenza due to other identified influenza virus** `MCC`
with the same other identified influenza virus pneumonia
CC Excl: See code: J09.X1

    J10.08 **Influenza due to other identified influenza**   `HIV` `MCC`
virus with other specified **pneumonia**
Code also other specified type of pneumonia
CC Excl: See code: J09.X1

J10.1 **Influenza due to other identified influenza virus with** other **respiratory manifestations**
Influenza due to other identified influenza virus NOS
Influenza due to other identified influenza virus with laryngitis
Influenza due to other identified influenza virus with pharyngitis
Influenza due to other identified influenza virus with upper respiratory symptoms
Use additional code for associated pleural effusion, if applicable (J91.8)
Use additional code for associated sinusitis, if applicable (J01.-)

J10.2 **Influenza due to other identified influenza virus with gastrointestinal manifestations**
Influenza due to other identified influenza virus gastroenteritis
EXCLUDES 1 'intestinal flu' [viral gastroenteritis] (A08.-)

☑5ᵗʰ **J10.8** **Influenza due to other identified influenza virus** with other **manifestations**

    J10.81 **Influenza due to other identified influenza virus** with encephalopathy

    J10.82 **Influenza due to other identified influenza virus** with myocarditis

    J10.83 **Influenza due to other identified influenza virus** with otitis media
Use additional code for any associated perforated tympanic membrane (H72.-)

    J10.89 **Influenza due to other identified influenza virus** with other manifestations
Use additional codes to identify the manifestations

☑4ᵗʰ **J11** **Influenza due to** unidentified **influenza virus**

☑5ᵗʰ **J11.0** **Influenza due to unidentified influenza virus with** pneumonia
Code also associated lung abscess, if applicable (J85.1)

    J11.00 **Influenza due to unidentified influenza virus**   `MCC`
with unspecified type **of pneumonia**
Influenza with pneumonia NOS
CC Excl: See code: J09.X1

☑ Additional Character Required   ☑x7ᵗʰ Placeholder Alert   Unacceptable PDx   Manifestation   Hospital Acquired Condition   *EXCLUDES 1* Not Coded Here   *EXCLUDES 2* Not Included Here

Chapter 10. Diseases of the Respiratory System

J11.08   **Influenza due to unidentified influenza virus** `MCC`
     with specified pneumonia
       Code also other specified type of pneumonia
       CC Excl: See code: J09.X1

J11.1   **Influenza due to unidentified influenza virus with other**
     respiratory manifestations
       Influenza NOS
       Influenzal laryngitis NOS
       Influenzal pharyngitis NOS
       Influenza with upper respiratory symptoms NOS
       Use additional code for associated pleural effusion, if applicable
         (J91.8)
       Use additional code for associated sinusitis, if applicable (J01.-)

J11.2   **Influenza due to unidentified influenza virus with**
     gastrointestinal manifestations
       Influenza gastroenteritis NOS
       EXCLUDES 1   'intestinal flu' [viral gastroenteritis] (A08.-)

✓5ᵗʰ **J11.8**   **Influenza due to unidentified influenza virus with other**
     manifestations

     J11.81   **Influenza due to unidentified influenza virus with**
         encephalopathy
         Influenzal encephalopathy NOS

     J11.82   **Influenza due to unidentified influenza virus with**
         myocarditis
         Influenzal myocarditis NOS

     J11.83   **Influenza due to unidentified influenza virus with**
         otitis media
         Influenzal otitis media NOS
         Use additional code for any associated perforated
           tympanic membrane (H72.-)

     J11.89   **Influenza due to unidentified influenza virus with**
         other manifestations
         Use additional codes to identify the manifestations

✓4ᵗʰ **J12**   **Viral pneumonia, not elsewhere classified**
     INCLUDES   bronchopneumonia due to viruses other than influenza
          viruses
     Code first associated influenza, if applicable (J09.X1, J10.0-, J11.0-)
     Code also associated abscess, if applicable (J85.1)
     EXCLUDES 1   aspiration pneumonia due to anesthesia during labor and
          delivery (O74.0)
         aspiration pneumonia due to anesthesia during pregnancy
          (O29)
         aspiration pneumonia due to anesthesia during puerperium
          (O89.0)
         aspiration pneumonia due to solids and liquids (J69.-)
         aspiration pneumonia NOS (J69.0)
         congenital pneumonia (P23.0)
         congenital rubella pneumonitis (P35.0)
         interstitial pneumonia NOS (J84.9)
         lipid pneumonia (J69.1)
         neonatal aspiration pneumonia (P24.-)
     AHA: 2013, 4Q, 118

> **CC Excl: For MCC codes in category J12, unless otherwise
> noted:** A15.0-A15.6, A15.8-A15.9, A17.9, A18.82, A18.84, A18.89,
> A20.2, A21.1, A22.1, A31.0, A37.01, A37.11, A37.81, A37.91, A42.0,
> A43.0, A48.1, B25.0, B39.0-B39.2, B44.0, B58.3, B59, B67.1, J09.X1-
> J09.X2, J10.00-J10.1, J11.00-J11.1, J12.0-J18.1, J18.8-J18.9, J22,
> J60-J70.4, J70.8-J70.9, J98.4, J98.8-J99, R91.1

J12.0   **Adenoviral pneumonia**   `MCC`

J12.1   **Respiratory syncytial virus pneumonia**   `MCC`

J12.2   **Parainfluenza virus pneumonia**   `MCC`

J12.3   **Human metapneumovirus pneumonia**   `HIV` `MCC`

✓5ᵗʰ **J12.8**   **Other viral pneumonia**

     J12.81   **Pneumonia due to SARS-associated**   `HIV` `MCC`
         coronavirus
         Severe acute respiratory syndrome NOS
         CC Excl: A15.0-A15.6, A15.8-A15.9, A17.9, A18.82,
         A18.84, A18.89, A21.2, A22.1, A31.0, A37.01, A37.11,
         A37.81, A37.91, A42.0, A43.0, A48.1, B25.0, B39.0-B39.2,
         B44.0, B58.3, B59, B67.1, J09.X1-J09.X2, J10.00-J10.1,
         J11.00-J11.1, J12.0-J18.1, J18.8-J18.9, J22, J44.9, J47.0-
         J70.4, J70.8-J70.9, J98.4, J98.8-J99, Q33.4, R91.1

     J12.89   **Other viral pneumonia**   `HIV` `MCC`

J12.9   **Viral pneumonia, unspecified**   `HIV` `MCC`

J13   **Pneumonia due to Streptococcus pneumoniae**   `HIV` `MCC`
     Bronchopneumonia due to S. pneumoniae
     Code first associated influenza, if applicable (J09.X1, J10.0-, J11.0-)
     Code also associated lung abscess, if applicable (J85.1)
     EXCLUDES 1   congenital pneumonia due to S. pneumoniae (P23.6)
         lobar pneumonia, unspecified organism (J18.1)
         pneumonia due to other streptococci (J15.3-J15.4)
     AHA: 2013, 4Q, 118
     CC Excl: See code: J09.X1

J14   **Pneumonia due to Hemophilus influenzae**   `HIV` `MCC`
     Bronchopneumonia due to H. influenzae
     Code first associated influenza, if applicable (J09.X1, J10.0-, J11.0-)
     Code also associated lung abscess, if applicable (J85.1)
     EXCLUDES 1   congenital pneumonia due to H. influenzae (P23.6)
     AHA: 2013, 4Q, 118
     CC Excl: See code: J09.X1

✓4ᵗʰ **J15**   **Bacterial pneumonia, not elsewhere classified**
     Bronchopneumonia due to bacteria other than S. pneumoniae and H.
       influenzae
     Code first associated influenza, if applicable (J09.X1, J10.0-, J11.0-)
     Code also associated lung abscess, if applicable (J85.1)
     EXCLUDES 1   chlamydial pneumonia (J16.0)
         congenital pneumonia (P23.-)
         Legionnaires' disease (A48.1)
         spirochetal pneumonia (A69.8)
     AHA: 2013, 4Q, 118

> **CC Excl: For MCC codes in category J15, unless otherwise
> noted:** See code: J09.X1

J15.0   **Pneumonia due to Klebsiella pneumoniae**   `HIV` `MCC`

J15.1   **Pneumonia due to Pseudomonas**   `HIV` `MCC`

✓5ᵗʰ **J15.2**   **Pneumonia due to staphylococcus**

     J15.20   **Pneumonia due to staphylococcus,**   `HIV` `MCC`
         unspecified

     ✓6ᵗʰ **J15.21**   **Pneumonia due to Staphylococcus aureus**   `HIV` `MCC`

         J15.211   **Pneumonia due to methicillin**   `HIV` `MCC`
            susceptible Staphylococcus aureus
            MSSA pneumonia
            Pneumonia due to Staphylococcus aureus
            NOS

         J15.212   **Pneumonia due to methicillin**   `HIV` `MCC`
            resistant Staphylococcus aureus

     J15.29   **Pneumonia due to other staphylococcus**   `HIV` `MCC`

J15.3   **Pneumonia due to streptococcus, group B**   `HIV` `MCC`

J15.4   **Pneumonia due to other streptococci**   `HIV` `MCC`
     EXCLUDES 1   pneumonia due to streptococcus, group B (J15.3)
         pneumonia due to Streptococcus pneumoniae (J13)

J15.5   **Pneumonia due to Escherichia coli**   `HIV` `MCC`

J15.6   **Pneumonia due to other aerobic Gram-negative**   `HIV` `MCC`
     bacteria
       Pneumonia due to Serratia marcescens

J15.7   **Pneumonia due to Mycoplasma pneumoniae**   `MCC`

J15.8   **Pneumonia due to other specified bacteria**   `HIV` `MCC`

J15.9   **Unspecified bacterial pneumonia**   `HIV` `MCC`
       Pneumonia due to gram-positive bacteria

✓4ᵗʰ **J16**   **Pneumonia due to other infectious organisms, not elsewhere**
     classified
     Code first associated influenza, if applicable (J09.X1, J10.0-, J11.0-)
     Code also associated lung abscess, if applicable (J85.1)
     EXCLUDES 1   congenital pneumonia (P23.-)
         ornithosis (A70)
         pneumocystosis (B59)
         pneumonia NOS (J18.9)
     AHA: 2013, 4Q, 118

J16.0   **Chlamydial pneumonia**   `MCC`
       CC Excl: See code: J09.X1

J16.8   **Pneumonia due to other specified infectious organisms**   `MCC`
       CC Excl: See code: J09.X1

Ⓝ Newborn: 0   Ⓟ Pediatric: 0-17   Ⓜ Maternity: 12-55   Ⓐ Adult: 15-124   `MCC` Major CC Condition   `PDxMCC` PDx acts as own MCC   `CC` CC Condition   `PDxCC` PDx acts as own CC

648   ICD-10-CM 2016

J17   *Pneumonia in diseases classified elsewhere*   `MCC`
> *Code first underlying disease, such as:*
> *Q fever (A78)*
> *rheumatic fever (I00)*
> *schistosomiasis (B65.0-B65.9)*
>   `EXCLUDES 1`   *candidial pneumonia (B37.1)*
> *chlamydial pneumonia (J16.0)*
> *gonorrheal pneumonia (A54.84)*
> *histoplasmosis pneumonia (B39.0-B39.2)*
> *measles pneumonia (B05.2)*
> *nocardiosis pneumonia (A43.0)*
> *pneumocystosis (B59)*
> *pneumonia due to Pneumocystis carinii (B59)*
> *pneumonia due to Pneumocystis jiroveci (B59)*
> *pneumonia in actinomycosis (A42.0)*
> *pneumonia in anthrax (A22.1)*
> *pneumonia in ascariasis (B77.81)*
> *pneumonia in aspergillosis (B44.0-B44.1)*
> *pneumonia in coccidioidomycosis (B38.0-B38.2)*
> *pneumonia in cytomegalovirus disease (B25.0)*
> *pneumonia in toxoplasmosis (B58.3)*
> *rubella pneumonia (B06.81)*
> *salmonella pneumonia (A02.22)*
> *spirochetal infection NEC with pneumonia (A69.8)*
> *tularemia pneumonia (A21.2)*
> *typhoid fever with pneumonia (A01.03)*
> *varicella pneumonia (B01.2)*
> *whooping cough with pneumonia (A37 with fifth-character 1)*

AHA: 2013, 4Q, 118
CC Excl: A15.0-A15.6, A15.8-A15.9, A17.9, A18.82, A18.84, A18.89, A21.2, A22.1, A31.0, A37.01, A37.11, A37.81, A37.91, A42.0, A43.0, A48.1, B25.0, B39.0-B39.2, B44.0, B58.3, B59, B67.1, J09.X1-J09.X2, J10.00-J10.1, J11.00-J11.1, J12.0-J12.3, J12.89-J18.1, J18.8-J18.9, J22, J44.9, J47.0-J70.4, J70.8-J70.9, J98.4, J98.8-J99, Q33.4, R91.1

✓4th **J18**   **Pneumonia, unspecified organism**
> *Code first associated influenza, if applicable (J09.X1, J10.0-, J11.0-)*
>   `EXCLUDES 1`   *abscess of lung with pneumonia (J85.1)*
> *aspiration pneumonia due to anesthesia during labor and delivery (O74.0)*
> *aspiration pneumonia due to anesthesia during pregnancy (O29)*
> *aspiration pneumonia due to anesthesia during puerperium (O89.0)*
> *aspiration pneumonia due to solids and liquids (J69.-)*
> *aspiration pneumonia NOS (J69.0)*
> *congenital pneumonia (P23.0)*
> *drug-induced interstitial lung disorder (J70.2-J70.4)*
> *interstitial pneumonia NOS (J84.9)*
> *lipid pneumonia (J69.1)*
> *neonatal aspiration pneumonia (P24.-)*
> *pneumonitis due to external agents (J67-J70)*
> *pneumonitis due to fumes and vapors (J68.0)*
> *usual interstitial pneumonia (J84.17)*

AHA: 2013, 4Q, 118

> **CC Excl: For CC/MCC codes in category J18, unless otherwise noted:** See code: J17

J18.0   **Bronchopneumonia, unspecified organism**   `MCC`
>   `EXCLUDES 1`   *hypostatic bronchopneumonia (J18.2)*
> *lipid pneumonia (J69.1)*
>   `EXCLUDES 2`   *acute bronchiolitis (J21.-)*
> *chronic bronchiolitis (J44.9)*

J18.1   **Lobar pneumonia, unspecified organism**   `HIV` `MCC`

J18.2   **Hypostatic pneumonia, unspecified organism**   `CC`
> Hypostatic bronchopneumonia
> Passive pneumonia
> **CC Excl:** J18.2, J22, J81.1, J98.4, J98.8-J99, R91.1

J18.8   **Other pneumonia, unspecified organism**   `HIV` `MCC`

J18.9   **Pneumonia, unspecified organism**   `HIV` `MCC`
> **AHA:** 2014, 3Q, 4; 2013, 4Q, 119; 2012, 4Q, 94

Other acute lower respiratory infections (J20-J22)

   `EXCLUDES 2`   *chronic obstructive pulmonary disease with acute lower respiratory infection (J44.0)*

✓4th **J20**   **Acute bronchitis**
>   `INCLUDES`   acute and subacute bronchitis (with) bronchospasm
> acute and subacute bronchitis (with) tracheitis
> acute and subacute bronchitis (with) tracheobronchitis, acute
> acute and subacute fibrinous bronchitis
> acute and subacute membranous bronchitis
> acute and subacute purulent bronchitis
> acute and subacute septic bronchitis
>   `EXCLUDES 1`   *bronchitis NOS (J40)*
> *tracheobronchitis NOS (J40)*
>   `EXCLUDES 2`   *acute bronchitis with bronchiectasis (J47.0)*
> *acute bronchitis with chronic obstructive asthma (J44.0)*
> *acute bronchitis with chronic obstructive pulmonary disease (J44.0)*
> *allergic bronchitis NOS (J45.909)*
> *bronchitis due to chemicals, fumes and vapors (J68.0)*
> *chronic bronchitis NOS (J42)*
> *chronic mucopurulent bronchitis (J41.1)*
> *chronic obstructive bronchitis (J44.-)*
> *chronic obstructive tracheobronchitis (J44.-)*
> *chronic simple bronchitis (J41.0)*
> *chronic tracheobronchitis (J42)*

J20.0   **Acute bronchitis due to Mycoplasma pneumoniae**

J20.1   **Acute bronchitis due to Hemophilus influenzae**

J20.2   **Acute bronchitis due to streptococcus**

J20.3   **Acute bronchitis due to coxsackievirus**

J20.4   **Acute bronchitis due to parainfluenza virus**

J20.5   **Acute bronchitis due to respiratory syncytial virus**

J20.6   **Acute bronchitis due to rhinovirus**

J20.7   **Acute bronchitis due to echovirus**

J20.8   **Acute bronchitis due to other specified organisms**

J20.9   **Acute bronchitis, unspecified**

✓4th **J21**   **Acute bronchiolitis**
> Acute bronchiolitis with bronchospasm
>   `EXCLUDES 2`   *respiratory bronchiolitis interstitial lung disease (J84.115)*

> **CC Excl: For CC codes in category J21, unless otherwise noted:** J20.0-J21.9

J21.0   **Acute bronchiolitis due to respiratory syncytial virus**   `CC`
> **CC Excl:** J21.0

J21.1   **Acute bronchiolitis due to human metapneumovirus**   `CC`

J21.8   **Acute bronchiolitis due to other specified organisms**   `CC`

J21.9   **Acute bronchiolitis, unspecified**   `CC`
> Bronchiolitis (acute)
>   `EXCLUDES 1`   *chronic bronchiolitis (J44.-)*

J22   **Unspecified acute lower respiratory infection**
> Acute (lower) respiratory (tract) infection NOS
>   `EXCLUDES 1`   *upper respiratory infection (acute) (J06.9)*

Other diseases of upper respiratory tract (J30-J39)

✓4th **J30**   **Vasomotor and allergic rhinitis**
>   `INCLUDES`   spasmodic rhinorrhea
>   `EXCLUDES 1`   *allergic rhinitis with asthma (bronchial) (J45.909)*
> *rhinitis NOS (J31.0)*

J30.0   **Vasomotor rhinitis**

J30.1   **Allergic rhinitis due to pollen**
> Allergy NOS due to pollen
> Hay fever
> Pollinosis

J30.2   **Other seasonal allergic rhinitis**

J30.5   **Allergic rhinitis due to food**

✓5th **J30.8**   **Other allergic rhinitis**

     J30.81   **Allergic rhinitis due to animal (cat) (dog) hair and dander**

     J30.89   **Other allergic rhinitis**
> Perennial allergic rhinitis

J30.9   **Allergic rhinitis, unspecified**

✓ Additional Character Required   ✓x7th Placeholder Alert   Unacceptable PDx   Manifestation   Hospital Acquired Condition   `EXCLUDES 1` Not Coded Here   `EXCLUDES 2` Not Included Here

ICD-10-CM 2016   **649**

✓4ᵗʰ J31 Chronic rhinitis, nasopharyngitis and pharyngitis

Use additional code to identify:
exposure to environmental tobacco smoke (Z77.22)
exposure to tobacco smoke in the perinatal period (P96.81)
history of tobacco use (Z87.891)
occupational exposure to environmental tobacco smoke (Z57.31)
tobacco dependence (F17.-)
tobacco use (Z72.Ø)

J31.Ø Chronic rhinitis
Atrophic rhinitis (chronic)
Granulomatous rhinitis (chronic)
Hypertrophic rhinitis (chronic)
Obstructive rhinitis (chronic)
Ozena
Purulent rhinitis (chronic)
Rhinitis (chronic) NOS
Ulcerative rhinitis (chronic)
EXCLUDES 1　allergic rhinitis (J30.1-J30.9)
vasomotor rhinitis (J30.Ø)

J31.1 Chronic nasopharyngitis
EXCLUDES 2　acute nasopharyngitis (J00)

J31.2 Chronic pharyngitis
Atrophic pharyngitis (chronic)
Chronic sore throat
Granular pharyngitis (chronic)
Hypertrophic pharyngitis (chronic)
EXCLUDES 2　acute pharyngitis (J02.9)

✓4ᵗʰ J32 Chronic sinusitis

INCLUDES　sinus abscess
sinus empyema
sinus infection
sinus suppuration

Use additional code to identify:
exposure to environmental tobacco smoke (Z77.22)
exposure to tobacco smoke in the perinatal period (P96.81)
history of tobacco use (Z87.891)
infectious agent (B95-B97)
occupational exposure to environmental tobacco smoke (Z57.31)
tobacco dependence (F17.-)
tobacco use (Z72.Ø)
EXCLUDES 2　acute sinusitis (J01.-)

J32.Ø Chronic maxillary sinusitis
Antritis (chronic)
Maxillary sinusitis NOS

J32.1 Chronic frontal sinusitis
Frontal sinusitis NOS

J32.2 Chronic ethmoidal sinusitis
Ethmoidal sinusitis NOS
EXCLUDES 1　Woakes' ethmoiditis (J33.1)

J32.3 Chronic sphenoidal sinusitis
Sphenoidal sinusitis NOS

J32.4 Chronic pansinusitis
Pansinusitis NOS

J32.8 Other chronic sinusitis
Sinusitis (chronic) involving more than one sinus but not pansinusitis

J32.9 Chronic sinusitis, unspecified
Sinusitis (chronic) NOS

✓4ᵗʰ J33 Nasal polyp

Use additional code to identify:
exposure to environmental tobacco smoke (Z77.22)
exposure to tobacco smoke in the perinatal period (P96.81)
history of tobacco use (Z87.891)
occupational exposure to environmental tobacco smoke (Z57.31)
tobacco dependence (F17.-)
tobacco use (Z72.Ø)
EXCLUDES 1　adenomatous polyps (D14.Ø)

J33.Ø Polyp of nasal cavity
Choanal polyp
Nasopharyngeal polyp

J33.1 Polypoid sinus degeneration
Woakes' syndrome or ethmoiditis

J33.8 Other polyp of sinus
Accessory polyp of sinus
Ethmoidal polyp of sinus
Maxillary polyp of sinus
Sphenoidal polyp of sinus

J33.9 Nasal polyp, unspecified

✓4ᵗʰ J34 Other and unspecified disorders of nose and nasal sinuses

EXCLUDES 2　varicose ulcer of nasal septum (I86.8)

J34.Ø Abscess, furuncle and carbuncle of nose
Cellulitis of nose　　　Ulceration of nose
Necrosis of nose

J34.1 Cyst and mucocele of nose and nasal sinus

J34.2 Deviated nasal septum
Deflection or deviation of septum (nasal) (acquired)
EXCLUDES 1　congenital deviated nasal septum (Q67.4)

J34.3 Hypertrophy of nasal turbinates

✓5ᵗʰ J34.8 Other specified disorders of nose and nasal sinuses

J34.81 Nasal mucositis (ulcerative)
Code also type of associated therapy, such as:
antineoplastic and immunosuppressive drugs (T45.1X-)
radiological procedure and radiotherapy (Y84.2)
EXCLUDES 2　gastrointestinal mucositis (ulcerative) (K92.81)
mucositis (ulcerative) of vagina and vulva (N76.81)
oral mucositis (ulcerative) (K12.3-)

J34.89 Other specified disorders of nose and nasal sinuses
Perforation of nasal septum NOS
Rhinolith

J34.9 Unspecified disorder of nose and nasal sinuses

✓4ᵗʰ J35 Chronic diseases of tonsils and adenoids

Use additional code to identify:
exposure to environmental tobacco smoke (Z77.22)
exposure to tobacco smoke in the perinatal period (P96.81)
history of tobacco use (Z87.891)
occupational exposure to environmental tobacco smoke (Z57.31)
tobacco dependence (F17.-)
tobacco use (Z72.Ø)

✓5ᵗʰ J35.Ø Chronic tonsillitis and adenoiditis
EXCLUDES 2　acute tonsillitis (J03.-)

J35.Ø1 Chronic tonsillitis

J35.Ø2 Chronic adenoiditis

J35.Ø3 Chronic tonsillitis and adenoiditis

J35.1 Hypertrophy of tonsils
Enlargement of tonsils
EXCLUDES 1　hypertrophy of tonsils with tonsillitis (J35.Ø-)

J35.2 Hypertrophy of adenoids
Enlargement of adenoids
EXCLUDES 1　hypertrophy of adenoids with adenoiditis (J35.Ø-)

J35.3 Hypertrophy of tonsils with hypertrophy of adenoids
EXCLUDES 1　hypertrophy of tonsils and adenoids with tonsillitis and adenoiditis (J35.Ø3)

J35.8 Other chronic diseases of tonsils and adenoids
Adenoid vegetations　　　　Tonsillar tag
Amygdalolith　　　　　　　Ulcer of tonsil
Calculus, tonsil
Cicatrix of tonsil (and adenoid)

J35.9 Chronic disease of tonsils and adenoids, unspecified
Disease (chronic) of tonsils and adenoids NOS

J36 Peritonsillar abscess　　　　　　　　　　　　　CC

INCLUDES　abscess of tonsil
peritonsillar cellulitis
quinsy
Use additional code (B95-B97) to identify infectious agent
EXCLUDES 1　acute tonsillitis (J03.-)
chronic tonsillitis (J35.Ø)
retropharyngeal abscess (J39.Ø)
tonsillitis NOS (J03.9-)
CC Excl: J22, J36, J98.8-J98.9

✓4ᵗʰ J37 Chronic laryngitis and laryngotracheitis

Use additional code to identify:
exposure to environmental tobacco smoke (Z77.22)
exposure to tobacco smoke in the perinatal period (P96.81)
history of tobacco use (Z87.891)
infectious agent (B95-B97)
occupational exposure to environmental tobacco smoke (Z57.31)
tobacco dependence (F17.-)
tobacco use (Z72.Ø)

J37.Ø Chronic laryngitis
Catarrhal laryngitis
Hypertrophic laryngitis
Sicca laryngitis
EXCLUDES 2　acute laryngitis (J04.Ø)
obstructive (acute) laryngitis (J05.Ø)

J37.1 **Chronic laryngotracheitis**
Laryngitis, chronic, with tracheitis (chronic)
Tracheitis, chronic, with laryngitis
EXCLUDES1 *chronic tracheitis (J42)*
EXCLUDES2 *acute laryngotracheitis (J04.2)*
acute tracheitis (J04.1)

✓4ᵗʰ **J38 Diseases of vocal cords and larynx, not elsewhere classified**
Use additional code to identify:
exposure to environmental tobacco smoke (Z77.22)
exposure to tobacco smoke in the perinatal period (P96.81)
history of tobacco use (Z87.891)
occupational exposure to environmental tobacco smoke (Z57.31)
tobacco dependence (F17.-)
tobacco use (Z72.0)
EXCLUDES1 *congenital laryngeal stridor (P28.89)*
obstructive laryngitis (acute) (J05.0)
postprocedural subglottic stenosis (J95.5)
stridor (R06.1)
ulcerative laryngitis (J04.0)

✓5ᵗʰ **J38.0 Paralysis of vocal cords and larynx**
Laryngoplegia
Paralysis of glottis

J38.00 **Paralysis of vocal cords and larynx, unspecified**
J38.01 **Paralysis of vocal cords and larynx, unilateral**
J38.02 **Paralysis of vocal cords and larynx, bilateral**

J38.1 **Polyp of vocal cord and larynx**
EXCLUDES1 *adenomatous polyps (D14.1)*

J38.2 **Nodules of vocal cords**
Chorditis (fibrinous)(nodosa)(tuberosa)
Singer's nodes
Teacher's nodes

J38.3 **Other diseases of vocal cords**
Abscess of vocal cords
Cellulitis of vocal cords
Granuloma of vocal cords
Leukokeratosis of vocal cords
Leukoplakia of vocal cords

J38.4 **Edema of larynx**
Edema (of) glottis
Subglottic edema
Supraglottic edema
EXCLUDES1 *acute obstructive laryngitis [croup] (J05.0)*
edematous laryngitis (J04.0)

J38.5 **Laryngeal spasm**
Laryngismus (stridulus)

J38.6 **Stenosis of larynx**

J38.7 **Other diseases of larynx**
Abscess of larynx   Pachyderma of larynx
Cellulitis of larynx   Perichondritis of larynx
Disease of larynx NOS   Ulcer of larynx
Necrosis of larynx

✓4ᵗʰ **J39 Other diseases of upper respiratory tract**
EXCLUDES1 *acute respiratory infection NOS (J22)*
acute upper respiratory infection (J06.9)
upper respiratory inflammation due to chemicals, gases, fumes or vapors (J68.2)

J39.0 **Retropharyngeal and parapharyngeal abscess** CC
Peripharyngeal abscess
EXCLUDES1 *peritonsillar abscess (J36)*
CC Excl: J22, J39.0-J39.1, J98.8-J98.9

J39.1 **Other abscess of pharynx** CC
Cellulitis of pharynx
Nasopharyngeal abscess
CC Excl: See code: J39.0

J39.2 **Other diseases of pharynx**
Cyst of pharynx
Edema of pharynx
EXCLUDES2 *chronic pharyngitis (J31.2)*
ulcerative pharyngitis (J02.9)

J39.3 **Upper respiratory tract hypersensitivity reaction, site unspecified**
EXCLUDES1 *hypersensitivity reaction of upper respiratory tract, such as:*
extrinsic allergic alveolitis (J67.9)
pneumoconiosis (J60-J67.9)

J39.8 **Other specified diseases of upper respiratory tract**
J39.9 **Disease of upper respiratory tract, unspecified**

Chronic lower respiratory diseases (J40-J47)
EXCLUDES1 *bronchitis due to chemicals, gases, fumes and vapors (J68.0)*
EXCLUDES2 *cystic fibrosis (E84.-)*

J40 Bronchitis, not specified as acute or chronic
Bronchitis NOS
Bronchitis with tracheitis NOS
Catarrhal bronchitis
Tracheobronchitis NOS
Use additional code to identify:
exposure to environmental tobacco smoke (Z77.22)
exposure to tobacco smoke in the perinatal period (P96.81)
history of tobacco use (Z87.891)
occupational exposure to environmental tobacco smoke (Z57.31)
tobacco dependence (F17.-)
tobacco use (Z72.0)
EXCLUDES1 *acute bronchitis (J20.-)*
allergic bronchitis NOS (J45.909)
asthmatic bronchitis NOS (J45.9-)
bronchitis due to chemicals, gases, fumes and vapors (J68.0)

✓4ᵗʰ **J41 Simple and mucopurulent chronic bronchitis**
Use additional code to identify:
exposure to environmental tobacco smoke (Z77.22)
exposure to tobacco smoke in the perinatal period (P96.81)
history of tobacco use (Z87.891)
occupational exposure to environmental tobacco smoke (Z57.31)
tobacco dependence (F17.-)
tobacco use (Z72.0)
EXCLUDES1 *chronic bronchitis NOS (J42)*
chronic obstructive bronchitis (J44.-)

J41.0 **Simple chronic bronchitis**
J41.1 **Mucopurulent chronic bronchitis**
J41.8 **Mixed simple and mucopurulent chronic bronchitis**

J42 Unspecified chronic bronchitis
Chronic bronchitis NOS
Chronic tracheitis
Chronic tracheobronchitis
Use additional code to identify:
exposure to environmental tobacco smoke (Z77.22)
exposure to tobacco smoke in the perinatal period (P96.81)
history of tobacco use (Z87.891)
occupational exposure to environmental tobacco smoke (Z57.31)
tobacco dependence (F17.-)
tobacco use (Z72.0)
EXCLUDES1 *chronic asthmatic bronchitis (J44.-)*
chronic bronchitis with airways obstruction (J44.-)
chronic emphysematous bronchitis (J44.-)
chronic obstructive pulmonary disease NOS (J44.9)
simple and mucopurulent chronic bronchitis (J41.-)

✓4ᵗʰ **J43 Emphysema**
Use additional code to identify:
exposure to environmental tobacco smoke (Z77.22)
history of tobacco use (Z87.891)
occupational exposure to environmental tobacco smoke (Z57.31)
tobacco dependence (F17.-)
tobacco use (Z72.0)
EXCLUDES1 *compensatory emphysema (J98.3)*
emphysema due to inhalation of chemicals, gases, fumes or vapors (J68.4)
emphysema with chronic (obstructive) bronchitis (J44.-)
emphysematous (obstructive) bronchitis (J44.-)
interstitial emphysema (J98.2)
mediastinal emphysema (J98.2)
neonatal interstitial emphysema (P25.0)
surgical (subcutaneous) emphysema (T81.82)
traumatic subcutaneous emphysema (T79.7)

J43.0 **Unilateral pulmonary emphysema [MacLeod's syndrome]**
Swyer-James syndrome
Unilateral emphysema
Unilateral hyperlucent lung
Unilateral pulmonary artery functional hypoplasia
Unilateral transparency of lung

J43.1 **Panlobular emphysema**
Panacinar emphysema

J43.2 **Centrilobular emphysema**
J43.8 **Other emphysema**
J43.9 **Emphysema, unspecified**
Bullous emphysema (lung)(pulmonary)
Emphysema (lung)(pulmonary) NOS
Emphysematous bleb
Vesicular emphysema (lung)(pulmonary)

Chapter 10. Diseases of the Respiratory System

✓4ᵗʰ J44   Other chronic obstructive pulmonary disease

     INCLUDES   asthma with chronic obstructive pulmonary disease
            chronic asthmatic (obstructive) bronchitis
            chronic bronchitis with airways obstruction
            chronic bronchitis with emphysema
            chronic emphysematous bronchitis
            chronic obstructive asthma
            chronic obstructive bronchitis
            chronic obstructive tracheobronchitis

     Code also type of asthma, if applicable (J45.-)
     Use additional code to identify:
        exposure to environmental tobacco smoke (Z77.22)
        history of tobacco use (Z87.891)
        occupational exposure to environmental tobacco smoke (Z57.31)
        tobacco dependence (F17.-)
        tobacco use (Z72.0)

     EXCLUDES 1   *bronchiectasis (J47.-)*
            chronic bronchitis NOS (J42)
            chronic simple and mucopurulent bronchitis (J41.-)
            chronic tracheitis (J42)
            chronic tracheobronchitis (J42)
            emphysema without chronic bronchitis (J43.-)
            lung diseases due to external agents (J60-J70)

     AHA: 2013, 4Q, 109

J44.0   Chronic obstructive pulmonary disease with acute lower   **CC**
         respiratory infection
         Use additional code to identify the infection
         CC Excl: J10.08, J41.1-J42, J44.0-J44.1

J44.1   Chronic obstructive pulmonary disease with (acute)   **CC**
         exacerbation
         Decompensated COPD
         Decompensated COPD with (acute) exacerbation
         EXCLUDES 2   *chronic obstructive pulmonary disease [COPD] with*
                    acute bronchitis (J44.0)
         CC Excl: See code: J44.0

J44.9   Chronic obstructive pulmonary disease, unspecified
         Chronic obstructive airway disease NOS
         Chronic obstructive lung disease NOS
         AHA: 2014, 4Q, 21; 2013, 4Q, 129

✓4ᵗʰ J45   Asthma

     INCLUDES   allergic (predominantly) asthma
            allergic bronchitis NOS
            allergic rhinitis with asthma
            atopic asthma
            extrinsic allergic asthma
            hay fever with asthma
            idiosyncratic asthma
            intrinsic nonallergic asthma
            nonallergic asthma

     Use additional code to identify:
        exposure to environmental tobacco smoke (Z77.22)
        exposure to tobacco smoke in the perinatal period (P96.81)
        history of tobacco use (Z87.891)
        occupational exposure to environmental tobacco smoke (Z57.31)
        tobacco dependence (F17.-)
        tobacco use (Z72.0)

     EXCLUDES 1   *detergent asthma (J69.8)*
            eosinophilic asthma (J82)
            lung diseases due to external agents (J60-J70)
            miner's asthma (J60)
            wheezing NOS (R06.2)
            wood asthma (J67.8)

     EXCLUDES 2   *asthma with chronic obstructive pulmonary disease (J44.9)*
            chronic asthmatic (obstructive) bronchitis (J44.9)
            chronic obstructive asthma (J44.9)

     CC Excl: For CC codes in category J45, unless otherwise noted:
     J10.08, J22, J45.998, J98.4, J98.8-J99, R91.1

✓5ᵗʰ J45.2   Mild intermittent asthma

     J45.20   Mild intermittent asthma, uncomplicated
            Mild intermittent asthma NOS

     J45.21   Mild intermittent asthma with (acute)   **CC**
            exacerbation

     J45.22   Mild intermittent asthma with status   **CC**
            asthmaticus

✓5ᵗʰ J45.3   Mild persistent asthma

     J45.30   Mild persistent asthma, uncomplicated
            Mild persistent asthma NOS

     J45.31   Mild persistent asthma with (acute) exacerbation   **CC**

     J45.32   Mild persistent asthma with status asthmaticus   **CC**

✓5ᵗʰ J45.4   Moderate persistent asthma

     J45.40   Moderate persistent asthma, uncomplicated
            Moderate persistent asthma NOS

     J45.41   Moderate persistent asthma with (acute)   **CC**
            exacerbation

     J45.42   Moderate persistent asthma with status   **CC**
            asthmaticus

✓5ᵗʰ J45.5   Severe persistent asthma

     J45.50   Severe persistent asthma, uncomplicated
            Severe persistent asthma NOS

     J45.51   Severe persistent asthma with (acute)   **CC**
            exacerbation

     J45.52   Severe persistent asthma with status   **CC**
            asthmaticus

✓5ᵗʰ J45.9   Other and unspecified asthma

     ✓6ᵗʰ J45.90   Unspecified asthma
            Asthmatic bronchitis NOS
            Childhood asthma NOS
            Late onset asthma

         J45.901   Unspecified asthma with (acute)   **CC**
                 exacerbation

         J45.902   Unspecified asthma with status   **CC**
                 asthmaticus

         J45.909   Unspecified asthma, uncomplicated
                 Asthma NOS

     ✓6ᵗʰ J45.99   Other asthma
         J45.990   Exercise induced bronchospasm
         J45.991   Cough variant asthma
         J45.998   Other asthma

✓4ᵗʰ J47   Bronchiectasis

     INCLUDES   bronchiolectasis

     Use additional code to identify:
        exposure to environmental tobacco smoke (Z77.22)
        exposure to tobacco smoke in the perinatal period (P96.81)
        history of tobacco use (Z87.891)
        occupational exposure to environmental tobacco smoke (Z57.31)
        tobacco dependence (F17.-)
        tobacco use (Z72.0)

     EXCLUDES 1   *congenital bronchiectasis (Q33.4)*
            tuberculous bronchiectasis (current disease) (A15.0)

J47.0   Bronchiectasis with acute lower respiratory infection   **CC**
         Bronchiectasis with acute bronchitis
         CC Excl: A17.9, A18.82, A18.84, A18.89, J09.X2, J10.08, J10.1, J11.1,
         J44.9, J47.0-J47.1, J68.1, J68.4-J68.9, Q33.4

J47.1   Bronchiectasis with (acute) exacerbation   **CC**
         CC Excl: See code: J47.0

J47.9   Bronchiectasis, uncomplicated
         Bronchiectasis NOS

Lung diseases due to external agents (J60-J70)

     EXCLUDES 2   *asthma (J45.-)*
            malignant neoplasm of bronchus and lung (C34.-)

J60   Coalworker's pneumoconiosis   **A**
     Anthracosilicosis
     Anthracosis
     Black lung disease
     Coalworker's lung
     EXCLUDES 1   *coalworker pneumoconiosis with tuberculosis, any type in A15*
            (J65)

J61   Pneumoconiosis due to asbestos and other mineral fibers   **A**
     Asbestosis
     EXCLUDES 1   *pleural plaque with asbestosis (J92.0)*
            pneumoconiosis with tuberculosis, any type in A15 (J65)

✓4ᵗʰ J62   Pneumoconiosis due to dust containing silica
     INCLUDES   silicotic fibrosis (massive) of lung
     EXCLUDES 1   *pneumoconiosis with tuberculosis, any type in A15 (J65)*

J62.0   Pneumoconiosis due to talc dust

J62.8   Pneumoconiosis due to other dust containing silica
         Silicosis NOS

✓4ᵗʰ J63   Pneumoconiosis due to other inorganic dusts
     EXCLUDES 1   *pneumoconiosis with tuberculosis, any type in A15 (J65)*

J63.0   Aluminosis (of lung)

J63.1   Bauxite fibrosis (of lung)

J63.2   Berylliosis

J63.3   Graphite fibrosis (of lung)

J63.4   Siderosis

J63.5   **Stannosis**

J63.6   **Pneumoconiosis due to other specified inorganic dusts**

J64   **Unspecified pneumoconiosis**
      EXCLUDES1   *pneumonoconiosis with tuberculosis, any type in A15 (J65)*

J65   **Pneumoconiosis associated with tuberculosis**
      Any condition in J60-J64 with tuberculosis, any type in A15
      Silicotuberculosis

✓4ᵗʰ **J66**   **Airway disease due to specific organic dust**
      EXCLUDES2   *allergic alveolitis (J67.-)*
               asbestosis (J61)
               bagassosis (J67.1)
               farmer's lung (J67.0)
               hypersensitivity pneumonitis due to organic dust (J67.-)
               reactive airways dysfunction syndrome (J68.3)

J66.0   **Byssinosis**
      Airway disease due to cotton dust

J66.1   **Flax-dressers' disease**

J66.2   **Cannabinosis**

J66.8   **Airway disease due to other specific organic dusts**

✓4ᵗʰ **J67**   **Hypersensitivity pneumonitis due to organic dust**
      INCLUDES   allergic alveolitis and pneumonitis due to inhaled organic dust and particles of fungal, actinomycetic or other origin
      EXCLUDES1   *pneumonitis due to inhalation of chemicals, gases, fumes or vapors (J68.0)*

      CC Excl: For CC codes in category J67, unless otherwise noted: A15.0-A15.6, A15.8-A15.9, A17.9, A18.82, A18.84, A18.89, A21.2, A22.1, A31.0, A37.01, A37.11, A37.81, A37.91, A42.0, A43.0, A48.1, B25.0, B39.0-B39.2, B44.0, B58.3, B59, B67.1, J09.X1-J09.X2, J10.00-J10.1, J11.00-J11.1, J12.0-J12.3, J12.89-J18.1, J18.8-J18.9, J22, J44.9, J47.0-J70.4, J70.8-J70.9, J98.4, J98.8-J99, Q33.4, R91.1

J67.0   **Farmer's lung**
      Harvester's lung
      Haymaker's lung
      Moldy hay disease

J67.1   **Bagassosis**
      Bagasse disease
      Bagasse pneumonitis

J67.2   **Bird fancier's lung**
      Budgerigar fancier's disease or lung
      Pigeon fancier's disease or lung

J67.3   **Suberosis**
      Corkhandler's disease or lung
      Corkworker's disease or lung

J67.4   **Maltworker's lung**
      Alveolitis due to Aspergillus clavatus

J67.5   **Mushroom-worker's lung**

J67.6   **Maple-bark-stripper's lung**
      Alveolitis due to Cryptostroma corticale
      Cryptostromosis

J67.7   **Air conditioner and humidifier lung**   CC
      Allergic alveolitis due to fungal, thermophilic actinomycetes and other organisms growing in ventilation [air conditioning] systems

J67.8   **Hypersensitivity pneumonitis due to other organic dusts**   CC
      Cheese-washer's lung
      Coffee-worker's lung
      Fish-meal worker's lung
      Furrier's lung
      Sequoiosis

J67.9   **Hypersensitivity pneumonitis due to unspecified organic dust**   CC
      Allergic alveolitis (extrinsic) NOS
      Hypersensitivity pneumonitis NOS

✓4ᵗʰ **J68**   **Respiratory conditions due to inhalation of chemicals, gases, fumes and vapors**
      Code first (T51-T65) to identify cause
      Use additional code to identify associated respiratory conditions, such as:
         acute respiratory failure (J96.0-)

      CC Excl: For CC/MCC codes in category J68, unless otherwise noted: See code: J67

J68.0   **Bronchitis and pneumonitis due to chemicals, gases, fumes and vapors**   CC
      Chemical bronchitis (acute)

J68.1   **Pulmonary edema due to chemicals, gases, fumes and vapors**   MCC
      Chemical pulmonary edema (acute) (chronic)
      EXCLUDES1   *pulmonary edema (acute) (chronic) NOS (J81.-)*

J68.2   **Upper respiratory inflammation due to chemicals, gases, fumes and vapors, not elsewhere classified**

J68.3   **Other acute and subacute respiratory conditions due to chemicals, gases, fumes and vapors**
      Reactive airways dysfunction syndrome

J68.4   **Chronic respiratory conditions due to chemicals, gases, fumes and vapors**
      Emphysema (diffuse) (chronic) due to inhalation of chemicals, gases, fumes and vapors
      Obliterative bronchiolitis (chronic) (subacute) due to inhalation of chemicals, gases, fumes and vapors
      Pulmonary fibrosis (chronic) due to inhalation of chemicals, gases, fumes and vapors
      EXCLUDES1   *chronic pulmonary edema due to chemicals, gases, fumes and vapors (J68.1)*

J68.8   **Other respiratory conditions due to chemicals, gases, fumes and vapors**

J68.9   **Unspecified respiratory condition due to chemicals, gases, fumes and vapors**

✓4ᵗʰ **J69**   **Pneumonitis due to solids and liquids**
      EXCLUDES1   *neonatal aspiration syndromes (P24.-)*
               postprocedural pneumonitis (J95.4)

      CC Excl: For MCC codes in category J69, unless otherwise noted: See code: J67

J69.0   **Pneumonitis due to inhalation of food and vomit**   MCC
      Aspiration pneumonia NOS
      Aspiration pneumonia (due to) food (regurgitated)
      Aspiration pneumonia (due to) gastric secretions
      Aspiration pneumonia (due to) milk
      Aspiration pneumonia (due to) vomit
      Code also any associated foreign body in respiratory tract (T17.-)
      EXCLUDES1   *chemical pneumonitis due to anesthesia (J95.4)*
               obstetric aspiration pneumonitis (O74.0)

J69.1   **Pneumonitis due to inhalation of oils and essences**   MCC
      Exogenous lipoid pneumonia
      Lipid pneumonia NOS
      Code first (T51-T65) to identify substance
      EXCLUDES1   *endogenous lipoid pneumonia (J84.89)*

J69.8   **Pneumonitis due to inhalation of other solids and liquids**   MCC
      Pneumonitis due to aspiration of blood
      Pneumonitis due to aspiration of detergent
      Code first (T51-T65) to identify substance

✓4ᵗʰ **J70**   **Respiratory conditions due to other external agents**

      CC Excl: For CC codes in category J70, unless otherwise noted: See code: J67

J70.0   **Acute pulmonary manifestations due to radiation**   CC
      Radiation pneumonitis
      Use additional code (W88-W90, X39.0-) to identify the external cause

J70.1   **Chronic and other pulmonary manifestations due to radiation**   CC
      Fibrosis of lung following radiation
      Use additional code (W88-W90, X39.0-) to identify the external cause

J70.2   **Acute drug-induced interstitial lung disorders**
      Use additional code for adverse effect, if applicable, to identify drug (T36-T50 with fifth or sixth character 5)
      EXCLUDES1   *interstitial pneumonia NOS (J84.9)*
               lymphoid interstitial pneumonia (J84.2)

J70.3   **Chronic drug-induced interstitial lung disorders**
      Use additional code for adverse effect, if applicable, to identify drug (T36-T50 with fifth or sixth character 5)
      EXCLUDES1   *interstitial pneumonia NOS (J84.9)*
               lymphoid interstitial pneumonia (J84.2)

J70.4   **Drug-induced interstitial lung disorders, unspecified**
      Use additional code for adverse effect, if applicable, to identify drug (T36-T50 with fifth or sixth character 5)
      EXCLUDES1   *interstitial pneumonia NOS (J84.9)*
               lymphoid interstitial pneumonia (J84.2)

J70.5   **Respiratory conditions due to smoke inhalation**
      Smoke inhalation NOS
      EXCLUDES1   *smoke inhalation due to chemicals, gases, fumes and vapors (J68.9)*
      AHA: 2013, 4Q, 121

✓ Additional Character Required   ✓x7ᵗʰ Placeholder Alert   Unacceptable PDx   Manifestation   Hospital Acquired Condition   EXCLUDES1 Not Coded Here   EXCLUDES2 Not Included Here

Chapter 10. Diseases of the Respiratory System

J70.8   Respiratory conditions due to other specified external agents
Code first (T51-T65) to identify the external agent

J70.9   Respiratory conditions due to unspecified external agent
Code first (T51-T65) to identify the external agent

Other respiratory diseases principally affecting the interstitium (J80-J84)

J80   Acute respiratory distress syndrome   CC
Acute respiratory distress syndrome in adult or child
Adult hyaline membrane disease
EXCLUDES 1   respiratory distress syndrome in newborn (perinatal) (P22.0)
CC Excl: J22, J80, J96.00-J96.92, J98.8-J98.9, R09.2

✓4ᵗʰ **J81   Pulmonary edema**
Use additional code to identify:
exposure to environmental tobacco smoke (Z77.22)
history of tobacco use (Z87.891)
occupational exposure to environmental tobacco smoke (Z57.31)
tobacco dependence (F17.-)
tobacco use (Z72.0)
EXCLUDES 1   chemical (acute) pulmonary edema (J68.1)
hypostatic pneumonia (J18.2)
passive pneumonia (J18.2)
pulmonary edema due to external agents (J60-J70)
pulmonary edema with heart disease NOS (I50.1)
pulmonary edema with heart failure (I50.1)

J81.0   Acute pulmonary edema   MCC
Acute edema of lung
CC Excl: I09.81, I50.9, J22, J81.0, J98.8-J98.9

J81.1   Chronic pulmonary edema   CC
Pulmonary congestion (chronic) (passive)
Pulmonary edema NOS
CC Excl: J18.2, J22, J81.1, J98.4, J98.8-J99, R91.1

J82   Pulmonary eosinophilia, not elsewhere classified   CC
Allergic pneumonia
Eosinophilic asthma
Eosinophilic pneumonia
Löffler's pneumonia
Tropical (pulmonary) eosinophilia NOS
EXCLUDES 1   pulmonary eosinophilia due to aspergillosis (B44.-)
pulmonary eosinophilia due to drugs (J70.2-J70.4)
pulmonary eosinophilia due to specified parasitic infection (B50-B83)
pulmonary eosinophilia due to systemic connective tissue disorders (M30-M36)
pulmonary infiltrate NOS (R91.8)
CC Excl: A15.0-A15.6, A15.8-A15.9, A17.9, A18.82, A18.84, A18.89, A20.2, A21.1, A22.1, A31.0, A37.01, A37.11, A37.81, A37.91, A42.0, A43.0, A48.1, B25.0, B39.0-B39.2, B44.0, B58.3, B59, B67.1, J09.X1-J09.X2, J10.00-J10.1, J11.00-J11.1, J12.0-J12.3, J12.89-J18.1, J18.8-J18.9, J22, J47.0-J70.4, J70.8-J70.9, J82, J98.4, J98.8-J99, Q33.4, R91.1

✓4ᵗʰ **J84   Other interstitial pulmonary diseases**
EXCLUDES 1   drug-induced interstitial lung disorders (J70.2-J70.4)
interstitial emphysema (J98.2)
lung diseases due to external agents (J60-J70)

✓5ᵗʰ **J84.0   Alveolar and parieto-alveolar conditions**

CC Excl: For CC codes in subcategory J84.0, unless otherwise noted: A15.0-A15.6, A15.8-A15.9, A17.9, A18.82, A18.84, A18.89, J22, J44.9, J47.0-J70.4, J70.8-J70.9, J84.01-J84.82, J84.89-J84.9, J98.4, J98.8-J99, Q33.4, R91.1

J84.01   Alveolar proteinosis   CC
J84.02   Pulmonary alveolar microlithiasis   CC
J84.03   *Idiopathic pulmonary hemosiderosis*   CC
Essential brown induration of lung
Code first underlying disease, such as:
disorders of iron metabolism (E83.1-)
EXCLUDES 1   acute idiopathic pulmonary hemorrhage in infants [AIPHI] (R04.81)

J84.09   Other alveolar and parieto-alveolar conditions   CC

✓5ᵗʰ **J84.1   Other interstitial pulmonary diseases with fibrosis**
EXCLUDES 1   pulmonary fibrosis (chronic) due to inhalation of chemicals, gases, fumes or vapors (J68.4)
pulmonary fibrosis (chronic) following radiation (J70.1)

CC Excl: For CC codes in subcategory J84.1, unless otherwise noted: See code: J84.0

J84.10   Pulmonary fibrosis, unspecified
Capillary fibrosis of lung
Cirrhosis of lung (chronic) NOS
Fibrosis of lung (atrophic) (chronic) (confluent) (massive) (perialveolar) (peribronchial) NOS
Induration of lung (chronic) NOS
Postinflammatory pulmonary fibrosis

✓6ᵗʰ **J84.11   Idiopathic interstitial pneumonia**
EXCLUDES 1   lymphoid interstitial pneumonia (J84.2)
pneumocystis pneumonia (B59)

J84.111   Idiopathic interstitial pneumonia, not otherwise specified

J84.112   Idiopathic pulmonary fibrosis
Cryptogenic fibrosing alveolitis
Idiopathic fibrosing alveolitis

J84.113   Idiopathic non-specific interstitial pneumonitis
EXCLUDES 1   non-specific interstitial pneumonia NOS, or due to known underlying cause (J84.89)

J84.114   Acute interstitial pneumonitis   CC
Hamman-Rich syndrome
EXCLUDES 1   pneumocystis pneumonia (B59)

J84.115   Respiratory bronchiolitis interstitial lung disease

J84.116   Cryptogenic organizing pneumonia   CC
EXCLUDES 1   organizing pneumonia NOS, or due to known underlying cause (J84.89)

J84.117   Desquamative interstitial pneumonia   CC

J84.17   *Other interstitial pulmonary diseases with fibrosis in diseases classified elsewhere*
Interstitial pneumonia (nonspecific) (usual) due to collagen vascular disease
Interstitial pneumonia (nonspecific) (usual) in diseases classified elsewhere
Organizing pneumonia due to collagen vascular disease
Organizing pneumonia in diseases classified elsewhere
Code first underlying disease, such as:
progressive systemic sclerosis (M34.0)
rheumatoid arthritis (M05.00-M06.9)
systemic lupus erythematosis (M32.0-M32.9)

J84.2   Lymphoid interstitial pneumonia   CC
Lymphoid interstitial pneumonitis
CC Excl: See code: J84.0

✓5ᵗʰ **J84.8   Other specified interstitial pulmonary diseases**
EXCLUDES 1   exogenous lipoid pneumonia (J69.1)
unspecified lipoid pneumonia (J69.1)

J84.81   Lymphangioleiomyomatosis   MCC ♀
Lymphangiomyomatosis
CC Excl: See code: J84.0

J84.82   Adult pulmonary Langerhans cell histiocytosis   CC A
Adult PLCH
CC Excl: See code: J84.0

J84.83   Surfactant mutations of the lung   MCC
CC Excl: J84.83-J84.848, P22.0-P28.5, P28.89-P29.2, P29.4, P29.89-P29.9, P84, P94.1-P94.9, P96.0, P96.3-P96.5, P96.82-P96.89

✓6ᵗʰ **J84.84   Other interstitial lung diseases of childhood**

CC Excl: For MCC codes in subcategory J84.84, unless otherwise noted: See code: J84.83

J84.841   Neuroendocrine cell hyperplasia of infancy   MCC

J84.842   Pulmonary interstitial glycogenosis   MCC

J84.843   Alveolar capillary dysplasia with vein misalignment   MCC

J84.848   Other interstitial lung diseases of childhood   MCC

N Newborn: 0   P Pediatric: 0-17   M Maternity: 12-55   A Adult: 15-124   MCC Major CC Condition   PDxMCC PDx acts as own MCC   CC CC Condition   PDxCC PDx acts as own CC

654   ICD-10-CM 2016

J84.89   **Other specified interstitial pulmonary diseases**
Endogenous lipoid pneumonia
Interstitial pneumonitis
Non-specific interstitial pneumonitis NOS
Organizing pneumonia due to known underlying cause
Organizing pneumonia NOS
Code first, if applicable:
   poisoning due to drug or toxin (T51-T65 with fifth or sixth character to indicate intent), for toxic pneumonopathy
   underlying cause of pneumonopathy, if known
Use additional code, for adverse effect, to identify drug (T36-T50 with fifth or sixth character 5), if drug-induced
   EXCLUDES 1   cryptogenic organizing pneumonia (J84.116)
     idiopathic non-specific interstitial pneumonitis (J84.113)
     lipoid pneumonia, exogenous or unspecified (J69.1)
     lymphoid interstitial pneumonia (J84.2)

J84.9   **Interstitial pulmonary disease, unspecified**   CC
Interstitial pneumonia NOS
CC Excl: See code: J84.0

Suppurative and necrotic conditions of the lower respiratory tract (J85-J86)

J85   **Abscess of lung and mediastinum**
Use additional code (B95-B97) to identify infectious agent.

J85.0   **Gangrene and necrosis of lung**   MCC
CC Excl: A06.5, A15.6, A15.8-A15.9, A17.9, A18.82, A18.84, A18.89, J22, J85.0-J85.2, J98.8-J98.9

J85.1   **Abscess of lung with pneumonia**   MCC
Code also the type of pneumonia
CC Excl: See code: J85.0

J85.2   **Abscess of lung without pneumonia**   MCC
Abscess of lung NOS
CC Excl: See code: J85.0

J85.3   **Abscess of mediastinum**   MCC
CC Excl: J22, J85.3, J98.8-J98.9

J86   **Pyothorax**
Use additional code (B95-B97) to identify infectious agent
  EXCLUDES 1   abscess of lung (J85.-)
     pyothorax due to tuberculosis (A15.6)

J86.0   **Pyothorax with fistula**   MCC
Bronchocutaneous fistula
Bronchopleural fistula
Hepatopleural fistula
Mediastinal fistula
Pleural fistula
Thoracic fistula
Any condition classifiable to J86.9 with fistula
CC Excl: J22-J86.9, J98.4, J98.8-J99, R91.1

J86.9   **Pyothorax without fistula**   MCC
Abscess of pleura
Abscess of thorax
Empyema (chest) (lung) (pleura)
Fibrinopurulent pleurisy
Purulent pleurisy
Pyopneumothorax
Septic pleurisy
Seropurulent pleurisy
Suppurative pleurisy
CC Excl: See code: J86.0

Other diseases of the pleura (J90-J94)

J90   **Pleural effusion, not elsewhere classified**   CC
Encysted pleurisy
Pleural effusion NOS
Pleurisy with effusion (exudative) (serous)
  EXCLUDES 1   chylous (pleural) effusion (J94.0)
     malignant pleural effusion (J91.0))
     pleurisy NOS (R09.1)
     tuberculous pleural effusion (A15.6)
CC Excl: A15.0-A15.6, A15.8-A15.9, A17.9, A18.82, A18.84, A18.89, J22, J90-J92.9, J94.0-J94.9, J98.4, J98.8-J99, R09.1, R91.1

J91   **Pleural effusion in conditions classified elsewhere**
  EXCLUDES 2   pleural effusion in heart failure (I50.-)
     pleural effusion in systemic lupus erythematosus (M32.13)

J91.0   **Malignant pleural effusion**   CC
Code first underlying neoplasm
CC Excl: C45.7-C45.9, C76.8, C78.2-C78.39, C79.89-C7A.00, C7A.098-C7B.00, C7B.09-C80.2, D49.81-D49.9, J90-J91.0, J94.0, J94.2

J91.8   **Pleural effusion in other conditions classified elsewhere**   CC
Code first underlying disease, such as:
   filariasis (B74.0-B74.9)
   influenza (J09.X2, J10.1, J11.1)
CC Excl: See code: J90

J92   **Pleural plaque**
INCLUDES   pleural thickening

J92.0   **Pleural plaque with presence of asbestos**

J92.9   **Pleural plaque without asbestos**
Pleural plaque NOS

J93   **Pneumothorax and air leak**
  EXCLUDES 1   congenital or perinatal pneumothorax (P25.1)
     postprocedural air leak (J95.812)
     postprocedural pneumothorax (J95.811)
     traumatic pneumothorax (S27.0)
     tuberculous (current disease) pneumothorax (A15.-)
     pyopneumothorax (J86.-)

CC Excl: For CC/MCC codes in category J93, unless otherwise noted: J22, J93.9, J95.811-J95.812, J98.4, J98.8-J99, R91.1

J93.0   **Spontaneous tension pneumothorax**   MCC

J93.1   **Other spontaneous pneumothorax**

J93.11   **Primary spontaneous pneumothorax**   CC

J93.12   **Secondary spontaneous pneumothorax**   CC
Code first underlying condition, such as:
   catamenial pneumothorax due to endometriosis (N80.8)
   cystic fibrosis (E84.-)
   eosinophilic pneumonia (J82)
   lymphangioleiomyomatosis (J84.81)
   malignant neoplasm of bronchus and lung (C34.-)
   Marfan's syndrome (Q87.4)
   pneumonia due to Pneumocystis carinii (B59)
   secondary malignant neoplasm of lung (C78.0-)
   spontaneous rupture of the esophagus (K22.3)

J93.8   **Other pneumothorax and air leak**

J93.81   **Chronic pneumothorax**   CC

J93.82   **Other air leak**   CC
Persistent air leak

J93.83   **Other pneumothorax**   CC
Acute pneumothorax
Spontaneous pneumothorax NOS

J93.9   **Pneumothorax, unspecified**   CC
Pneumothorax NOS

J94   **Other pleural conditions**
  EXCLUDES 1   pleurisy NOS (R09.1)
     traumatic hemopneumothorax (S27.2)
     traumatic hemothorax (S27.1)
     tuberculous pleural conditions (current disease) (A15.-)

J94.0   **Chylous effusion**   CC
Chyliform effusion
CC Excl: See code: J90

J94.1   **Fibrothorax**

J94.2   **Hemothorax**   CC
Hemopneumothorax
CC Excl: See code: J90

J94.8   **Other specified pleural conditions**   CC
Hydropneumothorax
Hydrothorax
CC Excl: No excl

J94.9   **Pleural condition, unspecified**

✔ Additional Character Required   ✔x7th Placeholder Alert   Unacceptable PDx   Manifestation   Hospital Acquired Condition   EXCLUDES 1 Not Coded Here   EXCLUDES 2 Not Included Here

ICD-10-CM 2016   655

Chapter 10. Diseases of the Respiratory System

Intraoperative and postprocedural complications and disorders of respiratory system, not elsewhere classified (J95)

✓4ᵗʰ J95 Intraoperative and postprocedural complications and disorders of respiratory system, not elsewhere classified

> *EXCLUDES 2* aspiration pneumonia (J69.-)
> emphysema (subcutaneous) resulting from a procedure (T81.82)
> hypostatic pneumonia (J18.2)
> pulmonary manifestations due to radiation (J70.0-J70.1)

✓5ᵗʰ J95.0 Tracheostomy complications

> **CC Excl: For CC codes in subcategory J95.0, unless otherwise noted:** J22, J39.8, J95.00-J95.09, J98.01-J98.09, J98.8-J98.9

J95.00   Unspecified tracheostomy complication `CC`

J95.01   Hemorrhage from tracheostomy stoma `CC`

J95.02   Infection of tracheostomy stoma `CC`
> Use additional code to identify type of infection, such as:
> cellulitis of neck (L03.8)
> sepsis (A40, A41-)

J95.03   Malfunction of tracheostomy stoma `CC`
> Mechanical complication of tracheostomy stoma
> Obstruction of tracheostomy airway
> Tracheal stenosis due to tracheostomy

J95.04   Tracheo-esophageal fistula following tracheostomy `CC`

J95.09   Other tracheostomy complication `CC`

J95.1 Acute pulmonary insufficiency following thoracic surgery `MCC`
> *EXCLUDES 2* functional disturbances following cardiac surgery (I97.0, I97.1-)
> **CC Excl:** J22, J95.3, J95.821-J95.822, J98.8-J98.9

J95.2 Acute pulmonary insufficiency following nonthoracic surgery `MCC`
> *EXCLUDES 2* functional disturbances following cardiac surgery (I97.0, I97.1-)
> **CC Excl:** See code: J95.1

J95.3 Chronic pulmonary insufficiency following surgery `MCC`
> *EXCLUDES 2* functional disturbances following cardiac surgery (I97.0, I97.1-)
> **CC Excl:** See code: J95.1

J95.4 Chemical pneumonitis due to anesthesia `CC`
> Mendelson's syndrome
> Postprocedural aspiration pneumonia
> Use additional code for adverse effect, if applicable, to identify drug (T41.- with fifth or sixth character 5)
> *EXCLUDES 1* aspiration pneumonitis due to anesthesia complicating labor and delivery (O74.0)
> aspiration pneumonitis due to anesthesia complicating pregnancy (O29)
> aspiration pneumonitis due to anesthesia complicating the puerperium (O89.01)
> **CC Excl:** D78.81-D78.89, E36.8, E89.810-E89.89, H59.011-H59.019, H59.031-H59.099, H59.811-H59.89, H95.811-H95.89, I97.3, J95.4-J95.5, J95.84, J95.851-J95.89, L76.81-L76.82, M96.89, N98.1-N98.9, T81.82XA, T81.89XA, T81.9XXA

J95.5 Postprocedural subglottic stenosis `CC`
> **CC Excl:** See code: J95.4

✓5ᵗʰ J95.6 Intraoperative hemorrhage and hematoma of a respiratory system organ or structure complicating a procedure
> *EXCLUDES 1* intraoperative hemorrhage and hematoma of a respiratory system organ or structure due to accidental puncture and laceration during procedure (J95.7-)

J95.61   Intraoperative hemorrhage and hematoma of a respiratory system organ or structure complicating a respiratory system procedure `CC`
> **CC Excl:** H95.811-H95.89, I85.01, I85.11, I97.3, J95.61-J95.62, J95.830-J95.831, K21.9, K22.8, K23-K25.0, K25.2, K25.4, K25.6, K26.0, K26.2, K26.4, K26.6, K27.0, K27.2, K27.4, K27.6, K28.0, K28.2, K28.4, K28.6, K29.01, K29.21, K29.31, K29.41, K29.51, K29.61, K29.71, K29.81, K29.91, K31.811, K55.21, K57.01, K57.11, K57.13, K57.21, K57.31, K57.33, K57.41, K57.51, K57.53, K57.81, K57.91, K57.93, K62.5, K92.0-K92.2, M96.89, N98.1-N98.9, P54.1-P54.3, T81.10XA, T81.11XA, T81.12XA, T81.19XA, T81.82XA, T81.89XA, T81.9XXA

J95.62   Intraoperative hemorrhage and hematoma of a respiratory system organ or structure complicating other procedure `CC`
> **CC Excl:** See code: J95.61

✓5ᵗʰ J95.7 Accidental puncture and laceration of a respiratory system organ or structure during a procedure
> *EXCLUDES 2* postprocedural pneumothorax (J95.811)

J95.71   Accidental puncture and laceration of a respiratory system organ or structure during a respiratory system procedure `CC`
> **CC Excl:** D78.11-D78.12, D78.81-D78.89, E36.11-E36.8, E89.810-E89.89, G96.11, G97.41-G97.49, H59.011-H59.019, H59.031-H59.099, H59.211-H59.229, H59.811-H59.89, H95.31-H95.32, H95.811-H95.89, I97.3, I97.51-I97.52, J95.71-J95.72, K91.71-K91.72, L76.11-L76.12, L76.81-L76.82, M96.820-M96.821, M96.89, N98.1-N98.9, N99.71-N99.72, T81.10XA, T81.11XA, T81.12XA, T81.19XA, T81.82XA, T81.89XA, T81.9XXA

J95.72   Accidental puncture and laceration of a respiratory system organ or structure during other procedure `CC`
> **CC Excl:** See code: J95.71

✓5ᵗʰ J95.8 Other intraoperative and postprocedural complications and disorders of respiratory system, not elsewhere classified

✓6ᵗʰ J95.81   Postprocedural pneumothorax and air leak

9 J95.811   Postprocedural pneumothorax `CC`
> **CC Excl:** J22, J93.9, J95.811-J95.812, J98.4, J98.8-J99, R91.1

J95.812   Postprocedural air leak `CC`
> **CC Excl:** See code: J95.811

✓6ᵗʰ J95.82   Postprocedural respiratory failure
> *EXCLUDES 1* respiratory failure in other conditions (J96.-)

J95.821   Acute postprocedural respiratory failure `MCC`
> Postprocedural respiratory failure NOS
> **CC Excl:** See code: J95.1

J95.822   Acute and chronic postprocedural respiratory failure `MCC`
> **CC Excl:** See code: J95.1

✓6ᵗʰ J95.83   Postprocedural hemorrhage and hematoma of a respiratory system organ or structure following a procedure

J95.830   Postprocedural hemorrhage and hematoma of a respiratory system organ or structure following a respiratory system procedure `CC`
> **CC Excl:** See code: J95.61

J95.831   Postprocedural hemorrhage and hematoma of a respiratory system organ or structure following other procedure `CC`
> **CC Excl:** See code: J95.61

J95.84   Transfusion-related acute lung injury (TRALI) `CC`
> **CC Excl:** See code: J95.4

✓6ᵗʰ J95.85   Complication of respirator [ventilator]

> **CC Excl: For CC codes in subcategory J95.85, unless otherwise noted:** See code: J95.4

J95.850   Mechanical complication of respirator `CC`
> *EXCLUDES 1* encounter for respirator [ventilator] dependence during power failure (Z99.12)
> **CC Excl:** J95.850, Z99.12, Z99.81-Z99.89

J95.851   Ventilator associated pneumonia `CC`
> Ventilator associated pneumonitis
> Use additional code to identify the organism, if known (B95.-, B96.-, B97.-)
> *EXCLUDES 1* ventilator lung in newborn (P27.8)

J95.859   Other complication of respirator [ventilator] `CC`

J95.88   Other intraoperative complications of respiratory system, not elsewhere classified `CC`
> **CC Excl:** See code: J95.4

---

9 HAC = as SDx not POA, in combination with one of the following procedure codes: 05H[M,N,P,Q]33Z or 0JH63XZ.

Ⓝ Newborn: 0   Ⓟ Pediatric: 0-17   Ⓜ Maternity: 12-55   Ⓐ Adult: 15-124   `MCC` Major CC Condition   `PDx MCC` PDx acts as own MCC   `CC` CC Condition   `PDx CC` PDx acts as own CC

656   ICD-10-CM 2016

J95.89   **Other postprocedural complications and disorders of respiratory system, not elsewhere classified**   `CC`

Use additional code to identify disorder, such as:
aspiration pneumonia (J69.-)
bacterial or viral pneumonia (J12-J18)

EXCLUDES 2   *acute pulmonary insufficiency following thoracic surgery (J95.1)*
postprocedural subglottic stenosis (J95.5)

CC Excl: See code: J95.4

Other diseases of the respiratory system (J96-J99)

☑4ᵗʰ   **J96**   **Respiratory failure, not elsewhere classified**

EXCLUDES 1   *acute respiratory distress syndrome (J80)*
cardiorespiratory failure (R09.2)
newborn respiratory distress syndrome (P22.0)
postprocedural respiratory failure (J95.82-)
respiratory arrest (R09.2)
respiratory arrest of newborn (P28.81)
respiratory failure of newborn (P28.5)

CC Excl: For CC/MCC codes in category J96, unless otherwise noted: J22, J80, J96.00-J96.92, J98.8-J98.9, R09.2

☑5ᵗʰ   **J96.0**   **Acute respiratory failure**

J96.00   **Acute respiratory failure, unspecified whether with hypoxia or hypercapnia**   `MCC`
AHA: 2013, 4Q, 121

J96.01   **Acute respiratory failure with hypoxia**   `MCC`

J96.02   **Acute respiratory failure with hypercapnia**   `MCC`

☑5ᵗʰ   **J96.1**   **Chronic respiratory failure**

J96.10   **Chronic respiratory failure, unspecified whether with hypoxia or hypercapnia**   `CC`
AHA: 2015, 1Q, 21

J96.11   **Chronic respiratory failure with hypoxia**   `CC`
AHA: 2013, 4Q, 129

J96.12   **Chronic respiratory failure with hypercapnia**   `CC`

☑5ᵗʰ   **J96.2**   **Acute and chronic respiratory failure**
Acute on chronic respiratory failure

J96.20   **Acute and chronic respiratory failure, unspecified whether with hypoxia or hypercapnia**   `MCC`

J96.21   **Acute and chronic respiratory failure with hypoxia**   `MCC`

J96.22   **Acute and chronic respiratory failure with hypercapnia**   `MCC`

☑5ᵗʰ   **J96.9**   **Respiratory failure, unspecified**

J96.90   **Respiratory failure, unspecified, unspecified whether with hypoxia or hypercapnia**   `MCC`

J96.91   **Respiratory failure, unspecified with hypoxia**   `MCC`

J96.92   **Respiratory failure, unspecified with hypercapnia**   `MCC`

☑4ᵗʰ   **J98**   **Other respiratory disorders**

Use additional code to identify:
exposure to environmental tobacco smoke (Z77.22)
exposure to tobacco smoke in the perinatal period (P96.81)
history of tobacco use (Z87.891)
occupational exposure to environmental tobacco smoke (Z57.31)
tobacco dependence (F17.-)
tobacco use (Z72.0)

EXCLUDES 1   *newborn apnea (P28.4)*
newborn sleep apnea (P28.3)

EXCLUDES 2   *apnea NOS (R06.81)*
sleep apnea (G47.3-)

☑5ᵗʰ   **J98.0**   **Diseases of bronchus, not elsewhere classified**

J98.01   **Acute bronchospasm**

EXCLUDES 1   *acute bronchiolitis with bronchospasm (J21.-)*
acute bronchitis with bronchospasm (J20.-)
asthma (J45.-)
exercise induced bronchospasm (J45.990)

J98.09   **Other diseases of bronchus, not elsewhere classified**
Broncholithiasis
Calcification of bronchus
Stenosis of bronchus
Tracheobronchial collapse
Tracheobronchial dyskinesia
Ulcer of bronchus

☑5ᵗʰ   **J98.1**   **Pulmonary collapse**

EXCLUDES 1   *therapeutic collapse of lung status (Z98.3)*

J98.11   **Atelectasis**   `CC`

EXCLUDES 1   *newborn atelectasis*
tuberculous atelectasis (current disease) (A15)

CC Excl: J22, J98.19, J98.8-J98.9

J98.19   **Other pulmonary collapse**   `CC`
CC Excl: See code: J98.11

J98.2   **Interstitial emphysema**
Mediastinal emphysema

EXCLUDES 1   *emphysema NOS (J43.9)*
emphysema in newborn (P25.0)
surgical emphysema (subcutaneous) (T81.82)
traumatic subcutaneous emphysema (T79.7)

J98.3   **Compensatory emphysema**

J98.4   **Other disorders of lung**
Calcification of lung
Cystic lung disease (acquired)
Lung disease NOS
Pulmolithiasis

EXCLUDES 1   *acute interstitial pneumonitis (J84.114)*
pulmonary insufficiency following surgery (J95.1-J95.2)

5   **J98.5**   **Diseases of mediastinum, not elsewhere classified**   `MCC`
Fibrosis of mediastinum
Hernia of mediastinum
Retraction of mediastinum
Mediastinitis

EXCLUDES 2   *abscess of mediastinum (J85.3)*

CC Excl: No excl

J98.6   **Disorders of diaphragm**
Diaphragmatitis
Paralysis of diaphragm
Relaxation of diaphragm

EXCLUDES 1   *congenital malformation of diaphragm NEC (Q79.1)*
congenital diaphragmatic hernia (Q79.0)

EXCLUDES 2   *diaphragmatic hernia (K44.-)*

J98.8   **Other specified respiratory disorders**

J98.9   **Respiratory disorder, unspecified**
Respiratory disease (chronic) NOS

J99   *Respiratory disorders in diseases classified elsewhere*

Code first underlying disease, such as:
amyloidosis (E85.-)
ankylosing spondylitis (M45)
congenital syphilis (A50.5)
cryoglobulinemia (D89.1)
early congenital syphilis (A50.0)
schistosomiasis (B65.0-B65.9)

EXCLUDES 1   *respiratory disorders in:*
amebiasis (A06.5)
blastomycosis (B40.0-B40.2)
candidiasis (B37.1)
coccidioidomycosis (B38.0-B38.2)
cystic fibrosis with pulmonary manifestations (E84.0)
dermatomyositis (M33.01, M33.11)
histoplasmosis (B39.0-B39.2)
late syphilis (A52.72, A52.73)
polymyositis (M33.21)
sicca syndrome (M35.02)
systemic lupus erythematosus (M32.13)
systemic sclerosis (M34.81)
Wegener's granulomatosis (M31.30-M31.31)

---

5   HAC = as SDx not POA, in combination with one of the following procedure codes: 021[0,1,2,3][0,4][9,A,J,K][3,8,9,C,F,W]; 021[0,1,2,3][0,4]Z[3,8,9,C,F].

☑ Additional Character Required   ✓x7ᵗʰ Placeholder Alert   Unacceptable PDx   Manifestation   Hospital Acquired Condition   *EXCLUDES 1* Not Coded Here   *EXCLUDES 2* Not Included Here

Chapter 11. Diseases of the Digestive System (KØØ–K95)

Chapter Specific Coding Guidelines and Examples
Reserved for future guideline expansion.

Chapter 11. Diseases of the Digestive System (K00-K95)

EXCLUDES 2   certain conditions originating in the perinatal period (P04-P96)
certain infectious and parasitic diseases (A00-B99)
complications of pregnancy, childbirth and the puerperium (O00-O9A)
congenital malformations, deformations and chromosomal abnormalities (Q00-Q99)
endocrine, nutritional and metabolic diseases (E00-E88)
injury, poisoning and certain other consequences of external causes (S00-T88)
neoplasms (C00-D49)
symptoms, signs and abnormal clinical and laboratory findings, not elsewhere classified (R00-R94)

This chapter contains the following blocks:
K00-K14   Diseases of oral cavity and salivary glands
K20-K31   Diseases of esophagus, stomach and duodenum
K35-K38   Diseases of appendix
K40-K46   Hernia
K50-K52   Noninfective enteritis and colitis
K55-K64   Other diseases of intestines
K65-K68   Diseases of peritoneum and retroperitoneum
K70-K77   Diseases of liver
K80-K87   Disorders of gallbladder, biliary tract and pancreas
K90-K95   Other diseases of the digestive system

Diseases of oral cavity and salivary glands (K00-K14)

✓4ᵗʰ **K00   Disorders of tooth development and eruption**
EXCLUDES 2   embedded and impacted teeth (K01.-)

K00.0   Anodontia
Hypodontia
Oligodontia
EXCLUDES 1   acquired absence of teeth (K08.1-)

K00.1   Supernumerary teeth
Distomolar
Fourth molar
Mesiodens
Paramolar
Supplementary teeth
EXCLUDES 2   supernumerary roots (K00.2)

K00.2   Abnormalities of size and form of teeth
Concrescence of teeth
Dens evaginatus
Dens in dente
Dens invaginatus
Enamel pearls
Fusion of teeth
Gemination of teeth
Macrodontia
Microdontia
Peg-shaped [conical] teeth
Supernumerary roots
Taurodontism
Tuberculum paramolare
EXCLUDES 1   abnormalities of teeth due to congenital syphilis (A50.5)
tuberculum Carabelli, which is regarded as a normal variation and should not be coded

K00.3   Mottled teeth
Dental fluorosis
Mottling of enamel
Nonfluoride enamel opacities
EXCLUDES 2   deposits [accretions] on teeth (K03.6)

K00.4   Disturbances in tooth formation
Aplasia and hypoplasia of cementum
Dilaceration of tooth
Enamel hypoplasia (neonatal) (postnatal) (prenatal)
Regional odontodysplasia
Turner's tooth
EXCLUDES 1   Hutchinson's teeth and mulberry molars in congenital syphilis (A50.5)
EXCLUDES 2   mottled teeth (K00.3)

K00.5   Hereditary disturbances in tooth structure, not elsewhere classified
Amelogenesis imperfecta
Dentinogenesis imperfecta
Odontogenesis imperfecta
Dentinal dysplasia
Shell teeth

K00.6   Disturbances in tooth eruption
Dentia praecox
Natal tooth
Neonatal tooth
Premature eruption of tooth
Premature shedding of primary [deciduous] tooth
Prenatal teeth
Retained [persistent] primary tooth
EXCLUDES 2   embedded and impacted teeth (K01.-)

K00.7   Teething syndrome

K00.8   Other disorders of tooth development
Color changes during tooth formation
Intrinsic staining of teeth NOS
EXCLUDES 2   posteruptive color changes (K03.7)

K00.9   Disorder of tooth development, unspecified
Disorder of odontogenesis NOS

✓4ᵗʰ **K01   Embedded and impacted teeth**
EXCLUDES 1   abnormal position of fully erupted teeth (M26.3-)

K01.0   Embedded teeth

K01.1   Impacted teeth

✓4ᵗʰ **K02   Dental caries**
Dental cavities
Tooth decay

K02.3   Arrested dental caries
Arrested coronal and root caries

✓5ᵗʰ **K02.5   Dental caries on pit and fissure surface**
Dental caries on chewing surface of tooth

K02.51   Dental caries on pit and fissure surface limited to enamel
White spot lesions [initial caries] on pit and fissure surface of tooth

K02.52   Dental caries on pit and fissure surface penetrating into dentin

K02.53   Dental caries on pit and fissure surface penetrating into pulp

✓5ᵗʰ **K02.6   Dental caries on smooth surface**

K02.61   Dental caries on smooth surface limited to enamel
White spot lesions [initial caries] on smooth surface of tooth

K02.62   Dental caries on smooth surface penetrating into dentin

K02.63   Dental caries on smooth surface penetrating into pulp

K02.7   Dental root caries

K02.9   Dental caries, unspecified

✓4ᵗʰ **K03   Other diseases of hard tissues of teeth**
EXCLUDES 2   bruxism (F45.8)
dental caries (K02.-)
teeth-grinding NOS (F45.8)

K03.0   Excessive attrition of teeth
Approximal wear of teeth
Occlusal wear of teeth

K03.1   Abrasion of teeth
Dentifrice abrasion of teeth
Habitual abrasion of teeth
Occupational abrasion of teeth
Ritual abrasion of teeth
Traditional abrasion of teeth
Wedge defect NOS

K03.2   Erosion of teeth
Erosion of teeth due to diet
Erosion of teeth due to drugs and medicaments
Erosion of teeth due to persistent vomiting
Erosion of teeth NOS
Idiopathic erosion of teeth
Occupational erosion of teeth

K03.3   Pathological resorption of teeth
Internal granuloma of pulp
Resorption of teeth (external)

K03.4   Hypercementosis
Cementation hyperplasia

K03.5   Ankylosis of teeth

Chapter 11. Diseases of the Digestive System

K03.6   Deposits [accretions] on teeth
Betel deposits [accretions] on teeth
Black deposits [accretions] on teeth
Extrinsic staining of teeth NOS
Green deposits [accretions] on teeth
Materia alba deposits [accretions] on teeth
Orange deposits [accretions] on teeth
Staining of teeth NOS
Subgingival dental calculus
Supragingival dental calculus
Tobacco deposits [accretions] on teeth

K03.7   Posteruptive color changes of dental hard tissues
EXCLUDES 2   deposits [accretions] on teeth (K03.6)

✓5th **K03.8   Other specified diseases of hard tissues of teeth**

K03.81   Cracked tooth
EXCLUDES 1   asymptomatic craze lines in enamel—omit code
broken or fractured tooth due to trauma (S02.5)

K03.89   Other specified diseases of hard tissues of teeth

K03.9   Disease of hard tissues of teeth, unspecified

✓4th **K04   Diseases of pulp and periapical tissues**

K04.0   Pulpitis   CC
Acute pulpitis
Chronic (hyperplastic) (ulcerative) pulpitis
Irreversible pulpitis
Reversible pulpitis
CC Excl: K00.0-K08.9, M26.00-M26.9, M27.61-M27.69

K04.1   Necrosis of pulp
Pulpal gangrene

K04.2   Pulp degeneration
Denticles
Pulpal calcifications
Pulpal stones

K04.3   Abnormal hard tissue formation in pulp
Secondary or irregular dentine

K04.4   Acute apical periodontitis of pulpal origin   CC
Acute apical periodontitis NOS
EXCLUDES 1   acute periodontitis (K05.2-)
CC Excl: See code: K04.0

K04.5   Chronic apical periodontitis
Apical or periapical granuloma
Apical periodontitis NOS
EXCLUDES 1   chronic periodontitis (K05.3-)

K04.6   Periapical abscess with sinus
Dental abscess with sinus
Dentoalveolar abscess with sinus

K04.7   Periapical abscess without sinus
Dental abscess without sinus
Dentoalveolar abscess without sinus
Periapical abscess without sinus

K04.8   Radicular cyst
Apical (periodontal) cyst
Periapical cyst
Residual radicular cyst
EXCLUDES 2   lateral periodontal cyst (K09.0)

✓5th **K04.9   Other and unspecified diseases of pulp and periapical tissues**

K04.90   Unspecified diseases of pulp and periapical tissues

K04.99   Other diseases of pulp and periapical tissues

✓4th **K05   Gingivitis and periodontal diseases**
Use additional code to identify:
alcohol abuse and dependence (F10.-)
exposure to environmental tobacco smoke (Z77.22)
exposure to tobacco smoke in the perinatal period (P96.81)
history of tobacco use (Z87.891)
occupational exposure to environmental tobacco smoke (Z57.31)
tobacco dependence (F17.-)
tobacco use (Z72.0)

✓5th **K05.0   Acute gingivitis**
EXCLUDES 1   acute necrotizing ulcerative gingivitis (A69.1)
herpesviral [herpes simplex] gingivostomatitis (B00.2)

K05.00   Acute gingivitis, plaque induced
Acute gingivitis NOS

K05.01   Acute gingivitis, non-plaque induced

✓5th **K05.1   Chronic gingivitis**
Desquamative gingivitis (chronic)
Gingivitis (chronic) NOS
Hyperplastic gingivitis (chronic)
Simple marginal gingivitis (chronic)
Ulcerative gingivitis (chronic)

K05.10   Chronic gingivitis, plaque induced
Chronic gingivitis NOS
Gingivitis NOS

K05.11   Chronic gingivitis, non-plaque induced

✓5th **K05.2   Aggressive periodontitis**
Acute pericoronitis
EXCLUDES 1   acute apical periodontitis (K04.4)
periapical abscess (K04.7)
periapical abscess with sinus (K04.6)

K05.20   Aggressive periodontitis, unspecified

K05.21   Aggressive periodontitis, localized
Periodontal abscess

K05.22   Aggressive periodontitis, generalized

✓5th **K05.3   Chronic periodontitis**
Chronic pericoronitis
Complex periodontitis
Periodontitis NOS
Simplex periodontitis
EXCLUDES 1   chronic apical periodontitis (K04.5)

K05.30   Chronic periodontitis, unspecified

K05.31   Chronic periodontitis, localized

K05.32   Chronic periodontitis, generalized

K05.4   Periodontosis
Juvenile periodontosis

K05.5   Other periodontal diseases
EXCLUDES 2   leukoplakia of gingiva (K13.21)

K05.6   Periodontal disease, unspecified

✓4th **K06   Other disorders of gingiva and edentulous alveolar ridge**
EXCLUDES 2   acute gingivitis (K05.0)
atrophy of edentulous alveolar ridge (K08.2)
chronic gingivitis (K05.1)
gingivitis NOS (K05.1)

K06.0   Gingival recession
Gingival recession (generalized) (localized) (postinfective) (postprocedural)

K06.1   Gingival enlargement
Gingival fibromatosis

K06.2   Gingival and edentulous alveolar ridge lesions associated with trauma
Irritative hyperplasia of edentulous ridge [denture hyperplasia]
Use additional code (Chapter 20) to identify external cause or denture status (Z97.2)

K06.8   Other specified disorders of gingiva and edentulous alveolar ridge
Fibrous epulis
Flabby alveolar ridge
Giant cell epulis
Peripheral giant cell granuloma of gingiva
Pyogenic granuloma of gingiva
EXCLUDES 2   gingival cyst (K09.0)

K06.9   Disorder of gingiva and edentulous alveolar ridge, unspecified

✓4th **K08   Other disorders of teeth and supporting structures**
EXCLUDES 2   dentofacial anomalies [including malocclusion] (M26.-)
disorders of jaw (M27.-)

K08.0   Exfoliation of teeth due to systemic causes
Code also underlying systemic condition

✓5th **K08.1   Complete loss of teeth**
Acquired loss of teeth, complete
EXCLUDES 1   congenital absence of teeth (K00.0)
exfoliation of teeth due to systemic causes (K08.0)
partial loss of teeth (K08.4-)

✓6th **K08.10   Complete loss of teeth, unspecified cause**

K08.101   Complete loss of teeth, unspecified cause, class I

K08.102   Complete loss of teeth, unspecified cause, class II

K08.103   Complete loss of teeth, unspecified cause, class III

K08.104   Complete loss of teeth, unspecified cause, class IV

N Newborn: 0   P Pediatric: 0-17   M Maternity: 12-55   A Adult: 15-124   MCC Major CC Condition   PDxMCC PDx acts as own MCC   CC CC Condition   PDxCC PDx acts as own CC

660   ICD-10-CM 2016

K08.109   **Complete loss of teeth, unspecified cause, unspecified class**
Edentulism NOS

✓6ᵗʰ K08.11   **Complete loss of teeth** due to trauma

K08.111   **Complete loss of teeth due to trauma, class I**

K08.112   **Complete loss of teeth due to trauma, class II**

K08.113   **Complete loss of teeth due to trauma, class III**

K08.114   **Complete loss of teeth due to trauma, class IV**

K08.119   **Complete loss of teeth due to trauma, unspecified class**

✓6ᵗʰ K08.12   **Complete loss of teeth due to** periodontal diseases

K08.121   **Complete loss of teeth due to periodontal diseases,** class I

K08.122   **Complete loss of teeth due to periodontal diseases,** class II

K08.123   **Complete loss of teeth due to periodontal diseases,** class III

K08.124   **Complete loss of teeth due to periodontal diseases,** class IV

K08.129   **Complete loss of teeth due to periodontal diseases,** unspecified class

✓6ᵗʰ K08.13   **Complete loss of teeth due to** caries

K08.131   **Complete loss of teeth due to caries,** class I

K08.132   **Complete loss of teeth due to caries, class II**

K08.133   **Complete loss of teeth due to caries, class III**

K08.134   **Complete loss of teeth due to caries, class IV**

K08.139   **Complete loss of teeth due to caries,** unspecified class

✓6ᵗʰ K08.19   **Complete loss of teeth due to** other specified cause

K08.191   **Complete loss of teeth due to other specified cause,** class I

K08.192   **Complete loss of teeth due to other specified cause,** class II

K08.193   **Complete loss of teeth due to other specified cause,** class III

K08.194   **Complete loss of teeth due to other specified cause,** class IV

K08.199   **Complete loss of teeth due to other specified cause,** unspecified class

✓5ᵗʰ K08.2   **Atrophy of edentulous alveolar ridge**

K08.20   Unspecified **atrophy of edentulous alveolar ridge**
Atrophy of the mandible NOS
Atrophy of the maxilla NOS

K08.21   Minimal **atrophy of the** mandible
Minimal atrophy of the edentulous mandible

K08.22   Moderate **atrophy of the** mandible
Moderate atrophy of the edentulous mandible

K08.23   Severe **atrophy of the** mandible
Severe atrophy of the edentulous mandible

K08.24   Minimal **atrophy of** maxilla
Minimal atrophy of the edentulous maxilla

K08.25   Moderate **atrophy of the** maxilla
Moderate atrophy of the edentulous maxilla

K08.26   Severe **atrophy of the** maxilla
Severe atrophy of the edentulous maxilla

K08.3   **Retained dental root**

✓5ᵗʰ K08.4   **Partial loss of teeth**
Acquired loss of teeth, partial
EXCLUDES 1 complete loss of teeth (K08.1-)
congenital absence of teeth (K00.0)
EXCLUDES 2 exfoliation of teeth due to systemic causes (K08.0)

✓6ᵗʰ K08.40   **Partial loss of teeth,** unspecified cause

K08.401   **Partial loss of teeth, unspecified cause,** class I

K08.402   **Partial loss of teeth, unspecified cause,** class II

K08.403   **Partial loss of teeth, unspecified cause,** class III

K08.404   **Partial loss of teeth, unspecified cause,** class IV

K08.409   **Partial loss of teeth, unspecified cause, unspecified class**
Tooth extraction status NOS

✓6ᵗʰ K08.41   **Partial loss of teeth due to** trauma

K08.411   **Partial loss of teeth due to trauma, class I**

K08.412   **Partial loss of teeth due to trauma, class II**

K08.413   **Partial loss of teeth due to trauma, class III**

K08.414   **Partial loss of teeth due to trauma, class IV**

K08.419   **Partial loss of teeth due to trauma, unspecified class**

✓6ᵗʰ K08.42   **Partial loss of teeth due to** periodontal diseases

K08.421   **Partial loss of teeth due to periodontal diseases,** class I

K08.422   **Partial loss of teeth due to periodontal diseases,** class II

K08.423   **Partial loss of teeth due to periodontal diseases,** class III

K08.424   **Partial loss of teeth due to periodontal diseases,** class IV

K08.429   **Partial loss of teeth due to periodontal diseases,** unspecified class

✓6ᵗʰ K08.43   **Partial loss of teeth due to** caries

K08.431   **Partial loss of teeth due to caries,** class I

K08.432   **Partial loss of teeth due to caries,** class II

K08.433   **Partial loss of teeth due to caries,** class III

K08.434   **Partial loss of teeth due to caries, class IV**

K08.439   **Partial loss of teeth due to caries, unspecified class**

✓6ᵗʰ K08.49   **Partial loss of teeth due to** other specified cause

K08.491   **Partial loss of teeth due to other specified cause, class I**

K08.492   **Partial loss of teeth due to other specified cause, class II**

K08.493   **Partial loss of teeth due to other specified cause, class III**

K08.494   **Partial loss of teeth due to other specified cause, class IV**

K08.499   **Partial loss of teeth due to other specified cause, unspecified class**

✓5ᵗʰ K08.5   **Unsatisfactory restoration of tooth**
Defective bridge, crown, filling
Defective dental restoration
EXCLUDES 1 dental restoration status (Z98.811)
EXCLUDES 2 endosseous dental implant failure (M27.6-)
unsatisfactory endodontic treatment (M27.5-)

K08.50   **Unsatisfactory restoration of tooth, unspecified**
Defective dental restoration NOS

K08.51   **Open restoration margins of tooth**
Dental restoration failure of marginal integrity
Open margin on tooth restoration
Poor gingival margin to tooth restoration

K08.52   **Unrepairable overhanging of dental restorative materials**
Overhanging of tooth restoration

✓6ᵗʰ K08.53   **Fractured dental restorative material**
EXCLUDES 1 cracked tooth (K03.81)
traumatic fracture of tooth (S02.5)

K08.530   **Fractured dental restorative material** without loss of material

K08.531   **Fractured dental restorative material** with loss of material

K08.539   **Fractured dental restorative material, unspecified**

K08.54   **Contour of existing restoration of tooth biologically incompatible with oral health**
Dental restoration failure of periodontal anatomical integrity
Unacceptable contours of existing restoration of tooth
Unacceptable morphology of existing restoration of tooth

K08.55   **Allergy to existing dental restorative material**
Use additional code to identify the specific type of allergy

✓ Additional Character Required   ✓x7ᵗʰ Placeholder Alert   Unacceptable PDx   Manifestation   Hospital Acquired Condition   **EXCLUDES 1** Not Coded Here   **EXCLUDES 2** Not Included Here

K08.56   **Poor aesthetic of existing restoration of tooth**
Dental restoration aesthetically inadequate or displeasing

K08.59   **Other unsatisfactory restoration of tooth**
Other defective dental restoration

K08.8   **Other specified disorders of teeth and supporting structures**
Enlargement of alveolar ridge NOS
Irregular alveolar process
Toothache NOS

K08.9   **Disorder of teeth and supporting structures, unspecified**

√4ᵗʰ **K09**   **Cysts of oral region, not elsewhere classified**
INCLUDES   lesions showing histological features both of aneurysmal cyst and of another fibro-osseous lesion
EXCLUDES 2   *cysts of jaw (M27.0-, M27.4-)*
radicular cyst (K04.8)

K09.0   **Developmental odontogenic cysts**
Dentigerous cyst
Eruption cyst
Follicular cyst
Gingival cyst
Lateral periodontal cyst
Primordial cyst
EXCLUDES 2   *keratocysts (D16.4, D16.5)*
odontogenic keratocystic tumors (D16.4, D16.5)

K09.1   **Developmental (nonodontogenic) cysts of oral region**
Cyst (of) incisive canal
Cyst (of) palatine of papilla
Globulomaxillary cyst
Median palatal cyst
Nasoalveolar cyst
Nasolabial cyst
Nasopalatine duct cyst

K09.8   **Other cysts of oral region, not elsewhere classified**
Dermoid cyst
Epidermoid cyst
Lymphoepithelial cyst
Epstein's pearl

K09.9   **Cyst of oral region, unspecified**

√4ᵗʰ **K11**   **Diseases of salivary glands**
Use additional code to identify:
alcohol abuse and dependence (F10.-)
exposure to environmental tobacco smoke (Z77.22)
exposure to tobacco smoke in the perinatal period (P96.81)
history of tobacco use (Z87.891)
occupational exposure to environmental tobacco smoke (Z57.31)
tobacco dependence (F17.-)
tobacco use (Z72.0)

K11.0   **Atrophy of salivary gland**

K11.1   **Hypertrophy of salivary gland**

√5ᵗʰ **K11.2**   **Sialoadenitis**
Parotitis
EXCLUDES 1   *epidemic parotitis (B26.-)*
mumps (B26.-)
uveoparotid fever [Heerfordt] (D86.89)

     K11.20   **Sialoadenitis, unspecified**

     K11.21   **Acute sialoadenitis**
EXCLUDES 1   *acute recurrent sialoadenitis (K11.22)*

     K11.22   **Acute recurrent sialoadenitis**

     K11.23   **Chronic sialoadenitis**

K11.3   **Abscess of salivary gland**   CC
CC Excl: K11.0-K11.9, K31.89-K31.9, K92.81, R68.2

K11.4   **Fistula of salivary gland**   CC
EXCLUDES 1   *congenital fistula of salivary gland (Q38.4)*
CC Excl: See code: K11.3

K11.5   **Sialolithiasis**
Calculus of salivary gland or duct
Stone of salivary gland or duct

K11.6   **Mucocele of salivary gland**
Mucous extravasation cyst of salivary gland
Mucous retention cyst of salivary gland
Ranula

K11.7   **Disturbances of salivary secretion**
Hypoptyalism
Ptyalism
Xerostomia
EXCLUDES 2   *dry mouth NOS (R68.2)*

K11.8   **Other diseases of salivary glands**
Benign lymphoepithelial lesion of salivary gland
Mikulicz' disease
Necrotizing sialometaplasia
Sialectasia
Stenosis of salivary duct
Stricture of salivary duct
EXCLUDES 1   *sicca syndrome [Sjögren] (M35.0-)*

K11.9   **Disease of salivary gland, unspecified**
Sialoadenopathy NOS

√4ᵗʰ **K12**   **Stomatitis and related lesions**
Use additional code to identify:
alcohol abuse and dependence (F10.-)
exposure to environmental tobacco smoke (Z77.22)
exposure to tobacco smoke in the perinatal period (P96.81)
history of tobacco use (Z87.891)
occupational exposure to environmental tobacco smoke (Z57.31)
tobacco dependence (F17.-)
tobacco use (Z72.0)
EXCLUDES 1   *cancrum oris (A69.0)*
cheilitis (K13.0)
gangrenous stomatitis (A69.0)
herpesviral [herpes simplex] gingivostomatitis (B00.2)
noma (A69.0)

K12.0   **Recurrent oral aphthae**
Aphthous stomatitis (major) (minor)
Bednar's aphthae
Periadenitis mucosa necrotica recurrens
Recurrent aphthous ulcer
Stomatitis herpetiformis

K12.1   **Other forms of stomatitis**
Stomatitis NOS
Denture stomatitis
Ulcerative stomatitis
Vesicular stomatitis
EXCLUDES 1   *acute necrotizing ulcerative stomatitis (A69.1)*
Vincent's stomatitis (A69.1)

K12.2   **Cellulitis and abscess of mouth**   CC
Cellulitis of mouth (floor)
Submandibular abscess
EXCLUDES 2   *abscess of salivary gland (K11.3)*
abscess of tongue (K14.0)
periapical abscess (K04.6-K04.7)
periodontal abscess (K05.21)
peritonsillar abscess (J36)
CC Excl: K12.1-K12.39, K14.0, K14.2

√5ᵗʰ **K12.3**   **Oral mucositis (ulcerative)**
Mucositis (oral) (oropharyneal)
EXCLUDES 2   *gastrointestinal mucositis (ulcerative) (K92.81)*
mucositis (ulcerative) of vagina and vulva (N76.81)
nasal mucositis (ulcerative) (J34.81)

     K12.30   **Oral mucositis (ulcerative), unspecified**

     K12.31   **Oral mucositis (ulcerative) due to antineoplastic therapy**
Use additional code for adverse effect, if applicable, to identify antineoplastic and immunosuppressive drugs (T45.1X5)
Use additional code for other antineoplastic therapy, such as:
radiological procedure and radiotherapy (Y84.2)

     K12.32   **Oral mucositis (ulcerative) due to other drugs**
Use additional code for adverse effect, if applicable, to identify drug (T36-T50 with fifth or sixth character 5)

     K12.33   **Oral mucositis (ulcerative) due to radiation**
Use additional external cause code (W88-W90, X39.0-) to identify cause

     K12.39   **Other oral mucositis (ulcerative)**
Viral oral mucositis (ulcerative)

☑4ᵗʰ K13 Other diseases of lip and oral mucosa

INCLUDES   epithelial disturbances of tongue

Use additional code to identify:
- alcohol abuse and dependence (F10.-)
- exposure to environmental tobacco smoke (Z77.22)
- exposure to tobacco smoke in the perinatal period (P96.81)
- history of tobacco use (Z87.891)
- occupational exposure to environmental tobacco smoke (Z57.31)
- tobacco dependence (F17.-)
- tobacco use (Z72.0)

EXCLUDES 2   certain disorders of gingiva and edentulous alveolar ridge (K05-K06)
- cysts of oral region (K09.-)
- diseases of tongue (K14.-)
- stomatitis and related lesions (K12.-)

K13.0 Diseases of lips
- Abscess of lips
- Angular cheilitis
- Cellulitis of lips
- Cheilitis NOS
- Cheilodynia
- Cheilosis
- Exfoliative cheilitis
- Fistula of lips
- Glandular cheilitis
- Hypertrophy of lips
- Perlèche NEC

EXCLUDES 1   ariboflavinosis (E53.0)
- cheilitis due to radiation-related disorders (L55-L59)
- congenital fistula of lips (Q38.0)
- congenital hypertrophy of lips (Q18.6)
- Perlèche due to candidiasis (B37.83)
- Perlèche due to riboflavin deficiency (E53.0)

K13.1 Cheek and lip biting

☑5ᵗʰ K13.2 Leukoplakia and other disturbances of oral epithelium, including tongue

EXCLUDES 1   carcinoma in situ of oral epithelium (D00.0-)
- hairy leukoplakia (K13.3)

K13.21 Leukoplakia of oral mucosa, including tongue
- Leukokeratosis of oral mucosa
- Leukoplakia of gingiva, lips, tongue

EXCLUDES 1   hairy leukoplakia (K13.3)
- leukokeratosis nicotina palati (K13.24)

K13.22 Minimal keratinized residual ridge mucosa
- Minimal keratinization of alveolar ridge mucosa

K13.23 Excessive keratinized residual ridge mucosa
- Excessive keratinization of alveolar ridge mucosa

K13.24 Leukokeratosis nicotina palati
- Smoker's palate

K13.29 Other disturbances of oral epithelium, including tongue
- Erythroplakia of mouth or tongue
- Focal epithelial hyperplasia of mouth or tongue
- Leukoedema of mouth or tongue
- Other oral epithelium disturbances

K13.3 Hairy leukoplakia

K13.4 Granuloma and granuloma-like lesions of oral mucosa
- Eosinophilic granuloma
- Granuloma pyogenicum
- Verrucous xanthoma

K13.5 Oral submucous fibrosis
- Submucous fibrosis of tongue

K13.6 Irritative hyperplasia of oral mucosa

EXCLUDES 2   irritative hyperplasia of edentulous ridge [denture hyperplasia] (K06.2)

☑5ᵗʰ K13.7 Other and unspecified lesions of oral mucosa

K13.70 Unspecified lesions of oral mucosa

K13.79 Other lesions of oral mucosa
- Focal oral mucinosis

☑4ᵗʰ K14 Diseases of tongue

Use additional code to identify:
- alcohol abuse and dependence (F10.-)
- exposure to environmental tobacco smoke (Z77.22)
- history of tobacco use (Z87.891)
- occupational exposure to environmental tobacco smoke (Z57.31)
- tobacco dependence (F17.-)
- tobacco use (Z72.0)

EXCLUDES 2   erythroplakia (K13.29)
- focal epithelial hyperplasia (K13.29)
- leukedema of tongue (K13.29)
- leukoplakia of tongue (K13.21)
- hairy leukoplakia (K13.3)
- macroglossia (congenital) (Q38.2)
- submucous fibrosis of tongue (K13.5)

K14.0 Glossitis
- Abscess of tongue
- Ulceration (traumatic) of tongue

EXCLUDES 1   atrophic glossitis (K14.4)

K14.1 Geographic tongue
- Benign migratory glossitis
- Glossitis areata exfoliativa

K14.2 Median rhomboid glossitis

K14.3 Hypertrophy of tongue papillae
- Black hairy tongue
- Coated tongue
- Hypertrophy of foliate papillae
- Lingua villosa nigra

K14.4 Atrophy of tongue papillae
- Atrophic glossitis

K14.5 Plicated tongue
- Fissured tongue
- Furrowed tongue
- Scrotal tongue

EXCLUDES 1   fissured tongue, congenital (Q38.3)

K14.6 Glossodynia
- Glossopyrosis
- Painful tongue

K14.8 Other diseases of tongue
- Atrophy of tongue
- Crenated tongue
- Enlargement of tongue
- Glossocele
- Glossoptosis
- Hypertrophy of tongue

K14.9 Disease of tongue, unspecified
- Glossopathy NOS

Diseases of esophagus, stomach and duodenum (K20-K31)

EXCLUDES 2   hiatus hernia (K44.-)

☑4ᵗʰ K20 Esophagitis

Use additional code to identify:
- alcohol abuse and dependence (F10.-)

EXCLUDES 1   erosion of esophagus (K22.1-)
- esophagitis with gastro-esophageal reflux disease (K21.0)
- reflux esophagitis (K21.0)
- ulcerative esophagitis (K22.1-)

EXCLUDES 2   eosinophilic gastritis or gastroenteritis (K52.81)

K20.0 Eosinophilic esophagitis

K20.8 Other esophagitis
- Abscess of esophagus

K20.9 Esophagitis, unspecified
- Esophagitis NOS

☑4ᵗʰ K21 Gastro-esophageal reflux disease

EXCLUDES 1   newborn esophageal reflux (P78.83)

K21.0 Gastro-esophageal reflux disease with esophagitis
- Reflux esophagitis

K21.9 Gastro-esophageal reflux disease without esophagitis
- Esophageal reflux NOS

☑4ᵗʰ K22 Other diseases of esophagus

EXCLUDES 2   esophageal varices (I85.-)

K22.0 Achalasia of cardia
- Achalasia NOS
- Cardiospasm

EXCLUDES 1   congenital cardiospasm (Q39.5)

☑ Additional Character Required   ☑×7ᵗʰ Placeholder Alert   Unacceptable PDx   Manifestation   Hospital Acquired Condition   EXCLUDES 1 Not Coded Here   EXCLUDES 2 Not Included Here

Chapter 11. Diseases of the Digestive System

K22.1–K27.9

✓5ᵗʰ **K22.1** **Ulcer of esophagus**
Barrett's ulcer
Erosion of esophagus
Fungal ulcer of esophagus
Peptic ulcer of esophagus
Ulcer of esophagus due to ingestion of chemicals
Ulcer of esophagus due to ingestion of drugs and medicaments
Ulcerative esophagitis
Code first poisoning due to drug or toxin, if applicable (T36-T65 with fifth or sixth character 1-4 or 6)
Use additional code for adverse effect, if applicable, to identify drug (T36-T50 with fifth or sixth character 5)
EXCLUDES 1   *Barrett's esophagus (K22.7-)*

     K22.10 **Ulcer of esophagus without bleeding**   CC
         Ulcer of esophagus NOS
         CC Excl: K22.11, K22.8-K23, K31.82

     K22.11 **Ulcer of esophagus with bleeding**   MCC
         EXCLUDES 2   *bleeding esophageal varices (I85.01, I85.11)*
         CC Excl: E16.4, I85.01, K22.10-K22.11, K22.6-K22.719, K25.0-K28.9, K29.01, K29.21, K29.31, K29.41, K29.51, K29.61, K29.71, K29.81, K29.91, K31.811, K31.89-K31.9, K55.21, K57.01, K57.11, K57.13, K57.21, K57.31, K57.33, K57.41, K57.51, K57.53, K57.81, K57.91, K57.93, K62.5, K92.0-K92.81

K22.2 **Esophageal obstruction**
Compression of esophagus
Constriction of esophagus
Stenosis of esophagus
Stricture of esophagus
EXCLUDES 1   *congenital stenosis or stricture of esophagus (Q39.3)*

K22.3 **Perforation of esophagus**   MCC
Rupture of esophagus
EXCLUDES 1   *traumatic perforation of (thoracic) esophagus (S27.8-)*
CC Excl: K21.9, K22.3, K22.6, K22.8-K23

K22.4 **Dyskinesia of esophagus**
Corkscrew esophagus
Diffuse esophageal spasm
Spasm of esophagus
EXCLUDES 1   *cardiospasm (K22.0)*

K22.5 **Diverticulum of esophagus, acquired**
Esophageal pouch, acquired
EXCLUDES 1   *diverticulum of esophagus (congenital) (Q39.6)*

K22.6 **Gastro-esophageal laceration-hemorrhage syndrome**   MCC
Mallory-Weiss syndrome
CC Excl: E16.4, I85.01, K21.9, K22.10-K22.11, K22.3, K22.6-K28.9, K29.01, K29.21, K29.31, K29.41, K29.51, K29.61, K29.71, K29.81, K29.91, K31.811, K55.21, K57.01, K57.11, K57.13, K57.21, K57.31, K57.33, K57.41, K57.51, K57.53, K57.81, K57.91, K57.93, K62.5, K92.0-K92.2

✓5ᵗʰ **K22.7** **Barrett's esophagus**
Barrett's disease
Barrett's syndrome
EXCLUDES 1   *Barrett's ulcer (K22.1)*
               malignant neoplasm of esophagus (C15.-)

     K22.70 **Barrett's esophagus without dysplasia**
         Barrett's esophagus NOS

     ✓6ᵗʰ **K22.71** **Barrett's esophagus with dysplasia**
         K22.710 **Barrett's esophagus with low grade dysplasia**
         K22.711 **Barrett's esophagus with high grade dysplasia**
         K22.719 **Barrett's esophagus with dysplasia, unspecified**

K22.8 **Other specified diseases of esophagus**
Hemorrhage of esophagus NOS
EXCLUDES 2   *esophageal varices (I85.-)*
              Paterson-Kelly syndrome (D50.1)

K22.9 **Disease of esophagus, unspecified**

K23 ***Disorders of esophagus in diseases classified elsewhere***
Code first underlying disease, such as:
congenital syphilis (A50.5)
EXCLUDES 1   *late syphilis (A52.79)*
              megaesophagus due to Chagas' disease (B57.31)
              tuberculosis (A18.83)

✓4ᵗʰ **K25** **Gastric ulcer**
INCLUDES   erosion (acute) of stomach
            pylorus ulcer (peptic)
            stomach ulcer (peptic)
Use additional code to identify:
alcohol abuse and dependence (F10.-)
EXCLUDES 1   *acute gastritis (K29.0-)*
              peptic ulcer NOS (K27.-)

CC Excl: For CC/MCC codes in category K25, unless otherwise noted: See code: K22.11

K25.0 **Acute gastric ulcer with hemorrhage**   MCC
K25.1 **Acute gastric ulcer with perforation**   MCC
K25.2 **Acute gastric ulcer with both hemorrhage and perforation**   MCC
K25.3 **Acute gastric ulcer without hemorrhage or perforation**   CC
K25.4 **Chronic or unspecified gastric ulcer with hemorrhage**   MCC
K25.5 **Chronic or unspecified gastric ulcer with perforation**   MCC
K25.6 **Chronic or unspecified gastric ulcer with both hemorrhage and perforation**   MCC
K25.7 **Chronic gastric ulcer without hemorrhage or perforation**
K25.9 **Gastric ulcer, unspecified as acute or chronic, without hemorrhage or perforation**

✓4ᵗʰ **K26** **Duodenal ulcer**
INCLUDES   erosion (acute) of duodenum
            duodenum ulcer (peptic)
            postpyloric ulcer (peptic)
Use additional code to identify:
alcohol abuse and dependence (F10.-)
EXCLUDES 1   *peptic ulcer NOS (K27.-)*

CC Excl: For CC/MCC codes in category K26, unless otherwise noted: E16.4, I85.01, K22.10-K22.11, K22.6-K22.719, K25.0-K28.9, K29.01, K29.21, K29.31, K29.41, K29.51, K29.61, K29.71, K29.81, K29.91, K31.5, K31.811, K31.89-K31.9, K55.21, K57.01, K57.11, K57.13, K57.21, K57.31, K57.33, K57.41, K57.51, K57.53, K57.81, K57.91, K57.93, K62.5, K92.0-K92.81

K26.0 **Acute duodenal ulcer with hemorrhage**   MCC
K26.1 **Acute duodenal ulcer with perforation**   MCC
K26.2 **Acute duodenal ulcer with both hemorrhage and perforation**   MCC
K26.3 **Acute duodenal ulcer without hemorrhage or perforation**   CC
     CC Excl: E16.4, I85.01, K22.6, K25.0-K28.9, K29.01, K29.21, K29.31, K29.41, K29.51, K29.61, K29.71, K29.81, K29.91, K31.5, K31.811, K31.82, K31.89-K31.9, K55.21, K57.01, K57.11, K57.13, K57.21, K57.31, K57.33, K57.41, K57.51, K57.53, K57.81, K57.91, K57.93, K62.5, K92.0-K92.81
K26.4 **Chronic or unspecified duodenal ulcer with hemorrhage**   MCC
K26.5 **Chronic or unspecified duodenal ulcer with perforation**   MCC
K26.6 **Chronic or unspecified duodenal ulcer with both hemorrhage and perforation**   MCC
K26.7 **Chronic duodenal ulcer without hemorrhage or perforation**
K26.9 **Duodenal ulcer, unspecified as acute or chronic, without hemorrhage or perforation**

✓4ᵗʰ **K27** **Peptic ulcer, site unspecified**
INCLUDES   gastroduodenal ulcer NOS
            peptic ulcer NOS
Use additional code to identify:
alcohol abuse and dependence (F10.-)
EXCLUDES 1   *peptic ulcer of newborn (P78.82)*

CC Excl: For CC/MCC codes in category K27, unless otherwise noted: See code: K26

K27.0 **Acute peptic ulcer, site unspecified, with hemorrhage**   MCC
K27.1 **Acute peptic ulcer, site unspecified, with perforation**   MCC
K27.2 **Acute peptic ulcer, site unspecified, with both hemorrhage and perforation**   MCC
K27.3 **Acute peptic ulcer, site unspecified, without hemorrhage or perforation**   CC
K27.4 **Chronic or unspecified peptic ulcer, site unspecified, with hemorrhage**   MCC
K27.5 **Chronic or unspecified peptic ulcer, site unspecified, with perforation**   MCC
K27.6 **Chronic or unspecified peptic ulcer, site unspecified, with both hemorrhage and perforation**   MCC
K27.7 **Chronic peptic ulcer, site unspecified, without hemorrhage or perforation**
K27.9 **Peptic ulcer, site unspecified, unspecified as acute or chronic, without hemorrhage or perforation**

N Newborn: 0   P Pediatric: 0-17   M Maternity: 12-55   A Adult: 15-124   MCC Major CC Condition   PDxMCC PDx acts as own MCC   CC CC Condition   PDxCC PDx acts as own CC

664   ICD-10-CM 2016

✓4th **K28　Gastrojejunal ulcer**
　　INCLUDES　anastomotic ulcer (peptic) or erosion
　　　　　　　gastrocolic ulcer (peptic) or erosion
　　　　　　　gastrointestinal ulcer (peptic) or erosion
　　　　　　　gastrojejunal ulcer (peptic) or erosion
　　　　　　　jejunal ulcer (peptic) or erosion
　　　　　　　marginal ulcer (peptic) or erosion
　　　　　　　stomal ulcer (peptic) or erosion
　　Use additional code to identify:
　　　alcohol abuse and dependence (F10.-)
　　EXCLUDES 1　primary ulcer of small intestine (K63.3)

　　CC Excl: For CC/MCC codes in category K28, unless otherwise
　　noted: See code: K22.11

K28.0　Acute gastrojejunal ulcer with hemorrhage　　MCC
K28.1　Acute gastrojejunal ulcer with perforation　　MCC
K28.2　Acute gastrojejunal ulcer with both hemorrhage and　　MCC
　　　　perforation
K28.3　Acute gastrojejunal ulcer without hemorrhage or　　CC
　　　　perforation
K28.4　Chronic or unspecified gastrojejunal ulcer with　　MCC
　　　　hemorrhage
K28.5　Chronic or unspecified gastrojejunal ulcer with　　MCC
　　　　perforation
K28.6　Chronic or unspecified gastrojejunal ulcer with both　　MCC
　　　　hemorrhage and perforation
K28.7　Chronic gastrojejunal ulcer without hemorrhage or
　　　　perforation
K28.9　Gastrojejunal ulcer, unspecified as acute or chronic, without
　　　　hemorrhage or perforation

✓4th **K29　Gastritis and duodenitis**
　　EXCLUDES 1　eosinophilic gastritis or gastroenteritis (K52.81)
　　　　　　　Zollinger-Ellison syndrome (E16.4)

　　CC Excl: For MCC codes in category K29, unless otherwise
　　noted: E16.4, I85.01, K22.10-K22.11, K22.6-K22.719, K25.0-K28.9,
　　K29.01, K29.21, K29.31, K29.41, K29.51, K29.61, K29.71, K29.81,
　　K29.91, K31.811, K55.21, K57.01, K57.11, K57.13, K57.21, K57.31,
　　K57.33, K57.41, K57.51, K57.53, K57.81, K57.91, K57.93, K62.5,
　　K92.0-K92.2

✓5th **K29.0**　Acute gastritis
　　　　Use additional code to identify:
　　　　　alcohol abuse and dependence (F10.-)
　　　　EXCLUDES 1　erosion (acute) of stomach (K25.-)
　　　　K29.00　Acute gastritis without bleeding
　　　　K29.01　Acute gastritis with bleeding　　MCC

✓5th **K29.2**　Alcoholic gastritis
　　　　Use additional code to identify:
　　　　　alcohol abuse and dependence (F10.-)
　　　　K29.20　Alcoholic gastritis without bleeding
　　　　K29.21　Alcoholic gastritis with bleeding　　MCC

✓5th **K29.3**　Chronic superficial gastritis
　　　　K29.30　Chronic superficial gastritis without bleeding
　　　　K29.31　Chronic superficial gastritis with bleeding　　MCC

✓5th **K29.4**　Chronic atrophic gastritis
　　　　Gastric atrophy
　　　　K29.40　Chronic atrophic gastritis without bleeding
　　　　K29.41　Chronic atrophic gastritis with bleeding　　MCC

✓5th **K29.5**　Unspecified chronic gastritis
　　　　Chronic antral gastritis
　　　　Chronic fundal gastritis
　　　　K29.50　Unspecified chronic gastritis without bleeding
　　　　K29.51　Unspecified chronic gastritis with bleeding　　MCC

✓5th **K29.6**　Other gastritis
　　　　Giant hypertrophic gastritis
　　　　Granulomatous gastritis
　　　　Ménétrier's disease
　　　　K29.60　Other gastritis without bleeding
　　　　K29.61　Other gastritis with bleeding　　MCC

✓5th **K29.7**　Gastritis, unspecified
　　　　K29.70　Gastritis, unspecified, without bleeding
　　　　K29.71　Gastritis, unspecified, with bleeding　　MCC

✓5th **K29.8**　Duodenitis
　　　　K29.80　Duodenitis without bleeding
　　　　K29.81　Duodenitis with bleeding　　MCC

✓5th **K29.9**　Gastroduodenitis, unspecified
　　　　K29.90　Gastroduodenitis, unspecified, without bleeding
　　　　K29.91　Gastroduodenitis, unspecified, with bleeding　　MCC

K30　Functional dyspepsia
　　Indigestion
　　EXCLUDES 1　dyspepsia NOS (R10.13)
　　　　　　　heartburn (R12)
　　　　　　　nervous dyspepsia (F45.8)
　　　　　　　neurotic dyspepsia (F45.8)
　　　　　　　psychogenic dyspepsia (F45.8)

✓4th **K31　Other diseases of stomach and duodenum**
　　INCLUDES　functional disorders of stomach
　　EXCLUDES 2　diabetic gastroparesis (E08.43, E09.43, E10.43, E11.43, E13.43)
　　　　　　　diverticulum of duodenum (K57.00-K57.13)

K31.0　Acute dilatation of stomach　　CC
　　　　Acute distention of stomach
　　　　CC Excl: K31.0
K31.1　Adult hypertrophic pyloric stenosis　　CC A
　　　　Pyloric stenosis NOS
　　　　EXCLUDES 1　congenital or infantile pyloric stenosis (Q40.0)
　　　　CC Excl: K30, K31.1, K31.5, K31.84, Q38.5, Q40.0, Q40.8-Q41.9,
　　　　Q43.4-Q43.9
K31.2　Hourglass stricture and stenosis of stomach
　　　　EXCLUDES 1　congenital hourglass stomach (Q40.2)
　　　　　　　　hourglass contraction of stomach (K31.89)
K31.3　Pylorospasm, not elsewhere classified
　　　　EXCLUDES 1　congenital or infantile pylorospasm (Q40.0)
　　　　　　　　neurotic pylorospasm (F45.8)
　　　　　　　　psychogenic pylorospasm (F45.8)
K31.4　Gastric diverticulum
　　　　EXCLUDES 1　congenital diverticulum of stomach (Q40.2)
K31.5　Obstruction of duodenum　　CC
　　　　Constriction of duodenum
　　　　Duodenal ileus (chronic)
　　　　Stenosis of duodenum
　　　　Stricture of duodenum
　　　　Volvulus of duodenum
　　　　EXCLUDES 1　congenital stenosis of duodenum (Q41.0)
　　　　CC Excl: K31.5, Q38.5, Q40.8-Q41.9, Q43.4-Q43.9
K31.6　Fistula of stomach and duodenum　　CC
　　　　Gastrocolic fistula
　　　　Gastrojejunocolic fistula
　　　　CC Excl: K31.6, Q38.5, Q40.8-Q40.9, Q43.4-Q43.9
K31.7　Polyp of stomach and duodenum
　　　　EXCLUDES 1　adenomatous polyp of stomach (D13.1)

✓5th **K31.8**　Other specified diseases of stomach and duodenum
　　✓6th **K31.81**　Angiodysplasia of stomach and duodenum
　　　　　　K31.811　Angiodysplasia of stomach and　　MCC
　　　　　　　　　　duodenum with bleeding
　　　　　　　　　　CC Excl: See code: K29
　　　　　　K31.819　Angiodysplasia of stomach and
　　　　　　　　　　duodenum without bleeding
　　　　　　　　　　Angiodysplasia of stomach and duodenum
　　　　　　　　　　NOS
　　　　K31.82　Dieulafoy lesion (hemorrhagic) of stomach and　　MCC
　　　　　　　　duodenum
　　　　　　EXCLUDES 2　Dieulafoy lesion of intestine (K63.81)
　　　　　　CC Excl: E16.4, I85.01, K22.10-K22.11, K22.6-K22.719,
　　　　　　K25.0-K28.9, K29.01, K29.21, K29.31, K29.41, K29.51,
　　　　　　K29.61, K29.71, K29.81, K29.91, K31.811, K31.82, K55.21,
　　　　　　K57.01, K57.11, K57.13, K57.21, K57.31, K57.33, K57.41,
　　　　　　K57.51, K57.53, K57.81, K57.91, K57.93, K62.5, K92.0-
　　　　　　K92.2
　　　　K31.83　Achlorhydria
　　　　K31.84　Gastroparesis
　　　　　　Gastroparalysis
　　　　　　Code first underlying disease, if known, such as:
　　　　　　　anorexia nervosa (F50.0-)
　　　　　　　diabetes mellitus (E08.43, E09.43, E10.43, E11.43,
　　　　　　　E13.43)
　　　　　　　scleroderma (M34.-)
　　　　　　AHA: 2013, 4Q, 114
　　　　K31.89　Other diseases of stomach and duodenum
K31.9　Disease of stomach and duodenum, unspecified

Diseases of appendix (K35-K38)

✓4ᵗʰ K35 Acute appendicitis

> **CC Excl: For CC/MCC codes in category K35, unless otherwise noted:** K31.89-K38.9, K92.81

K35.2 Acute appendicitis with generalized peritonitis `MCC`
Appendicitis (acute) with generalized (diffuse) peritonitis following rupture or perforation of appendix
Perforated appendix NOS
Ruptured appendix NOS

K35.3 Acute appendicitis with localized peritonitis `MCC`
Acute appendicitis with or without perforation or rupture NOS
Acute appendicitis with or without perforation or rupture with localized peritonitis
Acute appendicitis with peritoneal abscess

✓5ᵗʰ K35.8 Other and unspecified acute appendicitis

K35.80 Unspecified acute appendicitis `CC`
Acute appendicitis NOS
Acute appendicitis without (localized) (generalized) peritonitis

K35.89 Other acute appendicitis `CC`

K36 Other appendicitis
Chronic appendicitis
Recurrent appendicitis

K37 Unspecified appendicitis
> **EXCLUDES 1** unspecified appendicitis with peritonitis (K35.2-K35.3)

✓4ᵗʰ K38 Other diseases of appendix

K38.0 Hyperplasia of appendix

K38.1 Appendicular concretions
Fecalith of appendix
Stercolith of appendix

K38.2 Diverticulum of appendix

K38.3 Fistula of appendix

K38.8 Other specified diseases of appendix
Intussusception of appendix

K38.9 Disease of appendix, unspecified

Hernia (K40-K46)

> **NOTE** Hernia with both gangrene and obstruction is classified to hernia with gangrene.
> **INCLUDES** acquired hernia
> congenital [except diaphragmatic or hiatus] hernia
> recurrent hernia

✓4ᵗʰ K40 Inguinal hernia
> **INCLUDES** bubonocele
> direct inguinal hernia
> double inguinal hernia
> indirect inguinal hernia
> inguinal hernia NOS
> oblique inguinal hernia
> scrotal hernia

> **CC Excl: For CC/MCC codes in category K40, unless otherwise noted:** K31.89-K31.9, K40.00-K40.91, K45.0, K45.8-K46.0, K92.81

✓5ᵗʰ K40.0 Bilateral inguinal hernia, with obstruction, without gangrene
Inguinal hernia (bilateral) causing obstruction without gangrene
Incarcerated inguinal hernia (bilateral) without gangrene
Irreducible inguinal hernia (bilateral) without gangrene
Strangulated inguinal hernia (bilateral) without gangrene

K40.00 Bilateral inguinal hernia, with obstruction, without gangrene, not specified as recurrent `CC`
Bilateral inguinal hernia, with obstruction, without gangrene NOS

K40.01 Bilateral inguinal hernia, with obstruction, without gangrene, recurrent `CC`

✓5ᵗʰ K40.1 Bilateral inguinal hernia, with gangrene

K40.10 Bilateral inguinal hernia, with gangrene, not specified as recurrent `MCC`
Bilateral inguinal hernia, with gangrene NOS

K40.11 Bilateral inguinal hernia, with gangrene, recurrent `MCC`

✓5ᵗʰ K40.2 Bilateral inguinal hernia, without obstruction or gangrene

K40.20 Bilateral inguinal hernia, without obstruction or gangrene, not specified as recurrent
Bilateral inguinal hernia NOS

K40.21 Bilateral inguinal hernia, without obstruction or gangrene, recurrent

✓5ᵗʰ K40.3 Unilateral inguinal hernia, with obstruction, without gangrene
Inguinal hernia (unilateral) causing obstruction without gangrene
Incarcerated inguinal hernia (unilateral) without gangrene
Irreducible inguinal hernia (unilateral) without gangrene
Strangulated inguinal hernia (unilateral) without gangrene

K40.30 Unilateral inguinal hernia, with obstruction, without gangrene, not specified as recurrent `CC`
Inguinal hernia, with obstruction NOS
Unilateral inguinal hernia, with obstruction, without gangrene NOS

K40.31 Unilateral inguinal hernia, with obstruction, without gangrene, recurrent `CC`

✓5ᵗʰ K40.4 Unilateral inguinal hernia, with gangrene

K40.40 Unilateral inguinal hernia, with gangrene, not specified as recurrent `MCC`
Inguinal hernia with gangrene NOS
Unilateral inguinal hernia with gangrene NOS

K40.41 Unilateral inguinal hernia, with gangrene, recurrent `MCC`

✓5ᵗʰ K40.9 Unilateral inguinal hernia, without obstruction or gangrene

K40.90 Unilateral inguinal hernia, without obstruction or gangrene, not specified as recurrent
Inguinal hernia NOS
Unilateral inguinal hernia NOS

K40.91 Unilateral inguinal hernia, without obstruction or gangrene, recurrent

✓4ᵗʰ K41 Femoral hernia

> **CC Excl: For CC/MCC codes in category K41, unless otherwise noted:** K31.89-K31.9, K41.00-K41.91, K45.0, K45.8-K46.0, K92.81

✓5ᵗʰ K41.0 Bilateral femoral hernia, with obstruction, without gangrene
Femoral hernia (bilateral) causing obstruction, without gangrene
Incarcerated femoral hernia (bilateral), without gangrene
Irreducible femoral hernia (bilateral), without gangrene
Strangulated femoral hernia (bilateral), without gangrene

K41.00 Bilateral femoral hernia, with obstruction, without gangrene, not specified as recurrent `CC`
Bilateral femoral hernia, with obstruction, without gangrene NOS

K41.01 Bilateral femoral hernia, with obstruction, without gangrene, recurrent `CC`

✓5ᵗʰ K41.1 Bilateral femoral hernia, with gangrene

K41.10 Bilateral femoral hernia, with gangrene, not specified as recurrent `MCC`
Bilateral femoral hernia, with gangrene NOS
CC Excl: K31.89-K31.9, K41.10-K41.21, K41.40-K41.91, K45.0, K45.8-K46.0, K92.81

K41.11 Bilateral femoral hernia, with gangrene, recurrent `MCC`
CC Excl: See code: K41.10

✓5ᵗʰ K41.2 Bilateral femoral hernia, without obstruction or gangrene

K41.20 Bilateral femoral hernia, without obstruction or gangrene, not specified as recurrent
Bilateral femoral hernia NOS

K41.21 Bilateral femoral hernia, without obstruction or gangrene, recurrent

✓5ᵗʰ K41.3 Unilateral femoral hernia, with obstruction, without gangrene
Femoral hernia (unilateral) causing obstruction, without gangrene
Incarcerated femoral hernia (unilateral), without gangrene
Irreducible femoral hernia (unilateral), without gangrene
Strangulated femoral hernia (unilateral), without gangrene

K41.30 Unilateral femoral hernia, with obstruction, without gangrene, not specified as recurrent `CC`
Femoral hernia, with obstruction NOS
Unilateral femoral hernia, with obstruction NOS

K41.31 Unilateral femoral hernia, with obstruction, without gangrene, recurrent `CC`

✓5ᵗʰ K41.4 Unilateral femoral hernia, with gangrene

K41.40 Unilateral femoral hernia, with gangrene, not specified as recurrent `MCC`
Femoral hernia, with gangrene NOS
Unilateral femoral hernia, with gangrene NOS
CC Excl: See code: K41.10

Ⓝ Newborn: 0   Ⓟ Pediatric: 0-17   Ⓜ Maternity: 12-55   Ⓐ Adult: 15-124   `MCC` Major CC Condition   `PDxMCC` PDx acts as own MCC   `CC` CC Condition   `PDxCC` PDx acts as own CC

666

ICD-10-CM 2016

K41.41   **Unilateral femoral hernia, with gangrene, recurrent**   `MCC`
     CC Excl: See code: K41.10

☑5ᵗʰ **K41.9**   Unilateral **femoral hernia, without obstruction or gangrene**

K41.90   **Unilateral femoral hernia, without obstruction or gangrene, not specified as recurrent**
     Femoral hernia NOS
     Unilateral femoral hernia NOS

K41.91   **Unilateral femoral hernia, without obstruction or gangrene, recurrent**

☑4ᵗʰ **K42**   Umbilical **hernia**
    `INCLUDES`   paraumbilical hernia
    `EXCLUDES 1`   omphalocele (Q79.2)

K42.0   **Umbilical hernia with obstruction, without gangrene**   `CC`
     Umbilical hernia causing obstruction, without gangrene
     Incarcerated umbilical hernia, without gangrene
     Irreducible umbilical hernia, without gangrene
     Strangulated umbilical hernia, without gangrene
     CC Excl: K42.0-K42.1, K43.0, K43.1, K43.3-K43.4, K43.6-K43.7, K45.0, K45.8-K46.0

K42.1   **Umbilical hernia with gangrene**   `MCC`
     Gangrenous umbilical hernia
     CC Excl: K31.89-K31.9, K42.0-K43.0, K43.1, K43.2-K43.9, K45.0, K45.8-K46.0, K46.9, K92.81

K42.9   **Umbilical hernia without obstruction or gangrene**
     Umbilical hernia NOS

☑4ᵗʰ **K43**   Ventral **hernia**

K43.0   **Incisional hernia with obstruction, without gangrene**   `CC`
     Incisional hernia causing obstruction, without gangrene
     Incarcerated incisional hernia, without gangrene
     Irreducible incisional hernia, without gangrene
     Strangulated incisional hernia, without gangrene
     CC Excl: See code: K42.0

K43.1   **Incisional hernia with gangrene**   `MCC`
     Gangrenous incisional hernia
     CC Excl: See code: K42.1

K43.2   **Incisional hernia without obstruction or gangrene**
     Incisional hernia NOS

K43.3   **Parastomal hernia with obstruction, without gangrene**   `CC`
     Incarcerated parastomal hernia, without gangrene
     Irreducible parastomal hernia, without gangrene
     Parastomal hernia causing obstruction, without gangrene
     Strangulated parastomal hernia, without gangrene
     CC Excl: See code: K42.0

K43.4   **Parastomal hernia with gangrene**   `MCC`
     Gangrenous parastomal hernia
     CC Excl: See code: K42.1

K43.5   **Parastomal hernia without obstruction or gangrene**
     Parastomal hernia NOS

K43.6   **Other and unspecified ventral hernia with obstruction, without gangrene**   `CC`
     Epigastric hernia causing obstruction, without gangrene
     Hypogastric hernia causing obstruction, without gangrene
     Incarcerated epigastric hernia without gangrene
     Incarcerated hypogastric hernia without gangrene
     incarcerated midline hernia without gangrene
     Incarcerated spigelian hernia without gangrene
     Incarcerated subxiphoid hernia without gangrene
     Irreducible epigastric hernia without gangrene
     Irreducible hypogastric hernia without gangrene
     Irreducible midline hernia without gangrene
     Irreducible spigelian hernia without gangrene
     Irreducible subxiphoid hernia without gangrene
     Midline hernia causing obstruction, without gangrene
     Spigelian hernia causing obstruction, without gangrene
     Strangulated epigastric hernia without gangrene
     Strangulated hypogastric hernia without gangrene
     Strangulated midline hernia without gangrene
     Strangulated spigelian hernia without gangrene
     Strangulated subxiphoid hernia without gangrene
     Subxiphoid hernia causing obstruction, without gangrene
     CC Excl: See code: K42.0

K43.7   **Other and unspecified ventral hernia with gangrene**   `MCC`
     Any condition listed under K43.6 specified as gangrenous
     CC Excl: See code: K42.1

K43.9   **Ventral hernia without obstruction or gangrene**
     Epigastric hernia
     Ventral hernia NOS

☑4ᵗʰ **K44**   Diaphragmatic **hernia**
    `INCLUDES`   hiatus hernia (esophageal) (sliding)
          paraesophageal hernia
    `EXCLUDES 1`   congenital diaphragmatic hernia (Q79.0)
          congenital hiatus hernia (Q40.1)

K44.0   **Diaphragmatic hernia with obstruction, without gangrene**   `CC`
     Diaphragmatic hernia causing obstruction
     Incarcerated diaphragmatic hernia
     Irreducible diaphragmatic hernia
     Strangulated diaphragmatic hernia
     CC Excl: K44.0-K45.0, K45.8-K46.0

K44.1   **Diaphragmatic hernia with gangrene**   `MCC`
     Gangrenous diaphragmatic hernia
     CC Excl: See code: K44.0

K44.9   **Diaphragmatic hernia without obstruction or gangrene**
     Diaphragmatic hernia NOS

☑4ᵗʰ **K45**   Other abdominal **hernia**
    `INCLUDES`   abdominal hernia, specified site NEC
          lumbar hernia
          obturator hernia
          pudendal hernia
          retroperitoneal hernia
          sciatic hernia

K45.0   **Other specified abdominal hernia with obstruction, without gangrene**   `CC`
     Other specified abdominal hernia causing obstruction
     Other specified incarcerated abdominal hernia
     Other specified irreducible abdominal hernia
     Other specified strangulated abdominal hernia
     CC Excl: K40.00-K43.0, K43.1, K43.2-K43.9, K44.0-K46.9

K45.1   **Other specified abdominal hernia with gangrene**   `MCC`
     Any condition listed under K45 specified as gangrenous
     CC Excl: K31.89-K31.9, K40.00-K43.0, K43.1, K43.2-K43.9, K44.0-K46.9, K92.81

K45.8   **Other specified abdominal hernia without obstruction or gangrene**

☑4ᵗʰ **K46**   Unspecified abdominal **hernia**
    `INCLUDES`   enterocele
          epiplocele
          hernia NOS
          interstitial hernia
          intestinal hernia
          intra-abdominal hernia
    `EXCLUDES 1`   vaginal enterocele (N81.5)

K46.0   **Unspecified abdominal hernia with obstruction, without gangrene**   `CC`
     Unspecified abdominal hernia causing obstruction
     Unspecified incarcerated abdominal hernia
     Unspecified irreducible abdominal hernia
     Unspecified strangulated abdominal hernia
     CC Excl: See code: K45.0

K46.1   **Unspecified abdominal hernia with gangrene**   `MCC`
     Any condition listed under K46 specified as gangrenous
     CC Excl: See code: K45.1

K46.9   **Unspecified abdominal hernia without obstruction or gangrene**
     Abdominal hernia NOS

Noninfective enteritis and colitis (K50-K52)

    `INCLUDES`   noninfective inflammatory bowel disease
    `EXCLUDES 1`   irritable bowel syndrome (K58.-)
          megacolon (K59.3)

☑4ᵗʰ **K50**   Crohn's disease [regional enteritis]
    `INCLUDES`   granulomatous enteritis
    Use additional code to identify manifestations, such as:
      pyoderma gangrenosum (L88)
    `EXCLUDES 1`   ulcerative colitis (K51.-)
    AHA: 2012, 4Q, 104

> **CC Excl: For CC codes in category K50, unless otherwise noted:**
> K50.00-K51.919

☑5ᵗʰ **K50.0**   **Crohn's disease of small intestine**
     Crohn's disease [regional enteritis] of duodenum
     Crohn's disease [regional enteritis] of ileum
     Crohn's disease [regional enteritis] of jejunum
     Regional ileitis
     Terminal ileitis
     `EXCLUDES 1`   Crohn's disease of both small and large intestine (K50.8-)

    K50.00   **Crohn's disease of small intestine without complications**   `CC`

☑ Additional Character Required   ☑x7ᵗʰ Placeholder Alert   Unacceptable PDx   Manifestation   Hospital Acquired Condition   `EXCLUDES 1` Not Coded Here   `EXCLUDES 2` Not Included Here

ICD-10-CM 2016   667

✓6th **K50.01 Crohn's disease of small intestine with complications**

K50.011 Crohn's disease of small intestine with rectal bleeding CC

K50.012 Crohn's disease of small intestine with intestinal obstruction PDxCC CC

K50.013 Crohn's disease of small intestine with fistula PDxCC CC

K50.014 Crohn's disease of small intestine with abscess PDxCC CC
    AHA: 2012, 4Q, 104

K50.018 Crohn's disease of small intestine with other complication CC

K50.019 Crohn's disease of small intestine with unspecified complications CC

✓5th **K50.1 Crohn's disease of large intestine**
Crohn's disease [regional enteritis] of colon
Crohn's disease [regional enteritis] of large bowel
Crohn's disease [regional enteritis] of rectum
Granulomatous colitis
Regional colitis
EXCLUDES 1 *Crohn's disease of both small and large intestine (K50.8)*

K50.10 Crohn's disease of large intestine without complications CC

✓6th **K50.11 Crohn's disease of large intestine with complications**

K50.111 Crohn's disease of large intestine with rectal bleeding CC

K50.112 Crohn's disease of large intestine with intestinal obstruction PDxCC CC

K50.113 Crohn's disease of large intestine with fistula PDxCC CC

K50.114 Crohn's disease of large intestine with abscess PDxCC CC

K50.118 Crohn's disease of large intestine with other complication CC

K50.119 Crohn's disease of large intestine with unspecified complications CC

✓5th **K50.8 Crohn's disease of both small and large intestine**

K50.80 Crohn's disease of both small and large intestine without complications CC

✓6th **K50.81 Crohn's disease of both small and large intestine with complications**

K50.811 Crohn's disease of both small and large intestine with rectal bleeding CC

K50.812 Crohn's disease of both small and large intestine with intestinal obstruction PDxCC CC

K50.813 Crohn's disease of both small and large intestine with fistula PDxCC CC

K50.814 Crohn's disease of both small and large intestine with abscess PDxCC CC

K50.818 Crohn's disease of both small and large intestine with other complication CC

K50.819 Crohn's disease of both small and large intestine with unspecified complications CC

✓5th **K50.9 Crohn's disease, unspecified**

CC Excl: For CC codes in subcategory K50.9, unless otherwise noted: K50.00-K50.919

K50.90 Crohn's disease, unspecified, without complications CC
Crohn's disease NOS
Regional enteritis NOS

✓6th **K50.91 Crohn's disease, unspecified, with complications**

K50.911 Crohn's disease, unspecified, with rectal bleeding CC

K50.912 Crohn's disease, unspecified, with intestinal obstruction PDxCC CC

K50.913 Crohn's disease, unspecified, with fistula PDxCC CC

K50.914 Crohn's disease, unspecified, with abscess PDxCC CC

K50.918 Crohn's disease, unspecified, with other complication CC

K50.919 Crohn's disease, unspecified, with unspecified complications CC

✓4th **K51 Ulcerative colitis**
Use additional code to identify manifestations, such as:
pyoderma gangrenosum (L88)
EXCLUDES 1 *Crohn's disease [regional enteritis] (K50.-)*

CC Excl: For CC codes in category K51, unless otherwise noted: See code: K50.9

✓5th **K51.0 Ulcerative (chronic) pancolitis**
Backwash ileitis

K51.00 Ulcerative (chronic) pancolitis without complications CC
Ulcerative (chronic) pancolitis NOS

✓6th **K51.01 Ulcerative (chronic) pancolitis with complications**

K51.011 Ulcerative (chronic) pancolitis with rectal bleeding CC

K51.012 Ulcerative (chronic) pancolitis with intestinal obstruction PDxCC CC

K51.013 Ulcerative (chronic) pancolitis with fistula PDxCC CC

K51.014 Ulcerative (chronic) pancolitis with abscess PDxCC CC

K51.018 Ulcerative (chronic) pancolitis with other complication CC

K51.019 Ulcerative (chronic) pancolitis with unspecified complications CC

✓5th **K51.2 Ulcerative (chronic) proctitis**

K51.20 Ulcerative (chronic) proctitis without complications CC
Ulcerative (chronic) proctitis NOS

✓6th **K51.21 Ulcerative (chronic) proctitis with complications**

K51.211 Ulcerative (chronic) proctitis with rectal bleeding CC

K51.212 Ulcerative (chronic) proctitis with intestinal obstruction PDxCC CC

K51.213 Ulcerative (chronic) proctitis with fistula PDxCC CC

K51.214 Ulcerative (chronic) proctitis with abscess PDxCC CC

K51.218 Ulcerative (chronic) proctitis with other complication CC

K51.219 Ulcerative (chronic) proctitis with unspecified complications CC

✓5th **K51.3 Ulcerative (chronic) rectosigmoiditis**

K51.30 Ulcerative (chronic) rectosigmoiditis without complications CC
Ulcerative (chronic) rectosigmoiditis NOS

✓6th **K51.31 Ulcerative (chronic) rectosigmoiditis with complications**

K51.311 Ulcerative (chronic) rectosigmoiditis with rectal bleeding CC

K51.312 Ulcerative (chronic) rectosigmoiditis with intestinal obstruction PDxCC CC

K51.313 Ulcerative (chronic) rectosigmoiditis with fistula PDxCC CC

K51.314 Ulcerative (chronic) rectosigmoiditis with abscess PDxCC CC

K51.318 Ulcerative (chronic) rectosigmoiditis with other complication CC

K51.319 Ulcerative (chronic) rectosigmoiditis with unspecified complications CC

✓5th **K51.4 Inflammatory polyps of colon**
EXCLUDES 1 *adenomatous polyp of colon (D12.6)*
polyposis of colon (D12.6)
polyps of colon NOS (K63.5)

K51.40 Inflammatory polyps of colon without complications CC
Inflammatory polyps of colon NOS

✓6th **K51.41 Inflammatory polyps of colon with complications**

K51.411 Inflammatory polyps of colon with rectal bleeding CC

K51.412 Inflammatory polyps of colon with intestinal obstruction PDxCC CC

K51.413 Inflammatory polyps of colon with fistula PDxCC CC

K51.414 Inflammatory polyps of colon with abscess PDxCC CC

K51.418   **Inflammatory polyps of colon with other complication** `CC`

K51.419   **Inflammatory polyps of colon with unspecified complications** `CC`

√5ᵗʰ **K51.5**   **Left sided colitis**
Left hemicolitis

K51.50   **Left sided colitis** without complications `CC`
Left sided colitis NOS

√6ᵗʰ **K51.51**   **Left sided colitis** with complications

K51.511   **Left sided colitis with** rectal bleeding `CC`

K51.512   **Left sided colitis with** intestinal obstruction `PDxCC` `CC`

K51.513   **Left sided colitis with** fistula `PDxCC` `CC`

K51.514   **Left sided colitis with** abscess `PDxCC` `CC`

K51.518   **Left sided colitis with** other complication `CC`

K51.519   **Left sided colitis with** unspecified complications `CC`

√5ᵗʰ **K51.8**   **Other ulcerative colitis**

K51.80   **Other ulcerative colitis** without complications `CC`

√6ᵗʰ **K51.81**   **Other ulcerative colitis** with complications

K51.811   **Other ulcerative colitis with** rectal bleeding `CC`

K51.812   **Other ulcerative colitis with** intestinal obstruction `PDxCC` `CC`

K51.813   **Other ulcerative colitis with** fistula `PDxCC` `CC`

K51.814   **Other ulcerative colitis with** abscess `PDxCC` `CC`

K51.818   **Other ulcerative colitis with** other complication `CC`

K51.819   **Other ulcerative colitis with** unspecified complications `CC`

√5ᵗʰ **K51.9**   **Ulcerative colitis, unspecified**

> **CC Excl:** For CC codes in subcategory K51.9, unless otherwise noted: K51.00-K51.919

K51.90   **Ulcerative colitis, unspecified,** without complications `CC`

√6ᵗʰ **K51.91**   **Ulcerative colitis, unspecified,** with complications

K51.911   **Ulcerative colitis, unspecified with** rectal bleeding `CC`

K51.912   **Ulcerative colitis, unspecified with** intestinal obstruction `PDxCC` `CC`

K51.913   **Ulcerative colitis, unspecified with** fistula `PDxCC` `CC`

K51.914   **Ulcerative colitis, unspecified with** abscess `PDxCC` `CC`

K51.918   **Ulcerative colitis, unspecified with** other complication `CC`

K51.919   **Ulcerative colitis, unspecified with** unspecified complications `CC`

√4ᵗʰ **K52**   **Other and unspecified noninfective gastroenteritis and colitis**

K52.0   **Gastroenteritis and colitis due to** radiation `CC`
CC Excl: K52.0

K52.1   **Toxic gastroenteritis and colitis** `CC`
Drug-induced gastroenteritis and colitis
Code first (T51-T65) to identify toxic agent
Use additional code for adverse effect, if applicable, to identify drug (T36-T50 with fifth or sixth character 5)
CC Excl: K52.1

K52.2   **Allergic and dietetic gastroenteritis and colitis**
Food hypersensitivity gastroenteritis or colitis
Use additional code to identify type of food allergy (Z91.01-, Z91.02-)

√5ᵗʰ **K52.8**   **Other specified noninfective gastroenteritis and colitis**

K52.81   **Eosinophilic gastritis or gastroenteritis**
Eosinophilic enteritis
EXCLUDES 1   *eosinophilic esophagitis (K20.0)*

K52.82   **Eosinophilic colitis**

K52.89   **Other specified noninfective gastroenteritis and colitis**
Collagenous colitis
Lymphocytic colitis
Microscopic colitis (collagenous or lymphocytic)

K52.9   **Noninfective gastroenteritis and colitis, unspecified**
Colitis NOS   Ileitis NOS
Enteritis NOS   Jejunitis NOS
Gastroenteritis NOS   Sigmoiditis NOS
EXCLUDES 1   *diarrhea NOS (R19.7)*
functional diarrhea (K59.1)
infectious gastroenteritis and colitis NOS (A09)
neonatal diarrhea (noninfective) (P78.3)
psychogenic diarrhea (F45.8)

Other diseases of intestines (K55-K64)

√4ᵗʰ **K55**   **Vascular disorders of intestine**
EXCLUDES 1   *necrotizing enterocolitis of newborn (P77.-)*

K55.0   **Acute vascular disorders of intestine** `MCC`
Acute fulminant ischemic colitis
Acute intestinal infarction
Acute small intestine ischemia
Infarction of appendices epiploicae
Mesenteric (artery) (vein) embolism
Mesenteric (artery) (vein) infarction
Mesenteric (artery) (vein) thrombosis
Necrosis of intestine
Subacute ischemic colitis
CC Excl: K55.0-K55.1

K55.1   **Chronic vascular disorders of intestine** `CC`
Chronic ischemic colitis
Chronic ischemic enteritis
Chronic ischemic enterocolitis
Ischemic stricture of intestine
Mesenteric atherosclerosis
Mesenteric vascular insufficiency
CC Excl: K55.0-K55.1, K55.8-K55.9

√5ᵗʰ **K55.2**   **Angiodysplasia of colon**

K55.20   **Angiodysplasia of colon** without hemorrhage

K55.21   **Angiodysplasia of colon** with hemorrhage `MCC`
CC Excl: E16.4, I85.01, K22.10-K22.11, K22.6-K22.719, K25.0-K28.9, K29.01, K29.21, K29.31, K29.41, K29.51, K29.61, K29.71, K29.81, K29.91, K31.811, K55.21, K57.01, K57.11, K57.13, K57.21, K57.31, K57.33, K57.41, K57.51, K57.53, K57.81, K57.91, K57.93, K62.5, K92.0-K92.2

K55.8   **Other vascular disorders of intestine** `CC`
CC Excl: See code: K55.1

K55.9   **Vascular disorder of intestine,** unspecified `CC`
Ischemic colitis
Ischemic enteritis
Ischemic enterocolitis
CC Excl: See code: K55.1

√4ᵗʰ **K56**   **Paralytic ileus and intestinal obstruction without hernia**
EXCLUDES 1   *congenital stricture or stenosis of intestine (Q41-Q42)*
cystic fibrosis with meconium ileus (E84.11)
intestinal obstruction with hernia (K40-K46)
ischemic stricture of intestine (K55.1)
meconium ileus NOS (P76.0)
neonatal intestinal obstructions classifiable to P76-
obstruction of duodenum (K31.5)
postprocedural intestinal obstruction (K91.3)
stenosis of anus or rectum (K62.4)

> **CC Excl:** For CC/MCC codes in category K56, unless otherwise noted: K56.0-K56.3, K56.49-K56.7, K63.4, K63.89-K63.9, K92.89-K92.9, R11.13

K56.0   **Paralytic ileus** `CC`
Paralysis of bowel   Paralysis of intestine
Paralysis of colon
EXCLUDES 1   *gallstone ileus (K56.3)*
ileus NOS (K56.7)
obstructive ileus NOS (K56.69)

K56.1   **Intussusception** `CC`
Intussusception or invagination of bowel
Intussusception or invagination of colon
Intussusception or invagination of intestine
Intussusception or invagination of rectum
EXCLUDES 2   *intussusception of appendix (K38.8)*

K56.2   **Volvulus** `MCC`
Strangulation of colon or intestine
Torsion of colon or intestine
Twist of colon or intestine
EXCLUDES 2   *volvulus of duodenum (K31.5)*

K56.3   **Gallstone ileus** `CC`
Obstruction of intestine by gallstone

Chapter 11. Diseases of the Digestive System

√5ᵗʰ **K56.4 Other impaction of intestine**

K56.41 Fecal impaction
EXCLUDES 1 constipation (K59.0-)
incomplete defecation (R15.0)

K56.49 Other impaction of intestine `CC`

K56.5 Intestinal adhesions [bands] with obstruction (postprocedural) (postinfection) `CC`
Abdominal hernia due to adhesions with obstruction
Peritoneal adhesions [bands] with intestinal obstruction (postprocedural) (postinfection)

√5ᵗʰ **K56.6 Other and unspecified intestinal obstruction**

K56.60 Unspecified intestinal obstruction `CC`
Intestinal obstruction NOS
EXCLUDES 1 intestinal obstruction due to specified condition—code to condition

K56.69 Other intestinal obstruction `CC`
Enterostenosis NOS
Obstructive ileus NOS
Occlusion of colon or intestine NOS
Stenosis of colon or intestine NOS
Stricture of colon or intestine NOS
EXCLUDES 1 intestinal obstruction due to specified condition—code to condition

K56.7 Ileus, unspecified `CC`
EXCLUDES 1 obstructive ileus (K56.69)

√4ᵗʰ **K57 Diverticular disease of intestine**
EXCLUDES 1 congenital diverticulum of intestine (Q43.8)
Meckel's diverticulum (Q43.0)
EXCLUDES 2 diverticulum of appendix (K38.2)

CC Excl: For CC/MCC codes in category K57, unless otherwise noted: E16.4, I85.01, K22.10-K22.11, K22.6-K22.719, K25.0-K28.9, K29.01, K29.21, K29.31, K29.41, K29.51, K29.61, K29.71, K29.81, K29.91, K31.811, K55.21, K57.01, K57.11, K57.13, K57.21, K57.31, K57.33, K57.41, K57.51, K57.53, K57.81, K57.91, K57.93, K62.5, K92.0-K92.2

√5ᵗʰ **K57.0 Diverticulitis of small intestine with perforation and abscess**
Diverticulitis of small intestine with peritonitis
EXCLUDES 1 diverticulitis of both small and large intestine with perforation and abscess (K57.4-)

K57.00 Diverticulitis of small intestine with perforation and abscess without bleeding `PDxCC` `CC`
CC Excl: K57.00-K57.13

K57.01 Diverticulitis of small intestine with perforation and abscess with bleeding `PDxCC` `MCC`

√5ᵗʰ **K57.1 Diverticular disease of small intestine without perforation or abscess**
EXCLUDES 1 diverticular disease of both small and large intestine without perforation or abscess (K57.5-)

K57.10 Diverticulosis of small intestine without perforation or abscess without bleeding
Diverticular disease of small intestine NOS

K57.11 Diverticulosis of small intestine without perforation or abscess with bleeding `MCC`

K57.12 Diverticulitis of small intestine without perforation or abscess without bleeding `CC`
CC Excl: See code: K57.00

K57.13 Diverticulitis of small intestine without perforation or abscess with bleeding `MCC`

√5ᵗʰ **K57.2 Diverticulitis of large intestine with perforation and abscess**
Diverticulitis of colon with peritonitis
EXCLUDES 1 diverticulitis of both small and large intestine with perforation and abscess (K57.4-)

K57.20 Diverticulitis of large intestine with perforation and abscess without bleeding `PDxCC` `CC`
CC Excl: K57.20-K57.93

K57.21 Diverticulitis of large intestine with perforation and abscess with bleeding `PDxCC` `MCC`

√5ᵗʰ **K57.3 Diverticular disease of large intestine without perforation or abscess**
EXCLUDES 1 diverticular disease of both small and large intestine without perforation or abscess (K57.5-)

K57.30 Diverticulosis of large intestine without perforation or abscess without bleeding
Diverticular disease of colon NOS

K57.31 Diverticulosis of large intestine without perforation or abscess with bleeding `MCC`

K57.32 Diverticulitis of large intestine without perforation or abscess without bleeding `CC`
CC Excl: See code: K57.20

K57.33 Diverticulitis of large intestine without perforation or abscess with bleeding `MCC`

√5ᵗʰ **K57.4 Diverticulitis of both small and large intestine with perforation and abscess**
Diverticulitis of both small and large intestine with peritonitis

K57.40 Diverticulitis of both small and large intestine with perforation and abscess without bleeding `PDxCC` `CC`
CC Excl: See code: K57.20

K57.41 Diverticulitis of both small and large intestine with perforation and abscess with bleeding `PDxCC` `MCC`

√5ᵗʰ **K57.5 Diverticular disease of both small and large intestine without perforation or abscess**

K57.50 Diverticulosis of both small and large intestine without perforation or abscess without bleeding
Diverticular disease of both small and large intestine NOS

K57.51 Diverticulosis of both small and large intestine without perforation or abscess with bleeding `MCC`

K57.52 Diverticulitis of both small and large intestine without perforation or abscess without bleeding `PDxCC` `CC`
CC Excl: See code: K57.20

K57.53 Diverticulitis of both small and large intestine without perforation or abscess with bleeding `MCC`

√5ᵗʰ **K57.8 Diverticulitis of intestine, part unspecified, with perforation and abscess**
Diverticulitis of intestine NOS with peritonitis

K57.80 Diverticulitis of intestine, part unspecified, with perforation and abscess without bleeding `PDxCC` `CC`
CC Excl: See code: K57.20

K57.81 Diverticulitis of intestine, part unspecified, with perforation and abscess with bleeding `PDxCC` `MCC`

√5ᵗʰ **K57.9 Diverticular disease of intestine, part unspecified, without perforation or abscess**

K57.90 Diverticulosis of intestine, part unspecified, without perforation or abscess without bleeding
Diverticular disease of intestine NOS

K57.91 Diverticulosis of intestine, part unspecified, without perforation or abscess with bleeding `MCC`

K57.92 Diverticulitis of intestine, part unspecified, without perforation or abscess without bleeding `CC`
CC Excl: See code: K57.20

K57.93 Diverticulitis of intestine, part unspecified, without perforation or abscess with bleeding `MCC`

√4ᵗʰ **K58 Irritable bowel syndrome**
INCLUDES irritable colon
spastic colon

K58.0 Irritable bowel syndrome with diarrhea

K58.9 Irritable bowel syndrome without diarrhea
Irritable bowel syndrome NOS

√4ᵗʰ **K59 Other functional intestinal disorders**
EXCLUDES 1 change in bowel habit NOS (R19.4)
intestinal malabsorption (K90.-)
psychogenic intestinal disorders (F45.8)
EXCLUDES 2 functional disorders of stomach (K31.-)

√5ᵗʰ **K59.0 Constipation**
EXCLUDES 1 fecal impaction (K56.41)
incomplete defecation (R15.0)

K59.00 Constipation, unspecified

K59.01 Slow transit constipation

K59.02 Outlet dysfunction constipation

K59.09 Other constipation

K59.1 Functional diarrhea
EXCLUDES 1 diarrhea NOS (R19.7)
irritable bowel syndrome with diarrhea (K58.0)

K59.2 Neurogenic bowel, not elsewhere classified `CC`
CC Excl: K58.0-K58.9, K59.1-K59.9, K91.0-K91.1

K59.3 Megacolon, not elsewhere classified   `CC`
Dilatation of colon
Toxic megacolon
Code first (T51-T65) to identify toxic agent
> *EXCLUDES 1*   congenital megacolon (aganglionic) (Q43.1)
> megacolon (due to) (in) Chagas' disease (B57.32)
> megacolon (due to) (in) Clostridium difficile (A04.7)
> megacolon (due to) (in) Hirschsprung's disease (Q43.1)

CC Excl: See code: K59.2

K59.4 Anal spasm
Proctalgia fugax

K59.8 Other specified functional intestinal disorders
Atony of colon
Pseudo-obstruction (acute) (chronic) of intestine

K59.9 Functional intestinal disorder, unspecified

✓4th **K60 Fissure and fistula of anal and rectal regions**
> *EXCLUDES 1*   fissure and fistula of anal and rectal regions with abscess or
> cellulitis (K61.-)
> *EXCLUDES 2*   anal sphincter tear (healed) (nontraumatic) (old) (K62.81)

K60.0 Acute anal fissure

K60.1 Chronic anal fissure

K60.2 Anal fissure, unspecified

K60.3 Anal fistula

K60.4 Rectal fistula
Fistula of rectum to skin
> *EXCLUDES 1*   rectovaginal fistula (N82.3)
> vesicorectal fistual (N32.1)

K60.5 Anorectal fistula

✓4th **K61 Abscess of anal and rectal regions**
> INCLUDES   abscess of anal and rectal regions
> cellulitis of anal and rectal regions

CC Excl: For CC codes in category K61, unless otherwise
noted: K61.0-K61.4

K61.0 Anal abscess   `CC`
Perianal abscess
> *EXCLUDES 1*   intrasphincteric abscess (K61.4)

K61.1 Rectal abscess   `CC`
Perirectal abscess
> *EXCLUDES 1*   ischiorectal abscess (K61.3)

AHA: 2012, 4Q, 104

K61.2 Anorectal abscess   `CC`

K61.3 Ischiorectal abscess   `CC`
Abscess of ischiorectal fossa

K61.4 Intrasphincteric abscess   `CC`

✓4th **K62 Other diseases of anus and rectum**
> INCLUDES   anal canal
> *EXCLUDES 2*   colostomy and enterostomy malfunction (K94.0-, K94.1-)
> fecal incontinence (R15.-)
> hemorrhoids (K64.-)

K62.0 Anal polyp

K62.1 Rectal polyp
> *EXCLUDES 1*   adenomatous polyp (D12.8)

K62.2 Anal prolapse
Prolapse of anal canal

K62.3 Rectal prolapse
Prolapse of rectal mucosa

K62.4 Stenosis of anus and rectum
Stricture of anus (sphincter)

K62.5 Hemorrhage of anus and rectum   `CC`
> *EXCLUDES 1*   gastrointestinal bleeding NOS (K92.2)
> melena (K92.1)
> neonatal rectal hemorrhage (P54.2)

CC Excl: E16.4, I85.01, K22.10-K22.11, K22.6-K22.719, K25.0-K28.9,
K29.01, K29.21, K29.31, K29.41, K29.51, K29.61, K29.71, K29.81,
K29.91, K31.811, K55.21, K57.01, K57.11, K57.13, K57.21, K57.31,
K57.33, K57.41, K57.51, K57.53, K57.81, K57.91, K57.93, K62.5,
K92.0-K92.2

K62.6 Ulcer of anus and rectum   `CC`
Solitary ulcer of anus and rectum
Stercoral ulcer of anus and rectum
> *EXCLUDES 1*   fissure and fistula of anus and rectum (K60.-)
> ulcerative colitis (K51.-)

CC Excl: K62.6

K62.7 Radiation proctitis
Use additional code to identify the type of radiation (W90.-)

✓5th **K62.8 Other specified diseases of anus and rectum**
> *EXCLUDES 2*   ulcerative proctitis (K51.2)

K62.81 Anal sphincter tear (healed) (nontraumatic) (old)
Tear of anus, nontraumatic
Use additional code for any associated fecal
incontinence (R15.-)
> *EXCLUDES 2*   anal fissure (K60.-)
> anal sphincter tear (healed) (old)
> complicating delivery (O34.7-)
> traumatic tear of anal sphincter (S31.831)

K62.82 Dysplasia of anus
Anal intraepithelial neoplasia I and II (AIN I and II)
(histologically confirmed)
Dysplasia of anus NOS
Mild and moderate dysplasia of anus (histologically
confirmed)
> *EXCLUDES 1*   abnormal results from anal cytologic
> examination without histologic
> confirmation (R85.61-)
> anal intraepithelial neoplasia III (D01.3)
> carcinoma in situ of anus (D01.3)
> HGSIL of anus (R85.613)
> severe dysplasia of anus (D01.3)

K62.89 Other specified diseases of anus and rectum
Proctitis NOS
Use additional code for any associated fecal
incontinence (R15.-)

K62.9 Disease of anus and rectum, unspecified

✓4th **K63 Other diseases of intestine**

K63.0 Abscess of intestine   `CC`
> *EXCLUDES 1*   abscess of intestine with Crohn's disease (K50.014,
> K50.114, K50.814, K50.914)
> abscess of intestine with diverticular disease (K57.0,
> K57.2, K57.4, K57.8)
> abscess of intestine with ulcerative colitis (K51.014,
> K51.214, K51.314, K51.414, K51.514, K51.814,
> K51.914)
> *EXCLUDES 2*   abscess of anal and rectal regions (K61.-)
> abscess of appendix (K35.3)

CC Excl: K63.0

K63.1 Perforation of intestine (nontraumatic)   `MCC`
Perforation (nontraumatic) of rectum
> *EXCLUDES 1*   perforation (nontraumatic) of duodenum (K26.-)
> perforation (nontraumatic) of intestine with
> diverticular disease (K57.0, K57.2, K57.4, K57.8)
> *EXCLUDES 2*   perforation (nontraumatic) of appendix (K35.2, K35.3)

CC Excl: K63.1

K63.2 Fistula of intestine   `CC`
> *EXCLUDES 1*   fistula of duodenum (K31.6)
> fistula of intestine with Crohn's disease (K50.013,
> K50.113, K50.813, K50.913)
> fistula of intestine with ulcerative colitis (K51.013,
> K51.213, K51.313, K51.413, K51.513, K51.813,
> K51.913)
> *EXCLUDES 2*   fistula of anal and rectal regions (K60.-)
> fistula of appendix (K38.3)
> intestinal-genital fistula, female (N82.2-N82.4)
> vesicointestinal fistula (N32.1)

CC Excl: K63.2

K63.3 Ulcer of intestine   `CC`
Primary ulcer of small intestine
> *EXCLUDES 1*   duodenal ulcer (K26.-)
> gastrointestinal ulcer (K28.-)
> gastrojejunal ulcer (K28.-)
> jejunal ulcer (K28.-)
> peptic ulcer, site unspecified (K27.-)
> ulcer of intestine with perforation (K63.1)
> ulcer of anus or rectum (K62.6)
> ulcerative colitis (K51.-)

CC Excl: K63.3

K63.4 Enteroptosis

K63.5 Polyp of colon
> *EXCLUDES 1*   adenomatous polyp of colon (D12.6)
> inflammatory polyp of colon (K51.4-)
> polyposis of colon (D12.6)

✓ Additional Character Required   ✓x7th Placeholder Alert   Unacceptable PDx   Manifestation   Hospital Acquired Condition   *EXCLUDES 1* Not Coded Here   *EXCLUDES 2* Not Included Here

ICD-10-CM 2016   **671**

Chapter 11. Diseases of the Digestive System

✓5th **K63.8 Other specified diseases of intestine**

    K63.81 Dieulafoy lesion of intestine `MCC`
        EXCLUDES 2 Dieulafoy lesion of stomach and duodenum (K31.82)
        CC Excl: E16.4, I85.01, K22.10-K22.11, K22.6-K22.719, K25.0-K28.9, K29.01, K29.21, K29.31, K29.41, K29.51, K29.61, K29.71, K29.81, K29.91, K31.811, K55.21, K57.01, K57.11, K57.13, K57.21, K57.31, K57.33, K57.41, K57.51, K57.53, K57.81, K57.91, K57.93, K62.5, K63.81, K92.0-K92.2

    K63.89 Other specified diseases of intestine
        AHA: 2013, 2Q, 31

K63.9 Disease of intestine, unspecified

✓4th **K64 Hemorrhoids and perianal venous thrombosis**
    INCLUDES piles
    EXCLUDES 1 hemorrhoids complicating childbirth and the puerperium (O87.2)
             hemorrhoids complicating pregnancy (O22.4)

K64.0 First degree hemorrhoids
    Grade/stage I hemorrhoids
    Hemorrhoids (bleeding) without prolapse outside of anal canal

K64.1 Second degree hemorrhoids
    Grade/stage II hemorrhoids
    Hemorrhoids (bleeding) that prolapse with straining, but retract spontaneously

K64.2 Third degree hemorrhoids
    Grade/stage III hemorrhoids
    Hemorrhoids (bleeding) that prolapse with straining and require manual replacement back inside anal canal

K64.3 Fourth degree hemorrhoids
    Grade/stage IV hemorrhoids
    Hemorrhoids (bleeding) with prolapsed tissue that cannot be manually replaced

K64.4 Residual hemorrhoidal skin tags
    External hemorrhoids, NOS   Skin tags of anus

K64.5 Perianal venous thrombosis
    External hemorrhoids with thrombosis
    Perianal hematoma
    Thrombosed hemorrhoids NOS

K64.8 Other hemorrhoids
    Internal hemorrhoids, without mention of degree
    Prolapsed hemorrhoids, degree not specified

K64.9 Unspecified hemorrhoids
    Hemorrhoids (bleeding) NOS
    Hemorrhoids (bleeding) without mention of degree

Diseases of peritoneum and retroperitoneum (K65-K68)

✓4th **K65 Peritonitis**
    Use additional code (B95-B97), to identify infectious agent
    EXCLUDES 1 acute appendicitis with generalized peritonitis (K35.2)
             aseptic peritonitis (T81.6)
             benign paroxysmal peritonitis (E85.0)
             chemical peritonitis (T81.6)
             diverticulitis of both small and large intestine with peritonitis (K57.4-)
             diverticulitis of colon with peritonitis (K57.2-)
             diverticulitis of intestine, NOS, with peritonitis (K57.8-)
             diverticulitis of small intestine with peritonitis (K57.0-)
             gonococcal peritonitis (A54.85)
             neonatal peritonitis (P78.0-P78.1)
             pelvic peritonitis, female (N73.3-N73.5)
             periodic familial peritonitis (E85.0)
             peritonitis due to talc or other foreign substance (T81.6)
             peritonitis in chlamydia (A74.81)
             peritonitis in diphtheria (A36.89)
             peritonitis in syphilis (late) (A52.74)
             peritonitis in tuberculosis (A18.31)
             peritonitis with or following abortion or ectopic or molar pregnancy (O00-O07, O08.0)
             peritonitis with or following appendicitis (K35.-)
             peritonitis with or following diverticular disease of intestine (K57.-)
             puerperal peritonitis (O85)
             retroperitoneal infections (K68.-)

    CC Excl: For MCC codes in category K65, unless otherwise noted:
    K63.4, K63.89-K63.9, K65.0-K65.9, K67, K68.19-K68.9, K92.89-K92.9, R11.13

K65.0 Generalized (acute) peritonitis `MCC`
    Pelvic peritonitis (acute), male
    Subphrenic peritonitis (acute)
    Suppurative peritonitis (acute)

K65.1 Peritoneal abscess `MCC`
    Abdominopelvic abscess   Subdiaphragmatic abscess
    Abscess (of) omentum   Subhepatic abscess
    Abscess (of) peritoneum   Subphrenic abscess
    Mesenteric abscess
    Retrocecal abscess

K65.2 Spontaneous bacterial peritonitis `MCC`
    EXCLUDES 1 bacterial peritonitis NOS (K65.9)

K65.3 Choleperitonitis `MCC`
    Peritonitis due to bile

K65.4 Sclerosing mesenteritis `CC`
    Fat necrosis of peritoneum
    (Idiopathic) sclerosing mesenteric fibrosis
    Mesenteric lipodystrophy
    Mesenteric panniculitis
    Retractile mesenteritis

K65.8 Other peritonitis `MCC`
    Chronic proliferative peritonitis   Peritonitis due to urine

K65.9 Peritonitis, unspecified `MCC`
    Bacterial peritonitis NOS
    AHA: 2013, 2Q, 31

✓4th **K66 Other disorders of peritoneum**
    EXCLUDES 2 ascites (R18.-)
           peritoneal effusion (chronic) (R18.8)

K66.0 Peritoneal adhesions (postprocedural) (postinfection)
    Adhesions (of) abdominal (wall)   Adhesions (of) omentum
    Adhesions (of) diaphragm   Adhesions (of) stomach
    Adhesions (of) intestine   Adhesive bands
    Adhesions (of) male pelvis   Mesenteric adhesions
    EXCLUDES 1 female pelvic adhesions [bands] (N73.6)
           peritoneal adhesions with intestinal obstruction (K56.5)

K66.1 Hemoperitoneum `MCC`
    EXCLUDES 1 traumatic hemoperitoneum (S36.8-)
    CC Excl: K66.1

K66.8 Other specified disorders of peritoneum

K66.9 Disorder of peritoneum, unspecified

K67 Disorders of peritoneum in infectious diseases classified elsewhere `MCC`
    Code first underlying disease, such as:
        congenital syphilis (A50.0)
        helminthiasis (B65.0-B83.9)
    EXCLUDES 1 peritonitis in chlamydia (A74.81)
           peritonitis in diphtheria (A36.89)
           peritonitis in gonococcal (A54.85)
           peritonitis in syphilis (late) (A52.74)
           peritonitis in tuberculosis (A18.31)
    CC Excl: See code: K65

✓4th **K68 Disorders of retroperitoneum**

✓5th **K68.1 Retroperitoneal abscess**

    4, 6, 8 **K68.11 Postprocedural retroperitoneal abscess** `CC`
        CC Excl: D78.81-D78.89, E36.8, E89.810-E89.89, H59.011-H59.019, H59.031-H59.099, H59.811-H59.89, H95.811-H95.89, I97.3, K68.11, L76.81-L76.82, M96.89, N98.1-N98.9, T81.4XXA, T81.82XA, T81.89XA, T81.9XXA

    K68.12 Psoas muscle abscess `MCC`
        CC Excl: K68.12, M60.000-M60.19, M61.00-M61.19, M61.30-M61.59, M62.3, M62.50-M62.59, M62.89, M72.6

    K68.19 Other retroperitoneal abscess `MCC`
        CC Excl: See code: K65

K68.9 Other disorders of retroperitoneum `MCC`
    CC Excl: See code: K65

---

4 HAC = as SDx not POA, in combination with PDx E66.01 **AND** one of the following procedure codes: 0D16[0,4,8][7,J,K,Z][9,A,B,L] or 0DV64CZ.

6 HAC = as SDx not POA, in combination with one of the following procedure codes: 0RG[0,1,2,4,6,7,8,A][0,3,4][7,A,J,K,Z][0,1,J]; 0RG[E,F,G,H,J,K][0,3,4][4,7,J,K,Z]Z; 0RG[L,M][0,3,4][4,5,7,J,K,Z]Z; 0RQ[E,F,G,H,J,K,L,M][0,3,4,X]ZZ; 0RU[E,F,G,H,J,K,L,M][0,3,4][7,J,K]Z; 0SG[0,1,3][0,3,4][7,A,J,K,Z][0,1,J]; 0SG[7,8][0,3,4][4,7,J,K,Z]Z.

8 HAC = as SDx not POA, in combination with one of the following procedure codes: 02H43[J,K,M]Z; 02H[6,7]3[J,M]Z; 02H[K,L]3JZ; 02HN[0,3,4][J,M]Z; 02PA[0,3,4]MZ; 02PAXMZ; 02WA[0,3,4]MZ; 0JH[6,8][0,3][4,5,6,7,8,9,P]Z; 0JPT[0,3]PZ; 0JWT[0,3]PZ.

N Newborn: 0 P Pediatric: 0-17 M Maternity: 12-55 A Adult: 15-124 MCC Major CC Condition PDxMCC PDx acts as own MCC CC CC Condition PDxCC PDx acts as own CC

672   ICD-10-CM 2016

Diseases of liver (K70-K77)

EXCLUDES 1   *jaundice NOS (R17)*
EXCLUDES 2   *hemochromatosis (E83.11-)*
       Reye's syndrome (G93.7)
       viral hepatitis (B15-B19)
       Wilson's disease (E83.0)

✓4ᵗʰ K70   Alcoholic liver disease
Use additional code to identify:
alcohol abuse and dependence (F10.-)

K70.0   **Alcoholic fatty liver**   A

✓5ᵗʰ **K70.1**   **Alcoholic hepatitis**

     K70.10   **Alcoholic hepatitis without ascites**   A

     K70.11   **Alcoholic hepatitis with ascites**   A

K70.2   **Alcoholic fibrosis and sclerosis of liver**   A

✓5ᵗʰ **K70.3**   **Alcoholic cirrhosis of liver**
Alcoholic cirrhosis NOS

     K70.30   **Alcoholic cirrhosis of liver without ascites**   A

     K70.31   **Alcoholic cirrhosis of liver with ascites**   A

✓5ᵗʰ **K70.4**   **Alcoholic hepatic failure**
Acute alcoholic hepatic failure
Alcoholic hepatic failure NOS
Chronic alcoholic hepatic failure
Subacute alcoholic hepatic failure

     K70.40   **Alcoholic hepatic failure without coma**   A

     K70.41   **Alcoholic hepatic failure with coma**   PDx MCC   MCC   A
          CC Excl: K72.91, K76.5, K76.89-K76.9

K70.9   **Alcoholic liver disease, unspecified**   A

✓4ᵗʰ K71   Toxic liver disease
INCLUDES   drug-induced idiosyncratic (unpredictable) liver disease
         drug-induced toxic (predictable) liver disease

Code first poisoning due to drug or toxin, if applicable (T36-T65 with fifth or sixth character 1-4 or 6)
Use additional code for adverse effect, if applicable, to identify drug (T36-T50 with fifth or sixth character 5)

EXCLUDES 2   *alcoholic liver disease (K70.-)*
       Budd-Chiari syndrome (I82.0)

K71.0   **Toxic liver disease with cholestasis**
Cholestasis with hepatocyte injury
"Pure" cholestasis

✓5ᵗʰ **K71.1**   **Toxic liver disease with hepatic necrosis**
Hepatic failure (acute) (chronic) due to drugs

     K71.10   **Toxic liver disease with hepatic necrosis, without coma**

     K71.11   **Toxic liver disease with hepatic necrosis, with coma**   PDx MCC   MCC
          CC Excl: See code: K70.41

K71.2   **Toxic liver disease with acute hepatitis**

K71.3   **Toxic liver disease with chronic persistent hepatitis**

K71.4   **Toxic liver disease with chronic lobular hepatitis**

✓5ᵗʰ **K71.5**   **Toxic liver disease with chronic active hepatitis**
Toxic liver disease with lupoid hepatitis

     K71.50   **Toxic liver disease with chronic active hepatitis without ascites**

     K71.51   **Toxic liver disease with chronic active hepatitis with ascites**

K71.6   **Toxic liver disease with hepatitis, not elsewhere classified**

K71.7   **Toxic liver disease with fibrosis and cirrhosis of liver**

K71.8   **Toxic liver disease with other disorders of liver**
Toxic liver disease with focal nodular hyperplasia
Toxic liver disease with hepatic granulomas
Toxic liver disease with peliosis hepatis
Toxic liver disease with veno-occlusive disease of liver

K71.9   **Toxic liver disease, unspecified**

✓4ᵗʰ K72   Hepatic failure, not elsewhere classified
INCLUDES   acute hepatitis NEC, with hepatic failure
         fulminant hepatitis NEC, with hepatic failure
         hepatic encephalopathy NOS
         liver (cell) necrosis with hepatic failure
         malignant hepatitis NEC, with hepatic failure
         yellow liver atrophy or dystrophy

EXCLUDES 1   *alcoholic hepatic failure (K70.4)*
       hepatic failure with toxic liver disease (K71.1-)
       icterus of newborn (P55-P59)
       postprocedural hepatic failure (K91.82)
       viral hepatitis with hepatic coma (B15-B19)

EXCLUDES 2   *hepatic failure complicating abortion or ectopic or molar pregnancy (O00-O07, O08.8)*
       hepatic failure complicating pregnancy, childbirth and the puerperium (O26.6-)

✓5ᵗʰ **K72.0**   **Acute and subacute hepatic failure**
AHA: 2014, 2Q, 13

     K72.00   **Acute and subacute hepatic failure without coma**   MCC
          CC Excl: K72.00-K72.01, K76.2-K76.3, K76.5, K76.89-K76.9

     K72.01   **Acute and subacute hepatic failure with coma**   PDx MCC   MCC
          CC Excl: See code: K72.00

✓5ᵗʰ **K72.1**   **Chronic hepatic failure**

     K72.10   **Chronic hepatic failure without coma**

     K72.11   **Chronic hepatic failure with coma**   PDx MCC   MCC
          CC Excl: K72.91, K76.5, K76.89-K76.9

✓5ᵗʰ **K72.9**   **Hepatic failure, unspecified**

     K72.90   **Hepatic failure, unspecified without coma**
          CC Excl: No Excl

     K72.91   **Hepatic failure, unspecified with coma**   MCC
          Hepatic coma NOS
          CC Excl: K72.91-K76.5, K76.89-K76.9

✓4ᵗʰ K73   Chronic hepatitis, not elsewhere classified
EXCLUDES 1   *alcoholic hepatitis (chronic) (K70.1-)*
       drug-induced hepatitis (chronic) (K71.-)
       granulomatous hepatitis (chronic) NEC (K75.3)
       reactive, nonspecific hepatitis (chronic) (K75.2)
       viral hepatitis (chronic) (B15-B19)

K73.0   **Chronic persistent hepatitis, not elsewhere classified**

K73.1   **Chronic lobular hepatitis, not elsewhere classified**

K73.2   **Chronic active hepatitis, not elsewhere classified**

K73.8   **Other chronic hepatitis, not elsewhere classified**

K73.9   **Chronic hepatitis, unspecified**

✓4ᵗʰ K74   Fibrosis and cirrhosis of liver
Code also, if applicable, viral hepatitis (acute) (chronic) (B15-B19)
EXCLUDES 1   *alcoholic cirrhosis (of liver) (K70.3)*
       alcoholic fibrosis of liver (K70.2)
       cardiac sclerosis of liver (K76.1)
       cirrhosis (of liver) with toxic liver disease (K71.7)
       congenital cirrhosis (of liver) (P78.81)
       pigmentary cirrhosis (of liver) (E83.110)

K74.0   **Hepatic fibrosis**

K74.1   **Hepatic sclerosis**

K74.2   **Hepatic fibrosis with hepatic sclerosis**

K74.3   **Primary biliary cirrhosis**
Chronic nonsuppurative destructive cholangitis

K74.4   **Secondary biliary cirrhosis**

K74.5   **Biliary cirrhosis, unspecified**

✓5ᵗʰ **K74.6**   **Other and unspecified cirrhosis of liver**

     K74.60   **Unspecified cirrhosis of liver**
          Cirrhosis (of liver) NOS

     K74.69   **Other cirrhosis of liver**
          Cryptogenic cirrhosis (of liver)
          Macronodular cirrhosis (of liver)
          Micronodular cirrhosis (of liver)
          Mixed type cirrhosis (of liver)
          Portal cirrhosis (of liver)
          Postnecrotic cirrhosis (of liver)

✓ Additional Character Required   ✓x7ᵗʰ Placeholder Alert   Unacceptable PDx   Manifestation   Hospital Acquired Condition   EXCLUDES 1 Not Coded Here   EXCLUDES 2 Not Included Here

Chapter 11. Diseases of the Digestive System

✓4th K75 Other inflammatory liver diseases

EXCLUDES 2   *toxic liver disease (K71.-)*

K75.0 Abscess of liver   `MCC`
Cholangitic hepatic abscess
Hematogenic hepatic abscess
Hepatic abscess NOS
Lymphogenic hepatic abscess
Pylephlebitic hepatic abscess
EXCLUDES 1   *amebic liver abscess (A06.4)*
cholangitis without liver abscess (K83.0)
pylephlebitis without liver abscess (K75.1)
CC Excl: A06.4, K75.1, K76.5, K76.89-K76.9

K75.1 Phlebitis of portal vein   `MCC`
Pylephlebitis
EXCLUDES 1   *pylephlebitic liver abscess (K75.0)*
CC Excl: See code: K75.0

K75.2 Nonspecific reactive hepatitis
EXCLUDES 1   *acute or subacute hepatitis (K72.0-)*
chronic hepatitis NEC (K73.-)
viral hepatitis (B15-B19)

K75.3 Granulomatous hepatitis, not elsewhere classified
EXCLUDES 1   *acute or subacute hepatitis (K72.0-)*
chronic hepatitis NEC (K73.-)
viral hepatitis (B15-B19)

K75.4 Autoimmune hepatitis
Lupoid hepatitis NEC

✓5th K75.8 Other specified inflammatory liver diseases

K75.81 Nonalcoholic steatohepatitis (NASH)

K75.89 Other specified inflammatory liver diseases

K75.9 Inflammatory liver disease, unspecified
Hepatitis NOS
EXCLUDES 1   *acute or subacute hepatitis (K72.0-)*
chronic hepatitis NEC (K73.-)
viral hepatitis (B15-B19)

✓4th K76 Other diseases of liver

EXCLUDES 2   *alcoholic liver disease (K70.-)*
amyloid degeneration of liver (E85.-)
cystic disease of liver (congenital) (Q44.6)
hepatic vein thrombosis (I82.0)
hepatomegaly NOS (R16.0)
pigmentary cirrhosis (of liver) (E83.110)
portal vein thrombosis (I81)
toxic liver disease (K71.-)

K76.0 Fatty (change of) liver, not elsewhere classified
Nonalcoholic fatty liver disease (NAFLD)
EXCLUDES 1   *nonalcoholic steatohepatitis (NASH) (K75.81)*

K76.1 Chronic passive congestion of liver
Cardiac cirrhosis
Cardiac sclerosis

K76.2 Central hemorrhagic necrosis of liver   `MCC`
EXCLUDES 1   *liver necrosis with hepatic failure (K72.-)*
CC Excl: K72.00-K72.01, K76.2-K76.3, K76.5, K76.89-K76.9

K76.3 Infarction of liver   `MCC`
CC Excl: See code: K76.2

K76.4 Peliosis hepatis
Hepatic angiomatosis

K76.5 Hepatic veno-occlusive disease
EXCLUDES 1   *Budd-Chiari syndrome (I82.0)*

K76.6 Portal hypertension   `CC`
Use additional code for any associated complications, such as:
portal hypertensive gastropathy (K31.89)
CC Excl: K72.91-K76.6, K76.89-K76.9

K76.7 Hepatorenal syndrome   `MCC`
EXCLUDES 1   *hepatorenal syndrome following labor and delivery (O90.4)*
postprocedural hepatorenal syndrome (K91.82)
CC Excl: K76.5-K76.7, K76.89-K76.9

✓5th K76.8 Other specified diseases of liver

K76.81 Hepatopulmonary syndrome
Code first underlying liver disease, such as:
alcoholic cirrhosis of liver (K70.3-)
cirrhosis of liver without mention of alcohol (K74.6-)

K76.89 Other specified diseases of liver
Cyst (simple) of liver
Focal nodular hyperplasia of liver
Hepatoptosis

K76.9 Liver disease, unspecified

K77 Liver disorders in diseases classified elsewhere   `CC`
Code first underlying disease, such as:
amyloidosis (E85.-)
congenital syphilis (A50.0, A50.5)
congenital toxoplasmosis (P37.1)
schistosomiasis (B65.0-B65.9)
EXCLUDES 1   *alcoholic hepatitis (K70.1-)*
alcoholic liver disease (K70-.)
cytomegaloviral hepatitis (B25.1)
herpesviral [herpes simplex] hepatitis (B00.81)
infectious mononucleosis with liver disease (B27.0-B27.9 with .9)
mumps hepatitis (B26.81)
sarcoidosis with liver disease (D86.89)
secondary syphilis with liver disease (A51.45)
syphilis (late) with liver disease (A52.74)
toxoplasmosis (acquired) hepatitis (B58.1)
tuberculosis with liver disease (A18.83)
CC Excl: No Excl

Disorders of gallbladder, biliary tract and pancreas (K80-K87)

✓4th K80 Cholelithiasis
EXCLUDES 1   *retained cholelithiasis following cholecystectomy (K91.86)*

✓5th K80.0 Calculus of gallbladder with acute cholecystitis
Any condition listed in K80.2 with acute cholecystitis

K80.00 Calculus of gallbladder with acute cholecystitis without obstruction   `CC`
CC Excl: K80.00-K80.21, K80.40, K80.44, K80.62-K80.63, K80.66-K80.67, K80.80, K81.0-K81.9, K82.9, K83.5-K83.9, K87

K80.01 Calculus of gallbladder with acute cholecystitis with obstruction   `CC`
CC Excl: K80.00-K80.21, K80.62-K80.63, K80.66-K80.67, K80.80, K81.0-K81.9, K82.9, K83.5-K83.9, K87

✓5th K80.1 Calculus of gallbladder with other cholecystitis

CC Excl: For CC codes in subcategory K80.1, unless otherwise noted: See code: K80.01

K80.10 Calculus of gallbladder with chronic cholecystitis without obstruction   `CC`
Cholelithiasis with cholecystitis NOS

K80.11 Calculus of gallbladder with chronic cholecystitis with obstruction   `CC`

K80.12 Calculus of gallbladder with acute and chronic cholecystitis without obstruction   `CC`
CC Excl: See code: K80.00

K80.13 Calculus of gallbladder with acute and chronic cholecystitis with obstruction   `CC`

K80.18 Calculus of gallbladder with other cholecystitis without obstruction   `CC`

K80.19 Calculus of gallbladder with other cholecystitis with obstruction   `CC`

✓5th K80.2 Calculus of gallbladder without cholecystitis
Cholecystolithiasis without cholecystitis
Cholelithiasis (without cholecystitis)
Colic (recurrent) of gallbladder (without cholecystitis)
Gallstone (impacted) of cystic duct (without cholecystitis)
Gallstone (impacted) of gallbladder (without cholecystitis)

K80.20 Calculus of gallbladder without cholecystitis without obstruction

K80.21 Calculus of gallbladder without cholecystitis with obstruction   `CC`
CC Excl: See code: K80.01

✓5th K80.3 Calculus of bile duct with cholangitis
Any condition listed in K80.5 with cholangitis

CC Excl: For CC codes in subcategory K80.3, unless otherwise noted: K83.0, K83.5-K83.9, K87

K80.30 Calculus of bile duct with cholangitis, unspecified, without obstruction   `PDxCC` `CC`

K80.31 Calculus of bile duct with cholangitis, unspecified, with obstruction   `PDxCC` `CC`
CC Excl: K80.30-K80.71, K80.81-K81.9, K83.5-K83.9, K87

K80.32 Calculus of bile duct with acute cholangitis without obstruction   `PDxCC` `CC`

K80.33 Calculus of bile duct with acute cholangitis with obstruction   `PDxCC` `CC`
CC Excl: See code: K80.31

K80.34 Calculus of bile duct with chronic cholangitis without obstruction   `PDxCC` `CC`

`N` Newborn: 0   `P` Pediatric: 0-17   `M` Maternity: 12-55   `A` Adult: 15-124   `MCC` Major CC Condition   `PDxMCC` PDx acts as own MCC   `CC` CC Condition   `PDxCC` PDx acts as own CC

674   ICD-10-CM 2016

K80.35 Calculus of bile duct with **chronic cholangitis with obstruction** `PDxCC` `CC`
CC Excl: See code: K80.31

K80.36 Calculus of bile duct with **acute and chronic cholangitis without obstruction** `PDxCC` `CC`

K80.37 Calculus of bile duct with **acute and chronic cholangitis with obstruction** `PDxCC` `CC`
CC Excl: See code: K80.31

✓5th **K80.4** Calculus of **bile duct with cholecystitis**
Any condition listed in K80.5 with cholecystitis (with cholangitis)

CC Excl: For CC codes in subcategory K80.4, unless otherwise noted: K80.30-K80.71, K80.81-K81.9, K83.5-K83.9, K87

K80.40 Calculus of bile duct with cholecystitis, **unspecified, without obstruction** `CC`

K80.41 Calculus of bile duct with cholecystitis, **unspecified, with obstruction** `CC`

K80.42 Calculus of bile duct with **acute cholecystitis without obstruction** `CC`

K80.43 Calculus of bile duct with **acute cholecystitis with obstruction** `CC`

K80.44 Calculus of bile duct with **chronic cholecystitis without obstruction** `CC`

K80.45 Calculus of bile duct with **chronic cholecystitis with obstruction** `CC`

K80.46 Calculus of bile duct with **acute and chronic cholecystitis without obstruction** `CC`

K80.47 Calculus of bile duct with **acute and chronic cholecystitis with obstruction** `CC`

✓5th **K80.5** Calculus of **bile duct without cholangitis or cholecystitis**
Choledocholithiasis (without cholangitis or cholecystitis)
Gallstone (impacted) of bile duct NOS (without cholangitis or cholecystitis)
Gallstone (impacted) of common duct (without cholangitis or cholecystitis)
Gallstone (impacted) of hepatic duct (without cholangitis or cholecystitis)
Hepatic cholelithiasis (without cholangitis or cholecystitis)
Hepatic colic (recurrent) (without cholangitis or cholecystitis)

K80.50 Calculus of bile duct without cholangitis or cholecystitis **without obstruction**

K80.51 Calculus of bile duct without cholangitis or cholecystitis **with obstruction** `CC`
CC Excl: K80.30-K80.71, K80.81-K81.9, K83.5-K83.9, K87

✓5th **K80.6** Calculus of **gallbladder and bile duct with cholecystitis**

CC Excl: For CC codes in subcategory K80.6, unless otherwise noted: See code: K80.51

K80.60 Calculus of gallbladder and bile duct with **cholecystitis, unspecified, without obstruction** `CC`

K80.61 Calculus of gallbladder and bile duct with **cholecystitis, unspecified, with obstruction** `CC`

K80.62 Calculus of gallbladder and bile duct with **acute cholecystitis without obstruction** `CC`
CC Excl: K80.62-K80.63, K81.0-K81.9, K82.9, K83.5-K83.9, K87

K80.63 Calculus of gallbladder and bile duct with **acute cholecystitis with obstruction** `CC`
CC Excl: See code: K80.62

K80.64 Calculus of gallbladder and bile duct with **chronic cholecystitis without obstruction** `CC`

K80.65 Calculus of gallbladder and bile duct with **chronic cholecystitis with obstruction** `CC`

K80.66 Calculus of gallbladder and bile duct with **acute and chronic cholecystitis without obstruction** `CC`
CC Excl: K80.66-K80.67, K81.0-K81.9, K82.9, K83.5-K83.9, K87

K80.67 Calculus of gallbladder and bile duct with **acute and chronic cholecystitis with obstruction** `MCC`
CC Excl: See code: K80.66

✓5th **K80.7** Calculus of **gallbladder and bile duct without cholecystitis**

K80.70 Calculus of gallbladder and bile duct without **cholecystitis without obstruction**

K80.71 Calculus of gallbladder and bile duct without **cholecystitis with obstruction** `CC`
CC Excl: See code: K80.51

✓5th **K80.8** Other **cholelithiasis**

K80.80 Other cholelithiasis **without obstruction**

K80.81 Other **cholelithiasis with obstruction** `CC`
CC Excl: See code: K80.51

✓4th **K81** Cholecystitis
EXCLUDES 1 cholecystitis with cholelithiasis (K80.-)

K81.0 Acute cholecystitis `CC`
Abscess of gallbladder
Angiocholecystitis
Emphysematous (acute) cholecystitis
Empyema of gallbladder
Gangrene of gallbladder
Gangrenous cholecystitis
Suppurative cholecystitis
CC Excl: K80.00, K80.12, K80.62-K80.63, K80.66-K80.67, K81.0-K81.9, K82.9, K83.5-K83.9, K87

K81.1 Chronic cholecystitis

K81.2 Acute cholecystitis with chronic cholecystitis `CC`
CC Excl: K81.0-K81.9, K82.9, K83.5-K83.9, K87

K81.9 Cholecystitis, unspecified

✓4th **K82** Other diseases of gallbladder
EXCLUDES 1 nonvisualization of gallbladder (R93.2)
postcholecystectomy syndrome (K91.5)

CC Excl: For CC/MCC codes in category K82, unless otherwise noted: K82.0-K82.9, K83.5-K83.9, K87

K82.0 Obstruction of gallbladder `CC`
Occlusion of cystic duct or gallbladder without cholelithiasis
Stenosis of cystic duct or gallbladder without cholelithiasis
Stricture of cystic duct or gallbladder without cholelithiasis
EXCLUDES 1 obstruction of gallbladder with cholelithiasis (K80.-)

K82.1 Hydrops of gallbladder `CC`
Mucocele of gallbladder

K82.2 Perforation of gallbladder `MCC`
Rupture of cystic duct or gallbladder

K82.3 Fistula of gallbladder `CC`
Cholecystocolic fistula
Cholecystoduodenal fistula

K82.4 Cholesterolosis of gallbladder
Strawberry gallbladder
EXCLUDES 1 cholesterolosis of gallbladder with cholecystis (K81.-)
cholesterolosis of gallbladder with cholelithiasis (K80.-)

K82.8 Other specified diseases of gallbladder
Adhesions of cystic duct or gallbladder
Atrophy of cystic duct or gallbladder
Cyst of cystic duct or gallbladder
Dyskinesia of cystic duct or gallbladder
Hypertrophy of cystic duct or gallbladder
Nonfunctioning of cystic duct or gallbladder
Ulcer of cystic duct or gallbladder

K82.9 Disease of gallbladder, unspecified

✓4th **K83** Other diseases of biliary tract
EXCLUDES 1 postcholecystectomy syndrome (K91.5)
EXCLUDES 2 conditions involving the gallbladder (K81-K82)
conditions involving the cystic duct (K81-K82)

K83.0 Cholangitis `CC`
Ascending cholangitis | Sclerosing cholangitis
Cholangitis NOS | Secondary cholangitis
Primary cholangitis | Stenosing cholangitis
Recurrent cholangitis | Suppurative cholangitis
EXCLUDES 1 cholangitic liver abscess (K75.0)
cholangitis with choledocholithiasis (K80.3-, K80.4-)
chronic nonsuppurative destructive cholangitis (K74.3)
CC Excl: K83.0, K83.5-K83.9, K87

K83.1 Obstruction of bile duct `MCC`
Occlusion of bile duct without cholelithiasis
Stenosis of bile duct without cholelithiasis
Stricture of bile duct without cholelithiasis
EXCLUDES 1 congenital obstruction of bile duct (Q44.3)
obstruction of bile duct with cholelithiasis (K80.-)
CC Excl: K80.31, K80.33, K80.35, K80.37, K80.41, K80.43, K80.45, K80.47, K80.51, K80.81, K83.1, K83.5-K83.9, K87, Q44.2-Q44.3

K83.2 Perforation of bile duct `MCC`
Rupture of bile duct
CC Excl: K83.2-K83.3, K83.5-K83.9, K87

K83.3 Fistula of bile duct `CC`
Choledochoduodenal fistula
CC Excl: See code: K83.2

K83.4 Spasm of sphincter of Oddi

K83.5 Biliary cyst

✓ Additional Character Required ✓x7th Placeholder Alert Unacceptable PDx Manifestation Hospital Acquired Condition *EXCLUDES 1* Not Coded Here *EXCLUDES 2* Not Included Here

Chapter 11. Diseases of the Digestive System

K83.8　Other specified diseases of biliary tract
Adhesions of biliary tract　　　Hypertrophy of biliary tract
Atrophy of biliary tract　　　　Ulcer of biliary tract

K83.9　Disease of biliary tract, unspecified

√4ᵗʰ **K85　Acute pancreatitis**
Abscess of pancreas　　　　　Hemorrhagic pancreatitis
Acute necrosis of pancreas　　Infective necrosis of pancreas
Acute (recurrent) pancreatitis　Subacute pancreatitis
Gangrene of (gangrenous) pancreas　Suppurative pancreatitis

> **CC Excl: For MCC codes in category K85, unless otherwise noted:**
> B25.2, K86.1, K86.8-K86.9

K85.0　Idiopathic acute pancreatitis `MCC`

K85.1　Biliary acute pancreatitis `MCC`
Gallstone pancreatitis

K85.2　Alcohol induced acute pancreatitis `MCC`
EXCLUDES 2 alcohol induced chronic pancreatitis (K86.0)

K85.3　Drug induced acute pancreatitis `MCC`
Use additional code for adverse effect, if applicable, to identify drug (T36-T50 with fifth or sixth character 5)
Use additional code to identify drug abuse and dependence (F11. – F17.-)

K85.8　Other acute pancreatitis `MCC`

K85.9　Acute pancreatitis, unspecified `MCC`
Pancreatitis NOS

√4ᵗʰ **K86　Other diseases of pancreas**
EXCLUDES 2 fibrocystic disease of pancreas (E84.-)
islet cell tumor (of pancreas) (D13.7)
pancreatic steatorrhea (K90.3)

K86.0　Alcohol-induced chronic pancreatitis `CC`
Use additional code to identify:
alcohol abuse and dependence (F10.-)
EXCLUDES 2 alcohol induced acute pancreatitis (K85.2)
CC Excl: B25.2, E16.8, K85.0-K86.9

K86.1　Other chronic pancreatitis `CC`
Chronic pancreatitis NOS　　Recurrent chronic pancreatitis
Infectious chronic pancreatitis　Relapsing chronic pancreatitis
CC Excl: See code: K86.0

K86.2　Cyst of pancreas `CC`
CC Excl: K86.2-K86.9

K86.3　Pseudocyst of pancreas `CC`
CC Excl: See code: K86.2

K86.8　Other specified diseases of pancreas
Aseptic pancreatic necrosis　　Fibrosis of pancreas
Atrophy of pancreas　　　　　Pancreatic fat necrosis
Calculus of pancreas　　　　　Pancreatic infantilism
Cirrhosis of pancreas　　　　　Pancreatic necrosis NOS

K86.9　Disease of pancreas, unspecified

K87　*Disorders of gallbladder, biliary tract and pancreas in diseases classified elsewhere*
Code first underlying disease
EXCLUDES 1 cytomegaloviral pancreatitis (B25.2)
mumps pancreatitis (B26.3)
syphilitic gallbladder (A52.74)
syphilitic pancreas (A52.74)
tuberculosis of gallbladder (A18.83)
tuberculosis of pancreas (A18.83)

Other diseases of the digestive system (K90-K95)

√4ᵗʰ **K90　Intestinal malabsorption**
EXCLUDES 1 intestinal malabsorption following gastrointestinal surgery (K91.2)

> **CC Excl: For CC codes in category K90, unless otherwise noted:**
> E84.19, K90.0-K90.4, K90.89-K90.9, K91.2

K90.0　Celiac disease
Gluten-sensitive enteropathy
Idiopathic steatorrhea
Nontropical sprue
Use additional code for associated disorders including:
dermatitis herpetiformis (L13.0)
gluten ataxia (G32.81)

K90.1　Tropical sprue `CC`
Sprue NOS　　　　　　Tropical steatorrhea

K90.2　Blind loop syndrome, not elsewhere classified `CC`
Blind loop syndrome NOS
EXCLUDES 1 congenital blind loop syndrome (Q43.8)
postsurgical blind loop syndrome (K91.2)

K90.3　Pancreatic steatorrhea `CC`

K90.4　Malabsorption due to intolerance, not elsewhere classified `CC`
Malabsorption due to intolerance to carbohydrate
Malabsorption due to intolerance to fat
Malabsorption due to intolerance to protein
Malabsorption due to intolerance to starch
EXCLUDES 2 gluten-sensitive enteropathy (K90.0)
lactose intolerance (E73.-)

√5ᵗʰ **K90.8　Other intestinal malabsorption**

K90.81　Whipple's disease `CC`
CC Excl: K90.81

K90.89　Other intestinal malabsorption `CC`

K90.9　Intestinal malabsorption, unspecified `CC`

√4ᵗʰ **K91　Intraoperative and postprocedural complications and disorders of digestive system, not elsewhere classified**
EXCLUDES 2 complications of artificial opening of digestive system (K94.-)
complications of bariatric procedures (K95.-)
gastrojejunal ulcer (K28.-)
postprocedural (radiation) retroperitoneal abscess (K68.11)
radiation colitis (K52.0)
radiation gastroenteritis (K52.0)
radiation proctitis (K62.7)

K91.0　Vomiting following gastrointestinal surgery

K91.1　Postgastric surgery syndromes
Dumping syndrome
Postgastrectomy syndrome
Postvagotomy syndrome

K91.2　Postsurgical malabsorption, not elsewhere classified `CC`
Postsurgical blind loop syndrome
EXCLUDES 1 malabsorption osteomalacia in adults (M83.2)
malabsorption osteoporosis, postsurgical (M80.8-, M81.8)
CC Excl: K90.3-K90.4, K90.89-K90.9, K91.2

K91.3　Postprocedural intestinal obstruction `CC`
CC Excl: D78.81-D78.89, E36.8, E89.810-E89.89, H59.011-H59.019, H59.031-H59.099, H59.811-H59.89, H95.811-H95.89, I97.3, K91.3, K91.81-K91.83, K91.850-K91.89, K94.20-K95.89, L76.81-L76.82, M96.89, N98.1-N98.9, T81.710A, T81.82XA, T81.89XA, T81.9XXA

K91.5　Postcholecystectomy syndrome

√5ᵗʰ **K91.6　Intraoperative hemorrhage and hematoma of a digestive system organ or structure complicating a procedure**
EXCLUDES 1 intraoperative hemorrhage and hematoma of a digestive system organ or structure due to accidental puncture and laceration during a procedure (K91.7-)

K91.61　Intraoperative hemorrhage and hematoma of a digestive system organ or structure complicating a digestive sytem procedure `CC`
CC Excl: H95.811-H95.89, I85.01, I85.11, I97.3, K21.9, K22.8, K23-K25.0, K25.2, K25.4, K25.6, K26.0, K26.2, K26.4, K26.6, K27.0, K27.2, K27.4, K27.6, K28.0, K28.2, K28.4, K28.6, K29.01, K29.21, K29.31, K29.41, K29.51, K29.61, K29.71, K29.81, K29.91, K31.811, K55.21, K57.01, K57.11, K57.13, K57.21, K57.31, K57.33, K57.41, K57.51, K57.53, K57.81, K57.91, K57.93, K62.5, K91.61-K91.62, K91.840-K91.841, K92.0-K92.2, M96.89, N98.1-N98.9, P54.1-P54.3, T81.10XA, T81.11XA, T81.12XA, T81.19XA, T81.82XA, T81.89XA, T81.9XXA

K91.62　Intraoperative hemorrhage and hematoma of a digestive system organ or structure complicating other procedure `CC`
CC Excl: See code: K91.61

√5ᵗʰ **K91.7　Accidental puncture and laceration of a digestive system organ or structure during a procedure**

K91.71　Accidental puncture and laceration of a digestive system organ or structure during a digestive system procedure `CC`
CC Excl: D78.11-D78.12, D78.81-D78.89, E36.11-E36.8, E89.810-E89.89, G96.11, G97.41-G97.49, H59.011-H59.019, H59.031-H59.099, H59.211-H59.229, H59.811-H59.89, H95.31-H95.32, H95.811-H95.89, I97.3, I97.51-I97.52, J95.71-J95.72, K91.71-K91.72, L76.11-L76.12, L76.81-L76.82, M96.820-M96.821, M96.89, N98.1-N98.9, N99.71-N99.72, T81.82XA, T81.89XA, T81.9XXA

K91.72　Accidental puncture and laceration of a digestive system organ or structure during other procedure `CC`
CC Excl: See code: K91.71

√5ᵗʰ **K91.8　Other intraoperative and postprocedural complications and disorders of digestive system**

> **CC Excl: For CC codes in subcategory K91.8, unless otherwise noted:** See code: K91.3

Ⓝ Newborn: 0　Ⓟ Pediatric: 0-17　Ⓜ Maternity: 12-55　Ⓐ Adult: 15-124　`MCC` Major CC Condition　`PDxMCC` PDx acts as own MCC　`CC` CC Condition　`PDxCC` PDx acts as own CC

676　　　　　　　　　　　　　　　　　　　　　　　　　　　　　　　　　　　ICD-10-CM 2016

K91.81 Other intraoperative complications of digestive system `CC`

K91.82 Postprocedural hepatic failure `CC`

K91.83 Postprocedural hepatorenal syndrome `CC`

✓6ᵗʰ **K91.84** Postprocedural hemorrhage and hematoma of a digestive system organ or structure following a procedure

     K91.840 Postprocedural hemorrhage and hematoma of a digestive system organ or structure following a digestive system procedure `CC`
         CC Excl: See code: K91.61

     K91.841 Postprocedural hemorrhage and hematoma of a digestive system organ or structure following other procedure `CC`
         CC Excl: See code: K91.61

✓6ᵗʰ **K91.85** Complications of intestinal pouch

     K91.850 Pouchitis `CC`
         Inflammation of internal ileoanal pouch

     K91.858 Other complications of intestinal pouch `CC`

K91.86 Retained cholelithiasis following cholecystectomy `CC`

K91.89 Other postprocedural complications and disorders of digestive system `CC`
     Use additional code, if applicable, to further specify disorder
     EXCLUDES 2   postprocedural retroperitoneal abscess (K68.11)

✓4ᵗʰ **K92 Other diseases of digestive system**
     EXCLUDES 1   neonatal gastrointestinal hemorrhage (P54.0-P54.3)

K92.0 Hematemesis `CC`
     CC Excl: E16.4, I85.01, K22.10-K22.11, K22.6-K22.719, K25.0-K28.9, K29.01, K29.21, K29.31, K29.41, K29.51, K29.61, K29.71, K29.81, K29.91, K31.811, K55.21, K57.01, K57.11, K57.13, K57.21, K57.31, K57.33, K57.41, K57.51, K57.53, K57.81, K57.91, K57.93, K62.5, K92.0-K92.2

K92.1 Melena `CC`
     EXCLUDES 1   occult blood in feces (R19.5)
     CC Excl: See code: K92.0

K92.2 Gastrointestinal hemorrhage, unspecified `CC`
     Gastric hemorrhage NOS
     Intestinal hemorrhage NOS
     EXCLUDES 1   acute hemorrhagic gastritis (K29.01)
         hemorrhage of anus and rectum (K62.5)
         angiodysplasia of stomach with hemorrhage (K31.811)
         diverticular disease with hemorrhage (K57.-)
         gastritis and duodenitis with hemorrhage (K29.-)
         peptic ulcer with hemorrhage (K25-K28)
     CC Excl: See code: K92.0

✓5ᵗʰ **K92.8** Other specified diseases of the digestive system

     K92.81 Gastrointestinal mucositis (ulcerative) `CC`
     Code also type of associated therapy, such as:
         antineoplastic and immunosuppressive drugs (T45.1X-)
         radiological procedure and radiotherapy (Y84.2)
     EXCLUDES 2   mucositis (ulcerative) of vagina and vulva (N76.81)
         nasal mucositis (ulcerative) (J34.81)
         oral mucositis (ulcerative) (K12.3-)
     CC Excl: E16.4, I85.01, K22.10-K22.11, K22.6-K22.719, K25.0-K28.9, K29.01, K29.21, K29.31, K29.41, K29.51, K29.61, K29.71, K29.81, K29.91, K31.811, K31.89-K31.9, K55.21, K57.01, K57.11, K57.13, K57.21, K57.31, K57.33, K57.41, K57.51, K57.53, K57.81, K57.91, K57.93, K62.5, K92.0-K92.81

     K92.89 Other specified diseases of the digestive system

K92.9 Disease of digestive system, unspecified

✓4ᵗʰ **K94 Complications of artificial openings of the digestive system**

✓5ᵗʰ **K94.0** Colostomy complications

     K94.00 Colostomy complication, unspecified

     K94.01 Colostomy hemorrhage `CC`
         CC Excl: K94.00-K94.19

     K94.02 Colostomy infection `CC`
     Use additional code to specify type of infection, such as:
         cellulitis of abdominal wall (L03.311)
         sepsis (A40-, A41-)
     CC Excl: See code: K94.01

     K94.03 Colostomy malfunction `CC`
     Mechanical complication of colostomy
     CC Excl: D78.81-D78.89, E36.8, E89.810-E89.89, H59.011-H59.019, H59.031-H59.099, H59.811-H59.89, H95.811-H95.89, I97.3, K91.3, K91.81-K91.83, K91.850-K91.89, K94.00-K95.89, L76.81-L76.82, M96.89, N98.1-N98.9, T81.710A, T81.82XA, T81.89XA, T81.9XXA

     K94.09 Other complications of colostomy `CC`
         CC Excl: See code: K94.01

✓5ᵗʰ **K94.1** Enterostomy complications

     K94.10 Enterostomy complication, unspecified

     K94.11 Enterostomy hemorrhage `CC`
         CC Excl: See code: K94.01

     K94.12 Enterostomy infection `CC`
     Use additional code to specify type of infection, such as:
         cellulitis of abdominal wall (L03.311)
         sepsis (A40-, A41-)
     CC Excl: See code: K94.01

     K94.13 Enterostomy malfunction `CC`
     Mechanical complication of enterostomy
     CC Excl: See code: K94.03

     K94.19 Other complications of enterostomy `CC`
         CC Excl: See code: K94.01

✓5ᵗʰ **K94.2** Gastrostomy complications

     K94.20 Gastrostomy complication, unspecified

     K94.21 Gastrostomy hemorrhage

     K94.22 Gastrostomy infection `CC`
     Use additional code to specify type of infection, such as:
         cellulitis of abdominal wall (L03.311)
         sepsis (A40-, A41-)
     CC Excl: See code: K91.3

     K94.23 Gastrostomy malfunction `CC`
     Mechanical complication of gastrostomy
     CC Excl: See code: K91.3

     K94.29 Other complications of gastrostomy

✓5ᵗʰ **K94.3** Esophagostomy complications

     CC Excl: For CC codes in subcategory K94.3, unless otherwise noted: D78.81-D78.89, E36.8, E89.810-E89.89, H59.011-H59.019, H59.031-H59.099, H59.811-H59.89, H95.811-H95.89, I97.3, K91.3, K91.81-K91.83, K91.850-K91.89, K94.20-K95.89, L76.81-L76.82, M96.89, N98.1-N98.9, T81.710A, T81.82XA, T81.89XA, T81.9XXA

     K94.30 Esophagostomy complications, unspecified `CC`

     K94.31 Esophagostomy hemorrhage `CC`

     K94.32 Esophagostomy infection `CC`
     Use additional code to identify the infection

     K94.33 Esophagostomy malfunction `CC`
     Mechanical complication of esophagostomy

     K94.39 Other complications of esophagostomy `CC`

✓4ᵗʰ **K95 Complications of bariatric procedures**

     CC Excl: For CC codes in category K95, unless otherwise noted: See code: K94.3

✓5ᵗʰ **K95.0** Complications of gastric band procedure

     4 **K95.01** Infection due to gastric band procedure `CC`
     Use additional code to specify type of infection or organism, such as:
         bacterial and viral infectious agents (B95.-, B96.-)
         cellulitis of abdominal wall (L03.311)
         sepsis (A40.-, A41.-)

     K95.09 Other complications of gastric band procedure `CC`
     Use additional code, if applicable, to further specify complication

✓5ᵗʰ **K95.8** Complications of other bariatric procedure
     EXCLUDES 1   complications of gastric band surgery (K95.0-)

     4 **K95.81** Infection due to other bariatric procedure `CC`
     Use additional code to specify type of infection or organism, such as:
         bacterial and viral infectious agents (B95.-, B96.-)
         cellulitis of abdominal wall (L03.311)
         sepsis (A40.-, A41.-)

     K95.89 Other complications of other bariatric procedure `CC`
     Use additional code, if applicable, to further specify complication

---

4   HAC = as SDx not POA, in combination with PDx E66.01 **AND** one of the following procedure codes: 0D16[0,4,8][7,J,K,Z][9,A,B,L] or 0DV64CZ.

✓ Additional Character Required   ✓x7ᵗʰ Placeholder Alert   Unacceptable PDx   Manifestation   Hospital Acquired Condition   *EXCLUDES 1* Not Coded Here   *EXCLUDES 2* Not Included Here

Chapter 12. Diseases of the Skin and Subcutaneous Tissue (L00–L99)

Chapter Specific Guidelines with Coding Examples

The chapter specific guidelines from the ICD-10-CM Official Guidelines for Coding and Reporting have been provided below. Along with these guidelines are coding examples, contained in the shaded boxes, that have been developed to help illustrate the coding and/or sequencing guidance found in these guidelines.

a. Pressure ulcer stage codes

1) Pressure ulcer stages

Codes from category L89, Pressure ulcer, are combination codes that identify the site of the pressure ulcer as well as the stage of the ulcer.

The ICD-10-CM classifies pressure ulcer stages based on severity, which is designated by stages 1-4, unspecified stage and unstageable.

Assign as many codes from category L89 as needed to identify all the pressure ulcers the patient has, if applicable.

> Stage 4 pressure ulcer right heel, 9 x 10 cm that invades the muscle and fascia; stage 2 pressure ulcer of left elbow
>
> **L89.614   Pressure ulcer of right heel, stage 4**
>
> **L89.022   Pressure ulcer of left elbow, stage 2**
>
> *Explanation:* Patient has a right heel pressure ulcer documented as stage 4 and a left elbow pressure ulcer documented as stage 2. Combination codes from category L89 Pressure ulcer, identify the site of the pressure ulcer as well as the stage. Assign as many codes from category L89 as needed to identify all the pressure ulcers the patient has.

2) Unstageable pressure ulcers

Assignment of the code for unstageable pressure ulcer (L89.--0) should be based on the clinical documentation. These codes are used for pressure ulcers whose stage cannot be clinically determined (e.g., the ulcer is covered by eschar or has been treated with a skin or muscle graft) and pressure ulcers that are documented as deep tissue injury but not documented as due to trauma. This code should not be confused with the codes for unspecified stage (L89.--9). When there is no documentation regarding the stage of the pressure ulcer, assign the appropriate code for unspecified stage (L89.--9).

> Pressure ulcer of the right lower back documented as unstageable due to the presence of thick eschar covering the ulcer
>
> **L89.130   Pressure ulcer of right lower back, unstageable**
>
> *Explanation:* Codes for unstageable pressure ulcers are assigned when the stage cannot be clinically determined (e.g., the ulcer is covered by eschar or has been treated with a skin or muscle graft).

3) Documented pressure ulcer stage

Assignment of the pressure ulcer stage code should be guided by clinical documentation of the stage or documentation of the terms found in the Alphabetic Index. For clinical terms describing the stage that are not found in the Alphabetic Index, and there is no documentation of the stage, the provider should be queried.

> Left heel pressure ulcer with partial thickness skin loss involving the dermis
>
> **L89.622   Pressure ulcer of left heel, stage 2**
>
> *Explanation:* Code assignment for the pressure ulcer stage should be guided by either the clinical documentation of the stage or the documentation of terms found in the Alphabetic Index. The clinical documentation describing the left heel pressure ulcer "partial thickness skin loss involving the dermis" matches the ICD-10-CM index parenthetical description for stage 2 "(abrasion, blister, partial thickness skin loss involving epidermis and/or dermis)."

4) Patients admitted with pressure ulcers documented as healed

No code is assigned if the documentation states that the pressure ulcer is completely healed.

> Patient receiving follow-up examination of a completely healed pressure ulcer of the foot
>
> **Z09   Encounter for follow-up examination after completed treatment for conditions other than malignant neoplasm**
>
> **Z87.2   Personal history of diseases of the skin and subcutaneous tissue**
>
> *Explanation:* Assign only codes for the reason for the encounter and the personal history of the pressure ulcer. Personal history code Z87.2 includes conditions classifiable to L00–L99 such as pressure ulcer. No code is assigned for a pressure ulcer documented as completely healed.

5) Patients admitted with pressure ulcers documented as healing

Pressure ulcers described as healing should be assigned the appropriate pressure ulcer stage code based on the documentation in the medical record. If the documentation does not provide information about the stage of the healing pressure ulcer, assign the appropriate code for unspecified stage.

If the documentation is unclear as to whether the patient has a current (new) pressure ulcer or if the patient is being treated for a healing pressure ulcer, query the provider.

> Healing stage 2 sacral pressure ulcer
>
> **L89.152   Pressure ulcer of sacral region, stage 2**
>
> *Explanation:* Pressure ulcers described as healing should be assigned the appropriate code for the pressure ulcer stage as documented.

6) Patient admitted with pressure ulcer evolving into another stage during the admission

If a patient is admitted with a pressure ulcer at one stage and it progresses to a higher stage, assign the code for the highest stage reported for that site.

> Stage 3 right hip pressure ulcer worsened during admission to a stage 4 pressure ulcer
>
> **L89.214   Pressure ulcer of right hip, stage 4**
>
> *Explanation:* A pressure ulcer that progresses from a lower stage to a higher stage is assigned only the code for the highest stage reported for that site.

Chapter 12. Diseases of the Skin and Subcutaneous Tissue (L00-L99)

> EXCLUDES 2   certain conditions originating in the perinatal period (P04-P96)
> certain infectious and parasitic diseases (A00-B99)
> complications of pregnancy, childbirth and the puerperium (O00-O9A)
> congenital malformations, deformations, and chromosomal abnormalities (Q00-Q99)
> endocrine, nutritional and metabolic diseases (E00-E88)
> lipomelanotic reticulosis (I89.8)
> neoplasms (C00-D49)
> symptoms, signs and abnormal clinical and laboratory findings, not elsewhere classified (R00-R94)
> systemic connective tissue disorders (M30-M36)
> viral warts (B07.-)

This chapter contains the following blocks:

L00-L08   Infections of the skin and subcutaneous tissue
L10-L14   Bullous disorders
L20-L30   Dermatitis and eczema
L40-L45   Papulosquamous disorders
L49-L54   Urticaria and erythema
L55-L59   Radiation-related disorders of the skin and subcutaneous tissue
L60-L75   Disorders of skin appendages
L76   Intraoperative and postprocedural complications of skin and subcutaneous tissue
L80-L99   Other disorders of the skin and subcutaneous tissue

Infections of the skin and subcutaneous tissue (L00-L08)

Use additional code (B95-B97) to identify infectious agent

> EXCLUDES 2   hordeolum (H00.0)
> infective dermatitis (L30.3)
> local infections of skin classified in Chapter 1
> lupus panniculitis (L93.2)
> panniculitis NOS (M79.3)
> panniculitis of neck and back (M54.0-)
> Perlèche NOS (K13.0)
> Perlèche due to candidiasis (B37.0)
> Perlèche due to riboflavin deficiency (E53.0)
> pyogenic granuloma (L98.0)
> relapsing panniculitis [Weber-Christian] (M35.6)
> viral warts (B07.-)
> zoster (B02.-)

L00   Staphylococcal scalded skin syndrome
Ritter's disease
Use additional code to identify percentage of skin exfoliation (L49.-)

> EXCLUDES 1   bullous impetigo (L01.03)
> pemphigus neonatorum (L01.03)
> toxic epidermal necrolysis [Lyell] (L51.2)

✓4ᵗʰ **L01   Impetigo**

> EXCLUDES 1   impetigo herpetiformis (L40.1)

✓5ᵗʰ **L01.0   Impetigo**
Impetigo contagiosa   Impetigo vulgaris

L01.00   Impetigo, unspecified
Impetigo NOS

L01.01   Non-bullous impetigo

L01.02   Bockhart's impetigo
Impetigo follicularis
Perifolliculitis NOS
Superficial pustular perifolliculitis

L01.03   Bullous impetigo
Impetigo neonatorum   Pemphigus neonatorum

L01.09   Other impetigo
Ulcerative impetigo

L01.1   Impetiginization of other dermatoses

✓4ᵗʰ **L02   Cutaneous abscess, furuncle and carbuncle**
Use additional code to identify organism (B95-B96)

> EXCLUDES 2   abscess of anus and rectal regions (K61.-)
> abscess of female genital organs (external) (N76.4)
> abscess of male genital organs (external) (N48.2, N49-)

✓5ᵗʰ **L02.0   Cutaneous abscess, furuncle and carbuncle of face**

> EXCLUDES 2   abscess of ear, external (H60.0)
> abscess of eyelid (H00.0)
> abscess of head [any part, except face] (L02.8)
> abscess of lacrimal gland (H04.0)
> abscess of lacrimal passages (H04.3)
> abscess of mouth (K12.2)
> abscess of nose (J34.0)
> abscess of orbit (H05.0)
> submandibular abscess (K12.2)

L02.01   Cutaneous abscess of face   CC
CC Excl: No Excl

L02.02   Furuncle of face
Boil of face   Folliculitis of face

L02.03   Carbuncle of face

✓5ᵗʰ **L02.1   Cutaneous abscess, furuncle and carbuncle of neck**

L02.11   Cutaneous abscess of neck   CC
CC Excl: A17.9, A18.4, A18.82, A18.84, A18.89, A48.2-A48.4, A48.8-A49.9, B78.1, B95.0-B96.89, E83.2, L02.11, L02.811-L02.818, L02.91, L03.221-L03.222, L03.811-L03.91, L08.0, L08.81-L08.9, L44.8-L45, L73.2, L88, L92.8, L94.2, L94.4, L98.0, L98.3, L98.8, L99, Z16.10-Z16.39

L02.12   Furuncle of neck
Boil of neck   Folliculitis of neck

L02.13   Carbuncle of neck

✓5ᵗʰ **L02.2   Cutaneous abscess, furuncle and carbuncle of trunk**

> EXCLUDES 1   non-newborn omphalitis (L08.82)
> omphalitis of newborn (P38.-)

> EXCLUDES 2   abscess of breast (N61)
> abscess of buttocks (L02.3)
> abscess of female external genital organs (N76.4)
> abscess of hip (L02.4)
> abscess of male external genital organs (N48.2, N49-)

CC Excl: For CC codes in subcategory L02.2, unless otherwise noted: A17.9, A18.4, A18.82, A18.84, A18.89, A48.2-A48.4, A48.8-A49.9, B78.1, B95.0-B96.89, E83.2, L02.211-L02.219, L02.811-L02.818, L02.91, L03.311-L03.316, L03.319-L03.326, L03.329-L03.91, L08.0, L08.81-L08.9, L44.8-L45, L73.2, L88, L92.8, L94.2, L94.4, L98.0, L98.3, L98.8, L99, Z16.10-Z16.39

✓6ᵗʰ **L02.21   Cutaneous abscess of trunk**

L02.211   Cutaneous abscess of abdominal wall   CC

L02.212   Cutaneous abscess of back [any part, except buttock]   CC

L02.213   Cutaneous abscess of chest wall   CC

L02.214   Cutaneous abscess of groin   CC

L02.215   Cutaneous abscess of perineum   CC

L02.216   Cutaneous abscess of umbilicus   CC

L02.219   Cutaneous abscess of trunk, unspecified   CC

✓6ᵗʰ **L02.22   Furuncle of trunk**
Boil of trunk   Folliculitis of trunk

L02.221   Furuncle of abdominal wall

L02.222   Furuncle of back [any part, except buttock]

L02.223   Furuncle of chest wall

L02.224   Furuncle of groin

L02.225   Furuncle of perineum

L02.226   Furuncle of umbilicus

L02.229   Furuncle of trunk, unspecified

✓6ᵗʰ **L02.23   Carbuncle of trunk**

L02.231   Carbuncle of abdominal wall

L02.232   Carbuncle of back [any part, except buttock]

L02.233   Carbuncle of chest wall

L02.234   Carbuncle of groin

L02.235   Carbuncle of perineum

L02.236   Carbuncle of umbilicus

L02.239   Carbuncle of trunk, unspecified

✓5ᵗʰ **L02.3   Cutaneous abscess, furuncle and carbuncle of buttock**

> EXCLUDES 1   pilonidal cyst with abscess (L05.01)

L02.31   Cutaneous abscess of buttock   CC
Cutaneous abscess of gluteal region
CC Excl: A17.9, A18.4, A18.82, A18.84, A18.89, A48.2-A48.4, A48.8-A49.9, B78.1, B95.0-B96.89, E83.2, L02.31, L02.811-L02.818, L02.91, L03.317, L03.327, L03.811-L03.91, L08.0, L08.81-L08.9, L44.8-L45, L73.2, L88, L92.8, L94.2, L94.4, L98.0, L98.3, L98.8, L99, Z16.10-Z16.39

L02.32   Furuncle of buttock
Boil of buttock   Furuncle of gluteal region
Folliculitis of buttock

L02.33   Carbuncle of buttock
Carbuncle of gluteal region

☑ Additional Character Required   ✓x7ᵗʰ Placeholder Alert   Unacceptable PDx   Manifestation   Hospital Acquired Condition   EXCLUDES 1 Not Coded Here   EXCLUDES 2 Not Included Here

Chapter 12. Diseases of the Skin and Subcutaneous Tissue

L02.4–L03.029

✓5ᵗʰ **L02.4 Cutaneous abscess, furuncle and carbuncle of limb**

EXCLUDES 2   cutaneous abscess, furuncle and carbuncle of groin (L02.214, L02.224, L02.234)
cutaneous abscess, furuncle and carbuncle of hand (L02.5-)
cutaneous abscess, furuncle and carbuncle of foot (L02.6-)

CC Excl: For CC codes in subcategory L02.4, unless otherwise noted: A17.9, A18.4, A18.82, A18.84, A18.89, A48.2-A48.4, A48.8-A49.9, B78.1, B95.0-B96.89, E83.2, L02.411-L02.414, L02.811-L02.818, L02.91, L03.111-L03.114, L03.121-L03.124, L03.811-L03.91, L08.0, L08.81-L08.9, L44.8-L45, L73.2, L88, L92.8, L94.2, L94.4, L98.0, L98.3, L98.8, L99, Z16.10-Z16.39

✓6ᵗʰ **L02.41 Cutaneous abscess of limb**

     L02.411 Cutaneous abscess of right axilla   CC
     L02.412 Cutaneous abscess of left axilla   CC
     L02.413 Cutaneous abscess of right upper limb   CC
     L02.414 Cutaneous abscess of left upper limb   CC
     L02.415 Cutaneous abscess of right lower limb   CC

         CC Excl: A17.9-A18.4, A18.82, A18.84, A18.89, A48.2-A48.4, A48.8-A49.9, B78.1, B95.0-B96.89, E83.2, L02.415-L02.419, L02.811-L02.818, L02.91, L03.115-L03.119, L03.125-L03.129, L03.811-L03.91, L08.0, L08.81-L08.9, L44.8-L45, L73.2, L88, L92.8, L94.2, L94.4, L98.0, L98.3, L98.8, L99, Z16.10-Z16.39

     L02.416 Cutaneous abscess of left lower limb   CC
         CC Excl: See code: L02.415
     L02.419 Cutaneous abscess of limb, unspecified   CC
         CC Excl: See code: L02.415

✓6ᵗʰ **L02.42 Furuncle of limb**
     Boil of limb   Folliculitis of limb
     L02.421 Furuncle of right axilla
     L02.422 Furuncle of left axilla
     L02.423 Furuncle of right upper limb
     L02.424 Furuncle of left upper limb
     L02.425 Furuncle of right lower limb
     L02.426 Furuncle of left lower limb
     L02.429 Furuncle of limb, unspecified

✓6ᵗʰ **L02.43 Carbuncle of limb**
     L02.431 Carbuncle of right axilla
     L02.432 Carbuncle of left axilla
     L02.433 Carbuncle of right upper limb
     L02.434 Carbuncle of left upper limb
     L02.435 Carbuncle of right lower limb
     L02.436 Carbuncle of left lower limb
     L02.439 Carbuncle of limb, unspecified

✓5ᵗʰ **L02.5 Cutaneous abscess, furuncle and carbuncle of hand**

CC Excl: For CC codes in subcategory L02.5, unless otherwise noted: A17.9, A18.4, A18.82, A18.84, A18.89, A48.2-A48.4, A48.8-A49.9, B78.1, B95.0-B96.89, E83.2, L02.511-L02.519, L02.811-L02.818, L02.91, L03.811-L03.91, L08.0, L08.81-L08.9, L44.8-L45, L73.2, L88, L92.8, L94.2, L94.4, L98.0, L98.3, L98.8, L99, Z16.10-Z16.39

✓6ᵗʰ **L02.51 Cutaneous abscess of hand**
     L02.511 Cutaneous abscess of right hand   CC
     L02.512 Cutaneous abscess of left hand   CC
     L02.519 Cutaneous abscess of unspecified hand   CC

✓6ᵗʰ **L02.52 Furuncle hand**
     Boil of hand   Folliculitis of hand
     L02.521 Furuncle right hand
     L02.522 Furuncle left hand
     L02.529 Furuncle unspecified hand

✓6ᵗʰ **L02.53 Carbuncle of hand**
     L02.531 Carbuncle of right hand
     L02.532 Carbuncle of left hand
     L02.539 Carbuncle of unspecified hand

✓5ᵗʰ **L02.6 Cutaneous abscess, furuncle and carbuncle of foot**

CC Excl: For CC codes in subcategory L02.6, unless otherwise noted: A17.9, A18.4, A18.82, A18.84, A18.89, A48.2-A48.4, A48.8-A49.9, B78.1, B95.0-B96.89, E83.2, L02.611-L02.619, L02.811-L02.818, L02.91, L03.811-L03.91, L08.0, L08.81-L08.9, L44.8-L45, L73.2, L88, L92.8, L94.2, L94.4, L98.0, L98.3, L98.8, L99, Z16.10-Z16.39

✓6ᵗʰ **L02.61 Cutaneous abscess of foot**
     L02.611 Cutaneous abscess of right foot   CC
     L02.612 Cutaneous abscess of left foot   CC
     L02.619 Cutaneous abscess of unspecified foot   CC

✓6ᵗʰ **L02.62 Furuncle of foot**
     Boil of foot   Folliculitis of foot
     L02.621 Furuncle of right foot
     L02.622 Furuncle of left foot
     L02.629 Furuncle of unspecified foot

✓6ᵗʰ **L02.63 Carbuncle of foot**
     L02.631 Carbuncle of right foot
     L02.632 Carbuncle of left foot
     L02.639 Carbuncle of unspecified foot

✓5ᵗʰ **L02.8 Cutaneous abscess, furuncle and carbuncle of other sites**

✓6ᵗʰ **L02.81 Cutaneous abscess of other sites**
     L02.811 Cutaneous abscess of head [any part, except face]   CC
         CC Excl: A17.9, A18.4, A18.82, A18.84, A18.89, A48.2-A48.4, A48.8-A49.9, B78.1, B95.0-B96.89, E83.2, L02.811-L02.818, L02.91, L03.811-L03.91, L08.0, L08.81-L08.9, L44.8-L45, L73.2, L88, L92.8, L94.2, L94.4, L98.0, L98.3, L98.8, L99, Z16.10-Z16.39
     L02.818 Cutaneous abscess of other sites   CC
         CC Excl: See code: L02.811

✓6ᵗʰ **L02.82 Furuncle of other sites**
     Boil of other sites   Folliculitis of other sites
     L02.821 Furuncle of head [any part, except face]
     L02.828 Furuncle of other sites

✓6ᵗʰ **L02.83 Carbuncle of other sites**
     L02.831 Carbuncle of head [any part, except face]
     L02.838 Carbuncle of other sites

✓5ᵗʰ **L02.9 Cutaneous abscess, furuncle and carbuncle, unspecified**
     L02.91 Cutaneous abscess, unspecified   CC
         CC Excl: See code: L02.811
     L02.92 Furuncle, unspecified
         Boil NOS   Furunculosis NOS
     L02.93 Carbuncle, unspecified

✓4ᵗʰ **L03 Cellulitis and acute lymphangitis**

EXCLUDES 2   cellulitis of anal and rectal region (K61.-)
cellulitis of external auditory canal (H60.1)
cellulitis of eyelid (H00.03-)
cellulitis of external genital organs (N76.4)
cellulitis of lacrimal apparatus (H04.3)
cellulitis of male external genital organs (N48.2, N49-)
cellulitis of mouth (K12.2)
cellulitis of nose (J34.0)
eosinophilic cellulitis [Wells] (L98.3)
febrile neutrophilic dermatosis [Sweet] (L98.2)
lymphangitis (chronic) (subacute) (I89.1)

✓5ᵗʰ **L03.0 Cellulitis and acute lymphangitis of finger and toe**
     Infection of nail   Paronychia
     Onychia   Perionychia

✓6ᵗʰ **L03.01 Cellulitis of finger**
     Felon
     Whitlow
         EXCLUDES 1   herpetic whitlow (B00.89)
     L03.011 Cellulitis of right finger
     L03.012 Cellulitis of left finger
     L03.019 Cellulitis of unspecified finger

✓6ᵗʰ **L03.02 Acute lymphangitis of finger**
     Hangnail with lymphangitis of finger
     L03.021 Acute lymphangitis of right finger
     L03.022 Acute lymphangitis of left finger
     L03.029 Acute lymphangitis of unspecified finger

Ⓝ Newborn: 0   Ⓟ Pediatric: 0-17   Ⓜ Maternity: 12-55   Ⓐ Adult: 15-124   MCC Major CC Condition   PDxMCC PDx acts as own MCC   CC CC Condition   PDxCC PDx acts as own CC

680   ICD-10-CM 2016

✓6ᵗʰ **L03.03**   **Cellulitis** of toe
    L03.031   **Cellulitis of right** toe
    L03.032   **Cellulitis of left** toe
    L03.039   **Cellulitis of unspecified** toe

✓6ᵗʰ **L03.04**   **Acute lymphangitis of** toe
    Hangnail with lymphangitis of toe
    L03.041   **Acute lymphangitis of right** toe
    L03.042   **Acute lymphangitis of left** toe
    L03.049   **Acute lymphangitis of unspecified** toe

✓5ᵗʰ **L03.1**   **Cellulitis and acute lymphangitis of** other parts of limb

> **CC Excl: For CC codes in subcategory L03.1, unless otherwise noted:** A17.9, A18.4, A18.82, A18.84, A18.89, A48.2-A48.4, A48.8-A49.9, B78.1, B95.0-B96.89, E83.2, L02.411-L02.414, L02.811-L02.818, L02.91, L03.111-L03.114, L03.121-L03.124, L03.811-L03.91, L08.0, L08.81-L08.9, L44.8-L45, L73.2, L88, L92.8, L94.2, L94.4, L98.0, L98.3, L98.8, L99, Z16.10-Z16.39

✓6ᵗʰ **L03.11**   **Cellulitis of** other parts of limb
    EXCLUDES 2   cellulitis of fingers (L03.01-)
          cellulitis of toes (L03.03-)
          groin (L03.314)
    L03.111   **Cellulitis of right axilla**   CC
    L03.112   **Cellulitis of left axilla**   CC
    L03.113   **Cellulitis of right upper limb**   CC
    L03.114   **Cellulitis of left upper limb**   CC
    L03.115   **Cellulitis of right lower limb**   CC
          CC Excl: See code: L02.415
    L03.116   **Cellulitis of left lower limb**   CC
          CC Excl: See code: L02.415
    L03.119   **Cellulitis of unspecified part of limb**   CC
          CC Excl: See code: L02.415

✓6ᵗʰ **L03.12**   **Acute lymphangitis of** other parts of limb
    EXCLUDES 2   acute lymphangitis of fingers (L03.02-)
          acute lymphangitis of groin (L03.324)
          acute lymphangitis of toes (L03.04-)
    L03.121   **Acute lymphangitis of right axilla**   CC
    L03.122   **Acute lymphangitis of left axilla**   CC
    L03.123   **Acute lymphangitis of right upper limb**   CC
    L03.124   **Acute lymphangitis of left upper limb**   CC
    L03.125   **Acute lymphangitis of right lower limb**   CC
          CC Excl: See code: L02.415
    L03.126   **Acute lymphangitis of left lower limb**   CC
          CC Excl: See code: L02.415
    L03.129   **Acute lymphangitis of unspecified part of limb**   CC
          CC Excl: See code: L02.415

✓5ᵗʰ **L03.2**   **Cellulitis and acute lymphangitis of** face and neck

✓6ᵗʰ **L03.21**   **Cellulitis and acute lymphangitis of** face
    L03.211   **Cellulitis of face**   CC
          EXCLUDES 2   cellulitis of ear (H60.1-)
            cellulitis of eyelid (H00.03-)
            cellulitis of head (L03.811)
            cellulitis of lacrimal apparatus (H04.3)
            cellulitis of lip (K13.0)
            cellulitis of mouth (K12.2)
            cellulitis of nose (internal) (J34.0)
            cellulitis of orbit (H05.0)
            cellulitis of scalp (L03.811)
          AHA: 2013, 4Q, 123
          CC Excl: A17.9, A18.4, A18.82, A18.84, A18.89, A48.2-A48.4, A48.8-A49.9, B78.1, B95.0-B96.89, E83.2, L02.811-L02.818, L02.91, L03.211, L03.811-L03.91, L08.0, L08.81-L08.9, L44.8-L45, L73.2, L88, L92.8, L94.2, L94.4, L98.0, L98.3, L98.8, L99, Z16.10-Z16.39
    L03.212   **Acute lymphangitis of face**   CC
          CC Excl: No Excl

✓6ᵗʰ **L03.22**   **Cellulitis and acute lymphangitis of** neck
    L03.221   **Cellulitis of neck**   CC
          CC Excl: A17.9, A18.4, A18.82, A18.84, A18.89, A48.2-A48.4, A48.8-A49.9, B78.1, B95.0-B96.89, E83.2, L02.11, L02.811-L02.818, L02.91, L03.221-L03.222, L03.811-L03.91, L08.0, L08.81-L08.9, L44.8-L45, L73.2, L88, L92.8, L94.2, L94.4, L98.0, L98.3, L98.8, L99, Z16.10-Z16.39
    L03.222   **Acute lymphangitis of neck**   CC
          CC Excl: See code: L03.221

✓5ᵗʰ **L03.3**   **Cellulitis and acute lymphangitis of** trunk

> **CC Excl: For CC codes in subcategory L03.3, unless otherwise noted:** A17.9, A18.4, A18.82, A18.84, A18.89, A48.2-A48.4, A48.8-A49.9, B78.1, B95.0-B96.89, E83.2, L02.211-L02.219, L02.811-L02.818, L02.91, L03.311-L03.316, L03.319-L03.326, L03.329-L03.91, L08.0, L08.81-L08.9, L44.8-L45, L73.2, L88, L92.8, L94.2, L94.4, L98.0, L98.3, L98.8, L99, Z16.10-Z16.39

✓6ᵗʰ **L03.31**   **Cellulitis of** trunk
    EXCLUDES 2   cellulitis of anal and rectal regions (K61.-)
          cellulitis of breast NOS (N61)
          cellulitis of female external genital organs (N76.4)
          cellulitis of male external genital organs (N48.2, N49-)
          omphalitis of newborn (P38.-)
          puerperal cellulitis of breast (O91.2)
    L03.311   **Cellulitis of abdominal wall**   CC
          EXCLUDES 2   cellulitis of umbilicus (L03.316)
            cellulitis of groin (L03.314)
    L03.312   **Cellulitis of back [any part except buttock]**   CC
    L03.313   **Cellulitis of chest wall**   CC
    L03.314   **Cellulitis of groin**   CC
    L03.315   **Cellulitis of perineum**   CC
    L03.316   **Cellulitis of umbilicus**   CC
    L03.317   **Cellulitis of buttock**
          CC Excl: A17.9, A18.4, A18.82, A18.84, A18.89, A48.2-A48.4, A48.8-A49.9, B78.1, B95.0-B96.89, E83.2, L02.31, L02.811-L02.818, L02.91, L03.317, L03.327, L03.811-L03.91, L08.0, L08.81-L08.9, L44.8-L45, L73.2, L88, L92.8, L94.2, L94.4, L98.0, L98.3, L98.8, L99, Z16.10-Z16.39
    L03.319   **Cellulitis of trunk, unspecified**   CC

✓6ᵗʰ **L03.32**   **Acute lymphangitis of** trunk
    L03.321   **Acute lymphangitis of abdominal wall**   CC
    L03.322   **Acute lymphangitis of back [any part except buttock]**   CC
    L03.323   **Acute lymphangitis of chest wall**   CC
    L03.324   **Acute lymphangitis of groin**   CC
    L03.325   **Acute lymphangitis of perineum**   CC
    L03.326   **Acute lymphangitis of umbilicus**   CC
    L03.327   **Acute lymphangitis of buttock**   CC
          CC Excl: See code: L03.317
    L03.329   **Acute lymphangitis of trunk, unspecified**   CC

✓5ᵗʰ **L03.8**   **Cellulitis and acute lymphangitis of** other sites

> **CC Excl: For CC codes in subcategory L03.8, unless otherwise noted:** A17.9, A18.4, A18.82, A18.84, A18.89, A48.2-A48.4, A48.8-A49.9, B78.1, B95.0-B96.89, E83.2, L02.811-L02.818, L02.91, L03.811-L03.91, L08.0, L08.81-L08.9, L44.8-L45, L73.2, L88, L92.8, L94.2, L94.4, L98.0, L98.3, L98.8, L99, Z16.10-Z16.39

✓6ᵗʰ **L03.81**   **Cellulitis of** other sites
    L03.811   **Cellulitis of head [any part, except face]**   CC
          Cellulitis of scalp
          EXCLUDES 2   cellulitis of face (L03.211)
    L03.818   **Cellulitis of other sites**   CC

✓6ᵗʰ **L03.89**   **Acute lymphangitis of** other sites
    L03.891   **Acute lymphangitis of head [any part, except face]**   CC
    L03.898   **Acute lymphangitis of other sites**   CC

✓5ᵗʰ **L03.9**   **Cellulitis and acute lymphangitis, unspecified**

> **CC Excl: For CC codes in subcategory L03.9, unless otherwise noted:** See code: L03.8

    L03.90   **Cellulitis, unspecified**   CC
    L03.91   **Acute lymphangitis, unspecified**   CC
          EXCLUDES 1   lymphangitis NOS (I89.1)

✓ Additional Character Required   ✓x7ᵗʰ Placeholder Alert   Unacceptable PDx   Manifestation   Hospital Acquired Condition   *EXCLUDES 1* Not Coded Here   *EXCLUDES 2* Not Included Here

✓4ᵗʰ L04   Acute lymphadenitis

INCLUDES   abscess (acute) of lymph nodes, except mesenteric
acute lymphadenitis, except mesenteric

EXCLUDES 1   chronic or subacute lymphadenitis, except mesenteric (I88.1)
enlarged lymph nodes (R59.-)
human immunodeficiency virus [HIV] disease resulting in
generalized lymphadenopathy (B20)
lymphadenitis NOS (I88.9)
nonspecific mesenteric lymphadenitis (I88.0)

L04.0   Acute lymphadenitis of **face, head and neck**

L04.1   Acute lymphadenitis of **trunk**

L04.2   Acute lymphadenitis of **upper limb**
Acute lymphadenitis of axilla   Acute lymphadenitis of shoulder

L04.3   Acute lymphadenitis of **lower limb**
Acute lymphadenitis of hip
EXCLUDES 2   acute lymphadenitis of groin (L04.1)

L04.8   Acute lymphadenitis of **other sites**

L04.9   Acute lymphadenitis, **unspecified**

✓4ᵗʰ L05   Pilonidal cyst and sinus

✓5ᵗʰ L05.0   Pilonidal cyst and sinus **with abscess**

L05.01   Pilonidal **cyst** with abscess   `CC`
Parasacral dimple with abscess
Pilonidal abscess
Pilonidal dimple with abscess
Postanal dimple with abscess
CC Excl: L05.01-L05.92, L44.8-L45, L94.2, L94.4, L98.8, L99

L05.02   Pilonidal **sinus** with abscess   `CC`
Coccygeal fistula with abscess
Coccygeal sinus with abscess
Pilonidal fistula with abscess
CC Excl: See code: L05.01

✓5ᵗʰ L05.9   Pilonidal cyst and sinus **without abscess**

L05.91   Pilonidal **cyst** without abscess
Parasacral dimple   Postanal dimple
Pilonidal dimple   Pilonidal cyst NOS

L05.92   Pilonidal **sinus** without abscess
Coccygeal fistula
Coccygeal sinus without abscess
Pilonidal fistula

✓4ᵗʰ L08   Other local infections of skin and subcutaneous tissue

L08.0   Pyoderma
Dermatitis gangrenosa   Septic dermatitis
Purulent dermatitis   Suppurative dermatitis
EXCLUDES 1   pyoderma gangrenosum (L88)
pyoderma vegetans (L08.81)

L08.1   Erythrasma   `HIV` `CC`
CC Excl: A42.81-A42.9, A43.1-A43.9, B47.1, L08.1

✓5ᵗʰ L08.8   Other specified local infections of the skin and subcutaneous tissue

L08.81   Pyoderma vegetans
EXCLUDES 1   pyoderma gangrenosum (L88)
pyoderma NOS (L08.0)

L08.82   Omphalitis not of newborn
EXCLUDES 1   omphalitis of newborn (P38.-)

L08.89   Other specified local infections of the skin and subcutaneous tissue

L08.9   Local infection of the skin and subcutaneous tissue, unspecified

Bullous disorders (L10-L14)

EXCLUDES 1   benign familial pemphigus [Hailey-Hailey] (Q82.8)
staphylococcal scalded skin syndrome (L00)
toxic epidermal necrolysis [Lyell] (L51.2)

✓4ᵗʰ L10   Pemphigus

EXCLUDES 1   pemphigus neonatorum (L01.03)

CC Excl: For CC codes in category L10, unless otherwise noted:
L10.0-L10.9, L12.0-L12.1, L12.8-L12.9, L13.8-L14, L44.8-L45, L94.2, L94.4, L98.8, L99

L10.0   Pemphigus **vulgaris**   `CC`

L10.1   Pemphigus **vegetans**   `CC`

L10.2   Pemphigus **foliaceous**   `CC`

L10.3   Brazilian **pemphigus [fogo selvagem]**   `CC`

L10.4   Pemphigus **erythematosus**   `CC`
Senear-Usher syndrome

L10.5   Drug-induced **pemphigus**   `CC`
Use additional code for adverse effect, if applicable, to identify drug (T36-T50 with fifth or sixth character 5)

✓5ᵗʰ L10.8   Other pemphigus

L10.81   Paraneoplastic **pemphigus**   `CC`

L10.89   Other **pemphigus**   `CC`

L10.9   Pemphigus, **unspecified**

✓4ᵗʰ L11   Other acantholytic disorders

L11.0   Acquired keratosis follicularis
EXCLUDES 1   keratosis follicularis (congenital) [Darier-White] (Q82.8)

L11.1   Transient acantholytic dermatosis [Grover]

L11.8   Other specified acantholytic disorders

L11.9   Acantholytic disorder, unspecified

✓4ᵗʰ L12   Pemphigoid

EXCLUDES 1   herpes gestationis (O26.4-)
impetigo herpetiformis (L40.1)

CC Excl: For CC codes in category L12, unless otherwise noted:
See code: L10

L12.0   Bullous **pemphigoid**   `CC`

L12.1   Cicatricial **pemphigoid**
Benign mucous membrane pemphigoid

L12.2   Chronic **bullous disease of childhood**   `P`
Juvenile dermatitis herpetiformis

✓5ᵗʰ L12.3   Acquired epidermolysis bullosa

EXCLUDES 1   epidermolysis bullosa (congenital) (Q81.-)

L12.30   Acquired epidermolysis bullosa, unspecified   `CC`
CC Excl: L00, L12.30-L12.35, L26, L30.4, L44.8-L45, L51.0-L54, L71.0-L71.9, L92.0, L93.0-L93.2, L94.2, L94.4, L95.1, L98.2, L98.8, L99

L12.31   Epidermolysis bullosa due to drug   `CC`
Use additional code for adverse effect, if applicable, to identify drug (T36-T50 with fifth or sixth character 5)
CC Excl: See code: L12.30

L12.35   Other acquired epidermolysis bullosa   `CC`
CC Excl: See code: L12.30

L12.8   Other **pemphigoid**   `CC`

L12.9   Pemphigoid, **unspecified**   `CC`

✓4ᵗʰ L13   Other bullous disorders

L13.0   Dermatitis herpetiformis
Duhring's disease
Hydroa herpetiformis
EXCLUDES 1   juvenile dermatitis herpetiformis (L12.2)
senile dermatitis herpetiformis (L12.0)

L13.1   Subcorneal pustular dermatitis
Sneddon-Wilkinson disease

L13.8   Other specified bullous disorders

L13.9   Bullous disorder, unspecified

L14   *Bullous disorders in diseases classified elsewhere*
Code first underlying disease

Dermatitis and eczema (L20-L30)

NOTE   In this block the terms dermatitis and eczema are used synonymously and interchangeably.

EXCLUDES 2   chronic (childhood) granulomatous disease (D71)
dermatitis gangrenosa (L08.0)
dermatitis herpetiformis (L13.0)
dry skin dermatitis (L85.3)
factitial dermatitis (L98.1)
perioral dermatitis (L71.0)
radiation-related disorders of the skin and subcutaneous tissue (L55-L59)
stasis dermatitis (I83.1-I83.2)

✓4ᵗʰ L20   Atopic dermatitis

L20.0   Besnier's prurigo

✓5ᵗʰ L20.8   Other atopic dermatitis

EXCLUDES 2   circumscribed neurodermatitis (L28.0)

L20.81   Atopic neurodermatitis
Diffuse neurodermatitis

L20.82   Flexural eczema

L20.83   Infantile (acute) (chronic) eczema   `P`

L20.84   Intrinsic (allergic) eczema

L20.89   Other atopic dermatitis

L20.9   Atopic dermatitis, unspecified

N Newborn: 0   P Pediatric: 0-17   M Maternity: 12-55   A Adult: 15-124   **MCC** Major CC Condition   **PDxMCC** PDx acts as own MCC   `CC` CC Condition   **PDxCC** PDx acts as own CC

682   ICD-10-CM 2016

✓4ᵗʰ **L21   Seborrheic dermatitis**
> EXCLUDES 2   *infective dermatitis (L30.3)*
> *seborrheic keratosis (L82.-)*

   L21.0   Seborrhea capitis   P
> Cradle cap

   L21.1   Seborrheic infantile dermatitis   P

   L21.8   Other seborrheic dermatitis

   L21.9   Seborrheic dermatitis, unspecified
> Seborrhea NOS

L22   Diaper dermatitis
> Diaper erythema   Psoriasiform diaper rash
> Diaper rash

✓4ᵗʰ **L23   Allergic contact dermatitis**
> EXCLUDES 1   *allergy NOS (T78.40)*
> *contact dermatitis NOS (L25.9)*
> *dermatitis NOS (L30.9)*
> EXCLUDES 2   *dermatitis due to substances taken internally (L27.-)*
> *dermatitis of eyelid (H01.1-)*
> *diaper dermatitis (L22)*
> *eczema of external ear (H60.5-)*
> *irritant contact dermatitis (L24.-)*
> *perioral dermatitis (L71.0)*
> *radiation-related disorders of the skin and subcutaneous tissue (L55-L59)*

   L23.0   Allergic contact dermatitis due to metals
> Allergic contact dermatitis due to chromium
> Allergic contact dermatitis due to nickel

   L23.1   Allergic contact dermatitis due to adhesives

   L23.2   Allergic contact dermatitis due to cosmetics

   L23.3   Allergic contact dermatitis due to drugs in contact with skin
> Use additional code for adverse effect, if applicable, to identify drug (T36-T50 with fifth or sixth character 5)
> EXCLUDES 2   *dermatitis due to ingested drugs and medicaments (L27.0-L27.1)*

   L23.4   Allergic contact dermatitis due to dyes

   L23.5   Allergic contact dermatitis due to other chemical products
> Allergic contact dermatitis due to cement
> Allergic contact dermatitis due to insecticide
> Allergic contact dermatitis due to plastic
> Allergic contact dermatitis due to rubber

   L23.6   Allergic contact dermatitis due to food in contact with the skin
> EXCLUDES 2   *dermatitis due to ingested food (L27.2)*

   L23.7   Allergic contact dermatitis due to plants, except food
> EXCLUDES 2   *allergy NOS due to pollen (J30.1)*

   ✓5ᵗʰ **L23.8   Allergic contact dermatitis due to other agents**

      L23.81   Allergic contact dermatitis due to animal (cat) (dog) dander
> Allergic contact dermatitis due to animal (cat) (dog) hair

      L23.89   Allergic contact dermatitis due to other agents

   L23.9   Allergic contact dermatitis, unspecified cause
> Allergic contact eczema NOS

✓4ᵗʰ **L24   Irritant contact dermatitis**
> EXCLUDES 1   *allergy NOS (T78.40)*
> *contact dermatitis NOS (L25.9)*
> *dermatitis NOS (L30.9)*
> EXCLUDES 2   *allergic contact dermatitis (L23.-)*
> *dermatitis due to substances taken internally (L27.-)*
> *dermatitis of eyelid (H01.1-)*
> *diaper dermatitis (L22)*
> *eczema of external ear (H60.5-)*
> *perioral dermatitis (L71.0)*
> *radiation-related disorders of the skin and subcutaneous tissue (L55-L59)*

   L24.0   Irritant contact dermatitis due to detergents

   L24.1   Irritant contact dermatitis due to oils and greases

   L24.2   Irritant contact dermatitis due to solvents
> Irritant contact dermatitis due to chlorocompound
> Irritant contact dermatitis due to cyclohexane
> Irritant contact dermatitis due to ester
> Irritant contact dermatitis due to glycol
> Irritant contact dermatitis due to hydrocarbon
> Irritant contact dermatitis due to ketone

   L24.3   Irritant contact dermatitis due to cosmetics

   L24.4   Irritant contact dermatitis due to drugs in contact with skin
> Use additional code for adverse effect, if applicable, to identify drug (T36-T50 with fifth or sixth character 5)

   L24.5   Irritant contact dermatitis due to other chemical products
> Irritant contact dermatitis due to cement
> Irritant contact dermatitis due to insecticide
> Irritant contact dermatitis due to plastic
> Irritant contact dermatitis due to rubber

   L24.6   Irritant contact dermatitis due to food in contact with skin
> EXCLUDES 2   *dermatitis due to ingested food (L27.2)*

   L24.7   Irritant contact dermatitis due to plants, except food
> EXCLUDES 2   *allergy NOS to pollen (J30.1)*

   ✓5ᵗʰ **L24.8   Irritant contact dermatitis due to other agents**

      L24.81   Irritant contact dermatitis due to metals
> Irritant contact dermatitis due to chromium
> Irritant contact dermatitis due to nickel

      L24.89   Irritant contact dermatitis due to other agents
> Irritant contact dermatitis due to dyes

   L24.9   Irritant contact dermatitis, unspecified cause
> Irritant contact eczema NOS

✓4ᵗʰ **L25   Unspecified contact dermatitis**
> EXCLUDES 1   *allergic contact dermatitis (L23.-)*
> *allergy NOS (T78.40)*
> *dermatitis NOS (L30.9)*
> *irritant contact dermatitis (L24.-)*
> EXCLUDES 2   *dermatitis due to ingested substances (L27.-)*
> *dermatitis of eyelid (H01.1-)*
> *eczema of external ear (H60.5-)*
> *perioral dermatitis (L71.0)*
> *radiation-related disorders of the skin and subcutaneous tissue (L55-L59)*

   L25.0   Unspecified contact dermatitis due to cosmetics

   L25.1   Unspecified contact dermatitis due to drugs in contact with skin
> Use additional code for adverse effect, if applicable, to identify drug (T36-T50 with fifth or sixth character 5)
> EXCLUDES 2   *dermatitis due to ingested drugs and medicaments (L27.0-L27.1)*

   L25.2   Unspecified contact dermatitis due to dyes

   L25.3   Unspecified contact dermatitis due to other chemical products
> Unspecified contact dermatitis due to cement
> Unspecified contact dermatitis due to insecticide

   L25.4   Unspecified contact dermatitis due to food in contact with skin
> EXCLUDES 2   *dermatitis due to ingested food (L27.2)*

   L25.5   Unspecified contact dermatitis due to plants, except food
> EXCLUDES 1   *nettle rash (L50.9)*
> EXCLUDES 2   *allergy NOS due to pollen (J30.1)*

   L25.8   Unspecified contact dermatitis due to other agents

   L25.9   Unspecified contact dermatitis, unspecified cause
> Contact dermatitis (occupational) NOS
> Contact eczema (occupational) NOS

L26   Exfoliative dermatitis
> Hebra's pityriasis
> EXCLUDES 1   *Ritter's disease (L00)*

✓4ᵗʰ **L27   Dermatitis due to substances taken internally**
> EXCLUDES 1   *allergy NOS (T78.40)*
> EXCLUDES 2   *adverse food reaction, except dermatitis (T78.0-T78.1)*
> *contact dermatitis (L23-L25)*
> *drug photoallergic response (L56.1)*
> *drug phototoxic response (L56.0)*
> *urticaria (L50.-)*

   L27.0   Generalized skin eruption due to drugs and medicaments taken internally
> Use additional code for adverse effect, if applicable, to identify drug (T36-T50 with fifth or sixth character 5)

   L27.1   Localized skin eruption due to drugs and medicaments taken internally
> Use additional code for adverse effect, if applicable, to identify drug (T36-T50 with fifth or sixth character 5)

   L27.2   Dermatitis due to ingested food
> EXCLUDES 2   *dermatitis due to food in contact with skin (L23.6, L24.6, L25.4)*

   L27.8   Dermatitis due to other substances taken internally

   L27.9   Dermatitis due to unspecified substance taken internally

✓4ᵗʰ **L28   Lichen simplex chronicus and prurigo**

   L28.0   Lichen simplex chronicus
> Circumscribed neurodermatitis   Lichen NOS

   L28.1   Prurigo nodularis

✓ Additional Character Required   ✓x7ᵗʰ Placeholder Alert   Unacceptable PDx   Manifestation   Hospital Acquired Condition   EXCLUDES 1 Not Coded Here   EXCLUDES 2 Not Included Here

ICD-10-CM 2016   683

Chapter 12. Diseases of the Skin and Subcutaneous Tissue

L28.2 Other prurigo
Prurigo NOS   Prurigo mitis
Prurigo Hebra   Urticaria papulosa

√4ᵗʰ L29 Pruritus
EXCLUDES 1 neurotic excoriation (L98.1)
psychogenic pruritus (F45.8)

L29.0 Pruritus ani
L29.1 Pruritus scroti   ♂
L29.2 Pruritus vulvae   ♀
L29.3 Anogenital pruritus, unspecified
L29.8 Other pruritus
L29.9 Pruritus, unspecified
Itch NOS

√4ᵗʰ L30 Other and unspecified dermatitis
EXCLUDES 2 contact dermatitis (L23-L25)
dry skin dermatitis (L85.3)
small plaque parapsoriasis (L41.3)
stasis dermatitis (I83.1-.2)

L30.0 Nummular dermatitis
L30.1 Dyshidrosis [pompholyx]
L30.2 Cutaneous autosensitization
Candidid [levurid]   Eczematid
Dermatophytid
L30.3 Infective dermatitis
Infectious eczematoid dermatitis
L30.4 Erythema intertrigo
L30.5 Pityriasis alba
L30.8 Other specified dermatitis
L30.9 Dermatitis, unspecified
Eczema NOS

Papulosquamous disorders (L40-L45)

√4ᵗʰ L40 Psoriasis
L40.0 Psoriasis vulgaris
Nummular psoriasis   Plaque psoriasis
L40.1 Generalized pustular psoriasis
Impetigo herpetiformis   Von Zumbusch's disease
L40.2 Acrodermatitis continua
L40.3 Pustulosis palmaris et plantaris
L40.4 Guttate psoriasis
√5ᵗʰ L40.5 Arthropathic psoriasis
L40.50 Arthropathic psoriasis, unspecified
L40.51 Distal interphalangeal psoriatic arthropathy
L40.52 Psoriatic arthritis mutilans
L40.53 Psoriatic spondylitis
L40.54 Psoriatic juvenile arthropathy
L40.59 Other psoriatic arthropathy
L40.8 Other psoriasis
Flexural psoriasis
L40.9 Psoriasis, unspecified

√4ᵗʰ L41 Parapsoriasis
EXCLUDES 1 poikiloderma vasculare atrophicans (L94.5)
L41.0 Pityriasis lichenoides et varioliformis acuta
Mucha-Habermann disease
L41.1 Pityriasis lichenoides chronica
L41.3 Small plaque parapsoriasis
L41.4 Large plaque parapsoriasis
L41.5 Retiform parapsoriasis
L41.8 Other parapsoriasis
L41.9 Parapsoriasis, unspecified

L42 Pityriasis rosea

√4ᵗʰ L43 Lichen planus
EXCLUDES 1 lichen planopilaris (L66.1)
L43.0 Hypertrophic lichen planus
L43.1 Bullous lichen planus
L43.2 Lichenoid drug reaction
Use additional code for adverse effect, if applicable, to identify drug (T36-T50 with fifth or sixth character 5)
L43.3 Subacute (active) lichen planus
Lichen planus tropicus
L43.8 Other lichen planus
L43.9 Lichen planus, unspecified

√4ᵗʰ L44 Other papulosquamous disorders
L44.0 Pityriasis rubra pilaris
L44.1 Lichen nitidus
L44.2 Lichen striatus
L44.3 Lichen ruber moniliformis
L44.4 Infantile papular acrodermatitis [Gianotti-Crosti] P
L44.8 Other specified papulosquamous disorders
L44.9 Papulosquamous disorder, unspecified

L45 Papulosquamous disorders in diseases classified elsewhere
Code first underlying disease

Urticaria and erythema (L49-L54)
EXCLUDES 1 Lyme disease (A69.2-)
rosacea (L71.-)

√4ᵗʰ L49 Exfoliation due to erythematous conditions according to extent of body surface involved
Code first erythematous condition causing exfoliation, such as:
Ritter's disease (L00)
(Staphylococcal) scalded skin syndrom (L00)
Stevens-Johnson syndrome (L51.1)
Stevens-Johnson syndrome-toxic epidermal necrolysis overlap syndrome (L51.3)
toxic epidermal necrolysis (L51.2)

L49.0 Exfoliation due to erythematous condition involving less than 10 percent of body surface
Exfoliation due to erythematous condition NOS
L49.1 Exfoliation due to erythematous condition involving 10-19 percent of body surface
L49.2 Exfoliation due to erythematous condition involving 20-29 percent of body surface
L49.3 Exfoliation due to erythematous condition involving 30-39 percent of body surface CC
CC Excl: L49.3
L49.4 Exfoliation due to erythematous condition involving 40-49 percent of body surface CC
CC Excl: L49.4
L49.5 Exfoliation due to erythematous condition involving 50-59 percent of body surface CC
CC Excl: L49.5
L49.6 Exfoliation due to erythematous condition involving 60-69 percent of body surface CC
CC Excl: L49.6
L49.7 Exfoliation due to erythematous condition involving 70-79 percent of body surface CC
CC Excl: L49.7
L49.8 Exfoliation due to erythematous condition involving 80-89 percent of body surface CC
CC Excl: L49.8
L49.9 Exfoliation due to erythematous condition involving 90 or more percent of body surface CC
CC Excl: L49.9

√4ᵗʰ L50 Urticaria
EXCLUDES 1 allergic contact dermatitis (L23.-)
angioneurotic edema (T78.3)
giant urticaria (T78.3)
hereditary angio-edema (D84.1)
Quincke's edema (T78.3)
serum urticaria (T80.6-)
solar urticaria (L56.3)
urticaria neonatorum (P83.8)
urticaria papulosa (L28.2)
urticaria pigmentosa (Q82.2)
L50.0 Allergic urticaria
L50.1 Idiopathic urticaria
L50.2 Urticaria due to cold and heat
L50.3 Dermatographic urticaria
L50.4 Vibratory urticaria
L50.5 Cholinergic urticaria
L50.6 Contact urticaria
L50.8 Other urticaria
Chronic urticaria
Recurrent periodic urticaria
L50.9 Urticaria, unspecified

✓4ᵗʰ **L51**   **Erythema multiforme**

Use additional code for adverse effect, if applicable, to identify drug (T36-T50 with fifth or sixth character 5)

Use additional code to identify associated manifestations, such as:
arthropathy associated with dermatological disorders (M14.8-)
conjunctival edema (H11.42)
conjunctivitis (H10.22-)
corneal scars and opacities (H17.-)
corneal ulcer (H16.0-)
edema of eyelid (H02.84)
inflammation of eyelid (H01.8)
keratoconjunctivitis sicca (H16.22-)
mechanical lagophthalmos (H02.22-)
stomatitis (K12.-)
symblepharon (H11.23-)
Use additional code to identify percentage of skin exfoliation (L49.-)

EXCLUDES 1   staphylococcal scalded skin syndrome (L00)
Ritter's disease (L00)

L51.0   **Nonbullous erythema multiforme**

L51.1   **Stevens-Johnson syndrome**   CC
CC Excl: L00, L12.30-L12.35, L26, L30.4, L44.8-L45, L51.0-L54, L71.0-L71.9, L92.0, L93.0-L93.2, L94.2, L94.4, L95.1, L98.2, L98.8, L99

L51.2   **Toxic epidermal necrolysis [Lyell]**   CC
CC Excl: See code: L51.1

L51.3   **Stevens-Johnson syndrome-toxic epidermal necrolysis overlap syndrome**   CC
SJS-TEN overlap syndrome
CC Excl: See code: L51.1

L51.8   **Other erythema multiforme**

L51.9   **Erythema multiforme, unspecified**
Erythema iris
Erythema multiforme major NOS
Erythema multiforme minor NOS
Herpes iris

L52   **Erythema nodosum**
EXCLUDES 1   tuberculous erythema nodosum (A18.4)

✓4ᵗʰ **L53**   **Other erythematous conditions**
EXCLUDES 1   erythema ab igne (L59.0)
erythema due to external agents in contact with skin (L23-L25)
erythema intertrigo (L30.4)

CC Excl: For CC codes in category L53, unless otherwise noted:
L12.30-L12.35, L44.8-L45, L51.0-L53.3, L71.0-L71.9, L93.0-L93.2, L94.2, L94.4, L98.8, L99

L53.0   **Toxic erythema**   CC
Code first poisoning due to drug or toxin, if applicable (T36-T65 with fifth or sixth character 1-4 or 6)
Use additional code for adverse effect, if applicable, to identify drug (T36-T50 with fifth or sixth character 5)
EXCLUDES 1   neonatal erythema toxicum (P83.1)

L53.1   **Erythema annulare centrifugum**   CC

L53.2   **Erythema marginatum**   CC

L53.3   **Other chronic figurate erythema**   CC

L53.8   **Other specified erythematous conditions**

L53.9   **Erythematous condition, unspecified**
Erythema NOS
Erythroderma NOS

L54   **Erythema in diseases classified elsewhere**
Code first underlying disease

Radiation-related disorders of the skin and subcutaneous tissue (L55-L59)

✓4ᵗʰ **L55**   **Sunburn**

L55.0   **Sunburn of first degree**

L55.1   **Sunburn of second degree**

L55.2   **Sunburn of third degree**

L55.9   **Sunburn, unspecified**

✓4ᵗʰ **L56**   **Other acute skin changes due to ultraviolet radiation**
Use additional code to identify the source of the ultraviolet radiation (W89, X32)

L56.0   **Drug phototoxic response**
Use additional code for adverse effect, if applicable, to identify drug (T36-T50 with fifth or sixth character 5)

L56.1   **Drug photoallergic response**
Use additional code for adverse effect, if applicable, to identify drug (T36-T50 with fifth or sixth character 5)

L56.2   **Photocontact dermatitis [berloque dermatitis]**

L56.3   **Solar urticaria**

L56.4   **Polymorphous light eruption**

L56.5   **Disseminated superficial actinic porokeratosis (DSAP)**

L56.8   **Other specified acute skin changes due to ultraviolet radiation**

L56.9   **Acute skin change due to ultraviolet radiation, unspecified**

✓4ᵗʰ **L57**   **Skin changes due to chronic exposure to nonionizing radiation**
Use additional code to identify the source of the ultraviolet radiation (W89, X32)

L57.0   **Actinic keratosis**
Keratosis NOS
Senile keratosis
Solar keratosis

L57.1   **Actinic reticuloid**

L57.2   **Cutis rhomboidalis nuchae**

L57.3   **Poikiloderma of Civatte**

L57.4   **Cutis laxa senilis**
Elastosis senilis

L57.5   **Actinic granuloma**

L57.8   **Other skin changes due to chronic exposure to nonionizing radiation**
Farmer's skin
Sailor's skin
Solar dermatitis

L57.9   **Skin changes due to chronic exposure to nonionizing radiation, unspecified**

✓4ᵗʰ **L58**   **Radiodermatitis**
Use additional code to identify the source of the radiation (W88, W90)

L58.0   **Acute radiodermatitis**

L58.1   **Chronic radiodermatitis**

L58.9   **Radiodermatitis, unspecified**

✓4ᵗʰ **L59**   **Other disorders of skin and subcutaneous tissue related to radiation**

L59.0   **Erythema ab igne [dermatitis ab igne]**

L59.8   **Other specified disorders of the skin and subcutaneous tissue related to radiation**

L59.9   **Disorder of the skin and subcutaneous tissue related to radiation, unspecified**

Disorders of skin appendages (L60-L75)
EXCLUDES 1   congenital malformations of integument (Q84.-)

✓4ᵗʰ **L60**   **Nail disorders**
EXCLUDES 2   clubbing of nails (R68.3)
onychia and paronychia (L03.0-)

L60.0   **Ingrowing nail**

L60.1   **Onycholysis**

L60.2   **Onychogryphosis**

L60.3   **Nail dystrophy**

L60.4   **Beau's lines**

L60.5   **Yellow nail syndrome**

L60.8   **Other nail disorders**

L60.9   **Nail disorder, unspecified**

L62   **Nail disorders in diseases classified elsewhere**
Code first underlying disease, such as:
pachydermoperiostosis (M89.4-)

✓4ᵗʰ **L63**   **Alopecia areata**

L63.0   **Alopecia (capitis) totalis**

L63.1   **Alopecia universalis**

L63.2   **Ophiasis**

L63.8   **Other alopecia areata**

L63.9   **Alopecia areata, unspecified**

✓4ᵗʰ **L64**   **Androgenic alopecia**
INCLUDES   male-pattern baldness

L64.0   **Drug-induced androgenic alopecia**
Use additional code for adverse effect, if applicable, to identify drug (T36-T50 with fifth or sixth character 5)

L64.8   **Other androgenic alopecia**

L64.9   **Androgenic alopecia, unspecified**

✓ Additional Character Required   ✓x7ᵗʰ Placeholder Alert   Unacceptable PDx   Manifestation   Hospital Acquired Condition   **EXCLUDES 1** Not Coded Here   **EXCLUDES 2** Not Included Here

Chapter 12. Diseases of the Skin and Subcutaneous Tissue

✓4th **L65 Other nonscarring hair loss**
> Use additional code for adverse effect, if applicable, to identify drug (T36-T50 with fifth or sixth character 5)
> EXCLUDES 1   trichotillomania (F63.3)

L65.0   **Telogen effluvium**

L65.1   **Anagen effluvium**

L65.2   **Alopecia mucinosa**

L65.8   **Other specified nonscarring hair loss**

L65.9   **Nonscarring hair loss, unspecified**
> Alopecia NOS

✓4th **L66 Cicatricial alopecia [scarring hair loss]**

L66.0   **Pseudopelade**

L66.1   **Lichen planopilaris**
> Follicular lichen planus

L66.2   **Folliculitis decalvans**

L66.3   **Perifolliculitis capitis abscedens**

L66.4   **Folliculitis ulerythematosa reticulata**

L66.8   **Other cicatricial alopecia**
> AHA: 2015, 1Q, 19

L66.9   **Cicatricial alopecia, unspecified**

✓4th **L67 Hair color and hair shaft abnormalities**
> EXCLUDES 1   monilethrix (Q84.1)
> pili annulati (Q84.1)
> telogen effluvium (L65.0)

L67.0   **Trichorrhexis nodosa**

L67.1   **Variations in hair color**
> Canities
> Greyness, hair (premature)
> Heterochromia of hair
> Poliosis circumscripta, acquired
> Poliosis NOS

L67.8   **Other hair color and hair shaft abnormalities**
> Fragilitas crinium

L67.9   **Hair color and hair shaft abnormality, unspecified**

✓4th **L68 Hypertrichosis**
> INCLUDES   excess hair
> EXCLUDES 1   congenital hypertrichosis (Q84.2)
> persistent lanugo (Q84.2)

L68.0   **Hirsutism**

L68.1   **Acquired hypertrichosis lanuginosa**

L68.2   **Localized hypertrichosis**

L68.3   **Polytrichia**

L68.8   **Other hypertrichosis**

L68.9   **Hypertrichosis, unspecified**

✓4th **L70 Acne**
> EXCLUDES 2   acne keloid (L73.0)

L70.0   **Acne vulgaris**

L70.1   **Acne conglobata**

L70.2   **Acne varioliformis**
> Acne necrotica miliaris

L70.3   **Acne tropica**

L70.4   **Infantile acne**

L70.5   **Acné excoriée des jeunes filles**
> Picker's acne

L70.8   **Other acne**

L70.9   **Acne, unspecified**

✓4th **L71 Rosacea**
> Use additional code for adverse effect, if applicable, to identify drug (T36-T50 with fifth or sixth character 5)

L71.0   **Perioral dermatitis**

L71.1   **Rhinophyma**

L71.8   **Other rosacea**

L71.9   **Rosacea, unspecified**

✓4th **L72 Follicular cysts of skin and subcutaneous tissue**

L72.0   **Epidermal cyst**

✓5th L72.1   **Pilar and trichodermal cyst**

L72.11   **Pilar cyst**

L72.12   **Trichodermal cyst**
> Trichilemmal (proliferating) cyst

L72.2   **Steatocystoma multiplex**

L72.3   **Sebaceous cyst**
> EXCLUDES 2   pilar cyst (L72.11)
> trichilemmal (proliferating) cyst (L72.12)

L72.8   **Other follicular cysts of the skin and subcutaneous tissue**

L72.9   **Follicular cyst of the skin and subcutaneous tissue, unspecified**

✓4th **L73 Other follicular disorders**

L73.0   **Acne keloid**

L73.1   **Pseudofolliculitis barbae**

L73.2   **Hidradenitis suppurativa**

L73.8   **Other specified follicular disorders**
> Sycosis barbae

L73.9   **Follicular disorder, unspecified**

✓4th **L74 Eccrine sweat disorders**
> EXCLUDES 2   generalized hyperhidrosis (R61)

L74.0   **Miliaria rubra**

L74.1   **Miliaria crystallina**

L74.2   **Miliaria profunda**
> Miliaria tropicalis

L74.3   **Miliaria, unspecified**

L74.4   **Anhidrosis**
> Hypohidrosis

✓5th L74.5   **Focal hyperhidrosis**

✓6th L74.51   **Primary focal hyperhidrosis**

L74.510   **Primary focal hyperhidrosis, axilla**

L74.511   **Primary focal hyperhidrosis, face**

L74.512   **Primary focal hyperhidrosis, palms**

L74.513   **Primary focal hyperhidrosis, soles**

L74.519   **Primary focal hyperhidrosis, unspecified**

L74.52   **Secondary focal hyperhidrosis**
> Frey's syndrome

L74.8   **Other eccrine sweat disorders**

L74.9   **Eccrine sweat disorder, unspecified**
> Sweat gland disorder NOS

✓4th **L75 Apocrine sweat disorders**
> EXCLUDES 1   dyshidrosis (L30.1)
> hidradenitis suppurativa (L73.2)

L75.0   **Bromhidrosis**

L75.1   **Chromhidrosis**

L75.2   **Apocrine miliaria**
> Fox-Fordyce disease

L75.8   **Other apocrine sweat disorders**

L75.9   **Apocrine sweat disorder, unspecified**

Intraoperative and postprocedural complications of skin and subcutaneous tissue (L76)

✓4th **L76 Intraoperative and postprocedural complications of skin and subcutaneous tissue**

> **CC Excl: For CC codes in category L76, unless otherwise noted:**
> H95.811-H95.89, I85.01, I85.11, I97.3, K21.9, K22.8, K23-K25.0, K25.2, K25.4, K25.6, K26.0, K26.2, K26.4, K26.6, K27.0, K27.2, K27.4, K27.6, K28.0, K28.2, K28.4, K28.6, K29.01, K29.21, K29.31, K29.41, K29.51, K29.61, K29.71, K29.81, K29.91, K31.811, K55.21, K57.01, K57.11, K57.13, K57.21, K57.31, K57.33, K57.41, K57.51, K57.53, K57.81, K57.91, K57.93, K62.5, K92.0-K92.2, L76.01-L76.02, L76.21-L76.82, M96.89, N98.1-N98.9, P54.1-P54.3, T81.10XA, T81.11XA, T81.12XA, T81.19XA, T81.82XA, T81.89XA, T81.9XXA

✓5th L76.0   **Intraoperative hemorrhage and hematoma of skin and subcutaneous tissue complicating a procedure**
> EXCLUDES 1   intraoperative hemorrhage and hematoma of skin and subcutaneous tissue due to accidental puncture and laceration during a procedure (L76.1-)

L76.01   **Intraoperative hemorrhage and hematoma of skin and subcutaneous tissue complicating a dermatologic procedure**   CC

L76.02   **Intraoperative hemorrhage and hematoma of skin and subcutaneous tissue complicating other procedure**   CC

N Newborn: 0   P Pediatric: 0-17   M Maternity: 12-55   A Adult: 15-124   MCC Major CC Condition   PDxMCC PDx acts as own MCC   CC CC Condition   PDxCC PDx acts as own CC

686   ICD-10-CM 2016

✓5ᵗʰ **L76.1 Accidental puncture and laceration of skin and subcutaneous tissue during a procedure**

  L76.11 Accidental puncture and laceration of skin and subcutaneous tissue during a dermatologic procedure `CC`
    CC Excl: D78.11-D78.12, D78.81-D78.89, E36.11-E36.8, E89.810-E89.89, G96.11, G97.41, G97.48-G97.49, H59.011-H59.019, H59.031-H59.099, H59.211-H59.229, H59.811-H59.89, H95.31-H95.32, H95.811-H95.89, I97.3, I97.51-I97.52, J95.71-J95.72, K91.71-K91.72, L76.11-L76.12, L76.81-L76.82, M96.820-M96.821, M96.89, N98.1-N98.9, N99.71-N99.72, T81.82XA, T81.89XA, T81.9XXA

  L76.12 Accidental puncture and laceration of skin and subcutaneous tissue during other procedure `CC`
    CC Excl: See code: D76.11

✓5ᵗʰ **L76.2 Postprocedural hemorrhage and hematoma of skin and subcutaneous tissue following a procedure**

  L76.21 Postprocedural hemorrhage and hematoma of skin and subcutaneous tissue following a dermatologic procedure `CC`

  L76.22 Postprocedural hemorrhage and hematoma of skin and subcutaneous tissue following other procedure `CC`

✓5ᵗʰ **L76.8 Other intraoperative and postprocedural complications of skin and subcutaneous tissue**
  Use additional code, if applicable, to further specify disorder

  L76.81 Other intraoperative complications of skin and subcutaneous tissue

  L76.82 Other postprocedural complications of skin and subcutaneous tissue

Other disorders of the skin and subcutaneous tissue (L80-L99)

L80 Vitiligo
  EXCLUDES2 vitiligo of eyelids (H02.73-)
    vitiligo of vulva (N90.89)

✓4ᵗʰ **L81 Other disorders of pigmentation**
  EXCLUDES1 birthmark NOS (Q82.5)
    Peutz-Jeghers syndrome (Q85.8)
  EXCLUDES2 nevus—see Alphabetical Index

  L81.0 Postinflammatory hyperpigmentation
  L81.1 Chloasma
  L81.2 Freckles
  L81.3 Café au lait spots
  L81.4 Other melanin hyperpigmentation
    Lentigo
  L81.5 Leukoderma, not elsewhere classified
  L81.6 Other disorders of diminished melanin formation
  L81.7 Pigmented purpuric dermatosis
    Angioma serpiginosum
  L81.8 Other specified disorders of pigmentation
    Iron pigmentation   Tattoo pigmentation
  L81.9 Disorder of pigmentation, unspecified

✓4ᵗʰ **L82 Seborrheic keratosis**
  INCLUDES dermatosis papulosa nigra
    Leser-Trélat disease
  EXCLUDES2 seborrheic dermatitis (L21.-)

  L82.0 Inflamed seborrheic keratosis
  L82.1 Other seborrheic keratosis
    Seborrheic keratosis NOS

L83 Acanthosis nigricans
  Confluent and reticulated papillomatosis

L84 Corns and callosities
  Callus   Clavus

✓4ᵗʰ **L85 Other epidermal thickening**
  EXCLUDES2 hypertrophic disorders of the skin (L91.-)

  L85.0 Acquired ichthyosis
    EXCLUDES1 congenital ichthyosis (Q80.-)
  L85.1 Acquired keratosis [keratoderma] palmaris et plantaris
    EXCLUDES1 inherited keratosis palmaris et plantaris (Q82.8)
  L85.2 Keratosis punctata (palmaris et plantaris)
  L85.3 Xerosis cutis
    Dry skin dermatitis
  L85.8 Other specified epidermal thickening
    Cutaneous horn
  L85.9 Epidermal thickening, unspecified

L86 **Keratoderma in diseases classified elsewhere**
  Code first underlying disease, such as:
    Reiter's disease (M02.3-)
  EXCLUDES1 gonococcal keratoderma (A54.89)
    gonococcal keratosis (A54.89)
    keratoderma due to vitamin A deficiency (E50.8)
    keratosis due to vitamin A deficiency (E50.8)
    xeroderma due to vitamin A deficiency (E50.8)

✓4ᵗʰ **L87 Transepidermal elimination disorders**
  EXCLUDES1 granuloma annulare (perforating) (L92.0)

  L87.0 Keratosis follicularis et parafollicularis in cutem penetrans
    Hyperkeratosis follicularis penetrans
    Kyrle disease
  L87.1 Reactive perforating collagenosis
  L87.2 Elastosis perforans serpiginosa
  L87.8 Other transepidermal elimination disorders
  L87.9 Transepidermal elimination disorder, unspecified

L88 Pyoderma gangrenosum `CC`
  Phagedenic pyoderma
  EXCLUDES1 dermatitis gangrenosa (L08.0)
  CC Excl: L08.0, L08.81, L88

✓4ᵗʰ **L89 Pressure ulcer**
  Bed sore   Pressure area
  Decubitus ulcer   Pressure sore
  Plaster ulcer
  Code first any associated gangrene (I96)
  EXCLUDES2 decubitus (trophic) ulcer of cervix (uteri) (N86)
    diabetic ulcers (E08.621, E08.622, E09.621, E09.622, E10.621, E10.622, E11.621, E11.622, E13.621, E13.622)
    non-pressure chronic ulcer of skin (L97.-)
    skin infections (L00-L08)
    varicose ulcer (I83.0, I83.2)

  CC Excl: For MCC codes in category L89, unless otherwise noted: L89.000-L89.95, L97.101-L97.929, L98.411-L98.499

✓5ᵗʰ **L89.0 Pressure ulcer of elbow**

✓6ᵗʰ **L89.00 Pressure ulcer of unspecified elbow**
  L89.000 Pressure ulcer of unspecified elbow, unstageable
  L89.001 Pressure ulcer of unspecified elbow, stage 1
    Healing pressure ulcer of unspecified elbow, stage 1
    Pressure pre-ulcer skin changes limited to persistent focal edema, unspecified elbow
  L89.002 Pressure ulcer of unspecified elbow, stage 2
    Healing pressure ulcer of unspecified elbow, stage 2
    Pressure ulcer with abrasion, blister, partial thickness skin loss involving epidermis and/or dermis, unspecified elbow
  L89.003 Pressure ulcer of unspecified elbow, stage 3 `PDxMCC` `MCC`
    Healing pressure ulcer of unspecified elbow, stage 3
    Pressure ulcer with full thickness skin loss involving damage or necrosis of subcutaneous tissue, unspecified elbow
  L89.004 Pressure ulcer of unspecified elbow, stage 4 `PDxMCC` `MCC`
    Healing pressure ulcer of unspecified elbow, stage 4
    Pressure ulcer with necrosis of soft tissues through to underlying muscle, tendon, or bone, unspecified elbow
  L89.009 Pressure ulcer of unspecified elbow, unspecified stage
    Healing pressure ulcer of elbow NOS
    Healing pressure ulcer of unspecified elbow, unspecified stage

✓6ᵗʰ **L89.01 Pressure ulcer of right elbow**
  L89.010 Pressure ulcer of right elbow, unstageable
  L89.011 Pressure ulcer of right elbow, stage 1
    Healing pressure ulcer of right elbow, stage 1
    Pressure pre-ulcer skin changes limited to persistent focal edema, right elbow

---

✓ Additional Character Required   ✓x7ᵗʰ Placeholder Alert   Unacceptable PDx   Manifestation   Hospital Acquired Condition   EXCLUDES1 Not Coded Here   EXCLUDES2 Not Included Here

L89.012 Pressure ulcer of right elbow, stage 2
Healing pressure ulcer of right elbow, stage 2
Pressure ulcer with abrasion, blister, partial thickness skin loss involving epidermis and/or dermis, right elbow

L89.013 Pressure ulcer of right elbow, stage 3 `PDxMCC` `MCC`
Healing pressure ulcer of right elbow, stage 3
Pressure ulcer with full thickness skin loss involving damage or necrosis of subcutaneous tissue, right elbow

L89.014 Pressure ulcer of right elbow, stage 4 `PDxMCC` `MCC`
Healing pressure ulcer of right elbow, stage 4
Pressure ulcer with necrosis of soft tissues through to underlying muscle, tendon, or bone, right elbow

L89.019 Pressure ulcer of right elbow, unspecified stage
Healing pressure right of elbow NOS
Healing pressure ulcer of unspecified elbow, unspecified stage

✓6ᵗʰ **L89.02 Pressure ulcer of left elbow**

L89.020 Pressure ulcer of left elbow, unstageable

L89.021 Pressure ulcer of left elbow, stage 1
Healing pressure ulcer of left elbow, stage 1
Pressure pre-ulcer skin changes limited to persistent focal edema, left elbow

L89.022 Pressure ulcer of left elbow, stage 2
Healing pressure ulcer of left elbow, stage 2
Pressure ulcer with abrasion, blister, partial thickness skin loss involving epidermis and/or dermis, left elbow

L89.023 Pressure ulcer of left elbow, stage 3 `PDxMCC` `MCC`
Healing pressure ulcer of left elbow, stage 3
Pressure ulcer with full thickness skin loss involving damage or necrosis of subcutaneous tissue, left elbow

L89.024 Pressure ulcer of left elbow, stage 4 `PDxMCC` `MCC`
Healing pressure ulcer of left elbow, stage 4
Pressure ulcer with necrosis of soft tissues through to underlying muscle, tendon, or bone, left elbow

L89.029 Pressure ulcer of left elbow, unspecified stage
Healing pressure ulcer of left of elbow NOS
Healing pressure ulcer of unspecified elbow, unspecified stage

✓5ᵗʰ **L89.1 Pressure ulcer of back**

✓6ᵗʰ **L89.10 Pressure ulcer of unspecified part of back**

L89.100 Pressure ulcer of unspecified part of back, unstageable

L89.101 Pressure ulcer of unspecified part of back, stage 1
Healing pressure ulcer of unspecified part of back, stage 1
Pressure pre-ulcer skin changes limited to persistent focal edema, unspecified part of back

L89.102 Pressure ulcer of unspecified part of back, stage 2
Healing pressure ulcer of unspecified part of back, stage 2
Pressure ulcer with abrasion, blister, partial thickness skin loss involving epidermis and/or dermis, unspecified part of back

L89.103 Pressure ulcer of unspecified part of back, stage 3 `PDxMCC` `MCC`
Healing pressure ulcer of unspecified part of back, stage 3
Pressure ulcer with full thickness skin loss involving damage or necrosis of subcutaneous tissue, unspecified part of back

L89.104 Pressure ulcer of unspecified part of back, stage 4 `PDxMCC` `MCC`
Healing pressure ulcer of unspecified part of back, stage 4
Pressure ulcer with necrosis of soft tissues through to underlying muscle, tendon, or bone, unspecified part of back

L89.109 Pressure ulcer of unspecified part of back, unspecified stage
Healing pressure ulcer of unspecified part of back NOS
Healing pressure ulcer of unspecified part of back, unspecified stage

✓6ᵗʰ **L89.11 Pressure ulcer of right upper back**
Pressure ulcer of right shoulder blade

L89.110 Pressure ulcer of right upper back, unstageable

L89.111 Pressure ulcer of right upper back, stage 1
Healing pressure ulcer of right upper back, stage 1
Pressure pre-ulcer skin changes limited to persistent focal edema, right upper back

L89.112 Pressure ulcer of right upper back, stage 2
Healing pressure ulcer of right upper back, stage 2
Pressure ulcer with abrasion, blister, partial thickness skin loss involving epidermis and/or dermis, right upper back

L89.113 Pressure ulcer of right upper back, stage 3 `PDxMCC` `MCC`
Healing pressure ulcer of right upper back, stage 3
Pressure ulcer with full thickness skin loss involving damage or necrosis of subcutaneous tissue, right upper back

L89.114 Pressure ulcer of right upper back, stage 4 `PDxMCC` `MCC`
Healing pressure ulcer of right upper back, stage 4
Pressure ulcer with necrosis of soft tissues through to underlying muscle, tendon, or bone, right upper back

L89.119 Pressure ulcer of right upper back, unspecified stage
Healing pressure ulcer of right upper back NOS
Healing pressure ulcer of right upper back, unspecified stage

✓6ᵗʰ **L89.12 Pressure ulcer of left upper back**
Pressure ulcer of left shoulder blade

L89.120 Pressure ulcer of left upper back, unstageable

L89.121 Pressure ulcer of left upper back, stage 1
Healing pressure ulcer of left upper back, stage 1
Pressure pre-ulcer skin changes limited to persistent focal edema, left upper back

L89.122 Pressure ulcer of left upper back, stage 2
Healing pressure ulcer of left upper back, stage 2
Pressure ulcer with abrasion, blister, partial thickness skin loss involving epidermis and/or dermis, left upper back

L89.123 Pressure ulcer of left upper back, stage 3 `PDxMCC` `MCC`
Healing pressure ulcer of left upper back, stage 3
Pressure ulcer with full thickness skin loss involving damage or necrosis of subcutaneous tissue, left upper back

L89.124 Pressure ulcer of left upper back, stage 4 `PDxMCC` `MCC`
Healing pressure ulcer of left upper back, stage 4
Pressure ulcer with necrosis of soft tissues through to underlying muscle, tendon, or bone, left upper back

N Newborn: 0   P Pediatric: 0-17   M Maternity: 12-55   A Adult: 15-124   MCC Major CC Condition   PDxMCC PDx acts as own MCC   CC CC Condition   PDxCC PDx acts as own CC

688   ICD-10-CM 2016

L89.012–L89.124

L89.129 **Pressure ulcer of left upper back, unspecified stage**
　　Healing pressure ulcer of left upper back NOS
　　Healing pressure ulcer of left upper back, unspecified stage

✓6ᵗʰ **L89.13** **Pressure ulcer of right lower back**

L89.130 **Pressure ulcer of right lower back, unstageable**

L89.131 **Pressure ulcer of right lower back, stage 1**
　　Healing pressure ulcer of right lower back, stage 1
　　Pressure pre-ulcer skin changes limited to persistent focal edema, right lower back

L89.132 **Pressure ulcer of right lower back, stage 2**
　　Healing pressure ulcer of right lower back, stage 2
　　Pressure ulcer with abrasion, blister, partial thickness skin loss involving epidermis and/or dermis, right lower back

L89.133 **Pressure ulcer of right lower back, stage 3** `PDxMCC` `MCC`
　　Healing pressure ulcer of right lower back, stage 3
　　Pressure ulcer with full thickness skin loss involving damage or necrosis of subcutaneous tissue, right lower back

L89.134 **Pressure ulcer of right lower back, stage 4** `PDxMCC` `MCC`
　　Healing pressure ulcer of right lower back, stage 4
　　Pressure ulcer with necrosis of soft tissues through to underlying muscle, tendon, or bone, right lower back

L89.139 **Pressure ulcer of right lower back, unspecified stage**
　　Healing pressure ulcer of right lower back NOS
　　Healing pressure ulcer of right lower back, unspecified stage

✓6ᵗʰ **L89.14** **Pressure ulcer of left lower back**

L89.140 **Pressure ulcer of left lower back, unstageable**

L89.141 **Pressure ulcer of left lower back, stage 1**
　　Healing pressure ulcer of left lower back, stage 1
　　Pressure pre-ulcer skin changes limited to persistent focal edema, left lower back

L89.142 **Pressure ulcer of left lower back, stage 2**
　　Healing pressure ulcer of left lower back, stage 2
　　Pressure ulcer with abrasion, blister, partial thickness skin loss involving epidermis and/or dermis, left lower back

L89.143 **Pressure ulcer of left lower back, stage 3** `PDxMCC` `MCC`
　　Healing pressure ulcer of left lower back, stage 3
　　Pressure ulcer with full thickness skin loss involving damage or necrosis of subcutaneous tissue, left lower back

L89.144 **Pressure ulcer of left lower back, stage 4** `PDxMCC` `MCC`
　　Healing pressure ulcer of left lower back, stage 4
　　Pressure ulcer with necrosis of soft tissues through to underlying muscle, tendon, or bone, left lower back

L89.149 **Pressure ulcer of left lower back, unspecified stage**
　　Healing pressure *ulcer of left lower* back NOS
　　Healing pressure ulcer of left lower back, unspecified stage

✓6ᵗʰ **L89.15** **Pressure ulcer of sacral region**
　　Pressure ulcer of coccyx
　　Pressure ulcer of tailbone

L89.150 **Pressure ulcer of sacral region, unstageable**

L89.151 **Pressure ulcer of sacral region, stage 1**
　　Healing pressure ulcer of sacral region, stage 1
　　Pressure pre-ulcer skin changes limited to persistent focal edema, sacral region

L89.152 **Pressure ulcer of sacral region, stage 2**
　　Healing pressure ulcer of sacral region, stage 2
　　Pressure ulcer with abrasion, blister, partial thickness skin loss involving epidermis and/or dermis, sacral region

L89.153 **Pressure ulcer of sacral region, stage 3** `PDxMCC` `MCC`
　　Healing pressure ulcer of sacral region, stage 3
　　Pressure ulcer with full thickness skin loss involving damage or necrosis of subcutaneous tissue, sacral region

L89.154 **Pressure ulcer of sacral region, stage 4** `PDxMCC` `MCC`
　　Healing pressure ulcer of sacral region, stage 4
　　Pressure ulcer with necrosis of soft tissues through to underlying muscle, tendon, or bone, sacral region

L89.159 **Pressure ulcer of sacral region, unspecified stage**
　　Healing pressure ulcer of sacral region NOS
　　Healing pressure ulcer of sacral region, unspecified stage

✓5ᵗʰ **L89.2** **Pressure ulcer of hip**

✓6ᵗʰ **L89.20** **Pressure ulcer of unspecified hip**

L89.200 **Pressure ulcer of unspecified hip, unstageable**

L89.201 **Pressure ulcer of unspecified hip, stage 1**
　　Healing pressure ulcer of unspecified hip back, stage 1
　　Pressure pre-ulcer skin changes limited to persistent focal edema, unspecified hip

L89.202 **Pressure ulcer of unspecified hip, stage 2**
　　Healing pressure ulcer of unspecified hip, stage 2
　　Pressure ulcer with abrasion, blister, partial thickness skin loss involving epidermis and/or dermis, unspecified hip

L89.203 **Pressure ulcer of unspecified hip, stage 3** `PDxMCC` `MCC`
　　Healing pressure ulcer of unspecified hip, stage 3
　　Pressure ulcer with full thickness skin loss involving damage or necrosis of subcutaneous tissue, unspecified hip

L89.204 **Pressure ulcer of unspecified hip, stage 4** `PDxMCC` `MCC`
　　Healing pressure ulcer of unspecified hip, stage 4
　　Pressure ulcer with necrosis of soft tissues through to underlying muscle, tendon, or bone, unspecified hip

L89.209 **Pressure ulcer of unspecified hip, unspecified stage**
　　Healing pressure ulcer of unspecified hip NOS
　　Healing pressure ulcer of unspecified hip, unspecified stage

✓6ᵗʰ **L89.21** **Pressure ulcer of right hip**

L89.210 **Pressure ulcer of right hip, unstageable**

L89.211 **Pressure ulcer of right hip, stage 1**
　　Healing pressure ulcer of right hip back, stage 1
　　Pressure pre-ulcer skin changes limited to persistent focal edema, right hip

L89.212 **Pressure ulcer of right hip, stage 2**
　　Healing pressure ulcer of right hip, stage 2
　　Pressure ulcer with abrasion, blister, partial thickness skin loss involving epidermis and/or dermis, right hip

L89.213 **Pressure ulcer of right hip, stage 3** `PDxMCC` `MCC`
　　Healing pressure ulcer of right hip, stage 3
　　Pressure ulcer with full thickness skin loss involving damage or necrosis of subcutaneous tissue, right hip

✓ Additional Character Required　✓x7ᵗʰ Placeholder Alert　Unacceptable PDx　Manifestation　Hospital Acquired Condition　**EXCLUDES1** Not Coded Here　*EXCLUDES2* Not Included Here

ICD-10-CM 2016　　　　　　　　689

Chapter 12. Diseases of the Skin and Subcutaneous Tissue

L89.214   **Pressure ulcer of right hip, stage 4** `PDxMCC` `MCC`
> Healing pressure ulcer of right hip, stage 4
> Pressure ulcer with necrosis of soft tissues through to underlying muscle, tendon, or bone, right hip

L89.219   **Pressure ulcer of right hip, unspecified stage**
> Healing pressure ulcer of right hip NOS
> Healing pressure ulcer of right hip, unspecified stage

√6th **L89.22**   **Pressure ulcer of left hip**

L89.220   **Pressure ulcer of left hip, unstageable**

L89.221   **Pressure ulcer of left hip, stage 1**
> Healing pressure ulcer of left hip back, stage 1
> Pressure pre-ulcer skin changes limited to persistent focal edema, left hip

L89.222   **Pressure ulcer of left hip, stage 2**
> Healing pressure ulcer of left hip, stage 2
> Pressure ulcer with abrasion, blister, partial thickness skin loss involving epidermis and/or dermis, left hip

L89.223   **Pressure ulcer of left hip, stage 3** `PDxMCC` `MCC`
> Healing pressure ulcer of left hip, stage 3
> Pressure ulcer with full thickness skin loss involving damage or necrosis of subcutaneous tissue, left hip

L89.224   **Pressure ulcer of left hip, stage 4** `PDxMCC` `MCC`
> Healing pressure ulcer of left hip, stage 4
> Pressure ulcer with necrosis of soft tissues through to underlying muscle, tendon, or bone, left hip

L89.229   **Pressure ulcer of left hip, unspecified stage**
> Healing pressure ulcer of left hip NOS
> Healing pressure ulcer of left hip, unspecified stage

√5th **L89.3**   **Pressure ulcer of buttock**

√6th **L89.30**   **Pressure ulcer of unspecified buttock**

L89.300   **Pressure ulcer of unspecified buttock, unstageable**

L89.301   **Pressure ulcer of unspecified buttock, stage 1**
> Healing pressure ulcer of unspecified buttock, stage 1
> Pressure pre-ulcer skin changes limited to persistent focal edema, unspecified buttock

L89.302   **Pressure ulcer of unspecified buttock, stage 2**
> Healing pressure ulcer of unspecified buttock, stage 2
> Pressure ulcer with abrasion, blister, partial thickness skin loss involving epidermis and/or dermis, unspecified buttock

L89.303   **Pressure ulcer of unspecified buttock, stage 3** `PDxMCC` `MCC`
> Healing pressure ulcer of unspecified buttock, stage 3
> Pressure ulcer with full thickness skin loss involving damage or necrosis of subcutaneous tissue, unspecified buttock

L89.304   **Pressure ulcer of unspecified buttock, stage 4** `PDxMCC` `MCC`
> Healing pressure ulcer of unspecified buttock, stage 4
> Pressure ulcer with necrosis of soft tissues through to underlying muscle, tendon, or bone, unspecified buttock

L89.309   **Pressure ulcer of unspecified buttock, unspecified stage**
> Healing pressure ulcer of unspecified buttock NOS
> Healing pressure ulcer of unspecified buttock, unspecified stage

√6th **L89.31**   **Pressure ulcer of right buttock**

L89.310   **Pressure ulcer of right buttock, unstageable**

L89.311   **Pressure ulcer of right buttock, stage 1**
> Healing pressure ulcer of right buttock, stage 1
> Pressure pre-ulcer skin changes limited to persistent focal edema, right buttock

L89.312   **Pressure ulcer of right buttock, stage 2**
> Healing pressure ulcer of right buttock, stage 2
> Pressure ulcer with abrasion, blister, partial thickness skin loss involving epidermis and/or dermis, right buttock

L89.313   **Pressure ulcer of right buttock, stage 3** `PDxMCC` `MCC`
> Healing pressure ulcer of right buttock, stage 3
> Pressure ulcer with full thickness skin loss involving damage or necrosis of subcutaneous tissue, right buttock

L89.314   **Pressure ulcer of right buttock, stage 4** `PDxMCC` `MCC`
> Healing pressure ulcer of right buttock, stage 4
> Pressure ulcer with necrosis of soft tissues through to underlying muscle, tendon, or bone, right buttock

L89.319   **Pressure ulcer of right buttock, unspecified stage**
> Healing pressure ulcer of right buttock NOS
> Healing pressure ulcer of right buttock, unspecified stage

√6th **L89.32**   **Pressure ulcer of left buttock**

L89.320   **Pressure ulcer of left buttock, unstageable**

L89.321   **Pressure ulcer of left buttock, stage 1**
> Healing pressure ulcer of left buttock, stage 1
> Pressure pre-ulcer skin changes limited to persistent focal edema, left buttock

L89.322   **Pressure ulcer of left buttock, stage 2**
> Healing pressure ulcer of left buttock, stage 2
> Pressure ulcer with abrasion, blister, partial thickness skin loss involving epidermis and/or dermis, left buttock

L89.323   **Pressure ulcer of left buttock, stage 3** `PDxMCC` `MCC`
> Healing pressure ulcer of left buttock, stage 3
> Pressure ulcer with full thickness skin loss involving damage or necrosis of subcutaneous tissue, left buttock

L89.324   **Pressure ulcer of left buttock, stage 4** `PDxMCC` `MCC`
> Healing pressure ulcer of left buttock, stage 4
> Pressure ulcer with necrosis of soft tissues through to underlying muscle, tendon, or bone, left buttock

L89.329   **Pressure ulcer of left buttock, unspecified stage**
> Healing pressure ulcer of left buttock NOS
> Healing pressure ulcer of left buttock, unspecified stage

√5th **L89.4**   **Pressure ulcer of contiguous site of back, buttock and hip**

L89.40   **Pressure ulcer of contiguous site of back, buttock and hip, unspecified stage**
> Healing pressure ulcer of contiguous site of back, buttock and hip NOS
> Healing pressure ulcer of contiguous site of back, buttock and hip, unspecified stage

L89.41   **Pressure ulcer of contiguous site of back, buttock and hip, stage 1**
> Healing pressure ulcer of contiguous site of back, buttock and hip, stage 1
> Pressure pre-ulcer skin changes limited to persistent focal edema, contiguous site of back, buttock and hip

L89.42   **Pressure ulcer of contiguous site of back, buttock and hip, stage 2**
> Healing pressure ulcer of contiguous site of back, buttock and hip, stage 2
> Pressure ulcer with abrasion, blister, partial thickness skin loss involving epidermis and/or dermis, contiguous site of back, buttock and hip

N Newborn: 0   P Pediatric: 0-17   M Maternity: 12-55   A Adult: 15-124   MCC Major CC Condition   PDxMCC PDx acts as own MCC   CC CC Condition   PDxCC PDx acts as own CC

690   ICD-10-CM 2016

L89.43   **Pressure ulcer of contiguous site of back,** `PDxMCC` `MCC`
buttock and hip, stage 3
    Healing pressure ulcer of contiguous site of back,
      buttock and hip, stage 3
    Pressure ulcer with full thickness skin loss involving
      damage or necrosis of subcutaneous tissue,
      contiguous site of back, buttock and hip

L89.44   **Pressure ulcer of contiguous site of back,** `PDxMCC` `MCC`
buttock and hip, stage 4
    Healing pressure ulcer of contiguous site of back,
      buttock and hip, stage 4
    Pressure ulcer with necrosis of soft tissues through to
      underlying muscle, tendon, or bone, contiguous
      site of back, buttock and hip

L89.45   **Pressure ulcer of contiguous site of back, buttock**
and hip, unstageable

✓5ᵗʰ **L89.5**   **Pressure ulcer of ankle**

   ✓6ᵗʰ **L89.50**   **Pressure ulcer of unspecified ankle**

L89.500   **Pressure ulcer of unspecified ankle,**
unstageable

L89.501   **Pressure ulcer of unspecified ankle,**
stage 1
    Healing pressure ulcer of unspecified ankle,
      stage 1
    Pressure pre-ulcer skin changes limited to
      persistent focal edema, unspecified
      ankle

L89.502   **Pressure ulcer of unspecified ankle,**
stage 2
    Healing pressure ulcer of unspecified ankle,
      stage 2
    Pressure ulcer with abrasion, blister, partial
      thickness skin loss involving epidermis
      and/or dermis, unspecified ankle

L89.503   **Pressure ulcer of unspecified** `PDxMCC` `MCC`
ankle, stage 3
    Healing pressure ulcer of unspecified ankle,
      stage 3
    Pressure ulcer with full thickness skin loss
      involving damage or necrosis of
      subcutaneous tissue, unspecified
      ankle

L89.504   **Pressure ulcer of unspecified** `PDxMCC` `MCC`
ankle, stage 4
    Healing pressure ulcer of unspecified ankle,
      stage 4
    Pressure ulcer with necrosis of soft tissues
      through to underlying muscle,
      tendon, or bone, unspecified ankle

L89.509   **Pressure ulcer of unspecified ankle,**
unspecified stage
    Healing pressure ulcer of unspecified ankle
      NOS
    Healing pressure ulcer of unspecified ankle,
      unspecified stage

   ✓6ᵗʰ **L89.51**   **Pressure ulcer of right ankle**

L89.510   **Pressure ulcer of right ankle, unstageable**

L89.511   **Pressure ulcer of right ankle, stage 1**
    Healing pressure ulcer of right ankle,
      stage 1
    Pressure pre-ulcer skin changes limited to
      persistent focal edema, right ankle

L89.512   **Pressure ulcer of right ankle, stage 2**
    Healing pressure ulcer of right ankle,
      stage 2
    Pressure ulcer with abrasion, blister, partial
      thickness skin loss involving epidermis
      and/or dermis, right ankle

L89.513   **Pressure ulcer of right ankle,** `PDxMCC` `MCC`
stage 3
    Healing pressure ulcer of right ankle,
      stage 3
    Pressure ulcer with full thickness skin loss
      involving damage or necrosis of
      subcutaneous tissue, right ankle

L89.514   **Pressure ulcer of right ankle,** `PDxMCC` `MCC`
stage 4
    Healing pressure ulcer of right ankle,
      stage 4
    Pressure ulcer with necrosis of soft tissues
      through to underlying muscle,
      tendon, or bone, right ankle

L89.519   **Pressure ulcer of right ankle, unspecified**
stage
    Healing pressure ulcer of right ankle NOS
    Healing pressure ulcer of right ankle,
      unspecified stage

   ✓6ᵗʰ **L89.52**   **Pressure ulcer of left ankle**

L89.520   **Pressure ulcer of left ankle, unstageable**

L89.521   **Pressure ulcer of left ankle, stage 1**
    Healing pressure ulcer of left ankle, stage 1
    Pressure pre-ulcer skin changes limited to
      persistnt focal edema, left ankle

L89.522   **Pressure ulcer of left ankle, stage 2**
    Healing pressure ulcer of left ankle, stage 2
    Pressure ulcer with abrasion, blister, partial
      thickness skin loss involving epidermis
      and/or dermis, left ankle

L89.523   **Pressure ulcer of left ankle,** `PDxMCC` `MCC`
stage 3
    Healing pressure ulcer of left ankle, stage 3
    Pressure ulcer with full thickness skin loss
      involving damage or necrosis of
      subcutaneous tissue, left ankle

L89.524   **Pressure ulcer of left ankle,** `PDxMCC` `MCC`
stage 4
    Healing pressure ulcer of left ankle, stage 4
    Pressure ulcer with necrosis of soft tissues
      through to underlying muscle,
      tendon, or bone, left ankle

L89.529   **Pressure ulcer of left ankle, unspecified**
stage
    Healing pressure ulcer of left ankle NOS
    Healing pressure ulcer of left ankle,
      unspecified stage

✓5ᵗʰ **L89.6**   **Pressure ulcer of heel**

   ✓6ᵗʰ **L89.60**   **Pressure ulcer of unspecified heel**

L89.600   **Pressure ulcer of unspecified heel,**
unstageable

L89.601   **Pressure ulcer of unspecified heel, stage 1**
    Healing pressure ulcer of unspecified heel,
      stage 1
    Pressure pre-ulcer skin changes limited to
      persistent focal edema, unspecified
      heel

L89.602   **Pressure ulcer of unspecified heel, stage 2**
    Healing pressure ulcer of unspecified heel,
      stage 2
    Pressure ulcer with abrasion, blister, partial
      thickness skin loss involving epidermis
      and/or dermis, unspecified heel

L89.603   **Pressure ulcer of unspecified** `PDxMCC` `MCC`
heel, stage 3
    Healing pressure ulcer of unspecified heel,
      stage 3
    Pressure ulcer with full thickness skin loss
      involving damage or necrosis of
      subcutaneous tissue, unspecified heel

L89.604   **Pressure ulcer of unspecified** `PDxMCC` `MCC`
heel, stage 4
    Healing pressure ulcer of unspecified heel,
      stage 4
    Pressure ulcer with necrosis of soft tissues
      through to underlying muscle,
      tendon, or bone, unspecified heel

L89.609   **Pressure ulcer of unspecified heel,**
unspecified stage
    Healing pressure ulcer of unspecified heel
      NOS
    Healing pressure ulcer of unspecified heel,
      unspecified stage

   ✓6ᵗʰ **L89.61**   **Pressure ulcer of right heel**

L89.610   **Pressure ulcer of right heel, unstageable**

L89.611   **Pressure ulcer of right heel, stage 1**
    Healing pressure ulcer of right heel, stage 1
    Pressure pre-ulcer skin changes limited to
      persistent focal edema, right heel

L89.612   **Pressure ulcer of right heel, stage 2**
    Healing pressure ulcer of right heel, stage 2
    Pressure ulcer with abrasion, blister, partial
      thickness skin loss involving epidermis
      and/or dermis, right heel

✅ Additional Character Required   ✓x7ᵗʰ Placeholder Alert   Unacceptable PDx   Manifestation   Hospital Acquired Condition   **EXCLUDES 1** Not Coded Here   *EXCLUDES 2* Not Included Here

ICD-10-CM 2016   691

L89.613 Pressure ulcer of right heel, stage 3 `PDxMCC` `MCC`
Healing pressure ulcer of right heel, stage 3
Pressure ulcer with full thickness skin loss involving damage or necrosis of subcutaneous tissue, right heel

L89.614 Pressure ulcer of right heel, stage 4 `PDxMCC` `MCC`
Healing pressure ulcer of right heel, stage 4
Pressure ulcer with necrosis of soft tissues through to underlying muscle, tendon, or bone, right heel

L89.619 Pressure ulcer of right heel, unspecified stage
Healing pressure ulcer of right heel NOS
Healing pressure ulcer of unspecified heel, right stage

✓6ᵗʰ **L89.62 Pressure ulcer of left heel**

L89.62Ø Pressure ulcer of left heel, unstageable

L89.621 Pressure ulcer of left heel, stage 1
Healing pressure ulcer of left heel, stage 1
Pressure pre-ulcer skin changes limited to persistent focal edema, left heel

L89.622 Pressure ulcer of left heel, stage 2
Healing pressure ulcer of left heel, stage 2
Pressure ulcer with abrasion, blister, partial thickness skin loss involving epidermis and/or dermis, left heel

L89.623 Pressure ulcer of left heel, stage 3 `PDxMCC` `MCC`
Healing pressure ulcer of left heel, stage 3
Pressure ulcer with full thickness skin loss involving damage or necrosis of subcutaneous tissue, left heel

L89.624 Pressure ulcer of left heel, stage 4 `PDxMCC` `MCC`
Healing pressure ulcer of left heel, stage 4
Pressure ulcer with necrosis of soft tissues through to underlying muscle, tendon, or bone, left heel

L89.629 Pressure ulcer of left heel, unspecified stage
Healing pressure ulcer of left heel NOS
Healing pressure ulcer of left heel, unspecified stage

✓5ᵗʰ **L89.8 Pressure ulcer of other site**

✓6ᵗʰ **L89.81 Pressure ulcer of head**
Pressure ulcer of face

L89.81Ø Pressure ulcer of head, unstageable

L89.811 Pressure ulcer of head, stage 1
Healing pressure ulcer of head, stage 1
Pressure pre-ulcer skin changes limited to persistent focal edema, head

L89.812 Pressure ulcer of head, stage 2
Healing pressure ulcer of head, stage 2
Pressure ulcer with abrasion, blister, partial thickness skin loss involving epidermis and/or dermis, head

L89.813 Pressure ulcer of head, stage 3 `PDxMCC` `MCC`
Healing pressure ulcer of head, stage 3
Pressure ulcer with full thickness skin loss involving damage or necrosis of subcutaneous tissue, head

L89.814 Pressure ulcer of head, stage 4 `PDxMCC` `MCC`
Healing pressure ulcer of head, stage 4
Pressure ulcer with necrosis of soft tissues through to underlying muscle, tendon, or bone, head

L89.819 Pressure ulcer of head, unspecified stage
Healing pressure ulcer of head NOS
Healing pressure ulcer of head, unspecified stage

✓6ᵗʰ **L89.89 Pressure ulcer of other site**

L89.89Ø Pressure ulcer of other site, unstageable

L89.891 Pressure ulcer of other site, stage 1
Healing pressure ulcer of other site, stage 1
Pressure pre-ulcer skin changes limited to persistent focal edema, other site

L89.892 Pressure ulcer of other site, stage 2
Healing pressure ulcer of other site, stage 2
Pressure ulcer with abrasion, blister, partial thickness skin loss involving epidermis and/or dermis, other site

L89.893 Pressure ulcer of other site, stage 3 `PDxMCC` `MCC`
Healing pressure ulcer of other site, stage 3
Pressure ulcer with full thickness skin loss involving damage or necrosis of subcutaneous tissue, other site

L89.894 Pressure ulcer of other site, stage 4 `PDxMCC` `MCC`
Healing pressure ulcer of other site, stage 4
Pressure ulcer with necrosis of soft tissues through to underlying muscle, tendon, or bone, other site

L89.899 Pressure ulcer of other site, unspecified stage
Healing pressure ulcer of other site NOS
Healing pressure ulcer of other site, unspecified stage

✓5ᵗʰ **L89.9 Pressure ulcer of unspecified site**

L89.9Ø Pressure ulcer of unspecified site, unspecified stage
Healing pressure ulcer of unspecified site NOS
Healing pressure ulcer of unspecified site, unspecified stage

L89.91 Pressure ulcer of unspecified site, stage 1
Healing pressure ulcer of unspecified site, stage 1
Pressure pre-ulcer skin changes limited to persistent focal edema, unspecified site

L89.92 Pressure ulcer of unspecified site, stage 2
Healing pressure ulcer of unspecified site, stage 2
Pressure ulcer with abrasion, blister, partial thickness skin loss involving epidermis and/or dermis, unspecified site

L89.93 Pressure ulcer of unspecified site, stage 3 `PDxMCC` `MCC`
Healing pressure ulcer of unspecified site, stage 3
Pressure ulcer with full thickness skin loss involving damage or necrosis of subcutaneous tissue, unspecified site

L89.94 Pressure ulcer of unspecified site, stage 4 `PDxMCC` `MCC`
Healing pressure ulcer of unspecified site, stage 4
Pressure ulcer with necrosis of soft tissues through to underlying muscle, tendon, or bone, unspecified site

L89.95 Pressure ulcer of unspecified site, unstageable

✓4ᵗʰ **L90 Atrophic disorders of skin**

L90.Ø Lichen sclerosus et atrophicus
EXCLUDES 2 lichen sclerosus of external female genital organs (N90.4)
lichen sclerosus of external male genital organs (N48.0)

L90.1 Anetoderma of Schweninger-Buzzi

L90.2 Anetoderma of Jadassohn-Pellizzari

L90.3 Atrophoderma of Pasini and Pierini

L90.4 Acrodermatitis chronica atrophicans

L90.5 Scar conditions and fibrosis of skin
Adherent scar (skin)   Fibrosis of skin NOS
Cicatrix   Scar NOS
Disfigurement of skin due to scar
EXCLUDES 2 hypertrophic scar (L91.Ø)
keloid scar (L91.Ø)
AHA: 2015, 1Q, 19

L90.6 Striae atrophicae

L90.8 Other atrophic disorders of skin

L90.9 Atrophic disorder of skin, unspecified

✓4ᵗʰ **L91 Hypertrophic disorders of skin**

L91.Ø Hypertrophic scar
Keloid   Keloid scar
EXCLUDES 2 acne keloid (L73.Ø)
scar NOS (L90.5)

L91.8 Other hypertrophic disorders of the skin

L91.9 Hypertrophic disorder of the skin, unspecified

✓4ᵗʰ **L92 Granulomatous disorders of skin and subcutaneous tissue**
EXCLUDES 2 actinic granuloma (L57.5)

L92.Ø Granuloma annulare
Perforating granuloma annulare

N Newborn: 0 P Pediatric: 0-17 M Maternity: 12-55 A Adult: 15-124 MCC Major CC Condition PDxMCC PDx acts as own MCC CC CC Condition PDxCC PDx acts as own CC

692 ICD-10-CM 2016

L92.1 Necrobiosis lipoidica, not elsewhere classified
> EXCLUDES 1   *necrobiosis lipoidica associated with diabetes mellitus (E08-E13 with .620)*

L92.2 Granuloma faciale [eosinophilic granuloma of skin]

L92.3 Foreign body granuloma of the skin and subcutaneous tissue
> Use additional code to identify the type of retained foreign body (Z18.-)

L92.8 Other granulomatous disorders of the skin and subcutaneous tissue

L92.9 Granulomatous disorder of the skin and subcutaneous tissue, unspecified

✓4ᵗʰ L93 Lupus erythematosus
> Use additional code for adverse effect, if applicable, to identify drug (T36-T50 with fifth or sixth character 5)
> EXCLUDES 1   *lupus exedens (A18.4)*
> *lupus vulgaris (A18.4)*
> *scleroderma (M34.-)*
> *systemic lupus erythematosus (M32.-)*

L93.0 Discoid lupus erythematosus
> Lupus erythematosus NOS

L93.1 Subacute cutaneous lupus erythematosus

L93.2 Other local lupus erythematosus
> Lupus erythematosus profundus
> Lupus panniculitis

✓4ᵗʰ L94 Other localized connective tissue disorders
> EXCLUDES 1   *systemic connective tissue disorders (M30-M36)*

L94.0 Localized scleroderma [morphea]
> Circumscribed scleroderma

L94.1 Linear scleroderma
> En coup de sabre lesion

L94.2 Calcinosis cutis

L94.3 Sclerodactyly

L94.4 Gottron's papules

L94.5 Poikiloderma vasculare atrophicans

L94.6 Ainhum

L94.8 Other specified localized connective tissue disorders

L94.9 Localized connective tissue disorder, unspecified

✓4ᵗʰ L95 Vasculitis limited to skin, not elsewhere classified
> EXCLUDES 1   *angioma serpiginosum (L81.7)*
> *Henoch(-Schönlein) purpura (D69.0)*
> *hypersensitivity angiitis (M31.0)*
> *lupus panniculitis (L93.2)*
> *panniculitis NOS (M79.3)*
> *panniculitis of neck and back (M54.0-)*
> *polyarteritis nodosa (M30.0)*
> *relapsing panniculitis (M35.6)*
> *rheumatoid vasculitis (M05.2)*
> *serum sickness (T80.6-)*
> *urticaria (L50.-)*
> *Wegener's granulomatosis (M31.3-)*

L95.0 Livedoid vasculitis
> Atrophie blanche (en plaque)

L95.1 Erythema elevatum diutinum

L95.8 Other vasculitis limited to the skin

L95.9 Vasculitis limited to the skin, unspecified

✓4ᵗʰ L97 Non-pressure chronic ulcer of lower limb, not elsewhere classified
> INCLUDES   chronic ulcer of skin of lower limb NOS
> non-healing ulcer of skin
> non-infected sinus of skin
> trophic ulcer NOS
> tropical ulcer NOS
> ulcer of skin of lower limb NOS

Code first any associated underlying condition, such as:
> atherosclerosis of the lower extremities (I70.23-, I70.24-, I70.33-, I70.34-, I70.43-, I70.44-, I70.53-, I70.54-, I70.63-, I70.64-, I70.73-, I70.74-)
> chronic venous hypertension (I87.31-, I87.33-)
> diabetic ulcers (E08.621, E08.622, E09.621, E09.622, E10.621, E10.622, E11.621, E11.622, E13.621, E13.622)
> postphlebitic syndrome (I87.01-, I87.03-)
> postthrombotic syndrome (I87.01-, I87.03-)
> varicose ulcer (I83.0-, I83.2-)

Code first any associated gangrene (I96)
> EXCLUDES 2   *pressure ulcer (pressure area) (L89.-)*
> *skin infections (L00-L08)*
> *specific infections classified to A00-B99*

CC Excl: For CC codes in category L97, unless otherwise noted: I70.231-I70.25, L44.8-L45, L94.2, L94.4, L97.101-L97.929, L98.411-L98.499, L98.8, L99

✓5ᵗʰ L97.1 Non-pressure chronic ulcer of thigh

✓6ᵗʰ L97.10 Non-pressure chronic ulcer of unspecified thigh

L97.101 Non-pressure chronic ulcer of unspecified thigh limited to breakdown of skin   CC

L97.102 Non-pressure chronic ulcer of unspecified thigh with fat layer exposed   CC

L97.103 Non-pressure chronic ulcer of unspecified thigh with necrosis of muscle   CC

L97.104 Non-pressure chronic ulcer of unspecified thigh with necrosis of bone   CC

L97.109 Non-pressure chronic ulcer of unspecified thigh with unspecified severity   CC

✓6ᵗʰ L97.11 Non-pressure chronic ulcer of right thigh

L97.111 Non-pressure chronic ulcer of right thigh limited to breakdown of skin   CC

L97.112 Non-pressure chronic ulcer of right thigh with fat layer exposed   CC

L97.113 Non-pressure chronic ulcer of right thigh with necrosis of muscle   CC

L97.114 Non-pressure chronic ulcer of right thigh with necrosis of bone   CC

L97.119 Non-pressure chronic ulcer of right thigh with unspecified severity   CC

✓6ᵗʰ L97.12 Non-pressure chronic ulcer of left thigh

L97.121 Non-pressure chronic ulcer of left thigh limited to breakdown of skin   CC

L97.122 Non-pressure chronic ulcer of left thigh with fat layer exposed   CC

L97.123 Non-pressure chronic ulcer of left thigh with necrosis of muscle   CC

L97.124 Non-pressure chronic ulcer of left thigh with necrosis of bone   CC

L97.129 Non-pressure chronic ulcer of left thigh with unspecified severity   CC

✓5ᵗʰ L97.2 Non-pressure chronic ulcer of calf

✓6ᵗʰ L97.20 Non-pressure chronic ulcer of unspecified calf

L97.201 Non-pressure chronic ulcer of unspecified calf limited to breakdown of skin   CC

L97.202 Non-pressure chronic ulcer of unspecified calf with fat layer exposed   CC

L97.203 Non-pressure chronic ulcer of unspecified calf with necrosis of muscle   CC

L97.204 Non-pressure chronic ulcer of unspecified calf with necrosis of bone   CC

L97.209 Non-pressure chronic ulcer of unspecified calf with unspecified severity   CC

✓ Additional Character Required   ✓x7ᵗʰ Placeholder Alert   Unacceptable PDx   Manifestation   Hospital Acquired Condition   EXCLUDES 1 Not Coded Here   EXCLUDES 2 Not Included Here

ICD-10-CM 2016   693

√6ᵗʰ **L97.21** Non-pressure chronic ulcer of right calf

     L97.211 Non-pressure chronic ulcer of right calf limited to breakdown of skin `CC`

     L97.212 Non-pressure chronic ulcer of right calf with fat layer exposed `CC`

     L97.213 Non-pressure chronic ulcer of right calf with necrosis of muscle `CC`

     L97.214 Non-pressure chronic ulcer of right calf with necrosis of bone `CC`

     L97.219 Non-pressure chronic ulcer of right calf with unspecified severity `CC`

√6ᵗʰ **L97.22** Non-pressure chronic ulcer of left calf

     L97.221 Non-pressure chronic ulcer of left calf limited to breakdown of skin `CC`

     L97.222 Non-pressure chronic ulcer of left calf with fat layer exposed `CC`

     L97.223 Non-pressure chronic ulcer of left calf with necrosis of muscle `CC`

     L97.224 Non-pressure chronic ulcer of left calf with necrosis of bone `CC`

     L97.229 Non-pressure chronic ulcer of left calf with unspecified severity `CC`

√5ᵗʰ **L97.3** Non-pressure chronic ulcer of ankle

√6ᵗʰ **L97.30** Non-pressure chronic ulcer of unspecified ankle

     L97.301 Non-pressure chronic ulcer of unspecified ankle limited to breakdown of skin `CC`

     L97.302 Non-pressure chronic ulcer of unspecified ankle with fat layer exposed `CC`

     L97.303 Non-pressure chronic ulcer of unspecified ankle with necrosis of muscle `CC`

     L97.304 Non-pressure chronic ulcer of unspecified ankle with necrosis of bone `CC`

     L97.309 Non-pressure chronic ulcer of unspecified ankle with unspecified severity `CC`

√6ᵗʰ **L97.31** Non-pressure chronic ulcer of right ankle

     L97.311 Non-pressure chronic ulcer of right ankle limited to breakdown of skin `CC`

     L97.312 Non-pressure chronic ulcer of right ankle with fat layer exposed `CC`

     L97.313 Non-pressure chronic ulcer of right ankle with necrosis of muscle `CC`

     L97.314 Non-pressure chronic ulcer of right ankle with necrosis of bone `CC`

     L97.319 Non-pressure chronic ulcer of right ankle with unspecified severity `CC`

√6ᵗʰ **L97.32** Non-pressure chronic ulcer of left ankle

     L97.321 Non-pressure chronic ulcer of left ankle limited to breakdown of skin `CC`

     L97.322 Non-pressure chronic ulcer of left ankle with fat layer exposed `CC`

     L97.323 Non-pressure chronic ulcer of left ankle with necrosis of muscle `CC`

     L97.324 Non-pressure chronic ulcer of left ankle with necrosis of bone `CC`

     L97.329 Non-pressure chronic ulcer of left ankle with unspecified severity `CC`

√5ᵗʰ **L97.4** Non-pressure chronic ulcer of heel and midfoot
     Non-pressure chronic ulcer of plantar surface of midfoot

√6ᵗʰ **L97.40** Non-pressure chronic ulcer of unspecified heel and midfoot

     L97.401 Non-pressure chronic ulcer of unspecified heel and midfoot limited to breakdown of skin `CC`

     L97.402 Non-pressure chronic ulcer of unspecified heel and midfoot with fat layer exposed `CC`

     L97.403 Non-pressure chronic ulcer of unspecified heel and midfoot with necrosis of muscle `CC`

     L97.404 Non-pressure chronic ulcer of unspecified heel and midfoot with necrosis of bone `CC`

     L97.409 Non-pressure chronic ulcer of unspecified heel and midfoot with unspecified severity `CC`

√6ᵗʰ **L97.41** Non-pressure chronic ulcer of right heel and midfoot

     L97.411 Non-pressure chronic ulcer of right heel and midfoot limited to breakdown of skin `CC`

     L97.412 Non-pressure chronic ulcer of right heel and midfoot with fat layer exposed `CC`

     L97.413 Non-pressure chronic ulcer of right heel and midfoot with necrosis of muscle `CC`

     L97.414 Non-pressure chronic ulcer of right heel and midfoot with necrosis of bone `CC`

     L97.419 Non-pressure chronic ulcer of right heel and midfoot with unspecified severity `CC`

√6ᵗʰ **L97.42** Non-pressure chronic ulcer of left heel and midfoot

     L97.421 Non-pressure chronic ulcer of left heel and midfoot limited to breakdown of skin `CC`

     L97.422 Non-pressure chronic ulcer of left heel and midfoot with fat layer exposed `CC`

     L97.423 Non-pressure chronic ulcer of left heel and midfoot with necrosis of muscle `CC`

     L97.424 Non-pressure chronic ulcer of left heel and midfoot with necrosis of bone `CC`

     L97.429 Non-pressure chronic ulcer of left heel and midfoot with unspecified severity `CC`

√5ᵗʰ **L97.5** Non-pressure chronic ulcer of other part of foot
     Non-pressure chronic ulcer of toe

√6ᵗʰ **L97.50** Non-pressure chronic ulcer of other part of unspecified foot

     L97.501 Non-pressure chronic ulcer of other part of unspecified foot limited to breakdown of skin

     L97.502 Non-pressure chronic ulcer of other part of unspecified foot with fat layer exposed

     L97.503 Non-pressure chronic ulcer of other part of unspecified foot with necrosis of muscle

     L97.504 Non-pressure chronic ulcer of other part of unspecified foot with necrosis of bone

     L97.509 Non-pressure chronic ulcer of other part of unspecified foot with unspecified severity

√6ᵗʰ **L97.51** Non-pressure chronic ulcer of other part of right foot

     L97.511 Non-pressure chronic ulcer of other part of right foot limited to breakdown of skin

     L97.512 Non-pressure chronic ulcer of other part of right foot with fat layer exposed

     L97.513 Non-pressure chronic ulcer of other part of right foot with necrosis of muscle

     L97.514 Non-pressure chronic ulcer of other part of right foot with necrosis of bone

     L97.519 Non-pressure chronic ulcer of other part of right foot with unspecified severity

√6ᵗʰ **L97.52** Non-pressure chronic ulcer of other part of left foot

     L97.521 Non-pressure chronic ulcer of other part of left foot limited to breakdown of skin

     L97.522 Non-pressure chronic ulcer of other part of left foot with fat layer exposed

     L97.523 Non-pressure chronic ulcer of other part of left foot with necrosis of muscle

     L97.524 Non-pressure chronic ulcer of other part of left foot with necrosis of bone

     L97.529 Non-pressure chronic ulcer of other part of left foot with unspecified severity

√5ᵗʰ **L97.8** Non-pressure chronic ulcer of other part of lower leg

√6ᵗʰ **L97.80** Non-pressure chronic ulcer of other part of unspecified lower leg

     L97.801 Non-pressure chronic ulcer of other part of unspecified lower leg limited to breakdown of skin `CC`

     L97.802 Non-pressure chronic ulcer of other part of unspecified lower leg with fat layer exposed `CC`

     L97.803 Non-pressure chronic ulcer of other part of unspecified lower leg with necrosis of muscle `CC`

     L97.804 Non-pressure chronic ulcer of other part of unspecified lower leg with necrosis of bone `CC`

N Newborn: 0   P Pediatric: 0-17   M Maternity: 12-55   A Adult: 15-124   MCC Major CC Condition   PDxMCC PDx acts as own MCC   CC CC Condition   PDxCC PDx acts as own CC

694   ICD-10-CM 2016

L97.809   Non-pressure chronic ulcer of other part of unspecified lower leg with unspecified severity   `CC`

✓6ᵗʰ **L97.81**   Non-pressure chronic ulcer of other part of right lower leg

    L97.811   Non-pressure chronic ulcer of other part of right lower leg limited to breakdown of skin   `CC`

    L97.812   Non-pressure chronic ulcer of other part of right lower leg with fat layer exposed   `CC`

    L97.813   Non-pressure chronic ulcer of other part of right lower leg with necrosis of muscle   `CC`

    L97.814   Non-pressure chronic ulcer of other part of right lower leg with necrosis of bone   `CC`

    L97.819   Non-pressure chronic ulcer of other part of right lower leg with unspecified severity   `CC`

✓6ᵗʰ **L97.82**   Non-pressure chronic ulcer of other part of left lower leg

    L97.821   Non-pressure chronic ulcer of other part of left lower leg limited to breakdown of skin   `CC`

    L97.822   Non-pressure chronic ulcer of other part of left lower leg with fat layer exposed   `CC`

    L97.823   Non-pressure chronic ulcer of other part of left lower leg with necrosis of muscle   `CC`

    L97.824   Non-pressure chronic ulcer of other part of left lower leg with necrosis of bone   `CC`

    L97.829   Non-pressure chronic ulcer of other part of left lower leg with unspecified severity   `CC`

✓5ᵗʰ **L97.9**   Non-pressure chronic ulcer of unspecified part of lower leg

✓6ᵗʰ **L97.90**   Non-pressure chronic ulcer of unspecified part of unspecified lower leg

    L97.901   Non-pressure chronic ulcer of unspecified part of unspecified lower leg limited to breakdown of skin   `CC`

    L97.902   Non-pressure chronic ulcer of unspecified part of unspecified lower leg with fat layer exposed   `CC`

    L97.903   Non-pressure chronic ulcer of unspecified part of unspecified lower leg with necrosis of muscle   `CC`

    L97.904   Non-pressure chronic ulcer of unspecified part of unspecified lower leg with necrosis of bone   `CC`

    L97.909   Non-pressure chronic ulcer of unspecified part of unspecified lower leg with unspecified severity   `CC`

✓6ᵗʰ **L97.91**   Non-pressure chronic ulcer of unspecified part of right lower leg

    L97.911   Non-pressure chronic ulcer of unspecified part of right lower leg limited to breakdown of skin   `CC`

    L97.912   Non-pressure chronic ulcer of unspecified part of right lower leg with fat layer exposed   `CC`

    L97.913   Non-pressure chronic ulcer of unspecified part of right lower leg with necrosis of muscle   `CC`

    L97.914   Non-pressure chronic ulcer of unspecified part of right lower leg with necrosis of bone   `CC`

    L97.919   Non-pressure chronic ulcer of unspecified part of right lower leg with unspecified severity   `CC`

✓6ᵗʰ **L97.92**   Non-pressure chronic ulcer of unspecified part of left lower leg

    L97.921   Non-pressure chronic ulcer of unspecified part of left lower leg limited to breakdown of skin   `CC`

    L97.922   Non-pressure chronic ulcer of unspecified part of left lower leg with fat layer exposed   `CC`

    L97.923   Non-pressure chronic ulcer of unspecified part of left lower leg with necrosis of muscle   `CC`

    L97.924   Non-pressure chronic ulcer of unspecified part of left lower leg with necrosis of bone   `CC`

    L97.929   Non-pressure chronic ulcer of unspecified part of left lower leg with unspecified severity   `CC`

✓4ᵗʰ **L98**   **Other disorders of skin and subcutaneous tissue, not elsewhere classified**

L98.0   **Pyogenic granuloma**
> *EXCLUDES 2*   *pyogenic granuloma of gingiva (K06.8)*
> *pyogenic granuloma of maxillary alveolar ridge (K04.5)*
> *pyogenic granuloma of oral mucosa (K13.4)*

L98.1   **Factitial dermatitis**
Neurotic excoriation

L98.2   **Febrile neutrophilic dermatosis [Sweet]**

L98.3   **Eosinophilic cellulitis [Wells]**   `CC`
CC Excl: A17.9, A18.4, A18.82, A18.84, A18.89, A48.2-A48.4, A48.8-A49.9, B78.1, B95.0-B96.89, E83.2, L02.811-L02.818, L02.91, L03.811-L03.91, L08.0, L08.81-L08.9, L44.8-L45, L73.2, L88, L92.8, L94.2, L94.4, L98.0, L98.3, L98.8, L99, M00.011-M00.012, M00.021-M00.022, M00.031-M00.032, M00.041-M00.042, M00.051-M00.052, M00.061-M00.062, M00.071-M00.072, Z16.10-Z16.39

✓5ᵗʰ **L98.4**   **Non-pressure chronic ulcer of skin, not elsewhere classified**
Chronic ulcer of skin NOS   Ulcer of skin NOS
Tropical ulcer NOS
> *EXCLUDES 2*   *pressure ulcer (pressure area) (L89.-)*
> *gangrene (I96)*
> *skin infections (L00-L08)*
> *specific infections classified to A00-B99*
> *ulcer of lower limb NEC (L97.-)*
> *varicose ulcer (I83.0-I82.2)*

  ✓6ᵗʰ **L98.41**   Non-pressure chronic ulcer of buttock

    L98.411   Non-pressure chronic ulcer of buttock limited to breakdown of skin

    L98.412   Non-pressure chronic ulcer of buttock with fat layer exposed

    L98.413   Non-pressure chronic ulcer of buttock with necrosis of muscle

    L98.414   Non-pressure chronic ulcer of buttock with necrosis of bone

    L98.419   Non-pressure chronic ulcer of buttock with unspecified severity

  ✓6ᵗʰ **L98.42**   Non-pressure chronic ulcer of back

    L98.421   Non-pressure chronic ulcer of back limited to breakdown of skin

    L98.422   Non-pressure chronic ulcer of back with fat layer exposed

    L98.423   Non-pressure chronic ulcer of back with necrosis of muscle

    L98.424   Non-pressure chronic ulcer of back with necrosis of bone

    L98.429   Non-pressure chronic ulcer of back with unspecified severity

  ✓6ᵗʰ **L98.49**   Non-pressure chronic ulcer of skin of other sites
Non-pressure chronic ulcer of skin NOS

    L98.491   Non-pressure chronic ulcer of skin of other sites limited to breakdown of skin

    L98.492   Non-pressure chronic ulcer of skin of other sites with fat layer exposed

    L98.493   Non-pressure chronic ulcer of skin of other sites with necrosis of muscle

    L98.494   Non-pressure chronic ulcer of skin of other sites with necrosis of bone

    L98.499   Non-pressure chronic ulcer of skin of other sites with unspecified severity

L98.5   **Mucinosis of the skin**
Focal mucinosis   Reticular erythematous mucinosis
Lichen myxedematosus
> *EXCLUDES 1*   *focal oral mucinosis (K13.79)*
> *myxedema (E03.9)*

L98.6   **Other infiltrative disorders of the skin and subcutaneous tissue**
> *EXCLUDES 1*   *hyalinosis cutis et mucosae (E78.89)*

L98.8   **Other specified disorders of the skin and subcutaneous tissue**
AHA: 2013, 2Q, 32

L98.9   **Disorder of the skin and subcutaneous tissue, unspecified**

✓ Additional Character Required   ✓x7ᵗʰ Placeholder Alert   Unacceptable PDx   Manifestation   Hospital Acquired Condition   *EXCLUDES 1* Not Coded Here   *EXCLUDES 2* Not Included Here

L99 **Other disorders of skin and subcutaneous tissue in diseases classified elsewhere**

Code first underlying disease, such as:
amyloidosis (E85.-)

EXCLUDES 1   skin disorders in diabetes (E08-E13 with .62)
skin disorders in gonorrhea (A54.89)
skin disorders in syphilis (A51.31, A52.79)

Chapter 13. Diseases of the Musculoskeletal System and Connective Tissue (M00–M99)

Chapter Specific Guidelines with Coding Examples

The chapter specific guidelines from the ICD-10-CM Official Guidelines for Coding and Reporting have been provided below. Along with these guidelines are coding examples, contained in the shaded boxes, that have been developed to help illustrate the coding and/or sequencing guidance found in these guidelines.

a. Site and laterality

Most of the codes within Chapter 13 have site and laterality designations. The site represents the bone, joint or the muscle involved. For some conditions where more than one bone, joint or muscle is usually involved, such as osteoarthritis, there is a "multiple sites" code available. For categories where no multiple site code is provided and more than one bone, joint or muscle is involved, multiple codes should be used to indicate the different sites involved.

> Right elbow infective bursitis
>
> **M71.121   Other infective bursitis, right elbow**
>
> *Explanation:* Most of the codes within chapter 13 have site and laterality designations. The site represents the bone, joint, or the muscle involved.

> Rheumatoid arthritis of multiple sites without rheumatoid factor
>
> **M06.09   Rheumatoid arthritis without rheumatoid factor, multiple sites**
>
> *Explanation:* For some conditions where more than one bone, joint or muscle is usually involved, such as osteoarthritis, there is a "multiple sites" code available.

> Osteomyelitis of the fourth thoracic and second lumbar vertebrae
>
> **M46.24   Osteomyelitis of vertebra, thoracic region**
>
> **M46.26   Osteomyelitis of vertebra, lumbar region**
>
> *Explanation:* For categories without a multiple site code and more than one bone, joint, or muscle is involved, multiple codes should be used to indicate the different sites involved.

1) Bone versus joint

For certain conditions, the bone may be affected at the upper or lower end, (e.g., avascular necrosis of bone, M87, Osteoporosis, M80, M81). Though the portion of the bone affected may be at the joint, the site designation will be the bone, not the joint.

> Idiopathic avascular necrosis of the femoral head of the left hip joint
>
> **M87.052   Idiopathic aseptic necrosis of left femur**
>
> *Explanation:* For certain conditions such as avascular necrosis, the bone may be affected at the joint, but the site designation is the bone, not the joint.

b. Acute traumatic versus chronic or recurrent musculoskeletal conditions

Many musculoskeletal conditions are a result of previous injury or trauma to a site, or are recurrent conditions. Bone, joint or muscle conditions that are the result of a healed injury are usually found in chapter 13. Recurrent bone, joint or muscle conditions are also usually found in chapter 13. Any current, acute injury should be coded to the appropriate injury code from chapter 19. Chronic or recurrent conditions should generally be coded with a code from chapter 13. If it is difficult to determine from the documentation in the record which code is best to describe a condition, query the provider.

> Acute traumatic bucket handle tear of right medial meniscus
>
> **S83.211A   Bucket-handle tear of medial meniscus, current injury, right knee, initial encounter**
>
> *Explanation:* Any current, acute injury is not coded in chapter 13. It should instead be coded to the appropriate injury code from chapter 19.

> Old bucket handle tear of right medial meniscus
>
> **M23.203   Derangement of unspecified medial meniscus due to old tear or injury, right knee**
>
> *Explanation:* Chronic or recurrent conditions should generally be coded with a code from chapter 13.

c. Coding of Pathologic Fractures

7th character A is for use as long as the patient is receiving active treatment for the fracture. Examples of active treatment are: surgical treatment, emergency department encounter, evaluation and continuing treatment by the same or a different physician. While the patient may be seen by a new or different provider over the course of treatment for a pathological fracture, assignment of the 7th character is based on whether the patient is undergoing active treatment and not whether the provider is seeing the patient for the first time.

7th character, D is to be used for encounters after the patient has completed active treatment. The other 7th characters, listed under each subcategory in the Tabular List, are to be used for subsequent encounters for treatment of problems associated with the healing, such as malunions, nonunions, and sequelae.

Care for complications of surgical treatment for fracture repairs during the healing or recovery phase should be coded with the appropriate complication codes.

See Section I.C.19. Coding of traumatic fractures.

> Pathologic fracture of left foot, unknown cause, currently under active treatment by a follow-up provider
>
> **M84.475A   Pathological fracture, left foot, initial encounter for fracture**
>
> *Explanation:* Seventh character A is for use as long as the patient is receiving active treatment for a pathologic fracture. Examples of active treatment are surgical treatment, emergency department encounter, evaluation, and continuing treatment by the same or a different physician.
>
> The seventh character is based on whether the patient is undergoing active treatment and not whether the provider is seeing the patient for the first time.

d. Osteoporosis

Osteoporosis is a systemic condition, meaning that all bones of the musculoskeletal system are affected. Therefore, site is not a component of the codes under category M81, Osteoporosis without current pathological fracture. The site codes under category M80, Osteoporosis with current pathological fracture, identify the site of the fracture, not the osteoporosis.

1) Osteoporosis without pathological fracture

Category M81, Osteoporosis without current pathological fracture, is for use for patients with osteoporosis who do not currently have a pathologic fracture due to the osteoporosis, even if they have had a fracture in the past. For patients with a history of osteoporosis fractures, status code Z87.310, Personal history of (healed) osteoporosis fracture, should follow the code from M81.

> Age-related osteoporosis with healed osteoporotic fracture of the lumbar vertebra
>
> **M81.0   Age-related osteoporosis without current pathological fracture**
>
> **Z87.310   Personal history of (healed) osteoporosis fracture**
>
> *Explanation:* Category M81 is used for patients with osteoporosis who do not currently have a pathologic fracture due to the osteoporosis. To report a previous (healed) fracture, status code Z87.310 Personal history of (healed) osteoporosis fracture, should follow the code from M81.

2) Osteoporosis with current pathological fracture

Category M80, Osteoporosis with current pathological fracture, is for patients who have a current pathologic fracture at the time of an encounter. The codes under M80 identify the site of the fracture. A code from category M80, not a traumatic fracture code, should be used for any patient with known osteoporosis who suffers a fracture, even if the patient had a minor fall or trauma, if that fall or trauma would not usually break a normal, healthy bone.

> Disuse osteoporosis with current fracture of right shoulder sustained lifting a grocery bag, initial encounter
>
> **M80.811A   Other osteoporosis with current pathological fracture, right shoulder, initial encounter for fracture**
>
> *Explanation:* A code from category M80, not a traumatic fracture code, should be used for any patient with known osteoporosis who suffers a fracture, even if the patient had a minor fall or trauma, if that fall or trauma would not usually break a normal, healthy bone.

Muscle/Tendon Table

ICD-10-CM categorizes certain muscles and tendons in the upper and lower extremities by their action (e.g., extension, flexion), their anatomical location (e.g., posterior, anterior), and/or whether they are intrinsic or extrinsic to a certain anatomical area. The Muscle/Tendon Table is provided at the beginning of chapters 13 and 19 as a resource to help users when code selection depends on one or more of these characteristics. The categories and/or subcategories that relate to this table are identified by the icon ✦. Please note that this table is not all-inclusive, and proper code assignment should be based on the provider's documentation.

Body Region	Muscle	Extensor Tendon	Flexor Tendon	Other Tendon
Shoulder				
	Deltoid	Posterior deltoid	Anterior deltoid	
	Rotator cuff			
	Infraspinatus			Infraspinatus
	Subscapularis			Subscapularis
	Supraspinatus			Supraspinatus
	Teres minor			Teres minor
	Teres major	Teres major		
Upper arm				
	Anterior muscles			
	Biceps brachii — long head		Biceps brachii — long head	
	Biceps brachii — short head		Biceps brachii — short head	
	Brachialis		Brachialis	
	Coracobrachialis		Coracobrachialis	
	Posterior muscles			
	Triceps brachii	Triceps brachii		
Forearm				
	Anterior muscles			
	Flexors			
	Deep			
	Flexor digitorum profundus		Flexor digitorum profundus	
	Flexor pollicis longus		Flexor pollicis longus	
	Intermediate			
	Flexor digitorum superficialis		Flexor digitorum superficialis	
	Superficial			
	Flexor carpi radialis		Flexor carpi radialis	
	Flexor carpi ulnaris		Flexor carpi ulnaris	
	Palmaris longus		Palmaris longus	
	Pronators			
	Pronator quadratus			Pronator quadratus
	Pronator teres			Pronator teres
	Posterior muscles			
	Extensors			
	Deep			
	Abductor pollicis longus			Abductor pollicis longus
	Extensor indicis	Extensor indicis		
	Extensor pollicis brevis	Extensor pollicis brevis		
	Extensor pollicis longus	Extensor pollicis longus		
	Superficial			
	Brachioradialis			Brachioradialis
	Extensor carpi radialis brevis	Extensor carpi radialis brevis		
	Extensor carpi radialis longus	Extensor carpi radialis longus		
	Extensor carpi ulnaris	Extensor carpi ulnaris		
	Extensor digiti minimi	Extensor digiti minimi		
	Extensor digitorum	Extensor digitorum		
	Anconeus	Anconeus		
	Supinator			Supinator

Body Region	Muscle	Extensor Tendon	Flexor Tendon	Other Tendon
Hand				
Extrinsic — attach to a site in the forearm as well as a site in the hand with action related to hand movement at the wrist				
	Extensor carpi radialis brevis	Extensor carpi radialis brevis		
	Extensor carpi radialis longus	Extensor carpie radialis longus		
	Extensor carpi ulnaris	Extensor carpi ulnaris		
	Flexor carpi radialis		Flexor carpi radialis	
	Flexor carpi ulnaris		Flexor carpi ulnaris	
	Flexor digitorum superficialis		Flexor digitorum superficialis	
	Palmaris longus		Palmaris longus	
Extrinsic — attach to a site in the forearm as well as a site in the hand with action in the hand related to finger movement				
	Adductor pollicis longus			Adductor pollicis longus
	Extensor digiti minimi	Extensor digiti minimi		
	Extensor digitorum	Extensor digitorum		
	Extensor indicis	Extensor indicis		
	Flexor digitorum profundus		Flexor digitorum profundus	
	Flexor digitorum superficialis		Flexor digitorum superficialis	
Extrinsic — attach to a site in the forearm as well as a site in the hand with action in the hand related to thumb movement				
	Extensor pollicis brevis	Extensor pollicis brevis		
	Extensor pollicis longus	Extensor pollicis longus		
	Flexor pollicis longus		Flexor pollicis longus	
Intrinsic — found within the hand only				
	Adductor pollicis			Adductor pollicis
	Dorsal interossei	Dorsal interossei	Dorsal interossei	
	Lumbricals	Lumbricals	Lumbricals	
	Palmaris brevis			Palmaris brevis
	Palmar interossei	Palmar interossei	Palmar interossei	
	Hypothenar muscles			
	Abductor digiti minimi			Abductor digiti minimi
	Flexor digiti minimi brevis		Flexor digiti minimi brevis	
	Oppenens digiti minimi		Oppenens digiti minimi	
	Thenar muscles			
	Abductor pollicis brevis			Abductor pollicis brevis
	Flexor pollicis brevis		Flexor pollicis brevis	
	Oppenens pollicis		Oppenens pollicis	
Thigh				
	Anterior muscles			
	Iliopsoas		Iliopsoas	
	Pectineus		Pectineus	
	Quadriceps	Quadriceps		
	Rectus femoris	Rectus femoris — Extends knee	Rectus femoris — Flexes hip	
	Vastus intermedius	Vastus intermedius		
	Vastus lateralis	Vastus lateralis		
	Vastus medialis	Vastus medialis		
	Sartorius		Sartorius	
	Medial muscles			
	Adductor brevis			Adductor brevis
	Adductor longus			Adductor longus
	Adductor magnus			Adductor magnus
	Gracilis			Gracilis
	Obturator externus			Obturator externus
	Posterior muscles			
	Hamstring	Hamstring — Extends hip	Hamstring — Flexes knee	
	Biceps femoris	Biceps femoris	Biceps femoris	
	Semimembranosus	Semimembranosus	Semimembranosus	
	Semitendinosus	Semitendinosus	Semitendinosus	

Body Region	Muscle	Extensor Tendon	Flexor Tendon	Other Tendon
Lower leg				
	Anterior muscles			
	Extensor digitorum longus	Extensor digitorum longus		
	Extensor hallucis longus	Extensor hallucis longus		
	Fibularis (peroneus) tertius	Fibularis (peroneus) tertius		
	Tibialis anterior	Tibialis anterior		Tibialis anterior
	Lateral muscles			
	Fibularis (peroneus) brevis		Fibularis (peroneus) brevis	
	Fibularis (peroneus) longus		Fibularis (peroneus) longus	
	Posterior muscles			
	Deep			
	Flexor digitorum longus		Flexor digitorum longus	
	Flexor hallucis longus		Flexor hallucis longus	
	Popliteus		Popliteus	
	Tibialis posterior		Tibialis posterior	
	Superficial			
	Gastrocnemius		Gastrocnemius	
	Plantaris		Plantaris	
	Soleus		Soleus	
				Calcaneal (Achilles)
Ankle/Foot				
Extrinsic — attach to a site in the lower leg as well as a site in the foot with action related to foot movement at the ankle				
	Plantaris		Plantaris	
	Soleus		Soleus	
	Tibialis anterior	Tibialis anterior		
	Tibialis posterior		Tibialis posterior	
Extrinsic — attach to a site in the lower leg as well as a site in the foot with action in the foot related to toe movement				
	Extensor digitorum longus	Extensor digitorum longus		
	Extensor hallucis longus	Extensor hallicus longus		
	Flexor digitorum longus		Flexor digitorum longus	
	Flexor hallucis longus		Flexor hallucis longus	
Intrinsic — found within the ankle/foot only				
	Dorsal muscles			
	Extensor digitorum brevis	Extensor digitorum brevis		
	Extensor hallucis brevis	Extensor hallucis brevis		
	Plantar muscles			
	Abductor digiti minimi		Abductor digiti minimi	
	Abductor hallucis		Abductor hallucis	
	Dorsal interossei	Dorsal interossei	Dorsal interossei	
	Flexor digiti minimi brevis		Flexor digiti minimi brevis	
	Flexor digitorum brevis		Flexor digitorum brevis	
	Flexor hallucis brevis		Flexor hallucis brevis	
	Lumbricals	Lumbricals	Lumbricals	
	Quadratus plantae		Quadratus plantae	
	Plantar interossei	Plantar interossei	Plantar interossei	

Chapter 13. Diseases of the Musculoskeletal System and Connective Tissue (M00-M99)

NOTE Use an external cause code following the code for the musculoskeletal condition, if applicable, to identify the cause of the musculoskeletal condition.

EXCLUDES 2 arthropathic psoriasis (L40.5-)
certain conditions originating in the perinatal period (P04-P96)
certain infectious and parasitic diseases (A00-B99)
compartment syndrome (traumatic) (T79.A-)
complications of pregnancy, childbirth and the puerperium (O00-O9A)
congenital malformations, deformations, and chromosomal abnormalities (Q00-Q99)
endocrine, nutritional and metabolic diseases (E00-E88)
injury, poisoning and certain other consequences of external causes (S00-T88)
neoplasms (C00-D49)
symptoms, signs and abnormal clinical and laboratory findings, not elsewhere classified (R00-R94)

This chapter contains the following blocks:

M00-M02	Infectious arthropathies
M05-M14	Inflammatory polyarthropathies
M15-M19	Osteoarthritis
M20-M25	Other joint disorders
M26-M27	Dentofacial anomalies [including malocclusion] and other disorders of jaw
M30-M36	Systemic connective tissue disorders
M40-M43	Deforming dorsopathies
M45-M49	Spondylopathies
M50-M54	Other dorsopathies
M60-M63	Disorders of muscles
M65-M67	Disorders of synovium and tendon
M70-M79	Other soft tissue disorders
M80-M85	Disorders of bone density and structure
M86-M90	Other osteopathies
M91-M94	Chondropathies
M95	Other disorders of the musculoskeletal system and connective tissue
M96	Intraoperative and postprocedural complications and disorders of musculoskeletal system, not elsewhere classified
M99	Biomechanical lesions, not elsewhere classified

ARTHROPATHIES (M00-M25)

INCLUDES disorders affecting predominantly peripheral (limb) joints

Infectious arthropathies (M00-M02)

NOTE This block comprises arthropathies due to microbiological agents. Distinction is made between the following types of etiological relationship:

a) direct infection of joint, where organisms invade synovial tissue and microbial antigen is present in the joint;

b) indirect infection, which may be of two types: a reactive arthropathy, where microbial infection of the body is established but neither organisms nor antigens can be identified in the joint, and a postinfective arthropathy, where microbial antigen is present but recovery of an organism is inconstant and evidence of local multiplication is lacking.

✓4ᵗʰ **M00 Pyogenic arthritis**

✓5ᵗʰ **M00.0 Staphylococcal arthritis and polyarthritis**
Use additional code (B95.61-B95.8) to identify bacterial agent
EXCLUDES 2 infection and inflammatory reaction due to internal joint prosthesis (T84.5-)

M00.00 Staphylococcal arthritis, unspecified joint CC
CC Excl: A17.9, A18.02, A18.09, A18.82, A18.84, A18.89, A39.83-A39.84, A54.40, A54.42-A54.43, A54.82, A54.84, A54.89-A54.9, B06.82, M00.00-M02.30, M02.319, M02.329, M02.339, M02.349, M02.359, M02.369, M02.379-M02.9, M05.40-M05.59, M05.70-M06.09, M06.20-M06.39, M06.80-M07.69, M11.00-M11.9, M12.10-M15.0, M15.3-M15.9, M16.2-M16.9, M17.2-M17.9, M18.2-M18.9, M19.111-M19.93, M24.10-M24.176, M25.00, M25.08-M25.18, M25.40-M25.676, M25.80-M25.9, M35.2, M36.1-M36.4, R26.2, R29.4

✓6ᵗʰ **M00.01 Staphylococcal arthritis, shoulder**
M00.011 Staphylococcal arthritis, right shoulder CC
M00.012 Staphylococcal arthritis, left shoulder CC
M00.019 Staphylococcal arthritis, unspecified shoulder CC
CC Excl: A17.9, A18.02, A18.09, A18.82, A18.84, A18.89, A39.83-A39.84, A54.40, A54.42-A54.43, A54.82, A54.84, A54.89-A54.9, B06.82, M00.00-M00.019, M00.08-M00.119, M00.18-M00.219, M00.28-M00.819, M00.88-M01.X19, M01.X8-M02.119, M02.18-M02.30, M02.319, M02.38-M02.819, M02.88-M02.9, M05.40-M05.59, M05.70-M06.09, M06.20-M06.39, M06.80-M07.619, M07.68-M07.69, M11.00-M11.019, M11.08-M11.119, M11.18-M11.219, M11.28-M11.819, M11.88-M11.9, M12.10-M12.119, M12.18-M12.219, M12.28-M12.319, M12.38-M12.419, M12.48-M12.519, M12.58-M12.819, M12.88-M13.119, M13.80-M13.819, M13.88-M15.0, M15.3-M15.9, M19.011-M19.019, M19.111-M19.119, M19.211-M19.219, M19.90-M19.93, M24.10-M24.119, M25.00-M25.019, M25.08-M25.119, M25.18, M25.40-M25.419, M25.48-M25.519, M25.60-M25.619, M25.80-M25.819, M25.9, M35.2, M36.1-M36.4, R26.2

✓6ᵗʰ **M00.02 Staphylococcal arthritis, elbow**
M00.021 Staphylococcal arthritis, right elbow CC
M00.022 Staphylococcal arthritis, left elbow CC
M00.029 Staphylococcal arthritis, unspecified elbow CC
CC Excl: A17.9, A18.02, A18.09, A18.82, A18.84, A18.89, A39.83-A39.84, A54.40, A54.42-A54.43, A54.82, A54.84, A54.89-A54.9, B06.82, M00.00, M00.021-M00.029, M00.08-M00.10, M00.121-M00.129, M00.18-M00.20, M00.221-M00.229, M00.28-M00.80, M00.821-M00.829, M00.88-M01.X0, M01.X21-M01.X29, M01.X8, M01.X9, M02.00-M02.1, M02.121-M02.129, M02.18-M02.30, M02.329, M02.38-M02.80, M02.821-M02.829, M02.88-M02.9, M05.40-M05.59, M05.70-M06.09, M06.20-M06.39, M06.80-M07.60, M07.621-M07.629, M07.68-M07.69, M11.00, M11.021-M11.029, M11.08-M11.10, M11.121-M11.129, M11.18-M11.20, M11.221-M11.229, M11.28-M11.80, M11.821-M11.829, M11.88-M11.9, M12.10, M12.121-M12.129, M12.18-M12.20, M12.221-M12.229, M12.28-M12.30, M12.321-M12.329, M12.38-M12.40, M12.421-M12.429, M12.48-M12.50, M12.521-M12.529, M12.58-M12.80, M12.821-M12.829, M12.88-M13.10, M13.121-M13.129, M13.80, M13.821-M13.829, M13.88-M15.0, M15.3-M15.9, M19.021-M19.029, M19.121-M19.129, M19.221-M19.229, M19.90-M19.93, M24.10, M24.121-M24.129, M25.00, M25.021-M25.029, M25.08-M25.10, M25.121-M25.129, M25.18, M25.40, M25.421-M25.429, M25.48-M25.50, M25.521-M25.529, M25.60, M25.621-M25.629, M25.80, M25.821-M25.829, M25.9, M35.2, M36.1-M36.4, R26.2

Chapter 13. Diseases of the Musculoskeletal System and Connective Tissue

✓6ᵗʰ **M00.03 Staphylococcal arthritis, wrist**
Staphylococcal arthritis of carpal bones

    M00.031 Staphylococcal arthritis, right wrist `CC`

    M00.032 Staphylococcal arthritis, left wrist `CC`

    M00.039 Staphylococcal arthritis, unspecified wrist `CC`

        CC Excl: A17.9, A18.02, A18.09, A18.82, A18.84, A18.89, A39.83-A39.84, A54.40, A54.42-A54.43, A54.82, A54.84, A54.89-A54.9, B06.82, M00.00, M00.31-M00.039, M00.08-M00.10, M00.131-M00.139, M00.18-M00.20, M00.231-M00.239, M00.28-M00.80, M00.831-M00.839, M00.88-M01.X0, M01.X31-M01.X39, M01.X8-M02.10, M02.131-M02.139, M02.18-M02.30, M02.339, M02.38-M02.80, M02.831-M02.839, M02.88-M02.9, M05.40-M05.59, M05.70-M06.09, M06.20-M06.39, M06.80-M07.60, M07.631-M07.639, M07.68-M07.69, M11.00, M11.031-M11.039, M11.08-M11.10, M11.131-M11.139, M11.18-M11.20, M11.231-M11.239, M11.28-M11.80, M11.831-M11.839, M11.88-M11.9, M12.10, M12.131-M12.139, M12.18-M12.20, M12.231-M12.239, M12.28-M12.30, M12.331-M12.339, M12.38-M12.40, M12.431-M12.439, M12.48-M12.50, M12.531-M12.539, M12.58-M12.80, M12.831-M12.839, M12.88-M13.10, M13.131-M13.139, M13.80, M13.831-M13.839, M13.88-M15.0, M15.3-M15.9, M19.031-M19.039, M19.131-M19.139, M19.231-M19.239, M19.90-M19.93, M24.10, M24.131-M24.139, M25.00, M25.031-M25.039, M25.08-M25.10, M25.131-M25.139, M25.18, M25.40, M25.431-M25.439, M25.48-M25.50, M25.531-M25.539, M25.60, M25.631-M25.639, M25.80, M25.831-M25.839, M25.9, M35.2, M36.1-M36.4, R26.2

✓6ᵗʰ **M00.04 Staphylococcal arthritis, hand**
Staphylococcal arthritis of metacarpus and phalanges

    M00.041 Staphylococcal arthritis, right hand `CC`

    M00.042 Staphylococcal arthritis, left hand `CC`

    M00.049 Staphylococcal arthritis, unspecified hand `CC`

        CC Excl: A17.9, A18.02, A18.09, A18.82, A18.84, A18.89, A39.83-A39.84, A54.40, A54.42-A54.43, A54.82, A54.84, A54.89-A54.9, B06.82, M00.00, M.041-M00.049, M00.08-M00.10, M00.141-M00.149, M00.18-M00.20, M00.241-M00.249, M00.28-M00.80, M00.841-M00.849, M00.88-M01.X0, M01.X41-M01.X49, M01.X8-M02.10, M02.141-M02.149, M02.18-M02.30, M02.349, M02.38-M02.80, M02.841-M02.849, M02.88-M02.9, M05.40-M05.59, M05.70-M06.09, M06.20-M06.39, M06.80-M07.60, M07.641-M07.649, M07.68-M07.69, M11.00, M11.041-M11.049, M11.08-M11.10, M11.141-M11.149, M11.18-M11.20, M11.241-M11.249, M11.28-M11.80, M11.841-M11.849, M11.88-M11.9, M12.10, M12.141-M12.149, M12.18-M12.20, M12.241-M12.249, M12.28-M12.30, M12.341-M12.349, M12.38-M12.40, M12.441-M12.449, M12.48-M12.50, M12.541-M12.549, M12.58-M12.80, M12.841-M12.849, M12.88-M13.10, M13.141-M13.149, M13.80, M13.841-M13.849, M13.88-M15.9, M18.0-M18.9, M19.041-M19.049, M19.141-M19.149, M19.241-M19.249, M19.90-M19.93, M24.10, M24.141-M24.149, M25.00, M25.041-M25.049, M25.08-M25.10, M25.141-M25.149, M25.18, M25.40, M25.441-M25.449, M25.48-M25.50, M25.60, M25.641-M25.649, M25.80, M25.841-M25.849, M25.9, M35.2, M36.1-M36.4, R26.2

✓6ᵗʰ **M00.05 Staphylococcal arthritis, hip**

    M00.051 Staphylococcal arthritis, right hip `CC`

    M00.052 Staphylococcal arthritis, left hip `CC`

    M00.059 Staphylococcal arthritis, unspecified hip `CC`

        CC Excl: A17.9, A18.02, A18.09, A18.82, A18.84, A18.89, A39.83-A39.84, A54.40, A54.42-A54.43, A54.82, A54.84, A54.89-A54.9, B06.82, M00.00, M00.051-M00.059, M00.08-M00.10, M00.151-M00.159, M00.18-M00.20, M00.251-M00.259, M00.28-M00.80, M00.851-M00.859, M00.88-M01.X0, M01.X51-M01.X59, M01.X8-M02.10, M02.151-M02.159, M02.18-M02.30, M02.359, M02.38-M02.80, M02.851-M02.859, M02.88-M02.9, M05.40-M05.59, M05.70-M06.09, M06.20-M06.39, M06.80-M07.60, M07.651-M07.659, M07.68-M07.69, M11.00, M11.051-M11.059, M11.08-M11.10, M11.151-M11.159, M11.18-M11.20, M11.251-M11.259, M11.28-M11.80, M11.851-M11.859, M11.88-M11.9, M12.10, M12.151-M12.159, M12.18-M12.20, M12.251-M12.259, M12.28-M12.30, M12.351-M12.359, M12.38-M12.40, M12.451-M12.459, M12.48-M12.50, M12.551-M12.559, M12.58-M12.80, M12.851-M12.859, M12.88-M13.10, M13.151-M13.159, M13.80, M13.851-M13.859, M13.88-M15.0, M15.3-M16.9, M19.90-M19.93, M24.10, M24.151-M24.159, M25.00, M25.051-M25.059, M25.08-M25.10, M25.151-M25.159, M25.18, M25.40, M25.451-M25.459, M25.48-M25.50, M25.551-M25.559, M25.60, M25.651-M25.659, M25.80, M25.851-M25.859, M25.9, M35.2, M36.1-M36.4, R26.2, R29.4

✓6ᵗʰ **M00.06 Staphylococcal arthritis, knee**

    M00.061 Staphylococcal arthritis, right knee `CC`

    M00.062 Staphylococcal arthritis, left knee `CC`

    M00.069 Staphylococcal arthritis, unspecified knee `CC`

        CC Excl: A17.9, A18.02, A18.09, A18.82, A18.84, A18.89, A39.83-A39.84, A54.40, A54.42-A54.43, A54.82, A54.84, A54.89-A54.9, B06.82, M00.00, M00.61-M00.069, M00.08-M00.10, M00.161-M00.169, M00.18-M00.20, M00.261-M00.269, M00.28-M00.80, M00.861-M00.869, M00.88-M01.X0, M01.X61-M01.X69, M01.X8-M02.10, M02.161-M02.169, M02.18-M02.30, M02.369, M02.38-M02.80, M02.861-M02.869, M02.88-M02.9, M05.40-M05.59, M05.70-M06.09, M06.20-M06.39, M06.80-M07.60, M07.661-M07.669, M07.68-M07.69, M11.00, M11.061-M11.069, M11.08-M11.10, M11.161-M11.169, M11.18-M11.20, M11.261-M11.269, M11.28-M11.80, M11.861-M11.869, M11.88-M11.9, M12.10, M12.161-M12.169, M12.18-M12.20, M12.261-M12.269, M12.28-M12.30, M12.361-M12.369, M12.38-M12.40, M12.461-M12.469, M12.48-M12.50, M12.561-M12.569, M12.58-M12.80, M12.861-M12.869, M12.88-M13.10, M13.161-M13.169, M13.80, M13.861-M13.869, M13.88-M15.0, M15.3-M15.9, M17.0-M17.9, M19.90-M19.93, M24.10, M25.00, M25.061-M25.069, M25.08-M25.10, M25.161-M25.169, M25.18, M25.40, M25.461-M25.469, M25.48-M25.50, M25.561-M25.569, M25.60, M25.661-M25.669, M25.80, M25.861-M25.869, M25.9, M35.2, M36.1-M36.4, R26.2

Ⓝ Newborn: 0   Ⓟ Pediatric: 0-17   Ⓜ Maternity: 12-55   Ⓐ Adult: 15-124   `MCC` Major CC Condition   `PDxMCC` PDx acts as own MCC   `CC` CC Condition   `PDxCC` PDx acts as own CC

702   ICD-10-CM 2016

√6ᵗʰ M00.07 Staphylococcal arthritis, ankle and foot
Staphylococcal arthritis, tarsus, metatarsus and phalanges

    M00.071 Staphylococcal arthritis, right ankle and foot `CC`

    M00.072 Staphylococcal arthritis, left ankle and foot `CC`

    M00.079 Staphylococcal arthritis, unspecified ankle and foot `CC`
      CC Excl: A17.9, A18.02, A18.09, A18.82, A18.84, A18.89, A39.83-A39.84, A54.40, A54.42-A54.43, A54.82, A54.84, A54.89-A54.9, B06.82, M00.00, M00.071-M00.10, M00.171-M00.20, M00.271-M00.80, M00.871-M01.X0, M01.X71-M02.10, M02.171-M02.30, M02.379-M02.80, M02.871-M02.9, M05.40-M05.59, M05.70-M06.09, M06.20-M06.39, M06.80-M07.60, M07.671-M07.69, M11.00, M11.071-M11.10, M11.171-M11.20, M11.271-M11.80, M11.871-M11.9, M12.10, M12.171-M12.20, M12.271-M12.30, M12.371-M12.40, M12.471-M12.50, M12.571-M12.80, M12.871-M13.10, M13.171-M13.80, M13.871-M15.0, M15.3-M15.9, M19.071-M19.079, M19.171-M19.179, M19.271-M19.93, M24.10, M24.171-M24.176, M25.00, M25.071-M25.10, M25.171-M25.18, M25.40, M25.471-M25.50, M25.571-M25.60, M25.671-M25.676, M25.80, M25.871-M25.9, M35.2, M36.1-M36.4, R26.2

  M00.08 Staphylococcal arthritis, vertebrae `CC`
    CC Excl: A17.9, A18.02, A18.09, A18.82, A18.84, A18.89, A39.83-A39.84, A54.40, A54.42-A54.43, A54.82, A54.84, A54.89-A54.9, B06.82, M00.00-M02.30, M02.319, M02.329, M02.339, M02.349, M02.359, M02.369, M02.379-M02.9, M05.40-M05.59, M05.70-M06.09, M06.20-M06.39, M06.80-M07.69, M11.00-M11.9, M12.10-M15.0, M15.3-M15.9, M16.2-M16.9, M17.2-M17.9, M18.2-M18.9, M19.111-M19.93, M24.10-M24.176, M25.00, M25.08-M25.18, M25.40-M25.676, M25.80-M25.9, M35.2, M36.1-M36.4, R26.2, R29.4

  M00.09 Staphylococcal polyarthritis `CC`
    CC Excl: See code: M00.08

√5ᵗʰ M00.1 Pneumococcal arthritis and polyarthritis

  M00.10 Pneumococcal arthritis, unspecified joint `CC`
    CC Excl: See code: M00.08

  √6ᵗʰ M00.11 Pneumococcal arthritis, shoulder

    M00.111 Pneumococcal arthritis, right shoulder `CC`
      CC Excl: A17.9, A18.02, A18.09, A18.82, A18.84, A18.89, A39.83-A39.84, A54.40, A54.42-A54.43, A54.82, A54.84, A54.89-A54.9, B06.82, M00.00-M00.019, M00.08-M00.119, M00.18-M00.219, M00.28-M00.819, M00.88-M01.X19, M01.X8-M02.119, M02.18-M02.211

    M00.112 Pneumococcal arthritis, left shoulder `CC`
      CC Excl: See code: M00.111

    M00.119 Pneumococcal arthritis, unspecified shoulder `CC`
      CC Excl: See code: M00.111

√6ᵗʰ M00.12 Pneumococcal arthritis, elbow

  M00.121 Pneumococcal arthritis, right elbow `CC`
    CC Excl: A17.9, A18.02, A18.09, A18.82, A18.84, A18.89, A39.83-A39.84, A54.40, A54.42-A54.43, A54.82, A54.84, A54.89-A54.9, B06.82, M00.00, M00.021-M00.029, M00.08-M00.10, M00.121-M00.129, M00.18-M00.20, M00.221-M00.229, M00.28-M00.80, M00.821-M00.829, M00.88-M01.X0, M01.X21-M01.X29, M01.X8-M02.10, M02.121-M02.129, M02.18-M02.30, M02.329, M02.38-M02.80, M02.821-M02.829, M02.88-M02.9, M05.40-M05.59, M05.70-M06.09, M06.20-M06.39, M06.80-M07.60, M07.621-M07.629, M07.68-M07.69, M11.00, M11.021-M11.029, M11.08-M11.10, M11.121-M11.129, M11.18-M11.20, M11.221-M11.229, M11.28-M11.80, M11.821-M11.829, M11.88-M11.9, M12.10, M12.121-M12.129, M12.18-M12.20, M12.221-M12.229, M12.28-M12.30, M12.321-M12.329, M12.38-M12.40, M12.421-M12.429, M12.48-M12.50, M12.521-M12.529, M12.58-M12.80, M12.821-M12.829, M12.88-M13.10, M13.121-M13.129, M13.80, M13.821-M13.829, M13.88-M15.0, M15.3-M15.9, M19.021-M19.029, M19.121-M19.129, M19.221-M19.229, M19.90-M19.93, M24.10, M24.121-M24.129, M25.00, M25.021-M25.029, M25.08-M25.10, M25.121-M25.129, M25.18, M25.40, M25.421-M25.429, M25.48-M25.50, M25.521-M25.529, M25.60, M25.621-M25.629, M25.80, M25.821-M25.829, M25.9, M35.2, M36.1-M36.4, R26.2

  M00.122 Pneumococcal arthritis, left elbow `CC`
    CC Excl: See code: M00.121

  M00.129 Pneumococcal arthritis, unspecified elbow `CC`
    CC Excl: See code: M00.121

√6ᵗʰ M00.13 Pneumococcal arthritis, wrist
Pneumococcal arthritis of carpal bones

  M00.131 Pneumococcal arthritis, right wrist `CC`
    CC Excl: A17.9, A18.02, A18.09, A18.82, A18.84, A18.89, A39.83-A39.84, A54.40, A54.42-A54.43, A54.82, A54.84, A54.89-A54.9, B06.82, M00.00, M00.031-M00.039, M00.08-M00.10, M00.131-M00.139, M00.18-M00.20, M00.231-M00.239, M00.28-M00.80, M00.831-M00.839, M00.88-M01.X0, M01.X31-M01.X39, M01.X8-M02.10, M02.131-M02.139, M02.18-M02.30, M02.339, M02.38-M02.80, M02.831-M02.839, M02.88-M02.9, M05.40-M05.59, M05.70-M06.09, M06.20-M06.39, M06.80-M07.60, M07.631-M07.639, M07.68-M07.69, M11.00, M11.031-M11.039, M11.08-M11.10, M11.131-M11.139, M11.18-M11.20, M11.231-M11.239, M11.28-M11.80, M11.831-M11.839, M11.88-M11.9, M12.10, M12.131-M12.139, M12.18-M12.20, M12.231-M12.239, M12.28-M12.30, M12.331-M12.339, M12.38-M12.40, M12.431-M12.439, M12.48-M12.50, M12.531-M12.539, M12.58-M12.80, M12.831-M12.839, M12.88-M13.10, M13.131-M13.139, M13.80, M13.831-M13.839, M13.88-M15.0, M15.3-M15.9, M19.031-M19.039, M19.131-M19.139, M19.231-M19.239, M19.90-M19.93, M24.10, M24.131-M24.139, M25.00, M25.031-M25.039, M25.08-M25.10, M25.131-M25.139, M25.18, M25.40, M25.431-M25.439, M25.48-M25.50, M25.531-M25.539, M25.60, M25.631-M25.639, M25.80, M25.831-M25.839, M25.9, M35.2, M36.1-M36.4, R26.2

  M00.132 Pneumococcal arthritis, left wrist `CC`
    CC Excl: See code: M00.131

  M00.139 Pneumococcal arthritis, unspecified wrist `CC`
    CC Excl: See code: M00.131

☑ Additional Character Required   √x7ᵗʰ Placeholder Alert   Unacceptable PDx   Manifestation   Hospital Acquired Condition   **EXCLUDES 1** Not Coded Here   **EXCLUDES 2** Not Included Here

ICD-10-CM 2016   **703**

✓6th **M00.14 Pneumococcal arthritis, hand**
Pneumococcal arthritis of metacarpus and phalanges

M00.141 Pneumococcal arthritis, right hand CC
CC Excl: A17.9, A18.02, A18.09, A18.82,
A18.84, A18.89, A39.83-A39.84, A54.40,
A54.42-A54.43, A54.82, A54.84, A54.89-
A54.9, B06.82, M00.00, M00.041-M00.049,
M00.08-M00.10, M00.141-M00.149, M00.18-
M00.20, M00.241-M00.249, M00.28-M00.80,
M00.841-M00.849, M00.88-M01.X0,
M01.X41-M01.X49, M01.X8-M02.10,
M02.141-M02.149, M02.18-M02.30,
M02.349, M02.38-M02.80, M02.841-
M02.849, M02.88-M02.9, M05.40-M05.59,
M05.70-M06.09, M06.20-M06.39, M06.80-
M07.60, M07.641-M07.649, M07.68-M07.69,
M11.00, M11.041-M11.049, M11.08-M11.10,
M11.141-M11.149, M11.18-M11.20,
M11.241-M11.249, M11.28-M11.80,
M11.841-M11.849, M11.88-M11.9, M12.10,
M12.141-M12.149, M12.18-M12.20,
M12.241-M12.249, M12.28-M12.30,
M12.341-M12.349, M12.38-M12.40,
M12.441-M12.449, M12.48-M12.50,
M12.541-M12.549, M12.58-M12.80,
M12.841-M12.849, M12.88-M13.10,
M13.141-M13.149, M13.80, M13.841-
M13.849, M13.88-M15.9, M18.0-M18.9,
M19.041-M19.049, M19.141-M19.149,
M19.241-M19.249, M19.90-M19.93, M24.10,
M24.141-M24.149, M25.00, M25.041-
M25.049, M25.08-M25.10, M25.141-
M25.149, M25.18, M25.40, M25.441-
M25.449, M25.48-M25.50, M25.60, M25.641-
M25.649, M25.80, M25.841-M25.849, M25.9,
M35.2, M36.1-M36.4, R26.2

M00.142 Pneumococcal arthritis, left hand CC
CC Excl: See code: M00.141

M00.149 Pneumococcal arthritis, unspecified hand CC
CC Excl: See code: M00.141

✓6th **M00.15 Pneumococcal arthritis, hip**

M00.151 Pneumococcal arthritis, right hip CC
CC Excl: A17.9, A18.02, A18.09, A18.82,
A18.84, A18.89, A39.83-A39.84, A54.40,
A54.42-A54.43, A54.82, A54.84, A54.89-
A54.9, B06.82, M00.00, M00.051-M00.059,
M00.08-M00.10, M00.151-M00.159, M00.18-
M00.20, M00.251-M00.259, M00.28-M00.80,
M00.851-M00.859, M00.88-M01.X0,
M01.X51-M01.X59, M01.X8-M02.10,
M02.151-M02.159, M02.18-M02.30,
M02.359, M02.38-M02.80, M02.851-
M02.859, M02.88-M02.9, M05.40-M05.59,
M05.70-M06.09, M06.20-M06.39, M06.80-
M07.60, M07.651-M07.659, M07.68-M07.69,
M11.00, M11.051-M11.059, M11.08-M11.10,
M11.151-M11.159, M11.18-M11.20,
M11.251-M11.259, M11.28-M11.80,
M11.851-M11.859, M11.88-M11.9, M12.10,
M12.151-M12.159, M12.18-M12.20,
M12.251-M12.259, M12.28-M12.30,
M12.351-M12.359, M12.38-M12.40,
M12.451-M12.459, M12.48-M12.50,
M12.551-M12.559, M12.58-M12.80,
M12.851-M12.859, M12.88-M13.10,
M13.151-M13.159, M13.80, M13.851-
M13.859, M13.88-M15.0, M15.3-M16.9,
M19.90-M19.93, M24.10, M24.151-M24.159,
M25.00, M25.051-M25.059, M25.08-M25.10,
M25.151-M25.159, M25.18, M25.40,
M25.451-M25.459, M25.48-M25.50,
M25.551-M25.559, M25.60, M25.651-
M25.659, M25.80, M25.851-M25.859, M25.9,
M35.2, M36.1-M36.4, R26.2, R29.4

M00.152 Pneumococcal arthritis, left hip CC
CC Excl: See code: M00.151

M00.159 Pneumococcal arthritis, unspecified hip CC
CC Excl: See code: M00.151

✓6th **M00.16 Pneumococcal arthritis, knee**

M00.161 Pneumococcal arthritis, right knee CC
CC Excl: A17.9, A18.02, A18.09, A18.82,
A18.84, A18.89, A39.83-A39.84, A54.40,
A54.42-A54.43, A54.82, A54.84, A54.89-
A54.9, B06.82, M00.00, M00.061-M00.069,
M00.08-M00.10, M00.161-M00.169, M00.18-
M00.20, M00.261-M00.269, M00.28-M00.80,
M00.861-M00.869, M00.88-M01.X0,
M01.X61-M01.X69, M01.X8-M02.10, M02.161-
M02.169, M02.18-M02.30, M02.369, M02.38-
M02.80, M02.861-M02.869, M02.88-M02.9,
M05.40-M05.59, M05.70-M06.09, M06.20-
M06.39, M06.80-M07.60, M07.661-M07.669,
M07.68-M07.69, M11.00, M11.061-M11.069,
M11.08-M11.10, M11.161-M11.169, M11.18-
M11.20, M11.261-M11.269, M11.28-M11.80,
M11.861-M11.869, M11.88-M11.9, M12.10,
M12.161-M12.169, M12.18-M12.20, M12.261-
M12.269, M12.28-M12.30, M12.361-M12.369,
M12.38-M12.40, M12.461-M12.469, M12.48-
M12.50, M12.561-M12.569, M12.58-M12.80,
M12.861-M12.869, M12.88-M13.10, M13.161-
M13.169, M13.80, M13.861-M13.869, M13.88-
M15.0, M15.3-M15.9, M17.0-M17.9, M19.90-
M19.93, M24.10, M25.00, M25.061-M25.069,
M25.08-M25.10, M25.161-M25.169, M25.18,
M25.40, M25.461-M25.469, M25.48-M25.50,
M25.561-M25.569, M25.60, M25.661-
M25.669, M25.80, M25.861-M25.869, M25.9,
M35.2, M36.1-M36.4, R26.2

M00.162 Pneumococcal arthritis, left knee CC
CC Excl: See code: M00.161

M00.169 Pneumococcal arthritis, unspecified knee CC
CC Excl: See code: M00.161

✓6th **M00.17 Pneumococcal arthritis, ankle and foot**
Pneumococcal arthritis, tarsus, metatarsus and phalanges

M00.171 Pneumococcal arthritis, right ankle and foot CC
CC Excl: A17.9, A18.02, A18.09, A18.82,
A18.84, A18.89, A39.83-A39.84, A54.40,
A54.42-A54.43, A54.82, A54.84, A54.89-
A54.9, B06.82, M00.00, M00.071-M00.10,
M00.171-M00.20, M00.271-M00.80,
M00.871-M01.X0, M01.X71-M02.10,
M02.171-M02.30, M02.379-M02.80,
M02.871-M02.9, M05.40-M05.59, M05.70-
M06.09, M06.20-M06.39, M06.80-M07.60,
M07.671-M07.69, M11.00, M11.071-M11.10,
M11.171-M11.20, M11.271-M11.80, M11.871-
M11.9, M12.10, M12.171-M12.20, M12.271-
M12.30, M12.371-M12.40, M12.471-M12.50,
M12.571-M12.80, M12.871-M13.10, M13.171-
M13.80, M13.871-M15.0, M15.3-M15.9,
M19.071-M19.079, M19.171-M19.179,
M19.271-M19.93, M24.10, M24.171-M24.176,
M25.00, M25.071-M25.10, M25.171-M25.18,
M25.40, M25.471-M25.50, M25.571-M25.60,
M25.671-M25.676, M25.80, M25.871-M25.9,
M35.2, M36.1-M36.4, R26.2

M00.172 Pneumococcal arthritis, left ankle and foot CC
CC Excl: See code: M00.171

M00.179 Pneumococcal arthritis, unspecified ankle and foot CC
CC Excl: See code: M00.171

M00.18 Pneumococcal arthritis, vertebrae CC
CC Excl: A17.9, A18.02, A18.09, A18.82, A18.84, A18.89,
A39.83-A39.84, A54.40, A54.42-A54.43, A54.82, A54.84,
A54.89-A54.9, B06.82, M00.00-M02.30, M02.319,
M02.329, M02.339, M02.349, M02.359, M02.369,
M02.379-M02.9, M05.40-M05.59, M05.70-M06.09,
M06.20-M06.39, M06.80-M07.69, M11.00-M11.9,
M12.10-M15.0, M15.3-M15.9, M16.2-M16.9, M17.2-
M17.9, M18.2-M18.9, M19.111-M19.93, M24.10-
M24.176, M25.00, M25.08-M25.18, M25.40-M25.676,
M25.80-M25.9, M35.2, M36.1-M36.4, R26.2, R29.4

M00.19 Pneumococcal polyarthritis CC
CC Excl: See code: M00.18

✓5th **M00.2 Other streptococcal arthritis and polyarthritis**
Use additional code (B95.0-B95.2, B95.4-B95.5) to identify
bacterial agent

M00.20 Other streptococcal arthritis, unspecified joint CC
CC Excl: See code: M00.18

✓6th **M00.21 Other streptococcal arthritis, shoulder**

    M00.211 Other streptococcal arthritis, right shoulder [CC]
        CC Excl: A17.9, A18.02, A18.09, A18.82, A18.84, A18.89, A39.83-A39.84, A54.40, A54.42-A54.43, A54.82, A54.84, A54.89-A54.9, B06.82, M00.00-M00.019, M00.08-M00.119, M00.18-M00.219, M00.28-M00.819, M00.88-M01.X19, M01.X8-M02.119, M02.18-M02.211

    M00.212 Other streptococcal arthritis, left shoulder [CC]
        CC Excl: See code: M00.211

    M00.219 Other streptococcal arthritis, unspecified shoulder [CC]
        CC Excl: See code: M00.211

✓6th **M00.22 Other streptococcal arthritis, elbow**

    M00.221 Other streptococcal arthritis, right elbow [CC]
        CC Excl: A17.9, A18.02, A18.09, A18.82, A18.84, A18.89, A39.83-A39.84, A54.40, A54.42-A54.43, A54.82, A54.84, A54.89-A54.9, B06.82, M00.00, M00.021-M00.029, M00.08-M00.10, M00.121-M00.129, M00.18-M00.20, M00.221-M00.229, M00.28-M00.80, M00.821-M00.829, M00.88-M01.X0, M01.X21-M01.X29, M01.X8-M02.10, M02.121-M02.129, M02.18-M02.30, M02.329, M02.38-M02.80, M02.821-M02.829, M02.88-M02.9, M05.40-M05.59, M05.70-M06.09, M06.20-M06.39, M06.80-M07.60, M07.621-M07.629, M07.68-M07.69, M11.00, M11.021-M11.029, M11.08-M11.10, M11.121-M11.129, M11.18-M11.20, M11.221-M11.229, M11.28-M11.80, M11.821-M11.829, M11.88-M11.9, M12.10, M12.121-M12.129, M12.18-M12.20, M12.221-M12.229, M12.28-M12.30, M12.321-M12.329, M12.38-M12.40, M12.421-M12.429, M12.48-M12.50, M12.521-M12.529, M12.58-M12.80, M12.821-M12.829, M12.88-M13.10, M13.121-M13.129, M13.80, M13.821-M13.829, M13.88-M15.0, M15.3-M15.9, M19.021-M19.029, M19.121-M19.129, M19.221-M19.229, M19.90-M19.93, M24.10, M24.121-M24.129, M25.00, M25.021-M25.029, M25.08-M25.10, M25.121-M25.129, M25.18, M25.40, M25.421-M25.429, M25.48-M25.50, M25.521-M25.529, M25.60, M25.621-M25.629, M25.80, M25.821-M25.829, M25.9, M35.2, M36.1-M36.4, R26.2

    M00.222 Other streptococcal arthritis, left elbow [CC]
        CC Excl: See code: M00.221

    M00.229 Other streptococcal arthritis, unspecified elbow [CC]
        CC Excl: See code: M00.221

✓6th **M00.23 Other streptococcal arthritis, wrist**
    Other streptococcal arthritis of carpal bones

    M00.231 Other streptococcal arthritis, right wrist [CC]
        CC Excl: A17.9, A18.02, A18.09, A18.82, A18.84, A18.89, A39.83-A39.84, A54.40, A54.42-A54.43, A54.82, A54.84, A54.89-A54.9, B06.82, M00.00, M00.031-M00.039, M00.08-M00.10, M00.131-M00.139, M00.18-M00.20, M00.231-M00.239, M00.28-M00.80, M00.831-M00.839, M00.88-M01.X0, M01.X31-M01.X39, M01.X8-M02.10, M02.131-M02.139, M02.18-M02.30, M02.339, M02.38-M02.80, M02.831-M02.839, M02.88-M02.9, M05.40-M05.59, M05.70-M06.09, M06.20-M06.39, M06.80-M07.60, M07.631-M07.639, M07.68-M07.69, M11.00, M11.031-M11.039, M11.08-M11.10, M11.131-M11.139, M11.18-M11.20, M11.231-M11.239, M11.28-M11.80, M11.831-M11.839, M11.88-M11.9, M12.10, M12.131-M12.139, M12.18-M12.20, M12.231-M12.239, M12.28-M12.30, M12.331-M12.339, M12.38-M12.40, M12.431-M12.439, M12.48-M12.50, M12.531-M12.539, M12.58-M12.80, M12.831-M12.839, M12.88-M13.10, M13.131-M13.139, M13.80, M13.831-M13.839, M13.88-M15.0, M15.3-M15.9, M19.031-M19.039, M19.131-M19.139, M19.231-M19.239, M19.90-M19.93, M24.10, M24.131-M24.139, M25.00, M25.031-M25.039, M25.08-M25.10, M25.131-M25.139, M25.18, M25.40, M25.431-M25.439, M25.48-M25.50, M25.531-M25.539, M25.60, M25.631-M25.639, M25.80, M25.831-M25.839, M25.9, M35.2, M36.1-M36.4, R26.2

    M00.232 Other streptococcal arthritis, left wrist [CC]
        CC Excl: See code: M00.231

    M00.239 Other streptococcal arthritis, unspecified wrist [CC]
        CC Excl: See code: M00.231

✓6th **M00.24 Other streptococcal arthritis, hand**
    Other streptococcal arthritis metacarpus and phalanges

    M00.241 Other streptococcal arthritis, right hand [CC]
        CC Excl: A17.9, A18.02, A18.09, A18.82, A18.84, A18.89, A39.83-A39.84, A54.40, A54.42-A54.43, A54.82, A54.84, A54.89-A54.9, B06.82, M00.00, M00.041-M00.049, M00.08-M00.10, M00.141-M00.149, M00.18-M00.20, M00.241-M00.249, M00.28-M00.80, M00.841-M00.849, M00.88-M01.X0, M01.X41-M01.X49, M01.X8-M02.10, M02.141-M02.149, M02.18-M02.30, M02.349, M02.38-M02.80, M02.841-M02.849, M02.88-M02.9, M05.40-M05.59, M05.70-M06.09, M06.20-M06.39, M06.80-M07.60, M07.641-M07.649, M07.68-M07.69, M11.00, M11.041-M11.049, M11.08-M11.10, M11.141-M11.149, M11.18-M11.20, M11.241-M11.249, M11.28-M11.80, M11.841-M11.849, M11.88-M11.9, M12.10, M12.141-M12.149, M12.18-M12.20, M12.241-M12.249, M12.28-M12.30, M12.341-M12.349, M12.38-M12.40, M12.441-M12.449, M12.48-M12.50, M12.541-M12.549, M12.58-M12.80, M12.841-M12.849, M12.88-M13.10, M13.141-M13.149, M13.80, M13.841-M13.849, M13.88-M15.9, M18.0-M18.9, M19.041-M19.049, M19.141-M19.149, M19.241-M19.249, M19.90-M19.93, M24.10, M24.141-M24.149, M25.00, M25.041-M25.049, M25.08-M25.10, M25.141-M25.149, M25.18, M25.40, M25.441-M25.449, M25.48-M25.50, M25.60, M25.641-M25.649, M25.80, M25.841-M25.849, M25.9, M35.2, M36.1-M36.4, R26.2

    M00.242 Other streptococcal arthritis, left hand [CC]
        CC Excl: See code: M00.241

    M00.249 Other streptococcal arthritis, unspecified hand [CC]
        CC Excl: See code: M00.241

✓6th **M00.25 Other streptococcal arthritis, hip**

    M00.251 Other streptococcal arthritis, right hip [CC]
        CC Excl: A17.9, A18.02, A18.09, A18.82, A18.84, A18.89, A39.83-A39.84, A54.40, A54.42-A54.43, A54.82, A54.84, A54.89-A54.9, B06.82, M00.00, M00.051-M00.059, M00.08-M00.10, M00.151-M00.159, M00.18-M00.20, M00.251-M00.259, M00.28-M00.80, M00.851-M00.859, M00.88-M01.X0, M01.X51-M01.X59, M01.X8-M02.10, M02.151-M02.159, M02.18-M02.30, M02.359, M02.38-M02.80, M02.851-M02.859, M02.88-M02.9, M05.40-M05.59, M05.70-M06.09, M06.20-M06.39, M06.80-M07.60, M07.651-M07.659, M07.68-M07.69, M11.00, M11.051-M11.059, M11.08-M11.10, M11.151-M11.159, M11.18-M11.20, M11.251-M11.259, M11.28-M11.80, M11.851-M11.859, M11.88-M11.9, M12.10, M12.151-M12.159, M12.18-M12.20, M12.251-M12.259, M12.28-M12.30, M12.351-M12.359, M12.38-M12.40, M12.451-M12.459, M12.48-M12.50, M12.551-M12.559, M12.58-M12.80, M12.851-M12.859, M12.88-M13.10, M13.151-M13.159, M13.80, M13.851-M13.859, M13.88-M15.0, M15.3-M16.9, M19.90-M19.93, M24.10, M24.151-M24.159, M25.00, M25.051-M25.059, M25.08-M25.10, M25.151-M25.159, M25.18, M25.40, M25.451-M25.459, M25.48-M25.50, M25.551-M25.559, M25.60, M25.651-M25.659, M25.80, M25.851-M25.859, M25.9, M35.2, M36.1-M36.4, R26.2, R29.4

    M00.252 Other streptococcal arthritis, left hip [CC]
        CC Excl: See code: M00.251

    M00.259 Other streptococcal arthritis, unspecified hip [CC]
        CC Excl: See code: M00.251

✓ Additional Character Required   ✓x7th Placeholder Alert   Unacceptable PDx   Manifestation   Hospital Acquired Condition   **EXCLUDES 1** Not Coded Here   **EXCLUDES 2** Not Included Here

✓6ᵗʰ **M00.26 Other streptococcal arthritis, knee**

M00.261 Other streptococcal arthritis, right knee `CC`
CC Excl: A17.9, A18.02, A18.09, A18.82, A18.84, A18.89, A39.83-A39.84, A54.40, A54.42-A54.43, A54.82, A54.84, A54.89-A54.9, B06.82, M00.00, M00.061-M00.069, M00.08-M00.10, M00.161-M00.169, M00.18-M00.20, M00.261-M00.269, M00.28-M00.80, M00.861-M00.869, M00.88-M01.X0, M01.X61-M01.X69, M01.X8-M02.10, M02.161-M02.169, M02.18-M02.30, M02.369, M02.38-M02.80, M02.861-M02.869, M02.88-M02.9, M05.40-M05.59, M05.70-M06.09, M06.20-M06.39, M06.80-M07.60, M07.661-M07.669, M07.68-M07.69, M11.00, M11.061-M11.069, M11.08-M11.10, M11.161-M11.169, M11.18-M11.20, M11.261-M11.269, M11.28-M11.80, M11.861-M11.869, M11.88-M11.9, M12.10, M12.161-M12.169, M12.18-M12.20, M12.261-M12.269, M12.28-M12.30, M12.361-M12.369, M12.38-M12.40, M12.461-M12.469, M12.48-M12.50, M12.561-M12.569, M12.58-M12.80, M12.861-M12.869, M12.88-M13.10, M13.161-M13.169, M13.80, M13.861-M13.869, M13.88-M15.0, M15.3-M15.9, M17.0-M17.9, M19.90-M19.93, M24.10, M25.00, M25.061-M25.069, M25.08-M25.10, M25.161-M25.169, M25.18, M25.40, M25.461-M25.469, M25.48-M25.50, M25.561-M25.569, M25.60, M25.661-M25.669, M25.80, M25.861-M25.869, M25.9, M35.2, M36.1-M36.4, R26.2

M00.262 Other streptococcal arthritis, left knee `CC`
CC Excl: See code: M00.261

M00.269 Other streptococcal arthritis, unspecified knee `CC`
CC Excl: See code: M00.261

✓6ᵗʰ **M00.27 Other streptococcal arthritis, ankle and foot**
Other streptococcal arthritis, tarsus, metatarsus and phalanges

M00.271 Other streptococcal arthritis, right ankle and foot `CC`
CC Excl: A17.9, A18.02, A18.09, A18.82, A18.84, A18.89, A39.83-A39.84, A54.40, A54.42-A54.43, A54.82, A54.84, A54.89-A54.9, B06.82, M00.00, M00.071–M00.10, M00.171-M00.20, M00.271-M00.80, M00.871-M01.X0, M01.X71-M02.10, M02.171-M02.30, M02.379-M02.80, M02.871-M02.9, M05.40-M05.59, M05.70-M06.09, M06.20-M06.39, M06.80-M07.60, M07.671-M07.69, M11.00, M11.071-M11.10, M11.171-M11.20, M11.271-M11.80, M11.871-M11.9, M12.10, M12.171-M12.20, M12.271-M12.30, M12.371-M12.40, M12.471-M12.50, M12.571-M12.80, M12.871-M13.10, M13.171-M13.80, M13.871-M15.0, M15.3-M15.9, M19.071-M19.079, M19.171-M19.179, M19.271-M19.93, M24.10, M24.171-M24.176, M25.00, M25.071-M25.10, M25.171-M25.18, M25.40, M25.471-M25.50, M25.571-M25.60, M25.671-M25.676, M25.80, M25.871-M25.9, M35.2, M36.1-M36.4, R26.2

M00.272 Other streptococcal arthritis, left ankle and foot `CC`
CC Excl: See code: M00.271

M00.279 Other streptococcal arthritis, unspecified ankle and foot `CC`
CC Excl: See code: M00.271

M00.28 Other streptococcal arthritis, vertebrae `CC`
CC Excl: A17.9, A18.02, A18.09, A18.82, A18.84, A18.89, A39.83-A39.84, A54.40, A54.42-A54.43, A54.82, A54.84, A54.89-A54.9, B06.82, M00.00-M02.30, M02.319, M02.329, M02.339, M02.349, M02.359, M02.369, M02.379-M02.9, M05.40-M05.59, M05.70-M06.09, M06.20-M06.39, M06.80-M07.69, M11.00-M11.9, M12.10-M15.0, M15.3-M15.9, M16.2-M16.9, M17.2-M17.9, M18.2-M18.9, M19.111-M19.93, M24.10-M24.176, M25.00, M25.08-M25.18, M25.40-M25.676, M25.80-M25.9, M35.2, M36.1-M36.4, R26.2, R29.4

M00.29 Other streptococcal polyarthritis `CC`
CC Excl: See code: M00.28

✓5ᵗʰ **M00.8 Arthritis and polyarthritis due to other bacteria**
Use additional code (B96) to identify bacteria

M00.80 Arthritis due to other bacteria, unspecified joint `CC`
CC Excl: See code: M00.28

✓6ᵗʰ **M00.81 Arthritis due to other bacteria, shoulder**

M00.811 Arthritis due to other bacteria, right shoulder `CC`
CC Excl: A17.9, A18.02, A18.09, A18.82, A18.84, A18.89, A39.83-A39.84, A54.40, A54.42-A54.43, A54.82, A54.84, A54.89-A54.9, B06.82, M00.00-M00.019, M00.08-M00.119, M00.18-M00.219, M00.28-M00.819, M00.88-M01.X19, M01.X8-M02.119, M02.18-M02.211

M00.812 Arthritis due to other bacteria, left shoulder `CC`
CC Excl: See code: M00.811

M00.819 Arthritis due to other bacteria, unspecified shoulder `CC`
CC Excl: See code: M00.811

✓6ᵗʰ **M00.82 Arthritis due to other bacteria, elbow**

M00.821 Arthritis due to other bacteria, right elbow `CC`
CC Excl: A17.9, A18.02, A18.09, A18.82, A18.84, A18.89, A39.83-A39.84, A54.40, A54.42-A54.43, A54.82, A54.84, A54.89-A54.9, B06.82, M00.00, M00.021-M00.029, M00.08-M00.10, M00.121-M00.129, M00.18-M00.20, M00.221-M00.229, M00.28-M00.80, M00.821-M00.829, M00.88-M01.X0, M01.X21-M01.X29, M01.X8-M02.10, M02.121-M02.129, M02.18-M02.30, M02.329, M02.38-M02.80, M02.821-M02.829, M02.88-M02.9, M05.40-M05.59, M05.70-M06.09, M06.20-M06.39, M06.80-M07.60, M07.621-M07.629, M07.68-M07.69, M11.00, M11.021-M11.029, M11.08-M11.10, M11.121-M11.129, M11.18-M11.20, M11.221-M11.229, M11.28-M11.80, M11.821-M11.829, M11.88-M11.9, M12.10, M12.121-M12.129, M12.18-M12.20, M12.221-M12.229, M12.28-M12.30, M12.321-M12.329, M12.38-M12.40, M12.421-M12.429, M12.48-M12.50, M12.521-M12.529, M12.58-M12.80, M12.821-M12.829, M12.88-M13.10, M13.121-M13.129, M13.80, M13.821-M13.829, M13.88-M15.0, M15.3-M15.9, M19.021-M19.029, M19.121-M19.129, M19.221-M19.229, M19.90-M19.93, M24.10, M24.121-M24.129, M25.00, M25.021-M25.029, M25.08-M25.10, M25.121-M25.129, M25.18, M25.40, M25.421-M25.429, M25.48-M25.50, M25.521-M25.529, M25.60, M25.621-M25.629, M25.80, M25.821-M25.829, M25.9, M35.2, M36.1-M36.4, R26.2

M00.822 Arthritis due to other bacteria, left elbow `CC`
CC Excl: See code: M00.821

M00.829 Arthritis due to other bacteria, unspecified elbow `CC`
CC Excl: See code: M00.821

✓6ᵗʰ **M00.83 Arthritis due to other bacteria, wrist**
Arthritis due to other bacteria, carpal bones

M00.831 Arthritis due to other bacteria, right wrist `CC`
CC Excl: A17.9, A18.02, A18.09, A18.82, A18.84, A18.89, A39.83-A39.84, A54.40, A54.42-A54.43, A54.82, A54.84, A54.89-A54.9, B06.82, M00.00, M00.031-M00.039, M00.08-M00.10, M00.131-M00.139, M00.18-M00.20, M00.231-M00.239, M00.28-M00.80, M00.831-M00.839, M00.88-M01.X0, M01.X31-M01.X39, M01.X8-M02.10, M02.131-M02.139, M02.18-M02.30, M02.339, M02.38-M02.80, M02.831-M02.839, M02.88-M02.9, M05.40-M05.59, M05.70-M06.09, M06.20-M06.39, M06.80-M07.60, M07.631-M07.639, M07.68-M07.69, M11.00, M11.031-M11.039, M11.08-M11.10, M11.131-M11.139, M11.18-M11.20, M11.231-M11.239, M11.28-M11.80, M11.831-M11.839, M11.88-M11.9, M12.10, M12.131-M12.139, M12.18-M12.20, M12.231-M12.239, M12.28-M12.30, M12.331-M12.339, M12.38-M12.40, M12.431-M12.439, M12.48-M12.50, M12.531-M12.539, M12.58-M12.80, M12.831-M12.839, M12.88-M13.10, M13.131-M13.139, M13.80, M13.831-M13.839, M13.88-M15.0, M15.3-M15.9, M19.031-M19.039, M19.131-M19.139, M19.231-M19.239, M19.90-M19.93, M24.10, M24.131-M24.139, M25.00, M25.031-M25.039, M25.08-M25.10, M25.131-M25.139, M25.18, M25.40, M25.431-M25.439, M25.48-M25.50, M25.531-M25.539, M25.60, M25.631-M25.639, M25.80, M25.831-M25.839, M25.9, M35.2, M36.1-M36.4, R26.2

M00.832 **Arthritis due to other bacteria, left wrist** `CC`
    CC Excl: See code: M00.831

M00.839 **Arthritis due to other bacteria, unspecified wrist** `CC`
    CC Excl: See code: M00.831

✓6ᵗʰ **M00.84** **Arthritis due to other bacteria, hand**
    Arthritis due to other bacteria, metacarpus and phalanges

M00.841 **Arthritis due to other bacteria, right hand** `CC`
    CC Excl: A17.9, A18.02, A18.09, A18.82, A18.84, A18.89, A39.83-A39.84, A54.40, A54.42-A54.43, A54.82, A54.84, A54.89-A54.9, B06.82, M00.00, M00.041-M00.049, M00.08-M00.10, M00.141-M00.149, M00.18-M00.20, M00.241-M00.249, M00.28-M00.80, M00.841-M00.849, M00.88-M01.X0, M01.X41-M01.X49, M01.X8-M02.10, M02.141-M02.149, M02.18-M02.30, M02.349, M02.38-M02.80, M02.841-M02.849, M02.88-M02.9, M05.40-M05.59, M05.70-M06.09, M06.20-M06.39, M06.80-M07.60, M07.641-M07.649, M07.68-M07.69, M11.00, M11.041-M11.049, M11.08-M11.10, M11.141-M11.149, M11.18-M11.20, M11.241-M11.249, M11.28-M11.80, M11.841-M11.849, M11.88-M11.9, M12.10, M12.141-M12.149, M12.18-M12.20, M12.241-M12.249, M12.28-M12.30, M12.341-M12.349, M12.38-M12.40, M12.441-M12.449, M12.48-M12.50, M12.541-M12.549, M12.58-M12.80, M12.841-M12.849, M12.88-M13.10, M13.141-M13.149, M13.80, M13.841-M13.849, M13.88-M15.9, M18.0-M18.9, M19.041-M19.049, M19.141-M19.149, M19.241-M19.249, M19.90-M19.93, M24.10, M24.141-M24.149, M25.00, M25.041-M25.049, M25.08-M25.10, M25.141-M25.149, M25.18, M25.40, M25.441-M25.449, M25.48-M25.50, M25.60, M25.641-M25.649, M25.80, M25.841-M25.849, M25.9, M35.2, M36.1-M36.4, R26.2

M00.842 **Arthritis due to other bacteria, left hand** `CC`
    CC Excl: See code: M00.841

M00.849 **Arthritis due to other bacteria, unspecified hand** `CC`
    CC Excl: See code: M00.841

✓6ᵗʰ **M00.85** **Arthritis due to other bacteria, hip**

M00.851 **Arthritis due to other bacteria, right hip** `CC`
    CC Excl: A17.9, A18.02, A18.09, A18.82, A18.84, A18.89, A39.83-A39.84, A54.40, A54.42-A54.43, A54.82, A54.84, A54.89-A54.9, B06.82, M00.00, M00.051-M00.059, M00.08-M00.10, M00.151-M00.159, M00.18-M00.20, M00.251-M00.259, M00.28-M00.80, M00.851-M00.859, M00.88-M01.X0, M01.X51-M01.X59, M01.X8-M02.10, M02.151-M02.159, M02.18-M02.30, M02.359, M02.38-M02.80, M02.851-M02.859, M02.88-M02.9, M05.40-M05.59, M05.70-M06.09, M06.20-M06.39, M06.80-M07.60, M07.651-M07.659, M07.68-M07.69, M11.00, M11.051-M11.059, M11.08-M11.10, M11.151-M11.159, M11.18-M11.20, M11.251-M11.259, M11.28-M11.80, M11.851-M11.859, M11.88-M11.9, M12.10, M12.151-M12.159, M12.18-M12.20, M12.251-M12.259, M12.28-M12.30, M12.351-M12.359, M12.38-M12.40, M12.451-M12.459, M12.48-M12.50, M12.551-M12.559, M12.58-M12.80, M12.851-M12.859, M12.88-M13.10, M13.151-M13.159, M13.80, M13.851-M13.859, M13.88-M15.0, M15.3-M16.9, M19.90-M19.93, M24.10, M24.151-M24.159, M25.00, M25.051-M25.059, M25.08-M25.10, M25.151-M25.159, M25.18, M25.40, M25.451-M25.459, M25.48-M25.50, M25.551-M25.559, M25.60, M25.651-M25.659, M25.80, M25.851-M25.859, M25.9, M35.2, M36.1-M36.4, R26.2, R29.4

M00.852 **Arthritis due to other bacteria, left hip** `CC`
    CC Excl: See code: M00.851

M00.859 **Arthritis due to other bacteria, unspecified hip** `CC`
    CC Excl: See code: M00.851

✓6ᵗʰ **M00.86** **Arthritis due to other bacteria, knee**

M00.861 **Arthritis due to other bacteria, right knee** `CC`
    CC Excl: A17.9, A18.02, A18.09, A18.82, A18.84, A18.89, A39.83-A39.84, A54.40, A54.42-A54.43, A54.82, A54.84, A54.89-A54.9, B06.82, M00.00, M00.061-M00.069, M00.08-M00.10, M00.161-M00.169, M00.18-M00.20, M00.261-M00.269, M00.28-M00.80, M00.861-M00.869, M00.88-M01.X0, M01.X61-M01.X69, M01.X8-M02.10, M02.161-M02.169, M02.18-M02.30, M02.369, M02.38-M02.80, M02.861-M02.869, M02.88-M02.9, M05.40-M05.59, M05.70-M06.09, M06.20-M06.39, M06.80-M07.60, M07.661-M07.669, M07.68-M07.69, M11.00, M11.061-M11.069, M11.08-M11.10, M11.161-M11.169, M11.18-M11.20, M11.261-M11.269, M11.28-M11.80, M11.861-M11.869, M11.88-M11.9, M12.10, M12.161-M12.169, M12.18-M12.20, M12.261-M12.269, M12.28-M12.30, M12.361-M12.369, M12.38-M12.40, M12.461-M12.469, M12.48-M12.50, M12.561-M12.569, M12.58-M12.80, M12.861-M12.869, M12.88-M13.10, M13.161-M13.169, M13.80, M13.861-M13.869, M13.88-M15.0, M15.3-M15.9, M17.0-M17.9, M19.90-M19.93, M24.10, M25.00, M25.061-M25.069, M25.08-M25.10, M25.161-M25.169, M25.18, M25.40, M25.461-M25.469, M25.48-M25.50, M25.561-M25.569, M25.60, M25.661-M25.669, M25.80, M25.861-M25.869, M25.9, M35.2, M36.1-M36.4, R26.2

M00.862 **Arthritis due to other bacteria, left knee** `CC`
    CC Excl: See code: M00.861

M00.869 **Arthritis due to other bacteria, unspecified knee** `CC`
    CC Excl: See code: M00.861

✓6ᵗʰ **M00.87** **Arthritis due to other bacteria, ankle and foot**
    Arthritis due to other bacteria, tarsus, metatarsus, and phalanges

M00.871 **Arthritis due to other bacteria, right ankle and foot** `CC`
    CC Excl: A17.9, A18.02, A18.09, A18.82, A18.84, A18.89, A39.83-A39.84, A54.40, A54.42-A54.43, A54.82, A54.84, A54.89-A54.9, B06.82, M00.00, M00.071-M00.10, M00.171-M00.20, M00.271-M00.80, M00.871-M01.X0, M01.X71-M02.10, M02.171-M02.30, M02.379-M02.80, M02.871-M02.9, M05.40-M05.59, M05.70-M06.09, M06.20-M06.39, M06.80-M07.60, M07.671-M07.69, M11.00, M11.071-M11.10, M11.171-M11.20, M11.271-M11.80, M11.871-M11.9, M12.10, M12.171-M12.20, M12.271-M12.30, M12.371-M12.40, M12.471-M12.50, M12.571-M12.80, M12.871-M13.10, M13.171-M13.80, M13.871-M15.0, M15.3-M15.9, M19.071-M19.079, M19.171-M19.179, M19.271-M19.93, M24.10, M24.171-M24.176, M25.00, M25.071-M25.10, M25.171-M25.18, M25.40, M25.471-M25.50, M25.571-M25.60, M25.671-M25.676, M25.80, M25.871-M25.9, M35.2, M36.1-M36.4, R26.2

M00.872 **Arthritis due to other bacteria, left ankle and foot** `CC`
    CC Excl: See code: M00.871

M00.879 **Arthritis due to other bacteria, unspecified ankle and foot** `CC`
    CC Excl: See code: M00.871

M00.88 **Arthritis due to other bacteria, vertebrae** `CC`
    CC Excl: A17.9, A18.02, A18.09, A18.82, A18.84, A18.89, A39.83-A39.84, A54.40, A54.42-A54.43, A54.82, A54.84, A54.89-A54.9, B06.82, M00.00-M02.30, M02.319, M02.329, M02.339, M02.349, M02.359, M02.369, M02.379-M02.9, M05.40-M05.59, M05.70-M06.09, M06.20-M06.39, M06.80-M07.69, M11.00-M11.9, M12.10-M15.0, M15.3-M15.9, M16.2-M16.9, M17.2-M17.9, M18.2-M18.9, M19.111-M19.93, M24.10-M24.176, M25.00, M25.08-M25.18, M25.40-M25.676, M25.80-M25.9, M35.2, M36.1-M36.4, R26.2, R29.4

M00.89 **Polyarthritis due to other bacteria** `CC`
    CC Excl: See code: M00.88

M00.9 **Pyogenic arthritis, unspecified** `CC`
    Infective arthritis NOS
    CC Excl: See code: M00.88

✓ Additional Character Required ✓x7ᵗʰ Placeholder Alert Unacceptable PDx Manifestation Hospital Acquired Condition **EXCLUDES 1** Not Coded Here *EXCLUDES 2* Not Included Here

✓4ᵗʰ **M01 Direct infections of joint in infectious and parasitic diseases classified elsewhere**

Code first underlying disease, such as:
leprosy [Hansen's disease] (A30.-)
mycoses (B35-B49)
O'nyong-nyong fever (A92.1)
paratyphoid fever (A01.1-A01.4)

EXCLUDES 1   *arthropathy in Lyme disease (A69.23)*
gonococcal arthritis (A54.42)
meningococcal arthritis (A39.83)
mumps arthritis (B26.85)
postinfective arthropathy (M02.-)
postmeningococcal arthritis (A39.84)
reactive arthritis (M02.3)
rubella arthritis (B06.82)
sarcoidosis arthritis (D86.86)
typhoid fever arthritis (A01.04)
tuberculosis arthritis (A18.01-A18.02)

✓5ᵗʰ **M01.X Direct infection of joint in infectious and parasitic diseases classified elsewhere**

M01.X0   **Direct infection of unspecified joint in infectious and parasitic diseases classified elsewhere**   CC
CC Excl: A02.23, A17.9, A18.02, A18.09, A18.82, A18.84, A18.89, A39.83-A39.84, A54.40, A54.42-A54.43, A54.82, A54.84, A54.89-A54.9, B06.82, M00.00-M02.30, M02.319, M02.329, M02.339, M02.349, M02.359, M02.369, M02.379-M02.9, M05.40-M05.59, M05.70-M06.09, M06.20-M06.39, M06.80-M07.69, M11.00-M11.9, M12.10-M15.0, M15.3-M15.9, M16.2-M16.9, M17.2-M17.9, M18.2-M18.9, M19.111-M19.93, M24.10-M24.176, M25.00, M25.08-M25.18, M25.40-M25.676, M25.80-M25.9, M35.2, M36.1-M36.4, R29.4

✓6ᵗʰ **M01.X1 Direct infection of shoulder joint in infectious and parasitic diseases classified elsewhere**

M01.X11   **Direct infection of right shoulder in infectious and parasitic diseases classified elsewhere**   CC
CC Excl: A02.23, A17.9, A18.02, A18.09, A18.82, A18.84, A18.89, A39.83-A39.84, A54.40, A54.42-A54.43, A54.82, A54.84, A54.89-A54.9, B06.82, M00.00-M02.30, M02.319, M02.329, M02.339, M02.349, M02.359, M02.369, M02.379-M02.9, M05.40-M05.59, M05.70-M06.09, M06.20-M06.39, M06.80-M07.69, M11.00-M11.9, M12.10-M12.419

M01.X12   **Direct infection of left shoulder in infectious and parasitic diseases classified elsewhere**   CC
CC Excl: See code: M01.X11

M01.X19   **Direct infection of unspecified shoulder in infectious and parasitic diseases classified elsewhere**   CC
CC Excl: See code: M01.X11

✓6ᵗʰ **M01.X2 Direct infection of elbow in infectious and parasitic diseases classified elsewhere**

M01.X21   **Direct infection of right elbow in infectious and parasitic diseases classified elsewhere**   CC
CC Excl: See code: M01.X0

M01.X22   **Direct infection of left elbow in infectious and parasitic diseases classified elsewhere**   CC
CC Excl: See code: M01.X0

M01.X29   **Direct infection of unspecified elbow in infectious and parasitic diseases classified elsewhere**   CC
CC Excl: See code: M01.X0

✓6ᵗʰ **M01.X3 Direct infection of wrist in infectious and parasitic diseases classified elsewhere**
Direct infection of carpal bones in infectious and parasitic diseases classified elsewhere

M01.X31   **Direct infection of right wrist in infectious and parasitic diseases classified elsewhere**   CC
CC Excl: See code: M01.X0

M01.X32   **Direct infection of left wrist in infectious and parasitic diseases classified elsewhere**   CC
CC Excl: See code: M01.X0

M01.X39   **Direct infection of unspecified wrist in infectious and parasitic diseases classified elsewhere**   CC
CC Excl: See code: M01.X0

✓6ᵗʰ **M01.X4 Direct infection of hand in infectious and parasitic diseases classified elsewhere**
Direct infection of metacarpus and phalanges in infectious and parasitic diseases classified elsewhere

M01.X41   **Direct infection of right hand in infectious and parasitic diseases classified elsewhere**   CC
CC Excl: See code: M01.X0

M01.X42   **Direct infection of left hand in infectious and parasitic diseases classified elsewhere**   CC
CC Excl: See code: M01.X0

M01.X49   **Direct infection of unspecified hand in infectious and parasitic diseases classified elsewhere**   CC
CC Excl: See code: M01.X0

✓6ᵗʰ **M01.X5 Direct infection of hip in infectious and parasitic diseases classified elsewhere**

M01.X51   **Direct infection of right hip in infectious and parasitic diseases classified elsewhere**   CC
CC Excl: See code: M01.X0

M01.X52   **Direct infection of left hip in infectious and parasitic diseases classified elsewhere**   CC
CC Excl: See code: M01.X0

M01.X59   **Direct infection of unspecified hip in infectious and parasitic diseases classified elsewhere**   CC
CC Excl: See code: M01.X0

✓6ᵗʰ **M01.X6 Direct infection of knee in infectious and parasitic diseases classified elsewhere**

M01.X61   **Direct infection of right knee in infectious and parasitic diseases classified elsewhere**   CC
CC Excl: See code: M01.X0

M01.X62   **Direct infection of left knee in infectious and parasitic diseases classified elsewhere**   CC
CC Excl: See code: M01.X0

M01.X69   **Direct infection of unspecified knee in infectious and parasitic diseases classified elsewhere**   CC
CC Excl: See code: M01.X0

✓6ᵗʰ **M01.X7 Direct infection of ankle and foot in infectious and parasitic diseases classified elsewhere**
Direct infection of tarsus, metatarsus and phalanges in infectious and parasitic diseases classified elsewhere

M01.X71   **Direct infection of right ankle and foot in infectious and parasitic diseases classified elsewhere**   CC
CC Excl: See code: M01.X0

M01.X72   **Direct infection of left ankle and foot in infectious and parasitic diseases classified elsewhere**   CC
CC Excl: See code: M01.X0

M01.X79   **Direct infection of unspecified ankle and foot in infectious and parasitic diseases classified elsewhere**   CC
CC Excl: See code: M01.X0

M01.X8   **Direct infection of vertebrae in infectious and parasitic diseases classified elsewhere**   CC
CC Excl: See code: M01.X0

M01.X9   **Direct infection of multiple joints in infectious and parasitic diseases classified elsewhere**   CC
CC Excl: See code: M01.X0

✓4ᵗʰ M02 Postinfective and reactive arthropathies

Code first underlying disease, such as:
congenital syphilis [Clutton's joints] (A50.5)
enteritis due to Yersinia enterocolitica (A04.6)
infective endocarditis (I33.0)
viral hepatitis (B15-B19)

EXCLUDES 1   Behçet's disease (M35.2)
direct infections of joint in infectious and parasitic diseases
classified elsewhere (M01.-)
mumps arthritis (B26.85)
postmeningococcal arthritis (A39.84)
rheumatic fever (I00)
rubella arthritis (B06.82)
syphilis arthritis (late) (A52.77)
tabetic arthropathy [Charcôt's] (A52.16)

✓5ᵗʰ M02.0 Arthropathy following intestinal bypass

M02.00 Arthropathy following intestinal bypass, unspecified site

✓6ᵗʰ M02.01 Arthropathy following intestinal bypass, shoulder
- **M02.011 Arthropathy following intestinal bypass, right shoulder**
- **M02.012 Arthropathy following intestinal bypass, left shoulder**
- **M02.019 Arthropathy following intestinal bypass, unspecified shoulder**

✓6ᵗʰ M02.02 Arthropathy following intestinal bypass, elbow
- **M02.021 Arthropathy following intestinal bypass, right elbow**
- **M02.022 Arthropathy following intestinal bypass, left elbow**
- **M02.029 Arthropathy following intestinal bypass, unspecified elbow**

✓6ᵗʰ M02.03 Arthropathy following intestinal bypass, wrist
Arthropathy following intestinal bypass, carpal bones
- **M02.031 Arthropathy following intestinal bypass, right wrist**
- **M02.032 Arthropathy following intestinal bypass, left wrist**
- **M02.039 Arthropathy following intestinal bypass, unspecified wrist**

✓6ᵗʰ M02.04 Arthropathy following intestinal bypass, hand
Arthropathy following intestinal bypass, metacarpals and phalanges
- **M02.041 Arthropathy following intestinal bypass, right hand**
- **M02.042 Arthropathy following intestinal bypass, left hand**
- **M02.049 Arthropathy following intestinal bypass, unspecified hand**

✓6ᵗʰ M02.05 Arthropathy following intestinal bypass, hip
- **M02.051 Arthropathy following intestinal bypass, right hip**
- **M02.052 Arthropathy following intestinal bypass, left hip**
- **M02.059 Arthropathy following intestinal bypass, unspecified hip**

✓6ᵗʰ M02.06 Arthropathy following intestinal bypass, knee
- **M02.061 Arthropathy following intestinal bypass, right knee**
- **M02.062 Arthropathy following intestinal bypass, left knee**
- **M02.069 Arthropathy following intestinal bypass, unspecified knee**

✓6ᵗʰ M02.07 Arthropathy following intestinal bypass, ankle and foot
Arthropathy following intestinal bypass, tarsus, metatarsus and phalanges
- **M02.071 Arthropathy following intestinal bypass, right ankle and foot**
- **M02.072 Arthropathy following intestinal bypass, left ankle and foot**
- **M02.079 Arthropathy following intestinal bypass, unspecified ankle and foot**

M02.08 Arthropathy following intestinal bypass, vertebrae

M02.09 Arthropathy following intestinal bypass, multiple sites

✓5ᵗʰ M02.1 Postdysenteric arthropathy

M02.10 Postdysenteric arthropathy, unspecified site   CC
CC Excl: A02.23, A17.9, A18.02, A18.09, A18.82, A18.84, A18.89, A39.83-A39.84, A54.40, A54.42-A54.43, A54.82, A54.84, A54.89-A54.9, B06.82, M00.00-M02.30, M02.319, M02.329, M02.339, M02.349, M02.359, M02.369, M02.379-M02.9, M05.40-M05.59, M05.70-M06.09, M06.20-M06.39, M06.80-M07.69, M11.00-M11.9, M12.10-M15.0, M15.3-M15.9, M16.2-M16.9, M17.2-M17.9, M18.2-M18.9, M19.111-M19.93, M24.10-M24.176, M25.00, M25.08-M25.18, M25.40-M25.676, M25.80-M25.9, M35.2, M36.1-M36.4, R29.4

✓6ᵗʰ M02.11 Postdysenteric arthropathy, shoulder
- **M02.111 Postdysenteric arthropathy, right shoulder**   CC
  CC Excl: See code: M02.10
- **M02.112 Postdysenteric arthropathy, left shoulder**   CC
  CC Excl: See code: M02.10
- **M02.119 Postdysenteric arthropathy, unspecified shoulder**   CC
  CC Excl: See code: M02.10

✓6ᵗʰ M02.12 Postdysenteric arthropathy, elbow
- **M02.121 Postdysenteric arthropathy, right elbow**   CC
  CC Excl: See code: M02.10
- **M02.122 Postdysenteric arthropathy, left elbow**   CC
  CC Excl: See code: M02.10
- **M02.129 Postdysenteric arthropathy, unspecified elbow**   CC
  CC Excl: See code: M02.10

✓6ᵗʰ M02.13 Postdysenteric arthropathy, wrist
Postdysenteric arthropathy, carpal bones
- **M02.131 Postdysenteric arthropathy, right wrist**   CC
  CC Excl: See code: M02.10
- **M02.132 Postdysenteric arthropathy, left wrist**   CC
  CC Excl: See code: M02.10
- **M02.139 Postdysenteric arthropathy, unspecified wrist**   CC
  CC Excl: See code: M02.10

✓6ᵗʰ M02.14 Postdysenteric arthropathy, hand
Postdysenteric arthropathy, metacarpus and phalanges
- **M02.141 Postdysenteric arthropathy, right hand**   CC
  CC Excl: See code: M02.10
- **M02.142 Postdysenteric arthropathy, left hand**   CC
  CC Excl: See code: M02.10
- **M02.149 Postdysenteric arthropathy, unspecified hand**   CC
  CC Excl: See code: M02.10

✓6ᵗʰ M02.15 Postdysenteric arthropathy, hip
- **M02.151 Postdysenteric arthropathy, right hip**   CC
  CC Excl: See code: M02.10
- **M02.152 Postdysenteric arthropathy, left hip**   CC
  CC Excl: See code: M02.10
- **M02.159 Postdysenteric arthropathy, unspecified hip**   CC
  CC Excl: See code: M02.10

✓6ᵗʰ M02.16 Postdysenteric arthropathy, knee
- **M02.161 Postdysenteric arthropathy, right knee**   CC
  CC Excl: A02.23, A17.9, A18.02, A18.09, A18.82, A18.84, A18.89, A39.83-A39.84, A54.40, A54.42-A54.43, A54.82, A54.84, A54.89-A54.9, B06.82, M00.00-M02.30, M02.319, M02.329, M02.339, M02.349, M02.359, M02.369, M02.379-M02.9, M05.40-M05.59, M05.70-M06.09, M06.20-M06.39, M06.80-M07.69, M11.00-M11.9, M12.10-M12.179, M12.19-M15.0, M15.3-M15.9, M16.2-M16.9, M17.2-M17.9, M18.2-M18.9, M19.111-M19.93, M24.10-M24.176, M25.00, M25.08-M25.18, M25.40-M25.676, M25.80-M25.9, M35.2, M36.1-M36.4, R29.4
- **M02.162 Postdysenteric arthropathy, left knee**   CC
  CC Excl: See code: M02.161
- **M02.169 Postdysenteric arthropathy, unspecified knee**   CC
  CC Excl: See code: M02.161

✓ Additional Character Required   ✓x7ᵗʰ Placeholder Alert   Unacceptable PDx   Manifestation   Hospital Acquired Condition   EXCLUDES 1 Not Coded Here   EXCLUDES 2 Not Included Here

ICD-10-CM 2016   709

Chapter 13. Diseases of the Musculoskeletal System and Connective Tissue

M02–M02.169

✓6ᵗʰ **M02.17 Postdysenteric arthropathy, ankle and foot**
Postdysenteric arthropathy, tarsus, metatarsus and phalanges

     M02.171 Postdysenteric arthropathy, right ankle and foot CC
CC Excl: See code: M02.10

     M02.172 Postdysenteric arthropathy, left ankle and foot CC
CC Excl: See code: M02.10

     M02.179 Postdysenteric arthropathy, unspecified ankle and foot CC
CC Excl: See code: M02.10

M02.18 Postdysenteric arthropathy, vertebrae CC
CC Excl: A02.23, A17.9, A18.02, A18.09, A18.82, A18.84, A18.89, A39.83-A39.84, A54.40, A54.42-A54.43, A54.82, A54.84, A54.89-A54.9, B06.82, M00.00-M02.30, M02.319, M02.329, M02.349, M02.359, M02.369, M02.379-M02.9, M05.40-M05.59, M05.70-M06.39, M06.80-M07.69, M11.00-M11.9, M12.10-M15.0, M15.3-M15.9, M16.2-M16.9, M17.2-M17.9, M18.2-M18.9, M19.111-M19.93, M24.10-M24.176, M25.00, M25.08-M25.18, M25.40-M25.676, M25.80-M25.9, M35.2, M36.1-M36.4, R29.4

M02.19 Postdysenteric arthropathy, multiple sites CC
CC Excl: See code: M02.10

✓5ᵗʰ **M02.2 Postimmunization arthropathy**

M02.20 Postimmunization arthropathy, unspecified site

✓6ᵗʰ **M02.21 Postimmunization arthropathy, shoulder**
     M02.211 Postimmunization arthropathy, right shoulder
     M02.212 Postimmunization arthropathy, left shoulder
     M02.219 Postimmunization arthropathy, unspecified shoulder

✓6ᵗʰ **M02.22 Postimmunization arthropathy, elbow**
     M02.221 Postimmunization arthropathy, right elbow
     M02.222 Postimmunization arthropathy, left elbow
     M02.229 Postimmunization arthropathy, unspecified elbow

✓6ᵗʰ **M02.23 Postimmunization arthropathy, wrist**
Postimmunization arthropathy, carpal bones
     M02.231 Postimmunization arthropathy, right wrist
     M02.232 Postimmunization arthropathy, left wrist
     M02.239 Postimmunization arthropathy, unspecified wrist

✓6ᵗʰ **M02.24 Postimmunization arthropathy, hand**
Postimmunization arthropathy, metacarpus and phalanges
     M02.241 Postimmunization arthropathy, right hand
     M02.242 Postimmunization arthropathy, left hand
     M02.249 Postimmunization arthropathy, unspecified hand

✓6ᵗʰ **M02.25 Postimmunization arthropathy, hip**
     M02.251 Postimmunization arthropathy, right hip
     M02.252 Postimmunization arthropathy, left hip
     M02.259 Postimmunization arthropathy, unspecified hip

✓6ᵗʰ **M02.26 Postimmunization arthropathy, knee**
     M02.261 Postimmunization arthropathy, right knee
     M02.262 Postimmunization arthropathy, left knee
     M02.269 Postimmunization arthropathy, unspecified knee

✓6ᵗʰ **M02.27 Postimmunization arthropathy, ankle and foot**
Postimmunization arthropathy, tarsus, metatarsus and phalanges
     M02.271 Postimmunization arthropathy, right ankle and foot
     M02.272 Postimmunization arthropathy, left ankle and foot
     M02.279 Postimmunization arthropathy, unspecified ankle and foot

M02.28 Postimmunization arthropathy, vertebrae

M02.29 Postimmunization arthropathy, multiple sites

✓5ᵗʰ **M02.3 Reiter's disease**
Reactive arthritis

M02.30 Reiter's disease, unspecified site PDxCC CC
CC Excl: A02.23, A17.9, A18.02, A18.09, A18.82, A18.84, A18.89, A39.83-A39.84, A54.40, A54.42-A54.43, A54.82, A54.84, A54.89-A54.9, B06.82, M00.00-M02.30, M02.319, M02.329, M02.339, M02.349, M02.359, M02.369, M02.379-M02.9, M05.40-M05.59, M05.70-M06.09, M06.20-M06.39, M06.80-M07.69, M11.00-M11.9, M12.10-M15.0, M15.3-M15.9, M16.2-M16.9, M17.2-M17.9, M18.2-M18.9, M19.111-M19.93, M24.10-M24.176, M25.00, M25.08-M25.18, M25.40-M25.676, M25.80-M25.9, M35.2, M36.1-M36.4, R29.4

✓6ᵗʰ **M02.31 Reiter's disease, shoulder**
     M02.311 Reiter's disease, right shoulder PDxCC CC
CC Excl: See code: M02.30
     M02.312 Reiter's disease, left shoulder PDxCC CC
CC Excl: See code: M02.30
     M02.319 Reiter's disease, unspecified shoulder PDxCC CC
CC Excl: See code: M02.30

✓6ᵗʰ **M02.32 Reiter's disease, elbow**
     M02.321 Reiter's disease, right elbow PDxCC CC
CC Excl: See code: M02.30
     M02.322 Reiter's disease, left elbow PDxCC CC
CC Excl: See code: M02.30
     M02.329 Reiter's disease, unspecified elbow PDxCC CC
CC Excl: See code: M02.30

✓6ᵗʰ **M02.33 Reiter's disease, wrist**
Reiter's disease, carpal bones
     M02.331 Reiter's disease, right wrist PDxCC CC
CC Excl: See code: M02.30
     M02.332 Reiter's disease, left wrist PDxCC CC
CC Excl: See code: M02.30
     M02.339 Reiter's disease, unspecified wrist PDxCC CC
CC Excl: See code: M02.30

✓6ᵗʰ **M02.34 Reiter's disease, hand**
Reiter's disease, metacarpus and phalanges
     M02.341 Reiter's disease, right hand PDxCC CC
CC Excl: See code: M02.30
     M02.342 Reiter's disease, left hand PDxCC CC
CC Excl: See code: M02.30
     M02.349 Reiter's disease, unspecified hand PDxCC CC
CC Excl: See code: M02.30

✓6ᵗʰ **M02.35 Reiter's disease, hip**
     M02.351 Reiter's disease, right hip PDxCC CC
CC Excl: See code: M02.30
     M02.352 Reiter's disease, left hip PDxCC CC
CC Excl: See code: M02.30
     M02.359 Reiter's disease, unspecified hip PDxCC CC
CC Excl: See code: M02.30

✓6ᵗʰ **M02.36 Reiter's disease, knee**
     M02.361 Reiter's disease, right knee PDxCC CC
CC Excl: See code: M02.30
     M02.362 Reiter's disease, left knee PDxCC CC
CC Excl: See code: M02.30
     M02.369 Reiter's disease, unspecified knee PDxCC CC
CC Excl: See code: M02.30

✓6ᵗʰ **M02.37 Reiter's disease, ankle and foot**
Reiter's disease, tarsus, metatarsus and phalanges
     M02.371 Reiter's disease, right ankle and foot PDxCC CC
CC Excl: See code: M02.30
     M02.372 Reiter's disease, left ankle and foot PDxCC CC
CC Excl: See code: M02.30
     M02.379 Reiter's disease, unspecified ankle and foot PDxCC CC
CC Excl: See code: M02.30

M02.38 Reiter's disease, vertebrae PDxCC CC
CC Excl: See code: M02.30

M02.39 Reiter's disease, multiple sites PDxCC CC
CC Excl: See code: M02.30

✓5ᵗʰ **M02.8 Other reactive arthropathies**

M02.80 Other reactive arthropathies, unspecified site `CC`
CC Excl: See code: M02.30

✓6ᵗʰ **M02.81 Other reactive arthropathies, shoulder**

M02.811 Other reactive arthropathies, right shoulder `CC`
CC Excl: A02.23, A17.9, A18.02, A18.09, A18.82, A18.84, A18.89, A39.83-A39.84, A54.40, A54.42-A54.43, A54.82, A54.84, A54.89-A54.9, B06.82, M00.00, M00.019, M00.029, M00.039, M00.049, M00.059, M00.069, M00.079, M00.08-M02.30, M02.319, M02.329, M02.339, M02.349, M02.359, M02.369, M02.379-M02.9, M05.40-M05.59, M05.70-M06.09, M06.20-M06.39, M06.80-M07.69, M11.00-M11.9, M12.10-M12.419

M02.812 Other reactive arthropathies, left shoulder `CC`
CC Excl: See code: M02.811

M02.819 Other reactive arthropathies, unspecified shoulder `CC`
CC Excl: See code: M02.811

✓6ᵗʰ **M02.82 Other reactive arthropathies, elbow**

M02.821 Other reactive arthropathies, right elbow `CC`
CC Excl: A02.23, A17.9, A18.02, A18.09, A18.82, A18.84, A18.89, A39.83-A39.84, A54.40, A54.42-A54.43, A54.82, A54.84, A54.89-A54.9, B06.82, M00.00-M02.30, M02.319, M02.329, M02.339, M02.349, M02.359, M02.369, M02.379-M02.9, M05.40-M05.59, M05.70-M06.09, M06.20-M06.39, M06.80-M07.69, M11.00-M11.9, M12.10-M15.0, M15.3-M15.9, M16.2-M16.9, M17.2-M17.9, M18.2-M18.9, M19.111-M19.93, M24.10-M24.176, M25.00, M25.08-M25.18, M25.40-M25.676, M25.80-M25.9, M35.2, M36.1-M36.4, R29.4

M02.822 Other reactive arthropathies, left elbow `CC`
CC Excl: See code: M02.821

M02.829 Other reactive arthropathies, unspecified elbow `CC`
CC Excl: See code: M02.821

✓6ᵗʰ **M02.83 Other reactive arthropathies, wrist**
Other reactive arthropathies, carpal bones

M02.831 Other reactive arthropathies, right wrist `CC`
CC Excl: See code: M02.821

M02.832 Other reactive arthropathies, left wrist `CC`
CC Excl: See code: M02.821

M02.839 Other reactive arthropathies, unspecified wrist `CC`
CC Excl: See code: M02.821

✓6ᵗʰ **M02.84 Other reactive arthropathies, hand**
Other reactive arthropathies, metacarpus and phalanges

M02.841 Other reactive arthropathies, right hand `CC`
CC Excl: See code: M02.821

M02.842 Other reactive arthropathies, left hand `CC`
CC Excl: See code: M02.821

M02.849 Other reactive arthropathies, unspecified hand `CC`
CC Excl: See code: M02.821

✓6ᵗʰ **M02.85 Other reactive arthropathies, hip**

M02.851 Other reactive arthropathies, right hip `CC`
CC Excl: See code: M02.821

M02.852 Other reactive arthropathies, left hip `CC`
CC Excl: See code: M02.821

M02.859 Other reactive arthropathies, unspecified hip `CC`
CC Excl: See code: M02.821

✓6ᵗʰ **M02.86 Other reactive arthropathies, knee**

M02.861 Other reactive arthropathies, right knee `CC`
CC Excl: See code: M02.821

M02.862 Other reactive arthropathies, left knee `CC`
CC Excl: See code: M02.821

M02.869 Other reactive arthropathies, unspecified knee `CC`
CC Excl: See code: M02.821

✓6ᵗʰ **M02.87 Other reactive arthropathies, ankle and foot**
Other reactive arthropathies, tarsus, metatarsus and phalanges

M02.871 Other reactive arthropathies, right ankle and foot `CC`
CC Excl: See code: M02.821

M02.872 Other reactive arthropathies, left ankle and foot `CC`
CC Excl: See code: M02.821

M02.879 Other reactive arthropathies, unspecified ankle and foot `CC`
CC Excl: See code: M02.821

M02.88 *Other reactive arthropathies, vertebrae* `CC`
CC Excl: See code: M02.821

M02.89 *Other reactive arthropathies, multiple sites* `CC`
CC Excl: See code: M02.821

M02.9 *Reactive arthropathy, unspecified*

Inflammatory polyarthropathies (M05-M14)

✓4ᵗʰ **M05 Rheumatoid arthritis with rheumatoid factor**
EXCLUDES 1   *rheumatic fever (I00)*
juvenile rheumatoid arthritis (M08.-)
rheumatoid arthritis of spine (M45.-)

✓5ᵗʰ **M05.0 Felty's syndrome**
Rheumatoid arthritis with splenoadenomegaly and leukopenia

M05.00 Felty's syndrome, unspecified site

✓6ᵗʰ **M05.01 Felty's syndrome, shoulder**
M05.011 Felty's syndrome, right shoulder
M05.012 Felty's syndrome, left shoulder
M05.019 Felty's syndrome, unspecified shoulder

✓6ᵗʰ **M05.02 Felty's syndrome, elbow**
M05.021 Felty's syndrome, right elbow
M05.022 Felty's syndrome, left elbow
M05.029 Felty's syndrome, unspecified elbow

✓6ᵗʰ **M05.03 Felty's syndrome, wrist**
Felty's syndrome, carpal bones
M05.031 Felty's syndrome, right wrist
M05.032 Felty's syndrome, left wrist
M05.039 Felty's syndrome, unspecified wrist

✓6ᵗʰ **M05.04 Felty's syndrome, hand**
Felty's syndrome, metacarpus and phalanges
M05.041 Felty's syndrome, right hand
M05.042 Felty's syndrome, left hand
M05.049 Felty's syndrome, unspecified hand

✓6ᵗʰ **M05.05 Felty's syndrome, hip**
M05.051 Felty's syndrome, right hip
M05.052 Felty's syndrome, left hip
M05.059 Felty's syndrome, unspecified hip

✓6ᵗʰ **M05.06 Felty's syndrome, knee**
M05.061 Felty's syndrome, right knee
M05.062 Felty's syndrome, left knee
M05.069 Felty's syndrome, unspecified knee

✓6ᵗʰ **M05.07 Felty's syndrome, ankle and foot**
Felty's syndrome, tarsus, metatarsus and phalanges
M05.071 Felty's syndrome, right ankle and foot
M05.072 Felty's syndrome, left ankle and foot
M05.079 Felty's syndrome, unspecified ankle and foot

M05.09 Felty's syndrome, multiple sites

✓5ᵗʰ **M05.1 Rheumatoid lung disease with rheumatoid arthritis**
M05.10 Rheumatoid lung disease with rheumatoid arthritis of unspecified site

✓6ᵗʰ **M05.11 Rheumatoid lung disease with rheumatoid arthritis of shoulder**
M05.111 Rheumatoid lung disease with rheumatoid arthritis of right shoulder
M05.112 Rheumatoid lung disease with rheumatoid arthritis of left shoulder
M05.119 Rheumatoid lung disease with rheumatoid arthritis of unspecified shoulder

---

✓ Additional Character Required   ✓x7ᵗʰ Placeholder Alert   Unacceptable PDx   Manifestation   Hospital Acquired Condition   EXCLUDES 1 Not Coded Here   EXCLUDES 2 Not Included Here

Chapter 13. Diseases of the Musculoskeletal System and Connective Tissue

✓6ᵗʰ **M05.12 Rheumatoid lung disease with rheumatoid arthritis of elbow**
- **M05.121 Rheumatoid lung disease with rheumatoid arthritis of right elbow**
- **M05.122 Rheumatoid lung disease with rheumatoid arthritis of left elbow**
- **M05.129 Rheumatoid lung disease with rheumatoid arthritis of unspecified elbow**

✓6ᵗʰ **M05.13 Rheumatoid lung disease with rheumatoid arthritis of wrist**
Rheumatoid lung disease with rheumatoid arthritis, carpal bones
- **M05.131 Rheumatoid lung disease with rheumatoid arthritis of right wrist**
- **M05.132 Rheumatoid lung disease with rheumatoid arthritis of left wrist**
- **M05.139 Rheumatoid lung disease with rheumatoid arthritis of unspecified wrist**

✓6ᵗʰ **M05.14 Rheumatoid lung disease with rheumatoid arthritis of hand**
Rheumatoid lung disease with rheumatoid arthritis, metacarpus and phalanges
- **M05.141 Rheumatoid lung disease with rheumatoid arthritis of right hand**
- **M05.142 Rheumatoid lung disease with rheumatoid arthritis of left hand**
- **M05.149 Rheumatoid lung disease with rheumatoid arthritis of unspecified hand**

✓6ᵗʰ **M05.15 Rheumatoid lung disease with rheumatoid arthritis of hip**
- **M05.151 Rheumatoid lung disease with rheumatoid arthritis of right hip**
- **M05.152 Rheumatoid lung disease with rheumatoid arthritis of left hip**
- **M05.159 Rheumatoid lung disease with rheumatoid arthritis of unspecified hip**

✓6ᵗʰ **M05.16 Rheumatoid lung disease with rheumatoid arthritis of knee**
- **M05.161 Rheumatoid lung disease with rheumatoid arthritis of right knee**
- **M05.162 Rheumatoid lung disease with rheumatoid arthritis of left knee**
- **M05.169 Rheumatoid lung disease with rheumatoid arthritis of unspecified knee**

✓6ᵗʰ **M05.17 Rheumatoid lung disease with rheumatoid arthritis of ankle and foot**
Rheumatoid lung disease with rheumatoid arthritis, tarsus, metatarsus and phalanges
- **M05.171 Rheumatoid lung disease with rheumatoid arthritis of right ankle and foot**
- **M05.172 Rheumatoid lung disease with rheumatoid arthritis of left ankle and foot**
- **M05.179 Rheumatoid lung disease with rheumatoid arthritis of unspecified ankle and foot**

M05.19 Rheumatoid lung disease with rheumatoid arthritis of multiple sites

✓5ᵗʰ **M05.2 Rheumatoid vasculitis with rheumatoid arthritis**

M05.20 Rheumatoid vasculitis with rheumatoid arthritis of unspecified site

✓6ᵗʰ **M05.21 Rheumatoid vasculitis with rheumatoid arthritis of shoulder**
- **M05.211 Rheumatoid vasculitis with rheumatoid arthritis of right shoulder**
- **M05.212 Rheumatoid vasculitis with rheumatoid arthritis of left shoulder**
- **M05.219 Rheumatoid vasculitis with rheumatoid arthritis of unspecified shoulder**

✓6ᵗʰ **M05.22 Rheumatoid vasculitis with rheumatoid arthritis of elbow**
- **M05.221 Rheumatoid vasculitis with rheumatoid arthritis of right elbow**
- **M05.222 Rheumatoid vasculitis with rheumatoid arthritis of left elbow**
- **M05.229 Rheumatoid vasculitis with rheumatoid arthritis of unspecified elbow**

✓6ᵗʰ **M05.23 Rheumatoid vasculitis with rheumatoid arthritis of wrist**
Rheumatoid vasculitis with rheumatoid arthritis, carpal bones
- **M05.231 Rheumatoid vasculitis with rheumatoid arthritis of right wrist**
- **M05.232 Rheumatoid vasculitis with rheumatoid arthritis of left wrist**
- **M05.239 Rheumatoid vasculitis with rheumatoid arthritis of unspecified wrist**

✓6ᵗʰ **M05.24 Rheumatoid vasculitis with rheumatoid arthritis of hand**
Rheumatoid vasculitis with rheumatoid arthritis, metacarpus and phalanges
- **M05.241 Rheumatoid vasculitis with rheumatoid arthritis of right hand**
- **M05.242 Rheumatoid vasculitis with rheumatoid arthritis of left hand**
- **M05.249 Rheumatoid vasculitis with rheumatoid arthritis of unspecified hand**

✓6ᵗʰ **M05.25 Rheumatoid vasculitis with rheumatoid arthritis of hip**
- **M05.251 Rheumatoid vasculitis with rheumatoid arthritis of right hip**
- **M05.252 Rheumatoid vasculitis with rheumatoid arthritis of left hip**
- **M05.259 Rheumatoid vasculitis with rheumatoid arthritis of unspecified hip**

✓6ᵗʰ **M05.26 Rheumatoid vasculitis with rheumatoid arthritis of knee**
- **M05.261 Rheumatoid vasculitis with rheumatoid arthritis of right knee**
- **M05.262 Rheumatoid vasculitis with rheumatoid arthritis of left knee**
- **M05.269 Rheumatoid vasculitis with rheumatoid arthritis of unspecified knee**

✓6ᵗʰ **M05.27 Rheumatoid vasculitis with rheumatoid arthritis of ankle and foot**
Rheumatoid vasculitis with rheumatoid arthritis, tarsus, metatarsus and phalanges
- **M05.271 Rheumatoid vasculitis with rheumatoid arthritis of right ankle and foot**
- **M05.272 Rheumatoid vasculitis with rheumatoid arthritis of left ankle and foot**
- **M05.279 Rheumatoid vasculitis with rheumatoid arthritis of unspecified ankle and foot**

M05.29 Rheumatoid vasculitis with rheumatoid arthritis of multiple sites

✓5ᵗʰ **M05.3 Rheumatoid heart disease with rheumatoid arthritis**
Rheumatoid carditis   Rheumatoid myocarditis
Rheumatoid endocarditis   Rheumatoid pericarditis

M05.30 Rheumatoid heart disease with rheumatoid arthritis of unspecified site

✓6ᵗʰ **M05.31 Rheumatoid heart disease with rheumatoid arthritis of shoulder**
- **M05.311 Rheumatoid heart disease with rheumatoid arthritis of right shoulder**
- **M05.312 Rheumatoid heart disease with rheumatoid arthritis of left shoulder**
- **M05.319 Rheumatoid heart disease with rheumatoid arthritis of unspecified shoulder**

✓6ᵗʰ **M05.32 Rheumatoid heart disease with rheumatoid arthritis of elbow**
- **M05.321 Rheumatoid heart disease with rheumatoid arthritis of right elbow**
- **M05.322 Rheumatoid heart disease with rheumatoid arthritis of left elbow**
- **M05.329 Rheumatoid heart disease with rheumatoid arthritis of unspecified elbow**

✓6ᵗʰ **M05.33 Rheumatoid heart disease with rheumatoid arthritis of wrist**
Rheumatoid heart disease with rheumatoid arthritis, carpal bones
- **M05.331 Rheumatoid heart disease with rheumatoid arthritis of right wrist**
- **M05.332 Rheumatoid heart disease with rheumatoid arthritis of left wrist**

M05.339 **Rheumatoid heart disease with rheumatoid arthritis of** unspecified **wrist**

√6ᵗʰ **M05.34 Rheumatoid heart disease with rheumatoid arthritis of** hand
Rheumatoid heart disease with rheumatoid arthritis, metacarpus and phalanges

M05.341 **Rheumatoid heart disease with rheumatoid arthritis of** right **hand**

M05.342 **Rheumatoid heart disease with rheumatoid arthritis of** left **hand**

M05.349 **Rheumatoid heart disease with rheumatoid arthritis of** unspecified **hand**

√6ᵗʰ **M05.35 Rheumatoid heart disease with rheumatoid arthritis of** hip

M05.351 **Rheumatoid heart disease with rheumatoid arthritis of** right **hip**

M05.352 **Rheumatoid heart disease with rheumatoid arthritis of** left **hip**

M05.359 **Rheumatoid heart disease with rheumatoid arthritis of** unspecified **hip**

√6ᵗʰ **M05.36 Rheumatoid heart disease with rheumatoid arthritis of** knee

M05.361 **Rheumatoid heart disease with rheumatoid arthritis of** right **knee**

M05.362 **Rheumatoid heart disease with rheumatoid arthritis of** left **knee**

M05.369 **Rheumatoid heart disease with rheumatoid arthritis of** unspecified **knee**

√6ᵗʰ **M05.37 Rheumatoid heart disease with rheumatoid arthritis of** ankle and foot
Rheumatoid heart disease with rheumatoid arthritis, tarsus, metatarsus and phalanges

M05.371 **Rheumatoid heart disease with rheumatoid arthritis of** right **ankle and foot**

M05.372 **Rheumatoid heart disease with rheumatoid arthritis of** left **ankle and foot**

M05.379 **Rheumatoid heart disease with rheumatoid arthritis of** unspecified **ankle and foot**

M05.39 **Rheumatoid heart disease with rheumatoid arthritis of** multiple sites

√5ᵗʰ **M05.4 Rheumatoid** myopathy with rheumatoid arthritis

> **CC Excl: For all CC codes in subcategory M05.4, unless otherwise noted:** E08.40-E08.49, E08.618-E08.638, E08.649-E08.8, E09.40-E09.49, E09.618-E09.638, E09.649-E09.8, E10.40-E10.49, E10.618-E10.638, E10.649, E10.69-E10.8, E11.40-E11.49, E11.618-E11.638, E11.649, E11.69-E11.8, E13.40-E13.49, E13.618-E13.638, E13.649-E13.8, G32.89, G70.00-G72.3, G72.81-G73.7, G96.8-G96.9, G98.0-G98.8, G99.8

M05.40 **Rheumatoid myopathy with rheumatoid arthritis of** unspecified **site** PDxCC CC

√6ᵗʰ **M05.41 Rheumatoid myopathy with rheumatoid arthritis of** shoulder

M05.411 **Rheumatoid myopathy with rheumatoid arthritis of** right **shoulder** PDxCC CC

M05.412 **Rheumatoid myopathy with rheumatoid arthritis of** left **shoulder** PDxCC CC

M05.419 **Rheumatoid myopathy with rheumatoid arthritis of** unspecified **shoulder** PDxCC CC

√6ᵗʰ **M05.42 Rheumatoid myopathy with rheumatoid arthritis of** elbow

M05.421 **Rheumatoid myopathy with rheumatoid arthritis of** right **elbow** PDxCC CC

M05.422 **Rheumatoid myopathy with rheumatoid arthritis of** left **elbow** PDxCC CC

M05.429 **Rheumatoid myopathy with rheumatoid arthritis of** unspecified **elbow** PDxCC CC

√6ᵗʰ **M05.43 Rheumatoid myopathy with rheumatoid arthritis of** wrist
Rheumatoid myopathy with rheumatoid arthritis, carpal bones

M05.431 **Rheumatoid myopathy with rheumatoid arthritis of** right **wrist** PDxCC CC

M05.432 **Rheumatoid myopathy with rheumatoid arthritis of** left **wrist** PDxCC CC

M05.439 **Rheumatoid myopathy with rheumatoid arthritis of** unspecified **wrist** PDxCC CC

√6ᵗʰ **M05.44 Rheumatoid myopathy with rheumatoid arthritis of** hand
Rheumatoid myopathy with rheumatoid arthritis, metacarpus and phalanges

M05.441 **Rheumatoid myopathy with rheumatoid arthritis of** right **hand** PDxCC CC

M05.442 **Rheumatoid myopathy with rheumatoid arthritis of** left **hand** PDxCC CC

M05.449 **Rheumatoid myopathy with rheumatoid arthritis of** unspecified **hand** PDxCC CC

√6ᵗʰ **M05.45 Rheumatoid myopathy with rheumatoid arthritis of** hip

M05.451 **Rheumatoid myopathy with rheumatoid arthritis of** right **hip** PDxCC CC

M05.452 **Rheumatoid myopathy with rheumatoid arthritis of** left **hip** PDxCC CC

M05.459 **Rheumatoid myopathy with rheumatoid arthritis of** unspecified **hip** PDxCC CC

√6ᵗʰ **M05.46 Rheumatoid myopathy with rheumatoid arthritis of** knee

M05.461 **Rheumatoid myopathy with rheumatoid arthritis of** right **knee** PDxCC CC

M05.462 **Rheumatoid myopathy with rheumatoid arthritis of** left **knee** PDxCC CC

M05.469 **Rheumatoid myopathy with rheumatoid arthritis of** unspecified **knee** PDxCC CC

√6ᵗʰ **M05.47 Rheumatoid myopathy with rheumatoid arthritis of** ankle and foot
Rheumatoid myopathy with rheumatoid arthritis, tarsus, metatarsus and phalanges

M05.471 **Rheumatoid myopathy with rheumatoid arthritis of** right **ankle and foot** PDxCC CC

M05.472 **Rheumatoid myopathy with rheumatoid arthritis of** left **ankle and foot** PDxCC CC

M05.479 **Rheumatoid myopathy with rheumatoid arthritis of** unspecified **ankle and foot** PDxCC CC

M05.49 **Rheumatoid myopathy with rheumatoid arthritis of** multiple sites PDxCC CC

√5ᵗʰ **M05.5 Rheumatoid** polyneuropathy with rheumatoid arthritis

M05.50 **Rheumatoid polyneuropathy with rheumatoid arthritis of** unspecified **site**

√6ᵗʰ **M05.51 Rheumatoid polyneuropathy with rheumatoid arthritis of** shoulder

M05.511 **Rheumatoid polyneuropathy with rheumatoid arthritis of** right **shoulder**

M05.512 **Rheumatoid polyneuropathy with rheumatoid arthritis of** left **shoulder**

M05.519 **Rheumatoid polyneuropathy with rheumatoid arthritis of** unspecified **shoulder**

√6ᵗʰ **M05.52 Rheumatoid polyneuropathy with rheumatoid arthritis of** elbow

M05.521 **Rheumatoid polyneuropathy with rheumatoid arthritis of** right **elbow**

M05.522 **Rheumatoid polyneuropathy with rheumatoid arthritis of** left **elbow**

M05.529 **Rheumatoid polyneuropathy with rheumatoid arthritis of** unspecified **elbow**

√6ᵗʰ **M05.53 Rheumatoid polyneuropathy with rheumatoid arthritis of** wrist
Rheumatoid polyneuropathy with rheumatoid arthritis, carpal bones

M05.531 **Rheumatoid polyneuropathy with rheumatoid arthritis of** right **wrist**

M05.532 **Rheumatoid polyneuropathy with rheumatoid arthritis of** left **wrist**

M05.539 **Rheumatoid polyneuropathy with rheumatoid arthritis of** unspecified **wrist**

√6ᵗʰ **M05.54 Rheumatoid polyneuropathy with rheumatoid arthritis of** hand
Rheumatoid polyneuropathy with rheumatoid arthritis, metacarpus and phalanges

---

✔ Additional Character Required   √x7ᵗʰ Placeholder Alert   Unacceptable PDx   Manifestation   Hospital Acquired Condition   **EXCLUDES1** Not Coded Here   **EXCLUDES2** Not Included Here

M05.541   Rheumatoid polyneuropathy with rheumatoid arthritis of right hand

M05.542   Rheumatoid polyneuropathy with rheumatoid arthritis of left hand

M05.549   Rheumatoid polyneuropathy with rheumatoid arthritis of unspecified hand

✓6ᵗʰ M05.55   Rheumatoid polyneuropathy with rheumatoid arthritis of hip

M05.551   Rheumatoid polyneuropathy with rheumatoid arthritis of right hip

M05.552   Rheumatoid polyneuropathy with rheumatoid arthritis of left hip

M05.559   Rheumatoid polyneuropathy with rheumatoid arthritis of unspecified hip

✓6ᵗʰ M05.56   Rheumatoid polyneuropathy with rheumatoid arthritis of knee

M05.561   Rheumatoid polyneuropathy with rheumatoid arthritis of right knee

M05.562   Rheumatoid polyneuropathy with rheumatoid arthritis of left knee

M05.569   Rheumatoid polyneuropathy with rheumatoid arthritis of unspecified knee

✓6ᵗʰ M05.57   Rheumatoid polyneuropathy with rheumatoid arthritis of ankle and foot
Rheumatoid polyneuropathy with rheumatoid arthritis, tarsus, metatarsus and phalanges

M05.571   Rheumatoid polyneuropathy with rheumatoid arthritis of right ankle and foot

M05.572   Rheumatoid polyneuropathy with rheumatoid arthritis of left ankle and foot

M05.579   Rheumatoid polyneuropathy with rheumatoid arthritis of unspecified ankle and foot

M05.59   Rheumatoid polyneuropathy with rheumatoid arthritis of multiple sites

✓5ᵗʰ M05.6   Rheumatoid arthritis with involvement of other organs and systems

M05.60   Rheumatoid arthritis of unspecified site with involvement of other organs and systems

✓6ᵗʰ M05.61   Rheumatoid arthritis of shoulder with involvement of other organs and systems

M05.611   Rheumatoid arthritis of right shoulder with involvement of other organs and systems

M05.612   Rheumatoid arthritis of left shoulder with involvement of other organs and systems

M05.619   Rheumatoid arthritis of unspecified shoulder with involvement of other organs and systems

✓6ᵗʰ M05.62   Rheumatoid arthritis of elbow with involvement of other organs and systems

M05.621   Rheumatoid arthritis of right elbow with involvement of other organs and systems

M05.622   Rheumatoid arthritis of left elbow with involvement of other organs and systems

M05.629   Rheumatoid arthritis of unspecified elbow with involvement of other organs and systems

✓6ᵗʰ M05.63   Rheumatoid arthritis of wrist with involvement of other organs and systems
Rheumatoid arthritis of carpal bones with involvement of other organs and systems

M05.631   Rheumatoid arthritis of right wrist with involvement of other organs and systems

M05.632   Rheumatoid arthritis of left wrist with involvement of other organs and systems

M05.639   Rheumatoid arthritis of unspecified wrist with involvement of other organs and systems

✓6ᵗʰ M05.64   Rheumatoid arthritis of hand with involvement of other organs and systems
Rheumatoid arthritis of metacarpus and phalanges with involvement of other organs and systems

M05.641   Rheumatoid arthritis of right hand with involvement of other organs and systems

M05.642   Rheumatoid arthritis of left hand with involvement of other organs and systems

M05.649   Rheumatoid arthritis of unspecified hand with involvement of other organs and systems

✓6ᵗʰ M05.65   Rheumatoid arthritis of hip with involvement of other organs and systems

M05.651   Rheumatoid arthritis of right hip with involvement of other organs and systems

M05.652   Rheumatoid arthritis of left hip with involvement of other organs and systems

M05.659   Rheumatoid arthritis of unspecified hip with involvement of other organs and systems

✓6ᵗʰ M05.66   Rheumatoid arthritis of knee with involvement of other organs and systems

M05.661   Rheumatoid arthritis of right knee with involvement of other organs and systems

M05.662   Rheumatoid arthritis of left knee with involvement of other organs and systems

M05.669   Rheumatoid arthritis of unspecified knee with involvement of other organs and systems

✓6ᵗʰ M05.67   Rheumatoid arthritis of ankle and foot with involvement of other organs and systems
Rheumatoid arthritis of tarsus, metatarsus and phalanges with involvement of other organs and systems

M05.671   Rheumatoid arthritis of right ankle and foot with involvement of other organs and systems

M05.672   Rheumatoid arthritis of left ankle and foot with involvement of other organs and systems

M05.679   Rheumatoid arthritis of unspecified ankle and foot with involvement of other organs and systems

M05.69   Rheumatoid arthritis of multiple sites with involvement of other organs and systems

✓5ᵗʰ M05.7   Rheumatoid arthritis with rheumatoid factor without organ or systems involvement

M05.70   Rheumatoid arthritis with rheumatoid factor of unspecified site without organ or systems involvement

✓6ᵗʰ M05.71   Rheumatoid arthritis with rheumatoid factor of shoulder without organ or systems involvement

M05.711   Rheumatoid arthritis with rheumatoid factor of right shoulder without organ or systems involvement

M05.712   Rheumatoid arthritis with rheumatoid factor of left shoulder without organ or systems involvement

M05.719   Rheumatoid arthritis with rheumatoid factor of unspecified shoulder without organ or systems involvement

✓6ᵗʰ M05.72   Rheumatoid arthritis with rheumatoid factor of elbow without organ or systems involvement

M05.721   Rheumatoid arthritis with rheumatoid factor of right elbow without organ or systems involvement

M05.722   Rheumatoid arthritis with rheumatoid factor of left elbow without organ or systems involvement

M05.729   Rheumatoid arthritis with rheumatoid factor of unspecified elbow without organ or systems involvement

✓6ᵗʰ M05.73   Rheumatoid arthritis with rheumatoid factor of wrist without organ or systems involvement

M05.731   Rheumatoid arthritis with rheumatoid factor of right wrist without organ or systems involvement

M05.732   Rheumatoid arthritis with rheumatoid factor of left wrist without organ or systems involvement

M05.739   Rheumatoid arthritis with rheumatoid factor of unspecified wrist without organ or systems involvement

✓6ᵗʰ M05.74   Rheumatoid arthritis with rheumatoid factor of hand without organ or systems involvement

M05.741   Rheumatoid arthritis with rheumatoid factor of right hand without organ or systems involvement

Ⓝ Newborn: 0   Ⓟ Pediatric: 0-17   Ⓜ Maternity: 12-55   Ⓐ Adult: 15-124   MCC Major CC Condition   PDxMCC PDx acts as own MCC   CC CC Condition   PDxCC PDx acts as own CC

714   ICD-10-CM 2016

M05.742   Rheumatoid arthritis with rheumatoid factor of left hand without organ or systems involvement

M05.749   Rheumatoid arthritis with rheumatoid factor of unspecified hand without organ or systems involvement

✓6ᵗʰ   **M05.75**   Rheumatoid arthritis with rheumatoid factor of hip without organ or systems involvement

M05.751   Rheumatoid arthritis with rheumatoid factor of right hip without organ or systems involvement

M05.752   Rheumatoid arthritis with rheumatoid factor of left hip without organ or systems involvement

M05.759   Rheumatoid arthritis with rheumatoid factor of unspecified hip without organ or systems involvement

✓6ᵗʰ   **M05.76**   Rheumatoid arthritis with rheumatoid factor of knee without organ or systems involvement

M05.761   Rheumatoid arthritis with rheumatoid factor of right knee without organ or systems involvement

M05.762   Rheumatoid arthritis with rheumatoid factor of left knee without organ or systems involvement

M05.769   Rheumatoid arthritis with rheumatoid factor of unspecified knee without organ or systems involvement

✓6ᵗʰ   **M05.77**   Rheumatoid arthritis with rheumatoid factor of ankle and foot without organ or systems involvement

M05.771   Rheumatoid arthritis with rheumatoid factor of right ankle and foot without organ or systems involvement

M05.772   Rheumatoid arthritis with rheumatoid factor of left ankle and foot without organ or systems involvement

M05.779   Rheumatoid arthritis with rheumatoid factor of unspecified ankle and foot without organ or systems involvement

M05.79   Rheumatoid arthritis with rheumatoid factor of multiple sites without organ or systems involvement

✓5ᵗʰ   **M05.8**   Other rheumatoid arthritis with rheumatoid factor

M05.80   Other rheumatoid arthritis with rheumatoid factor of unspecified site

✓6ᵗʰ   **M05.81**   Other rheumatoid arthritis with rheumatoid factor of shoulder

M05.811   Other rheumatoid arthritis with rheumatoid factor of right shoulder

M05.812   Other rheumatoid arthritis with rheumatoid factor of left shoulder

M05.819   Other rheumatoid arthritis with rheumatoid factor of unspecified shoulder

✓6ᵗʰ   **M05.82**   Other rheumatoid arthritis with rheumatoid factor of elbow

M05.821   Other rheumatoid arthritis with rheumatoid factor of right elbow

M05.822   Other rheumatoid arthritis with rheumatoid factor of left elbow

M05.829   Other rheumatoid arthritis with rheumatoid factor of unspecified elbow

✓6ᵗʰ   **M05.83**   Other rheumatoid arthritis with rheumatoid factor of wrist

M05.831   Other rheumatoid arthritis with rheumatoid factor of right wrist

M05.832   Other rheumatoid arthritis with rheumatoid factor of left wrist

M05.839   Other rheumatoid arthritis with rheumatoid factor of unspecified wrist

✓6ᵗʰ   **M05.84**   Other rheumatoid arthritis with rheumatoid factor of hand

M05.841   Other rheumatoid arthritis with rheumatoid factor of right hand

M05.842   Other rheumatoid arthritis with rheumatoid factor of left hand

M05.849   Other rheumatoid arthritis with rheumatoid factor of unspecified hand

✓6ᵗʰ   **M05.85**   Other rheumatoid arthritis with rheumatoid factor of hip

M05.851   Other rheumatoid arthritis with rheumatoid factor of right hip

M05.852   Other rheumatoid arthritis with rheumatoid factor of left hip

M05.859   Other rheumatoid arthritis with rheumatoid factor of unspecified hip

✓6ᵗʰ   **M05.86**   Other rheumatoid arthritis with rheumatoid factor of knee

M05.861   Other rheumatoid arthritis with rheumatoid factor of right knee

M05.862   Other rheumatoid arthritis with rheumatoid factor of left knee

M05.869   Other rheumatoid arthritis with rheumatoid factor of unspecified knee

✓6ᵗʰ   **M05.87**   Other rheumatoid arthritis with rheumatoid factor of ankle and foot

M05.871   Other rheumatoid arthritis with rheumatoid factor of right ankle and foot

M05.872   Other rheumatoid arthritis with rheumatoid factor of left ankle and foot

M05.879   Other rheumatoid arthritis with rheumatoid factor of unspecified ankle and foot

M05.89   Other rheumatoid arthritis with rheumatoid factor of multiple sites

M05.9   Rheumatoid arthritis with rheumatoid factor, unspecified

✓4ᵗʰ   **M06**   **Other rheumatoid arthritis**

✓5ᵗʰ   **M06.0**   Rheumatoid arthritis without rheumatoid factor

M06.00   Rheumatoid arthritis without rheumatoid factor, unspecified site

✓6ᵗʰ   **M06.01**   Rheumatoid arthritis without rheumatoid factor, shoulder

M06.011   Rheumatoid arthritis without rheumatoid factor, right shoulder

M06.012   Rheumatoid arthritis without rheumatoid factor, left shoulder

M06.019   Rheumatoid arthritis without rheumatoid factor, unspecified shoulder

✓6ᵗʰ   **M06.02**   Rheumatoid arthritis without rheumatoid factor, elbow

M06.021   Rheumatoid arthritis without rheumatoid factor, right elbow

M06.022   Rheumatoid arthritis without rheumatoid factor, left elbow

M06.029   Rheumatoid arthritis without rheumatoid factor, unspecified elbow

✓6ᵗʰ   **M06.03**   Rheumatoid arthritis without rheumatoid factor, wrist

M06.031   Rheumatoid arthritis without rheumatoid factor, right wrist

M06.032   Rheumatoid arthritis without rheumatoid factor, left wrist

M06.039   Rheumatoid arthritis without rheumatoid factor, unspecified wrist

✓6ᵗʰ   **M06.04**   Rheumatoid arthritis without rheumatoid factor, hand

M06.041   Rheumatoid arthritis without rheumatoid factor, right hand

M06.042   Rheumatoid arthritis without rheumatoid factor, left hand

M06.049   Rheumatoid arthritis without rheumatoid factor, unspecified hand

✓6ᵗʰ   **M06.05**   Rheumatoid arthritis without rheumatoid factor, hip

M06.051   Rheumatoid arthritis without rheumatoid factor, right hip

M06.052   Rheumatoid arthritis without rheumatoid factor, left hip

M06.059   Rheumatoid arthritis without rheumatoid factor, unspecified hip

✓6ᵗʰ   **M06.06**   Rheumatoid arthritis without rheumatoid factor, knee

M06.061   Rheumatoid arthritis without rheumatoid factor, right knee

M06.062   Rheumatoid arthritis without rheumatoid factor, left knee

✓ Additional Character Required   ✓x7ᵗʰ Placeholder Alert   Unacceptable PDx   **Manifestation**   Hospital Acquired Condition   **EXCLUDES1** Not Coded Here   EXCLUDES2 Not Included Here

ICD-10-CM 2016   715

M06.069   Rheumatoid arthritis without rheumatoid factor, unspecified **knee**

✓6ᵗʰ   M06.07   Rheumatoid arthritis without rheumatoid factor, **ankle and foot**

M06.071   Rheumatoid arthritis without rheumatoid factor, right **ankle and foot**

M06.072   Rheumatoid arthritis without rheumatoid factor, left **ankle and foot**

M06.079   Rheumatoid arthritis without rheumatoid factor, unspecified **ankle and foot**

M06.08   Rheumatoid arthritis without rheumatoid factor, **vertebrae**

M06.09   Rheumatoid arthritis without rheumatoid factor, **multiple sites**

M06.1   Adult-onset Still's disease   Ⓐ

    EXCLUDES 1   *Still's disease NOS (M08.2-)*

✓5ᵗʰ   **M06.2   Rheumatoid bursitis**

M06.20   Rheumatoid bursitis, **unspecified site**

✓6ᵗʰ   M06.21   Rheumatoid bursitis, **shoulder**

M06.211   Rheumatoid bursitis, right **shoulder**

M06.212   Rheumatoid bursitis, left **shoulder**

M06.219   Rheumatoid bursitis, unspecified **shoulder**

✓6ᵗʰ   M06.22   Rheumatoid bursitis, **elbow**

M06.221   Rheumatoid bursitis, right **elbow**

M06.222   Rheumatoid bursitis, left **elbow**

M06.229   Rheumatoid bursitis, unspecified **elbow**

✓6ᵗʰ   M06.23   Rheumatoid bursitis, **wrist**

M06.231   Rheumatoid bursitis, right **wrist**

M06.232   Rheumatoid bursitis, left **wrist**

M06.239   Rheumatoid bursitis, unspecified **wrist**

✓6ᵗʰ   M06.24   Rheumatoid bursitis, **hand**

M06.241   Rheumatoid bursitis, right **hand**

M06.242   Rheumatoid bursitis, left **hand**

M06.249   Rheumatoid bursitis, unspecified **hand**

✓6ᵗʰ   M06.25   Rheumatoid bursitis, **hip**

M06.251   Rheumatoid bursitis, right **hip**

M06.252   Rheumatoid bursitis, left **hip**

M06.259   Rheumatoid bursitis, unspecified **hip**

✓6ᵗʰ   M06.26   Rheumatoid bursitis, **knee**

M06.261   Rheumatoid bursitis, right **knee**

M06.262   Rheumatoid bursitis, left **knee**

M06.269   Rheumatoid bursitis, unspecified **knee**

✓6ᵗʰ   M06.27   Rheumatoid bursitis, **ankle and foot**

M06.271   Rheumatoid bursitis, right **ankle and foot**

M06.272   Rheumatoid bursitis, left **ankle and foot**

M06.279   Rheumatoid bursitis, unspecified **ankle and foot**

M06.28   Rheumatoid bursitis, **vertebrae**

M06.29   Rheumatoid bursitis, **multiple sites**

✓5ᵗʰ   **M06.3   Rheumatoid nodule**

M06.30   Rheumatoid nodule, **unspecified site**

✓6ᵗʰ   M06.31   Rheumatoid nodule, **shoulder**

M06.311   Rheumatoid nodule, right **shoulder**

M06.312   Rheumatoid nodule, left **shoulder**

M06.319   Rheumatoid nodule, unspecified **shoulder**

✓6ᵗʰ   M06.32   Rheumatoid nodule, **elbow**

M06.321   Rheumatoid nodule, right **elbow**

M06.322   Rheumatoid nodule, left **elbow**

M06.329   Rheumatoid nodule, unspecified **elbow**

✓6ᵗʰ   M06.33   Rheumatoid nodule, **wrist**

M06.331   Rheumatoid nodule, right **wrist**

M06.332   Rheumatoid nodule, left **wrist**

M06.339   Rheumatoid nodule, unspecified **wrist**

✓6ᵗʰ   M06.34   Rheumatoid nodule, **hand**

M06.341   Rheumatoid nodule, right **hand**

M06.342   Rheumatoid nodule, left **hand**

M06.349   Rheumatoid nodule, unspecified **hand**

✓6ᵗʰ   M06.35   Rheumatoid nodule, **hip**

M06.351   Rheumatoid nodule, right **hip**

M06.352   Rheumatoid nodule, left **hip**

M06.359   Rheumatoid nodule, unspecified **hip**

✓6ᵗʰ   M06.36   Rheumatoid nodule, **knee**

M06.361   Rheumatoid nodule, right **knee**

M06.362   Rheumatoid nodule, left **knee**

M06.369   Rheumatoid nodule, unspecified **knee**

✓6ᵗʰ   M06.37   Rheumatoid nodule, **ankle and foot**

M06.371   Rheumatoid nodule, right **ankle and foot**

M06.372   Rheumatoid nodule, left **ankle and foot**

M06.379   Rheumatoid nodule, unspecified **ankle and foot**

M06.38   Rheumatoid nodule, **vertebrae**

M06.39   Rheumatoid nodule, **multiple sites**

M06.4   Inflammatory polyarthropathy

    EXCLUDES 1   *polyarthritis NOS (M13.0)*

✓5ᵗʰ   **M06.8   Other specified rheumatoid arthritis**

M06.80   Other specified rheumatoid arthritis, **unspecified site**

✓6ᵗʰ   M06.81   Other specified rheumatoid arthritis, **shoulder**

M06.811   Other specified rheumatoid arthritis, right **shoulder**

M06.812   Other specified rheumatoid arthritis, left **shoulder**

M06.819   Other specified rheumatoid arthritis, unspecified **shoulder**

✓6ᵗʰ   M06.82   Other specified rheumatoid arthritis, **elbow**

M06.821   Other specified rheumatoid arthritis, right **elbow**

M06.822   Other specified rheumatoid arthritis, left **elbow**

M06.829   Other specified rheumatoid arthritis, unspecified **elbow**

✓6ᵗʰ   M06.83   Other specified rheumatoid arthritis, **wrist**

M06.831   Other specified rheumatoid arthritis, right **wrist**

M06.832   Other specified rheumatoid arthritis, left **wrist**

M06.839   Other specified rheumatoid arthritis, unspecified **wrist**

✓6ᵗʰ   M06.84   Other specified rheumatoid arthritis, **hand**

M06.841   Other specified rheumatoid arthritis, right **hand**

M06.842   Other specified rheumatoid arthritis, left **hand**

M06.849   Other specified rheumatoid arthritis, unspecified **hand**

✓6ᵗʰ   M06.85   Other specified rheumatoid arthritis, **hip**

M06.851   Other specified rheumatoid arthritis, right **hip**

M06.852   Other specified rheumatoid arthritis, left **hip**

M06.859   Other specified rheumatoid arthritis, unspecified **hip**

✓6ᵗʰ   M06.86   Other specified rheumatoid arthritis, **knee**

M06.861   Other specified rheumatoid arthritis, right **knee**

M06.862   Other specified rheumatoid arthritis, left **knee**

M06.869   Other specified rheumatoid arthritis, unspecified **knee**

✓6ᵗʰ   M06.87   Other specified rheumatoid arthritis, **ankle and foot**

M06.871   Other specified rheumatoid arthritis, right **ankle and foot**

M06.872   Other specified rheumatoid arthritis, left **ankle and foot**

M06.879   Other specified rheumatoid arthritis, unspecified **ankle and foot**

M06.88   Other specified rheumatoid arthritis, **vertebrae**

M06.89   Other specified rheumatoid arthritis, **multiple sites**

M06.9   Rheumatoid arthritis, unspecified

✓4ᵗʰ   **M07   Enteropathic arthropathies**

    Code also associated enteropathy, such as:
    regional enteritis [Crohn's disease] (K50.-)
    ulcerative colitis (K51.-)

    EXCLUDES 1   *psoriatic arthropathies (L40.5-)*

✓5ᵗʰ   **M07.6   Enteropathic arthropathies**

M07.60   Enteropathic arthropathies, **unspecified site**

Ⓝ Newborn: 0   Ⓟ Pediatric: 0–17   Ⓜ Maternity: 12–55   Ⓐ Adult: 15–124   **MCC** Major CC Condition   **PDx MCC** PDx acts as own MCC   **CC** CC Condition   **PDx CC** PDx acts as own CC

716   ICD-10-CM 2016

✓6th **M07.61** **Enteropathic arthropathies,** shoulder
     M07.611 **Enteropathic arthropathies,** right shoulder
     M07.612 **Enteropathic arthropathies, left** shoulder
     M07.619 **Enteropathic arthropathies, unspecified** shoulder

✓6th **M07.62** **Enteropathic arthropathies,** elbow
     M07.621 **Enteropathic arthropathies, right** elbow
     M07.622 **Enteropathic arthropathies, left** elbow
     M07.629 **Enteropathic arthropathies, unspecified** elbow

✓6th **M07.63** **Enteropathic arthropathies,** wrist
     M07.631 **Enteropathic arthropathies, right** wrist
     M07.632 **Enteropathic arthropathies, left** wrist
     M07.639 **Enteropathic arthropathies, unspecified** wrist

✓6th **M07.64** **Enteropathic arthropathies,** hand
     M07.641 **Enteropathic arthropathies, right** hand
     M07.642 **Enteropathic arthropathies, left** hand
     M07.649 **Enteropathic arthropathies, unspecified** hand

✓6th **M07.65** **Enteropathic arthropathies,** hip
     M07.651 **Enteropathic arthropathies, right** hip
     M07.652 **Enteropathic arthropathies, left** hip
     M07.659 **Enteropathic arthropathies, unspecified** hip

✓6th **M07.66** **Enteropathic arthropathies,** knee
     M07.661 **Enteropathic arthropathies, right** knee
     M07.662 **Enteropathic arthropathies, left** knee
     M07.669 **Enteropathic arthropathies, unspecified** knee

✓6th **M07.67** **Enteropathic arthropathies,** ankle and foot
     M07.671 **Enteropathic arthropathies, right** ankle and foot
     M07.672 **Enteropathic arthropathies, left** ankle and foot
     M07.679 **Enteropathic arthropathies, unspecified** ankle and foot

     M07.68 **Enteropathic arthropathies,** vertebrae
     M07.69 **Enteropathic arthropathies,** multiple sites

✓4th **M08** **Juvenile arthritis**
Code also any associated underlying condition, such as:
     regional enteritis [Crohn's disease] (K50.-)
     ulcerative colitis (K51.-)
     EXCLUDES 1   arthropathy in Whipple's disease (M14.8)
             Felty's syndrome (M05.0)
             juvenile dermatomyositis (M33.0-)
             psoriatic juvenile arthropathy (L40.54)

✓5th **M08.0** **Unspecified juvenile** rheumatoid arthritis
Juvenile rheumatoid arthritis with or without rheumatoid factor
     M08.00 **Unspecified juvenile rheumatoid arthritis of** unspecified site

✓6th **M08.01** **Unspecified juvenile rheumatoid arthritis,** shoulder
     M08.011 **Unspecified juvenile rheumatoid arthritis, right** shoulder
     M08.012 **Unspecified juvenile rheumatoid arthritis, left** shoulder
     M08.019 **Unspecified juvenile rheumatoid arthritis, unspecified** shoulder

✓6th **M08.02** **Unspecified juvenile rheumatoid arthritis of** elbow
     M08.021 **Unspecified juvenile rheumatoid arthritis, right** elbow
     M08.022 **Unspecified juvenile rheumatoid arthritis, left** elbow
     M08.029 **Unspecified juvenile rheumatoid arthritis, unspecified** elbow

✓6th **M08.03** **Unspecified juvenile rheumatoid arthritis,** wrist
     M08.031 **Unspecified juvenile rheumatoid arthritis, right** wrist
     M08.032 **Unspecified juvenile rheumatoid arthritis, left** wrist
     M08.039 **Unspecified juvenile rheumatoid arthritis, unspecified** wrist

✓6th **M08.04** **Unspecified juvenile rheumatoid arthritis,** hand
     M08.041 **Unspecified juvenile rheumatoid arthritis, right** hand
     M08.042 **Unspecified juvenile rheumatoid arthritis, left** hand
     M08.049 **Unspecified juvenile rheumatoid arthritis, unspecified** hand

✓6th **M08.05** **Unspecified juvenile rheumatoid arthritis,** hip
     M08.051 **Unspecified juvenile rheumatoid arthritis, right** hip
     M08.052 **Unspecified juvenile rheumatoid arthritis, left** hip
     M08.059 **Unspecified juvenile rheumatoid arthritis, unspecified** hip

✓6th **M08.06** **Unspecified juvenile rheumatoid arthritis,** knee
     M08.061 **Unspecified juvenile rheumatoid arthritis, right** knee
     M08.062 **Unspecified juvenile rheumatoid arthritis, left** knee
     M08.069 **Unspecified juvenile rheumatoid arthritis, unspecified** knee

✓6th **M08.07** **Unspecified juvenile rheumatoid arthritis,** ankle and foot
     M08.071 **Unspecified juvenile rheumatoid arthritis, right** ankle and foot
     M08.072 **Unspecified juvenile rheumatoid arthritis, left** ankle and foot
     M08.079 **Unspecified juvenile rheumatoid arthritis, unspecified** ankle and foot

     M08.08 **Unspecified juvenile rheumatoid arthritis,** vertebrae
     M08.09 **Unspecified juvenile rheumatoid arthritis,** multiple sites

     M08.1 **Juvenile** ankylosing spondylitis
         EXCLUDES 1   ankylosing spondylitis in adults (M45.0-)

✓5th **M08.2** **Juvenile rheumatoid arthritis** with systemic onset
Still's disease NOS
         EXCLUDES 1   adult-onset Still's disease (M06.1-)

     M08.20 **Juvenile rheumatoid arthritis with systemic onset, unspecified site**

✓6th **M08.21** **Juvenile rheumatoid arthritis with systemic onset, shoulder**
     M08.211 **Juvenile rheumatoid arthritis with systemic onset, right shoulder**
     M08.212 **Juvenile rheumatoid arthritis with systemic onset, left shoulder**
     M08.219 **Juvenile rheumatoid arthritis with systemic onset, unspecified shoulder**

✓6th **M08.22** **Juvenile rheumatoid arthritis with systemic onset, elbow**
     M08.221 **Juvenile rheumatoid arthritis with systemic onset, right elbow**
     M08.222 **Juvenile rheumatoid arthritis with systemic onset, left elbow**
     M08.229 **Juvenile rheumatoid arthritis with systemic onset, unspecified elbow**

✓6th **M08.23** **Juvenile rheumatoid arthritis with systemic onset, wrist**
     M08.231 **Juvenile rheumatoid arthritis with systemic onset, right wrist**
     M08.232 **Juvenile rheumatoid arthritis with systemic onset, left wrist**
     M08.239 **Juvenile rheumatoid arthritis with systemic onset, unspecified wrist**

✓6th **M08.24** **Juvenile rheumatoid arthritis with systemic onset, hand**
     M08.241 **Juvenile rheumatoid arthritis with systemic onset, right hand**
     M08.242 **Juvenile rheumatoid arthritis with systemic onset, left hand**
     M08.249 **Juvenile rheumatoid arthritis with systemic onset, unspecified hand**

✓6th **M08.25** **Juvenile rheumatoid arthritis with systemic onset, hip**
     M08.251 **Juvenile rheumatoid arthritis with systemic onset, right hip**
     M08.252 **Juvenile rheumatoid arthritis with systemic onset, left hip**

M08.259 Juvenile rheumatoid arthritis with systemic onset, unspecified hip

✓6ᵗʰ **M08.26** Juvenile rheumatoid arthritis with systemic onset, knee

    M08.261 Juvenile rheumatoid arthritis with systemic onset, right knee

    M08.262 Juvenile rheumatoid arthritis with systemic onset, left knee

    M08.269 Juvenile rheumatoid arthritis with systemic onset, unspecified knee

✓6ᵗʰ **M08.27** Juvenile rheumatoid arthritis with systemic onset, ankle and foot

    M08.271 Juvenile rheumatoid arthritis with systemic onset, right ankle and foot

    M08.272 Juvenile rheumatoid arthritis with systemic onset, left ankle and foot

    M08.279 Juvenile rheumatoid arthritis with systemic onset, unspecified ankle and foot

M08.28 Juvenile rheumatoid arthritis with systemic onset, vertebrae

M08.29 Juvenile rheumatoid arthritis with systemic onset, multiple sites

M08.3 Juvenile rheumatoid polyarthritis (seronegative)

✓5ᵗʰ **M08.4** Pauciarticular juvenile rheumatoid arthritis

    M08.40 Pauciarticular juvenile rheumatoid arthritis, unspecified site

✓6ᵗʰ **M08.41** Pauciarticular juvenile rheumatoid arthritis, shoulder

    M08.411 Pauciarticular juvenile rheumatoid arthritis, right shoulder

    M08.412 Pauciarticular juvenile rheumatoid arthritis, left shoulder

    M08.419 Pauciarticular juvenile rheumatoid arthritis, unspecified shoulder

✓6ᵗʰ **M08.42** Pauciarticular juvenile rheumatoid arthritis, elbow

    M08.421 Pauciarticular juvenile rheumatoid arthritis, right elbow

    M08.422 Pauciarticular juvenile rheumatoid arthritis, left elbow

    M08.429 Pauciarticular juvenile rheumatoid arthritis, unspecified elbow

✓6ᵗʰ **M08.43** Pauciarticular juvenile rheumatoid arthritis, wrist

    M08.431 Pauciarticular juvenile rheumatoid arthritis, right wrist

    M08.432 Pauciarticular juvenile rheumatoid arthritis, left wrist

    M08.439 Pauciarticular juvenile rheumatoid arthritis, unspecified wrist

✓6ᵗʰ **M08.44** Pauciarticular juvenile rheumatoid arthritis, hand

    M08.441 Pauciarticular juvenile rheumatoid arthritis, right hand

    M08.442 Pauciarticular juvenile rheumatoid arthritis, left hand

    M08.449 Pauciarticular juvenile rheumatoid arthritis, unspecified hand

✓6ᵗʰ **M08.45** Pauciarticular juvenile rheumatoid arthritis, hip

    M08.451 Pauciarticular juvenile rheumatoid arthritis, right hip

    M08.452 Pauciarticular juvenile rheumatoid arthritis, left hip

    M08.459 Pauciarticular juvenile rheumatoid arthritis, unspecified hip

✓6ᵗʰ **M08.46** Pauciarticular juvenile rheumatoid arthritis, knee

    M08.461 Pauciarticular juvenile rheumatoid arthritis, right knee

    M08.462 Pauciarticular juvenile rheumatoid arthritis, left knee

    M08.469 Pauciarticular juvenile rheumatoid arthritis, unspecified knee

✓6ᵗʰ **M08.47** Pauciarticular juvenile rheumatoid arthritis, ankle and foot

    M08.471 Pauciarticular juvenile rheumatoid arthritis, right ankle and foot

    M08.472 Pauciarticular juvenile rheumatoid arthritis, left ankle and foot

    M08.479 Pauciarticular juvenile rheumatoid arthritis, unspecified ankle and foot

M08.48 Pauciarticular juvenile rheumatoid arthritis, vertebrae

✓5ᵗʰ **M08.8** Other juvenile arthritis

    M08.80 Other juvenile arthritis, unspecified site

✓6ᵗʰ **M08.81** Other juvenile arthritis, shoulder

    M08.811 Other juvenile arthritis, right shoulder

    M08.812 Other juvenile arthritis, left shoulder

    M08.819 Other juvenile arthritis, unspecified shoulder

✓6ᵗʰ **M08.82** Other juvenile arthritis, elbow

    M08.821 Other juvenile arthritis, right elbow

    M08.822 Other juvenile arthritis, left elbow

    M08.829 Other juvenile arthritis, unspecified elbow

✓6ᵗʰ **M08.83** Other juvenile arthritis, wrist

    M08.831 Other juvenile arthritis, right wrist

    M08.832 Other juvenile arthritis, left wrist

    M08.839 Other juvenile arthritis, unspecified wrist

✓6ᵗʰ **M08.84** Other juvenile arthritis, hand

    M08.841 Other juvenile arthritis, right hand

    M08.842 Other juvenile arthritis, left hand

    M08.849 Other juvenile arthritis, unspecified hand

✓6ᵗʰ **M08.85** Other juvenile arthritis, hip

    M08.851 Other juvenile arthritis, right hip

    M08.852 Other juvenile arthritis, left hip

    M08.859 Other juvenile arthritis, unspecified hip

✓6ᵗʰ **M08.86** Other juvenile arthritis, knee

    M08.861 Other juvenile arthritis, right knee

    M08.862 Other juvenile arthritis, left knee

    M08.869 Other juvenile arthritis, unspecified knee

✓6ᵗʰ **M08.87** Other juvenile arthritis, ankle and foot

    M08.871 Other juvenile arthritis, right ankle and foot

    M08.872 Other juvenile arthritis, left ankle and foot

    M08.879 Other juvenile arthritis, unspecified ankle and foot

M08.88 Other juvenile arthritis, other specified site
    Other juvenile arthritis, vertebrae

M08.89 Other juvenile arthritis, multiple sites

✓5ᵗʰ **M08.9** Juvenile arthritis, unspecified

    EXCLUDES 1   *juvenile rheumatoid arthritis, unspecified (M08.0-)*

    M08.90 Juvenile arthritis, unspecified, unspecified site

✓6ᵗʰ **M08.91** Juvenile arthritis, unspecified, shoulder

    M08.911 Juvenile arthritis, unspecified, right shoulder

    M08.912 Juvenile arthritis, unspecified, left shoulder

    M08.919 Juvenile arthritis, unspecified, unspecified shoulder

✓6ᵗʰ **M08.92** Juvenile arthritis, unspecified, elbow

    M08.921 Juvenile arthritis, unspecified, right elbow

    M08.922 Juvenile arthritis, unspecified, left elbow

    M08.929 Juvenile arthritis, unspecified, unspecified elbow

✓6ᵗʰ **M08.93** Juvenile arthritis, unspecified, wrist

    M08.931 Juvenile arthritis, unspecified, right wrist

    M08.932 Juvenile arthritis, unspecified, left wrist

    M08.939 Juvenile arthritis, unspecified, unspecified wrist

✓6ᵗʰ **M08.94** Juvenile arthritis, unspecified, hand

    M08.941 Juvenile arthritis, unspecified, right hand

    M08.942 Juvenile arthritis, unspecified, left hand

    M08.949 Juvenile arthritis, unspecified, unspecified hand

✓6ᵗʰ **M08.95** Juvenile arthritis, unspecified, hip

    M08.951 Juvenile arthritis, unspecified, right hip

    M08.952 Juvenile arthritis, unspecified, left hip

    M08.959 Juvenile arthritis, unspecified, unspecified hip

✓6ᵗʰ **M08.96** Juvenile arthritis, unspecified, knee

    M08.961 Juvenile arthritis, unspecified, right knee

    M08.962 Juvenile arthritis, unspecified, left knee

    M08.969 Juvenile arthritis, unspecified, unspecified knee

Ⓝ Newborn: 0   Ⓟ Pediatric: 0-17   Ⓜ Maternity: 12-55   Ⓐ Adult: 15-124   **MCC** Major CC Condition   **PDxMCC** PDx acts as own MCC   **CC** CC Condition   **PDxCC** PDx acts as own CC

718   ICD-10-CM 2016

✓6th **M08.97** Juvenile arthritis, unspecified, ankle and foot

     M08.971 Juvenile arthritis, unspecified, right ankle and foot

     M08.972 Juvenile arthritis, unspecified, left ankle and foot

     M08.979 Juvenile arthritis, unspecified, unspecified ankle and foot

     M08.98 Juvenile arthritis, unspecified, vertebrae

     M08.99 Juvenile arthritis, unspecified, multiple sites

✓4th **M1A Chronic gout**

     Use additional code to identify:

         autonomic neuropathy in diseases classified elsewhere (G99.0)

         calculus of urinary tract in diseases classified elsewhere (N22)

         cardiomyopathy in diseases classified elsewhere (I43)

         disorders of external ear in diseases classified elsewhere (H61.1-, H62.8-)

         disorders of iris and ciliary body in diseases classified elsewhere (H22)

         glomerular disorders in diseases classified elsewhere (N08)

     EXCLUDES 1   acute gout (M10.-)

              gout NOS (M10.-)

> The appropriate 7th character is to be added to each code from category M1A.
> 0   without tophus (tophi)
> 1   with tophus (tophi)

✓5th **M1A.0 Idiopathic chronic gout**

     Chronic gouty bursitis

     Primary chronic gout

     ✓x7th **M1A.00** Idiopathic chronic gout, unspecified site

     ✓6th **M1A.01** Idiopathic chronic gout, shoulder

         ✓7th **M1A.011** Idiopathic chronic gout, right shoulder

         ✓7th **M1A.012** Idiopathic chronic gout, left shoulder

         ✓7th **M1A.019** Idiopathic chronic gout, unspecified shoulder

     ✓6th **M1A.02** Idiopathic chronic gout, elbow

         ✓7th **M1A.021** Idiopathic chronic gout, right elbow

         ✓7th **M1A.022** Idiopathic chronic gout, left elbow

         ✓7th **M1A.029** Idiopathic chronic gout, unspecified elbow

     ✓6th **M1A.03** Idiopathic chronic gout, wrist

         ✓7th **M1A.031** Idiopathic chronic gout, right wrist

         ✓7th **M1A.032** Idiopathic chronic gout, left wrist

         ✓7th **M1A.039** Idiopathic chronic gout, unspecified wrist

     ✓6th **M1A.04** Idiopathic chronic gout, hand

         ✓7th **M1A.041** Idiopathic chronic gout, right hand

         ✓7th **M1A.042** Idiopathic chronic gout, left hand

         ✓7th **M1A.049** Idiopathic chronic gout, unspecified hand

     ✓6th **M1A.05** Idiopathic chronic gout, hip

         ✓7th **M1A.051** Idiopathic chronic gout, right hip

         ✓7th **M1A.052** Idiopathic chronic gout, left hip

         ✓7th **M1A.059** Idiopathic chronic gout, unspecified hip

     ✓6th **M1A.06** Idiopathic chronic gout, knee

         ✓7th **M1A.061** Idiopathic chronic gout, right knee

         ✓7th **M1A.062** Idiopathic chronic gout, left knee

         ✓7th **M1A.069** Idiopathic chronic gout, unspecified knee

     ✓6th **M1A.07** Idiopathic chronic gout, ankle and foot

         ✓7th **M1A.071** Idiopathic chronic gout, right ankle and foot

         ✓7th **M1A.072** Idiopathic chronic gout, left ankle and foot

         ✓7th **M1A.079** Idiopathic chronic gout, unspecified ankle and foot

     ✓x7th **M1A.08** Idiopathic chronic gout, vertebrae

     ✓x7th **M1A.09** Idiopathic chronic gout, multiple sites

✓5th **M1A.1 Lead-induced chronic gout**

     Code first toxic effects of lead and its compounds (T56.0-)

     ✓x7th **M1A.10** Lead-induced chronic gout, unspecified site

     ✓6th **M1A.11** Lead-induced chronic gout, shoulder

         ✓7th **M1A.111** Lead-induced chronic gout, right shoulder

         ✓7th **M1A.112** Lead-induced chronic gout, left shoulder

         ✓7th **M1A.119** Lead-induced chronic gout, unspecified shoulder

     ✓6th **M1A.12** Lead-induced chronic gout, elbow

         ✓7th **M1A.121** Lead-induced chronic gout, right elbow

         ✓7th **M1A.122** Lead-induced chronic gout, left elbow

         ✓7th **M1A.129** Lead-induced chronic gout, unspecified elbow

     ✓6th **M1A.13** Lead-induced chronic gout, wrist

         ✓7th **M1A.131** Lead-induced chronic gout, right wrist

         ✓7th **M1A.132** Lead-induced chronic gout, left wrist

         ✓7th **M1A.139** Lead-induced chronic gout, unspecified wrist

     ✓6th **M1A.14** Lead-induced chronic gout, hand

         ✓7th **M1A.141** Lead-induced chronic gout, right hand

         ✓7th **M1A.142** Lead-induced chronic gout, left hand

         ✓7th **M1A.149** Lead-induced chronic gout, unspecified hand

     ✓6th **M1A.15** Lead-induced chronic gout, hip

         ✓7th **M1A.151** Lead-induced chronic gout, right hip

         ✓7th **M1A.152** Lead-induced chronic gout, left hip

         ✓7th **M1A.159** Lead-induced chronic gout, unspecified hip

     ✓6th **M1A.16** Lead-induced chronic gout, knee

         ✓7th **M1A.161** Lead-induced chronic gout, right knee

         ✓7th **M1A.162** Lead-induced chronic gout, left knee

         ✓7th **M1A.169** Lead-induced chronic gout, unspecified knee

     ✓6th **M1A.17** Lead-induced chronic gout, ankle and foot

         ✓7th **M1A.171** Lead-induced chronic gout, right ankle and foot

         ✓7th **M1A.172** Lead-induced chronic gout, left ankle and foot

         ✓7th **M1A.179** Lead-induced chronic gout, unspecified ankle and foot

     ✓x7th **M1A.18** Lead-induced chronic gout, vertebrae

     ✓x7th **M1A.19** Lead-induced chronic gout, multiple sites

✓5th **M1A.2 Drug-induced chronic gout**

     Use additional code for adverse effect, if applicable, to identify drug (T36-T50 with fifth or sixth character 5)

     ✓x7th **M1A.20** Drug-induced chronic gout, unspecified site

     ✓6th **M1A.21** Drug-induced chronic gout, shoulder

         ✓7th **M1A.211** Drug-induced chronic gout, right shoulder

         ✓7th **M1A.212** Drug-induced chronic gout, left shoulder

         ✓7th **M1A.219** Drug-induced chronic gout, unspecified shoulder

     ✓6th **M1A.22** Drug-induced chronic gout, elbow

         ✓7th **M1A.221** Drug-induced chronic gout, right elbow

         ✓7th **M1A.222** Drug-induced chronic gout, left elbow

         ✓7th **M1A.229** Drug-induced chronic gout, unspecified elbow

     ✓6th **M1A.23** Drug-induced chronic gout, wrist

         ✓7th **M1A.231** Drug-induced chronic gout, right wrist

         ✓7th **M1A.232** Drug-induced chronic gout, left wrist

         ✓7th **M1A.239** Drug-induced chronic gout, unspecified wrist

     ✓6th **M1A.24** Drug-induced chronic gout, hand

         ✓7th **M1A.241** Drug-induced chronic gout, right hand

         ✓7th **M1A.242** Drug-induced chronic gout, left hand

         ✓7th **M1A.249** Drug-induced chronic gout, unspecified hand

     ✓6th **M1A.25** Drug-induced chronic gout, hip

         ✓7th **M1A.251** Drug-induced chronic gout, right hip

         ✓7th **M1A.252** Drug-induced chronic gout, left hip

         ✓7th **M1A.259** Drug-induced chronic gout, unspecified hip

     ✓6th **M1A.26** Drug-induced chronic gout, knee

         ✓7th **M1A.261** Drug-induced chronic gout, right knee

         ✓7th **M1A.262** Drug-induced chronic gout, left knee

         ✓7th **M1A.269** Drug-induced chronic gout, unspecified knee

---

✓ Additional Character Required   ✓x7th Placeholder Alert   Unacceptable PDx   Manifestation   Hospital Acquired Condition   **EXCLUDES 1** Not Coded Here   **EXCLUDES 2** Not Included Here

Chapter 13. Diseases of the Musculoskeletal System and Connective Tissue

√6ᵗʰ **M1A.27 Drug-induced chronic gout,** ankle and foot

    √7ᵗʰ **M1A.271 Drug-induced chronic gout, right** ankle and foot

    √7ᵗʰ **M1A.272 Drug-induced chronic gout, left** ankle and foot

    √7ᵗʰ **M1A.279 Drug-induced chronic gout,** unspecified ankle and foot

√x7ᵗʰ **M1A.28 Drug-induced chronic gout,** vertebrae

√x7ᵗʰ **M1A.29 Drug-induced chronic gout,** multiple sites

√5ᵗʰ **M1A.3 Chronic gout** due to renal impairment

    Code first associated renal disease

√x7ᵗʰ **M1A.30 Chronic gout due to renal impairment,** unspecified site

√6ᵗʰ **M1A.31 Chronic gout due to renal impairment,** shoulder

    √7ᵗʰ **M1A.311 Chronic gout due to renal impairment, right** shoulder

    √7ᵗʰ **M1A.312 Chronic gout due to renal impairment, left** shoulder

    √7ᵗʰ **M1A.319 Chronic gout due to renal impairment, unspecified** shoulder

√6ᵗʰ **M1A.32 Chronic gout due to renal impairment,** elbow

    √7ᵗʰ **M1A.321 Chronic gout due to renal impairment, right** elbow

    √7ᵗʰ **M1A.322 Chronic gout due to renal impairment, left** elbow

    √7ᵗʰ **M1A.329 Chronic gout due to renal impairment, unspecified** elbow

√6ᵗʰ **M1A.33 Chronic gout due to renal impairment,** wrist

    √7ᵗʰ **M1A.331 Chronic gout due to renal impairment, right** wrist

    √7ᵗʰ **M1A.332 Chronic gout due to renal impairment, left** wrist

    √7ᵗʰ **M1A.339 Chronic gout due to renal impairment, unspecified** wrist

√6ᵗʰ **M1A.34 Chronic gout due to renal impairment,** hand

    √7ᵗʰ **M1A.341 Chronic gout due to renal impairment, right** hand

    √7ᵗʰ **M1A.342 Chronic gout due to renal impairment, left** hand

    √7ᵗʰ **M1A.349 Chronic gout due to renal impairment, unspecified** hand

√6ᵗʰ **M1A.35 Chronic gout due to renal impairment,** hip

    √7ᵗʰ **M1A.351 Chronic gout due to renal impairment, right** hip

    √7ᵗʰ **M1A.352 Chronic gout due to renal impairment, left** hip

    √7ᵗʰ **M1A.359 Chronic gout due to renal impairment, unspecified** hip

√6ᵗʰ **M1A.36 Chronic gout due to renal impairment,** knee

    √7ᵗʰ **M1A.361 Chronic gout due to renal impairment, right** knee

    √7ᵗʰ **M1A.362 Chronic gout due to renal impairment, left** knee

    √7ᵗʰ **M1A.369 Chronic gout due to renal impairment, unspecified** knee

√6ᵗʰ **M1A.37 Chronic gout due to renal impairment,** ankle and foot

    √7ᵗʰ **M1A.371 Chronic gout due to renal impairment, right** ankle and foot

    √7ᵗʰ **M1A.372 Chronic gout due to renal impairment, left** ankle and foot

    √7ᵗʰ **M1A.379 Chronic gout due to renal impairment, unspecified** ankle and foot

√x7ᵗʰ **M1A.38 Chronic gout due to renal impairment,** vertebrae

√x7ᵗʰ **M1A.39 Chronic gout due to renal impairment,** multiple sites

√5ᵗʰ **M1A.4 Other secondary chronic gout**

    Code first associated condition

√x7ᵗʰ **M1A.40 Other secondary chronic gout,** unspecified site

√6ᵗʰ **M1A.41 Other secondary chronic gout,** shoulder

    √7ᵗʰ **M1A.411 Other secondary chronic gout, right** shoulder

    √7ᵗʰ **M1A.412 Other secondary chronic gout, left** shoulder

    √7ᵗʰ **M1A.419 Other secondary chronic gout,** unspecified shoulder

√6ᵗʰ **M1A.42 Other secondary chronic gout,** elbow

    √7ᵗʰ **M1A.421 Other secondary chronic gout, right** elbow

    √7ᵗʰ **M1A.422 Other secondary chronic gout, left** elbow

    √7ᵗʰ **M1A.429 Other secondary chronic gout, unspecified** elbow

√6ᵗʰ **M1A.43 Other secondary chronic gout,** wrist

    √7ᵗʰ **M1A.431 Other secondary chronic gout, right** wrist

    √7ᵗʰ **M1A.432 Other secondary chronic gout, left** wrist

    √7ᵗʰ **M1A.439 Other secondary chronic gout, unspecified** wrist

√6ᵗʰ **M1A.44 Other secondary chronic gout,** hand

    √7ᵗʰ **M1A.441 Other secondary chronic gout, right** hand

    √7ᵗʰ **M1A.442 Other secondary chronic gout, left** hand

    √7ᵗʰ **M1A.449 Other secondary chronic gout, unspecified** hand

√6ᵗʰ **M1A.45 Other secondary chronic gout,** hip

    √7ᵗʰ **M1A.451 Other secondary chronic gout, right** hip

    √7ᵗʰ **M1A.452 Other secondary chronic gout, left** hip

    √7ᵗʰ **M1A.459 Other secondary chronic gout, unspecified** hip

√6ᵗʰ **M1A.46 Other secondary chronic gout,** knee

    √7ᵗʰ **M1A.461 Other secondary chronic gout, right** knee

    √7ᵗʰ **M1A.462 Other secondary chronic gout, left** knee

    √7ᵗʰ **M1A.469 Other secondary chronic gout, unspecified** knee

√6ᵗʰ **M1A.47 Other secondary chronic gout,** ankle and foot

    √7ᵗʰ **M1A.471 Other secondary chronic gout, right** ankle and foot

    √7ᵗʰ **M1A.472 Other secondary chronic gout, left** ankle and foot

    √7ᵗʰ **M1A.479 Other secondary chronic gout,** unspecified ankle and foot

√x7ᵗʰ **M1A.48 Other secondary chronic gout,** vertebrae

√x7ᵗʰ **M1A.49 Other secondary chronic gout,** multiple sites

√x7ᵗʰ **M1A.9 Chronic gout,** unspecified

√4ᵗʰ **M10 Gout**

    Acute gout   Gout NOS
    Gout attack   Podagra
    Gout flare

    Use additional code to identify:
      autonomic neuropathy in diseases classified elsewhere (G99.0)
      calculus of urinary tract in diseases classified elsewhere (N22)
      cardiomyopathy in diseases classified elsewhere (I43)
      disorders of external ear in diseases classified elsewhere (H61.1-, H62.8-)
      disorders of iris and ciliary body in diseases classified elsewhere (H22)
      glomerular disorders in diseases classified elsewhere (N08)

    EXCLUDES 1   chronic gout (M1A.-)

√5ᵗʰ **M10.0 Idiopathic gout**

    Gouty bursitis
    Primary gout

    M10.00 Idiopathic gout, unspecified site

√6ᵗʰ **M10.01 Idiopathic gout,** shoulder

    M10.011 Idiopathic gout, right shoulder

    M10.012 Idiopathic gout, left shoulder

    M10.019 Idiopathic gout, unspecified shoulder

√6ᵗʰ **M10.02 Idiopathic gout,** elbow

    M10.021 Idiopathic gout, right elbow

    M10.022 Idiopathic gout, left elbow

    M10.029 Idiopathic gout, unspecified elbow

√6ᵗʰ **M10.03 Idiopathic gout,** wrist

    M10.031 Idiopathic gout, right wrist

    M10.032 Idiopathic gout, left wrist

    M10.039 Idiopathic gout, unspecified wrist

√6ᵗʰ **M10.04 Idiopathic gout,** hand

    M10.041 Idiopathic gout, right hand

    M10.042 Idiopathic gout, left hand

    M10.049 Idiopathic gout, unspecified hand

√6ᵗʰ **M10.05 Idiopathic gout,** hip

    M10.051 Idiopathic gout, right hip

N Newborn: 0   P Pediatric: 0-17   M Maternity: 12-55   A Adult: 15-124   MCC Major CC Condition   PDxMCC PDx acts as own MCC   CC CC Condition   PDxCC PDx acts as own CC

720   ICD-10-CM 2016

M10.052 Idiopathic gout, left hip
M10.059 Idiopathic gout, unspecified hip
√6ᵗʰ M10.06 Idiopathic gout, knee
M10.061 Idiopathic gout, right knee
M10.062 Idiopathic gout, left knee
M10.069 Idiopathic gout, unspecified knee
√6ᵗʰ M10.07 Idiopathic gout, ankle and foot
M10.071 Idiopathic gout, right ankle and foot
M10.072 Idiopathic gout, left ankle and foot
M10.079 Idiopathic gout, unspecified ankle and foot
M10.08 Idiopathic gout, vertebrae
M10.09 Idiopathic gout, multiple sites
√5ᵗʰ M10.1 Lead-induced gout
Code first toxic effects of lead and its compounds (T56.0-)
M10.10 Lead-induced gout, unspecified site
√6ᵗʰ M10.11 Lead-induced gout, shoulder
M10.111 Lead-induced gout, right shoulder
M10.112 Lead-induced gout, left shoulder
M10.119 Lead-induced gout, unspecified shoulder
√6ᵗʰ M10.12 Lead-induced gout, elbow
M10.121 Lead-induced gout, right elbow
M10.122 Lead-induced gout, left elbow
M10.129 Lead-induced gout, unspecified elbow
√6ᵗʰ M10.13 Lead-induced gout, wrist
M10.131 Lead-induced gout, right wrist
M10.132 Lead-induced gout, left wrist
M10.139 Lead-induced gout, unspecified wrist
√6ᵗʰ M10.14 Lead-induced gout, hand
M10.141 Lead-induced gout, right hand
M10.142 Lead-induced gout, left hand
M10.149 Lead-induced gout, unspecified hand
√6ᵗʰ M10.15 Lead-induced gout, hip
M10.151 Lead-induced gout, right hip
M10.152 Lead-induced gout, left hip
M10.159 Lead-induced gout, unspecified hip
√6ᵗʰ M10.16 Lead-induced gout, knee
M10.161 Lead-induced gout, right knee
M10.162 Lead-induced gout, left knee
M10.169 Lead-induced gout, unspecified knee
√6ᵗʰ M10.17 Lead-induced gout, ankle and foot
M10.171 Lead-induced gout, right ankle and foot
M10.172 Lead-induced gout, left ankle and foot
M10.179 Lead-induced gout, unspecified ankle and foot
M10.18 Lead-induced gout, vertebrae
M10.19 Lead-induced gout, multiple sites
√5ᵗʰ M10.2 Drug-induced gout
Use additional code for adverse effect, if applicable, to identify drug (T36-T50 with fifth or sixth character 5)
M10.20 Drug-induced gout, unspecified site
√6ᵗʰ M10.21 Drug-induced gout, shoulder
M10.211 Drug-induced gout, right shoulder
M10.212 Drug-induced gout, left shoulder
M10.219 Drug-induced gout, unspecified shoulder
√6ᵗʰ M10.22 Drug-induced gout, elbow
M10.221 Drug-induced gout, right elbow
M10.222 Drug-induced gout, left elbow
M10.229 Drug-induced gout, unspecified elbow
√6ᵗʰ M10.23 Drug-induced gout, wrist
M10.231 Drug-induced gout, right wrist
M10.232 Drug-induced gout, left wrist
M10.239 Drug-induced gout, unspecified wrist
√6ᵗʰ M10.24 Drug-induced gout, hand
M10.241 Drug-induced gout, right hand
M10.242 Drug-induced gout, left hand
M10.249 Drug-induced gout, unspecified hand
√6ᵗʰ M10.25 Drug-induced gout, hip
M10.251 Drug-induced gout, right hip
M10.252 Drug-induced gout, left hip
M10.259 Drug-induced gout, unspecified hip

√6ᵗʰ M10.26 Drug-induced gout, knee
M10.261 Drug-induced gout, right knee
M10.262 Drug-induced gout, left knee
M10.269 Drug-induced gout, unspecified knee
√6ᵗʰ M10.27 Drug-induced gout, ankle and foot
M10.271 Drug-induced gout, right ankle and foot
M10.272 Drug-induced gout, left ankle and foot
M10.279 Drug-induced gout, unspecified ankle and foot
M10.28 Drug-induced gout, vertebrae
M10.29 Drug-induced gout, multiple sites
√5ᵗʰ M10.3 Gout due to renal impairment
Code first associated renal disease
M10.30 Gout due to renal impairment, unspecified site
√6ᵗʰ M10.31 Gout due to renal impairment, shoulder
M10.311 Gout due to renal impairment, right shoulder
M10.312 Gout due to renal impairment, left shoulder
M10.319 Gout due to renal impairment, unspecified shoulder
√6ᵗʰ M10.32 Gout due to renal impairment, elbow
M10.321 Gout due to renal impairment, right elbow
M10.322 Gout due to renal impairment, left elbow
M10.329 Gout due to renal impairment, unspecified elbow
√6ᵗʰ M10.33 Gout due to renal impairment, wrist
M10.331 Gout due to renal impairment, right wrist
M10.332 Gout due to renal impairment, left wrist
M10.339 Gout due to renal impairment, unspecified wrist
√6ᵗʰ M10.34 Gout due to renal impairment, hand
M10.341 Gout due to renal impairment, right hand
M10.342 Gout due to renal impairment, left hand
M10.349 Gout due to renal impairment, unspecified hand
√6ᵗʰ M10.35 Gout due to renal impairment, hip
M10.351 Gout due to renal impairment, right hip
M10.352 Gout due to renal impairment, left hip
M10.359 Gout due to renal impairment, unspecified hip
√6ᵗʰ M10.36 Gout due to renal impairment, knee
M10.361 Gout due to renal impairment, right knee
M10.362 Gout due to renal impairment, left knee
M10.369 Gout due to renal impairment, unspecified knee
√6ᵗʰ M10.37 Gout due to renal impairment, ankle and foot
M10.371 Gout due to renal impairment, right ankle and foot
M10.372 Gout due to renal impairment, left ankle and foot
M10.379 Gout due to renal impairment, unspecified ankle and foot
M10.38 Gout due to renal impairment, vertebrae
M10.39 Gout due to renal impairment, multiple sites
√5ᵗʰ M10.4 Other secondary gout
Code first associated condition
M10.40 Other secondary gout, unspecified site
√6ᵗʰ M10.41 Other secondary gout, shoulder
M10.411 Other secondary gout, right shoulder
M10.412 Other secondary gout, left shoulder
M10.419 Other secondary gout, unspecified shoulder
√6ᵗʰ M10.42 Other secondary gout, elbow
M10.421 Other secondary gout, right elbow
M10.422 Other secondary gout, left elbow
M10.429 Other secondary gout, unspecified elbow
√6ᵗʰ M10.43 Other secondary gout, wrist
M10.431 Other secondary gout, right wrist
M10.432 Other secondary gout, left wrist
M10.439 Other secondary gout, unspecified wrist
√6ᵗʰ M10.44 Other secondary gout, hand
M10.441 Other secondary gout, right hand

✓ Additional Character Required   ✓x7ᵗʰ Placeholder Alert   Unacceptable PDx   Manifestation   Hospital Acquired Condition   **EXCLUDES 1** Not Coded Here   **EXCLUDES 2** Not Included Here

(Left margin: Chapter 13. Diseases of the Musculoskeletal System and Connective Tissue — M10.442–M11.27)

        M10.442   Other secondary gout, left hand
        M10.449   Other secondary gout, unspecified hand

√6ᵗʰ   M10.45   Other secondary gout, hip
        M10.451   Other secondary gout, right hip
        M10.452   Other secondary gout, left hip
        M10.459   Other secondary gout, unspecified hip

√6ᵗʰ   M10.46   Other secondary gout, knee
        M10.461   Other secondary gout, right knee
        M10.462   Other secondary gout, left knee
        M10.469   Other secondary gout, unspecified knee

√6ᵗʰ   M10.47   Other secondary gout, ankle and foot
        M10.471   Other secondary gout, right ankle and foot
        M10.472   Other secondary gout, left ankle and foot
        M10.479   Other secondary gout, unspecified ankle and foot

    M10.48   Other secondary gout, vertebrae
    M10.49   Other secondary gout, multiple sites

M10.9   Gout, unspecified
    Gout NOS

√4ᵗʰ   **M11   Other crystal arthropathies**

√5ᵗʰ   M11.0   Hydroxyapatite deposition disease
    M11.00   Hydroxyapatite deposition disease, unspecified site

√6ᵗʰ   M11.01   Hydroxyapatite deposition disease, shoulder
        M11.011   Hydroxyapatite deposition disease, right shoulder
        M11.012   Hydroxyapatite deposition disease, left shoulder
        M11.019   Hydroxyapatite deposition disease, unspecified shoulder

√6ᵗʰ   M11.02   Hydroxyapatite deposition disease, elbow
        M11.021   Hydroxyapatite deposition disease, right elbow
        M11.022   Hydroxyapatite deposition disease, left elbow
        M11.029   Hydroxyapatite deposition disease, unspecified elbow

√6ᵗʰ   M11.03   Hydroxyapatite deposition disease, wrist
        M11.031   Hydroxyapatite deposition disease, right wrist
        M11.032   Hydroxyapatite deposition disease, left wrist
        M11.039   Hydroxyapatite deposition disease, unspecified wrist

√6ᵗʰ   M11.04   Hydroxyapatite deposition disease, hand
        M11.041   Hydroxyapatite deposition disease, right hand
        M11.042   Hydroxyapatite deposition disease, left hand
        M11.049   Hydroxyapatite deposition disease, unspecified hand

√6ᵗʰ   M11.05   Hydroxyapatite deposition disease, hip
        M11.051   Hydroxyapatite deposition disease, right hip
        M11.052   Hydroxyapatite deposition disease, left hip
        M11.059   Hydroxyapatite deposition disease, unspecified hip

√6ᵗʰ   M11.06   Hydroxyapatite deposition disease, knee
        M11.061   Hydroxyapatite deposition disease, right knee
        M11.062   Hydroxyapatite deposition disease, left knee
        M11.069   Hydroxyapatite deposition disease, unspecified knee

√6ᵗʰ   M11.07   Hydroxyapatite deposition disease, ankle and foot
        M11.071   Hydroxyapatite deposition disease, right ankle and foot
        M11.072   Hydroxyapatite deposition disease, left ankle and foot
        M11.079   Hydroxyapatite deposition disease, unspecified ankle and foot

    M11.08   Hydroxyapatite deposition disease, vertebrae
    M11.09   Hydroxyapatite deposition disease, multiple sites

√5ᵗʰ   M11.1   Familial chondrocalcinosis
    M11.10   Familial chondrocalcinosis, unspecified site

√6ᵗʰ   M11.11   Familial chondrocalcinosis, shoulder
        M11.111   Familial chondrocalcinosis, right shoulder
        M11.112   Familial chondrocalcinosis, left shoulder
        M11.119   Familial chondrocalcinosis, unspecified shoulder

√6ᵗʰ   M11.12   Familial chondrocalcinosis, elbow
        M11.121   Familial chondrocalcinosis, right elbow
        M11.122   Familial chondrocalcinosis, left elbow
        M11.129   Familial chondrocalcinosis, unspecified elbow

√6ᵗʰ   M11.13   Familial chondrocalcinosis, wrist
        M11.131   Familial chondrocalcinosis, right wrist
        M11.132   Familial chondrocalcinosis, left wrist
        M11.139   Familial chondrocalcinosis, unspecified wrist

√6ᵗʰ   M11.14   Familial chondrocalcinosis, hand
        M11.141   Familial chondrocalcinosis, right hand
        M11.142   Familial chondrocalcinosis, left hand
        M11.149   Familial chondrocalcinosis, unspecified hand

√6ᵗʰ   M11.15   Familial chondrocalcinosis, hip
        M11.151   Familial chondrocalcinosis, right hip
        M11.152   Familial chondrocalcinosis, left hip
        M11.159   Familial chondrocalcinosis, unspecified hip

√6ᵗʰ   M11.16   Familial chondrocalcinosis, knee
        M11.161   Familial chondrocalcinosis, right knee
        M11.162   Familial chondrocalcinosis, left knee
        M11.169   Familial chondrocalcinosis, unspecified knee

√6ᵗʰ   M11.17   Familial chondrocalcinosis, ankle and foot
        M11.171   Familial chondrocalcinosis, right ankle and foot
        M11.172   Familial chondrocalcinosis, left ankle and foot
        M11.179   Familial chondrocalcinosis, unspecified ankle and foot

    M11.18   Familial chondrocalcinosis, vertebrae
    M11.19   Familial chondrocalcinosis, multiple sites

√5ᵗʰ   M11.2   Other chondrocalcinosis
    Chondrocalcinosis NOS
    M11.20   Other chondrocalcinosis, unspecified site

√6ᵗʰ   M11.21   Other chondrocalcinosis, shoulder
        M11.211   Other chondrocalcinosis, right shoulder
        M11.212   Other chondrocalcinosis, left shoulder
        M11.219   Other chondrocalcinosis, unspecified shoulder

√6ᵗʰ   M11.22   Other chondrocalcinosis, elbow
        M11.221   Other chondrocalcinosis, right elbow
        M11.222   Other chondrocalcinosis, left elbow
        M11.229   Other chondrocalcinosis, unspecified elbow

√6ᵗʰ   M11.23   Other chondrocalcinosis, wrist
        M11.231   Other chondrocalcinosis, right wrist
        M11.232   Other chondrocalcinosis, left wrist
        M11.239   Other chondrocalcinosis, unspecified wrist

√6ᵗʰ   M11.24   Other chondrocalcinosis, hand
        M11.241   Other chondrocalcinosis, right hand
        M11.242   Other chondrocalcinosis, left hand
        M11.249   Other chondrocalcinosis, unspecified hand

√6ᵗʰ   M11.25   Other chondrocalcinosis, hip
        M11.251   Other chondrocalcinosis, right hip
        M11.252   Other chondrocalcinosis, left hip
        M11.259   Other chondrocalcinosis, unspecified hip

√6ᵗʰ   M11.26   Other chondrocalcinosis, knee
        M11.261   Other chondrocalcinosis, right knee
        M11.262   Other chondrocalcinosis, left knee
        M11.269   Other chondrocalcinosis, unspecified knee

√6ᵗʰ   M11.27   Other chondrocalcinosis, ankle and foot

N Newborn: 0   P Pediatric: 0-17   M Maternity: 12-55   A Adult: 15-124   MCC Major CC Condition   PDxMCC PDx acts as own MCC   CC CC Condition   PDxCC PDx acts as own CC

722   ICD-10-CM 2016

M11.271   Other chondrocalcinosis, right ankle and foot

M11.272   Other chondrocalcinosis, left ankle and foot

M11.279   Other chondrocalcinosis, unspecified ankle and foot

M11.28   Other chondrocalcinosis, vertebrae

M11.29   Other chondrocalcinosis, multiple sites

√5th M11.8   Other specified crystal arthropathies

M11.80   Other specified crystal arthropathies, unspecified site

√6th M11.81   Other specified crystal arthropathies, shoulder

M11.811   Other specified crystal arthropathies, right shoulder

M11.812   Other specified crystal arthropathies, left shoulder

M11.819   Other specified crystal arthropathies, unspecified shoulder

√6th M11.82   Other specified crystal arthropathies, elbow

M11.821   Other specified crystal arthropathies, right elbow

M11.822   Other specified crystal arthropathies, left elbow

M11.829   Other specified crystal arthropathies, unspecified elbow

√6th M11.83   Other specified crystal arthropathies, wrist

M11.831   Other specified crystal arthropathies, right wrist

M11.832   Other specified crystal arthropathies, left wrist

M11.839   Other specified crystal arthropathies, unspecified wrist

√6th M11.84   Other specified crystal arthropathies, hand

M11.841   Other specified crystal arthropathies, right hand

M11.842   Other specified crystal arthropathies, left hand

M11.849   Other specified crystal arthropathies, unspecified hand

√6th M11.85   Other specified crystal arthropathies, hip

M11.851   Other specified crystal arthropathies, right hip

M11.852   Other specified crystal arthropathies, left hip

M11.859   Other specified crystal arthropathies, unspecified hip

√6th M11.86   Other specified crystal arthropathies, knee

M11.861   Other specified crystal arthropathies, right knee

M11.862   Other specified crystal arthropathies, left knee

M11.869   Other specified crystal arthropathies, unspecified knee

√6th M11.87   Other specified crystal arthropathies, ankle and foot

M11.871   Other specified crystal arthropathies, right ankle and foot

M11.872   Other specified crystal arthropathies, left ankle and foot

M11.879   Other specified crystal arthropathies, unspecified ankle and foot

M11.88   Other specified crystal arthropathies, vertebrae

M11.89   Other specified crystal arthropathies, multiple sites

M11.9   Crystal arthropathy, unspecified

√4th M12   Other and unspecified arthropathy

EXCLUDES 1   arthrosis (M15-M19)
cricoarytenoid arthropathy (J38.7)

√5th M12.0   Chronic postrheumatic arthropathy [Jaccoud]

M12.00   Chronic postrheumatic arthropathy [Jaccoud], unspecified site

√6th M12.01   Chronic postrheumatic arthropathy [Jaccoud], shoulder

M12.011   Chronic postrheumatic arthropathy [Jaccoud], right shoulder

M12.012   Chronic postrheumatic arthropathy [Jaccoud], left shoulder

M12.019   Chronic postrheumatic arthropathy [Jaccoud], unspecified shoulder

√6th M12.02   Chronic postrheumatic arthropathy [Jaccoud], elbow

M12.021   Chronic postrheumatic arthropathy [Jaccoud], right elbow

M12.022   Chronic postrheumatic arthropathy [Jaccoud], left elbow

M12.029   Chronic postrheumatic arthropathy [Jaccoud], unspecified elbow

√6th M12.03   Chronic postrheumatic arthropathy [Jaccoud], wrist

M12.031   Chronic postrheumatic arthropathy [Jaccoud], right wrist

M12.032   Chronic postrheumatic arthropathy [Jaccoud], left wrist

M12.039   Chronic postrheumatic arthropathy [Jaccoud], unspecified wrist

√6th M12.04   Chronic postrheumatic arthropathy [Jaccoud], hand

M12.041   Chronic postrheumatic arthropathy [Jaccoud], right hand

M12.042   Chronic postrheumatic arthropathy [Jaccoud], left hand

M12.049   Chronic postrheumatic arthropathy [Jaccoud], unspecified hand

√6th M12.05   Chronic postrheumatic arthropathy [Jaccoud], hip

M12.051   Chronic postrheumatic arthropathy [Jaccoud], right hip

M12.052   Chronic postrheumatic arthropathy [Jaccoud], left hip

M12.059   Chronic postrheumatic arthropathy [Jaccoud], unspecified hip

√6th M12.06   Chronic postrheumatic arthropathy [Jaccoud], knee

M12.061   Chronic postrheumatic arthropathy [Jaccoud], right knee

M12.062   Chronic postrheumatic arthropathy [Jaccoud], left knee

M12.069   Chronic postrheumatic arthropathy [Jaccoud], unspecified knee

√6th M12.07   Chronic postrheumatic arthropathy [Jaccoud], ankle and foot

M12.071   Chronic postrheumatic arthropathy [Jaccoud], right ankle and foot

M12.072   Chronic postrheumatic arthropathy [Jaccoud], left ankle and foot

M12.079   Chronic postrheumatic arthropathy [Jaccoud], unspecified ankle and foot

M12.08   Chronic postrheumatic arthropathy [Jaccoud], other specified site

Chronic postrheumatic arthropathy [Jaccoud], vertebrae

M12.09   Chronic postrheumatic arthropathy [Jaccoud], multiple sites

√5th M12.1   Kaschin-Beck disease

Osteochondroarthrosis deformans endemica

M12.10   Kaschin-Beck disease, unspecified site

√6th M12.11   Kaschin-Beck disease, shoulder

M12.111   Kaschin-Beck disease, right shoulder

M12.112   Kaschin-Beck disease, left shoulder

M12.119   Kaschin-Beck disease, unspecified shoulder

√6th M12.12   Kaschin-Beck disease, elbow

M12.121   Kaschin-Beck disease, right elbow

M12.122   Kaschin-Beck disease, left elbow

M12.129   Kaschin-Beck disease, unspecified elbow

√6th M12.13   Kaschin-Beck disease, wrist

M12.131   Kaschin-Beck disease, right wrist

M12.132   Kaschin-Beck disease, left wrist

M12.139   Kaschin-Beck disease, unspecified wrist

√6th M12.14   Kaschin-Beck disease, hand

M12.141   Kaschin-Beck disease, right hand

M12.142   Kaschin-Beck disease, left hand

M12.149   Kaschin-Beck disease, unspecified hand

√6th M12.15   Kaschin-Beck disease, hip

M12.151   Kaschin-Beck disease, right hip

M12.152   Kaschin-Beck disease, left hip

M12.159   Kaschin-Beck disease, unspecified hip

✔ Additional Character Required   ✔x7th Placeholder Alert   Unacceptable PDx   Manifestation   Hospital Acquired Condition   EXCLUDES 1 Not Coded Here   EXCLUDES 2 Not Included Here

ICD-10-CM 2016   723

✓6th **M12.16 Kaschin-Beck disease,** knee
    M12.161 Kaschin-Beck disease, right **knee**
    M12.162 Kaschin-Beck disease, left **knee**
    M12.169 Kaschin-Beck disease, unspecified **knee**

✓6th **M12.17 Kaschin-Beck disease, ankle and foot**
    M12.171 Kaschin-Beck disease, right **ankle and foot**
    M12.172 Kaschin-Beck disease, left **ankle and foot**
    M12.179 Kaschin-Beck disease, unspecified **ankle and foot**

M12.18 Kaschin-Beck disease, vertebrae
M12.19 Kaschin-Beck disease, multiple sites

✓5th **M12.2 Villonodular synovitis (pigmented)**
    M12.20 Villonodular synovitis (pigmented), unspecified site

✓6th **M12.21 Villonodular synovitis (pigmented),** shoulder
    M12.211 Villonodular synovitis (pigmented), right **shoulder**
    M12.212 Villonodular synovitis (pigmented), left **shoulder**
    M12.219 Villonodular synovitis (pigmented), unspecified **shoulder**

✓6th **M12.22 Villonodular synovitis (pigmented),** elbow
    M12.221 Villonodular synovitis (pigmented), right **elbow**
    M12.222 Villonodular synovitis (pigmented), left **elbow**
    M12.229 Villonodular synovitis (pigmented), unspecified **elbow**

✓6th **M12.23 Villonodular synovitis (pigmented),** wrist
    M12.231 Villonodular synovitis (pigmented), right **wrist**
    M12.232 Villonodular synovitis (pigmented), left **wrist**
    M12.239 Villonodular synovitis (pigmented), unspecified **wrist**

✓6th **M12.24 Villonodular synovitis (pigmented),** hand
    M12.241 Villonodular synovitis (pigmented), right **hand**
    M12.242 Villonodular synovitis (pigmented), left **hand**
    M12.249 Villonodular synovitis (pigmented), unspecified **hand**

✓6th **M12.25 Villonodular synovitis (pigmented),** hip
    M12.251 Villonodular synovitis (pigmented), right **hip**
    M12.252 Villonodular synovitis (pigmented), left **hip**
    M12.259 Villonodular synovitis (pigmented), unspecified **hip**

✓6th **M12.26 Villonodular synovitis (pigmented),** knee
    M12.261 Villonodular synovitis (pigmented), right **knee**
    M12.262 Villonodular synovitis (pigmented), left **knee**
    M12.269 Villonodular synovitis (pigmented), unspecified **knee**

✓6th **M12.27 Villonodular synovitis (pigmented), ankle and foot**
    M12.271 Villonodular synovitis (pigmented), right **ankle and foot**
    M12.272 Villonodular synovitis (pigmented), left **ankle and foot**
    M12.279 Villonodular synovitis (pigmented), unspecified **ankle and foot**

M12.28 Villonodular synovitis (pigmented), other specified site
    Villonodular synovitis (pigmented), vertebrae
M12.29 Villonodular synovitis (pigmented), multiple sites

✓5th **M12.3 Palindromic rheumatism**
    M12.30 Palindromic rheumatism, unspecified site

✓6th **M12.31 Palindromic rheumatism,** shoulder
    M12.311 Palindromic rheumatism, right **shoulder**
    M12.312 Palindromic rheumatism, left **shoulder**
    M12.319 Palindromic rheumatism, unspecified **shoulder**

✓6th **M12.32 Palindromic rheumatism,** elbow
    M12.321 Palindromic rheumatism, right **elbow**

    M12.322 Palindromic rheumatism, left **elbow**
    M12.329 Palindromic rheumatism, unspecified **elbow**

✓6th **M12.33 Palindromic rheumatism,** wrist
    M12.331 Palindromic rheumatism, right **wrist**
    M12.332 Palindromic rheumatism, left **wrist**
    M12.339 Palindromic rheumatism, unspecified **wrist**

✓6th **M12.34 Palindromic rheumatism,** hand
    M12.341 Palindromic rheumatism, right **hand**
    M12.342 Palindromic rheumatism, left **hand**
    M12.349 Palindromic rheumatism, unspecified **hand**

✓6th **M12.35 Palindromic rheumatism,** hip
    M12.351 Palindromic rheumatism, right **hip**
    M12.352 Palindromic rheumatism, left **hip**
    M12.359 Palindromic rheumatism, unspecified **hip**

✓6th **M12.36 Palindromic rheumatism,** knee
    M12.361 Palindromic rheumatism, right **knee**
    M12.362 Palindromic rheumatism, left **knee**
    M12.369 Palindromic rheumatism, unspecified **knee**

✓6th **M12.37 Palindromic rheumatism, ankle and foot**
    M12.371 Palindromic rheumatism, right **ankle and foot**
    M12.372 Palindromic rheumatism, left **ankle and foot**
    M12.379 Palindromic rheumatism, unspecified **ankle and foot**

M12.38 Palindromic rheumatism, other specified site
    Palindromic rheumatism, vertebrae
M12.39 Palindromic rheumatism, multiple sites

✓5th **M12.4 Intermittent hydrarthrosis**
    M12.40 Intermittent hydrarthrosis, unspecified site

✓6th **M12.41 Intermittent hydrarthrosis,** shoulder
    M12.411 Intermittent hydrarthrosis, right **shoulder**
    M12.412 Intermittent hydrarthrosis, left **shoulder**
    M12.419 Intermittent hydrarthrosis, unspecified **shoulder**

✓6th **M12.42 Intermittent hydrarthrosis,** elbow
    M12.421 Intermittent hydrarthrosis, right **elbow**
    M12.422 Intermittent hydrarthrosis, left **elbow**
    M12.429 Intermittent hydrarthrosis, unspecified **elbow**

✓6th **M12.43 Intermittent hydrarthrosis,** wrist
    M12.431 Intermittent hydrarthrosis, right **wrist**
    M12.432 Intermittent hydrarthrosis, left **wrist**
    M12.439 Intermittent hydrarthrosis, unspecified **wrist**

✓6th **M12.44 Intermittent hydrarthrosis,** hand
    M12.441 Intermittent hydrarthrosis, right **hand**
    M12.442 Intermittent hydrarthrosis, left **hand**
    M12.449 Intermittent hydrarthrosis, unspecified **hand**

✓6th **M12.45 Intermittent hydrarthrosis,** hip
    M12.451 Intermittent hydrarthrosis, right **hip**
    M12.452 Intermittent hydrarthrosis, left **hip**
    M12.459 Intermittent hydrarthrosis, unspecified **hip**

✓6th **M12.46 Intermittent hydrarthrosis,** knee
    M12.461 Intermittent hydrarthrosis, right **knee**
    M12.462 Intermittent hydrarthrosis, left **knee**
    M12.469 Intermittent hydrarthrosis, unspecified **knee**

✓6th **M12.47 Intermittent hydrarthrosis, ankle and foot**
    M12.471 Intermittent hydrarthrosis, right **ankle and foot**
    M12.472 Intermittent hydrarthrosis, left **ankle and foot**
    M12.479 Intermittent hydrarthrosis, unspecified **ankle and foot**

M12.48 Intermittent hydrarthrosis, other site
M12.49 Intermittent hydrarthrosis, multiple sites

N Newborn: 0   P Pediatric: 0-17   M Maternity: 12-55   A Adult: 15-124   MCC Major CC Condition   PDxMCC PDx acts as own MCC   CC CC Condition   PDxCC PDx acts as own CC

724   ICD-10-CM 2016

☑5ᵗʰ M12.5 Traumatic arthropathy

> **EXCLUDES 1**   *current injury–see Alphabetic Index*
> *post-traumatic osteoarthritis NOS (M19.1-)*
> *post-traumatic osteoarthritis of first carpometacarpal joint (M18.2-M18.3)*
> *post-traumatic osteoarthritis of hip (M16.4-M16.5)*
> *post-traumatic osteoarthritis of knee (M17.2-M17.3)*
> *post-traumatic osteoarthritis of other single joints (M19.1-)*

> **AHA:** 2015, 1Q, 17

M12.50 Traumatic arthropathy, unspecified site

☑6ᵗʰ M12.51 Traumatic arthropathy, shoulder
- **M12.511 Traumatic arthropathy,** right shoulder
- **M12.512 Traumatic arthropathy,** left shoulder
- **M12.519 Traumatic arthropathy,** unspecified shoulder

☑6ᵗʰ M12.52 Traumatic arthropathy, elbow
- **M12.521 Traumatic arthropathy,** right elbow
- **M12.522 Traumatic arthropathy,** left elbow
- **M12.529 Traumatic arthropathy,** unspecified elbow

☑6ᵗʰ M12.53 Traumatic arthropathy, wrist
- **M12.531 Traumatic arthropathy,** right wrist
- **M12.532 Traumatic arthropathy,** left wrist
- **M12.539 Traumatic arthropathy,** unspecified wrist

☑6ᵗʰ M12.54 Traumatic arthropathy, hand
- **M12.541 Traumatic arthropathy,** right hand
- **M12.542 Traumatic arthropathy,** left hand
- **M12.549 Traumatic arthropathy,** unspecified hand

☑6ᵗʰ M12.55 Traumatic arthropathy, hip
- **M12.551 Traumatic arthropathy,** right hip
- **M12.552 Traumatic arthropathy,** left hip
- **M12.559 Traumatic arthropathy,** unspecified hip

☑6ᵗʰ M12.56 Traumatic arthropathy, knee
- **M12.561 Traumatic arthropathy,** right knee
- **M12.562 Traumatic arthropathy,** left knee
- **M12.569 Traumatic arthropathy,** unspecified knee

☑6ᵗʰ M12.57 Traumatic arthropathy, ankle and foot
- **M12.571 Traumatic arthropathy,** right ankle and foot
- **M12.572 Traumatic arthropathy,** left ankle and foot
- **M12.579 Traumatic arthropathy,** unspecified ankle and foot

M12.58 Traumatic arthropathy, other specified site
> Traumatic arthropathy, vertebrae

M12.59 Traumatic arthropathy, multiple sites

☑5ᵗʰ M12.8 Other specific arthropathies, not elsewhere classified
> Transient arthropathy

M12.80 Other specific arthropathies, not elsewhere classified, unspecified site

☑6ᵗʰ M12.81 Other specific arthropathies, not elsewhere classified, shoulder
- **M12.811 Other specific arthropathies, not elsewhere classified,** right shoulder
- **M12.812 Other specific arthropathies, not elsewhere classified,** left shoulder
- **M12.819 Other specific arthropathies, not elsewhere classified,** unspecified shoulder

☑6ᵗʰ M12.82 Other specific arthropathies, not elsewhere classified, elbow
- **M12.821 Other specific arthropathies, not elsewhere classified,** right elbow
- **M12.822 Other specific arthropathies, not elsewhere classified,** left elbow
- **M12.829 Other specific arthropathies, not elsewhere classified,** unspecified elbow

☑6ᵗʰ M12.83 Other specific arthropathies, not elsewhere classified, wrist
- **M12.831 Other specific arthropathies, not elsewhere classified,** right wrist
- **M12.832 Other specific arthropathies, not elsewhere classified,** left wrist
- **M12.839 Other specific arthropathies, not elsewhere classified,** unspecified wrist

☑6ᵗʰ M12.84 Other specific arthropathies, not elsewhere classified, hand
- **M12.841 Other specific arthropathies, not elsewhere classified,** right hand
- **M12.842 Other specific arthropathies, not elsewhere classified,** left hand
- **M12.849 Other specific arthropathies, not elsewhere classified,** unspecified hand

☑6ᵗʰ M12.85 Other specific arthropathies, not elsewhere classified, hip
- **M12.851 Other specific arthropathies, not elsewhere classified,** right hip
- **M12.852 Other specific arthropathies, not elsewhere classified,** left hip
- **M12.859 Other specific arthropathies, not elsewhere classified,** unspecified hip

☑6ᵗʰ M12.86 Other specific arthropathies, not elsewhere classified, knee
- **M12.861 Other specific arthropathies, not elsewhere classified,** right knee
- **M12.862 Other specific arthropathies, not elsewhere classified,** left knee
- **M12.869 Other specific arthropathies, not elsewhere classified,** unspecified knee

☑6ᵗʰ M12.87 Other specific arthropathies, not elsewhere classified, ankle and foot
- **M12.871 Other specific arthropathies, not elsewhere classified,** right ankle and foot
- **M12.872 Other specific arthropathies, not elsewhere classified,** left ankle and foot
- **M12.879 Other specific arthropathies, not elsewhere classified,** unspecified ankle and foot

M12.88 Other specific arthropathies, not elsewhere classified, other specified site
> Other specific arthropathies, not elsewhere classified, vertebrae

M12.89 Other specific arthropathies, not elsewhere classified, multiple sites

M12.9 Arthropathy, unspecified

☑4ᵗʰ M13 Other arthritis

> **EXCLUDES 1**   *arthrosis (M15-M19)*
> *osteoarthritis (M15-M19)*

M13.0 Polyarthritis, unspecified

☑5ᵗʰ M13.1 Monoarthritis, not elsewhere classified

M13.10 Monoarthritis, not elsewhere classified, unspecified site

☑6ᵗʰ M13.11 Monoarthritis, not elsewhere classified, shoulder
- **M13.111 Monoarthritis, not elsewhere classified,** right shoulder
- **M13.112 Monoarthritis, not elsewhere classified,** left shoulder
- **M13.119 Monoarthritis, not elsewhere classified,** unspecified shoulder

☑6ᵗʰ M13.12 Monoarthritis, not elsewhere classified, elbow
- **M13.121 Monoarthritis, not elsewhere classified,** right elbow
- **M13.122 Monoarthritis, not elsewhere classified,** left elbow
- **M13.129 Monoarthritis, not elsewhere classified,** unspecified elbow

☑6ᵗʰ M13.13 Monoarthritis, not elsewhere classified, wrist
- **M13.131 Monoarthritis, not elsewhere classified,** right wrist
- **M13.132 Monoarthritis, not elsewhere classified,** left wrist
- **M13.139 Monoarthritis, not elsewhere classified,** unspecified wrist

☑6ᵗʰ M13.14 Monoarthritis, not elsewhere classified, hand
- **M13.141 Monoarthritis, not elsewhere classified,** right hand
- **M13.142 Monoarthritis, not elsewhere classified,** left hand
- **M13.149 Monoarthritis, not elsewhere classified,** unspecified hand

☑ Additional Character Required   ✔x7ᵗʰ Placeholder Alert   Unacceptable PDx   Manifestation   Hospital Acquired Condition   **EXCLUDES 1** Not Coded Here   **EXCLUDES 2** Not Included Here

ICD-10-CM 2016   725

✓6ᵗʰ **M13.15 Monoarthritis, not elsewhere classified,** hip

    M13.151 Monoarthritis, not elsewhere classified, right hip

    M13.152 Monoarthritis, not elsewhere classified, left hip

    M13.159 Monoarthritis, not elsewhere classified, unspecified hip

✓6ᵗʰ **M13.16 Monoarthritis, not elsewhere classified,** knee

    M13.161 Monoarthritis, not elsewhere classified, right knee

    M13.162 Monoarthritis, not elsewhere classified, left knee

    M13.169 Monoarthritis, not elsewhere classified, unspecified knee

✓6ᵗʰ **M13.17 Monoarthritis, not elsewhere classified,** ankle and foot

    M13.171 Monoarthritis, not elsewhere classified, right ankle and foot

    M13.172 Monoarthritis, not elsewhere classified, left ankle and foot

    M13.179 Monoarthritis, not elsewhere classified, unspecified ankle and foot

✓5ᵗʰ **M13.8 Other specified arthritis**
Allergic arthritis
> **EXCLUDES 1**   osteoarthritis (M15-M19)

    M13.80 Other specified arthritis, unspecified site

✓6ᵗʰ **M13.81 Other specified arthritis,** shoulder

    M13.811 Other specified arthritis, right shoulder

    M13.812 Other specified arthritis, left shoulder

    M13.819 Other specified arthritis, unspecified shoulder

✓6ᵗʰ **M13.82 Other specified arthritis,** elbow

    M13.821 Other specified arthritis, right elbow

    M13.822 Other specified arthritis, left elbow

    M13.829 Other specified arthritis, unspecified elbow

✓6ᵗʰ **M13.83 Other specified arthritis,** wrist

    M13.831 Other specified arthritis, right wrist

    M13.832 Other specified arthritis, left wrist

    M13.839 Other specified arthritis, unspecified wrist

✓6ᵗʰ **M13.84 Other specified arthritis,** hand

    M13.841 Other specified arthritis, right hand

    M13.842 Other specified arthritis, left hand

    M13.849 Other specified arthritis, unspecified hand

✓6ᵗʰ **M13.85 Other specified arthritis,** hip

    M13.851 Other specified arthritis, right hip

    M13.852 Other specified arthritis, left hip

    M13.859 Other specified arthritis, unspecified hip

✓6ᵗʰ **M13.86 Other specified arthritis,** knee

    M13.861 Other specified arthritis, right knee

    M13.862 Other specified arthritis, left knee

    M13.869 Other specified arthritis, unspecified knee

✓6ᵗʰ **M13.87 Other specified arthritis,** ankle and foot

    M13.871 Other specified arthritis, right ankle and foot

    M13.872 Other specified arthritis, left ankle and foot

    M13.879 Other specified arthritis, unspecified ankle and foot

    M13.88 Other specified arthritis, other site

    M13.89 Other specified arthritis, multiple sites

✓4ᵗʰ **M14 Arthropathies in other diseases classified elsewhere**
> **EXCLUDES 1**   arthropathy in:
>   diabetes mellitus (E08-E13 with .61-)
>   hematological disorders (M36.2-M36.3)
>   hypersensitivity reactions (M36.4)
>   neoplastic disease (M36.1)
>   neurosyphillis (A52.16)
>   sarcoidosis (D86.86)
>   enteropathic arthropathies (M07.-)
>   juvenile psoriatic arthropathy (L40.54)
>   lipoid dermatoarthritis (E78.81)

✓5ᵗʰ **M14.6 Charcôt's joint**
Neuropathic arthropathy
> **EXCLUDES 1**   Charcôt's joint in diabetes mellitus (E08-E13 with .610-)
>   Charcôt's joint in tabes dorsalis (A52.16)

    M14.60 Charcôt's joint, unspecified site

✓6ᵗʰ **M14.61 Charcôt's joint,** shoulder

    M14.611 Charcôt's joint, right shoulder

    M14.612 Charcôt's joint, left shoulder

    M14.619 Charcôt's joint, unspecified shoulder

✓6ᵗʰ **M14.62 Charcôt's joint,** elbow

    M14.621 Charcôt's joint, right elbow

    M14.622 Charcôt's joint, left elbow

    M14.629 Charcôt's joint, unspecified elbow

✓6ᵗʰ **M14.63 Charcôt's joint,** wrist

    M14.631 Charcôt's joint, right wrist

    M14.632 Charcôt's joint, left wrist

    M14.639 Charcôt's joint, unspecified wrist

✓6ᵗʰ **M14.64 Charcôt's joint,** hand

    M14.641 Charcôt's joint, right hand

    M14.642 Charcôt's joint, left hand

    M14.649 Charcôt's joint, unspecified hand

✓6ᵗʰ **M14.65 Charcôt's joint,** hip

    M14.651 Charcôt's joint, right hip

    M14.652 Charcôt's joint, left hip

    M14.659 Charcôt's joint, unspecified hip

✓6ᵗʰ **M14.66 Charcôt's joint,** knee

    M14.661 Charcôt's joint, right knee

    M14.662 Charcôt's joint, left knee

    M14.669 Charcôt's joint, unspecified knee

✓6ᵗʰ **M14.67 Charcôt's joint,** ankle and foot

    M14.671 Charcôt's joint, right ankle and foot

    M14.672 Charcôt's joint, left ankle and foot

    M14.679 Charcôt's joint, unspecified ankle and foot

    M14.68 Charcôt's joint, vertebrae

    M14.69 Charcôt's joint, multiple sites

✓5ᵗʰ **M14.8 Arthropathies in other specified diseases classified elsewhere**
Code first underlying disease, such as:
   amyloidosis (E85.-)
   erythema multiforme (L51.-)
   erythema nodosum (L52)
   hemochromatosis (E83.11-)
   hyperparathyroidism (E21.-)
   hypothyroidism (E00-E03)
   sickle-cell disorders (D57.-)
   thyrotoxicosis [hyperthyroidism] (E05.-)
   Whipple's disease (K90.81)

    M14.80 Arthropathies in other specified diseases classified elsewhere, unspecified site

✓6ᵗʰ **M14.81 Arthropathies in other specified diseases classified elsewhere,** shoulder

    M14.811 Arthropathies in other specified diseases classified elsewhere, right shoulder

    M14.812 Arthropathies in other specified diseases classified elsewhere, left shoulder

    M14.819 Arthropathies in other specified diseases classified elsewhere, unspecified shoulder

✓6ᵗʰ **M14.82 Arthropathies in other specified diseases classified elsewhere,** elbow

    M14.821 Arthropathies in other specified diseases classified elsewhere, right elbow

    M14.822 Arthropathies in other specified diseases classified elsewhere, left elbow

    M14.829 Arthropathies in other specified diseases classified elsewhere, unspecified elbow

✓6ᵗʰ **M14.83 Arthropathies in other specified diseases classified elsewhere,** wrist

    M14.831 Arthropathies in other specified diseases classified elsewhere, right wrist

    M14.832 Arthropathies in other specified diseases classified elsewhere, left wrist

    M14.839 Arthropathies in other specified diseases classified elsewhere, unspecified wrist

Ⓝ Newborn: 0   Ⓟ Pediatric: 0-17   Ⓜ Maternity: 12-55   Ⓐ Adult: 15-124   **MCC** Major CC Condition   **PDxMCC** PDx acts as own MCC   **CC** CC Condition   **PDxCC** PDx acts as own CC

726   ICD-10-CM 2016

√6ᵗʰ **M14.84 Arthropathies in other specified diseases classified elsewhere, hand**

    M14.841 Arthropathies in other specified diseases classified elsewhere, right hand

    M14.842 Arthropathies in other specified diseases classified elsewhere, left hand

    M14.849 Arthropathies in other specified diseases classified elsewhere, unspecified hand

√6ᵗʰ **M14.85 Arthropathies in other specified diseases classified elsewhere, hip**

    M14.851 Arthropathies in other specified diseases classified elsewhere, right hip

    M14.852 Arthropathies in other specified diseases classified elsewhere, left hip

    M14.859 Arthropathies in other specified diseases classified elsewhere, unspecified hip

√6ᵗʰ **M14.86 Arthropathies in other specified diseases classified elsewhere, knee**

    M14.861 Arthropathies in other specified diseases classified elsewhere, right knee

    M14.862 Arthropathies in other specified diseases classified elsewhere, left knee

    M14.869 Arthropathies in other specified diseases classified elsewhere, unspecified knee

√6ᵗʰ **M14.87 Arthropathies in other specified diseases classified elsewhere, ankle and foot**

    M14.871 Arthropathies in other specified diseases classified elsewhere, right ankle and foot

    M14.872 Arthropathies in other specified diseases classified elsewhere, left ankle and foot

    M14.879 Arthropathies in other specified diseases classified elsewhere, unspecified ankle and foot

    M14.88 Arthropathies in other specified diseases classified elsewhere, vertebrae

    M14.89 Arthropathies in other specified diseases classified elsewhere, multiple sites

Osteoarthritis (M15-M19)

EXCLUDES 2   *osteoarthritis of spine (M47.-)*

√4ᵗʰ **M15 Polyosteoarthritis**

    INCLUDES   arthritis of multiple sites

    EXCLUDES 1   *bilateral involvement of single joint (M16-M19)*

M15.0 Primary generalized (osteo)arthritis

M15.1 Heberden's nodes (with arthropathy)
    Interphalangeal distal osteoarthritis

M15.2 Bouchard's nodes (with arthropathy)
    Juxtaphalangeal distal osteoarthritis

M15.3 Secondary multiple arthritis
    Post-traumatic polyosteoarthritis

M15.4 Erosive (osteo)arthritis

M15.8 Other polyosteoarthritis

M15.9 Polyosteoarthritis, unspecified
    Generalized osteoarthritis NOS

√4ᵗʰ **M16 Osteoarthritis of hip**

M16.0 Bilateral primary osteoarthritis of hip

√5ᵗʰ **M16.1 Unilateral primary osteoarthritis of hip**
    Primary osteoarthritis of hip NOS

    M16.10 Unilateral primary osteoarthritis, unspecified hip

    M16.11 Unilateral primary osteoarthritis, right hip

    M16.12 Unilateral primary osteoarthritis, left hip

M16.2 Bilateral osteoarthritis resulting from hip dysplasia

√5ᵗʰ **M16.3 Unilateral osteoarthritis resulting from hip dysplasia**
    Dysplastic osteoarthritis of hip NOS

    M16.30 Unilateral osteoarthritis resulting from hip dysplasia, unspecified hip

    M16.31 Unilateral osteoarthritis resulting from hip dysplasia, right hip

    M16.32 Unilateral osteoarthritis resulting from hip dysplasia, left hip

M16.4 Bilateral post-traumatic osteoarthritis of hip

√5ᵗʰ **M16.5 Unilateral post-traumatic osteoarthritis of hip**
    Post-traumatic osteoarthritis of hip NOS

    M16.50 Unilateral post-traumatic osteoarthritis, unspecified hip

    M16.51 Unilateral post-traumatic osteoarthritis, right hip

    M16.52 Unilateral post-traumatic osteoarthritis, left hip

M16.6 Other bilateral secondary osteoarthritis of hip

M16.7 Other unilateral secondary osteoarthritis of hip
    Secondary osteoarthritis of hip NOS

M16.9 Osteoarthritis of hip, unspecified

√4ᵗʰ **M17 Osteoarthritis of knee**

M17.0 Bilateral primary osteoarthritis of knee

√5ᵗʰ **M17.1 Unilateral primary osteoarthritis of knee**
    Primary osteoarthritis of knee NOS

    M17.10 Unilateral primary osteoarthritis, unspecified knee

    M17.11 Unilateral primary osteoarthritis, right knee

    M17.12 Unilateral primary osteoarthritis, left knee

M17.2 Bilateral post-traumatic osteoarthritis of knee

√5ᵗʰ **M17.3 Unilateral post-traumatic osteoarthritis of knee**
    Post-traumatic osteoarthritis of knee NOS

    M17.30 Unilateral post-traumatic osteoarthritis, unspecified knee

    M17.31 Unilateral post-traumatic osteoarthritis, right knee

    M17.32 Unilateral post-traumatic osteoarthritis, left knee

M17.4 Other bilateral secondary osteoarthritis of knee

M17.5 Other unilateral secondary osteoarthritis of knee
    Secondary osteoarthritis of knee NOS

M17.9 Osteoarthritis of knee, unspecified

√4ᵗʰ **M18 Osteoarthritis of first carpometacarpal joint**

M18.0 Bilateral primary osteoarthritis of first carpometacarpal joints

√5ᵗʰ **M18.1 Unilateral primary osteoarthritis of first carpometacarpal joint**
    Primary osteoarthritis of first carpometacarpal joint NOS

    M18.10 Unilateral primary osteoarthritis of first carpometacarpal joint, unspecified hand

    M18.11 Unilateral primary osteoarthritis of first carpometacarpal joint, right hand

    M18.12 Unilateral primary osteoarthritis of first carpometacarpal joint, left hand

M18.2 Bilateral post-traumatic osteoarthritis of first carpometacarpal joints

√5ᵗʰ **M18.3 Unilateral post-traumatic osteoarthritis of first carpometacarpal joint**
    Post-traumatic osteoarthritis of first carpometacarpal joint NOS

    M18.30 Unilateral post-traumatic osteoarthritis of first carpometacarpal joint, unspecified hand

    M18.31 Unilateral post-traumatic osteoarthritis of first carpometacarpal joint, right hand

    M18.32 Unilateral post-traumatic osteoarthritis of first carpometacarpal joint, left hand

M18.4 Other bilateral secondary osteoarthritis of first carpometacarpal joints

√5ᵗʰ **M18.5 Other unilateral secondary osteoarthritis of first carpometacarpal joint**
    Secondary osteoarthritis of first carpometacarpal joint NOS

    M18.50 Other unilateral secondary osteoarthritis of first carpometacarpal joint, unspecified hand

    M18.51 Other unilateral secondary osteoarthritis of first carpometacarpal joint, right hand

    M18.52 Other unilateral secondary osteoarthritis of first carpometacarpal joint, left hand

M18.9 Osteoarthritis of first carpometacarpal joint, unspecified

√4ᵗʰ **M19 Other and unspecified osteoarthritis**

    EXCLUDES 1   *polyarthritis (M15.-)*

    EXCLUDES 2   *arthrosis of spine (M47.-)*
                  hallux rigidus (M20.2)
                   osteoarthritis of spine (M47.-)

√5ᵗʰ **M19.0 Primary osteoarthritis of other joints**

    √6ᵗʰ **M19.01 Primary osteoarthritis, shoulder**

        M19.011 Primary osteoarthritis, right shoulder

        M19.012 Primary osteoarthritis, left shoulder

        M19.019 Primary osteoarthritis, unspecified shoulder

    √6ᵗʰ **M19.02 Primary osteoarthritis, elbow**

        M19.021 Primary osteoarthritis, right elbow

        M19.022 Primary osteoarthritis, left elbow

        M19.029 Primary osteoarthritis, unspecified elbow

☑ Additional Character Required   √x7ᵗʰ Placeholder Alert   Unacceptable PDx   Manifestation   Hospital Acquired Condition   EXCLUDES 1 Not Coded Here   EXCLUDES 2 Not Included Here

ICD-10-CM 2016   727

✓6ᵗʰ **M19.03 Primary osteoarthritis, wrist**
　　M19.031 Primary osteoarthritis, right wrist
　　M19.032 Primary osteoarthritis, left wrist
　　M19.039 Primary osteoarthritis, unspecified wrist

✓6ᵗʰ **M19.04 Primary osteoarthritis, hand**
　　EXCLUDES 2　*primary osteoarthritis of first carpometacarpal joint (M18.0-, M18.1-)*
　　M19.041 Primary osteoarthritis, right hand
　　M19.042 Primary osteoarthritis, left hand
　　M19.049 Primary osteoarthritis, unspecified hand

✓6ᵗʰ **M19.07 Primary osteoarthritis ankle and foot**
　　M19.071 Primary osteoarthritis, right ankle and foot
　　M19.072 Primary osteoarthritis, left ankle and foot
　　M19.079 Primary osteoarthritis, unspecified ankle and foot

✓5ᵗʰ **M19.1 Post-traumatic osteoarthritis of other joints**

✓6ᵗʰ **M19.11 Post-traumatic osteoarthritis, shoulder**
　　M19.111 Post-traumatic osteoarthritis, right shoulder
　　M19.112 Post-traumatic osteoarthritis, left shoulder
　　M19.119 Post-traumatic osteoarthritis, unspecified shoulder

✓6ᵗʰ **M19.12 Post-traumatic osteoarthritis, elbow**
　　M19.121 Post-traumatic osteoarthritis, right elbow
　　M19.122 Post-traumatic osteoarthritis, left elbow
　　M19.129 Post-traumatic osteoarthritis, unspecified elbow

✓6ᵗʰ **M19.13 Post-traumatic osteoarthritis, wrist**
　　M19.131 Post-traumatic osteoarthritis, right wrist
　　M19.132 Post-traumatic osteoarthritis, left wrist
　　M19.139 Post-traumatic osteoarthritis, unspecified wrist

✓6ᵗʰ **M19.14 Post-traumatic osteoarthritis, hand**
　　EXCLUDES 2　*post-traumatic osteoarthritis of first carpometacarpal joint (M18.2-, M18.3-)*
　　M19.141 Post-traumatic osteoarthritis, right hand
　　M19.142 Post-traumatic osteoarthritis, left hand
　　M19.149 Post-traumatic osteoarthritis, unspecified hand

✓6ᵗʰ **M19.17 Post-traumatic osteoarthritis, ankle and foot**
　　M19.171 Post-traumatic osteoarthritis, right ankle and foot
　　M19.172 Post-traumatic osteoarthritis, left ankle and foot
　　M19.179 Post-traumatic osteoarthritis, unspecified ankle and foot

✓5ᵗʰ **M19.2 Secondary osteoarthritis of other joints**

✓6ᵗʰ **M19.21 Secondary osteoarthritis, shoulder**
　　M19.211 Secondary osteoarthritis, right shoulder
　　M19.212 Secondary osteoarthritis, left shoulder
　　M19.219 Secondary osteoarthritis, unspecified shoulder

✓6ᵗʰ **M19.22 Secondary osteoarthritis, elbow**
　　M19.221 Secondary osteoarthritis, right elbow
　　M19.222 Secondary osteoarthritis, left elbow
　　M19.229 Secondary osteoarthritis, unspecified elbow

✓6ᵗʰ **M19.23 Secondary osteoarthritis, wrist**
　　M19.231 Secondary osteoarthritis, right wrist
　　M19.232 Secondary osteoarthritis, left wrist
　　M19.239 Secondary osteoarthritis, unspecified wrist

✓6ᵗʰ **M19.24 Secondary osteoarthritis, hand**
　　M19.241 Secondary osteoarthritis, right hand
　　M19.242 Secondary osteoarthritis, left hand
　　M19.249 Secondary osteoarthritis, unspecified hand

✓6ᵗʰ **M19.27 Secondary osteoarthritis, ankle and foot**
　　M19.271 Secondary osteoarthritis, right ankle and foot
　　M19.272 Secondary osteoarthritis, left ankle and foot

M19.279 Secondary osteoarthritis, unspecified ankle and foot

✓5ᵗʰ **M19.9 Osteoarthritis, unspecified site**
　　M19.90 Unspecified osteoarthritis, unspecified site
　　　Arthrosis NOS
　　　Arthritis NOS
　　　Osteoarthritis NOS
　　M19.91 Primary osteoarthritis, unspecified site
　　　Primary osteoarthritis NOS
　　M19.92 Post-traumatic osteoarthritis, unspecified site
　　　Post-traumatic osteoarthritis NOS
　　M19.93 Secondary osteoarthritis, unspecified site
　　　Secondary osteoarthritis NOS

Other joint disorders (M20-M25)
EXCLUDES 2　*joints of the spine (M40-M54)*

✓4ᵗʰ **M20 Acquired deformities of fingers and toes**
　　EXCLUDES 1　*acquired absence of fingers and toes (Z89.-)*
　　　congenital absence of fingers and toes (Q71.3-, Q72.3-)
　　　congenital deformities and malformations of fingers and toes (Q66-, Q68-Q70, Q74-)

✓5ᵗʰ **M20.0 Deformity of finger(s)**
　　EXCLUDES 1　*clubbing of fingers (R68.3)*
　　　palmar fascial fibromatosis [Dupuytren] (M72.0)
　　　trigger finger (M65.3)

✓6ᵗʰ **M20.00 Unspecified deformity of finger(s)**
　　M20.001 Unspecified deformity of right finger(s)
　　M20.002 Unspecified deformity of left finger(s)
　　M20.009 Unspecified deformity of unspecified finger(s)

✓6ᵗʰ **M20.01 Mallet finger**
　　M20.011 Mallet finger of right finger(s)
　　M20.012 Mallet finger of left finger(s)
　　M20.019 Mallet finger of unspecified finger(s)

✓6ᵗʰ **M20.02 Boutonnière deformity**
　　M20.021 Boutonnière deformity of right finger(s)
　　M20.022 Boutonnière deformity of left finger(s)
　　M20.029 Boutonnière deformity of unspecified finger(s)

✓6ᵗʰ **M20.03 Swan-neck deformity**
　　M20.031 Swan-neck deformity of right finger(s)
　　M20.032 Swan-neck deformity of left finger(s)
　　M20.039 Swan-neck deformity of unspecified finger(s)

✓6ᵗʰ **M20.09 Other deformity of finger(s)**
　　M20.091 Other deformity of right finger(s)
　　M20.092 Other deformity of left finger(s)
　　M20.099 Other deformity of finger(s), unspecified finger(s)

✓5ᵗʰ **M20.1 Hallux valgus (acquired)**
　　Bunion
　　M20.10 Hallux valgus (acquired), unspecified foot
　　M20.11 Hallux valgus (acquired), right foot
　　M20.12 Hallux valgus (acquired), left foot

✓5ᵗʰ **M20.2 Hallux rigidus**
　　M20.20 Hallux rigidus, unspecified foot
　　M20.21 Hallux rigidus, right foot
　　M20.22 Hallux rigidus, left foot

✓5ᵗʰ **M20.3 Hallux varus (acquired)**
　　M20.30 Hallux varus (acquired), unspecified foot
　　M20.31 Hallux varus (acquired), right foot
　　M20.32 Hallux varus (acquired), left foot

✓5ᵗʰ **M20.4 Other hammer toe(s) (acquired)**
　　M20.40 Other hammer toe(s) (acquired), unspecified foot
　　M20.41 Other hammer toe(s) (acquired), right foot
　　M20.42 Other hammer toe(s) (acquired), left foot

✓5ᵗʰ **M20.5 Other deformities of toe(s) (acquired)**
　　✓6ᵗʰ **M20.5X Other deformities of toe(s) (acquired)**
　　　M20.5X1 Other deformities of toe(s) (acquired), right foot
　　　M20.5X2 Other deformities of toe(s) (acquired), left foot

N Newborn: 0　　P Pediatric: 0-17　　M Maternity: 12-55　　A Adult: 15-124　　MCC Major CC Condition　　PDxMCC PDx acts as own MCC　　CC CC Condition　　PDxCC PDx acts as own CC

M20.5X9   Other deformities of toe(s) (acquired), unspecified foot

✓5th **M20.6 Acquired deformities of toe(s), unspecified**

M20.60   Acquired deformities of toe(s), unspecified, unspecified foot

M20.61   Acquired deformities of toe(s), unspecified, right foot

M20.62   Acquired deformities of toe(s), unspecified, left foot

✓4th **M21 Other acquired deformities of limbs**

EXCLUDES 1   acquired absence of limb (Z89.-)
congenital absence of limbs (Q71-Q73)
congenital deformities and malformations of limbs (Q65-Q66, Q68-Q74)

EXCLUDES 2   acquired deformities of fingers or toes (M20.-)
coxa plana (M91.2)

✓5th **M21.0 Valgus deformity, not elsewhere classified**

EXCLUDES 1   metatarsus valgus (Q66.6)
talipes calcaneovalgus (Q66.4)

M21.00   Valgus deformity, not elsewhere classified, unspecified site

✓6th **M21.02 Valgus deformity, not elsewhere classified, elbow**
Cubitus valgus

M21.021   Valgus deformity, not elsewhere classified, right elbow

M21.022   Valgus deformity, not elsewhere classified, left elbow

M21.029   Valgus deformity, not elsewhere classified, unspecified elbow

✓6th **M21.05 Valgus deformity, not elsewhere classified, hip**

M21.051   Valgus deformity, not elsewhere classified, right hip

M21.052   Valgus deformity, not elsewhere classified, left hip

M21.059   Valgus deformity, not elsewhere classified, unspecified hip

✓6th **M21.06 Valgus deformity, not elsewhere classified, knee**
Genu valgum
Knock knee

M21.061   Valgus deformity, not elsewhere classified, right knee

M21.062   Valgus deformity, not elsewhere classified, left knee

M21.069   Valgus deformity, not elsewhere classified, unspecified knee

✓6th **M21.07 Valgus deformity, not elsewhere classified, ankle**

M21.071   Valgus deformity, not elsewhere classified, right ankle

M21.072   Valgus deformity, not elsewhere classified, left ankle

M21.079   Valgus deformity, not elsewhere classified, unspecified ankle

✓5th **M21.1 Varus deformity, not elsewhere classified**

EXCLUDES 1   metatarsus varus (Q66.2)
tibia vara (M92.5)

M21.10   Varus deformity, not elsewhere classified, unspecified site

✓6th **M21.12 Varus deformity, not elsewhere classified, elbow**
Cubitus varus, elbow

M21.121   Varus deformity, not elsewhere classified, right elbow

M21.122   Varus deformity, not elsewhere classified, left elbow

M21.129   Varus deformity, not elsewhere classified, unspecified elbow

✓6th **M21.15 Varus deformity, not elsewhere classified, hip**

M21.151   Varus deformity, not elsewhere classified, right hip

M21.152   Varus deformity, not elsewhere classified, left hip

M21.159   Varus deformity, not elsewhere classified, unspecified

✓6th **M21.16 Varus deformity, not elsewhere classified, knee**
Bow leg
Genu varum

M21.161   Varus deformity, not elsewhere classified, right knee

M21.162   Varus deformity, not elsewhere classified, left knee

M21.169   Varus deformity, not elsewhere classified, unspecified knee

✓6th **M21.17 Varus deformity, not elsewhere classified, ankle**

M21.171   Varus deformity, not elsewhere classified, right ankle

M21.172   Varus deformity, not elsewhere classified, left ankle

M21.179   Varus deformity, not elsewhere classified, unspecified ankle

✓5th **M21.2 Flexion deformity**

M21.20   Flexion deformity, unspecified site

✓6th **M21.21 Flexion deformity, shoulder**

M21.211   Flexion deformity, right shoulder

M21.212   Flexion deformity, left shoulder

M21.219   Flexion deformity, unspecified shoulder

✓6th **M21.22 Flexion deformity, elbow**

M21.221   Flexion deformity, right elbow

M21.222   Flexion deformity, left elbow

M21.229   Flexion deformity, unspecified elbow

✓6th **M21.23 Flexion deformity, wrist**

M21.231   Flexion deformity, right wrist

M21.232   Flexion deformity, left wrist

M21.239   Flexion deformity, unspecified wrist

✓6th **M21.24 Flexion deformity, finger joints**

M21.241   Flexion deformity, right finger joints

M21.242   Flexion deformity, left finger joints

M21.249   Flexion deformity, unspecified finger joints

✓6th **M21.25 Flexion deformity, hip**

M21.251   Flexion deformity, right hip

M21.252   Flexion deformity, left hip

M21.259   Flexion deformity, unspecified hip

✓6th **M21.26 Flexion deformity, knee**

M21.261   Flexion deformity, right knee

M21.262   Flexion deformity, left knee

M21.269   Flexion deformity, unspecified knee

✓6th **M21.27 Flexion deformity, ankle and toes**

M21.271   Flexion deformity, right ankle and toes

M21.272   Flexion deformity, left ankle and toes

M21.279   Flexion deformity, unspecified ankle and toes

✓5th **M21.3 Wrist or foot drop (acquired)**

✓6th **M21.33 Wrist drop (acquired)**

M21.331   Wrist drop, right wrist

M21.332   Wrist drop, left wrist

M21.339   Wrist drop, unspecified wrist

✓6th **M21.37 Foot drop (acquired)**

M21.371   Foot drop, right foot

M21.372   Foot drop, left foot

M21.379   Foot drop, unspecified foot

✓5th **M21.4 Flat foot [pes planus] (acquired)**

EXCLUDES 1   congenital pes planus (Q66.5-)

M21.40   Flat foot [pes planus] (acquired), unspecified foot

M21.41   Flat foot [pes planus] (acquired), right foot

M21.42   Flat foot [pes planus] (acquired), left foot

✓5th **M21.5 Acquired clawhand, clubhand, clawfoot and clubfoot**

EXCLUDES 1   clubfoot, not specified as acquired (Q66.89)

✓6th **M21.51 Acquired clawhand**

M21.511   Acquired clawhand, right hand

M21.512   Acquired clawhand, left hand

M21.519   Acquired clawhand, unspecified hand

✓6th **M21.52 Acquired clubhand**

M21.521   Acquired clubhand, right hand

M21.522   Acquired clubhand, left hand

M21.529   Acquired clubhand, unspecified hand

✓6th **M21.53 Acquired clawfoot**

M21.531   Acquired clawfoot, right foot

M21.532   Acquired clawfoot, left foot

M21.539   Acquired clawfoot, unspecified foot

✓ Additional Character Required   ✓x7th Placeholder Alert   Unacceptable PDx   Manifestation   Hospital Acquired Condition   EXCLUDES 1 Not Coded Here   EXCLUDES 2 Not Included Here

ICD-10-CM 2016   729

✓6ᵗʰ **M21.54 Acquired** clubfoot
     M21.541 Acquired clubfoot, right foot
     M21.542 Acquired clubfoot, left foot
     M21.549 Acquired clubfoot, unspecified foot

✓5ᵗʰ **M21.6 Other acquired deformities of foot**
     EXCLUDES 2   deformities of toe (acquired) (M20.1-M20.6)

     ✓6ᵗʰ **M21.6X Other acquired deformities of** foot
       M21.6X1 Other acquired deformities of right foot
       M21.6X2 Other acquired deformities of left foot
       M21.6X9 Other acquired deformities of unspecified foot

✓5ᵗʰ **M21.7 Unequal limb length (acquired)**
     NOTE   The site used should correspond to the shorter limb.
     M21.70 Unequal limb length (acquired), unspecified site

     ✓6ᵗʰ **M21.72 Unequal limb length (acquired), humerus**
       M21.721 Unequal limb length (acquired), right humerus
       M21.722 Unequal limb length (acquired), left humerus
       M21.729 Unequal limb length (acquired), unspecified humerus

     ✓6ᵗʰ **M21.73 Unequal limb length (acquired), ulna and radius**
       M21.731 Unequal limb length (acquired), right ulna
       M21.732 Unequal limb length (acquired), left ulna
       M21.733 Unequal limb length (acquired), right radius
       M21.734 Unequal limb length (acquired), left radius
       M21.739 Unequal limb length (acquired), unspecified ulna and radius

     ✓6ᵗʰ **M21.75 Unequal limb length (acquired), femur**
       M21.751 Unequal limb length (acquired), right femur
       M21.752 Unequal limb length (acquired), left femur
       M21.759 Unequal limb length (acquired), unspecified femur

     ✓6ᵗʰ **M21.76 Unequal limb length (acquired), tibia and fibula**
       M21.761 Unequal limb length (acquired), right tibia
       M21.762 Unequal limb length (acquired), left tibia
       M21.763 Unequal limb length (acquired), right fibula
       M21.764 Unequal limb length (acquired), left fibula
       M21.769 Unequal limb length (acquired), unspecified tibia and fibula

✓5ᵗʰ **M21.8 Other specified acquired deformities of limbs**
     EXCLUDES 2   coxa plana (M91.2)

     M21.80 Other specified acquired deformities of unspecified limb

     ✓6ᵗʰ **M21.82 Other specified acquired deformities of upper arm**
       M21.821 Other specified acquired deformities of right upper arm
       M21.822 Other specified acquired deformities of left upper arm
       M21.829 Other specified acquired deformities of unspecified upper arm

     ✓6ᵗʰ **M21.83 Other specified acquired deformities of forearm**
       M21.831 Other specified acquired deformities of right forearm
       M21.832 Other specified acquired deformities of left forearm
       M21.839 Other specified acquired deformities of unspecified forearm

     ✓6ᵗʰ **M21.85 Other specified acquired deformities of thigh**
       M21.851 Other specified acquired deformities of right thigh
       M21.852 Other specified acquired deformities of left thigh
       M21.859 Other specified acquired deformities of unspecified thigh

     ✓6ᵗʰ **M21.86 Other specified acquired deformities of lower leg**
       M21.861 Other specified acquired deformities of right lower leg
       M21.862 Other specified acquired deformities of left lower leg
       M21.869 Other specified acquired deformities of unspecified lower leg

✓5ᵗʰ **M21.9 Unspecified acquired deformity of limb and hand**
     M21.90 Unspecified acquired deformity of unspecified limb

     ✓6ᵗʰ **M21.92 Unspecified acquired deformity of upper arm**
       M21.921 Unspecified acquired deformity of right upper arm
       M21.922 Unspecified acquired deformity of left upper arm
       M21.929 Unspecified acquired deformity of unspecified upper arm

     ✓6ᵗʰ **M21.93 Unspecified acquired deformity of forearm**
       M21.931 Unspecified acquired deformity of right forearm
       M21.932 Unspecified acquired deformity of left forearm
       M21.939 Unspecified acquired deformity of unspecified forearm

     ✓6ᵗʰ **M21.94 Unspecified acquired deformity of hand**
       M21.941 Unspecified acquired deformity of hand, right hand
       M21.942 Unspecified acquired deformity of hand, left hand
       M21.949 Unspecified acquired deformity of hand, unspecified hand

     ✓6ᵗʰ **M21.95 Unspecified acquired deformity of thigh**
       M21.951 Unspecified acquired deformity of right thigh
       M21.952 Unspecified acquired deformity of left thigh
       M21.959 Unspecified acquired deformity of unspecified thigh

     ✓6ᵗʰ **M21.96 Unspecified acquired deformity of lower leg**
       M21.961 Unspecified acquired deformity of right lower leg
       M21.962 Unspecified acquired deformity of left lower leg
       M21.969 Unspecified acquired deformity of unspecified lower leg

✓4ᵗʰ **M22 Disorder of patella**
     EXCLUDES 1   traumatic dislocation of patella (S83.0-)

     ✓5ᵗʰ **M22.0 Recurrent dislocation of patella**
       M22.00 Recurrent dislocation of patella, unspecified knee
       M22.01 Recurrent dislocation of patella, right knee
       M22.02 Recurrent dislocation of patella, left knee

     ✓5ᵗʰ **M22.1 Recurrent subluxation of patella**
       Incomplete dislocation of patella
       M22.10 Recurrent subluxation of patella, unspecified knee
       M22.11 Recurrent subluxation of patella, right knee
       M22.12 Recurrent subluxation of patella, left knee

     ✓5ᵗʰ **M22.2 Patellofemoral disorders**
       ✓6ᵗʰ **M22.2X Patellofemoral disorders**
         M22.2X1 Patellofemoral disorders, right knee
         M22.2X2 Patellofemoral disorders, left knee
         M22.2X9 Patellofemoral disorders, unspecified knee

     ✓5ᵗʰ **M22.3 Other derangements of patella**
       ✓6ᵗʰ **M22.3X Other derangements of patella**
         M22.3X1 Other derangements of patella, right knee
         M22.3X2 Other derangements of patella, left knee
         M22.3X9 Other derangements of patella, unspecified knee

     ✓5ᵗʰ **M22.4 Chondromalacia patellae**
       M22.40 Chondromalacia patellae, unspecified knee
       M22.41 Chondromalacia patellae, right knee
       M22.42 Chondromalacia patellae, left knee

     ✓5ᵗʰ **M22.8 Other disorders of patella**
       ✓6ᵗʰ **M22.8X Other disorders of patella**
         M22.8X1 Other disorders of patella, right knee
         M22.8X2 Other disorders of patella, left knee
         M22.8X9 Other disorders of patella, unspecified knee

     ✓5ᵗʰ **M22.9 Unspecified disorder of patella**
       M22.90 Unspecified disorder of patella, unspecified knee
       M22.91 Unspecified disorder of patella, right knee

N Newborn: 0   P Pediatric: 0-17   M Maternity: 12-55   A Adult: 15-124   MCC Major CC Condition   PDx MCC PDx acts as own MCC   CC CC Condition   PDx CC PDx acts as own CC

730   ICD-10-CM 2016

M22.92   **Unspecified disorder of patella, left knee**

✓4ᵗʰ **M23 Internal derangement of knee**

> **EXCLUDES 1**   *ankylosis (M24.66)*
> *current injury—see injury of knee and lower leg (S80-S89)*
> *deformity of knee (M21.-)*
> *osteochondritis dissecans (M93.2)*
> *recurrent dislocation or subluxation of joints (M24.4)*
> *recurrent dislocation or subluxation of patella (M22.0-M22.1)*

✓5ᵗʰ **M23.0 Cystic meniscus**

  ✓6ᵗʰ **M23.00 Cystic meniscus, unspecified meniscus**
Cystic meniscus, unspecified lateral meniscus
Cystic meniscus, unspecified medial meniscus

    M23.000 **Cystic meniscus, unspecified lateral meniscus, right knee**
    M23.001 **Cystic meniscus, unspecified lateral meniscus, left knee**
    M23.002 **Cystic meniscus, unspecified lateral meniscus, unspecified knee**
    M23.003 **Cystic meniscus, unspecified medial meniscus, right knee**
    M23.004 **Cystic meniscus, unspecified medial meniscus, left knee**
    M23.005 **Cystic meniscus, unspecified medial meniscus, unspecified knee**
    M23.006 **Cystic meniscus, unspecified meniscus, right knee**
    M23.007 **Cystic meniscus, unspecified meniscus, left knee**
    M23.009 **Cystic meniscus, unspecified meniscus, unspecified knee**

  ✓6ᵗʰ **M23.01 Cystic meniscus, anterior horn of medial meniscus**
    M23.011 **Cystic meniscus, anterior horn of medial meniscus, right knee**
    M23.012 **Cystic meniscus, anterior horn of medial meniscus, left knee**
    M23.019 **Cystic meniscus, anterior horn of medial meniscus, unspecified knee**

  ✓6ᵗʰ **M23.02 Cystic meniscus, posterior horn of medial meniscus**
    M23.021 **Cystic meniscus, posterior horn of medial meniscus, right knee**
    M23.022 **Cystic meniscus, posterior horn of medial meniscus, left knee**
    M23.029 **Cystic meniscus, posterior horn of medial meniscus, unspecified knee**

  ✓6ᵗʰ **M23.03 Cystic meniscus, other medial meniscus**
    M23.031 **Cystic meniscus, other medial meniscus, right knee**
    M23.032 **Cystic meniscus, other medial meniscus, left knee**
    M23.039 **Cystic meniscus, other medial meniscus, unspecified knee**

  ✓6ᵗʰ **M23.04 Cystic meniscus, anterior horn of lateral meniscus**
    M23.041 **Cystic meniscus, anterior horn of lateral meniscus, right knee**
    M23.042 **Cystic meniscus, anterior horn of lateral meniscus, left knee**
    M23.049 **Cystic meniscus, anterior horn of lateral meniscus, unspecified knee**

  ✓6ᵗʰ **M23.05 Cystic meniscus, posterior horn of lateral meniscus**
    M23.051 **Cystic meniscus, posterior horn of lateral meniscus, right knee**
    M23.052 **Cystic meniscus, posterior horn of lateral meniscus, left knee**
    M23.059 **Cystic meniscus, posterior horn of lateral meniscus, unspecified knee**

  ✓6ᵗʰ **M23.06 Cystic meniscus, other lateral meniscus**
    M23.061 **Cystic meniscus, other lateral meniscus, right knee**
    M23.062 **Cystic meniscus, other lateral meniscus, left knee**
    M23.069 **Cystic meniscus, other lateral meniscus, unspecified knee**

✓5ᵗʰ **M23.2 Derangement of meniscus due to old tear or injury**
Old bucket-handle tear

  ✓6ᵗʰ **M23.20 Derangement of unspecified meniscus due to old tear or injury**
Derangement of unspecified lateral meniscus due to old tear or injury
Derangement of unspecified medial meniscus due to old tear or injury

    M23.200 **Derangement of unspecified lateral meniscus due to old tear or injury, right knee**
    M23.201 **Derangement of unspecified lateral meniscus due to old tear or injury, left knee**
    M23.202 **Derangement of unspecified lateral meniscus due to old tear or injury, unspecified knee**
    M23.203 **Derangement of unspecified medial meniscus due to old tear or injury, right knee**
    M23.204 **Derangement of unspecified medial meniscus due to old tear or injury, left knee**
    M23.205 **Derangement of unspecified medial meniscus due to old tear or injury, unspecified knee**
    M23.206 **Derangement of unspecified meniscus due to old tear or injury, right knee**
    M23.207 **Derangement of unspecified meniscus due to old tear or injury, left knee**
    M23.209 **Derangement of unspecified meniscus due to old tear or injury, unspecified knee**

  ✓6ᵗʰ **M23.21 Derangement of anterior horn of medial meniscus due to old tear or injury**
    M23.211 **Derangement of anterior horn of medial meniscus due to old tear or injury, right knee**
    M23.212 **Derangement of anterior horn of medial meniscus due to old tear or injury, left knee**
    M23.219 **Derangement of anterior horn of medial meniscus due to old tear or injury, unspecified knee**

  ✓6ᵗʰ **M23.22 Derangement of posterior horn of medial meniscus due to old tear or injury**
    M23.221 **Derangement of posterior horn of medial meniscus due to old tear or injury, right knee**
    M23.222 **Derangement of posterior horn of medial meniscus due to old tear or injury, left knee**
    M23.229 **Derangement of posterior horn of medial meniscus due to old tear or injury, unspecified knee**

  ✓6ᵗʰ **M23.23 Derangement of other medial meniscus due to old tear or injury**
    M23.231 **Derangement of other medial meniscus due to old tear or injury, right knee**
    M23.232 **Derangement of other medial meniscus due to old tear or injury, left knee**
    M23.239 **Derangement of other medial meniscus due to old tear or injury, unspecified knee**

  ✓6ᵗʰ **M23.24 Derangement of anterior horn of lateral meniscus due to old tear or injury**
    M23.241 **Derangement of anterior horn of lateral meniscus due to old tear or injury, right knee**
    M23.242 **Derangement of anterior horn of lateral meniscus due to old tear or injury, left knee**
    M23.249 **Derangement of anterior horn of lateral meniscus due to old tear or injury, unspecified knee**

  ✓6ᵗʰ **M23.25 Derangement of posterior horn of lateral meniscus due to old tear or injury**
    M23.251 **Derangement of posterior horn of lateral meniscus due to old tear or injury, right knee**

✓ Additional Character Required   ✓x7ᵗʰ Placeholder Alert   Unacceptable PDx   Manifestation   Hospital Acquired Condition   **EXCLUDES 1** Not Coded Here   **EXCLUDES 2** Not Included Here

ICD-10-CM 2016   731

M23.252 Derangement of posterior horn of lateral meniscus due to old tear or injury, left knee

M23.259 Derangement of posterior horn of lateral meniscus due to old tear or injury, unspecified knee

✓6ᵗʰ **M23.26** Derangement of other lateral meniscus due to old tear or injury

M23.261 Derangement of other lateral meniscus due to old tear or injury, right knee

M23.262 Derangement of other lateral meniscus due to old tear or injury, left knee

M23.269 Derangement of other lateral meniscus due to old tear or injury, unspecified knee

✓5ᵗʰ **M23.3** Other meniscus derangements
Degenerate meniscus
Detached meniscus
Retained meniscus

✓6ᵗʰ **M23.30** Other meniscus derangements, unspecified meniscus
Other meniscus derangements, unspecified lateral meniscus
Other meniscus derangements, unspecified medial meniscus

M23.300 Other meniscus derangements, unspecified lateral meniscus, right knee

M23.301 Other meniscus derangements, unspecified lateral meniscus, left knee

M23.302 Other meniscus derangements, unspecified lateral meniscus, unspecified knee

M23.303 Other meniscus derangements, unspecified medial meniscus, right knee

M23.304 Other meniscus derangements, unspecified medial meniscus, left knee

M23.305 Other meniscus derangements, unspecified medial meniscus, unspecified knee

M23.306 Other meniscus derangements, unspecified meniscus, right knee

M23.307 Other meniscus derangements, unspecified meniscus, left knee

M23.309 Other meniscus derangements, unspecified meniscus, unspecified knee

✓6ᵗʰ **M23.31** Other meniscus derangements, anterior horn of medial meniscus

M23.311 Other meniscus derangements, anterior horn of medial meniscus, right knee

M23.312 Other meniscus derangements, anterior horn of medial meniscus, left knee

M23.319 Other meniscus derangements, anterior horn of medial meniscus, unspecified knee

✓6ᵗʰ **M23.32** Other meniscus derangements, posterior horn of medial meniscus

M23.321 Other meniscus derangements, posterior horn of medial meniscus, right knee

M23.322 Other meniscus derangements, posterior horn of medial meniscus, left knee

M23.329 Other meniscus derangements, posterior horn of medial meniscus, unspecified knee

✓6ᵗʰ **M23.33** Other meniscus derangements, other medial meniscus

M23.331 Other meniscus derangements, other medial meniscus, right knee

M23.332 Other meniscus derangements, other medial meniscus, left knee

M23.339 Other meniscus derangements, other medial meniscus, unspecified knee

✓6ᵗʰ **M23.34** Other meniscus derangements, anterior horn of lateral meniscus

M23.341 Other meniscus derangements, anterior horn of lateral meniscus, right knee

M23.342 Other meniscus derangements, anterior horn of lateral meniscus, left knee

M23.349 Other meniscus derangements, anterior horn of lateral meniscus, unspecified knee

✓6ᵗʰ **M23.35** Other meniscus derangements, posterior horn of lateral meniscus

M23.351 Other meniscus derangements, posterior horn of lateral meniscus, right knee

M23.352 Other meniscus derangements, posterior horn of lateral meniscus, left knee

M23.359 Other meniscus derangements, posterior horn of lateral meniscus, unspecified knee

✓6ᵗʰ **M23.36** Other meniscus derangements, other lateral meniscus

M23.361 Other meniscus derangements, other lateral meniscus, right knee

M23.362 Other meniscus derangements, other lateral meniscus, left knee

M23.369 Other meniscus derangements, other lateral meniscus, unspecified knee

✓5ᵗʰ **M23.4** Loose body in knee

M23.40 Loose body in knee, unspecified knee

M23.41 Loose body in knee, right knee

M23.42 Loose body in knee, left knee

✓5ᵗʰ **M23.5** Chronic instability of knee

M23.50 Chronic instability of knee, unspecified knee

M23.51 Chronic instability of knee, right knee

M23.52 Chronic instability of knee, left knee

✓5ᵗʰ **M23.6** Other spontaneous disruption of ligament(s) of knee

✓6ᵗʰ **M23.60** Other spontaneous disruption of unspecified ligament of knee

M23.601 Other spontaneous disruption of unspecified ligament of right knee

M23.602 Other spontaneous disruption of unspecified ligament of left knee

M23.609 Other spontaneous disruption of unspecified ligament of unspecified knee

✓6ᵗʰ **M23.61** Other spontaneous disruption of anterior cruciate ligament of knee

M23.611 Other spontaneous disruption of anterior cruciate ligament of right knee

M23.612 Other spontaneous disruption of anterior cruciate ligament of left knee

M23.619 Other spontaneous disruption of anterior cruciate ligament of unspecified knee

✓6ᵗʰ **M23.62** Other spontaneous disruption of posterior cruciate ligament of knee

M23.621 Other spontaneous disruption of posterior cruciate ligament of right knee

M23.622 Other spontaneous disruption of posterior cruciate ligament of left knee

M23.629 Other spontaneous disruption of posterior cruciate ligament of unspecified knee

✓6ᵗʰ **M23.63** Other spontaneous disruption of medial collateral ligament of knee

M23.631 Other spontaneous disruption of medial collateral ligament of right knee

M23.632 Other spontaneous disruption of medial collateral ligament of left knee

M23.639 Other spontaneous disruption of medial collateral ligament of unspecified knee

✓6ᵗʰ **M23.64** Other spontaneous disruption of lateral collateral ligament of knee

M23.641 Other spontaneous disruption of lateral collateral ligament of right knee

M23.642 Other spontaneous disruption of lateral collateral ligament of left knee

M23.649 Other spontaneous disruption of lateral collateral ligament of unspecified knee

✓6ᵗʰ **M23.67** Other spontaneous disruption of capsular ligament of knee

M23.671 Other spontaneous disruption of capsular ligament of right knee

M23.672 Other spontaneous disruption of capsular ligament of left knee

M23.679 Other spontaneous disruption of capsular ligament of unspecified knee

Ⓝ Newborn: 0   Ⓟ Pediatric: 0-17   Ⓜ Maternity: 12-55   Ⓐ Adult: 15-124   **MCC** Major CC Condition   **PDxMCC** PDx acts as own MCC   **CC** CC Condition   **PDxCC** PDx acts as own CC

732   ICD-10-CM 2016

✓5ᵗʰ **M23.8 Other internal derangements of knee**
　　Laxity of ligament of knee
　　Snapping knee

　✓6ᵗʰ **M23.8X Other internal derangements of knee**
　　　M23.8X1 Other internal derangements of right knee
　　　M23.8X2 Other internal derangements of left knee
　　　M23.8X9 Other internal derangements of unspecified knee

✓5ᵗʰ **M23.9 Unspecified internal derangement of knee**
　　M23.90 Unspecified internal derangement of unspecified knee
　　M23.91 Unspecified internal derangement of right knee
　　M23.92 Unspecified internal derangement of left knee

✓4ᵗʰ **M24 Other specific joint derangements**
　EXCLUDES 1 current injury—see injury of joint by body region
　EXCLUDES 2 ganglion (M67.4)
　　　snapping knee (M23.8-)
　　　temporomandibular joint disorders (M26.6-)

✓5ᵗʰ **M24.0 Loose body in joint**
　EXCLUDES 2 loose body in knee (M23.4)

　　M24.00 Loose body in unspecified joint
　✓6ᵗʰ **M24.01 Loose body in** shoulder
　　　M24.011 Loose body in right **shoulder**
　　　M24.012 Loose body in left **shoulder**
　　　M24.019 Loose body in unspecified **shoulder**
　✓6ᵗʰ **M24.02 Loose body in** elbow
　　　M24.021 Loose body in right **elbow**
　　　M24.022 Loose body in left **elbow**
　　　M24.029 Loose body in unspecified **elbow**
　✓6ᵗʰ **M24.03 Loose body in** wrist
　　　M24.031 Loose body in right **wrist**
　　　M24.032 Loose body in left **wrist**
　　　M24.039 Loose body in unspecified **wrist**
　✓6ᵗʰ **M24.04 Loose body in** finger joints
　　　M24.041 Loose body in right **finger joint(s)**
　　　M24.042 Loose body in left **finger joint(s)**
　　　M24.049 Loose body in unspecified **finger joint(s)**
　✓6ᵗʰ **M24.05 Loose body in** hip
　　　M24.051 Loose body in right **hip**
　　　M24.052 Loose body in left **hip**
　　　M24.059 Loose body in unspecified **hip**
　✓6ᵗʰ **M24.07 Loose body in** ankle and toe joints
　　　M24.071 Loose body in right **ankle**
　　　M24.072 Loose body in left **ankle**
　　　M24.073 Loose body in unspecified **ankle**
　　　M24.074 Loose body in right **toe joint(s)**
　　　M24.075 Loose body in left **toe joint(s)**
　　　M24.076 Loose body in unspecified **toe joints**
　　M24.08 Loose body, other site

✓5ᵗʰ **M24.1 Other articular cartilage disorders**
　EXCLUDES 2 chondrocalcinosis (M11.1, M11.2-)
　　　internal derangement of knee (M23.-)
　　　metastatic calcification (E83.5)
　　　ochronosis (E70.2)

　　M24.10 Other articular cartilage disorders, unspecified site
　✓6ᵗʰ **M24.11 Other articular cartilage disorders,** shoulder
　　　M24.111 Other articular cartilage disorders, right **shoulder**
　　　M24.112 Other articular cartilage disorders, left **shoulder**
　　　M24.119 Other articular cartilage disorders, unspecified **shoulder**
　✓6ᵗʰ **M24.12 Other articular cartilage disorders,** elbow
　　　M24.121 Other articular cartilage disorders, right **elbow**
　　　M24.122 Other articular cartilage disorders, left **elbow**
　　　M24.129 Other articular cartilage disorders, unspecified **elbow**
　✓6ᵗʰ **M24.13 Other articular cartilage disorders,** wrist
　　　M24.131 Other articular cartilage disorders, right **wrist**
　　　M24.132 Other articular cartilage disorders, left **wrist**
　　　M24.139 Other articular cartilage disorders, unspecified **wrist**
　✓6ᵗʰ **M24.14 Other articular cartilage disorders,** hand
　　　M24.141 Other articular cartilage disorders, right **hand**
　　　M24.142 Other articular cartilage disorders, left **hand**
　　　M24.149 Other articular cartilage disorders, unspecified **hand**
　✓6ᵗʰ **M24.15 Other articular cartilage disorders,** hip
　　　M24.151 Other articular cartilage disorders, right **hip**
　　　M24.152 Other articular cartilage disorders, left **hip**
　　　M24.159 Other articular cartilage disorders, unspecified **hip**
　✓6ᵗʰ **M24.17 Other articular cartilage disorders,** ankle and foot
　　　M24.171 Other articular cartilage disorders, right **ankle**
　　　M24.172 Other articular cartilage disorders, left **ankle**
　　　M24.173 Other articular cartilage disorders, unspecified **ankle**
　　　M24.174 Other articular cartilage disorders, right **foot**
　　　M24.175 Other articular cartilage disorders, left **foot**
　　　M24.176 Other articular cartilage disorders, unspecified **foot**

✓5ᵗʰ **M24.2 Disorder of ligament**
　　Instability secondary to old ligament injury
　　Ligamentous laxity NOS
　EXCLUDES 1 familial ligamentous laxity (M35.7)
　EXCLUDES 2 internal derangement of knee (M23.5-M23.89)

　　M24.20 Disorder of ligament, unspecified site
　✓6ᵗʰ **M24.21 Disorder of ligament,** shoulder
　　　M24.211 Disorder of ligament, right **shoulder**
　　　M24.212 Disorder of ligament, left **shoulder**
　　　M24.219 Disorder of ligament, unspecified **shoulder**
　✓6ᵗʰ **M24.22 Disorder of ligament,** elbow
　　　M24.221 Disorder of ligament, right **elbow**
　　　M24.222 Disorder of ligament, left **elbow**
　　　M24.229 Disorder of ligament, unspecified **elbow**
　✓6ᵗʰ **M24.23 Disorder of ligament,** wrist
　　　M24.231 Disorder of ligament, right **wrist**
　　　M24.232 Disorder of ligament, left **wrist**
　　　M24.239 Disorder of ligament, unspecified **wrist**
　✓6ᵗʰ **M24.24 Disorder of ligament,** hand
　　　M24.241 Disorder of ligament, right **hand**
　　　M24.242 Disorder of ligament, left **hand**
　　　M24.249 Disorder of ligament, unspecified **hand**
　✓6ᵗʰ **M24.25 Disorder of ligament,** hip
　　　M24.251 Disorder of ligament, right **hip**
　　　M24.252 Disorder of ligament, left **hip**
　　　M24.259 Disorder of ligament, unspecified **hip**
　✓6ᵗʰ **M24.27 Disorder of ligament,** ankle and foot
　　　M24.271 Disorder of ligament, right **ankle**
　　　M24.272 Disorder of ligament, left **ankle**
　　　M24.273 Disorder of ligament, unspecified **ankle**
　　　M24.274 Disorder of ligament, right **foot**
　　　M24.275 Disorder of ligament, left **foot**
　　　M24.276 Disorder of ligament, unspecified **foot**
　　M24.28 Disorder of ligament, vertebrae

✓5ᵗʰ **M24.3 Pathological dislocation of joint, not elsewhere classified**
　EXCLUDES 1 congenital dislocation or displacement of joint—see congenital malformations and deformations of the musculoskeletal system (Q65-Q79)
　　　current injury—see injury of joints and ligaments by body region
　　　recurrent dislocation of joint (M24.4-)

　　M24.30 Pathological dislocation of unspecified joint, not elsewhere classified

✓ Additional Character Required　✓x7ᵗʰ Placeholder Alert　Unacceptable PDx　Manifestation　Hospital Acquired Condition　EXCLUDES 1 Not Coded Here　EXCLUDES 2 Not Included Here

ICD-10-CM 2016　　　　　　　　　　　　　　　　　　　　　　　　　　733

✓6th **M24.31 Pathological dislocation of** shoulder, **not elsewhere classified**
- M24.311 Pathological dislocation of right shoulder, not elsewhere classified
- M24.312 Pathological dislocation of left shoulder, not elsewhere classified
- M24.319 Pathological dislocation of unspecified shoulder, not elsewhere classified

✓6th **M24.32 Pathological dislocation of** elbow, **not elsewhere classified**
- M24.321 Pathological dislocation of right elbow, not elsewhere classified
- M24.322 Pathological dislocation of left elbow, not elsewhere classified
- M24.329 Pathological dislocation of unspecified elbow, not elsewhere classified

✓6th **M24.33 Pathological dislocation of** wrist, **not elsewhere classified**
- M24.331 Pathological dislocation of right wrist, not elsewhere classified
- M24.332 Pathological dislocation of left wrist, not elsewhere classified
- M24.339 Pathological dislocation of unspecified wrist, not elsewhere classified

✓6th **M24.34 Pathological dislocation of** hand, **not elsewhere classified**
- M24.341 Pathological dislocation of right hand, not elsewhere classified
- M24.342 Pathological dislocation of left hand, not elsewhere classified
- M24.349 Pathological dislocation of unspecified hand, not elsewhere classified

✓6th **M24.35 Pathological dislocation of** hip, **not elsewhere classified**
- M24.351 Pathological dislocation of right hip, not elsewhere classified
- M24.352 Pathological dislocation of left hip, not elsewhere classified
- M24.359 Pathological dislocation of unspecified hip, not elsewhere classified

✓6th **M24.36 Pathological dislocation of** knee, **not elsewhere classified**
- M24.361 Pathological dislocation of right knee, not elsewhere classified
- M24.362 Pathological dislocation of left knee, not elsewhere classified
- M24.369 Pathological dislocation of unspecified knee, not elsewhere classified

✓6th **M24.37 Pathological dislocation of** ankle and foot, **not elsewhere classified**
- M24.371 Pathological dislocation of right ankle, not elsewhere classified
- M24.372 Pathological dislocation of left ankle, not elsewhere classified
- M24.373 Pathological dislocation of unspecified ankle, not elsewhere classified
- M24.374 Pathological dislocation of right foot, not elsewhere classified
- M24.375 Pathological dislocation of left foot, not elsewhere classified
- M24.376 Pathological dislocation of unspecified foot, not elsewhere classified

✓5th **M24.4 Recurrent dislocation of joint**
Recurrent subluxation of joint
EXCLUDES 2 recurrent dislocation of patella (M22.0-M22.1)
recurrent vertebral dislocation (M43.3-, M43.4, M43.5-)
- **M24.40 Recurrent dislocation,** unspecified joint
- ✓6th **M24.41 Recurrent dislocation,** shoulder
  - M24.411 Recurrent dislocation, right shoulder
  - M24.412 Recurrent dislocation, left shoulder
  - M24.419 Recurrent dislocation, unspecified shoulder
- ✓6th **M24.42 Recurrent dislocation,** elbow
  - M24.421 Recurrent dislocation, right elbow
  - M24.422 Recurrent dislocation, left elbow
  - M24.429 Recurrent dislocation, unspecified elbow

✓6th **M24.43 Recurrent dislocation,** wrist
- M24.431 Recurrent dislocation, right wrist
- M24.432 Recurrent dislocation, left wrist
- M24.439 Recurrent dislocation, unspecified wrist

✓6th **M24.44 Recurrent dislocation,** hand and finger(s)
- M24.441 Recurrent dislocation, right hand
- M24.442 Recurrent dislocation, left hand
- M24.443 Recurrent dislocation, unspecified hand
- M24.444 Recurrent dislocation, right finger
- M24.445 Recurrent dislocation, left finger
- M24.446 Recurrent dislocation, unspecified finger

✓6th **M24.45 Recurrent dislocation,** hip
- M24.451 Recurrent dislocation, right hip
- M24.452 Recurrent dislocation, left hip
- M24.459 Recurrent dislocation, unspecified hip

✓6th **M24.46 Recurrent dislocation,** knee
- M24.461 Recurrent dislocation, right knee
- M24.462 Recurrent dislocation, left knee
- M24.469 Recurrent dislocation, unspecified knee

✓6th **M24.47 Recurrent dislocation,** ankle, foot and toes
- M24.471 Recurrent dislocation, right ankle
- M24.472 Recurrent dislocation, left ankle
- M24.473 Recurrent dislocation, unspecified ankle
- M24.474 Recurrent dislocation, right foot
- M24.475 Recurrent dislocation, left foot
- M24.476 Recurrent dislocation, unspecified foot
- M24.477 Recurrent dislocation, right toe(s)
- M24.478 Recurrent dislocation, left toe(s)
- M24.479 Recurrent dislocation, unspecified toe(s)

✓5th **M24.5 Contracture of joint**
EXCLUDES 1 contracture of muscle without contracture of joint (M62.4-)
contracture of tendon (sheath) without contracture of joint (M62.4-)
Dupuytren's contracture (M72.0)
EXCLUDES 2 acquired deformities of limbs (M20-M21)
- **M24.50 Contracture,** unspecified joint
- ✓6th **M24.51 Contracture,** shoulder
  - M24.511 Contracture, right shoulder
  - M24.512 Contracture, left shoulder
  - M24.519 Contracture, unspecified shoulder
- ✓6th **M24.52 Contracture,** elbow
  - M24.521 Contracture, right elbow
  - M24.522 Contracture, left elbow
  - M24.529 Contracture, unspecified elbow
- ✓6th **M24.53 Contracture,** wrist
  - M24.531 Contracture, right wrist
  - M24.532 Contracture, left wrist
  - M24.539 Contracture, unspecified wrist
- ✓6th **M24.54 Contracture,** hand
  - M24.541 Contracture, right hand
  - M24.542 Contracture, left hand
  - M24.549 Contracture, unspecified hand
- ✓6th **M24.55 Contracture,** hip
  - M24.551 Contracture, right hip
  - M24.552 Contracture, left hip
  - M24.559 Contracture, unspecified hip
- ✓6th **M24.56 Contracture,** knee
  - M24.561 Contracture, right knee
  - M24.562 Contracture, left knee
  - M24.569 Contracture, unspecified knee
- ✓6th **M24.57 Contracture,** ankle and foot
  - M24.571 Contracture, right ankle
  - M24.572 Contracture, left ankle
  - M24.573 Contracture, unspecified ankle
  - M24.574 Contracture, right foot
  - M24.575 Contracture, left foot
  - M24.576 Contracture, unspecified foot

✓5th **M24.6 Ankylosis of joint**
EXCLUDES 1 stiffness of joint without ankylosis (M25.6-)
EXCLUDES 2 spine (M43.2-)
- **M24.60 Ankylosis,** unspecified joint

√6th **M24.61 Ankylosis, shoulder**
    M24.611 Ankylosis, right shoulder
    M24.612 Ankylosis, left shoulder
    M24.619 Ankylosis, unspecified shoulder

√6th **M24.62 Ankylosis, elbow**
    M24.621 Ankylosis, right elbow
    M24.622 Ankylosis, left elbow
    M24.629 Ankylosis, unspecified elbow

√6th **M24.63 Ankylosis, wrist**
    M24.631 Ankylosis, right wrist
    M24.632 Ankylosis, left wrist
    M24.639 Ankylosis, unspecified wrist

√6th **M24.64 Ankylosis, hand**
    M24.641 Ankylosis, right hand
    M24.642 Ankylosis, left hand
    M24.649 Ankylosis, unspecified hand

√6th **M24.65 Ankylosis, hip**
    M24.651 Ankylosis, right hip
    M24.652 Ankylosis, left hip
    M24.659 Ankylosis, unspecified hip

√6th **M24.66 Ankylosis, knee**
    M24.661 Ankylosis, right knee
    M24.662 Ankylosis, left knee
    M24.669 Ankylosis, unspecified knee

√6th **M24.67 Ankylosis, ankle and foot**
    M24.671 Ankylosis, right ankle
    M24.672 Ankylosis, left ankle
    M24.673 Ankylosis, unspecified ankle
    M24.674 Ankylosis, right foot
    M24.675 Ankylosis, left foot
    M24.676 Ankylosis, unspecified foot

M24.7 Protrusio acetabuli

√5th **M24.8 Other specific joint derangements, not elsewhere classified**
    EXCLUDES 2   iliotibial band syndrome (M76.3)

    M24.80 Other specific joint derangements of unspecified joint, not elsewhere classified

√6th **M24.81 Other specific joint derangements of shoulder, not elsewhere classified**
    M24.811 Other specific joint derangements of right shoulder, not elsewhere classified
    M24.812 Other specific joint derangements of left shoulder, not elsewhere classified
    M24.819 Other specific joint derangements of unspecified shoulder, not elsewhere classified

√6th **M24.82 Other specific joint derangements of elbow, not elsewhere classified**
    M24.821 Other specific joint derangements of right elbow, not elsewhere classified
    M24.822 Other specific joint derangements of left elbow, not elsewhere classified
    M24.829 Other specific joint derangements of unspecified elbow, not elsewhere classified

√6th **M24.83 Other specific joint derangements of wrist, not elsewhere classified**
    M24.831 Other specific joint derangements of right wrist, not elsewhere classified
    M24.832 Other specific joint derangements of left wrist, not elsewhere classified
    M24.839 Other specific joint derangements of unspecified wrist, not elsewhere classified

√6th **M24.84 Other specific joint derangements of hand, not elsewhere classified**
    M24.841 Other specific joint derangements of right hand, not elsewhere classified
    M24.842 Other specific joint derangements of left hand, not elsewhere classified
    M24.849 Other specific joint derangements of unspecified hand, not elsewhere classified

√6th **M24.85 Other specific joint derangements of hip, not elsewhere classified**
    Irritable hip
    M24.851 Other specific joint derangements of right hip, not elsewhere classified

    M24.852 Other specific joint derangements of left hip, not elsewhere classified
    M24.859 Other specific joint derangements of unspecified hip, not elsewhere classified

√6th **M24.87 Other specific joint derangements of ankle and foot, not elsewhere classified**
    M24.871 Other specific joint derangements of right ankle, not elsewhere classified
    M24.872 Other specific joint derangements of left ankle, not elsewhere classified
    M24.873 Other specific joint derangements of unspecified ankle, not elsewhere classified
    M24.874 Other specific joint derangements of right foot, not elsewhere classified
    M24.875 Other specific joint derangements left foot, not elsewhere classified
    M24.876 Other specific joint derangements of unspecified foot, not elsewhere classified

M24.9 Joint derangement, unspecified

√4th **M25 Other joint disorder, not elsewhere classified**
    EXCLUDES 2   abnormality of gait and mobility (R26.-)
       acquired deformities of limb (M20-M21)
       calcification of bursa (M71.4-)
       calcification of shoulder (joint) (M75.3)
       calcification of tendon (M65.2-)
       difficulty in walking (R26.2)
       temporomandibular joint disorder (M26.6-)

√5th **M25.0 Hemarthrosis**
    EXCLUDES 1   current injury—see injury of joint by body region
       hemophilic arthropathy (M36.2)

    M25.00 Hemarthrosis, unspecified joint   CC
    CC Excl: M25.00-M25.08, T79.A11A, T79.A12A, T79.A19A, T79.A21A, T79.A22A, T79.A29A

√6th **M25.01 Hemarthrosis, shoulder**
    M25.011 Hemarthrosis, right shoulder   CC
    CC Excl: M25.00-M25.039, M25.08, T79.A11A, T79.A12A, T79.A19A
    M25.012 Hemarthrosis, left shoulder   CC
    CC Excl: See code: M25.011
    M25.019 Hemarthrosis, unspecified shoulder   CC
    CC Excl: See code: M25.011

√6th **M25.02 Hemarthrosis, elbow**
    M25.021 Hemarthrosis, right elbow   CC
    CC Excl: M25.00-M25.029, M25.08, T79.A11A, T79.A12A, T79.A19A
    M25.022 Hemarthrosis, left elbow   CC
    CC Excl: See code: M25.022
    M25.029 Hemarthrosis, unspecified elbow   CC
    CC Excl: See code: M25.022

√6th **M25.03 Hemarthrosis, wrist**
    M25.031 Hemarthrosis, right wrist   CC
    CC Excl: M25.00, M25.021-M25.049, M25.08, T79.A11-T79.A19 with 7th character A
    M25.032 Hemarthrosis, left wrist   CC
    CC Excl: See code: M25.031
    M25.039 Hemarthrosis, unspecified wrist   CC
    CC Excl: See code: M25.031

√6th **M25.04 Hemarthrosis, hand**
    M25.041 Hemarthrosis, right hand   CC
    CC Excl: M25.00, M25.031-M25.049, M25.08, T79.A11-T79.A19 with 7th character A
    M25.042 Hemarthrosis, left hand   CC
    CC Excl: See code: M25.041
    M25.049 Hemarthrosis, unspecified hand   CC
    CC Excl: See code: M25.041

√6th **M25.05 Hemarthrosis, hip**
    M25.051 Hemarthrosis, right hip   CC
    CC Excl: M25.00-M25.08, T79.A11A, T79.A12A, T79.A19A, T79.A21A, T79.A22A, T79.A29A
    M25.052 Hemarthrosis, left hip   CC
    CC Excl: See code: M25.051
    M25.059 Hemarthrosis, unspecified hip   CC
    CC Excl: See code: M25.051

√6th **M25.06 Hemarthrosis, knee**
    M25.061 Hemarthrosis, right knee   CC
    CC Excl: M25.00, M25.061-M25.08, T79.A21-T79.A29 with 7th character A

√ Additional Character Required   √x7th Placeholder Alert   Unacceptable PDx   Manifestation   Hospital Acquired Condition   *EXCLUDES 1* Not Coded Here   *EXCLUDES 2* Not Included Here

ICD-10-CM 2016   735

　　　　M25.062　Hemarthrosis, left knee `CC`
　　　　　　　CC Excl: See code: M25.061
　　　　M25.069　Hemarthrosis, unspecified knee `CC`
　　　　　　　CC Excl: See code: M25.061
　✓6th　M25.07　Hemarthrosis, ankle and foot
　　　　M25.071　Hemarthrosis, right ankle `CC`
　　　　　　　CC Excl: See code: M25.061
　　　　M25.072　Hemarthrosis, left ankle `CC`
　　　　　　　CC Excl: See code: M25.061
　　　　M25.073　Hemarthrosis, unspecified ankle `CC`
　　　　　　　CC Excl: See code: M25.061
　　　　M25.074　Hemarthrosis, right foot `CC`
　　　　　　　CC Excl: See code: M25.061
　　　　M25.075　Hemarthrosis, left foot `CC`
　　　　　　　CC Excl: See code: M25.061
　　　　M25.076　Hemarthrosis, unspecified foot `CC`
　　　　　　　CC Excl: See code: M25.061
　M25.08　Hemarthrosis, other specified site `CC`
　　　　Hemarthrosis, vertebrae
　　　　CC Excl: M25.00-M25.08, T79.A11A, T79.A12A,
　　　　T79.A19A, T79.A21A, T79.A22A, T79.A29A

✓5th　M25.1　Fistula of joint
　M25.10　Fistula, unspecified joint
　✓6th　M25.11　Fistula, shoulder
　　　　M25.111　Fistula, right shoulder
　　　　M25.112　Fistula, left shoulder
　　　　M25.119　Fistula, unspecified shoulder
　✓6th　M25.12　Fistula, elbow
　　　　M25.121　Fistula, right elbow
　　　　M25.122　Fistula, left elbow
　　　　M25.129　Fistula, unspecified elbow
　✓6th　M25.13　Fistula, wrist
　　　　M25.131　Fistula, right wrist
　　　　M25.132　Fistula, left wrist
　　　　M25.139　Fistula, unspecified wrist
　✓6th　M25.14　Fistula, hand
　　　　M25.141　Fistula, right hand
　　　　M25.142　Fistula, left hand
　　　　M25.149　Fistula, unspecified hand
　✓6th　M25.15　Fistula, hip
　　　　M25.151　Fistula, right hip
　　　　M25.152　Fistula, left hip
　　　　M25.159　Fistula, unspecified hip
　✓6th　M25.16　Fistula, knee
　　　　M25.161　Fistula, right knee
　　　　M25.162　Fistula, left knee
　　　　M25.169　Fistula, unspecified knee
　✓6th　M25.17　Fistula, ankle and foot
　　　　M25.171　Fistula, right ankle
　　　　M25.172　Fistula, left ankle
　　　　M25.173　Fistula, unspecified ankle
　　　　M25.174　Fistula, right foot
　　　　M25.175　Fistula, left foot
　　　　M25.176　Fistula, unspecified foot
　M25.18　Fistula, other specified site
　　　　Fistula, vertebrae

✓5th　M25.2　Flail joint
　M25.20　Flail joint, unspecified joint
　✓6th　M25.21　Flail joint, shoulder
　　　　M25.211　Flail joint, right shoulder
　　　　M25.212　Flail joint, left shoulder
　　　　M25.219　Flail joint, unspecified shoulder
　✓6th　M25.22　Flail joint, elbow
　　　　M25.221　Flail joint, right elbow
　　　　M25.222　Flail joint, left elbow
　　　　M25.229　Flail joint, unspecified elbow
　✓6th　M25.23　Flail joint, wrist
　　　　M25.231　Flail joint, right wrist
　　　　M25.232　Flail joint, left wrist
　　　　M25.239　Flail joint, unspecified wrist
　✓6th　M25.24　Flail joint, hand
　　　　M25.241　Flail joint, right hand
　　　　M25.242　Flail joint, left hand

　　　　M25.249　Flail joint, unspecified hand
　✓6th　M25.25　Flail joint, hip
　　　　M25.251　Flail joint, right hip
　　　　M25.252　Flail joint, left hip
　　　　M25.259　Flail joint, unspecified hip
　✓6th　M25.26　Flail joint, knee
　　　　M25.261　Flail joint, right knee
　　　　M25.262　Flail joint, left knee
　　　　M25.269　Flail joint, unspecified knee
　✓6th　M25.27　Flail joint, ankle and foot
　　　　M25.271　Flail joint, right ankle and foot
　　　　M25.272　Flail joint, left ankle and foot
　　　　M25.279　Flail joint, unspecified ankle and foot
　M25.28　Flail joint, other site

✓5th　M25.3　Other instability of joint
　　EXCLUDES 1　instability of joint secondary to old ligament injury
　　　　　(M24.2-)
　　　　　instability of joint secondary to removal of joint
　　　　　prosthesis (M96.8-)
　　EXCLUDES 2　spinal instabilities (M53.2-)
　M25.30　Other instability, unspecified joint
　✓6th　M25.31　Other instability, shoulder
　　　　M25.311　Other instability, right shoulder
　　　　M25.312　Other instability, left shoulder
　　　　M25.319　Other instability, unspecified shoulder
　✓6th　M25.32　Other instability, elbow
　　　　M25.321　Other instability, right elbow
　　　　M25.322　Other instability, left elbow
　　　　M25.329　Other instability, unspecified elbow
　✓6th　M25.33　Other instability, wrist
　　　　M25.331　Other instability, right wrist
　　　　M25.332　Other instability, left wrist
　　　　M25.339　Other instability, unspecified wrist
　✓6th　M25.34　Other instability, hand
　　　　M25.341　Other instability, right hand
　　　　M25.342　Other instability, left hand
　　　　M25.349　Other instability, unspecified hand
　✓6th　M25.35　Other instability, hip
　　　　M25.351　Other instability, right hip
　　　　M25.352　Other instability, left hip
　　　　M25.359　Other instability, unspecified hip
　✓6th　M25.36　Other instability, knee
　　　　M25.361　Other instability, right knee
　　　　M25.362　Other instability, left knee
　　　　M25.369　Other instability, unspecified knee
　✓6th　M25.37　Other instability, ankle and foot
　　　　M25.371　Other instability, right ankle
　　　　M25.372　Other instability, left ankle
　　　　M25.373　Other instability, unspecified ankle
　　　　M25.374　Other instability, right foot
　　　　M25.375　Other instability, left foot
　　　　M25.376　Other instability, unspecified foot

✓5th　M25.4　Effusion of joint
　　EXCLUDES 1　hydrarthrosis in yaws (A66.6)
　　　　　intermittent hydrarthrosis (M12.4-)
　　　　　other infective (teno)synovitis (M65.1-)
　M25.40　Effusion, unspecified joint
　✓6th　M25.41　Effusion, shoulder
　　　　M25.411　Effusion, right shoulder
　　　　M25.412　Effusion, left shoulder
　　　　M25.419　Effusion, unspecified shoulder
　✓6th　M25.42　Effusion, elbow
　　　　M25.421　Effusion, right elbow
　　　　M25.422　Effusion, left elbow
　　　　M25.429　Effusion, unspecified elbow
　✓6th　M25.43　Effusion, wrist
　　　　M25.431　Effusion, right wrist
　　　　M25.432　Effusion, left wrist
　　　　M25.439　Effusion, unspecified wrist
　✓6th　M25.44　Effusion, hand
　　　　M25.441　Effusion, right hand
　　　　M25.442　Effusion, left hand

M25.449　Effusion, unspecified hand

✓6ᵗʰ　M25.45　Effusion, hip
　　　　M25.451　Effusion, right hip
　　　　M25.452　Effusion, left hip
　　　　M25.459　Effusion, unspecified hip

✓6ᵗʰ　M25.46　Effusion, knee
　　　　M25.461　Effusion, right knee
　　　　M25.462　Effusion, left knee
　　　　M25.469　Effusion, unspecified knee

✓6ᵗʰ　M25.47　Effusion, ankle and foot
　　　　M25.471　Effusion, right ankle
　　　　M25.472　Effusion, left ankle
　　　　M25.473　Effusion, unspecified ankle
　　　　M25.474　Effusion, right foot
　　　　M25.475　Effusion, left foot
　　　　M25.476　Effusion, unspecified foot

　　　　M25.48　Effusion, other site

✓5ᵗʰ　M25.5　Pain in joint
　　　　EXCLUDES 2　pain in hand (M79.64-)
　　　　　　　　　　pain in fingers (M79.64-)
　　　　　　　　　　pain in foot (M79.67-)
　　　　　　　　　　pain in limb (M79.6-)
　　　　　　　　　　pain in toes (M79.67-)

　　　　M25.50　Pain in unspecified joint

✓6ᵗʰ　M25.51　Pain in shoulder
　　　　M25.511　Pain in right shoulder
　　　　M25.512　Pain in left shoulder
　　　　M25.519　Pain in unspecified shoulder

✓6ᵗʰ　M25.52　Pain in elbow
　　　　M25.521　Pain in right elbow
　　　　M25.522　Pain in left elbow
　　　　M25.529　Pain in unspecified elbow

✓6ᵗʰ　M25.53　Pain in wrist
　　　　M25.531　Pain in right wrist
　　　　M25.532　Pain in left wrist
　　　　M25.539　Pain in unspecified wrist

✓6ᵗʰ　M25.55　Pain in hip
　　　　M25.551　Pain in right hip
　　　　M25.552　Pain in left hip
　　　　M25.559　Pain in unspecified hip

✓6ᵗʰ　M25.56　Pain in knee
　　　　M25.561　Pain in right knee
　　　　M25.562　Pain in left knee
　　　　M25.569　Pain in unspecified knee

✓6ᵗʰ　M25.57　Pain in ankle and joints of foot
　　　　M25.571　Pain in right ankle and joints of right foot
　　　　M25.572　Pain in left ankle and joints of left foot
　　　　M25.579　Pain in unspecified ankle and joints of unspecified foot

✓5ᵗʰ　M25.6　Stiffness of joint, not elsewhere classified
　　　　EXCLUDES 1　ankylosis of joint (M24.6-)
　　　　　　　　　　contracture of joint (M24.5-)

　　　　M25.60　Stiffness of unspecified joint, not elsewhere classified

✓6ᵗʰ　M25.61　Stiffness of shoulder, not elsewhere classified
　　　　M25.611　Stiffness of right shoulder, not elsewhere classified
　　　　M25.612　Stiffness of left shoulder, not elsewhere classified
　　　　M25.619　Stiffness of unspecified shoulder, not elsewhere classified

✓6ᵗʰ　M25.62　Stiffness of elbow, not elsewhere classified
　　　　M25.621　Stiffness of right elbow, not elsewhere classified
　　　　M25.622　Stiffness of left elbow, not elsewhere classified
　　　　M25.629　Stiffness of unspecified elbow, not elsewhere classified

✓6ᵗʰ　M25.63　Stiffness of wrist, not elsewhere classified
　　　　M25.631　Stiffness of right wrist, not elsewhere classified
　　　　M25.632　Stiffness of left wrist, not elsewhere classified

　　　　M25.639　Stiffness of unspecified wrist, not elsewhere classified

✓6ᵗʰ　M25.64　Stiffness of hand, not elsewhere classified
　　　　M25.641　Stiffness of right hand, not elsewhere classified
　　　　M25.642　Stiffness of left hand, not elsewhere classified
　　　　M25.649　Stiffness of unspecified hand, not elsewhere classified

✓6ᵗʰ　M25.65　Stiffness of hip, not elsewhere classified
　　　　M25.651　Stiffness of right hip, not elsewhere classified
　　　　M25.652　Stiffness of left hip, not elsewhere classified
　　　　M25.659　Stiffness of unspecified hip, not elsewhere classified

✓6ᵗʰ　M25.66　Stiffness of knee, not elsewhere classified
　　　　M25.661　Stiffness of right knee, not elsewhere classified
　　　　M25.662　Stiffness of left knee, not elsewhere classified
　　　　M25.669　Stiffness of unspecified knee, not elsewhere classified

✓6ᵗʰ　M25.67　Stiffness of ankle and foot, not elsewhere classified
　　　　M25.671　Stiffness of right ankle, not elsewhere classified
　　　　M25.672　Stiffness of left ankle, not elsewhere classified
　　　　M25.673　Stiffness of unspecified ankle, not elsewhere classified
　　　　M25.674　Stiffness of right foot, not elsewhere classified
　　　　M25.675　Stiffness of left foot, not elsewhere classified
　　　　M25.676　Stiffness of unspecified foot, not elsewhere classified

✓5ᵗʰ　M25.7　Osteophyte
　　　　M25.70　Osteophyte, unspecified joint

✓6ᵗʰ　M25.71　Osteophyte, shoulder
　　　　M25.711　Osteophyte, right shoulder
　　　　M25.712　Osteophyte, left shoulder
　　　　M25.719　Osteophyte, unspecified shoulder

✓6ᵗʰ　M25.72　Osteophyte, elbow
　　　　M25.721　Osteophyte, right elbow
　　　　M25.722　Osteophyte, left elbow
　　　　M25.729　Osteophyte, unspecified elbow

✓6ᵗʰ　M25.73　Osteophyte, wrist
　　　　M25.731　Osteophyte, right wrist
　　　　M25.732　Osteophyte, left wrist
　　　　M25.739　Osteophyte, unspecified wrist

✓6ᵗʰ　M25.74　Osteophyte, hand
　　　　M25.741　Osteophyte, right hand
　　　　M25.742　Osteophyte, left hand
　　　　M25.749　Osteophyte, unspecified hand

✓6ᵗʰ　M25.75　Osteophyte, hip
　　　　M25.751　Osteophyte, right hip
　　　　M25.752　Osteophyte, left hip
　　　　M25.759　Osteophyte, unspecified hip

✓6ᵗʰ　M25.76　Osteophyte, knee
　　　　M25.761　Osteophyte, right knee
　　　　M25.762　Osteophyte, left knee
　　　　M25.769　Osteophyte, unspecified knee

✓6ᵗʰ　M25.77　Osteophyte, ankle and foot
　　　　M25.771　Osteophyte, right ankle
　　　　M25.772　Osteophyte, left ankle
　　　　M25.773　Osteophyte, unspecified ankle
　　　　M25.774　Osteophyte, right foot
　　　　M25.775　Osteophyte, left foot
　　　　M25.776　Osteophyte, unspecified foot

　　　　M25.78　Osteophyte, vertebrae

✓5ᵗʰ　M25.8　Other specified joint disorders
　　　　M25.80　Other specified joint disorders, unspecified joint

---

✓ Additional Character Required　✓x7ᵗʰ Placeholder Alert　Unacceptable PDx　Manifestation　Hospital Acquired Condition　EXCLUDES 1 Not Coded Here　EXCLUDES 2 Not Included Here

✓6ᵗʰ **M25.81 Other specified joint disorders, shoulder**
    M25.811 Other specified joint disorders, right shoulder
    M25.812 Other specified joint disorders, left shoulder
    M25.819 Other specified joint disorders, unspecified shoulder

✓6ᵗʰ **M25.82 Other specified joint disorders, elbow**
    M25.821 Other specified joint disorders, right elbow
    M25.822 Other specified joint disorders, left elbow
    M25.829 Other specified joint disorders, unspecified elbow

✓6ᵗʰ **M25.83 Other specified joint disorders, wrist**
    M25.831 Other specified joint disorders, right wrist
    M25.832 Other specified joint disorders, left wrist
    M25.839 Other specified joint disorders, unspecified wrist

✓6ᵗʰ **M25.84 Other specified joint disorders, hand**
    M25.841 Other specified joint disorders, right hand
    M25.842 Other specified joint disorders, left hand
    M25.849 Other specified joint disorders, unspecified hand

✓6ᵗʰ **M25.85 Other specified joint disorders, hip**
    AHA: 2014, 4Q, 25
    M25.851 Other specified joint disorders, right hip
    M25.852 Other specified joint disorders, left hip
    M25.859 Other specified joint disorders, unspecified hip

✓6ᵗʰ **M25.86 Other specified joint disorders, knee**
    M25.861 Other specified joint disorders, right knee
    M25.862 Other specified joint disorders, left knee
    M25.869 Other specified joint disorders, unspecified knee

✓6ᵗʰ **M25.87 Other specified joint disorders, ankle and foot**
    M25.871 Other specified joint disorders, right ankle and foot
    M25.872 Other specified joint disorders, left ankle and foot
    M25.879 Other specified joint disorders, unspecified ankle and foot

M25.9 Joint disorder, unspecified

Dentofacial anomalies [including malocclusion] and other disorders of jaw (M26-M27)

EXCLUDES 1   hemifacial atrophy or hypertrophy (Q67.4)
     unilateral condylar hyperplasia or hypoplasia (M27.8)

✓4ᵗʰ **M26 Dentofacial anomalies [including malocclusion]**
  ✓5ᵗʰ **M26.0 Major anomalies of jaw size**
    EXCLUDES 1   acromegaly (E22.0)
        Robin's syndrome (Q87.0)
    M26.00 Unspecified anomaly of jaw size
    M26.01 Maxillary hyperplasia
    M26.02 Maxillary hypoplasia
       AHA: 2014, 3Q, 23
    M26.03 Mandibular hyperplasia
    M26.04 Mandibular hypoplasia
    M26.05 Macrogenia
    M26.06 Microgenia
    M26.07 Excessive tuberosity of jaw
        Entire maxillary tuberosity
    M26.09 Other specified anomalies of jaw size

  ✓5ᵗʰ **M26.1 Anomalies of jaw-cranial base relationship**
    M26.10 Unspecified anomaly of jaw-cranial base relationship
    M26.11 Maxillary asymmetry
    M26.12 Other jaw asymmetry
    M26.19 Other specified anomalies of jaw-cranial base relationship

  ✓5ᵗʰ **M26.2 Anomalies of dental arch relationship**
    M26.20 Unspecified anomaly of dental arch relationship
  ✓6ᵗʰ **M26.21 Malocclusion, Angle's class**
    M26.211 Malocclusion, Angle's class I
        Neutro-occlusion

    M26.212 Malocclusion, Angle's class II
        Disto-occlusion Division I
        Disto-occlusion Division II
    M26.213 Malocclusion, Angle's class III
        Mesio-occlusion
    M26.219 Malocclusion, Angle's class, unspecified

  ✓6ᵗʰ **M26.22 Open occlusal relationship**
    M26.220 Open anterior occlusal relationship
        Anterior openbite
    M26.221 Open posterior occlusal relationship
        Posterior openbite

    M26.23 Excessive horizontal overlap
        Excessive horizontal overjet
    M26.24 Reverse articulation
        Crossbite (anterior) (posterior)
    M26.25 Anomalies of interarch distance
    M26.29 Other anomalies of dental arch relationship
        Midline deviation of dental arch
        Overbite (excessive) deep
        Overbite (excessive) horizontal
        Overbite (excessive) vertical
        Posterior lingual occlusion of mandibular teeth

  ✓5ᵗʰ **M26.3 Anomalies of tooth position of fully erupted tooth or teeth**
    EXCLUDES 2   embedded and impacted teeth (K01.-)
    M26.30 Unspecified anomaly of tooth position of fully erupted tooth or teeth
        Abnormal spacing of fully erupted tooth or teeth NOS
        Displacement of fully erupted tooth or teeth NOS
        Transposition of fully erupted tooth or teeth NOS
    M26.31 Crowding of fully erupted teeth
    M26.32 Excessive spacing of fully erupted teeth
        Diastema of fully erupted tooth or teeth NOS
    M26.33 Horizontal displacement of fully erupted tooth or teeth
        Tipped tooth or teeth
        Tipping of fully erupted tooth
    M26.34 Vertical displacement of fully erupted tooth or teeth
        Extruded tooth
        Infraeruption of tooth or teeth
        Supraeruption of tooth or teeth
    M26.35 Rotation of fully erupted tooth or teeth
    M26.36 Insufficient interocclusal distance of fully erupted teeth (ridge)
        Lack of adequate intermaxillary vertical dimension of fully erupted teeth
    M26.37 Excessive interocclusal distance of fully erupted teeth
        Excessive intermaxillary vertical dimension of fully erupted teeth
        Loss of occlusal vertical dimension of fully erupted teeth
    M26.39 Other anomalies of tooth position of fully erupted tooth or teeth

    M26.4 Malocclusion, unspecified

  ✓5ᵗʰ **M26.5 Dentofacial functional abnormalities**
    EXCLUDES 1   bruxism (F45.8)
        teeth-grinding NOS (F45.8)
    M26.50 Dentofacial functional abnormalities, unspecified
    M26.51 Abnormal jaw closure
    M26.52 Limited mandibular range of motion
    M26.53 Deviation in opening and closing of the mandible
    M26.54 Insufficient anterior guidance
        Insufficient anterior occlusal guidance
    M26.55 Centric occlusion maximum intercuspation discrepancy
       EXCLUDES 1   centric occlusion NOS (M26.59)
    M26.56 Non-working side interference
        Balancing side interference
    M26.57 Lack of posterior occlusal support
    M26.59 Other dentofacial functional abnormalities
        Centric occlusion (of teeth) NOS
        Malocclusion due to abnormal swallowing
        Malocclusion due to mouth breathing
        Malocclusion due to tongue, lip or finger habits

  ✓5ᵗʰ **M26.6 Temporomandibular joint disorders**
    EXCLUDES 2   current temporomandibular joint dislocation (S03.0)
        current temporomandibular joint sprain (S03.4)
    M26.60 Temporomandibular joint disorder, unspecified

M26.61 Adhesions and ankylosis of temporomandibular joint

M26.62 Arthralgia of temporomandibular joint

M26.63 Articular disc disorder of temporomandibular joint

M26.69 Other specified disorders of temporomandibular joint

✓5ᵗʰ **M26.7** Dental alveolar anomalies

M26.70 Unspecified alveolar anomaly

M26.71 Alveolar maxillary hyperplasia

M26.72 Alveolar mandibular hyperplasia

M26.73 Alveolar maxillary hypoplasia

M26.74 Alveolar mandibular hypoplasia

M26.79 Other specified alveolar anomalies

✓5ᵗʰ **M26.8** Other dentofacial anomalies

M26.81 Anterior soft tissue impingement
Anterior soft tissue impingement on teeth

M26.82 Posterior soft tissue impingement
Posterior soft tissue impingement on teeth

M26.89 Other dentofacial anomalies

M26.9 Dentofacial anomaly, unspecified

✓4ᵗʰ **M27 Other diseases of jaws**

M27.0 Developmental disorders of jaws
Latent bone cyst of jaw   Torus mandibularis
Stafne's cyst   Torus palatinus

M27.1 Giant cell granuloma, central
Giant cell granuloma NOS
EXCLUDES 1 peripheral giant cell granuloma (K06.8)

M27.2 Inflammatory conditions of jaws
Osteitis of jaw(s)
Osteomyelitis (neonatal) jaw(s)
Osteoradionecrosis jaw(s)
Periostitis jaw(s)
Sequestrum of jaw bone
Use additional code (W88-W90, X39.0) to identify radiation, if radiation-induced
EXCLUDES 2 osteonecrosis of jaw due to drug (M87.180)

M27.3 Alveolitis of jaws
Alveolar osteitis
Dry socket

✓5ᵗʰ **M27.4** Other and unspecified cysts of jaw
EXCLUDES 1 cysts of oral region (K09.-)
latent bone cyst of jaw (M27.0)
Stafne's cyst (M27.0)

M27.40 Unspecified cyst of jaw
Cyst of jaw NOS

M27.49 Other cysts of jaw
Aneurysmal cyst of jaw
Hemorrhagic cyst of jaw
Traumatic cyst of jaw

✓5ᵗʰ **M27.5** Periradicular pathology associated with previous endodontic treatment

M27.51 Perforation of root canal space due to endodontic treatment

M27.52 Endodontic overfill

M27.53 Endodontic underfill

M27.59 Other periradicular pathology associated with previous endodontic treatment

✓5ᵗʰ **M27.6** Endosseous dental implant failure

M27.61 Osseointegration failure of dental implant
Hemorrhagic complications of dental implant placement
Iatrogenic osseointegration failure of dental implant
Osseointegration failure of dental implant due to complications of systemic disease
Osseointegration failure of dental implant due to poor bone quality
Pre-integration failure of dental implant NOS
Pre-osseointegration failure of dental implant

M27.62 Post-osseointegration biological failure of dental implant
Failure of dental implant due to lack of attached gingiva
Failure of dental implant due to occlusal trauma (caused by poor prosthetic design)
Failure of dental implant due to parafunctional habits
Failure of dental implant due to periodontal infection (peri-implantitis)
Failure of dental implant due to poor oral hygiene
Iatrogenic post-osseointegration failure of dental implant
Post-osseointegration failure of dental implant due to complications of systemic disease

M27.63 Post-osseointegration mechanical failure of dental implant
Failure of dental prosthesis causing loss of dental implant
Fracture of dental implant
EXCLUDES 2 cracked tooth (K03.81)
fractured dental restorative material with loss of material (K08.531)
fractured dental restorative material without loss of material (K08.530)
fractured tooth (S02.5)

M27.69 Other endosseous dental implant failure
Dental implant failure NOS

M27.8 Other specified diseases of jaws
Cherubism
Exostosis
Fibrous dysplasia
Unilateral condylar hyperplasia
Unilateral condylar hypoplasia
EXCLUDES 1 jaw pain (R68.84)

M27.9 Disease of jaws, unspecified

Systemic connective tissue disorders (M30-M36)

INCLUDES autoimmune disease NOS
collagen (vascular) disease NOS
systemic autoimmune disease
systemic collagen (vascular) disease
EXCLUDES 1 autoimmune disease, single organ or single cell-type—code to relevant condition category

✓4ᵗʰ **M30 Polyarteritis nodosa and related conditions**
EXCLUDES 1 microscopic polyarteritis (M31.7)

M30.0 Polyarteritis nodosa   CC
CC Excl: E08.51-E08.59, E08.618-E08.638, E08.649-E08.8, E09.51-E09.59, E09.618-E09.638, E09.649-E09.8, E10.51-E10.59, E10.618-E10.638, E10.649, E10.69-E10.8, E11.51-E11.59, E11.618-E11.638, E11.649, E11.69-E11.8, E13.51-E13.59, E13.618-E13.638, E13.649-E13.8, I87.8-I87.9, I99.8-I99.9, M30.0-M31.7

M30.1 Polyarteritis with lung involvement [Churg-Strauss]   CC
Allergic granulomatous angiitis
CC Excl: See code: M30.0

M30.2 Juvenile polyarteritis   CC
CC Excl: See code: M30.0

M30.3 Mucocutaneous lymph node syndrome [Kawasaki]   CC
CC Excl: I87.8-I87.9, I99.8-I99.9, M30.0-M31.1, M31.30-M31.7

M30.8 Other conditions related to polyarteritis nodosa   CC
Polyangiitis overlap syndrome
CC Excl: See code: M30.0

✓4ᵗʰ **M31 Other necrotizing vasculopathies**

M31.0 Hypersensitivity angiitis   CC
Goodpasture's syndrome
CC Excl: See code: M30.0

M31.1 Thrombotic microangiopathy   MCC
Thrombotic thrombocytopenic purpura
CC Excl: See code: M30.0

M31.2 Lethal midline granuloma   CC
CC Excl: See code: M30.0

✓5ᵗʰ **M31.3** Wegener's granulomatosis
Necrotizing respiratory granulomatosis

M31.30 Wegener's granulomatosis without renal involvement   CC
Wegener's granulomatosis NOS
CC Excl: See code: M30.0

M31.31 Wegener's granulomatosis with renal involvement   CC
CC Excl: See code: M30.0

M31.4 Aortic arch syndrome [Takayasu]   CC
CC Excl: See code: M30.0

✓ Additional Character Required   ✓x7ᵗʰ Placeholder Alert   Unacceptable PDx   Manifestation   Hospital Acquired Condition   *EXCLUDES 1* Not Coded Here   *EXCLUDES 2* Not Included Here

M31.5 Giant cell arteritis with polymyalgia rheumatica

M31.6 Other giant cell arteritis

M31.7 Microscopic polyangiitis `CC`
Microscopic polyarteritis
EXCLUDES 1 *polyarteritis nodosa (M30.0)*
CC Excl: See code: M30.0

M31.8 Other specified necrotizing vasculopathies `CC`
Hypocomplementemic vasculitis
Septic vasculitis
CC Excl: I77.5, M31.8-M31.9

M31.9 Necrotizing vasculopathy, unspecified `CC`
CC Excl: See code: M31.8

✓4ᵗʰ **M32 Systemic lupus erythematosus (SLE)**
EXCLUDES 1 *lupus erythematosus (discoid) (NOS) (L93.0)*

M32.0 Drug-induced systemic lupus erythematosus
Use additional code for adverse effect, if applicable, to identify drug (T36-T50 with fifth or sixth character 5)

✓5ᵗʰ **M32.1 Systemic lupus erythematosus with organ or system involvement**

M32.10 Systemic lupus erythematosus, organ or system involvement unspecified

M32.11 Endocarditis in systemic lupus erythematosus `PDxCC` `CC`
Libman-Sacks disease
CC Excl: I38-I39, I87.8-I87.9, I99.8-I99.9

M32.12 Pericarditis in systemic lupus erythematosus `PDxCC` `CC`
Lupus pericarditis
CC Excl: I01.0, I09.2, I30.0-I30.9, I31.3-I32, I87.8-I87.9, I99.8-I99.9

M32.13 Lung involvement in systemic lupus erythematosus
Pleural effusion due to systemic lupus erythematosus

M32.14 Glomerular disease in systemic lupus erythematosus
Lupus renal disease NOS
AHA: 2013, 4Q, 125

M32.15 Tubulo-interstitial nephropathy in systemic lupus erythematosus

M32.19 Other organ or system involvement in systemic lupus erythematosus

M32.8 Other forms of systemic lupus erythematosus

M32.9 Systemic lupus erythematosus, unspecified
SLE NOS
Systemic lupus erythematosus NOS
Systemic lupus erythematosus without organ involvement

✓4ᵗʰ **M33 Dermatopolymyositis**

✓5ᵗʰ **M33.0 Juvenile dermatopolymyositis**

M33.00 Juvenile dermatopolymyositis, organ involvement unspecified `CC`
CC Excl: M33.00-M33.19, M33.90-M33.99, M36.0

M33.01 Juvenile dermatopolymyositis with respiratory involvement `CC`
CC Excl: See code: M33.00

M33.02 Juvenile dermatopolymyositis with myopathy `PDxCC` `CC`
CC Excl: E08.40-E08.49, E08.618-E08.638, E08.649-E08.8, E09.40-E09.49, E09.618-E09.638, E09.649-E09.8, E10.40-E10.49, E10.618-E10.638, E10.649, E10.69-E10.8, E11.40-E11.49, E11.618-E11.638, E11.649, E11.69-E11.8, E13.40-E13.49, E13.618-E13.638, E13.649-E13.8, G32.89, G70.00-G72.3, G72.81-G73.7, G96.8-G96.9, G98.0-G98.8, G99.8, M33.00-M33.19, M33.90-M33.99, M36.0

M33.09 Juvenile dermatopolymyositis with other organ involvement `CC`
CC Excl: See code: M33.00

✓5ᵗʰ **M33.1 Other dermatopolymyositis**

M33.10 Other dermatopolymyositis, organ involvement unspecified `CC`
CC Excl: See code: M33.00

M33.11 Other dermatopolymyositis with respiratory involvement `CC`
CC Excl: See code: M33.00

M33.12 Other dermatopolymyositis with myopathy `PDxCC` `CC`
CC Excl: See code: M33.02

M33.19 Other dermatopolymyositis with other organ involvement `CC`
CC Excl: See code: M33.00

✓5ᵗʰ **M33.2 Polymyositis**

M33.20 Polymyositis, organ involvement unspecified `CC`
CC Excl: M33.20-M33.29

M33.21 Polymyositis with respiratory involvement `CC`
CC Excl: See code: M33.20

M33.22 Polymyositis with myopathy `PDxCC` `CC`
CC Excl: E08.40-E08.49, E08.618-E08.638, E08.649-E08.8, E09.40-E09.49, E09.618-E09.638, E09.649-E09.8, E10.40-E10.49, E10.618-E10.638, E10.649, E10.69-E10.8, E11.40-E11.49, E11.618-E11.638, E11.649, E11.69-E11.8, E13.40-E13.49, E13.618-E13.638, E13.649-E13.8, G32.89, G70.00-G72.3, G72.81-G73.7, G96.8-G96.9, G98.0-G98.8, G99.8, M33.20-M33.29

M33.29 Polymyositis with other organ involvement `CC`
CC Excl: See code: M33.20

✓5ᵗʰ **M33.9 Dermatopolymyositis, unspecified**

M33.90 Dermatopolymyositis, unspecified, organ involvement unspecified `CC`
CC Excl: See code: M33.19

M33.91 Dermatopolymyositis, unspecified with respiratory involvement `CC`
CC Excl: See code: M33.19

M33.92 Dermatopolymyositis, unspecified with myopathy `PDxCC` `CC`
CC Excl: See code: M33.12

M33.99 Dermatopolymyositis, unspecified with other organ involvement `CC`
CC Excl: See code: M33.19

✓4ᵗʰ **M34 Systemic sclerosis [scleroderma]**
EXCLUDES 1 *circumscribed scleroderma (L94.0)*
neonatal scleroderma (P83.8)

M34.0 Progressive systemic sclerosis

M34.1 CR(E)ST syndrome
Combination of calcinosis, Raynaud's phenomenon, esophageal dysfunction, sclerodactyly, telangiectasia

M34.2 Systemic sclerosis induced by drug and chemical
Code first poisoning due to drug or toxin, if applicable (T36-T65 with fifth or sixth character 1-4 or 6)
Use additional code for adverse effect, if applicable, to identify drug (T36-T50 with fifth or sixth character 5)

✓5ᵗʰ **M34.8 Other forms of systemic sclerosis**

M34.81 Systemic sclerosis with lung involvement `PDxCC` `CC`
CC Excl: No excl

M34.82 Systemic sclerosis with myopathy `PDxCC` `CC`
CC Excl: E08.40-E08.49, E08.618-E08.638, E08.649-E08.8, E09.40-E09.49, E09.618-E09.638, E09.649-E09.8, E10.40-E10.49, E10.618-E10.638, E10.649, E10.69-E10.8, E11.40-E11.49, E11.618-E11.638, E11.649, E11.69-E11.8, E13.40-E13.49, E13.618-E13.638, E13.649-E13.8, G32.89, G70.00-G72.3, G72.81-G73.7, G96.8-G96.9, G98.0-G98.8, G99.8

M34.83 Systemic sclerosis with polyneuropathy

M34.89 Other systemic sclerosis

M34.9 Systemic sclerosis, unspecified

✓4ᵗʰ **M35 Other systemic involvement of connective tissue**
EXCLUDES 1 *reactive perforating collagenosis (L87.1)*

✓5ᵗʰ **M35.0 Sicca syndrome [Sjögren]**

M35.00 Sicca syndrome, unspecified

M35.01 Sicca syndrome with keratoconjunctivitis

M35.02 Sicca syndrome with lung involvement

M35.03 Sicca syndrome with myopathy `PDxCC` `CC`
CC Excl: See code M34.82

M35.04 Sicca syndrome with tubulo-interstitial nephropathy
Renal tubular acidosis in sicca syndrome

M35.09 Sicca syndrome with other organ involvement

M35.1 Other overlap syndromes `CC`
Mixed connective tissue disease
EXCLUDES 1 *polyangiitis overlap syndrome (M30.8)*
CC Excl: G72.41-G72.49, M35.1, M35.5, M35.8

M35.2 Behçet's disease `CC`
CC Excl: A02.23, A17.9, A18.02, A18.09, A18.82, A18.84, A18.89, A39.83-A39.84, A54.40, A54.42-A54.43, A54.82, A54.84, A54.89-A54.9, B06.82, M00.00, M00.019, M00.029, M00.039, M00.049, M00.059, M00.069, M00.079, M00.08-M02.30, M02.319, M02.329, M02.339, M02.349, M02.359, M02.369, M02.379-M02.9, M05.40-M05.59, M05.70-M06.09, M06.20-M06.39, M06.80-M07.69, M11.00-M11.9, M12.10-M15.0, M15.3-M15.9, M16.2-M16.9, M17.2-M17.9, M18.2-M18.9, M19.111-M19.93, M24.10-M24.176, M25.00, M25.08-M25.18, M25.40-M25.676, M25.80-M25.9, M35.2, M36.1-M36.4, R29.4

M35.3 Polymyalgia rheumatica
EXCLUDES 1 *polymyalgia rheumatica with giant cell arteritis (M31.5)*

M35.4 Diffuse (eosinophilic) fasciitis

M35.5 Multifocal fibrosclerosis CC
    CC Excl: G72.41-G72.49, M35.1, M35.5, M35.8

M35.6 Relapsing panniculitis [Weber-Christian]
    EXCLUDES 1   lupus panniculitis (L93.2)
                panniculitis NOS (M79.3-)

M35.7 Hypermobility syndrome
    Familial ligamentous laxity
    EXCLUDES 1   Ehlers-Danlos syndrome (Q79.6)
                ligamentous laxity, NOS (M24.2-)

M35.8 Other specified systemic involvement of connective tissue CC
    CC Excl: G72.41-G72.49, M35.1, M35.5, M35.8

M35.9 Systemic involvement of connective tissue, unspecified
    Autoimmune disease (systemic) NOS
    Collagen (vascular) disease NOS

√4th **M36 Systemic disorders of connective tissue in diseases classified elsewhere**
    EXCLUDES 2   arthropathies in diseases classified elsewhere (M14.-)

    M36.0 Dermato(poly)myositis in neoplastic disease CC
        Code first underlying neoplasm (C00-D49)
        CC Excl: M33.00-M33.19, M33.90-M33.99, M36.0

    M36.1 Arthropathy in neoplastic disease
        Code first underlying neoplasm, such as:
            leukemia (C91-C95)
            malignant histiocytosis (C96.A)
            multiple myeloma (C90.0)

    M36.2 Hemophilic arthropathy
        Hemarthrosis in hemophilic arthropathy
        Code first underlying disease, such as:
            factor VIII deficiency (D66)
               with vascular defect (D68.0)
            factor IX deficiency (D67)
            hemophilia (classical) (D66)
            hemophilia B (D67)
            hemophilia C (D68.1)

    M36.3 Arthropathy in other blood disorders

    M36.4 Arthropathy in hypersensitivity reactions classified elsewhere
        Code first underlying disease, such as:
            Henoch (-Schönlein) purpura (D69.0)
            serum sickness (T80.6-)

    M36.8 Systemic disorders of connective tissue in other diseases classified elsewhere
        Code first underlying disease, such as:
            alkaptonuria (E70.2)
            hypogammaglobulinemia (D80.-)
            ochronosis (E70.2)

DORSOPATHIES (M40-M54)

Deforming dorsopathies (M40-M43)

√4th **M40 Kyphosis and lordosis**
    EXCLUDES 1   congenital kyphosis and lordosis (Q76.4)
                kyphoscoliosis (M41.-)
                postprocedural kyphosis and lordosis (M96.-)

√5th **M40.0 Postural kyphosis**
        EXCLUDES 1   osteochondrosis of spine (M42.-)
    M40.00 Postural kyphosis, site unspecified
    M40.03 Postural kyphosis, cervicothoracic region
    M40.04 Postural kyphosis, thoracic region
    M40.05 Postural kyphosis, thoracolumbar region

√5th **M40.1 Other secondary kyphosis**
    M40.10 Other secondary kyphosis, site unspecified
    M40.12 Other secondary kyphosis, cervical region
    M40.13 Other secondary kyphosis, cervicothoracic region
    M40.14 Other secondary kyphosis, thoracic region
    M40.15 Other secondary kyphosis, thoracolumbar region

√5th **M40.2 Other and unspecified kyphosis**
    √6th **M40.20 Unspecified kyphosis**
        M40.202 Unspecified kyphosis, cervical region
        M40.203 Unspecified kyphosis, cervicothoracic region
        M40.204 Unspecified kyphosis, thoracic region
        M40.205 Unspecified kyphosis, thoracolumbar region
        M40.209 Unspecified kyphosis, site unspecified

√6th **M40.29 Other kyphosis**
    M40.292 Other kyphosis, cervical region
    M40.293 Other kyphosis, cervicothoracic region
    M40.294 Other kyphosis, thoracic region
    M40.295 Other kyphosis, thoracolumbar region
    M40.299 Other kyphosis, site unspecified

√5th **M40.3 Flatback syndrome**
    M40.30 Flatback syndrome, site unspecified
    M40.35 Flatback syndrome, thoracolumbar region
    M40.36 Flatback syndrome, lumbar region
    M40.37 Flatback syndrome, lumbosacral region

√5th **M40.4 Postural lordosis**
    Acquired lordosis
    M40.40 Postural lordosis, site unspecified
    M40.45 Postural lordosis, thoracolumbar region
    M40.46 Postural lordosis, lumbar region
    M40.47 Postural lordosis, lumbosacral region

√5th **M40.5 Lordosis, unspecified**
    M40.50 Lordosis, unspecified, site unspecified
    M40.55 Lordosis, unspecified, thoracolumbar region
    M40.56 Lordosis, unspecified, lumbar region
    M40.57 Lordosis, unspecified, lumbosacral region

√4th **M41 Scoliosis**
    INCLUDES   kyphoscoliosis
    EXCLUDES 1   congenital scoliosis due to bony malformation (Q76.3)
                congenital scoliosis NOS (Q67.5)
                kyphoscoliotic heart disease (I27.1)
                postprocedural scoliosis (M96.-)
                postural congenital scoliosis (Q67.5)

√5th **M41.0 Infantile idiopathic scoliosis**
    AHA: 2014, 4Q, 26
    M41.00 Infantile idiopathic scoliosis, site unspecified
    M41.02 Infantile idiopathic scoliosis, cervical region
    M41.03 Infantile idiopathic scoliosis, cervicothoracic region
    M41.04 Infantile idiopathic scoliosis, thoracic region
    M41.05 Infantile idiopathic scoliosis, thoracolumbar region
    M41.06 Infantile idiopathic scoliosis, lumbar region
    M41.07 Infantile idiopathic scoliosis, lumbosacral region
    M41.08 Infantile idiopathic scoliosis, sacral and sacrococcygeal region

√5th **M41.1 Juvenile and adolescent idiopathic scoliosis**
    √6th **M41.11 Juvenile idiopathic scoliosis**
        AHA: 2014, 4Q, 28
        M41.112 Juvenile idiopathic scoliosis, cervical region
        M41.113 Juvenile idiopathic scoliosis, cervicothoracic region
        M41.114 Juvenile idiopathic scoliosis, thoracic region
        M41.115 Juvenile idiopathic scoliosis, thoracolumbar region
        M41.116 Juvenile idiopathic scoliosis, lumbar region
        M41.117 Juvenile idiopathic scoliosis, lumbosacral region
        M41.119 Juvenile idiopathic scoliosis, site unspecified

    √6th **M41.12 Adolescent scoliosis**
        M41.122 Adolescent idiopathic scoliosis, cervical region
        M41.123 Adolescent idiopathic scoliosis, cervicothoracic region
        M41.124 Adolescent idiopathic scoliosis, thoracic region
        M41.125 Adolescent idiopathic scoliosis, thoracolumbar region
        M41.126 Adolescent idiopathic scoliosis, lumbar region
        M41.127 Adolescent idiopathic scoliosis, lumbosacral region
        M41.129 Adolescent idiopathic scoliosis, site unspecified

√5th **M41.2 Other idiopathic scoliosis**
    M41.20 Other idiopathic scoliosis, site unspecified

√ Additional Character Required   √x7th Placeholder Alert   Unacceptable PDx   Manifestation   Hospital Acquired Condition   *EXCLUDES 1* Not Coded Here   *EXCLUDES 2* Not Included Here

Chapter 13. Diseases of the Musculoskeletal System and Connective Tissue

M41.22   **Other idiopathic scoliosis, cervical region**

M41.23   **Other idiopathic scoliosis, cervicothoracic region**

M41.24   **Other idiopathic scoliosis, thoracic region**

M41.25   **Other idiopathic scoliosis, thoracolumbar region**

M41.26   **Other idiopathic scoliosis, lumbar region**

M41.27   **Other idiopathic scoliosis, lumbosacral region**

✓5ᵗʰ **M41.3 Thoracogenic scoliosis**

M41.30   **Thoracogenic scoliosis, site unspecified**

M41.34   **Thoracogenic scoliosis, thoracic region**

M41.35   **Thoracogenic scoliosis, thoracolumbar region**

✓5ᵗʰ **M41.4 Neuromuscular scoliosis**

Scoliosis secondary to cerebral palsy, Friedreich's ataxia, poliomyelitis and other neuromuscular disorders

Code also underlying condition

AHA: 2014, 4Q, 27

M41.40   **Neuromuscular scoliosis, site unspecified**

M41.41   **Neuromuscular scoliosis, occipito-atlanto-axial region**

M41.42   **Neuromuscular scoliosis, cervical region**

M41.43   **Neuromuscular scoliosis, cervicothoracic region**

M41.44   **Neuromuscular scoliosis, thoracic region**

M41.45   **Neuromuscular scoliosis, thoracolumbar region**

M41.46   **Neuromuscular scoliosis, lumbar region**

M41.47   **Neuromuscular scoliosis, lumbosacral region**

✓5ᵗʰ **M41.5 Other secondary scoliosis**

M41.50   **Other secondary scoliosis, site unspecified**

M41.52   **Other secondary scoliosis, cervical region**

M41.53   **Other secondary scoliosis, cervicothoracic region**

M41.54   **Other secondary scoliosis, thoracic region**

M41.55   **Other secondary scoliosis, thoracolumbar region**

M41.56   **Other secondary scoliosis, lumbar region**

M41.57   **Other secondary scoliosis, lumbosacral region**

✓5ᵗʰ **M41.8 Other forms of scoliosis**

M41.80   **Other forms of scoliosis, site unspecified**

M41.82   **Other forms of scoliosis, cervical region**

M41.83   **Other forms of scoliosis, cervicothoracic region**

M41.84   **Other forms of scoliosis, thoracic region**

M41.85   **Other forms of scoliosis, thoracolumbar region**

M41.86   **Other forms of scoliosis, lumbar region**

M41.87   **Other forms of scoliosis, lumbosacral region**

M41.9   **Scoliosis, unspecified**

✓4ᵗʰ **M42 Spinal osteochondrosis**

✓5ᵗʰ **M42.0 Juvenile osteochondrosis of spine**

Calvé's disease

Scheuermann's disease

EXCLUDES 1   *postural kyphosis (M40.0)*

M42.00   **Juvenile osteochondrosis of spine, site unspecified**

M42.01   **Juvenile osteochondrosis of spine, occipito-atlanto-axial region**

M42.02   **Juvenile osteochondrosis of spine, cervical region**

M42.03   **Juvenile osteochondrosis of spine, cervicothoracic region**

M42.04   **Juvenile osteochondrosis of spine, thoracic region**

M42.05   **Juvenile osteochondrosis of spine, thoracolumbar region**

M42.06   **Juvenile osteochondrosis of spine, lumbar region**

M42.07   **Juvenile osteochondrosis of spine, lumbosacral region**

M42.08   **Juvenile osteochondrosis of spine, sacral and sacrococcygeal region**

M42.09   **Juvenile osteochondrosis of spine, multiple sites in spine**

✓5ᵗʰ **M42.1 Adult osteochondrosis of spine**

M42.10   **Adult osteochondrosis of spine, site unspecified**   A

M42.11   **Adult osteochondrosis of spine, occipito-atlanto-axial region**   A

M42.12   **Adult osteochondrosis of spine, cervical region**   A

M42.13   **Adult osteochondrosis of spine, cervicothoracic region**   A

M42.14   **Adult osteochondrosis of spine, thoracic region**   A

M42.15   **Adult osteochondrosis of spine, thoracolumbar region**   A

M42.16   **Adult osteochondrosis of spine, lumbar region**   A

M42.17   **Adult osteochondrosis of spine, lumbosacral region**   A

M42.18   **Adult osteochondrosis of spine, sacral and sacrococcygeal region**   A

M42.19   **Adult osteochondrosis of spine, multiple sites in spine**   A

M42.9   **Spinal osteochondrosis, unspecified**

✓4ᵗʰ **M43 Other deforming dorsopathies**

EXCLUDES 1   *congenital spondylolysis and spondylolisthesis (Q76.2)*
hemivertebra (Q76.3-Q76.4)
Klippel-Feil syndrome (Q76.1)
lumbarization and sacralization (Q76.4)
platyspondylisis (Q76.4)
spina bifida occulta (Q76.0)
spinal curvature in osteoporosis (M80.-)
spinal curvature in Paget's disease of bone [osteitis deformans] (M88.-)

✓5ᵗʰ **M43.0 Spondylolysis**

EXCLUDES 1   *congenital spondylolysis (Q76.2)*
spondylolisthesis (M43.1)

M43.00   **Spondylolysis, site unspecified**

M43.01   **Spondylolysis, occipito-atlanto-axial region**

M43.02   **Spondylolysis, cervical region**

M43.03   **Spondylolysis, cervicothoracic region**

M43.04   **Spondylolysis, thoracic region**

M43.05   **Spondylolysis, thoracolumbar region**

M43.06   **Spondylolysis, lumbar region**

M43.07   **Spondylolysis, lumbosacral region**

M43.08   **Spondylolysis, sacral and sacrococcygeal region**

M43.09   **Spondylolysis, multiple sites in spine**

✓5ᵗʰ **M43.1 Spondylolisthesis**

EXCLUDES 1   *acute traumatic of lumbosacral region (S33.1)*
acute traumatic of sites other than lumbosacral— code to Fracture, vertebra, by region
congenital spondylolisthesis (Q76.2)

M43.10   **Spondylolisthesis, site unspecified**

M43.11   **Spondylolisthesis, occipito-atlanto-axial region**

M43.12   **Spondylolisthesis, cervical region**

M43.13   **Spondylolisthesis, cervicothoracic region**

M43.14   **Spondylolisthesis, thoracic region**

M43.15   **Spondylolisthesis, thoracolumbar region**

M43.16   **Spondylolisthesis, lumbar region**

M43.17   **Spondylolisthesis, lumbosacral region**

M43.18   **Spondylolisthesis, sacral and sacrococcygeal region**

M43.19   **Spondylolisthesis, multiple sites in spine**

✓5ᵗʰ **M43.2 Fusion of spine**

Ankylosis of spinal joint

EXCLUDES 1   *ankylosing spondylitis (M45.0-)*
congenital fusion of spine (Q76.4)

EXCLUDES 2   *arthrodesis status (Z98.1)*
pseudoarthrosis after fusion or arthrodesis (M96.0)

M43.20   **Fusion of spine, site unspecified**

M43.21   **Fusion of spine, occipito-atlanto-axial region**

M43.22   **Fusion of spine, cervical region**

M43.23   **Fusion of spine, cervicothoracic region**

M43.24   **Fusion of spine, thoracic region**

M43.25   **Fusion of spine, thoracolumbar region**

M43.26   **Fusion of spine, lumbar region**

M43.27   **Fusion of spine, lumbosacral region**

M43.28   **Fusion of spine, sacral and sacrococcygeal region**

M43.3   **Recurrent atlantoaxial dislocation with myelopathy**

M43.4   **Other recurrent atlantoaxial dislocation**

✓5ᵗʰ **M43.5 Other recurrent vertebral dislocation**

EXCLUDES 1   *biomechanical lesions NEC (M99.-)*

✓6ᵗʰ **M43.5X Other recurrent vertebral dislocation**

M43.5X2   **Other recurrent vertebral dislocation, cervical region**

M43.5X3   **Other recurrent vertebral dislocation, cervicothoracic region**

M43.5X4   **Other recurrent vertebral dislocation, thoracic region**

M43.5X5   **Other recurrent vertebral dislocation, thoracolumbar region**

N Newborn: 0   P Pediatric: 0-17   M Maternity: 12-55   A Adult: 15-124   MCC Major CC Condition   PDxMCC PDx acts as own MCC   CC CC Condition   PDxCC PDx acts as own CC

742   ICD-10-CM 2016

M43.5X6 Other recurrent vertebral dislocation, lumbar region

M43.5X7 Other recurrent vertebral dislocation, lumbosacral region

M43.5X8 Other recurrent vertebral dislocation, sacral and sacrococcygeal region

M43.5X9 Other recurrent vertebral dislocation, site unspecified

M43.6 Torticollis
EXCLUDES 1   congenital (sternomastoid) torticollis (Q68.0)
     current injury—see Injury, of spine, by body region
     ocular torticollis (R29.891)
     psychogenic torticollis (F45.8)
     spasmodic torticollis (G24.3)
     torticollis due to birth injury (P15.2)

✓5th M43.8 Other specified deforming dorsopathies
EXCLUDES 2   kyphosis and lordosis (M40.-)
     scoliosis (M41.-)

✓6th M43.8X Other specified deforming dorsopathies

M43.8X1 Other specified deforming dorsopathies, occipito-atlanto-axial region

M43.8X2 Other specified deforming dorsopathies, cervical region

M43.8X3 Other specified deforming dorsopathies, cervicothoracic region

M43.8X4 Other specified deforming dorsopathies, thoracic region

M43.8X5 Other specified deforming dorsopathies, thoracolumbar region

M43.8X6 Other specified deforming dorsopathies, lumbar region

M43.8X7 Other specified deforming dorsopathies, lumbosacral region

M43.8X8 Other specified deforming dorsopathies, sacral and sacrococcygeal region

M43.8X9 Other specified deforming dorsopathies, site unspecified

M43.9 Deforming dorsopathy, unspecified
Curvature of spine NOS

Spondylopathies (M45-M49)

✓4th M45 Ankylosing spondylitis
Rheumatoid arthritis of spine
EXCLUDES 1   arthropathy in Reiter's disease (M02.3-)
     juvenile (ankylosing) spondylitis (M08.1)
EXCLUDES 2   Behçet's disease (M35.2)

M45.0 Ankylosing spondylitis of multiple sites in spine

M45.1 Ankylosing spondylitis of occipito-atlanto-axial region

M45.2 Ankylosing spondylitis of cervical region

M45.3 Ankylosing spondylitis of cervicothoracic region

M45.4 Ankylosing spondylitis of thoracic region

M45.5 Ankylosing spondylitis of thoracolumbar region

M45.6 Ankylosing spondylitis lumbar region

M45.7 Ankylosing spondylitis of lumbosacral region

M45.8 Ankylosing spondylitis sacral and sacrococcygeal region

M45.9 Ankylosing spondylitis of unspecified sites in spine

✓4th M46 Other inflammatory spondylopathies

✓5th M46.0 Spinal enthesopathy
Disorder of ligamentous or muscular attachments of spine

M46.00 Spinal enthesopathy, site unspecified

M46.01 Spinal enthesopathy, occipito-atlanto-axial region

M46.02 Spinal enthesopathy, cervical region

M46.03 Spinal enthesopathy, cervicothoracic region

M46.04 Spinal enthesopathy, thoracic region

M46.05 Spinal enthesopathy, thoracolumbar region

M46.06 Spinal enthesopathy, lumbar region

M46.07 Spinal enthesopathy, lumbosacral region

M46.08 Spinal enthesopathy, sacral and sacrococcygeal region

M46.09 Spinal enthesopathy, multiple sites in spine

M46.1 Sacroiliitis, not elsewhere classified

✓5th M46.2 Osteomyelitis of vertebra

> **CC Excl:** For CC codes in subcategory M46.20, unless otherwise noted: A02.24, A17.9, A18.03-A18.09, A18.82, A18.84, A18.89, M46.20-M46.39, M86.00-M86.9

M46.20 Osteomyelitis of vertebra, site unspecified `CC`

M46.21 Osteomyelitis of vertebra, occipito-atlanto-axial region `CC`

M46.22 Osteomyelitis of vertebra, cervical region `CC`

M46.23 Osteomyelitis of vertebra, cervicothoracic region `CC`

M46.24 Osteomyelitis of vertebra, thoracic region `CC`

M46.25 Osteomyelitis of vertebra, thoracolumbar region `CC`

M46.26 Osteomyelitis of vertebra, lumbar region `CC`

M46.27 Osteomyelitis of vertebra, lumbosacral region `CC`

M46.28 Osteomyelitis of vertebra, sacral and sacrococcygeal region `CC`

✓5th M46.3 Infection of intervertebral disc (pyogenic)
Use additional code (B95-B97) to identify infectious agent

M46.30 Infection of intervertebral disc (pyogenic), site unspecified `CC`
     CC Excl: A17.9-A18.01, A18.03-A18.09, A18.82, A18.84, A18.89, M46.20-M46.39, M86.00-M86.9

M46.31 Infection of intervertebral disc (pyogenic), occipito-atlanto-axial region `CC`
     CC Excl: See code: M46.30

M46.32 Infection of intervertebral disc (pyogenic), cervical region `CC`
     CC Excl: See code: M46.30

M46.33 Infection of intervertebral disc (pyogenic), cervicothoracic region `CC`
     CC Excl: See code: M46.30

M46.34 Infection of intervertebral disc (pyogenic), thoracic region `CC`
     CC Excl: See code: M46.30

M46.35 Infection of intervertebral disc (pyogenic), thoracolumbar region `CC`
     CC Excl: See code: M46.30

M46.36 Infection of intervertebral disc (pyogenic), lumbar region `CC`
     CC Excl: See code: M46.30

M46.37 Infection of intervertebral disc (pyogenic), lumbosacral region `CC`
     CC Excl: See code: M46.30

M46.38 Infection of intervertebral disc (pyogenic), sacral and sacrococcygeal region `CC`
     CC Excl: See code: M46.30

M46.39 Infection of intervertebral disc (pyogenic), multiple sites in spine `CC`
     CC Excl: See code: M46.30

✓5th M46.4 Discitis, unspecified

M46.40 Discitis, unspecified, site unspecified

M46.41 Discitis, unspecified, occipito-atlanto-axial region

M46.42 Discitis, unspecified, cervical region

M46.43 Discitis, unspecified, cervicothoracic region

M46.44 Discitis, unspecified, thoracic region

M46.45 Discitis, unspecified, thoracolumbar region

M46.46 Discitis, unspecified, lumbar region

M46.47 Discitis, unspecified, lumbosacral region

M46.48 Discitis, unspecified, sacral and sacrococcygeal region

M46.49 Discitis, unspecified, multiple sites in spine

✓5th M46.5 Other infective spondylopathies

M46.50 Other infective spondylopathies, site unspecified

M46.51 Other infective spondylopathies, occipito-atlanto-axial region

M46.52 Other infective spondylopathies, cervical region

M46.53 Other infective spondylopathies, cervicothoracic region

M46.54 Other infective spondylopathies, thoracic region

M46.55 Other infective spondylopathies, thoracolumbar region

M46.56 Other infective spondylopathies, lumbar region

M46.57 Other infective spondylopathies, lumbosacral region

M46.58 Other infective spondylopathies, sacral and sacrococcygeal region

✓ Additional Character Required   ✓x7th Placeholder Alert   Unacceptable PDx   Manifestation   Hospital Acquired Condition   *EXCLUDES 1* Not Coded Here   *EXCLUDES 2* Not Included Here

ICD-10-CM 2016   743

Chapter 13. Diseases of the Musculoskeletal System and Connective Tissue

M46.59   Other infective spondylopathies, multiple sites in spine

✓5th **M46.8**   Other specified inflammatory spondylopathies

     M46.80   Other specified inflammatory spondylopathies, site unspecified

     M46.81   Other specified inflammatory spondylopathies, occipito-atlanto-axial region

     M46.82   Other specified inflammatory spondylopathies, cervical region

     M46.83   Other specified inflammatory spondylopathies, cervicothoracic region

     M46.84   Other specified inflammatory spondylopathies, thoracic region

     M46.85   Other specified inflammatory spondylopathies, thoracolumbar region

     M46.86   Other specified inflammatory spondylopathies, lumbar region

     M46.87   Other specified inflammatory spondylopathies, lumbosacral region

     M46.88   Other specified inflammatory spondylopathies, sacral and sacrococcygeal region

     M46.89   Other specified inflammatory spondylopathies, multiple sites in spine

✓5th **M46.9**   Unspecified inflammatory spondylopathy

     M46.90   Unspecified inflammatory spondylopathy, site unspecified

     M46.91   Unspecified inflammatory spondylopathy, occipito-atlanto-axial region

     M46.92   Unspecified inflammatory spondylopathy, cervical region

     M46.93   Unspecified inflammatory spondylopathy, cervicothoracic region

     M46.94   Unspecified inflammatory spondylopathy, thoracic region

     M46.95   Unspecified inflammatory spondylopathy, thoracolumbar region

     M46.96   Unspecified inflammatory spondylopathy, lumbar region

     M46.97   Unspecified inflammatory spondylopathy, lumbosacral region

     M46.98   Unspecified inflammatory spondylopathy, sacral and sacrococcygeal region

     M46.99   Unspecified inflammatory spondylopathy, multiple sites in spine

✓4th **M47**   **Spondylosis**

     INCLUDES   arthrosis or osteoarthritis of spine
              degeneration of facet joints

✓5th **M47.0**   Anterior spinal and vertebral artery compression syndromes

     ✓6th **M47.01**   Anterior spinal artery compression syndromes

         CC Excl: For CC codes in subcategory M47.01, unless otherwise noted: M47.011-M47.029, M47.11-M47.13, M47.21-M47.23, M47.811-M47.813, M47.891-M47.893

         M47.011   Anterior spinal artery compression syndromes, occipito-atlanto-axial region   CC

         M47.012   Anterior spinal artery compression syndromes, cervical region   CC

         M47.013   Anterior spinal artery compression syndromes, cervicothoracic region   CC

         M47.014   Anterior spinal artery compression syndromes, thoracic region   CC

         M47.015   Anterior spinal artery compression syndromes, thoracolumbar region   CC

         M47.016   Anterior spinal artery compression syndromes, lumbar region   CC

         M47.019   Anterior spinal artery compression syndromes, site unspecified   CC

     ✓6th **M47.02**   Vertebral artery compression syndromes

         M47.021   Vertebral artery compression syndromes, occipito-atlanto-axial region   CC

         M47.022   Vertebral artery compression syndromes, cervical region   CC

         M47.029   Vertebral artery compression syndromes, site unspecified   CC

✓5th **M47.1**   Other spondylosis with myelopathy
     Spondylogenic compression of spinal cord
     EXCLUDES 1   vertebral subluxation (M43.3-M43.5X9)

     M47.10   Other spondylosis with myelopathy, site unspecified   CC
         CC Excl: M25.78, M47.011-M47.16, M47.20-M47.9, M48.10-M48.38, M48.9

     M47.11   Other spondylosis with myelopathy, occipito-atlanto-axial region   CC
         CC Excl: M47.011-M47.029, M47.11-M47.13, M47.21-M47.23, M47.811-M47.813, M47.891-M47.893

     M47.12   Other spondylosis with myelopathy, cervical region   CC
         CC Excl: See code: M47.11

     M47.13   Other spondylosis with myelopathy, cervicothoracic region   CC
         CC Excl: See code: M47.11

     M47.14   Other spondylosis with myelopathy, thoracic region   CC
         CC Excl: M47.14-M47.15

     M47.15   Other spondylosis with myelopathy, thoracolumbar region   CC
         CC Excl: See code: M47.14

     M47.16   Other spondylosis with myelopathy, lumbar region   CC
         CC Excl: M46.40, M46.46-M46.49, M47.16, M47.26-M47.28, M47.816-M47.818, M47.896-M47.898, M51.06, M51.26-M51.27, M51.36-M51.37, M51.46-M51.47, M51.86-M51.9

✓5th **M47.2**   Other spondylosis with radiculopathy

     M47.20   Other spondylosis with radiculopathy, site unspecified

     M47.21   Other spondylosis with radiculopathy, occipito-atlanto-axial region

     M47.22   Other spondylosis with radiculopathy, cervical region

     M47.23   Other spondylosis with radiculopathy, cervicothoracic region

     M47.24   Other spondylosis with radiculopathy, thoracic region

     M47.25   Other spondylosis with radiculopathy, thoracolumbar region

     M47.26   Other spondylosis with radiculopathy, lumbar region

     M47.27   Other spondylosis with radiculopathy, lumbosacral region

     M47.28   Other spondylosis with radiculopathy, sacral and sacrococcygeal region

✓5th **M47.8**   Other spondylosis

     ✓6th **M47.81**   Spondylosis without myelopathy or radiculopathy

         M47.811   Spondylosis without myelopathy or radiculopathy, occipito-atlanto-axial region

         M47.812   Spondylosis without myelopathy or radiculopathy, cervical region

         M47.813   Spondylosis without myelopathy or radiculopathy, cervicothoracic region

         M47.814   Spondylosis without myelopathy or radiculopathy, thoracic region

         M47.815   Spondylosis without myelopathy or radiculopathy, thoracolumbar region

         M47.816   Spondylosis without myelopathy or radiculopathy, lumbar region

         M47.817   Spondylosis without myelopathy or radiculopathy, lumbosacral region

         M47.818   Spondylosis without myelopathy or radiculopathy, sacral and sacrococcygeal region

         M47.819   Spondylosis without myelopathy or radiculopathy, site unspecified

     ✓6th **M47.89**   Other spondylosis

         M47.891   Other spondylosis, occipito-atlanto-axial region

         M47.892   Other spondylosis, cervical region

         M47.893   Other spondylosis, cervicothoracic region

         M47.894   Other spondylosis, thoracic region

         M47.895   Other spondylosis, thoracolumbar region

         M47.896   Other spondylosis, lumbar region

         M47.897   Other spondylosis, lumbosacral region

N Newborn: 0   P Pediatric: 0-17   M Maternity: 12-55   A Adult: 15-124   MCC Major CC Condition   PDxMCC PDx acts as own MCC   CC CC Condition   PDxCC PDx acts as own CC

744   ICD-10-CM 2016

M47.898   **Other spondylosis,** sacral and sacrococcygeal **region**

M47.899   **Other spondylosis,** site unspecified

M47.9 Spondylosis, unspecified

✓4ᵗʰ **M48 Other spondylopathies**

✓5ᵗʰ **M48.0 Spinal stenosis**
Caudal stenosis

M48.00   **Spinal stenosis,** site unspecified

M48.01   **Spinal stenosis,** occipito-atlanto-axial **region**

M48.02   **Spinal stenosis,** cervical **region**

M48.03   **Spinal stenosis,** cervicothoracic **region**

M48.04   **Spinal stenosis,** thoracic **region**

M48.05   **Spinal stenosis,** thoracolumbar **region**

M48.06   **Spinal stenosis,** lumbar **region**

M48.07   **Spinal stenosis,** lumbosacral **region**

M48.08   **Spinal stenosis,** sacral and sacrococcygeal **region**

✓5ᵗʰ **M48.1 Ankylosing hyperostosis [Forestier]**
Diffuse idiopathic skeletal hyperostosis [DISH]

M48.10   **Ankylosing hyperostosis [Forestier],** site unspecified

M48.11   **Ankylosing hyperostosis [Forestier],** occipito-atlanto-axial **region**

M48.12   **Ankylosing hyperostosis [Forestier],** cervical **region**

M48.13   **Ankylosing hyperostosis [Forestier],** cervicothoracic **region**

M48.14   **Ankylosing hyperostosis [Forestier],** thoracic **region**

M48.15   **Ankylosing hyperostosis [Forestier],** thoracolumbar **region**

M48.16   **Ankylosing hyperostosis [Forestier],** lumbar **region**

M48.17   **Ankylosing hyperostosis [Forestier],** lumbosacral **region**

M48.18   **Ankylosing hyperostosis [Forestier],** sacral and sacrococcygeal **region**

M48.19   **Ankylosing hyperostosis [Forestier],** multiple sites **in spine**

✓5ᵗʰ **M48.2 Kissing spine**

M48.20   **Kissing spine,** site unspecified

M48.21   **Kissing spine,** occipito-atlanto-axial **region**

M48.22   **Kissing spine,** cervical **region**

M48.23   **Kissing spine,** cervicothoracic **region**

M48.24   **Kissing spine,** thoracic **region**

M48.25   **Kissing spine,** thoracolumbar **region**

M48.26   **Kissing spine,** lumbar **region**

M48.27   **Kissing spine,** lumbosacral **region**

✓5ᵗʰ **M48.3 Traumatic spondylopathy**

> **CC Excl: For CC codes in subcategory M48.3, unless otherwise noted:** M48.30-M48.38

M48.30   **Traumatic spondylopathy,** site unspecified   `CC`

M48.31   **Traumatic spondylopathy,** occipito-atlanto-axial **region**   `CC`

M48.32   **Traumatic spondylopathy,** cervical **region**   `CC`

M48.33   **Traumatic spondylopathy,** cervicothoracic **region**   `CC`

M48.34   **Traumatic spondylopathy,** thoracic **region**   `CC`

M48.35   **Traumatic spondylopathy,** thoracolumbar **region**   `CC`

M48.36   **Traumatic spondylopathy,** lumbar **region**   `CC`

M48.37   **Traumatic spondylopathy,** lumbosacral **region**   `CC`

M48.38   **Traumatic spondylopathy,** sacral and sacrococcygeal **region**   `CC`

✓5ᵗʰ **M48.4 Fatigue fracture of vertebra**
Stress fracture of vertebra

> **EXCLUDES 1**   *pathological fracture NOS (M84.4-)*
> *pathological fracture of vertebra due to neoplasm (M84.58)*
> *pathological fracture of vertebra due to other diagnosis (M84.68)*
> *pathological fracture of vertebra due to osteoporosis (M80.-)*
> *traumatic fracture of vertebrae (S12.0-S12.3-, S22.0-, S32.0-)*

> The appropriate 7th character is to be added to each code from subcategory M48.4.
> A   initial encounter for fracture
> D   subsequent encounter for fracture with routine healing
> G   subsequent encounter for fracture with delayed healing
> S   sequela of fracture

✓x7ᵗʰ   M48.40   **Fatigue fracture of vertebra,** site unspecified

✓x7ᵗʰ   M48.41   **Fatigue fracture of vertebra,** occipito-atlanto-axial **region**

✓x7ᵗʰ   M48.42   **Fatigue fracture of vertebra,** cervical **region**

✓x7ᵗʰ   M48.43   **Fatigue fracture of vertebra,** cervicothoracic **region**

✓x7ᵗʰ   M48.44   **Fatigue fracture of vertebra,** thoracic **region**

✓x7ᵗʰ   M48.45   **Fatigue fracture of vertebra,** thoracolumbar **region**

✓x7ᵗʰ   M48.46   **Fatigue fracture of vertebra,** lumbar **region**

✓x7ᵗʰ   M48.47   **Fatigue fracture of vertebra,** lumbosacral **region**

✓x7ᵗʰ   M48.48   **Fatigue fracture of vertebra,** sacral and sacrococcygeal **region**

✓5ᵗʰ **M48.5 Collapsed vertebra, not elsewhere classified**
Collapsed vertebra NOS
Wedging of vertebra NOS

> **EXCLUDES 1**   *current injury—see Injury of spine, by body region*
> *fatigue fracture of vertebra (M48.4)*
> *pathological fracture of vertebra due to neoplasm (M84.58)*
> *pathological fracture of vertebra due to other diagnosis (M84.68)*
> *pathological fracture of vertebra due to osteoporosis (M80.-)*
> *pathological fracture NOS (M84.4-)*
> *stress fracture of vertebra (M48.4-)*
> *traumatic fracture of vertebra (S12-, S22-, S32-)*

> The appropriate 7th character is to be added to each code from subcategory M48.5.
> A   initial encounter for fracture
> D   subsequent encounter for fracture with routine healing
> G   subsequent encounter for fracture with delayed healing
> S   sequela of fracture

> **CC Excl: For CC codes in subcategory M48.5 with 7th character A, unless otherwise noted:** M48.40X-M48.58X with 7th A, M80.00X-M84.68X with 7th A

✓x7ᵗʰ   M48.50   **Collapsed vertebra, not elsewhere classified,** site unspecified   `CC`

✓x7ᵗʰ   M48.51   **Collapsed vertebra, not elsewhere classified,** occipito-atlanto-axial **region**   `CC`

✓x7ᵗʰ   M48.52   **Collapsed vertebra, not elsewhere classified,** cervical **region**   `CC`

✓x7ᵗʰ   M48.53   **Collapsed vertebra, not elsewhere classified,** cervicothoracic **region**   `CC`

✓x7ᵗʰ   M48.54   **Collapsed vertebra, not elsewhere classified,** thoracic **region**   `CC`

✓x7ᵗʰ   M48.55   **Collapsed vertebra, not elsewhere classified,** thoracolumbar **region**   `CC`

✓x7ᵗʰ   M48.56   **Collapsed vertebra, not elsewhere classified,** lumbar **region**   `CC`

✓x7ᵗʰ   M48.57   **Collapsed vertebra, not elsewhere classified,** lumbosacral **region**   `CC`

✓x7ᵗʰ   M48.58   **Collapsed vertebra, not elsewhere classified,** sacral and sacrococcygeal **region**   `CC`

✓ Additional Character Required   ✓x7ᵗʰ Placeholder Alert   Unacceptable PDx   Manifestation   Hospital Acquired Condition   **EXCLUDES 1** Not Coded Here   *EXCLUDES 2* Not Included Here

✓5ᵗʰ **M48.8 Other specified spondylopathies**
Ossification of posterior longitudinal ligament

✓6ᵗʰ **M48.8X Other specified spondylopathies**

M48.8X1 Other specified spondylopathies, occipito-atlanto-axial region

M48.8X2 Other specified spondylopathies, cervical region

M48.8X3 Other specified spondylopathies, cervicothoracic region

M48.8X4 Other specified spondylopathies, thoracic region

M48.8X5 Other specified spondylopathies, thoracolumbar region

M48.8X6 Other specified spondylopathies, lumbar region

M48.8X7 Other specified spondylopathies, lumbosacral region

M48.8X8 Other specified spondylopathies, sacral and sacrococcygeal region

M48.8X9 Other specified spondylopathies, site unspecified

M48.9 Spondylopathy, unspecified

✓4ᵗʰ **M49 Spondylopathies in diseases classified elsewhere**
INCLUDES curvature of spine in diseases classified elsewhere
deformity of spine in diseases classified elsewhere
kyphosis in diseases classified elsewhere
scoliosis in diseases classified elsewhere
spondylopathy in diseases classified elsewhere

Code first underlying disease, such as:
brucellosis (A23.-)
Charcôt-Marie-Tooth disease (G60.0)
enterobacterial infections (A01-A04)
osteitis fibrosa cystica (E21.0)

EXCLUDES 1 *curvature of spine in tuberculosis [Pott's] (A18.01)*
enteropathic arthropathies (M07.-)
gonococcal spondylitis (A54.41)
neuropathic [tabes dorsalis] spondylitis (A52.11)
neuropathic spondylopathy in syringomyelia (G95.0)
neuropathic spondylopathy in tabes dorsalis (A52.11)
nonsyphilitic neuropathic spondylopathy NEC (G98.0)
spondylitis in syphilis (acquired) (A52.77)
tuberculous spondylitis (A18.01)
typhoid fever spondylitis (A01.05)

✓5ᵗʰ **M49.8 Spondylopathy in diseases classified elsewhere**

M49.80 *Spondylopathy in diseases classified elsewhere, site unspecified*

M49.81 *Spondylopathy in diseases classified elsewhere, occipito-atlanto-axial region*

M49.82 *Spondylopathy in diseases classified elsewhere, cervical region*

M49.83 *Spondylopathy in diseases classified elsewhere, cervicothoracic region*

M49.84 *Spondylopathy in diseases classified elsewhere, thoracic region*

M49.85 *Spondylopathy in diseases classified elsewhere, thoracolumbar region*

M49.86 *Spondylopathy in diseases classified elsewhere, lumbar region*

M49.87 *Spondylopathy in diseases classified elsewhere, lumbosacral region*

M49.88 *Spondylopathy in diseases classified elsewhere, sacral and sacrococcygeal region*

M49.89 *Spondylopathy in diseases classified elsewhere, multiple sites in spine*

Other dorsopathies (M50-M54)

EXCLUDES 1 *current injury—see injury of spine by body region*
discitis NOS (M46.4-)

✓4ᵗʰ **M50 Cervical disc disorders**
NOTE Code to the most superior level of disorder.
INCLUDES cervicothoracic disc disorders with cervicalgia
cervicothoracic disc disorders

✓5ᵗʰ **M50.0 Cervical disc disorder with myelopathy**

M50.00 Cervical disc disorder with myelopathy, unspecified cervical region CC
CC Excl: M50.00-M50.03, M50.20-M50.23

M50.01 Cervical disc disorder with myelopathy, high cervical region CC
C2-C3 disc disorder with myelopathy
C3-C4 disc disorder with myelopathy
CC Excl: See code: M50.00

M50.02 Cervical disc disorder with myelopathy, mid-cervical region CC
C4-C5 disc disorder with myelopathy
C5-C6 disc disorder with myelopathy
C6-C7 disc disorder with myelopathy
CC Excl: See code: M50.00

M50.03 Cervical disc disorder with myelopathy, cervicothoracic region CC
C7-T1 disc disorder with myelopathy
CC Excl: See code: M50.00

✓5ᵗʰ **M50.1 Cervical disc disorder with radiculopathy**
EXCLUDES 2 *brachial radiculitis NOS (M54.13)*

M50.10 Cervical disc disorder with radiculopathy, unspecified cervical region

M50.11 Cervical disc disorder with radiculopathy, high cervical region
C2-C3 disc disorder with radiculopathy
C3 radiculopathy due to disc disorder
C3-C4 disc disorder with radiculopathy
C4 radiculopathy due to disc disorder

M50.12 Cervical disc disorder with radiculopathy, mid-cervical region
C4-C5 disc disorder with radiculopathy
C5 radiculopathy due to disc disorder
C5-C6 disc disorder with radiculopathy
C6 radiculopathy due to disc disorder
C6-C7 disc disorder with radiculopathy
C7 radiculopathy due to disc disorder

M50.13 Cervical disc disorder with radiculopathy, cervicothoracic region
C7-T1 disc disorder with radiculopathy
C8 radiculopathy due to disc disorder

✓5ᵗʰ **M50.2 Other cervical disc displacement**

M50.20 Other cervical disc displacement, unspecified cervical region

M50.21 Other cervical disc displacement, high cervical region
Other C2-C3 cervical disc displacement
Other C3-C4 cervical disc displacement

M50.22 Other cervical disc displacement, mid-cervical region
Other C4-C5 cervical disc displacement
Other C5-C6 cervical disc displacement
Other C6-C7 cervical disc displacement

M50.23 Other cervical disc displacement, cervicothoracic region
Other C7-T1 cervical disc displacement

✓5ᵗʰ **M50.3 Other cervical disc degeneration**

M50.30 Other cervical disc degeneration, unspecified cervical region

M50.31 Other cervical disc degeneration, high cervical region
Other C2-C3 cervical disc degeneration
Other C3-C4 cervical disc degeneration

M50.32 Other cervical disc degeneration, mid-cervical region
Other C4-C5 cervical disc degeneration
Other C5-C6 cervical disc degeneration
Other C6-C7 cervical disc degeneration

M50.33 Other cervical disc degeneration, cervicothoracic region
Other C7-T1 cervical disc degeneration

✓5ᵗʰ **M50.8 Other cervical disc disorders**

M50.80 Other cervical disc disorders, unspecified cervical region

M50.81 Other cervical disc disorders, high cervical region
Other C2-C3 cervical disc disorders
Other C3-C4 cervical disc disorders

M50.82 Other cervical disc disorders, mid-cervical region
Other C4-C5 cervical disc disorders
Other C5-C6 cervical disc disorders
Other C6-C7 cervical disc disorders

M50.83 Other cervical disc disorders, cervicothoracic region
Other C7-T1 cervical disc disorders

✓5ᵗʰ **M50.9 Cervical disc disorder, unspecified**

    M50.90 Cervical disc disorder, unspecified, unspecified cervical region

    M50.91 Cervical disc disorder, unspecified, high cervical region
        C2-C3 cervical disc disorder, unspecified
        C3-C4 cervical disc disorder, unspecified

    M50.92 Cervical disc disorder, unspecified, mid-cervical region
        C4-C5 cervical disc disorder, unspecified
        C5-C6 cervical disc disorder, unspecified
        C6-C7 cervical disc disorder, unspecified

    M50.93 Cervical disc disorder, unspecified, cervicothoracic region
        C7-T1 cervical disc disorder, unspecified

✓4ᵗʰ **M51 Thoracic, thoracolumbar, and lumbosacral intervertebral disc disorders**
    EXCLUDES 2 cervical and cervicothoracic disc disorders (M50.-)
              sacral and sacrococcygeal disorders (M53.3)

✓5ᵗʰ **M51.0 Thoracic, thoracolumbar and lumbosacral intervertebral disc disorders with myelopathy**

    M51.04 Intervertebral disc disorders with myelopathy, thoracic region CC
        CC Excl: M51.04-M51.05, M51.24-M51.25

    M51.05 Intervertebral disc disorders with myelopathy, thoracolumbar region CC
        CC Excl: See code: M51.04

    M51.06 Intervertebral disc disorders with myelopathy, lumbar region CC
        CC Excl: M51.06, M51.24-M51.25

✓5ᵗʰ **M51.1 Thoracic, thoracolumbar and lumbosacral intervertebral disc disorders with radiculopathy**
    Sciatica due to intervertebral disc disorder
    EXCLUDES 1 lumbar radiculitis NOS (M54.16)
              sciatica NOS (M54.3)

    M51.14 Intervertebral disc disorders with radiculopathy, thoracic region

    M51.15 Intervertebral disc disorders with radiculopathy, thoracolumbar region

    M51.16 Intervertebral disc disorders with radiculopathy, lumbar region

    M51.17 Intervertebral disc disorders with radiculopathy, lumbosacral region

✓5ᵗʰ **M51.2 Other thoracic, thoracolumbar and lumbosacral intervertebral disc displacement**
    Lumbago due to displacement of intervertebral disc

    M51.24 Other intervertebral disc displacement, thoracic region

    M51.25 Other intervertebral disc displacement, thoracolumbar region

    M51.26 Other intervertebral disc displacement, lumbar region

    M51.27 Other intervertebral disc displacement, lumbosacral region

✓5ᵗʰ **M51.3 Other thoracic, thoracolumbar and lumbosacral intervertebral disc degeneration**
    AHA: 2013, 3Q, 22

    M51.34 Other intervertebral disc degeneration, thoracic region

    M51.35 Other intervertebral disc degeneration, thoracolumbar region

    M51.36 Other intervertebral disc degeneration, lumbar region

    M51.37 Other intervertebral disc degeneration, lumbosacral region

✓5ᵗʰ **M51.4 Schmorl's nodes**

    M51.44 Schmorl's nodes, thoracic region

    M51.45 Schmorl's nodes, thoracolumbar region

    M51.46 Schmorl's nodes, lumbar region

    M51.47 Schmorl's nodes, lumbosacral region

✓5ᵗʰ **M51.8 Other thoracic, thoracolumbar and lumbosacral intervertebral disc disorders**

    M51.84 Other intervertebral disc disorders, thoracic region

    M51.85 Other intervertebral disc disorders, thoracolumbar region

    M51.86 Other intervertebral disc disorders, lumbar region

    M51.87 Other intervertebral disc disorders, lumbosacral region

  M51.9 Unspecified thoracic, thoracolumbar and lumbosacral intervertebral disc disorder

✓4ᵗʰ **M53 Other and unspecified dorsopathies, not elsewhere classified**

  M53.0 Cervicocranial syndrome
    Posterior cervical sympathetic syndrome

  M53.1 Cervicobrachial syndrome
    EXCLUDES 2 cervical disc disorder (M50.-)
              thoracic outlet syndrome (G54.0)

✓5ᵗʰ **M53.2 Spinal instabilities**

  ✓6ᵗʰ **M53.2X Spinal instabilities**

    M53.2X1 Spinal instabilities, occipito-atlanto-axial region

    M53.2X2 Spinal instabilities, cervical region

    M53.2X3 Spinal instabilities, cervicothoracic region

    M53.2X4 Spinal instabilities, thoracic region

    M53.2X5 Spinal instabilities, thoracolumbar region

    M53.2X6 Spinal instabilities, lumbar region

    M53.2X7 Spinal instabilities, lumbosacral region

    M53.2X8 Spinal instabilities, sacral and sacrococcygeal region

    M53.2X9 Spinal instabilities, site unspecified

  M53.3 Sacrococcygeal disorders, not elsewhere classified
    Coccygodynia

✓5ᵗʰ **M53.8 Other specified dorsopathies**

    M53.80 Other specified dorsopathies, site unspecified

    M53.81 Other specified dorsopathies, occipito-atlanto-axial region

    M53.82 Other specified dorsopathies, cervical region

    M53.83 Other specified dorsopathies, cervicothoracic region

    M53.84 Other specified dorsopathies, thoracic region

    M53.85 Other specified dorsopathies, thoracolumbar region

    M53.86 Other specified dorsopathies, lumbar region

    M53.87 Other specified dorsopathies, lumbosacral region

    M53.88 Other specified dorsopathies, sacral and sacrococcygeal region

  M53.9 Dorsopathy, unspecified

✓4ᵗʰ **M54 Dorsalgia**
    EXCLUDES 1 psychogenic dorsalgia (F45.41)

✓5ᵗʰ **M54.0 Panniculitis affecting regions of neck and back**
    EXCLUDES 1 lupus panniculitis (L93.2)
              panniculitis NOS (M79.3)
              relapsing [Weber-Christian] panniculitis (M35.6)

    M54.00 Panniculitis affecting regions of neck and back, site unspecified

    M54.01 Panniculitis affecting regions of neck and back, occipito-atlanto-axial region

    M54.02 Panniculitis affecting regions of neck and back, cervical region

    M54.03 Panniculitis affecting regions of neck and back, cervicothoracic region

    M54.04 Panniculitis affecting regions of neck and back, thoracic region

    M54.05 Panniculitis affecting regions of neck and back, thoracolumbar region

    M54.06 Panniculitis affecting regions of neck and back, lumbar region

    M54.07 Panniculitis affecting regions of neck and back, lumbosacral region

    M54.08 Panniculitis affecting regions of neck and back, sacral and sacrococcygeal region

    M54.09 Panniculitis affecting regions, neck and back, multiple sites in spine

✓ Additional Character Required   ✓x7ᵗʰ Placeholder Alert   Unacceptable PDx   Manifestation   Hospital Acquired Condition   EXCLUDES 1 Not Coded Here   EXCLUDES 2 Not Included Here

√5ᵗʰ M54.1 Radiculopathy
Brachial neuritis or radiculitis NOS
Lumbar neuritis or radiculitis NOS
Lumbosacral neuritis or radiculitis NOS
Thoracic neuritis or radiculitis NOS
Radiculitis NOS
> **EXCLUDES 1**   neuralgia and neuritis NOS (M79.2)
> radiculopathy with cervical disc disorder (M50.1)
> radiculopathy with lumbar and other intervertebral
>   disc disorder (M51.1-)
> radiculopathy with spondylosis (M47.2-)

    M54.10 Radiculopathy, site unspecified
    M54.11 Radiculopathy, occipito-atlanto-axial region
    M54.12 Radiculopathy, cervical region
    M54.13 Radiculopathy, cervicothoracic region
    M54.14 Radiculopathy, thoracic region
    M54.15 Radiculopathy, thoracolumbar region
    M54.16 Radiculopathy, lumbar region
    M54.17 Radiculopathy, lumbosacral region
    M54.18 Radiculopathy, sacral and sacrococcygeal region

M54.2 Cervicalgia
> **EXCLUDES 1**   cervicalgia due to intervertebral cervical disc disorder
>   (M50.-)

√5ᵗʰ M54.3 Sciatica
> **EXCLUDES 1**   lesion of sciatic nerve (G57.0)
> sciatica due to intervertebral disc disorder (M51.1-)
> sciatica with lumbago (M54.4-)

    M54.30 Sciatica, unspecified side
    M54.31 Sciatica, right side
    M54.32 Sciatica, left side

√5ᵗʰ M54.4 Lumbago with sciatica
> **EXCLUDES 1**   lumbago with sciatica due to intervertebral disc
>   disorder (M51.1-)

    M54.40 Lumbago with sciatica, unspecified side
    M54.41 Lumbago with sciatica, right side
    M54.42 Lumbago with sciatica, left side

M54.5 Low back pain
Loin pain
Lumbago NOS
> **EXCLUDES 1**   low back strain (S39.012)
> lumbago due to intervertebral disc displacement
>   (M51.2-)
> lumbago with sciatica (M54.4-)

M54.6 Pain in thoracic spine
> **EXCLUDES 1**   pain in thoracic spine due to intervertebral disc disorder
>   (M51.-)

√5ᵗʰ M54.8 Other dorsalgia
> **EXCLUDES 1**   dorsalgia in thoracic region (M54.6)
> low back pain (M54.5)

    M54.81 Occipital neuralgia
    M54.89 Other dorsalgia

M54.9 Dorsalgia, unspecified
Backache NOS
Back pain NOS

SOFT TISSUE DISORDERS (M60-M79)

Disorders of muscles (M60-M63)

> **EXCLUDES 1**   dermatopolymyositis (M33.-)
> muscular dystrophies and myopathies (G71-G72)
> myopathy in amyloidosis (E85.-)
> myopathy in polyarteritis nodosa (M30.0)
> myopathy in rheumatoid arthritis (M05.32)
> myopathy in scleroderma (M34.-)
> myopathy in Sjögren's syndrome (M35.03)
> myopathy in systemic lupus erythematosus (M32.-)

√4ᵗʰ M60 Myositis
> **EXCLUDES 2**   inclusion body myositis [IBM] (G72.41)

√5ᵗʰ M60.0 Infective myositis
Tropical pyomyositis
Use additional code (B95-B97) to identify infectious agent

> **CC Excl: For CC codes in subcategory M60.0, unless otherwise noted:** K68.12, M60.000-M60.19, M61.00-M61.19, M61.30-M61.59, M62.3, M62.50-M62.59, M62.89, M72.6

√6ᵗʰ M60.00 Infective myositis, unspecified site
    M60.000 Infective myositis, unspecified right arm `CC`
      Infective myositis, right upper limb NOS
    M60.001 Infective myositis, unspecified left arm `CC`
      Infective myositis, left upper limb NOS
    M60.002 Infective myositis, unspecified arm `CC`
      Infective myositis, upper limb NOS
    M60.003 Infective myositis, unspecified right leg `CC`
      Infective myositis, right lower limb NOS
    M60.004 Infective myositis, unspecified left leg `CC`
      Infective myositis, left lower limb NOS
    M60.005 Infective myositis, unspecified leg `CC`
      Infective myositis, lower limb NOS
    M60.009 Infective myositis, unspecified site

√6ᵗʰ M60.01 Infective myositis, shoulder
    M60.011 Infective myositis, right shoulder `CC`
    M60.012 Infective myositis, left shoulder `CC`
    M60.019 Infective myositis, unspecified shoulder `CC`

√6ᵗʰ M60.02 Infective myositis, upper arm
    M60.021 Infective myositis, right upper arm `CC`
    M60.022 Infective myositis, left upper arm `CC`
    M60.029 Infective myositis, unspecified upper arm `CC`

√6ᵗʰ M60.03 Infective myositis, forearm
    M60.031 Infective myositis, right forearm `CC`
    M60.032 Infective myositis, left forearm `CC`
    M60.039 Infective myositis, unspecified forearm `CC`

√6ᵗʰ M60.04 Infective myositis, hand and fingers
    M60.041 Infective myositis, right hand `CC`
    M60.042 Infective myositis, left hand `CC`
    M60.043 Infective myositis, unspecified hand `CC`
    M60.044 Infective myositis, right finger(s) `CC`
    M60.045 Infective myositis, left finger(s) `CC`
    M60.046 Infective myositis, unspecified finger(s) `CC`

√6ᵗʰ M60.05 Infective myositis, thigh
    M60.051 Infective myositis, right thigh `CC`
    M60.052 Infective myositis, left thigh `CC`
    M60.059 Infective myositis, unspecified thigh `CC`

√6ᵗʰ M60.06 Infective myositis, lower leg
    M60.061 Infective myositis, right lower leg `CC`
    M60.062 Infective myositis, left lower leg `CC`
    M60.069 Infective myositis, unspecified lower leg `CC`

√6ᵗʰ M60.07 Infective myositis, ankle, foot and toes
    M60.070 Infective myositis, right ankle `CC`
    M60.071 Infective myositis, left ankle `CC`
    M60.072 Infective myositis, unspecified ankle `CC`
    M60.073 Infective myositis, right foot `CC`
    M60.074 Infective myositis, left foot `CC`
    M60.075 Infective myositis, unspecified foot `CC`
    M60.076 Infective myositis, right toe(s) `CC`
    M60.077 Infective myositis, left toe(s) `CC`
    M60.078 Infective myositis, unspecified toe(s) `CC`

    M60.08 Infective myositis, other site `CC`
    M60.09 Infective myositis, multiple sites `CC`

M60.1 Interstitial myositis
    M60.10 Interstitial myositis of unspecified site

√6ᵗʰ M60.11 Interstitial myositis, shoulder
    M60.111 Interstitial myositis, right shoulder
    M60.112 Interstitial myositis, left shoulder
    M60.119 Interstitial myositis, unspecified shoulder

√6ᵗʰ M60.12 Interstitial myositis, upper arm
    M60.121 Interstitial myositis, right upper arm
    M60.122 Interstitial myositis, left upper arm
    M60.129 Interstitial myositis, unspecified upper arm

√6ᵗʰ M60.13 Interstitial myositis, forearm
    M60.131 Interstitial myositis, right forearm

N Newborn: 0   P Pediatric: 0-17   M Maternity: 12-55   A Adult: 15-124   **MCC** Major CC Condition   **PDxMCC** PDx acts as own MCC   **CC** CC Condition   **PDxCC** PDx acts as own CC

748   ICD-10-CM 2016

M60.132   Interstitial myositis, left forearm

M60.139   Interstitial myositis, unspecified forearm

✓6ᵗʰ   M60.14   Interstitial myositis, hand

M60.141   Interstitial myositis, right hand

M60.142   Interstitial myositis, left hand

M60.149   Interstitial myositis, unspecified hand

✓6ᵗʰ   M60.15   Interstitial myositis, thigh

M60.151   Interstitial myositis, right thigh

M60.152   Interstitial myositis, left thigh

M60.159   Interstitial myositis, unspecified thigh

✓6ᵗʰ   M60.16   Interstitial myositis, lower leg

M60.161   Interstitial myositis, right lower leg

M60.162   Interstitial myositis, left lower leg

M60.169   Interstitial myositis, unspecified lower leg

✓6ᵗʰ   M60.17   Interstitial myositis, ankle and foot

M60.171   Interstitial myositis, right ankle and foot

M60.172   Interstitial myositis, left ankle and foot

M60.179   Interstitial myositis, unspecified ankle and foot

M60.18   Interstitial myositis, other site

M60.19   Interstitial myositis, multiple sites

✓5ᵗʰ   **M60.2   Foreign body granuloma of soft tissue, not elsewhere classified**

Use additional code to identify the type of retained foreign body (Z18.-)

EXCLUDES 1   foreign body granuloma of skin and subcutaneous tissue (L92.3)

M60.20   Foreign body granuloma of soft tissue, not elsewhere classified, unspecified site

✓6ᵗʰ   M60.21   Foreign body granuloma of soft tissue, not elsewhere classified, shoulder

M60.211   Foreign body granuloma of soft tissue, not elsewhere classified, right shoulder

M60.212   Foreign body granuloma of soft tissue, not elsewhere classified, left shoulder

M60.219   Foreign body granuloma of soft tissue, not elsewhere classified, unspecified shoulder

✓6ᵗʰ   M60.22   Foreign body granuloma of soft tissue, not elsewhere classified, upper arm

M60.221   Foreign body granuloma of soft tissue, not elsewhere classified, right upper arm

M60.222   Foreign body granuloma of soft tissue, not elsewhere classified, left upper arm

M60.229   Foreign body granuloma of soft tissue, not elsewhere classified, unspecified upper arm

✓6ᵗʰ   M60.23   Foreign body granuloma of soft tissue, not elsewhere classified, forearm

M60.231   Foreign body granuloma of soft tissue, not elsewhere classified, right forearm

M60.232   Foreign body granuloma of soft tissue, not elsewhere classified, left forearm

M60.239   Foreign body granuloma of soft tissue, not elsewhere classified, unspecified forearm

✓6ᵗʰ   M60.24   Foreign body granuloma of soft tissue, not elsewhere classified, hand

M60.241   Foreign body granuloma of soft tissue, not elsewhere classified, right hand

M60.242   Foreign body granuloma of soft tissue, not elsewhere classified, left hand

M60.249   Foreign body granuloma of soft tissue, not elsewhere classified, unspecified hand

✓6ᵗʰ   M60.25   Foreign body granuloma of soft tissue, not elsewhere classified, thigh

M60.251   Foreign body granuloma of soft tissue, not elsewhere classified, right thigh

M60.252   Foreign body granuloma of soft tissue, not elsewhere classified, left thigh

M60.259   Foreign body granuloma of soft tissue, not elsewhere classified, unspecified thigh

✓6ᵗʰ   M60.26   Foreign body granuloma of soft tissue, not elsewhere classified, lower leg

M60.261   Foreign body granuloma of soft tissue, not elsewhere classified, right lower leg

M60.262   Foreign body granuloma of soft tissue, not elsewhere classified, left lower leg

M60.269   Foreign body granuloma of soft tissue, not elsewhere classified, unspecified lower leg

✓6ᵗʰ   M60.27   Foreign body granuloma of soft tissue, not elsewhere classified, ankle and foot

M60.271   Foreign body granuloma of soft tissue, not elsewhere classified, right ankle and foot

M60.272   Foreign body granuloma of soft tissue, not elsewhere classified, left ankle and foot

M60.279   Foreign body granuloma of soft tissue, not elsewhere classified, unspecified ankle and foot

M60.28   Foreign body granuloma of soft tissue, not elsewhere classified, other site

✓5ᵗʰ   **M60.8   Other myositis**

M60.80   Other myositis, unspecified site

✓6ᵗʰ   M60.81   Other myositis shoulder

M60.811   Other myositis, right shoulder

M60.812   Other myositis, left shoulder

M60.819   Other myositis, unspecified shoulder

✓6ᵗʰ   M60.82   Other myositis, upper arm

M60.821   Other myositis, right upper arm

M60.822   Other myositis, left upper arm

M60.829   Other myositis, unspecified upper arm

✓6ᵗʰ   M60.83   Other myositis, forearm

M60.831   Other myositis, right forearm

M60.832   Other myositis, left forearm

M60.839   Other myositis, unspecified forearm

✓6ᵗʰ   M60.84   Other myositis, hand

M60.841   Other myositis, right hand

M60.842   Other myositis, left hand

M60.849   Other myositis, unspecified hand

✓6ᵗʰ   M60.85   Other myositis, thigh

M60.851   Other myositis, right thigh

M60.852   Other myositis, left thigh

M60.859   Other myositis, unspecified thigh

✓6ᵗʰ   M60.86   Other myositis, lower leg

M60.861   Other myositis, right lower leg

M60.862   Other myositis, left lower leg

M60.869   Other myositis, unspecified lower leg

✓6ᵗʰ   M60.87   Other myositis, ankle and foot

M60.871   Other myositis, right ankle and foot

M60.872   Other myositis, left ankle and foot

M60.879   Other myositis, unspecified ankle and foot

M60.88   Other myositis, other site

M60.89   Other myositis, multiple sites

M60.9   Myositis, unspecified

✓4ᵗʰ   **M61   Calcification and ossification of muscle**

✓5ᵗʰ   **M61.0   Myositis ossificans traumatica**

M61.00   Myositis ossificans traumatica, unspecified site

✓6ᵗʰ   M61.01   Myositis ossificans traumatica, shoulder

M61.011   Myositis ossificans traumatica, right shoulder

M61.012   Myositis ossificans traumatica, left shoulder

M61.019   Myositis ossificans traumatica, unspecified shoulder

✓6ᵗʰ   M61.02   Myositis ossificans traumatica, upper arm

M61.021   Myositis ossificans traumatica, right upper arm

M61.022   Myositis ossificans traumatica, left upper arm

M61.029   Myositis ossificans traumatica, unspecified upper arm

✓6ᵗʰ   M61.03   Myositis ossificans traumatica, forearm

M61.031   Myositis ossificans traumatica, right forearm

M61.032   Myositis ossificans traumatica, left forearm

M61.039   Myositis ossificans traumatica, unspecified forearm

✓6ᵗʰ   M61.04   Myositis ossificans traumatica, hand

M61.041   Myositis ossificans traumatica, right hand

M61.042   Myositis ossificans traumatica, left hand

✓ Additional Character Required   ✓x7ᵗʰ Placeholder Alert   Unacceptable PDx   Manifestation   Hospital Acquired Condition   EXCLUDES 1 Not Coded Here   EXCLUDES 2 Not Included Here

ICD-10-CM 2016   749

Chapter 13. Diseases of the Musculoskeletal System and Connective Tissue

M61.049–M61.29

M61.049   Myositis ossificans traumatica, unspecified **hand**

✓6ᵗʰ **M61.05**   Myositis ossificans traumatica, **thigh**

    M61.051   Myositis ossificans traumatica, **right** thigh

    M61.052   Myositis ossificans traumatica, **left** thigh

    M61.059   Myositis ossificans traumatica, unspecified **thigh**

✓6ᵗʰ **M61.06**   Myositis ossificans traumatica, **lower leg**

    M61.061   Myositis ossificans traumatica, **right** lower leg

    M61.062   Myositis ossificans traumatica, **left** lower leg

    M61.069   Myositis ossificans traumatica, unspecified **lower leg**

✓6ᵗʰ **M61.07**   Myositis ossificans traumatica, **ankle and foot**

    M61.071   Myositis ossificans traumatica, **right** ankle and foot

    M61.072   Myositis ossificans traumatica, **left** ankle and foot

    M61.079   Myositis ossificans traumatica, unspecified **ankle and foot**

M61.08   Myositis ossificans traumatica, **other site**

M61.09   Myositis ossificans traumatica, **multiple sites**

✓5ᵗʰ **M61.1**   **Myositis ossificans progressiva**
Fibrodysplasia ossificans progressiva

M61.10   Myositis ossificans progressiva, **unspecified site**

✓6ᵗʰ **M61.11**   Myositis ossificans progressiva, **shoulder**

    M61.111   Myositis ossificans progressiva, **right** shoulder

    M61.112   Myositis ossificans progressiva, **left** shoulder

    M61.119   Myositis ossificans progressiva, unspecified **shoulder**

✓6ᵗʰ **M61.12**   Myositis ossificans progressiva, **upper arm**

    M61.121   Myositis ossificans progressiva, **right** upper arm

    M61.122   Myositis ossificans progressiva, **left** upper arm

    M61.129   Myositis ossificans progressiva, unspecified **arm**

✓6ᵗʰ **M61.13**   Myositis ossificans progressiva, **forearm**

    M61.131   Myositis ossificans progressiva, **right** forearm

    M61.132   Myositis ossificans progressiva, **left** forearm

    M61.139   Myositis ossificans progressiva, unspecified **forearm**

✓6ᵗʰ **M61.14**   Myositis ossificans progressiva, **hand and finger(s)**

    M61.141   Myositis ossificans progressiva, **right hand**

    M61.142   Myositis ossificans progressiva, **left hand**

    M61.143   Myositis ossificans progressiva, unspecified **hand**

    M61.144   Myositis ossificans progressiva, **right finger(s)**

    M61.145   Myositis ossificans progressiva, **left finger(s)**

    M61.146   Myositis ossificans progressiva, unspecified **finger(s)**

✓6ᵗʰ **M61.15**   Myositis ossificans progressiva, **thigh**

    M61.151   Myositis ossificans progressiva, **right thigh**

    M61.152   Myositis ossificans progressiva, **left thigh**

    M61.159   Myositis ossificans progressiva, unspecified **thigh**

✓6ᵗʰ **M61.16**   Myositis ossificans progressiva, **lower leg**

    M61.161   Myositis ossificans progressiva, **right lower leg**

    M61.162   Myositis ossificans progressiva, **left lower leg**

    M61.169   Myositis ossificans progressiva, unspecified **lower leg**

✓6ᵗʰ **M61.17**   Myositis ossificans progressiva, **ankle, foot and toe(s)**

    M61.171   Myositis ossificans progressiva, **right ankle**

    M61.172   Myositis ossificans progressiva, **left ankle**

M61.173   Myositis ossificans progressiva, unspecified **ankle**

M61.174   Myositis ossificans progressiva, **right foot**

M61.175   Myositis ossificans progressiva, **left foot**

M61.176   Myositis ossificans progressiva, unspecified **foot**

M61.177   Myositis ossificans progressiva, **right toe(s)**

M61.178   Myositis ossificans progressiva, **left toe(s)**

M61.179   Myositis ossificans progressiva, unspecified **toe(s)**

M61.18   Myositis ossificans progressiva, **other site**

M61.19   Myositis ossificans progressiva, **multiple sites**

✓5ᵗʰ **M61.2**   **Paralytic calcification and ossification of muscle**
Myositis ossificans associated with quadriplegia or paraplegia

M61.20   Paralytic calcification and ossification of muscle, **unspecified site**

✓6ᵗʰ **M61.21**   Paralytic calcification and ossification of muscle, **shoulder**

    M61.211   Paralytic calcification and ossification of muscle, **right shoulder**

    M61.212   Paralytic calcification and ossification of muscle, **left shoulder**

    M61.219   Paralytic calcification and ossification of muscle, **unspecified shoulder**

✓6ᵗʰ **M61.22**   Paralytic calcification and ossification of muscle, **upper arm**

    M61.221   Paralytic calcification and ossification of muscle, **right upper arm**

    M61.222   Paralytic calcification and ossification of muscle, **left upper arm**

    M61.229   Paralytic calcification and ossification of muscle, **unspecified upper arm**

✓6ᵗʰ **M61.23**   Paralytic calcification and ossification of muscle, **forearm**

    M61.231   Paralytic calcification and ossification of muscle, **right forearm**

    M61.232   Paralytic calcification and ossification of muscle, **left forearm**

    M61.239   Paralytic calcification and ossification of muscle, **unspecified forearm**

✓6ᵗʰ **M61.24**   Paralytic calcification and ossification of muscle, **hand**

    M61.241   Paralytic calcification and ossification of muscle, **right hand**

    M61.242   Paralytic calcification and ossification of muscle, **left hand**

    M61.249   Paralytic calcification and ossification of muscle, **unspecified hand**

✓6ᵗʰ **M61.25**   Paralytic calcification and ossification of muscle, **thigh**

    M61.251   Paralytic calcification and ossification of muscle, **right thigh**

    M61.252   Paralytic calcification and ossification of muscle, **left thigh**

    M61.259   Paralytic calcification and ossification of muscle, **unspecified thigh**

✓6ᵗʰ **M61.26**   Paralytic calcification and ossification of muscle, **lower leg**

    M61.261   Paralytic calcification and ossification of muscle, **right lower leg**

    M61.262   Paralytic calcification and ossification of muscle, **left lower leg**

    M61.269   Paralytic calcification and ossification of muscle, **unspecified lower leg**

✓6ᵗʰ **M61.27**   Paralytic calcification and ossification of muscle, **ankle and foot**

    M61.271   Paralytic calcification and ossification of muscle, **right ankle and foot**

    M61.272   Paralytic calcification and ossification of muscle, **left ankle and foot**

    M61.279   Paralytic calcification and ossification of muscle, **unspecified ankle and foot**

M61.28   Paralytic calcification and ossification of muscle, **other site**

M61.29   Paralytic calcification and ossification of muscle, **multiple sites**

Ⓝ Newborn: 0   Ⓟ Pediatric: 0-17   Ⓜ Maternity: 12-55   Ⓐ Adult: 15-124   **MCC** Major CC Condition   **PDxMCC** PDx acts as own MCC   **CC** CC Condition   **PDxCC** PDx acts as own CC

750

ICD-10-CM 2016

✓5ᵗʰ **M61.3** Calcification and ossification of muscles associated with burns
     Myositis ossificans associated with burns

M61.3Ø Calcification and ossification of muscles associated with burns, unspecified site

✓6ᵗʰ **M61.31** Calcification and ossification of muscles associated with burns, shoulder

M61.311 Calcification and ossification of muscles associated with burns, right shoulder

M61.312 Calcification and ossification of muscles associated with burns, left shoulder

M61.319 Calcification and ossification of muscles associated with burns, unspecified shoulder

✓6ᵗʰ **M61.32** Calcification and ossification of muscles associated with burns, upper arm

M61.321 Calcification and ossification of muscles associated with burns, right upper arm

M61.322 Calcification and ossification of muscles associated with burns, left upper arm

M61.329 Calcification and ossification of muscles associated with burns, unspecified upper arm

✓6ᵗʰ **M61.33** Calcification and ossification of muscles associated with burns, forearm

M61.331 Calcification and ossification of muscles associated with burns, right forearm

M61.332 Calcification and ossification of muscles associated with burns, left forearm

M61.339 Calcification and ossification of muscles associated with burns, unspecified forearm

✓6ᵗʰ **M61.34** Calcification and ossification of muscles associated with burns, hand

M61.341 Calcification and ossification of muscles associated with burns, right hand

M61.342 Calcification and ossification of muscles associated with burns, left hand

M61.349 Calcification and ossification of muscles associated with burns, unspecified hand

✓6ᵗʰ **M61.35** Calcification and ossification of muscles associated with burns, thigh

M61.351 Calcification and ossification of muscles associated with burns, right thigh

M61.352 Calcification and ossification of muscles associated with burns, left thigh

M61.359 Calcification and ossification of muscles associated with burns, unspecified thigh

✓6ᵗʰ **M61.36** Calcification and ossification of muscles associated with burns, lower leg

M61.361 Calcification and ossification of muscles associated with burns, right lower leg

M61.362 Calcification and ossification of muscles associated with burns, left lower leg

M61.369 Calcification and ossification of muscles associated with burns, unspecified lower leg

✓6ᵗʰ **M61.37** Calcification and ossification of muscles associated with burns, ankle and foot

M61.371 Calcification and ossification of muscles associated with burns, right ankle and foot

M61.372 Calcification and ossification of muscles associated with burns, left ankle and foot

M61.379 Calcification and ossification of muscles associated with burns, unspecified ankle and foot

M61.38 Calcification and ossification of muscles associated with burns, other site

M61.39 Calcification and ossification of muscles associated with burns, multiple sites

✓5ᵗʰ **M61.4** Other calcification of muscle

> **EXCLUDES 1**   calcific tendinitis NOS (M65.2-)
>   calcific tendinitis of shoulder (M75.3)

M61.4Ø Other calcification of muscle, unspecified site

✓6ᵗʰ **M61.41** Other calcification of muscle, shoulder

M61.411 Other calcification of muscle, right shoulder

M61.412 Other calcification of muscle, left shoulder

M61.419 Other calcification of muscle, unspecified shoulder

✓6ᵗʰ **M61.42** Other calcification of muscle, upper arm

M61.421 Other calcification of muscle, right upper arm

M61.422 Other calcification of muscle, left upper arm

M61.429 Other calcification of muscle, unspecified upper arm

✓6ᵗʰ **M61.43** Other calcification of muscle, forearm

M61.431 Other calcification of muscle, right forearm

M61.432 Other calcification of muscle, left forearm

M61.439 Other calcification of muscle, unspecified forearm

✓6ᵗʰ **M61.44** Other calcification of muscle, hand

M61.441 Other calcification of muscle, right hand

M61.442 Other calcification of muscle, left hand

M61.449 Other calcification of muscle, unspecified hand

✓6ᵗʰ **M61.45** Other calcification of muscle, thigh

M61.451 Other calcification of muscle, right thigh

M61.452 Other calcification of muscle, left thigh

M61.459 Other calcification of muscle, unspecified thigh

✓6ᵗʰ **M61.46** Other calcification of muscle, lower leg

M61.461 Other calcification of muscle, right lower leg

M61.462 Other calcification of muscle, left lower leg

M61.469 Other calcification of muscle, unspecified lower leg

✓6ᵗʰ **M61.47** Other calcification of muscle, ankle and foot

M61.471 Other calcification of muscle, right ankle and foot

M61.472 Other calcification of muscle, left ankle and foot

M61.479 Other calcification of muscle, unspecified ankle and foot

M61.48 Other calcification of muscle, other site

M61.49 Other calcification of muscle, multiple sites

✓5ᵗʰ **M61.5** Other ossification of muscle

M61.5Ø Other ossification of muscle, unspecified site

✓6ᵗʰ **M61.51** Other ossification of muscle, shoulder

M61.511 Other ossification of muscle, right shoulder

M61.512 Other ossification of muscle, left shoulder

M61.519 Other ossification of muscle, unspecified shoulder

✓6ᵗʰ **M61.52** Other ossification of muscle, upper arm

M61.521 Other ossification of muscle, right upper arm

M61.522 Other ossification of muscle, left upper arm

M61.529 Other ossification of muscle, unspecified upper arm

✓6ᵗʰ **M61.53** Other ossification of muscle, forearm

M61.531 Other ossification of muscle, right forearm

M61.532 Other ossification of muscle, left forearm

M61.539 Other ossification of muscle, unspecified forearm

✓6ᵗʰ **M61.54** Other ossification of muscle, hand

M61.541 Other ossification of muscle, right hand

M61.542 Other ossification of muscle, left hand

M61.549 Other ossification of muscle, unspecified hand

✓6ᵗʰ **M61.55** Other ossification of muscle, thigh

M61.551 Other ossification of muscle, right thigh

M61.552 Other ossification of muscle, left thigh

M61.559 Other ossification of muscle, unspecified thigh

✓6ᵗʰ **M61.56** Other ossification of muscle, lower leg

M61.561 Other ossification of muscle, right lower leg

M61.562 Other ossification of muscle, left lower leg

✔ Additional Character Required   ✔x7ᵗʰ Placeholder Alert   Unacceptable PDx   **Manifestation**   Hospital Acquired Condition   **EXCLUDES 1** Not Coded Here   **EXCLUDES 2** Not Included Here

M61.569 **Other ossification of muscle**, unspecified lower leg

✓6ᵗʰ M61.57 **Other ossification of muscle**, ankle and foot

     M61.571 **Other ossification of muscle**, right ankle and foot

     M61.572 **Other ossification of muscle**, left ankle and foot

     M61.579 **Other ossification of muscle**, unspecified ankle and foot

M61.58 **Other ossification of muscle**, other site

M61.59 **Other ossification of muscle**, multiple sites

M61.9 **Calcification and ossification of muscle**, unspecified

✓4ᵗʰ **M62 Other disorders of muscle**

    EXCLUDES 1   *alcoholic myopathy (G72.1)*
                  cramp and spasm (R25.2)
                  drug-induced myopathy (G72.0)
                  myalgia (M79.1)
                  stiff-man syndrome (G25.82)

    EXCLUDES 2   *nontraumatic hematoma of muscle (M79.81)*

✓5ᵗʰ **M62.0 Separation of muscle (nontraumatic)**
      Diastasis of muscle

    EXCLUDES 1   *diastasis recti complicating pregnancy, labor and delivery (O71.8)*
                  traumatic separation of muscle—see strain of muscle by body region

M62.00 **Separation of muscle (nontraumatic)**, unspecified site

✓6ᵗʰ M62.01 **Separation of muscle (nontraumatic)**, shoulder

     M62.011 **Separation of muscle (nontraumatic)**, right shoulder

     M62.012 **Separation of muscle (nontraumatic)**, left shoulder

     M62.019 **Separation of muscle (nontraumatic)**, unspecified shoulder

✓6ᵗʰ M62.02 **Separation of muscle (nontraumatic)**, upper arm

     M62.021 **Separation of muscle (nontraumatic)**, right upper arm

     M62.022 **Separation of muscle (nontraumatic)**, left upper arm

     M62.029 **Separation of muscle (nontraumatic)**, unspecified upper arm

✓6ᵗʰ M62.03 **Separation of muscle (nontraumatic)**, forearm

     M62.031 **Separation of muscle (nontraumatic)**, right forearm

     M62.032 **Separation of muscle (nontraumatic)**, left forearm

     M62.039 **Separation of muscle (nontraumatic)**, unspecified forearm

✓6ᵗʰ M62.04 **Separation of muscle (nontraumatic)**, hand

     M62.041 **Separation of muscle (nontraumatic)**, right hand

     M62.042 **Separation of muscle (nontraumatic)**, left hand

     M62.049 **Separation of muscle (nontraumatic)**, unspecified hand

✓6ᵗʰ M62.05 **Separation of muscle (nontraumatic)**, thigh

     M62.051 **Separation of muscle (nontraumatic)**, right thigh

     M62.052 **Separation of muscle (nontraumatic)**, left thigh

     M62.059 **Separation of muscle (nontraumatic)**, unspecified thigh

✓6ᵗʰ M62.06 **Separation of muscle (nontraumatic)**, lower leg

     M62.061 **Separation of muscle (nontraumatic)**, right lower leg

     M62.062 **Separation of muscle (nontraumatic)**, left lower leg

     M62.069 **Separation of muscle (nontraumatic)**, unspecified lower leg

✓6ᵗʰ M62.07 **Separation of muscle (nontraumatic)**, ankle and foot

     M62.071 **Separation of muscle (nontraumatic)**, right ankle and foot

     M62.072 **Separation of muscle (nontraumatic)**, left ankle and foot

     M62.079 **Separation of muscle (nontraumatic)**, unspecified ankle and foot

M62.08 **Separation of muscle (nontraumatic)**, other site

✓5ᵗʰ **M62.1 Other rupture of muscle (nontraumatic)**

    EXCLUDES 1   *traumatic rupture of muscle—see strain of muscle by body region*

    EXCLUDES 2   *rupture of tendon (M66.-)*

M62.10 **Other rupture of muscle (nontraumatic)**, unspecified site

✓6ᵗʰ M62.11 **Other rupture of muscle (nontraumatic)**, shoulder

     M62.111 **Other rupture of muscle (nontraumatic)**, right shoulder

     M62.112 **Other rupture of muscle (nontraumatic)**, left shoulder

     M62.119 **Other rupture of muscle (nontraumatic)**, unspecified shoulder

✓6ᵗʰ M62.12 **Other rupture of muscle (nontraumatic)**, upper arm

     M62.121 **Other rupture of muscle (nontraumatic)**, right upper arm

     M62.122 **Other rupture of muscle (nontraumatic)**, left upper arm

     M62.129 **Other rupture of muscle (nontraumatic)**, unspecified upper arm

✓6ᵗʰ M62.13 **Other rupture of muscle (nontraumatic)**, forearm

     M62.131 **Other rupture of muscle (nontraumatic)**, right forearm

     M62.132 **Other rupture of muscle (nontraumatic)**, left forearm

     M62.139 **Other rupture of muscle (nontraumatic)**, unspecified forearm

✓6ᵗʰ M62.14 **Other rupture of muscle (nontraumatic)**, hand

     M62.141 **Other rupture of muscle (nontraumatic)**, right hand

     M62.142 **Other rupture of muscle (nontraumatic)**, left hand

     M62.149 **Other rupture of muscle (nontraumatic)**, unspecified hand

✓6ᵗʰ M62.15 **Other rupture of muscle (nontraumatic)**, thigh

     M62.151 **Other rupture of muscle (nontraumatic)**, right thigh

     M62.152 **Other rupture of muscle (nontraumatic)**, left thigh

     M62.159 **Other rupture of muscle (nontraumatic)**, unspecified thigh

✓6ᵗʰ M62.16 **Other rupture of muscle (nontraumatic)**, lower leg

     M62.161 **Other rupture of muscle (nontraumatic)**, right lower leg

     M62.162 **Other rupture of muscle (nontraumatic)**, left lower leg

     M62.169 **Other rupture of muscle (nontraumatic)**, unspecified lower leg

✓6ᵗʰ M62.17 **Other rupture of muscle (nontraumatic)**, ankle and foot

     M62.171 **Other rupture of muscle (nontraumatic)**, right ankle and foot

     M62.172 **Other rupture of muscle (nontraumatic)**, left ankle and foot

     M62.179 **Other rupture of muscle (nontraumatic)**, unspecified ankle and foot

M62.18 **Other rupture of muscle (nontraumatic)**, other site

✓5ᵗʰ **M62.2 Nontraumatic ischemic infarction of muscle**

    EXCLUDES 1   *compartment syndrome (traumatic) (T79.A-)*
                  nontraumatic compartment syndrome (M79.A-)
                  rhabdomyolysis (M62.82)
                  traumatic ischemia of muscle (T79.6)
                  Volkmann's ischemic contracture (T79.6)

M62.20 **Nontraumatic ischemic infarction of muscle**, unspecified site

✓6ᵗʰ M62.21 **Nontraumatic ischemic infarction of muscle**, shoulder

     M62.211 **Nontraumatic ischemic infarction of muscle**, right shoulder

     M62.212 **Nontraumatic ischemic infarction of muscle**, left shoulder

     M62.219 **Nontraumatic ischemic infarction of muscle**, unspecified shoulder

✓6ᵗʰ M62.22 **Nontraumatic ischemic infarction of muscle**, upper arm

     M62.221 **Nontraumatic ischemic infarction of muscle**, right upper arm

N Newborn: 0   P Pediatric: 0-17   M Maternity: 12-55   A Adult: 15-124   **MCC** Major CC Condition   **PDxMCC** PDx acts as own MCC   **CC** CC Condition   **PDxCC** PDx acts as own CC

752   ICD-10-CM 2016

M62.222   Nontraumatic ischemic infarction of muscle, **left upper arm**

M62.229   Nontraumatic ischemic infarction of muscle, **unspecified upper arm**

✓6ᵗʰ   **M62.23**   Nontraumatic ischemic infarction of muscle, **forearm**

M62.231   Nontraumatic ischemic infarction of muscle, **right forearm**

M62.232   Nontraumatic ischemic infarction of muscle, **left forearm**

M62.239   Nontraumatic ischemic infarction of muscle, **unspecified forearm**

✓6ᵗʰ   **M62.24**   Nontraumatic ischemic infarction of muscle, **hand**

M62.241   Nontraumatic ischemic infarction of muscle, **right hand**

M62.242   Nontraumatic ischemic infarction of muscle, **left hand**

M62.249   Nontraumatic ischemic infarction of muscle, **unspecified hand**

✓6ᵗʰ   **M62.25**   Nontraumatic ischemic infarction of muscle, **thigh**

M62.251   Nontraumatic ischemic infarction of muscle, **right thigh**

M62.252   Nontraumatic ischemic infarction of muscle, **left thigh**

M62.259   Nontraumatic ischemic infarction of muscle, **unspecified thigh**

✓6ᵗʰ   **M62.26**   Nontraumatic ischemic infarction of muscle, **lower leg**

M62.261   Nontraumatic ischemic infarction of muscle, **right lower leg**

M62.262   Nontraumatic ischemic infarction of muscle, **left lower leg**

M62.269   Nontraumatic ischemic infarction of muscle, **unspecified lower leg**

✓6ᵗʰ   **M62.27**   Nontraumatic ischemic infarction of muscle, **ankle and foot**

M62.271   Nontraumatic ischemic infarction of muscle, **right ankle and foot**

M62.272   Nontraumatic ischemic infarction of muscle, **left ankle and foot**

M62.279   Nontraumatic ischemic infarction of muscle, **unspecified ankle and foot**

M62.28   Nontraumatic ischemic infarction of muscle, **other site**

M62.3   Immobility syndrome (paraplegic)

✓5ᵗʰ   **M62.4**   Contracture of muscle

Contracture of tendon (sheath)

EXCLUDES 1   contracture of joint (M24.5-)

M62.40   Contracture of muscle, **unspecified site**

✓6ᵗʰ   **M62.41**   Contracture of muscle, **shoulder**

M62.411   Contracture of muscle, **right shoulder**

M62.412   Contracture of muscle, **left shoulder**

M62.419   Contracture of muscle, **unspecified shoulder**

✓6ᵗʰ   **M62.42**   Contracture of muscle, **upper arm**

M62.421   Contracture of muscle, **right upper arm**

M62.422   Contracture of muscle, **left upper arm**

M62.429   Contracture of muscle, **unspecified upper arm**

✓6ᵗʰ   **M62.43**   Contracture of muscle, **forearm**

M62.431   Contracture of muscle, **right forearm**

M62.432   Contracture of muscle, **left forearm**

M62.439   Contracture of muscle, **unspecified forearm**

✓6ᵗʰ   **M62.44**   Contracture of muscle, **hand**

M62.441   Contracture of muscle, **right hand**

M62.442   Contracture of muscle, **left hand**

M62.449   Contracture of muscle, **unspecified hand**

✓6ᵗʰ   **M62.45**   Contracture of muscle, **thigh**

M62.451   Contracture of muscle, **right thigh**

M62.452   Contracture of muscle, **left thigh**

M62.459   Contracture of muscle, **unspecified thigh**

✓6ᵗʰ   **M62.46**   Contracture of muscle, **lower leg**

M62.461   Contracture of muscle, **right lower leg**

M62.462   Contracture of muscle, **left lower leg**

M62.469   Contracture of muscle, **unspecified lower leg**

✓6ᵗʰ   **M62.47**   Contracture of muscle, **ankle and foot**

M62.471   Contracture of muscle, **right ankle and foot**

M62.472   Contracture of muscle, **left ankle and foot**

M62.479   Contracture of muscle, **unspecified ankle and foot**

M62.48   Contracture of muscle, **other site**

M62.49   Contracture of muscle, **multiple sites**

✓5ᵗʰ   **M62.5**   Muscle wasting and atrophy, not elsewhere classified

Disuse atrophy NEC

EXCLUDES 1   neuralgic amyotrophy (G54.5)
     progressive muscular atrophy (G12.29)

EXCLUDES 2   pelvic muscle wasting (N81.84)

M62.50   Muscle wasting and atrophy, not elsewhere classified, **unspecified site**

✓6ᵗʰ   **M62.51**   Muscle wasting and atrophy, not elsewhere classified, **shoulder**

M62.511   Muscle wasting and atrophy, not elsewhere classified, **right shoulder**

M62.512   Muscle wasting and atrophy, not elsewhere classified, **left shoulder**

M62.519   Muscle wasting and atrophy, not elsewhere classified, **unspecified shoulder**

✓6ᵗʰ   **M62.52**   Muscle wasting and atrophy, not elsewhere classified, **upper arm**

M62.521   Muscle wasting and atrophy, not elsewhere classified, **right upper arm**

M62.522   Muscle wasting and atrophy, not elsewhere classified, **left upper arm**

M62.529   Muscle wasting and atrophy, not elsewhere classified, **unspecified upper arm**

✓6ᵗʰ   **M62.53**   Muscle wasting and atrophy, not elsewhere classified, **forearm**

M62.531   Muscle wasting and atrophy, not elsewhere classified, **right forearm**

M62.532   Muscle wasting and atrophy, not elsewhere classified, **left forearm**

M62.539   Muscle wasting and atrophy, not elsewhere classified, **unspecified forearm**

✓6ᵗʰ   **M62.54**   Muscle wasting and atrophy, not elsewhere classified, **hand**

M62.541   Muscle wasting and atrophy, not elsewhere classified, **right hand**

M62.542   Muscle wasting and atrophy, not elsewhere classified, **left hand**

M62.549   Muscle wasting and atrophy, not elsewhere classified, **unspecified hand**

✓6ᵗʰ   **M62.55**   Muscle wasting and atrophy, not elsewhere classified, **thigh**

M62.551   Muscle wasting and atrophy, not elsewhere classified, **right thigh**

M62.552   Muscle wasting and atrophy, not elsewhere classified, **left thigh**

M62.559   Muscle wasting and atrophy, not elsewhere classified, **unspecified thigh**

✓6ᵗʰ   **M62.56**   Muscle wasting and atrophy, not elsewhere classified, **lower leg**

M62.561   Muscle wasting and atrophy, not elsewhere classified, **right lower leg**

M62.562   Muscle wasting and atrophy, not elsewhere classified, **left lower leg**

M62.569   Muscle wasting and atrophy, not elsewhere classified, **unspecified lower leg**

✓6ᵗʰ   **M62.57**   Muscle wasting and atrophy, not elsewhere classified, **ankle and foot**

M62.571   Muscle wasting and atrophy, not elsewhere classified, **right ankle and foot**

M62.572   Muscle wasting and atrophy, not elsewhere classified, **left ankle and foot**

M62.579   Muscle wasting and atrophy, not elsewhere classified, **unspecified ankle and foot**

M62.58   Muscle wasting and atrophy, not elsewhere classified, **other site**

✓ Additional Character Required   **✓×7ᵗʰ** Placeholder Alert   Unacceptable PDx   Manifestation   Hospital Acquired Condition   **EXCLUDES 1** Not Coded Here   **EXCLUDES 2** Not Included Here

M62.59   Muscle wasting and atrophy, not elsewhere classified, multiple sites

✓5ᵗʰ **M62.8**   Other specified disorders of muscle
> EXCLUDES 2   nontraumatic hematoma of muscle (M79.81)

M62.81   Muscle weakness (generalized)

M62.82   Rhabdomyolysis   CC
> EXCLUDES 1   traumatic rhabdomyolysis (T79.6)
> CC Excl: K68.12, M60.000–M60.19, M61.00–M61.19, M61.30–M61.59, M62.3, M62.50–M62.59, M62.82, M62.89, M72.6

✓6ᵗʰ **M62.83**   Muscle spasm

M62.830   Muscle spasm of back

M62.831   Muscle spasm of calf
> Charley-horse

M62.838   Other muscle spasm

M62.89   Other specified disorders of muscle
> Muscle (sheath) hernia

M62.9   Disorder of muscle, unspecified

✓4ᵗʰ **M63**   Disorders of muscle in diseases classified elsewhere
> Code first underlying disease, such as:
> leprosy (A30.-)
> neoplasm (C49-, C79.89, D21-, D48.1)
> schistosomiasis (B65.-)
> trichinellosis (B75)
> EXCLUDES 1   myopathy in cysticercosis (B69.81)
> myopathy in endocrine diseases (G73.7)
> myopathy in metabolic diseases (G73.7)
> myopathy in sarcoidosis (D86.87)
> myopathy in secondary syphilis (A51.49)
> myopathy in syphilis (late) (A52.78)
> myopathy in toxoplasmosis (B58.82)
> myopathy in tuberculosis (A18.09)

✓5ᵗʰ **M63.8**   Disorders of muscle in diseases classified elsewhere

M63.80   *Disorders of muscle in diseases classified elsewhere, unspecified site*

✓6ᵗʰ **M63.81**   Disorders of muscle in diseases classified elsewhere, shoulder

M63.811   *Disorders of muscle in diseases classified elsewhere, right shoulder*

M63.812   *Disorders of muscle in diseases classified elsewhere, left shoulder*

M63.819   *Disorders of muscle in diseases classified elsewhere, unspecified shoulder*

✓6ᵗʰ **M63.82**   Disorders of muscle in diseases classified elsewhere, upper arm

M63.821   *Disorders of muscle in diseases classified elsewhere, right upper arm*

M63.822   *Disorders of muscle in diseases classified elsewhere, left upper arm*

M63.829   *Disorders of muscle in diseases classified elsewhere, unspecified upper arm*

✓6ᵗʰ **M63.83**   Disorders of muscle in diseases classified elsewhere, forearm

M63.831   *Disorders of muscle in diseases classified elsewhere, right forearm*

M63.832   *Disorders of muscle in diseases classified elsewhere, left forearm*

M63.839   *Disorders of muscle in diseases classified elsewhere, unspecified forearm*

✓6ᵗʰ **M63.84**   Disorders of muscle in diseases classified elsewhere, hand

M63.841   *Disorders of muscle in diseases classified elsewhere, right hand*

M63.842   *Disorders of muscle in diseases classified elsewhere, left hand*

M63.849   *Disorders of muscle in diseases classified elsewhere, unspecified hand*

✓6ᵗʰ **M63.85**   Disorders of muscle in diseases classified elsewhere, thigh

M63.851   *Disorders of muscle in diseases classified elsewhere, right thigh*

M63.852   *Disorders of muscle in diseases classified elsewhere, left thigh*

M63.859   *Disorders of muscle in diseases classified elsewhere, unspecified thigh*

✓6ᵗʰ **M63.86**   Disorders of muscle in diseases classified elsewhere, lower leg

M63.861   *Disorders of muscle in diseases classified elsewhere, right lower leg*

M63.862   *Disorders of muscle in diseases classified elsewhere, left lower leg*

M63.869   *Disorders of muscle in diseases classified elsewhere, unspecified lower leg*

✓6ᵗʰ **M63.87**   Disorders of muscle in diseases classified elsewhere, ankle and foot

M63.871   *Disorders of muscle in diseases classified elsewhere, right ankle and foot*

M63.872   *Disorders of muscle in diseases classified elsewhere, left ankle and foot*

M63.879   *Disorders of muscle in diseases classified elsewhere, unspecified ankle and foot*

M63.88   *Disorders of muscle in diseases classified elsewhere, other site*

M63.89   *Disorders of muscle in diseases classified elsewhere, multiple sites*

Disorders of synovium and tendon (M65-M67)

✓4ᵗʰ **M65**   Synovitis and tenosynovitis
> EXCLUDES 1   chronic crepitant synovitis of hand and wrist (M70.0-)
> current injury—see injury of ligament or tendon by body region
> soft tissue disorders related to use, overuse and pressure (M70.-)

✓5ᵗʰ **M65.0**   Abscess of tendon sheath
> Use additional code (B95-B96) to identify bacterial agent.

M65.00   Abscess of tendon sheath, unspecified site

✓6ᵗʰ **M65.01**   Abscess of tendon sheath, shoulder

M65.011   Abscess of tendon sheath, right shoulder

M65.012   Abscess of tendon sheath, left shoulder

M65.019   Abscess of tendon sheath, unspecified shoulder

✓6ᵗʰ **M65.02**   Abscess of tendon sheath, upper arm

M65.021   Abscess of tendon sheath, right upper arm

M65.022   Abscess of tendon sheath, left upper arm

M65.029   Abscess of tendon sheath, unspecified upper arm

✓6ᵗʰ **M65.03**   Abscess of tendon sheath, forearm

M65.031   Abscess of tendon sheath, right forearm

M65.032   Abscess of tendon sheath, left forearm

M65.039   Abscess of tendon sheath, unspecified forearm

✓6ᵗʰ **M65.04**   Abscess of tendon sheath, hand

M65.041   Abscess of tendon sheath, right hand

M65.042   Abscess of tendon sheath, left hand

M65.049   Abscess of tendon sheath, unspecified hand

✓6ᵗʰ **M65.05**   Abscess of tendon sheath, thigh

M65.051   Abscess of tendon sheath, right thigh

M65.052   Abscess of tendon sheath, left thigh

M65.059   Abscess of tendon sheath, unspecified thigh

✓6ᵗʰ **M65.06**   Abscess of tendon sheath, lower leg

M65.061   Abscess of tendon sheath, right lower leg

M65.062   Abscess of tendon sheath, left lower leg

M65.069   Abscess of tendon sheath, unspecified lower leg

✓6ᵗʰ **M65.07**   Abscess of tendon sheath, ankle and foot

M65.071   Abscess of tendon sheath, right ankle and foot

M65.072   Abscess of tendon sheath, left ankle and foot

M65.079   Abscess of tendon sheath, unspecified ankle and foot

M65.08   Abscess of tendon sheath, other site

✓5ᵗʰ **M65.1**   Other infective (teno)synovitis

M65.10   Other infective (teno)synovitis, unspecified site

✓6ᵗʰ **M65.11**   Other infective (teno)synovitis, shoulder

M65.111   Other infective (teno)synovitis, right shoulder

M65.112   Other infective (teno)synovitis, left shoulder

N Newborn: 0   P Pediatric: 0-17   M Maternity: 12-55   A Adult: 15-124   MCC Major CC Condition   PDx MCC PDx acts as own MCC   CC CC Condition   PDx CC PDx acts as own CC

754   ICD-10-CM 2016

         M65.119   Other infective (teno)synovitis, unspecified **shoulder**

☑6ᵗʰ **M65.12**   Other infective (teno)synovitis, **elbow**
         M65.121   Other infective (teno)synovitis, **right elbow**
         M65.122   Other infective (teno)synovitis, **left elbow**
         M65.129   Other infective (teno)synovitis, unspecified **elbow**

☑6ᵗʰ **M65.13**   Other infective (teno)synovitis, **wrist**
         M65.131   Other infective (teno)synovitis, **right wrist**
         M65.132   Other infective (teno)synovitis, **left wrist**
         M65.139   Other infective (teno)synovitis, unspecified **wrist**

☑6ᵗʰ **M65.14**   Other infective (teno)synovitis, **hand**
         M65.141   Other infective (teno)synovitis, **right hand**
         M65.142   Other infective (teno)synovitis, **left hand**
         M65.149   Other infective (teno)synovitis, unspecified **hand**

☑6ᵗʰ **M65.15**   Other infective (teno)synovitis, **hip**
         M65.151   Other infective (teno)synovitis, **right hip**
         M65.152   Other infective (teno)synovitis, **left hip**
         M65.159   Other infective (teno)synovitis, unspecified **hip**

☑6ᵗʰ **M65.16**   Other infective (teno)synovitis, **knee**
         M65.161   Other infective (teno)synovitis, **right knee**
         M65.162   Other infective (teno)synovitis, **left knee**
         M65.169   Other infective (teno)synovitis, unspecified **knee**

☑6ᵗʰ **M65.17**   Other infective (teno)synovitis, **ankle and foot**
         M65.171   Other infective (teno)synovitis, **right ankle and foot**
         M65.172   Other infective (teno)synovitis, **left ankle and foot**
         M65.179   Other infective (teno)synovitis, unspecified **ankle and foot**

     M65.18   Other infective (teno)synovitis, **other site**
     M65.19   Other infective (teno)synovitis, **multiple sites**

☑5ᵗʰ **M65.2**   **Calcific tendinitis**
     EXCLUDES 1   tendinitis as classified in M75-M77
                  calcified tendinitis of shoulder (M75.3)

     M65.20   Calcific tendinitis, **unspecified site**

☑6ᵗʰ **M65.22**   Calcific tendinitis, **upper arm**
         M65.221   Calcific tendinitis, **right upper arm**
         M65.222   Calcific tendinitis, **left upper arm**
         M65.229   Calcific tendinitis, **unspecified upper arm**

☑6ᵗʰ **M65.23**   Calcific tendinitis, **forearm**
         M65.231   Calcific tendinitis, **right forearm**
         M65.232   Calcific tendinitis, **left forearm**
         M65.239   Calcific tendinitis, **unspecified forearm**

☑6ᵗʰ **M65.24**   Calcific tendinitis, **hand**
         M65.241   Calcific tendinitis, **right hand**
         M65.242   Calcific tendinitis, **left hand**
         M65.249   Calcific tendinitis, **unspecified hand**

☑6ᵗʰ **M65.25**   Calcific tendinitis, **thigh**
         M65.251   Calcific tendinitis, **right thigh**
         M65.252   Calcific tendinitis, **left thigh**
         M65.259   Calcific tendinitis, **unspecified thigh**

☑6ᵗʰ **M65.26**   Calcific tendinitis, **lower leg**
         M65.261   Calcific tendinitis, **right lower leg**
         M65.262   Calcific tendinitis, **left lower leg**
         M65.269   Calcific tendinitis, **unspecified lower leg**

☑6ᵗʰ **M65.27**   Calcific tendinitis, **ankle and foot**
         M65.271   Calcific tendinitis, **right ankle and foot**
         M65.272   Calcific tendinitis, **left ankle and foot**
         M65.279   Calcific tendinitis, **unspecified ankle and foot**

     M65.28   Calcific tendinitis, **other site**
     M65.29   Calcific tendinitis, **multiple sites**

     M65.3   **Trigger finger**
         Nodular tendinous disease
     M65.30   Trigger finger, **unspecified finger**

☑6ᵗʰ **M65.31**   Trigger **thumb**
         M65.311   Trigger thumb, **right thumb**
         M65.312   Trigger thumb, **left thumb**
         M65.319   Trigger thumb, unspecified **thumb**

☑6ᵗʰ **M65.32**   Trigger finger, **index finger**
         M65.321   Trigger finger, **right index finger**
         M65.322   Trigger finger, **left index finger**
         M65.329   Trigger finger, **unspecified index finger**

☑6ᵗʰ **M65.33**   Trigger finger, **middle finger**
         M65.331   Trigger finger, **right middle finger**
         M65.332   Trigger finger, **left middle finger**
         M65.339   Trigger finger, **unspecified middle finger**

☑6ᵗʰ **M65.34**   Trigger finger, **ring finger**
         M65.341   Trigger finger, **right ring finger**
         M65.342   Trigger finger, **left ring finger**
         M65.349   Trigger finger, **unspecified ring finger**

☑6ᵗʰ **M65.35**   Trigger finger, **little finger**
         M65.351   Trigger finger, **right little finger**
         M65.352   Trigger finger, **left little finger**
         M65.359   Trigger finger, **unspecified little finger**

     M65.4   **Radial styloid tenosynovitis [de Quervain]**

☑5ᵗʰ **M65.8**   **Other synovitis and tenosynovitis**
     M65.80   Other synovitis and tenosynovitis, **unspecified site**

☑6ᵗʰ **M65.81**   Other synovitis and tenosynovitis, **shoulder**
         M65.811   Other synovitis and tenosynovitis, **right shoulder**
         M65.812   Other synovitis and tenosynovitis, **left shoulder**
         M65.819   Other synovitis and tenosynovitis, unspecified **shoulder**

☑6ᵗʰ **M65.82**   Other synovitis and tenosynovitis, **upper arm**
         M65.821   Other synovitis and tenosynovitis, **right upper arm**
         M65.822   Other synovitis and tenosynovitis, **left upper arm**
         M65.829   Other synovitis and tenosynovitis, unspecified **upper arm**

☑6ᵗʰ **M65.83**   Other synovitis and tenosynovitis, **forearm**
         M65.831   Other synovitis and tenosynovitis, **right forearm**
         M65.832   Other synovitis and tenosynovitis, **left forearm**
         M65.839   Other synovitis and tenosynovitis, unspecified **forearm**

☑6ᵗʰ **M65.84**   Other synovitis and tenosynovitis, **hand**
         M65.841   Other synovitis and tenosynovitis, **right hand**
         M65.842   Other synovitis and tenosynovitis, **left hand**
         M65.849   Other synovitis and tenosynovitis, unspecified **hand**

☑6ᵗʰ **M65.85**   Other synovitis and tenosynovitis, **thigh**
         M65.851   Other synovitis and tenosynovitis, **right thigh**
         M65.852   Other synovitis and tenosynovitis, **left thigh**
         M65.859   Other synovitis and tenosynovitis, unspecified **thigh**

☑6ᵗʰ **M65.86**   Other synovitis and tenosynovitis, **lower leg**
         M65.861   Other synovitis and tenosynovitis, **right lower leg**
         M65.862   Other synovitis and tenosynovitis, **left lower leg**
         M65.869   Other synovitis and tenosynovitis, unspecified **lower leg**

☑6ᵗʰ **M65.87**   Other synovitis and tenosynovitis, **ankle and foot**
         M65.871   Other synovitis and tenosynovitis, **right ankle and foot**
         M65.872   Other synovitis and tenosynovitis, **left ankle and foot**
         M65.879   Other synovitis and tenosynovitis, unspecified **ankle and foot**

     M65.88   Other synovitis and tenosynovitis, **other site**
     M65.89   Other synovitis and tenosynovitis, **multiple sites**

     M65.9   **Synovitis and tenosynovitis, unspecified**

☑ Additional Character Required   ☑x7ᵗʰ Placeholder Alert   Unacceptable PDx   Manifestation   Hospital Acquired Condition   **EXCLUDES 1** Not Coded Here   **EXCLUDES 2** Not Included Here

√4ᵗʰ **M66 Spontaneous rupture of synovium and tendon**
> INCLUDES   rupture that occurs when a normal force is applied to tissues that are inferred to have less than normal strength
> EXCLUDES 2   rotator cuff syndrome (M75.1-)
> rupture where an abnormal force is applied to normal tissue—see injury of tendon by body region

M66.0 Rupture of popliteal cyst

√5ᵗʰ **M66.1 Rupture of synovium**
> Rupture of synovial cyst
> EXCLUDES 2   rupture of popliteal cyst (M66.0)

   M66.10 Rupture of synovium, unspecified joint

√6ᵗʰ **M66.11 Rupture of synovium, shoulder**
   M66.111 Rupture of synovium, right shoulder
   M66.112 Rupture of synovium, left shoulder
   M66.119 Rupture of synovium, unspecified shoulder

√6ᵗʰ **M66.12 Rupture of synovium, elbow**
   M66.121 Rupture of synovium, right elbow
   M66.122 Rupture of synovium, left elbow
   M66.129 Rupture of synovium, unspecified elbow

√6ᵗʰ **M66.13 Rupture of synovium, wrist**
   M66.131 Rupture of synovium, right wrist
   M66.132 Rupture of synovium, left wrist
   M66.139 Rupture of synovium, unspecified wrist

√6ᵗʰ **M66.14 Rupture of synovium, hand and fingers**
   M66.141 Rupture of synovium, right hand
   M66.142 Rupture of synovium, left hand
   M66.143 Rupture of synovium, unspecified hand
   M66.144 Rupture of synovium, right finger(s)
   M66.145 Rupture of synovium, left finger(s)
   M66.146 Rupture of synovium, unspecified finger(s)

√6ᵗʰ **M66.15 Rupture of synovium, hip**
   M66.151 Rupture of synovium, right hip
   M66.152 Rupture of synovium, left hip
   M66.159 Rupture of synovium, unspecified hip

√6ᵗʰ **M66.17 Rupture of synovium, ankle, foot and toes**
   M66.171 Rupture of synovium, right ankle
   M66.172 Rupture of synovium, left ankle
   M66.173 Rupture of synovium, unspecified ankle
   M66.174 Rupture of synovium, right foot
   M66.175 Rupture of synovium, left foot
   M66.176 Rupture of synovium, unspecified foot
   M66.177 Rupture of synovium, right toe(s)
   M66.178 Rupture of synovium, left toe(s)
   M66.179 Rupture of synovium, unspecified toe(s)

   M66.18 Rupture of synovium, other site

✦ √5ᵗʰ **M66.2 Spontaneous rupture of extensor tendons**

   M66.20 Spontaneous rupture of extensor tendons, unspecified site

√6ᵗʰ **M66.21 Spontaneous rupture of extensor tendons, shoulder**
   M66.211 Spontaneous rupture of extensor tendons, right shoulder
   M66.212 Spontaneous rupture of extensor tendons, left shoulder
   M66.219 Spontaneous rupture of extensor tendons, unspecified shoulder

√6ᵗʰ **M66.22 Spontaneous rupture of extensor tendons, upper arm**
   M66.221 Spontaneous rupture of extensor tendons, right upper arm
   M66.222 Spontaneous rupture of extensor tendons, left upper arm
   M66.229 Spontaneous rupture of extensor tendons, unspecified upper arm

√6ᵗʰ **M66.23 Spontaneous rupture of extensor tendons, forearm**
   M66.231 Spontaneous rupture of extensor tendons, right forearm
   M66.232 Spontaneous rupture of extensor tendons, left forearm
   M66.239 Spontaneous rupture of extensor tendons, unspecified forearm

√6ᵗʰ **M66.24 Spontaneous rupture of extensor tendons, hand**
   M66.241 Spontaneous rupture of extensor tendons, right hand
   M66.242 Spontaneous rupture of extensor tendons, left hand
   M66.249 Spontaneous rupture of extensor tendons, unspecified hand

√6ᵗʰ **M66.25 Spontaneous rupture of extensor tendons, thigh**
   M66.251 Spontaneous rupture of extensor tendons, right thigh
   M66.252 Spontaneous rupture of extensor tendons, left thigh
   M66.259 Spontaneous rupture of extensor tendons, unspecified thigh

√6ᵗʰ **M66.26 Spontaneous rupture of extensor tendons, lower leg**
   M66.261 Spontaneous rupture of extensor tendons, right lower leg
   M66.262 Spontaneous rupture of extensor tendons, left lower leg
   M66.269 Spontaneous rupture of extensor tendons, unspecified lower leg

√6ᵗʰ **M66.27 Spontaneous rupture of extensor tendons, ankle and foot**
   M66.271 Spontaneous rupture of extensor tendons, right ankle and foot
   M66.272 Spontaneous rupture of extensor tendons, left ankle and foot
   M66.279 Spontaneous rupture of extensor tendons, unspecified ankle and foot

   M66.28 Spontaneous rupture of extensor tendons, other site

   M66.29 Spontaneous rupture of extensor tendons, multiple sites

✦ √5ᵗʰ **M66.3 Spontaneous rupture of flexor tendons**

   M66.30 Spontaneous rupture of flexor tendons, unspecified site

√6ᵗʰ **M66.31 Spontaneous rupture of flexor tendons, shoulder**
   M66.311 Spontaneous rupture of flexor tendons, right shoulder
   M66.312 Spontaneous rupture of flexor tendons, left shoulder
   M66.319 Spontaneous rupture of flexor tendons, unspecified shoulder

√6ᵗʰ **M66.32 Spontaneous rupture of flexor tendons, upper arm**
   M66.321 Spontaneous rupture of flexor tendons, right upper arm
   M66.322 Spontaneous rupture of flexor tendons, left upper arm
   M66.329 Spontaneous rupture of flexor tendons, unspecified upper arm

√6ᵗʰ **M66.33 Spontaneous rupture of flexor tendons, forearm**
   M66.331 Spontaneous rupture of flexor tendons, right forearm
   M66.332 Spontaneous rupture of flexor tendons, left forearm
   M66.339 Spontaneous rupture of flexor tendons, unspecified forearm

√6ᵗʰ **M66.34 Spontaneous rupture of flexor tendons, hand**
   M66.341 Spontaneous rupture of flexor tendons, right hand
   M66.342 Spontaneous rupture of flexor tendons, left hand
   M66.349 Spontaneous rupture of flexor tendons, unspecified hand

√6ᵗʰ **M66.35 Spontaneous rupture of flexor tendons, thigh**
   M66.351 Spontaneous rupture of flexor tendons, right thigh
   M66.352 Spontaneous rupture of flexor tendons, left thigh
   M66.359 Spontaneous rupture of flexor tendons, unspecified thigh

√6ᵗʰ **M66.36 Spontaneous rupture of flexor tendons, lower leg**
   M66.361 Spontaneous rupture of flexor tendons, right lower leg

---

✦ Refer to the Muscle/Tendon Table at beginning of this chapter.

N Newborn: 0   P Pediatric: 0-17   M Maternity: 12-55   A Adult: 15-124   MCC Major CC Condition   PDxMCC PDx acts as own MCC   CC CC Condition   PDxCC PDx acts as own CC

756   ICD-10-CM 2016

M66.362 Spontaneous rupture of flexor tendons, left lower leg

M66.369 Spontaneous rupture of flexor tendons, unspecified lower leg

✓6ᵗʰ **M66.37** Spontaneous rupture of flexor tendons, ankle and foot

    M66.371 Spontaneous rupture of flexor tendons, right ankle and foot

    M66.372 Spontaneous rupture of flexor tendons, left ankle and foot

    M66.379 Spontaneous rupture of flexor tendons, unspecified ankle and foot

M66.38 Spontaneous rupture of flexor tendons, other site

M66.39 Spontaneous rupture of flexor tendons, multiple sites

✦ ✓5ᵗʰ **M66.8** Spontaneous rupture of other tendons

M66.80 Spontaneous rupture of other tendons, unspecified site

✓6ᵗʰ **M66.81** Spontaneous rupture of other tendons, shoulder

    M66.811 Spontaneous rupture of other tendons, right shoulder

    M66.812 Spontaneous rupture of other tendons, left shoulder

    M66.819 Spontaneous rupture of other tendons, unspecified shoulder

✓6ᵗʰ **M66.82** Spontaneous rupture of other tendons, upper arm

    M66.821 Spontaneous rupture of other tendons, right upper arm

    M66.822 Spontaneous rupture of other tendons, left upper arm

    M66.829 Spontaneous rupture of other tendons, unspecified upper arm

✓6ᵗʰ **M66.83** Spontaneous rupture of other tendons, forearm

    M66.831 Spontaneous rupture of other tendons, right forearm

    M66.832 Spontaneous rupture of other tendons, left forearm

    M66.839 Spontaneous rupture of other tendons, unspecified forearm

✓6ᵗʰ **M66.84** Spontaneous rupture of other tendons, hand

    M66.841 Spontaneous rupture of other tendons, right hand

    M66.842 Spontaneous rupture of other tendons, left hand

    M66.849 Spontaneous rupture of other tendons, unspecified hand

✓6ᵗʰ **M66.85** Spontaneous rupture of other tendons, thigh

    M66.851 Spontaneous rupture of other tendons, right thigh

    M66.852 Spontaneous rupture of other tendons, left thigh

    M66.859 Spontaneous rupture of other tendons, unspecified thigh

✓6ᵗʰ **M66.86** Spontaneous rupture of other tendons, lower leg

    M66.861 Spontaneous rupture of other tendons, right lower leg

    M66.862 Spontaneous rupture of other tendons, left lower leg

    M66.869 Spontaneous rupture of other tendons, unspecified lower leg

✓6ᵗʰ **M66.87** Spontaneous rupture of other tendons, ankle and foot

    M66.871 Spontaneous rupture of other tendons, right ankle and foot

    M66.872 Spontaneous rupture of other tendons, left ankle and foot

    M66.879 Spontaneous rupture of other tendons, unspecified ankle and foot

M66.88 Spontaneous rupture of other tendons, other

M66.89 Spontaneous rupture of other tendons, multiple sites

M66.9 Spontaneous rupture of unspecified tendon
Rupture at musculotendinous junction, nontraumatic

✓4ᵗʰ **M67** Other disorders of synovium and tendon
EXCLUDES 1 palmar fascial fibromatosis [Dupuytren] (M72.0)
tendinitis NOS (M77.9-)
xanthomatosis localized to tendons (E78.2)

✓5ᵗʰ **M67.0** Short Achilles tendon (acquired)

M67.00 Short Achilles tendon (acquired), unspecified ankle

M67.01 Short Achilles tendon (acquired), right ankle

M67.02 Short Achilles tendon (acquired), left ankle

✓5ᵗʰ **M67.2** Synovial hypertrophy, not elsewhere classified
EXCLUDES 1 villonodular synovitis (pigmented) (M12.2-)

M67.20 Synovial hypertrophy, not elsewhere classified, unspecified site

✓6ᵗʰ **M67.21** Synovial hypertrophy, not elsewhere classified, shoulder

    M67.211 Synovial hypertrophy, not elsewhere classified, right shoulder

    M67.212 Synovial hypertrophy, not elsewhere classified, left shoulder

    M67.219 Synovial hypertrophy, not elsewhere classified, unspecified shoulder

✓6ᵗʰ **M67.22** Synovial hypertrophy, not elsewhere classified, upper arm

    M67.221 Synovial hypertrophy, not elsewhere classified, right upper arm

    M67.222 Synovial hypertrophy, not elsewhere classified, left upper arm

    M67.229 Synovial hypertrophy, not elsewhere classified, unspecified upper arm

✓6ᵗʰ **M67.23** Synovial hypertrophy, not elsewhere classified, forearm

    M67.231 Synovial hypertrophy, not elsewhere classified, right forearm

    M67.232 Synovial hypertrophy, not elsewhere classified, left forearm

    M67.239 Synovial hypertrophy, not elsewhere classified, unspecified forearm

✓6ᵗʰ **M67.24** Synovial hypertrophy, not elsewhere classified, hand

    M67.241 Synovial hypertrophy, not elsewhere classified, right hand

    M67.242 Synovial hypertrophy, not elsewhere classified, left hand

    M67.249 Synovial hypertrophy, not elsewhere classified, unspecified hand

✓6ᵗʰ **M67.25** Synovial hypertrophy, not elsewhere classified, thigh

    M67.251 Synovial hypertrophy, not elsewhere classified, right thigh

    M67.252 Synovial hypertrophy, not elsewhere classified, left thigh

    M67.259 Synovial hypertrophy, not elsewhere classified, unspecified thigh

✓6ᵗʰ **M67.26** Synovial hypertrophy, not elsewhere classified, lower leg

    M67.261 Synovial hypertrophy, not elsewhere classified, right lower leg

    M67.262 Synovial hypertrophy, not elsewhere classified, left lower leg

    M67.269 Synovial hypertrophy, not elsewhere classified, unspecified lower leg

✓6ᵗʰ **M67.27** Synovial hypertrophy, not elsewhere classified, ankle and foot

    M67.271 Synovial hypertrophy, not elsewhere classified, right ankle and foot

    M67.272 Synovial hypertrophy, not elsewhere classified, left ankle and foot

    M67.279 Synovial hypertrophy, not elsewhere classified, unspecified ankle and foot

M67.28 Synovial hypertrophy, not elsewhere classified, other site

M67.29 Synovial hypertrophy, not elsewhere classified, multiple sites

✓5ᵗʰ **M67.3** Transient synovitis
Toxic synovitis
EXCLUDES 1 palindromic rheumatism (M12.3-)

M67.30 Transient synovitis, unspecified site

✦ Refer to the Muscle/Tendon Table at beginning of this chapter.

✓ Additional Character Required   ✓x7ᵗʰ Placeholder Alert   Unacceptable PDx   Manifestation   Hospital Acquired Condition   *EXCLUDES 1* Not Coded Here   *EXCLUDES 2* Not Included Here

✓6th **M67.31 Transient synovitis, shoulder**
     M67.311 Transient synovitis, right shoulder
     M67.312 Transient synovitis, left shoulder
     M67.319 Transient synovitis, unspecified shoulder

✓6th **M67.32 Transient synovitis, elbow**
     M67.321 Transient synovitis, right elbow
     M67.322 Transient synovitis, left elbow
     M67.329 Transient synovitis, unspecified elbow

✓6th **M67.33 Transient synovitis, wrist**
     M67.331 Transient synovitis, right wrist
     M67.332 Transient synovitis, left wrist
     M67.339 Transient synovitis, unspecified wrist

✓6th **M67.34 Transient synovitis, hand**
     M67.341 Transient synovitis, right hand
     M67.342 Transient synovitis, left hand
     M67.349 Transient synovitis, unspecified hand

✓6th **M67.35 Transient synovitis, hip**
     M67.351 Transient synovitis, right hip
     M67.352 Transient synovitis, left hip
     M67.359 Transient synovitis, unspecified hip

✓6th **M67.36 Transient synovitis, knee**
     M67.361 Transient synovitis, right knee
     M67.362 Transient synovitis, left knee
     M67.369 Transient synovitis, unspecified knee

✓6th **M67.37 Transient synovitis, ankle and foot**
     M67.371 Transient synovitis, right ankle and foot
     M67.372 Transient synovitis, left ankle and foot
     M67.379 Transient synovitis, unspecified ankle and foot

     M67.38 Transient synovitis, other site
     M67.39 Transient synovitis, multiple sites

✓5th **M67.4 Ganglion**
     Ganglion of joint or tendon (sheath)
     EXCLUDES 1 ganglion in yaws (A66.6)
     EXCLUDES 2 cyst of bursa (M71.2-M71.3)
         cyst of synovium (M71.2-M71.3)

     M67.40 Ganglion, unspecified site

✓6th **M67.41 Ganglion, shoulder**
     M67.411 Ganglion, right shoulder
     M67.412 Ganglion, left shoulder
     M67.419 Ganglion, unspecified shoulder

✓6th **M67.42 Ganglion, elbow**
     M67.421 Ganglion, right elbow
     M67.422 Ganglion, left elbow
     M67.429 Ganglion, unspecified elbow

✓6th **M67.43 Ganglion, wrist**
     M67.431 Ganglion, right wrist
     M67.432 Ganglion, left wrist
     M67.439 Ganglion, unspecified wrist

✓6th **M67.44 Ganglion, hand**
     M67.441 Ganglion, right hand
     M67.442 Ganglion, left hand
     M67.449 Ganglion, unspecified hand

✓6th **M67.45 Ganglion, hip**
     M67.451 Ganglion, right hip
     M67.452 Ganglion, left hip
     M67.459 Ganglion, unspecified hip

✓6th **M67.46 Ganglion, knee**
     M67.461 Ganglion, right knee
     M67.462 Ganglion, left knee
     M67.469 Ganglion, unspecified knee

✓6th **M67.47 Ganglion, ankle and foot**
     M67.471 Ganglion, right ankle and foot
     M67.472 Ganglion, left ankle and foot
     M67.479 Ganglion, unspecified ankle and foot

     M67.48 Ganglion, other site
     M67.49 Ganglion, multiple sites

✓5th **M67.5 Plica syndrome**
     Plica knee

     M67.50 Plica syndrome, unspecified knee
     M67.51 Plica syndrome, right knee

     M67.52 Plica syndrome, left knee

✓5th **M67.8 Other specified disorders of synovium and tendon**
     M67.80 Other specified disorders of synovium and tendon, unspecified site

✓6th **M67.81 Other specified disorders of synovium and tendon, shoulder**
     M67.811 Other specified disorders of synovium, right shoulder
     M67.812 Other specified disorders of synovium, left shoulder
     M67.813 Other specified disorders of tendon, right shoulder
     M67.814 Other specified disorders of tendon, left shoulder
     M67.819 Other specified disorders of synovium and tendon, unspecified shoulder

✓6th **M67.82 Other specified disorders of synovium and tendon, elbow**
     M67.821 Other specified disorders of synovium, right elbow
     M67.822 Other specified disorders of synovium, left elbow
     M67.823 Other specified disorders of tendon, right elbow
     M67.824 Other specified disorders of tendon, left elbow
     M67.829 Other specified disorders of synovium and tendon, unspecified elbow

✓6th **M67.83 Other specified disorders of synovium and tendon, wrist**
     M67.831 Other specified disorders of synovium, right wrist
     M67.832 Other specified disorders of synovium, left wrist
     M67.833 Other specified disorders of tendon, right wrist
     M67.834 Other specified disorders of tendon, left wrist
     M67.839 Other specified disorders of synovium and tendon, unspecified forearm

✓6th **M67.84 Other specified disorders of synovium and tendon, hand**
     M67.841 Other specified disorders of synovium, right hand
     M67.842 Other specified disorders of synovium, left hand
     M67.843 Other specified disorders of tendon, right hand
     M67.844 Other specified disorders of tendon, left hand
     M67.849 Other specified disorders of synovium and tendon, unspecified hand

✓6th **M67.85 Other specified disorders of synovium and tendon, hip**
     M67.851 Other specified disorders of synovium, right hip
     M67.852 Other specified disorders of synovium, left hip
     M67.853 Other specified disorders of tendon, right hip
     M67.854 Other specified disorders of tendon, left hip
     M67.859 Other specified disorders of synovium and tendon, unspecified hip

✓6th **M67.86 Other specified disorders of synovium and tendon, knee**
     M67.861 Other specified disorders of synovium, right knee
     M67.862 Other specified disorders of synovium, left knee
     M67.863 Other specified disorders of tendon, right knee
     M67.864 Other specified disorders of tendon, left knee
     M67.869 Other specified disorders of synovium and tendon, unspecified knee

N Newborn: 0   P Pediatric: 0-17   M Maternity: 12-55   A Adult: 15-124   MCC Major CC Condition   PDx MCC PDx acts as own MCC   CC CC Condition   PDx CC PDx acts as own CC

758   ICD-10-CM 2016

√6th **M67.87** **Other specified disorders of synovium and tendon, ankle and foot**
     M67.871 Other specified disorders of synovium, right ankle and foot
     M67.872 Other specified disorders of synovium, left ankle and foot
     M67.873 Other specified disorders of tendon, right ankle and foot
     M67.874 Other specified disorders of tendon, left ankle and foot
     M67.879 Other specified disorders of synovium and tendon, unspecified ankle and foot
   M67.88 Other specified disorders of synovium and tendon, other site
   M67.89 Other specified disorders of synovium and tendon, multiple sites

√5th **M67.9** **Unspecified disorder of synovium and tendon**
   M67.90 Unspecified disorder of synovium and tendon, unspecified site
   √6th **M67.91** **Unspecified disorder of synovium and tendon, shoulder**
     M67.911 Unspecified disorder of synovium and tendon, right shoulder
     M67.912 Unspecified disorder of synovium and tendon, left shoulder
     M67.919 Unspecified disorder of synovium and tendon, unspecified shoulder
   √6th **M67.92** **Unspecified disorder of synovium and tendon, upper arm**
     M67.921 Unspecified disorder of synovium and tendon, right upper arm
     M67.922 Unspecified disorder of synovium and tendon, left upper arm
     M67.929 Unspecified disorder of synovium and tendon, unspecified upper arm
   √6th **M67.93** **Unspecified disorder of synovium and tendon, forearm**
     M67.931 Unspecified disorder of synovium and tendon, right forearm
     M67.932 Unspecified disorder of synovium and tendon, left forearm
     M67.939 Unspecified disorder of synovium and tendon, unspecified forearm
   √6th **M67.94** **Unspecified disorder of synovium and tendon, hand**
     M67.941 Unspecified disorder of synovium and tendon, right hand
     M67.942 Unspecified disorder of synovium and tendon, left hand
     M67.949 Unspecified disorder of synovium and tendon, unspecified hand
   √6th **M67.95** **Unspecified disorder of synovium and tendon, thigh**
     M67.951 Unspecified disorder of synovium and tendon, right thigh
     M67.952 Unspecified disorder of synovium and tendon, left thigh
     M67.959 Unspecified disorder of synovium and tendon, unspecified thigh
   √6th **M67.96** **Unspecified disorder of synovium and tendon, lower leg**
     M67.961 Unspecified disorder of synovium and tendon, right lower leg
     M67.962 Unspecified disorder of synovium and tendon, left lower leg
     M67.969 Unspecified disorder of synovium and tendon, unspecified lower leg
   √6th **M67.97** **Unspecified disorder of synovium and tendon, ankle and foot**
     M67.971 Unspecified disorder of synovium and tendon, right ankle and foot
     M67.972 Unspecified disorder of synovium and tendon, left ankle and foot
     M67.979 Unspecified disorder of synovium and tendon, unspecified ankle and foot
   M67.98 Unspecified disorder of synovium and tendon, other site
   M67.99 Unspecified disorder of synovium and tendon, multiple sites

Other soft tissue disorders (M70-M79)

√4th **M70** **Soft tissue disorders related to use, overuse and pressure**
   INCLUDES   soft tissue disorders of occupational origin
   Use additional external cause code to identify activity causing disorder (Y93.-)
   EXCLUDES 1   bursitis NOS (M71.9-)
   EXCLUDES 2   bursitis of shoulder (M75.5)
     enthesopathies (M76-M77)
     pressure ulcer (pressure area) (L89.-)

√5th **M70.0** **Crepitant synovitis (acute) (chronic) of hand and wrist**
   √6th **M70.03** **Crepitant synovitis (acute) (chronic), wrist**
     M70.031 Crepitant synovitis (acute) (chronic), right wrist
     M70.032 Crepitant synovitis (acute) (chronic), left wrist
     M70.039 Crepitant synovitis (acute) (chronic), unspecified wrist
   √6th **M70.04** **Crepitant synovitis (acute) (chronic), hand**
     M70.041 Crepitant synovitis (acute) (chronic), right hand
     M70.042 Crepitant synovitis (acute) (chronic), left hand
     M70.049 Crepitant synovitis (acute) (chronic), unspecified hand

√5th **M70.1** **Bursitis of hand**
   M70.10 Bursitis, unspecified hand
   M70.11 Bursitis, right hand
   M70.12 Bursitis, left hand

√5th **M70.2** **Olecranon bursitis**
   M70.20 Olecranon bursitis, unspecified elbow
   M70.21 Olecranon bursitis, right elbow
   M70.22 Olecranon bursitis, left elbow

√5th **M70.3** **Other bursitis of elbow**
   M70.30 Other bursitis of elbow, unspecified elbow
   M70.31 Other bursitis of elbow, right elbow
   M70.32 Other bursitis of elbow, left elbow

√5th **M70.4** **Prepatellar bursitis**
   M70.40 Prepatellar bursitis, unspecified knee
   M70.41 Prepatellar bursitis, right knee
   M70.42 Prepatellar bursitis, left knee

√5th **M70.5** **Other bursitis of knee**
   M70.50 Other bursitis of knee, unspecified knee
   M70.51 Other bursitis of knee, right knee
   M70.52 Other bursitis of knee, left knee

√5th **M70.6** **Trochanteric bursitis**
   Trochanteric tendinitis
   M70.60 Trochanteric bursitis, unspecified hip
   M70.61 Trochanteric bursitis, right hip
   M70.62 Trochanteric bursitis, left hip

√5th **M70.7** **Other bursitis of hip**
   Ischial bursitis
   M70.70 Other bursitis of hip, unspecified hip
   M70.71 Other bursitis of hip, right hip
   M70.72 Other bursitis of hip, left hip

√5th **M70.8** **Other soft tissue disorders related to use, overuse and pressure**
   M70.80 Other soft tissue disorders related to use, overuse and pressure of unspecified site
   √6th **M70.81** **Other soft tissue disorders related to use, overuse and pressure of shoulder**
     M70.811 Other soft tissue disorders related to use, overuse and pressure, right shoulder
     M70.812 Other soft tissue disorders related to use, overuse and pressure, left shoulder
     M70.819 Other soft tissue disorders related to use, overuse and pressure, unspecified shoulder
   √6th **M70.82** **Other soft tissue disorders related to use, overuse and pressure of upper arm**
     M70.821 Other soft tissue disorders related to use, overuse and pressure, right upper arm
     M70.822 Other soft tissue disorders related to use, overuse and pressure, left upper arm

M70.829 Other soft tissue disorders related to use, overuse and pressure, unspecified upper arms

✓6ᵗʰ **M70.83** Other soft tissue disorders related to use, overuse and pressure of forearm

    M70.831 Other soft tissue disorders related to use, overuse and pressure, right forearm

    M70.832 Other soft tissue disorders related to use, overuse and pressure, left forearm

    M70.839 Other soft tissue disorders related to use, overuse and pressure, unspecified forearm

✓6ᵗʰ **M70.84** Other soft tissue disorders related to use, overuse and pressure of hand

    M70.841 Other soft tissue disorders related to use, overuse and pressure, right hand

    M70.842 Other soft tissue disorders related to use, overuse and pressure, left hand

    M70.849 Other soft tissue disorders related to use, overuse and pressure, unspecified hand

✓6ᵗʰ **M70.85** Other soft tissue disorders related to use, overuse and pressure of thigh

    M70.851 Other soft tissue disorders related to use, overuse and pressure, right thigh

    M70.852 Other soft tissue disorders related to use, overuse and pressure, left thigh

    M70.859 Other soft tissue disorders related to use, overuse and pressure, unspecified thigh

✓6ᵗʰ **M70.86** Other soft tissue disorders related to use, overuse and pressure lower leg

    M70.861 Other soft tissue disorders related to use, overuse and pressure, right lower leg

    M70.862 Other soft tissue disorders related to use, overuse and pressure, left lower leg

    M70.869 Other soft tissue disorders related to use, overuse and pressure, unspecified leg

✓6ᵗʰ **M70.87** Other soft tissue disorders related to use, overuse and pressure of ankle and foot

    M70.871 Other soft tissue disorders related to use, overuse and pressure, right ankle and foot

    M70.872 Other soft tissue disorders related to use, overuse and pressure, left ankle and foot

    M70.879 Other soft tissue disorders related to use, overuse and pressure, unspecified ankle and foot

M70.88 Other soft tissue disorders related to use, overuse and pressure other site

M70.89 Other soft tissue disorders related to use, overuse and pressure multiple sites

✓5ᵗʰ **M70.9** Unspecified soft tissue disorder related to use, overuse and pressure

M70.90 Unspecified soft tissue disorder related to use, overuse and pressure of unspecified site

✓6ᵗʰ **M70.91** Unspecified soft tissue disorder related to use, overuse and pressure of shoulder

    M70.911 Unspecified soft tissue disorder related to use, overuse and pressure, right shoulder

    M70.912 Unspecified soft tissue disorder related to use, overuse and pressure, left shoulder

    M70.919 Unspecified soft tissue disorder related to use, overuse and pressure, unspecified shoulder

✓6ᵗʰ **M70.92** Unspecified soft tissue disorder related to use, overuse and pressure of upper arm

    M70.921 Unspecified soft tissue disorder related to use, overuse and pressure, right upper arm

    M70.922 Unspecified soft tissue disorder related to use, overuse and pressure, left upper arm

    M70.929 Unspecified soft tissue disorder related to use, overuse and pressure, unspecified upper arm

✓6ᵗʰ **M70.93** Unspecified soft tissue disorder related to use, overuse and pressure of forearm

    M70.931 Unspecified soft tissue disorder related to use, overuse and pressure, right forearm

    M70.932 Unspecified soft tissue disorder related to use, overuse and pressure, left forearm

M70.939 Unspecified soft tissue disorder related to use, overuse and pressure, unspecified forearm

✓6ᵗʰ **M70.94** Unspecified soft tissue disorder related to use, overuse and pressure of hand

    M70.941 Unspecified soft tissue disorder related to use, overuse and pressure, right hand

    M70.942 Unspecified soft tissue disorder related to use, overuse and pressure, left hand

    M70.949 Unspecified soft tissue disorder related to use, overuse and pressure, unspecified hand

✓6ᵗʰ **M70.95** Unspecified soft tissue disorder related to use, overuse and pressure of thigh

    M70.951 Unspecified soft tissue disorder related to use, overuse and pressure, right thigh

    M70.952 Unspecified soft tissue disorder related to use, overuse and pressure, left thigh

    M70.959 Unspecified soft tissue disorder related to use, overuse and pressure, unspecified thigh

✓6ᵗʰ **M70.96** Unspecified soft tissue disorder related to use, overuse and pressure lower leg

    M70.961 Unspecified soft tissue disorder related to use, overuse and pressure, right lower leg

    M70.962 Unspecified soft tissue disorder related to use, overuse and pressure, left lower leg

    M70.969 Unspecified soft tissue disorder related to use, overuse and pressure, unspecified lower leg

✓6ᵗʰ **M70.97** Unspecified soft tissue disorder related to use, overuse and pressure of ankle and foot

    M70.971 Unspecified soft tissue disorder related to use, overuse and pressure, right ankle and foot

    M70.972 Unspecified soft tissue disorder related to use, overuse and pressure, left ankle and foot

    M70.979 Unspecified soft tissue disorder related to use, overuse and pressure, unspecified ankle and foot

M70.98 Unspecified soft tissue disorder related to use, overuse and pressure other

M70.99 Unspecified soft tissue disorder related to use, overuse and pressure multiple sites

✓4ᵗʰ **M71** **Other bursopathies**

    EXCLUDES 1   bunion (M20.1)
                 bursitis related to use, overuse or pressure (M70.-)
                  enthesopathies (M76-M77)

✓5ᵗʰ **M71.0** Abscess of bursa

    Use additional code (B95.-, B96.-) to identify causative organism

M71.00 Abscess of bursa, unspecified site

✓6ᵗʰ **M71.01** Abscess of bursa, shoulder

    M71.011 Abscess of bursa, right shoulder

    M71.012 Abscess of bursa, left shoulder

    M71.019 Abscess of bursa, unspecified shoulder

✓6ᵗʰ **M71.02** Abscess of bursa, elbow

    M71.021 Abscess of bursa, right elbow

    M71.022 Abscess of bursa, left elbow

    M71.029 Abscess of bursa, unspecified elbow

✓6ᵗʰ **M71.03** Abscess of bursa, wrist

    M71.031 Abscess of bursa, right wrist

    M71.032 Abscess of bursa, left wrist

    M71.039 Abscess of bursa, unspecified wrist

✓6ᵗʰ **M71.04** Abscess of bursa, hand

    M71.041 Abscess of bursa, right hand

    M71.042 Abscess of bursa, left hand

    M71.049 Abscess of bursa, unspecified hand

✓6ᵗʰ **M71.05** Abscess of bursa, hip

    M71.051 Abscess of bursa, right hip

    M71.052 Abscess of bursa, left hip

    M71.059 Abscess of bursa, unspecified hip

✓6ᵗʰ **M71.06** Abscess of bursa, knee

    M71.061 Abscess of bursa, right knee

    M71.062 Abscess of bursa, left knee

    M71.069 Abscess of bursa, unspecified knee

Ⓝ Newborn: 0   Ⓟ Pediatric: 0-17   Ⓜ Maternity: 12-55   Ⓐ Adult: 15-124   **MCC** Major CC Condition   **PDxMCC** PDx acts as own MCC   **CC** CC Condition   **PDxCC** PDx acts as own CC

760   ICD-10-CM 2016

  ✓6ᵗʰ **M71.07** **Abscess of bursa, ankle and foot**
    M71.071 **Abscess of bursa, right ankle and foot**
    M71.072 **Abscess of bursa, left ankle and foot**
    M71.079 **Abscess of bursa, unspecified ankle and foot**
  M71.08 **Abscess of bursa, other site**
  M71.09 **Abscess of bursa, multiple sites**

✓5ᵗʰ **M71.1** **Other infective bursitis**
  Use additional code (B95.-, B96.-) to identify causative organism
  M71.10 **Other infective bursitis, unspecified site**
  ✓6ᵗʰ **M71.11** **Other infective bursitis, shoulder**
    M71.111 **Other infective bursitis, right shoulder**
    M71.112 **Other infective bursitis, left shoulder**
    M71.119 **Other infective bursitis, unspecified shoulder**
  ✓6ᵗʰ **M71.12** **Other infective bursitis, elbow**
    M71.121 **Other infective bursitis, right elbow**
    M71.122 **Other infective bursitis, left elbow**
    M71.129 **Other infective bursitis, unspecified elbow**
  ✓6ᵗʰ **M71.13** **Other infective bursitis, wrist**
    M71.131 **Other infective bursitis, right wrist**
    M71.132 **Other infective bursitis, left wrist**
    M71.139 **Other infective bursitis, unspecified wrist**
  ✓6ᵗʰ **M71.14** **Other infective bursitis, hand**
    M71.141 **Other infective bursitis, right hand**
    M71.142 **Other infective bursitis, left hand**
    M71.149 **Other infective bursitis, unspecified hand**
  ✓6ᵗʰ **M71.15** **Other infective bursitis, hip**
    M71.151 **Other infective bursitis, right hip**
    M71.152 **Other infective bursitis, left hip**
    M71.159 **Other infective bursitis, unspecified hip**
  ✓6ᵗʰ **M71.16** **Other infective bursitis, knee**
    M71.161 **Other infective bursitis, right knee**
    M71.162 **Other infective bursitis, left knee**
    M71.169 **Other infective bursitis, unspecified knee**
  ✓6ᵗʰ **M71.17** **Other infective bursitis, ankle and foot**
    M71.171 **Other infective bursitis, right ankle and foot**
    M71.172 **Other infective bursitis, left ankle and foot**
    M71.179 **Other infective bursitis, unspecified ankle and foot**
  M71.18 **Other infective bursitis, other site**
  M71.19 **Other infective bursitis, multiple sites**

✓5ᵗʰ **M71.2** **Synovial cyst of popliteal space [Baker]**
  EXCLUDES 1 synovial cyst of popliteal space with rupture (M66.0)
  M71.20 **Synovial cyst of popliteal space [Baker], unspecified knee**
  M71.21 **Synovial cyst of popliteal space [Baker], right knee**
  M71.22 **Synovial cyst of popliteal space [Baker], left knee**

✓5ᵗʰ **M71.3** **Other bursal cyst**
  Synovial cyst NOS
  EXCLUDES 1 synovial cyst with rupture (M66.1-)
  M71.30 **Other bursal cyst, unspecified site**
  ✓6ᵗʰ **M71.31** **Other bursal cyst, shoulder**
    M71.311 **Other bursal cyst, right shoulder**
    M71.312 **Other bursal cyst, left shoulder**
    M71.319 **Other bursal cyst, unspecified shoulder**
  ✓6ᵗʰ **M71.32** **Other bursal cyst, elbow**
    M71.321 **Other bursal cyst, right elbow**
    M71.322 **Other bursal cyst, left elbow**
    M71.329 **Other bursal cyst, unspecified elbow**
  ✓6ᵗʰ **M71.33** **Other bursal cyst, wrist**
    M71.331 **Other bursal cyst, right wrist**
    M71.332 **Other bursal cyst, left wrist**
    M71.339 **Other bursal cyst, unspecified wrist**
  ✓6ᵗʰ **M71.34** **Other bursal cyst, hand**
    M71.341 **Other bursal cyst, right hand**
    M71.342 **Other bursal cyst, left hand**
    M71.349 **Other bursal cyst, unspecified hand**
  ✓6ᵗʰ **M71.35** **Other bursal cyst, hip**
    M71.351 **Other bursal cyst, right hip**
    M71.352 **Other bursal cyst, left hip**

    M71.359 **Other bursal cyst, unspecified hip**
  ✓6ᵗʰ **M71.37** **Other bursal cyst, ankle and foot**
    M71.371 **Other bursal cyst, right ankle and foot**
    M71.372 **Other bursal cyst, left ankle and foot**
    M71.379 **Other bursal cyst, unspecified ankle and foot**
  M71.38 **Other bursal cyst, other site**
  M71.39 **Other bursal cyst, multiple sites**

✓5ᵗʰ **M71.4** **Calcium deposit in bursa**
  EXCLUDES 2 calcium deposit in bursa of shoulder (M75.3)
  M71.40 **Calcium deposit in bursa, unspecified site**
  ✓6ᵗʰ **M71.42** **Calcium deposit in bursa, elbow**
    M71.421 **Calcium deposit in bursa, right elbow**
    M71.422 **Calcium deposit in bursa, left elbow**
    M71.429 **Calcium deposit in bursa, unspecified elbow**
  ✓6ᵗʰ **M71.43** **Calcium deposit in bursa, wrist**
    M71.431 **Calcium deposit in bursa, right wrist**
    M71.432 **Calcium deposit in bursa, left wrist**
    M71.439 **Calcium deposit in bursa, unspecified wrist**
  ✓6ᵗʰ **M71.44** **Calcium deposit in bursa, hand**
    M71.441 **Calcium deposit in bursa, right hand**
    M71.442 **Calcium deposit in bursa, left hand**
    M71.449 **Calcium deposit in bursa, unspecified hand**
  ✓6ᵗʰ **M71.45** **Calcium deposit in bursa, hip**
    M71.451 **Calcium deposit in bursa, right hip**
    M71.452 **Calcium deposit in bursa, left hip**
    M71.459 **Calcium deposit in bursa, unspecified hip**
  ✓6ᵗʰ **M71.46** **Calcium deposit in bursa, knee**
    M71.461 **Calcium deposit in bursa, right knee**
    M71.462 **Calcium deposit in bursa, left knee**
    M71.469 **Calcium deposit in bursa, unspecified knee**
  ✓6ᵗʰ **M71.47** **Calcium deposit in bursa, ankle and foot**
    M71.471 **Calcium deposit in bursa, right ankle and foot**
    M71.472 **Calcium deposit in bursa, left ankle and foot**
    M71.479 **Calcium deposit in bursa, unspecified ankle and foot**
  M71.48 **Calcium deposit in bursa, other site**
  M71.49 **Calcium deposit in bursa, multiple sites**

✓5ᵗʰ **M71.5** **Other bursitis, not elsewhere classified**
  EXCLUDES 1 bursitis NOS (M71.9-)
  EXCLUDES 2 bursitis of shoulder (M75.5)
    bursitis of tibial collateral [Pellegrini-Stieda] (M76.4)
  M71.50 **Other bursitis, not elsewhere classified, unspecified site**
  ✓6ᵗʰ **M71.52** **Other bursitis, not elsewhere classified, elbow**
    M71.521 **Other bursitis, not elsewhere classified, right elbow**
    M71.522 **Other bursitis, not elsewhere classified, left elbow**
    M71.529 **Other bursitis, not elsewhere classified, unspecified elbow**
  ✓6ᵗʰ **M71.53** **Other bursitis, not elsewhere classified, wrist**
    M71.531 **Other bursitis, not elsewhere classified, right wrist**
    M71.532 **Other bursitis, not elsewhere classified, left wrist**
    M71.539 **Other bursitis, not elsewhere classified, unspecified wrist**
  ✓6ᵗʰ **M71.54** **Other bursitis, not elsewhere classified, hand**
    M71.541 **Other bursitis, not elsewhere classified, right hand**
    M71.542 **Other bursitis, not elsewhere classified, left hand**
    M71.549 **Other bursitis, not elsewhere classified, unspecified hand**
  ✓6ᵗʰ **M71.55** **Other bursitis, not elsewhere classified, hip**
    M71.551 **Other bursitis, not elsewhere classified, right hip**

✓ Additional Character Required   ✓x7ᵗʰ Placeholder Alert   Unacceptable PDx   Manifestation   Hospital Acquired Condition   EXCLUDES 1 Not Coded Here   EXCLUDES 2 Not Included Here

M71.552   Other bursitis, not elsewhere classified, left hip

M71.559   Other bursitis, not elsewhere classified, unspecified hip

✓6ᵗʰ   **M71.56**   **Other bursitis, not elsewhere classified, knee**

M71.561   Other bursitis, not elsewhere classified, right knee

M71.562   Other bursitis, not elsewhere classified, left knee

M71.569   Other bursitis, not elsewhere classified, unspecified knee

✓6ᵗʰ   **M71.57**   **Other bursitis, not elsewhere classified, ankle and foot**

M71.571   Other bursitis, not elsewhere classified, right ankle and foot

M71.572   Other bursitis, not elsewhere classified, left ankle and foot

M71.579   Other bursitis, not elsewhere classified, unspecified ankle and foot

M71.58   Other bursitis, not elsewhere classified, other site

✓5ᵗʰ   **M71.8**   **Other specified bursopathies**

M71.80   Other specified bursopathies, unspecified site

✓6ᵗʰ   **M71.81**   **Other specified bursopathies, shoulder**

M71.811   Other specified bursopathies, right shoulder

M71.812   Other specified bursopathies, left shoulder

M71.819   Other specified bursopathies, unspecified shoulder

✓6ᵗʰ   **M71.82**   **Other specified bursopathies, elbow**

M71.821   Other specified bursopathies, right elbow

M71.822   Other specified bursopathies, left elbow

M71.829   Other specified bursopathies, unspecified elbow

✓6ᵗʰ   **M71.83**   **Other specified bursopathies, wrist**

M71.831   Other specified bursopathies, right wrist

M71.832   Other specified bursopathies, left wrist

M71.839   Other specified bursopathies, unspecified wrist

✓6ᵗʰ   **M71.84**   **Other specified bursopathies, hand**

M71.841   Other specified bursopathies, right hand

M71.842   Other specified bursopathies, left hand

M71.849   Other specified bursopathies, unspecified hand

✓6ᵗʰ   **M71.85**   **Other specified bursopathies, hip**

M71.851   Other specified bursopathies, right hip

M71.852   Other specified bursopathies, left hip

M71.859   Other specified bursopathies, unspecified hip

✓6ᵗʰ   **M71.86**   **Other specified bursopathies, knee**

M71.861   Other specified bursopathies, right knee

M71.862   Other specified bursopathies, left knee

M71.869   Other specified bursopathies, unspecified knee

✓6ᵗʰ   **M71.87**   **Other specified bursopathies, ankle and foot**

M71.871   Other specified bursopathies, right ankle and foot

M71.872   Other specified bursopathies, left ankle and foot

M71.879   Other specified bursopathies, unspecified ankle and foot

M71.88   Other specified bursopathies, other site

M71.89   Other specified bursopathies, multiple sites

M71.9   **Bursopathy, unspecified**
Bursitis NOS

✓4ᵗʰ   **M72**   **Fibroblastic disorders**

   EXCLUDES 2   retroperitoneal fibromatosis (D48.3)

M72.0   **Palmar fascial fibromatosis [Dupuytren]**   Ⓐ

M72.1   **Knuckle pads**

M72.2   **Plantar fascial fibromatosis**
Plantar fasciitis

M72.4   **Pseudosarcomatous fibromatosis**
Nodular fasciitis

M72.6   **Necrotizing fasciitis**   MCC
   Use additional code (B95.-, B96.-) to identify causative organism
   CC Excl: K68.12, M60.000-M60.19, M61.00-M61.19, M61.30-M61.59, M62.3, M62.50-M62.59, M62.89, M72.6

M72.8   **Other fibroblastic disorders**
Abscess of fascia
Fasciitis NEC
Other infective fasciitis
   Use additional code to (B95.-, B96.-) identify causative organism
   EXCLUDES 1   diffuse (eosinophilic) fasciitis (M35.4)
      necrotizing fasciitis (M72.6)
      nodular fasciitis (M72.4)
      perirenal fasciitis NOS (N13.5)
      perirenal fasciitis with infection (N13.6)
      plantar fasciitis (M72.2)

M72.9   **Fibroblastic disorder, unspecified**
Fasciitis NOS   Fibromatosis NOS

✓4ᵗʰ   **M75**   **Shoulder lesions**

   EXCLUDES 2   shoulder-hand syndrome (M89.0-)

✓5ᵗʰ   **M75.0**   **Adhesive capsulitis of shoulder**
Frozen shoulder
Periarthritis of shoulder

M75.00   Adhesive capsulitis of unspecified shoulder

M75.01   Adhesive capsulitis of right shoulder

M75.02   Adhesive capsulitis of left shoulder

✓5ᵗʰ   **M75.1**   **Rotator cuff tear or rupture, not specified as traumatic**
Rotator cuff syndrome
Supraspinatus syndrome
Supraspinatus tear or rupture, not specified as traumatic
   EXCLUDES 1   tear of rotator cuff, traumatic (S46.01-)

✓6ᵗʰ   **M75.10**   **Unspecified rotator cuff tear or rupture, not specified as traumatic**

M75.100   Unspecified rotator cuff tear or rupture of unspecified shoulder, not specified as traumatic

M75.101   Unspecified rotator cuff tear or rupture of right shoulder, not specified as traumatic

M75.102   Unspecified rotator cuff tear or rupture of left shoulder, not specified as traumatic

✓6ᵗʰ   **M75.11**   **Incomplete rotator cuff tear or rupture not specified as traumatic**

M75.110   Incomplete rotator cuff tear or rupture of unspecified shoulder, not specified as traumatic

M75.111   Incomplete rotator cuff tear or rupture of right shoulder, not specified as traumatic

M75.112   Incomplete rotator cuff tear or rupture of left shoulder, not specified as traumatic

✓6ᵗʰ   **M75.12**   **Complete rotator cuff tear or rupture not specified as traumatic**

M75.120   Complete rotator cuff tear or rupture of unspecified shoulder, not specified as traumatic

M75.121   Complete rotator cuff tear or rupture of right shoulder, not specified as traumatic

M75.122   Complete rotator cuff tear or rupture of left shoulder, not specified as traumatic

✓5ᵗʰ   **M75.2**   **Bicipital tendinitis**

M75.20   Bicipital tendinitis, unspecified shoulder

M75.21   Bicipital tendinitis, right shoulder

M75.22   Bicipital tendinitis, left shoulder

✓5ᵗʰ   **M75.3**   **Calcific tendinitis of shoulder**
Calcified bursa of shoulder

M75.30   Calcific tendinitis of unspecified shoulder

M75.31   Calcific tendinitis of right shoulder

M75.32   Calcific tendinitis of left shoulder

✓5ᵗʰ   **M75.4**   **Impingement syndrome of shoulder**

M75.40   Impingement syndrome of unspecified shoulder

M75.41   Impingement syndrome of right shoulder

M75.42   Impingement syndrome of left shoulder

✓5ᵗʰ   **M75.5**   **Bursitis of shoulder**

M75.50   Bursitis of unspecified shoulder

M75.51   Bursitis of right shoulder

M75.52   Bursitis of left shoulder

✓5ᵗʰ   **M75.8**   **Other shoulder lesions**

M75.80   Other shoulder lesions, unspecified shoulder

Ⓝ Newborn: 0   Ⓟ Pediatric: 0-17   Ⓜ Maternity: 12-55   Ⓐ Adult: 15-124   MCC Major CC Condition   PDxMCC PDx acts as own MCC   CC CC Condition   PDxCC PDx acts as own CC

762   ICD-10-CM 2016

M75.81   Other shoulder lesions, right shoulder

M75.82   Other shoulder lesions, left shoulder

✓5ᵗʰ   **M75.9   Shoulder lesion, unspecified**

    M75.90   Shoulder lesion, unspecified, unspecified shoulder

    M75.91   Shoulder lesion, unspecified, right shoulder

    M75.92   Shoulder lesion, unspecified, left shoulder

✓4ᵗʰ   **M76   Enthesopathies, lower limb, excluding foot**

    EXCLUDES 2   bursitis due to use, overuse and pressure (M70.-)

                enthesopathies of ankle and foot (M77.5-)

✓5ᵗʰ   **M76.0   Gluteal tendinitis**

    M76.00   Gluteal tendinitis, unspecified hip

    M76.01   Gluteal tendinitis, right hip

    M76.02   Gluteal tendinitis, left hip

✓5ᵗʰ   **M76.1   Psoas tendinitis**

    M76.10   Psoas tendinitis, unspecified hip

    M76.11   Psoas tendinitis, right hip

    M76.12   Psoas tendinitis, left hip

✓5ᵗʰ   **M76.2   Iliac crest spur**

    M76.20   Iliac crest spur, unspecified hip

    M76.21   Iliac crest spur, right hip

    M76.22   Iliac crest spur, left hip

✓5ᵗʰ   **M76.3   Iliotibial band syndrome**

    M76.30   Iliotibial band syndrome, unspecified leg

    M76.31   Iliotibial band syndrome, right leg

    M76.32   Iliotibial band syndrome, left leg

✓5ᵗʰ   **M76.4   Tibial collateral bursitis [Pellegrini-Stieda]**

    M76.40   Tibial collateral bursitis [Pellegrini-Stieda], unspecified leg

    M76.41   Tibial collateral bursitis [Pellegrini-Stieda], right leg

    M76.42   Tibial collateral bursitis [Pellegrini-Stieda], left leg

✓5ᵗʰ   **M76.5   Patellar tendinitis**

    M76.50   Patellar tendinitis, unspecified knee

    M76.51   Patellar tendinitis, right knee

    M76.52   Patellar tendinitis, left knee

✓5ᵗʰ   **M76.6   Achilles tendinitis**

    Achilles bursitis

    M76.60   Achilles tendinitis, unspecified leg

    M76.61   Achilles tendinitis, right leg

    M76.62   Achilles tendinitis, left leg

✓5ᵗʰ   **M76.7   Peroneal tendinitis**

    M76.70   Peroneal tendinitis, unspecified leg

    M76.71   Peroneal tendinitis, right leg

    M76.72   Peroneal tendinitis, left leg

✓5ᵗʰ   **M76.8   Other specified enthesopathies of lower limb, excluding foot**

    ✓6ᵗʰ   **M76.81   Anterior tibial syndrome**

       M76.811   Anterior tibial syndrome, right leg

       M76.812   Anterior tibial syndrome, left leg

       M76.819   Anterior tibial syndrome, unspecified leg

    ✓6ᵗʰ   **M76.82   Posterior tibial tendinitis**

       M76.821   Posterior tibial tendinitis, right leg

       M76.822   Posterior tibial tendinitis, left leg

       M76.829   Posterior tibial tendinitis, unspecified leg

    ✓6ᵗʰ   **M76.89   Other specified enthesopathies of lower limb, excluding foot**

       M76.891   Other specified enthesopathies of right lower limb, excluding foot

       M76.892   Other specified enthesopathies of left lower limb, excluding foot

       M76.899   Other specified enthesopathies of unspecified lower limb, excluding foot

    M76.9   Unspecified enthesopathy, lower limb, excluding foot

✓4ᵗʰ   **M77   Other enthesopathies**

    EXCLUDES 1   bursitis NOS (M71.9-)

    EXCLUDES 2   bursitis due to use, overuse and pressure (M70.-)

                osteophyte (M25.7)

                spinal enthesopathy (M46.0-)

✓5ᵗʰ   **M77.0   Medial epicondylitis**

    M77.00   Medial epicondylitis, unspecified elbow

    M77.01   Medial epicondylitis, right elbow

    M77.02   Medial epicondylitis, left elbow

✓5ᵗʰ   **M77.1   Lateral epicondylitis**

    Tennis elbow

    M77.10   Lateral epicondylitis, unspecified elbow

    M77.11   Lateral epicondylitis, right elbow

    M77.12   Lateral epicondylitis, left elbow

✓5ᵗʰ   **M77.2   Periarthritis of wrist**

    M77.20   Periarthritis, unspecified wrist

    M77.21   Periarthritis, right wrist

    M77.22   Periarthritis, left wrist

✓5ᵗʰ   **M77.3   Calcaneal spur**

    M77.30   Calcaneal spur, unspecified foot

    M77.31   Calcaneal spur, right foot

    M77.32   Calcaneal spur, left foot

✓5ᵗʰ   **M77.4   Metatarsalgia**

    EXCLUDES   Morton's metatarsalgia (G57.6)

    M77.40   Metatarsalgia, unspecified foot

    M77.41   Metatarsalgia, right foot

    M77.42   Metatarsalgia, left foot

✓5ᵗʰ   **M77.5   Other enthesopathy of foot**

    M77.50   Other enthesopathy of unspecified foot

    M77.51   Other enthesopathy of right foot

    M77.52   Other enthesopathy of left foot

    M77.8   Other enthesopathies, not elsewhere classified

    M77.9   Enthesopathy, unspecified

      Bone spur NOS   Periarthritis NOS

      Capsulitis NOS   Tendinitis NOS

✓4ᵗʰ   **M79   Other and unspecified soft tissue disorders, not elsewhere classified**

    EXCLUDES 1   psychogenic rheumatism (F45.8)

                soft tissue pain, psychogenic (F45.41)

    M79.0   Rheumatism, unspecified

    EXCLUDES 1   fibromyalgia (M79.7)

                palindromic rheumatism (M12.3-)

    M79.1   Myalgia

    Myofascial pain syndrome

    EXCLUDES 1   fibromyalgia (M79.7)

                myositis (M60.-)

    M79.2   Neuralgia and neuritis, unspecified

    EXCLUDES 1   brachial radiculitis NOS (M54.1)

                lumbosacral radiculitis NOS (M54.1)

                mononeuropathies (G56-G58)

                radiculitis NOS (M54.1)

                sciatica (M54.3-M54.4)

    M79.3   Panniculitis, unspecified

    EXCLUDES 1   lupus panniculitis (L93.2)

                neck and back panniculitis (M54.0-)

                relapsing [Weber-Christian] panniculitis (M35.6)

    M79.4   Hypertrophy of (infrapatellar) fat pad

    M79.5   Residual foreign body in soft tissue

    EXCLUDES 1   foreign body granuloma of skin and subcutaneous tissue (L92.3)

                foreign body granuloma of soft tissue (M60.2-)

✓5ᵗʰ   **M79.6   Pain in limb, hand, foot, fingers and toes**

    EXCLUDES 2   pain in joint (M25.5-)

    ✓6ᵗʰ   **M79.60   Pain in limb, unspecified**

       M79.601   Pain in right arm

         Pain in right upper limb NOS

       M79.602   Pain in left arm

         Pain in left upper limb NOS

       M79.603   Pain in arm, unspecified

         Pain in upper limb NOS

       M79.604   Pain in right leg

         Pain in right lower limb NOS

       M79.605   Pain in left leg

         Pain in left lower limb NOS

       M79.606   Pain in leg, unspecified

         Pain in lower limb NOS

       M79.609   Pain in unspecified limb

         Pain in limb NOS

    ✓6ᵗʰ   **M79.62   Pain in upper arm**

       Pain in axillary region

       M79.621   Pain in right upper arm

       M79.622   Pain in left upper arm

       M79.629   Pain in unspecified upper arm

✓ Additional Character Required   ✗×7ᵗʰ Placeholder Alert   Unacceptable PDx   Manifestation   Hospital Acquired Condition   EXCLUDES 1 Not Coded Here   EXCLUDES 2 Not Included Here

Chapter 13. Diseases of the Musculoskeletal System and Connective Tissue

M79.63–M80.029

√6th **M79.63 Pain in forearm**
- M79.631 Pain in right forearm
- M79.632 Pain in left forearm
- M79.639 Pain in unspecified forearm

√6th **M79.64 Pain in hand and fingers**
- M79.641 Pain in right hand
- M79.642 Pain in left hand
- M79.643 Pain in unspecified hand
- M79.644 Pain in right finger(s)
- M79.645 Pain in left finger(s)
- M79.646 Pain in unspecified finger(s)

√6th **M79.65 Pain in thigh**
- M79.651 Pain in right thigh
- M79.652 Pain in left thigh
- M79.659 Pain in unspecified thigh

√6th **M79.66 Pain in lower leg**
- M79.661 Pain in right lower leg
- M79.662 Pain in left lower leg
- M79.669 Pain in unspecified lower leg

√6th **M79.67 Pain in foot and toes**
- M79.671 Pain in right foot
- M79.672 Pain in left foot
- M79.673 Pain in unspecified foot
- M79.674 Pain in right toe(s)
- M79.675 Pain in left toe(s)
- M79.676 Pain in unspecified toe(s)

M79.7 Fibromyalgia
Fibromyositis   Myofibrositis
Fibrositis

√5th **M79.A Nontraumatic compartment syndrome**
Code first, if applicable, associated postprocedural complication
EXCLUDES 1   compartment syndrome NOS (T79.A-)
fibromyalgia (M79.7)
nontraumatic ischemic infarction of muscle (M62.2-)
traumatic compartment syndrome (T79.A-)

√6th **M79.A1 Nontraumatic compartment syndrome of upper extremity**
Nontraumatic compartment syndrome of shoulder, arm, forearm, wrist, hand, and fingers

CC Excl: M70.80-M70.99, M79.81-M79.9, R29.898, S45.301-S45.899 with 7th A, S55.201-S55.899 with 7th A, S65.801-S65.899 with 7th A

- M79.A11 Nontraumatic compartment syndrome of right upper extremity CC
- M79.A12 Nontraumatic compartment syndrome of left upper extremity CC
- M79.A19 Nontraumatic compartment syndrome of unspecified upper extremity CC

√6th **M79.A2 Nontraumatic compartment syndrome of lower extremity**
Nontraumatic compartment syndrome of hip, buttock, thigh, leg, foot, and toes

CC Excl: M70.80-M70.99, M79.81-M79.9, R29.898, S75.801-S75.899 with 7th A, S85.201-S85.299 with 7th A, S85.801-S85.899 with 7th A, S95.001-S95.099 with 7th A, S95.201-S95.899 with 7th A

- M79.A21 Nontraumatic compartment syndrome of right lower extremity CC
- M79.A22 Nontraumatic compartment syndrome of left lower extremity CC
- M79.A29 Nontraumatic compartment syndrome of unspecified lower extremity CC

M79.A3 Nontraumatic compartment syndrome of abdomen CC
CC Excl: S31.001 with 7th A, S31.011 with 7th A, S31.021 with 7th A, S31.031 with 7th A, S31.041 with 7th A, S31.051-S31.159 with 7th A, S31.600-S31.659 with 7th A, S31.831-S31.839 with 7th A, S36.00-S37.99 with 7th A, S38.3XX-S39.023 with 7th A, T14.90-T14.91, T79.8XX-T79.9XX with 7th A

M79.A9 Nontraumatic compartment syndrome of other sites CC
CC Excl: S31.001 with 7th A, S31.011 with 7th A, S31.021 with 7th A, S31.031 with 7th A, S31.041 with 7th A, S31.051 with 7th A, S31.600-S31.659 with 7th A, S36.81X-S36.899 with 7th A

√5th **M79.8 Other specified soft tissue disorders**

M79.81 Nontraumatic hematoma of soft tissue
Nontraumatic hematoma of muscle
Nontraumatic seroma of muscle and soft tissue

M79.89 Other specified soft tissue disorders
Polyalgia

M79.9 Soft tissue disorder, unspecified

OSTEOPATHIES AND CHONDROPATHIES (M80-M94)

Disorders of bone density and structure (M80-M85)

√4th **M80 Osteoporosis with current pathological fracture**
INCLUDES   osteoporosis with current fragility fracture
Use additional code to identify major osseous defect, if applicable (M89.7-)
EXCLUDES 1   collapsed vertebra NOS (M48.5)
pathological fracture NOS (M84.4)
wedging of vertebra NOS (M48.5)
EXCLUDES 2   personal history of (healed) osteoporosis fracture (Z87.310)

The appropriate 7th character is to be added to each code from category M80.
- A   initial encounter for fracture
- D   subsequent encounter for fracture with routine healing
- G   subsequent encounter for fracture with delayed healing
- K   subsequent encounter for fracture with nonunion
- P   subsequent encounter for fracture with malunion
- S   sequela

CC Excl: For codes M80, CC with 7th character A, unless otherwise noted: M48.40X-M48.58X with 7th A, M80.00X-M84.68X with 7th A
CC codes with 7th character K or P: M80.00X-M84.68X with 7th [K, P], S02.0XX-S02.92X with 7th K, S12.000-S12.691 with 7th K, S22.000-S22.9XX with 7th K, S32.000-S32.9XX with 7th K, S42.001-S42.92 with 7th [K, P], S49.001-S49.199 with 7th [K, P], S52.001-S52.92X with 7th [K, M, N, P, Q, R], S59.001-S59.299 with 7th [K, P], S62.001-S62.92X with 7th [K, P], S72.001-S72.92X with 7th [K, M, N, P, Q, R], S79.001-S79.199 with 7th [K, P], S82.001-S82.92X with 7th [K, M, N, P, Q, R], S89.001-S89.399 with 7th [K, P], S92.001-S92.919 with 7th [K, P]

√5th **M80.0 Age-related osteoporosis with current pathological fracture**
Involutional osteoporosis with current pathological fracture
Osteoporosis NOS with current pathological fracture
Postmenopausal osteoporosis with current pathological fracture
Senile osteoporosis with current pathological fracture

17 √x7th **M80.00 Age-related osteoporosis with current pathological fracture, unspecified site** CC A

√6th **M80.01 Age-related osteoporosis with current pathological fracture, shoulder**

17 √7th M80.011 Age-related osteoporosis with current pathological fracture, right shoulder CC A

17 √7th M80.012 Age-related osteoporosis with current pathological fracture, left shoulder CC A

17 √7th M80.019 Age-related osteoporosis with current pathological fracture, unspecified shoulder CC A

√6th **M80.02 Age-related osteoporosis with current pathological fracture, humerus**

17 √7th M80.021 Age-related osteoporosis with current pathological fracture, right humerus CC A

17 √7th M80.022 Age-related osteoporosis with current pathological fracture, left humerus CC A

17 √7th M80.029 Age-related osteoporosis with current pathological fracture, unspecified humerus CC A

---

17   CC only if an initial encounter (7th character A, B, or C – specific to category) OR a subsequent encounter for nonunion or malunion (7th character K, M, N, P, Q, or R – specific to category).

N Newborn: 0   P Pediatric: 0-17   M Maternity: 12-55   A Adult: 15-124   MCC Major CC Condition   PDxMCC PDx acts as own MCC   CC CC Condition   PDxCC PDx acts as own CC

764   ICD-10-CM 2016

√6ᵗʰ **M80.03 Age-related osteoporosis with current pathological fracture, forearm**
Age-related osteoporosis with current pathological fracture of wrist

17 √7ᵗʰ **M80.031 Age-related osteoporosis with current pathological fracture, right forearm** `CC` `A`

17 √7ᵗʰ **M80.032 Age-related osteoporosis with current pathological fracture, left forearm** `CC` `A`

17 √7ᵗʰ **M80.039 Age-related osteoporosis with current pathological fracture, unspecified forearm** `CC` `A`

√6ᵗʰ **M80.04 Age-related osteoporosis with current pathological fracture, hand**

17 √7ᵗʰ **M80.041 Age-related osteoporosis with current pathological fracture, right hand** `CC` `A`

17 √7ᵗʰ **M80.042 Age-related osteoporosis with current pathological fracture, left hand** `CC` `A`

17 √7ᵗʰ **M80.049 Age-related osteoporosis with current pathological fracture, unspecified hand** `CC` `A`

√6ᵗʰ **M80.05 Age-related osteoporosis with current pathological fracture, femur**
Age-related osteoporosis with current pathological fracture of hip

17 √7ᵗʰ **M80.051 Age-related osteoporosis with current pathological fracture, right femur** `CC` `A`

17 √7ᵗʰ **M80.052 Age-related osteoporosis with current pathological fracture, left femur** `CC` `A`

17 √7ᵗʰ **M80.059 Age-related osteoporosis with current pathological fracture, unspecified femur** `CC` `A`

√6ᵗʰ **M80.06 Age-related osteoporosis with current pathological fracture, lower leg**

17 √7ᵗʰ **M80.061 Age-related osteoporosis with current pathological fracture, right lower leg** `CC` `A`

17 √7ᵗʰ **M80.062 Age-related osteoporosis with current pathological fracture, left lower leg** `CC` `A`

17 √7ᵗʰ **M80.069 Age-related osteoporosis with current pathological fracture, unspecified lower leg** `CC` `A`

√6ᵗʰ **M80.07 Age-related osteoporosis with current pathological fracture, ankle and foot**

17 √7ᵗʰ **M80.071 Age-related osteoporosis with current pathological fracture, right ankle and foot** `CC` `A`

17 √7ᵗʰ **M80.072 Age-related osteoporosis with current pathological fracture, left ankle and foot** `CC` `A`

17 √7ᵗʰ **M80.079 Age-related osteoporosis with current pathological fracture, unspecified ankle and foot** `CC` `A`

17 √x7ᵗʰ **M80.08 Age-related osteoporosis with current pathological fracture, vertebra(e)** `CC` `A`

√5ᵗʰ **M80.8 Other osteoporosis with current pathological fracture**
Drug-induced osteoporosis with current pathological fracture
Idiopathic osteoporosis with current pathological fracture
Osteoporosis of disuse with current pathological fracture
Postoophorectomy osteoporosis with current pathological fracture
Postsurgical malabsorption osteoporosis with current pathological fracture
Post-traumatic osteoporosis with current pathological fracture
Use additional code for adverse effect, if applicable, to identify drug (T36-T50 with fifth or sixth character 5)

17 √x7ᵗʰ **M80.80 Other osteoporosis with current pathological fracture, unspecified site** `CC`

√6ᵗʰ **M80.81 Other osteoporosis with pathological fracture, shoulder**

17 √7ᵗʰ **M80.811 Other osteoporosis with current pathological fracture, right shoulder** `CC`

17 √7ᵗʰ **M80.812 Other osteoporosis with current pathological fracture, left shoulder** `CC`

17 √7ᵗʰ **M80.819 Other osteoporosis with current pathological fracture, unspecified shoulder** `CC`

√6ᵗʰ **M80.82 Other osteoporosis with current pathological fracture, humerus**

17 √7ᵗʰ **M80.821 Other osteoporosis with current pathological fracture, right humerus** `CC`

17 √7ᵗʰ **M80.822 Other osteoporosis with current pathological fracture, left humerus** `CC`

17 √7ᵗʰ **M80.829 Other osteoporosis with current pathological fracture, unspecified humerus** `CC`

√6ᵗʰ **M80.83 Other osteoporosis with current pathological fracture, forearm**
Other osteoporosis with current pathological fracture of wrist

17 √7ᵗʰ **M80.831 Other osteoporosis with current pathological fracture, right forearm** `CC`

17 √7ᵗʰ **M80.832 Other osteoporosis with current pathological fracture, left forearm** `CC`

17 √7ᵗʰ **M80.839 Other osteoporosis with current pathological fracture, unspecified forearm** `CC`

√6ᵗʰ **M80.84 Other osteoporosis with current pathological fracture, hand**

17 √7ᵗʰ **M80.841 Other osteoporosis with current pathological fracture, right hand** `CC`

17 √7ᵗʰ **M80.842 Other osteoporosis with current pathological fracture, left hand** `CC`

17 √7ᵗʰ **M80.849 Other osteoporosis with current pathological fracture, unspecified hand** `CC`

√6ᵗʰ **M80.85 Other osteoporosis with current pathological fracture, femur**
Other osteoporosis with current pathological fracture of hip

17 √7ᵗʰ **M80.851 Other osteoporosis with current pathological fracture, right femur** `CC`

17 √7ᵗʰ **M80.852 Other osteoporosis with current pathological fracture, left femur** `CC`

17 √7ᵗʰ **M80.859 Other osteoporosis with current pathological fracture, unspecified femur** `CC`

√6ᵗʰ **M80.86 Other osteoporosis with current pathological fracture, lower leg**

17 √7ᵗʰ **M80.861 Other osteoporosis with current pathological fracture, right lower leg** `CC`

17 √7ᵗʰ **M80.862 Other osteoporosis with current pathological fracture, left lower leg** `CC`

17 √7ᵗʰ **M80.869 Other osteoporosis with current pathological fracture, unspecified lower leg** `CC`

√6ᵗʰ **M80.87 Other osteoporosis with current pathological fracture, ankle and foot**

17 √7ᵗʰ **M80.871 Other osteoporosis with current pathological fracture, right ankle and foot** `CC`

17 √7ᵗʰ **M80.872 Other osteoporosis with current pathological fracture, left ankle and foot** `CC`

17 √7ᵗʰ **M80.879 Other osteoporosis with current pathological fracture, unspecified ankle and foot** `CC`

17 √x7ᵗʰ **M80.88 Other osteoporosis with current pathological fracture, vertebra(e)** `CC`

---

17 CC only if an initial encounter (7th character A, B, or C – specific to category) **OR** a subsequent encounter for nonunion or malunion (7th character K, M, N, P, Q, or R – specific to category).

☑ Additional Character Required   √x7ᵗʰ Placeholder Alert   Unacceptable PDx   Manifestation   Hospital Acquired Condition   *EXCLUDES 1* Not Coded Here   *EXCLUDES 2* Not Included Here

✓4ᵗʰ M81 Osteoporosis without current pathological fracture

Use additional code to identify:
major osseous defect, if applicable (M89.7-)
personal history of (healed) osteoporosis fracture, if applicable (Z87.310)

EXCLUDES 1 osteoporosis with current pathological fracture (M80.-)
Sudeck's atrophy (M89.0)

M81.0 Age-related osteoporosis without current pathological fracture　Ⓐ

Involutional osteoporosis without current pathological fracture
Osteoporosis NOS
Postmenopausal osteoporosis without current pathological fracture
Senile osteoporosis without current pathological fracture

M81.6 Localized osteoporosis [Lequesne]

EXCLUDES 1 Sudeck's atrophy (M89.0)

M81.8 Other osteoporosis without current pathological fracture

Drug-induced osteoporosis without current pathological fracture
Idiopathic osteoporosis without current pathological fracture
Osteoporosis of disuse without current pathological fracture
Postoophorectomy osteoporosis without current pathological fracture
Postsurgical malabsorption osteoporosis without current pathological fracture
Post-traumatic osteoporosis without current pathological fracture

Use additional code for adverse effect, if applicable, to identify drug (T36-T50 with fifth or sixth character 5)

✓4ᵗʰ M83 Adult osteomalacia

EXCLUDES 1 infantile and juvenile osteomalacia (E55.0)
renal osteodystrophy (N25.0)
rickets (active) (E55.0)
rickets (active) sequelae (E64.3)
vitamin D-resistant osteomalacia (E83.3)
vitamin D-resistant rickets (active) (E83.3)

M83.0 Puerperal osteomalacia　Ⓜ♀

M83.1 Senile osteomalacia　Ⓐ

M83.2 Adult osteomalacia due to malabsorption　Ⓐ

Postsurgical malabsorption osteomalacia in adults

M83.3 Adult osteomalacia due to malnutrition　Ⓐ

M83.4 Aluminum bone disease

M83.5 Other drug-induced osteomalacia in adults　Ⓐ

Use additional code for adverse effect, if applicable, to identify drug (T36-T50 with fifth or sixth character 5)

M83.8 Other adult osteomalacia　Ⓐ

M83.9 Adult osteomalacia, unspecified　Ⓐ

✓4ᵗʰ M84 Disorder of continuity of bone

EXCLUDES 2 traumatic fracture of bone-see fracture, by site

✓5ᵗʰ M84.3 Stress fracture

Fatigue fracture　　　Stress fracture NOS
March fracture　　　Stress reaction

Use additional external cause code(s) to identify the cause of the stress fracture

EXCLUDES 1 pathological fracture NOS (M84.4-)
pathological fracture due to osteoporosis (M80.-)
traumatic fracture (S12-, S22-, S32-, S42-, S52-, S62-, S72-, S82-, S92-)

EXCLUDES 2 personal history of (healed) stress (fatigue) fracture (Z87.312)
stress fracture of vertebra (M48.4-

> The appropriate 7th character is to be added to each code from subcategory M84.3.
> A　initial encounter for fracture
> D　subsequent encounter for fracture with routine healing
> G　subsequent encounter for fracture with delayed healing
> K　subsequent encounter for fracture with nonunion
> P　subsequent encounter for fracture with malunion
> S　sequela

> **CC Excl:** For CC codes in subcatagory M84.3, unless otherwise noted: For CC codes with 7th character K or P: M80.00X-M84.68X with 7th [K, P], S02.0XX-S02.92X with 7th K, S12.000-S12.691 with 7th K, S22.000-S22.9XX with 7th K, S32000-S32.9XX with 7th K, S42.001-S42.92X with 7th [K, P], S49.001-S49.199 with 7th [K, P], S52.001-S52.92X with 7th [K, M, N, P, Q, R], S59.001-S59.299 with 7th [K, P], S62.001-S62.92X with 7th [K, P], S72.001-S72.92X with 7th [K, M, N, P, Q, R], S79.001-S79.199 with 7th [K, P], S82.001-S82.92X with 7th [K, M, N, P, Q, R], S89.001-S89.399 with 7th [K, P], S92.001-S92.919 with 7th [K, P]

18 ✓x7ᵗʰ **M84.30** Stress fracture, unspecified site　CC

✓6ᵗʰ **M84.31** Stress fracture, shoulder
　18 ✓7ᵗʰ **M84.311** Stress fracture, right shoulder　CC
　18 ✓7ᵗʰ **M84.312** Stress fracture, left shoulder　CC
　18 ✓7ᵗʰ **M84.319** Stress fracture, unspecified shoulder　CC

✓6ᵗʰ **M84.32** Stress fracture, humerus
　18 ✓7ᵗʰ **M84.321** Stress fracture, right humerus　CC
　18 ✓7ᵗʰ **M84.322** Stress fracture, left humerus　CC
　18 ✓7ᵗʰ **M84.329** Stress fracture, unspecified humerus　CC

✓6ᵗʰ **M84.33** Stress fracture, ulna and radius
　18 ✓7ᵗʰ **M84.331** Stress fracture, right ulna　CC
　18 ✓7ᵗʰ **M84.332** Stress fracture, left ulna　CC
　18 ✓7ᵗʰ **M84.333** Stress fracture, right radius　CC
　18 ✓7ᵗʰ **M84.334** Stress fracture, left radius　CC
　18 ✓7ᵗʰ **M84.339** Stress fracture, unspecified ulna and radius

✓6ᵗʰ **M84.34** Stress fracture, hand and fingers
　18 ✓7ᵗʰ **M84.341** Stress fracture, right hand　CC
　18 ✓7ᵗʰ **M84.342** Stress fracture, left hand　CC
　18 ✓7ᵗʰ **M84.343** Stress fracture, unspecified hand　CC
　18 ✓7ᵗʰ **M84.344** Stress fracture, right finger(s)　CC
　18 ✓7ᵗʰ **M84.345** Stress fracture, left finger(s)　CC
　18 ✓7ᵗʰ **M84.346** Stress fracture, unspecified finger(s)　CC

✓6ᵗʰ **M84.35** Stress fracture, pelvis and femur
Stress fracture, hip
　18 ✓7ᵗʰ **M84.350** Stress fracture, pelvis　CC
　18 ✓7ᵗʰ **M84.351** Stress fracture, right femur　CC
　18 ✓7ᵗʰ **M84.352** Stress fracture, left femur　CC
　18 ✓7ᵗʰ **M84.353** Stress fracture, unspecified femur　CC
　18 ✓7ᵗʰ **M84.359** Stress fracture, hip, unspecified

✓6ᵗʰ **M84.36** Stress fracture, tibia and fibula
　18 ✓7ᵗʰ **M84.361** Stress fracture, right tibia　CC
　18 ✓7ᵗʰ **M84.362** Stress fracture, left tibia　CC
　18 ✓7ᵗʰ **M84.363** Stress fracture, right fibula　CC
　18 ✓7ᵗʰ **M84.364** Stress fracture, left fibula　CC
　18 ✓7ᵗʰ **M84.369** Stress fracture, unspecified tibia and fibula　CC

✓6ᵗʰ **M84.37** Stress fracture, ankle, foot and toes
　18 ✓7ᵗʰ **M84.371** Stress fracture, right ankle　CC
　18 ✓7ᵗʰ **M84.372** Stress fracture, left ankle　CC
　18 ✓7ᵗʰ **M84.373** Stress fracture, unspecified ankle　CC
　18 ✓7ᵗʰ **M84.374** Stress fracture, right foot　CC
　18 ✓7ᵗʰ **M84.375** Stress fracture, left foot　CC
　18 ✓7ᵗʰ **M84.376** Stress fracture, unspecified foot　CC
　18 ✓7ᵗʰ **M84.377** Stress fracture, right toe(s)　CC
　18 ✓7ᵗʰ **M84.378** Stress fracture, left toe(s)　CC
　18 ✓7ᵗʰ **M84.379** Stress fracture, unspecified toe(s)　CC

18 ✓x7ᵗʰ **M84.38** Stress fracture, other site　CC
EXCLUDES 2 stress fracture of vertebra (M48.4-)

---

18 CC only if a subsequent encounter for nonunion or malunion (7th character K, M, N, P, Q, or R – specific to category).

Ⓝ Newborn: 0　Ⓟ Pediatric: 0-17　Ⓜ Maternity: 12-55　Ⓐ Adult: 15-124　MCC Major CC Condition　PDxMCC PDx acts as own MCC　CC CC Condition　PDxCC PDx acts as own CC

766　　　　ICD-10-CM 2016

√5th **M84.4 Pathological fracture,** not elsewhere classified
Chronic fracture
Pathological fracture NOS

EXCLUDES 1   collapsed vertebra NEC (M48.5)
pathological fracture in neoplastic disease (M84.5-)
pathological fracture in osteoporosis (M80.-)
pathological fracture in other disease (M84.6-)
stress fracture (M84.3-)
traumatic fracture (S12.-, S22.-, S32.-, S42.-, S52.-, S62.-, S72.-, S82.-, S92.-)

EXCLUDES 2   personal history of (healed) pathological fracture (Z87.311)

The appropriate 7th character is to be added to each code from subcategory M84.4.
A   initial encounter for fracture
D   subsequent encounter for fracture with routine healing
G   subsequent encounter for fracture with delayed healing
K   subsequent encounter for fracture with nonunion
P   subsequent encounter for fracture with malunion
S   sequela

CC Excl: For codes M84.4, CC with 7th character A, unless otherwise noted: M48.40X-M48.58X with 7th A, M80.00X-M84.68X with 7th A
CC with 7th character K or P: M80.00X-M84.68X with 7th [K, P], S02.0XX-S02.92Xwith 7th K, S12.000-S12.691 with 7th K, S22.000-S22.9XX with 7th K, S32.000-S32.9XX with 7th K, S42.001-S42.92X with 7th [K, P], S49.001-S49.199 with 7th [K, P], S52.001-S52.92X with 7th [K, M, N, P, Q, R], S59.001-S59.299 with 7th [K, P], S62.001-S62.92X with 7th [K, P], S72.001-S72.92X with 7th [K, M, N, P, Q, R], S79.001-S79.199 with 7th [K, P], S82.001-S82.92X with 7th [K, M, N, P, Q, R], S89.001-S89.399 with 7th [K, P], S92.001-S92.919 with 7th [K, P]

17   √x7th   **M84.40 Pathological fracture,** unspecified site   CC

√6th   **M84.41 Pathological fracture,** shoulder
   17 √7th   **M84.411 Pathological fracture,** right shoulder   CC
   17 √7th   **M84.412 Pathological fracture,** left shoulder   CC
   17 √7th   **M84.419 Pathological fracture,** unspecified shoulder   CC

√6th   **M84.42 Pathological fracture,** humerus
   17 √7th   **M84.421 Pathological fracture,** right humerus   CC
   17 √7th   **M84.422 Pathological fracture,** left humerus   CC
   17 √7th   **M84.429 Pathological fracture,** unspecified humerus   CC

√6th   **M84.43 Pathological fracture,** ulna and radius
   17 √7th   **M84.431 Pathological fracture,** right ulna   CC
   17 √7th   **M84.432 Pathological fracture,** left ulna   CC
   17 √7th   **M84.433 Pathological fracture,** right radius   CC
   17 √7th   **M84.434 Pathological fracture,** left radius   CC
   17 √7th   **M84.439 Pathological fracture,** unspecified ulna and radius   CC

√6th   **M84.44 Pathological fracture,** hand and fingers
   17 √7th   **M84.441 Pathological fracture,** right hand   CC
   17 √7th   **M84.442 Pathological fracture,** left hand   CC
   17 √7th   **M84.443 Pathological fracture,** unspecified hand   CC
   17 √7th   **M84.444 Pathological fracture,** right finger(s)   CC
   17 √7th   **M84.445 Pathological fracture,** left finger(s)   CC
   17 √7th   **M84.446 Pathological fracture,** unspecified finger(s)   CC

√6th   **M84.45 Pathological fracture,** femur and pelvis
   17 √7th   **M84.451 Pathological fracture,** right femur   CC
   17 √7th   **M84.452 Pathological fracture,** left femur   CC
   17 √7th   **M84.453 Pathological fracture,** unspecified femur   CC
   17 √7th   **M84.454 Pathological fracture,** pelvis   CC
   17 √7th   **M84.459 Pathological fracture,** hip, unspecified   CC

√6th   **M84.46 Pathological fracture,** tibia and fibula
   17 √7th   **M84.461 Pathological fracture,** right tibia   CC
   17 √7th   **M84.462 Pathological fracture,** left tibia   CC
   17 √7th   **M84.463 Pathological fracture,** right fibula   CC
   17 √7th   **M84.464 Pathological fracture,** left fibula   CC

   17 √7th   **M84.469 Pathological fracture,** unspecified tibia and fibula   CC

√6th   **M84.47 Pathological fracture,** ankle, foot and toes
   17 √7th   **M84.471 Pathological fracture,** right ankle   CC
   17 √7th   **M84.472 Pathological fracture,** left ankle   CC
   17 √7th   **M84.473 Pathological fracture,** unspecified ankle   CC
   17 √7th   **M84.474 Pathological fracture,** right foot   CC
   17 √7th   **M84.475 Pathological fracture,** left foot   CC
   17 √7th   **M84.476 Pathological fracture,** unspecified foot   CC
   17 √7th   **M84.477 Pathological fracture,** right toe(s)   CC
   17 √7th   **M84.478 Pathological fracture,** left toe(s)   CC
   17 √7th   **M84.479 Pathological fracture,** unspecified toe(s)   CC

17   √x7th   **M84.48 Pathological fracture,** other site   CC

√5th   **M84.5 Pathological fracture in** neoplastic disease
Code also underlying neoplasm

The appropriate 7th character is to be added to each code from subcategory M84.5.
A   initial encounter for fracture
D   subsequent encounter for fracture with routine healing
G   subsequent encounter for fracture with delayed healing
K   subsequent encounter for fracture with nonunion
P   subsequent encounter for fracture with malunion
S   sequela

CC Excl: For codes M84.5, CC with 7th character A, unless otherwise noted: M48.40X-M48.58X with 7th A, M80.00X-M84.68X with 7th A
CC with 7th character K or P: M80.00X-M84.68X with 7th [K, P], S02.0XX-S02.92X with 7th K, S12.000-S12.691 with 7th K, S22.000-S22.9XX with 7th K, S32.000-S32.9XX with 7th K, S42.001-S42.92X with 7th [K, P], S49.001-S49.199 with 7th [K, P], S52.001-S52.92X with 7th [K, M, N, P, Q, R], S59.001-S59.299 with 7th [K, P], S62.001-S62.92X with 7th [K, P], S72.001-S72.92X with 7th [K, M, N, P, Q, R], S79.001-S79.199 with 7th [K, P], S82.001-S82.92X with 7th [K, M, N, P, Q, R], S89.001-S89.399 with 7th [K, P], S92.001-S92.919 with 7th [K, P]

17   √x7th   **M84.50 Pathological fracture in neoplastic disease,** unspecified site   CC

√6th   **M84.51 Pathological fracture in neoplastic disease,** shoulder
   17 √7th   **M84.511 Pathological fracture in neoplastic disease,** right shoulder   CC
   17 √7th   **M84.512 Pathological fracture in neoplastic disease,** left shoulder   CC
   17 √7th   **M84.519 Pathological fracture in neoplastic disease,** unspecified shoulder   CC

√6th   **M84.52 Pathological fracture in neoplastic disease,** humerus
   17 √7th   **M84.521 Pathological fracture in neoplastic disease,** right humerus   CC
   17 √7th   **M84.522 Pathological fracture in neoplastic disease,** left humerus   CC
   17 √7th   **M84.529 Pathological fracture in neoplastic disease,** unspecified humerus   CC

√6th   **M84.53 Pathological fracture in neoplastic disease,** ulna and radius
   17 √7th   **M84.531 Pathological fracture in neoplastic disease,** right ulna   CC
   17 √7th   **M84.532 Pathological fracture in neoplastic disease,** left ulna   CC
   17 √7th   **M84.533 Pathological fracture in neoplastic disease,** right radius   CC
   17 √7th   **M84.534 Pathological fracture in neoplastic disease,** left radius   CC
   17 √7th   **M84.539 Path**unspecified**ological fracture in neoplastic disease, ulna and radius**   CC

√6th   **M84.54 Pathological fracture in neoplastic disease,** hand
   17 √7th   **M84.541 Pathological fracture in neoplastic disease,** right hand   CC
   17 √7th   **M84.542 Pathological fracture in neoplastic disease,** left hand   CC
   17 √7th   **M84.549 Pathological fracture in neoplastic disease,** unspecified hand   CC

---

17   CC only if an initial encounter (7th character A, B, or C – specific to category) **OR** a subsequent encounter for nonunion or malunion (7th character K, M, N, P, Q, or R – specific to category).

✓ Additional Character Required   √x7th Placeholder Alert   Unacceptable PDx   Manifestation   Hospital Acquired Condition   *EXCLUDES 1* Not Coded Here   *EXCLUDES 2* Not Included Here

√6ᵗʰ **M84.55 Pathological fracture in neoplastic disease, pelvis and femur**

17 √7ᵗʰ   M84.550 Pathological fracture in neoplastic disease, pelvis   CC

17 √7ᵗʰ   M84.551 Pathological fracture in neoplastic disease, right femur   CC

17 √7ᵗʰ   M84.552 Pathological fracture in neoplastic disease, left femur   CC

17 √7ᵗʰ   M84.553 Pathological fracture in neoplastic disease, unspecified femur   CC

17 √7ᵗʰ   M84.559 Pathological fracture in neoplastic disease, hip, unspecified   CC

√6ᵗʰ **M84.56 Pathological fracture in neoplastic disease, tibia and fibula**

17 √7ᵗʰ   M84.561 Pathological fracture in neoplastic disease, right tibia   CC

17 √7ᵗʰ   M84.562 Pathological fracture in neoplastic disease, left tibia   CC

17 √7ᵗʰ   M84.563 Pathological fracture in neoplastic disease, right fibula   CC

17 √7ᵗʰ   M84.564 Pathological fracture in neoplastic disease, left fibula   CC

17 √7ᵗʰ   M84.569 Pathological fracture in neoplastic disease, unspecified tibia and fibula   CC

√6ᵗʰ **M84.57 Pathological fracture in neoplastic disease, ankle and foot**

17 √7ᵗʰ   M84.571 Pathological fracture in neoplastic disease, right ankle   CC

17 √7ᵗʰ   M84.572 Pathological fracture in neoplastic disease, left ankle   CC

17 √7ᵗʰ   M84.573 Pathological fracture in neoplastic disease, unspecified ankle   CC

17 √7ᵗʰ   M84.574 Pathological fracture in neoplastic disease, right foot   CC

17 √7ᵗʰ   M84.575 Pathological fracture in neoplastic disease, left foot   CC

17 √7ᵗʰ   M84.576 Pathological fracture in neoplastic disease, unspecified foot   CC

17 √x7ᵗʰ   M84.58 Pathological fracture in neoplastic disease, other specified site   CC
    Pathological fracture in neoplastic disease, vertebrae

√5ᵗʰ **M84.6 Pathological fracture in other disease**
    Code also underlying condition
    EXCLUDES 1 *pathological fracture in osteoporosis (M80.-)*

> The appropriate 7th character is to be added to each code from subcategory M84.6.
> A   initial encounter for fracture
> D   subsequent encounter for fracture with routine healing
> G   subsequent encounter for fracture with delayed healing
> K   subsequent encounter for fracture with nonunion
> P   subsequent encounter for fracture with malunion
> S   sequela

> **CC Excl: For codes M84.6, CC with 7th character A, unless otherwise noted:** M48.40X-M48.58X with 7th A, M80.00X-M84.68X with 7th A.
> **CC with 7th character K or P:** M80.00X-M84.68X with 7th [K, P], S02.0XX-S02.92X with 7th K, S12.000-S12.691 with 7th K, S22.000-S22.9XX with 7th K, S32.000-S32.9XX with 7th K, S42.001-S42.92X with 7th [K, P], S49.001-S49.199 with 7th [K, P], S52.001-S52.92X with 7th [K, M, N, P, Q, R], S59.001-S59.299 with 7th [K, P], S62.001-S62.92X with 7th [K, P], S72.001-S72.92X with 7th [K, M, N, P, Q, R], S79.001-S79.199 with 7th [K, P], S82.001-S82.92X with 7th [K, M, N, P, Q, R], S89.001-S89.399 with 7th [K, P], S92.001-S92.919 with 7th [K, P]

17 √x7ᵗʰ   M84.60 Pathological fracture in other disease, unspecified site   CC

√6ᵗʰ **M84.61 Pathological fracture in other disease, shoulder**

17 √7ᵗʰ   M84.611 Pathological fracture in other disease, right shoulder   CC

17 √7ᵗʰ   M84.612 Pathological fracture in other disease, left shoulder   CC

17 √7ᵗʰ   M84.619 Pathological fracture in other disease, unspecified shoulder   CC

√6ᵗʰ **M84.62 Pathological fracture in other disease, humerus**

17 √7ᵗʰ   M84.621 Pathological fracture in other disease, right humerus   CC

17 √7ᵗʰ   M84.622 Pathological fracture in other disease, left humerus   CC

17 √7ᵗʰ   M84.629 Pathological fracture in other disease, unspecified humerus

√6ᵗʰ **M84.63 Pathological fracture in other disease, ulna and radius**

17 √7ᵗʰ   M84.631 Pathological fracture in other disease, right ulna   CC

17 √7ᵗʰ   M84.632 Pathological fracture in other disease, left ulna   CC

17 √7ᵗʰ   M84.633 Pathological fracture in other disease, right radius   CC

17 √7ᵗʰ   M84.634 Pathological fracture in other disease, left radius   CC

17 √7ᵗʰ   M84.639 Pathological fracture in other disease, unspecified ulna and radius   CC

√6ᵗʰ **M84.64 Pathological fracture in other disease, hand**

17 √7ᵗʰ   M84.641 Pathological fracture in other disease, right hand   CC

17 √7ᵗʰ   M84.642 Pathological fracture in other disease, left hand   CC

17 √7ᵗʰ   M84.649 Pathological fracture in other disease, unspecified hand   CC

√6ᵗʰ **M84.65 Pathological fracture in other disease, pelvis and femur**

17 √7ᵗʰ   M84.650 Pathological fracture in other disease, pelvis   CC

17 √7ᵗʰ   M84.651 Pathological fracture in other disease, right femur   CC

17 √7ᵗʰ   M84.652 Pathological fracture in other disease, left femur   CC

17 √7ᵗʰ   M84.653 Pathological fracture in other disease, unspecified femur   CC

17 √7ᵗʰ   M84.659 Pathological fracture in other disease, hip, unspecified   CC

√6ᵗʰ **M84.66 Pathological fracture in other disease, tibia and fibula**

17 √7ᵗʰ   M84.661 Pathological fracture in other disease, right tibia   CC

17 √7ᵗʰ   M84.662 Pathological fracture in other disease, left tibia   CC

17 √7ᵗʰ   M84.663 Pathological fracture in other disease, right fibula   CC

17 √7ᵗʰ   M84.664 Pathological fracture in other disease, left fibula   CC

17 √7ᵗʰ   M84.669 Pathological fracture in other disease, unspecified tibia and fibula   CC

√6ᵗʰ **M84.67 Pathological fracture in other disease, ankle and foot**

17 √7ᵗʰ   M84.671 Pathological fracture in other disease, right ankle   CC

17 √7ᵗʰ   M84.672 Pathological fracture in other disease, left ankle   CC

17 √7ᵗʰ   M84.673 Pathological fracture in other disease, unspecified ankle   CC

17 √7ᵗʰ   M84.674 Pathological fracture in other disease, right foot   CC

17 √7ᵗʰ   M84.675 Pathological fracture in other disease, left foot   CC

17 √7ᵗʰ   M84.676 Pathological fracture in other disease, unspecified foot   CC

17 √x7ᵗʰ   M84.68 Pathological fracture in other disease, other site   CC

√5ᵗʰ **M84.8 Other disorders of continuity of bone**

    M84.80 Other disorders of continuity of bone, unspecified site

√6ᵗʰ **M84.81 Other disorders of continuity of bone, shoulder**

    M84.811 Other disorders of continuity of bone, right shoulder

    M84.812 Other disorders of continuity of bone, left shoulder

---

17   CC only if an initial encounter (7th character A, B, or C – specific to category) **OR** a subsequent encounter for nonunion or malunion (7th character K, M, N, P, Q, or R – specific to category).

Ⓝ Newborn: 0   Ⓟ Pediatric: 0-17   Ⓜ Maternity: 12-55   Ⓐ Adult: 15-124   **MCC** Major CC Condition   **PDxMCC** PDx acts as own MCC   **CC** CC Condition   **PDxCC** PDx acts as own CC

768   ICD-10-CM 2016

        M84.819   Other disorders of continuity of bone, unspecified shoulder

✓6ᵗʰ **M84.82** **Other disorders of continuity of bone, humerus**
        M84.821   Other disorders of continuity of bone, right humerus
        M84.822   Other disorders of continuity of bone, left humerus
        M84.829   Other disorders of continuity of bone, unspecified humerus

✓6ᵗʰ **M84.83** **Other disorders of continuity of bone, ulna and radius**
        M84.831   Other disorders of continuity of bone, right ulna
        M84.832   Other disorders of continuity of bone, left ulna
        M84.833   Other disorders of continuity of bone, right radius
        M84.834   Other disorders of continuity of bone, left radius
        M84.839   Other disorders of continuity of bone, unspecified ulna and radius

✓6ᵗʰ **M84.84** **Other disorders of continuity of bone, hand**
        M84.841   Other disorders of continuity of bone, right hand
        M84.842   Other disorders of continuity of bone, left hand
        M84.849   Other disorders of continuity of bone, unspecified hand

✓6ᵗʰ **M84.85** **Other disorders of continuity of bone, pelvic region and thigh**
        M84.851   Other disorders of continuity of bone, right pelvic region and thigh
        M84.852   Other disorders of continuity of bone, left pelvic region and thigh
        M84.859   Other disorders of continuity of bone, unspecified pelvic region and thigh

✓6ᵗʰ **M84.86** **Other disorders of continuity of bone, tibia and fibula**
        M84.861   Other disorders of continuity of bone, right tibia
        M84.862   Other disorders of continuity of bone, left tibia
        M84.863   Other disorders of continuity of bone, right fibula
        M84.864   Other disorders of continuity of bone, left fibula
        M84.869   Other disorders of continuity of bone, unspecified tibia and fibula

✓6ᵗʰ **M84.87** **Other disorders of continuity of bone, ankle and foot**
        M84.871   Other disorders of continuity of bone, right ankle and foot
        M84.872   Other disorders of continuity of bone, left ankle and foot
        M84.879   Other disorders of continuity of bone, unspecified ankle and foot

    M84.88 **Other disorders of continuity of bone, other site**

M84.9 **Disorder of continuity of bone, unspecified**

✓4ᵗʰ **M85** **Other disorders of bone density and structure**
      EXCLUDES 1 *osteogenesis imperfecta (Q78.0)*
                osteopetrosis (Q78.2)
                osteopoikilosis (Q78.8)
                polyostotic fibrous dysplasia (Q78.1)

✓5ᵗʰ **M85.0** **Fibrous dysplasia (monostotic)**
      EXCLUDES 2 *fibrous dysplasia of jaw (M27.8)*
    M85.00 **Fibrous dysplasia (monostotic), unspecified site**

✓6ᵗʰ **M85.01** **Fibrous dysplasia (monostotic), shoulder**
        M85.011   Fibrous dysplasia (monostotic), right shoulder
        M85.012   Fibrous dysplasia (monostotic), left shoulder
        M85.019   Fibrous dysplasia (monostotic), unspecified shoulder

✓6ᵗʰ **M85.02** **Fibrous dysplasia (monostotic), upper arm**
        M85.021   Fibrous dysplasia (monostotic), right upper arm
        M85.022   Fibrous dysplasia (monostotic), left upper arm
        M85.029   Fibrous dysplasia (monostotic), unspecified upper arm

✓6ᵗʰ **M85.03** **Fibrous dysplasia (monostotic), forearm**
        M85.031   Fibrous dysplasia (monostotic), right forearm
        M85.032   Fibrous dysplasia (monostotic), left forearm
        M85.039   Fibrous dysplasia (monostotic), unspecified forearm

✓6ᵗʰ **M85.04** **Fibrous dysplasia (monostotic), hand**
        M85.041   Fibrous dysplasia (monostotic), right hand
        M85.042   Fibrous dysplasia (monostotic), left hand
        M85.049   Fibrous dysplasia (monostotic), unspecified hand

✓6ᵗʰ **M85.05** **Fibrous dysplasia (monostotic), thigh**
        M85.051   Fibrous dysplasia (monostotic), right thigh
        M85.052   Fibrous dysplasia (monostotic), left thigh
        M85.059   Fibrous dysplasia (monostotic), unspecified thigh

✓6ᵗʰ **M85.06** **Fibrous dysplasia (monostotic), lower leg**
        M85.061   Fibrous dysplasia (monostotic), right lower leg
        M85.062   Fibrous dysplasia (monostotic), left lower leg
        M85.069   Fibrous dysplasia (monostotic), unspecified lower leg

✓6ᵗʰ **M85.07** **Fibrous dysplasia (monostotic), ankle and foot**
        M85.071   Fibrous dysplasia (monostotic), right ankle and foot
        M85.072   Fibrous dysplasia (monostotic), left ankle and foot
        M85.079   Fibrous dysplasia (monostotic), unspecified ankle and foot

    M85.08 **Fibrous dysplasia (monostotic), other site**
    M85.09 **Fibrous dysplasia (monostotic), multiple sites**

✓5ᵗʰ **M85.1** **Skeletal fluorosis**
    M85.10 **Skeletal fluorosis, unspecified site**

✓6ᵗʰ **M85.11** **Skeletal fluorosis, shoulder**
        M85.111   Skeletal fluorosis, right shoulder
        M85.112   Skeletal fluorosis, left shoulder
        M85.119   Skeletal fluorosis, unspecified shoulder

✓6ᵗʰ **M85.12** **Skeletal fluorosis, upper arm**
        M85.121   Skeletal fluorosis, right upper arm
        M85.122   Skeletal fluorosis, left upper arm
        M85.129   Skeletal fluorosis, unspecified upper arm

✓6ᵗʰ **M85.13** **Skeletal fluorosis, forearm**
        M85.131   Skeletal fluorosis, right forearm
        M85.132   Skeletal fluorosis, left forearm
        M85.139   Skeletal fluorosis, unspecified forearm

✓6ᵗʰ **M85.14** **Skeletal fluorosis, hand**
        M85.141   Skeletal fluorosis, right hand
        M85.142   Skeletal fluorosis, left hand
        M85.149   Skeletal fluorosis, unspecified hand

✓6ᵗʰ **M85.15** **Skeletal fluorosis, thigh**
        M85.151   Skeletal fluorosis, right thigh
        M85.152   Skeletal fluorosis, left thigh
        M85.159   Skeletal fluorosis, unspecified thigh

✓6ᵗʰ **M85.16** **Skeletal fluorosis, lower leg**
        M85.161   Skeletal fluorosis, right lower leg
        M85.162   Skeletal fluorosis, left lower leg
        M85.169   Skeletal fluorosis, unspecified lower leg

✓6ᵗʰ **M85.17** **Skeletal fluorosis, ankle and foot**
        M85.171   Skeletal fluorosis, right ankle and foot
        M85.172   Skeletal fluorosis, left ankle and foot
        M85.179   Skeletal fluorosis, unspecified ankle and foot

    M85.18 **Skeletal fluorosis, other site**
    M85.19 **Skeletal fluorosis, multiple sites**

M85.2 **Hyperostosis of skull**

✓5ᵗʰ **M85.3** **Osteitis condensans**
    M85.30 **Osteitis condensans, unspecified site**

✓ Additional Character Required   ✓x7ᵗʰ Placeholder Alert   Unacceptable PDx   Manifestation   Hospital Acquired Condition   **EXCLUDES 1** Not Coded Here   *EXCLUDES 2* Not Included Here

✓6ᵗʰ **M85.31 Osteitis condensans, shoulder**
       M85.311 Osteitis condensans, right shoulder
       M85.312 Osteitis condensans, left shoulder
       M85.319 Osteitis condensans, unspecified shoulder

✓6ᵗʰ **M85.32 Osteitis condensans, upper arm**
       M85.321 Osteitis condensans, right upper arm
       M85.322 Osteitis condensans, left upper arm
       M85.329 Osteitis condensans, unspecified upper arm

✓6ᵗʰ **M85.33 Osteitis condensans, forearm**
       M85.331 Osteitis condensans, right forearm
       M85.332 Osteitis condensans, left forearm
       M85.339 Osteitis condensans, unspecified forearm

✓6ᵗʰ **M85.34 Osteitis condensans, hand**
       M85.341 Osteitis condensans, right hand
       M85.342 Osteitis condensans, left hand
       M85.349 Osteitis condensans, unspecified hand

✓6ᵗʰ **M85.35 Osteitis condensans, thigh**
       M85.351 Osteitis condensans, right thigh
       M85.352 Osteitis condensans, left thigh
       M85.359 Osteitis condensans, unspecified thigh

✓6ᵗʰ **M85.36 Osteitis condensans, lower leg**
       M85.361 Osteitis condensans, right lower leg
       M85.362 Osteitis condensans, left lower leg
       M85.369 Osteitis condensans, unspecified lower leg

✓6ᵗʰ **M85.37 Osteitis condensans, ankle and foot**
       M85.371 Osteitis condensans, right ankle and foot
       M85.372 Osteitis condensans, left ankle and foot
       M85.379 Osteitis condensans, unspecified ankle and foot

     M85.38 Osteitis condensans, other site
     M85.39 Osteitis condensans, multiple sites

✓5ᵗʰ **M85.4 Solitary bone cyst**
       EXCLUDES 2   *solitary cyst of jaw (M27.4)*

     M85.40 Solitary bone cyst, unspecified site

✓6ᵗʰ **M85.41 Solitary bone cyst, shoulder**
       M85.411 Solitary bone cyst, right shoulder
       M85.412 Solitary bone cyst, left shoulder
       M85.419 Solitary bone cyst, unspecified shoulder

✓6ᵗʰ **M85.42 Solitary bone cyst, humerus**
       M85.421 Solitary bone cyst, right humerus
       M85.422 Solitary bone cyst, left humerus
       M85.429 Solitary bone cyst, unspecified humerus

✓6ᵗʰ **M85.43 Solitary bone cyst, ulna and radius**
       M85.431 Solitary bone cyst, right ulna and radius
       M85.432 Solitary bone cyst, left ulna and radius
       M85.439 Solitary bone cyst, unspecified ulna and radius

✓6ᵗʰ **M85.44 Solitary bone cyst, hand**
       M85.441 Solitary bone cyst, right hand
       M85.442 Solitary bone cyst, left hand
       M85.449 Solitary bone cyst, unspecified hand

✓6ᵗʰ **M85.45 Solitary bone cyst, pelvis**
       M85.451 Solitary bone cyst, right pelvis
       M85.452 Solitary bone cyst, left pelvis
       M85.459 Solitary bone cyst, unspecified pelvis

✓6ᵗʰ **M85.46 Solitary bone cyst, tibia and fibula**
       M85.461 Solitary bone cyst, right tibia and fibula
       M85.462 Solitary bone cyst, left tibia and fibula
       M85.469 Solitary bone cyst, unspecified tibia and fibula

✓6ᵗʰ **M85.47 Solitary bone cyst, ankle and foot**
       M85.471 Solitary bone cyst, right ankle and foot
       M85.472 Solitary bone cyst, left ankle and foot
       M85.479 Solitary bone cyst, unspecified ankle and foot

     M85.48 Solitary bone cyst, other site

✓5ᵗʰ **M85.5 Aneurysmal bone cyst**
       EXCLUDES 2   *aneurysmal cyst of jaw (M27.4)*

     M85.50 Aneurysmal bone cyst, unspecified site

✓6ᵗʰ **M85.51 Aneurysmal bone cyst, shoulder**
       M85.511 Aneurysmal bone cyst, right shoulder
       M85.512 Aneurysmal bone cyst, left shoulder
       M85.519 Aneurysmal bone cyst, unspecified shoulder

✓6ᵗʰ **M85.52 Aneurysmal bone cyst, upper arm**
       M85.521 Aneurysmal bone cyst, right upper arm
       M85.522 Aneurysmal bone cyst, left upper arm
       M85.529 Aneurysmal bone cyst, unspecified upper arm

✓6ᵗʰ **M85.53 Aneurysmal bone cyst, forearm**
       M85.531 Aneurysmal bone cyst, right forearm
       M85.532 Aneurysmal bone cyst, left forearm
       M85.539 Aneurysmal bone cyst, unspecified forearm

✓6ᵗʰ **M85.54 Aneurysmal bone cyst, hand**
       M85.541 Aneurysmal bone cyst, right hand
       M85.542 Aneurysmal bone cyst, left hand
       M85.549 Aneurysmal bone cyst, unspecified hand

✓6ᵗʰ **M85.55 Aneurysmal bone cyst, thigh**
       M85.551 Aneurysmal bone cyst, right thigh
       M85.552 Aneurysmal bone cyst, left thigh
       M85.559 Aneurysmal bone cyst, unspecified thigh

✓6ᵗʰ **M85.56 Aneurysmal bone cyst, lower leg**
       M85.561 Aneurysmal bone cyst, right lower leg
       M85.562 Aneurysmal bone cyst, left lower leg
       M85.569 Aneurysmal bone cyst, unspecified lower leg

✓6ᵗʰ **M85.57 Aneurysmal bone cyst, ankle and foot**
       M85.571 Aneurysmal bone cyst, right ankle and foot
       M85.572 Aneurysmal bone cyst, left ankle and foot
       M85.579 Aneurysmal bone cyst, unspecified ankle and foot

     M85.58 Aneurysmal bone cyst, other site
     M85.59 Aneurysmal bone cyst, multiple sites

✓5ᵗʰ **M85.6 Other cyst of bone**
       EXCLUDES 1   *cyst of jaw NEC (M27.4)*
               osteitis fibrosa cystica generalisata [von Recklinghausen's disease of bone] (E21.0)

     M85.60 Other cyst of bone, unspecified site

✓6ᵗʰ **M85.61 Other cyst of bone, shoulder**
       M85.611 Other cyst of bone, right shoulder
       M85.612 Other cyst of bone, left shoulder
       M85.619 Other cyst of bone, unspecified shoulder

✓6ᵗʰ **M85.62 Other cyst of bone, upper arm**
       M85.621 Other cyst of bone, right upper arm
       M85.622 Other cyst of bone, left upper arm
       M85.629 Other cyst of bone, unspecified upper arm

✓6ᵗʰ **M85.63 Other cyst of bone, forearm**
       M85.631 Other cyst of bone, right forearm
       M85.632 Other cyst of bone, left forearm
       M85.639 Other cyst of bone, unspecified forearm

✓6ᵗʰ **M85.64 Other cyst of bone, hand**
       M85.641 Other cyst of bone, right hand
       M85.642 Other cyst of bone, left hand
       M85.649 Other cyst of bone, unspecified hand

✓6ᵗʰ **M85.65 Other cyst of bone, thigh**
       M85.651 Other cyst of bone, right thigh
       M85.652 Other cyst of bone, left thigh
       M85.659 Other cyst of bone, unspecified thigh

✓6ᵗʰ **M85.66 Other cyst of bone, lower leg**
       M85.661 Other cyst of bone, right lower leg
       M85.662 Other cyst of bone, left lower leg
       M85.669 Other cyst of bone, unspecified lower leg

✓6ᵗʰ **M85.67 Other cyst of bone, ankle and foot**
       M85.671 Other cyst of bone, right ankle and foot
       M85.672 Other cyst of bone, left ankle and foot
       M85.679 Other cyst of bone, unspecified ankle and foot

     M85.68 Other cyst of bone, other site
     M85.69 Other cyst of bone, multiple sites

✓5ᵗʰ **M85.8 Other specified disorders of bone density and structure**
Hyperostosis of bones, except skull
Osteosclerosis, acquired

EXCLUDES 1 *diffuse idiopathic skeletal hyperostosis [DISH] (M48.1)*
osteosclerosis congenita (Q77.4)
osteosclerosis fragilitas (generalista) (Q78.2)
osteosclerosis myelofibrosis (D75.81)

M85.80 Other specified disorders of bone density and structure, unspecified site

✓6ᵗʰ **M85.81 Other specified disorders of bone density and structure, shoulder**

M85.811 Other specified disorders of bone density and structure, right shoulder

M85.812 Other specified disorders of bone density and structure, left shoulder

M85.819 Other specified disorders of bone density and structure, unspecified shoulder

✓6ᵗʰ **M85.82 Other specified disorders of bone density and structure, upper arm**

M85.821 Other specified disorders of bone density and structure, right upper arm

M85.822 Other specified disorders of bone density and structure, left upper arm

M85.829 Other specified disorders of bone density and structure, unspecified upper arm

✓6ᵗʰ **M85.83 Other specified disorders of bone density and structure, forearm**

M85.831 Other specified disorders of bone density and structure, right forearm

M85.832 Other specified disorders of bone density and structure, left forearm

M85.839 Other specified disorders of bone density and structure, unspecified forearm

✓6ᵗʰ **M85.84 Other specified disorders of bone density and structure, hand**

M85.841 Other specified disorders of bone density and structure, right hand

M85.842 Other specified disorders of bone density and structure, left hand

M85.849 Other specified disorders of bone density and structure, unspecified hand

✓6ᵗʰ **M85.85 Other specified disorders of bone density and structure, thigh**

M85.851 Other specified disorders of bone density and structure, right thigh

M85.852 Other specified disorders of bone density and structure, left thigh

M85.859 Other specified disorders of bone density and structure, unspecified thigh

✓6ᵗʰ **M85.86 Other specified disorders of bone density and structure, lower leg**

M85.861 Other specified disorders of bone density and structure, right lower leg

M85.862 Other specified disorders of bone density and structure, left lower leg

M85.869 Other specified disorders of bone density and structure, unspecified lower leg

✓6ᵗʰ **M85.87 Other specified disorders of bone density and structure, ankle and foot**

M85.871 Other specified disorders of bone density and structure, right ankle and foot

M85.872 Other specified disorders of bone density and structure, left ankle and foot

M85.879 Other specified disorders of bone density and structure, unspecified ankle and foot

M85.88 Other specified disorders of bone density and structure, other site

M85.89 Other specified disorders of bone density and structure, multiple sites

M85.9 Disorder of bone density and structure, unspecified

Other osteopathies (M86-M90)

EXCLUDES 1 *postprocedural osteopathies (M96.-)*

✓4ᵗʰ **M86 Osteomyelitis**
Use additional code (B95-B97) to identify infectious agent
Use additional code to identify major osseous defect, if applicable (M89.7-)

EXCLUDES 1 *osteomyelitis due to:*
echinococcus (B67.2)
gonococcus (A54.43)
salmonella (A02.24)

EXCLUDES 2 *ostemyelitis of:*
orbit (H05.0-)
petrous bone (H70.2-)
vertebra (M46.2-)

✓5ᵗʰ **M86.0 Acute hematogenous osteomyelitis**

M86.00 Acute hematogenous osteomyelitis, unspecified site CC
CC Excl: A17.9, A18.03-A18.09, A18.82, A18.84, A18.89, M46.20-M46.39, M86.00-M86.9

✓6ᵗʰ **M86.01 Acute hematogenous osteomyelitis, shoulder**

M86.011 Acute hematogenous osteomyelitis, right shoulder CC
CC Excl: A17.9, A18.03-A18.09, A18.82, A18.84, A18.89, M46.20-M46.39, M86.00, M86.08-M86.10, M86.18-M86.20, M86.28-M86.319, M86.38-M86.419, M86.48-M86.519, M86.58-M86.619, M86.68-M86.8X1, M86.8X8-M86.9

M86.012 Acute hematogenous osteomyelitis, left shoulder CC
CC Excl: See code: M86.011

M86.019 Acute hematogenous osteomyelitis, unspecified shoulder CC
CC Excl: See code: M86.011

✓6ᵗʰ **M86.02 Acute hematogenous osteomyelitis, humerus**

M86.021 Acute hematogenous osteomyelitis, right humerus CC
CC Excl: A17.9, A18.03-A18.09, A18.82, A18.84, A18.89, M46.20-M46.39, M86.00, M86.08-M86.10, M86.18-M86.20, M86.28-M86.30, M86.321-M86.329, M86.38-M86.40, M86.421-M86.429, M86.48-M86.50, M86.521-M86.529, M86.58-M86.60, M86.621-M86.629, M86.68-M86.8X0, M86.8X2, M86.8X8-M86.9

M86.022 Acute hematogenous osteomyelitis, left humerus CC
CC Excl: See code: M86.021

M86.029 Acute hematogenous osteomyelitis, unspecified humerus CC
CC Excl: See code: M86.021

✓6ᵗʰ **M86.03 Acute hematogenous osteomyelitis, radius and ulna**

M86.031 Acute hematogenous osteomyelitis, right radius and ulna CC
CC Excl: A17.9, A18.03-A18.09, A18.82, A18.84, A18.89, M46.20-M46.39, M86.00, M86.08-M86.10, M86.18-M86.20, M86.28-M86.30, M86.331-M86.339, M86.38-M86.40, M86.431-M86.439, M86.48-M86.50, M86.531-M86.539, M86.58-M86.60, M86.631-M86.639, M86.68-M86.8X0, M86.8X3, M86.8X8-M86.9

M86.032 Acute hematogenous osteomyelitis, left radius and ulna CC
CC Excl: See code: M86.031

M86.039 Acute hematogenous osteomyelitis, unspecified radius and ulna CC
CC Excl: See code: M86.031

✓6ᵗʰ **M86.04 Acute hematogenous osteomyelitis, hand**

M86.041 Acute hematogenous osteomyelitis, right hand CC
CC Excl: A17.9, A18.03-A18.09, A18.82, A18.84, A18.89, M46.20-M46.39, M86.00, M86.08-M86.10, M86.18-M86.20, M86.28-M86.30, M86.341-M86.349, M86.38-M86.40, M86.441-M86.449, M86.48-M86.50, M86.541-M86.549, M86.58-M86.60, M86.641-M86.649, M86.68-M86.8X0, M86.8X4, M86.8X8-M86.9

M86.042 Acute hematogenous osteomyelitis, left hand CC
CC Excl: See code: M86.041

M86.049 Acute hematogenous osteomyelitis, unspecified hand CC
CC Excl: See code: M86.041

✓ Additional Character Required   ✓x7ᵗʰ Placeholder Alert   Unacceptable PDx   Manifestation   Hospital Acquired Condition   **EXCLUDES 1** Not Coded Here   **EXCLUDES 2** Not Included Here

ICD-10-CM 2016   771

√6th **M86.05** **Acute hematogenous osteomyelitis, femur**

M86.051 **Acute hematogenous osteomyelitis,**   CC
right femur
CC Excl: A17.9, A18.03-A18.09, A18.82,
A18.84, A18.89, M46.20-M46.39, M86.00,
M86.08-M86.10, M86.18-M86.20, M86.28-
M86.30, M86.351-M86.359, M86.38-M86.40,
M86.451-M86.459, M86.48-M86.50,
M86.551-M86.559, M86.58-M86.60,
M86.651-M86.659, M86.68-M86.8X0,
M86.8X5, M86.8X8-M86.9

M86.052 **Acute hematogenous osteomyelitis,**   CC
left femur
CC Excl: See code: M86.051

M86.059 **Acute hematogenous osteomyelitis,**   CC
unspecified femur
CC Excl: See code: M86.051

√6th **M86.06** **Acute hematogenous osteomyelitis, tibia and fibula**

M86.061 **Acute hematogenous osteomyelitis,**   CC
right tibia and fibula
CC Excl: A17.9, A18.03-A18.09, A18.82,
A18.84, A18.89, M46.20-M46.39, M86.00,
M86.08-M86.10, M86.18-M86.20, M86.28-
M86.30, M86.361-M86.369, M86.38-M86.40,
M86.461-M86.469, M86.48-M86.50,
M86.561-M86.569, M86.58-M86.60,
M86.661-M86.669, M86.68-M86.8X0,
M86.8X6, M86.8X8-M86.9

M86.062 **Acute hematogenous osteomyelitis,**   CC
left tibia and fibula
CC Excl: See code: M86.061

M86.069 **Acute hematogenous osteomyelitis,**   CC
unspecified tibia and fibula
CC Excl: See code: M86.061

√6th **M86.07** **Acute hematogenous osteomyelitis, ankle and foot**

M86.071 **Acute hematogenous osteomyelitis,**   CC
right ankle and foot
CC Excl: A17.9, A18.03-A18.09, A18.82,
A18.84, A18.89, M46.20-M46.39, M86.00,
M86.08-M86.10, M86.18-M86.20, M86.28-
M86.30, M86.371-M86.40, M86.471-M86.50,
M86.571-M86.60, M86.671-M86.8X0,
M86.8X7-M86.9

M86.072 **Acute hematogenous osteomyelitis,**   CC
left ankle and foot
CC Excl: See code: M86.071

M86.079 **Acute hematogenous osteomyelitis,**   CC
unspecified ankle and foot
CC Excl: See code: M86.071

M86.08 **Acute hematogenous osteomyelitis, other sites**   CC
CC Excl: A17.9-A18.01, A18.03-A18.09, A18.82, A18.84,
A18.89, M46.20-M46.39, M86.00-M86.9

M86.09 **Acute hematogenous osteomyelitis, multiple**   CC
sites
CC Excl: A17.9, A18.03-A18.09, A18.82, A18.84, A18.89,
M46.20-M46.39, M86.00-M86.9

√5th **M86.1** **Other acute osteomyelitis**

M86.10 **Other acute osteomyelitis, unspecified site**   CC
CC Excl: See code: 86.09

√6th **M86.11** **Other acute osteomyelitis, shoulder**

M86.111 **Other acute osteomyelitis, right**   CC
shoulder
CC Excl: See code: M86.071

M86.112 **Other acute osteomyelitis, left**   CC
shoulder
CC Excl: See code: M86.071

M86.119 **Other acute osteomyelitis,**   CC
unspecified shoulder
CC Excl: See code: M86.071

√6th **M86.12** **Other acute osteomyelitis, humerus**

M86.121 **Other acute osteomyelitis, right**   CC
humerus
CC Excl: See code: M86.021

M86.122 **Other acute osteomyelitis, left**   CC
humerus
CC Excl: See code: M86.021

M86.129 **Other acute osteomyelitis,**   CC
unspecified humerus
CC Excl: See code: M86.021

√6th **M86.13** **Other acute osteomyelitis, radius and ulna**

M86.131 **Other acute osteomyelitis, right**   CC
radius and ulna
CC Excl: See code: M86.031

M86.132 **Other acute osteomyelitis, left**   CC
radius and ulna
CC Excl: See code: M86.031

M86.139 **Other acute osteomyelitis,**   CC
unspecified radius and ulna
CC Excl: See code: M86.031

√6th **M86.14** **Other acute osteomyelitis, hand**

M86.141 **Other acute osteomyelitis, right hand**   CC
CC Excl: See code: M86.041

M86.142 **Other acute osteomyelitis, left hand**   CC
CC Excl: See code: M86.041

M86.149 **Other acute osteomyelitis,**   CC
unspecified hand
CC Excl: See code: M86.041

√6th **M86.15** **Other acute osteomyelitis, femur**

M86.151 **Other acute osteomyelitis, right femur**   CC
CC Excl: See code: M86.051

M86.152 **Other acute osteomyelitis, left femur**   CC
CC Excl: See code: M86.051

M86.159 **Other acute osteomyelitis, unspecified**   CC
femur
CC Excl: See code: M86.051

√6th **M86.16** **Other acute osteomyelitis, tibia and fibula**

M86.161 **Other acute osteomyelitis, right tibia**   CC
and fibula
CC Excl: See code: M86.061

M86.162 **Other acute osteomyelitis, left tibia**   CC
and fibula
CC Excl: See code: M86.061

M86.169 **Other acute osteomyelitis,**   CC
unspecified tibia and fibula
CC Excl: See code: M86.061

√6th **M86.17** **Other acute osteomyelitis, ankle and foot**

M86.171 **Other acute osteomyelitis, right ankle**   CC
and foot
CC Excl: See code: M86.071

M86.172 **Other acute osteomyelitis, left ankle**   CC
and foot
CC Excl: See code: M86.071

M86.179 **Other acute osteomyelitis,**   CC
unspecified ankle and foot
CC Excl: See code: M86.071

M86.18 **Other acute osteomyelitis, other site**   CC
CC Excl: A17.9-A18.01, A18.03-A18.09, A18.82, A18.84,
A18.89, M46.20-M46.39, M86.00-M86.9

M86.19 **Other acute osteomyelitis, multiple sites**   CC
CC Excl: A17.9, A18.03-A18.09, A18.82, A18.84, A18.89,
M46.20-M46.39, M86.00-M86.9

√5th **M86.2** **Subacute osteomyelitis**

M86.20 **Subacute osteomyelitis, unspecified site**   CC
CC Excl: See code: M86.19

√6th **M86.21** **Subacute osteomyelitis, shoulder**

M86.211 **Subacute osteomyelitis, right**   CC
shoulder
CC Excl: A17.9, A18.03-A18.09, A18.82,
A18.84, A18.89, M46.20-M46.39, M86.00,
M86.08-M86.10, M86.18-M86.20, M86.28-
M86.319, M86.38-M86.419, M86.48-
M86.519, M86.58-M86.619, M86.68-
M86.8X1, M86.8X8-M86.9

M86.212 **Subacute osteomyelitis, left shoulder**   CC
CC Excl: See code: M86.211

M86.219 **Subacute osteomyelitis, unspecified**   CC
shoulder
CC Excl: See code: M86.211

√6th **M86.22** **Subacute osteomyelitis, humerus**

M86.221 **Subacute osteomyelitis, right**   CC
humerus
CC Excl: A17.9, A18.03-A18.09, A18.82,
A18.84, A18.89, M46.20-M46.39, M86.00,
M86.08-M86.10, M86.18-M86.20, M86.28-
M86.30, M86.321-M86.329, M86.38-M86.40,
M86.421-M86.429, M86.48-M86.50,
M86.521-M86.529, M86.58-M86.60,
M86.621-M86.629, M86.68-M86.8X0,
M86.8X2, M86.8X8-M86.9

M86.222 **Subacute osteomyelitis, left humerus**   CC
CC Excl: See code: M86.221

M86.229 **Subacute osteomyelitis, unspecified**   CC
humerus
CC Excl: See code: M86.221

N Newborn: 0   P Pediatric: 0-17   M Maternity: 12-55   A Adult: 15-124   MCC Major CC Condition   PDxMCC PDx acts as own MCC   CC CC Condition   PDxCC PDx acts as own CC

772   ICD-10-CM 2016

√6ᵗʰ **M86.23 Subacute osteomyelitis, radius and ulna**

    M86.231 Subacute osteomyelitis, right radius and ulna `CC`
        CC Excl: A17.9, A18.03-A18.09, A18.82, A18.84, A18.89, M46.20-M46.39, M86.00, M86.08-M86.10, M86.18-M86.20, M86.28-M86.30, M86.331-M86.339, M86.38-M86.40, M86.431-M86.439, M86.48-M86.50, M86.531-M86.539, M86.58-M86.60, M86.631-M86.639, M86.68-M86.8X0, M86.8X3, M86.8X8-M86.9

    M86.232 Subacute osteomyelitis, left radius and ulna `CC`
        CC Excl: See code: M86.231

    M86.239 Subacute osteomyelitis, unspecified radius and ulna `CC`
        CC Excl: See code: M86.231

√6ᵗʰ **M86.24 Subacute osteomyelitis, hand**

    M86.241 Subacute osteomyelitis, right hand `CC`
        CC Excl: A17.9, A18.03-A18.09, A18.82, A18.84, A18.89, M46.20-M46.39, M86.00, M86.08-M86.10, M86.18-M86.20, M86.28-M86.30, M86.341-M86.349, M86.38-M86.40, M86.441-M86.449, M86.48-M86.50, M86.541-M86.549, M86.58-M86.60, M86.641-M86.649, M86.68-M86.8X0, M86.8X4, M86.8X8-M86.9

    M86.242 Subacute osteomyelitis, left hand `CC`
        CC Excl: See code: M86.241

    M86.249 Subacute osteomyelitis, unspecified hand `CC`
        CC Excl: See code: M86.241

√6ᵗʰ **M86.25 Subacute osteomyelitis, femur**

    M86.251 Subacute osteomyelitis, right femur `CC`
        CC Excl: A17.9, A18.03-A18.09, A18.82, A18.84, A18.89, M46.20-M46.39, M86.00, M86.08-M86.10, M86.18-M86.20, M86.28-M86.30, M86.351-M86.359, M86.38-M86.40, M86.451-M86.459, M86.48-M86.50, M86.551-M86.559, M86.58-M86.60, M86.651-M86.659, M86.68-M86.8X0, M86.8X5, M86.8X8-M86.9

    M86.252 Subacute osteomyelitis, left femur `CC`
        CC Excl: See code: M86.251

    M86.259 Subacute osteomyelitis, unspecified femur `CC`
        CC Excl: See code: M86.251

√6ᵗʰ **M86.26 Subacute osteomyelitis, tibia and fibula**

    M86.261 Subacute osteomyelitis, right tibia and fibula `CC`
        CC Excl: A17.9, A18.03-A18.09, A18.82, A18.84, A18.89, M46.20-M46.39, M86.00, M86.08-M86.10, M86.18-M86.20, M86.28-M86.30, M86.361-M86.369, M86.38-M86.40, M86.461-M86.469, M86.48-M86.50, M86.561-M86.569, M86.58-M86.60, M86.661-M86.669, M86.68-M86.8X0, M86.8X6, M86.8X8-M86.9

    M86.262 Subacute osteomyelitis, left tibia and fibula `CC`
        CC Excl: See code: M86.261

    M86.269 Subacute osteomyelitis, unspecified tibia and fibula `CC`
        CC Excl: See code: M86.261

√6ᵗʰ **M86.27 Subacute osteomyelitis, ankle and foot**

    M86.271 Subacute osteomyelitis, right ankle and foot `CC`
        CC Excl: A17.9, A18.03-A18.09, A18.82, A18.84, A18.89, M46.20-M46.39, M86.00, M86.08-M86.10, M86.18-M86.20, M86.28-M86.30, M86.371-M86.40, M86.471-M86.50, M86.571-M86.60, M86.671-M86.8X0, M86.8X7-M86.9

    M86.272 Subacute osteomyelitis, left ankle and foot `CC`
        CC Excl: See code: M86.271

    M86.279 Subacute osteomyelitis, unspecified ankle and foot `CC`
        CC Excl: See code: M86.271

M86.28 Subacute osteomyelitis, other site `CC`
    CC Excl: A17.9-A18.01, A18.03-A18.09, A18.82, A18.84, A18.89, M46.20-M46.39, M86.00-M86.9

M86.29 Subacute osteomyelitis, multiple sites `CC`
    CC Excl: A17.9, A18.03-A18.09, A18.82, A18.84, A18.89, M46.20-M46.39, M86.00-M86.9

√5ᵗʰ **M86.3 Chronic multifocal osteomyelitis**

    M86.30 Chronic multifocal osteomyelitis, unspecified site `CC`
        CC Excl: M46.20-M46.39, M86.30-M86.9, M88.0-M88.9, M90.60-M90.69

√6ᵗʰ **M86.31 Chronic multifocal osteomyelitis, shoulder**

    M86.311 Chronic multifocal osteomyelitis, right shoulder `CC`
        CC Excl: A02.24, A17.9, A18.03-A18.09, A18.82, A18.84, A18.89, M46.20-M46.39, M86.00-M86.9

    M86.312 Chronic multifocal osteomyelitis, left shoulder `CC`
        CC Excl: See code: M86.311

    M86.319 Chronic multifocal osteomyelitis, unspecified shoulder `CC`
        CC Excl: See code: M86.311

√6ᵗʰ **M86.32 Chronic multifocal osteomyelitis, humerus**

    M86.321 Chronic multifocal osteomyelitis, right humerus `CC`
        CC Excl: See code: M86.311

    M86.322 Chronic multifocal osteomyelitis, left humerus `CC`
        CC Excl: See code: M86.311

    M86.329 Chronic multifocal osteomyelitis, unspecified humerus `CC`
        CC Excl: See code: M86.311

√6ᵗʰ **M86.33 Chronic multifocal osteomyelitis, radius and ulna**

    M86.331 Chronic multifocal osteomyelitis, right radius and ulna `CC`
        CC Excl: See code: M86.311

    M86.332 Chronic multifocal osteomyelitis, left radius and ulna `CC`
        CC Excl: See code: M86.311

    M86.339 Chronic multifocal osteomyelitis, unspecified radius and ulna `CC`
        CC Excl: See code: M86.311

√6ᵗʰ **M86.34 Chronic multifocal osteomyelitis, hand**

    M86.341 Chronic multifocal osteomyelitis, right hand `CC`
        CC Excl: See code: M86.311

    M86.342 Chronic multifocal osteomyelitis, left hand `CC`
        CC Excl: See code: M86.311

    M86.349 Chronic multifocal osteomyelitis, unspecified hand `CC`
        CC Excl: See code: M86.311

√6ᵗʰ **M86.35 Chronic multifocal osteomyelitis, femur**

    M86.351 Chronic multifocal osteomyelitis, right femur `CC`
        CC Excl: See code: M86.311

    M86.352 Chronic multifocal osteomyelitis, left femur `CC`
        CC Excl: See code: M86.311

    M86.359 Chronic multifocal osteomyelitis, unspecified femur `CC`
        CC Excl: See code: M86.311

√6ᵗʰ **M86.36 Chronic multifocal osteomyelitis, tibia and fibula**

    M86.361 Chronic multifocal osteomyelitis, right tibia and fibula `CC`
        CC Excl: See code: M86.311

    M86.362 Chronic multifocal osteomyelitis, left tibia and fibula `CC`
        CC Excl: See code: M86.311

    M86.369 Chronic multifocal osteomyelitis, unspecified tibia and fibula `CC`
        CC Excl: See code: M86.311

√6ᵗʰ **M86.37 Chronic multifocal osteomyelitis, ankle and foot**

    M86.371 Chronic multifocal osteomyelitis, right ankle and foot `CC`
        CC Excl: See code: M86.311

    M86.372 Chronic multifocal osteomyelitis, left ankle and foot `CC`
        CC Excl: See code: M86.311

    M86.379 Chronic multifocal osteomyelitis, unspecified ankle and foot `CC`
        CC Excl: See code: M86.311

    M86.38 Chronic multifocal osteomyelitis, other site `CC`
        CC Excl: See code: 86.311

    M86.39 Chronic multifocal osteomyelitis, multiple sites `CC`
        CC Excl: See code: 86.311

√ Additional Character Required   √x7ᵗʰ Placeholder Alert   Unacceptable PDx   Manifestation   Hospital Acquired Condition   **EXCLUDES1** Not Coded Here   **EXCLUDES2** Not Included Here

Chapter 13. Diseases of the Musculoskeletal System and Connective Tissue

M86.23–M86.39

Chapter 13. Diseases of the Musculoskeletal System and Connective Tissue

M86.4–M86.632

√5ᵗʰ **M86.4 Chronic osteomyelitis with draining sinus**

> **CC Excl: For CC codes in subcategory M86.4, M86.5, M86.6, M86.8, M86.9, unless otherwise noted:** A02.24, A17.9, A18.03-A18.09, A18.82, A18.84, A18.89, M46.20-M46.39, M86.00-M86.9

M86.40 Chronic osteomyelitis with draining sinus, unspecified site CC
> **CC Excl:** M46.20-M46.39, M86.30-M86.9, M88.0-M88.9, M90.60-M90.69

√6ᵗʰ **M86.41 Chronic osteomyelitis with draining sinus, shoulder**

M86.411 Chronic osteomyelitis with draining sinus, right shoulder CC

M86.412 Chronic osteomyelitis with draining sinus, left shoulder CC

M86.419 Chronic osteomyelitis with draining sinus, unspecified shoulder CC

√6ᵗʰ **M86.42 Chronic osteomyelitis with draining sinus, humerus**

M86.421 Chronic osteomyelitis with draining sinus, right humerus CC

M86.422 Chronic osteomyelitis with draining sinus, left humerus CC

M86.429 Chronic osteomyelitis with draining sinus, unspecified humerus CC

√6ᵗʰ **M86.43 Chronic osteomyelitis with draining sinus, radius and ulna**

M86.431 Chronic osteomyelitis with draining sinus, right radius and ulna CC

M86.432 Chronic osteomyelitis with draining sinus, left radius and ulna CC

M86.439 Chronic osteomyelitis with draining sinus, unspecified radius and ulna CC

√6ᵗʰ **M86.44 Chronic osteomyelitis with draining sinus, hand**

M86.441 Chronic osteomyelitis with draining sinus, right hand CC

M86.442 Chronic osteomyelitis with draining sinus, left hand CC

M86.449 Chronic osteomyelitis with draining sinus, unspecified hand CC

√6ᵗʰ **M86.45 Chronic osteomyelitis with draining sinus, femur**

M86.451 Chronic osteomyelitis with draining sinus, right femur CC

M86.452 Chronic osteomyelitis with draining sinus, left femur CC

M86.459 Chronic osteomyelitis with draining sinus, unspecified femur CC

√6ᵗʰ **M86.46 Chronic osteomyelitis with draining sinus, tibia and fibula**

M86.461 Chronic osteomyelitis with draining sinus, right tibia and fibula CC

M86.462 Chronic osteomyelitis with draining sinus, left tibia and fibula CC

M86.469 Chronic osteomyelitis with draining sinus, unspecified tibia and fibula CC

√6ᵗʰ **M86.47 Chronic osteomyelitis with draining sinus, ankle and foot**

M86.471 Chronic osteomyelitis with draining sinus, right ankle and foot CC

M86.472 Chronic osteomyelitis with draining sinus, left ankle and foot CC

M86.479 Chronic osteomyelitis with draining sinus, unspecified ankle and foot CC

M86.48 Chronic osteomyelitis with draining sinus, other site CC

M86.49 Chronic osteomyelitis with draining sinus, multiple sites CC

√5ᵗʰ **M86.5 Other chronic hematogenous osteomyelitis**

M86.50 Other chronic hematogenous osteomyelitis, unspecified site CC
> **CC Excl:** M46.20-M46.39, M86.30-M86.9, M88.0-M88.9, M90.60-M90.69

√6ᵗʰ **M86.51 Other chronic hematogenous osteomyelitis, shoulder**

M86.511 Other chronic hematogenous osteomyelitis, right shoulder CC

M86.512 Other chronic hematogenous osteomyelitis, left shoulder CC

M86.519 Other chronic hematogenous osteomyelitis, unspecified shoulder CC

√6ᵗʰ **M86.52 Other chronic hematogenous osteomyelitis, humerus**

M86.521 Other chronic hematogenous osteomyelitis, right humerus CC

M86.522 Other chronic hematogenous osteomyelitis, left humerus CC

M86.529 Other chronic hematogenous osteomyelitis, unspecified humerus CC

√6ᵗʰ **M86.53 Other chronic hematogenous osteomyelitis, radius and ulna**

M86.531 Other chronic hematogenous osteomyelitis, right radius and ulna CC

M86.532 Other chronic hematogenous osteomyelitis, left radius and ulna CC

M86.539 Other chronic hematogenous osteomyelitis, unspecified radius and ulna CC

√6ᵗʰ **M86.54 Other chronic hematogenous osteomyelitis, hand**

M86.541 Other chronic hematogenous osteomyelitis, right hand CC

M86.542 Other chronic hematogenous osteomyelitis, left hand CC

M86.549 Other chronic hematogenous osteomyelitis, unspecified hand CC

√6ᵗʰ **M86.55 Other chronic hematogenous osteomyelitis, femur**

M86.551 Other chronic hematogenous osteomyelitis, right femur CC

M86.552 Other chronic hematogenous osteomyelitis, left femur CC

M86.559 Other chronic hematogenous osteomyelitis, unspecified femur CC

√6ᵗʰ **M86.56 Other chronic hematogenous osteomyelitis, tibia and fibula**

M86.561 Other chronic hematogenous osteomyelitis, right tibia and fibula CC

M86.562 Other chronic hematogenous osteomyelitis, left tibia and fibula CC

M86.569 Other chronic hematogenous osteomyelitis, unspecified tibia and fibula CC

√6ᵗʰ **M86.57 Other chronic hematogenous osteomyelitis, ankle and foot**

M86.571 Other chronic hematogenous osteomyelitis, right ankle and foot CC

M86.572 Other chronic hematogenous osteomyelitis, left ankle and foot CC

M86.579 Other chronic hematogenous osteomyelitis, unspecified ankle and foot CC

M86.58 Other chronic hematogenous osteomyelitis, other site CC

M86.59 Other chronic hematogenous osteomyelitis, multiple sites CC

√5ᵗʰ **M86.6 Other chronic osteomyelitis**

M86.60 Other chronic osteomyelitis, unspecified site CC
> **CC Excl:** M46.20-M46.39, M86.30-M86.9, M88.0-M88.9, M90.60-M90.69

√6ᵗʰ **M86.61 Other chronic osteomyelitis, shoulder**

M86.611 Other chronic osteomyelitis, right shoulder CC

M86.612 Other chronic osteomyelitis, left shoulder CC

M86.619 Other chronic osteomyelitis, unspecified shoulder CC

√6ᵗʰ **M86.62 Other chronic osteomyelitis, humerus**

M86.621 Other chronic osteomyelitis, right humerus CC

M86.622 Other chronic osteomyelitis, left humerus CC

M86.629 Other chronic osteomyelitis, unspecified humerus CC

√6ᵗʰ **M86.63 Other chronic osteomyelitis, radius and ulna**

M86.631 Other chronic osteomyelitis, right radius and ulna CC

M86.632 Other chronic osteomyelitis, left radius and ulna CC

N Newborn: 0   P Pediatric: 0-17   M Maternity: 12-55   A Adult: 15-124   **MCC** Major CC Condition   **PDxMCC** PDx acts as own MCC   **CC** CC Condition   **PDxCC** PDx acts as own CC

774   ICD-10-CM 2016

M86.639 **Other chronic osteomyelitis, unspecified radius and ulna** `CC`

√6ᵗʰ **M86.64 Other chronic osteomyelitis, hand**

 M86.641 **Other chronic osteomyelitis, right hand** `CC`

 M86.642 **Other chronic osteomyelitis, left hand** `CC`

 M86.649 **Other chronic osteomyelitis, unspecified hand** `CC`

√6ᵗʰ **M86.65 Other chronic osteomyelitis, thigh**

 M86.651 **Other chronic osteomyelitis, right thigh** `CC`

 M86.652 **Other chronic osteomyelitis, left thigh** `CC`

 M86.659 **Other chronic osteomyelitis, unspecified thigh** `CC`

√6ᵗʰ **M86.66 Other chronic osteomyelitis, tibia and fibula**

 M86.661 **Other chronic osteomyelitis, right tibia and fibula** `CC`

 M86.662 **Other chronic osteomyelitis, left tibia and fibula** `CC`

 M86.669 **Other chronic osteomyelitis, unspecified tibia and fibula** `CC`

√6ᵗʰ **M86.67 Other chronic osteomyelitis, ankle and foot**

 M86.671 **Other chronic osteomyelitis, right ankle and foot** `CC`

 M86.672 **Other chronic osteomyelitis, left ankle and foot** `CC`

 M86.679 **Other chronic osteomyelitis, unspecified ankle and foot** `CC`

M86.68 **Other chronic osteomyelitis, other site** `CC`

M86.69 **Other chronic osteomyelitis, multiple sites** `CC`

√5ᵗʰ **M86.8 Other osteomyelitis**
 Brodie's abscess

√6ᵗʰ **M86.8X Other osteomyelitis**

 M86.8X0 **Other osteomyelitis, multiple sites** `CC`

 M86.8X1 **Other osteomyelitis, shoulder** `CC`

 M86.8X2 **Other osteomyelitis, upper arm** `CC`

 M86.8X3 **Other osteomyelitis, forearm** `CC`

 M86.8X4 **Other osteomyelitis, hand** `CC`

 M86.8X5 **Other osteomyelitis, thigh** `CC`

 M86.8X6 **Other osteomyelitis, lower leg** `CC`

 M86.8X7 **Other osteomyelitis, ankle and foot** `CC`

 M86.8X8 **Other osteomyelitis, other site** `CC`

 M86.8X9 **Other osteomyelitis, unspecified sites** `CC`
  CC Excl: M46.20-M46.39, M86.30-M86.9, M88.0-M88.9, M90.60-M90.69

M86.9 **Osteomyelitis, unspecified** `CC`
 Infection of bone NOS
 Periostitis without osteomyelitis
 CC Excl: See code: M86.8X9

√4ᵗʰ **M87 Osteonecrosis**
 INCLUDES avascular necrosis of bone
 Use additional code to identify major osseous defect, if applicable (M89.7-)
 EXCLUDES 1 juvenile osteonecrosis (M91-M92)
  osteochondropathies (M90-M93)

√5ᵗʰ **M87.0 Idiopathic aseptic necrosis of bone**

 M87.00 **Idiopathic aseptic necrosis of unspecified bone** `CC`
  CC Excl: M87.00-M87.9, M90.50-M90.59

√6ᵗʰ   M87.01 **Idiopathic aseptic necrosis of shoulder**
  Idiopathic aseptic necrosis of clavicle and scapula

  M87.011 **Idiopathic aseptic necrosis of right shoulder** `CC`
   CC Excl: M87.00-M87.050, M87.061-M87.073, M87.077-M87.146, M87.161-M87.173, M87.177-M87.250, M87.261-M87.273, M87.277-M87.346, M87.361-M87.373, M87.377-M87.849, M87.861-M87.873, M87.877-M87.9, M90.50-M90.549, M90.561-M90.59

  M87.012 **Idiopathic aseptic necrosis of left shoulder** `CC`
   CC Excl: See code: M87.011

  M87.019 **Idiopathic aseptic necrosis of unspecified shoulder** `CC`
   CC Excl: See code: M87.011

√6ᵗʰ **M87.02 Idiopathic aseptic necrosis of humerus**

 M87.021 **Idiopathic aseptic necrosis of right humerus** `CC`
  CC Excl: See code: M87.011

 M87.022 **Idiopathic aseptic necrosis of left humerus** `CC`
  CC Excl: See code: M87.011

 M87.029 **Idiopathic aseptic necrosis of unspecified humerus** `CC`
  CC Excl: See code: M87.011

√6ᵗʰ **M87.03 Idiopathic aseptic necrosis of radius, ulna and carpus**

 M87.031 **Idiopathic aseptic necrosis of right radius** `CC`
  CC Excl: M87.00-M87.9, M90.50-M90.59

 M87.032 **Idiopathic aseptic necrosis of left radius** `CC`
  CC Excl: See code: M87.31

 M87.033 **Idiopathic aseptic necrosis of unspecified radius** `CC`
  CC Excl: See code: M87.31

 M87.034 **Idiopathic aseptic necrosis of right ulna** `CC`
  CC Excl: See code: M87.31

 M87.035 **Idiopathic aseptic necrosis of left ulna** `CC`
  CC Excl: See code: M87.31

 M87.036 **Idiopathic aseptic necrosis of unspecified ulna** `CC`
  CC Excl: See code: M87.31

 M87.037 **Idiopathic aseptic necrosis of right carpus** `CC`
  CC Excl: See code: M87.31

 M87.038 **Idiopathic aseptic necrosis of left carpus** `CC`
  CC Excl: See code: M87.31

 M87.039 **Idiopathic aseptic necrosis of unspecified carpus** `CC`
  CC Excl: See code: M87.31

√6ᵗʰ **M87.04 Idiopathic aseptic necrosis of hand and fingers**
 Idiopathic aseptic necrosis of metacarpals and phalanges of hands

 M87.041 **Idiopathic aseptic necrosis of right hand** `CC`
  CC Excl: See code: M87.31

 M87.042 **Idiopathic aseptic necrosis of left hand** `CC`
  CC Excl: See code: M87.31

 M87.043 **Idiopathic aseptic necrosis of unspecified hand** `CC`
  CC Excl: See code: M87.31

 M87.044 **Idiopathic aseptic necrosis of right finger(s)** `CC`
  CC Excl: See code: M87.31

 M87.045 **Idiopathic aseptic necrosis of left finger(s)** `CC`
  CC Excl: See code: M87.31

 M87.046 **Idiopathic aseptic necrosis of unspecified finger(s)** `CC`
  CC Excl: See code: M87.31

√6ᵗʰ **M87.05 Idiopathic aseptic necrosis of pelvis and femur**

 M87.050 **Idiopathic aseptic necrosis of pelvis** `CC`
  CC Excl: See code: M87.31

 M87.051 **Idiopathic aseptic necrosis of right femur** `CC`
  CC Excl: M87.00, M87.031-M87.073, M87.077-M87.119, M87.131-M87.173, M87.177-M87.219, M87.231-M87.273, M87.277-M87.319, M87.331-M87.373, M87.377-M87.819, M87.831-M87.873, M87.877-M87.9, M90.50, M90.521-M90.59

 M87.052 **Idiopathic aseptic necrosis of left femur** `CC`
  CC Excl: See code: M87.051

 M87.059 **Idiopathic aseptic necrosis of unspecified femur** `CC`
  Idiopathic aseptic necrosis of hip NOS
  CC Excl: See code: M87.051

√6ᵗʰ **M87.06 Idiopathic aseptic necrosis of tibia and fibula**

 M87.061 **Idiopathic aseptic necrosis of right tibia** `CC`
  CC Excl: M87.00-M87.9, M90.50-M90.59

 M87.062 **Idiopathic aseptic necrosis of left tibia** `CC`
  CC Excl: See code: M87.61

M87.063 Idiopathic aseptic necrosis of unspecified tibia `CC`
CC Excl: See code: M87.61

M87.064 Idiopathic aseptic necrosis of right fibula `CC`
CC Excl: See code: M87.61

M87.065 Idiopathic aseptic necrosis of left fibula `CC`
CC Excl: See code: M87.61

M87.066 Idiopathic aseptic necrosis of unspecified fibula `CC`
CC Excl: See code: M87.61

√6ᵗʰ **M87.07 Idiopathic aseptic necrosis of ankle, foot and toes**
Idiopathic aseptic necrosis of metatarsus, tarsus, and phalanges of toes

M87.071 Idiopathic aseptic necrosis of right ankle `CC`
CC Excl: See code: M87.61

M87.072 Idiopathic aseptic necrosis of left ankle `CC`
CC Excl: See code: M87.61

M87.073 Idiopathic aseptic necrosis of unspecified ankle `CC`
CC Excl: See code: M87.61

M87.074 Idiopathic aseptic necrosis of right foot `CC`
CC Excl: M87.00, M87.031-M87.050, M87.061-M87.119, M87.131-M87.146, M87.161-M87.219, M87.231-M87.250, M87.261-M87.319, M87.331-M87.346, M87.361-M87.819, M87.831-M87.849, M87.861-M87.9, M90.50, M90.521-M90.549, M90.561-M90.59

M87.075 Idiopathic aseptic necrosis of left foot `CC`
CC Excl: See code: M87.074

M87.076 Idiopathic aseptic necrosis of unspecified foot `CC`
CC Excl: See code: M87.074

M87.077 Idiopathic aseptic necrosis of right toe(s) `CC`
CC Excl: M87.00-M87.9, M90.50-M90.59

M87.078 Idiopathic aseptic necrosis of left toe(s) `CC`
CC Excl: See code: M87.077

M87.079 Idiopathic aseptic necrosis of unspecified toe(s) `CC`
CC Excl: See code: M87.077

M87.08 Idiopathic aseptic necrosis of bone, other site `CC`
CC Excl: See code: M87.077

M87.09 Idiopathic aseptic necrosis of bone, multiple sites `CC`
CC Excl: See code: M87.077

√5ᵗʰ **M87.1 Osteonecrosis due to drugs**
Use additional code for adverse effect, if applicable, to identify drug (T36-T50 with fifth or sixth character 5)

M87.10 Osteonecrosis due to drugs, unspecified bone `CC`
CC Excl: See code: M87.00

√6ᵗʰ **M87.11 Osteonecrosis due to drugs, shoulder**

M87.111 Osteonecrosis due to drugs, right shoulder `CC`
CC Excl: See code: M87.77

M87.112 Osteonecrosis due to drugs, left shoulder `CC`
CC Excl: See code: M87.77

M87.119 Osteonecrosis due to drugs, unspecified shoulder `CC`
CC Excl: See code: M87.77

√6ᵗʰ **M87.12 Osteonecrosis due to drugs, humerus**

M87.121 Osteonecrosis due to drugs, right humerus `CC`
CC Excl: M87.00-M87.050, M87.061-M87.073, M87.077-M87.146, M87.161-M87.173, M87.177-M87.250, M87.261-M87.273, M87.277-M87.346, M87.361-M87.373, M87.377-M87.849, M87.861-M87.873, M87.877-M87.9, M90.50-M90.549, M90.561-M90.59

M87.122 Osteonecrosis due to drugs, left humerus `CC`
CC Excl: See code: M87.121

M87.129 Osteonecrosis due to drugs, unspecified humerus `CC`
CC Excl: See code: M87.121

√6ᵗʰ **M87.13 Osteonecrosis due to drugs of radius, ulna and carpus**

M87.131 Osteonecrosis due to drugs of right radius `CC`
CC Excl: See code: M87.077

M87.132 Osteonecrosis due to drugs of left radius `CC`
CC Excl: See code: M87.077

M87.133 Osteonecrosis due to drugs of unspecified radius `CC`
CC Excl: See code: M87.077

M87.134 Osteonecrosis due to drugs of right ulna `CC`
CC Excl: See code: M87.077

M87.135 Osteonecrosis due to drugs of left ulna `CC`
CC Excl: See code: M87.077

M87.136 Osteonecrosis due to drugs of unspecified ulna `CC`
CC Excl: See code: M87.077

M87.137 Osteonecrosis due to drugs of right carpus `CC`
CC Excl: See code: M87.077

M87.138 Osteonecrosis due to drugs of left carpus `CC`
CC Excl: See code: M87.077

M87.139 Osteonecrosis due to drugs of unspecified carpus `CC`
CC Excl: See code: M87.077

√6ᵗʰ **M87.14 Osteonecrosis due to drugs, hand and fingers**

M87.141 Osteonecrosis due to drugs, right hand `CC`
CC Excl: See code: M87.077

M87.142 Osteonecrosis due to drugs, left hand `CC`
CC Excl: See code: M87.077

M87.143 Osteonecrosis due to drugs, unspecified hand `CC`
CC Excl: See code: M87.077

M87.144 Osteonecrosis due to drugs, right finger(s) `CC`
CC Excl: See code: M87.077

M87.145 Osteonecrosis due to drugs, left finger(s) `CC`
CC Excl: See code: M87.077

M87.146 Osteonecrosis due to drugs, unspecified finger(s) `CC`
CC Excl: See code: M87.077

√6ᵗʰ **M87.15 Osteonecrosis due to drugs, pelvis and femur**

M87.150 Osteonecrosis due to drugs, pelvis `CC`
CC Excl: M87.00, M87.031-M87.073, M87.077-M87.119, M87.131-M87.173, M87.177-M87.219, M87.231-M87.273, M87.277-M87.319, M87.331-M87.373, M87.377-M87.819, M87.831-M87.873, M87.877-M87.9, M90.50, M90.521-M90.59

M87.151 Osteonecrosis due to drugs, right femur `CC`
CC Excl: See code: M87.150

M87.152 Osteonecrosis due to drugs, left femur `CC`
CC Excl: See code: M87.150

M87.159 Osteonecrosis due to drugs, unspecified femur `CC`
CC Excl: See code: M87.150

√6ᵗʰ **M87.16 Osteonecrosis due to drugs, tibia and fibula**

M87.161 Osteonecrosis due to drugs, right tibia `CC`
CC Excl: M87.00-M87.9, M90.50-M90.59

M87.162 Osteonecrosis due to drugs, left tibia `CC`
CC Excl: See code: M87.161

M87.163 Osteonecrosis due to drugs, unspecified tibia `CC`
CC Excl: See code: M87.161

M87.164 Osteonecrosis due to drugs, right fibula `CC`
CC Excl: See code: M87.161

M87.165 Osteonecrosis due to drugs, left fibula `CC`
CC Excl: See code: M87.161

M87.166 Osteonecrosis due to drugs, unspecified fibula `CC`
CC Excl: See code: M87.161

✓6ᵗʰ **M87.17 Osteonecrosis due to drugs, ankle, foot and toes**

  M87.171 Osteonecrosis due to drugs, right ankle CC
    CC Excl: See code: M87.161

  M87.172 Osteonecrosis due to drugs, left ankle CC
    CC Excl: See code: M87.161

  M87.173 Osteonecrosis due to drugs, unspecified ankle CC
    CC Excl: See code: M87.161

  M87.174 Osteonecrosis due to drugs, right foot CC
    CC Excl: M87.00, M87.031-M87.050, M87.061-M87.119, M87.131-M87.146, M87.161-M87.219, M87.231-M87.250, M87.261-M87.319, M87.331-M87.346, M87.361-M87.819, M87.831-M87.849, M87.861-M87.9, M90.50, M90.521-M90.549, M90.561-M90.59

  M87.175 Osteonecrosis due to drugs, left foot CC
    CC Excl: See code: M87.174

  M87.176 Osteonecrosis due to drugs, unspecified foot CC
    CC Excl: See code: M87.174

  M87.177 Osteonecrosis due to drugs, right toe(s) CC
    CC Excl: See code: M87.161

  M87.178 Osteonecrosis due to drugs, left toe(s) CC
    CC Excl: See code: M87.161

  M87.179 Osteonecrosis due to drugs, unspecified toe(s) CC
    CC Excl: See code: M87.161

✓6ᵗʰ **M87.18 Osteonecrosis due to drugs, other site**

  M87.180 Osteonecrosis due to drugs, jaw CC
    CC Excl: See code: M87.161

  M87.188 Osteonecrosis due to drugs, other site CC
    CC Excl: See code: M87.161

M87.19 Osteonecrosis due to drugs, multiple sites CC
  CC Excl: See code: M87.161

✓5ᵗʰ **M87.2 Osteonecrosis due to previous trauma**

M87.20 Osteonecrosis due to previous trauma, unspecified bone CC
  CC Excl: See code: M87.161

✓6ᵗʰ **M87.21 Osteonecrosis due to previous trauma, shoulder**

  M87.211 Osteonecrosis due to previous trauma, right shoulder CC
    CC Excl: See code: M87.161

  M87.212 Osteonecrosis due to previous trauma, left shoulder CC
    CC Excl: See code: M87.161

  M87.219 Osteonecrosis due to previous trauma, unspecified shoulder CC
    CC Excl: See code: M87.161

✓6ᵗʰ **M87.22 Osteonecrosis due to previous trauma, humerus**

  M87.221 Osteonecrosis due to previous trauma, right humerus CC
    CC Excl: M87.00-M87.050, M87.061-M87.073, M87.077-M87.146, M87.161-M87.173, M87.177-M87.250, M87.261-M87.273, M87.277-M87.346, M87.361-M87.373, M87.377-M87.849, M87.861-M87.873, M87.877-M87.9, M90.50-M90.549, M90.561-M90.59

  M87.222 Osteonecrosis due to previous trauma, left humerus CC
    CC Excl: See code: M87.221

  M87.229 Osteonecrosis due to previous trauma, unspecified humerus CC
    CC Excl: See code: M87.221

✓6ᵗʰ **M87.23 Osteonecrosis due to previous trauma of radius, ulna and carpus**

  M87.231 Osteonecrosis due to previous trauma of right radius CC
    CC Excl: See code: M87.161

  M87.232 Osteonecrosis due to previous trauma of left radius CC
    CC Excl: See code: M87.161

  M87.233 Osteonecrosis due to previous trauma of unspecified radius CC
    CC Excl: See code: M87.161

  M87.234 Osteonecrosis due to previous trauma of right ulna CC
    CC Excl: See code: M87.161

  M87.235 Osteonecrosis due to previous trauma of left ulna CC
    CC Excl: See code: M87.161

  M87.236 Osteonecrosis due to previous trauma of unspecified ulna CC
    CC Excl: See code: M87.161

  M87.237 Osteonecrosis due to previous trauma of right carpus CC
    CC Excl: See code: M87.161

  M87.238 Osteonecrosis due to previous trauma of left carpus CC
    CC Excl: See code: M87.161

  M87.239 Osteonecrosis due to previous trauma of unspecified carpus CC
    CC Excl: See code: M87.161

✓6ᵗʰ **M87.24 Osteonecrosis due to previous trauma, hand and fingers**

  M87.241 Osteonecrosis due to previous trauma, right hand CC
    CC Excl: See code: M87.161

  M87.242 Osteonecrosis due to previous trauma, left hand CC
    CC Excl: See code: M87.161

  M87.243 Osteonecrosis due to previous trauma, unspecified hand CC
    CC Excl: See code: M87.161

  M87.244 Osteonecrosis due to previous trauma, right finger(s) CC
    CC Excl: See code: M87.161

  M87.245 Osteonecrosis due to previous trauma, left finger(s) CC
    CC Excl: See code: M87.161

  M87.246 Osteonecrosis due to previous trauma, unspecified finger(s) CC
    CC Excl: See code: M87.161

✓6ᵗʰ **M87.25 Osteonecrosis due to previous trauma, pelvis and femur**

  M87.250 Osteonecrosis due to previous trauma, pelvis CC
    CC Excl: M87.00-M87.9, M90.50-M90.59

  M87.251 Osteonecrosis due to previous trauma, right femur CC
    CC Excl: M87.00, M87.031-M87.073, M87.077-M87.119, M87.131-M87.173, M87.177-M87.219, M87.231-M87.273, M87.277-M87.319, M87.331-M87.373, M87.377-M87.819, M87.831-M87.873, M87.877-M87.9, M90.50, M90.521-M90.59

  M87.252 Osteonecrosis due to previous trauma, left femur CC
    CC Excl: See code: M87.251

  M87.256 Osteonecrosis due to previous trauma, unspecified femur CC
    CC Excl: See code: M87.251

✓6ᵗʰ **M87.26 Osteonecrosis due to previous trauma, tibia and fibula**

  M87.261 Osteonecrosis due to previous trauma, right tibia CC
    CC Excl: See code: M87.250

  M87.262 Osteonecrosis due to previous trauma, left tibia CC
    CC Excl: See code: M87.250

  M87.263 Osteonecrosis due to previous trauma, unspecified tibia CC
    CC Excl: See code: M87.250

  M87.264 Osteonecrosis due to previous trauma, right fibula CC
    CC Excl: See code: M87.250

  M87.265 Osteonecrosis due to previous trauma, left fibula CC
    CC Excl: See code: M87.250

  M87.266 Osteonecrosis due to previous trauma, unspecified fibula CC
    CC Excl: See code: M87.250

✓6ᵗʰ **M87.27 Osteonecrosis due to previous trauma, ankle, foot and toes**

  M87.271 Osteonecrosis due to previous trauma, right ankle CC
    CC Excl: See code: M87.250

  M87.272 Osteonecrosis due to previous trauma, left ankle CC
    CC Excl: See code: M87.250

M87.273   **Osteonecrosis due to previous trauma, CC unspecified ankle**
CC Excl: See code: M87.250

M87.274   **Osteonecrosis due to previous trauma, CC right foot**
CC Excl: M87.00, M87.031-M87.050,
M87.061-M87.119, M87.131-M87.146,
M87.161-M87.219, M87.231-M87.250,
M87.261-M87.319, M87.331-M87.346,
M87.361-M87.819, M87.831-M87.849,
M87.861-M87.9, M90.50, M90.521-M90.549,
M90.561-M90.59

M87.275   **Osteonecrosis due to previous trauma, CC left foot**
CC Excl: See code: M87.274

M87.276   **Osteonecrosis due to previous trauma, CC unspecified foot**
CC Excl: See code: M87.274

M87.277   **Osteonecrosis due to previous trauma, CC right toe(s)**
CC Excl: See code: M87.250

M87.278   **Osteonecrosis due to previous trauma, CC left toe(s)**
CC Excl: See code: M87.250

M87.279   **Osteonecrosis due to previous trauma, CC unspecified toe(s)**
CC Excl: See code: M87.250

M87.28   **Osteonecrosis due to previous trauma, other site** CC
CC Excl: See code: M87.250

M87.29   **Osteonecrosis due to previous trauma, multiple** CC **sites**
CC Excl: See code: M87.250

☑5ᵗʰ   **M87.3**   **Other secondary osteonecrosis**

M87.30   **Other secondary osteonecrosis, unspecified bone** CC
CC Excl: M87.00-M87.9, M90.50-M90.59

☑6ᵗʰ   **M87.31**   **Other secondary osteonecrosis, shoulder**

M87.311   **Other secondary osteonecrosis, right** CC **shoulder**
CC Excl: See code: M87.30

M87.312   **Other secondary osteonecrosis, left** CC **shoulder**
CC Excl: See code: M87.30

M87.319   **Other secondary osteonecrosis,** CC **unspecified shoulder**
CC Excl: See code: M87.30

☑6ᵗʰ   **M87.32**   **Other secondary osteonecrosis, humerus**

M87.321   **Other secondary osteonecrosis, right** CC **humerus**
CC Excl: M87.00-M87.050, M87.061-
M87.073, M87.077-M87.146, M87.161-
M87.173, M87.177-M87.250, M87.261-
M87.273, M87.277-M87.346, M87.361-
M87.373, M87.377-M87.849, M87.861-
M87.873, M87.877-M87.9, M90.50-M90.549,
M90.561-M90.59

M87.322   **Other secondary osteonecrosis, left** CC **humerus**
CC Excl: See code: M87.321

M87.329   **Other secondary osteonecrosis,** CC **unspecified humerus**
CC Excl: See code: M87.321

☑6ᵗʰ   **M87.33**   **Other secondary osteonecrosis of radius, ulna and carpus**

M87.331   **Other secondary osteonecrosis of right** CC **radius**
CC Excl: See code: M87.30

M87.332   **Other secondary osteonecrosis of left** CC **radius**
CC Excl: See code: M87.30

M87.333   **Other secondary osteonecrosis of** CC **unspecified radius**
CC Excl: See code: M87.30

M87.334   **Other secondary osteonecrosis of right** CC **ulna**
CC Excl: See code: M87.30

M87.335   **Other secondary osteonecrosis of left** CC **ulna**
CC Excl: See code: M87.30

M87.336   **Other secondary osteonecrosis of** CC **unspecified ulna**
CC Excl: See code: M87.30

M87.337   **Other secondary osteonecrosis of right** CC **carpus**
CC Excl: See code: M87.30

M87.338   **Other secondary osteonecrosis of left** CC **carpus**
CC Excl: See code: M87.30

M87.339   **Other secondary osteonecrosis of** CC **unspecified carpus**
CC Excl: See code: M87.30

☑6ᵗʰ   **M87.34**   **Other secondary osteonecrosis, hand and fingers**

M87.341   **Other secondary osteonecrosis, right** CC **hand**
CC Excl: See code: M87.30

M87.342   **Other secondary osteonecrosis, left** CC **hand**
CC Excl: See code: M87.30

M87.343   **Other secondary osteonecrosis,** CC **unspecified hand**
CC Excl: See code: M87.30

M87.344   **Other secondary osteonecrosis, right** CC **finger(s)**
CC Excl: See code: M87.30

M87.345   **Other secondary osteonecrosis, left** CC **finger(s)**
CC Excl: See code: M87.30

M87.346   **Other secondary osteonecrosis,** CC **unspecified finger(s)**
CC Excl: See code: M87.30

☑6ᵗʰ   **M87.35**   **Other secondary osteonecrosis, pelvis and femur**

M87.350   **Other secondary osteonecrosis, pelvis** CC
CC Excl: M87.00, M87.031-M87.073,
M87.077-M87.119, M87.131-M87.173,
M87.177-M87.219, M87.231-M87.273,
M87.277-M87.319, M87.331-M87.373,
M87.377-M87.819, M87.831-M87.873,
M87.877-M87.9, M90.50, M90.521-M90.59

M87.351   **Other secondary osteonecrosis, right** CC **femur**
CC Excl: See code: M87.350

M87.352   **Other secondary osteonecrosis, left** CC **femur**
CC Excl: See code: M87.350

M87.353   **Other secondary osteonecrosis,** CC **unspecified femur**
CC Excl: See code: M87.350

☑6ᵗʰ   **M87.36**   **Other secondary osteonecrosis, tibia and fibula**

M87.361   **Other secondary osteonecrosis, right** CC **tibia**
CC Excl: M87.00-M87.9, M90.50-M90.59

M87.362   **Other secondary osteonecrosis, left** CC **tibia**
CC Excl: See code: M87.361

M87.363   **Other secondary osteonecrosis,** CC **unspecified tibia**
CC Excl: See code: M87.361

M87.364   **Other secondary osteonecrosis, right** CC **fibula**
CC Excl: See code: M87.361

M87.365   **Other secondary osteonecrosis, left** CC **fibula**
CC Excl: See code: M87.361

M87.366   **Other secondary osteonecrosis,** CC **unspecified fibula**
CC Excl: See code: M87.361

☑6ᵗʰ   **M87.37**   **Other secondary osteonecrosis, ankle and foot**

M87.371   **Other secondary osteonecrosis, right** CC **ankle**
CC Excl: See code: M87.361

M87.372   **Other secondary osteonecrosis, left** CC **ankle**
CC Excl: See code: M87.361

M87.373   **Other secondary osteonecrosis,** CC **unspecified ankle**
CC Excl: See code: M87.361

M87.374   **Other secondary osteonecrosis, right** CC **foot**
CC Excl: M87.00, M87.031-M87.050,
M87.061-M87.119, M87.131-M87.146,
M87.161-M87.219, M87.231-M87.250,
M87.261-M87.319, M87.331-M87.346,
M87.361-M87.819, M87.831-M87.849,
M87.861-M87.9, M90.50, M90.521-M90.549,
M90.561-M90.59

ℕ Newborn: 0   ℙ Pediatric: 0-17   𝕄 Maternity: 12-55   𝔸 Adult: 15-124   **MCC** Major CC Condition   **PDxMCC** PDx acts as own MCC   **CC** CC Condition   **PDxCC** PDx acts as own CC

778   ICD-10-CM 2016

M87.375 **Other secondary osteonecrosis, left foot** CC
     CC Excl: See code: M87.374

M87.376 **Other secondary osteonecrosis, unspecified foot** CC
     CC Excl: See code: M87.374

M87.377 **Other secondary osteonecrosis, right toe(s)** CC
     CC Excl: See code: M87.361

M87.378 **Other secondary osteonecrosis, left toe(s)** CC
     CC Excl: See code: M87.361

M87.379 **Other secondary osteonecrosis, unspecified toe(s)** CC
     CC Excl: See code: M87.361

M87.38 **Other secondary osteonecrosis, other site** CC
     CC Excl: See code: M87.361

M87.39 **Other secondary osteonecrosis, multiple sites** CC
     CC Excl: See code: M87.361

✓5ᵗʰ M87.8 **Other osteonecrosis**

M87.80 **Other osteonecrosis, unspecified bone** CC
     CC Excl: See code: M87.361

✓6ᵗʰ M87.81 **Other osteonecrosis, shoulder**

M87.811 **Other osteonecrosis, right shoulder** CC
     CC Excl: See code: M87.361

M87.812 **Other osteonecrosis, left shoulder** CC
     CC Excl: See code: M87.361

M87.819 **Other osteonecrosis, unspecified shoulder** CC
     CC Excl: See code: M87.361

✓6ᵗʰ M87.82 **Other osteonecrosis, humerus**

M87.821 **Other osteonecrosis, right humerus** CC
     CC Excl: M87.00-M87.050, M87.061-M87.073, M87.077-M87.146, M87.161-M87.173, M87.177-M87.250, M87.261-M87.273, M87.277-M87.346, M87.361-M87.373, M87.377-M87.819, M87.861-M87.873, M87.877-M87.9, M90.50-M90.549, M90.561-M90.59

M87.822 **Other osteonecrosis, left humerus** CC
     CC Excl: See code: M87.821

M87.829 **Other osteonecrosis, unspecified humerus** CC
     CC Excl: See code: M87.821

✓6ᵗʰ M87.83 **Other osteonecrosis of radius, ulna and carpus**

M87.831 **Other osteonecrosis of right radius** CC
     CC Excl: See code: M87.361

M87.832 **Other osteonecrosis of left radius** CC
     CC Excl: See code: M87.361

M87.833 **Other osteonecrosis of unspecified radius** CC
     CC Excl: See code: M87.361

M87.834 **Other osteonecrosis of right ulna** CC
     CC Excl: See code: M87.361

M87.835 **Other osteonecrosis of left ulna** CC
     CC Excl: See code: M87.361

M87.836 **Other osteonecrosis of unspecified ulna** CC
     CC Excl: See code: M87.361

M87.837 **Other osteonecrosis of right carpus** CC
     CC Excl: See code: M87.361

M87.838 **Other osteonecrosis of left carpus** CC
     CC Excl: See code: M87.361

M87.839 **Other osteonecrosis of unspecified carpus** CC
     CC Excl: See code: M87.361

✓6ᵗʰ M87.84 **Other osteonecrosis, hand and fingers**

M87.841 **Other osteonecrosis, right hand** CC
     CC Excl: See code: M87.361

M87.842 **Other osteonecrosis, left hand** CC
     CC Excl: See code: M87.361

M87.843 **Other osteonecrosis, unspecified hand** CC
     CC Excl: See code: M87.361

M87.844 **Other osteonecrosis, right finger(s)** CC
     CC Excl: See code: M87.361

M87.845 **Other osteonecrosis, left finger(s)** CC
     CC Excl: See code: M87.361

M87.849 **Other osteonecrosis, unspecified finger(s)** CC
     CC Excl: See code: M87.361

✓6ᵗʰ M87.85 **Other osteonecrosis, pelvis and femur**

M87.850 **Other osteonecrosis, pelvis** CC
     CC Excl: M87.00, M87.031-M87.073, M87.077-M87.119, M87.131-M87.173, M87.177-M87.219, M87.231-M87.273, M87.277-M87.319, M87.331-M87.373, M87.377-M87.819, M87.831-M87.873, M87.877-M87.9, M90.50, M90.521-M90.59

M87.851 **Other osteonecrosis, right femur** CC
     CC Excl: See code: M87.850

M87.852 **Other osteonecrosis, left femur** CC
     CC Excl: See code: M87.850

M87.859 **Other osteonecrosis, unspecified femur** CC
     CC Excl: See code: M87.850

✓6ᵗʰ M87.86 **Other osteonecrosis, tibia and fibula**

M87.861 **Other osteonecrosis, right tibia** CC
     CC Excl: See code: M87.361

M87.862 **Other osteonecrosis, left tibia** CC
     CC Excl: See code: M87.361

M87.863 **Other osteonecrosis, unspecified tibia** CC
     CC Excl: See code: M87.361

M87.864 **Other osteonecrosis, right fibula** CC
     CC Excl: See code: M87.361

M87.865 **Other osteonecrosis, left fibula** CC
     CC Excl: See code: M87.361

M87.869 **Other osteonecrosis, unspecified fibula** CC
     CC Excl: See code: M87.361

✓6ᵗʰ M87.87 **Other osteonecrosis, ankle, foot and toes**

M87.871 **Other osteonecrosis, right ankle** CC
     CC Excl: See code: M87.361

M87.872 **Other osteonecrosis, left ankle** CC
     CC Excl: See code: M87.361

M87.873 **Other osteonecrosis, unspecified ankle** CC
     CC Excl: See code: M87.361

M87.874 **Other osteonecrosis, right foot** CC
     CC Excl: M87.00, M87.031-M87.050, M87.061-M87.119, M87.131-M87.146, M87.161-M87.219, M87.231-M87.250, M87.261-M87.319, M87.331-M87.346, M87.361-M87.819, M87.831-M87.849, M87.861-M87.9, M90.50, M90.521-M90.549, M90.561-M90.59

M87.875 **Other osteonecrosis, left foot** CC
     CC Excl: See code: M87.874

M87.876 **Other osteonecrosis, unspecified foot** CC
     CC Excl: See code: M87.874

M87.877 **Other osteonecrosis, right toe(s)** CC
     CC Excl: See code: M87.361

M87.878 **Other osteonecrosis, left toe(s)** CC
     CC Excl: See code: M87.361

M87.879 **Other osteonecrosis, unspecified toe(s)** CC
     CC Excl: See code: M87.361

M87.88 **Other osteonecrosis, other site** CC
     CC Excl: See code: M87.361

M87.89 **Other osteonecrosis, multiple sites** CC
     CC Excl: See code: M87.361

M87.9 **Osteonecrosis, unspecified** CC
     Necrosis of bone NOS
     CC Excl: See code: M87.361

✓4ᵗʰ **M88 Osteitis deformans [Paget's disease of bone]**
     EXCLUDES 1 osteitis deformans in neoplastic disease (M90.6)

M88.0 **Osteitis deformans of skull**

M88.1 **Osteitis deformans of vertebrae**

✓5ᵗʰ M88.8 **Osteitis deformans of other bones**

✓6ᵗʰ M88.81 **Osteitis deformans of shoulder**

M88.811 **Osteitis deformans of right shoulder**

M88.812 **Osteitis deformans of left shoulder**

M88.819 **Osteitis deformans of unspecified shoulder**

✓6ᵗʰ M88.82 **Osteitis deformans of upper arm**

M88.821 **Osteitis deformans of right upper arm**

M88.822 **Osteitis deformans of left upper arm**

M88.829 **Osteitis deformans of unspecified upper arm**

✓6ᵗʰ M88.83 **Osteitis deformans of forearm**

M88.831 **Osteitis deformans of right forearm**

M88.832 **Osteitis deformans of left forearm**

M88.839 **Osteitis deformans of unspecified forearm**

✓ Additional Character Required   ✓x7ᵗʰ Placeholder Alert   Unacceptable PDx   Manifestation   Hospital Acquired Condition   **EXCLUDES 1** Not Coded Here   **EXCLUDES 2** Not Included Here

ICD-10-CM 2016   779

✓6th **M88.84 Osteitis deformans of hand**
M88.841 Osteitis deformans of right hand
M88.842 Osteitis deformans of left hand
M88.849 Osteitis deformans of unspecified hand

✓6th **M88.85 Osteitis deformans of thigh**
M88.851 Osteitis deformans of right thigh
M88.852 Osteitis deformans of left thigh
M88.859 Osteitis deformans of unspecified thigh

✓6th **M88.86 Osteitis deformans of lower leg**
M88.861 Osteitis deformans of right lower leg
M88.862 Osteitis deformans of left lower leg
M88.869 Osteitis deformans of unspecified lower leg

✓6th **M88.87 Osteitis deformans of ankle and foot**
M88.871 Osteitis deformans of right ankle and foot
M88.872 Osteitis deformans of left ankle and foot
M88.879 Osteitis deformans of unspecified ankle and foot

M88.88 Osteitis deformans of other bones
EXCLUDES 2 osteitis deformans of skull (M88.0)
osteitis deformans of vertebrae (M88.1)

M88.89 Osteitis deformans of multiple sites
M88.9 Osteitis deformans of unspecified bone

✓4th **M89 Other disorders of bone**
✓5th **M89.0 Algoneurodystrophy**
Shoulder-hand syndrome
Sudeck's atrophy
EXCLUDES 1 causalgia, lower limb (G57.7-)
causalgia, upper limb (G56.4-)
complex regional pain syndrome II, lower limb (G57.7-)
complex regional pain syndrome II, upper limb (G56.4-)
reflex sympathetic dystrophy (G90.5-)

M89.00 Algoneurodystrophy, unspecified site
✓6th **M89.01 Algoneurodystrophy, shoulder**
M89.011 Algoneurodystrophy, right shoulder
M89.012 Algoneurodystrophy, left shoulder
M89.019 Algoneurodystrophy, unspecified shoulder

✓6th **M89.02 Algoneurodystrophy, upper arm**
M89.021 Algoneurodystrophy, right upper arm
M89.022 Algoneurodystrophy, left upper arm
M89.029 Algoneurodystrophy, unspecified upper arm

✓6th **M89.03 Algoneurodystrophy, forearm**
M89.031 Algoneurodystrophy, right forearm
M89.032 Algoneurodystrophy, left forearm
M89.039 Algoneurodystrophy, unspecified forearm

✓6th **M89.04 Algoneurodystrophy, hand**
M89.041 Algoneurodystrophy, right hand
M89.042 Algoneurodystrophy, left hand
M89.049 Algoneurodystrophy, unspecified hand

✓6th **M89.05 Algoneurodystrophy, thigh**
M89.051 Algoneurodystrophy, right thigh
M89.052 Algoneurodystrophy, left thigh
M89.059 Algoneurodystrophy, unspecified thigh

✓6th **M89.06 Algoneurodystrophy, lower leg**
M89.061 Algoneurodystrophy, right lower leg
M89.062 Algoneurodystrophy, left lower leg
M89.069 Algoneurodystrophy, unspecified lower leg

✓6th **M89.07 Algoneurodystrophy, ankle and foot**
M89.071 Algoneurodystrophy, right ankle and foot
M89.072 Algoneurodystrophy, left ankle and foot
M89.079 Algoneurodystrophy, unspecified ankle and foot

M89.08 Algoneurodystrophy, other site
M89.09 Algoneurodystrophy, multiple sites

✓5th **M89.1 Physeal arrest**
Arrest of growth plate
Epiphyseal arrest
Growth plate arrest

✓6th **M89.12 Physeal arrest, humerus**

M89.121 Complete physeal arrest, right proximal humerus
M89.122 Complete physeal arrest, left proximal humerus
M89.123 Partial physeal arrest, right proximal humerus
M89.124 Partial physeal arrest, left proximal humerus
M89.125 Complete physeal arrest, right distal humerus
M89.126 Complete physeal arrest, left distal humerus
M89.127 Partial physeal arrest, right distal humerus
M89.128 Partial physeal arrest, left distal humerus
M89.129 Physeal arrest, humerus, unspecified

✓6th **M89.13 Physeal arrest, forearm**
M89.131 Complete physeal arrest, right distal radius
M89.132 Complete physeal arrest, left distal radius
M89.133 Partial physeal arrest, right distal radius
M89.134 Partial physeal arrest, left distal radius
M89.138 Other physeal arrest of forearm
M89.139 Physeal arrest, forearm, unspecified

✓6th **M89.15 Physeal arrest, femur**
M89.151 Complete physeal arrest, right proximal femur
M89.152 Complete physeal arrest, left proximal femur
M89.153 Partial physeal arrest, right proximal femur
M89.154 Partial physeal arrest, left proximal femur
M89.155 Complete physeal arrest, right distal femur
M89.156 Complete physeal arrest, left distal femur
M89.157 Partial physeal arrest, right distal femur
M89.158 Partial physeal arrest, left distal femur
M89.159 Physeal arrest, femur, unspecified

✓6th **M89.16 Physeal arrest, lower leg**
M89.160 Complete physeal arrest, right proximal tibia
M89.161 Complete physeal arrest, left proximal tibia
M89.162 Partial physeal arrest, right proximal tibia
M89.163 Partial physeal arrest, left proximal tibia
M89.164 Complete physeal arrest, right distal tibia
M89.165 Complete physeal arrest, left distal tibia
M89.166 Partial physeal arrest, right distal tibia
M89.167 Partial physeal arrest, left distal tibia
M89.168 Other physeal arrest of lower leg
M89.169 Physeal arrest, lower leg, unspecified

M89.18 Physeal arrest, other site

✓5th **M89.2 Other disorders of bone development and growth**
M89.20 Other disorders of bone development and growth, unspecified site
✓6th **M89.21 Other disorders of bone development and growth, shoulder**
M89.211 Other disorders of bone development and growth, right shoulder
M89.212 Other disorders of bone development and growth, left shoulder
M89.219 Other disorders of bone development and growth, unspecified shoulder

✓6th **M89.22 Other disorders of bone development and growth, humerus**
M89.221 Other disorders of bone development and growth, right humerus
M89.222 Other disorders of bone development and growth, left humerus
M89.229 Other disorders of bone development and growth, unspecified humerus

✓6th **M89.23 Other disorders of bone development and growth, ulna and radius**
M89.231 Other disorders of bone development and growth, right ulna

M89.232   **Other disorders of bone development and growth,** left **ulna**

M89.233   **Other disorders of bone development and growth,** right **radius**

M89.234   **Other disorders of bone development and growth,** left **radius**

M89.239   **Other disorders of bone development and growth,** unspecified **ulna and radius**

√6ᵗʰ   **M89.24**   **Other disorders of bone development and growth, hand**

M89.241   **Other disorders of bone development and growth,** right **hand**

M89.242   **Other disorders of bone development and growth,** left **hand**

M89.249   **Other disorders of bone development and growth,** unspecified **hand**

√6ᵗʰ   **M89.25**   **Other disorders of bone development and growth, femur**

M89.251   **Other disorders of bone development and growth,** right **femur**

M89.252   **Other disorders of bone development and growth,** left **femur**

M89.259   **Other disorders of bone development and growth,** unspecified **femur**

√6ᵗʰ   **M89.26**   **Other disorders of bone development and growth, tibia and fibula**

M89.261   **Other disorders of bone development and growth,** right **tibia**

M89.262   **Other disorders of bone development and growth,** left **tibia**

M89.263   **Other disorders of bone development and growth,** right **fibula**

M89.264   **Other disorders of bone development and growth,** left **fibula**

M89.269   **Other disorders of bone development and growth,** unspecified **lower leg**

√6ᵗʰ   **M89.27**   **Other disorders of bone development and growth, ankle and foot**

M89.271   **Other disorders of bone development and growth,** right **ankle and foot**

M89.272   **Other disorders of bone development and growth,** left **ankle and foot**

M89.279   **Other disorders of bone development and growth,** unspecified **ankle and foot**

M89.28   **Other disorders of bone development and growth, other site**

M89.29   **Other disorders of bone development and growth, multiple sites**

√5ᵗʰ   **M89.3**   **Hypertrophy of bone**

M89.30   **Hypertrophy of bone,** unspecified site

√6ᵗʰ   **M89.31**   **Hypertrophy of bone,** shoulder

M89.311   **Hypertrophy of bone,** right **shoulder**

M89.312   **Hypertrophy of bone,** left **shoulder**

M89.319   **Hypertrophy of bone,** unspecified **shoulder**

√6ᵗʰ   **M89.32**   **Hypertrophy of bone,** humerus

M89.321   **Hypertrophy of bone,** right **humerus**

M89.322   **Hypertrophy of bone,** left **humerus**

M89.329   **Hypertrophy of bone,** unspecified **humerus**

√6ᵗʰ   **M89.33**   **Hypertrophy of bone,** ulna and radius

M89.331   **Hypertrophy of bone,** right **ulna**

M89.332   **Hypertrophy of bone,** left **ulna**

M89.333   **Hypertrophy of bone,** right **radius**

M89.334   **Hypertrophy of bone,** left **radius**

M89.339   **Hypertrophy of bone,** unspecified **ulna and radius**

√6ᵗʰ   **M89.34**   **Hypertrophy of bone,** hand

M89.341   **Hypertrophy of bone,** right **hand**

M89.342   **Hypertrophy of bone,** left **hand**

M89.349   **Hypertrophy of bone,** unspecified **hand**

√6ᵗʰ   **M89.35**   **Hypertrophy of bone,** femur

M89.351   **Hypertrophy of bone,** right **femur**

M89.352   **Hypertrophy of bone,** left **femur**

M89.359   **Hypertrophy of bone,** unspecified **femur**

√6ᵗʰ   **M89.36**   **Hypertrophy of bone, tibia and fibula**

M89.361   **Hypertrophy of bone,** right **tibia**

M89.362   **Hypertrophy of bone,** left **tibia**

M89.363   **Hypertrophy of bone,** right **fibula**

M89.364   **Hypertrophy of bone,** left **fibula**

M89.369   **Hypertrophy of bone,** unspecified **tibia and fibula**

√6ᵗʰ   **M89.37**   **Hypertrophy of bone,** ankle and foot

M89.371   **Hypertrophy of bone,** right **ankle and foot**

M89.372   **Hypertrophy of bone,** left **ankle and foot**

M89.379   **Hypertrophy of bone,** unspecified **ankle and foot**

M89.38   **Hypertrophy of bone,** other site

M89.39   **Hypertrophy of bone,** multiple sites

√5ᵗʰ   **M89.4**   **Other hypertrophic osteoarthropathy**

Marie-Bamberger disease

Pachydermoperiostosis

M89.40   **Other hypertrophic osteoarthropathy,** unspecified site

√6ᵗʰ   **M89.41**   **Other hypertrophic osteoarthropathy,** shoulder

M89.411   **Other hypertrophic osteoarthropathy,** right **shoulder**

M89.412   **Other hypertrophic osteoarthropathy,** left **shoulder**

M89.419   **Other hypertrophic osteoarthropathy,** unspecified **shoulder**

√6ᵗʰ   **M89.42**   **Other hypertrophic osteoarthropathy,** upper arm

M89.421   **Other hypertrophic osteoarthropathy,** right **upper arm**

M89.422   **Other hypertrophic osteoarthropathy,** left **upper arm**

M89.429   **Other hypertrophic osteoarthropathy,** unspecified **upper arm**

√6ᵗʰ   **M89.43**   **Other hypertrophic osteoarthropathy,** forearm

M89.431   **Other hypertrophic osteoarthropathy,** right **forearm**

M89.432   **Other hypertrophic osteoarthropathy,** left **forearm**

M89.439   **Other hypertrophic osteoarthropathy,** unspecified **forearm**

√6ᵗʰ   **M89.44**   **Other hypertrophic osteoarthropathy,** hand

M89.441   **Other hypertrophic osteoarthropathy,** right **hand**

M89.442   **Other hypertrophic osteoarthropathy,** left **hand**

M89.449   **Other hypertrophic osteoarthropathy,** unspecified **hand**

√6ᵗʰ   **M89.45**   **Other hypertrophic osteoarthropathy,** thigh

M89.451   **Other hypertrophic osteoarthropathy,** right **thigh**

M89.452   **Other hypertrophic osteoarthropathy,** left **thigh**

M89.459   **Other hypertrophic osteoarthropathy,** unspecified **thigh**

√6ᵗʰ   **M89.46**   **Other hypertrophic osteoarthropathy,** lower leg

M89.461   **Other hypertrophic osteoarthropathy,** right **lower leg**

M89.462   **Other hypertrophic osteoarthropathy,** left **lower leg**

M89.469   **Other hypertrophic osteoarthropathy,** unspecified **lower leg**

√6ᵗʰ   **M89.47**   **Other hypertrophic osteoarthropathy,** ankle and foot

M89.471   **Other hypertrophic osteoarthropathy,** right **ankle and foot**

M89.472   **Other hypertrophic osteoarthropathy,** left **ankle and foot**

M89.479   **Other hypertrophic osteoarthropathy,** unspecified **ankle and foot**

M89.48   **Other hypertrophic osteoarthropathy,** other site

M89.49   **Other hypertrophic osteoarthropathy,** multiple sites

√5ᵗʰ   **M89.5**   **Osteolysis**

Use additional code to identify major osseous defect, if applicable (M89.7-)

EXCLUDES 2   *periprosthetic osteolysis of internal prosthetic joint (T84.05-)*

M89.50   **Osteolysis, unspecified site**

☑ Additional Character Required   √x7ᵗʰ Placeholder Alert   Unacceptable PDx   Manifestation   Hospital Acquired Condition   EXCLUDES 1 Not Coded Here   EXCLUDES 2 Not Included Here

ICD-10-CM 2016   781

Chapter 13. Diseases of the Musculoskeletal System and Connective Tissue

✓6th **M89.51 Osteolysis, shoulder**
    M89.511 Osteolysis, right shoulder
    M89.512 Osteolysis, left shoulder
    M89.519 Osteolysis, unspecified shoulder

✓6th **M89.52 Osteolysis, upper arm**
    M89.521 Osteolysis, right upper arm
    M89.522 Osteolysis, left upper arm
    M89.529 Osteolysis, unspecified upper arm

✓6th **M89.53 Osteolysis, forearm**
    M89.531 Osteolysis, right forearm
    M89.532 Osteolysis, left forearm
    M89.539 Osteolysis, unspecified forearm

✓6th **M89.54 Osteolysis, hand**
    M89.541 Osteolysis, right hand
    M89.542 Osteolysis, left hand
    M89.549 Osteolysis, unspecified hand

✓6th **M89.55 Osteolysis, thigh**
    M89.551 Osteolysis, right thigh
    M89.552 Osteolysis, left thigh
    M89.559 Osteolysis, unspecified thigh

✓6th **M89.56 Osteolysis, lower leg**
    M89.561 Osteolysis, right lower leg
    M89.562 Osteolysis, left lower leg
    M89.569 Osteolysis, unspecified lower leg

✓6th **M89.57 Osteolysis, ankle and foot**
    M89.571 Osteolysis, right ankle and foot
    M89.572 Osteolysis, left ankle and foot
    M89.579 Osteolysis, unspecified ankle and foot

M89.58 Osteolysis, other site

M89.59 Osteolysis, multiple sites

✓5th **M89.6 Osteopathy after poliomyelitis**
    Use additional code (B91) to identify previous poliomyelitis
    EXCLUDES 1   postpolio syndrome (G14)

    M89.60 Osteopathy after poliomyelitis, unspecified site

✓6th **M89.61 Osteopathy after poliomyelitis, shoulder**
    M89.611 Osteopathy after poliomyelitis, right shoulder
    M89.612 Osteopathy after poliomyelitis, left shoulder
    M89.619 Osteopathy after poliomyelitis, unspecified shoulder

✓6th **M89.62 Osteopathy after poliomyelitis, upper arm**
    M89.621 Osteopathy after poliomyelitis, right upper arm
    M89.622 Osteopathy after poliomyelitis, left upper arm
    M89.629 Osteopathy after poliomyelitis, unspecified upper arm

✓6th **M89.63 Osteopathy after poliomyelitis, forearm**
    M89.631 Osteopathy after poliomyelitis, right forearm
    M89.632 Osteopathy after poliomyelitis, left forearm
    M89.639 Osteopathy after poliomyelitis, unspecified forearm

✓6th **M89.64 Osteopathy after poliomyelitis, hand**
    M89.641 Osteopathy after poliomyelitis, right hand
    M89.642 Osteopathy after poliomyelitis, left hand
    M89.649 Osteopathy after poliomyelitis, unspecified hand

✓6th **M89.65 Osteopathy after poliomyelitis, thigh**
    M89.651 Osteopathy after poliomyelitis, right thigh
    M89.652 Osteopathy after poliomyelitis, left thigh
    M89.659 Osteopathy after poliomyelitis, unspecified thigh

✓6th **M89.66 Osteopathy after poliomyelitis, lower leg**
    M89.661 Osteopathy after poliomyelitis, right lower leg
    M89.662 Osteopathy after poliomyelitis, left lower leg
    M89.669 Osteopathy after poliomyelitis, unspecified lower leg

✓6th **M89.67 Osteopathy after poliomyelitis, ankle and foot**
    M89.671 Osteopathy after poliomyelitis, right ankle and foot
    M89.672 Osteopathy after poliomyelitis, left ankle and foot
    M89.679 Osteopathy after poliomyelitis, unspecified ankle and foot

M89.68 Osteopathy after poliomyelitis, other site

M89.69 Osteopathy after poliomyelitis, multiple sites

✓5th **M89.7 Major osseous defect**
    Code first underlying disease, if known, such as:
    aseptic necrosis of bone (M87.-)
    malignant neoplasm of bone (C40.-)
    osteolysis (M89.5)
    osteomyelitis (M86.-)
    osteonecrosis (M87.-)
    osteoporosis (M80.-, M81.-)
    periprosthetic osteolysis (T84.05-)

    M89.70 Major osseous defect, unspecified site

✓6th **M89.71 Major osseous defect, shoulder region**
    Major osseous defect clavicle or scapula
    M89.711 Major osseous defect, right shoulder region
    M89.712 Major osseous defect, left shoulder region
    M89.719 Major osseous defect, unspecified shoulder region

✓6th **M89.72 Major osseous defect, humerus**
    M89.721 Major osseous defect, right humerus
    M89.722 Major osseous defect, left humerus
    M89.729 Major osseous defect, unspecified humerus

✓6th **M89.73 Major osseous defect, forearm**
    Major osseous defect of radius and ulna
    M89.731 Major osseous defect, right forearm
    M89.732 Major osseous defect, left forearm
    M89.739 Major osseous defect, unspecified forearm

✓6th **M89.74 Major osseous defect, hand**
    Major osseous defect of carpus, fingers, metacarpus
    M89.741 Major osseous defect, right hand
    M89.742 Major osseous defect, left hand
    M89.749 Major osseous defect, unspecified hand

✓6th **M89.75 Major osseous defect, pelvic region and thigh**
    Major osseous defect of femur and pelvis
    M89.751 Major osseous defect, right pelvic region and thigh
    M89.752 Major osseous defect, left pelvic region and thigh
    M89.759 Major osseous defect, unspecified pelvic region and thigh

✓6th **M89.76 Major osseous defect, lower leg**
    Major osseous defect of fibula and tibia
    M89.761 Major osseous defect, right lower leg
    M89.762 Major osseous defect, left lower leg
    M89.769 Major osseous defect, unspecified lower leg

✓6th **M89.77 Major osseous defect, ankle and foot**
    Major osseous defect of metatarsus, tarsus, toes
    M89.771 Major osseous defect, right ankle and foot
    M89.772 Major osseous defect, left ankle and foot
    M89.779 Major osseous defect, unspecified ankle and foot

M89.78 Major osseous defect, other site

M89.79 Major osseous defect, multiple sites

✓5th **M89.8 Other specified disorders of bone**
    Infantile cortical hyperostoses
    Post-traumatic subperiosteal ossification

✓6th **M89.8X Other specified disorders of bone**
    M89.8X0 Other specified disorders of bone, multiple sites
    M89.8X1 Other specified disorders of bone, shoulder
    M89.8X2 Other specified disorders of bone, upper arm
    M89.8X3 Other specified disorders of bone, forearm
    M89.8X4 Other specified disorders of bone, hand
    M89.8X5 Other specified disorders of bone, thigh

N Newborn: 0   P Pediatric: 0-17   M Maternity: 12-55   A Adult: 15-124   MCC Major CC Condition   PDxMCC PDx acts as own MCC   CC CC Condition   PDxCC PDx acts as own CC

782   ICD-10-CM 2016

M89.8X6   **Other specified disorders of bone,** lower leg

M89.8X7   **Other specified disorders of bone,** ankle and foot

M89.8X8   **Other specified disorders of bone,** other site

M89.8X9   **Other specified disorders of bone,** unspecified site

M89.9   **Disorder of bone, unspecified**

✓4th **M90**   **Osteopathies in diseases classified elsewhere**

> **EXCLUDES 1**   *osteochondritis, osteomyelitis, and osteopathy (in):*
> *cryptococcosis (B45.3)*
> *diabetes mellitus (E08-E13 with .61-)*
> *gonococcal (A54.43)*
> *neurogenic syphilis (A52.11)*
> *renal osteodystrophy (N25.0)*
> *salmonellosis (A02.24)*
> *secondary syphilis (A51.46)*
> *syphilis (late) (A52.77)*

✓5th **M90.5**   **Osteonecrosis in diseases classified elsewhere**

> *Code first underlying disease, such as:*
> *caisson disease (T70.3)*
> *hemoglobinopathy (D50-D64)*

> **CC Excl: For CC codes in subcategory M90.5, unless otherwise noted: M87.00-M87.9, M90.50-M90.59**

M90.50   *Osteonecrosis in diseases classified elsewhere, unspecified site*   PDxCC CC

✓6th **M90.51**   **Osteonecrosis in diseases classified elsewhere, shoulder**

M90.511   *Osteonecrosis in diseases classified elsewhere, right shoulder*   PDxCC CC
> CC Excl: M87.00-M87.050, M87.061-M87.073, M87.077-M87.146, M87.161-M87.173, M87.177-M87.250, M87.261-M87.273, M87.277-M87.346, M87.361-M87.373, M87.377-M87.849, M87.861-M87.873, M87.877-M87.9, M90.50-M90.549, M90.561-M90.59

M90.512   *Osteonecrosis in diseases classified elsewhere, left shoulder*   PDxCC CC
> CC Excl: See code: M90.511

M90.519   *Osteonecrosis in diseases classified elsewhere, unspecified shoulder*   PDxCC CC
> CC Excl: See code: M90.511

✓6th **M90.52**   **Osteonecrosis in diseases classified elsewhere, upper arm**

M90.521   *Osteonecrosis in diseases classified elsewhere, right upper arm*   PDxCC CC

M90.522   *Osteonecrosis in diseases classified elsewhere, left upper arm*   PDxCC CC

M90.529   *Osteonecrosis in diseases classified elsewhere, unspecified upper arm*   PDxCC CC

✓6th **M90.53**   **Osteonecrosis in diseases classified elsewhere, forearm**

M90.531   *Osteonecrosis in diseases classified elsewhere, right forearm*   PDxCC CC

M90.532   *Osteonecrosis in diseases classified elsewhere, left forearm*   PDxCC CC

M90.539   *Osteonecrosis in diseases classified elsewhere, unspecified forearm*   PDxCC CC

✓6th **M90.54**   **Osteonecrosis in diseases classified elsewhere, hand**

M90.541   *Osteonecrosis in diseases classified elsewhere, right hand*   PDxCC CC

M90.542   *Osteonecrosis in diseases classified elsewhere, left hand*   PDxCC CC

M90.549   *Osteonecrosis in diseases classified elsewhere, unspecified hand*   PDxCC CC

✓6th **M90.55**   **Osteonecrosis in diseases classified elsewhere, thigh**

M90.551   *Osteonecrosis in diseases classified elsewhere, right thigh*   PDxCC CC
> CC Excl: M87.00, M87.031-M87.073, M87.077-M87.119, M87.131-M87.173, M87.177-M87.219, M87.231-M87.273, M87.277-M87.319, M87.331-M87.373, M87.377-M87.819, M87.831-M87.873, M87.877-M87.9, M90.50, M90.521-M90.59

M90.552   *Osteonecrosis in diseases classified elsewhere, left thigh*   PDxCC CC
> CC Excl: See code: M90.551

M90.559   *Osteonecrosis in diseases classified elsewhere, unspecified thigh*   PDxCC CC
> CC Excl: See code: M90.551

✓6th **M90.56**   **Osteonecrosis in diseases classified elsewhere, lower leg**

M90.561   *Osteonecrosis in diseases classified elsewhere, right lower leg*   PDxCC CC

M90.562   *Osteonecrosis in diseases classified elsewhere, left lower leg*   PDxCC CC

M90.569   *Osteonecrosis in diseases classified elsewhere, unspecified lower leg*   PDxCC CC

✓6th **M90.57**   **Osteonecrosis in diseases classified elsewhere, ankle and foot**

M90.571   *Osteonecrosis in diseases classified elsewhere, right ankle and foot*   PDxCC CC

M90.572   *Osteonecrosis in diseases classified elsewhere, left ankle and foot*   PDxCC CC

M90.579   *Osteonecrosis in diseases classified elsewhere, unspecified ankle and foot*   PDxCC CC

M90.58   *Osteonecrosis in diseases classified elsewhere, other site*   PDxCC CC

M90.59   *Osteonecrosis in diseases classified elsewhere, multiple sites*   PDxCC CC

✓5th **M90.6**   **Osteitis deformans in neoplastic diseases**

> *Osteitis deformans in malignant neoplasm of bone*
> *Code first the neoplasm (C40-, C41-)*
> **EXCLUDES 1**   *osteitis deformans [Paget's disease of bone] (M88.-)*

M90.60   *Osteitis deformans in neoplastic diseases, unspecified site*

✓6th **M90.61**   **Osteitis deformans in neoplastic diseases, shoulder**

M90.611   *Osteitis deformans in neoplastic diseases, right shoulder*

M90.612   *Osteitis deformans in neoplastic diseases, left shoulder*

M90.619   *Osteitis deformans in neoplastic diseases, unspecified shoulder*

✓6th **M90.62**   **Osteitis deformans in neoplastic diseases, upper arm**

M90.621   *Osteitis deformans in neoplastic diseases, right upper arm*

M90.622   *Osteitis deformans in neoplastic diseases, left upper arm*

M90.629   *Osteitis deformans in neoplastic diseases, unspecified upper arm*

✓6th **M90.63**   **Osteitis deformans in neoplastic diseases, forearm**

M90.631   *Osteitis deformans in neoplastic diseases, right forearm*

M90.632   *Osteitis deformans in neoplastic diseases, left forearm*

M90.639   *Osteitis deformans in neoplastic diseases, unspecified forearm*

✓6th **M90.64**   **Osteitis deformans in neoplastic diseases, hand**

M90.641   *Osteitis deformans in neoplastic diseases, right hand*

M90.642   *Osteitis deformans in neoplastic diseases, left hand*

M90.649   *Osteitis deformans in neoplastic diseases, unspecified hand*

✓6th **M90.65**   **Osteitis deformans in neoplastic diseases, thigh**

M90.651   *Osteitis deformans in neoplastic diseases, right thigh*

M90.652   *Osteitis deformans in neoplastic diseases, left thigh*

M90.659   *Osteitis deformans in neoplastic diseases, unspecified thigh*

✓6th **M90.66**   **Osteitis deformans in neoplastic diseases, lower leg**

M90.661   *Osteitis deformans in neoplastic diseases, right lower leg*

M90.662   *Osteitis deformans in neoplastic diseases, left lower leg*

✓ Additional Character Required   ✓x7th Placeholder Alert   Unacceptable PDx   Manifestation   Hospital Acquired Condition   EXCLUDES 1 Not Coded Here   EXCLUDES 2 Not Included Here

ICD-10-CM 2016   783

Chapter 13. Diseases of the Musculoskeletal System and Connective Tissue

M90.669   *Osteitis deformans in neoplastic diseases, unspecified lower leg*

✓6ᵗʰ M90.67 Osteitis deformans in neoplastic diseases, ankle and foot

M90.671   *Osteitis deformans in neoplastic diseases, right ankle and foot*

M90.672   *Osteitis deformans in neoplastic diseases, left ankle and foot*

M90.679   *Osteitis deformans in neoplastic diseases, unspecified ankle and foot*

M90.68   *Osteitis deformans in neoplastic diseases, other site*

M90.69   *Osteitis deformans in neoplastic diseases, multiple sites*

✓5ᵗʰ M90.8 Osteopathy in diseases classified elsewhere
   Code first underlying disease, such as:
      rickets (E55.0)
      vitamin-D-resistant rickets (E83.3)

M90.80   *Osteopathy in diseases classified elsewhere, unspecified site*

✓6ᵗʰ M90.81 Osteopathy in diseases classified elsewhere, shoulder

M90.811   *Osteopathy in diseases classified elsewhere, right shoulder*

M90.812   *Osteopathy in diseases classified elsewhere, left shoulder*

M90.819   *Osteopathy in diseases classified elsewhere, unspecified shoulder*

✓6ᵗʰ M90.82 Osteopathy in diseases classified elsewhere, upper arm

M90.821   *Osteopathy in diseases classified elsewhere, right upper arm*

M90.822   *Osteopathy in diseases classified elsewhere, left upper arm*

M90.829   *Osteopathy in diseases classified elsewhere, unspecified upper arm*

✓6ᵗʰ M90.83 Osteopathy in diseases classified elsewhere, forearm

M90.831   *Osteopathy in diseases classified elsewhere, right forearm*

M90.832   *Osteopathy in diseases classified elsewhere, left forearm*

M90.839   *Osteopathy in diseases classified elsewhere, unspecified forearm*

✓6ᵗʰ M90.84 Osteopathy in diseases classified elsewhere, hand

M90.841   *Osteopathy in diseases classified elsewhere, right hand*

M90.842   *Osteopathy in diseases classified elsewhere, left hand*

M90.849   *Osteopathy in diseases classified elsewhere, unspecified hand*

✓6ᵗʰ M90.85 Osteopathy in diseases classified elsewhere, thigh

M90.851   *Osteopathy in diseases classified elsewhere, right thigh*

M90.852   *Osteopathy in diseases classified elsewhere, left thigh*

M90.859   *Osteopathy in diseases classified elsewhere, unspecified thigh*

✓6ᵗʰ M90.86 Osteopathy in diseases classified elsewhere, lower leg

M90.861   *Osteopathy in diseases classified elsewhere, right lower leg*

M90.862   *Osteopathy in diseases classified elsewhere, left lower leg*

M90.869   *Osteopathy in diseases classified elsewhere, unspecified lower leg*

✓6ᵗʰ M90.87 Osteopathy in diseases classified elsewhere, ankle and foot

M90.871   *Osteopathy in diseases classified elsewhere, right ankle and foot*

M90.872   *Osteopathy in diseases classified elsewhere, left ankle and foot*

M90.879   *Osteopathy in diseases classified elsewhere, unspecified ankle and foot*

M90.88   *Osteopathy in diseases classified elsewhere, other site*

M90.89   *Osteopathy in diseases classified elsewhere, multiple sites*

Chondropathies (M91-M94)

EXCLUDES 1 *postprocedural chondropathies (M96.-)*

✓4ᵗʰ **M91 Juvenile osteochondrosis of hip and pelvis**
   EXCLUDES 1 *slipped upper femoral epiphysis (nontraumatic) (M93.0)*

M91.0 Juvenile osteochondrosis of pelvis
   Osteochondrosis (juvenile) of acetabulum
   Osteochondrosis (juvenile) of iliac crest [Buchanan]
   Osteochondrosis (juvenile) of ischiopubic synchondrosis [van Neck]
   Osteochondrosis (juvenile) of symphysis pubis [Pierson]

✓5ᵗʰ M91.1 Juvenile osteochondrosis of head of femur [Legg-Calvé-Perthes]

M91.10   Juvenile osteochondrosis of head of femur [Legg-Calvé-Perthes], unspecified leg

M91.11   Juvenile osteochondrosis of head of femur [Legg-Calvé-Perthes], right leg

M91.12   Juvenile osteochondrosis of head of femur [Legg-Calvé-Perthes], left leg

✓5ᵗʰ M91.2 Coxa plana
   Hip deformity due to previous juvenile osteochondrosis

M91.20   Coxa plana, unspecified hip

M91.21   Coxa plana, right hip

M91.22   Coxa plana, left hip

✓5ᵗʰ M91.3 Pseudocoxalgia

M91.30   Pseudocoxalgia, unspecified hip

M91.31   Pseudocoxalgia, right hip

M91.32   Pseudocoxalgia, left hip

✓5ᵗʰ M91.4 Coxa magna

M91.40   Coxa magna, unspecified hip

M91.41   Coxa magna, right hip

M91.42   Coxa magna, left hip

✓5ᵗʰ M91.8 Other juvenile osteochondrosis of hip and pelvis
   Juvenile osteochondrosis after reduction of congenital dislocation of hip

M91.80   Other juvenile osteochondrosis of hip and pelvis, unspecified leg

M91.81   Other juvenile osteochondrosis of hip and pelvis, right leg

M91.82   Other juvenile osteochondrosis of hip and pelvis, left leg

✓5ᵗʰ M91.9 Juvenile osteochondrosis of hip and pelvis, unspecified

M91.90   Juvenile osteochondrosis of hip and pelvis, unspecified, unspecified leg

M91.91   Juvenile osteochondrosis of hip and pelvis, unspecified, right leg

M91.92   Juvenile osteochondrosis of hip and pelvis, unspecified, left leg

✓4ᵗʰ **M92 Other juvenile osteochondrosis**

✓5ᵗʰ M92.0 Juvenile osteochondrosis of humerus
   Osteochondrosis (juvenile) of capitulum of humerus [Panner]
   Osteochondrosis (juvenile) of head of humerus [Haas]

M92.00   Juvenile osteochondrosis of humerus, unspecified arm

M92.01   Juvenile osteochondrosis of humerus, right arm

M92.02   Juvenile osteochondrosis of humerus, left arm

✓5ᵗʰ M92.1 Juvenile osteochondrosis of radius and ulna
   Osteochondrosis (juvenile) of lower ulna [Burns]
   Osteochondrosis (juvenile) of radial head [Brailsford]

M92.10   Juvenile osteochondrosis of radius and ulna, unspecified arm

M92.11   Juvenile osteochondrosis of radius and ulna, right arm

M92.12   Juvenile osteochondrosis of radius and ulna, left arm

✓5ᵗʰ M92.2 Juvenile osteochondrosis, hand

✓6ᵗʰ M92.20   Unspecified juvenile osteochondrosis, hand

M92.201   Unspecified juvenile osteochondrosis, right hand

M92.202   Unspecified juvenile osteochondrosis, left hand

M92.209   Unspecified juvenile osteochondrosis, unspecified hand

✓6ᵗʰ **M92.21** **Osteochondrosis (juvenile) of** carpal lunate **[Kienböck]**

     M92.211 Osteochondrosis (juvenile) of carpal lunate [Kienböck], right hand

     M92.212 Osteochondrosis (juvenile) of carpal lunate [Kienböck], left hand

     M92.219 Osteochondrosis (juvenile) of carpal lunate [Kienböck], unspecified hand

✓6ᵗʰ **M92.22** **Osteochondrosis (juvenile) of** metacarpal heads **[Mauclaire]**

     M92.221 Osteochondrosis (juvenile) of metacarpal heads [Mauclaire], right hand

     M92.222 Osteochondrosis (juvenile) of metacarpal heads [Mauclaire], left hand

     M92.229 Osteochondrosis (juvenile) of metacarpal heads [Mauclaire], unspecified hand

✓6ᵗʰ **M92.29** Other **juvenile osteochondrosis,** hand

     M92.291 Other juvenile osteochondrosis, right hand

     M92.292 Other juvenile osteochondrosis, left hand

     M92.299 Other juvenile osteochondrosis, unspecified hand

✓5ᵗʰ **M92.3** **Other juvenile osteochondrosis,** upper limb

     M92.30 Other juvenile osteochondrosis, unspecified upper limb

     M92.31 Other juvenile osteochondrosis, right upper limb

     M92.32 Other juvenile osteochondrosis, left upper limb

✓5ᵗʰ **M92.4** **Juvenile osteochondrosis of** patella

Osteochondrosis (juvenile) of primary patellar center [Köhler]
Osteochondrosis (juvenile) of secondary patellar centre [Sinding Larsen]

     M92.40 Juvenile osteochondrosis of patella, unspecified knee

     M92.41 Juvenile osteochondrosis of patella, right knee

     M92.42 Juvenile osteochondrosis of patella, left knee

✓5ᵗʰ **M92.5** **Juvenile osteochondrosis of** tibia and fibula

Osteochondrosis (juvenile) of proximal tibia [Blount]
Osteochondrosis (juvenile) of tibial tubercle [Osgood-Schlatter]
Tibia vara

     M92.50 Juvenile osteochondrosis of tibia and fibula, unspecified leg

     M92.51 Juvenile osteochondrosis of tibia and fibula, right leg

     M92.52 Juvenile osteochondrosis of tibia and fibula, left leg

✓5ᵗʰ **M92.6** **Juvenile osteochondrosis of** tarsus

Osteochondrosis (juvenile) of calcaneum [Sever]
Osteochondrosis (juvenile) of os tibiale externum [Haglund]
Osteochondrosis (juvenile) of talus [Diaz]
Osteochondrosis (juvenile) of tarsal navicular [Köhler]

     M92.60 Juvenile osteochondrosis of tarsus, unspecified ankle

     M92.61 Juvenile osteochondrosis of tarsus, right ankle

     M92.62 Juvenile osteochondrosis of tarsus, left ankle

✓5ᵗʰ **M92.7** **Juvenile osteochondrosis of** metatarsus

Osteochondrosis (juvenile) of fifth metatarsus [Iselin]
Osteochondrosis (juvenile) of second metatarsus [Freiberg]

     M92.70 Juvenile osteochondrosis of metatarsus, unspecified foot

     M92.71 Juvenile osteochondrosis of metatarsus, right foot

     M92.72 Juvenile osteochondrosis of metatarsus, left foot

M92.8 Other **specified juvenile osteochondrosis**

Calcaneal apophysitis

M92.9 **Juvenile osteochondrosis,** unspecified

Juvenile apophysitis NOS   Juvenile osteochondritis NOS
Juvenile epiphysitis NOS   Juvenile osteochondrosis NOS

✓4ᵗʰ **M93** **Other osteochondropathies**

   EXCLUDES 2   osteochondrosis of spine (M42.-)

✓5ᵗʰ **M93.0** **Slipped upper femoral epiphysis (nontraumatic)**

Use additional code for associated chondrolysis (M94.3)

✓6ᵗʰ **M93.00** Unspecified **slipped upper femoral epiphysis (nontraumatic)**

     M93.001 Unspecified slipped upper femoral epiphysis (nontraumatic), right hip

     M93.002 Unspecified slipped upper femoral epiphysis (nontraumatic), left hip

     M93.003 Unspecified slipped upper femoral epiphysis (nontraumatic), unspecified hip

✓6ᵗʰ **M93.01** Acute **slipped upper femoral epiphysis (nontraumatic)**

     M93.011 Acute slipped upper femoral epiphysis (nontraumatic), right hip

     M93.012 Acute slipped upper femoral epiphysis (nontraumatic), left hip

     M93.013 Acute slipped upper femoral epiphysis (nontraumatic), unspecified hip

✓6ᵗʰ **M93.02** Chronic **slipped upper femoral epiphysis (nontraumatic)**

     M93.021 Chronic slipped upper femoral epiphysis (nontraumatic), right hip

     M93.022 Chronic slipped upper femoral epiphysis (nontraumatic), left hip

     M93.023 Chronic slipped upper femoral epiphysis (nontraumatic), unspecified hip

✓6ᵗʰ **M93.03** Acute on chronic **slipped upper femoral epiphysis (nontraumatic)**

     M93.031 Acute on chronic slipped upper femoral epiphysis (nontraumatic), right hip

     M93.032 Acute on chronic slipped upper femoral epiphysis (nontraumatic), left hip

     M93.033 Acute on chronic slipped upper femoral epiphysis (nontraumatic), unspecified hip

M93.1 **Kienböck's disease of adults**   Ⓐ

Adult osteochondrosis of carpal lunates

✓5ᵗʰ **M93.2** **Osteochondritis dissecans**

     M93.20 Osteochondritis dissecans of unspecified site

✓6ᵗʰ **M93.21** Osteochondritis dissecans of shoulder

     M93.211 Osteochondritis dissecans, right shoulder

     M93.212 Osteochondritis dissecans, left shoulder

     M93.219 Osteochondritis dissecans, unspecified shoulder

✓6ᵗʰ **M93.22** Osteochondritis dissecans of elbow

     M93.221 Osteochondritis dissecans, right elbow

     M93.222 Osteochondritis dissecans, left elbow

     M93.229 Osteochondritis dissecans, unspecified elbow

✓6ᵗʰ **M93.23** Osteochondritis dissecans of wrist

     M93.231 Osteochondritis dissecans, right wrist

     M93.232 Osteochondritis dissecans, left wrist

     M93.239 Osteochondritis dissecans, unspecified wrist

✓6ᵗʰ **M93.24** Osteochondritis dissecans of joints of hand

     M93.241 Osteochondritis dissecans, joints of right hand

     M93.242 Osteochondritis dissecans, joints of left hand

     M93.249 Osteochondritis dissecans, joints of unspecified hand

✓6ᵗʰ **M93.25** Osteochondritis dissecans of hip

     M93.251 Osteochondritis dissecans, right hip

     M93.252 Osteochondritis dissecans, left hip

     M93.259 Osteochondritis dissecans, unspecified hip

✓6ᵗʰ **M93.26** Osteochondritis dissecans knee

     M93.261 Osteochondritis dissecans, right knee

     M93.262 Osteochondritis dissecans, left knee

     M93.269 Osteochondritis dissecans, unspecified knee

✓6ᵗʰ **M93.27** Osteochondritis dissecans of ankle and joints of foot

     M93.271 Osteochondritis dissecans, right ankle and joints of right foot

     M93.272 Osteochondritis dissecans, left ankle and joints of left foot

     M93.279 Osteochondritis dissecans, unspecified ankle and joints of foot

     M93.28 Osteochondritis dissecans other site

     M93.29 Osteochondritis dissecans multiple sites

✓5ᵗʰ **M93.8** **Other specified osteochondropathies**

     M93.80 Other specified osteochondropathies of unspecified site

✓ Additional Character Required   ✓x7ᵗʰ Placeholder Alert   Unacceptable PDx   ■ Manifestation   Hospital Acquired Condition   *EXCLUDES 1* Not Coded Here   *EXCLUDES 2* Not Included Here

ICD-10-CM 2016   785

✓6ᵗʰ **M93.81 Other specified osteochondropathies of** shoulder
- **M93.811 Other specified osteochondropathies, right** shoulder
- **M93.812 Other specified osteochondropathies, left** shoulder
- **M93.819 Other specified osteochondropathies, unspecified** shoulder

✓6ᵗʰ **M93.82 Other specified osteochondropathies of** upper arm
- **M93.821 Other specified osteochondropathies, right** upper arm
- **M93.822 Other specified osteochondropathies, left** upper arm
- **M93.829 Other specified osteochondropathies, unspecified** upper arm

✓6ᵗʰ **M93.83 Other specified osteochondropathies of** forearm
- **M93.831 Other specified osteochondropathies, right** forearm
- **M93.832 Other specified osteochondropathies, left** forearm
- **M93.839 Other specified osteochondropathies, unspecified** forearm

✓6ᵗʰ **M93.84 Other specified osteochondropathies of** hand
- **M93.841 Other specified osteochondropathies, right** hand
- **M93.842 Other specified osteochondropathies, left** hand
- **M93.849 Other specified osteochondropathies, unspecified** hand

✓6ᵗʰ **M93.85 Other specified osteochondropathies of** thigh
- **M93.851 Other specified osteochondropathies, right** thigh
- **M93.852 Other specified osteochondropathies, left** thigh
- **M93.859 Other specified osteochondropathies, unspecified** thigh

✓6ᵗʰ **M93.86 Other specified osteochondropathies** lower leg
- **M93.861 Other specified osteochondropathies, right** lower leg
- **M93.862 Other specified osteochondropathies, left** lower leg
- **M93.869 Other specified osteochondropathies, unspecified** lower leg

✓6ᵗʰ **M93.87 Other specified osteochondropathies of** ankle and foot
- **M93.871 Other specified osteochondropathies, right** ankle and foot
- **M93.872 Other specified osteochondropathies, left** ankle and foot
- **M93.879 Other specified osteochondropathies, unspecified** ankle and foot

M93.88 Other specified osteochondropathies other site

M93.89 Other specified osteochondropathies multiple sites

✓5ᵗʰ **M93.9 Osteochondropathy, unspecified**
Apophysitis NOS   Osteochondritis NOS
Epiphysitis NOS   Osteochondrosis NOS

- **M93.90 Osteochondropathy, unspecified of** unspecified site

✓6ᵗʰ **M93.91 Osteochondropathy, unspecified of** shoulder
- **M93.911 Osteochondropathy, unspecified, right** shoulder
- **M93.912 Osteochondropathy, unspecified, left** shoulder
- **M93.919 Osteochondropathy, unspecified, unspecified** shoulder

✓6ᵗʰ **M93.92 Osteochondropathy, unspecified of** upper arm
- **M93.921 Osteochondropathy, unspecified, right** upper arm
- **M93.922 Osteochondropathy, unspecified, left** upper arm
- **M93.929 Osteochondropathy, unspecified, unspecified** upper arm

✓6ᵗʰ **M93.93 Osteochondropathy, unspecified of** forearm
- **M93.931 Osteochondropathy, unspecified, right** forearm
- **M93.932 Osteochondropathy, unspecified, left** forearm
- **M93.939 Osteochondropathy, unspecified, unspecified** forearm

✓6ᵗʰ **M93.94 Osteochondropathy, unspecified of** hand
- **M93.941 Osteochondropathy, unspecified, right** hand
- **M93.942 Osteochondropathy, unspecified, left** hand
- **M93.949 Osteochondropathy, unspecified, unspecified** hand

✓6ᵗʰ **M93.95 Osteochondropathy, unspecified of** thigh
- **M93.951 Osteochondropathy, unspecified, right** thigh
- **M93.952 Osteochondropathy, unspecified, left** thigh
- **M93.959 Osteochondropathy, unspecified, unspecified** thigh

✓6ᵗʰ **M93.96 Osteochondropathy, unspecified** lower leg
- **M93.961 Osteochondropathy, unspecified, right** lower leg
- **M93.962 Osteochondropathy, unspecified, left** lower leg
- **M93.969 Osteochondropathy, unspecified, unspecified** lower leg

✓6ᵗʰ **M93.97 Osteochondropathy, unspecified of** ankle and foot
- **M93.971 Osteochondropathy, unspecified, right** ankle and foot
- **M93.972 Osteochondropathy, unspecified, left** ankle and foot
- **M93.979 Osteochondropathy, unspecified, unspecified** ankle and foot

M93.98 Osteochondropathy, unspecified other site

M93.99 Osteochondropathy, unspecified multiple sites

✓4ᵗʰ **M94 Other disorders of cartilage**

M94.0 Chondrocostal junction syndrome [Tietze]
Costochondritis

M94.1 Relapsing polychondritis

✓5ᵗʰ **M94.2 Chondromalacia**
EXCLUDES 1   chondromalacia patellae (M22.4)

- **M94.20 Chondromalacia, unspecified site**

✓6ᵗʰ **M94.21 Chondromalacia, shoulder**
- **M94.211 Chondromalacia, right shoulder**
- **M94.212 Chondromalacia, left shoulder**
- **M94.219 Chondromalacia, unspecified shoulder**

✓6ᵗʰ **M94.22 Chondromalacia, elbow**
- **M94.221 Chondromalacia, right elbow**
- **M94.222 Chondromalacia, left elbow**
- **M94.229 Chondromalacia, unspecified elbow**

✓6ᵗʰ **M94.23 Chondromalacia, wrist**
- **M94.231 Chondromalacia, right wrist**
- **M94.232 Chondromalacia, left wrist**
- **M94.239 Chondromalacia, unspecified wrist**

✓6ᵗʰ **M94.24 Chondromalacia, joints of hand**
- **M94.241 Chondromalacia, joints of right hand**
- **M94.242 Chondromalacia, joints of left hand**
- **M94.249 Chondromalacia, joints of unspecified hand**

✓6ᵗʰ **M94.25 Chondromalacia, hip**
- **M94.251 Chondromalacia, right hip**
- **M94.252 Chondromalacia, left hip**
- **M94.259 Chondromalacia, unspecified hip**

✓6ᵗʰ **M94.26 Chondromalacia, knee**
- **M94.261 Chondromalacia, right knee**
- **M94.262 Chondromalacia, left knee**
- **M94.269 Chondromalacia, unspecified knee**

✓6ᵗʰ **M94.27 Chondromalacia, ankle and joints of foot**
- **M94.271 Chondromalacia, right ankle and joints of right foot**
- **M94.272 Chondromalacia, left ankle and joints of left foot**
- **M94.279 Chondromalacia, unspecified ankle and joints of foot**

M94.28 Chondromalacia, other site

M94.29 Chondromalacia, multiple sites

☑5ᵗʰ **M94.3 Chondrolysis**
> Code first any associated slipped upper femoral epiphysis (nontraumatic) (M93.0-)

   ☑6ᵗʰ **M94.35 Chondrolysis, hip**
     M94.351 Chondrolysis, right hip
     M94.352 Chondrolysis, left hip
     M94.359 Chondrolysis, unspecified hip

☑5ᵗʰ **M94.8 Other specified disorders of cartilage**

   ☑6ᵗʰ **M94.8X Other specified disorders of cartilage**
     M94.8X0 Other specified disorders of cartilage, multiple sites
     M94.8X1 Other specified disorders of cartilage, shoulder
     M94.8X2 Other specified disorders of cartilage, upper arm
     M94.8X3 Other specified disorders of cartilage, forearm
     M94.8X4 Other specified disorders of cartilage, hand
     M94.8X5 Other specified disorders of cartilage, thigh
     M94.8X6 Other specified disorders of cartilage, lower leg
     M94.8X7 Other specified disorders of cartilage, ankle and foot
     M94.8X8 Other specified disorders of cartilage, other site
     M94.8X9 Other specified disorders of cartilage, unspecified sites

M94.9 Disorder of cartilage, unspecified

Other disorders of the musculoskeletal system and connective tissue (M95)

☑4ᵗʰ **M95 Other acquired deformities of musculoskeletal system and connective tissue**
> EXCLUDES 2   acquired absence of limbs and organs (Z89-Z90)
> acquired deformities of limbs (M20-M21)
> congenital malformations and deformations of the musculoskeletal system (Q65-Q79)
> deforming dorsopathies (M40-M43)
> dentofacial anomalies [including malocclusion] (M26.-)
> postprocedural musculoskeletal disorders (M96.-)

M95.0 Acquired deformity of nose
> EXCLUDES 2   deviated nasal septum (J34.2)

☑5ᵗʰ **M95.1 Cauliflower ear**
> EXCLUDES 2   other acquired deformities of ear (H61.1)

   M95.10 Cauliflower ear, unspecified ear
   M95.11 Cauliflower ear, right ear
   M95.12 Cauliflower ear, left ear

M95.2 Other acquired deformity of head

M95.3 Acquired deformity of neck

M95.4 Acquired deformity of chest and rib
> AHA: 2014, 4Q, 26-27

M95.5 Acquired deformity of pelvis
> EXCLUDES 1   maternal care for known or suspected disproportion (O33.-)

M95.8 Other specified acquired deformities of musculoskeletal system

M95.9 Acquired deformity of musculoskeletal system, unspecified

Intraoperative and postprocedural complications and disorders of musculoskeletal system, not elsewhere classified (M96)

☑4ᵗʰ **M96 Intraoperative and postprocedural complications and disorders of musculoskeletal system, not elsewhere classified**
> EXCLUDES 2   arthropathy following intestinal bypass (M02.0-)
> complications of internal orthopedic prosthetic devices, implants and grafts (T84.-)
> disorders associated with osteoporosis (M80)
> presence of functional implants and other devices (Z96-Z97)

M96.0 Pseudarthrosis after fusion or arthrodesis   CC
> CC Excl: No Excl

M96.1 Postlaminectomy syndrome, not elsewhere classified

M96.2 Postradiation kyphosis

M96.3 Postlaminectomy kyphosis

M96.4 Postsurgical lordosis

M96.5 Postradiation scoliosis

☑5ᵗʰ **M96.6 Fracture of bone following insertion of orthopedic implant, joint prosthesis, or bone plate**
> Intraoperative fracture of bone during insertion of orthopedic implant, joint prosthesis, or bone plate
> EXCLUDES 2   complication of internal orthopedic devices, implants or grafts (T84.-)

   ☑6ᵗʰ **M96.62 Fracture of humerus following insertion of orthopedic implant, joint prosthesis, or bone plate**
     M96.621 Fracture of humerus following insertion of orthopedic implant, joint prosthesis, or bone plate, right arm   CC
> CC Excl: D78.81-D78.89, E36.8, E89.810-E89.89, H59.011-H59.019, H59.031-H59.099, H59.811-H59.89, H95.811-H95.89, I97.3, L76.81-L76.82, M96.621-M96.69, M96.89, N98.1-N98.9, T84.010-T84.9XX with 7th A; T81.82XA, T81.89XA, T81.9XXA, T84.9

     M96.622 Fracture of humerus following insertion of orthopedic implant, joint prosthesis, or bone plate, left arm   CC
> CC Excl: See code: M96.621

     M96.629 Fracture of humerus following insertion of orthopedic implant, joint prosthesis, or bone plate, unspecified arm   CC
> CC Excl: See code: M96.621

   ☑6ᵗʰ **M96.63 Fracture of radius or ulna following insertion of orthopedic implant, joint prosthesis, or bone plate**
     M96.631 Fracture of radius or ulna following insertion of orthopedic implant, joint prosthesis, or bone plate, right arm   CC
> CC Excl: See code: M96.621

     M96.632 Fracture of radius or ulna following insertion of orthopedic implant, joint prosthesis, or bone plate, left arm   CC
> CC Excl: See code: M96.621

     M96.639 Fracture of radius or ulna following insertion of orthopedic implant, joint prosthesis, or bone plate, unspecified arm   CC
> CC Excl: See code: M96.621

   M96.65 Fracture of pelvis following insertion of orthopedic implant, joint prosthesis, or bone plate   CC
> CC Excl: See code: M96.621

☑6ᵗʰ **M96.66 Fracture of femur following insertion of orthopedic implant, joint prosthesis, or bone plate**
     M96.661 Fracture of femur following insertion of orthopedic implant, joint prosthesis, or bone plate, right leg   CC
> CC Excl: See code: M96.621

     M96.662 Fracture of femur following insertion of orthopedic implant, joint prosthesis, or bone plate, left leg   CC
> CC Excl: See code: M96.621

     M96.669 Fracture of femur following insertion of orthopedic implant, joint prosthesis, or bone plate, unspecified leg   CC
> CC Excl: See code: M96.621

☑6ᵗʰ **M96.67 Fracture of tibia or fibula following insertion of orthopedic implant, joint prosthesis, or bone plate**
     M96.671 Fracture of tibia or fibula following insertion of orthopedic implant, joint prosthesis, or bone plate, right leg   CC
> CC Excl: See code: M96.621

     M96.672 Fracture of tibia or fibula following insertion of orthopedic implant, joint prosthesis, or bone plate, left leg   CC
> CC Excl: See code: M96.621

     M96.679 Fracture of tibia or fibula following insertion of orthopedic implant, joint prosthesis, or bone plate, unspecified leg   CC
> CC Excl: See code: M96.621

   M96.69 Fracture of other bone following insertion of orthopedic implant, joint prosthesis, or bone plate   CC
> CC Excl: See code: M96.621

☑ Additional Character Required   ☑x7ᵗʰ Placeholder Alert   Unacceptable PDx   Manifestation   Hospital Acquired Condition   EXCLUDES 1 Not Coded Here   EXCLUDES 2 Not Included Here

ICD-10-CM 2016   787

✓5ᵗʰ M96.8 Other intraoperative and postprocedural complications and disorders of musculoskeletal system, not elsewhere classified

✓6ᵗʰ M96.81 Intraoperative hemorrhage and hematoma of a musculoskeletal structure complicating a procedure

> **EXCLUDES 1** intraoperative hemorrhage and hematoma of a musculoskeletal structure due to accidental puncture and laceration during a procedure (M96.82-)

M96.810 Intraoperative hemorrhage and hematoma of a musculoskeletal structure complicating a musculoskeletal system procedure `CC`

CC Excl: H95.811-H95.89, I85.01, I85.11, I97.3, K21.9, K22.8, K23-K25.0, K25.2, K25.4, K25.6, K26.0, K26.2, K26.4, K26.6, K27.0, K27.2, K27.4, K27.6, K28.0, K28.2, K28.4, K28.6, K29.01, K29.21, K29.31, K29.41, K29.51, K29.61, K29.71, K29.81, K29.91, K31.811, K55.21, K57.01, K57.11, K57.13, K57.21, K57.31, K57.33, K57.41, K57.51, K57.53, K57.81, K57.91, K57.93, K62.5, K92.0-K92.2, M96.810-M96.811, M96.830-M96.89, N98.1-N98.9, P54.1-P54.3, T81.10XA, T81.11XA, T81.12XA, T81.19XA, T81.82XA, T81.89XA, T81.9XXA

M96.811 Intraoperative hemorrhage and hematoma of a musculoskeletal structure complicating other procedure `CC`

CC Excl: See code: M96.810

✓6ᵗʰ M96.82 Accidental puncture and laceration of a musculoskeletal structure during a procedure

M96.820 Accidental puncture and laceration of a musculoskeletal structure during a musculoskeletal system procedure `CC`

CC Excl: D78.11-D78.12, D78.81-D78.89, E36.11-E36.8, E89.810-E89.89, G96.11, G97.41-G97.49, H59.011-H59.019, H59.031-H59.099, H59.211-H59.229, H59.811-H59.89, H95.31-H95.32, H95.811-H95.89, I97.3, I97.51-I97.52, J95.71-J95.72, K91.71-K91.72, L76.11-L76.12, L76.81-L76.82, M96.820-M96.821, M96.89, N98.1-N98.9, N99.71-N99.72, T81.82XA, T81.89XA, T81.9XXA

M96.821 Accidental puncture and laceration of a musculoskeletal structure during other procedure `CC`

CC Excl: See code: M96.820

✓6ᵗʰ M96.83 Postprocedural hemorrhage and hematoma of a musculoskeletal structure following a procedure

M96.830 Postprocedural hemorrhage and hematoma of a musculoskeletal structure following a musculoskeletal system procedure `CC`

CC Excl: See code: M96.810

M96.831 Postprocedural hemorrhage and hematoma of a musculoskeletal structure following other procedure `CC`

CC Excl: See code: M96.810

M96.89 Other intraoperative and postprocedural complications and disorders of the musculoskeletal system `CC`

Instability of joint secondary to removal of joint prosthesis

Use additional code, if applicable, to further specify disorder

CC Excl: D78.81-D78.89, E36.8, E89.810-E89.89, H59.011-H59.019, H59.031-H59.099, H59.811-H59.89, H95.811-H95.89, I97.3, L76.81-L76.82, M96.89, N98.1-N98.9, T81.82XA, T81.89XA, T81.9XXA

Biomechanical lesions, not elsewhere classified (M99)

✓4ᵗʰ M99 Biomechanical lesions, not elsewhere classified

> **NOTE** This category should not be used if the condition can be classified elsewhere.

✓5ᵗʰ M99.0 Segmental and somatic dysfunction

M99.00 Segmental and somatic dysfunction of head region

M99.01 Segmental and somatic dysfunction of cervical region

M99.02 Segmental and somatic dysfunction of thoracic region

M99.03 Segmental and somatic dysfunction of lumbar region

M99.04 Segmental and somatic dysfunction of sacral region

M99.05 Segmental and somatic dysfunction of pelvic region

M99.06 Segmental and somatic dysfunction of lower extremity

M99.07 Segmental and somatic dysfunction of upper extremity

M99.08 Segmental and somatic dysfunction of rib cage

M99.09 Segmental and somatic dysfunction of abdomen and other regions

✓5ᵗʰ M99.1 Subluxation complex (vertebral)

> **CC Excl:** For CC codes in subcategory M99.1, unless otherwise noted: M99.10-M99.11, S03.8XX-S03.9XX with 7th A, S12.000-S12.691 with 7th [A, B], S12.9XX-S13.4XX with 7th A, S13.8XXA, S14.0XX-S14.108 with 7th A, S14.111-S14.118 with 7th A, S14.121-S14.128 with 7th A, S14.131-S14.138 with 7th A, S14.141-S14.148 with 7th A, S14.151-S14.158 with 7th A, S16.1XX A, S29.011-S29.019 with 7th A, S38.3XX-S39.013 with 7th A, T14.90-T14.91, T79.A0X-T79.9XX with 7th A

M99.10 Subluxation complex (vertebral) of head region `CC`

M99.11 Subluxation complex (vertebral) of cervical region `CC`

M99.12 Subluxation complex (vertebral) of thoracic region

M99.13 Subluxation complex (vertebral) of lumbar region

M99.14 Subluxation complex (vertebral) of sacral region

M99.15 Subluxation complex (vertebral) of pelvic region

M99.16 Subluxation complex (vertebral) of lower extremity

M99.17 Subluxation complex (vertebral) of upper extremity

M99.18 Subluxation complex (vertebral) of rib cage `CC`

CC Excl: M99.18, S43.201-S43.226 with 7th character A

M99.19 Subluxation complex (vertebral) of abdomen and other regions

✓6ᵗʰ M99.2 Subluxation stenosis of neural canal

M99.20 Subluxation stenosis of neural canal of head region

M99.21 Subluxation stenosis of neural canal of cervical region

M99.22 Subluxation stenosis of neural canal of thoracic region

M99.23 Subluxation stenosis of neural canal of lumbar region

M99.24 Subluxation stenosis of neural canal of sacral region

M99.25 Subluxation stenosis of neural canal of pelvic region

M99.26 Subluxation stenosis of neural canal of lower extremity

M99.27 Subluxation stenosis of neural canal of upper extremity

M99.28 Subluxation stenosis of neural canal of rib cage

M99.29 Subluxation stenosis of neural canal of abdomen and other regions

✓5ᵗʰ M99.3 Osseous stenosis of neural canal

M99.30 Osseous stenosis of neural canal of head region

M99.31 Osseous stenosis of neural canal of cervical region

M99.32 Osseous stenosis of neural canal of thoracic region

M99.33 Osseous stenosis of neural canal of lumbar region

M99.34 Osseous stenosis of neural canal of sacral region

M99.35 Osseous stenosis of neural canal of pelvic region

M99.36 Osseous stenosis of neural canal of lower extremity

M99.37 Osseous stenosis of neural canal of upper extremity

M99.38 Osseous stenosis of neural canal of rib cage

M99.39 Osseous stenosis of neural canal of abdomen and other regions

✓5ᵗʰ M99.4 Connective tissue stenosis of neural canal

M99.40 Connective tissue stenosis of neural canal of head region

M99.41 Connective tissue stenosis of neural canal of cervical region

M99.42 Connective tissue stenosis of neural canal of thoracic region

M99.43 Connective tissue stenosis of neural canal of lumbar region

M99.44 Connective tissue stenosis of neural canal of sacral region

M99.45 Connective tissue stenosis of neural canal of pelvic region

M99.46 Connective tissue stenosis of neural canal of lower extremity

N Newborn: 0   P Pediatric: 0-17   M Maternity: 12-55   A Adult: 15-124   **MCC** Major CC Condition   **PDxMCC** PDx acts as own MCC   **CC** CC Condition   **PDxCC** PDx acts as own CC

788

ICD-10-CM 2016

M99.47   **Connective tissue stenosis of neural canal of** upper **extremity**

M99.48   **Connective tissue stenosis of neural canal of** rib cage

M99.49   **Connective tissue stenosis of neural canal of** abdomen and other **regions**

✓5ᵗʰ   M99.5   **Intervertebral disc stenosis of neural canal**

M99.50   **Intervertebral disc stenosis of neural canal of** head **region**

M99.51   **Intervertebral disc stenosis of neural canal of** cervical **region**

M99.52   **Intervertebral disc stenosis of neural canal of** thoracic **region**

M99.53   **Intervertebral disc stenosis of neural canal of** lumbar **region**

M99.54   **Intervertebral disc stenosis of neural canal of** sacral **region**

M99.55   **Intervertebral disc stenosis of neural canal of** pelvic **region**

M99.56   **Intervertebral disc stenosis of neural canal of** lower **extremity**

M99.57   **Intervertebral disc stenosis of neural canal of** upper **extremity**

M99.58   **Intervertebral disc stenosis of neural canal of** rib cage

M99.59   **Intervertebral disc stenosis of neural canal of** abdomen and other **regions**

✓5ᵗʰ   M99.6   **Osseous and subluxation stenosis of intervertebral foramina**

M99.60   **Osseous and subluxation stenosis of intervertebral foramina of** head **region**

M99.61   **Osseous and subluxation stenosis of intervertebral foramina of** cervical **region**

M99.62   **Osseous and subluxation stenosis of intervertebral foramina of** thoracic **region**

M99.63   **Osseous and subluxation stenosis of intervertebral foramina of** lumbar **region**

M99.64   **Osseous and subluxation stenosis of intervertebral foramina of** sacral **region**

M99.65   **Osseous and subluxation stenosis of intervertebral foramina of** pelvic **region**

M99.66   **Osseous and subluxation stenosis of intervertebral foramina of** lower **extremity**

M99.67   **Osseous and subluxation stenosis of intervertebral foramina of** upper **extremity**

M99.68   **Osseous and subluxation stenosis of intervertebral foramina of** rib cage

M99.69   **Osseous and subluxation stenosis of intervertebral foramina of** abdomen and other **regions**

✓5ᵗʰ   M99.7   **Connective tissue and disc stenosis of intervertebral foramina**

M99.70   **Connective tissue and disc stenosis of intervertebral foramina of** head **region**

M99.71   **Connective tissue and disc stenosis of intervertebral foramina of** cervical **region**

M99.72   **Connective tissue and disc stenosis of intervertebral foramina of** thoracic **region**

M99.73   **Connective tissue and disc stenosis of intervertebral foramina of** lumbar **region**

M99.74   **Connective tissue and disc stenosis of intervertebral foramina of** sacral **region**

M99.75   **Connective tissue and disc stenosis of intervertebral foramina of** pelvic **region**

M99.76   **Connective tissue and disc stenosis of intervertebral foramina of** lower **extremity**

M99.77   **Connective tissue and disc stenosis of intervertebral foramina of** upper **extremity**

M99.78   **Connective tissue and disc stenosis of intervertebral foramina of** rib cage

M99.79   **Connective tissue and disc stenosis of intervertebral foramina of** abdomen and other **regions**

✓5ᵗʰ   M99.8   **Other** biomechanical lesions

M99.80   **Other biomechanical lesions of** head **region**

M99.81   **Other biomechanical lesions of** cervical **region**

M99.82   **Other biomechanical lesions of** thoracic **region**

M99.83   **Other biomechanical lesions of** lumbar **region**

M99.84   **Other biomechanical lesions of** sacral **region**

M99.85   **Other biomechanical lesions of** pelvic **region**

M99.86   **Other biomechanical lesions of** lower **extremity**

M99.87   **Other biomechanical lesions of** upper **extremity**

M99.88   **Other biomechanical lesions of** rib cage

M99.89   **Other biomechanical lesions of** abdomen and other **regions**

M99.9   **Biomechanical lesion,** unspecified

✓ Additional Character Required   ✓x7ᵗʰ Placeholder Alert   Unacceptable PDx   Manifestation   Hospital Acquired Condition   **EXCLUDES 1** Not Coded Here   **EXCLUDES 2** Not Included Here

ICD-10-CM 2016   789

Chapter 14. Diseases of Genitourinary System (NØØ–N99)

Chapter Specific Guidelines with Coding Examples

The chapter specific guidelines from the ICD-10-CM Official Guidelines for Coding and Reporting have been provided below. Along with these guidelines are coding examples, contained in the shaded boxes, that have been developed to help illustrate the coding and/or sequencing guidance found in these guidelines.

a. Chronic kidney disease

1) Stages of chronic kidney disease (CKD)

The ICD-10-CM classifies CKD based on severity. The severity of CKD is designated by stages 1-5. Stage 2, code N18.2, equates to mild CKD; stage 3, code N18.3, equates to moderate CKD; and stage 4, code N18.4, equates to severe CKD. Code N18.6, End stage renal disease (ESRD), is assigned when the provider has documented end-stage-renal disease (ESRD).

If both a stage of CKD and ESRD are documented, assign code N18.6 only.

Stage 5 chronic kidney disease with ESRD requiring chronic dialysis

N18.6   **End stage renal disease**

Z99.2   **Dependence on renal dialysis**

Explanation: The diagnostic statement indicates the patient has chronic kidney disease, documented both as stage 5 and as ESRD requiring chronic dialysis. Code N18.6 End stage renal disease (ESRD), is assigned when the provider has documented end-stage-renal disease (ESRD). If both a stage of CKD and ESRD are documented, assign code N18.6 only.

---

2) Chronic kidney disease and kidney transplant status

Patients who have undergone kidney transplant may still have some form of chronic kidney disease (CKD) because the kidney transplant may not fully restore kidney function. Therefore, the presence of CKD alone does not constitute a transplant complication. Assign the appropriate N18 code for the patient's stage of CKD and code Z94.Ø, Kidney transplant status. If a transplant complication such as failure or rejection or other transplant complication is documented, see section I.C.19.g for information on coding complications of a kidney transplant. If the documentation is unclear as to whether the patient has a complication of the transplant, query the provider.

Patient with residual chronic kidney disease stage 1 after kidney transplant

N18.1   **Chronic kidney disease, stage 1**

Z94.Ø   **Kidney transplant status**

Explanation: Patients who have undergone kidney transplant may still have some form of chronic kidney disease (CKD) because the kidney transplant may not fully restore kidney function. The presence of CKD alone does not constitute a transplant complication. Assign the appropriate N18 code for the patient's stage of CKD and code Z94.0 Kidney transplant status.

---

3) Chronic kidney disease with other conditions

Patients with CKD may also suffer from other serious conditions, most commonly diabetes mellitus and hypertension. The sequencing of the CKD code in relationship to codes for other contributing conditions is based on the conventions in the Tabular List.

See I.C.9. Hypertensive chronic kidney disease.

See I.C.19. Chronic kidney disease and kidney transplant complications.

Type 1 diabetic chronic kidney disease, stage 2

E10.22   **Type 1 diabetes mellitus with diabetic chronic kidney disease**

N18.2   **Chronic kidney disease, stage 2 (mild)**

Explanation: Patients with CKD may also suffer from other serious conditions such as diabetes mellitus. The sequencing of the CKD code in relationship to codes for other contributing conditions is based on the conventions in the Tabular List. Diabetic CKD code E10.22 includes an instructional note to "Use additional code to identify stage of chronic kidney disease (N18.1–N18.6)," thus providing sequencing direction.

Chapter 14. Diseases of the Genitourinary System (N00-N99)

> EXCLUDES 2   certain conditions originating in the perinatal period (P04-P96)
> certain infectious and parasitic diseases (A00-B99)
> complications of pregnancy, childbirth and the puerperium (O00-O9A)
> congenital malformations, deformations and chromosomal abnormalities (Q00-Q99)
> endocrine, nutritional and metabolic diseases (E00-E88)
> injury, poisoning and certain other consequences of external causes (S00-T88)
> neoplasms (C00-D49)
> symptoms, signs and abnormal clinical and laboratory findings, not elsewhere classified (R00-R94)

This chapter contains the following blocks:

N00-N08	Glomerular diseases
N10-N16	Renal tubulo-interstitial diseases
N17-N19	Acute kidney failure and chronic kidney disease
N20-N23	Urolithiasis
N25-N29	Other disorders of kidney and ureter
N30-N39	Other diseases of the urinary system
N40-N53	Diseases of male genital organs
N60-N65	Disorders of breast
N70-N77	Inflammatory diseases of female pelvic organs
N80-N98	Noninflammatory disorders of female genital tract
N99	Intraoperative and postprocedural complications and disorders of genitourinary system, not elsewhere classified

Glomerular diseases (N00-N08)

Code also any associated kidney failure (N17-N19).

> EXCLUDES 1   hypertensive chronic kidney disease (I12.-)

✓4th **N00   Acute nephritic syndrome**

> INCLUDES   acute glomerular disease
> acute glomerulonephritis
> acute nephritis
>
> EXCLUDES 1   acute tubulo-interstitial nephritis (N10)
> nephritic syndrome NOS (N05.-)

CC Excl: For MCC codes in category N00, unless otherwise noted:
A17.9, A18.10-A18.11, A18.13, A18.82, A18.84, A18.89, A54.21, A54.29, A54.82, A54.84, A54.89-A54.9, A59.00, A59.8-A59.9, B37.41-B37.49, E08.21-E08.29, E08.618-E08.638, E08.649-E08.8, E09.21-E09.29, E09.618-E09.638, E09.649-E09.8, E10.21-E10.29, E10.618-E10.638, E10.649, E10.69-E10.8, E11.21-E11.29, E11.618-E11.638, E11.649, E11.69-E11.8, E13.21-E13.29, E13.618-E13.638, E13.649-E13.8, E88.3, M10.30-M10.39, N00.0-N11.0, N11.8-N13.39, N13.6, N14.0-N19, N25.0-N26.1, N26.9-N27.9, N28.1-N29, N36.41-N36.43, N36.8-N36.9, N39.8-N39.9, R31.0-R31.9

N00.0   Acute nephritic syndrome with minor glomerular abnormality   MCC
Acute nephritic syndrome with minimal change lesion

N00.1   Acute nephritic syndrome with focal and segmental glomerular lesions   MCC
Acute nephritic syndrome with focal and segmental hyalinosis
Acute nephritic syndrome with focal and segmental sclerosis
Acute nephritic syndrome with focal glomerulonephritis

N00.2   Acute nephritic syndrome with diffuse membranous glomerulonephritis   MCC

N00.3   Acute nephritic syndrome with diffuse mesangial proliferative glomerulonephritis   MCC

N00.4   Acute nephritic syndrome with diffuse endocapillary proliferative glomerulonephritis   MCC

N00.5   Acute nephritic syndrome with diffuse mesangiocapillary glomerulonephritis   MCC
Acute nephritic syndrome with membranoproliferative glomerulonephritis, types 1 and 3, or NOS

N00.6   Acute nephritic syndrome with dense deposit disease   MCC
Acute nephritic syndrome with membranoproliferative glomerulonephritis, type 2

N00.7   Acute nephritic syndrome with diffuse crescentic glomerulonephritis   MCC
Acute nephritic syndrome with extracapillary glomerulonephritis

N00.8   Acute nephritic syndrome with other morphologic changes   MCC
Acute nephritic syndrome with proliferative glomerulonephritis NOS
CC Excl: A17.9, A18.10-A18.11, A18.13, A18.82, A18.84, A18.89, A54.21, A54.29, A54.82, A54.84, A54.89-A54.9, A59.00, A59.8-A59.9, B37.41-B37.49, E08.21-E08.29, E09.21-E09.29, E88.3, M10.30-M10.39, N00.0-N11.0, N11.8-N13.39, N13.6, N14.0-N19, N25.0-N26.1, N26.9-N27.9, N28.1-N29, N36.41-N36.43, N36.8-N36.9, N39.8-N39.9, R31.0-R31.9

N00.9   Acute nephritic syndrome with unspecified morphologic changes   MCC

✓4th **N01   Rapidly progressive nephritic syndrome**

> INCLUDES   rapidly progressive glomerular disease
> rapidly progressive glomerulonephritis
> rapidly progressive nephritis
>
> EXCLUDES 1   nephritic syndrome NOS (N05.-)

CC Excl: For MCC codes in category N01, unless otherwise noted:
See code: N00

N01.0   Rapidly progressive nephritic syndrome with minor glomerular abnormality   MCC
Rapidly progressive nephritic syndrome with minimal change lesion

N01.1   Rapidly progressive nephritic syndrome with focal and segmental glomerular lesions   MCC
Rapidly progressive nephritic syndrome with focal and segmental hyalinosis
Rapidly progressive nephritic syndrome with focal and segmental sclerosis
Rapidly progressive nephritic syndrome with focal glomerulonephritis

N01.2   Rapidly progressive nephritic syndrome with diffuse membranous glomerulonephritis   MCC

N01.3   Rapidly progressive nephritic syndrome with diffuse mesangial proliferative glomerulonephritis   MCC

N01.4   Rapidly progressive nephritic syndrome with diffuse endocapillary proliferative glomerulonephritis   MCC

N01.5   Rapidly progressive nephritic syndrome with diffuse mesangiocapillary glomerulonephritis   MCC
Rapidly progressive nephritic syndrome with membranoproliferative glomerulonephritis, types 1 and 3, or NOS

N01.6   Rapidly progressive nephritic syndrome with dense deposit disease   MCC
Rapidly progressive nephritic syndrome with membranoproliferative glomerulonephritis, type 2

N01.7   Rapidly progressive nephritic syndrome with diffuse crescentic glomerulonephritis   MCC
Rapidly progressive nephritic syndrome with extracapillary glomerulonephritis

N01.8   Rapidly progressive nephritic syndrome with other morphologic changes   MCC
Rapidly progressive nephritic syndrome with proliferative glomerulonephritis NOS

N01.9   Rapidly progressive nephritic syndrome with unspecified morphologic changes   MCC

✓4th **N02   Recurrent and persistent hematuria**

> EXCLUDES 1   acute cystitis with hematuria (N30.01)
> hematuria NOS (R31.9)
> hematuria not associated with specified morphologic lesions (R31.-)

CC Excl: For CC codes in category N02, unless otherwise noted:
See code: N00

N02.0   Recurrent and persistent hematuria with minor glomerular abnormality   CC
Recurrent and persistent hematuria with minimal change lesion

N02.1   Recurrent and persistent hematuria with focal and segmental glomerular lesions   CC
Recurrent and persistent hematuria with focal and segmental hyalinosis
Recurrent and persistent hematuria with focal and segmental sclerosis
Recurrent and persistent hematuria with focal glomerulonephritis

N02.2   Recurrent and persistent hematuria with diffuse membranous glomerulonephritis   CC

N02.3   Recurrent and persistent hematuria with diffuse mesangial proliferative glomerulonephritis   CC

N02.4   Recurrent and persistent hematuria with diffuse endocapillary proliferative glomerulonephritis   CC

☑ Additional Character Required   ✓x7th Placeholder Alert   Unacceptable PDx   Manifestation   Hospital Acquired Condition   EXCLUDES 1 Not Coded Here   EXCLUDES 2 Not Included Here

ICD-10-CM 2016   791

N02.5 **Recurrent and persistent hematuria with** diffuse mesangiocapillary glomerulonephritis   `CC`
    Recurrent and persistent hematuria with membranoproliferative glomerulonephritis, types 1 and 3, or NOS

N02.6 **Recurrent and persistent hematuria with** dense deposit disease   `CC`
    Recurrent and persistent hematuria with membranoproliferative glomerulonephritis, type 2

N02.7 **Recurrent and persistent hematuria with** diffuse crescentic glomerulonephritis   `CC`
    Recurrent and persistent hematuria with extracapillary glomerulonephritis

N02.8 **Recurrent and persistent hematuria with** other morphologic changes   `CC`
    Recurrent and persistent hematuria with proliferative glomerulonephritis NOS
    CC Excl: A17.9, A18.10-A18.11, A18.13, A18.82, A18.84, A18.89, A54.21, A54.29, A54.82, A54.84, A54.89-A54.9, A59.00, A59.8-A59.9, B37.41-B37.49, E08.21-E08.29, E08.618-E08.638, E08.649-E08.8, E09.21-E09.29, E09.618-E09.638, E09.649-E09.8, E10.21-E10.29, E10.618-E10.638, E10.649, E10.69-E10.8, E11.21-E11.29, E11.618-E11.638, E11.649, E11.69-E11.8, E13.21-E13.29, E13.618-E13.638, E13.649-E13.8, M10.30-M10.39, N00.0-N11.0, N11.8-N13.39, N13.6, N14.0-N19, N25.0-N26.1, N26.9-N27.9, N28.1-N29, N36.41-N36.43, N36.8-N36.9, N39.8-N39.9, R31.0-R31.9

N02.9 **Recurrent and persistent hematuria with** unspecified morphologic changes   `CC`

✓4ᵗʰ N03 **Chronic** nephritic syndrome
   INCLUDES   chronic glomerular disease
         chronic glomerulonephritis
         chronic nephritis
   EXCLUDES 1   *chronic tubulo-interstitial nephritis (N11.-)*
         diffuse sclerosing glomerulonephritis (N05.8-)
         nephritic syndrome NOS (N05.-)

CC Excl: For CC codes in catagory N03, unless otherwise noted:
A17.9, A18.10-A18.11, A18.13, A18.82, A18.84, A18.89, A54.21, A54.29, A54.82, A54.84, A54.89-A54.9, A59.00, A59.8-A59.9, A98.5, B37.41-B37.49, E08.21-E08.29, E08.618-E08.638, E08.649-E08.8, E09.21-E09.29, E09.618-E09.638, E09.649-E09.8, E10.21-E10.29, E10.618-E10.638, E10.649, E10.69-E10.8, E11.21-E11.29, E11.618-E11.638, E11.649, E11.69-E11.8, E13.21-E13.29, E13.618-E13.638, E13.649-E13.8, E88.3, M10.30-M10.39, N00.0-N11.0, N11.8-N13.39, N13.6, N14.0-N17.9, N19, N25.0-N26.1, N26.9-N27.9, N28.1-N29, N36.41-N36.43, N36.8-N36.9, N39.8-N39.9, R31.0-R31.9

N03.0 **Chronic nephritic syndrome with** minor glomerular abnormality   `CC`
    Chronic nephritic syndrome with minimal change lesion

N03.1 **Chronic nephritic syndrome with** focal and segmental glomerular lesions   `CC`
    Chronic nephritic syndrome with focal and segmental hyalinosis
    Chronic nephritic syndrome with focal and segmental sclerosis
    Chronic nephritic syndrome with focal glomerulonephritis

N03.2 **Chronic nephritic syndrome with** diffuse membranous glomerulonephritis   `CC`

N03.3 **Chronic nephritic syndrome with** diffuse mesangial proliferative glomerulonephritis   `CC`

N03.4 **Chronic nephritic syndrome with** diffuse endocapillary proliferative glomerulonephritis   `CC`

N03.5 **Chronic nephritic syndrome with** diffuse mesangiocapillary glomerulonephritis   `CC`
    Chronic nephritic syndrome with membranoproliferative glomerulonephritis, types 1 and 3, or NOS

N03.6 **Chronic nephritic syndrome with** dense deposit disease   `CC`
    Chronic nephritic syndrome with membranoproliferative glomerulonephritis, type 2

N03.7 **Chronic nephritic syndrome with** diffuse crescentic glomerulonephritis   `CC`
    Chronic nephritic syndrome with extracapillary glomerulonephritis

N03.8 **Chronic nephritic syndrome with** other morphologic changes   `CC`
    Chronic nephritic syndrome with proliferative glomerulonephritis NOS

N03.9 **Chronic nephritic syndrome with** unspecified morphologic changes   `CC`

✓4ᵗʰ N04 **Nephrotic syndrome**
   INCLUDES   congenital nephrotic syndrome
         lipoid nephrosis

CC Excl: For CC codes in category N04, unless otherwise noted:
A17.9, A18.10-A18.11, A18.13, A18.82, A18.84, A18.89, A54.21, A54.29, A54.82, A54.84, A54.89-A54.9, A59.00, A59.8-A59.9, B37.41-B37.49, E08.21-E08.29, E08.618-E08.638, E08.649-E08.8, E09.21-E09.29, E09.618-E09.638, E09.649-E09.8, E10.21-E10.29, E10.618-E10.638, E10.649, E10.69-E10.8, E11.21-E11.29, E11.618-E11.638, E11.649, E11.69-E11.8, E13.21-E13.29, E13.618-E13.638, E13.649-E13.8, M10.30-M10.39, N00.0-N11.0, N11.8-N13.39, N13.6, N14.0-N19, N25.0-N26.1, N26.9-N27.9, N28.1-N29, N36.41-N36.43, N36.8-N36.9, N39.8-N39.9, R31.0-R31.9

N04.0 **Nephrotic syndrome with** minor glomerular abnormality   `CC`
    Nephrotic syndrome with minimal change lesion

N04.1 **Nephrotic syndrome with** focal and segmental glomerular lesions   `CC`
    Nephrotic syndrome with focal and segmental hyalinosis
    Nephrotic syndrome with focal and segmental sclerosis
    Nephrotic syndrome with focal glomerulonephritis

N04.2 **Nephrotic syndrome with** diffuse membranous glomerulonephritis   `CC`

N04.3 **Nephrotic syndrome with** diffuse mesangial proliferative glomerulonephritis   `CC`

N04.4 **Nephrotic syndrome with** diffuse endocapillary proliferative glomerulonephritis   `CC`

N04.5 **Nephrotic syndrome with** diffuse mesangiocapillary glomerulonephritis   `CC`
    Nephrotic syndrome with membranoproliferative glomerulonephritis, types 1 and 3, or NOS

N04.6 **Nephrotic syndrome with** dense deposit disease   `CC`
    Nephrotic syndrome with membranoproliferative glomerulonephritis, type 2

N04.7 **Nephrotic syndrome with** diffuse crescentic glomerulonephritis   `CC`
    Nephrotic syndrome with extracapillary glomerulonephritis
    CC Excl: A17.9, A18.10-A18.11, A18.13, A18.82, A18.84, A18.89, A54.21, A54.29, A54.82, A54.84, A54.89-A54.9, A59.00, A59.8-A59.9, B37.41-B37.49, E08.21-E08.29, E08.618-E08.638, E08.649-E08.8, E09.21-E09.29, E09.618-E09.638, E09.649-E09.8, E10.21-E10.29, E10.618-E10.638, E10.649, E10.69-E10.8, E11.21-E11.29, E11.618-E11.638, E11.649, E11.69-E11.8, E13.21-E13.29, E13.618-E13.638, E13.649-E13.8, E88.3, M10.30-M10.39, N00.0-N11.0, N11.8-N13.39, N13.6, N14.0-N19, N25.0-N26.1, N26.9-N27.9, N28.1-N29, N36.41-N36.43, N36.8-N36.9, N39.8-N39.9, R31.0-R31.9

N04.8 **Nephrotic syndrome with** other morphologic changes   `CC`
    Nephrotic syndrome with proliferative glomerulonephritis NOS
    CC Excl: See code: N04.7

N04.9 **Nephrotic syndrome with** unspecified morphologic changes   `CC`
    CC Excl: See code: N04.7

✓4ᵗʰ N05 **Unspecified** nephritic syndrome
   INCLUDES   glomerular disease NOS
         glomerulonephritis NOS
         nephritis NOS
         nephropathy NOS and renal disease NOS with morphological lesion specified in .0-.8
   EXCLUDES 1   *nephropathy NOS with no stated morphological lesion (N28.9)*
         renal disease NOS with no stated morphological lesion (N28.9)
         tubulo-interstitial nephritis NOS (N12)

CC Excl: For CC codes in category N05, unless otherwise noted:
A17.9, A18.10-A18.11, A18.13, A18.82, A18.84, A18.89, A54.21, A54.29, A54.82, A54.84, A54.89-A54.9, A59.00, A59.8-A59.9, A98.5, B37.41-B37.49, E08.21-E08.29, E08.618-E08.638, E08.649-E08.8, E09.21-E09.29, E09.618-E09.638, E09.649-E09.8, E10.21-E10.29, E10.618-E10.638, E10.649, E10.69-E10.8, E11.21-E11.29, E11.618-E11.638, E11.649, E11.69-E11.8, E13.21-E13.29, E13.618-E13.638, E13.649-E13.8, M10.30-M10.39, N00.0-N11.0, N11.8-N13.39, N13.6, N14.0-N17.9, N19, N25.0-N26.1, N26.9-N27.9, N28.1-N29, N36.41-N36.43, N36.8-N36.9, N39.8-N39.9, R31.0-R31.9

N05.0 **Unspecified nephritic syndrome with** minor glomerular abnormality
    Unspecified nephritic syndrome with minimal change lesion

N05.1 **Unspecified nephritic syndrome with** focal and segmental glomerular lesions
    Unspecified nephritic syndrome with focal and segmental hyalinosis
    Unspecified nephritic syndrome with focal and segmental sclerosis
    Unspecified nephritic syndrome with focal glomerulonephritis

N05.2 Unspecified nephritic syndrome with diffuse membranous glomerulonephritis `CC`

N05.3 Unspecified nephritic syndrome with diffuse mesangial proliferative glomerulonephritis `CC`

N05.4 Unspecified nephritic syndrome with diffuse endocapillary proliferative glomerulonephritis `CC`

N05.5 Unspecified nephritic syndrome with diffuse mesangiocapillary glomerulonephritis `CC`
Unspecified nephritic syndrome with membranoproliferative glomerulonephritis, types 1 and 3, or NOS

N05.6 Unspecified nephritic syndrome with dense deposit disease
Unspecified nephritic syndrome with membranoproliferative glomerulonephritis, type 2

N05.7 Unspecified nephritic syndrome with diffuse crescentic glomerulonephritis
Unspecified nephritic syndrome with extracapillary glomerulonephritis

N05.8 Unspecified nephritic syndrome with other morphologic changes
Unspecified nephritic syndrome with proliferative glomerulonephritis NOS

N05.9 Unspecified nephritic syndrome with unspecified morphologic changes

✓4ᵗʰ **N06 Isolated proteinuria with specified morphological lesion**
EXCLUDES 1   proteinuria not associated with specific morphologic lesions (R80.0)

CC Excl: For CC codes in category N06, unless otherwise noted:
See code: N03

N06.0 Isolated proteinuria with minor glomerular abnormality
Isolated proteinuria with minimal change lesion

N06.1 Isolated proteinuria with focal and segmental glomerular lesions
Isolated proteinuria with focal and segmental hyalinosis
Isolated proteinuria with focal and segmental sclerosis
Isolated proteinuria with focal glomerulonephritis

N06.2 Isolated proteinuria with diffuse membranous glomerulonephritis `CC`

N06.3 Isolated proteinuria with diffuse mesangial proliferative glomerulonephritis `CC`

N06.4 Isolated proteinuria with diffuse endocapillary proliferative glomerulonephritis `CC`

N06.5 Isolated proteinuria with diffuse mesangiocapillary glomerulonephritis `CC`
Isolated proteinuria with membranoproliferative glomerulonephritis, types 1 and 3, or NOS

N06.6 Isolated proteinuria with dense deposit disease
Isolated proteinuria with membranoproliferative glomerulonephritis, type 2

N06.7 Isolated proteinuria with diffuse crescentic glomerulonephritis
Isolated proteinuria with extracapillary glomerulonephritis

N06.8 Isolated proteinuria with other morphologic lesion
Isolated proteinuria with proliferative glomerulonephritis NOS

N06.9 Isolated proteinuria with unspecified morphologic lesion

✓4ᵗʰ **N07 Hereditary nephropathy, not elsewhere classified**
EXCLUDES 2   Alport's syndrome (Q87.81-)
hereditary amyloid nephropathy (E85.-)
nail patella syndrome (Q87.2)
non-neuropathic heredofamilial amyloidosis (E85.-)

CC Excl: For CC codes in category N07, unless otherwise noted:
A17.9, A18.10-A18.11, A18.13, A18.82, A18.84, A18.89, A54.21, A54.29, A54.82, A54.84, A54.89-A54.9, A59.00, A59.8-A59.9, A98.5, B37.41-B37.49, E08.21-E08.29, E08.618-E08.638, E08.649-E08.8, E09.21-E09.29, E09.618-E09.638, E09.649-E09.8, E10.21-E10.29, E10.618-E10.638, E10.649, E10.69-E10.8, E11.21-E11.29, E11.618-E11.638, E11.649, E11.69-E11.8, E13.21-E13.29, E13.618-E13.638, E13.649-E13.8, M10.30-M10.39, N00.0-N11.0, N11.8-N13.39, N13.6, N14.0-N17.9, N19, N25.0-N26.1, N26.9-N27.9, N28.1-N29, N36.41-N36.43, N36.8-N36.9, N39.8-N39.9, R31.0-R31.9

N07.0 Hereditary nephropathy, not elsewhere classified with minor glomerular abnormality
Hereditary nephropathy, not elsewhere classified with minimal change lesion

N07.1 Hereditary nephropathy, not elsewhere classified with focal and segmental glomerular lesions
Hereditary nephropathy, not elsewhere classified with focal and segmental hyalinosis
Hereditary nephropathy, not elsewhere classified with focal and segmental sclerosis
Hereditary nephropathy, not elsewhere classified with focal glomerulonephritis

N07.2 Hereditary nephropathy, not elsewhere classified with diffuse membranous glomerulonephritis `CC`

N07.3 Hereditary nephropathy, not elsewhere classified with diffuse mesangial proliferative glomerulonephritis `CC`

N07.4 Hereditary nephropathy, not elsewhere classified with diffuse endocapillary proliferative glomerulonephritis `CC`

N07.5 Hereditary nephropathy, not elsewhere classified with diffuse mesangiocapillary glomerulonephritis `CC`
Hereditary nephropathy, not elsewhere classified with membranoproliferative glomerulonephritis, types 1 and 3, or NOS

N07.6 Hereditary nephropathy, not elsewhere classified with dense deposit disease
Hereditary nephropathy, not elsewhere classified with membranoproliferative glomerulonephritis, type 2

N07.7 Hereditary nephropathy, not elsewhere classified with diffuse crescentic glomerulonephritis
Hereditary nephropathy, not elsewhere classified with extracapillary glomerulonephritis

N07.8 Hereditary nephropathy, not elsewhere classified with other morphologic lesions
Hereditary nephropathy, not elsewhere classified with proliferative glomerulonephritis NOS

N07.9 Hereditary nephropathy, not elsewhere classified with unspecified morphologic lesions

N08 Glomerular disorders in diseases classified elsewhere
Glomerulonephritis   Nephropathy
Nephritis
Code first underlying disease, such as:
  amyloidosis (E85.-)
  congenital syphilis (A50.5)
  cryoglobulinemia (D89.1)
  disseminated intravascular coagulation (D65)
  gout (M1A.-, M10.-)
  microscopic polyangiitis (M31.7)
  multiple myeloma (C90.0-)
  sepsis (A40.0-A41.9)
  sickle-cell disease (D57.0-D57.8)

EXCLUDES 1   glomerulonephritis, nephritis and nephropathy (in):
  antiglomerular basement membrane disease (M31.0)
  diabetes (E08-E13 with .21)
  gonococcal (A54.21)
  Goodpasture's syndrome (M31.0)
  hemolytic-uremic syndrome (D59.3)
  lupus (M32.14)
  mumps (B26.83)
  syphilis (A52.75)
  systemic lupus erythematosus (M32.14)
  Wegener's granulomatosis (M31.31)
pyelonephritis in diseases classified elsewhere (N16)
renal tubulo-interstitial disorders classified elsewhere (N16)

Renal tubulo-interstitial diseases (N10-N16)

INCLUDES   pyelonephritis
EXCLUDES 1   pyeloureteritis cystica (N28.85)

1 **N10 Acute tubulo-interstitial nephritis** `CC`
Acute infectious interstitial nephritis   Acute pyelonephritis
Hemoglobin nephrosis
Acute pyelitis   Myoglobin nephrosis
Use additional code (B95-B97), to identify infectious agent
CC Excl: A17.9, A18.10-A18.11, A18.13, A18.82, A18.84, A18.89, A54.21, A54.29, A54.82, A54.84, A54.89-A54.9, A59.00, A59.8-A59.9, B37.41-B37.49, E08.21-E08.29, E08.618-E08.638, E08.649-E08.8, E09.21-E09.29, E09.618-E09.638, E09.649-E09.8, E10.21-E10.29, E10.618-E10.638, E10.649, E10.69-E10.8, E11.21-E11.29, E11.618-E11.638, E11.649, E11.69-E11.8, E13.21-E13.29, E13.618-E13.638, E13.649-E13.8, M10.30-M10.39, N00.0-N11.0, N11.8-N13.39, N13.6, N14.0-N19, N25.0-N26.1, N26.9-N27.9, N28.1-N29, N36.41-N36.43, N36.8-N36.9, N39.0, N39.8-N39.9, R31.0-R31.9

---

1   HAC = as SDx not POA, in combination with SDx code T83.51XA also not POA.

✓ Additional Character Required   ✓x7ᵗʰ Placeholder Alert   Unacceptable PDx   Manifestation   Hospital Acquired Condition   EXCLUDES 1 Not Coded Here   EXCLUDES 2 Not Included Here

Chapter 14. Diseases of Genitourinary System

N11   **Chronic tubulo-interstitial nephritis**
   INCLUDES   chronic infectious interstitial nephritis
              chronic pyelitis
              chronic pyelonephritis
   Use additional code (B95-B97), to identify infectious agent

N11.0   **Nonobstructive reflux-associated chronic pyelonephritis**
   Pyelonephritis (chronic) associated with (vesicoureteral) reflux
   EXCLUDES 1   vesicoureteral reflux NOS (N13.70)

N11.1   **Chronic obstructive pyelonephritis**   PDxCC CC
   Pyelonephritis (chronic) associated with anomaly of pelviureteric junction
   Pyelonephritis (chronic) associated with anomaly of pyeloureteric junction
   Pyelonephritis (chronic) associated with crossing of vessel
   Pyelonephritis (chronic) associated with kinking of ureter
   Pyelonephritis (chronic) associated with obstruction of ureter
   Pyelonephritis (chronic) associated with stricture of pelviureteric junction
   Pyelonephritis (chronic) associated with stricture of ureter
   EXCLUDES 1   calculous pyelonephritis (N20.9)
               obstructive uropathy (N13.-)
   CC Excl: N11.1, N13.4-N13.5, N13.8-N13.9, N28.82, N28.89-N30.91, N32.89-N33, N36.41-N36.43, N36.8-N36.9, N39.0, N39.8-N39.9, Q62.4-Q62.8, Q64.10-Q64.19, Q64.8-Q64.9, R31.0-R31.9, Z90.6

N11.8   **Other chronic tubulo-interstitial nephritis**   CC
   Nonobstructive chronic pyelonephritis NOS
   CC Excl: A17.9, A18.10-A18.11, A18.13, A18.82, A18.84, A18.89, A54.21, A54.29, A54.82, A54.84, A54.89-A54.9, A59.00, A59.8-A59.9, A98.5, B37.41-B37.49, E08.21-E08.29, E08.618-E08.638, E08.649-E08.8, E09.21-E09.29, E09.618-E09.638, E09.649-E09.8, E10.21-E10.29, E10.618-E10.638, E10.649, E10.69-E10.8, E11.21-E11.29, E11.618-E11.638, E11.649, E11.69-E11.8, E13.21-E13.29, E13.618-E13.638, E13.649-E13.8, M10.30-M10.39, N00.0-N11.0, N11.8-N13.39, N13.6, N14.0-N17.9, N19, N25.0-N26.1, N26.9-N27.9, N28.1-N29, N36.41-N36.43, N36.8-N36.9, N39.8-N39.9, O23.01-O23.03, O23.11-O23.13, O23.21-O23.23, O23.31-O23.33, O23.41-O23.513, O23.521-O23.523, O23.591-O23.593, O23.91-O23.93, O86.11, O86.13-O86.29, R31.0-R31.9

¹ N11.9   **Chronic tubulo-interstitial nephritis, unspecified**   CC
   Chronic interstitial nephritis NOS
   Chronic pyelitis NOS
   Chronic pyelonephritis NOS
   CC Excl: A17.9, A18.10-A18.11, A18.13, A18.82, A18.84, A18.89, A54.21, A54.29, A54.82, A54.84, A54.89-A54.9, A59.00, A59.8-A59.9, B37.41-B37.49, E08.21-E08.29, E09.21-E09.29, M10.30-M10.39, N00.0-N11.0, N11.8-N13.39, N13.6, N14.0-N19, N25.0-N26.1, N26.9-N27.9, N28.1-N29, N36.41-N36.43, N36.8-N36.9, N39.0, N39.8-N39.9, R31.0-R31.9

¹ N12   **Tubulo-interstitial nephritis, not specified as acute or chronic**   CC
   Interstitial nephritis NOS
   Pyelitis NOS
   Pyelonephritis NOS
   EXCLUDES 1   calculous pyelonephritis (N20.9)
   CC Excl: See code: N11.9

N13   **Obstructive and reflux uropathy**
   EXCLUDES 2   calculus of kidney and ureter without hydronephrosis (N20.-)
               congenital obstructive defects of renal pelvis and ureter (Q62.0-Q62.3)
               hydronephrosis with ureteropelvic junction obstruction (Q62.1)
               obstructive pyelonephritis (N11.1)

   CC Excl: For CC codes in category N13, unless otherwise noted:
   See code: N11.9

N13.1   **Hydronephrosis with ureteral stricture, not elsewhere classified**   PDxCC CC
   EXCLUDES 1   hydronephrosis with ureteral stricture with infection (N13.6)

N13.2   **Hydronephrosis with renal and ureteral calculous obstruction**   PDxCC CC
   EXCLUDES 1   hydronephrosis with renal and ureteral calculous obstruction with infection (N13.6)

N13.3   **Other and unspecified hydronephrosis**
   EXCLUDES 1   hydronephrosis with infection (N13.6)

   N13.30   **Unspecified hydronephrosis**   CC
   N13.39   **Other hydronephrosis**   CC

N13.4   **Hydroureter**   CC
   EXCLUDES 1   congenital hydroureter (Q62.3-)
               hydroureter with infection (N13.6)
               vesicoureteral-reflux with hydroureter (N13.73-)
   CC Excl: N11.1, N13.4-N13.5, N13.8-N13.9, N28.82, N28.89-N30.91, N32.89-N33, N36.41-N36.43, N36.8-N36.9, N39.0, N39.8-N39.9, Q62.4-Q62.8, Q64.10-Q64.19, Q64.8-Q64.9, R31.0-R31.9

N13.5   **Crossing vessel and stricture of ureter without hydronephrosis**
   Kinking and stricture of ureter without hydronephrosis
   EXCLUDES 1   crossing vessel and stricture of ureter without hydronephrosis with infection (N13.6)

¹ N13.6   **Pyonephrosis**   CC
   Conditions in N13.1-N13.5 with infection
   Obstructive uropathy with infection
   Use additional code (B95-B97), to identify infectious agent

N13.7   **Vesicoureteral-reflux**
   EXCLUDES 1   reflux-associated pyelonephritis (N11.0)

   N13.70   **Vesicoureteral-reflux, unspecified**
      Vesicoureteral-reflux NOS

   N13.71   **Vesicoureteral-reflux without reflux nephropathy**

   N13.72   **Vesicoureteral-reflux with reflux nephropathy without hydroureter**
      N13.721   **Vesicoureteral-reflux with reflux nephropathy without hydroureter, unilateral**
      N13.722   **Vesicoureteral-reflux with reflux nephropathy without hydroureter, bilateral**
      N13.729   **Vesicoureteral-reflux with reflux nephropathy without hydroureter, unspecified**

   N13.73   **Vesicoureteral-reflux with reflux nephropathy with hydroureter**
      N13.731   **Vesicoureteral-reflux with reflux nephropathy with hydroureter, unilateral**
      N13.732   **Vesicoureteral-reflux with reflux nephropathy with hydroureter, bilateral**
      N13.739   **Vesicoureteral-reflux with reflux nephropathy with hydroureter, unspecified**

N13.8   **Other obstructive and reflux uropathy**   CC
   Urinary tract obstruction due to specified cause
   Code first, if applicable, any causal condition, such as: enlarged prostate (N40.1)
   CC Excl: See code: N11.1

N13.9   **Obstructive and reflux uropathy, unspecified**
   Urinary tract obstruction NOS

N14   **Drug- and heavy-metal-induced tubulo-interstitial and tubular conditions**
   Code first poisoning due to drug or toxin, if applicable (T36-T65 with fifth or sixth character 1-4 or 6)
   Use additional code for adverse effect, if applicable, to identify drug (T36-T50 with fifth or sixth character 5)

N14.0   **Analgesic nephropathy**
N14.1   **Nephropathy induced by other drugs, medicaments and biological substances**
N14.2   **Nephropathy induced by unspecified drug, medicament or biological substance**
N14.3   **Nephropathy induced by heavy metals**
N14.4   **Toxic nephropathy, not elsewhere classified**

N15   **Other renal tubulo-interstitial diseases**

N15.0   **Balkan nephropathy**
   Balkan endemic nephropathy

¹ N15.1   **Renal and perinephric abscess**   MCC
   CC Excl: A17.9, A18.10-A18.11, A18.13, A18.82, A18.84, A18.89, A54.21, A54.29, A54.82, A54.84, A54.89-A54.9, A59.00, A59.8-A59.9, B37.41-B37.49, E08.21-E08.29, E08.618-E08.638, E08.649-E08.8, E09.21-E09.29, E09.618-E09.638, E09.649-E09.8, E10.21-E10.29, E10.618-E10.638, E10.649, E10.69-E10.8, E11.21-E11.29, E11.618-E11.638, E11.649, E11.69-E11.8, E13.21-E13.29, E13.618-E13.638, E13.649-E13.8, M10.30-M10.39, N00.0-N11.0, N11.8-N13.39, N13.6, N14.0-N19, N25.0-N26.1, N26.9-N27.9, N28.1-N29, N36.41-N36.43, N36.8-N36.9, N39.0, N39.8-N39.9, R31.0-R31.9

N15.8   **Other specified renal tubulo-interstitial diseases**

N15.9   **Renal tubulo-interstitial disease, unspecified**
   Infection of kidney NOS
   EXCLUDES 1   urinary tract infection NOS (N39.0)

---

¹   HAC = as SDx not POA, in combination with SDx code T83.51XA also not POA.

 Newborn: 0   Pediatric: 0-17   Maternity: 12-55   Adult: 15-124   MCC Major CC Condition   PDxMCC PDx acts as own MCC   CC CC Condition   PDxCC PDx acts as own CC

794   ICD-10-CM 2016

N16 *Renal tubulo-interstitial disorders in diseases classified elsewhere*
Pyelonephritis
Tubulo-interstitial nephritis
Code first underlying disease, such as:
    brucellosis (A23.0-A23.9)
    cryoglobulinemia (D89.1)
    glycogen storage disease (E74.0)
    leukemia (C91-C95)
    lymphoma (C81.0-C85.9, C96.0-C96.9)
    multiple myeloma (C90.0-)
    sepsis (A40.0-A41.9)
    Wilson's disease (E83.0)
    EXCLUDES 1 diphtheritic pyelonephritis and tubulo-interstitial nephritis
        (A36.84)
        pyelonephritis and tubulo-interstitial nephritis in candidiasis
            (B37.49)
        pyelonephritis and tubulo-interstitial nephritis in cystinosis
            (E72.04)
        pyelonephritis and tubulo-interstitial nephritis in salmonella
            infection (A02.25)
        pyelonephritis and tubulo-interstitial nephritis in sarcoidosis
            (D86.84)
        pyelonephritis and tubulo-interstitial nephritis in sicca
            syndrome [Sjogren's] (M35.04)
        pyelonephritis and tubulo-interstitial nephritis in systemic lupus
            erythematosus (M32.15)
        pyelonephritis and tubulo-interstitial nephritis in toxoplasmosis
            (B58.83)
        renal tubular degeneration in diabetes (E08-E13 with .29)
        syphilitic pyelonephritis and tubulo-interstitial nephritis
            (A52.75)

Acute kidney failure and chronic kidney disease (N17-N19)

EXCLUDES 2 *congenital renal failure (P96.0)*
    drug- and heavy-metal-induced tubulo-interstitial and tubular
        conditions (N14.-)
    extrarenal uremia (R39.2)
    hemolytic-uremic syndrome (D59.3)
    hepatorenal syndrome (K76.7)
    postpartum hepatorenal syndrome (O90.4)
    posttraumatic renal failure (T79.5)
    prerenal uremia (R39.2)
    renal failure complicating abortion or ectopic or molar pregnancy (O00-
        O07, O08.4)
    renal failure following labor and delivery (O90.4)
    renal failure postprocedural (N99.0)

✓4ᵗʰ N17 Acute kidney failure
Code also associated underlying condition
    EXCLUDES 1 *posttraumatic renal failure (T79.5)*
AHA: 2013, 4Q, 124

> **CC Excl: For CC/MCC codes in category N17, unless otherwise
> noted:** E08.21-E08.29, E08.618-E08.638, E08.649-E08.8, E09.21-E09.29,
> E09.618-E09.638, E09.649-E09.8, E10.21-E10.29, E10.618-E10.638,
> E10.649, E10.69-E10.8, E11.21-E11.29, E11.618-E11.638, E11.649,
> E11.69-E11.8, E13.21-E13.29, E13.618-E13.638, E13.649-E13.8, E88.3,
> M10.30-M10.39, N00.0-N11.0, N11.8-N13.39, N13.6, N14.0-N19, N25.0-
> N26.1, N26.9-N27.9, N28.1-N29, N36.41-N36.43, N36.8-N36.9, N39.8-
> N39.9, Q60.0-Q62.39, Q63.0-Q63.9, Q64.8-Q64.9, R31.0-R31.9

N17.0 Acute kidney failure with tubular necrosis `MCC`
Acute tubular necrosis
Renal tubular necrosis
Tubular necrosis NOS

N17.1 Acute kidney failure with acute cortical necrosis `MCC`
Acute cortical necrosis
Cortical necrosis NOS
Renal cortical necrosis

N17.2 Acute kidney failure with medullary necrosis `MCC`
Medullary [papillary] necrosis NOS
Acute medullary [papillary] necrosis
Renal medullary [papillary] necrosis

N17.8 Other acute kidney failure `CC`
CC Excl: E08.21-E08.29, E08.618-E08.638, E08.649-E08.8, E09.21-
E09.29, E09.618-E09.638, E09.649-E09.8, E10.21-E10.29, E10.618-
E10.638, E10.649, E10.69-E10.8, E11.21-E11.29, E11.618-E11.638,
E11.649, E11.69-E11.8, E13.21-E13.29, E13.618-E13.638, E13.649-
E13.8, E88.3, M10.30-M10.39, N00.0-N11.0, N11.8-N13.39, N13.6,
N14.0-N19, N25.0-N26.1, N26.9-N27.9, N28.1-N29, N36.41-N36.43,
N36.8-N36.9, N39.8-N39.9, R31.0-R31.9

N17.9 Acute kidney failure, unspecified `CC`
Acute kidney injury (nontraumatic)
EXCLUDES 2 *traumatic kidney injury (S37.0-)*

✓4ᵗʰ N18 Chronic kidney disease (CKD)
Code first any associated:
    diabetic chronic kidney disease (E08.22, E09.22, E10.22, E11.22,
        E13.22)
    hypertensive chronic kidney disease (I12-, I13-)
Use additional code to identify kidney transplant status, if applicable,
    (Z94.0)
AHA: 2013, 1Q, 24

N18.1 Chronic kidney disease, stage 1

N18.2 Chronic kidney disease, stage 2 (mild)

N18.3 Chronic kidney disease, stage 3 (moderate)

N18.4 Chronic kidney disease, stage 4 (severe) `CC`
CC Excl: E08.21-E08.29, E08.618-E08.638, E08.649-E08.8, E09.21-
E09.29, E09.618-E09.638, E09.649-E09.8, E10.21-E10.29, E10.618-
E10.638, E10.649, E10.69-E10.8, E11.21-E11.29, E11.618-E11.638,
E11.649, E11.69-E11.8, E13.21-E13.29, E13.618-E13.638, E13.649-
E13.8, M10.30-M10.39, N00.0-N11.0, N11.8-N13.39, N13.6, N14.0-
N19, N25.0-N26.1, N26.9-N27.9, N28.1-N29, N36.41-N36.43, N36.8-
N36.9, N39.8-N39.9, Q60.0-Q62.39, Q63.0-Q63.9, Q64.8-Q64.9,
R31.0-R31.9

N18.5 Chronic kidney disease, stage 5 `CC`
EXCLUDES 1 *chronic kidney disease, stage 5 requiring chronic*
        dialysis (N18.6)
CC Excl: See code: N18.4

N18.6 End stage renal disease `MCC`
Chronic kidney disease requiring chronic dialysis
Use additional code to identify dialysis status (Z99.2)
AHA: 2013, 4Q, 124-125
CC Excl: E08.21-E08.29, E08.618-E08.638, E08.649-E08.8, E09.21-
E09.29, E09.618-E09.638, E09.649-E09.8, E10.21-E10.29, E10.618-
E10.638, E10.649, E10.69-E10.8, E11.21-E11.29, E11.618-E11.638,
E11.649, E11.69-E11.8, E13.21-E13.29, E13.618-E13.638, E13.649-
E13.8, I12.9, M10.30-M10.39, N00.0-N11.0, N11.8-N13.39, N13.6,
N14.0-N19, N25.0-N26.1, N26.9-N27.9, N28.1-N29, N36.41-N36.43,
N36.8-N36.9, N39.8-N39.9, Q60.0-Q62.39, Q63.0-Q63.9, Q64.8-
Q64.9, R31.0-R31.9

N18.9 Chronic kidney disease, unspecified
Chronic renal disease   Chronic renal insufficiency
Chronic renal failure NOS   Chronic uremia

N19 Unspecified kidney failure
Uremia NOS
EXCLUDES 1 *acute kidney failure (N17.-)*
        chronic kidney disease (N18.-)
        chronic uremia (N18.9)
        extrarenal uremia (R39.2)
        prerenal uremia (R39.2)
        renal insufficiency (acute) (N28.9)
        uremia of newborn (P96.0)

Urolithiasis (N20-N23)

✓4ᵗʰ N20 Calculus of kidney and ureter
Calculous pyelonephritis
EXCLUDES 1 *nephrocalcinosis (E83.5)*
        that with hydronephrosis (N13.2)

N20.0 Calculus of kidney
Nephrolithiasis NOS   Staghorn calculus
Renal calculus   Stone in kidney
Renal stone

N20.1 Calculus of ureter `CC`
Ureteric stone
CC Excl: N11.1, N13.4-N13.5, N13.8-N13.9, N20.0-N22, N28.82,
N28.89-N29, N36.41-N36.43, N36.8-N36.9, N39.8-N39.9, R31.0-
R31.9

N20.2 Calculus of kidney with calculus of ureter `CC`
CC Excl: See code: N20.1

N20.9 Urinary calculus, unspecified

✓4ᵗʰ N21 Calculus of lower urinary tract
Calculus of lower urinary tract with cystitis and urethritis

N21.0 Calculus in bladder
Calculus in diverticulum of bladder
Urinary bladder stone
EXCLUDES 2 *staghorn calculus (N20.0)*

N21.1 Calculus in urethra
EXCLUDES 2 *calculus of prostate (N42.0)*

N21.8 Other lower urinary tract calculus

N21.9 Calculus of lower urinary tract, unspecified
EXCLUDES 1 *calculus of urinary tract NOS (N20.9)*

Chapter 14. Diseases of Genitourinary System

N22   Calculus of urinary tract in diseases classified elsewhere
Code first underlying disease, such as:
gout (M1A.-, M10.-)
schistosomiasis (B65.0-B65.9)

N23   Unspecified renal colic

Other disorders of kidney and ureter (N25-N29)
EXCLUDES 2   disorders of kidney and ureter with urolithiasis (N20-N23)

✓4th N25   Disorders resulting from impaired renal tubular function
EXCLUDES 1   metabolic disorders classifiable to E70-E88

N25.0   Renal osteodystrophy
Azotemic osteodystrophy   Renal rickets
Phosphate-losing tubular disorders   Renal short stature

N25.1   Nephrogenic diabetes insipidus   CC
EXCLUDES 1   diabetes insipidus NOS (E23.2)
CC Excl: A17.9, A18.10-A18.11, A18.13, A18.82, A18.84, A18.89,
A54.21, A54.29, A54.82, A54.84, A54.89-A54.9, A59.00, A59.8-
A59.9, A98.5, B37.41-B37.49, E08.21-E08.29, E08.618-E08.638,
E08.649-E08.8, E09.21-E09.29, E09.618-E09.638, E09.649-E09.8,
E10.21-E10.29, E10.618-E10.638, E10.649, E10.69-E10.8, E11.21-
E11.29, E11.618-E11.638, E11.649, E11.69-E11.8, E13.21-E13.29,
E13.618-E13.638, E13.649-E13.8, M10.30-M10.39, N00.0-N11.0,
N11.8-N13.39, N13.6, N14.0-N17.9, N18.3-N18.6, N19, N25.0-
N26.1, N26.9-N27.9, N28.1-N29, N36.41-N36.43, N36.8-N36.9,
N39.8-N39.9, R31.0-R31.9

✓5th N25.8   Other disorders resulting from impaired renal tubular function

N25.81   Secondary hyperparathyroidism of renal origin   CC
EXCLUDES 1   secondary hyperparathyroidism, non-renal (E21.1)
CC Excl: A17.9, A18.10-A18.11, A18.13, A18.82, A18.84,
A18.89, A54.21, A54.29, A54.82, A54.84, A54.89-A54.9,
A59.00, A59.8-A59.9, A98.5, B37.41-B37.49, E08.21-
E08.29, E08.618-E08.638, E08.649-E08.8, E09.21-E09.29,
E09.618-E09.638, E09.649-E09.8, E10.21-E10.29,
E10.618-E10.638, E10.649, E10.69-E10.8, E11.21-E11.29,
E11.618-E11.638, E11.649, E11.69-E11.8, E13.21-E13.29,
E13.618-E13.638, E13.649-E13.8, M10.30-M10.39, N00.0-
N11.0, N11.8-N13.39, N13.6, N14.0-N17.9, N19, N25.0-
N25.1, N25.89-N26.1, N26.9-N27.9, N28.1-N29, N36.41-
N36.43, N36.8-N36.9, N39.8-N39.9, R31.0-R31.9

N25.89   Other disorders resulting from impaired renal tubular function
Hypokalemic nephropathy
Lightwood-Albright syndrome
Renal tubular acidosis NOS

N25.9   Disorder resulting from impaired renal tubular function, unspecified

✓4th N26   Unspecified contracted kidney
EXCLUDES 1   contracted kidney due to hypertension (I12.-)
diffuse sclerosing glomerulonephritis (N05.8-)
hypertensive nephrosclerosis (arteriolar) (arteriosclerotic) (I12.-)
small kidney of unknown cause (N27.-)

N26.1   Atrophy of kidney (terminal)

N26.2   Page kidney

N26.9   Renal sclerosis, unspecified

✓4th N27   Small kidney of unknown cause
INCLUDES   oligonephronia

N27.0   Small kidney, unilateral

N27.1   Small kidney, bilateral

N27.9   Small kidney, unspecified

✓4th N28   Other disorders of kidney and ureter, not elsewhere classified

N28.0   Ischemia and infarction of kidney   CC
Renal artery embolism   Renal artery thrombosis
Renal artery obstruction   Renal infarct
Renal artery occlusion
EXCLUDES 1   atherosclerosis of renal artery (extrarenal part) (I70.1)
congenital stenosis of renal artery (Q27.1)
Goldblatt's kidney (I70.1)
CC Excl: N13.70-N13.739, N28.0, N28.9-N29

N28.1   Cyst of kidney, acquired
Cyst (multiple)(solitary) of kidney, acquired
EXCLUDES 1   cystic kidney disease (congenital) (Q61.-)

✓5th N28.8   Other specified disorders of kidney and ureter
EXCLUDES 1   hydroureter (N13.4)
ureteric stricture with hydronephrosis (N13.1)
ureteric stricture without hydronephrosis (N13.5)

CC Excl: For CC codes in subcategory N28.8, unless
otherwise noted: A17.9, A18.10-A18.11, A18.13, A18.82,
A18.84, A18.89, A54.21, A54.29, A54.82, A54.84, A54.89-
A54.9, A59.00, A59.8-A59.9, B37.41-B37.49, E08.21-E08.29,
E09.21-E09.29, M10.30-M10.39, N00.0-N11.0, N11.8-
N13.39, N13.6, N14.0-N19, N25.0-N26.1, N26.9-N27.9,
N28.1-N29, N36.41-N36.43, N36.8-N36.9, N39.0, N39.8-
N39.9, R31.0-R31.9

N28.81   Hypertrophy of kidney

N28.82   Megaloureter

N28.83   Nephroptosis

1   **N28.84   Pyelitis cystica**   CC

1   **N28.85   Pyeloureteritis cystica**   CC

1   **N28.86   Ureteritis cystica**   CC

N28.89   Other specified disorders of kidney and ureter

N28.9   Disorder of kidney and ureter, unspecified
Nephropathy NOS
Renal disease (acute) NOS
Renal insufficiency (acute)
EXCLUDES 1   chronic renal insufficiency (N18.9)
unspecified nephritic syndrome (N05.-)

N29   Other disorders of kidney and ureter in diseases classified elsewhere
Code first underlying disease, such as:
amyloidosis (E85.-)
nephrocalcinosis (E83.5)
schistosomiasis (B65.0-B65.9)
EXCLUDES 1   disorders of kidney and ureter in:
cystinosis (E72.0)
gonorrhea (A54.21)
syphilis (A52.75)
tuberculosis (A18.11)

Other diseases of the urinary system (N30-N39)
EXCLUDES 1   urinary infection (complicating):
abortion or ectopic or molar pregnancy (O00-O07, O08.8)
pregnancy, childbirth and the puerperium (O23-, O75.3, O86.2-)

✓4th N30   Cystitis
Use additional code to identify infectious agent (B95-B97)
EXCLUDES 1   prostatocystitis (N41.3)

CC Excl: For CC codes in category N30, unless otherwise noted:
A17.9, A18.10, A18.12-A18.13, A18.82, A18.84, A18.89, A54.00-
A54.02, A54.09-A54.1, A54.82, A54.84, A54.89-A54.9, A59.00, A59.8-
A59.9, B37.41-B37.49, N11.1, N13.4-N13.5, N13.8-N13.9, N28.82,
N28.89-N30.91, N32.89-N33, N36.41-N36.43, N36.8-N36.9, N39.0,
N39.8-N39.9, R31.0-R31.9

✓5th N30.0   Acute cystitis
EXCLUDES 1   irradiation cystitis (N30.4-)
trigonitis (N30.3-)

1   **N30.00   Acute cystitis without hematuria**   CC

1   **N30.01   Acute cystitis with hematuria**   CC

✓5th N30.1   Interstitial cystitis (chronic)

N30.10   Interstitial cystitis (chronic) without hematuria

N30.11   Interstitial cystitis (chronic) with hematuria

✓5th N30.2   Other chronic cystitis

N30.20   Other chronic cystitis without hematuria

N30.21   Other chronic cystitis with hematuria

✓5th N30.3   Trigonitis
Urethrotrigonitis

N30.30   Trigonitis without hematuria

N30.31   Trigonitis with hematuria

✓5th N30.4   Irradiation cystitis

N30.40   Irradiation cystitis without hematuria   CC

N30.41   Irradiation cystitis with hematuria   CC

✓5th N30.8   Other cystitis
Abscess of bladder

N30.80   Other cystitis without hematuria

N30.81   Other cystitis with hematuria

---

1   HAC = as SDx not POA, in combination with SDx code T83.51XA also not POA.

N   Newborn: 0   P   Pediatric: 0-17   M   Maternity: 12-55   A   Adult: 15-124   MCC   Major CC Condition   PDxMCC   PDx acts as own MCC   CC   CC Condition   PDxCC   PDx acts as own CC

796   ICD-10-CM 2016

✓5ᵗʰ **N30.9 Cystitis, unspecified**
     N30.90 Cystitis, unspecified without hematuria
     N30.91 Cystitis, unspecified with hematuria

✓4ᵗʰ **N31 Neuromuscular dysfunction of bladder, not elsewhere classified**
     Use additional code to identify any associated urinary incontinence (N39.3-N39.4-)
     EXCLUDES 1   cord bladder NOS (G95.89)
           neurogenic bladder due to cauda equina syndrome (G83.4)
           neuromuscular dysfunction due to spinal cord lesion (G95.89)

    N31.0 Uninhibited neuropathic bladder, not elsewhere classified
    N31.1 Reflex neuropathic bladder, not elsewhere classified
    N31.2 Flaccid neuropathic bladder, not elsewhere classified
     Atonic (motor) (sensory) neuropathic bladder
     Autonomous neuropathic bladder
     Nonreflex neuropathic bladder

    N31.8 Other neuromuscular dysfunction of bladder
    N31.9 Neuromuscular dysfunction of bladder, unspecified
     Neurogenic bladder dysfunction NOS

✓4ᵗʰ **N32 Other disorders of bladder**
     EXCLUDES 2   calculus of bladder (N21.0)
           cystocele (N81.1-)
           hernia or prolapse of bladder, female (N81.1-)

    N32.0 Bladder-neck obstruction
     Bladder-neck stenosis (acquired)
     EXCLUDES 1   congenital bladder-neck obstruction (Q64.3-)

    N32.1 Vesicointestinal fistula   CC
     Vesicorectal fistula
     CC Excl: A54.00, A54.02, A54.09-A54.1, A54.82, A54.84, A54.89-A54.9, N32.1-N32.2, N32.89-N33, N36.41-N36.43, N36.8-N36.9, N39.8-N39.9, R30.0, R30.9-R31.9

    N32.2 Vesical fistula, not elsewhere classified   CC
     EXCLUDES 1   fistula between bladder and female genital tract (N82.0-N82.1)
     CC Excl: See code: N32.1

    N32.3 Diverticulum of bladder
     EXCLUDES 1   congenital diverticulum of bladder (Q64.6)
           diverticulitis of bladder (N30.8-)

✓5ᵗʰ **N32.8 Other specified disorders of bladder**
    N32.81 Overactive bladder
     Detrusor muscle hyperactivity
     EXCLUDES 1   frequent urination due to specified bladder condition—code to condition

    N32.89 Other specified disorders of bladder
     Bladder hemorrhage   Calcified bladder
     Bladder hypertrophy   Contracted bladder

    N32.9 Bladder disorder, unspecified

N33   *Bladder disorders in diseases classified elsewhere*
     Code first underlying disease, such as:
     schistosomiasis (B65.0-B65.9)
     EXCLUDES 1   bladder disorder in syphilis (A52.76)
           bladder disorder in tuberculosis (A18.12)
           candidal cystitis (B37.41)
           chlamydial cystitis (A56.01)
           cystitis in gonorrhea (A54.01)
           cystitis in neurogenic bladder (N31.-)
           diphtheritic cystitis (A36.85)
           neurogenic bladder (N31.-)
           syphilitic cystitis (A52.76)
           trichomonal cystitis (A59.03)

✓4ᵗʰ **N34 Urethritis and urethral syndrome**
     Use additional code (B95-B97), to identify infectious agent
     EXCLUDES 2   Reiter's disease (M02.3-)
           urethritis in diseases with a predominantly sexual mode of transmission (A50-A64)
           urethrotrigonitis (N30.3-)

   ¹ **N34.0 Urethral abscess**   CC
     Abscess (of) Cowper's gland
     Abscess (of) Littrés gland
     Abscess (of) urethral (gland)
     Periurethral abscess
     EXCLUDES 1   urethral caruncle (N36.2)
     CC Excl: A54.00, A54.02, A54.09-A54.1, A54.82, A54.84, A54.89-A54.9, A59.00, A59.03, A59.8-A59.9, B37.41-B37.49, N13.9, N34.0-N34.3, N35.111-N35.9, N36.41-N36.43, N36.8-N39.0, N39.8-N39.9, N44.1-N44.8, N47.6, N48.1-N48.9, N49.1-N49.9, N50.3-N50.8, N51, N53.11-N53.9, Q54.0-Q55.21, Q55.23-Q55.9, Q64.0, Q64.2-Q64.9, R30.0, R30.9-R31.9

    N34.1 Nonspecific urethritis
     Nongonococcal urethritis
     Nonvenereal urethritis

    N34.2 Other urethritis
     Meatitis, urethral   Ulcer of urethra (meatus)
     Postmenopausal urethritis   Urethritis NOS

    N34.3 Urethral syndrome, unspecified

✓4ᵗʰ **N35 Urethral stricture**
     EXCLUDES 1   congenital urethral stricture (Q64.3-)
           postprocedural urethral stricture (N99.1-)

✓5ᵗʰ **N35.0 Post-traumatic urethral stricture**
     Urethral stricture due to injury
     EXCLUDES 1   postprocedural urethral stricture (N99.1-)

✓6ᵗʰ **N35.01 Post-traumatic urethral stricture, male**
     N35.010 Post-traumatic urethral stricture, male, meatal   ♂
     N35.011 Post-traumatic bulbous urethral stricture
     N35.012 Post-traumatic membranous urethral stricture
     N35.013 Post-traumatic anterior urethral stricture
     N35.014 Post-traumatic urethral stricture, male, unspecified   ♂

✓6ᵗʰ **N35.02 Post-traumatic urethral stricture, female**
     N35.021 Urethral stricture due to childbirth   ♀
     N35.028 Other post-traumatic urethral stricture, female   ♀

✓5ᵗʰ **N35.1 Postinfective urethral stricture, not elsewhere classified**
     EXCLUDES 1   urethral stricture associated with schistosomiasis (B65-, N29)
           gonococcal urethral stricture (A54.01)
           syphilitic urethral stricture (A52.76)

✓6ᵗʰ **N35.11 Postinfective urethral stricture, not elsewhere classified, male**
     N35.111 Postinfective urethral stricture, not elsewhere classified, male, meatal   ♂
     N35.112 Postinfective bulbous urethral stricture, not elsewhere classified
     N35.113 Postinfective membranous urethral stricture, not elsewhere classified
     N35.114 Postinfective anterior urethral stricture, not elsewhere classified
     N35.119 Postinfective urethral stricture, not elsewhere classified, male, unspecified   ♂

    N35.12 Postinfective urethral stricture, not elsewhere classified, female   ♀

    N35.8 Other urethral stricture
     EXCLUDES 1   postprocedural urethral stricture (N99.1-)

    N35.9 Urethral stricture, unspecified

✓4ᵗʰ **N36 Other disorders of urethra**
    N36.0 Urethral fistula   CC
     Urethroperineal fistula   Urinary fistula NOS
     Urethrorectal fistula
     EXCLUDES 1   urethroscrotal fistula (N50.8)
           urethrovaginal fistula (N82.1)
           urethrovesicovaginal fistula (N82.1)
     CC Excl: N13.9, N34.0, N34.2-N36.43, N36.5-N37, N39.8-N39.9, N44.1-N44.8, N47.6, N48.1-N48.9, N49.1-N49.9, N50.3-N50.8, N51, N53.11-N53.9, N99.110-N99.12, Q54.0-Q55.21, Q55.23-Q55.9, Q64.0, Q64.8-Q64.9, R30.0, R30.9-R31.9

    N36.1 Urethral diverticulum
    N36.2 Urethral caruncle

✓5ᵗʰ **N36.4 Urethral functional and muscular disorders**
     Use additional code to identify associated urinary stress incontinence (N39.3)
    N36.41 Hypermobility of urethra
    N36.42 Intrinsic sphincter deficiency (ISD)
    N36.43 Combined hypermobility of urethra and intrinsic sphincter deficiency
    N36.44 Muscular disorders of urethra
     Bladder sphincter dyssynergy

    N36.5 Urethral false passage
    N36.8 Other specified disorders of urethra
    N36.9 Urethral disorder, unspecified

---

¹   HAC = as SDx not POA, in combination with SDx code T83.51XA also not POA.

✓ Additional Character Required   ✓7ᵗʰ Placeholder Alert   Unacceptable PDx   Manifestation   Hospital Acquired Condition   *EXCLUDES 1* Not Coded Here   *EXCLUDES 2* Not Included Here

Chapter 14. Diseases of Genitourinary System

N37 Urethral disorders in diseases classified elsewhere
Code first underlying disease
EXCLUDES 1 urethritis (in):
candidal infection (B37.41)
chlamydial (A56.01)
gonorrhea (A54.01)
syphilis (A52.76)
trichomonal infection (A59.03)
tuberculosis (A18.13)

✓4th N39 Other disorders of urinary system
EXCLUDES 2 hematuria NOS (R31.-)
recurrent or persistent hematuria (N02.-)
recurrent or persistent hematuria with specified morphological lesion (N02.-)
proteinuria NOS (R80.-)

1 N39.0 Urinary tract infection, site not specified CC
Use additional code (B95-B97), to identify infectious agent
EXCLUDES 1 candidiasis of urinary tract (B37.4-)
neonatal urinary tract infection (P39.3)
urinary tract infection of specified site, such as:
cystitis (N30.-)
urethritis (N34.-)
AHA: 2012, 4Q, 94
CC Excl: A54.82, A54.84, A54.89-A54.9, A59.00, A59.8-A59.9, B37.41-B37.49, N10, N11.9-N13.39, N13.6, N13.9, N15.1, N28.82, N28.84-N30.91, N34.1, N36.41-N36.43, N36.8-N36.9, N39.0, N39.8-N39.9, N99.511, R30.0, R30.9-R31.9, T83.51XA

N39.3 Stress incontinence (female) (male)
Code also any associated overactive bladder (N32.81)
EXCLUDES 1 mixed incontinence (N39.46)

✓5th N39.4 Other specified urinary incontinence
Code also any associated overactive bladder (N32.81)
EXCLUDES 1 enuresis NOS (R32)
functional urinary incontinence (R39.81)
urinary incontinence associated with cognitive impairment (R39.81)
urinary incontinence NOS (R32)
urinary incontinence of nonorganic origin (F98.0)

N39.41 Urge incontinence
EXCLUDES 1 mixed incontinence (N39.46)

N39.42 Incontinence without sensory awareness
N39.43 Post-void dribbling
N39.44 Nocturnal enuresis
N39.45 Continuous leakage
N39.46 Mixed incontinence
Urge and stress incontinence

✓6th N39.49 Other specified urinary incontinence
N39.490 Overflow incontinence
N39.498 Other specified urinary incontinence
Reflex incontinence
Total incontinence

N39.8 Other specified disorders of urinary system
N39.9 Disorder of urinary system, unspecified

Diseases of male genital organs (N40-N53)

✓4th N40 Enlarged prostate
Adenofibromatous hypertrophy of prostate
Benign hypertrophy of the prostate
Benign prostatic hyperplasia
Benign prostatic hypertrophy
BPH
Nodular prostate
Polyp of prostate
EXCLUDES 1 benign neoplasms of prostate (adenoma, benign) (fibroadenoma) (fibroma) (myoma) (D29.1)
EXCLUDES 2 malignant neoplasm of prostate (C61)

N40.0 Enlarged prostate without lower urinary tract symptoms A♂
Enlarged prostate NOS   Enlarged prostate without LUTS

N40.1 Enlarged prostate with lower urinary tract symptoms A♂
Enlarged prostate with LUTS
Use additional code for associated symptoms, when specified:
incomplete bladder emptying (R39.14)
nocturia (R35.1)
straining on urination (R39.16)
urinary frequency (R35.0)
urinary hesitancy (R39.11)
urinary incontinence (N39.4-)
urinary obstruction (N13.8)
urinary retention (R33.8)
urinary urgency (R39.15)
weak urinary stream (R39.12)

N40.2 Nodular prostate without lower urinary tract symptoms A♂
Nodular prostate without LUTS

N40.3 Nodular prostate with lower urinary tract symptoms A♂
Use additional code for associated symptoms, when specified:
incomplete bladder emptying (R39.14)
nocturia (R35.1)
straining on urination (R39.16)
urinary frequency (R35.0)
urinary hesitancy (R39.11)
urinary incontinence (N39.4-)
urinary obstruction (N13.8)
urinary retention (R33.8)
urinary urgency (R39.15)
weak urinary stream (R39.12)

✓4th N41 Inflammatory diseases of prostate
Use additional code (B95-B97), to identify infectious agent

N41.0 Acute prostatitis CC A♂
CC Excl: A18.14, A54.22, A54.82, A54.84, A54.89-A54.9, A59.00, A59.02, A59.8-A59.9, B37.41-B37.49, N40.0-N41.0, N41.1, N41.2-N42.9

N41.1 Chronic prostatitis A♂
N41.2 Abscess of prostate CC A♂
CC Excl: See code: N41.0

N41.3 Prostatocystitis A♂
N41.4 Granulomatous prostatitis A♂
N41.8 Other inflammatory diseases of prostate A♂
N41.9 Inflammatory disease of prostate, unspecified A♂
Prostatitis NOS

✓4th N42 Other and unspecified disorders of prostate
N42.0 Calculus of prostate A♂
Prostatic stone

N42.1 Congestion and hemorrhage of prostate A♂
EXCLUDES 1 enlarged prostate (N40.-)
hematuria (R31.-)
hyperplasia of prostate (N40.-)
inflammatory diseases of prostate (N41.-)

N42.3 Dysplasia of prostate ♂
Prostatic intraepithelial neoplasia I (PIN I)
Prostatic intraepithelial neoplasia II (PIN II)
EXCLUDES 1 prostatic intraepithelial neoplasia III (PIN III) (D07.5)

✓5th N42.8 Other specified disorders of prostate
N42.81 Prostatodynia syndrome A♂
Painful prostate syndrome
N42.82 Prostatosis syndrome A♂
N42.83 Cyst of prostate A♂
N42.89 Other specified disorders of prostate A♂
N42.9 Disorder of prostate, unspecified A♂

✓4th N43 Hydrocele and spermatocele
INCLUDES hydrocele of spermatic cord, testis or tunica vaginalis
EXCLUDES 1 congenital hydrocele (P83.5)

N43.0 Encysted hydrocele ♂
N43.1 Infected hydrocele CC♂
Use additional code (B95-B97), to identify infectious agent
CC Excl: A59.00, A59.8-A59.9, B37.41-B37.49, N43.0-N43.3

N43.2 Other hydrocele ♂
N43.3 Hydrocele, unspecified ♂
✓5th N43.4 Spermatocele of epididymis
Spermatic cyst
N43.40 Spermatocele of epididymis, unspecified ♂
N43.41 Spermatocele of epididymis, single ♂
N43.42 Spermatocele of epididymis, multiple ♂

✓4th N44 Noninflammatory disorders of testis

CC Excl: For CC codes in category N44, unless otherwise noted: N44.00-N44.04

✓5th N44.0 Torsion of testis
N44.00 Torsion of testis, unspecified CC♂
N44.01 Extravaginal torsion of spermatic cord CC♂
N44.02 Intravaginal torsion of spermatic cord CC♂
Torsion of spermatic cord NOS
N44.03 Torsion of appendix testis CC♂
N44.04 Torsion of appendix epididymis CC♂

---

1 HAC = as SDx not POA, in combination with SDx code T83.51XA also not POA.

N44.1 Cyst of tunica albuginea **testis** ♂

N44.2 Benign cyst **of testis** ♂

N44.8 Other **noninflammatory disorders of the testis** ♂

✓4th N45 **Orchitis and epididymitis**
Use additional code (B95-B97), to identify infectious agent

N45.1 **Epididymitis** ♂

N45.2 **Orchitis** ♂

N45.3 **Epididymo-orchitis** ♂

N45.4 Abscess **of epididymis or testis** CC ♂
CC Excl: A54.23, A54.82, A54.84, A54.89-A54.9, A59.00, A59.8-A59.9, B26.0, B37.41-B37.49, N45.1-N45.4

✓4th N46 **Male infertility**
EXCLUDES 1 vasectomy status (Z98.52)

✓5th N46.0 **Azoospermia**
Absolute male infertility
Male infertility due to germinal (cell) aplasia
Male infertility due to spermatogenic arrest (complete)

N46.01 Organic **azoospermia** A ♂
Azoospermia NOS

✓6th N46.02 **Azoospermia due to** extratesticular causes
Code also associated cause

N46.021 **Azoospermia due to** drug therapy A ♂

N46.022 **Azoospermia due to** infection A ♂

N46.023 **Azoospermia due to** obstruction of efferent ducts A ♂

N46.024 **Azoospermia due to** radiation A ♂

N46.025 **Azoospermia due to** systemic disease A ♂

N46.029 **Azoospermia due to** other extratesticular causes A ♂

✓5th N46.1 **Oligospermia**
Male infertility due to germinal cell desquamation
Male infertility due to hypospermatogenesis
Male infertility due to incomplete spermatogenic arrest

N46.11 Organic **oligospermia** A ♂
Oligospermia NOS

✓6th N46.12 **Oligospermia due to** extratesticular causes
Code also associated cause

N46.121 **Oligospermia due to** drug therapy A ♂

N46.122 **Oligospermia due to** infection A ♂

N46.123 **Oligospermia due to** obstruction of efferent ducts A ♂

N46.124 **Oligospermia due to** radiation A ♂

N46.125 **Oligospermia due to** systemic disease A ♂

N46.129 **Oligospermia due to** other extratesticular causes A ♂

N46.8 Other **male infertility** A ♂

N46.9 **Male infertility, unspecified** A ♂

✓4th N47 **Disorders of prepuce**

N47.0 **Adherent prepuce, newborn** N ♂

N47.1 **Phimosis** ♂

N47.2 **Paraphimosis** ♂

N47.3 **Deficient foreskin** ♂

N47.4 **Benign cyst of prepuce** ♂

N47.5 **Adhesions of prepuce and glans penis** ♂

N47.6 **Balanoposthitis** ♂
Use additional code (B95-B97), to identify infectious agent
EXCLUDES 1 balanitis (N48.1)

N47.7 Other **inflammatory diseases of prepuce** ♂
Use additional code (B95-B97), to identify infectious agent

N47.8 Other **disorders of prepuce** ♂

✓4th N48 **Other disorders of penis**

N48.0 **Leukoplakia of penis** ♂
Balanitis xerotica obliterans
Kraurosis of penis
Lichen sclerosus of external male genital organs
EXCLUDES 1 carcinoma in situ of penis (D07.4)

N48.1 **Balanitis** ♂
Use additional code (B95-B97), to identify infectious agent
EXCLUDES 1 amebic balanitis (A06.8)
balanitis xerotica obliterans (N48.0)
candidal balanitis (B37.42)
gonococcal balanitis (A54.23)
herpesviral [herpes simplex] balanitis (A60.01)

✓5th N48.2 Other **inflammatory disorders of penis**
Use additional code (B95-B97), to identify infectious agent
EXCLUDES 1 balanitis (N48.1)
balanitis xerotica obliterans (N48.0)
balanoposthitis (N47.6)

N48.21 **Abscess of corpus cavernosum and penis** ♂

N48.22 **Cellulitis of corpus cavernosum and penis** ♂

N48.29 Other **inflammatory disorders of penis** ♂

✓5th N48.3 **Priapism**
Painful erection
Code first underlying cause

CC Excl: For CC codes in subcategory N48.3, unless otherwise noted: N47.6, N48.0-N48.9, N52.01-N52.9

N48.30 **Priapism, unspecified** CC ♂

N48.31 **Priapism** due to trauma CC ♂

N48.32 *Priapism due to disease classified elsewhere* CC ♂

N48.33 **Priapism, drug-induced** CC ♂

N48.39 Other **priapism** CC ♂

N48.5 **Ulcer of penis** ♂

N48.6 **Induration penis plastica** ♂
Peyronie's disease
Plastic induration of penis

✓5th N48.8 Other **specified disorders of penis**

N48.81 **Thrombosis of superficial vein of penis** ♂

N48.82 **Acquired torsion of penis** ♂
Acquired torsion of penis NOS
EXCLUDES 1 congenital torsion of penis (Q55.63)

N48.83 **Acquired buried penis** ♂
EXCLUDES 1 congenital hidden penis (Q55.64)

N48.89 Other **specified disorders of penis** ♂

N48.9 **Disorder of penis, unspecified** ♂

✓4th N49 **Inflammatory disorders of male genital organs, not elsewhere classified**
Use additional code (B95-B97), to identify infectious agent
EXCLUDES 1 inflammation of penis (N48.1, N48.2-)
orchitis and epididymitis (N45.-)

N49.0 **Inflammatory disorders of** seminal vesicle ♂
Vesiculitis NOS

N49.1 **Inflammatory disorders of** spermatic cord, tunica vaginalis and vas deferens ♂
Vasitis

N49.2 **Inflammatory disorders of** scrotum ♂

N49.3 **Fournier gangrene** ♂

N49.8 **Inflammatory disorders of** other specified male genital organs ♂
Inflammation of multiple sites in male genital organs

N49.9 **Inflammatory disorder of** unspecified male genital organ ♂
Abscess of unspecified male genital organ
Boil of unspecified male genital organ
Carbuncle of unspecified male genital organ
Cellulitis of unspecified male genital organ

✓4th N50 **Other and unspecified disorders of male genital organs**
EXCLUDES 2 torsion of testis (N44.0-)

N50.0 **Atrophy of testis** ♂

N50.1 **Vascular disorders of male genital organs** ♂
Hematocele, NOS, of male genital organs
Hemorrhage of male genital organs
Thrombosis of male genital organs

N50.3 **Cyst of epididymis** ♂

N50.8 **Other specified disorders of male genital organs** ♂
Atrophy of scrotum, seminal vesicle, spermatic cord, tunica vaginalis and vas deferens
Chylocele, tunica vaginalis (nonfilarial) NOS
Edema of scrotum, seminal vesicle, spermatic cord, testis, tunica vaginalis and vas deferens
Hypertrophy of scrotum, seminal vesicle, spermatic cord, testis, tunica vaginalis and vas deferens
Stricture of spermatic cord, tunica vaginalis, and vas deferens
Ulcer of scrotum, seminal vesicle, spermatic cord, testis, tunica vaginalis and vas deferens
Urethroscrotal fistula

N50.9 **Disorder of male genital organs, unspecified** ♂

Chapter 14. Diseases of Genitourinary System

N51   Disorders of male genital organs in diseases classified elsewhere   ♂

Code first underlying disease, such as:
filariasis (B74.0–B74.9)

> EXCLUDES 1   amebic balanitis (A06.8)
> candidal balanitis (B37.42)
> gonococcal balanitis (A54.23)
> gonococcal prostatitis (A54.22)
> herpesviral [herpes simplex] balanitis (A60.01)
> trichomonal prostatitis (A59.02)
> tuberculous prostatitis (A18.14)

✓4th **N52   Male erectile dysfunction**

> EXCLUDES 1   psychogenic impotence (F52.21)

   ✓5th **N52.0   Vasculogenic erectile dysfunction**

     N52.01   Erectile dysfunction due to arterial insufficiency   A ♂

     N52.02   Corporo-venous occlusive erectile dysfunction   A ♂

     N52.03   Combined arterial insufficiency and corporo-venous occlusive erectile dysfunction   A ♂

   N52.1   Erectile dysfunction due to diseases classified elsewhere   A ♂

Code first underlying disease

   N52.2   Drug-induced erectile dysfunction   A ♂

   ✓5th **N52.3   Post-surgical erectile dysfunction**

     N52.31   Erectile dysfunction following radical prostatectomy   A ♂

     N52.32   Erectile dysfunction following radical cystectomy   A ♂

     N52.33   Erectile dysfunction following urethral surgery   A ♂

     N52.34   Erectile dysfunction following simple prostatectomy   A ♂

     N52.39   Other post-surgical erectile dysfunction   A ♂

   N52.8   Other male erectile dysfunction   A ♂

   N52.9   Male erectile dysfunction, unspecified   A ♂
Impotence NOS

✓4th **N53   Other male sexual dysfunction**

> EXCLUDES 1   psychogenic sexual dysfunction (F52.-)

   ✓5th **N53.1   Ejaculatory dysfunction**

> EXCLUDES 1   premature ejaculation (F52.4)

     N53.11   Retarded ejaculation   ♂

     N53.12   Painful ejaculation   ♂

     N53.13   Anejaculatory orgasm   ♂

     N53.14   Retrograde ejaculation   ♂

     N53.19   Other ejaculatory dysfunction   ♂
Ejaculatory dysfunction NOS

   N53.8   Other male sexual dysfunction   ♂

   N53.9   Unspecified male sexual dysfunction   ♂

Disorders of breast (N60-N65)

> EXCLUDES 1   disorders of breast associated with childbirth (O91-O92)

✓4th **N60   Benign mammary dysplasia**

> INCLUDES   fibrocystic mastopathy

   ✓5th **N60.0   Solitary cyst of breast**
Cyst of breast

     N60.01   Solitary cyst of right breast

     N60.02   Solitary cyst of left breast

     N60.09   Solitary cyst of unspecified breast

   ✓5th **N60.1   Diffuse cystic mastopathy**
Cystic breast
Fibrocystic disease of breast

> EXCLUDES 1   diffuse cystic mastopathy with epithelial proliferation (N60.3-)

     N60.11   Diffuse cystic mastopathy of right breast   A

     N60.12   Diffuse cystic mastopathy of left breast   A

     N60.19   Diffuse cystic mastopathy of unspecified breast   A

   ✓5th **N60.2   Fibroadenosis of breast**
Adenofibrosis of breast

> EXCLUDES 2   fibroadenoma of breast (D24.-)

     N60.21   Fibroadenosis of right breast

     N60.22   Fibroadenosis of left breast

     N60.29   Fibroadenosis of unspecified breast

   ✓5th **N60.3   Fibrosclerosis of breast**
Cystic mastopathy with epithelial proliferation

     N60.31   Fibrosclerosis of right breast

     N60.32   Fibrosclerosis of left breast

     N60.39   Fibrosclerosis of unspecified breast

   ✓5th **N60.4   Mammary duct ectasia**

     N60.41   Mammary duct ectasia of right breast

     N60.42   Mammary duct ectasia of left breast

     N60.49   Mammary duct ectasia of unspecified breast

   ✓5th **N60.8   Other benign mammary dysplasias**

     N60.81   Other benign mammary dysplasias of right breast

     N60.82   Other benign mammary dysplasias of left breast

     N60.89   Other benign mammary dysplasias of unspecified breast

   ✓5th **N60.9   Unspecified benign mammary dysplasia**

     N60.91   Unspecified benign mammary dysplasia of right breast

     N60.92   Unspecified benign mammary dysplasia of left breast

     N60.99   Unspecified benign mammary dysplasia of unspecified breast

N61   Inflammatory disorders of breast
Abscess (acute) (chronic) (nonpuerperal) of areola
Abscess (acute) (chronic) (nonpuerperal) of breast
Carbuncle of breast
Infective mastitis (acute) (subacute) (nonpuerperal)
Mastitis (acute) (subacute) (nonpuerperal) NOS

> EXCLUDES 1   inflammatory carcinoma of breast (C50.9)
> inflammatory disorder of breast associated with childbirth (O91.-)
> neonatal infective mastitis (P39.0)
> thrombophlebitis of breast [Mondor's disease] (I80.8)

N62   Hypertrophy of breast
Gynecomastia
Hypertrophy of breast NOS
Massive pubertal hypertrophy of breast

> EXCLUDES 1   breast engorgement of newborn (P83.4)
> disproportion of reconstructed breast (N65.1)

N63   Unspecified lump in breast
Nodule(s) NOS in breast

✓4th **N64   Other disorders of breast**

> EXCLUDES 2   mechanical complication of breast prosthesis and implant (T85.4-)

   N64.0   Fissure and fistula of nipple

   N64.1   Fat necrosis of breast
Fat necrosis (segmental) of breast
Code first breast necrosis due to breast graft (T85.89)

   N64.2   Atrophy of breast

   N64.3   Galactorrhea not associated with childbirth

   N64.4   Mastodynia

   ✓5th **N64.5   Other signs and symptoms in breast**

> EXCLUDES 2   abnormal findings on diagnostic imaging of breast (R92.-)

     N64.51   Induration of breast

     N64.52   Nipple discharge

> EXCLUDES 1   abnormal findings in nipple discharge (R89.-)

     N64.53   Retraction of nipple

     N64.59   Other signs and symptoms in breast

   ✓5th **N64.8   Other specified disorders of breast**

     N64.81   Ptosis of breast   A

> EXCLUDES 1   ptosis of native breast in relation to reconstructed breast (N65.1)

     N64.82   Hypoplasia of breast   A
Micromastia

> EXCLUDES 1   congenital absence of breast (Q83.0)
> hypoplasia of native breast in relation to reconstructed breast (N65.1)

     N64.89   Other specified disorders of breast
Galactocele
Subinvolution of breast (postlactational)

   N64.9   Disorder of breast, unspecified

N Newborn: 0   P Pediatric: 0-17   M Maternity: 12-55   A Adult: 15-124   MCC Major CC Condition   PDxMCC PDx acts as own MCC   CC CC Condition   PDxCC PDx acts as own CC

✅**4ᵗʰ N65 Deformity and disproportion of reconstructed breast**

    N65.0 Deformity of reconstructed breast   A
        Contour irregularity in reconstructed breast
        Excess tissue in reconstructed breast
        Misshapen reconstructed breast

    N65.1 Disproportion of reconstructed breast   A
        Breast asymmetry between native breast and reconstructed breast
        Disproportion between native breast and reconstructed breast

Inflammatory diseases of female pelvic organs (N70-N77)

EXCLUDES 1 *inflammatory diseases of female pelvic organs complicating:*
abortion or ectopic or molar pregnancy (O00-O07, O08.0)
pregnancy, childbirth and the puerperium (O23-, O75.3, O85, O86-)

✅**4ᵗʰ N70 Salpingitis and oophoritis**
    INCLUDES   abscess (of) fallopian tube
             abscess (of) ovary
             pyosalpinx
             salpingo-oophoritis
             tubo-ovarian abscess
             tubo-ovarian inflammatory disease
    Use additional code (B95-B97), to identify infectious agent
    EXCLUDES 1 *gonococcal infection (A54.24)*
              tuberculous infection (A18.17)

> **CC Excl: For CC codes in subcategory N70.0, unless otherwise noted:** A17.9, A18.10, A18.16-A18.18, A18.82, A18.84, A18.89, A54.03, A54.24, A54.82, A54.84, A54.89-A54.9, A59.00, A59.8-A59.9, B37.41-B37.49, N70.01-N71.9, N73.0-N74, N75.9, N76.5, N76.81-N76.89, N90.810-N90.818, N94.818-N94.9, N96, Q55.0-Q55.21, Q55.23-Q55.4, Q55.7-Q55.9

    ✅**5ᵗʰ N70.0 Acute salpingitis and oophoritis**
        N70.01 Acute salpingitis   CC ♀
        N70.02 Acute oophoritis   CC ♀
        N70.03 Acute salpingitis and oophoritis   CC ♀

    ✅**5ᵗʰ N70.1 Chronic salpingitis and oophoritis**
        Hydrosalpinx
        N70.11 Chronic salpingitis   ♀
        N70.12 Chronic oophoritis   ♀
        N70.13 Chronic salpingitis and oophoritis   ♀

    ✅**5ᵗʰ N70.9 Salpingitis and oophoritis, unspecified**
        N70.91 Salpingitis, unspecified   ♀
        N70.92 Oophoritis, unspecified   ♀
        N70.93 Salpingitis and oophoritis, unspecified   ♀

✅**4ᵗʰ N71 Inflammatory disease of uterus, except cervix**
    Endo (myo) metritis   Pyometra
    Metritis   Uterine abscess
    Myometritis
    Use additional code (B95-B97), to identify infectious agent
    EXCLUDES 1 *hyperplastic endometritis (N85.0-)*
              infection of uterus following delivery (O85, O86.-)

    N71.0 Acute inflammatory disease of uterus   CC ♀
> **CC Excl:** A17.9, A18.10, A18.16-A18.18, A18.82, A18.84, A18.89, A54.03, A54.24, A54.82, A54.84, A54.89-A54.9, A59.00, A59.8-A59.9, B37.41-B37.49, N70.01-N74, N75.9, N76.5, N76.81-N76.89, N85.8-N85.9, N90.810-N90.818, N94.818-N94.9, N96, Q55.0-Q55.21, Q55.23-Q55.4, Q55.7-Q55.9

    N71.1 Chronic inflammatory disease of uterus   ♀
    N71.9 Inflammatory disease of uterus, unspecified   ♀

N72 Inflammatory disease of cervix uteri   ♀
    Cervicitis (with or without erosion or ectropion)
    Endocervicitis (with or without erosion or ectropion)
    Exocervicitis (with or without erosion or ectropion)
    Use additional code (B95-B97), to identify infectious agent
    EXCLUDES 1 *erosion and ectropion of cervix without cervicitis (N86)*

✅**4ᵗʰ N73 Other female pelvic inflammatory diseases**
    Use additional code (B95-B97), to identify infectious agent

> **CC Excl: For CC/MCC codes in category N73, unless otherwise noted:** A17.9, A18.10, A18.16-A18.18, A18.82, A18.84, A18.89, A54.03, A54.24, A54.82, A54.84, A54.89-A54.9, A59.00, A59.8-A59.9, B37.41-B37.49, N70.01-N71.9, N73.0-N74, N75.9, N76.5, N76.81-N76.89, N90.810-N90.818, N94.818-N94.9, N96, Q55.0-Q55.21, Q55.23-Q55.4, Q55.7-Q55.9

    N73.0 Acute parametritis and pelvic cellulitis   CC ♀
        Abscess of broad ligament
        Abscess of parametrium
        Pelvic cellulitis, female

    N73.1 Chronic parametritis and pelvic cellulitis   ♀
        Any condition in N73.0 specified as chronic
        EXCLUDES 1 *tuberculous parametritis and pelvic cellulitis (A18.17)*

    N73.2 Unspecified parametritis and pelvic cellulitis   ♀
        Any condition in N73.0 unspecified whether acute or chronic

    N73.3 Female acute pelvic peritonitis   MCC ♀
    N73.4 Female chronic pelvic peritonitis   CC ♀
        EXCLUDES 1 *tuberculous pelvic (female) peritonitis (A18.17)*

    N73.5 Female pelvic peritonitis, unspecified   ♀
    N73.6 Female pelvic peritoneal adhesions (postinfective)   ♀
        EXCLUDES 2 *postprocedural pelvic peritoneal adhesions (N99.4)*
        AHA: 2014, 1Q, 6

    N73.8 Other specified female pelvic inflammatory diseases   ♀
    N73.9 Female pelvic inflammatory disease, unspecified   ♀
        Female pelvic infection or inflammation NOS

N74 *Female pelvic inflammatory disorders in diseases classified elsewhere*   ♀
    Code first underlying disease
    EXCLUDES 1 *chlamydial cervicitis (A56.02)*
             chlamydial pelvic inflammatory disease (A56.11)
             gonococcal cervicitis (A54.03)
             gonococcal pelvic inflammatory disease (A54.24)
             herpesviral [herpes simplex] cervicitis (A60.03)
             herpesviral [herpes simplex] pelvic inflammatory disease (A60.09)
             syphilitic cervicitis (A52.76)
             syphilitic pelvic inflammatory disease (A52.76)
             trichomonal cervicitis (A59.09)
             tuberculous cervicitis (A18.16)
             tuberculous pelvic inflammatory disease (A18.17)

✅**4ᵗʰ N75 Diseases of Bartholin's gland**
    N75.0 Cyst of Bartholin's gland   ♀
    N75.1 Abscess of Bartholin's gland   CC ♀
> **CC Excl:** A17.9, A18.10, A18.16-A18.18, A18.82, A18.84, A18.89, A59.00-A59.01, A59.8-A59.9, B37.3-B37.49, N75.0-N77.1, N84.3, N90.3, N90.6-N90.9, N94.810-N94.9, N96, Q55.0-Q55.21, Q55.23-Q55.4, Q55.7-Q55.9

    N75.8 Other diseases of Bartholin's gland   ♀
        Bartholinitis

    N75.9 Disease of Bartholin's gland, unspecified   ♀

✅**4ᵗʰ N76 Other inflammation of vagina and vulva**
    Use additional code (B95-B97), to identify infectious agent
    EXCLUDES 2 *senile (atrophic) vaginitis (N95.2)*
             vulvar vestibulitis (N94.810)

    N76.0 Acute vaginitis   ♀
        Acute vulvovaginitis
        Vaginitis NOS
        Vulvovaginitis NOS

    N76.1 Subacute and chronic vaginitis   ♀
        Chronic vulvovaginitis
        Subacute vulvovaginitis

    N76.2 Acute vulvitis   ♀
        Vulvitis NOS

    N76.3 Subacute and chronic vulvitis   ♀
    N76.4 Abscess of vulva   CC ♀
        Furuncle of vulva
        CC Excl: See code: N75.1

    N76.5 Ulceration of vagina   ♀
    N76.6 Ulceration of vulva   ♀

    ✅**5ᵗʰ N76.8 Other specified inflammation of vagina and vulva**
        N76.81 Mucositis (ulcerative) of vagina and vulva   CC ♀
            Code also type of associated therapy, such as:
                antineoplastic and immunosuppressive drugs (T45.1X-)
                radiological procedure and radiotherapy (Y84.2)
            EXCLUDES 2 *gastrointestinal mucositis (ulcerative) (K92.81)*
                nasal mucositis (ulcerative) (J34.81)
                oral mucositis (ulcerative) (K12.3-)
            CC Excl: N72, N75.9, N76.5, N76.81-N76.89

        N76.89 Other specified inflammation of vagina and vulva   ♀

✅ Additional Character Required   **√x7ᵗʰ** Placeholder Alert   Unacceptable PDx   Manifestation   Hospital Acquired Condition   **EXCLUDES 1** Not Coded Here   **EXCLUDES 2** Not Included Here

ICD-10-CM 2016   **801**

✓4ᵗʰ N77 Vulvovaginal ulceration and inflammation in diseases classified elsewhere

N77.0 Ulceration of vulva in diseases classified elsewhere ♀
Code first underlying disease, such as:
Behçet's disease (M35.2)
EXCLUDES 1 ulceration of vulva in gonococcal infection (A54.02)
ulceration of vulva in herpesviral [herpes simplex] infection (A60.04)
ulceration of vulva in syphilis (A51.0)
ulceration of vulva in tuberculosis (A18.18)

N77.1 Vaginitis, vulvitis and vulvovaginitis in diseases classified elsewhere ♀
Code first underlying disease, such as:
pinworm (B80)
EXCLUDES 1 candidal vulvovaginitis (B37.3)
chlamydial vulvovaginitis (A56.02)
gonococcal vulvovaginitis (A54.02)
herpesviral [herpes simplex] vulvovaginitis (A60.04)
trichomonal vulvovaginitis (A59.01)
tuberculous vulvovaginitis (A18.18)
vulvovaginitis in early syphilis (A51.0)
vulvovaginitis in late syphilis (A52.76)

Noninflammatory disorders of female genital tract (N80-N98)

✓4ᵗʰ N80 Endometriosis

N80.0 Endometriosis of uterus ♀
Adenomyosis
EXCLUDES 1 stromal endometriosis (D39.0)
N80.1 Endometriosis of ovary ♀
N80.2 Endometriosis of fallopian tube ♀
N80.3 Endometriosis of pelvic peritoneum ♀
N80.4 Endometriosis of rectovaginal septum and vagina ♀
N80.5 Endometriosis of intestine ♀
N80.6 Endometriosis in cutaneous scar ♀
N80.8 Other endometriosis ♀
N80.9 Endometriosis, unspecified ♀

✓4ᵗʰ N81 Female genital prolapse

EXCLUDES 1 genital prolapse complicating pregnancy, labor or delivery (O34.5-)
prolapse and hernia of ovary and fallopian tube (N83.4)
prolapse of vaginal vault after hysterectomy (N99.3)

N81.0 Urethrocele ♀
EXCLUDES 1 urethrocele with cystocele (N81.1-)
urethrocele with prolapse of uterus (N81.2-N81.4)

✓5ᵗʰ N81.1 Cystocele
Cystocele with urethrocele
Cystourethrocele
EXCLUDES 1 cystocele with prolapse of uterus (N81.2-N81.4)
N81.10 Cystocele, unspecified ♀
Prolapse of (anterior) vaginal wall NOS
N81.11 Cystocele, midline ♀
N81.12 Cystocele, lateral ♀
Paravaginal cystocele

N81.2 Incomplete uterovaginal prolapse ♀
First degree uterine prolapse
Prolapse of cervix NOS
Second degree uterine prolapse
EXCLUDES 1 cervical stump prolapse (N81.85)

N81.3 Complete uterovaginal prolapse ♀
Procidentia (uteri) NOS
Third degree uterine prolapse

N81.4 Uterovaginal prolapse, unspecified ♀
Prolapse of uterus NOS

N81.5 Vaginal enterocele ♀
EXCLUDES 1 enterocele with prolapse of uterus (N81.2-N81.4)

N81.6 Rectocele ♀
Prolapse of posterior vaginal wall
Use additional code for any associated fecal incontinence, if applicable (R15.-)
EXCLUDES 2 perineocele (N81.81)
rectal prolapse (K62.3)
rectocele with prolapse of uterus (N81.2-N81.4)

✓5ᵗʰ N81.8 Other female genital prolapse
N81.81 Perineocele ♀
N81.82 Incompetence or weakening of pubocervical tissue ♀
N81.83 Incompetence or weakening of rectovaginal tissue ♀
N81.84 Pelvic muscle wasting
Disuse atrophy of pelvic muscles and anal sphincter
N81.85 Cervical stump prolapse ♀
N81.89 Other female genital prolapse ♀
Deficient perineum
Old laceration of muscles of pelvic floor
N81.9 Female genital prolapse, unspecified ♀

✓4ᵗʰ N82 Fistulae involving female genital tract
EXCLUDES 1 vesicointestinal fistulae (N32.1)

CC Excl: For CC codes in category N82, unless otherwise noted: N82.0-N82.9

N82.0 Vesicovaginal fistula CC ♀
N82.1 Other female urinary-genital tract fistulae CC ♀
Cervicovesical fistula   Uteroureteric fistula
Ureterovaginal fistula   Uterovesical fistula
Urethrovaginal fistula
N82.2 Fistula of vagina to small intestine CC ♀
N82.3 Fistula of vagina to large intestine CC ♀
Rectovaginal fistula
N82.4 Other female intestinal-genital tract fistulae CC ♀
Intestinouterine fistula
N82.5 Female genital tract-skin fistulae CC ♀
Uterus to abdominal wall fistula
Vaginoperineal fistula
N82.8 Other female genital tract fistulae CC ♀
N82.9 Female genital tract fistula, unspecified CC ♀

✓4ᵗʰ N83 Noninflammatory disorders of ovary, fallopian tube and broad ligament
EXCLUDES 2 hydrosalpinx (N70.1-)

N83.0 Follicular cyst of ovary ♀
Cyst of graafian follicle
Hemorrhagic follicular cyst (of ovary)
N83.1 Corpus luteum cyst ♀
Hemorrhagic corpus luteum cyst
✓5ᵗʰ N83.2 Other and unspecified ovarian cysts
EXCLUDES 1 developmental ovarian cyst (Q50.1)
neoplastic ovarian cyst (D27.-)
polycystic ovarian syndrome (E28.2)
Stein-Leventhal syndrome (E28.2)
N83.20 Unspecified ovarian cysts ♀
N83.29 Other ovarian cysts ♀
Retention cyst of ovary
Simple cyst of ovary
✓5ᵗʰ N83.3 Acquired atrophy of ovary and fallopian tube
N83.31 Acquired atrophy of ovary ♀
N83.32 Acquired atrophy of fallopian tube ♀
N83.33 Acquired atrophy of ovary and fallopian tube ♀
N83.4 Prolapse and hernia of ovary and fallopian tube ♀
✓5ᵗʰ N83.5 Torsion of ovary, ovarian pedicle and fallopian tube
Torsion of accessory tube

CC Excl: For CC codes in subcategory N83.5, unless otherwise noted: N83.0-N83.9, N99.83

N83.51 Torsion of ovary and ovarian pedicle CC ♀
N83.52 Torsion of fallopian tube CC ♀
Torsion of hydatid of Morgagni
N83.53 Torsion of ovary, ovarian pedicle and fallopian tube CC ♀
N83.6 Hematosalpinx ♀
EXCLUDES 1 hematosalpinx (with) (in):
hematocolpos (N89.7)
hematometra (N85.7)
tubal pregnancy (O00.1)
N83.7 Hematoma of broad ligament ♀
N83.8 Other noninflammatory disorders of ovary, fallopian tube and broad ligament ♀
Broad ligament laceration syndrome [Allen-Masters]
N83.9 Noninflammatory disorder of ovary, fallopian tube and broad ligament, unspecified ♀

N Newborn: 0   P Pediatric: 0-17   M Maternity: 12-55   A Adult: 15-124   **MCC** Major CC Condition   **PDxMCC** PDx acts as own MCC   **CC** CC Condition   **PDxCC** PDx acts as own CC

✓4ᵗʰ **N84 Polyp of female genital tract**

     EXCLUDES 1   *adenomatous polyp (D28.-)*
                             placental polyp (O90.89)

     N84.0 Polyp of corpus uteri   ♀
         Polyp of endometrium
         Polyp of uterus NOS
         EXCLUDES 1 *polypoid endometrial hyperplasia (N85.0-)*

     N84.1 Polyp of cervix uteri   ♀
         Mucous polyp of cervix

     N84.2 Polyp of vagina   ♀

     N84.3 Polyp of vulva   ♀
         Polyp of labia

     N84.8 Polyp of other parts of female genital tract   ♀

     N84.9 Polyp of female genital tract, unspecified   ♀

✓4ᵗʰ **N85 Other noninflammatory disorders of uterus, except cervix**

     EXCLUDES 1   *endometriosis (N80.-)*
                           inflammatory diseases of uterus (N71.-)
                           noninflammatory disorders of cervix, except malposition (N86-N88)
                           polyp of corpus uteri (N84.0)
                           uterine prolapse (N81.-)

     ✓5ᵗʰ **N85.0 Endometrial hyperplasia**

         N85.00 Endometrial hyperplasia, unspecified   ♀
                 Hyperplasia (adenomatous) (cystic) (glandular) of
                       endometrium
                 Hyperplastic endometritis

         N85.01 Benign endometrial hyperplasia   ♀
                 Endometrial hyperplasia (complex) (simple) without
                       atypia

         N85.02 Endometrial intraepithelial neoplasia [EIN]   ♀
                 Endometrial hyperplasia with atypia
                 EXCLUDES 1 *malignant neoplasm of endometrium (with*
                                  endometrial intraepithelial neoplasia
                                  [EIN]) (C54.1)

     N85.2 Hypertrophy of uterus   ♀
         Bulky or enlarged uterus
         EXCLUDES 1 *puerperal hypertrophy of uterus (O90.89)*

     N85.3 Subinvolution of uterus   ♀
         EXCLUDES 1 *puerperal subinvolution of uterus (O90.89)*

     N85.4 Malposition of uterus   ♀
         Anteversion of uterus
         Retroflexion of uterus
         Retroversion of uterus
         EXCLUDES 1 *malposition of uterus complicating pregnancy, labor or*
                                delivery (O34.5-, O65.5)

     N85.5 Inversion of uterus   ♀
         EXCLUDES 1 *current obstetric trauma (O71.2)*
                                postpartum inversion of uterus (O71.2)

     N85.6 Intrauterine synechiae   ♀

     N85.7 Hematometra   ♀
         Hematosalpinx with hematometra
         EXCLUDES 1 *hematometra with hematocolpos (N89.7)*

     N85.8 Other specified noninflammatory disorders of uterus   ♀
         Atrophy of uterus, acquired
         Fibrosis of uterus NOS

     N85.9 Noninflammatory disorder of uterus, unspecified   ♀
         Disorder of uterus NOS

N86 Erosion and ectropion of cervix uteri   ♀
     Decubitus (trophic) ulcer of cervix
     Eversion of cervix
     EXCLUDES 1 *erosion and ectropion of cervix with cervicitis (N72)*

✓4ᵗʰ **N87 Dysplasia of cervix uteri**
     EXCLUDES 1 *abnormal results from cervical cytologic examination without*
                       histologic confirmation (R87.61-)
                       carcinoma in situ of cervix uteri (D06.-)
                       cervical intraepithelial neoplasia III [CIN III] (D06.-)
                       HGSIL of cervix (R87.613)
                       severe dysplasia of cervix uteri (D06.-)

     N87.0 Mild cervical dysplasia   ♀
         Cervical intraepithelial neoplasia I [CIN I]

     N87.1 Moderate cervical dysplasia   ♀
         Cervical intraepithelial neoplasia II [CIN II]

     N87.9 Dysplasia of cervix uteri, unspecified   ♀
         Anaplasia of cervix
         Cervical atypism
         Cervical dysplasia NOS

✓4ᵗʰ **N88 Other noninflammatory disorders of cervix uteri**
     EXCLUDES 2 *inflammatory disease of cervix (N72)*
                       polyp of cervix (N84.1)

     N88.0 Leukoplakia of cervix uteri   ♀

     N88.1 Old laceration of cervix uteri   ♀
         Adhesions of cervix
         EXCLUDES 1 *current obstetric trauma (O71.3)*

     N88.2 Stricture and stenosis of cervix uteri   ♀
         EXCLUDES 1 *stricture and stenosis of cervix uteri complicating labor*
                                (O65.5)

     N88.3 Incompetence of cervix uteri   ♀
         Investigation and management of (suspected) cervical
                 incompetence in a nonpregnant woman
         EXCLUDES 1 *cervical incompetence complicating pregnancy*
                                (O34.3-)

     N88.4 Hypertrophic elongation of cervix uteri   ♀

     N88.8 Other specified noninflammatory disorders of cervix uteri   ♀
         EXCLUDES 1 *current obstetric trauma (O71.3)*

     N88.9 Noninflammatory disorder of cervix uteri, unspecified   ♀

✓4ᵗʰ **N89 Other noninflammatory disorders of vagina**
     EXCLUDES 1 *abnormal results from vaginal cytologic examination without*
                       histologic confirmation (R87.62-)
                       carcinoma in situ of vagina (D07.2)
                       HGSIL of vagina (R87.623)
                       inflammation of vagina (N76.-)
                       senile (atrophic) vaginitis (N95.2)
                       severe dysplasia of vagina (D07.2)
                       trichomonal leukorrhea (A59.00)
                       vaginal intraepithelial neoplasia [VAIN], grade III (D07.2)

     N89.0 Mild vaginal dysplasia   ♀
         Vaginal intraepithelial neoplasia [VAIN], grade I

     N89.1 Moderate vaginal dysplasia   ♀
         Vaginal intraepithelial neoplasia [VAIN], grade II

     N89.3 Dysplasia of vagina, unspecified   ♀

     N89.4 Leukoplakia of vagina   ♀

     N89.5 Stricture and atresia of vagina   ♀
         Vaginal adhesions   Vaginal stenosis
         EXCLUDES 1 *congenital atresia or stricture (Q52.4)*
                                postprocedural adhesions of vagina (N99.2)

     N89.6 Tight hymenal ring   ♀
         Rigid hymen
         Tight introitus
         EXCLUDES 1 *imperforate hymen (Q52.3)*

     N89.7 Hematocolpos   ♀
         Hematocolpos with hematometra or hematosalpinx

     N89.8 Other specified noninflammatory disorders of vagina   ♀
         Leukorrhea NOS
         Old vaginal laceration
         Pessary ulcer of vagina
         EXCLUDES 1 *current obstetric trauma (O70-, O71.4, O71.7-O71.8)*
                                old laceration involving muscles of pelvic floor (N81.8)

     N89.9 Noninflammatory disorder of vagina, unspecified   ♀

✓4ᵗʰ **N90 Other noninflammatory disorders of vulva and perineum**
     EXCLUDES 1 *anogenital (venereal) warts (A63.0)*
                       carcinoma in situ of vulva (D07.1)
                       condyloma acuminatum (A63.0)
                       current obstetric trauma (O70-, O71.7-O71.8)
                       inflammation of vulva (N76.-)
                       severe dysplasia of vulva (D07.1)
                       vulvar intraepithelial neoplasm III [VIN III] (D07.1)

     N90.0 Mild vulvar dysplasia   ♀
         Vulvar intraepithelial neoplasia [VIN], grade I

     N90.1 Moderate vulvar dysplasia   ♀
         Vulvar intraepithelial neoplasia [VIN], grade II

     N90.3 Dysplasia of vulva, unspecified   ♀

     N90.4 Leukoplakia of vulva   ♀
         Dystrophy of vulva   Lichen sclerosus of external female
         Kraurosis of vulva   genital organs

     N90.5 Atrophy of vulva   ♀
         Stenosis of vulva

     N90.6 Hypertrophy of vulva   ♀
         Hypertrophy of labia

     N90.7 Vulvar cyst   ♀

Chapter 14. Diseases of Genitourinary System

N90.8–N97.9

✓5ᵗʰ **N90.8 Other specified noninflammatory disorders of vulva and perineum**

     ✓6ᵗʰ **N90.81 Female genital mutilation status**
        Female genital cutting status

        N90.810 Female genital mutilation status, unspecified ♀
           Female genital cutting status, unspecified
           Female genital mutilation status NOS

        N90.811 Female genital mutilation Type I status ♀
           Clitorectomy status
           Female genital cutting Type I status

        N90.812 Female genital mutilation Type II status ♀
           Clitorectomy with excision of labia minora status
           Female genital cutting Type II status

        N90.813 Female genital mutilation Type III status ♀
           Female genital cutting Type III status
           Infibulation status

        N90.818 Other female genital mutilation status ♀
           Female genital cutting Type IV status
           Female genital mutilation Type IV status
           Other female genital cutting status

     N90.89 Other specified noninflammatory disorders of vulva and perineum ♀
        Adhesions of vulva
        Hypertrophy of clitoris

N90.9 Noninflammatory disorder of vulva and perineum, unspecified ♀

✓4ᵗʰ **N91 Absent, scanty and rare menstruation**
     EXCLUDES 1   *ovarian dysfunction (E28.-)*

N91.0 Primary amenorrhea ♀
N91.1 Secondary amenorrhea ♀
N91.2 Amenorrhea, unspecified ♀
N91.3 Primary oligomenorrhea ♀
N91.4 Secondary oligomenorrhea ♀
N91.5 Oligomenorrhea, unspecified ♀
     Hypomenorrhea NOS

✓4ᵗʰ **N92 Excessive, frequent and irregular menstruation**
     EXCLUDES 1   *postmenopausal bleeding (N95.0)*
               precocious puberty (menstruation) (E30.1)

N92.0 Excessive and frequent menstruation with regular cycle ♀
     Heavy periods NOS
     Menorrhagia NOS
     Polymenorrhea

N92.1 Excessive and frequent menstruation with irregular cycle ♀
     Irregular intermenstrual bleeding
     Irregular, shortened intervals between menstrual bleeding
     Menometrorrhagia
     Metrorrhagia

N92.2 Excessive menstruation at puberty P ♀
     Excessive bleeding associated with onset of menstrual periods
     Pubertal menorrhagia
     Puberty bleeding

N92.3 Ovulation bleeding ♀
     Regular intermenstrual bleeding

N92.4 Excessive bleeding in the premenopausal period ♀
     Climacteric menorrhagia or metrorrhagia
     Menopausal menorrhagia or metrorrhagia
     Preclimacteric menorrhagia or metrorrhagia
     Premenopausal menorrhagia or metrorrhagia

N92.5 Other specified irregular menstruation ♀
N92.6 Irregular menstruation, unspecified ♀
     Irregular bleeding NOS
     Irregular periods NOS
     EXCLUDES 1   *irregular menstruation with:*
          lengthened intervals or scanty bleeding (N91.3-N91.5)
          shortened intervals or excessive bleeding (N92.1)

✓4ᵗʰ **N93 Other abnormal uterine and vaginal bleeding**
     EXCLUDES 1   *neonatal vaginal hemorrhage (P54.6)*
               precocious puberty (menstruation) (E30.1)
               pseudomenses (P54.6)

N93.0 Postcoital and contact bleeding ♀
N93.8 Other specified abnormal uterine and vaginal bleeding ♀
     Dysfunctional or functional uterine or vaginal bleeding NOS
N93.9 Abnormal uterine and vaginal bleeding, unspecified ♀

✓4ᵗʰ **N94 Pain and other conditions associated with female genital organs and menstrual cycle**

N94.0 Mittelschmerz ♀
N94.1 Dyspareunia ♀
     EXCLUDES 1   *psychogenic dyspareunia (F52.6)*

N94.2 Vaginismus ♀
     EXCLUDES 1   *psychogenic vaginismus (F52.5)*

N94.3 Premenstrual tension syndrome ♀
     Premenstrual dysphoric disorder
     Code also associated menstrual migraine (G43.82-, G43.83-)

N94.4 Primary dysmenorrhea ♀
N94.5 Secondary dysmenorrhea ♀
N94.6 Dysmenorrhea, unspecified ♀
     EXCLUDES 1   *psychogenic dysmenorrhea (F45.8)*

✓5ᵗʰ **N94.8 Other specified conditions associated with female genital organs and menstrual cycle**

     ✓6ᵗʰ **N94.81 Vulvodynia**
        N94.810 Vulvar vestibulitis ♀
        N94.818 Other vulvodynia ♀
        N94.819 Vulvodynia, unspecified ♀
           Vulvodynia NOS

     N94.89 Other specified conditions associated with female genital organs and menstrual cycle ♀

N94.9 Unspecified condition associated with female genital organs and menstrual cycle ♀

✓4ᵗʰ **N95 Menopausal and other perimenopausal disorders**
     Menopausal and other perimenopausal disorders due to naturally occurring (age-related) menopause and perimenopause
     EXCLUDES 1   *excessive bleeding in the premenopausal period (N92.4)*
          menopausal and perimenopausal disorders due to artificial or premature menopause (E89.4-, E28.31-)
          premature menopause (E28.31-)
     EXCLUDES 2   *postmenopausal osteoporosis (M81.0-)*
          postmenopausal osteoporosis with current pathological fracture (M80.0-)
          postmenopausal urethritis (N34.2)

N95.0 Postmenopausal bleeding ♀
N95.1 Menopausal and female climacteric states ♀
     Symptoms such as flushing, sleeplessness, headache, lack of concentration, associated with natural (age-related) menopause
     Use additional code for associated symptoms
     EXCLUDES 1   *asymptomatic menopausal state (Z78.0)*
          symptoms associated with artificial menopause (E89.41)
          symptoms associated with premature menopause (E28.310)

N95.2 Postmenopausal atrophic vaginitis ♀
     Senile (atrophic) vaginitis

N95.8 Other specified menopausal and perimenopausal disorders ♀
N95.9 Unspecified menopausal and perimenopausal disorder ♀

N96 Recurrent pregnancy loss ♀
     Investigation or care in a nonpregnant woman with history of recurrent pregnancy loss
     EXCLUDES 1   *recurrent pregnancy loss with current pregnancy (O26.2-)*

✓4ᵗʰ **N97 Female infertility**
     INCLUDES   inability to achieve a pregnancy
              sterility, female NOS
     EXCLUDES 1   *female infertility associated with:*
          hypopituitarism (E23.0)
          Stein-Leventhal syndrome (E28.2)
     EXCLUDES 2   *incompetence of cervix uteri (N88.3)*

N97.0 Female infertility associated with anovulation ♀
N97.1 Female infertility of tubal origin ♀
     Female infertility associated with congenital anomaly of tube
     Female infertility due to tubal block
     Female infertility due to tubal occlusion
     Female infertility due to tubal stenosis

N97.2 Female infertility of uterine origin ♀
     Female infertility associated with congenital anomaly of uterus
     Female infertility due to nonimplantation of ovum

N97.8 Female infertility of other origin ♀
N97.9 Female infertility, unspecified ♀

N Newborn: 0   P Pediatric: 0-17   M Maternity: 12-55   A Adult: 15-124   MCC Major CC Condition   PDxMCC PDx acts as own MCC   CC CC Condition   PDxCC PDx acts as own CC

804   ICD-10-CM 2016

☑4ᵗʰ **N98 Complications associated with artificial fertilization**

N98.0 Infection associated with artificial insemination   ᴄᴄ ♀
CC Excl: N98.0, T80.211A, T80.212A, T80.218A, T80.219A, T80.22XA, T80.29XA, T82.7XXA, T88.0XXA

N98.1 Hyperstimulation of ovaries   ᴄᴄ ♀
Hyperstimulation of ovaries NOS
Hyperstimulation of ovaries associated with induced ovulation
CC Excl: D78.81-D78.89, E36.8, E89.810-E89.89, H59.011-H59.019, H59.031-H59.099, H59.811-H59.89, H95.811-H95.89, I97.3, L76.81-L76.82, M96.89, N98.1-N98.9, T81.8[2,9]XA, T81.9XXA

N98.2 Complications of attempted introduction of fertilized ovum following in vitro fertilization   ᴄᴄ ♀
CC Excl: See code: N98.1

N98.3 Complications of attempted introduction of embryo in embryo transfer   ᴄᴄ ♀
CC Excl: See code: N98.1

N98.8 Other complications associated with artificial fertilization   ᴄᴄ ♀
CC Excl: See code: N98.1

N98.9 Complication associated with artificial fertilization, unspecified   ᴄᴄ ♀
CC Excl: See code: N98.1

Intraoperative and postprocedural complications and disorders of genitourinary system, not elsewhere classified (N99)

☑4ᵗʰ **N99 Intraoperative and postprocedural complications and disorders of genitourinary system, not elsewhere classified**
EXCLUDES 2   *irradiation cystitis (N30.4-)*
postoophorectomy osteoporosis with current pathological fracture (M80.8-)
postoophorectomy osteoporosis without current pathological fracture (M81.8)

N99.0 Postprocedural (acute) (chronic) kidney failure
Use additional code for type of kidney disease

☑5ᵗʰ **N99.1 Postprocedural urethral stricture**
Postcatheterization urethral stricture

☑6ᵗʰ **N99.11 Postprocedural urethral stricture, male**
N99.110 Postprocedural urethral stricture, male, ♂ meatal
N99.111 Postprocedural bulbous urethral stricture
N99.112 Postprocedural membranous urethral stricture
N99.113 Postprocedural anterior urethral stricture
N99.114 Postprocedural urethral stricture, male, ♂ unspecified

N99.12 Postprocedural urethral stricture, female   ♀

N99.2 Postprocedural adhesions of vagina   ♀

N99.3 Prolapse of vaginal vault after hysterectomy   ♀

N99.4 Postprocedural pelvic peritoneal adhesions
EXCLUDES 2   *pelvic peritoneal adhesions NOS (N73.6)*
postinfective pelvic peritoneal adhesions (N73.6)

☑5ᵗʰ **N99.5 Complications of stoma of urinary tract**
EXCLUDES 2   *mechanical complication of urinary (indwelling) catheter (T83.0-)*

☑6ᵗʰ **N99.51 Complication of cystostomy**
N99.510 Cystostomy hemorrhage   ᴄᴄ
CC Excl: D78.81-D78.89, E36.8, E89.810-E89.89, H59.011-H59.019, H59.031-H59.099, H59.811-H59.89, H95.811-H95.89, I97.3, L76.81-L76.82, M96.89, N32.89, N33, N98.1-N98.9, N99.510-N99.518, T81.82A, T81.89X-T81.9XX with 7th A, T83.010A, T83.020A, T83.030A, T83.090A, T83.110-T83.29X with 7th A, T83.410-T83.718 with 7th A, T83.728-T83.9XX with 7th A, T85.310-T85.311 with 7th A, T85.320-T85.321 with 7th A, T85.390-T85.391 with 7th A, T85.510-T85.9XX with 7th A, T86.820-T86.829, T86.842-T86.849

N99.511 Cystostomy infection   ᴄᴄ
CC Excl: D78.81-D78.89, E36.8, E89.810-E89.89, H59.011-H59.019, H59.031-H59.099, H59.811-H59.89, H95.811-H95.89, I97.3, L76.81-L76.82, M96.89, N32.89, N33, N39.0, N98.1-N98.9, N99.510-N99.518, T81.82A, T81.89X-T81.9XX with 7th A, T83.010A, T83.020A, T83.030A, T83.090A, T83.110-T83.29X with 7th A, T83.410-T83.718 with 7th A, T83.728-T83.9XX with 7th A, T85.310-T85.311 with 7th A, T85.320-T85.321 with 7th A, T85.390-T85.391 with 7th A, T85.510-T85.612 with 7th A, T85.614-T85.622 with 7th A, T85.624-T85.692 with 7th A, T85.694-T85.9XX with 7th A, T86.842-T86.849

N99.512 Cystostomy malfunction   ᴄᴄ
CC Excl: D78.81-D78.89, E36.8, E89.810-E89.89, H59.011-H59.019, H59.031-H59.099, H59.811-H59.89, H95.811-H95.89, I97.3, L76.81-L76.82, M96.89, N32.89, N33, N98.1-N98.9, N99.510-N99.518, T81.82XA, T81.89XA, T81.9XXA, T83.010A, T83.020A, T83.030A, T83.090A, T83.110A, T83.111A, T83.112A, T83.118A, T83.120A, T83.121A, T83.122A, T83.128A, T83.190A, T83.191A, T83.192A, T83.198A, T83.21XA, T83.22XA, T83.23XA, T83.29XA, T83.410A, T83.418A, T83.420A, T83.428A, T83.490A, T83.498A, T83.51XA, T83.59XA, T83.6XXA, T83.718A, T83.728A, T83.81XA, T83.82XA, T83.83XA, T83.84XA, T83.85XA, T83.86XA, T83.89XA, T83.9XXA

N99.518 Other cystostomy complication   ᴄᴄ
CC Excl: See code: N99.510

☑6ᵗʰ **N99.52 Complication of other external stoma of urinary tract**
N99.520 Hemorrhage of other external stoma of urinary tract
N99.521 Infection of other external stoma of urinary tract
N99.522 Malfunction of other external stoma of urinary tract
N99.528 Other complication of other external stoma of urinary tract

☑6ᵗʰ **N99.53 Complication of other stoma of urinary tract**
N99.530 Hemorrhage of other stoma of urinary tract
N99.531 Infection of other stoma of urinary tract
N99.532 Malfunction of other stoma of urinary tract
N99.538 Other complication of other stoma of urinary tract

☑5ᵗʰ **N99.6 Intraoperative hemorrhage and hematoma of a genitourinary system organ or structure complicating a procedure**
EXCLUDES 1   *intraoperative hemorrhage and hematoma of a genitourinary system organ or structure due to accidental puncture or laceration during a procedure (N99.7-)*

N99.61 Intraoperative hemorrhage and hematoma of a genitourinary system organ or structure complicating a genitourinary system procedure   ᴄᴄ
CC Excl: H95.811-H95.89, I85.01, I85.11, I97.3, K21.9, K22.8, K23-K25.0, K25.2, K25.4, K25.6, K26.0, K26.2, K26.4, K26.6, K27.0, K27.2, K27.4, K27.6, K28.0, K28.2, K28.4, K28.6, K29.01, K29.21, K29.31, K29.41, K29.51, K29.61, K29.71, K29.81, K29.91, K31.811, K55.21, K57.01, K57.11, K57.13, K57.21, K57.31, K57.33, K57.41, K57.51, K57.53, K57.81, K57.91, K57.93, K62.5, K92.0-K92.2, M96.89, N98.1-N98.9, N99.61-N99.62, N99.820-N99.821, P54.1-P54.3, T81.10XA, T81.11XA, T81.12XA, T81.19XA, T81.82XA, T81.89XA, T81.9XXA

N99.62 Intraoperative hemorrhage and hematoma of a genitourinary system organ or structure complicating other procedure   ᴄᴄ
CC Excl: See code: N99.61

☑ Additional Character Required   ☑x7ᵗʰ Placeholder Alert   Unacceptable PDx   Manifestation   Hospital Acquired Condition   *EXCLUDES 1* Not Coded Here   *EXCLUDES 2* Not Included Here

Chapter 14. Diseases of Genitourinary System

√5ᵗʰ **N99.7** **Accidental puncture and laceration of a genitourinary system organ or structure during a procedure**

    N99.71 **Accidental puncture and laceration of a genitourinary system organ or structure during a genitourinary system procedure**   CC
        CC Excl: D78.11-D78.12, D78.81-D78.89, E36.11-E36.8, E89.810-E89.89, G96.11, G97.41, G97.48-G97.49, H59.011-H59.019, H59.031-H59.099, H59.211-H59.229, H59.811-H59.89, H95.31-H95.32, H95.811-H95.89, I97.3, I97.51-I97.52, J95.71-J95.72, K91.71-K91.72, L76.11-L76.12, L76.81-L76.82, M96.820-M96.821, M96.89, N98.1-N98.9, N99.71-N99.72, T81.8[2,9]XA, T81.9XXA

    N99.72 **Accidental puncture and laceration of a genitourinary system organ or structure during other procedure**   CC
        CC Excl: See code: N99.71

√5ᵗʰ **N99.8** **Other intraoperative and postprocedural complications and disorders of genitourinary system**

    N99.81 **Other intraoperative complications of genitourinary system**

√6ᵗʰ **N99.82** **Postprocedural hemorrhage and hematoma of a genitourinary system organ or structure following a procedure**

    N99.820 **Postprocedural hemorrhage and hematoma of a genitourinary system organ or structure following a genitourinary system procedure**   CC
        CC Excl: See code: N99.61

    N99.821 **Postprocedural hemorrhage and hematoma of a genitourinary system organ or structure following other procedure**   CC
        CC Excl: See code: N99.61

    N99.83 **Residual ovary syndrome**   ♀

    N99.89 **Other postprocedural complications and disorders of genitourinary system**

N | Newborn: 0   P | Pediatric: 0-17   M | Maternity: 12-55   A | Adult: 15-124   **MCC** Major CC Condition   **PDxMCC** PDx acts as own MCC   **CC** CC Condition   **PDxCC** PDx acts as own CC

806

ICD-10-CM 2016

Chapter 15. Pregnancy, Childbirth, and the Puerperium (O00–O9A)

Chapter Specific Guidelines with Coding Examples

The chapter specific guidelines from the ICD-10-CM Official Guidelines for Coding and Reporting have been provided below. Along with these guidelines are coding examples, contained in the shaded boxes, that have been developed to help illustrate the coding and/or sequencing guidance found in these guidelines.

a. General rules for obstetric cases

1) Codes from chapter 15 and sequencing priority

Obstetric cases require codes from chapter 15, codes in the range O00-O9A, Pregnancy, Childbirth, and the Puerperium. Chapter 15 codes have sequencing priority over codes from other chapters. Additional codes from other chapters may be used in conjunction with chapter 15 codes to further specify conditions. Should the provider document that the pregnancy is incidental to the encounter, then code Z33.1, Pregnant state, incidental, should be used in place of any chapter 15 codes. It is the provider's responsibility to state that the condition being treated is not affecting the pregnancy.

Bladder abscess in pregnant patient at 25 weeks' gestation

O23.12   **Infections of bladder in pregnancy, second trimester**

N30.80   **Other cystitis without hematuria**

Z3A.25   **25 weeks gestation of pregnancy**

Explanation: The documentation does not indicate that the pregnancy is incidental or in any way unaffected by the bladder abscess; therefore, an obstetrics code should be sequenced first. An additional code was provided to identify the specific bladder condition as this information is not called out specifically in the obstetrics code.

---

2) Chapter 15 codes used only on the maternal record

Chapter 15 codes are to be used only on the maternal record, never on the record of the newborn.

3) Final character for trimester

The majority of codes in Chapter 15 have a final character indicating the trimester of pregnancy. The timeframes for the trimesters are indicated at the beginning of the chapter. If trimester is not a component of a code, it is because the condition always occurs in a specific trimester, or the concept of trimester of pregnancy is not applicable. Certain codes have characters for only certain trimesters because the condition does not occur in all trimesters, but it may occur in more than just one.

Assignment of the final character for trimester should be based on the provider's documentation of the trimester (or number of weeks) for the current admission/encounter. This applies to the assignment of trimester for pre-existing conditions as well as those that develop during or are due to the pregnancy. The provider's documentation of the number of weeks may be used to assign the appropriate code identifying the trimester.

Whenever delivery occurs during the current admission, and there is an "in childbirth" option for the obstetric complication being coded, the "in childbirth" code should be assigned.

Pregnant patient at 21 weeks' gestation admitted with excessive vomiting

O21.2   **Late vomiting of pregnancy**

Z3A.21   **21 weeks gestation of pregnancy**

Explanation: Category O21 classifies vomiting in pregnancy. Although code selection is based on whether the vomiting is before or after 20 completed weeks, these codes are not further classified by trimester. If vomiting only in the second trimester was documented, the provider should be queried for the specific week of gestation, as this will affect code selection.

---

4) Selection of trimester for inpatient admissions that encompass more than one trimester

In instances when a patient is admitted to a hospital for complications of pregnancy during one trimester and remains in the hospital into a subsequent trimester, the trimester character for the antepartum complication code should be assigned on the basis of the trimester when the complication developed, not the trimester of the discharge. If the condition developed prior to the current admission/encounter or represents a pre-existing condition, the trimester character for the trimester at the time of the admission/encounter should be assigned.

Patient admitted at 27 6/7 weeks' gestation for hemorrhaging from placenta previa; three days after admission at 28 1/7 weeks' gestation, she developed gestational hypertension

O44.12   **Placenta previa with hemorrhage, second trimester**

O13.3   **Gestational [pregnancy-induced] hypertension without significant proteinuria, third trimester**

Z3A.27   **27 weeks gestation of pregnancy**

Explanation: The patient presented with hemorrhaging from placenta previa while still in her 27th week, which falls within the second trimester. The gestational hypertension did not occur until three days after admission, putting the patient in her 28th week of pregnancy or what is considered to be the third trimester. The weeks of gestation captured by a code from category Z3A should represent only the gestational weeks upon admission.

---

5) Unspecified trimester

Each category that includes codes for trimester has a code for "unspecified trimester." The "unspecified trimester" code should rarely be used, such as when the documentation in the record is insufficient to determine the trimester and it is not possible to obtain clarification.

6) 7th character for fetus identification

Where applicable, a 7th character is to be assigned for certain categories (O31, O32, O33.3 - O33.6, O35, O36, O40, O41, O60.1, O60.2, O64, and O69) to identify the fetus for which the complication code applies.

Assign 7th character "0":

- For single gestations
- When the documentation in the record is insufficient to determine the fetus affected and it is not possible to obtain clarification.
- When it is not possible to clinically determine which fetus is affected.

Maternal patient with twin gestations is seen after ultrasound identifies fetus B to be in breech presentation

O32.1XX2   **Maternal care for breech presentation, fetus 2**

Explanation: The documentation indicates that although there are two fetuses, only one fetus is determined to be in breech presentation. Whether fetus 2 or fetus B is used, the coder can assign the seventh character of 2 to identify the second fetus as the one in breech.

---

b. Selection of OB principal or first-listed diagnosis

1) Routine outpatient prenatal visits

For routine outpatient prenatal visits when no complications are present, a code from category Z34, Encounter for supervision of normal pregnancy, should be used as the first-listed diagnosis. These codes should not be used in conjunction with chapter 15 codes.

2) Prenatal outpatient visits for high-risk patients

For routine prenatal outpatient visits for patients with high-risk pregnancies, a code from category O09, Supervision of high-risk pregnancy, should be used as the first-listed diagnosis. Secondary chapter 15 codes may be used in conjunction with these codes if appropriate.

3) Episodes when no delivery occurs

In episodes when no delivery occurs, the principal diagnosis should correspond to the principal complication of the pregnancy which necessitated the encounter. Should more than one complication exist, all of which are treated or monitored, any of the complications codes may be sequenced first.

4) When a delivery occurs

When a delivery occurs, the principal diagnosis should correspond to the main circumstances or complication of the delivery. In cases of cesarean delivery, the selection of the principal diagnosis should be the condition established after study that was responsible for the patient's admission. If the patient was admitted with a condition that resulted in the performance of a cesarean procedure, that condition should be selected as the principal diagnosis. If the reason for the admission/encounter was unrelated to the condition resulting in the cesarean delivery, the condition related to the reason for the admission/encounter should be selected as the principal diagnosis.

Maternal patient with diet-controlled gestational diabetes was admitted at 38 weeks' gestation in obstructed labor due to footling presentation; cesarean performed for the malpresentation

O64.8XX0	Obstructed labor due to other malposition and malpresentation, fetus not applicable or unspecified
O24.420	Gestational diabetes mellitus in childbirth, diet controlled
Z3A.38	38 weeks gestation of pregnancy
Z37.0	Single live birth

Explanation: The obstructed labor necessitated the cesarean procedure.

At 39 weeks' gestation, a maternal patient presents with hemorrhage with coagulation defect; the next day the patient goes into labor and eventually delivers via cesarean section due to arrested active phase of labor

O46.003	Antepartum hemorrhage with coagulation defect, unspecified, third trimester
O62.1	Secondary uterine inertia
Z3A.39	39 weeks gestation of pregnancy
Z37.0	Single live birth

Explanation: The patient was admitted because of the antepartum hemorrhage with coagulation defect. The arrested active phase, although the reason for the cesarean delivery, did not develop until later into the stay.

5) Outcome of delivery

A code from category Z37, Outcome of delivery, should be included on every maternal record when a delivery has occurred. These codes are not to be used on subsequent records or on the newborn record.

c. Pre-existing conditions versus conditions due to the pregnancy

Certain categories in Chapter 15 distinguish between conditions of the mother that existed prior to pregnancy (pre-existing) and those that are a direct result of pregnancy. When assigning codes from Chapter 15, it is important to assess if a condition was pre-existing prior to pregnancy or developed during or due to the pregnancy in order to assign the correct code.

Categories that do not distinguish between pre-existing and pregnancy-related conditions may be used for either. It is acceptable to use codes specifically for the puerperium with codes complicating pregnancy and childbirth if a condition arises postpartum during the delivery encounter.

d. Pre-existing hypertension in pregnancy

Category O10, Pre-existing hypertension complicating pregnancy, childbirth and the puerperium, includes codes for hypertensive heart and hypertensive chronic kidney disease. When assigning one of the O10 codes that includes hypertensive heart disease or hypertensive chronic kidney disease, it is necessary to add a secondary code from the appropriate hypertension category to specify the type of heart failure or chronic kidney disease.

See Section I.C.9. Hypertension.

e. Fetal conditions affecting the management of the mother

1) Codes from categories O35 and O36

Codes from categories O35, Maternal care for known or suspected fetal abnormality and damage, and O36, Maternal care for other fetal problems, are assigned only when the fetal condition is actually responsible for modifying the management of the mother, i.e., by requiring diagnostic studies, additional observation, special care, or termination of pregnancy. The fact that the fetal condition exists does not justify assigning a code from this series to the mother's record.

A patient is seen for spotting 15 weeks into her pregnancy; the doctors also suspect fetal hydrocephalus

O26.852	Spotting complicating pregnancy
Z3A.15	15 weeks gestation of pregnancy

Explanation: Whether the fetal hydrocephalus was suspected or confirmed, an additional code is not warranted for this condition as the documentation does not indicate that this fetal condition is in any way altering the management of the mother or complicating her pregnancy.

2) In utero surgery

In cases when surgery is performed on the fetus, a diagnosis code from category O35, Maternal care for known or suspected fetal abnormality and damage, should be assigned identifying the fetal condition. Assign the appropriate procedure code for the procedure performed.

No code from Chapter 16, the perinatal codes, should be used on the mother's record to identify fetal conditions. Surgery performed in utero on a fetus is still to be coded as an obstetric encounter.

f. HIV infection in pregnancy, childbirth and the puerperium

During pregnancy, childbirth or the puerperium, a patient admitted because of an HIV-related illness should receive a principal diagnosis from subcategory O98.7-, Human immunodeficiency [HIV] disease complicating pregnancy, childbirth and the puerperium, followed by the code(s) for the HIV-related illness(es).

Patients with asymptomatic HIV infection status admitted during pregnancy, childbirth, or the puerperium should receive codes of O98.7- and Z21, Asymptomatic human immunodeficiency virus [HIV] infection status.

A previously asymptomatic HIV patient who is 13 weeks pregnant is admitted with oral thrush

O98.711	Human immunodeficiency virus [HIV] disease complicating pregnancy, first trimester
B20	Human immunodeficiency virus [HIV] disease
B37.0	Candidal stomatitis
Z3A.13	13 weeks gestation of pregnancy

Explanation: Because oral thrush is an HIV-related condition, this patient is now considered to have HIV disease. An obstetrics code indicating that HIV is complicating the pregnancy is coded first, followed by B20 for HIV disease as well as a code for the oral thrush.

g. Diabetes mellitus in pregnancy

Diabetes mellitus is a significant complicating factor in pregnancy. Pregnant women who are diabetic should be assigned a code from category O24, Diabetes mellitus in pregnancy, childbirth, and the puerperium, first, followed by the appropriate diabetes code(s) (E08-E13) from Chapter 4.

h. Long term use of insulin

Code Z79.4, Long-term (current) use of insulin, should also be assigned if the diabetes mellitus is being treated with insulin.

i. Gestational (pregnancy induced) diabetes

Gestational (pregnancy induced) diabetes can occur during the second and third trimester of pregnancy in women who were not diabetic prior to pregnancy. Gestational diabetes can cause complications in the pregnancy similar to those of pre-existing diabetes mellitus. It also puts the woman at greater risk of developing diabetes after the pregnancy. Codes for gestational diabetes are in subcategory O24.4, Gestational diabetes mellitus. No other code from category O24, Diabetes mellitus in pregnancy, childbirth, and the puerperium, should be used with a code from O24.4.

The codes under subcategory O24.4 include diet controlled and insulin controlled. If a patient with gestational diabetes is treated with both diet and insulin, only the code for insulin-controlled is required.

Code Z79.4, Long-term (current) use of insulin, should not be assigned with codes from subcategory O24.4.

An abnormal glucose tolerance in pregnancy is assigned a code from subcategory O99.81, Abnormal glucose complicating pregnancy, childbirth, and the puerperium.

j. Sepsis and septic shock complicating abortion, pregnancy, childbirth and the puerperium

When assigning a chapter 15 code for sepsis complicating abortion, pregnancy, childbirth, and the puerperium, a code for the specific type of infection should be assigned as an additional diagnosis. If severe sepsis is present, a code from subcategory R65.2, Severe sepsis, and code(s) for associated organ dysfunction(s) should also be assigned as additional diagnoses.

Patient is seen several days after a miscarriage with sepsis; cultures return MSSA

O03.87	Sepsis following complete or unspecified spontaneous abortion
B95.61	Methicillin susceptible Staphylococcus aureus infection as the cause of diseases classified elsewhere

Explanation: The type of infection that caused this patient to become septic was methicillin susceptible *Staphylococcus aureus* (MSSA), which as a secondary code helps capture all aspects related to this patient's septic condition.

k. Puerperal sepsis

Code O85, Puerperal sepsis, should be assigned with a secondary code to identify the causal organism (e.g., for a bacterial infection, assign a code from category B95-B96, Bacterial infections in conditions classified elsewhere). A code from category A40, Streptococcal sepsis, or A41, Other sepsis, should not be used for puerperal sepsis. If applicable, use additional codes to identify severe sepsis (R65.2-) and any associated acute organ dysfunction.

l. Alcohol and tobacco use during pregnancy, childbirth and the puerperium

1) Alcohol use during pregnancy, childbirth and the puerperium

Codes under subcategory O99.31, Alcohol use complicating pregnancy, childbirth, and the puerperium, should be assigned for any pregnancy case when a mother uses alcohol during the pregnancy or postpartum. A secondary code from category F10, Alcohol related disorders, should also be assigned to identify manifestations of the alcohol use.

2) Tobacco use during pregnancy, childbirth and the puerperium

Codes under subcategory O99.33, Smoking (tobacco) complicating pregnancy, childbirth, and the puerperium, should be assigned for any pregnancy case when a mother uses any type of tobacco product during the pregnancy or postpartum. A secondary code from category F17, Nicotine dependence, should also be assigned to identify the type of nicotine dependence.

m. Poisoning, toxic effects, adverse effects and underdosing in a pregnant patient

A code from subcategory O9A.2, Injury, poisoning and certain other consequences of external causes complicating pregnancy, childbirth, and the puerperium, should be sequenced first, followed by the appropriate injury, poisoning, toxic effect, adverse effect or underdosing code, and then the additional code(s) that specifies the condition caused by the poisoning, toxic effect, adverse effect or underdosing.

See Section I.C.19. Adverse effects, poisoning, underdosing and toxic effects.

Patient admitted with accidental carbon monoxide poisoning from a gas heating implement; the patient is 18 weeks' pregnant

O9A.212	Injury, poisoning and certain other consequences of external causes complicating pregnancy, second trimester
T58.11XA	Toxic effect of carbon monoxide from utility gas, accidental (unintentional), initial encounter
Z3A.18	18 weeks gestation of pregnancy

Explanation: Although the carbon monoxide poisoning is the reason the patient was admitted, a code from the obstetrics chapter must be sequenced first. Chapter 15 codes have sequencing priority over codes from other chapters.

n. Normal delivery, code O80

1) Encounter for full term uncomplicated delivery

Code O80 should be assigned when a woman is admitted for a full-term normal delivery and delivers a single, healthy infant without any complications antepartum, during the delivery, or postpartum during the delivery episode. Code O80 is always a principal diagnosis. It is not to be used if any other code from chapter 15 is needed to describe a current complication of the antenatal, delivery, or perinatal period. Additional codes from other chapters may be used with code O80 if they are not related to or are in any way complicating the pregnancy.

2) Uncomplicated delivery with resolved antepartum complication

Code O80 may be used if the patient had a complication at some point during the pregnancy, but the complication is not present at the time of the admission for delivery.

Patient presents in labor at 39 weeks' gestation and delivers a healthy newborn; patient had abnormal glucose levels in her first trimester, which have since resolved

O80	Encounter for full-term uncomplicated delivery
Z37.0	Single live birth

Explanation: The abnormal glucose levels during the first trimester cannot be coded if they are not affecting the patient's current trimester. Without additional complications associated with the pregnancy, fetus, or mother, code O80 is appropriate.

3) Outcome of delivery for O80

Z37.0, Single live birth, is the only outcome of delivery code appropriate for use with O80.

o. The peripartum and postpartum periods

1) Peripartum and postpartum periods

The postpartum period begins immediately after delivery and continues for six weeks following delivery. The peripartum period is defined as the last month of pregnancy to five months postpartum.

2) Peripartum and postpartum complication

A postpartum complication is any complication occurring within the six-week period.

3) Pregnancy-related complications after 6 week period

Chapter 15 codes may also be used to describe pregnancy-related complications after the peripartum or postpartum period if the provider documents that a condition is pregnancy related.

Patient admitted for varicose veins. She had a baby boy three months ago; the varicose veins started to appear one month ago. The doctor attributes the patient's pregnancy as the cause of the varicose veins, which continue to be painful and bother the patient. She is seeking surgical relief.

O87.4	Varicose veins of the lower extremity in the puerperium

Explanation: Although the varicose veins occurred several months after the delivery of the newborn, the doctor attributed the varicose veins to pregnancy and therefore a code from chapter 15 is appropriate.

4) Admission for routine postpartum care following delivery outside hospital

When the mother delivers outside the hospital prior to admission and is admitted for routine postpartum care and no complications are noted, code Z39.0, Encounter for care and examination of mother immediately after delivery, should be assigned as the principal diagnosis.

5) Pregnancy associated cardiomyopathy

Pregnancy associated cardiomyopathy, code O90.3, is unique in that it may be diagnosed in the third trimester of pregnancy but may continue to progress months after delivery. For this reason, it is referred to as peripartum cardiomyopathy. Code O90.3 is only for use when the cardiomyopathy develops as a result of pregnancy in a woman who did not have pre-existing heart disease.

p. Code O94, Sequelae of complication of pregnancy, childbirth, and the puerperium

1) Code O94

Code O94, Sequelae of complication of pregnancy, childbirth, and the puerperium, is for use in those cases when an initial complication of a pregnancy develops a sequelae requiring care or treatment at a future date.

2) After the initial postpartum period

This code may be used at any time after the initial postpartum period.

3) Sequencing of code O94

This code, like all sequela codes, is to be sequenced following the code describing the sequelae of the complication.

q. Termination of pregnancy and spontaneous abortions

1) Abortion with liveborn fetus

When an attempted termination of pregnancy results in a liveborn fetus, assign code Z33.2, Encounter for elective termination of pregnancy and a code from category Z37, Outcome of Delivery.

2) Retained products of conception following an abortion

Subsequent encounters for retained products of conception following a spontaneous abortion or elective termination of pregnancy are assigned the appropriate code from category O03, Spontaneous abortion, or codes O07.4, Failed attempted termination of pregnancy without complication and Z33.2, Encounter for elective termination of pregnancy. This advice is appropriate even when the patient was discharged previously with a discharge diagnosis of complete abortion.

> Patient was seen two days ago for complete spontaneous abortion but returns today for urinary tract infection (UTI) with ultrasound showing retained products of conception
>
> **O03.38**   **Urinary tract infection following incomplete spontaneous abortion**
>
> *Explanation:* Although the diagnosis from the patient's previous stay indicated that the patient had a complete abortion, it is now determined that there were actually retained products of conception (POC). An abortion with retained POC is considered incomplete and in this case resulted in the patient developing a UTI.

3) Complications leading to abortion

Codes from Chapter 15 may be used as additional codes to identify any documented complications of the pregnancy in conjunction with codes in categories in O07 and O08.

r. Abuse in a pregnant patient

For suspected or confirmed cases of abuse of a pregnant patient, a code(s) from subcategories O9A.3, Physical abuse complicating pregnancy, childbirth, and the puerperium, O9A.4, Sexual abuse complicating pregnancy, childbirth, and the puerperium, and O9A.5, Psychological abuse complicating pregnancy, childbirth, and the puerperium, should be sequenced first, followed by the appropriate codes (if applicable) to identify any associated current injury due to physical abuse, sexual abuse, and the perpetrator of abuse.

See Section I.C.19. Adult and child abuse, neglect and other maltreatment.

Chapter 15. Pregnancy, Childbirth and the Puerperium (O00-O9A)

NOTE CODES FROM THIS CHAPTER ARE FOR USE ONLY ON MATERNAL RECORDS, NEVER ON NEWBORN RECORDS.

Codes from this chapter are for use for conditions related to or aggravated by the pregnancy, childbirth, or by the puerperium (maternal causes or obstetric causes).

NOTE Trimesters are counted from the first day of the last menstrual period. They are defined as follows:

1st trimester- less than 14 weeks Ø days
2nd trimester- 14 weeks Ø days to less than 28 weeks Ø days
3rd trimester- 28 weeks Ø days until delivery

Use additional code from category Z3A, Weeks of gestation, to identify the specific week of the pregnancy

EXCLUDES 1 *supervision of normal pregnancy (Z34.-)*
EXCLUDES 2 *mental and behavioral disorders associated with the puerperium (F53)*
dobstetrical tetanus (A34)
postpartum necrosis of pituitary gland (E23.Ø)
puerperal osteomalacia (M83.Ø)

AHA: 2014, 3Q, 17

This chapter contains the following blocks:

O00-O08   Pregnancy with abortive outcome
O09   Supervision of high risk pregnancy
O10-O16   Edema, proteinuria and hypertensive disorders in pregnancy, childbirth and the puerperium
O20-O29   Other maternal disorders predominantly related to pregnancy
O30-O48   Maternal care related to the fetus and amniotic cavity and possible delivery problems
O60-O77   Complications of labor and delivery
O80, O82   Encounter for delivery
O85-O92   Complications predominantly related to the puerperium
O94-O9A   Other obstetric conditions, not elsewhere classified

Pregnancy with abortive outcome (O00-O08)

EXCLUDES 1 *continuing pregnancy in multiple gestation after abortion of one fetus or more (O31.1-, O31.3-)*

✓4ᵗʰ O00 Ectopic pregnancy

INCLUDES ruptured ectopic pregnancy

Use additional code from category O08 to identify any associated complication

AHA: 2014, 3Q, 17

CC Excl: For CC codes in category O00, unless otherwise noted: O00.0-O00.9

O00.0 Abdominal pregnancy   CC M ♀
   EXCLUDES 1 *maternal care for viable fetus in abdominal pregnancy (O36.7-)*

O00.1 Tubal pregnancy   CC M ♀
   Fallopian pregnancy
   Rupture of (fallopian) tube due to pregnancy
   Tubal abortion

O00.2 Ovarian pregnancy   CC M ♀

O00.8 Other ectopic pregnancy   CC M ♀
   Cervical pregnancy   Intraligamentous pregnancy
   Cornual pregnancy   Mural pregnancy

O00.9 Ectopic pregnancy, unspecified   CC M ♀

✓4ᵗʰ O01 Hydatidiform mole

Use additional code from category O08 to identify any associated complication

   EXCLUDES 1 *chorioadenoma (destruens) (D39.2)*
     malignant hydatidiform mole (D39.2)

AHA: 2014, 3Q, 17

O01.0 Classical hydatidiform mole   M ♀
   Complete hydatidiform mole

O01.1 Incomplete and partial hydatidiform mole   M ♀

O01.9 Hydatidiform mole, unspecified   M ♀
   Trophoblastic disease NOS
   Vesicular mole NOS

✓4ᵗʰ O02 Other abnormal products of conception

Use additional code from category O08 to identify any associated complication

   EXCLUDES 1 *papyraceous fetus (O31.0-)*

AHA: 2014, 3Q, 17

O02.0 Blighted ovum and nonhydatidiform mole   M ♀
   Carneous mole   Molar pregnancy NEC
   Fleshy mole   Pathological ovum
   Intrauterine mole NOS

O02.1 Missed abortion   M ♀
   Early fetal death, before completion of 20 weeks of gestation, with retention of dead fetus
   EXCLUDES 1 *failed induced abortion (O07.-)*
     fetal death (intrauterine) (late) (O36.4)
     missed abortion with blighted ovum (O02.0)
     missed abortion with hydatidiform mole (O01.-)
     missed abortion with nonhydatidiform (O02.0)
     missed abortion with other abnormal products of conception (O02.8-)
     missed delivery (O36.4)
     stillbirth (P95)

✓5ᵗʰ O02.8 Other specified abnormal products of conception
   EXCLUDES 1 *abnormal products of conception with blighted ovum (O02.0)*
     abnormal products of conception with hydatidiform mole (O01.-)
     abnormal products of conception with nonhydatidiform mole (O02.0)

   O02.81 Inappropriate change in quantitative human chorionic gonadotropin (hCG) in early pregnancy   M ♀
     Biochemical pregnancy
     Chemical pregnancy
     Inappropriate level of quantitative human chorionic gonadotropin (hCG) for gestational age in early pregnancy

   O02.89 Other abnormal products of conception   M ♀

O02.9 Abnormal product of conception, unspecified   M ♀

✓4ᵗʰ O03 Spontaneous abortion
   NOTE Incomplete abortion includes retained products of conception following spontaneous abortion
   INCLUDES miscarriage

> **CC Excl: For CC/MCC codes in category O03, unless otherwise noted:** O03.0-O07.4, O20.0-O20.9, O25.10-O25.3, O26.10-O26.13, O26.30-O26.43, O26.63-O26.819, O26.841-O26.86, O26.891-O26.93, O29.011-O29.93, O35.7XX0-O35.7XX9, O44.00-O44.13, O45.8X1-O45.93, O75.4, O75.81, O75.89-O75.9, O80, O90.89, O99.111-O99.285, O99.330-O99.335, O99.350-O99.355, O99.511-O99.73, O99.820-O99.825, O99.840-O9A.53, Z33.2

O03.0 Genital tract and pelvic infection following incomplete spontaneous abortion   CC M ♀
   Endometritis following incomplete spontaneous abortion
   Oophoritis following incomplete spontaneous abortion
   Parametritis following incomplete spontaneous abortion
   Pelvic peritonitis following incomplete spontaneous abortion
   Salpingitis following incomplete spontaneous abortion
   Salpingo-oophoritis following incomplete spontaneous abortion
   EXCLUDES 1 *sepsis following incomplete spontaneous abortion (O03.37)*
     urinary tract infection following incomplete spontaneous abortion (O03.38)

O03.1 Delayed or excessive hemorrhage following incomplete spontaneous abortion   M ♀
   Afibrinogenemia following incomplete spontaneous abortion
   Defibrination syndrome following incomplete spontaneous abortion
   Hemolysis following incomplete spontaneous abortion
   Intravascular coagulation following incomplete spontaneous abortion

O03.2 Embolism following incomplete spontaneous abortion   MCC M ♀
   Air embolism following incomplete spontaneous abortion
   Amniotic fluid embolism following incomplete spontaneous abortion
   Blood-clot embolism following incomplete spontaneous abortion
   Embolism NOS following incomplete spontaneous abortion
   Fat embolism following incomplete spontaneous abortion
   Pulmonary embolism following incomplete spontaneous abortion
   Pyemic embolism following incomplete spontaneous abortion
   Septic or septicopyemic embolism following incomplete spontaneous abortion
   Soap embolism following incomplete spontaneous abortion

✓5ᵗʰ O03.3 Other and unspecified complications following incomplete spontaneous abortion

   O03.30 Unspecified complication following incomplete spontaneous abortion   CC M ♀

✓ Additional Character Required   ✓x7ᵗʰ Placeholder Alert   Unacceptable PDx   Manifestation   Hospital Acquired Condition   **EXCLUDES 1** Not Coded Here   **EXCLUDES 2** Not Included Here

ICD-10-CM 2016   811

O03.31   Shock following incomplete spontaneous abortion   MCC M♀
Circulatory collapse following incomplete spontaneous abortion
Shock (postprocedural) following incomplete spontaneous abortion
EXCLUDES 1 shock due to infection following incomplete spontaneous abortion (O03.37)

O03.32   Renal failure following incomplete spontaneous abortion   MCC M♀
Kidney failure (acute) following incomplete spontaneous abortion
Oliguria following incomplete spontaneous abortion
Renal shutdown following incomplete spontaneous abortion
Renal tubular necrosis following incomplete spontaneous abortion
Uremia following incomplete spontaneous abortion

O03.33   Metabolic disorder following incomplete spontaneous abortion   CC M♀

O03.34   Damage to pelvic organs following incomplete spontaneous abortion   CC M♀
Laceration, perforation, tear or chemical damage of bladder following incomplete spontaneous abortion
Laceration, perforation, tear or chemical damage of bowel following incomplete spontaneous abortion
Laceration, perforation, tear or chemical damage of broad ligament following incomplete spontaneous abortion
Laceration, perforation, tear or chemical damage of cervix following incomplete spontaneous abortion
Laceration, perforation, tear or chemical damage of periurethral tissue following incomplete spontaneous abortion
Laceration, perforation, tear or chemical damage of uterus following incomplete spontaneous abortion
Laceration, perforation, tear or chemical damage of vagina following incomplete spontaneous abortion

O03.35   Other venous complications following incomplete spontaneous abortion   CC M♀

O03.36   Cardiac arrest following incomplete spontaneous abortion   CC M♀

O03.37   Sepsis following incomplete spontaneous abortion   CC M♀
Use additional code to identify infectious agent (B95-B97)
Use additional code to identify severe sepsis, if applicable (R65.2-)
EXCLUDES 1 septic or septicopyemic embolism following incomplete spontaneous abortion (O03.2)

O03.38   Urinary tract infection following incomplete spontaneous abortion   CC M♀
Cystitis following incomplete spontaneous abortion

O03.39   Incomplete spontaneous abortion with other complications   CC M♀

O03.4   Incomplete spontaneous abortion without complication   M♀

O03.5   Genital tract and pelvic infection following complete or unspecified spontaneous abortion   CC M♀
Endometritis following complete or unspecified spontaneous abortion
Oophoritis following complete or unspecified spontaneous abortion
Parametritis following complete or unspecified spontaneous abortion
Pelvic peritonitis following complete or unspecified spontaneous abortion
Salpingitis following complete or unspecified spontaneous abortion
Salpingo-oophoritis following complete or unspecified spontaneous abortion
EXCLUDES 1 sepsis following complete or unspecified spontaneous abortion (O03.87)
urinary tract infection following complete or unspecified spontaneous abortion (O03.88)

O03.6   Delayed or excessive hemorrhage following complete or unspecified spontaneous abortion   M♀
Afibrinogenemia following complete or unspecified spontaneous abortion
Defibrination syndrome following complete or unspecified spontaneous abortion
Hemolysis following complete or unspecified spontaneous abortion
Intravascular coagulation following complete or unspecified spontaneous abortion

O03.7   Embolism following complete or unspecified spontaneous abortion   CC M♀
Air embolism following complete or unspecified spontaneous abortion
Amniotic fluid embolism following complete or unspecified spontaneous abortion
Blood-clot embolism following complete or unspecified spontaneous abortion
Embolism NOS following complete or unspecified spontaneous abortion
Fat embolism following complete or unspecified spontaneous abortion
Pulmonary embolism following complete or unspecified spontaneous abortion
Pyemic embolism following complete or unspecified spontaneous abortion
Septic or septicopyemic embolism following complete or unspecified spontaneous abortion
Soap embolism following complete or unspecified spontaneous abortion

√5ᵗʰ **O03.8   Other and unspecified complications following complete or unspecified spontaneous abortion**

O03.80   Unspecified complication following complete or unspecified spontaneous abortion   CC M♀

O03.81   Shock following complete or unspecified spontaneous abortion   MCC M♀
Circulatory collapse following complete or unspecified spontaneous abortion
Shock (postprocedural) following complete or unspecified spontaneous abortion
EXCLUDES 1 shock due to infection following complete or unspecified spontaneous abortion (O03.87)

O03.82   Renal failure following complete or unspecified spontaneous abortion   MCC M♀
Kidney failure (acute) following complete or unspecified spontaneous abortion
Oliguria following complete or unspecified spontaneous abortion
Renal shutdown following complete or unspecified spontaneous abortion
Renal tubular necrosis following complete or unspecified spontaneous abortion
Uremia following complete or unspecified spontaneous abortion

O03.83   Metabolic disorder following complete or unspecified spontaneous abortion   CC M♀

O03.84   Damage to pelvic organs following complete or unspecified spontaneous abortion   CC M♀
Laceration, perforation, tear or chemical damage of bladder following complete or unspecified spontaneous abortion
Laceration, perforation, tear or chemical damage of bowel following complete or unspecified spontaneous abortion
Laceration, perforation, tear or chemical damage of broad ligament following complete or unspecified spontaneous abortion
Laceration, perforation, tear or chemical damage of cervix following complete or unspecified spontaneous abortion
Laceration, perforation, tear or chemical damage of periurethral tissue following complete or unspecified spontaneous abortion
Laceration, perforation, tear or chemical damage of uterus following complete or unspecified spontaneous abortion
Laceration, perforation, tear or chemical damage of vagina following complete or unspecified spontaneous abortion

O03.85   Other venous complications following complete or unspecified spontaneous abortion   CC M♀

O03.86   Cardiac arrest following complete or unspecified spontaneous abortion   CC M♀

O03.87 **Sepsis following complete or unspecified** `CC` `M` `♀`
spontaneous abortion
Use additional code to identify infectious agent (B95-B97)
Use additional code to identify severe sepsis, if applicable (R65.2-)
EXCLUDES 1 *septic or septicopyemic embolism following complete or unspecified spontaneous abortion (O03.7)*

O03.88 **Urinary tract infection following complete or** `CC` `M` `♀`
unspecified spontaneous abortion
Cystitis following complete or unspecified spontaneous abortion

O03.89 **Complete or unspecified spontaneous** `CC` `M` `♀`
abortion with other complications

O03.9 **Complete or unspecified spontaneous abortion without** `M` `♀`
complication
Miscarriage NOS
Spontaneous abortion NOS

`✓4ᵗʰ` **O04** **Complications following (induced) termination of pregnancy**
INCLUDES complications following (induced) termination of pregnancy
EXCLUDES 1 encounter for elective termination of pregnancy, uncomplicated (Z33.2)
failed attempted termination of pregnancy (O07.-)

CC Excl: For CC/MCC codes in category O04, unless otherwise noted: See code: O03

O04.5 **Genital tract and pelvic infection following (induced)** `CC` `M` `♀`
termination of pregnancy
Endometritis following (induced) termination of pregnancy
Oophoritis following (induced) termination of pregnancy
Parametritis following (induced) termination of pregnancy
Pelvic peritonitis following (induced) termination of pregnancy
Salpingitis following (induced) termination of pregnancy
Salpingo-oophoritis following (induced) termination of pregnancy
EXCLUDES 1 *sepsis following (induced) termination of pregnancy (O04.87)*
urinary tract infection following (induced) termination of pregnancy (O04.88)

O04.6 **Delayed or excessive hemorrhage following (induced)** `M` `♀`
termination of pregnancy
Afibrinogenemia following (induced) termination of pregnancy
Defibrination syndrome following (induced) termination of pregnancy
Hemolysis following (induced) termination of pregnancy
Intravascular coagulation following (induced) termination of pregnancy

O04.7 **Embolism following (induced) termination of** `MCC` `M` `♀`
pregnancy
Air embolism following (induced) termination of pregnancy
Amniotic fluid embolism following (induced) termination of pregnancy
Blood-clot embolism following (induced) termination of pregnancy
Embolism NOS following (induced) termination of pregnancy
Fat embolism following (induced) termination of pregnancy
Pulmonary embolism following (induced) termination of pregnancy
Pyemic embolism following (induced) termination of pregnancy
Septic or septicopyemic embolism following (induced) termination of pregnancy
Soap embolism following (induced) termination of pregnancy

`✓5ᵗʰ` **O04.8** **(Induced) termination of pregnancy with other and**
unspecified complications

O04.80 **(Induced) termination of pregnancy with** `CC` `M` `♀`
unspecified complications

O04.81 **Shock following (induced) termination of** `MCC` `M` `♀`
pregnancy
Circulatory collapse following (induced) termination of pregnancy
Shock (postprocedural) following (induced) termination of pregnancy
EXCLUDES 1 *shock due to infection following (induced) termination of pregnancy (O04.87)*

O04.82 **Renal failure following (induced)** `MCC` `M` `♀`
termination of pregnancy
Kidney failure (acute) following (induced) termination of pregnancy
Oliguria following (induced) termination of pregnancy
Renal shutdown following (induced) termination of pregnancy
Renal tubular necrosis following (induced) termination of pregnancy
Uremia following (induced) termination of pregnancy

O04.83 **Metabolic disorder following (induced)** `CC` `M` `♀`
termination of pregnancy

O04.84 **Damage to pelvic organs following (induced)** `CC` `M` `♀`
termination of pregnancy
Laceration, perforation, tear or chemical damage of bladder following (induced) termination of pregnancy
Laceration, perforation, tear or chemical damage of bowel following (induced) termination of pregnancy
Laceration, perforation, tear or chemical damage of broad ligament following (induced) termination of pregnancy
Laceration, perforation, tear or chemical damage of cervix following (induced) termination of pregnancy
Laceration, perforation, tear or chemical damage of periurethral tissue following (induced) termination of pregnancy
Laceration, perforation, tear or chemical damage of uterus following (induced) termination of pregnancy
Laceration, perforation, tear or chemical damage of vagina following (induced) termination of pregnancy

O04.85 **Other venous complications following** `CC` `M` `♀`
(induced) termination of pregnancy

O04.86 **Cardiac arrest following (induced)** `CC` `M` `♀`
termination of pregnancy

O04.87 **Sepsis following (induced) termination of** `CC` `M` `♀`
pregnancy
Use additional code to identify infectious agent (B95-B97)
Use additional code to identify severe sepsis, if applicable (R65.2-)
EXCLUDES 1 *septic or septicopyemic embolism following (induced) termination of pregnancy (O04.7)*
CC Excl: O03.0–O07.4, O20.0–O20.9, O25.10–O25.3, O26.10–O26.13, O26.30–O26.43, O26.63–O26.819, O26.841–O26.86, O26.891–O26.93, O29.011–O29.93, O35.7X–O35.7X, O44.00–O44.13, O45.8X1–O45.93, O75.4, O75.81, O75.89–O75.9, O80, O90.89, O99.111–O99.285, O99.330–O99.335, O99.350–O99.355, O99.511–O99.73, O99.820–O99.825, O99.840–O9A.53, Z33.2

O04.88 **Urinary tract infection following (induced)** `CC` `M` `♀`
termination of pregnancy
Cystitis following (induced) termination of pregnancy
CC Excl: O03.0–O07.4, O20.0–O20.9, O25.10–O25.3, O26.10–O26.13, O26.30–O26.43, O26.63–O26.819, O26.841–O26.86, O26.891–O26.93, O29.011–O29.93, O35.7X–O35.7X, O44.00–O44.13, O45.8X1–O45.93, O75.4, O75.81, O75.89–O75.9, O80, O90.89, O99.111–O99.285, O99.330–O99.335, O99.350–O99.355, O99.511–O99.73, O99.820–O99.825, O99.840–O9A.53, Z33.2

O04.89 **(Induced) termination of pregnancy with** `CC` `M` `♀`
other complications
CC Excl: See code O04.88

Chapter 15. Pregnancy, Childbirth, and the Puerperium

✓4ᵗʰ **O07   Failed attempted termination of pregnancy**

> INCLUDES   failure of attempted induction of termination of pregnancy
> incomplete elective abortion
> EXCLUDES 1   *incomplete spontaneous abortion (O03.0-)*

O07.0   Genital tract and pelvic infection following failed CC M ♀
attempted termination of pregnancy

Endometritis following failed attempted termination of
pregnancy
Oophoritis following failed attempted termination of pregnancy
Parametritis following failed attempted termination of
pregnancy
Pelvic peritonitis following failed attempted termination of
pregnancy
Salpingitis following failed attempted termination of pregnancy
Salpingo-oophoritis following failed attempted termination of
pregnancy

> EXCLUDES 1   *sepsis following failed attempted termination of*
> *pregnancy (O07.37)*
> *urinary tract infection following failed attempted*
> *termination of pregnancy (O07.38)*

CC Excl: O03.0-O04.89, O07.1, O07.30, O07.35-O07.36, O07.38-
O07.4, O20.0-O20.9, O25.10-O25.3, O26.10-O26.13, O26.30-
O26.43, O26.63-O26.819, O26.841-O26.86, O26.891-O26.93,
O29.011-O29.93, O35.7XX0-O35.7XX9, O44.00-O44.13, O45.8X1-
O45.93, O75.4, O75.81, O75.89-O75.9, O80, O90.89, O99.111-
O99.285, O99.330-O99.335, O99.350-O99.355, O99.511-O99.73,
O99.820-O99.825, O99.840-O9A.53, Z33.2

O07.1   Delayed or excessive hemorrhage following failed CC M ♀
attempted termination of pregnancy

Afibrinogenemia following failed attempted termination of
pregnancy
Defibrination syndrome following failed attempted termination
of pregnancy
Hemolysis following failed attempted termination of pregnancy
Intravascular coagulation following failed attempted
termination of pregnancy

CC Excl: O03.0-O04.89, O07.1, O07.30, O07.35-O07.36, O07.38-
O07.4, O20.0-O20.9, O25.10-O25.3, O26.10-O26.13, O26.30-
O26.43, O26.63-O26.819, O26.841-O26.86, O26.891-O26.93,
O29.011-O29.93, O35.7XX0-O35.7XX9, O44.00-O44.13, O45.8X1-
O45.93, O75.4, O75.81, O75.89-O75.9, O80, O90.89, O99.111-
O99.285, O99.330-O99.335, O99.350-O99.355, O99.511-O99.73,
O99.820-O99.825, O99.840-O9A.53, Z33.2

O07.2   Embolism following failed attempted termination of MCC M ♀
pregnancy

Air embolism following failed attempted termination of
pregnancy
Amniotic fluid embolism following failed attempted termination
of pregnancy
Blood-clot embolism following failed attempted termination of
pregnancy
Embolism NOS following failed attempted termination of
pregnancy
Fat embolism following failed attempted termination of
pregnancy
Pulmonary embolism following failed attempted termination of
pregnancy
Pyemic embolism following failed attempted termination of
pregnancy
Septic or septicopyemic embolism following failed attempted
termination of pregnancy
Soap embolism following failed attempted termination of
pregnancy

CC Excl: O03.0-O04.89, O07.2-O07.30, O07.35-O07.36, O07.38-
O07.4, O20.0-O20.9, O25.10-O25.3, O26.10-O26.13, O26.30-
O26.43, O26.63-O26.819, O26.841-O26.86, O26.891-O26.93,
O29.011-O29.93, O35.7XX0-O35.7XX9, O44.00-O44.13, O45.8X1-
O45.93, O75.4, O75.81, O75.89-O75.9, O80, O90.89, O99.111-
O99.285, O99.330-O99.335, O99.350-O99.355, O99.511-O99.73,
O99.820-O99.825, O99.840-O9A.53, Z33.2

✓5ᵗʰ **O07.3   Failed attempted termination of pregnancy with other and**
unspecified complications

O07.30   Failed attempted termination of pregnancy CC M ♀
with unspecified complications

CC Excl: O03.0-O07.4, O20.0-O20.9, O25.10-O25.3,
O26.10-O26.13, O26.30-O26.43, O26.63-O26.819,
O26.841-O26.86, O26.891-O26.93, O29.011-O29.93,
O35.7X-O35.7X, O44.00-O44.13, O45.8X1-O45.93, O75.4,
O75.81, O75.89-O75.9, O80, O90.89, O99.111-O99.285,
O99.330-O99.335, O99.350-O99.355, O99.511-O99.73,
O99.820-O99.825, O99.840-O9A.53, Z33.2

O07.31   Shock following failed attempted MCC M ♀
termination of pregnancy

Circulatory collapse following failed attempted
termination of pregnancy
Shock (postprocedural) following failed attempted
termination of pregnancy

> EXCLUDES 1   *shock due to infection following failed*
> *attempted termination of pregnancy*
> *(O07.37)*

CC Excl: O03.0-O04.89, O07.30-O07.31, O07.33, O07.35-
O07.36, O07.38-O07.4, O20.0-O20.9, O25.10-O25.3,
O26.10-O26.13, O26.30-O26.43, O26.63-O26.819,
O26.841-O26.86, O26.891-O26.93, O29.011-O29.93,
O35.7XX0-O35.7XX9, O44.00-O44.13, O45.8X1-O45.93,
O75.4, O75.81, O75.89-O75.9, O80, O90.89, O99.111-
O99.285, O99.330-O99.335, O99.350-O99.355, O99.511-
O99.73, O99.820-O99.825, O99.840-O9A.53, Z33.2

O07.32   Renal failure following failed attempted MCC M ♀
termination of pregnancy

Kidney failure (acute) following failed attempted
termination of pregnancy
Oliguria following failed attempted termination of
pregnancy
Renal shutdown following failed attempted
termination of pregnancy
Renal tubular necrosis following failed attempted
termination of pregnancy
Uremia following failed attempted termination of
pregnancy

CC Excl: O03.0-O04.89, O07.30, O07.32, O07.35-O07.36,
O07.38-O07.4, O20.0-O20.9, O25.10-O25.3, O26.10-
O26.13, O26.30-O26.43, O26.63-O26.819, O26.841-
O26.86, O26.891-O26.93, O29.011-O29.93, O35.7XX0-
O35.7XX9, O44.00-O44.13, O45.8X1-O45.93, O75.4,
O75.81, O75.89-O75.9, O80, O90.89, O99.111-O99.285,
O99.330-O99.335, O99.350-O99.355, O99.511-O99.73,
O99.820-O99.825, O99.840-O9A.53, Z33.2

O07.33   Metabolic disorder following failed CC M ♀
attempted termination of pregnancy
CC Excl: See code: O07.30

O07.34   Damage to pelvic organs following failed CC M ♀
attempted termination of pregnancy

Laceration, perforation, tear or chemical damage of
bladder following failed attempted termination
of pregnancy
Laceration, perforation, tear or chemical damage of
bowel following failed attempted termination of
pregnancy
Laceration, perforation, tear or chemical damage of
broad ligament following failed attempted
termination of pregnancy
Laceration, perforation, tear or chemical damage of
cervix following failed attempted termination of
pregnancy
Laceration, perforation, tear or chemical damage of
periurethral tissue following failed attempted
termination of pregnancy
Laceration, perforation, tear or chemical damage of
uterus following failed attempted termination of
pregnancy
Laceration, perforation, tear or chemical damage of
vagina following failed attempted termination of
pregnancy

CC Excl: O03.0-O04.89, O07.30, O07.34-O07.36, O07.38-
O07.4, O20.0-O20.9, O25.10-O25.3, O26.10-O26.13,
O26.30-O26.43, O26.63-O26.819, O26.841-O26.86,
O26.891-O26.93, O29.011-O29.93, O35.7XX0-O35.7XX9,
O44.00-O44.13, O45.8X1-O45.93, O75.4, O75.81, O75.89-
O75.9, O80, O90.89, O99.111-O99.285, O99.330-
O99.335, O99.350-O99.355, O99.511-O99.73, O99.820-
O99.825, O99.840-O9A.53, Z33.2

O07.35   Other venous complications following failed CC M ♀
attempted termination of pregnancy
CC Excl: See code: O07.30

O07.36   Cardiac arrest following failed attempted CC M ♀
termination of pregnancy
CC Excl: See code: O07.30

Ⓝ Newborn: 0   Ⓟ Pediatric: 0-17   Ⓜ Maternity: 12-55   Ⓐ Adult: 15-124   MCC Major CC Condition   PDxMCC PDx acts as own MCC   CC CC Condition   PDxCC PDx acts as own CC

814   ICD-10-CM 2016

O07.37   **Sepsis following failed attempted**   `CC` `M`♀
termination of pregnancy
Use additional code to identify infectious agent (B95-B97)
Use additional code to identify severe sepsis, if applicable (R65.2-)
EXCLUDES 1   *septic or septicopyemic embolism following failed attempted termination of pregnancy (O07.2)*
CC Excl: O03.0-O07.0, O07.30, O07.35-O07.4, O20.0-O20.9, O25.10-O25.3, O26.10-O26.13, O26.30-O26.43, O26.63-O26.819, O26.841-O26.86, O26.891-O26.93, O29.011-O29.93, O35.7X-O35.7X, O44.00-O44.13, O45.8X1-O45.93, O75.4, O75.81, O75.89-O75.9, O80, O90.89, O99.111-O99.285, O99.330-O99.335, O99.350-O99.355, O99.511-O99.73, O99.820-O99.825, O99.840-O9A.53, Z33.2

O07.38   **Urinary tract infection following failed**   `CC` `M`♀
attempted termination of pregnancy
Cystitis following failed attempted termination of pregnancy
CC Excl: See code: O07.30

O07.39   **Failed attempted termination of pregnancy**   `CC` `M`♀
with other complications
CC Excl: See code: O07.30

O07.4   **Failed attempted termination of pregnancy** without   `M`♀
complication

✅4ᵗʰ **O08**   **Complications following ectopic and molar pregnancy**
This category is for use with categories O00-O02 to identify any associated complications

> **CC Excl: For CC/MCC codes in category O08, unless otherwise noted:** O08.2-O08.81, O08.83-O08.9, O20.0-O20.9, O25.10-O25.3, O26.10-O26.13, O26.30-O26.43, O26.63-O26.819, O26.841-O26.86, O26.891-O26.93, O29.011-O29.93, O35.7XX0-O35.7XX9, O44.00-O44.13, O45.8X1-O45.93, O75.4, O75.81, O75.89-O75.9, O80, O90.89, O99.111-O99.285, O99.330-O99.335, O99.350-O99.355, O99.511-O99.73, O99.820-O99.825, O99.840-O9A.53

O08.0   **Genital tract and pelvic infection following ectopic**   `CC` `M`♀
and molar pregnancy
Endometritis following ectopic and molar pregnancy
Oophoritis following ectopic and molar pregnancy
Parametritis following ectopic and molar pregnancy
Pelvic peritonitis following ectopic and molar pregnancy
Salpingitis following ectopic and molar pregnancy
Salpingo-oophoritis following ectopic and molar pregnancy
EXCLUDES 1   *sepsis following ectopic and molar pregnancy (O08.82)*
urinary tract infection (O08.83)
CC Excl: A34, O08.0, O08.2-O08.9, O20.0-O20.9, O25.10-O25.3, O26.10-O26.13, O26.30-O26.43, O26.63-O26.819, O26.841-O26.86, O26.891-O26.93, O29.011-O29.93, O35.7XX0-O35.7XX9, O44.00-O44.13, O45.8X1-O45.93, O75.4, O75.81, O75.89-O75.9, O80, O90.89, O99.111-O99.285, O99.330-O99.335, O99.350-O99.355, O99.511-O99.73, O99.820-O99.825, O99.840-O9A.53

O08.1   **Delayed or excessive hemorrhage following ectopic**   `CC` `M`♀
and molar pregnancy
Afibrinogenemia following ectopic and molar pregnancy
Defibrination syndrome following ectopic and molar pregnancy
Hemolysis following ectopic and molar pregnancy
Intravascular coagulation following ectopic and molar pregnancy
EXCLUDES 1   *delayed or excessive hemorrhage due to incomplete abortion (O03.1)*
CC Excl: O08.1-O08.81, O08.83-O08.9, O20.0-O20.9, O25.10-O25.3, O26.10-O26.13, O26.30-O26.43, O26.63-O26.819, O26.841-O26.86, O26.891-O26.93, O29.011-O29.93, O35.7XX0-O35.7XX9, O44.00-O44.13, O45.8X1-O45.93, O75.4, O75.81, O75.89-O75.9, O80, O90.89, O99.111-O99.285, O99.330-O99.335, O99.350-O99.355, O99.511-O99.73, O99.820-O99.825, O99.840-O9A.53

O08.2   **Embolism following ectopic and molar pregnancy**   `MCC` `M`♀
Air embolism following ectopic and molar pregnancy
Amniotic fluid embolism following ectopic and molar pregnancy
Blood-clot embolism following ectopic and molar pregnancy
Embolism NOS following ectopic and molar pregnancy
Fat embolism following ectopic and molar pregnancy
Pulmonary embolism following ectopic and molar pregnancy
Pyemic embolism following ectopic and molar pregnancy
Septic or septicopyemic embolism following ectopic and molar pregnancy
Soap embolism following ectopic and molar pregnancy

O08.3   **Shock following ectopic and molar pregnancy**   `MCC` `M`♀
Circulatory collapse following ectopic and molar pregnancy
Shock (postprocedural) following ectopic and molar pregnancy
EXCLUDES 1   *shock due to infection following ectopic and molar pregnancy (O08.82)*

O08.4   **Renal failure following ectopic and molar pregnancy**   `MCC` `M`♀
Kidney failure (acute) following ectopic and molar pregnancy
Oliguria following ectopic and molar pregnancy
Renal shutdown following ectopic and molar pregnancy
Renal tubular necrosis following ectopic and molar pregnancy
Uremia following ectopic and molar pregnancy

O08.5   **Metabolic disorders following an ectopic and molar**   `CC` `M`♀
pregnancy

O08.6   **Damage to pelvic organs and tissues following an**   `CC` `M`♀
ectopic and molar pregnancy
Laceration, perforation, tear or chemical damage of bladder following an ectopic and molar pregnancy
Laceration, perforation, tear or chemical damage of bowel following an ectopic and molar pregnancy
Laceration, perforation, tear or chemical damage of broad ligament following an ectopic and molar pregnancy
Laceration, perforation, tear or chemical damage of cervix following an ectopic and molar pregnancy
Laceration, perforation, tear or chemical damage of periurethral tissue following an ectopic and molar pregnancy
Laceration, perforation, tear or chemical damage of uterus following an ectopic and molar pregnancy
Laceration, perforation, tear or chemical damage of vagina following an ectopic and molar pregnancy

O08.7   **Other venous complications following an ectopic**   `CC` `M`♀
and molar pregnancy

✅5ᵗʰ **O08.8**   **Other complications following an ectopic and molar pregnancy**

O08.81   **Cardiac arrest following an ectopic and molar**   `CC` `M`♀
pregnancy

O08.82   **Sepsis following ectopic and molar pregnancy**   `CC` `M`♀
Use additional code to identify infectious agent (B95-B97)
Use additional code to identify severe sepsis, if applicable (R65.2-)
EXCLUDES 1   *septic or septicopyemic embolism following ectopic and molar pregnancy (O08.2)*
CC Excl: See code: O08.0

O08.83   **Urinary tract infection following an ectopic**   `CC` `M`♀
and molar pregnancy
Cystitis following an ectopic and molar pregnancy
CC Excl: O08.2-O08.81, O08.83-O08.9, O20.0-O20.9, O25.10-O25.3, O26.10-O26.13, O26.30-O26.43, O26.63-O26.819, O26.841-O26.86, O26.891-O26.93, O29.011-O29.93, O35.7XX0-O35.7XX9, O44.00-O44.13, O45.8X1-O45.93, O75.4, O75.81, O75.89-O75.9, O80, O90.89, O99.111-O99.285, O99.330-O99.335, O99.350-O99.355, O99.511-O99.73, O99.820-O99.825, O99.840-O9A.53

O08.89   **Other complications following an ectopic**   `CC` `M`♀
and molar pregnancy
CC Excl: See code: O08.83

O08.9   **Unspecified complication following an ectopic and**   `MCC` `M`♀
molar pregnancy
CC Excl: See code: O08.83

Supervision of high risk pregnancy (O09)

✅4ᵗʰ **O09**   **Supervision of high risk pregnancy**

✅5ᵗʰ **O09.0**   **Supervision of pregnancy with history of infertility**

O09.00   **Supervision of pregnancy with history of**   `M`♀
infertility, unspecified trimester

O09.01   **Supervision of pregnancy with history of**   `M`♀
infertility, first trimester

O09.02   **Supervision of pregnancy with history of**   `M`♀
infertility, second trimester

O09.03   **Supervision of pregnancy with history of**   `M`♀
infertility, third trimester

✅5ᵗʰ **O09.1**   **Supervision of pregnancy with history of ectopic or molar pregnancy**

O09.10   **Supervision of pregnancy with history of**   `M`♀
ectopic or molar pregnancy, unspecified trimester

O09.11   **Supervision of pregnancy with history of**   `M`♀
ectopic or molar pregnancy, first trimester

O09.12   **Supervision of pregnancy with history of**   `M`♀
ectopic or molar pregnancy, second trimester

O09.13   **Supervision of pregnancy with history of**   `M`♀
ectopic or molar pregnancy, third trimester

✓5ᵗʰ **O09.2** **Supervision of pregnancy with** other poor reproductive or obstetric history
> EXCLUDES 2   *pregnancy care for patient with history of recurrent pregnancy loss (O26.2-)*

  ✓6ᵗʰ **O09.21** **Supervision of pregnancy with history of** pre-term labor

     O09.211 **Supervision of pregnancy with history of pre-term labor,** first trimester   Ⓜ♀

     O09.212 **Supervision of pregnancy with history of pre-term labor,** second trimester   Ⓜ♀

     O09.213 **Supervision of pregnancy with history of pre-term labor,** third trimester   ♀

     O09.219 **Supervision of pregnancy with history of pre-term labor,** unspecified trimester   Ⓜ♀

  ✓6ᵗʰ **O09.29** **Supervision of pregnancy with** other poor reproductive or obstetric history
> Supervision of pregnancy with history of neonatal death
> Supervision of pregnancy with history of stillbirth

     O09.291 **Supervision of pregnancy with other poor reproductive or obstetric history,** first trimester   Ⓜ♀

     O09.292 **Supervision of pregnancy with other poor reproductive or obstetric history,** second trimester   ♀

     O09.293 **Supervision of pregnancy with other poor reproductive or obstetric history,** third trimester   ♀

     O09.299 **Supervision of pregnancy with other poor reproductive or obstetric history,** unspecified trimester   Ⓜ♀

✓5ᵗʰ **O09.3** **Supervision of pregnancy with** insufficient antenatal care
> Supervision of concealed pregnancy
> Supervision of hidden pregnancy

   O09.30 **Supervision of pregnancy with insufficient antenatal care,** unspecified trimester   Ⓜ♀

   O09.31 **Supervision of pregnancy with insufficient antenatal care,** first trimester   Ⓜ♀

   O09.32 **Supervision of pregnancy with insufficient antenatal care,** second trimester   Ⓜ♀

   O09.33 **Supervision of pregnancy with insufficient antenatal care,** third trimester   Ⓜ♀

✓5ᵗʰ **O09.4** **Supervision of pregnancy with** grand multiparity

   O09.40 **Supervision of pregnancy with grand multiparity,** unspecified trimester   Ⓜ♀

   O09.41 **Supervision of pregnancy with grand multiparity,** first trimester   Ⓜ♀

   O09.42 **Supervision of pregnancy with grand multiparity,** second trimester   Ⓜ♀

   O09.43 **Supervision of pregnancy with grand multiparity,** third trimester   Ⓜ♀

✓5ᵗʰ **O09.5** **Supervision of** elderly primigravida and multigravida
> Pregnancy for a female 35 years and older at expected date of delivery

  ✓6ᵗʰ **O09.51** **Supervision of** elderly primigravida

     O09.511 **Supervision of elderly primigravida,** first trimester   Ⓜ♀

     O09.512 **Supervision of elderly primigravida,** second trimester   Ⓜ♀

     O09.513 **Supervision of elderly primigravida,** third trimester   Ⓜ♀

     O09.519 **Supervision of elderly primigravida,** unspecified trimester   Ⓜ♀

  ✓6ᵗʰ **O09.52** **Supervision of** elderly multigravida

     O09.521 **Supervision of elderly multigravida,** first trimester   Ⓜ♀

     O09.522 **Supervision of elderly multigravida,** second trimester   Ⓜ♀

     O09.523 **Supervision of elderly multigravida,** third trimester   Ⓜ♀

     O09.529 **Supervision of elderly multigravida,** unspecified trimester   Ⓜ♀

✓5ᵗʰ **O09.6** **Supervision of** young primigravida and multigravida
> Supervision of pregnancy for a female less than 16 years old at expected date of delivery

  ✓6ᵗʰ **O09.61** **Supervision of young** primigravida

     O09.611 **Supervision of young primigravida,** first trimester   Ⓜ♀

     O09.612 **Supervision of young primigravida,** second trimester   Ⓜ♀

     O09.613 **Supervision of young primigravida,** third trimester   Ⓜ♀

     O09.619 **Supervision of young primigravida,** unspecified trimester   Ⓜ♀

  ✓6ᵗʰ **O09.62** **Supervision of young** multigravida

     O09.621 **Supervision of young multigravida,** first trimester   Ⓜ♀

     O09.622 **Supervision of young multigravida,** second trimester   Ⓜ♀

     O09.623 **Supervision of young multigravida,** third trimester   Ⓜ♀

     O09.629 **Supervision of young multigravida,** unspecified trimester   Ⓜ♀

✓5ᵗʰ **O09.7** **Supervision of high risk pregnancy due to** social problems

   O09.70 **Supervision of high risk pregnancy due to social problems,** unspecified trimester   Ⓜ♀

   O09.71 **Supervision of high risk pregnancy due to social problems,** first trimester   Ⓜ♀

   O09.72 **Supervision of high risk pregnancy due to social problems,** second trimester   Ⓜ♀

   O09.73 **Supervision of high risk pregnancy due to social problems,** third trimester   Ⓜ♀

✓5ᵗʰ **O09.8** **Supervision of** other high risk pregnancies

  ✓6ᵗʰ **O09.81** **Supervision of pregnancy resulting from assisted reproductive technology**
> Supervision of pregnancy resulting from in-vitro fertilization

     O09.811 **Supervision of pregnancy resulting from assisted reproductive technology,** first trimester   Ⓜ♀

     O09.812 **Supervision of pregnancy resulting from assisted reproductive technology,** second trimester   ♀

     O09.813 **Supervision of pregnancy resulting from assisted reproductive technology,** third trimester   Ⓜ♀

     O09.819 **Supervision of pregnancy resulting from assisted reproductive technology,** unspecified trimester   Ⓜ♀

  ✓6ᵗʰ **O09.82** **Supervision of pregnancy with history of in utero procedure during previous pregnancy**

     O09.821 **Supervision of pregnancy with history of in utero procedure during previous pregnancy,** first trimester   Ⓜ♀

     O09.822 **Supervision of pregnancy with history of in utero procedure during previous pregnancy,** second trimester   Ⓜ♀

     O09.823 **Supervision of pregnancy with history of in utero procedure during previous pregnancy,** third trimester   Ⓜ♀

     O09.829 **Supervision of pregnancy with history of in utero procedure during previous pregnancy,** unspecified trimester   Ⓜ♀
> EXCLUDES 1   *supervision of pregnancy affected by in utero procedure during current pregnancy (O35.7)*

  ✓6ᵗʰ **O09.89** **Supervision of** other high risk pregnancies

     O09.891 **Supervision of other high risk pregnancies,** first trimester   Ⓜ♀

     O09.892 **Supervision of other high risk pregnancies,** second trimester   Ⓜ♀

     O09.893 **Supervision of other high risk pregnancies,** third trimester   Ⓜ♀

     O09.899 **Supervision of other high risk pregnancies,** unspecified trimester   Ⓜ♀

✓5ᵗʰ **O09.9** **Supervision of high risk pregnancy, unspecified**

   O09.90 **Supervision of high risk pregnancy, unspecified,** unspecified trimester   Ⓜ♀

   O09.91 **Supervision of high risk pregnancy, unspecified,** first trimester   Ⓜ♀

   O09.92 **Supervision of high risk pregnancy, unspecified,** second trimester   Ⓜ♀

   O09.93 **Supervision of high risk pregnancy, unspecified,** third trimester   Ⓜ♀

Ⓝ Newborn: 0   Ⓟ Pediatric: 0-17   Ⓜ Maternity: 12-55   Ⓐ Adult: 15-124   MCC Major CC Condition   PDxMCC PDx acts as own MCC   CC CC Condition   PDxCC PDx acts as own CC

816   ICD-10-CM 2016

Edema, proteinuria and hypertensive disorders in pregnancy, childbirth and the puerperium (O10-O16)

✓4ᵗʰ O10 Pre-existing hypertension complicating pregnancy, childbirth and the puerperium

Pre-existing hypertension with pre-existing proteinuria complicating pregnancy, childbirth and the puerperium

EXCLUDES 2 *pre-existing hypertension with superimposed pre-eclampsia complicating pregnancy, childbirth and the puerperium (O11.-)*

CC Excl: For CC/MCC codes in category O10, unless otherwise noted: O10.011-O12.03, O12.20-O16.9, O25.10-O26.13, O26.30-O26.43, O26.63-O26.819, O26.841-O26.86, O26.891-O26.93, O29.011-O29.93, O35.7XX0-O35.7XX9, O75.4, O75.81, O75.89-O75.9, O80, O90.89, O99.111-O99.285, O99.330-O99.335, O99.350-O99.355, O99.511-O99.73, O99.820-O99.825, O99.840-O9A.53

✓5ᵗʰ O10.0 Pre-existing essential hypertension complicating pregnancy, childbirth and the puerperium

Any condition in I10 specified as a reason for obstetric care during pregnancy, childbirth or the puerperium

✓6ᵗʰ O10.01 Pre-existing essential hypertension complicating pregnancy

O10.011 Pre-existing essential hypertension complicating pregnancy, first trimester ᶜᶜ Ⓜ ♀

O10.012 Pre-existing essential hypertension complicating pregnancy, second trimester ᶜᶜ Ⓜ ♀

O10.013 Pre-existing essential hypertension complicating pregnancy, third trimester ᶜᶜ Ⓜ ♀

O10.019 Pre-existing essential hypertension complicating pregnancy, unspecified trimester Ⓜ ♀

O10.02 Pre-existing essential hypertension complicating childbirth ᶜᶜ Ⓜ ♀

O10.03 Pre-existing essential hypertension complicating the puerperium Ⓜ ♀

✓5ᵗʰ O10.1 Pre-existing hypertensive heart disease complicating pregnancy, childbirth and the puerperium

Any condition in I11 specified as a reason for obstetric care during pregnancy, childbirth or the puerperium

Use additional code from I11 to identify the type of hypertensive heart disease

✓6ᵗʰ O10.11 Pre-existing hypertensive heart disease complicating pregnancy

O10.111 Pre-existing hypertensive heart disease complicating pregnancy, first trimester Ⓜ ♀

O10.112 Pre-existing hypertensive heart disease complicating pregnancy, second trimester Ⓜ ♀

O10.113 Pre-existing hypertensive heart disease complicating pregnancy, third trimester Ⓜ ♀

O10.119 Pre-existing hypertensive heart disease complicating pregnancy, unspecified trimester Ⓜ ♀

O10.12 Pre-existing hypertensive heart disease complicating childbirth Ⓜ ♀

O10.13 Pre-existing hypertensive heart disease complicating the puerperium Ⓜ ♀

✓5ᵗʰ O10.2 Pre-existing hypertensive chronic kidney disease complicating pregnancy, childbirth and the puerperium

Any condition in I12 specified as a reason for obstetric care during pregnancy, childbirth or the puerperium

Use additional code from I12 to identify the type of hypertensive chronic kidney disease

✓6ᵗʰ O10.21 Pre-existing hypertensive chronic kidney disease complicating pregnancy

O10.211 Pre-existing hypertensive chronic kidney disease complicating pregnancy, first trimester Ⓜ ♀

O10.212 Pre-existing hypertensive chronic kidney disease complicating pregnancy, second trimester Ⓜ ♀

O10.213 Pre-existing hypertensive chronic kidney disease complicating pregnancy, third trimester Ⓜ ♀

O10.219 Pre-existing hypertensive chronic kidney disease complicating pregnancy, unspecified trimester Ⓜ ♀

O10.22 Pre-existing hypertensive chronic kidney disease complicating childbirth Ⓜ ♀

O10.23 Pre-existing hypertensive chronic kidney disease complicating the puerperium Ⓜ ♀

✓5ᵗʰ O10.3 Pre-existing hypertensive heart and chronic kidney disease complicating pregnancy, childbirth and the puerperium

Any condition in I13 specified as a reason for obstetric care during pregnancy, childbirth or the puerperium

Use additional code from I13 to identify the type of hypertensive heart and chronic kidney disease

✓6ᵗʰ O10.31 Pre-existing hypertensive heart and chronic kidney disease complicating pregnancy

O10.311 Pre-existing hypertensive heart and chronic kidney disease complicating pregnancy, first trimester Ⓜ ♀

O10.312 Pre-existing hypertensive heart and chronic kidney disease complicating pregnancy, second trimester Ⓜ ♀

O10.313 Pre-existing hypertensive heart and chronic kidney disease complicating pregnancy, third trimester Ⓜ ♀

O10.319 Pre-existing hypertensive heart and chronic kidney disease complicating pregnancy, unspecified trimester Ⓜ ♀

O10.32 Pre-existing hypertensive heart and chronic kidney disease complicating childbirth Ⓜ ♀

O10.33 Pre-existing hypertensive heart and chronic kidney disease complicating the puerperium Ⓜ ♀

✓5ᵗʰ O10.4 Pre-existing secondary hypertension complicating pregnancy, childbirth and the puerperium

Any condition in I15 specified as a reason for obstetric care during pregnancy, childbirth or the puerperium

Use additional code from I15 to identify the type of secondary hypertension

✓6ᵗʰ O10.41 Pre-existing secondary hypertension complicating pregnancy

O10.411 Pre-existing secondary hypertension complicating pregnancy, first trimester ᶜᶜ Ⓜ ♀

O10.412 Pre-existing secondary hypertension complicating pregnancy, second trimester ᶜᶜ Ⓜ ♀

O10.413 Pre-existing secondary hypertension complicating pregnancy, third trimester ᶜᶜ Ⓜ ♀

O10.419 Pre-existing secondary hypertension complicating pregnancy, unspecified trimester Ⓜ ♀

O10.42 Pre-existing secondary hypertension complicating childbirth ᴹᶜᶜ Ⓜ ♀

O10.43 Pre-existing secondary hypertension complicating the puerperium ᶜᶜ Ⓜ ♀

✓5ᵗʰ O10.9 Unspecified pre-existing hypertension complicating pregnancy, childbirth and the puerperium

✓6ᵗʰ O10.91 Unspecified pre-existing hypertension complicating pregnancy

O10.911 Unspecified pre-existing hypertension complicating pregnancy, first trimester ᶜᶜ Ⓜ ♀

O10.912 Unspecified pre-existing hypertension complicating pregnancy, second trimester ᶜᶜ Ⓜ ♀

O10.913 Unspecified pre-existing hypertension complicating pregnancy, third trimester ᶜᶜ Ⓜ ♀

O10.919 Unspecified pre-existing hypertension complicating pregnancy, unspecified trimester Ⓜ ♀

O10.92 Unspecified pre-existing hypertension complicating childbirth ᶜᶜ Ⓜ ♀

O10.93 Unspecified pre-existing hypertension complicating the puerperium Ⓜ ♀

☑ Additional Character Required   ✓x7ᵗʰ Placeholder Alert   Unacceptable PDx   Manifestation   Hospital Acquired Condition   *EXCLUDES 1* Not Coded Here   *EXCLUDES 2* Not Included Here

ICD-10-CM 2016   817

Chapter 15. Pregnancy, Childbirth, and the Puerperium

O11–O21.9

√4ᵗʰ **O11 Pre-existing hypertension with pre-eclampsia**
Conditions in O10 complicated by pre-eclampsia
Pre-eclampsia superimposed pre-existing hypertension
Use additional code from O10 to identify the type of hypertension

CC Excl: For MCC codes in category O11, unless otherwise noted:
See code: O10

O11.1 Pre-existing hypertension with pre-eclampsia, first trimester   MCC Mᵒ�

O11.2 Pre-existing hypertension with pre-eclampsia, second trimester   MCC M♀

O11.3 Pre-existing hypertension with pre-eclampsia, third trimester   MCC M♀

O11.9 Pre-existing hypertension with pre-eclampsia, unspecified trimester   M♀

√4ᵗʰ **O12 Gestational [pregnancy-induced] edema and proteinuria without hypertension**

CC Excl: For CC codes in category O12, unless otherwise noted:
O12.11–O12.13, O12.21–O12.23, O26.831–O26.833, O90.89

√5ᵗʰ **O12.0 Gestational edema**
O12.00 Gestational edema, unspecified trimester   M♀
O12.01 Gestational edema, first trimester   M♀
O12.02 Gestational edema, second trimester   M♀
O12.03 Gestational edema, third trimester   M♀

√5ᵗʰ **O12.1 Gestational proteinuria**
O12.10 Gestational proteinuria, unspecified trimester   M♀
O12.11 Gestational proteinuria, first trimester   CC M♀
O12.12 Gestational proteinuria, second trimester   CC M♀
O12.13 Gestational proteinuria, third trimester   CC M♀

√5ᵗʰ **O12.2 Gestational edema with proteinuria**
O12.20 Gestational edema with proteinuria, unspecified trimester   M♀
O12.21 Gestational edema with proteinuria, first trimester   PDx CC CC M♀
O12.22 Gestational edema with proteinuria, second trimester   PDx CC CC M♀
O12.23 Gestational edema with proteinuria, third trimester   PDx CC CC M♀

√4ᵗʰ **O13 Gestational [pregnancy-induced] hypertension without significant proteinuria**
INCLUDES gestational hypertension NOS

CC Excl: For CC codes in category O13, unless otherwise noted:
See code: O10

O13.1 Gestational [pregnancy-induced] hypertension without significant proteinuria, first trimester   M♀

O13.2 Gestational [pregnancy-induced] hypertension without significant proteinuria, second trimester   M♀

O13.3 Gestational [pregnancy-induced] hypertension without significant proteinuria, third trimester   M♀

O13.9 Gestational [pregnancy-induced] hypertension without significant proteinuria, unspecified trimester   M♀

√4ᵗʰ **O14 Pre-eclampsia**
EXCLUDES 1 pre-existing hypertension with pre-eclampsia (O11)

CC Excl: For CC codes in category O14, unless otherwise noted:
See code: O10

√5ᵗʰ **O14.0 Mild to moderate pre-eclampsia**
O14.00 Mild to moderate pre-eclampsia, unspecified trimester   M♀
O14.02 Mild to moderate pre-eclampsia, second trimester   CC M♀
O14.03 Mild to moderate pre-eclampsia, third trimester   CC M♀

√5ᵗʰ **O14.1 Severe pre-eclampsia**
EXCLUDES 1 HELLP syndrome (O14.2-)
O14.10 Severe pre-eclampsia, unspecified trimester   M♀
O14.12 Severe pre-eclampsia, second trimester   MCC M♀
O14.13 Severe pre-eclampsia, third trimester   MCC M♀

√5ᵗʰ **O14.2 HELLP syndrome**
Severe pre-eclampsia with hemolysis, elevated liver enzymes and low platelet count (HELLP)
O14.20 HELLP syndrome (HELLP), unspecified trimester   M♀
O14.22 HELLP syndrome (HELLP), second trimester   MCC M♀
O14.23 HELLP syndrome (HELLP), third trimester   MCC M♀

√5ᵗʰ **O14.9 Unspecified pre-eclampsia**
O14.90 Unspecified pre-eclampsia, unspecified trimester   M♀
O14.92 Unspecified pre-eclampsia, second trimester   CC M♀
O14.93 Unspecified pre-eclampsia, third trimester   CC M♀

√4ᵗʰ **O15 Eclampsia**
INCLUDES convulsions following conditions in O10-O14 and O16

CC Excl: For MCC codes in category O15, unless otherwise noted:
See code: O10

√5ᵗʰ **O15.0 Eclampsia in pregnancy**
O15.00 Eclampsia in pregnancy, unspecified trimester   M♀
O15.02 Eclampsia in pregnancy, second trimester   MCC M♀
O15.03 Eclampsia in pregnancy, third trimester   MCC M♀
O15.1 Eclampsia in labor   MCC M♀
O15.2 Eclampsia in the puerperium   MCC M♀
O15.9 Eclampsia, unspecified as to time period   M♀
Eclampsia NOS

√4ᵗʰ **O16 Unspecified maternal hypertension**

CC Excl: For CC codes in category O16, unless otherwise noted:
See code: O10

O16.1 Unspecified maternal hypertension, first trimester   CC M♀
O16.2 Unspecified maternal hypertension, second trimester   CC M♀
O16.3 Unspecified maternal hypertension, third trimester   CC M♀
O16.9 Unspecified maternal hypertension, unspecified trimester   M♀

Other maternal disorders predominantly related to pregnancy (O20-O29)

EXCLUDES 2 maternal care related to the fetus and amniotic cavity and possible delivery problems (O30-O48)
maternal diseases classifiable elsewhere but complicating pregnancy, labor and delivery, and the puerperium (O98-O99)

√4ᵗʰ **O20 Hemorrhage in early pregnancy**
Hemorrhage before completion of 20 weeks gestation
EXCLUDES 1 pregnancy with abortive outcome (O00-O08)
O20.0 Threatened abortion   CC M♀
Hemorrhage specified as due to threatened abortion
CC Excl: O20.0-O20.9, O25.10-O25.3, O26.10-O26.13, O26.30-O26.43, O26.63-O26.819, O26.841-O26.86, O26.891-O26.93, O29.011-O29.93, O35.7XX0-O35.7XX9, O44.00-O44.13, O75.4, O75.81, O75.89-O75.9, O80, O90.89, O99.111-O99.285, O99.330-O99.335, O99.350-O99.355, O99.511-O99.73, O99.820-O99.825, O99.840-O9A.53
O20.8 Other hemorrhage in early pregnancy   M♀
O20.9 Hemorrhage in early pregnancy, unspecified   CC M♀
CC Excl: See code: O20.0

√4ᵗʰ **O21 Excessive vomiting in pregnancy**
O21.0 Mild hyperemesis gravidarum   M♀
Hyperemesis gravidarum, mild or unspecified, starting before the end of the 20th week of gestation
O21.1 Hyperemesis gravidarum with metabolic disturbance   M♀
Hyperemesis gravidarum, starting before the end of the 20th week of gestation, with metabolic disturbance such as carbohydrate depletion
Hyperemesis gravidarum, starting before the end of the 20th week of gestation, with metabolic disturbance such as dehydration
Hyperemesis gravidarum, starting before the end of the 20th week of gestation, with metabolic disturbance such as electrolyte imbalance
O21.2 Late vomiting of pregnancy   M♀
Excessive vomiting starting after 20 completed weeks of gestation
O21.8 Other vomiting complicating pregnancy   M♀
Vomiting due to diseases classified elsewhere, complicating pregnancy
Use additional code to identify cause
O21.9 Vomiting of pregnancy, unspecified   M♀

Ⓝ Newborn: 0   Ⓟ Pediatric: 0-17   Ⓜ Maternity: 12-55   Ⓐ Adult: 15-124   MCC Major CC Condition   PDx MCC PDx acts as own MCC   CC CC Condition   PDx CC PDx acts as own CC

818   ICD-10-CM 2016

✓4ᵗʰ O22 Venous complications and hemorrhoids in pregnancy

EXCLUDES 1 venous complications of:
  abortion NOS (O03.9)
  ectopic or molar pregnancy (O08.7)
  failed attempted abortion (O07.35)
  induced abortion (O04.85)
  spontaneous abortion (O03.89)

EXCLUDES 2 obstetric pulmonary embolism (O88.-)
  venous complications and hemorrhoids of childbirth and the puerperium (O87.-)

CC Excl: For CC/MCC codes in category O22, unless otherwise noted: O22.20-O22.93, O25.10-O25.3, O26.10-O26.13, O26.30-O26.43, O26.63-O26.819, O26.841-O26.86, O26.891-O26.93, O29.011-O29.93, O35.7XX0-O35.7XX9, O75.4, O75.81, O75.89-O75.9, O80, O87.0-O87.3, O87.8-O87.9, O90.89, O99.111-O99.285, O99.330-O99.335, O99.350-O99.355, O99.511-O99.73, O99.820-O99.825, O99.840-O9A.53

✓5ᵗʰ O22.0 Varicose veins of lower extremity in pregnancy
Varicose veins NOS in pregnancy

  O22.00 Varicose veins of lower extremity in pregnancy, unspecified trimester M♀

  O22.01 Varicose veins of lower extremity in pregnancy, first trimester M♀

  O22.02 Varicose veins of lower extremity in pregnancy, second trimester M♀

  O22.03 Varicose veins of lower extremity in pregnancy, third trimester M♀

✓5ᵗʰ O22.1 Genital varices in pregnancy
Perineal varices in pregnancy
Vaginal varices in pregnancy
Vulval varices in pregnancy

  O22.10 Genital varices in pregnancy, unspecified trimester M♀

  O22.11 Genital varices in pregnancy, first trimester M♀

  O22.12 Genital varices in pregnancy, second trimester M♀

  O22.13 Genital varices in pregnancy, third trimester M♀

✓5ᵗʰ O22.2 Superficial thrombophlebitis in pregnancy
Phlebitis in pregnancy NOS
Thrombophlebitis of legs in pregnancy
Thrombosis in pregnancy NOS
Use additional code to identify the superficial thrombophlebitis (I80.0-)

  O22.20 Superficial thrombophlebitis in pregnancy, unspecified trimester CC M♀

  O22.21 Superficial thrombophlebitis in pregnancy, first trimester CC M♀

  O22.22 Superficial thrombophlebitis in pregnancy, second trimester CC M♀

  O22.23 Superficial thrombophlebitis in pregnancy, third trimester CC M♀

✓5ᵗʰ O22.3 Deep phlebothrombosis in pregnancy
Deep vein thrombosis, antepartum
Use additional code to identify the deep vein thrombosis (I82.4-, I82.5-, I82.62-, I82.72-)
Use additional code, if applicable, for associated long-term (current) use of anticoagulants (Z79.01)

  O22.30 Deep phlebothrombosis in pregnancy, unspecified trimester CC M♀

  O22.31 Deep phlebothrombosis in pregnancy, first trimester MCC M♀

  O22.32 Deep phlebothrombosis in pregnancy, second trimester MCC M♀

  O22.33 Deep phlebothrombosis in pregnancy, third trimester MCC M♀

✓5ᵗʰ O22.4 Hemorrhoids in pregnancy

  O22.40 Hemorrhoids in pregnancy, unspecified trimester CC M♀

  O22.41 Hemorrhoids in pregnancy, first trimester CC M♀

  O22.42 Hemorrhoids in pregnancy, second trimester CC M♀

  O22.43 Hemorrhoids in pregnancy, third trimester CC M♀

✓5ᵗʰ O22.5 Cerebral venous thrombosis in pregnancy
Cerebrovenous sinus thrombosis in pregnancy

  O22.50 Cerebral venous thrombosis in pregnancy, unspecified trimester CC M♀

  O22.51 Cerebral venous thrombosis in pregnancy, first trimester CC M♀

  O22.52 Cerebral venous thrombosis in pregnancy, second trimester CC M♀

  O22.53 Cerebral venous thrombosis in pregnancy, third trimester CC M♀

✓5ᵗʰ O22.8 Other venous complications in pregnancy

  ✓6ᵗʰ O22.8X Other venous complications in pregnancy

    O22.8X1 Other venous complications in pregnancy, first trimester CC M♀

    O22.8X2 Other venous complications in pregnancy, second trimester CC M♀

    O22.8X3 Other venous complications in pregnancy, third trimester CC M♀

    O22.8X9 Other venous complications in pregnancy, unspecified trimester CC M♀

✓5ᵗʰ O22.9 Venous complication in pregnancy, unspecified
Gestational phlebitis NOS
Gestational phlebopathy NOS
Gestational thrombosis NOS

  O22.90 Venous complication in pregnancy, unspecified, unspecified trimester CC M♀

  O22.91 Venous complication in pregnancy, unspecified, first trimester M♀

  O22.92 Venous complication in pregnancy, unspecified, second trimester M♀

  O22.93 Venous complication in pregnancy, unspecified, third trimester M♀

✓4ᵗʰ O23 Infections of genitourinary tract in pregnancy
Use additional code to identify organism (B95.-, B96.-)

EXCLUDES 2 gonococcal infections complicating pregnancy, childbirth and the puerperium (O98.2)
  infections with a predominantly sexual mode of transmission NOS complicating pregnancy, childbirth and the puerperium (O98.3)
  syphilis complicating pregnancy, childbirth and the puerperium (O98.1)
  tuberculosis of genitourinary system complicating pregnancy, childbirth and the puerperium (O98.0)
  venereal disease NOS complicating pregnancy, childbirth and the puerperium (O98.3)

CC Excl: For CC codes in category O23, unless otherwise noted: O23.00-O23.93, O25.10-O25.3, O26.10-O26.13, O26.30-O26.43, O26.63-O26.819, O26.841-O26.86, O26.891-O26.93, O29.011-O29.93, O35.7XX0-O35.7XX9, O75.4, O75.81, O75.89-O75.9, O80, O86.11, O86.13-O86.29, O90.89, O99.111-O99.285, O99.330-O99.335, O99.350-O99.355, O99.511-O99.73, O99.820-O99.825, O99.840-O9A.53

✓5ᵗʰ O23.0 Infections of kidney in pregnancy
Pyelonephritis in pregnancy

  O23.00 Infections of kidney in pregnancy, unspecified trimester M♀

  O23.01 Infections of kidney in pregnancy, first trimester CC M♀

  O23.02 Infections of kidney in pregnancy, second trimester CC M♀

  O23.03 Infections of kidney in pregnancy, third trimester CC M♀

✓5ᵗʰ O23.1 Infections of bladder in pregnancy

  O23.10 Infections of bladder in pregnancy, unspecified trimester M♀

  O23.11 Infections of bladder in pregnancy, first trimester CC M♀

  O23.12 Infections of bladder in pregnancy, second trimester CC M♀

  O23.13 Infections of bladder in pregnancy, third trimester CC M♀

✓5ᵗʰ O23.2 Infections of urethra in pregnancy

  O23.20 Infections of urethra in pregnancy, unspecified trimester M♀

  O23.21 Infections of urethra in pregnancy, first trimester CC M♀

  O23.22 Infections of urethra in pregnancy, second trimester CC M♀

  O23.23 Infections of urethra in pregnancy, third trimester CC M♀

✓5ᵗʰ O23.3 Infections of other parts of urinary tract in pregnancy

  O23.30 Infections of other parts of urinary tract in pregnancy, unspecified trimester M♀

  O23.31 Infections of other parts of urinary tract in pregnancy, first trimester CC M♀

✓ Additional Character Required   ✓x7ᵗʰ Placeholder Alert   Unacceptable PDx   Manifestation   Hospital Acquired Condition   *EXCLUDES 1* Not Coded Here   *EXCLUDES 2* Not Included Here

ICD-10-CM 2016   819

Chapter 15. Pregnancy, Childbirth, and the Puerperium

O23.32–O24.439

O23.32   **Infections of other parts of urinary tract in pregnancy, second trimester**   CC M♀

O23.33   **Infections of other parts of urinary tract in pregnancy, third trimester**   CC M♀

√5ᵗʰ **O23.4**   **Unspecified infection of urinary tract in pregnancy**

   O23.40   **Unspecified infection of urinary tract in pregnancy, unspecified trimester**   M♀

   O23.41   **Unspecified infection of urinary tract in pregnancy, first trimester**   CC M♀

   O23.42   **Unspecified infection of urinary tract in pregnancy, second trimester**   CC M♀

   O23.43   **Unspecified infection of urinary tract in pregnancy, third trimester**   CC M♀

√5ᵗʰ **O23.5**   **Infections of the genital tract in pregnancy**

   √6ᵗʰ **O23.51**   **Infection of cervix in pregnancy**

     O23.511   **Infections of cervix in pregnancy, first trimester**   CC M♀

     O23.512   **Infections of cervix in pregnancy, second trimester**   CC M♀

     O23.513   **Infections of cervix in pregnancy, third trimester**   CC M♀

     O23.519   **Infections of cervix in pregnancy, unspecified trimester**   M♀

   √6ᵗʰ **O23.52**   **Salpingo-oophoritis in pregnancy**
     Oophoritis in pregnancy
     Salpingitis in pregnancy

     O23.521   **Salpingo-oophoritis in pregnancy, first trimester**   CC M♀

     O23.522   **Salpingo-oophoritis in pregnancy, second trimester**   CC M♀

     O23.523   **Salpingo-oophoritis in pregnancy, third trimester**   CC M♀

     O23.529   **Salpingo-oophoritis in pregnancy, unspecified trimester**   M♀

   √6ᵗʰ **O23.59**   **Infection of other part of genital tract in pregnancy**

     O23.591   **Infection of other part of genital tract in pregnancy, first trimester**   CC M♀

     O23.592   **Infection of other part of genital tract in pregnancy, second trimester**   CC M♀

     O23.593   **Infection of other part of genital tract in pregnancy, third trimester**   CC M♀

     O23.599   **Infection of other part of genital tract in pregnancy, unspecified trimester**   M♀

√5ᵗʰ **O23.9**   **Unspecified genitourinary tract infection in pregnancy**
   Genitourinary tract infection in pregnancy NOS

   O23.90   **Unspecified genitourinary tract infection in pregnancy, unspecified trimester**   M♀

   O23.91   **Unspecified genitourinary tract infection in pregnancy, first trimester**   CC M♀

   O23.92   **Unspecified genitourinary tract infection in pregnancy, second trimester**   CC M♀

   O23.93   **Unspecified genitourinary tract infection in pregnancy, third trimester**   CC M♀

√4ᵗʰ **O24**   **Diabetes mellitus in pregnancy, childbirth, and the puerperium**

> **CC Excl:** For CC/MCC codes in category O24, unless otherwise noted: O24.011–O24.33, O24.811–O25.3, O26.10–O26.13, O26.30–O26.43, O26.63–O26.819, O26.841–O26.86, O26.891–O26.93, O29.011–O29.93, O35.7XX0–O35.7XX9, O75.4, O75.81, O75.89–O75.9, O80, O90.89, O99.111–O99.285, O99.330–O99.335, O99.350–O99.355, O99.511–O99.73, O99.820–O99.825, O99.840–O9A.53

√5ᵗʰ **O24.0**   **Pre-existing diabetes mellitus, type 1, in pregnancy, childbirth and the puerperium**
   Juvenile onset diabetes mellitus, in pregnancy, childbirth and the puerperium
   Ketosis-prone diabetes mellitus in pregnancy, childbirth and the puerperium
   Use additional code from category E10 to further identify any manifestations

   √6ᵗʰ **O24.01**   **Pre-existing diabetes mellitus, type 1, in pregnancy**

     O24.011   **Pre-existing diabetes mellitus, type 1, in pregnancy, first trimester**   CC M♀

     O24.012   **Pre-existing diabetes mellitus, type 1, in pregnancy, second trimester**   CC M♀

     O24.013   **Pre-existing diabetes mellitus, type 1, in pregnancy, third trimester**   CC M♀

     O24.019   **Pre-existing diabetes mellitus, type 1, in pregnancy, unspecified trimester**   CC M♀

   O24.02   **Pre-existing diabetes mellitus, type 1, in childbirth**   MCC M♀

   O24.03   **Pre-existing diabetes mellitus, type 1, in the puerperium**   CC M♀

√5ᵗʰ **O24.1**   **Pre-existing diabetes mellitus, type 2, in pregnancy, childbirth and the puerperium**
   Insulin-resistant diabetes mellitus in pregnancy, childbirth and the puerperium
   Use additional code (for):
     from category E11 to further identify any manifestations
     long-term (current) use of insulin (Z79.4)

   √6ᵗʰ **O24.11**   **Pre-existing diabetes mellitus, type 2, in pregnancy**

     O24.111   **Pre-existing diabetes mellitus, type 2, in pregnancy, first trimester**   CC M♀

     O24.112   **Pre-existing diabetes mellitus, type 2, in pregnancy, second trimester**   CC M♀

     O24.113   **Pre-existing diabetes mellitus, type 2, in pregnancy, third trimester**   CC M♀

     O24.119   **Pre-existing diabetes mellitus, type 2, in pregnancy, unspecified trimester**   CC M♀

   O24.12   **Pre-existing diabetes mellitus, type 2, in childbirth**   MCC M♀

   O24.13   **Pre-existing diabetes mellitus, type 2, in the puerperium**   CC M♀

√5ᵗʰ **O24.3**   **Unspecified pre-existing diabetes mellitus in pregnancy, childbirth and the puerperium**
   Use additional code (for):
     from category E11 to further identify any manifestation
     long-term (current) use of insulin (Z79.4)

   √6ᵗʰ **O24.31**   **Unspecified pre-existing diabetes mellitus in pregnancy**

     O24.311   **Unspecified pre-existing diabetes mellitus in pregnancy, first trimester**   CC M♀

     O24.312   **Unspecified pre-existing diabetes mellitus in pregnancy, second trimester**   CC M♀

     O24.313   **Unspecified pre-existing diabetes mellitus in pregnancy, third trimester**   CC M♀

     O24.319   **Unspecified pre-existing diabetes mellitus in pregnancy, unspecified trimester**   CC M♀

   O24.32   **Unspecified pre-existing diabetes mellitus in childbirth**   MCC M♀

   O24.33   **Unspecified pre-existing diabetes mellitus in the puerperium**   CC M♀

√5ᵗʰ **O24.4**   **Gestational diabetes mellitus**
   Diabetes mellitus arising in pregnancy
   Gestational diabetes mellitus NOS

   √6ᵗʰ **O24.41**   **Gestational diabetes mellitus in pregnancy**

     O24.410   **Gestational diabetes mellitus in pregnancy, diet controlled**   M♀

     O24.414   **Gestational diabetes mellitus in pregnancy, insulin controlled**   M♀

     O24.419   **Gestational diabetes mellitus in pregnancy, unspecified control**   M♀

   √6ᵗʰ **O24.42**   **Gestational diabetes mellitus in childbirth**

     O24.420   **Gestational diabetes mellitus in childbirth, diet controlled**   M♀

     O24.424   **Gestational diabetes mellitus in childbirth, insulin controlled**   M♀

     O24.429   **Gestational diabetes mellitus in childbirth, unspecified control**   M♀

   √6ᵗʰ **O24.43**   **Gestational diabetes mellitus in the puerperium**

     O24.430   **Gestational diabetes mellitus in the puerperium, diet controlled**   M♀

     O24.434   **Gestational diabetes mellitus in the puerperium, insulin controlled**   M♀

     O24.439   **Gestational diabetes mellitus in the puerperium, unspecified control**   M♀

Ⓝ Newborn: 0   Ⓟ Pediatric: 0-17   Ⓜ Maternity: 12-55   Ⓐ Adult: 15-124   MCC Major CC Condition   PDxMCC PDx acts as own MCC   CC CC Condition   PDxCC PDx acts as own CC

820

ICD-10-CM 2016

✓5ᵗʰ **O24.8** **Other pre-existing** diabetes mellitus in pregnancy, childbirth, and the puerperium
Use additional code (for):
    from categories E08, E09 and E13 to further identify any manifestation
    long-term (current) use of insulin (Z79.4)

  ✓6ᵗʰ **O24.81** **Other pre-existing diabetes mellitus in** pregnancy

    O24.811 Other pre-existing diabetes mellitus in pregnancy, first trimester   CC M ♀

    O24.812 Other pre-existing diabetes mellitus in pregnancy, second trimester   CC M ♀

    O24.813 Other pre-existing diabetes mellitus in pregnancy, third trimester   CC M ♀

    O24.819 Other pre-existing diabetes mellitus in pregnancy, unspecified trimester   CC M ♀

  O24.82 Other pre-existing diabetes mellitus in childbirth   MCC M ♀

  O24.83 Other pre-existing diabetes mellitus in the puerperium   CC M ♀

✓5ᵗʰ **O24.9** **Unspecified** diabetes mellitus in pregnancy, childbirth and the puerperium
Use additional code for long-term (current) use of insulin (Z79.4)

  ✓6ᵗʰ **O24.91** **Unspecified diabetes mellitus in** pregnancy

    O24.911 Unspecified diabetes mellitus in pregnancy, first trimester   CC M ♀

    O24.912 Unspecified diabetes mellitus in pregnancy, second trimester   CC M ♀

    O24.913 Unspecified diabetes mellitus in pregnancy, third trimester   CC M ♀

    O24.919 Unspecified diabetes mellitus in pregnancy, unspecified trimester   CC M ♀

  O24.92 Unspecified diabetes mellitus in childbirth   M ♀

  O24.93 Unspecified diabetes mellitus in the puerperium   CC M ♀

✓4ᵗʰ **O25** **Malnutrition** in pregnancy, childbirth and the puerperium

  ✓5ᵗʰ **O25.1** **Malnutrition in** pregnancy

    O25.10 Malnutrition in pregnancy, unspecified trimester M ♀

    O25.11 Malnutrition in pregnancy, first trimester   M ♀

    O25.12 Malnutrition in pregnancy, second trimester   M ♀

    O25.13 Malnutrition in pregnancy, third trimester   M ♀

  O25.2 Malnutrition in childbirth   M ♀

  O25.3 Malnutrition in the puerperium   M ♀

✓4ᵗʰ **O26** **Maternal care for other conditions predominantly related to pregnancy**

  ✓5ᵗʰ **O26.0** **Excessive weight gain in pregnancy**
EXCLUDES 2 gestational edema (O12.0, O12.2)

    O26.00 Excessive weight gain in pregnancy, unspecified trimester   M ♀

    O26.01 Excessive weight gain in pregnancy, first trimester   M ♀

    O26.02 Excessive weight gain in pregnancy, second trimester   M ♀

    O26.03 Excessive weight gain in pregnancy, third trimester   M ♀

  ✓5ᵗʰ **O26.1** **Low weight gain in pregnancy**

    O26.10 Low weight gain in pregnancy, unspecified trimester   M ♀

    O26.11 Low weight gain in pregnancy, first trimester   M ♀

    O26.12 Low weight gain in pregnancy, second trimester   M ♀

    O26.13 Low weight gain in pregnancy, third trimester   M ♀

  ✓5ᵗʰ **O26.2** **Pregnancy care for patient with recurrent pregnancy loss**

    CC Excl: For CC codes in subcategory O26.2, unless otherwise noted: O26.21-O26.23

    O26.20 Pregnancy care for patient with recurrent pregnancy loss, unspecified trimester   M ♀

    O26.21 Pregnancy care for patient with recurrent pregnancy loss, first trimester   M ♀

    O26.22 Pregnancy care for patient with recurrent pregnancy loss, second trimester   M ♀

    O26.23 Pregnancy care for patient with recurrent pregnancy loss, third trimester   M ♀

✓5ᵗʰ **O26.3** **Retained intrauterine contraceptive device in pregnancy**

  O26.30 Retained intrauterine contraceptive device in pregnancy, unspecified trimester   M ♀

  O26.31 Retained intrauterine contraceptive device in pregnancy, first trimester   M ♀

  O26.32 Retained intrauterine contraceptive device in pregnancy, second trimester   M ♀

  O26.33 Retained intrauterine contraceptive device in pregnancy, third trimester   M ♀

✓5ᵗʰ **O26.4** **Herpes gestationis**

  O26.40 Herpes gestationis, unspecified trimester   M ♀

  O26.41 Herpes gestationis, first trimester   M ♀

  O26.42 Herpes gestationis, second trimester   M ♀

  O26.43 Herpes gestationis, third trimester   M ♀

✓5ᵗʰ **O26.5** **Maternal hypotension syndrome**
Supine hypotensive syndrome

CC Excl: For MCC codes in subcategory O26.5, unless otherwise noted: O25.10-O25.3, O26.10-O26.13, O26.30-O26.43, O26.51-O26.53, O26.63-O26.819, O26.841-O26.86, O26.891-O26.93, O29.011-O29.93, O35.7XX0-O35.7XX9, O75.1, O75.4, O75.81, O75.89-O75.9, O80, O90.89, O99.111-O99.285, O99.330-O99.335, O99.350-O99.355, O99.511-O99.73, O99.820-O99.825, O99.840-O9A.53

  O26.50 Maternal hypotension syndrome, unspecified trimester   M ♀

  O26.51 Maternal hypotension syndrome, first trimester   M ♀

  O26.52 Maternal hypotension syndrome, second trimester   M ♀

  O26.53 Maternal hypotension syndrome, third trimester   M ♀

✓5ᵗʰ **O26.6** **Liver and biliary tract disorders in pregnancy, childbirth and the puerperium**
Use additional code to identify the specific disorder
EXCLUDES 2 hepatorenal syndrome following labor and delivery (O90.4)

CC Excl: For CC codes in subcategory O26.6, unless otherwise noted: O25.10-O25.3, O26.10-O26.13, O26.30-O26.43, O26.611-O26.819, O26.841-O26.86, O26.891-O26.93, O29.011-O29.93, O35.7XX0-O35.7XX9, O75.4, O75.81, O75.89-O75.9, O80, O90.89, O99.111-O99.285, O99.330-O99.335, O99.350-O99.355, O99.511-O99.73, O99.820-O99.825, O99.840-O9A.53

  ✓6ᵗʰ **O26.61** **Liver and biliary tract disorders in** pregnancy

    O26.611 Liver and biliary tract disorders in pregnancy, first trimester   CC M ♀

    O26.612 Liver and biliary tract disorders in pregnancy, second trimester   CC M ♀

    O26.613 Liver and biliary tract disorders in pregnancy, third trimester   CC M ♀

    O26.619 Liver and biliary tract disorders in pregnancy, unspecified trimester   M ♀

  O26.62 Liver and biliary tract disorders in childbirth   CC M ♀

  O26.63 Liver and biliary tract disorders in the puerperium   M ♀

✓5ᵗʰ **O26.7** **Subluxation of symphysis (pubis) in pregnancy, childbirth and the puerperium**
EXCLUDES 1 traumatic separation of symphysis (pubis) during childbirth (O71.6)

  ✓6ᵗʰ **O26.71** **Subluxation of symphysis (pubis) in pregnancy**

    O26.711 Subluxation of symphysis (pubis) in pregnancy, first trimester   M ♀

    O26.712 Subluxation of symphysis (pubis) in pregnancy, second trimester   M ♀

    O26.713 Subluxation of symphysis (pubis) in pregnancy, third trimester   M ♀

    O26.719 Subluxation of symphysis (pubis) in pregnancy, unspecified trimester   M ♀

  O26.72 Subluxation of symphysis (pubis) in childbirth   M ♀

  O26.73 Subluxation of symphysis (pubis) in the puerperium   M ♀

✓5ᵗʰ **O26.8** **Other specified pregnancy related conditions**

  ✓6ᵗʰ **O26.81** **Pregnancy related exhaustion and fatigue**

    O26.811 Pregnancy related exhaustion and fatigue, first trimester   M ♀

✓ Additional Character Required   ✓x7ᵗʰ Placeholder Alert   Unacceptable PDx   Manifestation   Hospital Acquired Condition   EXCLUDES 1 Not Coded Here   EXCLUDES 2 Not Included Here

Chapter 15. Pregnancy, Childbirth, and the Puerperium

O26.812–O29.099

    O26.812 Pregnancy related exhaustion and fatigue, second trimester M♀

    O26.813 Pregnancy related exhaustion and fatigue, third trimester M♀

    O26.819 Pregnancy related exhaustion and fatigue, unspecified trimester ♀

✓6ᵗʰ **O26.82 Pregnancy related peripheral neuritis**

    O26.821 Pregnancy related peripheral neuritis, first trimester M♀

    O26.822 Pregnancy related peripheral neuritis, second trimester M♀

    O26.823 Pregnancy related peripheral neuritis, third trimester M♀

    O26.829 Pregnancy related peripheral neuritis, unspecified trimester ♀

✓6ᵗʰ **O26.83 Pregnancy related renal disease**
> Use additional code to identify the specific disorder

> **CC Excl: For CC codes in subcategory O26.83, unless otherwise noted:** O12.11–O12.13, O12.21–O12.23, O26.831–O26.833, O90.89

    O26.831 Pregnancy related renal disease, first trimester CC M♀

    O26.832 Pregnancy related renal disease, second trimester CC M♀

    O26.833 Pregnancy related renal disease, third trimester CC M♀

    O26.839 Pregnancy related renal disease, unspecified trimester M♀

✓6ᵗʰ **O26.84 Uterine size-date discrepancy complicating pregnancy**
> *EXCLUDES 1* encounter for suspected problem with fetal growth ruled out (Z03.74)

    O26.841 Uterine size-date discrepancy, first trimester M♀

    O26.842 Uterine size-date discrepancy, second trimester M♀

    O26.843 Uterine size-date discrepancy, third trimester M♀

    O26.849 Uterine size-date discrepancy, unspecified trimester M♀

✓6ᵗʰ **O26.85 Spotting complicating pregnancy**

    O26.851 Spotting complicating pregnancy, first trimester M♀

    O26.852 Spotting complicating pregnancy, second trimester M♀

    O26.853 Spotting complicating pregnancy, third trimester M♀

    O26.859 Spotting complicating pregnancy, unspecified trimester M♀

O26.86 Pruritic urticarial papules and plaques of pregnancy (PUPPP) M♀
> Polymorphic eruption of pregnancy

✓6ᵗʰ **O26.87 Cervical shortening**
> *EXCLUDES 1* encounter for suspected cervical shortening ruled out (Z03.75)

> **CC Excl: For CC codes in subcategory O26.87, unless otherwise noted:** O26.872–O26.879, O34.31–O34.33

    O26.872 Cervical shortening, second trimester CC M♀

    O26.873 Cervical shortening, third trimester CC M♀

    O26.879 Cervical shortening, unspecified trimester CC M♀

✓6ᵗʰ **O26.89 Other specified pregnancy related conditions**

    O26.891 Other specified pregnancy related conditions, first trimester M♀

    O26.892 Other specified pregnancy related conditions, second trimester ♀

    O26.893 Other specified pregnancy related conditions, third trimester M♀

    O26.899 Other specified pregnancy related conditions, unspecified trimester M♀

✓5ᵗʰ **O26.9 Pregnancy related conditions, unspecified**

    O26.90 Pregnancy related conditions, unspecified, unspecified trimester M♀

    O26.91 Pregnancy related conditions, unspecified, first trimester M♀

    O26.92 Pregnancy related conditions, unspecified, second trimester M♀

    O26.93 Pregnancy related conditions, unspecified, third trimester M♀

✓4ᵗʰ **O28 Abnormal findings on antenatal screening of mother**
> *EXCLUDES 1* diagnostic findings classified elsewhere—see Alphabetical Index

O28.0 Abnormal hematological finding on antenatal screening of mother M♀

O28.1 Abnormal biochemical finding on antenatal screening of mother M♀

O28.2 Abnormal cytological finding on antenatal screening of mother M♀

O28.3 Abnormal ultrasonic finding on antenatal screening of mother M♀

O28.4 Abnormal radiological finding on antenatal screening of mother M♀

O28.5 Abnormal chromosomal and genetic finding on antenatal screening of mother M♀

O28.8 Other abnormal findings on antenatal screening of mother M♀

O28.9 Unspecified abnormal findings on antenatal screening of mother M♀

✓4ᵗʰ **O29 Complications of anesthesia during pregnancy**
> *INCLUDES* maternal complications arising from the administration of a general, regional or local anesthetic, analgesic or other sedation during pregnancy
> Use additional code, if necessary, to identify the complication
> *EXCLUDES 2* complications of anesthesia during labor and delivery (O74.-)
> complications of anesthesia during the puerperium (O89.-)

✓5ᵗʰ **O29.0 Pulmonary complications of anesthesia during pregnancy**

  ✓6ᵗʰ **O29.01 Aspiration pneumonitis due to anesthesia during pregnancy**
> Inhalation of stomach contents or secretions NOS due to anesthesia during pregnancy
> Mendelson's syndrome due to anesthesia during pregnancy

    O29.011 Aspiration pneumonitis due to anesthesia during pregnancy, first trimester M♀

    O29.012 Aspiration pneumonitis due to anesthesia during pregnancy, second trimester M♀

    O29.013 Aspiration pneumonitis due to anesthesia during pregnancy, third trimester M♀

    O29.019 Aspiration pneumonitis due to anesthesia during pregnancy, unspecified trimester M♀

  ✓6ᵗʰ **O29.02 Pressure collapse of lung due to anesthesia during pregnancy**

    O29.021 Pressure collapse of lung due to anesthesia during pregnancy, first trimester M♀

    O29.022 Pressure collapse of lung due to anesthesia during pregnancy, second trimester M♀

    O29.023 Pressure collapse of lung due to anesthesia during pregnancy, third trimester M♀

    O29.029 Pressure collapse of lung due to anesthesia during pregnancy, unspecified trimester M♀

  ✓6ᵗʰ **O29.09 Other pulmonary complications of anesthesia during pregnancy**

    O29.091 Other pulmonary complications of anesthesia during pregnancy, first trimester M♀

    O29.092 Other pulmonary complications of anesthesia during pregnancy, second trimester M♀

    O29.093 Other pulmonary complications of anesthesia during pregnancy, third trimester M♀

    O29.099 Other pulmonary complications of anesthesia during pregnancy, unspecified trimester M♀

N Newborn: 0   P Pediatric: 0-17   M Maternity: 12-55   A Adult: 15-124   MCC Major CC Condition   PDxMCC PDx acts as own MCC   CC CC Condition   PDxCC PDx acts as own CC

822   ICD-10-CM 2016

✓5ᵗʰ **O29.1** Cardiac complications of anesthesia during pregnancy

    ✓6ᵗʰ **O29.11** Cardiac arrest due to anesthesia during pregnancy

        O29.111 Cardiac arrest due to anesthesia during pregnancy, first trimester Ⓜ♀

        O29.112 Cardiac arrest due to anesthesia during pregnancy, second trimester Ⓜ♀

        O29.113 Cardiac arrest due to anesthesia during pregnancy, third trimester Ⓜ♀

        O29.119 Cardiac arrest due to anesthesia during pregnancy, unspecified trimester Ⓜ♀

    ✓6ᵗʰ **O29.12** Cardiac failure due to anesthesia during pregnancy

        O29.121 Cardiac failure due to anesthesia during pregnancy, first trimester Ⓜ♀

        O29.122 Cardiac failure due to anesthesia during pregnancy, second trimester Ⓜ♀

        O29.123 Cardiac failure due to anesthesia during pregnancy, third trimester Ⓜ♀

        O29.129 Cardiac failure due to anesthesia during pregnancy, unspecified trimester Ⓜ♀

    ✓6ᵗʰ **O29.19** Other cardiac complications of anesthesia during pregnancy

        O29.191 Other cardiac complications of anesthesia during pregnancy, first trimester Ⓜ♀

        O29.192 Other cardiac complications of anesthesia during pregnancy, second trimester Ⓜ♀

        O29.193 Other cardiac complications of anesthesia during pregnancy, third trimester Ⓜ♀

        O29.199 Other cardiac complications of anesthesia during pregnancy, unspecified trimester Ⓜ♀

✓5ᵗʰ **O29.2** Central nervous system complications of anesthesia during pregnancy

    ✓6ᵗʰ **O29.21** Cerebral anoxia due to anesthesia during pregnancy

        O29.211 Cerebral anoxia due to anesthesia during pregnancy, first trimester Ⓜ♀

        O29.212 Cerebral anoxia due to anesthesia during pregnancy, second trimester Ⓜ♀

        O29.213 Cerebral anoxia due to anesthesia during pregnancy, third trimester Ⓜ♀

        O29.219 Cerebral anoxia due to anesthesia during pregnancy, unspecified trimester Ⓜ♀

    ✓6ᵗʰ **O29.29** Other central nervous system complications of anesthesia during pregnancy

        O29.291 Other central nervous system complications of anesthesia during pregnancy, first trimester Ⓜ♀

        O29.292 Other central nervous system complications of anesthesia during pregnancy, second trimester Ⓜ♀

        O29.293 Other central nervous system complications of anesthesia during pregnancy, third trimester Ⓜ♀

        O29.299 Other central nervous system complications of anesthesia during pregnancy, unspecified trimester Ⓜ♀

✓5ᵗʰ **O29.3** Toxic reaction to local anesthesia during pregnancy

    ✓6ᵗʰ **O29.3X** Toxic reaction to local anesthesia during pregnancy

        O29.3X1 Toxic reaction to local anesthesia during pregnancy, first trimester Ⓜ♀

        O29.3X2 Toxic reaction to local anesthesia during pregnancy, second trimester Ⓜ♀

        O29.3X3 Toxic reaction to local anesthesia during pregnancy, third trimester Ⓜ♀

        O29.3X9 Toxic reaction to local anesthesia during pregnancy, unspecified trimester Ⓜ♀

✓5ᵗʰ **O29.4** Spinal and epidural anesthesia induced headache during pregnancy

    O29.40 Spinal and epidural anesthesia induced headache during pregnancy, unspecified trimester Ⓜ♀

    O29.41 Spinal and epidural anesthesia induced headache during pregnancy, first trimester Ⓜ♀

    O29.42 Spinal and epidural anesthesia induced headache during pregnancy, second trimester Ⓜ♀

    O29.43 Spinal and epidural anesthesia induced headache during pregnancy, third trimester Ⓜ♀

✓5ᵗʰ **O29.5** Other complications of spinal and epidural anesthesia during pregnancy

    ✓6ᵗʰ **O29.5X** Other complications of spinal and epidural anesthesia during pregnancy

        O29.5X1 Other complications of spinal and epidural anesthesia during pregnancy, first trimester Ⓜ♀

        O29.5X2 Other complications of spinal and epidural anesthesia during pregnancy, second trimester Ⓜ♀

        O29.5X3 Other complications of spinal and epidural anesthesia during pregnancy, third trimester Ⓜ♀

        O29.5X9 Other complications of spinal and epidural anesthesia during pregnancy, unspecified trimester Ⓜ♀

✓5ᵗʰ **O29.6** Failed or difficult intubation for anesthesia during pregnancy

    O29.60 Failed or difficult intubation for anesthesia during pregnancy, unspecified trimester Ⓜ♀

    O29.61 Failed or difficult intubation for anesthesia during pregnancy, first trimester Ⓜ♀

    O29.62 Failed or difficult intubation for anesthesia during pregnancy, second trimester Ⓜ♀

    O29.63 Failed or difficult intubation for anesthesia during pregnancy, third trimester Ⓜ♀

✓5ᵗʰ **O29.8** Other complications of anesthesia during pregnancy

    ✓6ᵗʰ **O29.8X** Other complications of anesthesia during pregnancy

        O29.8X1 Other complications of anesthesia during pregnancy, first trimester Ⓜ♀

        O29.8X2 Other complications of anesthesia during pregnancy, second trimester Ⓜ♀

        O29.8X3 Other complications of anesthesia during pregnancy, third trimester Ⓜ♀

        O29.8X9 Other complications of anesthesia during pregnancy, unspecified trimester Ⓜ♀

✓5ᵗʰ **O29.9** Unspecified complication of anesthesia during pregnancy

    O29.90 Unspecified complication of anesthesia during pregnancy, unspecified trimester Ⓜ♀

    O29.91 Unspecified complication of anesthesia during pregnancy, first trimester Ⓜ♀

    O29.92 Unspecified complication of anesthesia during pregnancy, second trimester Ⓜ♀

    O29.93 Unspecified complication of anesthesia during pregnancy, third trimester Ⓜ♀

Maternal care related to the fetus and amniotic cavity and possible delivery problems (O30-O48)

✓4ᵗʰ **O30 Multiple gestation**

Code also any complications specific to multiple gestation

CC Excl: For CC codes in category O30, unless otherwise noted:
O30.001-O30.019, O30.031-O30.93, O31.10X0-O31.23X9, O31.31X0-O32.9XX9, O80

✓5ᵗʰ **O30.0** Twin pregnancy

    ✓6ᵗʰ **O30.00** Twin pregnancy, unspecified number of placenta and unspecified number of amniotic sacs

        O30.001 Twin pregnancy, unspecified number of placenta and unspecified number of amniotic sacs, first trimester Ⓜ♀

        O30.002 Twin pregnancy, unspecified number of placenta and unspecified number of amniotic sacs, second trimester Ⓜ♀

        O30.003 Twin pregnancy, unspecified number of placenta and unspecified number of amniotic sacs, third trimester Ⓜ♀

        O30.009 Twin pregnancy, unspecified number of placenta and unspecified number of amniotic sacs, unspecified trimester Ⓜ♀

    ✓6ᵗʰ **O30.01** Twin pregnancy, monochorionic/monoamniotic

Twin pregnancy, one placenta, one amniotic sac

EXCLUDES 1 conjoined twins (O30.02-)

        O30.011 Twin pregnancy, monochorionic/ monoamniotic, first trimester Ⓜ♀

        O30.012 Twin pregnancy, monochorionic/ monoamniotic, second trimester Ⓜ♀

        O30.013 Twin pregnancy, monochorionic/ monoamniotic, third trimester Ⓜ♀

✔ Additional Character Required   ✔x7ᵗʰ Placeholder Alert   Unacceptable PDx   ▓ Manifestation   Hospital Acquired Condition   EXCLUDES 1 Not Coded Here   EXCLUDES 2 Not Included Here

ICD-10-CM 2016

823

Chapter 15. Pregnancy, Childbirth, and the Puerperium

O30.019 Twin pregnancy, monochorionic/monoamniotic, unspecified trimester Ⓜ♀

✓6ᵗʰ **O30.02** Conjoined twin pregnancy

O30.021 Conjoined twin pregnancy, first trimester Ⓜ♀

O30.022 Conjoined twin pregnancy, second trimester Ⓜ♀

O30.023 Conjoined twin pregnancy, third trimester Ⓜ♀

O30.029 Conjoined twin pregnancy, unspecified trimester Ⓜ♀

✓6ᵗʰ **O30.03** Twin pregnancy, monochorionic/diamniotic
Twin pregnancy, one placenta, two amniotic sacs

O30.031 Twin pregnancy, monochorionic/diamniotic, first trimester Ⓜ♀

O30.032 Twin pregnancy, monochorionic/diamniotic, second trimester Ⓜ♀

O30.033 Twin pregnancy, monochorionic/diamniotic, third trimester Ⓜ♀

O30.039 Twin pregnancy, monochorionic/diamniotic, unspecified trimester Ⓜ♀

✓6ᵗʰ **O30.04** Twin pregnancy, dichorionic/diamniotic
Twin pregnancy, two placentae, two amniotic sacs

O30.041 Twin pregnancy, dichorionic/diamniotic, first trimester Ⓜ♀

O30.042 Twin pregnancy, dichorionic/diamniotic, second trimester Ⓜ♀

O30.043 Twin pregnancy, dichorionic/diamniotic, third trimester Ⓜ♀

O30.049 Twin pregnancy, dichorionic/diamniotic, unspecified trimester Ⓜ♀

✓6ᵗʰ **O30.09** Twin pregnancy, unable to determine number of placenta and number of amniotic sacs

O30.091 Twin pregnancy, unable to determine number of placenta and number of amniotic sacs, first trimester Ⓜ♀

O30.092 Twin pregnancy, unable to determine number of placenta and number of amniotic sacs, second trimester Ⓜ♀

O30.093 Twin pregnancy, unable to determine number of placenta and number of amniotic sacs, third trimester Ⓜ♀

O30.099 Twin pregnancy, unable to determine number of placenta and number of amniotic sacs, unspecified trimester Ⓜ♀

✓5ᵗʰ **O30.1** Triplet pregnancy

✓6ᵗʰ **O30.10** Triplet pregnancy, unspecified number of placenta and unspecified number of amniotic sacs

O30.101 Triplet pregnancy, unspecified number of placenta and unspecified number of amniotic sacs, first trimester CC Ⓜ♀

O30.102 Triplet pregnancy, unspecified number of placenta and unspecified number of amniotic sacs, second trimester CC Ⓜ♀

O30.103 Triplet pregnancy, unspecified number of placenta and unspecified number of amniotic sacs, third trimester CC Ⓜ♀

O30.109 Triplet pregnancy, unspecified number of placenta and unspecified number of amniotic sacs, unspecified trimester Ⓜ♀

✓6ᵗʰ **O30.11** Triplet pregnancy with two or more monochorionic fetuses

O30.111 Triplet pregnancy with two or more monochorionic fetuses, first trimester CC Ⓜ♀

O30.112 Triplet pregnancy with two or more monochorionic fetuses, second trimester CC Ⓜ♀

O30.113 Triplet pregnancy with two or more monochorionic fetuses, third trimester CC Ⓜ♀

O30.119 Triplet pregnancy with two or more monochorionic fetuses, unspecified trimester Ⓜ♀

✓6ᵗʰ **O30.12** Triplet pregnancy with two or more monoamniotic fetuses

O30.121 Triplet pregnancy with two or more monoamniotic fetuses, first trimester CC Ⓜ♀

O30.122 Triplet pregnancy with two or more monoamniotic fetuses, second trimester CC Ⓜ♀

O30.123 Triplet pregnancy with two or more monoamniotic fetuses, third trimester CC Ⓜ♀

O30.129 Triplet pregnancy with two or more monoamniotic fetuses, unspecified trimester Ⓜ♀

✓6ᵗʰ **O30.19** Triplet pregnancy, unable to determine number of placenta and number of amniotic sacs

O30.191 Triplet pregnancy, unable to determine number of placenta and number of amniotic sacs, first trimester CC Ⓜ♀

O30.192 Triplet pregnancy, unable to determine number of placenta and number of amniotic sacs, second trimester CC Ⓜ♀

O30.193 Triplet pregnancy, unable to determine number of placenta and number of amniotic sacs, third trimester CC Ⓜ♀

O30.199 Triplet pregnancy, unable to determine number of placenta and number of amniotic sacs, unspecified trimester Ⓜ♀

✓6ᵗʰ **O30.2** Quadruplet pregnancy

✓6ᵗʰ **O30.20** Quadruplet pregnancy, unspecified number of placenta and unspecified number of amniotic sacs

O30.201 Quadruplet pregnancy, unspecified number of placenta and unspecified number of amniotic sacs, first trimester CC Ⓜ♀

O30.202 Quadruplet pregnancy, unspecified number of placenta and unspecified number of amniotic sacs, second trimester CC Ⓜ♀

O30.203 Quadruplet pregnancy, unspecified number of placenta and unspecified number of amniotic sacs, third trimester CC Ⓜ♀

O30.209 Quadruplet pregnancy, unspecified number of placenta and unspecified number of amniotic sacs, unspecified trimester Ⓜ♀

✓6ᵗʰ **O30.21** Quadruplet pregnancy with two or more monochorionic fetuses

O30.211 Quadruplet pregnancy with two or more monochorionic fetuses, first trimester CC Ⓜ♀

O30.212 Quadruplet pregnancy with two or more monochorionic fetuses, second trimester CC Ⓜ♀

O30.213 Quadruplet pregnancy with two or more monochorionic fetuses, third trimester CC Ⓜ♀

O30.219 Quadruplet pregnancy with two or more monochorionic fetuses, unspecified trimester Ⓜ♀

✓6ᵗʰ **O30.22** Quadruplet pregnancy with two or more monoamniotic fetuses

O30.221 Quadruplet pregnancy with two or more monoamniotic fetuses, first trimester CC Ⓜ♀

O30.222 Quadruplet pregnancy with two or more monoamniotic fetuses, second trimester CC Ⓜ♀

O30.223 Quadruplet pregnancy with two or more monoamniotic fetuses, third trimester CC Ⓜ♀

Ⓝ Newborn: 0   Ⓟ Pediatric: 0-17   Ⓜ Maternity: 12-55   Ⓐ Adult: 15-124   MCC Major CC Condition   PDxMCC PDx acts as own MCC   CC CC Condition   PDxCC PDx acts as own CC

824   ICD-10-CM 2016

O30.229 Quadruplet pregnancy with two or more monoamniotic fetuses, **unspecified trimester** Ⓜ♀

✓6th **O30.29** Quadruplet pregnancy, **unable to determine number of placenta and number of amniotic sacs**

O30.291 Quadruplet pregnancy, unable to determine number of placenta and number of amniotic sacs, **first trimester** ⒸⒸⓂ♀

O30.292 Quadruplet pregnancy, unable to determine number of placenta and number of amniotic sacs, **second trimester** ⒸⒸⓂ♀

O30.293 Quadruplet pregnancy, unable to determine number of placenta and number of amniotic sacs, **third trimester** ⒸⒸⓂ♀

O30.299 Quadruplet pregnancy, unable to determine number of placenta and number of amniotic sacs, **unspecified trimester** ⓂⓂ♀

✓5th **O30.8** Other **specified multiple gestation**
Multiple gestation pregnancy greater than quadruplets

✓6th **O30.80** Other specified multiple gestation, **unspecified number** of placenta and **unspecified number** of amniotic sacs

O30.801 Other specified multiple gestation, unspecified number of placenta and unspecified number of amniotic sacs, **first trimester** ⒸⒸⓂ♀

O30.802 Other specified multiple gestation, unspecified number of placenta and unspecified number of amniotic sacs, **second trimester** ⒸⒸⓂ♀

O30.803 Other specified multiple gestation, unspecified number of placenta and unspecified number of amniotic sacs, **third trimester** ⒸⒸⓂ♀

O30.809 Other specified multiple gestation, unspecified number of placenta and unspecified number of amniotic sacs, **unspecified trimester** ⓂⓂ♀

✓6th **O30.81** Other specified multiple gestation with **two or more monochorionic fetuses**

O30.811 Other specified multiple gestation with two or more monochorionic fetuses, **first trimester** ⒸⒸⓂ♀

O30.812 Other specified multiple gestation with two or more monochorionic fetuses, **second trimester** ⒸⒸⓂ♀

O30.813 Other specified multiple gestation with two or more monochorionic fetuses, **third trimester** ⒸⒸⓂ♀

O30.819 Other specified multiple gestation with two or more monochorionic fetuses, **unspecified trimester** ⓂⓂ♀

✓6th **O30.82** Other specified multiple gestation with **two or more monoamniotic fetuses**

O30.821 Other specified multiple gestation with two or more monoamniotic fetuses, **first trimester** ⒸⒸⓂ♀

O30.822 Other specified multiple gestation with two or more monoamniotic fetuses, **second trimester** ⒸⒸⓂ♀

O30.823 Other specified multiple gestation with two or more monoamniotic fetuses, **third trimester** ⒸⒸⓂ♀

O30.829 Other specified multiple gestation with two or more monoamniotic fetuses, **unspecified trimester** ⓂⓂ♀

✓6th **O30.89** Other **specified multiple gestation, unable to determine number** of placenta and number of amniotic sacs

O30.891 Other specified multiple gestation, unable to determine number of placenta and number of amniotic sacs, **first trimester** ⒸⒸⓂ♀

O30.892 Other specified multiple gestation, unable to determine number of placenta and number of amniotic sacs, **second trimester** ⒸⒸⓂ♀

O30.893 Other specified multiple gestation, unable to determine number of placenta and number of amniotic sacs, **third trimester** ⒸⒸⓂ♀

O30.899 Other specified multiple gestation, unable to determine number of placenta and number of amniotic sacs, **unspecified trimester** ⓂⓂ♀

✓5th **O30.9** Multiple **gestation, unspecified**
Multiple pregnancy NOS

O30.90 Multiple gestation, unspecified, **unspecified trimester** ⓂⓂ♀

O30.91 Multiple gestation, unspecified, **first trimester** ⓂⓂ♀

O30.92 Multiple gestation, unspecified, **second trimester** ⓂⓂ♀

O30.93 Multiple gestation, unspecified, **third trimester** ⓂⓂ♀

✓4th **O31** **Complications specific to multiple gestation**

EXCLUDES 2 *delayed delivery of second twin, triplet, etc. (O63.2)*
malpresentation of one fetus or more (O32.9)
placental transfusion syndromes (O43.0-)

AHA: 2012, 4Q, 107

One of the following 7th characters is to be assigned to each code under category O31. 7th character 0 is for single gestations and multiple gestations where the fetus is unspecified. 7th characters 1 through 9 are for cases of multiple gestations to identify the fetus for which the code applies. The appropriate code from category O30, Multiple gestation, must also be assigned when assigning a code from category O31 that has a 7th character of 1 through 9.

0	not applicable or unspecified	3	fetus 3
		4	fetus 4
1	fetus 1	5	fetus 5
2	fetus 2	9	other fetus

✓5th **O31.0** **Papyraceous fetus**
Fetus compressus

✓x7th **O31.00** **Papyraceous fetus, unspecified trimester** ⓂⓂ♀

✓x7th **O31.01** **Papyraceous fetus, first trimester** ⓂⓂ♀

✓x7th **O31.02** **Papyraceous fetus, second trimester** ⓂⓂ♀

✓x7th **O31.03** **Papyraceous fetus, third trimester** ⓂⓂ♀

✓5th **O31.1** **Continuing pregnancy after spontaneous abortion of one fetus or more**

✓x7th **O31.10** **Continuing pregnancy after spontaneous abortion of one fetus or more, unspecified trimester** ⓂⓂ♀

✓x7th **O31.11** **Continuing pregnancy after spontaneous abortion of one fetus or more, first trimester** ⓂⓂ♀

✓x7th **O31.12** **Continuing pregnancy after spontaneous abortion of one fetus or more, second trimester** ⓂⓂ♀

✓x7th **O31.13** **Continuing pregnancy after spontaneous abortion of one fetus or more, third trimester** ⓂⓂ♀

✓5th **O31.2** **Continuing pregnancy after intrauterine death of one fetus or more**

✓x7th **O31.20** **Continuing pregnancy after intrauterine death of one fetus or more, unspecified trimester** ⓂⓂ♀

✓x7th **O31.21** **Continuing pregnancy after intrauterine death of one fetus or more, first trimester** ⓂⓂ♀

✓x7th **O31.22** **Continuing pregnancy after intrauterine death of one fetus or more, second trimester** ⓂⓂ♀

✓x7th **O31.23** **Continuing pregnancy after intrauterine death of one fetus or more, third trimester** ⓂⓂ♀

✓5th **O31.3** **Continuing pregnancy after elective fetal reduction of one fetus or more**
Continuing pregnancy after selective termination of one fetus or more

✓x7th **O31.30** **Continuing pregnancy after elective fetal reduction of one fetus or more, unspecified trimester** ⓂⓂ♀

✓x7th **O31.31** **Continuing pregnancy after elective fetal reduction of one fetus or more, first trimester** ⓂⓂ♀

✓x7th **O31.32** **Continuing pregnancy after elective fetal reduction of one fetus or more, second trimester** ⓂⓂ♀

✓x7th **O31.33** **Continuing pregnancy after elective fetal reduction of one fetus or more, third trimester** ⓂⓂ♀

✓ Additional Character Required   ✓x7th Placeholder Alert   Unacceptable PDx   Manifestation   Hospital Acquired Condition   *EXCLUDES 1* Not Coded Here   *EXCLUDES 2* Not Included Here

ICD-10-CM 2016   825

√5ᵗʰ **O31.8 Other complications specific to multiple gestation**

√6ᵗʰ **O31.8X Other complications specific to multiple gestation**

> **CC Excl: For CC codes in subcategory O31.8X, unless otherwise noted:** See code: O30

√7ᵗʰ **O31.8X1 Other complications specific to multiple gestation, first trimester** CC M♀

√7ᵗʰ **O31.8X2 Other complications specific to multiple gestation, second trimester** CC M♀

√7ᵗʰ **O31.8X3 Other complications specific to multiple gestation, third trimester** CC M♀

√7ᵗʰ **O31.8X9 Other complications specific to multiple gestation, unspecified trimester** M♀

√4ᵗʰ **O32 Maternal care for malpresentation of fetus**
> INCLUDES the listed conditions as a reason for observation, hospitalization or other obstetric care of the mother, or for cesarean delivery before onset of labor
> EXCLUDES1 malpresentation of fetus with obstructed labor (O64.-)
> **AHA:** 2012, 4Q, 107

> One of the following 7th characters is to be assigned to each code under category O32. 7th character Ø is for single gestations and multiple gestations where the fetus is unspecified. 7th characters 1 through 9 are for cases of multiple gestations to identify the fetus for which the code applies. The appropriate code from category O30, Multiple gestation, must also be assigned when assigning a code from category O32 that has a 7th character of 1 through 9.
>
> | | | | |
> |---|---|---|---|
> | Ø | not applicable or unspecified | 3 | fetus 3 |
> | | | 4 | fetus 4 |
> | 1 | fetus 1 | 5 | fetus 5 |
> | 2 | fetus 2 | 9 | other fetus |

√x7ᵗʰ **O32.0 Maternal care for unstable lie** M♀

√x7ᵗʰ **O32.1 Maternal care for breech presentation** M♀
> Maternal care for buttocks presentation
> Maternal care for complete breech
> Maternal care for frank breech
> > EXCLUDES1 footling presentation (O32.8)
> > incomplete breech (O32.8)

√x7ᵗʰ **O32.2 Maternal care for transverse and oblique lie** M♀
> Maternal care for oblique presentation
> Maternal care for transverse presentation

√x7ᵗʰ **O32.3 Maternal care for face, brow and chin presentation** M♀

√x7ᵗʰ **O32.4 Maternal care for high head at term** M♀
> Maternal care for failure of head to enter pelvic brim

√x7ᵗʰ **O32.6 Maternal care for compound presentation** M♀

√x7ᵗʰ **O32.8 Maternal care for other malpresentation of fetus** M♀
> Maternal care for footling presentation
> Maternal care for incomplete breech

√x7ᵗʰ **O32.9 Maternal care for malpresentation of fetus, unspecified** M♀

√4ᵗʰ **O33 Maternal care for disproportion**
> INCLUDES the listed conditions as a reason for observation, hospitalization or other obstetric care of the mother, or for cesarean delivery before onset of labor
> EXCLUDES1 disproportion with obstructed labor (O65-O66)

O33.0 Maternal care for disproportion due to deformity of maternal pelvic bones CC M♀
> Maternal care for disproportion due to pelvic deformity causing disproportion NOS
> **CC Excl:** O33.0

O33.1 Maternal care for disproportion due to generally contracted pelvis M♀
> Maternal care for disproportion due to contracted pelvis NOS causing disproportion

O33.2 Maternal care for disproportion due to inlet contraction of pelvis M♀
> Maternal care for disproportion due to inlet contraction (pelvis) causing disproportion

√x7ᵗʰ **O33.3 Maternal care for disproportion due to outlet contraction of pelvis** M♀
> Maternal care for disproportion due to mid-cavity contraction (pelvis)
> Maternal care for disproportion due to outlet contraction (pelvis)

> One of the following 7th characters is to be assigned to code O33.3. 7th character Ø is for single gestations and multiple gestations where the fetus is unspecified. 7th characters 1 through 9 are for cases of multiple gestations to identify the fetus for which the code applies. The appropriate code from category O30, Multiple gestation, must also be assigned when assigning code O33.3 with a 7th character of 1 through 9.
>
> | | | | |
> |---|---|---|---|
> | Ø | not applicable or unspecified | 3 | fetus 3 |
> | | | 4 | fetus 4 |
> | 1 | fetus 1 | 5 | fetus 5 |
> | 2 | fetus 2 | 9 | other fetus |

√x7ᵗʰ **O33.4 Maternal care for disproportion of mixed maternal and fetal origin** M♀

> One of the following 7th characters is to be assigned to code O33.4. 7th character Ø is for single gestations and multiple gestations where the fetus is unspecified. 7th characters 1 through 9 are for cases of multiple gestations to identify the fetus for which the code applies. The appropriate code from category O30, Multiple gestation, must also be assigned when assigning code O33.4 with a 7th character of 1 through 9.
>
> | | | | |
> |---|---|---|---|
> | Ø | not applicable or unspecified | 3 | fetus 3 |
> | | | 4 | fetus 4 |
> | 1 | fetus 1 | 5 | fetus 5 |
> | 2 | fetus 2 | 9 | other fetus |

√x7ᵗʰ **O33.5 Maternal care for disproportion due to unusually large fetus** M♀
> Maternal care for disproportion due to disproportion of fetal origin with normally formed fetus
> Maternal care for disproportion due to fetal disproportion NOS

> One of the following 7th characters is to be assigned to code O33.5. 7th character Ø is for single gestations and multiple gestations where the fetus is unspecified. 7th characters 1 through 9 are for cases of multiple gestations to identify the fetus for which the code applies. The appropriate code from category O30, Multiple gestation, must also be assigned when assigning code O33.5 with a 7th character of 1 through 9.
>
> | | | | |
> |---|---|---|---|
> | Ø | not applicable or unspecified | 3 | fetus 3 |
> | | | 4 | fetus 4 |
> | 1 | fetus 1 | 5 | fetus 5 |
> | 2 | fetus 2 | 9 | other fetus |

√x7ᵗʰ **O33.6 Maternal care for disproportion due to hydrocephalic fetus** M♀

> One of the following 7th characters is to be assigned to code O33.6. 7th character Ø is for single gestations and multiple gestations where the fetus is unspecified. 7th characters 1 through 9 are for cases of multiple gestations to identify the fetus for which the code applies. The appropriate code from category O30, Multiple gestation, must also be assigned when assigning code O33.6 with a 7th character of 1 through 9.
>
> | | | | |
> |---|---|---|---|
> | Ø | not applicable or unspecified | 3 | fetus 3 |
> | | | 4 | fetus 4 |
> | 1 | fetus 1 | 5 | fetus 5 |
> | 2 | fetus 2 | 9 | other fetus |

O33.7 Maternal care for disproportion due to other fetal deformities M♀
> Maternal care for disproportion due to fetal ascites
> Maternal care for disproportion due to fetal hydrops
> Maternal care for disproportion due to fetal meningomyelocele
> Maternal care for disproportion due to fetal sacral teratoma
> Maternal care for disproportion due to fetal tumor
> > EXCLUDES1 obstructed labor due to other fetal deformities (O66.3)

O33.8 Maternal care for disproportion of other origin M♀

O33.9 Maternal care for disproportion, unspecified M♀
> Maternal care for disproportion due to cephalopelvic disproportion NOS
> Maternal care for disproportion due to fetopelvic disproportion NOS

N Newborn: 0   P Pediatric: 0-17   M Maternity: 12-55   A Adult: 15-124   MCC Major CC Condition   PDxMCC PDx acts as own MCC   CC CC Condition   PDxCC PDx acts as own CC

826

ICD-10-CM 2016

✓4ᵗʰ O34　Maternal care for abnormality of pelvic organs

> **INCLUDES**　the listed conditions as a reason for hospitalization or other obstetric care of the mother, or for cesarean delivery before onset of labor
> Code first any associated obstructed labor (O65.5)
> Use additional code for specific condition

✓5ᵗʰ O34.0　Maternal care for congenital malformation of uterus

O34.00　Maternal care for unspecified congenital malformation of uterus, unspecified trimester　Ⓜ♀

O34.01　Maternal care for unspecified congenital malformation of uterus, first trimester　Ⓜ♀

O34.02　Maternal care for unspecified congenital malformation of uterus, second trimester　Ⓜ♀

O34.03　Maternal care for unspecified congenital malformation of uterus, third trimester　Ⓜ♀

✓5ᵗʰ O34.1　Maternal care for benign tumor of corpus uteri

> **EXCLUDES 2**　maternal care for benign tumor of cervix (O34.4-)
> maternal care for malignant neoplasm of uterus (O9A.1-)

O34.10　Maternal care for benign tumor of corpus uteri, unspecified trimester　Ⓜ♀

O34.11　Maternal care for benign tumor of corpus uteri, first trimester　Ⓜ♀

O34.12　Maternal care for benign tumor of corpus uteri, second trimester　Ⓜ♀

O34.13　Maternal care for benign tumor of corpus uteri, third trimester　Ⓜ♀

✓5ᵗʰ O34.2　Maternal care due to uterine scar from previous surgery

O34.21　Maternal care for scar from previous cesarean delivery　Ⓜ♀

O34.29　Maternal care due to uterine scar from other previous surgery　Ⓜ♀

✓5ᵗʰ O34.3　Maternal care for cervical incompetence

Maternal care for cerclage with or without cervical incompetence
Maternal care for Shirodkar suture with or without cervical incompetence

> **CC Excl: For MCC codes in subcategory O34.3, unless otherwise noted:** O26.872-O26.879, O34.31-O34.33

O34.30　Maternal care for cervical incompetence, unspecified trimester　Ⓜ♀

O34.31　Maternal care for cervical incompetence, first trimester　MCC Ⓜ♀

O34.32　Maternal care for cervical incompetence, second trimester　MCC Ⓜ♀

O34.33　Maternal care for cervical incompetence, third trimester　MCC Ⓜ♀

✓5ᵗʰ O34.4　Maternal care for other abnormalities of cervix

O34.40　Maternal care for other abnormalities of cervix, unspecified trimester　Ⓜ♀

O34.41　Maternal care for other abnormalities of cervix, first trimester　Ⓜ♀

O34.42　Maternal care for other abnormalities of cervix, second trimester　Ⓜ♀

O34.43　Maternal care for other abnormalities of cervix, third trimester　Ⓜ♀

✓5ᵗʰ O34.5　Maternal care for other abnormalities of gravid uterus

✓6ᵗʰ O34.51　Maternal care for incarceration of gravid uterus

O34.511　Maternal care for incarceration of gravid uterus, first trimester　Ⓜ♀

O34.512　Maternal care for incarceration of gravid uterus, second trimester　Ⓜ♀

O34.513　Maternal care for incarceration of gravid uterus, third trimester　Ⓜ♀

O34.519　Maternal care for incarceration of gravid uterus, unspecified trimester　Ⓜ♀

✓6ᵗʰ O34.52　Maternal care for prolapse of gravid uterus

O34.521　Maternal care for prolapse of gravid uterus, first trimester　Ⓜ♀

O34.522　Maternal care for prolapse of gravid uterus, second trimester　Ⓜ♀

O34.523　Maternal care for prolapse of gravid uterus, third trimester　Ⓜ♀

O34.529　Maternal care for prolapse of gravid uterus, unspecified trimester　Ⓜ♀

✓6ᵗʰ O34.53　Maternal care for retroversion of gravid uterus

O34.531　Maternal care for retroversion of gravid uterus, first trimester　Ⓜ♀

O34.532　Maternal care for retroversion of gravid uterus, second trimester　Ⓜ♀

O34.533　Maternal care for retroversion of gravid uterus, third trimester　Ⓜ♀

O34.539　Maternal care for retroversion of gravid uterus, unspecified trimester　Ⓜ♀

✓6ᵗʰ O34.59　Maternal care for other abnormalities of gravid uterus

O34.591　Maternal care for other abnormalities of gravid uterus, first trimester　Ⓜ♀

O34.592　Maternal care for other abnormalities of gravid uterus, second trimester　Ⓜ♀

O34.593　Maternal care for other abnormalities of gravid uterus, third trimester　Ⓜ♀

O34.599　Maternal care for other abnormalities of gravid uterus, unspecified trimester　Ⓜ♀

✓5ᵗʰ O34.6　Maternal care for abnormality of vagina

> **EXCLUDES 2**　maternal care for vaginal varices in pregnancy (O22.1-)

O34.60　Maternal care for abnormality of vagina, unspecified trimester　Ⓜ♀

O34.61　Maternal care for abnormality of vagina, first trimester　Ⓜ♀

O34.62　Maternal care for abnormality of vagina, second trimester　Ⓜ♀

O34.63　Maternal care for abnormality of vagina, third trimester　Ⓜ♀

✓5ᵗʰ O34.7　Maternal care for abnormality of vulva and perineum

> **EXCLUDES 2**　maternal care for perineal and vulval varices in pregnancy (O22.1-)

O34.70　Maternal care for abnormality of vulva and perineum, unspecified trimester　Ⓜ♀

O34.71　Maternal care for abnormality of vulva and perineum, first trimester　Ⓜ♀

O34.72　Maternal care for abnormality of vulva and perineum, second trimester　Ⓜ♀

O34.73　Maternal care for abnormality of vulva and perineum, third trimester　Ⓜ♀

✓5ᵗʰ O34.8　Maternal care for other abnormalities of pelvic organs

O34.80　Maternal care for other abnormalities of pelvic organs, unspecified trimester　Ⓜ♀

O34.81　Maternal care for other abnormalities of pelvic organs, first trimester　Ⓜ♀

O34.82　Maternal care for other abnormalities of pelvic organs, second trimester　Ⓜ♀

O34.83　Maternal care for other abnormalities of pelvic organs, third trimester　Ⓜ♀

✓5ᵗʰ O34.9　Maternal care for abnormality of pelvic organ, unspecified

O34.90　Maternal care for abnormality of pelvic organ, unspecified, unspecified trimester　Ⓜ♀

O34.91　Maternal care for abnormality of pelvic organ, unspecified, first trimester　Ⓜ♀

O34.92　Maternal care for abnormality of pelvic organ, unspecified, second trimester　Ⓜ♀

O34.93　Maternal care for abnormality of pelvic organ, unspecified, third trimester　Ⓜ♀

✔ Additional Character Required　✔x7ᵗʰ Placeholder Alert　Unacceptable PDx　Manifestation　Hospital Acquired Condition　**EXCLUDES 1** Not Coded Here　**EXCLUDES 2** Not Included Here

ICD-10-CM 2016　　　　　827

Chapter 15. Pregnancy, Childbirth, and the Puerperium

✓4th O35 Maternal care for known or suspected fetal abnormality and damage

INCLUDES the listed conditions in the fetus as a reason for hospitalization or other obstetric care to the mother, or for termination of pregnancy

Code also any associated maternal condition

EXCLUDES 1 encounter for suspected maternal and fetal conditions ruled out (Z03.7-)

One of the following 7th characters is to be assigned to each code under category O35. 7th character 0 is for single gestations and multiple gestations where the fetus is unspecified. 7th characters 1 through 9 are for cases of multiple gestations to identify the fetus for which the code applies. The appropriate code from category O30, Multiple gestation, must also be assigned when assigning a code from category O35 that has a 7th character of 1 through 9.

0	not applicable or unspecified	3	fetus 3
		4	fetus 4
1	fetus 1	5	fetus 5
2	fetus 2	9	other fetus

✓x7th O35.0 Maternal care for (suspected) central nervous system malformation in fetus   M♀
Maternal care for fetal anencephaly
Maternal care for fetal hydrocephalus
Maternal care for fetal spina bifida
    EXCLUDES 2 chromosomal abnormality in fetus (O35.1)

✓x7th O35.1 Maternal care for (suspected) chromosomal abnormality in fetus   M♀

✓x7th O35.2 Maternal care for (suspected) hereditary disease in fetus   M♀
    EXCLUDES 2 chromosomal abnormality in fetus (O35.1)

✓x7th O35.3 Maternal care for (suspected) damage to fetus from viral disease in mother   M♀
Maternal care for damage to fetus from maternal cytomegalovirus infection
Maternal care for damage to fetus from maternal rubella

✓x7th O35.4 Maternal care for (suspected) damage to fetus from alcohol   M♀

✓x7th O35.5 Maternal care for (suspected) damage to fetus by drugs   M♀
Maternal care for damage to fetus from drug addiction

✓x7th O35.6 Maternal care for (suspected) damage to fetus by radiation   M♀

✓x7th O35.7 Maternal care for (suspected) damage to fetus by other medical procedures   M♀
Maternal care for damage to fetus by amniocentesis
Maternal care for damage to fetus by biopsy procedures
Maternal care for damage to fetus by hematological investigation
Maternal care for damage to fetus by intrauterine contraceptive device
Maternal care for damage to fetus by intrauterine surgery

✓x7th O35.8 Maternal care for other (suspected) fetal abnormality and damage   M♀
Maternal care for damage to fetus from maternal listeriosis
Maternal care for damage to fetus from maternal toxoplasmosis

✓x7th O35.9 Maternal care for (suspected) fetal abnormality and damage, unspecified   M♀

✓4th O36 Maternal care for other fetal problems

INCLUDES the listed conditions in the fetus as a reason for hospitalization or other obstetric care of the mother, or for termination of pregnancy

EXCLUDES 1 encounter for suspected maternal and fetal conditions ruled out (Z03.7-)
    placental transfusion syndromes (O43.0-)

EXCLUDES 2 labor and delivery complicated by fetal stress (O77.-)

One of the following 7th characters is to be assigned to each code under category O36. 7th character 0 is for single gestations and multiple gestations where the fetus is unspecified. 7th characters 1 through 9 are for cases of multiple gestations to identify the fetus for which the code applies. The appropriate code from category O30, Multiple gestation, must also be assigned when assigning a code from category O36 that has a 7th character of 1 through 9.

0	not applicable or unspecified	3	fetus 3
		4	fetus 4
1	fetus 1	5	fetus 5
2	fetus 2	9	other fetus

✓5th O36.0 Maternal care for rhesus isoimmunization
Maternal care for Rh incompatibility (with hydrops fetalis)

CC Excl: For CC codes in subcategory O36.0, unless otherwise noted: O36.0110-O36.0139, O36.0910-O36.0939

✓6th O36.01 Maternal care for anti-D [Rh] antibodies
AHA: 2014, 4Q, 17

✓7th O36.011 Maternal care for anti-D [Rh] antibodies, first trimester   CC M♀

✓7th O36.012 Maternal care for anti-D [Rh] antibodies, second trimester   CC M♀

✓7th O36.013 Maternal care for anti-D [Rh] antibodies, third trimester   CC M♀

✓7th O36.019 Maternal care for anti-D [Rh] antibodies, unspecified trimester   M♀

✓6th O36.09 Maternal care for other rhesus isoimmunization

✓7th O36.091 Maternal care for other rhesus isoimmunization, first trimester   CC M♀

✓7th O36.092 Maternal care for other rhesus isoimmunization, second trimester   CC M♀

✓7th O36.093 Maternal care for other rhesus isoimmunization, third trimester   CC M♀

✓7th O36.099 Maternal care for other rhesus isoimmunization, unspecified trimester   M♀

✓5th O36.1 Maternal care for other isoimmunization
Maternal care for ABO isoimmunization

✓6th O36.11 Maternal care for Anti-A sensitization
Maternal care for isoimmunization NOS (with hydrops fetalis)

✓7th O36.111 Maternal care for Anti-A sensitization, first trimester   M♀

✓7th O36.112 Maternal care for Anti-A sensitization, second trimester   M♀

✓7th O36.113 Maternal care for Anti-A sensitization, third trimester   M♀

✓7th O36.119 Maternal care for Anti-A sensitization, unspecified trimester   M♀

✓6th O36.19 Maternal care for other isoimmunization
Maternal care for Anti-B sensitization

✓7th O36.191 Maternal care for other isoimmunization, first trimester   M♀

✓7th O36.192 Maternal care for other isoimmunization, second trimester   M♀

✓7th O36.193 Maternal care for other isoimmunization, third trimester   M♀

✓7th O36.199 Maternal care for other isoimmunization, unspecified trimester   M♀

✓5th O36.2 Maternal care for hydrops fetalis
Maternal care for hydrops fetalis NOS
Maternal care for hydrops fetalis not associated with isoimmunization

EXCLUDES 1 hydrops fetalis associated with ABO isoimmunization (O36.1-)
    hydrops fetalis associated with rhesus isoimmunization (O36.0-)

✓x7th O36.20 Maternal care for hydrops fetalis, unspecified trimester   M♀

N Newborn: 0 P Pediatric: 0-17 M Maternity: 12-55 A Adult: 15-124 MCC Major CC Condition PDxMCC PDx acts as own MCC CC CC Condition PDxCC PDx acts as own CC

828   ICD-10-CM 2016

☑x7ᵗʰ **O36.21** **Maternal care for hydrops fetalis, first** M♀
trimester

☑x7ᵗʰ **O36.22** **Maternal care for hydrops fetalis, second** M♀
trimester

☑x7ᵗʰ **O36.23** **Maternal care for hydrops fetalis, third** M♀
trimester

☑x7ᵗʰ **O36.4** **Maternal care for intrauterine death** CC M♀
Maternal care for intrauterine fetal death NOS
Maternal care for intrauterine fetal death after completion of 20
weeks of gestation
Maternal care for late fetal death
Maternal care for missed delivery
EXCLUDES 1 *missed abortion (O02.1)*
stillbirth (P95)
CC Excl: O36.4XX0–O36.4XX9

☑5ᵗʰ **O36.5** **Maternal care for known or suspected poor fetal growth**

> **CC Excl: For CC codes in subcategory O36.5, unless**
> **otherwise noted:** O36.5110–O36.5139, O36.5910–
> O36.5939

☑6ᵗʰ **O36.51** **Maternal care for known or suspected placental**
insufficiency

☑7ᵗʰ **O36.511** **Maternal care for known or** M♀
suspected placental insufficiency, first
trimester

☑7ᵗʰ **O36.512** **Maternal care for known or** M♀
suspected placental insufficiency, second
trimester

☑7ᵗʰ **O36.513** **Maternal care for known or** M♀
suspected placental insufficiency, third
trimester

☑7ᵗʰ **O36.519** **Maternal care for known or suspected** M♀
placental insufficiency, unspecified
trimester

☑6ᵗʰ **O36.59** **Maternal care for other known or suspected poor**
fetal growth
Maternal care for known or suspected light-for-dates
NOS
Maternal care for known or suspected small-for-dates
NOS

☑7ᵗʰ **O36.591** **Maternal care for other known or** M♀
suspected poor fetal growth, first
trimester

☑7ᵗʰ **O36.592** **Maternal care for other known or** M♀
suspected poor fetal growth, second
trimester

☑7ᵗʰ **O36.593** **Maternal care for other known or** M♀
suspected poor fetal growth, third
trimester

☑7ᵗʰ **O36.599** **Maternal care for other known or** M♀
suspected poor fetal growth,
unspecified trimester

☑5ᵗʰ **O36.6** **Maternal care for excessive fetal growth**
Maternal care for known or suspected large-for-dates

☑x7ᵗʰ **O36.60** **Maternal care for excessive fetal growth,** M♀
unspecified trimester

☑x7ᵗʰ **O36.61** **Maternal care for excessive fetal growth,** M♀
first trimester

☑x7ᵗʰ **O36.62** **Maternal care for excessive fetal growth,** M♀
second trimester

☑x7ᵗʰ **O36.63** **Maternal care for excessive fetal growth,** M♀
third trimester

☑5ᵗʰ **O36.7** **Maternal care for viable fetus in abdominal pregnancy**

☑x7ᵗʰ **O36.70** **Maternal care for viable fetus in abdominal** M♀
pregnancy, unspecified trimester

☑x7ᵗʰ **O36.71** **Maternal care for viable fetus in abdominal** M♀
pregnancy, first trimester

☑x7ᵗʰ **O36.72** **Maternal care for viable fetus in abdominal** M♀
pregnancy, second trimester

☑x7ᵗʰ **O36.73** **Maternal care for viable fetus in abdominal** M♀
pregnancy, third trimester

☑5ᵗʰ **O36.8** **Maternal care for other specified fetal problems**

☑x7ᵗʰ **O36.80** **Pregnancy with inconclusive fetal viability** M♀
Encounter to determine fetal viability of pregnancy

☑6ᵗʰ **O36.81** **Decreased fetal movements**

☑7ᵗʰ **O36.812** **Decreased fetal movements, second** M♀
trimester

☑7ᵗʰ **O36.813** **Decreased fetal movements, third** M♀
trimester

☑7ᵗʰ **O36.819** **Decreased fetal movements,** M♀
unspecified trimester

☑6ᵗʰ **O36.82** **Fetal anemia and thrombocytopenia**

☑7ᵗʰ **O36.821** **Fetal anemia and thrombocytopenia,** M♀
first trimester

☑7ᵗʰ **O36.822** **Fetal anemia and thrombocytopenia,** M♀
second trimester

☑7ᵗʰ **O36.823** **Fetal anemia and thrombocytopenia,** M♀
third trimester

☑7ᵗʰ **O36.829** **Fetal anemia and thrombocytopenia,** M♀
unspecified trimester

☑6ᵗʰ **O36.89** **Maternal care for other specified fetal problems**

☑7ᵗʰ **O36.891** **Maternal care for other specified fetal** M♀
problems, first trimester

☑7ᵗʰ **O36.892** **Maternal care for other specified fetal** M♀
problems, second trimester

☑7ᵗʰ **O36.893** **Maternal care for other specified fetal** M♀
problems, third trimester

☑7ᵗʰ **O36.899** **Maternal care for other specified fetal** M♀
problems, unspecified trimester

☑5ᵗʰ **O36.9** **Maternal care for fetal problem, unspecified**

☑x7ᵗʰ **O36.90** **Maternal care for fetal problem, unspecified,** M♀
unspecified trimester

☑x7ᵗʰ **O36.91** **Maternal care for fetal problem, unspecified,** M♀
first trimester

☑x7ᵗʰ **O36.92** **Maternal care for fetal problem, unspecified,** M♀
second trimester

☑x7ᵗʰ **O36.93** **Maternal care for fetal problem, unspecified,** M♀
third trimester

☑4ᵗʰ **O40** **Polyhydramnios**
INCLUDES   Hydramnios
EXCLUDES 1 *encounter for suspected maternal and fetal conditions ruled out*
(Z03.7-)

> One of the following 7th characters is to be assigned to each code
> under category O40. 7th character 0 is for single gestations and
> multiple gestations where the fetus is unspecified. 7th characters 1
> through 9 are for cases of multiple gestations to identify the fetus
> for which the code applies. The appropriate code from category
> O30, Multiple gestation, must also be assigned when assigning a
> code from category O40 that has a 7th character of 1 through 9.
> | 0 | not applicable or | 3 | fetus 3 |
> | | unspecified | 4 | fetus 4 |
> | 1 | fetus 1 | 5 | fetus 5 |
> | 2 | fetus 2 | 9 | other fetus |

☑x7ᵗʰ **O40.1** **Polyhydramnios, first trimester** M♀

☑x7ᵗʰ **O40.2** **Polyhydramnios, second trimester** M♀

☑x7ᵗʰ **O40.3** **Polyhydramnios, third trimester** M♀

☑x7ᵗʰ **O40.9** **Polyhydramnios, unspecified trimester** M♀

☑4ᵗʰ **O41** **Other disorders of amniotic fluid and membranes**
EXCLUDES 1 *encounter for suspected maternal and fetal conditions ruled out*
(Z03.7-)

> One of the following 7th characters is to be assigned to each code
> under category O41. 7th character 0 is for single gestations and
> multiple gestations where the fetus is unspecified. 7th characters 1
> through 9 are for cases of multiple gestations to identify the fetus
> for which the code applies. The appropriate code from category
> O30, Multiple gestation, must also be assigned when assigning a
> code from category O41 that has a 7th character of 1 through 9.
> | 0 | not applicable or | 3 | fetus 3 |
> | | unspecified | 4 | fetus 4 |
> | 1 | fetus 1 | 5 | fetus 5 |
> | 2 | fetus 2 | 9 | other fetus |

☑5ᵗʰ **O41.0** **Oligohydramnios**
Oligohydramnios without rupture of membranes

> **CC Excl: For CC codes in subcategory O41.0, unless**
> **otherwise noted:** O41.01X0–O41.03X9

☑x7ᵗʰ **O41.00** **Oligohydramnios, unspecified trimester** M♀

☑x7ᵗʰ **O41.01** **Oligohydramnios, first trimester** CC M♀

☑x7ᵗʰ **O41.02** **Oligohydramnios, second trimester** CC M♀

☑x7ᵗʰ **O41.03** **Oligohydramnios, third trimester** CC M♀

☑ Additional Character Required   ☑x7ᵗʰ Placeholder Alert   Unacceptable PDx   Manifestation   Hospital Acquired Condition   EXCLUDES 1 Not Coded Here   EXCLUDES 2 Not Included Here

ICD-10-CM 2016

829

✓5th O41.1 Infection of amniotic sac and membranes

> **CC Excl: For MCC codes in subcategory O41.1, unless otherwise noted:** O41.1010-O41.1039, O41.1210-O41.1239, O41.1410-O41.1439

- **✓6th O41.10 Infection of amniotic sac and membranes, unspecified**
  - **✓7th O41.101 Infection of amniotic sac and membranes, unspecified, first trimester** MCC M♀
  - **✓7th O41.102 Infection of amniotic sac and membranes, unspecified, second trimester** MCC M♀
  - **✓7th O41.103 Infection of amniotic sac and membranes, unspecified, third trimester** MCC M♀
  - **✓7th O41.109 Infection of amniotic sac and membranes, unspecified, unspecified trimester** M♀
- **✓6th O41.12 Chorioamnionitis**
  - **✓7th O41.121 Chorioamnionitis, first trimester** MCC M♀
  - **✓7th O41.122 Chorioamnionitis, second trimester** MCC M♀
  - **✓7th O41.123 Chorioamnionitis, third trimester** MCC M♀
  - **✓7th O41.129 Chorioamnionitis, unspecified trimester** M♀
- **✓6th O41.14 Placentitis**
  - **✓7th O41.141 Placentitis, first trimester** MCC M♀
  - **✓7th O41.142 Placentitis, second trimester** MCC M♀
  - **✓7th O41.143 Placentitis, third trimester** MCC M♀
  - **✓7th O41.149 Placentitis, unspecified trimester** M♀

✓5th O41.8 Other specified disorders of amniotic fluid and membranes

> **CC Excl: For CC codes in subcategory O41.8, unless otherwise noted:** O41.8X10-O41.8X39

- **✓6th O41.8X Other specified disorders of amniotic fluid and membranes**
  - **✓7th O41.8X1 Other specified disorders of amniotic fluid and membranes, first trimester** M♀
  - **✓7th O41.8X2 Other specified disorders of amniotic fluid and membranes, second trimester** M♀
  - **✓7th O41.8X3 Other specified disorders of amniotic fluid and membranes, third trimester** M♀
  - **✓7th O41.8X9 Other specified disorders of amniotic fluid and membranes, unspecified trimester** M♀

✓5th O41.9 Disorder of amniotic fluid and membranes, unspecified

- **✓x7th O41.90 Disorder of amniotic fluid and membranes, unspecified, unspecified trimester** M♀
- **✓x7th O41.91 Disorder of amniotic fluid and membranes, unspecified, first trimester** M♀
- **✓x7th O41.92 Disorder of amniotic fluid and membranes, unspecified, second trimester** M♀
- **✓x7th O41.93 Disorder of amniotic fluid and membranes, unspecified, third trimester** M♀

✓4th O42 Premature rupture of membranes

✓5th O42.0 Premature rupture of membranes, onset of labor within 24 hours of rupture

- **O42.00 Premature rupture of membranes, onset of labor within 24 hours of rupture, unspecified weeks of gestation** M♀
- **✓6th O42.01 Preterm premature rupture of membranes, onset of labor within 24 hours of rupture**
  Premature rupture of membranes before 37 completed weeks of gestation
  - **O42.011 Preterm premature rupture of membranes, onset of labor within 24 hours of rupture, first trimester** M♀
  - **O42.012 Preterm premature rupture of membranes, onset of labor within 24 hours of rupture, second trimester** M♀
  - **O42.013 Preterm premature rupture of membranes, onset of labor within 24 hours of rupture, third trimester** M♀

  - **O42.019 Preterm premature rupture of membranes, onset of labor within 24 hours of rupture, unspecified trimester** M♀
- **O42.02 Full-term premature rupture of membranes, onset of labor within 24 hours of rupture** M♀
  Premature rupture of membranes after 37 completed weeks of gestation

✓5th O42.1 Premature rupture of membranes, onset of labor more than 24 hours following rupture

- **O42.10 Premature rupture of membranes, onset of labor more than 24 hours following rupture, unspecified weeks of gestation** M♀
- **✓6th O42.11 Preterm premature rupture of membranes, onset of labor more than 24 hours following rupture**
  Premature rupture of membranes before 37 completed weeks of gestation
  - **O42.111 Preterm premature rupture of membranes, onset of labor more than 24 hours following rupture, first trimester** M♀
  - **O42.112 Preterm premature rupture of membranes, onset of labor more than 24 hours following rupture, second trimester** M♀
  - **O42.113 Preterm premature rupture of membranes, onset of labor more than 24 hours following rupture, third trimester** M♀
  - **O42.119 Preterm premature rupture of membranes, onset of labor more than 24 hours following rupture, unspecified trimester** M♀
- **O42.12 Full-term premature rupture of membranes, onset of labor more than 24 hours following rupture** M♀
  Premature rupture of membranes after 37 completed weeks of gestation

✓5th O42.9 Premature rupture of membranes, unspecified as to length of time between rupture and onset of labor

- **O42.90 Premature rupture of membranes, unspecified as to length of time between rupture and onset of labor, unspecified weeks of gestation** M♀
- **✓6th O42.91 Preterm premature rupture of membranes, unspecified as to length of time between rupture and onset of labor**
  Premature rupture of membranes before 37 completed weeks of gestation
  - **O42.911 Preterm premature rupture of membranes, unspecified as to length of time between rupture and onset of labor, first trimester** M♀
  - **O42.912 Preterm premature rupture of membranes, unspecified as to length of time between rupture and onset of abor, second trimester** M♀
  - **O42.913 Preterm premature rupture of membranes, unspecified as to length of time between rupture and onset of labor, third trimester** M♀
  - **O42.919 Preterm premature rupture of membranes, unspecified as to length of time between rupture and onset of labor, unspecified trimester** M♀
- **O42.92 Full-term premature rupture of membranes, unspecified as to length of time between rupture and onset of labor** M♀
  Premature rupture of membranes after 37 completed weeks of gestation

---

N Newborn: 0   P Pediatric: 0-17   M Maternity: 12-55   A Adult: 15-124   MCC Major CC Condition   PDxMCC PDx acts as own MCC   CC CC Condition   PDxCC PDx acts as own CC

830   ICD-10-CM 2016

✓4th **O43 Placental disorders**

> EXCLUDES 2   *maternal care for poor fetal growth due to placental*
> *insufficiency (O36.5-)*
> *placenta previa (O44.-)*
> *placental polyp (O90.89)*
> *placentitis (O41.14-)*
> *premature separation of placenta [abruptio placentae] (O45.-)*

✓5th **O43.0 Placental transfusion syndromes**

  ✓6th **O43.01 Fetomaternal placental transfusion syndrome**
Maternofetal placental transfusion syndrome

    O43.011 Fetomaternal placental transfusion Ⓜ♀
syndrome, first trimester

    O43.012 Fetomaternal placental transfusion Ⓜ♀
syndrome, second trimester

    O43.013 Fetomaternal placental transfusion Ⓜ♀
syndrome, third trimester

    O43.019 Fetomaternal placental transfusion Ⓜ♀
syndrome, unspecified trimester

  ✓6th **O43.02 Fetus-to-fetus placental transfusion syndrome**

    O43.021 Fetus-to-fetus placental transfusion Ⓜ♀
syndrome, first trimester

    O43.022 Fetus-to-fetus placental transfusion Ⓜ♀
syndrome, second trimester

    O43.023 Fetus-to-fetus placental transfusion Ⓜ♀
syndrome, third trimester

    O43.029 Fetus-to-fetus placental transfusion Ⓜ♀
syndrome, unspecified trimester

✓5th **O43.1 Malformation of placenta**

  ✓6th **O43.10 Malformation of placenta, unspecified**
Abnormal placenta NOS

    O43.101 Malformation of placenta, Ⓜ♀
unspecified, first trimester

    O43.102 Malformation of placenta, Ⓜ♀
unspecified, second trimester

    O43.103 Malformation of placenta, Ⓜ♀
unspecified, third trimester

    O43.109 Malformation of placenta, Ⓜ♀
unspecified, unspecified trimester

  ✓6th **O43.11 Circumvallate placenta**

    O43.111 Circumvallate placenta, first trimester Ⓜ♀

    O43.112 Circumvallate placenta, second Ⓜ♀
trimester

    O43.113 Circumvallate placenta, third Ⓜ♀
trimester

    O43.119 Circumvallate placenta, unspecified Ⓜ♀
trimester

  ✓6th **O43.12 Velamentous insertion of umbilical cord**

    O43.121 Velamentous insertion of umbilical Ⓜ♀
cord, first trimester

    O43.122 Velamentous insertion of umbilical ♀
cord, second trimester

    O43.123 Velamentous insertion of umbilical Ⓜ♀
cord, third trimester

    O43.129 Velamentous insertion of umbilical Ⓜ♀
cord, unspecified trimester

  ✓6th **O43.19 Other malformation of placenta**

    O43.191 Other malformation of placenta, Ⓜ♀
first trimester

    O43.192 Other malformation of placenta, Ⓜ♀
second trimester

    O43.193 Other malformation of placenta, Ⓜ♀
third trimester

    O43.199 Other malformation of placenta, Ⓜ♀
unspecified trimester

✓5th **O43.2 Morbidly adherent placenta**
Code also associated third stage postpartum hemorrhage, if
applicable (O72.0)

> EXCLUDES 1   *retained placenta (O73.-)*

  ✓6th **O43.21 Placenta accreta**

    O43.211 Placenta accreta, first trimester Ⓜ♀

    O43.212 Placenta accreta, second trimester Ⓜ♀

    O43.213 Placenta accreta, third trimester Ⓜ♀

    O43.219 Placenta accreta, unspecified Ⓜ♀
trimester

  ✓6th **O43.22 Placenta increta**

    O43.221 Placenta increta, first trimester Ⓜ♀

    O43.222 Placenta increta, second trimester Ⓜ♀

    O43.223 Placenta increta, third trimester Ⓜ♀

    O43.229 Placenta increta, unspecified Ⓜ♀
trimester

  ✓6th **O43.23 Placenta percreta**

    O43.231 Placenta percreta, first trimester Ⓜ♀

    O43.232 Placenta percreta, second trimester Ⓜ♀

    O43.233 Placenta percreta, third trimester Ⓜ♀

    O43.239 Placenta percreta, unspecified Ⓜ♀
trimester

✓5th **O43.8 Other placental disorders**

  ✓6th **O43.81 Placental infarction**

    O43.811 Placental infarction, first trimester Ⓜ♀

    O43.812 Placental infarction, second trimester Ⓜ♀

    O43.813 Placental infarction, third trimester Ⓜ♀

    O43.819 Placental infarction, unspecified Ⓜ♀
trimester

  ✓6th **O43.89 Other placental disorders**
Placental dysfunction

    O43.891 Other placental disorders, first Ⓜ♀
trimester

    O43.892 Other placental disorders, second Ⓜ♀
trimester

    O43.893 Other placental disorders, third Ⓜ♀
trimester

    O43.899 Other placental disorders, Ⓜ♀
unspecified trimester

✓5th **O43.9 Unspecified placental disorder**

    O43.90 Unspecified placental disorder, unspecified Ⓜ♀
trimester

    O43.91 Unspecified placental disorder, first trimester Ⓜ♀

    O43.92 Unspecified placental disorder, second Ⓜ♀
trimester

    O43.93 Unspecified placental disorder, third trimester Ⓜ♀

✓4th **O44 Placenta previa**

> **CC Excl: For CC/MCC codes in category O44, unless otherwise**
> **noted:** O20.0-O20.9, O25.10-O25.3, O26.10-O26.13, O26.30-O26.43,
> O26.63-O26.819, O26.841-O26.86, O26.891-O26.93, O29.011-O29.93,
> O35.7XX0-O35.7XX9, O44.00-O44.13, O75.4, O75.81, O75.89-O75.9,
> O80, O90.89, O99.111-O99.285, O99.330-O99.335, O99.350-O99.355,
> O99.511-O99.73, O99.820-O99.825, O99.840-O9A.53

✓5th **O44.0 Placenta previa specified as without hemorrhage**
Low implantation of placenta specified as without hemorrhage

    O44.00 Placenta previa specified as without Ⓜ♀
hemorrhage, unspecified trimester

    O44.01 Placenta previa specified as without CC Ⓜ♀
hemorrhage, first trimester

    O44.02 Placenta previa specified as without CC Ⓜ♀
hemorrhage, second trimester

    O44.03 Placenta previa specified as without CC Ⓜ♀
hemorrhage, third trimester

✓5th **O44.1 Placenta previa with hemorrhage**
Low implantation of placenta, NOS or with hemorrhage
Marginal placenta previa, NOS or with hemorrhage
Partial placenta previa, NOS or with hemorrhage
Total placenta previa, NOS or with hemorrhage

> EXCLUDES 1   *labor and delivery complicated by hemorrhage from*
> *vasa previa (O69.4)*

    O44.10 Placenta previa with hemorrhage, unspecified Ⓜ♀
trimester

    O44.11 Placenta previa with hemorrhage, first MCC Ⓜ♀
trimester

    O44.12 Placenta previa with hemorrhage, second MCC Ⓜ♀
trimester

    O44.13 Placenta previa with hemorrhage, third MCC Ⓜ♀
trimester

✔ Additional Character Required   ✓x7th Placeholder Alert   Unacceptable PDx   Manifestation   Hospital Acquired Condition   EXCLUDES 1 Not Coded Here   EXCLUDES 2 Not Included Here

ICD-10-CM 2016   831

✓4th **O45 Premature separation of placenta [abruptio placentae]**

  ✓5th **O45.0 Premature separation of placenta with coagulation defect**

> **CC Excl: For MCC codes in subcategory O45.0, unless otherwise noted:** O25.10-O25.3, O26.10-O26.13, O26.30-O26.43, O26.63-O26.819, O26.841-O26.86, O26.891-O26.93, O29.011-O29.93, O35.7XX0-O35.7XX9, O45.001-O45.099, O46.001-O46.93, O67.0-O67.9, O75.4, O75.81, O75.89-O75.9, O80, O90.89, O99.111-O99.285, O99.330-O99.335, O99.350-O99.355, O99.511-O99.73, O99.820-O99.825, O99.840-O9A.53

    ✓6th **O45.00 Premature separation of placenta with coagulation defect, unspecified**

      O45.001 Premature separation of placenta MCC M♀ **with coagulation defect, unspecified, first trimester**

      O45.002 Premature separation of placenta MCC M♀ **with coagulation defect, unspecified, second trimester**

      O45.003 Premature separation of placenta MCC M♀ **with coagulation defect, unspecified, third trimester**

      O45.009 Premature separation of placenta M♀ **with coagulation defect, unspecified, unspecified trimester**

    ✓6th **O45.01 Premature separation of placenta with afibrinogenemia**

      Premature separation of placenta with hypofibrinogenemia

      O45.011 Premature separation of placenta MCC M♀ **with afibrinogenemia, first trimester**

      O45.012 Premature separation of placenta MCC M♀ **with afibrinogenemia, second trimester**

      O45.013 Premature separation of placenta MCC M♀ **with afibrinogenemia, third trimester**

      O45.019 Premature separation of placenta M♀ **with afibrinogenemia, unspecified trimester**

    ✓6th **O45.02 Premature separation of placenta with disseminated intravascular coagulation**

      O45.021 Premature separation of placenta MCC M♀ **with disseminated intravascular coagulation, first trimester**

      O45.022 Premature separation of placenta MCC M♀ **with disseminated intravascular coagulation, second trimester**

      O45.023 Premature separation of placenta MCC M♀ **with disseminated intravascular coagulation, third trimester**

      O45.029 Premature separation of placenta M♀ **with disseminated intravascular coagulation, unspecified trimester**

    ✓6th **O45.09 Premature separation of placenta with other coagulation defect**

      O45.091 Premature separation of placenta MCC M♀ **with other coagulation defect, first trimester**

      O45.092 Premature separation of placenta MCC M♀ **with other coagulation defect, second trimester**

      O45.093 Premature separation of placenta MCC M♀ **with other coagulation defect, third trimester**

      O45.099 Premature separation of placenta M♀ **with other coagulation defect, unspecified trimester**

  ✓5th **O45.8 Other premature separation of placenta**

> **CC Excl: For MCC codes in subcategory O45.8, unless otherwise noted:** O20.0-O20.9, O25.10-O25.3, O26.10-O26.13, O26.30-O26.43, O26.63-O26.819, O26.841-O26.86, O26.891-O26.93, O29.011-O29.93, O35.7XX0-O35.7XX9, O44.00-O44.13, O45.8X1-O45.8X3, O45.91-O45.93, O75.4, O75.81, O75.89-O75.9, O80, O90.89, O99.111-O99.285, O99.330-O99.335, O99.350-O99.355, O99.511-O99.73, O99.820-O99.825, O99.840-O9A.53

    ✓6th **O45.8X Other premature separation of placenta**

      O45.8X1 Other premature separation of MCC M♀ **placenta, first trimester**

      O45.8X2 Other premature separation of MCC M♀ **placenta, second trimester**

      O45.8X3 Other premature separation of MCC M♀ **placenta, third trimester**

      O45.8X9 Other premature separation of M♀ **placenta, unspecified trimester**

  ✓5th **O45.9 Premature separation of placenta, unspecified**

    Abruptio placentae NOS

> **CC Excl: For MCC codes in subcategory O45.9, unless otherwise noted:** See code: O45.8

    O45.90 Premature separation of placenta, unspecified, M♀ **unspecified trimester**

    O45.91 Premature separation of placenta, MCC M♀ **unspecified, first trimester**

    O45.92 Premature separation of placenta, MCC M♀ **unspecified, second trimester**

    O45.93 Premature separation of placenta, MCC M♀ **unspecified, third trimester**

✓4th **O46 Antepartum hemorrhage, not elsewhere classified**

  EXCLUDES 1 hemorrhage in early pregnancy (O20.-)
      intrapartum hemorrhage NEC (O67.-)
      placenta previa (O44.-)
      premature separation of placenta [abruptio placentae] (O45.-)

  ✓5th **O46.0 Antepartum hemorrhage with coagulation defect**

> **CC Excl: For MCC codes in subcategory O46.0, unless otherwise noted:** See code: O45.0

    ✓6th **O46.00 Antepartum hemorrhage with coagulation defect, unspecified**

      O46.001 Antepartum hemorrhage with MCC M♀ **coagulation defect, unspecified, first trimester**

      O46.002 Antepartum hemorrhage with MCC M♀ **coagulation defect, unspecified, second trimester**

      O46.003 Antepartum hemorrhage with MCC M♀ **coagulation defect, unspecified, third trimester**

      O46.009 Antepartum hemorrhage with M♀ **coagulation defect, unspecified, unspecified trimester**

    ✓6th **O46.01 Antepartum hemorrhage with afibrinogenemia**

      Antepartum hemorrhage with hypofibrinogenemia

      O46.011 Antepartum hemorrhage with MCC M♀ **afibrinogenemia, first trimester**

      O46.012 Antepartum hemorrhage with MCC M♀ **afibrinogenemia, second trimester**

      O46.013 Antepartum hemorrhage with MCC M♀ **afibrinogenemia, third trimester**

      O46.019 Antepartum hemorrhage with M♀ **afibrinogenemia, unspecified trimester**

    ✓6th **O46.02 Antepartum hemorrhage with disseminated intravascular coagulation**

      O46.021 Antepartum hemorrhage with MCC M♀ **disseminated intravascular coagulation, first trimester**

      O46.022 Antepartum hemorrhage with MCC M♀ **disseminated intravascular coagulation, second trimester**

      O46.023 Antepartum hemorrhage with MCC M♀ **disseminated intravascular coagulation, third trimester**

      O46.029 Antepartum hemorrhage with M♀ **disseminated intravascular coagulation, unspecified trimester**

    ✓6th **O46.09 Antepartum hemorrhage with other coagulation defect**

      O46.091 Antepartum hemorrhage with MCC M♀ **other coagulation defect, first trimester**

      O46.092 Antepartum hemorrhage with MCC M♀ **other coagulation defect, second trimester**

      O46.093 Antepartum hemorrhage with MCC M♀ **other coagulation defect, third trimester**

      O46.099 Antepartum hemorrhage with other M♀ **coagulation defect, unspecified trimester**

N Newborn: 0   P Pediatric: 0-17   M Maternity: 12-55   A Adult: 15-124   MCC Major CC Condition   PDxMCC PDx acts as own MCC   CC CC Condition   PDxCC PDx acts as own CC

832   ICD-10-CM 2016

√5ᵗʰ **O46.8 Other antepartum hemorrhage**

√6ᵗʰ **O46.8X Other antepartum hemorrhage**

O46.8X1 Other antepartum hemorrhage, first trimester M♀

O46.8X2 Other antepartum hemorrhage, second trimester M♀

O46.8X3 Other antepartum hemorrhage, third trimester M♀

O46.8X9 Other antepartum hemorrhage, unspecified trimester M♀

√5ᵗʰ **O46.9 Antepartum hemorrhage, unspecified**

O46.90 Antepartum hemorrhage, unspecified, unspecified trimester M♀

O46.91 Antepartum hemorrhage, unspecified, first trimester M♀

O46.92 Antepartum hemorrhage, unspecified, second trimester M♀

O46.93 Antepartum hemorrhage, unspecified, third trimester M♀

√4ᵗʰ **O47 False labor**

Braxton Hicks contractions   Threatened labor

EXCLUDES 1   *preterm labor (O60.-)*

CC Excl: For CC codes in category O47, unless otherwise noted:
O25.10–O25.3, O26.10–O26.13, O26.30–O26.43, O26.63–O26.819,
O26.841–O26.86, O26.891–O26.93, O29.011–O29.93, O35.7XX0–
O35.7XX9, O47.00–O47.9, O60.00–O60.23, O75.4, O75.81, O75.89–
O75.9, O80, O90.89, O99.111–O99.285, O99.330–O99.335, O99.350–
O99.355, O99.511–O99.73, O99.820–O99.825, O99.840–O9A.53

√5ᵗʰ **O47.0 False labor before 37 completed weeks of gestation**

O47.00 False labor before 37 completed weeks of gestation, unspecified trimester M♀

O47.02 False labor before 37 completed weeks of gestation, second trimester CC M♀

O47.03 False labor before 37 completed weeks of gestation, third trimester CC M♀

O47.1 False labor at or after 37 completed weeks of gestation CC M♀

O47.9 False labor, unspecified M♀

√4ᵗʰ **O48 Late pregnancy**

O48.0 Post-term pregnancy M♀

Pregnancy over 40 completed weeks to 42 completed weeks gestation

O48.1 Prolonged pregnancy M♀

Pregnancy which has advanced beyond 42 completed weeks gestation

Complications of labor and delivery (O60-O77)

√4ᵗʰ **O60 Preterm labor**

INCLUDES   onset (spontaneous) of labor before 37 completed weeks of gestation

EXCLUDES 1   *false labor (O47.0-)*
threatened labor NOS (O47.0-)

CC Excl: For CC/MCC codes in category O60, unless otherwise noted: See code: O47

√5ᵗʰ **O60.0 Preterm labor without delivery**

O60.00 Preterm labor without delivery, unspecified trimester M♀

O60.02 Preterm labor without delivery, second trimester MCC M♀

O60.03 Preterm labor without delivery, third trimester MCC M♀

√5ᵗʰ **O60.1 Preterm labor with preterm delivery**

One of the following 7th characters is to be assigned to each code under subcategory O60.1. 7th character 0 is for single gestations and multiple gestations where the fetus is unspecified. 7th characters 1 through 9 are for cases of multiple gestations to identify the fetus for which the code applies. The appropriate code from category O30, Multiple gestation, must also be assigned when assigning a code from subcategory O60.1 that has a 7th character of 1 through 9.

0	not applicable or unspecified	3	fetus 3
		4	fetus 4
1	fetus 1	5	fetus 5
2	fetus 2	9	other fetus

√x7ᵗʰ **O60.10 Preterm labor with preterm delivery, unspecified trimester** CC M♀

Preterm labor with delivery NOS

√x7ᵗʰ **O60.12 Preterm labor second trimester with preterm delivery second trimester** MCC M♀

√x7ᵗʰ **O60.13 Preterm labor second trimester with preterm delivery third trimester** MCC M♀

√x7ᵗʰ **O60.14 Preterm labor third trimester with preterm delivery third trimester** MCC M♀

√5ᵗʰ **O60.2 Term delivery with preterm labor**

One of the following 7th characters is to be assigned to each code under subcategory O60.2. 7th character 0 is for single gestations and multiple gestations where the fetus is unspecified. 7th characters 1 through 9 are for cases of multiple gestations to identify the fetus for which the code applies. The appropriate code from category O30, Multiple gestation, must also be assigned when assigning a code from subcategory O60.2 that has a 7th character of 1 through 9.

0	not applicable or unspecified	3	fetus 3
		4	fetus 4
1	fetus 1	5	fetus 5
2	fetus 2	9	other fetus

√x7ᵗʰ **O60.20 Term delivery with preterm labor, unspecified trimester** CC M♀

√x7ᵗʰ **O60.22 Term delivery with preterm labor, second trimester** MCC M♀

√x7ᵗʰ **O60.23 Term delivery with preterm labor, third trimester** MCC M♀

√4ᵗʰ **O61 Failed induction of labor**

O61.0 Failed medical induction of labor M♀

Failed induction (of labor) by oxytocin
Failed induction (of labor) by prostaglandins

O61.1 Failed instrumental induction of labor M♀

Failed mechanical induction (of labor)
Failed surgical induction (of labor)

O61.8 Other failed induction of labor M♀

O61.9 Failed induction of labor, unspecified M♀

√4ᵗʰ **O62 Abnormalities of forces of labor**

O62.0 Primary inadequate contractions M♀

Failure of cervical dilatation
Primary hypotonic uterine dysfunction
Uterine inertia during latent phase of labor

O62.1 Secondary uterine inertia M♀

Arrested active phase of labor
Secondary hypotonic uterine dysfunction

O62.2 Other uterine inertia M♀

Atony of uterus without hemorrhage	Poor contractions
Atony of uterus NOS	Slow slope active phase
Desultory labor	of labor
Hypotonic uterine dysfunction NOS	Uterine inertia NOS
Irregular labor	

EXCLUDES 1   *atony of uterus with hemorrhage (postpartum) (O72.1)*
postpartum atony of uterus without hemorrhage (O75.89)

O62.3 Precipitate labor M♀

O62.4 Hypertonic, incoordinate, and prolonged uterine contractions M♀

Cervical spasm	Incoordinate uterine action
Contraction ring dystocia	Tetanic contractions
Dyscoordinate labor	Uterine dystocia NOS
Hour-glass contraction of uterus	Uterine spasm
Hypertonic uterine dysfunction	

EXCLUDES 1   *dystocia (fetal) (maternal) NOS (O66.9)*

O62.8 Other abnormalities of forces of labor M♀

O62.9 Abnormality of forces of labor, unspecified M♀

✔ Additional Character Required   √x7ᵗʰ Placeholder Alert   Unacceptable PDx   Manifestation   Hospital Acquired Condition   EXCLUDES 1 Not Coded Here   EXCLUDES 2 Not Included Here

Chapter 15. Pregnancy, Childbirth, and the Puerperium

✓4ᵗʰ **O63 Long labor**

O63.0 Prolonged first stage (of labor)   M ♀

O63.1 Prolonged second stage (of labor)   M ♀

O63.2 Delayed delivery of second twin, triplet, etc.   M ♀

O63.9 Long labor, unspecified   CC M ♀
Prolonged labor NOS
CC Excl: O25.10-O25.3, O26.10-O26.13, O26.30-O26.43, O26.63-O26.819, O26.841-O26.86, O26.891-O26.93, O29.011-O29.93, O35.7XX0-O35.7XX9, O36.8120-O36.8199, O63.9, O71.00-O71.1, O71.5, O71.81, O71.89-O71.9, O75.4, O75.81, O75.89-O75.9, O80, O90.89, O99.111-O99.285, O99.330-O99.335, O99.350-O99.355, O99.511-O99.73, O99.820-O99.825, O99.840-O9A.53

✓4ᵗʰ **O64 Obstructed labor due to malposition and malpresentation of fetus**

One of the following 7th characters is to be assigned to each code under category O64. 7th character 0 is for single gestations and multiple gestations where the fetus is unspecified. 7th characters 1 through 9 are for cases of multiple gestations to identify the fetus for which the code applies. The appropriate code from category O30, Multiple gestation, must also be assigned when assigning a code from category O64 that has a 7th character of 1 through 9.

0	not applicable or unspecified	3	fetus 3
		4	fetus 4
1	fetus 1	5	fetus 5
2	fetus 2	9	other fetus

✓x7ᵗʰ **O64.0 Obstructed labor due to incomplete rotation of fetal head**   M ♀
Deep transverse arrest
Obstructed labor due to persistent occipitoiliac (position)
Obstructed labor due to persistent occipitoposterior (position)
Obstructed labor due to persistent occipitosacral (position)
Obstructed labor due to persistent occipitotransverse (position)

✓x7ᵗʰ **O64.1 Obstructed labor due to breech presentation**   M ♀
Obstructed labor due to buttocks presentation
Obstructed labor due to complete breech presentation
Obstructed labor due to frank breech presentation

✓x7ᵗʰ **O64.2 Obstructed labor due to face presentation**   M ♀
Obstructed labor due to chin presentation

✓x7ᵗʰ **O64.3 Obstructed labor due to brow presentation**   M ♀

✓x7ᵗʰ **O64.4 Obstructed labor due to shoulder presentation**   M ♀
Prolapsed arm
EXCLUDES 1 impacted shoulders (O66.0)
shoulder dystocia (O66.0)

✓x7ᵗʰ **O64.5 Obstructed labor due to compound presentation**   M ♀

✓x7ᵗʰ **O64.8 Obstructed labor due to other malposition and malpresentation**   M ♀
Obstructed labor due to footling presentation
Obstructed labor due to incomplete breech presentation

✓x7ᵗʰ **O64.9 Obstructed labor due to malposition and malpresentation, unspecified**   M ♀

✓4ᵗʰ **O65 Obstructed labor due to maternal pelvic abnormality**

O65.0 Obstructed labor due to deformed pelvis   M ♀

O65.1 Obstructed labor due to generally contracted pelvis   M ♀

O65.2 Obstructed labor due to pelvic inlet contraction   M ♀

O65.3 Obstructed labor due to pelvic outlet and mid-cavity contraction   M ♀

O65.4 Obstructed labor due to fetopelvic disproportion, unspecified   M ♀
EXCLUDES 1 dystocia due to abnormality of fetus (O66.2-O66.3)

O65.5 Obstructed labor due to abnormality of maternal pelvic organs   M ♀
Obstructed labor due to conditions listed in O34-
Use additional code to identify abnormality of pelvic organs (O34.-)

O65.8 Obstructed labor due to other maternal pelvic abnormalities   M ♀

O65.9 Obstructed labor due to maternal pelvic abnormality, unspecified   M ♀

✓4ᵗʰ **O66 Other obstructed labor**

O66.0 Obstructed labor due to shoulder dystocia   M ♀
Impacted shoulders

O66.1 Obstructed labor due to locked twins   M ♀

O66.2 Obstructed labor due to unusually large fetus   M ♀

O66.3 Obstructed labor due to other abnormalities of fetus   M ♀
Dystocia due to fetal ascites
Dystocia due to fetal hydrops
Dystocia due to fetal meningomyelocele
Dystocia due to fetal sacral teratoma
Dystocia due to fetal tumor
Dystocia due to hydrocephalic fetus
Use additional code to identify cause of obstruction

✓5ᵗʰ **O66.4 Failed trial of labor**

O66.40 Failed trial of labor, unspecified   M ♀

O66.41 Failed attempted vaginal birth after previous cesarean delivery   M ♀
Code first rupture of uterus, if applicable (O71.0-, O71.1)

O66.5 Attempted application of vacuum extractor and forceps   M ♀
Attempted application of vacuum or forceps, with subsequent delivery by forceps or cesarean delivery

O66.6 Obstructed labor due to other multiple fetuses   M ♀

O66.8 Other specified obstructed labor   M ♀
Use additional code to identify cause of obstruction

O66.9 Obstructed labor, unspecified   M ♀
Dystocia NOS   Maternal dystocia NOS
Fetal dystocia NOS

✓4ᵗʰ **O67 Labor and delivery complicated by intrapartum hemorrhage, not elsewhere classified**
EXCLUDES 1 antepartum hemorrhage NEC (O46.-)
placenta previa (O44.-)
premature separation of placenta [abruptio placentae] (O45.-)
EXCLUDES 2 postpartum hemorrhage (O72.-)

O67.0 Intrapartum hemorrhage with coagulation defect   MCC M ♀
Intrapartum hemorrhage (excessive) associated with afibrinogenemia
Intrapartum hemorrhage (excessive) associated with disseminated intravascular coagulation
Intrapartum hemorrhage (excessive) associated with hyperfibrinolysis
Intrapartum hemorrhage (excessive) associated with hypofibrinogenemia
CC Excl: O25.10-O25.3, O26.10-O26.13, O26.30-O26.43, O26.63-O26.819, O26.841-O26.86, O26.891-O26.93, O29.011-O29.93, O35.7X-O35.7X, O45.001-O45.099, O46.001-O46.93, O67.0-O67.9, O75.4, O75.81, O75.89-O75.9, O80, O90.89, O99.111-O99.285, O99.330-O99.335, O99.350-O99.355, O99.511-O99.73, O99.820-O99.825, O99.840-O9A.53

O67.8 Other intrapartum hemorrhage   M ♀
Excessive intrapartum hemorrhage

O67.9 Intrapartum hemorrhage, unspecified   M ♀

O68 Labor and delivery complicated by abnormality of fetal acid-base balance   CC M ♀
Fetal acidemia complicating labor and delivery
Fetal acidosis complicating labor and delivery
Fetal alkalosis complicating labor and delivery
Fetal metabolic acidemia complicating labor and delivery
EXCLUDES 1 fetal stress NOS (O77.9)
labor and delivery complicated by electrocardiographic evidence of fetal stress (O77.8)
labor and delivery complicated by ultrasonic evidence of fetal stress (O77.8)
EXCLUDES 2 abnormality in fetal heart rate or rhythm (O76)
labor and delivery complicated by meconium in amniotic fluid (O77.0)
CC Excl: O68-O76, P03.811

✓4ᵗʰ **O69 Labor and delivery complicated by umbilical cord complications**

One of the following 7th characters is to be assigned to each code under category O69. 7th character 0 is for single gestations and multiple gestations where the fetus is unspecified. 7th characters 1 through 9 are for cases of multiple gestations to identify the fetus for which the code applies. The appropriate code from category O30, Multiple gestation, must also be assigned when assigning a code from category O69 that has a 7th character of 1 through 9.

0	not applicable or unspecified	3	fetus 3
		4	fetus 4
1	fetus 1	5	fetus 5
2	fetus 2	9	other fetus

✓x7ᵗʰ **O69.0 Labor and delivery complicated by prolapse of cord**   M ♀

✓x7ᵗʰ **O69.1 Labor and delivery complicated by cord around neck, with compression**   M ♀
EXCLUDES 1 labor and delivery complicated by cord around neck, without compression (O69.81)

N Newborn: 0   P Pediatric: 0-17   M Maternity: 12-55   A Adult: 15-124   MCC Major CC Condition   PDxMCC PDx acts as own MCC   CC CC Condition   PDxCC PDx acts as own CC

834   ICD-10-CM 2016

✓x7ᵗʰ O69.2 Labor and delivery complicated by other cord entanglement, with compression Ⓜ♀
Labor and delivery complicated by compression of cord NOS
Labor and delivery complicated by entanglement of cords of twins in monoamniotic sac
Labor and delivery complicated by knot in cord
EXCLUDES 1   *labor and delivery complicated by other cord entanglement, without compression (O69.82)*

✓x7ᵗʰ O69.3 Labor and delivery complicated by short cord Ⓜ♀

✓x7ᵗʰ O69.4 Labor and delivery complicated by vasa previa Ⓜ♀
Labor and delivery complicated by hemorrhage from vasa previa

✓x7ᵗʰ O69.5 Labor and delivery complicated by vascular lesion of cord Ⓜ♀
Labor and delivery complicated by cord bruising
Labor and delivery complicated by cord hematoma
Labor and delivery complicated by thrombosis of umbilical vessels

✓5ᵗʰ O69.8 Labor and delivery complicated by other cord complications

   ✓x7ᵗʰ O69.81 Labor and delivery complicated by cord around neck, without compression Ⓜ♀

   ✓x7ᵗʰ O69.82 Labor and delivery complicated by other cord entanglement, without compression Ⓜ♀

   ✓x7ᵗʰ O69.89 Labor and delivery complicated by other cord complications Ⓜ♀

✓x7ᵗʰ O69.9 Labor and delivery complicated by cord complication, unspecified Ⓜ♀

✓4ᵗʰ O70 Perineal laceration during delivery
Episiotomy extended by laceration
EXCLUDES 1   *obstetric high vaginal laceration alone (O71.4)*

  O70.0 First degree perineal laceration during delivery Ⓜ♀
Perineal laceration, rupture or tear involving fourchette during delivery
Perineal laceration, rupture or tear involving labia during delivery
Perineal laceration, rupture or tear involving skin during delivery
Perineal laceration, rupture or tear involving vagina during delivery
Perineal laceration, rupture or tear involving vulva during delivery
Slight perineal laceration, rupture or tear during delivery

  O70.1 Second degree perineal laceration during delivery Ⓜ♀
Perineal laceration, rupture or tear during delivery as in O70.0, also involving pelvic floor
Perineal laceration, rupture or tear during delivery as in O70.0, also involving perineal muscles
Perineal laceration, rupture or tear during delivery as in O70.0, also involving vaginal muscles
EXCLUDES 1   *perineal laceration involving anal sphincter (O70.2)*

  O70.2 Third degree perineal laceration during delivery CC Ⓜ♀
Perineal laceration, rupture or tear during delivery as in O70.1, also involving anal sphincter
Perineal laceration, rupture or tear during delivery as in O70.1, also involving rectovaginal septum
Perineal laceration, rupture or tear during delivery as in O70.1, also involving sphincter NOS
EXCLUDES 1   *anal sphincter tear during delivery without third degree perineal laceration (O70.4)*
perineal laceration involving anal or rectal mucosa (O70.3)
CC Excl: O25.10-O25.3, O26.10-O26.13, O26.30-O26.43, O26.63-O26.819, O26.841-O26.86, O26.891-O26.93, O29.011-O29.93, O35.7XX0-O35.7XX9, O36.8120-O36.8199, O70.2, O70.4, O71.00-O71.1, O71.5, O71.81, O71.89-O71.9, O75.4, O75.81, O75.89-O75.9, O80, O90.89, O99.111-O99.285, O99.330-O99.335, O99.350-O99.355, O99.511-O99.73, O99.820-O99.825, O99.840-O9A.53

  O70.3 Fourth degree perineal laceration during delivery CC Ⓜ♀
Perineal laceration, rupture or tear during delivery as in O70.2, also involving anal mucosa
Perineal laceration, rupture or tear during delivery as in O70.2, also involving rectal mucosa
CC Excl: O25.10-O25.3, O26.10-O26.13, O26.30-O26.43, O26.63-O26.819, O26.841-O26.86, O26.891-O26.93, O29.011-O29.93, O35.7XX0-O35.7XX9, O36.8120-O36.8199, O70.3, O71.00-O71.1, O71.5, O71.81, O71.89-O71.9, O75.4, O75.81, O75.89-O75.9, O80, O90.89, O99.111-O99.285, O99.330-O99.335, O99.350-O99.355, O99.511-O99.73, O99.820-O99.825, O99.840-O9A.53

  O70.4 Anal sphincter tear complicating delivery, not associated with third degree laceration CC Ⓜ♀
EXCLUDES 1   *anal sphincter tear with third degree perineal laceration (O70.2)*
CC Excl: See code: O70.2

  O70.9 Perineal laceration during delivery, unspecified Ⓜ♀

✓4ᵗʰ O71 Other obstetric trauma
Obstetric damage from instruments

✓5ᵗʰ O71.0 Rupture of uterus (spontaneous) before onset of labor
EXCLUDES 1   *disruption of (current) cesarean delivery wound (O90.0)*
laceration of uterus, NEC (O71.81)

  O71.00 Rupture of uterus before onset of labor, unspecified trimester Ⓜ♀

  O71.02 Rupture of uterus before onset of labor, second trimester MCC Ⓜ♀
CC Excl: O25.10-O25.3, O26.10-O26.13, O26.30-O26.43, O26.63-O26.819, O26.841-O26.86, O26.891-O26.93, O29.011-O29.93, O35.7XX0-O35.7XX9, O36.8120-O36.8199, O71.00-O71.1, O71.5, O71.81, O71.89-O71.9, O75.4, O75.81, O75.89-O75.9, O80, O90.89, O99.111-O99.285, O99.330-O99.335, O99.350-O99.355, O99.511-O99.73, O99.820-O99.825, O99.840-O9A.53

  O71.03 Rupture of uterus before onset of labor, third trimester MCC Ⓜ♀
CC Excl: See code: O71.02

  O71.1 Rupture of uterus during labor MCC Ⓜ♀
Rupture of uterus not stated as occurring before onset of labor
EXCLUDES 1   *disruption of cesarean delivery wound (O90.0)*
laceration of uterus, NEC (O71.81)
CC Excl: See code: O71.02

  O71.2 Postpartum inversion of uterus CC Ⓜ♀
CC Excl: O25.10-O25.3, O26.10-O26.13, O26.30-O26.43, O26.63-O26.819, O26.841-O26.86, O26.891-O26.93, O29.011-O29.93, O35.7XX0-O35.7XX9, O36.8120-O36.8199, O71.00-O71.2, O71.5, O71.81, O71.89-O71.9, O75.4, O75.81, O75.89-O75.9, O80, O90.89, O99.111-O99.285, O99.330-O99.335, O99.350-O99.355, O99.511-O99.73, O99.820-O99.825, O99.840-O9A.53

  O71.3 Obstetric laceration of cervix CC Ⓜ♀
Annular detachment of cervix
CC Excl: O25.10-O25.3, O26.10-O26.13, O26.30-O26.43, O26.63-O26.819, O26.841-O26.86, O26.891-O26.93, O29.011-O29.93, O35.7XX0-O35.7XX9, O36.8120-O36.8199, O71.00-O71.1, O71.3, O71.5, O71.81, O71.89-O71.9, O75.4, O75.81, O75.89-O75.9, O80, O90.89, O99.111-O99.285, O99.330-O99.335, O99.350-O99.355, O99.511-O99.73, O99.820-O99.825, O99.840-O9A.53

  O71.4 Obstetric high vaginal laceration alone CC Ⓜ♀
Laceration of vaginal wall without perineal laceration
EXCLUDES 1   *obstetric high vaginal laceration with perineal laceration (O70.-)*
CC Excl: O25.10-O25.3, O26.10-O26.13, O26.30-O26.43, O26.63-O26.819, O26.841-O26.86, O26.891-O26.93, O29.011-O29.93, O35.7XX0-O35.7XX9, O36.8120-O36.8199, O71.00-O71.1, O71.4-O71.5, O71.81, O71.89-O71.9, O75.4, O75.81, O75.89-O75.9, O80, O90.89, O99.111-O99.285, O99.330-O99.335, O99.350-O99.355, O99.511-O99.73, O99.820-O99.825, O99.840-O9A.53

  O71.5 Other obstetric injury to pelvic organs CC Ⓜ♀
Obstetric injury to bladder
Obstetric injury to urethra
EXCLUDES 2   *obstetric periurethral trauma (O71.82)*
AHA: 2014, 4Q, 18
CC Excl: O25.10-O25.3, O26.10-O26.13, O26.30-O26.43, O26.63-O26.819, O26.841-O26.86, O26.891-O26.93, O29.011-O29.93, O35.7XX0-O35.7XX9, O36.8120-O36.8199, O71.00-O71.1, O71.5, O71.81, O71.89-O71.9, O75.4, O75.81, O75.89-O75.9, O80, O90.89, O99.111-O99.285, O99.330-O99.335, O99.350-O99.355, O99.511-O99.73, O99.820-O99.825, O99.840-O9A.53

  O71.6 Obstetric damage to pelvic joints and ligaments CC Ⓜ♀
Obstetric avulsion of inner symphyseal cartilage
Obstetric damage to coccyx
Obstetric traumatic separation of symphysis (pubis)
CC Excl: O25.10-O25.3, O26.10-O26.13, O26.30-O26.43, O26.63-O26.819, O26.841-O26.86, O26.891-O26.93, O29.011-O29.93, O35.7XX0-O35.7XX9, O36.8120-O36.8199, O71.00-O71.1, O71.5-O71.6, O71.81, O71.89-O71.9, O75.4, O75.81, O75.89-O75.9, O80, O90.89, O99.111-O99.285, O99.330-O99.335, O99.350-O99.355, O99.511-O99.73, O99.820-O99.825, O99.840-O9A.53

  O71.7 Obstetric hematoma of pelvis CC Ⓜ♀
Obstetric hematoma of perineum
Obstetric hematoma of vagina
Obstetric hematoma of vulva
CC Excl: O25.10-O25.3, O26.10-O26.13, O26.30-O26.43, O26.63-O26.819, O26.841-O26.86, O26.891-O26.93, O29.011-O29.93, O35.7XX0-O35.7XX9, O36.8120-O36.8199, O71.00-O71.1, O71.5, O71.7-O71.81, O71.89-O71.9, O75.4, O75.81, O75.89-O75.9, O80, O90.89, O99.111-O99.285, O99.330-O99.335, O99.350-O99.355, O99.511-O99.73, O99.820-O99.825, O99.840-O9A.53

✓5ᵗʰ O71.8 Other specified obstetric trauma

  O71.81 Laceration of uterus, not elsewhere classified Ⓜ♀

  O71.82 Other specified trauma to perineum and vulva Ⓜ♀
Obstetric periurethral trauma
AHA: 2014, 4Q, 18

✓ Additional Character Required   ✓x7ᵗʰ Placeholder Alert   Unacceptable PDx   Manifestation   Hospital Acquired Condition   EXCLUDES 1 Not Coded Here   EXCLUDES 2 Not Included Here

071.89   Other specified obstetric trauma   M ♀

071.9   Obstetric trauma, unspecified   M ♀

✔4ᵗʰ **072   Postpartum hemorrhage**

    INCLUDES   hemorrhage after delivery of fetus or infant

072.0   Third-stage hemorrhage   CC M ♀

    Hemorrhage associated with retained, trapped or adherent placenta

    Retained placenta NOS

    Code also type of adherent placenta (043.2-)

    CC Excl: 025.10-025.3, 026.10-026.13, 026.30-026.43, 026.63-026.819, 026.841-026.86, 026.891-026.93, 029.011-029.93, 035.7XX0-035.7XX9, 036.8120-036.8199, 071.00-071.1, 071.5, 071.81, 071.89-072.0, 075.4, 075.81, 075.89-075.9, 080, 090.89, 099.111-099.285, 099.330-099.335, 099.350-099.355, 099.511-099.73, 099.820-099.825, 099.840-09A.12

072.1   Other immediate postpartum hemorrhage   CC M ♀

    Hemorrhage following delivery of placenta

    Postpartum hemorrhage (atonic) NOS

    Uterine atony with hemorrhage

      EXCLUDES 1   uterine atony NOS (062.2)

         uterine atony without hemorrhage (062.2)

         postpartum atony of uterus without hemorrhage (075.89)

    CC Excl: 025.10-025.3, 026.10-026.13, 026.30-026.43, 026.63-026.819, 026.841-026.86, 026.891-026.93, 029.011-029.93, 035.7XX0-035.7XX9, 036.8120-036.8199, 071.00-071.1, 071.5, 071.81, 071.89-071.9, 072.1, 075.4, 075.81, 075.89-075.9, 080, 090.89, 099.111-099.285, 099.330-099.335, 099.350-099.355, 099.511-099.73, 099.820-099.825, 099.840-09A.53

072.2   Delayed and secondary postpartum hemorrhage   CC M ♀

    Hemorrhage associated with retained portions of placenta or membranes after the first 24 hours following delivery of placenta

    Retained products of conception NOS, following delivery

    CC Excl: 025.10-025.3, 026.10-026.13, 026.30-026.43, 026.63-026.819, 026.841-026.86, 026.891-026.93, 029.011-029.93, 035.7XX0-035.7XX9, 036.8120-036.8199, 071.00-071.1, 071.5, 071.81, 071.89-071.9, 072.2, 075.4, 075.81, 075.89-075.9, 080, 090.89, 099.111-099.285, 099.330-099.335, 099.350-099.355, 099.511-099.73, 099.820-099.825, 099.840-09A.53

072.3   Postpartum coagulation defects   M ♀

    Postpartum afibrinogenemia

    Postpartum fibrinolysis

✔4ᵗʰ **073   Retained placenta and membranes, without hemorrhage**

    EXCLUDES 1   placenta accreta (043.21-)

         placenta increta (043.22-)

         placenta percreta (043.23-)

073.0   Retained placenta without hemorrhage   M ♀

    Adherent placenta, without hemorrhage

    Trapped placenta without hemorrhage

073.1   Retained portions of placenta and membranes, without hemorrhage   M ♀

    Retained products of conception following delivery, without hemorrhage

✔4ᵗʰ **074   Complications of anesthesia during labor and delivery**

    INCLUDES   maternal complications arising from the administration of a general, regional or local anesthetic, analgesic or other sedation during labor and delivery

    Use additional code, if applicable, to identify specific complication

074.0   Aspiration pneumonitis due to anesthesia during labor and delivery   M ♀

    Inhalation of stomach contents or secretions NOS due to anesthesia during labor and delivery

    Mendelson's syndrome due to anesthesia during labor and delivery

074.1   Other pulmonary complications of anesthesia during labor and delivery   M ♀

074.2   Cardiac complications of anesthesia during labor and delivery   M ♀

074.3   Central nervous system complications of anesthesia during labor and delivery   M ♀

074.4   Toxic reaction to local anesthesia during labor and delivery   M ♀

074.5   Spinal and epidural anesthesia-induced headache during labor and delivery   M ♀

074.6   Other complications of spinal and epidural anesthesia during labor and delivery   M ♀

074.7   Failed or difficult intubation for anesthesia during labor and delivery   M ♀

074.8   Other complications of anesthesia during labor and delivery   M ♀

074.9   Complication of anesthesia during labor and delivery, unspecified   M ♀

✔4ᵗʰ **075   Other complications of labor and delivery, not elsewhere classified**

    EXCLUDES 2   puerperal (postpartum) infection (086.-)

         puerperal (postpartum) sepsis (085)

075.0   Maternal distress during labor and delivery   M ♀

075.1   Shock during or following labor and delivery   MCC M ♀

    Obstetric shock following labor and delivery

    CC Excl: 025.10-025.3, 026.10-026.13, 026.30-026.43, 026.63-026.819, 026.841-026.86, 026.891-026.93, 029.011-029.93, 035.7XX0-035.7XX9, 075.1, 075.4, 075.81, 075.89-075.9, 080, 090.89, 099.111-099.285, 099.330-099.335, 099.350-099.355, 099.511-099.73, 099.820-099.825, 099.840-09A.53

075.2   Pyrexia during labor, not elsewhere classified   CC M ♀

    CC Excl: 075.2

075.3   Other infection during labor   MCC M ♀

    Sepsis during labor

    Use additional code (B95-B97), to identify infectious agent

    CC Excl: 025.10-025.3, 026.10-026.13, 026.30-026.43, 026.63-026.819, 026.841-026.86, 026.891-026.93, 029.011-029.93, 035.7XX0-035.7XX9, 075.3-075.4, 075.81, 075.89-075.9, 080, 090.89, 099.111-099.285, 099.330-099.335, 099.350-099.355, 099.511-099.73, 099.820-099.825, 099.840-09A.53

075.4   Other complications of obstetric surgery and procedures   M ♀

    Cardiac arrest following obstetric surgery or procedures

    Cardiac failure following obstetric surgery or procedures

    Cerebral anoxia following obstetric surgery or procedures

    Pulmonary edema following obstetric surgery or procedures

    Use additional code to identify specific complication

      EXCLUDES 2   complications of anesthesia during labor and delivery (074.-)

         disruption of obstetrical (surgical) wound (090.0-090.1)

         hematoma of obstetrical (surgical) wound (090.2)

         infection of obstetrical (surgical) wound (086.0)

075.5   Delayed delivery after artificial rupture of membranes   M ♀

✔5ᵗʰ **075.8   Other specified complications of labor and delivery**

075.81   Maternal exhaustion complicating labor and delivery   M ♀

075.82   Onset (spontaneous) of labor after 37 completedweeks of gestation but before 39 completed weeks gestation, with delivery by (planned) cesarean section   M ♀

    Delivery by (planned) cesarean section occurring after 37 completed weeks of gestation but before 39 completed weeks gestation due to (spontaneous) onset of labor

    Code first to specify reason for planned cesarean section such as:

      cephalopelvic disproportion (normally formed fetus) (033.9)

      previous cesarean delivery (034.21)

075.89   Other specified complications of labor and delivery   M ♀

075.9   Complication of labor and delivery, unspecified   M ♀

076   Abnormality in fetal heart rate and rhythm complicating labor and delivery   M ♀

    Depressed fetal heart rate tones complicating labor and delivery

    Fetal bradycardia complicating labor and delivery

    Fetal heart rate abnormal variability complicating labor and delivery

    Fetal heart rate decelerations complicating labor and delivery

    Fetal heart rate irregularity complicating labor and delivery

    Fetal tachycardia complicating labor and delivery

    Non-reassuring fetal heart rate or rhythm complicating labor and delivery

      EXCLUDES 1   fetal stress NOS (077.9)

         labor and delivery complicated by electrocardiographic evidence of fetal stress (077.8)

         labor and delivery complicated by ultrasonic evidence of fetal stress (077.8)

      EXCLUDES 2   fetal metabolic acidemia (068)

         other fetal stress (077.0-077.1)

    AHA: 2013, 4Q, 118

✔4ᵗʰ **077   Other fetal stress complicating labor and delivery**

077.0   Labor and delivery complicated by meconium in amniotic fluid   M ♀

    AHA: 2013, 4Q, 117-118

077.1   Fetal stress in labor or delivery due to drug administration   M ♀

N Newborn: 0   P Pediatric: 0-17   M Maternity: 12-55   A Adult: 15-124   MCC Major CC Condition   PDxMCC PDx acts as own MCC   CC CC Condition   PDxCC PDx acts as own CC

O77.8 **Labor and delivery complicated by other evidence of fetal stress** M♀

Labor and delivery complicated by electrocardiographic evidence of fetal stress

Labor and delivery complicated by ultrasonic evidence of fetal stress

EXCLUDES 1　*abnormality in fetal heart rate or rhythm (O76)*
abnormality of fetal acid-base balance (O68)
fetal metabolic acidemia (O68)

O77.9 **Labor and delivery complicated by fetal stress, unspecified** M♀

EXCLUDES 1　*abnormality in fetal heart rate or rhythm (O76)*
abnormality of fetal acid-base balance (O68)
fetal metabolic acidemia (O68)

Encounter for delivery (O80, O82)

O80 **Encounter for full-term uncomplicated delivery** M♀

NOTE　Delivery requiring minimal or no assistance, with or without episiotomy, without fetal manipulation [e.g., rotation version] or instrumentation [forceps] of a spontaneous, cephalic, vaginal, full-term, single, live-born infant. This code is for use as a single diagnosis code and is not to be used with any other code from chapter 15.

Use additional code to indicate outcome of delivery (Z37.0)

AHA: 2014, 2Q, 9

O82 **Encounter for cesarean delivery without indication** M♀

Use additional code to indicate outcome of delivery (Z37.0)

Complications predominantly related to the puerperium (O85-O92)

EXCLUDES 2　*mental and behavioral disorders associated with the puerperium (F53)*
obstetrical tetanus (A34)
puerperal osteomalacia (M83.0)

O85 **Puerperal sepsis** MCC M♀

Postpartum sepsis
Puerperal peritonitis
Puerperal pyemia

Use additional code (B95-B97), to identify infectious agent

Use additional code (R65.2-) to identify severe sepsis, if applicable

EXCLUDES 1　*fever of unknown origin following delivery (O86.4)*
genital tract infection following delivery (O86.1-)
obstetric pyemic and septic embolism (O88.3-)
puerperal septic thrombophlebitis (O86.81)
urinary tract infection following delivery (O86.2-)

EXCLUDES 2　*sepsis during labor (O75.3)*

CC Excl: O25.10-O25.3, O26.10-O26.13, O26.30-O26.43, O26.63-O26.819, O26.841-O26.86, O26.891-O26.93, O29.011-O29.93, O35.7XX0-O35.7XX9, O75.4, O75.81, O75.89-O75.9, O80, O85, O86.12, O86.81-O86.89, O90.89, O99.111-O99.285, O99.330-O99.335, O99.350-O99.355, O99.511-O99.73, O99.820-O99.825, O99.840-O9A.53

✓4th **O86** **Other puerperal infections**

Use additional code (B95-B97), to identify infectious agent

EXCLUDES 2　*infection during labor (O75.3)*
obstetrical tetanus (A34)

CC Excl: For CC/MCC codes in category O86, unless otherwise noted: O23.00-O23.93, O25.10-O25.3, O26.10-O26.13, O26.30-O26.43, O26.63-O26.819, O26.841-O26.86, O26.891-O26.93, O29.011-O29.93, O35.7XX0-O35.7XX9, O75.4, O75.81, O75.89-O75.9, O80, O86.11, O86.13-O86.29, O90.89, O99.111-O99.285, O99.330-O99.335, O99.350-O99.355, O99.511-O99.73, O99.820-O99.825, O99.840-O9A.53

O86.0 **Infection of obstetric surgical wound** M♀

Infected cesarean delivery wound following delivery
Infected perineal repair following delivery

✓5th **O86.1** **Other infection of genital tract following delivery**

O86.11 **Cervicitis following delivery** CC M♀

O86.12 **Endometritis following delivery** CC M♀

CC Excl: O25.10-O25.3, O26.10-O26.13, O26.30-O26.43, O26.63-O26.819, O26.841-O26.86, O26.891-O26.93, O29.011-O29.93, O35.7XX0-O35.7XX9, O75.4, O75.81, O75.89-O75.9, O80, O85, O86.12, O86.81-O86.89, O90.89, O99.111-O99.285, O99.330-O99.335, O99.350-O99.355, O99.511-O99.73, O99.820-O99.825, O99.840-O9A.53

O86.13 **Vaginitis following delivery** CC M♀

O86.19 **Other infection of genital tract following delivery** CC M♀

✓5th **O86.2** **Urinary tract infection following delivery**

O86.20 **Urinary tract infection following delivery, unspecified** CC M♀

Puerperal urinary tract infection NOS

O86.21 **Infection of kidney following delivery** CC M♀

O86.22 **Infection of bladder following delivery** CC M♀

Infection of urethra following delivery

O86.29 **Other urinary tract infection following delivery** CC M♀

O86.4 **Pyrexia of unknown origin following delivery** CC M♀

Puerperal infection NOS following delivery
Puerperal pyrexia NOS following delivery

EXCLUDES 2　*pyrexia during labor (O75.2)*

CC Excl: O22.20-O22.93, O25.10-O25.3, O26.10-O26.13, O26.30-O26.43, O26.63-O26.819, O26.841-O26.86, O26.891-O26.93, O29.011-O29.93, O35.7XX0-O35.7XX9, O75.4, O75.81, O75.89-O75.9, O80, O86.4, O87.0-O87.3, O87.8-O87.9, O90.89, O99.111-O99.285, O99.330-O99.335, O99.350-O99.355, O99.511-O99.73, O99.820-O99.825, O99.840-O9A.53

✓5th **O86.8** **Other specified puerperal infections**

O86.81 **Puerperal septic thrombophlebitis** MCC M♀

CC Excl: See code: O85

O86.89 **Other specified puerperal infections** MCC M♀

CC Excl: See code: O85

✓4th **O87** **Venous complications and hemorrhoids in the puerperium**

Venous complications in labor, delivery and the puerperium

EXCLUDES 2　*obstetric embolism (O88.-)*
puerperal septic thrombophlebitis (O86.81)
venous complications in pregnancy (O22.-)

CC Excl: For CC/MCC codes in category O87, unless otherwise noted: O22.20-O22.93, O25.10-O25.3, O26.10-O26.13, O26.30-O26.43, O26.63-O26.819, O26.841-O26.86, O26.891-O26.93, O29.011-O29.93, O35.7XX0-O35.7XX9, O75.4, O75.81, O75.89-O75.9, O80, O87.0-O87.3, O87.8-O87.9, O90.89, O99.111-O99.285, O99.330-O99.335, O99.350-O99.355, O99.511-O99.73, O99.820-O99.825, O99.840-O9A.53

O87.0 **Superficial thrombophlebitis in the puerperium** CC M♀

Puerperal phlebitis NOS
Puerperal thrombosis NOS

O87.1 **Deep phlebothrombosis in the puerperium** MCC M♀

Deep vein thrombosis, postpartum
Pelvic thrombophlebitis, postpartum

Use additional code to identify the deep vein thrombosis (I82.4-, I82.5-, I82.62-. I82.72-)

Use additional code, if applicable, for associated long-term (current) use of anticoagulants (Z79.01)

O87.2 **Hemorrhoids in the puerperium** CC M♀

O87.3 **Cerebral venous thrombosis in the puerperium** CC M♀

Cerebrovenous sinus thrombosis in the puerperium

O87.4 **Varicose veins of lower extremity in the puerperium** M♀

O87.8 **Other venous complications in the puerperium** CC M♀

Genital varices in the puerperium

O87.9 **Venous complication in the puerperium, unspecified** M♀

Puerperal phlebopathy NOS

✓4th **O88** **Obstetric embolism**

EXCLUDES 1　*embolism complicating abortion NOS (O03.2)*
embolism complicating ectopic or molar pregnancy (O08.2)
embolism complicating failed attempted abortion (O07.2)
embolism complicating induced abortion (O04.7)
embolism complicating spontaneous abortion (O03.2, O03.7)

CC Excl: For CC/MCC codes in category O88, unless otherwise noted: O25.10-O25.3, O26.10-O26.13, O26.30-O26.43, O26.63-O26.819, O26.841-O26.86, O26.891-O26.93, O29.011-O29.93, O35.7XX0-O35.7XX9, O75.4, O75.81, O75.89-O75.9, O80, O88.011-O88.83, O90.89, O99.111-O99.285, O99.330-O99.335, O99.350-O99.355, O99.511-O99.73, O99.820-O99.825, O99.840-O9A.53

✓5th **O88.0** **Obstetric air embolism**

✓6th **O88.01** **Obstetric air embolism in pregnancy**

O88.011 **Air embolism in pregnancy, first trimester** MCC M♀

O88.012 **Air embolism in pregnancy, second trimester** MCC M♀

O88.013 **Air embolism in pregnancy, third trimester** MCC M♀

O88.019 **Air embolism in pregnancy, unspecified trimester** M♀

O88.02 **Air embolism in childbirth** MCC M♀

O88.03 **Air embolism in the puerperium** MCC M♀

✓5th **O88.1 Amniotic fluid embolism**
Anaphylactoid syndrome in pregnancy

    ✓6th **O88.11 Amniotic fluid embolism in** pregnancy

      O88.111 Amniotic fluid embolism in MCC M♀
pregnancy, **first trimester**

      O88.112 Amniotic fluid embolism in MCC M♀
pregnancy, **second trimester**

      O88.113 Amniotic fluid embolism in MCC M♀
pregnancy, **third trimester**

      O88.119 Amniotic fluid embolism in M♀
pregnancy, **unspecified trimester**

    O88.12 Amniotic fluid embolism in childbirth MCC M♀

    O88.13 Amniotic fluid embolism in the puerperium MCC M♀

✓5th **O88.2 Obstetric** thromboembolism

    ✓6th **O88.21 Thromboembolism in** pregnancy
Obstetric (pulmonary) embolism NOS

      O88.211 Thromboembolism in pregnancy, MCC M♀
first trimester

      O88.212 Thromboembolism in pregnancy, MCC M♀
second trimester

      O88.213 Thromboembolism in pregnancy, MCC M♀
third trimester

      O88.219 Thromboembolism in pregnancy, M♀
unspecified trimester

    O88.22 Thromboembolism in childbirth MCC M♀

    O88.23 Thromboembolism in the puerperium MCC M♀
Puerperal (pulmonary) embolism NOS

✓5th **O88.3 Obstetric** pyemic and septic embolism

    ✓6th **O88.31 Pyemic and septic embolism in** pregnancy

      O88.311 Pyemic and septic embolism in MCC M♀
pregnancy, **first trimester**

      O88.312 Pyemic and septic embolism in MCC M♀
pregnancy, **second trimester**

      O88.313 Pyemic and septic embolism in MCC M♀
pregnancy, **third trimester**

      O88.319 Pyemic and septic embolism in CC M♀
pregnancy, **unspecified trimester**

    O88.32 Pyemic and septic embolism in childbirth MCC M♀

    O88.33 Pyemic and septic embolism in the MCC M♀
puerperium

✓5th **O88.8 Other obstetric** embolism
Obstetric fat embolism

    ✓6th **O88.81 Other embolism in** pregnancy

      O88.811 Other embolism in pregnancy, MCC M♀
first trimester

      O88.812 Other embolism in pregnancy, MCC M♀
second trimester

      O88.813 Other embolism in pregnancy, MCC M♀
third trimester

      O88.819 Other embolism in pregnancy, M♀
unspecified trimester

    O88.82 Other embolism in childbirth MCC M♀

    O88.83 Other embolism in the puerperium MCC M♀

✓4th **O89 Complications of anesthesia during the puerperium**
INCLUDES   maternal complications arising from the administration of a general, regional or local anesthetic, analgesic or other sedation during the puerperium
Use additional code, if applicable, to identify specific complication

    ✓5th **O89.0 Pulmonary complications of anesthesia during the puerperium**

      O89.01 Aspiration pneumonitis due to anesthesia M♀
during the puerperium
Inhalation of stomach contents or secretions NOS due to anesthesia during the puerperium
Mendelson's syndrome due to anesthesia during the puerperium

      O89.09 Other pulmonary complications of anesthesia M♀
during the puerperium

    O89.1 Cardiac complications of anesthesia during the M♀
puerperium

    O89.2 Central nervous system complications of anesthesia M♀
during the puerperium

    O89.3 Toxic reaction to local anesthesia during the puerperium M♀

    O89.4 Spinal and epidural anesthesia-induced headache M♀
during the puerperium

    O89.5 Other complications of spinal and epidural anesthesia M♀
during the puerperium

    O89.6 Failed or difficult intubation for anesthesia during the M♀
puerperium

    O89.8 Other complications of anesthesia during the puerperium M♀

    O89.9 Complication of anesthesia during the puerperium, M♀
unspecified

✓4th **O90 Complications of the puerperium, not elsewhere classified**

    O90.0 Disruption of cesarean delivery wound M♀
Dehiscence of cesarean delivery wound
EXCLUDES 1   *rupture of uterus (spontaneous) before onset of labor (O71.0-)*
rupture of uterus during labor (O71.1)

    O90.1 Disruption of perineal obstetric wound M♀
Disruption of wound of episiotomy
Disruption of wound of perineal laceration
Secondary perineal tear

    O90.2 Hematoma of obstetric wound M♀

    O90.3 Peripartum cardiomyopathy MCC M♀
Conditions in I42- arising during pregnancy and the puerperium
EXCLUDES 1   *pre-existing heart disease complicating pregnancy and the puerperium (O99.4-)*
CC Excl: O25.10-O25.3, O26.10-O26.13, O26.30-O26.43, O26.63-O26.819, O26.841-O26.86, O26.891-O26.93, O29.011-O29.93, O35.7XX0-O35.7XX9, O75.4, O75.81, O75.89-O75.9, O80, O90.3, O90.89, O99.111-O99.285, O99.330-O99.335, O99.350-O99.73, O99.820-O99.825, O99.840-O9A.53

    O90.4 Postpartum acute kidney failure MCC M♀
Hepatorenal syndrome following labor and delivery
CC Excl: O25.10-O25.3, O26.10-O26.13, O26.30-O26.43, O26.63-O26.819, O26.841-O26.86, O26.891-O26.93, O29.011-O29.93, O35.7XX0-O35.7XX9, O75.4, O75.81, O75.89-O75.9, O80, O90.4, O90.89, O99.111-O99.285, O99.330-O99.335, O99.350-O99.355, O99.511-O99.73, O99.820-O99.825, O99.840-O9A.53

    O90.5 Postpartum thyroiditis M♀

    O90.6 Postpartum mood disturbance M♀
Postpartum blues
Postpartum dysphoria
Postpartum sadness
EXCLUDES 1   *postpartum depression (F53)*
puerperal psychosis (F53)

    ✓5th **O90.8 Other complications of the puerperium, not elsewhere classified**

      O90.81 Anemia of the puerperium M♀
Postpartum anemia NOS
EXCLUDES 1   *pre-existing anemia complicating the puerperium (O99.03)*

      O90.89 Other complications of the puerperium, not M♀
elsewhere classified
Placental polyp

    O90.9 Complication of the puerperium, unspecified M♀

✓4th **O91 Infections of breast associated with pregnancy, the puerperium and lactation**
Use additional code to identify infection

    ✓5th **O91.0 Infection of nipple associated with pregnancy, the puerperium and lactation**

      ✓6th **O91.01 Infection of nipple associated with** pregnancy
Gestational abscess of nipple

        O91.011 Infection of nipple associated with M♀
pregnancy, first trimester

        O91.012 Infection of nipple associated with M♀
pregnancy, second trimester

        O91.013 Infection of nipple associated with M♀
pregnancy, third trimester

        O91.019 Infection of nipple associated with M♀
pregnancy, unspecified trimester

      O91.02 Infection of nipple associated with the M♀
puerperium
Puerperal abscess of nipple

      O91.03 Infection of nipple associated with lactation M♀
Abscess of nipple associated with lactation

    ✓5th **O91.1 Abscess of breast associated with pregnancy, the puerperium and lactation**

      ✓6th **O91.11 Abscess of breast associated with** pregnancy
Gestational mammary abscess
Gestational purulent mastitis
Gestational subareolar abscess

        O91.111 Abscess of breast associated with M♀
pregnancy, first trimester

O91.112 **Abscess of breast associated with pregnancy, second trimester** Ⓜ♀

O91.113 **Abscess of breast associated with pregnancy, third trimester** Ⓜ♀

O91.119 **Abscess of breast associated with pregnancy, unspecified trimester** Ⓜ♀

O91.12 **Abscess of breast associated with the puerperium** Ⓜ♀
Puerperal mammary abscess
Puerperal purulent mastitis
Puerperal subareolar abscess

O91.13 **Abscess of breast associated with lactation** Ⓜ♀
Mammary abscess associated with lactation
Purulent mastitis associated with lactation
Subareolar abscess associated with lactation

✓5ᵗʰ O91.2 **Nonpurulent mastitis associated with pregnancy, the puerperium and lactation**

✓6ᵗʰ O91.21 **Nonpurulent mastitis associated with pregnancy**
Gestational interstitial mastitis
Gestational lymphangitis of breast
Gestational mastitis NOS
Gestational parenchymatous mastitis

O91.211 **Nonpurulent mastitis associated with pregnancy, first trimester** Ⓜ♀

O91.212 **Nonpurulent mastitis associated with pregnancy, second trimester** Ⓜ♀

O91.213 **Nonpurulent mastitis associated with pregnancy, third trimester** Ⓜ♀

O91.219 **Nonpurulent mastitis associated with pregnancy, unspecified trimester** Ⓜ♀

O91.22 **Nonpurulent mastitis associated with the puerperium** Ⓜ♀
Puerperal interstitial mastitis
Puerperal lymphangitis of breast
Puerperal mastitis NOS
Puerperal parenchymatous mastitis

O91.23 **Nonpurulent mastitis associated with lactation** Ⓜ♀
Interstitial mastitis associated with lactation
Lymphangitis of breast associated with lactation
Mastitis NOS associated with lactation
Parenchymatous mastitis associated with lactation

✓4ᵗʰ O92 **Other disorders of breast and disorders of lactation associated with pregnancy and the puerperium**

✓5ᵗʰ O92.0 **Retracted nipple associated with pregnancy, the puerperium, and lactation**

✓6ᵗʰ O92.01 **Retracted nipple associated with pregnancy**

O92.011 **Retracted nipple associated with pregnancy, first trimester** Ⓜ♀

O92.012 **Retracted nipple associated with pregnancy, second trimester** Ⓜ♀

O92.013 **Retracted nipple associated with pregnancy, third trimester** Ⓜ♀

O92.019 **Retracted nipple associated with pregnancy, unspecified trimester** Ⓜ♀

O92.02 **Retracted nipple associated with the puerperium** Ⓜ♀

O92.03 **Retracted nipple associated with lactation** Ⓜ♀

✓5ᵗʰ O92.1 **Cracked nipple associated with pregnancy, the puerperium, and lactation**
Fissure of nipple, gestational or puerperal

✓6ᵗʰ O92.11 **Cracked nipple associated with pregnancy**

O92.111 **Cracked nipple associated with pregnancy, first trimester** Ⓜ♀

O92.112 **Cracked nipple associated with pregnancy, second trimester** Ⓜ♀

O92.113 **Cracked nipple associated with pregnancy, third trimester** Ⓜ♀

O92.119 **Cracked nipple associated with pregnancy, unspecified trimester** Ⓜ♀

O92.12 **Cracked nipple associated with the puerperium** Ⓜ♀

O92.13 **Cracked nipple associated with lactation** Ⓜ♀

✓5ᵗʰ O92.2 **Other and unspecified disorders of breast associated with pregnancy and the puerperium**

O92.20 **Unspecified disorder of breast associated with pregnancy and the puerperium** Ⓜ♀

O92.29 **Other disorders of breast associated with pregnancy and the puerperium** Ⓜ♀

O92.3 **Agalactia** Ⓜ♀
Primary agalactia
EXCLUDES 1 *elective agalactia (O92.5)*
secondary agalactia (O92.5)
therapeutic agalactia (O92.5)

O92.4 **Hypogalactia** Ⓜ♀

O92.5 **Suppressed lactation** Ⓜ♀
Elective agalactia   Therapeutic agalactia
Secondary agalactia
EXCLUDES 1 *primary agalactia (O92.3)*

O92.6 **Galactorrhea** Ⓜ♀

✓5ᵗʰ O92.7 **Other and unspecified disorders of lactation**

O92.70 **Unspecified disorders of lactation** Ⓜ♀

O92.79 **Other disorders of lactation** Ⓜ♀
Puerperal galactocele

Other obstetric conditions, not elsewhere classified (O94-O9A)

O94 **Sequelae of complication of pregnancy, childbirth, and the puerperium** Ⓜ♀
NOTE This category is to be used to indicate conditions in O00-O77.-, O85-O94 and O98-O9A.- as the cause of late effects. The sequelae include conditions specified as such, or as late effects, which may occur at any time after the puerperium.
Code first condition resulting from (sequela) of complication of pregnancy, childbirth, and the puerperium

✓4ᵗʰ O98 **Maternal infectious and parasitic diseases classifiable elsewhere but complicating pregnancy, childbirth and the puerperium**
INCLUDES the listed conditions when complicating the pregnant state, when aggravated by the pregnancy, or as a reason for obstetric care
Use additional code (Chapter 1), to identify specific infectious or parasitic disease
EXCLUDES 2 *herpes gestationis (O26.4-)*
infectious carrier state (O99.82-, O99.83-)
obstetrical tetanus (A34)
puerperal infection (O86.-)
puerperal sepsis (O85)
when the reason for maternal care is that the disease is known or suspected to have affected the fetus (O35-O36)

✓5ᵗʰ O98.0 **Tuberculosis complicating pregnancy, childbirth and the puerperium**
Conditions in A15-A19

CC Excl: For CC codes in subcategory O98.0, unless otherwise noted: O25.10-O25.3, O26.10-O26.13, O26.30-O26.43, O26.63-O26.819, O26.841-O26.86, O26.891-O26.93, O29.011-O29.93, O35.7XX0-O35.7XX9, O75.4, O75.81, O75.89-O75.9, O80, O90.89, O98.011-O98.03, O99.111-O99.285, O99.330-O99.335, O99.350-O99.355, O99.511-O99.73, O99.820-O99.825, O99.840-O9A.53

✓6ᵗʰ O98.01 **Tuberculosis complicating pregnancy**

O98.011 **Tuberculosis complicating pregnancy, first trimester** CC Ⓜ♀

O98.012 **Tuberculosis complicating pregnancy, second trimester** CC Ⓜ♀

O98.013 **Tuberculosis complicating pregnancy, third trimester** CC Ⓜ♀

O98.019 **Tuberculosis complicating pregnancy, unspecified trimester** Ⓜ♀

O98.02 **Tuberculosis complicating childbirth** CC Ⓜ♀

O98.03 **Tuberculosis complicating the puerperium** CC Ⓜ♀

✓5ᵗʰ O98.1 **Syphilis complicating pregnancy, childbirth and the puerperium**
Conditions in A50-A53

CC Excl: For CC codes in subcategory O98.1, unless otherwise noted: O26.11-O26.13, O26.31-O26.33, O26.41-O26.43, O26.63-O26.713, O26.72-O26.813, O26.86, O26.891-O26.893, O26.90-O26.93, O29.011-O29.013, O29.021-O29.023, O29.091-O29.093, O29.111-O29.113, O29.121-O29.123, O29.191-O29.193, O29.211-O29.213, O29.291-O29.293, O29.3X1-O29.3X3, O29.41-O29.5X3, O29.61-O29.8X3, O29.91-O29.93, O35.7XX0-O35.7XX9, O98.111-O98.33, O99.351-O99.353, O99.355, O99.89

✓6ᵗʰ O98.11 **Syphilis complicating pregnancy**

O98.111 **Syphilis complicating pregnancy, first trimester** CC Ⓜ♀

O98.112 **Syphilis complicating pregnancy, second trimester** CC Ⓜ♀

O98.113 **Syphilis complicating pregnancy, third trimester** CC Ⓜ♀

Chapter 15. Pregnancy, Childbirth, and the Puerperium

O98.119 **Syphilis complicating pregnancy,** Ⓜ♀
unspecified trimester

O98.12 **Syphilis complicating childbirth** ᶜᶜ Ⓜ♀

O98.13 **Syphilis complicating the puerperium** ᶜᶜ Ⓜ♀

✓5ᵗʰ **O98.2** **Gonorrhea complicating pregnancy, childbirth and the puerperium**
Conditions in A54-

> **CC Excl: For CC codes in subcategory O98.2, unless otherwise noted:** See code: O98.1

✓6ᵗʰ **O98.21** **Gonorrhea complicating pregnancy**

O98.211 **Gonorrhea complicating** ᶜᶜ Ⓜ♀
pregnancy, first trimester

O98.212 **Gonorrhea complicating** ᶜᶜ Ⓜ♀
pregnancy, second trimester

O98.213 **Gonorrhea complicating** ᶜᶜ Ⓜ♀
pregnancy, third trimester

O98.219 **Gonorrhea complicating pregnancy,** Ⓜ♀
unspecified trimester

O98.22 **Gonorrhea complicating childbirth** ᶜᶜ Ⓜ♀

O98.23 **Gonorrhea complicating the puerperium** ᶜᶜ Ⓜ♀

✓5ᵗʰ **O98.3** **Other infections with a predominantly sexual mode of transmission complicating pregnancy, childbirth and the puerperium**
Conditions in A55-A64

> **CC Excl: For CC codes in subcategory O98.3, unless otherwise noted:** See code: O98.1

✓6ᵗʰ **O98.31** **Other infections with a predominantly sexual mode of transmission complicating pregnancy**

O98.311 **Other infections with a** ᶜᶜ Ⓜ♀
predominantly sexual mode of transmission complicating pregnancy, first trimester

O98.312 **Other infections with a** ᶜᶜ Ⓜ♀
predominantly sexual mode of transmission complicating pregnancy, second trimester

O98.313 **Other infections with a** ᶜᶜ Ⓜ♀
predominantly sexual mode of transmission complicating pregnancy, third trimester

O98.319 **Other infections with a** Ⓜ♀
predominantly sexual mode of transmission complicating pregnancy, unspecified trimester

O98.32 **Other infections with a predominantly sexual** ᶜᶜ Ⓜ♀
mode of transmission complicating childbirth

O98.33 **Other infections with a predominantly sexual** ᶜᶜ Ⓜ♀
mode of transmission complicating the puerperium

✓5ᵗʰ **O98.4** **Viral hepatitis complicating pregnancy, childbirth and the puerperium**
Conditions in B15-B19

> **CC Excl: For CC codes in subcategory O98.4, unless otherwise noted:** O98.411-O98.613, O98.711-O98.93, O99.830-O99.835

✓6ᵗʰ **O98.41** **Viral hepatitis complicating pregnancy**

O98.411 **Viral hepatitis complicating** ᶜᶜ Ⓜ♀
pregnancy, first trimester

O98.412 **Viral hepatitis complicating** ᶜᶜ Ⓜ♀
pregnancy, second trimester

O98.413 **Viral hepatitis complicating** ᶜᶜ Ⓜ♀
pregnancy, third trimester

O98.419 **Viral hepatitis complicating** Ⓜ♀
pregnancy, unspecified trimester

O98.42 **Viral hepatitis complicating childbirth** ᶜᶜ Ⓜ♀

O98.43 **Viral hepatitis complicating the puerperium** ᶜᶜ Ⓜ♀

✓5ᵗʰ **O98.5** **Other viral diseases complicating pregnancy, childbirth and the puerperium**
Conditions in A80-B09, B25-B34, R87.81-, R87.82-

> **EXCLUDES 1**   *human immunodeficiency virus [HIV] disease complicating pregnancy, childbirth and the puerperium (O98.7-)*

> **CC Excl: For CC codes in subcategory O98.5, unless otherwise noted:** See code: O98.4

✓6ᵗʰ **O98.51** **Other viral diseases complicating pregnancy**

O98.511 **Other viral diseases complicating** ᶜᶜ Ⓜ♀
pregnancy, first trimester

O98.512 **Other viral diseases complicating** ᶜᶜ Ⓜ♀
pregnancy, second trimester

O98.513 **Other viral diseases complicating** ᶜᶜ Ⓜ♀
pregnancy, third trimester

O98.519 **Other viral diseases complicating** Ⓜ♀
pregnancy, unspecified trimester

O98.52 **Other viral diseases complicating childbirth** ᶜᶜ Ⓜ♀

O98.53 **Other viral diseases complicating the** ᶜᶜ Ⓜ♀
puerperium

✓5ᵗʰ **O98.6** **Protozoal diseases complicating pregnancy, childbirth and the puerperium**
Conditions in B50-B64

> **CC Excl: For CC codes in subcategory O98.6, unless otherwise noted:** O25.10-O25.3, O26.10-O26.13, O26.30-O26.43, O26.63-O26.819, O26.841-O26.86, O26.891-O26.93, O29.011-O29.93, O35.7XX0-O35.7XX9, O75.4, O75.81, O75.89-O75.9, O80, O90.89, O98.411-O98.93, O99.111-O99.285, O99.330-O99.335, O99.350-O99.355, O99.511-O99.73, O99.820-O9A.53

✓6ᵗʰ **O98.61** **Protozoal diseases complicating pregnancy**

O98.611 **Protozoal diseases complicating** ᶜᶜ Ⓜ♀
pregnancy, first trimester

O98.612 **Protozoal diseases complicating** ᶜᶜ Ⓜ♀
pregnancy, second trimester

O98.613 **Protozoal diseases complicating** ᶜᶜ Ⓜ♀
pregnancy, third trimester

O98.619 **Protozoal diseases complicating** Ⓜ♀
pregnancy, unspecified trimester

O98.62 **Protozoal diseases complicating childbirth** ᶜᶜ Ⓜ♀
CC Excl: O25.10-O25.3, O26.10-O26.13, O26.30-O26.43, O26.63-O26.819, O26.841-O26.86, O26.891-O26.93, O29.011-O29.93, O35.7XX0-O35.7XX9, O75.4, O75.81, O75.89-O75.9, O80, O90.89, O98.611-O98.63, O99.111-O99.285, O99.330-O99.335, O99.350-O99.355, O99.511-O99.73, O99.820-O99.825, O99.840-O9A.53

O98.63 **Protozoal diseases complicating the** ᶜᶜ Ⓜ♀
puerperium
CC Excl: See code: O98.62

✓5ᵗʰ **O98.7** **Human immunodeficiency virus [HIV] disease complicating pregnancy, childbirth and the puerperium**
Use additional code to identify the type of HIV disease:
acquired immune deficiency syndrome (AIDS) (B20)
asymptomatic HIV status (Z21)
HIV positive NOS (Z21)
symptomatic HIV disease (B20)

> **CC Excl: For CC codes in subcategory O98.7, unless otherwise noted:** O98.411-O98.613, O98.711-O98.93, O99.830-O99.835

✓6ᵗʰ **O98.71** **Human immunodeficiency virus [HIV] disease complicating pregnancy**

O98.711 **Human immunodeficiency virus** ᶜᶜ Ⓜ♀
[HIV] disease complicating pregnancy, first trimester

O98.712 **Human immunodeficiency virus** ᶜᶜ Ⓜ♀
[HIV] disease complicating pregnancy, second trimester

O98.713 **Human immunodeficiency virus** ᶜᶜ Ⓜ♀
[HIV] disease complicating pregnancy, third trimester

O98.719 **Human immunodeficiency virus [HIV]** Ⓜ♀
disease complicating pregnancy, unspecified trimester

O98.72 **Human immunodeficiency virus [HIV]** ᶜᶜ Ⓜ♀
disease complicating childbirth

O98.73 **Human immunodeficiency virus [HIV]** ᶜᶜ Ⓜ♀
disease complicating the puerperium

✓5ᵗʰ **O98.8** **Other maternal infectious and parasitic diseases complicating pregnancy, childbirth and the puerperium**

> **CC Excl: For CC codes in subcategory O98.8, unless otherwise noted:** See code: O98.7

✓6ᵗʰ **O98.81** **Other maternal infectious and parasitic diseases complicating pregnancy**

O98.811 **Other maternal infectious and** ᶜᶜ Ⓜ♀
parasitic diseases complicating pregnancy, first trimester

O98.812 **Other maternal infectious and** ᶜᶜ Ⓜ♀
parasitic diseases complicating pregnancy, second trimester

Ⓝ Newborn: 0   Ⓟ Pediatric: 0-17   Ⓜ Maternity: 12-55   Ⓐ Adult: 15-124   ᴹᶜᶜ Major CC Condition   ᴾᴰˣᴹᶜᶜ PDx acts as own MCC   ᶜᶜ CC Condition   ᴾᴰˣᶜᶜ PDx acts as own CC

840   ICD-10-CM 2016

O98.813   Other maternal infectious and parasitic diseases complicating pregnancy, third trimester   CC M ♀

O98.819   Other maternal infectious and parasitic diseases complicating pregnancy, unspecified trimester   M ♀

O98.82   Other maternal infectious and parasitic diseases complicating childbirth   CC M ♀

O98.83   Other maternal infectious and parasitic diseases complicating the puerperium   CC M ♀

√5ᵗʰ **O98.9**   Unspecified maternal infectious and parasitic disease complicating pregnancy, childbirth and the puerperium

> **CC Excl:** For CC codes in subcategory O98.9, unless otherwise noted: See code: O98.7

√6ᵗʰ **O98.91**   Unspecified maternal infectious and parasitic disease complicating pregnancy

O98.911   Unspecified maternal infectious and parasitic disease complicating pregnancy, first trimester   CC M ♀

O98.912   Unspecified maternal infectious and parasitic disease complicating pregnancy, second trimester   CC M ♀

O98.913   Unspecified maternal infectious and parasitic disease complicating pregnancy, third trimester   CC M ♀

O98.919   Unspecified maternal infectious and parasitic disease complicating pregnancy, unspecified trimester   M ♀

O98.92   Unspecified maternal infectious and parasitic disease complicating childbirth   CC M ♀

O98.93   Unspecified maternal infectious and parasitic disease complicating the puerperium   CC M ♀

√4ᵗʰ **O99**   Other maternal diseases classifiable elsewhere but complicating pregnancy, childbirth and the puerperium

> INCLUDES   conditions which complicate the pregnant state, are aggravated by the pregnancy or are a main reason for obstetric care

Use additional code to identify specific condition

> EXCLUDES 2   when the reason for maternal care is that the condition is known or suspected to have affected the fetus (O35-O36)

√5ᵗʰ **O99.0**   Anemia complicating pregnancy, childbirth and the puerperium
Conditions in D50-D64

> EXCLUDES 1   anemia arising in the puerperium (O90.81)
> postpartum anemia NOS (O90.81)

√6ᵗʰ **O99.01**   Anemia complicating pregnancy

O99.011   Anemia complicating pregnancy, first trimester   M ♀

O99.012   Anemia complicating pregnancy, second trimester   M ♀

O99.013   Anemia complicating pregnancy, third trimester   M ♀

O99.019   Anemia complicating pregnancy, unspecified trimester   M ♀

O99.02   Anemia complicating childbirth   M ♀

O99.03   Anemia complicating the puerperium   M ♀

> EXCLUDES 1   postpartum anemia not pre-existing prior to delivery (O90.81)

√5ᵗʰ **O99.1**   Other diseases of the blood and blood-forming organs and certain disorders involving the immune mechanism complicating pregnancy, childbirth and the puerperium
Conditions in D65-D89

> EXCLUDES 2   hemorrhage with coagulation defects (O45.-, O46.0-, O67.0, O72.3)

> **CC Excl:** For CC codes in subcategory O99.1, unless otherwise noted: O25.11-O25.3, O99.281-O99.285, O99.511-O99.513, O99.52-O99.613, O99.62-O99.713, O99.72-O99.73, O99.820-O99.825, O9A.111-O9A.113, O9A.12-O9A.213, O9A.22-O9A.313, O9A.32-O9A.413, O9A.42-O9A.513, O9A.52-O9A.53

√6ᵗʰ **O99.11**   Other diseases of the blood and blood-forming organs and certain disorders involving the immune mechanism complicating pregnancy

O99.111   Other diseases of the blood and blood-forming organs and certain disorders involving the immune mechanism complicating pregnancy, first trimester   CC M ♀

O99.112   Other diseases of the blood and blood-forming organs and certain disorders involving the immune mechanism complicating pregnancy, second trimester   CC M ♀

O99.113   Other diseases of the blood and blood-forming organs and certain disorders involving the immune mechanism complicating pregnancy, third trimester   CC M ♀

O99.119   Other diseases of the blood and blood-forming organs and certain disorders involving the immune mechanism complicating pregnancy, unspecified trimester   CC M ♀

> **CC Excl:** O25.10-O99.280, O99.519, O99.619, O99.719, O9A.119, O9A.219, O9A.319, O9A.419, O9A.519

O99.12   Other diseases of the blood and blood-forming organs and certain disorders involving the immune mechanism complicating childbirth   CC M ♀

O99.13   Other diseases of the blood and blood-forming organs and certain disorders involving the immune mechanism complicating the puerperium   CC M ♀

√5ᵗʰ **O99.2**   Endocrine, nutritional and metabolic diseases complicating pregnancy, childbirth and the puerperium
Conditions in E00-E88

> EXCLUDES 2   diabetes mellitus (O24.-)
> malnutrition (O25.-)
> postpartum thyroiditis (O90.5)

√6ᵗʰ **O99.21**   Obesity complicating pregnancy, childbirth, and the puerperium
Use additional code to identify the type of obesity (E66.-)

O99.210   Obesity complicating pregnancy, unspecified trimester   M ♀

O99.211   Obesity complicating pregnancy, first trimester   M ♀

O99.212   Obesity complicating pregnancy, second trimester   M ♀

O99.213   Obesity complicating pregnancy, third trimester   M ♀

O99.214   Obesity complicating childbirth   M ♀

O99.215   Obesity complicating the puerperium   M ♀

√6ᵗʰ **O99.28**   Other endocrine, nutritional and metabolic diseases complicating pregnancy, childbirth and the puerperium

O99.280   Endocrine, nutritional and metabolic diseases complicating pregnancy, unspecified trimester   M ♀

O99.281   Endocrine, nutritional and metabolic diseases complicating pregnancy, first trimester   M ♀

O99.282   Endocrine, nutritional and metabolic diseases complicating pregnancy, second trimester   M ♀

O99.283   Endocrine, nutritional and metabolic diseases complicating pregnancy, third trimester   M ♀

O99.284   Endocrine, nutritional and metabolic diseases complicating childbirth   M ♀

O99.285   Endocrine, nutritional and metabolic diseases complicating the puerperium   M ♀

√5ᵗʰ **O99.3**   Mental disorders and diseases of the nervous system complicating pregnancy, childbirth and the puerperium

> **CC Excl:** For CC codes in subcategory O99.3, unless otherwise noted: O25.10-O25.3, O26.10-O26.13, O26.30-O26.43, O26.63-O26.819, O26.841-O26.86, O26.891-O26.93, O29.011-O29.93, O35.7XX0-O35.7XX9, O75.4, O75.81, O75.89-O75.9, O80, O90.89, O99.111-O99.285, O99.320-O99.335, O99.350-O99.355, O99.511-O99.73, O99.820-O99.825, O99.840-O9A.53

√6ᵗʰ **O99.31**   Alcohol use complicating pregnancy, childbirth, and the puerperium
Use additional code(s) from F10 to identify manifestations of the alcohol use

O99.310   Alcohol use complicating pregnancy, unspecified trimester   M ♀

√ Additional Character Required   √x7ᵗʰ Placeholder Alert   Unacceptable PDx   Manifestation   Hospital Acquired Condition   EXCLUDES 1 Not Coded Here   EXCLUDES 2 Not Included Here

O99.311 Alcohol use complicating pregnancy, first trimester Ⓜ♀

O99.312 Alcohol use complicating pregnancy, second trimester Ⓜ♀

O99.313 Alcohol use complicating pregnancy, third trimester Ⓜ♀

O99.314 Alcohol use complicating childbirth Ⓜ♀

O99.315 Alcohol use complicating the puerperium Ⓜ♀

√6ᵗʰ **O99.32 Drug use complicating pregnancy, childbirth, and the puerperium**
Use additional code(s) from F11-F16 and F18-F19 to identify manifestations of the drug use

O99.320 Drug use complicating pregnancy, unspecified trimester Ⓜ♀

O99.321 Drug use complicating pregnancy, first trimester ⒸⒸⓂ♀

O99.322 Drug use complicating pregnancy, second trimester ⒸⒸⓂ♀

O99.323 Drug use complicating pregnancy, third trimester ⒸⒸⓂ♀

O99.324 Drug use complicating childbirth ⒸⒸⓂ♀

O99.325 Drug use complicating the puerperium ⒸⒸⓂ♀

√6ᵗʰ **O99.33 Smoking (tobacco) complicating pregnancy, childbirth, and the puerperium**
Use additional code from F17 to identify type of tobacco

O99.330 Smoking (tobacco) complicating pregnancy, unspecified trimester Ⓜ♀

O99.331 Smoking (tobacco) complicating pregnancy, first trimester Ⓜ♀

O99.332 Smoking (tobacco) complicating pregnancy, second trimester Ⓜ♀

O99.333 Smoking (tobacco) complicating pregnancy, third trimester Ⓜ♀

O99.334 Smoking (tobacco) complicating childbirth Ⓜ♀

O99.335 Smoking (tobacco) complicating the puerperium Ⓜ♀

√6ᵗʰ **O99.34 Other mental disorders complicating pregnancy, childbirth, and the puerperium**
Conditions in F01-F09 and F20-F99
EXCLUDES 2 *postpartum mood disturbance (O90.6)*
postnatal psychosis (F53)
puerperal psychosis (F53)

O99.340 Other mental disorders complicating pregnancy, unspecified trimester Ⓜ♀

O99.341 Other mental disorders complicating pregnancy, first trimester Ⓜ♀

O99.342 Other mental disorders complicating pregnancy, second trimester Ⓜ♀

O99.343 Other mental disorders complicating pregnancy, third trimester Ⓜ♀

O99.344 Other mental disorders complicating childbirth Ⓜ♀

O99.345 Other mental disorders complicating the puerperium Ⓜ♀

√6ᵗʰ **O99.35 Diseases of the nervous system complicating pregnancy, childbirth, and the puerperium**
Conditions in G00-G99
EXCLUDES 2 *pregnancy related peripheral neuritis (O26.8-)*

O99.350 Diseases of the nervous system complicating pregnancy, unspecified trimester Ⓜ♀

O99.351 Diseases of the nervous system complicating pregnancy, first trimester Ⓜ♀

O99.352 Diseases of the nervous system complicating pregnancy, second trimester Ⓜ♀

O99.353 Diseases of the nervous system complicating pregnancy, third trimester Ⓜ♀

O99.354 Diseases of the nervous system complicating childbirth ⒸⒸⓂ♀
CC Excl: See code: O99.1

O99.355 Diseases of the nervous system complicating the puerperium ⒸⒸⓂ♀
CC Excl: See code: O99.1

√5ᵗʰ **O99.4 Diseases of the circulatory system complicating pregnancy, childbirth and the puerperium**
Conditions in I00-I99
EXCLUDES 1 *peripartum cardiomyopathy (O90.3)*
EXCLUDES 2 *hypertensive disorders (O10-O16)*
obstetric embolism (O88.-)
venous complications and cerebrovenous sinus thrombosis in labor, childbirth and the puerperium (O87.-)
venous complications and cerebrovenous sinus thrombosis in pregnancy (O22.-)

CC Excl: For CC codes in subcategory O99.4, unless otherwise noted: O25.10-O25.3, O26.10-O26.13, O26.30-O26.43, O26.63-O26.819, O26.841-O26.86, O26.891-O26.93, O29.011-O29.93, O35.7XX0-O35.7XX9, O75.4, O75.81, O75.89-O75.9, O80, O90.3, O90.89, O99.111-O99.285, O99.330-O99.335, O99.350-O99.73, O99.820-O99.825, O99.840-O9A.53

√6ᵗʰ **O99.41 Diseases of the circulatory system complicating pregnancy**

O99.411 Diseases of the circulatory system complicating pregnancy, first trimester ⒸⒸⓂ♀

O99.412 Diseases of the circulatory system complicating pregnancy, second trimester ⒸⒸⓂ♀

O99.413 Diseases of the circulatory system complicating pregnancy, third trimester ⒸⒸⓂ♀

O99.419 Diseases of the circulatory system complicating pregnancy, unspecified trimester Ⓜ♀

O99.42 Diseases of the circulatory system complicating childbirth ⓂⒸⒸⓂ♀
CC Excl: See code: O90.3

O99.43 Diseases of the circulatory system complicating the puerperium ⒸⒸⓂ♀

√5ᵗʰ **O99.5 Diseases of the respiratory system complicating pregnancy, childbirth and the puerperium**
Conditions in J00-J99

√6ᵗʰ **O99.51 Diseases of the respiratory system complicating pregnancy**

O99.511 Diseases of the respiratory system complicating pregnancy, first trimester Ⓜ♀

O99.512 Diseases of the respiratory system complicating pregnancy, second trimester Ⓜ♀

O99.513 Diseases of the respiratory system complicating pregnancy, third trimester Ⓜ♀

O99.519 Diseases of the respiratory system complicating pregnancy, unspecified trimester Ⓜ♀

O99.52 Diseases of the respiratory system complicating childbirth Ⓜ♀

O99.53 Diseases of the respiratory system complicating the puerperium Ⓜ♀

√5ᵗʰ **O99.6 Diseases of the digestive system complicating pregnancy, childbirth and the puerperium**
Conditions in K00-K93
EXCLUDES 2 *liver and biliary tract disorders in pregnancy, childbirth and the puerperium (O26.6-)*

√6ᵗʰ **O99.61 Diseases of the digestive system complicating pregnancy**

O99.611 Diseases of the digestive system complicating pregnancy, first trimester Ⓜ♀

O99.612 Diseases of the digestive system complicating pregnancy, second trimester Ⓜ♀

O99.613 Diseases of the digestive system complicating pregnancy, third trimester Ⓜ♀

O99.619 Diseases of the digestive system complicating pregnancy, unspecified trimester Ⓜ♀

O99.62   **Diseases of the digestive system complicating** M♀
childbirth

O99.63   **Diseases of the digestive system complicating** M♀
the puerperium

✓5ᵗʰ **O99.7**   **Diseases of the** skin and subcutaneous **tissue complicating**
pregnancy, childbirth and the puerperium
Conditions in L00-L99
EXCLUDES 2   *herpes gestationis (O26.4)*
pruritic urticarial papules and plaques of pregnancy
(PUPPP) (O26.86)

✓6ᵗʰ **O99.71**   **Diseases of the skin and subcutaneous tissue**
complicating pregnancy

O99.711   **Diseases of the skin and** M♀
subcutaneous tissue complicating
pregnancy, first trimester

O99.712   **Diseases of the skin and** M♀
subcutaneous tissue complicating
pregnancy, second trimester

O99.713   **Diseases of the skin and** M♀
subcutaneous tissue complicating
pregnancy, third trimester

O99.719   **Diseases of the skin and** M♀
subcutaneous tissue complicating
pregnancy, unspecified trimester

O99.72   **Diseases of the skin and subcutaneous tissue** M♀
complicating childbirth

O99.73   **Diseases of the skin and subcutaneous tissue** M♀
complicating the puerperium

✓5ᵗʰ **O99.8**   **Other** specified diseases and conditions complicating
pregnancy, childbirth and the puerperium
Conditions in D00-D48, H00-H95, M00-N99, and Q00-Q99
Use additional code to identify condition
EXCLUDES 2   *genitourinary infections in pregnancy (O23.-)*
infection of genitourinary tract following delivery
(O86.1-O86.3)
malignant neoplasm complicating pregnancy,
childbirth and the puerperium (O9A.1-)
maternal care for known or suspected abnormality of
maternal pelvic organs (O34.-)
postpartum acute kidney failure (O90.4)
traumatic injuries in pregnancy (O9A.2)

CC Excl: For CC codes in subcategory O99.8, unless
otherwise noted: O98.411-O98.613, O98.711-O98.93,
O99.830-O99.835

✓6ᵗʰ **O99.81**   Abnormal glucose **complicating pregnancy,**
childbirth and the puerperium
EXCLUDES 1   *gestational diabetes (O24.4-)*

O99.810   **Abnormal glucose complicating** M♀
pregnancy

O99.814   **Abnormal glucose complicating** M♀
childbirth

O99.815   **Abnormal glucose complicating the** M♀
puerperium

✓6ᵗʰ **O99.82**   Streptococcus B carrier state **complicating**
pregnancy, childbirth and the puerperium

O99.820   **Streptococcus B carrier state** M♀
complicating pregnancy

O99.824   **Streptococcus B carrier state** M♀
complicating childbirth

O99.825   **Streptococcus B carrier state** M♀
complicating the puerperium

✓6ᵗʰ **O99.83**   Other infection carrier state **complicating**
pregnancy, childbirth and the puerperium
Use additional code to identify the carrier state (Z22.-)

O99.830   **Other infection carrier state** CC M♀
complicating pregnancy

O99.834   **Other infection carrier state** CC M♀
complicating childbirth

O99.835   **Other infection carrier state** CC M♀
complicating the puerperium

✓6ᵗʰ **O99.84**   Bariatric surgery status **complicating pregnancy,**
childbirth and the puerperium
Gastric banding status complicating pregnancy,
childbirth and the puerperium
Gastric bypass status for obesity complicating
pregnancy, childbirth and the puerperium
Obesity surgery status complicating pregnancy,
childbirth and the puerperium

O99.840   **Bariatric surgery status complicating** M♀
pregnancy, unspecified trimester

O99.841   **Bariatric surgery status complicating** M♀
pregnancy, first trimester

O99.842   **Bariatric surgery status complicating** M♀
pregnancy, second trimester

O99.843   **Bariatric surgery status complicating** M♀
pregnancy, third trimester

O99.844   **Bariatric surgery status complicating** M♀
childbirth

O99.845   **Bariatric surgery status complicating** M♀
the puerperium

O99.89   Other specified diseases and conditions M♀
complicating pregnancy, childbirth and the
puerperium

✓4ᵗʰ **O9A**   **Maternal malignant neoplasms, traumatic injuries and abuse**
classifiable elsewhere but complicating pregnancy, childbirth
and the puerperium

✓5ᵗʰ **O9A.1**   Malignant neoplasm complicating pregnancy, childbirth and
the puerperium
Conditions in C00-C96
Use additional code to identify neoplasm
EXCLUDES 2   *maternal care for benign tumor of corpus uteri (O34.1-)*
maternal care for benign tumor of cervix (O34.4-)

✓6ᵗʰ **O9A.11**   **Malignant neoplasm complicating** pregnancy

O9A.111   **Malignant neoplasm complicating** M♀
pregnancy, first trimester

O9A.112   **Malignant neoplasm complicating** M♀
pregnancy, second trimester

O9A.113   **Malignant neoplasm complicating** M♀
pregnancy, third trimester

O9A.119   **Malignant neoplasm complicating** M♀
pregnancy, unspecified trimester

O9A.12   **Malignant neoplasm complicating** childbirth M♀

O9A.13   **Malignant neoplasm complicating the** M♀
puerperium

✓5ᵗʰ **O9A.2**   Injury, poisoning and certain other consequences of external
causes complicating pregnancy, childbirth and the
puerperium
Conditions in S00-T88, except T74 and T76
Use additional code(s) to identify the injury or poisoning
EXCLUDES 2   *physical, sexual and psychological abuse complicating*
pregnancy, childbirth and the puerperium
(O9A.3-, O9A.4-, O9A.5-)

✓6ᵗʰ **O9A.21**   **Injury, poisoning and certain other consequences of**
external causes complicating pregnancy

O9A.211   **Injury, poisoning and certain other** M♀
consequences of external causes
complicating pregnancy,
first trimester

O9A.212   **Injury, poisoning and certain other** M♀
consequences of external causes
complicating pregnancy,
second trimester

O9A.213   **Injury, poisoning and certain other** M♀
consequences of external causes
complicating pregnancy,
third trimester

O9A.219   **Injury, poisoning and certain other** M♀
consequences of external causes
complicating pregnancy, unspecified
trimester

O9A.22   **Injury, poisoning and certain other** M♀
consequences of external causes complicating
childbirth

O9A.23   **Injury, poisoning and certain other** M♀
consequences of external causes complicating the
puerperium

✓5ᵗʰ **O9A.3**   Physical abuse complicating pregnancy, childbirth and the
puerperium
Conditions in T74.11 or T76.11
Use additional code (if applicable):
to identify any associated current injury due to physical abuse
to identify the perpetrator of abuse (Y07.-)
EXCLUDES 2   *sexual abuse complicating pregnancy, childbirth and*
the puerperium (O9A.4)

✓6ᵗʰ **O9A.31**   **Physical abuse complicating** pregnancy

O9A.311   **Physical abuse complicating** M♀
pregnancy, first trimester

O9A.312   **Physical abuse complicating** M♀
pregnancy, second trimester

☑ Additional Character Required   ✓x7ᵗʰ Placeholder Alert   Unacceptable PDx   Manifestation   Hospital Acquired Condition   *EXCLUDES 1* Not Coded Here   *EXCLUDES 2* Not Included Here

ICD-10-CM 2016   843

O9A.313   **Physical abuse complicating**   Ⓜ♀
          pregnancy, third trimester

O9A.319   **Physical abuse complicating**   Ⓜ♀
          pregnancy, unspecified trimester

O9A.32   **Physical abuse complicating childbirth**   Ⓜ♀

O9A.33   **Physical abuse complicating the puerperium**   Ⓜ♀

√5ᵗʰ **O9A.4   Sexual abuse complicating pregnancy, childbirth and the**
          puerperium
          Conditions in T74.21 or T76.21
          Use additional code (if applicable):
             to identify any associated current injury due to sexual abuse
             to identify the perpetrator of abuse (Y07.-)

√6ᵗʰ **O9A.41   Sexual abuse complicating pregnancy**

O9A.411   **Sexual abuse complicating**   Ⓜ♀
          pregnancy, first trimester

O9A.412   **Sexual abuse complicating**   Ⓜ♀
          pregnancy, second trimester

O9A.413   **Sexual abuse complicating**   Ⓜ♀
          pregnancy, third trimester

O9A.419   **Sexual abuse complicating**   Ⓜ♀
          pregnancy, unspecified trimester

O9A.42   **Sexual abuse complicating childbirth**   Ⓜ♀

O9A.43   **Sexual abuse complicating the puerperium**   Ⓜ♀

√5ᵗʰ **O9A.5   Psychological abuse complicating pregnancy, childbirth and**
          the puerperium
          Conditions in T74.31 or T76.31
          Use additional code to identify the perpetrator of abuse (Y07.-)

√6ᵗʰ **O9A.51   Psychological abuse complicating pregnancy**

O9A.511   **Psychological abuse complicating**   Ⓜ♀
          pregnancy, first trimester

O9A.512   **Psychological abuse complicating**   Ⓜ♀
          pregnancy, second trimester

O9A.513   **Psychological abuse complicating**   Ⓜ♀
          pregnancy, third trimester

O9A.519   **Psychological abuse complicating**   Ⓜ♀
          pregnancy, unspecified trimester

O9A.52   **Psychological abuse complicating childbirth**   Ⓜ♀

O9A.53   **Psychological abuse complicating the**   Ⓜ♀
          puerperium

Chapter 16. Certain Conditions Originating in the Perinatal Period (P00–P96)

Chapter Specific Guidelines with Coding Examples

The chapter specific guidelines from the ICD-10-CM Official Guidelines for Coding and Reporting have been provided below. Along with these guidelines are coding examples, contained in the shaded boxes, that have been developed to help illustrate the coding and/or sequencing guidance found in these guidelines.

For coding and reporting purposes the perinatal period is defined as before birth through the 28th day following birth. The following guidelines are provided for reporting purposes

a. General Perinatal Rules

1) Use of chapter 16 codes

Codes in this chapter are <u>never</u> for use on the maternal record. Codes from Chapter 15, the obstetric chapter, are never permitted on the newborn record. Chapter 16 codes may be used throughout the life of the patient if the condition is still present.

2) Principal diagnosis for birth record

When coding the birth episode in a newborn record, assign a code from category Z38, Liveborn infants according to place of birth and type of delivery, as the principal diagnosis. A code from category Z38 is assigned only once, to a newborn at the time of birth. If a newborn is transferred to another institution, a code from category Z38 should not be used at the receiving hospital.

A code from category Z38 is used only on the newborn record, not on the mother's record.

> Newborn delivered via vaginal delivery in Rural Hospital A, experienced meconium aspiration resulting in pneumonia. Rural hospital A is not equipped to handle the extensive respiratory therapy this baby needs and transfers the patient to Metropolis Hospital B, where the pneumonia resolves and the newborn is eventually discharged.
>
> *Rural hospital A*
>
> **Z38.00**   **Single liveborn infant, delivered vaginally**
>
> **P24.01**   **Meconium aspiration with respiratory symptoms**
>
> *Metropolis hospital B*
>
> **P24.01**   **Meconium aspiration with respiratory symptoms**
>
> *Explanation:* A code from category Z38 is a one-time use only code. The hospital that actually delivered the newborn, in this case Rural Hospital A, can append a code from category Z38 but for the delivery admission only. Once the patient is transferred or discharged, the Z38 category no longer applies for that patient.
>
> The reason for the transfer to Metropolis hospital B was for the respiratory symptoms (pneumonia) the newborn was exhibiting secondary to aspirating meconium.

3) Use of codes from other chapters with codes from chapter 16

Codes from other chapters may be used with codes from chapter 16 if the codes from the other chapters provide more specific detail. Codes for signs and symptoms may be assigned when a definitive diagnosis has not been established. If the reason for the encounter is a perinatal condition, the code from chapter 16 should be sequenced first.

4) Use of chapter 16 codes after the perinatal period

Should a condition originate in the perinatal period, and continue throughout the life of the patient, the perinatal code should continue to be used regardless of the patient's age.

> A 7-year-old patient with history of birth injury that resulted in Erb's palsy is seen for subscapularis release
>
> **P14.0**   **Erb's paralysis due to birth injury**
>
> *Explanation:* Although in this instance Erb's palsy is specifically related to a birth injury, it has not resolved and continues to be a health concern. A perinatal code is appropriate even though this patient is beyond the perinatal period.

5) Birth process or community acquired conditions

If a newborn has a condition that may be either due to the birth process or community acquired and the documentation does not indicate which it is, the default is due to the birth process and the code from Chapter 16 should be used. If the condition is community-acquired, a code from Chapter 16 should not be assigned.

6) Code all clinically significant conditions

All clinically significant conditions noted on routine newborn examination should be coded. A condition is clinically significant if it requires:

- clinical evaluation; or
- therapeutic treatment; or
- diagnostic procedures; or
- extended length of hospital stay; or
- increased nursing care and/or monitoring; or
- has implications for future health care needs

Note: The perinatal guidelines listed above are the same as the general coding guidelines for "additional diagnoses", except for the final point regarding implications for future health care needs. Codes should be assigned for conditions that have been specified by the provider as having implications for future health care needs.

b. Observation and evaluation of newborns for suspected conditions not found

Reserved for future expansion

c. Coding additional perinatal diagnoses

1) Assigning codes for conditions that require treatment

Assign codes for conditions that require treatment or further investigation, prolong the length of stay, or require resource utilization.

2) Codes for conditions specified as having implications for future health care needs

Assign codes for conditions that have been specified by the provider as having implications for future health care needs.

Note: This guideline should not be used for adult patients.

> An abnormal noise was heard in the left hip of a post-term newborn during a physical examination. The pediatrician would like to follow the patient after discharge as a hip click can be an early sign of hip dysplasia. The newborn was delivered via cesarean at 41 weeks.
>
> **Z38.01**   **Single liveborn infant, delivered by cesarean**
>
> **P08.21**   **Post-term newborn**
>
> **R29.4**   **Clicking hip**
>
> *Explanation:* The abnormal hip noise or click is appended as a secondary diagnosis not only because it is an abnormal finding upon examination, but also due to its potential to be part of a bigger health issue. The hip dysplasia has not yet been diagnosed and does not warrant a code at this time.

d. Prematurity and fetal growth retardation

Providers utilize different criteria in determining prematurity. A code for prematurity should not be assigned unless it is documented. Assignment of codes in categories P05, Disorders of newborn related to slow fetal growth and fetal malnutrition, and P07, Disorders of newborn related to short gestation and low birth weight, not elsewhere classified, should be based on the recorded birth weight and estimated gestational age. Codes from category P05 should not be assigned with codes from category P07.

When both birth weight and gestational age are available, two codes from category P07 should be assigned, with the code for birth weight sequenced before the code for gestational age.

Chapter 16. Certain Conditions Originating in the Perinatal Period

e. Low birth weight and immaturity status

Codes from category P07, Disorders of newborn related to short gestation and low birth weight, not elsewhere classified, are for use for a child or adult who was premature or had a low birth weight as a newborn and this is affecting the patient's current health status.

See Section I.C.21. Factors influencing health status and contact with health services, Status.

> A 35-year-old patient, who weighed 659 grams at birth, is seen for heart disease documented as being a consequence of the low birth weight
>
> **I51.9**　　**Heart disease, unspecified**
>
> **P07.02**　　**Extremely low birth weight newborn, 500–749 grams**
>
> *Explanation:* A code from subcategories P07.0- and P07.1- is appropriate, regardless of the age of the patient, as long as the documentation provides a clear link between the patient's current illness and the low birth weight.

f. Bacterial Sepsis of Newborn

Category P36, Bacterial sepsis of newborn, includes congenital sepsis. If a perinate is documented as having sepsis without documentation of congenital or community acquired, the default is congenital and a code from category P36 should be assigned. If the P36 code includes the causal organism, an additional code from category B95, Streptococcus, Staphylococcus, and Enterococcus as the cause of diseases classified elsewhere, or B96, Other bacterial agents as the cause of diseases classified elsewhere, should not be assigned. If the P36 code does not include the causal organism, assign an additional code from category B96. If applicable, use additional codes to identify severe sepsis (R65.2-) and any associated acute organ dysfunction.

> A full-term infant develops severe sepsis 24 hours after discharge from the hospital and is readmitted; cultures identified *E. coli* as the infective agent
>
> **P36.4**　　**Sepsis of newborn due to Escherichia coli**
>
> **R65.20**　　**Severe sepsis without septic shock**
>
> *Explanation:* Even though this newborn was discharged and could have acquired *E. coli* from his/her external environment, due to the lack of documentation specifying specifically how this pathogen was acquired, the default is to code the *E. coli* sepsis as congenital. A code from chapter 1, "Certain Infectious and Parasitic Diseases," is not required because the perinatal sepsis code identifies both the sepsis and the bacteria causing the sepsis.

g. Stillbirth

Code P95, Stillbirth, is only for use in institutions that maintain separate records for stillbirths. No other code should be used with P95. Code P95 should not be used on the mother's record.

Chapter 16. Certain Conditions Originating in the Perinatal Period (P00-P96)

NOTE   Codes from this chapter are for use on newborn records only, never on maternal records.

INCLUDES   conditions that have their origin in the fetal or perinatal period (before birth through the first 28 days after birth) even if morbidity occurs later

EXCLUDES 2   congenital malformations, deformations and chromosomal abnormalities (Q00-Q99)
endocrine, nutritional and metabolic diseases (E00-E88)
injury, poisoning and certain other consequences of external causes (S00-T88)
neoplasms (C00-D49)
tetanus neonatorum (A33)

This chapter contains the following blocks:

P00-P04	Newborn affected by maternal factors and by complications of pregnancy, labor, and delivery
P05-P08	Disorders of newborn related to length of gestation and fetal growth
P09	Abnormal findings on neonatal screening
P10-P15	Birth trauma
P19-P29	Respiratory and cardiovascular disorders specific to the perinatal period
P35-P39	Infections specific to the perinatal period
P50-P61	Hemorrhagic and hematological disorders of newborn
P70-P74	Transitory endocrine and metabolic disorders specific to newborn
P76-P78	Digestive system disorders of newborn
P80-P83	Conditions involving the integument and temperature regulation of newborn
P84	Other problems with newborn
P90-P96	Other disorders originating in the perinatal period

Newborn affected by maternal factors and by complications of pregnancy, labor, and delivery (P00-P04)

NOTE   These codes are for use when the listed maternal conditions are specified as the cause of confirmed morbidity or potential morbidity which have their origin in the perinatal period (before birth through the first 28 days after birth). Codes from these categories are also for use for newborns who are suspected of having an abnormal condition resulting from exposure from the mother or the birth process, but without signs or symptoms, and, which after examination and observation, is found not to exist. These codes may be used even if treatment is begun for a suspected condition that is ruled out.

✓4ᵗʰ P00   Newborn (suspected to be) affected by maternal conditions that may be unrelated to present pregnancy
Code first any current condition in newborn
EXCLUDES 2   newborn (suspected to be) affected by maternal complications of pregnancy (P01.-)
newborn affected by maternal endocrine and metabolic disorders (P70-P74)
newborn affected by noxious substances transmitted via placenta or breast milk (P04.-)

P00.0   Newborn (suspected to be) affected by maternal hypertensive disorders N
Newborn (suspected to be) affected by maternal conditions classifiable to O10-O11, O13-O16

P00.1   Newborn (suspected to be) affected by maternal renal and urinary tract diseases N
Newborn (suspected to be) affected by maternal conditions classifiable to N00-N39

P00.2   Newborn (suspected to be) affected by maternal infectious and parasitic diseases N
Newborn (suspected to be) affected by maternal infectious disease classifiable to A00-B99, J09 and J10
EXCLUDES 1   infections specific to the perinatal period (P35-P39)
maternal genital tract or other localized infections (P00.8)

P00.3   Newborn (suspected to be) affected by other maternal circulatory and respiratory diseases N
Newborn (suspected to be) affected by maternal conditions classifiable to I00-I99, J00-J99, Q20-Q34 and not included in P00.0, P00.2

P00.4   Newborn (suspected to be) affected by maternal nutritional disorders N
Newborn (suspected to be) affected by maternal disorders classifiable to E40-E64
Maternal malnutrition NOS

P00.5   Newborn (suspected to be) affected by maternal injury N
Newborn (suspected to be) affected by maternal conditions classifiable to O9A.2-

P00.6   Newborn (suspected to be) affected by surgical procedure on mother N
Newborn (suspected to be) affected by amniocentesis
EXCLUDES 1   Cesarean delivery for present delivery (P03.4)
damage to placenta from amniocentesis, Cesarean delivery or surgical induction (P02.1)
previous surgery to uterus or pelvic organs (P03.89)
EXCLUDES 2   newborn affected by complication of (fetal) intrauterine procedure (P96.5)

P00.7   Newborn (suspected to be) affected by other medical procedures on mother, not elsewhere classified
Newborn (suspected to be) affected by radiation to mother
EXCLUDES 1   damage to placenta from amniocentesis, cesarean delivery or surgical induction (P02.1)
newborn affected by other complications of labor and delivery (P03.-)

✓5ᵗʰ P00.8   Newborn (suspected to be) affected by other maternal conditions

   P00.81   Newborn (suspected to be) affected by periodontal disease in mother N

   P00.89   Newborn (suspected to be) affected by other maternal conditions N
Newborn (suspected to be) affected by conditions classifiable to T80-T88
Newborn (suspected to be) affected by maternal genital tract or other localized infections
Newborn (suspected to be) affected by maternal systemic lupus erythematosus

P00.9   Newborn (suspected to be) affected by unspecified maternal condition N

✓4ᵗʰ P01   Newborn (suspected to be) affected by maternal complications of pregnancy N
Code first any current condition in newborn

P01.0   Newborn (suspected to be) affected by incompetent cervix N

P01.1   Newborn (suspected to be) affected by premature rupture of membranes N

P01.2   Newborn (suspected to be) affected by oligohydramnios N
EXCLUDES 1   oligohydramnios due to premature rupture of membranes (P01.1)

P01.3   Newborn (suspected to be) affected by polyhydramnios N
Newborn (suspected to be) affected by hydramnios

P01.4   Newborn (suspected to be) affected by ectopic pregnancy N
Newborn (suspected to be) affected by abdominal pregnancy

P01.5   Newborn (suspected to be) affected by multiple pregnancy N
Newborn (suspected to be) affected by triplet (pregnancy)
Newborn (suspected to be) affected by twin (pregnancy)

P01.6   Newborn (suspected to be) affected by maternal death N

P01.7   Newborn (suspected to be) affected by malpresentation before labor N
Newborn (suspected to be) affected by breech presentation before labor
Newborn (suspected to be) affected by external version before labor
Newborn (suspected to be) affected by face presentation before labor
Newborn (suspected to be) affected by transverse lie before labor
Newborn (suspected to be) affected by unstable lie before labor

P01.8   Newborn (suspected to be) affected by other maternal complications of pregnancy N

P01.9   Newborn (suspected to be) affected by maternal complication of pregnancy, unspecified N

✓4ᵗʰ P02   Newborn (suspected to be) affected by complications of placenta, cord and membranes N
Code first any current condition in newborn

P02.0   Newborn (suspected to be) affected by placenta previa N

P02.1   Newborn (suspected to be) affected by other forms of placental separation and hemorrhage N
Newborn (suspected to be) affected by abruptio placenta
Newborn (suspected to be) affected by accidental hemorrhage
Newborn (suspected to be) affected by antepartum hemorrhage
Newborn (suspected to be) affected by damage to placenta from amniocentesis, cesarean delivery or surgical induction
Newborn (suspected to be) affected by maternal blood loss
Newborn (suspected to be) affected by premature separation of placenta

✓5ᵗʰ P02.2   Newborn (suspected to be) affected by other and unspecified morphological and functional abnormalities of placenta

   P02.20   Newborn (suspected to be) affected by unspecified morphological and functional abnormalities of placenta N

☑ Additional Character Required   ✓x7ᵗʰ Placeholder Alert   Unacceptable PDx   Manifestation   Hospital Acquired Condition   **EXCLUDES 1** Not Coded Here   **EXCLUDES 2** Not Included Here

Chapter 16. Certain Conditions Originating in the Perinatal Period

P02.29 **Newborn (suspected to be) affected by** other morphological and functional **abnormalities of placenta** N
    Newborn (suspected to be) affected by placental dysfunction
    Newborn (suspected to be) affected by placental infarction
    Newborn (suspected to be) affected by placental insufficiency

P02.3 **Newborn (suspected to be) affected by** placental **transfusion syndromes** N
    Newborn (suspected to be) affected by placental and cord abnormalities resulting in twin-to-twin or other transplacental transfusion

P02.4 **Newborn (suspected to be) affected by** prolapsed cord N

P02.5 **Newborn (suspected to be) affected by** other compression of umbilical cord N
    Newborn (suspected to be) affected by umbilical cord (tightly) around neck
    Newborn (suspected to be) affected by entanglement of umbilical cord
    Newborn (suspected to be) affected by knot in umbilical cord

✓5ᵗʰ **P02.6** **Newborn (suspected to be) affected by** other and unspecified conditions of umbilical cord

  P02.60 **Newborn (suspected to be) affected by** unspecified conditions of umbilical cord N

  P02.69 **Newborn (suspected to be) affected by** other conditions of umbilical cord N
    Newborn (suspected to be) affected by short umbilical cord
    Newborn (suspected to be) affected by vasa previa
    EXCLUDES 1 *newborn affected by single umbilical artery (Q27.0)*

P02.7 **Newborn (suspected to be) affected by** chorioamnionitis N
    Newborn (suspected to be) affected by amnionitis
    Newborn (suspected to be) affected by membranitis
    Newborn (suspected to be) affected by placentitis

P02.8 **Newborn (suspected to be) affected by** other abnormalities of membranes N

P02.9 **Newborn (suspected to be) affected by** abnormality of membranes, unspecified N

✓4ᵗʰ **P03** **Newborn (suspected to be) affected by other complications of labor and delivery**
    Code first any current condition in newborn

P03.0 **Newborn (suspected to be) affected by** breech delivery and extraction N

P03.1 **Newborn (suspected to be) affected by** other malpresentation, malposition and disproportion **during labor and delivery** N
    Newborn (suspected to be) affected by contracted pelvis
    Newborn (suspected to be) affected by conditions classifiable to O64-O66
    Newborn (suspected to be) affected by persistent occipitoposterior
    Newborn (suspected to be) affected by transverse lie

P03.2 **Newborn (suspected to be) affected by** forceps delivery N

P03.3 **Newborn (suspected to be) affected by** delivery by vacuum extractor [**ventouse**] N

P03.4 **Newborn (suspected to be) affected by** Cesarean delivery N

P03.5 **Newborn (suspected to be) affected by** precipitate delivery N
    Newborn (suspected to be) affected by rapid second stage

P03.6 **Newborn (suspected to be) affected by** abnormal uterine contractions N
    Newborn (suspected to be) affected by conditions classifiable to O62-, except O62.3
    Newborn (suspected to be) affected by hypertonic labor
    Newborn (suspected to be) affected by uterine inertia

✓5ᵗʰ **P03.8** **Newborn (suspected to be) affected by** other specified complications of labor and delivery

  ✓6ᵗʰ **P03.81** **Newborn (suspected to be) affected by** abnormality in fetal (intrauterine) heart rate or rhythm
    EXCLUDES 1 *neonatal cardiac dysrhythmia (P29.1-)*

    P03.810 **Newborn (suspected to be) affected by** abnormality in fetal (intrauterine) heart rate or rhythm before the onset of labor N

    P03.811 **Newborn (suspected to be) affected by** abnormality in fetal (intrauterine) heart rate or rhythm during labor N

    P03.819 **Newborn (suspected to be) affected by** abnormality in fetal (intrauterine) heart rate or rhythm, unspecified as to time of onset N

  P03.82 **Meconium passage during delivery** N
    EXCLUDES 1 *meconium aspiration (P24.00, P24.01)*
    meconium staining (P96.83)

  P03.89 **Newborn (suspected to be) affected by** other specified complications of labor and delivery N
    Newborn (suspected to be) affected by abnormality of maternal soft tissues
    Newborn (suspected to be) affected by conditions classifiable to O60-O75 and by procedures used in labor and delivery not included in P02- and P03.0-P03.6
    Newborn (suspected to be) affected by induction of labor

P03.9 **Newborn (suspected to be) affected by** complication of labor and delivery, unspecified N

✓4ᵗʰ **P04** **Newborn (suspected to be) affected by** noxious substances transmitted via placenta or breast milk
    INCLUDES nonteratogenic effects of substances transmitted via placenta
    EXCLUDES 2 *congenital malformations (Q00-Q99)*
    neonatal jaundice from excessive hemolysis due to drugs or toxins transmitted from mother (P58.4)
    newborn in contact with and (suspected) exposures hazardous to health not transmitted via placenta or breast milk (Z77.-)

P04.0 **Newborn (suspected to be) affected by maternal** anesthesia and analgesia **in pregnancy, labor and delivery** N
    Newborn (suspected to be) affected by reactions and intoxications from maternal opiates and tranquilizers administered during labor and delivery

P04.1 **Newborn (suspected to be) affected by** other maternal medication N
    Newborn (suspected to be) affected by cancer chemotherapy
    Newborn (suspected to be) affected by cytotoxic drugs
    EXCLUDES 1 *dysmorphism due to warfarin (Q86.2)*
    fetal hydantoin syndrome (Q86.1)
    maternal use of drugs of addiction (P04.4-)

P04.2 **Newborn (suspected to be) affected by maternal** use of tobacco N
    Newborn (suspected to be) affected by exposure in utero to tobacco smoke
    EXCLUDES 2 *newborn exposure to environmental tobacco smoke (P96.81)*

P04.3 **Newborn (suspected to be) affected by maternal** use of alcohol N
    EXCLUDES 1 *fetal alcohol syndrome (Q86.0)*

✓5ᵗʰ **P04.4** **Newborn (suspected to be) affected by maternal use of** drugs of addiction

  P04.41 **Newborn (suspected to be) affected by maternal use of cocaine** N
    "Crack baby"

  P04.49 **Newborn (suspected to be) affected by maternal use of other drugs of addiction** N
    EXCLUDES 2 *newborn (suspected to be) affected by maternal anesthesia and analgesia (P04.0)*
    withdrawal symptoms from maternal use of drugs of addiction (P96.1)

P04.5 **Newborn (suspected to be) affected by maternal use of nutritional chemical substances** N

P04.6 **Newborn (suspected to be) affected by maternal exposure to environmental chemical substances** N

P04.8 **Newborn (suspected to be) affected by other maternal noxious substances** N

P04.9 **Newborn (suspected to be) affected by maternal noxious substance, unspecified** N

Disorders of newborn related to length of gestation and fetal growth (P05-P08)

✓4ᵗʰ **P05** **Disorders of newborn related to slow fetal growth and fetal malnutrition**

✓5ᵗʰ **P05.0** **Newborn light for gestational age**
    Newborn light-for-dates

  P05.00 **Newborn light for gestational age, unspecified weight** N

P05.01 Newborn light for gestational age, less than 500 grams

P05.02 Newborn light for gestational age, 500-749 grams

P05.03 Newborn light for gestational age, 750-999 grams

P05.04 Newborn light for gestational age, 1000-1249 grams

P05.05 Newborn light for gestational age, 1250-1499 grams

P05.06 Newborn light for gestational age, 1500-1749 grams

P05.07 Newborn light for gestational age, 1750-1999 grams

P05.08 Newborn light for gestational age, 2000-2499 grams

√5ᵗʰ P05.1 Newborn small for gestational age
Newborn small-and-light-for-dates
Newborn small-for-dates

P05.10 Newborn small for gestational age, unspecified weight

P05.11 Newborn small for gestational age, less than 500 grams

P05.12 Newborn small for gestational age, 500-749 grams

P05.13 Newborn small for gestational age, 750-999 grams

P05.14 Newborn small for gestational age, 1000-1249 grams

P05.15 Newborn small for gestational age, 1250-1499 grams

P05.16 Newborn small for gestational age, 1500-1749 grams

P05.17 Newborn small for gestational age, 1750-1999 grams

P05.18 Newborn small for gestational age, 2000-2499 grams

P05.2 Newborn affected by fetal (intrauterine) malnutrition not light or small for gestational age
Infant, not light or small for gestational age, showing signs of fetal malnutrition, such as dry, peeling skin and loss of subcutaneous tissue
EXCLUDES1 newborn affected by fetal malnutrition with light for gestational age (P05.0-)
newborn affected by fetal malnutrition with small for gestational age (P05.1-)

P05.9 Newborn affected by slow intrauterine growth, unspecified
Newborn affected by fetal growth retardation NOS

√4ᵗʰ P07 Disorders of newborn related to short gestation and low birth weight, not elsewhere classified
NOTE When both birth weight and gestational age of the newborn are available, both should be coded with birth weight sequenced before gestational age
INCLUDES the listed conditions, without further specification, as the cause of morbidity or additional care, in newborn
EXCLUDES1 low birth weight due to slow fetal growth and fetal malnutrition (P05.-)

√5ᵗʰ P07.0 Extremely low birth weight newborn
Newborn birth weight 999 g. or less

P07.00 Extremely low birth weight newborn, unspecified weight

P07.01 Extremely low birth weight newborn, less than 500 grams

P07.02 Extremely low birth weight newborn, 500-749 grams

P07.03 Extremely low birth weight newborn, 750-999 grams

√5ᵗʰ P07.1 Other low birth weight newborn
Newborn birth weight 1000-2499 g.

P07.10 Other low birth weight newborn, unspecified weight

P07.14 Other low birth weight newborn, 1000-1249 grams

P07.15 Other low birth weight newborn, 1250-1499 grams

P07.16 Other low birth weight newborn, 1500-1749 grams

P07.17 Other low birth weight newborn, 1750-1999 grams

P07.18 Other low birth weight newborn, 2000-2499 grams

√5ᵗʰ P07.2 Extreme immaturity of newborn
Less than 28 completed weeks (less than 196 completed days) of gestation.

P07.20 Extreme immaturity of newborn, unspecified weeks of gestation
Gestational age less than 28 completed weeks NOS

P07.21 Extreme immaturity of newborn, gestational age less than 23 completed weeks
Extreme immaturity of newborn, gestational age less than 23 weeks, 0 days

P07.22 Extreme immaturity of newborn, gestational age 23 completed weeks
Extreme immaturity of newborn, gestational age 23 weeks, 0 days through 23 weeks, 6 days

P07.23 Extreme immaturity of newborn, gestational age 24 completed weeks
Extreme immaturity of newborn, gestational age 24 weeks, 0 days through 24 weeks, 6 days

P07.24 Extreme immaturity of newborn, gestational age 25 completed weeks
Extreme immaturity of newborn, gestational age 25 weeks, 0 days through 25 weeks, 6 days

P07.25 Extreme immaturity of newborn, gestational age 26 completed weeks
Extreme immaturity of newborn, gestational age 26 weeks, 0 days through 26 weeks, 6 days

P07.26 Extreme immaturity of newborn, gestational age 27 completed weeks
Extreme immaturity of newborn, gestational age 27 weeks, 0 days through 27 weeks, 6 days

√5ᵗʰ P07.3 Preterm [premature] newborn [other]
28 completed weeks or more but less than 37 completed weeks (196 completed days but less than 259 completed days) of gestation
Prematurity NOS

P07.30 Preterm newborn, unspecified weeks of gestation

P07.31 Preterm newborn, gestational age 28 completed weeks
Preterm newborn, gestational age 28 weeks, 0 days through 28 weeks, 6 days

P07.32 Preterm newborn, gestational age 29 completed weeks
Preterm newborn, gestational age 29 weeks, 0 days through 29 weeks, 6 days

P07.33 Preterm newborn, gestational age 30 completed weeks
Preterm newborn, gestational age 30 weeks, 0 days through 30 weeks, 6 days

P07.34 Preterm newborn, gestational age 31 completed weeks
Preterm newborn, gestational age 31 weeks, 0 days through 31 weeks, 6 days

P07.35 Preterm newborn, gestational age 32 completed weeks
Preterm newborn, gestational age 32 weeks, 0 days through 32 weeks, 6 days

P07.36 Preterm newborn, gestational age 33 completed weeks
Preterm newborn, gestational age 33 weeks, 0 days through 33 weeks, 6 days

P07.37 Preterm newborn, gestational age 34 completed weeks
Preterm newborn, gestational age 34 weeks, 0 days through 34 weeks, 6 days

P07.38 Preterm newborn, gestational age 35 completed weeks
Preterm newborn, gestational age 35 weeks, 0 days through 35 weeks, 6 days

P07.39 Preterm newborn, gestational age 36 completed weeks
Preterm newborn, gestational age 36 weeks, 0 days through 36 weeks, 6 days

☑4ᵗʰ P08 Disorders of newborn related to long gestation and high birth weight

NOTE When both birth weight and gestational age of the newborn are available, priority of assignment should be given to birth weight

INCLUDES the listed conditions, without further specification, as causes of morbidity or additional care, in newborn

P08.0 Exceptionally large newborn baby   N
Usually implies a birth weight of 4500 g. or more
EXCLUDES 1 syndrome of infant of diabetic mother (P70.1)
syndrome of infant of mother with gestational diabetes (P70.0)

P08.1 Other heavy for gestational age newborn   N
Other newborn heavy- or large-for-dates regardless of period of gestation
Usually implies a birth weight of 4000 g. to 4499 g.
EXCLUDES 1 newborn with a birth weight of 4500 or more (P08.0)
syndrome of infant of diabetic mother (P70.1)
syndrome of infant of mother with gestational diabetes (P70.0).

☑5ᵗʰ **P08.2 Late newborn, not heavy for gestational age**
AHA: 2014, 1Q, 14

P08.21 Post-term newborn   N
Newborn with gestation period over 40 completed weeks to 42 completed weeks

P08.22 Prolonged gestation of newborn   N
Newborn with gestation period over 42 completed weeks (294 days or more), not heavy- or large-for-dates.
Postmaturity NOS

Abnormal findings on neonatal screening (P09)

P09 Abnormal findings on neonatal screening   N
Use additional code to identify signs, symptoms and conditions associated with the screening
EXCLUDES 2 nonspecific serologic evidence of human immunodeficiency virus [HIV] (R75)

Birth trauma (P10-P15)

☑4ᵗʰ P10 Intracranial laceration and hemorrhage due to birth injury
EXCLUDES 1 intracranial hemorrhage of newborn NOS (P52.9)
intracranial hemorrhage of newborn due to anoxia or hypoxia (P52.-)
nontraumatic intracranial hemorrhage of newborn (P52.-)

P10.0 Subdural hemorrhage due to birth injury   MCC N
Subdural hematoma (localized) due to birth injury
EXCLUDES 1 subdural hemorrhage accompanying tentorial tear (P10.4)
CC Excl: P10.0-P10.1, P10.4-P11.2, P11.9, P15.0-P15.9, P29.0-P29.2, P29.4, P29.89-P29.9, P52.4, P52.6-P52.9, P94.1-P94.9, P96.0, P96.3-P96.5, P96.82-P96.89

P10.1 Cerebral hemorrhage due to birth injury   MCC N
CC Excl: See code P10.0

P10.2 Intraventricular hemorrhage due to birth injury   CC N
CC Excl: P10.2-P10.3, P29.0-P29.2, P29.4, P29.89-P29.9, P50.0-P50.9, P52.0-P52.3, P52.5, P53-P54.0, P54.6-P54.9, P60-P61.9, P94.1-P94.9, P96.0, P96.3-P96.5, P96.82-P96.89

P10.3 Subarachnoid hemorrhage due to birth injury   MCC N
CC Excl: P10.2-P10.3, P29.0-P29.2, P29.4, P29.89-P29.9, P50.0-P50.9, P52.0-P52.3, P52.5, P53-P54.0, P54.6-P54.9, P60-P61.9, P91.2, P94.1-P94.9, P96.0, P96.3-P96.5, P96.82-P96.89

P10.4 Tentorial tear due to birth injury   MCC N
CC Excl: See code P10.0

P10.8 Other intracranial lacerations and hemorrhages due to birth injury   MCC N
CC Excl: See code P10.0

P10.9 Unspecified intracranial laceration and hemorrhage due to birth injury   MCC N
CC Excl: See code P10.0

☑4ᵗʰ P11 Other birth injuries to central nervous system

P11.0 Cerebral edema due to birth injury   MCC N
CC Excl: See code P10.0

P11.1 Other specified brain damage due to birth injury   N

P11.2 Unspecified brain damage due to birth injury   MCC N
CC Excl: See code P10.0

P11.3 Birth injury to facial nerve   N
Facial palsy due to birth injury

P11.4 Birth injury to other cranial nerves   N

P11.5 Birth injury to spine and spinal cord   N
Fracture of spine due to birth injury

P11.9 Birth injury to central nervous system, unspecified   MCC N
CC Excl: See code P10.0

☑4ᵗʰ P12 Birth injury to scalp

P12.0 Cephalhematoma due to birth injury   N

P12.1 Chignon (from vacuum extraction) due to birth injury   N

P12.2 Epicranial subaponeurotic hemorrhage due to birth injury   CC N
Subgaleal hemorrhage
CC Excl: P10.0-P10.1, P10.4-P11.2, P11.9, P12.2, P15.0-P15.9, P29.0-P29.2, P29.4, P29.89-P29.9, P52.4, P52.6-P52.9, P94.1-P94.9, P96.0, P96.3-P96.5, P96.82-P96.89

P12.3 Bruising of scalp due to birth injury   N

P12.4 Injury of scalp of newborn due to monitoring equipment   N
Sampling incision of scalp of newborn
Scalp clip (electrode) injury of newborn

☑5ᵗʰ **P12.8 Other birth injuries to scalp**

P12.81 Caput succedaneum   N

P12.89 Other birth injuries to scalp   N

P12.9 Birth injury to scalp, unspecified   N

☑4ᵗʰ P13 Birth injury to skeleton
EXCLUDES 2 birth injury to spine (P11.5)

P13.0 Fracture of skull due to birth injury   N

P13.1 Other birth injuries to skull   N
EXCLUDES 1 cephalhematoma (P12.0)

P13.2 Birth injury to femur   N

P13.3 Birth injury to other long bones   N

P13.4 Fracture of clavicle due to birth injury   N

P13.8 Birth injuries to other parts of skeleton   N

P13.9 Birth injury to skeleton, unspecified   N

☑4ᵗʰ P14 Birth injury to peripheral nervous system

P14.0 Erb's paralysis due to birth injury   N

P14.1 Klumpke's paralysis due to birth injury   N

P14.2 Phrenic nerve paralysis due to birth injury   N

P14.3 Other brachial plexus birth injuries   N

P14.8 Birth injuries to other parts of peripheral nervous system   N

P14.9 Birth injury to peripheral nervous system, unspecified   N

☑4ᵗʰ P15 Other birth injuries

P15.0 Birth injury to liver   N
Rupture of liver due to birth injury

P15.1 Birth injury to spleen   N
Rupture of spleen due to birth injury

P15.2 Sternomastoid injury due to birth injury   N

P15.3 Birth injury to eye   N
Subconjunctival hemorrhage due to birth injury
Traumatic glaucoma due to birth injury

P15.4 Birth injury to face   N
Facial congestion due to birth injury

P15.5 Birth injury to external genitalia   N

P15.6 Subcutaneous fat necrosis due to birth injury   N

P15.8 Other specified birth injuries   N

P15.9 Birth injury, unspecified   N

Respiratory and cardiovascular disorders specific to the perinatal period (P19-P29)

☑4ᵗʰ P19 Metabolic acidemia in newborn
Metabolic acidemia in newborn

P19.0 Metabolic acidemia in newborn first noted before onset of labor   N

P19.1 Metabolic acidemia in newborn first noted during labor   N

P19.2 Metabolic acidemia noted at birth   N

P19.9 Metabolic acidemia, unspecified   N

√4ᵗʰ **P22 Respiratory distress of newborn**
> **EXCLUDES 1**   *respiratory arrest of newborn (P28.81)*
> *respiratory failure of newborn NOS (P28.5)*

P22.0 Respiratory distress syndrome of newborn   MCC N
Cardiorespiratory distress syndrome of newborn
Hyaline membrane disease
Idiopathic respiratory distress syndrome [IRDS or RDS] of newborn
Pulmonary hypoperfusion syndrome
Respiratory distress syndrome, type I
CC Excl: J84.83-J84.848, P22.0-P28.5, P28.89-P29.2, P29.4, P29.89-P29.9, P84, P94.1-P94.9, P96.0, P96.3-P96.5, P96.82-P96.89

P22.1 Transient tachypnea of newborn   N
Idiopathic tachypnea of newborn
Respiratory distress syndrome, type II
Wet lung syndrome

P22.8 Other respiratory distress of newborn   N

P22.9 Respiratory distress of newborn, unspecified   N

√4ᵗʰ **P23 Congenital pneumonia**
> **INCLUDES**   infective pneumonia acquired in utero or during birth
> **EXCLUDES 1**   *neonatal pneumonia resulting from aspiration (P24.-)*

> **CC Excl: For MCC codes in subcategory P23, unless otherwise noted:** J84.83-J84.848, P22.0-P28.5, P28.89-P29.2, P29.4, P29.89-P29.9, P84, P94.1-P94.9, P96.0, P96.3-P96.5, P96.82-P96.89

P23.0 Congenital pneumonia due to viral agent   MCC N
Use additional code (B97) to identify organism
> **EXCLUDES 1**   *congenital rubella pneumonitis (P35.0)*

P23.1 Congenital pneumonia due to Chlamydia   MCC N

P23.2 Congenital pneumonia due to staphylococcus   MCC N

P23.3 Congenital pneumonia due to streptococcus, group B   MCC N

P23.4 Congenital pneumonia due to Escherichia coli   MCC N

P23.5 Congenital pneumonia due to Pseudomonas   MCC N

P23.6 Congenital pneumonia due to other bacterial agents   MCC N
Congenital pneumonia due to Hemophilus influenzae
Congenital pneumonia due to Klebsiella pneumoniae
Congenital pneumonia due to Mycoplasma
Congenital pneumonia due to Streptococcus, except group B
Use additional code (B95-B96) to identify organism

P23.8 Congenital pneumonia due to other organisms   MCC N

P23.9 Congenital pneumonia, unspecified   MCC N

√4ᵗʰ **P24 Neonatal aspiration**
> **INCLUDES**   aspiration in utero and during delivery

√5ᵗʰ **P24.0 Meconium aspiration**
> **EXCLUDES 1**   *meconium passage (without aspiration) during delivery (P03.82)*
> *meconium staining (P96.83)*

P24.00 Meconium aspiration without respiratory symptoms   N
Meconium aspiration NOS

P24.01 Meconium aspiration with respiratory symptoms   MCC N
Meconium aspiration pneumonia
Meconium aspiration pneumonitis
Meconium aspiration syndrome NOS
Use additional code to identify any secondary pulmonary hypertension, if applicable (I27.2)
CC Excl: See code P23

√5ᵗʰ **P24.1 Neonatal aspiration of (clear) amniotic fluid and mucus**
Neonatal aspiration of liquor (amnii)

P24.10 Neonatal aspiration of (clear) amniotic fluid and mucus without respiratory symptoms   N
Neonatal aspiration of amniotic fluid and mucus NOS

P24.11 Neonatal aspiration of (clear) amniotic fluid and mucus with respiratory symptoms   MCC N
Neonatal aspiration of amniotic fluid and mucus with pneumonia
Neonatal aspiration of amniotic fluid and mucus with pneumonitis
Use additional code to identify any secondary pulmonary hypertension, if applicable (I27.2)
CC Excl: See code P23

√5ᵗʰ **P24.2 Neonatal aspiration of blood**

P24.20 Neonatal aspiration of blood without respiratory symptoms   N
Neonatal aspiration of blood NOS

P24.21 Neonatal aspiration of blood with respiratory symptoms   MCC N
Neonatal aspiration of blood with pneumonia
Neonatal aspiration of blood with pneumonitis
Use additional code to identify any secondary pulmonary hypertension, if applicable (I27.2)
CC Excl: See code P23

√5ᵗʰ **P24.3 Neonatal aspiration of milk and regurgitated food**
Neonatal aspiration of stomach contents

P24.30 Neonatal aspiration of milk and regurgitated food without respiratory symptoms   N
Neonatal aspiration of milk and regurgitated food NOS

P24.31 Neonatal aspiration of milk and regurgitated food with respiratory symptoms   MCC N
Neonatal aspiration of milk and regurgitated food with pneumonia
Neonatal aspiration of milk and regurgitated food with pneumonitis
Use additional code to identify any secondary pulmonary hypertension, if applicable (I27.2)
CC Excl: See code P23

√5ᵗʰ **P24.8 Other neonatal aspiration**

P24.80 Other neonatal aspiration without respiratory symptoms   N
Neonatal aspiration NEC

P24.81 Other neonatal aspiration with respiratory symptoms   MCC N
Neonatal aspiration pneumonia NEC
Neonatal aspiration with pneumonitis NEC
Neonatal aspiration with pneumonia NOS
Neonatal aspiration with pneumonitis NOS
Use additional code to identify any secondary pulmonary hypertension, if applicable (I27.2)
CC Excl: See code P23

P24.9 Neonatal aspiration, unspecified   N

√4ᵗʰ **P25 Interstitial emphysema and related conditions originating in the perinatal period**

> **CC Excl: For MCC codes in subcategory P25, unless otherwise noted:** J84.83-J84.848, P22.0-P28.5, P28.89-P29.2, P29.4, P29.89-P29.9, P84, P94.1-P94.9, P96.0, P96.3-P96.5, P96.82-P96.89

P25.0 Interstitial emphysema originating in the perinatal period   MCC N

P25.1 Pneumothorax originating in the perinatal period   MCC N

P25.2 Pneumomediastinum originating in the perinatal period   MCC N

P25.3 Pneumopericardium originating in the perinatal period   MCC N

P25.8 Other conditions related to interstitial emphysema originating in the perinatal period   MCC N

√4ᵗʰ **P26 Pulmonary hemorrhage originating in the perinatal period**
> **EXCLUDES 1**   *acute idiopathic hemorrhage in infants over 28 days old (R04.81)*

> **CC Excl: For MCC codes in subcategory P26, unless otherwise noted:** J84.83-J84.848, P22.0-P28.5, P28.89-P29.2, P29.4, P29.89-P29.9, P84, P94.1-P94.9, P96.0, P96.3-P96.5, P96.82-P96.89

P26.0 Tracheobronchial hemorrhage originating in the perinatal period   MCC N

P26.1 Massive pulmonary hemorrhage originating in the perinatal period   MCC N

P26.8 Other pulmonary hemorrhages originating in the perinatal period   MCC N

P26.9 Unspecified pulmonary hemorrhage originating in the perinatal period   MCC N

√4ᵗʰ **P27 Chronic respiratory disease originating in the perinatal period**
> **EXCLUDES 1**   *respiratory distress of newborn (P22.0-P22.9)*

> **CC Excl: For MCC codes in subcategory P27, unless otherwise noted:** J84.83-J84.848, P22.0-P28.5, P28.89-P29.2, P29.4, P29.89-P29.9, P84, P94.1-P94.9, P96.0, P96.3-P96.5, P96.82-P96.89

P27.0 Wilson-Mikity syndrome   MCC
Pulmonary dysmaturity

P27.1 Bronchopulmonary dysplasia originating in the perinatal period   MCC

P27.8 Other chronic respiratory diseases originating in the perinatal period   MCC
Congenital pulmonary fibrosis   Ventilator lung in newborn

P27.9 Unspecified chronic respiratory disease originating in the perinatal period   MCC

☑ Additional Character Required   √x7ᵗʰ Placeholder Alert   Unacceptable PDx   Manifestation   Hospital Acquired Condition   **EXCLUDES 1** Not Coded Here   **EXCLUDES 2** Not Included Here

Chapter 16. Certain Conditions Originating in the Perinatal Period

✓4th **P28 Other respiratory conditions originating in the perinatal period**
> EXCLUDES 1 *congenital malformations of the respiratory system (Q30-Q34)*

P28.0 Primary atelectasis of newborn   cc N
> Primary failure to expand terminal respiratory units
> Pulmonary hypoplasia associated with short gestation
> Pulmonary immaturity NOS
> **CC Excl:** See code P27

✓5th **P28.1 Other and unspecified atelectasis of newborn**

     P28.10 Unspecified atelectasis of newborn   cc N
> Atelectasis of newborn NOS
> **CC Excl:** See code P27

     P28.11 Resorption atelectasis without respiratory distress syndrome   cc N
>> EXCLUDES 1 *resorption atelectasis with respiratory distress syndrome (P22.0)*
> **CC Excl:** See code P27

     P28.19 Other atelectasis of newborn   cc N
> Partial atelectasis of newborn
> Secondary atelectasis of newborn
> **CC Excl:** See code P27

P28.2 Cyanotic attacks of newborn   cc N
> EXCLUDES 1 *apnea of newborn (P28.3-P28.4)*
> **CC Excl:** P22.8-P22.9, P28.2-P28.4, P28.81-P28.9, R06.81, R23.0

P28.3 Primary sleep apnea of newborn   cc N
> Central sleep apnea of newborn
> Obstructive sleep apnea of newborn
> Sleep apnea of newborn NOS
> **CC Excl:** P22.8-P22.9, P28.2, P28.4, P28.81-P28.9, R06.81

P28.4 Other apnea of newborn   cc N
> Apnea of prematurity
> Obstructive apnea of newborn
> EXCLUDES 1 *obstructive sleep apnea of newborn (P28.3)*
> **CC Excl:** P22.8-P22.9, P28.2-P28.4, P28.81-P28.9, R06.81

P28.5 Respiratory failure of newborn   MCC N
> EXCLUDES 1 *respiratory arrest of newborn (P28.81)*
>   *respiratory distress of newborn (P22.0-)*
> **CC Excl:** See code P27

✓5th **P28.8 Other specified respiratory conditions of newborn**

     P28.81 Respiratory arrest of newborn   MCC N
> **CC Excl:** P22.1-P22.9, P24.00, P24.10, P24.20, P24.30, P24.80, Code P28.2-P28.5, P28.89-P28.9, P29.81, R06.81, R09.2

     P28.89 Other specified respiratory conditions of newborn   N
> Congenital laryngeal stridor
> Sniffles in newborn
> Snuffles in newborn
> EXCLUDES 1 *early congenital syphilitic rhinitis (A50.05)*

P28.9 Respiratory condition of newborn, unspecified   N
> Respiratory depression in newborn

✓4th **P29 Cardiovascular disorders originating in the perinatal period**
> EXCLUDES 1 *congenital malformations of the circulatory system (Q20-Q28)*

P29.0 Neonatal cardiac failure

✓5th **P29.1 Neonatal cardiac dysrhythmia**

     P29.11 Neonatal tachycardia   N

     P29.12 Neonatal bradycardia   N

P29.2 Neonatal hypertension   N

P29.3 Persistent fetal circulation   MCC N
> Delayed closure of ductus arteriosus
> (Persistent) pulmonary hypertension of newborn
> **CC Excl:** I27.0, I27.2-I27.81, I27.89-I27.9

P29.4 Transient myocardial ischemia in newborn   N

✓5th **P29.8 Other cardiovascular disorders originating in the perinatal period**

     P29.81 Cardiac arrest of newborn   MCC N
> **CC Excl:** P29.81

     P29.89 Other cardiovascular disorders originating in the perinatal period   N
> **AHA:** 2014, 4Q, 23

P29.9 Cardiovascular disorder originating in the perinatal period, unspecified   N

Infections specific to the perinatal period (P35-P39)

Infections acquired in utero, during birth via the umbilicus, or during the first 28 days after birth

> EXCLUDES 2 *asymptomatic human immunodeficiency virus [HIV] infection status (Z21)*
> *congenital gonococcal infection (A54.-)*
> *congenital pneumonia (P23.-)*
> *congenital syphilis (A50.-)*
> *human immunodeficiency virus [HIV] disease (B20)*
> *infant botulism (A48.51)*
> *infectious diseases not specific to the perinatal period (A00-B99, J09, J10-)*
> *intestinal infectious disease (A00-A09)*
> *laboratory evidence of human immunodeficiency virus [HIV] (R75)*
> *tetanus neonatorum (A33)*

✓4th **P35 Congenital viral diseases**
> INCLUDES infections acquired in utero or during birth

P35.0 Congenital rubella syndrome   cc N
> Congenital rubella pneumonitis
> **CC Excl:** P29.0-P29.2, P29.4, P29.89-P35.9, P37.0-P37.4, P37.8-P37.9, P94.1-P94.9, P96.0, P96.3-P96.5, P96.82-P96.89

P35.1 Congenital cytomegalovirus infection   MCC N
> **CC Excl:** See code P35.0

P35.2 Congenital herpesviral [herpes simplex] infection   MCC N
> **CC Excl:** A17.82, A28.1, A50.42, A52.14, A75.9, A79.9, A81.1, A81.82-A81.89, A83.0-A85.8, A87.2, A88.0, A88.8, A92.1-A92.8, A93.0, B00.4, B00.82, B01.11-B01.12, B04, B06.01, B08.09, B08.20-B08.22, B08.60-B08.79, B09-B10.09, B26.2, B27.00-B27.99, B33.1, B45.0, B45.2-B45.9, B54, B58.2, B75, B97.10, B97.21, G04.00-G04.01, G04.31, G04.81-G05.4, G37.0, G37.4-G37.5, H66.40-H66.43, J09.X3-J09.X9, J10.2-J10.89, J11.2-J11.89, L44.4, M1A.10X0-M1A.19X1, M32.0-M32.9, P35.2-P35.9, P37.0-P37.4, P37.8-P37.9, T56.0X1A, T56.0X2A, T56.0X3A, T56.0X4A

P35.3 Congenital viral hepatitis   MCC N
> **CC Excl:** See code P35.2

P35.8 Other congenital viral diseases   MCC N
> Congenital varicella [chickenpox]
> **CC Excl:** See code P35.2

P35.9 Congenital viral disease, unspecified   MCC N
> **CC Excl:** See code P35.2

✓4th **P36 Bacterial sepsis of newborn**
> INCLUDES congenital sepsis
> Use additional code(s), if applicable, to identify severe sepsis (R65.2-) and associated acute organ dysfunction(s)

> **CC Excl: For MCC codes in subcategory P36, unless otherwise noted:** P29.0-P29.2, P29.4, P29.89-P29.9, P36.0-P36.9, P37.5, P38.1-P39.9, P53, P60-P61.9, P94.1-P94.9, P96.0, P96.3-P96.5, P96.82-P96.89

P36.0 Sepsis of newborn due to streptococcus, group B   MCC N

✓5th **P36.1 Sepsis of newborn due to other and unspecified streptococci**

     P36.10 Sepsis of newborn due to unspecified streptococci   MCC N

     P36.19 Sepsis of newborn due to other streptococci   MCC N

P36.2 Sepsis of newborn due to Staphylococcus aureus   MCC N

✓5th **P36.3 Sepsis of newborn due to other and unspecified staphylococci**

     P36.30 Sepsis of newborn due to unspecified staphylococci   MCC N

     P36.39 Sepsis of newborn due to other staphylococci   MCC N

P36.4 Sepsis of newborn due to Escherichia coli   MCC N

P36.5 Sepsis of newborn due to anaerobes   MCC N

P36.8 Other bacterial sepsis of newborn   MCC N
> Use additional code from category B96 to identify organism

P36.9 Bacterial sepsis of newborn, unspecified   MCC N

N Newborn: 0   P Pediatric: 0-17   M Maternity: 12-55   A Adult: 15-124   MCC Major CC Condition   PDxMCC PDx acts as own MCC   CC CC Condition   PDxCC PDx acts as own CC

852   ICD-10-CM 2016

✓4ᵗʰ **P37 Other congenital infectious and parasitic diseases**

     EXCLUDES 2   congenital syphilis (A50.-)
              infectious neonatal diarrhea (A00-A09)
              necrotizing enterocolitis in newborn (P77.-)
              noninfectious neonatal diarrhea (P78.3)
              ophthalmia neonatorum due to gonococcus (A54.31)
              tetanus neonatorum (A33)

> **CC Excl: For MCC codes in subcategory P37, unless otherwise noted:** A17.82, A28.1, A50.42, A52.14, A75.9, A79.9, A81.1, A81.82-A81.89, A83.0-A85.8, A87.2, A88.0, A88.8, A92.1-A92.8, A93.0, B00.4, B00.82, B01.11-B01.12, B04, B06.01, B08.09, B08.20-B08.22, B08.60-B08.79, B09-B10.09, B26.2, B27.00-B27.99, B33.1, B45.0, B45.2-B45.9, B54, B58.2, B75, B97.10, B97.21, G04.00-G04.01, G04.31, G04.81-G05.4, G37.0, G37.4-G37.5, H66.40-H66.43, J09.X3-J09.X9, J10.2-J10.89, J11.2-J11.89, L44.4, M1A.10X0-M1A.19X1, M32.0-M32.9, P35.2-P35.9, P37.0-P37.4, P37.8-P37.9, T56.0X1A, T56.0X2A, T56.0X3A, T56.0X4A

     P37.0 Congenital tuberculosis   `MCC` `N`

     P37.1 Congenital toxoplasmosis   `MCC` `N`
         Hydrocephalus due to congenital toxoplasmosis

     P37.2 Neonatal (disseminated) listeriosis   `MCC` `N`

     P37.3 Congenital falciparum malaria   `MCC` `N`

     P37.4 Other congenital malaria   `MCC` `N`

     P37.5 Neonatal candidiasis   `N`

     P37.8 Other specified congenital infectious and parasitic diseases   `MCC` `N`

     P37.9 Congenital infectious or parasitic disease, unspecified   `MCC` `N`

✓4ᵗʰ **P38 Omphalitis of newborn**

     EXCLUDES 1   omphalitis not of newborn (L08.82)
              tetanus omphalitis (A33)
              umbilical hemorrhage of newborn (P51.-)

     P38.1 Omphalitis with mild hemorrhage   `CC` `N`
         CC Excl: P39.2-P39.9

     P38.9 Omphalitis without hemorrhage   `CC` `N`
         Omphalitis of newborn NOS
         CC Excl: See code P38.1

✓4ᵗʰ **P39 Other infections specific to the perinatal period**
     Use additional code to identify organism or specific infection

     P39.0 Neonatal infective mastitis   `CC` `N`
         EXCLUDES 1   breast engorgement of newborn (P83.4)
                   noninfective mastitis of newborn (P83.4)
         CC Excl: See code P38.1

     P39.1 Neonatal conjunctivitis and dacryocystitis   `N`
         Neonatal chlamydial conjunctivitis
         Ophthalmia neonatorum NOS
         EXCLUDES 1   gonococcal conjunctivitis (A54.31)

     P39.2 Intra-amniotic infection affecting newborn, not elsewhere classified   `CC` `N`
         CC Excl: A02.1, A20.7, A22.7, A39.2-A39.4, A40.9-A41.9, A42.7, A48.2, A48.4, A48.8-A49.9, B00.7, B92, B94.2-B96.89, P39.2-P39.9, P95, P96.9, R78.81

     P39.3 Neonatal urinary tract infection   `CC` `N`
         CC Excl: A49.9, N10-N11.0, N11.8-N12, N13.6, N15.1, N28.82, N28.84-N30.31, N30.80-N30.91, N36.9, N39.0, N39.9, N99.511, P39.2, P39.4-P39.9, R30.0, R30.9, T83.51XA

     P39.4 Neonatal skin infection   `CC` `N`
         Neonatal pyoderma
         EXCLUDES 1   pemphigus neonatorum (L00)
                   staphylococcal scalded skin syndrome (L00)
         CC Excl: See code P39.2

     P39.8 Other specified infections specific to the perinatal period   `CC` `N`
         CC Excl: See code P39.2

     P39.9 Infection specific to the perinatal period, unspecified   `CC` `N`
         CC Excl: See code P39.2

Hemorrhagic and hematological disorders of newborn (P50-P61)

     EXCLUDES 1   congenital stenosis and stricture of bile ducts (Q44.3)
              Crigler-Najjar syndrome (E80.5)
              Dubin-Johnson syndrome (E80.6)
              Gilbert syndrome (E80.4)
              hereditary hemolytic anemias (D55-D58)

✓4ᵗʰ **P50 Newborn affected by intrauterine (fetal) blood loss**
     EXCLUDES 1   congenital anemia from intrauterine (fetal) blood loss (P61.3)

     P50.0 Newborn affected by intrauterine (fetal) blood loss from vasa previa   `N`

     P50.1 Newborn affected by intrauterine (fetal) blood loss from ruptured cord   `N`

     P50.2 Newborn affected by intrauterine (fetal) blood loss from placenta   `N`

     P50.3 Newborn affected by hemorrhage into co-twin   `N`

     P50.4 Newborn affected by hemorrhage into maternal circulation   `N`

     P50.5 Newborn affected by intrauterine (fetal) blood loss from cut end of co-twin's cord   `N`

     P50.8 Newborn affected by other intrauterine (fetal) blood loss   `N`

     P50.9 Newborn affected by intrauterine (fetal) blood loss, unspecified   `N`
         Newborn affected by fetal hemorrhage NOS

✓4ᵗʰ **P51 Umbilical hemorrhage of newborn**
     EXCLUDES 1   omphalitis with mild hemorrhage (P38.1)
              umbilical hemorrhage from cut end of co-twins cord (P50.5)

     P51.0 Massive umbilical hemorrhage of newborn   `N`

     P51.8 Other umbilical hemorrhages of newborn   `N`
         Slipped umbilical ligature NOS

     P51.9 Umbilical hemorrhage of newborn, unspecified   `N`

✓4ᵗʰ **P52 Intracranial nontraumatic hemorrhage of newborn**
     Intracranial hemorrhage due to anoxia or hypoxia
     EXCLUDES 1   intracranial hemorrhage due to birth injury (P10.-)
              intracranial hemorrhage due to other injury (S06.-)

     P52.0 Intraventricular (nontraumatic) hemorrhage, grade 1, of newborn   `CC` `N`
         Subependymal hemorrhage (without intraventricular extension)
         Bleeding into germinal matrix
         CC Excl: P10.2-P10.3, P29.0-P29.2, P29.4, P29.89-P29.9, P50.0-P50.9, P52.0-P52.3, P52.5, P53-P54.0, P54.6-P54.9, P60-P61.9, P94.1-P94.9, P96.0, P96.3-P96.5, P96.82-P96.89

     P52.1 Intraventricular (nontraumatic) hemorrhage, grade 2, of newborn   `CC` `N`
         Subependymal hemorrhage with intraventricular extension
         Bleeding into ventricle
         CC Excl: See code P52.0

✓5ᵗʰ   **P52.2 Intraventricular (nontraumatic) hemorrhage, grade 3 and grade 4, of newborn**

         P52.21 Intraventricular (nontraumatic) hemorrhage, grade 3, of newborn   `MCC` `N`
              Subependymal hemorrhage with intraventricular extension with enlargement of ventricle
              CC Excl: See code P52.0

         P52.22 Intraventricular (nontraumatic) hemorrhage, grade 4, of newborn   `MCC` `N`
              Bleeding into cerebral cortex
              Subependymal hemorrhage with intracerebral extension
              CC Excl: See code P52.0

     P52.3 Unspecified intraventricular (nontraumatic) hemorrhage of newborn   `CC` `N`
         CC Excl: See code P52.0

     P52.4 Intracerebral (nontraumatic) hemorrhage of newborn   `MCC` `N`
         CC Excl: P10.0-P10.1, P10.4-P11.2, P11.9, P15.0-P15.9, P29.0-P29.2, P29.4, P29.89-P29.9, P52.4, P52.6-P52.9, P94.1-P94.9, P96.0, P96.3-P96.5, P96.82-P96.89

     P52.5 Subarachnoid (nontraumatic) hemorrhage of newborn   `MCC` `N`
         CC Excl: P10.2-P10.3, P29.0-P29.2, P29.4, P29.89-P29.9, P50.0-P50.9, P52.0-P52.3, P52.5, P53-P54.0, P54.6-P54.9, P60-P61.9, P91.2, P94.1-P94.9, P96.0, P96.3-P96.5, P96.82-P96.89

     P52.6 Cerebellar (nontraumatic) and posterior fossa hemorrhage of newborn   `MCC` `N`
         CC Excl: See code P52.4

     P52.8 Other intracranial (nontraumatic) hemorrhages of newborn   `MCC` `N`
         CC Excl: See code P52.4

     P52.9 Intracranial (nontraumatic) hemorrhage of newborn, unspecified   `MCC` `N`
         CC Excl: See code P52.4

P53 Hemorrhagic disease of newborn   `CC` `N`
     Vitamin K deficiency of newborn
     CC Excl: P29.0-P29.2, P29.4, P29.89-P29.9, P53, P60-P61.9, P94.1-P94.9, P96.0, P96.3-P96.5, P96.82-P96.89

✓4ᵗʰ **P54 Other neonatal hemorrhages**
     EXCLUDES 1   newborn affected by (intrauterine) blood loss (P50.-)
              pulmonary hemorrhage originating in the perinatal period (P26.-)

     P54.0 Neonatal hematemesis   `N`
         EXCLUDES 1   neonatal hematemesis due to swallowed maternal blood (P78.2)

P54.1 Neonatal melena `MCC` `N`
> **EXCLUDES 1**   neonatal melena due to swallowed maternal blood (P78.2)
> **CC Excl:** P29.0-P29.2, P29.4, P29.89-P29.9, P50.0-P50.9, P53-P54.4, P54.6-P54.9, P60-P61.9, P94.1-P94.9, P96.0, P96.3-P96.5, P96.82-P96.89

P54.2 Neonatal rectal hemorrhage `MCC` `N`
> **CC Excl:** See code P54.1

P54.3 Other neonatal gastrointestinal hemorrhage `MCC` `N`
> **CC Excl:** See code P54.1

P54.4 Neonatal adrenal hemorrhage `CC` `N`
> **CC Excl:** See code P54.1

P54.5 Neonatal cutaneous hemorrhage `N`
> Neonatal bruising   Neonatal petechiae
> Neonatal ecchymoses   Neonatal superficial hematomata
> **EXCLUDES 2**   bruising of scalp due to birth injury (P12.3)
>   cephalhematoma due to birth injury (P12.0)

P54.6 Neonatal vaginal hemorrhage `N` ♀
> Neonatal pseudomenses

P54.8 Other specified neonatal hemorrhages `N`

P54.9 Neonatal hemorrhage, unspecified `N`

✓4ᵗʰ **P55 Hemolytic disease of newborn**

P55.0 Rh isoimmunization of newborn `N`

P55.1 ABO isoimmunization of newborn `N`

P55.8 Other hemolytic diseases of newborn `N`

P55.9 Hemolytic disease of newborn, unspecified `N`

✓4ᵗʰ **P56 Hydrops fetalis due to hemolytic disease**
> **EXCLUDES 1**   hydrops fetalis NOS (P83.2)

P56.0 Hydrops fetalis due to isoimmunization `MCC` `N`
> **CC Excl:** P29.0-P29.2, P29.4, P29.89-P29.9, P55.0-P57.0, P94.1-P94.9, P96.0, P96.3-P96.5, P96.82-P96.89

✓5ᵗʰ **P56.9 Hydrops fetalis due to other and unspecified hemolytic disease**

> **P56.90 Hydrops fetalis due to unspecified hemolytic disease** `MCC` `N`
> > **CC Excl:** See code P56.0

> **P56.99 Hydrops fetalis due to other hemolytic disease** `MCC` `N`
> > **CC Excl:** See code P56.0

✓4ᵗʰ **P57 Kernicterus**

P57.0 Kernicterus due to isoimmunization `MCC` `N`
> **CC Excl:** See code P56.0

P57.8 Other specified kernicterus `MCC` `N`
> **EXCLUDES 1**   Crigler-Najjar syndrome (E80.5)
> **CC Excl:** P29.0-P29.2, P29.4, P29.89-P29.9, P57.8-P59.9, P94.1-P94.9, P96.0, P96.3-P96.5, P96.82-P96.89

P57.9 Kernicterus, unspecified `MCC` `N`
> **CC Excl:** See code P57.8

✓4ᵗʰ **P58 Neonatal jaundice due to other excessive hemolysis**
> **EXCLUDES 1**   jaundice due to isoimmunization (P55-P57)

P58.0 Neonatal jaundice due to bruising `N`

P58.1 Neonatal jaundice due to bleeding `N`

P58.2 Neonatal jaundice due to infection `N`

P58.3 Neonatal jaundice due to polycythemia `N`

✓5ᵗʰ **P58.4 Neonatal jaundice due to drugs or toxins transmitted from mother or given to newborn**
> Code first poisoning due to drug or toxin, if applicable (T36-T65 with fifth or sixth character 1-4 or 6)
> Use additional code for adverse effect, if applicable, to identify drug (T36-T50 with fifth or sixth character 5)

> **P58.41 Neonatal jaundice due to drugs or toxins transmitted from mother** `N`

> **P58.42 Neonatal jaundice due to drugs or toxins given to newborn** `N`

P58.5 Neonatal jaundice due to swallowed maternal blood `N`

P58.8 Neonatal jaundice due to other specified excessive hemolysis `N`

P58.9 Neonatal jaundice due to excessive hemolysis, unspecified `N`

✓4ᵗʰ **P59 Neonatal jaundice from other and unspecified causes**
> **EXCLUDES 1**   jaundice due to inborn errors of metabolism (E70-E88)
>   kernicterus (P57.-)

P59.0 Neonatal jaundice associated with preterm delivery `N`
> Hyperbilirubinemia of prematurity
> Jaundice due to delayed conjugation associated with preterm delivery

P59.1 Inspissated bile syndrome `MCC` `N`
> **CC Excl:** See code P57.8

✓5ᵗʰ **P59.2 Neonatal jaundice from other and unspecified hepatocellular damage**
> **EXCLUDES 1**   congenital viral hepatitis (P35.3)

> **P59.20 Neonatal jaundice from unspecified hepatocellular damage** `MCC` `N`
> > **CC Excl:** See code P57.8

> **P59.29 Neonatal jaundice from other hepatocellular damage** `MCC` `N`
> > Neonatal giant cell hepatitis
> > Neonatal (idiopathic) hepatitis
> > **CC Excl:** See code P57.8

P59.3 Neonatal jaundice from breast milk inhibitor `N`

P59.8 Neonatal jaundice from other specified causes `N`

P59.9 Neonatal jaundice, unspecified `N`
> Neonatal physiological jaundice (intense)(prolonged) NOS

P60 Disseminated intravascular coagulation of newborn `MCC` `N`
> Defibrination syndrome of newborn
> **CC Excl:** P29.0-P29.2, P29.4, P29.89-P29.9, P53, P60-P61.9, P94.1-P94.9, P96.0, P96.3-P96.5, P96.82-P96.89

✓4ᵗʰ **P61 Other perinatal hematological disorders**
> **EXCLUDES 1**   transient hypogammaglobulinemia of infancy (D80.7)

P61.0 Transient neonatal thrombocytopenia `MCC` `N`
> Neonatal thrombocytopenia due to exchange transfusion
> Neonatal thrombocytopenia due to idiopathic maternal thrombocytopenia
> Neonatal thrombocytopenia due to isoimmunization
> **CC Excl:** See code P60

P61.1 Polycythemia neonatorum `N`

P61.2 Anemia of prematurity `CC` `N`
> **CC Excl:** D50.0-D55.9, D56.4, D57.00-D57.3, D57.80-D64.9, D75.9, P61.2-P61.4

P61.3 Congenital anemia from fetal blood loss `CC` `N`
> **CC Excl:** See code P61.2

P61.4 Other congenital anemias, not elsewhere classified `CC` `N`
> Congenital anemia NOS
> **CC Excl:** See code P61.2

P61.5 Transient neonatal neutropenia `MCC` `N`
> **EXCLUDES 1**   congenital neutropenia (nontransient) (D70.0)
> **CC Excl:** D50.1-D53.9, D56.4, D57.00-D57.20, D57.3, D57.811-D57.819, D58.2, D59.0-D59.1, D59.3, D60.0-D61.9, D63.0-D64.9, D75.9, P61.5, P61.8-P61.9

P61.6 Other transient neonatal disorders of coagulation `CC` `N`
> **CC Excl:** P29.0-P29.2, P29.4, P29.89-P29.9, P53, P60-P61.9, P94.1-P94.9, P96.0, P96.3-P96.5, P96.82-P96.89

P61.8 Other specified perinatal hematological disorders `N`

P61.9 Perinatal hematological disorder, unspecified `N`

Transitory endocrine and metabolic disorders specific to newborn (P70-P74)

> **INCLUDES**   transitory endocrine and metabolic disturbances caused by the infant's response to maternal endocrine and metabolic factors, or its adjustment to extrauterine environment

✓4ᵗʰ **P70 Transitory disorders of carbohydrate metabolism specific to newborn**

P70.0 Syndrome of infant of mother with gestational diabetes `N`
> Newborn (with hypoglycemia) affected by maternal gestational diabetes
> **EXCLUDES 1**   newborn (with hypoglycemia) affected by maternal (pre-existing) diabetes mellitus (P70.1)
>   syndrome of infant of a diabetic mother (P70.1)

P70.1 Syndrome of infant of a diabetic mother `N`
> Newborn (with hypoglycemia) affected by maternal (pre-existing) diabetes mellitus
> **EXCLUDES 1**   newborn (with hypoglycemia) affected by maternal gestational diabetes (P70.0)
>   syndrome of infant of mother with gestational diabetes (P70.0)

P70.2 Neonatal diabetes mellitus `CC` `N`
> **CC Excl:** P29.0-P29.2, P29.4, P29.89-P29.9, P70.0-P70.4, P70.9-P71.9, P72.1, P72.9-P74.4, P74.9, P94.0-P94.9, P96.0, P96.3-P96.5, P96.82-P96.89

P70.3 Iatrogenic neonatal hypoglycemia `N`

P70.4 Other neonatal hypoglycemia `N`
> Transitory neonatal hypoglycemia

P70.8 Other transitory disorders of carbohydrate metabolism of newborn `CC` `N`
> **CC Excl:** P70.0-P70.4, P70.9-P71.9, P72.1, P72.9-P74.4, P74.9, P94.0

`N` Newborn: 0   `P` Pediatric: 0-17   `M` Maternity: 12-55   `A` Adult: 15-124   `MCC` Major CC Condition   `PDxMCC` PDx acts as own MCC   `CC` CC Condition   `PDxCC` PDx acts as own CC

P70.9   **Transitory disorder of carbohydrate metabolism of newborn**, unspecified   N

☑4ᵗʰ **P71   Transitory neonatal disorders of calcium and magnesium metabolism**

> **CC Excl:** For CC codes in subcategory P71, unless otherwise noted: P29.0-P29.2, P29.4, P29.89-P29.9, P70.0-P70.4, P70.9-P71.9, P72.1, P72.9-P74.4, P74.9, P94.0-P94.9, P96.0, P96.3-P96.5, P96.82-P96.89

P71.0   **Cow's milk hypocalcemia** in newborn   CC N

P71.1   **Other** neonatal **hypocalcemia**   CC N
> *EXCLUDES 1*   neonatal hypoparathyroidism (P71.4)

P71.2   **Neonatal** hypomagnesemia   CC N

P71.3   **Neonatal tetany without calcium or magnesium deficiency**
> Neonatal tetany NOS

P71.4   **Transitory neonatal** hypoparathyroidism   CC N

P71.8   **Other** transitory neonatal **disorders of calcium and magnesium metabolism**   CC N

P71.9   **Transitory neonatal disorder of calcium and magnesium metabolism**, unspecified   CC N

☑4ᵗʰ **P72   Other transitory neonatal** endocrine **disorders**
> *EXCLUDES 1*   congenital hypothyroidism with or without goiter (E03.0-E03.1)
> dyshormogenetic goiter (E07.1)
> Pendred's syndrome (E07.1)

> **CC Excl:** For CC codes in subcategory P72, unless otherwise noted: P70.0-P70.4, P70.9-P71.9, P72.1, P72.9-P74.4, P74.9, P94.0

P72.0   **Neonatal goiter, not elsewhere classified**   CC N
> Transitory congenital goiter with normal functioning

P72.1   **Transitory** neonatal **hyperthyroidism**   CC N
> Neonatal thyrotoxicosis
> **CC Excl:** P29.0-P29.2, P29.4, P29.89-P29.9, P70.0-P70.4, P70.9-P71.9, P72.1, P72.9-P74.4, P74.9, P94.0-P94.9, P96.0, P96.3-P96.5, P96.82-P96.89

P72.2   **Other** transitory neonatal **disorders of thyroid function, not elsewhere classified**   CC N
> Transitory neonatal hypothyroidism

P72.8   **Other specified transitory neonatal endocrine disorders**   CC N

P72.9   **Transitory neonatal endocrine disorder**, unspecified   N

☑4ᵗʰ **P74   Other transitory neonatal** electrolyte and metabolic **disturbances**

P74.0   **Late metabolic acidosis of newborn**   MCC N
> *EXCLUDES 1*   (fetal) metabolic acidosis of newborn (P19)
> **CC Excl:** P29.0-P29.2, P29.4, P29.89-P29.9, P70.0-P70.4, P70.9-P71.9, P72.1, P72.9-P74.4, P74.9, P94.0-P94.9, P96.0, P96.3-P96.5, P96.82-P96.89

P74.1   **Dehydration** of newborn   N

P74.2   **Disturbances of** sodium balance **of newborn**   N

P74.3   **Disturbances of** potassium balance **of newborn**   N

P74.4   **Other transitory electrolyte disturbances of newborn**   N

P74.5   **Transitory** tyrosinemia **of newborn**   CC N
> **CC Excl:** P70.0-P70.4, P70.9-P71.9, P72.1, P72.9-P74.4, P74.9, P94.0

P74.6   **Transitory** hyperammonemia **of newborn**   CC N
> **CC Excl:** See code: P70.8

P74.8   **Other** transitory metabolic **disturbances of newborn**   CC N
> Amino-acid metabolic disorders described as transitory
> **CC Excl:** See code: P70.8

P74.9   **Transitory metabolic disturbance of newborn**, unspecified   N

Digestive system disorders of newborn (P76-P78)

☑4ᵗʰ **P76   Other intestinal obstruction of newborn**

P76.0   **Meconium plug syndrome**   N
> Meconium ileus NOS
> *EXCLUDES 1*   meconium ileus in cystic fibrosis (E84.11)

P76.1   **Transitory ileus of newborn**   CC N
> *EXCLUDES 1*   Hirschsprung's disease (Q43.1)
> **CC Excl:** P76.0-P78.9

P76.2   **Intestinal obstruction due to inspissated milk**   N

P76.8   **Other specified intestinal obstruction of newborn**   N
> *EXCLUDES 1*   intestinal obstruction classifiable to K56-

P76.9   **Intestinal obstruction of newborn**, unspecified   N

☑4ᵗʰ **P77   Necrotizing enterocolitis of newborn**

P77.1   **Stage 1 necrotizing enterocolitis in newborn**   MCC N
> Necrotizing enterocolitis without pneumatosis, without perforation
> **CC Excl:** P29.0-P29.2, P29.4, P29.89-P29.9, P76.0-P78.9, P94.1-P94.9, P96.0, P96.3-P96.5, P96.82-P96.89

P77.2   **Stage 2 necrotizing enterocolitis in newborn**   MCC N
> Necrotizing enterocolitis with pneumatosis, without perforation
> **CC Excl:** See code P77.1

P77.3   **Stage 3 necrotizing enterocolitis in newborn**   MCC N
> Necrotizing enterocolitis with perforation
> Necrotizing enterocolitis with pneumatosis and perforation
> **CC Excl:** See code P77.1

P77.9   **Necrotizing enterocolitis in newborn**, unspecified   MCC N
> Necrotizing enterocolitis in newborn, NOS
> **CC Excl:** See code P77.1

☑4ᵗʰ **P78   Other perinatal digestive system disorders**
> *EXCLUDES 1*   cystic fibrosis (E84.0-E84.9)
> neonatal gastrointestinal hemorrhages (P54.0-P54.3)

P78.0   **Perinatal intestinal perforation**   MCC N
> Meconium peritonitis
> **CC Excl:** See code P77.1

P78.1   **Other neonatal peritonitis**   N
> Neonatal peritonitis NOS

P78.2   **Neonatal hematemesis and melena due to swallowed maternal blood**   N

P78.3   **Noninfective neonatal diarrhea**   N
> Neonatal diarrhea NOS

☑5ᵗʰ P78.8   **Other specified perinatal digestive system disorders**

P78.81   **Congenital cirrhosis (of liver)**   N

P78.82   **Peptic ulcer of newborn**   N

P78.83   **Newborn esophageal reflux**   N
> Neonatal esophageal reflux

P78.89   **Other specified perinatal digestive system disorders**   N

P78.9   **Perinatal digestive system disorder**, unspecified   N

Conditions involving the integument and temperature regulation of newborn (P80-P83)

☑4ᵗʰ **P80   Hypothermia of newborn**

P80.0   **Cold injury syndrome**   N
> Severe and usually chronic hypothermia associated with a pink flushed appearance, edema and neurological and biochemical abnormalities.
> *EXCLUDES 1*   mild hypothermia of newborn (P80.8)

P80.8   **Other hypothermia of newborn**   N
> Mild hypothermia of newborn

P80.9   **Hypothermia of newborn**, unspecified   N

☑4ᵗʰ **P81   Other disturbances of temperature regulation of newborn**

P81.0   **Environmental hyperthermia of newborn**   N

P81.8   **Other specified disturbances of temperature regulation of newborn**   N

P81.9   **Disturbance of temperature regulation of newborn, unspecified**   N
> Fever of newborn NOS

☑4ᵗʰ **P83   Other conditions of integument specific to newborn**
> *EXCLUDES 1*   congenital malformations of skin and integument (Q80-Q84)
> hydrops fetalis due to hemolytic disease (P56.-)
> neonatal skin infection (P39.4)
> staphylococcal scalded skin syndrome (L00)
> *EXCLUDES 2*   cradle cap (L21.0)
> diaper [napkin] dermatitis (L22)

P83.0   **Sclerema neonatorum**   CC N
> **CC Excl:** P83.0, P83.30-P83.39

P83.1   **Neonatal erythema toxicum**   N

P83.2   **Hydrops fetalis not due to hemolytic disease**   MCC N
> Hydrops fetalis NOS
> **CC Excl:** P29.0-P29.2, P29.4, P29.89-P29.9, P83.2, P94.1-P94.9, P96.0, P96.3-P96.5, P96.82-P96.89

☑5ᵗʰ P83.3   **Other and unspecified edema specific to newborn**

P83.30   **Unspecified edema specific to newborn**   CC N
> **CC Excl:** P80.0-P83.0, P83.30-P83.39

P83.39   **Other edema specific to newborn**   CC N
> **CC Excl:** See code P83.30

P83.4   **Breast engorgement of newborn**   N
> Noninfective mastitis of newborn

☑ Additional Character Required   ✗7ᵗʰ Placeholder Alert   Unacceptable PDx   Manifestation   Hospital Acquired Condition   *EXCLUDES 1* Not Coded Here   *EXCLUDES 2* Not Included Here

P83.5   **Congenital hydrocele**   ♂

P83.6   **Umbilical polyp of newborn**   N

P83.8   **Other specified conditions of integument specific to newborn**   N
> Bronze baby syndrome   Urticaria neonatorum
> Neonatal scleroderma

P83.9   **Condition of the integument specific to newborn, unspecified**   N

Other problems with newborn (P84)

P84   **Other problems with newborn**   N
> Acidemia of newborn   Hypoxemia of newborn
> Acidosis of newborn   Hypoxia of newborn NOS
> Anoxia of newborn NOS   Mixed metabolic and respiratory
> Asphyxia of newborn NOS   acidosis of newborn
> Hypercapnia of newborn
>
> *EXCLUDES 1*   intracranial hemorrhage due to anoxia or hypoxia (P52.-)
>   hypoxic ischemic encephalopathy [HIE] (P91.6-)
>   late metabolic acidosis of newborn (P74.0)
>
> **CC Excl:** No Excl

Other disorders originating in the perinatal period (P90–P96)

P90   **Convulsions of newborn**   MCC N
> *EXCLUDES 1*   benign myoclonic epilepsy in infancy (G40.3-)
>   benign neonatal convulsions (familial) (G40.3-)
>
> **CC Excl:** P29.0-P29.2, P29.4, P29.89-P29.9, P90, P91.8-P91.9, P94.1-P94.9, P96.0, P96.3-P96.5, P96.82-P96.89

✓4th **P91**   **Other disturbances of cerebral status of newborn**

   P91.0   **Neonatal cerebral ischemia**   MCC N
> **CC Excl:** P90-P91.1, P91.3-P91.5, P91.8-P91.9

   P91.1   **Acquired periventricular cysts of newborn**   MCC N
> **CC Excl:** See code P91.0

   P91.2   **Neonatal cerebral leukomalacia**   MCC N
> Periventricular leukomalacia
> **CC Excl:** P10.2-P10.3, P29.0-P29.2, P29.4, P29.89-P29.9, P50.0-P50.9, P52.0-P52.3, P52.5, P53-P54.0, P54.6-P54.9, P60-P61.9, P91.2, P94.1-P94.9, P96.0, P96.3-P96.5, P96.82-P96.89

   P91.3   **Neonatal cerebral irritability**   MCC N
> **CC Excl:** See code P91.0

   P91.4   **Neonatal cerebral depression**   MCC N
> **CC Excl:** See code P91.0

   P91.5   **Neonatal coma**   MCC N
> **CC Excl:** See code P91.0

✓5th   **P91.6**   **Hypoxic ischemic encephalopathy [HIE]**

     P91.60   **Hypoxic ischemic encephalopathy [HIE], unspecified**   CC N
> **CC Excl:** P84, P91.60-P91.63

     P91.61   **Mild hypoxic ischemic encephalopathy [HIE]**   CC N
> **CC Excl:** See code P91.60

     P91.62   **Moderate hypoxic ischemic encephalopathy [HIE]**   CC N
> **CC Excl:** See code P91.60

     P91.63   **Severe hypoxic ischemic encephalopathy [HIE]**   MCC N
> **CC Excl:** See code P91.60

   P91.8   **Other specified disturbances of cerebral status of newborn**   N

   P91.9   **Disturbance of cerebral status of newborn, unspecified**   N

✓4th **P92**   **Feeding problems of newborn**
> *EXCLUDES 1*   feeding problems in child over 28 days old (R63.3)

✓5th   **P92.0**   **Vomiting of newborn**
> *EXCLUDES 1*   vomiting of child over 28 days old (R11.-)

     P92.01   **Bilious vomiting of newborn**   MCC N
> *EXCLUDES 1*   bilious vomiting in child over 28 days old (R11.14)
> **CC Excl:** P92.01-P92.09

     P92.09   **Other vomiting of newborn**   N
> *EXCLUDES 1*   regurgitation of food in newborn (P92.1)

   P92.1   **Regurgitation and rumination of newborn**   N

   P92.2   **Slow feeding of newborn**   N

   P92.3   **Underfeeding of newborn**   N

   P92.4   **Overfeeding of newborn**   N

   P92.5   **Neonatal difficulty in feeding at breast**   N

   P92.6   **Failure to thrive in newborn**   N
> *EXCLUDES 1*   failure to thrive in child over 28 days old (R62.51)

   P92.8   **Other feeding problems of newborn**   N

   P92.9   **Feeding problem of newborn, unspecified**   N

✓4th **P93**   **Reactions and intoxications due to drugs administered to newborn**
> **INCLUDES**   reactions and intoxications due to drugs administered to fetus affecting newborn
>
> *EXCLUDES 1*   jaundice due to drugs or toxins transmitted from mother or given to newborn (P58.4-)
>   reactions and intoxications from maternal opiates, tranquilizers and other medication (P04.0-P04.1, P04.4)
>   withdrawal symptoms from maternal use of drugs of addiction (P96.1)
>   withdrawal symptoms from therapeutic use of drugs in newborn (P96.2)

   P93.0   **Grey baby syndrome**   CC N
> Grey syndrome from chloramphenicol administration in newborn
> **CC Excl:** P93.0-P93.8, P96.1-P96.2

   P93.8   **Other reactions and intoxications due to drugs administered to newborn**   CC N
> Use additional code for adverse effect, if applicable, to identify drug (T36-T50 with fifth or sixth character 5)
> **CC Excl:** See code P93.0

✓4th **P94**   **Disorders of muscle tone of newborn**

   P94.0   **Transient neonatal myasthenia gravis**   CC N
> *EXCLUDES 1*   myasthenia gravis (G70.0)
> **CC Excl:** P29.0-P29.2, P29.4, P29.89-P29.9, P70.0-P70.4, P70.9-P71.9, P72.1, P72.9-P74.4, P74.9, P94.0-P94.9, P96.0, P96.3-P96.5, P96.82-P96.89

   P94.1   **Congenital hypertonia**   N

   P94.2   **Congenital hypotonia**   N
> Floppy baby syndrome, unspecified

   P94.8   **Other disorders of muscle tone of newborn**   N

   P94.9   **Disorder of muscle tone of newborn, unspecified**   N

P95   **Stillbirth**   N
> Deadborn fetus NOS
> Fetal death of unspecified cause
> Stillbirth NOS
>
> *EXCLUDES 1*   maternal care for intrauterine death (O36.4)
>   missed abortion (O02.1)
>   outcome of delivery, stillbirth (Z37.1, Z37.3, Z37.4, Z37.7)

✓4th **P96**   **Other conditions originating in the perinatal period**

   P96.0   **Congenital renal failure**   N
> Uremia of newborn

   P96.1   **Neonatal withdrawal symptoms from maternal use of drugs of addiction**   CC N
> Drug withdrawal syndrome in infant of dependent mother
> Neonatal abstinence syndrome
>
> *EXCLUDES 1*   reactions and intoxications from maternal opiates and tranquilizers administered during labor and delivery (P04.0)
>
> **CC Excl:** P93.0-P93.8, P96.1-P96.2

   P96.2   **Withdrawal symptoms from therapeutic use of drugs in newborn**   CC N
> **CC Excl:** See code P96.1

   P96.3   **Wide cranial sutures of newborn**   N
> Neonatal craniotabes

   P96.5   **Complication to newborn due to (fetal) intrauterine procedure**   N
> *EXCLUDES 2*   newborn (suspected to be) affected by amniocentesis (P00.6)

✓5th   **P96.8**   **Other specified conditions originating in the perinatal period**

     P96.81   **Exposure to (parental) (environmental) tobacco smoke in the perinatal period**
> *EXCLUDES 2*   newborn affected by in utero exposure to tobacco (P04.2)
>   exposure to environmental tobacco smoke after the perinatal period (Z77.22)

     P96.82   **Delayed separation of umbilical cord**   N

     P96.83   **Meconium staining**   N
> *EXCLUDES 1*   meconium aspiration (P24.00, P24.01)
>   meconium passage during delivery (P03.82)

     P96.89   **Other specified conditions originating in the perinatal period**   N
> Use additional code to specify condition

   P96.9   **Condition originating in the perinatal period, unspecified**   N
> Congenital debility NOS

N Newborn: 0   P Pediatric: 0-17   M Maternity: 12-55   A Adult: 15-124   MCC Major CC Condition   PDxMCC PDx acts as own MCC   CC CC Condition   PDxCC PDx acts as own CC

856   ICD-10-CM 2016

Chapter 17. Congenital Malformations, Deformations, and Chromosomal Abnormalities (Q00–Q99)

Chapter Specific Guidelines with Coding Examples

The chapter specific guidelines from the ICD-10-CM Official Guidelines for Coding and Reporting have been provided below. Along with these guidelines are coding examples, contained in the shaded boxes, that have been developed to help illustrate the coding and/or sequencing guidance found in these guidelines.

Assign an appropriate code(s) from categories Q00-Q99, Congenital malformations, deformations, and chromosomal abnormalities when a malformation/deformation or chromosomal abnormality is documented. A malformation/deformation/or chromosomal abnormality may be the principal/first-listed diagnosis on a record or a secondary diagnosis.

When a malformation/deformation/or chromosomal abnormality does not have a unique code assignment, assign additional code(s) for any manifestations that may be present.

When the code assignment specifically identifies the malformation/deformation/or chromosomal abnormality, manifestations that are an inherent component of the anomaly should not be coded separately. Additional codes should be assigned for manifestations that are not an inherent component.

8-day-old infant with tetralogy of Fallot and pulmonary stenosis

Q21.3   **Tetralogy of Fallot**

Explanation: Pulmonary stenosis is inherent in the disease process of tetralogy of Fallot. When the code assignment specifically identifies the malformation/deformation/or chromosomal abnormality, manifestations that are inherent components of the anomaly should not be coded separately.

7-month-old infant with Down syndrome and common atrioventricular canal

Q90.9   **Down syndrome, unspecified**

Q21.2   **Atrioventricular septal defect**

Explanation: While a common atrioventricular canal is often associated with patients with Down syndrome, this manifestation is not an inherent component and may be reported separately. When the code assignment specifically identifies the anomaly, manifestations that are inherent components of the condition should not be coded separately. Additional codes should be assigned for manifestations that are not inherent components.

Codes from Chapter 17 may be used throughout the life of the patient. If a congenital malformation or deformity has been corrected, a personal history code should be used to identify the history of the malformation or deformity. Although present at birth, malformation/deformation/or chromosomal abnormality may not be identified until later in life. Whenever the condition is diagnosed by the physician, it is appropriate to assign a code from codes Q00-Q99. For the birth admission, the appropriate code from category Z38, Liveborn infants, according to place of birth and type of delivery, should be sequenced as the principal diagnosis, followed by any congenital anomaly codes, Q00- Q99.

Three-year-old with history of corrected ventricular septal defect

Z87.74   **Personal history of (corrected) congenital malformations of heart and circulatory system**

Explanation: If a congenital malformation or deformity has been corrected, a personal history code should be used to identify the history of the malformation or deformity.

Forty-year-old man with headaches diagnosed with congenital arteriovenous malformation by brain scan

Q28.2   **Arteriovenous malformation of cerebral vessels**

Explanation: Although present at birth, malformations may not be identified until later in life. Whenever the condition is diagnosed by the physician, it is appropriate to assign a code from the range Q00–Q99.

Newborn with anencephaly delivered vaginally in hospital

Z38.00   **Single liveborn infant, delivered vaginally**

Q00.0   **Anencephaly**

Explanation: For the birth admission, the appropriate code from category Z38 Liveborn infants, according to place of birth and type of delivery, should be sequenced as the principal diagnosis, followed by any congenital anomaly codes, Q00–Q99.

Chapter 17. Congenital Malformations, Deformations and Chromosomal Abnormalities (Q00-Q99)

NOTE Codes from this chapter are not for use on maternal or fetal records.

EXCLUDES 2 inborn errors of metabolism (E70-E88)

This chapter contains the following blocks:

Q00-Q07 Congenital malformations of the nervous system
Q10-Q18 Congenital malformations of eye, ear, face and neck
Q20-Q28 Congenital malformations of the circulatory system
Q30-Q34 Congenital malformations of the respiratory system
Q35-Q37 Cleft lip and cleft palate
Q38-Q45 Other congenital malformations of the digestive system
Q50-Q56 Congenital malformations of genital organs
Q60-Q64 Congenital malformations of the urinary system
Q65-Q79 Congenital malformations and deformations of the musculoskeletal system
Q80-Q89 Other congenital malformations
Q90-Q99 Chromosomal abnormalities, not elsewhere classified

Congenital malformations of the nervous system (Q00-Q07)

✓4ᵗʰ Q00 Anencephaly and similar malformations

> **CC Excl: For MCC codes in category Q00, unless otherwise noted:** Q00.0-Q00.2

  Q00.0 Anencephaly   MCC
    Acephaly
    Acrania
    Amyelencephaly
    Hemianencephaly
    Hemicephaly

  Q00.1 Craniorachischisis   MCC

  Q00.2 Iniencephaly   MCC

✓4ᵗʰ Q01 Encephalocele
  INCLUDES Arnold-Chiari syndrome, type III
      encephalocystocele
      encephalomyelocele
      hydroencephalocele
      hydromeningocele, cranial
      meningocele, cerebral
      meningoencephalocele
  EXCLUDES 1 Meckel-Gruber syndrome (Q61.9)

> **CC Excl: For CC codes in category Q01, unless otherwise noted:** Q01.0-Q02, Q04.0-Q04.8

  Q01.0 Frontal encephalocele   CC

  Q01.1 Nasofrontal encephalocele   CC

  Q01.2 Occipital encephalocele   CC

  Q01.8 Encephalocele of other sites   CC

  Q01.9 Encephalocele, unspecified   CC

Q02 Microcephaly
  INCLUDES hydromicrocephaly
      micrencephalon
  EXCLUDES 1 Meckel-Gruber syndrome (Q61.9)

✓4ᵗʰ Q03 Congenital hydrocephalus
  INCLUDES hydrocephalus in newborn
  EXCLUDES 1 Arnold-Chiari syndrome, type II (Q07.0-)
      acquired hydrocephalus (G91.-)
      hydrocephalus due to congenital toxoplasmosis (P37.1)
      hydrocephalus with spina bifida (Q05.0-Q05.4)

  Q03.0 Malformations of aqueduct of Sylvius
    Anomaly of aqueduct of Sylvius
    Obstruction of aqueduct of Sylvius, congenital
    Stenosis of aqueduct of Sylvius

  Q03.1 Atresia of foramina of Magendie and Luschka
    Dandy-Walker syndrome

  Q03.8 Other congenital hydrocephalus

  Q03.9 Congenital hydrocephalus, unspecified

✓4ᵗʰ Q04 Other congenital malformations of brain
  EXCLUDES 1 cyclopia (Q87.0)
      macrocephaly (Q75.3)

> **CC Excl: For MCC codes in category Q04, unless otherwise noted:** See code: Q01

  Q04.0 Congenital malformations of corpus callosum   MCC
    Agenesis of corpus callosum

  Q04.1 Arhinencephaly   MCC

  Q04.2 Holoprosencephaly   MCC

  Q04.3 Other reduction deformities of brain   MCC
    Absence of part of brain
    Agenesis of part of brain
    Agyria
    Aplasia of part of brain
    Hydranencephaly
    Hypoplasia of part of brain
    Lissencephaly
    Microgyria
    Pachygyria
    EXCLUDES 1 congenital malformations of corpus callosum (Q04.0)

  Q04.4 Septo-optic dysplasia of brain   CC
    CC Excl: Q04.4-Q04.8

  Q04.5 Megalencephaly   CC
    CC Excl: See code: Q04.4

  Q04.6 Congenital cerebral cysts   CC
    Porencephaly
    Schizencephaly
    EXCLUDES 1 acquired porencephalic cyst (G93.0)
    CC Excl: See code: Q04.4

  Q04.8 Other specified congenital malformations of brain   CC
    Arnold-Chiari syndrome, type IV
    Macrogyria
    CC Excl: See code: Q04.4

  Q04.9 Congenital malformation of brain, unspecified
    Congenital anomaly NOS of brain
    Congenital deformity NOS of brain
    Congenital disease or lesion NOS of brain
    Multiple anomalies NOS of brain, congenital

✓4ᵗʰ Q05 Spina bifida
    Hydromeningocele (spinal)
    Meningocele (spinal)
    Meningomyelocele
    Myelocele
    Myelomeningocele
    Rachischisis
    Spina bifida (aperta)(cystica)
    Syringomyelocele
  Use additional code for any associated paraplegia (paraparesis) (G82.2-)
  EXCLUDES 1 Arnold-Chiari syndrome, type II (Q07.0-)
      spina bifida occulta (Q76.0)

> **CC Excl: For CC codes in category Q05, unless otherwise noted:** E78.71-E78.72, G90.1, Q05.0-Q06.1, Q06.3, Q06.8-Q07.9, Q87.1-Q87.89, Q89.7-Q89.8, Q99.2

  Q05.0 Cervical spina bifida with hydrocephalus   CC

  Q05.1 Thoracic spina bifida with hydrocephalus   CC
    Dorsal spina bifida with hydrocephalus
    Thoracolumbar spina bifida with hydrocephalus

  Q05.2 Lumbar spina bifida with hydrocephalus   CC
    Lumbosacral spina bifida with hydrocephalus

  Q05.3 Sacral spina bifida with hydrocephalus   CC

  Q05.4 Unspecified spina bifida with hydrocephalus   CC

  Q05.5 Cervical spina bifida without hydrocephalus

  Q05.6 Thoracic spina bifida without hydrocephalus
    Dorsal spina bifida NOS
    Thoracolumbar spina bifida NOS

  Q05.7 Lumbar spina bifida without hydrocephalus
    Lumbosacral spina bifida NOS

  Q05.8 Sacral spina bifida without hydrocephalus

  Q05.9 Spina bifida, unspecified

✓4ᵗʰ Q06 Other congenital malformations of spinal cord

  Q06.0 Amyelia

  Q06.1 Hypoplasia and dysplasia of spinal cord
    Atelomyelia
    Myelatelia
    Myelodysplasia of spinal cord

  Q06.2 Diastematomyelia

  Q06.3 Other congenital cauda equina malformations

  Q06.4 Hydromyelia
    Hydrorachis

  Q06.8 Other specified congenital malformations of spinal cord

  Q06.9 Congenital malformation of spinal cord, unspecified
    Congenital anomaly NOS of spinal cord
    Congenital deformity NOS of spinal cord
    Congenital disease or lesion NOS of spinal cord

N Newborn: 0   **P** Pediatric: 0-17   **M** Maternity: 12-55   **A** Adult: 15-124   **MCC** Major CC Condition   **PDxMCC** PDx acts as own MCC   **CC** CC Condition   **PDxCC** PDx acts as own CC

858   ICD-10-CM 2016

✓4ᵗʰ Q07 Other congenital malformations of nervous system

> *EXCLUDES 2*   *congenital central alveolar hypoventilation syndrome (G47.35)*
> *familial dysautonomia [Riley-Day] (G90.1)*
> *neurofibromatosis (nonmalignant) (Q85.0-)*

> **CC Excl: For CC codes in category Q07, unless otherwise noted:** See code: Q05.0

✓5ᵗʰ Q07.0 Arnold-Chiari syndrome
Arnold-Chiari syndrome, type II
> *EXCLUDES 1*   *Arnold-Chiari syndrome, type III (Q01.-)*
> *Arnold-Chiari syndrome, type IV (Q04.8)*

   Q07.00 Arnold-Chiari syndrome without spina bifida or hydrocephalus

   Q07.01 Arnold-Chiari syndrome with spina bifida

   Q07.02 Arnold-Chiari syndrome with hydrocephalus   `CC`

   Q07.03 Arnold-Chiari syndrome with spina bifida and hydrocephalus   `CC`

Q07.8 Other specified congenital malformations of nervous system
Agenesis of nerve
Displacement of brachial plexus
Jaw-winking syndrome
Marcus Gunn's syndrome

Q07.9 Congenital malformation of nervous system, unspecified
Congenital anomaly NOS of nervous system
Congenital deformity NOS of nervous system
Congenital disease or lesion NOS of nervous system

Congenital malformations of eye, ear, face and neck (Q10-Q18)

> *EXCLUDES 2*   *cleft lip and cleft palate (Q35-Q37)*
> *congenital malformation of cervical spine (Q05.0, Q05.5, Q67.5, Q76.0-Q76.4)*
> *congenital malformation of larynx (Q31.-)*
> *congenital malformation of lip NEC (Q38.0)*
> *congenital malformation of nose (Q30.-)*
> *congenital malformation of parathyroid gland (Q89.2)*
> *congenital malformation of thyroid gland (Q89.2)*

✓4ᵗʰ Q10 Congenital malformations of eyelid, lacrimal apparatus and orbit

> *EXCLUDES 1*   *cryptophthalmos NOS (Q11.2)*
> *cryptophthalmos syndrome (Q87.0)*

Q10.0 Congenital ptosis

Q10.1 Congenital ectropion

Q10.2 Congenital entropion

Q10.3 Other congenital malformations of eyelid
Ablepharon
Blepharophimosis, congenital
Coloboma of eyelid
Congenital absence or agenesis of cilia
Congenital absence or agenesis of eyelid
Congenital accessory eyelid
Congenital accessory eye muscle
Congenital malformation of eyelid NOS

Q10.4 Absence and agenesis of lacrimal apparatus
Congenital absence of punctum lacrimale

Q10.5 Congenital stenosis and stricture of lacrimal duct

Q10.6 Other congenital malformations of lacrimal apparatus
Congenital malformation of lacrimal apparatus NOS

Q10.7 Congenital malformation of orbit

✓4ᵗʰ Q11 Anophthalmos, microphthalmos and macrophthalmos

Q11.0 Cystic eyeball

Q11.1 Other anophthalmos
Anophthalmos NOS
Agenesis of eye
Aplasia of eye

Q11.2 Microphthalmos
Cryptophthalmos NOS
Dysplasia of eye
Hypoplasia of eye
Rudimentary eye
> *EXCLUDES 1*   *cryptophthalmos syndrome (Q87.0)*

Q11.3 Macrophthalmos
> *EXCLUDES 1*   *macrophthalmos in congenital glaucoma (Q15.0)*

✓4ᵗʰ Q12 Congenital lens malformations

Q12.0 Congenital cataract

Q12.1 Congenital displaced lens

Q12.2 Coloboma of lens

Q12.3 Congenital aphakia

Q12.4 Spherophakia

Q12.8 Other congenital lens malformations
Microphakia

Q12.9 Congenital lens malformation, unspecified

✓4ᵗʰ Q13 Congenital malformations of anterior segment of eye

Q13.0 Coloboma of iris
Coloboma NOS

Q13.1 Absence of iris
Aniridia
Use additional code for associated glaucoma (H42)

Q13.2 Other congenital malformations of iris
Anisocoria, congenital
Atresia of pupil
Congenital malformation of iris NOS
Corectopia

Q13.3 Congenital corneal opacity

Q13.4 Other congenital corneal malformations
Congenital malformation of cornea NOS
Microcornea
Peter's anomaly

Q13.5 Blue sclera

✓5ᵗʰ Q13.8 Other congenital malformations of anterior segment of eye

   Q13.81 Rieger's anomaly
Use additional code for associated glaucoma (H42)

   Q13.89 Other congenital malformations of anterior segment of eye

Q13.9 Congenital malformation of anterior segment of eye, unspecified

✓4ᵗʰ Q14 Congenital malformations of posterior segment of eye

> *EXCLUDES 2*   *optic nerve hypoplasia (H47.03-)*

Q14.0 Congenital malformation of vitreous humor
Congenital vitreous opacity

Q14.1 Congenital malformation of retina
Congenital retinal aneurysm

Q14.2 Congenital malformation of optic disc
Coloboma of optic disc

Q14.3 Congenital malformation of choroid

Q14.8 Other congenital malformations of posterior segment of eye
Coloboma of the fundus

Q14.9 Congenital malformation of posterior segment of eye, unspecified

✓4ᵗʰ Q15 Other congenital malformations of eye

> *EXCLUDES 1*   *congenital nystagmus (H55.01)*
> *ocular albinism (E70.31-)*
> *optic nerve hypoplasia (H47.03-)*
> *retinitis pigmentosa (H35.52)*

Q15.0 Congenital glaucoma
Axenfeld's anomaly
Buphthalmos
Glaucoma of childhood
Glaucoma of newborn
Hydrophthalmos
Keratoglobus, congenital, with glaucoma
Macrocornea with glaucoma
Macrophthalmos in congenital glaucoma
Megalocornea with glaucoma

Q15.8 Other specified congenital malformations of eye

Q15.9 Congenital malformation of eye, unspecified
Congenital anomaly of eye
Congenital deformity of eye

✓4ᵗʰ Q16 Congenital malformations of ear causing impairment of hearing

> *EXCLUDES 1*   *congenital deafness (H90.-)*

Q16.0 Congenital absence of (ear) auricle

Q16.1 Congenital absence, atresia and stricture of auditory canal (external)
Congenital atresia or stricture of osseous meatus

Q16.2 Absence of eustachian tube

Q16.3 Congenital malformation of ear ossicles
Congenital fusion of ear ossicles

Q16.4 Other congenital malformations of middle ear
Congenital malformation of middle ear NOS

Q16.5 Congenital malformation of inner ear
Congenital anomaly of membranous labyrinth
Congenital anomaly of organ of Corti

Q16.9 Congenital malformation of ear causing impairment of hearing, unspecified
Congenital absence of ear NOS

✓ Additional Character Required   ✓x7ᵗʰ Placeholder Alert   Unacceptable PDx   Manifestation   Hospital Acquired Condition   *EXCLUDES 1* Not Coded Here   *EXCLUDES 2* Not Included Here

☑4ᵗʰ Q17 Other congenital malformations of ear

> **EXCLUDES 1** congenital malformations of ear with impairment of hearing (Q16.0–Q16.9)
> preauricular sinus (Q18.1)

Q17.0 Accessory auricle
Accessory tragus
Polyotia
Preauricular appendage or tag
Supernumerary ear
Supernumerary lobule

Q17.1 Macrotia

Q17.2 Microtia

Q17.3 Other misshapen ear
Pointed ear

Q17.4 Misplaced ear
Low-set ears
> **EXCLUDES 1** cervical auricle (Q18.2)

Q17.5 Prominent ear
Bat ear

Q17.8 Other specified congenital malformations of ear
Congenital absence of lobe of ear

Q17.9 Congenital malformation of ear, unspecified
Congenital anomaly of ear NOS

☑4ᵗʰ Q18 Other congenital malformations of face and neck

> **EXCLUDES 1** cleft lip and cleft palate (Q35-Q37)
> conditions classified to Q67.0-Q67.4
> congenital malformations of skull and face bones (Q75.-)
> cyclopia (Q87.0)
> dentofacial anomalies [including malocclusion] (M26.-)
> malformation syndromes affecting facial appearance (Q87.0)
> persistent thyroglossal duct (Q89.2)

Q18.0 Sinus, fistula and cyst of branchial cleft
Branchial vestige

Q18.1 Preauricular sinus and cyst
Fistula of auricle, congenital
Cervicoaural fistula

Q18.2 Other branchial cleft malformations
Branchial cleft malformation NOS
Cervical auricle
Otocephaly

Q18.3 Webbing of neck
Pterygium colli

Q18.4 Macrostomia

Q18.5 Microstomia

Q18.6 Macrocheilia
Hypertrophy of lip, congenital

Q18.7 Microcheilia

Q18.8 Other specified congenital malformations of face and neck
Medial cyst of face and neck
Medial fistula of face and neck
Medial sinus of face and neck

Q18.9 Congenital malformation of face and neck, unspecified
Congenital anomaly NOS of face and neck

Congenital malformations of the circulatory system (Q20-Q28)

☑4ᵗʰ Q20 Congenital malformations of cardiac chambers and connections

> **EXCLUDES 1** dextrocardia with situs inversus (Q89.3)
> mirror-image atrial arrangement with situs inversus (Q89.3)

> **CC Excl: For CC/MCC codes in category Q20, unless otherwise noted:** E78.71-E78.72, I23.0-I23.3, I23.6-I23.8, I51.0, P29.3, Q20.0-Q21.9, Q23.8-Q23.9, Q24.8-Q24.9, Q27.30, Q27.4, Q28.0-Q28.1, Q28.8-Q28.9, Q87.1-Q87.89, Q89.7-Q89.8, Q99.2

Q20.0 Common arterial trunk `MCC`
Persistent truncus arteriosus
> **EXCLUDES 1** aortic septal defect (Q21.4)

Q20.1 Double outlet right ventricle `MCC`
Taussig-Bing syndrome

Q20.2 Double outlet left ventricle `MCC`

Q20.3 Discordant ventriculoarterial connection `MCC`
Dextrotransposition of aorta
Transposition of great vessels (complete)

Q20.4 Double inlet ventricle `MCC`
Common ventricle
Cor triloculare biatriatum
Single ventricle

Q20.5 Discordant atrioventricular connection `CC`
Corrected transposition
Levotransposition
Ventricular inversion

Q20.6 Isomerism of atrial appendages
Isomerism of atrial appendages with asplenia or polysplenia

Q20.8 Other congenital malformations of cardiac chambers and connections
Cor binoculare

Q20.9 Congenital malformation of cardiac chambers and connections, unspecified

☑4ᵗʰ Q21 Congenital malformations of cardiac septa

> **EXCLUDES 1** acquired cardiac septal defect (I51.0)

> **CC Excl: For CC/MCC codes in category Q 21, unless otherwise noted:** See code Q20.0

Q21.0 Ventricular septal defect `CC`
Roger's disease

Q21.1 Atrial septal defect `CC`
Coronary sinus defect
Patent or persistent foramen ovale
Patent or persistent ostium secundum defect (type II)
Patent or persistent sinus venosus defect
CC Excl: E78.71-E78.72, I23.0-I23.3, I23.6-I23.8, I51.0, Q20.0-Q20.9, Q21.1-Q21.9, Q23.8-Q23.9, Q24.8-Q24.9, Q27.30, Q27.4, Q28.0-Q28.1, Q28.8-Q28.9, Q87.2-Q87.3, Q87.5-Q87.89, Q89.7-Q89.8

Q21.2 Atrioventricular septal defect `CC`
Common atrioventricular canal
Endocardial cushion defect
Ostium primum atrial septal defect (type I)

Q21.3 Tetralogy of Fallot `MCC`
Ventricular septal defect with pulmonary stenosis or atresia, dextroposition of aorta and hypertrophy of right ventricle.
AHA: 2014, 3Q, 16

Q21.4 Aortopulmonary septal defect
Aortic septal defect
Aortopulmonary window

Q21.8 Other congenital malformations of cardiac septa
Eisenmenger's defect
Pentalogy of Fallot
> **EXCLUDES 1** Eisenmenger's complex (I27.8)
> Eisenmenger's syndrome (I27.8)

Q21.9 Congenital malformation of cardiac septum, unspecified
Septal (heart) defect NOS

☑4ᵗʰ Q22 Congenital malformations of pulmonary and tricuspid valves

Q22.0 Pulmonary valve atresia `MCC`
CC Excl: E78.71-E78.72, P29.3, Q20.9, Q22.0-Q22.3, Q23.8-Q23.9, Q24.8-Q24.9, Q27.30, Q27.4, Q28.0-Q28.1, Q28.8-Q28.9, Q87.1-Q87.89, Q89.7-Q89.8, Q99.2

Q22.1 Congenital pulmonary valve stenosis `CC`
CC Excl: See code: Q22.0

Q22.2 Congenital pulmonary valve insufficiency `CC`
Congenital pulmonary valve regurgitation
CC Excl: E78.71-E78.72, Q20.9, Q22.0-Q22.3, Q23.8-Q23.9, Q24.8-Q24.9, Q27.30, Q27.4, Q28.0-Q28.1, Q28.8-Q28.9, Q87.2-Q87.3, Q87.5-Q87.89, Q89.7-Q89.8

Q22.3 Other congenital malformations of pulmonary valve `CC`
Congenital malformation of pulmonary valve NOS
Supernumerary cusps of pulmonary valve
CC Excl: See code: Q22.2

Q22.4 Congenital tricuspid stenosis `MCC`
Congenital tricuspid atresia
CC Excl: E78.71-E78.72, P29.3, Q20.9, Q22.4-Q23.9, Q24.8-Q24.9, Q27.30, Q27.4, Q28.0-Q28.1, Q28.8-Q28.9, Q87.1-Q87.89, Q89.7-Q89.8, Q99.2

Q22.5 Ebstein's anomaly `MCC`
CC Excl: See code: Q22.4

Q22.6 Hypoplastic right heart syndrome `MCC`
CC Excl: See code: Q22.4

Q22.8 Other congenital malformations of tricuspid valve `MCC`
CC Excl: See code: Q22.4

Q22.9 Congenital malformation of tricuspid valve, unspecified `MCC`
CC Excl: See code: Q22.4

N Newborn: 0   **P** Pediatric: 0-17   **M** Maternity: 12-55   **A** Adult: 15-124   **MCC** Major CC Condition   **PDxMCC** PDx acts as own MCC   **CC** CC Condition   **PDxCC** PDx acts as own CC

860   ICD-10-CM 2016

☑4ᵗʰ **Q23 Congenital malformations of aortic and mitral valves**

> **CC Excl: For CC/MCC codes in category Q23, unless otherwise noted:** See code: Q22.4

 Q23.0 Congenital stenosis of aortic valve   `CC`
   Congenital aortic atresia
   Congenital aortic stenosis NOS
   > **EXCLUDES 1** congenital stenosis of aortic valve in hypoplastic left heart syndrome (Q23.4)
   > congenital subaortic stenosis (Q24.4)
   > supravalvular aortic stenosis (congenital) (Q25.3)

 Q23.1 Congenital insufficiency of aortic valve   `CC`
   Bicuspid aortic valve
   Congenital aortic insufficiency

 Q23.2 Congenital mitral stenosis   `CC`
   Congenital mitral atresia

 Q23.3 Congenital mitral insufficiency   `CC`

 Q23.4 Hypoplastic left heart syndrome   `MCC`

 Q23.8 Other congenital malformations of aortic and mitral valves

 Q23.9 Congenital malformation of aortic and mitral valves, unspecified

☑4ᵗʰ **Q24 Other congenital malformations of heart**
   > **EXCLUDES 1** endocardial fibroelastosis (I42.4)

 Q24.0 Dextrocardia   `CC`
   > **EXCLUDES 1** dextrocardia with situs inversus (Q89.3)
   > isomerism of atrial appendages (with asplenia or polysplenia) (Q20.6)
   > mirror-image atrial arrangement with situs inversus (Q89.3)
   CC Excl: E78.71-E78.72, Q20.9, Q23.8-Q24.4, Q24.8-Q24.9, Q27.30, Q27.4, Q28.0-Q28.1, Q28.8-Q28.9, Q87.2-Q87.3, Q87.5-Q87.89, Q89.7-Q89.8

 Q24.1 Levocardia   `CC`
   CC Excl: See code: Q24.0

 Q24.2 Cor triatriatum   `MCC`
   CC Excl: E78.71-E78.72, P29.3, Q20.9, Q23.8-Q23.9, Q24.2-Q24.4, Q24.8-Q24.9, Q27.30, Q27.4, Q28.0-Q28.1, Q28.8-Q28.9, Q87.1-Q87.89, Q89.7-Q89.8, Q99.2

 Q24.3 Pulmonary infundibular stenosis   `CC`
   Subvalvular pulmonic stenosis
   CC Excl: See code: Q24.2

 Q24.4 Congenital subaortic stenosis   `MCC`
   CC Excl: See code: Q24.2

 Q24.5 Malformation of coronary vessels   `CC`
   Congenital coronary (artery) aneurysm
   CC Excl: Q20.9-Q23.9, Q24.5, Q24.8-Q24.9

 Q24.6 Congenital heart block   `MCC`
   CC Excl: E78.71-E78.72, P29.3, Q20.9, Q23.8-Q23.9, Q24.6-Q24.9, Q27.30, Q27.4, Q28.0-Q28.1, Q28.8-Q28.9, Q87.1-Q87.89, Q89.7-Q89.8, Q99.2

 Q24.8 Other specified congenital malformations of heart
   Congenital diverticulum of left ventricle
   Congenital malformation of myocardium
   Congenital malformation of pericardium
   Malposition of heart
   Uhl's disease

 Q24.9 Congenital malformation of heart, unspecified
   Congenital anomaly of heart
   Congenital disease of heart

☑4ᵗʰ **Q25 Congenital malformations of great arteries**

 Q25.0 Patent ductus arteriosus   `CC`
   Patent ductus Botallo
   Persistent ductus arteriosus
   CC Excl: Q25.0, Q27.30, Q27.4, Q28.0-Q28.1, Q28.8

 Q25.1 Coarctation of aorta   `CC`
   Coarctation of aorta (preductal) (postductal)
   CC Excl: E78.71-E78.72, Q25.1-Q25.3, Q27.30, Q27.4, Q28.0-Q28.1, Q28.8-Q28.9, Q87.2-Q87.3, Q87.5-Q87.89, Q89.7-Q89.8

 Q25.2 Atresia of aorta   `CC`
   CC Excl: E78.71-E78.72, P29.3, Q25.1-Q25.3, Q27.30, Q27.4, Q28.0-Q28.1, Q28.8-Q28.9, Q87.1-Q87.89, Q89.7-Q89.8, Q99.2

 Q25.3 Supravalvular aortic stenosis   `CC`
   > **EXCLUDES 1** congenital aortic stenosis NOS (Q23.0)
   > congenital stenosis of aortic valve (Q23.0)
   CC Excl: See code: Q25.2

 Q25.4 Other congenital malformations of aorta   `CC`
   Absence of aorta
   Aneurysm of sinus of Valsalva (ruptured)
   Aplasia of aorta
   Congenital aneurysm of aorta
   Congenital malformations of aorta
   Congenital dilatation of aorta
   Double aortic arch [vascular ring of aorta]
   Hypoplasia of aorta
   Persistent convolutions of aortic arch
   Persistent right aortic arch
   > **EXCLUDES 1** hypoplasia of aorta in hypoplastic left heart syndrome (Q23.4)
   CC Excl: E78.71-E78.72, Q25.1-Q25.4, Q25.8-Q25.9, Q27.30, Q27.4, Q28.0-Q28.1, Q28.8-Q28.9, Q87.2-Q87.3, Q87.5-Q87.89, Q89.7-Q89.8

 Q25.5 Atresia of pulmonary artery   `MCC`
   CC Excl: Q25.5-Q25.79, Q27.30, Q27.4, Q28.0-Q28.1, Q28.8-Q28.9

 Q25.6 Stenosis of pulmonary artery   `MCC`
   Supravalvular pulmonary stenosis
   CC Excl: See code: Q25.5

☑5ᵗʰ **Q25.7 Other congenital malformations of pulmonary artery**

> **CC Excl: For CC codes in subcategory Q25.7, unless otherwise noted:** See code: Q25.5

  Q25.71 Coarctation of pulmonary artery   `MCC`

  Q25.72 Congenital pulmonary arteriovenous malformation   `MCC`
   Congenital pulmonary arteriovenous aneurysm

  Q25.79 Other congenital malformations of pulmonary artery   `MCC`
   Aberrant pulmonary artery
   Agenesis of pulmonary artery
   Congenital aneurysm of pulmonary artery
   Congenital anomaly of pulmonary artery
   Hypoplasia of pulmonary artery

 Q25.8 Other congenital malformations of other great arteries   `CC`
   CC Excl: See code: Q25.4

 Q25.9 Congenital malformation of great arteries, unspecified   `CC`
   CC Excl: See code: Q25.4

☑4ᵗʰ **Q26 Congenital malformations of great veins**

 Q26.0 Congenital stenosis of vena cava   `CC`
   Congenital stenosis of vena cava (inferior)(superior)
   CC Excl: Q26.0-Q26.1, Q26.8, Q27.30, Q27.4, Q28.0-Q28.1, Q28.8-Q28.9

 Q26.1 Persistent left superior vena cava   `CC`
   CC Excl: See code: Q26.0

 Q26.2 Total anomalous pulmonary venous connection   `CC`
   Total anomalous pulmonary venous return [TAPVR], subdiaphragmatic
   Total anomalous pulmonary venous return [TAPVR], supradiaphragmatic
   CC Excl: Q26.2, Q27.30, Q27.4, Q28.0-Q28.1, Q28.8-Q28.9

 Q26.3 Partial anomalous pulmonary venous connection   `CC`
   Partial anomalous pulmonary venous return
   CC Excl: Q26.3-Q26.4, Q27.30, Q27.4, Q28.0-Q28.1, Q28.8-Q28.9

 Q26.4 Anomalous pulmonary venous connection, unspecified   `CC`
   CC Excl: See code: Q26.3

 Q26.5 Anomalous portal venous connection

 Q26.6 Portal vein-hepatic artery fistula

 Q26.8 Other congenital malformations of great veins   `CC`
   Absence of vena cava (inferior) (superior)
   Azygos continuation of inferior vena cava
   Persistent left posterior cardinal vein
   Scimitar syndrome
   CC Excl: See code: Q26.0

 Q26.9 Congenital malformation of great vein, unspecified   `CC`
   Congenital anomaly of vena cava (inferior) (superior) NOS
   CC Excl: Q26.9-Q27.30, Q27.4, Q28.0-Q28.1, Q28.8-Q28.9

☑4ᵗʰ **Q27 Other congenital malformations of peripheral vascular system**
   > **EXCLUDES 2** anomalies of cerebral and precerebral vessels (Q28.0-Q28.3)
   > anomalies of coronary vessels (Q24.5)
   > anomalies of pulmonary artery (Q25.5-Q25.7)
   > congenital retinal aneurysm (Q14.1)
   > hemangioma and lymphangioma (D18.-)

 Q27.0 Congenital absence and hypoplasia of umbilical artery
   Single umbilical artery

 Q27.1 Congenital renal artery stenosis

 Q27.2 Other congenital malformations of renal artery
   Congenital malformation of renal artery NOS
   Multiple renal arteries

☑ Additional Character Required   ☑Ⓧ⁷ᵗʰ Placeholder Alert   Unacceptable PDx   Manifestation   Hospital Acquired Condition   **EXCLUDES 1** Not Coded Here   **EXCLUDES 2** Not Included Here

✓5ᵗʰ Q27.3 Arteriovenous malformation (peripheral)
Arteriovenous aneurysm
  EXCLUDES 1 acquired arteriovenous aneurysm (I77.0)
  EXCLUDES 2 arteriovenous malformation of cerebral vessels (Q28.2)
                arteriovenous malformation of precerebral vessels
                (Q28.0)

  Q27.30 Arteriovenous malformation, site unspecified `CC`
    CC Excl: Q20.0–Q20.8, Q21.0–Q21.9, Q27.30, Q27.4,
    Q28.0–Q28.1, Q28.8

  Q27.31 Arteriovenous malformation of vessel of upper limb

  Q27.32 Arteriovenous malformation of vessel of lower limb

  Q27.33 Arteriovenous malformation of digestive system vessel

  Q27.34 Arteriovenous malformation of renal vessel

  Q27.39 Arteriovenous malformation, other site

Q27.4 Congenital phlebectasia `CC`
  CC Excl: See code: Q27.30

Q27.8 Other specified congenital malformations of peripheral vascular system
Absence of peripheral vascular system
Atresia of peripheral vascular system
Congenital aneurysm (peripheral)
Congenital stricture, artery
Congenital varix
  EXCLUDES 1 arteriovenous malformation (Q27.3-)

Q27.9 Congenital malformation of peripheral vascular system, unspecified
Anomaly of artery or vein NOS

✓4ᵗʰ Q28 Other congenital malformations of circulatory system
  EXCLUDES 1 congenital aneurysm NOS (Q27.8)
                congenital coronary aneurysm (Q24.5)
                ruptured cerebral arteriovenous malformation (I60.8)
                ruptured malformation of precerebral vessels (I72.0)
  EXCLUDES 2 congenital peripheral aneurysm (Q27.8)
                congenital pulmonary aneurysm (Q25.79)
                congenital retinal aneurysm (Q14.1)

  CC Excl: For CC/MCC codes in category Q28, unless otherwise
  noted: See code: Q27.30

  Q28.0 Arteriovenous malformation of precerebral vessels `CC`
  Congenital arteriovenous precerebral aneurysm (nonruptured)

  Q28.1 Other malformations of precerebral vessels `CC`
  Congenital malformation of precerebral vessels NOS
  Congenital precerebral aneurysm (nonruptured)

  Q28.2 Arteriovenous malformation of cerebral vessels `MCC`
  Arteriovenous malformation of brain NOS
  Congenital arteriovenous cerebral aneurysm (nonruptured)
    CC Excl: Q27.30, Q27.4, Q28.0–Q28.9

  Q28.3 Other malformations of cerebral vessels `MCC`
  Congenital cerebral aneurysm (nonruptured)
  Congenital malformation of cerebral vessels NOS
  Developmental venous anomaly
    CC Excl: See code: Q28.2

  Q28.8 Other specified congenital malformations of circulatory system `CC`
  Congenital aneurysm, specified site NEC
  Spinal vessel anomaly
    CC Excl: Q20.0–Q20.8, Q21.0–Q21.9, Q27.30, Q27.4, Q28.0–Q28.1,
    Q28.8

  Q28.9 Congenital malformation of circulatory system, unspecified `CC`
    CC Excl: Q20.0–Q28.9

Congenital malformations of the respiratory system (Q30–Q34)

✓4ᵗʰ Q30 Congenital malformations of nose
  EXCLUDES 1 congenital deviation of nasal septum (Q67.4)

  Q30.0 Choanal atresia
  Atresia of nares (anterior) (posterior)
  Congenital stenosis of nares (anterior) (posterior)

  Q30.1 Agenesis and underdevelopment of nose
  Congenital absent of nose

  Q30.2 Fissured, notched and cleft nose

  Q30.3 Congenital perforated nasal septum

  Q30.8 Other congenital malformations of nose
  Accessory nose
  Congenital anomaly of nasal sinus wall

  Q30.9 Congenital malformation of nose, unspecified

✓4ᵗʰ Q31 Congenital malformations of larynx
  EXCLUDES 1 congenital laryngeal stridor NOS (P28.89)

  CC Excl: For CC codes in category Q31, unless otherwise noted:
  J39.8, J45.990, J98.09, Q31.1–Q32.4, Q34.0–Q34.9

  Q31.0 Web of larynx
  Glottic web of larynx
  Subglottic web of larynx
  Web of larynx NOS

  Q31.1 Congenital subglottic stenosis `CC`

  Q31.2 Laryngeal hypoplasia `CC`

  Q31.3 Laryngocele `CC`

  Q31.5 Congenital laryngomalacia `CC`

  Q31.8 Other congenital malformations of larynx `CC`
  Absence of larynx
  Agenesis of larynx
  Atresia of larynx
  Congenital cleft thyroid cartilage
  Congenital fissure of epiglottis
  Congenital stenosis of larynx NEC
  Posterior cleft of cricoid cartilage

  Q31.9 Congenital malformation of larynx, unspecified `CC`

✓4ᵗʰ Q32 Congenital malformations of trachea and bronchus
  EXCLUDES 1 congenital bronchiectasis (Q33.4)

  CC Excl: For CC codes in category Q32, unless otherwise noted:
  See code: Q31

  Q32.0 Congenital tracheomalacia `CC`

  Q32.1 Other congenital malformations of trachea `CC`
  Atresia of trachea
  Congenital anomaly of tracheal cartilage
  Congenital dilatation of trachea
  Congenital malformation of trachea
  Congenital stenosis of trachea
  Congenital tracheocele

  Q32.2 Congenital bronchomalacia `CC`

  Q32.3 Congenital stenosis of bronchus `CC`

  Q32.4 Other congenital malformations of bronchus `CC`
  Absence of bronchus
  Agenesis of bronchus
  Atresia of bronchus
  Congenital diverticulum of bronchus
  Congenital malformation of bronchus NOS

✓4ᵗʰ Q33 Congenital malformations of lung

  CC Excl: For CC/MCC codes in category Q33, unless otherwise
  noted: Q33.0–Q34.9

  Q33.0 Congenital cystic lung `CC`
  Congenital cystic lung disease
  Congenital honeycomb lung
  Congenital polycystic lung disease
    EXCLUDES 1 cystic fibrosis (E84.0)
                  cystic lung disease, acquired or unspecified (J98.4)

  Q33.1 Accessory lobe of lung
  Azygos lobe (fissured), lung

  Q33.2 Sequestration of lung `MCC`

  Q33.3 Agenesis of lung `MCC`
  Congenital absence of lung (lobe)

  Q33.4 Congenital bronchiectasis `CC`
    CC Excl: J44.9, J47.0–J47.9, J68.1, J68.4–J68.9, Q33.4

  Q33.5 Ectopic tissue in lung

  Q33.6 Congenital hypoplasia and dysplasia of lung `MCC`
    EXCLUDES 1 pulmonary hypoplasia associated with short gestation
                  (P28.0)
    CC Excl: Q33.0–Q34.9

  Q33.8 Other congenital malformations of lung

  Q33.9 Congenital malformation of lung, unspecified

✓4ᵗʰ Q34 Other congenital malformations of respiratory system
  EXCLUDES 2 congenital central alveolar hypoventilation syndrome (G47.35)

  Q34.0 Anomaly of pleura

  Q34.1 Congenital cyst of mediastinum

  Q34.8 Other specified congenital malformations of respiratory system
  Atresia of nasopharynx

  Q34.9 Congenital malformation of respiratory system, unspecified
  Congenital absence of respiratory system
  Congenital anomaly of respiratory system NOS

N Newborn: 0   P Pediatric: 0-17   M Maternity: 12-55   A Adult: 15-124   MCC Major CC Condition   PDxMCC PDx acts as own MCC   CC CC Condition   PDxCC PDx acts as own CC

862
ICD-10-CM 2016

Cleft lip and cleft palate (Q35-Q37)

Use additional code to identify associated malformation of the nose (Q30.2)

EXCLUDES 1   Robin's syndrome (Q87.0)

✓4ᵗʰ Q35 Cleft palate

     INCLUDES   fissure of palate
                   palatoschisis

     EXCLUDES 1   cleft palate with cleft lip (Q37.-)

     Q35.1 Cleft hard palate

     Q35.3 Cleft soft palate

     Q35.5 Cleft hard palate with cleft soft palate

     Q35.7 Cleft uvula

     Q35.9 Cleft palate, unspecified
         Cleft palate NOS

✓4ᵗʰ Q36 Cleft lip

     Cheiloschisis
     Congenital fissure of lip
     Harelip
     Labium leporinum

     EXCLUDES 1   cleft lip with cleft palate (Q37.-)

     Q36.0 Cleft lip, bilateral

     Q36.1 Cleft lip, median

     Q36.9 Cleft lip, unilateral
         Cleft lip NOS

✓4ᵗʰ Q37 Cleft palate with cleft lip

     Cheilopalatoschisis

     Q37.0 Cleft hard palate with bilateral cleft lip

     Q37.1 Cleft hard palate with unilateral cleft lip
         Cleft hard palate with cleft lip NOS

     Q37.2 Cleft soft palate with bilateral cleft lip

     Q37.3 Cleft soft palate with unilateral cleft lip
         Cleft soft palate with cleft lip NOS

     Q37.4 Cleft hard and soft palate with bilateral cleft lip

     Q37.5 Cleft hard and soft palate with unilateral cleft lip
         Cleft hard and soft palate with cleft lip NOS

     Q37.8 Unspecified cleft palate with bilateral cleft lip

     Q37.9 Unspecified cleft palate with unilateral cleft lip
         Cleft palate with cleft lip NOS

Other congenital malformations of the digestive system (Q38-Q45)

✓4ᵗʰ Q38 Other congenital malformations of tongue, mouth and pharynx

     EXCLUDES 1   dentofacial anomalies (M26.-)
                 macrostomia (Q18.4)
                 microstomia (Q18.5)

     Q38.0 Congenital malformations of lips, not elsewhere classified
         Congenital fistula of lip
         Congenital malformation of lip NOS
         Van der Woude's syndrome

         EXCLUDES 1   cleft lip (Q36.-)
                     cleft lip with cleft palate (Q37.-)
                     macrocheilia (Q18.6)
                     microcheilia (Q18.7)

     Q38.1 Ankyloglossia
         Tongue tie

     Q38.2 Macroglossia
         Congenital hypertrophy of tongue

     Q38.3 Other congenital malformations of tongue
         Aglossia
         Bifid tongue
         Congenital adhesion of tongue
         Congenital fissure of tongue
         Congenital malformation of tongue NOS
         Double tongue
         Hypoglossia
         Hypoplasia of tongue
         Microglossia

     Q38.4 Congenital malformations of salivary glands and ducts
         Atresia of salivary glands and ducts
         Congenital absence of salivary glands and ducts
         Congenital accessory salivary glands and ducts
         Congenital fistula of salivary gland

     Q38.5 Congenital malformations of palate, not elsewhere classified
         Congenital absence of uvula
         Congenital malformation of palate NOS
         Congenital high arched palate

         EXCLUDES 1   cleft palate (Q35.-)
                     cleft palate with cleft lip (Q37.-)

     Q38.6 Other congenital malformations of mouth
         Congenital malformation of mouth NOS

     Q38.7 Congenital pharyngeal pouch
         Congenital diverticulum of pharynx

         EXCLUDES 1   pharyngeal pouch syndrome (D82.1)

     Q38.8 Other congenital malformations of pharynx
         Congenital malformation of pharynx NOS
         Imperforate pharynx

✓4ᵗʰ Q39 Congenital malformations of esophagus

     CC Excl: For CC/MCC codes in category Q39, unless otherwise noted: Q39.0-Q39.9, Q45.8-Q45.9

     Q39.0 Atresia of esophagus without fistula   MCC
         Atresia of esophagus NOS

     Q39.1 Atresia of esophagus with tracheo-esophageal fistula   MCC
         Atresia of esophagus with broncho-esophageal fistula

     Q39.2 Congenital tracheo-esophageal fistula without atresia   MCC
         Congenital tracheo-esophageal fistula NOS

     Q39.3 Congenital stenosis and stricture of esophagus   MCC

     Q39.4 Esophageal web   MCC

     Q39.5 Congenital dilatation of esophagus   CC
         Congenital cardiospasm
         CC Excl: Q39.5-Q39.9, Q45.8-Q45.9

     Q39.6 Congenital diverticulum of esophagus   CC
         Congenital esophageal pouch
         CC Excl: See code: Q39.5

     Q39.8 Other congenital malformations of esophagus   CC
         Congenital absence of esophagus
         Congenital displacement of esophagus
         Congenital duplication of esophagus
         CC Excl: See code: Q39.5

     Q39.9 Congenital malformation of esophagus, unspecified   CC
         CC Excl: See code: Q39.5

✓4ᵗʰ Q40 Other congenital malformations of upper alimentary tract

     Q40.0 Congenital hypertrophic pyloric stenosis
         Congenital or infantile constriction
         Congenital or infantile hypertrophy
         Congenital or infantile spasm
         Congenital or infantile stenosis
         Congenital or infantile stricture

     Q40.1 Congenital hiatus hernia
         Congenital displacement of cardia through esophageal hiatus

         EXCLUDES 1   congenital diaphragmatic hernia (Q79.0)

     Q40.2 Other specified congenital malformations of stomach
         Congenital displacement of stomach
         Congenital diverticulum of stomach
         Congenital hourglass stomach
         Congenital duplication of stomach
         Megalogastria
         Microgastria

     Q40.3 Congenital malformation of stomach, unspecified

     Q40.8 Other specified congenital malformations of upper alimentary tract

     Q40.9 Congenital malformation of upper alimentary tract, unspecified
         Congenital anomaly of upper alimentary tract
         Congenital deformity of upper alimentary tract

✓4ᵗʰ Q41 Congenital absence, atresia and stenosis of small intestine

     Congenital obstruction, occlusion or stricture of small intestine or intestine NOS

     EXCLUDES 1   cystic fibrosis with intestinal manifestation (E84.11)
                 meconium ileus NOS (without cystic fibrosis) (P76.0)

     CC Excl: For CC codes in category Q41, unless otherwise noted: Q41.0-Q41.9, Q45.8-Q45.9

     Q41.0 Congenital absence, atresia and stenosis of duodenum   CC

     Q41.1 Congenital absence, atresia and stenosis of jejunum   CC
         Apple peel syndrome
         Imperforate jejunum

     Q41.2 Congenital absence, atresia and stenosis of ileum   CC

     Q41.8 Congenital absence, atresia and stenosis of other specified parts of small intestine   CC

     Q41.9 Congenital absence, atresia and stenosis of small intestine, part unspecified   CC
         Congenital absence, atresia and stenosis of intestine NOS

✓ Additional Character Required   ✓x7ᵗʰ Placeholder Alert   Unacceptable PDx   Manifestation   Hospital Acquired Condition   **EXCLUDES 1** Not Coded Here   **EXCLUDES 2** Not Included Here

Chapter 17. Congenital Malformations, Deformations, and Chromosomal Abnormalities

Q42–Q51.0

☑4ᵗʰ **Q42 Congenital absence, atresia and stenosis of large intestine**
Congenital obstruction, occlusion and stricture of large intestine

CC Excl: For CC codes in category Q42, unless otherwise noted:
Q42.0-Q42.9, Q45.8-Q45.9

Q42.0 Congenital absence, atresia and stenosis of rectum with fistula   CC

Q42.1 Congenital absence, atresia and stenosis of rectum without fistula   CC
Imperforate rectum

Q42.2 Congenital absence, atresia and stenosis of anus with fistula   CC

Q42.3 Congenital absence, atresia and stenosis of anus without fistula   CC
Imperforate anus

Q42.8 Congenital absence, atresia and stenosis of other parts of large intestine   CC

Q42.9 Congenital absence, atresia and stenosis of large intestine, part unspecified   CC

☑4ᵗʰ **Q43 Other congenital malformations of intestine**

CC Excl: For CC codes in category Q43, unless otherwise noted:
Q41.0-Q43.9

Q43.0 Meckel's diverticulum (displaced) (hypertrophic)
Persistent omphalomesenteric duct
Persistent vitelline duct

Q43.1 Hirschsprung's disease   CC
Aganglionosis
Congenital (aganglionic) megacolon
CC Excl: Q43.1-Q43.2, Q45.8-Q45.9

Q43.2 Other congenital functional disorders of colon   CC
Congenital dilatation of colon
CC Excl: See code: Q43.1

Q43.3 Congenital malformations of intestinal fixation   CC
Congenital omental, anomalous adhesions [bands]
Congenital peritoneal adhesions [bands]
Incomplete rotation of cecum and colon
Insufficient rotation of cecum and colon
Jackson's membrane
Malrotation of colon
Rotation failure of cecum and colon
Universal mesentery
CC Excl: Q43.3-Q43.9

Q43.4 Duplication of intestine   CC

Q43.5 Ectopic anus   CC

Q43.6 Congenital fistula of rectum and anus   CC
EXCLUDES 1   *congenital fistula of anus with absence, atresia and stenosis (Q42.2)*
congenital fistula of rectum with absence, atresia and stenosis (Q42.0)
congenital rectovaginal fistula (Q52.2)
congenital urethrorectal fistula (Q64.73)
pilonidal fistula or sinus (L05.-)

Q43.7 Persistent cloaca   CC
Cloaca NOS

Q43.8 Other specified congenital malformations of intestine   CC
Congenital blind loop syndrome
Congenital diverticulitis, colon
Congenital diverticulum, intestine
Dolichocolon
Megaloappendix
Megaloduodenum
Microcolon
Transposition of appendix
Transposition of colon
Transposition of intestine
AHA: 2013, 2Q, 31

Q43.9 Congenital malformation of intestine, unspecified   CC

☑4ᵗʰ **Q44 Congenital malformations of gallbladder, bile ducts and liver**

CC Excl: For CC/MCC codes in category Q44, unless otherwise noted: Q44.0-Q44.7

Q44.0 Agenesis, aplasia and hypoplasia of gallbladder   CC
Congenital absence of gallbladder

Q44.1 Other congenital malformations of gallbladder   CC
Congenital malformation of gallbladder NOS
Intrahepatic gallbladder

Q44.2 Atresia of bile ducts   MCC
CC Excl: Q44.2-Q44.3, Q45.8-Q45.9

Q44.3 Congenital stenosis and stricture of bile ducts   MCC
CC Excl: See code: Q44.2

Q44.4 Choledochal cyst   CC

Q44.5 Other congenital malformations of bile ducts   CC
Accessory hepatic duct
Biliary duct duplication
Congenital malformation of bile duct NOS
Cystic duct duplication

Q44.6 Cystic disease of liver   CC
Fibrocystic disease of liver
CC Excl: Q44.0-Q44.1, Q44.4-Q44.7

Q44.7 Other congenital malformations of liver   CC
Accessory liver
Alagille's syndrome
Congenital absence of liver
Congenital hepatomegaly
Congenital malformation of liver NOS

☑4ᵗʰ **Q45 Other congenital malformations of digestive system**
EXCLUDES 2   *congenital diaphragmatic hernia (Q79.0)*
congenital hiatus hernia (Q40.1)

CC Excl: For CC/MCC codes in category Q45, unless otherwise noted: Q45.0-Q45.9

Q45.0 Agenesis, aplasia and hypoplasia of pancreas   CC
Congenital absence of pancreas

Q45.1 Annular pancreas   CC

Q45.2 Congenital pancreatic cyst   CC

Q45.3 Other congenital malformations of pancreas and pancreatic duct   CC
Accessory pancreas
Congenital malformation of pancreas or pancreatic duct NOS
EXCLUDES 1   *congenital diabetes mellitus (E10.-)*
cystic fibrosis (E84.0-E84.9)
fibrocystic disease of pancreas (E84.-)
neonatal diabetes mellitus (P70.2)

Q45.8 Other specified congenital malformations of digestive system
Absence (complete) (partial) of alimentary tract NOS
Duplication of digestive system
Malposition, congenital of digestive system

Q45.9 Congenital malformation of digestive system, unspecified
Congenital anomaly of digestive system
Congenital deformity of digestive system

Congenital malformations of genital organs (Q50-Q56)
EXCLUDES 1   *androgen insensitivity syndrome (E34.5-)*
syndromes associated with anomalies in the number and form of chromosomes (Q90-Q99)

☑4ᵗʰ **Q50 Congenital malformations of ovaries, fallopian tubes and broad ligaments**

☑5ᵗʰ **Q50.0 Congenital absence of ovary**
EXCLUDES 1   *Turner's syndrome (Q96.-)*

Q50.01 Congenital absence of ovary, unilateral   ♀

Q50.02 Congenital absence of ovary, bilateral   ♀

Q50.1 Developmental ovarian cyst   ♀

Q50.2 Congenital torsion of ovary   ♀

☑5ᵗʰ **Q50.3 Other congenital malformations of ovary**

Q50.31 Accessory ovary   ♀

Q50.32 Ovarian streak   ♀
46, XX with streak gonads

Q50.39 Other congenital malformation of ovary   ♀
Congenital malformation of ovary NOS

Q50.4 Embryonic cyst of fallopian tube   ♀
Fimbrial cyst

Q50.5 Embryonic cyst of broad ligament   ♀
Epoophoron cyst
Parovarian cyst

Q50.6 Other congenital malformations of fallopian tube and broad ligament   ♀
Absence of fallopian tube and broad ligament
Accessory fallopian tube and broad ligament
Atresia of fallopian tube and broad ligament
Congenital malformation of fallopian tube or broad ligament NOS

☑4ᵗʰ **Q51 Congenital malformations of uterus and cervix**

Q51.0 Agenesis and aplasia of uterus   ♀
Congenital absence of uterus

Ⓝ Newborn: 0   Ⓟ Pediatric: 0-17   Ⓜ Maternity: 12-55   Ⓐ Adult: 15-124   **MCC** Major CC Condition   **PDxMCC** PDx acts as own MCC   **CC** CC Condition   **PDxCC** PDx acts as own CC

☑5ᵗʰ **Q51.1** **Doubling** of uterus with doubling of cervix and vagina
- **Q51.10** **Doubling of uterus with doubling of cervix and vagina** without obstruction ♀
  Doubling of uterus with doubling of cervix and vagina NOS
- **Q51.11** **Doubling of uterus with doubling of cervix and vagina** with obstruction ♀

Q51.2 **Other doubling of uterus** ♀
  Doubling of uterus NOS
  Septate uterus, complete or partial

Q51.3 **Bicornate uterus** ♀
  Bicornate uterus, complete or partial

Q51.4 **Unicornate uterus** ♀
  Unicornate uterus with or without a separate uterine horn
  Uterus with only one functioning horn

Q51.5 **Agenesis and aplasia of cervix** ♀
  Congenital absence of cervix

Q51.6 **Embryonic cyst of cervix** ♀

Q51.7 **Congenital fistulae between uterus and digestive and urinary tracts** ♀

☑5ᵗʰ **Q51.8** **Other congenital malformations of uterus and cervix**
- ☑6ᵗʰ **Q51.81** **Other congenital malformations of uterus**
  - **Q51.810** **Arcuate uterus** ♀
    Arcuatus uterus
  - **Q51.811** **Hypoplasia of uterus** ♀
  - **Q51.818** **Other congenital malformations of uterus** ♀
    Müllerian anomaly of uterus NEC
- ☑6ᵗʰ **Q51.82** **Other congenital malformations of cervix**
  - **Q51.820** **Cervical duplication** ♀
  - **Q51.821** **Hypoplasia of cervix** ♀
  - **Q51.828** **Other congenital malformations of cervix** ♀

Q51.9 **Congenital malformation of uterus and cervix, unspecified** ♀

☑4ᵗʰ **Q52** **Other congenital malformations of female genitalia**
Q52.0 **Congenital absence of vagina** ♀
  Vaginal agenesis, total or partial

☑5ᵗʰ **Q52.1** **Doubling of vagina**
  EXCLUDES 1 doubling of vagina with doubling of uterus and cervix (Q51.1-)
- **Q52.10** **Doubling of vagina, unspecified** ♀
  Septate vagina NOS
- **Q52.11** **Transverse vaginal septum** ♀
- **Q52.12** **Longitudinal vaginal septum** ♀
  Longitudinal vaginal septum with or without obstruction

Q52.2 **Congenital rectovaginal fistula** ♀
  EXCLUDES 1 cloaca (Q43.7)

Q52.3 **Imperforate hymen** ♀

Q52.4 **Other congenital malformations of vagina** ♀
  Canal of Nuck cyst, congenital
  Congenital malformation of vagina NOS
  Embryonic vaginal cyst
  Gartner's duct cyst

Q52.5 **Fusion of labia** ♀

Q52.6 **Congenital malformation of clitoris** ♀

☑5ᵗʰ **Q52.7** **Other and unspecified congenital malformations of vulva**
- **Q52.70** **Unspecified congenital malformations of vulva** ♀
  Congenital malformation of vulva NOS
- **Q52.71** **Congenital absence of vulva** ♀
- **Q52.79** **Other congenital malformations of vulva** ♀
  Congenital cyst of vulva

Q52.8 **Other specified congenital malformations of female genitalia** ♀

Q52.9 **Congenital malformation of female genitalia, unspecified** ♀

☑4ᵗʰ **Q53** **Undescended and ectopic testicle**
☑5ᵗʰ **Q53.0** **Ectopic testis**
- **Q53.00** **Ectopic testis, unspecified** ♂
- **Q53.01** **Ectopic testis, unilateral** ♂
- **Q53.02** **Ectopic testes, bilateral** ♂

☑5ᵗʰ **Q53.1** **Undescended testicle, unilateral**
- **Q53.10** **Unspecified undescended testicle, unilateral** ♂
- **Q53.11** **Abdominal testis, unilateral** ♂

- **Q53.12** **Ectopic perineal testis, unilateral** ♂

☑5ᵗʰ **Q53.2** **Undescended testicle, bilateral**
- **Q53.20** **Undescended testicle, unspecified, bilateral** ♂
- **Q53.21** **Abdominal testis, bilateral** ♂
- **Q53.22** **Ectopic perineal testis, bilateral** ♂

Q53.9 **Undescended testicle, unspecified** ♂
  Cryptorchism NOS

☑4ᵗʰ **Q54** **Hypospadias**
  EXCLUDES 1 epispadias (Q64.0)
Q54.0 **Hypospadias, balanic**
  Hypospadias, coronal
  Hypospadias, glandular
Q54.1 **Hypospadias, penile** ♂
Q54.2 **Hypospadias, penoscrotal** ♂
Q54.3 **Hypospadias, perineal** ♂
Q54.4 **Congenital chordee**
  Chordee without hypospadias
Q54.8 **Other hypospadias**
  Hypospadias with intersex state
Q54.9 **Hypospadias, unspecified** ♂

☑4ᵗʰ **Q55** **Other congenital malformations of male genital organs**
  EXCLUDES 1 congenital hydrocele (P83.5)
  hypospadias (Q54.-)
Q55.0 **Absence and aplasia of testis** ♂
  Monorchism
Q55.1 **Hypoplasia of testis and scrotum** ♂
  Fusion of testes
☑5ᵗʰ **Q55.2** **Other and unspecified congenital malformations of testis and scrotum**
- **Q55.20** **Unspecified congenital malformations of testis and scrotum** ♂
  Congenital malformation of testis or scrotum NOS
- **Q55.21** **Polyorchism** ♂
- **Q55.22** **Retractile testis** ♂
- **Q55.23** **Scrotal transposition** ♂
- **Q55.29** **Other congenital malformations of testis and scrotum** ♂

Q55.3 **Atresia of vas deferens** ♂
  Code first any associated cystic fibrosis (E84.-)
Q55.4 **Other congenital malformations of vas deferens, epididymis, seminal vesicles and prostate** ♂
  Absence or aplasia of prostate
  Absence or aplasia of spermatic cord
  Congenital malformation of vas deferens, epididymis, seminal vesicles or prostate NOS

Q55.5 **Congenital absence and aplasia of penis** ♂
☑5ᵗʰ **Q55.6** **Other congenital malformations of penis**
- **Q55.61** **Curvature of penis (lateral)** ♂
- **Q55.62** **Hypoplasia of penis** ♂
  Micropenis
- **Q55.63** **Congenital torsion of penis** ♂
  EXCLUDES 1 acquired torsion of penis (N48.82)
- **Q55.64** **Hidden penis** ♂
  Buried penis
  Concealed penis
  EXCLUDES 1 acquired buried penis (N48.83)
- **Q55.69** **Other congenital malformation of penis** ♂
  Congenital malformation of penis NOS

Q55.7 **Congenital vasocutaneous fistula** ♂
Q55.8 **Other specified congenital malformations of male genital organs** ♂
Q55.9 **Congenital malformation of male genital organ, unspecified** ♂
  Congenital anomaly of male genital organ
  Congenital deformity of male genital organ

☑4ᵗʰ **Q56** **Indeterminate sex and pseudohermaphroditism**
  EXCLUDES 1 46, XX true hermaphrodite (Q99.1)
  androgen insensitivity syndrome (E34.5-)
  chimera 46, XX/46, XY true hermaphrodite (Q99.0)
  female pseudohermaphroditism with adrenocortical disorder (E25.-)
  pseudohermaphroditism with specified chromosomal anomaly (Q96-Q99)
  pure gonadal dysgenesis (Q99.1)
Q56.0 **Hermaphroditism, not elsewhere classified**
  Ovotestis

☑ Additional Character Required   ☑xᵗʰ Placeholder Alert   Unacceptable PDx   Manifestation   Hospital Acquired Condition   *EXCLUDES 1* Not Coded Here   *EXCLUDES 2* Not Included Here

Q56.1   **Male pseudohermaphroditism, not elsewhere classified**   ♂
: 46, XY with streak gonads
: Male pseudohermaphroditism NOS

Q56.2   **Female pseudohermaphroditism, not elsewhere classified**   ♀
: Female pseudohermaphroditism NOS

Q56.3   **Pseudohermaphroditism, unspecified**

Q56.4   **Indeterminate sex, unspecified**
: Ambiguous genitalia

Congenital malformations of the urinary system (Q60-Q64)

√4ᵗʰ **Q60**   **Renal agenesis and other reduction defects of kidney**
: Congenital absence of kidney
: Congenital atrophy of kidney
: Infantile atrophy of kidney

> **CC Excl: For CC codes in category Q60, unless otherwise noted:** N13.9, Q60.0-Q60.6

Q60.0   **Renal agenesis, unilateral**   CC

Q60.1   **Renal agenesis, bilateral**   CC

Q60.2   **Renal agenesis, unspecified**   CC

Q60.3   **Renal hypoplasia, unilateral**   CC

Q60.4   **Renal hypoplasia, bilateral**   CC

Q60.5   **Renal hypoplasia, unspecified**   CC

Q60.6   **Potter's syndrome**   CC

√4ᵗʰ **Q61**   **Cystic kidney disease**
: **EXCLUDES 1**   *acquired cyst of kidney (N28.1)*
:   *Potter's syndrome (Q60.6)*

√5ᵗʰ **Q61.0**   **Congenital renal cyst**

     Q61.00   **Congenital renal cyst, unspecified**   CC
: Cyst of kidney NOS (congenital)
: **CC Excl:** N13.9, Q61.00, Q61.9

     Q61.01   **Congenital single renal cyst**   CC
: **CC Excl:** N13.9, Q61.01

     Q61.02   **Congenital multiple renal cysts**   CC
: **CC Excl:** N13.9, Q61.02, Q61.5-Q61.8

√6ᵗʰ **Q61.1**   **Polycystic kidney, infantile type**
: Polycystic kidney, autosomal recessive

     Q61.11   **Cystic dilatation of collecting ducts**   CC
: **CC Excl:** N13.9, Q61.11-Q61.3

     Q61.19   **Other polycystic kidney, infantile type**   CC
: **CC Excl:** See code: Q61.11

Q61.2   **Polycystic kidney, adult type**   CC
: Polycystic kidney, autosomal dominant
: **CC Excl:** See code: Q61.11

Q61.3   **Polycystic kidney, unspecified**   CC
: **CC Excl:** See code: Q61.11

Q61.4   **Renal dysplasia**   CC
: Multicystic dysplastic kidney
: Multicystic kidney (development)
: Multicystic kidney disease
: Multicystic renal dysplasia
: **EXCLUDES 1** *polycystic kidney disease (Q61.11-Q61.3)*
: **CC Excl:** N13.9, Q61.4

Q61.5   **Medullary cystic kidney**   CC
: Nephronopthisis
: Sponge kidney NOS
: **CC Excl:** See code: Q61.02

Q61.8   **Other cystic kidney diseases**   CC
: Fibrocystic kidney
: Fibrocystic renal degeneration or disease
: **CC Excl:** See code: Q61.02

Q61.9   **Cystic kidney disease, unspecified**   CC
: Meckel-Gruber syndrome
: **CC Excl:** See code: Q61.00

√4ᵗʰ **Q62**   **Congenital obstructive defects of renal pelvis and congenital malformations of ureter**

> **CC Excl: For CC codes in category Q62, unless otherwise noted:** N13.9, Q62.0-Q62.2, Q62.39

Q62.0   **Congenital hydronephrosis**   CC

√5ᵗʰ **Q62.1**   **Congenital occlusion of ureter**
: Atresia and stenosis of ureter

     Q62.10   **Congenital occlusion of ureter, unspecified**   CC

     Q62.11   **Congenital occlusion of ureteropelvic junction**   CC

     Q62.12   **Congenital occlusion of ureterovesical orifice**   CC

Q62.2   **Congenital megaureter**   CC
: Congenital dilatation of ureter

√5ᵗʰ **Q62.3**   **Other obstructive defects of renal pelvis and ureter**

     Q62.31   **Congenital ureterocele, orthotopic**   CC

     Q62.32   **Cecoureterocele**   CC
: Ectopic ureterocele

     Q62.39   **Other obstructive defects of renal pelvis and ureter**   CC
: Ureteropelvic junction obstruction NOS

Q62.4   **Agenesis of ureter**
: Congenital absence ureter

Q62.5   **Duplication of ureter**
: Accessory ureter
: Double ureter

√5ᵗʰ **Q62.6**   **Malposition of ureter**

     Q62.60   **Malposition of ureter, unspecified**

     Q62.61   **Deviation of ureter**

     Q62.62   **Displacement of ureter**

     Q62.63   **Anomalous implantation of ureter**
: Ectopia of ureter
: Ectopic ureter

     Q62.69   **Other malposition of ureter**

Q62.7   **Congenital vesico-uretero-renal reflux**

Q62.8   **Other congenital malformations of ureter**
: Anomaly of ureter NOS

√4ᵗʰ **Q63**   **Other congenital malformations of kidney**
: **EXCLUDES 1** *congenital nephrotic syndrome (N04.-)*

Q63.0   **Accessory kidney**

Q63.1   **Lobulated, fused and horseshoe kidney**

Q63.2   **Ectopic kidney**
: Congenital displaced kidney
: Malrotation of kidney

Q63.3   **Hyperplastic and giant kidney**
: Compensatory hypertrophy of kidney

Q63.8   **Other specified congenital malformations of kidney**
: Congenital renal calculi

Q63.9   **Congenital malformation of kidney, unspecified**

√4ᵗʰ **Q64**   **Other congenital malformations of urinary system**

Q64.0   **Epispadias**   ♂
: **EXCLUDES 1** *hypospadias (Q54.-)*

√5ᵗʰ **Q64.1**   **Exstrophy of urinary bladder**

> **CC Excl: For CC codes in subcategory Q64.1, unless otherwise noted:** N13.9, Q64.10-Q64.19, Q64.8-Q64.9

     Q64.10   **Exstrophy of urinary bladder, unspecified**   CC
: Ectopia vesicae

     Q64.11   **Supravesical fissure of urinary bladder**   CC

     Q64.12   **Cloacal extrophy of urinary bladder**   CC

     Q64.19   **Other exstrophy of urinary bladder**   CC
: Extroversion of bladder

Q64.2   **Congenital posterior urethral valves**   CC
: **CC Excl:** N13.9, Q64.2-Q64.39, Q64.8-Q64.9

√5ᵗʰ **Q64.3**   **Other atresia and stenosis of urethra and bladder neck**

> **CC Excl: For CC codes in subcategory Q64.3, unless otherwise noted:** See code: Q64.2

     Q64.31   **Congenital bladder neck obstruction**   CC
: Congenital obstruction of vesicourethral orifice

     Q64.32   **Congenital stricture of urethra**   CC

     Q64.33   **Congenital stricture of urinary meatus**   CC

     Q64.39   **Other atresia and stenosis of urethra and bladder neck**   CC
: Atresia and stenosis of urethra and bladder neck NOS

Q64.4   **Malformation of urachus**
: Cyst of urachus
: Patent urachus
: Prolapse of urachus

Q64.5   **Congenital absence of bladder and urethra**

Q64.6   **Congenital diverticulum of bladder**

√5ᵗʰ **Q64.7**   **Other and unspecified congenital malformations of bladder and urethra**
: **EXCLUDES 1** *congenital prolapse of bladder (mucosa) (Q79.4)*

     Q64.70   **Unspecified congenital malformation of bladder and urethra**
: Malformation of bladder or urethra NOS

     Q64.71   **Congenital prolapse of urethra**

     Q64.72   **Congenital prolapse of urinary meatus**

N Newborn: 0   P Pediatric: 0-17   M Maternity: 12-55   A Adult: 15-124   MCC Major CC Condition   PDxMCC PDx acts as own MCC   CC CC Condition   PDxCC PDx acts as own CC

866   ICD-10-CM 2016

Q64.73 Congenital urethrorectal fistula

Q64.74 Double urethra

Q64.75 Double urinary meatus

Q64.79 Other congenital malformations of bladder and urethra

Q64.8 Other specified congenital malformations of urinary system

Q64.9 Congenital malformation of urinary system, unspecified
Congenital anomaly NOS of urinary system
Congenital deformity NOS of urinary system

Congenital malformations and deformations of the musculoskeletal system (Q65-Q79)

✓4ᵗʰ **Q65** **Congenital deformities of hip**
    EXCLUDES1   clicking hip (R29.4)

✓5ᵗʰ **Q65.0** Congenital dislocation of hip, unilateral

    Q65.00 Congenital dislocation of unspecified hip, unilateral

    Q65.01 Congenital dislocation of right hip, unilateral

    Q65.02 Congenital dislocation of left hip, unilateral

Q65.1 Congenital dislocation of hip, bilateral

Q65.2 Congenital dislocation of hip, unspecified

✓5ᵗʰ **Q65.3** Congenital partial dislocation of hip, unilateral

    Q65.30 Congenital partial dislocation of unspecified hip, unilateral

    Q65.31 Congenital partial dislocation of right hip, unilateral

    Q65.32 Congenital partial dislocation of left hip, unilateral

Q65.4 Congenital partial dislocation of hip, bilateral

Q65.5 Congenital partial dislocation of hip, unspecified

Q65.6 Congenital unstable hip
Congenital dislocatable hip

✓5ᵗʰ **Q65.8** Other congenital deformities of hip

    Q65.81 Congenital coxa valga

    Q65.82 Congenital coxa vara

    Q65.89 Other specified congenital deformities of hip
Anteversion of femoral neck
Congenital acetabular dysplasia

Q65.9 Congenital deformity of hip, unspecified

✓4ᵗʰ **Q66** **Congenital deformities of feet**
    EXCLUDES1   reduction defects of feet (Q72.-)
                valgus deformities (acquired) (M21.0-)
                varus deformities (acquired) (M21.1-)

Q66.0 Congenital talipes equinovarus

Q66.1 Congenital talipes calcaneovarus

Q66.2 Congenital metatarsus (primus) varus

Q66.3 Other congenital varus deformities of feet
Hallux varus, congenital

Q66.4 Congenital talipes calcaneovalgus

✓5ᵗʰ **Q66.5** Congenital pes planus
Congenital flat foot
Congenital rigid flat foot
Congenital spastic (everted) flat foot
    EXCLUDES1   pes planus, acquired (M21.4)

    Q66.50 Congenital pes planus, unspecified foot

    Q66.51 Congenital pes planus, right foot

    Q66.52 Congenital pes planus, left foot

Q66.6 Other congenital valgus deformities of feet
Congenital metatarsus valgus

Q66.7 Congenital pes cavus

✓5ᵗʰ **Q66.8** Other congenital deformities of feet

    Q66.80 Congenital vertical talus deformity, unspecified foot

    Q66.81 Congenital vertical talus deformity, right foot

    Q66.82 Congenital vertical talus deformity, left foot

    Q66.89 Other specified congenital deformities of feet
Congenital asymmetric talipes
Congenital clubfoot NOS
Congenital talipes NOS
Congenital tarsal coalition
Hammer toe, congenital

Q66.9 Congenital deformity of feet, unspecified

✓4ᵗʰ **Q67** **Congenital musculoskeletal deformities of head, face, spine and chest**
    EXCLUDES1   congenital malformation syndromes classified to Q87-
                Potter's syndrome (Q60.6)

Q67.0 Congenital facial asymmetry

Q67.1 Congenital compression facies

Q67.2 Dolichocephaly

Q67.3 Plagiocephaly

Q67.4 Other congenital deformities of skull, face and jaw
Congenital depressions in skull
Congenital hemifacial atrophy or hypertrophy
Deviation of nasal septum, congenital
Squashed or bent nose, congenital
    EXCLUDES1   dentofacial anomalies [including malocclusion] (M26.-)
                syphilitic saddle nose (A50.5)

Q67.5 Congenital deformity of spine   [CC]
Congenital postural scoliosis
Congenital scoliosis NOS
    EXCLUDES1   infantile idiopathic scoliosis (M41.0)
                scoliosis due to congenital bony malformation (Q76.3)
    AHA: 2014, 4Q, 26
    CC Excl: Q67.5, Q76.3, Q76.425-Q76.429

Q67.6 Pectus excavatum
Congenital funnel chest

Q67.7 Pectus carinatum
Congenital pigeon chest

Q67.8 Other congenital deformities of chest   [CC]
Congenital deformity of chest wall NOS
    CC Excl: Q67.6-Q67.8, Q68.1, Q74.3

✓4ᵗʰ **Q68** **Other congenital musculoskeletal deformities**
    EXCLUDES1   reduction defects of limb(s) (Q71-Q73)
    EXCLUDES2   congenital myotonic chondrodystrophy (G71.13)

Q68.0 Congenital deformity of sternocleidomastoid muscle
Congenital contracture of sternocleidomastoid (muscle)
Congenital (sternomastoid) torticollis
Sternomastoid tumor (congenital)

Q68.1 Congenital deformity of finger(s) and hand   [CC]
Congenital clubfinger
Spade-like hand (congenital)
    CC Excl: See code: Q67.8

Q68.2 Congenital deformity of knee
Congenital dislocation of knee   Congenital genu recurvatum

Q68.3 Congenital bowing of femur
    EXCLUDES1   anteversion of femur (neck) (Q65.89)

Q68.4 Congenital bowing of tibia and fibula

Q68.5 Congenital bowing of long bones of leg, unspecified

Q68.6 Discoid meniscus

Q68.8 Other specified congenital musculoskeletal deformities
Congenital deformity of clavicle
Congenital deformity of elbow
Congenital deformity of forearm
Congenital deformity of scapula
Congenital deformity of wrist
Congenital dislocation of elbow
Congenital dislocation of shoulder
Congenital dislocation of wrist

✓4ᵗʰ **Q69** **Polydactyly**

Q69.0 Accessory finger(s)

Q69.1 Accessory thumb(s)

Q69.2 Accessory toe(s)
Accessory hallux

Q69.9 Polydactyly, unspecified
Supernumerary digit(s) NOS

✓4ᵗʰ **Q70** **Syndactyly**

✓5ᵗʰ **Q70.0** Fused fingers
Complex syndactyly of fingers with synostosis

    Q70.00 Fused fingers, unspecified hand

    Q70.01 Fused fingers, right hand

    Q70.02 Fused fingers, left hand

    Q70.03 Fused fingers, bilateral

✓5ᵗʰ **Q70.1** Webbed fingers
Simple syndactyly of fingers without synostosis

    Q70.10 Webbed fingers, unspecified hand

    Q70.11 Webbed fingers, right hand

    Q70.12 Webbed fingers, left hand

    Q70.13 Webbed fingers, bilateral

✓5ᵗʰ **Q70.2** Fused toes
Complex syndactyly of toes with synostosis

    Q70.20 Fused toes, unspecified foot

    Q70.21 Fused toes, right foot

    Q70.22 Fused toes, left foot

☑ Additional Character Required   ✓x7ᵗʰ Placeholder Alert   Unacceptable PDx   Manifestation   Hospital Acquired Condition   EXCLUDES1 Not Coded Here   EXCLUDES2 Not Included Here

ICD-10-CM 2016   867

Q70.23 Fused toes, bilateral

✓5ᵗʰ **Q70.3 Webbed toes**
Simple syndactyly of toes without synostosis
Q70.30 Webbed toes, unspecified **foot**
Q70.31 Webbed toes, right **foot**
Q70.32 Webbed toes, left **foot**
Q70.33 Webbed toes, bilateral

Q70.4 Polysyndactyly, unspecified
EXCLUDES 1 specified syndactyly of hand and feet—code to specified conditions (Q70.0-Q70.3-)

Q70.9 Syndactyly, unspecified
Symphalangy NOS

✓4ᵗʰ **Q71 Reduction defects of** upper limb
✓5ᵗʰ **Q71.0 Congenital** complete absence **of upper limb**
Q71.00 Congenital complete absence of unspecified **upper limb**
Q71.01 Congenital complete absence of right **upper limb**
Q71.02 Congenital complete absence of left **upper limb**
Q71.03 Congenital complete absence of upper limb, bilateral

✓5ᵗʰ **Q71.1 Congenital** absence of upper arm and forearm with hand present
Q71.10 Congenital absence of unspecified **upper arm and forearm with hand present**
Q71.11 Congenital absence of right **upper arm and forearm with hand present**
Q71.12 Congenital absence of left **upper arm and forearm with hand present**
Q71.13 Congenital absence of upper arm and forearm with hand present, bilateral

✓5ᵗʰ **Q71.2 Congenital** absence of both forearm and hand
Q71.20 Congenital absence of both forearm and hand, unspecified **upper limb**
Q71.21 Congenital absence of both forearm and hand, right **upper limb**
Q71.22 Congenital absence of both forearm and hand, left **upper limb**
Q71.23 Congenital absence of both forearm and hand, bilateral

✓5ᵗʰ **Q71.3 Congenital** absence of hand and finger
Q71.30 Congenital absence of unspecified **hand and finger**
Q71.31 Congenital absence of right **hand and finger**
Q71.32 Congenital absence of left **hand and finger**
Q71.33 Congenital absence of hand and finger, bilateral

✓5ᵗʰ **Q71.4 Longitudinal reduction defect of** radius
Clubhand (congenital)
Radial clubhand
Q71.40 Longitudinal reduction defect of unspecified **radius**
Q71.41 Longitudinal reduction defect of right **radius**
Q71.42 Longitudinal reduction defect of left **radius**
Q71.43 Longitudinal reduction defect of radius, bilateral

✓5ᵗʰ **Q71.5 Longitudinal reduction defect of** ulna
Q71.50 Longitudinal reduction defect of unspecified **ulna**
Q71.51 Longitudinal reduction defect of right **ulna**
Q71.52 Longitudinal reduction defect of left **ulna**
Q71.53 Longitudinal reduction defect of ulna, bilateral

✓5ᵗʰ **Q71.6 Lobster-claw hand**
Q71.60 Lobster-claw hand, unspecified **hand**
Q71.61 Lobster-claw right **hand**
Q71.62 Lobster-claw left **hand**
Q71.63 Lobster-claw hand, bilateral

✓5ᵗʰ **Q71.8 Other reduction defects of** upper limb
✓6ᵗʰ **Q71.81 Congenital** shortening **of upper limb**
Q71.811 Congenital shortening of right **upper limb**
Q71.812 Congenital shortening of left **upper limb**
Q71.813 Congenital shortening of upper limb, bilateral
Q71.819 Congenital shortening of unspecified **upper limb**
✓6ᵗʰ **Q71.89 Other reduction defects of upper limb**
Q71.891 Other reduction defects of right **upper limb**
Q71.892 Other reduction defects of left **upper limb**

Q71.893 Other reduction defects of upper limb, bilateral
Q71.899 Other reduction defects of unspecified **upper limb**

✓5ᵗʰ **Q71.9 Unspecified** reduction defect of upper limb
Q71.90 Unspecified reduction defect of unspecified **upper limb**
Q71.91 Unspecified reduction defect of right **upper limb**
Q71.92 Unspecified reduction defect of left **upper limb**
Q71.93 Unspecified reduction defect of upper limb, bilateral

✓4ᵗʰ **Q72 Reduction defects of** lower limb
✓5ᵗʰ **Q72.0 Congenital** complete absence **of lower limb**
Q72.00 Congenital complete absence of unspecified **lower limb**
Q72.01 Congenital complete absence of right **lower limb**
Q72.02 Congenital complete absence of left **lower limb**
Q72.03 Congenital complete absence of lower limb, bilateral

✓5ᵗʰ **Q72.1 Congenital** absence of thigh and lower leg with foot present
Q72.10 Congenital absence of unspecified **thigh and lower leg with foot present**
Q72.11 Congenital absence of right **thigh and lower leg with foot present**
Q72.12 Congenital absence of left **thigh and lower leg with foot present**
Q72.13 Congenital absence of thigh and lower leg with foot present, bilateral

✓5ᵗʰ **Q72.2 Congenital** absence of both lower leg and foot
Q72.20 Congenital absence of both lower leg and foot, unspecified **lower limb**
Q72.21 Congenital absence of both lower leg and foot, right **lower limb**
Q72.22 Congenital absence of both lower leg and foot, left **lower limb**
Q72.23 Congenital absence of both lower leg and foot, bilateral

✓5ᵗʰ **Q72.3 Congenital** absence of foot and toe(s)
Q72.30 Congenital absence of unspecified **foot and toe(s)**
Q72.31 Congenital absence of right **foot and toe(s)**
Q72.32 Congenital absence of left **foot and toe(s)**
Q72.33 Congenital absence of foot and toe(s), bilateral

✓5ᵗʰ **Q72.4 Longitudinal reduction defect of** femur
Proximal femoral focal deficiency
Q72.40 Longitudinal reduction defect of unspecified **femur**
Q72.41 Longitudinal reduction defect of right **femur**
Q72.42 Longitudinal reduction defect of left **femur**
Q72.43 Longitudinal reduction defect of femur, bilateral

✓5ᵗʰ **Q72.5 Longitudinal reduction defect of** tibia
Q72.50 Longitudinal reduction defect of unspecified **tibia**
Q72.51 Longitudinal reduction defect of right **tibia**
Q72.52 Longitudinal reduction defect of left **tibia**
Q72.53 Longitudinal reduction defect of tibia, bilateral

✓5ᵗʰ **Q72.6 Longitudinal reduction defect of** fibula
Q72.60 Longitudinal reduction defect of unspecified **fibula**
Q72.61 Longitudinal reduction defect of right **fibula**
Q72.62 Longitudinal reduction defect of left **fibula**
Q72.63 Longitudinal reduction defect of fibula, bilateral

✓5ᵗʰ **Q72.7 Split foot**
Q72.70 Split foot, unspecified **lower limb**
Q72.71 Split foot, right **lower limb**
Q72.72 Split foot, left **lower limb**
Q72.73 Split foot, bilateral

✓5ᵗʰ **Q72.8 Other reduction defects of** lower limb
✓6ᵗʰ **Q72.81 Congenital** shortening **of lower limb**
Q72.811 Congenital shortening of right **lower limb**
Q72.812 Congenital shortening of left **lower limb**
Q72.813 Congenital shortening of lower limb, bilateral
Q72.819 Congenital shortening of unspecified **lower limb**
✓6ᵗʰ **Q72.89 Other reduction defects of lower limb**
Q72.891 Other reduction defects of right **lower limb**

Q72.892   **Other reduction defects of** left **lower limb**

Q72.893   **Other reduction defects of lower limb,** bilateral

Q72.899   **Other reduction defects of** unspecified **lower limb**

✓5ᵗʰ   **Q72.9**   Unspecified **reduction defect of lower limb**

Q72.90   **Unspecified reduction defect of** unspecified **lower limb**

Q72.91   **Unspecified reduction defect of** right **lower limb**

Q72.92   **Unspecified reduction defect of** left **lower limb**

Q72.93   **Unspecified reduction defect of lower limb,** bilateral

✓4ᵗʰ   **Q73**   **Reduction defects of** unspecified **limb**

Q73.0   **Congenital** absence **of unspecified limb(s)**
Amelia NOS

Q73.1   Phocomelia, **unspecified limb(s)**
Phocomelia NOS

Q73.8   Other **reduction defects of unspecified limb(s)**
Longitudinal reduction deformity of unspecified limb(s)
Ectromelia of limb NOS
Hemimelia of limb NOS
Reduction defect of limb NOS

✓4ᵗʰ   **Q74**   Other **congenital malformations of limb(s)**
EXCLUDES 1   *polydactyly (Q69.-)*
reduction defect of limb (Q71-Q73)
syndactyly (Q70.-)

Q74.0   **Other congenital malformations of** upper limb(s), **including shoulder girdle**
Accessory carpal bones
Cleidocranial dysostosis
Congenital pseudarthrosis of clavicle
Macrodactylia (fingers)
Madelung's deformity
Radioulnar synostosis
Sprengel's deformity
Triphalangeal thumb

Q74.1   **Congenital malformation of** knee
Congenital absence of patella
Congenital dislocation of patella
Congenital genu valgum
Congenital genu varum
Rudimentary patella
EXCLUDES 1   *congenital dislocation of knee (Q68.2)*
congenital genu recurvatum (Q68.2)
nail patella syndrome (Q87.2)

Q74.2   **Other congenital malformations of** lower limb(s), **including pelvic girdle**
Congenital fusion of sacroiliac joint
Congenital malformation of ankle joint
Congenital malformation of sacroiliac joint
EXCLUDES 1   *anteversion of femur (neck) (Q65.89)*

Q74.3   **Arthrogryposis multiplex congenita**   CC
CC Excl: Q67.5, Q76.3, Q76.425-Q76.429

Q74.8   **Other** specified **congenital malformations of limb(s)**

Q74.9   Unspecified **congenital malformation of limb(s)**
Congenital anomaly of limb(s) NOS

✓4ᵗʰ   **Q75**   Other **congenital malformations of** skull and face bones
EXCLUDES 1   *congenital malformation of face NOS (Q18.-)*
congenital malformation syndromes classified to Q87.-
dentofacial anomalies [including malocclusion] (M26.-)
musculoskeletal deformities of head and face (Q67.0-Q67.4)
skull defects associated with congenital anomalies of brain such as:
anencephaly (Q00.0)
encephalocele (Q01.-)
hydrocephalus (Q03.-)
microcephaly (Q02)

Q75.0   **Craniosynostosis**
Acrocephaly
Imperfect fusion of skull
Oxycephaly
Trigonocephaly

Q75.1   **Craniofacial dysostosis**
Crouzon's disease

Q75.2   **Hypertelorism**

Q75.3   **Macrocephaly**

Q75.4   **Mandibulofacial dysostosis**
Franceschetti syndrome
Treacher Collins syndrome

Q75.5   **Oculomandibular dysostosis**

Q75.8   **Other specified congenital malformations of skull and face bones**
Absence of skull bone, congenital
Congenital deformity of forehead
Platybasia

Q75.9   **Congenital malformation of skull and face bones, unspecified**
Congenital anomaly of face bones NOS
Congenital anomaly of skull NOS

✓4ᵗʰ   **Q76**   **Congenital malformations of** spine and bony thorax
EXCLUDES 1   *congenital musculoskeletal deformities of spine and chest (Q67.5-Q67.8)*

Q76.0   **Spina bifida occulta**
EXCLUDES 1   *meningocele (spinal) (Q05.-)*
spina bifida (aperta) (cystica) (Q05.-)

Q76.1   **Klippel-Feil syndrome**
Cervical fusion syndrome

Q76.2   **Congenital spondylolisthesis**
Congenital spondylolysis
EXCLUDES 1   *spondylolisthesis (acquired) (M43.1-)*
spondylolysis (acquired) (M43.0-)

Q76.3   **Congenital scoliosis due to congenital bony malformation**   CC
Hemivertebra fusion or failure of segmentation with scoliosis
CC Excl: See code: Q67.5

✓5ᵗʰ   **Q76.4**   **Other congenital malformations of spine, not associated with scoliosis**

> CC Excl: For CC codes in subcategory Q76.4, unless otherwise noted: Q67.5, Q76.3, Q76.425-Q76.429

✓6ᵗʰ   **Q76.41**   **Congenital** kyphosis

Q76.411   **Congenital kyphosis,** occipito-atlanto-axial **region**

Q76.412   **Congenital kyphosis,** cervical **region**

Q76.413   **Congenital kyphosis,** cervicothoracic **region**

Q76.414   **Congenital kyphosis,** thoracic **region**

Q76.415   **Congenital kyphosis,** thoracolumbar **region**

Q76.419   **Congenital kyphosis,** unspecified **region**

✓6ᵗʰ   **Q76.42**   **Congenital** lordosis

Q76.425   **Congenital lordosis,** thoracolumbar **region**   CC

Q76.426   **Congenital lordosis,** lumbar **region**   CC

Q76.427   **Congenital lordosis,** lumbosacral **region**   CC

Q76.428   **Congenital lordosis,** sacral and sacrococcygeal **region**   CC

Q76.429   **Congenital lordosis,** unspecified **region**   CC

Q76.49   Other **congenital malformations of spine, not associated with scoliosis**
Congenital absence of vertebra NOS
Congenital fusion of spine NOS
Congenital malformation of lumbosacral (joint) (region) NOS
Congenital malformation of spine NOS
Hemivertebra NOS
Malformation of spine NOS
Platyspondylisis NOS
Supernumerary vertebra NOS

Q76.5   Cervical rib
Supernumerary rib in cervical region

Q76.6   Other **congenital malformations of** ribs   CC
Accessory rib
Congenital absence of rib
Congenital fusion of ribs
Congenital malformation of ribs NOS
EXCLUDES 1   *short rib syndrome (Q77.2)*
CC Excl: Q76.5-Q76.9, Q77.2

Q76.7   **Congenital malformation of** sternum   CC
Congenital absence of sternum
Sternum bifidum
CC Excl: See code: Q76.6

Q76.8   Other **congenital malformations of** bony thorax   CC
CC Excl: See code: Q76.6

Q76.9   **Congenital malformation of** bony thorax, unspecified   CC
CC Excl: See code: Q76.6b

✓ Additional Character Required   ✓x7ᵗʰ Placeholder Alert   Unacceptable PDx   Manifestation   Hospital Acquired Condition   *EXCLUDES 1* Not Coded Here   *EXCLUDES 2* Not Included Here

Q77 Osteochondrodysplasia with defects of growth of tubular bones and spine

EXCLUDES 1   mucopolysaccharidosis (E76.0-E76.3)
EXCLUDES 2   congenital myotonic chondrodystrophy (G71.13)

Q77.0 Achondrogenesis
Hypochondrogenesis

Q77.1 Thanatophoric short stature

Q77.2 Short rib syndrome `CC`
Asphyxiating thoracic dysplasia [Jeune]
CC Excl: Q76.5-Q76.9, Q77.2

Q77.3 Chondrodysplasia punctata
EXCLUDES 1   Rhizomelic chondrodysplasia punctata (E71.43)

Q77.4 Achondroplasia
Hypochondroplasia
Osteosclerosis congenita

Q77.5 Diastrophic dysplasia

Q77.6 Chondroectodermal dysplasia
Ellis-van Creveld syndrome

Q77.7 Spondyloepiphyseal dysplasia

Q77.8 Other osteochondrodysplasia with defects of growth of tubular bones and spine

Q77.9 Osteochondrodysplasia with defects of growth of tubular bones and spine, unspecified

☑4ᵗʰ Q78 Other osteochondrodysplasias
EXCLUDES 2   congenital myotonic chondrodystrophy (G71.13)

Q78.0 Osteogenesis imperfecta `CC`
Fragilitas ossium
Osteopsathyrosis
CC Excl: Q77.3, Q77.6, Q78.0-Q78.3, Q78.5-Q78.9

Q78.1 Polyostotic fibrous dysplasia
Albright(-McCune)(-Sternberg) syndrome

Q78.2 Osteopetrosis `CC`
Albers-Schönberg syndrome
Osteosclerosis NOS
CC Excl: See code: Q78.0

Q78.3 Progressive diaphyseal dysplasia
Camurati-Engelmann syndrome

Q78.4 Enchondromatosis
Maffucci's syndrome
Ollier's disease

Q78.5 Metaphyseal dysplasia
Pyle's syndrome

Q78.6 Multiple congenital exostoses
Diaphyseal aclasis

Q78.8 Other specified osteochondrodysplasias
Osteopoikilosis

Q78.9 Osteochondrodysplasia, unspecified
Chondrodystrophy NOS
Osteodystrophy NOS

☑4ᵗʰ Q79 Congenital malformations of musculoskeletal system, not elsewhere classified
EXCLUDES 2   congenital (sternomastoid) torticollis (Q68.0)

CC Excl: For CC/MCC codes in category Q79, unless otherwise noted: Q79.2-Q79.59

Q79.0 Congenital diaphragmatic hernia `MCC`
EXCLUDES 1   congenital hiatus hernia (Q40.1)
CC Excl: Q40.1-Q79.1

Q79.1 Other congenital malformations of diaphragm `MCC`
Absence of diaphragm
Congenital malformation of diaphragm NOS
Eventration of diaphragm
CC Excl: See code: Q79.0

Q79.2 Exomphalos `MCC`
Omphalocele
EXCLUDES 1   umbilical hernia (K42.-)

Q79.3 Gastroschisis `MCC`

Q79.4 Prune belly syndrome `MCC`
Congenital prolapse of bladder mucosa
Eagle-Barrett syndrome

☑5ᵗʰ Q79.5 Other congenital malformations of abdominal wall
EXCLUDES 1   umbilical hernia (K42.-)

Q79.51 Congenital hernia of bladder `MCC`

Q79.59 Other congenital malformations of abdominal wall `MCC`

Q79.6 Ehlers-Danlos syndrome `CC`
CC Excl: Q79.6

Q79.8 Other congenital malformations of musculoskeletal system
Absence of muscle
Absence of tendon
Accessory muscle
Amyotrophia congenita
Congenital constricting bands
Congenital shortening of tendon
Poland syndrome

Q79.9 Congenital malformation of musculoskeletal system, unspecified
Congenital anomaly of musculoskeletal system NOS
Congenital deformity of musculoskeletal system NOS

Other congenital malformations (Q80-Q89)

☑4ᵗʰ Q80 Congenital ichthyosis
EXCLUDES 1   Refsum's disease (G60.1)

Q80.0 Ichthyosis vulgaris

Q80.1 X-linked ichthyosis

Q80.2 Lamellar ichthyosis
Collodion baby

Q80.3 Congenital bullous ichthyosiform erythroderma

Q80.4 Harlequin fetus

Q80.8 Other congenital ichthyosis

Q80.9 Congenital ichthyosis, unspecified

☑4ᵗʰ Q81 Epidermolysis bullosa

Q81.0 Epidermolysis bullosa simplex
EXCLUDES 1   Cockayne's syndrome (Q87.1)

Q81.1 Epidermolysis bullosa letalis
Herlitz' syndrome

Q81.2 Epidermolysis bullosa dystrophica

Q81.8 Other epidermolysis bullosa

Q81.9 Epidermolysis bullosa, unspecified

☑4ᵗʰ Q82 Other congenital malformations of skin
EXCLUDES 1   acrodermatitis enteropathica (E83.2)
congenital erythropoietic porphyria (E80.0)
pilonidal cyst or sinus (L05.-)
Sturge-Weber (-Dimitri) syndrome (Q85.8)

Q82.0 Hereditary lymphedema

Q82.1 Xeroderma pigmentosum

Q82.2 Mastocytosis
Urticaria pigmentosa
EXCLUDES 1   malignant mastocytosis (C96.2)

Q82.3 Incontinentia pigmenti

Q82.4 Ectodermal dysplasia (anhidrotic)
EXCLUDES 1   Ellis-van Creveld syndrome (Q77.6)

Q82.5 Congenital non-neoplastic nevus
Birthmark NOS
Flammeus Nevus
Portwine Nevus
Sanguineous Nevus
Strawberry Nevus
Vascular Nevus NOS
Verrucous Nevus
EXCLUDES 2   araneus nevus (I78.1)
café au lait spots (L81.3)
lentigo (L81.4)
melanocytic nevus (D22.-)
nevus NOS (D22.-)
pigmented nevus (D22.-)
spider nevus (I78.1)
stellar nevus (I78.1)

Q82.8 Other specified congenital malformations of skin
Abnormal palmar creases
Accessory skin tags
Benign familial pemphigus [Hailey-Hailey]
Congenital poikiloderma
Cutis laxa (hyperelastica)
Dermatoglyphic anomalies
Inherited keratosis palmaris et plantaris
Keratosis follicularis [Darier-White]
EXCLUDES 1   Ehlers-Danlos syndrome (Q79.6)

Q82.9 Congenital malformation of skin, unspecified

☑4ᵗʰ Q83 Congenital malformations of breast
EXCLUDES 2   absence of pectoral muscle (Q79.8)
hypoplasia of breast (N64.82)
micromastia (N64.82)

Q83.0 Congenital absence of breast with absent nipple

ℕ Newborn: 0   ℙ Pediatric: 0-17   Ⅿ Maternity: 12-55   Ⓐ Adult: 15-124   `MCC` Major CC Condition   `PDxMCC` PDx acts as own MCC   `CC` CC Condition   `PDxCC` PDx acts as own CC

870   ICD-10-CM 2016

Q83.1 Accessory breast
Supernumerary breast

Q83.2 Absent nipple

Q83.3 Accessory nipple
Supernumerary nipple

Q83.8 Other congenital malformations of breast

Q83.9 Congenital malformation of breast, unspecified

✓4ᵗʰ **Q84 Other congenital malformations of integument**

Q84.0 Congenital alopecia
Congenital atrichosis

Q84.1 Congenital morphological disturbances of hair, not elsewhere classified
Beaded hair
Monilethrix
Pili annulati
EXCLUDES 1 Menkes' kinky hair syndrome (E83.0)

Q84.2 Other congenital malformations of hair
Congenital hypertrichosis
Congenital malformation of hair NOS
Persistent lanugo

Q84.3 Anonychia
EXCLUDES 1 nail patella syndrome (Q87.2)

Q84.4 Congenital leukonychia

Q84.5 Enlarged and hypertrophic nails
Congenital onychauxis
Pachyonychia

Q84.6 Other congenital malformations of nails
Congenital clubnail
Congenital koilonychia
Congenital malformation of nail NOS

Q84.8 Other specified congenital malformations of integument
Aplasia cutis congenita

Q84.9 Congenital malformation of integument, unspecified
Congenital anomaly of integument NOS
Congenital deformity of integument NOS

✓4ᵗʰ **Q85 Phakomatoses, not elsewhere classified**
EXCLUDES 1 ataxia telangiectasia [Louis-Bar] (G11.3)
familial dysautonomia [Riley-Day] (G90.1)

✓5ᵗʰ **Q85.0 Neurofibromatosis (nonmalignant)**

Q85.00 Neurofibromatosis, unspecified

Q85.01 Neurofibromatosis, type 1
Von Recklinghausen disease

Q85.02 Neurofibromatosis, type 2
Acoustic neurofibromatosis

Q85.03 Schwannomatosis

Q85.09 Other neurofibromatosis

Q85.1 Tuberous sclerosis   CC
Bourneville's disease
Epiloia
CC Excl: Q85.1-Q85.9, Q89.7, Q89.9

Q85.8 Other phakomatoses, not elsewhere classified   CC
Peutz-Jeghers Syndrome
Sturge-Weber(-Dimitri) syndrome
von Hippel-Lindau syndrome
EXCLUDES 1 Meckel-Gruber syndrome (Q61.9)
CC Excl: Q85.8-Q85.9, Q89.9

Q85.9 Phakomatosis, unspecified   CC
Hamartosis NOS
CC Excl: See code: Q85.8

✓4ᵗʰ **Q86 Congenital malformation syndromes due to known exogenous causes, not elsewhere classified**
EXCLUDES 2 iodine-deficiency-related hypothyroidism (E00-E02)
nonteratogenic effects of substances transmitted via placenta or breast milk (P04.-)

Q86.0 Fetal alcohol syndrome (dysmorphic)

Q86.1 Fetal hydantoin syndrome   N
Meadow's syndrome

Q86.2 Dysmorphism due to warfarin

Q86.8 Other congenital malformation syndromes due to known exogenous causes

✓4ᵗʰ **Q87 Other specified congenital malformation syndromes affecting multiple systems**
Use additional code(s) to identify all associated manifestations

Q87.0 Congenital malformation syndromes predominantly affecting facial appearance
Acrocephalopolysyndactyly
Acrocephalosyndactyly [Apert]
Cryptophthalmos syndrome
Cyclopia
Goldenhar syndrome
Moebius syndrome
Oro-facial-digital syndrome
Robin syndrome
Whistling face

Q87.1 Congenital malformation syndromes predominantly associated with short stature   CC
Aarskog syndrome
Cockayne syndrome
De Lange syndrome
Dubowitz syndrome
Noonan syndrome
Prader-Willi syndrome
Robinow-Silverman-Smith syndrome
Russell-Silver syndrome
Seckel syndrome
EXCLUDES 1 Ellis-van Creveld syndrome (Q77.6)
Smith-Lemli-Opitz syndrome (E78.72)
CC Excl: E78.71-E78.72, Q85.8-Q85.9, Q87.1-Q87.89, Q89.7-Q89.9, Q99.2

Q87.2 Congenital malformation syndromes predominantly involving limbs   CC
Holt-Oram syndrome
Klippel-Trenaunay-Weber syndrome
Nail patella syndrome
Rubinstein-Taybi syndrome
Sirenomelia syndrome
Thrombocytopenia with absent radius [TAR] syndrome
VATER syndrome
CC Excl: E78.71-E78.72, Q87.1-Q87.89, Q89.8, Q99.2

Q87.3 Congenital malformation syndromes involving early overgrowth   CC
Beckwith-Wiedemann syndrome
Sotos syndrome
Weaver syndrome
CC Excl: See code: Q87.2

✓5ᵗʰ **Q87.4 Marfan's syndrome**

CC Excl: For CC codes in subcategory Q87.4, unless otherwise noted: See code: Q87.1

Q87.40 Marfan's syndrome, unspecified   CC

✓6ᵗʰ **Q87.41 Marfan's syndrome with cardiovascular manifestations**

Q87.410 Marfan's syndrome with aortic dilation   CC

Q87.418 Marfan's syndrome with other cardiovascular manifestations   CC

Q87.42 Marfan's syndrome with ocular manifestations   CC

Q87.43 Marfan's syndrome with skeletal manifestation   CC

Q87.5 Other congenital malformation syndromes with other skeletal changes
CC Excl: See code: Q87.2

✓5ᵗʰ **Q87.8 Other specified congenital malformation syndromes, not elsewhere classified**
EXCLUDES 1 Zellweger syndrome (E71.510)

Q87.81 Alport syndrome   CC
Use additional code to identify stage of chronic kidney disease (N18.1-N18.6)
CC Excl: See code: Q87.2

Q87.89 Other specified congenital malformation syndromes, not elsewhere classified   CC
Laurence-Moon (-Bardet)-Biedl syndrome
CC Excl: See code: Q87.2

✓4ᵗʰ **Q89 Other congenital malformations, not elsewhere classified**

✓5ᵗʰ **Q89.0 Congenital absence and malformations of spleen**
EXCLUDES 1 isomerism of atrial appendages (with asplenia or polysplenia) (Q20.6)

Q89.01 Asplenia (congenital)   CC
CC Excl: Q89.01-Q89.09, Q89.9

Q89.09 Congenital malformations of spleen   CC
Congenital splenomegaly
CC Excl: See code: Q89.01

☑ Additional Character Required   ✓7ᵗʰ Placeholder Alert   Unacceptable PDx   Manifestation   Hospital Acquired Condition   EXCLUDES 1 Not Coded Here   EXCLUDES 2 Not Included Here

Q89.1 Congenital malformations of adrenal gland
> EXCLUDES 1 adrenogenital disorders (E25.-)
> congenital adrenal hyperplasia (E25.0)

Q89.2 Congenital malformations of other endocrine glands
Congenital malformation of parathyroid or thyroid gland
Persistent thyroglossal duct
Thyroglossal cyst
> EXCLUDES 1 congenital goiter (E03.0)
> congenital hypothyroidism (E03.1)

Q89.3 Situs inversus   CC
Dextrocardia with situs inversus
Mirror-image atrial arrangement with situs inversus
Situs inversus or transversus abdominalis
Situs inversus or transversus thoracis
Transposition of abdominal viscera
Transposition of thoracic viscera
> EXCLUDES 1 dextrocardia NOS (Q24.0)

CC Excl: Q89.3, Q89.7, Q89.9

Q89.4 Conjoined twins   MCC
Craniopagus
Dicephaly
Pygopagus
Thoracopagus
CC Excl: Q89.4-Q89.7, Q89.9

Q89.7 Multiple congenital malformations, not elsewhere classified   CC
Multiple congenital anomalies NOS
Multiple congenital deformities NOS
> EXCLUDES 1 congenital malformation syndromes affecting multiple systems (Q87.-)

CC Excl: See code: Q89.3

Q89.8 Other specified congenital malformations   CC
Use additional code(s) to identify all associated manifestations
CC Excl: E78.71-E78.72, Q87.1-Q87.89, Q89.8, Q99.2

Q89.9 Congenital malformation, unspecified
Congenital anomaly NOS
Congenital deformity NOS

Chromosomal abnormalities, not elsewhere classified (Q90-Q99)
> EXCLUDES 2 mitochondrial metabolic disorders (E88.4-)

✓4ᵗʰ Q90 Down syndrome
Use additional code(s) to identify any associated physical conditions and degree of intellectual disabilities (F70-F79)

Q90.0 Trisomy 21, nonmosaicism (meiotic nondisjunction)

Q90.1 Trisomy 21, mosaicism (mitotic nondisjunction)

Q90.2 Trisomy 21, translocation

Q90.9 Down syndrome, unspecified
Trisomy 21 NOS

✓4ᵗʰ Q91 Trisomy 18 and Trisomy 13

> CC Excl: For CC codes in category Q91, unless otherwise noted: Q90.0-Q99.1, Q99.8-Q99.9

Q91.0 Trisomy 18, nonmosaicism (meiotic nondisjunction)   CC

Q91.1 Trisomy 18, mosaicism (mitotic nondisjunction)   CC

Q91.2 Trisomy 18, translocation   CC

Q91.3 Trisomy 18, unspecified   CC

Q91.4 Trisomy 13, nonmosaicism (meiotic nondisjunction)   CC

Q91.5 Trisomy 13, mosaicism (mitotic nondisjunction)   CC

Q91.6 Trisomy 13, translocation   CC

Q91.7 Trisomy 13, unspecified   CC

✓4ᵗʰ Q92 Other trisomies and partial trisomies of the autosomes, not elsewhere classified
> INCLUDES unbalanced translocations and insertions
> EXCLUDES 1 trisomies of chromosomes 13, 18, 21 (Q90-Q91)

Q92.0 Whole chromosome trisomy, nonmosaicism (meiotic nondisjunction)

Q92.1 Whole chromosome trisomy, mosaicism (mitotic nondisjunction)

Q92.2 Partial trisomy
Less than whole arm duplicated
Whole arm or more duplicated
> EXCLUDES 1 partial trisomy due to unbalanced translocation (Q92.5)

Q92.5 Duplications with other complex rearrangements
Partial trisomy due to unbalanced translocations
Code also any associated deletions due to unbalanced translocations, inversions and insertions (Q93.7)

✓5ᵗʰ Q92.6 Marker chromosomes
Trisomies due to dicentrics
Trisomies due to extra rings
Trisomies due to isochromosomes
Individual with marker heterochromatin

Q92.61 Marker chromosomes in normal individual

Q92.62 Marker chromosomes in abnormal individual

Q92.7 Triploidy and polyploidy

Q92.8 Other specified trisomies and partial trisomies of autosomes
Duplications identified by fluorescence in situ hybridization (FISH)
Duplications identified by in situ hybridization (ISH)
Duplications seen only at prometaphase

Q92.9 Trisomy and partial trisomy of autosomes, unspecified

✓4ᵗʰ Q93 Monosomies and deletions from the autosomes, not elsewhere classified

> CC Excl: For CC/MCC codes in category Q93, unless otherwise noted: Q90.0-Q93.2, Q93.4, Q93.81-Q93.88, Q95.0-Q99.1, Q99.8-Q99.9

Q93.0 Whole chromosome monosomy, nonmosaicism (meiotic nondisjunction)

Q93.1 Whole chromosome monosomy, mosaicism (mitotic nondisjunction)

Q93.2 Chromosome replaced with ring, dicentric or isochromosome

Q93.3 Deletion of short arm of chromosome 4   CC
Wolff-Hirschorn syndrome

Q93.4 Deletion of short arm of chromosome 5   CC
Cri-du-chat syndrome
CC Excl: Q90.0-Q93.3, Q93.5-Q99.1, Q99.8-Q99.9

Q93.5 Other deletions of part of a chromosome   CC
Angelman syndrome

Q93.7 Deletions with other complex rearrangements   CC
Deletions due to unbalanced translocations, inversions and insertions
Code also any associated duplications due to unbalanced translocations, inversions and insertions (Q92.5)

✓5ᵗʰ Q93.8 Other deletions from the autosomes

Q93.81 Velo-cardio-facial syndrome   MCC
Deletion 22q11.2
CC Excl: Q90.0-Q93.7, Q93.88-Q99.1, Q99.8-Q99.9

Q93.88 Other microdeletions   CC
Miller-Dieker syndrome
Smith-Magenis syndrome
CC Excl: Q90.0-Q93.81, Q93.89-Q99.1, Q99.8-Q99.9

Q93.89 Other deletions from the autosomes   CC
Deletions identified by fluorescence in situ hybridization (FISH)
Deletions identified by in situ hybridization (ISH)
Deletions seen only at prometaphase

Q93.9 Deletion from autosomes, unspecified   CC

✓4ᵗʰ Q95 Balanced rearrangements and structural markers, not elsewhere classified
> INCLUDES Robertsonian and balanced reciprocal translocations and insertions

Q95.0 Balanced translocation and insertion in normal individual

Q95.1 Chromosome inversion in normal individual

Q95.2 Balanced autosomal rearrangement in abnormal individual

Q95.3 Balanced sex/autosomal rearrangement in abnormal individual

Q95.5 Individual with autosomal fragile site

Q95.8 Other balanced rearrangements and structural markers

Q95.9 Balanced rearrangement and structural marker, unspecified

✓4ᵗʰ Q96 Turner's syndrome
> EXCLUDES 1 Noonan syndrome (Q87.1)

Q96.0 Karyotype 45, X   ♀

Q96.1 Karyotype 46, X iso (Xq)   ♀
Karyotype 46, isochromosome Xq

Q96.2 Karyotype 46, X with abnormal sex chromosome, except iso (Xq)   ♀
Karyotype 46, X with abnormal sex chromosome, except isochromosome Xq

Q96.3 Mosaicism, 45, X/46, XX or XY   ♀

Q96.4 Mosaicism, 45, X/other cell line(s) with abnormal sex chromosome   ♀

Q96.8 Other variants of Turner's syndrome   ♀

Q96.9 Turner's syndrome, unspecified   ♀

N Newborn: 0   P Pediatric: 0-17   M Maternity: 12-55   A Adult: 15-124   MCC Major CC Condition   PDxMCC PDx acts as own MCC   CC CC Condition   PDxCC PDx acts as own CC

872   ICD-10-CM 2016

✓4ᵗʰ **Q97 Other sex chromosome abnormalities, female phenotype, not elsewhere classified**
> **EXCLUDES 1** *Turner's syndrome (Q96.-)*

Q97.0 Karyotype 47, XXX ♀
Q97.1 Female with more than three X chromosomes ♀
Q97.2 Mosaicism, lines with various numbers of X chromosomes ♀
Q97.3 Female with 46, XY karyotype ♀
Q97.8 Other specified sex chromosome abnormalities, female phenotype ♀
Q97.9 Sex chromosome abnormality, female phenotype, unspecified ♀

✓4ᵗʰ **Q98 Other sex chromosome abnormalities, male phenotype, not elsewhere classified**

Q98.0 Klinefelter syndrome karyotype 47, XXY ♂
Q98.1 Klinefelter syndrome, male with more than two X chromosomes ♂
Q98.3 Other male with 46, XX karyotype ♂
Q98.4 Klinefelter syndrome, unspecified ♂
Q98.5 Karyotype 47, XYY
Q98.6 Male with structurally abnormal sex chromosome ♂
Q98.7 Male with sex chromosome mosaicism ♂
Q98.8 Other specified sex chromosome abnormalities, male phenotype ♂
Q98.9 Sex chromosome abnormality, male phenotype, unspecified ♂

✓4ᵗʰ **Q99 Other chromosome abnormalities, not elsewhere classified**

Q99.0 Chimera 46, XX/46, XY
Chimera 46, XX/46, XY true hermaphrodite
Q99.1 46, XX true hermaphrodite
46, XX with streak gonads
46, XY with streak gonads
Pure gonadal dysgenesis
Q99.2 Fragile X chromosome
Fragile X syndrome
Q99.8 Other specified chromosome abnormalities
Q99.9 Chromosomal abnormality, unspecified

Chapter 18. Symptoms, Signs, and Abnormal Clinical and Laboratory Findings, Not Elsewhere Classified (R00–R99)

Chapter Specific Guidelines with Coding Examples

The chapter specific guidelines from the ICD-10-CM Official Guidelines for Coding and Reporting have been provided below. Along with these guidelines are coding examples, contained in the shaded boxes, that have been developed to help illustrate the coding and/or sequencing guidance found in these guidelines.

Chapter 18 includes symptoms, signs, abnormal results of clinical or other investigative procedures, and ill-defined conditions regarding which no diagnosis classifiable elsewhere is recorded. Signs and symptoms that point to a specific diagnosis have been assigned to a category in other chapters of the classification.

a. Use of symptom codes

Codes that describe symptoms and signs are acceptable for reporting purposes when a related definitive diagnosis has not been established (confirmed) by the provider.

Chest pain of unknown origin

R07.9   Chest pain, unspecified

Explanation: Codes that describe symptoms such as chest pain are acceptable for reporting purposes when the provider has not established (confirmed) a related definitive diagnosis.

---

b. Use of a symptom code with a definitive diagnosis code

Codes for signs and symptoms may be reported in addition to a related definitive diagnosis when the sign or symptom is not routinely associated with that diagnosis, such as the various signs and symptoms associated with complex syndromes. The definitive diagnosis code should be sequenced before the symptom code.

Signs or symptoms that are associated routinely with a disease process should not be assigned as additional codes, unless otherwise instructed by the classification.

Pneumonia with hemoptysis

J18.9   Pneumonia, unspecified organism

R04.2   Hemoptysis

Explanation: Codes for signs and symptoms may be reported in addition to a related definitive diagnosis when the sign or symptom is not routinely associated with that diagnosis.

Abdominal pain due to acute appendicitis

K35.80   Unspecified acute appendicitis

Explanation: Codes for signs or symptoms routinely associated with a disease process should not be assigned unless the classification instructs otherwise.

---

c. Combination codes that include symptoms

ICD-10-CM contains a number of combination codes that identify both the definitive diagnosis and common symptoms of that diagnosis. When using one of these combination codes, an additional code should not be assigned for the symptom.

Acute gastritis with hemorrhage

K29.01   Acute gastritis with bleeding

Explanation: When a combination code identifies both the definitive diagnosis and the symptom, an additional code should not be assigned for the symptom.

---

d. Repeated falls

Code R29.6, Repeated falls, is for use for encounters when a patient has recently fallen and the reason for the fall is being investigated.

Code Z91.81, History of falling, is for use when a patient has fallen in the past and is at risk for future falls. When appropriate, both codes R29.6 and Z91.81 may be assigned together.

e. Coma scale

The coma scale codes (R40.2-) can be used in conjunction with traumatic brain injury codes, acute cerebrovascular disease or sequelae of cerebrovascular disease codes. These codes are primarily for use by trauma registries, but they may be used in any setting where this information is collected. The coma scale codes should be sequenced after the diagnosis code(s).

These codes, one from each subcategory, are needed to complete the scale. The 7th character indicates when the scale was recorded. The 7th character should match for all three codes.

At a minimum, report the initial score documented on presentation at your facility. This may be a score from the emergency medicine technician (EMT) or in the emergency department. If desired, a facility may choose to capture multiple coma scale scores.

Assign code R40.24, Glasgow coma scale, total score, when only the total score is documented in the medical record and not the individual score(s).

23-year-old man found down after unknown injury with skull fracture and with concussion and loss of consciousness of unknown duration. EMS evaluated the patient in the field and reported the individual Glasgow coma scores:

Eye opening response—3: eyes open to speech

Verbal response—4: confused but coherent speech

Motor response—6: obeys commands fully

S02.0XXA   Fracture of vault of skull, initial encounter for closed fracture

S06.0X9A   Concussion with loss of consciousness of unspecified duration, initial encounter

R40.2131   Coma scale, eyes open, to sound, in the field [EMT or ambulance]

R40.2241   Coma scale, best verbal response, confused conversation, in the field [EMT or ambulance]

R40.2361   Coma scale, best motor response, obeys commands, in the field [EMT or ambulance]

Explanation: When individual scores for the Glasgow coma scale are documented, one code from each category is needed to complete the scale. The seventh character indicates when the scale was recorded and should match for all three codes. Assign code R40.24 Glasgow coma scale, total score, when only the total and not the individual score(s) is documented in the medical record.

---

f. Functional quadriplegia

Functional quadriplegia (code R53.2) is the lack of ability to use one's limbs or to ambulate due to extreme debility. It is not associated with neurologic deficit or injury, and code R53.2 should not be used for cases of neurologic quadriplegia. It should only be assigned if functional quadriplegia is specifically documented in the medical record.

g. SIRS due to non-infectious process

The systemic inflammatory response syndrome (SIRS) can develop as a result of certain non-infectious disease processes, such as trauma, malignant neoplasm, or pancreatitis. When SIRS is documented with a noninfectious condition, and no subsequent infection is documented, the code for the underlying condition, such as an injury, should be assigned, followed by code R65.10, Systemic inflammatory response syndrome (SIRS) of non-infectious origin without acute organ dysfunction, or code R65.11, Systemic inflammatory response syndrome (SIRS) of non-infectious origin with acute organ dysfunction. If an associated acute organ dysfunction is documented, the appropriate code(s) for the specific type of organ dysfunction(s) should be assigned in addition to code R65.11. If acute organ dysfunction is documented, but it cannot be determined if the acute organ dysfunction is associated with SIRS or due to another condition (e.g., directly due to the trauma), the provider should be queried.

Systemic inflammatory response syndrome (SIRS) due to acute gallstone pancreatitis

K85.1   Biliary acute pancreatitis

R65.10   Systemic inflammatory response syndrome (SIRS) of noninfectious origin without acute organ dysfunction

Explanation: When SIRS is documented with a noninfectious condition without subsequent infection documented, the code for the underlying condition such as pancreatitis should be assigned followed by the appropriate code for SIRS of noninfectious origin, either with or without associated organ dysfunction.

h. Death NOS

Code R99, Ill-defined and unknown cause of mortality, is only for use in the very limited circumstance when a patient who has already died is brought into an emergency department or other healthcare facility and is pronounced dead upon arrival. It does not represent the discharge disposition of death.

Chapter 18. Symptoms, Signs and Abnormal Clinical and Laboratory Findings, Not Elsewhere Classified (R00-R99)

NOTE This chapter includes symptoms, signs, abnormal results of clinical or other investigative procedures, and ill-defined conditions regarding which no diagnosis classifiable elsewhere is recorded.

Signs and symptoms that point rather definitely to a given diagnosis have been assigned to a category in other chapters of the classification. In general, categories in this chapter include the less well-defined conditions and symptoms that, without the necessary study of the case to establish a final diagnosis, point perhaps equally to two or more diseases or to two or more systems of the body. Practically all categories in the chapter could be designated "not otherwise specified", "unknown etiology" or "transient". The Alphabetical Index should be consulted to determine which symptoms and signs are to be allocated here and which to other chapters. The residual subcategories, numbered .8, are generally provided for other relevant symptoms that cannot be allocated elsewhere in the classification.

The conditions and signs or symptoms included in categories R00-R94 consist of:

(a)   cases for which no more specific diagnosis can be made even after all the facts bearing on the case have been investigated;

(b)   signs or symptoms existing at the time of initial encounter that proved to be transient and whose causes could not be determined;

(c)   provisional diagnosis in a patient who failed to return for further investigation or care;

(d)   cases referred elsewhere for investigation or treatment before the diagnosis was made;

(e)   cases in which a more precise diagnosis was not available for any other reason;

(f)   certain symptoms, for which supplementary information is provided, that represent important problems in medical care in their own right.

EXCLUDES 2 *abnormal findings on antenatal screening of mother (O28.-)*
certain conditions originating in the perinatal period (P04-P96)
signs and symptoms classified in the body system chapters
signs and symptoms of breast (N63, N64.5)

This chapter contains the following blocks:

R00-R09	Symptoms and signs involving the circulatory and respiratory systems
R10-R19	Symptoms and signs involving the digestive system and abdomen
R20-R23	Symptoms and signs involving the skin and subcutaneous tissue
R25-R29	Symptoms and signs involving the nervous and musculoskeletal systems
R30-R39	Symptoms and signs involving the genitourinary system
R40-R46	Symptoms and signs involving cognition, perception, emotional state and behavior
R47-R49	Symptoms and signs involving speech and voice
R50-R69	General symptoms and signs
R70-R79	Abnormal findings on examination of blood, without diagnosis
R80-R82	Abnormal findings on examination of urine, without diagnosis
R83-R89	Abnormal findings on examination of other body fluids, substances and tissues, without diagnosis
R90-R94	Abnormal findings on diagnostic imaging and in function studies, without diagnosis
R97	Abnormal tumor markers
R99	Ill-defined and unknown cause of mortality

Symptoms and signs involving the circulatory and respiratory systems (R00-R09)

✓4ᵗʰ **R00 Abnormalities of heart beat**
   EXCLUDES 1 *abnormalities originating in the perinatal period (P29.1-)*
           specified arrhythmias (I47-I49)

   R00.0 Tachycardia, unspecified
     Rapid heart beat
     Sinoauricular tachycardia NOS
     Sinus [sinusal] tachycardia NOS
     EXCLUDES 1 *neonatal tachycardia (P29.11)*
           paroxysmal tachycardia (I47.-)

   R00.1 Bradycardia, unspecified
     Sinoatrial bradycardia
     Sinus bradycardia
     Slow heart beat
     Vagal bradycardia
     Use additional code for adverse effect, if applicable, to identify drug (T36-T50 with fifth or sixth character 5)
     EXCLUDES 1 *neonatal bradycardia (P29.12)*

   R00.2 Palpitations
     Awareness of heart beat

   R00.8 Other abnormalities of heart beat

   R00.9 Unspecified abnormalities of heart beat

✓4ᵗʰ **R01 Cardiac murmurs and other cardiac sounds**
   EXCLUDES 1 *cardiac murmurs and sounds originating in the perinatal period (P29.8)*

   R01.0 Benign and innocent cardiac murmurs
     Functional cardiac murmur

   R01.1 Cardiac murmur, unspecified
     Cardiac bruit NOS
     Heart murmur NOS

   R01.2 Other cardiac sounds
     Cardiac dullness, increased or decreased
     Precordial friction

✓4ᵗʰ **R03 Abnormal blood-pressure reading, without diagnosis**

   13 **R03.0 Elevated blood-pressure reading, without diagnosis of hypertension**
     NOTE This category is to be used to record an episode of elevated blood pressure in a patient in whom no formal diagnosis of hypertension has been made, or as an isolated incidental finding.

   R03.1 Nonspecific low blood-pressure reading
     EXCLUDES 1 *hypotension (I95.-)*
           maternal hypotension syndrome (O26.5-)
           neurogenic orthostatic hypotension (G90.3)

✓4ᵗʰ **R04 Hemorrhage from respiratory passages**

   CC Excl: For CC codes in category Q93, unless otherwise noted: R04.2-R04.9, R09.3, R68.13

   R04.0 Epistaxis
     Hemorrhage from nose
     Nosebleed

   R04.1 Hemorrhage from throat
     EXCLUDES 2 *hemoptysis (R04.2)*

   R04.2 Hemoptysis   CC
     Blood-stained sputum
     Cough with hemorrhage
     AHA: 2013, 4Q, 118

✓5ᵗʰ **R04.8 Hemorrhage from other sites in respiratory passages**
     R04.81 Acute idiopathic pulmonary hemorrhage in infants   CC P
       AIPHI
       Acute idiopathic hemorrhage in infants over 28 days old
       EXCLUDES 1 *perinatal pulmonary hemorrhage (P26.-)*
            von Willebrand's disease (D68.0)

     R04.89 Hemorrhage from other sites in respiratory passages   CC
       Pulmonary hemorrhage NOS

   R04.9 Hemorrhage from respiratory passages, unspecified   CC

R05 Cough
   EXCLUDES 1 *cough with hemorrhage (R04.2)*
           smoker's cough (J41.0)

✓4ᵗʰ **R06 Abnormalities of breathing**
   EXCLUDES 1 *acute respiratory distress syndrome (J80)*
           respiratory arrest (R09.2)
           respiratory arrest of newborn (P28.81)
           respiratory distress syndrome of newborn (P22.-)
           respiratory failure (J96.-)
           respiratory failure of newborn (P28.5)

✓5ᵗʰ **R06.0 Dyspnea**
     EXCLUDES 1 *tachypnea NOS (R06.82)*
           transient tachypnea of newborn (P22.1)

     R06.00 Dyspnea, unspecified
     R06.01 Orthopnea
     R06.02 Shortness of breath
     R06.09 Other forms of dyspnea

---

13 Questionable admission when used as PDx.

Ⓝ Newborn: 0   Ⓟ Pediatric: 0-17   Ⓜ Maternity: 12-55   Ⓐ Adult: 15-124   MCC Major CC Condition   PDxMCC PDx acts as own MCC   CC CC Condition   PDxCC PDx acts as own CC

876   ICD-10-CM 2016

R06.1 **Stridor**
  EXCLUDES 1 *congenital laryngeal stridor (P28.89)*
              laryngismus (stridulus) (J38.5)

R06.2 **Wheezing**
  EXCLUDES 1 *asthma (J45.-)*

R06.3 **Periodic breathing**   CC
  Cheyne-Stokes breathing
  CC Excl: J22, J80, J96.00-J96.92, J98.8-J98.9, R06.3, R06.81, R09.2

R06.4 **Hyperventilation**
  EXCLUDES 1 *psychogenic hyperventilation (F45.8)*

R06.5 **Mouth breathing**
  EXCLUDES 2 *dry mouth NOS (R68.2)*

R06.6 **Hiccough**
  EXCLUDES 1 *psychogenic hiccough (F45.8)*

R06.7 **Sneezing**

✓5ᵗʰ R06.8 **Other abnormalities of breathing**
  R06.81 **Apnea, not elsewhere classified**
    Apnea NOS
    EXCLUDES 1 *apnea (of) newborn (P28.4)*
                sleep apnea (G47.3-)
                sleep apnea of newborn (primary) (P28.3)

  R06.82 **Tachypnea, not elsewhere classified**
    Tachypnea NOS
    EXCLUDES 1 *transitory tachypnea of newborn (P22.1)*

  R06.83 **Snoring**

  R06.89 **Other abnormalities of breathing**
    Breath-holding (spells)
    Sighing

R06.9 **Unspecified abnormalities of breathing**

✓4ᵗʰ **R07 Pain in throat and chest**
  EXCLUDES 1 *epidemic myalgia (B33.0)*
  EXCLUDES 2 *jaw pain (R68.84)*
              pain in breast (N64.4)

  R07.0 **Pain in throat**
    EXCLUDES 1 *chronic sore throat (J31.2)*
                sore throat (acute) NOS (J02.9)
    EXCLUDES 2 *dysphagia (R13.1-)*
                pain in neck (M54.2)

  R07.1 **Chest pain on breathing**
    Painful respiration

  R07.2 **Precordial pain**

✓5ᵗʰ R07.8 **Other chest pain**
  R07.81 **Pleurodynia**
    Pleurodynia NOS
    EXCLUDES 1 *epidemic pleurodynia (B33.0)*

  R07.82 **Intercostal pain**

  R07.89 **Other chest pain**
    Anterior chest-wall pain NOS

  R07.9 **Chest pain, unspecified**

✓4ᵗʰ **R09 Other symptoms and signs involving the circulatory and respiratory system**
  EXCLUDES 1 *acute respiratory distress syndrome (J80)*
              respiratory arrest of newborn (P28.81)
              respiratory distress syndrome of newborn (P22.0)
              respiratory failure (J96.-)
              respiratory failure of newborn (P28.5)

✓5ᵗʰ R09.0 **Asphyxia and hypoxemia**
  EXCLUDES 1 *asphyxia due to carbon monoxide (T58.-)*
              asphyxia due to foreign body in respiratory tract (T17.-)
              birth (intrauterine) asphyxia (P84)
              hypercapnia (R06.4)
              hyperventilation (R06.4)
              traumatic asphyxia (T71.-)

  R09.01 **Asphyxia**   CC
    CC Excl: G89.0-G89.4, J80, J96.00-J96.92, R09.01-R09.02, R09.2, R41.0-R41.3, R41.82, R41.9, R44.8-R44.9, R45.83-R45.84, R46.0-R46.89, R52, R68.0-R68.19, R68.81-R68.83, R68.89-R69

  R09.02 **Hypoxemia**

  R09.1 **Pleurisy**
    EXCLUDES 1 *pleurisy with effusion (J90)*

10 R09.2 **Respiratory arrest**   MCC
  Cardiorespiratory failure
  EXCLUDES 1 *cardiac arrest (I46.-)*
              respiratory arrest of newborn (P28.81)
              respiratory distress of newborn (P22.0)
              respiratory failure (J96.-)
              respiratory failure of newborn (P28.5)
              respiratory insufficiency (R06.89)
              respiratory insufficiency of newborn (P28.5)
  CC Excl: See code: R09.01

R09.3 **Abnormal sputum**
  Abnormal amount of sputum
  Abnormal color of sputum
  Abnormal odor of sputum
  Excessive sputum
  EXCLUDES 1 *blood-stained sputum (R04.2)*

✓5ᵗʰ R09.8 **Other specified symptoms and signs involving the circulatory and respiratory systems**
  R09.81 **Nasal congestion**

  R09.82 **Postnasal drip**

  R09.89 **Other specified symptoms and signs involving the circulatory and respiratory systems**
    Abnormal chest percussion
    Bruit (arterial)
    Chest tympany
    Choking sensation
    Feeling of foreign body in throat
    Friction sounds in chest
    Rales
    Weak pulse
    EXCLUDES 2 *foreign body in throat (T17.2-)*
                wheezing (R06.2)

Symptoms and signs involving the digestive system and abdomen (R10-R19)

  EXCLUDES 1 *congenital or infantile pylorospasm (Q40.0)*
              gastrointestinal hemorrhage (K92.0-K92.2)
              intestinal obstruction (K56.-)
              newborn gastrointestinal hemorrhage (P54.0-P54.3)
              newborn intestinal obstruction (P76.-)
              pylorospasm (K31.3)
              signs and symptoms involving the urinary system (R30-R39)
              symptoms referable to female genital organs (N94.-)
              symptoms referable to male genital organs male (N48-N50)

✓4ᵗʰ **R10 Abdominal and pelvic pain**
  EXCLUDES 1 *renal colic (N23)*
  EXCLUDES 2 *dorsalgia (M54.-)*
              flatulence and related conditions (R14.-)

  R10.0 **Acute abdomen**
    Severe abdominal pain (generalized) (with abdominal rigidity)
    EXCLUDES 1 *abdominal rigidity NOS (R19.3)*
                generalized abdominal pain NOS (R10.84)
                localized abdominal pain (R10.1-R10.3-)

✓5ᵗʰ R10.1 **Pain localized to upper abdomen**
  R10.10 **Upper abdominal pain, unspecified**
  R10.11 **Right upper quadrant pain**
  R10.12 **Left upper quadrant pain**
  R10.13 **Epigastric pain**
    Dyspepsia
    EXCLUDES 1 *functional dyspepsia (K30)*

  R10.2 **Pelvic and perineal pain**
    EXCLUDES 1 *vulvodynia (N94.81)*

✓5ᵗʰ R10.3 **Pain localized to other parts of lower abdomen**
  R10.30 **Lower abdominal pain, unspecified**
  R10.31 **Right lower quadrant pain**
  R10.32 **Left lower quadrant pain**
  R10.33 **Periumbilical pain**

✓5ᵗʰ R10.8 **Other abdominal pain**
  ✓6ᵗʰ R10.81 **Abdominal tenderness**
    Abdominal tenderness NOS
    R10.811 **Right upper quadrant abdominal tenderness**
    R10.812 **Left upper quadrant abdominal tenderness**
    R10.813 **Right lower quadrant abdominal tenderness**

---

10 MCC only if patient is discharged alive.

✓ Additional Character Required   ✓x7ᵗʰ Placeholder Alert   Unacceptable PDx   Manifestation   Hospital Acquired Condition   EXCLUDES 1 Not Coded Here   EXCLUDES 2 Not Included Here

Chapter 18. Symptoms, Signs, and Abnormal Clinical and Laboratory Findings, Not Elsewhere Classified

R10.814–R19.12

R10.814   **Left lower** quadrant abdominal tenderness

R10.815   **Periumbilic** abdominal tenderness

R10.816   **Epigastric** abdominal tenderness

R10.817   **Generalized** abdominal tenderness

R10.819   **Abdominal tenderness, unspecified** site

✓6th **R10.82**   Rebound abdominal tenderness

R10.821   **Right upper** quadrant rebound abdominal tenderness

R10.822   **Left upper** quadrant rebound abdominal tenderness

R10.823   **Right lower** quadrant rebound abdominal tenderness

R10.824   **Left lower** quadrant rebound abdominal tenderness

R10.825   **Periumbilic** rebound abdominal tenderness

R10.826   **Epigastric** rebound abdominal tenderness

R10.827   **Generalized** rebound abdominal tenderness

R10.829   **Rebound abdominal tenderness, unspecified** site

R10.83   Colic   P
    Colic NOS
    Infantile colic
    EXCLUDES 1   *colic in adult and child over 12 months old (R10.84)*

R10.84   **Generalized** abdominal pain
    EXCLUDES 1   *generalized abdominal pain associated with acute abdomen (R10.0)*

R10.9   **Unspecified** abdominal pain

✓4th **R11**   **Nausea and vomiting**
    EXCLUDES 1   *cyclical vomiting associated with migraine (G43.A-)*
           excessive vomiting in pregnancy (O21.-)
           hematemesis (K92.0)
           neonatal hematemesis (P54.0)
           newborn vomiting (P92.0-)
           psychogenic vomiting (F50.8)
           vomiting associated with bulimia nervosa (F50.2)
           vomiting following gastrointestinal surgery (K91.0)

R11.0   **Nausea**
    Nausea NOS   Nausea without vomiting

✓5th **R11.1**   Vomiting

R11.10   **Vomiting, unspecified**
    Vomiting NOS

R11.11   **Vomiting without nausea**

R11.12   **Projectile vomiting**

R11.13   **Vomiting of fecal matter**

R11.14   **Bilious vomiting**
    Bilious emesis

R11.2   **Nausea with vomiting, unspecified**
    Persistent nausea with vomiting NOS

R12   **Heartburn**
    EXCLUDES 1   *dyspepsia NOS (R10.13)*
           functional dyspepsia (K30)

✓4th **R13**   **Aphagia and dysphagia**

R13.0   **Aphagia**
    Inability to swallow
    EXCLUDES 1   *psychogenic aphagia (F50.9)*

✓5th **R13.1**   Dysphagia
    Code first, if applicable, dysphagia following cerebrovascular disease (I69. with final characters -91)
    EXCLUDES 1   *psychogenic dysphagia (F45.8)*

R13.10   **Dysphagia, unspecified**
    Difficulty in swallowing NOS

R13.11   **Dysphagia, oral phase**

R13.12   **Dysphagia, oropharyngeal phase**

R13.13   **Dysphagia, pharyngeal phase**

R13.14   **Dysphagia, pharyngoesophageal phase**

R13.19   **Other dysphagia**
    Cervical dysphagia
    Neurogenic dysphagia

✓4th **R14**   **Flatulence and related conditions**
    EXCLUDES 1   *psychogenic aerophagy (F45.8)*

R14.0   **Abdominal distension (gaseous)**
    Bloating
    Tympanites (abdominal) (intestinal)

R14.1   **Gas pain**

R14.2   **Eructation**

R14.3   **Flatulence**

✓4th **R15**   **Fecal incontinence**
    Encopresis NOS
    EXCLUDES 1   *fecal incontinence of nonorganic origin (F98.1)*

R15.0   **Incomplete defecation**
    EXCLUDES 1   *constipation (K59.0-)*
           fecal impaction (K56.41)

R15.1   **Fecal smearing**
    Fecal soiling

R15.2   **Fecal urgency**

R15.9   **Full incontinence of feces**
    Fecal incontinence NOS

✓4th **R16**   **Hepatomegaly and splenomegaly, not elsewhere classified**

R16.0   **Hepatomegaly, not elsewhere classified**
    Hepatomegaly NOS

R16.1   **Splenomegaly, not elsewhere classified**
    Splenomegaly NOS

R16.2   **Hepatomegaly with splenomegaly, not elsewhere classified**
    Hepatosplenomegaly NOS

R17   **Unspecified jaundice**   CC
    EXCLUDES 1   *neonatal jaundice (P55, P57-P59)*
    CC Excl: P57.8-P59.9, R17, R23.8-R23.9

✓4th **R18**   **Ascites**
    INCLUDES   *fluid in peritoneal cavity*
    EXCLUDES 1   *ascites in alcoholic cirrhosis (K70.31)*
           ascites in alcoholic hepatitis (K70.11)
           ascites in toxic liver disease with chronic active hepatitis (K71.51)

R18.0   **Malignant ascites**   CC
    Code first malignancy, such as:
      malignant neoplasm of ovary (C56.-)
      secondary malignant neoplasm of retroperitoneum and peritoneum (C78.6)
    CC Excl: G89.0-G89.4, R18.0-R19.09, R19.30-R19.37, R41.0-R41.3, R41.82, R41.9, R44.8-R44.9, R45.83-R45.84, R46.0-R46.89, R52, R68.0-R68.19, R68.81-R68.83, R68.89-R69

R18.8   **Other ascites**   CC
    Ascites NOS
    Peritoneal effusion (chronic)
    CC Excl: See code: R18.0

✓4th **R19**   **Other symptoms and signs involving the digestive system and abdomen**
    EXCLUDES 1   *acute abdomen (R10.0)*

✓5th **R19.0**   Intra-abdominal and pelvic swelling, mass and lump
    EXCLUDES 1   *abdominal distension (gaseous) (R14.-)*
           ascites (R18.-)

R19.00   **Intra-abdominal and pelvic swelling, mass and lump, unspecified** site

R19.01   **Right upper quadrant abdominal swelling, mass and lump**

R19.02   **Left upper quadrant abdominal swelling, mass and lump**

R19.03   **Right lower quadrant abdominal swelling, mass and lump**

R19.04   **Left lower quadrant abdominal swelling, mass and lump**

R19.05   **Periumbilic swelling, mass or lump**
    Diffuse or generalized umbilical swelling or mass

R19.06   **Epigastric swelling, mass or lump**

R19.07   **Generalized intra-abdominal and pelvic swelling, mass and lump**
    Diffuse or generalized intra-abdominal swelling or mass NOS
    Diffuse or generalized pelvic swelling or mass NOS

R19.09   **Other intra-abdominal and pelvic swelling, mass and lump**

✓5th **R19.1**   Abnormal bowel sounds

R19.11   **Absent bowel sounds**

R19.12   **Hyperactive bowel sounds**

N Newborn: 0   P Pediatric: 0-17   M Maternity: 12-55   A Adult: 15-124   MCC Major CC Condition   PDxMCC PDx acts as own MCC   CC CC Condition   PDxCC PDx acts as own CC

878   ICD-10-CM 2016

R19.15 **Other abnormal bowel sounds**
Abnormal bowel sounds NOS

R19.2 Visible peristalsis
Hyperperistalsis

☑5ᵗʰ **R19.3 Abdominal rigidity**
EXCLUDES 1 abdominal rigidity with severe abdominal pain (R10.0)

R19.30 **Abdominal rigidity, unspecified site**
R19.31 **Right upper quadrant abdominal rigidity**
R19.32 **Left upper quadrant abdominal rigidity**
R19.33 **Right lower quadrant abdominal rigidity**
R19.34 **Left lower quadrant abdominal rigidity**
R19.35 **Periumbilic abdominal rigidity**
R19.36 **Epigastric abdominal rigidity**
R19.37 **Generalized abdominal rigidity**

R19.4 Change in bowel habit
EXCLUDES 1 constipation (K59.0-)
functional diarrhea (K59.1)

R19.5 Other fecal abnormalities
Abnormal stool color
Bulky stools
Mucus in stools
Occult blood in feces
Occult blood in stools
EXCLUDES 1 melena (K92.1)
neonatal melena (P54.1)

R19.6 Halitosis

R19.7 Diarrhea, unspecified
Diarrhea NOS
EXCLUDES 1 functional diarrhea (K59.1)
neonatal diarrhea (P78.3)
psychogenic diarrhea (F45.8)

R19.8 Other specified symptoms and signs involving the digestive system and abdomen

Symptoms and signs involving the skin and subcutaneous tissue (R20-R23)

EXCLUDES 2 symptoms relating to breast (N64.4-N64.5)

☑4ᵗʰ **R20 Disturbances of skin sensation**
EXCLUDES 1 dissociative anesthesia and sensory loss (F44.6)
psychogenic disturbances (F45.8)

R20.0 Anesthesia of skin

R20.1 Hypoesthesia of skin

R20.2 Paresthesia of skin
Formication
Pins and needles
Tingling skin
EXCLUDES 1 acroparesthesia (I73.8)

R20.3 Hyperesthesia

R20.8 Other disturbances of skin sensation

R20.9 Unspecified disturbances of skin sensation

R21 Rash and other nonspecific skin eruption
Rash NOS
EXCLUDES 1 specified type of rash—code to condition
vesicular eruption (R23.8)

☑4ᵗʰ **R22 Localized swelling, mass and lump of skin and subcutaneous tissue**
Subcutaneous nodules (localized)(superficial)
EXCLUDES 1 abnormal findings on diagnostic imaging (R90-R93)
edema (R60.-)
enlarged lymph nodes (R59.-)
localized adiposity (E65)
swelling of joint (M25.4-)

R22.0 Localized swelling, mass and lump, head

R22.1 Localized swelling, mass and lump, neck

R22.2 Localized swelling, mass and lump, trunk
EXCLUDES 1 intra-abdominal or pelvic mass and lump (R19.0-)
intra-abdominal or pelvic swelling (R19.0-)
EXCLUDES 2 breast mass and lump (N63)

☑5ᵗʰ **R22.3 Localized swelling, mass and lump, upper limb**
R22.30 **Localized swelling, mass and lump, unspecified upper limb**
R22.31 **Localized swelling, mass and lump, right upper limb**
R22.32 **Localized swelling, mass and lump, left upper limb**
R22.33 **Localized swelling, mass and lump, upper limb, bilateral**

☑5ᵗʰ **R22.4 Localized swelling, mass and lump, lower limb**
R22.40 **Localized swelling, mass and lump, unspecified lower limb**
R22.41 **Localized swelling, mass and lump, right lower limb**
R22.42 **Localized swelling, mass and lump, left lower limb**
R22.43 **Localized swelling, mass and lump, lower limb, bilateral**

R22.9 Localized swelling, mass and lump, unspecified

☑4ᵗʰ **R23 Other skin changes**
R23.0 Cyanosis
EXCLUDES 1 acrocyanosis (I73.8)
cyanotic attacks of newborn (P28.2)

R23.1 Pallor
Clammy skin

R23.2 Flushing
Excessive blushing
Code first, if applicable, menopausal and female climacteric states (N95.1)

R23.3 Spontaneous ecchymoses
Petechiae
EXCLUDES 1 ecchymoses of newborn (P54.5)
purpura (D69.-)

R23.4 Changes in skin texture
Desquamation of skin
Induration of skin
Scaling of skin
EXCLUDES 1 epidermal thickening NOS (L85.9)

R23.8 Other skin changes

R23.9 Unspecified skin changes

Symptoms and signs involving the nervous and musculoskeletal systems (R25-R29)

☑4ᵗʰ **R25 Abnormal involuntary movements**
EXCLUDES 1 specific movement disorders (G20-G26)
stereotyped movement disorders (F98.4)
tic disorders (F95.-)

R25.0 Abnormal head movements

R25.1 Tremor, unspecified
EXCLUDES 1 chorea NOS (G25.5)
essential tremor (G25.0)
hysterical tremor (F44.4)
intention tremor (G25.2)

R25.2 Cramp and spasm
EXCLUDES 2 carpopedal spasm (R29.0)
charley-horse (M62.831)
infantile spasms (G40.4-)
muscle spasm of back (M62.830)
muscle spasm of calf (M62.831)

R25.3 Fasciculation
Twitching NOS

R25.8 Other abnormal involuntary movements

R25.9 Unspecified abnormal involuntary movements

☑4ᵗʰ **R26 Abnormalities of gait and mobility**
EXCLUDES 1 ataxia NOS (R27.0)
hereditary ataxia (G11.-)
locomotor (syphilitic) ataxia (A52.11)
immobility syndrome (paraplegic) (M62.3)

R26.0 Ataxic gait
Staggering gait

R26.1 Paralytic gait
Spastic gait

R26.2 Difficulty in walking, not elsewhere classified
EXCLUDES 1 falling (R29.6)
unsteadiness on feet (R26.81)

☑5ᵗʰ **R26.8 Other abnormalities of gait and mobility**
R26.81 **Unsteadiness on feet**
R26.89 **Other abnormalities of gait and mobility**

R26.9 Unspecified abnormalities of gait and mobility

☑4ᵗʰ **R27 Other lack of coordination**
EXCLUDES 1 ataxic gait (R26.0)
hereditary ataxia (G11.-)
vertigo NOS (R42)

R27.0 Ataxia, unspecified
EXCLUDES 1 ataxia following cerebrovascular disease (I69. with final characters -93)

Chapter 18. Symptoms, Signs, and Abnormal Clinical and Laboratory Findings, Not Elsewhere Classified

R27.8   Other lack of coordination

R27.9   Unspecified lack of coordination

✓4ᵗʰ R29   **Other symptoms and signs involving the nervous and musculoskeletal systems**

    R29.0   **Tetany**   CC

        Carpopedal spasm

        EXCLUDES 1   *hysterical tetany (F44.5)*

                 neonatal tetany (P71.3)

                 parathyroid tetany (E20.9)

                 post-thyroidectomy tetany (E89.2)

        CC Excl: A33, A35, G10-G11.2, G11.4, G20-G25.79, G25.82-G26, G32.81, G80.3, G81.10-G81.14, G89.0-G89.4, G90.3, R29.0, R41.0-R41.3, R41.82, R41.9, R44.8-R44.9, R45.83-R45.84, R46.0-R46.89, R52, R68.0-R68.19, R68.81-R68.83, R68.89-R69

    R29.1   **Meningismus**   CC

        CC Excl: R29.1, R29.810

    R29.2   **Abnormal reflex**

        EXCLUDES 2   *abnormal pupillary reflex (H57.0)*

                 hyperactive gag reflex (J39.2)

                 vasovagal reaction or syncope (R55)

    R29.3   **Abnormal posture**

    R29.4   **Clicking hip**

        EXCLUDES 1   *congenital deformities of hip (Q65.-)*

    R29.5   **Transient paralysis**   CC

        Code first any associated spinal cord injury (S14.0, S14.1-, S24.0, S24.1-, S34.0-, S34.1-)

        EXCLUDES 1   *transient ischemic attack (G45.9)*

        CC Excl: R29.5, R29.810

    R29.6   **Repeated falls**

        Falling

        Tendency to fall

        EXCLUDES 2   *at risk for falling (Z91.81)*

                 history of falling (Z91.81)

    ✓5ᵗʰ R29.8   **Other symptoms and signs involving the nervous and musculoskeletal systems**

       ✓6ᵗʰ R29.81   **Other symptoms and signs involving the nervous system**

            R29.810   **Facial weakness**

                Facial droop

                EXCLUDES 1   *Bell's palsy (G51.0)*

                           facial weakness following cerebrovascular disease (I69. with final characters -92)

            R29.818   **Other symptoms and signs involving the nervous system**

       ✓6ᵗʰ R29.89   **Other symptoms and signs involving the musculoskeletal system**

                EXCLUDES 2   *pain in limb (M79.6-)*

            R29.890   **Loss of height**

                EXCLUDES 1   *osteoporosis (M80-M81)*

            R29.891   **Ocular torticollis**

                EXCLUDES 1   *congenital (sternomastoid) torticollis Q68.0*

                           psychogenic torticollis (F45.8)

                           spasmodic torticollis (G24.3)

                           torticollis due to birth injury (P15.8)

                           torticollis NOS M43.6

            R29.898   **Other symptoms and signs involving the musculoskeletal system**

    ✓5ᵗʰ R29.9   **Unspecified symptoms and signs involving the nervous and musculoskeletal systems**

       R29.90   **Unspecified symptoms and signs involving the nervous system**

       R29.91   **Unspecified symptoms and signs involving the musculoskeletal system**

Symptoms and signs involving the genitourinary system (R30-R39)

✓4ᵗʰ R30   **Pain associated with micturition**

        EXCLUDES 1   *psychogenic pain associated with micturition (F45.8)*

    R30.0   **Dysuria**

        Strangury

    R30.1   **Vesical tenesmus**

    R30.9   **Painful micturition, unspecified**

        Painful urination NOS

✓4ᵗʰ R31   **Hematuria**

        EXCLUDES 1   *hematuria included with underlying conditions, such as:*

                 acute cystitis with hematuria (N30.01)

                 recurrent and persistent hematuria in glomerular diseases (N02.-)

    R31.0   **Gross hematuria**

    R31.1   **Benign essential microscopic hematuria**

    R31.2   **Other microscopic hematuria**

    R31.9   **Hematuria, unspecified**

R32   **Unspecified urinary incontinence**

        Enuresis NOS

        EXCLUDES 1   *functional urinary incontinence (R39.81)*

                 nonorganic enuresis (F98.0)

                 stress incontinence and other specified urinary incontinence (N39.3-N39.4-)

                 urinary incontinence associated with cognitive impairment (R39.81)

✓4ᵗʰ R33   **Retention of urine**

        EXCLUDES 1   *psychogenic retention of urine (F45.8)*

    R33.0   **Drug induced retention of urine**

        Use additional code for adverse effect, if applicable, to identify drug (T36-T50 with fifth or sixth character 5)

    R33.8   **Other retention of urine**

        Code first, if applicable, any causal condition, such as: enlarged prostate (N40.1)

    R33.9   **Retention of urine, unspecified**

R34   **Anuria and oliguria**

        EXCLUDES 1   *anuria and oliguria complicating abortion or ectopic or molar pregnancy (O00-O07, O08.4)*

                 anuria and oliguria complicating pregnancy (O26.83-)

                 anuria and oliguria complicating the puerperium (O90.4)

✓4ᵗʰ R35   **Polyuria**

        Code first, if applicable, any causal condition, such as: enlarged prostate (N40.1)

        EXCLUDES 1   *psychogenic polyuria (F45.8)*

    R35.0   **Frequency of micturition**

    R35.1   **Nocturia**

    R35.8   **Other polyuria**

        Polyuria NOS

✓4ᵗʰ R36   **Urethral discharge**

    R36.0   **Urethral discharge without blood**

    R36.1   **Hematospermia**   ♂

    R36.9   **Urethral discharge, unspecified**

        Penile discharge NOS

        Urethrorrhea

R37   **Sexual dysfunction, unspecified**

✓4ᵗʰ R39   **Other and unspecified symptoms and signs involving the genitourinary system**

    R39.0   **Extravasation of urine**   CC

        CC Excl: R30.1, R39.0, R39.2-R39.9

    ✓5ᵗʰ R39.1   **Other difficulties with micturition**

        Code first, if applicable, any causal condition, such as: enlarged prostate (N40.1)

       R39.11   **Hesitancy of micturition**

       R39.12   **Poor urinary stream**

            Weak urinary steam

       R39.13   **Splitting of urinary stream**

       R39.14   **Feeling of incomplete bladder emptying**

       R39.15   **Urgency of urination**

            EXCLUDES 1   *urge incontinence (N39.41, N39.46)*

       R39.16   **Straining to void**

       R39.19   **Other difficulties with micturition**

    R39.2   **Extrarenal uremia**

        Prerenal uremia

        EXCLUDES 1   *uremia NOS (N19)*

    ✓5ᵗʰ R39.8   **Other symptoms and signs involving the genitourinary system**

       R39.81   **Functional urinary incontinence**

            Urinary incontinence due to cognitive impairment, or severe physical disability or immobility

            EXCLUDES 1   *stress incontinence and other specified urinary incontinence (N39.3-N39.4-)*

                        urinary incontinence NOS (R32)

Ⓝ Newborn: 0   Ⓟ Pediatric: 0-17   Ⓜ Maternity: 12-55   Ⓐ Adult: 15-124   **MCC** Major CC Condition   **PDxMCC** PDx acts as own MCC   **CC** CC Condition   **PDxCC** PDx acts as own CC

880

ICD-10-CM 2016

R39.89   Other symptoms and signs involving the genitourinary system

R39.9   Unspecified symptoms and signs involving the genitourinary system

Symptoms and signs involving cognition, perception, emotional state and behavior (R40-R46)

EXCLUDES1   symptoms and signs constituting part of a pattern of mental disorder (F01-F99)

☑4th R40   Somnolence, stupor and coma

EXCLUDES1   neonatal coma (P91.5)
somnolence, stupor and coma in diabetes (E08-E13)
somnolence, stupor and coma in hepatic failure (K72.-)
somnolence, stupor and coma in hypoglycemia (nondiabetic) (E15)

R40.0   Somnolence
Drowsiness
EXCLUDES1   coma (R40.2-)

R40.1   Stupor
Catatonic stupor
Semicoma
EXCLUDES1   catatonic schizophrenia (F20.2)
coma (R40.2-)
depressive stupor (F31-F33)
dissociative stupor (F44.2)
manic stupor (F30.2)

☑5th R40.2   Coma
Code first any associated:
fracture of skull (S02.-)
intracranial injury (S06.-)
NOTE   One code from subcategories R40.21-R40.23 is required to complete the coma scale
AHA: 2014, 1Q, 19

CC Excl: For MCC codes in subcategory R40.2, unless otherwise noted: B15.0-B19.9, E03.5, E08.00-E08.59, E08.618-E09.59, E09.618-E10.59, E10.618-E10.649, E10.69-E11.59, E11.618-E11.649, E11.69-E13.59, E13.618-E16.2, E89.1, G32.89, G89.0-G89.4, G93.81-G93.9, G96.8-G96.9, G98.0-G98.8, G99.8, I60.00-I62.9, K72.91, R40.0-R40.2124, R40.2210-R40.2224, R40.2310-R40.2324, R40.2340-R40.2344, R40.3-R41.3, R41.82, R41.9-R42, R44.8-R44.9, R45.83-R45.84, R46.0-R46.89, R52, R55, R68.0-R68.19, R68.81-R68.83, R68.89-R69, S02.0XX-S02.19X with 7th character [A, B], S02.91X-S02.91X with 7th character [A, B], S06.0X0-S06.9X9 with 7th character A

R40.20   Unspecified coma   MCC
Coma NOS
Unconsciousness NOS

☑6th R40.21   Coma scale, eyes open

The following appropriate 7th character is to be added to subcategory R40.21-.
0   unspecified time
1   in the field [EMT or ambulance]
2   at arrival to emergency department
3   at hospital admission
4   24 hours or more after hospital admission

☑7th R40.211   Coma scale, eyes open, never   MCC
☑7th R40.212   Coma scale, eyes open, to pain   MCC
☑7th R40.213   Coma scale, eyes open, to sound
☑7th R40.214   Coma scale, eyes open, spontaneous

☑6th R40.22   Coma scale, best verbal response

The following appropriate 7th character is to be added to subcategory R40.22-.
0   unspecified time
1   in the field [EMT or ambulance]
2   at arrival to emergency department
3   at hospital admission
4   24 hours or more after hospital admission

☑7th R40.221   Coma scale, best verbal response, none   MCC
☑7th R40.222   Coma scale, best verbal response, incomprehensible words   MCC
☑7th R40.223   Coma scale, best verbal response, inappropriate words
☑7th R40.224   Coma scale, best verbal response, confused conversation

☑7th R40.225   Coma scale, best verbal response, oriented

☑6th R40.23   Coma scale, best motor response

The following appropriate 7th character is to be added to subcategory R40.23-.
0   unspecified time
1   in the field [EMT or ambulance]
2   at arrival to emergency department
3   at hospital admission
4   24 hours or more after hospital admission

☑7th R40.231   Coma scale, best motor response, none   MCC
☑7th R40.232   Coma scale, best motor response, extension   MCC
☑7th R40.233   Coma scale, best motor response, abnormal
☑7th R40.234   Coma scale, best motor response, flexion withdrawal   MCC
☑7th R40.235   Coma scale, best motor response, localizes pain
☑7th R40.236   Coma scale, best motor response, obeys commands

☑6th R40.24   Glasgow coma scale, total score
Use codes R40.21- through R40.23- only when the individual score(s) are documented

R40.241   Glasgow coma scale score 13-15
R40.242   Glasgow coma scale score 9-12
R40.243   Glasgow coma scale score 3-8
R40.244   Other coma, without documented Glasgow coma scale score, or with partial score reported

R40.3   Persistent vegetative state   CC
CC Excl: See code: R40.2

R40.4   Transient alteration of awareness

☑4th R41   Other symptoms and signs involving cognitive functions and awareness
EXCLUDES1   dissociative [conversion] disorders (F44.-)
mild cognitive impairment, so stated (G31.84)

R41.0   Disorientation, unspecified
Confusion NOS
Delirium NOS

R41.1   Anterograde amnesia

R41.2   Retrograde amnesia

R41.3   Other amnesia
Amnesia NOS
Memory loss NOS
EXCLUDES1   amnestic disorder due to known physiologic condition (F04)
amnestic syndrome due to psychoactive substance use (F10-F19 with 5th character .6)
mild memory disturbance due to known physiological condition (F06.8)
transient global amnesia (G45.4)

R41.4   Neurologic neglect syndrome   CC
Asomatognosia
Hemi-akinesia
Hemi-inattention
Hemispatial neglect
Left-sided neglect
Sensory neglect
Visuospatial neglect
EXCLUDES1   visuospatial deficit (R41.842)
CC Excl: R29.3, R29.6-R29.890, R29.90-R29.91, R41.4

☑5th R41.8   Other symptoms and signs involving cognitive functions and awareness

R41.81   Age-related cognitive decline   A
Senility NOS

R41.82   Altered mental status, unspecified
Change in mental status NOS
EXCLUDES1   altered level of consciousness (R40.-)
altered mental status due to known condition—code to condition
delirium NOS (R41.0)
AHA: 2012, 4Q, 97

R41.83   Borderline intellectual functioning
IQ level 71 to 84
EXCLUDES1   intellectual disabilities (F70-F79)

Chapter 18. Symptoms, Signs, and Abnormal Clinical and Laboratory Findings, Not Elsewhere Classified

R41.84–R48.9

✓6th **R41.84 Other specified cognitive deficit**

R41.840 Attention and concentration deficit
EXCLUDES 1 attention-deficit hyperactivity disorders (F90.-)

R41.841 Cognitive communication deficit

R41.842 Visuospatial deficit

R41.843 Psychomotor deficit

R41.844 Frontal lobe and executive function deficit

R41.89 Other symptoms and signs involving cognitive functions and awareness
Anosognosia

R41.9 Unspecified symptoms and signs involving cognitive functions and awareness

R42 Dizziness and giddiness
Light-headedness
Vertigo NOS
EXCLUDES 1 vertiginous syndromes (H81.-)
vertigo from infrasound (T75.23)

✓4th **R43 Disturbances of smell and taste**

R43.0 Anosmia

R43.1 Parosmia

R43.2 Parageusia

R43.8 Other disturbances of smell and taste
Mixed disturbance of smell and taste

R43.9 Unspecified disturbances of smell and taste

✓4th **R44 Other symptoms and signs involving general sensations and perceptions**
EXCLUDES 1 alcoholic hallucinations (F1.5)
hallucinations in drug psychosis (F11-F19 with .5)
hallucinations in mood disorders with psychotic symptoms (F30.2, F31.5, F32.3, F33.3)
hallucinations in schizophrenia, schizotypal and delusional disorders (F20-F29)
EXCLUDES 2 disturbances of skin sensation (R20.-)

CC Excl: For CC codes in category R44, unless otherwise noted:
G89.0-G89.4, R41.0-R41.3, R41.82, R41.9-R42, R44.0, R44.2-R44.9, R45.83-R45.84, R46.0-R46.89, R52, R68.0-R68.19, R68.81-R68.83, R68.89-R69

R44.0 Auditory hallucinations CC

R44.1 Visual hallucinations

R44.2 Other hallucinations CC

R44.3 Hallucinations, unspecified CC

R44.8 Other symptoms and signs involving general sensations and perceptions

R44.9 Unspecified symptoms and signs involving general sensations and perceptions

✓4th **R45 Symptoms and signs involving emotional state**

R45.0 Nervousness
Nervous tension

R45.1 Restlessness and agitation

R45.2 Unhappiness

R45.3 Demoralization and apathy
EXCLUDES 1 anhedonia (R45.84)

R45.4 Irritability and anger

R45.5 Hostility

R45.6 Violent behavior

R45.7 State of emotional shock and stress, unspecified

✓5th **R45.8 Other symptoms and signs involving emotional state**

R45.81 Low self-esteem

R45.82 Worries

R45.83 Excessive crying of child, adolescent or adult
EXCLUDES 1 excessive crying of infant (baby) R68.11

R45.84 Anhedonia

✓6th **R45.85 Homicidal and suicidal ideations**
EXCLUDES 1 suicide attempt (T14.91)

R45.850 Homicidal ideations

R45.851 Suicidal ideations CC
CC Excl: F05

R45.86 Emotional lability

R45.87 Impulsiveness

R45.89 Other symptoms and signs involving emotional state

✓4th **R46 Symptoms and signs involving appearance and behavior**
EXCLUDES 1 appearance and behavior in schizophrenia, schizotypal and delusional disorders (F20-F29)
mental and behavioral disorders (F01-F99)

R46.0 Very low level of personal hygiene

R46.1 Bizarre personal appearance

R46.2 Strange and inexplicable behavior

R46.3 Overactivity

R46.4 Slowness and poor responsiveness
EXCLUDES 1 stupor (R40.1)

R46.5 Suspiciousness and marked evasiveness

R46.6 Undue concern and preoccupation with stressful events

R46.7 Verbosity and circumstantial detail obscuring reason for contact

✓5th **R46.8 Other symptoms and signs involving appearance and behavior**

R46.81 Obsessive-compulsive behavior
EXCLUDES 1 obsessive-compulsive disorder (F42)

R46.89 Other symptoms and signs involving appearance and behavior

Symptoms and signs involving speech and voice (R47-R49)

✓4th **R47 Speech disturbances, not elsewhere classified**
EXCLUDES 1 autism (F84.0)
cluttering (F80.81)
specific developmental disorders of speech and language (F80.-)
stuttering (F80.81)

✓5th **R47.0 Dysphasia and aphasia**

R47.01 Aphasia CC
EXCLUDES 1 aphasia following cerebrovascular disease (I69. with final characters -20)
progressive isolated aphasia (G31.01)
CC Excl: F80.1, F80.81, I62.00-I66.9, R47.01-R47.9, R49.0-R49.9

R47.02 Dysphasia
EXCLUDES 1 dysphasia following cerebrovascular disease (I69. with final characters -21)

R47.1 Dysarthria and anarthria
EXCLUDES 1 dysarthria following cerebrovascular disease (I69. with final characters -22)

✓5th **R47.8 Other speech disturbances**
EXCLUDES 1 dysarthria following cerebrovascular disease (I69. with final characters -28)

R47.81 Slurred speech

R47.82 Fluency disorder in conditions classified elsewhere
Stuttering in conditions classified elsewhere
Code first underlying disease or condition, such as:
Parkinson's disease (G20)
EXCLUDES 1 adult onset fluency disorder (F98.5)
childhood onset fluency disorder (F80.81)
fluency disorder (stuttering) following cerebrovascular disease (I69. with final characters-23)

R47.89 Other speech disturbances

R47.9 Unspecified speech disturbances

✓4th **R48 Dyslexia and other symbolic dysfunctions, not elsewhere classified**
EXCLUDES 1 specific developmental disorders of scholastic skills (F81.-)

R48.0 Dyslexia and alexia

R48.1 Agnosia
Astereognosia (astereognosis)
Autotopagnosia
EXCLUDES 1 visual object agnosia (R48.3)

R48.2 Apraxia
EXCLUDES 1 apraxia following cerebrovascular disease (I69. with final characters -90)

R48.3 Visual agnosia
Prosopagnosia
Simultanagnosia (asimultagnosia)

R48.8 Other symbolic dysfunctions
Acalculia
Agraphia

R48.9 Unspecified symbolic dysfunctions

N Newborn: 0   P Pediatric: 0-17   M Maternity: 12-55   A Adult: 15-124   MCC Major CC Condition   PDxMCC PDx acts as own MCC   CC CC Condition   PDxCC PDx acts as own CC

882
ICD-10-CM 2016

✔4ᵗʰ **R49 Voice and resonance disorders**
> **EXCLUDES 1** *psychogenic voice and resonance disorders (F44.4)*

R49.0 Dysphonia
Hoarseness

R49.1 Aphonia
Loss of voice

✔5ᵗʰ **R49.2 Hypernasality and hyponasality**

R49.21 Hypernasality

R49.22 Hyponasality

R49.8 Other voice and resonance disorders

R49.9 Unspecified voice and resonance disorder
Change in voice NOS
Resonance disorder NOS

General symptoms and signs (R50-R69)

✔4ᵗʰ **R50 Fever of other and unknown origin**
> **EXCLUDES 1** *chills without fever (R68.83)*
> *febrile convulsions (R56.0-)*
> *fever of unknown origin during labor (O75.2)*
> *fever of unknown origin in newborn (P81.9)*
> *hypothermia due to illness (R68.0)*
> *malignant hyperthermia due to anesthesia (T88.3)*
> *puerperal pyrexia NOS (O86.4)*

R50.2 Drug induced fever
Use additional code for adverse effect, if applicable, to identify drug (T36-T50 with fifth or sixth character 5)
> **EXCLUDES 1** *postvaccination (postimmunization) fever (R50.83)*

✔5ᵗʰ **R50.8 Other specified fever**

R50.81 Fever presenting with conditions classified elsewhere
Code first underlying condition when associated fever is present, such as with:
leukemia (C91-C95)
neutropenia (D70.-)
sickle-cell disease (D57.-)
AHA: 2014, 4Q, 22

R50.82 Postprocedural fever
> **EXCLUDES 1** *postprocedural infection (T81.4)*
> *posttransfusion fever (R50.84)*
> *postvaccination (postimmunization) fever (R50.83)*

R50.83 Postvaccination fever
Postimmunization fever

R50.84 Febrile nonhemolytic transfusion reaction
FNHTR
Posttransfusion fever

R50.9 Fever, unspecified
Fever NOS	Hyperpyrexia NOS
Fever of unknown origin [FUO]	Persistent fever
Fever with chills	Pyrexia NOS
Fever with rigors	

R51 Headache
Facial pain NOS
> **EXCLUDES 1** *atypical face pain (G50.1)*
> *migraine and other headache syndromes (G43-G44)*
> *trigeminal neuralgia (G50.0)*

R52 Pain, unspecified
Acute pain NOS
Generalized pain NOS
Pain NOS
> **EXCLUDES 1** *acute and chronic pain, not elsewhere classified (G89.-)*
> *localized pain, unspecified type—code to pain by site, such as:*
> *abdomen pain (R10.-)*
> *back pain (M54.9)*
> *breast pain (N64.4)*
> *chest pain (R07.1-R07.9)*
> *ear pain (H92.0-)*
> *eye pain (H57.1)*
> *headache (R51)*
> *joint pain (M25.5-)*
> *limb pain (M79.6-)*
> *lumbar region pain (M54.5)*
> *pelvic and perineal pain (R10.2)*
> *renal colic (N23)*
> *shoulder pain (M25.51-)*
> *spine pain (M54.-)*
> *throat pain (R07.0)*
> *tongue pain (K14.6)*
> *tooth pain (K08.8)*
> *pain disorders exclusively related to psychological factors (F45.41)*

✔4ᵗʰ **R53 Malaise and fatigue**

R53.0 Neoplastic (malignant) related fatigue
Code first associated neoplasm

R53.1 Weakness
Asthenia NOS
> **EXCLUDES 1** *age-related weakness (R54)*
> *muscle weakness (M62.8-)*
> *senile asthenia (R54)*

AHA: 2015, 1Q, 25

R53.2 Functional quadriplegia   MCC
Complete immobility due to severe physical disability or frailty
> **EXCLUDES 1** *frailty NOS (R54)*
> *hysterical paralysis (F44.4)*
> *immobility syndrome (M62.3)*
> *neurologic quadriplegia (G82.5-)*
> *quadriplegia (G82.50)*

CC Excl: E08.40-E08.49, E08.618-E08.638, E08.649-E08.8, E09.40-E09.49, E09.618-E09.638, E09.649-E09.8, E10.40-E10.49, E10.618-E10.638, E10.649, E10.69-E10.8, E11.40-E11.49, E11.618-E11.638, E11.649, E11.69-E11.8, E13.40-E13.49, E13.618-E13.638, E13.649-E13.8, G04.1, G32.89, G80.0-G80.2, G80.4-G83.9, G90.1, G93.81, G93.89-G93.9, G96.8-G96.9, G98.0-G98.8, G99.8, Q06.0-Q06.1, Q06.3, Q06.8-Q06.9, Q07.8-Q07.9, R53.2

✔5ᵗʰ **R53.8 Other malaise and fatigue**
> **EXCLUDES 1** *combat exhaustion and fatigue (F43.0)*
> *congenital debility (P96.9)*
> *exhaustion and fatigue due to depressive episode (F32.-)*
> *exhaustion and fatigue due to excessive exertion (T73.3)*
> *exhaustion and fatigue due to exposure (T73.2)*
> *exhaustion and fatigue due to heat (T67.-)*
> *exhaustion and fatigue due to pregnancy (O26.8-)*
> *exhaustion and fatigue due to recurrent depressive episode (F33)*
> *exhaustion and fatigue due to senile debility (R54)*

R53.81 Other malaise
Chronic debility	Malaise NOS
Debility NOS	Nervous debility
General physical deterioration	
> **EXCLUDES 1** *age-related physical debility (R54)*

R53.82 Chronic fatigue, unspecified
Chronic fatigue syndrome NOS
> **EXCLUDES 1** *postviral fatigue syndrome (G93.3)*

R53.83 Other fatigue
Fatigue NOS	Lethargy
Lack of energy	Tiredness

R54 Age-related physical debility   A
Frailty	Senile asthenia
Old age	Senile debility
Senescence	
> **EXCLUDES 1** *age-related cognitive decline (R41.81)*
> *senile psychosis (F03)*
> *senility NOS (R41.81)*

R55 Syncope and collapse
Blackout	Vasovagal attack
Fainting	
> **EXCLUDES 1** *cardiogenic shock (R57.0)*
> *carotid sinus syncope (G90.01)*
> *heat syncope (T67.1)*
> *neurocirculatory asthenia (F45.8)*
> *neurogenic orthostatic hypotension (G90.3)*
> *orthostatic hypotension (I95.1)*
> *postprocedural shock (T81.1-)*
> *psychogenic syncope (F48.8)*
> *shock NOS (R57.9)*
> *shock complicating or following abortion or ectopic or molar pregnancy (O00-O07, O08.3)*
> *shock complicating or following labor and delivery (O75.1)*
> *Stokes-Adams attack (I45.9)*
> *unconsciousness NOS (R40.2-)*

✔ Additional Character Required   ✔x7ᵗʰ Placeholder Alert   Unacceptable PDx   Manifestation   Hospital Acquired Condition   **EXCLUDES 1** Not Coded Here   **EXCLUDES 2** Not Included Here

☑4th **R56** **Convulsions, not elsewhere classified**
> **EXCLUDES 1** dissociative convulsions and seizures (F44.5)
> epileptic convulsions and seizures (G40.-)
> newborn convulsions and seizures (P90)

☑5th **R56.0** **Febrile convulsions**

R56.00 **Simple febrile convulsions** CC
Febrile convulsion NOS
Febrile seizure NOS
CC Excl: G32.89, G40.001-G40.919, G89.0-G89.4, G93.81, G93.89-G93.9, G96.8-G96.9, G98.0-G98.8, G99.8, P90, P91.8-P91.9, R41.0-R41.3, R41.82, R41.9, R44.8-R44.9, R45.83-R45.84, R46.0-R46.89, R52, R56.00-R56.9, R68.0-R68.19, R68.81-R68.83, R68.89-R69

R56.01 **Complex febrile convulsions** CC
Atypical febrile seizure
Complex febrile seizure
Complicated febrile seizure
> **EXCLUDES 1** status epilepticus (G40.901)
CC Excl: See code: R56.00

R56.1 **Post traumatic seizures** CC
> **EXCLUDES 1** post traumatic epilepsy (G40.-)
CC Excl: E08.40-E08.49, E09.40-E09.49, E10.40-E10.49, E11.40-E11.49, E13.40-E13.49, G32.89, G40.001-G40.509, G40.801-G40.804, G40.811-G40.814, G40.821-G40.B19, G93.81, G93.89-G93.9, G96.8-G96.9, G98.0-G98.8, G99.8, R56.1

R56.9 **Unspecified convulsions**
Convulsion disorder
Fit NOS
Recurrent convulsions
Seizure(s) (convulsive) NOS

☑4th **R57** **Shock, not elsewhere classified**
> **EXCLUDES 1** anaphylactic shock NOS (T78.2)
> anaphylactic reaction or shock due to adverse food reaction (T78.0-)
> anaphylactic shock due to adverse effect of correct drug or medicament properly administered (T88.6)
> anaphylactic shock due to serum (T80.5-)
> anesthetic shock (T88.3)
> electric shock (T75.4)
> obstetric shock (O75.1)
> postprocedural shock (T81.1-)
> psychic shock (F43.0)
> septic shock (R65.21)
> shock complicating or following ectopic or molar pregnancy (O00-O07, O08.3)
> shock due to lightning (T75.01)
> traumatic shock (T79.4)
> toxic shock syndrome (A48.3)

CC Excl: For CC/MCC codes in category R57, unless otherwise noted: G89.0-G89.4, R09.89, R41.0-R41.3, R41.82, R41.9, R44.8-R44.9, R45.83-R45.84, R46.0-R46.89, R52, R57.0-R57.9, R65.21-R68.19, R68.81-R68.83, R68.89-R69

10 **R57.0** **Cardiogenic shock** MCC
10 **R57.1** **Hypovolemic shock** MCC
10 **R57.8** **Other shock** MCC
R57.9 **Shock, unspecified** CC
Failure of peripheral circulation NOS

R58 **Hemorrhage, not elsewhere classified**
Hemorrhage NOS
> **EXCLUDES 1** hemorrhage included with underlying conditions, such as:
> acute duodenal ulcer with hemorrhage (K26.0)
> acute gastritis with bleeding (K29.01)
> ulcerative enterocolitis with rectal bleeding (K51.01)

☑4th **R59** **Enlarged lymph nodes**
> **INCLUDES** swollen glands
> **EXCLUDES 1** acute lymphadenitis (L04.-)
> chronic lymphadenitis (I88.1)
> lymphadenitis NOS (I88.9)
> mesenteric (acute) (chronic) lymphadenitis (I88.0)

R59.0 **Localized enlarged lymph nodes**
R59.1 **Generalized enlarged lymph nodes**
Lymphadenopathy NOS
R59.9 **Enlarged lymph nodes, unspecified**

☑4th **R60** **Edema, not elsewhere classified**
> **EXCLUDES 1** angioneurotic edema (T78.3)
> ascites (R18.-)
> cerebral edema (G93.6)
> cerebral edema due to birth injury (P11.0)
> edema of larynx (J38.4)
> edema of nasopharynx (J39.2)
> edema of pharynx (J39.2)
> gestational edema (O12.0-)
> hereditary edema (Q82.0)
> hydrops fetalis NOS (P83.2)
> hydrothorax (J94.8)
> nutritional edema (E40-E46)
> hydrops fetalis NOS (P83.2)
> newborn edema (P83.3)
> pulmonary edema (J81.-)

R60.0 **Localized edema**
R60.1 **Generalized edema**
R60.9 **Edema, unspecified**
Fluid retention NOS

R61 **Generalized hyperhidrosis**
Excessive sweating
Night sweats
Secondary hyperhidrosis
Code first, if applicable, menopausal and female climacteric states (N95.1)
> **EXCLUDES 1** focal (primary) (secondary) hyperhidrosis (L74.5-)
> Frey's syndrome (L74.52)
> localized (primary) (secondary) hyperhidrosis (L74.5-)

☑4th **R62** **Lack of expected normal physiological development in childhood and adults**
> **EXCLUDES 1** delayed puberty (E30.0)
> gonadal dysgenesis (Q99.1)
> hypopituitarism (E23.0)

R62.0 **Delayed milestone in childhood** P
Delayed attainment of expected physiological developmental stage
Late talker
Late walker

☑5th **R62.5** **Other and unspecified lack of expected normal physiological development in childhood**
> **EXCLUDES 1** HIV disease resulting in failure to thrive (B20)
> physical retardation due to malnutrition (E45)

R62.50 **Unspecified lack of expected normal physiological development in childhood** P
Infantilism NOS

R62.51 **Failure to thrive (child)** P
Failure to gain weight
> **EXCLUDES 1** failure to thrive in child under 28 days old (P92.6)

R62.52 **Short stature (child)** P
Lack of growth
Physical retardation
Short stature NOS
> **EXCLUDES 1** short stature due to endocrine disorder (E34.3)

R62.59 **Other lack of expected normal physiological development in childhood** P

R62.7 **Adult failure to thrive** A

☑4th **R63** **Symptoms and signs concerning food and fluid intake**
> **EXCLUDES 1** bulimia NOS (F50.2)
> eating disorders of nonorganic origin (F50.-)
> malnutrition (E40-E46)

R63.0 **Anorexia**
Loss of appetite
> **EXCLUDES 1** anorexia nervosa (F50.0-)
> loss of appetite of nonorganic origin (F50.8)

R63.1 **Polydipsia**
Excessive thirst

R63.2 **Polyphagia**
Excessive eating
Hyperalimentation NOS

R63.3 **Feeding difficulties**
Feeding problem (elderly) (infant) NOS
> **EXCLUDES 1** feeding problems of newborn (P92.-)
> infant feeding disorder of nonorganic origin (F98.2-)

R63.4 **Abnormal weight loss**

---

10 MCC = only if patient is discharged alive.

R63.5 Abnormal weight gain
> *EXCLUDES 1* excessive weight gain in pregnancy (O26.0-)
> obesity (E66.-)

R63.6 Underweight
> Use additional code to identify body mass index (BMI), if known (Z68.-)
> *EXCLUDES 1* abnormal weight loss (R63.4)
> anorexia nervosa (F50.0-)
> malnutrition (E40-E46)

R63.8 Other symptoms and signs concerning food and fluid intake

R64 Cachexia `CC`
> Wasting syndrome
> Code first underlying condition, if known
> *EXCLUDES 1* abnormal weight loss (R63.4)
> nutritional marasmus (E41)
> **CC Excl:** G89.0-G89.4, R41.0-R41.3, R41.82, R41.9, R44.8-R44.9, R45.83-R45.84, R46.0-R46.89, R52, R64, R68.0-R68.19, R68.81-R68.83, R68.89-R69

√4ᵗʰ R65 Symptoms and signs specifically associated with systemic inflammation and infection
> **CC Excl: For CC/MCC codes in category R65, unless otherwise noted:** A02.1, A20.7, A22.7, A26.7, A32.7, A39.2-A39.4, A40.0-A40.1, A40.8-A41.9, A42.7, A48.2-A48.4, A48.8-A49.9, A54.86, B00.7, B37.7, B92, B94.2-B96.89, R65.10-R65.20, M00.011-M00.012, M00.021-M00.022, M00.031-M00.032, M00.041-M00.042, M00.051-M00.052, M00.061-M00.062, M00.071-M00.072, Z16.10-Z16.39

√5ᵗʰ R65.1 Systemic inflammatory response syndrome [SIRS] of non-infectious origin
> Code first underlying condition, such as:
> heatstroke (T67.0)
> injury and trauma (S00-T88)
> *EXCLUDES 1* sepsis—code to infection
> severe sepsis (R65.2)

> **R65.10 Systemic inflammatory response syndrome [SIRS] of non-infectious origin without acute organ dysfunction** `CC`
> Systemic inflammatory response syndrome (SIRS) NOS

> **R65.11 Systemic inflammatory response syndrome [SIRS] of non-infectious origin with acute organ dysfunction** `MCC`
> Use additional code to identify specific acute organ dysfunction, such as:
> acute kidney failure (N17.-)
> acute respiratory failure (J96.0-)
> critical illness myopathy (G72.81)
> critical illness polyneuropathy (G62.81)
> disseminated intravascular coagulopathy [DIC] (D65)
> encephalopathy (metabolic) (septic) (G93.41)
> hepatic failure (K72.0-)

√5ᵗʰ R65.2 Severe sepsis
> Infection with associated acute organ dysfunction
> Sepsis with acute organ dysfunction
> Sepsis with multiple organ dysfunction
> Systemic inflammatory response syndrome due to infectious process with acute organ dysfunction
> Code first underlying infection, such as:
> infection following a procedure (T81.4)
> infections following infusion, transfusion and therapeutic injection (T80.2-)
> puerperal sepsis (O85)
> sepsis following complete or unspecified spontaneous abortion (O03.87)
> sepsis following ectopic and molar pregnancy (O08.82)
> sepsis following incomplete spontaneous abortion (O03.37)
> sepsis following (induced) termination of pregnancy (O04.87)
> sepsis NOS (A41.9)
> Use additional code to identify specific acute organ dysfunction, such as:
> acute kidney failure (N17.-)
> acute respiratory failure (J96.0-)
> critical illness myopathy (G72.81)
> critical illness polyneuropathy (G62.81)
> disseminated intravascular coagulopathy [DIC] (D65)
> encephalopathy (metabolic) (septic) (G93.41)
> hepatic failure (K72.0-)

> **R65.20 Severe sepsis without septic shock** `MCC`
> Severe sepsis NOS
> **AHA:** 2013, 4Q, 119

> **R65.21 Severe sepsis with septic shock** `PDx MCC` `MCC`
> **CC Excl:** G89.0-G89.4, R09.89, R41.0-R41.3, R41.82, R41.9, R44.8-R44.9, R45.83-R45.84, R46.0-R46.89, R52, R57.0-R57.9, R65.21-R68.19, R68.81-R68.83, R68.89-R69

√4ᵗʰ R68 Other general symptoms and signs
> **R68.0 Hypothermia, not associated with low environmental temperature**
> *EXCLUDES 1* hypothermia due to anesthesia (T88.51)
> hypothermia due to low environmental temperature (T68)
> hypothermia NOS (accidental) (T68)
> newborn hypothermia (P80.-)

√5ᵗʰ R68.1 Nonspecific symptoms peculiar to infancy
> *EXCLUDES 1* colic, infantile (R10.83)
> neonatal cerebral irritability (P91.3)
> teething syndrome (K00.7)

> **R68.11 Excessive crying of infant (baby)** `P`
> *EXCLUDES 1* excessive crying of child, adolescent, or adult (R45.83)

> **R68.12 Fussy infant (baby)** `P`
> Irritable infant

> **R68.13 Apparent life threatening event in infant [ALTE]** `P`
> Apparent life threatening event in newborn
> Code first confirmed diagnosis, if known
> Use additional code(s) for associated signs and symptoms if no confirmed diagnosis established, or if signs and symptoms are not associated routinely with confirmed diagnosis, or provide additional information for cause of ALTE

> **R68.19 Other nonspecific symptoms peculiar to infancy** `P`

> **R68.2 Dry mouth, unspecified**
> *EXCLUDES 1* dry mouth due to dehydration (E86.0)
> dry mouth due to sicca syndrome [Sjögren] (M35.0-)
> salivary gland hyposecretion (K11.7)

> **R68.3 Clubbing of fingers**
> Clubbing of nails
> *EXCLUDES 1* congenital clubfinger (Q68.1)

√5ᵗʰ R68.8 Other general symptoms and signs
> **R68.81 Early satiety**
> **R68.82 Decreased libido** `A`
> Decreased sexual desire
> **R68.83 Chills (without fever)**
> Chills NOS
> *EXCLUDES 1* chills with fever (R50.9)
> **R68.84 Jaw pain**
> Mandibular pain
> Maxilla pain
> *EXCLUDES 1* temporomandibular joint arthralgia (M26.62)
> **R68.89 Other general symptoms and signs**

R69 Illness, unspecified
> Unknown and unspecified cases of morbidity

Abnormal findings on examination of blood, without diagnosis (R70-R79)
> *EXCLUDES 1* abnormalities (of)(on):
> abnormal findings on antenatal screening of mother (O28.-)
> coagulation hemorrhagic disorders (D65-D68)
> lipids (E78.-)
> platelets and thrombocytes (D69.-)
> white blood cells classified elsewhere (D70-D72)
> diagnostic abnormal findings classified elsewhere—see Alphabetical Index
> hemorrhagic and hematological disorders of newborn (P50-P61)

√4ᵗʰ R70 Elevated erythrocyte sedimentation rate and abnormality of plasma viscosity
> **R70.0 Elevated erythrocyte sedimentation rate**
> **R70.1 Abnormal plasma viscosity**

√4ᵗʰ R71 Abnormality of red blood cells
> *EXCLUDES 1* anemias (D50-D64)
> anemia of premature infant (P61.2)
> benign (familial) polycythemia (D75.0)
> congenital anemias (P61.2-P61.4)
> newborn anemia due to isoimmunization (P55.-)
> polycythemia neonatorum (P61.1)
> polycythemia NOS (D75.1)
> polycythemia vera (D45)
> secondary polycythemia (D75.1)

> **R71.0 Precipitous drop in hematocrit** `CC`
> Drop (precipitous) in hemoglobin
> Drop in hematocrit
> **CC Excl:** D62, D64.4-D64.9

✔ Additional Character Required   ✔x7ᵗʰ Placeholder Alert   Unacceptable PDx   `Manifestation`   `Hospital Acquired Condition`   *EXCLUDES 1* Not Coded Here   *EXCLUDES 2* Not Included Here

Chapter 18. Symptoms, Signs, and Abnormal Clinical and Laboratory Findings, Not Elsewhere Classified

R71.8   Other abnormality of red blood cells
Abnormal red-cell morphology NOS   Anisocytosis
Abnormal red-cell volume NOS   Poikilocytosis

✓4ᵗʰ R73   Elevated blood glucose level
> EXCLUDES 1   diabetes mellitus (E08-E13)
> diabetes mellitus in pregnancy, childbirth and the puerperium (O24.-)
> neonatal disorders (P70.0-P70.2)
> postsurgical hypoinsulinemia (E89.1)

✓5ᵗʰ R73.0   Abnormal glucose
> EXCLUDES 1   abnormal glucose in pregnancy (O99.81-)
> diabetes mellitus (E08-E13)
> dysmetabolic syndrome X (E88.81)
> gestational diabetes (O24.4-)
> glycosuria (R81)
> hypoglycemia (E16.2)

    R73.01   Impaired fasting glucose
        Elevated fasting glucose

    R73.02   Impaired glucose tolerance (oral)
        Elevated glucose tolerance

    R73.09   Other abnormal glucose
        Abnormal glucose NOS
        Abnormal non-fasting glucose tolerance
        Latent diabetes
        Prediabetes

R73.9   Hyperglycemia, unspecified

✓4ᵗʰ R74   Abnormal serum enzyme levels
R74.0   Nonspecific elevation of levels of transaminase and lactic acid dehydrogenase [LDH]

R74.8   Abnormal levels of other serum enzymes
Abnormal level of acid phosphatase
Abnormal level of alkaline phosphatase
Abnormal level of amylase
Abnormal level of lipase [triacylglycerol lipase]

R74.9   Abnormal serum enzyme level, unspecified

R75   Inconclusive laboratory evidence of human immunodeficiency virus [HIV]
Nonconclusive HIV-test finding in infants
> EXCLUDES 1   asymptomatic human immunodeficiency virus [HIV] infection status (Z21)
> human immunodeficiency virus [HIV] disease (B20)

✓4ᵗʰ R76   Other abnormal immunological findings in serum
R76.0   Raised antibody titer
> EXCLUDES 1   isoimmunization in pregnancy (O36.0-O36.1)
> isoimmunization affecting newborn (P55.-)

✓5ᵗʰ R76.1   Nonspecific reaction to test for tuberculosis
    R76.11   Nonspecific reaction to tuberculin skin test without active tuberculosis
        Abnormal result of Mantoux test
        PPD positive
        Tuberculin (skin test) positive
        Tuberculin (skin test) reactor
>   EXCLUDES 1   nonspecific reaction to cell mediated immunity measurement of gamma interferon antigen response without active tuberculosis (R76.12)

    R76.12   Nonspecific reaction to cell mediated immunity measurement of gamma interferon antigen response without active tuberculosis
        Nonspecific reaction to QuantiFERON-TB test (QFT) without active tuberculosis
>   EXCLUDES 1   nonspecific reaction to tuberculin skin test without active tuberculosis (R76.11)
> positive tuberculin skin test (R76.11)

R76.8   Other specified abnormal immunological findings in serum
Raised level of immunoglobulins NOS

R76.9   Abnormal immunological finding in serum, unspecified

✓4ᵗʰ R77   Other abnormalities of plasma proteins
> EXCLUDES 1   disorders of plasma-protein metabolism (E88.0)

R77.0   Abnormality of albumin
R77.1   Abnormality of globulin
Hyperglobulinemia NOS
R77.2   Abnormality of alphafetoprotein
R77.8   Other specified abnormalities of plasma proteins
R77.9   Abnormality of plasma protein, unspecified

✓4ᵗʰ R78   Findings of drugs and other substances, not normally found in blood
Use additional code to identify any retained foreign body, if applicable (Z18.-)
> EXCLUDES 1   mental or behavioral disorders due to psychoactive substance use (F10-F19)

R78.0   Finding of alcohol in blood
Use additional external cause code (Y90.-), for detail regarding alcohol level

R78.1   Finding of opiate drug in blood
R78.2   Finding of cocaine in blood
R78.3   Finding of hallucinogen in blood
R78.4   Finding of other drugs of addictive potential in blood
R78.5   Finding of other psychotropic drug in blood
R78.6   Finding of steroid agent in blood

✓5ᵗʰ R78.7   Finding of abnormal level of heavy metals in blood
    R78.71   Abnormal lead level in blood
>   EXCLUDES 1   lead poisoning (T56.0-)
    R78.79   Finding of abnormal level of heavy metals in blood

✓5ᵗʰ R78.8   Finding of other specified substances, not normally found in blood
    R78.81   Bacteremia   CC
>   EXCLUDES 1   sepsis—code to specified infection (A00-B99)
        CC Excl: B34.9, E07.81, G89.0-G89.4, R41.0-R41.3, R41.82, R41.9, R44.8-R44.9, R45.83-R45.84, R46.0-R46.89, R52, R68.0-R68.19, R68.81-R68.83, R68.89-R69, R70.1, R77.0-R77.9, R78.1-R78.6, R78.81, R78.9, R79.1-R79.89, R97.2

    R78.89   Finding of other specified substances, not normally found in blood
        Finding of abnormal level of lithium in blood

R78.9   Finding of unspecified substance, not normally found in blood

✓4ᵗʰ R79   Other abnormal findings of blood chemistry
Use additional code to identify any retained foreign body, if applicable (Z18.-)
> EXCLUDES 1   abnormality of fluid, electrolyte or acid-base balance (E86-E87)
> asymptomatic hyperuricemia (E79.0)
> hyperglycemia NOS (R73.9)
> hypoglycemia NOS (E16.2)
> neonatal hypoglycemia (P70.3-P70.4)
> specific findings indicating disorder of amino-acid metabolism (E70-E72)
> specific findings indicating disorder of carbohydrate metabolism (E73-E74)
> specific findings indicating disorder of lipid metabolism (E75.-)

R79.0   Abnormal level of blood mineral
Abnormal blood level of cobalt
Abnormal blood level of copper
Abnormal blood level of iron
Abnormal blood level of magnesium
Abnormal blood level of mineral NEC
Abnormal blood level of zinc
> EXCLUDES 1   abnormal level of lithium (R78.89)
> disorders of mineral metabolism (E83.-)
> neonatal hypomagnesemia (P71.2)
> nutritional mineral deficiency (E58-E61)

R79.1   Abnormal coagulation profile
Abnormal or prolonged bleeding time
Abnormal or prolonged coagulation time
Abnormal or prolonged partial thromboplastin time [PTT]
Abnormal or prolonged prothrombin time [PT]
> EXCLUDES 1   coagulation defects (D68.-)

✓5ᵗʰ R79.8   Other specified abnormal findings of blood chemistry
    R79.81   Abnormal blood-gas level
    R79.82   Elevated C-reactive protein [CRP]
    R79.89   Other specified abnormal findings of blood chemistry

R79.9   Abnormal finding of blood chemistry, unspecified

N Newborn: 0   P Pediatric: 0-17   M Maternity: 12-55   A Adult: 15-124   MCC Major CC Condition   PDxMCC PDx acts as own MCC   CC CC Condition   PDxCC PDx acts as own CC

886   ICD-10-CM 2016

Abnormal findings on examination of urine, without diagnosis (R80-R82)

> *EXCLUDES 1*   *abnormal findings on antenatal screening of mother (O28.-)*
> *diagnostic abnormal findings classified elsewhere—see Alphabetical Index*
> *specific findings indicating disorder of amino-acid metabolism (E70-E72)*

✓4ᵗʰ R80 Proteinuria
> *EXCLUDES 1*   *gestational proteinuria (O12.1-)*

R80.0 Isolated proteinuria
Idiopathic proteinuria
> *EXCLUDES 1*   *isolated proteinuria with specific morphological lesion (N06.-)*

R80.1 Persistent proteinuria, unspecified

R80.2 Orthostatic proteinuria, unspecified
Postural proteinuria

R80.3 Bence Jones proteinuria

R80.8 Other proteinuria

R80.9 Proteinuria, unspecified
Albuminuria NOS

R81 Glycosuria
> *EXCLUDES 1*   *renal glycosuria (E74.8)*

✓4ᵗʰ R82 Other and unspecified abnormal findings in urine
Chromoabnormalities in urine
Use additional code to identify any retained foreign body, if applicable (Z18.-)
> *EXCLUDES 2*   *hematuria (R31.-)*

R82.0 Chyluria   `CC`
> *EXCLUDES 1*   *filarial chyluria (B74.-)*
> **CC Excl:** G89.0-G89.4, R41.0-R41.3, R41.82, R41.9, R44.8-R44.9, R45.83-R45.84, R46.0-R46.89, R52, R68.0-R68.19, R68.81-R68.83, R68.89-R69, R82.0, R82.5-R82.99

R82.1 Myoglobinuria   `CC`
> **CC Excl:** G89.0-G89.4, R41.0-R41.3, R41.82, R41.9, R44.8-R44.9, R45.83-R45.84, R46.0-R46.89, R52, R68.0-R68.19, R68.81-R68.83, R68.89-R69, R82.1, R82.3, R82.5-R82.99

R82.2 Biliuria

R82.3 Hemoglobinuria
> *EXCLUDES 1*   *hemoglobinuria due to hemolysis from external causes NEC (D59.6)*
> *hemoglobinuria due to paroxysmal nocturnal [Marchiafava-Micheli] (D59.5)*

R82.4 Acetonuria
Ketonuria

R82.5 Elevated urine levels of drugs, medicaments and biological substances
Elevated urine levels of catecholamines
Elevated urine levels of indoleacetic acid
Elevated urine levels of 17-ketosteroids
Elevated urine levels of steroids

R82.6 Abnormal urine levels of substances chiefly nonmedicinal as to source
Abnormal urine level of heavy metals

R82.7 Abnormal findings on microbiological examination of urine
Positive culture findings of urine
> *EXCLUDES 1*   *colonization status (Z22.-)*

R82.8 Abnormal findings on cytological and histological examination of urine

✓5ᵗʰ R82.9 Other and unspecified abnormal findings in urine
R82.90 Unspecified abnormal findings in urine

R82.91 Other chromoabnormalities of urine
Chromoconversion (dipstick)
Idiopathic dipstick converts positive for blood with no cellular forms in sediment
> *EXCLUDES 1*   *hemoglobinuria (R82.3)*
> *myoglobinuria (R82.1)*

R82.99 Other abnormal findings in urine
Cells and casts in urine
Crystalluria
Melanuria

Abnormal findings on examination of other body fluids, substances and tissues, without diagnosis (R83-R89)

> *EXCLUDES 1*   *abnormal findings on antenatal screening of mother (O28.-)*
> *diagnostic abnormal findings classified elsewhere—see Alphabetical Index*
> *EXCLUDES 2*   *abnormal findings on examination of blood, without diagnosis (R70-R79)*
> *abnormal findings on examination of urine, without diagnosis (R80-R82)*
> *abnormal tumor markers (R97.-)*

✓4ᵗʰ R83 Abnormal findings in cerebrospinal fluid
R83.0 Abnormal level of enzymes in cerebrospinal fluid

R83.1 Abnormal level of hormones in cerebrospinal fluid

R83.2 Abnormal level of other drugs, medicaments and biological substances in cerebrospinal fluid

R83.3 Abnormal level of substances chiefly nonmedicinal as to source in cerebrospinal fluid

R83.4 Abnormal immunological findings in cerebrospinal fluid

R83.5 Abnormal microbiological findings in cerebrospinal fluid
Positive culture findings in cerebrospinal fluid
> *EXCLUDES 1*   *colonization status (Z22.-)*

R83.6 Abnormal cytological findings in cerebrospinal fluid

R83.8 Other abnormal findings in cerebrospinal fluid
Abnormal chromosomal findings in cerebrospinal fluid

R83.9 Unspecified abnormal finding in cerebrospinal fluid

✓4ᵗʰ R84 Abnormal findings in specimens from respiratory organs and thorax
Abnormal findings in bronchial washings
Abnormal findings in nasal secretions
Abnormal findings in pleural fluid
Abnormal findings in sputum
Abnormal findings in throat scrapings
> *EXCLUDES 1*   *blood-stained sputum (R04.2)*

R84.0 Abnormal level of enzymes in specimens from respiratory organs and thorax

R84.1 Abnormal level of hormones in specimens from respiratory organs and thorax

R84.2 Abnormal level of other drugs, medicaments and biological substances in specimens from respiratory organs and thorax

R84.3 Abnormal level of substances chiefly nonmedicinal as to source in specimens from respiratory organs and thorax

R84.4 Abnormal immunological findings in specimens from respiratory organs and thorax

R84.5 Abnormal microbiological findings in specimens from respiratory organs and thorax
Positive culture findings in specimens from respiratory organs and thorax
> *EXCLUDES 1*   *colonization status (Z22.-)*

R84.6 Abnormal cytological findings in specimens from respiratory organs and thorax

R84.7 Abnormal histological findings in specimens from respiratory organs and thorax

R84.8 Other abnormal findings in specimens from respiratory organs and thorax
Abnormal chromosomal findings in specimens from respiratory organs and thorax

R84.9 Unspecified abnormal finding in specimens from respiratory organs and thorax

✓4ᵗʰ R85 Abnormal findings in specimens from digestive organs and abdominal cavity
> *INCLUDES*   *abnormal findings in peritoneal fluid*
> *abnormal findings in saliva*
> *EXCLUDES 1*   *cloudy peritoneal dialysis effluent (R88.0)*
> *fecal abnormalities (R19.5)*

R85.0 Abnormal level of enzymes in specimens from digestive organs and abdominal cavity

R85.1 Abnormal level of hormones in specimens from digestive organs and abdominal cavity

R85.2 Abnormal level of other drugs, medicaments and biological substances in specimens from digestive organs and abdominal cavity

R85.3 Abnormal level of substances chiefly nonmedicinal as to source in specimens from digestive organs and abdominal cavity

R85.4 Abnormal immunological findings in specimens from digestive organs and abdominal cavity

✓ Additional Character Required   ✓x7ᵗʰ Placeholder Alert   Unacceptable PDx   Manifestation   Hospital Acquired Condition   *EXCLUDES 1* Not Coded Here   *EXCLUDES 2* Not Included Here

ICD-10-CM 2016   **887**

R85.5 **Abnormal microbiological findings in specimens from digestive organs and abdominal cavity**
Positive culture findings in specimens from digestive organs and abdominal cavity
EXCLUDES 1 colonization status (Z22.-)

R85.6 **Abnormal cytological findings in specimens from digestive organs and abdominal cavity**

R85.61 **Abnormal cytologic smear of anus**
EXCLUDES 1 abnormal cytological findings in specimens from other digestive organs and abdominal cavity (R85.69)
anal intraepithelial neoplasia I [AIN I] (K62.82)
anal intraepithelial neoplasia II [AIN II] (K62.82)
anal intraepithelial neoplasia III [AIN III] (D01.3)
carcinoma in situ of anus (histologically confirmed) (D01.3)
dysplasia (mild) (moderate) of anus (histologically confirmed) (K62.82)
severe dysplasia of anus (histologically confirmed) (D01.3)
EXCLUDES 2 anal high risk human papillomavirus (HPV) DNA test positive (R85.81)
anal low risk human papillomavirus (HPV) DNA test positive (R85.82)

R85.610 **Atypical squamous cells of undetermined significance on cytologic smear of anus [ASC-US]**

R85.611 **Atypical squamous cells cannot exclude high grade squamous intraepithelial lesion on cytologic smear of anus [ASC-H]**

R85.612 **Low grade squamous intraepithelial lesion on cytologic smear of anus [LGSIL]**

R85.613 **High grade squamous intraepithelial lesion on cytologic smear of anus [HGSIL]**

R85.614 **Cytologic evidence of malignancy on smear of anus**

R85.615 **Unsatisfactory cytologic smear of anus**
Inadequate sample of cytologic smear of anus

R85.616 **Satisfactory anal smear but lacking transformation zone**

R85.618 **Other abnormal cytological findings on specimens from anus**

R85.619 **Unspecified abnormal cytological findings in specimens from anus**
Abnormal anal cytology NOS
Atypical glandular cells of anus NOS

R85.69 **Abnormal cytological findings in specimens from other digestive organs and abdominal cavity**

R85.7 **Abnormal histological findings in specimens from digestive organs and abdominal cavity**

R85.8 **Other abnormal findings in specimens from digestive organs and abdominal cavity**

R85.81 **Anal high risk human papillomavirus [HPV] DNA test positive**
EXCLUDES 1 anogenital warts due to human papillomavirus (HPV) (A63.0)
condyloma acuminatum (A63.0)

R85.82 **Anal low risk human papillomavirus [HPV] DNA test positive**
Use additional code for associated human papillomavirus (B97.7)

R85.89 **Other abnormal findings in specimens from digestive organs and abdominal cavity**
Abnormal chromosomal findings in specimens from digestive organs and abdominal cavity

R85.9 **Unspecified abnormal finding in specimens from digestive organs and abdominal cavity**

R86 **Abnormal findings in specimens from male genital organs**
INCLUDES abnormal findings in prostatic secretions
abnormal findings in semen, seminal fluid
abnormal spermatozoa
EXCLUDES 1 azoospermia (N46.0-)
oligospermia (N46.1-)

R86.0 **Abnormal level of enzymes in specimens from male genital organs** ♂

R86.1 **Abnormal level of hormones in specimens from male genital organs** ♂

R86.2 **Abnormal level of other drugs, medicaments and biological substances in specimens from male genital organs** ♂

R86.3 **Abnormal level of substances chiefly nonmedicinal as to source in specimens from male genital organs** ♂

R86.4 **Abnormal immunological findings in specimens from male genital organs** ♂

R86.5 **Abnormal microbiological findings in specimens from male genital organs** ♂
Positive culture findings in specimens from male genital organs
EXCLUDES 1 colonization status (Z22.-)

R86.6 **Abnormal cytological findings in specimens from male genital organs** ♂

R86.7 **Abnormal histological findings in specimens from male genital organs** ♂

R86.8 **Other abnormal findings in specimens from male genital organs** ♂
Abnormal chromosomal findings in specimens from male genital organs

R86.9 **Unspecified abnormal finding in specimens from male genital organs** ♂

R87 **Abnormal findings in specimens from female genital organs**
Abnormal findings in secretion and smears from cervix uteri
Abnormal findings in secretion and smears from vagina
Abnormal findings in secretion and smears from vulva

R87.0 **Abnormal level of enzymes in specimens from female genital organs** ♀

R87.1 **Abnormal level of hormones in specimens from female genital organs** ♀

R87.2 **Abnormal level of other drugs, medicaments and biological substances in specimens from female genital organs** ♀

R87.3 **Abnormal level of substances chiefly nonmedicinal as to source in specimens from female genital organs** ♀

R87.4 **Abnormal immunological findings in specimens from female genital organs** ♀

R87.5 **Abnormal microbiological findings in specimens from female genital organs** ♀
Positive culture findings in specimens from female genital organs
EXCLUDES 1 colonization status (Z22.-)

R87.6 **Abnormal cytological findings in specimens from female genital organs**

R87.61 **Abnormal cytological findings in specimens from cervix uteri**
EXCLUDES 1 abnormal cytological findings in specimens from other female genital organs (R87.69)
abnormal cytological findings in specimens from vagina (R87.62-)
carcinoma in situ of cervix uteri (histologically confirmed) (D06.-)
cervical intraepithelial neoplasia I [CIN I] (N87.0)
cervical intraepithelial neoplasia II [CIN II] (N87.1)
cervical intraepithelial neoplasia III [CIN III] (D06.-)
dysplasia (mild) (moderate) of cervix uteri (histologically confirmed) (N87.-)
severe dysplasia of cervix uteri (histologically confirmed) (D06.-)
EXCLUDES 2 cervical high risk human papillomavirus (HPV) DNA test positive (R87.810)
cervical low risk human papillomavirus (HPV) DNA test positive (R87.820)

R87.610 **Atypical squamous cells of undetermined significance on cytologic smear of cervix [ASC-US]** ♀

R87.611 **Atypical squamous cells cannot exclude high grade squamous intraepithelial lesion on cytologic smear of cervix [ASC-H]** ♀

R87.612 **Low grade squamous intraepithelial lesion on cytologic smear of cervix [LGSIL]** ♀

R87.613 **High grade squamous intraepithelial lesion on cytologic smear of cervix [HGSIL]** ♀

R87.614 **Cytologic evidence of malignancy on smear of cervix** ♀

R87.615   **Unsatisfactory cytologic smear of cervix**   ♀
>> Inadequate sample of cytologic smear of cervix

R87.616   **Satisfactory cervical smear but lacking transformation zone**   ♀

R87.618   **Other abnormal cytological findings on specimens from cervix uteri**   ♀

R87.619   **Unspecified abnormal cytological findings in specimens from cervix uteri**   ♀
>> Abnormal cervical cytology NOS
>> Abnormal Papanicolaou smear of cervix NOS
>> Abnormal thin preparation smear of cervix NOS
>> Atypical endocervical cells of cervix NOS
>> Atypical endometrial cells of cervix NOS
>> Atypical glandular cells of cervix NOS

✓6ᵗʰ **R87.62**   **Abnormal cytological findings in specimens from vagina**
> Use additional code to identify acquired absence of uterus and cervix, if applicable (Z90.71-)
> *EXCLUDES 1*   *abnormal cytological findings in specimens from cervix uteri (R87.61-)*
>> *abnormal cytological findings in specimens from other female genital organs (R87.69)*
>> *carcinoma in situ of vagina (histologically confirmed) (D07.2)*
>> *dysplasia (mild) (moderate) of vagina (histologically confirmed) (N89.-)*
>> *severe dysplasia of vagina (histologically confirmed) (D07.2)*
>> *vaginal intraepithelial neoplasia I [VAIN I] (N89.0)*
>> *vaginal intraepithelial neoplasia II [VAIN II] (N89.1)*
>> *vaginal intraepithelial neoplasia III [VAIN III] (D07.2)*
> *EXCLUDES 2*   *vaginal high risk human papillomavirus (HPV) DNA test positive (R87.811)*
>> *vaginal low risk human papillomavirus (HPV) DNA test positive (R87.821)*

R87.620   **Atypical squamous cells of undetermined significance on cytologic smear of vagina [ASC-US]**   ♀

R87.621   **Atypical squamous cells cannot exclude high grade squamous intraepithelial lesion on cytologic smear of vagina [ASC-H]**   ♀

R87.622   **Low grade squamous intraepithelial lesion on cytologic smear of vagina [LGSIL]**   ♀

R87.623   **High grade squamous intraepithelial lesion on cytologic smear of vagina [HGSIL]**   ♀

R87.624   **Cytologic evidence of malignancy on smear of vagina**   ♀

R87.625   **Unsatisfactory cytologic smear of vagina**   ♀
>> Inadequate sample of cytologic smear of vagina

R87.628   **Other abnormal cytological findings on specimens from vagina**   ♀

R87.629   **Unspecified abnormal cytological findings in specimens from vagina**   ♀
>> Abnormal Papanicolaou smear of vagina NOS
>> Abnormal thin preparation smear of vagina NOS
>> Abnormal vaginal cytology NOS
>> Atypical endocervical cells of vagina NOS
>> Atypical endometrial cells of vagina NOS
>> Atypical glandular cells of vagina NOS

R87.69   **Abnormal cytological findings in specimens from other female genital organs**   ♀
>> Abnormal cytological findings in specimens from female genital organs NOS
> *EXCLUDES 1*   *dysplasia of vulva (histologically confirmed) (N90.0-N90.3)*

R87.7   **Abnormal histological findings in specimens from female genital organs**   ♀
> *EXCLUDES 1*   *carcinoma in situ (histologically confirmed) of female genital organs (D06-D07.3)*
>> *cervical intraepithelial neoplasia I [CIN I] (N87.0)*
>> *cervical intraepithelial neoplasia II [CIN II] (N87.1)*
>> *cervical intraepithelial neoplasia III [CIN III] (D06.-)*
>> *dysplasia (mild) (moderate) of cervix uteri (histologically confirmed) (N87.-)*
>> *dysplasia (mild) (moderate) of vagina (histologically confirmed) (N89.-)*
>> *severe dysplasia of cervix uteri (histologically confirmed) (D06.-)*
>> *severe dysplasia of vagina (histologically confirmed) (D07.2)*
>> *vaginal intraepithelial neoplasia I [VAIN I] (N89.0)*
>> *vaginal intraepithelial neoplasia II [VAIN II] (N89.1)*
>> *vaginal intraepithelial neoplasia III [VAIN III] (D07.2)*

✓5ᵗʰ **R87.8**   **Other abnormal findings in specimens from female genital organs**

✓6ᵗʰ **R87.81**   **High risk human papillomavirus [HPV] DNA test positive from female genital organs**
> *EXCLUDES 1*   *anogenital warts due to human papillomavirus (HPV) (A63.0)*
>> *condyloma acuminatum (A63.0)*

R87.810   **Cervical high risk human papillomavirus [HPV] DNA test positive**   ♀

R87.811   **Vaginal high risk human papillomavirus [HPV] DNA test positive**   ♀

✓6ᵗʰ **R87.82**   **Low risk human papillomavirus [HPV] DNA test positive from female genital organs**
> Use additional code for associated human papillomavirus (B97.7)

R87.820   **Cervical low risk human papillomavirus [HPV] DNA test positive**   ♀

R87.821   **Vaginal low risk human papillomavirus [HPV] DNA test positive**   ♀

R87.89   **Other abnormal findings in specimens from female genital organs**   ♀
>> Abnormal chromosomal findings in specimens from female genital organs

R87.9   **Unspecified abnormal finding in specimens from female genital organs**   ♀

✓4ᵗʰ **R88**   **Abnormal findings in other body fluids and substances**

R88.0   **Cloudy (hemodialysis) (peritoneal) dialysis effluent**

R88.8   **Abnormal findings in other body fluids and substances**

✓4ᵗʰ **R89**   **Abnormal findings in specimens from other organs, systems and tissues**
> *INCLUDES*   abnormal findings in nipple discharge
>> abnormal findings in synovial fluid
>> abnormal findings in wound secretions

R89.0   **Abnormal level of enzymes in specimens from other organs, systems and tissues**

R89.1   **Abnormal level of hormones in specimens from other organs, systems and tissues**

R89.2   **Abnormal level of other drugs, medicaments and biological substances in specimens from other organs, systems and tissues**

R89.3   **Abnormal level of substances chiefly nonmedicinal as to source in specimens from other organs, systems and tissues**

R89.4   **Abnormal immunological findings in specimens from other organs, systems and tissues**

R89.5   **Abnormal microbiological findings in specimens from other organs, systems and tissues**
>> Positive culture findings in specimens from other organs, systems and tissues
> *EXCLUDES 1*   *colonization status (Z22.-)*

R89.6   **Abnormal cytological findings in specimens from other organs, systems and tissues**

R89.7   **Abnormal histological findings in specimens from other organs, systems and tissues**

R89.8   **Other abnormal findings in specimens from other organs, systems and tissues**
>> Abnormal chromosomal findings in specimens from other organs, systems and tissues

---

✓ Additional Character Required   ✓x7ᵗʰ Placeholder Alert   Unacceptable PDx   Manifestation   Hospital Acquired Condition   *EXCLUDES 1* Not Coded Here   *EXCLUDES 2* Not Included Here

R89.9 **Unspecified** abnormal finding in specimens from other organs, systems and tissues

Abnormal findings on diagnostic imaging and in function studies, without diagnosis (R90-R94)

INCLUDES nonspecific abnormal findings on diagnostic imaging by computerized axial tomography [CAT scan]
nonspecific abnormal findings on diagnostic imaging by magnetic resonance imaging [MRI][NMR]
nonspecific abnormal findings on diagnostic imaging by positron emission tomography [PET scan]
nonspecific abnormal findings on diagnostic imaging by thermography
nonspecific abnormal findings on diagnostic imaging by ultrasound [echogram]
nonspecific abnormal findings on diagnostic imaging by X-ray examination

EXCLUDES 1 abnormal findings on antenatal screening of mother (O28.-)
diagnostic abnormal findings classified elsewhere—see Alphabetical Index

✓4ᵗʰ **R90 Abnormal findings on** diagnostic imaging of central nervous system

R90.0 **Intracranial** space-occupying lesion found on diagnostic imaging of central nervous system

✓5ᵗʰ **R90.8 Other abnormal findings on diagnostic imaging of** central nervous system

R90.81 Abnormal echoencephalogram

R90.82 White matter disease, unspecified

R90.89 Other abnormal findings on diagnostic imaging of central nervous system
Other cerebrovascular abnormality found on diagnostic imaging of central nervous system

✓4ᵗʰ **R91 Abnormal findings on diagnostic imaging of** lung

R91.1 Solitary pulmonary nodule
Coin lesion lung
Solitary pulmonary nodule, subsegmental branch of the bronchial tree

R91.8 Other nonspecific abnormal finding of lung field
Lung mass NOS found on diagnostic imaging of lung
Pulmonary infiltrate NOS
Shadow, lung

✓4ᵗʰ **R92 Abnormal and inconclusive findings on diagnostic imaging of breast**

R92.0 Mammographic microcalcification **found on diagnostic imaging of breast**
EXCLUDES 2 mammographic calcification (calculus) found on diagnostic imaging of breast (R92.1)

R92.1 Mammographic calcification **found on diagnostic imaging of breast**
Mammographic calculus found on diagnostic imaging of breast

R92.2 Inconclusive mammogram
Dense breasts NOS
Inconclusive mammogram NEC
Inconclusive mammography due to dense breasts
Inconclusive mammography NEC
AHA: 2015, 1Q, 24

R92.8 Other abnormal and inconclusive findings on diagnostic imaging of breast

✓4ᵗʰ **R93 Abnormal findings on diagnostic imaging of** other body structures

R93.0 Abnormal findings on diagnostic imaging of skull and head, **not elsewhere classified**
EXCLUDES 1 intracranial space-occupying lesion found on diagnostic imaging (R90.0)

R93.1 Abnormal findings on diagnostic imaging of heart and coronary **circulation**
Abnormal echocardiogram NOS
Abnormal heart shadow

R93.2 Abnormal findings on diagnostic imaging of liver and biliary **tract**
Nonvisualization of gallbladder

R93.3 Abnormal findings on diagnostic imaging of other parts of **digestive tract**

R93.4 Abnormal findings on diagnostic imaging of urinary organs
Filling defect of bladder found on diagnostic imaging
Filling defect of kidney found on diagnostic imaging
Filling defect of ureter found on diagnostic imaging
EXCLUDES 1 hypertrophy of kidney (N28.81)

R93.5 Abnormal findings on diagnostic imaging of other abdominal regions, including retroperitoneum

R93.6 Abnormal findings on diagnostic imaging of limbs
EXCLUDES 2 abnormal finding in skin and subcutaneous tissue (R93.8)

R93.7 Abnormal findings on diagnostic imaging of other parts of musculoskeletal system
EXCLUDES 2 abnormal findings on diagnostic imaging of skull (R93.0)

R93.8 Abnormal findings on diagnostic imaging of other specified body structures
Abnormal finding by radioisotope localization of placenta
Abnormal radiological finding in skin and subcutaneous tissue
Mediastinal shift

R93.9 Diagnostic imaging inconclusive due to excess body fat of patient

✓4ᵗʰ **R94 Abnormal results of function studies**
INCLUDES abnormal results of radionuclide [radioisotope] uptake studies
abnormal results of scintigraphy

✓5ᵗʰ **R94.0 Abnormal results of function studies of** central nervous system

R94.01 Abnormal electroencephalogram [EEG]

R94.02 Abnormal brain scan

R94.09 Abnormal results of other function studies **of central nervous system**

✓5ᵗʰ **R94.1 Abnormal results of function studies of** peripheral nervous system and special senses

✓6ᵗʰ **R94.11 Abnormal results of function studies of** eye

R94.110 Abnormal electro-oculogram [EOG]

R94.111 Abnormal electroretinogram [ERG]
Abnormal retinal function study

R94.112 Abnormal visually evoked potential [VEP]

R94.113 Abnormal oculomotor **study**

R94.118 Abnormal results of other **function studies of eye**

✓6ᵗʰ **R94.12 Abnormal results of function studies of** ear and other special senses

R94.120 Abnormal auditory **function study**

R94.121 Abnormal vestibular **function study**

R94.128 Abnormal results of other **function studies of ear and other special senses**

✓6ᵗʰ **R94.13 Abnormal results of function studies of** peripheral nervous system

R94.130 Abnormal response to nerve stimulation, **unspecified**

R94.131 Abnormal electromyogram [EMG]
EXCLUDES 1 electromyogram of eye (R94.113)

R94.138 Abnormal results of other **function studies of peripheral nervous system**

R94.2 Abnormal results of pulmonary function **studies**
Reduced ventilatory capacity
Reduced vital capacity

✓5ᵗʰ **R94.3 Abnormal results of** cardiovascular function **studies**

R94.30 Abnormal result of cardiovascular function study, unspecified

R94.31 Abnormal electrocardiogram [ECG] [EKG]
EXCLUDES 1 long QT syndrome (I45.81)

R94.39 Abnormal result of other **cardiovascular function study**
Abnormal electrophysiological intracardiac studies
Abnormal phonocardiogram
Abnormal vectorcardiogram

R94.4 Abnormal results of kidney function **studies**
Abnormal renal function test

R94.5 Abnormal results of liver function **studies**

R94.6 Abnormal results of thyroid function **studies**

R94.7 Abnormal results of other endocrine function **studies**
EXCLUDES 2 abnormal glucose (R73.0-)

R94.8 Abnormal results of function studies of other organs and **systems**
Abnormal basal metabolic rate [BMR]
Abnormal bladder function test
Abnormal splenic function test

Abnormal tumor markers (R97)

✓4ᵗʰ **R97   Abnormal tumor markers**
Elevated tumor associated antigens [TAA]
Elevated tumor specific antigens [TSA]

R97.0   Elevated carcinoembryonic antigen [CEA]

R97.1   Elevated cancer antigen 125 [CA 125]   ♀

13 **R97.2   Elevated prostate specific antigen [PSA]**   🅰♂

R97.8   Other abnormal tumor markers

Ill-defined and unknown cause of mortality (R99)

R99   Ill-defined and unknown cause of mortality
Death (unexplained) NOS
Unspecified cause of mortality

---

13 Questionable admission when used as PDx.

✓ Additional Character Required   ✓x7ᵗʰ Placeholder Alert   Unacceptable PDx   Manifestation   Hospital Acquired Condition   *EXCLUDES 1* Not Coded Here   *EXCLUDES 2* Not Included Here

Chapter 19. Injury, Poisoning, and Certain Other Consequences of External Causes (S00–T88)

Chapter Specific Guidelines with Coding Examples

The chapter specific guidelines from the ICD-10-CM Official Guidelines for Coding and Reporting have been provided below. Along with these guidelines are coding examples, contained in the shaded boxes, that have been developed to help illustrate the coding and/or sequencing guidance found in these guidelines.

a. Application of 7th Characters in Chapter 19

Most categories in chapter 19 have a 7th character requirement for each applicable code. Most categories in this chapter have three 7th character values (with the exception of fractures): A, initial encounter, D, subsequent encounter and S, sequela. Categories for traumatic fractures have additional 7th character values. While the patient may be seen by a new or different provider over the course of treatment for an injury, assignment of the 7th character is based on whether the patient is undergoing active treatment and not whether the provider is seeing the patient for the first time.

For complication codes, active treatment refers to treatment for the condition described by the code, even though it may be related to an earlier precipitating problem. For example, code T84.50XA, Infection and inflammatory reaction due to unspecified internal joint prosthesis, initial encounter, is used when active treatment is provided for the infection, even though the condition relates to the prosthetic device, implant or graft that was placed at a previous encounter.

7th character "A", initial encounter is used while the patient is receiving active treatment for the condition. Examples of active treatment are: surgical treatment, emergency department encounter, and evaluation and continuing treatment by the same or a different physician.

> Patient admitted after fall from a skateboard onto the sidewalk, x-rays identify a nondisplaced fracture to the distal pole of the right scaphoid bone. The patient is placed in a cast.
>
> **S62.014A**   **Nondisplaced fracture of distal pole of navicular [scaphoid] bone of right wrist, initial encounter for closed fracture**
>
> **V00.131A**   **Fall from skateboard, initial encounter**
>
> **Y92.480**   **Sidewalk as the place of occurrence of the external cause**
>
> **Y93.51**   **Activity, roller skating (inline) and skateboarding**
>
> **Y99.8**   **Other external cause status**
>
> *Explanation:* This fracture would be coded with a seventh character A for initial encounter because the patient received x-rays to identify the site of the fracture and treatment was rendered; this would be considered active treatment.

7th character "D" subsequent encounter is used for encounters after the patient has received active treatment of the condition and is receiving routine care for the condition during the healing or recovery phase. Examples of subsequent care are: cast change or removal, an x-ray to check healing status of fracture, removal of external or internal fixation device, medication adjustment, other aftercare and follow up visits following treatment of the injury or condition.

> Patient admitted after fall from a skateboard onto the sidewalk resulted in casting of the right arm. X-rays are taken to evaluate how well the nondisplaced fracture to the distal pole of the right scaphoid bone is healing. The physician feels the fracture is healing appropriately; no adjustments to the cast are made.
>
> **S62.014D**   **Nondisplaced fracture of distal pole of navicular [scaphoid] bone of right wrist, subsequent encounter for fracture with routine healing**
>
> **V00.131D**   **Fall from skateboard, subsequent encounter**
>
> *Explanation:* This fracture would be coded with a seventh character D for subsequent encounter, whether the same physician who provided the initial cast application or a different physician is now seeing the patient. Although the patient received x-rays, the intent of the x-rays was to assess how the fracture was healing. There was no active treatment rendered and the visit is therefore considered a subsequent encounter.

The aftercare Z codes should not be used for aftercare for conditions such as injuries or poisonings, where 7th characters are provided to identify subsequent care. For example, for aftercare of an injury, assign the acute injury code with the 7th character "D" (subsequent encounter).

7th character "S", sequela, is for use for complications or conditions that arise as a direct result of a condition, such as scar formation after a burn. The scars are sequelae of the burn. When using 7th character "S", it is necessary to use both the injury code that precipitated the sequela and the code for the sequela itself. The "S" is added only to the injury code, not the sequela code. The 7th character "S" identifies the injury responsible for the sequela. The specific type of sequela (e.g. scar) is sequenced first, followed by the injury code.

See Section I.B.10 Sequelae, (Late Effects)

> Patient with a history of a nondisplaced fracture to the distal pole of the right scaphoid bone due to a fall from a skateboard is admitted for evaluation of arthritis to the right wrist that has developed as a consequence of the traumatic fracture.
>
> **M12.531**   **Traumatic arthropathy, right wrist**
>
> **S62.014S**   **Nondisplaced fracture of distal pole of navicular [scaphoid] bone of right wrist, sequela**
>
> **V00.131S**   **Fall from skateboard, sequela**
>
> *Explanation:* The code identifying the specific sequela condition (traumatic arthritis) should be coded first followed by the injury that instigated the development of the sequela (fracture). The scaphoid fracture injury code is given a 7th character S for sequela to represent its role as the inciting injury. The fracture has healed and is not being managed or treated on this admit and therefore is not applicable as a first listed or principal diagnosis. However, it is directly related to the development of the arthritis and should be appended as a secondary code to signify this cause and effect relationship.

b. Coding of injuries

When coding injuries, assign separate codes for each injury unless a combination code is provided, in which case the combination code is assigned. Code T07, Unspecified multiple injuries should not be assigned in the inpatient setting unless information for a more specific code is not available. Traumatic injury codes (S00-T14.9) are not to be used for normal, healing surgical wounds or to identify complications of surgical wounds.

> 11-year-old girl fell from her horse, resulting in a laceration to her right forearm with several large pieces of wooden fragments embedded in the wound as well as abrasions to her right ear; in addition, her right shoulder was dislocated
>
> **S43.004A**   **Unspecified dislocation of right shoulder joint, initial encounter**
>
> **S51.821A**   **Laceration with foreign body of right forearm, initial encounter**
>
> **S00.411A**   **Abrasion of right ear, initial encounter**
>
> **V80.010A**   **Animal-rider injured by fall from or being thrown from horse in noncollision accident, initial encounter**
>
> **Y93.52**   **Activity, horseback riding**
>
> *Explanation:* Each separate injury should be reported. The patient's injury to the forearm is reported with one combination code that captures both the laceration and the foreign body.

The code for the most serious injury, as determined by the provider and the focus of treatment, is sequenced first.

1) Superficial injuries

Superficial injuries such as abrasions or contusions are not coded when associated with more severe injuries of the same site.

2) Primary injury with damage to nerves/blood vessels

When a primary injury results in minor damage to peripheral nerves or blood vessels, the primary injury is sequenced first with additional code(s) for injuries to nerves and spinal cord (such as category S04), and/or injury to blood vessels (such as category S15). When the primary injury is to the blood vessels or nerves, that injury should be sequenced first.

c. Coding of traumatic fractures

The principles of multiple coding of injuries should be followed in coding fractures. Fractures of specified sites are coded individually by site in accordance with both the provisions within categories S02, S12, S22, S32, S42, S49, S52, S59, S62, S72, S79, S82, S89, and S92 and the level of detail furnished by medical record content.

A fracture not indicated as open or closed should be coded to closed. A fracture not indicated whether displaced or not displaced should be coded to displaced.

More specific guidelines are as follows:

1) Initial vs. Subsequent Encounter for Fractures

Traumatic fractures are coded using the appropriate 7th character for initial encounter (A, B, C) while the patient is receiving active treatment for the fracture. Examples of active treatment are: surgical treatment, emergency department encounter, and evaluation and continuing (ongoing) treatment by the same or different physician. The appropriate 7th character for initial encounter should also be assigned for a patient who delayed seeking treatment for the fracture or nonunion.

Fractures are coded using the appropriate 7th character for subsequent care for encounters after the patient has completed active treatment of the fracture and is receiving routine care for the fracture during the healing or recovery phase. Examples of fracture aftercare are: cast change or removal, an x-ray to check healing status of fracture, removal of external or internal fixation device, medication adjustment, and follow-up visits following fracture treatment.

Care for complications of surgical treatment for fracture repairs during the healing or recovery phase should be coded with the appropriate complication codes.

Care of complications of fractures, such as malunion and nonunion, should be reported with the appropriate 7th character for subsequent care with nonunion (K, M, N,) or subsequent care with malunion (P, Q, R).

Malunion/nonunion: The appropriate 7th character for initial encounter should also be assigned for a patient who delayed seeking treatment for the fracture or nonunion.

> Female patient fell during a hiking excursion almost six months ago and until recently did not feel she needed to seek medical attention for her left ankle pain; x-rays show nonunion of lateral malleolus and surgery has been scheduled
>
> **S82.862A** **Displaced Maisonneuve's fracture of left leg, initial encounter for closed fracture**
>
> **W01.0XXA** **Fall on same level from slipping, tripping and stumbling without subsequent striking against object, initial encounter**
>
> **Y92.821** **Forest as place of occurrence of the external cause**
>
> **Y93.01** **Activity, walking, marching and hiking**
>
> **Y99.8** **Other external cause status**
>
> *Explanation:* A seventh character of A is used for the lateral malleolus nonunion fracture to signify that the fracture is receiving active treatment. The delayed care for the fracture has resulted in a nonunion, but capturing the nonunion in the seventh character is trumped by the provision of active care.

A code from category M80, not a traumatic fracture code, should be used for any patient with known osteoporosis who suffers a fracture, even if the patient had a minor fall or trauma, if that fall or trauma would not usually break a normal, healthy bone.

See Section I.C.13. Osteoporosis.

The aftercare Z codes should not be used for aftercare for traumatic fractures. For aftercare of a traumatic fracture, assign the acute fracture code with the appropriate 7th character.

2) Multiple fractures sequencing

Multiple fractures are sequenced in accordance with the severity of the fracture.

d. Coding of burns and corrosions

The ICD-10-CM makes a distinction between burns and corrosions. The burn codes are for thermal burns, except sunburns, that come from a heat source, such as a fire or hot appliance. The burn codes are also for burns resulting from electricity and radiation. Corrosions are burns due to chemicals. The guidelines are the same for burns and corrosions.

Current burns (T20-T25) are classified by depth, extent and by agent (X code). Burns are classified by depth as first degree (erythema), second degree (blistering), and third degree (full-thickness involvement). Burns of the eye and internal organs (T26-T28) are classified by site, but not by degree.

1) Sequencing of burn and related condition codes

Sequence first the code that reflects the highest degree of burn when more than one burn is present.

a. When the reason for the admission or encounter is for treatment of external multiple burns, sequence first the code that reflects the burn of the highest degree.

b. When a patient has both internal and external burns, the circumstances of admission govern the selection of the principal diagnosis or first-listed diagnosis.

c. When a patient is admitted for burn injuries and other related conditions such as smoke inhalation and/or respiratory failure, the circumstances of admission govern the selection of the principal or first-listed diagnosis.

> Patient admitted with minor first-degree burns to multiple sites of her right and left hands as well as severe smoke inhalation. While she was sleeping at home, a candle on her dresser lit the bedroom curtains on fire.
>
> **T59.811A** **Toxic effect of smoke, accidental (unintentional), initial encounter**
>
> **J70.5** **Respiratory conditions due to smoke inhalation**
>
> **T23.191A** **Burn of first degree of multiple sites of right wrist and hand, initial encounter**
>
> **T23.192A** **Burn of first degree of multiple sites of left wrist and hand, initial encounter**
>
> **X08.8XXA** **Exposure to other specified smoke, fire and flames, initial encounter**
>
> **Y92.003** **Bedroom of unspecified non-institutional (private) residence as the place of occurrence of the external cause**
>
> **Y93.84** **Activity, sleeping**
>
> *Explanation:* Based on the documentation, the inhalation injury is more severe than the first-degree burns and is sequenced first. The burns to the hands are appended as secondary diagnoses.

2) Burns of the same local site

Classify burns of the same local site (three-character category level, T20-T28) but of different degrees to the subcategory identifying the highest degree recorded in the diagnosis.

> 10-year-old male patient is admitted for third-degree burns of his right palm and second-degree burns of multiple right fingers; right thumb not affected
>
> **T23.351A** **Burn of third degree of right palm, initial encounter**
>
> *Explanation:* Although there is a code for second-degree burns of multiple fingers, not including the thumb (T23.131-), this code falls in the same three-digit category that the third-degree burn of the right palm falls under, category T23. Only the subcategory identifying the highest degree is captured when different burn degrees are classified to a single category.

> Patient is admitted with third-degree burns of the scalp as well as second-degree burns to the back of the right hand
>
> **T20.35XA** **Burn of third degree of scalp [any part], initial encounter**
>
> **T23.261A** **Burn of second degree of back of right hand, initial encounter**
>
> *Explanation:* Since burns to the hand and scalp are classified to two different three-digit categories, both burns may be reported as they represent distinct sites.

3) Non-healing burns

Non-healing burns are coded as acute burns.

Necrosis of burned skin should be coded as a non-healed burn.

4) Infected burn

For any documented infected burn site, use an additional code for the infection.

5) Assign separate codes for each burn site

When coding burns, assign separate codes for each burn site. Category T30, Burn and corrosion, body region unspecified is extremely vague and should rarely be used.

6) Burns and Corrosions Classified According to Extent of Body Surface Involved

Assign codes from category T31, Burns classified according to extent of body surface involved, or T32, Corrosions classified according to extent of body surface involved, when the site of the burn is not specified or when there is a need for additional data. It is advisable to use category T31 as additional coding when needed to provide data for evaluating burn mortality, such as that needed by burn units. It is also advisable to use category T31 as an additional code for reporting purposes when there is mention of a third-degree burn involving 20 percent or more of the body surface.

Categories T31 and T32 are based on the classic "rule of nines" in estimating body surface involved: head and neck are assigned nine percent, each arm nine percent, each leg 18 percent, the anterior trunk 18 percent, posterior trunk 18 percent, and genitalia one percent. Providers may change these percentage assignments where necessary to accommodate infants and children who have proportionately larger heads than adults, and patients who have large buttocks, thighs, or abdomen that involve burns.

> Patient seen for dressing change after he accidentally spilled acetic acid on himself two days ago. The second-degree burns to his right thigh, covering about 3 percent of his body surface, are healing appropriately.
>
> **T54.2X1D**   **Toxic effect of corrosive acids and acid-like substances, accidental (unintentional), subsequent encounter**
>
> **T24.611D**   **Corrosion of second degree of right thigh, subsequent encounter**
>
> **T32.0**   **Corrosions involving less than 10% of body surface**
>
> *Explanation:* Code T32.0 provides additional information as to how much of the patient's body was affected by the corrosive substance.

7) Encounters for treatment of sequela of burns

Encounters for the treatment of the late effects of burns or corrosions (i.e., scars or joint contractures) should be coded with a burn or corrosion code with the 7th character "S" for sequela.

8) Sequelae with a late effect code and current burn

When appropriate, both a code for a current burn or corrosion with 7th character "A" or "D" and a burn or corrosion code with 7th character "S" may be assigned on the same record (when both a current burn and sequelae of an old burn exist). Burns and corrosions do not heal at the same rate and a current healing wound may still exist with sequela of a healed burn or corrosion.

See Section I.B.10 Sequela (Late Effects)

> Female patient seen for second-degree burn to the left ear; she also has significant scarring on her left elbow from a third-degree burn from childhood
>
> **T20.212A**   **Burn of second degree of left ear [any part, except ear drum], initial encounter**
>
> **L90.5**   **Scar conditions and fibrosis of skin**
>
> **T22.322S**   **Burn of third degree of left elbow, sequela**
>
> *Explanation:* The patient is being seen for management of a current second-degree burn, which is reflected in the code by appending the seventh character of A, indicating active treatment or management of this burn. The elbow scarring is a sequela of a previous third-degree burn. The sequela condition precedes the original burn injury, which is appended with a seventh character of S.

9) Use of an external cause code with burns and corrosions

An external cause code should be used with burns and corrosions to identify the source and intent of the burn, as well as the place where it occurred.

e. Adverse effects, poisoning, underdosing and toxic effects

Codes in categories T36-T65 are combination codes that include the substance that was taken as well as the intent. No additional external cause code is required for poisonings, toxic effects, adverse effects and underdosing codes.

1) Do not code directly from the Table of Drugs

Do not code directly from the Table of Drugs and Chemicals. Always refer back to the Tabular List.

2) Use as many codes as necessary to describe

Use as many codes as necessary to describe completely all drugs, medicinal or biological substances.

3) If the same code would describe the causative agent

If the same code would describe the causative agent for more than one adverse reaction, poisoning, toxic effect or underdosing, assign the code only once.

4) If two or more drugs, medicinal or biological substances

If two or more drugs, medicinal or biological substances are reported, code each individually unless a combination code is listed in the Table of Drugs and Chemicals.

5) The occurrence of drug toxicity is classified in ICD-10-CM as follows:

(a) Adverse effect

When coding an adverse effect of a drug that has been correctly prescribed and properly administered, assign the appropriate code for the nature of the adverse effect followed by the appropriate code for the adverse effect of the drug (T36-T50). The code for the drug should have a 5th or 6th character "5" (for example T36.0X5-) Examples of the nature of an adverse effect are tachycardia, delirium, gastrointestinal hemorrhaging, vomiting, hypokalemia, hepatitis, renal failure, or respiratory failure.

> Patient seen for stomach pain and jaundice, indicated by physician as possible side-effects of Inderal, recently started for hypertension. Inderal was discontinued and the patient switched to Atenolol instead.
>
> **R10.9**   **Unspecified abdominal pain**
>
> **R17**   **Unspecified jaundice**
>
> **T44.7X5A**   **Adverse effect of beta-adrenoreceptor antagonists, initial encounter**
>
> **I10**   **Essential (primary) hypertension**
>
> *Explanation:* The side-effects caused by the drug are listed first, followed by the code for the adverse effect of the drug to capture the specific drug that was used.

(b) Poisoning

When coding a poisoning or reaction to the improper use of a medication (e.g., overdose, wrong substance given or taken in error, wrong route of administration), first assign the appropriate code from categories T36-T50. The poisoning codes have an associated intent as their 5th or 6th character (accidental, intentional self-harm, assault and undetermined. Use additional code(s) for all manifestations of poisonings.

If there is also a diagnosis of abuse or dependence of the substance, the abuse or dependence is assigned as an additional code.

Examples of poisoning include:

(i) Error was made in drug prescription

Errors made in drug prescription or in the administration of the drug by provider, nurse, patient, or other person.

(ii) Overdose of a drug intentionally taken

If an overdose of a drug was intentionally taken or administered and resulted in drug toxicity, it would be coded as a poisoning.

(iii) Nonprescribed drug taken with correctly prescribed and properly administered drug

If a nonprescribed drug or medicinal agent was taken in combination with a correctly prescribed and properly administered drug, any drug toxicity or other reaction resulting from the interaction of the two drugs would be classified as a poisoning.

(iv) Interaction of drug(s) and alcohol

When a reaction results from the interaction of a drug(s) and alcohol, this would be classified as poisoning.

See Section I.C.4. if poisoning is the result of insulin pump malfunctions.

(c) Underdosing

Underdosing refers to taking less of a medication than is prescribed by a provider or a manufacturer's instruction. For underdosing, assign the code from categories T36-T50 (fifth or sixth character "6").

Codes for underdosing should never be assigned as principal or first-listed codes. If a patient has a relapse or exacerbation of the medical condition for which the drug is prescribed because of the reduction in dose, then the medical condition itself should be coded.

Noncompliance (Z91.12-, Z91.13-) or complication of care (Y63.6-Y63.9) codes are to be used with an underdosing code to indicate intent, if known.

> Patient admitted for atrial fibrillation with history of chronic atrial fibrillation for which she is prescribed amiodarone. Financial concerns have left the patient unable to pay for her prescriptions and she has been skipping her amiodarone dose every other day to offset the cost.
>
> **I48.2**   **Chronic atrial fibrillation**
>
> **T46.2X6A**   **Underdosing of other antidysrhythmic drugs, initial encounter**
>
> **Z91.12Ø**   **Patient's intentional underdosing of medication regimen due to financial hardship**
>
> *Explanation:* By skipping her amiodarone pill every other day, the patient's atrial fibrillation returned. The condition for which the drug was being taken is reported first, followed by an underdosing code to show that the patient was not adhering to her prescription regiment. The Z code helps elaborate on the patient's social and/or economic circumstances that led to the patient taking less then what she was prescribed.

(d) Toxic effects

When a harmful substance is ingested or comes in contact with a person, this is classified as a toxic effect. The toxic effect codes are in categories T51-T65.

Toxic effect codes have an associated intent: accidental, intentional self-harm, assault and undetermined.

f. Adult and child abuse, neglect and other maltreatment

Sequence first the appropriate code from categories T74.- (Adult and child abuse, neglect and other maltreatment, confirmed) or T76.- (Adult and child abuse, neglect and other maltreatment, suspected) for abuse, neglect and other maltreatment, followed by any accompanying mental health or injury code(s).

If the documentation in the medical record states abuse or neglect it is coded as confirmed (T74.-). It is coded as suspected if it is documented as suspected (T76.-).

For cases of confirmed abuse or neglect an external cause code from the assault section (X92-Y08) should be added to identify the cause of any physical injuries. A perpetrator code (Y07) should be added when the perpetrator of the abuse is known. For suspected cases of abuse or neglect, do not report external cause or perpetrator code.

If a suspected case of abuse, neglect or mistreatment is ruled out during an encounter code Z04.71, Encounter for examination and observation following alleged physical adult abuse, ruled out, or code Z04.72, Encounter for examination and observation following alleged child physical abuse, ruled out, should be used, not a code from T76.

If a suspected case of alleged rape or sexual abuse is ruled out during an encounter code Z04.41, Encounter for examination and observation following alleged physical adult abuse, ruled out, or code Z04.42, Encounter for examination and observation following alleged rape or sexual abuse, ruled out, should be used, not a code from T76.

See Section I.C.15. Abuse in a pregnant patient.

g. Complications of care

1) General guidelines for complications of care
(a) Documentation of complications of care

See Section I.B.16. for information on documentation of complications of care.

2) Pain due to medical devices

Pain associated with devices, implants or grafts left in a surgical site (for example painful hip prosthesis) is assigned to the appropriate code(s) found in Chapter 19, Injury, poisoning, and certain other consequences of external causes. Specific codes for pain due to medical devices are found in the T code section of the ICD-10-CM. Use additional code(s) from category G89 to identify acute or chronic pain due to presence of the device, implant or graft (G89.18 or G89.28).

> Chronic left breast pain secondary to breast implant
>
> **T85.84XA**   **Pain due to internal prosthetic devices, implants and grafts, not elsewhere classified, initial encounter**
>
> **N64.4**   **Mastodynia**
>
> **G89.28**   **Other chronic postprocedural pain**
>
> *Explanation:* As the pain is a complication related to the breast implant, the complication code is sequenced first. The T code does not describe the site or type of pain, so additional codes may be appended to indicate that the patient is experiencing chronic pain in the breast.

3) Transplant complications
(a) Transplant complications other than kidney

Codes under category T86, Complications of transplanted organs and tissues, are for use for both complications and rejection of transplanted organs. A transplant complication code is only assigned if the complication affects the function of the transplanted organ. Two codes are required to fully describe a transplant complication: the appropriate code from category T86 and a secondary code that identifies the complication.

Pre-existing conditions or conditions that develop after the transplant are not coded as complications unless they affect the function of the transplanted organs.

See I.C.21. for transplant organ removal status

See I.C.2. for malignant neoplasm associated with transplanted organ.

(b) Kidney transplant complications

Patients who have undergone kidney transplant may still have some form of chronic kidney disease (CKD) because the kidney transplant may not fully restore kidney function. Code T86.1- should be assigned for documented complications of a kidney transplant, such as transplant failure or rejection or other transplant complication. Code T86.1- should not be assigned for post kidney transplant patients who have chronic kidney (CKD) unless a transplant complication such as transplant failure or rejection is documented. If the documentation is unclear as to whether the patient has a complication of the transplant, query the provider.

Conditions that affect the function of the transplanted kidney, other than CKD, should be assigned a code from subcategory T86.1, Complications of transplanted organ, Kidney, and a secondary code that identifies the complication.

For patients with CKD following a kidney transplant, but who do not have a complication such as failure or rejection, *see section I.C.14. Chronic kidney disease and kidney transplant status.*

> Patient seen for chronic kidney disease stage 2; history of successful kidney transplant with no complications identified
>
> **N18.2**   **Chronic kidney disease, stage 2 (mild)**
>
> **Z94.Ø**   **Kidney transplant status**
>
> *Explanation:* This patient's stage 2 CKD is not indicated as being due to the transplanted kidney but instead is just the residual disease the patient had prior to the transplant.

4) Complication codes that include the external cause

As with certain other T codes, some of the complications of care codes have the external cause included in the code. The code includes the nature of the complication as well as the type of procedure that caused the complication. No external cause code indicating the type of procedure is necessary for these codes.

5) Complications of care codes within the body system chapters

Intraoperative and postprocedural complication codes are found within the body system chapters with codes specific to the organs and structures of that body system. These codes should be sequenced first, followed by a code(s) for the specific complication, if applicable.

> During a spinal fusion procedure, the surgeon inadvertently punctured the dura. The midline durotomy was repaired, and the fusion procedure was completed.
>
> **G97.41**   **Accidental puncture or laceration of dura during a procedure**
>
> *Explanation:* The accidental durotomy is not coded to an injury code in chapter 19 but instead is categorized to the nervous system chapter.

Muscle/Tendon Table

ICD-10-CM categorizes certain muscles and tendons in the upper and lower extremities by their action (e.g., extension, flexion), their anatomical location (e.g., posterior, anterior), and/or whether they are intrinsic or extrinsic to a certain anatomical area. The Muscle/Tendon Table is provided at the beginning of chapters 13 and 19 as a resource to help users when code selection depends on one or more of these characteristics. The categories and/or subcategories that relate to this table are identified by the icon ✦. Please note that this table is not all-inclusive, and proper code assignment should be based on the provider's documentation.

Body Region	Muscle	Extensor Tendon	Flexor Tendon	Other Tendon
Shoulder				
	Deltoid	Posterior deltoid	Anterior deltoid	
	Rotator cuff			
	Infraspinatus			Infraspinatus
	Subscapularis			Subscapularis
	Supraspinatus			Supraspinatus
	Teres minor			Teres minor
	Teres major	Teres major		
Upper arm				
	Anterior muscles			
	Biceps brachii — long head		Biceps brachii — long head	
	Biceps brachii — short head		Biceps brachii — short head	
	Brachialis		Brachialis	
	Coracobrachialis		Coracobrachialis	
	Posterior muscles			
	Triceps brachii	Triceps brachii		
Forearm				
	Anterior muscles			
	Flexors			
	Deep			
	Flexor digitorum profundus		Flexor digitorum profundus	
	Flexor pollicis longus		Flexor pollicis longus	
	Intermediate			
	Flexor digitorum superficialis		Flexor digitorum superficialis	
	Superficial			
	Flexor carpi radialis		Flexor carpi radialis	
	Flexor carpi ulnaris		Flexor carpi ulnaris	
	Palmaris longus		Palmaris longus	
	Pronators			
	Pronator quadratus			Pronator quadratus
	Pronator teres			Pronator teres
	Posterior muscles			
	Extensors			
	Deep			
	Abductor pollicis longus			Abductor pollicis longus
	Extensor indicis	Extensor indicis		
	Extensor pollicis brevis	Extensor pollicis brevis		
	Extensor pollicis longus	Extensor pollicis longus		
	Superficial			
	Brachioradialis			Brachioradialis
	Extensor carpi radialis brevis	Extensor carpi radialis brevis		
	Extensor carpi radialis longus	Extensor carpi radialis longus		
	Extensor carpi ulnaris	Extensor carpi ulnaris		
	Extensor digiti minimi	Extensor digiti minimi		
	Extensor digitorum	Extensor digitorum		
	Anconeus	Anconeus		
	Supinator			Supinator

Body Region	Muscle	Extensor Tendon	Flexor Tendon	Other Tendon
Hand				
Extrinsic — attach to a site in the forearm as well as a site in the hand with action related to hand movement at the wrist				
	Extensor carpi radialis brevis	Extensor carpi radialis brevis		
	Extensor carpi radialis longus	Extensor carpie radialis longus		
	Extensor carpi ulnaris	Extensor carpi ulnaris		
	Flexor carpi radialis		Flexor carpi radialis	
	Flexor carpi ulnaris		Flexor carpi ulnaris	
	Flexor digitorum superficialis		Flexor digitorum superficialis	
	Palmaris longus		Palmaris longus	
Extrinsic — attach to a site in the forearm as well as a site in the hand with action in the hand related to finger movement				
	Adductor pollicis longus			Adductor pollicis longus
	Extensor digiti minimi	Extensor digiti minimi		
	Extensor digitorum	Extensor digitorum		
	Extensor indicis	Extensor indicis		
	Flexor digitorum profundus		Flexor digitorum profundus	
	Flexor digitorum superficialis		Flexor digitorum superficialis	
Extrinsic — attach to a site in the forearm as well as a site in the hand with action in the hand related to thumb movement				
	Extensor pollicis brevis	Extensor pollicis brevis		
	Extensor pollicis longus	Extensor pollicis longus		
	Flexor pollicis longus		Flexor pollicis longus	
Intrinsic — found within the hand only				
	Adductor pollicis			Adductor pollicis
	Dorsal interossei	Dorsal interossei	Dorsal interossei	
	Lumbricals	Lumbricals	Lumbricals	
	Palmaris brevis			Palmaris brevis
	Palmar interossei	Palmar interossei	Palmar interossei	
	Hypothenar muscles			
	Abductor digiti minimi			Abductor digiti minimi
	Flexor digiti minimi brevis		Flexor digiti minimi brevis	
	Oppenens digiti minimi		Oppenens digiti minimi	
	Thenar muscles			
	Abductor pollicis brevis			Abductor pollicis brevis
	Flexor pollicis brevis		Flexor pollicis brevis	
	Oppenens pollicis		Oppenens pollicis	
Thigh				
	Anterior muscles			
	Iliopsoas		Iliopsoas	
	Pectineus		Pectineus	
	Quadriceps	Quadriceps		
	Rectus femoris	Rectus femoris — Extends knee	Rectus femoris — Flexes hip	
	Vastus intermedius	Vastus intermedius		
	Vastus lateralis	Vastus lateralis		
	Vastus medialis	Vastus medialis		
	Sartorius		Sartorius	
	Medial muscles			
	Adductor brevis			Adductor brevis
	Adductor longus			Adductor longus
	Adductor magnus			Adductor magnus
	Gracilis			Gracilis
	Obturator externus			Obturator externus
	Posterior muscles			
	Hamstring	Hamstring — Extends hip	Hamstring — Flexes knee	
	Biceps femoris	Biceps femoris	Biceps femoris	
	Semimembranosus	Semimembranosus	Semimembranosus	
	Semitendinosus	Semitendinosus	Semitendinosus	

Chapter 19. Injury, Poisoning, and Certain Other Consequences of External

Body Region	Muscle	Extensor Tendon	Flexor Tendon	Other Tendon
Lower leg				
	Anterior muscles			
	Extensor digitorum longus	Extensor digitorum longus		
	Extensor hallucis longus	Extensor hallucis longus		
	Fibularis (peroneus) tertius	Fibularis (peroneus) tertius		
	Tibialis anterior	Tibialis anterior		Tibialis anterior
	Lateral muscles			
	Fibularis (peroneus) brevis		Fibularis (peroneus) brevis	
	Fibularis (peroneus) longus		Fibularis (peroneus) longus	
	Posterior muscles			
	Deep			
	Flexor digitorum longus		Flexor digitorum longus	
	Flexor hallucis longus		Flexor hallucis longus	
	Popliteus		Popliteus	
	Tibialis posterior		Tibialis posterior	
	Superficial			
	Gastrocnemius		Gastrocnemius	
	Plantaris		Plantaris	
	Soleus		Soleus	
				Calcaneal (Achilles)
Ankle/Foot				
Extrinsic — attach to a site in the lower leg as well as a site in the foot with action related to foot movement at the ankle				
	Plantaris		Plantaris	
	Soleus		Soleus	
	Tibialis anterior	Tibialis anterior		
	Tibialis posterior		Tibialis posterior	
Extrinsic — attach to a site in the lower leg as well as a site in the foot with action in the foot related to toe movement				
	Extensor digitorum longus	Extensor digitorum longus		
	Extensor hallicus longus	Extensor hallicus longus		
	Flexor digitorum longus		Flexor digitorum longus	
	Flexor hallucis longus		Flexor hallucis longus	
Intrinsic — found within the ankle/foot only				
	Dorsal muscles			
	Extensor digitorum brevis	Extensor digitorum brevis		
	Extensor hallucis brevis	Extensor hallucis brevis		
	Plantar muscles			
	Abductor digiti minimi		Abductor digiti minimi	
	Abductor hallucis		Abductor hallucis	
	Dorsal interossei	Dorsal interossei	Dorsal interossei	
	Flexor digiti minimi brevis		Flexor digiti minimi brevis	
	Flexor digitorum brevis		Flexor digitorum brevis	
	Flexor hallucis brevis		Flexor hallucis brevis	
	Lumbricals	Lumbricals	Lumbricals	
	Quadratus plantae		Quadratus plantae	
	Plantar interossei	Plantar interossei	Plantar interossei	

Chapter 19. Injury, Poisoning and Certain Other Consequences of External Causes (S00-T88)

NOTE   Use secondary code(s) from Chapter 20, External causes of morbidity, to indicate cause of injury. Codes within the T section that include the external cause do not require an additional external cause code.

Use additional code to identify any retained foreign body, if applicable (Z18.-)

EXCLUDES 1   birth trauma (P10-P15)
         obstetric trauma (O70-O71)

NOTE   The chapter uses the S-section for coding different types of injuries related to single body regions and the T-section to cover injuries to unspecified body regions as well as poisoning and certain other consequences of external causes.

AHA: 2015, 1Q, 3-21

This chapter contains the following blocks:

S00-S09   Injuries to the head
S10-S19   Injuries to the neck
S20-S29   Injuries to the thorax
S30-S39   Injuries to the abdomen, lower back, lumbar spine, pelvis and external genitals
S40-S49   Injuries to the shoulder and upper arm
S50-S59   Injuries to the elbow and forearm
S60-S69   Injuries to the wrist, hand and fingers
S70-S79   Injuries to the hip and thigh
S80-S89   Injuries to the knee and lower leg
S90-S99   Injuries to the ankle and foot
T07   Injuries involving multiple body regions
T14   Injury of unspecified body region
T15-T19   Effects of foreign body entering through natural orifice
T20-T25   Burns and corrosions of external body surface, specified by site
T26-T28   Burns and corrosions confined to eye and internal organs
T30-T32   Burns and corrosions of multiple and unspecified body regions
T33-T34   Frostbite
T36-T50   Poisoning by, adverse effect of and underdosing of drugs, medicaments and biological substances
T51-T65   Toxic effects of substances chiefly nonmedicinal as to source
T66-T78   Other and unspecified effects of external causes
T79   Certain early complications of trauma
T80-T88   Complications of surgical and medical care, not elsewhere classified

Injuries to the head (S00-S09)

INCLUDES   injuries of ear
         injuries of eye
         injuries of face [any part]
         injuries of gum
         injuries of jaw
         injuries of oral cavity
         injuries of palate
         injuries of periocular area
         injuries of scalp
         injuries of temporomandibular joint area
         injuries of tongue
         injuries of tooth

Code also for any associated infection

EXCLUDES 2   burns and corrosions (T20-T32)
         effects of foreign body in ear (T16)
         effects of foreign body in larynx (T17.3)
         effects of foreign body in mouth NOS (T18.0)
         effects of foreign body in nose (T17.0-T17.1)
         effects of foreign body in pharynx (T17.2)
         effects of foreign body on external eye (T15.-)
         frostbite (T33-T34)
         insect bite or sting, venomous (T63.4)

S00   **Superficial injury of head**
     EXCLUDES 1   diffuse cerebral contusion (S06.2-)
           focal cerebral contusion (S06.3-)
           injury of eye and orbit (S05.-)
           open wound of head (S01.-)

The appropriate 7th is to be added to each code from category S00.
A   initial encounter
D   subsequent encounter
S   sequela

S00.0   **Superficial injury of scalp**
   S00.00   Unspecified superficial injury of scalp
   S00.01   Abrasion of scalp
   S00.02   Blister (nonthermal) of scalp
   S00.03   Contusion of scalp
       Bruise of scalp
       Hematoma of scalp

S00.04   External constriction of part of scalp
S00.05   Superficial foreign body of scalp
     Splinter in the scalp
S00.06   Insect bite (nonvenomous) of scalp
S00.07   Other superficial bite of scalp
     EXCLUDES 1   open bite of scalp (S01.05)

S00.1   **Contusion of eyelid and periocular area**
     Black eye
     EXCLUDES 2   contusion of eyeball and orbital tissues (S05.1)
   S00.10   Contusion of unspecified eyelid and periocular area
   S00.11   Contusion of right eyelid and periocular area
   S00.12   Contusion of left eyelid and periocular area

S00.2   **Other and unspecified superficial injuries of eyelid and periocular area**
     EXCLUDES 2   superficial injury of conjunctiva and cornea (S05.0-)
   S00.20   Unspecified superficial injury of eyelid and periocular area
     S00.201   Unspecified superficial injury of right eyelid and periocular area
     S00.202   Unspecified superficial injury of left eyelid and periocular area
     S00.209   Unspecified superficial injury of unspecified eyelid and periocular area
   S00.21   Abrasion of eyelid and periocular area
     S00.211   Abrasion of right eyelid and periocular area
     S00.212   Abrasion of left eyelid and periocular area
     S00.219   Abrasion of unspecified eyelid and periocular area
   S00.22   Blister (nonthermal) of eyelid and periocular area
     S00.221   Blister (nonthermal) of right eyelid and periocular area
     S00.222   Blister (nonthermal) of left eyelid and periocular area
     S00.229   Blister (nonthermal) of unspecified eyelid and periocular area
   S00.24   External constriction of eyelid and periocular area
     S00.241   External constriction of right eyelid and periocular area
     S00.242   External constriction of left eyelid and periocular area
     S00.249   External constriction of unspecified eyelid and periocular area
   S00.25   Superficial foreign body of eyelid and periocular area
     Splinter of eyelid and periocular area
     EXCLUDES 2   retained foreign body in eyelid (H02.81-)
     S00.251   Superficial foreign body of right eyelid and periocular area
     S00.252   Superficial foreign body of left eyelid and periocular area
     S00.259   Superficial foreign body of unspecified eyelid and periocular area
   S00.26   Insect bite (nonvenomous) of eyelid and periocular area
     S00.261   Insect bite (nonvenomous) of right eyelid and periocular area
     S00.262   Insect bite (nonvenomous) of left eyelid and periocular area
     S00.269   Insect bite (nonvenomous) of unspecified eyelid and periocular area
   S00.27   Other superficial bite of eyelid and periocular area
     EXCLUDES 1   open bite of eyelid and periocular area (S01.15)
     S00.271   Other superficial bite of right eyelid and periocular area
     S00.272   Other superficial bite of left eyelid and periocular area
     S00.279   Other superficial bite of unspecified eyelid and periocular area

S00.3   **Superficial injury of nose**
   S00.30   Unspecified superficial injury of nose
   S00.31   Abrasion of nose

✓ Additional Character Required   Placeholder Alert   Unacceptable PDx   Manifestation   Hospital Acquired Condition   **EXCLUDES 1** Not Coded Here   **EXCLUDES 2** Not Included Here

ICD-10-CM 2016   899

√x7ᵗʰ **S00.32** **Blister** (nonthermal) **of nose**

√x7ᵗʰ **S00.33** **Contusion of nose**
Bruise of nose
Hematoma of nose

√x7ᵗʰ **S00.34** **External constriction of nose**

√x7ᵗʰ **S00.35** **Superficial foreign body of nose**
Splinter in the nose

√x7ᵗʰ **S00.36** **Insect bite** (nonvenomous) **of nose**

√x7ᵗʰ **S00.37** **Other superficial bite of nose**
EXCLUDES 1 *open bite of nose (S01.25)*

√5ᵗʰ **S00.4** **Superficial injury of ear**

√6ᵗʰ **S00.40** **Unspecified superficial injury of ear**

√7ᵗʰ **S00.401** **Unspecified superficial injury of right ear**

√7ᵗʰ **S00.402** **Unspecified superficial injury of left ear**

√7ᵗʰ **S00.409** **Unspecified superficial injury of unspecified ear**

√6ᵗʰ **S00.41** **Abrasion of ear**

√7ᵗʰ **S00.411** **Abrasion of right ear**

√7ᵗʰ **S00.412** **Abrasion of left ear**

√7ᵗʰ **S00.419** **Abrasion of unspecified ear**

√6ᵗʰ **S00.42** **Blister** (nonthermal) **of ear**

√7ᵗʰ **S00.421** **Blister** (nonthermal) **of right ear**

√7ᵗʰ **S00.422** **Blister** (nonthermal) **of left ear**

√7ᵗʰ **S00.429** **Blister** (nonthermal) **of unspecified ear**

√6ᵗʰ **S00.43** **Contusion of ear**
Bruise of ear
Hematoma of ear

√7ᵗʰ **S00.431** **Contusion of right ear**

√7ᵗʰ **S00.432** **Contusion of left ear**

√7ᵗʰ **S00.439** **Contusion of unspecified ear**

√6ᵗʰ **S00.44** **External constriction of ear**

√7ᵗʰ **S00.441** **External constriction of right ear**

√7ᵗʰ **S00.442** **External constriction of left ear**

√7ᵗʰ **S00.449** **External constriction of unspecified ear**

√6ᵗʰ **S00.45** **Superficial foreign body of ear**
Splinter in the ear

√7ᵗʰ **S00.451** **Superficial foreign body of right ear**

√7ᵗʰ **S00.452** **Superficial foreign body of left ear**

√7ᵗʰ **S00.459** **Superficial foreign body of unspecified ear**

√6ᵗʰ **S00.46** **Insect bite** (nonvenomous) **of ear**

√7ᵗʰ **S00.461** **Insect bite** (nonvenomous) **of right ear**

√7ᵗʰ **S00.462** **Insect bite** (nonvenomous) **of left ear**

√7ᵗʰ **S00.469** **Insect bite** (nonvenomous) **of unspecified ear**

√6ᵗʰ **S00.47** **Other superficial bite of ear**
EXCLUDES 1 *open bite of ear (S01.35)*

√7ᵗʰ **S00.471** **Other superficial bite of right ear**

√7ᵗʰ **S00.472** **Other superficial bite of left ear**

√7ᵗʰ **S00.479** **Other superficial bite of unspecified ear**

√5ᵗʰ **S00.5** **Superficial injury of lip and oral cavity**

√6ᵗʰ **S00.50** **Unspecified superficial injury of lip and oral cavity**

√7ᵗʰ **S00.501** **Unspecified superficial injury of lip**

√7ᵗʰ **S00.502** **Unspecified superficial injury of oral cavity**

√6ᵗʰ **S00.51** **Abrasion of lip and oral cavity**

√7ᵗʰ **S00.511** **Abrasion of lip**

√7ᵗʰ **S00.512** **Abrasion of oral cavity**

√6ᵗʰ **S00.52** **Blister** (nonthermal) **of lip and oral cavity**

√7ᵗʰ **S00.521** **Blister** (nonthermal) **of lip**

√7ᵗʰ **S00.522** **Blister** (nonthermal) **of oral cavity**

√6ᵗʰ **S00.53** **Contusion of lip and oral cavity**

√7ᵗʰ **S00.531** **Contusion of lip**
Bruise of lip
Hematoma of oral cavity

√7ᵗʰ **S00.532** **Contusion of oral cavity**
Bruise of lip
Hematoma of oral cavity

√6ᵗʰ **S00.54** **External constriction of lip and oral cavity**

√7ᵗʰ **S00.541** **External constriction of lip**

√7ᵗʰ **S00.542** **External constriction of oral cavity**

√6ᵗʰ **S00.55** **Superficial foreign body of lip and oral cavity**

√7ᵗʰ **S00.551** **Superficial foreign body of lip**
Splinter of lip and oral cavity

√7ᵗʰ **S00.552** **Superficial foreign body of oral cavity**
Splinter of lip and oral cavity

√6ᵗʰ **S00.56** **Insect bite** (nonvenomous) **of lip and oral cavity**

√7ᵗʰ **S00.561** **Insect bite** (nonvenomous) **of lip**

√7ᵗʰ **S00.562** **Insect bite** (nonvenomous) **of oral cavity**

√6ᵗʰ **S00.57** **Other superficial bite of lip and oral cavity**

√7ᵗʰ **S00.571** **Other superficial bite of lip**
EXCLUDES 1 *open bite of lip (S01.551)*

√7ᵗʰ **S00.572** **Other superficial bite of oral cavity**
EXCLUDES 1 *open bite of oral cavity (S01.552)*

√5ᵗʰ **S00.8** **Superficial injury of other parts of head**

√x7ᵗʰ **S00.80** **Unspecified superficial injury of other part of head**

√x7ᵗʰ **S00.81** **Abrasion of other part of head**

√x7ᵗʰ **S00.82** **Blister** (nonthermal) **of other part of head**

√x7ᵗʰ **S00.83** **Contusion of other part of head**
Bruise of other part of head
Hematoma of other part of head

√x7ᵗʰ **S00.84** **External constriction of other part of head**

√x7ᵗʰ **S00.85** **Superficial foreign body of other part of head**
Splinter in other part of head

√x7ᵗʰ **S00.86** **Insect bite** (nonvenomous) **of other part of head**

√x7ᵗʰ **S00.87** **Other superficial bite of other part of head**
EXCLUDES 1 *open bite of other part of head (S01.85)*

√5ᵗʰ **S00.9** **Superficial injury of unspecified part of head**

√x7ᵗʰ **S00.90** **Unspecified superficial injury of unspecified part of head**

√x7ᵗʰ **S00.91** **Abrasion of unspecified part of head**

√x7ᵗʰ **S00.92** **Blister** (nonthermal) **of unspecified part of head**

√x7ᵗʰ **S00.93** **Contusion of unspecified part of head**
Bruise of head
Hematoma of head

√x7ᵗʰ **S00.94** **External constriction of unspecified part of head**

√x7ᵗʰ **S00.95** **Superficial foreign body of unspecified part of head**
Splinter of head

√x7ᵗʰ **S00.96** **Insect bite** (nonvenomous) **of unspecified part of head**

√x7ᵗʰ **S00.97** **Other superficial bite of unspecified part of head**
EXCLUDES 1 *open bite of head (S01.95)*

√4ᵗʰ **S01** **Open wound of head**
Code also any associated:
injury of cranial nerve (S04.-)
injury of muscle and tendon of head (S09.1-)
intracranial injury (S06.-)
wound infection
EXCLUDES 1 *open skull fracture (S02- with 7th B)*
EXCLUDES 2 *injury of eye and orbit (S05.-)*
traumatic amputation of part of head (S08.-)

The appropriate 7th is to be added to each code from category S01.
A　initial encounter
D　subsequent encounter
S　sequela

√5ᵗʰ **S01.0** **Open wound of scalp**
EXCLUDES 1 *avulsion of scalp (S08.0)*

√x7ᵗʰ **S01.00** **Unspecified open wound of scalp**

√x7ᵗʰ **S01.01** **Laceration without foreign body of scalp**

√x7ᵗʰ **S01.02** **Laceration with foreign body of scalp**

√x7ᵗʰ **S01.03** **Puncture wound without foreign body of scalp**

√x7ᵗʰ **S01.04** **Puncture wound with foreign body of scalp**

√x7ᵗʰ **S01.05** **Open bite of scalp**
Bite of scalp NOS
EXCLUDES 1 *superficial bite of scalp (S00.06, S00.07-)*

N Newborn: 0　P Pediatric: 0-17　M Maternity: 12-55　A Adult: 15-124　MCC Major CC Condition　PDxMCC PDx acts as own MCC　CC CC Condition　PDxCC PDx acts as own CC

900

ICD-10-CM 2016

Chapter 19. Injury, Poisoning, and Certain Other Consequences of External Causes

✓5ᵗʰ S01.1 Open wound of eyelid and periocular area
Open wound of eyelid and periocular area with or without involvement of lacrimal passages

> **CC Excl:** For CC codes in subcategory S01.1, unless otherwise noted: CC with 7th character A: S01.101-S01.159 with 7th A, S05.20X-S05.8X9 with 7th A, S05.91X-S05.92X with 7th A, S38.3XXA, T14.90-T14.91, T79.A0X-T79.9XX with 7th A

     ✓6ᵗʰ S01.10 Unspecified open wound of eyelid and periocular area
         ✓7ᵗʰ S01.101 Unspecified open wound of right eyelid and periocular area `CC`
         ✓7ᵗʰ S01.102 Unspecified open wound of left eyelid and periocular area `CC`
         ✓7ᵗʰ S01.109 Unspecified open wound of unspecified eyelid and periocular area `CC`

     ✓6ᵗʰ S01.11 Laceration without foreign body of eyelid and periocular area
         ✓7ᵗʰ S01.111 Laceration without foreign body of right eyelid and periocular area
         ✓7ᵗʰ S01.112 Laceration without foreign body of left eyelid and periocular area
         ✓7ᵗʰ S01.119 Laceration without foreign body of unspecified eyelid and periocular area

     ✓6ᵗʰ S01.12 Laceration with foreign body of eyelid and periocular area
         ✓7ᵗʰ S01.121 Laceration with foreign body of right eyelid and periocular area
         ✓7ᵗʰ S01.122 Laceration with foreign body of left eyelid and periocular area
         ✓7ᵗʰ S01.129 Laceration with foreign body of unspecified eyelid and periocular area

     ✓6ᵗʰ S01.13 Puncture wound without foreign body of eyelid and periocular area
         ✓7ᵗʰ S01.131 Puncture wound without foreign body of right eyelid and periocular area
         ✓7ᵗʰ S01.132 Puncture wound without foreign body of left eyelid and periocular area
         ✓7ᵗʰ S01.139 Puncture wound without foreign body of unspecified eyelid and periocular area

     ✓6ᵗʰ S01.14 Puncture wound with foreign body of eyelid and periocular area
         ✓7ᵗʰ S01.141 Puncture wound with foreign body of right eyelid and periocular area
         ✓7ᵗʰ S01.142 Puncture wound with foreign body of left eyelid and periocular area
         ✓7ᵗʰ S01.149 Puncture wound with foreign body of unspecified eyelid and periocular area

     ✓6ᵗʰ S01.15 Open bite of eyelid and periocular area
Bite of eyelid and periocular area NOS
> **EXCLUDES 1** superficial bite of eyelid and periocular area (S00.26, S00.27)

         ✓7ᵗʰ S01.151 Open bite of right eyelid and periocular area
         ✓7ᵗʰ S01.152 Open bite of left eyelid and periocular area
         ✓7ᵗʰ S01.159 Open bite of unspecified eyelid and periocular area

✓5ᵗʰ S01.2 Open wound of nose
     ✓x7ᵗʰ S01.20 Unspecified open wound of nose
     ✓x7ᵗʰ S01.21 Laceration without foreign body of nose
     ✓x7ᵗʰ S01.22 Laceration with foreign body of nose
     ✓x7ᵗʰ S01.23 Puncture wound without foreign body of nose
     ✓x7ᵗʰ S01.24 Puncture wound with foreign body of nose
     ✓x7ᵗʰ S01.25 Open bite of nose
Bite of nose NOS
> **EXCLUDES 1** superficial bite of nose (S00.36, S00.37)

✓5ᵗʰ S01.3 Open wound of ear
     ✓6ᵗʰ S01.30 Unspecified open wound of ear
         ✓7ᵗʰ S01.301 Unspecified open wound of right ear
         ✓7ᵗʰ S01.302 Unspecified open wound of left ear
         ✓7ᵗʰ S01.309 Unspecified open wound of unspecified ear

     ✓6ᵗʰ S01.31 Laceration without foreign body of ear
         ✓7ᵗʰ S01.311 Laceration without foreign body of right ear
         ✓7ᵗʰ S01.312 Laceration without foreign body of left ear
         ✓7ᵗʰ S01.319 Laceration without foreign body of unspecified ear

     ✓6ᵗʰ S01.32 Laceration with foreign body of ear
         ✓7ᵗʰ S01.321 Laceration with foreign body of right ear
         ✓7ᵗʰ S01.322 Laceration with foreign body of left ear
         ✓7ᵗʰ S01.329 Laceration with foreign body of unspecified ear

     ✓6ᵗʰ S01.33 Puncture wound without foreign body of ear
         ✓7ᵗʰ S01.331 Puncture wound without foreign body of right ear
         ✓7ᵗʰ S01.332 Puncture wound without foreign body of left ear
         ✓7ᵗʰ S01.339 Puncture wound without foreign body of unspecified ear

     ✓6ᵗʰ S01.34 Puncture wound with foreign body of ear
         ✓7ᵗʰ S01.341 Puncture wound with foreign body of right ear
         ✓7ᵗʰ S01.342 Puncture wound with foreign body of left ear
         ✓7ᵗʰ S01.349 Puncture wound with foreign body of unspecified ear

     ✓6ᵗʰ S01.35 Open bite of ear
Bite of ear NOS
> **EXCLUDES 1** superficial bite of ear (S00.46, S00.47)

         ✓7ᵗʰ S01.351 Open bite of right ear
         ✓7ᵗʰ S01.352 Open bite of left ear
         ✓7ᵗʰ S01.359 Open bite of unspecified ear

✓5ᵗʰ S01.4 Open wound of cheek and temporomandibular area
     ✓6ᵗʰ S01.40 Unspecified open wound of cheek and temporomandibular area
         ✓7ᵗʰ S01.401 Unspecified open wound of right cheek and temporomandibular area
         ✓7ᵗʰ S01.402 Unspecified open wound of left cheek and temporomandibular area
         ✓7ᵗʰ S01.409 Unspecified open wound of unspecified cheek and temporomandibular area

     ✓6ᵗʰ S01.41 Laceration without foreign body of cheek and temporomandibular area
         ✓7ᵗʰ S01.411 Laceration without foreign body of right cheek and temporomandibular area
         ✓7ᵗʰ S01.412 Laceration without foreign body of left cheek and temporomandibular area
         ✓7ᵗʰ S01.419 Laceration without foreign body of unspecified cheek and temporomandibular area

     ✓6ᵗʰ S01.42 Laceration with foreign body of cheek and temporomandibular area
         ✓7ᵗʰ S01.421 Laceration with foreign body of right cheek and temporomandibular area
         ✓7ᵗʰ S01.422 Laceration with foreign body of left cheek and temporomandibular area
         ✓7ᵗʰ S01.429 Laceration with foreign body of unspecified cheek and temporomandibular area

     ✓6ᵗʰ S01.43 Puncture wound without foreign body of cheek and temporomandibular area
         ✓7ᵗʰ S01.431 Puncture wound without foreign body of right cheek and temporomandibular area
         ✓7ᵗʰ S01.432 Puncture wound without foreign body of left cheek and temporomandibular area
         ✓7ᵗʰ S01.439 Puncture wound without foreign body of unspecified cheek and temporomandibular area

     ✓6ᵗʰ S01.44 Puncture wound with foreign body of cheek and temporomandibular area
         ✓7ᵗʰ S01.441 Puncture wound with foreign body of right cheek and temporomandibular area
         ✓7ᵗʰ S01.442 Puncture wound with foreign body of left cheek and temporomandibular area

---

✓ Additional Character Required   ✓x7ᵗʰ Placeholder Alert   Unacceptable PDx   Manifestation   Hospital Acquired Condition   **EXCLUDES 1** Not Coded Here   **EXCLUDES 2** Not Included Here

✓7ᵗʰ **S01.449** **Puncture wound with foreign body of unspecified cheek and temporomandibular area**

✓6ᵗʰ **S01.45** **Open bite of cheek and temporomandibular area**
Bite of cheek and temporomandibular area NOS
EXCLUDES 2   *superficial bite of cheek and temporomandibular area (S00.86, S00.87)*

     ✓7ᵗʰ **S01.451** **Open bite of right cheek and temporomandibular area**

     ✓7ᵗʰ **S01.452** **Open bite of left cheek and temporomandibular area**

     ✓7ᵗʰ **S01.459** **Open bite of unspecified cheek and temporomandibular area**

✓5ᵗʰ **S01.5** **Open wound of lip and oral cavity**
EXCLUDES 2   *tooth dislocation (S03.2)*
               tooth fracture (S02.5)

   ✓6ᵗʰ **S01.50** **Unspecified open wound of lip and oral cavity**

     ✓7ᵗʰ **S01.501** **Unspecified open wound of lip**

     ✓7ᵗʰ **S01.502** **Unspecified open wound of oral cavity**

   ✓6ᵗʰ **S01.51** **Laceration of lip and oral cavity without foreign body**

     ✓7ᵗʰ **S01.511** **Laceration without foreign body of lip**

     ✓7ᵗʰ **S01.512** **Laceration without foreign body of oral cavity**

   ✓6ᵗʰ **S01.52** **Laceration of lip and oral cavity with foreign body**

     ✓7ᵗʰ **S01.521** **Laceration with foreign body of lip**

     ✓7ᵗʰ **S01.522** **Laceration with foreign body of oral cavity**

   ✓6ᵗʰ **S01.53** **Puncture wound of lip and oral cavity without foreign body**

     ✓7ᵗʰ **S01.531** **Puncture wound without foreign body of lip**

     ✓7ᵗʰ **S01.532** **Puncture wound without foreign body of oral cavity**

   ✓6ᵗʰ **S01.54** **Puncture wound of lip and oral cavity with foreign body**

     ✓7ᵗʰ **S01.541** **Puncture wound with foreign body of lip**

     ✓7ᵗʰ **S01.542** **Puncture wound with foreign body of oral cavity**

   ✓6ᵗʰ **S01.55** **Open bite of lip and oral cavity**

     ✓7ᵗʰ **S01.551** **Open bite of lip**
Bite of lip NOS
EXCLUDES 1   *superficial bite of lip (S00.571)*

     ✓7ᵗʰ **S01.552** **Open bite of oral cavity**
Bite of oral cavity NOS
EXCLUDES 1   *superficial bite of oral cavity (S00.572)*

✓5ᵗʰ **S01.8** **Open wound of other parts of head**

   ✓x7ᵗʰ **S01.80** **Unspecified open wound of other part of head**

   ✓x7ᵗʰ **S01.81** **Laceration without foreign body of other part of head**

   ✓x7ᵗʰ **S01.82** **Laceration with foreign body of other part of head**

   ✓x7ᵗʰ **S01.83** **Puncture wound without foreign body of other part of head**

   ✓x7ᵗʰ **S01.84** **Puncture wound with foreign body of other part of head**

   ✓x7ᵗʰ **S01.85** **Open bite of other part of head**
Bite of other part of head NOS
EXCLUDES 1   *superficial bite of other part of head (S00.85)*

✓5ᵗʰ **S01.9** **Open wound of unspecified part of head**

   ✓x7ᵗʰ **S01.90** **Unspecified open wound of unspecified part of head**

   ✓x7ᵗʰ **S01.91** **Laceration without foreign body of unspecified part of head**

   ✓x7ᵗʰ **S01.92** **Laceration with foreign body of unspecified part of head**

   ✓x7ᵗʰ **S01.93** **Puncture wound without foreign body of unspecified part of head**

   ✓x7ᵗʰ **S01.94** **Puncture wound with foreign body of unspecified part of head**

   ✓x7ᵗʰ **S01.95** **Open bite of unspecified part of head**
Bite of head NOS
EXCLUDES 1   *superficial bite of head NOS (S00.97)*

✓4ᵗʰ **S02** **Fracture of skull and facial bones**
NOTE   A fracture not indicated as open or closed should be coded to closed.
Code also any associated intracranial injury (S06.-).

The appropriate 7th is to be added to each code from category S02.
A   initial encounter for closed fracture
B   initial encounter for open fracture
D   subsequent encounter for fracture with routine healing
G   subsequent encounter for fracture with delayed healing
K   subsequent encounter for fracture with nonunion
S   sequela

7,16,19 ✓x7ᵗʰ **S02.0** **Fracture of vault of skull**   MCC CC
Fracture of frontal bone
Fracture of parietal bone

CC Excl: For CC/MCC codes in subcategory S02.0, unless otherwise noted: CC with 7th character A or MCC with 7th character B: S01.90X–S02.92X with 7th A, S06.0X0–S07.9XX with 7th A, S08.89X–S09.19X with 7th A, S09.8XX–S09.90X with 7th A, S09.92X–S09.93X with 7th A, S16.8XX–S19.9XX with 7th A, S38.3XX with 7th A, T14.90–T14.91, T79.A0X–T79.9XX with 7th A
CC with 7th character K: M80.00X–M84.68X with 7th [K, P], S02.0XX–S02.92X with 7th K, S12.000–S12.691 with 7th K, S22.000–S22.9XX with 7th K, S32.000–S32.9XX with 7th K, S42.001–S42.92X with 7th [K, P], S49.001–S49.199 with 7th [K, P], S52.001–S52.92X with 7th [K, M, N, P, Q, R], S59.001–S59.299 with 7th [K, P], S62.001–S62.92X with 7th [K, P], S72.001–S72.92X with 7th [K, M, N, P, Q, R], S79.001–S79.199 with 7th [K, P], S82.001–S82.92X with 7th [K, M, N, P, Q, R], S89.001–S89.399 with 7th [K, P], S92.001–S92.919 with 7th [K, P]

✓5ᵗʰ **S02.1** **Fracture of base of skull**
EXCLUDES 1   *orbit NOS (S02.8)*
EXCLUDES 2   *orbital floor (S02.3-)*

CC Excl: For CC codes in subcategory S02.1, unless otherwise noted: CC with 7th character A or MCC with 7th character B: S01.90X–S02.92X with 7th A, S06.0X0–S07.9XX with 7th A, S08.89X–S09.19X with 7th A, S09.8XX–S09.90X with 7th A, S09.92X–S09.93X with 7th A, S16.8XX–S19.9XX with 7th A, S38.3XXA, T14.90–T14.91, T79.A0X–T79.9XX with 7th A
CC with 7th character K: M80.00X–M84.68X with 7th [K, P], S02.0XX–S02.92X with 7th K, S12.000–S12.691 with 7th K, S22.000–S22.9XX with 7th K, S32.000–S32.9XX with 7th K, S42.001–S42.92X with 7th [K, P], S49.001–S49.199 with 7th [K, P], S52.001–S52.92X with 7th [K, M, N, P, Q, R], S59.001–S59.299 with 7th [K, P], S62.001–S62.92X with 7th [K, P], S72.001–S72.92X with 7th [K, M, N, P, Q, R], S79.001–S79.199 with 7th [K, P], S82.001–S82.92X with 7th [K, M, N, P, Q, R], S89.001–S89.399 with 7th [K, P], S92.001–S92.919 with 7th [K, P]

7,16,19 ✓x7ᵗʰ **S02.10** **Unspecified fracture of base of skull**   MCC CC

   ✓6ᵗʰ **S02.11** **Fracture of occiput**

7,16,19 ✓7ᵗʰ **S02.110** **Type I occipital condyle fracture**   MCC CC

7,16,19 ✓7ᵗʰ **S02.111** **Type II occipital condyle fracture**   MCC CC

7,16,19 ✓7ᵗʰ **S02.112** **Type III occipital condyle fracture**   MCC CC

7,16,19 ✓7ᵗʰ **S02.113** **Unspecified occipital condyle fracture**   MCC CC

7,16,19 ✓7ᵗʰ **S02.118** **Other fracture of occiput**   MCC CC

7,16,19 ✓7ᵗʰ **S02.119** **Unspecified fracture of occiput**   MCC CC

7,16,19 ✓x7ᵗʰ **S02.19** **Other fracture of base of skull**   MCC CC
Fracture of anterior fossa of base of skull
Fracture of ethmoid sinus
Fracture of frontal sinus
Fracture of middle fossa of base of skull
Fracture of orbital roof
Fracture of posterior fossa of base of skull
Fracture of sphenoid
Fracture of temporal bone

---

7   HAC = Initial encounter only (7th character A, B or C) and not POA.
16 MCC only if an open fracture (7th character B or C – specific to category).
19 CC only if an initial encounter for a closed fracture (7th character A) **OR** a subsequent encounter for nonunion or malunion (7th character K, M, N, P, Q, or R – specific to category).

7,20 ✓x7th **S02.2** **Fracture of nasal bones** `CC`

CC Excl: CC with 7th character B: S01.90X-S02.92X with 7th A, S06.0X0-S07.9XX with 7th A, S08.89-S09.19X with 7th A, S09.8XX-S09.90X with 7th A, S09.92X-S09.93X with 7th A, S16.8XX-S19.9XX with 7th A, S38.3XXA, T14.90-T14.91, T79.A0X-T79.9XX with 7th A
CC Excl: CC with 7th character K: M80.00X-M84.68X with 7th [K, P], S02.0XX-S02.92X with 7th K, S12.000-S12.691 with 7th K, S22.000-S22.9XX with 7th K, S32.000-S32.9XX with 7th K, S42.001-S42.92X with 7th [K, P], S49.001-S49.199 with 7th [K, P], S52.001-S52.92X with 7th [K, M, N, P, Q, R], S59.001-S59.299 with 7th [K, P], S62.001-S62.92X with 7th [K, P], S72.001-S72.92X with 7th [K, M, N, P, Q, R], S79.001-S79.199 with 7th [K, P], S82.001-S82.92X with 7th [K, M, N, P, Q, R], S89.001-S89.399 with 7th [K, P], S92.001-S92.919 with 7th [K, P]

7,17 ✓x7th **S02.3** **Fracture of orbital floor** `CC`

EXCLUDES 1   orbit NOS (S02.8)
EXCLUDES 2   orbital roof (S02.1-)

CC Excl: CC with 7th character A or B: S01.90X-S02.92X with 7th A, S06.0X0-S07.9XX with 7th A, S08.89X-S09.19X with 7th A, S09.8XX-S09.90X with 7th A, S09.92X-S09.93X with 7th A, S16.8XX-S19.9XX with 7th A, S38.3XXA, T14.90-T14.91, T79.A0X-T79.9XX with 7th A
CC with 7th character K: M80.00X-M84.68X with 7th [K, P], S02.0XX-S02.92X with 7th K, S12.000-S12.691 with 7th K, S22.000-S22.9XX with 7th K, S32.000-S32.9XX with 7th K, S42.001-S42.92X with 7th [K, P], S49.001-S49.199 with 7th [K, P], S52.001-S52.92X with 7th [K, M, N, P, Q, R], S59.001-S59.299 with 7th [K, P], S62.001-S62.92X with 7th [K, P], S72.001-S72.92X with 7th [K, M, N, P, Q, R], S79.001-S79.199 with 7th [K, P], S82.001-S82.92X with 7th [K, M, N, P, Q, R], S89.001-S89.399 with 7th [K, P], S92.001-S92.919 with 7th [K, P]

✓5th **S02.4** **Fracture of malar, maxillary and zygoma bones**

Fracture of superior maxilla
Fracture of upper jaw (bone)
Fracture of zygomatic process of temporal bone

CC Excl: For CC codes in subcategory S02.4, unless otherwise noted: CC with 7th character A or B: S01.90X-S03.0XX with 7th A, S06.0X0-S07.9XX with 7th A, S08.89X-S09.19X with 7th A, S09.8XX-S09.90X with 7th A, S09.92X-S09.93X with 7th A, S16.8XX-S19.9XX with 7th A, S38.3XA, T14.90-T14.91, T79.A0X-T79.9XX with 7th A
CC with 7th character K: M80.00X-M84.68X with 7th [K, P], S02.0XX-S02.92X with 7th K, S12.000-S12.691 with 7th K, S22.000-S22.9XX with 7th K, S32.000-S32.9XX with 7th K, S42.001-S42.92X with 7th [K, P], S49.001-S49.199 with 7th [K, P], S52.001-S52.92X with 7th [K, M, N, P, Q, R], S59.001-S59.299 with 7th [K, P], S62.001-S62.92X with 7th [K, P], S72.001-S72.92X with 7th [K, M, N, P, Q, R], S79.001-S79.199 with 7th [K, P], S82.001-S82.92X with 7th [K, M, N, P, Q, R], S89.001-S89.399 with 7th [K, P], S92.001-S92.919 with 7th [K, P]

✓6th **S02.40** **Fracture of malar, maxillary and zygoma bones, unspecified**

7,17 ✓7th **S02.400** **Malar fracture unspecified** `CC`
7,17 ✓7th **S02.401** **Maxillary fracture, unspecified** `CC`
7,17 ✓7th **S02.402** **Zygomatic fracture, unspecified** `CC`

✓6th **S02.41** **LeFort fracture**

7,17 ✓7th **S02.411** **LeFort I fracture** `CC`
7,17 ✓7th **S02.412** **LeFort II fracture** `CC`
7,17 ✓7th **S02.413** **LeFort III fracture** `CC`

7,17 ✓x7th **S02.42** **Fracture of alveolus of maxilla** `CC`

CC Excl: CC with 7th character A or B: S01.90X-S02.92X with 7th A, S06.0X0-S07.9XX with 7th A, S08.89X-S09.19X with 7th A, S09.8XX-S09.90X with 7th A, S09.92X-S09.93X with 7th A, S16.8XX-S19.9XX with 7th A, S38.3XXA, T14.90-T14.91, T79.A0X-T79.9XX with 7th A
CC with 7th character K: M80.00X-M84.68X with 7th [K, P], S02.0XX-S02.92X with 7th K, S12.000-S12.691 with 7th K, S22.000-S22.9XX with 7th K, S32.000-S32.9XX with 7th K, S42.001-S42.92X with 7th [K, P], S49.001-S49.199 with 7th [K, P], S52.001-S52.92X with 7th [K, M, N, P, Q, R], S59.001-S59.299 with 7th [K, P], S62.001-S62.92X with 7th [K, P], S72.001-S72.92X with 7th [K, M, N, P, Q, R], S79.001-S79.199 with 7th [K, P], S82.001-S82.92X with 7th [K, M, N, P, Q, R], S89.001-S89.399 with 7th [K, P], S92.001-S92.919 with 7th [K, P]

18 ✓x7th **S02.5** **Fracture of tooth (traumatic)** `CC`

Broken tooth
EXCLUDES 1   cracked tooth (nontraumatic) (K03.81)
CC Excl: CC with 7th character K: See Code: S02.42

✓5th **S02.6** **Fracture of mandible**

Fracture of lower jaw (bone)

CC Excl: For CC codes in subcategory S02.6, unless otherwise noted: CC with 7th character A or B: S01.90X-S03.0XX with 7th A, S06.0X0-S07.9XX with 7th A, S08.89-S09.19X with 7th A, S09.8XX-S09.90X with 7th A, S09.92X-S09.93X with 7th A, S16.8XX-S19.9XX with 7th A, S38.3XXA, T14.90-T14.91, T79.A0X-T79.9XX with 7th A
CC with 7th character K: M80.00X-M84.68X with 7th [K, P], S02.0XX-S02.92X with 7th K, S12.000-S12.691 with 7th K, S22.000-S22.9XX with 7th K, S32.000-S32.9XX with 7th K, S42.001-S42.92X with 7th [K, P], S49.001-S49.199 with 7th [K, P], S52.001-S52.92X with 7th [K, M, N, P, Q, R], S59.001-S59.299 with 7th [K, P], S62.001-S62.92X with 7th [K, P], S72.001-S72.92X with 7th [K, M, N, P, Q, R], S79.001-S79.199 with 7th [K, P], S82.001-S82.92X with 7th [K, M, N, P, Q, R], S89.001-S89.399 with 7th [K, P], S92.001-S92.919 with 7th [K, P]

✓6th **S02.60** **Fracture of mandible, unspecified**

7,17 ✓7th **S02.600** **Fracture of unspecified part of body of mandible** `CC`
7,17 ✓7th **S02.609** **Fracture of mandible, unspecified** `CC`

7,17 ✓x7th **S02.61** **Fracture of condylar process of mandible** `CC`
7,17 ✓x7th **S02.62** **Fracture of subcondylar process of mandible** `CC`
7,17 ✓x7th **S02.63** **Fracture of coronoid process of mandible** `CC`
7,17 ✓x7th **S02.64** **Fracture of ramus of mandible** `CC`
7,17 ✓x7th **S02.65** **Fracture of angle of mandible** `CC`
7,17 ✓x7th **S02.66** **Fracture of symphysis of mandible** `CC`
7,17 ✓x7th **S02.67** **Fracture of alveolus of mandible** `CC`
7,17 ✓x7th **S02.69** **Fracture of mandible of other specified site** `CC`

7,17 ✓x7th **S02.8** **Fractures of other specified skull and facial bones** `CC`

Fracture of orbit NOS
Fracture of palate
EXCLUDES 1   fracture of orbital floor (S02.3-)
        fracture of orbital roof (S02.1-)
CC Excl: CC with 7th character A or B: S01.90X-S02.92X with 7th A, S06.0X0-S07.9XX with 7th A, S08.89X-S09.19X with 7th A, S09.8XX-S09.90X with 7th A, S09.92X-S09.93X with 7th A, S16.8XX-S19.9XX with 7th A, S38.3XXA, T14.90-T14.91, T79.A0X-T79.9XX with 7th A
CC with 7th character K: M80.00X-M84.68X with 7th [K, P], S02.0XX-S02.92X with 7th K, S12.000-S12.691 with 7th K, S22.000-S22.9XX with 7th K, S32.000-S32.9XX with 7th K, S42.001-S42.92X with 7th [K, P], S49.001-S49.199 with 7th [K, P], S52.001-S52.92X with 7th [K, M, N, P, Q, R], S59.001-S59.299 with 7th [K, P], S62.001-S62.92X with 7th [K, P], S72.001-S72.92X with 7th [K, M, N, P, Q, R], S79.001-S79.199 with 7th [K, P], S82.001-S82.92X with 7th [K, M, N, P, Q, R], S89.001-S89.399 with 7th [K, P], S92.001-S92.919 with 7th [K, P]

✓5th **S02.9** **Fracture of unspecified skull and facial bones**

CC Excl: For CC codes in subcategory S02.9, unless otherwise noted: CC with 7th character A or MCC with 7th character B: S01.90X-S02.92X with 7th A, S06.0X0-S07.9XX with 7th A, S08.89X-S09.19X with 7th A, S09.8XX-S09.90X with 7th A, S09.92X-S09.93X with 7th A, S16.8XX-S19.9XX with 7th A, S38.3XXA, T14.90-T14.91, T79.A0X-T79.9XX with 7th A
CC with 7th character K: M80.00X-M84.68X with 7th [K, P], S02.0XX-S02.92X with 7th K, S12.000-S12.691 with 7th K, S22.000-S22.9XX with 7th K, S32.000-S32.9XX with 7th K, S42.001-S42.92X with 7th [K, P], S49.001-S49.199 with 7th [K, P], S52.001-S52.92X with 7th [K, M, N, P, Q, R], S59.001-S59.299 with 7th [K, P], S62.001-S62.92X with 7th [K, P], S72.001-S72.92X with 7th [K, M, N, P, Q, R], S79.001-S79.199 with 7th [K, P], S82.001-S82.92X with 7th [K, M, N, P, Q, R], S89.001-S89.399 with 7th [K, P], S92.001-S92.919 with 7th [K, P]

7,16,19 ✓x7th **S02.91** **Unspecified fracture of skull** `MCC` `CC`
7,17 ✓x7th **S02.92** **Unspecified fracture of facial bones** `CC`

---

7   HAC = Initial encounter only (7th character A, B or C) and not POA.
16   MCC only if an open fracture (7th character B or C – specific to category).
17   CC only if an initial encounter (7th character A, B, or C – specific to category) OR a subsequent encounter for nonunion or malunion (7th character K, M, N, P, Q, or R – specific to category).
18   CC only if a subsequent encounter for nonunion or malunion (7th character K, M, N, P, Q, or R – specific to category).
19   CC only if an initial encounter for a closed fracture (7th character A) OR a subsequent encounter for nonunion or malunion (7th character K, M, N, P, Q, or R – specific to category).
20   CC only if an initial encounter for an open fracture (7th character B or C – specific to category) OR a subsequent encounter for nonunion or malunion (7th character K, M, N, P, Q, or R– specific to category).

✓ Additional Character Required   ✓x7th Placeholder Alert   Unacceptable PDx   Manifestation   Hospital Acquired Condition   EXCLUDES 1 Not Coded Here   EXCLUDES 2 Not Included Here

√4ᵗʰ **S03 Dislocation and sprain of joints and ligaments of head**

INCLUDES avulsion of joint (capsule) or ligament of head
laceration of cartilage, joint (capsule) or ligament of head
sprain of cartilage, joint (capsule) or ligament of head
traumatic hemarthrosis of joint or ligament of head
traumatic rupture of joint or ligament of head
traumatic subluxation of joint or ligament of head
traumatic tear of joint or ligament of head

Code also any associated open wound

EXCLUDES 2 *strain of muscle or tendon of head (S09.1)*

The appropriate 7th is to be added to each code from category S03.
A   initial encounter
D   subsequent encounter
S   sequela

√x7ᵗʰ **S03.0 Dislocation of jaw**
Dislocation of jaw (cartilage) (meniscus)
Dislocation of mandible
Dislocation of temporomandibular (joint)

√x7ᵗʰ **S03.1 Dislocation of septal cartilage of nose**

√x7ᵗʰ **S03.2 Dislocation of tooth**

√x7ᵗʰ **S03.4 Sprain of jaw**
Sprain of temporomandibular (joint) (ligament)

√x7ᵗʰ **S03.8 Sprain of joints and ligaments of other parts of head**

√x7ᵗʰ **S03.9 Sprain of joints and ligaments of unspecified parts of head**

√4ᵗʰ **S04 Injury of cranial nerve**
The selection of side should be based on the side of the body being affected
Code first any associated intracranial injury (S06.-)
Code also any associated:
     open wound of head (S01.-)
     skull fracture (S02.-)

The appropriate 7th is to be added to each code from category S04.
A   initial encounter
D   subsequent encounter
S   sequela

√5ᵗʰ **S04.0 Injury of optic nerve and pathways**
Use additional code to identify any visual field defect or blindness (H53.4-, H54)

CC Excl: For CC codes in subcategory S04.0, unless otherwise noted: CC with 7th character A: S04.011-S04.9XX with 7th A

√6ᵗʰ **S04.01 Injury of optic nerve**
Injury of 2nd cranial nerve
   √7ᵗʰ **S04.011 Injury of optic nerve, right eye** CC
   √7ᵗʰ **S04.012 Injury of optic nerve, left eye** CC
   √7ᵗʰ **S04.019 Injury of optic nerve, unspecified eye** CC
     Injury of optic nerve NOS

√x7ᵗʰ **S04.02 Injury of optic chiasm** CC

√6ᵗʰ **S04.03 Injury of optic tract and pathways**
Injury of optic radiation
   √7ᵗʰ **S04.031 Injury of optic tract and pathways, right eye** CC
   √7ᵗʰ **S04.032 Injury of optic tract and pathways, left eye** CC
   √7ᵗʰ **S04.039 Injury of optic tract and pathways, unspecified eye** CC
     Injury of optic tract and pathways NOS

√6ᵗʰ **S04.04 Injury of visual cortex**
   √7ᵗʰ **S04.041 Injury of visual cortex, right eye** CC
   √7ᵗʰ **S04.042 Injury of visual cortex, left eye** CC
   √7ᵗʰ **S04.049 Injury of visual cortex, unspecified eye** CC
     Injury of visual cortex NOS

√5ᵗʰ **S04.1 Injury of oculomotor nerve**
Injury of 3rd cranial nerve

CC Excl: For CC codes in subcategory S04.1, unless otherwise noted: CC with 7th character A: S04.10X-S04.12X with 7th A, S04.811-S04.9XX with 7th A

√x7ᵗʰ **S04.10 Injury of oculomotor nerve, unspecified side** CC
√x7ᵗʰ **S04.11 Injury of oculomotor nerve, right side** CC
√x7ᵗʰ **S04.12 Injury of oculomotor nerve, left side** CC

√5ᵗʰ **S04.2 Injury of trochlear nerve**
Injury of 4th cranial nerve

CC Excl: For CC codes in subcategory S04.2, unless otherwise noted: CC with 7th character A: S04.20X-S04.22X with 7th A, S04.811-S04.9XX with 7th A

√x7ᵗʰ **S04.20 Injury of trochlear nerve, unspecified side** CC
√x7ᵗʰ **S04.21 Injury of trochlear nerve, right side** CC
√x7ᵗʰ **S04.22 Injury of trochlear nerve, left side** CC

√5ᵗʰ **S04.3 Injury of trigeminal nerve**
Injury of 5th cranial nerve

CC Excl: For CC codes in subcategory S04.3, unless otherwise noted: CC with 7th character A: S04.30X-S04.32X with 7th A, S04.811-S04.9XX with 7th A

√x7ᵗʰ **S04.30 Injury of trigeminal nerve, unspecified side** CC
√x7ᵗʰ **S04.31 Injury of trigeminal nerve, right side** CC
√x7ᵗʰ **S04.32 Injury of trigeminal nerve, left side** CC

√5ᵗʰ **S04.4 Injury of abducent nerve**
Injury of 6th cranial nerve

CC Excl: For CC codes in subcategory S04.4, unless otherwise noted: CC with 7th character A: S04.40X-S04.42X with 7th A, S04.811-S04.9XX with 7th A

√x7ᵗʰ **S04.40 Injury of abducent nerve, unspecified side** CC
√x7ᵗʰ **S04.41 Injury of abducent nerve, right side** CC
√x7ᵗʰ **S04.42 Injury of abducent nerve, left side** CC

√5ᵗʰ **S04.5 Injury of facial nerve**
Injury of 7th cranial nerve

CC Excl: For CC codes in subcategory S04.5, unless otherwise noted: CC with 7th character A: S04.50X-S04.52X with 7th A, S04.811-S04.9XX with 7th A

√x7ᵗʰ **S04.50 Injury of facial nerve, unspecified side** CC
√x7ᵗʰ **S04.51 Injury of facial nerve, right side** CC
√x7ᵗʰ **S04.52 Injury of facial nerve, left side** CC

√5ᵗʰ **S04.6 Injury of acoustic nerve**
Injury of auditory nerve
Injury of 8th cranial nerve

CC Excl: For CC codes in subcategory S04.6, unless otherwise noted: CC with 7th character A: S04.60X-S04.62X with 7th A, S04.811-S04.9XX with 7th A

√x7ᵗʰ **S04.60 Injury of acoustic nerve, unspecified side** CC
√x7ᵗʰ **S04.61 Injury of acoustic nerve, right side** CC
√x7ᵗʰ **S04.62 Injury of acoustic nerve, left side** CC

√5ᵗʰ **S04.7 Injury of accessory nerve**
Injury of 11th cranial nerve

CC Excl: For CC codes in subcategory S04.7 unless otherwise noted: S04.70X-S04.9XX with 7th A

√x7ᵗʰ **S04.70 Injury of accessory nerve, unspecified side** CC
√x7ᵗʰ **S04.71 Injury of accessory nerve, right side** CC
√x7ᵗʰ **S04.72 Injury of accessory nerve, left side** CC

√5ᵗʰ **S04.8 Injury of other cranial nerves**

CC Excl: For CC codes in subcategory S04.8, unless otherwise noted: CC with 7th character A: S04.811-S04.9XX with 7th A

√6ᵗʰ **S04.81 Injury of olfactory [1st] nerve**
   √7ᵗʰ **S04.811 Injury of olfactory [1st] nerve, right side** CC
   √7ᵗʰ **S04.812 Injury of olfactory [1st] nerve, left side** CC
   √7ᵗʰ **S04.819 Injury of olfactory [1st] nerve, unspecified side** CC

√6ᵗʰ **S04.89 Injury of other cranial nerves**
Injury of vagus [10th] nerve
   √7ᵗʰ **S04.891 Injury of other cranial nerves, right side** CC
   √7ᵗʰ **S04.892 Injury of other cranial nerves, left side** CC
   √7ᵗʰ **S04.899 Injury of other cranial nerves, unspecified side** CC

√x7ᵗʰ **S04.9 Injury of unspecified cranial nerve** CC
CC Excl: CC with 7th character A: S04.8[1,9][1,2,9]A, S04.9XXA

Ⓝ Newborn: 0   Ⓟ Pediatric: 0-17   Ⓜ Maternity: 12-55   Ⓐ Adult: 15-124   MCC Major CC Condition   PDxMCC PDx acts as own MCC   CC CC Condition   PDxCC PDx acts as own CC

✓4ᵗʰ **S05** **Injury of eye and orbit**
Open wound of eye and orbit
EXCLUDES 2   2nd cranial [optic] nerve injury (S04.0-)
3rd cranial [oculomotor] nerve injury (S04.1-)
open wound of eyelid and periocular area (S01.1-)
orbital bone fracture (S02.1-, S02.3-, S02.8-)
superficial injury of eyelid (S00.1-S00.2)

The appropriate 7th is to be added to each code from category S05.
A   initial encounter
D   subsequent encounter
S   sequela

CC Excl: For CC codes in category S05, unless otherwise noted:
CC with 7th character A: S01.101-S01.159 with 7th A, S05.20X-
S05.8X9 with 7th A, S05.91X-S05.92X with 7th A, S38.3XXA, T14.90-
T14.91, T79.A0X-T79.9XX with 7th A

✓5ᵗʰ **S05.0** **Injury of conjunctiva and corneal abrasion without foreign body**
EXCLUDES 1   foreign body in conjunctival sac (T15.1)
foreign body in cornea (T15.0)

✓x7ᵗʰ **S05.00** **Injury of conjunctiva and corneal abrasion without foreign body, unspecified eye**

✓x7ᵗʰ **S05.01** **Injury of conjunctiva and corneal abrasion without foreign body, right eye**

✓x7ᵗʰ **S05.02** **Injury of conjunctiva and corneal abrasion without foreign body, left eye**

✓5ᵗʰ **S05.1** **Contusion of eyeball and orbital tissues**
Traumatic hyphema
EXCLUDES 2   black eye NOS (S00.1)
contusion of eyelid and periocular area (S00.1)

✓x7ᵗʰ **S05.10** **Contusion of eyeball and orbital tissues, unspecified eye**

✓x7ᵗʰ **S05.11** **Contusion of eyeball and orbital tissues, right eye**

✓x7ᵗʰ **S05.12** **Contusion of eyeball and orbital tissues, left eye**

✓5ᵗʰ **S05.2** **Ocular laceration and rupture with prolapse or loss of intraocular tissue**

✓x7ᵗʰ **S05.20** **Ocular laceration and rupture with prolapse or loss of intraocular tissue, unspecified eye** `CC`

✓x7ᵗʰ **S05.21** **Ocular laceration and rupture with prolapse or loss of intraocular tissue, right eye** `CC`

✓x7ᵗʰ **S05.22** **Ocular laceration and rupture with prolapse or loss of intraocular tissue, left eye** `CC`

✓5ᵗʰ **S05.3** **Ocular laceration without prolapse or loss of intraocular tissue**
Laceration of eye NOS

✓x7ᵗʰ **S05.30** **Ocular laceration without prolapse or loss of intraocular tissue, unspecified eye** `CC`

✓x7ᵗʰ **S05.31** **Ocular laceration without prolapse or loss of intraocular tissue, right eye** `CC`

✓x7ᵗʰ **S05.32** **Ocular laceration without prolapse or loss of intraocular tissue, left eye** `CC`

✓5ᵗʰ **S05.4** **Penetrating wound of orbit with or without foreign body**
EXCLUDES 2   retained (old) foreign body following penetrating wound in orbit (H05.5-)

✓x7ᵗʰ **S05.40** **Penetrating wound of orbit with or without foreign body, unspecified eye** `CC`

✓x7ᵗʰ **S05.41** **Penetrating wound of orbit with or without foreign body, right eye** `CC`

✓x7ᵗʰ **S05.42** **Penetrating wound of orbit with or without foreign body, left eye** `CC`

✓5ᵗʰ **S05.5** **Penetrating wound with foreign body of eyeball**
EXCLUDES 2   retained (old) intraocular foreign body (H44.6-, H44.7)

CC Excl: CC with 7th character A: S01.101-S01.159 with
7th A, S05.20X-S05.8X9 with 7th A, S05.91X-S05.92X with 7th
A, S38.3XXA, T14.90-T14.91, T79.8XX-T79.9XX with 7th A

✓x7ᵗʰ **S05.50** **Penetrating wound with foreign body of unspecified eyeball** `CC`

✓x7ᵗʰ **S05.51** **Penetrating wound with foreign body of right eyeball** `CC`

✓x7ᵗʰ **S05.52** **Penetrating wound with foreign body of left eyeball** `CC`

✓5ᵗʰ **S05.6** **Penetrating wound without foreign body of eyeball**
Ocular penetration NOS

✓x7ᵗʰ **S05.60** **Penetrating wound without foreign body of unspecified eyeball**

✓x7ᵗʰ **S05.61** **Penetrating wound without foreign body of right eyeball**

✓x7ᵗʰ **S05.62** **Penetrating wound without foreign body of left eyeball**

✓5ᵗʰ **S05.7** **Avulsion of eye**
Traumatic enucleation

✓x7ᵗʰ **S05.70** **Avulsion of unspecified eye** `CC`

✓x7ᵗʰ **S05.71** **Avulsion of right eye** `CC`

✓x7ᵗʰ **S05.72** **Avulsion of left eye** `CC`

✓5ᵗʰ **S05.8** **Other injuries of eye and orbit**
Lacrimal duct injury

✓6ᵗʰ **S05.8X** **Other injuries of eye and orbit**

✓7ᵗʰ **S05.8X1** **Other injuries of right eye and orbit** `CC`

✓7ᵗʰ **S05.8X2** **Other injuries of left eye and orbit** `CC`

✓7ᵗʰ **S05.8X9** **Other injuries of unspecified eye and orbit** `CC`

✓5ᵗʰ **S05.9** **Unspecified injury of eye and orbit**
Injury of eye NOS

✓x7ᵗʰ **S05.90** **Unspecified injury of unspecified eye and orbit**

✓x7ᵗʰ **S05.91** **Unspecified injury of right eye and orbit** `CC`

✓x7ᵗʰ **S05.92** **Unspecified injury of left eye and orbit** `CC`

✓4ᵗʰ **S06** **Intracranial injury**
Traumatic brain injury
Code also any associated:
open wound of head (S01.-)
skull fracture (S02.-)
EXCLUDES 1   head injury NOS (S09.90)

The appropriate 7th is to be added to each code from category S06.
A   initial encounter
D   subsequent encounter
S   sequela

For CC/MCC codes in category S06, unless otherwise noted: CC
or MCC as indicated with 7th A: S01.90X-S02.92X with 7th A,
S06.0X0-S07.9XX with 7th A, S08.89X-S09.19X with 7th A, S09.8X-
S09.90X with 7th A, S09.92X-S09.93X with 7th A, S16.8XX-S19.9XX
with 7th A, S38.3XXA, T14.90-T14.91, T79.A0X-T79.9XX with 7th A

✓5ᵗʰ **S06.0** **Concussion**
Commotio cerebri
EXCLUDES 1   concussion with other intracranial injuries classified in category S06—code to specified intracranial injury

✓6ᵗʰ **S06.0X** **Concussion**

✓7ᵗʰ **S06.0X0** **Concussion without loss of consciousness**

7 ✓7ᵗʰ **S06.0X1** **Concussion with loss of consciousness of 30 minutes or less** `CC`

7 ✓7ᵗʰ **S06.0X2** **Concussion with loss of consciousness of 31 minutes to 59 minutes** `CC`

7 ✓7ᵗʰ **S06.0X3** **Concussion with loss of consciousness of 1 hour to 5 hours 59 minutes** `CC`

7 ✓7ᵗʰ **S06.0X4** **Concussion with loss of consciousness of 6 hours to 24 hours** `CC`

7 ✓7ᵗʰ **S06.0X5** **Concussion with loss of consciousness greater than 24 hours with return to pre-existing conscious level** `CC`

7 ✓7ᵗʰ **S06.0X6** **Concussion with loss of consciousness greater than 24 hours without return to pre-existing conscious level with patient surviving** `MCC`

7 ✓7ᵗʰ **S06.0X7** **Concussion with loss of consciousness of any duration with death due to brain injury prior to regaining consciousness** `CC`

7 ✓7ᵗʰ **S06.0X8** **Concussion with loss of consciousness of any duration with death due to other cause prior to regaining consciousness** `CC`

7 ✓7ᵗʰ **S06.0X9** **Concussion with loss of consciousness of unspecified duration** `CC`
Concussion NOS

---

7   HAC = Initial encounter only (7th character A, B or C) and not POA.

✓ Additional Character Required   ✓x7ᵗʰ Placeholder Alert   Unacceptable PDx   Manifestation   Hospital Acquired Condition   *EXCLUDES 1* Not Coded Here   *EXCLUDES 2* Not Included Here

Chapter 19. Injury, Poisoning, and Certain Other Consequences of External Causes

S06.1–S06.313

√5ᵗʰ **S06.1 Traumatic cerebral edema**
Diffuse traumatic cerebral edema
Focal traumatic cerebral edema

√6ᵗʰ **S06.1X Traumatic cerebral edema**

√7ᵗʰ **S06.1X0 Traumatic cerebral edema** PDxMCC MCC
without loss of consciousness
CC Excl: CC with 7th character A: G93.6, G93.82

7 √7ᵗʰ **S06.1X1 Traumatic cerebral edema** PDxMCC MCC
with loss of consciousness of 30 minutes or less
CC Excl: MCC with 7th character A: G93.6, G93.82, S01.90X-S01.95X with 7th A, S02.0XX-S02.19X with 7th [A, B, S], S02.2XX-S02.8XX with 7th S, S02.91X with 7th [A, B, S], S02.92XS, S06.0X0-S07.9XX with 7th A, S08.89XA, S09.10X-S09.19X with 7th A, S09.8XXA, S09.90XA, S02.92X-S09.93X with 7th A, S16.8XX-S19.9XX with 7th A, S38.3XXA, T14.90-T14.91, T79.A0X-T79.9XX with 7th A

7 √7ᵗʰ **S06.1X2 Traumatic cerebral edema** PDxMCC MCC
with loss of consciousness of 31 minutes to 59 minutes
CC Excl: See code: S06.1X1

7 √7ᵗʰ **S06.1X3 Traumatic cerebral edema** PDxMCC MCC
with loss of consciousness of 1 hour to 5 hours 59 minutes
CC Excl: See code: S06.1X1

7 √7ᵗʰ **S06.1X4 Traumatic cerebral edema** PDxMCC MCC
with loss of consciousness of 6 hours to 24 hours
CC Excl: See code: S06.1X1

7 √7ᵗʰ **S06.1X5 Traumatic cerebral edema** PDxMCC MCC
with loss of consciousness greater than 24 hours with return to pre-existing conscious level
CC Excl: See code: S06.1X1

7 √7ᵗʰ **S06.1X6 Traumatic cerebral edema** PDxMCC MCC
with loss of consciousness greater than 24 hours without return to pre-existing conscious level with patient surviving
CC Excl: MCC with 7th character A: S01.90X-S01.95X with 7th A, S02.0XX-S02.19X with 7th [A, B, S], S02.2XX-S02.8XX with 7th S, S02.91X with 7th [A, B, S], S02.92XS, S06.0X0-S07.9XX with 7th A, S08.89XA, S09.10X-S09.19X with 7th A, S09.8XXA, S09.90XA, S09.92X-S09.93X with 7th A, S16.8XX-S19.9XX with 7th A, S38.3XXA, T14.90-T14.91, T79.A0X-T79.9XX with 7th A

7 √7ᵗʰ **S06.1X7 Traumatic cerebral edema** PDxMCC MCC
with loss of consciousness of any duration with death due to brain injury prior to regaining consciousness
CC Excl: See code: S06.1X6

7 √7ᵗʰ **S06.1X8 Traumatic cerebral edema** PDxMCC MCC
with loss of consciousness of any duration with death due to other cause prior to regaining consciousness
CC Excl: See code: S06.1X6

7 √7ᵗʰ **S06.1X9 Traumatic cerebral edema** PDxMCC MCC
with loss of consciousness of unspecified duration
Traumatic cerebral edema NOS
CC Excl: See code: S06.1X6

√5ᵗʰ **S06.2 Diffuse traumatic brain injury**
Diffuse axonal brain injury
EXCLUDES1 traumatic diffuse cerebral edema (S06.1X-)

√6ᵗʰ **S06.2X Diffuse traumatic brain injury**

√7ᵗʰ **S06.2X0 Diffuse traumatic brain injury without loss of consciousness**

7 √7ᵗʰ **S06.2X1 Diffuse traumatic brain injury with loss of consciousness of 30 minutes or less** CC

7 √7ᵗʰ **S06.2X2 Diffuse traumatic brain injury with loss of consciousness of 31 minutes to 59 minutes** CC

7 √7ᵗʰ **S06.2X3 Diffuse traumatic brain injury with loss of consciousness of 1 hour to 5 hours 59 minutes** CC

7 √7ᵗʰ **S06.2X4 Diffuse traumatic brain injury with loss of consciousness of 6 hours to 24 hours** CC

7 √7ᵗʰ **S06.2X5 Diffuse traumatic brain injury with loss of consciousness greater than 24 hours with return to pre-existing conscious levels** CC

7 √7ᵗʰ **S06.2X6 Diffuse traumatic brain injury with loss of consciousness greater than 24 hours without return to pre-existing conscious level with patient surviving** MCC

7 √7ᵗʰ **S06.2X7 Diffuse traumatic brain injury with loss of consciousness of any duration with death due to brain injury prior to regaining consciousness** MCC

7 √7ᵗʰ **S06.2X8 Diffuse traumatic brain injury with loss of consciousness of any duration with death due to other cause prior to regaining consciousness** MCC

7 √7ᵗʰ **S06.2X9 Diffuse traumatic brain injury with loss of consciousness of unspecified duration** CC
Diffuse traumatic brain injury NOS

√5ᵗʰ **S06.3 Focal traumatic brain injury**
EXCLUDES1 any condition classifiable to S06.4-S06.6
focal cerebral edema (S06.1)

√6ᵗʰ **S06.30 Unspecified focal traumatic brain injury**

√7ᵗʰ **S06.300 Unspecified focal traumatic brain injury without loss of consciousness**

7 √7ᵗʰ **S06.301 Unspecified focal traumatic brain injury with loss of consciousness of 30 minutes or less** CC

7 √7ᵗʰ **S06.302 Unspecified focal traumatic brain injury with loss of consciousness of 31 minutes to 59 minutes** CC

7 √7ᵗʰ **S06.303 Unspecified focal traumatic brain injury with loss of consciousness of 1 hour to 5 hours 59 minutes** CC

7 √7ᵗʰ **S06.304 Unspecified focal traumatic brain injury with loss of consciousness of 6 hours to 24 hours** CC

7 √7ᵗʰ **S06.305 Unspecified focal traumatic brain injury with loss of consciousness greater than 24 hours with return to pre-existing conscious level** CC

7 √7ᵗʰ **S06.306 Unspecified focal traumatic brain injury with loss of consciousness greater than 24 hours without return to pre-existing conscious level with patient surviving** MCC

7 √7ᵗʰ **S06.307 Unspecified focal traumatic brain injury with loss of consciousness of any duration with death due to brain injury prior to regaining consciousness** MCC

7 √7ᵗʰ **S06.308 Unspecified focal traumatic brain injury with loss of consciousness of any duration with death due to other cause prior to regaining consciousness** MCC

7 √7ᵗʰ **S06.309 Unspecified focal traumatic brain injury with loss of consciousness of unspecified duration** CC
Unspecified focal traumatic brain injury NOS

√6ᵗʰ **S06.31 Contusion and laceration of right cerebrum**

7 √7ᵗʰ **S06.310 Contusion and laceration of right cerebrum without loss of consciousness** MCC

7 √7ᵗʰ **S06.311 Contusion and laceration of right cerebrum with loss of consciousness of 30 minutes or less** MCC

7 √7ᵗʰ **S06.312 Contusion and laceration of right cerebrum with loss of consciousness of 31 minutes to 59 minutes** MCC

7 √7ᵗʰ **S06.313 Contusion and laceration of right cerebrum with loss of consciousness of 1 hour to 5 hours 59 minutes** MCC

---

7   HAC = Initial encounter only (7th character A, B or C) and not POA.

N Newborn: 0   P Pediatric: 0-17   M Maternity: 12-55   A Adult: 15-124   MCC Major CC Condition   PDxMCC PDx acts as own MCC   CC CC Condition   PDxCC PDx acts as own CC

906   ICD-10-CM 2016

7 √7ᵗʰ **S06.314 Contusion and laceration of right cerebrum with loss of consciousness of 6 hours to 24 hours** MCC

7 √7ᵗʰ **S06.315 Contusion and laceration of right cerebrum with loss of consciousness greater than 24 hours with return to pre-existing conscious level** MCC

7 √7ᵗʰ **S06.316 Contusion and laceration of right cerebrum with loss of consciousness greater than 24 hours without return to pre-existing conscious level with patient surviving** MCC

7 √7ᵗʰ **S06.317 Contusion and laceration of right cerebrum with loss of consciousness of any duration with death due to brain injury prior to regaining consciousness** MCC

7 √7ᵗʰ **S06.318 Contusion and laceration of right cerebrum with loss of consciousness of any duration with death due to other cause prior to regaining consciousness** MCC

7 √7ᵗʰ **S06.319 Contusion and laceration of right cerebrum with loss of consciousness of unspecified duration** MCC
Contusion and laceration of right cerebrum NOS

√6ᵗʰ **S06.32 Contusion and laceration of left cerebrum**

7 √7ᵗʰ **S06.320 Contusion and laceration of left cerebrum without loss of consciousness** MCC

7 √7ᵗʰ **S06.321 Contusion and laceration of left cerebrum with loss of consciousness of 30 minutes or less** MCC

7 √7ᵗʰ **S06.322 Contusion and laceration of left cerebrum with loss of consciousness of 31 minutes to 59 minutes** MCC

7 √7ᵗʰ **S06.323 Contusion and laceration of left cerebrum with loss of consciousness of 1 hour to 5 hours 59 minutes** MCC

7 √7ᵗʰ **S06.324 Contusion and laceration of left cerebrum with loss of consciousness of 6 hours to 24 hours** MCC

7 √7ᵗʰ **S06.325 Contusion and laceration of left cerebrum with loss of consciousness greater than 24 hours with return to pre-existing conscious level** MCC

7 √7ᵗʰ **S06.326 Contusion and laceration of left cerebrum with loss of consciousness greater than 24 hours without return to pre-existing conscious level with patient surviving** MCC

7 √7ᵗʰ **S06.327 Contusion and laceration of left cerebrum with loss of consciousness of any duration with death due to brain injury prior to regaining consciousness** MCC

7 √7ᵗʰ **S06.328 Contusion and laceration of left cerebrum with loss of consciousness of any duration with death due to other cause prior to regaining consciousness** MCC

7 √7ᵗʰ **S06.329 Contusion and laceration of left cerebrum with loss of consciousness of unspecified duration** MCC
Contusion and laceration of left cerebrum NOS

√6ᵗʰ **S06.33 Contusion and laceration of cerebrum, unspecified**

7 √7ᵗʰ **S06.330 Contusion and laceration of cerebrum, unspecified, without loss of consciousness** MCC

7 √7ᵗʰ **S06.331 Contusion and laceration of cerebrum, unspecified, with loss of consciousness of 30 minutes or less** MCC

7 √7ᵗʰ **S06.332 Contusion and laceration of cerebrum, unspecified, with loss of consciousness of 31 minutes to 59 minutes** MCC

7 √7ᵗʰ **S06.333 Contusion and laceration of cerebrum, unspecified, with loss of consciousness of 1 hour to 5 hours 59 minutes** MCC

7 √7ᵗʰ **S06.334 Contusion and laceration of cerebrum, unspecified, with loss of consciousness of 6 hours to 24 hours** MCC

7 √7ᵗʰ **S06.335 Contusion and laceration of cerebrum, unspecified, with loss of consciousness greater than 24 hours with return to pre-existing conscious level** MCC

7 √7ᵗʰ **S06.336 Contusion and laceration of cerebrum, unspecified, with loss of consciousness greater than 24 hours without return to pre-existing conscious level with patient surviving** MCC

7 √7ᵗʰ **S06.337 Contusion and laceration of cerebrum, unspecified, with loss of consciousness of any duration with death due to brain injury prior to regaining consciousness** MCC

7 √7ᵗʰ **S06.338 Contusion and laceration of cerebrum, unspecified, with loss of consciousness of any duration with death due to other cause prior to regaining consciousness** MCC

7 √7ᵗʰ **S06.339 Contusion and laceration of cerebrum, unspecified, with loss of consciousness of unspecified duration** MCC
Contusion and laceration of cerebrum NOS

√6ᵗʰ **S06.34 Traumatic hemorrhage of right cerebrum**
Traumatic intracerebral hemorrhage and hematoma of right cerebrum

7 √7ᵗʰ **S06.340 Traumatic hemorrhage of right cerebrum without loss of consciousness** MCC

7 √7ᵗʰ **S06.341 Traumatic hemorrhage of right cerebrum with loss of consciousness of 30 minutes or less** MCC

7 √7ᵗʰ **S06.342 Traumatic hemorrhage of right cerebrum with loss of consciousness of 31 minutes to 59 minutes** MCC

7 √7ᵗʰ **S06.343 Traumatic hemorrhage of right cerebrum with loss of consciousness of 1 hours to 5 hours 59 minutes** MCC

7 √7ᵗʰ **S06.344 Traumatic hemorrhage of right cerebrum with loss of consciousness of 6 hours to 24 hours** MCC

7 √7ᵗʰ **S06.345 Traumatic hemorrhage of right cerebrum with loss of consciousness greater than 24 hours with return to pre-existing conscious level** MCC

7 √7ᵗʰ **S06.346 Traumatic hemorrhage of right cerebrum with loss of consciousness greater than 24 hours without return to pre-existing conscious level with patient surviving** MCC

7 √7ᵗʰ **S06.347 Traumatic hemorrhage of right cerebrum with loss of consciousness of any duration with death due to brain injury prior to regaining consciousness** MCC

7 √7ᵗʰ **S06.348 Traumatic hemorrhage of right cerebrum with loss of consciousness of any duration with death due to other cause prior to regaining consciousness** MCC

7 √7ᵗʰ **S06.349 Traumatic hemorrhage of right cerebrum with loss of consciousness of unspecified duration** MCC
Traumatic hemorrhage of right cerebrum NOS

√6ᵗʰ **S06.35 Traumatic hemorrhage of left cerebrum**
Traumatic intracerebral hemorrhage and hematoma of left cerebrum

7 √7ᵗʰ **S06.350 Traumatic hemorrhage of left cerebrum without loss of consciousness** MCC

7 √7ᵗʰ **S06.351 Traumatic hemorrhage of left cerebrum with loss of consciousness of 30 minutes or less** MCC

7   HAC = Initial encounter only (7th character A, B or C) and not POA.

✔ Additional Character Required   √x7ᵗʰ Placeholder Alert   Unacceptable PDx   Manifestation   Hospital Acquired Condition   EXCLUDES 1 Not Coded Here   EXCLUDES 2 Not Included Here
ICD-10-CM 2016   907

7 ✓7ᵗʰ **S06.352** Traumatic hemorrhage of left cerebrum with loss of consciousness of 31 minutes to 59 minutes   `MCC`

7 ✓7ᵗʰ **S06.353** Traumatic hemorrhage of left cerebrum with loss of consciousness of 1 hours to 5 hours 59 minutes   `MCC`

7 ✓7ᵗʰ **S06.354** Traumatic hemorrhage of left cerebrum with loss of consciousness of 6 hours to 24 hours   `MCC`

7 ✓7ᵗʰ **S06.355** Traumatic hemorrhage of left cerebrum with loss of consciousness greater than 24 hours with return to pre-existing conscious level   `MCC`

7 ✓7ᵗʰ **S06.356** Traumatic hemorrhage of left cerebrum with loss of consciousness greater than 24 hours without return to pre-existing conscious level with patient surviving   `MCC`

7 ✓7ᵗʰ **S06.357** Traumatic hemorrhage of left cerebrum with loss of consciousness of any duration with death due to brain injury prior to regaining consciousness   `MCC`

7 ✓7ᵗʰ **S06.358** Traumatic hemorrhage of left cerebrum with loss of consciousness of any duration with death due to other cause prior to regaining consciousness   `MCC`

7 ✓7ᵗʰ **S06.359** Traumatic hemorrhage of left cerebrum with loss of consciousness of unspecified duration   `MCC`
> Traumatic hemorrhage of left cerebrum NOS

✓6ᵗʰ **S06.36** Traumatic hemorrhage of cerebrum, unspecified
> Traumatic intracerebral hemorrhage and hematoma, unspecified

7 ✓7ᵗʰ **S06.360** Traumatic hemorrhage of cerebrum, unspecified, without loss of consciousness   `MCC`

7 ✓7ᵗʰ **S06.361** Traumatic hemorrhage of cerebrum, unspecified, with loss of consciousness of 30 minutes or less   `MCC`

7 ✓7ᵗʰ **S06.362** Traumatic hemorrhage of cerebrum, unspecified, with loss of consciousness of 31 minutes to 59 minutes   `MCC`

7 ✓7ᵗʰ **S06.363** Traumatic hemorrhage of cerebrum, unspecified, with loss of consciousness of 1 hours to 5 hours 59 minutes   `MCC`

7 ✓7ᵗʰ **S06.364** Traumatic hemorrhage of cerebrum, unspecified, with loss of consciousness of 6 hours to 24 hours   `MCC`

7 ✓7ᵗʰ **S06.365** Traumatic hemorrhage of cerebrum, unspecified, with loss of consciousness greater than 24 hours with return to pre-existing conscious level   `MCC`

7 ✓7ᵗʰ **S06.366** Traumatic hemorrhage of cerebrum, unspecified, with loss of consciousness greater than 24 hours without return to pre-existing conscious level with patient surviving   `MCC`

7 ✓7ᵗʰ **S06.367** Traumatic hemorrhage of cerebrum, unspecified, with loss of consciousness of any duration with death due to brain injury prior to regaining consciousness   `MCC`

7 ✓7ᵗʰ **S06.368** Traumatic hemorrhage of cerebrum, unspecified, with loss of consciousness of any duration with death due to other cause prior to regaining consciousness   `MCC`

7 ✓7ᵗʰ **S06.369** Traumatic hemorrhage of cerebrum, unspecified, with loss of consciousness of unspecified duration   `MCC`
> Traumatic hemorrhage of cerebrum NOS

✓6ᵗʰ **S06.37** Contusion, laceration, and hemorrhage of cerebellum

7 ✓7ᵗʰ **S06.370** Contusion, laceration, and hemorrhage of cerebellum without loss of consciousness   `MCC`
> **CC Excl:** No Excl

7 ✓7ᵗʰ **S06.371** Contusion, laceration, and hemorrhage of cerebellum with loss of consciousness of 30 minutes or less   `CC`

7 ✓7ᵗʰ **S06.372** Contusion, laceration, and hemorrhage of cerebellum with loss of consciousness of 31 minutes to 59 minutes   `CC`

7 ✓7ᵗʰ **S06.373** Contusion, laceration, and hemorrhage of cerebellum with loss of consciousness of 1 hour to 5 hours 59 minutes   `CC`

7 ✓7ᵗʰ **S06.374** Contusion, laceration, and hemorrhage of cerebellum with loss of consciousness of 6 hours to 24 hours   `CC`

7 ✓7ᵗʰ **S06.375** Contusion, laceration, and hemorrhage of cerebellum with loss of consciousness greater than 24 hours with return to pre-existing conscious level   `CC`

7 ✓7ᵗʰ **S06.376** Contusion, laceration, and hemorrhage of cerebellum with loss of consciousness greater than 24 hours without return to pre-existing conscious level with patient surviving   `MCC`

7 ✓7ᵗʰ **S06.377** Contusion, laceration, and hemorrhage of cerebellum with loss of consciousness of any duration with death due to brain injury prior to regaining consciousness   `MCC`

7 ✓7ᵗʰ **S06.378** Contusion, laceration, and hemorrhage of cerebellum with loss of consciousness of any duration with death due to other cause prior to regaining consciousness   `MCC`

7 ✓7ᵗʰ **S06.379** Contusion, laceration, and hemorrhage of cerebellum with loss of consciousness of unspecified duration   `CC`
> Contusion, laceration, and hemorrhage of cerebellum NOS

✓6ᵗʰ **S06.38** Contusion, laceration, and hemorrhage of brainstem

7 ✓7ᵗʰ **S06.380** Contusion, laceration, and hemorrhage of brainstem without loss of consciousness   `MCC`
> **CC Excl:** No Excl

7 ✓7ᵗʰ **S06.381** Contusion, laceration, and hemorrhage of brainstem with loss of consciousness of 30 minutes or less   `CC`

7 ✓7ᵗʰ **S06.382** Contusion, laceration, and hemorrhage of brainstem with loss of consciousness of 31 minutes to 59 minutes   `CC`

7 ✓7ᵗʰ **S06.383** Contusion, laceration, and hemorrhage of brainstem with loss of consciousness of 1 hour to 5 hours 59 minutes   `CC`

7 ✓7ᵗʰ **S06.384** Contusion, laceration, and hemorrhage of brainstem with loss of consciousness of 6 hours to 24 hours   `CC`

7 ✓7ᵗʰ **S06.385** Contusion, laceration, and hemorrhage of brainstem with loss of consciousness greater than 24 hours with return to pre-existing conscious level   `CC`

7 ✓7ᵗʰ **S06.386** Contusion, laceration, and hemorrhage of brainstem with loss of consciousness greater than 24 hours without return to pre-existing conscious level with patient surviving   `MCC`

7 ✓7ᵗʰ **S06.387** Contusion, laceration, and hemorrhage of brainstem with loss of consciousness of any duration with death due to brain injury prior to regaining consciousness   `MCC`

7 ✓7ᵗʰ **S06.388** Contusion, laceration, and hemorrhage of brainstem with loss of consciousness of any duration with death due to other cause prior to regaining consciousness   `MCC`

---

7 HAC = Initial encounter only (7th character A, B or C) and not POA.

Ⓝ Newborn: 0   Ⓟ Pediatric: 0-17   Ⓜ Maternity: 12-55   Ⓐ Adult: 15-124   `MCC` Major CC Condition   `PDxMCC` PDx acts as own MCC   `CC` CC Condition   `PDxCC` PDx acts as own CC

908   ICD-10-CM 2016

7 ✓7th **S06.389** **Contusion, laceration, and hemorrhage of brainstem with loss of consciousness of unspecified duration** `CC`
Contusion, laceration, and hemorrhage of brainstem NOS

✓5th **S06.4** **Epidural hemorrhage**
Extradural hemorrhage NOS
Extradural hemorrhage (traumatic)

✓6th **S06.4X** **Epidural hemorrhage**

7 ✓7th **S06.4X0** **Epidural hemorrhage without loss of consciousness** `MCC`

7 ✓7th **S06.4X1** **Epidural hemorrhage with loss of consciousness of 30 minutes or less** `MCC`

7 ✓7th **S06.4X2** **Epidural hemorrhage with loss of consciousness of 31 minutes to 59 minutes** `MCC`

7 ✓7th **S06.4X3** **Epidural hemorrhage with loss of consciousness of 1 hour to 5 hours 59 minutes** `MCC`

7 ✓7th **S06.4X4** **Epidural hemorrhage with loss of consciousness of 6 hours to 24 hours** `MCC`

7 ✓7th **S06.4X5** **Epidural hemorrhage with loss of consciousness greater than 24 hours with return to pre-existing conscious level** `MCC`

7 ✓7th **S06.4X6** **Epidural hemorrhage with loss of consciousness greater than 24 hours without return to pre-existing conscious level with patient surviving** `MCC`

7 ✓7th **S06.4X7** **Epidural hemorrhage with loss of consciousness of any duration with death due to brain injury prior to regaining consciousness** `MCC`

7 ✓7th **S06.4X8** **Epidural hemorrhage with loss of consciousness of any duration with death due to other causes prior to regaining consciousness** `MCC`

7 ✓7th **S06.4X9** **Epidural hemorrhage with loss of consciousness of unspecified duration** `MCC`
Epidural hemorrhage NOS

✓5th **S06.5** **Traumatic subdural hemorrhage**

✓6th **S06.5X** **Traumatic subdural hemorrhage**

7 ✓7th **S06.5X0** **Traumatic subdural hemorrhage without loss of consciousness** `MCC`

7 ✓7th **S06.5X1** **Traumatic subdural hemorrhage with loss of consciousness of 30 minutes or less** `MCC`

7 ✓7th **S06.5X2** **Traumatic subdural hemorrhage with loss of consciousness of 31 minutes to 59 minutes** `MCC`

7 ✓7th **S06.5X3** **Traumatic subdural hemorrhage with loss of consciousness of 1 hour to 5 hours 59 minutes** `MCC`

7 ✓7th **S06.5X4** **Traumatic subdural hemorrhage with loss of consciousness of 6 hours to 24 hours** `MCC`

7 ✓7th **S06.5X5** **Traumatic subdural hemorrhage with loss of consciousness greater than 24 hours with return to pre-existing conscious level** `MCC`

7 ✓7th **S06.5X6** **Traumatic subdural hemorrhage with loss of consciousness greater than 24 hours without return to pre-existing conscious level with patient surviving** `MCC`

7 ✓7th **S06.5X7** **Traumatic subdural hemorrhage with loss of consciousness of any duration with death due to brain injury before regaining consciousness** `MCC`

7 ✓7th **S06.5X8** **Traumatic subdural hemorrhage with loss of consciousness of any duration with death due to other cause before regaining consciousness** `MCC`

7 ✓7th **S06.5X9** **Traumatic subdural hemorrhage with loss of consciousness of unspecified duration** `MCC`
Traumatic subdural hemorrhage NOS

✓5th **S06.6** **Traumatic subarachnoid hemorrhage**

✓6th **S06.6X** **Traumatic subarachnoid hemorrhage**

7 ✓7th **S06.6X0** **Traumatic subarachnoid hemorrhage without loss of consciousness** `MCC`

7 ✓7th **S06.6X1** **Traumatic subarachnoid hemorrhage with loss of consciousness of 30 minutes or less** `MCC`

7 ✓7th **S06.6X2** **Traumatic subarachnoid hemorrhage with loss of consciousness of 31 minutes to 59 minutes** `MCC`

7 ✓7th **S06.6X3** **Traumatic subarachnoid hemorrhage with loss of consciousness of 1 hour to 5 hours 59 minutes** `MCC`

7 ✓7th **S06.6X4** **Traumatic subarachnoid hemorrhage with loss of consciousness of 6 hours to 24 hours** `MCC`

7 ✓7th **S06.6X5** **Traumatic subarachnoid hemorrhage with loss of consciousness greater than 24 hours with return to pre-existing conscious level** `MCC`

7 ✓7th **S06.6X6** **Traumatic subarachnoid hemorrhage with loss of consciousness greater than 24 hours without return to pre-existing conscious level with patient surviving** `MCC`

7 ✓7th **S06.6X7** **Traumatic subarachnoid hemorrhage with loss of consciousness of any duration with death due to brain injury prior to regaining consciousness** `MCC`

7 ✓7th **S06.6X8** **Traumatic subarachnoid hemorrhage with loss of consciousness of any duration with death due to other cause prior to regaining consciousness** `MCC`

7 ✓7th **S06.6X9** **Traumatic subarachnoid hemorrhage with loss of consciousness of unspecified duration** `MCC`
Traumatic subarachnoid hemorrhage NOS

✓5th **S06.8** **Other specified intracranial injuries**

✓6th **S06.81** **Injury of right internal carotid artery, intracranial portion, not elsewhere classified**

✓7th **S06.810** **Injury of right internal carotid artery, intracranial portion, not elsewhere classified without loss of consciousness**

7 ✓7th **S06.811** **Injury of right internal carotid artery, intracranial portion, not elsewhere classified with loss of consciousness of 30 minutes or less** `CC`

7 ✓7th **S06.812** **Injury of right internal carotid artery, intracranial portion, not elsewhere classified with loss of consciousness of 31 minutes to 59 minutes** `CC`

7 ✓7th **S06.813** **Injury of right internal carotid artery, intracranial portion, not elsewhere classified with loss of consciousness of 1 hour to 5 hours 59 minutes** `CC`

7 ✓7th **S06.814** **Injury of right internal carotid artery, intracranial portion, not elsewhere classified with loss of consciousness of 6 hours to 24 hours** `CC`

7 ✓7th **S06.815** **Injury of right internal carotid artery, intracranial portion, not elsewhere classified with loss of consciousness greater than 24 hours with return to pre-existing conscious level** `CC`

7 ✓7th **S06.816** **Injury of right internal carotid artery, intracranial portion, not elsewhere classified with loss of consciousness greater than 24 hours without return to pre-existing conscious level with patient surviving** `MCC`

7 ✓7th **S06.817** **Injury of right internal carotid artery, intracranial portion, not elsewhere classified with loss of consciousness of any duration with death due to brain injury prior to regaining consciousness** `MCC`

---

7 HAC = Initial encounter only (7th character A, B or C) and not POA.

7 ✓7ᵗʰ **S06.818** **Injury of right internal carotid artery, intracranial portion, not elsewhere classified with loss of consciousness of any duration with death due to other cause prior to regaining consciousness** `MCC`

7 ✓7ᵗʰ **S06.819** **Injury of right internal carotid artery, intracranial portion, not elsewhere classified with loss of consciousness of unspecified duration** `CC`
> Injury of right internal carotid artery, intracranial portion, not elsewhere classified NOS

✓6ᵗʰ **S06.82** **Injury of left internal carotid artery, intracranial portion, not elsewhere classified**

   ✓7ᵗʰ **S06.820** **Injury of left internal carotid artery, intracranial portion, not elsewhere classified without loss of consciousness**

7 ✓7ᵗʰ **S06.821** **Injury of left internal carotid artery, intracranial portion, not elsewhere classified with loss of consciousness of 30 minutes or less** `CC`

7 ✓7ᵗʰ **S06.822** **Injury of left internal carotid artery, intracranial portion, not elsewhere classified with loss of consciousness of 31 minutes to 59 minutes** `CC`

7 ✓7ᵗʰ **S06.823** **Injury of left internal carotid artery, intracranial portion, not elsewhere classified with loss of consciousness of 1 hour to 5 hours 59 minutes** `CC`

7 ✓7ᵗʰ **S06.824** **Injury of left internal carotid artery, intracranial portion, not elsewhere classified with loss of consciousness of 6 hours to 24 hours** `CC`

7 ✓7ᵗʰ **S06.825** **Injury of left internal carotid artery, intracranial portion, not elsewhere classified with loss of consciousness greater than 24 hours with return to pre-existing conscious level** `CC`

7 ✓7ᵗʰ **S06.826** **Injury of left internal carotid artery, intracranial portion, not elsewhere classified with loss of consciousness greater than 24 hours without return to pre-existing conscious level with patient surviving** `MCC`

7 ✓7ᵗʰ **S06.827** **Injury of left internal carotid artery, intracranial portion, not elsewhere classified with loss of consciousness of any duration with death due to brain injury prior to regaining consciousness** `MCC`

7 ✓7ᵗʰ **S06.828** **Injury of left internal carotid artery, intracranial portion, not elsewhere classified with loss of consciousness of any duration with death due to other cause prior to regaining consciousness** `MCC`

7 ✓7ᵗʰ **S06.829** **Injury of left internal carotid artery, intracranial portion, not elsewhere classified with loss of consciousness of unspecified duration** `CC`
> Injury of left internal carotid artery, intracranial portion, not elsewhere classified NOS

✓6ᵗʰ **S06.89** **Other specified intracranial injury**

   ✓7ᵗʰ **S06.890** **Other specified intracranial injury without loss of consciousness**

7 ✓7ᵗʰ **S06.891** **Other specified intracranial injury with loss of consciousness of 30 minutes or less** `CC`

7 ✓7ᵗʰ **S06.892** **Other specified intracranial injury with loss of consciousness of 31 minutes to 59 minutes** `CC`

7 ✓7ᵗʰ **S06.893** **Other specified intracranial injury with loss of consciousness of 1 hour to 5 hours 59 minutes** `CC`

7 ✓7ᵗʰ **S06.894** **Other specified intracranial injury with loss of consciousness of 6 hours to 24 hours** `CC`

7 ✓7ᵗʰ **S06.895** **Other specified intracranial injury with loss of consciousness greater than 24 hours with return to pre-existing conscious level** `CC`

7 ✓7ᵗʰ **S06.896** **Other specified intracranial injury with loss of consciousness greater than 24 hours without return to pre-existing conscious level with patient surviving** `MCC`

7 ✓7ᵗʰ **S06.897** **Other specified intracranial injury with loss of consciousness of any duration with death due to brain injury prior to regaining consciousness** `MCC`

7 ✓7ᵗʰ **S06.898** **Other specified intracranial injury with loss of consciousness of any duration with death due to other cause prior to regaining consciousness** `MCC`

7 ✓7ᵗʰ **S06.899** **Other specified intracranial injury with loss of consciousness of unspecified duration** `CC`

✓5ᵗʰ **S06.9** **Unspecified intracranial injury**
> Brain injury NOS
> Head injury NOS with loss of consciousness
> **EXCLUDES 1**   head injury NOS (S09.90)

✓6ᵗʰ **S06.9X** **Unspecified intracranial injury**

   ✓7ᵗʰ **S06.9X0** **Unspecified intracranial injury without loss of consciousness**

7 ✓7ᵗʰ **S06.9X1** **Unspecified intracranial injury with loss of consciousness of 30 minutes or less** `CC`

7 ✓7ᵗʰ **S06.9X2** **Unspecified intracranial injury with loss of consciousness of 31 minutes to 59 minutes** `CC`

7 ✓7ᵗʰ **S06.9X3** **Unspecified intracranial injury with loss of consciousness of 1 hour to 5 hours 59 minutes** `CC`

7 ✓7ᵗʰ **S06.9X4** **Unspecified intracranial injury with loss of consciousness of 6 hours to 24 hours** `CC`

7 ✓7ᵗʰ **S06.9X5** **Unspecified intracranial injury with loss of consciousness greater than 24 hours with return to pre-existing conscious level** `CC`

7 ✓7ᵗʰ **S06.9X6** **Unspecified intracranial injury with loss of consciousness greater than 24 hours without return to pre-existing conscious level with patient surviving** `MCC`

7 ✓7ᵗʰ **S06.9X7** **Unspecified intracranial injury with loss of consciousness of any duration with death due to brain injury prior to regaining consciousness** `MCC`

7 ✓7ᵗʰ **S06.9X8** **Unspecified intracranial injury with loss of consciousness of any duration with death due to other cause prior to regaining consciousness** `MCC`

7 ✓7ᵗʰ **S06.9X9** **Unspecified intracranial injury with loss of consciousness of unspecified duration** `CC`

✓4ᵗʰ **S07** **Crushing injury of head**
> Use additional code for all associated injuries, such as:
>   intracranial injuries (S06.-)
>   skull fractures (S02.-)

> The appropriate 7th is to be added to each code from category S07.
> A   initial encounter
> D   subsequent encounter
> S   sequela

> **For CC/MCC codes in category S07, unless otherwise noted: CC with 7th character A:** S01.90X–S02.92X with 7th A, S07.0XX–S07.9XX with 7th A, S08.89X–S09.19X with 7th A, S09.8XX–S09.90X with 7th A, S09.92X–S09.93X with 7th A, S16.8XX–S19.9XX with 7th A, T14.90–T14.91, T79.A0X–T79.9XX with 7th A

7 ✓x7ᵗʰ **S07.0** **Crushing injury of face** `CC`

7 ✓x7ᵗʰ **S07.1** **Crushing injury of skull** `CC`

7 ✓x7ᵗʰ **S07.8** **Crushing injury of other parts of head** `CC`

7 ✓x7ᵗʰ **S07.9** **Crushing injury of head, part unspecified** `CC`

---

7   HAC = Initial encounter only (7th character A, B or C) and not POA.

N Newborn: 0   P Pediatric: 0-17   M Maternity: 12-55   A Adult: 15-124   `MCC` Major CC Condition   `PDxMCC` PDx acts as own MCC   `CC` CC Condition   `PDxCC` PDx acts as own CC

910   ICD-10-CM 2016

✓4th **S08 Avulsion and traumatic amputation of part of head**

> NOTE   An amputation not identified as partial or complete should be coded to complete

> The appropriate 7th is to be added to each code from category S08.
> A   initial encounter
> D   subsequent encounter
> S   sequela

✓x7th **S08.0 Avulsion** of scalp

✓5th **S08.1 Traumatic amputation of** ear

    ✓6th **S08.11 Complete traumatic amputation of** ear

       ✓7th **S08.111 Complete traumatic amputation of right ear**

       ✓7th **S08.112 Complete traumatic amputation of left ear**

       ✓7th **S08.119 Complete traumatic amputation of unspecified ear**

    ✓6th **S08.12 Partial traumatic amputation of** ear

       ✓7th **S08.121 Partial traumatic amputation of right ear**

       ✓7th **S08.122 Partial traumatic amputation of left ear**

       ✓7th **S08.129 Partial traumatic amputation of unspecified ear**

✓5th **S08.8 Traumatic amputation of** other parts of head

    ✓6th **S08.81 Traumatic amputation of** nose

       ✓7th **S08.811 Complete traumatic amputation of nose**

       ✓7th **S08.812 Partial traumatic amputation of nose**

    ✓x7th **S08.89 Traumatic amputation of** other parts of head

✓4th **S09 Other and unspecified injuries of head**

> The appropriate 7th is to be added to each code from category S09.
> A   initial encounter
> D   subsequent encounter
> S   sequela

✓x7th **S09.0 Injury of** blood vessels of head, not elsewhere classified   CC

> EXCLUDES1   injury of cerebral blood vessels (S06.-)
> injury of precerebral blood vessels (S15.-)
> **CC Excl: CC with 7th character A:** S09.0XX with 7th A, S15.101-S15.199 with 7th A, S15.8XX-S15.9XX with 7th A, T14.90-T14.91, T79.A0X-T79.9XX with 7th A

✓5th **S09.1 Injury of** muscle and tendon of head

> Code also any associated open wound (S01.-)
> EXCLUDES2   sprain to joints and ligament of head (S03.9)

    ✓x7th **S09.10 Unspecified injury of muscle and tendon of head**
       Injury of muscle and tendon of head NOS

    ✓x7th **S09.11 Strain of muscle and tendon of head**

    ✓x7th **S09.12 Laceration of muscle and tendon of head**

    ✓x7th **S09.19 Other specified injury of muscle and tendon of head**

✓5th **S09.2 Traumatic rupture of** ear drum

> EXCLUDES1   traumatic rupture of ear drum due to blast injury (S09.31-)

> **CC Excl: For CC codes in subcategory S09.2, unless otherwise noted: CC with 7th character A:** S01.301-S01.359 with 7th A, S08.111-S08.129 with 7th A, S09.20X-S09.399 with 7th A, S09.91XA, S38.3XXA, T14.90-T14.91, T79.8XX-T79.9XX with 7th A

    ✓x7th **S09.20 Traumatic rupture of unspecified ear drum**   CC

    ✓x7th **S09.21 Traumatic rupture of right ear drum**   CC

    ✓x7th **S09.22 Traumatic rupture of left ear drum**   CC

✓5th **S09.3 Other specified and unspecified injury of middle and inner ear**

> EXCLUDES1   injury to ear NOS (S09.91-)
> EXCLUDES2   injury to external ear (S00.4-, S01.3-, S08.1-)

> **CC Excl: For CC codes in subcategory S09.3, unless otherwise noted: CC with 7th character A:** S01.301-S01.359 with 7th A, S08.111-S08.129 with 7th A, S09.20X-S09.399 with 7th A, S09.91X with 7th A, S38.3XXA, T14.90-T14.91, T79.8XX-T79.9XX with 7th A

    ✓6th **S09.30 Unspecified injury of** middle and inner ear

       ✓7th **S09.301 Unspecified injury of right middle and inner ear**   CC

       ✓7th **S09.302 Unspecified injury of left middle and inner ear**   CC

       ✓7th **S09.309 Unspecified injury of unspecified middle and inner ear**   CC

    ✓6th **S09.31 Primary blast injury of** ear
       Blast injury of ear NOS

       ✓7th **S09.311 Primary blast injury of right ear**   CC

       ✓7th **S09.312 Primary blast injury of left ear**   CC

       ✓7th **S09.313 Primary blast injury of ear, bilateral**   CC

       ✓7th **S09.319 Primary blast injury of unspecified ear**   CC

    ✓6th **S09.39 Other specified injury of middle and inner ear**
       Secondary blast injury to ear

       ✓7th **S09.391 Other specified injury of right middle and inner ear**   CC

       ✓7th **S09.392 Other specified injury of left middle and inner ear**   CC

       ✓7th **S09.399 Other specified injury of unspecified middle and inner ear**   CC

✓x7th **S09.8 Other specified injuries of head**

✓5th **S09.9 Unspecified injury of face and head**

    ✓x7th **S09.90 Unspecified injury of head**
       Head injury NOS
> EXCLUDES1   brain injury NOS (S06.9-)
> head injury NOS with loss of consciousness (S06.9-)
> intracranial injury NOS (S06.9-)

    ✓x7th **S09.91 Unspecified injury of ear**
       Injury of ear NOS

    ✓x7th **S09.92 Unspecified injury of nose**
       Injury of nose NOS

    ✓x7th **S09.93 Unspecified injury of face**
       Injury of face NOS

Injuries to the neck (S10-S19)

INCLUDES   injuries of nape
         injuries of supraclavicular region
         injuries of throat

EXCLUDES2   burns and corrosions (T20-T32)
         effects of foreign body in esophagus (T18.1)
         effects of foreign body in larynx (T17.3)
         effects of foreign body in pharynx (T17.2)
         effects of foreign body in trachea (T17.4)
         frostbite (T33-T34)
         insect bite or sting, venomous (T63.4)

✓4th **S10 Superficial injury of neck**

> The appropriate 7th is to be added to each code from category S10.
> A   initial encounter
> D   subsequent encounter
> S   sequela

✓x7th **S10.0 Contusion of throat**

| Contusion of cervical esophagus | Contusion of pharynx |
| Contusion of larynx | Contusion of trachea |

✓5th **S10.1 Other and unspecified superficial injuries of throat**

    ✓x7th **S10.10 Unspecified superficial injuries of throat**

    ✓x7th **S10.11 Abrasion of throat**

    ✓x7th **S10.12 Blister (nonthermal) of throat**

    ✓x7th **S10.14 External constriction of part of throat**

    ✓x7th **S10.15 Superficial foreign body of throat**
       Splinter in the throat

    ✓x7th **S10.16 Insect bite (nonvenomous) of throat**

    ✓x7th **S10.17 Other superficial bite of throat**
> EXCLUDES1   open bite of throat (S11.85)

✓5th **S10.8 Superficial injury of other specified parts of neck**

    ✓x7th **S10.80 Unspecified superficial injury of other specified part of neck**

    ✓x7th **S10.81 Abrasion of other specified part of neck**

    ✓x7th **S10.82 Blister (nonthermal) of other specified part of neck**

    ✓x7th **S10.83 Contusion of other specified part of neck**

    ✓x7th **S10.84 External constriction of other specified part of neck**

    ✓x7th **S10.85 Superficial foreign body of other specified part of neck**
       Splinter in other specified part of neck

    ✓x7th **S10.86 Insect bite of other specified part of neck**

    ✓x7th **S10.87 Other superficial bite of other specified part of neck**
> EXCLUDES1   open bite of other specified parts of neck (S11.85)

✓ Additional Character Required   ✓x7th Placeholder Alert   Unacceptable PDx   Manifestation   Hospital Acquired Condition   EXCLUDES1 Not Coded Here   EXCLUDES2 Not Included Here

√5ᵗʰ **S10.9**   **Superficial injury of** unspecified **part of neck**

√x7ᵗʰ   **S10.90**   **Unspecified superficial injury of unspecified part of** neck

√x7ᵗʰ   **S10.91**   **Abrasion of unspecified part of neck**

√x7ᵗʰ   **S10.92**   **Blister (nonthermal) of unspecified part of neck**

√x7ᵗʰ   **S10.93**   **Contusion of unspecified part of neck**

√x7ᵗʰ   **S10.94**   **External constriction of unspecified part of neck**

√x7ᵗʰ   **S10.95**   **Superficial foreign body of unspecified part of neck**

√x7ᵗʰ   **S10.96**   **Insect bite of unspecified part of neck**

√x7ᵗʰ   **S10.97**   **Other superficial bite of unspecified part of neck**

√4ᵗʰ **S11**   **Open wound of neck**

Code also any associated:
spinal cord injury (S14.0, S14.1-)
wound infection

EXCLUDES 2   *open fracture of vertebra (S12- with 7th B)*

The appropriate 7th is to be added to each code from category S11.
A   initial encounter
D   subsequent encounter
S   sequela

√5ᵗʰ **S11.0**   **Open wound of larynx and trachea**

CC Excl: For MCC codes in subcategory S11.0, unless otherwise noted: MCC with 7th character A: S11.011-S11.039 with 7th A, S11.80X-S11.95X with 7th A, S13.4XXA, S13.8XXA, S16.1XX-S16.2XX with 7th A, S38.3XXA, T14.90-T14.91, T79.A0X-T79.9XX with 7th A

√6ᵗʰ   **S11.01**   **Open wound of** larynx

EXCLUDES 2   *open wound of vocal cord (S11.03)*

√7ᵗʰ   **S11.011**   **Laceration without foreign body of larynx**   MCC

√7ᵗʰ   **S11.012**   **Laceration with foreign body of larynx**   MCC

√7ᵗʰ   **S11.013**   **Puncture wound without foreign body of larynx**   MCC

√7ᵗʰ   **S11.014**   **Puncture wound with foreign body of larynx**   MCC

√7ᵗʰ   **S11.015**   **Open bite of larynx**   MCC
Bite of larynx NOS

√7ᵗʰ   **S11.019**   **Unspecified open wound of larynx**   MCC

√6ᵗʰ   **S11.02**   **Open wound of** trachea
Open wound of cervical trachea
Open wound of trachea NOS

EXCLUDES 2   *open wound of thoracic trachea (S27.5-)*

√7ᵗʰ   **S11.021**   **Laceration without foreign body of trachea**   MCC

√7ᵗʰ   **S11.022**   **Laceration with foreign body of trachea**   MCC

√7ᵗʰ   **S11.023**   **Puncture wound without foreign body of trachea**   MCC

√7ᵗʰ   **S11.024**   **Puncture wound with foreign body of trachea**   MCC

√7ᵗʰ   **S11.025**   **Open bite of trachea**   MCC
Bite of trachea NOS

√7ᵗʰ   **S11.029**   **Unspecified open wound of trachea**   MCC

√6ᵗʰ   **S11.03**   **Open wound of** vocal cord

√7ᵗʰ   **S11.031**   **Laceration without foreign body of vocal cord**   MCC

√7ᵗʰ   **S11.032**   **Laceration with foreign body of vocal cord**   MCC

√7ᵗʰ   **S11.033**   **Puncture wound without foreign body of vocal cord**   MCC

√7ᵗʰ   **S11.034**   **Puncture wound with foreign body of vocal cord**   MCC

√7ᵗʰ   **S11.035**   **Open bite of vocal cord**   MCC
Bite of vocal cord NOS

√7ᵗʰ   **S11.039**   **Unspecified open wound of vocal cord**   MCC

√5ᵗʰ **S11.1**   **Open wound of** thyroid gland

CC Excl: For CC codes in subcategory S11.1, unless otherwise noted: CC with 7th character A: S11.1X-S11.15X with 7th A, S11.80X-S11.95X with 7th A, S13.4XXA, S13.8XXA, S16.1XX-S16.2XX with 7th A, S38.3XXA, T14.90-T14.91, T79.8XX-T79.9XX with 7th A

√x7ᵗʰ   **S11.10**   **Unspecified open wound of thyroid gland**   CC

√x7ᵗʰ   **S11.11**   **Laceration without foreign body of thyroid gland**   CC

√x7ᵗʰ   **S11.12**   **Laceration with foreign body of thyroid gland**   CC
CC Excl: CC with 7th character A: S11.10-S11.15 with 7th A, S11.80-S11.95 with 7th A, S13.4XXA, S13.8XXA, S16.1X-S16.2X with 7th A, S38.3XXA, T14.90-T14.91, T79.A0X-T79.9XX with 7th A

√x7ᵗʰ   **S11.13**   **Puncture wound without foreign body of thyroid gland**   CC

√x7ᵗʰ   **S11.14**   **Puncture wound with foreign body of thyroid gland**   CC
CC Excl: See code: S11.12

√x7ᵗʰ   **S11.15**   **Open bite of thyroid gland**   CC
Bite of thyroid gland NOS

√5ᵗʰ **S11.2**   **Open wound of pharynx and cervical esophagus**

EXCLUDES 1   *open wound of esophagus NOS (S27.8-)*

CC Excl: For CC codes in subcategory S11.2, unless otherwise noted: CC with 7th character A: S11.20X-S11.95X with 7th A, S13.4XXA, S13.8XXA, S16.1XX-S16.2XX with 7th A, S38.3XXA, T14.90-T14.91, T79.8XX-T79.9XX with 7th A

√x7ᵗʰ   **S11.20**   **Unspecified open wound of pharynx and cervical esophagus**   CC

√x7ᵗʰ   **S11.21**   **Laceration without foreign body of pharynx and cervical esophagus**   CC

√x7ᵗʰ   **S11.22**   **Laceration with foreign body of pharynx and cervical esophagus**   CC
CC Excl: CC with 7th character A: S11.20X-S11.95X with 7th A, S13.4XXA, S13.8XXA, S16.1XX-S16.2XX with 7th A, S38.3XXA, T14.90-T14.91, T79.A0X-T79.9XX with 7th A

√x7ᵗʰ   **S11.23**   **Puncture wound without foreign body of pharynx and cervical esophagus**   CC

√x7ᵗʰ   **S11.24**   **Puncture wound with foreign body of pharynx and cervical esophagus**   CC
CC Excl: CC with 7th character A: See Code: S11.22

√x7ᵗʰ   **S11.25**   **Open bite of pharynx and cervical esophagus**   CC
Bite of pharynx and cervical esophagus NOS

√5ᵗʰ **S11.8**   **Open wound of** other specified parts of neck

√x7ᵗʰ   **S11.80**   **Unspecified open wound of other specified part of neck**

√x7ᵗʰ   **S11.81**   **Laceration without foreign body of other specified part of neck**

√x7ᵗʰ   **S11.82**   **Laceration with foreign body of other specified part of neck**

√x7ᵗʰ   **S11.83**   **Puncture wound without foreign body of other specified part of neck**

√x7ᵗʰ   **S11.84**   **Puncture wound with foreign body of other specified part of neck**

√x7ᵗʰ   **S11.85**   **Open bite of other specified part of neck**
Bite of other specified part of neck NOS

EXCLUDES 1   *superficial bite of other specified part of neck (S10.87)*

√x7ᵗʰ   **S11.89**   **Other open wound of other specified part of neck**

√5ᵗʰ **S11.9**   **Open wound of** unspecified **part of neck**

√x7ᵗʰ   **S11.90**   **Unspecified open wound of unspecified part of neck**

√x7ᵗʰ   **S11.91**   **Laceration without foreign body of unspecified part of neck**

√x7ᵗʰ   **S11.92**   **Laceration with foreign body of unspecified part of neck**

√x7ᵗʰ   **S11.93**   **Puncture wound without foreign body of unspecified part of neck**

√x7ᵗʰ   **S11.94**   **Puncture wound with foreign body of unspecified part of neck**

√x7ᵗʰ   **S11.95**   **Open bite of unspecified part of neck**
Bite of neck NOS

EXCLUDES 1   *superficial bite of neck (S10.97)*

Ⓝ Newborn: 0   Ⓟ Pediatric: 0-17   Ⓜ Maternity: 12-55   Ⓐ Adult: 15-124   **MCC** Major CC Condition   **PDxMCC** PDx acts as own MCC   **CC** CC Condition   **PDxCC** PDx acts as own CC

912   ICD-10-CM 2016

✓4ᵗʰ S12 Fracture of cervical vertebra and other parts of neck

> **NOTE**   A fracture not indicated as nondisplaced or displaced should be classified to displaced.
> A fracture not indicated as open or closed should be coded to closed.
>
> **INCLUDES**   fracture of cervical neural arch
> fracture of cervical spine
> fracture of cervical spinous process
> fracture of cervical transverse process
> fracture of cervical vertebral arch
> fracture of neck

Code first any associated cervical spinal cord injury (S14.0, S14.1-)

> The appropriate 7th is to be added to all codes from subcategories S12.0-S12.6.
> A   initial encounter for closed fracture
> B   initial encounter for open fracture
> D   subsequent encounter for fracture with routine healing
> G   subsequent encounter for fracture with delayed healing
> K   subsequent encounter for fracture with nonunion
> S   sequela

✓5ᵗʰ S12.0 Fracture of first cervical vertebra
    Atlas

> **For CC/MCC codes in subcategory S12.0, unless otherwise noted: CC with 7th character A or MCC with 7th character B:** M48.40X-M48.58X with 7th S, M80.08XS, M80.88XS, M84.350XS, M84.454S, M84.550S, M84.58XS, M84.650S, M99.10-M99.11, M99.15-M99.17, M99.19, S03.8XX-S03.9XX with 7th A, S12.000-S13.4XX with 7th [A, B, S], S13.8XX-S14.159 with 7th A, S16.1XXA, S22.000-S22.9XX with 7th S, S23.20X-S23.29X with 7th A, S23.9XXA, S24.109A, S24.119A, S24.139A, S24.149A, S24.159A, S29.001-S29.019 with 7th A, S29.091-S29.9XX with 7th A, S32.000-S32.9XX with 7th S, S33.30X-S33.39X with 7th A, S33.9XXA, S38.1XXA, S38.3XX-S39.013 with 7th A, S39.091-S39.94X with 7th A, T14.90-T14.91, T79.A0X-T79.9XX with 7th A
> **CC with 7th character K:** M80.00X-M84.68X with 7th [K, P], S02.0XX-S02.92X with 7th K, S12.000-S12.691 with 7th K, S22.000-S22.9XX with 7th K, S32.000-S32.9XX with 7th K, S42.001-S42.92X with 7th [K, P], S49.001-S49.199 with 7th [K, P], S52.001-S52.92X with 7th [K, M, N, P, Q, R], S59.001-S59.299 with 7th [K, P], S62.001-S62.92X with 7th [K, P], S72.001-S72.92X with 7th [K, M, N, P, Q, R], S79.001-S79.199 with 7th [K, P], S82.001-S82.92X with 7th [K, M, N, P, Q, R], S89.001-S89.399 with 7th [K, P], S92.001-S92.919 with 7th [K, P]

    ✓6ᵗʰ S12.00 Unspecified fracture of first cervical vertebra
      7,16,19 ✓7ᵗʰ **S12.000 Unspecified displaced fracture of first cervical vertebra** `MCC` `CC`
      7,16,19 ✓7ᵗʰ **S12.001 Unspecified nondisplaced fracture of first cervical vertebra** `MCC` `CC`
    7,16,19 ✓x7ᵗʰ **S12.01 Stable burst fracture of first cervical vertebra** `MCC` `CC`
    7,16,19 ✓x7ᵗʰ **S12.02 Unstable burst fracture of first cervical vertebra** `MCC` `CC`
    ✓6ᵗʰ S12.03 Posterior arch fracture of first cervical vertebra
      7,16,19 ✓7ᵗʰ **S12.030 Displaced posterior arch fracture of first cervical vertebra** `MCC` `CC`
      7,16,19 ✓7ᵗʰ **S12.031 Nondisplaced posterior arch fracture of first cervical vertebra** `MCC` `CC`
    ✓6ᵗʰ S12.04 Lateral mass fracture of first cervical vertebra
      7,16,19 ✓7ᵗʰ **S12.040 Displaced lateral mass fracture of first cervical vertebra** `MCC` `CC`
      7,16,19 ✓7ᵗʰ **S12.041 Nondisplaced lateral mass fracture of first cervical vertebra** `MCC` `CC`
    ✓6ᵗʰ S12.09 Other fracture of first cervical vertebra
      7,16,19 ✓7ᵗʰ **S12.090 Other displaced fracture of first cervical vertebra** `MCC` `CC`
      7,16,19 ✓7ᵗʰ **S12.091 Other nondisplaced fracture of first cervical vertebra** `MCC` `CC`

✓5ᵗʰ S12.1 Fracture of second cervical vertebra
    Axis
    ✓6ᵗʰ S12.10 Unspecified fracture of second cervical vertebra
      7,16,19 ✓7ᵗʰ **S12.100 Unspecified displaced fracture of second cervical vertebra** `MCC` `CC`
      7,16,19 ✓7ᵗʰ **S12.101 Unspecified nondisplaced fracture of second cervical vertebra** `MCC` `CC`

    ✓6ᵗʰ S12.11 Type II dens fracture
      7,16,19 ✓7ᵗʰ **S12.110 Anterior displaced Type II dens fracture** `MCC` `CC`
      7,16,19 ✓7ᵗʰ **S12.111 Posterior displaced Type II dens fracture** `MCC` `CC`
      7,16,19 ✓7ᵗʰ **S12.112 Nondisplaced Type II dens fracture** `MCC` `CC`
    ✓6ᵗʰ S12.12 Other dens fracture
      7,16,19 ✓7ᵗʰ **S12.120 Other displaced dens fracture** `MCC` `CC`
      7,16,19 ✓7ᵗʰ **S12.121 Other nondisplaced dens fracture** `MCC` `CC`
    ✓6ᵗʰ S12.13 Unspecified traumatic spondylolisthesis of second cervical vertebra
      7,16,19 ✓7ᵗʰ **S12.130 Unspecified traumatic displaced spondylolisthesis of second cervical vertebra** `MCC` `CC`
      7,16,19 ✓7ᵗʰ **S12.131 Unspecified traumatic nondisplaced spondylolisthesis of second cervical vertebra** `MCC` `CC`
    7,16,19 ✓x7ᵗʰ **S12.14 Type III traumatic spondylolisthesis of second cervical vertebra** `MCC` `CC`
    ✓6ᵗʰ S12.15 Other traumatic spondylolisthesis of second cervical vertebra
      7,16,19 ✓7ᵗʰ **S12.150 Other traumatic displaced spondylolisthesis of second cervical vertebra** `MCC` `CC`
      7,16,19 ✓7ᵗʰ **S12.151 Other traumatic nondisplaced spondylolisthesis of second cervical vertebra** `MCC` `CC`
    ✓6ᵗʰ S12.19 Other fracture of second cervical vertebra
      7,16,19 ✓7ᵗʰ **S12.190 Other displaced fracture of second cervical vertebra** `MCC` `CC`
      7,16,19 ✓7ᵗʰ **S12.191 Other nondisplaced fracture of second cervical vertebra** `MCC` `CC`

✓5ᵗʰ S12.2 Fracture of third cervical vertebra
    ✓6ᵗʰ S12.20 Unspecified fracture of third cervical vertebra
      7,16,19 ✓7ᵗʰ **S12.200 Unspecified displaced fracture of third cervical vertebra** `MCC` `CC`
      7,16,19 ✓7ᵗʰ **S12.201 Unspecified nondisplaced fracture of third cervical vertebra** `MCC` `CC`
    ✓6ᵗʰ S12.23 Unspecified traumatic spondylolisthesis of third cervical vertebra
      7,16,19 ✓7ᵗʰ **S12.230 Unspecified traumatic displaced spondylolisthesis of third cervical vertebra** `MCC` `CC`
      7,16,19 ✓7ᵗʰ **S12.231 Unspecified traumatic nondisplaced spondylolisthesis of third cervical vertebra** `MCC` `CC`
    7,16,19 ✓x7ᵗʰ **S12.24 Type III traumatic spondylolisthesis of third cervical vertebra** `MCC` `CC`
    ✓6ᵗʰ S12.25 Other traumatic spondylolisthesis of third cervical vertebra
      7,16,19 ✓7ᵗʰ **S12.250 Other traumatic displaced spondylolisthesis of third cervical vertebra** `MCC` `CC`
      7,16,19 ✓7ᵗʰ **S12.251 Other traumatic nondisplaced spondylolisthesis of third cervical vertebra** `MCC` `CC`
    ✓6ᵗʰ S12.29 Other fracture of third cervical vertebra
      7,16,19 ✓7ᵗʰ **S12.290 Other displaced fracture of third cervical vertebra** `MCC` `CC`
      7,16,19 ✓7ᵗʰ **S12.291 Other nondisplaced fracture of third cervical vertebra** `MCC` `CC`

✓5ᵗʰ S12.3 Fracture of fourth cervical vertebra
    ✓6ᵗʰ S12.30 Unspecified fracture of fourth cervical vertebra
      7,16,19 ✓7ᵗʰ **S12.300 Unspecified displaced fracture of fourth cervical vertebra** `MCC` `CC`
      7,16,19 ✓7ᵗʰ **S12.301 Unspecified nondisplaced fracture of fourth cervical vertebra** `MCC` `CC`

---

7   HAC = Initial encounter only (7th character A, B or C) and not POA.
16   MCC only if an open fracture (7th character B or C – specific to category).
19   CC only if an initial encounter for a closed fracture (7th character A) **OR** a subsequent encounter for nonunion or malunion (7th character K, M, N, P, Q, or R – specific to category).

✓ Additional Character Required   ✓x7ᵗʰ Placeholder Alert   Unacceptable PDx   Manifestation   Hospital Acquired Condition   **EXCLUDES 1** Not Coded Here   **EXCLUDES 2** Not Included Here

✓6th **S12.33** Unspecified traumatic spondylolisthesis of fourth cervical vertebra

7,16,19 ✓7th **S12.330** Unspecified traumatic displaced spondylolisthesis of fourth cervical vertebra `MCC` `CC`

7,16,19 ✓7th **S12.331** Unspecified traumatic nondisplaced spondylolisthesis of fourth cervical vertebra `MCC` `CC`

7,16,19 ✓x7th **S12.34** Type III traumatic spondylolisthesis of fourth cervical vertebra `MCC` `CC`

✓6th **S12.35** Other traumatic spondylolisthesis of fourth cervical vertebra

7,16,19 ✓7th **S12.350** Other traumatic displaced spondylolisthesis of fourth cervical vertebra `MCC` `CC`

7,16,19 ✓7th **S12.351** Other traumatic nondisplaced spondylolisthesis of fourth cervical vertebra `MCC` `CC`

✓6th **S12.39** Other fracture of fourth cervical vertebra

7,16,19 ✓7th **S12.390** Other displaced fracture of fourth cervical vertebra `MCC` `CC`

7,16,19 ✓7th **S12.391** Other nondisplaced fracture of fourth cervical vertebra `MCC` `CC`

✓5th **S12.4** Fracture of fifth cervical vertebra

✓6th **S12.40** Unspecified fracture of fifth cervical vertebra

7,16,19 ✓7th **S12.400** Unspecified displaced fracture of fifth cervical vertebra `MCC` `CC`

7,16,19 ✓7th **S12.401** Unspecified nondisplaced fracture of fifth cervical vertebra `MCC` `CC`

✓6th **S12.43** Unspecified traumatic spondylolisthesis of fifth cervical vertebra

7,16,19 ✓7th **S12.430** Unspecified traumatic displaced spondylolisthesis of fifth cervical vertebra `MCC` `CC`

7,16,19 ✓7th **S12.431** Unspecified traumatic nondisplaced spondylolisthesis of fifth cervical vertebra `MCC` `CC`

7,16,19 ✓x7th **S12.44** Type III traumatic spondylolisthesis of fifth cervical vertebra `MCC` `CC`

✓6th **S12.45** Other traumatic spondylolisthesis of fifth cervical vertebra

7,16,19 ✓7th **S12.450** Other traumatic displaced spondylolisthesis of fifth cervical vertebra `MCC` `CC`

7,16,19 ✓7th **S12.451** Other traumatic nondisplaced spondylolisthesis of fifth cervical vertebra `MCC` `CC`

✓6th **S12.49** Other fracture of fifth cervical vertebra

7,16,19 ✓7th **S12.490** Other displaced fracture of fifth cervical vertebra `MCC` `CC`

7,16,19 ✓7th **S12.491** Other nondisplaced fracture of fifth cervical vertebra `MCC` `CC`

✓5th **S12.5** Fracture of sixth cervical vertebra

✓6th **S12.50** Unspecified fracture of sixth cervical vertebra

7,16,19 ✓7th **S12.500** Unspecified displaced fracture of sixth cervical vertebra `MCC` `CC`

7,16,19 ✓7th **S12.501** Unspecified nondisplaced fracture of sixth cervical vertebra `MCC` `CC`

✓6th **S12.53** Unspecified traumatic spondylolisthesis of sixth cervical vertebra

7,16,19 ✓7th **S12.530** Unspecified traumatic displaced spondylolisthesis of sixth cervical vertebra `MCC` `CC`

7,16,19 ✓7th **S12.531** Unspecified traumatic nondisplaced spondylolisthesis of sixth cervical vertebra `MCC` `CC`

7,16,19 ✓x7th **S12.54** Type III traumatic spondylolisthesis of sixth cervical vertebra `MCC` `CC`

✓6th **S12.55** Other traumatic spondylolisthesis of sixth cervical vertebra

7,16,19 ✓7th **S12.550** Other traumatic displaced spondylolisthesis of sixth cervical vertebra `MCC` `CC`

7,16,19 ✓7th **S12.551** Other traumatic nondisplaced spondylolisthesis of sixth cervical vertebra `MCC`

✓6th **S12.59** Other fracture of sixth cervical vertebra

7,16,19 ✓7th **S12.590** Other displaced fracture of sixth cervical vertebra `MCC` `CC`

7,16,19 ✓7th **S12.591** Other nondisplaced fracture of sixth cervical vertebra `MCC` `CC`

✓5th **S12.6** Fracture of seventh cervical vertebra

✓6th **S12.60** Unspecified fracture of seventh cervical vertebra

7,16,19 **S12.600** Unspecified displaced fracture of seventh cervical vertebra `MCC` `CC`

7,16,19 **S12.601** Unspecified nondisplaced fracture of seventh cervical vertebra `MCC` `CC`

✓6th **S12.63** Unspecified traumatic spondylolisthesis of seventh cervical vertebra

7,16,19 ✓7th **S12.630** Unspecified traumatic displaced spondylolisthesis of seventh cervical vertebra `MCC` `CC`

7,16,19 ✓7th **S12.631** Unspecified traumatic nondisplaced spondylolisthesis of seventh cervical vertebra `MCC` `CC`

7,16,19 ✓x7th **S12.64** Type III traumatic spondylolisthesis of seventh cervical vertebra `MCC` `CC`

✓6th **S12.65** Other traumatic spondylolisthesis of seventh cervical vertebra

7,16,19 ✓7th **S12.650** Other traumatic displaced spondylolisthesis of seventh cervical vertebra `MCC` `CC`

7,16,19 ✓7th **S12.651** Other traumatic nondisplaced spondylolisthesis of seventh cervical vertebra `MCC` `CC`

✓6th **S12.69** Other fracture of seventh cervical vertebra

7,16,19 ✓7th **S12.690** Other displaced fracture of seventh cervical vertebra `MCC` `CC`

7,16,19 ✓7th **S12.691** Other nondisplaced fracture of seventh cervical vertebra `MCC` `CC`

7 ✓x7th **S12.8** Fracture of other parts of neck `MCC`

Hyoid bone   Thyroid cartilage
Larynx   Trachea

The appropriate 7th is to be added to code S12.8.
A   initial encounter
D   subsequent encounter
S   sequela

CC Excl: MCC with 7th character A: S03.8XX-S03.9XX with 7th A, S12.8XX with 7th A, S29.011-S29.019 with 7th A, S38.3XX-S39.013 with 7th A, T14.90-T14.91, T79.A0X-T79.9XX with 7th A

7 ✓x7th **S12.9** Fracture of neck, unspecified `CC`

Fracture of cervical spine NOS   Fracture of neck NOS
Fracture of cervical vertebra NOS

The appropriate 7th is to be added to code S12.9.
A   initial encounter
D   subsequent encounter
S   sequela

CC Excl: M48.40X-M48.58X with 7th S, M80.08XS, M80.88XS, M84.350S, M84.454S, M84.550S, M84.58XS, M84.650S, M99.10-M99.11, M99.15-M99.17, M99.19, S03.8XX-S03.9XX with 7th A, S12.000-S13.4XX with 7th [A, B, S], S13.8XX-S14.159 with 7th A, S16.1XXA, S22.000-S22.9XX with 7th S, S23.20X-S23.29X with 7th A, S23.9XXA, S24.109A, S24.119A, S24.139A, S24.149A, S24.159A, S29.001-S29.019 with 7th A, S29.091-S29.9XX with 7th A, S32.000-S32.9XX with 7th S, S33.30X-S33.39X with 7th A, S33.9XXA, S38.1XXA, S38.3XX-S39.013 with 7th A, S39.091-S39.94X with 7th A, T14.90-T14.91, T79.A0X-T79.9XX with 7th A

---

7 HAC = Initial encounter only (7th character A, B or C) and not POA.
16 MCC only if an open fracture (7th character B or C – specific to category).
19 CC only if an initial encounter for a closed fracture (7th character A) OR a subsequent encounter for nonunion or malunion (7th character K, M, N, P, Q, or R – specific to category).

N Newborn: 0   P Pediatric: 0-17   M Maternity: 12-55   A Adult: 15-124   `MCC` Major CC Condition   `PDxMCC` PDx acts as own MCC   `CC` CC Condition   `PDxCC` PDx acts as own CC

914   ICD-10-CM 2016

✓4ᵗʰ S13   Dislocation and sprain of joints and ligaments at neck level

     INCLUDES   avulsion of joint or ligament at neck level
                     laceration of cartilage, joint or ligament at neck level
                     sprain of cartilage, joint or ligament at neck level
                     traumatic hemarthrosis of joint or ligament at neck level
                     traumatic rupture of joint or ligament at neck level
                     traumatic subluxation of joint or ligament at neck level
                     traumatic tear of joint or ligament at neck level

     Code also any associated open wound
     EXCLUDES 2   *strain of muscle or tendon at neck level (S16.1)*

     The appropriate 7th is to be added to each code from category S13.
     A   initial encounter
     D   subsequent encounter
     S   sequela

7   **✓x7ᵗʰ S13.0   Traumatic rupture of cervical intervertebral disc**   CC
     EXCLUDES 1   *rupture or displacement (nontraumatic) of cervical intervertebral disc NOS (M50.-)*
     CC Excl: CC with 7th character A: M99.10-M99.11, S03.8XX-S03.9XX with 7th A, S12.000-S12.691 with 7th [A, B], S12.9XX-S13.4XX with 7th A, S13.8XXA, S14.0XX-S14.108 with 7th A, S14.111-S14.118 with 7th A, S14.121-S14.128 with 7th A, S14.131-S14.138 with 7th A, S14.141-S14.148 with 7th A, S14.151-S14.158 with 7th A, S16.1XXA, S29.011-S29.019 with 7th A, S38.3XX-S39.013 with 7th A, T14.90-T14.91, T79.A0X-T79.9XX with 7th A

     ✓5ᵗʰ S13.1   Subluxation and dislocation of cervical vertebrae
         Code also any associated:
            open wound of neck (S11.-)
            spinal cord injury (S14.1-)
         EXCLUDES 2   *fracture of cervical vertebrae (S12.0--S12.3-)*
         CC Excl: For codes in subcategory S13.1, unless otherwise noted: See code: S13.0

         ✓6ᵗʰ S13.10   Subluxation and dislocation of unspecified cervical vertebrae

            7   **✓7ᵗʰ S13.100   Subluxation of unspecified cervical vertebrae**   CC

            7   **✓7ᵗʰ S13.101   Dislocation of unspecified cervical vertebrae**   CC

         ✓6ᵗʰ S13.11   Subluxation and dislocation of C0/C1 cervical vertebrae
            Subluxation and dislocation of atlantooccipital joint
            Subluxation and dislocation of atloidooccipital joint
            Subluxation and dislocation of occipitoatloid joint

            7   **✓7ᵗʰ S13.110   Subluxation of C0/C1 cervical vertebrae**   CC

            7   **✓7ᵗʰ S13.111   Dislocation of C0/C1 cervical vertebrae**   CC

         ✓6ᵗʰ S13.12   Subluxation and dislocation of C1/C2 cervical vertebrae
            Subluxation and dislocation of atlantoaxial joint

            7   **✓7ᵗʰ S13.120   Subluxation of C1/C2 cervical vertebrae**   CC

            7   **✓7ᵗʰ S13.121   Dislocation of C1/C2 cervical vertebrae**   CC

         ✓6ᵗʰ S13.13   Subluxation and dislocation of C2/C3 cervical vertebrae

            7   **✓7ᵗʰ S13.130   Subluxation of C2/C3 cervical vertebrae**   CC

            7   **✓7ᵗʰ S13.131   Dislocation of C2/C3 cervical vertebrae**   CC

         ✓6ᵗʰ S13.14   Subluxation and dislocation of C3/C4 cervical vertebrae

            7   **✓7ᵗʰ S13.140   Subluxation of C3/C4 cervical vertebrae**   CC

            7   **✓7ᵗʰ S13.141   Dislocation of C3/C4 cervical vertebrae**   CC

         ✓6ᵗʰ S13.15   Subluxation and dislocation of C4/C5 cervical vertebrae

            7   **✓7ᵗʰ S13.150   Subluxation of C4/C5 cervical vertebrae**   CC

            7   **✓7ᵗʰ S13.151   Dislocation of C4/C5 cervical vertebrae**   CC

         ✓6ᵗʰ S13.16   Subluxation and dislocation of C5/C6 cervical vertebrae

            7   **✓7ᵗʰ S13.160   Subluxation of C5/C6 cervical vertebrae**   CC

            7   **✓7ᵗʰ S13.161   Dislocation of C5/C6 cervical vertebrae**   CC

         ✓6ᵗʰ S13.17   Subluxation and dislocation of C6/C7 cervical vertebrae

            7   **✓7ᵗʰ S13.170   Subluxation of C6/C7 cervical vertebrae**   CC

            7   **✓7ᵗʰ S13.171   Dislocation of C6/C7 cervical vertebrae**   CC

         ✓6ᵗʰ S13.18   Subluxation and dislocation of C7/T1 cervical vertebrae

            7   **✓7ᵗʰ S13.180   Subluxation of C7/T1 cervical vertebrae**   CC

            7   **✓7ᵗʰ S13.181   Dislocation of C7/T1 cervical vertebrae**   CC

     ✓5ᵗʰ S13.2   Dislocation of other and unspecified parts of neck
         CC Excl: For codes in subcategory S13.2, unless otherwise noted: See code: S13.0

         7   **S13.20   Dislocation of unspecified parts of neck**   CC

         7   **S13.29   Dislocation of other parts of neck**   CC

     ✓x7ᵗʰ S13.4   Sprain of ligaments of cervical spine
         Sprain of anterior longitudinal (ligament), cervical
         Sprain of atlanto-axial (joints)
         Sprain of atlanto-occipital (joints)
         Whiplash injury of cervical spine

     ✓x7ᵗʰ S13.5   Sprain of thyroid region
         Sprain of cricoarytenoid (joint) (ligament)
         Sprain of cricothyroid (joint) (ligament)
         Sprain of thyroid cartilage

     ✓x7ᵗʰ S13.8   Sprain of joints and ligaments of other parts of neck

     ✓x7ᵗʰ S13.9   Sprain of joints and ligaments of unspecified parts of neck

✓4ᵗʰ S14   Injury of nerves and spinal cord at neck level
     NOTE   Code to highest level of cervical cord injury.
     Code also any associated:
         fracture of cervical vertebra (S12.0- – S12.6-)
         open wound of neck (S11.-)
         transient paralysis (R29.5)

     The appropriate 7th is to be added to each code from category S14.
     A   initial encounter
     D   subsequent encounter
     S   sequela

     CC Excl: For MCC codes in category S14, unless otherwise noted:
     MCC with 7th character A: M48.40X-M48.58X with 7th S, M80.08XS, M80.88XS, M84.350S, M84.454S, M84.550S, M84.58XS, M84.650S, M99.10-M99.11, M99.15-M99.17, M99.19, S03.1XXA, S12.000-S13.29X with 7th [A, B, S], S13.9XX-S14.159 with 7th A, S22.000-S22.9XX with 7th S, S23.20X-S23.29X with 7th A, S23.9XA, S24.109XA, S24.119A, S24.139A, S24.149A, S24.159A, S29.001-S29.009 with 7th A, S29.091-S29.9XX with 7th A, S32.000-S32.9XX with 7th S, S33.30X-S33.39X with 7th A, S33.9XXA, S38.1XX, S39.001-S39.003 with 7th A, S39.091-S39.94X with 7th A, T14.90-T14.91, T79.A0X-T79.9XX with 7th A

     ✓x7ᵗʰ S14.0   Concussion and edema of cervical spinal cord   MCC

     ✓5ᵗʰ S14.1   Other and unspecified injuries of cervical spinal cord

         ✓6ᵗʰ S14.10   Unspecified injury of cervical spinal cord

            7   **✓7ᵗʰ S14.101   Unspecified injury at C1 level of cervical spinal cord**   MCC

            7   **✓7ᵗʰ S14.102   Unspecified injury at C2 level of cervical spinal cord**   MCC

            7   **✓7ᵗʰ S14.103   Unspecified injury at C3 level of cervical spinal cord**   MCC

            7   **✓7ᵗʰ S14.104   Unspecified injury at C4 level of cervical spinal cord**   MCC

            7   **✓7ᵗʰ S14.105   Unspecified injury at C5 level of cervical spinal cord**   MCC

            7   **✓7ᵗʰ S14.106   Unspecified injury at C6 level of cervical spinal cord**   MCC

            7   **✓7ᵗʰ S14.107   Unspecified injury at C7 level of cervical spinal cord**   MCC

            ✓7ᵗʰ S14.108   Unspecified injury at C8 level of cervical spinal cord   MCC

            7   **✓7ᵗʰ S14.109   Unspecified injury at unspecified level of cervical spinal cord**
                Injury of cervical spinal cord NOS
                CC Excl: No excl

         ✓6ᵗʰ S14.11   Complete lesion of cervical spinal cord

            7   **✓7ᵗʰ S14.111   Complete lesion at C1 level of cervical spinal cord**   MCC

---

7   HAC = Initial encounter only (7th character A, B or C) and not POA.

✓ Additional Character Required   ✓x7ᵗʰ Placeholder Alert   Unacceptable PDx   Manifestation   Hospital Acquired Condition   **EXCLUDES 1** Not Coded Here   **EXCLUDES 2** Not Included Here

7 ✓7ᵗʰ **S14.112** **Complete lesion at C2 level of cervical spinal cord**   `MCC`

7 ✓7ᵗʰ **S14.113** **Complete lesion at C3 level of cervical spinal cord**   `MCC`

7 ✓7ᵗʰ **S14.114** **Complete lesion at C4 level of cervical spinal cord**   `MCC`

7 ✓7ᵗʰ **S14.115** **Complete lesion at C5 level of cervical spinal cord**   `MCC`

7 ✓7ᵗʰ **S14.116** **Complete lesion at C6 level of cervical spinal cord**   `MCC`

7 ✓7ᵗʰ **S14.117** **Complete lesion at C7 level of cervical spinal cord**   `MCC`

✓7ᵗʰ **S14.118** **Complete lesion at C8 level of cervical spinal cord**   `MCC`

✓7ᵗʰ **S14.119** **Complete lesion at unspecified level of cervical spinal cord**

✓6ᵗʰ **S14.12** Central cord syndrome of cervical spinal cord

7 ✓7ᵗʰ **S14.121** **Central cord syndrome at C1 level of cervical spinal cord**   `MCC`

7 ✓7ᵗʰ **S14.122** **Central cord syndrome at C2 level of cervical spinal cord**   `MCC`

7 ✓7ᵗʰ **S14.123** **Central cord syndrome at C3 level of cervical spinal cord**   `MCC`

7 ✓7ᵗʰ **S14.124** **Central cord syndrome at C4 level of cervical spinal cord**   `MCC`

7 ✓7ᵗʰ **S14.125** **Central cord syndrome at C5 level of cervical spinal cord**   `MCC`

7 ✓7ᵗʰ **S14.126** **Central cord syndrome at C6 level of cervical spinal cord**   `MCC`

7 ✓7ᵗʰ **S14.127** **Central cord syndrome at C7 level of cervical spinal cord**   `MCC`

✓7ᵗʰ **S14.128** **Central cord syndrome at C8 level of cervical spinal cord**   `MCC`

✓7ᵗʰ **S14.129** **Central cord syndrome at unspecified level of cervical spinal cord**

✓6ᵗʰ **S14.13** Anterior cord syndrome of cervical spinal cord

7 ✓7ᵗʰ **S14.131** **Anterior cord syndrome at C1 level of cervical spinal cord**   `MCC`

7 ✓7ᵗʰ **S14.132** **Anterior cord syndrome at C2 level of cervical spinal cord**   `MCC`

7 ✓7ᵗʰ **S14.133** **Anterior cord syndrome at C3 level of cervical spinal cord**   `MCC`

7 ✓7ᵗʰ **S14.134** **Anterior cord syndrome at C4 level of cervical spinal cord**   `MCC`

7 ✓7ᵗʰ **S14.135** **Anterior cord syndrome at C5 level of cervical spinal cord**   `MCC`

7 ✓7ᵗʰ **S14.136** **Anterior cord syndrome at C6 level of cervical spinal cord**   `MCC`

7 ✓7ᵗʰ **S14.137** **Anterior cord syndrome at C7 level of cervical spinal cord**   `MCC`

✓7ᵗʰ **S14.138** **Anterior cord syndrome at C8 level of cervical spinal cord**   `MCC`

✓7ᵗʰ **S14.139** **Anterior cord syndrome at unspecified level of cervical spinal cord**

✓6ᵗʰ **S14.14** Brown-Séquard syndrome of cervical spinal cord

✓7ᵗʰ **S14.141** **Brown-Séquard syndrome at C1 level of cervical spinal cord**   `MCC`

✓7ᵗʰ **S14.142** **Brown-Séquard syndrome at C2 level of cervical spinal cord**   `MCC`

✓7ᵗʰ **S14.143** **Brown-Séquard syndrome at C3 level of cervical spinal cord**   `MCC`

✓7ᵗʰ **S14.144** **Brown-Séquard syndrome at C4 level of cervical spinal cord**   `MCC`

✓7ᵗʰ **S14.145** **Brown-Séquard syndrome at C5 level of cervical spinal cord**   `MCC`

✓7ᵗʰ **S14.146** **Brown-Séquard syndrome at C6 level of cervical spinal cord**   `MCC`

✓7ᵗʰ **S14.147** **Brown-Séquard syndrome at C7 level of cervical spinal cord**   `MCC`

✓7ᵗʰ **S14.148** **Brown-Séquard syndrome at C8 level of cervical spinal cord**   `MCC`

✓7ᵗʰ **S14.149** **Brown-Séquard syndrome at unspecified level of cervical spinal cord**

✓6ᵗʰ **S14.15** **Other incomplete lesions of cervical spinal cord**
Incomplete lesion of cervical spinal cord NOS
Posterior cord syndrome of cervical spinal cord

7 ✓7ᵗʰ **S14.151** **Other incomplete lesion at C1 level of cervical spinal cord**   `MCC`

7 ✓7ᵗʰ **S14.152** **Other incomplete lesion at C2 level of cervical spinal cord**   `MCC`

7 ✓7ᵗʰ **S14.153** **Other incomplete lesion at C3 level of cervical spinal cord**   `MCC`

7 ✓7ᵗʰ **S14.154** **Other incomplete lesion at C4 level of cervical spinal cord**   `MCC`

7 ✓7ᵗʰ **S14.155** **Other incomplete lesion at C5 level of cervical spinal cord**   `MCC`

7 ✓7ᵗʰ **S14.156** **Other incomplete lesion at C6 level of cervical spinal cord**   `MCC`

7 ✓7ᵗʰ **S14.157** **Other incomplete lesion at C7 level of cervical spinal cord**   `MCC`

✓7ᵗʰ **S14.158** **Other incomplete lesion at C8 level of cervical spinal cord**   `MCC`

✓7ᵗʰ **S14.159** **Other incomplete lesion at unspecified level of cervical spinal cord**

✓x7ᵗʰ **S14.2** **Injury of nerve root of cervical spine**

✓x7ᵗʰ **S14.3** **Injury of brachial plexus**

✓x7ᵗʰ **S14.4** **Injury of peripheral nerves of neck**

✓x7ᵗʰ **S14.5** **Injury of cervical sympathetic nerves**

✓x7ᵗʰ **S14.8** **Injury of other specified nerves of neck**

✓x7ᵗʰ **S14.9** **Injury of unspecified nerves of neck**

✓4ᵗʰ **S15** **Injury of blood vessels at neck level**
Code also any associated open wound (S11.-)

> The appropriate 7th is to be added to each code from category S15.
> A   initial encounter
> D   subsequent encounter
> S   sequela

> **CC Excl:** For CC codes in subcategory S15, unless otherwise noted: CC with 7th character A: S09.0XXA, S15.009A, S15.029A, S15.099-S15.199 with 7th A, S15.8XX-S15.9XX with 7th A, T14.90-T14.91, T79.A0X-T79.9XX with 7th A

✓5ᵗʰ **S15.0** **Injury of carotid artery of neck**
Injury of carotid artery (common) (external) (internal, extracranial portion)
Injury of carotid artery NOS
> **EXCLUDES 1** injury of internal carotid artery, intracranial portion (S06.8)

✓6ᵗʰ **S15.00** **Unspecified injury of carotid artery**

✓7ᵗʰ **S15.001** **Unspecified injury of right carotid artery**   `CC`

✓7ᵗʰ **S15.002** **Unspecified injury of left carotid artery**   `CC`

✓7ᵗʰ **S15.009** **Unspecified injury of unspecified carotid artery**   `CC`

✓6ᵗʰ **S15.01** **Minor laceration of carotid artery**
Incomplete transection of carotid artery
Laceration of carotid artery NOS
Superficial laceration of carotid artery

✓7ᵗʰ **S15.011** **Minor laceration of right carotid artery**   `CC`

✓7ᵗʰ **S15.012** **Minor laceration of left carotid artery**   `CC`

✓7ᵗʰ **S15.019** **Minor laceration of unspecified carotid artery**   `CC`

✓6ᵗʰ **S15.02** **Major laceration of carotid artery**
Complete transection of carotid artery
Traumatic rupture of carotid artery

✓7ᵗʰ **S15.021** **Major laceration of right carotid artery**   `CC`

✓7ᵗʰ **S15.022** **Major laceration of left carotid artery**   `CC`

✓7ᵗʰ **S15.029** **Major laceration of unspecified carotid artery**   `CC`

✓6ᵗʰ **S15.09** **Other specified injury of carotid artery**

✓7ᵗʰ **S15.091** **Other specified injury of right carotid artery**   `CC`

✓7ᵗʰ **S15.092** **Other specified injury of left carotid artery**   `CC`

✓7ᵗʰ **S15.099** **Other specified injury of unspecified carotid artery**   `CC`

---

7   HAC = Initial encounter only (7th character A, B or C) and not POA.

Ⓝ Newborn: 0   Ⓟ Pediatric: 0-17   Ⓜ Maternity: 12-55   Ⓐ Adult: 15-124   `MCC` Major CC Condition   `PDxMCC` PDx acts as own MCC   `CC` CC Condition   `PDxCC` PDx acts as own CC

916
ICD-10-CM 2016

✓5ᵗʰ **S15.1   Injury of** vertebral artery

> **CC Excl: For CC codes in subcategory S15.1, unless otherwise noted:** CC with 7th character A: S09.0XXA, S15.101-S15.199 with 7th A, S15.8XX-S15.9XX with 7th A, T14.90-T14.91, T79.A0X-T79.9XX with 7th A

> ✓6ᵗʰ **S15.10   Unspecified injury of** vertebral artery
>> ✓7ᵗʰ **S15.101   Unspecified injury of** right vertebral artery `CC`
>> ✓7ᵗʰ **S15.102   Unspecified injury of** left vertebral artery `CC`
>> ✓7ᵗʰ **S15.109   Unspecified injury of** unspecified vertebral artery `CC`
>
> ✓6ᵗʰ **S15.11   Minor laceration of** vertebral artery
>> Incomplete transection of vertebral artery
>> Laceration of vertebral artery NOS
>> Superficial laceration of vertebral artery
>> ✓7ᵗʰ **S15.111   Minor laceration of** right vertebral artery `CC`
>> ✓7ᵗʰ **S15.112   Minor laceration of** left vertebral artery `CC`
>> ✓7ᵗʰ **S15.119   Minor laceration of** unspecified vertebral artery `CC`
>
> ✓6ᵗʰ **S15.12   Major laceration of** vertebral artery
>> Complete transection of vertebral artery
>> Traumatic rupture of vertebral artery
>> ✓7ᵗʰ **S15.121   Major laceration of** right vertebral artery `CC`
>> ✓7ᵗʰ **S15.122   Major laceration of** left vertebral artery `CC`
>> ✓7ᵗʰ **S15.129   Major laceration of** unspecified vertebral artery `CC`
>
> ✓6ᵗʰ **S15.19   Other specified injury of** vertebral artery
>> ✓7ᵗʰ **S15.191   Other specified injury of** right vertebral artery `CC`
>> ✓7ᵗʰ **S15.192   Other specified injury of** left vertebral artery `CC`
>> ✓7ᵗʰ **S15.199   Other specified injury of** unspecified vertebral artery `CC`

✓5ᵗʰ **S15.2   Injury of** external jugular vein

> **CC Excl: For CC codes in subcategory S15.2, unless otherwise noted:** See code: S15.1

> ✓6ᵗʰ **S15.20   Unspecified injury of** external jugular vein
>> ✓7ᵗʰ **S15.201   Unspecified injury of** right external jugular vein `CC`
>> ✓7ᵗʰ **S15.202   Unspecified injury of** left external jugular vein `CC`
>> ✓7ᵗʰ **S15.209   Unspecified injury of** unspecified external jugular vein `CC`
>
> ✓6ᵗʰ **S15.21   Minor laceration of** external jugular vein
>> Incomplete transection of external jugular vein
>> Laceration of external jugular vein NOS
>> Superficial laceration of external jugular vein
>> ✓7ᵗʰ **S15.211   Minor laceration of** right external jugular vein `CC`
>> ✓7ᵗʰ **S15.212   Minor laceration of** left external jugular vein `CC`
>> ✓7ᵗʰ **S15.219   Minor laceration of** unspecified external jugular vein `CC`
>
> ✓6ᵗʰ **S15.22   Major laceration of** external jugular vein
>> Complete transection of external jugular vein
>> Traumatic rupture of external jugular vein
>> ✓7ᵗʰ **S15.221   Major laceration of** right external jugular vein `CC`
>> ✓7ᵗʰ **S15.222   Major laceration of** left external jugular vein `CC`
>> ✓7ᵗʰ **S15.229   Major laceration of** unspecified external jugular vein `CC`
>
> ✓6ᵗʰ **S15.29   Other specified injury of** external jugular vein
>> ✓7ᵗʰ **S15.291   Other specified injury of** right external jugular vein `CC`
>> ✓7ᵗʰ **S15.292   Other specified injury of** left external jugular vein `CC`
>> ✓7ᵗʰ **S15.299   Other specified injury of** unspecified external jugular vein `CC`

✓5ᵗʰ **S15.3   Injury of** internal jugular vein

> **CC Excl: For CC codes in subcategory S15.3, unless otherwise noted:** See code: S15.1

> ✓6ᵗʰ **S15.30   Unspecified injury of** internal jugular vein
>> ✓7ᵗʰ **S15.301   Unspecified injury of** right internal jugular vein `CC`
>> ✓7ᵗʰ **S15.302   Unspecified injury of** left internal jugular vein `CC`
>> ✓7ᵗʰ **S15.309   Unspecified injury of** unspecified internal jugular vein `CC`
>
> ✓6ᵗʰ **S15.31   Minor laceration of** internal jugular vein
>> Incomplete transection of internal jugular vein
>> Laceration of internal jugular vein NOS
>> Superficial laceration of internal jugular vein
>> ✓7ᵗʰ **S15.311   Minor laceration of** right internal jugular vein `CC`
>> ✓7ᵗʰ **S15.312   Minor laceration of** left internal jugular vein `CC`
>> ✓7ᵗʰ **S15.319   Minor laceration of** unspecified internal jugular vein `CC`
>
> ✓6ᵗʰ **S15.32   Major laceration of** internal jugular vein
>> Complete transection of internal jugular vein
>> Traumatic rupture of internal jugular vein
>> ✓7ᵗʰ **S15.321   Major laceration of** right internal jugular vein `CC`
>> ✓7ᵗʰ **S15.322   Major laceration of** left internal jugular vein `CC`
>> ✓7ᵗʰ **S15.329   Major laceration of** unspecified internal jugular vein `CC`
>
> ✓6ᵗʰ **S15.39   Other specified injury of** internal jugular vein
>> ✓7ᵗʰ **S15.391   Other specified injury of** right internal jugular vein `CC`
>> ✓7ᵗʰ **S15.392   Other specified injury of** left internal jugular vein `CC`
>> ✓7ᵗʰ **S15.399   Other specified injury of** unspecified internal jugular vein `CC`

✓x7ᵗʰ **S15.8   Injury of other specified blood vessels at neck level** `CC`
> **CC Excl:** See code: S15.1

✓x7ᵗʰ **S15.9   Injury of unspecified blood vessel at neck level** `CC`
> **CC Excl:** See code: S15.1

✓4ᵗʰ **S16   Injury of muscle, fascia and tendon at neck level**
> Code also any associated open wound (S11.-)
> *EXCLUDES 2*   sprain of joint or ligament at neck level (S13.9)

> The appropriate 7th is to be added to each code from category S16.
> A   initial encounter
> D   subsequent encounter
> S   sequela

✓x7ᵗʰ **S16.1   Strain of muscle, fascia and tendon at neck level**

✓x7ᵗʰ **S16.2   Laceration of muscle, fascia and tendon at neck level**

✓x7ᵗʰ **S16.8   Other specified injury of muscle, fascia and tendon at neck level**

✓x7ᵗʰ **S16.9   Unspecified injury of muscle, fascia and tendon at neck level**

✓4ᵗʰ **S17   Crushing injury of neck**
> Use additional code for all associated injuries, such as:
> injury of blood vessels (S15.-)
> open wound of neck (S11.-)
> spinal cord injury (S14.0, S14.1-)
> vertebral fracture (S12.0- – S12.3-)

> The appropriate 7th is to be added to each code from category S17.
> A   initial encounter
> D   subsequent encounter
> S   sequela

> **CC Excl: For CC codes in category S17, unless otherwise noted:** CC with 7th character A: S01.90X-S02.92X with 7th A, S07.0XX-S07.9XX with 7th A, S08.89X-S09.19X with 7th A, S09.8XX-S09.90X with 7th A, S09.92X-S09.93X with 7th A, S16.8XX-S19.9XX with 7th A, T14.90-T14.91, T79.A0X-T79.9XX with 7th A

7 ✓x7ᵗʰ **S17.0   Crushing injury of larynx and trachea** `CC`

7 ✓x7ᵗʰ **S17.8   Crushing injury of other specified parts of neck** `CC`

7 ✓x7ᵗʰ **S17.9   Crushing injury of neck, part unspecified** `CC`

---

7   HAC = Initial encounter only (7th character A, B or C) and not POA.

✓ Additional Character Required   ✓x7ᵗʰ Placeholder Alert   Unacceptable PDx   Manifestation   Hospital Acquired Condition   *EXCLUDES 1* Not Coded Here   *EXCLUDES 2* Not Included Here

Chapter 19. Injury, Poisoning, and Certain Other Consequences of External Causes

✓4ᵗʰ **S19 Other specified and unspecified injuries of neck**

> The appropriate 7th is to be added to each code from category S19.
> A   initial encounter
> D   subsequent encounter
> S   sequela

   ✓5ᵗʰ **S19.8 Other specified injuries of neck**

     ✓x7ᵗʰ **S19.80 Other specified injuries of unspecified part of neck**

     ✓x7ᵗʰ **S19.81 Other specified injuries of larynx**

     ✓x7ᵗʰ **S19.82 Other specified injuries of cervical trachea**
         EXCLUDES 2   *other specified injury of thoracic trachea (S27.5-)*

     ✓x7ᵗʰ **S19.83 Other specified injuries of vocal cord**

     ✓x7ᵗʰ **S19.84 Other specified injuries of thyroid gland**

     ✓x7ᵗʰ **S19.85 Other specified injuries of pharynx and cervical esophagus**

     ✓x7ᵗʰ **S19.89 Other specified injuries of other specified part of neck**

   ✓x7ᵗʰ **S19.9 Unspecified injury of neck**

Injuries to the thorax (S20-S29)

INCLUDES   injuries of breast
         injuries of chest (wall)
         injuries of interscapular area
EXCLUDES 2   *burns and corrosions (T20-T32)*
         effects of foreign body in bronchus (T17.5)
         effects of foreign body in esophagus (T18.1)
         effects of foreign body in lung (T17.8)
         effects of foreign body in trachea (T17.4)
         frostbite (T33-T34)
         injuries of axilla
         injuries of clavicle
         injuries of scapular region
         injuries of shoulder
         insect bite or sting, venomous (T63.4)

✓4ᵗʰ **S20 Superficial injury of thorax**

> The appropriate 7th is to be added to each code from category S20.
> A   initial encounter
> D   subsequent encounter
> S   sequela

   ✓5ᵗʰ **S20.0 Contusion of breast**

     ✓x7ᵗʰ **S20.00 Contusion of breast, unspecified breast**

     ✓x7ᵗʰ **S20.01 Contusion of right breast**

     ✓x7ᵗʰ **S20.02 Contusion of left breast**

   ✓5ᵗʰ **S20.1 Other and unspecified superficial injuries of breast**

     ✓6ᵗʰ **S20.10 Unspecified superficial injuries of breast**

        ✓7ᵗʰ **S20.101 Unspecified superficial injuries of breast, right breast**

        ✓7ᵗʰ **S20.102 Unspecified superficial injuries of breast, left breast**

        ✓7ᵗʰ **S20.109 Unspecified superficial injuries of breast, unspecified breast**

     ✓6ᵗʰ **S20.11 Abrasion of breast**

        ✓7ᵗʰ **S20.111 Abrasion of breast, right breast**

        ✓7ᵗʰ **S20.112 Abrasion of breast, left breast**

        ✓7ᵗʰ **S20.119 Abrasion of breast, unspecified breast**

     ✓6ᵗʰ **S20.12 Blister (nonthermal) of breast**

        ✓7ᵗʰ **S20.121 Blister (nonthermal) of breast, right breast**

        ✓7ᵗʰ **S20.122 Blister (nonthermal) of breast, left breast**

        ✓7ᵗʰ **S20.129 Blister (nonthermal) of breast, unspecified breast**

     ✓6ᵗʰ **S20.14 External constriction of part of breast**

        ✓7ᵗʰ **S20.141 External constriction of part of breast, right breast**

        ✓7ᵗʰ **S20.142 External constriction of part of breast, left breast**

        ✓7ᵗʰ **S20.149 External constriction of part of breast, unspecified breast**

     ✓6ᵗʰ **S20.15 Superficial foreign body of breast**
        Splinter in the breast

        ✓7ᵗʰ **S20.151 Superficial foreign body of breast, right breast**

        ✓7ᵗʰ **S20.152 Superficial foreign body of breast, left breast**

        ✓7ᵗʰ **S20.159 Superficial foreign body of breast, unspecified breast**

     ✓6ᵗʰ **S20.16 Insect bite (nonvenomous) of breast**

        ✓7ᵗʰ **S20.161 Insect bite (nonvenomous) of breast, right breast**

        ✓7ᵗʰ **S20.162 Insect bite (nonvenomous) of breast, left breast**

        ✓7ᵗʰ **S20.169 Insect bite (nonvenomous) of breast, unspecified breast**

     ✓6ᵗʰ **S20.17 Other superficial bite of breast**
        EXCLUDES 1   *open bite of breast (S21.05-)*

        ✓7ᵗʰ **S20.171 Other superficial bite of breast, right breast**

        ✓7ᵗʰ **S20.172 Other superficial bite of breast, left breast**

        ✓7ᵗʰ **S20.179 Other superficial bite of breast, unspecified breast**

   ✓5ᵗʰ **S20.2 Contusion of thorax**

     ✓x7ᵗʰ **S20.20 Contusion of thorax, unspecified**

     ✓6ᵗʰ **S20.21 Contusion of front wall of thorax**

        ✓7ᵗʰ **S20.211 Contusion of right front wall of thorax**

        ✓7ᵗʰ **S20.212 Contusion of left front wall of thorax**

        ✓7ᵗʰ **S20.219 Contusion of unspecified front wall of thorax**

     ✓6ᵗʰ **S20.22 Contusion of back wall of thorax**

        ✓7ᵗʰ **S20.221 Contusion of right back wall of thorax**

        ✓7ᵗʰ **S20.222 Contusion of left back wall of thorax**

        ✓7ᵗʰ **S20.229 Contusion of unspecified back wall of thorax**

   ✓5ᵗʰ **S20.3 Other and unspecified superficial injuries of front wall of thorax**

     ✓6ᵗʰ **S20.30 Unspecified superficial injuries of front wall of thorax**

        ✓7ᵗʰ **S20.301 Unspecified superficial injuries of right front wall of thorax**

        ✓7ᵗʰ **S20.302 Unspecified superficial injuries of left front wall of thorax**

        ✓7ᵗʰ **S20.309 Unspecified superficial injuries of unspecified front wall of thorax**

     ✓6ᵗʰ **S20.31 Abrasion of front wall of thorax**

        ✓7ᵗʰ **S20.311 Abrasion of right front wall of thorax**

        ✓7ᵗʰ **S20.312 Abrasion of left front wall of thorax**

        ✓7ᵗʰ **S20.319 Abrasion of unspecified front wall of thorax**

     ✓6ᵗʰ **S20.32 Blister (nonthermal) of front wall of thorax**

        ✓7ᵗʰ **S20.321 Blister (nonthermal) of right front wall of thorax**

        ✓7ᵗʰ **S20.322 Blister (nonthermal) of left front wall of thorax**

        ✓7ᵗʰ **S20.329 Blister (nonthermal) of unspecified front wall of thorax**

     ✓6ᵗʰ **S20.34 External constriction of front wall of thorax**

        ✓7ᵗʰ **S20.341 External constriction of right front wall of thorax**

        ✓7ᵗʰ **S20.342 External constriction of left front wall of thorax**

        ✓7ᵗʰ **S20.349 External constriction of unspecified front wall of thorax**

     ✓6ᵗʰ **S20.35 Superficial foreign body of front wall of thorax**
        Splinter in front wall of thorax

        ✓7ᵗʰ **S20.351 Superficial foreign body of right front wall of thorax**

        ✓7ᵗʰ **S20.352 Superficial foreign body of left front wall of thorax**

        ✓7ᵗʰ **S20.359 Superficial foreign body of unspecified front wall of thorax**

     ✓6ᵗʰ **S20.36 Insect bite (nonvenomous) of front wall of thorax**

        ✓7ᵗʰ **S20.361 Insect bite (nonvenomous) of right front wall of thorax**

        ✓7ᵗʰ **S20.362 Insect bite (nonvenomous) of left front wall of thorax**

N Newborn: 0   P Pediatric: 0-17   M Maternity: 12-55   A Adult: 15-124   MCC Major CC Condition   PDxMCC PDx acts as own MCC   CC CC Condition   PDxCC PDx acts as own CC

918

ICD-10-CM 2016

✓7th **S20.369** Insect bite (nonvenomous) of unspecified front wall of thorax

✓6th **S20.37** Other superficial bite of front wall of thorax
  EXCLUDES 1 open bite of front wall of thorax (S21.14)

  ✓7th **S20.371** Other superficial bite of right front wall of thorax

  ✓7th **S20.372** Other superficial bite of left front wall of thorax

  ✓7th **S20.379** Other superficial bite of unspecified front wall of thorax

✓5th **S20.4** Other and unspecified superficial injuries of back wall of thorax

  ✓6th **S20.40** Unspecified superficial injuries of back wall of thorax

    ✓7th **S20.401** Unspecified superficial injuries of right back wall of thorax

    ✓7th **S20.402** Unspecified superficial injuries of left back wall of thorax

    ✓7th **S20.409** Unspecified superficial injuries of unspecified back wall of thorax

  ✓6th **S20.41** Abrasion of back wall of thorax

    ✓7th **S20.411** Abrasion of right back wall of thorax

    ✓7th **S20.412** Abrasion of left back wall of thorax

    ✓7th **S20.419** Abrasion of unspecified back wall of thorax

  ✓6th **S20.42** Blister (nonthermal) of back wall of thorax

    ✓7th **S20.421** Blister (nonthermal) of right back wall of thorax

    ✓7th **S20.422** Blister (nonthermal) of left back wall of thorax

    ✓7th **S20.429** Blister (nonthermal) of unspecified back wall of thorax

  ✓6th **S20.44** External constriction of back wall of thorax

    ✓7th **S20.441** External constriction of right back wall of thorax

    ✓7th **S20.442** External constriction of left back wall of thorax

    ✓7th **S20.449** External constriction of unspecified back wall of thorax

  ✓6th **S20.45** Superficial foreign body of back wall of thorax
    Splinter of back wall of thorax

    ✓7th **S20.451** Superficial foreign body of right back wall of thorax

    ✓7th **S20.452** Superficial foreign body of left back wall of thorax

    ✓7th **S20.459** Superficial foreign body of unspecified back wall of thorax

  ✓6th **S20.46** Insect bite (nonvenomous) of back wall of thorax

    ✓7th **S20.461** Insect bite (nonvenomous) of right back wall of thorax

    ✓7th **S20.462** Insect bite (nonvenomous) of left back wall of thorax

    ✓7th **S20.469** Insect bite (nonvenomous) of unspecified back wall of thorax

  ✓6th **S20.47** Other superficial bite of back wall of thorax
    EXCLUDES 1 open bite of back wall of thorax (S21.24)

    ✓7th **S20.471** Other superficial bite of right back wall of thorax

    ✓7th **S20.472** Other superficial bite of left back wall of thorax

    ✓7th **S20.479** Other superficial bite of unspecified back wall of thorax

✓5th **S20.9** Superficial injury of unspecified parts of thorax
  EXCLUDES 1 contusion of thorax NOS (S20.20)

  ✓x7th **S20.90** Unspecified superficial injury of unspecified parts of thorax
    Superficial injury of thoracic wall NOS

  ✓x7th **S20.91** Abrasion of unspecified parts of thorax

  ✓x7th **S20.92** Blister (nonthermal) of unspecified parts of thorax

  ✓x7th **S20.94** External constriction of unspecified parts of thorax

  ✓x7th **S20.95** Superficial foreign body of unspecified parts of thorax
    Splinter in thorax NOS

✓x7th **S20.96** Insect bite (nonvenomous) of unspecified parts of thorax

✓x7th **S20.97** Other superficial bite of unspecified parts of thorax
  EXCLUDES 1 open bite of thorax NOS (S21.95)

✓4th **S21** **Open wound of thorax**
  Code also any associated injury, such as:
    injury of heart (S26.-)
    injury of intrathoracic organs (S27.-)
    rib fracture (S22.3-, S22.4-)
    spinal cord injury (S24.0-, S24.1-)
    traumatic hemopneumothorax (S27.3)
    traumatic hemothorax (S27.1)
    traumatic pneumothorax (S27.0)
    wound infection
  EXCLUDES 1 traumatic amputation (partial) of thorax (S28.1)

  The appropriate 7th is to be added to each code from category S21.
  A   initial encounter
  D   subsequent encounter
  S   sequela

✓5th **S21.0** Open wound of breast

  ✓6th **S21.00** Unspecified open wound of breast

    ✓7th **S21.001** Unspecified open wound of right breast

    ✓7th **S21.002** Unspecified open wound of left breast

    ✓7th **S21.009** Unspecified open wound of unspecified breast

  ✓6th **S21.01** Laceration without foreign body of breast

    ✓7th **S21.011** Laceration without foreign body of right breast

    ✓7th **S21.012** Laceration without foreign body of left breast

    ✓7th **S21.019** Laceration without foreign body of unspecified breast

  ✓6th **S21.02** Laceration with foreign body of breast

    ✓7th **S21.021** Laceration with foreign body of right breast

    ✓7th **S21.022** Laceration with foreign body of left breast

    ✓7th **S21.029** Laceration with foreign body of unspecified breast

  ✓6th **S21.03** Puncture wound without foreign body of breast

    ✓7th **S21.031** Puncture wound without foreign body of right breast

    ✓7th **S21.032** Puncture wound without foreign body of left breast

    ✓7th **S21.039** Puncture wound without foreign body of unspecified breast

  ✓6th **S21.04** Puncture wound with foreign body of breast

    ✓7th **S21.041** Puncture wound with foreign body of right breast

    ✓7th **S21.042** Puncture wound with foreign body of left breast

    ✓7th **S21.049** Puncture wound with foreign body of unspecified breast

  ✓6th **S21.05** Open bite of breast
    Bite of breast NOS
    EXCLUDES 1 superficial bite of breast (S20.17)

    ✓7th **S21.051** Open bite of right breast

    ✓7th **S21.052** Open bite of left breast

    ✓7th **S21.059** Open bite of unspecified breast

✓5th **S21.1** Open wound of front wall of thorax without penetration into thoracic cavity
  Open wound of chest without penetration into thoracic cavity

  CC Excl: For CC codes in subcategory S21.1, unless otherwise noted: CC with 7th character A: S21.101-S21.159 with 7th A, S21.301-S21.95 with 7th A, S23.3XXA, S23.8XXA, S27.50X-S27.69X with 7th A, S27.892-S27.9XX with 7th A, S28.1XXA, S29.021A, S29.029A, S38.3XXA, T14.90-T14.91, T79.7XX-T79.9XX with 7th A

  ✓6th **S21.10** Unspecified open wound of front wall of thorax without penetration into thoracic cavity

    ✓7th **S21.101** Unspecified open wound of right front wall of thorax without penetration into thoracic cavity **CC**

    ✓7th **S21.102** Unspecified open wound of left front wall of thorax without penetration into thoracic cavity **CC**

✓ Additional Character Required   ✓x7th Placeholder Alert   Unacceptable PDx   ■ Manifestation   Hospital Acquired Condition   *EXCLUDES 1* Not Coded Here   *EXCLUDES 2* Not Included Here

ICD-10-CM 2016

919

Chapter 19. Injury, Poisoning, and Certain Other Consequences of External Causes

✓7ᵗʰ **S21.109** Unspecified open wound of unspecified front wall of thorax without penetration into thoracic cavity CC

✓6ᵗʰ **S21.11** Laceration without foreign body of front wall of thorax without penetration into thoracic cavity

     ✓7ᵗʰ **S21.111** Laceration without foreign body of right front wall of thorax without penetration into thoracic cavity CC

     ✓7ᵗʰ **S21.112** Laceration without foreign body of left front wall of thorax without penetration into thoracic cavity CC

     ✓7ᵗʰ **S21.119** Laceration without foreign body of unspecified front wall of thorax without penetration into thoracic cavity CC

✓6ᵗʰ **S21.12** Laceration with foreign body of front wall of thorax without penetration into thoracic cavity

     ✓7ᵗʰ **S21.121** Laceration with foreign body of right front wall of thorax without penetration into thoracic cavity CC

     ✓7ᵗʰ **S21.122** Laceration with foreign body of left front wall of thorax without penetration into thoracic cavity CC

     ✓7ᵗʰ **S21.129** Laceration with foreign body of unspecified front wall of thorax without penetration into thoracic cavity CC

✓6ᵗʰ **S21.13** Puncture wound without foreign body of front wall of thorax without penetration into thoracic cavity

     ✓7ᵗʰ **S21.131** Puncture wound without foreign body of right front wall of thorax without penetration into thoracic cavity CC

     ✓7ᵗʰ **S21.132** Puncture wound without foreign body of left front wall of thorax without penetration into thoracic cavity CC

     ✓7ᵗʰ **S21.139** Puncture wound without foreign body of unspecified front wall of thorax without penetration into thoracic cavity CC

✓6ᵗʰ **S21.14** Puncture wound with foreign body of front wall of thorax without penetration into thoracic cavity

     ✓7ᵗʰ **S21.141** Puncture wound with foreign body of right front wall of thorax without penetration into thoracic cavity CC

     ✓7ᵗʰ **S21.142** Puncture wound with foreign body of left front wall of thorax without penetration into thoracic cavity CC

     ✓7ᵗʰ **S21.149** Puncture wound with foreign body of unspecified front wall of thorax without penetration into thoracic cavity CC

✓6ᵗʰ **S21.15** Open bite of front wall of thorax without penetration into thoracic cavity
     Bite of front wall of thorax NOS
     EXCLUDES 1   *superficial bite of front wall of thorax (S20.37)*

     ✓7ᵗʰ **S21.151** Open bite of right front wall of thorax without penetration into thoracic cavity CC

     ✓7ᵗʰ **S21.152** Open bite of left front wall of thorax without penetration into thoracic cavity CC

     ✓7ᵗʰ **S21.159** Open bite of unspecified front wall of thorax without penetration into thoracic cavity CC

✓5ᵗʰ **S21.2** Open wound of back wall of thorax without penetration into thoracic cavity

     ✓6ᵗʰ **S21.20** Unspecified open wound of back wall of thorax without penetration into thoracic cavity

       ✓7ᵗʰ **S21.201** Unspecified open wound of right back wall of thorax without penetration into thoracic cavity

       ✓7ᵗʰ **S21.202** Unspecified open wound of left back wall of thorax without penetration into thoracic cavity

       ✓7ᵗʰ **S21.209** Unspecified open wound of unspecified back wall of thorax without penetration into thoracic cavity

     ✓6ᵗʰ **S21.21** Laceration without foreign body of back wall of thorax without penetration into thoracic cavity

       ✓7ᵗʰ **S21.211** Laceration without foreign body of right back wall of thorax without penetration into thoracic cavity

     ✓7ᵗʰ **S21.212** Laceration without foreign body of left back wall of thorax without penetration into thoracic cavity

     ✓7ᵗʰ **S21.219** Laceration without foreign body of unspecified back wall of thorax without penetration into thoracic cavity

✓6ᵗʰ **S21.22** Laceration with foreign body of back wall of thorax without penetration into thoracic cavity

     ✓7ᵗʰ **S21.221** Laceration with foreign body of right back wall of thorax without penetration into thoracic cavity

     ✓7ᵗʰ **S21.222** Laceration with foreign body of left back wall of thorax without penetration into thoracic cavity

     ✓7ᵗʰ **S21.229** Laceration with foreign body of unspecified back wall of thorax without penetration into thoracic cavity

✓6ᵗʰ **S21.23** Puncture wound without foreign body of back wall of thorax without penetration into thoracic cavity

     ✓7ᵗʰ **S21.231** Puncture wound without foreign body of right back wall of thorax without penetration into thoracic cavity

     ✓7ᵗʰ **S21.232** Puncture wound without foreign body of left back wall of thorax without penetration into thoracic cavity

     ✓7ᵗʰ **S21.239** Puncture wound without foreign body of unspecified back wall of thorax without penetration into thoracic cavity

✓6ᵗʰ **S21.24** Puncture wound with foreign body of back wall of thorax without penetration into thoracic cavity

     ✓7ᵗʰ **S21.241** Puncture wound with foreign body of right back wall of thorax without penetration into thoracic cavity

     ✓7ᵗʰ **S21.242** Puncture wound with foreign body of left back wall of thorax without penetration into thoracic cavity

     ✓7ᵗʰ **S21.249** Puncture wound with foreign body of unspecified back wall of thorax without penetration into thoracic cavity

✓6ᵗʰ **S21.25** Open bite of back wall of thorax without penetration into thoracic cavity
     Bite of back wall of thorax NOS
     EXCLUDES 1   *superficial bite of back wall of thorax (S20.47)*

     ✓7ᵗʰ **S21.251** Open bite of right back wall of thorax without penetration into thoracic cavity

     ✓7ᵗʰ **S21.252** Open bite of left back wall of thorax without penetration into thoracic cavity

     ✓7ᵗʰ **S21.259** Open bite of unspecified back wall of thorax without penetration into thoracic cavity

✓5ᵗʰ **S21.3** Open wound of front wall of thorax with penetration into thoracic cavity
     Open wound of chest with penetration into thoracic cavity

> **CC Excl: For MCC codes in subcategory S21.3, unless otherwise noted: MCC with 7th character A:** S21.101-S21.159 with 7th A, S21.301-S21.95X with 7th A, S27.50X-S27.69X with 7th A, S27.892-S27.9XX with 7th A, S28.1XXA, S29.021A, S29.029A, S38.3XXA, T14.90-T14.91, T79.7XX-T79.9XX with 7th A

✓6ᵗʰ **S21.30** Unspecified open wound of front wall of thorax with penetration into thoracic cavity

     ✓7ᵗʰ **S21.301** Unspecified open wound of right front wall of thorax with penetration into thoracic cavity MCC

     ✓7ᵗʰ **S21.302** Unspecified open wound of left front wall of thorax with penetration into thoracic cavity MCC

     ✓7ᵗʰ **S21.309** Unspecified open wound of unspecified front wall of thorax with penetration into thoracic cavity MCC
       CC Excl: S21.101-S21.159 with 7th A, S21.301-S21.95 with 7th A, S27.0XX-S27.309 with 7th A, S27.329A, S27.339A, S27.409 with 7th A, S27.50X-S27.803 with 7th A, S27.892-S27.9XX with 7th A, S28.1XXA, S29.021A, S29.029A, S38.3XXA, T14.90-T14.91, T79.7XX-T79.9XX with 7th A

N Newborn: 0   P Pediatric: 0-17   M Maternity: 12-55   A Adult: 15-124   MCC Major CC Condition   PDxMCC PDx acts as own MCC   CC CC Condition   PDxCC PDx acts as own CC

920   ICD-10-CM 2016

√6ᵗʰ **S21.31** **Laceration without foreign body of front wall of thorax with penetration into thoracic cavity**

     √7ᵗʰ **S21.311** Laceration without foreign body of right front wall of thorax with penetration into thoracic cavity   MCC

     √7ᵗʰ **S21.312** Laceration without foreign body of left front wall of thorax with penetration into thoracic cavity   MCC

     √7ᵗʰ **S21.319** Laceration without foreign body of unspecified front wall of thorax with penetration into thoracic cavity   MCC

√6ᵗʰ **S21.32** **Laceration with foreign body of front wall of thorax with penetration into thoracic cavity**

     √7ᵗʰ **S21.321** Laceration with foreign body of right front wall of thorax with penetration into thoracic cavity   MCC

     √7ᵗʰ **S21.322** Laceration with foreign body of left front wall of thorax with penetration into thoracic cavity   MCC

     √7ᵗʰ **S21.329** Laceration with foreign body of unspecified front wall of thorax with penetration into thoracic cavity   MCC

√6ᵗʰ **S21.33** **Puncture wound without foreign body of front wall of thorax with penetration into thoracic cavity**

     √7ᵗʰ **S21.331** Puncture wound without foreign body of right front wall of thorax with penetration into thoracic cavity   MCC

     √7ᵗʰ **S21.332** Puncture wound without foreign body of left front wall of thorax with penetration into thoracic cavity   MCC

     √7ᵗʰ **S21.339** Puncture wound without foreign body of unspecified front wall of thorax with penetration into thoracic cavity   MCC

√6ᵗʰ **S21.34** **Puncture wound with foreign body of front wall of thorax with penetration into thoracic cavity**

     √7ᵗʰ **S21.341** Puncture wound with foreign body of right front wall of thorax with penetration into thoracic cavity   MCC

     √7ᵗʰ **S21.342** Puncture wound with foreign body of left front wall of thorax with penetration into thoracic cavity   MCC

     √7ᵗʰ **S21.349** Puncture wound with foreign body of unspecified front wall of thorax with penetration into thoracic cavity   MCC

√6ᵗʰ **S21.35** **Open bite of front wall of thorax with penetration into thoracic cavity**
     EXCLUDES 1   *superficial bite of front wall of thorax (S20.37)*

     √7ᵗʰ **S21.351** Open bite of right front wall of thorax with penetration into thoracic cavity   MCC

     √7ᵗʰ **S21.352** Open bite of left front wall of thorax with penetration into thoracic cavity   MCC

     √7ᵗʰ **S21.359** Open bite of unspecified front wall of thorax with penetration into thoracic cavity   MCC

√5ᵗʰ **S21.4** **Open wound of back wall of thorax with penetration into thoracic cavity**

> **CC Excl: For MCC codes in subcategory S21.4, unless otherwise noted: MCC with 7th character A:** See code: S21.3

√6ᵗʰ **S21.40** **Unspecified open wound of back wall of thorax with penetration into thoracic cavity**

     √7ᵗʰ **S21.401** Unspecified open wound of right back wall of thorax with penetration into thoracic cavity   MCC

     √7ᵗʰ **S21.402** Unspecified open wound of left back wall of thorax with penetration into thoracic cavity   MCC

     √7ᵗʰ **S21.409** Unspecified open wound of unspecified back wall of thorax with penetration into thoracic cavity   MCC

√6ᵗʰ **S21.41** **Laceration without foreign body of back wall of thorax with penetration into thoracic cavity**

     √7ᵗʰ **S21.411** Laceration without foreign body of right back wall of thorax with penetration into thoracic cavity   MCC

     √7ᵗʰ **S21.412** Laceration without foreign body of left back wall of thorax with penetration into thoracic cavity   MCC

     √7ᵗʰ **S21.419** Laceration without foreign body of unspecified back wall of thorax with penetration into thoracic cavity   MCC

√6ᵗʰ **S21.42** **Laceration with foreign body of back wall of thorax with penetration into thoracic cavity**

     √7ᵗʰ **S21.421** Laceration with foreign body of right back wall of thorax with penetration into thoracic cavity   MCC

     √7ᵗʰ **S21.422** Laceration with foreign body of left back wall of thorax with penetration into thoracic cavity   MCC

     √7ᵗʰ **S21.429** Laceration with foreign body of unspecified back wall of thorax with penetration into thoracic cavity   MCC

√6ᵗʰ **S21.43** **Puncture wound without foreign body of back wall of thorax with penetration into thoracic cavity**

     √7ᵗʰ **S21.431** Puncture wound without foreign body of right back wall of thorax with penetration into thoracic cavity   MCC

     √7ᵗʰ **S21.432** Puncture wound without foreign body of left back wall of thorax with penetration into thoracic cavity   MCC

     √7ᵗʰ **S21.439** Puncture wound without foreign body of unspecified back wall of thorax with penetration into thoracic cavity   MCC

√6ᵗʰ **S21.44** **Puncture wound with foreign body of back wall of thorax with penetration into thoracic cavity**

     √7ᵗʰ **S21.441** Puncture wound with foreign body of right back wall of thorax with penetration into thoracic cavity   MCC

     √7ᵗʰ **S21.442** Puncture wound with foreign body of left back wall of thorax with penetration into thoracic cavity   MCC

     √7ᵗʰ **S21.449** Puncture wound with foreign body of unspecified back wall of thorax with penetration into thoracic cavity   MCC

√6ᵗʰ **S21.45** **Open bite of back wall of thorax with penetration into thoracic cavity**
     Bite of back wall of thorax NOS
     EXCLUDES 1   *superficial bite of back wall of thorax (S20.47)*

     √7ᵗʰ **S21.451** Open bite of right back wall of thorax with penetration into thoracic cavity   MCC

     √7ᵗʰ **S21.452** Open bite of left back wall of thorax with penetration into thoracic cavity   MCC

     √7ᵗʰ **S21.459** Open bite of unspecified back wall of thorax with penetration into thoracic cavity   MCC

√5ᵗʰ **S21.9** **Open wound of unspecified part of thorax**
     Open wound of thoracic wall NOS

> **CC Excl: For CC codes in subcategory S21.9, unless otherwise noted: CC with 7th character A:** S21.101-S21.159 with 7th A, S21.301-S21.95X with 7th A, S23.3XXA, S23.8XXA, S27.50X-S27.69X with 7th A, S27.892-S27.9XX with 7th A, S28.1XXA, S29.021A, S29.029A, S38.3XXA, T14.90-T14.91, T79.7XX-T79.9XX with 7th A

√x7ᵗʰ **S21.90** Unspecified open wound of unspecified part of thorax   CC

√x7ᵗʰ **S21.91** Laceration without foreign body of unspecified part of thorax   CC

√x7ᵗʰ **S21.92** Laceration with foreign body of unspecified part of thorax   CC

√x7ᵗʰ **S21.93** Puncture wound without foreign body of unspecified part of thorax   CC

√x7ᵗʰ **S21.94** Puncture wound with foreign body of unspecified part of thorax   CC

√x7ᵗʰ **S21.95** Open bite of unspecified part of thorax   CC
     EXCLUDES 1   *superficial bite of thorax (S20.97)*

☑ Additional Character Required   √x7ᵗʰ Placeholder Alert   Unacceptable PDx   Manifestation   Hospital Acquired Condition   **EXCLUDES 1** Not Coded Here   **EXCLUDES 2** Not Included Here

ICD-10-CM 2016   921

Chapter 19. Injury, Poisoning, and Certain Other Consequences of External Causes

✓4th **S22   Fracture of rib(s), sternum and thoracic spine**

NOTE   A fracture not indicated as nondisplaced or displaced should be coded to displaced.
A fracture not indicated as open or closed should be coded to closed.

INCLUDES   fracture of thoracic neural arch
fracture of thoracic spinous process
fracture of thoracic transverse process
fracture of thoracic vertebra
fracture of thoracic vertebral arch

Code first any associated:
injury of intrathoracic organ (S27.-)
spinal cord injury (S24.0-, S24.1-)

EXCLUDES 1   transection of thorax (S28.1)

EXCLUDES 2   fracture of clavicle (S42.0-)
fracture of scapula (S42.1-)

The appropriate 7th is to be added to each code from category S22.
A   initial encounter for closed fracture
B   initial encounter for open fracture
D   subsequent encounter for fracture with routine healing
G   subsequent encounter for fracture with delayed healing
K   subsequent encounter for fracture with nonunion
S   sequela

✓6th **S22.0   Fracture of thoracic vertebra**

CC Excl: For CC/MCC codes in subcategory S22.0, unless otherwise noted: CC with 7th character A or MCC with 7th character B: M48.40X-M48.58X with 7th S, M80.08XS, M80.88XS, M84.350S, M84.454S, M84.550S, M84.58S, M84.650S, M99.12, M99.15-M99.17, M99.19, S03.1XXA, S03.8XX-S03.9XX with 7th A, S12.000-S12.9XX with 7th S, S13.9XXA, S14.109A, S14.119A, S14.129 A, S14.139A, S14.149A, S14.159A, S22.000-S23.3XX with 7th [A, B, S], S23.8XX-S24.159 with 7th A, S29.001-S29.019 with 7th A, S29.091-S29.9XX with 7th A, S32.000-S32.9XX with 7th S, S33.30X-S33.39X with 7th A, S33.9XA, S38.1XXA, S38.3XX-S39.013 with 7th A, S39.091-S39.94X with 7th A, T14.90-T14.91, T79.A0X-T79.9XX with 7th A

CC with 7th character K: M80.00X-M84.68X with 7th [K, P], S02.0XX-S02.92X with 7th K, S12.000-S12.691 with 7th K, S22.000-S22.9XX with 7th K, S32.000-S32.9XX with 7th K, S42.001-S42.92X with 7th [K, P], S49.001-S49.199 with 7th [K, P], S52.001-S52.92X with 7th [K, M, N, P, Q, R], S59.001-S59.299 with 7th [K, P], S62.001-S62.92X with 7th [K, P], S72.001-S72.92X with 7th [K, M, N, P, Q, R], S79.001-S79.199 with 7th [K, P], S82.001-S82.92X with 7th [K, M, N, P, Q, R], S89.001-S89.399 with 7th [K, P], S92.001-S92.919 with 7th [K, P]

✓6th **S22.00   Fracture of unspecified thoracic vertebra**

7,16,19 ✓7th   **S22.000   Wedge compression fracture of unspecified thoracic vertebra**   MCC CC

7,16,19 ✓7th   **S22.001   Stable burst fracture of unspecified thoracic vertebra**   MCC CC

7,16,19 ✓7th   **S22.002   Unstable burst fracture of unspecified thoracic vertebra**   MCC CC

7,16,19 ✓7th   **S22.008   Other fracture of unspecified thoracic vertebra**   MCC CC

7,16,19 ✓7th   **S22.009   Unspecified fracture of unspecified thoracic vertebra**   MCC CC

✓6th **S22.01   Fracture of first thoracic vertebra**

7,16,19 ✓7th   **S22.010   Wedge compression fracture of first thoracic vertebra**   MCC CC

7,16,19 ✓7th   **S22.011   Stable burst fracture of first thoracic vertebra**   MCC CC

7,16,19 ✓7th   **S22.012   Unstable burst fracture of first thoracic vertebra**   MCC CC

7,16,19 ✓7th   **S22.018   Other fracture of first thoracic vertebra**   MCC CC

7,16,19 ✓7th   **S22.019   Unspecified fracture of first thoracic vertebra**   MCC CC

✓6th **S22.02   Fracture of second thoracic vertebra**

7,16,19 ✓7th   **S22.020   Wedge compression fracture of second thoracic vertebra**   MCC CC

7,16,19 ✓7th   **S22.021   Stable burst fracture of second thoracic vertebra**   MCC CC

7,16,19 ✓7th   **S22.022   Unstable burst fracture of second thoracic vertebra**   MCC CC

7,16,19 ✓7th   **S22.028   Other fracture of second thoracic vertebra**   MCC CC

7,16,19 ✓7th   **S22.029   Unspecified fracture of second thoracic vertebra**   MCC CC

✓6th **S22.03   Fracture of third thoracic vertebra**

7,16,19 ✓7th   **S22.030   Wedge compression fracture of third thoracic vertebra**   MCC CC

7,16,19 ✓7th   **S22.031   Stable burst fracture of third thoracic vertebra**   MCC CC

7,16,19 ✓7th   **S22.032   Unstable burst fracture of third thoracic vertebra**   MCC CC

7,16,19 ✓7th   **S22.038   Other fracture of third thoracic vertebra**   MCC CC

7,16,19 ✓7th   **S22.039   Unspecified fracture of third thoracic vertebra**   MCC CC

✓6th **S22.04   Fracture of fourth thoracic vertebra**

7,16,19 ✓7th   **S22.040   Wedge compression fracture of fourth thoracic vertebra**   MCC CC

7,16,19 ✓7th   **S22.041   Stable burst fracture of fourth thoracic vertebra**   MCC CC

7,16,19 ✓7th   **S22.042   Unstable burst fracture of fourth thoracic vertebra**   MCC CC

7,16,19 ✓7th   **S22.048   Other fracture of fourth thoracic vertebra**   MCC CC

7,16,19 ✓7th   **S22.049   Unspecified fracture of fourth thoracic vertebra**   MCC CC

✓6th **S22.05   Fracture of T5-T6 vertebra**

7,16,19 ✓7th   **S22.050   Wedge compression fracture of T5-T6 vertebra**   MCC CC

7,16,19 ✓7th   **S22.051   Stable burst fracture of T5-T6 vertebra**   MCC CC

7,16,19 ✓7th   **S22.052   Unstable burst fracture of T5-T6 vertebra**   MCC CC

7,16,19 ✓7th   **S22.058   Other fracture of T5-T6 vertebra**   MCC CC

7,16,19 ✓7th   **S22.059   Unspecified fracture of T5-T6 vertebra**   MCC CC

✓6th **S22.06   Fracture of T7-T8 vertebra**

7,16,19 ✓7th   **S22.060   Wedge compression fracture of T7-T8 vertebra**   MCC CC

7,16,19 ✓7th   **S22.061   Stable burst fracture of T7-T8 vertebra**   MCC CC

7,16,19 ✓7th   **S22.062   Unstable burst fracture of T7-T8 vertebra**   MCC CC

7,16,19 ✓7th   **S22.068   Other fracture of T7-T8 thoracic vertebra**   MCC CC

7,16,19 ✓7th   **S22.069   Unspecified fracture of T7-T8 vertebra**   MCC CC

✓6th **S22.07   Fracture of T9-T10 vertebra**

7,16,19 ✓7th   **S22.070   Wedge compression fracture of T9-T10 vertebra**   MCC CC

7,16,19 ✓7th   **S22.071   Stable burst fracture of T9-T10 vertebra**   MCC CC

7,16,19 ✓7th   **S22.072   Unstable burst fracture of T9-T10 vertebra**   MCC CC

7,16,19 ✓7th   **S22.078   Other fracture of T9-T10 vertebra**   MCC CC

7,16,19 ✓7th   **S22.079   Unspecified fracture of T9-T10 vertebra**   MCC CC

✓6th **S22.08   Fracture of T11-T12 vertebra**

7,16,19 ✓7th   **S22.080   Wedge compression fracture of T11-T12 vertebra**   MCC CC

7,16,19 ✓7th   **S22.081   Stable burst fracture of T11-T12 vertebra**   MCC CC

7,16,19 ✓7th   **S22.082   Unstable burst fracture of T11-T12 vertebra**   MCC CC

7,16,19 ✓7th   **S22.088   Other fracture of T11-T12 vertebra**   MCC CC

7,16,19 ✓7th   **S22.089   Unspecified fracture of T11-T12 vertebra**   MCC CC

---

7   HAC = Initial encounter only (7th character A, B or C) and not POA.
16   MCC only if an open fracture (7th character B or C – specific to category).
19   CC only if an initial encounter for a closed fracture (7th character A) **OR** a subsequent encounter for nonunion or malunion (7th character K, M, N, P, Q, or R – specific to category).

N Newborn: 0   P Pediatric: 0-17   M Maternity: 12-55   A Adult: 15-124   MCC Major CC Condition   PDxMCC PDx acts as own MCC   CC CC Condition   PDxCC PDx acts as own CC

√5th **S22.2 Fracture of sternum**

> **CC Excl: For CC/MCC codes in subcategory S22.2, unless otherwise noted: CC with 7th character A or MCC with 7th character B:** S03.8XX-S03.9XX with 7th A, S22.20X-S22.24X with 7th [A, B], S22.5XX-S22.5XX with 7th [A, B], S29.011-S29.019 with 7th A, S38.3XX-S39.013 with 7th A, T14.90-T14.91, T79.A0X-T79.9XX with 7th A
> **CC with 7th character K:** M80.00X-M84.68X with 7th [K, P], S02.0XX-S02.92X with 7th K, S12.000-S12.691 with 7th K, S22.000-S22.9XX with 7th K, S32.000-S32.9XX with 7th K, S42.001-S42.92X with 7th [K, P], S49.001-S49.199 with 7th [K, P], S52.001-S52.92X with 7th [K, M, N, P, Q, R], S59.001-S59.299 with 7th [K, P], S62.001-S62.92X with 7th [K, P], S72.001-S72.92X with 7th [K, M, N, P, Q, R], S79.001-S79.199 with 7th [K, P], S82.001-S82.92X with 7th [K, M, N, P, Q, R], S89.001-S89.399 with 7th [K, P], S92.001-S92.919 with 7th [K, P]

7,16,19 √x7th **S22.20 Unspecified fracture of sternum** `MCC` `CC`

7,16,19 √x7th **S22.21 Fracture of manubrium** `MCC` `CC`

7,16,19 √x7th **S22.22 Fracture of body of sternum** `MCC` `CC`

7,16,19 √x7th **S22.23 Sternal manubrial dissociation** `MCC` `CC`

7,16,19 √x7th **S22.24 Fracture of xiphoid process** `MCC` `CC`

√5th **S22.3 Fracture of one rib**

> **CC Excl: For CC/MCC codes in subcategory S22.3, unless otherwise noted: CC with 7th character A or MCC with 7th character B:** S03.8XX-S03.9XXwith 7th A, S22.20X-S22.5XX with 7th [A, B], S29.011-S29.019 with 7th A, S38.3XX-S39.013 with 7th A, T14.90-T14.91, T79.A0X-T79.9XX with 7th A
> **CC with 7th character K:** M80.00X-M84.68X with 7th [K, P], S02.0XX-S02.92X with 7th K, S12.000-S12.691 with 7th K, S22.000-S22.9XX with 7th K, S32.000-S32.9XX with 7th K, S42.001-S42.92X with 7th [K, P], S49.001-S49.199 with 7th [K, P], S52.001-S52.92X with 7th [K, M, N, P, Q, R], S59.001-S59.299 with 7th [K, P], S62.001-S62.92X with 7th [K, P], S72.001-S72.92X with 7th [K, M, N, P, Q, R], S79.001-S79.199 with 7th [K, P], S82.001-S82.92X with 7th [K, M, N, P, Q, R], S89.001-S89.399 with 7th [K, P], S92.001-S92.919 with 7th [K, P]

7,16,19 √x7th **S22.31 Fracture of one rib, right side** `MCC` `CC`

7,16,19 √x7th **S22.32 Fracture of one rib, left side** `MCC` `CC`

7,16,19 √x7th **S22.39 Fracture of one rib, unspecified side** `MCC` `CC`

√5th **S22.4 Multiple fractures of ribs**
Fractures of two or more ribs
EXCLUDES 1 flail chest (S22.5-)

> **CC Excl: For CC/MCC codes in subcategory S22.4, unless otherwise noted: CC with 7th character A or MCC with 7th character B:** S03.8XX-S03.9XX with 7th A, S22.31X-S22.5XX with 7th [A, B], S29.011-S29.019 with 7th A, S38.3XX-S39.013 with 7th A, T14.90-T14.91, T79.9XX with 7th A
> **CC with 7th character K:** M80.00X-M84.68X with 7th [K, P], S02.0XX-S02.92X with 7th K, S12.000-S12.691 with 7th K, S22.000-S22.9XX with 7th K, S32.000-S32.9XX with 7th K, S42.001-S42.92X with 7th [K, P], S49.001-S49.199 with 7th [K, P], S52.001-S52.92X with 7th [K, M, N, P, Q, R], S59.001-S59.299 with 7th [K, P], S62.001-S62.92X with 7th [K, P], S72.001-S72.92X with 7th [K, M, N, P, Q, R], S79.001-S79.199 with 7th [K, P], S82.001-S82.92X with 7th [K, M, N, P, Q, R], S89.001-S89.399 with 7th [K, P], S92.001-S92.919 with 7th [K, P]

7,16,19 √x7th **S22.41 Multiple fractures of ribs, right side** `MCC` `CC`

7,16,19 √x7th **S22.42 Multiple fractures of ribs, left side** `MCC` `CC`

7,16,19 √x7th **S22.43 Multiple fractures of ribs, bilateral** `MCC` `CC`

7,16,19 √x7th **S22.49 Multiple fractures of ribs, unspecified side** `MCC` `CC`
    CC Excl: No excl for codes with 7th B

7,18 √x7th **S22.5 Flail chest** `MCC` `CC`

> **CC Excl: For CC/MCC codes in subcategory S22.5, unless otherwise noted: CC with 7th character A or MCC with 7th character B:** S03.8XX-S03.9XX with 7th A, S22.20X-S22.5XX with 7th [A, B], S29.011-S29.019 with 7th A, S38.3XX-S39.013 with 7th A, T14.90-T14.91, T79.A0X-T79.9XX with 7th A
> **CC with 7th character K:** M80.00X-M80.88X[K,P], M84.30X-M84.68X[K,P], S02.0X-S02.92X[K], S12.000-S12.691[K], S22.000-S22.9X[K], S32.0[0-4][0-2,8-9]K, S32.050K

7,16,19 √x7th **S22.9 Fracture of bony thorax, part unspecified** `MCC` `CC`

> **CC Excl: For CC/MCC codes in subcategory S22.9, unless otherwise noted: CC with 7th character A or MCC with 7th character B:** M80.00X-M80.01X9 with 7th A, M80.041-M80.049 with 7th A, M80.80X-M80.819 with 7th A, M80.841-M80.849 with 7th A, M84.40X-M84.419 with 7th A, M84.441-M84.446 with 7th A, M84.454A, M84.474-M84.519 with 7th A, M84.541-M84.550 with 7th A, M84.574-M84.576 with 7th A, M84.60X-M84.619 with 7th A, M84.641-M84.650 with 7th A, M84.674-M84.68X with 7th A, S03.8XX-S03.9XX with 7th A, S22.9XX-S22.9XX with 7th [A, B], S29.011-S29.019 with 7th A, S32.301-S32.811 with 7th [A, B], S32.89X-S32.9XX with 7th [A, B], S33.4XXA, S33.6XX-S33.8XX with 7th A, S38.3XX-S39.013 with 7th A, S73.001-S73.199 with 7th A, S76.001-S76.019 with 7th A, S76.091-S76.119 with 7th A, S76.191-S76.219 with 7th A, S76.291-S76.319 with 7th A, S76.391-S76.819 with 7th A, S76.891-S76.919 with 7th A, S76.991-S76.999 with 7th A, S79.811-S79.929 with 7th A, T14.90-T14.91, T79.A9X-T79.9XX with 7th A
> **CC with 7th character K:** M80.00X-M84.68X with 7th [K, P], S02.0XX-S02.92X with 7th K, S12.000-S12.691 with 7th K, S22.000-S22.9XX with 7th K, S32.000-S32.9XX with 7th K, S42.001-S42.92X with 7th [K, P], S49.001-S49.199 with 7th [K, P], S52.001-S52.92X with 7th [K, M, N, P, Q, R], S59.001-S59.299 with 7th [K, P], S62.001-S62.92X with 7th [K, P], S72.001-S72.92X with 7th [K, M, N, P, Q, R], S79.001-S79.199 with 7th [K, P], S82.001-S82.92X with 7th [K, M, N, P, Q, R], S89.001-S89.399 with 7th [K, P], S92.001-S92.919 with 7th [K, P]

√4th **S23 Dislocation and sprain of joints and ligaments of thorax**
> **INCLUDES** avulsion of joint or ligament of thorax
> laceration of cartilage, joint or ligament of thorax
> sprain of cartilage, joint or ligament of thorax
> traumatic hemarthrosis of joint or ligament of thorax
> traumatic rupture of joint or ligament of thorax
> traumatic subluxation of joint or ligament of thorax
> traumatic tear of joint or ligament of thorax
>
> Code also any associated open wound
> **EXCLUDES 2** dislocation, sprain of sternoclavicular joint (S43.2, S43.6)
> strain of muscle or tendon of thorax (S29.01-)

> The appropriate 7th is to be added to each code from category S23.
> A   initial encounter
> D   subsequent encounter
> S   sequela

√x7th **S23.0 Traumatic rupture of thoracic intervertebral disc**
> **EXCLUDES 1** rupture or displacement (nontraumatic) of thoracic intervertebral disc NOS (M51- with fifth character 4)

√5th **S23.1 Subluxation and dislocation of thoracic vertebra**
> Code also any associated
> open wound of thorax (S21.-)
> spinal cord injury (S24.0-, S24.1-)
> **EXCLUDES 2** fracture of thoracic vertebrae (S22.0-)

   √6th **S23.10 Subluxation and dislocation of unspecified thoracic vertebra**
     √7th **S23.100 Subluxation of unspecified thoracic vertebra**
     √7th **S23.101 Dislocation of unspecified thoracic vertebra**

   √6th **S23.11 Subluxation and dislocation of T1/T2 thoracic vertebra**
     √7th **S23.110 Subluxation of T1/T2 thoracic vertebra**
     √7th **S23.111 Dislocation of T1/T2 thoracic vertebra**

   √6th **S23.12 Subluxation and dislocation of T2/T3-T3/T4 thoracic vertebra**
     √7th **S23.120 Subluxation of T2/T3 thoracic vertebra**
     √7th **S23.121 Dislocation of T2/T3 thoracic vertebra**
     √7th **S23.122 Subluxation of T3/T4 thoracic vertebra**
     √7th **S23.123 Dislocation of T3/T4 thoracic vertebra**

   √6th **S23.13 Subluxation and dislocation of T4/T5-T5/T6 thoracic vertebra**
     √7th **S23.130 Subluxation of T4/T5 thoracic vertebra**
     √7th **S23.131 Dislocation of T4/T5 thoracic vertebra**
     √7th **S23.132 Subluxation of T5/T6 thoracic vertebra**
     √7th **S23.133 Dislocation of T5/T6 thoracic vertebra**

---

7   HAC = Initial encounter only (7th character A, B or C) and not POA.
16   MCC only if an open fracture (7th character B or C – specific to category).
18   CC only if a subsequent encounter for nonunion or malunion (7th character K, M, N, P, Q, or R – specific to category).
19   CC only if an initial encounter for a closed fracture (7th character A) **OR** a subsequent encounter for nonunion or malunion (7th character K, M, N, P, Q, or R – specific to category).

✔ Additional Character Required   √x7th Placeholder Alert   Unacceptable PDx   Manifestation   Hospital Acquired Condition   **EXCLUDES 1** Not Coded Here   EXCLUDES 2 Not Included Here

Chapter 19. Injury, Poisoning, and Certain Other Consequences of External Causes

✓6th **S23.14** **Subluxation and dislocation of** T6/T7-T7/T8 **thoracic vertebra**

  ✓7th **S23.140** **Subluxation of** T6/T7 **thoracic vertebra**

  ✓7th **S23.141** **Dislocation of** T6/T7 **thoracic vertebra**

  ✓7th **S23.142** **Subluxation of** T7/T8 **thoracic vertebra**

  ✓7th **S23.143** **Dislocation of** T7/T8 **thoracic vertebra**

✓6th **S23.15** **Subluxation and dislocation of** T8/T9-T9/T10 **thoracic vertebra**

  ✓7th **S23.150** **Subluxation of** T8/T9 **thoracic vertebra**

  ✓7th **S23.151** **Dislocation of** T8/T9 **thoracic vertebra**

  ✓7th **S23.152** **Subluxation of** T9/T10 **thoracic vertebra**

  ✓7th **S23.153** **Dislocation of** T9/T10 **thoracic vertebra**

✓6th **S23.16** **Subluxation and dislocation of** T10/T11-T11/T12 **thoracic vertebra**

  ✓7th **S23.160** **Subluxation of** T10/T11 **thoracic vertebra**

  ✓7th **S23.161** **Dislocation of** T10/T11 **thoracic vertebra**

  ✓7th **S23.162** **Subluxation of** T11/T12 **thoracic vertebra**

  ✓7th **S23.163** **Dislocation of** T11/T12 **thoracic vertebra**

✓6th **S23.17** **Subluxation and dislocation of** T12/L1 **thoracic vertebra**

  ✓7th **S23.170** **Subluxation of** T12/L1 **thoracic vertebra**

  ✓7th **S23.171** **Dislocation of** T12/L1 **thoracic vertebra**

✓5th **S23.2** **Dislocation of other and unspecified parts of thorax**

  ✓x7th **S23.20** **Dislocation of unspecified part of thorax**

  ✓x7th **S23.29** **Dislocation of other parts of thorax**

✓x7th **S23.3** **Sprain of ligaments of thoracic spine**

✓5th **S23.4** **Sprain of ribs and sternum**

  ✓x7th **S23.41** **Sprain of ribs**

  ✓6th **S23.42** **Sprain of sternum**

    ✓7th **S23.420** **Sprain of sternoclavicular (joint) (ligament)**

    ✓7th **S23.421** **Sprain of chondrosternal joint**

    ✓7th **S23.428** **Other sprain of sternum**

    ✓7th **S23.429** **Unspecified sprain of sternum**

✓x7th **S23.8** **Sprain of other specified parts of thorax**

✓x7th **S23.9** **Sprain of unspecified parts of thorax**

✓4th **S24** **Injury of nerves and spinal cord at thorax level**

  NOTE   Code to highest level of thoracic spinal cord injury. Injuries to the spinal cord (S24.0 and S24.1) refer to the cord level and not bone level injury, and can affect nerve roots at and below the level given.

  Code also any associated:
    fracture of thoracic vertebra (S22.0-)
    open wound of thorax (S21.-)
    transient paralysis (R29.5)

  EXCLUDES 2   injury of brachial plexus (S14.3)

  The appropriate 7th is to be added to each code from category S24.
  A   initial encounter
  D   subsequent encounter
  S   sequela

  CC Excl: For MCC codes in category S24 unless otherwise noted: MCC with 7th character A: M48.40X-M48.58X with 7th S, M80.08XS, M80.88XS, M84.350S, M84.454S, M84.550S, M84.58S, M84.650S, M99.15-M99.17, M99.19, S03.1XXA, S12.000-S12.9XX with 7th S, S13.9XXA, S14.109A, S14.119A, S14.129A, S14.139A, S14.149A, S14.159A, S22.000-S22.9XX with 7th S, S23.20X-S23.29X with 7th A, S23.9XX-S24.159 with 7th A, S29.001-S29.009 with 7th A, S29.091-S29.9XX with 7th A, S32.000-S32.9XX with 7th S, S33.30X-S33.39X with 7th A, S33.9XXA, S38.1XXA, S39.001-S39.003 with 7th A, S39.091-S39.94X with 7th A, T14.90-T14.91, T79.A0X-T79.9XX with 7th A

  ✓x7th **S24.0** **Concussion and edema of thoracic spinal cord**   MCC

  ✓5th **S24.1** **Other and unspecified injuries of thoracic spinal cord**

    ✓6th **S24.10** **Unspecified injury of thoracic spinal cord**

      7 ✓7th **S24.101** **Unspecified injury at** T1 **level of thoracic spinal cord**   MCC

      7 ✓7th **S24.102** **Unspecified injury at** T2-T6 **level of thoracic spinal cord**   MCC

      7 ✓7th **S24.103** **Unspecified injury at** T7-T10 **level of thoracic spinal cord**   MCC

      7 ✓7th **S24.104** **Unspecified injury at** T11-T12 **level thoracic spinal cord**   MCC

      7 ✓7th **S24.109** **Unspecified injury at** unspecified **level of thoracic spinal cord**
        Injury of thoracic spinal cord NOS

    ✓6th **S24.11** **Complete lesion of thoracic spinal cord**

      7 ✓7th **S24.111** **Complete lesion at** T1 **level of thoracic spinal cord**   MCC

      7 ✓7th **S24.112** **Complete lesion at** T2-T6 **level of thoracic spinal cord**   MCC

      7 ✓7th **S24.113** **Complete lesion at** T7-T10 **level of thoracic spinal cord**   MCC

      7 ✓7th **S24.114** **Complete lesion at** T11-T12 **level of thoracic spinal cord**   MCC

      ✓7th **S24.119** **Complete lesion at** unspecified **level of thoracic spinal cord**

    ✓6th **S24.13** **Anterior cord syndrome of thoracic spinal cord**

      7 ✓7th **S24.131** **Anterior cord syndrome at** T1 **level of thoracic spinal cord**   MCC

      7 ✓7th **S24.132** **Anterior cord syndrome at** T2-T6 **level of thoracic spinal cord**   MCC

      7 ✓7th **S24.133** **Anterior cord syndrome at** T7-T10 **level of thoracic spinal cord**   MCC

      7 ✓7th **S24.134** **Anterior cord syndrome at** T11-T12 **level of thoracic spinal cord**   MCC

      ✓7th **S24.139** **Anterior cord syndrome at** unspecified **level of thoracic spinal cord**

    ✓6th **S24.14** **Brown-Séquard syndrome of thoracic spinal cord**

      ✓7th **S24.141** **Brown-Séquard syndrome at** T1 **level of thoracic spinal cord**   MCC

      ✓7th **S24.142** **Brown-Séquard syndrome at** T2-T6 **level of thoracic spinal cord**   MCC

      ✓7th **S24.143** **Brown-Séquard syndrome at** T7-T10 **level of thoracic spinal cord**   MCC

      ✓7th **S24.144** **Brown-Séquard syndrome at** T11-T12 **level of thoracic spinal cord**   MCC

      ✓7th **S24.149** **Brown-Séquard syndrome at** unspecified **level of thoracic spinal cord**

    ✓6th **S24.15** **Other incomplete lesions of thoracic spinal cord**
      Incomplete lesion of thoracic spinal cord NOS
      Posterior cord syndrome of thoracic spinal cord

      7 ✓7th **S24.151** **Other incomplete lesion at** T1 **level of thoracic spinal cord**   MCC

      7 ✓7th **S24.152** **Other incomplete lesion at** T2-T6 **level of thoracic spinal cord**   MCC

      7 ✓7th **S24.153** **Other incomplete lesion at** T7-T10 **level of thoracic spinal cord**   MCC

      7 ✓7th **S24.154** **Other incomplete lesion at** T11-T12 **level of thoracic spinal cord**   MCC

      ✓7th **S24.159** **Other incomplete lesion at** unspecified **level of thoracic spinal cord**

  ✓x7th **S24.2** **Injury of nerve root of thoracic spine**

  ✓x7th **S24.3** **Injury of peripheral nerves of thorax**

  ✓x7th **S24.4** **Injury of thoracic sympathetic nervous system**
    Injury of cardiac plexus   Injury of stellate ganglion
    Injury of esophageal plexus   Injury of thoracic sympathetic
    Injury of pulmonary plexus   ganglion

  ✓x7th **S24.8** **Injury of other specified nerves of thorax**

  ✓x7th **S24.9** **Injury of unspecified nerve of thorax**

✓4th **S25** **Injury of blood vessels of thorax**
  Code also any associated open wound (S21.-)

  The appropriate 7th is to be added to each code from category S25.
  A   initial encounter
  D   subsequent encounter
  S   sequela

  ✓5th **S25.0** **Injury of thoracic aorta**
    Injury of aorta NOS

    CC Excl: For MCC codes in subcategory S25.0, unless otherwise noted: MCC with 7th character A: S25.00X-S25.09X with 7th A, T14.90-T14.91, T79.A0X-T79.9XX with 7th A

  ✓x7th **S25.00** **Unspecified injury of thoracic aorta**   MCC

  ✓x7th **S25.01** **Minor laceration of thoracic aorta**   MCC
    Incomplete transection of thoracic aorta
    Laceration of thoracic aorta NOS
    Superficial laceration of thoracic aorta

7   HAC = Initial encounter only (7th character A, B or C) and not POA.

N Newborn: 0   P Pediatric: 0-17   M Maternity: 12-55   A Adult: 15-124   MCC Major CC Condition   PDxMCC PDx acts as own MCC   CC CC Condition   PDxCC PDx acts as own CC

924   ICD-10-CM 2016

√x7ᵗʰ S25.02 Major laceration of thoracic aorta `MCC`
   Complete transection of thoracic aorta
   Traumatic rupture of thoracic aorta

√x7ᵗʰ S25.09 Other specified injury of thoracic aorta `MCC`

√5ᵗʰ S25.1 Injury of innominate or subclavian artery

> CC Excl: For MCC codes in subcategory S25.1, unless otherwise noted: MCC with 7th character A: S25.101-S25.199 with 7th A, T14.90-T14.91, T79.A0X-T79.9XX with 7th A

√6ᵗʰ S25.10 Unspecified injury of innominate or subclavian artery

  √7ᵗʰ S25.101 Unspecified injury of right innominate or subclavian artery `MCC`

  √7ᵗʰ S25.102 Unspecified injury of left innominate or subclavian artery `MCC`

  √7ᵗʰ S25.109 Unspecified injury of unspecified innominate or subclavian artery `MCC`

√6ᵗʰ S25.11 Minor laceration of innominate or subclavian artery
   Incomplete transection of innominate or subclavian artery
   Laceration of innominate or subclavian artery NOS
   Superficial laceration of innominate or subclavian artery

  √7ᵗʰ S25.111 Minor laceration of right innominate or subclavian artery `MCC`

  √7ᵗʰ S25.112 Minor laceration of left innominate or subclavian artery `MCC`

  √7ᵗʰ S25.119 Minor laceration of unspecified innominate or subclavian artery `MCC`

√6ᵗʰ S25.12 Major laceration of innominate or subclavian artery
   Complete transection of innominate or subclavian artery
   Traumatic rupture of innominate or subclavian artery

  √7ᵗʰ S25.121 Major laceration of right innominate or subclavian artery `MCC`

  √7ᵗʰ S25.122 Major laceration of left innominate or subclavian artery `MCC`

  √7ᵗʰ S25.129 Major laceration of unspecified innominate or subclavian artery `MCC`

√6ᵗʰ S25.19 Other specified injury of innominate or subclavian artery

  √7ᵗʰ S25.191 Other specified injury of right innominate or subclavian artery `MCC`

  √7ᵗʰ S25.192 Other specified injury of left innominate or subclavian artery `MCC`

  √7ᵗʰ S25.199 Other specified injury of unspecified innominate or subclavian artery `MCC`

√5ᵗʰ S25.2 Injury of superior vena cava
   Injury of vena cava NOS

> CC Excl: For MCC codes in subcategory S25.2, unless otherwise noted: MCC with 7th character A: S25.20X-S25.29X with 7th A, T14.90-T14.91, T79.A0X-T79.9XX with 7th A

√x7ᵗʰ S25.20 Unspecified injury of superior vena cava `MCC`

√x7ᵗʰ S25.21 Minor laceration of superior vena cava `MCC`
   Incomplete transection of superior vena cava
   Laceration of superior vena cava NOS
   Superficial laceration of superior vena cava

√x7ᵗʰ S25.22 Major laceration of superior vena cava `MCC`
   Complete transection of superior vena cava
   Traumatic rupture of superior vena cava

√x7ᵗʰ S25.29 Other specified injury of superior vena cava `MCC`

√5ᵗʰ S25.3 Injury of innominate or subclavian vein

> CC Excl: For MCC codes in subcategory S25.3, unless otherwise noted: MCC with 7th character A: S25.301-S25.399 with 7th A, T14.90-T14.91, T79.A0X-T79.9XX with 7th A

√6ᵗʰ S25.30 Unspecified injury of innominate or subclavian vein
  √7ᵗʰ S25.301 Unspecified injury of right innominate or subclavian vein `MCC`
  √7ᵗʰ S25.302 Unspecified injury of left innominate or subclavian vein `MCC`
  √7ᵗʰ S25.309 Unspecified injury of unspecified innominate or subclavian vein `MCC`

√6ᵗʰ S25.31 Minor laceration of innominate or subclavian vein
   Incomplete transection of innominate or subclavian vein
   Laceration of innominate or subclavian vein NOS
   Superficial laceration of innominate or subclavian vein

  √7ᵗʰ S25.311 Minor laceration of right innominate or subclavian vein `MCC`
  √7ᵗʰ S25.312 Minor laceration of left innominate or subclavian vein `MCC`
  √7ᵗʰ S25.319 Minor laceration of unspecified innominate or subclavian vein `MCC`

√6ᵗʰ S25.32 Major laceration of innominate or subclavian vein
   Complete transection of innominate or subclavian vein
   Traumatic rupture of innominate or subclavian vein

  √7ᵗʰ S25.321 Major laceration of right innominate or subclavian vein `MCC`
  √7ᵗʰ S25.322 Major laceration of left innominate or subclavian vein `MCC`
  √7ᵗʰ S25.329 Major laceration of unspecified innominate or subclavian vein `MCC`

√6ᵗʰ S25.39 Other specified injury of innominate or subclavian vein
  √7ᵗʰ S25.391 Other specified injury of right innominate or subclavian vein `MCC`
  √7ᵗʰ S25.392 Other specified injury of left innominate or subclavian vein `MCC`
  √7ᵗʰ S25.399 Other specified injury of unspecified innominate or subclavian vein `MCC`

√5ᵗʰ S25.4 Injury of pulmonary blood vessels

> CC Excl: For MCC codes in subcategory S25.4, unless otherwise noted: MCC with 7th character A: S25.401-S25.499 with 7th A, T14.90-T14.91, T79.A0X-T79.9XX with 7th A

√6ᵗʰ S25.40 Unspecified injury of pulmonary blood vessels
  √7ᵗʰ S25.401 Unspecified injury of right pulmonary blood vessels `MCC`
  √7ᵗʰ S25.402 Unspecified injury of left pulmonary blood vessels `MCC`
  √7ᵗʰ S25.409 Unspecified injury of unspecified pulmonary blood vessels `MCC`

√6ᵗʰ S25.41 Minor laceration of pulmonary blood vessels
   Incomplete transection of pulmonary blood vessels
   Laceration of pulmonary blood vessels NOS
   Superficial laceration of pulmonary blood vessels

  √7ᵗʰ S25.411 Minor laceration of right pulmonary blood vessels `MCC`
  √7ᵗʰ S25.412 Minor laceration of left pulmonary blood vessels `MCC`
  √7ᵗʰ S25.419 Minor laceration of unspecified pulmonary blood vessels `MCC`

√6ᵗʰ S25.42 Major laceration of pulmonary blood vessels
   Complete transection of pulmonary blood vessels
   Traumatic rupture of pulmonary blood vessels

  √7ᵗʰ S25.421 Major laceration of right pulmonary blood vessels `MCC`
  √7ᵗʰ S25.422 Major laceration of left pulmonary blood vessels `MCC`
  √7ᵗʰ S25.429 Major laceration of unspecified pulmonary blood vessels `MCC`

√6ᵗʰ S25.49 Other specified injury of pulmonary blood vessels
  √7ᵗʰ S25.491 Other specified injury of right pulmonary blood vessels `MCC`
  √7ᵗʰ S25.492 Other specified injury of left pulmonary blood vessels `MCC`
  √7ᵗʰ S25.499 Other specified injury of unspecified pulmonary blood vessels `MCC`

√5ᵗʰ S25.5 Injury of intercostal blood vessels

> CC Excl: For CC codes in subcategory S25.5, unless otherwise noted: CC with 7th character A: S25.501-S25.899 with 7th A

√6ᵗʰ S25.50 Unspecified injury of intercostal blood vessels
  √7ᵗʰ S25.501 Unspecified injury of intercostal blood vessels, right side `CC`
  √7ᵗʰ S25.502 Unspecified injury of intercostal blood vessels, left side `CC`
  √7ᵗʰ S25.509 Unspecified injury of intercostal blood vessels, unspecified side `CC`

√6ᵗʰ **S25.51 Laceration of intercostal blood vessels**

    √7ᵗʰ **S25.511 Laceration of intercostal blood vessels, right side** `CC`

    √7ᵗʰ **S25.512 Laceration of intercostal blood vessels, left side** `CC`

    √7ᵗʰ **S25.519 Laceration of intercostal blood vessels, unspecified side** `CC`

√6ᵗʰ **S25.59 Other specified injury of intercostal blood vessels**

    √7ᵗʰ **S25.591 Other specified injury of intercostal blood vessels, right side** `CC`

    √7ᵗʰ **S25.592 Other specified injury of intercostal blood vessels, left side** `CC`

    √7ᵗʰ **S25.599 Other specified injury of intercostal blood vessels, unspecified side** `CC`

√5ᵗʰ **S25.8 Injury of other blood vessels of thorax**
Injury of azygos vein
Injury of mammary artery or vein

> **CC Excl:** For CC codes in subcategory S25.8, unless otherwise noted: CC with 7th character A: S25.00X–S25.99X with 7th A

√6ᵗʰ **S25.80 Unspecified injury of other blood vessels of thorax**

    √7ᵗʰ **S25.801 Unspecified injury of other blood vessels of thorax, right side** `CC`

    √7ᵗʰ **S25.802 Unspecified injury of other blood vessels of thorax, left side** `CC`

    √7ᵗʰ **S25.809 Unspecified injury of other blood vessels of thorax, unspecified side** `CC`

√6ᵗʰ **S25.81 Laceration of other blood vessels of thorax**

    √7ᵗʰ **S25.811 Laceration of other blood vessels of thorax, right side** `CC`

    √7ᵗʰ **S25.812 Laceration of other blood vessels of thorax, left side** `CC`

    √7ᵗʰ **S25.819 Laceration of other blood vessels of thorax, unspecified side** `CC`

√6ᵗʰ **S25.89 Other specified injury of other blood vessels of thorax**

    √7ᵗʰ **S25.891 Other specified injury of other blood vessels of thorax, right side** `CC`

    √7ᵗʰ **S25.892 Other specified injury of other blood vessels of thorax, left side** `CC`

    √7ᵗʰ **S25.899 Other specified injury of other blood vessels of thorax, unspecified side** `CC`

√5ᵗʰ **S25.9 Injury of unspecified blood vessel of thorax**

> **CC Excl:** For CC codes in subcategory S25.9, unless otherwise noted: See code: S25.8

√x7ᵗʰ **S25.90 Unspecified injury of unspecified blood vessel of thorax** `CC`

√x7ᵗʰ **S25.91 Laceration of unspecified blood vessel of thorax** `CC`

√x7ᵗʰ **S25.99 Other specified injury of unspecified blood vessel of thorax** `CC`

√4ᵗʰ **S26 Injury of heart**
Code also any associated:
  open wound of thorax (S21.-)
  traumatic hemopneumothorax (S27.2)
  traumatic hemothorax (S27.1)
  traumatic pneumothorax (S27.0)

> The appropriate 7th is to be added to each code from category S26.
> A   initial encounter
> D   subsequent encounter
> S   sequela

√5ᵗʰ **S26.0 Injury of heart with hemopericardium**

√x7ᵗʰ **S26.00 Unspecified injury of heart with hemopericardium** `CC`
CC Excl: CC with 7th character A: S21.301–S21.459 with 7th A, S26.00X–S26.99X with 7th A, S27.50X–S27.69X with 7th A, S27.892–S27.9XX with 7th A, T14.90–T14.91

√x7ᵗʰ **S26.01 Contusion of heart with hemopericardium** `CC`
CC Excl: CC with 7th character A: S21.101–S21.159 with 7th A, S21.301–S21.95X with 7th A, S26.00X–S26.99X with 7th A, S27.50X–S27.69X with 7th A, S27.892–S27.9XX with 7th A, S28.1XXA, S29.021A, S29.029A, S38.3XXA, T14.90–T14.91, T79.7XX–T79.9XX with 7th A

√6ᵗʰ **S26.02 Laceration of heart with hemopericardium**

    √7ᵗʰ **S26.020 Mild laceration of heart with hemopericardium** `MCC`
    Laceration of heart without penetration of heart chamber
    CC Excl: See code: S26.01

    √7ᵗʰ **S26.021 Moderate laceration of heart with hemopericardium** `MCC`
    Laceration of heart with penetration of heart chamber
    CC Excl: See code: S26.01

    √7ᵗʰ **S26.022 Major laceration of heart with hemopericardium** `MCC`
    Laceration of heart with penetration of multiple heart chambers
    CC Excl: See code: S26.01

√x7ᵗʰ **S26.09 Other injury of heart with hemopericardium** `CC`
CC Excl: CC with 7th character A: S21.301–S21.459 with 7th A, S26.00X–S26.99X with 7th A, S27.50X–S27.69X with 7th A, S27.892–S27.9X with 7th A, T14.90–T14.91

√5ᵗʰ **S26.1 Injury of heart without hemopericardium**

√x7ᵗʰ **S26.10 Unspecified injury of heart without hemopericardium** `CC`
CC Excl: See code: S26.09

√x7ᵗʰ **S26.11 Contusion of heart without hemopericardium** `CC`
CC Excl: CC with 7th character A: S21.101–S21.159 with 7th A, S21.301–S21.95X with 7th A, S26.00X–S26.99X with 7th A, S27.50X–S27.69X with 7th A, S27.892–S27.9XX with 7th A, S28.1XXA, S29.021A, S29.029A, S38.3XXA, T14.90–T14.91, T79.7XX–T79.9XX with 7th A

√x7ᵗʰ **S26.12 Laceration of heart without hemopericardium** `MCC`
CC Excl: MCC with 7th character A: See code: S26.11

√x7ᵗʰ **S26.19 Other injury of heart without hemopericardium** `CC`
CC Excl: CC with 7th character A: S21.301–S21.459 with 7th A, S26.00X–S26.99X with 7th A, S27.50X–S27.69X with 7th A, S27.892–S27.9XX with 7th A, T14.90–T14.91

√5ᵗʰ **S26.9 Injury of heart, unspecified with or without hemopericardium**

√x7ᵗʰ **S26.90 Unspecified injury of heart, unspecified with or without hemopericardium** `CC`
CC Excl: See code: S26.19

√x7ᵗʰ **S26.91 Contusion of heart, unspecified with or without hemopericardium** `CC`
CC Excl: CC with 7th character A: S21.101–S21.159 with 7th A, S21.301–S21.95 with 7th A, S26.00X–S26.99X with 7th A, S27.50X–S27.69X with 7th A, S27.892–S27.9XX with 7th A, S28.1XX with 7th A, S29.021 with 7th A, S29.029A, S38.3XX with 7th A, T14.90–T14.91, T79.7XX–T79.9XX with 7th A

√x7ᵗʰ **S26.92 Laceration of heart, unspecified with or without hemopericardium** `MCC`
Laceration of heart NOS
CC Excl: See code: S26.91

√x7ᵗʰ **S26.99 Other injury of heart, unspecified with or without hemopericardium** `CC`
CC Excl: CC with 7th character A: S21.301–S21.459 with 7th A, S26.00X–S26.99X with 7th A, S27.50X–S27.69X with 7th A, S27.892–S27.9X with 7th A, T14.90–T14.91

√4ᵗʰ **S27 Injury of other and unspecified intrathoracic organs**
Code also any associated open wound of thorax (S21.-)
EXCLUDES 2 injury of cervical esophagus (S10–S19)
      injury of trachea (cervical) (S10–S19)

> The appropriate 7th is to be added to each code from category S27.
> A   initial encounter
> D   subsequent encounter
> S   sequela

√x7ᵗʰ **S27.0 Traumatic pneumothorax** `CC`
EXCLUDES 1 spontaneous pneumothorax (J93.-)
CC Excl: CC with 7th character A: S21.101–S21.159 with 7th A, S21.301–S21.95X with 7th A, S27.0XX–S27.399 with 7th A, S27.50X–S27.69X with 7th A, S27.892–S27.9XXA, S28.1XXA, S29.021A, S29.029A, S38.3XXA, T14.90–T14.91, T79.7XX–T79.9XX with 7th A

√x7ᵗʰ **S27.1 Traumatic hemothorax** `MCC`
CC Excl: MCC with 7th character A: See code: S27.0

√x7ᵗʰ **S27.2 Traumatic hemopneumothorax** `MCC`
CC Excl: MCC with 7th character A: See code: S27.0

N Newborn: 0   P Pediatric: 0-17   M Maternity: 12-55   A Adult: 15-124   MCC Major CC Condition   PDxMCC PDx acts as own MCC   CC CC Condition   PDxCC PDx acts as own CC

926   ICD-10-CM 2016

√5ᵗʰ **S27.3**   **Other and unspecified injuries of lung**

> **CC Excl: For CC codes in subcategory S27.3, unless otherwise noted: CC with 7th character A:** S21.101-S21.159 with 7th A, S21.301-S21.95X with 7th A, S27.301-S27.399 with 7th A, S27.50X-S27.69X with 7th A, S27.892-S27.9XX with 7th A, S28.1XXA, S29.021A, S29.029A, S38.3XXA, T14.90-T14.91, T79.7XX-T79.9XX with 7th A

√6ᵗʰ **S27.30**   **Unspecified injury of lung**

√7ᵗʰ   **S27.301**   **Unspecified injury of lung, unilateral**   CC

√7ᵗʰ   **S27.302**   **Unspecified injury of lung, bilateral**   CC

√7ᵗʰ   **S27.309**   **Unspecified injury of lung, unspecified**   CC

√6ᵗʰ **S27.31**   **Primary blast injury of lung**
Blast injury of lung NOS

√7ᵗʰ   **S27.311**   **Primary blast injury of lung, unilateral**   CC

√7ᵗʰ   **S27.312**   **Primary blast injury of lung, bilateral**   CC

√7ᵗʰ   **S27.319**   **Primary blast injury of lung, unspecified**   CC

S27.32   **Contusion of lung**

√7ᵗʰ   **S27.321**   **Contusion of lung, unilateral**   CC

√7ᵗʰ   **S27.322**   **Contusion of lung, bilateral**   CC

√7ᵗʰ   **S27.329**   **Contusion of lung, unspecified**   CC

√6ᵗʰ **S27.33**   **Laceration of lung**

√7ᵗʰ   **S27.331**   **Laceration of lung, unilateral**   MCC
> **CC Excl: MCC with 7th character A:** S21.101-S21.159 with 7th A, S21.301-S21.95X with 7th A, S27.301-S27.399 with 7th A, S27.50X-S27.69X with 7th A, S27.892-S27.9XX with 7th A, S28.1XXA, S29.021A, S29.029A, S38.3XXA, T14.90-T14.91, T79.7XX-T79.9XX with 7th A

√7ᵗʰ   **S27.332**   **Laceration of lung, bilateral**   MCC
> **CC Excl:** See code: S27.331

√7ᵗʰ   **S27.339**   **Laceration of lung, unspecified**   MCC
> **CC Excl:** See code: S27.331

√6ᵗʰ **S27.39**   **Other injuries of lung**
Secondary blast injury of lung

√7ᵗʰ   **S27.391**   **Other injuries of lung, unilateral**   CC

√7ᵗʰ   **S27.392**   **Other injuries of lung, bilateral**   CC

√7ᵗʰ   **S27.399**   **Other injuries of lung, unspecified**   CC

√5ᵗʰ **S27.4**   **Injury of bronchus**

> **CC Excl: For MCC codes in subcategory S27.4, unless otherwise noted: MCC with 7th character A:** S21.101-S21.159 with 7th A, S21.301-S21.95X with 7th A, S27.401-S27.69X with 7th A, S27.892-S27.9XX with 7th A, S28.1XXA, S29.021XA, S29.029XA, S38.3XXA, T14.90-T14.91, T79.7XX-T79.9XX with 7th A

√6ᵗʰ **S27.40**   **Unspecified injury of bronchus**

√7ᵗʰ   **S27.401**   **Unspecified injury of bronchus, unilateral**   MCC

√7ᵗʰ   **S27.402**   **Unspecified injury of bronchus, bilateral**   MCC

√7ᵗʰ   **S27.409**   **Unspecified injury of bronchus, unspecified**   MCC

√6ᵗʰ **S27.41**   **Primary blast injury of bronchus**
Blast injury of bronchus NOS

√7ᵗʰ   **S27.411**   **Primary blast injury of bronchus, unilateral**   MCC

√7ᵗʰ   **S27.412**   **Primary blast injury of bronchus, bilateral**   MCC

√7ᵗʰ   **S27.419**   **Primary blast injury of bronchus, unspecified**   MCC

√6ᵗʰ **S27.42**   **Contusion of bronchus**

√7ᵗʰ   **S27.421**   **Contusion of bronchus, unilateral**   MCC

√7ᵗʰ   **S27.422**   **Contusion of bronchus, bilateral**   MCC

√7ᵗʰ   **S27.429**   **Contusion of bronchus, unspecified**   MCC

√6ᵗʰ **S27.43**   **Laceration of bronchus**

√7ᵗʰ   **S27.431**   **Laceration of bronchus, unilateral**   MCC

√7ᵗʰ   **S27.432**   **Laceration of bronchus, bilateral**   MCC

√7ᵗʰ   **S27.439**   **Laceration of bronchus, unspecified**   MCC

√6ᵗʰ **S27.49**   **Other injury of bronchus**
Secondary blast injury of bronchus

√7ᵗʰ   **S27.491**   **Other injury of bronchus, unilateral**   MCC

√7ᵗʰ   **S27.492**   **Other injury of bronchus, bilateral**   MCC

√7ᵗʰ   **S27.499**   **Other injury of bronchus, unspecified**   MCC

√5ᵗʰ **S27.5**   **Injury of thoracic trachea**

> **CC Excl: For CC codes in subcategory S27.5, unless otherwise noted: CC with 7th character A:** S21.101-S21.159 with 7th A, S21.301-S21.95X with 7th A, S27.50X-S27.69X with 7th A, S27.892-S27.9XX with 7th A, S28.1XXA, S29.021 with 7th A, S29.029A, S38.3XXA, T14.90-T14.91, T79.7XX-T79.9XX with 7th A

√x7ᵗʰ   **S27.50**   **Unspecified injury of thoracic trachea**   CC

√x7ᵗʰ   **S27.51**   **Primary blast injury of thoracic trachea**   CC
Blast injury of thoracic trachea NOS

√x7ᵗʰ   **S27.52**   **Contusion of thoracic trachea**   CC

√x7ᵗʰ   **S27.53**   **Laceration of thoracic trachea**   CC

√x7ᵗʰ   **S27.59**   **Other injury of thoracic trachea**   CC
Secondary blast injury of thoracic trachea

√5ᵗʰ **S27.6**   **Injury of pleura**

> **CC Excl: For CC codes in subcategory S27.6, unless otherwise noted:** See code: S27.5

√x7ᵗʰ   **S27.60**   **Unspecified injury of pleura**   CC

√x7ᵗʰ   **S27.63**   **Laceration of pleura**   CC

√x7ᵗʰ   **S27.69**   **Other injury of pleura**   CC

√5ᵗʰ **S27.8**   **Injury of other specified intrathoracic organs**

√6ᵗʰ **S27.80**   **Injury of diaphragm**

> **CC Excl: For CC/MCC codes in subcategory S27.80, unless otherwise noted: CC with 7th character A:** S21.101-S21.159 with 7th A, S21.301-S21.95 with 7th A, S27.50X-S27.809 with 7th A, S27.892-S27.9XX with 7th A, S28.1XXA, S29.021A, S29.029A, S38.3XXA, T14.90-T14.91, T79.7XX-T79.9XX with 7th A

√7ᵗʰ   **S27.802**   **Contusion of diaphragm**   CC

√7ᵗʰ   **S27.803**   **Laceration of diaphragm**   CC

√7ᵗʰ   **S27.808**   **Other injury of diaphragm**   CC

√7ᵗʰ   **S27.809**   **Unspecified injury of diaphragm**   CC

√6ᵗʰ **S27.81**   **Injury of esophagus (thoracic part)**

√7ᵗʰ   **S27.812**   **Contusion of esophagus (thoracic part)**   MCC
> **CC Excl: MCC with 7th character A:** S21.101-S21.159 with 7th A, S21.301-S21.95 with 7th A, S27.50X-S27.69X with 7th A, S27.812-S27.9XX with 7th A, S28.1XXA, S29.021A, S29.029A, S38.3XXA, T14.90-T14.91, T79.7XX-T79.9XX with 7th A

√7ᵗʰ   **S27.813**   **Laceration of esophagus (thoracic part)**   MCC
> **CC Excl:** See code: S27.812

√7ᵗʰ   **S27.818**   **Other injury of esophagus (thoracic part)**   MCC
> **CC Excl:** See code: S27.812

√7ᵗʰ   **S27.819**   **Unspecified injury of esophagus (thoracic part)**   MCC
> **CC Excl:** See code: S27.812

√6ᵗʰ **S27.89**   **Injury of other specified intrathoracic organs**
Injury of lymphatic thoracic duct
Injury of thymus gland

> **CC Excl: For CC codes in subcategory S27.89, unless otherwise noted: CC with 7th character A:** S21.101-S21.159 with 7th A, S21.301-S21.95X with 7th A, S27.50X-S27.69X with 7th A, S27.892-S27.9XX with 7th A, S28.1XXA, S29.021A, S29.029A, S38.3XXA, T14.90-T14.91, T79.7XX-T79.9XX with 7th A

√7ᵗʰ   **S27.892**   **Contusion of other specified intrathoracic organs**   CC

√7ᵗʰ   **S27.893**   **Laceration of other specified intrathoracic organs**   CC

√7ᵗʰ   **S27.898**   **Other injury of other specified intrathoracic organs**   CC

√7ᵗʰ   **S27.899**   **Unspecified injury of other specified intrathoracic organs**   CC

√x7ᵗʰ **S27.9**   **Injury of unspecified intrathoracic organ**   CC
> **CC Excl: CC with 7th character A:** S21.101-S21.159 with 7th A, S21.301-S21.95X with 7th A, S27.50X-S27.69X with 7th A, S27.892-S27.9XX with 7th A, S28.1XXA, S29.021A, S29.029A, S38.3XXA, T14.90-T14.91, T79.7XX-T79.9XX with 7th A

✔ Additional Character Required   √x7ᵗʰ Placeholder Alert   Unacceptable PDx   Manifestation   Hospital Acquired Condition   **EXCLUDES 1** Not Coded Here   **EXCLUDES 2** Not Included Here

✓4th S28　Crushing injury of thorax, and traumatic amputation of part of thorax

The appropriate 7th is to be added to each code from category S28.
A　initial encounter
D　subsequent encounter
S　sequela

✓x7th S28.0　Crushed chest
Use additional code for all associated injuries
EXCLUDES 1 flail chest (S22.5)

✓x7th S28.1　Traumatic amputation (partial) of part of thorax, except breast　CC
CC Excl: CC with 7th character A: S21.101-S21.159 with 7th A, S21.301-S21.95X with 7th A, S23.3XA, S23.8XA, S27.50X-S27.69X with 7th A, S27.892-S27.9XX with 7th A, S28.1XXA, S29.021A, S29.029A, S38.3XXA, T14.90-T14.91, T79.7XX-T79.9XX with 7th A

✓5th S28.2　Traumatic amputation of breast

  ✓6th S28.21　Complete traumatic amputation of breast
  Traumatic amputation of breast NOS

    ✓7th S28.211　Complete traumatic amputation of right breast

    ✓7th S28.212　Complete traumatic amputation of left breast

    ✓7th S28.219　Complete traumatic amputation of unspecified breast

  ✓6th S28.22　Partial traumatic amputation of breast

    ✓7th S28.221　Partial traumatic amputation of right breast

    ✓7th S28.222　Partial traumatic amputation of left breast

    ✓7th S28.229　Partial traumatic amputation of unspecified breast

✓4th S29　Other and unspecified injuries of thorax

Code also any associated open wound (S21.-)

The appropriate 7th is to be added to each code from category S29.
A　initial encounter
D　subsequent encounter
S　sequela

✓5th S29.0　Injury of muscle and tendon at thorax level

  ✓6th S29.00　Unspecified injury of muscle and tendon of thorax

    ✓7th S29.001　Unspecified injury of muscle and tendon of front wall of thorax

    ✓7th S29.002　Unspecified injury of muscle and tendon of back wall of thorax

    ✓7th S29.009　Unspecified injury of muscle and tendon of unspecified wall of thorax

  ✓6th S29.01　Strain of muscle and tendon of thorax

    ✓7th S29.011　Strain of muscle and tendon of front wall of thorax

    ✓7th S29.012　Strain of muscle and tendon of back wall of thorax

    ✓7th S29.019　Strain of muscle and tendon of unspecified wall of thorax

  ✓6th S29.02　Laceration of muscle and tendon of thorax

    ✓7th S29.021　Laceration of muscle and tendon of front wall of thorax　CC
    CC Excl: See code: S28.1

    ✓7th S29.022　Laceration of muscle and tendon of back wall of thorax

    ✓7th S29.029　Laceration of muscle and tendon of unspecified wall of thorax　CC
    CC Excl: See code: S28.1

  ✓6th S29.09　Other injury of muscle and tendon of thorax

    ✓7th S29.091　Other injury of muscle and tendon of front wall of thorax

    ✓7th S29.092　Other injury of muscle and tendon of back wall of thorax

    ✓7th S29.099　Other injury of muscle and tendon of unspecified wall of thorax

✓x7th S29.8　Other specified injuries of thorax

✓x7th S29.9　Unspecified injury of thorax

Injuries to the abdomen, lower back, lumbar spine, pelvis and external genitals (S30-S39)

INCLUDES　injuries to the abdominal wall
injuries to the anus
injuries to the buttock
injuries to the external genitalia
injuries to the flank
injuries to the groin

EXCLUDES 2　burns and corrosions (T20-T32)
effects of foreign body in anus and rectum (T18.5)
effects of foreign body in genitourinary tract (T19.-)
effects of foreign body in stomach, small intestine and colon (T18.2-T18.4)
frostbite (T33-T34)
insect bite or sting, venomous (T63.4)

✓4th S30　Superficial injury of abdomen, lower back, pelvis and external genitals

EXCLUDES 2　superficial injury of hip (S70.-)

The appropriate 7th is to be added to each code from category S30.
A　initial encounter
D　subsequent encounter
S　sequela

✓x7th S30.0　Contusion of lower back and pelvis
Contusion of buttock

✓x7th S30.1　Contusion of abdominal wall
Contusion of flank
Contusion of groin

✓5th S30.2　Contusion of external genital organs

  ✓6th S30.20　Contusion of unspecified external genital organ

    ✓7th S30.201　Contusion of unspecified external genital organ, male　♂

    ✓7th S30.202　Contusion of unspecified external genital organ, female　♀

  ✓x7th S30.21　Contusion of penis　♂

  ✓x7th S30.22　Contusion of scrotum and testes　♂

  ✓x7th S30.23　Contusion of vagina and vulva　♀

✓x7th S30.3　Contusion of anus

✓5th S30.8　Other superficial injuries of abdomen, lower back, pelvis and external genitals

  ✓6th S30.81　Abrasion of abdomen, lower back, pelvis and external genitals

    ✓7th S30.810　Abrasion of lower back and pelvis

    ✓7th S30.811　Abrasion of abdominal wall

    ✓7th S30.812　Abrasion of penis　♂

    ✓7th S30.813　Abrasion of scrotum and testes　♂

    ✓7th S30.814　Abrasion of vagina and vulva　♀

    ✓7th S30.815　Abrasion of unspecified external genital organs, male　♂

    ✓7th S30.816　Abrasion of unspecified external genital organs, female　♀

    ✓7th S30.817　Abrasion of anus

  ✓6th S30.82　Blister (nonthermal) of abdomen, lower back, pelvis and external genitals

    ✓7th S30.820　Blister (nonthermal) of lower back and pelvis

    ✓7th S30.821　Blister (nonthermal) of abdominal wall

    ✓7th S30.822　Blister (nonthermal) of penis　♂

    ✓7th S30.823　Blister (nonthermal) of scrotum and testes　♂

    ✓7th S30.824　Blister (nonthermal) of vagina and vulva　♀

    ✓7th S30.825　Blister (nonthermal) of unspecified external genital organs, male　♂

    ✓7th S30.826　Blister (nonthermal) of unspecified external genital organs, female　♀

    ✓7th S30.827　Blister (nonthermal) of anus

  ✓6th S30.84　External constriction of abdomen, lower back, pelvis and external genitals

    ✓7th S30.840　External constriction of lower back and pelvis

    ✓7th S30.841　External constriction of abdominal wall

√7ᵗʰ **S30.842** **External constriction of** penis ♂
Hair tourniquet syndrome of penis
Use additional cause code to identify the
constricting item (W49.0-)

√7ᵗʰ **S30.843** **External constriction of** scrotum ♂
and testes

√7ᵗʰ **S30.844** **External constriction of** ♀
vagina and vulva

√7ᵗʰ **S30.845** **External constriction of** unspecified ♂
external genital organs, male

√7ᵗʰ **S30.846** **External constriction of unspecified** ♀
external genital organs, female

√6ᵗʰ **S30.85** **Superficial** foreign body **of abdomen, lower back,
pelvis and external genitals**
Splinter in the abdomen, lower back, pelvis and
external genitals

√7ᵗʰ **S30.850** **Superficial foreign body of** lower back and
pelvis

√7ᵗʰ **S30.851** **Superficial foreign body of** abdominal
wall

√7ᵗʰ **S30.852** **Superficial foreign body of** penis ♂

√7ᵗʰ **S30.853** **Superficial foreign body of** scrotum ♂
and testes

√7ᵗʰ **S30.854** **Superficial foreign body of** vagina ♀
and vulva

√7ᵗʰ **S30.855** **Superficial foreign body of** unspecified ♂
external genital organs, male

√7ᵗʰ **S30.856** **Superficial foreign body of** unspecified ♀
external genital organs, female

√7ᵗʰ **S30.857** **Superficial foreign body of** anus

√6ᵗʰ **S30.86** **Insect bite (nonvenomous) of abdomen, lower back,
pelvis and external genitals**

√7ᵗʰ **S30.860** **Insect bite (nonvenomous) of** lower back
and pelvis

√7ᵗʰ **S30.861** **Insect bite (nonvenomous) of** abdominal
wall

√7ᵗʰ **S30.862** **Insect bite (nonvenomous) of** penis ♂

√7ᵗʰ **S30.863** **Insect bite (nonvenomous) of** scrotum ♂
and testes

√7ᵗʰ **S30.864** **Insect bite (nonvenomous) of** vagina ♀
and vulva

√7ᵗʰ **S30.865** **Insect bite (nonvenomous) of** ♂
**unspecified external genital
organs, male**

√7ᵗʰ **S30.866** **Insect bite (nonvenomous) of** ♀
**unspecified external genital
organs, female**

√7ᵗʰ **S30.867** **Insect bite (nonvenomous) of** anus

√6ᵗʰ **S30.87** **Other superficial** bite **of abdomen, lower back, pelvis
and external genitals**
EXCLUDES 1 *open bite of abdomen, lower back, pelvis and
external genitals (S31.05, S31.15,
S31.25, S31.35, S31.45, S31.55)*

√7ᵗʰ **S30.870** **Other superficial bite of** lower back and
pelvis

√7ᵗʰ **S30.871** **Other superficial bite of** abdominal wall

√7ᵗʰ **S30.872** **Other superficial bite of** penis ♂

√7ᵗʰ **S30.873** **Other superficial bite of** scrotum ♂
and testes

√7ᵗʰ **S30.874** **Other superficial bite of** vagina ♀
and vulva

√7ᵗʰ **S30.875** **Other superficial bite of** unspecified ♂
external genital organs, male

√7ᵗʰ **S30.876** **Other superficial bite of** unspecified ♀
external genital organs, female

√7ᵗʰ **S30.877** **Other superficial bite of** anus

√5ᵗʰ **S30.9** **Unspecified superficial injury of abdomen, lower back, pelvis
and external genitals**

√x7ᵗʰ **S30.91** **Unspecified superficial injury of** lower back and
pelvis

√x7ᵗʰ **S30.92** **Unspecified superficial injury of** abdominal wall

√x7ᵗʰ **S30.93** **Unspecified superficial injury of** penis ♂

√x7ᵗʰ **S30.94** **Unspecified superficial injury of** scrotum ♂
and testes

√x7ᵗʰ **S30.95** **Unspecified superficial injury of** vagina ♀
and vulva

√x7ᵗʰ **S30.96** **Unspecified superficial injury of** unspecified ♂
external genital organs, male

√x7ᵗʰ **S30.97** **Unspecified superficial injury of** unspecified ♀
external genital organs, female

√x7ᵗʰ **S30.98** **Unspecified superficial injury of** anus

√4ᵗʰ **S31** **Open wound of abdomen, lower back, pelvis and external
genitals**
Code also any associated:
spinal cord injury (S24.0, S24.1-, S34.0-, S34.1-)
wound infection
EXCLUDES 1 *traumatic amputation of part of abdomen, lower back and
pelvis (S38.2-, S38.3)*
EXCLUDES 2 *open wound of hip (S71.00-S71.02)*
open fracture of pelvis (S32.1- – S32.9 with 7th B)

The appropriate 7th is to be added to each code from category S31.
A   initial encounter
D   subsequent encounter
S   sequela

√5ᵗʰ **S31.0** **Open wound of** lower back and pelvis

√6ᵗʰ **S31.00** **Unspecified open wound of lower back and pelvis**

√7ᵗʰ **S31.000** **Unspecified open wound of lower back
and pelvis without penetration into
retroperitoneum**
Unspecified open wound of lower back and
pelvis NOS

√7ᵗʰ **S31.001** **Unspecified open wound of lower** [MCC]
**back and pelvis with penetration into
retroperitoneum**
CC Excl: CC with 7th character A: S31.001A,
S31.011A, S31.021, S31.031A, S31.041A,
S31.051-S31.159 with 7th A, S31.600-
S31.659 with 7th A, S31.831-S31.839 with
7th A, S36.81X-S36.99X with 7th A, S38.3XX-
S39.023 with 7th A, T14.90-T14.91, T79.A0X-
T79.9XX with 7th A

√6ᵗʰ **S31.01** **Laceration without foreign body of lower back and
pelvis**

√7ᵗʰ **S31.010** **Laceration without foreign body of lower
back and pelvis without penetration into
retroperitoneum**
Laceration without foreign body of lower
back and pelvis NOS

√7ᵗʰ **S31.011** **Laceration without foreign body of** [MCC]
**lower back and pelvis with penetration
into retroperitoneum**
CC Excl: See code: S30.001

√6ᵗʰ **S31.02** **Laceration with foreign body of lower back and
pelvis**

√7ᵗʰ **S31.020** **Laceration with foreign body of lower
back and pelvis without penetration into
retroperitoneum**
Laceration with foreign body of lower back
and pelvis NOS

√7ᵗʰ **S31.021** **Laceration with foreign body of lower** [MCC]
**back and pelvis with penetration into
retroperitoneum**
CC Excl: See code: S30.001

√6ᵗʰ **S31.03** **Puncture wound without foreign body of lower back
and pelvis**

√7ᵗʰ **S31.030** **Puncture wound without foreign body of
lower back and pelvis without penetration
into retroperitoneum**
Puncture wound without foreign body of
lower back and pelvis NOS

√7ᵗʰ **S31.031** **Puncture wound without foreign** [MCC]
**body of lower back and pelvis with
penetration into retroperitoneum**
CC Excl: See code: S30.001

√6ᵗʰ **S31.04** **Puncture wound with foreign body of lower back
and pelvis**

√7ᵗʰ **S31.040** **Puncture wound with foreign body of
lower back and pelvis without penetration
into retroperitoneum**
Puncture wound with foreign body of
lower back and pelvis NOS

Chapter 19. Injury, Poisoning, and Certain Other Consequences of External Causes

S31.041–S31.153

✓7ᵗʰ **S31.041**   **Puncture wound with foreign body** **MCC** **of lower back and pelvis with penetration into retroperitoneum**
    CC Excl: See code: S30.001

✓6ᵗʰ **S31.05**   **Open bite of lower back and pelvis**
    Bite of lower back and pelvis NOS
    EXCLUDES 1   *superficial bite of lower back and pelvis (S30.860, S30.870)*

    ✓7ᵗʰ **S31.050**   **Open bite of lower back and pelvis without penetration into retroperitoneum**
      Open bite of lower back and pelvis NOS

    ✓7ᵗʰ **S31.051**   **Open bite of lower back and pelvis** **MCC** **with penetration into retroperitoneum**
      CC Excl: See code: S30.001

✓5ᵗʰ **S31.1**   **Open wound of abdominal wall without penetration into peritoneal cavity**
    Open wound of abdominal wall NOS
    EXCLUDES 2   *open wound of abdominal wall with penetration into peritoneal cavity (S31.6-)*

   ✓6ᵗʰ **S31.10**   **Unspecified open wound of abdominal wall without penetration into peritoneal cavity**

    ✓7ᵗʰ **S31.100**   **Unspecified open wound of abdominal wall, right upper quadrant without penetration into peritoneal cavity**

    ✓7ᵗʰ **S31.101**   **Unspecified open wound of abdominal wall, left upper quadrant without penetration into peritoneal cavity**

    ✓7ᵗʰ **S31.102**   **Unspecified open wound of abdominal wall, epigastric region without penetration into peritoneal cavity**

    ✓7ᵗʰ **S31.103**   **Unspecified open wound of abdominal wall, right lower quadrant without penetration into peritoneal cavity**

    ✓7ᵗʰ **S31.104**   **Unspecified open wound of abdominal wall, left lower quadrant without penetration into peritoneal cavity**

    ✓7ᵗʰ **S31.105**   **Unspecified open wound of abdominal wall, periumbilic region without penetration into peritoneal cavity**

    ✓7ᵗʰ **S31.109**   **Unspecified open wound of abdominal wall, unspecified quadrant without penetration into peritoneal cavity**
      Unspecified open wound of abdominal wall NOS

   ✓6ᵗʰ **S31.11**   **Laceration without foreign body of abdominal wall without penetration into peritoneal cavity**

    ✓7ᵗʰ **S31.110**   **Laceration without foreign body of abdominal wall, right upper quadrant without penetration into peritoneal cavity**

    ✓7ᵗʰ **S31.111**   **Laceration without foreign body of abdominal wall, left upper quadrant without penetration into peritoneal cavity**

    ✓7ᵗʰ **S31.112**   **Laceration without foreign body of abdominal wall, epigastric region without penetration into peritoneal cavity**

    ✓7ᵗʰ **S31.113**   **Laceration without foreign body of abdominal wall, right lower quadrant without penetration into peritoneal cavity**

    ✓7ᵗʰ **S31.114**   **Laceration without foreign body of abdominal wall, left lower quadrant without penetration into peritoneal cavity**

    ✓7ᵗʰ **S31.115**   **Laceration without foreign body of abdominal wall, periumbilic region without penetration into peritoneal cavity**

    ✓7ᵗʰ **S31.119**   **Laceration without foreign body of abdominal wall, unspecified quadrant without penetration into peritoneal cavity**

   ✓6ᵗʰ **S31.12**   **Laceration with foreign body of abdominal wall without penetration into peritoneal cavity**

    ✓7ᵗʰ **S31.120**   **Laceration of abdominal wall with foreign body, right upper quadrant without penetration into peritoneal cavity**

    ✓7ᵗʰ **S31.121**   **Laceration of abdominal wall with foreign body, left upper quadrant without penetration into peritoneal cavity**

    ✓7ᵗʰ **S31.122**   **Laceration of abdominal wall with foreign body, epigastric region without penetration into peritoneal cavity**

    ✓7ᵗʰ **S31.123**   **Laceration of abdominal wall with foreign body, right lower quadrant without penetration into peritoneal cavity**

    ✓7ᵗʰ **S31.124**   **Laceration of abdominal wall with foreign body, left lower quadrant without penetration into peritoneal cavity**

    ✓7ᵗʰ **S31.125**   **Laceration of abdominal wall with foreign body, periumbilic region without penetration into peritoneal cavity**

    ✓7ᵗʰ **S31.129**   **Laceration of abdominal wall with foreign body, unspecified quadrant without penetration into peritoneal cavity**

   ✓6ᵗʰ **S31.13**   **Puncture wound of abdominal wall without foreign body without penetration into peritoneal cavity**

    ✓7ᵗʰ **S31.130**   **Puncture wound of abdominal wall without foreign body, right upper quadrant without penetration into peritoneal cavity**

    ✓7ᵗʰ **S31.131**   **Puncture wound of abdominal wall without foreign body, left upper quadrant without penetration into peritoneal cavity**

    ✓7ᵗʰ **S31.132**   **Puncture wound of abdominal wall without foreign body, epigastric region without penetration into peritoneal cavity**

    ✓7ᵗʰ **S31.133**   **Puncture wound of abdominal wall without foreign body, right lower quadrant without penetration into peritoneal cavity**

    ✓7ᵗʰ **S31.134**   **Puncture wound of abdominal wall without foreign body, left lower quadrant without penetration into peritoneal cavity**

    ✓7ᵗʰ **S31.135**   **Puncture wound of abdominal wall without foreign body, periumbilic region without penetration into peritoneal cavity**

    ✓7ᵗʰ **S31.139**   **Puncture wound of abdominal wall without foreign body, unspecified quadrant without penetration into peritoneal cavity**

   ✓6ᵗʰ **S31.14**   **Puncture wound of abdominal wall with foreign body without penetration into peritoneal cavity**

    ✓7ᵗʰ **S31.140**   **Puncture wound of abdominal wall with foreign body, right upper quadrant without penetration into peritoneal cavity**

    ✓7ᵗʰ **S31.141**   **Puncture wound of abdominal wall with foreign body, left upper quadrant without penetration into peritoneal cavity**

    ✓7ᵗʰ **S31.142**   **Puncture wound of abdominal wall with foreign body, epigastric region without penetration into peritoneal cavity**

    ✓7ᵗʰ **S31.143**   **Puncture wound of abdominal wall with foreign body, right lower quadrant without penetration into peritoneal cavity**

    ✓7ᵗʰ **S31.144**   **Puncture wound of abdominal wall with foreign body, left lower quadrant without penetration into peritoneal cavity**

    ✓7ᵗʰ **S31.145**   **Puncture wound of abdominal wall with foreign body, periumbilic region without penetration into peritoneal cavity**

    ✓7ᵗʰ **S31.149**   **Puncture wound of abdominal wall with foreign body, unspecified quadrant without penetration into peritoneal cavity**

   ✓6ᵗʰ **S31.15**   **Open bite of abdominal wall without penetration into peritoneal cavity**
    Bite of abdominal wall NOS
    EXCLUDES 1   *superficial bite of abdominal wall (S30.871)*

    ✓7ᵗʰ **S31.150**   **Open bite of abdominal wall, right upper quadrant without penetration into peritoneal cavity**

    ✓7ᵗʰ **S31.151**   **Open bite of abdominal wall, left upper quadrant without penetration into peritoneal cavity**

    ✓7ᵗʰ **S31.152**   **Open bite of abdominal wall, epigastric region without penetration into peritoneal cavity**

    ✓7ᵗʰ **S31.153**   **Open bite of abdominal wall, right lower quadrant without penetration into peritoneal cavity**

Ⓝ Newborn: 0   Ⓟ Pediatric: 0-17   Ⓜ Maternity: 12-55   Ⓐ Adult: 15-124   **MCC** Major CC Condition   **PDxMCC** PDx acts as own MCC   **CC** CC Condition   **PDxCC** PDx acts as own CC

930   ICD-10-CM 2016

√7th **S31.154** Open bite of abdominal wall, left lower quadrant without penetration into peritoneal cavity

√7th **S31.155** Open bite of abdominal wall, periumbilic region without penetration into peritoneal cavity

√7th **S31.159** Open bite of abdominal wall, unspecified quadrant without penetration into peritoneal cavity

√5th **S31.2** Open wound of penis

√x7th **S31.20** Unspecified open wound of penis ♂

√x7th **S31.21** Laceration without foreign body of penis ♂

√x7th **S31.22** Laceration with foreign body of penis ♂

√x7th **S31.23** Puncture wound without foreign body of penis ♂

√x7th **S31.24** Puncture wound with foreign body of penis ♂

√x7th **S31.25** Open bite of penis ♂
Bite of penis NOS
EXCLUDES 1 superficial bite of penis (S30.862, S30.872)

√5th **S31.3** Open wound of scrotum and testes

√x7th **S31.30** Unspecified open wound of scrotum and testes ♂

√x7th **S31.31** Laceration without foreign body of scrotum and testes ♂

√x7th **S31.32** Laceration with foreign body of scrotum and testes ♂

√x7th **S31.33** Puncture wound without foreign body of scrotum and testes ♂

√x7th **S31.34** Puncture wound with foreign body of scrotum and testes ♂

√x7th **S31.35** Open bite of scrotum and testes ♂
Bite of scrotum and testes NOS
EXCLUDES 1 superficial bite of scrotum and testes (S30.863, S30.873)

√5th **S31.4** Open wound of vagina and vulva
EXCLUDES 1 injury to vagina and vulva during delivery (O70-, O71.4)

√x7th **S31.40** Unspecified open wound of vagina and vulva ♀

√x7th **S31.41** Laceration without foreign body of vagina and vulva ♀

√x7th **S31.42** Laceration with foreign body of vagina and vulva ♀

√x7th **S31.43** Puncture wound without foreign body of vagina and vulva ♀

√x7th **S31.44** Puncture wound with foreign body of vagina and vulva ♀

√x7th **S31.45** Open bite of vagina and vulva ♀
Bite of vagina and vulva NOS
EXCLUDES 1 superficial bite of vagina and vulva (S30.864, S30.874)

√5th **S31.5** Open wound of unspecified external genital organs
EXCLUDES 1 traumatic amputation of external genital organs (S38.21, S38.22)

√6th **S31.50** Unspecified open wound of unspecified external genital organs

√7th **S31.501** Unspecified open wound of unspecified ♂ external genital organs, male

√7th **S31.502** Unspecified open wound of unspecified ♀ external genital organs, female

√6th **S31.51** Laceration without foreign body of unspecified external genital organs

√7th **S31.511** Laceration without foreign body of ♂ unspecified external genital organs, male

√7th **S31.512** Laceration without foreign body of ♀ unspecified external genital organs, female

√6th **S31.52** Laceration with foreign body of unspecified external genital organs

√7th **S31.521** Laceration with foreign body of ♂ unspecified external genital organs, male

√7th **S31.522** Laceration with foreign body of ♀ unspecified external genital organs, female

√6th **S31.53** Puncture wound without foreign body of unspecified external genital organs

√7th **S31.531** Puncture wound without foreign body ♂ of unspecified external genital organs, male

√7th **S31.532** Puncture wound without foreign body ♀ of unspecified external genital organs, female

√6th **S31.54** Puncture wound with foreign body of unspecified external genital organs

√7th **S31.541** Puncture wound with foreign body of ♂ unspecified external genital organs, male

√7th **S31.542** Puncture wound with foreign body of ♀ unspecified external genital organs, female

√6th **S31.55** Open bite of unspecified external genital organs
Bite of unspecified external genital organs NOS
EXCLUDES 1 superficial bite of unspecified external genital organs (S30.865, S30.866, S30.875, S30.876)

√7th **S31.551** Open bite of unspecified external ♂ genital organs, male

√7th **S31.552** Open bite of unspecified external ♀ genital organs, female

√5th **S31.6** Open wound of abdominal wall with penetration into peritoneal cavity

CC Excl: For MCC codes in category S31.6, unless otherwise noted: MCC with 7th character A: S31.001A, S31.011A, S31.021, S31.031A, S31.041A, S31.051-S31.159 with 7th A, S31.600-S31.659 with 7th A, S31.831-S31.839 with 7th A, S36.81X-S36.99X with 7th A, S38.3XX-S39.023 with 7th A, T14.90-T14.91, T79.A0X-T79.9XX with 7th A

√6th **S31.60** Unspecified open wound of abdominal wall with penetration into peritoneal cavity

√7th **S31.600** Unspecified open wound of ☒MCC abdominal wall, right upper quadrant with penetration into peritoneal cavity

√7th **S31.601** Unspecified open wound of ☒MCC abdominal wall, left upper quadrant with penetration into peritoneal cavity

√7th **S31.602** Unspecified open wound of ☒MCC abdominal wall, epigastric region with penetration into peritoneal cavity

√7th **S31.603** Unspecified open wound of ☒MCC abdominal wall, right lower quadrant with penetration into peritoneal cavity

√7th **S31.604** Unspecified open wound of ☒MCC abdominal wall, left lower quadrant with penetration into peritoneal cavity

√7th **S31.605** Unspecified open wound of ☒MCC abdominal wall, periumbilic region with penetration into peritoneal cavity

√7th **S31.609** Unspecified open wound of ☒MCC abdominal wall, unspecified quadrant with penetration into peritoneal cavity

√6th **S31.61** Laceration without foreign body of abdominal wall with penetration into peritoneal cavity

√7th **S31.610** Laceration without foreign body of ☒MCC abdominal wall, right upper quadrant with penetration into peritoneal cavity

√7th **S31.611** Laceration without foreign body of ☒MCC abdominal wall, left upper quadrant with penetration into peritoneal cavity

√7th **S31.612** Laceration without foreign body of ☒MCC abdominal wall, epigastric region with penetration into peritoneal cavity

√7th **S31.613** Laceration without foreign body of ☒MCC abdominal wall, right lower quadrant with penetration into peritoneal cavity

√7th **S31.614** Laceration without foreign body of ☒MCC abdominal wall, left lower quadrant with penetration into peritoneal cavity

√7th **S31.615** Laceration without foreign body of ☒MCC abdominal wall, periumbilic region with penetration into peritoneal cavity

√7th **S31.619** Laceration without foreign body of ☒MCC abdominal wall, unspecified quadrant with penetration into peritoneal cavity

☑ Additional Character Required   √x7th Placeholder Alert   Unacceptable PDx   Manifestation   Hospital Acquired Condition   *EXCLUDES 1* Not Coded Here   *EXCLUDES 2* Not Included Here

ICD-10-CM 2016   931

Chapter 19. Injury, Poisoning, and Certain Other Consequences of External Causes

√6ᵗʰ **S31.62** **Laceration with foreign body of abdominal wall with penetration into peritoneal cavity**

√7ᵗʰ **S31.620** Laceration with foreign body of abdominal wall, **right upper quadrant** with penetration into peritoneal cavity `MCC`

√7ᵗʰ **S31.621** Laceration with foreign body of abdominal wall, **left upper quadrant** with penetration into peritoneal cavity `MCC`

√7ᵗʰ **S31.622** Laceration with foreign body of abdominal wall, **epigastric region** with penetration into peritoneal cavity `MCC`

√7ᵗʰ **S31.623** Laceration with foreign body of abdominal wall, **right lower quadrant** with penetration into peritoneal cavity `MCC`

√7ᵗʰ **S31.624** Laceration with foreign body of abdominal wall, **left lower quadrant** with penetration into peritoneal cavity `MCC`

√7ᵗʰ **S31.625** Laceration with foreign body of abdominal wall, **periumbilic region** with penetration into peritoneal cavity `MCC`

√7ᵗʰ **S31.629** Laceration with foreign body of abdominal wall, **unspecified quadrant** with penetration into peritoneal cavity `MCC`

√6ᵗʰ **S31.63** **Puncture wound without foreign body of abdominal wall with penetration into peritoneal cavity**

√7ᵗʰ **S31.630** Puncture wound without foreign body of abdominal wall, **right upper quadrant** with penetration into peritoneal cavity `MCC`

√7ᵗʰ **S31.631** Puncture wound without foreign body of abdominal wall, **left upper quadrant** with penetration into peritoneal cavity `MCC`

√7ᵗʰ **S31.632** Puncture wound without foreign body of abdominal wall, **epigastric region** with penetration into peritoneal cavity `MCC`

√7ᵗʰ **S31.633** Puncture wound without foreign body of abdominal wall, **right lower quadrant** with penetration into peritoneal cavity `MCC`

√7ᵗʰ **S31.634** Puncture wound without foreign body of abdominal wall, **left lower quadrant** with penetration into peritoneal cavity `MCC`

√7ᵗʰ **S31.635** Puncture wound without foreign body of abdominal wall, **periumbilic region** with penetration into peritoneal cavity `MCC`

√7ᵗʰ **S31.639** Puncture wound without foreign body of abdominal wall, **unspecified quadrant** with penetration into peritoneal cavity `MCC`

√6ᵗʰ **S31.64** **Puncture wound with foreign body of abdominal wall with penetration into peritoneal cavity**

√7ᵗʰ **S31.640** Puncture wound with foreign body of abdominal wall, **right upper quadrant** with penetration into peritoneal cavity `MCC`

√7ᵗʰ **S31.641** Puncture wound with foreign body of abdominal wall, **left upper quadrant** with penetration into peritoneal cavity `MCC`

√7ᵗʰ **S31.642** Puncture wound with foreign body of abdominal wall, **epigastric region** with penetration into peritoneal cavity `MCC`

√7ᵗʰ **S31.643** Puncture wound with foreign body of abdominal wall, **right lower quadrant** with penetration into peritoneal cavity `MCC`

√7ᵗʰ **S31.644** Puncture wound with foreign body of abdominal wall, **left lower quadrant** with penetration into peritoneal cavity `MCC`

√7ᵗʰ **S31.645** Puncture wound with foreign body of abdominal wall, **periumbilic region** with penetration into peritoneal cavity `MCC`

√7ᵗʰ **S31.649** Puncture wound with foreign body of abdominal wall, **unspecified quadrant** with penetration into peritoneal cavity `MCC`

√6ᵗʰ **S31.65** **Open bite of abdominal wall with penetration into peritoneal cavity**

EXCLUDES 1 *superficial bite of abdominal wall (S30.861, S30.871)*

√7ᵗʰ **S31.650** Open bite of abdominal wall, **right upper quadrant** with penetration into peritoneal cavity `MCC`

√7ᵗʰ **S31.651** Open bite of abdominal wall, **left upper quadrant** with penetration into peritoneal cavity `MCC`

√7ᵗʰ **S31.652** Open bite of abdominal wall, **epigastric region** with penetration into peritoneal cavity `MCC`

√7ᵗʰ **S31.653** Open bite of abdominal wall, **right lower quadrant** with penetration into peritoneal cavity `MCC`

√7ᵗʰ **S31.654** Open bite of abdominal wall, **left lower quadrant** with penetration into peritoneal cavity `MCC`

√7ᵗʰ **S31.655** Open bite of abdominal wall, **periumbilic region** with penetration into peritoneal cavity `MCC`

√7ᵗʰ **S31.659** Open bite of abdominal wall, **unspecified quadrant** with penetration into peritoneal cavity `MCC`

√5ᵗʰ **S31.8** **Open wound of other parts of abdomen, lower back and pelvis**

√6ᵗʰ **S31.80** **Open wound of unspecified buttock**

√7ᵗʰ **S31.801** Laceration without foreign body of unspecified buttock

√7ᵗʰ **S31.802** Laceration with foreign body of unspecified buttock

√7ᵗʰ **S31.803** Puncture wound without foreign body of unspecified buttock

√7ᵗʰ **S31.804** Puncture wound with foreign body of unspecified buttock

√7ᵗʰ **S31.805** Open bite of unspecified buttock
Bite of buttock NOS
EXCLUDES 1 *superficial bite of buttock (S30.870)*

√7ᵗʰ **S31.809** Unspecified open wound of unspecified buttock

√6ᵗʰ **S31.81** **Open wound of right buttock**

√7ᵗʰ **S31.811** Laceration without foreign body of right buttock

√7ᵗʰ **S31.812** Laceration with foreign body of right buttock

√7ᵗʰ **S31.813** Puncture wound without foreign body of right buttock

√7ᵗʰ **S31.814** Puncture wound with foreign body of right buttock

√7ᵗʰ **S31.815** Open bite of right buttock
Bite of right buttock NOS
EXCLUDES 1 *superficial bite of buttock (S30.870)*

√7ᵗʰ **S31.819** Unspecified open wound of right buttock

√6ᵗʰ **S31.82** **Open wound of left buttock**

√7ᵗʰ **S31.821** Laceration without foreign body of left buttock

√7ᵗʰ **S31.822** Laceration with foreign body of left buttock

√7ᵗʰ **S31.823** Puncture wound without foreign body of left buttock

√7ᵗʰ **S31.824** Puncture wound with foreign body of left buttock

√7ᵗʰ **S31.825** Open bite of left buttock
Bite of left buttock NOS
EXCLUDES 1 *superficial bite of buttock (S30.870)*

√7ᵗʰ **S31.829** Unspecified open wound of left buttock

√6ᵗʰ **S31.83** **Open wound of anus**

√7ᵗʰ **S31.831** Laceration without foreign body of anus

√7ᵗʰ **S31.832** Laceration with foreign body of anus

√7ᵗʰ **S31.833** Puncture wound without foreign body of anus

Ⓝ Newborn: 0   Ⓟ Pediatric: 0-17   Ⓜ Maternity: 12-55   Ⓐ Adult: 15-124   `MCC` Major CC Condition   `PDxMCC` PDx acts as own MCC   `CC` CC Condition   `PDxCC` PDx acts as own CC

932   ICD-10-CM 2016

√7ᵗʰ **S31.834** Puncture wound with foreign body of anus

√7ᵗʰ **S31.835** Open bite of anus
Bite of anus NOS
EXCLUDES 1 superficial bite of anus (S30.877)

√7ᵗʰ **S31.839** Unspecified open wound of anus

√4ᵗʰ S32 Fracture of lumbar spine and pelvis

NOTE A fracture not indicated as displaced or nondisplaced should be coded to displaced.
A fracture not indicated as opened or closed should be coded to closed.

INCLUDES fracture of lumbosacral neural arch
fracture of lumbosacral spinous process
fracture of lumbosacral transverse process
fracture of lumbosacral vertebra
fracture of lumbosacral vertebral arch

Code first any associated spinal cord and spinal nerve injury (S34.-)

EXCLUDES 1 transection of abdomen (S38.3)
EXCLUDES 2 fracture of hip NOS (S72.0-)

AHA: 2012, 4Q, 93

The appropriate 7th is to be added to each code from category S32.
A   initial encounter for closed fracture
B   initial encounter for open fracture
D   subsequent encounter for fracture with routine healing
G   subsequent encounter for fracture with delayed healing
K   subsequent encounter for fracture with nonunion
S   sequela

√5ᵗʰ S32.0 Fracture of lumbar vertebra
Fracture of lumbar spine NOS

CC Excl: For CC/MCC codes in subcategory S32.0, unless otherwise noted: CC with 7th character A or MCC with 7th character B: M48.40X-M48.58X with 7th S, M80.08XS, M80.88XS, M84.350S, M84.454S, M84.550S, M84.58XS, M84.650S, M99.13, M99.15-M99.17, M99.19, S03.8XX-S03.9XX with 7th A, S12.000-S12.9XX with 7th S, S13.9XXA, S14.109A, S14.119A, S14.129A, S14.139A, S14.149A, S14.159A, S22.000-S22.9XX with 7th S, S23.20X-S23.29X with 7th A, S23.9XXA, S24.109A, S24.119A, S24.139A, S24.149A, S24.159A, S29.001-S29.019 with 7th A, S29.091-S29.9XX with 7th A, S32.000-S33.39X with 7th [A, B, S], S33.5XXA, S33.9XX-S34.01X with 7th A, S34.101-S34.129 with 7th A, S38.1XXA, S38.3XX-S39.013 with 7th A, S39.091-S39.94X with 7th A, T14.90-T14.91, T79.A0X-T79.9XX with 7th A

CC with 7th character K: M80.00X-M84.68X with 7th [K, P], S02.0XX-S02.92X with 7th K, S12.000-S12.691 with 7th K, S22.000-S22.9XX with 7th K, S32.000-S32.9XX with 7th K, S42.001-S42.92X with 7th [K, P], S49.001-S49.199 with 7th [K, P], S52.001-S52.92X with 7th [K, M, N, P, Q, R], S59.001-S59.299 with 7th [K, P], S62.001-S62.92X with 7th [K, P], S72.001-S72.92X with 7th [K, M, N, P, Q, R], S79.001-S79.199 with 7th [K, P], S82.001-S82.92X with 7th [K, M, N, P, Q, R], S89.001-S89.399 with 7th [K, P], S92.001-S92.919 with 7th [K, P]

√6ᵗʰ S32.00 Fracture of unspecified lumbar vertebra

7,16,19 √7ᵗʰ **S32.000** Wedge compression fracture of unspecified lumbar vertebra   MCC CC

7,16,19 √7ᵗʰ **S32.001** Stable burst fracture of unspecified lumbar vertebra   MCC CC

7,16,19 √7ᵗʰ **S32.002** Unstable burst fracture of unspecified lumbar vertebra   MCC CC

7,16,19 √7ᵗʰ **S32.008** Other fracture of unspecified lumbar vertebra   MCC CC

7,16,19 √7ᵗʰ **S32.009** Unspecified fracture of unspecified lumbar vertebra   MCC CC

√6ᵗʰ S32.01 Fracture of first lumbar vertebra

7,16,19 √7ᵗʰ **S32.010** Wedge compression fracture of first lumbar vertebra   MCC CC

7,16,19 √7ᵗʰ **S32.011** Stable burst fracture of first lumbar vertebra   MCC CC

7,16,19 √7ᵗʰ **S32.012** Unstable burst fracture of first lumbar vertebra   MCC CC

7,16,19 √7ᵗʰ **S32.018** Other fracture of first lumbar vertebra   MCC CC

7,16,19 √7ᵗʰ **S32.019** Unspecified fracture of first lumbar vertebra   MCC CC

√6ᵗʰ S32.02 Fracture of second lumbar vertebra

7,16,19 √7ᵗʰ **S32.020** Wedge compression fracture of second lumbar vertebra   MCC CC

7,16,19 √7ᵗʰ **S32.021** Stable burst fracture of second lumbar vertebra   MCC CC

7,16,19 √7ᵗʰ **S32.022** Unstable burst fracture of second lumbar vertebra   MCC CC

7,16,19 √7ᵗʰ **S32.028** Other fracture of second lumbar vertebra   MCC CC

7,16,19 √7ᵗʰ **S32.029** Unspecified fracture of second lumbar vertebra   MCC CC

√6ᵗʰ S32.03 Fracture of third lumbar vertebra

7,16,19 √7ᵗʰ **S32.030** Wedge compression fracture of third lumbar vertebra   MCC CC

7,16,19 √7ᵗʰ **S32.031** Stable burst fracture of third lumbar vertebra   MCC CC

7,16,19 √7ᵗʰ **S32.032** Unstable burst fracture of third lumbar vertebra   MCC CC

7,16,19 √7ᵗʰ **S32.038** Other fracture of third lumbar vertebra   MCC CC

7,16,19 √7ᵗʰ **S32.039** Unspecified fracture of third lumbar vertebra   MCC CC

√6ᵗʰ S32.04 Fracture of fourth lumbar vertebra

7,16,19 √7ᵗʰ **S32.040** Wedge compression fracture of fourth lumbar vertebra   MCC CC

7,16,19 √7ᵗʰ **S32.041** Stable burst fracture of fourth lumbar vertebra   MCC CC

7,16,19 √7ᵗʰ **S32.042** Unstable burst fracture of fourth lumbar vertebra   MCC CC

7,16,19 √7ᵗʰ **S32.048** Other fracture of fourth lumbar vertebra   MCC CC

7,16,19 √7ᵗʰ **S32.049** Unspecified fracture of fourth lumbar vertebra   MCC CC

√6ᵗʰ S32.05 Fracture of fifth lumbar vertebra

7,16,19 √7ᵗʰ **S32.050** Wedge compression fracture of fifth lumbar vertebra   MCC CC

7,16,19 √7ᵗʰ **S32.051** Stable burst fracture of fifth lumbar vertebra   MCC CC

7,16,19 √7ᵗʰ **S32.052** Unstable burst fracture of fifth lumbar vertebra   MCC CC

7,16,19 √7ᵗʰ **S32.058** Other fracture of fifth lumbar vertebra   MCC CC

7,16,19 √7ᵗʰ **S32.059** Unspecified fracture of fifth lumbar vertebra   MCC CC

√5ᵗʰ S32.1 Fracture of sacrum

NOTE For vertical fractures, code to most medial fracture extension.
Use two codes if both a vertical and transverse fracture are present.

Code also any associated fracture of pelvic ring (S32.8-)

CC Excl: For CC/MCC codes in subcategory S32.1, unless otherwise noted: CC with 7th character A or MCC with 7th character B: M48.40X-M48.58X with 7th S, M80.08XS, M80.88XS, M84.350S, M84.454S, M84.550S, M84.58XS, M84.650S, M99.14-M99.17, M99.19, S03.8XX-S03.9XX with 7th A, S12.000-S12.9XX with 7th S, S13.9XXA, S14.109A, S14.119, S14.129A, S14.139A, S14.149 A, S14.159A, S22.000-S22.9XX with 7th S, S23.20X-S23.29X with 7th A, S23.9XXA, S24.109A, S24.119A, S24.139A, S24.149 A, S24.159A, S29.001-S29.019 with 7th A, S29.091-S29.9XX with 7th A, S32.000-S32.9XX with 7th S, S33.2XX-S33.4XX with 7th A, S33.6XX-S34.02X with 7th A, S34.131-S34.139 with 7th A, S34.3XX with 7th A, S38.1XX with 7th A, S38.3XX-S39.013 with 7th A, S39.091-S39.94X A, T14.90-T14.91, T79.A0X-T79.9XX with 7th A

CC with 7th character K: M80.00X-M84.68X with 7th [K, P], S02.0XX-S02.92X with 7th K, S12.000-S12.691 with 7th K, S22.000-S22.9XX with 7th K, S32.000-S32.9XX with 7th K, S42.001-S42.92X with 7th [K, P], S49.001-S49.199 with 7th [K, P], S52.001-S52.92X with 7th [K, M, N, P, Q, R], S59.001-S59.299 with 7th [K, P], S62.001-S62.92X with 7th [K, P], S72.001-S72.92X with 7th [K, M, N, P, Q, R], S79.001-S79.199 with 7th [K, P], S82.001-S82.92X with 7th [K, M, N, P, Q, R], S89.001-S89.399 with 7th [K, P], S92.001-S92.919 with 7th [K, P]

7,16,19 √x7ᵗʰ **S32.10** Unspecified fracture of sacrum   MCC CC

---

7   HAC = Initial encounter only (7th character A, B or C) and not POA.
16   MCC only if an open fracture (7th character B or C – specific to category).
19   CC only if an initial encounter for a closed fracture (7th character A) **OR** a subsequent encounter for nonunion or malunion (7th character K, M, N, P, Q, or R – specific to category).

√ Additional Character Required   √x7ᵗʰ Placeholder Alert   Unacceptable PDx   Manifestation   Hospital Acquired Condition   **EXCLUDES 1** Not Coded Here   **EXCLUDES 2** Not Included Here

√6ᵗʰ S32.11 Zone I fracture of sacrum
Vertical sacral ala fracture of sacrum

7,16,19 √7ᵗʰ S32.110 **Nondisplaced Zone I fracture of sacrum** `MCC` `CC`

7,16,19 √7ᵗʰ S32.111 **Minimally displaced Zone I fracture of sacrum** `MCC` `CC`

7,16,19 √7ᵗʰ S32.112 **Severely displaced Zone I fracture of sacrum** `MCC` `CC`

7,16,19 √7ᵗʰ S32.119 **Unspecified Zone I fracture of sacrum** `MCC` `CC`

√6ᵗʰ S32.12 Zone II fracture of sacrum
Vertical foraminal region fracture of sacrum

7,16,19 √7ᵗʰ S32.120 **Nondisplaced Zone II fracture of sacrum** `MCC` `CC`

7,16,19 √7ᵗʰ S32.121 **Minimally displaced Zone II fracture of sacrum** `MCC` `CC`

7,16,19 √7ᵗʰ S32.122 **Severely displaced Zone II fracture of sacrum** `MCC` `CC`

7,16,19 √7ᵗʰ S32.129 **Unspecified Zone II fracture of sacrum** `MCC` `CC`

√6ᵗʰ S32.13 Zone III fracture of sacrum
Vertical fracture into spinal canal region of sacrum

7,16,19 √7ᵗʰ S32.130 **Nondisplaced Zone III fracture of sacrum** `MCC` `CC`

7,16,19 √7ᵗʰ S32.131 **Minimally displaced Zone III fracture of sacrum** `MCC` `CC`

7,16,19 √7ᵗʰ S32.132 **Severely displaced Zone III fracture of sacrum** `MCC` `CC`

7,16,19 √7ᵗʰ S32.139 **Unspecified Zone III fracture of sacrum** `MCC` `CC`

7,16,19 √x7ᵗʰ S32.14 **Type 1 fracture of sacrum** `MCC` `CC`
Transverse flexion fracture of sacrum without displacement

7,16,19 √x7ᵗʰ S32.15 **Type 2 fracture of sacrum** `MCC` `CC`
Transverse flexion fracture of sacrum with posterior displacement

7,16,19 √x7ᵗʰ S32.16 **Type 3 fracture of sacrum** `MCC` `CC`
Transverse extension fracture of sacrum with anterior displacement

7,16,19 √x7ᵗʰ S32.17 **Type 4 fracture of sacrum** `MCC` `CC`
Transverse segmental comminution of upper sacrum

7,16,19 √x7ᵗʰ S32.19 **Other fracture of sacrum** `MCC` `CC`

7,16,19 √x7ᵗʰ S32.2 **Fracture of coccyx** `MCC` `CC`
CC Excl: See code: S32.1

√5ᵗʰ S32.3 Fracture of ilium

EXCLUDES 1 *fracture of ilium with associated disruption of pelvic ring (S32.8-)*

CC Excl: For CC/MCC codes in subcategory S32.3, unless otherwise noted: CC with 7th character A: M80.00X-M80.019 with 7th A, M80.041-M80.049 with 7th A, M80.80X-M80.819 with 7th A, M80.841-M80.849 with 7th A, M84.40X-M84.419 with 7th A, M84.441-M84.446 with 7th A, M84.454 with 7th A, M84.474-M84.519 with 7th A, M84.541-M84.550 with 7th A, M84.574-M84.576 with 7th A, M84.60X-M84.619 with 7th A, M84.641-M84.650 with 7th A, M84.674-M84.68X with 7th A, S03.8XX-S03.9XX with 7th A, S22.9XX-S22.9XX with 7th [A, B], S29.011-S29.019 with 7th A, S32.301-S32.811 with 7th [A, B], S32.89X-S32.9XX with 7th [A, B], S33.4XX with 7th A, S33.6XX-S33.8XX with 7th A, S38.3XX-S39.013 with 7th A, S73.001-S73.199 with 7th A, S76.001-S76.019 with 7th A, S76.091-S76.119 with 7th A, S76.191-S76.219 with 7th A, S76.291-S76.319 with 7th A, S76.391-S76.819 with 7th A, S76.891-S76.919 with 7th A, S76.991-S76.999 with 7th A, S79.811-S79.929 with 7th A, T14.90-T14.91, T79.A9X-T79.9XX with 7th A
MCC with 7th character B: M48.40X-M48.58X with 7th A, M80.00X-M84.68X with 7th A, S03.8XX-S03.9XX with 7th A, S22.9XX-S22.9XX with 7th [A, B], S29.011-S29.019 with 7th A, S32.301-S32.399 with 7th [A, B], S32.810-S32.811 with 7th [A, B], S32.89X-S32.9XX with 7th [A, B], S33.4XX with 7th A, S33.6XX-S33.8XX with 7th A, S38.3XX-S39.013 with 7th A, S73.001-S73.199 with 7th A, S76.001-S76.019 with 7th A, S76.091-S76.119 with 7th A, S76.191-S76.219 with 7th A, S76.291-S76.319 with 7th A, S76.391-S76.819 with 7th A, S76.891-S76.919 with 7th A, S76.991-S76.999 with 7th A, S79.811-S79.929 with 7th A, T14.90-T14.91, T79.A0X-T79.9XX with 7th A
CC with 7th character K: M80.00X-M84.68X with 7th [K, P], S02.0XX-S02.92X with 7th K, S12.000-S12.691 with 7th K, S22.000-S22.9XX with 7th K, S32.000-S32.9XX with 7th K, S42.001-S42.92X with 7th [K, P], S49.001-S49.199 with 7th [K, P], S52.001-S52.92X with 7th [K, M, N, P, Q, R], S59.001-S59.299 with 7th [K, P], S62.001-S62.92X with 7th [K, P], S72.001-S72.92X with 7th [K, M, N, P, Q, R], S79.001-S79.199 with 7th [K, P], S82.001-S82.92X with 7th [K, M, N, P, Q, R], S89.001-S89.399 with 7th [K, P], S92.001-S92.919 with 7th [K, P]

√6ᵗʰ S32.30 Unspecified fracture of ilium

7,16,19 √7ᵗʰ S32.301 **Unspecified fracture of right ilium** `MCC` `CC`

7,16,19 √7ᵗʰ S32.302 **Unspecified fracture of left ilium** `MCC` `CC`

7,16,19 √7ᵗʰ S32.309 **Unspecified fracture of unspecified ilium** `MCC` `CC`

√6ᵗʰ S32.31 Avulsion fracture of ilium

7,16,19 √7ᵗʰ S32.311 **Displaced avulsion fracture of right ilium** `MCC` `CC`

7,16,19 √7ᵗʰ S32.312 **Displaced avulsion fracture of left ilium** `MCC` `CC`

7,16,19 √7ᵗʰ S32.313 **Displaced avulsion fracture of unspecified ilium** `MCC` `CC`

7,16,19 √7ᵗʰ S32.314 **Nondisplaced avulsion fracture of right ilium** `MCC` `CC`

7,16,19 √7ᵗʰ S32.315 **Nondisplaced avulsion fracture of left ilium** `MCC` `CC`

7,16,19 √7ᵗʰ S32.316 **Nondisplaced avulsion fracture of unspecified ilium** `MCC` `CC`

√6ᵗʰ S32.39 Other fracture of ilium

7,16,19 √7ᵗʰ S32.391 **Other fracture of right ilium** `MCC` `CC`

7,16,19 √7ᵗʰ S32.392 **Other fracture of left ilium** `MCC` `CC`

7,16,19 √7ᵗʰ S32.399 **Other fracture of unspecified ilium** `MCC` `CC`

---

7 HAC = Initial encounter only (7th character A, B or C) and not POA.
16 MCC only if an open fracture (7th character B or C – specific to category).
19 CC only if an initial encounter for a closed fracture (7th character A) **OR** a subsequent encounter for nonunion or malunion (7th character K, M, N, P, Q, or R – specific to category).

✓5ᵗʰ **S32.4 Fracture of acetabulum**

Code also any associated fracture of pelvic ring (S32.8-)

CC Excl: For CC/MCC codes in subcategory S32.4, unless otherwise noted: MCC with 7th character A: M48.40X-M48.58X with 7th A, M80.00X-M84.68X with 7th A, S03.8XX-S03.9XX with 7th A, S22.9XX-S22.9XX with 7th [A, B], S29.011-S29.019 with 7th A, S32.401-S32.499 with 7th [A, B], S32.810-S32.811 with 7th [A, B], S32.89X-S32.9XX with 7th [A, B], S33.4XX with 7th A, S33.6XX-S33.8XX with 7th A, S38.3XX-S39.013 with 7th A, S73.001-S73.199 with 7th A, S76.001-S76.019 with 7th A, S76.091-S76.119 with 7th A, S76.191-S76.219 with 7th A, S76.291-S76.319 with 7th A, S76.391-S76.819 with 7th A, S76.891-S76.919 with 7th A, S76.991-S76.999 with 7th A, S79.811-S79.929 with 7th A, T14.90-T14.91, T79.A0X-T79.9XX with 7th A

MCC with 7th character B: S03.8XX-S03.9XX with 7th A, S22.9XX-S22.9XX with 7th [A, B], S29.011-S29.019 with 7th A, S32.401-S32.499 with 7th [A, B], S32.810-S32.811 with 7th [A, B], S32.89X-S32.9XX with 7th [A, B], S33.4XX with 7th A, S33.6XX-S33.8XX with 7th A, S38.3XX-S39.013 with 7th A, S73.001-S73.199 with 7th A, S76.001-S76.019 with 7th A, S76.091-S76.119 with 7th A, S76.191-S76.219 with 7th A, S76.291-S76.319 with 7th A, S76.391-S76.819 with 7th A, S76.891-S76.919 with 7th A, S76.991-S76.999 with 7th A, S79.811-S79.929 with 7th A, T14.90-T14.91, T79.A0X-T79.9XX with 7th A

CC with 7th character K: M80.00X-M84.68X with 7th [K, P], S02.0XX-S02.92X with 7th K, S12.000-S12.691 with 7th K, S22.000-S22.9XX with 7th K, S32.000-S32.9XX with 7th K, S42.001-S42.92X with 7th [K, P], S49.001-S49.199 with 7th [K, P], S52.001-S52.92X with 7th [K, M, N, P, Q, R], S59.001-S59.299 with 7th [K, P], S62.001-S62.92X with 7th [K, P], S72.001-S72.92X with 7th [K, M, N, P, Q, R], S79.001-S79.199 with 7th [K, P], S82.001-S82.92X with 7th [K, M, N, P, Q, R], S89.001-S89.399 with 7th [K, P], S92.001-S92.919 with 7th [K, P]

✓6ᵗʰ **S32.40 Unspecified fracture of acetabulum**

7,18 ✓7ᵗʰ **S32.401 Unspecified fracture of right acetabulum** `MCC` `CC`

7,18 ✓7ᵗʰ **S32.402 Unspecified fracture of left acetabulum** `MCC` `CC`

7,18 ✓7ᵗʰ **S32.409 Unspecified fracture of unspecified acetabulum** `MCC` `CC`

✓6ᵗʰ **S32.41 Fracture of anterior wall of acetabulum**

7,18 ✓7ᵗʰ **S32.411 Displaced fracture of anterior wall of right acetabulum** `MCC` `CC`

7,18 ✓7ᵗʰ **S32.412 Displaced fracture of anterior wall of left acetabulum** `MCC` `CC`

7,18 ✓7ᵗʰ **S32.413 Displaced fracture of anterior wall of unspecified acetabulum** `MCC` `CC`

7,18 ✓7ᵗʰ **S32.414 Nondisplaced fracture of anterior wall of right acetabulum** `MCC` `CC`

7,18 ✓7ᵗʰ **S32.415 Nondisplaced fracture of anterior wall of left acetabulum** `MCC` `CC`

7,18 ✓7ᵗʰ **S32.416 Nondisplaced fracture of anterior wall of unspecified acetabulum** `MCC` `CC`

✓6ᵗʰ **S32.42 Fracture of posterior wall of acetabulum**

7,18 ✓7ᵗʰ **S32.421 Displaced fracture of posterior wall of right acetabulum** `MCC` `CC`

7,18 ✓7ᵗʰ **S32.422 Displaced fracture of posterior wall of left acetabulum** `MCC` `CC`

7,18 ✓7ᵗʰ **S32.423 Displaced fracture of posterior wall of unspecified acetabulum** `MCC` `CC`

7,18 ✓7ᵗʰ **S32.424 Nondisplaced fracture of posterior wall of right acetabulum** `MCC` `CC`

7,18 ✓7ᵗʰ **S32.425 Nondisplaced fracture of posterior wall of left acetabulum** `MCC` `CC`

7,18 ✓7ᵗʰ **S32.426 Nondisplaced fracture of posterior wall of unspecified acetabulum** `MCC` `CC`

✓6ᵗʰ **S32.43 Fracture of anterior column [iliopubic] of acetabulum**

7,18 ✓7ᵗʰ **S32.431 Displaced fracture of anterior column [iliopubic] of right acetabulum** `MCC` `CC`

7,18 ✓7ᵗʰ **S32.432 Displaced fracture of anterior column [iliopubic] of left acetabulum** `MCC` `CC`

7,18 ✓7ᵗʰ **S32.433 Displaced fracture of anterior column [iliopubic] of unspecified acetabulum** `MCC` `CC`

7,18 ✓7ᵗʰ **S32.434 Nondisplaced fracture of anterior column [iliopubic] of right acetabulum** `MCC` `CC`

7,18 ✓7ᵗʰ **S32.435 Nondisplaced fracture of anterior column [iliopubic] of left acetabulum** `MCC` `CC`

7,18 ✓7ᵗʰ **S32.436 Nondisplaced fracture of anterior column [iliopubic] of unspecified acetabulum** `MCC` `CC`

✓6ᵗʰ **S32.44 Fracture of posterior column [ilioischial] of acetabulum**

7,18 ✓7ᵗʰ **S32.441 Displaced fracture of posterior column [ilioischial] of right acetabulum** `MCC` `CC`

7,18 ✓7ᵗʰ **S32.442 Displaced fracture of posterior column [ilioischial] of left acetabulum** `MCC` `CC`

7,18 ✓7ᵗʰ **S32.443 Displaced fracture of posterior column [ilioischial] of unspecified acetabulum** `MCC` `CC`

7,18 ✓7ᵗʰ **S32.444 Nondisplaced fracture of posterior column [ilioischial] of right acetabulum** `MCC` `CC`

7,18 ✓7ᵗʰ **S32.445 Nondisplaced fracture of posterior column [ilioischial] of left acetabulum** `MCC` `CC`

7,18 ✓7ᵗʰ **S32.446 Nondisplaced fracture of posterior column [ilioischial] of unspecified acetabulum** `MCC` `CC`

✓6ᵗʰ **S32.45 Transverse fracture of acetabulum**

7,18 ✓7ᵗʰ **S32.451 Displaced transverse fracture of right acetabulum** `MCC` `CC`

7,18 ✓7ᵗʰ **S32.452 Displaced transverse fracture of left acetabulum** `MCC` `CC`

7,18 ✓7ᵗʰ **S32.453 Displaced transverse fracture of unspecified acetabulum** `MCC` `CC`

7,18 ✓7ᵗʰ **S32.454 Nondisplaced transverse fracture of right acetabulum** `MCC` `CC`

7,18 ✓7ᵗʰ **S32.455 Nondisplaced transverse fracture of left acetabulum** `MCC` `CC`

7,18 ✓7ᵗʰ **S32.456 Nondisplaced transverse fracture of unspecified acetabulum** `MCC` `CC`

✓6ᵗʰ **S32.46 Associated transverse-posterior fracture of acetabulum**

7,18 ✓7ᵗʰ **S32.461 Displaced associated transverse-posterior fracture of right acetabulum** `MCC` `CC`

7,18 ✓7ᵗʰ **S32.462 Displaced associated transverse-posterior fracture of left acetabulum** `MCC` `CC`

7,18 ✓7ᵗʰ **S32.463 Displaced associated transverse-posterior fracture of unspecified acetabulum** `MCC` `CC`

7,18 ✓7ᵗʰ **S32.464 Nondisplaced associated transverse-posterior fracture of right acetabulum** `MCC` `CC`

7,18 ✓7ᵗʰ **S32.465 Nondisplaced associated transverse-posterior fracture of left acetabulum** `MCC` `CC`

7,18 ✓7ᵗʰ **S32.466 Nondisplaced associated transverse-posterior fracture of unspecified acetabulum** `MCC` `CC`

✓6ᵗʰ **S32.47 Fracture of medial wall of acetabulum**

7,18 ✓7ᵗʰ **S32.471 Displaced fracture of medial wall of right acetabulum** `MCC` `CC`

7,18 ✓7ᵗʰ **S32.472 Displaced fracture of medial wall of left acetabulum** `MCC` `CC`

7,18 ✓7ᵗʰ **S32.473 Displaced fracture of medial wall of unspecified acetabulum** `MCC` `CC`

7,18 ✓7ᵗʰ **S32.474 Nondisplaced fracture of medial wall of right acetabulum** `MCC` `CC`

7,18 ✓7ᵗʰ **S32.475 Nondisplaced fracture of medial wall of left acetabulum** `MCC` `CC`

7,18 ✓7ᵗʰ **S32.476 Nondisplaced fracture of medial wall of unspecified acetabulum** `MCC` `CC`

---

7 HAC = Initial encounter only (7th character A, B or C) and not POA.
18 CC only if a subsequent encounter for nonunion or malunion (7th character K, M, N, P, Q, or R – specific to category).

✔ Additional Character Required   ✔x7ᵗʰ Placeholder Alert   Unacceptable PDx   Manifestation   Hospital Acquired Condition   **EXCLUDES 1** Not Coded Here   **EXCLUDES 2** Not Included Here

Chapter 19. Injury, Poisoning, and Certain Other Consequences of External Causes

√6ᵗʰ **S32.48**   Dome fracture of acetabulum

7,18 √7ᵗʰ **S32.481**   **Displaced dome fracture of right acetabulum**   MCC CC

7,18 √7ᵗʰ **S32.482**   **Displaced dome fracture of left acetabulum**   MCC CC

7,18 √7ᵗʰ **S32.483**   **Displaced dome fracture of unspecified acetabulum**   MCC CC

7,18 √7ᵗʰ **S32.484**   **Nondisplaced dome fracture of right acetabulum**   MCC CC

7,18 √7ᵗʰ **S32.485**   **Nondisplaced dome fracture of left acetabulum**   MCC CC

7,18 √7ᵗʰ **S32.486**   **Nondisplaced dome fracture of unspecified acetabulum**   MCC CC

√6ᵗʰ **S32.49**   Other specified fracture of acetabulum

7,18 √7ᵗʰ **S32.491**   **Other specified fracture of right acetabulum**   MCC CC

7,18 √7ᵗʰ **S32.492**   **Other specified fracture of left acetabulum**   MCC CC

7,18 √7ᵗʰ **S32.499**   **Other specified fracture of unspecified acetabulum**   MCC CC

√5ᵗʰ **S32.5**   **Fracture of pubis**

EXCLUDES 1   fracture of pubis with associated disruption of pelvic ring (S32.8-)

CC Excl: For CC/MCC codes in subcategory S32.5, unless otherwise noted: CC with 7th character A or MCC with 7th character B: M48.40X-M48.58X with 7th A, M80.00X-M84.68X with 7th A, S03.8XX-S03.9XX with 7th A, S22.9XX-S22.9XX with 7th [A, B], S29.011-S29.019 with 7th A, S32.501-S32.599 with 7th [A, B], S32.810-S32.811 with 7th [A, B], S32.89X-S32.9XX with 7th [A, B], S33.4XXA, S33.6XX-S33.8XX with 7th A, S38.3X-S39.013 with 7th A, S73.001-S73.199 with 7th A, S76.001-S76.019 with 7th A, S76.091-S76.119 with 7th A, S76.191-S76.219 A, S76.291-S76.319 with 7th A, S76.391-S76.819 with 7th A, S76.891-S76.919 with 7th A, S76.991-S76.999 with 7th A, S79.811-S79.929 with 7th A, T14.90-T14.91, T79.A0X-T79.9XX with 7th A

CC with 7th character K: M80.00X-M84.68X with 7th [K, P], S02.0XX-S02.92X with 7th K, S12.000-S12.691 with 7th K, S22.000-S22.9XX with 7th K, S32.000-S32.9XX with 7th K, S42.001-S42.92X with 7th [K, P], S49.001-S49.199 with 7th [K, P], S52.001-S52.92X with 7th [K, M, N, P, Q, R], S59.001-S59.299 with 7th [K, P], S62.001-S62.92X with 7th [K, P], S72.001-S72.92X with 7th [K, M, N, P, Q, R], S79.001-S79.199 with 7th [K, P], S82.001-S82.92X with 7th [K, M, N, P, Q, R], S89.001-S89.399 with 7th [K, P], S92.001-S92.919 with 7th [K, P]

√6ᵗʰ **S32.50**   Unspecified fracture of pubis

7,16,19 √7ᵗʰ **S32.501**   **Unspecified fracture of right pubis**   MCC CC

7,16,19 √7ᵗʰ **S32.502**   **Unspecified fracture of left pubis**   MCC CC

7,16,19 √7ᵗʰ **S32.509**   **Unspecified fracture of unspecified pubis**   MCC CC

√6ᵗʰ **S32.51**   Fracture of superior rim of pubis

7,16,19 √7ᵗʰ **S32.511**   **Fracture of superior rim of right pubis**   MCC CC

7,16,19 √7ᵗʰ **S32.512**   **Fracture of superior rim of left pubis**   MCC CC

7,16,19 √7ᵗʰ **S32.519**   **Fracture of superior rim of unspecified pubis**   MCC CC

√6ᵗʰ **S32.59**   Other specified fracture of pubis

7,16,19 √7ᵗʰ **S32.591**   **Other specified fracture of right pubis**   MCC CC

7,16,19 √7ᵗʰ **S32.592**   **Other specified fracture of left pubis**   MCC CC

7,16,19 √7ᵗʰ **S32.599**   **Other specified fracture of unspecified pubis**   MCC CC

√5ᵗʰ **S32.6**   **Fracture of ischium**

EXCLUDES 1   fracture of ischium with associated disruption of pelvic ring (S32.8-)

CC Excl: For CC/MCC codes in subcategory S32.6, unless otherwise noted: CC with 7th character A: S32.601-S32.699 with 7th A

MCC with 7th character B: M48.40X-M48.58X with 7th A, M80.00X-M84.68X with 7th A, S03.8XX-S03.9XX with 7th A, S22.9XX-S22.9XX with 7th [A, B], S29.011-S29.019 with 7th A, S32.601-S32.811 with 7th [A, B], S32.89X-S32.9XX with 7th [A, B], S33.4XX with 7th A, S33.6XX-S33.8XX with 7th A, S38.3XX-S39.013 with 7th A, S73.001-S73.199 with 7th A, S76.001-S76.019 with 7th A, S76.091-S76.119 with 7th A, S76.191-S76.219 with 7th A, S76.291-S76.319 with 7th A, S76.391-S76.819 with 7th A, S76.891-S76.919 with 7th A, S76.991-S76.999 with 7th A, S79.811-S79.929 with 7th A, T14.90-T14.91, T79.A0X-T79.9XX with 7th A

CC with 7th character K: M80.00X-M84.68X with 7th [K, P], S02.0XX-S02.92X with 7th K, S12.000-S12.691 with 7th K, S22.000-S22.9XX with 7th K, S32.000-S32.9XX with 7th K, S42.001-S42.92X with 7th [K, P], S49.001-S49.199 with 7th [K, P], S52.001-S52.92X with 7th [K, M, N, P, Q, R], S59.001-S59.299 with 7th [K, P], S62.001-S62.92X with 7th [K, P], S72.001-S72.92X with 7th [K, M, N, P, Q, R], S79.001-S79.199 with 7th [K, P], S82.001-S82.92X with 7th [K, M, N, P, Q, R], S89.001-S89.399 with 7th [K, P], S92.001-S92.919 with 7th [K, P]

√6ᵗʰ **S32.60**   Unspecified fracture of ischium

7,16,19 √7ᵗʰ **S32.601**   **Unspecified fracture of right ischium**   MCC CC

7,16,19 √7ᵗʰ **S32.602**   **Unspecified fracture of left ischium**   MCC CC

7,16,19 √7ᵗʰ **S32.609**   **Unspecified fracture of unspecified ischium**   MCC CC

√6ᵗʰ **S32.61**   Avulsion fracture of ischium

7,16,19 √7ᵗʰ **S32.611**   **Displaced avulsion fracture of right ischium**   MCC CC

7,16,19 √7ᵗʰ **S32.612**   **Displaced avulsion fracture of left ischium**   MCC CC

7,16,19 √7ᵗʰ **S32.613**   **Displaced avulsion fracture of unspecified ischium**   MCC CC

7,16,19 √7ᵗʰ **S32.614**   **Nondisplaced avulsion fracture of right ischium**   MCC CC

7,16,19 √7ᵗʰ **S32.615**   **Nondisplaced avulsion fracture of left ischium**   MCC CC

7,16,19 √7ᵗʰ **S32.616**   **Nondisplaced avulsion fracture of unspecified ischium**   MCC CC

√6ᵗʰ **S32.69**   Other specified fracture of ischium

7,16,19 √7ᵗʰ **S32.691**   **Other specified fracture of right ischium**   MCC CC

7,16,19 √7ᵗʰ **S32.692**   **Other specified fracture of left ischium**   MCC CC

7,16,19 √7ᵗʰ **S32.699**   **Other specified fracture of unspecified ischium**   MCC CC

---

7   HAC = Initial encounter only (7th character A, B or C) and not POA.
16   MCC only if an open fracture (7th character B or C – specific to category).
18   CC only if a subsequent encounter for nonunion or malunion (7th character K, M, N, P, Q, or R – specific to category).
19   CC only if an initial encounter for a closed fracture (7th character A) **OR** a subsequent encounter for nonunion or malunion (7th character K, M, N, P, Q, or R – specific to category).

N Newborn: 0   P Pediatric: 0-17   M Maternity: 12-55   A Adult: 15-124   MCC Major CC Condition   PDxMCC PDx acts as own MCC   CC CC Condition   PDxCC PDx acts as own CC

☑5ᵗʰ S32.8 Fracture of other parts of pelvis
Code also any associated:
fracture of acetabulum (S32.4-)
sacral fracture (S32.1-)

☑6ᵗʰ S32.81 Multiple fractures of pelvis with disruption of pelvic ring
Multiple pelvic fractures with disruption of pelvic circle

CC Excl: For CC/MCC codes in subcategory S32.81, unless otherwise noted: CC with 7th character A or MCC with 7th character B: M48.40X-M48.58X with 7th A, M80.00X-M84.68X with 7th A, S03.8XX-S03.9XX with 7th A, S22.9XX-S22.9XX with 7th [A, B], S29.011-S29.019 with 7th A, S32.301-S32.811 with 7th [A, B], S32.89X-S32.9XX with 7th [A, B], S33.4XX with 7th A, S33.6XX-S33.8XX with 7th A, S38.3XX-S39.013 with 7th A, S73.001-S73.199 with 7th A, S76.001-S76.019 with 7th A, S76.091-S76.119 with 7th A, S76.191-S76.219 with 7th A, S76.291-S76.319 with 7th A, S76.391-S76.819 with 7th A, S76.891-S76.919 with 7th A, S76.991-S76.999 with 7th A, S79.811-S79.929 with 7th A, T14.90-T14.91, T79.A0X-T79.9XX with 7th A
CC with 7th character K: M80.00X-M84.68X with 7th [K, P], S02.0XX-S02.92X with 7th K, S12.000-S12.691 with 7th K, S22.000-S22.9XX with 7th K, S32.000-S32.9XX with 7th K, S42.001-S42.92X with 7th [K, P], S49.001-S49.199 with 7th [K, P], S52.001-S52.92X with 7th [K, M, N, P, Q, R], S59.001-S59.299 with 7th [K, P], S62.001-S62.92X with 7th [K, P], S72.001-S72.92X with 7th [K, M, N, P, Q, R], S79.001-S79.199 with 7th [K, P], S82.001-S82.92X with 7th [K, M, N, P, Q, R], S89.001-S89.399 with 7th [K, P], S92.001-S92.919 with 7th [K, P]

7,16,19 ☑7ᵗʰ **S32.810 Multiple fractures of pelvis with stable disruption of pelvic ring** MCC CC

7,16,19 ☑7ᵗʰ **S32.811 Multiple fractures of pelvis with unstable disruption of pelvic ring** MCC CC

7,16,19 ✓ₓ7ᵗʰ **S32.82 Multiple fractures of pelvis without disruption of pelvic ring** MCC CC
Multiple pelvic fractures without disruption of pelvic circle
CC Excl: CC with 7th character A or MCC with 7th character B: S32.89 with 7th A
CC with 7th character K: M80.00X-M84.68X with 7th [K, P], S02.0XX-S02.92X with 7th K, S12.000-S12.691 with 7th K, S22.000-S22.9XX with 7th K, S32.000-S32.9XX with 7th K, S42.001-S42.92X with 7th [K, P], S49.001-S49.199 with 7th [K, P], S52.001-S52.92X with 7th [K, M, N, P, Q, R], S59.001-S59.299 with 7th [K, P], S62.001-S62.92X with 7th [K, P], S72.001-S72.92X with 7th [K, M, N, P, Q, R], S79.001-S79.199 with 7th [K, P], S82.001-S82.92X with 7th [K, M, N, P, Q, R], S89.001-S89.399 with 7th [K, P], S92.001-S92.919 with 7th [K, P]

7,16,19 ✓ₓ7ᵗʰ **S32.89 Fracture of other parts of pelvis** MCC CC
CC Excl: CC with 7th character A or MCC with 7th character B: M48.40X-M48.58X with 7th A, M80.00X-M84.68X with 7th A, S03.8XX-S03.9XX with 7th A, S22.9XX-S22.9XX with 7th [A, B], S29.011-S29.019 with 7th A, S32.301-S32.9XX with 7th [A, B], S33.4XX with 7th A, S33.6XX-S33.8XX with 7th A, S38.3X-S39.013 with 7th A, S73.001-S73.199 with 7th A, S76.001-S76.019 with 7th A, S76.091-S76.119 with 7th A, S76.191-S76.219 with 7th A, S76.291-S76.319 with 7th A, S76.391-S76.819 with 7th A, S76.891-S76.919 with 7th A, S76.991-S76.999 with 7th A, S79.811-S79.929 with 7th A, T14.90-T14.91, T79.A0X-T79.9XX with 7th A
CC with 7th character K: M80.00X-M84.68X with 7th [K, P], S02.0XX-S02.92X with 7th K, S12.000-S12.691 with 7th K, S22.000-S22.9XX with 7th K, S32.000-S32.9XX with 7th K, S42.001-S42.92X with 7th [K, P], S49.001-S49.199 with 7th [K, P], S52.001-S52.92X with 7th [K, M, N, P, Q, R], S59.001-S59.299 with 7th [K, P], S62.001-S62.92X with 7th [K, M, N, P, Q, R], S72.001-S72.92X with 7th [K, M, N, P, Q, R], S79.001-S79.199 with 7th [K, P], S82.001-S82.92X with 7th [K, M, N, P, Q, R], S89.001-S89.399 with 7th [K, P], S92.001-S92.919 with 7th [K, P]

7,16,19 ✓ₓ7ᵗʰ **S32.9 Fracture of unspecified parts of lumbosacral spine and pelvis** MCC CC
Fracture of lumbosacral spine NOS
Fracture of pelvis NOS
AHA: 2012, 4Q, 93
CC Excl: See code: S32.81

☑4ᵗʰ S33 Dislocation and sprain of joints and ligaments of lumbar spine and pelvis
INCLUDES avulsion of joint or ligament of lumbar spine and pelvis
laceration of cartilage, joint or ligament of lumbar spine and pelvis
sprain of cartilage, joint or ligament of lumbar spine and pelvis
traumatic hemarthrosis of joint or ligament of lumbar spine and pelvis
traumatic rupture of joint or ligament of lumbar spine and pelvis
traumatic subluxation of joint or ligament of lumbar spine and pelvis
traumatic tear of joint or ligament of lumbar spine and pelvis
Code also any associated open wound
EXCLUDES 1 nontraumatic rupture or displacement of lumbar intervertebral disc NOS (M51.-)
obstetric damage to pelvic joints and ligaments (O71.6)
EXCLUDES 2 dislocation and sprain of joints and ligaments of hip (S73.-)
strain of muscle of lower back and pelvis (S39.01-)

The appropriate 7th is to be added to each code from category S33.
A   initial encounter
D   subsequent encounter
S   sequela

✓ₓ7ᵗʰ S33.0 Traumatic rupture of lumbar intervertebral disc
EXCLUDES 1 rupture or displacement (nontraumatic) of lumbar intervertebral disc NOS (M51- with fifth character 6)

☑5ᵗʰ S33.1 Subluxation and dislocation of lumbar vertebra
Code also any associated:
open wound of abdomen, lower back and pelvis (S31)
spinal cord injury (S24.0, S24.1-, S34.0-, S34.1-)
EXCLUDES 2 fracture of lumbar vertebrae (S32.0-)

☑6ᵗʰ S33.10 Subluxation and dislocation of unspecified lumbar vertebra
☑7ᵗʰ S33.100 Subluxation of unspecified lumbar vertebra
☑7ᵗʰ S33.101 Dislocation of unspecified lumbar vertebra

☑6ᵗʰ S33.11 Subluxation and dislocation of L1/L2 lumbar vertebra
☑7ᵗʰ S33.110 Subluxation of L1/L2 lumbar vertebra
☑7ᵗʰ S33.111 Dislocation of L1/L2 lumbar vertebra

☑6ᵗʰ S33.12 Subluxation and dislocation of L2/L3 lumbar vertebra
☑7ᵗʰ S33.120 Subluxation of L2/L3 lumbar vertebra
☑7ᵗʰ S33.121 Dislocation of L2/L3 lumbar vertebra

☑6ᵗʰ S33.13 Subluxation and dislocation of L3/L4 lumbar vertebra
☑7ᵗʰ S33.130 Subluxation of L3/L4 lumbar vertebra
☑7ᵗʰ S33.131 Dislocation of L3/L4 lumbar vertebra

☑6ᵗʰ S33.14 Subluxation and dislocation of L4/L5 lumbar vertebra
☑7ᵗʰ S33.140 Subluxation of L4/L5 lumbar vertebra
☑7ᵗʰ S33.141 Dislocation of L4/L5 lumbar vertebra

✓ₓ7ᵗʰ S33.2 Dislocation of sacroiliac and sacrococcygeal joint

☑5ᵗʰ S33.3 Dislocation of other and unspecified parts of lumbar spine and pelvis
✓ₓ7ᵗʰ S33.30 Dislocation of unspecified parts of lumbar spine and pelvis
✓ₓ7ᵗʰ S33.39 Dislocation of other parts of lumbar spine and pelvis

✓ₓ7ᵗʰ S33.4 Traumatic rupture of symphysis pubis
✓ₓ7ᵗʰ S33.5 Sprain of ligaments of lumbar spine
✓ₓ7ᵗʰ S33.6 Sprain of sacroiliac joint
✓ₓ7ᵗʰ S33.8 Sprain of other parts of lumbar spine and pelvis
✓ₓ7ᵗʰ S33.9 Sprain of unspecified parts of lumbar spine and pelvis

---

7 HAC = Initial encounter only (7th character A, B or C) and not POA.
16 MCC only if an open fracture (7th character B or C – specific to category).
19 CC only if an initial encounter for a closed fracture (7th character A) **OR** a subsequent encounter for nonunion or malunion (7th character K, M, N, P, Q, or R – specific to category).

☑ Additional Character Required   ✓ₓ7ᵗʰ Placeholder Alert   Unacceptable PDx   Manifestation   Hospital Acquired Condition   EXCLUDES1 Not Coded Here   EXCLUDES2 Not Included Here

✓4ᵗʰ S34 Injury of lumbar and sacral spinal cord and nerves at abdomen, lower back and pelvis level

> **NOTE** Code to highest level of lumbar cord injury.
> Injuries to the spinal cord (S34.0 and S34.1) refer to the cord level and not bone level injury, and can affect nerve roots at and below the level given.

Code also any associated:
fracture of vertebra (S22.0-, S32.0-)
open wound of abdomen, lower back and pelvis (S31.-)
transient paralysis (R29.5)

> The appropriate 7th is to be added to each code from category S34.
> A   initial encounter
> D   subsequent encounter
> S   sequela

✓5ᵗʰ S34.0 Concussion and edema of lumbar and sacral spinal cord

✓x7ᵗʰ S34.01 Concussion and edema of lumbar spinal cord
CC Excl: MCC with 7th character A: M48.40X-M48.58X with 7th S, M80.08XS, M80.88XS, M84.350S, M84.454S, M84.550S, M84.58XS, M84.650S, M99.15-M99.17, M99.19, S03.1XXA, S12.000-S12.9XX with 7th S, S13.9XXA, S14.109A, S14.119A, S14.129A, S14.139A, S14.149A, S14.159A, S22.000-S22.9X with 7th S, S23.20X-S23.29X with 7th A, S23.9XXA, S24.109A, S24.119A, S24.139A, S24.149A, S24.159A, S29.001-S29.009 with 7th A, S29.091-S29.9XX with 7th A, S32.000-S32.9XX with 7th S, S33.30X-S33.39X with 7th A, S33.9XX-S34.01X with 7th A, S34.101-S34.129 with 7th A, S38.1XA, S39.001-S39.003 with 7th A, S39.091-S39.94X with 7th A, T14.90-T14.91, T79.A0X-T79.9XX with 7th A

✓x7ᵗʰ S34.02 Concussion and edema of sacral spinal cord MCC
Concussion and edema of conus medullaris
CC Excl: MCC with 7th character A: M48.40X-M48.58X with 7th S, M80.08XS, M80.88XS, M84.350S, M84.454S, M84.550S, M84.58XS, M84.650S, M99.15-M99.17, M99.19, S03.1XXA, S12.000-S12.9XX with 7th S, S13.9XXA, S14.109A, S14.119A, S14.129A, S14.139A, S14.149A, S14.159A, S22.000-S22.9XX with 7th S, S23.20X-S23.29X with 7th A, S23.9XA, S24.109A, S24.119A, S24.139A, S24.149A, S24.159A, S29.001-S29.009 with 7th A, S29.091-S29.9XX with 7th A, S32.000-S32.9XX with 7th S, S33.30X-S33.39X with 7th A, S33.9XX-S34.02X with 7th A, S34.131-S34.139 with 7th A, S34.3XXA, S38.1XA, S39.001-S39.003 with 7th A, S39.091-S39.94X with 7th A, T14.90-T14.91, T79.A0X-T79.9XX with 7th A

✓5ᵗʰ S34.1 Other and unspecified injury of lumbar and sacral spinal cord

✓6ᵗʰ S34.10 Unspecified injury to lumbar spinal cord

> CC Excl: For MCC codes in subcategory S34.10, unless otherwise noted: MCC with 7th character A: M48.40X-M48.58X with 7th S, M80.08XS, M80.88XS, M84.350S, M84.454S, M84.550S, M84.58XS, M84.650S, M99.15-M99.17, M99.19, S03.1XXA, S12.000-S12.9XX with 7th S, S13.9XXA, S14.109A, S14.119A, S14.129A, S14.139A, S14.149A, S14.159A, S22.000-S22.9XX with 7th S, S23.20X-S23.29X with 7th A, S23.9XA, S24.109A, S24.119A, S24.139A, S24.149A, S24.159A, S29.001-S29.009 with 7th A, S29.091-S29.9XX with 7th A, S32.000-S32.9XX with 7th S, S33.30X-S33.39X with 7th A, S33.9XX-S34.01X with 7th A, S34.101-S34.129 with 7th A, S38.1XA, S39.001-S39.003 with 7th A, S39.091-S39.94X with 7th A, T14.90-T14.91, T79.A0X-T79.9XX with 7th A

7 ✓7ᵗʰ S34.101 **Unspecified injury to L1 level of lumbar spinal cord** MCC

7 ✓7ᵗʰ S34.102 **Unspecified injury to L2 level of lumbar spinal cord** MCC

7 ✓7ᵗʰ S34.103 **Unspecified injury to L3 level of lumbar spinal cord** MCC

7 ✓7ᵗʰ S34.104 **Unspecified injury to L4 level of lumbar spinal cord** MCC

7 ✓7ᵗʰ S34.105 **Unspecified injury to L5 level of lumbar spinal cord** MCC

7 ✓7ᵗʰ S34.109 **Unspecified injury to unspecified level of lumbar spinal cord** MCC

✓6ᵗʰ S34.11 Complete lesion of lumbar spinal cord

> CC Excl: For MCC codes in subcategory S34.11, unless otherwise noted: See code: S34.10

7 ✓7ᵗʰ S34.111 **Complete lesion of L1 level of lumbar spinal cord** MCC

7 ✓7ᵗʰ S34.112 **Complete lesion of L2 level of lumbar spinal cord** MCC

7 ✓7ᵗʰ S34.113 **Complete lesion of L3 level of lumbar spinal cord** MCC

7 ✓7ᵗʰ S34.114 **Complete lesion of L4 level of lumbar spinal cord** MCC

7 ✓7ᵗʰ S34.115 **Complete lesion of L5 level of lumbar spinal cord** MCC

7 ✓7ᵗʰ S34.119 **Complete lesion of unspecified level of lumbar spinal cord** MCC

✓6ᵗʰ S34.12 Incomplete lesion of lumbar spinal cord

> CC Excl: For MCC codes in subcategory S34.12, unless otherwise noted: See code: S34.10

7 ✓7ᵗʰ S34.121 **Incomplete lesion of L1 level of lumbar spinal cord** MCC

7 ✓7ᵗʰ S34.122 **Incomplete lesion of L2 level of lumbar spinal cord** MCC

7 ✓7ᵗʰ S34.123 **Incomplete lesion of L3 level of lumbar spinal cord** MCC

7 ✓7ᵗʰ S34.124 **Incomplete lesion of L4 level of lumbar spinal cord** MCC

7 ✓7ᵗʰ S34.125 **Incomplete lesion of L5 level of lumbar spinal cord** MCC

7 ✓7ᵗʰ S34.129 **Incomplete lesion of unspecified level of lumbar spinal cord** MCC

✓6ᵗʰ S34.13 Other and unspecified injury to sacral spinal cord
Other injury to conus medullaris

> CC Excl: For MCC codes in subcategory S34.13, unless otherwise noted: MCC with 7th character A: M48.40X-M48.58X with 7th S, M80.08XS, M80.88XS, M84.350S, M84.454S, M84.550S, M84.58XS, M84.650S, M99.15-M99.17, M99.19, S03.1XXA, S12.000-S12.9XX with 7th S, S13.9XXA, S14.109A, S14.119A, S14.129A, S14.139A, S14.149A, S14.159A, S22.000-S22.9XX with 7th S, S23.20X-S23.29X with 7th A, S23.9XXA, S24.109A, S24.119A, S24.139A, S24.149A, S24.159A, S29.001-S29.009 with 7th A, S29.091-S29.9XX with 7th A, S32.000-S32.9XX with 7th S, S33.30X-S33.39X with 7th A, S33.9XX-S34.02X with 7th A, S34.131-S34.139 with 7th A, S34.3XXA, S38.1XA, S39.001-S39.003 with 7th A, S39.091-S39.94X with 7th A, T14.90-T14.91, T79.A0X-T79.9XX with 7th A

7 ✓7ᵗʰ S34.131 **Complete lesion of sacral spinal cord** MCC
Complete lesion of conus medullaris

7 ✓7ᵗʰ S34.132 **Incomplete lesion of sacral spinal cord** MCC
Incomplete lesion of conus medullaris

7 ✓7ᵗʰ S34.139 **Unspecified injury to sacral spinal cord** MCC
Unspecified injury of conus medullaris

✓5ᵗʰ S34.2 Injury of nerve root of lumbar and sacral spine

✓x7ᵗʰ S34.21 Injury of nerve root of lumbar spine

✓x7ᵗʰ S34.22 Injury of nerve root of sacral spine

7 ✓x7ᵗʰ **S34.3 Injury of cauda equina** MCC
CC Excl: See code: S34.13

✓x7ᵗʰ S34.4 Injury of lumbosacral plexus

✓x7ᵗʰ S34.5 Injury of lumbar, sacral and pelvic sympathetic nerves
Injury of celiac ganglion or plexus
Injury of hypogastric plexus
Injury of mesenteric plexus (inferior) (superior)
Injury of splanchnic nerve

✓x7ᵗʰ S34.6 Injury of peripheral nerve(s) at abdomen, lower back and pelvis level

✓x7ᵗʰ S34.8 Injury of other nerves at abdomen, lower back and pelvis level

✓x7ᵗʰ S34.9 Injury of unspecified nerves at abdomen, lower back and pelvis level

---

7   HAC = Initial encounter only (7th character A, B or C) and not POA.

Ⓝ Newborn: 0   Ⓟ Pediatric: 0-17   Ⓜ Maternity: 12-55   Ⓐ Adult: 15-124   MCC Major CC Condition   PDxMCC PDx acts as own MCC   CC CC Condition   PDxCC PDx acts as own CC

938   ICD-10-CM 2016

☑️4th **S35 Injury of blood vessels at abdomen, lower back and pelvis level**
Code also any associated open wound (S31.-)

The appropriate 7th is to be added to each code from category S35.
A   initial encounter
D   subsequent encounter
S   sequela

☑️5th **S35.0 Injury of abdominal aorta**
EXCLUDES 1 injury of aorta NOS (S25.0)

CC Excl: For MCC codes in subcategory S35.0, unless otherwise noted: MCC with 7th character A: S35.00X-S35.09X with 7th A, S35.8X1-S35.99X with 7th A, T14.90-T14.91, T79.A0X-T79.9XX with 7th A

☑️x7th **S35.00 Unspecified injury of abdominal aorta**   `MCC`
☑️x7th **S35.01 Minor laceration of abdominal aorta**   `MCC`
Incomplete transection of abdominal aorta
Laceration of abdominal aorta NOS
Superficial laceration of abdominal aorta

☑️x7th **S35.02 Major laceration of abdominal aorta**   `MCC`
Complete transection of abdominal aorta
Traumatic rupture of abdominal aorta

☑️x7th **S35.09 Other injury of abdominal aorta**   `MCC`

☑️5th **S35.1 Injury of inferior vena cava**
Injury of hepatic vein
EXCLUDES 1 injury of vena cava NOS (S25.2)

CC Excl: For MCC codes in subcategory S35.1, unless otherwise noted: MCC with 7th character A: S35.10X-S35.19X with 7th A, S35.8X1-S35.99X with 7th A, T14.90-T14.91, T79.A0X-T79.9XX with 7th A

☑️x7th **S35.10 Unspecified injury of inferior vena cava**   `MCC`
☑️x7th **S35.11 Minor laceration of inferior vena cava**   `MCC`
Incomplete transection of inferior vena cava
Laceration of inferior vena cava NOS
Superficial laceration of inferior vena cava

☑️x7th **S35.12 Major laceration of inferior vena cava**   `MCC`
Complete transection of inferior vena cava
Traumatic rupture of inferior vena cava

☑️x7th **S35.19 Other injury of inferior vena cava**   `MCC`

☑️5th **S35.2 Injury of celiac or mesenteric artery and branches**
☑️6th **S35.21 Injury of celiac artery**

CC Excl: For MCC codes in subcategory S35.21, unless otherwise noted: MCC with 7th character A: S35.211-S35.219 with 7th A, S35.8X1-S35.99X with 7th A, T14.90-T14.91, T79.A0X-T79.9XX with 7th A

☑️7th **S35.211 Minor laceration of celiac artery**   `MCC`
Incomplete transection of celiac artery
Laceration of celiac artery NOS
Superficial laceration of celiac artery

☑️7th **S35.212 Major laceration of celiac artery**   `MCC`
Complete transection of celiac artery
Traumatic rupture of celiac artery

☑️7th **S35.218 Other injury of celiac artery**   `MCC`
☑️7th **S35.219 Unspecified injury of celiac artery**   `MCC`

☑️6th **S35.22 Injury of superior mesenteric artery**

CC Excl: For MCC codes in subcategory S35.22, unless otherwise noted: MCC with 7th character A: S35.221-S35.229 with 7th A, S35.8X1-S35.99X with 7th A, T14.90-T14.91, T79.A0X-T79.9XX with 7th A

☑️7th **S35.221 Minor laceration of superior mesenteric artery**   `MCC`
Incomplete transection of superior mesenteric artery
Laceration of superior mesenteric artery NOS
Superficial laceration of superior mesenteric artery

☑️7th **S35.222 Major laceration of superior mesenteric artery**   `MCC`
Complete transection of superior mesenteric artery
Traumatic rupture of superior mesenteric artery

☑️7th **S35.228 Other injury of superior mesenteric artery**   `MCC`

☑️7th **S35.229 Unspecified injury of superior mesenteric artery**   `MCC`

☑️6th **S35.23 Injury of inferior mesenteric artery**

CC Excl: For MCC codes in subcategory S35.23, unless otherwise noted: MCC with 7th character A: S35.231-S35.239 with 7th A, S35.8X1-S35.99X with 7th A, T14.90-T14.91, T79.A0X-T79.9XX with 7th A

☑️7th **S35.231 Minor laceration of inferior mesenteric artery**   `MCC`
Incomplete transection of inferior mesenteric artery
Laceration of inferior mesenteric artery NOS
Superficial laceration of inferior mesenteric artery

☑️7th **S35.232 Major laceration of inferior mesenteric artery**   `MCC`
Complete transection of inferior mesenteric artery
Traumatic rupture of inferior mesenteric artery

☑️7th **S35.238 Other injury of inferior mesenteric artery**   `MCC`

☑️7th **S35.239 Unspecified injury of inferior mesenteric artery**   `MCC`

☑️6th **S35.29 Injury of branches of celiac and mesenteric artery**
Injury of gastric artery
Injury of gastroduodenal artery
Injury of hepatic artery
Injury of splenic artery

☑️7th **S35.291 Minor laceration of branches of celiac and mesenteric artery**   `MCC`
Incomplete transection of branches of celiac and mesenteric artery
Laceration of branches of celiac and mesenteric artery NOS
Superficial laceration of branches of celiac and mesenteric artery
CC Excl: MCC with 7th character A: S35.291A, S35.8X1-S35.99X with 7th A, T14.90-T14.91, T79.A0X with 7th A, T79.A3X-T79.9XX with 7th A

☑️7th **S35.292 Major laceration of branches of celiac and mesenteric artery**   `MCC`
Complete transection of branches of celiac and mesenteric artery
Traumatic rupture of branches of celiac and mesenteric artery
CC Excl: MCC with 7th character A: S35.292-S35.298 with 7th A, S35.8X1-S35.99X with 7th A, T14.90-T14.91, T79.A0X-T79.9XX with 7th A

☑️7th **S35.298 Other injury of branches of celiac and mesenteric artery**   `MCC`
CC Excl: See code: S35.292

☑️7th **S35.299 Unspecified injury of branches of celiac and mesenteric artery**   `MCC`
CC Excl: MCC with 7th character A: S35.299A, S35.8X1-S35.99X with 7th A, T14.90-T14.91, T79.A0X-T79.9XX with 7th A

☑️5th **S35.3 Injury of portal or splenic vein and branches**
☑️6th **S35.31 Injury of portal vein**

CC Excl: For MCC codes in subcategory S35.31, unless otherwise noted: MCC with 7th character A: S35.311-S35.319 with 7th A, S35.8X1-S35.99X with 7th A, T14.90-T14.91, T79.A0X-T79.9XX with 7th A

☑️7th **S35.311 Laceration of portal vein**   `MCC`
☑️7th **S35.318 Other specified injury of portal vein**   `MCC`
☑️7th **S35.319 Unspecified injury of portal vein**   `MCC`

☑️6th **S35.32 Injury of splenic vein**

CC Excl: For MCC codes in subcategory S35.32, unless otherwise noted: MCC with 7th character A: S35.321-S35.329 with 7th A, S35.8X1-S35.99X with 7th A, T14.90-T14.91, T79.A0X-T79.9XX with 7th A

☑️7th **S35.321 Laceration of splenic vein**   `MCC`
☑️7th **S35.328 Other specified injury of splenic vein**   `MCC`

Chapter 19. Injury, Poisoning, and Certain Other Consequences of External Causes

S35–S35.328

Chapter 19. Injury, Poisoning, and Certain Other Consequences of External Causes

S35.329–S35.8X8

✓7ᵗʰ **S35.329** Unspecified **injury of splenic vein** `MCC`

✓6ᵗʰ **S35.33** Injury of **superior mesenteric vein**

> **CC Excl:** For MCC codes in subcategory S35.33, unless otherwise noted: MCC with 7th character A: S35.331-S35.339 with 7th A, S35.8X1-S35.99X with 7th A, T14.90-T14.91, T79.A0X-T79.9XX with 7th A

✓7ᵗʰ **S35.331** Laceration **of superior mesenteric vein** `MCC`

✓7ᵗʰ **S35.338** Other specified **injury of superior mesenteric vein** `MCC`

✓7ᵗʰ **S35.339** Unspecified **injury of superior mesenteric vein** `MCC`

✓6ᵗʰ **S35.34** Injury of **inferior mesenteric vein**

> **CC Excl:** For MCC codes in subcategory S35.34, unless otherwise noted: MCC with 7th character A: S35.341-S35.349 with 7th A, S35.8X1-S35.99X with 7th A, T14.90-T14.91, T79.A0X-T79.9XX with 7th A

✓7ᵗʰ **S35.341** Laceration **of inferior mesenteric vein** `MCC`

✓7ᵗʰ **S35.348** Other specified **injury of inferior mesenteric vein** `MCC`

✓7ᵗʰ **S35.349** Unspecified **injury of inferior mesenteric vein** `MCC`

✓5ᵗʰ **S35.4** Injury of **renal blood vessels**

✓6ᵗʰ **S35.40** Unspecified **injury of renal blood vessel**

✓7ᵗʰ **S35.401** Unspecified **injury of** right **renal artery** `MCC`
> **CC Excl:** MCC with 7th character A: S35.401-S35.403 with 7th A, S35.411-S35.413 with 7th A, S35.491-S35.493 with 7th A, S35.8X1-S35.99X with 7th A, T14.90-T14.91, T79.A0X-T79.9XX with 7th A

✓7ᵗʰ **S35.402** Unspecified **injury of** left **renal artery** `MCC`
> **CC Excl:** See code: S35.401

✓7ᵗʰ **S35.403** Unspecified **injury of** unspecified **renal artery** `MCC`
> **CC Excl:** See code: S35.401

✓7ᵗʰ **S35.404** Unspecified **injury of** right **renal vein** `MCC`
> **CC Excl:** MCC with 7th character A: S35.404-S35.406 with 7th A, S35.414-S35.416 with 7th A, S35.494-S35.496 with 7th A, S35.8X1-S35.99X with 7th A, T14.90-T14.91, T79.A0X-T79.9XX with 7th A

✓7ᵗʰ **S35.405** Unspecified **injury of** left **renal vein** `MCC`
> **CC Excl:** See code: S35.404

✓7ᵗʰ **S35.406** Unspecified **injury of** unspecified **renal vein** `MCC`
> **CC Excl:** See code: S35.404

✓6ᵗʰ **S35.41** Laceration **of renal blood vessel**

✓7ᵗʰ **S35.411** Laceration **of** right **renal artery** `MCC`
> **CC Excl:** MCC with 7th character A: S35.401-S35.403 with 7th A, S35.411-S35.413 with 7th A, S35.491-S35.493 with 7th A, S35.8X1-S35.99X with 7th A, T14.90-T14.91, T79.A0X-T79.9XX with 7th A

✓7ᵗʰ **S35.412** Laceration **of** left **renal artery** `MCC`
> **CC Excl:** See code: S35.411

✓7ᵗʰ **S35.413** Laceration **of** unspecified **renal artery** `MCC`
> **CC Excl:** See code: S35.411

✓7ᵗʰ **S35.414** Laceration **of** right **renal vein** `MCC`
> **CC Excl:** MCC with 7th character A: S35.404-S35.406 with 7th A, S35.414-S35.416 with 7th A, S35.494-S35.496 with 7th A, S35.8X1-S35.99X with 7th A, T14.90-T14.91, T79.A0X-T79.9XX with 7th A

✓7ᵗʰ **S35.415** Laceration **of** left **renal vein** `MCC`
> **CC Excl:** See code: S35.414

✓7ᵗʰ **S35.416** Laceration **of** unspecified **renal vein** `MCC`
> **CC Excl:** See code: S35.414

✓6ᵗʰ **S35.49** Other specified **injury of renal blood vessel**

✓7ᵗʰ **S35.491** Other specified **injury of** right **renal artery** `MCC`
> **CC Excl:** MCC with 7th character A: S35.401-S35.403 with 7th A, S35.411-S35.413 with 7th A, S35.491-S35.493 with 7th A, S35.8X1-S35.99X with 7th A, T14.90-T14.91, T79.A0X-T79.9XX with 7th A

✓7ᵗʰ **S35.492** Other specified **injury of** left **renal artery** `MCC`
> **CC Excl:** See code: S35.491

✓7ᵗʰ **S35.493** Other specified **injury of** unspecified **renal artery** `MCC`
> **CC Excl:** See code: S35.491

✓7ᵗʰ **S35.494** Other specified **injury of** right **renal vein** `MCC`
> **CC Excl:** MCC with 7th character A: S35.404-S35.406 with 7th A, S35.414-S35.416 with 7th A, S35.494-S35.496 with 7th A, S35.8X1-S35.99X with 7th A, T14.90-T14.91, T79.A0X-T79.9XX with 7th A

✓7ᵗʰ **S35.495** Other specified **injury of** left **renal vein** `MCC`
> **CC Excl:** See code: S35.494

✓7ᵗʰ **S35.496** Other specified **injury of** unspecified **renal vein** `MCC`
> **CC Excl:** See code: S35.494

✓5ᵗʰ **S35.5** Injury of **iliac blood vessels**

✓×7ᵗʰ **S35.50** Injury of **unspecified iliac blood vessel(s)** `MCC`
> **CC Excl:** MCC with 7th character A: S35.50X-S35.516 with 7th A, S35.59X-S35.99X with 7th A, T14.90-T14.91, T79.A0X-T79.9XX with 7th A

✓6ᵗʰ **S35.51** Injury of **iliac artery or vein**
Injury of hypogastric artery or vein

✓7ᵗʰ **S35.511** Injury of **right iliac artery** `MCC`
> **CC Excl:** MCC with 7th character A: S35.50X-S35.513 with 7th A, S35.59X-S35.99X with 7th A, T14.90-T14.91, T79.A0X-T79.9XX with 7th A

✓7ᵗʰ **S35.512** Injury of **left iliac artery** `MCC`
> **CC Excl:** See code: S35.511

✓7ᵗʰ **S35.513** Injury of **unspecified iliac artery** `MCC`
> **CC Excl:** See code: S35.511

✓7ᵗʰ **S35.514** Injury of **right iliac vein** `MCC`
> **CC Excl:** MCC with 7th character A: S35.50X-S35.516 with 7th A, S35.59X-S35.99X with 7th A, T14.90-T14.91, T79.A0X-T79.9XX with 7th A

✓7ᵗʰ **S35.515** Injury of **left iliac vein** `MCC`
> **CC Excl:** See code: S35.514

✓7ᵗʰ **S35.516** Injury of **unspecified iliac vein** `MCC`
> **CC Excl:** See code: S35.514

✓6ᵗʰ **S35.53** Injury of **uterine artery or vein**

✓7ᵗʰ **S35.531** Injury of **right uterine artery** `CC` ♀
> **CC Excl:** CC with 7th character A: S 35.50X with 7th A, S35.531-S35.99X with 7th A, T14.90-T14.91, T79.A0X with 7th A, T79.A3X-T79.9XX with 7th A

✓7ᵗʰ **S35.532** Injury of **left uterine artery** `CC` ♀
> **CC Excl:** See code: S35.531

✓7ᵗʰ **S35.533** Injury of **unspecified uterine artery** `CC` ♀
> **CC Excl:** See code: S35.531

✓7ᵗʰ **S35.534** Injury of **right uterine vein** `CC` ♀
> **CC Excl:** MCC with 7th character A: S35.50X with 7th A, S35.534-S35.99X with 7th A, T14.90-T14.91, T79.A0X with 7th A, T79.A3X-T79.9XX with 7th A

✓7ᵗʰ **S35.535** Injury of **left uterine vein** `CC` ♀
> **CC Excl:** See code: S35.534

✓7ᵗʰ **S35.536** Injury of **unspecified uterine vein** `CC` ♀
> **CC Excl:** See code: S35.534

✓×7ᵗʰ **S35.59** Injury of **other iliac blood vessels** `MCC`
> **CC Excl:** MCC with 7th character A: S35.50X-S35.516 with 7th A, S35.59X-S35.99X with 7th A, T14.90-T14.91, T79.A0X-T79.9XX with 7th A

✓5ᵗʰ **S35.8** Injury of **other blood vessels at abdomen, lower back and pelvis level**
Injury of ovarian artery or vein

✓6ᵗʰ **S35.8X** Injury of **other blood vessels at abdomen, lower back and pelvis level**

> **CC Excl:** For CC codes in subcategory S35.8X, unless otherwise noted: CC with 7th character A: S35.8X1-S35.99X with 7th A, T14.90-T14.91, T79.A0X with 7th A, T79.A3X-T79.9XX with 7th A

✓7ᵗʰ **S35.8X1** Laceration **of other blood vessels at abdomen, lower back and pelvis level** `CC`

✓7ᵗʰ **S35.8X8** Other specified **injury of other blood vessels at abdomen, lower back and pelvis level** `CC`

Ⓝ Newborn: 0   Ⓟ Pediatric: 0-17   Ⓜ Maternity: 12-55   Ⓐ Adult: 15-124   `MCC` Major CC Condition   `PDxMCC` PDx acts as own MCC   `CC` CC Condition   `PDxCC` PDx acts as own CC

940   ICD-10-CM 2016

☑7ᵗʰ **S35.8X9**   Unspecified **injury of other blood vessels at abdomen, lower back and pelvis level**   CC

☑5ᵗʰ **S35.9**   Injury of unspecified **blood vessel at abdomen, lower back and pelvis level**

CC Excl: For CC codes in subcategory S35.9: CC with 7th character A: S35.00-S35.99X with 7th A, T14.90-T14.91, T79.A0X with 7th A, T79.A3X-T79.9XX with 7th A

☑x7ᵗʰ **S35.90**   Unspecified **injury of unspecified blood vessel at abdomen, lower back and pelvis level**   CC

☑x7ᵗʰ **S35.91**   Laceration **of unspecified blood vessel at abdomen, lower back and pelvis level**   CC

☑x7ᵗʰ **S35.99**   Other specified **injury of unspecified blood vessel at abdomen, lower back and pelvis level**   CC

☑4ᵗʰ **S36**   **Injury of intra-abdominal organs**
Code also any associated open wound (S31.-)

The appropriate 7th is to be added to each code from category S36.
A   initial encounter
D   subsequent encounter
S   sequela

☑5ᵗʰ **S36.0**   **Injury of** spleen

CC Excl: For CC/MCC codes in subcategory S36.0, unless otherwise noted: CC or MCC as indicated with 7th A: S31.001A, S31.011A, S31.021A, S31.031A, S31.041A, S31.051-S31.159 with 7th A, S31.600-S31.659 with 7th A, S31.831-S31.839 with 7th A, S36.00X-S36.09X with 7th A, S36.81X-S36.99X with 7th A, S38.3XX-S39.023 with 7th A, T14.90-T14.91, T79.A0X-T79.9XX with 7th A

☑x7ᵗʰ **S36.00**   Unspecified **injury of spleen**   CC

☑6ᵗʰ **S36.02**   Contusion **of spleen**

☑7ᵗʰ **S36.020**   Minor **contusion of spleen**   CC
Contusion of spleen less than 2 cm

☑7ᵗʰ **S36.021**   Major **contusion of spleen**   CC
Contusion of spleen greater than 2 cm

☑7ᵗʰ **S36.029**   Unspecified **contusion of spleen**   CC

☑6ᵗʰ **S36.03**   Laceration **of spleen**

☑7ᵗʰ **S36.030**   Superficial (capsular) **laceration of spleen**   CC
Laceration of spleen less than 1cm
Minor laceration of spleen

☑7ᵗʰ **S36.031**   Moderate **laceration of spleen**   MCC
Laceration of spleen 1 to 3 cm

☑7ᵗʰ **S36.032**   Major **laceration of spleen**   MCC
Avulsion of spleen
Laceration of spleen greater than 3 cm
Massive laceration of spleen
Multiple moderate lacerations of spleen
Stellate laceration of spleen

☑7ᵗʰ **S36.039**   Unspecified **laceration of spleen**   CC

☑x7ᵗʰ **S36.09**   Other **injury of spleen**   CC

☑5ᵗʰ **S36.1**   **Injury of liver and gallbladder and bile duct**

☑6ᵗʰ **S36.11**   Injury of liver

CC Excl: For CC/MCC codes in subcategory S36.11, unless otherwise noted: CC or MCC as indicated with 7th A: S31.001A, S31.011A, S31.021A, S31.031A, S31.041A, S31.051-S31.159 with 7th A, S31.600-S31.659 with 7th A, S31.831-S31.839 with 7th A, S36.112-S36.119 with 7th A, S36.81X-S36.99X with 7th A, S38.3XX-S39.023 with 7th A, T14.90-T14.91, T79.A0X-T79.9XX with 7th A

☑7ᵗʰ **S36.112**   Contusion **of liver**   CC

☑7ᵗʰ **S36.113**   Laceration **of liver, unspecified degree**   CC

☑7ᵗʰ **S36.114**   Minor **laceration of liver**   CC
Laceration involving capsule only, or, without significant involvement of hepatic parenchyma [i.e., less than 1cm deep]

☑7ᵗʰ **S36.115**   Moderate **laceration of liver**   MCC
Laceration involving parenchyma but without major disruption of parenchyma [i.e., less than 10 cm long and less than 3 cm deep]

☑7ᵗʰ **S36.116**   Major **laceration of liver**   MCC
Laceration with significant disruption of hepatic parenchyma [i.e., greater than 10 cm long and 3 cm deep]
Multiple moderate lacerations, with or without hematoma
Stellate laceration of liver

☑7ᵗʰ **S36.118**   Other **injury of liver**   CC

☑7ᵗʰ **S36.119**   Unspecified **injury of liver**   CC

☑6ᵗʰ **S36.12**   Injury of **gallbladder**

CC Excl: For CC codes in subcategory S36.12, unless otherwise noted: CC with 7th character A: S31.001A, S31.011A, S31.021A, S31.031A, S31.041A, S31.051-S31.159 with 7th A, S31.600-S31.659 with 7th A, S31.831-S31.839 with 7th A, S36.122-S36.13X with 7th A, S36.81X-S36.99X with 7th A, S38.3XX-S39.023 with 7th A, T14.90-T14.91, T79.A0X-T79.9XX with 7th A

☑7ᵗʰ **S36.122**   Contusion **of gallbladder**   CC

☑7ᵗʰ **S36.123**   Laceration **of gallbladder**   CC

☑7ᵗʰ **S36.128**   Other **injury of gallbladder**   CC

☑7ᵗʰ **S36.129**   Unspecified **injury of gallbladder**   CC

☑x7ᵗʰ **S36.13**   Injury of **bile duct**   CC
CC Excl: See code: S36.12

☑5ᵗʰ **S36.2**   **Injury of** pancreas

CC Excl: For CC codes in subcategory S36.2, unless otherwise noted: CC with 7th character A: M79.A3, S31.001A, S31.011A, S31.021A, S31.031A, S31.041A, S31.051-S31.159 with 7th A, S31.600-S31.659 with 7th A, S31.831-S31.839 with 7th A, S36.200-S36.299 with 7th A, S36.81X-S36.99X with 7th A, S38.3XX-S39.023 with 7th A, T14.90-T14.91, T79.A3X-T79.9XX with 7th A

☑6ᵗʰ **S36.20**   Unspecified **injury of pancreas**

☑7ᵗʰ **S36.200**   Unspecified **injury of head of pancreas**   CC

☑7ᵗʰ **S36.201**   Unspecified **injury of body of pancreas**   CC

☑7ᵗʰ **S36.202**   Unspecified **injury of tail of pancreas**   CC

☑7ᵗʰ **S36.209**   Unspecified **injury of unspecified part of pancreas**   CC

☑6ᵗʰ **S36.22**   Contusion **of pancreas**

☑7ᵗʰ **S36.220**   Contusion of **head of pancreas**   CC

☑7ᵗʰ **S36.221**   Contusion of **body of pancreas**   CC

☑7ᵗʰ **S36.222**   Contusion of **tail of pancreas**   CC

☑7ᵗʰ **S36.229**   Contusion of **unspecified part of pancreas**   CC

☑6ᵗʰ **S36.23**   Laceration **of pancreas, unspecified degree**

☑7ᵗʰ **S36.230**   Laceration of **head of pancreas, unspecified degree**   CC

☑7ᵗʰ **S36.231**   Laceration of **body of pancreas, unspecified degree**   CC

☑7ᵗʰ **S36.232**   Laceration of **tail of pancreas, unspecified degree**   CC

☑7ᵗʰ **S36.239**   Laceration of **unspecified part of pancreas, unspecified degree**   CC

☑6ᵗʰ **S36.24**   Minor **laceration of pancreas**

☑7ᵗʰ **S36.240**   Minor **laceration of head of pancreas**   CC

☑7ᵗʰ **S36.241**   Minor **laceration of body of pancreas**   CC

☑7ᵗʰ **S36.242**   Minor **laceration of tail of pancreas**   CC

☑7ᵗʰ **S36.249**   Minor **laceration of unspecified part of pancreas**   CC

☑6ᵗʰ **S36.25**   Moderate **laceration of pancreas**

☑7ᵗʰ **S36.250**   Moderate **laceration of head of pancreas**   CC

☑7ᵗʰ **S36.251**   Moderate **laceration of body of pancreas**   CC

☑7ᵗʰ **S36.252**   Moderate **laceration of tail of pancreas**   CC

☑7ᵗʰ **S36.259**   Moderate **laceration of unspecified part of pancreas**   CC

☑6ᵗʰ **S36.26**   Major **laceration of pancreas**

☑7ᵗʰ **S36.260**   Major **laceration of head of pancreas**   CC

☑7ᵗʰ **S36.261**   Major **laceration of body of pancreas**   CC

☑7ᵗʰ **S36.262**   Major **laceration of tail of pancreas**   CC

☑7ᵗʰ **S36.269**   Major **laceration of unspecified part of pancreas**   CC

☑ Additional Character Required   ☑x7ᵗʰ Placeholder Alert   Unacceptable PDx   Manifestation   Hospital Acquired Condition   EXCLUDES 1 Not Coded Here   EXCLUDES 2 Not Included Here

ICD-10-CM 2016   941

√6th **S36.29** Other injury of pancreas
- √7th **S36.290** Other injury of head of pancreas ᴄᴄ
- √7th **S36.291** Other injury of body of pancreas ᴄᴄ
- √7th **S36.292** Other injury of tail of pancreas ᴄᴄ
- √7th **S36.299** Other injury of unspecified part of pancreas ᴄᴄ

√5th **S36.3** Injury of stomach

> **CC Excl: For CC codes in subcategory S36.3, unless otherwise noted: CC with 7th character A:** M79.A3, S31.001A, S31.011A, S31.021A, S31.031A, S31.041A, S31.051-S31.159 with 7th A, S31.600-S31.659 with 7th A, S31.831-S31.839 with 7th A, S36.30X-S36.39X with 7th A, S36.81X-S36.99X with 7th A, S38.3XX-S39.023 with 7th A, T14.90-T14.91, T79.A3X-T79.9XX with 7th A

√x7th **S36.30** Unspecified injury of stomach ᴄᴄ
√x7th **S36.32** Contusion of stomach ᴄᴄ
√x7th **S36.33** Laceration of stomach ᴄᴄ
√x7th **S36.39** Other injury of stomach ᴄᴄ

√5th **S36.4** Injury of small intestine

> **CC Excl: For CC codes in subcategory S36.4, unless otherwise noted: CC with 7th character A:** M79.A3, S31.001A, S31.011A, S31.021A, S31.031A, S31.041A, S31.051-S31.159 with 7th A, S31.600-S31.659 with 7th A, S31.831-S31.839 with 7th A, S36.400-S36.499 with 7th A, S36.81X-S36.99X with 7th A, S38.3XX-S39.023 with 7th A, T14.90-T14.91, T79.A3X-T79.9XX with 7th A

√6th **S36.40** Unspecified injury of small intestine
- √7th **S36.400** Unspecified injury of duodenum ᴄᴄ
- √7th **S36.408** Unspecified injury of other part of small intestine ᴄᴄ
- √7th **S36.409** Unspecified injury of unspecified part of small intestine ᴄᴄ

√6th **S36.41** Primary blast injury of small intestine
Blast injury of small intestine NOS
- √7th **S36.410** Primary blast injury of duodenum ᴄᴄ
- √7th **S36.418** Primary blast injury of other part of small intestine ᴄᴄ
- √7th **S36.419** Primary blast injury of unspecified part of small intestine ᴄᴄ

√6th **S36.42** Contusion of small intestine
- √7th **S36.420** Contusion of duodenum ᴄᴄ
- √7th **S36.428** Contusion of other part of small intestine ᴄᴄ
- √7th **S36.429** Contusion of unspecified part of small intestine ᴄᴄ

√6th **S36.43** Laceration of small intestine
- √7th **S36.430** Laceration of duodenum ᴄᴄ
- √7th **S36.438** Laceration of other part of small intestine ᴄᴄ
- √7th **S36.439** Laceration of unspecified part of small intestine ᴄᴄ

√6th **S36.49** Other injury of small intestine
- √7th **S36.490** Other injury of duodenum ᴄᴄ
- √7th **S36.498** Other injury of other part of small intestine ᴄᴄ
- √7th **S36.499** Other injury of unspecified part of small intestine ᴄᴄ

√5th **S36.5** Injury of colon
> *EXCLUDES 2* injury of rectum (S36.6-)

> **CC Excl: For CC/MCC codes in subcategory S36.5, unless otherwise noted: CC with 7th character A:** M79.A3, S31.001A, S31.011A, S31.021A, S31.031A, S31.041A, S31.051-S31.159 with 7th A, S31.600-S31.659 with 7th A, S31.831-S31.839 with 7th A, S36.500-S36.99X with 7th A, S38.3XX-S39.023 with 7th A, T14.90-T14.91, T79.A3X-T79.9XX with 7th A

√6th **S36.50** Unspecified injury of colon
- √7th **S36.500** Unspecified injury of ascending [right] colon ᴄᴄ
- √7th **S36.501** Unspecified injury of transverse colon ᴄᴄ
- √7th **S36.502** Unspecified injury of descending [left] colon ᴄᴄ
- √7th **S36.503** Unspecified injury of sigmoid colon ᴄᴄ

- √7th **S36.508** Unspecified injury of other part of colon ᴄᴄ
- √7th **S36.509** Unspecified injury of unspecified part of colon ᴄᴄ

√6th **S36.51** Primary blast injury of colon
Blast injury of colon NOS
- √7th **S36.510** Primary blast injury of ascending [right] colon ᴄᴄ
- √7th **S36.511** Primary blast injury of transverse colon ᴄᴄ
- √7th **S36.512** Primary blast injury of descending [left] colon ᴄᴄ
- √7th **S36.513** Primary blast injury of sigmoid colon ᴄᴄ
- √7th **S36.518** Primary blast injury of other part of colon ᴄᴄ
- √7th **S36.519** Primary blast injury of unspecified part of colon ᴄᴄ

√6th **S36.52** Contusion of colon
- √7th **S36.520** Contusion of ascending [right] colon ᴄᴄ
- √7th **S36.521** Contusion of transverse colon ᴄᴄ
- √7th **S36.522** Contusion of descending [left] colon ᴄᴄ
- √7th **S36.523** Contusion of sigmoid colon ᴄᴄ
- √7th **S36.528** Contusion of other part of colon ᴄᴄ
- √7th **S36.529** Contusion of unspecified part of colon ᴄᴄ

√6th **S36.53** Laceration of colon
- √7th **S36.530** Laceration of ascending [right] colon ᴄᴄ
- √7th **S36.531** Laceration of transverse colon ᴄᴄ
- √7th **S36.532** Laceration of descending [left] colon ᴄᴄ
- √7th **S36.533** Laceration of sigmoid colon ᴄᴄ
- √7th **S36.538** Laceration of other part of colon ᴄᴄ
- √7th **S36.539** Laceration of unspecified part of colon ᴄᴄ

√6th **S36.59** Other injury of colon
Secondary blast injury of colon
- √7th **S36.590** Other injury of ascending [right] colon ᴄᴄ
- √7th **S36.591** Other injury of transverse colon ᴄᴄ
- √7th **S36.592** Other injury of descending [left] colon ᴄᴄ
- √7th **S36.593** Other injury of sigmoid colon ᴄᴄ
- √7th **S36.598** Other injury of other part of colon ᴄᴄ
- √7th **S36.599** Other injury of unspecified part of colon ᴄᴄ

√5th **S36.6** Injury of rectum

> **CC Excl: For CC codes in subcategory S36.6, unless otherwise noted: CC with 7th character A: See Code:** S86.5

√x7th **S36.60** Unspecified injury of rectum ᴄᴄ
√x7th **S36.61** Primary blast injury of rectum ᴄᴄ
Blast injury of rectum NOS
√x7th **S36.62** Contusion of rectum ᴄᴄ
√x7th **S36.63** Laceration of rectum ᴄᴄ
√x7th **S36.69** Other injury of rectum ᴄᴄ
Secondary blast injury of rectum

√5th **S36.8** Injury of other intra-abdominal organs

> **CC Excl: For CC codes in subcategory S36.8, unless otherwise noted: CC with 7th character A:** S31.001A, S31.011A, S31.021A, S31.031A, S31.041A, S31.051-S31.159 with 7th A, S31.600-S31.659 with 7th A, S31.831-S31.839 with 7th A, S36.81X-S36.99X with 7th A, S38.3XX-S39.023 with 7th A, T14.90-T14.91, T79.A0X-T79.9XX with 7th A

√x7th **S36.81** Injury of peritoneum ᴄᴄ
√6th **S36.89** Injury of other intra-abdominal organs
Injury of retroperitoneum
- √7th **S36.892** Contusion of other intra-abdominal organs ᴄᴄ
- √7th **S36.893** Laceration of other intra-abdominal organs ᴄᴄ
- √7th **S36.898** Other injury of other intra-abdominal organs ᴄᴄ
- √7th **S36.899** Unspecified injury of other intra-abdominal organs ᴄᴄ

Ⓝ Newborn: 0   Ⓟ Pediatric: 0-17   Ⓜ Maternity: 12-55   Ⓐ Adult: 15-124   ᴹᶜᶜ Major CC Condition   ᴾᴰˣᴹᶜᶜ PDx acts as own MCC   ᴄᴄ CC Condition   ᴾᴰˣᶜᶜ PDx acts as own CC

942   ICD-10-CM 2016

√5ᵗʰ **S36.9** **Injury of unspecified intra-abdominal organ**

> **CC Excl: For CC codes in subcategory S36.9, unless otherwise noted: CC with 7th character A: See Code: S36.8**

√x7ᵗʰ **S36.90** **Unspecified** injury of unspecified intra-abdominal organ   CC

√x7ᵗʰ **S36.92** **Contusion** of unspecified intra-abdominal organ   CC

√x7ᵗʰ **S36.93** **Laceration** of unspecified intra-abdominal organ   CC

√x7ᵗʰ **S36.99** **Other** injury of unspecified intra-abdominal organ   CC

√4ᵗʰ **S37** **Injury of urinary and pelvic organs**
Code also any associated open wound (S31.-)
> EXCLUDES 1   obstetric trauma to pelvic organs (O71.-)
> EXCLUDES 2   injury of peritoneum (S36.81)
> injury of retroperitoneum (S36.89-)

> The appropriate 7th is to be added to each code from category S37.
> A   initial encounter
> D   subsequent encounter
> S   sequela

√5ᵗʰ **S37.0** **Injury of** kidney
> EXCLUDES 2   acute kidney injury (nontraumatic) (N17.9)

> **CC Excl: For CC/MCC codes in subcategory S37.0, unless otherwise noted: CC or MCC as indicated with 7th A:** S31.001A, S31.011A, S31.021A, S31.031A, S31.041A, S31.051-S31.159 with 7th A, S31.600-S31.659 with 7th A, S31.831-S31.839 with 7th A, S36.81X-S37.099 with 7th A, S38.3XX-S39.023 with 7th A, T14.90-T14.91, T79.A0X-T79.9XX with 7th A

√6ᵗʰ **S37.00** **Unspecified** injury of kidney

√7ᵗʰ **S37.001** **Unspecified injury of** right **kidney**   CC

√7ᵗʰ **S37.002** **Unspecified injury of** left **kidney**   CC

√7ᵗʰ **S37.009** **Unspecified injury of** unspecified **kidney**   CC

√6ᵗʰ **S37.01** **Minor contusion** of kidney
Contusion of kidney less than 2 cm
Contusion of kidney NOS

√7ᵗʰ **S37.011** **Minor contusion of** right **kidney**   CC

√7ᵗʰ **S37.012** **Minor contusion of** left **kidney**   CC

√7ᵗʰ **S37.019** **Minor contusion of** unspecified **kidney**   CC

√6ᵗʰ **S37.02** **Major contusion** of kidney
Contusion of kidney greater than 2 cm

√7ᵗʰ **S37.021** **Major contusion of** right **kidney**   CC

√7ᵗʰ **S37.022** **Major contusion of** left **kidney**   CC

√7ᵗʰ **S37.029** **Major contusion of** unspecified **kidney**   CC

√6ᵗʰ **S37.03** **Laceration** of kidney, **unspecified** degree

√7ᵗʰ **S37.031** **Laceration of** right **kidney, unspecified degree**   CC

√7ᵗʰ **S37.032** **Laceration of** left **kidney, unspecified degree**   CC

√7ᵗʰ **S37.039** **Laceration of** unspecified **kidney, unspecified degree**   CC

√6ᵗʰ **S37.04** **Minor laceration** of kidney
Laceration of kidney less than 1 cm

√7ᵗʰ **S37.041** **Minor laceration of** right **kidney**   CC

√7ᵗʰ **S37.042** **Minor laceration of** left **kidney**   CC

√7ᵗʰ **S37.049** **Minor laceration of** unspecified **kidney**   CC

√6ᵗʰ **S37.05** **Moderate laceration** of kidney
Laceration of kidney 1 to 3 cm

√7ᵗʰ **S37.051** **Moderate laceration of** right **kidney**   CC

√7ᵗʰ **S37.052** **Moderate laceration of** left **kidney**   CC

√7ᵗʰ **S37.059** **Moderate laceration of** unspecified **kidney**   CC

√6ᵗʰ **S37.06** **Major laceration** of kidney
Avulsion of kidney
Laceration of kidney greater than 3 cm
Massive laceration of kidney
Multiple moderate lacerations of kidney
Stellate laceration of kidney

√7ᵗʰ **S37.061** **Major laceration of** right **kidney**   MCC

√7ᵗʰ **S37.062** **Major laceration of** left **kidney**   MCC

√7ᵗʰ **S37.069** **Major laceration of** unspecified **kidney**   MCC

√6ᵗʰ **S37.09** **Other** injury of kidney

√7ᵗʰ **S37.091** **Other injury of** right **kidney**   MCC

√7ᵗʰ **S37.092** **Other injury of** left **kidney**   MCC

√7ᵗʰ **S37.099** **Other injury of** unspecified **kidney**   MCC

√5ᵗʰ **S37.1** **Injury of** ureter

> **CC Excl: For CC codes in subcategory S37.1, unless otherwise noted: CC with 7th character A:** S31.001A, S31.011A, S31.021A, S31.031A, S31.041A, S31.051-S31.159 with 7th A, S31.600-S31.659 with 7th A, S31.831-S31.839 with 7th A, S36.81X-S37.099 with 7th A, S38.3XX-S39.023 with 7th A, T14.90-T14.91, T79.A0X-T79.9XX with 7th A

√x7ᵗʰ **S37.10** **Unspecified** injury of ureter   CC

√x7ᵗʰ **S37.12** **Contusion** of ureter   CC

√x7ᵗʰ **S37.13** **Laceration** of ureter   CC

√x7ᵗʰ **S37.19** **Other** injury of ureter   CC

√5ᵗʰ **S37.2** **Injury of** bladder

> **CC Excl: For CC codes in subcategory S37.2, unless otherwise noted: CC with 7th character A:** S31.001A, S31.011A, S31.021A, S31.031A, S31.041A, S31.051-S31.159 with 7th A, S31.600-S31.659 with 7th A, S31.831-S31.839 with 7th A, S36.81X-S36.99X with 7th A, S37.20-S37.599 with 7th A, S37.822-S37.99 with 7th A, S38.3XX-S39.023 with 7th A, T14.90-T14.91, T79.A0X-T79.9XX with 7th A

√x7ᵗʰ **S37.20** **Unspecified** injury of bladder   CC

√x7ᵗʰ **S37.22** **Contusion** of bladder   CC

√x7ᵗʰ **S37.23** **Laceration** of bladder   CC

√x7ᵗʰ **S37.29** **Other** injury of bladder   CC

√5ᵗʰ **S37.3** **Injury of** urethra

> **CC Excl: For CC codes in subcategory S37.3, unless otherwise noted: See code: S37.2**

√x7ᵗʰ **S37.30** **Unspecified** injury of urethra   CC

√x7ᵗʰ **S37.32** **Contusion** of urethra   CC

√x7ᵗʰ **S37.33** **Laceration** of urethra   CC

√x7ᵗʰ **S37.39** **Other** injury of urethra   CC

√5ᵗʰ **S37.4** **Injury of** ovary

√6ᵗʰ **S37.40** **Unspecified** injury of ovary

√7ᵗʰ **S37.401** **Unspecified injury of ovary,** unilateral   ♀

√7ᵗʰ **S37.402** **Unspecified injury of ovary,** bilateral   ♀

√7ᵗʰ **S37.409** **Unspecified injury of ovary,** unspecified   ♀

√6ᵗʰ **S37.42** **Contusion** of ovary

√7ᵗʰ **S37.421** **Contusion of ovary,** unilateral   ♀

√7ᵗʰ **S37.422** **Contusion of ovary,** bilateral   ♀

√7ᵗʰ **S37.429** **Contusion of ovary,** unspecified   ♀

√6ᵗʰ **S37.43** **Laceration** of ovary

√7ᵗʰ **S37.431** **Laceration of ovary,** unilateral   ♀

√7ᵗʰ **S37.432** **Laceration of ovary,** bilateral   ♀

√7ᵗʰ **S37.439** **Laceration of ovary,** unspecified   ♀

√6ᵗʰ **S37.49** **Other** injury of ovary

√7ᵗʰ **S37.491** **Other injury of ovary,** unilateral   ♀

√7ᵗʰ **S37.492** **Other injury of ovary,** bilateral   ♀

√7ᵗʰ **S37.499** **Other injury of ovary,** unspecified   ♀

√5ᵗʰ **S37.5** **Injury of** fallopian tube

S37.50 **Unspecified** injury of fallopian tube

√7ᵗʰ **S37.501** **Unspecified injury of fallopian tube,** unilateral   ♀

√7ᵗʰ **S37.502** **Unspecified injury of fallopian tube,** bilateral   ♀

√7ᵗʰ **S37.509** **Unspecified injury of fallopian tube,** unspecified   ♀

√6ᵗʰ **S37.51** **Primary blast injury** of fallopian tube
Blast injury of fallopian tube NOS

√7ᵗʰ **S37.511** **Primary blast injury of fallopian tube,** unilateral   ♀

√7ᵗʰ **S37.512** **Primary blast injury of fallopian tube,** bilateral   ♀

√7ᵗʰ **S37.519** **Primary blast injury of fallopian tube,** unspecified   ♀

√6ᵗʰ **S37.52** **Contusion** of fallopian tube

√7ᵗʰ **S37.521** **Contusion of fallopian tube,** unilateral   ♀

√7ᵗʰ **S37.522** **Contusion of fallopian tube,** bilateral   ♀

☑ Additional Character Required   √x7ᵗʰ Placeholder Alert   Unacceptable PDx   Manifestation   Hospital Acquired Condition   EXCLUDES 1 Not Coded Here   EXCLUDES 2 Not Included Here

Chapter 19. Injury, Poisoning, and Certain Other Consequences of External Causes

☑7ᵗʰ **S37.529** Contusion of fallopian tube, unspecified ♀

☑6ᵗʰ **S37.53** Laceration of fallopian tube

     ☑7ᵗʰ **S37.531** Laceration of fallopian tube, unilateral ♀

     ☑7ᵗʰ **S37.532** Laceration of fallopian tube, bilateral ♀

     ☑7ᵗʰ **S37.539** Laceration of fallopian tube, unspecified ♀

☑6ᵗʰ **S37.59** Other injury of fallopian tube
     Secondary blast injury of fallopian tube

     ☑7ᵗʰ **S37.591** Other injury of fallopian tube, unilateral ♀

     ☑7ᵗʰ **S37.592** Other injury of fallopian tube, bilateral ♀

     ☑7ᵗʰ **S37.599** Other injury of fallopian tube, unspecified ♀

☑5ᵗʰ **S37.6** Injury of uterus
     EXCLUDES 1   injury to gravid uterus (O9A.2-)
               injury to uterus during delivery (O71.-)

     CC Excl: For CC codes in subcategory S37.6, unless otherwise noted: CC with 7th character A: S31.001A, S31.011A, S31.021A, S31.031A, S31.041A, S31.051-S31.159 with 7th A, S31.600-S31.659 with 7th A, S31.831-S31.839 with 7th A, S36.81X-S36.99X with 7th A, S37.401-S37.69X with 7th A, S37.822-S37.99X with 7th A, S38.3XX-S39.023 with 7th A, T14.90-T14.91, T79.A0X-T79.9XX with 7th A

     ☑x7ᵗʰ **S37.60** Unspecified injury of uterus   CC ♀

     ☑x7ᵗʰ **S37.62** Contusion of uterus   CC ♀

     ☑x7ᵗʰ **S37.63** Laceration of uterus   CC ♀

     ☑x7ᵗʰ **S37.69** Other injury of uterus   CC ♀

☑5ᵗʰ **S37.8** Injury of other urinary and pelvic organs

☑6ᵗʰ **S37.81** Injury of adrenal gland

     CC Excl: For CC codes in subcategory S37.81, unless otherwise noted: CC with 7th character A: S31.001A, S31.011A, S31.021A, S31.031A, S31.041A, S31.051-S31.159 with 7th A, S31.600-S31.659 with 7th A, S31.831-S31.839 with 7th A, S36.81X-S36.99X with 7th A, S37.812-S37.819 with 7th A, S38.3XX-S39.023 with 7th A, T14.90-T14.91, T79.A0X-T79.9XX with 7th A

     ☑7ᵗʰ **S37.812** Contusion of adrenal gland   CC

     ☑7ᵗʰ **S37.813** Laceration of adrenal gland   CC

     ☑7ᵗʰ **S37.818** Other injury of adrenal gland   CC

     ☑7ᵗʰ **S37.819** Unspecified injury of adrenal gland   CC

☑6ᵗʰ **S37.82** Injury of prostate

     ☑7ᵗʰ **S37.822** Contusion of prostate ♂

     ☑7ᵗʰ **S37.823** Laceration of prostate ♂

     ☑7ᵗʰ **S37.828** Other injury of prostate ♂

     ☑7ᵗʰ **S37.829** Unspecified injury of prostate ♂

☑6ᵗʰ **S37.89** Injury of other urinary and pelvic organ

     CC Excl: For CC codes in subcategory S37.89, unless otherwise noted: CC with 7th character A: S31.001A, S31.011A, S31.021A, S31.031A, S31.041A, S31.051-S31.159 with 7th A, S31.600-S31.659 with 7th A, S31.831-S31.839 with 7th A, S36.81X-S36.99X with 7th A, S37.401-S37.599 with 7th A, S37.822-S37.99X with 7th A, S38.3X-S39.023 with 7th A, T14.90-T14.91, T79.A0X-T79.9XX with 7th A

     ☑7ᵗʰ **S37.892** Contusion of other urinary and pelvic organ   CC

     ☑7ᵗʰ **S37.893** Laceration of other urinary and pelvic organ   CC

     ☑7ᵗʰ **S37.898** Other injury of other urinary and pelvic organ   CC

     ☑7ᵗʰ **S37.899** Unspecified injury of other urinary and pelvic organ   CC

☑5ᵗʰ **S37.9** Injury of unspecified urinary and pelvic organ

     CC Excl: For CC codes in subcategory S37.9, unless otherwise noted: CC with 7th character A: See code: S37.89

     ☑x7ᵗʰ **S37.90** Unspecified injury of unspecified urinary and pelvic organ   CC

     ☑x7ᵗʰ **S37.92** Contusion of unspecified urinary and pelvic organ   CC

     ☑x7ᵗʰ **S37.93** Laceration of unspecified urinary and pelvic organ   CC

☑x7ᵗʰ **S37.99** Other injury of unspecified urinary and pelvic organ   CC

☑4ᵗʰ **S38** Crushing injury and traumatic amputation of abdomen, lower back, pelvis and external genitals
     NOTE An amputation not identified as partial or complete should be coded to complete.

     The appropriate 7th is to be added to each code from category S38.
     A   initial encounter
     D   subsequent encounter
     S   sequela

☑5ᵗʰ **S38.0** Crushing injury of external genital organs
     Use additional code for any associated injuries

     ☑6ᵗʰ **S38.00** Crushing injury of unspecified external genital organs

         ☑7ᵗʰ **S38.001** Crushing injury of unspecified external genital organs, male ♂

         ☑7ᵗʰ **S38.002** Crushing injury of unspecified external genital organs, female ♀

     ☑x7ᵗʰ **S38.01** Crushing injury of penis ♂

     ☑x7ᵗʰ **S38.02** Crushing injury of scrotum and testis ♂

     ☑x7ᵗʰ **S38.03** Crushing injury of vulva ♀

☑x7ᵗʰ **S38.1** Crushing injury of abdomen, lower back, and pelvis
     Use additional code for all associated injuries, such as:
         fracture of thoracic or lumbar spine and pelvis (S22.0-, S32-)
         injury to intra-abdominal organs (S36.-)
         injury to urinary and pelvic organs (S37.-)
         open wound of abdominal wall (S31.-)
         spinal cord injury (S34.0, S34.1-)
     EXCLUDES 2   crushing injury of external genital organs (S38.0-)

☑5ᵗʰ **S38.2** Traumatic amputation of external genital organs

     ☑6ᵗʰ **S38.21** Traumatic amputation of female external genital organs
         Traumatic amputation of clitoris
         Traumatic amputation of labium (majus) (minus)
         Traumatic amputation of vulva

         ☑7ᵗʰ **S38.211** Complete traumatic amputation of female external genital organs ♀

         ☑7ᵗʰ **S38.212** Partial traumatic amputation of female external genital organs ♀

     ☑6ᵗʰ **S38.22** Traumatic amputation of penis

         ☑7ᵗʰ **S38.221** Complete traumatic amputation of penis ♂

         ☑7ᵗʰ **S38.222** Partial traumatic amputation of penis ♂

     ☑6ᵗʰ **S38.23** Traumatic amputation of scrotum and testis

         ☑7ᵗʰ **S38.231** Complete traumatic amputation of scrotum and testis ♂

         ☑7ᵗʰ **S38.232** Partial traumatic amputation of scrotum and testis ♂

☑x7ᵗʰ **S38.3** Transection (partial) of abdomen

☑4ᵗʰ **S39** Other and unspecified injuries of abdomen, lower back, pelvis and external genitals
     Code also any associated open wound (S31.-)
     EXCLUDES 2   sprain of joints and ligaments of lumbar spine and pelvis (S33.-)

     The appropriate 7th is to be added to each code from category S39.
     A   initial encounter
     D   subsequent encounter
     S   sequela

☑5ᵗʰ **S39.0** Injury of muscle, fascia and tendon of abdomen, lower back and pelvis

     ☑6ᵗʰ **S39.00** Unspecified injury of muscle, fascia and tendon of abdomen, lower back and pelvis

         ☑7ᵗʰ **S39.001** Unspecified injury of muscle, fascia and tendon of abdomen

         ☑7ᵗʰ **S39.002** Unspecified injury of muscle, fascia and tendon of lower back

         ☑7ᵗʰ **S39.003** Unspecified injury of muscle, fascia and tendon of pelvis

     ☑6ᵗʰ **S39.01** Strain of muscle, fascia and tendon of abdomen, lower back and pelvis

         ☑7ᵗʰ **S39.011** Strain of muscle, fascia and tendon of abdomen

         ☑7ᵗʰ **S39.012** Strain of muscle, fascia and tendon of lower back

    ✓7ᵗʰ **S39.013**   Strain of muscle, fascia and tendon of pelvis

  ✓6ᵗʰ **S39.02**   Laceration of muscle, fascia and tendon of abdomen, lower back and pelvis

    ✓7ᵗʰ **S39.021**   Laceration of muscle, fascia and tendon of abdomen

    ✓7ᵗʰ **S39.022**   Laceration of muscle, fascia and tendon of lower back

    ✓7ᵗʰ **S39.023**   Laceration of muscle, fascia and tendon of pelvis

  ✓6ᵗʰ **S39.09**   Other injury of muscle, fascia and tendon of abdomen, lower back and pelvis

    ✓7ᵗʰ **S39.091**   Other injury of muscle, fascia and tendon of abdomen

    ✓7ᵗʰ **S39.092**   Other injury of muscle, fascia and tendon of lower back

    ✓7ᵗʰ **S39.093**   Other injury of muscle, fascia and tendon of pelvis

✓5ᵗʰ **S39.8**   Other specified injuries of abdomen, lower back, pelvis and external genitals

  ✓x7ᵗʰ **S39.81**   Other specified injuries of abdomen

  ✓x7ᵗʰ **S39.82**   Other specified injuries of lower back

  ✓x7ᵗʰ **S39.83**   Other specified injuries of pelvis

  ✓6ᵗʰ **S39.84**   Other specified injuries of external genitals

    ✓7ᵗʰ **S39.840**   Fracture of corpus cavernosum penis   ♂

    ✓7ᵗʰ **S39.848**   Other specified injuries of external genitals

✓5ᵗʰ **S39.9**   Unspecified injury of abdomen, lower back, pelvis and external genitals

  ✓x7ᵗʰ **S39.91**   Unspecified injury of abdomen

  ✓x7ᵗʰ **S39.92**   Unspecified injury of lower back

  ✓x7ᵗʰ **S39.93**   Unspecified injury of pelvis

  ✓x7ᵗʰ **S39.94**   Unspecified injury of external genitals

Injuries to the shoulder and upper arm (S40-S49)

INCLUDES   injuries of axilla
            injuries of scapular region
EXCLUDES 2   burns and corrosions (T20-T32)
            frostbite (T33-T34)
            injuries of elbow (S50-S59)
            insect bite or sting, venomous (T63.4)

✓4ᵗʰ **S40**   **Superficial injury of shoulder and upper arm**

> The appropriate 7th is to be added to each code from category S40.
> A   initial encounter
> D   subsequent encounter
> S   sequela

✓5ᵗʰ **S40.0**   Contusion of shoulder and upper arm

  ✓6ᵗʰ **S40.01**   Contusion of shoulder

    ✓7ᵗʰ **S40.011**   Contusion of right shoulder

    ✓7ᵗʰ **S40.012**   Contusion of left shoulder

    ✓7ᵗʰ **S40.019**   Contusion of unspecified shoulder

  ✓6ᵗʰ **S40.02**   Contusion of upper arm

    ✓7ᵗʰ **S40.021**   Contusion of right upper arm

    ✓7ᵗʰ **S40.022**   Contusion of left upper arm

    ✓7ᵗʰ **S40.029**   Contusion of unspecified upper arm

✓5ᵗʰ **S40.2**   Other superficial injuries of shoulder

  ✓6ᵗʰ **S40.21**   Abrasion of shoulder

    ✓7ᵗʰ **S40.211**   Abrasion of right shoulder

    ✓7ᵗʰ **S40.212**   Abrasion of left shoulder

    ✓7ᵗʰ **S40.219**   Abrasion of unspecified shoulder

  ✓6ᵗʰ **S40.22**   Blister (nonthermal) of shoulder

    ✓7ᵗʰ **S40.221**   Blister (nonthermal) of right shoulder

    ✓7ᵗʰ **S40.222**   Blister (nonthermal) of left shoulder

    ✓7ᵗʰ **S40.229**   Blister (nonthermal) of unspecified shoulder

  ✓6ᵗʰ **S40.24**   External constriction of shoulder

    ✓7ᵗʰ **S40.241**   External constriction of right shoulder

    ✓7ᵗʰ **S40.242**   External constriction of left shoulder

    ✓7ᵗʰ **S40.249**   External constriction of unspecified shoulder

  ✓6ᵗʰ **S40.25**   Superficial foreign body of shoulder
       Splinter in the shoulder

    ✓7ᵗʰ **S40.251**   Superficial foreign body of right shoulder

    ✓7ᵗʰ **S40.252**   Superficial foreign body of left shoulder

    ✓7ᵗʰ **S40.259**   Superficial foreign body of unspecified shoulder

  ✓6ᵗʰ **S40.26**   Insect bite (nonvenomous) of shoulder

    ✓7ᵗʰ **S40.261**   Insect bite (nonvenomous) of right shoulder

    ✓7ᵗʰ **S40.262**   Insect bite (nonvenomous) of left shoulder

    ✓7ᵗʰ **S40.269**   Insect bite (nonvenomous) of unspecified shoulder

  ✓6ᵗʰ **S40.27**   Other superficial bite of shoulder
     EXCLUDES 1   open bite of shoulder (S41.05)

    ✓7ᵗʰ **S40.271**   Other superficial bite of right shoulder

    ✓7ᵗʰ **S40.272**   Other superficial bite of left shoulder

    ✓7ᵗʰ **S40.279**   Other superficial bite of unspecified shoulder

✓5ᵗʰ **S40.8**   Other superficial injuries of upper arm

  ✓6ᵗʰ **S40.81**   Abrasion of upper arm

    ✓7ᵗʰ **S40.811**   Abrasion of right upper arm

    ✓7ᵗʰ **S40.812**   Abrasion of left upper arm

    ✓7ᵗʰ **S40.819**   Abrasion of unspecified upper arm

  ✓6ᵗʰ **S40.82**   Blister (nonthermal) of upper arm

    ✓7ᵗʰ **S40.821**   Blister (nonthermal) of right upper arm

    ✓7ᵗʰ **S40.822**   Blister (nonthermal) of left upper arm

    ✓7ᵗʰ **S40.829**   Blister (nonthermal) of unspecified upper arm

  ✓6ᵗʰ **S40.84**   External constriction of upper arm

    ✓7ᵗʰ **S40.841**   External constriction of right upper arm

    ✓7ᵗʰ **S40.842**   External constriction of left upper arm

    ✓7ᵗʰ **S40.849**   External constriction of unspecified upper arm

  ✓6ᵗʰ **S40.85**   Superficial foreign body of upper arm
       Splinter in the upper arm

    ✓7ᵗʰ **S40.851**   Superficial foreign body of right upper arm

    ✓7ᵗʰ **S40.852**   Superficial foreign body of left upper arm

    ✓7ᵗʰ **S40.859**   Superficial foreign body of unspecified upper arm

  ✓6ᵗʰ **S40.86**   Insect bite (nonvenomous) of upper arm

    ✓7ᵗʰ **S40.861**   Insect bite (nonvenomous) of right upper arm

    ✓7ᵗʰ **S40.862**   Insect bite (nonvenomous) of left upper arm

    ✓7ᵗʰ **S40.869**   Insect bite (nonvenomous) of unspecified upper arm

  ✓6ᵗʰ **S40.87**   Other superficial bite of upper arm
     EXCLUDES 1   open bite of upper arm (S41.14)
     EXCLUDES 2   other superficial bite of shoulder (S40.27-)

    ✓7ᵗʰ **S40.871**   Other superficial bite of right upper arm

    ✓7ᵗʰ **S40.872**   Other superficial bite of left upper arm

    ✓7ᵗʰ **S40.879**   Other superficial bite of unspecified upper arm

✓5ᵗʰ **S40.9**   Unspecified superficial injury of shoulder and upper arm

  ✓6ᵗʰ **S40.91**   Unspecified superficial injury of shoulder

    ✓7ᵗʰ **S40.911**   Unspecified superficial injury of right shoulder

    ✓7ᵗʰ **S40.912**   Unspecified superficial injury of left shoulder

    ✓7ᵗʰ **S40.919**   Unspecified superficial injury of unspecified shoulder

  ✓6ᵗʰ **S40.92**   Unspecified superficial injury of upper arm

    ✓7ᵗʰ **S40.921**   Unspecified superficial injury of right upper arm

    ✓7ᵗʰ **S40.922**   Unspecified superficial injury of left upper arm

    ✓7ᵗʰ **S40.929**   Unspecified superficial injury of unspecified upper arm

✓ Additional Character Required   ✓x7ᵗʰ Placeholder Alert   Unacceptable PDx   Manifestation   Hospital Acquired Condition   EXCLUDES 1 Not Coded Here   EXCLUDES 2 Not Included Here

ICD-10-CM 2016   945

√4th S41   Open wound of shoulder and upper arm

Code also any associated wound infection

EXCLUDES 1   *traumatic amputation of shoulder and upper arm (S48.-)*

EXCLUDES 2   *open fracture of shoulder and upper arm (S42.- with 7th character B or C)*

The appropriate 7th is to be added to each code from category S41.
A   initial encounter
D   subsequent encounter
S   sequela

√5th S41.0   Open wound of shoulder

   √6th S41.00   Unspecified open wound of shoulder

     √7th   S41.001   Unspecified open wound of right shoulder

     √7th   S41.002   Unspecified open wound of left shoulder

     √7th   S41.009   Unspecified open wound of unspecified shoulder

   √6th S41.01   Laceration without foreign body of shoulder

     √7th   S41.011   Laceration without foreign body of right shoulder

     √7th   S41.012   Laceration without foreign body of left shoulder

     √7th   S41.019   Laceration without foreign body of unspecified shoulder

   √6th S41.02   Laceration with foreign body of shoulder

     √7th   S41.021   Laceration with foreign body of right shoulder

     √7th   S41.022   Laceration with foreign body of left shoulder

     √7th   S41.029   Laceration with foreign body of unspecified shoulder

   √6th S41.03   Puncture wound without foreign body of shoulder

     √7th   S41.031   Puncture wound without foreign body of right shoulder

     √7th   S41.032   Puncture wound without foreign body of left shoulder

     √7th   S41.039   Puncture wound without foreign body of unspecified shoulder

   √6th S41.04   Puncture wound with foreign body of shoulder

     √7th   S41.041   Puncture wound with foreign body of right shoulder

     √7th   S41.042   Puncture wound with foreign body of left shoulder

     √7th   S41.049   Puncture wound with foreign body of unspecified shoulder

   √6th S41.05   Open bite of shoulder

Bite of shoulder NOS

EXCLUDES 1   *superficial bite of shoulder (S40.27)*

     √7th   S41.051   Open bite of right shoulder

     √7th   S41.052   Open bite of left shoulder

     √7th   S41.059   Open bite of unspecified shoulder

√5th S41.1   Open wound of upper arm

   √6th S41.10   Unspecified open wound of upper arm

     √7th   S41.101   Unspecified open wound of right upper arm

     √7th   S41.102   Unspecified open wound of left upper arm

     √7th   S41.109   Unspecified open wound of unspecified upper arm

   √6th S41.11   Laceration without foreign body of upper arm

     √7th   S41.111   Laceration without foreign body of right upper arm

     √7th   S41.112   Laceration without foreign body of left upper arm

     √7th   S41.119   Laceration without foreign body of unspecified upper arm

   √6th S41.12   Laceration with foreign body of upper arm

     √7th   S41.121   Laceration with foreign body of right upper arm

     √7th   S41.122   Laceration with foreign body of left upper arm

     √7th   S41.129   Laceration with foreign body of unspecified upper arm

√6th S41.13   Puncture wound without foreign body of upper arm

     √7th   S41.131   Puncture wound without foreign body of right upper arm

     √7th   S41.132   Puncture wound without foreign body of left upper arm

     √7th   S41.139   Puncture wound without foreign body of unspecified upper arm

√6th S41.14   Puncture wound with foreign body of upper arm

     √7th   S41.141   Puncture wound with foreign body of right upper arm

     √7th   S41.142   Puncture wound with foreign body of left upper arm

     √7th   S41.149   Puncture wound with foreign body of unspecified upper arm

√6th S41.15   Open bite of upper arm

Bite of upper arm NOS

EXCLUDES 1   *superficial bite of upper arm (S40.87)*

     √7th   S41.151   Open bite of right upper arm

     √7th   S41.152   Open bite of left upper arm

     √7th   S41.159   Open bite of unspecified upper arm

√4th S42   Fracture of shoulder and upper arm

NOTE   A fracture not indicated as displaced or nondisplaced should be coded to displaced.
A fracture not indicated as open or closed should be coded to closed.

EXCLUDES 1   *traumatic amputation of shoulder and upper arm (S48.-)*

The appropriate 7th is to be added to all codes from category S42 [unless otherwise indicated].
A   initial encounter for closed fracture
B   initial encounter for open fracture
D   subsequent encounter for fracture with routine healing
G   subsequent encounter for fracture with delayed healing
K   subsequent encounter for fracture with nonunion
P   subsequent encounter for fracture with malunion
S   sequela

√5th S42.0   Fracture of clavicle

CC Excl: For CC/MCC codes in subcategory S42.0, unless otherwise noted: CC with 7th character B: S42.001–S42.036 with 7th [A, B], S62.90XB
CC with 7th character K or P: M80.00X–M84.68X with 7th [K, P], S02.0XX–S02.92X with 7th K, S12.000–S12.691 with 7th K, S22.000–S22.9XX with 7th K, S32.000–S32.9XX with 7th K, S42.001–S42.92X with 7th [K, P], S49.001–S49.199 with 7th [K, P], S52.001–S52.92X with 7th [K, M, N, P, Q, R], S59.001–S59.299 with 7th [K, P], S62.001–S62.92X with 7th [K, P], S72.001–S72.92X with 7th [K, M, N, P, Q, R], S79.001–S79.199 with 7th [K, P], S82.001–S82.92X with 7th [K, M, N, P, Q, R], S89.001–S89.399 with 7th [K, P], S92.001–S92.919 with 7th [K, P]

   √6th S42.00   Fracture of unspecified part of clavicle

     15,20 √7th   S42.001   **Fracture of unspecified part of right clavicle**   CC

     15,20 √7th   S42.002   **Fracture of unspecified part of left clavicle**   CC

     15,20 √7th   S42.009   **Fracture of unspecified part of unspecified clavicle**   CC
       AHA: 2012, 4Q, 93

   √6th S42.01   Fracture of sternal end of clavicle

     15,20 √7th   S42.011   **Anterior displaced fracture of sternal end of right clavicle**   CC

     15,20 √7th   S42.012   **Anterior displaced fracture of sternal end of left clavicle**   CC

     15,20 √7th   S42.013   **Anterior displaced fracture of sternal end of unspecified clavicle**   CC
       Displaced fracture of sternal end of clavicle NOS

     15,20 √7th   S42.014   **Posterior displaced fracture of sternal end of right clavicle**   CC

     15,20 √7th   S42.015   **Posterior displaced fracture of sternal end of left clavicle**   CC

     15,20 √7th   S42.016   **Posterior displaced fracture of sternal end of unspecified clavicle**   CC

     15,20 √7th   S42.017   **Nondisplaced fracture of sternal end of right clavicle**   CC

---

15 HAC = Initial encounter for open fracture only (7th character B or C – specific to category) and not POA.

20 CC only if an initial encounter for an open fracture (7th character B or C) **OR** a subsequent encounter for nonunion or malunion (7th character K, M, N, P, Q, or R – specific to category).

N Newborn: 0   P Pediatric: 0-17   M Maternity: 12-55   A Adult: 15-124   **MCC** Major CC Condition   **PDxMCC** PDx acts as own MCC   **CC** CC Condition   **PDxCC** PDx acts as own CC

946   ICD-10-CM 2016

15,20 √7th **S42.018** Nondisplaced **fracture of sternal end** of **left** clavicle   CC

15,20 √7th **S42.019** Nondisplaced **fracture of sternal end of unspecified** clavicle   CC

√6th **S42.02** Fracture of **shaft of clavicle**

15,20 √7th **S42.021** Displaced **fracture of shaft of right** clavicle   CC

15,20 √7th **S42.022** Displaced **fracture of shaft of left** clavicle   CC

15,20 √7th **S42.023** Displaced **fracture of shaft of unspecified** clavicle   CC

15,20 √7th **S42.024** Nondisplaced **fracture of shaft of right** clavicle   CC

15,20 √7th **S42.025** Nondisplaced **fracture of shaft of left** clavicle   CC

15,20 √7th **S42.026** Nondisplaced **fracture of shaft of unspecified** clavicle   CC

√6th **S42.03** Fracture of **lateral end of clavicle**
Fracture of acromial end of clavicle

15,20 √7th **S42.031** Displaced **fracture of lateral end of right** clavicle   CC

15,20 √7th **S42.032** Displaced **fracture of lateral end of left** clavicle   CC

15,20 √7th **S42.033** Displaced **fracture of lateral end of unspecified** clavicle   CC

15,20 √7th **S42.034** Nondisplaced **fracture of lateral end of right** clavicle   CC

15,20 √7th **S42.035** Nondisplaced **fracture of lateral end of left** clavicle   CC

15,20 √7th **S42.036** Nondisplaced **fracture of lateral end of unspecified** clavicle   CC

√5th **S42.1** Fracture of **scapula**

> **CC Excl: For CC/MCC codes in subcatagory S42.1, unless otherwise noted:** S42.101-S42.199 with 7th [A, B], S62.90XB
> **CC with 7th character K or P:** M80.00X-M84.68X with 7th [K, P], S02.0XX-S02.92X with 7th K, S12.000-S12.691 with 7th K, S22.000-S22.9XX with 7th K, S32.000-S32.9XX with 7th K, S42.001-S42.92X with 7th [K, P], S49.001-S49.199 with 7th [K, P], S52.001-S52.92X with 7th [K, M, N, P, Q, R], S59.001-S59.299 with 7th [K, P], S62.001-S62.92X with 7th [K, P], S72.001-S72.92X with 7th [K, M, N, P, Q, R], S79.001-S79.199 with 7th [K, P], S82.001-S82.92X with 7th [K, M, N, P, Q, R], S89.001-S89.399 with 7th [K, P], S92.001-S92.919 with 7th[K, P]

√6th **S42.10** Fracture of **unspecified part of scapula**

15,20 √7th **S42.101** Fracture of unspecified part of scapula, **right shoulder**   CC

15,20 √7th **S42.102** Fracture of unspecified part of scapula, **left shoulder**   CC

15,20 √7th **S42.109** Fracture of unspecified part of scapula, **unspecified shoulder**   CC

√6th **S42.11** Fracture of **body of scapula**

15,20 √7th **S42.111** Displaced **fracture of body of scapula, right shoulder**   CC

15,20 √7th **S42.112** Displaced **fracture of body of scapula, left shoulder**   CC

15,20 √7th **S42.113** Displaced **fracture of body of scapula, unspecified shoulder**   CC

15,20 √7th **S42.114** Nondisplaced **fracture of body of scapula, right shoulder**   CC

15,20 √7th **S42.115** Nondisplaced **fracture of body of scapula, left shoulder**   CC

15,20 √7th **S42.116** Nondisplaced **fracture of body of scapula, unspecified shoulder**   CC

√6th **S42.12** Fracture of **acromial process**

15,20 √7th **S42.121** Displaced **fracture of acromial process, right shoulder**   CC

15,20 √7th **S42.122** Displaced **fracture of acromial process, left shoulder**   CC

15,20 √7th **S42.123** Displaced **fracture of acromial process, unspecified shoulder**   CC

15,20 √7th **S42.124** Nondisplaced **fracture of acromial process, right shoulder**   CC

15,20 √7th **S42.125** Nondisplaced **fracture of acromial process, left shoulder**   CC

15,20 √7th **S42.126** Nondisplaced **fracture of acromial process, unspecified shoulder**   CC

√6th **S42.13** Fracture of **coracoid process**

15,20 √7th **S42.131** Displaced **fracture of coracoid process, right shoulder**   CC

15,20 √7th **S42.132** Displaced **fracture of coracoid process, left shoulder**   CC

15,20 √7th **S42.133** Displaced **fracture of coracoid process, unspecified shoulder**   CC

15,20 √7th **S42.134** Nondisplaced **fracture of coracoid process, right shoulder**   CC

15,20 √7th **S42.135** Nondisplaced **fracture of coracoid process, left shoulder**   CC

15,20 √7th **S42.136** Nondisplaced **fracture of coracoid process, unspecified shoulder**   CC

√6th **S42.14** Fracture of **glenoid cavity of scapula**

15,20 √7th **S42.141** Displaced **fracture of glenoid cavity of scapula, right shoulder**   CC

15,20 √7th **S42.142** Displaced **fracture of glenoid cavity of scapula, left shoulder**   CC

15,20 √7th **S42.143** Displaced **fracture of glenoid cavity of scapula, unspecified shoulder**   CC

15,20 √7th **S42.144** Nondisplaced **fracture of glenoid cavity of scapula, right shoulder**   CC

15,20 √7th **S42.145** Nondisplaced **fracture of glenoid cavity of scapula, left shoulder**   CC

15,20 √7th **S42.146** Nondisplaced **fracture of glenoid cavity of scapula, unspecified shoulder**   CC

√6th **S42.15** Fracture of **neck of scapula**

15,20 √7th **S42.151** Displaced **fracture of neck of scapula, right shoulder**   CC

15,20 √7th **S42.152** Displaced **fracture of neck of scapula, left shoulder**   CC

15,20 √7th **S42.153** Displaced **fracture of neck of scapula, unspecified shoulder**   CC

15,20 √7th **S42.154** Nondisplaced **fracture of neck of scapula, right shoulder**   CC

15,20 √7th **S42.155** Nondisplaced **fracture of neck of scapula, left shoulder**   CC

15,20 √7th **S42.156** Nondisplaced **fracture of neck of scapula, unspecified shoulder**   CC

√6th **S42.19** Fracture of **other part of scapula**

15,20 √7th **S42.191** Fracture of other part of scapula, **right shoulder**   CC

15,20 √7th **S42.192** Fracture of other part of scapula, **left shoulder**   CC

15,20 √7th **S42.199** Fracture of other part of scapula, **unspecified shoulder**   CC

---

15 HAC = Initial encounter for open fracture only (7th character B or C – specific to category) and not POA.
20 CC only if an initial encounter for an open fracture (7th character B or C) **OR** a subsequent encounter for nonunion or malunion (7th character K, M, N, P, Q, or R – specific to category).

☑ Additional Character Required   √x7th Placeholder Alert   Unacceptable PDx   Manifestation   Hospital Acquired Condition   *EXCLUDES 1* Not Coded Here   *EXCLUDES 2* Not Included Here

Chapter 19. Injury, Poisoning, and Certain Other Consequences of External Causes *(side margin)*

S42.2–S42.254 *(side margin)*

✓5ᵗʰ **S42.2** **Fracture of upper end of humerus**
Fracture of proximal end of humerus
EXCLUDES 2 *fracture of shaft of humerus (S42.3-)*
physeal fracture of upper end of humerus (S49.0-)

✓6ᵗʰ **S42.20** **Unspecified fracture of upper end of humerus**

7,16,19 ✓7ᵗʰ **S42.201** **Unspecified fracture of upper end of right humerus** MCC CC
CC Excl: CC with 7th character A: S42.201-S42.271 with 7th [A, B], S42.279-S42.311 with 7th A, S42.319-S42.481 with 7th A, S42.489-S42.92X with 7th A, S49.001 with 7th A, S49.009-S49.011 with 7th A, S49.019-S49.021 with 7th A, S49.029-S49.031 with 7th A, S49.039-S49.041 with 7th A, S49.049-S49.091 with 7th A, S49.099-S49.101 with 7th A, S49.109-S49.111 with 7th A, S49.119-S49.121 with 7th A, S49.129-S49.131 with 7th A, S49.139-S49.141 with 7th A, S49.149-S49.191 with 7th A, S49.199A
MCC with 7th character B: S42.201-S42.266 with 7th B, S42.291-S42.92X with 7th B, S49.101-S49.199 with 7th A, S62.90XB
CC with 7th character K or P: M80.00X-M84.68X with 7th [K, P], S02.0XX-S02.92X with 7th K, S12.000-S12.691 with 7th K, S22.000-S22.9XX with 7th K, S32.000-S32.9XX with 7th K, S42.001-S42.92X with 7th [K, P], S49.001-S49.199 with 7th [K, P], S52.001-S52.92X with 7th [K, M, N, P, Q, R], S59.001-S59.299 with 7th [K, P], S62.001-S62.92X with 7th [K, P], S72.001-S72.92X with 7th [K, M, N, P, Q, R], S79.001-S79.199 with 7th [K, P], S82.001-S82.92X with 7th [K, M, N, P, Q, R], S89.001-S89.399 with 7th [K, P], S92.001-S92.919 with 7th [K, P]

7,16,19 ✓7ᵗʰ **S42.202** **Unspecified fracture of upper end of left humerus** MCC CC
CC Excl: CC with 7th character A: S42.201-S42.266 with 7th B, S42.272-S42.309 with 7th A, S42.312-S42.476 with 7th A, S42.482-S42.92X with 7th A, S49.002-S49.009 with 7th A, S49.012-S49.019 with 7th A, S49.022-S49.029 with 7th A, S49.032-S49.039 with 7th A, S49.042-S49.049 with 7th A, S49.092-S49.099 with 7th A, S49.102-S49.109 with 7th A, S49.112-S49.119 with 7th A, S49.122-S49.129 with 7th A, S49.132-S49.139 with 7th A, S49.142-S49.149 with 7th A, S49.192-S49.199 with 7th A
MCC with 7th character B: MCC Excl: S42.201-S42.266 with 7th B, S42.291-S42.92X with 7th B, S49.101-S49.199 with 7th A, S62.90XB
CC with 7th character K or P: CC Excl: M80.00X-M84.68X with 7th [K, P], S02.0XX-S02.92X with 7th K, S12.000-S12.691 with 7th K, S22.000-S22.9XX with 7th K, S32.000-S32.9XX with 7th K, S42.001-S42.92X with 7th [K, P], S49.001-S49.199 with 7th [K, P], S52.001-S52.92X with 7th [K, M, N, P, Q, R], S59.001-S59.299 with 7th [K, P], S62.001-S62.92X with 7th [K, P], S72.001-S72.92X with 7th [K, M, N, P, Q, R], S79.001-S79.199 with 7th [K, P], S82.001-S82.92X with 7th [K, M, N, P, Q, R], S89.001-S89.399 with 7th [K, P], S92.001-S92.919 with 7th [K, P]

7,16,19 ✓7ᵗʰ **S42.209** **Unspecified fracture of upper end of unspecified humerus** MCC CC
CC Excl: CC with 7th character A: S42.201-S42.92X with 7th [A, B], S49.001-S49.199 with 7th A
MCC with 7th character B: S42.201-S42.266 with 7th B, S42.291-S42.92X with 7th B, S49.101-S49.199 with 7th A, S62.90XB
CC with 7th character K or P: M80.00X-M84.68X with 7th [K, P], S02.0XX-S02.92X with 7th K, S12.000-S12.691 with 7th K, S22.000-S22.9XX with 7th K, S32.000-S32.9XX with 7th K, S42.001-S42.92X with 7th [K, P], S49.001-S49.199 with 7th [K, P], S52.001-S52.92X with 7th [K, M, N, P, Q, R], S59.001-S59.299 with 7th [K, P], S62.001-S62.92X with 7th [K, P], S72.001-S72.92X with 7th [K, M, N, P, Q, R], S79.001-S79.199 with 7th [K, P], S82.001-S82.92X with 7th [K, M, N, P, Q, R], S89.001-S89.399 with 7th [K, P], S92.001-S92.919 with 7th [K, P]

✓6ᵗʰ **S42.21** **Unspecified fracture of surgical neck of humerus**
Fracture of neck of humerus NOS

7,16,19 ✓7ᵗʰ **S42.211** **Unspecified displaced fracture of surgical neck of right humerus** MCC CC
CC Excl: See code: S42.201

7,16,19 ✓7ᵗʰ **S42.212** **Unspecified displaced fracture of surgical neck of left humerus** MCC CC
CC Excl: See code: S42.202

7,16,19 ✓7ᵗʰ **S42.213** **Unspecified displaced fracture of surgical neck of unspecified humerus** MCC CC
CC Excl: See code: S42.209

7,16,19 ✓7ᵗʰ **S42.214** **Unspecified nondisplaced fracture of surgical neck of right humerus** MCC CC
CC Excl: See code: S42.201

7,16,19 ✓7ᵗʰ **S42.215** **Unspecified nondisplaced fracture of surgical neck of left humerus** MCC CC
CC Excl: See code: S42.202

7,16,19 ✓7ᵗʰ **S42.216** **Unspecified nondisplaced fracture of surgical neck of unspecified humerus** MCC CC
CC Excl: Se code: S42.209

✓6ᵗʰ **S42.22** **2-part fracture of surgical neck of humerus**

7,16,19 ✓7ᵗʰ **S42.221** **2-part displaced fracture of surgical neck of right humerus** MCC CC
CC Excl: See code: S42.201

7,16,19 ✓7ᵗʰ **S42.222** **2-part displaced fracture of surgical neck of left humerus** MCC CC
CC Excl: See code: S42.202

7,16,19 ✓7ᵗʰ **S42.223** **2-part displaced fracture of surgical neck of unspecified humerus** MCC CC
CC Excl: See code: S42.209

7,16,19 ✓7ᵗʰ **S42.224** **2-part nondisplaced fracture of surgical neck of right humerus** MCC CC
CC Excl: See code: S42.201

7,16,19 ✓7ᵗʰ **S42.225** **2-part nondisplaced fracture of surgical neck of left humerus** MCC CC
CC Excl: See code: S42.202

7,16,19 ✓7ᵗʰ **S42.226** **2-part nondisplaced fracture of surgical neck of unspecified humerus** MCC CC
CC Excl: See code: S42.209

✓6ᵗʰ **S42.23** **3-part fracture of surgical neck of humerus**

7,16,19 ✓7ᵗʰ **S42.231** **3-part fracture of surgical neck of right humerus** MCC CC
CC Excl: See code: S42.201

7,16,19 ✓7ᵗʰ **S42.232** **3-part fracture of surgical neck of left humerus** MCC CC
CC Excl: See code: S42.202

7,16,19 ✓7ᵗʰ **S42.239** **3-part fracture of surgical neck of unspecified humerus** MCC CC
CC Excl: See code: S42.209

✓6ᵗʰ **S42.24** **4-part fracture of surgical neck of humerus**

7,16,19 ✓7ᵗʰ **S42.241** **4-part fracture of surgical neck of right humerus** MCC CC
CC Excl: See code: S42.201

7,16,19 ✓7ᵗʰ **S42.242** **4-part fracture of surgical neck of left humerus** MCC CC
CC Excl: See code: S42.202

7,16,19 ✓7ᵗʰ **S42.249** **4-part fracture of surgical neck of unspecified humerus** MCC CC
CC Excl: See code: S42.209

✓6ᵗʰ **S42.25** **Fracture of greater tuberosity of humerus**

7,16,19 ✓7ᵗʰ **S42.251** **Displaced fracture of greater tuberosity of right humerus** MCC CC
CC Excl: See code: S42.201

7,16,19 ✓7ᵗʰ **S42.252** **Displaced fracture of greater tuberosity of left humerus** MCC CC
CC Excl: See code: S42.202

7,16,19 ✓7ᵗʰ **S42.253** **Displaced fracture of greater tuberosity of unspecified humerus** MCC CC
CC Excl: See code: S42.209

7,16,19 ✓7ᵗʰ **S42.254** **Nondisplaced fracture of greater tuberosity of right humerus** MCC CC
CC Excl: See code: S42.201

---

7   HAC = Initial encounter only (7th character A, B or C) and not POA.
16   MCC only if an open fracture (7th character B or C – specific to category).
19   CC only if an initial encounter for a closed fracture (7th character A) **OR** a subsequent encounter for nonunion or malunion (7th character K, M, N, P, Q, or R – specific to category).

7,16,19 ✓7ᵗʰ **S42.255** **Nondisplaced fracture of greater** `MCC` `CC`
tuberosity of left humerus
CC Excl: See code: S42.202

7,16,19 ✓7ᵗʰ **S42.256** **Nondisplaced fracture of greater** `MCC` `CC`
tuberosity of unspecified humerus
CC Excl: See code: S42.209

✓6ᵗʰ **S42.26** **Fracture of lesser tuberosity of humerus**

7,16,19 ✓7ᵗʰ **S42.261** **Displaced fracture of lesser** `MCC` `CC`
tuberosity of right humerus
CC Excl: See code: S42.201

7,16,19 ✓7ᵗʰ **S42.262** **Displaced fracture of lesser** `MCC` `CC`
tuberosity of left humerus
CC Excl: See code: S42.202

7,16,19 ✓7ᵗʰ **S42.263** **Displaced fracture of lesser** `MCC` `CC`
tuberosity of unspecified humerus
CC Excl: See code: S42.209

7,16,19 ✓7ᵗʰ **S42.264** **Nondisplaced fracture of lesser** `MCC` `CC`
tuberosity of right humerus
CC Excl: See code: S42.201

7,16,19 ✓7ᵗʰ **S42.265** **Nondisplaced fracture of lesser** `MCC` `CC`
tuberosity of left humerus
CC Excl: See code: S42.202

7,16,19 ✓7ᵗʰ **S42.266** **Nondisplaced fracture of lesser** `MCC` `CC`
tuberosity of unspecified humerus
CC Excl: See code: S42.209

✓6ᵗʰ **S42.27** **Torus fracture of upper end of humerus**

> The appropriate 7th is to be added to all codes in
> subcategory S42.27.
> A   initial encounter for closed fracture
> D   subsequent encounter for fracture with
>   routine healing
> G   subsequent encounter for fracture with
>   delayed healing
> K   subsequent encounter for fracture with
>   nonunion
> P   subsequent encounter for fracture with
>   malunion
> S   sequela

7,19 ✓7ᵗʰ **S42.271** **Torus fracture of upper end of right** `CC`
humerus
CC Excl: See code: S42.201

7,19 ✓7ᵗʰ **S42.272** **Torus fracture of upper end of left** `CC`
humerus
CC Excl: See code: S42.202

7,19 ✓7ᵗʰ **S42.279** **Torus fracture of upper end of** `CC`
unspecified humerus
CC Excl: See code: S42.209

✓6ᵗʰ **S42.29** **Other fracture of upper end of humerus**
Fracture of anatomical neck of humerus
Fracture of articular head of humerus

7,16,19 ✓7ᵗʰ **S42.291** **Other displaced fracture of upper** `MCC` `CC`
end of right humerus
CC Excl: See code: S42.201

7,16,19 ✓7ᵗʰ **S42.292** **Other displaced fracture of upper** `MCC` `CC`
end of left humerus
CC Excl: See code: S42.202

7,16,19 ✓7ᵗʰ **S42.293** **Other displaced fracture of upper** `MCC` `CC`
end of unspecified humerus
CC Excl: See code: S42.209

7,16,19 ✓7ᵗʰ **S42.294** **Other nondisplaced fracture of** `MCC` `CC`
upper end of right humerus
CC Excl: See code: S42.201

7,16,19 ✓7ᵗʰ **S42.295** **Other nondisplaced fracture of** `MCC` `CC`
upper end of left humerus
CC Excl: See code: S42.202

7,16,19 ✓7ᵗʰ **S42.296** **Other nondisplaced fracture of** `MCC` `CC`
upper end of unspecified humerus
CC Excl: See code: S42.209

✓5ᵗʰ **S42.3** **Fracture of shaft of humerus**
Fracture of humerus NOS
Fracture of upper arm NOS
EXCLUDES 2   physeal fractures of upper end of humerus (S49.0-)
         physeal fractures of lower end of humerus (S49.1-)

✓6ᵗʰ **S42.30** **Unspecified fracture of shaft of humerus**

7,16,19 ✓7ᵗʰ **S42.301** **Unspecified fracture of shaft of** `MCC` `CC`
humerus, right arm
CC Excl: See code: S42.201

7,16,19 ✓7ᵗʰ **S42.302** **Unspecified fracture of shaft of** `MCC` `CC`
humerus, left arm
CC Excl: See code: S42.202

7,16,19 ✓7ᵗʰ **S42.309** **Unspecified fracture of shaft of** `MCC` `CC`
humerus, unspecified arm
CC Excl: See code: S42.209

✓6ᵗʰ **S42.31** **Greenstick fracture of shaft of humerus**

> The appropriate 7th is to be added to all codes in
> subcategory S42.31.
> A   initial encounter for closed fracture
> D   subsequent encounter for fracture with
>   routine healing
> G   subsequent encounter for fracture with
>   delayed healing
> K   subsequent encounter for fracture with
>   nonunion
> P   subsequent encounter for fracture with
>   malunion
> S   sequela

7,19 ✓7ᵗʰ **S42.311** **Greenstick fracture of shaft of** `CC`
humerus, right arm
CC Excl: CC with 7th character A: S42.311A,
S42.319-S42.321 with 7th A, S42.323-
S42.324 with 7th A, S42.326-S42.331 with
7th A, S42.333-S42.334 with 7th A, S42.336-
S42.341 with 7th A, S42.343-S42.344 with
7th A, S42.346-S42.351 with 7th A, S42.353-
S42.354 with 7th A, S42.356-S42.361 with
7th A, S42.363-S42.364 with 7th A, S42.366-
S42.391 with 7th A, S42.399A
CC with 7th character K or P: M80.00X-
M84.68X with 7th [K, P], S02.0XX-S02.92X
with 7th K, S12.000-S12.691 with 7th K,
S22.000-S22.9XX with 7th K, S32.000-
S32.9XX with 7th K, S42.001-S42.92X with
7th [K, P], S49.001-S49.199 with 7th [K, P],
S52.001-S52.92X with 7th [K, M, N, P, Q, R],
S59.001-S59.299 with 7th [K, P], S62.001-
S62.92X with 7th [K, P], S72.001-S72.92X
with 7th [K, M, N, P, Q, R], S79.001-S79.199
with 7th [K, P], S82.001-S82.92X with 7th [K,
M, N, P, Q, R], S89.001-S89.399 with 7th [K, P],
S92.001-S92.919 with 7th [K, P]

7,19 ✓7ᵗʰ **S42.312** **Greenstick fracture of shaft of** `CC`
humerus, left arm
CC Excl: CC with 7th character A: S42.312-
S42.319 with 7th A, S42.322-S42.323 with
7th A, S42.325-S42.326 with 7th A, S42.332-
S42.333 with 7th A, S42.335-S42.336 with
7th A, S42.342-S42.343 with 7th A, S42.345-
S42.346 with 7th A, S42.352-S42.353 with
7th A, S42.355-S42.356 with 7th A, S42.362-
S42.363 with 7th A, S42.365-S42.366 with
7th A, S42.392-S42.399 with 7th A
CC with 7th character K or P: M80.00X-
M84.68X with 7th [K, P], S02.0XX-S02.92X
with 7th K, S12.000-S12.691 with 7th K,
S22.000-S22.9XX with 7th K, S32.000-
S32.9XX with 7th K, S42.001-S42.92X with
7th [K, P], S49.001-S49.199 with 7th [K, P],
S52.001-S52.92X with 7th [K, M, N, P, Q, R],
S59.001-S59.299 with 7th [K, P], S62.001-
S62.92X with 7th [K, P], S72.001-S72.92X
with 7th [K, M, N, P, Q, R], S79.001-S79.199
with 7th [K, P], S82.001-S82.92X with 7th [K,
M, N, P, Q, R], S89.001-S89.399 with 7th [K, P],
S92.001-S92.919 with 7th [K, P]

---

7   HAC = Initial encounter only (7th character A, B or C) and not POA.
16   MCC only if an open fracture (7th character B or C – specific to category).
19   CC only if an initial encounter for a closed fracture (7th character A) **OR** a subsequent encounter for nonunion or malunion (7th character K, M, N, P, Q, or R – specific to category).

✅ Additional Character Required   ✓x7ᵗʰ Placeholder Alert   Unacceptable PDx   Manifestation   Hospital Acquired Condition   *EXCLUDES 1* Not Coded Here   *EXCLUDES 2* Not Included Here

7,19 ✓7ᵗʰ **S42.319 Greenstick fracture of shaft of humerus, unspecified arm** CC
    CC Excl: CC with 7th character A: S42.311-S42.399 with 7th A
    CC with 7th character K or P: M80.00X-M84.68X with 7th [K, P], S02.0XX-S02.92X with 7th K, S12.000-S12.691 with 7th K, S22.000-S22.9XX with 7th K, S32.000-S32.9XX with 7th K, S42.001-S42.92X with 7th [K, P], S49.001-S49.199 with 7th [K, P], S52.001-S52.92X with 7th [K, M, N, P, Q, R], S59.001-S59.299 with 7th [K, P], S62.001-S62.92X with 7th [K, P], S72.001-S72.92X with 7th [K, M, N, P, Q, R], S79.001-S79.199 with 7th [K, P], S82.001-S82.92X with 7th [K, M, N, P, Q, R], S89.001-S89.399 with 7th [K, P], S92.001-S92.919 with 7th [K, P]

✓6ᵗʰ **S42.32 Transverse** fracture of shaft of humerus

7,16,19 ✓7ᵗʰ **S42.321 Displaced transverse fracture of shaft of humerus, right arm** MCC CC
    CC Excl: CC with 7th character A: S42.311 with 7th A, S42.319-S42.321 with 7th A, S42.323-S42.324 with 7th A, S42.326-S42.331 with 7th A, S42.333-S42.334 with 7th A, S42.336-S42.341 with 7th A, S42.343-S42.344 with 7th A, S42.346-S42.351 with 7th A, S42.353-S42.354 with 7th A, S42.356-S42.361 with 7th A, S42.363-S42.364 with 7th A, S42.366-S42.391 with 7th A, S42.399A
    MCC with 7th character B: S42.201-S42.266 with 7th B, S42.291-S42.92X with 7th B, S49.101-S49.199 with 7th A, S62.90XB
    CC with 7th character K or P: M80.00X-M84.68X with 7th [K, P], S02.0XX-S02.92X with 7th K, S12.000-S12.691 with 7th K, S22.000-S22.9XX with 7th K, S32.000-S32.9XX with 7th K, S42.001-S42.92X with 7th [K, P], S49.001-S49.199 with 7th [K, P], S52.001-S52.92X with 7th [K, M, N, P, Q, R], S59.001-S59.299 with 7th [K, P], S62.001-S62.92X with 7th [K, P], S72.001-S72.92X with 7th [K, M, N, P, Q, R], S79.001-S79.199 with 7th [K, P], S82.001-S82.92X with 7th [K, M, N, P, Q, R], S89.001-S89.399 with 7th [K, P], S92.001-S92.919 with 7th [K, P]

7,16,19 ✓7ᵗʰ **S42.322 Displaced transverse fracture of shaft of humerus, left arm** MCC CC
    CC Excl: CC with 7th character A: S42.312-S42.319 with 7th A, S42.322-S42.323 with 7th A, S42.325-S42.326 with 7th A, S42.332-S42.333 with 7th A, S42.335-S42.336 with 7th A, S42.342-S42.343 with 7th A, S42.345-S42.346 with 7th A, S42.352-S42.353 with 7th A, S42.355-S42.356 with 7th A, S42.362-S42.363 with 7th A, S42.365-S42.366 with 7th A, S42.392-S42.399 with 7th A
    MCC with 7th character B: S42.201-S42.266 with 7th B, S42.291-S42.92X with 7th B, S49.101-S49.199 with 7th A, S62.90XB
    CC with 7th character K or P: M80.00X-M84.68X with 7th [K, P], S02.0XX-S02.92X with 7th K, S12.000-S12.691 with 7th K, S22.000-S22.9XX with 7th K, S32.000-S32.9XX with 7th K, S42.001-S42.92X with 7th [K, P], S49.001-S49.199 with 7th [K, P], S52.001-S52.92X with 7th [K, M, N, P, Q, R], S59.001-S59.299 with 7th [K, P], S62.001-S62.92X with 7th [K, P], S72.001-S72.92X with 7th [K, M, N, P, Q, R], S79.001-S79.199 with 7th [K, P], S82.001-S82.92X with 7th [K, M, N, P, Q, R], S89.001-S89.399 with 7th [K, P], S92.001-S92.919 with 7th [K, P]

7,16,19 ✓7ᵗʰ **S42.323 Displaced transverse fracture of shaft of humerus, unspecified arm** MCC CC
    CC Excl: CC with 7th character A: S42.311-S42.399 with 7th A
    MCC with 7th character B: S42.201-S42.266 with 7th B, S42.291-S42.92X with 7th B, S49.101-S49.199 with 7th A, S62.90XB

7,16,19 ✓7ᵗʰ **S42.324 Nondisplaced transverse fracture of shaft of humerus, right arm** MCC CC
    CC Excl: See code: S42.321

7,16,19 ✓7ᵗʰ **S42.325 Nondisplaced transverse fracture of shaft of humerus, left arm** MCC CC
    CC Excl: See code: S42.322

7,16,19 ✓7ᵗʰ **S42.326 Nondisplaced transverse fracture of shaft of humerus, unspecified arm** MCC CC
    CC Excl: See code: S42.323

✓6ᵗʰ **S42.33 Oblique** fracture of shaft of humerus

7,16,19 ✓7ᵗʰ **S42.331 Displaced oblique fracture of shaft of humerus, right arm** MCC CC
    CC Excl: See code: S42.321

7,16,19 ✓7ᵗʰ **S42.332 Displaced oblique fracture of shaft of humerus, left arm** MCC CC
    CC Excl: See code: S42.322

7,16,19 ✓7ᵗʰ **S42.333 Displaced oblique fracture of shaft of humerus, unspecified arm** MCC CC
    CC Excl: See code: S42.323

7,16,19 ✓7ᵗʰ **S42.334 Nondisplaced oblique fracture of shaft of humerus, right arm** MCC CC
    CC Excl: See code: S42.321

7,16,19 ✓7ᵗʰ **S42.335 Nondisplaced oblique fracture of shaft of humerus, left arm** MCC CC
    CC Excl: See code: S42.322

7,16,19 ✓7ᵗʰ **S42.336 Nondisplaced oblique fracture of shaft of humerus, unspecified arm** MCC CC
    CC Excl: See code: S42.323

✓6ᵗʰ **S42.34 Spiral** fracture of shaft of humerus

7,16,19 ✓7ᵗʰ **S42.341 Displaced spiral fracture of shaft of humerus, right arm** MCC CC
    CC Excl: See code: S42.321

7,16,19 ✓7ᵗʰ **S42.342 Displaced spiral fracture of shaft of humerus, left arm** MCC CC
    CC Excl: See code: S42.322

7,16,19 ✓7ᵗʰ **S42.343 Displaced spiral fracture of shaft of humerus, unspecified arm** MCC CC
    CC Excl: See code: S42.323

7,16,19 ✓7ᵗʰ **S42.344 Nondisplaced spiral fracture of shaft of humerus, right arm** MCC CC
    CC Excl: See code: S42.321

7,16,19 ✓7ᵗʰ **S42.345 Nondisplaced spiral fracture of shaft of humerus, left arm** MCC CC
    CC Excl: See code: S42.322

7,16,19 ✓7ᵗʰ **S42.346 Nondisplaced spiral fracture of shaft of humerus, unspecified arm** MCC CC
    CC Excl: See code: S42.323

✓6ᵗʰ **S42.35 Comminuted** fracture of shaft of humerus

7,16,19 ✓7ᵗʰ **S42.351 Displaced comminuted fracture of shaft of humerus, right arm** MCC CC
    CC Excl: See code: S42.321

7,16,19 ✓7ᵗʰ **S42.352 Displaced comminuted fracture of shaft of humerus, left arm** MCC CC
    CC Excl: See code: S42.322

7,16,19 ✓7ᵗʰ **S42.353 Displaced comminuted fracture of shaft of humerus, unspecified arm** MCC CC
    CC Excl: See code: S42.323

7,16,19 ✓7ᵗʰ **S42.354 Nondisplaced comminuted fracture of shaft of humerus, right arm** MCC CC
    CC Excl: See code: S42.321

7,16,19 ✓7ᵗʰ **S42.355 Nondisplaced comminuted fracture of shaft of humerus, left arm** MCC CC
    CC Excl: See code: S42.322

7,16,19 ✓7ᵗʰ **S42.356 Nondisplaced comminuted fracture of shaft of humerus, unspecified arm** MCC CC
    CC Excl: See code: S42.323

✓6ᵗʰ **S42.36 Segmental** fracture of shaft of humerus

7,16,19 ✓7ᵗʰ **S42.361 Displaced segmental fracture of shaft of humerus, right arm** MCC CC
    CC Excl: See code: S42.321

7,16,19 ✓7ᵗʰ **S42.362 Displaced segmental fracture of shaft of humerus, left arm** MCC CC
    CC Excl: See code: S42.322

7,16,19 ✓7ᵗʰ **S42.363 Displaced segmental fracture of shaft of humerus, unspecified arm** MCC CC
    CC Excl: See code: S42.323

7,16,19 ✓7ᵗʰ **S42.364 Nondisplaced segmental fracture of shaft of humerus, right arm** MCC CC
    CC Excl: See code: S42.321

7,16,19 ✓7ᵗʰ **S42.365 Nondisplaced segmental fracture of shaft of humerus, left arm** MCC CC
    CC Excl: See code: S42.322

---

7 HAC = Initial encounter only (7th character A, B or C) and not POA.
16 MCC only if an open fracture (7th character B or C – specific to category).
19 CC only if an initial encounter for a closed fracture (7th character A) **OR** a subsequent encounter for nonunion or malunion (7th character K, M, N, P, Q, or R – specific to category).

Ⓝ Newborn: 0   Ⓟ Pediatric: 0-17   Ⓜ Maternity: 12-55   Ⓐ Adult: 15-124   MCC Major CC Condition   PDxMCC PDx acts as own MCC   CC CC Condition   PDxCC PDx acts as own CC

7,16,19 ✓7ᵗʰ **S42.366** **Nondisplaced** segmental fracture of shaft of humerus, **unspecified** arm   MCC CC
> CC Excl: See code: S42.323

✓6ᵗʰ **S42.39** **Other** fracture of shaft of humerus

7,16,19 ✓7ᵗʰ **S42.391** **Other** fracture of shaft of **right** humerus   MCC CC
> CC Excl: See code: S42.321

7,16,19 ✓7ᵗʰ **S42.392** **Other** fracture of shaft of **left** humerus   MCC CC
> CC Excl: See code: S42.322

7,16,19 ✓7ᵗʰ **S42.399** **Other** fracture of shaft of **unspecified humerus**   MCC CC
> CC Excl: See code: S42.323

✓5ᵗʰ **S42.4** **Fracture of lower end of humerus**
Fracture of distal end of humerus
> EXCLUDES 2   *fracture of shaft of humerus (S42.3-)*
> *physeal fracture of lower end of humerus (S49.1-)*

✓6ᵗʰ **S42.40** **Unspecified** fracture of lower end of humerus
Fracture of elbow NOS

7,16,19 ✓7ᵗʰ **S42.401** **Unspecified fracture of lower end of right humerus**   MCC CC
> CC Excl: CC with 7th character A: S42.201-S42.271 with 7th [A, B], S42.279-S42.311 with 7th A, S42.319-S42.481 with 7th A, S42.489-S42.92X with 7th A, S49.001A, S49.009-S49.011 with 7th A, S49.019-S49.021 with 7th A, S49.029-S49.031 with 7th A, S49.039-S49.041 with 7th A, S49.049-S49.091 with 7th A, S49.099-S49.101 with 7th A, S49.109-S49.111 with 7th A, S49.119-S49.121 with 7th A, S49.129-S49.131 with 7th A, S49.139-S49.141 with 7th A, S49.149-S49.191 with 7th A, S49.199A
> MCC with 7th character B: S42.201-S42.266 with 7th B, S42.291-S42.92X with 7th B, S49.101-S49.199 with 7th A, S62.9XB
> CC with 7th character K or P: M80.00X-M84.68X with 7th [K, P], S02.0XX-S02.92X with 7th K, S12.000-S12.691 with 7th K, S22.000-S22.9XX with 7th K, S32.000-S32.9XX with 7th K, S42.001-S42.92X with 7th [K, P], S49.001-S49.199 with 7th [K, P], S52.001-S52.92X with 7th [K, M, N, P, Q, R], S59.001-S59.299 with 7th [K, P], S62.001-S62.92X with 7th [K, P], S72.001-S72.92X with 7th [K, M, N, P, Q, R], S79.001-S79.199 with 7th [K, P], S82.001-S82.92X with 7th [K, M, N, P, Q, R], S89.001-S89.399 with 7th [K, P], S92.001-S92.919 with 7th [K, P]

7,16,19 ✓7ᵗʰ **S42.402** **Unspecified fracture of lower end of left humerus**   MCC CC
> CC Excl: CC with 7th character A: S42.201-S42.266 with 7th B, S42.272-S42.309 with 7th A, S42.312-S42.476 with 7th A, S42.482-S42.92X with 7th A, S49.002-S49.009 with 7th A, S49.012-S49.019 with 7th A, S49.022-S49.029 with 7th A, S49.032-S49.039 with 7th A, S49.042-S49.049 with 7th A, S49.092-S49.099 with 7th A, S49.102-S49.109 with 7th A, S49.112-S49.119 with 7th A, S49.122-S49.129 with 7th A, S49.132-S49.139 with 7th A, S49.142-S49.149 with 7th A, S49.192-S49.199 with 7th A
> MCC with 7th character B: S42.201-S42.266 with 7th B, S42.291-S42.92X with 7th B, S49.101-S49.199 with 7th A, S62.90XB
> CC with 7th character K or P: M80.00X-M84.68X with 7th [K, P], S02.0XX-S02.92X with 7th K, S12.000-S12.691 with 7th K, S22.000-S22.9XX with 7th K, S32.000-S32.9XX with 7th K, S42.001-S42.92X with 7th [K, P], S49.001-S49.199 with 7th [K, P], S52.001-S52.92X with 7th [K, M, N, P, Q, R], S59.001-S59.299 with 7th [K, P], S62.001-S62.92X with 7th [K, P], S72.001-S72.92X with 7th [K, M, N, P, Q, R], S79.001-S79.199 with 7th [K, P], S82.001-S82.92X with 7th [K, M, N, P, Q, R], S89.001-S89.399 with 7th [K, P], S92.001-S92.919 with 7th [K, P]

7,16,19 ✓7ᵗʰ **S42.409** **Unspecified fracture of lower end of unspecified humerus**   MCC CC
> CC Excl: CC with 7th character A: S42.201-S42.92X with 7th [A, B], S49.001-S49.199 with 7th A
> MCC with 7th character B: S42.201-S42.266 with 7th B, S42.291-S42.92X with 7th B, S49.101-S49.199 with 7th A, S62.90XB
> CC with 7th character K or P: M80.00X-M84.68X with 7th [K, P], S02.0XX-S02.92X with 7th K, S12.000-S12.691 with 7th K, S22.000-S22.9XX with 7th K, S32.000-S32.9XX with 7th K, S42.001-S42.92X with 7th [K, P], S49.001-S49.199 with 7th [K, P], S52.001-S52.92X with 7th [K, M, N, P, Q, R], S59.001-S59.299 with 7th [K, P], S62.001-S62.92X with 7th [K, P], S72.001-S72.92X with 7th [K, M, N, P, Q, R], S79.001-S79.199 with 7th [K, P], S82.001-S82.92X with 7th [K, M, N, P, Q, R], S89.001-S89.399 with 7th [K, P], S92.001-S92.919 with 7th [K, P]

✓6ᵗʰ **S42.41** **Simple supracondylar fracture without intercondylar fracture of humerus**

7,16,19 ✓7ᵗʰ **S42.411** **Displaced simple supracondylar fracture without intercondylar fracture of right humerus**   MCC CC
> CC Excl: See code: S42.401

7,16,19 ✓7ᵗʰ **S42.412** **Displaced simple supracondylar fracture without intercondylar fracture of left humerus**   MCC CC
> CC Excl: See code: S42.402

7,16,19 ✓7ᵗʰ **S42.413** **Displaced simple supracondylar fracture without intercondylar fracture of unspecified humerus**   MCC CC
> CC Excl: See code: S42.409

7,16,19 ✓7ᵗʰ **S42.414** **Nondisplaced simple supracondylar fracture without intercondylar fracture of right humerus**   MCC CC
> CC Excl: See code: S42.401

7,16,19 ✓7ᵗʰ **S42.415** **Nondisplaced simple supracondylar fracture without intercondylar fracture of left humerus**   MCC CC
> CC Excl: See code: S42.402

7,16,19 ✓7ᵗʰ **S42.416** **Nondisplaced simple supracondylar fracture without intercondylar fracture of unspecified humerus**   MCC CC
> CC Excl: See code: S42.409

✓6ᵗʰ **S42.42** **Comminuted supracondylar fracture without intercondylar fracture of humerus**

7,16,19 ✓7ᵗʰ **S42.421** **Displaced comminuted supracondylar fracture without intercondylar fracture of right humerus**   MCC CC
> CC Excl: See code: S42.401

7,16,19 ✓7ᵗʰ **S42.422** **Displaced comminuted supracondylar fracture without intercondylar fracture of left humerus**   MCC CC
> CC Excl: See code: S42.402

7,16,19 ✓7ᵗʰ **S42.423** **Displaced comminuted supracondylar fracture without intercondylar fracture of unspecified humerus**   MCC CC
> CC Excl: See code: S42.409

7,16,19 ✓7ᵗʰ **S42.424** **Nondisplaced comminuted supracondylar fracture without intercondylar fracture of right humerus**   MCC CC
> CC Excl: See code: S42.401

7,16,19 ✓7ᵗʰ **S42.425** **Nondisplaced comminuted supracondylar fracture without intercondylar fracture of left humerus**   MCC CC
> CC Excl: See code: S42.402

7,16,19 ✓7ᵗʰ **S42.426** **Nondisplaced comminuted supracondylar fracture without intercondylar fracture of unspecified humerus**   MCC CC
> CC Excl: See code: S42.409

---

7   HAC = Initial encounter only (7th character A, B or C) and not POA.
16   MCC only if an open fracture (7th character B or C – specific to category).
19   CC only if an initial encounter for a closed fracture (7th character A) **OR** a subsequent encounter for nonunion or malunion (7th character K, M, N, P, Q, or R – specific to category).

✓ Additional Character Required   ✓x7ᵗʰ Placeholder Alert   Unacceptable PDx   Manifestation   Hospital Acquired Condition   **EXCLUDES1** Not Coded Here   **EXCLUDES2** Not Included Here

Chapter 19. Injury, Poisoning, and Certain Other Consequences of External Causes *(side margin)*

S42.43–S42.481 *(side margin)*

✓6ᵗʰ **S42.43**   Fracture (avulsion) of lateral epicondyle of humerus

7,16,19 ✓7ᵗʰ **S42.431**   Displaced fracture (avulsion) of lateral epicondyle of right humerus   MCC CC
CC Excl: See code: S42.401

7,16,19 ✓7ᵗʰ **S42.432**   Displaced fracture (avulsion) of lateral epicondyle of left humerus   MCC CC
CC Excl: See code: S42.402

7,16,19 ✓7ᵗʰ **S42.433**   Displaced fracture (avulsion) of lateral epicondyle of unspecified humerus   MCC CC
CC Excl: See code: S42.409

7,16,19 ✓7ᵗʰ **S42.434**   Nondisplaced fracture (avulsion) of lateral epicondyle of right humerus   MCC CC
CC Excl: See code: S42.401

7,16,19 ✓7ᵗʰ **S42.435**   Nondisplaced fracture (avulsion) of lateral epicondyle of left humerus   MCC CC
CC Excl: See code: S42.402

7,16,19 ✓7ᵗʰ **S42.436**   Nondisplaced fracture (avulsion) of lateral epicondyle of unspecified humerus   MCC CC
CC Excl: See code: S42.409

✓6ᵗʰ **S42.44**   Fracture (avulsion) of medial epicondyle of humerus

7,16,19 ✓7ᵗʰ **S42.441**   Displaced fracture (avulsion) of medial epicondyle of right humerus   MCC CC
CC Excl: See code: S42.401

7,16,19 ✓7ᵗʰ **S42.442**   Displaced fracture (avulsion) of medial epicondyle of left humerus   MCC CC
CC Excl: See code: S42.402

7,16,19 ✓7ᵗʰ **S42.443**   Displaced fracture (avulsion) of medial epicondyle of unspecified humerus   MCC CC
CC Excl: See code: S42.409

7,16,19 ✓7ᵗʰ **S42.444**   Nondisplaced fracture (avulsion) of medial epicondyle of right humerus   MCC CC
CC Excl: See code: S42.401

7,16,19 ✓7ᵗʰ **S42.445**   Nondisplaced fracture (avulsion) of medial epicondyle of left humerus   MCC CC
CC Excl: See code: S42.402

7,16,19 ✓7ᵗʰ **S42.446**   Nondisplaced fracture (avulsion) medial epicondyle of unspecified of humerus   MCC CC
CC Excl: See code: S42.409

7,16,19 ✓7ᵗʰ **S42.447**   Incarcerated fracture (avulsion) of medial epicondyle of right humerus   MCC CC
CC Excl: See code: S42.401

7,16,19 ✓7ᵗʰ **S42.448**   Incarcerated fracture (avulsion) of medial epicondyle of left humerus   MCC CC
CC Excl: See code: S42.402

7,16,19 ✓7ᵗʰ **S42.449**   Incarcerated fracture (avulsion) of medial epicondyle of unspecified humerus   MCC CC
CC Excl: See code: S42.409

✓6ᵗʰ **S42.45**   Fracture of lateral condyle of humerus
Fracture of capitellum of humerus

7,16,19 ✓7ᵗʰ **S42.451**   Displaced fracture of lateral condyle of right humerus   MCC CC
CC Excl: See code: S42.401

7,16,19 ✓7ᵗʰ **S42.452**   Displaced fracture of lateral condyle of left humerus   MCC CC
CC Excl: See code: S42.402

7,16,19 ✓7ᵗʰ **S42.453**   Displaced fracture of lateral condyle of unspecified humerus   MCC CC
CC Excl: See code: S42.409

7,16,19 ✓7ᵗʰ **S42.454**   Nondisplaced fracture of lateral condyle of right humerus   MCC CC
CC Excl: See code: S42.401

7,16,19 ✓7ᵗʰ **S42.455**   Nondisplaced fracture of lateral condyle of left humerus   MCC CC
CC Excl: See code: S42.402

7,16,19 ✓7ᵗʰ **S42.456**   Nondisplaced fracture of lateral condyle of unspecified humerus   MCC CC
CC Excl: See code: S42.409

✓6ᵗʰ **S42.46**   Fracture of medial condyle of humerus
Trochlea fracture of humerus

7,16,19 ✓7ᵗʰ **S42.461**   Displaced fracture of medial condyle of right humerus   MCC CC
CC Excl: See code: S42.401

7,16,19 ✓7ᵗʰ **S42.462**   Displaced fracture of medial condyle of left humerus   MCC CC
CC Excl: See code: S42.402

7,16,19 ✓7ᵗʰ **S42.463**   Displaced fracture of medial condyle of unspecified humerus   MCC CC
CC Excl: See code: S42.409

7,16,19 ✓7ᵗʰ **S42.464**   Nondisplaced fracture of medial condyle of right humerus   MCC CC
CC Excl: See code: S42.401

7,16,19 ✓7ᵗʰ **S42.465**   Nondisplaced fracture of medial condyle of left humerus   MCC CC
CC Excl: See code: S42.402

7,16,19 ✓7ᵗʰ **S42.466**   Nondisplaced fracture of medial condyle of unspecified humerus   MCC CC
CC Excl: See code: S42.409

✓6ᵗʰ **S42.47**   Transcondylar fracture of humerus

7,16,19 ✓7ᵗʰ **S42.471**   Displaced transcondylar fracture of right humerus   MCC CC
CC Excl: See code: S42.401

7,16,19 ✓7ᵗʰ **S42.472**   Displaced transcondylar fracture of left humerus   MCC CC
CC Excl: See code: S42.402

7,16,19 ✓7ᵗʰ **S42.473**   Displaced transcondylar fracture of unspecified humerus   MCC CC
CC Excl: See code: S42.409

7,16,19 ✓7ᵗʰ **S42.474**   Nondisplaced transcondylar fracture of right humerus   MCC CC
CC Excl: See code: S42.401

7,16,19 ✓7ᵗʰ **S42.475**   Nondisplaced transcondylar fracture of left humerus   MCC CC
CC Excl: See code: S42.402

7,16,19 ✓7ᵗʰ **S42.476**   Nondisplaced transcondylar fracture of unspecified humerus   MCC CC
CC Excl: See code: S42.409

✓6ᵗʰ **S42.48**   Torus fracture of lower end of humerus

> The appropriate 7th is to be added to all codes in subcategory S42.48.
> A   initial encounter for closed fracture
> D   subsequent encounter for fracture with routine healing
> G   subsequent encounter for fracture with delayed healing
> K   subsequent encounter for fracture with nonunion
> P   subsequent encounter for fracture with malunion
> S   sequela

7,19 ✓7ᵗʰ **S42.481**   Torus fracture of lower end of right humerus   CC
CC Excl: CC with 7th character A: S42.201-S42.271 with 7th [A, B], S42.279-S42.311 with 7th A, S42.319-S42.481 with 7th A, S42.489-S42.92X with 7th A, S49.001A, S49.009-S49.011 with 7th A, S49.019-S49.021 with 7th A, S49.029-S49.031 with 7th A, S49.039-S49.041 with 7th A, S49.049-S49.091 with 7th A, S49.099-S49.101 with 7th A, S49.109-S49.111 with 7th A, S49.119-S49.121 with 7th A, S49.129-S49.131 with 7th A, S49.139-S49.141 with 7th A, S49.149-S49.191 with 7th A, S49.199A
CC Excl: with 7th K or P: M80.00X-M84.68X with 7th [K, P], S02.0XX-S02.92X with 7th K, S12.000-S12.691 with 7th K, S22.000-S22.9XX with 7th K, S32.000-S32.9XX with 7th K, S42.001-S42.92X with 7th [K, P], S49.001-S49.199 with 7th [K, P], S52.001-S52.92X with 7th [K, M, N, P, Q, R], S59.001-S59.299 with 7th [K, P], S62.001-S62.92X with 7th [K, P], S72.001-S72.92X with 7th [K, M, N, P, Q, R], S79.001-S79.199 with 7th [K, P], S82.001-S82.92X with 7th [K, M, N, P, Q, R], S89.001-S89.399 with 7th [K, P], S92.001-S92.919 with 7th [K, P]

---

7   HAC = Initial encounter only (7th character A, B or C) and not POA.
16   MCC only if an open fracture (7th character B or C – specific to category).
19   CC only if an initial encounter for a closed fracture (7th character A) **OR** a subsequent encounter for nonunion or malunion (7th character K, M, N, P, Q, or R – specific to category).

N Newborn: 0   P Pediatric: 0-17   M Maternity: 12-55   A Adult: 15-124   MCC Major CC Condition   PDxMCC PDx acts as own MCC   CC CC Condition   PDxCC PDx acts as own CC

7,19 ✓7ᵗʰ **S42.482** **Torus fracture of lower end of left humerus** `CC`
> **CC Excl: CC with 7th character A:** S42.201-S42.266 with 7th B, S42.272-S42.309 with 7th A, S42.312-S42.476 with 7th A, S42.482-S42.92X with 7th A, S49.002-S49.009 with 7th A, S49.012-S49.019 with 7th A, S49.022-S49.029 with 7th A, S49.032-S49.039 with 7th A, S49.042-S49.049 with 7th A, S49.092-S49.099 with 7th A, S49.102-S49.109 with 7th A, S49.112-S49.119 with 7th A, S49.122-S49.129 with 7th A, S49.132-S49.139 with 7th A, S49.142-S49.149 with 7th A, S49.192-S49.199 with 7th A
> **CC Excl: with 7th K or P:** M80.00X-M84.68X with 7th [K, P], S02.0XX-S02.92X with 7th K, S12.000-S12.691 with 7th K, S22.000-S22.9XX with 7th K, S32.000-S32.9XX with 7th K, S42.001-S42.92X with 7th [K, P], S49.001-S49.199 with 7th [K, P], S52.001-S52.92X with 7th [K, M, N, P, Q, R], S59.001-S59.299 with 7th [K, P], S62.001-S62.92X with 7th [K, P], S72.001-S72.92X with 7th [K, M, N, P, Q, R], S79.001-S79.199 with 7th [K, P], S82.001-S82.92X with 7th [K, M, N, P, Q, R], S89.001-S89.399 with 7th [K, P], S92.001-S92.919 with 7th [K, P]

7,19 ✓7ᵗʰ **S42.489** **Torus fracture of lower end of unspecified humerus** `CC`
> **CC Excl: CC with 7th character A:** S42.201-S42.92X with 7th [A, B], S49.001-S49.199 with 7th A
> **CC Excl: CC with 7th character K or P:** M80.00X-M84.68X with 7th [K, P], S02.0XX-S02.92X with 7th K, S12.000-S12.691 with 7th K, S22.000-S22.9XX with 7th K, S32.000-S32.9XX with 7th K, S42.001-S42.92X with 7th [K, P], S49.001-S49.199 with 7th [K, P], S52.001-S52.92X with 7th [K, M, N, P, Q, R], S59.001-S59.299 with 7th [K, P], S62.001-S62.92X with 7th [K, P], S72.001-S72.92X with 7th [K, M, N, P, Q, R], S79.001-S79.199 with 7th [K, P], S82.001-S82.92X with 7th [K, M, N, P, Q, R], S89.001-S89.399 with 7th [K, P], S92.001-S92.919 with 7th [K, P]

✓6ᵗʰ **S42.49** **Other fracture of lower end of humerus**

7,16,19 ✓7ᵗʰ **S42.491** **Other displaced fracture of lower end of right humerus** `MCC` `CC`
> **CC Excl:** See code: S42.401

7,16,19 ✓7ᵗʰ **S42.492** **Other displaced fracture of lower end of left humerus** `MCC` `CC`
> **CC Excl:** See code: S42.402

7,16,19 ✓7ᵗʰ **S42.493** **Other displaced fracture of lower end of unspecified humerus** `MCC` `CC`
> **CC Excl:** See code: S42.409

7,16,19 ✓7ᵗʰ **S42.494** **Other nondisplaced fracture of lower end of right humerus** `MCC` `CC`
> **CC Excl:** See code: S42.401

7,16,19 ✓7ᵗʰ **S42.495** **Other nondisplaced fracture of lower end of left humerus** `MCC` `CC`
> **CC Excl:** See code: S42.402

7,16,19 ✓7ᵗʰ **S42.496** **Other nondisplaced fracture of lower end of unspecified humerus** `MCC` `CC`
> **CC Excl:** See code: S42.409

✓5ᵗʰ **S42.9** **Fracture of shoulder girdle, part unspecified**
> Fracture of shoulder NOS

7,16,19 ✓x7ᵗʰ **S42.90** **Fracture of unspecified shoulder girdle, part unspecified** `MCC` `CC`
> **CC Excl:** See code: S42.409

7,16,19 ✓x7ᵗʰ **S42.91** **Fracture of right shoulder girdle, part unspecified** `MCC` `CC`
> **CC Excl:** See code: S42.409

7,16,19 ✓x7ᵗʰ **S42.92** **Fracture of left shoulder girdle, part unspecified** `MCC` `CC`
> **CC Excl:** See code: S42.409

✓4ᵗʰ **S43** **Dislocation and sprain of joints and ligaments of shoulder girdle**
> **INCLUDES** avulsion of joint or ligament of shoulder girdle
> laceration of cartilage, joint or ligament of shoulder girdle
> sprain of cartilage, joint or ligament of shoulder girdle
> traumatic hemarthrosis of joint or ligament of shoulder girdle
> traumatic rupture of joint or ligament of shoulder girdle
> traumatic subluxation of joint or ligament of shoulder girdle
> traumatic tear of joint or ligament of shoulder girdle

Code also any associated open wound
> **EXCLUDES 2** *strain of muscle, fascia and tendon of shoulder and upper arm (S46.-)*

> The appropriate 7th is to be added to each code from category S43.
> A   initial encounter
> D   subsequent encounter
> S   sequela

✓5ᵗʰ **S43.0** **Subluxation and dislocation of shoulder joint**
> Dislocation of glenohumeral joint
> Subluxation of glenohumeral joint

✓6ᵗʰ **S43.00** **Unspecified subluxation and dislocation of shoulder joint**
> Dislocation of humerus NOS
> Subluxation of humerus NOS

   ✓7ᵗʰ **S43.001** **Unspecified subluxation of right shoulder joint**

   ✓7ᵗʰ **S43.002** **Unspecified subluxation of left shoulder joint**

   ✓7ᵗʰ **S43.003** **Unspecified subluxation of unspecified shoulder joint**

   ✓7ᵗʰ **S43.004** **Unspecified dislocation of right shoulder joint**

   ✓7ᵗʰ **S43.005** **Unspecified dislocation of left shoulder joint**

   ✓7ᵗʰ **S43.006** **Unspecified dislocation of unspecified shoulder joint**

✓6ᵗʰ **S43.01** **Anterior subluxation and dislocation of humerus**

   ✓7ᵗʰ **S43.011** **Anterior subluxation of right humerus**

   ✓7ᵗʰ **S43.012** **Anterior subluxation of left humerus**

   ✓7ᵗʰ **S43.013** **Anterior subluxation of unspecified humerus**

   ✓7ᵗʰ **S43.014** **Anterior dislocation of right humerus**

   ✓7ᵗʰ **S43.015** **Anterior dislocation of left humerus**

   ✓7ᵗʰ **S43.016** **Anterior dislocation of unspecified humerus**

✓6ᵗʰ **S43.02** **Posterior subluxation and dislocation of humerus**

   ✓7ᵗʰ **S43.021** **Posterior subluxation of right humerus**

   ✓7ᵗʰ **S43.022** **Posterior subluxation of left humerus**

   ✓7ᵗʰ **S43.023** **Posterior subluxation of unspecified humerus**

   ✓7ᵗʰ **S43.024** **Posterior dislocation of right humerus**

   ✓7ᵗʰ **S43.025** **Posterior dislocation of left humerus**

   ✓7ᵗʰ **S43.026** **Posterior dislocation of unspecified humerus**

✓6ᵗʰ **S43.03** **Inferior subluxation and dislocation of humerus**

   ✓7ᵗʰ **S43.031** **Inferior subluxation of right humerus**

   ✓7ᵗʰ **S43.032** **Inferior subluxation of left humerus**

   ✓7ᵗʰ **S43.033** **Inferior subluxation of unspecified humerus**

   ✓7ᵗʰ **S43.034** **Inferior dislocation of right humerus**

   ✓7ᵗʰ **S43.035** **Inferior dislocation of left humerus**

   ✓7ᵗʰ **S43.036** **Inferior dislocation of unspecified humerus**

✓6ᵗʰ **S43.08** **Other subluxation and dislocation of shoulder joint**

   ✓7ᵗʰ **S43.081** **Other subluxation of right shoulder joint**

   ✓7ᵗʰ **S43.082** **Other subluxation of left shoulder joint**

   ✓7ᵗʰ **S43.083** **Other subluxation of unspecified shoulder joint**

   ✓7ᵗʰ **S43.084** **Other dislocation of right shoulder joint**

   ✓7ᵗʰ **S43.085** **Other dislocation of left shoulder joint**

   ✓7ᵗʰ **S43.086** **Other dislocation of unspecified shoulder joint**

---

7   HAC = Initial encounter only (7th character A, B or C) and not POA.
16   MCC only if an open fracture (7th character B or C – specific to category).
19   CC only if an initial encounter for a closed fracture (7th character A) **OR** a subsequent encounter for nonunion or malunion (7th character K, M, N, P, Q, or R – specific to category).

✓ Additional Character Required   ✓x7ᵗʰ Placeholder Alert   Unacceptable PDx   Manifestation   Hospital Acquired Condition   **EXCLUDES 1** Not Coded Here   **EXCLUDES 2** Not Included Here

√5ᵗʰ **S43.1 Subluxation and dislocation of acromioclavicular joint**

√6ᵗʰ **S43.10 Unspecified dislocation of acromioclavicular joint**

√7ᵗʰ **S43.101 Unspecified dislocation of right acromioclavicular joint**

√7ᵗʰ **S43.102 Unspecified dislocation of left acromioclavicular joint**

√7ᵗʰ **S43.109 Unspecified dislocation of unspecified acromioclavicular joint**

√6ᵗʰ **S43.11 Subluxation of acromioclavicular joint**

√7ᵗʰ **S43.111 Subluxation of right acromioclavicular joint**

√7ᵗʰ **S43.112 Subluxation of left acromioclavicular joint**

√7ᵗʰ **S43.119 Subluxation of unspecified acromioclavicular joint**

√6ᵗʰ **S43.12 Dislocation of acromioclavicular joint, 100%-200% displacement**

√7ᵗʰ **S43.121 Dislocation of right acromioclavicular joint, 100%-200% displacement**

√7ᵗʰ **S43.122 Dislocation of left acromioclavicular joint, 100%-200% displacement**

√7ᵗʰ **S43.129 Dislocation of unspecified acromioclavicular joint, 100%-200% displacement**

√6ᵗʰ **S43.13 Dislocation of acromioclavicular joint, greater than 200% displacement**

√7ᵗʰ **S43.131 Dislocation of right acromioclavicular joint, greater than 200% displacement**

√7ᵗʰ **S43.132 Dislocation of left acromioclavicular joint, greater than 200% displacement**

√7ᵗʰ **S43.139 Dislocation of unspecified acromioclavicular joint, greater than 200% displacement**

√6ᵗʰ **S43.14 Inferior dislocation of acromioclavicular joint**

√7ᵗʰ **S43.141 Inferior dislocation of right acromioclavicular joint**

√7ᵗʰ **S43.142 Inferior dislocation of left acromioclavicular joint**

√7ᵗʰ **S43.149 Inferior dislocation of unspecified acromioclavicular joint**

√6ᵗʰ **S43.15 Posterior dislocation of acromioclavicular joint**

√7ᵗʰ **S43.151 Posterior dislocation of right acromioclavicular joint**

√7ᵗʰ **S43.152 Posterior dislocation of left acromioclavicular joint**

√7ᵗʰ **S43.159 Posterior dislocation of unspecified acromioclavicular joint**

√5ᵗʰ **S43.2 Subluxation and dislocation of sternoclavicular joint**

√6ᵗʰ **S43.20 Unspecified subluxation and dislocation of sternoclavicular joint**

7 √7ᵗʰ **S43.201 Unspecified subluxation of right sternoclavicular joint**   CC
CC Excl: CC with 7th character A: M99.18, S43.201 with 7th A, S43.203-S43.204 with 7th A, S43.206-S43.211 with 7th A, S43.213-S43.214 with 7th A, S43.216-S43.221 with 7th A, S43.223-S43.224 with 7th A, S43.226A

7 √7ᵗʰ **S43.202 Unspecified subluxation of left sternoclavicular joint**   CC
CC Excl: CC with 7th character A: M99.18, S43.202-S43.203 with 7th A, S43.205-S43.206 with 7th A, S43.212-S43.213 with 7th A, S43.215-S43.216 with 7th A, S43.222-S43.223 with 7th A, S43.225-S43.226 with 7th A

7 √7ᵗʰ **S43.203 Unspecified subluxation of unspecified sternoclavicular joint**   CC
CC Excl: CC with 7th character A: M99.18, S43.201-S43.226 with 7th A

7 √7ᵗʰ **S43.204 Unspecified dislocation of right sternoclavicular joint**   CC
CC Excl: See code: S43.201

7 √7ᵗʰ **S43.205 Unspecified dislocation of left sternoclavicular joint**   CC
CC Excl: See code: S43.202

7 √7ᵗʰ **S43.206 Unspecified dislocation of unspecified sternoclavicular joint**   CC
CC Excl: See code: S43.203

√6ᵗʰ **S43.21 Anterior subluxation and dislocation of sternoclavicular joint**

7 √7ᵗʰ **S43.211 Anterior subluxation of right sternoclavicular joint**   CC
CC Excl: See code: S43.201

7 √7ᵗʰ **S43.212 Anterior subluxation of left sternoclavicular joint**   CC
CC Excl: See code: S43.202

7 √7ᵗʰ **S43.213 Anterior subluxation of unspecified sternoclavicular joint**   CC
CC Excl: See code: S43.203

7 √7ᵗʰ **S43.214 Anterior dislocation of right sternoclavicular joint**   CC
CC Excl: See code: S43.201

7 √7ᵗʰ **S43.215 Anterior dislocation of left sternoclavicular joint**   CC
CC Excl: See code: S43.202

7 √7ᵗʰ **S43.216 Anterior dislocation of unspecified sternoclavicular joint**   CC
CC Excl: See code: S43.203

√6ᵗʰ **S43.22 Posterior subluxation and dislocation of sternoclavicular joint**

7 √7ᵗʰ **S43.221 Posterior subluxation of right sternoclavicular joint**   CC
CC Excl: See code: S43.201

7 √7ᵗʰ **S43.222 Posterior subluxation of left sternoclavicular joint**   CC
CC Excl: See code: S43.202

7 √7ᵗʰ **S43.223 Posterior subluxation of unspecified sternoclavicular joint**   CC
CC Excl: See code: S43.203

7 √7ᵗʰ **S43.224 Posterior dislocation of right sternoclavicular joint**   CC
CC Excl: See code: S43.201

7 √7ᵗʰ **S43.225 Posterior dislocation of left sternoclavicular joint**   CC
CC Excl: See code: S43.202

7 √7ᵗʰ **S43.226 Posterior dislocation of unspecified sternoclavicular joint**   CC
CC Excl: See code: S43.203

√5ᵗʰ **S43.3 Subluxation and dislocation of other and unspecified parts of shoulder girdle**

√6ᵗʰ **S43.30 Subluxation and dislocation of unspecified parts of shoulder girdle**
Dislocation of shoulder girdle NOS
Subluxation of shoulder girdle NOS

√7ᵗʰ **S43.301 Subluxation of unspecified parts of right shoulder girdle**

√7ᵗʰ **S43.302 Subluxation of unspecified parts of left shoulder girdle**

√7ᵗʰ **S43.303 Subluxation of unspecified parts of unspecified shoulder girdle**

√7ᵗʰ **S43.304 Dislocation of unspecified parts of right shoulder girdle**

√7ᵗʰ **S43.305 Dislocation of unspecified parts of left shoulder girdle**

√7ᵗʰ **S43.306 Dislocation of unspecified parts of unspecified shoulder girdle**

√6ᵗʰ **S43.31 Subluxation and dislocation of scapula**

√7ᵗʰ **S43.311 Subluxation of right scapula**

√7ᵗʰ **S43.312 Subluxation of left scapula**

√7ᵗʰ **S43.313 Subluxation of unspecified scapula**

√7ᵗʰ **S43.314 Dislocation of right scapula**

√7ᵗʰ **S43.315 Dislocation of left scapula**

√7ᵗʰ **S43.316 Dislocation of unspecified scapula**

√6ᵗʰ **S43.39 Subluxation and dislocation of other parts of shoulder girdle**

√7ᵗʰ **S43.391 Subluxation of other parts of right shoulder girdle**

√7ᵗʰ **S43.392 Subluxation of other parts of left shoulder girdle**

√7ᵗʰ **S43.393 Subluxation of other parts of unspecified shoulder girdle**

√7ᵗʰ **S43.394 Dislocation of other parts of right shoulder girdle**

---

7   HAC = Initial encounter only (7th character A, B or C) and not POA.

N Newborn: 0   P Pediatric: 0-17   M Maternity: 12-55   A Adult: 15-124   **MCC** Major CC Condition   **PDxMCC** PDx acts as own MCC   **CC** CC Condition   **PDxCC** PDx acts as own CC

954   ICD-10-CM 2016

√7ᵗʰ **S43.395** Dislocation of other parts of left shoulder girdle

√7ᵗʰ **S43.396** Dislocation of other parts of unspecified shoulder girdle

√5ᵗʰ **S43.4 Sprain of shoulder joint**

     √6ᵗʰ **S43.40** Unspecified sprain of shoulder joint

        √7ᵗʰ **S43.401** Unspecified sprain of right shoulder joint

        √7ᵗʰ **S43.402** Unspecified sprain of left shoulder joint

        √7ᵗʰ **S43.409** Unspecified sprain of unspecified shoulder joint

     √6ᵗʰ **S43.41** Sprain of coracohumeral (ligament)

        √7ᵗʰ **S43.411** Sprain of right coracohumeral (ligament)

        √7ᵗʰ **S43.412** Sprain of left coracohumeral (ligament)

        √7ᵗʰ **S43.419** Sprain of unspecified coracohumeral (ligament)

     √6ᵗʰ **S43.42** Sprain of rotator cuff capsule

        EXCLUDES 1 *rotator cuff syndrome (complete) (incomplete), not specified as traumatic (M75.1-)*

        EXCLUDES 2 *injury of tendon of rotator cuff (S46.0-)*

        √7ᵗʰ **S43.421** Sprain of right rotator cuff capsule

        √7ᵗʰ **S43.422** Sprain of left rotator cuff capsule

        √7ᵗʰ **S43.429** Sprain of unspecified rotator cuff capsule

     √6ᵗʰ **S43.43** Superior glenoid labrum lesion
          SLAP lesion

        √7ᵗʰ **S43.431** Superior glenoid labrum lesion of right shoulder

        √7ᵗʰ **S43.432** Superior glenoid labrum lesion of left shoulder

        √7ᵗʰ **S43.439** Superior glenoid labrum lesion of unspecified shoulder

     √6ᵗʰ **S43.49** Other sprain of shoulder joint

        √7ᵗʰ **S43.491** Other sprain of right shoulder joint

        √7ᵗʰ **S43.492** Other sprain of left shoulder joint

        √7ᵗʰ **S43.499** Other sprain of unspecified shoulder joint

√5ᵗʰ **S43.5 Sprain of acromioclavicular joint**
     Sprain of acromioclavicular ligament

     √x7ᵗʰ **S43.50** Sprain of unspecified acromioclavicular joint

     √x7ᵗʰ **S43.51** Sprain of right acromioclavicular joint

     √x7ᵗʰ **S43.52** Sprain of left acromioclavicular joint

√5ᵗʰ **S43.6 Sprain of sternoclavicular joint**

     √x7ᵗʰ **S43.60** Sprain of unspecified sternoclavicular joint

     √x7ᵗʰ **S43.61** Sprain of right sternoclavicular joint

     √x7ᵗʰ **S43.62** Sprain of left sternoclavicular joint

√5ᵗʰ **S43.8 Sprain of other specified parts of shoulder girdle**

     √x7ᵗʰ **S43.80** Sprain of other specified parts of unspecified shoulder girdle

     √x7ᵗʰ **S43.81** Sprain of other specified parts of right shoulder girdle

     √x7ᵗʰ **S43.82** Sprain of other specified parts of left shoulder girdle

√5ᵗʰ **S43.9 Sprain of unspecified parts of shoulder girdle**

     √x7ᵗʰ **S43.90** Sprain of unspecified parts of unspecified shoulder girdle
          Sprain of shoulder girdle NOS

     √x7ᵗʰ **S43.91** Sprain of unspecified parts of right shoulder girdle

     √x7ᵗʰ **S43.92** Sprain of unspecified parts of left shoulder girdle

√4ᵗʰ **S44 Injury of nerves at shoulder and upper arm level**
     Code also any associated open wound (S41.-)
     EXCLUDES 2 *injury of brachial plexus (S14.3-)*

     The appropriate 7th is to be added to each code from category S44.
     A   initial encounter
     D   subsequent encounter
     S   sequela

     √5ᵗʰ **S44.0 Injury of ulnar nerve at upper arm level**
        EXCLUDES 1 *ulnar nerve NOS (S54.0)*

        √x7ᵗʰ **S44.00** Injury of ulnar nerve at upper arm level, unspecified arm

        √x7ᵗʰ **S44.01** Injury of ulnar nerve at upper arm level, right arm

        √x7ᵗʰ **S44.02** Injury of ulnar nerve at upper arm level, left arm

√5ᵗʰ **S44.1 Injury of median nerve at upper arm level**
     EXCLUDES 1 *median nerve NOS (S54.1)*

     √x7ᵗʰ **S44.10** Injury of median nerve at upper arm level, unspecified arm

     √x7ᵗʰ **S44.11** Injury of median nerve at upper arm level, right arm

     √x7ᵗʰ **S44.12** Injury of median nerve at upper arm level, left arm

√5ᵗʰ **S44.2 Injury of radial nerve at upper arm level**
     EXCLUDES 1 *radial nerve NOS (S54.2)*

     √x7ᵗʰ **S44.20** Injury of radial nerve at upper arm level, unspecified arm

     √x7ᵗʰ **S44.21** Injury of radial nerve at upper arm level, right arm

     √x7ᵗʰ **S44.22** Injury of radial nerve at upper arm level, left arm

√5ᵗʰ **S44.3 Injury of axillary nerve**

     √x7ᵗʰ **S44.30** Injury of axillary nerve, unspecified arm

     √x7ᵗʰ **S44.31** Injury of axillary nerve, right arm

     √x7ᵗʰ **S44.32** Injury of axillary nerve, left arm

√5ᵗʰ **S44.4 Injury of musculocutaneous nerve**

     √x7ᵗʰ **S44.40** Injury of musculocutaneous nerve, unspecified arm

     √x7ᵗʰ **S44.41** Injury of musculocutaneous nerve, right arm

     √x7ᵗʰ **S44.42** Injury of musculocutaneous nerve, left arm

√5ᵗʰ **S44.5 Injury of cutaneous sensory nerve at shoulder and upper arm level**

     √x7ᵗʰ **S44.50** Injury of cutaneous sensory nerve at shoulder and upper arm level, unspecified arm

     √x7ᵗʰ **S44.51** Injury of cutaneous sensory nerve at shoulder and upper arm level, right arm

     √x7ᵗʰ **S44.52** Injury of cutaneous sensory nerve at shoulder and upper arm level, left arm

√5ᵗʰ **S44.8 Injury of other nerves at shoulder and upper arm level**

     √6ᵗʰ **S44.8X** Injury of other nerves at shoulder and upper arm level

        √7ᵗʰ **S44.8X1** Injury of other nerves at shoulder and upper arm level, right arm

        √7ᵗʰ **S44.8X2** Injury of other nerves at shoulder and upper arm level, left arm

        √7ᵗʰ **S44.8X9** Injury of other nerves at shoulder and upper arm level, unspecified arm

√5ᵗʰ **S44.9 Injury of unspecified nerve at shoulder and upper arm level**

     √x7ᵗʰ **S44.90** Injury of unspecified nerve at shoulder and upper arm level, unspecified arm

     √x7ᵗʰ **S44.91** Injury of unspecified nerve at shoulder and upper arm level, right arm

     √x7ᵗʰ **S44.92** Injury of unspecified nerve at shoulder and upper arm level, left arm

√4ᵗʰ **S45 Injury of blood vessels at shoulder and upper arm level**
     Code also any associated open wound (S41.-)
     EXCLUDES 2 *injury of subclavian artery (S25.1)*
                injury of subclavian vein (S25.3)

     The appropriate 7th is to be added to each code from category S45.
     A   initial encounter
     D   subsequent encounter
     S   sequela

     √5ᵗʰ **S45.0 Injury of axillary artery**

        √6ᵗʰ **S45.00** Unspecified injury of axillary artery

        √7ᵗʰ **S45.001** Unspecified injury of axillary artery, right side   **MCC**
          CC Excl: MCC with 7th character A:
          S45.001A, S45.009-S45.011 with 7th A, S45.019-S45.091 with 7th A, S45.099A, S45.301A, S45.309-S45.311 with 7th A, S45.319-S45.391 with 7th A, S45.399-S45.801 with 7th A, S45.809-S45.811 with 7th A, S45.819-S45.891 with 7th A, S45.899-S45.901 with 7th A, S45.909-S45.911 with 7th A, S45.919-S45.991 with 7th A, S45.999A, S55.201A, S55.209-S55.211 with 7th A, S55.219-S55.291 with 7th A, S55.299-S55.801 with 7th A, S55.809-S55.811 with 7th A, S55.819-S55.891 with 7th A, S55.899-S55.901 with 7th A, S55.909-S55.911 with 7th A, S55.919-S55.991 with 7th A, S55.999A, S65.801A, S65.809-S65.811 with 7th A, S65.819-S65.891 with 7th A, S65.899-S65.901 with 7th A, S65.909-S65.911 with 7th A, S65.919-S65.991 with 7th A, S65.999A

✓ Additional Character Required   √x7ᵗʰ Placeholder Alert   Unacceptable PDx   **Manifestation**   Hospital Acquired Condition   **EXCLUDES 1** Not Coded Here   **EXCLUDES 2** Not Included Here

ICD-10-CM 2016   **955**

√7ᵗʰ **S45.002** **Unspecified injury of axillary artery, left side** MCC
CC Excl: MCC with 7th character A:
S45.002-S45.009 with 7th A, S45.012-
S45.019 with 7th A, S45.092-S45.099 with
7th A, S45.302-S45.309 with 7th A, S45.312-
S45.319 with 7th A, S45.392-S45.399 with
7th A, S45.802-S45.809 with 7th A, S45.812-
S45.819 with 7th A, S45.892-S45.899 with
7th A, S45.902-S45.909 with 7th A, S45.912-
S45.919 with 7th A, S45.992-S45.999 with
7th A, S55.202-S55.209 with 7th A, S55.212-
S55.219 with 7th A, S55.292-S55.299 with
7th A, S55.802-S55.809 with 7th A, S55.812-
S55.819 with 7th A, S55.892-S55.899 with
7th A, S55.902-S55.909 with 7th A, S55.912-
S55.919 with 7th A, S55.992-S55.999 with
7th A, S65.802-S65.809 with 7th A, S65.812-
S65.819 with 7th A, S65.892-S65.899 with
7th A, S65.902-S65.909 with 7th A, S65.912-
S65.919 with 7th A, S65.992-S65.999 with
7th A

√7ᵗʰ **S45.009** **Unspecified injury of axillary artery, unspecified side** MCC
CC Excl: MCC with 7th character A:
S45.001-S45.099 with 7th A, S45.301-
S45.999 with 7th A, S55.201-S55.999 with
7th A, S65.801-S65.999 with 7th A

√6ᵗʰ **S45.01** **Laceration of axillary artery**

√7ᵗʰ **S45.011** **Laceration of axillary artery, right side** MCC
CC Excl: MCC with 7th character A:
S45.001A, S45.009-S45.011 with 7th A,
S45.019-S45.091 with 7th A, S45.099A,
S45.301A, S45.309-S45.311 with 7th A,
S45.319-S45.391 with 7th A, S45.399-
S45.801 with 7th A, S45.809-S45.811 with
7th A, S45.819-S45.891 with 7th A, S45.899-
S45.901 with 7th A, S45.909-S45.911 with
7th A, S45.919-S45.991 with 7th A, S45.999A,
S55.201A, S55.209-S55.211 with 7th A,
S55.219-S55.291 with 7th A, S55.299-
S55.801 with 7th A, S55.809-S55.811 with
7th A, S55.819-S55.891 with 7th A, S55.899-
S55.901 with 7th A, S55.909-S55.911 with
7th A, S55.919-S55.991 with 7th A, S55.999
with 7th A, S65.801A, S65.809-S65.811 with
7th A, S65.819-S65.891 with 7th A, S65.899-
S65.901 with 7th A, S65.909-S65.911 with
7th A, S65.919-S65.991 with 7th A, S65.999A

√7ᵗʰ **S45.012** **Laceration of axillary artery, left side** MCC
CC Excl: MCC with 7th character A:
S45.002-S45.009 with 7th A, S45.012-S45.019
with 7th A, S45.092-S45.099 with 7th A,
S45.302-S45.309 with 7th A, S45.312-S45.319
with 7th A, S45.392-S45.399 with 7th A,
S45.802-S45.809 with 7th A, S45.812-S45.819
with 7th A, S45.892-S45.899 with 7th A,
S45.902-S45.909 with 7th A, S45.912-S45.919
with 7th A, S45.992-S45.999 with 7th A,
S55.202-S55.209 with 7th A, S55.212-S55.219
with 7th A, S55.292-S55.299 with 7th A,
S55.802-S55.809 with 7th A, S55.812-S55.819
with 7th A, S55.892-S55.899 with 7th A,
S55.902-S55.909 with 7th A, S55.912-S55.919
with 7th A, S55.992-S55.999 with 7th A,
S65.802-S65.809 with 7th A, S65.812-S65.819
with 7th A, S65.892-S65.899 with 7th A,
S65.902-S65.909 with 7th A, S65.912-S65.919
with 7th A, S65.992-S65.999 with 7th A

√7ᵗʰ **S45.019** **Laceration of axillary artery, unspecified side** MCC
CC Excl: MCC with 7th character A:
S45.001-S45.099 with 7th A, S45.301-
S45.999 with 7th A, S55.201-S55.999 with
7th A, S65.801-S65.999 with 7th A

√6ᵗʰ **S45.09** **Other specified injury of axillary artery**

√7ᵗʰ **S45.091** **Other specified injury of axillary artery, right side** MCC
CC Excl: MCC with 7th character A:
S45.001A, S45.009-S45.011 with 7th A,
S45.019-S45.091 with 7th A, S45.099A,
S45.301A, S45.309-S45.311 with 7th A,
S45.319-S45.391 with 7th A, S45.399-
S45.801 with 7th A, S45.809-S45.811 with
7th A, S45.819-S45.891 with 7th A, S45.899-
S45.901 with 7th A, S45.909-S45.911 with
7th A, S45.919-S45.991 with 7th A, S45.999A,
S55.201A, S55.209-S55.211 with 7th A,
S55.219-S55.291 with 7th A, S55.299-
S55.801 with 7th A, S55.809-S55.811 with
7th A, S55.819-S55.891 with 7th A, S55.899-
S55.901 with 7th A, S55.909-S55.911 with
7th A, S55.919-S55.991 with 7th A, S55.999A,
S65.801A, S65.809-S65.811 with 7th A,
S65.819-S65.891 with 7th A, S65.899-
S65.901 with 7th A, S65.909-S65.911 with
7th A, S65.919-S65.991 with 7th A, S65.999A

√7ᵗʰ **S45.092** **Other specified injury of axillary artery, left side** MCC
CC Excl: MCC with 7th character A:
S45.002-S45.009 with 7th A, S45.012-S45.019
with 7th A, S45.092-S45.099 with 7th A,
S45.302-S45.309 with 7th A, S45.312-S45.319
with 7th A, S45.392-S45.399 with 7th A,
S45.802-S45.809 with 7th A, S45.812-S45.819
with 7th A, S45.892-S45.899 with 7th A,
S45.902-S45.909 with 7th A, S45.912-S45.919
with 7th A, S45.992-S45.999 with 7th A,
S55.202-S55.209 with 7th A, S55.212-S55.219
with 7th A, S55.292-S55.299 with 7th A,
S55.802-S55.809 with 7th A, S55.812-S55.819
with 7th A, S55.892-S55.899 with 7th A,
S55.902-S55.909 with 7th A, S55.912-S55.919
with 7th A, S55.992-S55.999 with 7th A,
S65.802-S65.809 with 7th A, S65.812-S65.819
with 7th A, S65.892-S65.899 with 7th A,
S65.902-S65.909 with 7th A, S65.912-S65.919
with 7th A, S65.992-S65.999 with 7th A

√7ᵗʰ **S45.099** **Other specified injury of axillary artery, unspecified side** MCC
CC Excl:MCC with 7th character A:
S45.001-S45.099 with 7th A, S45.301-
S45.999 with 7th A, S55.201-S55.999 with
7th A, S65.801-S65.999 with 7th A

√5ᵗʰ **S45.1** **Injury of brachial artery**

√6ᵗʰ **S45.10** **Unspecified injury of brachial artery**

√7ᵗʰ **S45.101** **Unspecified injury of brachial artery, right side** CC
CC Excl: CC with 7th character A: S45.101
with 7th A, S45.109-S45.111 with 7th A,
S45.119-S45.191 with 7th A, S45.199-
S45.201 with 7th A, S45.209-S45.211 with
7th A, S45.219-S45.291 with 7th A, S45.299-
S45.301 with 7th A, S45.309-S45.311 with
7th A, S45.319-S45.391 with 7th A, S45.399-
S45.801 with 7th A, S45.809-S45.811 with
7th A, S45.819-S45.891 with 7th A, S45.899-
S45.901 with 7th A, S45.909-S45.911 with
7th A, S45.919-S45.991 with 7th A, S45.999
with 7th A, S55.201 with 7th A, S55.209-
S55.211 with 7th A, S55.219-S55.291 with
7th A, S55.299-S55.801 with 7th A, S55.809-
S55.811 with 7th A, S55.819-S55.891 with
7th A, S55.899-S55.901 with 7th A, S55.909-
S55.911 with 7th A, S55.919-S55.991 with
7th A, S55.999 with 7th A, S65.801 with 7th
A, S65.809-S65.811 with 7th A, S65.819-
S65.891 with 7th A, S65.899-S65.901 with
7th A, S65.909-S65.911 with 7th A, S65.919-
S65.991 with 7th A, S65.999A

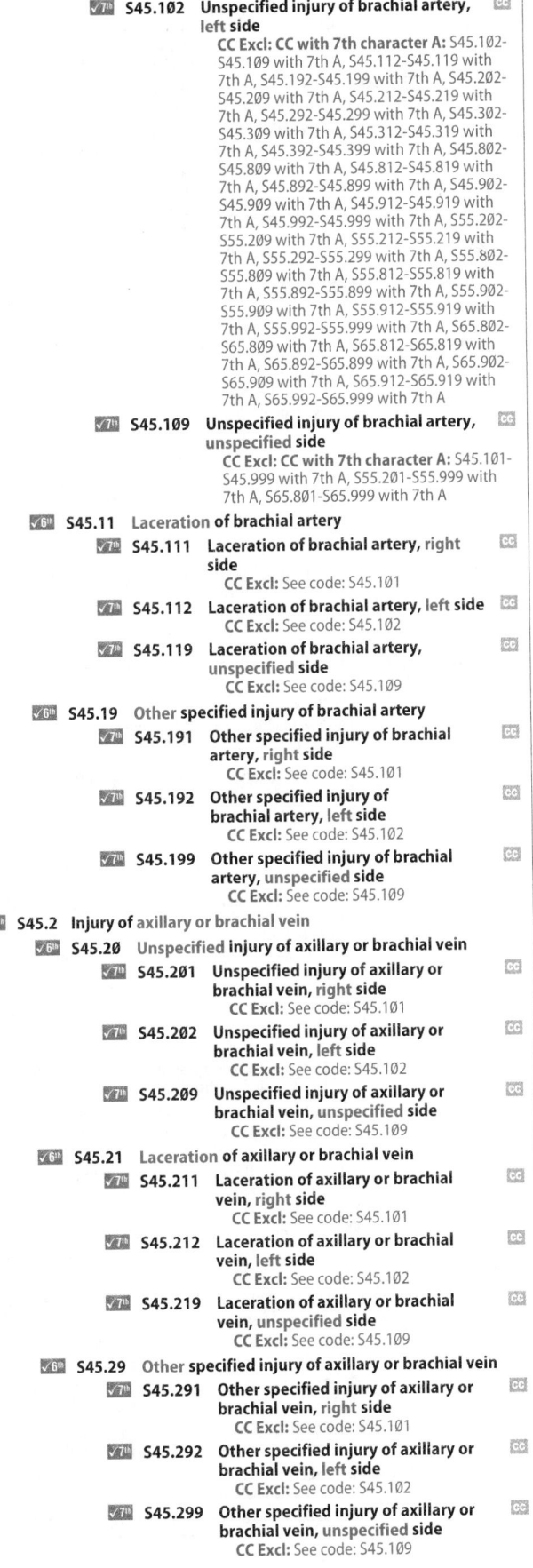

√7ᵗʰ S45.102 Unspecified injury of brachial artery, left side **CC**
  CC Excl: CC with 7th character A: S45.102-S45.109 with 7th A, S45.112-S45.119 with 7th A, S45.192-S45.199 with 7th A, S45.202-S45.209 with 7th A, S45.212-S45.219 with 7th A, S45.292-S45.299 with 7th A, S45.302-S45.309 with 7th A, S45.312-S45.319 with 7th A, S45.392-S45.399 with 7th A, S45.802-S45.809 with 7th A, S45.812-S45.819 with 7th A, S45.892-S45.899 with 7th A, S45.902-S45.909 with 7th A, S45.912-S45.919 with 7th A, S45.992-S45.999 with 7th A, S55.202-S55.209 with 7th A, S55.212-S55.219 with 7th A, S55.292-S55.299 with 7th A, S55.802-S55.809 with 7th A, S55.812-S55.819 with 7th A, S55.892-S55.899 with 7th A, S55.902-S55.909 with 7th A, S55.912-S55.919 with 7th A, S55.992-S55.999 with 7th A, S65.802-S65.809 with 7th A, S65.812-S65.819 with 7th A, S65.892-S65.899 with 7th A, S65.902-S65.909 with 7th A, S65.912-S65.919 with 7th A, S65.992-S65.999 with 7th A

√7ᵗʰ S45.109 Unspecified injury of brachial artery, unspecified side **CC**
  CC Excl: CC with 7th character A: S45.101-S45.999 with 7th A, S55.201-S55.999 with 7th A, S65.801-S65.999 with 7th A

√6ᵗʰ S45.11 Laceration of brachial artery
  √7ᵗʰ S45.111 Laceration of brachial artery, right side **CC**
    CC Excl: See code: S45.101
  √7ᵗʰ S45.112 Laceration of brachial artery, left side **CC**
    CC Excl: See code: S45.102
  √7ᵗʰ S45.119 Laceration of brachial artery, unspecified side **CC**
    CC Excl: See code: S45.109

√6ᵗʰ S45.19 Other specified injury of brachial artery
  √7ᵗʰ S45.191 Other specified injury of brachial artery, right side **CC**
    CC Excl: See code: S45.101
  √7ᵗʰ S45.192 Other specified injury of brachial artery, left side **CC**
    CC Excl: See code: S45.102
  √7ᵗʰ S45.199 Other specified injury of brachial artery, unspecified side **CC**
    CC Excl: See code: S45.109

√5ᵗʰ S45.2 Injury of axillary or brachial vein
  √6ᵗʰ S45.20 Unspecified injury of axillary or brachial vein
    √7ᵗʰ S45.201 Unspecified injury of axillary or brachial vein, right side **CC**
      CC Excl: See code: S45.101
    √7ᵗʰ S45.202 Unspecified injury of axillary or brachial vein, left side **CC**
      CC Excl: See code: S45.102
    √7ᵗʰ S45.209 Unspecified injury of axillary or brachial vein, unspecified side **CC**
      CC Excl: See code: S45.109

  √6ᵗʰ S45.21 Laceration of axillary or brachial vein
    √7ᵗʰ S45.211 Laceration of axillary or brachial vein, right side **CC**
      CC Excl: See code: S45.101
    √7ᵗʰ S45.212 Laceration of axillary or brachial vein, left side **CC**
      CC Excl: See code: S45.102
    √7ᵗʰ S45.219 Laceration of axillary or brachial vein, unspecified side **CC**
      CC Excl: See code: S45.109

  √6ᵗʰ S45.29 Other specified injury of axillary or brachial vein
    √7ᵗʰ S45.291 Other specified injury of axillary or brachial vein, right side **CC**
      CC Excl: See code: S45.101
    √7ᵗʰ S45.292 Other specified injury of axillary or brachial vein, left side **CC**
      CC Excl: See code: S45.102
    √7ᵗʰ S45.299 Other specified injury of axillary or brachial vein, unspecified side **CC**
      CC Excl: See code: S45.109

√5ᵗʰ S45.3 Injury of superficial vein at shoulder and upper arm level
  √6ᵗʰ S45.30 Unspecified injury of superficial vein at shoulder and upper arm level
    √7ᵗʰ S45.301 Unspecified injury of superficial vein at shoulder and upper arm level, right arm **CC**
      CC Excl: CC with 7th character A: S45.309-S45.311 with 7th A, S45.319-S45.391 with 7th A, S45.399-S45.801 with 7th A, S45.809-S45.811 with 7th A, S45.819-S45.891 with 7th A, S45.899-S45.901 with 7th A, S45.909-S45.911 with 7th A, S45.919-S45.991 with 7th A, S45.999 with 7th A, S55.001A, S55.009-S55.011 with 7th A, S55.019-S55.091 with 7th A, S55.099 with 7th A, S55.201 with 7th A, S55.209-S55.211 with 7th A, S55.219-S55.291 with 7th A, S55.299-S55.801 with 7th A, S55.809-S55.811 with 7th A, S55.819-S55.891 with 7th A, S55.899-S55.901 with 7th A, S55.909-S55.911 with 7th A, S55.919-S55.991 with 7th A, S55.999 with 7th A, S65.001 with 7th A, S65.009-S65.011 with 7th A, S65.019-S65.091 with 7th A, S65.099 with 7th A, S65.201 with 7th A, S65.209-S65.211 with 7th A, S65.219-S65.291 with 7th A, S65.299-S65.301 with 7th A, S65.309-S65.311 with 7th A, S65.319-S65.391 with 7th A, S65.399-S65.401 with 7th A, S65.409-S65.411 with 7th A, S65.419-S65.491 with 7th A, S65.499-S65.500 with 7th A, S65.502 with 7th A, S65.504 with 7th A, S65.506 with 7th A, S65.508-S65.510 with 7th A, S65.512 with 7th A, S65.514 with 7th A, S65.516 with 7th A, S65.518-S65.590A, S65.592A, S65.594 A, S65.596A, S65.598-S65.801 with 7th A, S65.809-S65.811 with 7th A, S65.819-S65.891 with 7th A, S65.899-S65.901 with 7th A, S65.909-S65.911 with 7th A, S65.919-S65.991 with 7th A, S65.999A

    √7ᵗʰ S45.302 Unspecified injury of superficial vein at shoulder and upper arm level, left arm **CC**
      CC Excl: CC with 7th character A: S45.302-S45.309 with 7th A, S45.312-S45.319 with 7th A, S45.392-S45.399 with 7th A, S45.802-S45.809 with 7th A, S45.812-S45.819 with 7th A, S45.892-S45.899 with 7th A, S45.902-S45.909 with 7th A, S45.912-S45.919 with 7th A, S45.992-S45.999 with 7th A, S55.002-S55.009 with 7th A, S55.012-S55.019 with 7th A, S55.092-S55.099 with 7th A, S55.202-S55.209 with 7th A, S55.212-S55.219 with 7th A, S55.292-S55.299 with 7th A, S55.802-S55.809 with 7th A, S55.812-S55.819 with 7th A, S55.892-S55.899 with 7th A, S55.902-S55.909 with 7th A, S55.912-S55.919 with 7th A, S55.992-S55.999 with 7th A, S65.002-S65.009 with 7th A, S65.012-S65.019 with 7th A, S65.092-S65.099 with 7th A, S65.202-S65.209 with 7th A, S65.212-S65.219 with 7th A, S65.292-S65.299 with 7th A, S65.302-S65.309 with 7th A, S65.312-S65.319 with 7th A, S65.392-S65.399 with 7th A, S65.402-S65.409 with 7th A, S65.412-S65.419 with 7th A, S65.492-S65.499 with 7th A, S65.501A, S65.503A, S65.505A, S65.507-S65.509 with 7th A, S65.511A, S65.513A, S65.515 A, S65.517-S65.519 with 7th A, S65.591A, S65.593 A, S65.595A, S65.597-S65.599 with 7th A, S65.802-S65.809 with 7th A, S65.812-S65.819 with 7th A, S65.892-S65.899 with 7th A, S65.902-S65.909 with 7th A, S65.912-S65.919 with 7th A, S65.992-S65.999 with 7th A

    √7ᵗʰ S45.309 Unspecified injury of superficial vein at shoulder and upper arm level, unspecified arm **CC**
      CC Excl: CC with 7th character A: S45.301-S45.999 with 7th A, S55.001-S55.099 with 7th A, S55.201-S55.999 with 7th A, S65.001-S65.099 with 7th A, S65.201-S65.999 A

  √6ᵗʰ S45.31 Laceration of superficial vein at shoulder and upper arm level
    √7ᵗʰ S45.311 Laceration of superficial vein at shoulder and upper arm level, right arm **CC**
      CC Excl: See code: S45.301

☑ Additional Character Required √x7ᵗʰ Placeholder Alert Unacceptable PDx Manifestation Hospital Acquired Condition **EXCLUDES 1** Not Coded Here **EXCLUDES 2** Not Included Here

ICD-10-CM 2016

957

✓7th S45.312 Laceration of superficial vein at shoulder and upper arm level, left arm   CC
CC Excl: See code: S45.302

✓7th S45.319 Laceration of superficial vein at shoulder and upper arm level, unspecified arm   CC
CC Excl: See code: S45.309

✓6th S45.39 Other specified injury of superficial vein at shoulder and upper arm level

✓7th S45.391 Other specified injury of superficial vein at shoulder and upper arm level, right arm   CC
CC Excl: See code: S45.301

✓7th S45.392 Other specified injury of superficial vein at shoulder and upper arm level, left arm   CC
CC Excl: See code: S45.302

✓7th S45.399 Other specified injury of superficial vein at shoulder and upper arm level, unspecified arm   CC
CC Excl: See code: S45.309

✓5th S45.8 Injury of other specified blood vessels at shoulder and upper arm level

✓6th S45.80 Unspecified injury of other specified blood vessels at shoulder and upper arm level

✓7th S45.801 Unspecified injury of other specified blood vessels at shoulder and upper arm level, right arm   CC
CC Excl: See code: S45.301

✓7th S45.802 Unspecified injury of other specified blood vessels at shoulder and upper arm level, left arm   CC
CC Excl: See code: S45.302

✓7th S45.809 Unspecified injury of other specified blood vessels at shoulder and upper arm level, unspecified arm   CC
CC Excl: See code: S45.309

✓6th S45.81 Laceration of other specified blood vessels at shoulder and upper arm level

✓7th S45.811 Laceration of other specified blood vessels at shoulder and upper arm level, right arm   CC
CC Excl: See code: S45.301

✓7th S45.812 Laceration of other specified blood vessels at shoulder and upper arm level, left arm   CC
CC Excl: See code: S45.302

✓7th S45.819 Laceration of other specified blood vessels at shoulder and upper arm level, unspecified arm   CC
CC Excl: See code: S45.309

✓6th S45.89 Other specified injury of other specified blood vessels at shoulder and upper arm level

✓7th S45.891 Other specified injury of other specified blood vessels at shoulder and upper arm level, right arm   CC
CC Excl: See code: S45.301

✓7th S45.892 Other specified injury of other specified blood vessels at shoulder and upper arm level, left arm   CC
CC Excl: See code: S45.302

✓7th S45.899 Other specified injury of other specified blood vessels at shoulder and upper arm level, unspecified arm   CC
CC Excl: See code: S45.309

✓5th S45.9 Injury of unspecified blood vessel at shoulder and upper arm level

✓6th S45.90 Unspecified injury of unspecified blood vessel at shoulder and upper arm level

✓7th S45.901 Unspecified injury of unspecified blood vessel at shoulder and upper arm level, right arm   CC
CC Excl: See code: S45.301

✓7th S45.902 Unspecified injury of unspecified blood vessel at shoulder and upper arm level, left arm   CC
CC Excl: See code: S45.302

✓7th S45.909 Unspecified injury of unspecified blood vessel at shoulder and upper arm level, unspecified arm   CC
CC Excl: See code: S45.309

✓6th S45.91 Laceration of unspecified blood vessel at shoulder and upper arm level

✓7th S45.911 Laceration of unspecified blood vessel at shoulder and upper arm level, right arm   CC
CC Excl: See code: S45.301

✓7th S45.912 Laceration of unspecified blood vessel at shoulder and upper arm level, left arm   CC
CC Excl: See code: S45.302

✓7th S45.919 Laceration of unspecified blood vessel at shoulder and upper arm level, unspecified arm   CC
CC Excl: See code: S45.309

✓6th S45.99 Other specified injury of unspecified blood vessel at shoulder and upper arm level

✓7th S45.991 Other specified injury of unspecified blood vessel at shoulder and upper arm level, right arm   CC
CC Excl: See code: S45.301

✓7th S45.992 Other specified injury of unspecified blood vessel at shoulder and upper arm level, left arm   CC
CC Excl: See code: S45.302

✓7th S45.999 Other specified injury of unspecified blood vessel at shoulder and upper arm level, unspecified arm   CC
CC Excl: See code: S45.309

✦ ✓4th S46 Injury of muscle, fascia and tendon at shoulder and upper arm level

Code also any associated open wound (S41.-)

EXCLUDES 2   injury of muscle, fascia and tendon at elbow (S56.-)
sprain of joints and ligaments of shoulder girdle (S43.9)

The appropriate 7th is to be added to each code from category S46.
A   initial encounter
D   subsequent encounter
S   sequela

✓5th S46.0 Injury of muscle(s) and tendon(s) of the rotator cuff of shoulder

CC Excl: For CC codes in subcategory S46.0, unless otherwise noted: CC with 7th character A: S41.001A, S41.009-S41.011 with 7th A, S41.019-S41.021 with 7th A, S41.029-S41.031 with 7th A, S41.039-S41.041 with 7th A, S41.049-S41.051 with 7th A, S41.059-S41.101 with 7th A, S41.109-S41.111 with 7th A, S41.119-S41.121 with 7th A, S41.129-S41.131 with 7th A, S41.139-S41.141 with 7th A, S41.149-S41.151 with 7th A, S41.159 A, S46.021A, S46.029A, S46.121A, S46.129A, S46.221A, S46.229A, S46.321A, S46.329A, S46.821A, S46.829A, S46.921A, S46.929A

✓6th S46.00 Unspecified injury of muscle(s) and tendon(s) of the rotator cuff of shoulder

✓7th S46.001 Unspecified injury of muscle(s) and tendon(s) of the rotator cuff of right shoulder

✓7th S46.002 Unspecified injury of muscle(s) and tendon(s) of the rotator cuff of left shoulder

✓7th S46.009 Unspecified injury of muscle(s) and tendon(s) of the rotator cuff of unspecified shoulder

✓6th S46.01 Strain of muscle(s) and tendon(s) of the rotator cuff of shoulder

✓7th S46.011 Strain of muscle(s) and tendon(s) of the rotator cuff of right shoulder

✓7th S46.012 Strain of muscle(s) and tendon(s) of the rotator cuff of left shoulder

✓7th S46.019 Strain of muscle(s) and tendon(s) of the rotator cuff of unspecified shoulder

✓6th S46.02 Laceration of muscle(s) and tendon(s) of the rotator cuff of shoulder

✓7th S46.021 Laceration of muscle(s) and tendon(s) of the rotator cuff of right shoulder   CC

✓7th S46.022 Laceration of muscle(s) and tendon(s) of the rotator cuff of left shoulder   CC

✦ Refer to the Muscle/Tendon Table at beginning of this chapter.

√7ᵗʰ **S46.029** Laceration of muscle(s) and tendon(s) of the rotator cuff of unspecified shoulder   CC

√6ᵗʰ **S46.09** Other injury of muscle(s) and tendon(s) of the rotator cuff of shoulder

√7ᵗʰ **S46.091** Other injury of muscle(s) and tendon(s) of the rotator cuff of right shoulder

√7ᵗʰ **S46.092** Other injury of muscle(s) and tendon(s) of the rotator cuff of left shoulder

√7ᵗʰ **S46.099** Other injury of muscle(s) and tendon(s) of the rotator cuff of unspecified shoulder

√5ᵗʰ **S46.1** Injury of muscle, fascia and tendon of long head of biceps

√6ᵗʰ **S46.10** Unspecified injury of muscle, fascia and tendon of long head of biceps

√7ᵗʰ **S46.101** Unspecified injury of muscle, fascia and tendon of long head of biceps, right arm

√7ᵗʰ **S46.102** Unspecified injury of muscle, fascia and tendon of long head of biceps, left arm

√7ᵗʰ **S46.109** Unspecified injury of muscle, fascia and tendon of long head of biceps, unspecified arm

√6ᵗʰ **S46.11** Strain of muscle, fascia and tendon of long head of biceps

√7ᵗʰ **S46.111** Strain of muscle, fascia and tendon of long head of biceps, right arm

√7ᵗʰ **S46.112** Strain of muscle, fascia and tendon of long head of biceps, left arm

√7ᵗʰ **S46.119** Strain of muscle, fascia and tendon of long head of biceps, unspecified arm

√6ᵗʰ **S46.12** Laceration of muscle, fascia and tendon of long head of biceps

√7ᵗʰ **S46.121** Laceration of muscle, fascia and tendon of long head of biceps, right arm   CC
CC Excl: CC with 7th character A: S41.001A, S41.009-S41.011 with 7th A, S41.019-S41.021 with 7th A, S41.029-S41.031 with 7th A, S41.039-S41.041 with 7th A, S41.049-S41.051 with 7th A, S41.059-S41.101 with 7th A, S41.109-S41.111 with 7th A, S41.119-S41.121 with 7th A, S41.129-S41.131 with 7th A, S41.139-S41.141 with 7th A, S41.149-S41.151 with 7th A, S41.159A, S46.021A, S46.029A, S46.121A, S46.129A, S46.221A, S46.229 A, S46.321A, S46.329A, S46.821A, S46.829A, S46.921A, S46.929A

√7ᵗʰ **S46.122** Laceration of muscle, fascia and tendon of long head of biceps, left arm   CC
CC Excl: CC with 7th character A: S41.002-S41.009 with 7th A, S41.012-S41.019 with 7th A, S41.022-S41.029 with 7th A, S41.032-S41.039 with 7th A, S41.042-S41.049 with 7th A, S41.052-S41.059 with 7th A, S41.102-S41.109 with 7th A, S41.112-S41.119 with 7th A, S41.122-S41.129 with 7th A, S41.132-S41.139 with 7th A, S41.142-S41.149 with 7th A, S41.152-S41.159 with 7th A, S46.022-S46.029 with 7th A, S46.122-S46.129 with 7th A, S46.222-S46.229 with 7th A, S46.322-S46.329 with 7th A, S46.822-S46.829 with 7th A, S46.922-S46.929 with 7th A

√7ᵗʰ **S46.129** Laceration of muscle, fascia and tendon of long head of biceps, unspecified arm   CC
CC Excl: CC with 7th character A: S41.001-S41.159 with 7th A, S46.021-S46.029 with 7th A, S46.121-S46.129 with 7th A, S46.221-S46.229 with 7th A, S46.321-S46.329 with 7th A, S46.821-S46.829 with 7th A, S46.921-S46.929 with 7th A

√6ᵗʰ **S46.19** Other injury of muscle, fascia and tendon of long head of biceps

√7ᵗʰ **S46.191** Other injury of muscle, fascia and tendon of long head of biceps, right arm

√7ᵗʰ **S46.192** Other injury of muscle, fascia and tendon of long head of biceps, left arm

√7ᵗʰ **S46.199** Other injury of muscle, fascia and tendon of long head of biceps, unspecified arm

√5ᵗʰ **S46.2** Injury of muscle, fascia and tendon of other parts of biceps

√6ᵗʰ **S46.20** Unspecified injury of muscle, fascia and tendon of other parts of biceps

√7ᵗʰ **S46.201** Unspecified injury of muscle, fascia and tendon of other parts of biceps, right arm

√7ᵗʰ **S46.202** Unspecified injury of muscle, fascia and tendon of other parts of biceps, left arm

√7ᵗʰ **S46.209** Unspecified injury of muscle, fascia and tendon of other parts of biceps, unspecified arm

√6ᵗʰ **S46.21** Strain of muscle, fascia and tendon of other parts of biceps

√7ᵗʰ **S46.211** Strain of muscle, fascia and tendon of other parts of biceps, right arm

√7ᵗʰ **S46.212** Strain of muscle, fascia and tendon of other parts of biceps, left arm

√7ᵗʰ **S46.219** Strain of muscle, fascia and tendon of other parts of biceps, unspecified arm

√6ᵗʰ **S46.22** Laceration of muscle, fascia and tendon of other parts of biceps

√7ᵗʰ **S46.221** Laceration of muscle, fascia and tendon of other parts of biceps, right arm   CC
CC Excl: CC with 7th character A: See code: S46.121

√7ᵗʰ **S46.222** Laceration of muscle, fascia and tendon of other parts of biceps, left arm   CC
CC Excl: CC with 7th character A: See code: S46.122

√7ᵗʰ **S46.229** Laceration of muscle, fascia and tendon of other parts of biceps, unspecified arm   CC
CC Excl: CC with 7th character A: See code: S46.129

√6ᵗʰ **S46.29** Other injury of muscle, fascia and tendon of other parts of biceps

√7ᵗʰ **S46.291** Other injury of muscle, fascia and tendon of other parts of biceps, right arm

√7ᵗʰ **S46.292** Other injury of muscle, fascia and tendon of other parts of biceps, left arm

√7ᵗʰ **S46.299** Other injury of muscle, fascia and tendon of other parts of biceps, unspecified arm

√5ᵗʰ **S46.3** Injury of muscle, fascia and tendon of triceps

√6ᵗʰ **S46.30** Unspecified injury of muscle, fascia and tendon of triceps

√7ᵗʰ **S46.301** Unspecified injury of muscle, fascia and tendon of triceps, right arm

√7ᵗʰ **S46.302** Unspecified injury of muscle, fascia and tendon of triceps, left arm

√7ᵗʰ **S46.309** Unspecified injury of muscle, fascia and tendon of triceps, unspecified arm

√6ᵗʰ **S46.31** Strain of muscle, fascia and tendon of triceps

√7ᵗʰ **S46.311** Strain of muscle, fascia and tendon of triceps, right arm

√7ᵗʰ **S46.312** Strain of muscle, fascia and tendon of triceps, left arm

√7ᵗʰ **S46.319** Strain of muscle, fascia and tendon of triceps, unspecified arm

√6ᵗʰ **S46.32** Laceration of muscle, fascia and tendon of triceps

√7ᵗʰ **S46.321** Laceration of muscle, fascia and tendon of triceps, right arm   CC
CC Excl: CC with 7th character A: See code: S46.121

√7ᵗʰ **S46.322** Laceration of muscle, fascia and tendon of triceps, left arm   CC
CC Excl: CC with 7th character A: See code: S46.122

√7ᵗʰ **S46.329** Laceration of muscle, fascia and tendon of triceps, unspecified arm   CC
CC Excl: CC with 7th character A: See code: S46.129

√6ᵗʰ **S46.39** Other injury of muscle, fascia and tendon of triceps

√7ᵗʰ **S46.391** Other injury of muscle, fascia and tendon of triceps, right arm

√7ᵗʰ **S46.392** Other injury of muscle, fascia and tendon of triceps, left arm

✔ Additional Character Required   ✔x7ᵗʰ Placeholder Alert   Unacceptable PDx   Manifestation   Hospital Acquired Condition   **EXCLUDES 1** Not Coded Here   **EXCLUDES 2** Not Included Here

ICD-10-CM 2016   959

✓7ᵗʰ **S46.399**   **Other injury of muscle, fascia and tendon of triceps, unspecified arm**

✓5ᵗʰ **S46.8**   **Injury of other muscles, fascia and tendons at shoulder and upper arm level**

    ✓6ᵗʰ **S46.80**   **Unspecified injury of other muscles, fascia and tendons at shoulder and upper arm level**

       ✓7ᵗʰ **S46.801**   Unspecified injury of other muscles, fascia and tendons at shoulder and upper arm level, right arm

       ✓7ᵗʰ **S46.802**   Unspecified injury of other muscles, fascia and tendons at shoulder and upper arm level, left arm

       ✓7ᵗʰ **S46.809**   Unspecified injury of other muscles, fascia and tendons at shoulder and upper arm level, unspecified arm

    ✓6ᵗʰ **S46.81**   **Strain of other muscles, fascia and tendons at shoulder and upper arm level**

       ✓7ᵗʰ **S46.811**   Strain of other muscles, fascia and tendons at shoulder and upper arm level, right arm

       ✓7ᵗʰ **S46.812**   Strain of other muscles, fascia and tendons at shoulder and upper arm level, left arm

       ✓7ᵗʰ **S46.819**   Strain of other muscles, fascia and tendons at shoulder and upper arm level, unspecified arm

    ✓6ᵗʰ **S46.82**   **Laceration of other muscles, fascia and tendons at shoulder and upper arm level**

       ✓7ᵗʰ **S46.821**   Laceration of other muscles, fascia and tendons at shoulder and upper arm level, right arm   CC
          CC Excl: CC with 7th character A: See code: S46.121

       ✓7ᵗʰ **S46.822**   Laceration of other muscles, fascia and tendons at shoulder and upper arm level, left arm   CC
          CC Excl: CC with 7th character A: See code: S46.122

       ✓7ᵗʰ **S46.829**   Laceration of other muscles, fascia and tendons at shoulder and upper arm level, unspecified arm   CC
          CC Excl: CC with 7th character A: See code: S46.129

    ✓6ᵗʰ **S46.89**   **Other injury of other muscles, fascia and tendons at shoulder and upper arm level**

       ✓7ᵗʰ **S46.891**   Other injury of other muscles, fascia and tendons at shoulder and upper arm level, right arm

       ✓7ᵗʰ **S46.892**   Other injury of other muscles, fascia and tendons at shoulder and upper arm level, left arm

       ✓7ᵗʰ **S46.899**   Other injury of other muscles, fascia and tendons at shoulder and upper arm level, unspecified arm

✓5ᵗʰ **S46.9**   **Injury of unspecified muscle, fascia and tendon at shoulder and upper arm level**

    ✓6ᵗʰ **S46.90**   **Unspecified injury of unspecified muscle, fascia and tendon at shoulder and upper arm level**

       ✓7ᵗʰ **S46.901**   Unspecified injury of unspecified muscle, fascia and tendon at shoulder and upper arm level, right arm

       ✓7ᵗʰ **S46.902**   Unspecified injury of unspecified muscle, fascia and tendon at shoulder and upper arm level, left arm

       ✓7ᵗʰ **S46.909**   Unspecified injury of unspecified muscle, fascia and tendon at shoulder and upper arm level, unspecified arm

    ✓6ᵗʰ **S46.91**   **Strain of unspecified muscle, fascia and tendon at shoulder and upper arm level**

       ✓7ᵗʰ **S46.911**   Strain of unspecified muscle, fascia and tendon at shoulder and upper arm level, right arm

       ✓7ᵗʰ **S46.912**   Strain of unspecified muscle, fascia and tendon at shoulder and upper arm level, left arm

       ✓7ᵗʰ **S46.919**   Strain of unspecified muscle, fascia and tendon at shoulder and upper arm level, unspecified arm

    ✓6ᵗʰ **S46.92**   **Laceration of unspecified muscle, fascia and tendon at shoulder and upper arm level**

       ✓7ᵗʰ **S46.921**   Laceration of unspecified muscle, fascia and tendon at shoulder and upper arm level, right arm   CC
          CC Excl: CC with 7th character A: See code: S46.121

       ✓7ᵗʰ **S46.922**   Laceration of unspecified muscle, fascia and tendon at shoulder and upper arm level, left arm   CC
          CC Excl: CC with 7th character A: See code: S46.122

       ✓7ᵗʰ **S46.929**   Laceration of unspecified muscle, fascia and tendon at shoulder and upper arm level, unspecified arm   CC
          CC Excl: CC with 7th character A: See code: S46.129

    ✓6ᵗʰ **S46.99**   **Other injury of unspecified muscle, fascia and tendon at shoulder and upper arm level**

       ✓7ᵗʰ **S46.991**   Other injury of unspecified muscle, fascia and tendon at shoulder and upper arm level, right arm

       ✓7ᵗʰ **S46.992**   Other injury of unspecified muscle, fascia and tendon at shoulder and upper arm level, left arm

       ✓7ᵗʰ **S46.999**   Other injury of unspecified muscle, fascia and tendon at shoulder and upper arm level, unspecified arm

✓4ᵗʰ **S47**   **Crushing injury of shoulder and upper arm**

    Use additional code for all associated injuries

    EXCLUDES 2   crushing injury of elbow (S57.0-)

    The appropriate 7th is to be added to each code from category S47.
    A   initial encounter
    D   subsequent encounter
    S   sequela

✓x7ᵗʰ **S47.1**   **Crushing injury of right shoulder and upper arm**

✓x7ᵗʰ **S47.2**   **Crushing injury of left shoulder and upper arm**

✓x7ᵗʰ **S47.9**   **Crushing injury of shoulder and upper arm, unspecified arm**

✓4ᵗʰ **S48**   **Traumatic amputation of shoulder and upper arm**

    NOTE   An amputation not identified as partial or complete should be coded to complete.

    EXCLUDES 1   traumatic amputation at elbow level (S58.0)

    The appropriate 7th is to be added to each code from category S48.
    A   initial encounter
    D   subsequent encounter
    S   sequela

✓5ᵗʰ **S48.0**   **Traumatic amputation at shoulder joint**

    ✓6ᵗʰ **S48.01**   **Complete traumatic amputation at shoulder joint**

       ✓7ᵗʰ **S48.011**   Complete traumatic amputation at right shoulder joint   CC
          CC Excl: CC with 7th character A: S41.001A, S41.009-S41.011 with 7th A, S41.019-S41.021 with 7th A, S41.029-S41.031 with 7th A, S41.039-S41.041 with 7th A, S41.049-S41.051 with 7th A, S41.059-S41.101 with 7th A, S41.109-S41.111 with 7th A, S41.119-S41.121 with 7th A, S41.129-S41.131 with 7th A, S41.139-S41.141 with 7th A, S41.149-S41.151 with 7th A, S41.159A, S46.021A, S46.029A, S46.121A, S46.129A, S46.221A, S46.229A, S46.321A, S46.329A, S46.821A, S46.829A, S46.921A, S46.929A, S48.011A, S48.019-S48.021 with 7th A, S48.029-S48.111 with 7th A, S48.119-S48.121 with 7th A, S48.129-S48.911 with 7th A, S48.919-S48.921 with 7th A, S48.929A, S51.001A, S51.009-S51.011 with 7th A, S51.019-S51.021 with 7th A, S51.029-S51.031 with 7th A, S51.039-S51.041 with 7th A, S51.049-S51.051 with 7th A, S51.059-S51.801 with 7th A, S51.809-S51.811 with 7th A, S51.819-S51.821 with 7th A, S51.829-S51.831 with 7th A, S51.839-S51.841 with 7th A, S51.849-S51.851 with 7th A, S51.859 with 7th A, S56.021A, S56.029A, S56.121A, S56.123A, S56.125A, S56.127A, S56.129A, S56.221A, S56.229A, S56.321A, S56.329A, S56.421A, S56.423A, S56.425A, S56.427A, S56.429A, S56.521A, S56.529A, S56.821A, S56.829A, S56.921A, S56.929A, S58.011A, S58.019-S58.021 with 7th A, S58.029-S58.111 with

N Newborn: 0   P Pediatric: 0-17   M Maternity: 12-55   A Adult: 15-124   **MCC** Major CC Condition   **PDxMCC** PDx acts as own MCC   **CC** CC Condition   **PDxCC** PDx acts as own CC

960   ICD-10-CM 2016

7th A, S58.119-S58.121 with 7th A, S58.129-S58.911 with 7th A, S58.919-S58.921 with 7th A, S58.929A, S61.001A, S61.009-S61.011 with 7th A, S61.019-S61.021 with 7th A, S61.029-S61.031 with 7th A, S61.039-S61.041 with 7th A, S61.049-S61.051 with 7th A, S61.059-S61.101 with 7th A, S61.109-S61.111 with 7th A, S61.119-S61.121 with 7th A, S61.129-S61.131 with 7th A, S61.139-S61.141 with 7th A, S61.149-S61.151 with 7th A, S61.159-S61.200 with 7th A, S61.202A, S61.204A, S61.206A, S61.208-S61.210 with 7th A, S61.212A, S61.214A, S61.216A, S61.218-S61.220 with 7th A, S61.222A, S61.224A, S61.226A, S61.228-S61.230 with 7th A, S61.232A, S61.234A, S61.236 A, S61.238-S61.240 with 7th A, S61.242A, S61.244A, S61.246A, S61.248-S61.250 with 7th A, S61.252A, S61.254A, S61.256A, S61.258-S61.300 with 7th A, S61.302A, S61.304A, S61.306A, S61.308-S61.310 with 7th A, S61.312A, S61.314A, S61.316A, S61.318-S61.320 with 7th A, S61.322A, S61.324 A, S61.326A, S61.328-S61.330 with 7th A, S61.332A, S61.334A, S61.336A, S61.338-S61.340 with 7th A, S61.342 A, S61.344A, S61.346A, S61.348-S61.350 with 7th A, S61.352A, S61.354A, S61.356A, S61.358-S61.401 with 7th A, S61.409-S61.411 with 7th A, S61.419-S61.421 with 7th A, S61.429-S61.431 with 7th A, S61.439-S61.441 with 7th A, S61.449-S61.451 with 7th A, S61.459-S61.501 with 7th A, S61.509-S61.511 with 7th A, S61.519-S61.521 with 7th A, S61.529-S61.531 with 7th A, S61.539-S61.541 with 7th A, S61.549-S61.551 with 7th A, S61.559A, S66.021A, S66.029A, S66.120A, S66.122A, S66.124A, S66.126A, S66.128-S66.129 with 7th A, S66.221A, S66.229A, S66.320A, S66.322A, S66.324A, S66.326A, S66.328-S66.329 with 7th A, S66.421A, S66.429A, S66.520A, S66.522A, S66.524A, S66.526A, S66.528-S66.529 with 7th A, S66.821A, S66.829A, S66.921A, S66.929A, S68.011A, S68.019-S68.021 with 7th A, S68.029-S68.110 with 7th A, S68.112A, S68.114A, S68.116A, S68.118-S68.120 with 7th A, S68.122A, S68.124A, S68.126A, S68.128-S68.411 with 7th A, S68.419-S68.421 with 7th A, S68.429-S68.511 with 7th A, S68.519-S68.521 with 7th A, S68.529-S68.610 with 7th A, S68.612A, S68.614A, S68.616A, S68.618-S68.620 with 7th A, S68.622A, S68.624A, S68.626A, S68.628-S68.711 with 7th A, S68.719-S68.721 with 7th A, S68.729A, T14.90-T14.91, T79.A0X-T79.9XX with 7th A

√7th **S48.012**   **Complete traumatic amputation at left shoulder joint**   CC
  CC Excl: CC with 7th character A: S41.002-S41.009 with 7th A, S41.012-S41.019 with 7th A, S41.022-S41.029 with 7th A, S41.032-S41.039 with 7th A, S41.042-S41.049 with 7th A, S41.052-S41.059 with 7th A, S41.102-S41.109 with 7th A, S41.112-S41.119 with 7th A, S41.122-S41.129 with 7th A, S41.132-S41.139 with 7th A, S41.142-S41.149 with 7th A, S41.152-S41.159 with 7th A, S46.022-S46.029 with 7th A, S46.122-S46.129 with 7th A, S46.222-S46.229 with 7th A, S46.322-S46.329 with 7th A, S46.822-S46.829 with 7th A, S46.922-S46.929 with 7th A, S48.012-S48.019 with 7th A, S48.022-S48.029 with 7th A, S48.112-S48.119 with 7th A, S48.122-S48.129 with 7th A, S48.912-S48.919 with 7th A, S48.922-S48.929 with 7th A, S51.002-S51.009 with 7th A, S51.012-S51.019 with 7th A, S51.022-S51.029 with 7th A, S51.032-S51.039 with 7th A, S51.042-S51.049 with 7th A, S51.052-S51.059 with 7th A, S51.802-S51.809 with 7th A, S51.812-S51.819 with 7th A, S51.822-S51.829 with 7th A, S51.832-S51.839 with 7th A, S51.842-S51.849 with 7th A, S51.852-S51.859 with 7th A, S56.022-S56.029A, S56.122A, S56.124A, S56.126A, S56.128-S56.129 with 7th A, S56.222-S56.229 with 7th A, S56.322-S56.329 with 7th A, S56.422A, S56.424A, S56.426 A, S56.428-S56.429 with 7th A, S56.522-S56.529 with 7th A, S56.822-S56.829 with 7th A, S56.922-S56.929 with 7th A, S58.012-S58.019 with 7th A, S58.022-S58.029 with

7th A, S58.112-S58.119 with 7th A, S58.122-S58.129 with 7th A, S58.912-S58.919 with 7th A, S58.922-S58.929 with 7th A, S61.002-S61.009 with 7th A, S61.012-S61.019 with 7th A, S61.022-S61.029 with 7th A, S61.032-S61.039 with 7th A, S61.042-S61.049 with 7th A, S61.052-S61.059 with 7th A, S61.102-S61.109 with 7th A, S61.112-S61.119 with 7th A, S61.122-S61.129 with 7th A, S61.132-S61.139 with 7th A, S61.142-S61.149 with 7th A, S61.152-S61.159 with 7th A, S61.201 with 7th A, S61.203A, S61.205A, S61.207-S61.209 with 7th A, S61.211A, S61.213A, S61.215A, S61.217-S61.219 with 7th A, S61.221A, S61.223A, S61.225A, S61.227-S61.229 with 7th A, S61.231A, S61.233A, S61.235A, S61.237-S61.239 with 7th A, S61.241A, S61.243A, S61.245A, S61.247-S61.249 with 7th A, S61.251A, S61.253A, S61.255A, S61.257-S61.259 with 7th A, S61.301A, S61.303A, S61.305A, S61.307-S61.309 with 7th A, S61.311A, S61.313A, S61.315A, S61.317-S61.319 with 7th A, S61.321A, S61.323A, S61.325A, S61.327-S61.329 with 7th A, S61.331A, S61.333A, S61.335A, S61.337-S61.339 with 7th A, S61.341 with 7th A, S61.343A, S61.345A, S61.347-S61.349 with 7th A, S61.351A, S61.353A, S61.355A, S61.357-S61.359 with 7th A, S61.402-S61.409 with 7th A, S61.412-S61.419 with 7th A, S61.422-S61.429 with 7th A, S61.432-S61.439 with 7th A, S61.442-S61.449 with 7th A, S61.452-S61.459 with 7th A, S61.502-S61.509 with 7th A, S61.512-S61.519 with 7th A, S61.522-S61.529 with 7th A, S61.532-S61.539 with 7th A, S61.542-S61.549 with 7th A, S61.552-S61.559 with 7th A, S66.022-S66.029 with 7th A, S66.121A, S66.123A, S66.125A, S66.127-S66.129 with 7th A, S66.222-S66.229 with 7th A, S66.321A, S66.323A, S66.325A, S66.327-S66.329 with 7th A, S66.422-S66.429 with 7th A, S66.521A, S66.523A, S66.525A, S66.527-S66.529 with 7th A, S66.822-S66.829 with 7th A, S66.922-S66.929 with 7th A, S68.012-S68.019 with 7th A, S68.022-S68.029 with 7th A, S68.111A, S68.113A, S68.115A, S68.117-S68.119 with 7th A, S68.121 A, S68.123A, S68.125A, S68.127-S68.129 with 7th A, S68.412-S68.419A, S68.422-S68.429 with 7th A, S68.512-S68.519 with 7th A, S68.522-S68.529 with 7th A, S68.611A, S68.613A, S68.615 with 7th A, S68.617-S68.619 with 7th A, S68.621A, S68.623A, S68.625A, S68.627-S68.629 with 7th A, S68.712-S68.719 with 7th A, S68.722-S68.729 with 7th A, T14.90-T14.91, T79.A0X-T79.9XX with 7th A

√7th **S48.019**   **Complete traumatic amputation at unspecified shoulder joint**   CC
  CC Excl: CC with 7th character A: S41.001-S41.159 with 7th A, S46.021-S46.029 with 7th A, S46.121-S46.129 with 7th A, S46.221-S46.229 with 7th A, S46.321-S46.329 with 7th A, S46.821-S46.829 with 7th A, S46.921-S46.929 with 7th A, S48.011-S48.929 with 7th A, S51.001-S51.859 with 7th A, S56.021-S56.029 with 7th A, S56.121-S56.129 with 7th A, S56.221-S56.229 with 7th A, S56.321-S56.329 with 7th A, S56.421-S56.429 with 7th A, S56.521-S56.529 with 7th A, S56.821-S56.829 with 7th A, S56.921-S56.929 with 7th A, S58.011-S58.929 with 7th A, S61.001-S61.559 with 7th A, S66.021-S66.029 with 7th A, S66.120-S66.129 with 7th A, S66.221-S66.229 with 7th A, S66.320-S66.329 with 7th A, S66.421-S66.429 with 7th A, S66.520-S66.529 with 7th A, S66.821-S66.829 with 7th A, S66.921-S66.929 with 7th A, S68.011-S68.729 with 7th A, T14.90-T14.91, T79.A0X-T79.9XX with 7th A

√6th **S48.02**   **Partial traumatic amputation at shoulder joint**

√7th **S48.021**   **Partial traumatic amputation at right shoulder joint**   CC
  CC Excl: CC with 7th character A: See code: S48.011

√7th **S48.022**   **Partial traumatic amputation at left shoulder joint**   CC
  CC Excl: CC with 7th character A: See code: S48.012

☑ Additional Character Required   ☑x7th Placeholder Alert   Unacceptable PDx   Manifestation   Hospital Acquired Condition   **EXCLUDES 1** Not Coded Here   **EXCLUDES 2** Not Included Here

✓7ᵗʰ **S48.029** **Partial traumatic amputation at unspecified shoulder joint**   CC
     CC Excl: CC with 7th character A: See code: S48.019

✓5ᵗʰ **S48.1** **Traumatic amputation at level between shoulder and elbow**

   ✓6ᵗʰ **S48.11** **Complete traumatic amputation at level between shoulder and elbow**

     ✓7ᵗʰ **S48.111** **Complete traumatic amputation at level between right shoulder and elbow**   CC
       CC Excl: CC with 7th character A: See code: S48.011

     ✓7ᵗʰ **S48.112** **Complete traumatic amputation at level between left shoulder and elbow**   CC
       CC Excl: CC with 7th character A: See code: S48.012

     ✓7ᵗʰ **S48.119** **Complete traumatic amputation at level between unspecified shoulder and elbow**   CC
       CC Excl: CC with 7th character A: See code: S48.019

   ✓6ᵗʰ **S48.12** **Partial traumatic amputation at level between shoulder and elbow**

     ✓7ᵗʰ **S48.121** **Partial traumatic amputation at level between right shoulder and elbow**   CC

     ✓7ᵗʰ **S48.122** **Partial traumatic amputation at level between left shoulder and elbow**   CC

     ✓7ᵗʰ **S48.129** **Partial traumatic amputation at level between unspecified shoulder and elbow**   CC

✓5ᵗʰ **S48.9** **Traumatic amputation of shoulder and upper arm, level unspecified**

   ✓6ᵗʰ **S48.91** **Complete traumatic amputation of shoulder and upper arm, level unspecified**

     ✓7ᵗʰ **S48.911** **Complete traumatic amputation of right shoulder and upper arm, level unspecified**   CC
       CC Excl: CC with 7th character A: See code: S48.011

     ✓7ᵗʰ **S48.912** **Complete traumatic amputation of left shoulder and upper arm, level unspecified**   CC
       CC Excl: CC with 7th character A: See code: S48.012

     ✓7ᵗʰ **S48.919** **Complete traumatic amputation of unspecified shoulder and upper arm, level unspecified**   CC
       CC Excl: CC with 7th character A: See code: S48.019

   ✓6ᵗʰ **S48.92** **Partial traumatic amputation of shoulder and upper arm, level unspecified**

     ✓7ᵗʰ **S48.921** **Partial traumatic amputation of right shoulder and upper arm, level unspecified**   CC
       CC Excl: CC with 7th character A: See code: S48.011

     ✓7ᵗʰ **S48.922** **Partial traumatic amputation of left shoulder and upper arm, level unspecified**   CC
       CC Excl: CC with 7th character A: See code: S48.012

     ✓7ᵗʰ **S48.929** **Partial traumatic amputation of unspecified shoulder and upper arm, level unspecified**   CC
       CC Excl: CC with 7th character A: See code: S48.019

✓4ᵗʰ **S49** **Other and unspecified injuries of shoulder and upper arm**

> The appropriate 7th is to be added to each code from subcategories S49.0 and S49.1.
> A   initial encounter for closed fracture
> D   subsequent encounter for fracture with routine healing
> G   subsequent encounter for fracture with delayed healing
> K   subsequent encounter for fracture with nonunion
> P   subsequent encounter for fracture with malunion
> S   sequela

✓5ᵗʰ **S49.0** **Physeal fracture of upper end of humerus**

   ✓6ᵗʰ **S49.00** **Unspecified physeal fracture of upper end of humerus**

7,19 ✓7ᵗʰ **S49.001** **Unspecified physeal fracture of upper end of humerus, right arm**   CC
     CC Excl: CC with 7th character A: S42.201-S42.271 with 7th [A, B], S42.279-S42.311 with 7th A, S42.319-S42.481 with 7th A, S42.489-S42.92X with 7th A, S49.001A, S49.009-S49.011 with 7th A, S49.019-S49.021 with 7th A, S49.029-S49.031 with 7th A, S49.039-S49.041 with 7th A, S49.049-S49.091 with 7th A, S49.099-S49.101 with 7th A, S49.109-S49.111 with 7th A, S49.119-S49.121 with 7th A, S49.129-S49.131 with 7th A, S49.139-S49.141 A, S49.149-S49.191 with 7th A, S49.199A
     CC with 7th character K or P: M80.00X-M84.68X with 7th [K, P], S02.0XX-S02.92X with 7th K, S12.000-S12.691 with 7th K, S22.000-S22.9XX with 7th K, S32.000-S32.9XX with 7th K, S42.001-S42.92X with 7th [K, P], S49.001-S49.199 with 7th [K, P], S52.001-S52.92X with 7th [K, M, N, P, Q, R], S59.001-S59.299 with 7th [K, P], S62.001-S62.92X with 7th [K, P], S72.001-S72.92X with 7th [K, M, N, P, Q, R], S79.001-S79.199 with 7th [K, P], S82.001-S82.92X with 7th [K, M, N, P, Q, R], S89.001-S89.399 with 7th [K, P], S92.001-S92.919 with 7th [K, P]

7,19 ✓7ᵗʰ **S49.002** **Unspecified physeal fracture of upper end of humerus, left arm**   CC
     CC Excl: CC with 7th character A: S42.201-S42.266 with 7th B, S42.272-S42.309 with 7th A, S42.312-S42.476 with 7th A, S42.482-S42.92X with 7th A, S49.002-S49.009 with 7th A, S49.012-S49.019 with 7th A, S49.022-S49.029 with 7th A, S49.032-S49.039 with 7th A, S49.042-S49.049 with 7th A, S49.092-S49.099 with 7th A, S49.102-S49.109 with 7th A, S49.112-S49.119 with 7th A, S49.122-S49.129 with 7th A, S49.132-S49.139 with 7th A, S49.142-S49.149 with 7th A, S49.192-S49.199 with 7th A
     CC with 7th character K or P: M80.00X-M84.68X with 7th [K, P], S02.0XX-S02.92X with 7th K, S12.000-S12.691 with 7th K, S22.000-S22.9XX with 7th K, S32.000-S32.9XX with 7th K, S42.001-S42.92X with 7th [K, P], S49.001-S49.199 with 7th [K, P], S52.001-S52.92X with 7th [K, M, N, P, Q, R], S59.001-S59.299 with 7th [K, P], S62.001-S62.92X with 7th [K, P], S72.001-S72.92X with 7th [K, M, N, P, Q, R], S79.001-S79.199 with 7th [K, P], S82.001-S82.92X with 7th [K, M, N, P, Q, R], S89.001-S89.399 with 7th [K, P], S92.001-S92.919 with 7th [K, P]

7,19 ✓7ᵗʰ **S49.009** **Unspecified physeal fracture of upper end of humerus, unspecified arm**   CC
     CC Excl: CC with 7th character A: S42.201-S42.92X with 7th [A, B], S49.001-S49.199 with 7th A
     CC with 7th character K or P: M80.00X-M84.68X with 7th [K, P], S02.0XX-S02.92X with 7th K, S12.000-S12.691 with 7th K, S22.000-S22.9XX with 7th K, S32.000-S32.9XX with 7th K, S42.001-S42.92X with 7th [K, P], S49.001-S49.199 with 7th [K, P], S52.001-S52.92X with 7th [K, M, N, P, Q, R], S59.001-S59.299 with 7th [K, P], S62.001-S62.92X with 7th [K, P], S72.001-S72.92X with 7th [K, M, N, P, Q, R], S79.001-S79.199 with 7th [K, P], S82.001-S82.92X with 7th [K, M, N, P, Q, R], S89.001-S89.399 with 7th [K, P], S92.001-S92.919 with 7th [K, P]

   ✓6ᵗʰ **S49.01** **Salter-Harris Type I physeal fracture of upper end of humerus**

7,19 ✓7ᵗʰ **S49.011** **Salter-Harris Type I physeal fracture of upper end of humerus, right arm**   CC
     CC Excl: See code: S49.001

7,19 ✓7ᵗʰ **S49.012** **Salter-Harris Type I physeal fracture of upper end of humerus, left arm**   CC
     CC Excl: See code: S49.002

7,19 ✓7ᵗʰ **S49.019** **Salter-Harris Type I physeal fracture of upper end of humerus, unspecified arm**   CC
     CC Excl: See code: S49.009

---

7   HAC = Initial encounter only (7th character A, B or C) and not POA.
19   CC only if an initial encounter for a closed fracture (7th character A) **OR** a subsequent encounter for nonunion or malunion (7th character K, M, N, P, Q, or R – specific to category).

N Newborn: 0   **P** Pediatric: 0-17   **M** Maternity: 12-55   **A** Adult: 15-124   **MCC** Major CC Condition   **PDxMCC** PDx acts as own MCC   **CC** CC Condition   **PDxCC** PDx acts as own CC

✓6ᵗʰ S49.02   Salter-Harris Type II physeal fracture of upper end of humerus

    7,19 ✓7ᵗʰ **S49.021**   **Salter-Harris Type II physeal fracture of upper end of humerus, right arm**   CC
       CC Excl: See code: S49.001

    7,19 ✓7ᵗʰ **S49.022**   **Salter-Harris Type II physeal fracture of upper end of humerus, left arm**   CC
       CC Excl: See code: S49.002

    7,19 ✓7ᵗʰ **S49.029**   **Salter-Harris Type II physeal fracture of upper end of humerus, unspecified arm**   CC
       CC Excl: See code: S49.009

✓6ᵗʰ S49.03   Salter-Harris Type III physeal fracture of upper end of humerus

    7,19 ✓7ᵗʰ **S49.031**   **Salter-Harris Type III physeal fracture of upper end of humerus, right arm**   CC
       CC Excl: See code: S49.001

    7,19 ✓7ᵗʰ **S49.032**   **Salter-Harris Type III physeal fracture of upper end of humerus, left arm**   CC
       CC Excl: See code: S49.002

    7,19 ✓7ᵗʰ **S49.039**   **Salter-Harris Type III physeal fracture of upper end of humerus, unspecified arm**   CC
       CC Excl: See code: S49.009

✓6ᵗʰ S49.04   Salter-Harris Type IV physeal fracture of upper end of humerus

    7,19 ✓7ᵗʰ **S49.041**   **Salter-Harris Type IV physeal fracture of upper end of humerus, right arm**   CC
       CC Excl: See code: S49.001

    7,19 ✓7ᵗʰ **S49.042**   **Salter-Harris Type IV physeal fracture of upper end of humerus, left arm**   CC
       CC Excl: See code: S49.002

    7,19 ✓7ᵗʰ **S49.049**   **Salter-Harris Type IV physeal fracture of upper end of humerus, unspecified arm**   CC
       CC Excl: See code: S49.009

✓6ᵗʰ S49.09   Other physeal fracture of upper end of humerus

    7,19 ✓7ᵗʰ **S49.091**   **Other physeal fracture of upper end of humerus, right arm**   CC
       CC Excl: See code: S49.001

    7,19 ✓7ᵗʰ **S49.092**   **Other physeal fracture of upper end of humerus, left arm**   CC
       CC Excl: See code: S49.002

    7,19 ✓7ᵗʰ **S49.099**   **Other physeal fracture of upper end of humerus, unspecified arm**   CC
       CC Excl: See code: S49.009

✓5ᵗʰ S49.1   Physeal fracture of lower end of humerus

   ✓6ᵗʰ S49.10   Unspecified physeal fracture of lower end of humerus

    7,19 ✓7ᵗʰ **S49.101**   **Unspecified physeal fracture of lower end of humerus, right arm**   CC
       CC Excl: See code: S49.001

    7,19 ✓7ᵗʰ **S49.102**   **Unspecified physeal fracture of lower end of humerus, left arm**   CC
       CC Excl: See code: S49.002

    7,19 ✓7ᵗʰ **S49.109**   **Unspecified physeal fracture of lower end of humerus, unspecified arm**   CC
       CC Excl: See code: S49.009

   ✓6ᵗʰ S49.11   Salter-Harris Type I physeal fracture of lower end of humerus

    7,19 ✓7ᵗʰ **S49.111**   **Salter-Harris Type I physeal fracture of lower end of humerus, right arm**   CC
       CC Excl: See code: S49.001

    7,19 ✓7ᵗʰ **S49.112**   **Salter-Harris Type I physeal fracture of lower end of humerus, left arm**   CC
       CC Excl: See code: S49.002

    7,19 ✓7ᵗʰ **S49.119**   **Salter-Harris Type I physeal fracture of lower end of humerus, unspecified arm**   CC
       CC Excl: See code: S49.009

   ✓6ᵗʰ S49.12   Salter-Harris Type II physeal fracture of lower end of humerus

    7,19 ✓7ᵗʰ **S49.121**   **Salter-Harris Type II physeal fracture of lower end of humerus, right arm**   CC
       CC Excl: See code: S49.001

    7,19 ✓7ᵗʰ **S49.122**   **Salter-Harris Type II physeal fracture of lower end of humerus, left arm**   CC
       CC Excl: See code: S49.002

    7,19 ✓7ᵗʰ **S49.129**   **Salter-Harris Type II physeal fracture of lower end of humerus, unspecified arm**   CC
       CC Excl: See code: S49.009

   ✓6ᵗʰ S49.13   Salter Harris Type III physeal fracture of lower end of humerus

    7,19 ✓7ᵗʰ **S49.131**   **Salter Harris Type III physeal fracture of lower end of humerus, right arm**   CC
       CC Excl: See code: S49.001

    7,19 ✓7ᵗʰ **S49.132**   **Salter Harris Type III physeal fracture of lower end of humerus, left arm**   CC
       CC Excl: See code: S49.002

    7,19 ✓7ᵗʰ **S49.139**   **Salter-Harris Type III physeal fracture of lower end of humerus, unspecified arm**   CC
       CC Excl: See code: S49.009

   ✓6ᵗʰ S49.14   Salter-Harris Type IV physeal fracture of lower end of humerus

    7,19 ✓7ᵗʰ **S49.141**   **Salter-Harris Type IV physeal fracture of lower end of humerus, right arm**   CC
       CC Excl: See code: S49.001

    7,19 ✓7ᵗʰ **S49.142**   **Salter-Harris Type IV physeal fracture of lower end of humerus, left arm**   CC
       CC Excl: See code: S49.002

    7,19 ✓7ᵗʰ **S49.149**   **Salter-Harris Type IV physeal fracture of lower end of humerus, unspecified arm**   CC
       CC Excl: See code: S49.009

   ✓6ᵗʰ S49.19   Other physeal fracture of lower end of humerus

    7,19 ✓7ᵗʰ **S49.191**   **Other physeal fracture of lower end of humerus, right arm**   CC
       CC Excl: See code: S49.001

    7,19 ✓7ᵗʰ **S49.192**   **Other physeal fracture of lower end of humerus, left arm**   CC
       CC Excl: See code: S49.002

    7,19 ✓7ᵗʰ **S49.199**   **Other physeal fracture of lower end of humerus, unspecified arm**   CC
       CC Excl: See code: S49.009

✓5ᵗʰ S49.8   Other specified injuries of shoulder and upper arm

> The appropriate 7th is to be added to each code in subcategory S49.8.
> A   initial encounter
> D   subsequent encounter
> S   sequela

   ✓x7ᵗʰ **S49.80**   **Other specified injuries of shoulder and upper arm, unspecified arm**

   ✓x7ᵗʰ **S49.81**   **Other specified injuries of right shoulder and upper arm**

   ✓x7ᵗʰ **S49.82**   **Other specified injuries of left shoulder and upper arm**

✓5ᵗʰ S49.9   Unspecified injury of shoulder and upper arm

> The appropriate 7th is to be added to each code in subcategory S49.9.
> A   initial encounter
> D   subsequent encounter
> S   sequela

   ✓x7ᵗʰ **S49.90**   **Unspecified injury of shoulder and upper arm, unspecified arm**

   ✓x7ᵗʰ **S49.91**   **Unspecified injury of right shoulder and upper arm**

   ✓x7ᵗʰ **S49.92**   **Unspecified injury of left shoulder and upper arm**

Injuries to the elbow and forearm (S50-S59)

EXCLUDES 2   burns and corrosions (T20-T32)
          frostbite (T33-T34)
          injuries of wrist and hand (S60-S69)
          insect bite or sting, venomous (T63.4)

✓4ᵗʰ S50   **Superficial injury of elbow and forearm**

EXCLUDES 2   superficial injury of wrist and hand (S60.-)

> The appropriate 7th is to be added to each code from category S50.
> A   initial encounter
> D   subsequent encounter
> S   sequela

   ✓5ᵗʰ S50.0   Contusion of elbow

    ✓x7ᵗʰ **S50.00**   **Contusion of unspecified elbow**

---

7   HAC = Initial encounter only (7th character A, B or C) and not POA.
19   CC only if an initial encounter for a closed fracture (7th character A) **OR** a subsequent encounter for nonunion or malunion (7th character K, M, N, P, Q, or R – specific to category).

✓ Additional Character Required   ✓x7ᵗʰ Placeholder Alert   Unacceptable PDx   Manifestation   Hospital Acquired Condition   *EXCLUDES 1* Not Coded Here   *EXCLUDES 2* Not Included Here

✓x7th **S50.01**   Contusion of right elbow
✓x7th **S50.02**   Contusion of left elbow
✓5th **S50.1**   Contusion of forearm
     ✓x7th **S50.10**   Contusion of unspecified forearm
     ✓x7th **S50.11**   Contusion of right forearm
     ✓x7th **S50.12**   Contusion of left forearm
✓5th **S50.3**   Other superficial injuries of elbow
     ✓6th **S50.31**   Abrasion of elbow
         ✓7th **S50.311**   Abrasion of right elbow
         ✓7th **S50.312**   Abrasion of left elbow
         ✓7th **S50.319**   Abrasion of unspecified elbow
     ✓6th **S50.32**   Blister (nonthermal) of elbow
         ✓7th **S50.321**   Blister (nonthermal) of right elbow
         ✓7th **S50.322**   Blister (nonthermal) of left elbow
         ✓7th **S50.329**   Blister (nonthermal) of unspecified elbow
     ✓6th **S50.34**   External constriction of elbow
         ✓7th **S50.341**   External constriction of right elbow
         ✓7th **S50.342**   External constriction of left elbow
         ✓7th **S50.349**   External constriction of unspecified elbow
     ✓6th **S50.35**   Superficial foreign body of elbow
         Splinter in the elbow
         ✓7th **S50.351**   Superficial foreign body of right elbow
         ✓7th **S50.352**   Superficial foreign body of left elbow
         ✓7th **S50.359**   Superficial foreign body of unspecified elbow
     ✓6th **S50.36**   Insect bite (nonvenomous) of elbow
         ✓7th **S50.361**   Insect bite (nonvenomous) of right elbow
         ✓7th **S50.362**   Insect bite (nonvenomous) of left elbow
         ✓7th **S50.369**   Insect bite (nonvenomous) of unspecified elbow
     ✓6th **S50.37**   Other superficial bite of elbow
         EXCLUDES 1   open bite of elbow (S51.04)
         ✓7th **S50.371**   Other superficial bite of right elbow
         ✓7th **S50.372**   Other superficial bite of left elbow
         ✓7th **S50.379**   Other superficial bite of unspecified elbow
✓5th **S50.8**   Other superficial injuries of forearm
     ✓6th **S50.81**   Abrasion of forearm
         ✓7th **S50.811**   Abrasion of right forearm
         ✓7th **S50.812**   Abrasion of left forearm
         ✓7th **S50.819**   Abrasion of unspecified forearm
     ✓6th **S50.82**   Blister (nonthermal) of forearm
         ✓7th **S50.821**   Blister (nonthermal) of right forearm
         ✓7th **S50.822**   Blister (nonthermal) of left forearm
         ✓7th **S50.829**   Blister (nonthermal) of unspecified forearm
     ✓6th **S50.84**   External constriction of forearm
         ✓7th **S50.841**   External constriction of right forearm
         ✓7th **S50.842**   External constriction of left forearm
         ✓7th **S50.849**   External constriction of unspecified forearm
     ✓6th **S50.85**   Superficial foreign body of forearm
         Splinter in the forearm
         ✓7th **S50.851**   Superficial foreign body of right forearm
         ✓7th **S50.852**   Superficial foreign body of left forearm
         ✓7th **S50.859**   Superficial foreign body of unspecified forearm
     ✓6th **S50.86**   Insect bite (nonvenomous) of forearm
         ✓7th **S50.861**   Insect bite (nonvenomous) of right forearm
         ✓7th **S50.862**   Insect bite (nonvenomous) of left forearm
         ✓7th **S50.869**   Insect bite (nonvenomous) of unspecified forearm
     ✓6th **S50.87**   Other superficial bite of forearm
         EXCLUDES 1   open bite of forearm (S51.84)
         ✓7th **S50.871**   Other superficial bite of right forearm
         ✓7th **S50.872**   Other superficial bite of left forearm
         ✓7th **S50.879**   Other superficial bite of unspecified forearm

✓5th **S50.9**   Unspecified superficial injury of elbow and forearm
     ✓6th **S50.90**   Unspecified superficial injury of elbow
         ✓7th **S50.901**   Unspecified superficial injury of right elbow
         ✓7th **S50.902**   Unspecified superficial injury of left elbow
         ✓7th **S50.909**   Unspecified superficial injury of unspecified elbow
     ✓6th **S50.91**   Unspecified superficial injury of forearm
         ✓7th **S50.911**   Unspecified superficial injury of right forearm
         ✓7th **S50.912**   Unspecified superficial injury of left forearm
         ✓7th **S50.919**   Unspecified superficial injury of unspecified forearm

✓4th **S51**   **Open wound of elbow and forearm**
     Code also any associated wound infection
     EXCLUDES 1   open fracture of elbow and forearm (S52- with open fracture 7th character)
         traumatic amputation of elbow and forearm (S58.-)
     EXCLUDES 2   open wound of wrist and hand (S61.-)

     The appropriate 7th is to be added to each code from category S51.
     A   initial encounter
     D   subsequent encounter
     S   sequela

✓5th **S51.0**   Open wound of elbow
     ✓6th **S51.00**   Unspecified open wound of elbow
         ✓7th **S51.001**   Unspecified open wound of right elbow
             AHA: 2012, 4Q, 108
         ✓7th **S51.002**   Unspecified open wound of left elbow
         ✓7th **S51.009**   Unspecified open wound of unspecified elbow
             Open wound of elbow NOS
     ✓6th **S51.01**   Laceration without foreign body of elbow
         ✓7th **S51.011**   Laceration without foreign body of right elbow
         ✓7th **S51.012**   Laceration without foreign body of left elbow
         ✓7th **S51.019**   Laceration without foreign body of unspecified elbow
     ✓6th **S51.02**   Laceration with foreign body of elbow
         ✓7th **S51.021**   Laceration with foreign body of right elbow
         ✓7th **S51.022**   Laceration with foreign body of left elbow
         ✓7th **S51.029**   Laceration with foreign body of unspecified elbow
     ✓6th **S51.03**   Puncture wound without foreign body of elbow
         ✓7th **S51.031**   Puncture wound without foreign body of right elbow
         ✓7th **S51.032**   Puncture wound without foreign body of left elbow
         ✓7th **S51.039**   Puncture wound without foreign body of unspecified elbow
     ✓6th **S51.04**   Puncture wound with foreign body of elbow
         ✓7th **S51.041**   Puncture wound with foreign body of right elbow
         ✓7th **S51.042**   Puncture wound with foreign body of left elbow
         ✓7th **S51.049**   Puncture wound with foreign body of unspecified elbow
     ✓6th **S51.05**   Open bite of elbow
         Bite of elbow NOS
         EXCLUDES 1   superficial bite of elbow (S50.36, S50.37)
         ✓7th **S51.051**   Open bite, right elbow
         ✓7th **S51.052**   Open bite, left elbow
         ✓7th **S51.059**   Open bite, unspecified elbow
✓5th **S51.8**   Open wound of forearm
     EXCLUDES 2   open wound of elbow (S51.0-)
     ✓6th **S51.80**   Unspecified open wound of forearm
         ✓7th **S51.801**   Unspecified open wound of right forearm
         ✓7th **S51.802**   Unspecified open wound of left forearm
         ✓7th **S51.809**   Unspecified open wound of unspecified forearm
             Open wound of forearm NOS

N Newborn: 0   P Pediatric: 0-17   M Maternity: 12-55   A Adult: 15-124   **MCC** Major CC Condition   **PDxMCC** PDx acts as own MCC   **CC** CC Condition   **PDxCC** PDx acts as own CC

√6ᵗʰ **S51.81** Laceration without foreign body of forearm

    √7ᵗʰ **S51.811** Laceration without foreign body of right forearm

    √7ᵗʰ **S51.812** Laceration without foreign body of left forearm

    √7ᵗʰ **S51.819** Laceration without foreign body of unspecified forearm

√6ᵗʰ **S51.82** Laceration with foreign body of forearm

    √7ᵗʰ **S51.821** Laceration with foreign body of right forearm

    √7ᵗʰ **S51.822** Laceration with foreign body of left forearm

    √7ᵗʰ **S51.829** Laceration with foreign body of unspecified forearm

√6ᵗʰ **S51.83** Puncture wound without foreign body of forearm

    √7ᵗʰ **S51.831** Puncture wound without foreign body of right forearm

    √7ᵗʰ **S51.832** Puncture wound without foreign body of left forearm

    √7ᵗʰ **S51.839** Puncture wound without foreign body of unspecified forearm

√6ᵗʰ **S51.84** Puncture wound with foreign body of forearm

    √7ᵗʰ **S51.841** Puncture wound with foreign body of right forearm

    √7ᵗʰ **S51.842** Puncture wound with foreign body of left forearm

    √7ᵗʰ **S51.849** Puncture wound with foreign body of unspecified forearm

√6ᵗʰ **S51.85** Open bite of forearm

    Bite of forearm NOS

    EXCLUDES 1 *superficial bite of forearm (S50.86, S50.87)*

    √7ᵗʰ **S51.851** Open bite of right forearm

    √7ᵗʰ **S51.852** Open bite of left forearm

    √7ᵗʰ **S51.859** Open bite of unspecified forearm

√4ᵗʰ **S52** **Fracture of forearm**

    NOTE A fracture not indicated as displaced or nondisplaced should be coded to displaced.

    A fracture not indicated as open or closed should be coded to closed.

    The open fracture designations are based on the Gustilo open fracture classification.

    EXCLUDES 1 *traumatic amputation of forearm (S58.-)*

    EXCLUDES 2 *fracture at wrist and hand level (S62.-)*

The appropriate 7th is to be added to all codes from category S52 [unless otherwise indicated].

A   initial encounter for closed fracture

B   initial encounter for open fracture type I or II

     initial encounter for open fracture NOS

C   initial encounter for open fracture type IIIA, IIIB, or IIIC

D   subsequent encounter for closed fracture with routine healing

E   subsequent encounter for open fracture type I or II with routine healing

F   subsequent encounter for open fracture type IIIA, IIIB, or IIIC with routine healing

G   subsequent encounter for closed fracture with delayed healing

H   subsequent encounter for open fracture type I or II with delayed healing

J   subsequent encounter for open fracture type IIIA, IIIB, or IIIC with delayed healing

K   subsequent encounter for closed fracture with nonunion

M   subsequent encounter for open fracture type I or II with nonunion

N   subsequent encounter for open fracture type IIIA, IIIB, or IIIC with nonunion

P   subsequent encounter for closed fracture with malunion

Q   subsequent encounter for open fracture type I or II with malunion

R   subsequent encounter for open fracture type IIIA, IIIB, or IIIC with malunion

S   sequela

√6ᵗʰ **S52.0** Fracture of upper end of ulna

    Fracture of proximal end of ulna

    EXCLUDES 2 *fracture of elbow NOS (S42.40-)*

          fractures of shaft of ulna (S52.2-)

√6ᵗʰ **S52.00** Unspecified fracture of upper end of ulna

    CC Excl: For CC/MCC codes in subcategory S52.00: MCC with 7th character B or C: S52.001-S52.009 with 7th [B, C], S52.021-S52.109 with 7th [B, C], S52.121-S52.516 with 7th [B, C], S52.531-S52.616 with 7th [A, B, C], S52.691-S52.92X with 7th [A, B, C], S59.001-S59.099 with 7th A, S59.201-S59.299 with 7th A, S62.90XB **CC with 7th character K, M, N, P, Q, or R:** M80.00X-M84.68X with 7th [K, P], S02.0XX-S02.92X with 7th K, S12.000-S12.691 with 7th K, S22.000-S22.9XX with 7th K, S32.000-S32.9XX with 7th K, S42.001-S42.92X with 7th [K, P], S49.001-S49.199 with 7th [K, P], S52.001-S52.92X with 7th [K, M, N, P, Q, R], S59.001-S59.299 with 7th [K, P], S62.001-S62.92X with 7th [K, P], S72.001-S72.92X with 7th [K, M, N, P, Q, R], S79.001-S79.199 with 7th [K, P], S82.001-S82.92X with 7th [K, M, N, P, Q, R], S89.001-S89.399 with 7th [K, P], S92.001-S92.919 with 7th [K, P]

15,16,18 √7ᵗʰ **S52.001** Unspecified fracture of upper end of right ulna   MCC CC

15,16,18 √7ᵗʰ **S52.002** Unspecified fracture of upper end of left ulna   MCC CC

15,16,18 √7ᵗʰ **S52.009** Unspecified fracture of upper end of unspecified ulna   MCC CC

√6ᵗʰ **S52.01** Torus fracture of upper end of ulna

The appropriate 7th is to be added to all codes in subcategory S52.01.

A   initial encounter for closed fracture

D   subsequent encounter for fracture with routine healing

G   subsequent encounter for fracture with delayed healing

K   subsequent encounter for fracture with nonunion

P   subsequent encounter for fracture with malunion

S   sequela

7,19 √7ᵗʰ **S52.011** Torus fracture of upper end of right ulna   CC

    CC Excl: CC with 7th character A: S52.001-S52.011 with 7th [A, B, C], S52.019-S52.111 with 7th A, S52.119-S52.211 with 7th A, S52.219-S52.311 with 7th A, S52.319-S52.521 with 7th A, S52.529-S52.621 with 7th A, S52.629-S52.92X with 7th A, S59.001A, S59.009-S59.011 with 7th A, S59.019-S59.021 with 7th A, S59.029-S59.031 with 7th A, S59.039-S59.041 with 7th A, S59.049-S59.091 with 7th A, S59.099-S59.101 with 7th A, S59.109-S59.111 with 7th A, S59.119-S59.121 with 7th A, S59.129-S59.131 with 7th A, S59.139-S59.141 with 7th A, S59.149-S59.191 with 7th A, S59.199-S59.201 with 7th A, S59.209-S59.211 with 7th A, S59.219-S59.221 with 7th A, S59.229-S59.231 with 7th A, S59.239-S59.241 with 7th A, S59.249-S59.291 with 7th A, S59.299A **CC with 7th character K or P:** M80.00X-M84.68X with 7th [K, P], S02.0XX-S02.92X with 7th K, S12.000-S12.691 with 7th K, S22.000-S22.9XX with 7th K, S32.000-S32.9XX with 7th K, S42.001-S42.92X with 7th [K, P], S49.001-S49.199 with 7th [K, P], S52.001-S52.92X with 7th [K, M, N, P, Q, R], S59.001-S59.299 with 7th [K, P], S62.001-S62.92X with 7th [K, P], S72.001-S72.92X with 7th [K, M, N, P, Q, R], S79.001-S79.199 with 7th [K, P], S82.001-S82.92X with 7th [K, M, N, P, Q, R], S89.001-S89.399 with 7th [K, P], S92.001-S92.919 with 7th [K, P]

---

7   HAC = Initial encounter only (7th character A, B or C) and not POA.

15   HAC = Initial encounter for open fracture only (7th character B or C – specific to category) and not POA.

16   MCC only if an open fracture (7th character B or C – specific to category).

18   CC only if a subsequent encounter for nonunion or malunion (7th character K, M, N, P, Q, or R – specific to category).

19   CC only if an initial encounter for a closed fracture (7th character A) **OR** a subsequent encounter for nonunion or malunion (7th character K, M, N, P, Q, or R – specific to category).

√ Additional Character Required   √x7ᵗʰ Placeholder Alert   Unacceptable PDx   Manifestation   Hospital Acquired Condition   **EXCLUDES 1** Not Coded Here   **EXCLUDES 2** Not Included Here

7,19 ✓7th **S52.012** **Torus fracture of upper end of left ulna**   CC

CC Excl: CC with 7th character A: S52.001-S52.009 with 7th [B, C], S52.012-S52.109 with 7th A, S52.112-S52.209 with 7th A, S52.212-S52.309 with 7th A, S52.312-S52.516 with 7th A, S52.522-S52.616 with 7th A, S52.622-S52.92X with 7th A, S59.002-S59.009 with 7th A, S59.012-S59.019 with 7th A, S59.022-S59.029 with 7th A, S59.032-S59.039 with 7th A, S59.042-S59.049 with 7th A, S59.092-S59.099 with 7th A, S59.102-S59.109 with 7th A, S59.112-S59.119 with 7th A, S59.122-S59.129 with 7th A, S59.132-S59.139 with 7th A, S59.142-S59.149 with 7th A, S59.192-S59.199 with 7th A, S59.202-S59.209 with 7th A, S59.212-S59.219 with 7th A, S59.222-S59.229 with 7th A, S59.232-S59.239 with 7th A, S59.242-S59.249 with 7th A, S59.292-S59.299 with 7th A

CC with 7th character K or P: M80.00X-M84.68X with 7th [K, P], S02.0XX-S02.92X with 7th K, S12.000-S12.691 with 7th K, S22.000-S22.9XX with 7th K, S32.000-S32.9XX with 7th K, S42.001-S42.92X with 7th [K, P], S49.001-S49.199 with 7th [K, P], S52.001-S52.92X with 7th [K, M, N, P, Q, R], S59.001-S59.299 with 7th [K, P], S62.001-S62.92X with 7th [K, P], S72.001-S72.92X with 7th [K, M, N, P, Q, R], S79.001-S79.199 with 7th [K, P], S82.001-S82.92X with 7th [K, M, N, P, Q, R], S89.001-S89.399 with 7th [K, P], S92.001-S92.919 with 7th [K, P]

7,19 ✓7th **S52.019** **Torus fracture of upper end of unspecified ulna**   CC

CC Excl: CC with 7th character A: S52.001-S52.92X with 7th [A, B, C], S59.001-S59.299 with 7th A

CC with 7th character K or P: M80.00X-M84.68X with 7th [K, P], S02.0XX-S02.92X with 7th K, S12.000-S12.691 with 7th K, S22.000-S22.9XX with 7th K, S32.000-S32.9XX with 7th K, S42.001-S42.92X with 7th [K, P], S49.001-S49.199 with 7th [K, P], S52.001-S52.92X with 7th [K, M, N, P, Q, R], S59.001-S59.299 with 7th [K, P], S62.001-S62.92X with 7th [K, P], S72.001-S72.92X with 7th [K, M, N, P, Q, R], S79.001-S79.199 with 7th [K, P], S82.001-S82.92X with 7th [K, M, N, P, Q, R], S89.001-S89.399 with 7th [K, P], S92.001-S92.919 with 7th [K, P]

✓6th **S52.02** **Fracture of olecranon process without intraarticular extension of ulna**

CC Excl: For CC/MCC codes in subcatagory S52.02, unless otherwise noted: MCC with 7th character B or C: S52.001-S52.009 with 7th [B, C], S52.021-S52.109 with 7th [B, C], S52.121-S52.516 with 7th [B, C], S52.531-S52.616 with 7th [B, C], S52.691-S52.92X with 7th [A, B, C], S59.001-S59.099 with 7th A, S59.201-S59.299 with 7th A, S62.90XB

CC with 7th character K, M, N, P, Q, or R: M80.00X-M84.68X with 7th [K, P], S02.0XX-S02.92X with 7th K, S12.000-S12.691 with 7th K, S22.000-S22.9XX with 7th K, S32.000-S32.9XX with 7th K, S42.001-S42.92X with 7th [K, P], S49.001-S49.199 with 7th [K, P], S52.001-S52.92X with 7th [K, M, N, P, Q, R], S59.001-S59.299 with 7th [K, P], S62.001-S62.92X with 7th [K, P], S72.001-S72.92X with 7th [K, M, N, P, Q, R], S79.001-S79.199 with 7th [K, P], S82.001-S82.92X with 7th [K, M, N, P, Q, R], S89.001-S89.399 with 7th [K, P], S92.001-S92.919 with 7th [K, P]

15,16,18 ✓7th **S52.021** **Displaced fracture of olecranon process without intraarticular extension of right ulna**   MCC CC

15,16,18 ✓7th **S52.022** **Displaced fracture of olecranon process without intraarticular extension of left ulna**   MCC CC

15,16,18 ✓7th **S52.023** **Displaced fracture of olecranon process without intraarticular extension of unspecified ulna**   MCC CC

15,16,18 ✓7th **S52.024** **Nondisplaced fracture of olecranon process without intraarticular extension of right ulna**   MCC CC

15,16,18 ✓7th **S52.025** **Nondisplaced fracture of olecranon process without intraarticular extension of left ulna**   MCC CC

15,16,18 ✓7th **S52.026** **Nondisplaced fracture of olecranon process without intra-articular extension of unspecified ulna**   MCC CC

✓6th **S52.03** **Fracture of olecranon process with intraarticular extension of ulna**

CC Excl: For CC/MCC codes in subcatagory S52.03, unless otherwise noted: MCC with 7th character B or C: S52.001-S52.009 with 7th [B, C], S52.021-S52.109 with 7th [B, C], S52.121-S52.516 with 7th [B, C], S52.531-S52.616 with 7th [B, C], S52.691-S52.92 with 7th [A, B, C], S59.001-S59.099 with 7th A, S59.201-S59.299 with 7th A, S62.90X with 7th B

CC with 7th character K, M, N, P, Q, or R: M80.00X-M84.68X with 7th [K, P], S02.0XX-S02.92X with 7th K, S12.000-S12.691 with 7th K, S22.000-S22.9XX with 7th K, S32.000-S32.9XX with 7th K, S42.001-S42.92X with 7th [K, P], S49.001-S49.199 with 7th [K, P], S52.001-S52.92X with 7th [K, M, N, P, Q, R], S59.001-S59.299 with 7th [K, P], S62.001-S62.92X with 7th [K, P], S72.001-S72.92X with 7th [K, M, N, P, Q, R], S79.001-S79.199 with 7th [K, P], S82.001-S82.92X with 7th [K, M, N, P, Q, R], S89.001-S89.399 with 7th [K, P], S92.001-S92.919 with 7th [K, P]

15,16,18 ✓7th **S52.031** **Displaced fracture of olecranon process with intraarticular extension of right ulna**   MCC CC

15,16,18 ✓7th **S52.032** **Displaced fracture of olecranon process with intraarticular extension of left ulna**   MCC CC

15,16,18 ✓7th **S52.033** **Displaced fracture of olecranon process with intraarticular extension of unspecified ulna**   MCC CC

15,16,18 ✓7th **S52.034** **Nondisplaced fracture of olecranon process with intraarticular extension of right ulna**   MCC CC

15,16,18 ✓7th **S52.035** **Nondisplaced fracture of olecranon process with intraarticular extension of left ulna**   MCC CC

15,16,18 ✓7th **S52.036** **Nondisplaced fracture of olecranon process with intraarticular extension of unspecified ulna**   MCC CC

✓6th **S52.04** **Fracture of coronoid process of ulna**

CC Excl: For CC/MCC codes in subcatagory S52.04, unless otherwise noted: MCC with 7th character B or C: S52.001-S52.009 with 7th [B, C], S52.021-S52.109 with 7th [B, C], S52.121-S52.516 with 7th [B, C], S52.531-S52.616 with 7th [A, B, C], S52.691-S52.92X with 7th [A, B, C], S59.001-S59.099 with 7th A, S59.201-S59.299 with 7th A, S62.90XB

CC with 7th character K, M, N, P, Q, or R: M80.00X-M84.68X with 7th [K, P], S02.0XX-S02.92X with 7th K, S12.000-S12.691 with 7th K, S22.000-S22.9XX with 7th K, S32.000-S32.9XX with 7th K, S42.001-S42.92X with 7th [K, P], S49.001-S49.199 with 7th [K, P], S52.001-S52.92X with 7th [K, M, N, P, Q, R], S59.001-S59.299 with 7th [K, P], S62.001-S62.92X with 7th [K, P], S72.001-S72.92X with 7th [K, M, N, P, Q, R], S79.001-S79.199 with 7th [K, P], S82.001-S82.92X with 7th [K, M, N, P, Q, R], S89.001-S89.399 with 7th [K, P], S92.001-S92.919 with 7th [K, P]

15,16,18 ✓7th **S52.041** **Displaced fracture of coronoid process of right ulna**   MCC CC

15,16,18 ✓7th **S52.042** **Displaced fracture of coronoid process of left ulna**   MCC CC

15,16,18 ✓7th **S52.043** **Displaced fracture of coronoid process of unspecified ulna**   MCC CC

---

7   HAC = Initial encounter only (7th character A, B or C) and not POA.
15   HAC = Initial encounter for open fracture only (7th character B or C – specific to category) and not POA.
16   MCC only if an open fracture (7th character B or C – specific to category).
18   CC only if a subsequent encounter for nonunion or malunion (7th character K, M, N, P, Q, or R – specific to category).
19   CC only if an initial encounter for a closed fracture (7th character A) OR a subsequent encounter for nonunion or malunion (7th character K, M, N, P, Q, or R – specific to category).

N Newborn: 0   P Pediatric: 0-17   M Maternity: 12-55   A Adult: 15-124   MCC Major CC Condition   PDxMCC PDx acts as own MCC   CC CC Condition   PDxCC PDx acts as own CC

966   ICD-10-CM 2016

15,16,18 ✓7ᵗʰ **S52.044** **Nondisplaced** fracture of coronoid process of **right** ulna   `MCC` `CC`

15,16,18 ✓7ᵗʰ **S52.045** **Nondisplaced** fracture of coronoid process of **left** ulna   `MCC` `CC`

15,16,18 ✓7ᵗʰ **S52.046** **Nondisplaced** fracture of coronoid process of **unspecified** ulna   `MCC` `CC`

✓6ᵗʰ **S52.09** Other fracture of upper end of ulna

CC Excl: For CC/MCC codes in subcatagory S52.09, unless otherwise noted: MCC with 7th character B or C: S52.001-S52.009 with 7th [B, C], S52.021-S52.109 with 7th [B, C], S52.121-S52.516 with 7th [B, C], S52.531-S52.616 with 7th [A, B, C], S52.691-S52.92X with 7th [A, B, C], S59.001-S59.099 with 7th A, S59.201-S59.299 with 7th A, S62.90XB

CC with 7th character K, M, N, P, Q, or R: M80.00X-M84.68X with 7th [K, P], S02.0XX-S02.92X with 7th K, S12.000-S12.691 with 7th K, S22.000-S22.9XX with 7th K, S32.000-S32.9XX with 7th K, S42.001-S42.92X with 7th [K, P], S49.001-S49.199 with 7th [K, P], S52.001-S52.92X with 7th [K, M, N, P, Q, R], S59.001-S59.299 with 7th [K, P], S62.001-S62.92X with 7th [K, P], S72.001-S72.92X with 7th [K, M, N, P, Q, R], S79.001-S79.199 with 7th [K, P], S82.001-S82.92X with 7th [K, M, N, P, Q, R], S89.001-S89.399 with 7th [K, P], S92.001-S92.919 with 7th [K, P]

15,16,18 ✓7ᵗʰ **S52.091** **Other fracture of upper end of right ulna**   `MCC` `CC`

15,16,18 ✓7ᵗʰ **S52.092** **Other fracture of upper end of left ulna**   `MCC` `CC`

15,16,18 ✓7ᵗʰ **S52.099** **Other fracture of upper end of unspecified ulna**   `MCC` `CC`

✓6ᵗʰ **S52.1** Fracture of upper end of radius
Fracture of proximal end of radius
EXCLUDES 2 *physeal fractures of upper end of radius (S59.2-)*
fracture of shaft of radius (S52.3-)

✓6ᵗʰ **S52.10** Unspecified fracture of upper end of radius

CC Excl: For CC/MCC codes in subcatagory S52.10, unless otherwise noted: MCC with 7th character B or C: S52.001-S52.009 with 7th [B, C], S52.021-S52.109 with 7th [B, C], S52.121-S52.516 with 7th [B, C], S52.531-S52.616 with 7th [A, B, C], S52.691-S52.92X with 7th [A, B, C], S59.001-S59.099 with 7th A, S59.201-S59.299 with 7th A, S62.90XB

CC with 7th character K, M, N, P, Q, or R: M80.00X-M84.68X with 7th [K, P], S02.0XX-S02.92X with 7th K, S12.000-S12.691 with 7th K, S22.000-S22.9XX with 7th K, S32.000-S32.9XX with 7th K, S42.001-S42.92X with 7th [K, P], S49.001-S49.199 with 7th [K, P], S52.001-S52.92X with 7th [K, M, N, P, Q, R], S59.001-S59.299 with 7th [K, P], S62.001-S62.92X with 7th [K, P], S72.001-S72.92X with 7th [K, M, N, P, Q, R], S79.001-S79.199 with 7th [K, P], S82.001-S82.92X with 7th [K, M, N, P, Q, R], S89.001-S89.399 with 7th [K, P], S92.001-S92.919 with 7th [K, P]

15,16,18 ✓7ᵗʰ **S52.101** **Unspecified fracture of upper end of right radius**   `MCC` `CC`

15,16,18 ✓7ᵗʰ **S52.102** **Unspecified fracture of upper end of left radius**   `MCC` `CC`

15,16,18 ✓7ᵗʰ **S52.109** **Unspecified fracture of upper end of unspecified radius**   `MCC` `CC`

✓6ᵗʰ **S52.11** Torus fracture of upper end of radius

The appropriate 7th is to be added to all codes in subcategory S52.11.
A   initial encounter for closed fracture
D   subsequent encounter for fracture with routine healing
G   subsequent encounter for fracture with delayed healing
K   subsequent encounter for fracture with nonunion
P   subsequent encounter for fracture with malunion
S   sequela

7,19 ✓7ᵗʰ **S52.111** **Torus fracture of upper end of right radius**   `CC`

CC Excl: CC with 7th character A: S52.001-S52.011 with 7th [A, B, C], S52.019-S52.111 with 7th A, S52.119-S52.211 with 7th A, S52.219-S52.311 with 7th A, S52.319-S52.521 with 7th A, S52.529-S52.621 with 7th A, S52.629-S52.92X with 7th A, S59.001 with 7th A, S59.009-S59.011 with 7th A, S59.019-S59.021 with 7th A, S59.029-S59.031 with 7th A, S59.039-S59.041 with 7th A, S59.049-S59.091 with 7th A, S59.099-S59.101 with 7th A, S59.109-S59.111 with 7th A, S59.119-S59.121 with 7th A, S59.129-S59.131 with 7th A, S59.139-S59.141 with 7th A, S59.149-S59.191 with 7th A, S59.199-S59.201 with 7th A, S59.209-S59.211 with 7th A, S59.219-S59.221 with 7th A, S59.229-S59.231 with 7th A, S59.239-S59.241 with 7th A, S59.249-S59.291 with 7th A, S59.299A

CC with 7th character K, P: M80.00X-M84.68X with 7th [K, P], S02.0XX-S02.92X with 7th K, S12.000-S12.691 with 7th K, S22.000-S22.9XX with 7th K, S32.000-S32.9XX with 7th K, S42.001-S42.92X with 7th [K, P], S49.001-S49.199 with 7th [K, P], S52.001-S52.92X with 7th [K, M, N, P, Q, R], S59.001-S59.299 with 7th [K, P], S62.001-S62.92X with 7th [K, P], S72.001-S72.92X with 7th [K, M, N, P, Q, R], S79.001-S79.199 with 7th [K, P], S82.001-S82.92X with 7th [K, M, N, P, Q, R], S89.001-S89.399 with 7th [K, P], S92.001-S92.919 with 7th [K, P]

7,19 ✓7ᵗʰ **S52.112** **Torus fracture of upper end of left radius**   `CC`

CC Excl: CC with 7th character A: S52.001-S52.009 with 7th [B, C], S52.012-S52.109 with 7th A, S52.112-S52.209 with 7th A, S52.212-S52.309 with 7th A, S52.312-S52.516 with 7th A, S52.522-S52.616 with 7th A, S52.622-S52.92X with 7th A, S59.002-S59.009 with 7th A, S59.012-S59.019 with 7th A, S59.022-S59.029 with 7th A, S59.032-S59.039 with 7th A, S59.042-S59.049 with 7th A, S59.092-S59.099 with 7th A, S59.102-S59.109 with 7th A, S59.112-S59.119 with 7th A, S59.122-S59.129 with 7th A, S59.132-S59.139 with 7th A, S59.142-S59.149 with 7th A, S59.192-S59.199 with 7th A, S59.202-S59.209 with 7th A, S59.212-S59.219 with 7th A, S59.222-S59.229 with 7th A, S59.232-S59.239 with 7th A, S59.242-S59.249 with 7th A, S59.292-S59.299 with 7th A

CC with 7th character K or P: M80.00X-M84.68X with 7th [K, P], S02.0XX-S02.92X with 7th K, S12.000-S12.691 with 7th K, S22.000-S22.9XX with 7th K, S32.000-S32.9XX with 7th K, S42.001-S42.92X with 7th [K, P], S49.001-S49.199 with 7th [K, P], S52.001-S52.92X with 7th [K, M, N, P, Q, R], S59.001-S59.299 with 7th [K, P], S62.001-S62.92X with 7th [K, P], S72.001-S72.92X with 7th [K, M, N, P, Q, R], S79.001-S79.199 with 7th [K, P], S82.001-S82.92X with 7th [K, M, N, P, Q, R], S89.001-S89.399 with 7th [K, P], S92.001-S92.919 with 7th [K, P]

---

7   HAC = Initial encounter only (7th character A, B or C) and not POA.
15 HAC = Initial encounter for open fracture only (7th character B or C – specific to category) and not POA.
16 MCC only if an open fracture (7th character B or C – specific to category).
18 CC only if a subsequent encounter for nonunion or malunion (7th character K, M, N, P, Q, or R – specific to category).
19 CC only if an initial encounter for a closed fracture (7th character A) **OR** a subsequent encounter for nonunion or malunion (7th character K, M, N, P, Q, or R – specific to category).

✓ Additional Character Required   ✓x7ᵗʰ Placeholder Alert   Unacceptable PDx   Manifestation   Hospital Acquired Condition   *EXCLUDES 1* Not Coded Here   *EXCLUDES 2* Not Included Here

7,19 ✓7th **S52.119** **Torus fracture of upper end of unspecified radius** `CC`

CC Excl: CC with 7th character A: S52.001-S52.92X with 7th [A, B, C], S59.001-S59.299 with 7th A

CC Excl: CC with 7th character K or P: M80.00X-M84.68X with 7th [K, P], S02.0XX-S02.92X with 7th K, S12.000-S12.691 with 7th K, S22.000-S22.9XX with 7th K, S32.000-S32.9XX with 7th K, S42.001-S42.92X with 7th [K, P], S49.001-S49.199 with 7th [K, P], S52.001-S52.92X with 7th [K, M, N, P, Q, R], S59.001-S59.299 with 7th [K, P], S62.001-S62.92X with 7th [K, P], S72.001-S72.92X with 7th [K, M, N, P, Q, R], S79.001-S79.199 with 7th [K, P], S82.001-S82.92X with 7th [K, M, N, P, Q, R], S89.001-S89.399 with 7th [K, P], S92.001-S92.919 with 7th [K, P]

✓6th **S52.12** **Fracture of head of radius**

CC Excl: For CC/MCC codes in subcatagory S52.12: See code: S52.10

15,16,18 ✓7th **S52.121** **Displaced fracture of head of right radius** `MCC` `CC`

15,16,18 ✓7th **S52.122** **Displaced fracture of head of left radius** `MCC` `CC`

15,16,18 ✓7th **S52.123** **Displaced fracture of head of unspecified radius** `MCC` `CC`

15,16,18 ✓7th **S52.124** **Nondisplaced fracture of head of right radius** `MCC` `CC`

15,16,18 ✓7th **S52.125** **Nondisplaced fracture of head of left radius** `MCC` `CC`

15,16,18 ✓7th **S52.126** **Nondisplaced fracture of head of unspecified radius** `MCC` `CC`

✓6th **S52.13** **Fracture of neck of radius**

CC Excl: For CC/MCC codes in subcatagory S52.13: See code: S52.10

15,16,18 ✓7th **S52.131** **Displaced fracture of neck of right radius** `MCC` `CC`

15,16,18 ✓7th **S52.132** **Displaced fracture of neck of left radius** `MCC` `CC`

15,16,18 ✓7th **S52.133** **Displaced fracture of neck of unspecified radius** `MCC` `CC`

15,16,18 ✓7th **S52.134** **Nondisplaced fracture of neck of right radius** `MCC` `CC`

15,16,18 ✓7th **S52.135** **Nondisplaced fracture of neck of left radius** `MCC` `CC`

15,16,18 ✓7th **S52.136** **Nondisplaced fracture of neck of unspecified radius** `MCC` `CC`

✓6th **S52.18** **Other fracture of upper end of radius**

CC Excl: For CC/MCC codes in subcatagory S52.18: See code: S52.10

15,16,18 ✓7th **S52.181** **Other fracture of upper end of right radius** `MCC` `CC`

15,16,18 ✓7th **S52.182** **Other fracture of upper end of left radius** `MCC` `CC`

15,16,18 ✓7th **S52.189** **Other fracture of upper end of unspecified radius** `MCC` `CC`

✓5th **S52.2** **Fracture of shaft of ulna**

✓6th **S52.20** **Unspecified fracture of shaft of ulna**
Fracture of ulna NOS

7,16,19 ✓7th **S52.201** **Unspecified fracture of shaft of right ulna** `MCC` `CC`

CC Excl: CC with 7th character A: S52.001-S52.011 with 7th [A, B, C], S52.019-S52.111 with 7th A, S52.119-S52.211 with 7th A, S52.219-S52.311 with 7th A, S52.319-S52.521 with 7th A, S52.529-S52.621 with 7th A, S52.629-S52.92X with 7th A, S59.001A, S59.009-S59.011 with 7th A, S59.019-S59.021 with 7th A, S59.029-S59.031 with 7th A, S59.039-S59.041 with 7th A, S59.049-S59.091 with 7th A, S59.099-S59.101 with 7th A, S59.109-S59.111 with 7th A, S59.119-S59.121 with 7th A, S59.129-S59.131 with 7th A, S59.139-S59.141 with 7th A, S59.149-S59.191 with 7th A, S59.199-S59.201 with 7th A, S59.209-S59.211 with 7th A, S59.219-S59.221 with 7th A, S59.229-S59.231 with 7th A, S59.239-S59.241 with 7th A, S59.249-S59.291 with 7th A, S59.299A

MCC with 7th character B or C: S52.001-S52.009 with 7th [B, C], S52.021-S52.109 with 7th [B, C], S52.121-S52.516 with 7th [B, C], S52.531-S52.616 with 7th [A, B, C], S52.691-S52.92X with 7th [A, B, C], S59.001-S59.099 with 7th A, S59.201-S59.299 with 7th A, S62.90XB

MCC with 7th character K, M, N, P, Q or R: M80.00X-M84.68X with 7th [K, P], S02.0XX-S02.92X with 7th K, S12.000-S12.691 with 7th K, S22.000-S22.9XX with 7th K, S32.000-S32.9XX with 7th K, S42.001-S42.92X with 7th [K, P], S49.001-S49.199 with 7th [K, P], S52.001-S52.92X with 7th [K, M, N, P, Q, R], S59.001-S59.299 with 7th [K, P], S62.001-S62.92X with 7th [K, P], S72.001-S72.92X with 7th [K, M, N, P, Q, R], S79.001-S79.199 with 7th [K, P], S82.001-S82.92X with 7th [K, M, N, P, Q, R], S89.001-S89.399 with 7th [K, P], S92.001-S92.919 with 7th [K, P]

7,16,19 ✓7th **S52.202** **Unspecified fracture of shaft of left ulna** `MCC` `CC`

CC Excl: CC with 7th character A: S52.001-S52.009 with 7th [B, C], S52.012-S52.109 with 7th A, S52.112-S52.209 with 7th A, S52.212-S52.309 with 7th A, S52.312-S52.516 with 7th A, S52.522-S52.616 with 7th A, S52.622-S52.92X with 7th A, S59.002-S59.009 with 7th A, S59.012-S59.019 with 7th A, S59.022-S59.029 with 7th A, S59.032-S59.039 with 7th A, S59.042-S59.049 with 7th A, S59.092-S59.099 with 7th A, S59.102-S59.109 with 7th A, S59.112-S59.119 with 7th A, S59.122-S59.129 with 7th A, S59.132-S59.139 with 7th A, S59.142-S59.149 with 7th A, S59.192-S59.199 with 7th A, S59.202-S59.209 with 7th A, S59.212-S59.219 with 7th A, S59.222-S59.229 with 7th A, S59.232-S59.239 with 7th A, S59.242-S59.249 with 7th A, S59.292-S59.299 with 7th A

MCC with 7th character B or C: S52.001-S52.009 with 7th [B, C], S52.021-S52.109 with 7th [B, C], S52.121-S52.516 with 7th [B, C], S52.531-S52.616 with 7th [A, B, C], S52.691-S52.92X with 7th [A, B, C], S59.001-S59.099 with 7th A, S59.201-S59.299 with 7th A, S62.90X with 7th B

MCC with 7th character K, M, N, P, Q or R: M80.00X-M84.68X with 7th [K, P], S02.0XX-S02.92X with 7th K, S12.000-S12.691 with 7th K, S22.000-S22.9XX with 7th K, S32.000-S32.9XX with 7th K, S42.001-S42.92X with 7th [K, P], S49.001-S49.199 with 7th [K, P], S52.001-S52.92X with 7th [K, M, N, P, Q, R], S59.001-S59.299 with 7th [K, P], S62.001-S62.92X with 7th [K, P], S72.001-S72.92X with 7th [K, M, N, P, Q, R], S79.001-S79.199 with 7th [K, P], S82.001-S82.92X with 7th [K, M, N, P, Q, R], S89.001-S89.399 with 7th [K, P], S92.001-S92.919 with 7th [K, P]

---

7 HAC = Initial encounter only (7th character A, B or C) and not POA.
15 HAC = Initial encounter for open fracture only (7th character B or C – specific to category) and not POA.
16 MCC only if an open fracture (7th character B or C – specific to category).
18 CC only if a subsequent encounter for nonunion or malunion (7th character K, M, N, P, Q, or R – specific to category).
19 CC only if an initial encounter for a closed fracture (7th character A) **OR** a subsequent encounter for nonunion or malunion (7th character K, M, N, P, Q, or R – specific to category).

`N` Newborn: 0   `P` Pediatric: 0-17   `M` Maternity: 12-55   `A` Adult: 15-124   `MCC` Major CC Condition   `PDxMCC` PDx acts as own MCC   `CC` CC Condition   `PDxCC` PDx acts as own CC

968   ICD-10-CM 2016

7,16,19 ✓7ᵗʰ **S52.209 Unspecified fracture of shaft of unspecified ulna** MCC CC

CC Excl: CC with 7th character A: S52.001-S52.92X with 7th [A, B, C], S59.001-S59.299 with 7th A
MCC with 7th character B or C: S52.001-S52.009 with 7th [B, C], S52.021-S52.109 with 7th [B, C], S52.121-S52.516 with 7th [B, C], S52.531-S52.616 with 7th [A, B, C], S52.691-S52.92X with 7th [A, B, C], S59.001-S59.099 with 7th A, S59.201-S59.299 with 7th A, S62.90XB
MCC with 7th character K, M, N, P, Q or R: M80.00X-M84.68X with 7th [K, P], S02.0XX-S02.92X with 7th K, S12.000-S12.691 with 7th K, S22.000-S22.9XX with 7th K, S32.000-S32.9XX with 7th K, S42.001-S42.92X with 7th [K, P], S49.001-S49.199 with 7th [K, P], S52.001-S52.92X with 7th [K, M, N, P, Q, R], S59.001-S59.299 with 7th [K, P], S62.001-S62.92X with 7th [K, P], S72.001-S72.92X with 7th [K, M, N, P, Q, R], S79.001-S79.199 with 7th [K, P], S82.001-S82.92X with 7th [K, M, N, P, Q, R], S89.001-S89.399 with 7th [K, P], S92.001-S92.919 with 7th [K, P]

✓6ᵗʰ **S52.21 Greenstick fracture of shaft of ulna**

The appropriate 7th is to be added to all codes in subcategory S52.21.
A   initial encounter for closed fracture
D   subsequent encounter for fracture with routine healing
G   subsequent encounter for fracture with delayed healing
K   subsequent encounter for fracture with nonunion
P   subsequent encounter for fracture with malunion
S   sequela

7,19 ✓7ᵗʰ **S52.211 Greenstick fracture of shaft of right ulna** CC

CC Excl: CC with 7th character A: S52.001-S52.011 with 7th [A, B, C], S52.019-S52.111 with 7th A, S52.119-S52.211 with 7th A, S52.219-S52.311 with 7th A, S52.319-S52.521 with 7th A, S52.529-S52.621 with 7th A, S52.629-S52.92X with 7th A, S59.001 with 7th A, S59.009-S59.011 with 7th A, S59.019-S59.021 with 7th A, S59.029-S59.031 with 7th A, S59.039-S59.041 with 7th A, S59.049-S59.091 with 7th A, S59.099-S59.101 with 7th A, S59.109-S59.111 with 7th A, S59.119-S59.121 with 7th A, S59.129-S59.131 with 7th A, S59.139-S59.141 with 7th A, S59.149-S59.191 with 7th A, S59.199-S59.201 with 7th A, S59.209-S59.211 with 7th A, S59.219-S59.221 with 7th A, S59.229-S59.231 with 7th A, S59.239-S59.241 with 7th A, S59.249-S59.291 with 7th A, S59.299A
CC with 7th character K or P: M80.00X-M84.68X with 7th [K, P], S02.0XX-S02.92X with 7th K, S12.000-S12.691 with 7th K, S22.000-S22.9XX with 7th K, S32.000-S32.9XX with 7th K, S42.001-S42.92X with 7th [K, P], S49.001-S49.199 with 7th [K, P], S52.001-S52.92X with 7th [K, M, N, P, Q, R], S59.001-S59.299 with 7th [K, P], S62.001-S62.92X with 7th [K, P], S72.001-S72.92X with 7th [K, M, N, P, Q, R], S79.001-S79.199 with 7th [K, P], S82.001-S82.92X with 7th [K, M, N, P, Q, R], S89.001-S89.399 with 7th [K, P], S92.001-S92.919 with 7th [K, P]

7,19 ✓7ᵗʰ **S52.212 Greenstick fracture of shaft of left ulna** CC

CC Excl: CC with 7th character A: S52.001-S52.009 with 7th [B, C], S52.012-S52.109 with 7th A, S52.112-S52.209 with 7th A, S52.212-S52.309 with 7th A, S52.312-S52.516 with 7th A, S52.522-S52.616 with 7th A, S52.622-S52.92X with 7th A, S59.002-S59.009 with 7th A, S59.012-S59.019 with 7th A, S59.022-S59.029 with 7th A, S59.032-S59.039 with 7th A, S59.042-S59.049 with 7th A, S59.092-S59.099 with 7th A, S59.102-S59.109 with 7th A, S59.112-S59.119 with 7th A, S59.122-S59.129 with 7th A, S59.132-S59.139 with 7th A, S59.142-S59.149 with 7th A, S59.192-S59.199 with 7th A, S59.202-S59.209 with 7th A, S59.212-S59.219 with 7th A, S59.222-S59.229 with 7th A, S59.232-S59.239 with 7th A, S59.242-S59.249 with 7th A, S59.292-S59.299 with 7th A
CC with 7th character K or P: M80.00X-M84.68X with 7th [K, P], S02.0XX-S02.92X with 7th K, S12.000-S12.691 with 7th K, S22.000-S22.9XX with 7th K, S32.000-S32.9XX with 7th K, S42.001-S42.92X with 7th [K, P], S49.001-S49.199 with 7th [K, P], S52.001-S52.92X with 7th [K, M, N, P, Q, R], S59.001-S59.299 with 7th [K, P], S62.001-S62.92X with 7th [K, P], S72.001-S72.92X with 7th [K, M, N, P, Q, R], S79.001-S79.199 with 7th [K, P], S82.001-S82.92X with 7th [K, M, N, P, Q, R], S89.001-S89.399 with 7th [K, P], S92.001-S92.919 with 7th [K, P]

7,19 ✓7ᵗʰ **S52.219 Greenstick fracture of shaft of unspecified ulna** CC

CC Excl: CC with 7th character A: S52.001-S52.92X with 7th [A, B, C], S59.001-S59.299 with 7th A
CC with 7th character K or P: M80.00X-M84.68X with 7th [K, P], S02.0XX-S02.92X with 7th K, S12.000-S12.691 with 7th K, S22.000-S22.9XX with 7th K, S32.000-S32.9XX with 7th K, S42.001-S42.92X with 7th [K, P], S49.001-S49.199 with 7th [K, P], S52.001-S52.92X with 7th [K, M, N, P, Q, R], S59.001-S59.299 with 7th [K, P], S62.001-S62.92X with 7th [K, P], S72.001-S72.92X with 7th [K, M, N, P, Q, R], S79.001-S79.199 with 7th [K, P], S82.001-S82.92X with 7th [K, M, N, P, Q, R], S89.001-S89.399 with 7th [K, P], S92.001-S92.919 with 7th [K, P]

✓6ᵗʰ **S52.22 Transverse fracture of shaft of ulna**

7,16,19 ✓7ᵗʰ **S52.221 Displaced transverse fracture of shaft of right ulna** MCC CC
CC Excl: See code: S52.201

7,16,19 ✓7ᵗʰ **S52.222 Displaced transverse fracture of shaft of left ulna** MCC CC
CC Excl: See code: S52.202

7,16,19 ✓7ᵗʰ **S52.223 Displaced transverse fracture of shaft of unspecified ulna** MCC CC
CC Excl: See code: S52.209

7,16,19 ✓7ᵗʰ **S52.224 Nondisplaced transverse fracture of shaft of right ulna** MCC CC
CC Excl: See code: S52.201

7,16,19 ✓7ᵗʰ **S52.225 Nondisplaced transverse fracture of shaft of left ulna** MCC CC
CC Excl: See code: S52.202

7,16,19 ✓7ᵗʰ **S52.226 Nondisplaced transverse fracture of shaft of unspecified ulna** MCC CC
CC Excl: See code: S52.209

✓6ᵗʰ **S52.23 Oblique fracture of shaft of ulna**

7,16,19 ✓7ᵗʰ **S52.231 Displaced oblique fracture of shaft of right ulna** MCC CC
CC Excl: See code: S52.201

7,16,19 ✓7ᵗʰ **S52.232 Displaced oblique fracture of shaft of left ulna** MCC CC
CC Excl: See code: S52.202

7,16,19 ✓7ᵗʰ **S52.233 Displaced oblique fracture of shaft of unspecified ulna** MCC CC
CC Excl: See code: S52.209

7,16,19 ✓7ᵗʰ **S52.234 Nondisplaced oblique fracture of shaft of right ulna** MCC CC
CC Excl: See code: S52.201

---

7   HAC = Initial encounter only (7th character A, B or C) and not POA.
16   MCC only if an open fracture (7th character B or C – specific to category).
19   CC only if an initial encounter for a closed fracture (7th character A) **OR** a subsequent encounter for nonunion or malunion (7th character K, M, N, P, Q, or R – specific to category).

✓ Additional Character Required   ✓x7ᵗʰ Placeholder Alert   Unacceptable PDx   Manifestation   Hospital Acquired Condition   *EXCLUDES 1* Not Coded Here   *EXCLUDES 2* Not Included Here

7,16,19 ✓7th **S52.235** **Nondisplaced oblique fracture of shaft of left ulna** MCC CC
CC Excl: See code: S52.202

7,16,19 ✓7th **S52.236** **Nondisplaced oblique fracture of shaft of unspecified ulna** MCC CC
CC Excl: See code: S52.209

✓6th **S52.24** Spiral fracture of shaft of ulna

7,16,19 ✓7th **S52.241** **Displaced spiral fracture of shaft of ulna, right arm** MCC CC
CC Excl: See code: S52.201

7,16,19 ✓7th **S52.242** **Displaced spiral fracture of shaft of ulna, left arm** MCC CC
CC Excl: See code: S52.202

7,16,19 ✓7th **S52.243** **Displaced spiral fracture of shaft of ulna, unspecified arm** MCC CC
CC Excl: See code: S52.209

7,16,19 ✓7th **S52.244** **Nondisplaced spiral fracture of shaft of ulna, right arm** MCC CC
CC Excl: See code: S52.201

7,16,19 ✓7th **S52.245** **Nondisplaced spiral fracture of shaft of ulna, left arm** MCC CC
CC Excl: See code: S52.202

7,16,19 ✓7th **S52.246** **Nondisplaced spiral fracture of shaft of ulna, unspecified arm** MCC CC
CC Excl: See code: S52.209

✓6th **S52.25** Comminuted fracture of shaft of ulna

7,16,19 ✓7th **S52.251** **Displaced comminuted fracture of shaft of ulna, right arm** MCC CC
CC Excl: See code: S52.201

7,16,19 ✓7th **S52.252** **Displaced comminuted fracture of shaft of ulna, left arm** MCC CC
CC Excl: See code: S52.202

7,16,19 ✓7th **S52.253** **Displaced comminuted fracture of shaft of ulna, unspecified arm** MCC CC
CC Excl: See code: S52.209

7,16,19 ✓7th **S52.254** **Nondisplaced comminuted fracture of shaft of ulna, right arm** MCC CC
CC Excl: See code: S52.201

7,16,19 ✓7th **S52.255** **Nondisplaced comminuted fracture of shaft of ulna, left arm** MCC CC
CC Excl: See code: S52.202

7,16,19 ✓7th **S52.256** **Nondisplaced comminuted fracture of shaft of ulna, unspecified arm** MCC CC
CC Excl: See code: S52.209

✓6th **S52.26** Segmental fracture of shaft of ulna

7,16,19 ✓7th **S52.261** **Displaced segmental fracture of shaft of ulna, right arm** MCC CC
CC Excl: See code: S52.201

7,16,19 ✓7th **S52.262** **Displaced segmental fracture of shaft of ulna, left arm** MCC CC
CC Excl: See code: S52.202

7,16,19 ✓7th **S52.263** **Displaced segmental fracture of shaft of ulna, unspecified arm** MCC CC
CC Excl: See code: S52.209

7,16,19 ✓7th **S52.264** **Nondisplaced segmental fracture of shaft of ulna, right arm** MCC CC
CC Excl: See code: S52.201

7,16,19 ✓7th **S52.265** **Nondisplaced segmental fracture of shaft of ulna, left arm** MCC CC
CC Excl: See code: S52.202

7,16,19 ✓7th **S52.266** **Nondisplaced segmental fracture of shaft of ulna, unspecified arm** MCC CC
CC Excl: See code: S52.209

✓6th **S52.27** Monteggia's fracture of ulna
Fracture of upper shaft of ulna with dislocation of radial head

15,16,18 ✓7th **S52.271** **Monteggia's fracture of right ulna** MCC CC
CC Excl: See code: S52.201

15,16,18 ✓7th **S52.272** **Monteggia's fracture of left ulna** MCC CC
CC Excl: See code: S52.202

15,16,18 ✓7th **S52.279** **Monteggia's fracture of unspecified ulna** MCC CC
CC Excl: See code: S52.209

✓6th **S52.28** Bent bone of ulna

7,16,19 ✓7th **S52.281** **Bent bone of right ulna** MCC CC
CC Excl: See code: S52.201

7,16,19 ✓7th **S52.282** **Bent bone of left ulna** MCC CC
CC Excl: See code: S52.202

7,16,19 ✓7th **S52.283** **Bent bone of unspecified ulna** MCC CC
CC Excl: See code: S52.209

✓6th **S52.29** Other fracture of shaft of ulna

7,16,19 ✓7th **S52.291** **Other fracture of shaft of right ulna** MCC CC
CC Excl: See code: S52.201

7,16,19 ✓7th **S52.292** **Other fracture of shaft of left ulna** MCC CC
CC Excl: See code: S52.202

7,16,19 ✓7th **S52.299** **Other fracture of shaft of unspecified ulna** MCC CC
CC Excl: See code: S52.209

✓5th **S52.3** Fracture of shaft of radius

✓6th **S52.30** Unspecified fracture of shaft of radius

7,16,19 ✓7th **S52.301** **Unspecified fracture of shaft of right radius** MCC CC
CC Excl: See Code: S52.201

7,16,19 ✓7th **S52.302** **Unspecified fracture of shaft of left radius** MCC CC
CC Excl: See Code: S52.202

7,16,19 ✓7th **S52.309** **Unspecified fracture of shaft of unspecified radius** MCC CC
CC Excl: See Code: S52.209

✓6th **S52.31** Greenstick fracture of shaft of radius

> The appropriate 7th is to be added to all codes in subcategory S52.31.
> A   initial encounter for closed fracture
> D   subsequent encounter for fracture with routine healing
> G   subsequent encounter for fracture with delayed healing
> K   subsequent encounter for fracture with nonunion
> P   subsequent encounter for fracture with malunion
> S   sequela

7,19 ✓7th **S52.311** **Greenstick fracture of shaft of radius, right arm** CC
CC Excl: CC with 7th character A: S52.001-S52.011 with 7th [A, B, C], S52.019-S52.111 with 7th A, S52.119-S52.211 with 7th A, S52.219-S52.311 with 7th A, S52.319-S52.521 with 7th A, S52.529-S52.621 with 7th A, S52.629-S52.92X with 7th A, S59.001 with 7th A, S59.009-S59.011 with 7th A, S59.019-S59.021 with 7th A, S59.029-S59.031 with 7th A, S59.039-S59.041 with 7th A, S59.049-S59.091 with 7th A, S59.099-S59.101 with 7th A, S59.109-S59.111 with 7th A, S59.119-S59.121 with 7th A, S59.129-S59.131 with 7th A, S59.139-S59.141 with 7th A, S59.149-S59.191 with 7th A, S59.199-S59.201 with 7th A, S59.209-S59.211 with 7th A, S59.219-S59.221 with 7th A, S59.229-S59.231 with 7th A, S59.239-S59.241 with 7th A, S59.249-S59.291 with 7th A, S59.299A
CC with 7th character K or P: M80.00X-M84.68X with 7th [K, P], S02.0XX-S02.92X with 7th K, S12.000-S12.691 with 7th K, S22.000-S22.9XX with 7th K, S32.000-S32.9XX with 7th K, S42.001-S42.92X with 7th [K, P], S49.001-S49.199 with 7th [K, P], S52.001-S52.92X with 7th [K, M, N, P, Q, R], S59.001-S59.299 with 7th [K, P], S62.001-S62.92X with 7th [K, P], S72.001-S72.92X with 7th [K, M, N, P, Q, R], S79.001-S79.199 with 7th [K, P], S82.001-S82.92X with 7th [K, M, N, P, Q, R], S89.001-S89.399 with 7th [K, P], S92.001-S92.919 with 7th [K, P]

---

7   HAC = Initial encounter only (7th character A, B or C) and not POA.
15   HAC = Initial encounter for open fracture only (7th character B or C – specific to category) and not POA.
16   MCC only if an open fracture (7th character B or C – specific to category).
18   CC only if a subsequent encounter for nonunion or malunion (7th character K, M, N, P, Q, or R – specific to category).
19   CC only if an initial encounter for a closed fracture (7th character A) **OR** a subsequent encounter for nonunion or malunion (7th character K, M, N, P, Q, or R – specific to category).

N Newborn: 0   P Pediatric: 0-17   M Maternity: 12-55   A Adult: 15-124   MCC Major CC Condition   PDxMCC PDx acts as own MCC   CC CC Condition   PDxCC PDx acts as own CC

7,19 ✓7th **S52.312 Greenstick fracture of shaft of radius, left arm**
CC Excl: CC with 7th character A: S52.001-S52.009 with 7th [B, C], S52.012-S52.109 with 7th A, S52.112-S52.209 with 7th A, S52.212-S52.309 with 7th A, S52.312-S52.516 with 7th A, S52.522-S52.616 with 7th A, S52.622-S52.92X with 7th A, S59.002-S59.009 with 7th A, S59.012-S59.019 with 7th A, S59.022-S59.029 with 7th A, S59.032-S59.039 with 7th A, S59.042-S59.049 with 7th A, S59.092-S59.099 with 7th A, S59.102-S59.109 with 7th A, S59.112-S59.119 with 7th A, S59.122-S59.129 with 7th A, S59.132-S59.139 with 7th A, S59.142-S59.149 with 7th A, S59.192-S59.199 with 7th A, S59.202-S59.209 with 7th A, S59.212-S59.219 with 7th A, S59.222-S59.229 with 7th A, S59.232-S59.239 with 7th A, S59.242-S59.249 with 7th A, S59.292-S59.299 with 7th A
CC with 7th character K or P: M80.00X-M84.68X with 7th [K, P], S02.0XX-S02.92X with 7th K, S12.000-S12.691 with 7th K, S22.000-S22.9XX with 7th K, S32.000-S32.9XX with 7th K, S42.001-S42.92X with 7th [K, P], S49.001-S49.199 with 7th [K, P], S52.001-S52.92X with 7th [K, M, N, P, Q, R], S59.001-S59.299 with 7th [K, P], S62.001-S62.92X with 7th [K, P], S72.001-S72.92X with 7th [K, M, N, P, Q, R], S79.001-S79.199 with 7th [K, P], S82.001-S82.92X with 7th [K, M, N, P, Q, R], S89.001-S89.399 with 7th [K, P], S92.001-S92.919 with 7th [K, P]

7,19 ✓7th **S52.319 Greenstick fracture of shaft of radius, unspecified arm**
CC Excl: CC with 7th character A: S52.001-S52.92X with 7th [A, B, C], S59.001-S59.299 with 7th A
CC with 7th character K or P: M80.00X-M84.68X with 7th [K, P], S02.0XX-S02.92X with 7th K, S12.000-S12.691 with 7th K, S22.000-S22.9XX with 7th K, S32.000-S32.9XX with 7th K, S42.001-S42.92X with 7th [K, P], S49.001-S49.199 with 7th [K, P], S52.001-S52.92X with 7th [K, M, N, P, Q, R], S59.001-S59.299 with 7th [K, P], S62.001-S62.92X with 7th [K, P], S72.001-S72.92X with 7th [K, M, N, P, Q, R], S79.001-S79.199 with 7th [K, P], S82.001-S82.92X with 7th [K, M, N, P, Q, R], S89.001-S89.399 with 7th [K, P], S92.001-S92.919 with 7th [K, P]

✓6th **S52.32 Transverse fracture of shaft of radius**

7,16,19 ✓7th **S52.321 Displaced transverse fracture of shaft of right radius** MCC CC
CC Excl: See code: S52.201

7,16,19 ✓7th **S52.322 Displaced transverse fracture of shaft of left radius** MCC CC
CC Excl: See code: S52.202

7,16,19 ✓7th **S52.323 Displaced transverse fracture of shaft of unspecified radius** MCC CC
CC Excl: See code: S52.209

7,16,19 ✓7th **S52.324 Nondisplaced transverse fracture of shaft of right radius** MCC CC
CC Excl: See code: S52.201

7,16,19 ✓7th **S52.325 Nondisplaced transverse fracture of shaft of left radius** MCC CC
CC Excl: See code: S52.202

7,16,19 ✓7th **S52.326 Nondisplaced transverse fracture of shaft of unspecified radius** MCC CC
CC Excl: See code: S52.209

✓6th **S52.33 Oblique fracture of shaft of radius**

7,16,19 ✓7th **S52.331 Displaced oblique fracture of shaft of right radius** MCC CC
CC Excl: See code: S52.201

7,16,19 ✓7th **S52.332 Displaced oblique fracture of shaft of left radius** MCC CC
CC Excl: See code: S52.202

7,16,19 ✓7th **S52.333 Displaced oblique fracture of shaft of unspecified radius** MCC CC
CC Excl: See code: S52.209

7,16,19 ✓7th **S52.334 Nondisplaced oblique fracture of shaft of right radius** MCC CC
CC Excl: See code: S52.201

7,16,19 ✓7th **S52.335 Nondisplaced oblique fracture of shaft of left radius** MCC CC
CC Excl: See code: S52.202

7,16,19 ✓7th **S52.336 Nondisplaced oblique fracture of shaft of unspecified radius** MCC CC
CC Excl: See code: S52.209

✓6th **S52.34 Spiral fracture of shaft of radius**

7,16,19 ✓7th **S52.341 Displaced spiral fracture of shaft of radius, right arm** MCC CC
CC Excl: See code: S52.201

7,16,19 ✓7th **S52.342 Displaced spiral fracture of shaft of radius, left arm** MCC CC
CC Excl: See code: S52.202

7,16,19 ✓7th **S52.343 Displaced spiral fracture of shaft of radius, unspecified arm** MCC CC
CC Excl: See code: S52.209

7,16,19 ✓7th **S52.344 Nondisplaced spiral fracture of shaft of radius, right arm** MCC CC
CC Excl: See code: S52.201

7,16,19 ✓7th **S52.345 Nondisplaced spiral fracture of shaft of radius, left arm** MCC CC
CC Excl: See code: S52.202

7,16,19 ✓7th **S52.346 Nondisplaced spiral fracture of shaft of radius, unspecified arm** MCC CC
CC Excl: See code: S52.209

✓6th **S52.35 Comminuted fracture of shaft of radius**

7,16,19 ✓7th **S52.351 Displaced comminuted fracture of shaft of radius, right arm** MCC CC
CC Excl: See code: S52.201

7,16,19 ✓7th **S52.352 Displaced comminuted fracture of shaft of radius, left arm** MCC CC
CC Excl: See code: S52.202

7,16,19 ✓7th **S52.353 Displaced comminuted fracture sof haft of radius, unspecified arm** MCC CC
CC Excl: See code: S52.209

7,16,19 ✓7th **S52.354 Nondisplaced comminuted fracture of shaft of radius, right arm** MCC CC
CC Excl: See code: S52.201

7,16,19 ✓7th **S52.355 Nondisplaced comminuted fracture of shaft of radius, left arm** MCC CC
CC Excl: See code: S52.202

7,16,19 ✓7th **S52.356 Nondisplaced comminuted fracture of shaft of radius, unspecified arm** MCC CC
CC Excl: See code: S52.209

✓6th **S52.36 Segmental fracture of shaft of radius**

7,16,19 ✓7th **S52.361 Displaced segmental fracture of shaft of radius, right arm** MCC CC
CC Excl: See code: S52.201

7,16,19 ✓7th **S52.362 Displaced segmental fracture of shaft of radius, left arm** MCC CC
CC Excl: See code: S52.202

7,16,19 ✓7th **S52.363 Displaced segmental fracture of shaft of radius, unspecified arm** MCC CC
CC Excl: See code: S52.209

7,16,19 ✓7th **S52.364 Nondisplaced segmental fracture of shaft of radius, right arm** MCC CC
CC Excl: See code: S52.201

7,16,19 ✓7th **S52.365 Nondisplaced segmental fracture of shaft of radius, left arm** MCC CC
CC Excl: See code: S52.202

7,16,19 ✓7th **S52.366 Nondisplaced segmental fracture of shaft of radius, unspecified arm** MCC CC
CC Excl: See code: S52.209

✓6th **S52.37 Galeazzi's fracture**
Fracture of lower shaft of radius with radioulnar joint dislocation

7,16,19 ✓7th **S52.371 Galeazzi's fracture of right radius** MCC CC
CC Excl: See code: S52.201

7,16,19 ✓7th **S52.372 Galeazzi's fracture of left radius** MCC CC
CC Excl: See code: S52.202

7,16,19 ✓7th **S52.379 Galeazzi's fracture of unspecified radius** MCC CC
CC Excl: See code: S52.209

---

7   HAC = Initial encounter only (7th character A, B or C) and not POA.
16   MCC only if an open fracture (7th character B or C – specific to category).
19   CC only if an initial encounter for a closed fracture (7th character A) **OR** a subsequent encounter for nonunion or malunion (7th character K, M, N, P, Q, or R – specific to category).

✓ Additional Character Required   ✓x7th Placeholder Alert   Unacceptable PDx   Manifestation   Hospital Acquired Condition   *EXCLUDES 1* Not Coded Here   *EXCLUDES 2* Not Included Here

√6ᵗʰ **S52.38**   Bent bone **of radius**

7,16,19 √7ᵗʰ **S52.381**   Bent bone **of right radius**   MCC CC
CC Excl: See code: S52.201

7,16,19 √7ᵗʰ **S52.382**   Bent bone **of left radius**   MCC CC
CC Excl: See code: S52.202

7,16,19 √7ᵗʰ **S52.389**   Bent bone **of unspecified radius**   MCC CC
CC Excl: See code: S52.209

√6ᵗʰ **S52.39**   Other **fracture of shaft of radius**

7,16,19 √7ᵗʰ **S52.391**   Other **fracture of shaft of radius, right arm**   MCC CC
CC Excl: See code: S52.201

7,16,19 √7ᵗʰ **S52.392**   Other **fracture of shaft of radius, left arm**   MCC CC
CC Excl: See code: S52.202

7,16,19 √7ᵗʰ **S52.399**   Other **fracture of shaft of radius, unspecified arm**   MCC CC
CC Excl: See code: S52.209

√5ᵗʰ **S52.5**   Fracture **of lower end of radius**
Fracture of distal end of radius
EXCLUDES 2   physeal fractures of lower end of radius (S59.2-)

√6ᵗʰ **S52.50**   Unspecified **fracture of the lower end of radius**

7,16,19 √7ᵗʰ **S52.501**   Unspecified **fracture of the lower end of right radius**   MCC CC
CC Excl: See code: S52.201

7,16,19 √7ᵗʰ **S52.502**   Unspecified **fracture of the lower end of left radius**   MCC CC
CC Excl: See code: S52.202

7,16,19 √7ᵗʰ **S52.509**   Unspecified **fracture of the lower end of unspecified radius**   MCC CC
CC Excl: See code: S52.209

√6ᵗʰ **S52.51**   Fracture **of radial styloid process**

7,16,19 √7ᵗʰ **S52.511**   Displaced **fracture of right radial styloid process**   MCC CC
CC Excl: See code: S52.201

7,16,19 √7ᵗʰ **S52.512**   Displaced **fracture of left radial styloid process**   MCC CC
CC Excl: See code: S52.202

7,16,19 √7ᵗʰ **S52.513**   Displaced **fracture of unspecified radial styloid process**   MCC CC
CC Excl: See code: S52.209

7,16,19 √7ᵗʰ **S52.514**   Nondisplaced **fracture of right radial styloid process**   MCC CC
CC Excl: See code: S52.201

7,16,19 √7ᵗʰ **S52.515**   Nondisplaced **fracture of left radial styloid process**   MCC CC
CC Excl: See code: S52.202

7,16,19 √7ᵗʰ **S52.516**   Nondisplaced **fracture of unspecified radial styloid process**   MCC CC
CC Excl: See code: S52.209

√6ᵗʰ **S52.52**   Torus **fracture of lower end of radius**

> The appropriate 7th is to be added to all codes in subcategory S52.52.
> A   initial encounter for closed fracture
> D   subsequent encounter for fracture with routine healing
> G   subsequent encounter for fracture with delayed healing
> K   subsequent encounter for fracture with nonunion
> P   subsequent encounter for fracture with malunion
> S   sequela

7,19 √7ᵗʰ **S52.521**   Torus **fracture of lower end of right radius**   CC
CC Excl: CC with 7th character A: S52.001-S52.011 with 7th [A, B, C], S52.019-S52.111 with 7th A, S52.119-S52.211 with 7th A, S52.219-S52.311 with 7th A, S52.319-S52.521 with 7th A, S52.529-S52.621 with 7th A, S52.629-S52.92X with 7th A, S59.001 with 7th A, S59.009-S59.011 with 7th A, S59.019-S59.021 with 7th A, S59.029-S59.031 with 7th A, S59.039-S59.041 with 7th A, S59.049-S59.091 with 7th A, S59.099-S59.101 with 7th A, S59.109-S59.111 with 7th A, S59.119-S59.121 with 7th A, S59.129-S59.131 with 7th A, S59.139-S59.141 with 7th A, S59.149-S59.191 with 7th A, S59.199-S59.201 with 7th A, S59.209-S59.211 with 7th A, S59.219-S59.221 with 7th A, S59.229-S59.231 with 7th A, S59.239-S59.241 with 7th A, S59.249-S59.291 with 7th A, S59.299A
CC with 7th character K or P: M80.00X-M84.68X with 7th [K, P], S02.0XX-S02.92X with 7th K, S12.000-S12.691 with 7th K, S22.000-S22.9XX with 7th K, S32.000-S32.9XX with 7th K, S42.001-S42.92X with 7th [K, P], S49.001-S49.199 with 7th [K, P], S52.001-S52.92X with 7th [K, M, N, P, Q, R], S59.001-S59.299 with 7th [K, P], S62.001-S62.92X with 7th [K, P], S72.001-S72.92X with 7th [K, M, N, P, Q, R], S79.001-S79.199 with 7th [K, P], S82.001-S82.92X with 7th [K, M, N, P, Q, R], S89.001-S89.399 with 7th [K, P], S92.001-S92.919 with 7th [K, P]

7,19 √7ᵗʰ **S52.522**   Torus **fracture of lower end of left radius**   CC
CC Excl: CC with 7th character A: S52.001-S52.009 with 7th [B, C], S52.012-S52.109 with 7th A, S52.112-S52.209 with 7th A, S52.212-S52.309 with 7th A, S52.312-S52.516 with 7th A, S52.522-S52.616 with 7th A, S52.622-S52.92X with 7th A, S59.002-S59.009 with 7th A, S59.012-S59.019 with 7th A, S59.022-S59.029 with 7th A, S59.032-S59.039 with 7th A, S59.042-S59.049 with 7th A, S59.092-S59.099 with 7th A, S59.102-S59.109 with 7th A, S59.112-S59.119 with 7th A, S59.122-S59.129 with 7th A, S59.132-S59.139 with 7th A, S59.142-S59.149 with 7th A, S59.192-S59.199 with 7th A, S59.202-S59.209 with 7th A, S59.212-S59.219 with 7th A, S59.222-S59.229 with 7th A, S59.232-S59.239 with 7th A, S59.242-S59.249 with 7th A, S59.292-S59.299 with 7th A
CC with 7th character K or P: M80.00X-M84.68X with 7th [K, P], S02.0XX-S02.92X with 7th K, S12.000-S12.691 with 7th K, S22.000-S22.9XX with 7th K, S32.000-S32.9XX with 7th K, S42.001-S42.92X with 7th [K, P], S49.001-S49.199 with 7th [K, P], S52.001-S52.92X with 7th [K, M, N, P, Q, R], S59.001-S59.299 with 7th [K, P], S62.001-S62.92X with 7th [K, P], S72.001-S72.92X with 7th [K, M, N, P, Q, R], S79.001-S79.199 with 7th [K, P], S82.001-S82.92X with 7th [K, M, N, P, Q, R], S89.001-S89.399 with 7th [K, P], S92.001-S92.919 with 7th [K, P]

7,19 √7ᵗʰ **S52.529**   Torus **fracture of lower end of unspecified radius**   CC
CC Excl: See code: S52.209

√6ᵗʰ **S52.53**   Colles' **fracture**

7,16,19 √7ᵗʰ **S52.531**   Colles' **fracture of right radius**   MCC CC
CC Excl: See code: S52.201

7,16,19 √7ᵗʰ **S52.532**   Colles' **fracture of left radius**   MCC CC
CC Excl: See code: S52.202

7,16,19 √7ᵗʰ **S52.539**   Colles' **fracture of unspecified radius**   MCC CC
CC Excl: See code: S52.209

√6ᵗʰ **S52.54**   Smith's **fracture**

7,16,19 √7ᵗʰ **S52.541**   Smith's **fracture of right radius**   MCC CC
CC Excl: See code: S52.201

7,16,19 √7ᵗʰ **S52.542**   Smith's **fracture of left radius**   MCC CC
CC Excl: See code: S52.202

7,16,19 √7ᵗʰ **S52.549**   Smith's **fracture of unspecified radius**   MCC CC
CC Excl: See code: S52.209

---

7   HAC = Initial encounter only (7th character A, B or C) and not POA.
16   MCC only if an open fracture (7th character B or C – specific to category).
19   CC only if an initial encounter for a closed fracture (7th character A) **OR** a subsequent encounter for nonunion or malunion (7th character K, M, N, P, Q, or R – specific to category).

N Newborn: 0   P Pediatric: 0-17   M Maternity: 12-55   A Adult: 15-124   MCC Major CC Condition   PDxMCC PDx acts as own MCC   CC CC Condition   PDxCC PDx acts as own CC

✓6ᵗʰ **S52.55**   Other extraarticular **fracture of lower end of radius**

7,16,19 ✓7ᵗʰ **S52.551**   **Other extraarticular fracture of lower end of right radius**   MCC CC
CC Excl: See code: S52.201

7,16,19 ✓7ᵗʰ **S52.552**   **Other extraarticular fracture of lower end of left radius**   MCC CC
CC Excl: See code: S52.202

7,16,19 ✓7ᵗʰ **S52.559**   **Other extraarticular fracture of lower end of unspecified radius**   MCC CC
CC Excl: See code: S52.209

✓6ᵗʰ **S52.56**   **Barton's fracture**

7,16,19 ✓7ᵗʰ **S52.561**   **Barton's fracture of right radius**   MCC CC
CC Excl: See code: S52.201

7,16,19 ✓7ᵗʰ **S52.562**   **Barton's fracture of left radius**   MCC CC
CC Excl: See code: S52.202

7,16,19 ✓7ᵗʰ **S52.569**   **Barton's fracture of unspecified radius**   MCC CC
CC Excl: See code: S52.209

✓6ᵗʰ **S52.57**   Other intraarticular **fracture of lower end of radius**

7,16,19 ✓7ᵗʰ **S52.571**   **Other intraarticular fracture of lower end of right radius**   MCC CC
CC Excl: See code: S52.201

7,16,19 ✓7ᵗʰ **S52.572**   **Other intraarticular fracture of lower end of left radius**   MCC CC
CC Excl: See code: S52.202

7,16,19 ✓7ᵗʰ **S52.579**   **Other intraarticular fracture of lower end of unspecified radius**   MCC CC
CC Excl: See code: S52.209

✓6ᵗʰ **S52.59**   Other fractures of lower end of radius

7,16,19 ✓7ᵗʰ **S52.591**   **Other fractures of lower end of right radius**   MCC CC
CC Excl: See code: S52.201

7,16,19 ✓7ᵗʰ **S52.592**   **Other fractures of lower end of left radius**   MCC CC
CC Excl: See code: S52.202

7,16,19 ✓7ᵗʰ **S52.599**   **Other fractures of lower end of unspecified radius**   MCC CC
CC Excl: See code: S52.209

✓5ᵗʰ **S52.6**   Fracture of lower end of ulna

✓6ᵗʰ **S52.60**   Unspecified **fracture of lower end of ulna**

7,16,19 ✓7ᵗʰ **S52.601**   **Unspecified fracture of lower end of right ulna**   MCC CC
CC Excl: See code: S52.201

7,16,19 ✓7ᵗʰ **S52.602**   **Unspecified fracture of lower end of left ulna**   MCC CC
CC Excl: See code: S52.202

7,16,19 ✓7ᵗʰ **S52.609**   **Unspecified fracture of lower end of unspecified ulna**   MCC CC
CC Excl: See code: S52.209

✓6ᵗʰ **S52.61**   Fracture of ulna styloid process

7,16,19 ✓7ᵗʰ **S52.611**   **Displaced fracture of right ulna styloid process**   MCC CC
CC Excl: See code: S52.201

7,16,19 ✓7ᵗʰ **S52.612**   **Displaced fracture of left ulna styloid process**   MCC CC
CC Excl: See code: S52.202

7,16,19 ✓7ᵗʰ **S52.613**   **Displaced fracture of unspecified ulna styloid process**   MCC CC
CC Excl: See code: S52.209

7,16,19 ✓7ᵗʰ **S52.614**   **Nondisplaced fracture of right ulna styloid process**   MCC CC
CC Excl: See code: S52.201

7,16,19 ✓7ᵗʰ **S52.615**   **Nondisplaced fracture of left ulna styloid process**   MCC CC
CC Excl: See code: S52.202

7,16,19 ✓7ᵗʰ **S52.616**   **Nondisplaced fracture of unspecified ulna styloid process**   MCC CC
CC Excl: See code: S52.209

✓6ᵗʰ **S52.62**   Torus **fracture of lower end of ulna**

> The appropriate 7th is to be added to all codes in subcategory S52.62.
> A   initial encounter for closed fracture
> D   subsequent encounter for fracture with routine healing
> G   subsequent encounter for fracture with delayed healing
> K   subsequent encounter for fracture with nonunion
> P   subsequent encounter for fracture with malunion
> S   sequela

7,19 ✓7ᵗʰ **S52.621**   **Torus fracture of lower end of right ulna**   CC
CC Excl: **CC with 7th character A:** S52.001-S52.011 with 7th [A, B, C], S52.019-S52.111 with 7th A, S52.119-S52.211 with 7th A, S52.219-S52.311 with 7th A, S52.319-S52.521 with 7th A, S52.529-S52.621 with 7th A, S52.629-S52.92X with 7th A, S59.001 with 7th A, S59.009-S59.011 with 7th A, S59.019-S59.021 with 7th A, S59.029-S59.031 with 7th A, S59.039-S59.041 with 7th A, S59.049-S59.091 with 7th A, S59.099-S59.101 with 7th A, S59.109-S59.111 with 7th A, S59.119-S59.121 with 7th A, S59.129-S59.131 with 7th A, S59.139-S59.141 with 7th A, S59.149-S59.191 with 7th A, S59.199-S59.201 with 7th A, S59.209-S59.211 with 7th A, S59.219-S59.221 with 7th A, S59.229-S59.231 with 7th A, S59.239-S59.241 with 7th A, S59.249-S59.291 with 7th A, S59.299A
CC with 7th character K or P: M80.00X-M84.68X with 7th [K, P], S02.0XX-S02.92X with 7th K, S12.000-S12.691 with 7th K, S22.000-S22.9XX with 7th K, S32.000-S32.9XX with 7th K, S42.001-S42.92X with 7th [K, P], S49.001-S49.199 with 7th [K, P], S52.001-S52.92X with 7th [K, M, N, P, Q, R], S59.001-S59.299 with 7th [K, P], S62.001-S62.92X with 7th [K, P], S72.001-S72.92X with 7th [K, M, N, P, Q, R], S79.001-S79.199 with 7th [K, P], S82.001-S82.92X with 7th [K, M, N, P, Q, R], S89.001-S89.399 with 7th [K, P], S92.001-S92.919 with 7th [K, P]

7,19 ✓7ᵗʰ **S52.622**   **Torus fracture of lower end of left ulna**   CC
CC Excl: **CC with 7th character A:** S52.001-S52.009 with 7th [B, C], S52.012-S52.109 with 7th A, S52.112-S52.209 with 7th A, S52.212-S52.309 with 7th A, S52.312-S52.516 with 7th A, S52.522-S52.616 with 7th A, S52.622-S52.92X with 7th A, S59.002-S59.009 with 7th A, S59.012-S59.019 with 7th A, S59.022-S59.029 with 7th A, S59.032-S59.039 with 7th A, S59.042-S59.049 with 7th A, S59.092-S59.099 with 7th A, S59.102-S59.109 with 7th A, S59.112-S59.119 with 7th A, S59.122-S59.129 with 7th A, S59.132-S59.139 with 7th A, S59.142-S59.149 with 7th A, S59.192-S59.199 with 7th A, S59.202-S59.209 with 7th A, S59.212-S59.219 with 7th A, S59.222-S59.229 with 7th A, S59.232-S59.239 with 7th A, S59.242-S59.249 with 7th A, S59.292-S59.299 with 7th A
CC with 7th character K or P: M80.00X-M84.68X with 7th [K, P], S02.0XX-S02.92X with 7th K, S12.000-S12.691 with 7th K, S22.000-S22.9XX with 7th K, S32.000-S32.9XX with 7th K, S42.001-S42.92X with 7th [K, P], S49.001-S49.199 with 7th [K, P], S52.001-S52.92X with 7th [K, M, N, P, Q, R], S59.001-S59.299 with 7th [K, P], S62.001-S62.92X with 7th [K, P], S72.001-S72.92X with 7th [K, M, N, P, Q, R], S79.001-S79.199 with 7th [K, P], S82.001-S82.92X with 7th [K, M, N, P, Q, R], S89.001-S89.399 with 7th [K, P], S92.001-S92.919 with 7th [K, P]

---

7   HAC = Initial encounter only (7th character A, B or C) and not POA.
16   MCC only if an open fracture (7th character B or C – specific to category).
19   CC only if an initial encounter for a closed fracture (7th character A) **OR** a subsequent encounter for nonunion or malunion (7th character K, M, N, P, Q, or R – specific to category).

✔ Additional Character Required   ✓x7ᵗʰ Placeholder Alert   Unacceptable PDx   Manifestation   Hospital Acquired Condition   *EXCLUDES 1* Not Coded Here   *EXCLUDES 2* Not Included Here

7,19 √7ᵗʰ **S52.629** **Torus fracture of lower end of** CC
unspecified ulna
CC Excl: CC with 7th character A: S52.001-
S52.92X with 7th [A, B, C], S59.001-S59.299
with 7th A
CC with 7th character K or P: M80.00X-
M84.68X with 7th [K, P], S02.0XX-S02.92X
with 7th K, S12.000-S12.691 with 7th K,
S22.000-S22.9XX with 7th K, S32.000-
S32.9XX with 7th K, S42.001-S42.92X with
7th [K, P], S49.001-S49.199 with 7th [K, P],
S52.001-S52.92X with 7th [K, M, N, P, Q, R],
S59.001-S59.299 with 7th [K, P], S62.001-
S62.92X with 7th [K, P], S72.001-S72.92X
with 7th [K, M, N, P, Q, R], S79.001-S79.199
with 7th [K, P], S82.001-S82.92X with 7th [K,
M, N, P, Q, R], S89.001-S89.399 with 7th [K, P],
S92.001-S92.919 with 7th [K, P]

√6ᵗʰ **S52.69** **Other fracture of lower end of ulna**

7,16,19 √7ᵗʰ **S52.691** **Other fracture of lower end of** MCC CC
right ulna
CC Excl: See code: S52.201

7,16,19 √7ᵗʰ **S52.692** **Other fracture of lower end of** MCC CC
left ulna
CC Excl: See code: S52.202

7,16,19 √7ᵗʰ **S52.699** **Other fracture of lower end of** MCC CC
unspecified ulna
CC Excl: See code: S52.209

√5ᵗʰ **S52.9** **Unspecified fracture of forearm**

7,16,19 √x7ᵗʰ **S52.90** **Unspecified fracture of unspecified forearm** MCC CC
CC Excl: CC with 7th character A: S52.001-S52.92X
with 7th [A, B, C], S59.001-S59.299 with 7th A
MCC with 7th character B or C: S52.001-S52.009 with
7th [B, C], S52.021-S52.109 with 7th [B, C], S52.121-
S52.516 with 7th [B, C], S52.531-S52.616 with 7th [A, B,
C], S52.691-S52.92X with 7th [A, B, C], S59.001-S59.099
with 7th A, S59.201-S59.299 with 7th A, S62.90XB
CC with 7th character K, M, N, P, Q or R: M80.00X-
M84.68X with 7th [K, P], S02.0XX-S02.92X with 7th K,
S12.000-S12.691 with 7th K, S22.000-S22.9XX with 7th K,
S32.000-S32.9XX with 7th K, S42.001-S42.92X with 7th
[K, P], S49.001-S49.199 with 7th [K, P], S52.001-S52.92X
with 7th [K, M, N, P, Q, R], S59.001-S59.299 with 7th [K,
P], S62.001-S62.92X with 7th [K, P], S72.001-S72.92X
with 7th [K, M, N, P, Q, R], S79.001-S79.199 with 7th [K,
P], S82.001-S82.92X with 7th [K, M, N, P, Q, R], S89.001-
S89.399 with 7th [K, P], S92.001-S92.919 with 7th [K, P]

7,16,19 √x7ᵗʰ **S52.91** **Unspecified fracture of right forearm** MCC CC
CC Excl: See code: S52.90

7,16,19 √x7ᵗʰ **S52.92** **Unspecified fracture of left forearm** MCC CC
CC Excl: See code: S52.90

√4ᵗʰ **S53** **Dislocation and sprain of joints and ligaments of elbow**
INCLUDES   avulsion of joint or ligament of elbow
laceration of cartilage, joint or ligament of elbow
sprain of cartilage, joint or ligament of elbow
traumatic hemarthrosis of joint or ligament of elbow
traumatic rupture of joint or ligament of elbow
traumatic subluxation of joint or ligament of elbow
traumatic tear of joint or ligament of elbow
Code also any associated open wound
EXCLUDES 2   strain of muscle, fascia and tendon at forearm level (S56.-)

The appropriate 7th is to be added to each code from category S53.
A   initial encounter
D   subsequent encounter
S   sequela

√5ᵗʰ **S53.0** **Subluxation and dislocation of radial head**
Dislocation of radiohumeral joint
Subluxation of radiohumeral joint
EXCLUDES 1   Monteggia's fracture-dislocation (S52.27-)

√6ᵗʰ **S53.00** **Unspecified subluxation and dislocation of radial
head**

√7ᵗʰ **S53.001** **Unspecified subluxation of right radial
head**

√7ᵗʰ **S53.002** **Unspecified subluxation of left radial head**

√7ᵗʰ **S53.003** **Unspecified subluxation of unspecified
radial head**

√7ᵗʰ **S53.004** **Unspecified dislocation of right radial
head**

√7ᵗʰ **S53.005** **Unspecified dislocation of left radial head**

√7ᵗʰ **S53.006** **Unspecified dislocation of unspecified
radial head**

√6ᵗʰ **S53.01** **Anterior subluxation and dislocation of radial head**
Anteriomedial subluxation and dislocation of radial
head

√7ᵗʰ **S53.011** **Anterior subluxation of right radial head**

√7ᵗʰ **S53.012** **Anterior subluxation of left radial head**

√7ᵗʰ **S53.013** **Anterior subluxation of unspecified radial
head**

√7ᵗʰ **S53.014** **Anterior dislocation of right radial head**

√7ᵗʰ **S53.015** **Anterior dislocation of left radial head**

√7ᵗʰ **S53.016** **Anterior dislocation of unspecified radial
head**

√6ᵗʰ **S53.02** **Posterior subluxation and dislocation of radial head**
Posteriolateral subluxation and dislocation of radial
head

√7ᵗʰ **S53.021** **Posterior subluxation of right radial head**

√7ᵗʰ **S53.022** **Posterior subluxation of left radial head**

√7ᵗʰ **S53.023** **Posterior subluxation of unspecified
radial head**

√7ᵗʰ **S53.024** **Posterior dislocation of right radial head**

√7ᵗʰ **S53.025** **Posterior dislocation of left radial head**

√7ᵗʰ **S53.026** **Posterior dislocation of unspecified radial
head**

√6ᵗʰ **S53.03** **Nursemaid's elbow**

√7ᵗʰ **S53.031** **Nursemaid's elbow, right elbow**

√7ᵗʰ **S53.032** **Nursemaid's elbow, left elbow**

√7ᵗʰ **S53.033** **Nursemaid's elbow, unspecified elbow**

√6ᵗʰ **S53.09** **Other subluxation and dislocation of radial head**

√7ᵗʰ **S53.091** **Other subluxation of right radial head**

√7ᵗʰ **S53.092** **Other subluxation of left radial head**

√7ᵗʰ **S53.093** **Other subluxation of unspecified radial
head**

√7ᵗʰ **S53.094** **Other dislocation of right radial head**

√7ᵗʰ **S53.095** **Other dislocation of left radial head**

√7ᵗʰ **S53.096** **Other dislocation of unspecified radial
head**

√5ᵗʰ **S53.1** **Subluxation and dislocation of ulnohumeral joint**
Subluxation and dislocation of elbow NOS
EXCLUDES 1   dislocation of radial head alone (S53.0-)

√6ᵗʰ **S53.10** **Unspecified subluxation and dislocation of
ulnohumeral joint**

√7ᵗʰ **S53.101** **Unspecified subluxation of right
ulnohumeral joint**

√7ᵗʰ **S53.102** **Unspecified subluxation of left
ulnohumeral joint**

√7ᵗʰ **S53.103** **Unspecified subluxation of unspecified
ulnohumeral joint**

√7ᵗʰ **S53.104** **Unspecified dislocation of right
ulnohumeral joint**

√7ᵗʰ **S53.105** **Unspecified dislocation of left
ulnohumeral joint**

√7ᵗʰ **S53.106** **Unspecified dislocation of unspecified
ulnohumeral joint**

√6ᵗʰ **S53.11** **Anterior subluxation and dislocation of ulnohumeral
joint**

√7ᵗʰ **S53.111** **Anterior subluxation of right ulnohumeral
joint**

√7ᵗʰ **S53.112** **Anterior subluxation of left ulnohumeral
joint**

√7ᵗʰ **S53.113** **Anterior subluxation of unspecified
ulnohumeral joint**

√7ᵗʰ **S53.114** **Anterior dislocation of right ulnohumeral
joint**
AHA: 2012, 4Q, 108

√7ᵗʰ **S53.115** **Anterior dislocation of left ulnohumeral
joint**

√7ᵗʰ **S53.116** **Anterior dislocation of unspecified
ulnohumeral joint**

---

7   HAC = Initial encounter only (7th character A, B or C) and not POA.
16   MCC only if an open fracture (7th character B or C – specific to category).
19   CC only if an initial encounter for a closed fracture (7th character A) **OR** a subsequent encounter for nonunion or malunion (7th character K, M, N, P, Q, or R – specific to category).

N Newborn: 0   P Pediatric: 0-17   M Maternity: 12-55   A Adult: 15-124   MCC Major CC Condition   PDx MCC PDx acts as own MCC   CC CC Condition   PDx CC PDx acts as own CC

✓6ᵗʰ **S53.12** Posterior subluxation and dislocation of ulnohumeral joint

    ✓7ᵗʰ **S53.121** Posterior subluxation of right ulnohumeral joint

    ✓7ᵗʰ **S53.122** Posterior subluxation of left ulnohumeral joint

    ✓7ᵗʰ **S53.123** Posterior subluxation of unspecified ulnohumeral joint

    ✓7ᵗʰ **S53.124** Posterior dislocation of right ulnohumeral joint

    ✓7ᵗʰ **S53.125** Posterior dislocation of left ulnohumeral joint

    ✓7ᵗʰ **S53.126** Posterior dislocation of unspecified ulnohumeral joint

✓6ᵗʰ **S53.13** Medial subluxation and dislocation of ulnohumeral joint

    ✓7ᵗʰ **S53.131** Medial subluxation of right ulnohumeral joint

    ✓7ᵗʰ **S53.132** Medial subluxation of left ulnohumeral joint

    ✓7ᵗʰ **S53.133** Medial subluxation of unspecified ulnohumeral joint

    ✓7ᵗʰ **S53.134** Medial dislocation of right ulnohumeral joint

    ✓7ᵗʰ **S53.135** Medial dislocation of left ulnohumeral joint

    ✓7ᵗʰ **S53.136** Medial dislocation of unspecified ulnohumeral joint

✓6ᵗʰ **S53.14** Lateral subluxation and dislocation of ulnohumeral joint

    ✓7ᵗʰ **S53.141** Lateral subluxation of right ulnohumeral joint

    ✓7ᵗʰ **S53.142** Lateral subluxation of left ulnohumeral joint

    ✓7ᵗʰ **S53.143** Lateral subluxation of unspecified ulnohumeral joint

    ✓7ᵗʰ **S53.144** Lateral dislocation of right ulnohumeral joint

    ✓7ᵗʰ **S53.145** Lateral dislocation of left ulnohumeral joint

    ✓7ᵗʰ **S53.146** Lateral dislocation of unspecified ulnohumeral joint

✓6ᵗʰ **S53.19** Other subluxation and dislocation of ulnohumeral joint

    ✓7ᵗʰ **S53.191** Other subluxation of right ulnohumeral joint

    ✓7ᵗʰ **S53.192** Other subluxation of left ulnohumeral joint

    ✓7ᵗʰ **S53.193** Other subluxation of unspecified ulnohumeral joint

    ✓7ᵗʰ **S53.194** Other dislocation of right ulnohumeral joint

    ✓7ᵗʰ **S53.195** Other dislocation of left ulnohumeral joint

    ✓7ᵗʰ **S53.196** Other dislocation of unspecified ulnohumeral joint

✓5ᵗʰ **S53.2** Traumatic rupture of radial collateral ligament

    EXCLUDES 1   *sprain of radial collateral ligament NOS (S53.43-)*

    ✓x7ᵗʰ **S53.20** Traumatic rupture of unspecified radial collateral ligament

    ✓x7ᵗʰ **S53.21** Traumatic rupture of right radial collateral ligament

    ✓x7ᵗʰ **S53.22** Traumatic rupture of left radial collateral ligament

✓5ᵗʰ **S53.3** Traumatic rupture of ulnar collateral ligament

    EXCLUDES 1   *sprain of ulnar collateral ligament (S53.44-)*

    ✓x7ᵗʰ **S53.30** Traumatic rupture of unspecified ulnar collateral ligament

    ✓x7ᵗʰ **S53.31** Traumatic rupture of right ulnar collateral ligament

    ✓x7ᵗʰ **S53.32** Traumatic rupture of left ulnar collateral ligament

✓5ᵗʰ **S53.4** Sprain of elbow

    EXCLUDES 2   *traumatic rupture of radial collateral ligament (S53.2-)*
          traumatic rupture of ulnar collateral ligament (S53.3-)

    ✓6ᵗʰ **S53.40** Unspecified sprain of elbow

       ✓7ᵗʰ **S53.401** Unspecified sprain of right elbow

       ✓7ᵗʰ **S53.402** Unspecified sprain of left elbow

       ✓7ᵗʰ **S53.409** Unspecified sprain of unspecified elbow
           Sprain of elbow NOS

    ✓6ᵗʰ **S53.41** Radiohumeral (joint) sprain

       ✓7ᵗʰ **S53.411** Radiohumeral (joint) sprain of right elbow

       ✓7ᵗʰ **S53.412** Radiohumeral (joint) sprain of left elbow

       ✓7ᵗʰ **S53.419** Radiohumeral (joint) sprain of unspecified elbow

    ✓6ᵗʰ **S53.42** Ulnohumeral (joint) sprain

       ✓7ᵗʰ **S53.421** Ulnohumeral (joint) sprain of right elbow

       ✓7ᵗʰ **S53.422** Ulnohumeral (joint) sprain of left elbow

       ✓7ᵗʰ **S53.429** Ulnohumeral (joint) sprain of unspecified elbow

    ✓6ᵗʰ **S53.43** Radial collateral ligament sprain

       ✓7ᵗʰ **S53.431** Radial collateral ligament sprain of right elbow

       ✓7ᵗʰ **S53.432** Radial collateral ligament sprain of left elbow

       ✓7ᵗʰ **S53.439** Radial collateral ligament sprain of unspecified elbow

    ✓6ᵗʰ **S53.44** Ulnar collateral ligament sprain

       ✓7ᵗʰ **S53.441** Ulnar collateral ligament sprain of right elbow

       ✓7ᵗʰ **S53.442** Ulnar collateral ligament sprain of left elbow

       ✓7ᵗʰ **S53.449** Ulnar collateral ligament sprain of unspecified elbow

    ✓6ᵗʰ **S53.49** Other sprain of elbow

       ✓7ᵗʰ **S53.491** Other sprain of right elbow

       ✓7ᵗʰ **S53.492** Other sprain of left elbow

       ✓7ᵗʰ **S53.499** Other sprain of unspecified elbow

✓4ᵗʰ **S54 Injury of nerves at forearm level**

    Code also any associated open wound (S51.-)

    EXCLUDES 2   *injury of nerves at wrist and hand level (S64.-)*

> The appropriate 7th is to be added to each code from category S54.
> A   initial encounter
> D   subsequent encounter
> S   sequela

✓5ᵗʰ **S54.0** Injury of ulnar nerve at forearm level
       Injury of ulnar nerve NOS

    ✓x7ᵗʰ **S54.00** Injury of ulnar nerve at forearm level, unspecified arm

    ✓x7ᵗʰ **S54.01** Injury of ulnar nerve at forearm level, right arm

    ✓x7ᵗʰ **S54.02** Injury of ulnar nerve at forearm level, left arm

✓5ᵗʰ **S54.1** Injury of median nerve at forearm level
       Injury of median nerve NOS

    ✓x7ᵗʰ **S54.10** Injury of median nerve at forearm level, unspecified arm

    ✓x7ᵗʰ **S54.11** Injury of median nerve at forearm level, right arm

    ✓x7ᵗʰ **S54.12** Injury of median nerve at forearm level, left arm

✓5ᵗʰ **S54.2** Injury of radial nerve at forearm level
       Injury of radial nerve NOS

    ✓x7ᵗʰ **S54.20** Injury of radial nerve at forearm level, unspecified arm

    ✓x7ᵗʰ **S54.21** Injury of radial nerve at forearm level, right arm

    ✓x7ᵗʰ **S54.22** Injury of radial nerve at forearm level, left arm

✓5ᵗʰ **S54.3** Injury of cutaneous sensory nerve at forearm level

    ✓x7ᵗʰ **S54.30** Injury of cutaneous sensory nerve at forearm level, unspecified arm

    ✓x7ᵗʰ **S54.31** Injury of cutaneous sensory nerve at forearm level, right arm

    ✓x7ᵗʰ **S54.32** Injury of cutaneous sensory nerve at forearm level, left arm

✓5ᵗʰ **S54.8** Injury of other nerves at forearm level

    ✓6ᵗʰ **S54.8X** Unspecified injury of other nerves at forearm level

       ✓7ᵗʰ **S54.8X1** Unspecified injury of other nerves at forearm level, right arm

       ✓7ᵗʰ **S54.8X2** Unspecified injury of other nerves at forearm level, left arm

       ✓7ᵗʰ **S54.8X9** Unspecified injury of other nerves at forearm level, unspecified arm

✓5ᵗʰ **S54.9** Injury of unspecified nerve at forearm level

✓ Additional Character Required   ✓x7ᵗʰ Placeholder Alert   Unacceptable PDx   ▪ Manifestation   Hospital Acquired Condition   EXCLUDES 1 Not Coded Here   EXCLUDES 2 Not Included Here

ICD-10-CM 2016   975

√x7th S54.90 Injury of unspecified nerve at forearm level, unspecified arm

√x7th S54.91 Injury of unspecified nerve at forearm level, right arm

√x7th S54.92 Injury of unspecified nerve at forearm level, left arm

√4th S55 **Injury of blood vessels at forearm level**
Code also any associated open wound (S51.-)
EXCLUDES 2 injury of blood vessels at wrist and hand level (S65.-)
injury of brachial vessels (S45.1-S45.2)

The appropriate 7th is to be added to each code from category S55.
A   initial encounter
D   subsequent encounter
S   sequela

√5th S55.0 **Injury of ulnar artery at forearm level**

√6th S55.00 **Unspecified injury of ulnar artery at forearm level**

√7th S55.001 **Unspecified injury of ulnar artery at forearm level, right arm** CC
CC Excl: CC with 7th character A: S45.301A, S45.309-S45.311 with 7th A, S45.319-S45.391 with 7th A, S45.399-S45.801 with 7th A, S45.809-S45.811 with 7th A, S45.819-S45.891 with 7th A, S45.899-S45.901 with 7th A, S45.909-S45.911 with 7th A, S45.919-S45.991 with 7th A, S45.999 with 7th A, S55.001A, S55.009-S55.011 with 7th A, S55.019-S55.091 with 7th A, S55.099 A, S55.201 with 7th A, S55.209-S55.211 with 7th A, S55.219-S55.291 with 7th A, S55.299-S55.801 with 7th A, S55.809-S55.811 with 7th A, S55.819-S55.891 with 7th A, S55.899-S55.901 with 7th A, S55.909-S55.911 with 7th A, S55.919-S55.991 with 7th A, S55.999 with 7th A, S65.001 with 7th A, S65.009-S65.011 with 7th A, S65.019-S65.091 with 7th A, S65.099A, S65.801A, S65.809-S65.811 with 7th A, S65.819-S65.891 with 7th A, S65.899-S65.901 with 7th A, S65.909-S65.911 with 7th A, S65.919-S65.991 with 7th A, S65.999A

√7th S55.002 **Unspecified injury of ulnar artery at forearm level, left arm** CC
CC Excl: CC with 7th character A: S45.302-S45.309 with 7th A, S45.312-S45.319 with 7th A, S45.392-S45.399 with 7th A, S45.802-S45.809 with 7th A, S45.812-S45.819 with 7th A, S45.892-S45.899 with 7th A, S45.902-S45.909 with 7th A, S45.912-S45.919 with 7th A, S45.992-S45.999 with 7th A, S55.002-S55.009 with 7th A, S55.012-S55.019 with 7th A, S55.092-S55.099 with 7th A, S55.202-S55.209 with 7th A, S55.212-S55.219 with 7th A, S55.292-S55.299 with 7th A, S55.802-S55.809 with 7th A, S55.812-S55.819 with 7th A, S55.892-S55.899 with 7th A, S55.902-S55.909 with 7th A, S55.912-S55.919 with 7th A, S55.992-S55.999 with 7th A, S65.002-S65.009 with 7th A, S65.012-S65.019 with 7th A, S65.092-S65.099 with 7th A, S65.802-S65.809 with 7th A, S65.812-S65.819 with 7th A, S65.892-S65.899 with 7th A, S65.902-S65.909 with 7th A, S65.912-S65.919 with 7th A, S65.992-S65.999 with 7th A

√7th S55.009 **Unspecified injury of ulnar artery at forearm level, unspecified arm** CC
CC Excl: CC with 7th character A: S45.301-S45.999 with 7th A, S55.001-S55.099 with 7th A, S55.201-S55.999 with 7th A, S65.001-S65.099 with 7th A, S65.801-S65.999 with 7th A

√6th S55.01 **Laceration of ulnar artery at forearm level**

√7th S55.011 **Laceration of ulnar artery at forearm level, right arm** CC
CC Excl: See code: S55.001

√7th S55.012 **Laceration of ulnar artery at forearm level, left arm** CC
CC Excl: See code: S55.002

√7th S55.019 **Laceration of ulnar artery at forearm level, unspecified arm** CC
CC Excl: See code: S55.009

√6th S55.09 **Other specified injury of ulnar artery at forearm level**

√7th S55.091 **Other specified injury of ulnar artery at forearm level, right arm** CC
CC Excl: See code: S55.001

√7th S55.092 **Other specified injury of ulnar artery at forearm level, left arm** CC
CC Excl: See code: S55.002

√7th S55.099 **Other specified injury of ulnar artery at forearm level, unspecified arm** CC
CC Excl: See code: S55.009

√5th S55.1 **Injury of radial artery at forearm level**

√6th S55.10 **Unspecified injury of radial artery at forearm level**

√7th S55.101 **Unspecified injury of radial artery at forearm level, right arm** CC
CC Excl: CC with 7th character A: S45.301 with 7th A, S45.309-S45.311 with 7th A, S45.319-S45.391 with 7th A, S45.399-S45.801 with 7th A, S45.809-S45.811 with 7th A, S45.819-S45.891 with 7th A, S45.899-S45.901 with 7th A, S45.909-S45.911 with 7th A, S45.919-S45.991 with 7th A, S45.999 with 7th A, S55.101 with 7th A, S55.109-S55.111 with 7th A, S55.119-S55.191 with 7th A, S55.199-S55.201 with 7th A, S55.209-S55.211 with 7th A, S55.219-S55.291 with 7th A, S55.299-S55.801 with 7th A, S55.809-S55.811 with 7th A, S55.819-S55.891 with 7th A, S55.899-S55.901 with 7th A, S55.909-S55.911 with 7th A, S55.919-S55.991 with 7th A, S55.999 with 7th A, S65.101 with 7th A, S65.109-S65.111 with 7th A, S65.119-S65.191 with 7th A, S65.199 with 7th A, S65.801 with 7th A, S65.809-S65.811 with 7th A, S65.819-S65.891 with 7th A, S65.899-S65.901 with 7th A, S65.909-S65.911 with 7th A, S65.919-S65.991 with 7th A, S65.999A

√7th S55.102 **Unspecified injury of radial artery at forearm level, left arm** CC
CC Excl: CC with 7th character A: S45.302-S45.309 with 7th A, S45.312-S45.319 with 7th A, S45.392-S45.399 with 7th A, S45.802-S45.809 with 7th A, S45.812-S45.819 with 7th A, S45.892-S45.899 with 7th A, S45.902-S45.909 with 7th A, S45.912-S45.919 with 7th A, S45.992-S45.999 with 7th A, S55.102-S55.109 with 7th A, S55.112-S55.119 with 7th A, S55.192-S55.199 with 7th A, S55.202-S55.209 with 7th A, S55.212-S55.219 with 7th A, S55.292-S55.299 with 7th A, S55.802-S55.809 with 7th A, S55.812-S55.819 with 7th A, S55.892-S55.899 with 7th A, S55.902-S55.909 with 7th A, S55.912-S55.919 with 7th A, S55.992-S55.999 with 7th A, S65.102-S65.109 with 7th A, S65.112-S65.119 with 7th A, S65.192-S65.199 with 7th A, S65.802-S65.809 with 7th A, S65.812-S65.819 with 7th A, S65.892-S65.899 with 7th A, S65.902-S65.909 with 7th A, S65.912-S65.919 with 7th A, S65.992-S65.999 with 7th A

√7th S55.109 **Unspecified injury of radial artery at forearm level, unspecified arm** CC
CC Excl: CC with 7th character A: S45.301-S45.999 with 7th A, S55.101-S55.999 with 7th A, S65.101-S65.199 with 7th A, S65.801-S65.999 with 7th A

√6th S55.11 **Laceration of radial artery at forearm level**

√7th S55.111 **Laceration of radial artery at forearm level, right arm** CC
CC Excl: See code: S55.101

√7th S55.112 **Laceration of radial artery at forearm level, left arm** CC
CC Excl: See code: S55.102

√7th S55.119 **Laceration of radial artery at forearm level, unspecified arm** CC
CC Excl: See code: S55.109

√6th S55.19 **Other specified injury of radial artery at forearm level**

√7th S55.191 **Other specified injury of radial artery at forearm level, right arm** CC
CC Excl: See code: S55.101

√7th S55.192 **Other specified injury of radial artery at forearm level, left arm** CC
CC Excl: See code: S55.102

√7th S55.199 **Other specified injury of radial artery at forearm level, unspecified arm** CC
CC Excl: See code: S55.109

N Newborn: 0   P Pediatric: 0-17   M Maternity: 12-55   A Adult: 15-124   **MCC** Major CC Condition   **PDxMCC** PDx acts as own MCC   CC CC Condition   **PDxCC** PDx acts as own CC

976   ICD-10-CM 2016

√5ᵗʰ **S55.2** Injury of vein at forearm level

  √6ᵗʰ **S55.20** Unspecified injury of vein at forearm level

    √7ᵗʰ **S55.201** Unspecified injury of vein at forearm level, right arm `CC`
      CC Excl: CC with 7th character A: S45.301A, S45.309-S45.311 with 7th A, S45.319-S45.391 with 7th A, S45.399-S45.801 with 7th A, S45.809-S45.811 with 7th A, S45.819-S45.891 with 7th A, S45.899-S45.901 with 7th A, S45.909-S45.911 with 7th A, S45.919-S45.991 with 7th A, S45.999 with 7th A, S55.001 with 7th A, S55.009-S55.011 with 7th A, S55.019-S55.091 with 7th A, S55.099A, S55.201A, S55.209-S55.211 with 7th A, S55.219-S55.291 with 7th A, S55.299-S55.801 with 7th A, S55.809-S55.811 with 7th A, S55.819-S55.891 with 7th A, S55.899-S55.901 with 7th A, S55.909-S55.911 with 7th A, S55.919-S55.991 with 7th A, S55.999A, S65.001 A, S65.009-S65.011 with 7th A, S65.019-S65.091 with 7th A, S65.099A, S65.201A, S65.209-S65.211 with 7th A, S65.219-S65.291 with 7th A, S65.299-S65.301 with 7th A, S65.309-S65.311 with 7th A, S65.319-S65.391 with 7th A, S65.399-S65.401 with 7th A, S65.409-S65.411 with 7th A, S65.419-S65.491 with 7th A, S65.499-S65.500A, S65.502A, S65.504A, S65.506A, S65.508-S65.510 with 7th A, S65.512A, S65.514A, S65.516A, S65.518-S65.590 with 7th A, S65.592A, S65.594A, S65.596A, S65.598-S65.801 with 7th A, S65.809-S65.811 with 7th A, S65.819-S65.891 with 7th A, S65.899-S65.901 with 7th A, S65.909-S65.911 with 7th A, S65.919-S65.991 with 7th A, S65.999A

    √7ᵗʰ **S55.202** Unspecified injury of vein at forearm level, left arm `CC`
      CC Excl: CC with 7th character A: S45.302-S45.309 with 7th A, S45.312-S45.319 with 7th A, S45.392-S45.399 with 7th A, S45.802-S45.809 with 7th A, S45.812-S45.819 with 7th A, S45.892-S45.899 with 7th A, S45.902-S45.909 with 7th A, S45.912-S45.919 with 7th A, S45.992-S45.999 with 7th A, S55.002-S55.009 with 7th A, S55.012-S55.019 with 7th A, S55.092-S55.099 with 7th A, S55.202-S55.209 with 7th A, S55.212-S55.219 with 7th A, S55.292-S55.299 with 7th A, S55.802-S55.809 with 7th A, S55.812-S55.819 with 7th A, S55.892-S55.899 with 7th A, S55.902-S55.909 with 7th A, S55.912-S55.919 with 7th A, S55.992-S55.999 with 7th A, S65.002-S65.009 with 7th A, S65.012-S65.019 with 7th A, S65.092-S65.099 with 7th A, S65.202-S65.209 with 7th A, S65.212-S65.219 with 7th A, S65.292-S65.299 with 7th A, S65.302-S65.309 with 7th A, S65.312-S65.319 with 7th A, S65.392-S65.399 with 7th A, S65.402-S65.409 with 7th A, S65.412-S65.419 with 7th A, S65.492-S65.499 with 7th A, S65.501 with 7th A, S65.503 with 7th A, S65.505 with 7th A, S65.507-S65.509 with 7th A, S65.511 with 7th A, S65.513 with 7th A, S65.515 with 7th A, S65.517-S65.519 with 7th A, S65.591 with 7th A, S65.593 with 7th A, S65.595 with 7th A, S65.597-S65.599 with 7th A, S65.802-S65.809 with 7th A, S65.812-S65.819 with 7th A, S65.892-S65.899 with 7th A, S65.902-S65.909 with 7th A, S65.912-S65.919 with 7th A, S65.992-S65.999 with 7th A

    √7ᵗʰ **S55.209** Unspecified injury of vein at forearm level, unspecified arm `CC`
      CC Excl: CC with 7th character A: S45.301-S45.999 with 7th A, S55.001-S55.099 with 7th A, S55.201-S55.999 with 7th A, S65.001-S65.099 with 7th A, S65.201-S65.999 with 7th A

  √6ᵗʰ **S55.21** Laceration of vein at forearm level

    √7ᵗʰ **S55.211** Laceration of vein at forearm level, right arm `CC`
      CC Excl: See code: S55.201

    √7ᵗʰ **S55.212** Laceration of vein at forearm level, left arm `CC`
      CC Excl: See code: S55.202

    √7ᵗʰ **S55.219** Laceration of vein at forearm level, unspecified arm `CC`
      CC Excl: See code: S55.209

  √6ᵗʰ **S55.29** Other specified injury of vein at forearm level

    √7ᵗʰ **S55.291** Other specified injury of vein at forearm level, right arm `CC`
      CC Excl: See code: S55.201

    √7ᵗʰ **S55.292** Other specified injury of vein at forearm level, left arm `CC`
      CC Excl: See code: S55.202

    √7ᵗʰ **S55.299** Other specified injury of vein at forearm level, unspecified arm `CC`
      CC Excl: See code: S55.209

√5ᵗʰ **S55.8** Injury of other blood vessels at forearm level

  √6ᵗʰ **S55.80** Unspecified injury of other blood vessels at forearm level

    √7ᵗʰ **S55.801** Unspecified injury of other blood vessels at forearm level, right arm `CC`
      CC Excl: See code: S55.201

    √7ᵗʰ **S55.802** Unspecified injury of other blood vessels at forearm level, left arm `CC`
      CC Excl: See code: S55.202

    √7ᵗʰ **S55.809** Unspecified injury of other blood vessels at forearm level, unspecified arm `CC`
      CC Excl: See code: S55.209

  √6ᵗʰ **S55.81** Laceration of other blood vessels at forearm level

    √7ᵗʰ **S55.811** Laceration of other blood vessels at forearm level, right arm `CC`
      CC Excl: See code: S55.201

    √7ᵗʰ **S55.812** Laceration of other blood vessels at forearm level, left arm `CC`
      CC Excl: See code: S55.202

    √7ᵗʰ **S55.819** Laceration of other blood vessels at forearm level, unspecified arm `CC`
      CC Excl: See code: S55.209

  √6ᵗʰ **S55.89** Other specified injury of other blood vessels at forearm level

    √7ᵗʰ **S55.891** Other specified injury of other blood vessels at forearm level, right arm `CC`
      CC Excl: See code: S55.201

    √7ᵗʰ **S55.892** Other specified injury of other blood vessels at forearm level, left arm `CC`
      CC Excl: See code: S55.202

    √7ᵗʰ **S55.899** Other specified injury of other blood vessels at forearm level, unspecified arm `CC`
      CC Excl: See code: S55.209

√5ᵗʰ **S55.9** Injury of unspecified blood vessel at forearm level

  √6ᵗʰ **S55.90** Unspecified injury of unspecified blood vessel at forearm level

    √7ᵗʰ **S55.901** Unspecified injury of unspecified blood vessel at forearm level, right arm `CC`
      CC Excl: See code: S55.201

    √7ᵗʰ **S55.902** Unspecified injury of unspecified blood vessel at forearm level, left arm `CC`
      CC Excl: See code: S55.202

    √7ᵗʰ **S55.909** Unspecified injury of unspecified blood vessel at forearm level, unspecified arm `CC`
      CC Excl: See code: S55.209

  √6ᵗʰ **S55.91** Laceration of unspecified blood vessel at forearm level

    √7ᵗʰ **S55.911** Laceration of unspecified blood vessel at forearm level, right arm `CC`
      CC Excl: See code: S55.201

    √7ᵗʰ **S55.912** Laceration of unspecified blood vessel at forearm level, left arm `CC`
      CC Excl: See code: S55.202

    √7ᵗʰ **S55.919** Laceration of unspecified blood vessel at forearm level, unspecified arm `CC`
      CC Excl: See code: S55.209

  √6ᵗʰ **S55.99** Other specified injury of unspecified blood vessel at forearm level

    √7ᵗʰ **S55.991** Other specified injury of unspecified blood vessel at forearm level, right arm `CC`
      CC Excl: See code: S55.201

    √7ᵗʰ **S55.992** Other specified injury of unspecified blood vessel at forearm level, left arm `CC`
      CC Excl: See code: S55.202

    √7ᵗʰ **S55.999** Other specified injury of unspecified blood vessel at forearm level, unspecified arm `CC`
      CC Excl: See code: S55.209

✔ Additional Character Required ✔x7ᵗʰ Placeholder Alert Unacceptable PDx Manifestation Hospital Acquired Condition **EXCLUDES 1** Not Coded Here *EXCLUDES 2* Not Included Here

✦ ✓4th **S56 Injury of muscle, fascia and tendon at forearm level**

Code also any associated open wound (S51.-)

EXCLUDES 2   injury of muscle, fascia and tendon at or below wrist (S66.-)
sprain of joints and ligaments of elbow (S53.4-)

The appropriate 7th is to be added to each code from category S56.
A   initial encounter
D   subsequent encounter
S   sequela

✓5th **S56.0 Injury of flexor muscle, fascia and tendon of thumb at forearm level**

✓6th **S56.00 Unspecified injury of flexor muscle, fascia and tendon of thumb at forearm level**

✓7th **S56.001 Unspecified injury of flexor muscle, fascia and tendon of right thumb at forearm level**

✓7th **S56.002 Unspecified injury of flexor muscle, fascia and tendon of left thumb at forearm level**

✓7th **S56.009 Unspecified injury of flexor muscle, fascia and tendon of unspecified thumb at forearm level**

✓6th **S56.01 Strain of flexor muscle, fascia and tendon of thumb at forearm level**

✓7th **S56.011 Strain of flexor muscle, fascia and tendon of right thumb at forearm level**

✓7th **S56.012 Strain of flexor muscle, fascia and tendon of left thumb at forearm level**

✓7th **S56.019 Strain of flexor muscle, fascia and tendon of unspecified thumb at forearm level**

✓6th **S56.02 Laceration of flexor muscle, fascia and tendon of thumb at forearm level**

✓7th **S56.021 Laceration of flexor muscle, fascia and tendon of right thumb at forearm level** CC

CC Excl: CC with 7th character A: S51.001A, S51.009-S51.011 with 7th A, S51.019-S51.021 with 7th A, S51.029-S51.031 with 7th A, S51.039-S51.041 with 7th A, S51.049-S51.051 with 7th A, S51.059-S51.801 with 7th A, S51.809-S51.811 with 7th A, S51.819-S51.821 with 7th A, S51.829-S51.831 with 7th A, S51.839-S51.841 with 7th A, S51.849-S51.851 with 7th A, S51.859A, S56.021A, S56.029 A, S56.121A, S56.123A, S56.125A, S56.127A, S56.129 A, S56.221 A, S56.229A, S56.321A, S56.329A, S56.421A, S56.423A, S56.425A, S56.427A, S56.429A, S56.521A, S56.529A, S56.821A, S56.829A, S56.921 A, S56.929A, S61.501A, S61.509-S61.511 with 7th A, S61.519-S61.521 with 7th A, S61.529-S61.531 with 7th A, S61.539-S61.541 with 7th A, S61.549-S61.551 with 7th A, S61.559A

✓7th **S56.022 Laceration of flexor muscle, fascia and tendon of left thumb at forearm level** CC

CC Excl: CC with 7th character A: S51.002-S51.009 with 7th A, S51.012-S51.019 with 7th A, S51.022-S51.029 with 7th A, S51.032-S51.039 with 7th A, S51.042-S51.049 with 7th A, S51.052-S51.059 with 7th A, S51.802-S51.809 with 7th A, S51.812-S51.819 with 7th A, S51.822-S51.829 with 7th A, S51.832-S51.839 with 7th A, S51.842-S51.849 with 7th A, S51.852-S51.859 with 7th A, S56.022-S56.029 with 7th A, S56.122A, S56.124A, S56.126A, S56.128-S56.129 with 7th A, S56.222-S56.229 with 7th A, S56.322-S56.329 with 7th A, S56.422A, S56.424 A, S56.426A, S56.428-S56.429 with 7th A, S56.522-S56.529 with 7th A, S56.822-S56.829 with 7th A, S56.922-S56.929 with 7th A, S61.502-S61.509 with 7th A, S61.512-S61.519 with 7th A, S61.522-S61.529 with 7th A, S61.532-S61.539 with 7th A, S61.542-S61.549 with 7th A, S61.552-S61.559 with 7th A

✓7th **S56.029 Laceration of flexor muscle, fascia and tendon of unspecified thumb at forearm level** CC

CC Excl: CC with 7th character A: S51.001-S51.859 with 7th A, S56.021-S56.029 with 7th A, S56.121-S56.129 with 7th A, S56.221-S56.229 with 7th A, S56.321-S56.329 with 7th A, S56.421-S56.429 with 7th A, S56.521-S56.529 with 7th A, S56.821-S56.829 with 7th A, S56.921-S56.929 with 7th A, S61.501-S61.559 with 7th A

✓6th **S56.09 Other injury of flexor muscle, fascia and tendon of thumb at forearm level**

✓7th **S56.091 Other injury of flexor muscle, fascia and tendon of right thumb at forearm level**

✓7th **S56.092 Other injury of flexor muscle, fascia and tendon of left thumb at forearm level**

✓7th **S56.099 Other injury of flexor muscle, fascia and tendon of unspecified thumb at forearm level**

✓6th **S56.1 Injury of flexor muscle, fascia and tendon of other and unspecified finger at forearm level**

✓6th **S56.10 Unspecified injury of flexor muscle, fascia and tendon of other and unspecified finger at forearm level**

✓7th **S56.101 Unspecified injury of flexor muscle, fascia and tendon of right index finger at forearm level**

✓7th **S56.102 Unspecified injury of flexor muscle, fascia and tendon of left index finger at forearm level**

✓7th **S56.103 Unspecified injury of flexor muscle, fascia and tendon of right middle finger at forearm level**

✓7th **S56.104 Unspecified injury of flexor muscle, fascia and tendon of left middle finger at forearm level**

✓7th **S56.105 Unspecified injury of flexor muscle, fascia and tendon of right ring finger at forearm level**

✓7th **S56.106 Unspecified injury of flexor muscle, fascia and tendon of left ring finger at forearm level**

✓7th **S56.107 Unspecified injury of flexor muscle, fascia and tendon of right little finger at forearm level**

✓7th **S56.108 Unspecified injury of flexor muscle, fascia and tendon of left little finger at forearm level**

✓7th **S56.109 Unspecified injury of flexor muscle, fascia and tendon of unspecified finger at forearm level**

✓6th **S56.11 Strain of flexor muscle, fascia and tendon of other and unspecified finger at forearm level**

✓7th **S56.111 Strain of flexor muscle, fascia and tendon of right index finger at forearm level**

✓7th **S56.112 Strain of flexor muscle, fascia and tendon of left index finger at forearm level**

✓7th **S56.113 Strain of flexor muscle, fascia and tendon of right middle finger at forearm level**

✓7th **S56.114 Strain of flexor muscle, fascia and tendon of left middle finger at forearm level**

✓7th **S56.115 Strain of flexor muscle, fascia and tendon of right ring finger at forearm level**

✓7th **S56.116 Strain of flexor muscle, fascia and tendon of left ring finger at forearm level**

✓7th **S56.117 Strain of flexor muscle, fascia and tendon of right little finger at forearm level**

✓7th **S56.118 Strain of flexor muscle, fascia and tendon of left little finger at forearm level**

✓7th **S56.119 Strain of flexor muscle, fascia and tendon of finger of unspecified finger at forearm level**

✦ Refer to the Muscle/Tendon Table at beginning of this chapter.

N Newborn: 0   P Pediatric: 0-17   M Maternity: 12-55   A Adult: 15-124   MCC Major CC Condition   PDxMCC PDx acts as own MCC   CC CC Condition   PDxCC PDx acts as own CC

978   ICD-10-CM 2016

√6ᵗʰ **S56.12** **Laceration of flexor muscle, fascia and tendon of other and unspecified finger at forearm level**

     √7ᵗʰ **S56.121** **Laceration of flexor muscle, fascia and tendon of right index finger at forearm level** CC
         CC Excl: See code: S56.021

     √7ᵗʰ **S56.122** **Laceration of flexor muscle, fascia and tendon of left index finger at forearm level** CC
         CC Excl: See code: S56.022

     √7ᵗʰ **S56.123** **Laceration of flexor muscle, fascia and tendon of right middle finger at forearm level** CC
         CC Excl: See code: S56.021

     √7ᵗʰ **S56.124** **Laceration of flexor muscle, fascia and tendon of left middle finger at forearm level** CC
         CC Excl: See code: S56.022

     √7ᵗʰ **S56.125** **Laceration of flexor muscle, fascia and tendon of right ring finger at forearm level** CC
         CC Excl: See code: S56.021

     √7ᵗʰ **S56.126** **Laceration of flexor muscle, fascia and tendon of left ring finger at forearm level** CC
         CC Excl: See code: S56.022

     √7ᵗʰ **S56.127** **Laceration of flexor muscle, fascia and tendon of right little finger at forearm level** CC
         CC Excl: See code: S56.021

     √7ᵗʰ **S56.128** **Laceration of flexor muscle, fascia and tendon of left little finger at forearm level** CC
         CC Excl: See code: S56.022

     √7ᵗʰ **S56.129** **Laceration of flexor muscle, fascia and tendon of unspecified finger at forearm level** CC
         CC Excl: See code: S56.029

√6ᵗʰ **S56.19** **Other injury of flexor muscle, fascia and tendon of other and unspecified finger at forearm level**

     √7ᵗʰ **S56.191** **Other injury of flexor muscle, fascia and tendon of right index finger at forearm level**

     √7ᵗʰ **S56.192** **Other injury of flexor muscle, fascia and tendon of left index finger at forearm level**

     √7ᵗʰ **S56.193** **Other injury of flexor muscle, fascia and tendon of right middle finger at forearm level**

     √7ᵗʰ **S56.194** **Other injury of flexor muscle, fascia and tendon of left middle finger at forearm level**

     √7ᵗʰ **S56.195** **Other injury of flexor muscle, fascia and tendon of right ring finger at forearm level**

     √7ᵗʰ **S56.196** **Other injury of flexor muscle, fascia and tendon of left ring finger at forearm level**

     √7ᵗʰ **S56.197** **Other injury of flexor muscle, fascia and tendon of right little finger at forearm level**

     √7ᵗʰ **S56.198** **Other injury of flexor muscle, fascia and tendon of left little finger at forearm level**

     √7ᵗʰ **S56.199** **Other injury of flexor muscle, fascia and tendon of unspecified finger at forearm level**

√5ᵗʰ **S56.2** **Injury of other flexor muscle, fascia and tendon at forearm level**

√6ᵗʰ **S56.20** **Unspecified injury of other flexor muscle, fascia and tendon at forearm level**

     √7ᵗʰ **S56.201** **Unspecified injury of other flexor muscle, fascia and tendon at forearm level, right arm**

     √7ᵗʰ **S56.202** **Unspecified injury of other flexor muscle, fascia and tendon at forearm level, left arm**

     √7ᵗʰ **S56.209** **Unspecified injury of other flexor muscle, fascia and tendon at forearm level, unspecified arm**

√6ᵗʰ **S56.21** **Strain of other flexor muscle, fascia and tendon at forearm level**

     √7ᵗʰ **S56.211** **Strain of other flexor muscle, fascia and tendon at forearm level, right arm**

     √7ᵗʰ **S56.212** **Strain of other flexor muscle, fascia and tendon at forearm level, left arm**

     √7ᵗʰ **S56.219** **Strain of other flexor muscle, fascia and tendon at forearm level, unspecified arm**

√6ᵗʰ **S56.22** **Laceration of other flexor muscle, fascia and tendon at forearm level**

     √7ᵗʰ **S56.221** **Laceration of other flexor muscle, fascia and tendon at forearm level, right arm** CC
         CC Excl: See code: S56.021

     √7ᵗʰ **S56.222** **Laceration of other flexor muscle, fascia and tendon at forearm level, left arm** CC
         CC Excl: See code: S56.022

     √7ᵗʰ **S56.229** **Laceration of other flexor muscle, fascia and tendon at forearm level, unspecified arm** CC
         CC Excl: See code: S56.029

√6ᵗʰ **S56.29** **Other injury of other flexor muscle, fascia and tendon at forearm level**

     √7ᵗʰ **S56.291** **Other injury of other flexor muscle, fascia and tendon at forearm level, right arm**

     √7ᵗʰ **S56.292** **Other injury of other flexor muscle, fascia and tendon at forearm level, left arm**

     √7ᵗʰ **S56.299** **Other injury of other flexor muscle, fascia and tendon at forearm level, unspecified arm**

√5ᵗʰ **S56.3** **Injury of extensor or abductor muscles, fascia and tendons of thumb at forearm level**

√6ᵗʰ **S56.30** **Unspecified injury of extensor or abductor muscles, fascia and tendons of thumb at forearm level**

     √7ᵗʰ **S56.301** **Unspecified injury of extensor or abductor muscles, fascia and tendons of right thumb at forearm level**

     √7ᵗʰ **S56.302** **Unspecified injury of extensor or abductor muscles, fascia and tendons of left thumb at forearm level**

     √7ᵗʰ **S56.309** **Unspecified injury of extensor or abductor muscles, fascia and tendons of unspecified thumb at forearm level**

√6ᵗʰ **S56.31** **Strain of extensor or abductor muscles, fascia and tendons of thumb at forearm level**

     √7ᵗʰ **S56.311** **Strain of extensor or abductor muscles, fascia and tendons of right thumb at forearm level**

     √7ᵗʰ **S56.312** **Strain of extensor or abductor muscles, fascia and tendons of left thumb at forearm level**

     √7ᵗʰ **S56.319** **Strain of extensor or abductor muscles, fascia and tendons of unspecified thumb at forearm level**

√6ᵗʰ **S56.32** **Laceration of extensor or abductor muscles, fascia and tendons of thumb at forearm level**

     √7ᵗʰ **S56.321** **Laceration of extensor or abductor muscles, fascia and tendons of right thumb at forearm level** CC
         CC Excl: See code: S56.021

     √7ᵗʰ **S56.322** **Laceration of extensor or abductor muscles, fascia and tendons of left thumb at forearm level** CC
         CC Excl: See code: S56.022

     √7ᵗʰ **S56.329** **Laceration of extensor or abductor muscles, fascia and tendons of unspecified thumb at forearm level** CC
         CC Excl: See code: S56.029

√6ᵗʰ **S56.39** **Other injury of extensor or abductor muscles, fascia and tendons of thumb at forearm level**

     √7ᵗʰ **S56.391** **Other injury of extensor or abductor muscles, fascia and tendons of right thumb at forearm level**

     √7ᵗʰ **S56.392** **Other injury of extensor or abductor muscles, fascia and tendons of left thumb at forearm level**

√ Additional Character Required   √x7ᵗʰ Placeholder Alert   Unacceptable PDx   Manifestation   Hospital Acquired Condition   *EXCLUDES 1* Not Coded Here   *EXCLUDES 2* Not Included Here

√7ᵗʰ **S56.399** Other injury of extensor or abductor muscles, fascia and tendons of unspecified thumb at forearm level

√5ᵗʰ **S56.4** Injury of extensor muscle, fascia and tendon of other and unspecified finger at forearm level

√6ᵗʰ **S56.40** Unspecified injury of extensor muscle, fascia and tendon of other and unspecified finger at forearm level

√7ᵗʰ **S56.401** Unspecified injury of extensor muscle, fascia and tendon of right index finger at forearm level

√7ᵗʰ **S56.402** Unspecified injury of extensor muscle, fascia and tendon of left index finger at forearm level

√7ᵗʰ **S56.403** Unspecified injury of extensor muscle, fascia and tendon of right middle finger at forearm level

√7ᵗʰ **S56.404** Unspecified injury of extensor muscle, fascia and tendon of left middle finger at forearm level

√7ᵗʰ **S56.405** Unspecified injury of extensor muscle, fascia and tendon of right ring finger at forearm level

√7ᵗʰ **S56.406** Unspecified injury of extensor muscle, fascia and tendon of left ring finger at forearm level

√7ᵗʰ **S56.407** Unspecified injury of extensor muscle, fascia and tendon of right little finger at forearm level

√7ᵗʰ **S56.408** Unspecified injury of extensor muscle, fascia and tendon of left little finger at forearm level

√7ᵗʰ **S56.409** Unspecified injury of extensor muscle, fascia and tendon of unspecified finger at forearm level

√6ᵗʰ **S56.41** Strain of extensor muscle, fascia and tendon of other and unspecified finger at forearm level

√7ᵗʰ **S56.411** Strain of extensor muscle, fascia and tendon of right index finger at forearm level

√7ᵗʰ **S56.412** Strain of extensor muscle, fascia and tendon of left index finger at forearm level

√7ᵗʰ **S56.413** Strain of extensor muscle, fascia and tendon of right middle finger at forearm level

√7ᵗʰ **S56.414** Strain of extensor muscle, fascia and tendon of left middle finger at forearm level

√7ᵗʰ **S56.415** Strain of extensor muscle, fascia and tendon of right ring finger at forearm level

√7ᵗʰ **S56.416** Strain of extensor muscle, fascia and tendon of left ring finger at forearm level

√7ᵗʰ **S56.417** Strain of extensor muscle, fascia and tendon of right little finger at forearm level

√7ᵗʰ **S56.418** Strain of extensor muscle, fascia and tendon of left little finger at forearm level

√7ᵗʰ **S56.419** Strain of extensor muscle, fascia and tendon of finger, unspecified finger at forearm level

√6ᵗʰ **S56.42** Laceration of extensor muscle, fascia and tendon of other and unspecified finger at forearm level

√7ᵗʰ **S56.421** Laceration of extensor muscle, fascia and tendon of right index finger at forearm level   CC
     CC Excl: See code: S56.021

√7ᵗʰ **S56.422** Laceration of extensor muscle, fascia and tendon of left index finger at forearm level   CC
     CC Excl: See code: S56.022

√7ᵗʰ **S56.423** Laceration of extensor muscle, fascia and tendon of right middle finger at forearm level   CC
     CC Excl: See code: S56.021

√7ᵗʰ **S56.424** Laceration of extensor muscle, fascia and tendon of left middle finger at forearm level   CC
     CC Excl: See code: S56.022

√7ᵗʰ **S56.425** Laceration of extensor muscle, fascia and tendon of right ring finger at forearm level   CC
     CC Excl: See code: S56.021

√7ᵗʰ **S56.426** Laceration of extensor muscle, fascia and tendon of left ring finger at forearm level   CC
     CC Excl: See code: S56.022

√7ᵗʰ **S56.427** Laceration of extensor muscle, fascia and tendon of right little finger at forearm level   CC
     CC Excl: See code: S56.021

√7ᵗʰ **S56.428** Laceration of extensor muscle, fascia and tendon of left little finger at forearm level   CC
     CC Excl: See code: S56.022

√7ᵗʰ **S56.429** Laceration of extensor muscle, fascia and tendon of unspecified finger at forearm level   CC
     CC Excl: See code: S56.029

√6ᵗʰ **S56.49** Other injury of extensor muscle, fascia and tendon of other and unspecified finger at forearm level

√7ᵗʰ **S56.491** Other injury of extensor muscle, fascia and tendon of right index finger at forearm level

√7ᵗʰ **S56.492** Other injury of extensor muscle, fascia and tendon of left index finger at forearm level

√7ᵗʰ **S56.493** Other injury of extensor muscle, fascia and tendon of right middle finger at forearm level

√7ᵗʰ **S56.494** Other injury of extensor muscle, fascia and tendon of left middle finger at forearm level

√7ᵗʰ **S56.495** Other injury of extensor muscle, fascia and tendon of right ring finger at forearm level

√7ᵗʰ **S56.496** Other injury of extensor muscle, fascia and tendon of left ring finger at forearm level

√7ᵗʰ **S56.497** Other injury of extensor muscle, fascia and tendon of right little finger at forearm level

√7ᵗʰ **S56.498** Other injury of extensor muscle, fascia and tendon of left little finger at forearm level

√7ᵗʰ **S56.499** Other injury of extensor muscle, fascia and tendon of unspecified finger at forearm level

√5ᵗʰ **S56.5** Injury of other extensor muscle, fascia and tendon at forearm level

√6ᵗʰ **S56.50** Unspecified injury of other extensor muscle, fascia and tendon at forearm level

√7ᵗʰ **S56.501** Unspecified injury of other extensor muscle, fascia and tendon at forearm level, right arm

√7ᵗʰ **S56.502** Unspecified injury of other extensor muscle, fascia and tendon at forearm level, left arm

√7ᵗʰ **S56.509** Unspecified injury of other extensor muscle, fascia and tendon at forearm level, unspecified arm

√6ᵗʰ **S56.51** Strain of other extensor muscle, fascia and tendon at forearm level

√7ᵗʰ **S56.511** Strain of other extensor muscle, fascia and tendon at forearm level, right arm

√7ᵗʰ **S56.512** Strain of other extensor muscle, fascia and tendon at forearm level, left arm

√7ᵗʰ **S56.519** Strain of other extensor muscle, fascia and tendon at forearm level, unspecified arm

√6ᵗʰ **S56.52** Laceration of other extensor muscle, fascia and tendon at forearm level

√7ᵗʰ **S56.521** Laceration of other extensor muscle, fascia and tendon at forearm level, right arm   CC
     CC Excl: See code: S56.021

√7ᵗʰ **S56.522** Laceration of other extensor muscle, fascia and tendon at forearm level, left arm   CC
     CC Excl: See code: S56.022

🅝 Newborn: 0   🅟 Pediatric: 0-17   🅜 Maternity: 12-55   🅐 Adult: 15-124   **MCC** Major CC Condition   **PDx MCC** PDx acts as own MCC   **CC** CC Condition   **PDx CC** PDx acts as own CC

980   ICD-10-CM 2016

√7ᵗʰ **S56.529** **Laceration of other extensor muscle,** `CC`
fascia and tendon at forearm level,
unspecified arm
CC Excl: See code: S56.029

√6ᵗʰ **S56.59** **Other injury of other extensor muscle, fascia and**
tendon at forearm level

√7ᵗʰ **S56.591** **Other injury of other extensor muscle,**
fascia and tendon at forearm level, right
arm

√7ᵗʰ **S56.592** **Other injury of other extensor muscle,**
fascia and tendon at forearm level, left
arm

√7ᵗʰ **S56.599** **Other injury of other extensor muscle,**
fascia and tendon at forearm level,
unspecified arm

√5ᵗʰ **S56.8** **Injury of** other muscles, fascia and tendons at forearm level

√6ᵗʰ **S56.80** **Unspecified injury of other muscles, fascia and**
tendons at forearm level

√7ᵗʰ **S56.801** **Unspecified injury of other muscles, fascia**
and tendons at forearm level, right arm

√7ᵗʰ **S56.802** **Unspecified injury of other muscles, fascia**
and tendons at forearm level, left arm

√7ᵗʰ **S56.809** **Unspecified injury of other muscles, fascia**
and tendons at forearm level, unspecified
arm

√6ᵗʰ **S56.81** **Strain of other muscles, fascia and tendons at**
forearm level

√7ᵗʰ **S56.811** **Strain of other muscles, fascia and**
tendons at forearm level, right arm

√7ᵗʰ **S56.812** **Strain of other muscles, fascia and**
tendons at forearm level, left arm

√7ᵗʰ **S56.819** **Strain of other muscles, fascia and**
tendons at forearm level, unspecified arm

√6ᵗʰ **S56.82** **Laceration of other muscles, fascia and tendons at**
forearm level

√7ᵗʰ **S56.821** **Laceration of other muscles, fascia** `CC`
and tendons at forearm level, right arm
CC Excl: See code: S56.021

√7ᵗʰ **S56.822** **Laceration of other muscles, fascia** `CC`
and tendons at forearm level, left arm
CC Excl: See code: S56.022

√7ᵗʰ **S56.829** **Laceration of other muscles, fascia** `CC`
and tendons at forearm level,
unspecified arm
CC Excl: See code: S56.029

√6ᵗʰ **S56.89** **Other injury of other muscles, fascia and tendons at**
forearm level

√7ᵗʰ **S56.891** **Other injury of other muscles, fascia**
and tendons at forearm level, right
arm

√7ᵗʰ **S56.892** **Other injury of other muscles, fascia**
and tendons at forearm level, left arm

√7ᵗʰ **S56.899** **Other injury of other muscles, fascia and**
tendons at forearm level, unspecified arm

√5ᵗʰ **S56.9** **Injury of** unspecified muscles, fascia and tendons at forearm
level

√6ᵗʰ **S56.90** **Unspecified injury of unspecified muscles, fascia and**
tendons at forearm level

√7ᵗʰ **S56.901** **Unspecified injury of unspecified muscles,**
fascia and tendons at forearm level, right
arm

√7ᵗʰ **S56.902** **Unspecified injury of unspecified muscles,**
fascia and tendons at forearm level, left
arm

√7ᵗʰ **S56.909** **Unspecified injury of unspecified muscles,**
fascia and tendons at forearm level,
unspecified arm

√6ᵗʰ **S56.91** **Strain of unspecified muscles, fascia and tendons at**
forearm level

√7ᵗʰ **S56.911** **Strain of unspecified muscles, fascia and**
tendons at forearm level, right arm

√7ᵗʰ **S56.912** **Strain of unspecified muscles, fascia and**
tendons at forearm level, left arm

√7ᵗʰ **S56.919** **Strain of unspecified muscles, fascia and**
tendons at forearm level, unspecified arm

√6ᵗʰ **S56.92** **Laceration of unspecified muscles, fascia and**
tendons at forearm level

√7ᵗʰ **S56.921** **Laceration of unspecified muscles,** `CC`
fascia and tendons at forearm level,
right arm
CC Excl: See code: S56.021

√7ᵗʰ **S56.922** **Laceration of unspecified muscles,** `CC`
fascia and tendons at forearm level,
left arm
CC Excl: See code: S56.022

√7ᵗʰ **S56.929** **Laceration of unspecified muscles,** `CC`
fascia and tendons at forearm level,
unspecified arm
CC Excl: See code: S56.029

√6ᵗʰ **S56.99** **Other injury of unspecified muscles, fascia and**
tendons at forearm level

√7ᵗʰ **S56.991** **Other injury of unspecified muscles, fascia**
and tendons at forearm level, right arm

√7ᵗʰ **S56.992** **Other injury of unspecified muscles, fascia**
and tendons at forearm level, left arm

√7ᵗʰ **S56.999** **Other injury of unspecified muscles, fascia**
and tendons at forearm level, unspecified
arm

√4ᵗʰ **S57** **Crushing injury of elbow and forearm**
Use additional code(s) for all associated injuries
EXCLUDES 2 crushing injury of wrist and hand (S67.-)

The appropriate 7th is to be added to each code from category S57.
A   initial encounter
D   subsequent encounter
S   sequela

√5ᵗʰ **S57.0** **Crushing injury of** elbow

√x7ᵗʰ **S57.00** **Crushing injury of** unspecified elbow

√x7ᵗʰ **S57.01** **Crushing injury of** right elbow

√x7ᵗʰ **S57.02** **Crushing injury of** left elbow

√5ᵗʰ **S57.8** **Crushing injury of** forearm

√x7ᵗʰ **S57.80** **Crushing injury of** unspecified forearm

√x7ᵗʰ **S57.81** **Crushing injury of** right forearm

√x7ᵗʰ **S57.82** **Crushing injury of** left forearm

☑ Additional Character Required   √x7ᵗʰ Placeholder Alert   Unacceptable PDx   Manifestation   Hospital Acquired Condition   **EXCLUDES 1** Not Coded Here   **EXCLUDES 2** Not Included Here

ICD-10-CM 2016   981

Chapter 19. Injury, Poisoning, and Certain Other Consequences of External Causes

S58–S58.012

√4th **S58**   **Traumatic amputation of elbow and forearm**

> **NOTE**   An amputation not identified as partial or complete should be coded to complete.
>
> **EXCLUDES 1**   *traumatic amputation of wrist and hand (S68.-)*

The appropriate 7th is to be added to each code from category S58.
A   initial encounter
D   subsequent encounter
S   sequela

√5th **S58.0**   **Traumatic amputation at elbow level**

√6th   **S58.01**   **Complete traumatic amputation at elbow level**

√7th   **S58.011**   **Complete traumatic amputation at elbow level, right arm**   CC

CC Excl: CC with 7th character A: S41.001 with 7th A, S41.009-S41.011 with 7th A, S41.019-S41.021 with 7th A, S41.029-S41.031 with 7th A, S41.039-S41.041 with 7th A, S41.049-S41.051 with 7th A, S41.059-S41.101 with 7th A, S41.109-S41.111 with 7th A, S41.119-S41.121 with 7th A, S41.129-S41.131 with 7th A, S41.139-S41.141 with 7th A, S41.149-S41.151 with 7th A, S41.159A, S46.021A, S46.029A, S46.121A, S46.129A, S46.221A, S46.229A, S46.321A, S46.329A, S46.821A, S46.829A, S46.921A, S46.929A, S48.011A, S48.019-S48.021 with 7th A, S48.029-S48.111 with 7th A, S48.119-S48.121 with 7th A, S48.129-S48.911 with 7th A, S48.919-S48.921 with 7th A, S48.929A, S51.001A, S51.009-S51.011 with 7th A, S51.019-S51.021 with 7th A, S51.029-S51.031 with 7th A, S51.039-S51.041 with 7th A, S51.049-S51.051 with 7th A, S51.059-S51.801 with 7th A, S51.809-S51.811 with 7th A, S51.819-S51.821 with 7th A, S51.829-S51.831 with 7th A, S51.839-S51.841 with 7th A, S51.849-S51.851 with 7th A, S51.859A, S56.021A, S56.029A, S56.121A, S56.123A, S56.125A, S56.127A, S56.129A, S56.221A, S56.229A, S56.321A, S56.329A, S56.421A, S56.423A, S56.425 with 7th A, S56.427 with 7th A, S56.429 with 7th A, S56.521 with 7th A, S56.529 with 7th A, S56.821 with 7th A, S56.829 with 7th A, S56.921 with 7th A, S56.929 with 7th A, S58.011 with 7th A, S58.019-S58.021 with 7th A, S58.029-S58.111 with 7th A, S58.119-S58.121 with 7th A, S58.129-S58.911 with 7th A, S58.919-S58.921 with 7th A, S58.929 with 7th A, S61.001 with 7th A, S61.009-S61.011 with 7th A, S61.019-S61.021 with 7th A, S61.029-S61.031 with 7th A, S61.039-S61.041 with 7th A, S61.049-S61.051 with 7th A, S61.059-S61.101 with 7th A, S61.109-S61.111 with 7th A, S61.119-S61.121 with 7th A, S61.129-S61.131 with 7th A, S61.139-S61.141 with 7th A, S61.149-S61.151 with 7th A, S61.159-S61.200 with 7th A, S61.202 with 7th A, S61.204 with 7th A, S61.206 with 7th A, S61.208-S61.210 with 7th A, S61.212 with 7th A, S61.214 with 7th A, S61.216 with 7th A, S61.218-S61.220 with 7th A, S61.222 with 7th A, S61.224 with 7th A, S61.226 with 7th A, S61.228-S61.230 with 7th A, S61.232 with 7th A, S61.234 with 7th A, S61.236 with 7th A, S61.238-S61.240 with 7th A, S61.242 with 7th A, S61.244 with 7th A, S61.246 with 7th A, S61.248-S61.250 with 7th A, S61.252 with 7th A, S61.254 with 7th A, S61.256 with 7th A, S61.258-S61.300 with 7th A, S61.302 with 7th A, S61.304 with 7th A, S61.306 with 7th A, S61.308-S61.310 with 7th A, S61.312 with 7th A, S61.314 with 7th A, S61.316 with 7th A, S61.318-S61.320 with 7th A, S61.322 with 7th A, S61.324 with 7th A, S61.326 with 7th A, S61.328-S61.330 with 7th A, S61.332 with 7th A, S61.334 with 7th A, S61.336 with 7th A, S61.338-S61.340 with 7th A, S61.342 with 7th A, S61.344 with 7th A, S61.346 with 7th A, S61.348-S61.350 with 7th A, S61.352 with 7th A, S61.354 with 7th A, S61.356 with 7th A, S61.358-S61.401 with 7th A, S61.409-S61.411 with 7th A, S61.419-S61.421 with 7th A, S61.429-S61.431 with 7th A, S61.439-S61.441 with 7th A, S61.449-S61.451 with 7th A, S61.459-S61.501 with 7th A, S61.509-S61.511 with 7th A, S61.519-S61.521 with 7th A, S61.529-S61.531 with 7th A, S61.539-S61.541 with 7th A, S61.549-S61.551 with 7th A, S61.559 with 7th A, S66.021 with 7th

A, S66.029 with 7th A, S66.120 with 7th A, S66.122 with 7th A, S66.124 with 7th A, S66.126 with 7th A, S66.128-S66.129 with 7th A, S66.221 with 7th A, S66.229 with 7th A, S66.320 with 7th A, S66.322 with 7th A, S66.324 with 7th A, S66.326 with 7th A, S66.328-S66.329 with 7th A, S66.421 with 7th A, S66.429 with 7th A, S66.520 with 7th A, S66.522 with 7th A, S66.524 with 7th A, S66.526 with 7th A, S66.528-S66.529 with 7th A, S66.821 with 7th A, S66.829 with 7th A, S66.921 with 7th A, S66.929 with 7th A, S68.011 with 7th A, S68.019-S68.021 with 7th A, S68.029-S68.110 with 7th A, S68.112 with 7th A, S68.114 with 7th A, S68.116 with 7th A, S68.118-S68.120 with 7th A, S68.122 with 7th A, S68.124 with 7th A, S68.126 with 7th A, S68.128-S68.411 with 7th A, S68.419-S68.421 with 7th A, S68.429-S68.511 with 7th A, S68.519-S68.521 with 7th A, S68.529-S68.610 with 7th A, S68.612 with 7th A, S68.614 with 7th A, S68.616 with 7th A, S68.618-S68.620 with 7th A, S68.622A, S68.624A, S68.626A, S68.628-S68.711 with 7th A, S68.719-S68.721 with 7th A, S68.729A, T14.90-T14.91, T79.A0X-T79.9XX with 7th A

√7th   **S58.012**   **Complete traumatic amputation at elbow level, left arm**   CC

CC Excl: CC with 7th character A: S41.002-S41.009 with 7th A, S41.012-S41.019 with 7th A, S41.022-S41.029 with 7th A, S41.032-S41.039 with 7th A, S41.042-S41.049 with 7th A, S41.052-S41.059 with 7th A, S41.102-S41.109 with 7th A, S41.112-S41.119 with 7th A, S41.122-S41.129 with 7th A, S41.132-S41.139 with 7th A, S41.142-S41.149 with 7th A, S41.152-S41.159 with 7th A, S46.022-S46.029 with 7th A, S46.122-S46.129 with 7th A, S46.222-S46.229 with 7th A, S46.322-S46.329 with 7th A, S46.822-S46.829 with 7th A, S46.922-S46.929 with 7th A, S48.012-S48.019 with 7th A, S48.022-S48.029 with 7th A, S48.112-S48.119 with 7th A, S48.122-S48.129 with 7th A, S48.912-S48.919 with 7th A, S48.922-S48.929 with 7th A, S51.002-S51.009 with 7th A, S51.012-S51.019 with 7th A, S51.022-S51.029 with 7th A, S51.032-S51.039 with 7th A, S51.042-S51.049 with 7th A, S51.052-S51.059 with 7th A, S51.802-S51.809 with 7th A, S51.812-S51.819 with 7th A, S51.822-S51.829 with 7th A, S51.832-S51.839 with 7th A, S51.842-S51.849 with 7th A, S51.852-S51.859 with 7th A, S56.022-S56.029 with 7th A, S56.122A, S56.124A, S56.126A, S56.128-S56.129 with 7th A, S56.222-S56.229 with 7th A, S56.322-S56.329 with 7th A, S56.422 with 7th A, S56.424A, S56.426A, S56.428-S56.429 with 7th A, S56.522-S56.529 with 7th A, S56.822-S56.829 with 7th A, S56.922-S56.929 with 7th A, S58.012-S58.019 with 7th A, S58.022-S58.029 with 7th A, S58.112-S58.119 with 7th A, S58.122-S58.129 with 7th A, S58.912-S58.919 with 7th A, S58.922-S58.929 with 7th A, S61.002-S61.009 with 7th A, S61.012-S61.019 with 7th A, S61.022-S61.029 with 7th A, S61.032-S61.039 with 7th A, S61.042-S61.049 with 7th A, S61.052-S61.059 with 7th A, S61.102-S61.109 with 7th A, S61.112-S61.119 with 7th A, S61.122-S61.129 with 7th A, S61.132-S61.139 with 7th A, S61.142-S61.149 with 7th A, S61.152-S61.159 with 7th A, S61.201A, S61.203A, S61.205A, S61.207-S61.209 with 7th A, S61.211A, S61.213A, S61.215A, S61.217-S61.219 with 7th A, S61.221A, S61.223A, S61.225A, S61.227-S61.229 with 7th A, S61.231A, S61.233A, S61.235A, S61.237-S61.239 with 7th A, S61.241A, S61.243A, S61.245A, S61.247-S61.249 with 7th A, S61.251A, S61.253A, S61.255 with 7th A, S61.257-S61.259 with 7th A, S61.301A, S61.303A, S61.305A, S61.307-S61.309 with 7th A, S61.311A, S61.313A, S61.315A, S61.317-S61.319A, S61.321A, S61.323A, S61.325A, S61.327-S61.329 with 7th A, S61.331A, S61.333A, S61.335 with 7th A, S61.337-S61.339 with 7th A, S61.341A, S61.343A, S61.345A, S61.347-S61.349 with 7th A, S61.351A, S61.353A, S61.355A, S61.357-S61.359 with 7th A, S61.402-S61.409 with 7th A, S61.412-S61.419 with 7th A, S61.422-

N Newborn: 0   P Pediatric: 0-17   M Maternity: 12-55   A Adult: 15-124   MCC Major CC Condition   PDxMCC PDx acts as own MCC   CC CC Condition   PDxCC PDx acts as own CC

982

ICD-10-CM 2016

S61.429 with 7th A, S61.432-S61.439 with 7th A, S61.442-S61.449 with 7th A, S61.452-S61.459 with 7th A, S61.502-S61.509 with 7th A, S61.512-S61.519 with 7th A, S61.522-S61.529 with 7th A, S61.532-S61.539 with 7th A, S61.542-S61.549 with 7th A, S61.552-S61.559 with 7th A, S66.022-S66.029 with 7th A, S66.121 character A, S66.123A, S66.125A, S66.127-S66.129 with 7th A, S66.222-S66.229 with 7th A, S66.321A, S66.323A, S66.325A, S66.327-S66.329 with 7th A, S66.422-S66.429 with 7th A, S66.521A, S66.523A, S66.525A, S66.527-S66.529 with 7th A, S66.822-S66.829 with 7th A, S66.922-S66.929 with 7th A, S68.012-S68.019 with 7th A, S68.022-S68.029 with 7th A, S68.111A, S68.113A, S68.115A, S68.117-S68.119A, S68.121A, S68.123A, S68.125A, S68.127-S68.129 with 7th A, S68.412-S68.419 with 7th A, S68.422-S68.429 with 7th A, S68.512-S68.519 with 7th A, S68.522-S68.529 with 7th A, S68.611A, S68.613, S68.615A, S68.617-S68.619 with 7th A, S68.621A, S68.623A, S68.625A, S68.627-S68.629 with 7th A, S68.712-S68.719 with 7th A, S68.722-S68.729 with 7th A, T14.90-T14.91, T79.A0X-T79.9XX with 7th A

√7ᵗʰ **S58.019 Complete traumatic amputation at** `CC`
elbow level, unspecified arm
CC Excl: CC with 7th character A: S41.001-S41.159 with 7th A, S46.021-S46.029 with 7th A, S46.121-S46.129 with 7th A, S46.229 with 7th A, S46.321-S46.329 with 7th A, S46.821-S46.829 with 7th A, S46.921-S46.929 with 7th A, S48.011-S48.929 with 7th A, S51.001-S51.859 with 7th A, S56.021-S56.029 with 7th A, S56.121-S56.129 with 7th A, S56.221-S56.229 with 7th A, S56.321-S56.329 with 7th A, S56.421-S56.429 with 7th A, S56.521-S56.529 with 7th A, S56.821-S56.829 with 7th A, S56.921-S56.929 with 7th A, S58.011-S58.929 with 7th A, S61.001-S61.559 with 7th A, S66.021-S66.029 with 7th A, S66.120-S66.129 with 7th A, S66.221-S66.229 with 7th A, S66.320-S66.329 with 7th A, S66.421-S66.429 with 7th A, S66.520-S66.529 with 7th A, S66.821-S66.829 with 7th A, S66.921-S66.929 with 7th A, S68.011-S68.729 with 7th A, T14.90-T14.91, T79.A0X-T79.9XX with 7th A

√6ᵗʰ **S58.02 Partial traumatic amputation at elbow level**

√7ᵗʰ **S58.021 Partial traumatic amputation at elbow** `CC`
level, right arm
CC Excl: See code: S58.011

√7ᵗʰ **S58.022 Partial traumatic amputation at elbow** `CC`
level, left arm
CC Excl: See code: S58.012

√7ᵗʰ **S58.029 Partial traumatic amputation at elbow** `CC`
level, unspecified arm
CC Excl: See code: S58.019

√5ᵗʰ **S58.1 Traumatic amputation at level between elbow and wrist**

√6ᵗʰ **S58.11 Complete traumatic amputation at level between elbow and wrist**

√7ᵗʰ **S58.111 Complete traumatic amputation at** `CC`
level between elbow and wrist, right arm
CC Excl: See code: S58.011

√7ᵗʰ **S58.112 Complete traumatic amputation at** `CC`
level between elbow and wrist, left arm
CC Excl: See code: S58.012

√7ᵗʰ **S58.119 Complete traumatic amputation at** `CC`
level between elbow and wrist, unspecified arm
CC Excl: See code: S58.019

√6ᵗʰ **S58.12 Partial traumatic amputation at level between elbow and wrist**

√7ᵗʰ **S58.121 Partial traumatic amputation at level** `CC`
between elbow and wrist, right arm
CC Excl: See code: S58.011

√7ᵗʰ **S58.122 Partial traumatic amputation at level** `CC`
between elbow and wrist, left arm
CC Excl: See code: S58.012

√7ᵗʰ **S58.129 Partial traumatic amputation at level** `CC`
between elbow and wrist, unspecified arm
CC Excl: See code: S58.019

√5ᵗʰ **S58.9 Traumatic amputation of forearm, level unspecified**
EXCLUDES 1 *traumatic amputation of wrist (S68.-)*

√6ᵗʰ **S58.91 Complete traumatic amputation of forearm, level unspecified**

√7ᵗʰ **S58.911 Complete traumatic amputation of** `CC`
right forearm, level unspecified
CC Excl: See code: S58.011

√7ᵗʰ **S58.912 Complete traumatic amputation of** `CC`
left forearm, level unspecified
CC Excl: See code: S58.012

√7ᵗʰ **S58.919 Complete traumatic amputation of** `CC`
unspecified forearm, level unspecified
CC Excl: See code: S58.019

√6ᵗʰ **S58.92 Partial traumatic amputation of forearm, level unspecified**

√7ᵗʰ **S58.921 Partial traumatic amputation of right** `CC`
forearm, level unspecified

√7ᵗʰ **S58.922 Partial traumatic amputation of left** `CC`
forearm, level unspecified

√7ᵗʰ **S58.929 Partial traumatic amputation of** `CC`
unspecified forearm, level unspecified

√4ᵗʰ **S59 Other and unspecified injuries of elbow and forearm**
EXCLUDES 2 *other and unspecified injuries of wrist and hand (S69.-)*

The appropriate 7th is to be added to each code from subcategories S59.0, S59.1, and S59.2.
A   initial encounter for closed fracture
D   subsequent encounter for fracture with routine healing
G   subsequent encounter for fracture with delayed healing
K   subsequent encounter for fracture with nonunion
P   subsequent encounter for fracture with malunion
S   sequela

√5ᵗʰ **S59.0 Physeal fracture of lower end of ulna**

√6ᵗʰ **S59.00 Unspecified physeal fracture of lower end of ulna**

7,19 √7ᵗʰ **S59.001 Unspecified physeal fracture of lower** `CC`
end of ulna, right arm
CC Excl: CC with 7th character A: S52.001-S52.011 with 7th [A, B, C], S52.019-S52.111 with 7th A, S52.119-S52.211 with 7th A, S52.219-S52.311 with 7th A, S52.319-S52.521 with 7th A, S52.529-S52.621 with 7th A, S52.629-S52.92X with 7th A, S59.001A, S59.009-S59.011 with 7th A, S59.019-S59.021 with 7th A, S59.029-S59.031 with 7th A, S59.039-S59.041 with 7th A, S59.049-S59.091 with 7th A, S59.099-S59.101 with 7th A, S59.109-S59.111 with 7th A, S59.119-S59.121 with 7th A, S59.129-S59.131 with 7th A, S59.139-S59.141 with 7th A, S59.149-S59.191 with 7th A, S59.199-S59.201 with 7th A, S59.209-S59.211 with 7th A, S59.219-S59.221 with 7th A, S59.229-S59.231 with 7th A, S59.239-S59.241 with 7th A, S59.249-S59.291 with 7th A, S59.299A
CC with 7th character K or P: M80.00X-M84.68X with 7th [K, P], S02.0XX-S02.92X with 7th K, S12.000-S12.691 with 7th K, S22.000-S22.9XX with 7th K, S32.000-S32.9XX with 7th K, S42.001-S42.92X with 7th [K, P], S49.001-S49.199 with 7th [K, P], S52.001-S52.92X with 7th [K, M, N, P, Q, R], S59.001-S59.299 with 7th [K, P], S62.001-S62.92X with 7th [K, P], S72.001-S72.92X with 7th [K, M, N, P, Q, R], S79.001-S79.199 with 7th [K, P], S82.001-S82.92X with 7th [K, M, N, P, Q, R], S89.001-S89.399 with 7th [K, P], S92.001-S92.919 with 7th [K, P]

---

7   HAC = Initial encounter only (7th character A, B or C) and not POA.
19   CC only if an initial encounter for a closed fracture (7th character A) **OR** a subsequent encounter for nonunion or malunion (7th character K, M, N, P, Q, or R – specific to category).

☑ Additional Character Required   ✓x7ᵗʰ Placeholder Alert   Unacceptable PDx   Manifestation   Hospital Acquired Condition   EXCLUDES 1 Not Coded Here   EXCLUDES 2 Not Included Here

ICD-10-CM 2016   983

7,19 √7th **S59.002 Unspecified physeal fracture of lower end of ulna, left arm** CC
CC Excl: CC with 7th character A: S52.001-S52.009 with 7th [B, C], S52.012-S52.109 with 7th A, S52.112-S52.209 with 7th A, S52.212-S52.309 with 7th A, S52.312-S52.516 with 7th A, S52.522-S52.616 with 7th A, S52.622-S52.92X with 7th A, S59.002-S59.009 with 7th A, S59.012-S59.019 with 7th A, S59.022-S59.029 with 7th A, S59.032-S59.039 with 7th A, S59.042-S59.049 with 7th A, S59.092-S59.099 with 7th A, S59.102-S59.109 with 7th A, S59.112-S59.119 with 7th A, S59.122-S59.129 with 7th A, S59.132-S59.139 with 7th A, S59.142-S59.149 with 7th A, S59.192-S59.199 with 7th A, S59.202-S59.209 with 7th A, S59.212-S59.219 with 7th A, S59.222-S59.229 with 7th A, S59.232-S59.239 with 7th A, S59.242-S59.249 with 7th A, S59.292-S59.299 with 7th A
CC with 7th character K or P: M80.00X-M84.68X with 7th [K, P], S02.0XX-S02.92X with 7th K, S12.000-S12.691 with 7th K, S22.000-S22.9XX with 7th K, S32.000-S32.9XX with 7th K, S42.001-S42.92X with 7th [K, P], S49.001-S49.199 with 7th [K, P], S52.001-S52.92X with 7th [K, M, N, P, Q, R], S59.001-S59.299 with 7th [K, P], S62.001-S62.92X with 7th [K, P], S72.001-S72.92X with 7th [K, M, N, P, Q, R], S79.001-S79.199 with 7th [K, P], S82.001-S82.92X with 7th [K, M, N, P, Q, R], S89.001-S89.399 with 7th [K, P], S92.001-S92.919 with 7th [K, P]

7,19 √7th **S59.009 Unspecified physeal fracture of lower end of ulna, unspecified arm** CC
CC Excl: CC with 7th character A: S52.001-S52.92X with 7th [A, B, C], S59.001-S59.299 with 7th A
CC with 7th character K or P: M80.00X-M84.68X with 7th [K, P], S02.0XX-S02.92X with 7th K, S12.000-S12.691 with 7th K, S22.000-S22.9XX with 7th K, S32.000-S32.9XX with 7th K, S42.001-S42.92X with 7th [K, P], S49.001-S49.199 with 7th [K, P], S52.001-S52.92X with 7th [K, M, N, P, Q, R], S59.001-S59.299 with 7th [K, P], S62.001-S62.92X with 7th [K, P], S72.001-S72.92X with 7th [K, M, N, P, Q, R], S79.001-S79.199 with 7th [K, P], S82.001-S82.92X with 7th [K, M, N, P, Q, R], S89.001-S89.399 with 7th [K, P], S92.001-S92.919 with 7th [K, P]

√6th **S59.01 Salter-Harris Type I physeal fracture of lower end of ulna**

7,19 √7th **S59.011 Salter-Harris Type I physeal fracture of lower end of ulna, right arm** CC
CC Excl: See code: S59.001

7,19 √7th **S59.012 Salter-Harris Type I physeal fracture of lower end of ulna, left arm** CC
CC Excl: See code: S59.002

7,19 √7th **S59.019 Salter-Harris Type I physeal fracture of lower end of ulna, unspecified arm** CC
CC Excl: See code: S59.009

√6th **S59.02 Salter-Harris Type II physeal fracture of lower end of ulna**

7,19 √7th **S59.021 Salter-Harris Type II physeal fracture of lower end of ulna, right arm** CC
CC Excl: See code: S59.001

7,19 √7th **S59.022 Salter-Harris Type II physeal fracture of lower end of ulna, left arm** CC
CC Excl: See code: S59.002

7,19 √7th **S59.029 Salter-Harris Type II physeal fracture of lower end of ulna, unspecified arm** CC
CC Excl: See code: S59.009

√6th **S59.03 Salter-Harris Type III physeal fracture of lower end of ulna**

7,19 √7th **S59.031 Salter-Harris Type III physeal fracture of lower end of ulna, right arm** CC
CC Excl: See code: S59.001

7,19 √7th **S59.032 Salter-Harris Type III physeal fracture of lower end of ulna, left arm** CC
CC Excl: See code: S59.002

7,19 √7th **S59.039 Salter-Harris Type III physeal fracture of lower end of ulna, unspecified arm**

CC Excl: See code: S59.009

√6th **S59.04 Salter-Harris Type IV physeal fracture of lower end of ulna**

7,19 √7th **S59.041 Salter-Harris Type IV physeal fracture of lower end of ulna, right arm** CC
CC Excl: See code: S59.001

7,19 √7th **S59.042 Salter-Harris Type IV physeal fracture of lower end of ulna, left arm** CC
CC Excl: See code: S59.002

7,19 √7th **S59.049 Salter-Harris Type IV physeal fracture of lower end of ulna, unspecified arm** CC
CC Excl: See code: S59.009

√6th **S59.09 Other physeal fracture of lower end of ulna**

7,19 √7th **S59.091 Other physeal fracture of lower end of ulna, right arm** CC
CC Excl: See code: S59.001

7,19 √7th **S59.092 Other physeal fracture of lower end of ulna, left arm** CC
CC Excl: See code: S59.002

7,19 √7th **S59.099 Other physeal fracture of lower end of ulna, unspecified arm** CC
CC Excl: See code: S59.009

√5th **S59.1 Physeal fracture of upper end of radius**

CC Excl: For CC/MCC codes in subcategory S59.1 with 7th K or P: See Code: S59.009

√6th **S59.10 Unspecified physeal fracture of upper end of radius**

18 √7th **S59.101 Unspecified physeal fracture of upper end of radius, right arm** CC

18 √7th **S59.102 Unspecified physeal fracture of upper end of radius, left arm** CC

18 √7th **S59.109 Unspecified physeal fracture of upper end of radius, unspecified arm** CC

√6th **S59.11 Salter-Harris Type I physeal fracture of upper end of radius**

18 √7th **S59.111 Salter-Harris Type I physeal fracture of upper end of radius, right arm** CC

18 √7th **S59.112 Salter-Harris Type I physeal fracture of upper end of radius, left arm** CC

18 √7th **S59.119 Salter-Harris Type I physeal fracture of upper end of radius, unspecified arm** CC

√6th **S59.12 Salter-Harris Type II physeal fracture of upper end of radius**

18 √7th **S59.121 Salter-Harris Type II physeal fracture of upper end of radius, right arm** CC

18 √7th **S59.122 Salter-Harris Type II physeal fracture of upper end of radius, left arm** CC

18 √7th **S59.129 Salter-Harris Type II physeal fracture of upper end of radius, unspecified arm** CC

√6th **S59.13 Salter-Harris Type III physeal fracture of upper end of radius**

18 √7th **S59.131 Salter-Harris Type III physeal fracture of upper end of radius, right arm** CC

18 √7th **S59.132 Salter-Harris Type III physeal fracture of upper end of radius, left arm** CC

18 √7th **S59.139 Salter-Harris Type III physeal fracture of upper end of radius, unspecified arm** CC

√6th **S59.14 Salter-Harris Type IV physeal fracture of upper end of radius**

18 √7th **S59.141 Salter-Harris Type IV physeal fracture of upper end of radius, right arm** CC

18 √7th **S59.142 Salter-Harris Type IV physeal fracture of upper end of radius, left arm** CC

18 √7th **S59.149 Salter-Harris Type IV physeal fracture of upper end of radius, unspecified arm** CC

√6th **S59.19 Other physeal fracture of upper end of radius**

18 √7th **S59.191 Other physeal fracture of upper end of radius, right arm** CC

18 √7th **S59.192 Other physeal fracture of upper end of radius, left arm** CC

18 √7th **S59.199 Other physeal fracture of upper end of radius, unspecified arm** CC

---

7   HAC = Initial encounter only (7th character A, B or C) and not POA.
18   CC only if a subsequent encounter for nonunion or malunion (7th character K, M, N, P, Q, or R – specific to category).
19   CC only if an initial encounter for a closed fracture (7th character A) **OR** a subsequent encounter for nonunion or malunion (7th character K, M, N, P, Q, or R – specific to category).

✓5ᵗʰ **S59.2**   **Physeal fracture of lower end of radius**

  ✓6ᵗʰ **S59.20**   **Unspecified physeal fracture of lower end of radius**

    7,19 ✓7ᵗʰ **S59.201**   **Unspecified physeal fracture of lower end of radius, right arm**   CC

CC Excl: CC with 7th character A: S52.001-S52.011 with 7th [A, B, C], S52.019-S52.111 with 7th A, S52.119-S52.211 with 7th A, S52.219-S52.311 with 7th A, S52.319-S52.521 with 7th A, S52.529-S52.621 with 7th A, S52.629-S52.92X with 7th A, S59.001A, S59.009-S59.011 with 7th A, S59.019-S59.021 with 7th A, S59.029-S59.031 with 7th A, S59.039-S59.041 with 7th A, S59.049-S59.091 with 7th A, S59.099-S59.101 with 7th A, S59.109-S59.111 with 7th A, S59.119-S59.121 with 7th A, S59.129-S59.131 with 7th A, S59.139-S59.141 with 7th A, S59.149-S59.191 with 7th A, S59.199-S59.201 with 7th A, S59.209-S59.211 with 7th A, S59.219-S59.221 with 7th A, S59.229-S59.231 with 7th A, S59.239-S59.241 with 7th A, S59.249-S59.291 with 7th A, S59.299A

CC with 7th character K or P: M80.00X-M84.68X with 7th [K, P], S02.0XX-S02.92X with 7th K, S12.000-S12.691 with 7th K, S22.000-S22.9XX with 7th K, S32.000-S32.9XX with 7th K, S42.001-S42.92X with 7th [K, P], S49.001-S49.199 with 7th [K, P], S52.001-S52.92X with 7th [K, M, N, P, Q, R], S59.001-S59.299 with 7th [K, P], S62.001-S62.92X with 7th [K, P], S72.001-S72.92X with 7th [K, M, N, P, Q, R], S79.001-S79.199 with 7th [K, P], S82.001-S82.92X with 7th [K, M, N, P, Q, R], S89.001-S89.399 with 7th [K, P], S92.001-S92.919 with 7th [K, P]

    7,19 ✓7ᵗʰ **S59.202**   **Unspecified physeal fracture of lower end of radius, left arm**   CC

CC Excl: CC with 7th character A: S52.001-S52.009 with 7th [B, C], S52.012-S52.109 with 7th A, S52.112-S52.209 with 7th A, S52.212-S52.309 with 7th A, S52.312-S52.516 with 7th A, S52.522-S52.616 with 7th A, S52.622-S52.92X with 7th A, S59.002-S59.009 with 7th A, S59.012-S59.019 with 7th A, S59.022-S59.029 with 7th A, S59.032-S59.039 with 7th A, S59.042-S59.049 with 7th A, S59.092-S59.099 with 7th A, S59.102-S59.109 with 7th A, S59.112-S59.119 with 7th A, S59.122-S59.129 with 7th A, S59.132-S59.139 with 7th A, S59.142-S59.149 with 7th A, S59.192-S59.199 with 7th A, S59.202-S59.209 with 7th A, S59.212-S59.219 with 7th A, S59.222-S59.229 with 7th A, S59.232-S59.239 with 7th A, S59.242-S59.249 with 7th A, S59.292-S59.299 with 7th A

CC with 7th character K or P: M80.00X-M84.68X with 7th [K, P], S02.0XX-S02.92X with 7th K, S12.000-S12.691 with 7th K, S22.000-S22.9XX with 7th K, S32.000-S32.9XX with 7th K, S42.001-S42.92X with 7th [K, P], S49.001-S49.199 with 7th [K, P], S52.001-S52.92X with 7th [K, M, N, P, Q, R], S59.001-S59.299 with 7th [K, P], S62.001-S62.92X with 7th [K, P], S72.001-S72.92X with 7th [K, M, N, P, Q, R], S79.001-S79.199 with 7th [K, P], S82.001-S82.92X with 7th [K, M, N, P, Q, R], S89.001-S89.399 with 7th [K, P], S92.001-S92.919 with 7th [K, P]

    7,19 ✓7ᵗʰ **S59.209**   **Unspecified physeal fracture of lower end of radius, unspecified arm**   CC

CC Excl: CC with 7th character A: S52.001-S52.92X with 7th [A, B, C], S59.001-S59.299 with 7th A

CC with 7th character K or P: M80.00X-M84.68X with 7th [K, P], S02.0XX-S02.92X with 7th K, S12.000-S12.691 with 7th K, S22.000-S22.9XX with 7th K, S32.000-S32.9XX with 7th K, S42.001-S42.92X with 7th [K, P], S49.001-S49.199 with 7th [K, P], S52.001-S52.92X with 7th [K, M, N, P, Q, R], S59.001-S59.299 with 7th [K, P], S62.001-S62.92X with 7th [K, P], S72.001-S72.92X with 7th [K, M, N, P, Q, R], S79.001-S79.199 with 7th [K, P], S82.001-S82.92X with 7th [K, M, N, P, Q, R], S89.001-S89.399 with 7th [K, P], S92.001-S92.919 with 7th [K, P]

  ✓6ᵗʰ **S59.21**   **Salter-Harris Type I physeal fracture of lower end of radius**

    7,19 ✓7ᵗʰ **S59.211**   **Salter-Harris Type I physeal fracture of lower end of radius, right arm**   CC
      CC Excl: See code: S59.201

    7,19 ✓7ᵗʰ **S59.212**   **Salter-Harris Type I physeal fracture of lower end of radius, left arm**   CC
      CC Excl: See code: S59.202

    7,19 ✓7ᵗʰ **S59.219**   **Salter-Harris Type I physeal fracture of lower end of radius, unspecified arm**   CC
      CC Excl: See code: S59.209

  ✓6ᵗʰ **S59.22**   **Salter-Harris Type II physeal fracture of lower end of radius**

    7,19 ✓7ᵗʰ **S59.221**   **Salter-Harris Type II physeal fracture of lower end of radius, right arm**   CC
      CC Excl: See code: S59.201

    7,19 ✓7ᵗʰ **S59.222**   **Salter-Harris Type II physeal fracture | of lower end of radius, left arm**   CC
      CC Excl: See code: S59.202

    7,19 ✓7ᵗʰ **S59.229**   **Salter-Harris Type II physeal fracture of lower end of radius, unspecified arm**   CC
      CC Excl: See code: S59.209

  ✓6ᵗʰ **S59.23**   **Salter-Harris Type III physeal fracture of lower end of radius**

    7,19 ✓7ᵗʰ **S59.231**   **Salter-Harris Type III physeal fracture of lower end of radius, right arm**   CC
      CC Excl: See code: S59.201

    7,19 ✓7ᵗʰ **S59.232**   **Salter-Harris Type III physeal fracture of lower end of radius, left arm**   CC
      CC Excl: See code: S59.202

    7,19 ✓7ᵗʰ **S59.239**   **Salter-Harris Type III physeal fracture of lower end of radius, unspecified arm**   CC
      CC Excl: See code: S59.209

  ✓6ᵗʰ **S59.24**   **Salter-Harris Type IV physeal fracture of lower end of radius**

    7,19 ✓7ᵗʰ **S59.241**   **Salter-Harris Type IV physeal fracture of lower end of radius, right arm**   CC
      CC Excl: See code: S59.201

    7,19 ✓7ᵗʰ **S59.242**   **Salter-Harris Type IV physeal fracture of lower end of radius, left arm**   CC
      CC Excl: See code: S59.202

    7,19 ✓7ᵗʰ **S59.249**   **Salter-Harris Type IV physeal fracture of lower end of radius, unspecified arm**   CC
      CC Excl: See code: S59.209

  ✓6ᵗʰ **S59.29**   **Other physeal fracture of lower end of radius**

    7,19 ✓7ᵗʰ **S59.291**   **Other physeal fracture of lower end of radius, right arm**   CC
      CC Excl: See code: S59.201

    7,19 ✓7ᵗʰ **S59.292**   **Other physeal fracture of lower end of radius, left arm**   CC
      CC Excl: See code: S59.202

    7,19 ✓7ᵗʰ **S59.299**   **Other physeal fracture of lower end of radius, unspecified arm**   CC
      CC Excl: See code: S59.209

✓5ᵗʰ **S59.8**   **Other specified injuries of elbow and forearm**

> The appropriate 7th is to be added to each code in subcategory S59.8.
> A   initial encounter
> D   subsequent encounter
> S   sequela

  ✓6ᵗʰ **S59.80**   **Other specified injuries of elbow**

    ✓7ᵗʰ **S59.801**   **Other specified injuries of right elbow**

    ✓7ᵗʰ **S59.802**   **Other specified injuries of left elbow**

    ✓7ᵗʰ **S59.809**   **Other specified injuries of unspecified elbow**

  ✓6ᵗʰ **S59.81**   **Other specified injuries of forearm**

    ✓7ᵗʰ **S59.811**   **Other specified injuries right forearm**

    ✓7ᵗʰ **S59.812**   **Other specified injuries left forearm**

    ✓7ᵗʰ **S59.819**   **Other specified injuries unspecified forearm**

---

7   HAC = Initial encounter only (7th character A, B or C) and not POA.
19   CC only if an initial encounter for a closed fracture (7th character A) **OR** a subsequent encounter for nonunion or malunion (7th character K, M, N, P, Q, or R – specific to category).

✓ Additional Character Required   ✓x7ᵗʰ Placeholder Alert   Unacceptable PDx   Manifestation   Hospital Acquired Condition   **EXCLUDES 1** Not Coded Here   **EXCLUDES 2** Not Included Here

√5th **S59.9** Unspecified injury of elbow and forearm

> The appropriate 7th is to be added to each code in subcategory S59.9.
> A   initial encounter
> D   subsequent encounter
> S   sequela

√6th **S59.90** Unspecified injury of elbow

√7th **S59.901** Unspecified injury of right elbow

√7th **S59.902** Unspecified injury of left elbow

√7th **S59.909** Unspecified injury of unspecified elbow

√6th **S59.91** Unspecified injury of forearm

√7th **S59.911** Unspecified injury of right forearm

√7th **S59.912** Unspecified injury of left forearm

√7th **S59.919** Unspecified injury of unspecified forearm

Injuries to the wrist, hand and fingers (S60-S69)

EXCLUDES 2　burns and corrosions (T20-T32)
frostbite (T33-T34)
insect bite or sting, venomous (T63.4)

√4th **S60** Superficial injury of wrist, hand and fingers

> The appropriate 7th is to be added to each code from category S60.
> A   initial encounter
> D   subsequent encounter
> S   sequela

√5th **S60.0** Contusion of finger without damage to nail

EXCLUDES 1　contusion involving nail (matrix) (S60.1)

√x7th **S60.00** Contusion of unspecified finger without damage to nail
Contusion of finger(s) NOS

√6th **S60.01** Contusion of thumb without damage to nail

√7th **S60.011** Contusion of right thumb without damage to nail

√7th **S60.012** Contusion of left thumb without damage to nail

√7th **S60.019** Contusion of unspecified thumb without damage to nail

√6th **S60.02** Contusion of index finger without damage to nail

√7th **S60.021** Contusion of right index finger without damage to nail

√7th **S60.022** Contusion of left index finger without damage to nail

√7th **S60.029** Contusion of unspecified index finger without damage to nail

√6th **S60.03** Contusion of middle finger without damage to nail

√7th **S60.031** Contusion of right middle finger without damage to nail

√7th **S60.032** Contusion of left middle finger without damage to nail

√7th **S60.039** Contusion of unspecified middle finger without damage to nail

√6th **S60.04** Contusion of ring finger without damage to nail

√7th **S60.041** Contusion of right ring finger without damage to nail

√7th **S60.042** Contusion of left ring finger without damage to nail

√7th **S60.049** Contusion of unspecified ring finger without damage to nail

√6th **S60.05** Contusion of little finger without damage to nail

√7th **S60.051** Contusion of right little finger without damage to nail

√7th **S60.052** Contusion of left little finger without damage to nail

√7th **S60.059** Contusion of unspecified little finger without damage to nail

√5th **S60.1** Contusion of finger with damage to nail

√x7th **S60.10** Contusion of unspecified finger with damage to nail

√6th **S60.11** Contusion of thumb with damage to nail

√7th **S60.111** Contusion of right thumb with damage to nail

√7th **S60.112** Contusion of left thumb with damage to nail

√7th **S60.119** Contusion of unspecified thumb with damage to nail

√6th **S60.12** Contusion of index finger with damage to nail

√7th **S60.121** Contusion of right index finger with damage to nail

√7th **S60.122** Contusion of left index finger with damage to nail

√7th **S60.129** Contusion of unspecified index finger with damage to nail

√6th **S60.13** Contusion of middle finger with damage to nail

√7th **S60.131** Contusion of right middle finger with damage to nail

√7th **S60.132** Contusion of left middle finger with damage to nail

√7th **S60.139** Contusion of unspecified middle finger with damage to nail

√6th **S60.14** Contusion of ring finger with damage to nail

√7th **S60.141** Contusion of right ring finger with damage to nail

√7th **S60.142** Contusion of left ring finger with damage to nail

√7th **S60.149** Contusion of unspecified ring finger with damage to nail

√6th **S60.15** Contusion of little finger with damage to nail

√7th **S60.151** Contusion of right little finger with damage to nail

√7th **S60.152** Contusion of left little finger with damage to nail

√7th **S60.159** Contusion of unspecified little finger with damage to nail

√5th **S60.2** Contusion of wrist and hand

EXCLUDES 2　contusion of fingers (S60.0-, S60.1-)

√6th **S60.21** Contusion of wrist

√7th **S60.211** Contusion of right wrist

√7th **S60.212** Contusion of left wrist

√7th **S60.219** Contusion of unspecified wrist

√6th **S60.22** Contusion of hand

√7th **S60.221** Contusion of right hand

√7th **S60.222** Contusion of left hand

√7th **S60.229** Contusion of unspecified hand

√5th **S60.3** Other superficial injuries of thumb

√6th **S60.31** Abrasion of thumb

√7th **S60.311** Abrasion of right thumb

√7th **S60.312** Abrasion of left thumb

√7th **S60.319** Abrasion of unspecified thumb

√6th **S60.32** Blister (nonthermal) of thumb

√7th **S60.321** Blister (nonthermal) of right thumb

√7th **S60.322** Blister (nonthermal) of left thumb

√7th **S60.329** Blister (nonthermal) of unspecified thumb

√6th **S60.34** External constriction of thumb
Hair tourniquet syndrome of thumb
Use additional cause code to identify the constricting item (W49.0-)

√7th **S60.341** External constriction of right thumb

√7th **S60.342** External constriction of left thumb

√7th **S60.349** External constriction of unspecified thumb

√6th **S60.35** Superficial foreign body of thumb
Splinter in the thumb

√7th **S60.351** Superficial foreign body of right thumb

√7th **S60.352** Superficial foreign body of left thumb

√7th **S60.359** Superficial foreign body of unspecified thumb

√6th **S60.36** Insect bite (nonvenomous) of thumb

√7th **S60.361** Insect bite (nonvenomous) of right thumb

√7th **S60.362** Insect bite (nonvenomous) of left thumb

√7th **S60.369** Insect bite (nonvenomous) of unspecified thumb

√6th **S60.37** Other superficial bite of thumb

EXCLUDES 1　open bite of thumb (S61.05-, S61.15-)

√7th **S60.371** Other superficial bite of right thumb

N Newborn: 0　P Pediatric: 0-17　M Maternity: 12-55　A Adult: 15-124　MCC Major CC Condition　PDx MCC PDx acts as own MCC　CC CC Condition　PDx CC PDx acts as own CC

986

ICD-10-CM 2016

☑7ᵗʰ **S60.372** Other superficial bite of left thumb

☑7ᵗʰ **S60.379** Other superficial bite of unspecified thumb

☑6ᵗʰ **S60.39** Other superficial injuries of thumb

☑7ᵗʰ **S60.391** Other superficial injuries of right thumb

☑7ᵗʰ **S60.392** Other superficial injuries of left thumb

☑7ᵗʰ **S60.399** Other superficial injuries of unspecified thumb

☑5ᵗʰ **S60.4** Other superficial injuries of other fingers

☑6ᵗʰ **S60.41** Abrasion of fingers

☑7ᵗʰ **S60.410** Abrasion of right index finger

☑7ᵗʰ **S60.411** Abrasion of left index finger

☑7ᵗʰ **S60.412** Abrasion of right middle finger

☑7ᵗʰ **S60.413** Abrasion of left middle finger

☑7ᵗʰ **S60.414** Abrasion of right ring finger

☑7ᵗʰ **S60.415** Abrasion of left ring finger

☑7ᵗʰ **S60.416** Abrasion of right little finger

☑7ᵗʰ **S60.417** Abrasion of left little finger

☑7ᵗʰ **S60.418** Abrasion of other finger
Abrasion of specified finger with unspecified laterality

☑7ᵗʰ **S60.419** Abrasion of unspecified finger

☑6ᵗʰ **S60.42** Blister (nonthermal) of fingers

☑7ᵗʰ **S60.420** Blister (nonthermal) of right index finger

☑7ᵗʰ **S60.421** Blister (nonthermal) of left index finger

☑7ᵗʰ **S60.422** Blister (nonthermal) of right middle finger

☑7ᵗʰ **S60.423** Blister (nonthermal) of left middle finger

☑7ᵗʰ **S60.424** Blister (nonthermal) of right ring finger

☑7ᵗʰ **S60.425** Blister (nonthermal) of left ring finger

☑7ᵗʰ **S60.426** Blister (nonthermal) of right little finger

☑7ᵗʰ **S60.427** Blister (nonthermal) of left little finger

☑7ᵗʰ **S60.428** Blister (nonthermal) of other finger
Blister (nonthermal) of specified finger with unspecified laterality

☑7ᵗʰ **S60.429** Blister (nonthermal) of unspecified finger

☑6ᵗʰ **S60.44** External constriction of fingers
Hair tourniquet syndrome of finger
Use additional cause code to identify the constricting item (W49.0-)

☑7ᵗʰ **S60.440** External constriction of right index finger

☑7ᵗʰ **S60.441** External constriction of left index finger

☑7ᵗʰ **S60.442** External constriction of right middle finger

☑7ᵗʰ **S60.443** External constriction of left middle finger

☑7ᵗʰ **S60.444** External constriction of right ring finger

☑7ᵗʰ **S60.445** External constriction of left ring finger

☑7ᵗʰ **S60.446** External constriction of right little finger

☑7ᵗʰ **S60.447** External constriction of left little finger

☑7ᵗʰ **S60.448** External constriction of other finger
External constriction of specified finger with unspecified laterality

☑7ᵗʰ **S60.449** External constriction of unspecified finger

☑6ᵗʰ **S60.45** Superficial foreign body of fingers
Splinter in the finger(s)

☑7ᵗʰ **S60.450** Superficial foreign body of right index finger

☑7ᵗʰ **S60.451** Superficial foreign body of left index finger

☑7ᵗʰ **S60.452** Superficial foreign body of right middle finger

☑7ᵗʰ **S60.453** Superficial foreign body of left middle finger

☑7ᵗʰ **S60.454** Superficial foreign body of right ring finger

☑7ᵗʰ **S60.455** Superficial foreign body of left ring finger

☑7ᵗʰ **S60.456** Superficial foreign body of right little finger

☑7ᵗʰ **S60.457** Superficial foreign body of left little finger

☑7ᵗʰ **S60.458** Superficial foreign body of other finger
Superficial foreign body of specified finger with unspecified laterality

☑7ᵗʰ **S60.459** Superficial foreign body of unspecified finger

☑6ᵗʰ **S60.46** Insect bite (nonvenomous) of fingers

☑7ᵗʰ **S60.460** Insect bite (nonvenomous) of right index finger

☑7ᵗʰ **S60.461** Insect bite (nonvenomous) of left index finger

☑7ᵗʰ **S60.462** Insect bite (nonvenomous) of right middle finger

☑7ᵗʰ **S60.463** Insect bite (nonvenomous) of left middle finger

☑7ᵗʰ **S60.464** Insect bite (nonvenomous) of right ring finger

☑7ᵗʰ **S60.465** Insect bite (nonvenomous) of left ring finger

☑7ᵗʰ **S60.466** Insect bite (nonvenomous) of right little finger

☑7ᵗʰ **S60.467** Insect bite (nonvenomous) of left little finger

☑7ᵗʰ **S60.468** Insect bite (nonvenomous) of other finger
Insect bite (nonvenomous) of specified finger with unspecified laterality

☑7ᵗʰ **S60.469** Insect bite (nonvenomous) of unspecified finger

☑6ᵗʰ **S60.47** Other superficial bite of fingers
EXCLUDES 1 open bite of fingers (S61.25-, S61.35-)

☑7ᵗʰ **S60.470** Other superficial bite of right index finger

☑7ᵗʰ **S60.471** Other superficial bite of left index finger

☑7ᵗʰ **S60.472** Other superficial bite of right middle finger

☑7ᵗʰ **S60.473** Other superficial bite of left middle finger

☑7ᵗʰ **S60.474** Other superficial bite of right ring finger

☑7ᵗʰ **S60.475** Other superficial bite of left ring finger

☑7ᵗʰ **S60.476** Other superficial bite of right little finger

☑7ᵗʰ **S60.477** Other superficial bite of left little finger

☑7ᵗʰ **S60.478** Other superficial bite of other finger
Other superficial bite of specified finger with unspecified laterality

☑7ᵗʰ **S60.479** Other superficial bite of unspecified finger

☑5ᵗʰ **S60.5** Other superficial injuries of hand
EXCLUDES 2 superficial injuries of fingers (S60.3-, S60.4-)

☑6ᵗʰ **S60.51** Abrasion of hand

☑7ᵗʰ **S60.511** Abrasion of right hand

☑7ᵗʰ **S60.512** Abrasion of left hand

☑7ᵗʰ **S60.519** Abrasion of unspecified hand

☑6ᵗʰ **S60.52** Blister (nonthermal) of hand

☑7ᵗʰ **S60.521** Blister (nonthermal) of right hand

☑7ᵗʰ **S60.522** Blister (nonthermal) of left hand

☑7ᵗʰ **S60.529** Blister (nonthermal) of unspecified hand

☑6ᵗʰ **S60.54** External constriction of hand

☑7ᵗʰ **S60.541** External constriction of right hand

☑7ᵗʰ **S60.542** External constriction of left hand

☑7ᵗʰ **S60.549** External constriction of unspecified hand

☑6ᵗʰ **S60.55** Superficial foreign body of hand
Splinter in the hand

☑7ᵗʰ **S60.551** Superficial foreign body of right hand

☑7ᵗʰ **S60.552** Superficial foreign body of left hand

☑7ᵗʰ **S60.559** Superficial foreign body of unspecified hand

☑6ᵗʰ **S60.56** Insect bite (nonvenomous) of hand

☑7ᵗʰ **S60.561** Insect bite (nonvenomous) of right hand

☑7ᵗʰ **S60.562** Insect bite (nonvenomous) of left hand

☑7ᵗʰ **S60.569** Insect bite (nonvenomous) of unspecified hand

☑6ᵗʰ **S60.57** Other superficial bite of hand
EXCLUDES 1 open bite of hand (S61.45-)

☑7ᵗʰ **S60.571** Other superficial bite of hand of right hand

☑7ᵗʰ **S60.572** Other superficial bite of hand of left hand

☑7ᵗʰ **S60.579** Other superficial bite of hand of unspecified hand

☑ Additional Character Required   ☑7ˣ Placeholder Alert   Unacceptable PDx   Manifestation   Hospital Acquired Condition   **EXCLUDES 1** Not Coded Here   **EXCLUDES 2** Not Included Here

ICD-10-CM 2016   987

Chapter 19. Injury, Poisoning, and Certain Other Consequences of External Causes

✓5th **S60.8** **Other superficial injuries of wrist**

  ✓6th **S60.81** **Abrasion of wrist**

    ✓7th **S60.811** **Abrasion of right wrist**

    ✓7th **S60.812** **Abrasion of left wrist**

    ✓7th **S60.819** **Abrasion of unspecified wrist**

  ✓6th **S60.82** **Blister (nonthermal) of wrist**

    ✓7th **S60.821** **Blister (nonthermal) of right wrist**

    ✓7th **S60.822** **Blister (nonthermal) of left wrist**

    ✓7th **S60.829** **Blister (nonthermal) of unspecified wrist**

  ✓6th **S60.84** **External constriction of wrist**

    ✓7th **S60.841** **External constriction of right wrist**

    ✓7th **S60.842** **External constriction of left wrist**

    ✓7th **S60.849** **External constriction of unspecified wrist**

  ✓6th **S60.85** **Superficial foreign body of wrist**
    Splinter in the wrist

    ✓7th **S60.851** **Superficial foreign body of right wrist**

    ✓7th **S60.852** **Superficial foreign body of left wrist**

    ✓7th **S60.859** **Superficial foreign body of unspecified wrist**

  ✓6th **S60.86** **Insect bite (nonvenomous) of wrist**

    ✓7th **S60.861** **Insect bite (nonvenomous) of right wrist**

    ✓7th **S60.862** **Insect bite (nonvenomous) of left wrist**

    ✓7th **S60.869** **Insect bite (nonvenomous) of unspecified wrist**

  ✓6th **S60.87** **Other superficial bite of wrist**
    EXCLUDES 1 *open bite of wrist (S61.55)*

    ✓7th **S60.871** **Other superficial bite of right wrist**

    ✓7th **S60.872** **Other superficial bite of left wrist**

    ✓7th **S60.879** **Other superficial bite of unspecified wrist**

✓5th **S60.9** **Unspecified superficial injury of wrist, hand and fingers**

  ✓6th **S60.91** **Unspecified superficial injury of wrist**

    ✓7th **S60.911** **Unspecified superficial injury of right wrist**

    ✓7th **S60.912** **Unspecified superficial injury of left wrist**

    ✓7th **S60.919** **Unspecified superficial injury of unspecified wrist**

  ✓6th **S60.92** **Unspecified superficial injury of hand**

    ✓7th **S60.921** **Unspecified superficial injury of right hand**

    ✓7th **S60.922** **Unspecified superficial injury of left hand**

    ✓7th **S60.929** **Unspecified superficial injury of unspecified hand**

  ✓6th **S60.93** **Unspecified superficial injury of thumb**

    ✓7th **S60.931** **Unspecified superficial injury of right thumb**

    ✓7th **S60.932** **Unspecified superficial injury of left thumb**

    ✓7th **S60.939** **Unspecified superficial injury of unspecified thumb**

  ✓6th **S60.94** **Unspecified superficial injury of other fingers**

    ✓7th **S60.940** **Unspecified superficial injury of right index finger**

    ✓7th **S60.941** **Unspecified superficial injury of left index finger**

    ✓7th **S60.942** **Unspecified superficial injury of right middle finger**

    ✓7th **S60.943** **Unspecified superficial injury of left middle finger**

    ✓7th **S60.944** **Unspecified superficial injury of right ring finger**

    ✓7th **S60.945** **Unspecified superficial injury of left ring finger**

    ✓7th **S60.946** **Unspecified superficial injury of right little finger**

    ✓7th **S60.947** **Unspecified superficial injury of left little finger**

    ✓7th **S60.948** **Unspecified superficial injury of other finger**
    Unspecified superficial injury of specified finger with unspecified laterality

    ✓7th **S60.949** **Unspecified superficial injury of unspecified finger**

✓4th **S61** **Open wound of wrist, hand and fingers**
  Code also any associated wound infection
  EXCLUDES 1 *open fracture of wrist, hand and finger (S62- with 7th character B)*
    traumatic amputation of wrist and hand (S68.-)

  The appropriate 7th is to be added to each code from category S61.
  A   initial encounter
  D   subsequent encounter
  S   sequela

  ✓5th **S61.0** **Open wound of thumb without damage to nail**
    EXCLUDES 1 *open wound of thumb with damage to nail (S61.1-)*

    ✓6th **S61.00** **Unspecified open wound of thumb without damage to nail**

      ✓7th **S61.001** **Unspecified open wound of right thumb without damage to nail**

      ✓7th **S61.002** **Unspecified open wound of left thumb without damage to nail**

      ✓7th **S61.009** **Unspecified open wound of unspecified thumb without damage to nail**

    ✓6th **S61.01** **Laceration without foreign body of thumb without damage to nail**

      ✓7th **S61.011** **Laceration without foreign body of right thumb without damage to nail**

      ✓7th **S61.012** **Laceration without foreign body of left thumb without damage to nail**

      ✓7th **S61.019** **Laceration without foreign body of unspecified thumb without damage to nail**

    ✓6th **S61.02** **Laceration with foreign body of thumb without damage to nail**

      ✓7th **S61.021** **Laceration with foreign body of right thumb without damage to nail**

      ✓7th **S61.022** **Laceration with foreign body of left thumb without damage to nail**

      ✓7th **S61.029** **Laceration with foreign body of unspecified thumb without damage to nail**

    ✓6th **S61.03** **Puncture wound without foreign body of thumb without damage to nail**

      ✓7th **S61.031** **Puncture wound without foreign body of right thumb without damage to nail**

      ✓7th **S61.032** **Puncture wound without foreign body of left thumb without damage to nail**

      ✓7th **S61.039** **Puncture wound without foreign body of unspecified thumb without damage to nail**

    ✓6th **S61.04** **Puncture wound with foreign body of thumb without damage to nail**

      ✓7th **S61.041** **Puncture wound with foreign body of right thumb without damage to nail**

      ✓7th **S61.042** **Puncture wound with foreign body of left thumb without damage to nail**

      ✓7th **S61.049** **Puncture wound with foreign body of unspecified thumb without damage to nail**

    ✓6th **S61.05** **Open bite of thumb without damage to nail**
      Bite of thumb NOS
      EXCLUDES 1 *superficial bite of thumb (S60.36-, S60.37-)*

      ✓7th **S61.051** **Open bite of right thumb without damage to nail**

      ✓7th **S61.052** **Open bite of left thumb without damage to nail**

      ✓7th **S61.059** **Open bite of unspecified thumb without damage to nail**

  ✓5th **S61.1** **Open wound of thumb with damage to nail**

    ✓6th **S61.10** **Unspecified open wound of thumb with damage to nail**

      ✓7th **S61.101** **Unspecified open wound of right thumb with damage to nail**

      ✓7th **S61.102** **Unspecified open wound of left thumb with damage to nail**

      ✓7th **S61.109** **Unspecified open wound of unspecified thumb with damage to nail**

N Newborn: 0   P Pediatric: 0-17   M Maternity: 12-55   A Adult: 15-124   MCC Major CC Condition   PDxMCC PDx acts as own MCC   CC CC Condition   PDxCC PDx acts as own CC

988

ICD-10-CM 2016

✓6th **S61.11** Laceration without foreign body of thumb with damage to nail

     ✓7th **S61.111** Laceration without foreign body of right thumb with damage to nail

     ✓7th **S61.112** Laceration without foreign body of left thumb with damage to nail

     ✓7th **S61.119** Laceration without foreign body of unspecified thumb with damage to nail

✓6th **S61.12** Laceration with foreign body of thumb with damage to nail

     ✓7th **S61.121** Laceration with foreign body of right thumb with damage to nail

     ✓7th **S61.122** Laceration with foreign body of left thumb with damage to nail

     ✓7th **S61.129** Laceration with foreign body of unspecified thumb with damage to nail

✓6th **S61.13** Puncture wound without foreign body of thumb with damage to nail

     ✓7th **S61.131** Puncture wound without foreign body of right thumb with damage to nail

     ✓7th **S61.132** Puncture wound without foreign body of left thumb with damage to nail

     ✓7th **S61.139** Puncture wound without foreign body of unspecified thumb with damage to nail

✓6th **S61.14** Puncture wound with foreign body of thumb with damage to nail

     ✓7th **S61.141** Puncture wound with foreign body of right thumb with damage to nail

     ✓7th **S61.142** Puncture wound with foreign body of left thumb with damage to nail

     ✓7th **S61.149** Puncture wound with foreign body of unspecified thumb with damage to nail

✓6th **S61.15** Open bite of thumb with damage to nail
     Bite of thumb with damage to nail NOS
     EXCLUDES 1 superficial bite of thumb (S60.36-, S60.37-)

     ✓7th **S61.151** Open bite of right thumb with damage to nail

     ✓7th **S61.152** Open bite of left thumb with damage to nail

     ✓7th **S61.159** Open bite of unspecified thumb with damage to nail

✓5th **S61.2** Open wound of other finger without damage to nail
     EXCLUDES 1 open wound of finger involving nail (matrix) (S61.3-)
     EXCLUDES 2 open wound of thumb without damage to nail (S61.0-)

     ✓6th **S61.20** Unspecified open wound of other finger without damage to nail

       ✓7th **S61.200** Unspecified open wound of right index finger without damage to nail

       ✓7th **S61.201** Unspecified open wound of left index finger without damage to nail

       ✓7th **S61.202** Unspecified open wound of right middle finger without damage to nail

       ✓7th **S61.203** Unspecified open wound of left middle finger without damage to nail

       ✓7th **S61.204** Unspecified open wound of right ring finger without damage to nail

       ✓7th **S61.205** Unspecified open wound of left ring finger without damage to nail

       ✓7th **S61.206** Unspecified open wound of right little finger without damage to nail

       ✓7th **S61.207** Unspecified open wound of left little finger without damage to nail

       ✓7th **S61.208** Unspecified open wound of other finger without damage to nail
         Unspecified open wound of specified finger with unspecified laterality without damage to nail

       ✓7th **S61.209** Unspecified open wound of unspecified finger without damage to nail

     ✓6th **S61.21** Laceration without foreign body of finger without damage to nail

       ✓7th **S61.210** Laceration without foreign body of right index finger without damage to nail

       ✓7th **S61.211** Laceration without foreign body of left index finger without damage to nail

     ✓7th **S61.212** Laceration without foreign body of right middle finger without damage to nail

     ✓7th **S61.213** Laceration without foreign body of left middle finger without damage to nail

     ✓7th **S61.214** Laceration without foreign body of right ring finger without damage to nail

     ✓7th **S61.215** Laceration without foreign body of left ring finger without damage to nail

     ✓7th **S61.216** Laceration without foreign body of right little finger without damage to nail

     ✓7th **S61.217** Laceration without foreign body of left little finger without damage to nail

     ✓7th **S61.218** Laceration without foreign body of other finger without damage to nail
       Laceration without foreign body of specified finger with unspecified laterality without damage to nail

     ✓7th **S61.219** Laceration without foreign body of unspecified finger without damage to nail

✓6th **S61.22** Laceration with foreign body of finger without damage to nail

     ✓7th **S61.220** Laceration with foreign body of right index finger without damage to nail

     ✓7th **S61.221** Laceration with foreign body of left index finger without damage to nail

     ✓7th **S61.222** Laceration with foreign body of right middle finger without damage to nail

     ✓7th **S61.223** Laceration with foreign body of left middle finger without damage to nail

     ✓7th **S61.224** Laceration with foreign body of right ring finger without damage to nail

     ✓7th **S61.225** Laceration with foreign body of left ring finger without damage to nail

     ✓7th **S61.226** Laceration with foreign body of right little finger without damage to nail

     ✓7th **S61.227** Laceration with foreign body of left little finger without damage to nail

     ✓7th **S61.228** Laceration with foreign body of other finger without damage to nail
       Laceration with foreign body of specified finger with unspecified laterality without damage to nail

     ✓7th **S61.229** Laceration with foreign body of unspecified finger without damage to nail

✓6th **S61.23** Puncture wound without foreign body of finger without damage to nail

     ✓7th **S61.230** Puncture wound without foreign body of right index finger without damage to nail

     ✓7th **S61.231** Puncture wound without foreign body of left index finger without damage to nail

     ✓7th **S61.232** Puncture wound without foreign body of right middle finger without damage to nail

     ✓7th **S61.233** Puncture wound without foreign body of left middle finger without damage to nail

     ✓7th **S61.234** Puncture wound without foreign body of right ring finger without damage to nail

     ✓7th **S61.235** Puncture wound without foreign body of left ring finger without damage to nail

     ✓7th **S61.236** Puncture wound without foreign body of right little finger without damage to nail

     ✓7th **S61.237** Puncture wound without foreign body of left little finger without damage to nail

     ✓7th **S61.238** Puncture wound without foreign body of other finger without damage to nail
       Puncture wound without foreign body of specified finger with unspecified laterality without damage to nail

     ✓7th **S61.239** Puncture wound without foreign body of unspecified finger without damage to nail

✓6th **S61.24** Puncture wound with foreign body of finger without damage to nail

     ✓7th **S61.240** Puncture wound with foreign body of right index finger without damage to nail

     ✓7th **S61.241** Puncture wound with foreign body of left index finger without damage to nail

✓ Additional Character Required   ✓x7th Placeholder Alert   Unacceptable PDx   Manifestation   Hospital Acquired Condition   **EXCLUDES 1** Not Coded Here   **EXCLUDES 2** Not Included Here

ICD-10-CM 2016   989

Chapter 19. Injury, Poisoning, and Certain Other Consequences of External Causes

√7ᵗʰ **S61.242** Puncture wound with foreign body of right middle finger without damage to nail

√7ᵗʰ **S61.243** Puncture wound with foreign body of left middle finger without damage to nail

√7ᵗʰ **S61.244** Puncture wound with foreign body of right ring finger without damage to nail

√7ᵗʰ **S61.245** Puncture wound with foreign body of left ring finger without damage to nail

√7ᵗʰ **S61.246** Puncture wound with foreign body of right little finger without damage to nail

√7ᵗʰ **S61.247** Puncture wound with foreign body of left little finger without damage to nail

√7ᵗʰ **S61.248** Puncture wound with foreign body of other finger without damage to nail
Puncture wound with foreign body of specified finger with unspecified laterality without damage to nail

√7ᵗʰ **S61.249** Puncture wound with foreign body of unspecified finger without damage to nail

√6ᵗʰ **S61.25** Open bite of finger without damage to nail
Bite of finger without damage to nail NOS
EXCLUDES 1 *superficial bite of finger (S60.46-, S60.47-)*

√7ᵗʰ **S61.250** Open bite of right index finger without damage to nail

√7ᵗʰ **S61.251** Open bite of left index finger without damage to nail

√7ᵗʰ **S61.252** Open bite of right middle finger without damage to nail

√7ᵗʰ **S61.253** Open bite of left middle finger without damage to nail

√7ᵗʰ **S61.254** Open bite of right ring finger without damage to nail

√7ᵗʰ **S61.255** Open bite of left ring finger without damage to nail

√7ᵗʰ **S61.256** Open bite of right little finger without damage to nail

√7ᵗʰ **S61.257** Open bite of left little finger without damage to nail

√7ᵗʰ **S61.258** Open bite of other finger without damage to nail
Open bite of specified finger with unspecified laterality without damage to nail

√7ᵗʰ **S61.259** Open bite of unspecified finger without damage to nail

√5ᵗʰ **S61.3** Open wound of other finger with damage to nail

√6ᵗʰ **S61.30** Unspecified open wound of finger with damage to nail

√7ᵗʰ **S61.300** Unspecified open wound of right index finger with damage to nail

√7ᵗʰ **S61.301** Unspecified open wound of left index finger with damage to nail

√7ᵗʰ **S61.302** Unspecified open wound of right middle finger with damage to nail

√7ᵗʰ **S61.303** Unspecified open wound of left middle finger with damage to nail

√7ᵗʰ **S61.304** Unspecified open wound of right ring finger with damage to nail

√7ᵗʰ **S61.305** Unspecified open wound of left ring finger with damage to nail

√7ᵗʰ **S61.306** Unspecified open wound of right little finger with damage to nail

√7ᵗʰ **S61.307** Unspecified open wound of left little finger with damage to nail

√7ᵗʰ **S61.308** Unspecified open wound of other finger with damage to nail
Unspecified open wound of specified finger with unspecified laterality with damage to nail

√7ᵗʰ **S61.309** Unspecified open wound of unspecified finger with damage to nail

√6ᵗʰ **S61.31** Laceration without foreign body of finger with damage to nail

√7ᵗʰ **S61.310** Laceration without foreign body of right index finger with damage to nail

√7ᵗʰ **S61.311** Laceration without foreign body of left index finger with damage to nail

√7ᵗʰ **S61.312** Laceration without foreign body of right middle finger with damage to nail

√7ᵗʰ **S61.313** Laceration without foreign body of left middle finger with damage to nail

√7ᵗʰ **S61.314** Laceration without foreign body of right ring finger with damage to nail

√7ᵗʰ **S61.315** Laceration without foreign body of left ring finger with damage to nail

√7ᵗʰ **S61.316** Laceration without foreign body of right little finger with damage to nail

√7ᵗʰ **S61.317** Laceration without foreign body of left little finger with damage to nail

√7ᵗʰ **S61.318** Laceration without foreign body of other finger with damage to nail
Laceration without foreign body of specified finger with unspecified laterality with damage to nail

√7ᵗʰ **S61.319** Laceration without foreign body of unspecified finger with damage to nail

√6ᵗʰ **S61.32** Laceration with foreign body of finger with damage to nail

√7ᵗʰ **S61.320** Laceration with foreign body of right index finger with damage to nail

√7ᵗʰ **S61.321** Laceration with foreign body of left index finger with damage to nail

√7ᵗʰ **S61.322** Laceration with foreign body of right middle finger with damage to nail

√7ᵗʰ **S61.323** Laceration with foreign body of left middle finger with damage to nail

√7ᵗʰ **S61.324** Laceration with foreign body of right ring finger with damage to nail

√7ᵗʰ **S61.325** Laceration with foreign body of left ring finger with damage to nail

√7ᵗʰ **S61.326** Laceration with foreign body of right little finger with damage to nail

√7ᵗʰ **S61.327** Laceration with foreign body of left little finger with damage to nail

√7ᵗʰ **S61.328** Laceration with foreign body of other finger with damage to nail
Laceration with foreign body of specified finger with unspecified laterality with damage to nail

√7ᵗʰ **S61.329** Laceration with foreign body of unspecified finger with damage to nail

√6ᵗʰ **S61.33** Puncture wound without foreign body of finger with damage to nail

√7ᵗʰ **S61.330** Puncture wound without foreign body of right index finger with damage to nail

√7ᵗʰ **S61.331** Puncture wound without foreign body of left index finger with damage to nail

√7ᵗʰ **S61.332** Puncture wound without foreign body of right middle finger with damage to nail

√7ᵗʰ **S61.333** Puncture wound without foreign body of left middle finger with damage to nail

√7ᵗʰ **S61.334** Puncture wound without foreign body of right ring finger with damage to nail

√7ᵗʰ **S61.335** Puncture wound without foreign body of left ring finger with damage to nail

√7ᵗʰ **S61.336** Puncture wound without foreign body of right little finger with damage to nail

√7ᵗʰ **S61.337** Puncture wound without foreign body of left little finger with damage to nail

√7ᵗʰ **S61.338** Puncture wound without foreign body of other finger with damage to nail
Puncture wound without foreign body of specified finger with unspecified laterality with damage to nail

√7ᵗʰ **S61.339** Puncture wound without foreign body of unspecified finger with damage to nail

√6ᵗʰ **S61.34** Puncture wound with foreign body of finger with damage to nail

√7ᵗʰ **S61.340** Puncture wound with foreign body of right index finger with damage to nail

√7ᵗʰ **S61.341** Puncture wound with foreign body of left index finger with damage to nail

---

N Newborn: 0   P Pediatric: 0-17   M Maternity: 12-55   A Adult: 15-124   **MCC** Major CC Condition   **PDxMCC** PDx acts as own MCC   **CC** CC Condition   **PDxCC** PDx acts as own CC

√7ᵗʰ **S61.342** **Puncture wound with foreign body of right middle finger with damage to nail**

√7ᵗʰ **S61.343** **Puncture wound with foreign body of left middle finger with damage to nail**

√7ᵗʰ **S61.344** **Puncture wound with foreign body of right ring finger with damage to nail**

√7ᵗʰ **S61.345** **Puncture wound with foreign body of left ring finger with damage to nail**

√7ᵗʰ **S61.346** **Puncture wound with foreign body of right little finger with damage to nail**

√7ᵗʰ **S61.347** **Puncture wound with foreign body of left little finger with damage to nail**

√7ᵗʰ **S61.348** **Puncture wound with foreign body of other finger with damage to nail**
Puncture wound with foreign body of specified finger with unspecified laterality with damage to nail

√7ᵗʰ **S61.349** **Puncture wound with foreign body of unspecified finger with damage to nail**

√6ᵗʰ **S61.35** **Open bite of finger with damage to nail**
Bite of finger with damage to nail NOS
EXCLUDES 1 *superficial bite of finger (S60.46-, S60.47-)*

√7ᵗʰ **S61.350** **Open bite of right index finger with damage to nail**

√7ᵗʰ **S61.351** **Open bite of left index finger with damage to nail**

√7ᵗʰ **S61.352** **Open bite of right middle finger with damage to nail**

√7ᵗʰ **S61.353** **Open bite of left middle finger with damage to nail**

√7ᵗʰ **S61.354** **Open bite of right ring finger with damage to nail**

√7ᵗʰ **S61.355** **Open bite of left ring finger with damage to nail**

√7ᵗʰ **S61.356** **Open bite of right little finger with damage to nail**

√7ᵗʰ **S61.357** **Open bite of left little finger with damage to nail**

√7ᵗʰ **S61.358** **Open bite of other finger with damage to nail**
Open bite of specified finger with unspecified laterality with damage to nail

√7ᵗʰ **S61.359** **Open bite of unspecified finger with damage to nail**

√5ᵗʰ **S61.4** **Open wound of hand**

√6ᵗʰ **S61.40** **Unspecified open wound of hand**

√7ᵗʰ **S61.401** **Unspecified open wound of right hand**

√7ᵗʰ **S61.402** **Unspecified open wound of left hand**

√7ᵗʰ **S61.409** **Unspecified open wound of unspecified hand**

√6ᵗʰ **S61.41** **Laceration without foreign body of hand**

√7ᵗʰ **S61.411** **Laceration without foreign body of right hand**

√7ᵗʰ **S61.412** **Laceration without foreign body of left hand**

√7ᵗʰ **S61.419** **Laceration without foreign body of unspecified hand**

√6ᵗʰ **S61.42** **Laceration with foreign body of hand**

√7ᵗʰ **S61.421** **Laceration with foreign body of right hand**

√7ᵗʰ **S61.422** **Laceration with foreign body of left hand**

√7ᵗʰ **S61.429** **Laceration with foreign body of unspecified hand**

√6ᵗʰ **S61.43** **Puncture wound without foreign body of hand**

√7ᵗʰ **S61.431** **Puncture wound without foreign body of right hand**

√7ᵗʰ **S61.432** **Puncture wound without foreign body of left hand**

√7ᵗʰ **S61.439** **Puncture wound without foreign body of unspecified hand**

√6ᵗʰ **S61.44** **Puncture wound with foreign body of hand**

√7ᵗʰ **S61.441** **Puncture wound with foreign body of right hand**

√7ᵗʰ **S61.442** **Puncture wound with foreign body of left hand**

√7ᵗʰ **S61.449** **Puncture wound with foreign body of unspecified hand**

√6ᵗʰ **S61.45** **Open bite of hand**
Bite of hand NOS
EXCLUDES 1 *superficial bite of hand (S60.56-, S60.57-)*

√7ᵗʰ **S61.451** **Open bite of right hand**

√7ᵗʰ **S61.452** **Open bite of left hand**

√7ᵗʰ **S61.459** **Open bite of unspecified hand**

√5ᵗʰ **S61.5** **Open wound of wrist**

√6ᵗʰ **S61.50** **Unspecified open wound of wrist**

√7ᵗʰ **S61.501** **Unspecified open wound of right wrist**

√7ᵗʰ **S61.502** **Unspecified open wound of left wrist**

√7ᵗʰ **S61.509** **Unspecified open wound of unspecified wrist**

√6ᵗʰ **S61.51** **Laceration without foreign body of wrist**

√7ᵗʰ **S61.511** **Laceration without foreign body of right wrist**

√7ᵗʰ **S61.512** **Laceration without foreign body of left wrist**

√7ᵗʰ **S61.519** **Laceration without foreign body of unspecified wrist**

√6ᵗʰ **S61.52** **Laceration with foreign body of wrist**

√7ᵗʰ **S61.521** **Laceration with foreign body of right wrist**

√7ᵗʰ **S61.522** **Laceration with foreign body of left wrist**

√7ᵗʰ **S61.529** **Laceration with foreign body of unspecified wrist**

√6ᵗʰ **S61.53** **Puncture wound without foreign body of wrist**

√7ᵗʰ **S61.531** **Puncture wound without foreign body of right wrist**

√7ᵗʰ **S61.532** **Puncture wound without foreign body of left wrist**

√7ᵗʰ **S61.539** **Puncture wound without foreign body of unspecified wrist**

√6ᵗʰ **S61.54** **Puncture wound with foreign body of wrist**

√7ᵗʰ **S61.541** **Puncture wound with foreign body of right wrist**

√7ᵗʰ **S61.542** **Puncture wound with foreign body of left wrist**

√7ᵗʰ **S61.549** **Puncture wound with foreign body of unspecified wrist**

√6ᵗʰ **S61.55** **Open bite of wrist**
Bite of wrist NOS
EXCLUDES 1 *superficial bite of wrist (S60.86-, S60.87-)*

√7ᵗʰ **S61.551** **Open bite of right wrist**

√7ᵗʰ **S61.552** **Open bite of left wrist**

√7ᵗʰ **S61.559** **Open bite of unspecified wrist**

✅ Additional Character Required   √x7ᵗʰ Placeholder Alert   Unacceptable PDx   Manifestation   Hospital Acquired Condition   **EXCLUDES 1** Not Coded Here   **EXCLUDES 2** Not Included Here

Chapter 19. Injury, Poisoning, and Certain Other Consequences of External Causes *(side margin)*

S62.135 *(side margin)*

✔4th S62 Fracture at wrist and hand level

NOTE   A fracture not indicated as displaced or nondisplaced should be coded to displaced.
A fracture not indicated as open or closed should be coded to closed.

EXCLUDES 1   *traumatic amputation of wrist and hand (S68.-)*
EXCLUDES 2   *fracture of distal parts of ulna and radius (S52.-)*

The appropriate 7th is to be added to each code from category S62.
A   initial encounter for closed fracture
B   initial encounter for open fracture
D   subsequent encounter for fracture with routine healing
G   subsequent encounter for fracture with delayed healing
K   subsequent encounter for fracture with nonunion
P   subsequent encounter for fracture with malunion
S   sequela

✔5th S62.0 Fracture of navicular [scaphoid] bone of wrist

CC Excl: For CC codes in subcategory S62.0, unless otherwise noted: CC with 7th character B: S62.001-S62.186 with 7th [A, B]
CC with 7th character K or P: M80.00X-M84.68X with 7th [K, P], S02.0XX-S02.92X with 7th K, S12.000-S12.691 with 7th K, S22.000-S22.9XX with 7th K, S32.000-S32.9XX with 7th K, S42.001-S42.92X with 7th [K, P], S49.001-S49.199 with 7th [K, P], S52.001-S52.92X with 7th [K, M, N, P, Q, R], S59.001-S59.299 with 7th [K, P], S62.001-S62.92X with 7th [K, P], S72.001-S72.92X with 7th [K, M, N, P, Q, R], S79.001-S79.199 with 7th [K, P], S82.001-S82.92X with 7th [K, M, N, P, Q, R], S89.001-S89.399 with 7th [K, P], S92.001-S92.919 with 7th [K, P]

✔6th S62.00 Unspecified fracture of navicular [scaphoid] bone of wrist

15,20 ✔7th **S62.001**   **Unspecified fracture of navicular [scaphoid] bone of right wrist**   CC

15,20 ✔7th **S62.002**   **Unspecified fracture of navicular [scaphoid] bone of left wrist**   CC
     AHA: 2012, 4Q, 106

15,20 ✔7th **S62.009**   **Unspecified fracture of navicular [scaphoid] bone of unspecified wrist**   CC

✔6th S62.01 Fracture of distal pole of navicular [scaphoid] bone of wrist

Fracture of volar tuberosity of navicular [scaphoid] bone of wrist

15,20 ✔7th **S62.011**   **Displaced fracture of distal pole of navicular [scaphoid] bone of right wrist**   CC

15,20 ✔7th **S62.012**   **Displaced fracture of distal pole of navicular [scaphoid] bone of left wrist**   CC

15,20 ✔7th **S62.013**   **Displaced fracture of distal pole of navicular [scaphoid] bone of unspecified wrist**   CC

15,20 ✔7th **S62.014**   **Nondisplaced fracture of distal pole of navicular [scaphoid] bone of right wrist**   CC

15,20 ✔7th **S62.015**   **Nondisplaced fracture of distal pole of navicular [scaphoid] bone of left wrist**   CC

15,20 ✔7th **S62.016**   **Nondisplaced fracture of distal pole of navicular [scaphoid] bone of unspecified wrist**   CC

✔6th S62.02 Fracture of middle third of navicular [scaphoid] bone of wrist

15,20 ✔7th **S62.021**   **Displaced fracture of middle third of navicular [scaphoid] bone of right wrist**   CC

15,20 ✔7th **S62.022**   **Displaced fracture of middle third of navicular [scaphoid] bone of left wrist**   CC

15,20 ✔7th **S62.023**   **Displaced fracture of middle third of navicular [scaphoid] bone of unspecified wrist**   CC

15,20 ✔7th **S62.024**   **Nondisplaced fracture of middle third of navicular [scaphoid] bone of right wrist**   CC

15,20 ✔7th **S62.025**   **Nondisplaced fracture of middle third of navicular [scaphoid] bone of left wrist**   CC

15,20 ✔7th **S62.026**   **Nondisplaced fracture of middle third of navicular [scaphoid] bone of unspecified wrist**   CC

✔6th S62.03 Fracture of proximal third of navicular [scaphoid] bone of wrist

15,20 ✔7th **S62.031**   **Displaced fracture of proximal third of navicular [scaphoid] bone of right wrist**   CC

15,20 ✔7th **S62.032**   **Displaced fracture of proximal third of navicular [scaphoid] bone of left wrist**   CC

15,20 ✔7th **S62.033**   **Displaced fracture of proximal third of navicular [scaphoid] bone of unspecified wrist**   CC

15,20 ✔7th **S62.034**   **Nondisplaced fracture of proximal third of navicular [scaphoid] bone of right wrist**   CC

15,20 ✔7th **S62.035**   **Nondisplaced fracture of proximal third of navicular [scaphoid] bone of left wrist**   CC

15,20 ✔7th **S62.036**   **Nondisplaced fracture of proximal third of navicular [scaphoid] bone of unspecified wrist**   CC

✔5th S62.1 Fracture of other and unspecified carpal bone(s)

EXCLUDES 2   *fracture of scaphoid of wrist (S62.0-)*

S62.1 CC Excl: For CC codes in subcategory S62.1, unless otherwise noted: See code: S62.0

✔6th S62.10 Fracture of unspecified carpal bone

Fracture of wrist NOS

15,20 ✔7th **S62.101**   **Fracture of unspecified carpal bone, right wrist**   CC

15,20 ✔7th **S62.102**   **Fracture of unspecified carpal bone, left wrist**   CC
     AHA: 2012, 4Q, 95

15,20 ✔7th **S62.109**   **Fracture of unspecified carpal bone, unspecified wrist**   CC

✔6th S62.11 Fracture of triquetrum [cuneiform] bone of wrist

15,20 ✔7th **S62.111**   **Displaced fracture of triquetrum [cuneiform] bone, right wrist**   CC

15,20 ✔7th **S62.112**   **Displaced fracture of triquetrum [cuneiform] bone, left wrist**   CC

15,20 ✔7th **S62.113**   **Displaced fracture of triquetrum [cuneiform] bone, unspecified wrist**   CC

15,20 ✔7th **S62.114**   **Nondisplaced fracture of triquetrum [cuneiform] bone, right wrist**   CC

15,20 ✔7th **S62.115**   **Nondisplaced fracture of triquetrum [cuneiform] bone, left wrist**   CC

15,20 ✔7th **S62.116**   **Nondisplaced fracture of triquetrum [cuneiform] bone, unspecified wrist**   CC

✔6th S62.12 Fracture of lunate [semilunar]

15,20 ✔7th **S62.121**   **Displaced fracture of lunate [semilunar], right wrist**   CC

15,20 ✔7th **S62.122**   **Displaced fracture of lunate [semilunar], left wrist**   CC

15,20 ✔7th **S62.123**   **Displaced fracture of lunate [semilunar], unspecified wrist**   CC

15,20 ✔7th **S62.124**   **Nondisplaced fracture of lunate [semilunar], right wrist**   CC

15,20 ✔7th **S62.125**   **Nondisplaced fracture of lunate [semilunar], left wrist**   CC

15,20 ✔7th **S62.126**   **Nondisplaced fracture of lunate [semilunar], unspecified wrist**   CC

✔6th S62.13 Fracture of capitate [os magnum] bone

15,20 ✔7th **S62.131**   **Displaced fracture of capitate [os magnum] bone, right wrist**   CC

15,20 ✔7th **S62.132**   **Displaced fracture of capitate [os magnum] bone, left wrist**   CC

15,20 ✔7th **S62.133**   **Displaced fracture of capitate [os magnum] bone, unspecified wrist**   CC

15,20 ✔7th **S62.134**   **Nondisplaced fracture of capitate [os magnum] bone, right wrist**   CC

15,20 ✔7th **S62.135**   **Nondisplaced fracture of capitate [os magnum] bone, left wrist**   CC

---

15 HAC = Initial encounter for open fracture only (7th character B or C – specific to category) and not POA.
20 CC only if an initial encounter for an open fracture (7th character B or C – specific to category) **OR** a subsequent encounter for nonunion or malunion (7th character K, M, N, P, Q, or R – specific to category).

N Newborn: 0   P Pediatric: 0-17   M Maternity: 12-55   A Adult: 15-124   MCC Major CC Condition   PDxMCC PDx acts as own MCC   CC CC Condition   PDxCC PDx acts as own CC

992   ICD-10-CM 2016

15,20 ✓7ᵗʰ **S62.136** Nondisplaced fracture of capitate [os magnum] bone, unspecified wrist `CC`

✓6ᵗʰ **S62.14** Fracture of body of hamate [unciform] bone
Fracture of hamate [unciform] bone NOS

   15,20 ✓7ᵗʰ **S62.141** Displaced fracture of body of hamate [unciform] bone, right wrist `CC`

   15,20 ✓7ᵗʰ **S62.142** Displaced fracture of body of hamate [unciform] bone, left wrist `CC`

   15,20 ✓7ᵗʰ **S62.143** Displaced fracture of body of hamate [unciform] bone, unspecified wrist `CC`

   15,20 ✓7ᵗʰ **S62.144** Nondisplaced fracture of body of hamate [unciform] bone, right wrist `CC`

   15,20 ✓7ᵗʰ **S62.145** Nondisplaced fracture of body of hamate [unciform] bone, left wrist `CC`

   15,20 ✓7ᵗʰ **S62.146** Nondisplaced fracture of body of hamate [unciform] bone, unspecified wrist `CC`

✓6ᵗʰ **S62.15** Fracture of hook process of hamate [unciform] bone
Fracture of unciform process of hamate [unciform] bone

   15,20 ✓7ᵗʰ **S62.151** Displaced fracture of hook process of hamate [unciform] bone, right wrist `CC`

   15,20 ✓7ᵗʰ **S62.152** Displaced fracture of hook process of hamate [unciform] bone, left wrist `CC`

   15,20 ✓7ᵗʰ **S62.153** Displaced fracture of hook process of hamate [unciform] bone, unspecified wrist `CC`

   15,20 ✓7ᵗʰ **S62.154** Nondisplaced fracture of hook process of hamate [unciform] bone, right wrist `CC`

   15,20 ✓7ᵗʰ **S62.155** Nondisplaced fracture of hook process of hamate [unciform] bone, left wrist `CC`

   15,20 ✓7ᵗʰ **S62.156** Nondisplaced fracture of hook process of hamate [unciform] bone, unspecified wrist `CC`

✓6ᵗʰ **S62.16** Fracture of pisiform

   15,20 ✓7ᵗʰ **S62.161** Displaced fracture of pisiform, right wrist `CC`

   15,20 ✓7ᵗʰ **S62.162** Displaced fracture of pisiform, left wrist `CC`

   15,20 ✓7ᵗʰ **S62.163** Displaced fracture of pisiform, unspecified wrist `CC`

   15,20 ✓7ᵗʰ **S62.164** Nondisplaced fracture of pisiform, right wrist `CC`

   15,20 ✓7ᵗʰ **S62.165** Nondisplaced fracture of pisiform, left wrist `CC`

   15,20 ✓7ᵗʰ **S62.166** Nondisplaced fracture of pisiform, unspecified wrist `CC`

✓6ᵗʰ **S62.17** Fracture of trapezium [larger multangular]

   15,20 ✓7ᵗʰ **S62.171** Displaced fracture of trapezium [larger multangular], right wrist `CC`

   15,20 ✓7ᵗʰ **S62.172** Displaced fracture of trapezium [larger multangular], left wrist `CC`

   15,20 ✓7ᵗʰ **S62.173** Displaced fracture of trapezium [larger multangular], unspecified wrist `CC`

   15,20 ✓7ᵗʰ **S62.174** Nondisplaced fracture of trapezium [larger multangular], right wrist `CC`

   15,20 ✓7ᵗʰ **S62.175** Nondisplaced fracture of trapezium [larger multangular], left wrist `CC`

   15,20 ✓7ᵗʰ **S62.176** Nondisplaced fracture of trapezium [larger multangular], unspecified wrist `CC`

✓6ᵗʰ **S62.18** Fracture of trapezoid [smaller multangular]

   15,20 ✓7ᵗʰ **S62.181** Displaced fracture of trapezoid [smaller multangular], right wrist `CC`

   15,20 ✓7ᵗʰ **S62.182** Displaced fracture of trapezoid [smaller multangular], left wrist `CC`

   15,20 ✓7ᵗʰ **S62.183** Displaced fracture of trapezoid [smaller multangular], unspecified wrist `CC`

   15,20 ✓7ᵗʰ **S62.184** Nondisplaced fracture of trapezoid [smaller multangular], right wrist `CC`

15,20 ✓7ᵗʰ **S62.185** Nondisplaced fracture of trapezoid [smaller multangular], left wrist `CC`

15,20 ✓7ᵗʰ **S62.186** Nondisplaced fracture of trapezoid [smaller multangular], unspecified wrist `CC`

✓5ᵗʰ **S62.2** Fracture of first metacarpal bone

> **S62.2 CC Excl: For CC codes in subcategory S62.2, unless otherwise noted: CC with 7th character B:** S62.201-S62.399 with 7th [A, B], S62.90X with 7th A
> **CC with 7th character K or P:** M80.00X-M84.68X with 7th [K, P], S02.0XX-S02.92X with 7th K, S12.000-S12.691 with 7th K, S22.000-S22.9XX with 7th K, S32.000-S32.9XX with 7th K, S42.001-S42.92X with 7th [K, P], S49.001-S49.199 with 7th [K, P], S52.001-S52.92X with 7th [K, M, N, P, Q, R], S59.001-S59.299 with 7th [K, P], S62.001-S62.92X with 7th [K, P], S72.001-S72.92X with 7th [K, M, N, P, Q, R], S79.001-S79.199 with 7th [K, P], S82.001-S82.92X with 7th [K, M, N, P, Q, R], S89.001-S89.399 with 7th [K, P], S92.001-S92.919 with 7th [K, P]

✓6ᵗʰ **S62.20** Unspecified fracture of first metacarpal bone

   15,20 ✓7ᵗʰ **S62.201** Unspecified fracture of first metacarpal bone, right hand `CC`

   15,20 ✓7ᵗʰ **S62.202** Unspecified fracture of first metacarpal bone, left hand `CC`

   15,20 ✓7ᵗʰ **S62.209** Unspecified fracture of first metacarpal bone, unspecified hand `CC`

✓6ᵗʰ **S62.21** Bennett's fracture

   15,20 ✓7ᵗʰ **S62.211** Bennett's fracture, right hand `CC`

   15,20 ✓7ᵗʰ **S62.212** Bennett's fracture, left hand `CC`

   15,20 ✓7ᵗʰ **S62.213** Bennett's fracture, unspecified hand `CC`

✓6ᵗʰ **S62.22** Rolando's fracture

   15,20 ✓7ᵗʰ **S62.221** Displaced Rolando's fracture, right hand `CC`

   15,20 ✓7ᵗʰ **S62.222** Displaced Rolando's fracture, left hand `CC`

   15,20 ✓7ᵗʰ **S62.223** Displaced Rolando's fracture, unspecified hand `CC`

   15,20 ✓7ᵗʰ **S62.224** Nondisplaced Rolando's fracture, right hand `CC`

   15,20 ✓7ᵗʰ **S62.225** Nondisplaced Rolando's fracture, left hand `CC`

   15,20 ✓7ᵗʰ **S62.226** Nondisplaced Rolando's fracture, unspecified hand `CC`

✓6ᵗʰ **S62.23** Other fracture of base of first metacarpal bone

   15,20 ✓7ᵗʰ **S62.231** Other displaced fracture of base of first metacarpal bone, right hand `CC`

   15,20 ✓7ᵗʰ **S62.232** Other displaced fracture of base of first metacarpal bone, left hand `CC`

   15,20 ✓7ᵗʰ **S62.233** Other displaced fracture of base of first metacarpal bone, unspecified hand `CC`

   15,20 ✓7ᵗʰ **S62.234** Other nondisplaced fracture of base of first metacarpal bone, right hand `CC`

   15,20 ✓7ᵗʰ **S62.235** Other nondisplaced fracture of base of first metacarpal bone, left hand `CC`

   15,20 ✓7ᵗʰ **S62.236** Other nondisplaced fracture of base of first metacarpal bone, unspecified hand `CC`

✓6ᵗʰ **S62.24** Fracture of shaft of first metacarpal bone

   15,20 ✓7ᵗʰ **S62.241** Displaced fracture of shaft of first metacarpal bone, right hand `CC`

   15,20 ✓7ᵗʰ **S62.242** Displaced fracture of shaft of first metacarpal bone, left hand `CC`

   15,20 ✓7ᵗʰ **S62.243** Displaced fracture of shaft of first metacarpal bone, unspecified hand `CC`

   15,20 ✓7ᵗʰ **S62.244** Nondisplaced fracture of shaft of first metacarpal bone, right hand `CC`

   15,20 ✓7ᵗʰ **S62.245** Nondisplaced fracture of shaft of first metacarpal bone, left hand `CC`

   15,20 ✓7ᵗʰ **S62.246** Nondisplaced fracture of shaft of first metacarpal bone, unspecified hand `CC`

✓6ᵗʰ **S62.25** Fracture of neck of first metacarpal bone

   15,20 ✓7ᵗʰ **S62.251** Displaced fracture of neck of first metacarpal bone, right hand `CC`

---

15 HAC = Initial encounter for open fracture only (7th character B or C – specific to category) and not POA.
20 CC only if an initial encounter for an open fracture (7th character B or C– specific to category) **OR** a subsequent encounter for nonunion or malunion (7th character K, M, N, P, Q, or R – specific to category).

✓ Additional Character Required   ✓ₓ7ᵗʰ Placeholder Alert   Unacceptable PDx   Manifestation   Hospital Acquired Condition   **EXCLUDES 1** Not Coded Here   **EXCLUDES 2** Not Included Here

15,20 ✓7th **S62.252** **Displaced fracture of neck of first metacarpal bone, left hand** CC

15,20 ✓7th **S62.253** **Displaced fracture of neck of first metacarpal bone, unspecified hand**

15,20 ✓7th **S62.254** **Nondisplaced fracture of neck of first metacarpal bone, right hand** CC

15,20 ✓7th **S62.255** **Nondisplaced fracture of neck of first metacarpal bone, left hand**

15,20 ✓7th **S62.256** **Nondisplaced fracture of neck of first metacarpal bone, unspecified hand** CC

✓6th **S62.29** **Other fracture of first metacarpal bone**

15,20 ✓7th **S62.291** **Other fracture of first metacarpal bone, right hand** CC

15,20 ✓7th **S62.292** **Other fracture of first metacarpal bone, left hand** CC

15,20 ✓7th **S62.299** **Other fracture of first metacarpal bone, unspecified hand** CC

✓5th **S62.3** **Fracture of other and unspecified metacarpal bone**
> EXCLUDES2   *fracture of first metacarpal bone (S62.2-)*
>
> **CC Excl: For CC codes in subcategory S62.3, unless otherwise noted: See code: S62.2**

✓6th **S62.30** **Unspecified fracture of other metacarpal bone**

15,20 ✓7th **S62.300** **Unspecified fracture of second metacarpal bone, right hand** CC

15,20 ✓7th **S62.301** **Unspecified fracture of second metacarpal bone, left hand** CC

15,20 ✓7th **S62.302** **Unspecified fracture of third metacarpal bone, right hand** CC

15,20 ✓7th **S62.303** **Unspecified fracture of third metacarpal bone, left hand** CC

15,20 ✓7th **S62.304** **Unspecified fracture of fourth metacarpal bone, right hand** CC

15,20 ✓7th **S62.305** **Unspecified fracture of fourth metacarpal bone, left hand** CC

15,20 ✓7th **S62.306** **Unspecified fracture of fifth metacarpal bone, right hand** CC

15,20 ✓7th **S62.307** **Unspecified fracture of fifth metacarpal bone, left hand** CC

15,20 ✓7th **S62.308** **Unspecified fracture of other metacarpal bone** CC
> Unspecified fracture of specified metacarpal bone with unspecified laterality

15,20 ✓7th **S62.309** **Unspecified fracture of unspecified metacarpal bone** CC

✓6th **S62.31** **Displaced fracture of base of other metacarpal bone**

15,20 ✓7th **S62.310** **Displaced fracture of base of second metacarpal bone, right hand** CC

15,20 ✓7th **S62.311** **Displaced fracture of base of second metacarpal bone, left hand** CC

15,20 ✓7th **S62.312** **Displaced fracture of base of third metacarpal bone, right hand** CC

15,20 ✓7th **S62.313** **Displaced fracture of base of third metacarpal bone, left hand** CC

15,20 ✓7th **S62.314** **Displaced fracture of base of fourth metacarpal bone, right hand** CC

15,20 ✓7th **S62.315** **Displaced fracture of base of fourth metacarpal bone, left hand** CC

15,20 ✓7th **S62.316** **Displaced fracture of base of fifth metacarpal bone, right hand** CC

15,20 ✓7th **S62.317** **Displaced fracture of base of fifth metacarpal bone, left hand** CC

15,20 ✓7th **S62.318** **Displaced fracture of base of other metacarpal bone** CC
> Displaced fracture of base of specified metacarpal bone with unspecified laterality

15,20 ✓7th **S62.319** **Displaced fracture of base of unspecified metacarpal bone** CC

✓6th **S62.32** **Displaced fracture of shaft of other metacarpal bone**

15,20 ✓7th **S62.320** **Displaced fracture of shaft of second metacarpal bone, right hand** CC

15,20 ✓7th **S62.321** **Displaced fracture of shaft of second metacarpal bone, left hand** CC

15,20 ✓7th **S62.322** **Displaced fracture of shaft of third metacarpal bone, right hand** CC

15,20 ✓7th **S62.323** **Displaced fracture of shaft of third metacarpal bone, left hand** CC

15,20 ✓7th **S62.324** **Displaced fracture of shaft of fourth metacarpal bone, right hand** CC

15,20 ✓7th **S62.325** **Displaced fracture of shaft of fourth metacarpal bone, left hand** CC

15,20 ✓7th **S62.326** **Displaced fracture of shaft of fifth metacarpal bone, right hand** CC

15,20 ✓7th **S62.327** **Displaced fracture of shaft of fifth metacarpal bone, left hand** CC

15,20 ✓7th **S62.328** **Displaced fracture of shaft of other metacarpal bone** CC
> Displaced fracture of shaft of specified metacarpal bone with unspecified laterality

15,20 ✓7th **S62.329** **Displaced fracture of shaft of unspecified metacarpal bone** CC

✓6th **S62.33** **Displaced fracture of neck of other metacarpal bone**

15,20 ✓7th **S62.330** **Displaced fracture of neck of second metacarpal bone, right hand** CC

15,20 ✓7th **S62.331** **Displaced fracture of neck of second metacarpal bone, left hand** CC

15,20 ✓7th **S62.332** **Displaced fracture of neck of third metacarpal bone, right hand** CC

15,20 ✓7th **S62.333** **Displaced fracture of neck of third metacarpal bone, left hand** CC

15,20 ✓7th **S62.334** **Displaced fracture of neck of fourth metacarpal bone, right hand** CC

15,20 ✓7th **S62.335** **Displaced fracture of neck of fourth metacarpal bone, left hand** CC

15,20 ✓7th **S62.336** **Displaced fracture of neck of fifth metacarpal bone, right hand** CC

15,20 ✓7th **S62.337** **Displaced fracture of neck of fifth metacarpal bone, left hand** CC

15,20 ✓7th **S62.338** **Displaced fracture of neck of other metacarpal bone** CC
> Displaced fracture of neck of specified metacarpal bone with unspecified laterality

15,20 ✓7th **S62.339** **Displaced fracture of neck of unspecified metacarpal bone** CC

✓6th **S62.34** **Nondisplaced fracture of base of other metacarpal bone**

15,20 ✓7th **S62.340** **Nondisplaced fracture of base of second metacarpal bone, right hand** CC

15,20 ✓7th **S62.341** **Nondisplaced fracture of base of second metacarpal bone, left hand** CC

15,20 ✓7th **S62.342** **Nondisplaced fracture of base of third metacarpal bone, right hand** CC

15,20 ✓7th **S62.343** **Nondisplaced fracture of base of third metacarpal bone, left hand** CC

15,20 ✓7th **S62.344** **Nondisplaced fracture of base of fourth metacarpal bone, right hand** CC

15,20 ✓7th **S62.345** **Nondisplaced fracture of base of fourth metacarpal bone, left hand** CC

15,20 ✓7th **S62.346** **Nondisplaced fracture of base of fifth metacarpal bone, right hand** CC

15,20 ✓7th **S62.347** **Nondisplaced fracture of base of fifth metacarpal bone, left hand** CC

15,20 ✓7th **S62.348** **Nondisplaced fracture of base of other metacarpal bone** CC
> Nondisplaced fracture of base of specified metacarpal bone with unspecified laterality

15,20 ✓7th **S62.349** **Nondisplaced fracture of base of unspecified metacarpal bone** CC

✓6th **S62.35** **Nondisplaced fracture of shaft of other metacarpal bone**

15,20 ✓7th **S62.350** **Nondisplaced fracture of shaft of second metacarpal bone, right hand** CC

---

15 HAC = Initial encounter for open fracture only (7th character B or C – specific to category) and not POA.

20 CC only if an initial encounter for an open fracture (7th character B or C– specific to category) **OR** a subsequent encounter for nonunion or malunion (7th character K, M, N, P, Q, or R – specific to category).

Ⓝ Newborn: 0   Ⓟ Pediatric: 0-17   Ⓜ Maternity: 12-55   Ⓐ Adult: 15-124   **MCC** Major CC Condition   **PDxMCC** PDx acts as own MCC   **CC** CC Condition   **PDxCC** PDx acts as own CC

994   ICD-10-CM 2016

15,20 √7ᵗʰ **S62.351 Nondisplaced fracture of shaft of second metacarpal bone, left hand** CC

15,20 √7ᵗʰ **S62.352 Nondisplaced fracture of shaft of third metacarpal bone, right hand** CC

15,20 √7ᵗʰ **S62.353 Nondisplaced fracture of shaft of third metacarpal bone, left hand** CC

15,20 √7ᵗʰ **S62.354 Nondisplaced fracture of shaft of fourth metacarpal bone, right hand** CC

15,20 √7ᵗʰ **S62.355 Nondisplaced fracture of shaft of fourth metacarpal bone, left hand** CC

15,20 √7ᵗʰ **S62.356 Nondisplaced fracture of shaft of fifth metacarpal bone, right hand** CC

15,20 √7ᵗʰ **S62.357 Nondisplaced fracture of shaft of fifth metacarpal bone, left hand** CC

15,20 √7ᵗʰ **S62.358 Nondisplaced fracture of shaft of other metacarpal bone** CC
    Nondisplaced fracture of shaft of specified metacarpal bone with unspecified laterality

15,20 √7ᵗʰ **S62.359 Nondisplaced fracture of shaft of unspecified metacarpal bone** CC

√6ᵗʰ **S62.36 Nondisplaced fracture of neck of other metacarpal bone**

15,20 √7ᵗʰ **S62.360 Nondisplaced fracture of neck of second metacarpal bone, right hand** CC

15,20 √7ᵗʰ **S62.361 Nondisplaced fracture of neck of second metacarpal bone, left hand** CC

15,20 √7ᵗʰ **S62.362 Nondisplaced fracture of neck of third metacarpal bone, right hand** CC

15,20 √7ᵗʰ **S62.363 Nondisplaced fracture of neck of third metacarpal bone, left hand** CC

15,20 √7ᵗʰ **S62.364 Nondisplaced fracture of neck of fourth metacarpal bone, right hand** CC

15,20 √7ᵗʰ **S62.365 Nondisplaced fracture of neck of fourth metacarpal bone, left hand** CC

15,20 √7ᵗʰ **S62.366 Nondisplaced fracture of neck of fifth metacarpal bone, right hand** CC

15,20 √7ᵗʰ **S62.367 Nondisplaced fracture of neck of fifth metacarpal bone, left hand** CC

15,20 √7ᵗʰ **S62.368 Nondisplaced fracture of neck of other metacarpal bone** CC
    Nondisplaced fracture of neck of specified metacarpal bone with unspecified laterality

15,20 √7ᵗʰ **S62.369 Nondisplaced fracture of neck of unspecified metacarpal bone** CC

√6ᵗʰ **S62.39 Other fracture of other metacarpal bone**

15,20 √7ᵗʰ **S62.390 Other fracture of second metacarpal bone, right hand** CC

15,20 √7ᵗʰ **S62.391 Other fracture of second metacarpal bone, left hand** CC

15,20 √7ᵗʰ **S62.392 Other fracture of third metacarpal bone, right hand** CC

15,20 √7ᵗʰ **S62.393 Other fracture of third metacarpal bone, left hand** CC

15,20 √7ᵗʰ **S62.394 Other fracture of fourth metacarpal bone, right hand** CC

15,20 √7ᵗʰ **S62.395 Other fracture of fourth metacarpal bone, left hand** CC

15,20 √7ᵗʰ **S62.396 Other fracture of fifth metacarpal bone, right hand** CC

15,20 √7ᵗʰ **S62.397 Other fracture of fifth metacarpal bone, left hand** CC

15,20 √7ᵗʰ **S62.398 Other fracture of other metacarpal bone** CC
    Other fracture of specified metacarpal bone with unspecified laterality

15,20 √7ᵗʰ **S62.399 Other fracture of unspecified metacarpal bone** CC

√5ᵗʰ **S62.5 Fracture of thumb**

> **CC Excl:** For CC codes in subcategory S62.5, unless otherwise noted: CC CC with 7th character B: S62.501-S62.92X with 7th [A, B]
> **CC CC with 7th character K or P:** M80.00X-M84.68X with 7th [K, P], S02.0XX-S02.92X with 7th K, S12.000-S12.691 with 7th K, S22.000-S22.9XX with 7th K, S32.000-S32.9XX with 7th K, S42.001-S42.92X with 7th [K, P], S49.001-S49.199 with 7th [K, P], S52.001-S52.92X with 7th [K, M, N, P, Q, R], S59.001-S59.299 with 7th [K, P], S62.001-S62.92X with 7th [K, P], S72.001-S72.92X with 7th [K, M, N, P, Q, R], S79.001-S79.199 with 7th [K, P], S82.001-S82.92X with 7th [K, M, N, P, Q, R], S89.001-S89.399 with 7th [K, P], S92.001-S92.919 with 7th [K, P]

√6ᵗʰ **S62.50 Fracture of unspecified phalanx of thumb**

15,20 √7ᵗʰ **S62.501 Fracture of unspecified phalanx of right thumb** CC

15,20 √7ᵗʰ **S62.502 Fracture of unspecified phalanx of left thumb** CC

15,20 √7ᵗʰ **S62.509 Fracture of unspecified phalanx of unspecified thumb** CC

√6ᵗʰ **S62.51 Fracture of proximal phalanx of thumb**

15,20 √7ᵗʰ **S62.511 Displaced fracture of proximal phalanx of right thumb** CC

15,20 √7ᵗʰ **S62.512 Displaced fracture of proximal phalanx of left thumb** CC

15,20 √7ᵗʰ **S62.513 Displaced fracture of proximal phalanx of unspecified thumb** CC

15,20 √7ᵗʰ **S62.514 Nondisplaced fracture of proximal phalanx of right thumb** CC

15,20 √7ᵗʰ **S62.515 Nondisplaced fracture of proximal phalanx of left thumb** CC

15,20 √7ᵗʰ **S62.516 Nondisplaced fracture of proximal phalanx of unspecified thumb** CC

√6ᵗʰ **S62.52 Fracture of distal phalanx of thumb**

15,20 √7ᵗʰ **S62.521 Displaced fracture of distal phalanx of right thumb** CC

15,20 √7ᵗʰ **S62.522 Displaced fracture of distal phalanx of left thumb** CC

15,20 √7ᵗʰ **S62.523 Displaced fracture of distal phalanx of unspecified thumb** CC

15,20 √7ᵗʰ **S62.524 Nondisplaced fracture of distal phalanx of right thumb** CC

15,20 √7ᵗʰ **S62.525 Nondisplaced fracture of distal phalanx of left thumb** CC

15,20 √7ᵗʰ **S62.526 Nondisplaced fracture of distal phalanx of unspecified thumb** CC

√5ᵗʰ **S62.6 Fracture of other and unspecified finger(s)**
    EXCLUDES 2   *fracture of thumb (S62.5-)*

> **CC Excl:** For CC codes in subcategory S62.6, unless otherwise noted: See code: S62.2

√6ᵗʰ **S62.60 Fracture of unspecified phalanx of finger**

15,20 √7ᵗʰ **S62.600 Fracture of unspecified phalanx of right index finger** CC

15,20 √7ᵗʰ **S62.601 Fracture of unspecified phalanx of left index finger** CC

15,20 √7ᵗʰ **S62.602 Fracture of unspecified phalanx of right middle finger** CC

15,20 √7ᵗʰ **S62.603 Fracture of unspecified phalanx of left middle finger** CC

15,20 √7ᵗʰ **S62.604 Fracture of unspecified phalanx of right ring finger** CC

15,20 √7ᵗʰ **S62.605 Fracture of unspecified phalanx of left ring finger** CC

15,20 √7ᵗʰ **S62.606 Fracture of unspecified phalanx of right little finger** CC

15,20 √7ᵗʰ **S62.607 Fracture of unspecified phalanx of left little finger** CC

15,20 √7ᵗʰ **S62.608 Fracture of unspecified phalanx of other finger** CC
    Fracture of unspecified phalanx of specified finger with unspecified laterality

---

15 HAC = Initial encounter for open fracture only (7th character B or C – specific to category) and not POA.
20 CC only if an initial encounter for an open fracture (7th character B or C– specific to category) OR a subsequent encounter for nonunion or malunion (7th character K, M, N, P, Q, or R – specific to category).

☑ Additional Character Required   ✗x7ᵗʰ Placeholder Alert   Unacceptable PDx   Manifestation   Hospital Acquired Condition   EXCLUDES 1 Not Coded Here   EXCLUDES 2 Not Included Here

Chapter 19. Injury, Poisoning, and Certain Other Consequences of External Causes

S62.609–S62.669

15,20 ✓7th **S62.609 Fracture of unspecified phalanx of unspecified finger** CC

✓6th **S62.61 Displaced fracture of proximal phalanx of finger**

15,20 ✓7th **S62.610 Displaced fracture of proximal phalanx of right index finger** CC

15,20 ✓7th **S62.611 Displaced fracture of proximal phalanx of left index finger** CC

15,20 ✓7th **S62.612 Displaced fracture of proximal phalanx of right middle finger** CC

15,20 ✓7th **S62.613 Displaced fracture of proximal phalanx of left middle finger** CC

15,20 ✓7th **S62.614 Displaced fracture of proximal phalanx of right ring finger** CC

15,20 ✓7th **S62.615 Displaced fracture of proximal phalanx of left ring finger** CC

15,20 ✓7th **S62.616 Displaced fracture of proximal phalanx of right little finger** CC

15,20 ✓7th **S62.617 Displaced fracture of proximal phalanx of left little finger** CC

15,20 ✓7th **S62.618 Displaced fracture of proximal phalanx of other finger** CC
     Displaced fracture of proximal phalanx of specified finger with unspecified laterality

15,20 ✓7th **S62.619 Displaced fracture of proximal phalanx of unspecified finger** CC

✓6th **S62.62 Displaced fracture of medial phalanx of finger**

15,20 ✓7th **S62.620 Displaced fracture of medial phalanx of right index finger** CC

15,20 ✓7th **S62.621 Displaced fracture of medial phalanx of left index finger** CC

15,20 ✓7th **S62.622 Displaced fracture of medial phalanx of right middle finger** CC

15,20 ✓7th **S62.623 Displaced fracture of medial phalanx of left middle finger** CC

15,20 ✓7th **S62.624 Displaced fracture of medial phalanx of right ring finger** CC

15,20 ✓7th **S62.625 Displaced fracture of medial phalanx of left ring finger** CC

15,20 ✓7th **S62.626 Displaced fracture of medial phalanx of right little finger** CC

15,20 ✓7th **S62.627 Displaced fracture of medial phalanx of left little finger** CC

15,20 ✓7th **S62.628 Displaced fracture of medial phalanx of other finger** CC
     Displaced fracture of medial phalanx of specified finger with unspecified laterality

15,20 ✓7th **S62.629 Displaced fracture of medial phalanx of unspecified finger** CC

✓6th **S62.63 Displaced fracture of distal phalanx of finger**

15,20 ✓7th **S62.630 Displaced fracture of distal phalanx of right index finger** CC

15,20 ✓7th **S62.631 Displaced fracture of distal phalanx of left index finger** CC

15,20 ✓7th **S62.632 Displaced fracture of distal phalanx of right middle finger** CC

15,20 ✓7th **S62.633 Displaced fracture of distal phalanx of left middle finger** CC

15,20 ✓7th **S62.634 Displaced fracture of distal phalanx of right ring finger** CC

15,20 ✓7th **S62.635 Displaced fracture of distal phalanx of left ring finger** CC

15,20 ✓7th **S62.636 Displaced fracture of distal phalanx of right little finger** CC

15,20 ✓7th **S62.637 Displaced fracture of distal phalanx of left little finger** CC

15,20 ✓7th **S62.638 Displaced fracture of distal phalanx of other finger** CC
     Displaced fracture of distal phalanx of specified finger with unspecified laterality

15,20 ✓7th **S62.639 Displaced fracture of distal phalanx of unspecified finger** CC

✓6th **S62.64 Nondisplaced fracture of proximal phalanx of finger**

15,20 ✓7th **S62.640 Nondisplaced fracture of proximal phalanx of right index finger** CC

15,20 ✓7th **S62.641 Nondisplaced fracture of proximal phalanx of left index finger** CC

15,20 ✓7th **S62.642 Nondisplaced fracture of proximal phalanx of right middle finger** CC

15,20 ✓7th **S62.643 Nondisplaced fracture of proximal phalanx of left middle finger** CC

15,20 ✓7th **S62.644 Nondisplaced fracture of proximal phalanx of right ring finger** CC

15,20 ✓7th **S62.645 Nondisplaced fracture of proximal phalanx of left ring finger** CC

15,20 ✓7th **S62.646 Nondisplaced fracture of proximal phalanx of right little finger** CC

15,20 ✓7th **S62.647 Nondisplaced fracture of proximal phalanx of left little finger** CC

15,20 ✓7th **S62.648 Nondisplaced fracture of proximal phalanx of other finger** CC
     Nondisplaced fracture of proximal phalanx of specified finger with unspecified laterality

15,20 ✓7th **S62.649 Nondisplaced fracture of proximal phalanx of unspecified finger** CC

✓6th **S62.65 Nondisplaced fracture of medial phalanx of finger**

15,20 ✓7th **S62.650 Nondisplaced fracture of medial phalanx of right index finger** CC

15,20 ✓7th **S62.651 Nondisplaced fracture of medial phalanx of left index finger** CC

15,20 ✓7th **S62.652 Nondisplaced fracture of medial phalanx of right middle finger** CC

15,20 ✓7th **S62.653 Nondisplaced fracture of medial phalanx of left middle finger** CC

15,20 ✓7th **S62.654 Nondisplaced fracture of medial phalanx of right ring finger** CC

15,20 ✓7th **S62.655 Nondisplaced fracture of medial phalanx of left ring finger** CC

15,20 ✓7th **S62.656 Nondisplaced fracture of medial phalanx of right little finger** CC

15,20 ✓7th **S62.657 Nondisplaced fracture of medial phalanx of left little finger** CC

15,20 ✓7th **S62.658 Nondisplaced fracture of medial phalanx of other finger** CC
     Nondisplaced fracture of medial phalanx of specified finger with unspecified laterality

15,20 ✓7th **S62.659 Nondisplaced fracture of medial phalanx of unspecified finger** CC

✓6th **S62.66 Nondisplaced fracture of distal phalanx of finger**

15,20 ✓7th **S62.660 Nondisplaced fracture of distal phalanx of right index finger** CC

15,20 ✓7th **S62.661 Nondisplaced fracture of distal phalanx of left index finger** CC

15,20 ✓7th **S62.662 Nondisplaced fracture of distal phalanx of right middle finger** CC

15,20 ✓7th **S62.663 Nondisplaced fracture of distal phalanx of left middle finger** CC

15,20 ✓7th **S62.664 Nondisplaced fracture of distal phalanx of right ring finger** CC

15,20 ✓7th **S62.665 Nondisplaced fracture of distal phalanx of left ring finger** CC

15,20 ✓7th **S62.666 Nondisplaced fracture of distal phalanx of right little finger** CC

15,20 ✓7th **S62.667 Nondisplaced fracture of distal phalanx of left little finger** CC

15,20 ✓7th **S62.668 Nondisplaced fracture of distal phalanx of other finger** CC
     Nondisplaced fracture of distal phalanx of specified finger with unspecified laterality

15,20 ✓7th **S62.669 Nondisplaced fracture of distal phalanx of unspecified finger** CC

---

15 HAC = Initial encounter for open fracture only (7th character B or C – specific to category) and not POA.

20 CC only if an initial encounter for an open fracture (7th character B or C– specific to category) **OR** a subsequent encounter for nonunion or malunion (7th character K, M, N, P, Q, or R – specific to category).

Ⓝ Newborn: 0   Ⓟ Pediatric: 0-17   Ⓜ Maternity: 12-55   Ⓐ Adult: 15-124   MCC Major CC Condition   PDxMCC PDx acts as own MCC   CC CC Condition   PDxCC PDx acts as own CC

✓5ᵗʰ **S62.9**   Unspecified fracture of wrist and hand

15,20 ✓x7ᵗʰ **S62.90**   **Unspecified fracture of unspecified wrist and hand**   CC
CC Excl: CC CC with 7th character B: S42.201-S42.92X with 7th [A, B], S49.001-S49.199 with 7th A, S52.001-S52.009 with 7th [A, B, C], S52.021-S52.109 with 7th [A, B, C], S52.121-S52.516 with 7th [A, B, C], S52.531-S52.616 with 7th [A, B, C], S52.691-S52.92X with 7th [A, B, C], S59.001-S59.299 with 7th A, S62.001-S62.92X with 7th [A, B]
CC CC with 7th character K or P: M80.00X-M84.68X with 7th [K, P], S02.0XX-S02.92X with 7th K, S12.000-S12.691 with 7th K, S22.000-S22.9XX with 7th K, S32.000-S32.9XX with 7th K, S42.001-S42.92X with 7th [K, P], S49.001-S49.199 with 7th [K, P], S52.001-S52.92X with 7th [K, M, N, P, Q, R], S59.001-S59.299 with 7th [K, P], S62.001-S62.92X with 7th [K, P], S72.001-S72.92X with 7th [K, M, N, P, Q, R], S79.001-S79.199 with 7th [K, P], S82.001-S82.92X with 7th [K, M, N, P, Q, R], S89.001-S89.399 with 7th [K, P], S92.001-S92.919 with 7th [K, P]

15,20 ✓x7ᵗʰ **S62.91**   **Unspecified fracture of right wrist and hand**   CC
CC Excl: CC CC with 7th character B: S62.501-S62.92X with 7th [A, B]
CC CC with 7th character K or P: M80.00X-M84.68X with 7th [K, P], S02.0XX-S02.92X with 7th K, S12.000-S12.691 with 7th K, S22.000-S22.9XX with 7th K, S32.000-S32.9XX with 7th K, S42.001-S42.92X with 7th [K, P], S49.001-S49.199 with 7th [K, P], S52.001-S52.92X with 7th [K, M, N, P, Q, R], S59.001-S59.299 with 7th [K, P], S62.001-S62.92X with 7th [K, P], S72.001-S72.92X with 7th [K, M, N, P, Q, R], S79.001-S79.199 with 7th [K, P], S82.001-S82.92X with 7th [K, M, N, P, Q, R], S89.001-S89.399 with 7th [K, P], S92.001-S92.919 with 7th [K, P]

15,20 ✓x7ᵗʰ **S62.92**   **Unspecified fracture of left wrist and hand**   CC
CC Excl: See code: S62.91

✓4ᵗʰ **S63**   **Dislocation and sprain of joints and ligaments at wrist and hand level**
INCLUDES   avulsion of joint or ligament at wrist and hand level
laceration of cartilage, joint or ligament at wrist and hand level
sprain of cartilage, joint or ligament at wrist and hand level
traumatic hemarthrosis of joint or ligament at wrist and hand level
traumatic rupture of joint or ligament at wrist and hand level
traumatic subluxation of joint or ligament at wrist and hand level
traumatic tear of joint or ligament at wrist and hand level
Code also any associated open wound
EXCLUDES 2   strain of muscle, fascia and tendon of wrist and hand (S66.-)

The appropriate 7th character is to be added to each code from category S63.
A   initial encounter
D   subsequent encounter
S   sequela

✓5ᵗʰ **S63.0**   **Subluxation and dislocation of wrist and hand joints**

✓6ᵗʰ **S63.00**   **Unspecified subluxation and dislocation of wrist and hand**
Dislocation of carpal bone NOS
Dislocation of distal end of radius NOS
Subluxation of carpal bone NOS
Subluxation of distal end of radius NOS

✓7ᵗʰ **S63.001**   Unspecified subluxation of right wrist and hand

✓7ᵗʰ **S63.002**   Unspecified subluxation of left wrist and hand

✓7ᵗʰ **S63.003**   Unspecified subluxation of unspecified wrist and hand

✓7ᵗʰ **S63.004**   Unspecified dislocation of right wrist and hand

✓7ᵗʰ **S63.005**   Unspecified dislocation of left wrist and hand

✓7ᵗʰ **S63.006**   Unspecified dislocation of unspecified wrist and hand

✓6ᵗʰ **S63.01**   **Subluxation and dislocation of distal radioulnar joint**

✓7ᵗʰ **S63.011**   Subluxation of distal radioulnar joint of right wrist

✓7ᵗʰ **S63.012**   Subluxation of distal radioulnar joint of left wrist

✓7ᵗʰ **S63.013**   Subluxation of distal radioulnar joint of unspecified wrist

✓7ᵗʰ **S63.014**   Dislocation of distal radioulnar joint of right wrist

✓7ᵗʰ **S63.015**   Dislocation of distal radioulnar joint of left wrist

✓7ᵗʰ **S63.016**   Dislocation of distal radioulnar joint of unspecified wrist

✓6ᵗʰ **S63.02**   **Subluxation and dislocation of radiocarpal joint**

✓7ᵗʰ **S63.021**   Subluxation of radiocarpal joint of right wrist

✓7ᵗʰ **S63.022**   Subluxation of radiocarpal joint of left wrist

✓7ᵗʰ **S63.023**   Subluxation of radiocarpal joint of unspecified wrist

✓7ᵗʰ **S63.024**   Dislocation of radiocarpal joint of right wrist

✓7ᵗʰ **S63.025**   Dislocation of radiocarpal joint of left wrist

✓7ᵗʰ **S63.026**   Dislocation of radiocarpal joint of unspecified wrist

✓6ᵗʰ **S63.03**   **Subluxation and dislocation of midcarpal joint**

✓7ᵗʰ **S63.031**   Subluxation of midcarpal joint of right wrist

✓7ᵗʰ **S63.032**   Subluxation of midcarpal joint of left wrist

✓7ᵗʰ **S63.033**   Subluxation of midcarpal joint of unspecified wrist

✓7ᵗʰ **S63.034**   Dislocation of midcarpal joint of right wrist

✓7ᵗʰ **S63.035**   Dislocation of midcarpal joint of left wrist

✓7ᵗʰ **S63.036**   Dislocation of midcarpal joint of unspecified wrist

✓6ᵗʰ **S63.04**   **Subluxation and dislocation of carpometacarpal joint of thumb**
EXCLUDES 2   interphalangeal subluxation and dislocation of thumb (S63.1-)

✓7ᵗʰ **S63.041**   Subluxation of carpometacarpal joint of right thumb

✓7ᵗʰ **S63.042**   Subluxation of carpometacarpal joint of left thumb

✓7ᵗʰ **S63.043**   Subluxation of carpometacarpal joint of unspecified thumb

✓7ᵗʰ **S63.044**   Dislocation of carpometacarpal joint of right thumb

✓7ᵗʰ **S63.045**   Dislocation of carpometacarpal joint of left thumb

✓7ᵗʰ **S63.046**   Dislocation of carpometacarpal joint of unspecified thumb

✓6ᵗʰ **S63.05**   **Subluxation and dislocation of other carpometacarpal joint**
EXCLUDES 2   subluxation and dislocation of carpometacarpal joint of thumb (S63.04-)

✓7ᵗʰ **S63.051**   Subluxation of other carpometacarpal joint of right hand

✓7ᵗʰ **S63.052**   Subluxation of other carpometacarpal joint of left hand

✓7ᵗʰ **S63.053**   Subluxation of other carpometacarpal joint of unspecified hand

✓7ᵗʰ **S63.054**   Dislocation of other carpometacarpal joint of right hand

✓7ᵗʰ **S63.055**   Dislocation of other carpometacarpal joint of left hand

✓7ᵗʰ **S63.056**   Dislocation of other carpometacarpal joint of unspecified hand

✓6ᵗʰ **S63.06**   **Subluxation and dislocation of metacarpal (bone), proximal end**

✓7ᵗʰ **S63.061**   Subluxation of metacarpal (bone), proximal end of right hand

✓7ᵗʰ **S63.062**   Subluxation of metacarpal (bone), proximal end of left hand

✓7ᵗʰ **S63.063**   Subluxation of metacarpal (bone), proximal end of unspecified hand

---

15   HAC = Initial encounter for open fracture only (7th character B or C – specific to category) and not POA.
20   CC only if an initial encounter for an open fracture (7th character B or C– specific to category) **OR** a subsequent encounter for nonunion or malunion (7th character K, M, N, P, Q, or R – specific to category).

✓ Additional Character Required   ✓x7ᵗʰ Placeholder Alert   Unacceptable PDx   Manifestation   Hospital Acquired Condition   EXCLUDES 1 Not Coded Here   EXCLUDES 2 Not Included Here

√7ᵗʰ **S63.064** Dislocation of metacarpal (bone), proximal end of right hand

√7ᵗʰ **S63.065** Dislocation of metacarpal (bone), proximal end of left hand

√7ᵗʰ **S63.066** Dislocation of metacarpal (bone), proximal end of unspecified hand

√6ᵗʰ **S63.07 Subluxation and dislocation of distal end of ulna**

√7ᵗʰ **S63.071 Subluxation of distal end of right ulna**

√7ᵗʰ **S63.072 Subluxation of distal end of left ulna**

√7ᵗʰ **S63.073 Subluxation of distal end of unspecified ulna**

√7ᵗʰ **S63.074 Dislocation of distal end of right ulna**

√7ᵗʰ **S63.075 Dislocation of distal end of left ulna**

√7ᵗʰ **S63.076 Dislocation of distal end of unspecified ulna**

√6ᵗʰ **S63.09 Other subluxation and dislocation of wrist and hand**

√7ᵗʰ **S63.091 Other subluxation of right wrist and hand**

√7ᵗʰ **S63.092 Other subluxation of left wrist and hand**

√7ᵗʰ **S63.093 Other subluxation of unspecified wrist and hand**

√7ᵗʰ **S63.094 Other dislocation of right wrist and hand**

√7ᵗʰ **S63.095 Other dislocation of left wrist and hand**

√7ᵗʰ **S63.096 Other dislocation of unspecified wrist and hand**

√5ᵗʰ **S63.1 Subluxation and dislocation of thumb**

√6ᵗʰ **S63.10 Unspecified subluxation and dislocation of thumb**

√7ᵗʰ **S63.101 Unspecified subluxation of right thumb**

√7ᵗʰ **S63.102 Unspecified subluxation of left thumb**

√7ᵗʰ **S63.103 Unspecified subluxation of unspecified thumb**

√7ᵗʰ **S63.104 Unspecified dislocation of right thumb**

√7ᵗʰ **S63.105 Unspecified dislocation of left thumb**

√7ᵗʰ **S63.106 Unspecified dislocation of unspecified thumb**

√6ᵗʰ **S63.11 Subluxation and dislocation of metacarpophalangeal joint of thumb**

√7ᵗʰ **S63.111 Subluxation of metacarpophalangeal joint of right thumb**

√7ᵗʰ **S63.112 Subluxation of metacarpophalangeal joint of left thumb**

√7ᵗʰ **S63.113 Subluxation of metacarpophalangeal joint of unspecified thumb**

√7ᵗʰ **S63.114 Dislocation of metacarpophalangeal joint of right thumb**

√7ᵗʰ **S63.115 Dislocation of metacarpophalangeal joint of left thumb**

√7ᵗʰ **S63.116 Dislocation of metacarpophalangeal joint of unspecified thumb**

√6ᵗʰ **S63.12 Subluxation and dislocation of unspecified interphalangeal joint of thumb**

√7ᵗʰ **S63.121 Subluxation of unspecified interphalangeal joint of right thumb**

√7ᵗʰ **S63.122 Subluxation of unspecified interphalangeal joint of left thumb**

√7ᵗʰ **S63.123 Subluxation of unspecified interphalangeal joint of unspecified thumb**

√7ᵗʰ **S63.124 Dislocation of unspecified interphalangeal joint of right thumb**

√7ᵗʰ **S63.125 Dislocation of unspecified interphalangeal joint of left thumb**

√7ᵗʰ **S63.126 Dislocation of unspecified interphalangeal joint of unspecified thumb**

√6ᵗʰ **S63.13 Subluxation and dislocation of proximal interphalangeal joint of thumb**

√7ᵗʰ **S63.131 Subluxation of proximal interphalangeal joint of right thumb**

√7ᵗʰ **S63.132 Subluxation of proximal interphalangeal joint of left thumb**

√7ᵗʰ **S63.133 Subluxation of proximal interphalangeal joint of unspecified thumb**

√7ᵗʰ **S63.134 Dislocation of proximal interphalangeal joint of right thumb**

√7ᵗʰ **S63.135 Dislocation of proximal interphalangeal joint of left thumb**

√7ᵗʰ **S63.136 Dislocation of proximal interphalangeal joint of unspecified thumb**

√6ᵗʰ **S63.14 Subluxation and dislocation of distal interphalangeal joint of thumb**

√7ᵗʰ **S63.141 Subluxation of distal interphalangeal joint of right thumb**

√7ᵗʰ **S63.142 Subluxation of distal interphalangeal joint of left thumb**

√7ᵗʰ **S63.143 Subluxation of distal interphalangeal joint of unspecified thumb**

√7ᵗʰ **S63.144 Dislocation of distal interphalangeal joint of right thumb**

√7ᵗʰ **S63.145 Dislocation of distal interphalangeal joint of left thumb**

√7ᵗʰ **S63.146 Dislocation of distal interphalangeal joint of unspecified thumb**

√5ᵗʰ **S63.2 Subluxation and dislocation of other finger(s)**

EXCLUDES 2   subluxation and dislocation of thumb (S63.1-)

√6ᵗʰ **S63.20 Unspecified subluxation of other finger**

√7ᵗʰ **S63.200 Unspecified subluxation of right index finger**

√7ᵗʰ **S63.201 Unspecified subluxation of left index finger**

√7ᵗʰ **S63.202 Unspecified subluxation of right middle finger**

√7ᵗʰ **S63.203 Unspecified subluxation of left middle finger**

√7ᵗʰ **S63.204 Unspecified subluxation of right ring finger**

√7ᵗʰ **S63.205 Unspecified subluxation of left ring finger**

√7ᵗʰ **S63.206 Unspecified subluxation of right little finger**

√7ᵗʰ **S63.207 Unspecified subluxation of left little finger**

√7ᵗʰ **S63.208 Unspecified subluxation of other finger**
Unspecified subluxation of specified finger with unspecified laterality

√7ᵗʰ **S63.209 Unspecified subluxation of unspecified finger**

√6ᵗʰ **S63.21 Subluxation of metacarpophalangeal joint of finger**

√7ᵗʰ **S63.210 Subluxation of metacarpophalangeal joint of right index finger**

√7ᵗʰ **S63.211 Subluxation of metacarpophalangeal joint of left index finger**

√7ᵗʰ **S63.212 Subluxation of metacarpophalangeal joint of right middle finger**

√7ᵗʰ **S63.213 Subluxation of metacarpophalangeal joint of left middle finger**

√7ᵗʰ **S63.214 Subluxation of metacarpophalangeal joint of right ring finger**

√7ᵗʰ **S63.215 Subluxation of metacarpophalangeal joint of left ring finger**

√7ᵗʰ **S63.216 Subluxation of metacarpophalangeal joint of right little finger**

√7ᵗʰ **S63.217 Subluxation of metacarpophalangeal joint of left little finger**

√7ᵗʰ **S63.218 Subluxation of metacarpophalangeal joint of other finger**
Subluxation of metacarpophalangeal joint of specified finger with unspecified laterality

√7ᵗʰ **S63.219 Subluxation of metacarpophalangeal joint of unspecified finger**

√6ᵗʰ **S63.22 Subluxation of unspecified interphalangeal joint of finger**

√7ᵗʰ **S63.220 Subluxation of unspecified interphalangeal joint of right index finger**

√7ᵗʰ **S63.221 Subluxation of unspecified interphalangeal joint of left index finger**

√7ᵗʰ **S63.222 Subluxation of unspecified interphalangeal joint of right middle finger**

√7ᵗʰ **S63.223 Subluxation of unspecified interphalangeal joint of left middle finger**

Ⓝ Newborn: 0   Ⓟ Pediatric: 0-17   Ⓜ Maternity: 12-55   Ⓐ Adult: 15-124   **MCC** Major CC Condition   **PDxMCC** PDx acts as own MCC   **CC** CC Condition   **PDxCC** PDx acts as own CC

998   ICD-10-CM 2016

√7ᵗʰ **S63.224 Subluxation of unspecified interphalangeal joint of** right ring **finger**

√7ᵗʰ **S63.225 Subluxation of unspecified interphalangeal joint of** left ring **finger**

√7ᵗʰ **S63.226 Subluxation of unspecified interphalangeal joint of** right little **finger**

√7ᵗʰ **S63.227 Subluxation of unspecified interphalangeal joint of** left little **finger**

√7ᵗʰ **S63.228 Subluxation of unspecified interphalangeal joint of** other **finger**
Subluxation of unspecified interphalangeal joint of specified finger with unspecified laterality

√7ᵗʰ **S63.229 Subluxation of unspecified inter-phalangeal joint of** unspecified **finger**

√6ᵗʰ **S63.23 Subluxation of** proximal interphalangeal **joint of finger**

√7ᵗʰ **S63.230 Subluxation of proximal interphalangeal joint of** right index **finger**

√7ᵗʰ **S63.231 Subluxation of proximal interphalangeal joint of** left index **finger**

√7ᵗʰ **S63.232 Subluxation of proximal interphalangeal joint of** right middle **finger**

√7ᵗʰ **S63.233 Subluxation of proximal interphalangeal joint of** left middle **finger**

√7ᵗʰ **S63.234 Subluxation of proximal interphalangeal joint of** right ring **finger**

√7ᵗʰ **S63.235 Subluxation of proximal interphalangeal joint of** left ring **finger**

√7ᵗʰ **S63.236 Subluxation of proximal interphalangeal joint of** right little **finger**

√7ᵗʰ **S63.237 Subluxation of proximal interphalangeal joint of** left little **finger**

√7ᵗʰ **S63.238 Subluxation of proximal interphalangeal joint of** other **finger**
Subluxation of proximal interphalangeal joint of specified finger with unspecified laterality

√7ᵗʰ **S63.239 Subluxation of proximal interphalangeal joint of** unspecified **finger**

√6ᵗʰ **S63.24 Subluxation of** distal interphalangeal **joint of finger**

√7ᵗʰ **S63.240 Subluxation of distal interphalangeal joint of** right index **finger**

√7ᵗʰ **S63.241 Subluxation of distal interphalangeal joint of** left index **finger**

√7ᵗʰ **S63.242 Subluxation of distal interphalangeal joint of** right middle **finger**

√7ᵗʰ **S63.243 Subluxation of distal interphalangeal joint of** left middle **finger**

√7ᵗʰ **S63.244 Subluxation of distal interphalangeal joint of** right ring **finger**

√7ᵗʰ **S63.245 Subluxation of distal interphalangeal joint of** left ring **finger**

√7ᵗʰ **S63.246 Subluxation of distal interphalangeal joint of** right little **finger**

√7ᵗʰ **S63.247 Subluxation of distal interphalangeal joint of** left little **finger**

√7ᵗʰ **S63.248 Subluxation of distal interphalangeal joint of** other **finger**
Subluxation of distal interphalangeal joint of specified finger with unspecified laterality

√7ᵗʰ **S63.249 Subluxation of distal interphalangeal joint of** unspecified **finger**

√6ᵗʰ **S63.25 Unspecified dislocation of** other **finger**

√7ᵗʰ **S63.250 Unspecified dislocation of** right index **finger**

√7ᵗʰ **S63.251 Unspecified dislocation of** left index **finger**

√7ᵗʰ **S63.252 Unspecified dislocation of** right middle **finger**

√7ᵗʰ **S63.253 Unspecified dislocation of** left middle **finger**

√7ᵗʰ **S63.254 Unspecified dislocation of** right ring **finger**

√7ᵗʰ **S63.255 Unspecified dislocation of** left ring **finger**

√7ᵗʰ **S63.256 Unspecified dislocation of** right little **finger**

√7ᵗʰ **S63.257 Unspecified dislocation of** left little **finger**

√7ᵗʰ **S63.258 Unspecified dislocation of** other **finger**
Unspecified dislocation of specified finger with unspecified laterality

√7ᵗʰ **S63.259 Unspecified dislocation of** unspecified **finger**
Unspecified dislocation of specified finger with unspecified laterality

√6ᵗʰ **S63.26 Dislocation of** metacarpophalangeal **joint of finger**

√7ᵗʰ **S63.260 Dislocation of metacarpophalangeal joint of** right index **finger**

√7ᵗʰ **S63.261 Dislocation of metacarpophalangeal joint of** left index **finger**

√7ᵗʰ **S63.262 Dislocation of metacarpophalangeal joint of** right middle **finger**

√7ᵗʰ **S63.263 Dislocation of metacarpophalangeal joint of** left middle **finger**

√7ᵗʰ **S63.264 Dislocation of metacarpophalangeal joint of** right ring **finger**

√7ᵗʰ **S63.265 Dislocation of metacarpophalangeal joint of** left ring **finger**

√7ᵗʰ **S63.266 Dislocation of metacarpophalangeal joint of** right little **finger**

√7ᵗʰ **S63.267 Dislocation of metacarpophalangeal joint of** left little **finger**

√7ᵗʰ **S63.268 Dislocation of metacarpophalangeal joint of** other **finger**
Dislocation of metacarpophalangeal joint of specified finger with unspecified laterality

√7ᵗʰ **S63.269 Dislocation of metacarpophalangeal joint of** unspecified **finger**

√6ᵗʰ **S63.27 Dislocation of** unspecified interphalangeal **joint of finger**

√7ᵗʰ **S63.270 Dislocation of unspecified interphalangeal joint of** right index **finger**

√7ᵗʰ **S63.271 Dislocation of unspecified interphalangeal joint of** left index **finger**

√7ᵗʰ **S63.272 Dislocation of unspecified interphalangeal joint of** right middle **finger**

√7ᵗʰ **S63.273 Dislocation of unspecified interphalangeal joint of** left middle **finger**

√7ᵗʰ **S63.274 Dislocation of unspecified interphalangeal joint of** right ring **finger**

√7ᵗʰ **S63.275 Dislocation of unspecified interphalangeal joint of** left ring **finger**

√7ᵗʰ **S63.276 Dislocation of unspecified interphalangeal joint of** right little **finger**

√7ᵗʰ **S63.277 Dislocation of unspecified interphalangeal joint of** left little **finger**

√7ᵗʰ **S63.278 Dislocation of unspecified interphalangeal joint of** other **finger**
Dislocation of unspecified interphalangeal joint of specified finger with unspecified laterality

√7ᵗʰ **S63.279 Dislocation of unspecified interphalangeal joint of** unspecified **finger**
Dislocation of unspecified interphalangeal joint of specified finger without specified laterality

√6ᵗʰ **S63.28 Dislocation of** proximal interphalangeal **joint of finger**

√7ᵗʰ **S63.280 Dislocation of proximal interphalangeal joint of right index finger**

√7ᵗʰ **S63.281 Dislocation of proximal interphalangeal joint of left index finger**

√7ᵗʰ **S63.282 Dislocation of proximal interphalangeal joint of right middle finger**

√7ᵗʰ **S63.283 Dislocation of proximal interphalangeal joint of left middle finger**

√7ᵗʰ **S63.284 Dislocation of proximal interphalangeal joint of right ring finger**

√7ᵗʰ **S63.285 Dislocation of proximal interphalangeal joint of left ring finger**

√7ᵗʰ **S63.286 Dislocation of proximal interphalangeal joint of right little finger**

☑ Additional Character Required   ☑ₓ7ᵗʰ Placeholder Alert   Unacceptable PDx   Manifestation   Hospital Acquired Condition   *EXCLUDES 1* Not Coded Here   *EXCLUDES 2* Not Included Here

✓7ᵗʰ **S63.287 Dislocation of proximal interphalangeal joint of** left little **finger**

✓7ᵗʰ **S63.288 Dislocation of proximal interphalangeal joint of** other **finger**
> Dislocation of proximal interphalangeal joint of specified finger with unspecified laterality

✓7ᵗʰ **S63.289 Dislocation of proximal interphalangeal joint of** unspecified **finger**

✓6ᵗʰ **S63.29 Dislocation of** distal interphalangeal joint **of finger**

✓7ᵗʰ **S63.290 Dislocation of distal interphalangeal joint of** right index **finger**

✓7ᵗʰ **S63.291 Dislocation of distal interphalangeal joint of** left index **finger**

✓7ᵗʰ **S63.292 Dislocation of distal interphalangeal joint of** right middle **finger**

✓7ᵗʰ **S63.293 Dislocation of distal interphalangeal joint of** left middle **finger**

✓7ᵗʰ **S63.294 Dislocation of distal interphalangeal joint of** right ring **finger**

✓7ᵗʰ **S63.295 Dislocation of distal interphalangeal joint of** left ring **finger**

✓7ᵗʰ **S63.296 Dislocation of distal interphalangeal joint of** right little **finger**

✓7ᵗʰ **S63.297 Dislocation of distal interphalangeal joint of** left little **finger**

✓7ᵗʰ **S63.298 Dislocation of distal interphalangeal joint of** other **finger**
> Dislocation of distal interphalangeal joint of specified finger with unspecified laterality

✓7ᵗʰ **S63.299 Dislocation of distal interphalangeal joint of** unspecified **finger**

✓5ᵗʰ **S63.3 Traumatic rupture of** ligament of wrist

✓6ᵗʰ **S63.30 Traumatic rupture of** unspecified ligament **of wrist**

✓7ᵗʰ **S63.301 Traumatic rupture of unspecified ligament of** right wrist

✓7ᵗʰ **S63.302 Traumatic rupture of unspecified ligament of** left wrist

✓7ᵗʰ **S63.309 Traumatic rupture of unspecified ligament of** unspecified wrist

✓6ᵗʰ **S63.31 Traumatic rupture of** collateral ligament **of wrist**

✓7ᵗʰ **S63.311 Traumatic rupture of collateral ligament of** right wrist

✓7ᵗʰ **S63.312 Traumatic rupture of collateral ligament of** left wrist

✓7ᵗʰ **S63.319 Traumatic rupture of collateral ligament of** unspecified wrist

✓6ᵗʰ **S63.32 Traumatic rupture of** radiocarpal ligament

✓7ᵗʰ **S63.321 Traumatic rupture of** right radiocarpal ligament

✓7ᵗʰ **S63.322 Traumatic rupture of** left radiocarpal ligament

✓7ᵗʰ **S63.329 Traumatic rupture of** unspecified radiocarpal ligament

✓6ᵗʰ **S63.33 Traumatic rupture of** ulnocarpal (palmar) ligament

✓7ᵗʰ **S63.331 Traumatic rupture of** right ulnocarpal (palmar) ligament

✓7ᵗʰ **S63.332 Traumatic rupture of** left ulnocarpal (palmar) ligament

✓7ᵗʰ **S63.339 Traumatic rupture of** unspecified ulnocarpal (palmar) ligament

✓6ᵗʰ **S63.39 Traumatic rupture of** other ligament **of wrist**

✓7ᵗʰ **S63.391 Traumatic rupture of other ligament of** right wrist

✓7ᵗʰ **S63.392 Traumatic rupture of other ligament of** left wrist

✓7ᵗʰ **S63.399 Traumatic rupture of other ligament of** unspecified wrist

✓5ᵗʰ **S63.4 Traumatic rupture of ligament of finger at** metacarpophalangeal and interphalangeal joint(s)

✓6ᵗʰ **S63.40 Traumatic rupture of** unspecified ligament of finger at metacarpophalangeal and interphalangeal joint

✓7ᵗʰ **S63.400 Traumatic rupture of unspecified ligament of** right index **finger at metacarpophalangeal and interphalangeal joint**

✓7ᵗʰ **S63.401 Traumatic rupture of unspecified ligament of** left index **finger at metacarpophalangeal and interphalangeal joint**

✓7ᵗʰ **S63.402 Traumatic rupture of unspecified ligament of** right middle **finger at metacarpophalangeal and interphalangeal joint**

✓7ᵗʰ **S63.403 Traumatic rupture of unspecified ligament of** left middle **finger at metacarpophalangeal and interphalangeal joint**

✓7ᵗʰ **S63.404 Traumatic rupture of unspecified ligament of** right ring **finger at metacarpophalangeal and interphalangeal joint**

✓7ᵗʰ **S63.405 Traumatic rupture of unspecified ligament of** left ring **finger at metacarpophalangeal and interphalangeal joint**

✓7ᵗʰ **S63.406 Traumatic rupture of unspecified ligament of** right little **finger at metacarpophalangeal and interphalangeal joint**

✓7ᵗʰ **S63.407 Traumatic rupture of unspecified ligament of** left little **finger at metacarpophalangeal and interphalangeal joint**

✓7ᵗʰ **S63.408 Traumatic rupture of unspecified ligament of** other **finger at metacarpophalangeal and interphalangeal joint**
> Traumatic rupture of unspecified ligament of specified finger with unspecified laterality at metacarpophalangeal and interphalangeal joint

✓7ᵗʰ **S63.409 Traumatic rupture of unspecified ligament of** unspecified **finger at metacarpophalangeal and interphalangeal joint**

✓6ᵗʰ **S63.41 Traumatic rupture of** collateral ligament **of finger at** metacarpophalangeal and interphalangeal joint

✓7ᵗʰ **S63.410 Traumatic rupture of collateral ligament of** right index **finger at metacarpophalangeal and interphalangeal joint**

✓7ᵗʰ **S63.411 Traumatic rupture of collateral ligament of** left index **finger at metacarpophalangeal and interphalangeal joint**

✓7ᵗʰ **S63.412 Traumatic rupture of collateral ligament of** right middle **finger at metacarpophalangeal and interphalangeal joint**

✓7ᵗʰ **S63.413 Traumatic rupture of collateral ligament of** left middle **finger at metacarpophalangeal and interphalangeal joint**

✓7ᵗʰ **S63.414 Traumatic rupture of collateral ligament of** right ring **finger at metacarpophalangeal and interphalangeal joint**

✓7ᵗʰ **S63.415 Traumatic rupture of collateral ligament of** left ring **finger at metacarpophalangeal and interphalangeal joint**

✓7ᵗʰ **S63.416 Traumatic rupture of collateral ligament of** right little **finger at metacarpophalangeal and interphalangeal joint**

✓7ᵗʰ **S63.417 Traumatic rupture of collateral ligament of** left little **finger at metacarpophalangeal and interphalangeal joint**

N Newborn: 0   P Pediatric: 0-17   M Maternity: 12-55   A Adult: 15-124   **MCC** Major CC Condition   **PDxMCC** PDx acts as own MCC   **CC** CC Condition   **PDxCC** PDx acts as own CC

1000   ICD-10-CM 2016

✓7ᵗʰ **S63.418** **Traumatic rupture of collateral ligament of** other **finger at metacarpophalangeal and interphalangeal joint**
Traumatic rupture of collateral ligament of specified finger with unspecified laterality at metacarpophalangeal and interphalangeal joint

✓7ᵗʰ **S63.419** **Traumatic rupture of collateral ligament of** unspecified **finger at metacarpophalangeal and interphalangeal joint**

✓6ᵗʰ **S63.42** **Traumatic rupture of** palmar ligament **of finger at metacarpophalangeal and interphalangeal joint**

✓7ᵗʰ **S63.420** **Traumatic rupture of palmar ligament of** right index **finger at metacarpophalangeal and interphalangeal joint**

✓7ᵗʰ **S63.421** **Traumatic rupture of palmar ligament of** left index **finger at metacarpophalangeal and interphalangeal joint**

✓7ᵗʰ **S63.422** **Traumatic rupture of palmar ligament of** right middle **finger at metacarpophalangeal and interphalangeal joint**

✓7ᵗʰ **S63.423** **Traumatic rupture of palmar ligament of** left middle **finger at metacarpophalangeal and interphalangeal joint**

✓7ᵗʰ **S63.424** **Traumatic rupture of palmar ligament of** right ring **finger at metacarpophalangeal and interphalangeal joint**

✓7ᵗʰ **S63.425** **Traumatic rupture of palmar ligament of** left ring **finger at metacarpophalangeal and interphalangeal joint**

✓7ᵗʰ **S63.426** **Traumatic rupture of palmar ligament of** right little **finger at metacarpophalangeal and interphalangeal joint**

✓7ᵗʰ **S63.427** **Traumatic rupture of palmar ligament of** left little **finger at metacarpophalangeal and interphalangeal joint**

✓7ᵗʰ **S63.428** **Traumatic rupture of palmar ligament of** other **finger at metacarpophalangeal and interphalangeal joint**
Traumatic rupture of palmar ligament of specified finger with unspecified laterality at metacarpophalangeal and interphalangeal joint

✓7ᵗʰ **S63.429** **Traumatic rupture of palmar ligament of** unspecified **finger at metacarpophalangeal and interphalangeal joint**

✓6ᵗʰ **S63.43** **Traumatic rupture of** volar plate **of finger at metacarpophalangeal and interphalangeal joint**

✓7ᵗʰ **S63.430** **Traumatic rupture of volar plate of** right index **finger at metacarpophalangeal and interphalangeal joint**

✓7ᵗʰ **S63.431** **Traumatic rupture of volar plate of** left index **finger at metacarpophalangeal and interphalangeal joint**

✓7ᵗʰ **S63.432** **Traumatic rupture of volar plate of** right middle **finger at metacarpophalangeal and interphalangeal joint**

✓7ᵗʰ **S63.433** **Traumatic rupture of volar plate of** left middle **finger at metacarpophalangeal and interphalangeal joint**

✓7ᵗʰ **S63.434** **Traumatic rupture of volar plate of** right ring **finger at metacarpophalangeal and interphalangeal joint**

✓7ᵗʰ **S63.435** **Traumatic rupture of volar plate of** left ring **finger at metacarpophalangeal and interphalangeal joint**

✓7ᵗʰ **S63.436** **Traumatic rupture of volar plate of** right little **finger at metacarpophalangeal and interphalangeal joint**

✓7ᵗʰ **S63.437** **Traumatic rupture of volar plate of** left little **finger at metacarpophalangeal and interphalangeal joint**

✓7ᵗʰ **S63.438** **Traumatic rupture of volar plate of** other **finger at metacarpophalangeal and interphalangeal joint**
Traumatic rupture of volar plate of specified finger with unspecified laterality at metacarpophalangeal and interphalangeal joint

✓7ᵗʰ **S63.439** **Traumatic rupture of volar plate of** unspecified **finger at metacarpophalangeal and interphalangeal joint**

✓6ᵗʰ **S63.49** **Traumatic rupture of** other ligament **of finger at metacarpophalangeal and interphalangeal joint**

✓7ᵗʰ **S63.490** **Traumatic rupture of other ligament of** right index **finger at metacarpophalangeal and interphalangeal joint**

✓7ᵗʰ **S63.491** **Traumatic rupture of other ligament of** left index **finger at metacarpophalangeal and interphalangeal joint**

✓7ᵗʰ **S63.492** **Traumatic rupture of other ligament of** right middle **finger at metacarpophalangeal and interphalangeal joint**

✓7ᵗʰ **S63.493** **Traumatic rupture of other ligament of** left middle **finger at metacarpophalangeal and interphalangeal joint**

✓7ᵗʰ **S63.494** **Traumatic rupture of other ligament of** right ring **finger at metacarpophalangeal and interphalangeal joint**

✓7ᵗʰ **S63.495** **Traumatic rupture of other ligament of** left ring **finger at metacarpophalangeal and interphalangeal joint**

✓7ᵗʰ **S63.496** **Traumatic rupture of other ligament of** right little **finger at metacarpophalangeal and interphalangeal joint**

✓7ᵗʰ **S63.497** **Traumatic rupture of other ligament of** left little **finger at metacarpophalangeal and interphalangeal joint**

✓7ᵗʰ **S63.498** **Traumatic rupture of other ligament of** other **finger at metacarpophalangeal and interphalangeal joint**
Traumatic rupture of ligament of specified finger with unspecified laterality at metacarpophalangeal and interphalangeal joint

✓7ᵗʰ **S63.499** **Traumatic rupture of other ligament of** unspecified **finger at metacarpophalangeal and interphalangeal joint**

✓5ᵗʰ **S63.5** **Other and unspecified** sprain of wrist

✓6ᵗʰ **S63.50** **Unspecified sprain of wrist**

✓7ᵗʰ **S63.501** **Unspecified sprain of** right **wrist**

✓7ᵗʰ **S63.502** **Unspecified sprain of** left **wrist**

✓7ᵗʰ **S63.509** **Unspecified sprain of** unspecified **wrist**

✓6ᵗʰ **S63.51** **Sprain of** carpal **(joint)**

✓7ᵗʰ **S63.511** **Sprain of carpal joint of** right **wrist**

✓7ᵗʰ **S63.512** **Sprain of carpal joint of** left **wrist**

✓7ᵗʰ **S63.519** **Sprain of carpal joint of** unspecified **wrist**

✓6ᵗʰ **S63.52** **Sprain of** radiocarpal **joint**
EXCLUDES 1 traumatic rupture of radiocarpal ligament (S63.32-)

✓7ᵗʰ **S63.521** **Sprain of radiocarpal joint of** right **wrist**

✓7ᵗʰ **S63.522** **Sprain of radiocarpal joint of** left **wrist**

✓7ᵗʰ **S63.529** **Sprain of radiocarpal joint of** unspecified **wrist**

✓6ᵗʰ **S63.59** **Other specified sprain of wrist**

✓7ᵗʰ **S63.591** **Other specified sprain of** right **wrist**

✓7ᵗʰ **S63.592** **Other specified sprain of** left **wrist**

✓7ᵗʰ **S63.599** **Other specified sprain of** unspecified **wrist**

✓5ᵗʰ **S63.6** **Other and unspecified sprain of finger(s)**
EXCLUDES 1 traumatic rupture of ligament of finger at metacarpophalangeal and interphalangeal joint(s) (S63.4-)

✓6ᵗʰ **S63.60** **Unspecified sprain of** thumb

✓7ᵗʰ **S63.601** **Unspecified sprain of** right **thumb**

✔ Additional Character Required   ✓ₓ7ᵗʰ Placeholder Alert   Unacceptable PDx   Manifestation   Hospital Acquired Condition   **EXCLUDES 1** Not Coded Here   **EXCLUDES 2** Not Included Here

√7ᵗʰ **S63.602** Unspecified sprain of left thumb
√7ᵗʰ **S63.609** Unspecified sprain of unspecified thumb
√6ᵗʰ **S63.61** Unspecified sprain of other and unspecified finger(s)
  √7ᵗʰ **S63.610** Unspecified sprain of right index finger
  √7ᵗʰ **S63.611** Unspecified sprain of left index finger
  √7ᵗʰ **S63.612** Unspecified sprain of right middle finger
  √7ᵗʰ **S63.613** Unspecified sprain of left middle finger
  √7ᵗʰ **S63.614** Unspecified sprain of right ring finger
  √7ᵗʰ **S63.615** Unspecified sprain of left ring finger
  √7ᵗʰ **S63.616** Unspecified sprain of right little finger
  √7ᵗʰ **S63.617** Unspecified sprain of left little finger
  √7ᵗʰ **S63.618** Unspecified sprain of other finger
    Unspecified sprain of specified finger with unspecified laterality
  √7ᵗʰ **S63.619** Unspecified sprain of unspecified finger
√6ᵗʰ **S63.62** Sprain of interphalangeal joint of thumb
  √7ᵗʰ **S63.621** Sprain of interphalangeal joint of right thumb
  √7ᵗʰ **S63.622** Sprain of interphalangeal joint of left thumb
  √7ᵗʰ **S63.629** Sprain of interphalangeal joint of unspecified thumb
√6ᵗʰ **S63.63** Sprain of interphalangeal joint of other and unspecified finger(s)
  √7ᵗʰ **S63.630** Sprain of interphalangeal joint of right index finger
  √7ᵗʰ **S63.631** Sprain of interphalangeal joint of left index finger
  √7ᵗʰ **S63.632** Sprain of interphalangeal joint of right middle finger
  √7ᵗʰ **S63.633** Sprain of interphalangeal joint of left middle finger
  √7ᵗʰ **S63.634** Sprain of interphalangeal joint of right ring finger
  √7ᵗʰ **S63.635** Sprain of interphalangeal joint of left ring finger
  √7ᵗʰ **S63.636** Sprain of interphalangeal joint of right little finger
  √7ᵗʰ **S63.637** Sprain of interphalangeal joint of left little finger
  √7ᵗʰ **S63.638** Sprain of interphalangeal joint of other finger
  √7ᵗʰ **S63.639** Sprain of interphalangeal joint of unspecified finger
√6ᵗʰ **S63.64** Sprain of metacarpophalangeal joint of thumb
  √7ᵗʰ **S63.641** Sprain of metacarpophalangeal joint of right thumb
  √7ᵗʰ **S63.642** Sprain of metacarpophalangeal joint of left thumb
  √7ᵗʰ **S63.649** Sprain of metacarpophalangeal joint of unspecified thumb
√6ᵗʰ **S63.65** Sprain of metacarpophalangeal joint of other and unspecified finger(s)
  √7ᵗʰ **S63.650** Sprain of metacarpophalangeal joint of right index finger
  √7ᵗʰ **S63.651** Sprain of metacarpophalangeal joint of left index finger
  √7ᵗʰ **S63.652** Sprain of metacarpophalangeal joint of right middle finger
  √7ᵗʰ **S63.653** Sprain of metacarpophalangeal joint of left middle finger
  √7ᵗʰ **S63.654** Sprain of metacarpophalangeal joint of right ring finger
  √7ᵗʰ **S63.655** Sprain of metacarpophalangeal joint of left ring finger
  √7ᵗʰ **S63.656** Sprain of metacarpophalangeal joint of right little finger
  √7ᵗʰ **S63.657** Sprain of metacarpophalangeal joint of left little finger
  √7ᵗʰ **S63.658** Sprain of metacarpophalangeal joint of other finger
    Sprain of metacarpophalangeal joint of specified finger with unspecified laterality

√7ᵗʰ **S63.659** Sprain of metacarpophalangeal joint of unspecified finger
√6ᵗʰ **S63.68** Other sprain of thumb
  √7ᵗʰ **S63.681** Other sprain of right thumb
  √7ᵗʰ **S63.682** Other sprain of left thumb
  √7ᵗʰ **S63.689** Other sprain of unspecified thumb
√6ᵗʰ **S63.69** Other sprain of other and unspecified finger(s)
  √7ᵗʰ **S63.690** Other sprain of right index finger
  √7ᵗʰ **S63.691** Other sprain of left index finger
  √7ᵗʰ **S63.692** Other sprain of right middle finger
  √7ᵗʰ **S63.693** Other sprain of left middle finger
  √7ᵗʰ **S63.694** Other sprain of right ring finger
  √7ᵗʰ **S63.695** Other sprain of left ring finger
  √7ᵗʰ **S63.696** Other sprain of right little finger
  √7ᵗʰ **S63.697** Other sprain of left little finger
  √7ᵗʰ **S63.698** Other sprain of other finger
    Other sprain of specified finger with unspecified laterality
  √7ᵗʰ **S63.699** Other sprain of unspecified finger
√5ᵗʰ **S63.8** Sprain of other part of wrist and hand
  √6ᵗʰ **S63.8X** Sprain of other part of wrist and hand
    √7ᵗʰ **S63.8X1** Sprain of other part of right wrist and hand
    √7ᵗʰ **S63.8X2** Sprain of other part of left wrist and hand
    √7ᵗʰ **S63.8X9** Sprain of other part of unspecified wrist and hand
√5ᵗʰ **S63.9** Sprain of unspecified part of wrist and hand
  √x7ᵗʰ **S63.90** Sprain of unspecified part of unspecified wrist and hand
  √x7ᵗʰ **S63.91** Sprain of unspecified part of right wrist and hand
  √x7ᵗʰ **S63.92** Sprain of unspecified part of left wrist and hand

√4ᵗʰ **S64** **Injury of nerves at wrist and hand level**
Code also any associated open wound (S61.-)

The appropriate 7th character is to be added to each code from category S64.
A   initial encounter
D   subsequent encounter
S   sequela

√6ᵗʰ **S64.0** Injury of ulnar nerve at wrist and hand level
  √x7ᵗʰ **S64.00** Injury of ulnar nerve at wrist and hand level of unspecified arm
  √x7ᵗʰ **S64.01** Injury of ulnar nerve at wrist and hand level of right arm
  √x7ᵗʰ **S64.02** Injury of ulnar nerve at wrist and hand level of left arm
√5ᵗʰ **S64.1** Injury of median nerve at wrist and hand level
  √x7ᵗʰ **S64.10** Injury of median nerve at wrist and hand level of unspecified arm
  √x7ᵗʰ **S64.11** Injury of median nerve at wrist and hand level of right arm
  √x7ᵗʰ **S64.12** Injury of median nerve at wrist and hand level of left arm
√5ᵗʰ **S64.2** Injury of radial nerve at wrist and hand level
  √x7ᵗʰ **S64.20** Injury of radial nerve at wrist and hand level of unspecified arm
  √x7ᵗʰ **S64.21** Injury of radial nerve at wrist and hand level of right arm
  √x7ᵗʰ **S64.22** Injury of radial nerve at wrist and hand level of left arm
√5ᵗʰ **S64.3** Injury of digital nerve of thumb
  √x7ᵗʰ **S64.30** Injury of digital nerve of unspecified thumb
  √x7ᵗʰ **S64.31** Injury of digital nerve of right thumb
  √x7ᵗʰ **S64.32** Injury of digital nerve of left thumb
√5ᵗʰ **S64.4** Injury of digital nerve of other and unspecified finger
  √x7ᵗʰ **S64.40** Injury of digital nerve of unspecified finger
  √6ᵗʰ **S64.49** Injury of digital nerve of other finger
    √7ᵗʰ **S64.490** Injury of digital nerve of right index finger
    √7ᵗʰ **S64.491** Injury of digital nerve of left index finger
    √7ᵗʰ **S64.492** Injury of digital nerve of right middle finger

☑7ᵗʰ **S64.493 Injury of digital nerve of left middle finger**

☑7ᵗʰ **S64.494 Injury of digital nerve of right ring finger**

☑7ᵗʰ **S64.495 Injury of digital nerve of left ring finger**

☑7ᵗʰ **S64.496 Injury of digital nerve of right little finger**

☑7ᵗʰ **S64.497 Injury of digital nerve of left little finger**

☑7ᵗʰ **S64.498 Injury of digital nerve of other finger**
Injury of digital nerve of specified finger with unspecified laterality

☑5ᵗʰ **S64.8 Injury of other nerves at wrist and hand level**

☑6ᵗʰ **S64.8X Injury of other nerves at wrist and hand level**

☑7ᵗʰ **S64.8X1 Injury of other nerves at wrist and hand level of right arm**

☑7ᵗʰ **S64.8X2 Injury of other nerves at wrist and hand level of left arm**

☑7ᵗʰ **S64.8X9 Injury of other nerves at wrist and hand level of unspecified arm**

☑5ᵗʰ **S64.9 Injury of unspecified nerve at wrist and hand level**

☑x7ᵗʰ **S64.90 Injury of unspecified nerve at wrist and hand level of unspecified arm**

☑x7ᵗʰ **S64.91 Injury of unspecified nerve at wrist and hand level of right arm**

☑x7ᵗʰ **S64.92 Injury of unspecified nerve at wrist and hand level of left arm**

☑4ᵗʰ **S65 Injury of blood vessels at wrist and hand level**
Code also any associated open wound (S61.-)

> The appropriate 7th character is to be added to each code from category S65.
> A initial encounter
> D subsequent encounter
> S sequela

☑5ᵗʰ **S65.0 Injury of ulnar artery at wrist and hand level**

☑6ᵗʰ **S65.00 Unspecified injury of ulnar artery at wrist and hand level**

☑7ᵗʰ **S65.001 Unspecified injury of ulnar artery at wrist and hand level of right arm** `CC`
CC Excl: CC CC with 7th character A: S45.301A, S45.309-S45.311 with 7th A, S45.319-S45.391 with 7th A, S45.399-S45.801 with 7th A, S45.809-S45.811 with 7th A, S45.819-S45.891 with 7th A, S45.899-S45.901 with 7th A, S45.909-S45.911 with 7th A, S45.919-S45.991 with 7th A, S45.999A, S55.001A, S55.009-S55.011 with 7th A, S55.019-S55.091 with 7th A, S55.099A, S55.201A, S55.209-S55.211 with 7th A, S55.219-S55.291 with 7th A, S55.299-S55.801 with 7th A, S55.809-S55.811 with 7th A, S55.819-S55.891 with 7th A, S55.899-S55.901 with 7th A, S55.909-S55.911 with 7th A, S55.919-S55.991 with 7th A, S55.999A, S65.001A, S65.009-S65.011 with 7th A, S65.019-S65.091 with 7th A, S65.099A, S65.801A, S65.809-S65.811 with 7th A, S65.819-S65.891 with 7th A, S65.899-S65.901 with 7th A, S65.909-S65.911 with 7th A, S65.919-S65.991 with 7th A, S65.999A

☑7ᵗʰ **S65.002 Unspecified injury of ulnar artery at wrist and hand level of left arm** `CC`
CC Excl: CC CC with 7th character A: S45.302-S45.309 with 7th A, S45.312-S45.319 with 7th A, S45.392-S45.399 with 7th A, S45.802-S45.809 with 7th A, S45.812-S45.819 with 7th A, S45.892-S45.899 with 7th A, S45.902-S45.909 with 7th A, S45.912-S45.919 with 7th A, S45.992-S45.999 with 7th A, S55.002-S55.009 with 7th A, S55.012-S55.019 with 7th A, S55.092-S55.099 with 7th A, S55.202-S55.209 with 7th A, S55.212-S55.219 with 7th A, S55.292-S55.299 with 7th A, S55.802-S55.809 with 7th A, S55.812-S55.819 with 7th A, S55.892-S55.899 with 7th A, S55.902-S55.909 with 7th A, S55.912-S55.919 with 7th A, S55.992-S55.999 with 7th A, S65.002-S65.009 with 7th A, S65.012-S65.019 with 7th A, S65.092-S65.099 with 7th A, S65.802-S65.809 with 7th A, S65.812-S65.819 with 7th A, S65.892-S65.899 with 7th A, S65.902-S65.909 with 7th A, S65.912-S65.919 with 7th A, S65.992-S65.999 with 7th A

☑7ᵗʰ **S65.009 Unspecified injury of ulnar artery at wrist and hand level of unspecified arm** `CC`
CC Excl: CC CC with 7th character A: S45.301-S45.999 with 7th A, S55.001-S55.099 with 7th A, S55.201-S55.999 with 7th A, S65.001-S65.099 with 7th A, S65.801-S65.999 with 7th A

☑6ᵗʰ **S65.01 Laceration of ulnar artery at wrist and hand level**

☑7ᵗʰ **S65.011 Laceration of ulnar artery at wrist and hand level of right arm** `CC`
CC Excl: CC CC with 7th character A: See code: S65.001

☑7ᵗʰ **S65.012 Laceration of ulnar artery at wrist and hand level of left arm** `CC`
CC Excl: CC CC with 7th character A: See code: S65.002

☑7ᵗʰ **S65.019 Laceration of ulnar artery at wrist and hand level of unspecified arm** `CC`
CC Excl: CC CC with 7th character A: See code: S65.009

☑6ᵗʰ **S65.09 Other specified injury of ulnar artery at wrist and hand level**

☑7ᵗʰ **S65.091 Other specified injury of ulnar artery at wrist and hand level of right arm** `CC`
CC Excl: CC CC with 7th character A: See code: S65.001

☑7ᵗʰ **S65.092 Other specified injury of ulnar artery at wrist and hand level of left arm** `CC`
CC Excl: CC CC with 7th character A: See code: S65.002

☑7ᵗʰ **S65.099 Other specified injury of ulnar artery at wrist and hand level of unspecified arm** `CC`
CC Excl: CC CC with 7th character A: See code: S65.009

☑5ᵗʰ **S65.1 Injury of radial artery at wrist and hand level**

☑6ᵗʰ **S65.10 Unspecified injury of radial artery at wrist and hand level**

☑7ᵗʰ **S65.101 Unspecified injury of radial artery at wrist and hand level of right arm** `CC`
CC Excl: CC CC with 7th character A: S45.301 A, S45.309-S45.311 with 7th A, S45.319-S45.391 with 7th A, S45.399-S45.801 with 7th A, S45.809-S45.811 with 7th A, S45.819-S45.891 with 7th A, S45.899-S45.901 with 7th A, S45.909-S45.911 with 7th A, S45.919-S45.991 with 7th A, S45.999A, S55.101A, S55.109-S55.111 with 7th A, S55.119-S55.191 with 7th A, S55.199-S55.201 with 7th A, S55.209-S55.211 with 7th A, S55.219-S55.291 with 7th A, S55.299-S55.801 with 7th A, S55.809-S55.811 with 7th A, S55.819-S55.891 with 7th A, S55.899-S55.901 with 7th A, S55.909-S55.911 with 7th A, S55.919-S55.991 with 7th A, S55.999A, S65.101A, S65.109-S65.111 with 7th A, S65.119-S65.191 with 7th A, S65.199A, S65.801 with 7th A, S65.809-S65.811 with 7th A, S65.819-S65.891 with 7th A, S65.899-S65.901 with 7th A, S65.909-S65.911 with 7th A, S65.919-S65.991 with 7th A, S65.999A

☑7ᵗʰ **S65.102 Unspecified injury of radial artery at wrist and hand level of left arm** `CC`
CC Excl: CC CC with 7th character A: S45.302-S45.309 with 7th A, S45.312-S45.319 with 7th A, S45.392-S45.399 with 7th A, S45.802-S45.809 with 7th A, S45.812-S45.819 with 7th A, S45.892-S45.899 with 7th A, S45.902-S45.909 with 7th A, S45.912-S45.919 with 7th A, S45.992-S45.999 with 7th A, S55.102-S55.109 with 7th A, S55.112-S55.119 with 7th A, S55.192-S55.199 with 7th A, S55.202-S55.209 with 7th A, S55.212-S55.219 with 7th A, S55.292-S55.299 with 7th A, S55.802-S55.809 with 7th A, S55.812-S55.819 with 7th A, S55.892-S55.899 with 7th A, S55.902-S55.909 with 7th A, S55.912-S55.919 with 7th A, S55.992-S55.999 with 7th A, S65.102-S65.109 with 7th A, S65.112-S65.119 with 7th A, S65.192-S65.199 with 7th A, S65.802-S65.809 with 7th A, S65.812-S65.819 with 7th A, S65.892-S65.899 with 7th A, S65.902-S65.909 with 7th A, S65.912-S65.919 with 7th A, S65.992-S65.999 with 7th A

✓7ᵗʰ **S65.109 Unspecified injury of radial artery at** `CC`
wrist and hand level of unspecified arm
CC Excl: CC CC with 7th character A:
S45.301-S45.301-S45.999 with 7th A,
S55.101-S55.999 with 7th A, S65.101-
S65.199 with 7th A, S65.801-S65.999 with
7th A

✓6ᵗʰ **S65.11 Laceration of radial artery at wrist and hand level**

✓7ᵗʰ **S65.111 Laceration of radial artery at wrist** `CC`
and hand level of right arm
CC Excl: CC CC with 7th character A: See
code: S65.101

✓7ᵗʰ **S65.112 Laceration of radial artery at wrist** `CC`
and hand level of left arm
CC Excl: CC CC with 7th character A: See
code: S65.102

✓7ᵗʰ **S65.119 Laceration of radial artery at wrist** `CC`
and hand level of unspecified arm
CC Excl: CC CC with 7th character A: See
code: S65.109

✓6ᵗʰ **S65.19 Other specified injury of radial artery at wrist and hand level**

✓7ᵗʰ **S65.191 Other specified injury of radial artery** `CC`
at wrist and hand level of right arm
CC Excl: CC CC with 7th character A: See
code: S65.101

✓7ᵗʰ **S65.192 Other specified injury of radial artery** `CC`
at wrist and hand level of left arm
CC Excl: CC CC with 7th character A: See
code: S65.102

✓7ᵗʰ **S65.199 Other specified injury of radial artery** `CC`
**at wrist and hand level of unspecified
arm**
CC Excl: CC CC with 7th character A: See
code: S65.109

✓5ᵗʰ **S65.2 Injury of superficial palmar arch**

✓6ᵗʰ **S65.20 Unspecified injury of superficial palmar arch**

✓7ᵗʰ **S65.201 Unspecified injury of superficial** `CC`
palmar arch of right hand
CC Excl: CC CC with 7th character A:
S45.301A, S45.309-S45.311 with 7th A,
S45.319-S45.391 with 7th A, S45.399-
S45.801 with 7th A, S45.809-S45.811 with
7th A, S45.819-S45.891 with 7th A, S45.899-
S45.901 with 7th A, S45.909-S45.911 with
7th A, S45.919-S45.991 with 7th A, S45.999A,
S55.201A, S55.209-S55.211 with 7th A,
S55.219-S55.291 with 7th A, S55.299-
S55.801 with 7th A, S55.809-S55.811 with
7th A, S55.819-S55.891 with 7th A, S55.899-
S55.901 with 7th A, S55.909-S55.911 with
7th A, S55.919-S55.991 with 7th A, S55.999A,
S65.201A, S65.209-S65.211 with 7th A,
S65.219-S65.291 with 7th A, S65.299-
S65.301 with 7th A, S65.309-S65.311 with
7th A, S65.319-S65.391 with 7th A, S65.399A,
S65.801A, S65.809-S65.811 with 7th A,
S65.819-S65.891 with 7th A, S65.899-
S65.901 with 7th A, S65.909-S65.911 with
7th A, S65.919-S65.991 with 7th A, S65.999A

✓7ᵗʰ **S65.202 Unspecified injury of superficial** `CC`
palmar arch of left hand
CC Excl: CC CC with 7th character A:
S45.302-S45.309 with 7th A, S45.312-
S45.319 with 7th A, S45.392-S45.399 with
7th A, S45.802-S45.809 with 7th A, S45.812-
S45.819 with 7th A, S45.892-S45.899 with
7th A, S45.902-S45.909 with 7th A, S45.912-
S45.919 with 7th A, S45.992-S45.999 with
7th A, S55.202-S55.209 with 7th A, S55.212-
S55.219 with 7th A, S55.292-S55.299 with
7th A, S55.802-S55.809 with 7th A, S55.812-
S55.819 with 7th A, S55.892-S55.899 with
7th A, S55.902-S55.909 with 7th A, S55.912-
S55.919 with 7th A, S55.992-S55.999 with
7th A, S65.202-S65.209 with 7th A, S65.212-
S65.219 with 7th A, S65.292-S65.299 with
7th A, S65.302-S65.309 with 7th A, S65.312-
S65.319 with 7th A, S65.392-S65.399 with
7th A, S65.802-S65.809 with 7th A, S65.812-
S65.819 with 7th A, S65.892-S65.899 with
7th A, S65.902-S65.909 with 7th A, S65.912-
S65.919 with 7th A, S65.992-S65.999 with
7th A

✓7ᵗʰ **S65.209 Unspecified injury of superficial** `CC`
palmar arch of unspecified hand
CC Excl: CC CC with 7th character A:
S45.301-S45.999 with 7th A, S55.201-
S55.999 with 7th A, S65.201-S65.399 with
7th A, S65.801-S65.999 with 7th A

✓6ᵗʰ **S65.21 Laceration of superficial palmar arch**

✓7ᵗʰ **S65.211 Laceration of superficial palmar** `CC`
arch of right hand
CC Excl: CC CC with 7th character A: See
code: S65.201

✓7ᵗʰ **S65.212 Laceration of superficial palmar** `CC`
arch of left hand
CC Excl: CC CC with 7th character A: See
code: S65.202

✓7ᵗʰ **S65.219 Laceration of superficial palmar** `CC`
arch of unspecified hand
CC Excl: CC CC with 7th character A: See
code: S65.209

✓6ᵗʰ **S65.29 Other specified injury of superficial palmar arch**

✓7ᵗʰ **S65.291 Other specified injury of superficial** `CC`
palmar arch of right hand
CC Excl: CC CC with 7th character A: See
code: S65.201

✓7ᵗʰ **S65.292 Other specified injury of superficial** `CC`
palmar arch of left hand
CC Excl: CC CC with 7th character A: See
code: S65.202

✓7ᵗʰ **S65.299 Other specified injury of superficial** `CC`
palmar arch of unspecified hand
CC Excl: CC CC with 7th character A: See
code: S65.209

✓5ᵗʰ **S65.3 Injury of deep palmar arch**

✓6ᵗʰ **S65.30 Unspecified injury of deep palmar arch**

✓7ᵗʰ **S65.301 Unspecified injury of deep palmar** `CC`
arch of right hand
CC Excl: CC CC with 7th character A: See
code: S65.201

✓7ᵗʰ **S65.302 Unspecified injury of deep palmar** `CC`
arch of left hand
CC Excl: CC CC with 7th character A: See
code: S65.202

✓7ᵗʰ **S65.309 Unspecified injury of deep palmar** `CC`
arch of unspecified hand
CC Excl: CC CC with 7th character A: See
code: S65.209

✓6ᵗʰ **S65.31 Laceration of deep palmar arch**

✓7ᵗʰ **S65.311 Laceration of deep palmar arch of** `CC`
right hand
CC Excl: CC CC with 7th character A: See
code: S65.201

✓7ᵗʰ **S65.312 Laceration of deep palmar arch of** `CC`
left hand
CC Excl: CC CC with 7th character A: See
code: S65.202

✓7ᵗʰ **S65.319 Laceration of deep palmar arch of** `CC`
unspecified hand
CC Excl: CC with 7th character A: See code:
S65.209

✓6ᵗʰ **S65.39 Other specified injury of deep palmar arch**

✓7ᵗʰ **S65.391 Other specified injury of deep palmar** `CC`
arch of right hand
CC Excl: CC with 7th character A: See code:
S65.201

✓7ᵗʰ **S65.392 Other specified injury of deep palmar** `CC`
arch of left hand
CC Excl: CC with 7th character A: See code:
S65.202

✓7ᵗʰ **S65.399 Other specified injury of deep palmar** `CC`
arch of unspecified hand
CC Excl: CC with 7th character A: See code:
S65.209

Ⓝ Newborn: 0   Ⓟ Pediatric: 0-17   Ⓜ Maternity: 12-55   Ⓐ Adult: 15-124   `MCC` Major CC Condition   `PDxMCC` PDx acts as own MCC   `CC` CC Condition   `PDxCC` PDx acts as own CC

1004   ICD-10-CM 2016

√5ᵗʰ **S65.4 Injury of blood vessel of thumb**

√6ᵗʰ **S65.40 Unspecified injury of blood vessel of thumb**

√7ᵗʰ **S65.401 Unspecified injury of blood vessel of right thumb** CC
CC Excl: CC with 7th character A: S45.301A, S45.309-S45.311 with 7th A, S45.319-S45.391 with 7th A, S45.399-S45.801 with 7th A, S45.809-S45.811 with 7th A, S45.819-S45.891 with 7th A, S45.899-S45.901 with 7th A, S45.909-S45.911 with 7th A, S45.919-S45.991 with 7th A, S45.999A, S55.201A, S55.209-S55.211 with 7th A, S55.219-S55.291 with 7th A, S55.299-S55.801 with 7th A, S55.809-S55.811 with 7th A, S55.819-S55.891 with 7th A, S55.899-S55.901 with 7th A, S55.909-S55.911 with 7th A, S55.919-S55.991 with 7th A, S55.999A, S65.401A, S65.409-S65.411 with 7th A, S65.419-S65.491 with 7th A, S65.499-S65.500 with 7th A, S65.502 A, S65.504A, S65.506A, S65.508-S65.510 with 7th A, S65.512A, S65.514A, S65.516A, S65.518-S65.590 with 7th A, S65.592A, S65.594A, S65.596 A, S65.598-S65.801 with 7th A, S65.809-S65.811 with 7th A, S65.819-S65.891 with 7th A, S65.899-S65.901 with 7th A, S65.909-S65.911 with 7th A, S65.919-S65.991 with 7th A, S65.999A

√7ᵗʰ **S65.402 Unspecified injury of blood vessel of left thumb** CC
CC Excl: CC with 7th character A: S45.302-S45.309 with 7th A, S45.312-S45.319 with 7th A, S45.392-S45.399 with 7th A, S45.802-S45.809 with 7th A, S45.812-S45.819 with 7th A, S45.892-S45.899 with 7th A, S45.902-S45.909 with 7th A, S45.912-S45.919 with 7th A, S45.992-S45.999 with 7th A, S55.202-S55.209 with 7th A, S55.212-S55.219 with 7th A, S55.292-S55.299 with 7th A, S55.802-S55.809 with 7th A, S55.812-S55.819 with 7th A, S55.892-S55.899 with 7th A, S55.902-S55.909 with 7th A, S55.912-S55.919 with 7th A, S55.992-S55.999 with 7th A, S65.402-S65.409 with 7th A, S65.412-S65.419 with 7th A, S65.492-S65.499 with 7th A, S65.501A, S65.503A, S65.505A, S65.507-S65.509 with 7th A, S65.511A, S65.513A, S65.515A, S65.517-S65.519 with 7th A, S65.591A, S65.593A, S65.595A, S65.597-S65.599 with 7th A, S65.802-S65.809 with 7th A, S65.812-S65.819 with 7th A, S65.892-S65.899 with 7th A, S65.902-S65.909 with 7th A, S65.912-S65.919 with 7th A, S65.992-S65.999 with 7th A

√7ᵗʰ **S65.409 Unspecified injury of blood vessel of unspecified thumb** CC
CC Excl: CC with 7th character A: S45.301-S45.999 with 7th A, S55.201-S55.999 with 7th A, S65.401-S65.999 with 7th A

√6ᵗʰ **S65.41 Laceration of blood vessel of thumb**

√7ᵗʰ **S65.411 Laceration of blood vessel of right thumb** CC
CC Excl: CC with 7th character A: See code: S65.401

√7ᵗʰ **S65.412 Laceration of blood vessel of left thumb** CC
CC Excl: CC with 7th character A: See code: S65.402

√7ᵗʰ **S65.419 Laceration of blood vessel of unspecified thumb** CC
CC Excl: CC with 7th character A: See code: S65.409

√6ᵗʰ **S65.49 Other specified injury of blood vessel of thumb**

√7ᵗʰ **S65.491 Other specified injury of blood vessel of right thumb** CC
CC Excl: CC with 7th character A: See code: S65.401

√7ᵗʰ **S65.492 Other specified injury of blood vessel of left thumb** CC
CC Excl: CC with 7th character A: See code: S65.402

√7ᵗʰ **S65.499 Other specified injury of blood vessel of unspecified thumb** CC
CC Excl: CC with 7th character A: See code: S65.409

√5ᵗʰ **S65.5 Injury of blood vessel of other and unspecified finger**

√6ᵗʰ **S65.50 Unspecified injury of blood vessel of other and unspecified finger**

√7ᵗʰ **S65.500 Unspecified injury of blood vessel of right index finger** CC
CC Excl: CC with 7th character A: See code: S65.401

√7ᵗʰ **S65.501 Unspecified injury of blood vessel of left index finger** CC
CC Excl: CC with 7th character A: See code: S65.402

√7ᵗʰ **S65.502 Unspecified injury of blood vessel of right middle finger** CC
CC Excl: CC with 7th character A: See code: S65.401

√7ᵗʰ **S65.503 Unspecified injury of blood vessel of left middle finger** CC
CC Excl: CC with 7th character A: See code: S65.402

√7ᵗʰ **S65.504 Unspecified injury of blood vessel of right ring finger** CC
CC Excl: CC with 7th character A: See code: S65.401

√7ᵗʰ **S65.505 Unspecified injury of blood vessel of left ring finger** CC
CC Excl: CC with 7th character A: See code: S65.402

√7ᵗʰ **S65.506 Unspecified injury of blood vessel of right little finger** CC
CC Excl: CC with 7th character A: See code: S65.401

√7ᵗʰ **S65.507 Unspecified injury of blood vessel of left little finger** CC
CC Excl: CC with 7th character A: See code: S65.402

√7ᵗʰ **S65.508 Unspecified injury of blood vessel of other finger** CC
Unspecified injury of blood vessel of specified finger with unspecified laterality
CC Excl: CC with 7th character A: See code: S65.409

√7ᵗʰ **S65.509 Unspecified injury of blood vessel of unspecified finger** CC
CC Excl: CC with 7th character A: See code: S65.409

√6ᵗʰ **S65.51 Laceration of blood vessel of other and unspecified finger**

√7ᵗʰ **S65.510 Laceration of blood vessel of right index finger** CC
CC Excl: CC with 7th character A: See code: S65.401

√7ᵗʰ **S65.511 Laceration of blood vessel of left index finger** CC
CC Excl: CC with 7th character A: See code: S65.402

√7ᵗʰ **S65.512 Laceration of blood vessel of right middle finger** CC
CC Excl: CC with 7th character A: See code: S65.401

√7ᵗʰ **S65.513 Laceration of blood vessel of left middle finger** CC
CC Excl: CC with 7th character A: See code: S65.402

√7ᵗʰ **S65.514 Laceration of blood vessel of right ring finger** CC
CC Excl: CC with 7th character A: See code: S65.401

√7ᵗʰ **S65.515 Laceration of blood vessel of left ring finger** CC
CC Excl: CC with 7th character A: See code: S65.402

√7ᵗʰ **S65.516 Laceration of blood vessel of right little finger** CC
CC Excl: CC with 7th character A: See code: S65.401

√7ᵗʰ **S65.517 Laceration of blood vessel of left little finger** CC
CC Excl: CC with 7th character A: See code: S65.402

✔ Additional Character Required   √x7ᵗʰ Placeholder Alert   Unacceptable PDx   Manifestation   Hospital Acquired Condition   *EXCLUDES 1* Not Coded Here   *EXCLUDES 2* Not Included Here

ICD-10-CM 2016   1005

√7ᵗʰ **S65.518** **Laceration of blood vessel of** other **finger** CC
Laceration of blood vessel of specified finger with unspecified laterality
CC Excl: CC with 7th character A: See code: S65.409

√7ᵗʰ **S65.519** **Laceration of blood vessel of** unspecified **finger** CC
CC Excl: CC with 7th character A: See code: S65.409

√6ᵗʰ **S65.59** **Other** specified injury of blood vessel of other and unspecified finger

√7ᵗʰ **S65.590** **Other specified injury of blood vessel of** right index **finger** CC
CC Excl: CC with 7th character A: See code: S65.401

√7ᵗʰ **S65.591** **Other specified injury of blood vessel of** left index **finger** CC
CC Excl: CC with 7th character A: See code: S65.402

√7ᵗʰ **S65.592** **Other specified injury of blood vessel of** right middle **finger** CC
CC Excl: CC with 7th character A: See code: S65.401

√7ᵗʰ **S65.593** **Other specified injury of blood vessel of** left middle **finger** CC
CC Excl: CC with 7th character A: See code: S65.402

√7ᵗʰ **S65.594** **Other specified injury of blood vessel of** right ring **finger** CC
CC Excl: CC with 7th character A: See code: S65.401

√7ᵗʰ **S65.595** **Other specified injury of blood vessel of** left ring **finger** CC
CC Excl: CC with 7th character A: See code: S65.402

√7ᵗʰ **S65.596** **Other specified injury of blood vessel of** right little **finger** CC
CC Excl: CC with 7th character A: See code: S65.401

√7ᵗʰ **S65.597** **Other specified injury of blood vessel of** left little **finger** CC
CC Excl: CC with 7th character A: See code: S65.402

√7ᵗʰ **S65.598** **Other specified injury of blood vessel of** other **finger** CC
Other specified injury of blood vessel of specified finger with unspecified laterality
CC Excl: CC with 7th character A: See code: S65.409

√7ᵗʰ **S65.599** **Other specified injury of blood vessel of** unspecified **finger** CC
CC Excl: CC with 7th character A: See code: S65.409

√5ᵗʰ **S65.8** **Injury of other blood vessels at** wrist and hand level

√6ᵗʰ **S65.80** **Unspecified** injury of other blood vessels at wrist and hand level

√7ᵗʰ **S65.801** **Unspecified injury of other blood vessels at wrist and hand level of** right **arm** CC
CC Excl: CC with 7th character A: S45.301A, S45.309-S45.311 with 7th A, S45.319-S45.391 with 7th A, S45.399-S45.801 with 7th A, S45.809-S45.811 with 7th A, S45.819-S45.891 with 7th A, S45.899-S45.901 with 7th A, S45.909-S45.911 with 7th A, S45.919-S45.991 with 7th A, S45.999A, S55.001A, S55.009-S55.011 with 7th A, S55.019-S55.091 with 7th A, S55.099A, S55.201A, S55.209-S55.211 with 7th A, S55.219-S55.291 with 7th A, S55.299-S55.801 with 7th A, S55.809-S55.811 with 7th A, S55.819-S55.891 with 7th A, S55.899-S55.901 with 7th A, S55.909-S55.911 with 7th A, S55.919-S55.991 with 7th A, S55.999A, S65.001A, S65.009-S65.011 with 7th A, S65.019-S65.091 with 7th A, S65.099A, S65.201A, S65.209-S65.211 with 7th A, S65.219-S65.291 with 7th A, S65.299-S65.301 with 7th A, S65.309-S65.311 with 7th A, S65.319-S65.391 with 7th A, S65.399-S65.401 with 7th A, S65.409-S65.411 with 7th A, S65.419-S65.491 with 7th A, S65.499-S65.500 with 7th A, S65.502A, S65.504A, S65.506A, S65.508-S65.510 with 7th A, S65.512A,

S65.514A, S65.516A, S65.518-S65.590 with 7th A, S65.592A, S65.594A, S65.596A, S65.598-S65.801 with 7th A, S65.809-S65.811 with 7th A, S65.819-S65.891 with 7th A, S65.899-S65.901 with 7th A, S65.909-S65.911 with 7th A, S65.919-S65.991 with 7th A, S65.999 with 7th A

√7ᵗʰ **S65.802** **Unspecified injury of other blood vessels at wrist and hand level of** left **arm** CC
CC Excl: CC with 7th character A: S45.302-S45.309 with 7th A, S45.312-S45.319 with 7th A, S45.392-S45.399 with 7th A, S45.802-S45.809 with 7th A, S45.812-S45.819 with 7th A, S45.892-S45.899 with 7th A, S45.902-S45.909 with 7th A, S45.912-S45.919 with 7th A, S45.992-S45.999 with 7th A, S55.002-S55.009 with 7th A, S55.012-S55.019 with 7th A, S55.092-S55.099 with 7th A, S55.202-S55.209 with 7th A, S55.212-S55.219 with 7th A, S55.292-S55.299 with 7th A, S55.802-S55.809 with 7th A, S55.812-S55.819 with 7th A, S55.892-S55.899 with 7th A, S55.902-S55.909 with 7th A, S55.912-S55.919 with 7th A, S55.992-S55.999 with 7th A, S65.002-S65.009 with 7th A, S65.012-S65.019 with 7th A, S65.092-S65.099 with 7th A, S65.202-S65.209 with 7th A, S65.212-S65.219 with 7th A, S65.292-S65.299 with 7th A, S65.302-S65.309 with 7th A, S65.312-S65.319 with 7th A, S65.392-S65.399 with 7th A, S65.402-S65.409 with 7th A, S65.412-S65.419 with 7th A, S65.492-S65.499 with 7th A, S65.501A, S65.503A, S65.505A, S65.507-S65.509 with 7th A, S65.511A, S65.513A, S65.515A, S65.517-S65.519 with 7th A, S65.591A, S65.593A, S65.595A, S65.597-S65.599 with 7th A, S65.802-S65.809 with 7th A, S65.812-S65.819 with 7th A, S65.892-S65.899 with 7th A, S65.902-S65.909 with 7th A, S65.912-S65.919 with 7th A, S65.992-S65.999 with 7th A

√7ᵗʰ **S65.809** **Unspecified injury of other blood vessels at wrist and hand level of** unspecified **arm** CC
CC Excl: CC with 7th character A: S45.301-S45.999 with 7th A, S55.001-S55.099 with 7th A, S55.201-S55.999 with 7th A, S65.001-S65.099 with 7th A, S65.201-S65.999 with 7th A

√6ᵗʰ **S65.81** **Laceration** of other blood vessels at wrist and hand level

√7ᵗʰ **S65.811** **Laceration of other blood vessels at wrist and hand level of** right **arm** CC
CC Excl: CC with 7th character A: See code: S65.801

√7ᵗʰ **S65.812** **Laceration of other blood vessels at wrist and hand level of** left **arm** CC
CC Excl: CC with 7th character A: See code: S65.802

√7ᵗʰ **S65.819** **Laceration of other blood vessels at wrist and hand level of** unspecified **arm** CC
CC Excl: CC with 7th character A: See code: S65.809

√6ᵗʰ **S65.89** **Other** specified injury of other blood vessels at wrist and hand level

√7ᵗʰ **S65.891** **Other specified injury of other blood vessels at wrist and hand level of** right **arm** CC
CC Excl: CC with 7th character A: See code: S65.801

√7ᵗʰ **S65.892** **Other specified injury of other blood vessels at wrist and hand level of** left **arm** CC
CC Excl: CC with 7th character A: See code: S65.802

√7ᵗʰ **S65.899** **Other specified injury of other blood vessels at wrist and hand level of** unspecified **arm** CC
CC Excl: CC with 7th character A: See code: S65.809

√5ᵗʰ **S65.9** **Injury of unspecified blood vessel at** wrist and hand level

√6ᵗʰ   **S65.90**   Unspecified **injury of unspecified blood vessel at wrist and hand level**

√7ᵗʰ   **S65.901**   **Unspecified injury of unspecified blood vessel at wrist and hand level of** right **arm**   `CC`
CC Excl: CC with 7th character A: See code: S65.801

√7ᵗʰ   **S65.902**   **Unspecified injury of unspecified blood vessel at wrist and hand level of** left **arm**   `CC`
CC Excl: CC with 7th character A: See code: S65.802

√7ᵗʰ   **S65.909**   **Unspecified injury of unspecified blood vessel at wrist and hand level of** unspecified **arm**   `CC`
CC Excl: CC with 7th character A: See code: S65.809

√6ᵗʰ   **S65.91**   Laceration **of unspecified blood vessel at wrist and hand level**

√7ᵗʰ   **S65.911**   **Laceration of unspecified blood vessel at wrist and hand level of** right **arm**   `CC`
CC Excl: CC with 7th character A: See code: S65.801

√7ᵗʰ   **S65.912**   **Laceration of unspecified blood vessel at wrist and hand level of** left **arm**   `CC`
CC Excl: CC with 7th character A: See code: S65.802

√7ᵗʰ   **S65.919**   **Laceration of unspecified blood vessel at wrist and hand level of** unspecified **arm**   `CC`
CC Excl: CC with 7th character A: See code: S65.809

√6ᵗʰ   **S65.99**   Other **specified injury of unspecified blood vessel at wrist and hand level**

√7ᵗʰ   **S65.991**   **Other specified injury of unspecified blood vessel at wrist and hand of** right **arm**   `CC`
CC Excl: CC with 7th character A: See code: S65.801

√7ᵗʰ   **S65.992**   **Other specified injury of unspecified blood vessel at wrist and hand of** left **arm**   `CC`
CC Excl: CC with 7th character A: See code: S65.802

√7ᵗʰ   **S65.999**   **Other specified injury of unspecified blood vessel at wrist and hand of** unspecified **arm**   `CC`
CC Excl: CC with 7th character A: See code: S65.809

✦ √4ᵗʰ **S66 Injury of muscle, fascia and tendon at wrist and hand level**
Code also any associated open wound (S61.-)
EXCLUDES 2   *sprain of joints and ligaments of wrist and hand (S63.-)*

The appropriate 7th character is to be added to each code from category S66.
A   initial encounter
D   subsequent encounter
S   sequela

√5ᵗʰ **S66.0** **Injury of** long flexor **muscle, fascia and tendon of** thumb **at wrist and hand level**

√6ᵗʰ   **S66.00**   Unspecified **injury of long flexor muscle, fascia and tendon of thumb at wrist and hand level**

√7ᵗʰ   **S66.001**   **Unspecified injury of long flexor muscle, fascia and tendon of** right **thumb at wrist and hand level**

√7ᵗʰ   **S66.002**   **Unspecified injury of long flexor muscle, fascia and tendon of** left **thumb at wrist and hand level**

√7ᵗʰ   **S66.009**   **Unspecified injury of long flexor muscle, fascia and tendon of** unspecified **thumb at wrist and hand level**

√6ᵗʰ   **S66.01**   Strain **of long flexor muscle, fascia and tendon of thumb at wrist and hand level**

√7ᵗʰ   **S66.011**   **Strain of long flexor muscle, fascia and tendon of** right **thumb at wrist and hand level**

√7ᵗʰ   **S66.012**   **Strain of long flexor muscle, fascia and tendon of** left **thumb at wrist and hand level**

√7ᵗʰ   **S66.019**   **Strain of long flexor muscle, fascia and tendon of** unspecified **thumb at wrist and hand level**

√6ᵗʰ   **S66.02**   Laceration **of long flexor muscle, fascia and tendon of thumb at wrist and hand level**

√7ᵗʰ   **S66.021**   **Laceration of long flexor muscle, fascia and tendon of** right **thumb at wrist and hand level**   `CC`
CC Excl: CC with 7th character A: S61.401A, S61.409-S61.411 with 7th A, S61.419-S61.421 with 7th A, S61.429-S61.431 with 7th A, S61.439-S61.441 with 7th A, S61.449-S61.451 with 7th A, S61.459A, S66.021A, S66.029A, S66.120A, S66.122A, S66.124A, S66.126A, S66.128-S66.129 with 7th A, S66.221A, S66.229A, S66.320A, S66.322A, S66.324A, S66.326A, S66.328-S66.329 with 7th A, S66.421A, S66.429A, S66.520A, S66.522A, S66.524A, S66.526A, S66.528-S66.529 with 7th A, S66.821A, S66.829A, S66.921A, S66.929 with 7th A

√7ᵗʰ   **S66.022**   **Laceration of long flexor muscle, fascia and tendon of** left **thumb at wrist and hand level**   `CC`
CC Excl: CC with 7th character A: S61.402-S61.409 with 7th A, S61.412-S61.419 with 7th A, S61.422-S61.429 with 7th A, S61.432-S61.439 with 7th A, S61.442-S61.449 with 7th A, S61.452-S61.459 with 7th A, S66.022-S66.029 with 7th A, S66.121A, S66.123A, S66.125A, S66.127-S66.129 with 7th A, S66.222-S66.229 with 7th A, S66.321A, S66.323A, S66.325A, S66.327-S66.329 with 7th A, S66.422-S66.429 with 7th A, S66.521A, S66.523A, S66.525A, S66.527-S66.529 with 7th A, S66.822-S66.829 with 7th A, S66.922-S66.929 with 7th A

√7ᵗʰ   **S66.029**   **Laceration of long flexor muscle, fascia and tendon of** unspecified **thumb at wrist and hand level**   `CC`
CC Excl: CC with 7th character A: S61.401-S61.459 with 7th A, S66.021-S66.029 with 7th A, S66.120-S66.129 with 7th A, S66.221-S66.229 with 7th A, S66.320-S66.329 with 7th A, S66.421-S66.429 with 7th A, S66.520-S66.529 with 7th A, S66.821-S66.829 with 7th A, S66.921-S66.929 with 7th A

√6ᵗʰ   **S66.09**   Other **specified injury of long flexor muscle, fascia and tendon of thumb at wrist and hand level**

√7ᵗʰ   **S66.091**   **Other specified injury of long flexor muscle, fascia and tendon of** right **thumb at wrist and hand level**

√7ᵗʰ   **S66.092**   **Other specified injury of long flexor muscle, fascia and tendon of** left **thumb at wrist and hand level**

√7ᵗʰ   **S66.099**   **Other specified injury of long flexor muscle, fascia and tendon of** unspecified **thumb at wrist and hand level**

√5ᵗʰ **S66.1** **Injury of** flexor muscle, fascia and tendon of other and unspecified **finger at wrist and hand level**
EXCLUDES 2   *Injury of long flexor muscle, fascia and tendon of thumb at wrist and hand level (S66.0-)*

√6ᵗʰ   **S66.10**   Unspecified **injury of flexor muscle, fascia and tendon of other and unspecified finger at wrist and hand level**

√7ᵗʰ   **S66.100**   **Unspecified injury of flexor muscle, fascia and tendon of** right index **finger at wrist and hand level**

√7ᵗʰ   **S66.101**   **Unspecified injury of flexor muscle, fascia and tendon of** left index **finger at wrist and hand level**

√7ᵗʰ   **S66.102**   **Unspecified injury of flexor muscle, fascia and tendon of** right middle **finger at wrist and hand level**

√7ᵗʰ   **S66.103**   **Unspecified injury of flexor muscle, fascia and tendon of** left middle **finger at wrist and hand level**

✦   Refer to the Muscle/Tendon Table at beginning of this chapter.

✔ Additional Character Required   √ₓ7ᵗʰ Placeholder Alert   Unacceptable PDx   Manifestation   Hospital Acquired Condition   *EXCLUDES 1* Not Coded Here   *EXCLUDES 2* Not Included Here

√7th S66.104 Unspecified injury of flexor muscle, fascia and tendon of right ring finger at wrist and hand level

√7th S66.105 Unspecified injury of flexor muscle, fascia and tendon of left ring finger at wrist and hand level

√7th S66.106 Unspecified injury of flexor muscle, fascia and tendon of right little finger at wrist and hand level

√7th S66.107 Unspecified injury of flexor muscle, fascia and tendon of left little finger at wrist and hand level

√7th S66.108 Unspecified injury of flexor muscle, fascia and tendon of other finger at wrist and hand level

Unspecified injury of flexor muscle, fascia and tendon of specified finger with unspecified laterality at wrist and hand level

√7th S66.109 Unspecified injury of flexor muscle, fascia and tendon of unspecified finger at wrist and hand level

√6th S66.11 Strain of flexor muscle, fascia and tendon of other and unspecified finger at wrist and hand level

√7th S66.110 Strain of flexor muscle, fascia and tendon of right index finger at wrist and hand level

√7th S66.111 Strain of flexor muscle, fascia and tendon of left index finger at wrist and hand level

√7th S66.112 Strain of flexor muscle, fascia and tendon of right middle finger at wrist and hand level

√7th S66.113 Strain of flexor muscle, fascia and tendon of left middle finger at wrist and hand level

√7th S66.114 Strain of flexor muscle, fascia and tendon of right ring finger at wrist and hand level

√7th S66.115 Strain of flexor muscle, fascia and tendon of left ring finger at wrist and hand level

√7th S66.116 Strain of flexor muscle, fascia and tendon of right little finger at wrist and hand level

√7th S66.117 Strain of flexor muscle, fascia and tendon of left little finger at wrist and hand level

√7th S66.118 Strain of flexor muscle, fascia and tendon of other finger at wrist and hand level

Strain of flexor muscle, fascia and tendon of specified finger with unspecified laterality at wrist and hand level

√7th S66.119 Strain of flexor muscle, fascia and tendon of unspecified finger at wrist and hand level

√6th S66.12 Laceration of flexor muscle, fascia and tendon of other and unspecified finger at wrist and hand level

√7th S66.120 Laceration of flexor muscle, fascia and tendon of right index finger at wrist and hand level   CC

CC Excl: CC with 7th character A: See code: S66.021

√7th S66.121 Laceration of flexor muscle, fascia and tendon of left index finger at wrist and hand level   CC

CC Excl: CC with 7th character A: See code: S66.022

√7th S66.122 Laceration of flexor muscle, fascia and tendon of right middle finger at wrist and hand level   CC

CC Excl: CC with 7th character A: See code: S66.021

√7th S66.123 Laceration of flexor muscle, fascia and tendon of left middle finger at wrist and hand level   CC

CC Excl: CC with 7th character A: See code: S66.022

√7th S66.124 Laceration of flexor muscle, fascia and tendon of right ring finger at wrist and hand level   CC

CC Excl: CC with 7th character A: See code: S66.021

√7th S66.125 Laceration of flexor muscle, fascia and tendon of left ring finger at wrist and hand level   CC

CC Excl: CC with 7th character A: See code: S66.022

√7th S66.126 Laceration of flexor muscle, fascia and tendon of right little finger at wrist and hand level   CC

CC Excl: CC with 7th character A: See code: S66.021

√7th S66.127 Laceration of flexor muscle, fascia and tendon of left little finger at wrist and hand level   CC

CC Excl: CC with 7th character A: See code: S66.022

√7th S66.128 Laceration of flexor muscle, fascia and tendon of other finger at wrist and hand level   CC

Laceration of flexor muscle, fascia and tendon of specified finger with unspecified laterality at wrist and hand level

CC Excl: CC with 7th character A: See code: S66.029

√7th S66.129 Laceration of flexor muscle, fascia and tendon of unspecified finger at wrist and hand level   CC

CC Excl: CC with 7th character A: See code: S66.029

√6th S66.19 Other injury of flexor muscle, fascia and tendon of other and unspecified finger at wrist and hand level

√7th S66.190 Other injury of flexor muscle, fascia and tendon of right index finger at wrist and hand level

√7th S66.191 Other injury of flexor muscle, fascia and tendon of left index finger at wrist and hand level

√7th S66.192 Other injury of flexor muscle, fascia and tendon of right middle finger at wrist and hand level

√7th S66.193 Other injury of flexor muscle, fascia and tendon of left middle finger at wrist and hand level

√7th S66.194 Other injury of flexor muscle, fascia and tendon of right ring finger at wrist and hand level

√7th S66.195 Other injury of flexor muscle, fascia and tendon of left ring finger at wrist and hand level

√7th S66.196 Other injury of flexor muscle, fascia and tendon of right little finger at wrist and hand level

√7th S66.197 Other injury of flexor muscle, fascia and tendon of left little finger at wrist and hand level

√7th S66.198 Other injury of flexor muscle, fascia and tendon of other finger at wrist and hand level

Other injury of flexor muscle, fascia and tendon of specified finger with unspecified laterality at wrist and hand level

√7th S66.199 Other injury of flexor muscle, fascia and tendon of unspecified finger at wrist and hand level

√5th S66.2 Injury of extensor muscle, fascia and tendon of thumb at wrist and hand level

√6th S66.20 Unspecified injury of extensor muscle, fascia and tendon of thumb at wrist and hand level

√7th S66.201 Unspecified injury of extensor muscle, fascia and tendon of right thumb at wrist and hand level

√7th S66.202 Unspecified injury of extensor muscle, fascia and tendon of left thumb at wrist and hand level

√7th S66.209 Unspecified injury of extensor muscle, fascia and tendon of unspecified thumb at wrist and hand level

---

✓6ᵗʰ **S66.21** **Strain** of extensor muscle, fascia and tendon of thumb at wrist and hand level

    ✓7ᵗʰ **S66.211** Strain of extensor muscle, fascia and tendon of **right** thumb at wrist and hand level

    ✓7ᵗʰ **S66.212** Strain of extensor muscle, fascia and tendon of **left** thumb at wrist and hand level

    ✓7ᵗʰ **S66.219** Strain of extensor muscle, fascia and tendon of **unspecified** thumb at wrist and hand level

✓6ᵗʰ **S66.22** **Laceration** of extensor muscle, fascia and tendon of thumb at wrist and hand level

    ✓7ᵗʰ **S66.221** Laceration of extensor muscle, fascia and tendon of **right** thumb at wrist and hand level   [CC]
       CC Excl: CC with 7th character A: See code: S66.021

    ✓7ᵗʰ **S66.222** Laceration of extensor muscle, fascia and tendon of **left** thumb at wrist and hand level   [CC]
       CC Excl: CC with 7th character A: See code: S66.022

    ✓7ᵗʰ **S66.229** Laceration of extensor muscle, fascia and tendon of **unspecified** thumb at wrist and hand level   [CC]
       CC Excl: CC with 7th character A: See code: S66.029

✓6ᵗʰ **S66.29** **Other specified** injury of extensor muscle, fascia and tendon of thumb at wrist and hand level

    ✓7ᵗʰ **S66.291** Other specified injury of extensor muscle, fascia and tendon of **right** thumb at wrist and hand level

    ✓7ᵗʰ **S66.292** Other specified injury of extensor muscle, fascia and tendon of **left** thumb at wrist and hand level

    ✓7ᵗʰ **S66.299** Other specified injury of extensor muscle, fascia and tendon of **unspecified** thumb at wrist and hand level

✓5ᵗʰ **S66.3** **Injury** of extensor muscle, fascia and tendon of **other and unspecified** finger at wrist and hand level

    EXCLUDES 2 *Injury of extensor muscle, fascia and tendon of thumb at wrist and hand level (S66.2-)*

✓6ᵗʰ **S66.30** **Unspecified** injury of extensor muscle, fascia and tendon of other and unspecified finger at wrist and hand level

    ✓7ᵗʰ **S66.300** Unspecified injury of extensor muscle, fascia and tendon of **right index** finger at wrist and hand level

    ✓7ᵗʰ **S66.301** Unspecified injury of extensor muscle, fascia and tendon of **left index** finger at wrist and hand level

    ✓7ᵗʰ **S66.302** Unspecified injury of extensor muscle, fascia and tendon of **right middle** finger at wrist and hand level

    ✓7ᵗʰ **S66.303** Unspecified injury of extensor muscle, fascia and tendon of **left middle** finger at wrist and hand level

    ✓7ᵗʰ **S66.304** Unspecified injury of extensor muscle, fascia and tendon of **right ring** finger at wrist and hand level

    ✓7ᵗʰ **S66.305** Unspecified injury of extensor muscle, fascia and tendon of **left ring** finger at wrist and hand level

    ✓7ᵗʰ **S66.306** Unspecified injury of extensor muscle, fascia and tendon of **right little** finger at wrist and hand level

    ✓7ᵗʰ **S66.307** Unspecified injury of extensor muscle, fascia and tendon of **left little** finger at wrist and hand level

    ✓7ᵗʰ **S66.308** Unspecified injury of extensor muscle, fascia and tendon of **other** finger at wrist and hand level
       Unspecified injury of extensor muscle, fascia and tendon of specified finger with unspecified laterality at wrist and hand level

    ✓7ᵗʰ **S66.309** Unspecified injury of extensor muscle, fascia and tendon of **unspecified** finger at wrist and hand level

✓6ᵗʰ **S66.31** **Strain** of extensor muscle, fascia and tendon of other and unspecified finger at wrist and hand level

    ✓7ᵗʰ **S66.310** Strain of extensor muscle, fascia and tendon of **right index** finger at wrist and hand level

    ✓7ᵗʰ **S66.311** Strain of extensor muscle, fascia and tendon of **left index** finger at wrist and hand level

    ✓7ᵗʰ **S66.312** Strain of extensor muscle, fascia and tendon of **right middle** finger at wrist and hand level

    ✓7ᵗʰ **S66.313** Strain of extensor muscle, fascia and tendon of **left middle** finger at wrist and hand level

    ✓7ᵗʰ **S66.314** Strain of extensor muscle, fascia and tendon of **right ring** finger at wrist and hand level

    ✓7ᵗʰ **S66.315** Strain of extensor muscle, fascia and tendon of **left ring** finger at wrist and hand level

    ✓7ᵗʰ **S66.316** Strain of extensor muscle, fascia and tendon of **right little** finger at wrist and hand level

    ✓7ᵗʰ **S66.317** Strain of extensor muscle, fascia and tendon of **left little** finger at wrist and hand level

    ✓7ᵗʰ **S66.318** Strain of extensor muscle, fascia and tendon of **other** finger at wrist and hand level
       Strain of extensor muscle, fascia and tendon of specified finger with unspecified laterality at wrist and hand level

    ✓7ᵗʰ **S66.319** Strain of extensor muscle, fascia and tendon of **unspecified** finger at wrist and hand level

✓6ᵗʰ **S66.32** **Laceration** of extensor muscle, fascia and tendon of other and unspecified finger at wrist and hand level

    ✓7ᵗʰ **S66.320** Laceration of extensor muscle, fascia and tendon of **right index** finger at wrist and hand level   [CC]
       CC Excl: CC with 7th character A: See code: S66.021

    ✓7ᵗʰ **S66.321** Laceration of extensor muscle, fascia and tendon of **left index** finger at wrist and hand level   [CC]
       CC Excl: CC with 7th character A: See code: S66.022

    ✓7ᵗʰ **S66.322** Laceration of extensor muscle, fascia and tendon of **right middle** finger at wrist and hand level   [CC]
       CC Excl: CC with 7th character A: See code: S66.021

    ✓7ᵗʰ **S66.323** Laceration of extensor muscle, fascia and tendon of **left middle** finger at wrist and hand level   [CC]
       CC Excl: CC with 7th character A: See code: S66.022

    ✓7ᵗʰ **S66.324** Laceration of extensor muscle, fascia and tendon of **right ring** finger at wrist and hand level   [CC]
       CC Excl: CC with 7th character A: See code: S66.021

    ✓7ᵗʰ **S66.325** Laceration of extensor muscle, fascia and tendon of **left ring** finger at wrist and hand level   [CC]
       CC Excl: CC with 7th character A: See code: S66.022

    ✓7ᵗʰ **S66.326** Laceration of extensor muscle, fascia and tendon of **right little** finger at wrist and hand level   [CC]
       CC Excl: CC with 7th character A: See code: S66.021

    ✓7ᵗʰ **S66.327** Laceration of extensor muscle, fascia and tendon of **left little** finger at wrist and hand level   [CC]
       CC Excl: CC with 7th character A: See code: S66.022

✓ Additional Character Required   ✓x7ᵗʰ Placeholder Alert   Unacceptable PDx   Manifestation   Hospital Acquired Condition   **EXCLUDES 1** Not Coded Here   **EXCLUDES 2** Not Included Here

ICD-10-CM 2016   1009

✓7ᵗʰ S66.328 Laceration of extensor muscle, fascia and tendon of other finger at wrist and hand level CC

> Laceration of extensor muscle, fascia and tendon of specified finger with unspecified laterality at wrist and hand level
>
> **CC Excl: CC with 7th character A:** See code: S66.029

✓7ᵗʰ S66.329 Laceration of extensor muscle, fascia and tendon of unspecified finger at wrist and hand level CC

> **CC Excl: CC with 7th character A:** See code: S66.029

✓6ᵗʰ S66.39 Other injury of extensor muscle, fascia and tendon of other and unspecified finger at wrist and hand level

✓7ᵗʰ S66.390 Other injury of extensor muscle, fascia and tendon of right index finger at wrist and hand level

✓7ᵗʰ S66.391 Other injury of extensor muscle, fascia and tendon of left index finger at wrist and hand level

✓7ᵗʰ S66.392 Other injury of extensor muscle, fascia and tendon of right middle finger at wrist and hand level

✓7ᵗʰ S66.393 Other injury of extensor muscle, fascia and tendon of left middle finger at wrist and hand level

✓7ᵗʰ S66.394 Other injury of extensor muscle, fascia and tendon of right ring finger at wrist and hand level

✓7ᵗʰ S66.395 Other injury of extensor muscle, fascia and tendon of left ring finger at wrist and hand level

✓7ᵗʰ S66.396 Other injury of extensor muscle, fascia and tendon of right little finger at wrist and hand level

✓7ᵗʰ S66.397 Other injury of extensor muscle, fascia and tendon of left little finger at wrist and hand level

✓7ᵗʰ S66.398 Other injury of extensor muscle, fascia and tendon of other finger at wrist and hand level

> Other injury of extensor muscle, fascia and tendon of specified finger with unspecified laterality at wrist and hand level

✓7ᵗʰ S66.399 Other injury of extensor muscle, fascia and tendon of unspecified finger at wrist and hand level

✓5ᵗʰ S66.4 Injury of intrinsic muscle, fascia and tendon of thumb at wrist and hand level

✓6ᵗʰ S66.40 Unspecified injury of intrinsic muscle, fascia and tendon of thumb at wrist and hand level

✓7ᵗʰ S66.401 Unspecified injury of intrinsic muscle, fascia and tendon of right thumb at wrist and hand level

✓7ᵗʰ S66.402 Unspecified injury of intrinsic muscle, fascia and tendon of left thumb at wrist and hand level

✓7ᵗʰ S66.409 Unspecified injury of intrinsic muscle, fascia and tendon of unspecified thumb at wrist and hand level

✓6ᵗʰ S66.41 Strain of intrinsic muscle, fascia and tendon of thumb at wrist and hand level

✓7ᵗʰ S66.411 Strain of intrinsic muscle, fascia and tendon of right thumb at wrist and hand level

✓7ᵗʰ S66.412 Strain of intrinsic muscle, fascia and tendon of left thumb at wrist and hand level

✓7ᵗʰ S66.419 Strain of intrinsic muscle, fascia and tendon of unspecified thumb at wrist and hand level

✓6ᵗʰ S66.42 Laceration of intrinsic muscle, fascia and tendon of thumb at wrist and hand level

✓7ᵗʰ S66.421 Laceration of intrinsic muscle, fascia and tendon of right thumb at wrist and hand level CC

> **CC Excl: CC with 7th character A:** See code: S66.021

✓7ᵗʰ S66.422 Laceration of intrinsic muscle, fascia and tendon of left thumb at wrist and hand level CC

> **CC Excl: CC with 7th character A:** See code: S66.022

✓7ᵗʰ S66.429 Laceration of intrinsic muscle, fascia and tendon of unspecified thumb at wrist and hand level CC

> **CC Excl: CC with 7th character A:** See code: S66.029

✓6ᵗʰ S66.49 Other specified injury of intrinsic muscle, fascia and tendon of thumb at wrist and hand level

✓7ᵗʰ S66.491 Other specified injury of intrinsic muscle, fascia and tendon of right thumb at wrist and hand level

✓7ᵗʰ S66.492 Other specified injury of intrinsic muscle, fascia and tendon of left thumb at wrist and hand level

✓7ᵗʰ S66.499 Other specified injury of intrinsic muscle, fascia and tendon of unspecified thumb at wrist and hand level

✓5ᵗʰ S66.5 Injury of intrinsic muscle, fascia and tendon of other and unspecified finger at wrist and hand level

> EXCLUDES 2   injury of intrinsic muscle, fascia and tendon of thumb at wrist and hand level (S66.4-)

✓6ᵗʰ S66.50 Unspecified injury of intrinsic muscle, fascia and tendon of other and unspecified finger at wrist and hand level

✓7ᵗʰ S66.500 Unspecified injury of intrinsic muscle, fascia and tendon of right index finger at wrist and hand level

✓7ᵗʰ S66.501 Unspecified injury of intrinsic muscle, fascia and tendon of left index finger at wrist and hand level

✓7ᵗʰ S66.502 Unspecified injury of intrinsic muscle, fascia and tendon of right middle finger at wrist and hand level

✓7ᵗʰ S66.503 Unspecified injury of intrinsic muscle, fascia and tendon of left middle finger at wrist and hand level

✓7ᵗʰ S66.504 Unspecified injury of intrinsic muscle, fascia and tendon of right ring finger at wrist and hand level

✓7ᵗʰ S66.505 Unspecified injury of intrinsic muscle, fascia and tendon of left ring finger at wrist and hand level

✓7ᵗʰ S66.506 Unspecified injury of intrinsic muscle, fascia and tendon of right little finger at wrist and hand level

✓7ᵗʰ S66.507 Unspecified injury of intrinsic muscle, fascia and tendon of left little finger at wrist and hand level

✓7ᵗʰ S66.508 Unspecified injury of intrinsic muscle, fascia and tendon of other finger at wrist and hand level

> Unspecified injury of intrinsic muscle, fascia and tendon of specified finger with unspecified laterality at wrist and hand level

✓7ᵗʰ S66.509 Unspecified injury of intrinsic muscle, fascia and tendon of unspecified finger at wrist and hand level

✓6ᵗʰ S66.51 Strain of intrinsic muscle, fascia and tendon of other and unspecified finger at wrist and hand level

✓7ᵗʰ S66.510 Strain of intrinsic muscle, fascia and tendon of right index finger at wrist and hand level

✓7ᵗʰ S66.511 Strain of intrinsic muscle, fascia and tendon of left index finger at wrist and hand level

✓7ᵗʰ S66.512 Strain of intrinsic muscle, fascia and tendon of right middle finger at wrist and hand level

Ⓝ Newborn: 0   Ⓟ Pediatric: 0-17   Ⓜ Maternity: 12-55   Ⓐ Adult: 15-124   **MCC** Major CC Condition   **PDxMCC** PDx acts as own MCC   **CC** CC Condition   **PDxCC** PDx acts as own CC

1010   ICD-10-CM 2016

✓7ᵗʰ **S66.513** **Strain of intrinsic muscle, fascia and tendon of** left middle **finger at wrist and hand level**

✓7ᵗʰ **S66.514** **Strain of intrinsic muscle, fascia and tendon of** right ring **finger at wrist and hand level**

✓7ᵗʰ **S66.515** **Strain of intrinsic muscle, fascia and tendon of** left ring **finger at wrist and hand level**

✓7ᵗʰ **S66.516** **Strain of intrinsic muscle, fascia and tendon of** right little **finger at wrist and hand level**

✓7ᵗʰ **S66.517** **Strain of intrinsic muscle, fascia and tendon of** left little **finger at wrist and hand level**

✓7ᵗʰ **S66.518** **Strain of intrinsic muscle, fascia and tendon of** other **finger at wrist and hand level**
Strain of intrinsic muscle, fascia and tendon of specified finger with unspecified laterality at wrist and hand level

✓7ᵗʰ **S66.519** **Strain of intrinsic muscle, fascia and tendon of** unspecified **finger at wrist and hand level**

✓6ᵗʰ **S66.52** **Laceration of intrinsic muscle, fascia and tendon of other and unspecified finger at wrist and hand level**

✓7ᵗʰ **S66.520** **Laceration of intrinsic muscle, fascia and tendon of** right index **finger at wrist and hand level** CC
CC Excl: CC with 7th character A: See code: S66.021

✓7ᵗʰ **S66.521** **Laceration of intrinsic muscle, fascia and tendon of** left index **finger at wrist and hand level** CC
CC Excl: CC with 7th character A: See code: S66.022

✓7ᵗʰ **S66.522** **Laceration of intrinsic muscle, fascia and tendon of** right middle **finger at wrist and hand level** CC
CC Excl: CC with 7th character A: See code: S66.021

✓7ᵗʰ **S66.523** **Laceration of intrinsic muscle, fascia and tendon of** left middle **finger at wrist and hand level** CC
CC Excl: CC with 7th character A: See code: S66.022

✓7ᵗʰ **S66.524** **Laceration of intrinsic muscle, fascia and tendon of** right ring **finger at wrist and hand level** CC
CC Excl: CC with 7th character A: See code: S66.021

✓7ᵗʰ **S66.525** **Laceration of intrinsic muscle, fascia and tendon of** left ring **finger at wrist and hand level** CC
CC Excl: CC with 7th character A: See code: S66.022

✓7ᵗʰ **S66.526** **Laceration of intrinsic muscle, fascia and tendon of** right little **finger at wrist and hand level** CC
CC Excl: CC with 7th character A: See code: S66.021

✓7ᵗʰ **S66.527** **Laceration of intrinsic muscle, fascia and tendon of** left little **finger at wrist and hand level** CC
CC Excl: CC with 7th character A: See code: S66.022

✓7ᵗʰ **S66.528** **Laceration of intrinsic muscle, fascia and tendon of** other **finger at wrist and hand level** CC
Laceration of intrinsic muscle, fascia and tendon of specified finger with unspecified laterality at wrist and hand level
CC Excl: CC with 7th character A: See code: S66.029

✓7ᵗʰ **S66.529** **Laceration of intrinsic muscle, fascia and tendon of** unspecified **finger at wrist and hand level** CC
CC Excl: CC with 7th character A: See code: S66.029

✓6ᵗʰ **S66.59** **Other injury of intrinsic muscle, fascia and tendon of other and unspecified finger at wrist and hand level**

✓7ᵗʰ **S66.590** **Other injury of intrinsic muscle, fascia and tendon of** right index **finger at wrist and hand level**

✓7ᵗʰ **S66.591** **Other injury of intrinsic muscle, fascia and tendon of** left index **finger at wrist and hand level**

✓7ᵗʰ **S66.592** **Other injury of intrinsic muscle, fascia and tendon of** right middle **finger at wrist and hand level**

✓7ᵗʰ **S66.593** **Other injury of intrinsic muscle, fascia and tendon of** left middle **finger at wrist and hand level**

✓7ᵗʰ **S66.594** **Other injury of intrinsic muscle, fascia and tendon of** right ring **finger at wrist and hand level**

✓7ᵗʰ **S66.595** **Other injury of intrinsic muscle, fascia and tendon of** left ring **finger at wrist and hand level**

✓7ᵗʰ **S66.596** **Other injury of intrinsic muscle, fascia and tendon of** right little **finger at wrist and hand level**

✓7ᵗʰ **S66.597** **Other injury of intrinsic muscle, fascia and tendon of** left little **finger at wrist and hand level**

✓7ᵗʰ **S66.598** **Other injury of intrinsic muscle, fascia and tendon of** other **finger at wrist and hand level**
Other injury of intrinsic muscle, fascia and tendon of specified finger with unspecified laterality at wrist and hand level

✓7ᵗʰ **S66.599** **Other injury of intrinsic muscle, fascia and tendon of** unspecified **finger at wrist and hand level**

✓5ᵗʰ **S66.8** **Injury of** other specified muscles, **fascia and tendons at wrist and hand level**

✓6ᵗʰ **S66.80** **Unspecified injury of other specified muscles, fascia and tendons at wrist and hand level**

✓7ᵗʰ **S66.801** **Unspecified injury of other specified muscles, fascia and tendons at wrist and hand level,** right **hand**

✓7ᵗʰ **S66.802** **Unspecified injury of other specified muscles, fascia and tendons at wrist and hand level,** left **hand**

✓7ᵗʰ **S66.809** **Unspecified injury of other specified muscles, fascia and tendons at wrist and hand level,** unspecified **hand**

✓6ᵗʰ **S66.81** **Strain of other specified muscles, fascia and tendons at wrist and hand level**

✓7ᵗʰ **S66.811** **Strain of other specified muscles, fascia and tendons at wrist and hand level,** right **hand**

✓7ᵗʰ **S66.812** **Strain of other specified muscles, fascia and tendons at wrist and hand level,** left **hand**

✓7ᵗʰ **S66.819** **Strain of other specified muscles, fascia and tendons at wrist and hand level,** unspecified **hand**

✓6ᵗʰ **S66.82** **Laceration of other specified muscles, fascia and tendons at wrist and hand level**

✓7ᵗʰ **S66.821** **Laceration of other specified muscles, fascia and tendons at wrist and hand level,** right **hand** CC
CC Excl: CC with 7th character A: See code: S66.021

✓7ᵗʰ **S66.822** **Laceration of other specified muscles, fascia and tendons at wrist and hand level,** left **hand** CC
CC Excl: CC with 7th character A: See code: S66.022

✓7ᵗʰ **S66.829** **Laceration of other specified muscles, fascia and tendons at wrist and hand level,** unspecified **hand** CC
CC Excl: CC with 7th character A: See code: S66.029

✓ Additional Character Required   ✗x7ᵗʰ Placeholder Alert   Unacceptable PDx   Manifestation   Hospital Acquired Condition   *EXCLUDES 1* Not Coded Here   *EXCLUDES 2* Not Included Here

√6ᵗʰ **S66.89 Other injury of other specified muscles, fascia and tendons at wrist and hand level**

    √7ᵗʰ **S66.891 Other injury of other specified muscles, fascia and tendons at wrist and hand level, right hand**

    √7ᵗʰ **S66.892 Other injury of other specified muscles, fascia and tendons at wrist and hand level, left hand**

    √7ᵗʰ **S66.899 Other injury of other specified muscles, fascia and tendons at wrist and hand level, unspecified hand**

√5ᵗʰ **S66.9 Injury of unspecified muscle, fascia and tendon at wrist and hand level**

   √6ᵗʰ **S66.90 Unspecified injury of unspecified muscle, fascia and tendon at wrist and hand level**

    √7ᵗʰ **S66.901 Unspecified injury of unspecified muscle, fascia and tendon at wrist and hand level, right hand**

    √7ᵗʰ **S66.902 Unspecified injury of unspecified muscle, fascia and tendon at wrist and hand level, left hand**

    √7ᵗʰ **S66.909 Unspecified injury of unspecified muscle, fascia and tendon at wrist and hand level, unspecified hand**

   √6ᵗʰ **S66.91 Strain of unspecified muscle, fascia and tendon at wrist and hand level**

    √7ᵗʰ **S66.911 Strain of unspecified muscle, fascia and tendon at wrist and hand level, right hand**

    √7ᵗʰ **S66.912 Strain of unspecified muscle, fascia and tendon at wrist and hand level, left hand**

    √7ᵗʰ **S66.919 Strain of unspecified muscle, fascia and tendon at wrist and hand level, unspecified hand**

   √6ᵗʰ **S66.92 Laceration of unspecified muscle, fascia and tendon at wrist and hand level**

    √7ᵗʰ **S66.921 Laceration of unspecified muscle, fascia and tendon at wrist and hand level, right hand**   `CC`
       CC Excl: CC with 7th character A: See code: S66.021

    √7ᵗʰ **S66.922 Laceration of unspecified muscle, fascia and tendon at wrist and hand level, left hand**   `CC`
       CC Excl: CC with 7th character A: See code: S66.022

    √7ᵗʰ **S66.929 Laceration of unspecified muscle, fascia and tendon at wrist and hand level, unspecified hand**   `CC`
       CC Excl: CC with 7th character A: See code: S66.029

   √6ᵗʰ **S66.99 Other injury of unspecified muscle, fascia and tendon at wrist and hand level**

    √7ᵗʰ **S66.991 Other injury of unspecified muscle, fascia and tendon at wrist and hand level, right hand**

    √7ᵗʰ **S66.992 Other injury of unspecified muscle, fascia and tendon at wrist and hand level, left hand**

    √7ᵗʰ **S66.999 Other injury of unspecified muscle, fascia and tendon at wrist and hand level, unspecified hand**

√4ᵗʰ **S67 Crushing injury of wrist, hand and fingers**
   Use additional code for all associated injuries, such as:
   fracture of wrist and hand (S62.-)
   open wound of wrist and hand (S61.-)

   The appropriate 7th character is to be added to each code from category S67.
   A   initial encounter
   D   subsequent encounter
   S   sequela

√5ᵗʰ **S67.0 Crushing injury of thumb**

   √x7ᵗʰ **S67.00 Crushing injury of unspecified thumb**

   √x7ᵗʰ **S67.01 Crushing injury of right thumb**

   √x7ᵗʰ **S67.02 Crushing injury of left thumb**

√5ᵗʰ **S67.1 Crushing injury of other and unspecified finger(s)**
   EXCLUDES 2   crushing injury of thumb (S67.0-)

   √x7ᵗʰ **S67.10 Crushing injury of unspecified finger(s)**

√6ᵗʰ **S67.19 Crushing injury of other finger(s)**

   √7ᵗʰ **S67.190 Crushing injury of right index finger**

   √7ᵗʰ **S67.191 Crushing injury of left index finger**

   √7ᵗʰ **S67.192 Crushing injury of right middle finger**

   √7ᵗʰ **S67.193 Crushing injury of left middle finger**

   √7ᵗʰ **S67.194 Crushing injury of right ring finger**

   √7ᵗʰ **S67.195 Crushing injury of left ring finger**

   √7ᵗʰ **S67.196 Crushing injury of right little finger**

   √7ᵗʰ **S67.197 Crushing injury of left little finger**

   √7ᵗʰ **S67.198 Crushing injury of other finger**
       Crushing injury of specified finger with unspecified laterality

√5ᵗʰ **S67.2 Crushing injury of hand**
   EXCLUDES 2   crushing injury of fingers (S67.1-)
       crushing injury of thumb (S67.0-)

   √x7ᵗʰ **S67.20 Crushing injury of unspecified hand**

   √x7ᵗʰ **S67.21 Crushing injury of right hand**

   √x7ᵗʰ **S67.22 Crushing injury of left hand**

√5ᵗʰ **S67.3 Crushing injury of wrist**

   √x7ᵗʰ **S67.30 Crushing injury of unspecified wrist**

   √x7ᵗʰ **S67.31 Crushing injury of right wrist**

   √x7ᵗʰ **S67.32 Crushing injury of left wrist**

√5ᵗʰ **S67.4 Crushing injury of wrist and hand**
   EXCLUDES 1   crushing injury of hand alone (S67.2-)
       crushing injury of wrist alone (S67.3-)
   EXCLUDES 2   crushing injury of fingers (S67.1-)
       crushing injury of thumb (S67.0-)

   √x7ᵗʰ **S67.40 Crushing injury of unspecified wrist and hand**

   √x7ᵗʰ **S67.41 Crushing injury of right wrist and hand**

   √x7ᵗʰ **S67.42 Crushing injury of left wrist and hand**

√5ᵗʰ **S67.9 Crushing injury of unspecified part(s) of wrist, hand and fingers**

   √x7ᵗʰ **S67.90 Crushing injury of unspecified part(s) of unspecified wrist, hand and fingers**

   √x7ᵗʰ **S67.91 Crushing injury of unspecified part(s) of right wrist, hand and fingers**

   √x7ᵗʰ **S67.92 Crushing injury of unspecified part(s) of left wrist, hand and fingers**

√4ᵗʰ **S68 Traumatic amputation of wrist, hand and fingers**
   NOTE   An amputation not identified as partial or complete should be coded to complete.

   The appropriate 7th character is to be added to each code from category S68.
   A   initial encounter
   D   subsequent encounter
   S   sequela

√5ᵗʰ **S68.0 Traumatic metacarpophalangeal amputation of thumb**
   Traumatic amputation of thumb NOS

   √6ᵗʰ **S68.01 Complete traumatic metacarpophalangeal amputation of thumb**

    √7ᵗʰ **S68.011 Complete traumatic metacarpophalangeal amputation of right thumb**

    √7ᵗʰ **S68.012 Complete traumatic metacarpophalangeal amputation of left thumb**

    √7ᵗʰ **S68.019 Complete traumatic metacarpophalangeal amputation of unspecified thumb**

   √6ᵗʰ **S68.02 Partial traumatic metacarpophalangeal amputation of thumb**

    √7ᵗʰ **S68.021 Partial traumatic metacarpophalangeal amputation of right thumb**

    √7ᵗʰ **S68.022 Partial traumatic metacarpophalangeal amputation of left thumb**

    √7ᵗʰ **S68.029 Partial traumatic metacarpophalangeal amputation of unspecified thumb**

N Newborn: 0   P Pediatric: 0-17   M Maternity: 12-55   A Adult: 15-124   MCC Major CC Condition   PDxMCC PDx acts as own MCC   CC CC Condition   PDxCC PDx acts as own CC

1012   ICD-10-CM 2016

√5ᵗʰ S68.1 Traumatic metacarpophalangeal amputation of other and unspecified finger
Traumatic amputation of finger NOS
     EXCLUDES 2   traumatic metacarpophalangeal amputation of thumb (S68.0-)

   √6ᵗʰ S68.11 Complete traumatic metacarpophalangeal amputation of other and unspecified finger

     √7ᵗʰ **S68.110** Complete traumatic metacarpophalangeal amputation of right index finger

     √7ᵗʰ **S68.111** Complete traumatic metacarpophalangeal amputation of left index finger

     √7ᵗʰ **S68.112** Complete traumatic metacarpophalangeal amputation of right middle finger

     √7ᵗʰ **S68.113** Complete traumatic metacarpophalangeal amputation of left middle finger

     √7ᵗʰ **S68.114** Complete traumatic metacarpophalangeal amputation of right ring finger

     √7ᵗʰ **S68.115** Complete traumatic metacarpophalangeal amputation of left ring finger

     √7ᵗʰ **S68.116** Complete traumatic metacarpophalangeal amputation of right little finger

     √7ᵗʰ **S68.117** Complete traumatic metacarpophalangeal amputation of left little finger

     √7ᵗʰ **S68.118** Complete traumatic metacarpophalangeal amputation of other finger
         Complete traumatic metacarpophalangeal amputation of specified finger with unspecified laterality

     √7ᵗʰ **S68.119** Complete traumatic metacarpophalangeal amputation of unspecified finger

   √6ᵗʰ S68.12 Partial traumatic metacarpophalangeal amputation of other and unspecified finger

     √7ᵗʰ **S68.120** Partial traumatic metacarpophalangeal amputation of right index finger

     √7ᵗʰ **S68.121** Partial traumatic metacarpophalangeal amputation of left index finger

     √7ᵗʰ **S68.122** Partial traumatic metacarpophalangeal amputation of right middle finger

     √7ᵗʰ **S68.123** Partial traumatic metacarpophalangeal amputation of left middle finger

     √7ᵗʰ **S68.124** Partial traumatic metacarpophalangeal amputation of right ring finger

     √7ᵗʰ **S68.125** Partial traumatic metacarpophalangeal amputation of left ring finger

     √7ᵗʰ **S68.126** Partial traumatic metacarpophalangeal amputation of right little finger

     √7ᵗʰ **S68.127** Partial traumatic metacarpophalangeal amputation of left little finger

     √7ᵗʰ **S68.128** Partial traumatic metacarpophalangeal amputation of other finger
         Partial traumatic metacarpophalangeal amputation of specified finger with unspecified laterality

     √7ᵗʰ **S68.129** Partial traumatic metacarpophalangeal amputation of unspecified finger

√5ᵗʰ S68.4 Traumatic amputation of hand at wrist level
Traumatic amputation of hand NOS
Traumatic amputation of wrist

   √6ᵗʰ S68.41 Complete traumatic amputation of hand at wrist level

     √7ᵗʰ **S68.411** Complete traumatic amputation of   **CC**
right hand at wrist level
     CC Excl: CC with 7th character A: S41.001A, S41.009-S41.011 with 7th A, S41.019-S41.021 with 7th A, S41.029-S41.031 with 7th A, S41.039-S41.041 with 7th A, S41.049-S41.051 with 7th A, S41.059-S41.101 with 7th A, S41.109-S41.111 with 7th A, S41.119-S41.121 with 7th A, S41.129-S41.131 with

7th A, S41.139-S41.141 with 7th A, S41.149-S41.151 with 7th A, S41.159A, S46.021A, S46.029A, S46.121A, S46.129A, S46.221A, S46.229A, S46.321A, S46.329A, S46.821A, S46.829A, S46.921A, S46.929 A, S48.011A, S48.019-S48.021 with 7th A, S48.029-S48.111 with 7th A, S48.119-S48.121 with 7th A, S48.129-S48.911 with 7th A, S48.919-S48.921 with 7th A, S48.929A, S51.001A, S51.009-S51.011 with 7th A, S51.019-S51.021 with 7th A, S51.029-S51.031 with 7th A, S51.039-S51.041 with 7th A, S51.049-S51.051 with 7th A, S51.059-S51.801 with 7th A, S51.809-S51.811 with 7th A, S51.819-S51.821 with 7th A, S51.829-S51.831 with 7th A, S51.839-S51.841 with 7th A, S51.849-S51.851A, S51.859A, S56.021A, S56.029A, S56.121A, S56.123A, S56.125A, S56.127A, S56.129A, S56.221A, S56.229A, S56.321A, S56.329A, S56.421A, S56.423A, S56.425A, S56.427A, S56.429A, S56.521A, S56.529A, S56.821A, S56.921 with 7th A, S56.929 with 7th A, S58.011 with 7th A, S58.019-S58.021 with 7th A, S58.029-S58.111 with 7th A, S58.119-S58.121 with 7th A, S58.129-S58.911 with 7th A, S58.919-S58.921 with 7th A, S58.929 with 7th A, S61.001 with 7th A, S61.009-S61.011 with 7th A, S61.019-S61.021 with 7th A, S61.029-S61.031 with 7th A, S61.039-S61.041 with 7th A, S61.049-S61.051 with 7th A, S61.059-S61.101 with 7th A, S61.109-S61.111 with 7th A, S61.119-S61.121 with 7th A, S61.129-S61.131 with 7th A, S61.139-S61.141 with 7th A, S61.149-S61.151 with 7th A, S61.159-S61.200 with 7th A, S61.202A, S61.204A, S61.206A, S61.208-S61.210 with 7th A, S61.212A, S61.214A, S61.216A, S61.218-S61.220 with 7th A, S61.222A, S61.224A, S61.226A, S61.228-S61.230 with 7th A, S61.232A, S61.234A, S61.236A, S61.238-S61.240 with 7th A, S61.242A, S61.244A, S61.246A, S61.248-S61.250 with 7th A, S61.252A, S61.254A, S61.256A, S61.258-S61.300A, S61.302A, S61.304A, S61.306A, S61.308-S61.310 with 7th A, S61.312A, S61.314A, S61.316A, S61.318-S61.320 with 7th A, S61.322A, S61.324A, S61.326A, S61.328-S61.330 with 7th A, S61.332A, S61.334A, S61.336A, S61.338-S61.340 with 7th A, S61.342A, S61.344A, S61.346A, S61.348-S61.350 with 7th A, S61.352A, S61.354A, S61.356A, S61.358-S61.401 with 7th A, S61.409-S61.411 with 7th A, S61.419-S61.421 with 7th A, S61.429-S61.431 with 7th A, S61.439-S61.441 with 7th A, S61.449-S61.451 with 7th A, S61.459-S61.501 with 7th A, S61.509-S61.511 with 7th A, S61.519-S61.521 with 7th A, S61.529-S61.531 with 7th A, S61.539-S61.541 with 7th A, S61.549-S61.551 with 7th A, S61.559A, S66.021A, S66.029A, S66.120A, S66.122A, S66.124A, S66.126A, S66.128-S66.129 with 7th A, S66.221A, S66.229A, S66.320A, S66.322A, S66.324A, S66.326A, S66.328-S66.329 with 7th A, S66.421A, S66.429A, S66.520A, S66.522A, S66.524A, S66.526A, S66.528-S66.529 with 7th A, S66.821A, S66.829A, S66.921A, S66.929A, S68.011A, S68.019-S68.021 with 7th A, S68.029-S68.110 with 7th A, S68.112A, S68.114A, S68.116A, S68.118-S68.120 with 7th A, S68.122A, S68.124A, S68.126A, S68.128-S68.411 with 7th A, S68.419-S68.421 with 7th A, S68.429-S68.511 with 7th A, S68.519-S68.521 with 7th A, S68.529-S68.610 with 7th A, S68.612A, S68.614A, S68.616A, S68.618-S68.620 with 7th A, S68.622A, S68.624A, S68.626A, S68.628-S68.711 with 7th A, S68.719-S68.721 with 7th A, S68.729A, T14.90-T14.91, T79.A0X-T79.9XX with 7th A

✓ Additional Character Required   ✓x7ᵗʰ Placeholder Alert   Unacceptable PDx   Manifestation   Hospital Acquired Condition   EXCLUDES 1 Not Coded Here   EXCLUDES 2 Not Included Here

ICD-10-CM 2016   1013

✓7th **S68.412 Complete traumatic amputation of left hand at wrist level** CC

CC Excl: CC with 7th character A: S41.002-S41.009 with 7th A, S41.012-S41.019 with 7th A, S41.022-S41.029 with 7th A, S41.032-S41.039 with 7th A, S41.042-S41.049 with 7th A, S41.052-S41.059 with 7th A, S41.102-S41.109 with 7th A, S41.112-S41.119 with 7th A, S41.122-S41.129 with 7th A, S41.132-S41.139 with 7th A, S41.142-S41.149 with 7th A, S41.152-S41.159 with 7th A, S46.022-S46.029 with 7th A, S46.122-S46.129 with 7th A, S46.222-S46.229 with 7th A, S46.322-S46.329 with 7th A, S46.822-S46.829 with 7th A, S46.922-S46.929 with 7th A, S48.012-S48.019 with 7th A, S48.022-S48.029 with 7th A, S48.112-S48.119 with 7th A, S48.122-S48.129 with 7th A, S48.912-S48.919 with 7th A, S48.922-S48.929 with 7th A, S51.002-S51.009 with 7th A, S51.012-S51.019 with 7th A, S51.022-S51.029 with 7th A, S51.032-S51.039 with 7th A, S51.042-S51.049 with 7th A, S51.052-S51.059 with 7th A, S51.802-S51.809 with 7th A, S51.812-S51.819 with 7th A, S51.822-S51.829 with 7th A, S51.832-S51.839 with 7th A, S51.842-S51.849 with 7th A, S51.852-S51.859 with 7th A, S56.022-S56.029 with 7th A, S56.122A, S56.124 A, S56.126A, S56.128-S56.129 with 7th A, S56.222-S56.229 with 7th A, S56.322-S56.329 with 7th A, S56.422A, S56.424A, S56.426A, S56.428-S56.429 with 7th A, S56.522-S56.529 with 7th A, S56.822-S56.829 with 7th A, S56.922-S56.929 with 7th A, S58.012-S58.019 with 7th A, S58.022-S58.029 with 7th A, S58.112-S58.119 with 7th A, S58.122-S58.129 with 7th A, S58.912-S58.919 with 7th A, S58.922-S58.929 with 7th A, S61.002-S61.009 with 7th A, S61.012-S61.019 with 7th A, S61.022-S61.029 with 7th A, S61.032-S61.039 with 7th A, S61.042-S61.049 with 7th A, S61.052-S61.059 with 7th A, S61.102-S61.109 with 7th A, S61.112-S61.119 with 7th A, S61.122-S61.129 with 7th A, S61.132-S61.139 with 7th A, S61.142-S61.149 with 7th A, S61.152-S61.159 with 7th A, S61.201A, S61.203A, S61.205A, S61.207-S61.209 with 7th A, S61.211A, S61.213A, S61.215A, S61.217-S61.219 with 7th A, S61.221A, S61.223A, S61.225A, S61.227-S61.229 with 7th A, S61.231A, S61.233A, S61.235A, S61.237-S61.239 with 7th A, S61.241A, S61.243A, S61.245 A, S61.247-S61.249 with 7th A, S61.251A, S61.253 A, S61.255A, S61.257-S61.259 with 7th A, S61.301 A, S61.303A, S61.305A, S61.307-S61.309 with 7th A, S61.311A, S61.313A, S61.315A, S61.317-S61.319 with 7th A, S61.321A, S61.323A, S61.325 A, S61.327-S61.329 with 7th A, S61.331A, S61.333A, S61.335A, S61.337-S61.339 with 7th A, S61.341A, S61.343A, S61.345A, S61.347-S61.349 with 7th A, S61.351A, S61.353A, S61.355A, S61.357-S61.359 with 7th A, S61.402-S61.409 with 7th A, S61.412-S61.419 with 7th A, S61.422-S61.429 with 7th A, S61.432-S61.439 with 7th A, S61.442-S61.449 with 7th A, S61.452-S61.459 with 7th A, S61.502-S61.509 with 7th A, S61.512-S61.519 with 7th A, S61.522-S61.529 with 7th A, S61.532-S61.539 with 7th A, S61.542-S61.549 with 7th A, S61.552-S61.559 with 7th A, S66.022-S66.029 with 7th A, S66.121A, S66.123A, S66.125A, S66.127-S66.129 with 7th A, S66.222-S66.229 with 7th A, S66.321A, S66.323A, S66.325A, S66.327-S66.329 with 7th A, S66.422-S66.429 with 7th A, S66.521A, S66.523A, S66.525A, S66.527-S66.529 with 7th A, S66.822-S66.829 with 7th A, S66.922-S66.929 with 7th A, S68.012-S68.019 with 7th A, S68.022-S68.029 with 7th A, S68.111A, S68.113A, S68.115A, S68.117-S68.119 with 7th A, S68.121A, S68.123A, S68.125A, S68.127-S68.129 with 7th A, S68.412-S68.419 with 7th A, S68.422-S68.429 with 7th A, S68.512-S68.519 with 7th A, S68.522-S68.529 with 7th A, S68.611A, S68.613A, S68.615A, S68.617-S68.619 with 7th A, S68.621A, S68.623A, S68.625A, S68.627-S68.629 with 7th A, S68.712-S68.719 with 7th A, S68.722-S68.729 with 7th A, T14.90-T14.91, T79.A0X-T79.9XX with 7th A

✓7th **S68.419 Complete traumatic amputation of unspecified hand at wrist level** CC

CC Excl: CC with 7th character A: S41.001-S41.159 with 7th A, S46.021-S46.029 with 7th A, S46.121-S46.129 with 7th A, S46.221-S46.229 with 7th A, S46.321-S46.329 with 7th A, S46.821-S46.829 with 7th A, S46.921-S46.929 with 7th A, S48.011-S48.929 with 7th A, S51.001-S51.859 with 7th A, S56.021-S56.029 with 7th A, S56.121-S56.129 with 7th A, S56.221-S56.229 with 7th A, S56.321-S56.329 with 7th A, S56.421-S56.429 with 7th A, S56.521-S56.529 with 7th A, S56.821-S56.829 with 7th A, S56.921-S56.929 with 7th A, S58.011-S58.929 with 7th A, S61.001-S61.559 with 7th A, S66.021-S66.029 with 7th A, S66.120-S66.129 with 7th A, S66.221-S66.229 with 7th A, S66.320-S66.329 with 7th A, S66.421-S66.429 with 7th A, S66.520-S66.529 with 7th A, S66.821-S66.829 with 7th A, S66.921-S66.929 with 7th A, S68.011-S68.729 with 7th A, T14.90-T14.91, T79.A0X-T79.9XX with 7th A

✓6th **S68.42 Partial traumatic amputation of hand at wrist level**

✓7th **S68.421 Partial traumatic amputation of right hand at wrist level** CC

CC Excl: CC with 7th character A: See code: S68.411

✓7th **S68.422 Partial traumatic amputation of left hand at wrist level** CC

CC Excl: CC with 7th character A: See code: S68.412

✓7th **S68.429 Partial traumatic amputation of unspecified hand at wrist level** CC

CC Excl: CC with 7th character A: See code: S68.419

✓5th **S68.5 Traumatic transphalangeal amputation of thumb**

Traumatic interphalangeal joint amputation of thumb

✓6th **S68.51 Complete traumatic transphalangeal amputation of thumb**

✓7th **S68.511 Complete traumatic transphalangeal amputation of right thumb**

✓7th **S68.512 Complete traumatic transphalangeal amputation of left thumb**

✓7th **S68.519 Complete traumatic transphalangeal amputation of unspecified thumb**

✓6th **S68.52 Partial traumatic transphalangeal amputation of thumb**

✓7th **S68.521 Partial traumatic transphalangeal amputation of right thumb**

✓7th **S68.522 Partial traumatic transphalangeal amputation of left thumb**

✓7th **S68.529 Partial traumatic transphalangeal amputation of unspecified thumb**

✓5th **S68.6 Traumatic transphalangeal amputation of other and unspecified finger**

✓6th **S68.61 Complete traumatic transphalangeal amputation of other and unspecified finger(s)**

✓7th **S68.610 Complete traumatic transphalangeal amputation of right index finger**

✓7th **S68.611 Complete traumatic transphalangeal amputation of left index finger**

✓7th **S68.612 Complete traumatic transphalangeal amputation of right middle finger**

✓7th **S68.613 Complete traumatic transphalangeal amputation of left middle finger**

✓7th **S68.614 Complete traumatic transphalangeal amputation of right ring finger**

✓7th **S68.615 Complete traumatic transphalangeal amputation of left ring finger**

✓7th **S68.616 Complete traumatic transphalangeal amputation of right little finger**

✓7th **S68.617 Complete traumatic transphalangeal amputation of left little finger**

✓7th **S68.618 Complete traumatic transphalangeal amputation of other finger**

Complete traumatic transphalangeal amputation of specified finger with unspecified laterality

✓7th **S68.619 Complete traumatic transphalangeal amputation of unspecified finger**

N Newborn: 0   P Pediatric: 0-17   M Maternity: 12-55   A Adult: 15-124   MCC Major CC Condition   PDxMCC PDx acts as own MCC   CC CC Condition   PDxCC PDx acts as own CC

1014

ICD-10-CM 2016

Chapter 19. Injury, Poisoning, and Certain Other Consequences of External Causes

√6ᵗʰ **S68.62** Partial traumatic transphalangeal amputation of other and unspecified finger

√7ᵗʰ **S68.620** Partial traumatic transphalangeal amputation of right index finger

√7ᵗʰ **S68.621** Partial traumatic transphalangeal amputation of left index finger

√7ᵗʰ **S68.622** Partial traumatic transphalangeal amputation of right middle finger

√7ᵗʰ **S68.623** Partial traumatic transphalangeal amputation of left middle finger

√7ᵗʰ **S68.624** Partial traumatic transphalangeal amputation of right ring finger

√7ᵗʰ **S68.625** Partial traumatic transphalangeal amputation of left ring finger

√7ᵗʰ **S68.626** Partial traumatic transphalangeal amputation of right little finger

√7ᵗʰ **S68.627** Partial traumatic transphalangeal amputation of left little finger

√7ᵗʰ **S68.628** Partial traumatic transphalangeal amputation of other finger

Partial traumatic transphalangeal amputation of specified finger with unspecified laterality

√7ᵗʰ **S68.629** Partial traumatic transphalangeal amputation of unspecified finger

√5ᵗʰ **S68.7** Traumatic transmetacarpal amputation of hand

√6ᵗʰ **S68.71** Complete traumatic transmetacarpal amputation of hand

√7ᵗʰ **S68.711** Complete traumatic transmetacarpal amputation of right hand   `CC`
  CC Excl: CC with 7th character A: See code: S68.411

√7ᵗʰ **S68.712** Complete traumatic transmetacarpal amputation of left hand   `CC`
  CC Excl: CC with 7th character A: See code: S68.412

√7ᵗʰ **S68.719** Complete traumatic transmetacarpal amputation of unspecified hand   `CC`
  CC Excl: CC with 7th character A: See code: S68.419

√6ᵗʰ **S68.72** Partial traumatic transmetacarpal amputation of hand

√7ᵗʰ **S68.721** Partial traumatic transmetacarpal amputation of right hand   `CC`
  CC Excl: CC with 7th character A: See code: S68.411

√7ᵗʰ **S68.722** Partial traumatic transmetacarpal amputation of left hand   `CC`
  CC Excl: CC with 7th character A: See code: S68.412

√7ᵗʰ **S68.729** Partial traumatic transmetacarpal amputation of unspecified hand   `CC`
  CC Excl: CC with 7th character A: See code: S68.419

√4ᵗʰ **S69** Other and unspecified injuries of wrist, hand and finger(s)

> The appropriate 7th character is to be added to each code from category S69.
> A   initial encounter
> D   subsequent encounter
> S   sequela

√5ᵗʰ **S69.8** Other specified injuries of wrist, hand and finger(s)

√x7ᵗʰ **S69.80** Other specified injuries of unspecified wrist, hand and finger(s)

√x7ᵗʰ **S69.81** Other specified injuries of right wrist, hand and finger(s)

√x7ᵗʰ **S69.82** Other specified injuries of left wrist, hand and finger(s)

√5ᵗʰ **S69.9** Unspecified injury of wrist, hand and finger(s)

√x7ᵗʰ **S69.90** Unspecified injury of unspecified wrist, hand and finger(s)

√x7ᵗʰ **S69.91** Unspecified injury of right wrist, hand and finger(s)

√x7ᵗʰ **S69.92** Unspecified injury of left wrist, hand and finger(s)

Injuries to the hip and thigh (S70-S79)

EXCLUDES 2   burns and corrosions (T20-T32)
frostbite (T33-T34)
snake bite (T63.0-)
venomous insect bite or sting (T63.4-)

√4ᵗʰ **S70** Superficial injury of hip and thigh

> The appropriate 7th character is to be added to each code from category S70.
> A   initial encounter
> D   subsequent encounter
> S   sequela

√5ᵗʰ **S70.0** Contusion of hip

√x7ᵗʰ **S70.00** Contusion of unspecified hip

√x7ᵗʰ **S70.01** Contusion of right hip

√x7ᵗʰ **S70.02** Contusion of left hip

√5ᵗʰ **S70.1** Contusion of thigh

√x7ᵗʰ **S70.10** Contusion of unspecified thigh

√x7ᵗʰ **S70.11** Contusion of right thigh

√x7ᵗʰ **S70.12** Contusion of left thigh

√5ᵗʰ **S70.2** Other superficial injuries of hip

√6ᵗʰ **S70.21** Abrasion of hip

√7ᵗʰ **S70.211** Abrasion, right hip

√7ᵗʰ **S70.212** Abrasion, left hip

√7ᵗʰ **S70.219** Abrasion, unspecified hip

√6ᵗʰ **S70.22** Blister (nonthermal) of hip

√7ᵗʰ **S70.221** Blister (nonthermal), right hip

√7ᵗʰ **S70.222** Blister (nonthermal), left hip

√7ᵗʰ **S70.229** Blister (nonthermal), unspecified hip

√6ᵗʰ **S70.24** External constriction of hip

√7ᵗʰ **S70.241** External constriction, right hip

√7ᵗʰ **S70.242** External constriction, left hip

√7ᵗʰ **S70.249** External constriction, unspecified hip

√6ᵗʰ **S70.25** Superficial foreign body of hip
Splinter in the hip

√7ᵗʰ **S70.251** Superficial foreign body, right hip

√7ᵗʰ **S70.252** Superficial foreign body, left hip

√7ᵗʰ **S70.259** Superficial foreign body, unspecified hip

√6ᵗʰ **S70.26** Insect bite (nonvenomous) of hip

√7ᵗʰ **S70.261** Insect bite (nonvenomous), right hip

√7ᵗʰ **S70.262** Insect bite (nonvenomous), left hip

√7ᵗʰ **S70.269** Insect bite (nonvenomous), unspecified hip

√6ᵗʰ **S70.27** Other superficial bite of hip
EXCLUDES 1   open bite of hip (S71.05-)

√7ᵗʰ **S70.271** Other superficial bite of hip, right hip

√7ᵗʰ **S70.272** Other superficial bite of hip, left hip

√7ᵗʰ **S70.279** Other superficial bite of hip, unspecified hip

√6ᵗʰ **S70.3** Other superficial injuries of thigh

√6ᵗʰ **S70.31** Abrasion of thigh

√7ᵗʰ **S70.311** Abrasion, right thigh

√7ᵗʰ **S70.312** Abrasion, left thigh

√7ᵗʰ **S70.319** Abrasion, unspecified thigh

√6ᵗʰ **S70.32** Blister (nonthermal) of thigh

√7ᵗʰ **S70.321** Blister (nonthermal), right thigh

√7ᵗʰ **S70.322** Blister (nonthermal), left thigh

√7ᵗʰ **S70.329** Blister (nonthermal), unspecified thigh

√6ᵗʰ **S70.34** External constriction of thigh

√7ᵗʰ **S70.341** External constriction, right thigh

√7ᵗʰ **S70.342** External constriction, left thigh

√7ᵗʰ **S70.349** External constriction, unspecified thigh

√6ᵗʰ **S70.35** Superficial foreign body of thigh
Splinter in the thigh

√7ᵗʰ **S70.351** Superficial foreign body, right thigh

√7ᵗʰ **S70.352** Superficial foreign body, left thigh

√7ᵗʰ **S70.359** Superficial foreign body, unspecified thigh

✔ Additional Character Required   √x7ᵗʰ Placeholder Alert   Unacceptable PDx   Manifestation   Hospital Acquired Condition   *EXCLUDES 1* Not Coded Here   *EXCLUDES 2* Not Included Here

ICD-10-CM 2016   1015

√6ᵗʰ S70.36 Insect bite (nonvenomous) of thigh

     √7ᵗʰ S70.361 Insect bite (nonvenomous), right thigh

     √7ᵗʰ S70.362 Insect bite (nonvenomous), left thigh

     √7ᵗʰ S70.369 Insect bite (nonvenomous), unspecified thigh

√6ᵗʰ S70.37 Other superficial bite of thigh

     EXCLUDES 1   *open bite of thigh (S71.15)*

     √7ᵗʰ S70.371 Other superficial bite of right thigh

     √7ᵗʰ S70.372 Other superficial bite of left thigh

     √7ᵗʰ S70.379 Other superficial bite of unspecified thigh

√5ᵗʰ S70.9 Unspecified superficial injury of hip and thigh

√6ᵗʰ S70.91 Unspecified superficial injury of hip

     √7ᵗʰ S70.911 Unspecified superficial injury of right hip

     √7ᵗʰ S70.912 Unspecified superficial injury of left hip

     √7ᵗʰ S70.919 Unspecified superficial injury of unspecified hip

√6ᵗʰ S70.92 Unspecified superficial injury of thigh

     √7ᵗʰ S70.921 Unspecified superficial injury of right thigh

     √7ᵗʰ S70.922 Unspecified superficial injury of left thigh

     √7ᵗʰ S70.929 Unspecified superficial injury of unspecified thigh

√4ᵗʰ S71 Open wound of hip and thigh

Code also any associated wound infection

EXCLUDES 1   *open fracture of hip and thigh (S72.-)*
     traumatic amputation of hip and thigh (S78.-)

EXCLUDES 2   *bite of venomous animal (T63.-)*
     open wound of ankle, foot and toes (S91.-)
     open wound of knee and lower leg (S81.-)

> The appropriate 7th character is to be added to each code from category S71.
> A   initial encounter
> D   subsequent encounter
> S   sequela

√5ᵗʰ S71.0 Open wound of hip

√6ᵗʰ S71.00 Unspecified open wound of hip

     √7ᵗʰ S71.001 Unspecified open wound, right hip

     √7ᵗʰ S71.002 Unspecified open wound, left hip

     √7ᵗʰ S71.009 Unspecified open wound, unspecified hip

√6ᵗʰ S71.01 Laceration without foreign body of hip

     √7ᵗʰ S71.011 Laceration without foreign body, right hip

     √7ᵗʰ S71.012 Laceration without foreign body, left hip

     √7ᵗʰ S71.019 Laceration without foreign body, unspecified hip

√6ᵗʰ S71.02 Laceration with foreign body of hip

     √7ᵗʰ S71.021 Laceration with foreign body, right hip

     √7ᵗʰ S71.022 Laceration with foreign body, left hip

     √7ᵗʰ S71.029 Laceration with foreign body, unspecified hip

√6ᵗʰ S71.03 Puncture wound without foreign body of hip

     √7ᵗʰ S71.031 Puncture wound without foreign body, right hip

     √7ᵗʰ S71.032 Puncture wound without foreign body, left hip

     √7ᵗʰ S71.039 Puncture wound without foreign body, unspecified hip

√6ᵗʰ S71.04 Puncture wound with foreign body of hip

     √7ᵗʰ S71.041 Puncture wound with foreign body, right hip

     √7ᵗʰ S71.042 Puncture wound with foreign body, left hip

     √7ᵗʰ S71.049 Puncture wound with foreign body, unspecified hip

√6ᵗʰ S71.05 Open bite of hip

     Bite of hip NOS

     EXCLUDES 1   *superficial bite of hip (S70.26, S70.27)*

     √7ᵗʰ S71.051 Open bite, right hip

     √7ᵗʰ S71.052 Open bite, left hip

     √7ᵗʰ S71.059 Open bite, unspecified hip

√5ᵗʰ S71.1 Open wound of thigh

√6ᵗʰ S71.10 Unspecified open wound of thigh

     √7ᵗʰ S71.101 Unspecified open wound, right thigh

     √7ᵗʰ S71.102 Unspecified open wound, left thigh

     √7ᵗʰ S71.109 Unspecified open wound, unspecified thigh

√6ᵗʰ S71.11 Laceration without foreign body of thigh

     √7ᵗʰ S71.111 Laceration without foreign body, right thigh

     √7ᵗʰ S71.112 Laceration without foreign body, left thigh

     √7ᵗʰ S71.119 Laceration without foreign body, unspecified thigh

√6ᵗʰ S71.12 Laceration with foreign body of thigh

     √7ᵗʰ S71.121 Laceration with foreign body, right thigh

     √7ᵗʰ S71.122 Laceration with foreign body, left thigh

     √7ᵗʰ S71.129 Laceration with foreign body, unspecified thigh

√6ᵗʰ S71.13 Puncture wound without foreign body of thigh

     √7ᵗʰ S71.131 Puncture wound without foreign body, right thigh

     √7ᵗʰ S71.132 Puncture wound without foreign body, left thigh

     √7ᵗʰ S71.139 Puncture wound without foreign body, unspecified thigh

√6ᵗʰ S71.14 Puncture wound with foreign body of thigh

     √7ᵗʰ S71.141 Puncture wound with foreign body, right thigh

     √7ᵗʰ S71.142 Puncture wound with foreign body, left thigh

     √7ᵗʰ S71.149 Puncture wound with foreign body, unspecified thigh

√6ᵗʰ S71.15 Open bite of thigh

     Bite of thigh NOS

     EXCLUDES 1   *superficial bite of thigh (S70.37-)*

     √7ᵗʰ S71.151 Open bite, right thigh

     √7ᵗʰ S71.152 Open bite, left thigh

     √7ᵗʰ S71.159 Open bite, unspecified thigh

√4ᵗʰ S72 Fracture of femur

NOTE   A fracture not indicated as displaced or nondisplaced should be coded to displaced.
The open fracture designations are based on the Gustilo open fracture classification A fracture not indicated as open or closed should be coded to closed.

EXCLUDES 1   *traumatic amputation of hip and thigh (S78.-)*

EXCLUDES 2   *fracture of foot (S92.-)*
     fracture of lower leg and ankle (S82.-)
     periprosthetic fracture of prosthetic implant of hip (T84.040, T84.041)

AHA: 2015, 1Q, 17; 2013, 4Q, 128

> The appropriate 7th character is to be added to all codes from category S72 [unless otherwise indicated].
> A   initial encounter for closed fracture
> B   initial encounter for open fracture type I or II
>   initial encounter for open fracture NOS
> C   initial encounter for open fracture type IIIA, IIIB, or IIIC
> D   subsequent encounter for closed fracture with routine healing
> E   subsequent encounter for open fracture type I or II with routine healing
> F   subsequent encounter for open fracture type IIIA, IIIB, or IIIC with routine healing
> G   subsequent encounter for closed fracture with delayed healing
> H   subsequent encounter for open fracture type I or II with delayed healing
> J   subsequent encounter for open fracture type IIIA, IIIB, or IIIC with delayed healing
> K   subsequent encounter for closed fracture with nonunion
> M   subsequent encounter for open fracture type I or II with nonunion
> N   subsequent encounter for open fracture type IIIA, IIIB, or IIIC with nonunion
> P   subsequent encounter for closed fracture with malunion
> Q   subsequent encounter for open fracture type I or II with malunion
> R   subsequent encounter for open fracture type IIIA, IIIB, or IIIC with malunion
> S   sequela

N Newborn: 0   P Pediatric: 0-17   M Maternity: 12-55   A Adult: 15-124   MCC Major CC Condition   PDxMCC PDx acts as own MCC   CC CC Condition   PDxCC PDx acts as own CC

1016   ICD-10-CM 2016

√5th S72.0 Fracture of head and neck of femur

    EXCLUDES 2   physeal fracture of upper end of femur (S79.0-)

√6th S72.00 Fracture of unspecified part of neck of femur
Fracture of hip NOS
Fracture of neck of femur NOS

7,18 **√7th S72.001 Fracture of unspecified part of**   MCC CC
neck of right femur
CC Excl: MCC with 7th A: M48.40X–M48.58X
with 7th A, M80.00X–M84.68X with 7th A,
S03.8XX–S03.9XX with 7th A, S29.011–
S29.019 with 7th A, S38.3XX–S39.013 with
7th A, S72.001–S72.471 with 7th [A, B, C],
S72.479–S72.92X with 7th A, S73.101A,
S73.109–S73.111 with 7th A, S73.119–
S73.121 with 7th A, S73.129–S73.191 with
7th A, S73.199A, S76.001A, S76.009–S76.011
with 7th A, S76.019A, S76.091A, S76.099–
S76.101 with 7th A, S76.109–S76.111 with
7th A, S76.119A, S76.191A, S76.199–S76.201
with 7th A, S76.209–S76.211 with 7th A,
S76.219A, S76.291A, S76.299–S76.301 with
7th A, S76.309–S76.311 with 7th A, S76.319A,
S76.391A, S76.399–S76.801 with 7th A,
S76.809–S76.811 with 7th A, S76.819A,
S76.891A, S76.899–S76.901 with 7th A,
S76.909–S76.911 with 7th A, S76.919A,
S76.991A, S76.999A, S79.001A, S79.009–
S79.011 with 7th A, S79.019–S79.091 with
7th A, S79.099–S79.101 with 7th A, S79.109–
S79.111 with 7th A, S79.119–S79.121 with
7th A, S79.129–S79.131 with 7th A, S79.139–
S79.141 with 7th A, S79.149 with 7th A, S79.191 with
7th A, S79.199–S79.811 with 7th A, S79.819–
S79.821 with 7th A, S79.829–S79.911 with
7th A, S79.919–S79.921 with 7th A, S79.929A,
S82.90X–S82.92X with 7th [A, B, C], T14.90–
T14.91, T79.A0X–T79.9XX with 7th A
MCC with 7th B or C: M48.40X–M48.58X
with 7th A, M80.00X–M84.68X with 7th A,
S03.8XX–S03.9XX with 7th A, S29.011–
S29.019 with 7th A, S38.3XX–S39.013 with
7th A, S72.001–S72.92X with 7th [A, B, C],
S73.101–S73.199 with 7th A, S76.001–
S76.019 with 7th A, S76.091–S76.119 with
7th A, S76.191–S76.219 with 7th A, S76.291–
S76.319 with 7th A, S76.391–S76.819 with
7th A, S76.891–S76.919 with 7th A, S76.991–
S76.999 with 7th A, S79.001–S79.929 with
7th A, S82.90X–S82.92X with 7th [A, B, C],
T14.90–T14.91, T79.A0X–T79.9XX with 7th A
CC with 7th character K, M, N, P, Q or R:
M80.00X–M84.68X with 7th [K, P], S02.0XX–
S02.92X with 7th K, S12.000–S12.691 with
7th K, S22.000–S22.9XX with 7th K, S32.000–
S32.9XX with 7th K, S42.001–S42.92X with
7th [K, P], S49.001–S49.199 with 7th [K, P],
S52.001–S52.92X with 7th [K, M, N, P, Q, R],
S59.001–S59.299 with 7th [K, P], S62.001–
S62.92X with 7th [K, P], S72.001–S72.92X
with 7th [K, M, N, P, Q, R], S79.001–S79.199
with 7th [K, P], S82.001–S82.92X with 7th [K,
M, N, P, Q, R], S89.001–S89.399 with 7th [K, P],
S92.001–S92.919 with 7th [K, P]

7,18 **√7th S72.002 Fracture of unspecified part of**   MCC CC
neck of left femur
CC Excl: MCC with 7th A: M48.40X–M48.58X
with 7th A, M80.00X–M84.68X with 7th A,
S03.8XX–S03.9XX with 7th A, S29.011–
S29.019 with 7th A, S38.3XX–S39.013 with
7th A, S72.001–S72.466 with 7th [B, C],
S72.472–S72.92X with 7th A, S73.102–
S73.109 with 7th A, S73.112–S73.119 with
7th A, S73.122–S73.129 with 7th A, S73.192–
S73.199 with 7th A, S76.002–S76.009 with
7th A, S76.012–S76.019 with 7th A, S76.092–
S76.099 with 7th A, S76.102–S76.109 with
7th A, S76.112–S76.119 with 7th A, S76.192–
S76.199 with 7th A, S76.202–S76.209 with
7th A, S76.212–S76.219 with 7th A, S76.292–
S76.299 with 7th A, S76.302–S76.309 with
7th A, S76.312–S76.319 with 7th A, S76.392–
S76.399 with 7th A, S76.802–S76.809 with
7th A, S76.812–S76.819 with 7th A, S76.892–
S76.899 with 7th A, S76.902–S76.909 with
7th A, S76.912–S76.919 with 7th A, S76.992–
S76.999 with 7th A, S79.002–S79.009 with
7th A, S79.012–S79.019 with 7th A, S79.092–
S79.099 with 7th A, S79.102–S79.109 with

7th A, S79.112–S79.119 with 7th A, S79.122–
S79.129 with 7th A, S79.132–S79.139 with
7th A, S79.142–S79.149 with 7th A, S79.192–
S79.199 with 7th A, S79.812–S79.819 with
7th A, S79.822–S79.829 with 7th A, S79.912–
S79.919 with 7th A, S79.922–S79.929 with
7th A, S82.90X–S82.92 with 7th [A, B, C],
T14.90–T14.91, T79.A0X–T79.9XX with 7th A
MCC with 7th B or C: M48.40X–M48.58X
with 7th A, M80.00X–M84.68X with 7th A,
S03.8XX–S03.9XX with 7th A, S29.011–
S29.019 with 7th A, S38.3XX–S39.013 with
7th A, S72.001–S72.92X with 7th [A, B, C],
S73.101–S73.199 with 7th A, S76.001–
S76.019 with 7th A, S76.091–S76.119 with
7th A, S76.191–S76.219 with 7th A, S76.291–
S76.319 with 7th A, S76.391–S76.819 with
7th A, S76.891–S76.919 with 7th A, S76.991–
S76.999 with 7th A, S79.001–S79.929 with
7th A, S82.90X–S82.92X with 7th [A, B, C],
T14.90–T14.91, T79.A0X–T79.9XX with 7th A
CC with 7th character K, M, N, P, Q or R:
M80.00X–M84.68X with 7th [K, P], S02.0XX–
S02.92X with 7th K, S12.000–S12.691 with
7th K, S22.000–S22.9XX with 7th K, S32.000–
S32.9XX with 7th K, S42.001–S42.92X with
7th [K, P], S49.001–S49.199 with 7th [K, P],
S52.001–S52.92X with 7th [K, M, N, P, Q, R],
S59.001–S59.299 with 7th [K, P], S62.001–
S62.92X with 7th [K, P], S72.001–S72.92X
with 7th [K, M, N, P, Q, R], S79.001–S79.199
with 7th [K, P], S82.001–S82.92X with 7th [K,
M, N, P, Q, R], S89.001–S89.399 with 7th [K, P],
S92.001–S92.919 with 7th [K, P]

7,18 **√7th S72.009 Fracture of unspecified part of**   MCC CC
neck of unspecified femur
CC Excl: MCC with 7th A, B or C: M48.40X–
M48.58X with 7th A, M80.00X–M84.68X with
7th A, S03.8XX–S03.9X with 7th A, S29.011–
S29.019 with 7th A, S38.3XX–S39.013 with
7th A, S72.001–S72.92X with 7th [A, B, C],
S73.101–S73.199 with 7th A, S76.001–
S76.019 with 7th A, S76.091–S76.119 with
7th A, S76.191–S76.219 with 7th A, S76.291–
S76.319 with 7th A, S76.391–S76.819 with
7th A, S76.891–S76.919 with 7th A, S76.991–
S76.999 with 7th A, S79.001–S79.929 with
7th A, S82.90X–S82.92X with 7th [A, B, C],
T14.90–T14.91, T79.A0X–T79.9XX with 7th A
CC with 7th character K, M, N, P, Q or R:
M80.00X–M84.68X with 7th [K, P], S02.0XX–
S02.92X with 7th K, S12.000–S12.691 with
7th K, S22.000–S22.9XX with 7th K, S32.000–
S32.9XX with 7th K, S42.001–S42.92X with
7th [K, P], S49.001–S49.199 with 7th [K, P],
S52.001–S52.92X with 7th [K, M, N, P, Q, R],
S59.001–S59.299 with 7th [K, P], S62.001–
S62.92X with 7th [K, P], S72.001–S72.92X
with 7th [K, M, N, P, Q, R], S79.001–S79.199
with 7th [K, P], S82.001–S82.92X with 7th [K,
M, N, P, Q, R], S89.001–S89.399 with 7th [K, P],
S92.001–S92.919 with 7th [K, P]

√6th S72.01 Unspecified intracapsular fracture of femur
Subcapital fracture of femur

7,18 **√7th S72.011 Unspecified intracapsular**   MCC CC
fracture of right femur
CC Excl: See code: S72.001

7,18 **√7th S72.012 Unspecified intracapsular**   MCC CC
fracture of left femur
CC Excl: See code: S72.002

7,18 **√7th S72.019 Unspecified intracapsular**   MCC CC
fracture of unspecified femur
CC Excl: See code: S72.009

√6th S72.02 Fracture of epiphysis (separation) (upper) of femur
Transepiphyseal fracture of femur

    EXCLUDES 1   capital femoral epiphyseal fracture
(pediatric) of femur (S79.01-)
Salter-Harris Type I physeal fracture of upper
end of femur (S79.01-)

7,18 **√7th S72.021 Displaced fracture of epiphysis**   MCC CC
(separation) (upper) of right femur
CC Excl: See code: S72.001

7,18 **√7th S72.022 Displaced fracture of epiphysis**   MCC CC
(separation) (upper) of left femur
CC Excl: See code: S72.002

---

7   HAC = Initial encounter only (7th character A, B or C) and not POA.
18   CC only if a subsequent encounter for nonunion or malunion (7th character K, M, N, P, Q, or R).

✔ Additional Character Required   ✔x7th Placeholder Alert   Unacceptable PDx   Manifestation   Hospital Acquired Condition   *EXCLUDES 1* Not Coded Here   *EXCLUDES 2* Not Included Here

ICD-10-CM 2016   1017

Chapter 19. Injury, Poisoning, and Certain Other Consequences of External Causes

7,18 √7ᵗʰ **S72.023** **Displaced fracture of epiphysis (separation) (upper) of unspecified femur** MCC CC
CC Excl: See code: S72.009

7,18 √7ᵗʰ **S72.024** **Nondisplaced fracture of epiphysis (separation) (upper) of right femur** MCC CC
CC Excl: See code: S72.001

7,18 √7ᵗʰ **S72.025** **Nondisplaced fracture of epiphysis (separation) (upper) of left femur** MCC CC
CC Excl: See code: S72.002

7,18 √7ᵗʰ **S72.026** **Nondisplaced fracture of epiphysis (separation) (upper) of unspecified femur** MCC CC
CC Excl: See code: S72.009

√6ᵗʰ **S72.03** **Midcervical fracture of femur**
Transcervical fracture of femur NOS

7,18 √7ᵗʰ **S72.031** **Displaced midcervical fracture of right femur** MCC CC
CC Excl: See code: S72.001

7,18 √7ᵗʰ **S72.032** **Displaced midcervical fracture of left femur** MCC CC
CC Excl: See code: S72.002

7,18 √7ᵗʰ **S72.033** **Displaced midcervical fracture of unspecified femur** MCC CC
CC Excl: See code: S72.009

7,18 √7ᵗʰ **S72.034** **Nondisplaced midcervical fracture of right femur** MCC CC
CC Excl: See code: S72.001

7,18 √7ᵗʰ **S72.035** **Nondisplaced midcervical fracture of left femur** MCC CC
CC Excl: See code: S72.002

7,18 √7ᵗʰ **S72.036** **Nondisplaced midcervical fracture of unspecified femur** MCC CC
CC Excl: See code: S72.009

√6ᵗʰ **S72.04** **Fracture of base of neck of femur**
Cervicotrochanteric fracture of femur

7,18 √7ᵗʰ **S72.041** **Displaced fracture of base of neck of right femur** MCC CC
CC Excl: See code: S72.001

7,18 √7ᵗʰ **S72.042** **Displaced fracture of base of neck of left femur** MCC CC
CC Excl: See code: S72.002

7,18 √7ᵗʰ **S72.043** **Displaced fracture of base of neck of unspecified femur** MCC CC
CC Excl: See code: S72.009

7,18 √7ᵗʰ **S72.044** **Nondisplaced fracture of base of neck of right femur** MCC CC
CC Excl: See code: S72.001

7,18 √7ᵗʰ **S72.045** **Nondisplaced fracture of base of neck of left femur** MCC CC
CC Excl: See code: S72.002

7,18 √7ᵗʰ **S72.046** **Nondisplaced fracture of base of neck of unspecified femur** MCC CC
CC Excl: See code: S72.009

√6ᵗʰ **S72.05** **Unspecified fracture of head of femur**
Fracture of head of femur NOS

7,18 √7ᵗʰ **S72.051** **Unspecified fracture of head of right femur** MCC CC
CC Excl: See code: S72.001

7,18 √7ᵗʰ **S72.052** **Unspecified fracture of head of left femur** MCC CC
CC Excl: See code: S72.002

7,18 √7ᵗʰ **S72.059** **Unspecified fracture of head of unspecified femur** MCC CC
CC Excl: See code: S72.009

√6ᵗʰ **S72.06** **Articular fracture of head of femur**

7,18 √7ᵗʰ **S72.061** **Displaced articular fracture of head of right femur** MCC CC
CC Excl: See code: S72.001

7,18 √7ᵗʰ **S72.062** **Displaced articular fracture of head of left femur** MCC CC
CC Excl: See code: S72.002

7,18 √7ᵗʰ **S72.063** **Displaced articular fracture of head of unspecified femur** MCC CC
CC Excl: See code: S72.009

7,18 √7ᵗʰ **S72.064** **Nondisplaced articular fracture of head of right femur** MCC CC
CC Excl: See code: S72.001

7,18 √7ᵗʰ **S72.065** **Nondisplaced articular fracture of head of left femur** MCC CC
CC Excl: See code: S72.002

7,18 √7ᵗʰ **S72.066** **Nondisplaced articular fracture of head of unspecified femur** MCC CC
CC Excl: See code: S72.009

√6ᵗʰ **S72.09** **Other fracture of head and neck of femur**

7,18 √7ᵗʰ **S72.091** **Other fracture of head and neck of right femur** MCC CC
CC Excl: See code: S72.001

7,18 √7ᵗʰ **S72.092** **Other fracture of head and neck of left femur** MCC CC
CC Excl: See code: S72.002

7,18 √7ᵗʰ **S72.099** **Other fracture of head and neck of unspecified femur** MCC CC
CC Excl: See code: S72.009

√5ᵗʰ **S72.1** **Pertrochanteric fracture**

√6ᵗʰ **S72.10** **Unspecified trochanteric fracture of femur**
Fracture of trochanter NOS

7,18 √7ᵗʰ **S72.101** **Unspecified trochanteric fracture of right femur** MCC CC
CC Excl: See code: S72.001

7,18 √7ᵗʰ **S72.102** **Unspecified trochanteric fracture of left femur** MCC CC
CC Excl: See code: S72.002

7,18 √7ᵗʰ **S72.109** **Unspecified trochanteric fracture of unspecified femur** MCC CC
CC Excl: See code: S72.009

√6ᵗʰ **S72.11** **Fracture of greater trochanter of femur**

7,18 √7ᵗʰ **S72.111** **Displaced fracture of greater trochanter of right femur** MCC CC
CC Excl: See code: S72.001

7,18 √7ᵗʰ **S72.112** **Displaced fracture of greater trochanter of left femur** MCC CC
CC Excl: See code: S72.002

7,18 √7ᵗʰ **S72.113** **Displaced fracture of greater trochanter of unspecified femur** MCC CC
CC Excl: See code: S72.009

7,18 √7ᵗʰ **S72.114** **Nondisplaced fracture of greater trochanter of right femur** MCC CC
CC Excl: See code: S72.001

7,18 √7ᵗʰ **S72.115** **Nondisplaced fracture of greater trochanter of left femur** MCC CC
CC Excl: See code: S72.002

7,18 √7ᵗʰ **S72.116** **Nondisplaced fracture of greater trochanter of unspecified femur** MCC CC
CC Excl: See code: S72.009

√6ᵗʰ **S72.12** **Fracture of lesser trochanter of femur**

7,18 √7ᵗʰ **S72.121** **Displaced fracture of lesser trochanter of right femur** MCC CC
CC Excl: See code: S72.001

7,18 √7ᵗʰ **S72.122** **Displaced fracture of lesser trochanter of left femur** MCC CC
CC Excl: See code: S72.002

7,18 √7ᵗʰ **S72.123** **Displaced fracture of lesser trochanter of unspecified femur** MCC CC
CC Excl: See code: S72.009

7,18 √7ᵗʰ **S72.124** **Nondisplaced fracture of lesser trochanter of right femur** MCC CC
CC Excl: See code: S72.001

7,18 √7ᵗʰ **S72.125** **Nondisplaced fracture of lesser trochanter of left femur** MCC CC
CC Excl: See code: S72.002

7,18 √7ᵗʰ **S72.126** **Nondisplaced fracture of lesser trochanter of unspecified femur** MCC CC
CC Excl: See code: S72.009

---

7   HAC = Initial encounter only (7th character A, B or C) and not POA.
18   CC only if a subsequent encounter for nonunion or malunion (7th character K, M, N, P, Q, or R).

√6th **S72.13**   **Apophyseal fracture of femur**

     EXCLUDES1   *chronic (nontraumatic) slipped upper femoral epiphysis (M93.0-)*

7,18 √7th   **S72.131**   **Displaced apophyseal fracture of right femur**   MCC CC
     CC Excl: See code: S72.001

7,18 √7th   **S72.132**   **Displaced apophyseal fracture of left femur**   MCC CC
     CC Excl: See code: S72.002

7,18 √7th   **S72.133**   **Displaced apophyseal fracture of unspecified femur**   MCC CC
     CC Excl: See code: S72.009

7,18 √7th   **S72.134**   **Nondisplaced apophyseal fracture of right femur**   MCC CC
     CC Excl: See code: S72.001

7,18 √7th   **S72.135**   **Nondisplaced apophyseal fractureof left femur**   MCC CC
     CC Excl: See code: S72.002

7,18 √7th   **S72.136**   **Nondisplaced apophyseal fracture of unspecified femur**   MCC CC
     CC Excl: See code: S72.009

√6th **S72.14**   **Intertrochanteric fracture of femur**

7,18 √7th   **S72.141**   **Displaced intertrochanteric fracture of right femur**   MCC CC
     CC Excl: See code: S72.001

7,18 √7th   **S72.142**   **Displaced intertrochanteric fracture of left femur**   MCC CC
     CC Excl: See code: S72.002

7,18 √7th   **S72.143**   **Displaced intertrochanteric fracture of unspecified femur**   MCC CC
     CC Excl: See code: S72.009

7,18 √7th   **S72.144**   **Nondisplaced intertrochanteric fracture of right femur**   MCC CC
     CC Excl: See code: S72.001

7,18 √7th   **S72.145**   **Nondisplaced intertrochanteric fracture of left femur**   MCC CC
     CC Excl: See code: S72.002

7,18 √7th   **S72.146**   **Nondisplaced intertrochanteric fracture of unspecified femur**   MCC CC
     CC Excl: See code: S72.009

√5th **S72.2**   **Subtrochanteric fracture of femur**

7,18 √x7th   **S72.21**   **Displaced subtrochanteric fracture of right femur**   MCC CC
     CC Excl: See code: S72.001

7,18 √x7th   **S72.22**   **Displaced subtrochanteric fracture of left femur**   MCC CC
     CC Excl: See code: S72.002

7,18 √x7th   **S72.23**   **Displaced subtrochanteric fracture of unspecified femur**   MCC CC
     CC Excl: See code: S72.009

7,18 √x7th   **S72.24**   **Nondisplaced subtrochanteric fracture of right femur**   MCC CC
     CC Excl: See code: S72.001

7,18 √x7th   **S72.25**   **Nondisplaced subtrochanteric fracture of left femur**   MCC CC
     CC Excl: See code: S72.002

7,18 √x7th   **S72.26**   **Nondisplaced subtrochanteric fracture of unspecified femur**   MCC CC
     CC Excl: See code: S72.009

√5th **S72.3**   **Fracture of shaft of femur**

√6th **S72.30**   **Unspecified fracture of shaft of femur**

7,18 √7th   **S72.301**   **Unspecified fracture of shaft of right femur**   MCC CC
     CC Excl: See code: S72.001

7,18 √7th   **S72.302**   **Unspecified fracture of shaft of left femur**   MCC CC
     CC Excl: See code: S72.002

7,18 √7th   **S72.309**   **Unspecified fracture of shaft of unspecified femur**   MCC CC
     CC Excl: See code: S72.009

√6th **S72.32**   **Transverse fracture of shaft of femur**

7,18 √7th   **S72.321**   **Displaced transverse fracture of shaft of right femur**   MCC CC
     CC Excl: See code: S72.001

7,18 √7th   **S72.322**   **Displaced transverse fracture of shaft of left femur**   MCC CC
     CC Excl: See code: S72.002

7,18 √7th   **S72.323**   **Displaced transverse fracture of shaft of unspecified femur**   MCC CC
     CC Excl: See code: S72.009

7,18 √7th   **S72.324**   **Nondisplaced transverse fracture of shaft of right femur**   MCC CC
     CC Excl: See code: S72.001

7,18 √7th   **S72.325**   **Nondisplaced transverse fracture of shaft of left femur**   MCC CC
     CC Excl: See code: S72.002

7,18 √7th   **S72.326**   **Nondisplaced transverse fracture of shaft of unspecified femur**   MCC CC
     CC Excl: See code: S72.009

√6th **S72.33**   **Oblique fracture of shaft of femur**

7,18 √7th   **S72.331**   **Displaced oblique fracture of shaft of right femur**   MCC CC
     CC Excl: See code: S72.001

7,18 √7th   **S72.332**   **Displaced oblique fracture of shaft of left femur**   MCC CC
     CC Excl: See code: S72.002

7,18 √7th   **S72.333**   **Displaced oblique fracture of shaft of unspecified femur**   MCC CC
     CC Excl: See code: S72.009

7,18 √7th   **S72.334**   **Nondisplaced oblique fracture of shaft of right femur**   MCC CC
     CC Excl: See code: S72.001

7,18 √7th   **S72.335**   **Nondisplaced oblique fracture of shaft of left femur**   MCC CC
     CC Excl: See code: S72.002

7,18 √7th   **S72.336**   **Nondisplaced oblique fracture of shaft of unspecified femur**   MCC CC
     CC Excl: See code: S72.009

√6th **S72.34**   **Spiral fracture of shaft of femur**

7,18 √7th   **S72.341**   **Displaced spiral fracture of shaft of right femur**   MCC CC
     CC Excl: See code: S72.001

7,18 √7th   **S72.342**   **Displaced spiral fracture of shaft of left femur**   MCC CC
     CC Excl: See code: S72.002

7,18 √7th   **S72.343**   **Displaced spiral fracture of shaft of unspecified femur**   MCC CC
     CC Excl: See code: S72.009

7,18 √7th   **S72.344**   **Nondisplaced spiral fracture of shaft of right femur**   MCC CC
     CC Excl: See code: S72.001

7,18 √7th   **S72.345**   **Nondisplaced spiral fracture of shaft of left femur**   MCC CC
     CC Excl: See code: S72.002

7,18 √7th   **S72.346**   **Nondisplaced spiral fracture of shaft of unspecified femur**   MCC CC
     CC Excl: See code: S72.009

√6th **S72.35**   **Comminuted fracture of shaft of femur**

7,18 √7th   **S72.351**   **Displaced comminuted fracture of shaft of right femur**   MCC CC
     CC Excl: See code: S72.001

7,18 √7th   **S72.352**   **Displaced comminuted fracture of shaft of left femur**   MCC CC
     CC Excl: See code: S72.002

7,18 √7th   **S72.353**   **Displaced comminuted fracture of shaft of unspecified femur**   MCC CC
     CC Excl: See code: S72.009

7,18 √7th   **S72.354**   **Nondisplaced comminuted fracture of shaft of right femur**   MCC CC
     CC Excl: See code: S72.001

7,18 √7th   **S72.355**   **Nondisplaced comminuted fracture of shaft of left femur**   MCC CC
     CC Excl: See code: S72.002

7,18 √7th   **S72.356**   **Nondisplaced comminuted fracture of shaft of unspecified femur**   MCC CC
     CC Excl: See code: S72.009

√6th **S72.36**   **Segmental fracture of shaft of femur**

7,18 √7th   **S72.361**   **Displaced segmental fracture of shaft of right femur**   MCC CC
     CC Excl: See code: S72.001

7,18 √7th   **S72.362**   **Displaced segmental fracture of shaft of left femur**   MCC CC
     CC Excl: See code: S72.002

---

7   HAC = Initial encounter only (7th character A, B or C) and not POA.
18   CC only if a subsequent encounter for nonunion or malunion (7th character K, M, N, P, Q, or R).

√ Additional Character Required   √x7th Placeholder Alert   Unacceptable PDx   Manifestation   Hospital Acquired Condition   EXCLUDES1 Not Coded Here   EXCLUDES2 Not Included Here

7,18 ✓7th **S72.363** **Displaced segmental fracture of shaft of unspecified femur** MCC CC
CC Excl: See code: S72.009

7,18 ✓7th **S72.364** **Nondisplaced segmental fracture of shaft of right femur** MCC CC
CC Excl: See code: S72.001

7,18 ✓7th **S72.365** **Nondisplaced segmental fracture of shaft of left femur** MCC CC
CC Excl: See code: S72.002

7,18 ✓7th **S72.366** **Nondisplaced segmental fracture of shaft of unspecified femur** MCC CC
CC Excl: See code: S72.009

✓6th **S72.39** **Other fracture of shaft of femur**

7,18 ✓7th **S72.391** **Other fracture of shaft of right femur** MCC CC
CC Excl: See code: S72.001

7,18 ✓7th **S72.392** **Other fracture of shaft of left femur** MCC CC
CC Excl: See code: S72.002

7,18 ✓7th **S72.399** **Other fracture of shaft of unspecified femur** MCC CC
CC Excl: See code: S72.00

✓5th **S72.4** **Fracture of lower end of femur**
Fracture of distal end of femur
EXCLUDES 2 *fracture of shaft of femur (S72.3-)*
physeal fracture of lower end of femur (S79.1-)

✓6th **S72.40** **Unspecified fracture of lower end of femur**

7,16,19 ✓7th **S72.401** **Unspecified fracture of lower end of right femur** MCC CC
CC Excl: CC with 7th character A: M80.00X-M80.019 with 7th A, M80.041-M80.059 with 7th A, M80.80X-M80.819 with 7th A, M80.841-M80.859 with 7th A, M84.40X-M84.419 with 7th A, M84.441-M84.459 with 7th A, M84.474-M84.519 with 7th A, M84.541-M84.559 with 7th A, M84.574-M84.576 with 7th A, M84.60X-M84.619 with 7th A, M84.641-M84.659 with 7th A, M84.674-M84.68X with 7th A, S03.8XX-S03.9XX with 7th A, S29.011-S29.019 with 7th A, S38.3XX-S39.013 with 7th A, S72.001-S72.471 with 7th [A, B, C], S72.479-S72.92X with 7th A, S73.101A, S73.109-S73.111 with 7th A, S73.119-S73.121 with 7th A, S73.129-S73.191 with 7th A, S73.199A, S76.001A, S76.009-S76.011 with 7th A, S76.019A, S76.091A, S76.099-S76.101 with 7th A, S76.109-S76.111 with 7th A, S76.119A, S76.191A, S76.199-S76.201 with 7th A, S76.209-S76.211 with 7th A, S76.219 with 7th A, S76.291A, S76.299-S76.301 with 7th A, S76.309-S76.311 with 7th A, S76.319A, S76.391A, S76.399-S76.801 with 7th A, S76.809-S76.811 with 7th A, S76.819A, S76.891A, S76.899-S76.901 with 7th A, S76.909-S76.911 with 7th A, S76.919A, S76.991A, S76.999A, S79.001A, S79.009-S79.011 with 7th A, S79.019-S79.091 with 7th A, S79.099-S79.101 with 7th A, S79.109-S79.111 with 7th A, S79.119-S79.121 with 7th A, S79.129-S79.131 with 7th A, S79.139-S79.141 with 7th A, S79.149-S79.191 with 7th A, S79.199-S79.811 with 7th A, S79.819-S79.821 with 7th A, S79.829-S79.911 with 7th A, S79.919-S79.921 with 7th A, S79.929A, S82.90-S82.92X with 7th [A, B, C], T14.90-T14.91, T79.A9X-T79.9XX with 7th A
MCC with 7th B or C: M80.00X-M80.019 with 7th A, M80.041-M80.059 with 7th A, M80.80X-M80.819 with 7th A, M80.841-M80.859 with 7th A, M84.40X-M84.419 with 7th A, M84.441-M84.459 with 7th A, M84.474-M84.519 with 7th A, M84.541-M84.559 with 7th A, M84.574-M84.576 with 7th A, M84.60X-M84.619 with 7th A, M84.641-M84.659 with 7th A, M84.674-M84.68X with 7th A, S03.8XX-S03.9XX with 7th A, S29.011-S29.019 with 7th A, S38.3XX-S39.013 with 7th A, S72.001-S72.92X with 7th [A, B, C], S73.101-S73.199 with 7th A, S76.001-S76.019 with 7th A, S76.091-S76.119 with 7th A, S76.191-S76.219 with 7th A, S76.291-

S76.319 with 7th A, S76.391-S76.819 with 7th A, S76.891-S76.919 with 7th A, S76.991-S76.999 with 7th A, S79.001-S79.929 with 7th A, S82.90X-S82.92X with 7th [A, B, C], T14.90-T14.91, T79.A9X-T79.9XX with 7th A
CC with 7th character K, M, N, P, Q or R: M80.00X-M84.68X with 7th [K, P], S02.0XX-S02.92X with 7th K, S12.000-S12.691 with 7th K, S22.000-S22.9XX with 7th K, S32.000-S32.9XX with 7th K, S42.001-S42.92X with 7th [K, P], S49.001-S49.199 with 7th [K, P], S52.001-S52.92X with 7th [K, M, N, P, Q, R], S59.001-S59.299 with 7th [K, P], S62.001-S62.92X with 7th [K, P], S72.001-S72.92X with 7th [K, M, N, P, Q, R], S79.001-S79.199 with 7th [K, P], S82.001-S82.92X with 7th [K, M, N, P, Q, R], S89.001-S89.399 with 7th [K, P], S92.001-S92.919 with 7th [K, P]

7,16,19 ✓7th **S72.402** **Unspecified fracture of lower end of left femur** MCC CC
CC Excl: CC with 7th character A: M80.00X-M80.019 with 7th A, M80.041-M80.059 with 7th A, M80.80X-M80.819 with 7th A, M80.841-M80.859 with 7th A, M84.40X-M84.419 with 7th A, M84.441-M84.459 with 7th A, M84.474-M84.519 with 7th A, M84.541-M84.559 with 7th A, M84.574-M84.576 with 7th A, M84.60X-M84.619 with 7th A, M84.641-M84.659 with 7th A, M84.674-M84.68 with 7th A, S03.8XX-S03.9XX with 7th A, S29.011-S29.019 with 7th A, S38.3XX-S39.013 with 7th A, S72.001-S72.466 with 7th [B, C], S72.472-S72.92X with 7th A, S73.102-S73.109 with 7th A, S73.112-S73.119 with 7th A, S73.122-S73.129 with 7th A, S73.192-S73.199 with 7th A, S76.002-S76.009 with 7th A, S76.012-S76.019 with 7th A, S76.092-S76.099 with 7th A, S76.102-S76.109 with 7th A, S76.112-S76.119 with 7th A, S76.192-S76.199 with 7th A, S76.202-S76.209 with 7th A, S76.212-S76.219 with 7th A, S76.292-S76.299 with 7th A, S76.302-S76.309 with 7th A, S76.312-S76.319 with 7th A, S76.392-S76.399 with 7th A, S76.802-S76.809 with 7th A, S76.812-S76.819 with 7th A, S76.892-S76.899 with 7th A, S76.902-S76.909 with 7th A, S76.912-S76.919 with 7th A, S76.992-S76.999 with 7th A, S79.002-S79.009 with 7th A, S79.012-S79.019 with 7th A, S79.092-S79.099 with 7th A, S79.102-S79.109 with 7th A, S79.112-S79.119 with 7th A, S79.122-S79.129 with 7th A, S79.132-S79.139 with 7th A, S79.142-S79.149 with 7th A, S79.192-S79.199 with 7th A, S79.812-S79.819 with 7th A, S79.822-S79.829 with 7th A, S79.912-S79.919 with 7th A, S79.922-S79.929 with 7th A, S82.90X-S82.92X with 7th [A, B, C], T14.90-T14.91, T79.A9X-T79.9XX with 7th A
MCC with 7th B or C: M80.00X-M80.019 with 7th A, M80.041-M80.059 with 7th A, M80.80X-M80.819 with 7th A, M80.841-M80.859 with 7th A, M84.40X-M84.419 with 7th A, M84.441-M84.459 with 7th A, M84.474-M84.519 with 7th A, M84.541-M84.559 with 7th A, M84.574-M84.576 with 7th A, M84.60X-M84.619 with 7th A, M84.641-M84.659 with 7th A, M84.674-M84.68X with 7th A, S03.8XX-S03.9XX with 7th A, S29.011-S29.019 with 7th A, S38.3XX-S39.013 with 7th A, S72.001-S72.92X with 7th [A, B, C], S73.101-S73.199 with 7th A, S76.001-S76.019 with 7th A, S76.091-S76.119 with 7th A, S76.191-S76.219 with 7th A, S76.291-S76.319 with 7th A, S76.391-S76.819 with 7th A, S76.891-S76.919 with 7th A, S76.991-S76.999 with 7th A, S79.001-S79.929 with 7th A, S82.90-S82.92X with 7th [A, B, C], T14.90-T14.91, T79.A9X-T79.9XX with 7th A
CC with 7th character K, M, N, P, Q or R: M80.00X-M84.68X with 7th [K, P], S02.0XX-S02.92X with 7th K, S12.000-S12.691 with 7th K, S22.000-S22.9XX with 7th K, S32.000-S32.9XX with 7th K, S42.001-S42.92X with 7th [K, P], S49.001-S49.199 with 7th [K, P], S52.001-S52.92X with 7th [K, M, N, P, Q, R], S59.001-S59.299 with 7th [K, P], S62.001-S62.92X with 7th [K, P], S72.001-S72.92X

---

7   HAC = Initial encounter only (7th character A, B or C) and not POA.
16   MCC only if an open fracture (7th character B or C).
18   CC only if a subsequent encounter for nonunion or malunion (7th character K, M, N, P, Q, or R).
19   CC only if an initial encounter for a closed fracture (7th character A) **OR** a subsequent encounter for nonunion or malunion (7th character K, M, N, P, Q, or R – specific to category).

N Newborn: 0   P Pediatric: 0-17   M Maternity: 12-55   A Adult: 15-124   MCC Major CC Condition   PDxMCC PDx acts as own MCC   CC CC Condition   PDxCC PDx acts as own CC

1020   ICD-10-CM 2016

with 7th [K, M, N, P, Q, R], S79.001-S79.199
with 7th [K, P], S82.001-S82.92X with 7th [K,
M, N, P, Q, R], S89.001-S89.399 with 7th [K, P],
S92.001-S92.919 with 7th [K, P]

7,16,19 √7ᵗʰ **S72.409　Unspecified fracture of lower end**　MCC CC
of unspecified femur
CC Excl: CC with 7th character A, MCC with
7th B or C: M80.00X-M80.019 with 7th A,
M80.041-M80.059 with 7th A, M80.80X-
M80.819 with 7th A, M80.841-M80.859 with
7th A, M84.40X-M84.419 with 7th A,
M84.441-M84.459 with 7th A, M84.474-
M84.519 with 7th A, M84.541-M84.559 with
7th A, M84.574-M84.576 with 7th A,
M84.60X-M84.619 with 7th A, M84.641-
M84.659 with 7th A, M84.674-M84.68 with
7th A, S03.8XX-S03.9XX with 7th A, S29.011-
S29.019 with 7th A, S38.3XX-S39.013 with
7th A, S72.001-S72.92X with 7th [A, B, C],
S73.101-S73.199 with 7th A, S76.001-
S76.019 with 7th A, S76.091-S76.119 with
7th A, S76.191-S76.219 with 7th A, S76.291-
S76.319 with 7th A, S76.391-S76.819 with
7th A, S76.891-S76.919 with 7th A, S76.991-
S76.999 with 7th A, S79.001-S79.929 with
7th A, S82.90X-S82.92X with 7th [A, B, C],
T14.90-T14.91, T79.A9X-T79.9XX with 7th A
CC with 7th character K, M, N, P, Q or R:
M80.00X-M84.68X with 7th [K, P], S02.0XX-
S02.92X with 7th K, S12.000-S12.691 with
7th K, S22.000-S22.9XX with 7th K, S32.000-
S32.9XX with 7th K, S42.001-S42.92X with
7th [K, P], S49.001-S49.199 with 7th [K, P],
S52.001-S52.92X with 7th [K, M, N, P, Q, R],
S59.001-S59.299 with 7th [K, P], S62.001-
S62.92X with 7th [K, P], S72.001-S72.92X
with 7th [K, M, N, P, Q, R], S79.001-S79.199
with 7th [K, P], S82.001-S82.92X with 7th [K,
M, N, P, Q, R], S89.001-S89.399 with 7th [K, P],
S92.001-S92.919 with 7th [K, P]

√6ᵗʰ **S72.41　Unspecified condyle fracture of lower end of femur**
Condyle fracture of femur NOS

7,16,19 √7ᵗʰ **S72.411　Displaced unspecified condyle**　MCC CC
fracture of lower end of right femur
CC Excl: See code: S72.401

7,16,19 √7ᵗʰ **S72.412　Displaced unspecified condyle**　MCC CC
fracture of lower end of left femur
CC Excl: See code: S72.402

7,16,19 √7ᵗʰ **S72.413　Displaced unspecified condyle**　MCC CC
fracture of lower end of
unspecified femur
CC Excl: See code: S72.409

7,16,19 √7ᵗʰ **S72.414　Nondisplaced unspecified condyle**　MCC CC
fracture of lower end of right femur
CC Excl: See code: S72.401

7,16,19 √7ᵗʰ **S72.415　Nondisplaced unspecified condyle**　MCC CC
fracture of lower end of left femur
CC Excl: See code: S72.402

7,16,19 √7ᵗʰ **S72.416　Nondisplaced unspecified**　MCC CC
condyle fracture of lower end of
unspecified femur
CC Excl: See code: S72.409

√6ᵗʰ **S72.42　Fracture of lateral condyle of femur**

7,16,19 √7ᵗʰ **S72.421　Displaced fracture of lateral**　MCC CC
condyle of right femur
CC Excl: See code: S72.401

7,16,19 √7ᵗʰ **S72.422　Displaced fracture of lateral**　MCC CC
condyle of left femur
CC Excl: See code: S72.402

7,16,19 √7ᵗʰ **S72.423　Displaced fracture of lateral**　MCC CC
condyle of unspecified femur
CC Excl: See code: S72.409

7,16,19 √7ᵗʰ **S72.424　Nondisplaced fracture of lateral**　MCC CC
condyle of right femur
CC Excl: See code: S72.401

7,16,19 √7ᵗʰ **S72.425　Nondisplaced fracture of lateral**　MCC CC
condyle of left femur
CC Excl: See code: S72.402

7,16,19 √7ᵗʰ **S72.426　Nondisplaced fracture of lateral**　MCC CC
condyle of unspecified femur
CC Excl: See code: S72.409

√6ᵗʰ **S72.43　Fracture of medial condyle of femur**

7,16,19 √7ᵗʰ **S72.431　Displaced fracture of medial**　MCC CC
condyle of right femur
CC Excl: See code: S72.401

7,16,19 √7ᵗʰ **S72.432　Displaced fracture of medial**　MCC CC
condyle of left femur
CC Excl: See code: S72.402

7,16,19 √7ᵗʰ **S72.433　Displaced fracture of medial**　MCC CC
condyle of unspecified femur
CC Excl: See code: S72.409

7,16,19 √7ᵗʰ **S72.434　Nondisplaced fracture of medial**　MCC CC
condyle of right femur
CC Excl: See code: S72.401

7,16,19 √7ᵗʰ **S72.435　Nondisplaced fracture of medial**　MCC CC
condyle of left femur
CC Excl: See code: S72.402

7,16,19 √7ᵗʰ **S72.436　Nondisplaced fracture of medial**　MCC CC
condyle of unspecified femur
CC Excl: See code: S72.409

√6ᵗʰ **S72.44　Fracture of lower epiphysis (separation) of femur**
EXCLUDES 1　*Salter-Harris Type I physeal fracture of lower*
end of femur (S79.11-)

7,16,19 √7ᵗʰ **S72.441　Displaced fracture of lower**　MCC CC
epiphysis (separation) of
right femur
CC Excl: See code: S72.401

7,16,19 √7ᵗʰ **S72.442　Displaced fracture of lower**　MCC CC
epiphysis (separation) of left
femur
CC Excl: See code: S72.402

7,16,19 √7ᵗʰ **S72.443　Displaced fracture of lower**　MCC CC
epiphysis (separation) of
unspecified femur
CC Excl: See code: S72.409

7,16,19 √7ᵗʰ **S72.444　Nondisplaced fracture of lower**　MCC CC
epiphysis (separation) of right femur
CC Excl: See code: S72.401

7,16,19 √7ᵗʰ **S72.445　Nondisplaced fracture of lower**　MCC CC
epiphysis (separation) of left femur
CC Excl: See code: S72.402

7,16,19 √7ᵗʰ **S72.446　Nondisplaced fracture of lower**　MCC CC
epiphysis (separation) of
unspecified femur
CC Excl: See code: S72.409

√6ᵗʰ **S72.45　Supracondylar fracture without intracondylar**
extension of lower end of femur
Supracondylar fracture of lower end of femur NOS
EXCLUDES 1　*supracondylar fracture with intracondylar*
extension of lower end of femur
(S72.46-)

7,16,19 √7ᵗʰ **S72.451　Displaced supracondylar fracture**　MCC CC
without intracondylar extension
of lower end of right femur
CC Excl: See code: S72.401

7,16,19 √7ᵗʰ **S72.452　Displaced supracondylar fracture**　MCC CC
without intracondylar extension
of lower end of left femur
CC Excl: See code: S72.402

7,16,19 √7ᵗʰ **S72.453　Displaced supracondylar fracture**　MCC CC
without intracondylar extension
of lower end of unspecified femur
CC Excl: See code: S72.409

7,16,19 √7ᵗʰ **S72.454　Nondisplaced supracondylar**　MCC CC
fracture without intracondylar
extension of lower end of right
femur
CC Excl: See code: S72.401

7,16,19 √7ᵗʰ **S72.455　Nondisplaced supracondylar**　MCC CC
fracture without intracondylar
extension of lower end of left
femur
CC Excl: See code: S72.402

7,16,19 √7ᵗʰ **S72.456　Nondisplaced supracondylar**　MCC CC
fracture without intracondylar
extension of lower end of
unspecified femur
CC Excl: See code: S72.409

7　HAC = Initial encounter only (7th character A, B or C) and not POA.
16　MCC only if an open fracture (7th character B or C).
19　CC only if an initial encounter for a closed fracture (7th character A) **OR** a subsequent encounter for nonunion or malunion (7th character K, M, N, P, Q, or R – specific to category).

✅ Additional Character Required　√x7ᵗʰ Placeholder Alert　Unacceptable PDx　Manifestation　Hospital Acquired Condition　EXCLUDES 1 Not Coded Here　EXCLUDES 2 Not Included Here

√6ᵗʰ **S72.46**   Supracondylar **fracture with intracondylar extension** of lower end of femur

> EXCLUDES 1   *supracondylar fracture without intracondylar extension of lower end of femur (S72.45-)*

7,16,19 √7ᵗʰ **S72.461**   **Displaced** supracondylar fracture   MCC CC
with intracondylar extension of lower end of **right** femur
CC Excl: See code: S72.401

7,16,19 √7ᵗʰ **S72.462**   **Displaced** supracondylar fracture   MCC CC
with intracondylar extension of lower end of **left** femur
CC Excl: See code: S72.402

7,16,19 √7ᵗʰ **S72.463**   **Displaced** supracondylar fracture   MCC CC
with intracondylar extension of lower end of **unspecified** femur
CC Excl: See code: S72.409

7,16,19 √7ᵗʰ **S72.464**   **Nondisplaced** supracondylar   MCC CC
fracture with intracondylar extension of lower end of **right** femur
CC Excl: See code: S72.401

7,16,19 √7ᵗʰ **S72.465**   **Nondisplaced** supracondylar   MCC CC
fracture with intracondylar extension of lower end of **left** femur
CC Excl: See code: S72.402

7,16,19 √7ᵗʰ **S72.466**   **Nondisplaced** supracondylar   MCC CC
fracture with intracondylar extension of lower end of **unspecified** femur
CC Excl: See code: S72.409

√6ᵗʰ **S72.47**   Torus **fracture of lower end of femur**

> The appropriate 7th character is to be added to all codes in subcategory S72.47.
> A   initial encounter for closed fracture
> D   subsequent encounter for fracture with routine healing
> G   subsequent encounter for fracture with delayed healing
> K   subsequent encounter for fracture with nonunion
> P   subsequent encounter for fracture with malunion
> S   sequela

7,19 √7ᵗʰ **S72.471**   **Torus fracture of lower end of**   CC
right femur
CC Excl: CC with 7th character A: M80.00X-M80.019 with 7th A, M80.041-M80.059 with 7th A, M80.80X-M80.819 with 7th A, M80.841-M80.859 with 7th A, M84.40X-M84.419 with 7th A, M84.441-M84.459 with 7th A, M84.474-M84.519 with 7th A, M84.541-M84.559 with 7th A, M84.574-M84.576 with 7th A, M84.60X-M84.619 with 7th A, M84.641-M84.659 with 7th A, M84.674-M84.68X with 7th A, S03.8XX-S03.9XX with 7th A, S29.011-S29.019 with 7th A, S38.3X-S39.013 with 7th A, S72.001-S72.471 with 7th [A, B, C], S72.479-S72.92X with 7th A, S73.101 with 7th A, S73.109-S73.111 with 7th A, S73.119-S73.121 with 7th A, S73.129-S73.191 with 7th A, S73.199 with 7th A, S76.001 with 7th A, S76.009-S76.011 with 7th A, S76.019A, S76.091A, S76.099-S76.101 with 7th A, S76.109-S76.111 with 7th A, S76.119A, S76.191A, S76.199-S76.201 with 7th A, S76.209-S76.211 with 7th A, S76.219A, S76.291 A, S76.299-S76.301 with 7th A, S76.309-S76.311 with 7th A, S76.319A, S76.391A, S76.399-S76.801 with 7th A, S76.809-S76.811 with 7th A, S76.819A, S76.891A, S76.899-S76.901 with 7th A, S76.909-S76.911 with 7th A, S76.919A, S76.991A, S76.999A, S79.001A, S79.009-S79.011 with 7th A, S79.019-S79.091 with 7th A, S79.099-S79.101 with 7th A, S79.109-S79.111 with 7th A, S79.119-S79.121 with 7th A, S79.129-S79.131 with 7th A, S79.139-S79.141 with 7th A, S79.149-S79.191 with 7th A, S79.199-S79.811 with 7th A, S79.819-S79.821 with 7th A, S79.829-S79.911 with 7th A, S79.919-S79.921 with 7th A, S79.929A, S82.90X-S82.92X with 7th [A, B, C], T14.90-T14.91, T79.A9X-T79.9XX with 7th A

CC Excl: CC with 7th character K or P:
M80.00X-M84.68X with 7th [K, P], S02.0XX-S02.92X with 7th K, S12.000-S12.691 with 7th K, S22.000-S22.9XX with 7th K, S32.000-S32.9XX with 7th K, S42.001-S42.92X with 7th [K, P], S49.001-S49.199 with 7th [K, P], S52.001-S52.92X with 7th [K, M, N, P, Q, R], S59.001-S59.299 with 7th [K, P], S62.001-S62.92X with 7th [K, P], S72.001-S72.92X with 7th [K, M, N, P, Q, R], S79.001-S79.199 with 7th [K, P], S82.001-S82.92X with 7th [K, M, N, P, Q, R], S89.001-S89.399 with 7th [K, P], S92.001-S92.919 with 7th [K, P]

7,19 √7ᵗʰ **S72.472**   **Torus fracture of lower end of**   CC
left femur
CC Excl: CC with 7th character A: M80.00X-M80.019 with 7th A, M80.041-M80.059 with 7th A, M80.80X-M80.819 with 7th A, M80.841-M80.859 with 7th A, M84.40X-M84.419 with 7th A, M84.441-M84.459 with 7th A, M84.474-M84.519 with 7th A, M84.541-M84.559 with 7th A, M84.574-M84.576 with 7th A, M84.60X-M84.619 with 7th A, M84.641-M84.659 with 7th A, M84.674-M84.68 with 7th A, S03.8XX-S03.9XX with 7th A, S29.011-S29.019 with 7th A, S38.3XX-S39.013 with 7th A, S72.001-S72.466 with 7th [B, C], S72.472-S72.92X with 7th A, S73.102-S73.109 with 7th A, S73.112-S73.119 with 7th A, S73.122-S73.129 with 7th A, S73.192-S73.199 with 7th A, S76.002-S76.009 with 7th A, S76.012-S76.019 with 7th A, S76.092-S76.099 with 7th A, S76.102-S76.109 with 7th A, S76.112-S76.119 with 7th A, S76.192-S76.199 with 7th A, S76.202-S76.209 with 7th A, S76.212-S76.219 with 7th A, S76.292-S76.299 with 7th A, S76.302-S76.309 with 7th A, S76.312-S76.319 with 7th A, S76.392-S76.399 with 7th A, S76.802-S76.809 with 7th A, S76.812-S76.819 with 7th A, S76.892-S76.899 with 7th A, S76.902-S76.909 with 7th A, S76.912-S76.919 with 7th A, S76.992-S76.999 with 7th A, S79.002-S79.009 with 7th A, S79.012-S79.019 with 7th A, S79.092-S79.099 with 7th A, S79.102-S79.109 with 7th A, S79.112-S79.119 with 7th A, S79.122-S79.129 with 7th A, S79.132-S79.139 with 7th A, S79.142-S79.149 with 7th A, S79.192-S79.199 with 7th A, S79.812-S79.819 with 7th A, S79.822-S79.829 with 7th A, S79.912-S79.919 with 7th A, S79.922-S79.929 with 7th A, S82.90X-S82.92X with 7th [A, B, C], T14.90-T14.91, T79.A9X-T79.9XX with 7th A

CC Excl: CC with 7th character K or P:
M80.00X-M84.68X with 7th [K, P], S02.0XX-S02.92X with 7th K, S12.000-S12.691 with 7th K, S22.000-S22.9XX with 7th K, S32.000-S32.9XX with 7th K, S42.001-S42.92X with 7th [K, P], S49.001-S49.199 with 7th [K, P], S52.001-S52.92X with 7th [K, M, N, P, Q, R], S59.001-S59.299 with 7th [K, P], S62.001-S62.92X with 7th [K, P], S72.001-S72.92X with 7th [K, M, N, P, Q, R], S79.001-S79.199 with 7th [K, P], S82.001-S82.92X with 7th [K, M, N, P, Q, R], S89.001-S89.399 with 7th [K, P], S92.001-S92.919 with 7th [K, P]

7,19 √7ᵗʰ **S72.479**   **Torus fracture of lower end of**   CC
unspecified femur
CC Excl: CC with 7th character A: M80.00X-M80.019 with 7th A, M80.041-M80.059 with 7th A, M80.80X-M80.819 with 7th A, M80.841- M80.859 with 7th A, M84.40X-M84.419 with 7th A, M84.441-M84.459 with 7th A, M84.474-M84.519 with 7th A, M84.541-M84.559 with 7th A, M84.574-M84.576 with 7th A, M84.60X-M84.619 with 7th A, M84.641-M84.659 with 7th A, M84.674-M84.68X with 7th A, S03.8XX-S03.9XX with 7th A, S29.011-S29.019 with 7th A, S38.3XX-S39.013 with 7th A, S72.001-S72.471 with 7th [A, B, C], S72.479-S72.92X with 7th A, S73.101A, S73.109-S73.111 with 7th A, S73.119-S73.121 with 7th A, S73.129-S73.191 with 7th A, S73.199A, S76.001A, S76.009-S76.011 with 7th A, S76.019A, S76.091A, S76.099-S76.101 with 7th A, S76.109-S76.111 with 7th A, S76.119A, S76.191A, S76.199-S76.201 with

---

7   HAC = Initial encounter only (7th character A, B or C) and not POA.
16   MCC only if an open fracture (7th character B or C).
19   CC only if an initial encounter for a closed fracture (7th character A) **OR** a subsequent encounter for nonunion or malunion (7th character K, M, N, P, Q, or R – specific to category).

N Newborn: 0   P Pediatric: 0-17   M Maternity: 12-55   A Adult: 15-124   MCC Major CC Condition   PDxMCC PDx acts as own MCC   CC CC Condition   PDxCC PDx acts as own CC

7th A, S76.209-S76.211 with 7th A, S76.219A, S76.291A, S76.299-S76.301 with 7th A, S76.309-S76.311 with 7th A, S76.319A, S76.391A, S76.399-S76.801 with 7th A, S76.809-S76.811 with 7th A, S76.819A, S76.891A, S76.899-S76.901 with 7th A, S76.909-S76.911 with 7th A, S76.919A, S76.991A, S76.999A, S79.001A, S79.009-S79.011 with 7th A, S79.019-S79.091 with 7th A, S79.099-S79.101 with 7th A, S79.109-S79.111 with 7th A, S79.119-S79.121 with 7th A, S79.129-S79.131 with 7th A, S79.139-S79.141 with 7th A, S79.149-S79.191 with 7th A, S79.199-S79.811 with 7th A, S79.819-S79.821 with 7th A, S79.829-S79.911 with 7th A, S79.919-S79.921 with 7th A, S79.929A, S82.90X-S82.92X with 7th [A, B, C], T14.90-T14.91, T79.A9X-T79.9XX with 7th A

CC with 7th character K or P: M80.00X-M84.68X with 7th [K, P], S02.0XX-S02.92X with 7th K, S12.000-S12.691 with 7th K, S22.000-S22.9XX with 7th K, S32.000-S32.9XX with 7th K, S42.001-S42.92X with 7th [K, P], S49.001-S49.199 with 7th [K, P], S52.001-S52.92X with 7th [K, M, N, P, Q, R], S59.001-S59.299 with 7th [K, P], S62.001-S62.92X with 7th [K, P], S72.001-S72.92X with 7th [K, M, N, P, Q, R], S79.001-S79.199 with 7th [K, P], S82.001-S82.92X with 7th [K, M, N, P, Q, R], S89.001-S89.399 with 7th [K, P], S92.001-S92.919 with 7th [K, P]

√6th **S72.49** Other **fracture of lower end of femur**

7,16,19 √7th **S72.491** Other fracture of lower end of right femur   MCC CC

CC Excl: CC for codes with 7th A: M80.00X-M80.019 with 7th A, M80.041-M80.059 with 7th A, M80.80X-M80.819 with 7th A, M80.841-M80.859 with 7th A, M84.40X-M84.419 with 7th A, M84.441-M84.459 with 7th A, M84.474-M84.519 with 7th A, M84.541-M84.559 with 7th A, M84.574-M84.576 with 7th A, M84.60X-M84.619 with 7th A, M84.641-M84.659 with 7th A, M84.674-M84.68 with 7th A, S03.8XX-S03.9XX with 7th A, S29.011-S29.019 with 7th A, S38.3XX-S39.013 with 7th A, S72.001-S72.471 with 7th [A, B, C], S72.479-S72.92X with 7th A, S73.101 with 7th A, S73.109-S73.111 with 7th A, S73.119-S73.121 with 7th A, S73.129-S73.191 with 7th A, S73.199A, S76.001A, S76.009-S76.011 with 7th A, S76.019A, S76.091A, S76.099-S76.101 with 7th A, S76.109-S76.111 with 7th A, S76.119 A, S76.191A, S76.199-S76.201 with 7th A, S76.209-S76.211 with 7th A, S76.219A, S76.291A, S76.299-S76.301 with 7th A, S76.309-S76.311 with 7th A, S76.319A, S76.391A, S76.399-S76.801 with 7th A, S76.809-S76.811 with 7th A, S76.819A, S76.891A, S76.899-S76.901 with 7th A, S76.909-S76.911 with 7th A, S76.919A, S76.991A, S76.999A, S79.001A, S79.009-S79.011 with 7th A, S79.019-S79.091 with 7th A, S79.099-S79.101 with 7th A, S79.109-S79.111 with 7th A, S79.119-S79.121 with 7th A, S79.129-S79.131 with 7th A, S79.139-S79.141 with 7th A, S79.149-S79.191 with 7th A, S79.199-S79.811 with 7th A, S79.819-S79.821 with 7th A, S79.829-S79.911 with 7th A, S79.919-S79.921 with 7th A, S79.929A, S82.90-S82.92 with 7th [A, B, C], T14.90-T14.91, T79.A9X-T79.9XX with 7th A

MCC for codes with 7th B or C: M80.00X-M80.019 with 7th A, M80.041-M80.059 with 7th A, M80.80X-M80.819 with 7th A, M80.841-M80.859 with 7th A, M84.40X-M84.419 with 7th A, M84.441-M84.459 with 7th A, M84.474-M84.519 with 7th A, M84.541-M84.559 with 7th A, M84.574-M84.576 with 7th A, M84.60X-M84.619 with 7th A, M84.641-M84.659 with 7th A, M84.674-M84.68 with 7th A, S03.8XX-S03.9XX with 7th A, S29.011-S29.019 with 7th A, S38.3XX-S39.013 with 7th A, S72.491-S72.499 with 7th [B, C], S73.101-S73.199 with 7th A, S76.001-S76.019 with 7th A, S76.091-S76.119 with 7th A, S76.191-S76.219 with 7th A, S76.291-S76.319 with 7th A, S76.391-S76.819 with 7th A, S76.891-S76.919 with 7th A, S76.991-S76.999 with 7th A, S79.811-

S79.929 with 7th A, S82.001-S82.099 with 7th [A, B, C], S82.90X-S82.92X with 7th [A, B, C], T14.90-T14.91, T79.A9X-T79.9XX with 7th A

CC for codes with 7th K, M, N, P, Q or R: M80.00X-M84.68X with 7th [K, P], S02.0XX-S02.92X with 7th K, S12.000-S12.691 with 7th K, S22.000-S22.9XX with 7th K, S32.000-S32.9XX with 7th K, S42.001-S42.92X with 7th [K, P], S49.001-S49.199 with 7th [K, P], S52.001-S52.92X with 7th [K, M, N, P, Q, R], S59.001-S59.299 with 7th [K, P], S62.001-S62.92X with 7th [K, P], S72.001-S72.92X with 7th [K, M, N, P, Q, R], S79.001-S79.199 with 7th [K, P], S82.001-S82.92X with 7th [K, M, N, P, Q, R], S89.001-S89.399 with 7th [K, P], S92.001-S92.919 with 7th [K, P]

7,16,19 √7th **S72.492** Other fracture of lower end of left femur   MCC CC

CC Excl: CC for codes with 7th A: M80.00X-M80.019 with 7th A, M80.041-M80.059 with 7th A, M80.80X-M80.819 with 7th A, M80.841-M80.859 with 7th A, M84.40X-M84.419 with 7th A, M84.441-M84.459 with 7th A, M84.474-M84.519 with 7th A, M84.541-M84.559 with 7th A, M84.574-M84.576 with 7th A, M84.60X-M84.619 with 7th A, M84.641-M84.659 with 7th A, M84.674-M84.68 with 7th A, S03.8XX-S03.9XX with 7th A, S29.011-S29.019 with 7th A, S38.3XX-S39.013 with 7th A, S72.001-S72.466 with 7th [B, C], S72.472-S72.92X with 7th A, S73.102-S73.109 with 7th A, S73.112-S73.119 with 7th A, S73.122-S73.129 with 7th A, S73.192-S73.199 with 7th A, S76.002-S76.009 with 7th A, S76.012-S76.019 with 7th A, S76.092-S76.099 with 7th A, S76.102-S76.109 with 7th A, S76.112-S76.119 with 7th A, S76.192-S76.199 with 7th A, S76.202-S76.209 with 7th A, S76.212-S76.219 with 7th A, S76.292-S76.299 with 7th A, S76.302-S76.309 with 7th A, S76.312-S76.319 with 7th A, S76.392-S76.399 with 7th A, S76.802-S76.809 with 7th A, S76.812-S76.819 with 7th A, S76.892-S76.899 with 7th A, S76.902-S76.909 with 7th A, S76.912-S76.919 with 7th A, S76.992-S76.999 with 7th A, S79.002-S79.009 with 7th A, S79.012-S79.019 with 7th A, S79.092-S79.099 with 7th A, S79.102-S79.109 with 7th A, S79.112-S79.119 with 7th A, S79.122-S79.129 with 7th A, S79.132-S79.139 with 7th A, S79.142-S79.149 with 7th A, S79.192-S79.199 with 7th A, S79.812-S79.819 with 7th A, S79.822-S79.829 with 7th A, S79.912-S79.919 with 7th A, S79.922-S79.929 with 7th A, S82.90X-S82.92X with 7th [A, B, C], T14.90-T14.91, T79.A9X-T79.9XX with 7th A

MCC for codes with 7th B or C: M80.00X-M80.019 with 7th A, M80.041-M80.059 with 7th A, M80.80X-M80.819 with 7th A, M80.841-M80.859 with 7th A, M84.40X-M84.419 with 7th A, M84.441-M84.459 with 7th A, M84.474-M84.519 with 7th A, M84.541-M84.559 with 7th A, M84.574-M84.576 with 7th A, M84.60X-M84.619 with 7th A, M84.641-M84.659 with 7th A, M84.674-M84.68 with 7th A, S03.8XX-S03.9XX with 7th A, S29.011-S29.019 with 7th A, S38.3X-S39.013 with 7th A, S72.491-S72.499 with 7th [B, C], S73.101-S73.199 with 7th A, S76.001-S76.019 with 7th A, S76.091-S76.119 with 7th A, S76.191-S76.219 with 7th A, S76.291-S76.319 with 7th A, S76.391-S76.819 with 7th A, S76.891-S76.919 with 7th A, S76.991-S76.999 with 7th A, S79.811-S79.929 with 7th A, S82.001-S82.099 with 7th [A, B, C], S82.90X-S82.92X with 7th [A, B, C], T14.90-T14.91, T79.A9X-T79.9XX with 7th A

CC for codes with 7th K, M, N, P, Q or R: M80.00X-M84.68 with 7th [K, P], S02.0XX-S02.92X with 7th K, S12.000-S12.691 with 7th K, S22.000-S22.9XX with 7th K, S32.000-S32.9XX with 7th K, S42.001-S42.92X with 7th [K, P], S49.001-S49.199 with 7th [K, P], S52.001-S52.92X with 7th [K, M, N, P, Q, R], S59.001-S59.299 with 7th [K, P], S62.001-S62.92X with 7th [K, P], S72.001-S72.92X with 7th [K, M, N, P, Q, R], S79.001-S79.199 with 7th [K, P], S82.001-S82.92X with 7th [K, M, N, P, Q, R], S89.001-S89.399 with 7th [K, P], S92.001-S92.919 with 7th [K, P]

---

7 HAC = Initial encounter only (7th character A, B or C) and not POA.
16 MCC only if an open fracture (7th character B or C).
19 CC only if an initial encounter for a closed fracture (7th character A) **OR** a subsequent encounter for nonunion or malunion (7th character K, M, N, P, Q, or R – specific to category).

✔ Additional Character Required   √x7th Placeholder Alert   Unacceptable PDx   Manifestation   Hospital Acquired Condition   EXCLUDES 1 Not Coded Here   EXCLUDES 2 Not Included Here

7,16,19 ✓7th **S72.499** **Other fracture of lower end of** MCC CC
unspecified femur
CC Excl: CC for codes with 7th A: M80.00X-
M80.019 with 7th A, M80.041-M80.059 with
7th A, M80.80X-M80.819 with 7th A,
M80.841-M80.859 with 7th A, M84.40X-
M84.419 with 7th A, M84.441-M84.459 with
7th A, M84.474-M84.519 with 7th A,
M84.541-M84.559 with 7th A, M84.574-
M84.576 with 7th A, M84.60X-M84.619 with
7th A, M84.641-M84.659 with 7th A,
M84.674-M84.68 with 7th A, S03.8XX-
S03.9XX with 7th A, S29.011-S29.019 with
7th A, S38.3XX-S39.013 with 7th A, S72.001-
S72.92X with 7th [A, B, C], S73.101-S73.199
with 7th A, S76.001-S76.019 with 7th A,
S76.091-S76.119 with 7th A, S76.191-
S76.219 with 7th A, S76.291-S76.319 with
7th A, S76.391-S76.819 with 7th A, S76.891-
S76.919 with 7th A, S76.991-S76.999 with
7th A, S79.001-S79.929 with 7th A, S82.90X-
S82.92X with 7th [A, B, C], T14.90-T14.91,
T79.A9X-T79.9XX with 7th A
MCC for codes with 7th B or C: M80.00X-
M80.019 with 7th A, M80.041-M80.059 with
7th A, M80.80X-M80.819 with 7th A,
M80.841-M80.859 with 7th A, M84.40X-
M84.419 with 7th A, M84.441-M84.459 with
7th A, M84.474-M84.519 with 7th A,
M84.541-M84.559 with 7th A, M84.574-
M84.576 with 7th A, M84.60X-M84.619 with
7th A, M84.641-M84.659 with 7th A,
M84.674-M84.68X with 7th A, S03.8XX-
S03.9XX with 7th A, S29.011-S29.019 with
7th A, S38.3XX-S39.013 with 7th A, S72.491-
S72.499 with 7th [B, C], S73.101-S73.199 with
7th A, S76.001-S76.019 with 7th A, S76.091-
S76.119 with 7th A, S76.191-S76.219 with
7th A, S76.291-S76.319 with 7th A, S76.391-
S76.819 with 7th A, S76.891-S76.919 with
7th A, S76.991-S76.999 with 7th A, S79.811-
S79.929 with 7th A, S82.001-S82.099 with
7th [A, B, C], S82.90X-S82.92X with 7th [A, B,
C], T14.90-T14.91, T79.A9X-T79.9XX with 7th
A
CC for codes with 7th K, M, N, P, Q or R:
M80.00X-M84.68X with 7th [K, P], S02.0XX-
S02.92X with 7th K, S12.000-S12.691 with
7th K, S22.000-S22.9XX with 7th K, S32.000-
S32.9XX with 7th K, S42.001-S42.92X with
7th [K, P], S49.001-S49.199 with 7th [K, P],
S52.001-S52.92X with 7th [K, M, N, P, Q, R],
S59.001-S59.299 with 7th [K, P], S62.001-
S62.92X with 7th [K, P], S72.001-S72.92X
with 7th [K, M, N, P, Q, R], S79.001-S79.199
with 7th [K, P], S82.001-S82.92X with 7th [K,
M, N, P, Q, R], S89.001-S89.399 with 7th [K, P],
S92.001-S92.919 with 7th [K, P]

✓5th **S72.8** **Other fracture of femur**

✓6th **S72.8X** **Other fracture of femur**

**CC Excl: For CC/MCC codes in subcategory
S72.8X, unless otherwise noted: MCC with 7th
A,B or C:** M48.40X-M48.58X with 7th A, M80.00X-
M84.68X with 7th A, S03.8XX-S03.9XX with 7th A,
S29.011-S29.019 with 7th A, S38.3XX-S39.013 with
7th A, S72.001-S72.92X with 7th [A, B, C], S73.101-
S73.199 with 7th A, S76.001-S76.019 with 7th A,
S76.091-S76.119 with 7th A, S76.191-S76.219 with
7th A, S76.291-S76.319 with 7th A, S76.391-
S76.819 with 7th A, S76.891-S76.919 with 7th A,
S76.991-S76.999 with 7th A, S79.001-S79.929 with
7th A, S82.90X-S82.92X with 7th [A, B, C], T14.90-
T14.91, T79.A0X-T79.9XX with 7th A
CC with 7th character K, M, N, P, Q or R:
M80.00X-M84.68X with 7th [K, P], S02.0XX-S02.92X
with 7th K, S12.000-S12.691 with 7th K, S22.000-
S22.9XX with 7th K, S32.000-S32.9XX with 7th K,
S42.001-S42.92X with 7th [K, P], S49.001-S49.199
with 7th [K, P], S52.001-S52.92X with 7th [K, M, N,
P, Q, R], S59.001-S59.299 with 7th [K, P], S62.001-
S62.92X with 7th [K, P], S72.001-S72.92X with 7th
[K, M, N, P, Q, R], S79.001-S79.199 with 7th [K, P],
S82.001-S82.92X with 7th [K, M, N, P, Q, R],
S89.001-S89.399 with 7th [K, P], S92.001-S92.919
with 7th [K, P]K

7,18 ✓7th **S72.8X1** **Other fracture of right femur** MCC CC
7,18 ✓7th **S72.8X2** **Other fracture of left femur** MCC CC
7,18 ✓7th **S72.8X9** **Other fracture of unspecified** MCC CC
femur

✓5th **S72.9** **Unspecified fracture of femur**
Fracture of thigh NOS
Fracture of upper leg NOS
EXCLUDES 1 fracture of hip NOS (S72.00-, S72.01-)

7,18 ✓x7th **S72.90** **Unspecified fracture of unspecified femur** MCC CC
AHA: 2012, 4Q, 93
CC Excl: See code: S72.8X

7,18 ✓x7th **S72.91** **Unspecified fracture of right femur** MCC CC
CC Excl: See code: S72.8X

7,18 ✓x7th **S72.92** **Unspecified fracture of left femur** MCC CC
CC Excl: See code: S72.8X

✓4th **S73** **Dislocation and sprain of joint and ligaments of hip**
INCLUDES avulsion of joint or ligament of hip
laceration of cartilage, joint or ligament of hip
sprain of cartilage, joint or ligament of hip
traumatic hemarthrosis of joint or ligament of hip
traumatic rupture of joint or ligament of hip
traumatic subluxation of joint or ligament of hip
traumatic tear of joint or ligament of hip
Code also any associated open wound
EXCLUDES 2 strain of muscle, fascia and tendon of hip and thigh (S76.-)

The appropriate 7th character is to be added to each code from
category S73.
A   initial encounter
D   subsequent encounter
S   sequela

✓5th **S73.0** **Subluxation and dislocation of hip**
EXCLUDES 2 dislocation and subluxation of hip prosthesis (T84.020,
T84.021)

✓6th **S73.00** **Unspecified subluxation and dislocation of hip**
Dislocation of hip NOS
Subluxation of hip NOS

7 ✓7th **S73.001** **Unspecified subluxation of right hip** CC
CC Excl: CC with 7th character A: M99.16-
M99.17, M99.19, S03.1XXA, S33.30X-S33.39X
with 7th A, S73.001A, S73.003-S73.004 with
7th A, S73.006A, S73.041A, S73.043-S73.044
with 7th A, S73.046A

7 ✓7th **S73.002** **Unspecified subluxation of left hip** CC
CC Excl: CC with 7th character A: M99.16-
M99.17, M99.19, S03.1XXA, S33.30X-S33.39X
with 7th A, S73.002-S73.003 with 7th A,
S73.005-S73.006 with 7th A, S73.042-
S73.043 with 7th A, S73.045-S73.046 with
7th A

7 ✓7th **S73.003** **Unspecified subluxation of**
unspecified hip CC
CC Excl: CC with 7th character A: M99.16-
M99.17, M99.19, S03.1XXA, S33.30X-S33.39X
with 7th A, S73.001-S73.006 with 7th A,
S73.041-S73.046 with 7th A

7 ✓7th **S73.004** **Unspecified dislocation of right hip** CC
CC Excl: See code: S73.001

7 ✓7th **S73.005** **Unspecified dislocation of left hip** CC
CC Excl: See code: S73.002

7 ✓7th **S73.006** **Unspecified dislocation of**
unspecified hip CC
CC Excl: See code: S73.003

✓6th **S73.01** **Posterior subluxation and dislocation of hip**

7 ✓7th **S73.011** **Posterior subluxation of right hip** CC
CC Excl: CC with 7th character A: M99.16-
M99.17, M99.19, S03.1XXA, S33.30X-S33.39X
with 7th A, S73.011 with 7th A, S73.013-
S73.014 with 7th A, S73.016 with 7th A

7 ✓7th **S73.012** **Posterior subluxation of left hip** CC
CC Excl: CC with 7th character A: M99.16-
M99.17, M99.19, S03.1XXA, S33.30X-S33.39X
with 7th A, S73.012-S73.013 with 7th A,
S73.015-S73.016 with 7th A

---

7 HAC = Initial encounter only (7th character A, B or C) and not POA.
16 MCC only if an open fracture (7th character B or C).
18 CC only if a subsequent encounter for nonunion or malunion (7th character K, M, N, P, Q, or R).
19 CC only if an initial encounter for a closed fracture (7th character A) **OR** a subsequent encounter for nonunion or malunion (7th character K, M, N, P, Q, or R – specific to category).

N Newborn: 0   P Pediatric: 0-17   M Maternity: 12-55   A Adult: 15-124   MCC Major CC Condition   PDxMCC PDx acts as own MCC   CC CC Condition   PDxCC PDx acts as own CC

7 √7ᵗʰ **S73.013** **Posterior subluxation of unspecified hip**   CC
CC Excl: CC with 7th character A:M99.16-M99.17, M99.19, S03.1XXA, S33.30X-S33.39X with 7th A, S73.011-S73.016 with 7th A

7 √7ᵗʰ **S73.014** **Posterior dislocation of right hip**   CC
CC Excl: See code: S73.011

7 √7ᵗʰ **S73.015** **Posterior dislocation of left hip**   CC
CC Excl: See code: S73.012

7 √7ᵗʰ **S73.016** **Posterior dislocation of unspecified hip**   CC
CC Excl: See code: S73.013

√6ᵗʰ **S73.02** Obturator subluxation and dislocation of hip

7 √7ᵗʰ **S73.021** **Obturator subluxation of right hip**   CC
CC Excl: CC with 7th character A: M99.16-M99.17, M99.19, S03.1XXA, S33.30X-S33.39X with 7th A, S73.021A, S73.023-S73.024 with 7th A, S73.026A

7 √7ᵗʰ **S73.022** **Obturator subluxation of left hip**   CC
CC Excl: CC with 7th character A: M99.16-M99.17, M99.19, S03.1XXA, S33.30X-S33.39X with 7th A, S73.022-S73.023 with 7th A, S73.025-S73.026 with 7th A

7 √7ᵗʰ **S73.023** **Obturator subluxation of unspecified hip**   CC
CC Excl: CC with 7th character A: M99.16-M99.17, M99.19, S03.1XXA, S33.30X-S33.39X with 7th A, S73.021-S73.026 with 7th A

7 √7ᵗʰ **S73.024** **Obturator dislocation of right hip**   CC
CC Excl:See code: S73.021

7 √7ᵗʰ **S73.025** **Obturator dislocation of left hip**   CC
CC Excl: See code: S73.022

7 √7ᵗʰ **S73.026** **Obturator dislocation of unspecified hip**   CC
CC Excl: See code: S73.023

√6ᵗʰ **S73.03** Other anterior dislocation of hip

7 √7ᵗʰ **S73.031** **Other anterior subluxation of right hip**   CC
CC Excl: CC with 7th character A: M99.16-M99.17, M99.19, S03.1XXA, S33.30X-S33.39X with 7th A, S73.031A, S73.033-S73.034 with 7th A, S73.036A

7 √7ᵗʰ **S73.032** **Other anterior subluxation of left hip**   CC
CC Excl: CC with 7th character AM99.16-M99.17, M99.19, S03.1XXA, S33.30X-S33.39X with 7th A, S73.032-S73.033 with 7th A, S73.035-S73.036 with 7th A

7 √7ᵗʰ **S73.033** **Other anterior subluxation of unspecified hip**   CC
CC Excl: CC with 7th character A: M99.16-M99.17, M99.19, S03.1XXA, S33.30X-S33.39X with 7th A, S73.031-S73.036 with 7th A

7 √7ᵗʰ **S73.034** **Other anterior dislocation of right hip**   CC
CC Excl:See code: S73.031

7 √7ᵗʰ **S73.035** **Other anterior dislocation of left hip**   CC
CC Excl: See code: S73.032

7 √7ᵗʰ **S73.036** **Other anterior dislocation of unspecified hip**   CC
CC Excl: See code: S73.033

√6ᵗʰ **S73.04** Central dislocation of hip

7 √7ᵗʰ **S73.041** **Central subluxation of right hip**   CC
CC Excl: See code: S73.001

7 √7ᵗʰ **S73.042** **Central subluxation of left hip**   CC
CC Excl: See code: S73.002

7 √7ᵗʰ **S73.043** **Central subluxation of unspecified hip**   CC
CC Excl: See code: S73.003

7 √7ᵗʰ **S73.044** **Central dislocation of right hip**   CC
CC Excl: See code: S73.001

7 √7ᵗʰ **S73.045** **Central dislocation of left hip**   CC
CC Excl: See code: S73.002

7 √7ᵗʰ **S73.046** **Central dislocation of unspecified hip**   CC
CC Excl: See code: S73.003

√5ᵗʰ **S73.1** Sprain of hip
AHA: 2014, 4Q, 25

√6ᵗʰ **S73.10** Unspecified sprain of hip

√7ᵗʰ **S73.101** Unspecified sprain of right hip

√7ᵗʰ **S73.102** Unspecified sprain of left hip

√7ᵗʰ **S73.109** Unspecified sprain of unspecified hip

√6ᵗʰ **S73.11** Iliofemoral ligament sprain of hip

√7ᵗʰ **S73.111** Iliofemoral ligament sprain of right hip

√7ᵗʰ **S73.112** Iliofemoral ligament sprain of left hip

√7ᵗʰ **S73.119** Iliofemoral ligament sprain of unspecified hip

√6ᵗʰ **S73.12** Ischiocapsular (ligament) sprain of hip

√7ᵗʰ **S73.121** Ischiocapsular ligament sprain of right hip

√7ᵗʰ **S73.122** Ischiocapsular ligament sprain of left hip

√7ᵗʰ **S73.129** Ischiocapsular ligament sprain of unspecified hip

√6ᵗʰ **S73.19** Other sprain of hip

√7ᵗʰ **S73.191** Other sprain of right hip

√7ᵗʰ **S73.192** Other sprain of left hip

√7ᵗʰ **S73.199** Other sprain of unspecified hip

√4ᵗʰ **S74** **Injury of nerves at hip and thigh level**
Code also any associated open wound (S71.-)
EXCLUDES 2   injury of nerves at ankle and foot level (S94.-)
injury of nerves at lower leg level (S84.-)

The appropriate 7th character is to be added to each code from category S74.
A   initial encounter
D   subsequent encounter
S   sequela

√5ᵗʰ **S74.0** **Injury of sciatic nerve at hip and thigh level**

√x7ᵗʰ **S74.00** Injury of sciatic nerve at hip and thigh level, unspecified leg

√x7ᵗʰ **S74.01** Injury of sciatic nerve at hip and thigh level, right leg

√x7ᵗʰ **S74.02** Injury of sciatic nerve at hip and thigh level, left leg

√5ᵗʰ **S74.1** **Injury of femoral nerve at hip and thigh level**

√x7ᵗʰ **S74.10** Injury of femoral nerve at hip and thigh level, unspecified leg

√x7ᵗʰ **S74.11** Injury of femoral nerve at hip and thigh level, right leg

√x7ᵗʰ **S74.12** Injury of femoral nerve at hip and thigh level, left leg

√5ᵗʰ **S74.2** **Injury of cutaneous sensory nerve at hip and thigh level**

√x7ᵗʰ **S74.20** Injury of cutaneous sensory nerve at hip and thigh level, unspecified leg

√x7ᵗʰ **S74.21** Injury of cutaneous sensory nerve at hip and high level, right leg

√x7ᵗʰ **S74.22** Injury of cutaneous sensory nerve at hip and thigh level, left leg

√5ᵗʰ **S74.8** **Injury of other nerves at hip and thigh level**

√6ᵗʰ **S74.8X** Injury of other nerves at hip and thigh level

√7ᵗʰ **S74.8X1** Injury of other nerves at hip and thigh level, right leg

√7ᵗʰ **S74.8X2** Injury of other nerves at hip and thigh level, left leg

√7ᵗʰ **S74.8X9** Injury of other nerves at hip and thigh level, unspecified leg

√5ᵗʰ **S74.9** **Injury of unspecified nerve at hip and thigh level**

√x7ᵗʰ **S74.90** Injury of unspecified nerve at hip and thigh level, unspecified leg

√x7ᵗʰ **S74.91** Injury of unspecified nerve at hip and thigh level, right leg

√x7ᵗʰ **S74.92** Injury of unspecified nerve at hip and thigh level, left leg

---

7   HAC = Initial encounter only (7th character A, B or C) and not POA.

✔ Additional Character Required   √x7ᵗʰ Placeholder Alert   Unacceptable PDx   Manifestation   Hospital Acquired Condition   *EXCLUDES 1* Not Coded Here   *EXCLUDES 2* Not Included Here

✓4ᵗʰ **S75** **Injury of blood vessels at hip and thigh level**

Code also any associated open wound (S71.-)

EXCLUDES 2   injury of blood vessels at lower leg level (S85.-)

injury of popliteal artery (S85.0)

The appropriate 7th character is to be added to each code from category S75.

A   initial encounter

D   subsequent encounter

S   sequela

✓5ᵗʰ **S75.0** **Injury of femoral artery**

✓6ᵗʰ   **S75.00**   **Unspecified injury of femoral artery**

✓7ᵗʰ   **S75.001**   **Unspecified injury of femoral artery, right leg** MCC

CC Excl: MCC with 7th A: S75.001A, S75.009-S75.011 with 7th A, S75.019-S75.021 with 7th A, S75.029-S75.091 with 7th A, S75.099 A, S75.801A, S75.809-S75.811 with 7th A, S75.819-S75.891 with 7th A, S75.899-S75.901 with 7th A, S75.909-S75.911 with 7th A, S75.919-S75.991 with 7th A, S75.999A, S85.201A, S85.209-S85.211 with 7th A, S85.219-S85.291 with 7th A, S85.299A, S85.801A, S85.809-S85.811 with 7th A, S85.819-S85.891 with 7th A, S85.899-S85.901 with 7th A, S85.909-S85.911 with 7th A, S85.919-S85.991 with 7th A, S85.999A, S95.001A, S95.009-S95.011 with 7th A, S95.019-S95.091 with 7th A, S95.099A, S95.201A, S95.209-S95.211 with 7th A, S95.219-S95.291 with 7th A, S95.299-S95.801 with 7th A, S95.809-S95.811 with 7th A, S95.819-S95.891 with 7th A, S95.899-S95.901 with 7th A, S95.909-S95.911 with 7th A, S95.919-S95.991 with 7th A, S95.999A

✓7ᵗʰ   **S75.002**   **Unspecified injury of femoral artery, left leg** MCC

CC Excl: MCC with 7th A: S75.002-S75.009 with 7th A, S75.012-S75.019 with 7th A, S75.022-S75.029 with 7th A, S75.092-S75.099 with 7th A, S75.802-S75.809 with 7th A, S75.812-S75.819 with 7th A, S75.892-S75.899 with 7th A, S75.902-S75.909 with 7th A, S75.912-S75.919 with 7th A, S75.992-S75.999 with 7th A, S85.202-S85.209 with 7th A, S85.212-S85.219 with 7th A, S85.292-S85.299 with 7th A, S85.802-S85.809 with 7th A, S85.812-S85.819 with 7th A, S85.892-S85.899 with 7th A, S85.902-S85.909 with 7th A, S85.912-S85.919 with 7th A, S85.992-S85.999 with 7th A, S95.002-S95.009 with 7th A, S95.012-S95.019 with 7th A, S95.092-S95.099 with 7th A, S95.202-S95.209 with 7th A, S95.212-S95.219 with 7th A, S95.292-S95.299 with 7th A, S95.802-S95.809 with 7th A, S95.812-S95.819 with 7th A, S95.892-S95.899 with 7th A, S95.902-S95.909 with 7th A, S95.912-S95.919 with 7th A, S95.992-S95.999 with 7th A

✓7ᵗʰ   **S75.009**   **Unspecified injury of femoral artery, unspecified leg** MCC

CC Excl: MCC with 7th A: S75.001-S75.099 with 7th A, S75.801-S75.999 with 7th A, S85.201-S85.299 with 7th A, S85.801-S85.999 with 7th A, S95.001-S95.099 with 7th A, S95.201-S95.999 with 7th A

✓6ᵗʰ   **S75.01**   **Minor laceration of femoral artery**

Incomplete transection of femoral artery

Laceration of femoral artery NOS

Superficial laceration of femoral artery

✓7ᵗʰ   **S75.011**   **Minor laceration of femoral artery, right leg** MCC

CC Excl: See code: S75.001

✓7ᵗʰ   **S75.012**   **Minor laceration of femoral artery, left leg** MCC

CC Excl: See code: S75.002

✓7ᵗʰ   **S75.019**   **Minor laceration of femoral artery, unspecified leg** MCC

CC Excl: See code: S75.009

✓6ᵗʰ   **S75.02**   **Major laceration of femoral artery**

Complete transection of femoral artery

Traumatic rupture of femoral artery

✓7ᵗʰ   **S75.021**   **Major laceration of femoral artery, right leg** MCC

CC Excl: See code: S75.001

✓7ᵗʰ   **S75.022**   **Major laceration of femoral artery, left leg** MCC

CC Excl: See code: S75.002

✓7ᵗʰ   **S75.029**   **Major laceration of femoral artery, unspecified leg** MCC

CC Excl: See code: S75.009

✓6ᵗʰ   **S75.09**   **Other specified injury of femoral artery**

✓7ᵗʰ   **S75.091**   **Other specified injury of femoral artery, right leg** MCC

CC Excl: See code: S75.001

✓7ᵗʰ   **S75.092**   **Other specified injury of femoral artery, left leg** MCC

CC Excl: See code: S75.002

✓7ᵗʰ   **S75.099**   **Other specified injury of femoral artery, unspecified leg** MCC

CC Excl: See code: S75.009

✓5ᵗʰ **S75.1** **Injury of femoral vein at hip and thigh level**

✓6ᵗʰ   **S75.10**   **Unspecified injury of femoral vein at hip and thigh level**

✓7ᵗʰ   **S75.101**   **Unspecified injury of femoral vein at hip and thigh level, right leg** MCC

CC Excl: MCC with 7th A: S75.101A, S75.109-S75.111 with 7th A, S75.119-S75.121 with 7th A, S75.129-S75.191 with 7th A, S75.199A, S75.801A, S75.809-S75.811 with 7th A, S75.819-S75.891 with 7th A, S75.899-S75.901 with 7th A, S75.909-S75.911 with 7th A, S75.919-S75.991 with 7th A, S75.999 with 7th A, S85.201A, S85.209-S85.211 with 7th A, S85.219-S85.291 with 7th A, S85.299A, S85.801A, S85.809-S85.811 with 7th A, S85.819-S85.891 with 7th A, S85.899-S85.901 with 7th A, S85.909-S85.911 with 7th A, S85.919-S85.991 with 7th A, S85.999A, S95.001A, S95.009-S95.011 with 7th A, S95.019-S95.091 with 7th A, S95.099A, S95.201A, S95.209-S95.211 with 7th A, S95.219-S95.291 with 7th A, S95.299-S95.801 with 7th A, S95.809-S95.811 with 7th A, S95.819-S95.891 with 7th A, S95.899-S95.901 with 7th A, S95.909-S95.911 with 7th A, S95.919-S95.991 with 7th A, S95.999A

✓7ᵗʰ   **S75.102**   **Unspecified injury of femoral vein at hip and thigh level, left leg** MCC

CC Excl: MCC with 7th A: S75.102-S75.109 with 7th A, S75.112-S75.119 with 7th A, S75.122-S75.129 with 7th A, S75.192-S75.199 with 7th A, S75.802-S75.809 with 7th A, S75.812-S75.819 with 7th A, S75.892-S75.899 with 7th A, S75.902-S75.909 with 7th A, S75.912-S75.919 with 7th A, S75.992-S75.999 with 7th A, S85.202-S85.209 with 7th A, S85.212-S85.219 with 7th A, S85.292-S85.299 with 7th A, S85.802-S85.809 with 7th A, S85.812-S85.819 with 7th A, S85.892-S85.899 with 7th A, S85.902-S85.909 with 7th A, S85.912-S85.919 with 7th A, S85.992-S85.999 with 7th A, S95.002-S95.009 with 7th A, S95.012-S95.019 with 7th A, S95.092-S95.099 with 7th A, S95.202-S95.209 with 7th A, S95.212-S95.219 with 7th A, S95.292-S95.299 with 7th A, S95.802-S95.809 with 7th A, S95.812-S95.819 with 7th A, S95.892-S95.899 with 7th A, S95.902-S95.909 with 7th A, S95.912-S95.919 with 7th A, S95.992-S95.999 with 7th A

✓7ᵗʰ   **S75.109**   **Unspecified injury of femoral vein at hip and thigh level, unspecified leg** MCC

CC Excl: MCC with 7th A: S75.101-S75.199 with 7th A, S75.801-S75.999 with 7th A, S85.201-S85.299 with 7th A, S85.801-S85.999 with 7th A, S95.001-S95.099 with 7th A, S95.201-S95.999 with 7th A

✓6ᵗʰ   **S75.11**   **Minor laceration of femoral vein at hip and thigh level**

Incomplete transection of femoral vein at hip and thigh level

Laceration of femoral vein at hip and thigh level NOS

Superficial laceration of femoral vein at hip and thigh level

✓7ᵗʰ   **S75.111**   **Minor laceration of femoral vein at hip and thigh level, right leg** MCC

CC Excl: See code: S75.101

N Newborn: 0   P Pediatric: 0-17   M Maternity: 12-55   A Adult: 15-124   MCC Major CC Condition   PDxMCC PDx acts as own MCC   CC CC Condition   PDxCC PDx acts as own CC

1026

ICD-10-CM 2016

S75-S75.111

√7ᵗʰ **S75.112** **Minor laceration of femoral vein at**   MCC
hip and thigh level, left leg
CC Excl: See code: S75.102

√7ᵗʰ **S75.119** **Minor laceration of femoral vein at**   MCC
hip and thigh level, unspecified leg
CC Excl: See code: S75.109

√6ᵗʰ **S75.12** **Major laceration of femoral vein at hip and thigh**
level
Complete transection of femoral vein at hip and thigh
level
Traumatic rupture of femoral vein at hip and thigh
level

√7ᵗʰ **S75.121** **Major laceration of femoral vein at**   MCC
hip and thigh level, right leg
CC Excl: See code: S75.101

√7ᵗʰ **S75.122** **Major laceration of femoral vein at**   MCC
hip and thigh level, left leg
CC Excl: See code: S75.102

√7ᵗʰ **S75.129** **Major laceration of femoral vein at**   MCC
hip and thigh level, unspecified leg
CC Excl: See code: S75.109

√6ᵗʰ **S75.19** **Other specified injury of femoral vein at hip and**
thigh level

√7ᵗʰ **S75.191** **Other specified injury of femoral vein**   MCC
at hip and thigh level, right leg
CC Excl: See code: S75.101

√7ᵗʰ **S75.192** **Other specified injury of femoral vein**   MCC
at hip and thigh level, left leg
CC Excl: See code: S75.102

√7ᵗʰ **S75.199** **Other specified injury of femoral vein**   MCC
at hip and thigh level, unspecified leg
CC Excl: See code: S75.109

√5ᵗʰ **S75.2** **Injury of greater saphenous vein at hip and thigh level**
EXCLUDES 1   greater saphenous vein NOS (S85.3)

√6ᵗʰ **S75.20** **Unspecified injury of greater saphenous vein at hip**
and thigh level

√7ᵗʰ **S75.201** **Unspecified injury of greater**   CC
saphenous vein at hip and thigh
level, right leg
CC Excl: CC with 7th character A: S75.201A,
S75.209-S75.211 with 7th A, S75.219-
S75.221 with 7th A, S75.229-S75.291 with
7th A, S75.299-S75.801 with 7th A, S75.809-
S75.811 with 7th A, S75.819-S75.891 with
7th A, S75.899-S75.901 with 7th A, S75.909-
S75.911 with 7th A, S75.919-S75.991 with
7th A, S75.999A, S85.201A, S85.209-S85.211
with 7th A, S85.219-S85.291 with 7th A,
S85.299-S85.301 with 7th A, S85.309-
S85.311 with 7th A, S85.319-S85.391 with
7th A, S85.399-S85.401 with 7th A, S85.409-
S85.411 with 7th A, S85.419-S85.491 with
7th A, S85.499A, S85.801A, S85.809-S85.811
with 7th A, S85.819-S85.891 with 7th A,
S85.899-S85.901 with 7th A, S85.909-
S85.911 with 7th A, S85.919-S85.991 with
7th A, S85.999A, S95.001A, S95.009-S95.011
with 7th A, S95.019-S95.091 with 7th A,
S95.099A, S95.201A, S95.209-S95.211 with
7th A, S95.219-S95.291 with 7th A, S95.299-
S95.801 with 7th A, S95.809-S95.811 with
7th A, S95.819-S95.891 with 7th A, S95.899-
S95.901 with 7th A, S95.909-S95.911 with
7th A, S95.919-S95.991 with 7th A, S95.999A

√7ᵗʰ **S75.202** **Unspecified injury of greater**   CC
saphenous vein at hip and thigh level,
left leg
CC Excl: CC with 7th character A: S75.202-
S75.209 with 7th A, S75.212-S75.219 with
7th A, S75.222-S75.229 with 7th A, S75.292-
S75.299 with 7th A, S75.802-S75.809 with
7th A, S75.812-S75.819 with 7th A, S75.892-
S75.899 with 7th A, S75.902-S75.909 with
7th A, S75.912-S75.919 with 7th A, S75.992-
S75.999 with 7th A, S85.202-S85.209 with
7th A, S85.212-S85.219 with 7th A, S85.292-
S85.299 with 7th A, S85.302-S85.309 with
7th A, S85.312-S85.319 with 7th A, S85.392-
S85.399 with 7th A, S85.402-S85.409 with
7th A, S85.412-S85.419 with 7th A, S85.492-
S85.499 with 7th A, S85.802-S85.809 with
7th A, S85.812-S85.819 with 7th A, S85.892-
S85.899 with 7th A, S85.902-S85.909 with
7th A, S85.912-S85.919 with 7th A, S85.992-
S85.999 with 7th A, S95.002-S95.009 with
7th A, S95.012-S95.019 with 7th A, S95.092-

S95.099 with 7th A, S95.202-S95.209 with
7th A, S95.212-S95.219 with 7th A, S95.292-
S95.299 with 7th A, S95.802-S95.809 with
7th A, S95.812-S95.819 with 7th A, S95.892-
S95.899 with 7th A, S95.902-S95.909 with
7th A, S95.912-S95.919 with 7th A, S95.992-
S95.999 with 7th A

√7ᵗʰ **S75.209** **Unspecified injury of greater**   CC
saphenous vein at hip and thigh
level, unspecified leg
CC Excl: CC with 7th character A: S75.201-
S75.999 with 7th A, S85.201-S85.499 with
7th A, S85.801-S85.999 with 7th A, S95.001-
S95.099 with 7th A, S95.201-S95.999 with
7th A

√6ᵗʰ **S75.21** **Minor laceration of greater saphenous vein at hip**
and thigh level
Incomplete transection of greater saphenous vein at
hip and thigh level
Laceration of greater saphenous vein at hip and thigh
level NOS
Superficial laceration of greater saphenous vein at hip
and thigh level

√7ᵗʰ **S75.211** **Minor laceration of greater saphenous**   CC
vein at hip and thigh level, right leg
CC Excl: See code: S75.201

√7ᵗʰ **S75.212** **Minor laceration of greater saphenous**   CC
vein at hip and thigh level, left leg
CC Excl: See code: S75.202

√7ᵗʰ **S75.219** **Minor laceration of greater saphenous**   CC
vein at hip and thigh level,
unspecified leg
CC Excl: See code: S75.209

√6ᵗʰ **S75.22** **Major laceration of greater saphenous vein at hip**
and thigh level
Complete transection of greater saphenous vein at hip
and thigh level
Traumatic rupture of greater saphenous vein at hip
and thigh level

√7ᵗʰ **S75.221** **Major laceration of greater saphenous**   CC
vein at hip and thigh level, right leg
CC Excl: See code: S75.201

√7ᵗʰ **S75.222** **Major laceration of greater saphenous**   CC
vein at hip and thigh level, left leg
CC Excl: See code: S75.202

√7ᵗʰ **S75.229** **Major laceration of greater saphenous**   CC
vein at hip and thigh level,
unspecified leg
CC Excl: See code: S75.209

√6ᵗʰ **S75.29** **Other specified injury of greater saphenous vein at**
hip and thigh level

√7ᵗʰ **S75.291** **Other specified injury of greater**   CC
saphenous vein at hip and thigh
level, right leg
CC Excl: See code: S75.201

√7ᵗʰ **S75.292** **Other specified injury of greater**   CC
saphenous vein at hip and thigh
level, left leg
CC Excl: See code: S75.202

√7ᵗʰ **S75.299** **Other specified injury of greater**   CC
saphenous vein at hip and thigh level,
unspecified leg
CC Excl: See code: S75.209

√5ᵗʰ **S75.8** **Injury of other blood vessels at hip and thigh level**

√6ᵗʰ **S75.80** **Unspecified injury of other blood vessels at hip and**
thigh level

√7ᵗʰ **S75.801** **Unspecified injury of other blood**   CC
vessels at hip and thigh level, right leg
CC Excl: CC with 7th character A: M79.A21-
M79.A29, S75.001 with 7th A, S75.009-
S75.011 with 7th A, S75.019-S75.021 with
7th A, S75.029-S75.091 with 7th A, S75.099-
S75.101 with 7th A, S75.109-S75.111 with
7th A, S75.119-S75.121 with 7th A, S75.129-
S75.191 with 7th A, S75.199-S75.201 with
7th A, S75.209-S75.211 with 7th A, S75.219-
S75.221 with 7th A, S75.229-S75.291 with
7th A, S75.299-S75.801 with 7th A, S75.809-
S75.811 with 7th A, S75.819-S75.891 with
7th A, S75.899-S75.901 with 7th A, S75.909-
S75.911 with 7th A, S75.919-S75.991 with
7th A, S75.999A, S85.001A, S85.009-S85.011
with 7th A, S85.019-S85.091 with 7th A,
S85.099-S85.101 with 7th A, S85.109-

√ Additional Character Required   √x7ᵗʰ Placeholder Alert   Unacceptable PDx   Manifestation   Hospital Acquired Condition   **EXCLUDES 1** Not Coded Here   **EXCLUDES 2** Not Included Here

ICD-10-CM 2016   1027

Chapter 19. Injury, Poisoning, and Certain Other Consequences of External Causes

S85.111 with 7th A, S85.119-S85.121 with 7th A, S85.129-S85.131 with 7th A, S85.139-S85.141 with 7th A, S85.149-S85.151 with 7th A, S85.159-S85.161 with 7th A, S85.169-S85.171 with 7th A, S85.179-S85.181 with 7th A, S85.189-S85.201 with 7th A, S85.209-S85.211 with 7th A, S85.219-S85.291 with 7th A, S85.299-S85.301 with 7th A, S85.309-S85.311 with 7th A, S85.319-S85.391 with 7th A, S85.399-S85.401 with 7th A, S85.409-S85.411 with 7th A, S85.419-S85.491 with 7th A, S85.499-S85.501 with 7th A, S85.509-S85.511 with 7th A, S85.519-S85.591 with 7th A, S85.599-S85.801 with 7th A, S85.809-S85.811 with 7th A, S85.819-S85.891 with 7th A, S85.899-S85.901 with 7th A, S85.909-S85.911 with 7th A, S85.919-S85.991 with 7th A, S85.999A, S95.001A, S95.009-S95.011 with 7th A, S95.019-S95.091 with 7th A, S95.099-S95.101 with 7th A, S95.109-S95.111 with 7th A, S95.119-S95.191 with 7th A, S95.199-S95.201 with 7th A, S95.209-S95.211 with 7th A, S95.219-S95.291 with 7th A, S95.299-S95.801 with 7th A, S95.809-S95.811 with 7th A, S95.819-S95.891 with 7th A, S95.899-S95.901 with 7th A, S95.909-S95.911 with 7th A, S95.919-S95.991 with 7th A, S95.999A

✓7th **S75.802**   **Unspecified injury of other blood vessels at hip and thigh level, left leg**   CC
CC Excl: CC with 7th character A: M79.A21-M79.A29, S75.002-S75.009 with 7th A, S75.012-S75.019 with 7th A, S75.022-S75.029 with 7th A, S75.092-S75.099 with 7th A, S75.102-S75.109 with 7th A, S75.112-S75.119 with 7th A, S75.122-S75.129 with 7th A, S75.192-S75.199 with 7th A, S75.202-S75.209 with 7th A, S75.212-S75.219 with 7th A, S75.222-S75.229 with 7th A, S75.292-S75.299 with 7th A, S75.802-S75.809 with 7th A, S75.812-S75.819 with 7th A, S75.892-S75.899 with 7th A, S75.902-S75.909 with 7th A, S75.912-S75.919 with 7th A, S75.992-S75.999 with 7th A, S85.002-S85.009 with 7th A, S85.012-S85.019 with 7th A, S85.092-S85.099 with 7th A, S85.102-S85.109 with 7th A, S85.112-S85.119 with 7th A, S85.122-S85.129 with 7th A, S85.132-S85.139 with 7th A, S85.142-S85.149 with 7th A, S85.152-S85.159 with 7th A, S85.162-S85.169 with 7th A, S85.172-S85.179 with 7th A, S85.182-S85.189 with 7th A, S85.202-S85.209 with 7th A, S85.212-S85.219 with 7th A, S85.292-S85.299 with 7th A, S85.302-S85.309 with 7th A, S85.312-S85.319 with 7th A, S85.392-S85.399 with 7th A, S85.402-S85.409 with 7th A, S85.412-S85.419 with 7th A, S85.492-S85.499 with 7th A, S85.502-S85.509 with 7th A, S85.512-S85.519 with 7th A, S85.592-S85.599 with 7th A, S85.802-S85.809 with 7th A, S85.812-S85.819 with 7th A, S85.892-S85.899 with 7th A, S85.902-S85.909 with 7th A, S85.912-S85.919 with 7th A, S85.992-S85.999 with 7th A, S95.002-S95.009 with 7th A, S95.012-S95.019 with 7th A, S95.092-S95.099 with 7th A, S95.102-S95.109 with 7th A, S95.112-S95.119 with 7th A, S95.192-S95.199 with 7th A, S95.202-S95.209 with 7th A, S95.212-S95.219 with 7th A, S95.292-S95.299 with 7th A, S95.802-S95.809 with 7th A, S95.812-S95.819 with 7th A, S95.892-S95.899 with 7th A, S95.902-S95.909 with 7th A, S95.912-S95.919 with 7th A, S95.992-S95.999 with 7th A

✓7th **S75.809**   **Unspecified injury of other blood vessels at hip and thigh level, unspecified leg**   CC
CC Excl: CC with 7th character A: M79.A21-M79.A29, S75.001-S75.999 with 7th A, S85.001-S85.999 with 7th A, S95.001-S95.999 with 7th A

✓6th **S75.81**   **Laceration of other blood vessels at hip and thigh level**

✓7th **S75.811**   **Laceration of other blood vessels at hip and thigh level, right leg**   CC
CC Excl: See code: S75.801

✓7th **S75.812**   **Laceration of other blood vessels at hip and thigh level, left leg**   CC
CC Excl: See code: S75.802

✓7th **S75.819**   **Laceration of other blood vessels at hip and thigh level, unspecified leg**   CC
CC Excl: See code: S75.809

✓6th **S75.89**   **Other specified injury of other blood vessels at hip and thigh level**

✓7th **S75.891**   **Other specified injury of other blood vessels at hip and thigh level, right leg**   CC
CC Excl: See code: S75.801

✓7th **S75.892**   **Other specified injury of other blood vessels at hip and thigh level, left leg**   CC
CC Excl: See code: S75.802

✓7th **S75.899**   **Other specified injury of other blood vessels at hip and thigh level, unspecified leg**   CC
CC Excl: See code: S75.809

✓5th **S75.9**   **Injury of unspecified blood vessel at hip and thigh level**

✓6th **S75.90**   **Unspecified injury of unspecified blood vessel at hip and thigh level**

✓7th **S75.901**   **Unspecified injury of unspecified blood vessel at hip and thigh level, right leg**   CC
CC Excl: See code: S75.801

✓7th **S75.902**   **Unspecified injury of unspecified blood vessel at hip and thigh level, left leg**   CC
CC Excl: See code: S75.802

✓7th **S75.909**   **Unspecified injury of unspecified blood vessel at hip and thigh level, unspecified leg**   CC
CC Excl: See code: S75.809

✓6th **S75.91**   **Laceration of unspecified blood vessel at hip and thigh level**

✓7th **S75.911**   **Laceration of unspecified blood vessel at hip and thigh level, right leg**   CC
CC Excl: See code: S75.801

✓7th **S75.912**   **Laceration of unspecified blood vessel at hip and thigh level, left leg**   CC
CC Excl: See code: S75.802

✓7th **S75.919**   **Laceration of unspecified blood vessel at hip and thigh level, unspecified leg**   CC
CC Excl: See code: S75.809

✓6th **S75.99**   **Other specified injury of unspecified blood vessel at hip and thigh level**

✓7th **S75.991**   **Other specified injury of unspecified blood vessel at hip and thigh level, right leg**   CC
CC Excl: See code: S75.801

✓7th **S75.992**   **Other specified injury of unspecified blood vessel at hip and thigh level, left leg**   CC
CC Excl: See code: S75.802

✓7th **S75.999**   **Other specified injury of unspecified blood vessel at hip and thigh level, unspecified leg**   CC
CC Excl: See code: S75.809

✦ ✓4th **S76 Injury of muscle, fascia and tendon at hip and thigh level**
Code also any associated open wound (S71.-)
EXCLUDES 2   injury of muscle, fascia and tendon at lower leg level (S86)
sprain of joint and ligament of hip (S73.1)

The appropriate 7th character is to be added to each code from category S76.
A   initial encounter
D   subsequent encounter
S   sequela

✓5th **S76.0**   **Injury of muscle, fascia and tendon of hip**

✓6th **S76.00**   **Unspecified injury of muscle, fascia and tendon of hip**

✓7th **S76.001**   **Unspecified injury of muscle, fascia and tendon of right hip**

✓7th **S76.002**   **Unspecified injury of muscle, fascia and tendon of left hip**

✓7th **S76.009**   **Unspecified injury of muscle, fascia and tendon of unspecified hip**

✓6th **S76.01**   **Strain of muscle, fascia and tendon of hip**

✓7th **S76.011**   **Strain of muscle, fascia and tendon of right hip**

✓7th **S76.012**   **Strain of muscle, fascia and tendon of left hip**

✦ Refer to the Muscle/Tendon Table at beginning of this chapter.

N Newborn: 0   P Pediatric: 0-17   M Maternity: 12-55   A Adult: 15-124   MCC Major CC Condition   PDxMCC PDx acts as own MCC   CC CC Condition   PDxCC PDx acts as own CC

√7ᵗʰ **S76.019   Strain of muscle, fascia and tendon of unspecified hip**

√6ᵗʰ **S76.02   Laceration of muscle, fascia and tendon of hip**

√7ᵗʰ **S76.021   Laceration of muscle, fascia and tendon of right hip** CC
CC Excl: CC with 7th character A: S71.001A, S71.009-S71.011 with 7th A, S71.019-S71.021 with 7th A, S71.029-S71.031 with 7th A, S71.039-S71.041 with 7th A, S71.049-S71.051 with 7th A, S71.059-S71.101 with 7th A, S71.109-S71.111 with 7th A, S71.119-S71.121 with 7th A, S71.129-S71.131 with 7th A, S71.139-S71.141 with 7th A, S71.149-S71.151 with 7th A, S71.159 with 7th A, S76.021 with 7th A, S76.029A, S76.121A, S76.129A, S76.221A, S76.229A, S76.321A, S76.329A, S76.821A, S76.829A, S76.921A, S76.929A

√7ᵗʰ **S76.022   Laceration of muscle, fascia and tendon of left hip** CC
CC Excl: CC with 7th character A: S71.002-S71.009 with 7th A, S71.012-S71.019 with 7th A, S71.022-S71.029 with 7th A, S71.032-S71.039 with 7th A, S71.042-S71.049 with 7th A, S71.052-S71.059 with 7th A, S71.102-S71.109 with 7th A, S71.112-S71.119 with 7th A, S71.122-S71.129 with 7th A, S71.132-S71.139 with 7th A, S71.142-S71.149 with 7th A, S71.152-S71.159 with 7th A, S76.022-S76.029 with 7th A, S76.122-S76.129 with 7th A, S76.222-S76.229 with 7th A, S76.322-S76.329 with 7th A, S76.822-S76.829 with 7th A, S76.922-S76.929 with 7th A

√7ᵗʰ **S76.029   Laceration of muscle, fascia and tendon of unspecified hip** CC
CC Excl: CC with 7th character A: S71.001-S71.159 with 7th A, S76.021-S76.029 with 7th A, S76.121-S76.129 with 7th A, S76.221-S76.229 with 7th A, S76.321-S76.329 with 7th A, S76.821-S76.829 with 7th A, S76.921-S76.929 with 7th A

√6ᵗʰ **S76.09   Other specified injury of muscle, fascia and tendon of hip**

√7ᵗʰ **S76.091   Other specified injury of muscle, fascia and tendon of right hip**

√7ᵗʰ **S76.092   Other specified injury of muscle, fascia and tendon of left hip**

√7ᵗʰ **S76.099   Other specified injury of muscle, fascia and tendon of unspecified hip**

√5ᵗʰ **S76.1   Injury of quadriceps muscle, fascia and tendon**
Injury of patellar ligament (tendon)

√6ᵗʰ **S76.10   Unspecified injury of quadriceps muscle, fascia and tendon**

√7ᵗʰ **S76.101   Unspecified injury of right quadriceps muscle, fascia and tendon**

√7ᵗʰ **S76.102   Unspecified injury of left quadriceps muscle, fascia and tendon**

√7ᵗʰ **S76.109   Unspecified injury of unspecified quadriceps muscle, fascia and tendon**

√6ᵗʰ **S76.11   Strain of quadriceps muscle, fascia and tendon**

√7ᵗʰ **S76.111   Strain of right quadriceps muscle, fascia and tendon**

√7ᵗʰ **S76.112   Strain of left quadriceps muscle, fascia and tendon**

√7ᵗʰ **S76.119   Strain of unspecified quadriceps muscle, fascia and tendon**

√6ᵗʰ **S76.12   Laceration of quadriceps muscle, fascia and tendon**

√7ᵗʰ **S76.121   Laceration of right quadriceps muscle, fascia and tendon** CC
CC Excl: See code: S76.021

√7ᵗʰ **S76.122   Laceration of left quadriceps muscle, fascia and tendon** CC
CC Excl: See code: S76.022

√7ᵗʰ **S76.129   Laceration of unspecified quadriceps muscle, fascia and tendon** CC
CC Excl: See code: S76.029

√6ᵗʰ **S76.19   Other specified injury of quadriceps muscle, fascia and tendon**

√7ᵗʰ **S76.191   Other specified injury of right quadriceps muscle, fascia and tendon**

√7ᵗʰ **S76.192   Other specified injury of left quadriceps muscle, fascia and tendon**

√7ᵗʰ **S76.199   Other specified injury of unspecified quadriceps muscle, fascia and tendon**

√5ᵗʰ **S76.2   Injury of adductor muscle, fascia and tendon of thigh**

√6ᵗʰ **S76.20   Unspecified injury of adductor muscle, fascia and tendon of thigh**

√7ᵗʰ **S76.201   Unspecified injury of adductor muscle, fascia and tendon of right thigh**

√7ᵗʰ **S76.202   Unspecified injury of adductor muscle, fascia and tendon of left thigh**

√7ᵗʰ **S76.209   Unspecified injury of adductor muscle, fascia and tendon of unspecified thigh**

√6ᵗʰ **S76.21   Strain of adductor muscle, fascia and tendon of thigh**

√7ᵗʰ **S76.211   Strain of adductor muscle, fascia and tendon of right thigh**

√7ᵗʰ **S76.212   Strain of adductor muscle, fascia and tendon of left thigh**

√7ᵗʰ **S76.219   Strain of adductor muscle, fascia and tendon of unspecified thigh**

√6ᵗʰ **S76.22   Laceration of adductor muscle, fascia and tendon of thigh**

√7ᵗʰ **S76.221   Laceration of adductor muscle, fascia and tendon of right thigh** CC
CC Excl: See code: S76.021

√7ᵗʰ **S76.222   Laceration of adductor muscle, fascia and tendon of left thigh** CC
CC Excl: See code: S76.022

√7ᵗʰ **S76.229   Laceration of adductor muscle, fascia and tendon of unspecified thigh** CC
CC Excl: See code: S76.029

√6ᵗʰ **S76.29   Other injury of adductor muscle, fascia and tendon of thigh**

√7ᵗʰ **S76.291   Other injury of adductor muscle, fascia and tendon of right thigh**

√7ᵗʰ **S76.292   Other injury of adductor muscle, fascia and tendon of left thigh**

√7ᵗʰ **S76.299   Other injury of adductor muscle, fascia and tendon of unspecified thigh**

√5ᵗʰ **S76.3   Injury of muscle, fascia and tendon of the posterior muscle group at thigh level**

√6ᵗʰ **S76.30   Unspecified injury of muscle, fascia and tendon of the posterior muscle group at thigh level**

√7ᵗʰ **S76.301   Unspecified injury of muscle, fascia and tendon of the posterior muscle group at thigh level, right thigh**

√7ᵗʰ **S76.302   Unspecified injury of muscle, fascia and tendon of the posterior muscle group at thigh level, left thigh**

√7ᵗʰ **S76.309   Unspecified injury of muscle, fascia and tendon of the posterior muscle group at thigh level, unspecified thigh**

√6ᵗʰ **S76.31   Strain of muscle, fascia and tendon of the posterior muscle group at thigh level**

√7ᵗʰ **S76.311   Strain of muscle, fascia and tendon of the posterior muscle group at thigh level, right thigh**

√7ᵗʰ **S76.312   Strain of muscle, fascia and tendon of the posterior muscle group at thigh level, left thigh**

√7ᵗʰ **S76.319   Strain of muscle, fascia and tendon of the posterior muscle group at thigh level, unspecified thigh**

√6ᵗʰ **S76.32   Laceration of muscle, fascia and tendon of the posterior muscle group at thigh level**

√7ᵗʰ **S76.321   Laceration of muscle, fascia and tendon of the posterior muscle group at thigh level, right thigh** CC
CC Excl: See code: S76.021

√7ᵗʰ **S76.322   Laceration of muscle, fascia and tendon of the posterior muscle group at thigh level, left thigh** CC
CC Excl: See code: S76.022

✓7th **S76.329** Laceration of muscle, fascia and tendon of the posterior muscle group at thigh level, unspecified thigh   CC
> CC Excl: See code: S76.029

✓6th **S76.39** Other specified injury of muscle, fascia and tendon of the posterior muscle group at thigh level

     ✓7th **S76.391** Other specified injury of muscle, fascia and tendon of the posterior muscle group at thigh level, right thigh

     ✓7th **S76.392** Other specified injury of muscle, fascia and tendon of the posterior muscle group at thigh level, left thigh

     ✓7th **S76.399** Other specified injury of muscle, fascia and tendon of the posterior muscle group at thigh level, unspecified thigh

✓5th **S76.8** Injury of other specified muscles, fascia and tendons at thigh level

     ✓6th **S76.80** Unspecified injury of other specified muscles, fascia and tendons at thigh level

       ✓7th **S76.801** Unspecified injury of other specified muscles, fascia and tendons at thigh level, right thigh

       ✓7th **S76.802** Unspecified injury of other specified muscles, fascia and tendons at thigh level, left thigh

       ✓7th **S76.809** Unspecified injury of other specified muscles, fascia and tendons at thigh level, unspecified thigh

     ✓6th **S76.81** Strain of other specified muscles, fascia and tendons at thigh level

       ✓7th **S76.811** Strain of other specified muscles, fascia and tendons at thigh level, right thigh

       ✓7th **S76.812** Strain of other specified muscles, fascia and tendons at thigh level, left thigh

       ✓7th **S76.819** Strain of other specified muscles, fascia and tendons at thigh level, unspecified thigh

     ✓6th **S76.82** Laceration of other specified muscles, fascia and tendons at thigh level

       ✓7th **S76.821** Laceration of other specified muscles, fascia and tendons at thigh level, right thigh   CC
> CC Excl: See code: S76.021

       ✓7th **S76.822** Laceration of other specified muscles, fascia and tendons at thigh level, left thigh   CC
> CC Excl: See code: S76.022

       ✓7th **S76.829** Laceration of other specified muscles, fascia and tendons at thigh level, unspecified thigh   CC
> CC Excl: See code: S76.029

     ✓6th **S76.89** Other injury of other specified muscles, fascia and tendons at thigh level

       ✓7th **S76.891** Other injury of other specified muscles, fascia and tendons at thigh level, right thigh

       ✓7th **S76.892** Other injury of other specified muscles, fascia and tendons at thigh level, left thigh

       ✓7th **S76.899** Other injury of other specified muscles, fascia and tendons at thigh level, unspecified thigh

✓5th **S76.9** Injury of unspecified muscles, fascia and tendons at thigh level

     ✓6th **S76.90** Unspecified injury of unspecified muscles, fascia and tendons at thigh level

       ✓7th **S76.901** Unspecified injury of unspecified muscles, fascia and tendons at thigh level, right thigh

       ✓7th **S76.902** Unspecified injury of unspecified muscles, fascia and tendons at thigh level, left thigh

       ✓7th **S76.909** Unspecified injury of unspecified muscles, fascia and tendons at thigh level, unspecified thigh

✓6th **S76.91** Strain of unspecified muscles, fascia and tendons at thigh level

     ✓7th **S76.911** Strain of unspecified muscles, fascia and tendons at thigh level, right thigh

     ✓7th **S76.912** Strain of unspecified muscles, fascia and tendons at thigh level, left thigh

     ✓7th **S76.919** Strain of unspecified muscles, fascia and tendons at thigh level, unspecified thigh

✓6th **S76.92** Laceration of unspecified muscles, fascia and tendons at thigh level

     ✓7th **S76.921** Laceration of unspecified muscles, fascia and tendons at thigh level, right thigh   CC
> CC Excl: See code: S76.021

     ✓7th **S76.922** Laceration of unspecified muscles, fascia and tendons at thigh level, left thigh   CC
> CC Excl: See code: S76.022

     ✓7th **S76.929** Laceration of unspecified muscles, fascia and tendons at thigh level, unspecified thigh   CC
> CC Excl: See code: S76.029

✓6th **S76.99** Other specified injury of unspecified muscles, fascia and tendons at thigh level

     ✓7th **S76.991** Other specified injury of unspecified muscles, fascia and tendons at thigh level, right thigh

     ✓7th **S76.992** Other specified injury of unspecified muscles, fascia and tendons at thigh level, left thigh

     ✓7th **S76.999** Other specified injury of unspecified muscles, fascia and tendons at thigh level, unspecified thigh

✓4th **S77** **Crushing injury of hip and thigh**
Use additional code(s) for all associated injuries
EXCLUDES 2   crushing injury of ankle and foot (S97.-)
          crushing injury of lower leg (S87.-)

> The appropriate 7th character is to be added to each code from category S77.
> A   initial encounter
> D   subsequent encounter
> S   sequela

✓5th **S77.0** Crushing injury of hip

> CC Excl: For CC codes in subcategory S77.0, unless otherwise noted: CC with 7th character A: S77.00X-S77.02X with 7th A, S77.20X-S77.22X with 7th A

7 ✓x7th **S77.00** Crushing injury of unspecified hip   CC
7 ✓x7th **S77.01** Crushing injury of right hip   CC
7 ✓x7th **S77.02** Crushing injury of left hip   CC

✓5th **S77.1** Crushing injury of thigh

> CC Excl: For CC codes in subcategory S77.1, unless otherwise noted: CC with 7th character A: S77.00X-S77.02X with 7th A, S77.20X-S77.22X with 7th A

7 ✓x7th **S77.10** Crushing injury of unspecified thigh   CC
7 ✓x7th **S77.11** Crushing injury of right thigh   CC
7 ✓x7th **S77.12** Crushing injury of left thigh   CC

✓5th **S77.2** Crushing injury of hip with thigh

   ✓x7th **S77.20** Crushing injury of unspecified hip with thigh
   ✓x7th **S77.21** Crushing injury of right hip with thigh
   ✓x7th **S77.22** Crushing injury of left hip with thigh

---

7   HAC = Initial encounter only (7th character A, B or C) and not POA.

N Newborn: 0   P Pediatric: 0-17   M Maternity: 12-55   A Adult: 15-124   MCC Major CC Condition   PDxMCC PDx acts as own MCC   CC CC Condition   PDxCC PDx acts as own CC

1030   ICD-10-CM 2016

✓4ᵗʰ S78   Traumatic amputation of hip and thigh

> **NOTE**   An amputation not identified as partial or complete should be coded to complete.
>
> **EXCLUDES1**   *traumatic amputation of knee (S88.0-)*

> The appropriate 7th character is to be added to each code from category S78.
> A   initial encounter
> D   subsequent encounter
> S   sequela

✓5ᵗʰ S78.0   Traumatic amputation at hip joint

✓6ᵗʰ S78.01   Complete traumatic amputation at hip joint

✓7ᵗʰ S78.011   Complete traumatic amputation at right hip joint   CC

CC Excl: CC with 7th character A: S71.001A, S71.009-S71.011 with 7th A, S71.019-S71.021 with 7th A, S71.029-S71.031 with 7th A, S71.039-S71.041 with 7th A, S71.049-S71.051 with 7th A, S71.059-S71.101 with 7th A, S71.109-S71.111 with 7th A, S71.119-S71.121 with 7th A, S71.129-S71.131 with 7th A, S71.139-S71.141 with 7th A, S71.149-S71.151 with 7th A, S71.159A, S76.021A, S76.029A, S76.121A, S76.129A, S76.221 A, S76.229A, S76.321A, S76.329A, S76.821A, S76.829A, S76.921A, S76.929A, S78.011A, S78.019-S78.021 with 7th A, S78.029-S78.111 with 7th A, S78.119-S78.121 with 7th A, S78.129-S78.911 with 7th A, S78.919-S78.921 with 7th A, S78.929A, S81.001A, S81.009-S81.011 with 7th A, S81.019-S81.021 with 7th A, S81.029-S81.031 with 7th A, S81.039-S81.041 with 7th A, S81.049-S81.051 with 7th A, S81.059-S81.801 with 7th A, S81.809-S81.811 with 7th A, S81.819-S81.821 with 7th A, S81.829-S81.831 with 7th A, S81.839-S81.841 with 7th A, S81.849-S81.851 with 7th A, S81.859A, S88.129-S98.131 with 7th A, S98.139-S98.141 with 7th A, S98.149-S98.211 with 7th A, S98.219-S98.221 with 7th A, S98.229-S98.311 with 7th A, S98.319-S98.321 with 7th A, S98.329-S98.911 with 7th A, S98.919-S98.921 with 7th A, S98.929 A, T14.90-T14.91, T79.A0X-T79.9XX with 7th A

✓7ᵗʰ S78.012   Complete traumatic amputation at left hip joint   CC

CC Excl: CC with 7th character A: S71.002-S71.009 with 7th A, S71.012-S71.019 with 7th A, S71.022-S71.029 with 7th A, S71.032-S71.039 with 7th A, S71.042-S71.049 with 7th A, S71.052-S71.059 with 7th A, S71.102-S71.109 with 7th A, S71.112-S71.119 with 7th A, S71.122-S71.129 with 7th A, S71.132-S71.139 with 7th A, S71.142-S71.149 with 7th A, S71.152-S71.159 with 7th A, S76.022-S76.029 with 7th A, S76.122-S76.129 with 7th A, S76.222-S76.229 with 7th A, S76.322-S76.329 with 7th A, S76.822-S76.829 with 7th A, S76.922-S76.929 with 7th A, S78.012-S78.019 with 7th A, S78.022-S78.029 with 7th A, S78.112-S78.119 with 7th A, S78.122-S78.129 with 7th A, S78.912-S78.919 with 7th A, S78.922-S78.929 with 7th A, S81.002-S81.009 with 7th A, S81.012-S81.019 with 7th A, S81.022-S81.029 with 7th A, S81.032-S81.039 with 7th A, S81.042-S81.049 with 7th A, S81.052-S81.059 with 7th A, S81.802-S81.809 with 7th A, S81.812-S81.819 with 7th A, S81.822-S81.829 with 7th A, S81.832-S81.839 with 7th A, S81.842-S81.849 with 7th A, S81.852-S81.859 with 7th A, S86.022-S86.029 with 7th A, S86.122-S86.129 with 7th A, S86.222-S86.229 with 7th A, S86.322-S86.329 with 7th A, S86.822-S86.829 with 7th A, S86.922-S86.929 with 7th A, S88.012-S88.019 with 7th A, S88.022-S88.029 with 7th A, S88.112-S88.119 with 7th A, S88.122-S88.129 with 7th A, S88.912-S88.919 with 7th A, S88.922-S88.929 with 7th A, S91.002-S91.009 with 7th A, S91.012-S91.019 with 7th A, S91.022-S91.029 with 7th A, S91.032-S91.039 with 7th A, S91.042-S91.049 with 7th A, S91.052-S91.059 with 7th A, S91.102-S91.103 with 7th A, S91.105-S91.109 with 7th A, S91.112-S91.113 with 7th A, S91.115-S91.119 with 7th A, S91.122-S91.123 with 7th A, S91.125-S91.129 with 7th A, S91.132-S91.133 with 7th A, S91.135-S91.139 with 7th A, S91.142-S91.143 with 7th A, S91.145-

S91.149 with 7th A, S91.152-S91.153 with 7th A, S91.155-S91.159 with 7th A, S91.202-S91.203 with 7th A, S91.205-S91.209 with 7th A, S91.212-S91.213 with 7th A, S91.215-S91.219 with 7th A, S91.222-S91.223 with 7th A, S91.225-S91.229 with 7th A, S91.232-S91.233 with 7th A, S91.235-S91.239 with 7th A, S91.242-S91.243 with 7th A, S91.245-S91.249 with 7th A, S91.252-S91.253 with 7th A, S91.255-S91.259 with 7th A, S91.302-S91.309 with 7th A, S91.312-S91.319 with 7th A, S91.322-S91.329 with 7th A, S91.332-S91.339 with 7th A, S91.342-S91.349 with 7th A, S91.352-S91.359 with 7th A, S96.022-S96.029 with 7th A, S96.122-S96.129 with 7th A, S96.222-S96.229 with 7th A, S96.822-S96.829 with 7th A, S96.922-S96.929 with 7th A, S98.012-S98.019 with 7th A, S98.022-S98.029 with 7th A, S98.112-S98.119 with 7th A, S98.122-S98.129 with 7th A, S98.132-S98.139 with 7th A, S98.142-S98.149 with 7th A, S98.212-S98.219 with 7th A, S98.222-S98.229 with 7th A, S98.312-S98.319 with 7th A, S98.322-S98.329 with 7th A, S98.912-S98.919 with 7th A, S98.922-S98.929 with 7th A, T14.90-T14.91, T79.A0X-T79.9XX with 7th A

✓7ᵗʰ S78.019   Complete traumatic amputation at unspecified hip joint   CC

CC Excl: CC with 7th character A: S71.001-S71.159 with 7th A, S76.021-S76.029 with 7th A, S76.121-S76.129 with 7th A, S76.221-S76.229 with 7th A, S76.321-S76.329 with 7th A, S76.821-S76.829 with 7th A, S76.921-S76.929 with 7th A, S78.011-S78.929 with 7th A, S81.001-S81.859 with 7th A, S86.021-S86.029 with 7th A, S86.121-S86.129 with 7th A, S86.221-S86.229 with 7th A, S86.321-S86.329 with 7th A, S86.821-S86.829 with 7th A, S86.921-S86.929 with 7th A, S88.011-S88.929 with 7th A, S91.001-S91.359 with 7th A, S96.021-S96.029 with 7th A, S96.121-S96.129 with 7th A, S96.221-S96.229 with 7th A, S96.821-S96.829 with 7th A, S96.921-S96.929 with 7th A, S98.011-S98.929 with 7th A, T14.90-T14.91, T79.A0X-T79.9XX with 7th A

✓6ᵗʰ S78.02   Partial traumatic amputation at hip joint

✓7ᵗʰ S78.021   Partial traumatic amputation at right hip joint   CC

CC Excl: See code: S78.011

✓7ᵗʰ S78.022   Partial traumatic amputation at left hip joint   CC

CC Excl: See code: S78.012

✓7ᵗʰ S78.029   Partial traumatic amputation at unspecified hip joint   CC

CC Excl: See code: S78.019

✓5ᵗʰ S78.1   Traumatic amputation at level between hip and knee

> **EXCLUDES1**   *traumatic amputation of knee (S88.0-)*

✓6ᵗʰ S78.11   Complete traumatic amputation at level between hip and knee

✓7ᵗʰ S78.111   Complete traumatic amputation at level between right hip and knee   CC

CC Excl: See code: S78.011

✓7ᵗʰ S78.112   Complete traumatic amputation at level between left hip and knee   CC

CC Excl: See code: S78.012

✓7ᵗʰ S78.119   Complete traumatic amputation at level between unspecified hip and knee   CC

CC Excl: See code: S78.019

✓6ᵗʰ S78.12   Partial traumatic amputation at level between hip and knee

✓7ᵗʰ S78.121   Partial traumatic amputation at level between right hip and knee   CC

CC Excl: See code: S78.011

✓7ᵗʰ S78.122   Partial traumatic amputation at level between left hip and knee   CC

CC Excl: See code: S78.012

✓7ᵗʰ S78.129   Partial traumatic amputation at level between unspecified hip and knee   CC

CC Excl: See code: S78.019

✓ Additional Character Required   ✓x7ᵗʰ Placeholder Alert   Unacceptable PDx   Manifestation   Hospital Acquired Condition   **EXCLUDES1** Not Coded Here   **EXCLUDES2** Not Included Here

✓5ᵗʰ **S78.9 Traumatic amputation** of hip and thigh, level unspecified

✓6ᵗʰ **S78.91 Complete traumatic amputation of hip and thigh, level unspecified**

✓7ᵗʰ **S78.911 Complete traumatic amputation of right hip and thigh, level unspecified** CC
CC Excl: See code: S78.011

✓7ᵗʰ **S78.912 Complete traumatic amputation of left hip and thigh, level unspecified** CC
CC Excl: See code: S78.012

✓7ᵗʰ **S78.919 Complete traumatic amputation of unspecified hip and thigh, level unspecified** CC
CC Excl: See code: S78.019

✓6ᵗʰ **S78.92 Partial traumatic amputation of hip and thigh, level unspecified**

✓7ᵗʰ **S78.921 Partial traumatic amputation of right hip and thigh, level unspecified** CC
CC Excl: See code: S78.011

✓7ᵗʰ **S78.922 Partial traumatic amputation of left hip and thigh, level unspecified** CC
CC Excl: See code: S78.012

✓7ᵗʰ **S78.929 Partial traumatic amputation of unspecified hip and thigh, level unspecified** CC
CC Excl: See code: S78.019

✓4ᵗʰ **S79 Other and unspecified injuries of hip and thigh**

✓5ᵗʰ **S79.0 Physeal fracture** of upper end of femur
NOTE A fracture not indicated as open or closed should be coded to closed.
EXCLUDES 1 apophyseal fracture of upper end of femur (S72.13-)
nontraumatic slipped upper femoral epiphysis (M93.0-)

The appropriate 7th character is to be added to each code from subcategory S79.0.
A initial encounter for closed fracture
D subsequent encounter for fracture with routine healing
G subsequent encounter for fracture with delayed healing
K subsequent encounter for fracture with nonunion
P subsequent encounter for fracture with malunion
S sequela

✓6ᵗʰ **S79.00 Unspecified physeal fracture of upper end of femur**

7,18 ✓7ᵗʰ **S79.001 Unspecified physeal fracture of upper end of right femur** MCC CC
CC Excl: MCC with 7th A: M48.40X-M48.58X with 7th A, M80.00X-M84.68X with 7th A, S03.8XX-S03.9XX with 7th A, S29.011-S29.019 with 7th A, S38.3XX-S39.013 with 7th A, S72.001-S72.471 with 7th [A, B, C], S72.479-S72.92X with 7th A, S73.101A, S73.109-S73.111 with 7th A, S73.119-S73.121 with 7th A, S73.129-S73.191 with 7th A, S73.199A, S76.001 A, S76.009-S76.011 with 7th A, S76.019A, S76.091A, S76.099-S76.101 with 7th A, S76.109-S76.111 with 7th A, S76.119A, S76.191A, S76.199-S76.201 with 7th A, S76.209-S76.211 with 7th A, S76.219A, S76.291A, S76.299-S76.301 with 7th A, S76.309-S76.311 with 7th A, S76.319A, S76.391A, S76.399-S76.801 with 7th A, S76.809-S76.811 with 7th A, S76.819 A, S76.891A, S76.899-S76.901 with 7th A, S76.909-S76.911 with 7th A, S76.919A, S76.991A, S76.999A, S79.001A, S79.009-S79.011 with 7th A, S79.019-S79.091 with 7th A, S79.099-S79.101 with 7th A, S79.109-S79.111 with 7th A, S79.119-S79.121 with 7th A, S79.129-S79.131 with 7th A, S79.139-S79.141 with 7th A, S79.149-S79.191 with 7th A, S79.199-S79.811 with 7th A, S79.819-S79.821 with 7th A, S79.829-S79.911 with 7th A, S79.919-S79.921 with 7th A, S79.929 with 7th A, S82.90X-S82.92X with 7th [A, B, C], T14.90-T14.91, T79.A0X-T79.9XX with 7th A
CC Excl: CC with 7th character K or P: M80.00X-M84.68X with 7th [K, P], S02.0XX-S02.92X with 7th K, S12.000-S12.691 with 7th K, S22.000-S22.9XX with 7th K, S32.000-S32.9XX with 7th K, S42.001-S42.92X with 7th [K, P], S49.001-S49.199 with 7th [K, P], S52.001-S52.92X with 7th [K, M, N, P, Q, R], S59.001-S59.299 with 7th [K, P], S62.001-S62.92X with 7th [K, P], S72.001-S72.92X with 7th [K, M, N, P, Q, R], S79.001-S79.199 with 7th [K, P], S82.001-S82.92X with 7th [K, M, N, P, Q, R], S89.001-S89.399 with 7th [K, P], S92.001-S92.919 with 7th [K, P]

7,18 ✓7ᵗʰ **S79.002 Unspecified physeal fracture of upper end of left femur** MCC CC
CC Excl: MCC with 7th A: M48.40X-M48.58X with 7th A, M80.00X-M84.68X with 7th A, S03.8XX-S03.9XX with 7th A, S29.011-S29.019 with 7th A, S38.3XX-S39.013 with 7th A, S72.001-S72.466 with 7th [B, C], S72.472-S72.92X with 7th A, S73.102-S73.109 with 7th A, S73.112-S73.119 with 7th A, S73.122-S73.129 with 7th A, S73.192-S73.199 with 7th A, S76.002-S76.009 with 7th A, S76.012-S76.019 with 7th A, S76.092-S76.099 with 7th A, S76.102-S76.109 with 7th A, S76.112-S76.119 with 7th A, S76.192-S76.199 with 7th A, S76.202-S76.209 with 7th A, S76.212-S76.219 with 7th A, S76.292-S76.299 with 7th A, S76.302-S76.309 with 7th A, S76.312-S76.319 with 7th A, S76.392-S76.399 with 7th A, S76.802-S76.809 with 7th A, S76.812-S76.819 with 7th A, S76.892-S76.899 with 7th A, S76.902-S76.909 with 7th A, S76.912-S76.919 with 7th A, S76.992-S76.999 with 7th A, S79.002-S79.009 with 7th A, S79.012-S79.019 with 7th A, S79.092-S79.099 with 7th A, S79.102-S79.109 with 7th A, S79.112-S79.119 with 7th A, S79.122-S79.129 with 7th A, S79.132-S79.139 with 7th A, S79.142-S79.149 with 7th A, S79.192-S79.199 with 7th A, S79.812-S79.819 with 7th A, S79.822-S79.829 with 7th A, S79.912-S79.919 with 7th A, S79.922-S79.929 with 7th A, S82.90X-S82.92X with 7th [A, B, C], T14.90-T14.91, T79.A0X-T79.9XX with 7th A
CC Excl: CC with 7th character K or P: M80.00X-M84.68X with 7th [K, P], S02.0XX-S02.92X with 7th K, S12.000-S12.691 with 7th K, S22.000-S22.9XX with 7th K, S32.000-S32.9XX with 7th K, S42.001-S42.92X with 7th [K, P], S49.001-S49.199 with 7th [K, P], S52.001-S52.92X with 7th [K, M, N, P, Q, R], S59.001-S59.299 with 7th [K, P], S62.001-S62.92X with 7th [K, P], S72.001-S72.92X with 7th [K, M, N, P, Q, R], S79.001-S79.199 with 7th [K, P], S82.001-S82.92X with 7th [K, M, N, P, Q, R], S89.001-S89.399 with 7th [K, P], S92.001-S92.919 with 7th [K, P]

7,18 ✓7ᵗʰ **S79.009 Unspecified physeal fracture of upper end of unspecified femur** MCC CC
CC Excl: MCC with 7th A: M48.40X-M48.58X with 7th A, M80.00X-M84.68X with 7th A, S03.8XX-S03.9XX with 7th A, S29.011-S29.019 with 7th A, S38.3XX-S39.013 with 7th A, S72.001-S72.92X with 7th [A, B, C], S73.101-S73.199 with 7th A, S76.001-S76.019 with 7th A, S76.091-S76.119 with 7th A, S76.191-S76.219 with 7th A, S76.291-S76.319 with 7th A, S76.391-S76.819 with 7th A, S76.891-S76.919 with 7th A, S76.991-S76.999 with 7th A, S79.001-S79.929 with 7th A, S82.90X-S82.92X with 7th [A, B, C], T14.90-T14.91, T79.A0X-T79.9XX with 7th A
CC Excl: CC with 7th character K or P: M80.00X-M84.68X with 7th [K, P], S02.0XX-S02.92X with 7th K, S12.000-S12.691 with 7th K, S22.000-S22.9XX with 7th K, S32.000-S32.9XX with 7th K, S42.001-S42.92X with 7th [K, P], S49.001-S49.199 with 7th [K, P], S52.001-S52.92X with 7th [K, M, N, P, Q, R], S59.001-S59.299 with 7th [K, P], S62.001-S62.92X with 7th [K, P], S72.001-S72.92X with 7th [K, M, N, P, Q, R], S79.001-S79.199 with 7th [K, P], S82.001-S82.92X with 7th [K, M, N, P, Q, R], S89.001-S89.399 with 7th [K, P], S92.001-S92.919 with 7th [K, P]

7 HAC = Initial encounter only (7th character A, B or C) and not POA.
18 CC only if a subsequent encounter for nonunion or malunion (7th character K, M, N, P, Q, or R – specific to category).

N Newborn: 0   P Pediatric: 0-17   M Maternity: 12-55   A Adult: 15-124   MCC Major CC Condition   PDxMCC PDx acts as own MCC   CC CC Condition   PDxCC PDx acts as own CC

1032   ICD-10-CM 2016

√6ᵗʰ **S79.01** **Salter-Harris Type I physeal fracture of upper end of femur**
> Acute on chronic slipped capital femoral epiphysis (traumatic)
> Acute slipped capital femoral epiphysis (traumatic)
> Capital femoral epiphyseal fracture
> *EXCLUDES 1*   *chronic slipped upper femoral epiphysis (nontraumatic) (M93.02-)*

7,18 √7ᵗʰ **S79.011** **Salter-Harris Type I physeal fracture of upper end of right femur**   MCC CC
> CC Excl: See code: S79.001

7,18 √7ᵗʰ **S79.012** **Salter-Harris Type I physeal fracture of upper end of left femur**   MCC CC
> CC Excl: See code: S79.002

7,18 √7ᵗʰ **S79.019** **Salter-Harris Type I physeal fracture of upper end of unspecified femur**   MCC CC
> CC Excl: See code: S79.009

√6ᵗʰ **S79.09** **Other physeal fracture of upper end of femur**

7,18 √7ᵗʰ **S79.091** **Other physeal fracture of upper end of right femur**   MCC CC
> CC Excl: See code: S79.001

7,18 √7ᵗʰ **S79.092** **Other physeal fracture of upper end of left femur**   MCC CC
> CC Excl: See code: S79.002

7,18 √7ᵗʰ **S79.099** **Other physeal fracture of upper end of unspecified femur**   MCC CC
> CC Excl: See code: S79.009

√5ᵗʰ **S79.1** **Physeal fracture of lower end of femur**
> **NOTE**   A fracture not indicated as open or closed should be coded to closed.

> The appropriate 7th character is to be added to each code from subcategory S79.1.
> A   initial encounter for closed fracture
> D   subsequent encounter for fracture with routine healing
> G   subsequent encounter for fracture with delayed healing
> K   subsequent encounter for fracture with nonunion
> P   subsequent encounter for fracture with malunion
> S   sequela

√6ᵗʰ **S79.10** **Unspecified physeal fracture of lower end of femur**

7,19 √7ᵗʰ **S79.101** **Unspecified physeal fracture of lower end of right femur**   CC
> CC Excl: CC with 7th character A: M80.00X-M80.019 with 7th A, M80.041-M80.059 with 7th A, M80.80X-M80.819 with 7th A, M80.841-M80.859 with 7th A, M84.40X-M84.419 with 7th A, M84.441-M84.459 with 7th A, M84.474-M84.519 with 7th A, M84.541-M84.559 with 7th A, M84.574-M84.576 with 7th A, M84.60X-M84.619 with 7th A, M84.641-M84.659 with 7th A, M84.674-M84.68X with 7th A, S03.8XX-S03.9XX with 7th A, S29.011-S29.019 with 7th A, S38.3XX-S39.013 with 7th A, S72.001-S72.471 with 7th [A, B, C], S72.479-S72.92X with 7th A, S73.101A, S73.109-S73.111 with 7th A, S73.119-S73.121 with 7th A, S73.129-S73.191 with 7th A, S73.199A, S76.001A, S76.009-S76.011 with 7th A, S76.019A, S76.091A, S76.099-S76.101 with 7th A, S76.109-S76.111 with 7th A, S76.119 with 7th A, S76.191A, S76.199-S76.201 with 7th A, S76.209-S76.211 with 7th A, S76.219A, S76.291A, S76.299-S76.301 with 7th A, S76.309-S76.311 with 7th A, S76.319A, S76.391A, S76.399-S76.801 with 7th A, S76.809-S76.811 with 7th A, S76.819 with 7th A, S76.891A, S76.899-S76.901 with 7th A, S76.909-S76.911 with 7th A, S76.919A, S76.991A, S76.999A, S79.001A, S79.009-S79.011 with 7th A, S79.019-S79.091 with 7th A, S79.099-S79.101 with 7th A, S79.109-S79.111 with 7th A, S79.119-S79.121 with 7th A, S79.129-S79.131 with 7th A, S79.139-S79.141 with 7th A, S79.149-S79.191 with 7th A, S79.199-S79.811 with 7th A, S79.819-S79.821 with 7th A, S79.829-S79.911 with 7th A, S79.919-S79.921 with 7th A, S79.929 with 7th A, S82.90X-S82.92X with 7th [A, B,

C], T14.90-T14.91, T79.A9X-T79.9XX with 7th A
> CC Excl: CC with 7th character K or P: M80.00X-M84.68 with 7th [K, P], S02.0XX-S02.92X with 7th K, S12.000-S12.691 with 7th K, S22.000-S22.9XX with 7th K, S32.000-S32.9XX with 7th K, S42.001-S42.92X with 7th [K, P], S49.001-S49.199 with 7th [K, P], S52.001-S52.92X with 7th [K, M, N, P, Q, R], S59.001-S59.299 with 7th [K, P], S62.001-S62.92X with 7th [K, P], S72.001-S72.92X with 7th [K, M, N, P, Q, R], S79.001-S79.199 with 7th [K, P], S82.001-S82.92X with 7th [K, M, N, P, Q, R], S89.001-S89.399 with 7th [K, P], S92.001-S92.919 with 7th [K, P]

7,19 √7ᵗʰ **S79.102** **Unspecified physeal fracture of lower end of left femur**   CC
> CC Excl: CC with 7th character A: M80.00X-M80.019 with 7th A, M80.041-M80.059 with 7th A, M80.80X-M80.819 with 7th A, M80.841-M80.859 with 7th A, M84.40X-M84.419 with 7th A, M84.441-M84.459 with 7th A, M84.474-M84.519 with 7th A, M84.541-M84.559 with 7th A, M84.574-M84.576 with 7th A, M84.60X-M84.619 with 7th A, M84.641-M84.659 with 7th A, M84.674-M84.68X with 7th A, S03.8XX-S03.9XX with 7th A, S29.011-S29.019 with 7th A, S38.3XX-S39.013 with 7th A, S72.001-S72.466 with 7th [B, C], S72.472-S72.92 with 7th A, S73.102-S73.109 with 7th A, S73.112-S73.119 with 7th A, S73.122-S73.129 with 7th A, S73.192-S73.199 with 7th A, S76.002-S76.009 with 7th A, S76.012-S76.019 with 7th A, S76.092-S76.099 with 7th A, S76.102-S76.109 with 7th A, S76.112-S76.119 with 7th A, S76.192-S76.199 with 7th A, S76.202-S76.209 with 7th A, S76.212-S76.219 with 7th A, S76.292-S76.299 with 7th A, S76.302-S76.309 with 7th A, S76.312-S76.319 with 7th A, S76.392-S76.399 with 7th A, S76.802-S76.809 with 7th A, S76.812-S76.819 with 7th A, S76.892-S76.899 with 7th A, S76.902-S76.909 with 7th A, S76.912-S76.919 with 7th A, S76.992-S76.999 with 7th A, S79.002-S79.009 with 7th A, S79.012-S79.019 with 7th A, S79.092-S79.099 with 7th A, S79.102-S79.109 with 7th A, S79.112-S79.119 with 7th A, S79.122-S79.129 with 7th A, S79.132-S79.139 with 7th A, S79.142-S79.149 with 7th A, S79.192-S79.199 with 7th A, S79.812-S79.819 with 7th A, S79.822-S79.829 with 7th A, S79.912-S79.919 with 7th A, S79.922-S79.929 with 7th A, S82.90X-S82.92X with 7th [A, B, C], T14.90-T14.91, T79.A9X-T79.9XX with 7th A
> CC Excl: CC with 7th character K or P: M80.00X-M84.68X with 7th [K, P], S02.0XX-S02.92X with 7th K, S12.000-S12.691 with 7th K, S22.000-S22.9XX with 7th K, S32.000-S32.9XX with 7th K, S42.001-S42.92X with 7th [K, P], S49.001-S49.199 with 7th [K, P], S52.001-S52.92X with 7th [K, M, N, P, Q, R], S59.001-S59.299 with 7th [K, P], S62.001-S62.92X with 7th [K, P], S72.001-S72.92X with 7th [K, M, N, P, Q, R], S79.001-S79.199 with 7th [K, P], S82.001-S82.92X with 7th [K, M, N, P, Q, R], S89.001-S89.399 with 7th [K, P], S92.001-S92.919 with 7th [K, P]

---

7   HAC = Initial encounter only (7th character A, B or C) and not POA.
18   CC only if a subsequent encounter for nonunion or malunion (7th character K, M, N, P, Q, or R – specific to category).
19   CC only if an initial encounter for a closed fracture (7th character A) **OR** a subsequent encounter for nonunion or malunion (7th character K, M, N, P, Q, or R – specific to category).

☑ Additional Character Required   √x7ᵗʰ Placeholder Alert   Unacceptable PDx   Manifestation   Hospital Acquired Condition   *EXCLUDES 1* Not Coded Here   *EXCLUDES 2* Not Included Here

Chapter 19. Injury, Poisoning, and Certain Other Consequences of External Causes

7,19 √7ᵗʰ **S79.109 Unspecified physeal fracture of lower end of unspecified femur** CC
CC Excl: CC with 7th character A: M80.00X-M80.019 with 7th A, M80.041-M80.059 with 7th A, M80.80X-M80.819 with 7th A, M80.841-M80.859 with 7th A, M84.40X-M84.419 with 7th A, M84.441-M84.459 with 7th A, M84.474-M84.519 with 7th A, M84.541-M84.559 with 7th A, M84.574-M84.576 with 7th A, M84.60X-M84.619 with 7th A, M84.641-M84.659 with 7th A, M84.674-M84.68X with 7th A, S03.8XX-S03.9XX with 7th A, S29.011-S29.019 with 7th A, S38.3XX-S39.013 with 7th A, S72.001-S72.92 with 7th [A, B, C], S73.101-S73.199 with 7th A, S76.001-S76.019 with 7th A, S76.091-S76.119 with 7th A, S76.191-S76.219 with 7th A, S76.291-S76.319 with 7th A, S76.391-S76.819 with 7th A, S76.891-S76.919 with 7th A, S76.991-S76.999 with 7th A, S79.001-S79.929 with 7th A, S82.90X-S82.92X with 7th [A, B, C], T14.90-T14.91, T79.A9X-T79.9XX with 7th A
CC Excl: CC with 7th character K or P: M80.00X-M84.68 with 7th [K, P], S02.0XX-S02.92X with 7th K, S12.000-S12.691 with 7th K, S22.000-S22.9XX with 7th K, S32.000-S32.9XX with 7th K, S42.001-S42.92X with 7th [K, P], S49.001-S49.199 with 7th [K, P], S52.001-S52.92X with 7th [K, M, N, P, Q, R], S59.001-S59.299 with 7th [K, P], S62.001-S62.92X with 7th [K, P], S72.001-S72.92X with 7th [K, M, N, P, Q, R], S79.001-S79.199 with 7th [K, P], S82.001-S82.92X with 7th [K, M, N, P, Q, R], S89.001-S89.399 with 7th [K, P], S92.001-S92.919 with 7th [K, P]

√6ᵗʰ **S79.11 Salter-Harris Type I physeal fracture of lower end of femur**

7,19 √7ᵗʰ **S79.111 Salter-Harris Type I physeal fracture of lower end of right femur** CC
CC Excl: See code: S79.101

7,19 √7ᵗʰ **S79.112 Salter-Harris Type I physeal fracture of lower end of left femur** CC
CC Excl: See code: S79.102

7,19 √7ᵗʰ **S79.119 Salter-Harris Type I physeal fracture of lower end of unspecified femur** CC
CC Excl: See code: S79.109

√6ᵗʰ **S79.12 Salter-Harris Type II physeal fracture of lower end of femur**

7,19 √7ᵗʰ **S79.121 Salter-Harris Type II physeal fracture of lower end of right femur** CC
CC Excl: See code: S79.101

7,19 √7ᵗʰ **S79.122 Salter-Harris Type II physeal fracture of lower end of left femur** CC
CC Excl: See code: S79.102

7,19 √7ᵗʰ **S79.129 Salter-Harris Type II physeal fracture of lower end of unspecified femur** CC
CC Excl: See code: S79.109

√6ᵗʰ **S79.13 Salter-Harris Type III physeal fracture of lower end of femur**

7,19 √7ᵗʰ **S79.131 Salter-Harris Type III physeal fracture of lower end of right femur** CC
CC Excl: See code: S79.101

7,19 √7ᵗʰ **S79.132 Salter-Harris Type III physeal fracture of lower end of left femur** CC
CC Excl: See code: S79.102

7,19 √7ᵗʰ **S79.139 Salter-Harris Type III physeal fracture of lower end of unspecified femur** CC
CC Excl: See code: S79.109

√6ᵗʰ **S79.14 Salter-Harris Type IV physeal fracture of lower end of femur**

7,19 √7ᵗʰ **S79.141 Salter-Harris Type IV physeal fracture of lower end of right femur** CC
CC Excl: See code: S79.101

7,19 √7ᵗʰ **S79.142 Salter-Harris Type IV physeal fracture of lower end of left femur** CC
CC Excl: See code: S79.102

7,19 √7ᵗʰ **S79.149 Salter-Harris Type IV physeal fracture of lower end of unspecified femur** CC
CC Excl: See code: S79.109

√6ᵗʰ **S79.19 Other physeal fracture of lower end of femur**

7,19 √7ᵗʰ **S79.191 Other physeal fracture of lower end of right femur** CC
CC Excl: See code: S79.101

7,19 √7ᵗʰ **S79.192 Other physeal fracture of lower end of left femur** CC
CC Excl: See code: S79.102

7,19 √7ᵗʰ **S79.199 Other physeal fracture of lower end of unspecified femur** CC
CC Excl: See code: S79.109

√5ᵗʰ **S79.8 Other specified injuries of hip and thigh**

The appropriate 7th character is to be added to each code in subcategory S79.8.
A   initial encounter
D   subsequent encounter
S   sequela

√6ᵗʰ **S79.81 Other specified injuries of hip**
√7ᵗʰ **S79.811 Other specified injuries of right hip**
√7ᵗʰ **S79.812 Other specified injuries of left hip**
√7ᵗʰ **S79.819 Other specified injuries of unspecified hip**

√6ᵗʰ **S79.82 Other specified injuries of thigh**
√7ᵗʰ **S79.821 Other specified injuries of right thigh**
√7ᵗʰ **S79.822 Other specified injuries of left thigh**
√7ᵗʰ **S79.829 Other specified injuries of unspecified thigh**

√5ᵗʰ **S79.9 Unspecified injury of hip and thigh**

The appropriate 7th character is to be added to each code in subcategory S79.9.
A   initial encounter
D   subsequent encounter
S   sequela

√6ᵗʰ **S79.91 Unspecified injury of hip**
√7ᵗʰ **S79.911 Unspecified injury of right hip**
√7ᵗʰ **S79.912 Unspecified injury of left hip**
√7ᵗʰ **S79.919 Unspecified injury of unspecified hip**

√6ᵗʰ **S79.92 Unspecified injury of thigh**
√7ᵗʰ **S79.921 Unspecified injury of right thigh**
√7ᵗʰ **S79.922 Unspecified injury of left thigh**
√7ᵗʰ **S79.929 Unspecified injury of unspecified thigh**

Injuries to the knee and lower leg (S80-S89)

EXCLUDES 2   burns and corrosions (T20-T32)
     frostbite (T33-T34)
     injuries of ankle and foot, except fracture of ankle and malleolus (S90-S99)
     insect bite or sting, venomous (T63.4)

√4ᵗʰ **S80 Superficial injury of knee and lower leg**
EXCLUDES 2   superficial injury of ankle and foot (S90.-)

The appropriate 7th character is to be added to each code from category S80.
A   initial encounter
D   subsequent encounter
S   sequela

√5ᵗʰ **S80.0 Contusion of knee**
√x7ᵗʰ **S80.00 Contusion of unspecified knee**
√x7ᵗʰ **S80.01 Contusion of right knee**
√x7ᵗʰ **S80.02 Contusion of left knee**

√5ᵗʰ **S80.1 Contusion of lower leg**
√x7ᵗʰ **S80.10 Contusion of unspecified lower leg**
√x7ᵗʰ **S80.11 Contusion of right lower leg**
√x7ᵗʰ **S80.12 Contusion of left lower leg**

√5ᵗʰ **S80.2 Other superficial injuries of knee**
√6ᵗʰ **S80.21 Abrasion of knee**
√7ᵗʰ **S80.211 Abrasion, right knee**
√7ᵗʰ **S80.212 Abrasion, left knee**
√7ᵗʰ **S80.219 Abrasion, unspecified knee**

---

7   HAC = Initial encounter only (7th character A, B or C) and not POA.
19   CC only if an initial encounter for a closed fracture (7th character A) **OR** a subsequent encounter for nonunion or malunion (7th character K, M, N, P, Q, or R – specific to category).

N Newborn: 0   P Pediatric: 0-17   M Maternity: 12-55   A Adult: 15-124   MCC Major CC Condition   PDxMCC PDx acts as own MCC   CC CC Condition   PDxCC PDx acts as own CC

1034   ICD-10-CM 2016

√6ᵗʰ **S80.22 Blister (nonthermal) of knee**
  √7ᵗʰ **S80.221 Blister (nonthermal), right knee**
  √7ᵗʰ **S80.222 Blister (nonthermal), left knee**
  √7ᵗʰ **S80.229 Blister (nonthermal), unspecified knee**
√6ᵗʰ **S80.24 External constriction of knee**
  √7ᵗʰ **S80.241 External constriction, right knee**
  √7ᵗʰ **S80.242 External constriction, left knee**
  √7ᵗʰ **S80.249 External constriction, unspecified knee**
√6ᵗʰ **S80.25 Superficial foreign body of knee**
    Splinter in the knee
  √7ᵗʰ **S80.251 Superficial foreign body, right knee**
  √7ᵗʰ **S80.252 Superficial foreign body, left knee**
  √7ᵗʰ **S80.259 Superficial foreign body, unspecified knee**
√6ᵗʰ **S80.26 Insect bite (nonvenomous) of knee**
  √7ᵗʰ **S80.261 Insect bite (nonvenomous), right knee**
  √7ᵗʰ **S80.262 Insect bite (nonvenomous), left knee**
  √7ᵗʰ **S80.269 Insect bite (nonvenomous), unspecified knee**
√6ᵗʰ **S80.27 Other superficial bite of knee**
    EXCLUDES 1 *open bite of knee (S81.05-)*
  √7ᵗʰ **S80.271 Other superficial bite of right knee**
  √7ᵗʰ **S80.272 Other superficial bite of left knee**
  √7ᵗʰ **S80.279 Other superficial bite of unspecified knee**
√5ᵗʰ **S80.8 Other superficial injuries of lower leg**
  √6ᵗʰ **S80.81 Abrasion of lower leg**
    √7ᵗʰ **S80.811 Abrasion, right lower leg**
    √7ᵗʰ **S80.812 Abrasion, left lower leg**
    √7ᵗʰ **S80.819 Abrasion, unspecified lower leg**
  √6ᵗʰ **S80.82 Blister (nonthermal) of lower leg**
    √7ᵗʰ **S80.821 Blister (nonthermal), right lower leg**
    √7ᵗʰ **S80.822 Blister (nonthermal), left lower leg**
    √7ᵗʰ **S80.829 Blister (nonthermal), unspecified lower leg**
  √6ᵗʰ **S80.84 External constriction of lower leg**
    √7ᵗʰ **S80.841 External constriction, right lower leg**
    √7ᵗʰ **S80.842 External constriction, left lower leg**
    √7ᵗʰ **S80.849 External constriction, unspecified lower leg**
  √6ᵗʰ **S80.85 Superficial foreign body of lower leg**
    Splinter in the lower leg
    √7ᵗʰ **S80.851 Superficial foreign body, right lower leg**
    √7ᵗʰ **S80.852 Superficial foreign body, left lower leg**
    √7ᵗʰ **S80.859 Superficial foreign body, unspecified lower leg**
  √6ᵗʰ **S80.86 Insect bite (nonvenomous) of lower leg**
    √7ᵗʰ **S80.861 Insect bite (nonvenomous), right lower leg**
    √7ᵗʰ **S80.862 Insect bite (nonvenomous), left lower leg**
    √7ᵗʰ **S80.869 Insect bite (nonvenomous), unspecified lower leg**
  √6ᵗʰ **S80.87 Other superficial bite of lower leg**
    EXCLUDES 1 *open bite of lower leg (S81.85-)*
    √7ᵗʰ **S80.871 Other superficial bite, right lower leg**
    √7ᵗʰ **S80.872 Other superficial bite, left lower leg**
    √7ᵗʰ **S80.879 Other superficial bite, unspecified lower leg**
√5ᵗʰ **S80.9 Unspecified superficial injury of knee and lower leg**
  √6ᵗʰ **S80.91 Unspecified superficial injury of knee**
    √7ᵗʰ **S80.911 Unspecified superficial injury of right knee**
    √7ᵗʰ **S80.912 Unspecified superficial injury of left knee**
    √7ᵗʰ **S80.919 Unspecified superficial injury of unspecified knee**
  √6ᵗʰ **S80.92 Unspecified superficial injury of lower leg**
    √7ᵗʰ **S80.921 Unspecified superficial injury of right lower leg**
    √7ᵗʰ **S80.922 Unspecified superficial injury of left lower leg**
    √7ᵗʰ **S80.929 Unspecified superficial injury of unspecified lower leg**

√4ᵗʰ **S81 Open wound of knee and lower leg**
  Code also any associated wound infection
  EXCLUDES 1 *open fracture of knee and lower leg (S82.-)*
         traumatic amputation of lower leg (S88.-)
  EXCLUDES 2 *open wound of ankle and foot (S91.-)*

  The appropriate 7th character is to be added to each code from category S81.
  A   initial encounter
  D   subsequent encounter
  S   sequela

  √5ᵗʰ **S81.0 Open wound of knee**
    √6ᵗʰ **S81.00 Unspecified open wound of knee**
      √7ᵗʰ **S81.001 Unspecified open wound, right knee**
      √7ᵗʰ **S81.002 Unspecified open wound, left knee**
      √7ᵗʰ **S81.009 Unspecified open wound, unspecified knee**
    √6ᵗʰ **S81.01 Laceration without foreign body of knee**
      √7ᵗʰ **S81.011 Laceration without foreign body, right knee**
      √7ᵗʰ **S81.012 Laceration without foreign body, left knee**
      √7ᵗʰ **S81.019 Laceration without foreign body, unspecified knee**
    √6ᵗʰ **S81.02 Laceration with foreign body of knee**
      √7ᵗʰ **S81.021 Laceration with foreign body, right knee**
      √7ᵗʰ **S81.022 Laceration with foreign body, left knee**
      √7ᵗʰ **S81.029 Laceration with foreign body, unspecified knee**
    √6ᵗʰ **S81.03 Puncture wound without foreign body of knee**
      √7ᵗʰ **S81.031 Puncture wound without foreign body, right knee**
      √7ᵗʰ **S81.032 Puncture wound without foreign body, left knee**
      √7ᵗʰ **S81.039 Puncture wound without foreign body, unspecified knee**
    √6ᵗʰ **S81.04 Puncture wound with foreign body of knee**
      √7ᵗʰ **S81.041 Puncture wound with foreign body, right knee**
      √7ᵗʰ **S81.042 Puncture wound with foreign body, left knee**
      √7ᵗʰ **S81.049 Puncture wound with foreign body, unspecified knee**
    √6ᵗʰ **S81.05 Open bite of knee**
      Bite of knee NOS
      EXCLUDES 1 *superficial bite of knee (S80.27-)*
      √7ᵗʰ **S81.051 Open bite, right knee**
      √7ᵗʰ **S81.052 Open bite, left knee**
      √7ᵗʰ **S81.059 Open bite, unspecified knee**
  √5ᵗʰ **S81.8 Open wound of lower leg**
    √6ᵗʰ **S81.80 Unspecified open wound of lower leg**
      √7ᵗʰ **S81.801 Unspecified open wound, right lower leg**
      √7ᵗʰ **S81.802 Unspecified open wound, left lower leg**
      √7ᵗʰ **S81.809 Unspecified open wound, unspecified lower leg**
    √6ᵗʰ **S81.81 Laceration without foreign body of lower leg**
      √7ᵗʰ **S81.811 Laceration without foreign body, right lower leg**
      √7ᵗʰ **S81.812 Laceration without foreign body, left lower leg**
      √7ᵗʰ **S81.819 Laceration without foreign body, unspecified lower leg**
    √6ᵗʰ **S81.82 Laceration with foreign body of lower leg**
      √7ᵗʰ **S81.821 Laceration with foreign body, right lower leg**
      √7ᵗʰ **S81.822 Laceration with foreign body, left lower leg**
      √7ᵗʰ **S81.829 Laceration with foreign body, unspecified lower leg**
    √6ᵗʰ **S81.83 Puncture wound without foreign body of lower leg**
      √7ᵗʰ **S81.831 Puncture wound without foreign body, right lower leg**
      √7ᵗʰ **S81.832 Puncture wound without foreign body, left lower leg**

√7ᵗʰ S81.839   **Puncture wound without foreign body, unspecified lower leg**

√6ᵗʰ S81.84   **Puncture wound with foreign body of lower leg**

√7ᵗʰ S81.841   **Puncture wound with foreign body, right lower leg**

√7ᵗʰ S81.842   **Puncture wound with foreign body, left lower leg**

√7ᵗʰ S81.849   **Puncture wound with foreign body, unspecified lower leg**

√6ᵗʰ S81.85   **Open bite of lower leg**
Bite of lower leg NOS
EXCLUDES 1   superficial bite of lower leg (S80.86-, S80.87-)

√7ᵗʰ S81.851   **Open bite, right lower leg**

√7ᵗʰ S81.852   **Open bite, left lower leg**

√7ᵗʰ S81.859   **Open bite, unspecified lower leg**

√4ᵗʰ S82   **Fracture of lower leg, including ankle**
NOTE   A fracture not indicated as displaced or nondisplaced should be coded to displaced.
A fracture not designated as open or closed should be coded to closed.
The open fracture designations are based on the Gustilo open fracture classification.
INCLUDES   fracture of malleolus
EXCLUDES 1   traumatic amputation of lower leg (S88.-)
EXCLUDES 2   fracture of foot, except ankle (S92.-)
periprosthetic fracture of prosthetic implant of knee (T84.042, T84.043)

The appropriate 7th character is to be added to all codes from category S82 [unless otherwise indicated].
A   initial encounter for closed fracture
B   initial encounter for open fracture type I or II
    initial encounter for open fracture NOS
C   initial encounter for open fracture type IIIA, IIIB, or IIIC
D   subsequent encounter for closed fracture with routine healing
E   subsequent encounter for open fracture type I or II with routine healing
F   subsequent encounter for open fracture type IIIA, IIIB, or IIIC with routine healing
G   subsequent encounter for closed fracture with delayed healing
H   subsequent encounter for open fracture type I or II with delayed healing
J   subsequent encounter for open fracture type IIIA, IIIB or IIIC with delayed healing
K   subsequent encounter for closed fracture with nonunion
M   subsequent encounter for open fracture type I or II with nonunion
N   subsequent encounter for open fracture type IIIA, IIIB or IIIC with nonunion
P   subsequent encounter for closed fracture with malunion
Q   subsequent encounter for open fracture type I or II with malunion
R   subsequent encounter for open fracture type IIIA, IIIB or IIIC with malunion
S   sequela

√5ᵗʰ S82.0   **Fracture of patella**
Knee cap

√6ᵗʰ S82.00   **Unspecified fracture of patella**

7,17 **√7ᵗʰ S82.001**   **Unspecified fracture of right patella**   CC
CC Excl: CC with 7th character A: S82.001-S82.099 with 7th [A, B, C]
CC with 7th character B or C: M80.00X-M80.019 with 7th A, M80.041-M80.049 with 7th A, M80.80X-M80.819 with 7th A, M80.841-M80.849 with 7th A, M84.40X-M84.419 with 7th A, M84.441-M84.446 with 7th A, M84.454 with 7th A, M84.474-M84.519 with 7th A, M84.541-M84.550 with 7th A, M84.574-M84.576 with 7th A, M84.60X-M84.619 with 7th A, M84.641-M84.650 with 7th A, M84.674-M84.68X with 7th A, S03.8XX-S03.9XX with 7th A, S29.011-S29.019 with 7th A, S38.3XX-S39.013 with 7th A, S73.101-S73.199 with 7th A, S76.001-S76.019 with 7th A, S76.091-S76.119 with 7th A, S76.191-S76.219 with 7th A, S76.291-S76.319 with 7th A, S76.391-S76.819 with 7th A, S76.891-S76.919 with 7th A, S76.991-S76.999 with 7th A, S79.811-S79.929 with 7th A, S82.001-S82.156 with 7th [B, C], S82.191-S82.299 with 7th [A, B, C],
S82.401-S82.499 with 7th [A, B, C], S82.831-S82.839 with 7th [A, B, C], S82.861-S82.866 with 7th [A, B, C], S82.90X-S82.92X with 7th [A, B, C], S89.001-S89.099 with 7th A, S89.201-S89.299 with 7th A, T14.90-T14.91, T79.A9X-T79.9XX with 7th A
CC Excl: CC with 7th character K, M, N, P, Q or R: M80.00X-M84.68 with 7th [K, P], S02.0XX-S02.92X with 7th K, S12.000-S12.691 with 7th K, S22.000-S22.9XX with 7th K, S32.000-S32.9XX with 7th K, S42.001-S42.92X with 7th [K, P], S49.001-S49.199 with 7th [K, P], S52.001-S52.92X with 7th [K, M, N, P, Q, R], S59.001-S59.299 with 7th [K, P], S62.001-S62.92X with 7th [K, P], S72.001-S72.92X with 7th [K, M, N, P, Q, R], S79.001-S79.199 with 7th [K, P], S82.001-S82.92X with 7th [K, M, N, P, Q, R], S89.001-S89.399 with 7th [K, P], S92.001-S92.919 with 7th [K, P]

7,17 **√7ᵗʰ S82.002**   **Unspecified fracture of left patella**   CC
CC Excl: CC with 7th character A: S82.001-S82.099 with 7th [B, C]
CC with 7th character B or C: M80.00X-M80.019 with 7th A, M80.041-M80.049 with 7th A, M80.80X-M80.819 with 7th A, M80.841-M80.849 with 7th A, M84.40X-M84.419 with 7th A, M84.441-M84.446 with 7th A, M84.454 with 7th A, M84.474-M84.519 with 7th A, M84.541-M84.550 with 7th A, M84.574-M84.576 with 7th A, M84.60X-M84.619 with 7th A, M84.641-M84.650 with 7th A, M84.674-M84.68 with 7th A, S03.8XX-S03.9XX with 7th A, S29.011-S29.019 with 7th A, S38.3X-S39.013 with 7th A, S73.101-S73.199 with 7th A, S76.001-S76.019 with 7th A, S76.091-S76.119 with 7th A, S76.191-S76.219 with 7th A, S76.291-S76.319 with 7th A, S76.391-S76.819 with 7th A, S76.891-S76.919 with 7th A, S76.991-S76.999 with 7th A, S79.811-S79.929 with 7th A, S82.001-S82.156 with 7th [B, C], S82.191-S82.299 with 7th [A, B, C], S82.401-S82.499 with 7th [A, B, C], S82.831-S82.839 with 7th [A, B, C], S82.861-S82.866 with 7th [A, B, C], S82.90X-S82.92X with 7th [A, B, C], S89.001-S89.099 with 7th A, S89.201-S89.299 with 7th A, T14.90-T14.91, T79.A9X-T79.9XX with 7th A
CC Excl: CC with 7th character K, M, N, P, Q or R: M80.00X-M84.68X with 7th [K, P], S02.0XX-S02.92X with 7th K, S12.000-S12.691 with 7th K, S22.000-S22.9XX with 7th K, S32.000-S32.9XX with 7th K, S42.001-S42.92X with 7th [K, P], S49.001-S49.199 with 7th [K, P], S52.001-S52.92X with 7th [K, M, N, P, Q, R], S59.001-S59.299 with 7th [K, P], S62.001-S62.92X with 7th [K, P], S72.001-S72.92X with 7th [K, M, N, P, Q, R], S79.001-S79.199 with 7th [K, P], S82.001-S82.92X with 7th [K, M, N, P, Q, R], S89.001-S89.399 with 7th [K, P], S92.001-S92.919 with 7th [K, P]

7,17 **√7ᵗʰ S82.009**   **Unspecified fracture of unspecified patella**   CC
CC Excl: CC with 7th character A: S82.001-S82.099 with 7th [A, B, C]
CC with 7th character B or C: M80.00X-M80.019 with 7th A, M80.041-M80.049 with 7th A, M80.80X-M80.819 with 7th A, M80.841-M80.849 with 7th A, M84.40X-M84.419 with 7th A, M84.441-M84.446 with 7th A, M84.454 with 7th A, M84.474-M84.519 with 7th A, M84.541-M84.550 with 7th A, M84.574-M84.576 with 7th A, M84.60X-M84.619 with 7th A, M84.641-M84.650 with 7th A, M84.674-M84.68X with 7th A, S03.8XX-S03.9XX with 7th A, S29.011-S29.019 with 7th A, S38.3XX-S39.013 with 7th A, S73.101-S73.199 with 7th A, S76.001-S76.019 with 7th A, S76.091-S76.119 with 7th A, S76.191-S76.219 with 7th A, S76.291-S76.319 with 7th A, S76.391-S76.819 with 7th A, S76.891-S76.919 with 7th A, S76.991-S76.999 with 7th A, S79.811-S79.929 with 7th A, S82.001-S82.156 with 7th [B, C], S82.191-S82.299 with 7th [A, B, C], S82.401-S82.499 with 7th [A, B, C], S82.831-S82.839 with 7th [A, B, C], S82.861-S82.866 with 7th [A, B, C], S82.90X-S82.92X with 7th [A, B, C], S89.001-S89.099 with 7th A, S89.201-S89.299 with 7th A, T14.90-T14.91, T79.A9X-T79.9XX with 7th A

---

7   HAC = Initial encounter only (7th character A, B or C) and not POA.
17   CC only if an initial encounter (7th character A, B or C) **OR** a subsequent encounter for nonunion or malunion (7th character K, M, N, P, Q, or R).

CC Excl: CC with 7th character K, M, N, P, Q or R: M80.00X-M84.68 with 7th [K, P], S02.0XX-S02.92X with 7th K, S12.000-S12.691 with 7th K, S22.000-S22.9XX with 7th K, S32.000-S32.9XX with 7th K, S42.001-S42.92X with 7th [K, P], S49.001-S49.199 with 7th [K, P], S52.001-S52.92X with 7th [K, M, N, P, Q, R], S59.001-S59.299 with 7th [K, P], S62.001-S62.92X with 7th [K, P], S72.001-S72.92X with 7th [K, M, N, P, Q, R], S79.001-S79.199 with 7th [K, P], S82.001-S82.92X with 7th [K, M, N, P, Q, R], S89.001-S89.399 with 7th [K, P], S92.001-S92.919 with 7th [K, P]

√6th **S82.01 Osteochondral fracture of patella**

7,17 √7th **S82.011 Displaced osteochondral fracture of right patella** CC
CC Excl: See code: S82.001

7,17 √7th **S82.012 Displaced osteochondral fracture of left patella** CC
CC Excl: See code: S82.002

7,17 √7th **S82.013 Displaced osteochondral fracture of unspecified patella** CC
CC Excl: See code: S82.009

7,17 √7th **S82.014 Nondisplaced osteochondral fracture of right patella** CC
CC Excl: See code: S82.001

7,17 √7th **S82.015 Nondisplaced osteochondral fracture of left patella** CC
CC Excl: See code: S82.002

7,17 √7th **S82.016 Nondisplaced osteochondral fracture of unspecified patella** CC
CC Excl: See code: S82.009

√6th **S82.02 Longitudinal fracture of patella**

7,17 √7th **S82.021 Displaced longitudinal fracture of right patella** CC
CC Excl: See code: S82.001

7,17 √7th **S82.022 Displaced longitudinal fracture of left patella** CC
CC Excl: See code: S82.002

7,17 √7th **S82.023 Displaced longitudinal fracture of unspecified patella** CC
CC Excl: See code: S82.009

7,17 √7th **S82.024 Nondisplaced longitudinal fracture of right patella** CC
CC Excl: See code: S82.001

7,17 √7th **S82.025 Nondisplaced longitudinal fracture of left patella** CC
CC Excl: See code: S82.002

7,17 √7th **S82.026 Nondisplaced longitudinal fracture of unspecified patella** CC
CC Excl: See code: S82.009

√6th **S82.03 Transverse fracture of patella**

7,17 √7th **S82.031 Displaced transverse fracture of right patella** CC
CC Excl: See code: S82.001

7,17 √7th **S82.032 Displaced transverse fracture of left patella** CC
CC Excl: See code: S82.002

7,17 √7th **S82.033 Displaced transverse fracture of unspecified patella** CC
CC Excl: See code: S82.009

7,17 √7th **S82.034 Nondisplaced transverse fracture of right patella** CC
CC Excl: See code: S82.001

7,17 √7th **S82.035 Nondisplaced transverse fracture of left patella** CC
CC Excl: See code: S82.002

7,17 √7th **S82.036 Nondisplaced transverse fracture of unspecified patella** CC
CC Excl: See code: S82.009

√6th **S82.04 Comminuted fracture of patella**

7,17 √7th **S82.041 Displaced comminuted fracture of right patella** CC
CC Excl: See code: S82.001

7,17 √7th **S82.042 Displaced comminuted fracture of left patella** CC
CC Excl: See code: S82.002

7,17 √7th **S82.043 Displaced comminuted fracture of unspecified patella** CC
CC Excl: See code: S82.009

7,17 √7th **S82.044 Nondisplaced comminuted fracture of right patella** CC
CC Excl: See code: S82.001

7,17 √7th **S82.045 Nondisplaced comminuted fracture of left patella** CC
CC Excl: See code: S82.002

7,17 √7th **S82.046 Nondisplaced comminuted fracture of unspecified patella** CC
CC Excl: See code: S82.009

√6th **S82.09 Other fracture of patella**

7,17 √7th **S82.091 Other fracture of right patella** CC
CC Excl: See code: S82.001

7,17 √7th **S82.092 Other fracture of left patella** CC
CC Excl: See code: S82.002

7,17 √7th **S82.099 Other fracture of unspecified patella** CC
CC Excl: See code: S82.009

√5th **S82.1 Fracture of upper end of tibia**
Fracture of proximal end of tibia
EXCLUDES2 *fracture of shaft of tibia (S82.2-)*
physeal fracture of upper end of tibia (S89.0-)

√6th **S82.10 Unspecified fracture of upper end of tibia**

7,16,19 √7th **S82.101 Unspecified fracture of upper end of right tibia** MCC CC
CC Excl: CC with 7th character A: M80.00X-M80.019 with 7th A, M80.041-M80.049 with 7th A, M80.061-M80.079 with 7th A, M80.80X-M80.819 with 7th A, M80.841-M80.849 with 7th A, M80.861-M80.879 with 7th A, M84.40X-M84.419 with 7th A, M84.441-M84.446 with 7th A, M84.454 with 7th A, M84.461-M84.519 with 7th A, M84.541-M84.550 with 7th A, M84.561-M84.576 with 7th A, M84.60X-M84.619 with 7th A, M84.641-M84.650 with 7th A, M84.661-M84.68X with 7th A, S03.8XX-S03.9XX with 7th A, S29.011-S29.019 with 7th A, S38.3XX-S39.013 with 7th A, S73.101A, S73.109-S73.111 with 7th A, S73.119-S73.121 with 7th A, S73.129-S73.191 with 7th A, S73.199A, S76.001A, S76.009-S76.011 with 7th A, S76.019A, S76.091A, S76.099-S76.101 with 7th A, S76.109-S76.111 with 7th A, S76.119A, S76.191A, S76.199-S76.201 with 7th A, S76.209-S76.211 with 7th A, S76.219A, S76.291A, S76.299-S76.301 with 7th A, S76.309-S76.311 with 7th A, S76.319A, S76.391A, S76.399-S76.801 with 7th A, S76.809-S76.811 with 7th A, S76.819A, S76.891A, S76.899-S76.901 with 7th A, S76.909-S76.911 with 7th A, S76.919A, S76.991A, S76.999A, S79.811A, S79.819-S79.821 with 7th A, S79.829-S79.911 with 7th A, S79.919-S79.921 with 7th A, S79.929A, S82.101-S82.156 with 7th [A, B, C], S82.191-S82.299 with 7th [A, B, C], S82.401-S82.499 with 7th [A, B, C], S82.831-S82.839 with 7th [A, B, C], S82.861-S82.866 with 7th [A, B, C], S82.90X-S82.92X with 7th [A, B, C], S89.001A, S89.009-S89.011 with 7th A, S89.019-S89.021 with 7th A, S89.029-S89.031 with 7th A, S89.039-S89.041 with 7th A, S89.049-S89.091 with 7th A, S89.099A, S89.201A, S89.209-S89.211 with 7th A, S89.219-S89.221 with 7th A, S89.229-S89.291 with 7th A, S89.299A, T14.90-T14.91, T79.A9X-T79.9XX with 7th A
MCC with 7th B or C: M80.00X-M80.019 with 7th A, M80.041-M80.049 with 7th A, M80.061-M80.079 with 7th A, M80.80X-M80.819 with 7th A, M80.841-M80.849 with 7th A, M80.861-M80.879 with 7th A, M84.40X-M84.419 with 7th A, M84.441-M84.446 with 7th A, M84.454 with 7th A, M84.461-M84.519 with 7th A, M84.541-M84.550 with 7th A, M84.561-M84.576 with 7th A, M84.60X-M84.619 with 7th A, M84.641-M84.650 with 7th A, M84.661-M84.68X with 7th A, S03.8XX-S03.9XX with 7th A, S29.011-S29.019 with 7th A, S38.3X-S39.013 with 7th A, S73.101-S73.199 with 7th A, S76.001-S76.019 with 7th A, S76.091-

---

7 HAC = Initial encounter only (7th character A, B or C) and not POA.
16 MCC only if an open fracture (7th character B or C).
17 CC only if an initial encounter (7th character A, B or C) **OR** a subsequent encounter for nonunion or malunion (7th character K, M, N, P, Q, or R).
19 CC only if an initial encounter for a closed fracture (7th character A) **OR** a subsequent encounter for nonunion or malunion (7th character K, M, N, P, Q, or R).

☑ Additional Character Required   √x7th Placeholder Alert   Unacceptable PDx   Manifestation   Hospital Acquired Condition   EXCLUDES1 Not Coded Here   EXCLUDES2 Not Included Here

ICD-10-CM 2016   1037

S82.01–S82.101

S76.119 with 7th A, S76.191-S76.219 with 7th A, S76.291-S76.319 with 7th A, S76.391-S76.819 with 7th A, S76.891-S76.919 with 7th A, S76.991-S76.999 with 7th A, S79.811-S79.929 with 7th A, S82.101-S82.156 with 7th [A, B, C], S82.191-S82.299 with 7th [A, B, C], S82.401-S82.499 with 7th [A, B, C], S82.831-S82.839 with 7th [A, B, C], S82.861-S82.866 with 7th [A, B, C], S82.90X-S82.92X with 7th [A, B, C], S89.001-S89.099 with 7th A, S89.201-S89.299 with 7th A, T14.90-T14.91, T79.A9X-T79.9XX with 7th A

CC with 7th character K, M, N, P, Q or R: M80.00X-M84.68X with 7th [K, P], S02.0XX-S02.92X with 7th K, S12.000-S12.691 with 7th K, S22.000-S22.9XX with 7th K, S32.000-S32.9XX with 7th K, S42.001-S42.92X with 7th [K, P], S49.001-S49.199 with 7th [K, P], S52.001-S52.92X with 7th [K, M, N, P, Q, R], S59.001-S59.299 with 7th [K, P], S62.001-S62.92X with 7th [K, P], S72.001-S72.92X with 7th [K, M, N, P, Q, R], S79.001-S79.199 with 7th [K, P], S82.001-S82.92X with 7th [K, M, N, P, Q, R], S89.001-S89.399 with 7th [K, P], S92.001-S92.919 with 7th [K, P]

7,16,19 ✓7ᵗʰ **S82.102** **Unspecified fracture of upper end of left tibia** `MCC` `CC`

CC Excl: CC with 7th character A: M80.00X-M80.019 with 7th A, M80.041-M80.049 with 7th A, M80.061-M80.079 with 7th A, M80.80X-M80.819 with 7th A, M80.841-M80.849 with 7th A, M80.861-M80.879 with 7th A, M84.40X-M84.419 with 7th A, M84.441-M84.446 with 7th A, M84.454 with 7th A, M84.461-M84.519 with 7th A, M84.541-M84.550 with 7th A, M84.561-M84.576 with 7th A, M84.60X-M84.619 with 7th A, M84.641-M84.650 with 7th A, M84.661-M84.68 with 7th A, S03.8XX-S03.9XX with 7th A, S29.011-S29.019 with 7th A, S38.3XX-S39.013 with 7th A, S73.102-S73.109 with 7th A, S73.112-S73.119 with 7th A, S73.122-S73.129 with 7th A, S73.192-S73.199 with 7th A, S76.002-S76.009 with 7th A, S76.012-S76.019 with 7th A, S76.092-S76.099 with 7th A, S76.102-S76.109 with 7th A, S76.112-S76.119 with 7th A, S76.192-S76.199 with 7th A, S76.202-S76.209 with 7th A, S76.212-S76.219 with 7th A, S76.292-S76.299 with 7th A, S76.302-S76.309 with 7th A, S76.312-S76.319 with 7th A, S76.392-S76.399 with 7th A, S76.802-S76.809 with 7th A, S76.812-S76.819 with 7th A, S76.892-S76.899 with 7th A, S76.902-S76.909 with 7th A, S76.912-S76.919 with 7th A, S76.992-S76.999 with 7th A, S79.812-S79.819 with 7th A, S79.822-S79.829 with 7th A, S79.912-S79.919 with 7th A, S79.922-S79.929 with 7th A, S82.101-S82.156 with 7th [B, C], S82.191-S82.299 with 7th [B, C], S82.401-S82.499 with 7th [B, C], S82.831-S82.839 with 7th [B, C], S82.861-S82.866 with 7th [B, C], S82.90X-S82.92X with 7th [A, B, C], S89.002-S89.009 with 7th A, S89.012-S89.019 with 7th A, S89.022-S89.029 with 7th A, S89.032-S89.039 with 7th A, S89.042-S89.049 with 7th A, S89.092-S89.099 with 7th A, S89.202-S89.209 with 7th A, S89.212-S89.219 with 7th A, S89.222-S89.229 with 7th A, S89.292-S89.299 with 7th A, T14.90-T14.91, T79.A9X-T79.9XX with 7th A

CC with 7th character K, M, N, P, Q or R: M80.00X-M84.68 with 7th [K, P], S02.0XX-S02.92X with 7th K, S12.000-S12.691 with 7th K, S22.000-S22.9XX with 7th K, S32.000-S32.9XX with 7th K, S42.001-S42.92X with 7th [K, P], S49.001-S49.199 with 7th [K, P], S52.001-S52.92X with 7th [K, M, N, P, Q, R], S59.001-S59.299 with 7th [K, P], S62.001-S62.92X with 7th [K, P], S72.001-S72.92X with 7th [K, M, N, P, Q, R], S79.001-S79.199 with 7th [K, P], S82.001-S82.92X with 7th [K, M, N, P, Q, R], S89.001-S89.399 with 7th [K, P], S92.001-S92.919 with 7th [K, P]

7,16,19 ✓7ᵗʰ **S82.109** **Unspecified fracture of upper end of unspecified tibia** `MCC` `CC`

CC Excl: CC with 7th character A: M80.00X-M80.019 with 7th A, M80.041-M80.049 with 7th A, M80.061-M80.079 with 7th A, M80.80X-M80.819 with 7th A, M80.841-M80.849 with 7th A, M80.861-M80.879 with 7th A, M84.40X-M84.419 with 7th A, M84.441-M84.446 with 7th A, M84.454 with 7th A, M84.461-M84.519 with 7th A, M84.541-M84.550 with 7th A, M84.561-M84.576 with 7th A, M84.60X-M84.619 with 7th A, M84.641-M84.650 with 7th A, M84.661-M84.68 with 7th A, S03.8XX-S03.9XX with 7th A, S29.011-S29.019 with 7th A, S38.3XX-S39.013 with 7th A, S73.101-S73.199 with 7th A, S76.001-S76.019 with 7th A, S76.091-S76.119 with 7th A, S76.191-S76.219 with 7th A, S76.291-S76.319 with 7th A, S76.391-S76.819 with 7th A, S76.891-S76.919 with 7th A, S76.991-S76.999 with 7th A, S79.811-S79.929 with 7th A, S82.101-S82.156 with 7th [A, B, C], S82.191-S82.299 with 7th [A, B, C], S82.401-S82.499 with 7th [A, B, C], S82.831-S82.839 with 7th [A, B, C], S82.861-S82.866 with 7th [A, B, C], S82.90X-S82.92X with 7th [A, B, C], S89.001-S89.099 with 7th A, S89.201-S89.299 with 7th A, T14.90-T14.91, T79.A9X-T79.9XX with 7th A

CC with 7th character K, M, N, P, Q or R: M80.00X-M84.68 with 7th [K, P], S02.0XX-S02.92X with 7th K, S12.000-S12.691 with 7th K, S22.000-S22.9XX with 7th K, S32.000-S32.9XX with 7th K, S42.001-S42.92X with 7th [K, P], S49.001-S49.199 with 7th [K, P], S52.001-S52.92X with 7th [K, M, N, P, Q, R], S59.001-S59.299 with 7th [K, P], S62.001-S62.92X with 7th [K, P], S72.001-S72.92X with 7th [K, M, N, P, Q, R], S79.001-S79.199 with 7th [K, P], S82.001-S82.92X with 7th [K, M, N, P, Q, R], S89.001-S89.399 with 7th [K, P], S92.001-S92.919 with 7th [K, P]

✓6ᵗʰ **S82.11** **Fracture of tibial spine**

7,16,19 ✓7ᵗʰ **S82.111** **Displaced fracture of right tibial spine** `MCC` `CC`
CC Excl: See code: S82.101

7,16,19 ✓7ᵗʰ **S82.112** **Displaced fracture of left tibial spine** `MCC` `CC`
CC Excl: See code: S82.102

7,16,19 ✓7ᵗʰ **S82.113** **Displaced fracture of unspecified tibial spine** `MCC` `CC`
CC Excl: See code: S82.109

7,16,19 ✓7ᵗʰ **S82.114** **Nondisplaced fracture of right tibial spine** `MCC` `CC`
CC Excl: See code: S82.101

7,16,19 ✓7ᵗʰ **S82.115** **Nondisplaced fracture of left tibial spine** `MCC` `CC`
CC Excl: See code: S82.102

7,16,19 ✓7ᵗʰ **S82.116** **Nondisplaced fracture of unspecified tibial spine** `MCC` `CC`
CC Excl: See code: S82.109

✓6ᵗʰ **S82.12** **Fracture of lateral condyle of tibia**

7,16,19 ✓7ᵗʰ **S82.121** **Displaced fracture of lateral condyle of right tibia** `MCC` `CC`
CC Excl: See code: S82.101

7,16,19 ✓7ᵗʰ **S82.122** **Displaced fracture of lateral condyle of left tibia** `MCC` `CC`
CC Excl: See code: S82.102

7,16,19 ✓7ᵗʰ **S82.123** **Displaced fracture of lateral condyle of unspecified tibia** `MCC` `CC`
CC Excl: See code: S82.109

7,16,19 ✓7ᵗʰ **S82.124** **Nondisplaced fracture of lateral condyle of right tibia** `MCC` `CC`
CC Excl: See code: S82.101

7,16,19 ✓7ᵗʰ **S82.125** **Nondisplaced fracture of lateral condyle of left tibia** `MCC` `CC`
CC Excl: See code: S82.102

7,16,19 ✓7ᵗʰ **S82.126** **Nondisplaced fracture of lateral condyle of unspecified tibia** `MCC` `CC`
CC Excl: See code: S82.109

---

7 HAC = Initial encounter only (7th character A, B or C) and not POA.
16 MCC only if an open fracture (7th character B or C).
19 CC only if an initial encounter for a closed fracture (7th character A) **OR** a subsequent encounter for nonunion or malunion (7th character K, M, N, P, Q, or R).

Ⓝ Newborn: 0 Ⓟ Pediatric: 0-17 Ⓜ Maternity: 12-55 Ⓐ Adult: 15-124 `MCC` Major CC Condition `PDxMCC` PDx acts as own MCC `CC` CC Condition `PDxCC` PDx acts as own CC

✓6ᵗʰ **S82.13** Fracture of medial condyle of tibia

7,16,19 ✓7ᵗʰ **S82.131** **Displaced fracture of medial condyle of right tibia** MCC CC
CC Excl: See code: S82.101

7,16,19 ✓7ᵗʰ **S82.132** **Displaced fracture of medial condyle of left tibia** MCC CC
CC Excl: See code: S82.102

7,16,19 ✓7ᵗʰ **S82.133** **Displaced fracture of medial condyle of unspecified tibia** MCC CC
CC Excl: See code: S82.109

7,16,19 ✓7ᵗʰ **S82.134** **Nondisplaced fracture of medial condyle of right tibia** MCC CC
CC Excl: See code: S82.101

7,16,19 ✓7ᵗʰ **S82.135** **Nondisplaced fracture of medial condyle of left tibia** MCC CC
CC Excl: See code: S82.102

7,16,19 ✓7ᵗʰ **S82.136** **Nondisplaced fracture of medial condyle of unspecified tibia** MCC CC
CC Excl: See code: S82.109

✓6ᵗʰ **S82.14** Bicondylar fracture of tibia
Fracture of tibial plateau NOS

7,16,19 ✓7ᵗʰ **S82.141** **Displaced bicondylar fracture of right tibia** MCC CC
CC Excl: See code: S82.101

7,16,19 ✓7ᵗʰ **S82.142** **Displaced bicondylar fracture of left tibia** MCC CC
CC Excl: See code: S82.102

7,16,19 ✓7ᵗʰ **S82.143** **Displaced bicondylar fracture of unspecified tibia** MCC CC
CC Excl: See code: S82.109

7,16,19 ✓7ᵗʰ **S82.144** **Nondisplaced bicondylar fracture of right tibia** MCC CC
CC Excl: See code: S82.101

7,16,19 ✓7ᵗʰ **S82.145** **Nondisplaced bicondylar fracture of left tibia** MCC CC
CC Excl: See code: S82.102

7,16,19 ✓7ᵗʰ **S82.146** **Nondisplaced bicondylar fracture of unspecified tibia** MCC CC
CC Excl: See code: S82.109

✓6ᵗʰ **S82.15** Fracture of tibial tuberosity

7,16,19 ✓7ᵗʰ **S82.151** **Displaced fracture of right tibial tuberosity** MCC CC
CC Excl: See code: S82.101

7,16,19 ✓7ᵗʰ **S82.152** **Displaced fracture of left tibial tuberosity** MCC CC
CC Excl: See code: S82.102

7,16,19 ✓7ᵗʰ **S82.153** **Displaced fracture of unspecified tibial tuberosity** MCC CC
CC Excl: See code: S82.109

7,16,19 ✓7ᵗʰ **S82.154** **Nondisplaced fracture of right tibial tuberosity** MCC CC
CC Excl: See code: S82.101

7,16,19 ✓7ᵗʰ **S82.155** **Nondisplaced fracture of left tibial tuberosity** MCC CC
CC Excl: See code: S82.102

7,16,19 ✓7ᵗʰ **S82.156** **Nondisplaced fracture of unspecified tibial tuberosity** MCC CC
CC Excl: See code: S82.109

✓6ᵗʰ **S82.16** Torus fracture of upper end of tibia

The appropriate 7th character is to be added to all codes in subcategory S82.16.
A   initial encounter for closed fracture
D   subsequent encounter for fracture with routine healing
G   subsequent encounter for fracture with delayed healing
K   subsequent encounter for fracture with nonunion
P   subsequent encounter for fracture with malunion
S   sequela

7,19 ✓7ᵗʰ **S82.161** **Torus fracture of upper end of right tibia** CC
CC Excl: CC with 7th character A: S82.101-S82.161 with 7th [A, B, C], S82.169-S82.299 with 7th A, S82.311A, S82.319A, S82.401-S82.811 with 7th [A, B, C], S82.819-S82.821

with 7th A, S82.829-S82.839 with 7th A, S82.861-S82.866 with 7th [A, B, C], S89.001A, S89.009-S89.011 with 7th A, S89.019-S89.021 with 7th A, S89.029-S89.031 with 7th A, S89.039-S89.041 with 7th A, S89.049-S89.091 with 7th A, S89.099A, S89.201A, S89.209-S89.211 with 7th A, S89.219-S89.221 with 7th A, S89.229-S89.291 with 7th A, S89.299A
CC with 7th character K or P: M80.00X-M84.68X with 7th [K, P], S02.0XX-S02.92X with 7th K, S12.000-S12.691 with 7th K, S22.000-S22.9XX with 7th K, S32.000-S32.9XX with 7th K, S42.001-S42.92X with 7th [K, P], S49.001-S49.199 with 7th [K, P], S52.001-S52.92X with 7th [K, M, N, P, Q, R], S59.001-S59.299 with 7th [K, P], S62.001-S62.92X with 7th [K, P], S72.001-S72.92X with 7th [K, M, N, P, Q, R], S79.001-S79.199 with 7th [K, P], S82.001-S82.92X with 7th [K, M, N, P, Q, R], S89.001-S89.399 with 7th [K, P], S92.001-S92.919 with 7th [K, P]

7,19 ✓7ᵗʰ **S82.162** **Torus fracture of upper end of left tibia** CC
CC Excl: CC with 7th character A: S82.101-S82.156 with 7th [B, C], S82.162-S82.299 with 7th A, S82.312-S82.319 with 7th A, S82.401-S82.499 with 7th [B, C], S82.812-S82.819 with 7th A, S82.822-S82.839 with 7th A, S82.861-S82.866 with 7th [B, C], S89.002-S89.009 with 7th A, S89.012-S89.019 with 7th A, S89.022-S89.029 with 7th A, S89.032-S89.039 with 7th A, S89.042-S89.049 with 7th A, S89.092-S89.099 with 7th A, S89.202-S89.209 with 7th A, S89.212-S89.219 with 7th A, S89.222-S89.229 with 7th A, S89.292-S89.299 with 7th A
CC with 7th character K or P: M80.00X-M84.68X with 7th [K, P], S02.0XX-S02.92X with 7th K, S12.000-S12.691 with 7th K, S22.000-S22.9XX with 7th K, S32.000-S32.9XX with 7th K, S42.001-S42.92X with 7th [K, P], S49.001-S49.199 with 7th [K, P], S52.001-S52.92X with 7th [K, M, N, P, Q, R], S59.001-S59.299 with 7th [K, P], S62.001-S62.92X with 7th [K, P], S72.001-S72.92X with 7th [K, M, N, P, Q, R], S79.001-S79.199 with 7th [K, P], S82.001-S82.92X with 7th [K, M, N, P, Q, R], S89.001-S89.399 with 7th [K, P], S92.001-S92.919 with 7th [K, P]

7,19 ✓7ᵗʰ **S82.169** **Torus fracture of upper end of unspecified tibia** CC
CC Excl: CC with 7th character A: S82.101-S82.299 with 7th [A, B, C], S82.311-S82.319 with 7th A, S82.401-S82.839 with 7th [A, B, C], S82.861-S82.866 with 7th [A, B, C], S89.001-S89.099 with 7th A, S89.201-S89.299 with 7th A
CC with 7th character K or P: M80.00X-M84.68X with 7th [K, P], S02.0XX-S02.92X with 7th K, S12.000-S12.691 with 7th K, S22.000-S22.9XX with 7th K, S32.000-S32.9XX with 7th K, S42.001-S42.92X with 7th [K, P], S49.001-S49.199 with 7th [K, P], S52.001-S52.92X with 7th [K, M, N, P, Q, R], S59.001-S59.299 with 7th [K, P], S62.001-S62.92X with 7th [K, P], S72.001-S72.92X with 7th [K, M, N, P, Q, R], S79.001-S79.199 with 7th [K, P], S82.001-S82.92X with 7th [K, M, N, P, Q, R], S89.001-S89.399 with 7th [K, P], S92.001-S92.919 with 7th [K, P]

✓6ᵗʰ **S82.19** Other fracture of upper end of tibia

7,16,19 ✓7ᵗʰ **S82.191** **Other fracture of upper end of right tibia** MCC CC
CC Excl: See code: S82.101

7,16,19 ✓7ᵗʰ **S82.192** **Other fracture of upper end of left tibia** MCC CC
CC Excl: See code: S82.102

7,16,19 ✓7ᵗʰ **S82.199** **Other fracture of upper end of unspecified tibia** MCC CC
CC Excl: See code: S82.109

---

7   HAC = Initial encounter only (7th character A, B or C) and not POA.
16 MCC only if an open fracture (7th character B or C).
19 CC only if an initial encounter for a closed fracture (7th character A) **OR** a subsequent encounter for nonunion or malunion (7th character K, M, N, P, Q, or R).

✓ Additional Character Required   ✓x7ᵗʰ Placeholder Alert   Unacceptable PDx   Manifestation   Hospital Acquired Condition   EXCLUDES 1 Not Coded Here   EXCLUDES 2 Not Included Here

✓5ᵗʰ S82.2 Fracture of shaft of tibia

    ✓6ᵗʰ S82.20 Unspecified fracture of shaft of tibia
        Fracture of tibia NOS

        7,16,19 ✓7ᵗʰ **S82.201 Unspecified fracture of shaft of right tibia**   `MCC` `CC`

            CC Excl: CC with 7th character A: M80.00X-M80.019 with 7th A, M80.041-M80.049 with 7th A, M80.061-M80.079 with 7th A, M80.80X-M80.819 with 7th A, M80.841-M80.849 with 7th A, M80.861-M80.879 with 7th A, M84.40X-M84.419 with 7th A, M84.441-M84.446 with 7th A, M84.454 with 7th A, M84.461-M84.519 with 7th A, M84.541-M84.550 with 7th A, M84.561-M84.576 with 7th A, M84.60X-M84.619 with 7th A, M84.641-M84.650 with 7th A, M84.661-M84.68 with 7th A, S03.8XX-S03.9XX with 7th A, S29.011-S29.019 with 7th A, S38.3XX-S39.013 with 7th A, S73.101A, S73.109-S73.111 with 7th A, S73.119-S73.121 with 7th A, S73.129-S73.191 with 7th A, S73.199A, S76.001A, S76.009-S76.011 with 7th A, S76.019A, S76.091A, S76.099-S76.101 with 7th A, S76.109-S76.111 with 7th A, S76.119A, S76.191A, S76.199-S76.201 with 7th A, S76.209-S76.211 with 7th A, S76.219A, S76.291A, S76.299-S76.301 with 7th A, S76.309-S76.311 with 7th A, S76.319A, S76.391A, S76.399-S76.801 with 7th A, S76.809-S76.811 with 7th A, S76.819A, S76.891A, S76.899-S76.901 with 7th A, S76.909-S76.911 with 7th A, S76.919A, S76.991A, S76.999A, S79.811A, S79.819-S79.821 with 7th A, S79.829-S79.911 with 7th A, S79.919-S79.921 with 7th A, S79.929A, S82.101-S82.161 with 7th [A, B, C], S82.169-S82.299 with 7th A, S82.311 with 7th A, S82.319 with 7th A, S82.401-S82.811 with 7th [A, B, C], S82.819-S82.821 with 7th A, S82.829-S82.839 with 7th A, S82.861-S82.866 with 7th [A, B, C], S82.90X-S82.92X with 7th [A, B, C], S89.001A, S89.009-S89.011 with 7th A, S89.019-S89.021 with 7th A, S89.029-S89.031 with 7th A, S89.039-S89.041 with 7th A, S89.049-S89.091 with 7th A, S89.099A, S89.201A, S89.209-S89.211 with 7th A, S89.219-S89.221 with 7th A, S89.229-S89.291 with 7th A, S89.299A, T14.90-T14.91, T79.A9X-T79.9XX with 7th A

            MCC with 7th B or C: M80.00X-M80.019 with 7th A, M80.041-M80.049 with 7th A, M80.061-M80.079 with 7th A, M80.80X-M80.819 with 7th A, M80.841-M80.849 with 7th A, M80.861-M80.879 with 7th A, M84.40X-M84.419 with 7th A, M84.441-M84.446 with 7th A, M84.454 with 7th A, M84.461-M84.519 with 7th A, M84.541-M84.550 with 7th A, M84.561-M84.576 with 7th A, M84.60X-M84.619 with 7th A, M84.641-M84.650 with 7th A, M84.661-M84.68 with 7th A, S03.8X-S03.9X with 7th A, S29.011-S29.019 with 7th A, S38.3XX-S39.013 with 7th A, S73.101-S73.199 with 7th A, S76.001-S76.019 with 7th A, S76.091-S76.119 with 7th A, S76.191-S76.219 with 7th A, S76.291-S76.319 with 7th A, S76.391-S76.819 with 7th A, S76.891-S76.919 with 7th A, S76.991-S76.999 with 7th A, S79.811-S79.929 with 7th A, S82.101-S82.156 with 7th [A, B, C], S82.191-S82.299 with 7th [A, B, C], S82.401-S82.499 with 7th [A, B, C], S82.831-S82.839 with 7th [A, B, C], S82.861-S82.866 with 7th [A, B, C], S82.90X-S82.92X with 7th [A, B, C], S89.001-S89.099 with 7th A, S89.201-S89.299 with 7th A, T14.90-T14.91, T79.A9X-T79.9XX with 7th A

            CC with 7th character K, M, N, P, Q or R: M80.00X-M84.68X with 7th [K, P], S02.0XX-S02.92X with 7th K, S12.000-S12.691 with 7th K, S22.000-S22.9XX with 7th K, S32.000-S32.9XX with 7th K, S42.001-S42.92X with 7th [K, P], S49.001-S49.199 with 7th [K, P], S52.001-S52.92X with 7th [K, M, N, P, Q, R], S59.001-S59.299 with 7th [K, P], S62.001-S62.92X with 7th [K, P], S72.001-S72.92X with 7th [K, M, N, P, Q, R], S79.001-S79.199 with 7th [K, P], S82.001-S82.92X with 7th [K, M, N, P, Q, R], S89.001-S89.399 with 7th [K, P], S92.001-S92.919 with 7th [K, P]

7,16,19 ✓7ᵗʰ **S82.202 Unspecified fracture of shaft of left tibia**   `MCC` `CC`
      CC Excl: See code: S82.192

7,16,19 ✓7ᵗʰ **S82.209 Unspecified fracture of shaft of unspecified tibia**   `MCC` `CC`
      CC Excl: See code: S82.199

✓6ᵗʰ S82.22 Transverse fracture of shaft of tibia

7,16,19 ✓7ᵗʰ **S82.221 Displaced transverse fracture of shaft of right tibia**   `MCC` `CC`
      CC Excl: See code: S82.191

7,16,19 ✓7ᵗʰ **S82.222 Displaced transverse fracture of shaft of left tibia**   `MCC` `CC`
      CC Excl: See code: S82.192

7,16,19 ✓7ᵗʰ **S82.223 Displaced transverse fracture of shaft of unspecified tibia**   `MCC` `CC`
      CC Excl: See code: S82.199

7,16,19 ✓7ᵗʰ **S82.224 Nondisplaced transverse fracture of shaft of right tibia**   `MCC` `CC`
      CC Excl: See code: S82.191

7,16,19 ✓7ᵗʰ **S82.225 Nondisplaced transverse fracture of shaft of left tibia**   `MCC` `CC`
      CC Excl: See code: S82.192

7,16,19 ✓7ᵗʰ **S82.226 Nondisplaced transverse fracture of shaft of unspecified tibia**   `MCC` `CC`
      CC Excl: See code: S82.199

✓6ᵗʰ S82.23 Oblique fracture of shaft of tibia

7,16,19 ✓7ᵗʰ **S82.231 Displaced oblique fracture of shaft of right tibia**   `MCC` `CC`
      CC Excl: See code: S82.191

7,16,19 ✓7ᵗʰ **S82.232 Displaced oblique fracture of shaft of left tibia**   `MCC` `CC`
      CC Excl: See code: S82.192

7,16,19 ✓7ᵗʰ **S82.233 Displaced oblique fracture of shaft of unspecified tibia**   `MCC` `CC`
      CC Excl: See code: S82.199

7,16,19 ✓7ᵗʰ **S82.234 Nondisplaced oblique fracture of shaft of right tibia**   `MCC` `CC`
      CC Excl: See code: S82.191

7,16,19 ✓7ᵗʰ **S82.235 Nondisplaced oblique fracture of shaft of left tibia**   `MCC` `CC`
      CC Excl: See code: S82.192

7,16,19 ✓7ᵗʰ **S82.236 Nondisplaced oblique fracture of shaft of unspecified tibia**   `MCC` `CC`
      CC Excl: See code: S82.199

✓6ᵗʰ S82.24 Spiral fracture of shaft of tibia
    Toddler fracture

7,16,19 ✓7ᵗʰ **S82.241 Displaced spiral fracture of shaft of right tibia**   `MCC` `CC`
      CC Excl: See code: S82.191

7,16,19 ✓7ᵗʰ **S82.242 Displaced spiral fracture of shaft of left tibia**   `MCC` `CC`
      CC Excl: See code: S82.192

7,16,19 ✓7ᵗʰ **S82.243 Displaced spiral fracture of shaft of unspecified tibia**   `MCC` `CC`
      CC Excl: See code: S82.199

7,16,19 ✓7ᵗʰ **S82.244 Nondisplaced spiral fracture of shaft of right tibia**   `MCC` `CC`
      CC Excl: See code: S82.191

7,16,19 ✓7ᵗʰ **S82.245 Nondisplaced spiral fracture of shaft of left tibia**   `MCC` `CC`
      CC Excl: See code: S82.192

7,16,19 ✓7ᵗʰ **S82.246 Nondisplaced spiral fracture of shaft of unspecified tibia**   `MCC` `CC`
      CC Excl: See code: S82.199

✓6ᵗʰ S82.25 Comminuted fracture of shaft of tibia

7,16,19 ✓7ᵗʰ **S82.251 Displaced comminuted fracture of shaft of right tibia**   `MCC` `CC`
      CC Excl: See code: S82.191

7,16,19 ✓7ᵗʰ **S82.252 Displaced comminuted fracture of shaft of left tibia**   `MCC` `CC`
      CC Excl: See code: S82.192

7,16,19 ✓7ᵗʰ **S82.253 Displaced comminuted fracture of shaft of unspecified tibia**   `MCC` `CC`
      CC Excl: See code: S82.199

7,16,19 ✓7ᵗʰ **S82.254 Nondisplaced comminuted fracture of shaft of right tibia**   `MCC` `CC`
      CC Excl: See code: S82.191

---

7   HAC = Initial encounter only (7th character A, B or C) and not POA.
16   MCC only if an open fracture (7th character B or C).
19   CC only if an initial encounter for a closed fracture (7th character A) **OR** a subsequent encounter for nonunion or malunion (7th character K, M, N, P, Q, or R).

7,16,19 ✓7ᵗʰ **S82.255** Nondisplaced comminuted fracture of shaft of left tibia   MCC CC
     CC Excl: See code: S82.192

7,16,19 ✓7ᵗʰ **S82.256** Nondisplaced comminuted fracture of shaft of unspecified tibia   MCC CC
     CC Excl: See code: S82.199

✓6ᵗʰ **S82.26** Segmental fracture of shaft of tibia

7,16,19 ✓7ᵗʰ **S82.261** Displaced segmental fracture of shaft of right tibia   MCC CC
     CC Excl: See code: S82.191

7,16,19 ✓7ᵗʰ **S82.262** Displaced segmental fracture of shaft of left tibia   MCC CC
     CC Excl: See code: S82.192

7,16,19 ✓7ᵗʰ **S82.263** Displaced segmental fracture of shaft of unspecified tibia   MCC CC
     CC Excl: See code: S82.199

7,16,19 ✓7ᵗʰ **S82.264** Nondisplaced segmental fracture of shaft of right tibia   MCC CC
     CC Excl: See code: S82.191

7,16,19 ✓7ᵗʰ **S82.265** Nondisplaced segmental fracture of shaft of left tibia   MCC CC
     CC Excl: See code: S82.192

7,16,19 ✓7ᵗʰ **S82.266** Nondisplaced segmental fracture of shaft of unspecified tibia   MCC CC
     CC Excl: See code: S82.199

✓6ᵗʰ **S82.29** Other fracture of shaft of tibia

7,16,19 ✓7ᵗʰ **S82.291** Other fracture of shaft of right tibia   MCC CC
     CC Excl: See code: S82.191

7,16,19 ✓7ᵗʰ **S82.292** Other fracture of shaft of left tibia   MCC CC
     CC Excl: See code: S82.192

7,16,19 ✓7ᵗʰ **S82.299** Other fracture of shaft of unspecified tibia   MCC CC
     CC Excl: See code: S82.199

✓5ᵗʰ **S82.3** Fracture of lower end of tibia
     EXCLUDES 1   bimalleolar fracture of lower leg (S82.84-)
             fracture of medial malleolus alone (S82.5-)
             Maisonneuve's fracture (S82.86-)
             pilon fracture of distal tibia (S82.87-)
             trimalleolar fractures of lower leg (S82.85-)

✓6ᵗʰ **S82.30** Unspecified fracture of lower end of tibia

CC Excl: For CC codes in subcategory S82.30, unless otherwise noted: CC with 7th character B or C: M80.00X-M80.019 with 7th A, M80.041-M80.049 with 7th A, M80.061-M80.079 with 7th A, M80.80X-M80.819 with 7th A, M80.841-M80.849 with 7th A, M80.861-M80.879 with 7th A, M84.40X-M84.419 with 7th A, M84.441-M84.446 with 7th A, M84.454 with 7th A, M84.461-M84.519 with 7th A, M84.541-M84.550 with 7th A, M84.561-M84.576 with 7th A, M84.60X-M84.619 with 7th A, M84.641-M84.650 with 7th A, M84.661-M84.68 with 7th A, S03.8XX-S03.9XX with 7th A, S29.011-S29.019 with 7th A, S38.3XX-S39.013 with 7th A, S73.101-S73.199 with 7th A, S76.001-S76.019 with 7th A, S76.091-S76.119 with 7th A, S76.191-S76.219 with 7th A, S76.291-S76.319 with 7th A, S76.391-S76.819 with 7th A, S76.891-S76.919 with 7th A, S76.991-S76.999 with 7th A, S79.811-S79.929 with 7th A, S82.301-S82.309 with 7th [A, B, C], S82.391-S82.399 with 7th [A, B, C], S82.51X-S82.66X with 7th [B, C], S82.841-S82.856 with 7th [A, B, C], S82.871-S82.92X with 7th [B, C], S89.101-S89.199 with 7th A, S89.301-S89.399 with 7th A, T14.90-T14.91, T79.A9X-T79.9XX with 7th A
CC with 7th character K, M, N, P, Q or R: M80.00X-M84.68X with 7th [K, P], S02.0XX-S02.92X with 7th K, S12.000-S12.691 with 7th K, S22.000-S22.9XX with 7th K, S32.000-S32.9XX with 7th K, S42.001-S42.92X with 7th [K, P], S49.001-S49.199 with 7th [K, P], S52.001-S52.92X with 7th [K, M, N, P, Q, R], S59.001-S59.299 with 7th [K, P], S62.001-S62.92X with 7th [K, P], S72.001-S72.92X with 7th [K, M, N, P, Q, R], S79.001-S79.199 with 7th [K, P], S82.001-S82.92X with 7th [K, M, N, P, Q, R], S89.001-S89.399 with 7th [K, P], S92.001-S92.919 with 7th [K, P]

15,20 ✓7ᵗʰ **S82.301** Unspecified fracture of lower end of right tibia   CC

15,20 ✓7ᵗʰ **S82.302** Unspecified fracture of lower end of left tibia   CC

15,20 ✓7ᵗʰ **S82.309** Unspecified fracture of lower end of unspecified tibia   CC

✓6ᵗʰ **S82.31** Torus fracture of lower end of tibia

The appropriate 7th character is to be added to all codes in subcategory S82.31.
A   initial encounter for closed fracture
D   subsequent encounter for fracture with routine healing
G   subsequent encounter for fracture with delayed healing
K   subsequent encounter for fracture with nonunion
P   subsequent encounter for fracture with malunion
S   sequela

7,19 ✓7ᵗʰ **S82.311** Torus fracture of lower end of right tibia   CC

CC Excl: CC with 7th character A: S82.101-S82.161 with 7th [A, B, C], S82.169-S82.299 with 7th A, S82.311 with 7th A, S82.319 with 7th A, S82.401-S82.811 with 7th [A, B, C], S82.819-S82.821 with 7th A, S82.829-S82.839 with 7th A, S82.861-S82.866 with 7th [A, B, C], S89.001 with 7th A, S89.009-S89.011 with 7th A, S89.019-S89.021 with 7th A, S89.029-S89.031 with 7th A, S89.039-S89.041 with 7th A, S89.049-S89.091 with 7th A, S89.099A, S89.201A, S89.209-S89.211 with 7th A, S89.219-S89.221 with 7th A, S89.229-S89.291 with 7th A, S89.299A
CC with 7th character K or P: M80.00X-M84.68X with 7th [K, P], S02.0XX-S02.92X with 7th K, S12.000-S12.691 with 7th K, S22.000-S22.9XX with 7th K, S32.000-S32.9XX with 7th K, S42.001-S42.92X with 7th [K, P], S49.001-S49.199 with 7th [K, P], S52.001-S52.92X with 7th [K, M, N, P, Q, R], S59.001-S59.299 with 7th [K, P], S62.001-S62.92X with 7th [K, P], S72.001-S72.92X with 7th [K, M, N, P, Q, R], S79.001-S79.199 with 7th [K, P], S82.001-S82.92X with 7th [K, M, N, P, Q, R], S89.001-S89.399 with 7th [K, P], S92.001-S92.919 with 7th [K, P]

7,19 ✓7ᵗʰ **S82.312** Torus fracture of lower end of left tibia   CC

CC Excl: CC with 7th character A: S82.101-S82.156 with 7th [B, C], S82.162-S82.299 with 7th A, S82.312-S82.319 with 7th A, S82.401-S82.499 with 7th [B, C], S82.812-S82.819 with 7th A, S82.822-S82.839 with 7th A, S82.861-S82.866 with 7th [B, C], S89.002-S89.009 with 7th A, S89.012-S89.019 with 7th A, S89.022-S89.029 with 7th A, S89.032-S89.039 with 7th A, S89.042-S89.049 with 7th A, S89.092-S89.099 with 7th A, S89.202-S89.209 with 7th A, S89.212-S89.219 with 7th A, S89.222-S89.229 with 7th A, S89.292-S89.299 with 7th A
CC with 7th character K or P: M80.00X-M84.68X with 7th [K, P], S02.0XX-S02.92X with 7th K, S12.000-S12.691 with 7th K, S22.000-S22.9XX with 7th K, S32.000-S32.9XX with 7th K, S42.001-S42.92X with 7th [K, P], S49.001-S49.199 with 7th [K, P], S52.001-S52.92X with 7th [K, M, N, P, Q, R], S59.001-S59.299 with 7th [K, P], S62.001-S62.92X with 7th [K, P], S72.001-S72.92X with 7th [K, M, N, P, Q, R], S79.001-S79.199 with 7th [K, P], S82.001-S82.92X with 7th [K, M, N, P, Q, R], S89.001-S89.399 with 7th [K, P], S92.001-S92.919 with 7th [K, P]

---

7   HAC = Initial encounter only (7th character A, B or C) and not POA.
15   HAC = Initial encounter for open fracture only (7th character B or C) and not POA.
16   MCC only if an open fracture (7th character B or C).
19   CC only if an initial encounter for a closed fracture (7th character A) **OR** a subsequent encounter for nonunion or malunion (7th character K, M, N, P, Q, or R).
20   CC only if an initial encounter for an open fracture (7th character B or C) **OR** a subsequent encounter for nonunion or malunion (7th character K, M, N, P, Q, or R).

✓ Additional Character Required   ✓x7ᵗʰ Placeholder Alert   Unacceptable PDx   Manifestation   Hospital Acquired Condition   EXCLUDES 1 Not Coded Here   EXCLUDES 2 Not Included Here

7,19 √7ᵗʰ **S82.319** **Torus fracture of lower end of unspecified tibia** CC

    CC Excl: CC with 7th character A: S82.101-S82.299 with 7th [A, B, C], S82.311-S82.319 with 7th A, S82.401-S82.839 with 7th [A, B, C], S82.861-S82.866 with 7th [A, B, C], S89.001-S89.099 with 7th A, S89.201-S89.299 with 7th A

    CC with 7th character K or P: M80.00X-M84.68X with 7th [K, P], S02.0XX-S02.92X with 7th K, S12.000-S12.691 with 7th K, S22.000-S22.9XX with 7th K, S32.000-S32.9XX with 7th [K, P], S42.001-S42.92X with 7th [K, P], S49.001-S49.199 with 7th [K, P], S52.001-S52.92X with 7th [K, M, N, P, Q, R], S59.001-S59.299 with 7th [K, P], S62.001-S62.92X with 7th [K, P], S72.001-S72.92X with 7th [K, M, N, P, Q, R], S79.001-S79.199 with 7th [K, P], S82.001-S82.92X with 7th [K, M, N, P, Q, R], S89.001-S89.399 with 7th [K, P], S92.001-S92.919 with 7th [K, P]

√6ᵗʰ **S82.39** **Other fracture of lower end of tibia**
    AHA: 2015, 1Q, 25

    CC Excl: For CC codes in subcategory S82.39, unless otherwise noted: See code: S82.30

15,20 √7ᵗʰ **S82.391** **Other fracture of lower end of right tibia** CC

15,20 √7ᵗʰ **S82.392** **Other fracture of lower end of left tibia** CC

15,20 √7ᵗʰ **S82.399** **Other fracture of lower end of unspecified tibia** CC

√5ᵗʰ **S82.4** **Fracture of shaft of fibula**
    EXCLUDES 2 fracture of lateral malleolus alone (S82.6-)

    CC Excl: For CC codes in subcategory S82.4, unless otherwise noted: MCC for codes with 7th B or C: M80.00X-M80.019 with 7th A, M80.041-M80.049 with 7th A, M80.061-M80.079 with 7th A, M80.80X-M80.819 with 7th A, M80.841-M80.849 with 7th A, M80.861-M80.879 with 7th A, M84.40X-M84.419 with 7th A, M84.441-M84.446 with 7th A, M84.454 with 7th A, M84.461-M84.519 with 7th A, M84.541-M84.550 with 7th A, M84.561-M84.576 with 7th A, M84.60X-M84.619 with 7th A, M84.641-M84.650 with 7th A, M84.661-M84.68 with 7th A, S03.8XX-S03.9XX with 7th A, S29.011-S29.019 with 7th A, S38.3XX-S39.013 with 7th A, S73.101-S73.199 with 7th A, S76.001-S76.019 with 7th A, S76.091-S76.119 with 7th A, S76.191-S76.219 with 7th A, S76.291-S76.319 with 7th A, S76.391-S76.819 with 7th A, S76.891-S76.919 with 7th A, S76.991-S76.999 with 7th A, S79.811-S79.929 with 7th A, S82.101-S82.156 with 7th [A, B, C], S82.191-S82.299 with 7th [A, B, C], S82.401-S82.499 with 7th [A, B, C], S82.831-S82.839 with 7th [A, B, C], S82.861-S82.866 with 7th [A, B, C], S82.90X-S82.92X with 7th [A, B, C], S89.001-S89.099 with 7th A, S89.201-S89.299 with 7th A, T14.90-T14.91, T79.A9X-T79.9XX with 7th A

    CC with 7th character K, M, N, P, Q or R: M80.00X-M84.68X with 7th [K, P], S02.0XX-S02.92X with 7th K, S12.000-S12.691 with 7th K, S22.000-S22.9XX with 7th K, S32.000-S32.9XX with 7th K, S42.001-S42.92X with 7th [K, P], S49.001-S49.199 with 7th [K, P], S52.001-S52.92X with 7th [K, M, N, P, Q, R], S59.001-S59.299 with 7th [K, P], S62.001-S62.92X with 7th [K, P], S72.001-S72.92X with 7th [K, M, N, P, Q, R], S79.001-S79.199 with 7th [K, P], S82.001-S82.92X with 7th [K, M, N, P, Q, R], S89.001-S89.399 with 7th [K, P], S92.001-S92.919 with 7th [K, P]

√6ᵗʰ **S82.40** **Unspecified fracture of shaft of fibula**

15,16,18 √7ᵗʰ **S82.401** **Unspecified fracture of shaft of right fibula** MCC CC

15,16,18 √7ᵗʰ **S82.402** **Unspecified fracture of shaft of left fibula** MCC CC

15,16,18 √7ᵗʰ **S82.409** **Unspecified fracture of shaft of unspecified fibula** MCC CC

√6ᵗʰ **S82.42** **Transverse fracture of shaft of fibula**

15,16,18 √7ᵗʰ **S82.421** **Displaced transverse fracture of shaft of right fibula** MCC CC

15,16,18 √7ᵗʰ **S82.422** **Displaced transverse fracture of shaft of left fibula** MCC CC

15,16,18 √7ᵗʰ **S82.423** **Displaced transverse fracture of shaft of unspecified fibula** MCC CC

15,16,18 √7ᵗʰ **S82.424** **Nondisplaced transverse fracture of shaft of right fibula** MCC CC

15,16,18 √7ᵗʰ **S82.425** **Nondisplaced transverse fracture of shaft of left fibula** MCC CC

15,16,18 √7ᵗʰ **S82.426** **Nondisplaced transverse fracture of shaft of unspecified fibula** MCC CC

√6ᵗʰ **S82.43** **Oblique fracture of shaft of fibula**

15,16,18 √7ᵗʰ **S82.431** **Displaced oblique fracture of shaft of right fibula** MCC CC

15,16,18 √7ᵗʰ **S82.432** **Displaced oblique fracture of shaft of left fibula** MCC CC

15,16,18 √7ᵗʰ **S82.433** **Displaced oblique fracture of shaft of unspecified fibula** MCC CC

15,16,18 √7ᵗʰ **S82.434** **Nondisplaced oblique fracture of shaft of right fibula** MCC CC

15,16,18 √7ᵗʰ **S82.435** **Nondisplaced oblique fracture of shaft of left fibula** MCC CC

15,16,18 √7ᵗʰ **S82.436** **Nondisplaced oblique fracture of shaft of unspecified fibula** MCC CC

√6ᵗʰ **S82.44** **Spiral fracture of shaft of fibula**

15,16,18 √7ᵗʰ **S82.441** **Displaced spiral fracture of shaft of right fibula** MCC CC

15,16,18 √7ᵗʰ **S82.442** **Displaced spiral fracture of shaft of left fibula** MCC CC

15,16,18 √7ᵗʰ **S82.443** **Displaced spiral fracture of shaft of unspecified fibula** MCC CC

15,16,18 √7ᵗʰ **S82.444** **Nondisplaced spiral fracture of shaft of right fibula** MCC CC

15,16,18 √7ᵗʰ **S82.445** **Nondisplaced spiral fracture of shaft of left fibula** MCC CC

15,16,18 √7ᵗʰ **S82.446** **Nondisplaced spiral fracture of sahft of unspecified fibula** MCC CC

√6ᵗʰ **S82.45** **Comminuted fracture of shaft of fibula**

15,16,18 √7ᵗʰ **S82.451** **Displaced comminuted fracture of shaft of right fibula** MCC CC

15,16,18 √7ᵗʰ **S82.452** **Displaced comminuted fracture of shaft of left fibula** MCC CC

15,16,18 √7ᵗʰ **S82.453** **Displaced comminuted fracture of shaft of unspecified fibula** MCC CC

15,16,18 √7ᵗʰ **S82.454** **Nondisplaced comminuted fracture of shaft of right fibula** MCC CC

15,16,18 √7ᵗʰ **S82.455** **Nondisplaced comminuted fracture of shaft of left fibula** MCC CC

15,16,18 √7ᵗʰ **S82.456** **Nondisplaced comminuted fracture of shaft of unspecified fibula** MCC CC

√6ᵗʰ **S82.46** **Segmental fracture of shaft of fibula**

15,16,18 √7ᵗʰ **S82.461** **Displaced segmental fracture of shaft of right fibula** MCC CC

15,16,18 √7ᵗʰ **S82.462** **Displaced segmental fracture of shaft of left fibula** MCC CC

15,16,18 √7ᵗʰ **S82.463** **Displaced segmental fracture of shaft of unspecified fibula** MCC CC

15,16,18 √7ᵗʰ **S82.464** **Nondisplaced segmental fracture of shaft of right fibula** MCC CC

15,16,18 √7ᵗʰ **S82.465** **Nondisplaced segmental fracture of shaft of left fibula** MCC CC

15,16,18 √7ᵗʰ **S82.466** **Nondisplaced segmental fracture of shaft of unspecified fibula** MCC CC

√6ᵗʰ **S82.49** **Other fracture of shaft of fibula**

15,16,18 √7ᵗʰ **S82.491** **Other fracture of shaft of right fibula** MCC CC

15,16,18 √7ᵗʰ **S82.492** **Other fracture of shaft of left fibula** MCC CC

15,16,18 √7ᵗʰ **S82.499** **Other fracture of shaft of unspecified fibula** MCC CC

---

7   HAC = Initial encounter only (7th character A, B or C) and not POA.
15   HAC = Initial encounter for open fracture only (7th character B or C) and not POA.
16   MCC only if an open fracture (7th character B or C).
18   CC only if a subsequent encounter for nonunion or malunion (7th character K, M, N, P, Q, or R).
19   CC only if an initial encounter for a closed fracture (7th character A) **OR** a subsequent encounter for nonunion or malunion (7th character K, M, N, P, Q, or R).
20   CC only if an initial encounter for an open fracture (7th character B or C) **OR** a subsequent encounter for nonunion or malunion (7th character K, M, N, P, Q, or R).

Ⓝ Newborn: 0   Ⓟ Pediatric: 0-17   Ⓜ Maternity: 12-55   Ⓐ Adult: 15-124   MCC Major CC Condition   PDxMCC PDx acts as own MCC   CC CC Condition   PDxCC PDx acts as own CC

✓5ᵗʰ **S82.5 Fracture of** medial malleolus

EXCLUDES 1 *pilon fracture of distal tibia (S82.87-)*
Salter-Harris type III of lower end of tibia (S89.13-)
Salter-Harris type IV of lower end of tibia (S89.14-)

CC Excl: For CC codes in subcategory S82.5, unless otherwise noted: CC with 7th character B or C: M80.00X-M80.019 with 7th A, M80.041-M80.049 with 7th A, M80.061-M80.079 with 7th A, M80.80X-M80.819 with 7th A, M80.841-M80.849 with 7th A, M80.861-M80.879 with 7th A, M84.40X-M84.419 with 7th A, M84.441-M84.446 with 7th A, M84.454 with 7th A, M84.461-M84.519 with 7th A, M84.541-M84.550 with 7th A, M84.561-M84.576 with 7th A, M84.60X-M84.619 with 7th A, M84.641-M84.650 with 7th A, M84.661-M84.68X with 7th A, S03.8XX-S03.9XX with 7th A, S29.011-S29.019 with 7th A, S38.3XX-S39.013 with 7th A, S73.101-S73.199 with 7th A, S76.001-S76.019 with 7th A, S76.091-S76.119 with 7th A, S76.191-S76.219 with 7th A, S76.291-S76.319 with 7th A, S76.391-S76.819 with 7th A, S76.891-S76.919 with 7th A, S76.991-S76.999 with 7th A, S79.811-S79.929 with 7th A, S82.301-S82.309 with 7th [A, B, C], S82.391-S82.399 with 7th [A, B, C], S82.51X-S82.66X with 7th [B, C], S82.841-S82.856 with 7th [A, B, C], S82.871-S82.92X with 7th [B, C], S89.101-S89.199 with 7th A, S89.301-S89.399 with 7th A, T14.90-T14.91, T79.A9X-T79.9XX with 7th A

CC with 7th character K, M, N, P, Q or R: M80.00X-M84.68X with 7th [K, P], S02.0XX-S02.92X with 7th K, S12.000-S12.691 with 7th K, S22.000-S22.9XX with 7th K, S32.000-S32.9XX with 7th K, S42.001-S42.92X with 7th [K, P], S49.001-S49.199 with 7th [K, P], S52.001-S52.92X with 7th [K, M, N, P, Q, R], S59.001-S59.299 with 7th [K, P], S62.001-S62.92X with 7th [K, P], S72.001-S72.92X with 7th [K, M, N, P, Q, R], S79.001-S79.199 with 7th [K, P], S82.001-S82.92X with 7th [K, M, N, P, Q, R], S89.001-S89.399 with 7th [K, P], S92.001-S92.919 with 7th [K, P]

15,20 ✓x7ᵗʰ **S82.51 Displaced fracture of medial malleolus of right tibia**   CC

15,20 ✓x7ᵗʰ **S82.52 Displaced fracture of medial malleolus of left tibia**   CC

15,20 ✓x7ᵗʰ **S82.53 Displaced fracture of medial malleolus of unspecified tibia**   CC

15,20 ✓x7ᵗʰ **S82.54 Nondisplaced fracture of medial malleolus of right tibia**   CC

15,20 ✓x7ᵗʰ **S82.55 Nondisplaced fracture of medial malleolus of left tibia**   CC

15,20 ✓x7ᵗʰ **S82.56 Nondisplaced fracture of medial malleolus of unspecified tibia**   CC

✓5ᵗʰ **S82.6 Fracture of** lateral malleolus

EXCLUDES 1 *pilon fracture of distal tibia (S82.87-)*

CC Excl: For CC codes in subcategory S82.6, unless otherwise noted: CC with 7th character B or C: M80.00X-M80.019 with 7th A, M80.041-M80.049 with 7th A, M80.061-M80.079 with 7th A, M80.80X-M80.819 with 7th A, M80.841-M80.849 with 7th A, M80.861-M80.879 with 7th A, M84.40X-M84.419 with 7th A, M84.441-M84.446 with 7th A, M84.454 with 7th A, M84.461-M84.519 with 7th A, M84.541-M84.550 with 7th A, M84.561-M84.576 with 7th A, M84.60X-M84.619 with 7th A, M84.641-M84.650 with 7th A, M84.661-M84.68X with 7th A, S03.8XX-S03.9XX with 7th A, S29.011-S29.019 with 7th A, S38.3XX-S39.013 with 7th A, S73.101-S73.199 with 7th A, S76.001-S76.019 with 7th A, S76.091-S76.119 with 7th A, S76.191-S76.219 with 7th A, S76.291-S76.319 with 7th A, S76.391-S76.819 with 7th A, S76.891-S76.919 with 7th A, S76.991-S76.999 with 7th A, S79.811-S79.929 with 7th A, S82.301-S82.309 with 7th [A, B, C], S82.391-S82.399 with 7th [A, B, C], S82.51X-S82.66X with 7th [B, C], S82.841-S82.856 with 7th [A, B, C], S82.871-S82.92X with 7th [B, C], S89.101-S89.199 with 7th A, S89.301-S89.399 with 7th A, T14.90-T14.91, T79.A9X-T79.9XX with 7th A

CC with 7th character K, M, N, P, Q or R: M80.00X-M84.68X with 7th [K, P], S02.0XX-S02.92X with 7th K, S12.000-S12.691 with 7th K, S22.000-S22.9XX with 7th K, S32.000-S32.9XX with 7th K, S42.001-S42.92X with 7th [K, P], S49.001-S49.199 with 7th [K, P], S52.001-S52.92X with 7th [K, M, N, P, Q, R], S59.001-S59.299 with 7th [K, P], S62.001-S62.92X with 7th [K, P], S72.001-S72.92X with 7th [K, M, N, P, Q, R], S79.001-S79.199 with 7th [K, P], S82.001-S82.92X with 7th [K, M, N, P, Q, R], S89.001-S89.399 with 7th [K, P], S92.001-S92.919 with 7th [K, P]

15,20 ✓x7ᵗʰ **S82.61 Displaced fracture of lateral malleolus of right fibula**   CC

15,20 ✓x7ᵗʰ **S82.62 Displaced fracture of lateral malleolus of left fibula**   CC

15,20 ✓x7ᵗʰ **S82.63 Displaced fracture of lateral malleolus of unspecified fibula**   CC

15,20 ✓x7ᵗʰ **S82.64 Nondisplaced fracture of lateral malleolus of right fibula**   CC

15,20 ✓x7ᵗʰ **S82.65 Nondisplaced fracture of lateral malleolus of left fibula**   CC

15,20 ✓x7ᵗʰ **S82.66 Nondisplaced fracture of lateral malleolus of unspecified fibula**   CC

✓5ᵗʰ **S82.8 Other fractures of** lower leg

✓6ᵗʰ **S82.81 Torus fracture of** upper end of fibula

The appropriate 7th character is to be added to all codes in subcategory S82.81.
A   initial encounter for closed fracture
D   subsequent encounter for fracture with routine healing
G   subsequent encounter for fracture with delayed healing
K   subsequent encounter for fracture wit nonunion
P   subsequent encounter for fracture with malunion
S   sequela

CC Excl: For codes in subcatgory S82.81, unless otherwise noted: CC with 7th character K or P: See code S82.6

18 ✓7ᵗʰ **S82.811 Torus fracture of upper end of right fibula**   CC

18 ✓7ᵗʰ **S82.812 Torus fracture of upper end of left fibula**   CC

18 ✓7ᵗʰ **S82.819 Torus fracture of upper end of unspecified fibula**   CC

✓6ᵗʰ **S82.82 Torus fracture of** lower end of fibula

The appropriate 7th character is to be added to all codes in subcategory S82.82.
A   initial encounter for closed fracture
D   subsequent encounter for fracture with routine healing
G   subsequent encounter for fracture with delayed healing
K   subsequent encounter for fracture with nonunion
P   subsequent encounter for fracture with malunion
S   sequela

CC Excl: For codes in subcatgory S82.82, unless otherwise noted: CC with 7th character K or P: See code: S82.6

18 ✓7ᵗʰ **S82.821 Torus fracture of lower end of right fibula**   CC

18 ✓7ᵗʰ **S82.822 Torus fracture of lower end of left fibula**   CC

18 ✓7ᵗʰ **S82.829 Torus fracture of lower end of unspecified fibula**   CC

---

15 HAC = Initial encounter for open fracture only (7th character B or C) and not POA.
18 CC only if a subsequent encounter for nonunion or malunion (7th character K, M, N, P, Q, or R).
20 CC only if an initial encounter for an open fracture (7th character B or C) **OR** a subsequent encounter for nonunion or malunion (7th character K, M, N, P, Q, or R).

✓ Additional Character Required   ✓x7ᵗʰ Placeholder Alert   Unacceptable PDx   Manifestation   Hospital Acquired Condition   **EXCLUDES 1** Not Coded Here   **EXCLUDES 2** Not Included Here

√6ᵗʰ **S82.83**   **Other fracture of upper and lower end of fibula**
AHA: 2015, 1Q, 25

> **CC Excl:** For codes in subcatgory S82.83, unless otherwise noted: MCC with 7th B or C: M80.00X-M80.019 with 7th A, M80.041-M80.049 with 7th A, M80.061-M80.079 with 7th A, M80.80X-M80.819 with 7th A, M80.841-M80.849 with 7th A, M80.861-M80.879 with 7th A, M84.40X-M84.419 with 7th A, M84.441-M84.446 with 7th A, M84.454 with 7th A, M84.461-M84.519 with 7th A, M84.541-M84.550 with 7th A, M84.561-M84.576 with 7th A, M84.60X-M84.619 with 7th A, M84.641-M84.650 with 7th A, M84.661-M84.68X with 7th A, S03.8XX-S03.9XX with 7th A, S29.011-S29.019 with 7th A, S38.3XX-S39.013 with 7th A, S73.101-S73.199 with 7th A, S76.001-S76.019 with 7th A, S76.091-S76.119 with 7th A, S76.191-S76.219 with 7th A, S76.291-S76.319 with 7th A, S76.391-S76.819 with 7th A, S76.891-S76.919 with 7th A, S76.991-S76.999 with 7th A, S79.811-S79.929 with 7th A, S82.101-S82.156 with 7th [A, B, C], S82.191-S82.299 with 7th [A, B, C], S82.401-S82.499 with 7th [A, B, C], S82.831-S82.839 with 7th [A, B, C], S82.861-S82.866 with 7th [A, B, C], S82.90X-S82.92X with 7th [A, B, C], S89.001-S89.099 with 7th A, S89.201-S89.299 with 7th A, T14.90-T14.91, T79.A9X-T79.9XX with 7th A
>
> **CC with 7th character K, M, N, P, Q or R:** M80.00X-M84.68X with 7th [K, P], S02.0XX-S02.92X with 7th [K, P], S12.000-S12.691 with 7th K, S22.000-S22.9XX with 7th K, S32.000-S32.9XX with 7th K, S42.001-S42.92X with 7th [K, P], S49.001-S49.199 with 7th [K, P], S52.001-S52.92X with 7th [K, M, N, P, Q, R], S59.001-S59.299 with 7th [K, P], S62.001-S62.92X with 7th [K, P], S72.001-S72.92X with 7th [K, M, N, P, Q, R], S79.001-S79.199 with 7th [K, P], S82.001-S82.92X with 7th [K, M, N, P, Q, R], S89.001-S89.399 with 7th [K, P], S92.001-S92.919 with 7th [K, P]

15,16,18 √7ᵗʰ **S82.831**   **Other fracture of upper and lower end of right fibula**   MCC CC

15,16,18 √7ᵗʰ **S82.832**   **Other fracture of upper and lower end of left fibula**   MCC CC

15,16,18 √7ᵗʰ **S82.839**   **Other fracture of upper and lower end of unspecified fibula**   MCC CC

√6ᵗʰ **S82.84**   **Bimalleolar fracture of lower leg**

> **CC Excl:** For codes in subcatgory S82.84, unless otherwise noted: CC with 7th character B or C: M80.00X-M80.019 with 7th A, M80.041-M80.049 with 7th A, M80.061-M80.079 with 7th A, M80.80X-M80.819 with 7th A, M80.841-M80.849 with 7th A, M80.861-M80.879 with 7th A, M84.40X-M84.419 with 7th A, M84.441-M84.446 with 7th A, M84.454 with 7th A, M84.461-M84.519 with 7th A, M84.541-M84.550 with 7th A, M84.561-M84.576 with 7th A, M84.60X-M84.619 with 7th A, M84.641-M84.650 with 7th A, M84.661-M84.68 with 7th A, S03.8XX-S03.9XX with 7th A, S29.011-S29.019 with 7th A, S38.3XX-S39.013 with 7th A, S73.101-S73.199 with 7th A, S76.001-S76.019 with 7th A, S76.091-S76.119 with 7th A, S76.191-S76.219 with 7th A, S76.291-S76.319 with 7th A, S76.391-S76.819 with 7th A, S76.891-S76.919 with 7th A, S76.991-S76.999 with 7th A, S79.811-S79.929 with 7th A, S82.301-S82.309 with 7th [A, B, C], S82.391-S82.399 with 7th [A, B, C], S82.51X-S82.66X with 7th [B, C], S82.841-S82.856 with 7th [A, B, C], S82.871-S82.92X with 7th [B, C], S89.101-S89.199 with 7th A, S89.301-S89.399 with 7th A, T14.90-T14.91, T79.A9X-T79.9XX with 7th A
>
> **CC with 7th character K, M, N, P, Q or R:** M80.00X-M84.68X with 7th [K, P], S02.0XX-S02.92X with 7th K, S12.000-S12.691 with 7th K, S22.000-S22.9XX with 7th K, S32.000-S32.9XX with 7th K, S42.001-S42.92X with 7th [K, P], S49.001-S49.199 with 7th [K, P], S52.001-S52.92X with 7th [K, M, N, P, Q, R], S59.001-S59.299 with 7th [K, P], S62.001-S62.92X with 7th [K, P], S72.001-S72.92X with 7th [K, M, N, P, Q, R], S79.001-S79.199 with 7th [K, P], S82.001-S82.92X with 7th [K, M, N, P, Q, R], S89.001-S89.399 with 7th [K, P], S92.001-S92.919 with 7th [K, P]

15,20 √7ᵗʰ **S82.841**   **Displaced bimalleolar fracture of right lower leg**   CC

15,20 √7ᵗʰ **S82.842**   **Displaced bimalleolar fracture of left lower leg**   CC

15,20 √7ᵗʰ **S82.843**   **Displaced bimalleolar fracture of unspecified lower leg**   CC

15,20 √7ᵗʰ **S82.844**   **Nondisplaced bimalleolar fracture of right lower leg**   CC

15,20 √7ᵗʰ **S82.845**   **Nondisplaced bimalleolar fracture of left lower leg**   CC

15,20 √7ᵗʰ **S82.846**   **Nondisplaced bimalleolar fracture of unspecified lower leg**   CC

√6ᵗʰ **S82.85**   **Trimalleolar fracture of lower leg**

> **CC Excl:** For codes in subcatgory S82.85, unless otherwise noted: See code: S82.84

15,20 √7ᵗʰ **S82.851**   **Displaced trimalleolar fracture of right lower leg**   CC

15,20 √7ᵗʰ **S82.852**   **Displaced trimalleolar fracture of left lower leg**   CC

15,20 √7ᵗʰ **S82.853**   **Displaced trimalleolar fracture of unspecified lower leg**   CC

15,20 √7ᵗʰ **S82.854**   **Nondisplaced trimalleolar fracture of right lower leg**   CC

15,20 √7ᵗʰ **S82.855**   **Nondisplaced trimalleolar fracture of left lower leg**   CC

15,20 √7ᵗʰ **S82.856**   **Nondisplaced trimalleolar fracture of unspecified lower leg**   CC

√6ᵗʰ **S82.86**   **Maisonneuve's fracture**

> **CC Excl:** For codes in subcatgory S82.86, unless otherwise noted: See code: S82.84

15,16,18 √7ᵗʰ **S82.861**   **Displaced Maisonneuve's fracture of right leg**   MCC CC

15,16,18 √7ᵗʰ **S82.862**   **Displaced Maisonneuve's fracture of left leg**   MCC CC

15,16,18 √7ᵗʰ **S82.863**   **Displaced Maisonneuve's fracture of unspecified leg**   MCC CC

15,16,18 √7ᵗʰ **S82.864**   **Nondisplaced Maisonneuve's fracture of right leg**   MCC CC

15,16,18 √7ᵗʰ **S82.865**   **Nondisplaced Maisonneuve's fracture of left leg**   MCC CC

15,16,18 √7ᵗʰ **S82.866**   **Nondisplaced Maisonneuve's fracture of unspecified leg**   MCC CC

√6ᵗʰ **S82.87**   **Pilon fracture of tibia**

> **CC Excl:** For codes in subcatgory S82.87, unless otherwise noted: See code: S82.85

15,20 √7ᵗʰ **S82.871**   **Displaced pilon fracture of right tibia**   CC

15,20 √7ᵗʰ **S82.872**   **Displaced pilon fracture of left tibia**   CC

15,20 √7ᵗʰ **S82.873**   **Displaced pilon fracture of unspecified tibia**   CC

15,20 √7ᵗʰ **S82.874**   **Nondisplaced pilon fracture of right tibia**   CC

15,20 √7ᵗʰ **S82.875**   **Nondisplaced pilon fracture of left tibia**   CC

15,20 √7ᵗʰ **S82.876**   **Nondisplaced pilon fracture of unspecified tibia**   CC

√6ᵗʰ **S82.89**   **Other fractures of lower leg**
Fracture of ankle NOS

> **CC Excl:** For codes in subcatgory S82.89, unless otherwise noted: See code: S82.84

15,20 √7ᵗʰ **S82.891**   **Other fracture of right lower leg**   CC

15,20 √7ᵗʰ **S82.892**   **Other fracture of left lower leg**   CC

15,20 √7ᵗʰ **S82.899**   **Other fracture of unspecified lower leg**   CC

---

15 HAC = Initial encounter for open fracture only (7th character B or C) and not POA.
16 MCC only if an open fracture (7th character B or C).
18 CC only if a subsequent encounter for nonunion or malunion (7th character K, M, N, P, Q, or R).
20 CC only if an initial encounter for an open fracture (7th character B or C) **OR** a subsequent encounter for nonunion or malunion (7th character K, M, N, P, Q, or R).

✓5ᵗʰ **S82.9**   Unspecified **fracture of lower leg**

> **CC Excl: For codes in subcatgory S82.9, unless otherwise noted: CC with 7th character B or C:** See code: S82.84

15,20 ✓x7ᵗʰ **S82.90**   **Unspecified fracture of** unspecified **lower leg**   CC

15,20 ✓x7ᵗʰ **S82.91**   **Unspecified fracture of** right **lower leg**   CC

15,20 ✓x7ᵗʰ **S82.92**   **Unspecified fracture of** left **lower leg**   CC

✓4ᵗʰ **S83**   **Dislocation and sprain of joints and ligaments of knee**

> INCLUDES   avulsion of joint or ligament of knee
> laceration of cartilage, joint or ligament of knee
> sprain of cartilage, joint or ligament of knee
> traumatic hemarthrosis of joint or ligament of knee
> traumatic rupture of joint or ligament of knee
> traumatic subluxation of joint or ligament of knee
> traumatic tear of joint or ligament of knee

Code also any associated open wound

> EXCLUDES 1   derangement of patella (M22.0-M22.3)
> injury of patellar ligament (tendon) (S76.1-)
> internal derangement of knee (M23.-)
> old dislocation of knee (M24.36)
> pathological dislocation of knee (M24.36)
> recurrent dislocation of knee (M22.0)

> EXCLUDES 2   strain of muscle, fascia and tendon of lower leg (S86.-)

> The appropriate 7th character is to be added to each code from category S83.
> A   initial encounter
> D   subsequent encounter
> S   sequela

✓5ᵗʰ **S83.0**   **Subluxation and dislocation of** patella

  ✓6ᵗʰ **S83.00**   **Unspecified subluxation and dislocation of patella**

    ✓7ᵗʰ **S83.001**   **Unspecified** subluxation of right **patella**

    ✓7ᵗʰ **S83.002**   **Unspecified** subluxation of left **patella**

    ✓7ᵗʰ **S83.003**   **Unspecified** subluxation of unspecified **patella**

    ✓7ᵗʰ **S83.004**   **Unspecified** dislocation of right **patella**

    ✓7ᵗʰ **S83.005**   **Unspecified** dislocation of left **patella**

    ✓7ᵗʰ **S83.006**   **Unspecified** dislocation of unspecified **patella**

  ✓6ᵗʰ **S83.01**   **Lateral subluxation and dislocation of patella**

    ✓7ᵗʰ **S83.011**   **Lateral** subluxation of right **patella**

    ✓7ᵗʰ **S83.012**   **Lateral** subluxation of left **patella**

    ✓7ᵗʰ **S83.013**   **Lateral** subluxation of unspecified **patella**

    ✓7ᵗʰ **S83.014**   **Lateral** dislocation of right **patella**

    ✓7ᵗʰ **S83.015**   **Lateral** dislocation of left **patella**

    ✓7ᵗʰ **S83.016**   **Lateral** dislocation of unspecified **patella**

  ✓6ᵗʰ **S83.09**   **Other subluxation and dislocation of patella**

    ✓7ᵗʰ **S83.091**   **Other** subluxation of right **patella**

    ✓7ᵗʰ **S83.092**   **Other** subluxation of left **patella**

    ✓7ᵗʰ **S83.093**   **Other** subluxation of unspecified **patella**

    ✓7ᵗʰ **S83.094**   **Other** dislocation of right **patella**

    ✓7ᵗʰ **S83.095**   **Other** dislocation of left **patella**

    ✓7ᵗʰ **S83.096**   **Other** dislocation of unspecified **patella**

✓5ᵗʰ **S83.1**   **Subluxation and dislocation of knee**

> EXCLUDES 2   instability of knee prosthesis (T84.022, T84.023)

  ✓6ᵗʰ **S83.10**   **Unspecified subluxation and dislocation of knee**

    ✓7ᵗʰ **S83.101**   **Unspecified** subluxation of right **knee**

    ✓7ᵗʰ **S83.102**   **Unspecified** subluxation of left **knee**

    ✓7ᵗʰ **S83.103**   **Unspecified** subluxation of unspecified **knee**

    ✓7ᵗʰ **S83.104**   **Unspecified** dislocation of right **knee**

    ✓7ᵗʰ **S83.105**   **Unspecified** dislocation of left **knee**

    ✓7ᵗʰ **S83.106**   **Unspecified** dislocation of unspecified **knee**

  ✓6ᵗʰ **S83.11**   **Anterior subluxation and dislocation of proximal end of tibia**

> Posterior subluxation and dislocation of distal end of femur

    ✓7ᵗʰ **S83.111**   **Anterior** subluxation of proximal end of tibia, right **knee**

    ✓7ᵗʰ **S83.112**   **Anterior** subluxation of proximal end of tibia, left **knee**

    ✓7ᵗʰ **S83.113**   **Anterior** subluxation of proximal end of tibia, unspecified **knee**

    ✓7ᵗʰ **S83.114**   **Anterior** dislocation of proximal end of tibia, right **knee**

    ✓7ᵗʰ **S83.115**   **Anterior** dislocation of proximal end of tibia, left **knee**

    ✓7ᵗʰ **S83.116**   **Anterior** dislocation of proximal end of tibia, unspecified **knee**

  ✓6ᵗʰ **S83.12**   **Posterior subluxation and dislocation of proximal end of tibia**

> Anterior dislocation of distal end of femur

    ✓7ᵗʰ **S83.121**   **Posterior** subluxation of proximal end of tibia, right **knee**

    ✓7ᵗʰ **S83.122**   **Posterior** subluxation of proximal end of tibia, left **knee**

    ✓7ᵗʰ **S83.123**   **Posterior** subluxation of proximal end of tibia, unspecified **knee**

    ✓7ᵗʰ **S83.124**   **Posterior** dislocation of proximal end of tibia, right **knee**

    ✓7ᵗʰ **S83.125**   **Posterior** dislocation of proximal end of tibia, left **knee**

    ✓7ᵗʰ **S83.126**   **Posterior** dislocation of proximal end of tibia, unspecified **knee**

  ✓6ᵗʰ **S83.13**   **Medial subluxation and dislocation of proximal end of tibia**

    ✓7ᵗʰ **S83.131**   **Medial** subluxation of proximal end of tibia, right **knee**

    ✓7ᵗʰ **S83.132**   **Medial** subluxation of proximal end of tibia, left **knee**

    ✓7ᵗʰ **S83.133**   **Medial** subluxation of proximal end of tibia, unspecified **knee**

    ✓7ᵗʰ **S83.134**   **Medial** dislocation of proximal end of tibia, right **knee**

    ✓7ᵗʰ **S83.135**   **Medial** dislocation of proximal end of tibia, left **knee**

    ✓7ᵗʰ **S83.136**   **Medial** dislocation of proximal end of tibia, unspecified **knee**

  ✓6ᵗʰ **S83.14**   **Lateral subluxation and dislocation of proximal end of tibia**

    ✓7ᵗʰ **S83.141**   **Lateral** subluxation of proximal end of tibia, right **knee**

    ✓7ᵗʰ **S83.142**   **Lateral** subluxation of proximal end of tibia, left **knee**

    ✓7ᵗʰ **S83.143**   **Lateral** subluxation of proximal end of tibia, unspecified **knee**

    ✓7ᵗʰ **S83.144**   **Lateral** dislocation of proximal end of tibia, right **knee**

    ✓7ᵗʰ **S83.145**   **Lateral** dislocation of proximal end of tibia, left **knee**

    ✓7ᵗʰ **S83.146**   **Lateral** dislocation of proximal end of tibia, unspecified **knee**

  ✓6ᵗʰ **S83.19**   **Other subluxation and dislocation of knee**

    ✓7ᵗʰ **S83.191**   **Other** subluxation of right **knee**

    ✓7ᵗʰ **S83.192**   **Other** subluxation of left **knee**

    ✓7ᵗʰ **S83.193**   **Other** subluxation of unspecified **knee**

    ✓7ᵗʰ **S83.194**   **Other** dislocation of right **knee**

    ✓7ᵗʰ **S83.195**   **Other** dislocation of left **knee**

    ✓7ᵗʰ **S83.196**   **Other** dislocation of unspecified **knee**

✓5ᵗʰ **S83.2**   **Tear of meniscus, current injury**

> EXCLUDES 1   old bucket-handle tear (M23.2)

  ✓6ᵗʰ **S83.20**   **Tear of unspecified meniscus, current injury**

> Tear of meniscus of knee NOS

    ✓7ᵗʰ **S83.200**   **Bucket-handle tear of unspecified meniscus, current injury,** right **knee**

    ✓7ᵗʰ **S83.201**   **Bucket-handle tear of unspecified meniscus, current injury,** left **knee**

    ✓7ᵗʰ **S83.202**   **Bucket-handle tear of unspecified meniscus, current injury,** unspecified **knee**

    ✓7ᵗʰ **S83.203**   **Other tear of unspecified meniscus, current injury,** right **knee**

---

15 HAC = Initial encounter for open fracture only (7th character B or C) and not POA.
20 CC only if an initial encounter for an open fracture (7th character B or C) **OR** a subsequent encounter for nonunion or malunion (7th character K, M, N, P, Q, or R).

✓ Additional Character Required   ✓x7ᵗʰ Placeholder Alert   Unacceptable PDx   Manifestation   Hospital Acquired Condition   EXCLUDES 1 Not Coded Here   EXCLUDES 2 Not Included Here

✓7ᵗʰ **S83.204** Other tear of unspecified meniscus, current injury, **left** knee

✓7ᵗʰ **S83.205** Other tear of unspecified meniscus, current injury, **unspecified** knee

✓7ᵗʰ **S83.206** Unspecified tear of unspecified meniscus, current injury, **right** knee

✓7ᵗʰ **S83.207** Unspecified tear of unspecified meniscus, current injury, **left** knee

✓7ᵗʰ **S83.209** Unspecified tear of unspecified meniscus, current injury, **unspecified** knee

✓6ᵗʰ **S83.21** Bucket-handle tear of **medial** meniscus, current injury

   ✓7ᵗʰ **S83.211** Bucket-handle tear of medial meniscus, current injury, **right** knee

   ✓7ᵗʰ **S83.212** Bucket-handle tear of medial meniscus, current injury, **left** knee

   ✓7ᵗʰ **S83.219** Bucket-handle tear of medial meniscus, current injury, **unspecified** knee

✓6ᵗʰ **S83.22** Peripheral tear of **medial** meniscus, current injury

   ✓7ᵗʰ **S83.221** Peripheral tear of medial meniscus, current injury, **right** knee

   ✓7ᵗʰ **S83.222** Peripheral tear of medial meniscus, current injury, **left** knee

   ✓7ᵗʰ **S83.229** Peripheral tear of medial meniscus, current injury, **unspecified** knee

✓6ᵗʰ **S83.23** Complex tear of **medial** meniscus, current injury

   ✓7ᵗʰ **S83.231** Complex tear of medial meniscus, current injury, **right** knee

   ✓7ᵗʰ **S83.232** Complex tear of medial meniscus, current injury, **left** knee

   ✓7ᵗʰ **S83.239** Complex tear of medial meniscus, current injury, **unspecified** knee

✓6ᵗʰ **S83.24** Other tear of **medial** meniscus, current injury

   ✓7ᵗʰ **S83.241** Other tear of medial meniscus, current injury, **right** knee

   ✓7ᵗʰ **S83.242** Other tear of medial meniscus, current injury, **left** knee

   ✓7ᵗʰ **S83.249** Other tear of medial meniscus, current injury, **unspecified** knee

✓6ᵗʰ **S83.25** Bucket-handle tear of **lateral** meniscus, current injury

   ✓7ᵗʰ **S83.251** Bucket-handle tear of lateral meniscus, current injury, **right** knee

   ✓7ᵗʰ **S83.252** Bucket-handle tear of lateral meniscus, current injury, **left** knee

   ✓7ᵗʰ **S83.259** Bucket-handle tear of lateral meniscus, current injury, **unspecified** knee

✓6ᵗʰ **S83.26** Peripheral tear of **lateral** meniscus, current injury

   ✓7ᵗʰ **S83.261** Peripheral tear of lateral meniscus, current injury, **right** knee

   ✓7ᵗʰ **S83.262** Peripheral tear of lateral meniscus, current injury, **left** knee

   ✓7ᵗʰ **S83.269** Peripheral tear of lateral meniscus, current injury, **unspecified** knee

✓6ᵗʰ **S83.27** Complex tear of **lateral** meniscus, current injury

   ✓7ᵗʰ **S83.271** Complex tear of lateral meniscus, current injury, **right** knee

   ✓7ᵗʰ **S83.272** Complex tear of lateral meniscus, current injury, **left** knee

   ✓7ᵗʰ **S83.279** Complex tear of lateral meniscus, current injury, **unspecified** knee

✓6ᵗʰ **S83.28** Other tear of **lateral** meniscus, current injury

   ✓7ᵗʰ **S83.281** Other tear of lateral meniscus, current injury, **right** knee

   ✓7ᵗʰ **S83.282** Other tear of lateral meniscus, current injury, **left** knee

   ✓7ᵗʰ **S83.289** Other tear of lateral meniscus, current injury, **unspecified** knee

✓5ᵗʰ **S83.3** Tear of articular cartilage of knee, current

   ✓×7ᵗʰ **S83.30** Tear of articular cartilage of **unspecified** knee, current

   ✓×7ᵗʰ **S83.31** Tear of articular cartilage of **right** knee, current

   ✓×7ᵗʰ **S83.32** Tear of articular cartilage of **left** knee, current

✓5ᵗʰ **S83.4** Sprain of **collateral ligament** of knee

   ✓6ᵗʰ **S83.40** Sprain of **unspecified** collateral ligament of knee

     ✓7ᵗʰ **S83.401** Sprain of unspecified collateral ligament of **right** knee

     ✓7ᵗʰ **S83.402** Sprain of unspecified collateral ligament of **left** knee

     ✓7ᵗʰ **S83.409** Sprain of unspecified collateral ligament of **unspecified** knee

   ✓6ᵗʰ **S83.41** Sprain of **medial** collateral ligament of knee
       Sprain of tibial collateral ligament

     ✓7ᵗʰ **S83.411** Sprain of medial collateral ligament of **right** knee

     ✓7ᵗʰ **S83.412** Sprain of medial collateral ligament of **left** knee

     ✓7ᵗʰ **S83.419** Sprain of medial collateral ligament of **unspecified** knee

   ✓6ᵗʰ **S83.42** Sprain of **lateral** collateral ligament of knee
       Sprain of fibular collateral ligament

     ✓7ᵗʰ **S83.421** Sprain of lateral collateral ligament of **right** knee

     ✓7ᵗʰ **S83.422** Sprain of lateral collateral ligament of **left** knee

     ✓7ᵗʰ **S83.429** Sprain of lateral collateral ligament of **unspecified** knee

✓5ᵗʰ **S83.5** Sprain of **cruciate ligament** of knee

   ✓6ᵗʰ **S83.50** Sprain of **unspecified** cruciate ligament of knee

     ✓7ᵗʰ **S83.501** Sprain of unspecified cruciate ligament of **right** knee

     ✓7ᵗʰ **S83.502** Sprain of unspecified cruciate ligament of **left** knee

     ✓7ᵗʰ **S83.509** Sprain of unspecified cruciate ligament of **unspecified** knee

   ✓6ᵗʰ **S83.51** Sprain of **anterior** cruciate ligament of knee

     ✓7ᵗʰ **S83.511** Sprain of anterior cruciate ligament of **right** knee

     ✓7ᵗʰ **S83.512** Sprain of anterior cruciate ligament of **left** knee

     ✓7ᵗʰ **S83.519** Sprain of anterior cruciate ligament of **unspecified** knee

   ✓6ᵗʰ **S83.52** Sprain of **posterior** cruciate ligament of knee

     ✓7ᵗʰ **S83.521** Sprain of posterior cruciate ligament of **right** knee

     ✓7ᵗʰ **S83.522** Sprain of posterior cruciate ligament of **left** knee

     ✓7ᵗʰ **S83.529** Sprain of posterior cruciate ligament of **unspecified** knee

✓5ᵗʰ **S83.6** Sprain of the **superior tibiofibular** joint and ligament

   ✓×7ᵗʰ **S83.60** Sprain of the superior tibiofibular joint and ligament, **unspecified** knee

   ✓×7ᵗʰ **S83.61** Sprain of the superior tibiofibular joint and ligament, **right** knee

   ✓×7ᵗʰ **S83.62** Sprain of the superior tibiofibular joint and ligament, **left** knee

✓5ᵗʰ **S83.8** Sprain of **other** specified parts of knee

   ✓6ᵗʰ **S83.8X** Sprain of other specified parts of knee

     ✓7ᵗʰ **S83.8X1** Sprain of other specified parts of **right** knee

     ✓7ᵗʰ **S83.8X2** Sprain of other specified parts of **left** knee

     ✓7ᵗʰ **S83.8X9** Sprain of other specified parts of **unspecified** knee

✓5ᵗʰ **S83.9** Sprain of **unspecified** site of knee

   ✓×7ᵗʰ **S83.90** Sprain of unspecified site of **unspecified** knee

   ✓×7ᵗʰ **S83.91** Sprain of unspecified site of **right** knee

   ✓×7ᵗʰ **S83.92** Sprain of unspecified site of **left** knee

---

Ⓝ Newborn: 0   Ⓟ Pediatric: 0-17   Ⓜ Maternity: 12-55   Ⓐ Adult: 15-124   **MCC** Major CC Condition   **PDx MCC** PDx acts as own MCC   **CC** CC Condition   **PDx CC** PDx acts as own CC

1046   ICD-10-CM 2016

✓4ᵗʰ **S84   Injury of nerves at lower leg level**
Code also any associated open wound (S81.-)
EXCLUDES 2 *injury of nerves at ankle and foot level (S94.-)*

> The appropriate 7th character is to be added to each code from category S84.
> A   initial encounter
> D   subsequent encounter
> S   sequela

✓5ᵗʰ **S84.0   Injury of tibial nerve at lower leg level**
   ✓x7ᵗʰ **S84.00   Injury of tibial nerve at lower leg level, unspecified leg**
   ✓x7ᵗʰ **S84.01   Injury of tibial nerve at lower leg level, right leg**
   ✓x7ᵗʰ **S84.02   Injury of tibial nerve at lower leg level, left leg**

✓5ᵗʰ **S84.1   Injury of peroneal nerve at lower leg level**
   ✓x7ᵗʰ **S84.10   Injury of peroneal nerve at lower leg level, unspecified leg**
   ✓x7ᵗʰ **S84.11   Injury of peroneal nerve at lower leg level, right leg**
   ✓x7ᵗʰ **S84.12   Injury of peroneal nerve at lower leg level, left leg**

✓5ᵗʰ **S84.2   Injury of cutaneous sensory nerve at lower leg level**
   ✓x7ᵗʰ **S84.20   Injury of cutaneous sensory nerve at lower leg level, unspecified leg**
   ✓x7ᵗʰ **S84.21   Injury of cutaneous sensory nerve at lower leg level, right leg**
   ✓x7ᵗʰ **S84.22   Injury of cutaneous sensory nerve at lower leg level, left leg**

✓5ᵗʰ **S84.8   Injury of other nerves at lower leg level**
   ✓6ᵗʰ **S84.80   Injury of other nerves at lower leg level**
     ✓7ᵗʰ **S84.801   Injury of other nerves at lower leg level, right leg**
     ✓7ᵗʰ **S84.802   Injury of other nerves at lower leg level, left leg**
     ✓7ᵗʰ **S84.809   Injury of other nerves at lower leg level, unspecified leg**

✓5ᵗʰ **S84.9   Injury of unspecified nerve at lower leg level**
   ✓x7ᵗʰ **S84.90   Injury of unspecified nerve at lower leg level, unspecified leg**
   ✓x7ᵗʰ **S84.91   Injury of unspecified nerve at lower leg level, right leg**
   ✓x7ᵗʰ **S84.92   Injury of unspecified nerve at lower leg level, left leg**

✓4ᵗʰ **S85   Injury of blood vessels at lower leg level**
Code also any associated open wound (S81.-)
EXCLUDES 2 *injury of blood vessels at ankle and foot level (S95.-)*

> The appropriate 7th character is to be added to each code from category S85.
> A   initial encounter
> D   subsequent encounter
> S   sequela

✓5ᵗʰ **S85.0   Injury of popliteal artery**
   ✓6ᵗʰ **S85.00   Unspecified injury of popliteal artery**
     ✓7ᵗʰ **S85.001   Unspecified injury of popliteal artery, right leg** MCC
     CC Excl: MCC with 7th character A: S75.801 with 7th A, S75.809-S75.811 with 7th A, S75.819-S75.891 with 7th A, S75.899-S75.901 with 7th A, S75.909-S75.911 with 7th A, S75.919-S75.991 with 7th A, S75.999A, S85.001A, S85.009-S85.011 with 7th A, S85.019-S85.091 with 7th A, S85.099A, S85.201A, S85.209-S85.211 with 7th A, S85.219-S85.291 with 7th A, S85.299A, S85.801A, S85.809-S85.811 with 7th A, S85.819-S85.891 with 7th A, S85.899-S85.901 with 7th A, S85.909-S85.911 with 7th A, S85.919-S85.991 with 7th A, S85.999A, S95.001A, S95.009-S95.011 with 7th A, S95.019-S95.091 with 7th A, S95.099A, S95.201A, S95.209-S95.211 with 7th A, S95.219-S95.291 with 7th A, S95.299-S95.801 with 7th A, S95.809-S95.811 with 7th A, S95.819-S95.891 with 7th A, S95.899-S95.901 with 7th A, S95.909-S95.911 with 7th A, S95.919-S95.991 with 7th A, S95.999 with 7th A

     ✓7ᵗʰ **S85.002   Unspecified injury of popliteal artery, left leg** MCC
     CC Excl: MCC with 7th character A: S75.802-S75.809 with 7th A, S75.812-S75.819 with 7th A, S75.892-S75.899 with 7th A, S75.902-S75.909 with 7th A, S75.912-S75.919 with 7th A, S75.992-S75.999 with 7th A, S85.002-S85.009 with 7th A, S85.012-S85.019 with 7th A, S85.092-S85.099 with 7th A, S85.202-S85.209 with 7th A, S85.212-S85.219 with 7th A, S85.292-S85.299 with 7th A, S85.802-S85.809 with 7th A, S85.812-S85.819 with 7th A, S85.892-S85.899 with 7th A, S85.902-S85.909 with 7th A, S85.912-S85.919 with 7th A, S85.992-S85.999 with 7th A, S95.002-S95.009 with 7th A, S95.012-S95.019 with 7th A, S95.092-S95.099 with 7th A, S95.202-S95.209 with 7th A, S95.212-S95.219 with 7th A, S95.292-S95.299 with 7th A, S95.802-S95.809 with 7th A, S95.812-S95.819 with 7th A, S95.892-S95.899 with 7th A, S95.902-S95.909 with 7th A, S95.912-S95.919 with 7th A, S95.992-S95.999 with 7th A

     ✓7ᵗʰ **S85.009   Unspecified injury of popliteal artery, unspecified leg** MCC
     CC Excl: MCC with 7th character A: S75.801-S75.999 with 7th A, S85.001-S85.099 with 7th A, S85.201-S85.299 with 7th A, S85.801-S85.999 with 7th A, S95.001-S95.099 with 7th A, S95.201-S95.999 with 7th A

   ✓6ᵗʰ **S85.01   Laceration of popliteal artery**
     ✓7ᵗʰ **S85.011   Laceration of popliteal artery, right leg** MCC
     CC Excl: See code: S85.001
     ✓7ᵗʰ **S85.012   Laceration of popliteal artery, left leg** MCC
     CC Excl: See code: S85.002
     ✓7ᵗʰ **S85.019   Laceration of popliteal artery, unspecified leg** MCC
     CC Excl: See code: S85.009

   ✓6ᵗʰ **S85.09   Other specified injury of popliteal artery**
     ✓7ᵗʰ **S85.091   Other specified injury of popliteal artery, right leg** MCC
     CC Excl: See code: S85.001
     ✓7ᵗʰ **S85.092   Other specified injury of popliteal artery, left leg** MCC
     CC Excl: See code: S85.002
     ✓7ᵗʰ **S85.099   Other specified injury of popliteal artery, unspecified leg** MCC
     CC Excl: See code: S85.009

✓5ᵗʰ **S85.1   Injury of tibial artery**
   ✓6ᵗʰ **S85.10   Unspecified injury of unspecified tibial artery**
     Injury of tibial artery NOS
     ✓7ᵗʰ **S85.101   Unspecified injury of unspecified tibial artery, right leg** CC
     CC Excl: CC with 7th character A: S75.801 with 7th A, S75.809-S75.811 with 7th A, S75.819-S75.891 with 7th A, S75.899-S75.901 with 7th A, S75.909-S75.911 with 7th A, S75.919-S75.991 with 7th A, S75.999A, S85.101A, S85.109-S85.111 with 7th A, S85.119-S85.121 with 7th A, S85.129A, S85.201A, S85.209-S85.211 with 7th A, S85.219-S85.291 with 7th A, S85.299 with 7th A, S85.801A, S85.809-S85.811 with 7th A, S85.819-S85.891 with 7th A, S85.899-S85.901 with 7th A, S85.909-S85.911 with 7th A, S85.919-S85.991 with 7th A, S85.999A, S95.001A, S95.009-S95.011 with 7th A, S95.019-S95.091 with 7th A, S95.099A, S95.201A, S95.209-S95.211 with 7th A, S95.219-S95.291 with 7th A, S95.299-S95.801 with 7th A, S95.809-S95.811 with 7th A, S95.819-S95.891 with 7th A, S95.899-S95.901 with 7th A, S95.909-S95.911 with 7th A, S95.919-S95.991 with 7th A, S95.999

✓ Additional Character Required   ✓x7ᵗʰ Placeholder Alert   Unacceptable PDx   Manifestation   Hospital Acquired Condition   EXCLUDES 1 Not Coded Here   EXCLUDES 2 Not Included Here

ICD-10-CM 2016   1047

S84–S85.101

Chapter 19. Injury, Poisoning, and Certain Other Consequences of External Causes

√7ᵗʰ **S85.102 Unspecified injury of unspecified tibial** CC
artery, left leg
CC Excl: CC with 7th character A: S75.802-
S75.809 with 7th A, S75.812-S75.819 with
7th A, S75.892-S75.899 with 7th A, S75.902-
S75.909 with 7th A, S75.912-S75.919 with
7th A, S75.992-S75.999 with 7th A, S85.102-
S85.109 with 7th A, S85.112-S85.119 with
7th A, S85.122-S85.129 with 7th A, S85.202-
S85.209 with 7th A, S85.212-S85.219 with
7th A, S85.292-S85.299 with 7th A, S85.802-
S85.809 with 7th A, S85.812-S85.819 with
7th A, S85.892-S85.899 with 7th A, S85.902-
S85.909 with 7th A, S85.912-S85.919 with
7th A, S85.992-S85.999 with 7th A, S95.002-
S95.009 with 7th A, S95.012-S95.019 with
7th A, S95.092-S95.099 with 7th A, S95.202-
S95.209 with 7th A, S95.212-S95.219 with
7th A, S95.292-S95.299 with 7th A, S95.802-
S95.809 with 7th A, S95.812-S95.819 with
7th A, S95.892-S95.899 with 7th A, S95.902-
S95.909 with 7th A, S95.912-S95.919 with
7th A, S95.992-S95.999 with 7th A

√7ᵗʰ **S85.109 Unspecified injury of unspecified tibial** CC
artery, unspecified leg
CC Excl: CC with 7th character A: S75.801-
S75.999 with 7th A, S85.101-S85.129 with
7th A, S85.201-S85.299 with 7th A, S85.801-
S85.999 with 7th A, S95.001-S95.099 with
7th A, S95.201-S95.999 with 7th A

√6ᵗʰ **S85.11 Laceration of unspecified tibial artery**

√7ᵗʰ **S85.111 Laceration of unspecified tibial artery,** CC
right leg
CC Excl: See code: S85.101

√7ᵗʰ **S85.112 Laceration of unspecified tibial artery,** CC
left leg
CC Excl: See code: S85.102

√7ᵗʰ **S85.119 Laceration of unspecified tibial artery,** CC
unspecified leg
CC Excl: See code: S85.109

√6ᵗʰ **S85.12 Other specified injury of unspecified tibial artery**

√7ᵗʰ **S85.121 Other specified injury of unspecified** CC
tibial artery, right leg
CC Excl: See code: S85.101

√7ᵗʰ **S85.122 Other specified injury of unspecified** CC
tibial artery, left leg
CC Excl: See code: S85.102

√7ᵗʰ **S85.129 Other specified injury of unspecified** CC
tibial artery, unspecified leg
CC Excl: See code: S85.109

√6ᵗʰ **S85.13 Unspecified injury of anterior tibial artery**

√7ᵗʰ **S85.131 Unspecified injury of anterior tibial** CC
artery, right leg
CC Excl: CC with 7th character A: S75.801
with 7th A, S75.809-S75.811 with 7th A,
S75.819-S75.891 with 7th A, S75.899-
S75.901 with 7th A, S75.909-S75.911 with
7th A, S75.919-S75.991 with 7th A, S75.999A,
S85.131A, S85.139-S85.141 with 7th A,
S85.149-S85.151 with 7th A, S85.159A,
S85.201A, S85.209-S85.211 with 7th A,
S85.219-S85.291 with 7th A, S85.299A,
S85.801A, S85.809-S85.811 with 7th A,
S85.819-S85.891 with 7th A, S85.899-
S85.901 with 7th A, S85.909-S85.911 with
7th A, S85.919-S85.991 with 7th A, S85.999A,
S95.001A, S95.009-S95.011 with 7th A,
S95.019-S95.091 with 7th A, S95.099A,
S95.201A, S95.209-S95.211 with 7th A,
S95.219-S95.291 with 7th A, S95.299-
S95.801 with 7th A, S95.809-S95.811 with
7th A, S95.819-S95.891 with 7th A, S95.899-
S95.901 with 7th A, S95.909-S95.911 with
7th A, S95.919-S95.991 with 7th A, S95.999
with 7th A

√7ᵗʰ **S85.132 Unspecified injury of anterior tibial** CC
artery, left leg
CC Excl: CC with 7th character A: S75.802-
S75.809 with 7th A, S75.812-S75.819 with
7th A, S75.892-S75.899 with 7th A, S75.902-
S75.909 with 7th A, S75.912-S75.919 with
7th A, S75.992-S75.999 with 7th A, S85.132-
S85.139 with 7th A, S85.142-S85.149 with
7th A, S85.152-S85.159 with 7th A, S85.202-
S85.209 with 7th A, S85.212-S85.219 with
7th A, S85.292-S85.299 with 7th A, S85.802-
S85.809 with 7th A, S85.812-S85.819 with
7th A, S85.892-S85.899 with 7th A, S85.902-
S85.909 with 7th A, S85.912-S85.919 with
7th A, S85.992-S85.999 with 7th A, S95.002-
S95.009 with 7th A, S95.012-S95.019 with
7th A, S95.092-S95.099 with 7th A, S95.202-
S95.209 with 7th A, S95.212-S95.219 with
7th A, S95.292-S95.299 with 7th A, S95.802-
S95.809 with 7th A, S95.812-S95.819 with
7th A, S95.892-S95.899 with 7th A, S95.902-
S95.909 with 7th A, S95.912-S95.919 with
7th A, S95.992-S95.999 with 7th A

√7ᵗʰ **S85.139 Unspecified injury of anterior tibial** CC
artery, unspecified leg
CC Excl: CC with 7th character A: S75.801-
S75.999 with 7th A, S85.131-S85.159 with
7th A, S85.201-S85.299 with 7th A, S85.801-
S85.999 with 7th A, S95.001-S95.099 with
7th A, S95.201-S95.999 with 7th A

√6ᵗʰ **S85.14 Laceration of anterior tibial artery**

√7ᵗʰ **S85.141 Laceration of anterior tibial artery,** CC
right leg
CC Excl: See code: S85.131

√7ᵗʰ **S85.142 Laceration of anterior tibial artery,** CC
left leg
CC Excl: See code: S85.132

√7ᵗʰ **S85.149 Laceration of anterior tibial artery,** CC
unspecified leg
CC Excl: See code: S85.139

√6ᵗʰ **S85.15 Other specified injury of anterior tibial artery**

√7ᵗʰ **S85.151 Other specified injury of anterior** CC
tibial artery, right leg
CC Excl: See code: S85.131

√7ᵗʰ **S85.152 Other specified injury of anterior** CC
tibial artery, left leg
CC Excl: See code: S85.132

√7ᵗʰ **S85.159 Other specified injury of anterior** CC
tibial artery, unspecified leg
CC Excl: See code: S85.139

√6ᵗʰ **S85.16 Unspecified injury of posterior tibial artery**

√7ᵗʰ **S85.161 Unspecified injury of posterior tibial** CC
artery, right leg
CC Excl: CC with 7th character A: S75.801
with 7th A, S75.809-S75.811 with 7th A,
S75.819-S75.891 with 7th A, S75.899-
S75.901 with 7th A, S75.909-S75.911 with
7th A, S75.919-S75.991 with 7th A, S75.999
with 7th A, S85.161 with 7th A, S85.169-
S85.171 with 7th A, S85.179-S85.181 with
7th A, S85.189-S85.201 with 7th A, S85.209-
S85.211 with 7th A, S85.219-S85.291 with
7th A, S85.299A, S85.801A, S85.809-S85.811
with 7th A, S85.819-S85.891 with 7th A,
S85.899-S85.901 with 7th A, S85.909-
S85.911 with 7th A, S85.919-S85.991 with
7th A, S85.999A, S95.001A, S95.009-S95.011
with 7th A, S95.019-S95.091 with 7th A,
S95.099A, S95.201A, S95.209-S95.211 with
7th A, S95.219-S95.291 with 7th A, S95.299-
S95.801 with 7th A, S95.809-S95.811 with
7th A, S95.819-S95.891 with 7th A, S95.899-
S95.901 with 7th A, S95.909-S95.911 with
7th A, S95.919-S95.991 with 7th A, S95.999
with 7th A

Ⓝ Newborn: 0   Ⓟ Pediatric: 0-17   Ⓜ Maternity: 12-55   Ⓐ Adult: 15-124   ᴹᶜᶜ Major CC Condition   ᴾᴰˣᴹᶜᶜ PDx acts as own MCC   ᶜᶜ CC Condition   ᴾᴰˣᶜᶜ PDx acts as own CC

1048   ICD-10-CM 2016

✓7ᵗʰ **S85.162** **Unspecified injury of posterior tibial artery, left leg** CC
CC Excl: CC with 7th character A: S75.802-S75.809 with 7th A, S75.812-S75.819 with 7th A, S75.892-S75.899 with 7th A, S75.902-S75.909 with 7th A, S75.912-S75.919 with 7th A, S75.992-S75.999 with 7th A, S85.162-S85.169 with 7th A, S85.172-S85.179 with 7th A, S85.182-S85.189 with 7th A, S85.202-S85.209 with 7th A, S85.212-S85.219 with 7th A, S85.292-S85.299 with 7th A, S85.802-S85.809 with 7th A, S85.812-S85.819 with 7th A, S85.892-S85.899 with 7th A, S85.902-S85.909 with 7th A, S85.912-S85.919 with 7th A, S85.992-S85.999 with 7th A, S95.002-S95.009 with 7th A, S95.012-S95.019 with 7th A, S95.092-S95.099 with 7th A, S95.202-S95.209 with 7th A, S95.212-S95.219 with 7th A, S95.292-S95.299 with 7th A, S95.802-S95.809 with 7th A, S95.812-S95.819 with 7th A, S95.892-S95.899 with 7th A, S95.902-S95.909 with 7th A, S95.912-S95.919 with 7th A, S95.992-S95.999 with 7th A

✓7ᵗʰ **S85.169** **Unspecified injury of posterior tibial artery, unspecified leg** CC
CC Excl: CC with 7th character A: S75.801-S75.999 with 7th A, S85.161-S85.299 with 7th A, S85.801-S85.999 with 7th A, S95.001-S95.099 with 7th A, S95.201-S95.999 with 7th A

✓6ᵗʰ **S85.17** **Laceration of posterior tibial artery**

✓7ᵗʰ **S85.171** **Laceration of posterior tibial artery, right leg** CC
CC Excl: See code: S85.161

✓7ᵗʰ **S85.172** **Laceration of posterior tibial artery, left leg** CC
CC Excl: See code: S85.162

✓7ᵗʰ **S85.179** **Laceration of posterior tibial artery, unspecified leg** CC
CC Excl: See code: S85.169

✓6ᵗʰ **S85.18** **Other specified injury of posterior tibial artery**

✓7ᵗʰ **S85.181** **Other specified injury of posterior tibial artery, right leg** CC
CC Excl: See code: S85.161

✓7ᵗʰ **S85.182** **Other specified injury of posterior tibial artery, left leg** CC
CC Excl: See code: S85.162

✓7ᵗʰ **S85.189** **Other specified injury of posterior tibial artery, unspecified leg** CC
CC Excl: See code: S85.169

✓5ᵗʰ **S85.2** **Injury of peroneal artery**

✓6ᵗʰ **S85.20** **Unspecified injury of peroneal artery**

✓7ᵗʰ **S85.201** **Unspecified injury of peroneal artery, right leg** CC
CC Excl: CC with 7th character A: M79.A21-M79.A29, S75.001 with 7th A, S75.009-S75.011 with 7th A, S75.019-S75.021 with 7th A, S75.029-S75.091 with 7th A, S75.099-S75.101 with 7th A, S75.109-S75.111 with 7th A, S75.119-S75.121 with 7th A, S75.129-S75.191 with 7th A, S75.199-S75.201 with 7th A, S75.209-S75.211 with 7th A, S75.219-S75.221 with 7th A, S75.229-S75.291 with 7th A, S75.299-S75.801 with 7th A, S75.809-S75.811 with 7th A, S75.819-S75.891 with 7th A, S75.899-S75.901 with 7th A, S75.909-S75.911 with 7th A, S75.919-S75.991 with 7th A, S75.999A, S85.001A, S85.009-S85.011 with 7th A, S85.019-S85.091 with 7th A, S85.099-S85.101 with 7th A, S85.109-S85.111 with 7th A, S85.119-S85.121 with 7th A, S85.129-S85.131 with 7th A, S85.139-S85.141 with 7th A, S85.149-S85.151 with 7th A, S85.159-S85.161 with 7th A, S85.169-S85.171 with 7th A, S85.179-S85.181 with 7th A, S85.189-S85.201 with 7th A, S85.209-S85.211 with 7th A, S85.219-S85.291 with 7th A, S85.299-S85.301 with 7th A, S85.309-S85.311 with 7th A, S85.319-S85.391 with 7th A, S85.399-S85.401 with 7th A, S85.409-S85.411 with 7th A, S85.419-S85.491 with 7th A, S85.499-S85.501 with 7th A, S85.509-S85.511 with 7th A, S85.519-S85.591 with 7th A, S85.599-S85.801 with 7th A, S85.809-S85.811 with 7th A, S85.819-S85.891 with 7th A, S85.899-S85.901 with 7th A, S85.909-S85.911 with 7th A, S85.919-S85.991 with 7th A, S85.999 with 7th A, S95.001 with 7th A, S95.009-S95.011 with 7th A, S95.019-S95.091 with 7th A, S95.099-S95.101 with 7th A, S95.109-S95.111 with 7th A, S95.119-S95.191 with 7th A, S95.199-S95.201 with 7th A, S95.209-S95.211 with 7th A, S95.219-S95.291 with 7th A, S95.299-S95.801 with 7th A, S95.809-S95.811 with 7th A, S95.819-S95.891 with 7th A, S95.899-S95.901 with 7th A, S95.909-S95.911 with 7th A, S95.919-S95.991 with 7th A, S95.999 with 7th A

✓7ᵗʰ **S85.202** **Unspecified injury of peroneal artery, left leg** CC
CC Excl: CC with 7th character A: M79.A21-M79.A29, S75.002-S75.009 with 7th A, S75.012-S75.019 with 7th A, S75.022-S75.029 with 7th A, S75.092-S75.099 with 7th A, S75.102-S75.109 with 7th A, S75.112-S75.119 with 7th A, S75.122-S75.129 with 7th A, S75.192-S75.199 with 7th A, S75.202-S75.209 with 7th A, S75.212-S75.219 with 7th A, S75.222-S75.229 with 7th A, S75.292-S75.299 with 7th A, S75.802-S75.809 with 7th A, S75.812-S75.819 with 7th A, S75.892-S75.899 with 7th A, S75.902-S75.909 with 7th A, S75.912-S75.919 with 7th A, S75.992-S75.999A, S85.002-S85.009 with 7th A, S85.012-S85.019 with 7th A, S85.092-S85.099 with 7th A, S85.102-S85.109 with 7th A, S85.112-S85.119 with 7th A, S85.122-S85.129 with 7th A, S85.132-S85.139 with 7th A, S85.142-S85.149 with 7th A, S85.152-S85.159 with 7th A, S85.162-S85.169 with 7th A, S85.172-S85.179 with 7th A, S85.182-S85.189 with 7th A, S85.202-S85.209 with 7th A, S85.212-S85.219 with 7th A, S85.292-S85.299 with 7th A, S85.302-S85.309 with 7th A, S85.312-S85.319 with 7th A, S85.392-S85.399 with 7th A, S85.402-S85.409 with 7th A, S85.412-S85.419 with 7th A, S85.492-S85.499 with 7th A, S85.502-S85.509 with 7th A, S85.512-S85.519 with 7th A, S85.592-S85.599 with 7th A, S85.802-S85.809 with 7th A, S85.812-S85.819 with 7th A, S85.892-S85.899 with 7th A, S85.902-S85.909 with 7th A, S85.912-S85.919 with 7th A, S85.992-S85.999 with 7th A, S95.002-S95.009 with 7th A, S95.012-S95.019 with 7th A, S95.092-S95.099 with 7th A, S95.102-S95.109 with 7th A, S95.112-S95.119 with 7th A, S95.192-S95.199 with 7th A, S95.202-S95.209 with 7th A, S95.212-S95.219 with 7th A, S95.292-S95.299 with 7th A, S95.802-S95.809 with 7th A, S95.812-S95.819 with 7th A, S95.892-S95.899 with 7th A, S95.902-S95.909 with 7th A, S95.912-S95.919 with 7th A, S95.992-S95.999 with 7th A

✓7ᵗʰ **S85.209** **Unspecified injury of peroneal artery, unspecified leg** CC
CC Excl: CC with 7th character A: M79.A21-M79.A29, S75.001-S75.999 with 7th A, S85.001-S85.999 with 7th A, S95.001-S95.999 with 7th A

✓6ᵗʰ **S85.21** **Laceration of peroneal artery**

✓7ᵗʰ **S85.211** **Laceration of peroneal artery, right leg** CC
CC Excl: See code: S85.201

✓7ᵗʰ **S85.212** **Laceration of peroneal artery, left leg** CC
CC Excl: See code: S85.202

✓7ᵗʰ **S85.219** **Laceration of peroneal artery, unspecified leg** CC
CC Excl: See code: S85.209

✓6ᵗʰ **S85.29** **Other specified injury of peroneal artery**

✓7ᵗʰ **S85.291** **Other specified injury of peroneal artery, right leg** CC
CC Excl: See code: S85.201

✓7ᵗʰ **S85.292** **Other specified injury of peroneal artery, left leg** CC
CC Excl: See code: S85.202

✓7ᵗʰ **S85.299** **Other specified injury of peroneal artery, unspecified leg** CC
CC Excl: See code: S85.209

√5ᵗʰ **S85.3** **Injury of greater saphenous vein at lower leg level**
Injury of greater saphenous vein NOS
Injury of saphenous vein NOS

  √6ᵗʰ **S85.30** **Unspecified injury of greater saphenous vein at lower leg level**

    √7ᵗʰ **S85.301** **Unspecified injury of greater saphenous vein at lower leg level, right leg** `CC`
CC Excl: CC with 7th character A: S75.201 with 7th A, S75.209-S75.211 with 7th A, S75.219-S75.221 with 7th A, S75.229-S75.291 with 7th A, S75.299-S75.801 with 7th A, S75.809-S75.811 with 7th A, S75.819-S75.891 with 7th A, S75.899-S75.901 with 7th A, S75.909-S75.911 with 7th A, S75.919-S75.991 with 7th A, S75.999A, S85.201A, S85.209-S85.211 with 7th A, S85.219-S85.291 with 7th A, S85.299-S85.301 with 7th A, S85.309-S85.311 with 7th A, S85.319-S85.391 with 7th A, S85.399-S85.401 with 7th A, S85.409-S85.411 with 7th A, S85.419-S85.491 with 7th A, S85.499 with 7th A, S85.801 with 7th A, S85.809-S85.811 with 7th A, S85.819-S85.891 with 7th A, S85.899-S85.901 with 7th A, S85.909-S85.911 with 7th A, S85.919-S85.991 with 7th A, S85.999A, S95.001A, S95.009-S95.011 with 7th A, S95.019-S95.091 with 7th A, S95.099A, S95.201A, S95.209-S95.211 with 7th A, S95.219-S95.291 with 7th A, S95.299-S95.801 with 7th A, S95.809-S95.811 with 7th A, S95.819-S95.891 with 7th A, S95.899-S95.901 with 7th A, S95.909-S95.911 with 7th A, S95.919-S95.991 with 7th A, S95.999 with 7th A

    √7ᵗʰ **S85.302** **Unspecified injury of greater saphenous vein at lower leg level, left leg** `CC`
CC Excl: CC with 7th character A: S75.202-S75.209 with 7th A, S75.212-S75.219 with 7th A, S75.222-S75.229 with 7th A, S75.292-S75.299 with 7th A, S75.802-S75.809 with 7th A, S75.812-S75.819 with 7th A, S75.892-S75.899 with 7th A, S75.902-S75.909 with 7th A, S75.912-S75.919 with 7th A, S75.992-S75.999 with 7th A, S85.202-S85.209 with 7th A, S85.212-S85.219 with 7th A, S85.292-S85.299 with 7th A, S85.302-S85.309 with 7th A, S85.312-S85.319 with 7th A, S85.392-S85.399 with 7th A, S85.402-S85.409 with 7th A, S85.412-S85.419 with 7th A, S85.492-S85.499 with 7th A, S85.802-S85.809 with 7th A, S85.812-S85.819 with 7th A, S85.892-S85.899 with 7th A, S85.902-S85.909 with 7th A, S85.912-S85.919 with 7th A, S85.992-S85.999 with 7th A, S95.002-S95.009 with 7th A, S95.012-S95.019 with 7th A, S95.092-S95.099 with 7th A, S95.202-S95.209 with 7th A, S95.212-S95.219 with 7th A, S95.292-S95.299 with 7th A, S95.802-S95.809 with 7th A, S95.812-S95.819 with 7th A, S95.892-S95.899 with 7th A, S95.902-S95.909 with 7th A, S95.912-S95.919 with 7th A, S95.992-S95.999 with 7th A

    √7ᵗʰ **S85.309** **Unspecified injury of greater saphenous vein at lower leg level, unspecified leg** `CC`
CC Excl: CC with 7th character A: S75.201-S75.999 with 7th A, S85.201-S85.499 with 7th A, S85.801-S85.999 with 7th A, S95.001-S95.099 with 7th A, S95.201-S95.999 with 7th A

  √6ᵗʰ **S85.31** **Laceration of greater saphenous vein at lower leg level**

    √7ᵗʰ **S85.311** **Laceration of greater saphenous vein at lower leg level, right leg** `CC`
CC Excl: See code: S85.301

    √7ᵗʰ **S85.312** **Laceration of greater saphenous vein at lower leg level, left leg** `CC`
CC Excl: See code: S85.302

    √7ᵗʰ **S85.319** **Laceration of greater saphenous vein at lower leg level, unspecified leg** `CC`
CC Excl: See code: S85.309

  √6ᵗʰ **S85.39** **Other specified injury of greater saphenous vein at lower leg level**

    √7ᵗʰ **S85.391** **Other specified injury of greater saphenous vein at lower leg level, right leg** `CC`
CC Excl: See code: S85.301

    √7ᵗʰ **S85.392** **Other specified injury of greater saphenous vein at lower leg level, left leg** `CC`
CC Excl: See code: S85.302

    √7ᵗʰ **S85.399** **Other specified injury of greater saphenous vein at lower leg level, unspecified leg** `CC`
CC Excl: See code: S85.309

√5ᵗʰ **S85.4** **Injury of lesser saphenous vein at lower leg level**

  √6ᵗʰ **S85.40** **Unspecified injury of lesser saphenous vein at lower leg level**

    √7ᵗʰ **S85.401** **Unspecified injury of lesser saphenous vein at lower leg level, right leg** `CC`
CC Excl: See code: S85.301

    √7ᵗʰ **S85.402** **Unspecified injury of lesser saphenous vein at lower leg level, left leg** `CC`
CC Excl: See code: S85.302

    √7ᵗʰ **S85.409** **Unspecified injury of lesser saphenous vein at lower leg level, unspecified leg** `CC`
CC Excl: See code: S85.309

  √6ᵗʰ **S85.41** **Laceration of lesser saphenous vein at lower leg level**

    √7ᵗʰ **S85.411** **Laceration of lesser saphenous vein at lower leg level, right leg** `CC`
CC Excl: See code: S85.301

    √7ᵗʰ **S85.412** **Laceration of lesser saphenous vein at lower leg level, left leg** `CC`
CC Excl: See code: S85.302

    √7ᵗʰ **S85.419** **Laceration of lesser saphenous vein at lower leg level, unspecified leg** `CC`
CC Excl: See code: S85.309

  √6ᵗʰ **S85.49** **Other specified injury of lesser saphenous vein at lower leg level**

    √7ᵗʰ **S85.491** **Other specified injury of lesser saphenous vein at lower leg level, right leg** `CC`
CC Excl: See code: S85.301

    √7ᵗʰ **S85.492** **Other specified injury of lesser saphenous vein at lower leg level, left leg** `CC`
CC Excl: See code: S85.302

    √7ᵗʰ **S85.499** **Other specified injury of lesser saphenous vein at lower leg level, unspecified leg** `CC`
CC Excl: See code: S85.309

√5ᵗʰ **S85.5** **Injury of popliteal vein**

  √6ᵗʰ **S85.50** **Unspecified injury of popliteal vein**

    √7ᵗʰ **S85.501** **Unspecified injury of popliteal vein, right leg** `MCC`
CC Excl: MCC with 7th A: S75.801 with 7th A, S75.809-S75.811 with 7th A, S75.819-S75.891 with 7th A, S75.899-S75.901 with 7th A, S75.909-S75.911 with 7th A, S75.919-S75.991 with 7th A, S75.999 with 7th A, S85.201 with 7th A, S85.209-S85.211 with 7th A, S85.219-S85.291 with 7th A, S85.299A, S85.501A, S85.509-S85.511 with 7th A, S85.519-S85.591 with 7th A, S85.599-S85.801 with 7th A, S85.809-S85.811 with 7th A, S85.819-S85.891 with 7th A, S85.899-S85.901 with 7th A, S85.909-S85.911 with 7th A, S85.919-S85.991 with 7th A, S85.999A, S95.001A, S95.009-S95.011 with 7th A, S95.019-S95.091 with 7th A, S95.099 with 7th A, S95.201 with 7th A, S95.209-S95.211 with 7th A, S95.219-S95.291 with 7th A, S95.299-S95.801 with 7th A, S95.809-S95.811 with 7th A, S95.819-S95.891 with 7th A, S95.899-S95.901 with 7th A, S95.909-S95.911 with 7th A, S95.919-S95.991 with 7th A, S95.999 with 7th A

N Newborn: 0   P Pediatric: 0-17   M Maternity: 12-55   A Adult: 15-124   **MCC** Major CC Condition   **PDxMCC** PDx acts as own MCC   **CC** CC Condition   **PDxCC** PDx acts as own CC

1050   ICD-10-CM 2016

√7ᵗʰ **S85.502** **Unspecified injury of popliteal vein, left leg** `MCC`
CC Excl: MCC with 7th A: S75.802-S75.809 with 7th A, S75.812-S75.819 with 7th A, S75.892-S75.899 with 7th A, S75.902-S75.909 with 7th A, S75.912-S75.919 with 7th A, S75.992-S75.999 with 7th A, S85.202-S85.209 with 7th A, S85.212-S85.219 with 7th A, S85.292-S85.299 with 7th A, S85.502-S85.509 with 7th A, S85.512-S85.519 with 7th A, S85.592-S85.599 with 7th A, S85.802-S85.809 with 7th A, S85.812-S85.819 with 7th A, S85.892-S85.899 with 7th A, S85.902-S85.909 with 7th A, S85.912-S85.919 with 7th A, S85.992-S85.999 with 7th A, S95.002-S95.009 with 7th A, S95.012-S95.019 with 7th A, S95.092-S95.099 with 7th A, S95.202-S95.209 with 7th A, S95.212-S95.219 with 7th A, S95.292-S95.299 with 7th A, S95.802-S95.809 with 7th A, S95.812-S95.819 with 7th A, S95.892-S95.899 with 7th A, S95.902-S95.909 with 7th A, S95.912-S95.919 with 7th A, S95.992-S95.999 with 7th A

√7ᵗʰ **S85.509** **Unspecified injury of popliteal vein, unspecified leg** `MCC`
CC Excl: MCC with 7th A: S75.801-S75.999 with 7th A, S85.201-S85.299 with 7th A, S85.501-S85.999 with 7th A, S95.001-S95.099 with 7th A, S95.201-S95.999 with 7th A

√6ᵗʰ **S85.51** **Laceration of popliteal vein**

√7ᵗʰ **S85.511** **Laceration of popliteal vein, right leg** `MCC`
CC Excl: See code: S85.501

√7ᵗʰ **S85.512** **Laceration of popliteal vein, left leg** `MCC`
CC Excl: See code: S85.502

√7ᵗʰ **S85.519** **Laceration of popliteal vein, unspecified leg** `MCC`
CC Excl: See code: S85.509

√6ᵗʰ **S85.59** **Other specified injury of popliteal vein**

√7ᵗʰ **S85.591** **Other specified injury of popliteal vein, right leg** `MCC`
CC Excl: See code: S85.501

√7ᵗʰ **S85.592** **Other specified injury of popliteal vein, left leg** `MCC`
CC Excl: See code: S85.502

√7ᵗʰ **S85.599** **Other specified injury of popliteal vein, unspecified leg** `MCC`
CC Excl: See code: S85.509

√5ᵗʰ **S85.8** **Injury of other blood vessels at lower leg level**

√6ᵗʰ **S85.80** **Unspecified injury of other blood vessels at lower leg level**

√7ᵗʰ **S85.801** **Unspecified injury of other blood vessels at lower leg level, right leg** `CC`
CC Excl: CC with 7th character A: See code: S85.501

√7ᵗʰ **S85.802** **Unspecified injury of other blood vessels at lower leg level, left leg** `CC`
CC Excl: CC with 7th character A: See code: S85.502

√7ᵗʰ **S85.809** **Unspecified injury of other blood vessels at lower leg level, unspecified leg** `CC`
CC Excl: CC with 7th character A: See code: S85.509

√6ᵗʰ **S85.81** **Laceration of other blood vessels at lower leg level**

√7ᵗʰ **S85.811** **Laceration of other blood vessels at lower leg level, right leg** `CC`
CC Excl: CC with 7th character A: See code: S85.501

√7ᵗʰ **S85.812** **Laceration of other blood vessels at lower leg level, left leg** `CC`
CC Excl: CC with 7th character A: See code: S85.502

√7ᵗʰ **S85.819** **Laceration of other blood vessels at lower leg level, unspecified leg** `CC`
CC Excl: CC with 7th character A: See code: S85.509

√6ᵗʰ **S85.89** **Other specified injury of other blood vessels at lower leg level**

√7ᵗʰ **S85.891** **Other specified injury of other blood vessels at lower leg level, right leg** `CC`
CC Excl: CC with 7th character A: See code: S85.501

√7ᵗʰ **S85.892** **Other specified injury of other blood vessels at lower leg level, left leg** `CC`
CC Excl: CC with 7th character A: See code: S85.502

√7ᵗʰ **S85.899** **Other specified injury of other blood vessels at lower leg level, unspecified leg** `CC`
CC Excl: CC with 7th character A: See code: S85.509

√5ᵗʰ **S85.9** **Injury of unspecified blood vessel at lower leg level**

√6ᵗʰ **S85.90** **Unspecified injury of unspecified blood vessel at lower leg level**

√7ᵗʰ **S85.901** **Unspecified injury of unspecified blood vessel at lower leg level, right leg** `CC`
CC Excl: See code: S85.501

√7ᵗʰ **S85.902** **Unspecified injury of unspecified blood vessel at lower leg level, left leg** `CC`
CC Excl: See code: S85.502

√7ᵗʰ **S85.909** **Unspecified injury of unspecified blood vessel at lower leg level, unspecified leg** `CC`
CC Excl: See code: S85.509

√6ᵗʰ **S85.91** **Laceration of unspecified blood vessel at lower leg level**

√7ᵗʰ **S85.911** **Laceration of unspecified blood vessel at lower leg level, right leg** `CC`
CC Excl: See code: S85.501

√7ᵗʰ **S85.912** **Laceration of unspecified blood vessel at lower leg level, left leg** `CC`
CC Excl: See code: S85.502

√7ᵗʰ **S85.919** **Laceration of unspecified blood vessel at lower leg level, unspecified leg** `CC`
CC Excl: See code: S85.509

√6ᵗʰ **S85.99** **Other specified injury of unspecified blood vessel at lower leg level**

√7ᵗʰ **S85.991** **Other specified injury of unspecified blood vessel at lower leg level, right leg** `CC`
CC Excl: See code: S85.501

√7ᵗʰ **S85.992** **Other specified injury of unspecified blood vessel at lower leg level, left leg** `CC`
CC Excl: See code: S85.502

√7ᵗʰ **S85.999** **Other specified injury of unspecified blood vessel at lower leg level, unspecified leg** `CC`
CC Excl: See code: S85.509

✦ √4ᵗʰ **S86 Injury of muscle, fascia and tendon at lower leg level**
Code also any associated open wound (S81.-)
EXCLUDES 2   injury of muscle, fascia and tendon at ankle (S96.-)
injury of patellar ligament (tendon) (S76.1-)
sprain of joints and ligaments of knee (S83.-)

The appropriate 7th character is to be added to each code from category S86.
A   initial encounter
D   subsequent encounter
S   sequela

√5ᵗʰ **S86.0** **Injury of Achilles tendon**

√6ᵗʰ **S86.00** **Unspecified injury of Achilles tendon**

√7ᵗʰ **S86.001** **Unspecified injury of right Achilles tendon**

√7ᵗʰ **S86.002** **Unspecified injury of left Achilles tendon**

√7ᵗʰ **S86.009** **Unspecified injury of unspecified Achilles tendon**

√6ᵗʰ **S86.01** **Strain of Achilles tendon**

√7ᵗʰ **S86.011** **Strain of right Achilles tendon**

√7ᵗʰ **S86.012** **Strain of left Achilles tendon**

√7ᵗʰ **S86.019** **Strain of unspecified Achilles tendon**

✦   Refer to the Muscle/Tendon Table at beginning of this chapter.

√6ᵗʰ **S86.02** **Laceration of Achilles tendon**

√7ᵗʰ **S86.021** **Laceration of right Achilles tendon** CC
CC Excl: CC with 7th character A: S81.001
with 7th A, S81.009-S81.011 with 7th A,
S81.019-S81.021 with 7th A, S81.029-
S81.031 with 7th A, S81.039-S81.041 with
7th A, S81.049-S81.051 with 7th A, S81.059-
S81.801 with 7th A, S81.809-S81.811 with
7th A, S81.819-S81.821 with 7th A, S81.829-
S81.831 with 7th A, S81.839-S81.841 with
7th A, S81.849-S81.851 with 7th A, S81.859A,
S86.021A, S86.029A, S86.121A, S86.129A,
S86.221A, S86.229A, S86.321A, S86.329A,
S86.821A, S86.829A, S86.921A, S86.929A,
S91.001A, S91.009-S91.011 with 7th A,
S91.019-S91.021 with 7th A, S91.029-
S91.031 with 7th A, S91.039-S91.041 with
7th A, S91.049-S91.051 with 7th A, S91.059A,
S96.021A, S96.029A, S96.121A, S96.129A,
S96.221A, S96.229A, S96.821A, S96.829A,
S96.921A, S96.929A

√7ᵗʰ **S86.022** **Laceration of left Achilles tendon** CC
CC Excl: CC with 7th character A: S81.002-
S81.009 with 7th A, S81.012-S81.019 with
7th A, S81.022-S81.029 with 7th A, S81.032-
S81.039 with 7th A, S81.042-S81.049 with
7th A, S81.052-S81.059 with 7th A, S81.802-
S81.809 with 7th A, S81.812-S81.819 with
7th A, S81.822-S81.829 with 7th A, S81.832-
S81.839 with 7th A, S81.842-S81.849 with
7th A, S81.852-S81.859 with 7th A, S86.022-
S86.029 with 7th A, S86.122-S86.129 with
7th A, S86.222-S86.229 with 7th A, S86.322-
S86.329 with 7th A, S86.822-S86.829 with
7th A, S86.922-S86.929 with 7th A, S91.002-
S91.009 with 7th A, S91.012-S91.019 with
7th A, S91.022-S91.029 with 7th A, S91.032-
S91.039 with 7th A, S91.042-S91.049 with
7th A, S91.052-S91.059 with 7th A, S96.022-
S96.029 with 7th A, S96.122-S96.129 with
7th A, S96.222-S96.229 with 7th A, S96.822-
S96.829 with 7th A, S96.922-S96.929 with
7th A

√7ᵗʰ **S86.029** **Laceration of unspecified Achilles tendon** CC
CC Excl: CC with 7th character A: S81.001-
S81.859 with 7th A, S86.021-S86.029 with
7th A, S86.121-S86.129 with 7th A, S86.221-
S86.229 with 7th A, S86.321-S86.329 with
7th A, S86.821-S86.829 with 7th A, S86.921-
S86.929 with 7th A, S91.001-S91.059 with
7th A, S96.021-S96.029 with 7th A, S96.121-
S96.129 with 7th A, S96.221-S96.229 with
7th A, S96.821-S96.829 with 7th A, S96.921-
S96.929 with 7th A

√6ᵗʰ **S86.09** **Other specified injury of Achilles tendon**

√7ᵗʰ **S86.091** **Other specified injury of right Achilles tendon**

√7ᵗʰ **S86.092** **Other specified injury of left Achilles tendon**

√7ᵗʰ **S86.099** **Other specified injury of unspecified Achilles tendon**

√5ᵗʰ **S86.1** **Injury of other muscle(s) and tendon(s) of posterior muscle group at lower leg level**

√6ᵗʰ **S86.10** **Unspecified injury of other muscle(s) and tendon(s) of posterior muscle group at lower leg level**

√7ᵗʰ **S86.101** **Unspecified injury of other muscle(s) and tendon(s) of posterior muscle group at lower leg level, right leg**

√7ᵗʰ **S86.102** **Unspecified injury of other muscle(s) and tendon(s) of posterior muscle group at lower leg level, left leg**

√7ᵗʰ **S86.109** **Unspecified injury of other muscle(s) and tendon(s) of posterior muscle group at lower leg level, unspecified leg**

√6ᵗʰ **S86.11** **Strain of other muscle(s) and tendon(s) of posterior muscle group at lower leg level**

√7ᵗʰ **S86.111** **Strain of other muscle(s) and tendon(s) of posterior muscle group at lower leg level, right leg**

√7ᵗʰ **S86.112** **Strain of other muscle(s) and tendon(s) of posterior muscle group at lower leg level, left leg**

√7ᵗʰ **S86.119** **Strain of other muscle(s) and tendon(s) of posterior muscle group at lower leg level, unspecified leg**

√6ᵗʰ **S86.12** **Laceration of other muscle(s) and tendon(s) of posterior muscle group at lower leg level**

√7ᵗʰ **S86.121** **Laceration of other muscle(s) and tendon(s) of posterior muscle group at lower leg level, right leg** CC
CC Excl: See code: S86.021

√7ᵗʰ **S86.122** **Laceration of other muscle(s) and tendon(s) of posterior muscle group at lower leg level, left leg** CC
CC Excl: See code: S86.022

√7ᵗʰ **S86.129** **Laceration of other muscle(s) and tendon(s) of posterior muscle group at lower leg level, unspecified leg** CC
CC Excl: See code: S86.029

√6ᵗʰ **S86.19** **Other injury of other muscle(s) and tendon(s) of posterior muscle group at lower leg level**

√7ᵗʰ **S86.191** **Other injury of other muscle(s) and tendon(s) of posterior muscle group at lower leg level, right leg**

√7ᵗʰ **S86.192** **Other injury of other muscle(s) and tendon(s) of posterior muscle group at lower leg level, left leg**

√7ᵗʰ **S86.199** **Other injury of other muscle(s) and tendon(s) of posterior muscle group at lower leg level, unspecified leg**

√5ᵗʰ **S86.2** **Injury of muscle(s) and tendon(s) of anterior muscle group at lower leg level**

√6ᵗʰ **S86.20** **Unspecified injury of muscle(s) and tendon(s) of anterior muscle group at lower leg level**

√7ᵗʰ **S86.201** **Unspecified injury of muscle(s) and tendon(s) of anterior muscle group at lower leg level, right leg**

√7ᵗʰ **S86.202** **Unspecified injury of muscle(s) and tendon(s) of anterior muscle group at lower leg level, left leg**

√7ᵗʰ **S86.209** **Unspecified injury of muscle(s) and tendon(s) of anterior muscle group at lower leg level, unspecified leg**

√6ᵗʰ **S86.21** **Strain of muscle(s) and tendon(s) of anterior muscle group at lower leg level**

√7ᵗʰ **S86.211** **Strain of muscle(s) and tendon(s) of anterior muscle group at lower leg level, right leg**

√7ᵗʰ **S86.212** **Strain of muscle(s) and tendon(s) of anterior muscle group at lower leg level, left leg**

√7ᵗʰ **S86.219** **Strain of muscle(s) and tendon(s) of anterior muscle group at lower leg level, unspecified leg**

√6ᵗʰ **S86.22** **Laceration of muscle(s) and tendon(s) of anterior muscle group at lower leg level**

√7ᵗʰ **S86.221** **Laceration of muscle(s) and tendon(s) of anterior muscle group at lower leg level, right leg** CC
CC Excl: See code: S86.021

√7ᵗʰ **S86.222** **Laceration of muscle(s) and tendon(s) of anterior muscle group at lower leg level, left leg** CC
CC Excl: See code: S86.022

√7ᵗʰ **S86.229** **Laceration of muscle(s) and tendon(s) of anterior muscle group at lower leg level, unspecified leg** CC
CC Excl: See code: S86.029

√6ᵗʰ **S86.29** **Other injury of muscle(s) and tendon(s) of anterior muscle group at lower leg level**

√7ᵗʰ **S86.291** **Other injury of muscle(s) and tendon(s) of anterior muscle group at lower leg level, right leg**

√7ᵗʰ **S86.292** **Other injury of muscle(s) and tendon(s) of anterior muscle group at lower leg level, left leg**

√7ᵗʰ **S86.299** **Other injury of muscle(s) and tendon(s) of anterior muscle group at lower leg level, unspecified leg**

Ⓝ Newborn: 0   Ⓟ Pediatric: 0-17   Ⓜ Maternity: 12-55   Ⓐ Adult: 15-124   **MCC** Major CC Condition   **PDxMCC** PDx acts as own MCC   **CC** CC Condition   **PDxCC** PDx acts as own CC

1052   ICD-10-CM 2016

☑5ᵗʰ **S86.3** Injury of muscle(s) and tendon(s) of peroneal muscle group at lower leg level

     ☑6ᵗʰ **S86.30** Unspecified injury of muscle(s) and tendon(s) of peroneal muscle group at lower leg level

         ☑7ᵗʰ **S86.301** Unspecified injury of muscle(s) and tendon(s) of peroneal muscle group at lower leg level, **right leg**

         ☑7ᵗʰ **S86.302** Unspecified injury of muscle(s) and tendon(s) of peroneal muscle group at lower leg level, **left leg**

         ☑7ᵗʰ **S86.309** Unspecified injury of muscle(s) and tendon(s) of peroneal muscle group at lower leg level, **unspecified leg**

     ☑6ᵗʰ **S86.31** Strain of muscle(s) and tendon(s) of peroneal muscle group at lower leg level

         ☑7ᵗʰ **S86.311** Strain of muscle(s) and tendon(s) of peroneal muscle group at lower leg level, **right leg**

         ☑7ᵗʰ **S86.312** Strain of muscle(s) and tendon(s) of peroneal muscle group at lower leg level, **left leg**

         ☑7ᵗʰ **S86.319** Strain of muscle(s) and tendon(s) of peroneal muscle group at lower leg level, **unspecified leg**

     ☑6ᵗʰ **S86.32** Laceration of muscle(s) and tendon(s) of peroneal muscle group at lower leg level

         ☑7ᵗʰ **S86.321** Laceration of muscle(s) and tendon(s) of peroneal muscle group at lower leg level, **right leg**   CC
            CC Excl: See code: S86.021

         ☑7ᵗʰ **S86.322** Laceration of muscle(s) and tendon(s) of peroneal muscle group at lower leg level, **left leg**   CC
            CC Excl: See code: S86.022

         ☑7ᵗʰ **S86.329** Laceration of muscle(s) and tendon(s) of peroneal muscle group at lower leg level, **unspecified leg**   CC
            CC Excl: See code: S86.029

     ☑6ᵗʰ **S86.39** Other injury of muscle(s) and tendon(s) of peroneal muscle group at lower leg level

         ☑7ᵗʰ **S86.391** Other injury of muscle(s) and tendon(s) of peroneal muscle group at lower leg level, **right leg**

         ☑7ᵗʰ **S86.392** Other injury of muscle(s) and tendon(s) of peroneal muscle group at lower leg level, **left leg**

         ☑7ᵗʰ **S86.399** Other injury of muscle(s) and tendon(s) of peroneal muscle group at lower leg level, **unspecified leg**

☑5ᵗʰ **S86.8** Injury of other muscles and tendons at lower leg level

     ☑6ᵗʰ **S86.80** Unspecified injury of other muscles and tendons at lower leg level

         ☑7ᵗʰ **S86.801** Unspecified injury of other muscle(s) and tendon(s) at lower leg level, **right leg**

         ☑7ᵗʰ **S86.802** Unspecified injury of other muscle(s) and tendon(s) at lower leg level, **left leg**

         ☑7ᵗʰ **S86.809** Unspecified injury of other muscle(s) and tendon(s) at lower leg level, **unspecified leg**

     ☑6ᵗʰ **S86.81** Strain of other muscles and tendons at lower leg level

         ☑7ᵗʰ **S86.811** Strain of other muscle(s) and tendon(s) at lower leg level, **right leg**

         ☑7ᵗʰ **S86.812** Strain of other muscle(s) and tendon(s) at lower leg level, **left leg**

         ☑7ᵗʰ **S86.819** Strain of other muscle(s) and tendon(s) at lower leg level, **unspecified leg**

     ☑6ᵗʰ **S86.82** Laceration of other muscles and tendons at lower leg level

         ☑7ᵗʰ **S86.821** Laceration of other muscle(s) and tendon(s) at lower leg level, **right leg**   CC
            CC Excl: See code: S86.021

         ☑7ᵗʰ **S86.822** Laceration of other muscle(s) and tendon(s) at lower leg level, **left leg**   CC
            CC Excl: See code: S86.022

         ☑7ᵗʰ **S86.829** Laceration of other muscle(s) and tendon(s) at lower leg level, **unspecified leg**   CC
            CC Excl: See code: S86.029

     ☑6ᵗʰ **S86.89** Other injury of other muscles and tendons at lower leg level

         ☑7ᵗʰ **S86.891** Other injury of other muscle(s) and tendon(s) at lower leg level, **right leg**

         ☑7ᵗʰ **S86.892** Other injury of other muscle(s) and tendon(s) at lower leg level, **left leg**

         ☑7ᵗʰ **S86.899** Other injury of other muscle(s) and tendon(s) at lower leg level, **unspecified leg**

☑5ᵗʰ **S86.9** Injury of **unspecified** muscle and tendon at lower leg level

     ☑6ᵗʰ **S86.90** Unspecified injury of unspecified muscle and tendon at lower leg level

         ☑7ᵗʰ **S86.901** Unspecified injury of unspecified muscle(s) and tendon(s) at lower leg level, **right leg**

         ☑7ᵗʰ **S86.902** Unspecified injury of unspecified muscle(s) and tendon(s) at lower leg level, **left leg**

         ☑7ᵗʰ **S86.909** Unspecified injury of unspecified muscle(s) and tendon(s) at lower leg level, **unspecified leg**

     ☑6ᵗʰ **S86.91** Strain of unspecified muscle and tendon at lower leg level

         ☑7ᵗʰ **S86.911** Strain of unspecified muscle(s) and tendon(s) at lower leg level, **right leg**

         ☑7ᵗʰ **S86.912** Strain of unspecified muscle(s) and tendon(s) at lower leg level, **left leg**

         ☑7ᵗʰ **S86.919** Strain of unspecified muscle(s) and tendon(s) at lower leg level, **unspecified leg**

     ☑6ᵗʰ **S86.92** Laceration of unspecified muscle and tendon at lower leg level

         ☑7ᵗʰ **S86.921** Laceration of unspecified muscle(s) and tendon(s) at lower leg level, **right leg**   CC
            CC Excl: See code: S86.021

         ☑7ᵗʰ **S86.922** Laceration of unspecified muscle(s) and tendon(s) at lower leg level, **left leg**   CC
            CC Excl: See code: S86.022

         ☑7ᵗʰ **S86.929** Laceration of unspecified muscle(s) and tendon(s) at lower leg level, **unspecified leg**   CC
            CC Excl: See code: S86.029

     ☑6ᵗʰ **S86.99** Other injury of unspecified muscle and tendon at lower leg level

         ☑7ᵗʰ **S86.991** Other injury of unspecified muscle(s) and tendon(s) at lower leg level, **right leg**

         ☑7ᵗʰ **S86.992** Other injury of unspecified muscle(s) and tendon(s) at lower leg level, **left leg**

         ☑7ᵗʰ **S86.999** Other injury of unspecified muscle(s) and tendon(s) at lower leg level, **unspecified leg**

☑4ᵗʰ **S87** **Crushing injury of lower leg**

     Use additional code(s) for all associated injuries

     EXCLUDES 2   crushing injury of ankle and foot (S97.-)

> The appropriate 7th character is to be added to each code from category S87.
> A   initial encounter
> D   subsequent encounter
> S   sequela

     ☑5ᵗʰ **S87.0** Crushing injury of knee

         ☑x7ᵗʰ **S87.00** Crushing injury of **unspecified** knee

         ☑x7ᵗʰ **S87.01** Crushing injury of **right** knee

         ☑x7ᵗʰ **S87.02** Crushing injury of **left** knee

     ☑5ᵗʰ **S87.8** Crushing injury of **lower leg**

         ☑x7ᵗʰ **S87.80** Crushing injury of **unspecified** lower leg

         ☑x7ᵗʰ **S87.81** Crushing injury of **right** lower leg

         ☑x7ᵗʰ **S87.82** Crushing injury of **left** lower leg

---

☑ Additional Character Required   ☑x7ᵗʰ Placeholder Alert   Unacceptable PDx   Manifestation   Hospital Acquired Condition   *EXCLUDES 1* Not Coded Here   *EXCLUDES 2* Not Included Here

√4ᵗʰ **S88** **Traumatic amputation of lower leg**

> **NOTE** An amputation not identified as partial or complete should be coded to complete.
>
> *EXCLUDES 1* *traumatic amputation of ankle and foot (S98.-)*

> The appropriate 7th character is to be added to each code from category S88.
> A   initial encounter
> D   subsequent encounter
> S   sequela

√5ᵗʰ **S88.0** **Traumatic amputation at knee level**

√6ᵗʰ   **S88.01**   **Complete traumatic amputation at knee level**

√7ᵗʰ   **S88.011**   **Complete traumatic amputation at knee level, right lower leg**   **CC**

CC Excl: CC with 7th character A: S71.001 with 7th A, S71.009-S71.011 with 7th A, S71.019-S71.021 with 7th A, S71.029-S71.031 with 7th A, S71.039-S71.041 with 7th A, S71.049-S71.051 with 7th A, S71.059-S71.101 with 7th A, S71.109-S71.111 with 7th A, S71.119-S71.121 with 7th A, S71.129-S71.131 with 7th A, S71.139-S71.141 with 7th A, S71.149-S71.151 with 7th A, S71.159A, S76.021A, S76.029A, S76.121 A, S76.129A, S76.221A, S76.229A, S76.321A, S76.329A, S76.821A, S76.829A, S76.921A, S76.929A, S78.011A, S78.019-S78.021 with 7th A, S78.029-S78.111 with 7th A, S78.119-S78.121 with 7th A, S78.129-S78.911 with 7th A, S78.919-S78.921 with 7th A, S78.929A, S81.001A, S81.009-S81.011 with 7th A, S81.019-S81.021 with 7th A, S81.029-S81.031 with 7th A, S81.039-S81.041 with 7th A, S81.049-S81.051 with 7th A, S81.059-S81.801 with 7th A, S81.809-S81.811 with 7th A, S81.819-S81.821 with 7th A, S81.829-S81.831 with 7th A, S81.839-S81.841 with 7th A, S81.849-S81.851 with 7th A, S81.859 with 7th A, S86.021A, S86.029A, S86.121A, S86.129A, S86.221A, S86.229A, S86.321A, S86.329A, S86.821A, S86.829A, S86.921A, S86.929A, S88.011A, S88.019-S88.021 with 7th A, S88.029-S88.111 with 7th A, S88.119-S88.121 with 7th A, S88.129-S88.911 with 7th A, S88.919-S88.921 with 7th A, S88.929A, S91.001A, S91.009-S91.011 with 7th A, S91.019-S91.021 with 7th A, S91.029-S91.031 with 7th A, S91.039-S91.041 with 7th A, S91.049-S91.051 with 7th A, S91.059-S91.101 with 7th A, S91.103-S91.104 with 7th A, S91.106-S91.111 with 7th A, S91.113-S91.114 with 7th A, S91.116-S91.121 with 7th A, S91.123-S91.124 with 7th A, S91.126-S91.131 with 7th A, S91.133-S91.134 with 7th A, S91.136-S91.141 with 7th A, S91.143-S91.144 with 7th A, S91.146-S91.151 with 7th A, S91.153-S91.154 with 7th A, S91.156-S91.201 with 7th A, S91.203-S91.204 with 7th A, S91.206-S91.211 with 7th A, S91.213-S91.214 with 7th A, S91.216-S91.221 with 7th A, S91.223-S91.224 with 7th A, S91.226-S91.231 with 7th A, S91.233-S91.234 with 7th A, S91.236-S91.241 with 7th A, S91.243-S91.244 with 7th A, S91.246-S91.251 with 7th A, S91.253-S91.254 with 7th A, S91.256-S91.301 with 7th A, S91.309-S91.311 with 7th A, S91.319-S91.321 with 7th A, S91.329-S91.331 with 7th A, S91.339-S91.341 with 7th A, S91.349-S91.351 with 7th A, S91.359A, S96.021A, S96.029A, S96.121A, S96.129A, S96.221A, S96.229A, S96.821A, S96.829A, S96.921A, S96.929A, S98.011A, S98.019-S98.021 with 7th A, S98.029-S98.111 with 7th A, S98.119-S98.121 with 7th A, S98.122-S98.129 with 7th A, S98.131-S98.139 with 7th A, S98.142-S98.149 with 7th A, S98.212-S98.219 with 7th A, S98.222-S98.229 with 7th A, S98.312-S98.319 with 7th A, S98.322-S98.329 with 7th A, S98.912-S98.919 with 7th A, S98.922-S98.929 with 7th A, T14.90-T14.91, T79.A0X-T79.9XX with 7th A

√7ᵗʰ   **S88.012**   **Complete traumatic amputation at knee level, left lower leg**   **CC**

CC Excl: CC with 7th character A: S71.002-S71.009 with 7th A, S71.012-S71.019 with 7th A, S71.022-S71.029 with 7th A, S71.032-S71.039 with 7th A, S71.042-S71.049 with 7th A, S71.052-S71.059 with 7th A, S71.102-S71.109 with 7th A, S71.112-S71.119 with 7th A, S71.122-S71.129 with 7th A, S71.132-S71.139 with 7th A, S71.142-S71.149 with 7th A, S71.152-S71.159 with 7th A, S76.022-S76.029 with 7th A, S76.122-S76.129 with 7th A, S76.222-S76.229 with 7th A, S76.322-S76.329 with 7th A, S76.822-S76.829 with 7th A, S76.922-S76.929 with 7th A, S78.012-S78.019 with 7th A, S78.022-S78.029 with 7th A, S78.112-S78.119 with 7th A, S78.122-S78.129 with 7th A, S78.912-S78.919 with 7th A, S78.922-S78.929 with 7th A, S81.002-S81.009 with 7th A, S81.012-S81.019 with 7th A, S81.022-S81.029 with 7th A, S81.032-S81.039 with 7th A, S81.042-S81.049 with 7th A, S81.052-S81.059 with 7th A, S81.802-S81.809 with 7th A, S81.812-S81.819 with 7th A, S81.822-S81.829 with 7th A, S81.832-S81.839 with 7th A, S81.842-S81.849 with 7th A, S81.852-S81.859 with 7th A, S86.022-S86.029 with 7th A, S86.122-S86.129 with 7th A, S86.222-S86.229 with 7th A, S86.322-S86.329 with 7th A, S86.822-S86.829 with 7th A, S86.922-S86.929 with 7th A, S88.012-S88.019 with 7th A, S88.022-S88.029 with 7th A, S88.112-S88.119 with 7th A, S88.122-S88.129 with 7th A, S88.912-S88.919 with 7th A, S88.922-S88.929 with 7th A, S91.002-S91.009 with 7th A, S91.012-S91.019 with 7th A, S91.022-S91.029 with 7th A, S91.032-S91.039 with 7th A, S91.042-S91.049 with 7th A, S91.052-S91.059 with 7th A, S91.102-S91.103 with 7th A, S91.105-S91.109 with 7th A, S91.112-S91.113 with 7th A, S91.115-S91.119 with 7th A, S91.122-S91.123 with 7th A, S91.125-S91.129 with 7th A, S91.132-S91.133 with 7th A, S91.135-S91.139 with 7th A, S91.142-S91.143 with 7th A, S91.145-S91.149 with 7th A, S91.152-S91.153 with 7th A, S91.155-S91.159 with 7th A, S91.202-S91.203 with 7th A, S91.205-S91.209 with 7th A, S91.212-S91.213 with 7th A, S91.215-S91.219 with 7th A, S91.222-S91.223 with 7th A, S91.225-S91.229 with 7th A, S91.232-S91.233 with 7th A, S91.235-S91.239 with 7th A, S91.242-S91.243 with 7th A, S91.245-S91.249 with 7th A, S91.252-S91.253 with 7th A, S91.255-S91.259 with 7th A, S91.302-S91.309 with 7th A, S91.312-S91.319 with 7th A, S91.322-S91.329 with 7th A, S91.332-S91.339 with 7th A, S91.342-S91.349 with 7th A, S91.352-S91.359 with 7th A, S96.022-S96.029 with 7th A, S96.122-S96.129 with 7th A, S96.222-S96.229 with 7th A, S96.822-S96.829 with 7th A, S96.922-S96.929 with 7th A, S98.012-S98.019 with 7th A, S98.022-S98.029 with 7th A, S98.112-S98.119 with 7th A, S98.122-S98.129 with 7th A, S98.132-S98.139 with 7th A, S98.142-S98.149 with 7th A, S98.212-S98.219 with 7th A, S98.222-S98.229 with 7th A, S98.312-S98.319 with 7th A, S98.322-S98.329 with 7th A, S98.912-S98.919 with 7th A, S98.922-S98.929 with 7th A, T14.90-T14.91, T79.A0X-T79.9XX with 7th A

√7ᵗʰ   **S88.019**   **Complete traumatic amputation at knee level, unspecified lower leg**   **CC**

CC Excl: CC with 7th character A: S71.001-S71.159 with 7th A, S76.021-S76.029 with 7th A, S76.121-S76.129 with 7th A, S76.221-S76.229 with 7th A, S76.321-S76.329 with 7th A, S76.821-S76.829 with 7th A, S76.921-S76.929 with 7th A, S78.011-S78.929 with 7th A, S81.001-S81.859 with 7th A, S86.021-S86.029 with 7th A, S86.121-S86.129 with 7th A, S86.221-S86.229 with 7th A, S86.321-S86.329 with 7th A, S86.821-S86.829 with 7th A, S86.921-S86.929 with 7th A, S88.011-S88.929 with 7th A, S91.001-S91.359 with 7th A, S96.021-S96.029 with 7th A, S96.121-S96.129 with 7th A, S96.221-S96.229 with 7th A, S96.821-S96.829 with 7th A, S96.921-S96.929 with 7th A, S98.011-S98.929 with 7th A, T14.90-T14.91, T79.A0X-T79.9XX with 7th A

N Newborn: 0   P Pediatric: 0-17   M Maternity: 12-55   A Adult: 15-124   MCC Major CC Condition   PDxMCC PDx acts as own MCC   CC CC Condition   PDxCC PDx acts as own CC

1054   ICD-10-CM 2016

S88–S88.019

✓6ᵗʰ **S88.02** Partial traumatic amputation at knee level

    ✓7ᵗʰ **S88.021** **Partial traumatic amputation at knee level, right lower leg** `CC`
        CC Excl: See code: S88.011

    ✓7ᵗʰ **S88.022** **Partial traumatic amputation at knee level, left lower leg** `CC`
        CC Excl: See code: S88.012

    ✓7ᵗʰ **S88.029** **Partial traumatic amputation at knee level, unspecified lower leg** `CC`
        CC Excl: See code: S88.019

✓5ᵗʰ **S88.1** Traumatic amputation at level between knee and ankle

  ✓6ᵗʰ **S88.11** Complete traumatic amputation at level between knee and ankle

    ✓7ᵗʰ **S88.111** **Complete traumatic amputation at levelbetween knee and ankle, right lower leg** `CC`
        CC Excl: See code: S88.011

    ✓7ᵗʰ **S88.112** **Complete traumatic amputation at level between knee and ankle, left lower leg** `CC`
        CC Excl: See code: S88.012

    ✓7ᵗʰ **S88.119** **Complete traumatic amputation at level between knee and ankle, unspecified lower leg** `CC`
        CC Excl: See code: S88.019

  ✓6ᵗʰ **S88.12** Partial traumatic amputation at level between knee and ankle

    ✓7ᵗʰ **S88.121** **Partial traumatic amputation at level between knee and ankle, right lower leg** `CC`
        CC Excl: See code: S88.011

    ✓7ᵗʰ **S88.122** **Partial traumatic amputation at levelbetween knee and ankle, left lower leg** `CC`
        CC Excl: See code: S88.012

    ✓7ᵗʰ **S88.129** **Partial traumatic amputation at level between knee and ankle, unspecified lower leg** `CC`
        CC Excl: See code: S88.019

✓5ᵗʰ **S88.9** Traumatic amputation of lower leg, level unspecified

  ✓6ᵗʰ **S88.91** Complete traumatic amputation of lower leg, level unspecified

    ✓7ᵗʰ **S88.911** **Complete traumatic amputation of right lower leg, level unspecified** `CC`
        CC Excl: See code: S88.011

    ✓7ᵗʰ **S88.912** **Complete traumatic amputation of left lower leg, level unspecified** `CC`
        CC Excl: See code: S88.012

    ✓7ᵗʰ **S88.919** **Complete traumatic amputation of unspecified lower leg, level unspecified** `CC`
        CC Excl: See code: S88.019

  ✓6ᵗʰ **S88.92** Partial traumatic amputation of lower leg, level unspecified

    ✓7ᵗʰ **S88.921** **Partial traumatic amputation of right lower leg, level unspecified** `CC`
        CC Excl: See code: S88.011

    ✓7ᵗʰ **S88.922** **Partial traumatic amputation of left lower leg, level unspecified** `CC`
        CC Excl: See code: S88.012

    ✓7ᵗʰ **S88.929** **Partial traumatic amputation of unspecified lower leg, level unspecified** `CC`
        CC Excl: See code: S88.019

✓4ᵗʰ **S89** **Other and unspecified injuries of lower leg**

    NOTE A fracture not indicated as open or closed should be coded to closed.

    EXCLUDES 2   other and unspecified injuries of ankle and foot (S99.-)

    The appropriate 7th character is to be added to each code from subcategories S89.0, S89.1, S89.2, and S89.3.
    A   initial encounter for closed fracture
    D   subsequent encounter for fracture with routine healing
    G   subsequent encounter for fracture with delayed healing
    K   subsequent encounter for fracture with nonunion
    P   subsequent encounter for fracture with malunion
    S   sequela

✓5ᵗʰ **S89.0** Physeal fracture of upper end of tibia

  ✓6ᵗʰ **S89.00** Unspecified physeal fracture of upper end of tibia

    7,19 ✓7ᵗʰ **S89.001** **Unspecified physeal fracture of upper end of right tibia** `CC`

    CC Excl: CC with 7th character A: M80.00X-M80.019 with 7th A, M80.041-M80.049 with 7th A, M80.061-M80.079 with 7th A, M80.80X-M80.819 with 7th A, M80.841-M80.849 with 7th A, M80.861-M80.879 with 7th A, M84.40X-M84.419 with 7th A, M84.441-M84.446 with 7th A, M84.454 with 7th A, M84.461-M84.519 with 7th A, M84.541-M84.550 with 7th A, M84.561-M84.576 with 7th A, M84.60X-M84.619 with 7th A, M84.641-M84.650 with 7th A, M84.661-M84.68X with 7th A, S03.8XX-S03.9XX with 7th A, S29.011-S29.019 with 7th A, S38.3XX-S39.013 with 7th A, S73.101A, S73.109-S73.111 with 7th A, S73.119-S73.121 with 7th A, S73.129-S73.191 with 7th A, S73.199A, S76.001A, S76.009-S76.011 with 7th A, S76.019A, S76.091A, S76.099-S76.101 with 7th A, S76.109-S76.111 with 7th A, S76.119A, S76.191A, S76.199-S76.201 with 7th A, S76.209-S76.211 with 7th A, S76.219A, S76.291A, S76.299-S76.301 with 7th A, S76.309-S76.311 with 7th A, S76.319A, S76.391A, S76.399-S76.801 with 7th A, S76.809-S76.811 with 7th A, S76.819A, S76.891A, S76.899-S76.901 with 7th A, S76.909-S76.911 with 7th A, S76.919A, S76.991A, S76.999A, S79.811A, S79.819-S79.821 with 7th A, S79.829-S79.911 with 7th A, S79.919-S79.921 with 7th A, S79.929A, S82.101-S82.156 with 7th [A, B, C], S82.191-S82.299 with 7th [A, B, C], S82.401-S82.499 with 7th [A, B, C], S82.831-S82.839 with 7th [A, B, C], S82.861-S82.866 with 7th [A, B, C], S82.90X-S82.92X with 7th [A, B, C], S89.001 with 7th A, S89.009-S89.011 with 7th A, S89.019-S89.021 with 7th A, S89.029-S89.031 with 7th A, S89.039-S89.041 with 7th A, S89.049-S89.091 with 7th A, S89.099A, S89.201A, S89.209-S89.211 with 7th A, S89.219-S89.221 with 7th A, S89.229-S89.291 with 7th A, S89.299A, T14.90-T14.91, T79.A9X-T79.9XX with 7th A
    CC with 7th character K or P: M80.00X-M84.68X with 7th [K, P], S02.0XX-S02.92X with 7th K, S12.000-S12.691 with 7th K, S22.000-S22.9XX with 7th K, S32.000-S32.9XX with 7th K, S42.001-S42.92X with 7th [K, P], S49.001-S49.199 with 7th [K, P], S52.001-S52.92X with 7th [K, M, N, P, Q, R], S59.001-S59.299 with 7th [K, P], S62.001-S62.92X with 7th [K, P], S72.001-S72.92X with 7th [K, M, N, P, Q, R], S79.001-S79.199 with 7th [K, P], S82.001-S82.92X with 7th [K, M, N, P, Q, R], S89.001-S89.399 with 7th [K, P], S92.001-S92.919 with 7th [K, P]

---

7   HAC = Initial encounter only (7th character A, B or C) and not POA.
19   CC only if an initial encounter for a closed fracture (7th character A) **OR** a subsequent encounter for nonunion or malunion (7th character K, M, N, P, Q, or R– specific to category).

✔ Additional Character Required   ✔x7ᵗʰ Placeholder Alert   <u>Unacceptable PDx</u>   <u>Manifestation</u>   Hospital Acquired Condition   *EXCLUDES 1* Not Coded Here   *EXCLUDES 2* Not Included Here

7,19 ✓7th **S89.002** **Unspecified physeal fracture of upper end of left tibia** `CC`

CC Excl: CC with 7th character A: M80.00X-M80.019 with 7th A, M80.041-M80.049 with 7th A, M80.061-M80.079 with 7th A, M80.80X-M80.819 with 7th A, M80.841-M80.849 with 7th A, M80.861-M80.879 with 7th A, M84.40X-M84.419 with 7th A, M84.441-M84.446 with 7th A, M84.454 with 7th A, M84.461-M84.519 with 7th A, M84.541-M84.550 with 7th A, M84.561-M84.576 with 7th A, M84.60X-M84.619 with 7th A, M84.641-M84.650 with 7th A, M84.661-M84.68X with 7th A, S03.8XX-S03.9XX with 7th A, S29.011-S29.019 with 7th A, S38.3XX-S39.013 with 7th A, S73.102-S73.109 with 7th A, S73.112-S73.119 with 7th A, S73.122-S73.129 with 7th A, S73.192-S73.199 with 7th A, S76.002-S76.009 with 7th A, S76.012-S76.019 with 7th A, S76.092-S76.099 with 7th A, S76.102-S76.109 with 7th A, S76.112-S76.119 with 7th A, S76.192-S76.199 with 7th A, S76.202-S76.209 with 7th A, S76.212-S76.219 with 7th A, S76.292-S76.299 with 7th A, S76.302-S76.309 with 7th A, S76.312-S76.319 with 7th A, S76.392-S76.399 with 7th A, S76.802-S76.809 with 7th A, S76.812-S76.819 with 7th A, S76.892-S76.899 with 7th A, S76.902-S76.909 with 7th A, S76.912-S76.919 with 7th A, S76.992-S76.999 with 7th A, S79.812-S79.819 with 7th A, S79.822-S79.829 with 7th A, S79.912-S79.919 with 7th A, S79.922-S79.929 with 7th A, S82.101-S82.156 with 7th [B, C], S82.191-S82.299 with 7th [B, C], S82.401-S82.499 with 7th [B, C], S82.831-S82.839 with 7th [B, C], S82.861-S82.866 with 7th [B, C], S82.90X-S82.92X with 7th [A, B, C], S89.002-S89.009 with 7th A, S89.012-S89.019 with 7th A, S89.022-S89.029 with 7th A, S89.032-S89.039 with 7th A, S89.042-S89.049 with 7th A, S89.092-S89.099 with 7th A, S89.202-S89.209 with 7th A, S89.212-S89.219 with 7th A, S89.222-S89.229 with 7th A, S89.292-S89.299 with 7th A, T14.90-T14.91, T79.A9X-T79.9XX with 7th A

CC with 7th character K or P: M80.00X-M84.68X with 7th [K, P], S02.0XX-S02.92X with 7th K, S12.000-S12.691 with 7th K, S22.000-S22.9XX with 7th K, S32.000-S32.9XX with 7th K, S42.001-S42.92X with 7th [K, P], S49.001-S49.199 with 7th [K, P], S52.001-S52.92X with 7th [K, M, N, P, Q, R], S59.001-S59.299 with 7th [K, P], S62.001-S62.92X with 7th [K, P], S72.001-S72.92X with 7th [K, M, N, P, Q, R], S79.001-S79.199 with 7th [K, P], S82.001-S82.92X with 7th [K, M, N, P, Q, R], S89.001-S89.399 with 7th [K, P], S92.001-S92.919 with 7th [K, P]

7,19 ✓7th **S89.009** **Unspecified physeal fracture of upper end of unspecified tibia** `CC`

CC Excl: CC with 7th character A: M80.00X-M80.019 with 7th A, M80.041-M80.049 with 7th A, M80.061-M80.079 with 7th A, M80.80X-M80.819 with 7th A, M80.841-M80.849 with 7th A, M80.861-M80.879 with 7th A, M84.40X-M84.419 with 7th A, M84.441-M84.446 with 7th A, M84.454 with 7th A, M84.461-M84.519 with 7th A, M84.541-M84.550 with 7th A, M84.561-M84.576 with 7th A, M84.60X-M84.619 with 7th A, M84.641-M84.650 with 7th A, M84.661-M84.68X with 7th A, S03.8XX-S03.9XX with 7th A, S29.011-S29.019 with 7th A, S38.3XX-S39.013 with 7th A, S73.101-S73.199 with 7th A, S76.001-S76.019 with 7th A, S76.091-S76.119 with 7th A, S76.191-S76.219 with 7th A, S76.291-S76.319 with 7th A, S76.391-S76.819 with 7th A, S76.891-S76.919 with 7th A, S76.991-S76.999 with 7th A, S79.811-S79.929 with 7th A, S82.101-S82.156 with 7th [A, B, C], S82.191-S82.299 with 7th [A, B, C], S82.401-S82.499 with 7th [A, B, C], S82.831-S82.839 with 7th [A, B, C], S82.861-S82.866 with 7th [A, B, C], S82.90X-S82.92X with 7th [A, B, C], S89.001-S89.099 with 7th A, S89.201-S89.299 with 7th A, T14.90-T14.91, T79.A9X-T79.9XX with 7th A

CC with 7th character K or P: M80.00X-M84.68X with 7th [K, P], S02.0XX-S02.92X with 7th K, S12.000-S12.691 with 7th K, S22.000-S22.9XX with 7th K, S32.000-S32.9XX with 7th K, S42.001-S42.92X with 7th [K, P], S49.001-S49.199 with 7th [K, P], S52.001-S52.92X with 7th [K, M, N, P, Q, R], S59.001-S59.299 with 7th [K, P], S62.001-S62.92X with 7th [K, P], S72.001-S72.92X with 7th [K, M, N, P, Q, R], S79.001-S79.199 with 7th [K, P], S82.001-S82.92X with 7th [K, M, N, P, Q, R], S89.001-S89.399 with 7th [K, P], S92.001-S92.919 with 7th [K, P]

✓6th **S89.01** Salter-Harris Type I physeal fracture of upper end of tibia

    7,19 ✓7th **S89.011** **Salter-Harris Type I physeal fracture of upper end of right tibia** `CC`
      CC Excl: See code: S89.001

    7,19 ✓7th **S89.012** **Salter-Harris Type I physeal fracture of upper end of left tibia** `CC`
      CC Excl: See code: S89.002

    7,19 ✓7th **S89.019** **Salter-Harris Type I physeal fracture of upper end of unspecified tibia** `CC`
      CC Excl: See code: S89.009

✓6th **S89.02** Salter-Harris Type II physeal fracture of upper end of tibia

    7,19 ✓7th **S89.021** **Salter-Harris Type II physeal fracture of upper end of right tibia** `CC`
      CC Excl: See code: S89.001

    7,19 ✓7th **S89.022** **Salter-Harris Type II physeal fracture of upper end of left tibia** `CC`
      CC Excl: See code: S89.002

    7,19 ✓7th **S89.029** **Salter-Harris Type II physeal fracture of upper end of unspecified tibia** `CC`
      CC Excl: See code: S89.009

✓6th **S89.03** Salter-Harris Type III physeal fracture of upper end of tibia

    7,19 ✓7th **S89.031** **Salter-Harris Type III physeal fracture of upper end of right tibia** `CC`
      CC Excl: See code: S89.001

    7,19 ✓7th **S89.032** **Salter-Harris Type III physeal fracture of upper end of left tibia** `CC`
      CC Excl: See code: S89.002

    7,19 ✓7th **S89.039** **Salter-Harris Type III physeal fracture of upper end of unspecified tibia** `CC`
      CC Excl: See code: S89.009

✓6th **S89.04** Salter-Harris Type IV physeal fracture of upper end of tibia

    7,19 ✓7th **S89.041** **Salter-Harris Type IV physeal fracture of upper end of right tibia** `CC`
      CC Excl: See code: S89.001

    7,19 ✓7th **S89.042** **Salter-Harris Type IV physeal fracture of upper end of left tibia** `CC`
      CC Excl: See code: S89.002

---

7 HAC = Initial encounter only (7th character A, B or C) and not POA.

19 CC only if an initial encounter for a closed fracture (7th character A) **OR** a subsequent encounter for nonunion or malunion (7th character K, M, N, P, Q, or R– specific to category).

N Newborn: 0   P Pediatric: 0-17   M Maternity: 12-55   A Adult: 15-124   **MCC** Major CC Condition   **PDxMCC** PDx acts as own MCC   **CC** CC Condition   **PDxCC** PDx acts as own CC

7,19 ✓7th **S89.049** **Salter-Harris Type IV physeal fracture** **of upper end of unspecified tibia** CC
        CC Excl: See code: S89.009

✓6th **S89.09** Other physeal fracture of upper end of tibia

   7,19 ✓7th **S89.091** **Other physeal fracture of upper end** **of right tibia** CC
        CC Excl: See code: S89.001

   7,19 ✓7th **S89.092** **Other physeal fracture of upper end** **of left tibia** CC
        CC Excl: See code: S89.002

   7,19 ✓7th **S89.099** **Other physeal fracture of upper end** **of unspecified tibia** CC
        CC Excl: See code: S89.009

✓5th **S89.1** Physeal fracture of lower end of tibia

> **CC Excl: For CC codes in subcategory S89.1, unless otherwise noted: CC with 7th character K or P:** M80.00X-M80.019 with 7th A, M80.041-M80.049 with 7th A, M80.061-M80.079 with 7th A, M80.80X-M80.819 with 7th A, M80.841-M80.849 with 7th A, M80.861-M80.879 with 7th A, M84.40X-M84.419 with 7th A, M84.441-M84.446 with 7th A, M84.454 with 7th A, M84.461-M84.519 with 7th A, M84.541-M84.550 with 7th A, M84.561-M84.576 with 7th A, M84.60X-M84.619 with 7th A, M84.641-M84.650 with 7th A, M84.661-M84.68X with 7th A, S03.8XX-S03.9XX with 7th A, S29.011-S29.019 with 7th A, S38.3XX-S39.013 with 7th A, S73.101-S73.199 with 7th A, S76.001-S76.019 with 7th A, S76.091-S76.119 with 7th A, S76.191-S76.219 with 7th A, S76.291-S76.319 with 7th A, S76.391-S76.819 with 7th A, S76.891-S76.919 with 7th A, S76.991-S76.999 with 7th A, S79.811-S79.929 with 7th A, S82.101-S82.156 with 7th [A, B, C], S82.191-S82.299 with 7th [A, B, C], S82.401-S82.499 with 7th [A, B, C], S82.831-S82.839 with 7th [A, B, C], S82.861-S82.866 with 7th [A, B, C], S82.90X-S82.92X with 7th [A, B, C], S89.001-S89.099 with 7th A, S89.201-S89.299 with 7th A, T14.90-T14.91, T79.A9X-T79.9XX with 7th A

✓6th **S89.10** Unspecified physeal fracture of lower end of tibia

   18 ✓7th **S89.101** **Unspecified physeal fracture of lower** **end of right tibia** CC

   18 ✓7th **S89.102** **Unspecified physeal fracture of lower** **end of left tibia** CC

   18 ✓7th **S89.109** **Unspecified physeal fracture of lower** **end of unspecified tibia** CC

✓6th **S89.11** Salter-Harris Type I physeal fracture of ower end of tibia

   18 ✓7th **S89.111** **Salter-Harris Type I physeal fracture of** **lower end of right tibia** CC

   18 ✓7th **S89.112** **Salter-Harris Type I physeal fracture** **oflower end of left tibia** CC

   18 ✓7th **S89.119** **Salter-Harris Type I physeal fracture** **of lower end of unspecified tibia** CC

✓6th **S89.12** Salter-Harris Type II physeal fracture of lower end of tibia

   18 ✓7th **S89.121** **Salter-Harris Type II physeal fracture** **of lower end of right tibia** CC

   18 ✓7th **S89.122** **Salter-Harris Type II physeal fracture** **of lower end of left tibia** CC

   18 ✓7th **S89.129** **Salter-Harris Type II physeal fracture** **of lower end of unspecified tibia** CC

✓6th **S89.13** Salter-Harris Type III physeal fracture of lower end of tibia

> **EXCLUDES 1** *fracture of medial malleolus (adult) (S82.5-)*

   18 ✓7th **S89.131** **Salter-Harris Type III physeal fracture** **of lower end of right tibia** CC

   18 ✓7th **S89.132** **Salter-Harris Type III physeal fracture** **of lower end of left tibia** CC

   18 ✓7th **S89.139** **Salter-Harris Type III physeal fracture** **of lower end of unspecified tibia** CC

✓6th **S89.14** Salter-Harris Type IV physeal fracture of lower end of tibia

> **EXCLUDES 1** *fracture of medial malleolus (adult) (S82.5-)*

   18 ✓7th **S89.141** **Salter-Harris Type IV physeal fracture** **oflower end of right tibia** CC

   18 ✓7th **S89.142** **Salter-Harris Type IV physeal fracture** **of lower end of left tibia** CC

   18 ✓7th **S89.149** **Salter-Harris Type IV physeal fracture** **of lower end of unspecified tibia** CC

   18 ✓6th **S89.19** Other physeal fracture of lower end of tibia

   18 ✓7th **S89.191** **Other physeal fracture of lower end** **of right tibia** CC

   18 ✓7th **S89.192** **Other physeal fracture of lower end** **of left tibia** CC

   18 ✓7th **S89.199** **Other physeal fracture of lower end** **of unspecified tibia** CC

✓5th **S89.2** Physeal fracture of upper end of fibula

> **CC Excl: For CC codes in subcategory S89.2, unless otherwise noted:** See code: S89.1

✓6th **S89.20** Unspecified physeal fracture of upper end of fibula

   18 ✓7th **S89.201** **Unspecified physeal fracture of upper** **end of right fibula** CC

   18 ✓7th **S89.202** **Unspecified physeal fracture of upper** **end of left fibula** CC

   18 ✓7th **S89.209** **Unspecified physeal fracture of upper** **end of unspecified fibula** CC

✓6th **S89.21** Salter-Harris Type I physeal fracture of upper end of fibula

   18 ✓7th **S89.211** **Salter-Harris Type I physeal fracture** **of upper end of right fibula** CC

   18 ✓7th **S89.212** **Salter-Harris Type I physeal fracture** **of upper end of left fibula** CC

   18 ✓7th **S89.219** **Salter-Harris Type I physeal fracture** **of upper end of unspecified fibula** CC

✓6th **S89.22** Salter-Harris Type II physeal fracture of upper end of fibula

   18 ✓7th **S89.221** **Salter-Harris Type II physeal fracture** **of upper end of right fibula** CC

   18 ✓7th **S89.222** **Salter-Harris Type II physeal fracture** **of upper end of left fibula** CC

   18 ✓7th **S89.229** **Salter-Harris Type II physeal fracture** **of upper end of unspecified fibula** CC

✓6th **S89.29** Other physeal fracture of upper end of fibula

   18 ✓7th **S89.291** **Other physeal fracture of upper end** **of right fibula** CC

   18 ✓7th **S89.292** **Other physeal fracture of upper end** **of left fibula** CC

   18 ✓7th **S89.299** **Other physeal fracture of upper end** **of unspecified fibula** CC

✓5th **S89.3** Physeal fracture of lower end of fibula

> **CC Excl: For CC codes in subcategory S89.3, unless otherwise noted:** See code: S89.1

✓6th **S89.30** Unspecified physeal fracture of lower end of fibula

   18 ✓7th **S89.301** **Unspecified physeal fracture of lower** **end of right fibula** CC

   18 ✓7th **S89.302** **Unspecified physeal fracture of lower** **end of left fibula** CC

   18 ✓7th **S89.309** **Unspecified physeal fracture of lower** **end of unspecified fibula** CC

✓6th **S89.31** Salter-Harris Type I physeal fracture of lower end of fibula

   18 ✓7th **S89.311** **Salter-Harris Type I physeal fracture** **of lower end of right fibula** CC

   18 ✓7th **S89.312** **Salter-Harris Type I physeal fracture** **of lower end of left fibula** CC

   18 ✓7th **S89.319** **Salter-Harris Type I physeal fracture** **of lower end of unspecified fibula** CC

✓6th **S89.32** Salter-Harris Type II physeal fracture of lower end of fibula

   18 ✓7th **S89.321** **Salter-Harris Type II physeal fracture** **of lower end of right fibula** CC

   18 ✓7th **S89.322** **Salter-Harris Type II physeal fracture** **of lower end of left fibula** CC

   18 ✓7th **S89.329** **Salter-Harris Type II physeal fracture** **of lower end of unspecified fibula** CC

---

7   HAC = Initial encounter only (7th character A, B or C) and not POA.
18   CC only if a subsequent encounter for nonunion or malunion (7th character K, M, N, P, Q, or R – specific to category).
19   CC only if an initial encounter for a closed fracture (7th character A) **OR** a subsequent encounter for nonunion or malunion (7th character K, M, N, P, Q, or R– specific to category).

✔ Additional Character Required   ✔x7th Placeholder Alert   Unacceptable PDx   Manifestation   Hospital Acquired Condition   **EXCLUDES 1** Not Coded Here   **EXCLUDES 2** Not Included Here

✓6ᵗʰ **S89.39** Other physeal fracture of lower end of fibula

18 ✓7ᵗʰ **S89.391** Other physeal fracture of lower end of right fibula `CC`

18 ✓7ᵗʰ **S89.392** Other physeal fracture of lower end of left fibula `CC`

18 ✓7ᵗʰ **S89.399** Other physeal fracture of lower end of unspecified fibula `CC`

✓5ᵗʰ **S89.8** Other specified injuries of lower leg

> The appropriate 7th character is to be added to each code in subcategory S89.8.
> A   initial encounter
> D   subsequent encounter
> S   sequela

✓x7ᵗʰ **S89.80** Other specified injuries of unspecified lower leg

✓x7ᵗʰ **S89.81** Other specified injuries of right lower leg

✓x7ᵗʰ **S89.82** Other specified injuries of left lower leg

✓5ᵗʰ **S89.9** Unspecified injury of lower leg

> The appropriate 7th character is to be added to each code in subcategory S89.9.
> A   initial encounter
> D   subsequent encounter
> S   sequela

✓x7ᵗʰ **S89.90** Unspecified injury of unspecified lower leg

✓x7ᵗʰ **S89.91** Unspecified injury of right lower leg

✓x7ᵗʰ **S89.92** Unspecified injury of left lower leg

Injuries to the ankle and foot (S90-S99)

EXCLUDES2   burns and corrosions (T20-T32)
fracture of ankle and malleolus (S82.-)
frostbite (T33-T34)
insect bite or sting, venomous (T63.4)

✓4ᵗʰ **S90** Superficial injury of ankle, foot and toes

> The appropriate 7th character is to be added to each code from category S90.
> A   initial encounter
> D   subsequent encounter
> S   sequela

✓5ᵗʰ **S90.0** Contusion of ankle

✓x7ᵗʰ **S90.00** Contusion of unspecified ankle

✓x7ᵗʰ **S90.01** Contusion of right ankle

✓x7ᵗʰ **S90.02** Contusion of left ankle

✓5ᵗʰ **S90.1** Contusion of toe without damage to nail

✓6ᵗʰ **S90.11** Contusion of great toe without damage to nail

✓7ᵗʰ **S90.111** Contusion of right great toe without damage to nail

✓7ᵗʰ **S90.112** Contusion of left great toe without damage to nail

✓7ᵗʰ **S90.119** Contusion of unspecified great toe without damage to nail

✓6ᵗʰ **S90.12** Contusion of lesser toe without damage to nail

✓7ᵗʰ **S90.121** Contusion of right lesser toe(s) without damage to nail

✓7ᵗʰ **S90.122** Contusion of left lesser toe(s) without damage to nail

✓7ᵗʰ **S90.129** Contusion of unspecified lesser toe(s) without damage to nail
Contusion of toe NOS

✓5ᵗʰ **S90.2** Contusion of toe with damage to nail

✓6ᵗʰ **S90.21** Contusion of great toe with damage to nail

✓7ᵗʰ **S90.211** Contusion of right great toe with damage to nail

✓7ᵗʰ **S90.212** Contusion of left great toe with damage to nail

✓7ᵗʰ **S90.219** Contusion of unspecified great toe with damage to nail

✓6ᵗʰ **S90.22** Contusion of lesser toe with damage to nail

✓7ᵗʰ **S90.221** Contusion of right lesser toe(s) with damage to nail

✓7ᵗʰ **S90.222** Contusion of left lesser toe(s) with damage to nail

✓7ᵗʰ **S90.229** Contusion of unspecified lesser toe(s) with damage to nail

✓5ᵗʰ **S90.3** Contusion of foot
EXCLUDES2   contusion of toes (S90.1-, S90.2-)

✓x7ᵗʰ **S90.30** Contusion of unspecified foot
Contusion of foot NOS

✓x7ᵗʰ **S90.31** Contusion of right foot

✓x7ᵗʰ **S90.32** Contusion of left foot

✓5ᵗʰ **S90.4** Other superficial injuries of toe

✓6ᵗʰ **S90.41** Abrasion of toe

✓7ᵗʰ **S90.411** Abrasion, right great toe

✓7ᵗʰ **S90.412** Abrasion, left great toe

✓7ᵗʰ **S90.413** Abrasion, unspecified great toe

✓7ᵗʰ **S90.414** Abrasion, right lesser toe(s)

✓7ᵗʰ **S90.415** Abrasion, left lesser toe(s)

✓7ᵗʰ **S90.416** Abrasion, unspecified lesser toe(s)

✓6ᵗʰ **S90.42** Blister (nonthermal) of toe

✓7ᵗʰ **S90.421** Blister (nonthermal), right great toe

✓7ᵗʰ **S90.422** Blister (nonthermal), left great toe

✓7ᵗʰ **S90.423** Blister (nonthermal), unspecified great toe

✓7ᵗʰ **S90.424** Blister (nonthermal), right lesser toe(s)

✓7ᵗʰ **S90.425** Blister (nonthermal), left lesser toe(s)

✓7ᵗʰ **S90.426** Blister (nonthermal), unspecified lesser toe(s)

✓6ᵗʰ **S90.44** External constriction of toe
Hair tourniquet syndrome of toe

✓7ᵗʰ **S90.441** External constriction, right great toe

✓7ᵗʰ **S90.442** External constriction, left great toe

✓7ᵗʰ **S90.443** External constriction, unspecified great toe

✓7ᵗʰ **S90.444** External constriction, right lesser toe(s)

✓7ᵗʰ **S90.445** External constriction, left lesser toe(s)

✓7ᵗʰ **S90.446** External constriction, unspecified lesser toe(s)

✓6ᵗʰ **S90.45** Superficial foreign body of toe
Splinter in the toe

✓7ᵗʰ **S90.451** Superficial foreign body, right great toe

✓7ᵗʰ **S90.452** Superficial foreign body, left great toe

✓7ᵗʰ **S90.453** Superficial foreign body, unspecified great toe

✓7ᵗʰ **S90.454** Superficial foreign body, right lesser toe(s)

✓7ᵗʰ **S90.455** Superficial foreign body, left lesser toe(s)

✓7ᵗʰ **S90.456** Superficial foreign body, unspecified lesser toe(s)

✓6ᵗʰ **S90.46** Insect bite (nonvenomous) of toe

✓7ᵗʰ **S90.461** Insect bite (nonvenomous), right great toe

✓7ᵗʰ **S90.462** Insect bite (nonvenomous), left great toe

✓7ᵗʰ **S90.463** Insect bite (nonvenomous), unspecified great toe

✓7ᵗʰ **S90.464** Insect bite (nonvenomous), right lesser toe(s)

✓7ᵗʰ **S90.465** Insect bite (nonvenomous), left lesser toe(s)

✓7ᵗʰ **S90.466** Insect bite (nonvenomous), unspecified lesser toe(s)

✓6ᵗʰ **S90.47** Other superficial bite of toe
EXCLUDES1   open bite of toe (S91.15-, S91.25-)

✓7ᵗʰ **S90.471** Other superficial bite of right great toe

✓7ᵗʰ **S90.472** Other superficial bite of left great toe

✓7ᵗʰ **S90.473** Other superficial bite of unspecified great toe

✓7ᵗʰ **S90.474** Other superficial bite of right lesser toe(s)

✓7ᵗʰ **S90.475** Other superficial bite of left lesser toe(s)

✓7ᵗʰ **S90.476** Other superficial bite of unspecified lesser toe(s)

✓5ᵗʰ **S90.5** Other superficial injuries of ankle

✓6ᵗʰ **S90.51** Abrasion of ankle

✓7ᵗʰ **S90.511** Abrasion, right ankle

---

18 CC only if a subsequent encounter for nonunion or malunion (7th character K, M, N, P, Q, or R – specific to category).

N Newborn: 0   P Pediatric: 0-17   M Maternity: 12-55   A Adult: 15-124   MCC Major CC Condition   PDxMCC PDx acts as own MCC   CC CC Condition   PDxCC PDx acts as own CC

1058   ICD-10-CM 2016

√7th S90.512   Abrasion, left ankle
√7th S90.519   Abrasion, unspecified ankle
√6th S90.52   Blister (nonthermal) of ankle
√7th S90.521   Blister (nonthermal), right ankle
√7th S90.522   Blister (nonthermal), left ankle
√7th S90.529   Blister (nonthermal), unspecified ankle
√6th S90.54   External constriction of ankle
√7th S90.541   External constriction, right ankle
√7th S90.542   External constriction, left ankle
√7th S90.549   External constriction, unspecified ankle
√6th S90.55   Superficial foreign body of ankle
Splinter in the ankle
√7th S90.551   Superficial foreign body, right ankle
√7th S90.552   Superficial foreign body, left ankle
√7th S90.559   Superficial foreign body, unspecified ankle
√6th S90.56   Insect bite (nonvenomous) of ankle
√7th S90.561   Insect bite (nonvenomous), right ankle
√7th S90.562   Insect bite (nonvenomous), left ankle
√7th S90.569   Insect bite (nonvenomous), unspecified ankle
√6th S90.57   Other superficial bite of ankle
EXCLUDES 1 open bite of ankle (S91.05-)
√7th S90.571   Other superficial bite of ankle, right ankle
√7th S90.572   Other superficial bite of ankle, left ankle
√7th S90.579   Other superficial bite of ankle, unspecified ankle
√5th S90.8   Other superficial injuries of foot
√6th S90.81   Abrasion of foot
√7th S90.811   Abrasion, right foot
√7th S90.812   Abrasion, left foot
√7th S90.819   Abrasion, unspecified foot
√6th S90.82   Blister (nonthermal) of foot
√7th S90.821   Blister (nonthermal), right foot
√7th S90.822   Blister (nonthermal), left foot
√7th S90.829   Blister (nonthermal), unspecified foot
√6th S90.84   External constriction of foot
√7th S90.841   External constriction, right foot
√7th S90.842   External constriction, left foot
√7th S90.849   External constriction, unspecified foot
√6th S90.85   Superficial foreign body of foot
Splinter in the foot
√7th S90.851   Superficial foreign body, right foot
√7th S90.852   Superficial foreign body, left foot
√7th S90.859   Superficial foreign body, unspecified foot
√6th S90.86   Insect bite (nonvenomous) of foot
√7th S90.861   Insect bite (nonvenomous), right foot
√7th S90.862   Insect bite (nonvenomous), left foot
√7th S90.869   Insect bite (nonvenomous), unspecified foot
√6th S90.87   Other superficial bite of foot
EXCLUDES 1 open bite of foot (S91.35-)
√7th S90.871   Other superficial bite of right foot
√7th S90.872   Other superficial bite of left foot
√7th S90.879   Other superficial bite of unspecified foot
√5th S90.9   Unspecified superficial injury of ankle, foot and toe
√6th S90.91   Unspecified superficial injury of ankle
√7th S90.911   Unspecified superficial injury of right ankle
√7th S90.912   Unspecified superficial injury of left ankle
√7th S90.919   Unspecified superficial injury of unspecified ankle
√6th S90.92   Unspecified superficial injury of foot
√7th S90.921   Unspecified superficial injury of right foot
√7th S90.922   Unspecified superficial injury of left foot
√7th S90.929   Unspecified superficial injury of unspecified foot

√6th S90.93   Unspecified superficial injury of toes
√7th S90.931   Unspecified superficial injury of right great toe
√7th S90.932   Unspecified superficial injury of left great toe
√7th S90.933   Unspecified superficial injury of unspecified great toe
√7th S90.934   Unspecified superficial injury of right lesser toe(s)
√7th S90.935   Unspecified superficial injury of left lesser toe(s)
√7th S90.936   Unspecified superficial injury of unspecified lesser toe(s)

√4th S91   Open wound of ankle, foot and toes
Code also any associated wound infection
EXCLUDES 1 open fracture of ankle, foot and toes (S92-with 7th B)
traumatic amputation of ankle and foot (S98.-)

The appropriate 7th character is to be added to each code from category S91.
A   initial encounter
D   subsequent encounter
S   sequela

√5th S91.0   Open wound of ankle
√6th S91.00   Unspecified open wound of ankle
√7th S91.001   Unspecified open wound, right ankle
√7th S91.002   Unspecified open wound, left ankle
√7th S91.009   Unspecified open wound, unspecified ankle
√6th S91.01   Laceration without foreign body of ankle
√7th S91.011   Laceration without foreign body, right ankle
√7th S91.012   Laceration without foreign body, left ankle
√7th S91.019   Laceration without foreign body, unspecified ankle
√6th S91.02   Laceration with foreign body of ankle
√7th S91.021   Laceration with foreign body, right ankle
√7th S91.022   Laceration with foreign body, left ankle
√7th S91.029   Laceration with foreign body, unspecified ankle
√6th S91.03   Puncture wound without foreign body of ankle
√7th S91.031   Puncture wound without foreign body, right ankle
√7th S91.032   Puncture wound without foreign body, left ankle
√7th S91.039   Puncture wound without foreign body, unspecified ankle
√6th S91.04   Puncture wound with foreign body of ankle
√7th S91.041   Puncture wound with foreign body, right ankle
√7th S91.042   Puncture wound with foreign body, left ankle
√7th S91.049   Puncture wound with foreign body, unspecified ankle
√6th S91.05   Open bite of ankle
EXCLUDES 1 superficial bite of ankle (S90.56-, S90.57-)
√7th S91.051   Open bite, right ankle
√7th S91.052   Open bite, left ankle
√7th S91.059   Open bite, unspecified ankle
√5th S91.1   Open wound of toe without damage to nail
√6th S91.10   Unspecified open wound of toe without damage to nail
√7th S91.101   Unspecified open wound of right great toe without damage to nail
√7th S91.102   Unspecified open wound of left great toe without damage to nail
√7th S91.103   Unspecified open wound of unspecified great toe without damage to nail
√7th S91.104   Unspecified open wound of right lesser toe(s) without damage to nail
√7th S91.105   Unspecified open wound of left lesser toe(s) without damage to nail

√7ᵗʰ **S91.106** Unspecified open wound of unspecified lesser toe(s) without damage to nail

√7ᵗʰ **S91.109** Unspecified open wound of unspecified toe(s) without damage to nail

√6ᵗʰ **S91.11** Laceration without foreign body of toe without damage to nail

√7ᵗʰ **S91.111** Laceration without foreign body of right great toe without damage to nail

√7ᵗʰ **S91.112** Laceration without foreign body of left great toe without damage to nail

√7ᵗʰ **S91.113** Laceration without foreign body of unspecified great toe without damage to nail

√7ᵗʰ **S91.114** Laceration without foreign body of right lesser toe(s) without damage to nail

√7ᵗʰ **S91.115** Laceration without foreign body of left lesser toe(s) without damage to nail

√7ᵗʰ **S91.116** Laceration without foreign body of unspecified lesser toe(s) without damage to nail

√7ᵗʰ **S91.119** Laceration without foreign body of unspecified toe without damage to nail

√6ᵗʰ **S91.12** Laceration with foreign body of toe without damage to nail

√7ᵗʰ **S91.121** Laceration with foreign body of right great toe without damage to nail

√7ᵗʰ **S91.122** Laceration with foreign body of left great toe without damage to nail

√7ᵗʰ **S91.123** Laceration with foreign body of unspecified great toe without damage to nail

√7ᵗʰ **S91.124** Laceration with foreign body of right lesser toe(s) without damage to nail

√7ᵗʰ **S91.125** Laceration with foreign body of left lesser toe(s) without damage to nail

√7ᵗʰ **S91.126** Laceration with foreign body of unspecified lesser toe(s) without damage to nail

√7ᵗʰ **S91.129** Laceration with foreign body of unspecified toe(s) without damage to nail

√6ᵗʰ **S91.13** Puncture wound without foreign body of toe without damage to nail

√7ᵗʰ **S91.131** Puncture wound without foreign body of right great toe without damage to nail

√7ᵗʰ **S91.132** Puncture wound without foreign body of left great toe without damage to nail

√7ᵗʰ **S91.133** Puncture wound without foreign body of unspecified great toe without damage to nail

√7ᵗʰ **S91.134** Puncture wound without foreign body of right lesser toe(s) without damage to nail

√7ᵗʰ **S91.135** Puncture wound without foreign body of left lesser toe(s) without damage to nail

√7ᵗʰ **S91.136** Puncture wound without foreign body of unspecified lesser toe(s) without damage to nail

√7ᵗʰ **S91.139** Puncture wound without foreign body of unspecified toe(s) without damage to nail

√6ᵗʰ **S91.14** Puncture wound with foreign body of toe without damage to nail

√7ᵗʰ **S91.141** Puncture wound with foreign body of right great toe without damage to nail

√7ᵗʰ **S91.142** Puncture wound with foreign body of left great toe without damage to nail

√7ᵗʰ **S91.143** Puncture wound with foreign body of unspecified great toe without damage to nail

√7ᵗʰ **S91.144** Puncture wound with foreign body of right lesser toe(s) without damage to nail

√7ᵗʰ **S91.145** Puncture wound with foreign body of left lesser toe(s) without damage to nail

√7ᵗʰ **S91.146** Puncture wound with foreign body of unspecified lesser toe(s) without damage to nail

√7ᵗʰ **S91.149** Puncture wound with foreign body of unspecified toe(s) without damage to nail

√6ᵗʰ **S91.15** Open bite of toe without damage to nail
Bite of toe NOS
EXCLUDES 1 *superficial bite of toe (S90.46-, S90.47-)*

√7ᵗʰ **S91.151** Open bite of right great toe without damage to nail

√7ᵗʰ **S91.152** Open bite of left great toe without damage to nail

√7ᵗʰ **S91.153** Open bite of unspecified great toe without damage to nail

√7ᵗʰ **S91.154** Open bite of right lesser toe(s) without damage to nail

√7ᵗʰ **S91.155** Open bite of left lesser toe(s) without damage to nail

√7ᵗʰ **S91.156** Open bite of unspecified lesser toe(s) without damage to nail

√7ᵗʰ **S91.159** Open bite of unspecified toe(s) without damage to nail

√5ᵗʰ **S91.2** Open wound of toe with damage to nail

√6ᵗʰ **S91.20** Unspecified open wound of toe with damage to nail

√7ᵗʰ **S91.201** Unspecified open wound of right great toe with damage to nail

√7ᵗʰ **S91.202** Unspecified open wound of left great toe with damage to nail

√7ᵗʰ **S91.203** Unspecified open wound of unspecified great toe with damage to nail

√7ᵗʰ **S91.204** Unspecified open wound of right lesser toe(s) with damage to nail

√7ᵗʰ **S91.205** Unspecified open wound of left lesser toe(s) with damage to nail

√7ᵗʰ **S91.206** Unspecified open wound of unspecified lesser toe(s) with damage to nail

√7ᵗʰ **S91.209** Unspecified open wound of unspecified toe(s) with damage to nail

√6ᵗʰ **S91.21** Laceration without foreign body of toe with damage to nail

√7ᵗʰ **S91.211** Laceration without foreign body of right great toe with damage to nail

√7ᵗʰ **S91.212** Laceration without foreign body of left great toe with damage to nail

√7ᵗʰ **S91.213** Laceration without foreign body of unspecified great toe with damage to nail

√7ᵗʰ **S91.214** Laceration without foreign body of right lesser toe(s) with damage to nail

√7ᵗʰ **S91.215** Laceration without foreign body of left lesser toe(s) with damage to nail

√7ᵗʰ **S91.216** Laceration without foreign body of unspecified lesser toe(s) with damage to nail

√7ᵗʰ **S91.219** Laceration without foreign body of unspecified toe(s) with damage to nail

√6ᵗʰ **S91.22** Laceration with foreign body of toe with damage to nail

√7ᵗʰ **S91.221** Laceration with foreign body of right great toe with damage to nail

√7ᵗʰ **S91.222** Laceration with foreign body of left great toe with damage to nail

√7ᵗʰ **S91.223** Laceration with foreign body of unspecified great toe with damage to nail

√7ᵗʰ **S91.224** Laceration with foreign body of right lesser toe(s) with damage to nail

√7ᵗʰ **S91.225** Laceration with foreign body of left lesser toe(s) with damage to nail

√7ᵗʰ **S91.226** Laceration with foreign body of unspecified lesser toe(s) with damage to nail

√7ᵗʰ **S91.229** Laceration with foreign body of unspecified toe(s) with damage to nail

√6ᵗʰ **S91.23** Puncture wound without foreign body of toe with damage to nail

√7ᵗʰ **S91.231** Puncture wound without foreign body of right great toe with damage to nail

√7ᵗʰ **S91.232** Puncture wound without foreign body of left great toe with damage to nail

√7ᵗʰ **S91.233** Puncture wound without foreign body of unspecified great toe with damage to nail

---

Ⓝ Newborn: 0   Ⓟ Pediatric: 0-17   Ⓜ Maternity: 12-55   Ⓐ Adult: 15-124   **MCC** Major CC Condition   **PDxMCC** PDx acts as own MCC   **CC** CC Condition   **PDxCC** PDx acts as own CC

1060   ICD-10-CM 2016

√7ᵗʰ **S91.234** **Puncture wound without foreign body of right lesser toe(s) with damage to nail**

√7ᵗʰ **S91.235** **Puncture wound without foreign body of left lesser toe(s) with damage to nail**

√7ᵗʰ **S91.236** **Puncture wound without foreign body of unspecified lesser toe(s) with damage to nail**

√7ᵗʰ **S91.239** **Puncture wound without foreign body of unspecified toe(s) with damage to nail**

√6ᵗʰ **S91.24** **Puncture wound with foreign body of toe with damage to nail**

√7ᵗʰ **S91.241** **Puncture wound with foreign body of right great toe with damage to nail**

√7ᵗʰ **S91.242** **Puncture wound with foreign body of left great toe with damage to nail**

√7ᵗʰ **S91.243** **Puncture wound with foreign body of unspecified great toe with damage to nail**

√7ᵗʰ **S91.244** **Puncture wound with foreign body of right lesser toe(s) with damage to nail**

√7ᵗʰ **S91.245** **Puncture wound with foreign body of left lesser toe(s) with damage to nail**

√7ᵗʰ **S91.246** **Puncture wound with foreign body of unspecified lesser toe(s) with damage to nail**

√7ᵗʰ **S91.249** **Puncture wound with foreign body of unspecified toe(s) with damage to nail**

√6ᵗʰ **S91.25** **Open bite of toe with damage to nail**
Bite of toe with damage to nail NOS
EXCLUDES 1 *superficial bite of toe (S90.46-, S90.47-)*

√7ᵗʰ **S91.251** **Open bite of right great toe with damage to nail**

√7ᵗʰ **S91.252** **Open bite of left great toe with damage to nail**

√7ᵗʰ **S91.253** **Open bite of unspecified great toe with damage to nail**

√7ᵗʰ **S91.254** **Open bite of right lesser toe(s) with damage to nail**

√7ᵗʰ **S91.255** **Open bite of left lesser toe(s) with damage to nail**

√7ᵗʰ **S91.256** **Open bite of unspecified lesser toe(s) with damage to nail**

√7ᵗʰ **S91.259** **Open bite of unspecified toe(s) with damage to nail**

√5ᵗʰ **S91.3** **Open wound of foot**

√6ᵗʰ **S91.30** **Unspecified open wound of foot**

√7ᵗʰ **S91.301** **Unspecified open wound, right foot**

√7ᵗʰ **S91.302** **Unspecified open wound, left foot**

√7ᵗʰ **S91.309** **Unspecified open wound, unspecified foot**

√6ᵗʰ **S91.31** **Laceration without foreign body of foot**

√7ᵗʰ **S91.311** **Laceration without foreign body, right foot**

√7ᵗʰ **S91.312** **Laceration without foreign body, left foot**

√7ᵗʰ **S91.319** **Laceration without foreign body, unspecified foot**

√6ᵗʰ **S91.32** **Laceration with foreign body of foot**

√7ᵗʰ **S91.321** **Laceration with foreign body, right foot**

√7ᵗʰ **S91.322** **Laceration with foreign body, left foot**

√7ᵗʰ **S91.329** **Laceration with foreign body, unspecified foot**

√6ᵗʰ **S91.33** **Puncture wound without foreign body of foot**

√7ᵗʰ **S91.331** **Puncture wound without foreign body, right foot**

√7ᵗʰ **S91.332** **Puncture wound without foreign body, left foot**

√7ᵗʰ **S91.339** **Puncture wound without foreign body, unspecified foot**

√6ᵗʰ **S91.34** **Puncture wound with foreign body of foot**

√7ᵗʰ **S91.341** **Puncture wound with foreign body, right foot**

√7ᵗʰ **S91.342** **Puncture wound with foreign body, left foot**

√7ᵗʰ **S91.349** **Puncture wound with foreign body, unspecified foot**

√6ᵗʰ **S91.35** **Open bite of foot**
EXCLUDES 1 *superficial bite of foot (S90.86-, S90.87-)*

√7ᵗʰ **S91.351** **Open bite, right foot**

√7ᵗʰ **S91.352** **Open bite, left foot**

√7ᵗʰ **S91.359** **Open bite, unspecified foot**

√4ᵗʰ **S92** **Fracture of foot and toe, except ankle**
NOTE A fracture not indicated as displaced or nondisplaced should be coded to displaced.
A fracture not indicated as open or closed should be coded to closed.
EXCLUDES 1 *traumatic amputation of ankle and foot (S98.-)*
EXCLUDES 2 *fracture of ankle (S82.-)*
fracture of malleolus (S82.-)

The appropriate 7th character is to be added to each code from category S92.
A   initial encounter for closed fracture
B   initial encounter for open fracture
D   subsequent encounter for fracture with routine healing
G   subsequent encounter for fracture with delayed healing
K   subsequent encounter for fracture with nonunion
P   subsequent encounter for fracture with malunion
S   sequela

√5ᵗʰ **S92.0** **Fracture of calcaneus**
Heel bone
Os calcis

CC Excl: For CC codes in subcategory S92.0, unless otherwise noted: CC with 7th character B: M80.00X-M80.019 with 7th A, M80.041-M80.049 with 7th A, M80.061-M80.079 with 7th A, M80.80X-M80.819 with 7th A, M80.841-M80.849 with 7th A, M80.861-M80.879 with 7th A, M84.40X-M84.419 with 7th A, M84.441-M84.446 with 7th A, M84.454 with 7th A, M84.461-M84.519 with 7th A, M84.541-M84.550 with 7th A, M84.561-M84.576 with 7th A, M84.60X-M84.619 with 7th A, M84.641-M84.650 with 7th A, M84.661-M84.68X with 7th A, S03.8XX-S03.9XX with 7th A, S29.011-S29.019 with 7th A, S38.3XX-S39.013 with 7th A, S73.101-S73.199 with 7th A, S76.001-S76.019 with 7th A, S76.091-S76.119 with 7th A, S76.191-S76.219 with 7th A, S76.291-S76.319 with 7th A, S76.391-S76.819 with 7th A, S76.891-S76.919 with 7th A, S76.991-S76.999 with 7th A, S79.811-S79.929 with 7th A, S82.90X-S82.92X with 7th [A, B, C], S92.001-S92.356 with 7th B, S92.901-S92.909 with 7th [A, B], T14.90-T14.91, T79.A9X-T79.9XX with 7th A
CC with 7th character K or P: M80.00X-M84.68X with 7th [K, P], S02.0XX-S02.92X with 7th K, S12.000-S12.691 with 7th K, S22.000-S22.9XX with 7th K, S32.000-S32.9XX with 7th K, S42.001-S42.92X with 7th [K, P], S49.001-S49.199 with 7th [K, P], S52.001-S52.92X with 7th [K, M, N, P, Q, R], S59.001-S59.299 with 7th [K, P], S62.001-S62.92X with 7th [K, P], S72.001-S72.92X with 7th [K, M, N, P, Q, R], S79.001-S79.199 with 7th [K, P], S82.001-S82.92X with 7th [K, M, N, P, Q, R], S89.001-S89.399 with 7th [K, P], S92.001-S92.919 with 7th [K, P]

√6ᵗʰ **S92.00** **Unspecified fracture of calcaneus**

15,20 √7ᵗʰ **S92.001** **Unspecified fracture of right calcaneus**   CC

15,20 √7ᵗʰ **S92.002** **Unspecified fracture of left calcaneus**   CC

15,20 √7ᵗʰ **S92.009** **Unspecified fracture of unspecified calcaneus**   CC

√6ᵗʰ **S92.01** **Fracture of body of calcaneus**

15,20 √7ᵗʰ **S92.011** **Displaced fracture of body of right calcaneus**   CC

15,20 √7ᵗʰ **S92.012** **Displaced fracture of body of left calcaneus**   CC

15,20 √7ᵗʰ **S92.013** **Displaced fracture of body of unspecified calcaneus**   CC

15,20 √7ᵗʰ **S92.014** **Nondisplaced fracture of body of right calcaneus**   CC

15,20 √7ᵗʰ **S92.015** **Nondisplaced fracture of body of left calcaneus**   CC

15,20 √7ᵗʰ **S92.016** **Nondisplaced fracture of body of unspecified calcaneus**   CC

---

15 HAC = Initial encounter for open fracture only (7th character B or C – specific to category) and not POA.
20 CC only if an initial encounter for an open fracture (7th character B or C – specific to category) **OR** a subsequent encounter for nonunion or malunion (7th character K, M, N, P, Q, or R – specific to category).

☑ Additional Character Required   √x7ᵗʰ Placeholder Alert   Unacceptable PDx   Manifestation   Hospital Acquired Condition   **EXCLUDES 1** Not Coded Here   **EXCLUDES 2** Not Included Here

Chapter 19. Injury, Poisoning, and Certain Other Consequences of External Causes

S92.02–S92.141

✓6th **S92.02**   **Fracture of** anterior process of calcaneus

15,20 ✓7th **S92.021**   **Displaced fracture of anterior process of right calcaneus**   CC

15,20 ✓7th **S92.022**   **Displaced fracture of anterior process of left calcaneus**   CC

15,20 ✓7th **S92.023**   **Displaced fracture of anterior process of unspecified calcaneus**   CC

15,20 ✓7th **S92.024**   **Nondisplaced fracture of anterior process of right calcaneus**   CC

15,20 ✓7th **S92.025**   **Nondisplaced fracture of anterior process of left calcaneus**   CC

15,20 ✓7th **S92.026**   **Nondisplaced fracture of anterior process of unspecified calcaneus**   CC

✓6th **S92.03**   Avulsion **fracture of** tuberosity of calcaneus

15,20 ✓7th **S92.031**   **Displaced avulsion fracture of tuberosity of right calcaneus**   CC

15,20 ✓7th **S92.032**   **Displaced avulsion fracture of tuberosity of left calcaneus**   CC

15,20 ✓7th **S92.033**   **Displaced avulsion fracture of tuberosity of unspecified calcaneus**   CC

15,20 ✓7th **S92.034**   **Nondisplaced avulsion fracture of tuberosity of right calcaneus**   CC

15,20 ✓7th **S92.035**   **Nondisplaced avulsion fracture of tuberosity of left calcaneus**   CC

15,20 ✓7th **S92.036**   **Nondisplaced avulsion fracture of tuberosity of unspecified calcaneus**   CC

✓6th **S92.04**   Other **fracture of** tuberosity of calcaneus

15,20 ✓7th **S92.041**   **Displaced other fracture of tuberosity of right calcaneus**   CC

15,20 ✓7th **S92.042**   **Displaced other fracture of tuberosity of left calcaneus**   CC

15,20 ✓7th **S92.043**   **Displaced other fracture of tuberosity of unspecified calcaneus**   CC

15,20 ✓7th **S92.044**   **Nondisplaced other fracture of tuberosity of right calcaneus**   CC

15,20 ✓7th **S92.045**   **Nondisplaced other fracture of tuberosity of left calcaneus**   CC

15,20 ✓7th **S92.046**   **Nondisplaced other fracture of tuberosity of unspecified calcaneus**   CC

✓6th **S92.05**   Other extraarticular **fracture of** calcaneus

15,20 ✓7th **S92.051**   **Displaced other extraarticular fracture of right calcaneus**   CC

15,20 ✓7th **S92.052**   **Displaced other extraarticular fracture of left calcaneus**   CC

15,20 ✓7th **S92.053**   **Displaced other extraarticular fracture of unspecified calcaneus**   CC

15,20 ✓7th **S92.054**   **Nondisplaced other extraarticular fracture of right calcaneus**   CC

15,20 ✓7th **S92.055**   **Nondisplaced other extraarticular fracture of left calcaneus**   CC

15,20 ✓7th **S92.056**   **Nondisplaced other extraarticular fracture of unspecified calcaneus**   CC

✓6th **S92.06**   Intraarticular **fracture of** calcaneus

15,20 ✓7th **S92.061**   **Displaced intraarticular fracture of right calcaneus**   CC

15,20 ✓7th **S92.062**   **Displaced intraarticular fracture of left calcaneus**   CC

15,20 ✓7th **S92.063**   **Displaced intraarticular fracture of unspecified calcaneus**   CC

15,20 ✓7th **S92.064**   **Nondisplaced intraarticular fracture of right calcaneus**   CC

15,20 ✓7th **S92.065**   **Nondisplaced intraarticular fracture of left calcaneus**   CC

15,20 ✓7th **S92.066**   **Nondisplaced intraarticular fracture of unspecified calcaneus**   CC

✓5th **S92.1**   **Fracture of** talus
Astragalus

> **CC Excl: For CC codes in subcategory S92.1, unless otherwise noted: CC with 7th character B:** M80.00X-M80.019 with 7th A, M80.041-M80.049 with 7th A, M80.80X-M80.819 with 7th A, M84.441-M84.446 with 7th A, M84.40X-M84.419 with 7th A, M84.441-M84.446 with 7th A, M84.454 with 7th A, M84.474-M84.519 with 7th A, M84.541-M84.550 with 7th A, M84.574-M84.576 with 7th A, M84.60X-M84.619 with 7th A, M84.641-M84.650 with 7th A, M84.674-M84.68X with 7th A, S03.8XX-S03.9XX with 7th A, S29.011-S29.019 with 7th A, S38.3XX-S39.013 with 7th A, S73.101-S73.199 with 7th A, S76.001-S76.019 with 7th A, S76.091-S76.119 with 7th A, S76.191-S76.219 with 7th A, S76.291-S76.319 with 7th A, S76.391-S76.819 with 7th A, S76.891-S76.919 with 7th A, S76.991-S76.999 with 7th A, S79.811-S79.929 with 7th A, S82.90X-S82.92X with 7th [A, B, C], S92.001-S92.356 with 7th B, S92.901-S92.909 with 7th [A, B], T14.90-T14.91, T79.A9X-T79.9XX with 7th A
>
> **CC with 7th character K or P:** M80.00X-M84.68X with 7th [K, P], S02.0XX-S02.92X with 7th K, S12.000-S12.691 with 7th K, S22.000-S22.9XX with 7th K, S32.000-S32.9XX with 7th K, S42.001-S42.92X with 7th [K, P], S49.001-S49.199 with 7th [K, P], S52.001-S52.92X with 7th [K, M, N, P, Q, R], S59.001-S59.299 with 7th [K, P], S62.001-S62.92X with 7th [K, P], S72.001-S72.92X with 7th [K, M, N, P, Q, R], S79.001-S79.199 with 7th [K, P], S82.001-S82.92X with 7th [K, M, N, P, Q, R], S89.001-S89.399 with 7th [K, P], S92.001-S92.919 with 7th [K, P]

✓6th **S92.10**   Unspecified **fracture of** talus

15,20 ✓7th **S92.101**   **Unspecified fracture of right talus**   CC

15,20 ✓7th **S92.102**   **Unspecified fracture of left talus**   CC

15,20 ✓7th **S92.109**   **Unspecified fracture of unspecified talus**   CC

✓6th **S92.11**   **Fracture of** neck of talus

15,20 ✓7th **S92.111**   **Displaced fracture of neck of right talus**   CC

15,20 ✓7th **S92.112**   **Displaced fracture of neck of left talus**   CC

15,20 ✓7th **S92.113**   **Displaced fracture of neck of unspecified talus**   CC

15,20 ✓7th **S92.114**   **Nondisplaced fracture of neck of right talus**   CC

15,20 ✓7th **S92.115**   **Nondisplaced fracture of neck of left talus**   CC

15,20 ✓7th **S92.116**   **Nondisplaced fracture of neck of unspecified talus**   CC

✓6th **S92.12**   **Fracture of** body of talus

15,20 ✓7th **S92.121**   **Displaced fracture of body of right talus**   CC

15,20 ✓7th **S92.122**   **Displaced fracture of body of left talus**   CC

15,20 ✓7th **S92.123**   **Displaced fracture of body of unspecified talus**   CC

15,20 ✓7th **S92.124**   **Nondisplaced fracture of body of right talus**   CC

15,20 ✓7th **S92.125**   **Nondisplaced fracture of body of left talus**   CC

15,20 ✓7th **S92.126**   **Nondisplaced fracture of body of unspecified talus**   CC

✓6th **S92.13**   **Fracture of** posterior process of talus

15,20 ✓7th **S92.131**   **Displaced fracture of posterior process of right talus**   CC

15,20 ✓7th **S92.132**   **Displaced fracture of posterior process of left talus**   CC

15,20 ✓7th **S92.133**   **Displaced fracture of posterior process of unspecified talus**   CC

15,20 ✓7th **S92.134**   **Nondisplaced fracture of posterior process of right talus**   CC

15,20 ✓7th **S92.135**   **Nondisplaced fracture of posterior process of left talus**   CC

15,20 ✓7th **S92.136**   **Nondisplaced fracture of posterior process of unspecified talus**   CC

✓6th **S92.14**   **Dome fracture of** talus

> **EXCLUDES 1**   osteochondritis dissecans (M93.2)

15,20 ✓7th **S92.141**   **Displaced dome fracture of right talus**   CC

---

15 HAC = Initial encounter for open fracture only (7th character B or C – specific to category) and not POA.

20 CC only if an initial encounter for an open fracture (7th character B or C) **OR** a subsequent encounter for nonunion or malunion (7th character K, M, N, P, Q, or R – specific to category).

N Newborn: 0   P Pediatric: 0-17   M Maternity: 12-55   A Adult: 15-124   **MCC** Major CC Condition   **PDxMCC** PDx acts as own MCC   **CC** CC Condition   **PDxCC** PDx acts as own CC

1062   ICD-10-CM 2016

15,20 ✓7ᵗʰ **S92.142** Displaced dome fracture of left talus   CC

15,20 ✓7ᵗʰ **S92.143** Displaced dome fracture of unspecified talus   CC

15,20 ✓7ᵗʰ **S92.144** Nondisplaced dome fracture of right talus   CC

15,20 ✓7ᵗʰ **S92.145** Nondisplaced dome fracture of left talus   CC

15,20 ✓7ᵗʰ **S92.146** Nondisplaced dome fracture of unspecified talus   CC

✓6ᵗʰ **S92.15** Avulsion fracture (chip fracture) of talus

15,20 ✓7ᵗʰ **S92.151** Displaced avulsion fracture (chip fracture) of right talus   CC

15,20 ✓7ᵗʰ **S92.152** Displaced avulsion fracture (chip fracture) of left talus   CC

15,20 ✓7ᵗʰ **S92.153** Displaced avulsion fracture (chip fracture) of unspecified talus   CC

15,20 ✓7ᵗʰ **S92.154** Nondisplaced avulsion fracture (chip fracture) of right talus   CC

15,20 ✓7ᵗʰ **S92.155** Nondisplaced avulsion fracture (chip fracture) of left talus   CC

15,20 ✓7ᵗʰ **S92.156** Nondisplaced avulsion fracture (chip fracture) of unspecified talus   CC

✓6ᵗʰ **S92.19** Other fracture of talus

15,20 ✓7ᵗʰ **S92.191** Other fracture of right talus   CC

15,20 ✓7ᵗʰ **S92.192** Other fracture of left talus   CC

15,20 ✓7ᵗʰ **S92.199** Other fracture of unspecified talus   CC

✓5ᵗʰ **S92.2** Fracture of other and unspecified tarsal bone(s)

> **CC Excl: For CC codes in subcategory S92.2, unless otherwise noted:** See code: S92.1

✓6ᵗʰ **S92.20** Fracture of unspecified tarsal bone(s)

> **CC Excl: For CC codes in subcategory S92.20, unless otherwise noted: CC with 7th character B:** S92.001–S92.919 with 7th [A, B]
> **CC with 7th character K or P:** M80.00X–M84.68X with 7th [K, P], S02.0XX–S02.92X with 7th K, S12.000–S12.691 with 7th K, S22.000–S22.9XX with 7th K, S32.000–S32.9XX with 7th K, S42.001–S42.92X with 7th [K, P], S49.001–S49.199 with 7th [K, P], S52.001–S52.92X with 7th [K, M, N, P, Q, R], S59.001–S59.299 with 7th [K, P], S62.001–S62.92X with 7th [K, P], S72.001–S72.92X with 7th [K, M, N, P, Q, R], S79.001–S79.199 with 7th [K, P], S82.001–S82.92X with 7th [K, M, N, P, Q, R], S89.001–S89.399 with 7th [K, P], S92.001–S92.919 with 7th [K, P]

15,20 ✓7ᵗʰ **S92.201** Fracture of unspecified tarsal bone(s) of right foot   CC

15,20 ✓7ᵗʰ **S92.202** Fracture of unspecified tarsal bone(s) of left foot   CC

15,20 ✓7ᵗʰ **S92.209** Fracture of unspecified tarsal bone(s) of unspecified foot   CC

✓6ᵗʰ **S92.21** Fracture of cuboid bone

15,20 ✓7ᵗʰ **S92.211** Displaced fracture of cuboid bone of right foot   CC

15,20 ✓7ᵗʰ **S92.212** Displaced fracture of cuboid bone of left foot   CC

15,20 ✓7ᵗʰ **S92.213** Displaced fracture of cuboid bone of unspecified foot   CC

15,20 ✓7ᵗʰ **S92.214** Nondisplaced fracture of cuboid bone of right foot   CC

15,20 ✓7ᵗʰ **S92.215** Nondisplaced fracture of cuboid bone of left foot   CC

15,20 ✓7ᵗʰ **S92.216** Nondisplaced fracture of cuboid bone of unspecified foot   CC

✓6ᵗʰ **S92.22** Fracture of lateral cuneiform

15,20 ✓7ᵗʰ **S92.221** Displaced fracture of lateral cuneiform of right foot   CC

15,20 ✓7ᵗʰ **S92.222** Displaced fracture of lateral cuneiform of left foot   CC

15,20 ✓7ᵗʰ **S92.223** Displaced fracture of lateral cuneiform of unspecified foot   CC

15,20 ✓7ᵗʰ **S92.224** Nondisplaced fracture of lateral cuneiform of right foot   CC

15,20 ✓7ᵗʰ **S92.225** Nondisplaced fracture of lateral cuneiform of left foot   CC

15,20 ✓7ᵗʰ **S92.226** Nondisplaced fracture of lateral cuneiform of unspecified foot   CC

✓6ᵗʰ **S92.23** Fracture of intermediate cuneiform

15,20 ✓7ᵗʰ **S92.231** Displaced fracture of intermediate cuneiform of right foot   CC

15,20 ✓7ᵗʰ **S92.232** Displaced fracture of intermediate cuneiform of left foot   CC

15,20 ✓7ᵗʰ **S92.233** Displaced fracture of intermediate cuneiform of unspecified foot   CC

15,20 ✓7ᵗʰ **S92.234** Nondisplaced fracture of intermediate cuneiform of right foot   CC

15,20 ✓7ᵗʰ **S92.235** Nondisplaced fracture of intermediate cuneiform of left foot   CC

15,20 ✓7ᵗʰ **S92.236** Nondisplaced fracture of intermediate cuneiform of unspecified foot   CC

✓6ᵗʰ **S92.24** Fracture of medial cuneiform

15,20 ✓7ᵗʰ **S92.241** Displaced fracture of medial cuneiform of right foot   CC

15,20 ✓7ᵗʰ **S92.242** Displaced fracture of medial cuneiform of left foot   CC

15,20 ✓7ᵗʰ **S92.243** Displaced fracture of medial cuneiform of unspecified foot   CC

15,20 ✓7ᵗʰ **S92.244** Nondisplaced fracture of medial cuneiform of right foot   CC

15,20 ✓7ᵗʰ **S92.245** Nondisplaced fracture of medial cuneiform of left foot   CC

15,20 ✓7ᵗʰ **S92.246** Nondisplaced fracture of medial cuneiform of unspecified foot   CC

✓6ᵗʰ **S92.25** Fracture of navicular [scaphoid] of foot

15,20 ✓7ᵗʰ **S92.251** Displaced fracture of navicular [scaphoid] of right foot   CC

15,20 ✓7ᵗʰ **S92.252** Displaced fracture of navicular [scaphoid] of left foot   CC

15,20 ✓7ᵗʰ **S92.253** Displaced fracture of navicular [scaphoid] of unspecified foot   CC

15,20 ✓7ᵗʰ **S92.254** Nondisplaced fracture of navicular [scaphoid] of right foot   CC

15,20 ✓7ᵗʰ **S92.255** Nondisplaced fracture of navicular [scaphoid] of left foot   CC

15,20 ✓7ᵗʰ **S92.256** Nondisplaced fracture of navicular [scaphoid] of unspecified foot   CC

✓5ᵗʰ **S92.3** Fracture of metatarsal bone(s)

> **CC Excl: For CC codes in subcategory S92.3, unless otherwise noted:** See code: S92.1

✓6ᵗʰ **S92.30** Fracture of unspecified metatarsal bone(s)

15,20 ✓7ᵗʰ **S92.301** Fracture of unspecified metatarsal bone(s), right foot   CC

15,20 ✓7ᵗʰ **S92.302** Fracture of unspecified metatarsal bone(s), left foot   CC

15,20 ✓7ᵗʰ **S92.309** Fracture of unspecified metatarsal bone(s), unspecified foot   CC

✓6ᵗʰ **S92.31** Fracture of first metatarsal bone

15,20 ✓7ᵗʰ **S92.311** Displaced fracture of first metatarsal bone, right foot   CC

15,20 ✓7ᵗʰ **S92.312** Displaced fracture of first metatarsal bone, left foot   CC

15,20 ✓7ᵗʰ **S92.313** Displaced fracture of first metatarsal bone, unspecified foot   CC

15,20 ✓7ᵗʰ **S92.314** Nondisplaced fracture of first metatarsal bone, right foot   CC

15,20 ✓7ᵗʰ **S92.315** Nondisplaced fracture of first metatarsal bone, left foot   CC

15,20 ✓7ᵗʰ **S92.316** Nondisplaced fracture of first metatarsal bone, unspecified foot   CC

✓6ᵗʰ **S92.32** Fracture of second metatarsal bone

15,20 ✓7ᵗʰ **S92.321** Displaced fracture of second metatarsal bone, right foot   CC

15,20 ✓7ᵗʰ **S92.322** Displaced fracture of second metatarsal bone, left foot   CC

---

15 HAC = Initial encounter for open fracture only (7th character B or C – specific to category) and not POA.
20 CC only if an initial encounter for an open fracture (7th character B or C – specific to category) **OR** a subsequent encounter for nonunion or malunion (7th character K, M, N, P, Q, or R – specific to category).

✓ Additional Character Required   ✓x7ᵗʰ Placeholder Alert   Unacceptable PDx   Manifestation   Hospital Acquired Condition   *EXCLUDES 1* Not Coded Here   *EXCLUDES 2* Not Included Here

15,20 ✓7ᵗʰ **S92.323** Displaced **fracture of second metatarsal bone, unspecified** foot   CC

15,20 ✓7ᵗʰ **S92.324** Nondisplaced **fracture of second metatarsal bone, right** foot   CC

15,20 ✓7ᵗʰ **S92.325** Nondisplaced **fracture of second metatarsal bone, left** foot   CC

15,20 ✓7ᵗʰ **S92.326** Nondisplaced **fracture of second metatarsal bone, unspecified** foot   CC

✓6ᵗʰ **S92.33** Fracture of **third** metatarsal bone

15,20 ✓7ᵗʰ **S92.331** Displaced **fracture of third metatarsal bone, right** foot   CC

15,20 ✓7ᵗʰ **S92.332** Displaced **fracture of third metatarsal bone, left** foot   CC

15,20 ✓7ᵗʰ **S92.333** Displaced **fracture of third metatarsal bone, unspecified** foot   CC

15,20 ✓7ᵗʰ **S92.334** Nondisplaced **fracture of third metatarsal bone, right** foot   CC

15,20 ✓7ᵗʰ **S92.335** Nondisplaced **fracture of third metatarsal bone, left** foot   CC

15,20 ✓7ᵗʰ **S92.336** Nondisplaced **fracture of third metatarsal bone, unspecified** foot   CC

✓6ᵗʰ **S92.34** Fracture of **fourth** metatarsal bone

15,20 ✓7ᵗʰ **S92.341** Displaced **fracture of fourth metatarsal bone, right** foot   CC

15,20 ✓7ᵗʰ **S92.342** Displaced **fracture of fourth metatarsal bone, left** foot   CC

15,20 ✓7ᵗʰ **S92.343** Displaced **fracture of fourth metatarsal bone, unspecified** foot   CC

15,20 ✓7ᵗʰ **S92.344** Nondisplaced **fracture of fourth metatarsal bone, right** foot   CC

15,20 ✓7ᵗʰ **S92.345** Nondisplaced **fracture of fourth metatarsal bone, left** foot   CC

15,20 ✓7ᵗʰ **S92.346** Nondisplaced **fracture of fourth metatarsal bone, unspecified** foot   CC

✓6ᵗʰ **S92.35** Fracture of **fifth** metatarsal bone

15,20 ✓7ᵗʰ **S92.351** Displaced **fracture of fifth metatarsal bone, right** foot   CC

15,20 ✓7ᵗʰ **S92.352** Displaced **fracture of fifth metatarsal bone, left** foot   CC

15,20 ✓7ᵗʰ **S92.353** Displaced **fracture of fifth metatarsal bone, unspecified** foot   CC

15,20 ✓7ᵗʰ **S92.354** Nondisplaced **fracture of fifth metatarsal bone, right** foot   CC

15,20 ✓7ᵗʰ **S92.355** Nondisplaced **fracture of fifth metatarsal bone, left** foot   CC

15,20 ✓7ᵗʰ **S92.356** Nondisplaced **fracture of fifth metatarsal bone, unspecified** foot   CC

✓5ᵗʰ **S92.4** Fracture of **great toe**

> **CC Excl: For CC codes in subcategory S92.4, unless otherwise noted:** CC with 7th character K or P: M80.00X-M84.68X with 7th [K, P], S02.0XX-S02.92X with 7th K, S12.000-S12.691 with 7th K, S22.000-S22.9XX with 7th K, S32.000-S32.9XX with 7th K, S42.001-S42.92X with 7th [K, P], S49.001-S49.199 with 7th [K, P], S52.001-S52.92X with 7th [K, M, N, P, Q, R], S59.001-S59.299 with 7th [K, P], S62.001-S62.92X with 7th [K, P], S72.001-S72.92X with 7th [K, M, N, P, Q, R], S79.001-S79.199 with 7th [K, P], S82.001-S82.92X with 7th [K, M, N, P, Q, R], S89.001-S89.399 with 7th [K, P], S92.001-S92.919 with 7th [K, P]

✓6ᵗʰ **S92.40** Unspecified **fracture of great toe**

18 ✓7ᵗʰ **S92.401** Displaced **unspecified fracture of right great** toe   CC

18 ✓7ᵗʰ **S92.402** Displaced **unspecified fracture of left great** toe   CC

18 ✓7ᵗʰ **S92.403** Displaced **unspecified fracture of unspecified great** toe   CC

18 ✓7ᵗʰ **S92.404** Nondisplaced **unspecified fracture of right great** toe   CC

18 ✓7ᵗʰ **S92.405** Nondisplaced **unspecified fracture of left great** toe   CC

18 ✓7ᵗʰ **S92.406** Nondisplaced **unspecified fracture of unspecified great** toe   CC

✓6ᵗʰ **S92.41** Fracture of **proximal phalanx of great toe**

18 ✓7ᵗʰ **S92.411** Displaced **fracture of proximal phalanx of right great** toe   CC

18 ✓7ᵗʰ **S92.412** Displaced **fracture of proximal phalanx of left great** toe   CC

18 ✓7ᵗʰ **S92.413** Displaced **fracture of proximal phalanx of unspecified great** toe   CC

18 ✓7ᵗʰ **S92.414** Nondisplaced **fracture of proximal phalanx of right great** toe   CC

18 ✓7ᵗʰ **S92.415** Nondisplaced **fracture of proximal phalanx of left great** toe   CC

18 ✓7ᵗʰ **S92.416** Nondisplaced **fracture of proximal phalanx of unspecified great** toe   CC

✓6ᵗʰ **S92.42** Fracture of **distal phalanx of great toe**

18 ✓7ᵗʰ **S92.421** Displaced **fracture of distal phalanx of right great** toe   CC

18 ✓7ᵗʰ **S92.422** Displaced **fracture of distal phalanx of left great** toe   CC

18 ✓7ᵗʰ **S92.423** Displaced **fracture of distal phalanx of unspecified great** toe   CC

18 ✓7ᵗʰ **S92.424** Nondisplaced **fracture of distal phalanx of right great** toe   CC

18 ✓7ᵗʰ **S92.425** Nondisplaced **fracture of distal phalanx of left great** toe   CC

18 ✓7ᵗʰ **S92.426** Nondisplaced **fracture of distal phalanx of unspecified great** toe   CC

✓6ᵗʰ **S92.49** Other **fracture of great toe**

18 ✓7ᵗʰ **S92.491** Other **fracture of right great** toe   CC

18 ✓7ᵗʰ **S92.492** Other **fracture of left great** toe   CC

18 ✓7ᵗʰ **S92.499** Other **fracture of unspecified great** toe   CC

✓5ᵗʰ **S92.5** Fracture of **lesser toe(s)**

> **CC Excl: For CC codes in subcategory S92.5, unless otherwise noted:** See code: S92.4

✓6ᵗʰ **S92.50** Unspecified **fracture of lesser toe(s)**

18 ✓7ᵗʰ **S92.501** Displaced **unspecified fracture of right lesser** toe(s)   CC

18 ✓7ᵗʰ **S92.502** Displaced **unspecified fracture of left lesser** toe(s)   CC

18 ✓7ᵗʰ **S92.503** Displaced **unspecified fracture of unspecified lesser** toe(s)   CC

18 ✓7ᵗʰ **S92.504** Nondisplaced **unspecified fracture of right lesser** toe(s)   CC

18 ✓7ᵗʰ **S92.505** Nondisplaced **unspecified fracture of left lesser** toe(s)   CC

18 ✓7ᵗʰ **S92.506** Nondisplaced **unspecified fracture of unspecified lesser** toe(s)   CC

✓6ᵗʰ **S92.51** Fracture of **proximal phalanx of lesser toe(s)**

18 ✓7ᵗʰ **S92.511** Displaced **fracture of proximal phalanx of right lesser** toe(s)   CC

18 ✓7ᵗʰ **S92.512** Displaced **fracture of proximal phalanx of left lesser** toe(s)   CC

18 ✓7ᵗʰ **S92.513** Displaced **fracture of proximal phalanx of unspecified lesser** toe(s)   CC

18 ✓7ᵗʰ **S92.514** Nondisplaced **fracture of proximal phalanx of right lesser** toe(s)   CC

18 ✓7ᵗʰ **S92.515** Nondisplaced **fracture of proximal phalanx of left lesser** toe(s)   CC

18 ✓7ᵗʰ **S92.516** Nondisplaced **fracture of proximal phalanx of unspecified lesser** toe(s)   CC

✓6ᵗʰ **S92.52** Fracture of **medial phalanx of lesser toe(s)**

18 ✓7ᵗʰ **S92.521** Displaced **fracture of medial phalanx of right lesser** toe(s)   CC

18 ✓7ᵗʰ **S92.522** Displaced **fracture of medial phalanx of left lesser** toe(s)   CC

18 ✓7ᵗʰ **S92.523** Displaced **fracture of medial phalanx of unspecified lesser** toe(s)   CC

18 ✓7ᵗʰ **S92.524** Nondisplaced **fracture of medial phalanx of right lesser** toe(s)   CC

18 ✓7ᵗʰ **S92.525** Nondisplaced **fracture of medial phalanx of left lesser** toe(s)   CC

18 ✓7ᵗʰ **S92.526** Nondisplaced **fracture of medial phalanx of unspecified lesser** toe(s)   CC

---

15 HAC = Initial encounter for open fracture only (7th character B or C – specific to category) and not POA.

18 CC only if a subsequent encounter for nonunion or malunion (7th character K, M, N, P, Q, or R – specific to category).

20 CC only if an initial encounter for an open fracture (7th character B or C – specific to category) **OR** a subsequent encounter for nonunion or malunion (7th character K, M, N, P, Q, or R – specific to category).

Ⓝ Newborn: 0   Ⓟ Pediatric: 0-17   Ⓜ Maternity: 12-55   Ⓐ Adult: 15-124   **MCC** Major CC Condition   **PDxMCC** PDx acts as own MCC   **CC** CC Condition   **PDxCC** PDx acts as own CC

√6th	**S92.53**	**Fracture of** distal phalanx **of lesser toe(s)**	
18 √7th	**S92.531**	**Displaced fracture of distal phalanx of** right lesser **toe(s)**	CC
18 √7th	**S92.532**	**Displaced fracture of distal phalanx of** left lesser **toe(s)**	CC
18 √7th	**S92.533**	**Displaced fracture of distal phalanx of** unspecified lesser **toe(s)**	CC
18 √7th	**S92.534**	**Nondisplaced fracture of distal phalanx of** right lesser **toe(s)**	CC
18 √7th	**S92.535**	**Nondisplaced fracture of distal phalanx of** left lesser **toe(s)**	CC
18 √7th	**S92.536**	**Nondisplaced fracture of distal phalanx of** unspecified lesser **toe(s)**	CC

√6th	**S92.59**	**Other fracture of lesser toe(s)**	
18 √7th	**S92.591**	**Other fracture of** right lesser **toe(s)**	CC
18 √7th	**S92.592**	**Other fracture of** left lesser **toe(s)**	CC
18 √7th	**S92.599**	**Other fracture of** unspecified lesser **toe(s)**	CC

√5th **S92.9 Unspecified** fracture of foot and toe

√6th **S92.90 Unspecified fracture of** foot

CC Excl: For CC codes in subcategory S92.90, unless otherwise noted: **CC with 7th character B:** S92.001-S92.919 with 7th [A, B]
CC with 7th character K or P: M80.00X-M84.68X with 7th [K, P], S02.0XX-S02.92X with 7th K, S12.000-S12.691 with 7th K, S22.000-S22.9XX with 7th K, S32.000-S32.9XX with 7th K, S42.001-S42.92X with 7th [K, P], S49.001-S49.199 with 7th [K, P], S52.001-S52.92X with 7th [K, M, N, P, Q, R], S59.001-S59.299 with 7th [K, P], S62.001-S62.92X with 7th [K, P], S72.001-S72.92X with 7th [K, M, N, P, Q, R], S79.001-S79.199 with 7th [K, P], S82.001-S82.92X with 7th [K, M, N, P, Q, R], S89.001-S89.399 with 7th [K, P], S92.001-S92.919 with 7th [K, P]

15,20 √7th	**S92.901**	**Unspecified fracture of** right foot	CC
15,20 √7th	**S92.902**	**Unspecified fracture of** left foot	CC
15,20 √7th	**S92.909**	**Unspecified fracture of** unspecified foot	CC

√6th **S92.91 Unspecified fracture of** toe

CC Excl: For CC codes in subcategory S92.91, unless otherwise noted: See code: S92.90

18 √7th	**S92.911**	**Unspecified fracture of** right **toe(s)**	CC
18 √7th	**S92.912**	**Unspecified fracture of** left **toe(s)**	CC
18 √7th	**S92.919**	**Unspecified fracture of** unspecified **toe(s)**	CC

√4th **S93 Dislocation and sprain of joints and ligaments at ankle, foot and toe level**

INCLUDES   avulsion of joint or ligament of ankle, foot and toe
laceration of cartilage, joint or ligament of ankle, foot and toe
sprain of cartilage, joint or ligament of ankle, foot and toe
traumatic hemarthrosis of joint or ligament of ankle, foot and toe
traumatic rupture of joint or ligament of ankle, foot and toe
traumatic subluxation of joint or ligament of ankle, foot and toe
traumatic tear of joint or ligament of ankle, foot and toe

Code also any associated open wound

EXCLUDES 2   strain of muscle and tendon of ankle and foot (S96.-)

The appropriate 7th character is to be added to each code from category S93.
A   initial encounter
D   subsequent encounter
S   sequela

√5th **S93.0 Subluxation and dislocation of** ankle joint
Subluxation and dislocation of astragalus
Subluxation and dislocation of fibula, lower end
Subluxation and dislocation of talus
Subluxation and dislocation of tibia, lower end

√x 7th	**S93.01**	**Subluxation of** right ankle joint
√x 7th	**S93.02**	**Subluxation of** left ankle joint
√x 7th	**S93.03**	**Subluxation of** unspecified ankle joint
√x 7th	**S93.04**	**Dislocation of** right ankle joint

√x 7th	**S93.05**	**Dislocation of** left ankle joint
√x 7th	**S93.06**	**Dislocation of** unspecified ankle joint

√5th **S93.1 Subluxation and dislocation of** toe

√6th **S93.10 Unspecified subluxation and dislocation of toe**
Dislocation of toe NOS
Subluxation of toe NOS

√7th	**S93.101**	**Unspecified** subluxation **of** right **toe(s)**
√7th	**S93.102**	**Unspecified** subluxation **of** left **toe(s)**
√7th	**S93.103**	**Unspecified** subluxation **of** unspecified **toe(s)**
√7th	**S93.104**	**Unspecified** dislocation **of** right **toe(s)**
√7th	**S93.105**	**Unspecified** dislocation **of** left **toe(s)**
√7th	**S93.106**	**Unspecified** dislocation **of** unspecified **toe(s)**

√6th **S93.11 Dislocation of** interphalangeal joint

√7th	**S93.111**	**Dislocation of interphalangeal joint of right great** toe
√7th	**S93.112**	**Dislocation of interphalangeal joint of left great** toe
√7th	**S93.113**	**Dislocation of interphalangeal joint of unspecified great** toe
√7th	**S93.114**	**Dislocation of interphalangeal joint of** right lesser **toe(s)**
√7th	**S93.115**	**Dislocation of interphalangeal joint of** left lesser **toe(s)**
√7th	**S93.116**	**Dislocation of interphalangeal joint of** unspecified lesser **toe(s)**
√7th	**S93.119**	**Dislocation of interphalangeal joint of** unspecified **toe(s)**

√6th **S93.12 Dislocation of** metatarsophalangeal joint

√7th	**S93.121**	**Dislocation of metatarsophalangeal joint of** right great **toe**
√7th	**S93.122**	**Dislocation of metatarsophalangeal joint of** left great **toe**
√7th	**S93.123**	**Dislocation of metatarsophalangeal joint of** unspecified great **toe**
√7th	**S93.124**	**Dislocation of metatarsophalangeal joint of** right lesser **toe(s)**
√7th	**S93.125**	**Dislocation of metatarsophalangeal joint of** left lesser **toe(s)**
√7th	**S93.126**	**Dislocation of metatarsophalangeal joint of** unspecified lesser **toe(s)**
√7th	**S93.129**	**Dislocation of metatarsophalangeal joint of** unspecified **toe(s)**

√6th **S93.13 Subluxation of** interphalangeal joint

√7th	**S93.131**	**Subluxation of interphalangeal joint of** right great **toe**
√7th	**S93.132**	**Subluxation of interphalangeal joint of** left great **toe**
√7th	**S93.133**	**Subluxation of interphalangeal joint of** unspecified great **toe**
√7th	**S93.134**	**Subluxation of interphalangeal joint of** right lesser **toe(s)**
√7th	**S93.135**	**Subluxation of interphalangeal joint of** left lesser **toe(s)**
√7th	**S93.136**	**Subluxation of interphalangeal joint of** unspecified lesser **toe(s)**
√7th	**S93.139**	**Subluxation of interphalangeal joint of** unspecified **toe(s)**

√6th **S93.14 Subluxation of** metatarsophalangeal joint

√7th	**S93.141**	**Subluxation of metatarsophalangeal joint of** right great **toe**
√7th	**S93.142**	**Subluxation of metatarsophalangeal joint of** left great **toe**
√7th	**S93.143**	**Subluxation of metatarsophalangeal joint of** unspecified great **toe**
√7th	**S93.144**	**Subluxation of metatarsophalangeal joint of** right lesser **toe(s)**
√7th	**S93.145**	**Subluxation of metatarsophalangeal joint of** left lesser **toe(s)**

15 HAC = Initial encounter for open fracture only (7th character B or C – specific to category) and not POA.
18 CC only if a subsequent encounter for nonunion or malunion (7th character K, M, N, P, Q, or R – specific to category).
20 CC only if an initial encounter for an open fracture (7th character B or C – specific to category) **OR** a subsequent encounter for nonunion or malunion (7th character K, M, N, P, Q, or R – specific to category).

☑ Additional Character Required   √x 7th Placeholder Alert   Unacceptable PDx   Manifestation   Hospital Acquired Condition   EXCLUDES 1 Not Coded Here   EXCLUDES 2 Not Included Here

√7ᵗʰ **S93.146** Subluxation of metatarsophalangeal joint of unspecified lesser toe(s)

√7ᵗʰ **S93.149** Subluxation of metatarsophalangeal joint of unspecified toe(s)

√5ᵗʰ **S93.3** Subluxation and dislocation of foot
> EXCLUDES 2   *dislocation of toe (S93.1-)*

√6ᵗʰ **S93.30** Unspecified subluxation and dislocation of foot
Dislocation of foot NOS
Subluxation of foot NOS

√7ᵗʰ **S93.301** Unspecified subluxation of right foot

√7ᵗʰ **S93.302** Unspecified subluxation of left foot

√7ᵗʰ **S93.303** Unspecified subluxation of unspecified foot

√7ᵗʰ **S93.304** Unspecified dislocation of right foot

√7ᵗʰ **S93.305** Unspecified dislocation of left foot

√7ᵗʰ **S93.306** Unspecified dislocation of unspecified foot

√6ᵗʰ **S93.31** Subluxation and dislocation of tarsal joint

√7ᵗʰ **S93.311** Subluxation of tarsal joint of right foot

√7ᵗʰ **S93.312** Subluxation of tarsal joint of left foot

√7ᵗʰ **S93.313** Subluxation of tarsal joint of unspecified foot

√7ᵗʰ **S93.314** Dislocation of tarsal joint of right foot

√7ᵗʰ **S93.315** Dislocation of tarsal joint of left foot

√7ᵗʰ **S93.316** Dislocation of tarsal joint of unspecified foot

√6ᵗʰ **S93.32** Subluxation and dislocation of tarsometatarsal joint

√7ᵗʰ **S93.321** Subluxation of tarsometatarsal joint of right foot

√7ᵗʰ **S93.322** Subluxation of tarsometatarsal joint of left foot

√7ᵗʰ **S93.323** Subluxation of tarsometatarsal joint of unspecified foot

√7ᵗʰ **S93.324** Dislocation of tarsometatarsal joint of right foot

√7ᵗʰ **S93.325** Dislocation of tarsometatarsal joint of left foot

√7ᵗʰ **S93.326** Dislocation of tarsometatarsal joint of unspecified foot

√6ᵗʰ **S93.33** Other subluxation and dislocation of foot

√7ᵗʰ **S93.331** Other subluxation of right foot

√7ᵗʰ **S93.332** Other subluxation of left foot

√7ᵗʰ **S93.333** Other subluxation of unspecified foot

√7ᵗʰ **S93.334** Other dislocation of right foot

√7ᵗʰ **S93.335** Other dislocation of left foot

√7ᵗʰ **S93.336** Other dislocation of unspecified foot

√5ᵗʰ **S93.4** Sprain of ankle
> EXCLUDES 2   *injury of Achilles tendon (S86.0-)*

√6ᵗʰ **S93.40** Sprain of unspecified ligament of ankle
Sprain of ankle NOS
Sprained ankle NOS

√7ᵗʰ **S93.401** Sprain of unspecified ligament of right ankle

√7ᵗʰ **S93.402** Sprain of unspecified ligament of left ankle

√7ᵗʰ **S93.409** Sprain of unspecified ligament of unspecified ankle

√6ᵗʰ **S93.41** Sprain of calcaneofibular ligament

√7ᵗʰ **S93.411** Sprain of calcaneofibular ligament of right ankle

√7ᵗʰ **S93.412** Sprain of calcaneofibular ligament of left ankle

√7ᵗʰ **S93.419** Sprain of calcaneofibular ligament of unspecified ankle

√6ᵗʰ **S93.42** Sprain of deltoid ligament

√7ᵗʰ **S93.421** Sprain of deltoid ligament of right ankle

√7ᵗʰ **S93.422** Sprain of deltoid ligament of left ankle

√7ᵗʰ **S93.429** Sprain of deltoid ligament of unspecified ankle

√6ᵗʰ **S93.43** Sprain of tibiofibular ligament

√7ᵗʰ **S93.431** Sprain of tibiofibular ligament of right ankle

√7ᵗʰ **S93.432** Sprain of tibiofibular ligament of left ankle

√7ᵗʰ **S93.439** Sprain of tibiofibular ligament of unspecified ankle

√6ᵗʰ **S93.49** Sprain of other ligament of ankle
Sprain of internal collateral ligament
Sprain of talofibular ligament

√7ᵗʰ **S93.491** Sprain of other ligament of right ankle

√7ᵗʰ **S93.492** Sprain of other ligament of left ankle

√7ᵗʰ **S93.499** Sprain of other ligament of unspecified ankle

√5ᵗʰ **S93.5** Sprain of toe

√6ᵗʰ **S93.50** Unspecified sprain of toe

√7ᵗʰ **S93.501** Unspecified sprain of right great toe

√7ᵗʰ **S93.502** Unspecified sprain of left great toe

√7ᵗʰ **S93.503** Unspecified sprain of unspecified great toe

√7ᵗʰ **S93.504** Unspecified sprain of right lesser toe(s)

√7ᵗʰ **S93.505** Unspecified sprain of left lesser toe(s)

√7ᵗʰ **S93.506** Unspecified sprain of unspecified lesser toe(s)

√7ᵗʰ **S93.509** Unspecified sprain of unspecified toe(s)

√6ᵗʰ **S93.51** Sprain of interphalangeal joint of toe

√7ᵗʰ **S93.511** Sprain of interphalangeal joint of right great toe

√7ᵗʰ **S93.512** Sprain of interphalangeal joint of left great toe

√7ᵗʰ **S93.513** Sprain of interphalangeal joint of unspecified great toe

√7ᵗʰ **S93.514** Sprain of interphalangeal joint of right lesser toe(s)

√7ᵗʰ **S93.515** Sprain of interphalangeal joint of left lesser toe(s)

√7ᵗʰ **S93.516** Sprain of interphalangeal joint of unspecified lesser toe(s)

√7ᵗʰ **S93.519** Sprain of interphalangeal joint of unspecified toe(s)

√6ᵗʰ **S93.52** Sprain of metatarsophalangeal joint of toe

√7ᵗʰ **S93.521** Sprain of metatarsophalangeal joint of right great toe

√7ᵗʰ **S93.522** Sprain of metatarsophalangeal joint of left great toe

√7ᵗʰ **S93.523** Sprain of metatarsophalangeal joint of unspecified great toe

√7ᵗʰ **S93.524** Sprain of metatarsophalangeal joint of right lesser toe(s)

√7ᵗʰ **S93.525** Sprain of metatarsophalangeal joint of left lesser toe(s)

√7ᵗʰ **S93.526** Sprain of metatarsophalangeal joint of unspecified lesser toe(s)

√7ᵗʰ **S93.529** Sprain of metatarsophalangeal joint of unspecified toe(s)

√5ᵗʰ **S93.6** Sprain of foot
> EXCLUDES 2   *sprain of metatarsophalangeal joint of toe (S93.52-)*
> *sprain of toe (S93.5-)*

√6ᵗʰ **S93.60** Unspecified sprain of foot

√7ᵗʰ **S93.601** Unspecified sprain of right foot

√7ᵗʰ **S93.602** Unspecified sprain of left foot

√7ᵗʰ **S93.609** Unspecified sprain of unspecified foot

√6ᵗʰ **S93.61** Sprain of tarsal ligament of foot

√7ᵗʰ **S93.611** Sprain of tarsal ligament of right foot

√7ᵗʰ **S93.612** Sprain of tarsal ligament of left foot

√7ᵗʰ **S93.619** Sprain of tarsal ligament of unspecified foot

√6ᵗʰ **S93.62** Sprain of tarsometatarsal ligament of foot

√7ᵗʰ **S93.621** Sprain of tarsometatarsal ligament of right foot

√7ᵗʰ **S93.622** Sprain of tarsometatarsal ligament of left foot

√7ᵗʰ **S93.629** Sprain of tarsometatarsal ligament of unspecified foot

√6ᵗʰ **S93.69** Other sprain of foot

√7ᵗʰ **S93.691** Other sprain of right foot

Ⓝ Newborn: 0   Ⓟ Pediatric: 0-17   Ⓜ Maternity: 12-55   Ⓐ Adult: 15-124   MCC Major CC Condition   PDxMCC PDx acts as own MCC   CC CC Condition   PDxCC PDx acts as own CC

1066   ICD-10-CM 2016

✓7ᵗʰ   **S93.692**   Other sprain of left foot

✓7ᵗʰ   **S93.699**   Other sprain of unspecified foot

✓4ᵗʰ **S94**   **Injury of nerves at ankle and foot level**
Code also any associated open wound (S91.-)

> The appropriate 7th character is to be added to each code from category S94.
> A   initial encounter
> D   subsequent encounter
> S   sequela

✓5ᵗʰ   **S94.0**   **Injury of lateral plantar nerve**

✓ₓ7ᵗʰ   **S94.00**   Injury of lateral plantar nerve, unspecified leg

✓ₓ7ᵗʰ   **S94.01**   Injury of lateral plantar nerve, right leg

✓ₓ7ᵗʰ   **S94.02**   Injury of lateral plantar nerve, left leg

✓5ᵗʰ   **S94.1**   **Injury of medial plantar nerve**

✓ₓ7ᵗʰ   **S94.10**   Injury of medial plantar nerve, unspecified leg

✓ₓ7ᵗʰ   **S94.11**   Injury of medial plantar nerve, right leg

✓ₓ7ᵗʰ   **S94.12**   Injury of medial plantar nerve, left leg

✓5ᵗʰ   **S94.2**   **Injury of deep peroneal nerve at ankle and foot level**
Injury of terminal, lateral branch of deep peroneal nerve

✓ₓ7ᵗʰ   **S94.20**   Injury of deep peroneal nerve at ankle and foot level, unspecified leg

✓ₓ7ᵗʰ   **S94.21**   Injury of deep peroneal nerve at ankle and foot level, right leg

✓ₓ7ᵗʰ   **S94.22**   Injury of deep peroneal nerve at ankle and foot level, left leg

✓5ᵗʰ   **S94.3**   **Injury of cutaneous sensory nerve at ankle and foot level**

✓ₓ7ᵗʰ   **S94.30**   Injury of cutaneous sensory nerve at ankle and foot level, unspecified leg

✓ₓ7ᵗʰ   **S94.31**   Injury of cutaneous sensory nerve at ankle and foot level, right leg

✓ₓ7ᵗʰ   **S94.32**   Injury of cutaneous sensory nerve at ankle and foot level, left leg

✓5ᵗʰ   **S94.8**   **Injury of other nerves at ankle and foot level**

✓6ᵗʰ   **S94.8X**   Injury of other nerves at ankle and foot level

✓7ᵗʰ   **S94.8X1**   Injury of other nerves at ankle and foot level, right leg

✓7ᵗʰ   **S94.8X2**   Injury of other nerves at ankle and foot level, left leg

✓7ᵗʰ   **S94.8X9**   Injury of other nerves at ankle and foot level, unspecified leg

✓5ᵗʰ   **S94.9**   **Injury of unspecified nerve at ankle and foot level**

✓ₓ7ᵗʰ   **S94.90**   Injury of unspecified nerve at ankle and foot level, unspecified leg

✓ₓ7ᵗʰ   **S94.91**   Injury of unspecified nerve at ankle and foot level, right leg

✓ₓ7ᵗʰ   **S94.92**   Injury of unspecified nerve at ankle and foot level, left leg

✓4ᵗʰ **S95**   **Injury of blood vessels at ankle and foot level**
Code also any associated open wound (S91.-)
EXCLUDES 2   injury of posterior tibial artery and vein (S85.1-, S85.8-)

> The appropriate 7th character is to be added to each code from category S95.
> A   initial encounter
> D   subsequent encounter
> S   sequela

✓5ᵗʰ   **S95.0**   **Injury of dorsal artery of foot**

✓6ᵗʰ   **S95.00**   Unspecified injury of dorsal artery of foot

✓7ᵗʰ   **S95.001**   Unspecified injury of dorsal artery of right foot   CC
CC Excl: CC with 7th character A: M79.A21-M79.A29, S75.001 with 7th A, S75.009-S75.011 with 7th A, S75.019-S75.021 with 7th A, S75.029-S75.091 with 7th A, S75.099-S75.101 with 7th A, S75.109-S75.111 with 7th A, S75.119-S75.121 with 7th A, S75.129-S75.191 with 7th A, S75.199-S75.201 with 7th A, S75.209-S75.211 with 7th A, S75.219-S75.221 with 7th A, S75.229-S75.291 with 7th A, S75.299-S75.801 with 7th A, S75.809-S75.811 with 7th A, S75.819-S75.891 with 7th A, S75.899-S75.901 with 7th A, S75.909-S75.911 with 7th A, S75.919-S75.991 with 7th A, S75.999A, S85.001A, S85.009-S85.011 with 7th A, S85.019-S85.091 with 7th A,

S85.099-S85.101 with 7th A, S85.109-S85.111 with 7th A, S85.119-S85.121 with 7th A, S85.129-S85.131 with 7th A, S85.139-S85.141 with 7th A, S85.149-S85.151 with 7th A, S85.159-S85.161 with 7th A, S85.169-S85.171 with 7th A, S85.179-S85.181 with 7th A, S85.189-S85.201 with 7th A, S85.209-S85.211 with 7th A, S85.219-S85.291 with 7th A, S85.299-S85.301 with 7th A, S85.309-S85.311 with 7th A, S85.319-S85.391 with 7th A, S85.399-S85.401 with 7th A, S85.409-S85.411 with 7th A, S85.419-S85.491 with 7th A, S85.499-S85.501 with 7th A, S85.509-S85.511 with 7th A, S85.519-S85.591 with 7th A, S85.599-S85.801 with 7th A, S85.809-S85.811 with 7th A, S85.819-S85.891 with 7th A, S85.899-S85.901 with 7th A, S85.909-S85.911 with 7th A, S85.919-S85.991 with 7th A, S85.999A, S95.001A, S95.009-S95.011 with 7th A, S95.019-S95.091 with 7th A, S95.099-S95.101 with 7th A, S95.109-S95.111 with 7th A, S95.119-S95.191 with 7th A, S95.199-S95.201 with 7th A, S95.209-S95.211 with 7th A, S95.219-S95.291 with 7th A, S95.299-S95.801 with 7th A, S95.809-S95.811 with 7th A, S95.819-S95.891 with 7th A, S95.899-S95.901 with 7th A, S95.909-S95.911 with 7th A, S95.919-S95.991 with 7th A, S95.999A

✓7ᵗʰ   **S95.002**   Unspecified injury of dorsal artery of left foot   CC
CC Excl: CC with 7th character A: M79.A21-M79.A29, S75.002-S75.009 with 7th A, S75.012-S75.019 with 7th A, S75.022-S75.029 with 7th A, S75.092-S75.099 with 7th A, S75.102-S75.109 with 7th A, S75.112-S75.119 with 7th A, S75.122-S75.129 with 7th A, S75.192-S75.199 with 7th A, S75.202-S75.209 with 7th A, S75.212-S75.219 with 7th A, S75.222-S75.229 with 7th A, S75.292-S75.299 with 7th A, S75.802-S75.809 with 7th A, S75.812-S75.819 with 7th A, S75.892-S75.899 with 7th A, S75.902-S75.909 with 7th A, S75.912-S75.919 with 7th A, S75.992-S75.999 with 7th A, S85.002-S85.009 with 7th A, S85.012-S85.019 with 7th A, S85.092-S85.099 with 7th A, S85.102-S85.109 with 7th A, S85.112-S85.119 with 7th A, S85.122-S85.129 with 7th A, S85.132-S85.139 with 7th A, S85.142-S85.149 with 7th A, S85.152-S85.159 with 7th A, S85.162-S85.169 with 7th A, S85.172-S85.179 with 7th A, S85.182-S85.189 with 7th A, S85.202-S85.209 with 7th A, S85.212-S85.219 with 7th A, S85.292-S85.299 with 7th A, S85.302-S85.309 with 7th A, S85.312-S85.319 with 7th A, S85.392-S85.399 with 7th A, S85.402-S85.409 with 7th A, S85.412-S85.419 with 7th A, S85.492-S85.499 with 7th A, S85.502-S85.509 with 7th A, S85.512-S85.519 with 7th A, S85.592-S85.599 with 7th A, S85.802-S85.809 with 7th A, S85.812-S85.819 with 7th A, S85.892-S85.899 with 7th A, S85.902-S85.909 with 7th A, S85.912-S85.919 with 7th A, S85.992-S85.999 with 7th A, S95.002-S95.009 with 7th A, S95.012-S95.019 with 7th A, S95.092-S95.099 with 7th A, S95.102-S95.109 with 7th A, S95.112-S95.119 with 7th A, S95.192-S95.199 with 7th A, S95.202-S95.209 with 7th A, S95.212-S95.219 with 7th A, S95.292-S95.299 with 7th A, S95.802-S95.809 with 7th A, S95.812-S95.819 with 7th A, S95.892-S95.899 with 7th A, S95.902-S95.909 with 7th A, S95.912-S95.919 with 7th A, S95.992-S95.999 with 7th A

✓7ᵗʰ   **S95.009**   Unspecified injury of dorsal artery of unspecified foot   CC
CC Excl: CC with 7th character A: M79.A21-M79.A29, S75.001-S75.999 with 7th A, S85.001-S85.999 with 7th A, S95.001-S95.999 with 7th A

√6ᵗʰ **S95.01** Laceration of dorsal artery of foot

√7ᵗʰ **S95.011** Laceration of dorsal artery of right foot [CC]
CC Excl: M79.A21-M79.A29, S75.001 with 7th A, S75.009-S75.011 with 7th A, S75.019-S75.021 with 7th A, S75.029-S75.091 with 7th A, S75.099-S75.101 with 7th A, S75.109-S75.111 with 7th A, S75.119-S75.121 with 7th A, S75.129-S75.191 with 7th A, S75.199-S75.201 with 7th A, S75.209-S75.211 with 7th A, S75.219-S75.221 with 7th A, S75.229-S75.291 with 7th A, S75.299-S75.801 with 7th A, S75.809-S75.811 with 7th A, S75.819-S75.891 with 7th A, S75.899-S75.901 with 7th A, S75.909-S75.911 with 7th A, S75.919-S75.991 with 7th A, S75.999 with 7th A, S85.001 with 7th A, S85.009-S85.011 with 7th A, S85.019-S85.091 with 7th A, S85.099-S85.101 with 7th A, S85.109-S85.111 with 7th A, S85.119-S85.121 with 7th A, S85.129-S85.131 with 7th A, S85.139-S85.141 with 7th A, S85.149-S85.151 with 7th A, S85.159-S85.161 with 7th A, S85.169-S85.171 with 7th A, S85.179-S85.181 with 7th A, S85.189-S85.201 with 7th A, S85.209-S85.211 with 7th A, S85.219-S85.291 with 7th A, S85.299-S85.301 with 7th A, S85.309-S85.311 with 7th A, S85.319-S85.391 with 7th A, S85.399-S85.401 with 7th A, S85.409-S85.411 with 7th A, S85.419-S85.491 with 7th A, S85.499-S85.501 with 7th A, S85.509-S85.511 with 7th A, S85.519-S85.591 with 7th A, S85.599-S85.801 with 7th A, S85.809-S85.811 with 7th A, S85.819-S85.891 with 7th A, S85.899-S85.901 with 7th A, S85.909-S85.911 with 7th A, S85.919-S85.991 with 7th A, S85.999A, S95.001A, S95.009-S95.011 with 7th A, S95.019-S95.091 with 7th A, S95.099-S95.101 with 7th A, S95.109-S95.111 with 7th A, S95.119-S95.191 with 7th A, S95.199-S95.201 with 7th A, S95.209-S95.211 with 7th A, S95.219-S95.291 with 7th A, S95.299-S95.801 with 7th A, S95.809-S95.811 with 7th A, S95.819-S95.891 with 7th A, S95.899-S95.901 with 7th A, S95.909-S95.911 with 7th A, S95.919-S95.991 with 7th A, S95.999 with 7th A

√7ᵗʰ **S95.012** Laceration of dorsal artery of left foot [CC]
CC Excl: M79.A21-M79.A29, S75.002-S75.009 with 7th A, S75.012-S75.019 with 7th A, S75.022-S75.029 with 7th A, S75.092-S75.099 with 7th A, S75.102-S75.109 with 7th A, S75.112-S75.119 with 7th A, S75.122-S75.129 with 7th A, S75.192-S75.199 with 7th A, S75.202-S75.209 with 7th A, S75.212-S75.219 with 7th A, S75.222-S75.229 with 7th A, S75.292-S75.299 with 7th A, S75.802-S75.809 with 7th A, S75.812-S75.819 with 7th A, S75.892-S75.899 with 7th A, S75.902-S75.909 with 7th A, S75.912-S75.919 with 7th A, S75.992-S75.999 with 7th A, S85.002-S85.009 with 7th A, S85.012-S85.019 with 7th A, S85.092-S85.099 with 7th A, S85.102-S85.109 with 7th A, S85.112-S85.119 with 7th A, S85.122-S85.129 with 7th A, S85.132-S85.139 with 7th A, S85.142-S85.149 with 7th A, S85.152-S85.159 with 7th A, S85.162-S85.169 with 7th A, S85.172-S85.179 with 7th A, S85.182-S85.189 with 7th A, S85.202-S85.209 with 7th A, S85.212-S85.219 with 7th A, S85.292-S85.299 with 7th A, S85.302-S85.309 with 7th A, S85.312-S85.319 with 7th A, S85.392-S85.399 with 7th A, S85.402-S85.409 with 7th A, S85.412-S85.419 with 7th A, S85.492-S85.499 with 7th A, S85.502-S85.509 with 7th A, S85.512-S85.519 with 7th A, S85.592-S85.599 with 7th A, S85.802-S85.809 with 7th A, S85.812-S85.819 with 7th A, S85.892-S85.899 with 7th A, S85.902-S85.909 with 7th A, S85.912-S85.919 with 7th A, S85.992-S85.999 with 7th A, S95.002-S95.009 with 7th A, S95.012-S95.019 with 7th A, S95.092-S95.099 with 7th A, S95.102-S95.109 with 7th A, S95.112-S95.119 with 7th A, S95.192-S95.199 with 7th A, S95.202-S95.209 with 7th A, S95.212-S95.219 with 7th A, S95.292-S95.299 with 7th A, S95.802-S95.809 with 7th A, S95.812-S95.819 with 7th A, S95.892-S95.899 with 7th A, S95.902-S95.909 with 7th A, S95.912-S95.919 with 7th A, S95.992-S95.999 with 7th A

√7ᵗʰ **S95.019** Laceration of dorsal artery of unspecified foot [CC]
CC Excl: M79.A21-M79.A29, S75.001-S75.999 with 7th A, S85.001-S85.999 with 7th A, S95.001-S95.999 with 7th A

√6ᵗʰ **S95.09** Other specified injury of dorsal artery of foot

√7ᵗʰ **S95.091** Other specified injury of dorsal artery of right foot [CC]
CC Excl: See code: S95.001

√7ᵗʰ **S95.092** Other specified injury of dorsal artery of left foot [CC]
CC Excl: See code: S95.002

√7ᵗʰ **S95.099** Other specified injury of dorsal artery of unspecified foot [CC]
CC Excl: See code: S95.009

√5ᵗʰ **S95.1** Injury of plantar artery of foot

√6ᵗʰ **S95.10** Unspecified injury of plantar artery of foot

√7ᵗʰ **S95.101** Unspecified injury of plantar artery of right foot [CC]
CC Excl: CC with 7th character A: S75.801 with 7th A, S75.809-S75.811 with 7th A, S75.819-S75.891 with 7th A, S75.899-S75.901 with 7th A, S75.909-S75.911 with 7th A, S75.919-S75.991 with 7th A, S75.999 with 7th A, S85.201 with 7th A, S85.209-S85.211 with 7th A, S85.219-S85.291 with 7th A, S85.299 with 7th A, S85.801 with 7th A, S85.809-S85.811 with 7th A, S85.819-S85.891 with 7th A, S85.899-S85.901 with 7th A, S85.909-S85.911 with 7th A, S85.919-S85.991 with 7th A, S85.999 with 7th A, S95.001 with 7th A, S95.009-S95.011 with 7th A, S95.019-S95.091 with 7th A, S95.099-S95.101 with 7th A, S95.109-S95.111 with 7th A, S95.119-S95.191 with 7th A, S95.199-S95.201 with 7th A, S95.209-S95.211 with 7th A, S95.219-S95.291 with 7th A, S95.299-S95.801 with 7th A, S95.809-S95.811 with 7th A, S95.819-S95.891 with 7th A, S95.899-S95.901 with 7th A, S95.909-S95.911 with 7th A, S95.919-S95.991 with 7th A, S95.999 with 7th A

√7ᵗʰ **S95.102** Unspecified injury of plantar artery of left foot [CC]
CC Excl: CC with 7th character A: S75.802-S75.809 with 7th A, S75.812-S75.819 with 7th A, S75.892-S75.899 with 7th A, S75.902-S75.909 with 7th A, S75.912-S75.919 with 7th A, S75.992-S75.999 with 7th A, S85.202-S85.209 with 7th A, S85.212-S85.219 with 7th A, S85.292-S85.299 with 7th A, S85.802-S85.809 with 7th A, S85.812-S85.819 with 7th A, S85.892-S85.899 with 7th A, S85.902-S85.909 with 7th A, S85.912-S85.919 with 7th A, S85.992-S85.999 with 7th A, S95.002-S95.009 with 7th A, S95.012-S95.019 with 7th A, S95.092-S95.099 with 7th A, S95.102-S95.109 with 7th A, S95.112-S95.119 with 7th A, S95.192-S95.199 with 7th A, S95.202-S95.209 with 7th A, S95.212-S95.219 with 7th A, S95.292-S95.299 with 7th A, S95.802-S95.809 with 7th A, S95.812-S95.819 with 7th A, S95.892-S95.899 with 7th A, S95.902-S95.909 with 7th A, S95.912-S95.919 with 7th A, S95.992-S95.999 with 7th A

√7ᵗʰ **S95.109** Unspecified injury of plantar artery of unspecified foot [CC]
CC Excl: CC with 7th character A: S75.801-S75.999 with 7th A, S85.201-S85.299 with 7th A, S85.801-S85.999 with 7th A, S95.001-S95.999 with 7th A

√6ᵗʰ **S95.11** Laceration of plantar artery of foot

√7ᵗʰ **S95.111** Laceration of plantar artery of right foot [CC]
CC Excl: See code: S95.101

√7ᵗʰ **S95.112** Laceration of plantar artery of left foot [CC]
CC Excl: See code: S95.102

√7ᵗʰ **S95.119** Laceration of plantar artery of unspecified foot [CC]
CC Excl: See code: S95.109

√6ᵗʰ **S95.19** Other specified injury of plantar artery of foot

√7ᵗʰ **S95.191** Other specified injury of plantar artery of right foot [CC]
CC Excl: See code: S95.101

N Newborn: 0   P Pediatric: 0-17   M Maternity: 12-55   A Adult: 15-124   MCC Major CC Condition   PDxMCC PDx acts as own MCC   CC CC Condition   PDxCC PDx acts as own CC

1068   ICD-10-CM 2016

✓7ᵗʰ **S95.192** **Other specified injury of plantar artery of left foot**   `CC`
CC Excl: See code: S95.102

✓7ᵗʰ **S95.199** **Other specified injury of plantar artery of unspecified foot**   `CC`
CC Excl: See code: S95.109

✓5ᵗʰ **S95.2** **Injury of dorsal vein of foot**

   ✓6ᵗʰ **S95.20** **Unspecified injury of dorsal vein of foot**

     ✓7ᵗʰ **S95.201** **Unspecified injury of dorsal vein of right foot**   `CC`
CC Excl: See code: S95.001

     ✓7ᵗʰ **S95.202** **Unspecified injury of dorsal vein of left foot**   `CC`
CC Excl: See code: S95.002

     ✓7ᵗʰ **S95.209** **Unspecified injury of dorsal vein of unspecified foot**   `CC`
CC Excl: See code: S95.009

   ✓6ᵗʰ **S95.21** **Laceration of dorsal vein of foot**

     ✓7ᵗʰ **S95.211** **Laceration of dorsal vein of right foot**   `CC`
CC Excl: See code: S95.001

     ✓7ᵗʰ **S95.212** **Laceration of dorsal vein of left foot**   `CC`
CC Excl: See code: S95.002

     ✓7ᵗʰ **S95.219** **Laceration of dorsal vein of unspecified foot**   `CC`
CC Excl: See code: S95.009

   ✓6ᵗʰ **S95.29** **Other specified injury of dorsal vein of foot**

     ✓7ᵗʰ **S95.291** **Other specified injury of dorsal vein of right foot**   `CC`
CC Excl: See code: S95.001

     ✓7ᵗʰ **S95.292** **Other specified injury of dorsal vein of left foot**   `CC`
CC Excl: See code: S95.002

     ✓7ᵗʰ **S95.299** **Other specified injury of dorsal vein of unspecified foot**   `CC`
CC Excl: See code: S95.009

✓5ᵗʰ **S95.8** **Injury of other blood vessels at ankle and foot level**

   ✓6ᵗʰ **S95.80** **Unspecified injury of other blood vessels at ankle and foot level**

     ✓7ᵗʰ **S95.801** **Unspecified injury of other blood vessels at ankle and foot level, right leg**   `CC`
CC Excl: See code: S95.001

     ✓7ᵗʰ **S95.802** **Unspecified injury of other blood vessels at ankle and foot level, left leg**   `CC`
CC Excl: See code: S95.002

     ✓7ᵗʰ **S95.809** **Unspecified injury of other blood vessels at ankle and foot level, unspecified leg**   `CC`
CC Excl: See code: S95.009

   ✓6ᵗʰ **S95.81** **Laceration of other blood vessels at ankle and foot level**

     ✓7ᵗʰ **S95.811** **Laceration of other blood vessels at ankle and foot level, right leg**   `CC`
CC Excl: See code: S95.001

     ✓7ᵗʰ **S95.812** **Laceration of other blood vessels at ankle and foot level, left leg**   `CC`
CC Excl: See code: S95.002

     ✓7ᵗʰ **S95.819** **Laceration of other blood vessels at ankle and foot level, unspecified leg**   `CC`
CC Excl: See code: S95.009

   ✓6ᵗʰ **S95.89** **Other specified injury of other blood vessels at ankle and foot level**

     ✓7ᵗʰ **S95.891** **Other specified injury of other blood vessels at ankle and foot level, right leg**   `CC`
CC Excl: See code: S95.001

     ✓7ᵗʰ **S95.892** **Other specified injury of other blood vessels at ankle and foot level, left leg**   `CC`
CC Excl: See code: S95.002

     ✓7ᵗʰ **S95.899** **Other specified injury of other blood vessels at ankle and foot level, unspecified leg**   `CC`
CC Excl: See code: S95.009

✓5ᵗʰ **S95.9** **Injury of unspecified blood vessel at ankle and foot level**

   ✓6ᵗʰ **S95.90** **Unspecified injury of unspecified blood vessel at ankle and foot level**

     ✓7ᵗʰ **S95.901** **Unspecified injury of unspecified blood vessel at ankle and foot level, right leg**   `CC`
CC Excl: See code: S95.001

     ✓7ᵗʰ **S95.902** **Unspecified injury of unspecified blood vessel at ankle and foot level, left leg**   `CC`
CC Excl: See code: S95.002

     ✓7ᵗʰ **S95.909** **Unspecified injury of unspecified blood vessel at ankle and foot level, unspecified leg**   `CC`
CC Excl: See code: S95.009

   ✓6ᵗʰ **S95.91** **Laceration of unspecified blood vessel at ankle and foot level**

     ✓7ᵗʰ **S95.911** **Laceration of unspecified blood vessel at ankle and foot level, right leg**   `CC`
CC Excl: See code: S95.001

     ✓7ᵗʰ **S95.912** **Laceration of unspecified blood vessel at ankle and foot level, left leg**   `CC`
CC Excl: See code: S95.002

     ✓7ᵗʰ **S95.919** **Laceration of unspecified blood vessel at ankle and foot level, unspecified leg**   `CC`
CC Excl: See code: S95.009

   ✓6ᵗʰ **S95.99** **Other specified injury of unspecified blood vessel at ankle and foot level**

     ✓7ᵗʰ **S95.991** **Other specified injury of unspecified blood vessel at ankle and foot level, right leg**   `CC`
CC Excl: See code: S95.001

     ✓7ᵗʰ **S95.992** **Other specified injury of unspecified blood vessel at ankle and foot level, left leg**   `CC`
CC Excl: See code: S95.002

     ✓7ᵗʰ **S95.999** **Other specified injury of unspecified blood vessel at ankle and foot level, unspecified leg**   `CC`
CC Excl: See code: S95.009

✦ ✓4ᵗʰ **S96 Injury of muscle and tendon at ankle and foot level**

Code also any associated open wound (S91.-)

EXCLUDES 2   injury of Achilles tendon (S86.0-)
           sprain of joints and ligaments of ankle and foot (S93.-)

> The appropriate 7th character is to be added to each code from category S96.
> A   initial encounter
> D   subsequent encounter
> S   sequela

✓5ᵗʰ **S96.0** **Injury of muscle and tendon of long flexor muscle of toe at ankle and foot level**

   ✓6ᵗʰ **S96.00** **Unspecified injury of muscle and tendon of long flexor muscle of toe at ankle and foot level**

     ✓7ᵗʰ **S96.001** **Unspecified injury of muscle and tendon of long flexor muscle of toe at ankle and foot level, right foot**

     ✓7ᵗʰ **S96.002** **Unspecified injury of muscle and tendon of long flexor muscle of toe at ankle and foot level, left foot**

     ✓7ᵗʰ **S96.009** **Unspecified injury of muscle and tendon of long flexor muscle of toe at ankle and foot level, unspecified foot**

   ✓6ᵗʰ **S96.01** **Strain of muscle and tendon of long flexor muscle of toe at ankle and foot level**

     ✓7ᵗʰ **S96.011** **Strain of muscle and tendon of long flexor muscle of toe at ankle and foot level, right foot**

     ✓7ᵗʰ **S96.012** **Strain of muscle and tendon of long flexor muscle of toe at ankle and foot level, left foot**

     ✓7ᵗʰ **S96.019** **Strain of muscle and tendon of long flexor muscle of toe at ankle and foot level, unspecified foot**

✦   Refer to the Muscle/Tendon Table at beginning of this chapter.

✓ Additional Character Required   ✓×7ᵗʰ Placeholder Alert   Unacceptable PDx   Manifestation   Hospital Acquired Condition   **EXCLUDES 1** Not Coded Here   **EXCLUDES 2** Not Included Here

ICD-10-CM 2016   1069

✓6ᵗʰ **S96.02** Laceration of muscle and tendon of long flexor muscle of toe at ankle and foot level

     ✓7ᵗʰ **S96.021** Laceration of muscle and tendon of long flexor muscle of toe at ankle and foot level, right foot   CC

         CC Excl: CC with 7th character A: S81.001A, S81.009-S81.011 with 7th A, S81.019-S81.021 with 7th A, S81.029-S81.031 with 7th A, S81.039-S81.041 with 7th A, S81.049-S81.051 with 7th A, S81.059-S81.801 with 7th A, S81.809-S81.811 with 7th A, S81.819-S81.821 with 7th A, S81.829-S81.831 with 7th A, S81.839-S81.841 with 7th A, S81.849-S81.851 with 7th A, S81.859A, S86.021A, S86.029 with 7th A, S86.121A, S86.129A, S86.221A, S86.229A, S86.321A, S86.329A, S86.821A, S86.829A, S86.921A, S86.929A, S91.001A, S91.009-S91.011 with 7th A, S91.019-S91.021 with 7th A, S91.029-S91.031 with 7th A, S91.039-S91.041 with 7th A, S91.049-S91.051 with 7th A, S91.059A, S96.021A, S96.029A, S96.121A, S96.129A, S96.221A, S96.229A, S96.821A, S96.829A, S96.921A, S96.929A

     ✓7ᵗʰ **S96.022** Laceration of muscle and tendon of long flexor muscle of toe at ankle and foot level, left foot   CC

         CC Excl: CC with 7th character A: S81.002-S81.009 with 7th A, S81.012-S81.019 with 7th A, S81.022-S81.029 with 7th A, S81.032-S81.039 with 7th A, S81.042-S81.049 with 7th A, S81.052-S81.059 with 7th A, S81.802-S81.809 with 7th A, S81.812-S81.819 with 7th A, S81.822-S81.829 with 7th A, S81.832-S81.839 with 7th A, S81.842-S81.849 with 7th A, S81.852-S81.859 with 7th A, S86.022-S86.029 with 7th A, S86.122-S86.129 with 7th A, S86.222-S86.229 with 7th A, S86.322-S86.329 with 7th A, S86.822-S86.829 with 7th A, S86.922-S86.929 with 7th A, S91.002-S91.009 with 7th A, S91.012-S91.019 with 7th A, S91.022-S91.029 with 7th A, S91.032-S91.039 with 7th A, S91.042-S91.049 with 7th A, S91.052-S91.059 with 7th A, S96.022-S96.029 with 7th A, S96.122-S96.129 with 7th A, S96.222-S96.229 with 7th A, S96.822-S96.829 with 7th A, S96.922-S96.929 with 7th A

     ✓7ᵗʰ **S96.029** Laceration of muscle and tendon of long flexor muscle of toe at ankle and foot level, unspecified foot   CC

         CC Excl: CC with 7th character A: S81.001-S81.859 with 7th A, S86.021-S86.029 with 7th A, S86.121-S86.129 with 7th A, S86.221-S86.229 with 7th A, S86.321-S86.329 with 7th A, S86.821-S86.829 with 7th A, S86.921-S86.929 with 7th A, S91.001-S91.059 with 7th A, S96.021-S96.029 with 7th A, S96.121-S96.129 with 7th A, S96.221-S96.229 with 7th A, S96.821-S96.829 with 7th A, S96.921-S96.929 with 7th A

✓6ᵗʰ **S96.09** Other injury of muscle and tendon of long flexor muscle of toe at ankle and foot level

     ✓7ᵗʰ **S96.091** Other injury of muscle and tendon of long flexor muscle of toe at ankle and foot level, right foot

     ✓7ᵗʰ **S96.092** Other injury of muscle and tendon of long flexor muscle of toe at ankle and foot level, left foot

     ✓7ᵗʰ **S96.099** Other injury of muscle and tendon of long flexor muscle of toe at ankle and foot level, unspecified foot

✓5ᵗʰ **S96.1** Injury of muscle and tendon of long extensor muscle of toe at ankle and foot level

✓6ᵗʰ **S96.10** Unspecified injury of muscle and tendon of long extensor muscle of toe at ankle and foot level

     ✓7ᵗʰ **S96.101** Unspecified injury of muscle and tendon of long extensor muscle of toe at ankle and foot level, right foot

     ✓7ᵗʰ **S96.102** Unspecified injury of muscle and tendon of long extensor muscle of toe at ankle and foot level, left foot

     ✓7ᵗʰ **S96.109** Unspecified injury of muscle and tendon of long extensor muscle of toe at ankle and foot level, unspecified foot

✓6ᵗʰ **S96.11** Strain of muscle and tendon of long extensor muscle of toe at ankle and foot level

     ✓7ᵗʰ **S96.111** Strain of muscle and tendon of long extensor muscle of toe at ankle and foot level, right foot

     ✓7ᵗʰ **S96.112** Strain of muscle and tendon of long extensor muscle of toe at ankle and foot level, left foot

     ✓7ᵗʰ **S96.119** Strain of muscle and tendon of long extensor muscle of toe at ankle and foot level, unspecified foot

✓6ᵗʰ **S96.12** Laceration of muscle and tendon of long extensor muscle of toe at ankle and foot level

     ✓7ᵗʰ **S96.121** Laceration of muscle and tendon of long extensor muscle of toe at ankle and foot level, right foot   CC

         CC Excl: See code: S95.021

     ✓7ᵗʰ **S96.122** Laceration of muscle and tendon of long extensor muscle of toe at ankle and foot level, left foot   CC

         CC Excl: See code: S95.022

     ✓7ᵗʰ **S96.129** Laceration of muscle and tendon of long extensor muscle of toe at ankle and foot level, unspecified foot   CC

         CC Excl: See code: S95.029

✓6ᵗʰ **S96.19** Other specified injury of muscle and tendon of long extensor muscle of toe at ankle and foot level

     ✓7ᵗʰ **S96.191** Other specified injury of muscle and tendon of long extensor muscle of toe at ankle and foot level, right foot

     ✓7ᵗʰ **S96.192** Other specified injury of muscle and tendon of long extensor muscle of toe at ankle and foot level, left foot

     ✓7ᵗʰ **S96.199** Other specified injury of muscle and tendon of long extensor muscle of toe at ankle and foot level, unspecified foot

✓5ᵗʰ **S96.2** Injury of intrinsic muscle and tendon at ankle and foot level

✓6ᵗʰ **S96.20** Unspecified injury of intrinsic muscle and tendon at ankle and foot level

     ✓7ᵗʰ **S96.201** Unspecified injury of intrinsic muscle and tendon at ankle and foot level, right foot

     ✓7ᵗʰ **S96.202** Unspecified injury of intrinsic muscle and tendon at ankle and foot level, left foot

     ✓7ᵗʰ **S96.209** Unspecified injury of intrinsic muscle and tendon at ankle and foot level, unspecified foot

✓6ᵗʰ **S96.21** Strain of intrinsic muscle and tendon at ankle and foot level

     ✓7ᵗʰ **S96.211** Strain of intrinsic muscle and tendon at ankle and foot level, right foot

     ✓7ᵗʰ **S96.212** Strain of intrinsic muscle and tendon at ankle and foot level, left foot

     ✓7ᵗʰ **S96.219** Strain of intrinsic muscle and tendon at ankle and foot level, unspecified foot

✓6ᵗʰ **S96.22** Laceration of intrinsic muscle and tendon at ankle and foot level

     ✓7ᵗʰ **S96.221** Laceration of intrinsic muscle and tendon at ankle and foot level, right foot   CC

         CC Excl: See code: S95.021

     ✓7ᵗʰ **S96.222** Laceration of intrinsic muscle and tendon at ankle and foot level, left foot   CC

         CC Excl: See code: S95.022

     ✓7ᵗʰ **S96.229** Laceration of intrinsic muscle and tendon at ankle and foot level, unspecified foot   CC

         CC Excl: See code: S95.029

✓6ᵗʰ **S96.29** Other specified injury of intrinsic muscle and tendon at ankle and foot level

     ✓7ᵗʰ **S96.291** Other specified injury of intrinsic muscle and tendon at ankle and foot level, right foot

     ✓7ᵗʰ **S96.292** Other specified injury of intrinsic muscle and tendon at ankle and foot level, left foot

✓7ᵗʰ **S96.299** Other specified injury of intrinsic muscle and tendon at ankle and foot level, unspecified foot

✓5ᵗʰ **S96.8** Injury of other specified muscles and tendons at ankle and foot level

  ✓6ᵗʰ **S96.80** Unspecified injury of other specified muscles and tendons at ankle and foot level

    ✓7ᵗʰ **S96.801** Unspecified injury of other specified muscles and tendons at ankle and foot level, right foot

    ✓7ᵗʰ **S96.802** Unspecified injury of other specified muscles and tendons at ankle and foot level, left foot

    ✓7ᵗʰ **S96.809** Unspecified injury of other specified muscles and tendons at ankle and foot level, unspecified foot

  ✓6ᵗʰ **S96.81** Strain of other specified muscles and tendons at ankle and foot level

    ✓7ᵗʰ **S96.811** Strain of other specified muscles and tendons at ankle and foot level, right foot

    ✓7ᵗʰ **S96.812** Strain of other specified muscles and tendons at ankle and foot level, left foot

    ✓7ᵗʰ **S96.819** Strain of other specified muscles and tendons at ankle and foot level, unspecified foot

  ✓6ᵗʰ **S96.82** Laceration of other specified muscles and tendons at ankle and foot level

    ✓7ᵗʰ **S96.821** Laceration of other specified muscles and tendons at ankle and foot level, right foot   CC
        CC Excl: See code: S95.021

    ✓7ᵗʰ **S96.822** Laceration of other specified muscles and tendons at ankle and foot level, left foot   CC
        CC Excl: See code: S95.022

    ✓7ᵗʰ **S96.829** Laceration of other specified muscles and tendons at ankle and foot level, unspecified foot   CC
        CC Excl: See code: S95.029

  ✓6ᵗʰ **S96.89** Other specified injury of other specified muscles and tendons at ankle and foot level

    ✓7ᵗʰ **S96.891** Other specified injury of other specified muscles and tendons at ankle and foot level, right foot

    ✓7ᵗʰ **S96.892** Other specified injury of other specified muscles and tendons at ankle and foot level, left foot

    ✓7ᵗʰ **S96.899** Other specified injury of other specified muscles and tendons at ankle and foot level, unspecified foot

✓5ᵗʰ **S96.9** Injury of unspecified muscle and tendon at ankle and foot level

  ✓6ᵗʰ **S96.90** Unspecified injury of unspecified muscle and tendon at ankle and foot level

    ✓7ᵗʰ **S96.901** Unspecified injury of unspecified muscle and tendon at ankle and foot level, right foot

    ✓7ᵗʰ **S96.902** Unspecified injury of unspecified muscle and tendon at ankle and foot level, left foot

    ✓7ᵗʰ **S96.909** Unspecified injury of unspecified muscle and tendon at ankle and foot level, unspecified foot

  ✓6ᵗʰ **S96.91** Strain of unspecified muscle and tendon at ankle and foot level

    ✓7ᵗʰ **S96.911** Strain of unspecified muscle and tendon at ankle and foot level, right foot

    ✓7ᵗʰ **S96.912** Strain of unspecified muscle and tendon at ankle and foot level, left foot

    ✓7ᵗʰ **S96.919** Strain of unspecified muscle and tendon at ankle and foot level, unspecified foot

  ✓6ᵗʰ **S96.92** Laceration of unspecified muscle and tendon at ankle and foot level

    ✓7ᵗʰ **S96.921** Laceration of unspecified muscle and tendon at ankle and foot level, right foot   CC
        CC Excl: See code: S95.021

    ✓7ᵗʰ **S96.922** Laceration of unspecified muscle and tendon at ankle and foot level, left foot   CC
        CC Excl: See code: S95.022

    ✓7ᵗʰ **S96.929** Laceration of unspecified muscle and tendon at ankle and foot level, unspecified foot   CC
        CC Excl: See code: S95.029

  ✓6ᵗʰ **S96.99** Other specified injury of unspecified muscle and tendon at ankle and foot level

    ✓7ᵗʰ **S96.991** Other specified injury of unspecified muscle and tendon at ankle and foot level, right foot

    ✓7ᵗʰ **S96.992** Other specified injury of unspecified muscle and tendon at ankle and foot level, left foot

    ✓7ᵗʰ **S96.999** Other specified injury of unspecified muscle and tendon at ankle and foot level, unspecified foot

✓4ᵗʰ **S97** **Crushing injury of ankle and foot**
Use additional code(s) for all associated injuries

> The appropriate 7th character is to be added to each code from category S97.
> A   initial encounter
> D   subsequent encounter
> S   sequela

✓5ᵗʰ **S97.0** Crushing injury of ankle

  ✓x7ᵗʰ **S97.00** Crushing injury of unspecified ankle

  ✓x7ᵗʰ **S97.01** Crushing injury of right ankle

  ✓x7ᵗʰ **S97.02** Crushing injury of left ankle

✓5ᵗʰ **S97.1** Crushing injury of toe

  ✓6ᵗʰ **S97.10** Crushing injury of unspecified toe(s)

    ✓7ᵗʰ **S97.101** Crushing injury of unspecified right toe(s)

    ✓7ᵗʰ **S97.102** Crushing injury of unspecified left toe(s)

    ✓7ᵗʰ **S97.109** Crushing injury of unspecified toe(s)
        Crushing injury of toe NOS

  ✓6ᵗʰ **S97.11** Crushing injury of great toe

    ✓7ᵗʰ **S97.111** Crushing injury of right great toe

    ✓7ᵗʰ **S97.112** Crushing injury of left great toe

    ✓7ᵗʰ **S97.119** Crushing injury of unspecified great toe

  ✓6ᵗʰ **S97.12** Crushing injury of lesser toe(s)

    ✓7ᵗʰ **S97.121** Crushing injury of right lesser toe(s)

    ✓7ᵗʰ **S97.122** Crushing injury of left lesser toe(s)

    ✓7ᵗʰ **S97.129** Crushing injury of unspecified lesser toe(s)

✓5ᵗʰ **S97.8** Crushing injury of foot

  ✓x7ᵗʰ **S97.80** Crushing injury of unspecified foot
        Crushing injury of foot NOS

  ✓x7ᵗʰ **S97.81** Crushing injury of right foot

  ✓x7ᵗʰ **S97.82** Crushing injury of left foot

✓ Additional Character Required ✓x7ᵗʰ Placeholder Alert Unacceptable PDx Manifestation Hospital Acquired Condition EXCLUDES 1 Not Coded Here EXCLUDES 2 Not Included Here

✓4ᵗʰ **S98   Traumatic amputation of ankle and foot**

An amputation not identified as partial or complete should be coded to complete

The appropriate 7th character is to be added to each code from category S98.
A   initial encounter
D   subsequent encounter
S   sequela

✓5ᵗʰ **S98.0   Traumatic amputation of foot at ankle level**

✓6ᵗʰ **S98.01   Complete traumatic amputation of foot at ankle level**

✓7ᵗʰ **S98.011   Complete traumatic amputation of right foot at ankle level** CC

CC Excl: CC with 7th character A: S71.001 with 7th A, S71.009-S71.011 with 7th A, S71.019-S71.021 with 7th A, S71.029-S71.031 with 7th A, S71.039-S71.041 with 7th A, S71.049-S71.051 with 7th A, S71.059-S71.101 with 7th A, S71.109-S71.111 with 7th A, S71.119-S71.121 with 7th A, S71.129-S71.131 with 7th A, S71.139-S71.141 with 7th A, S71.149-S71.151 with 7th A, S71.159 with 7th A, S76.021 with 7th A, S76.029 with 7th A, S76.121 with 7th A, S76.129 with 7th A, S76.221 with 7th A, S76.229 with 7th A, S76.321 with 7th A, S76.329 with 7th A, S76.821 with 7th A, S76.829 with 7th A, S76.921 with 7th A, S76.929 with 7th A, S78.011 with 7th A, S78.019-S78.021 with 7th A, S78.029-S78.111 with 7th A, S78.119-S78.121 with 7th A, S78.129-S78.911 with 7th A, S78.919-S78.921 with 7th A, S78.929 with 7th A, S81.001 with 7th A, S81.009-S81.011 with 7th A, S81.019-S81.021 with 7th A, S81.029-S81.031 with 7th A, S81.039-S81.041 with 7th A, S81.049-S81.051 with 7th A, S81.059-S81.801 with 7th A, S81.809-S81.811 with 7th A, S81.819-S81.821 with 7th A, S81.829-S81.831 with 7th A, S81.839-S81.841 with 7th A, S81.849-S81.851 with 7th A, S81.859 with 7th A, S86.021 with 7th A, S86.029 with 7th A, S86.121 with 7th A, S86.129 with 7th A, S86.221 with 7th A, S86.229 with 7th A, S86.321 with 7th A, S86.329 with 7th A, S86.821 with 7th A, S86.829 with 7th A, S86.921 with 7th A, S86.929 with 7th A, S88.011 with 7th A, S88.019-S88.021 with 7th A, S88.029-S88.111 with 7th A, S88.119-S88.121 with 7th A, S88.129-S88.911 with 7th A, S88.919-S88.921 with 7th A, S88.929 with 7th A, S91.001 with 7th A, S91.009-S91.011 with 7th A, S91.019-S91.021 with 7th A, S91.029-S91.031 with 7th A, S91.039-S91.041 with 7th A, S91.049-S91.051 with 7th A, S91.059-S91.101 with 7th A, S91.103-S91.104 with 7th A, S91.106-S91.111 with 7th A, S91.113-S91.114 with 7th A, S91.116-S91.121 with 7th A, S91.123-S91.124 with 7th A, S91.126-S91.131 with 7th A, S91.133-S91.134 with 7th A, S91.136-S91.141 with 7th A, S91.143-S91.144 with 7th A, S91.146-S91.151 with 7th A, S91.153-S91.154 with 7th A, S91.156-S91.201 with 7th A, S91.203-S91.204 with 7th A, S91.206-S91.211 with 7th A, S91.213-S91.214 with 7th A, S91.216-S91.221 with 7th A, S91.223-S91.224 with 7th A, S91.226-S91.231 with 7th A, S91.233-S91.234 with 7th A, S91.236-S91.241 with 7th A, S91.243-S91.244 with 7th A, S91.246-S91.251 with 7th A, S91.253-S91.254 with 7th A, S91.256-S91.301 with 7th A, S91.309-S91.311 with 7th A, S91.319-S91.321 with 7th A, S91.329-S91.331 with 7th A, S91.339-S91.341 with 7th A, S91.349-S91.351 with 7th A, S91.359 with 7th A, S96.021 with 7th A, S96.029 with 7th A, S96.121 with 7th A, S96.129 with 7th A, S96.221 with 7th A, S96.229 with 7th A, S96.821 with 7th A, S96.829 with 7th A, S96.921 with 7th A, S96.929 with 7th A, S98.011 with 7th A, S98.019-S98.021 with 7th A, S98.029-S98.111 with 7th A, S98.119-S98.121 with 7th A

✓7ᵗʰ **S98.012   Complete traumatic amputation of left foot at ankle level** CC

CC Excl: CC with 7th character A: S71.002-S71.009 with 7th A, S71.012-S71.019 with 7th A, S71.022-S71.029 with 7th A, S71.032-S71.039 with 7th A, S71.042-S71.049 with 7th A, S71.052-S71.059 with 7th A, S71.102-S71.109 with 7th A, S71.112-S71.119 with 7th A, S71.122-S71.129 with 7th A, S71.132-S71.139 with 7th A, S71.142-S71.149 with 7th A, S71.152-S71.159 with 7th A, S76.022-S76.029 with 7th A, S76.122-S76.129 with 7th A, S76.222-S76.229 with 7th A, S76.322-S76.329 with 7th A, S76.822-S76.829 with 7th A, S76.922-S76.929 with 7th A, S78.012-S78.019 with 7th A, S78.022-S78.029 with 7th A, S78.112-S78.119 with 7th A, S78.122-S78.129 with 7th A, S78.912-S78.919 with 7th A, S78.922-S78.929 with 7th A, S81.002-S81.009 with 7th A, S81.012-S81.019 with 7th A, S81.022-S81.029 with 7th A, S81.032-S81.039 with 7th A, S81.042-S81.049 with 7th A, S81.052-S81.059 with 7th A, S81.802-S81.809 with 7th A, S81.812-S81.819 with 7th A, S81.822-S81.829 with 7th A, S81.832-S81.839 with 7th A, S81.842-S81.849 with 7th A, S81.852-S81.859 with 7th A, S86.022-S86.029 with 7th A, S86.122-S86.129 with 7th A, S86.222-S86.229 with 7th A, S86.322-S86.329 with 7th A, S86.822-S86.829 with 7th A, S86.922-S86.929 with 7th A, S88.012-S88.019 with 7th A, S88.022-S88.029 with 7th A, S88.112-S88.119 with 7th A, S88.122-S88.129 with 7th A, S88.912-S88.919 with 7th A, S88.922-S88.929 with 7th A, S91.002-S91.009 with 7th A, S91.012-S91.019 with 7th A, S91.022-S91.029 with 7th A, S91.032-S91.039 with 7th A, S91.042-S91.049 with 7th A, S91.052-S91.059 with 7th A, S91.102-S91.103 with 7th A, S91.105-S91.109 with 7th A, S91.112-S91.113 with 7th A, S91.115-S91.119 with 7th A, S91.122-S91.123 with 7th A, S91.125-S91.129 with 7th A, S91.132-S91.133 with 7th A, S91.135-S91.139 with 7th A, S91.142-S91.143 with 7th A, S91.145-S91.149 with 7th A, S91.152-S91.153 with 7th A, S91.155-S91.159 with 7th A, S91.202-S91.203 with 7th A, S91.205-S91.209 with 7th A, S91.212-S91.213 with 7th A, S91.215-S91.219 with 7th A, S91.222-S91.223 with 7th A, S91.225-S91.229 with 7th A, S91.232-S91.233 with 7th A, S91.235-S91.239 with 7th A, S91.242-S91.243 with 7th A, S91.245-S91.249 with 7th A, S91.252-S91.253 with 7th A, S91.255-S91.259 with 7th A, S91.302-S91.309 with 7th A, S91.312-S91.319 with 7th A, S91.322-S91.329 with 7th A, S91.332-S91.339 with 7th A, S91.342-S91.349 with 7th A, S91.352-S91.359 with 7th A, S96.022-S96.029 with 7th A, S96.122-S96.129 with 7th A, S96.222-S96.229 with 7th A, S96.822-S96.829 with 7th A, S96.922-S96.929 with 7th A, S98.012-S98.019 with 7th A, S98.022-S98.029 with 7th A, S98.112-S98.119 with 7th A, S98.122-S98.129 with 7th A, S98.132-S98.139 with 7th A, S98.142-S98.149 with 7th A, S98.212-S98.219 with 7th A, S98.222-S98.229 with 7th A, S98.312-S98.319 with 7th A, S98.322-S98.329 with 7th A, S98.912-S98.919 with 7th A, S98.922-S98.929 with 7th A, T14.90-T14.91, T79.A0X-T79.9XX with 7th A

✓7ᵗʰ **S98.019   Complete traumatic amputation of unspecified foot at ankle level** CC

CC Excl: CC with 7th character A: S71.001-S71.159 with 7th A, S76.021-S76.029 with 7th A, S76.121-S76.129 with 7th A, S76.221-S76.229 with 7th A, S76.321-S76.329 with 7th A, S76.821-S76.829 with 7th A, S76.921-S76.929 with 7th A, S78.011-S78.929 with 7th A, S81.001-S81.859 with 7th A, S86.021-S86.029 with 7th A, S86.121-S86.129 with 7th A, S86.221-S86.229 with 7th A, S86.321-S86.329 with 7th A, S86.821-S86.829 with 7th A, S86.921-S86.929 with 7th A, S88.011-S88.929 with 7th A, S91.001-S91.359 with 7th A, S96.021-S96.029 with 7th A, S96.121-S96.129 with 7th A, S96.221-S96.229 with 7th A, S96.821-S96.829 with 7th A, S96.921-S96.929 with 7th A, S98.011-S98.929 with 7th A, T14.90-T14.91, T79.A0X-T79.9XX with 7th A

Ⓝ Newborn: 0   Ⓟ Pediatric: 0-17   Ⓜ Maternity: 12-55   Ⓐ Adult: 15-124   MCC Major CC Condition   PDxMCC PDx acts as own MCC   CC CC Condition   PDxCC PDx acts as own CC

1072   ICD-10-CM 2016

√6ᵗʰ **S98.02** Partial **traumatic amputation of foot at ankle level**

√7ᵗʰ **S98.021** **Partial traumatic amputation of right foot at ankle level** CC
CC Excl: See code: S98.011

√7ᵗʰ **S98.022** **Partial traumatic amputation of left foot at ankle level** CC
CC Excl: See code: S98.012

√7ᵗʰ **S98.029** **Partial traumatic amputation of unspecified foot at ankle level** CC
CC Excl: See code: S98.019

√5ᵗʰ **S98.1** **Traumatic amputation of one toe**

√6ᵗʰ **S98.11** Complete **traumatic amputation of great toe**

√7ᵗʰ **S98.111** **Complete traumatic amputation of right great toe**

√7ᵗʰ **S98.112** **Complete traumatic amputation of left great toe**

√7ᵗʰ **S98.119** **Complete traumatic amputation of unspecified great toe**

√6ᵗʰ **S98.12** Partial **traumatic amputation of great toe**

√7ᵗʰ **S98.121** **Partial traumatic amputation of right great toe**

√7ᵗʰ **S98.122** **Partial traumatic amputation of left great toe**

√7ᵗʰ **S98.129** **Partial traumatic amputation of unspecified great toe**

√6ᵗʰ **S98.13** Complete **traumatic amputation of one lesser toe**
Traumatic amputation of toe NOS

√7ᵗʰ **S98.131** **Complete traumatic amputation of one right lesser toe**

√7ᵗʰ **S98.132** **Complete traumatic amputation of one left lesser toe**

√7ᵗʰ **S98.139** **Complete traumatic amputation of one unspecified lesser toe**

√6ᵗʰ **S98.14** Partial **traumatic amputation of one lesser toe**

√7ᵗʰ **S98.141** **Partial traumatic amputation of one right lesser toe**

√7ᵗʰ **S98.142** **Partial traumatic amputation of one left lesser toe**

√7ᵗʰ **S98.149** **Partial traumatic amputation of one unspecified lesser toe**

√5ᵗʰ **S98.2** **Traumatic amputation of two or more lesser toes**

√6ᵗʰ **S98.21** Complete **traumatic amputation of two or more lesser toes**

√7ᵗʰ **S98.211** **Complete traumatic amputation of two or more right lesser toes**

√7ᵗʰ **S98.212** **Complete traumatic amputation of two or more left lesser toes**

√7ᵗʰ **S98.219** **Complete traumatic amputation of two or more unspecified lesser toes**

√6ᵗʰ **S98.22** Partial **traumatic amputation of two or more lesser toes**

√7ᵗʰ **S98.221** **Partial traumatic amputation of two or more right lesser toes**

√7ᵗʰ **S98.222** **Partial traumatic amputation of two or more left lesser toes**

√7ᵗʰ **S98.229** **Partial traumatic amputation of two or more unspecified lesser toes**

√5ᵗʰ **S98.3** **Traumatic amputation of midfoot**

√6ᵗʰ **S98.31** Complete **traumatic amputation of midfoot**

√7ᵗʰ **S98.311** **Complete traumatic amputation of right midfoot** CC
CC Excl: See code: S98.011

√7ᵗʰ **S98.312** **Complete traumatic amputation of left midfoot** CC
CC Excl: See code: S98.012

√7ᵗʰ **S98.319** **Complete traumatic amputation of unspecified midfoot** CC
CC Excl: See code: S98.019

√6ᵗʰ **S98.32** Partial **traumatic amputation of midfoot**

√7ᵗʰ **S98.321** **Partial traumatic amputation of right midfoot** CC
CC Excl: See code: S98.011

√7ᵗʰ **S98.322** **Partial traumatic amputation of left midfoot** CC
CC Excl: See code: S98.012

√7ᵗʰ **S98.329** **Partial traumatic amputation of unspecified midfoot** CC
CC Excl: See code: S98.019

√5ᵗʰ **S98.9** **Traumatic amputation of foot, level unspecified**

√6ᵗʰ **S98.91** Complete **traumatic amputation of foot, level unspecified**

√7ᵗʰ **S98.911** **Complete traumatic amputation of right foot, level unspecified** CC
CC Excl: See code: S98.011

√7ᵗʰ **S98.912** **Complete traumatic amputation of left foot, level unspecified** CC
CC Excl: See code: S98.012

√7ᵗʰ **S98.919** **Complete traumatic amputation of unspecified foot, level unspecified** CC
CC Excl: See code: S98.019

√6ᵗʰ **S98.92** Partial **traumatic amputation of foot, level unspecified**

√7ᵗʰ **S98.921** **Partial traumatic amputation of right foot, level unspecified** CC
CC Excl: See code: S98.011

√7ᵗʰ **S98.922** **Partial traumatic amputation of left foot, level unspecified** CC
CC Excl: See code: S98.012

√7ᵗʰ **S98.929** **Partial traumatic amputation of unspecified foot, level unspecified** CC
CC Excl: See code: S98.019

√4ᵗʰ **S99** **Other and unspecified injuries of ankle and foot**

The appropriate 7th character is to be added to each code from category S99.
A   initial encounter
D   subsequent encounter
S   sequela

√5ᵗʰ **S99.8** **Other specified injuries of ankle and foot**

√6ᵗʰ **S99.81** **Other specified injuries of ankle**

√7ᵗʰ **S99.811** **Other specified injuries of right ankle**

√7ᵗʰ **S99.812** **Other specified injuries of left ankle**

√7ᵗʰ **S99.819** **Other specified injuries of unspecified ankle**

√6ᵗʰ **S99.82** **Other specified injuries of foot**

√7ᵗʰ **S99.821** **Other specified injuries of right foot**

√7ᵗʰ **S99.822** **Other specified injuries of left foot**

√7ᵗʰ **S99.829** **Other specified injuries of unspecified foot**

√5ᵗʰ **S99.9** **Unspecified injury of ankle and foot**

√6ᵗʰ **S99.91** **Unspecified injury of ankle**

√7ᵗʰ **S99.911** **Unspecified injury of right ankle**

√7ᵗʰ **S99.912** **Unspecified injury of left ankle**

√7ᵗʰ **S99.919** **Unspecified injury of unspecified ankle**

√6ᵗʰ **S99.92** **Unspecified injury of foot**

√7ᵗʰ **S99.921** **Unspecified injury of right foot**

√7ᵗʰ **S99.922** **Unspecified injury of left foot**

√7ᵗʰ **S99.929** **Unspecified injury of unspecified foot**

Injury, Poisoning And Certain Other Consequences Of External Causes (T07-T88)

Injuries involving multiple body regions (T07)

EXCLUDES 1 *burns and corrosions (T20-T32)*
frostbite (T33-T34)
insect bite or sting, venomous (T63.4)
sunburn (L55.-)

T07 **Unspecified multiple injuries**
EXCLUDES 1 *injury NOS (T14)*

Injury of unspecified body region (T14)

√4ᵗʰ **T14** **Injury of unspecified body region**
EXCLUDES 1 *multiple unspecified injuries (T07)*

T14.8 **Other injury of unspecified body region**
Abrasion NOS
Contusion NOS
Crush injury NOS
Fracture NOS
Skin injury NOS
Vascular injury NOS

✓ Additional Character Required √xꜞᵗʰ Placeholder Alert Unacceptable PDx Manifestation Hospital Acquired Condition **EXCLUDES 1** Not Coded Here **EXCLUDES 2** Not Included Here

ICD-10-CM 2016

1073

Chapter 19. Injury, Poisoning, and Certain Other Consequences of External Causes

T14.9–T17.500

√5ᵗʰ **T14.9** **Unspecified injury**

T14.90 **Injury, unspecified**
Injury NOS

T14.91 **Suicide attempt**
Attempted suicide NOS

Effects of foreign body entering through natural orifice (T15-T19)

EXCLUDES 2   *foreign body accidentally left in operation wound (T81.5-)*
foreign body in penetrating wound—See open wound by body region
residual foreign body in soft tissue (M79.5)
splinter, without open wound—See superficial injury by body region

√4ᵗʰ **T15** **Foreign body on external eye**

EXCLUDES 2   *foreign body in penetrating wound of orbit and eye ball (S05.4-, S05.5-)*
open wound of eyelid and periocular area (S01.1-)
retained foreign body in eyelid (H02.8-)
retained (old) foreign body in penetrating wound of orbit and eye ball (H05.5-, H44.6-, H44.7-)
superficial foreign body of eyelid and periocular area (S00.25-)

The appropriate 7th character is to be added to each code from category T15.
A   initial encounter
D   subsequent encounter
S   sequela

√5ᵗʰ **T15.0** **Foreign body in cornea**

√x7ᵗʰ **T15.00** **Foreign body in cornea, unspecified eye**

√x7ᵗʰ **T15.01** **Foreign body in cornea, right eye**

√x7ᵗʰ **T15.02** **Foreign body in cornea, left eye**

√5ᵗʰ **T15.1** **Foreign body in conjunctival sac**

√x7ᵗʰ **T15.10** **Foreign body in conjunctival sac, unspecified eye**

√x7ᵗʰ **T15.11** **Foreign body in conjunctival sac, right eye**

√x7ᵗʰ **T15.12** **Foreign body in conjunctival sac, left eye**

√5ᵗʰ **T15.8** **Foreign body in other and multiple parts of external eye**
Foreign body in lacrimal punctum

√x7ᵗʰ **T15.80** **Foreign body in other and multiple parts of external eye, unspecified eye**

√x7ᵗʰ **T15.81** **Foreign body in other and multiple parts of external eye, right eye**

√x7ᵗʰ **T15.82** **Foreign body in other and multiple parts of external eye, left eye**

√5ᵗʰ **T15.9** **Foreign body on external eye, part unspecified**

√x7ᵗʰ **T15.90** **Foreign body on external eye, part unspecified, unspecified eye**

√x7ᵗʰ **T15.91** **Foreign body on external eye, part unspecified, right eye**

√x7ᵗʰ **T15.92** **Foreign body on external eye, part unspecified, left eye**

√4ᵗʰ **T16** **Foreign body in ear**
Foreign body in auditory canal

The appropriate 7th character is to be added to each code from category T16.
A   initial encounter
D   subsequent encounter
S   sequela

√x7ᵗʰ **T16.1** **Foreign body in right ear**

√x7ᵗʰ **T16.2** **Foreign body in left ear**

√x7ᵗʰ **T16.9** **Foreign body in ear, unspecified ear**

√4ᵗʰ **T17** **Foreign body in respiratory tract**

The appropriate 7th character is to be added to each code from category T17.
A   initial encounter
D   subsequent encounter
S   sequela

√x7ᵗʰ **T17.0** **Foreign body in nasal sinus**

√x7ᵗʰ **T17.1** **Foreign body in nostril**
Foreign body in nose NOS

√5ᵗʰ **T17.2** **Foreign body in pharynx**
Foreign body in nasopharynx   Foreign body in throat NOS

√6ᵗʰ **T17.20** **Unspecified foreign body in pharynx**

√7ᵗʰ **T17.200** **Unspecified foreign body in pharynx causing asphyxiation**

√7ᵗʰ **T17.208** **Unspecified foreign body in pharynx causing other injury**

√6ᵗʰ **T17.21** **Gastric contents in pharynx**
Aspiration of gastric contents into pharynx
Vomitus in pharynx

√7ᵗʰ **T17.210** **Gastric contents in pharynx causing asphyxiation**

√7ᵗʰ **T17.218** **Gastric contents in pharynx causing other injury**

√6ᵗʰ **T17.22** **Food in pharynx**
Bones in pharynx   Seeds in pharynx

√7ᵗʰ **T17.220** **Food in pharynx causing asphyxiation**

√7ᵗʰ **T17.228** **Food in pharynx causing other injury**

√6ᵗʰ **T17.29** **Other foreign object in pharynx**

√7ᵗʰ **T17.290** **Other foreign object in pharynx causing asphyxiation**

√7ᵗʰ **T17.298** **Other foreign object in pharynx causing other injury**

√5ᵗʰ **T17.3** **Foreign body in larynx**

√6ᵗʰ **T17.30** **Unspecified foreign body in larynx**

√7ᵗʰ **T17.300** **Unspecified foreign body in larynx causing asphyxiation**

√7ᵗʰ **T17.308** **Unspecified foreign body in larynx causing other injury**

√6ᵗʰ **T17.31** **Gastric contents in larynx**
Aspiration of gastric contents into larynx
Vomitus in larynx

√7ᵗʰ **T17.310** **Gastric contents in larynx causing asphyxiation**

√7ᵗʰ **T17.318** **Gastric contents in larynx causing other injury**

√6ᵗʰ **T17.32** **Food in larynx**
Bones in larynx   Seeds in larynx

√7ᵗʰ **T17.320** **Food in larynx causing asphyxiation**

√7ᵗʰ **T17.328** **Food in larynx causing other injury**

√6ᵗʰ **T17.39** **Other foreign object in larynx**

√7ᵗʰ **T17.390** **Other foreign object in larynx causing asphyxiation**

√7ᵗʰ **T17.398** **Other foreign object in larynx causing other injury**

√5ᵗʰ **T17.4** **Foreign body in trachea**

CC Excl: For CC codes in subcategory T17.4: CC with 7th character A, unless otherwise noted: T17.400-T17.498 with 7th A

√6ᵗʰ **T17.40** **Unspecified foreign body in trachea**

√7ᵗʰ **T17.400** **Unspecified foreign body in trachea causing asphyxiation** CC

√7ᵗʰ **T17.408** **Unspecified foreign body in trachea causing other injury** CC

√6ᵗʰ **T17.41** **Gastric contents in trachea**
Aspiration of gastric contents into trachea
Vomitus in trachea

√7ᵗʰ **T17.410** **Gastric contents in trachea causing asphyxiation** CC

√7ᵗʰ **T17.418** **Gastric contents in trachea causing other injury** CC

√6ᵗʰ **T17.42** **Food in trachea**
Bones in trachea   Seeds in trachea

√7ᵗʰ **T17.420** **Food in trachea causing asphyxiation** CC

√7ᵗʰ **T17.428** **Food in trachea causing other injury** CC

√6ᵗʰ **T17.49** **Other foreign object in trachea**

√7ᵗʰ **T17.490** **Other foreign object in trachea causing asphyxiation** CC

√7ᵗʰ **T17.498** **Other foreign object in trachea causing other injury** CC

√5ᵗʰ **T17.5** **Foreign body in bronchus**

CC Excl: For CC codes in subcategory T17.5: CC with 7th character A, unless otherwise noted: T17.400-T17.998 with 7th A

√6ᵗʰ **T17.50** **Unspecified foreign body in bronchus**

√7ᵗʰ **T17.500** **Unspecified foreign body in bronchus causing asphyxiation** CC

Ⓝ Newborn: 0   Ⓟ Pediatric: 0-17   Ⓜ Maternity: 12-55   Ⓐ Adult: 15-124   MCC Major CC Condition   PDxMCC PDx acts as own MCC   CC CC Condition   PDxCC PDx acts as own CC

1074   ICD-10-CM 2016

√7ᵗʰ **T17.508 Unspecified foreign body in** `CC`
bronchus causing other injury

√6ᵗʰ **T17.51 Gastric contents in bronchus**
Aspiration of gastric contents into bronchus
Vomitus in bronchus

√7ᵗʰ **T17.510 Gastric contents in bronchus** causing `CC`
asphyxiation

√7ᵗʰ **T17.518 Gastric contents in bronchus** causing `CC`
other injury

√6ᵗʰ **T17.52 Food in bronchus**
Bones in bronchus   Seeds in bronchus

√7ᵗʰ **T17.520 Food in bronchus** causing `CC`
asphyxiation

√7ᵗʰ **T17.528 Food in bronchus** causing other injury `CC`

√6ᵗʰ **T17.59 Other foreign object in bronchus**

√7ᵗʰ **T17.590 Other foreign object in bronchus** `CC`
causing asphyxiation

√7ᵗʰ **T17.598 Other foreign object in bronchus** `CC`
causing other injury

√5ᵗʰ **T17.8 Foreign body in other parts of respiratory tract**
Foreign body in bronchioles   Foreign body in lung

CC Excl: For CC codes in subcategory T17.8: CC with 7th
character A, unless otherwise noted: See code: T17.5

√6ᵗʰ **T17.80 Unspecified foreign body in other parts of**
respiratory tract

√7ᵗʰ **T17.800 Unspecified foreign body in other** `CC`
parts of respiratory tract causing
asphyxiation

√7ᵗʰ **T17.808 Unspecified foreign body in other** `CC`
parts of respiratory tract causing other
injury

√6ᵗʰ **T17.81 Gastric contents in other parts of respiratory tract**
Aspiration of gastric contents into other parts of
respiratory tract
Vomitus in other parts of respiratory tract

√7ᵗʰ **T17.810 Gastric contents in other parts of** `CC`
respiratory tract causing asphyxiation

√7ᵗʰ **T17.818 Gastric contents in other parts of** `CC`
respiratory tract causing other injury

√6ᵗʰ **T17.82 Food in other parts of respiratory tract**
Bones in other parts of respiratory tract
Seeds in other parts of respiratory tract

√7ᵗʰ **T17.820 Food in other parts of respiratory** `CC`
tract causing asphyxiation

√7ᵗʰ **T17.828 Food in other parts of respiratory** `CC`
tract causing other injury

√6ᵗʰ **T17.89 Other foreign object in other parts of respiratory**
tract

√7ᵗʰ **T17.890 Other foreign object in other parts of** `CC`
respiratory tract causing asphyxiation

√7ᵗʰ **T17.898 Other foreign object in other parts of** `CC`
respiratory tract causing other injury

√5ᵗʰ **T17.9 Foreign body in respiratory tract, part unspecified**

√6ᵗʰ **T17.90 Unspecified foreign body in respiratory tract, part**
unspecified

√7ᵗʰ **T17.900 Unspecified foreign body in respiratory**
tract, part unspecified causing
asphyxiation

√7ᵗʰ **T17.908 Unspecified foreign body in respiratory**
tract, part unspecified causing other
injury

√6ᵗʰ **T17.91 Gastric contents in respiratory tract, part**
unspecified
Aspiration of gastric contents into respiratory tract,
part unspecified
Vomitus in trachea respiratory tract, part unspecified

√7ᵗʰ **T17.910 Gastric contents in respiratory tract,**
part unspecified causing asphyxiation

√7ᵗʰ **T17.918 Gastric contents in respiratory tract,**
part unspecified causing other injury

√6ᵗʰ **T17.92 Food in respiratory tract, part unspecified**
Bones in respiratory tract, part unspecified
Seeds in respiratory tract, part unspecified

√7ᵗʰ **T17.920 Food in respiratory tract, part unspecified**
causing asphyxiation

√7ᵗʰ **T17.928 Food in respiratory tract, part unspecified**
causing other injury

√6ᵗʰ **T17.99 Other foreign object in respiratory tract, part**
unspecified

√7ᵗʰ **T17.990 Other foreign object in respiratory tract,**
part unspecified in causing asphyxiation

√7ᵗʰ **T17.998 Other foreign object in respiratory tract,**
part unspecified causing other injury

√4ᵗʰ **T18 Foreign body in alimentary tract**
EXCLUDES 2   foreign body in pharynx (T17.2-)

The appropriate 7th character is to be added to each code from
category T18.
A   initial encounter
D   subsequent encounter
S   sequela

√x7ᵗʰ **T18.0 Foreign body in** mouth

√5ᵗʰ **T18.1 Foreign body in** esophagus
EXCLUDES 2   foreign body in respiratory tract (T17.-)

√6ᵗʰ **T18.10 Unspecified foreign body in esophagus**

√7ᵗʰ **T18.100 Unspecified foreign body in esophagus**
causing compression of trachea
Unspecified foreign body in esophagus
causing obstruction of respiration

√7ᵗʰ **T18.108 Unspecified foreign body in esophagus**
causing other injury

√6ᵗʰ **T18.11 Gastric contents in esophagus**
Vomitus in esophagus

√7ᵗʰ **T18.110 Gastric contents in esophagus** causing
compression of trachea
Gastric contents in esophagus causing
obstruction of respiration

√7ᵗʰ **T18.118 Gastric contents in esophagus** causing
other injury

√6ᵗʰ **T18.12 Food in esophagus**
Bones in esophagus   Seeds in esophagus

√7ᵗʰ **T18.120 Food in esophagus** causing compression
of trachea
Food in esophagus causing obstruction of
respiration

√7ᵗʰ **T18.128 Food in esophagus** causing other injury

√6ᵗʰ **T18.19 Other foreign object in esophagus**
AHA: 2015, 1Q, 23

√7ᵗʰ **T18.190 Other foreign object in esophagus**
causing compression of trachea
Other foreign body in esophagus causing
obstruction of respiration

√7ᵗʰ **T18.198 Other foreign object in esophagus**
causing other injury

√x7ᵗʰ **T18.2 Foreign body in** stomach

√x7ᵗʰ **T18.3 Foreign body in** small intestine

√x7ᵗʰ **T18.4 Foreign body in** colon

√x7ᵗʰ **T18.5 Foreign body in** anus and rectum
Foreign body in rectosigmoid (junction)

√x7ᵗʰ **T18.8 Foreign body in** other parts of alimentary tract

√x7ᵗʰ **T18.9 Foreign body of alimentary tract,** part unspecified
Foreign body in digestive system NOS
Swallowed foreign body NOS

√4ᵗʰ **T19 Foreign body in genitourinary tract**
EXCLUDES 2   complications due to implanted mesh (T83.7-)
     mechanical complications of contraceptive device (intrauterine)
     (vaginal) (T83.3-)
     presence of contraceptive device (intrauterine) (vaginal) (Z97.5)

The appropriate 7th character is to be added to each code from
category T19.
A   initial encounter
D   subsequent encounter
S   sequela

√x7ᵗʰ **T19.0 Foreign body in** urethra

√x7ᵗʰ **T19.1 Foreign body in** bladder

√x7ᵗʰ **T19.2 Foreign body in** vulva and vagina   ♀

√x7ᵗʰ **T19.3 Foreign body in** uterus   ♀

√x7ᵗʰ **T19.4 Foreign body in** penis   ♂

√x7ᵗʰ **T19.8 Foreign body in** other parts of genitourinary tract

√ Additional Character Required   √x7ᵗʰ Placeholder Alert   Unacceptable PDx   Manifestation   Hospital Acquired Condition   EXCLUDES 1 Not Coded Here   EXCLUDES 2 Not Included Here

√x 7ᵗʰ **T19.9**   **Foreign body in genitourinary tract, part unspecified**

Burns and corrosions (T20-T32)

INCLUDES   burns (thermal) from electrical heating appliances
burns (thermal) from electricity
burns (thermal) from flame
burns (thermal) from friction
burns (thermal) from hot air and hot gases
burns (thermal) from hot objects
burns (thermal) from lightning
burns (thermal) from radiation
chemical burn [corrosion] (external) (internal)
scalds

EXCLUDES 2   *erythema [dermatitis] ab igne (L59.0)*
radiation-related disorders of the skin and subcutaneous tissue (L55-L59)
sunburn (L55.-)

Burns and corrosions of external body surface, specified by site (T20-T25)

INCLUDES   burns and corrosions of first degree [erythema]
burns and corrosions of second degree [blisters] [epidermal loss]
burns and corrosions of third degree [deep necrosis of underlying tissue] [full-thickness skin loss]

Use additional code from category T31 or T32 to identify extent of body surface involved

√4ᵗʰ **T20**   **Burn and corrosion of head, face, and neck**

EXCLUDES 2   *burn and corrosion of ear drum (T28.41, T28.91)*
burn and corrosion of eye and adnexa (T26.-)
burn and corrosion of mouth and pharynx (T28.0)

AHA: 2015, 1Q, 18-19

> The appropriate 7th character is to be added to each code from category T20.
> A   initial encounter
> D   subsequent encounter
> S   sequela

√5ᵗʰ **T20.0**   **Burn of unspecified degree of head, face, and neck**
Use additional external cause code to identify the source, place and intent of the burn (X00-X19, X75-X77, X96-X98, Y92)

√x 7ᵗʰ **T20.00**   **Burn of unspecified degree of head, face, and neck, unspecified site**

√6ᵗʰ **T20.01**   **Burn of unspecified degree of ear [any part, except ear drum]**
EXCLUDES 2   *burn of ear drum (T28.41-)*

√7ᵗʰ **T20.011**   **Burn of unspecified degree of right ear [any part, except ear drum]**

√7ᵗʰ **T20.012**   **Burn of unspecified degree of left ear [any part, except ear drum]**

√7ᵗʰ **T20.019**   **Burn of unspecified degree of unspecified ear [any part, except ear drum]**

√x 7ᵗʰ **T20.02**   **Burn of unspecified degree of lip(s)**

√x 7ᵗʰ **T20.03**   **Burn of unspecified degree of chin**

√x 7ᵗʰ **T20.04**   **Burn of unspecified degree of nose (septum)**

√x 7ᵗʰ **T20.05**   **Burn of unspecified degree of scalp [any part]**

√x 7ᵗʰ **T20.06**   **Burn of unspecified degree of forehead and cheek**

√x 7ᵗʰ **T20.07**   **Burn of unspecified degree of neck**

√x 7ᵗʰ **T20.09**   **Burn of unspecified degree of multiple sites of head, face, and neck**

√5ᵗʰ **T20.1**   **Burn of first degree of head, face, and neck**
Use additional external cause code to identify the source, place and intent of the burn (X00-X19, X75-X77, X96-X98, Y92)

√x 7ᵗʰ **T20.10**   **Burn of first degree of head, face, and neck, unspecified site**

√6ᵗʰ **T20.11**   **Burn of first degree of ear [any part, except ear drum]**
EXCLUDES 2   *burn of ear drum (T28.41-)*

√7ᵗʰ **T20.111**   **Burn of first degree of right ear [any part, except ear drum]**

√7ᵗʰ **T20.112**   **Burn of first degree of left ear [any part, except ear drum]**

√7ᵗʰ **T20.119**   **Burn of first degree of unspecified ear [any part, except ear drum]**

√x 7ᵗʰ **T20.12**   **Burn of first degree of lip(s)**

√x 7ᵗʰ **T20.13**   **Burn of first degree of chin**

√x 7ᵗʰ **T20.14**   **Burn of first degree of nose (septum)**

√x 7ᵗʰ **T20.15**   **Burn of first degree of scalp [any part]**

√x 7ᵗʰ **T20.16**   **Burn of first degree of forehead and cheek**

√x 7ᵗʰ **T20.17**   **Burn of first degree of neck**

√x 7ᵗʰ **T20.19**   **Burn of first degree of multiple sites of head, face, and neck**

√5ᵗʰ **T20.2**   **Burn of second degree of head, face, and neck**
Use additional external cause code to identify the source, place and intent of the burn (X00-X19, X75-X77, X96-X98, Y92)

√x 7ᵗʰ **T20.20**   **Burn of second degree of head, face, and neck, unspecified site**

√6ᵗʰ **T20.21**   **Burn of second degree of ear [any part, except ear drum]**
EXCLUDES 2   *burn of ear drum (T28.41-)*

√7ᵗʰ **T20.211**   **Burn of second degree of right ear [any part, except ear drum]**

√7ᵗʰ **T20.212**   **Burn of second degree of left ear [any part, except ear drum]**

√7ᵗʰ **T20.219**   **Burn of second degree of unspecified ear [any part, except ear drum]**

√x 7ᵗʰ **T20.22**   **Burn of second degree of lip(s)**

√x 7ᵗʰ **T20.23**   **Burn of second degree of chin**

√x 7ᵗʰ **T20.24**   **Burn of second degree of nose (septum)**

√x 7ᵗʰ **T20.25**   **Burn of second degree of scalp [any part]**

√x 7ᵗʰ **T20.26**   **Burn of second degree of forehead and cheek**

√x 7ᵗʰ **T20.27**   **Burn of second degree of neck**

√x 7ᵗʰ **T20.29**   **Burn of second degree of multiple sites of head, face, and neck**

√5ᵗʰ **T20.3**   **Burn of third degree of head, face, and neck**
Use additional external cause code to identify the source, place and intent of the burn (X00-X19, X75-X77, X96-X98, Y92)

7   √x 7ᵗʰ **T20.30**   **Burn of third degree of head, face, and neck, unspecified site**   CC
CC Excl: CC with 7th character A: T20.30XA, T20.39XA, T20.70XA, T20.79XA

√6ᵗʰ **T20.31**   **Burn of third degree of ear [any part, except ear drum]**
EXCLUDES 2   *burn of ear drum (T28.41-)*
AHA: 2015, 1Q, 18

7   √7ᵗʰ **T20.311**   **Burn of third degree of right ear [any part, except ear drum]**   CC
CC Excl: CC with 7th character A: T20.311-T20.319 with 7th A , T20.39XA, T20.711-T20.719 with 7th A, T20.79XA

7   √7ᵗʰ **T20.312**   **Burn of third degree of left ear [any part, except ear drum]**   CC
CC Excl: See code: T20.311

7   √7ᵗʰ **T20.319**   **Burn of third degree of unspecified ear [any part, except ear drum]**   CC
CC Excl: See code: T20.311

7   √x 7ᵗʰ **T20.32**   **Burn of third degree of lip(s)**   CC
CC Excl: CC with 7th character A: T20.32XA,T20.39XA,T20.72XA,T20.79XA

7   √x 7ᵗʰ **T20.33**   **Burn of third degree of chin**   CC
CC Excl: CC with 7th character A:T20.33XA,T20.39XA,T20.73XA,T20.79XA

7   √x 7ᵗʰ **T20.34**   **Burn of third degree of nose (septum)**   CC
CC Excl: CC with 7th character A: T20.34XA,T20.39XA,T20.74XA,T20.79XA

7   √x 7ᵗʰ **T20.35**   **Burn of third degree of scalp [any part]**   CC
CC Excl: CC with 7th character A: T20.35XA,T20.39XA,T20.75XA,T20.79XA

7   √x 7ᵗʰ **T20.36**   **Burn of third degree of forehead and cheek**   CC
CC Excl: CC with 7th character A: T20.36XA,T20.39XA,T20.76XA,T20.79XA

7   √x 7ᵗʰ **T20.37**   **Burn of third degree of neck**   CC
CC Excl: CC with 7th character A:T20.37XA,T20.39XA,T20.77XA,T20.79XA

7   √x 7ᵗʰ **T20.39**   **Burn of third degree of multiple sites of head, face, and neck**   CC
CC Excl: CC with 7th character A:T20.30X-T20.39X with 7th A, T20.70X-T20.79X with 7th A

---

7   HAC = Initial encounter only (7th character A, B or C) and not POA.

Ⓝ Newborn: 0   Ⓟ Pediatric: 0-17   Ⓜ Maternity: 12-55   Ⓐ Adult: 15-124   MCC Major CC Condition   PDxMCC PDx acts as own MCC   CC CC Condition   PDxCC PDx acts as own CC

1076

ICD-10-CM 2016

✓5ᵗʰ **T20.4** **Corrosion of unspecified degree of head, face, and neck**
Code first (T51-T65) to identify chemical and intent
Use additional external cause code to identify place (Y92)

    ✓x7ᵗʰ **T20.40** **Corrosion of unspecified degree of head, face, and neck, unspecified site**

    ✓6ᵗʰ **T20.41** **Corrosion of unspecified degree of ear [any part, except ear drum]**
EXCLUDES 2   corrosion of ear drum (T28.91-)

        ✓7ᵗʰ **T20.411** **Corrosion of unspecified degree of right ear [any part, except ear drum]**

        ✓7ᵗʰ **T20.412** **Corrosion of unspecified degree of left ear [any part, except ear drum]**

        ✓7ᵗʰ **T20.419** **Corrosion of unspecified degree of unspecified ear [any part, except ear drum]**

    ✓x7ᵗʰ **T20.42** **Corrosion of unspecified degree of lip(s)**

    ✓x7ᵗʰ **T20.43** **Corrosion of unspecified degree of chin**

    ✓x7ᵗʰ **T20.44** **Corrosion of unspecified degree of nose (septum)**

    ✓x7ᵗʰ **T20.45** **Corrosion of unspecified degree of scalp [any part]**

    ✓x7ᵗʰ **T20.46** **Corrosion of unspecified degree of forehead and cheek**

    ✓x7ᵗʰ **T20.47** **Corrosion of unspecified degree of neck**

    ✓x7ᵗʰ **T20.49** **Corrosion of unspecified degree of multiple sites of head, face, and neck**

✓5ᵗʰ **T20.5** **Corrosion of first degree of head, face, and neck**
Code first (T51-T65) to identify chemical and intent
Use additional external cause code to identify place (Y92)

    ✓x7ᵗʰ **T20.50** **Corrosion of first degree of head, face, and neck, unspecified site**

    ✓6ᵗʰ **T20.51** **Corrosion of first degree of ear [any part, except ear drum]**
EXCLUDES 2   corrosion of ear drum (T28.91-)

        ✓7ᵗʰ **T20.511** **Corrosion of first degree of right ear [any part, except ear drum]**

        ✓7ᵗʰ **T20.512** **Corrosion of first degree of left ear [any part, except ear drum]**

        ✓7ᵗʰ **T20.519** **Corrosion of first degree of unspecified ear [any part, except ear drum]**

    ✓x7ᵗʰ **T20.52** **Corrosion of first degree of lip(s)**

    ✓x7ᵗʰ **T20.53** **Corrosion of first degree of chin**

    ✓x7ᵗʰ **T20.54** **Corrosion of first degree of nose (septum)**

    ✓x7ᵗʰ **T20.55** **Corrosion of first degree of scalp [any part]**

    ✓x7ᵗʰ **T20.56** **Corrosion of first degree of forehead and cheek**

    ✓x7ᵗʰ **T20.57** **Corrosion of first degree of neck**

    ✓x7ᵗʰ **T20.59** **Corrosion of first degree of multiple sites of head, face, and neck**

✓5ᵗʰ **T20.6** **Corrosion of second degree of head, face, and neck**
Code first (T51-T65) to identify chemical and intent
Use additional external cause code to identify place (Y92)

    ✓x7ᵗʰ **T20.60** **Corrosion of second degree of head, face, and neck, unspecified site**

    ✓6ᵗʰ **T20.61** **Corrosion of second degree of ear [any part, except ear drum]**
EXCLUDES 2   corrosion of ear drum (T28.91-)

        ✓7ᵗʰ **T20.611** **Corrosion of second degree of right ear [any part, except ear drum]**

        ✓7ᵗʰ **T20.612** **Corrosion of second degree of left ear [any part, except ear drum]**

        ✓7ᵗʰ **T20.619** **Corrosion of second degree of unspecified ear [any part, except ear drum]**

    ✓x7ᵗʰ **T20.62** **Corrosion of second degree of lip(s)**

    ✓x7ᵗʰ **T20.63** **Corrosion of second degree of chin**

    ✓x7ᵗʰ **T20.64** **Corrosion of second degree of nose (septum)**

    ✓x7ᵗʰ **T20.65** **Corrosion of second degree of scalp [any part]**

    ✓x7ᵗʰ **T20.66** **Corrosion of second degree of forehead and cheek**

    ✓x7ᵗʰ **T20.67** **Corrosion of second degree of neck**

    ✓x7ᵗʰ **T20.69** **Corrosion of second degree of multiple sites of head, face, and neck**

✓5ᵗʰ **T20.7** **Corrosion of third degree of head, face, and neck**
Code first (T51-T65) to identify chemical and intent
Use additional external cause code to identify place (Y92)

    7 ✓x7ᵗʰ **T20.70** **Corrosion of third degree of head, face, and neck, unspecified site**   CC
CC Excl: CC with 7th character A:T20.30XA, T20.39XA, T20.70XA, T20.79XA

    ✓6ᵗʰ **T20.71** **Corrosion of third degree of ear [any part, except ear drum]**
EXCLUDES 2   corrosion of ear drum (T28.91-)

        7 ✓7ᵗʰ **T20.711** **Corrosion of third degree of right ear [any part, except ear drum]**   CC
CC Excl: CC with 7th character A: T20.311-T20.319 with 7th A, T20.39XA, T20.711-T20.719 with 7th A, T20.79XA

        7 ✓7ᵗʰ **T20.712** **Corrosion of third degree of left ear [any part, except ear drum]**   CC
CC Excl: See code: T20.711

        7 ✓7ᵗʰ **T20.719** **Corrosion of third degree of unspecified ear [any part, except ear drum]**   CC
CC Excl: See code: T20.711

    7 ✓x7ᵗʰ **T20.72** **Corrosion of third degree of lip(s)**   CC
CC Excl: CC with 7th character A: See code: T20.32

    7 ✓x7ᵗʰ **T20.73** **Corrosion of third degree of chin**   CC
CC Excl: CC with 7th character A: See code: T20.33

    7 ✓x7ᵗʰ **T20.74** **Corrosion of third degree of nose (septum)**   CC
CC Excl: CC with 7th character A: See code: T20.34

    7 ✓x7ᵗʰ **T20.75** **Corrosion of third degree of scalp [any part]**   CC
CC Excl: CC with 7th character A: See code: T20.35

    7 ✓x7ᵗʰ **T20.76** **Corrosion of third degree of forehead and cheek**   CC
CC Excl: CC with 7th character A: See code: T20.36

    7 ✓x7ᵗʰ **T20.77** **Corrosion of third degree of neck**   CC
CC Excl: CC with 7th character A: See code: T20.37

    7 ✓x7ᵗʰ **T20.79** **Corrosion of third degree of multiple sites of head, face, and neck**   CC
CC Excl: CC with 7th character A: See code: T20.39

✓4ᵗʰ **T21** **Burn and corrosion of trunk**
Burns and corrosion of hip region
EXCLUDES 2   burns and corrosion of:
         axilla (T22- with fifth character 4)
         scapular region (T22- with fifth character 6)
         shoulder (T22.- with fifth character 5)

The appropriate 7th character is to be added to each code from category T21.
A   initial encounter
D   subsequent encounter
S   sequela

✓5ᵗʰ **T21.0** **Burn of unspecified degree of trunk**
Use additional external cause code to identify the source, place and intent of the burn (X00-X19, X75-X77, X96-X98, Y92)

    ✓x7ᵗʰ **T21.00** **Burn of unspecified degree of trunk, unspecified site**

    ✓x7ᵗʰ **T21.01** **Burn of unspecified degree of chest wall**
Burn of of unspecified degree of breast

    ✓x7ᵗʰ **T21.02** **Burn of unspecified degree of abdominal wall**
Burn of unspecified degree of flank
Burn of unspecified degree of groin

    ✓x7ᵗʰ **T21.03** **Burn of unspecified degree of upper back**
Burn of unspecified degree of interscapular region

    ✓x7ᵗʰ **T21.04** **Burn of unspecified degree of lower back**

    ✓x7ᵗʰ **T21.05** **Burn of unspecified degree of buttock**
Burn of unspecified degree of anus

    ✓x7ᵗʰ **T21.06** **Burn of unspecified degree of male genital region** ♂
Burn of unspecified degree of penis
Burn of unspecified degree of scrotum
Burn of unspecified degree of testis

    ✓x7ᵗʰ **T21.07** **Burn of unspecified degree of female genital region** ♀
Burn of unspecified degree of labium (majus) (minus)
Burn of unspecified degree of perineum
Burn of unspecified degree of vulva
EXCLUDES 2   burn of vagina (T28.3)

    ✓x7ᵗʰ **T21.09** **Burn of unspecified degree of other site of trunk**

7   HAC = Initial encounter only (7th character A, B or C) and not POA.

✓ Additional Character Required   ✓x7ᵗʰ Placeholder Alert   Unacceptable PDx   Manifestation   Hospital Acquired Condition   *EXCLUDES 1* Not Coded Here   *EXCLUDES 2* Not Included Here

ICD-10-CM 2016   1077

T21.1 Burn of first degree of trunk
Use additional external cause code to identify the source, place and intent of the burn (X00-X19, X75-X77, X96-X98, Y92)

T21.10 Burn of first degree of trunk, unspecified site

T21.11 Burn of first degree of chest wall
Burn of first degree of breast

T21.12 Burn of first degree of abdominal wall
Burn of first degree of flank
Burn of first degree of groin

T21.13 Burn of first degree of upper back
Burn of first degree of interscapular region

T21.14 Burn of first degree of lower back

T21.15 Burn of first degree of buttock
Burn of first degree of anus

T21.16 Burn of first degree of male genital region ♂
Burn of first degree of penis
Burn of first degree of scrotum
Burn of first degree of testis

T21.17 Burn of first degree of female genital region ♀
Burn of first degree of labium (majus) (minus)
Burn of first degree of perineum
Burn of first degree of vulva
EXCLUDES 2 burn of vagina (T28.3)

T21.19 Burn of first degree of other site of trunk

T21.2 Burn of second degree of trunk
Use additional external cause code to identify the source, place and intent of the burn (X00-X19, X75-X77, X96-X98, Y92)

T21.20 Burn of second degree of trunk, unspecified site

T21.21 Burn of second degree of chest wall
Burn of second degree of breast

T21.22 Burn of second degree of abdominal wall
Burn of second degree of flank
Burn of second degree of groin

T21.23 Burn of second degree of upper back
Burn of second degree of interscapular region

T21.24 Burn of second degree of lower back

T21.25 Burn of second degree of buttock
Burn of second degree of anus

T21.26 Burn of second degree of male genital region ♂
Burn of second degree of penis
Burn of second degree of scrotum
Burn of second degree of testis

T21.27 Burn of second degree of female genital region ♀
Burn of second degree of labium (majus) (minus)
Burn of second degree of perineum
Burn of second degree of vulva
EXCLUDES 2 burn of vagina (T28.3)

T21.29 Burn of second degree of other site of trunk

T21.3 Burn of third degree of trunk
Use additional external cause code to identify the source, place and intent of the burn (X00-X19, X75-X77, X96-X98, Y92)

7 **T21.30 Burn of third degree of trunk, unspecified site** CC
CC Excl: CC with 7th character A:
T21.30XA,T21.39XA,T21.70XA,T21.79XA

7 **T21.31 Burn of third degree of chest wall** CC
Burn of third degree of breast
CC Excl: CC with 7th character A:
T21.30XA,T21.31XA,T21.39XA,T21.71XA,T21.79XA

7 **T21.32 Burn of third degree of abdominal wall** CC
Burn of third degree of flank
Burn of third degree of groin
CC Excl: CC with 7th character A:
T21.30XA,T21.32XA,T21.39XA,T21.72XA,T21.79XA

7 **T21.33 Burn of third degree of upper back** CC
Burn of third degree of interscapular region
CC Excl: CC with 7th character A: T2130XA,T2133-
T2135 with 7th A, T2139XA, T2170XA,T2173-T2175 with
7th A,T2179XA

7 **T21.34 Burn of third degree of lower back** CC
CC Excl: See code: T21.133

7 **T21.35 Burn of third degree of buttock** CC
Burn of third degree of anus
CC Excl: See code: T21.133

7 **T21.36 Burn of third degree of male genital region** CC ♂
Burn of third degree of penis
Burn of third degree of scrotum
Burn of third degree of testis
CC Excl: CC with 7th character A:
T21.30XA,T21.36XA,T21.37XA,T21.39XA,T21.70XA,T21.7
6XA,T21.77XA,T21.79XA

7 **T21.37 Burn of third degree of female genital region** CC ♀
Burn of third degree of labium (majus) (minus)
Burn of third degree of perineum
Burn of third degree of vulva
EXCLUDES 2 burn of vagina (T28.3)
CC Excl: See code: T21.136

7 **T21.39 Burn of third degree of other site of trunk** CC
CC Excl: CC with 7th character A: T22.30X-T22.312
with 7th A, T22.319A, T22.391-T22.399 with 7th A,
T22.70X-T22.719 with 7th A, T22.791-T22.799 with 7th
A

T21.4 Corrosion of unspecified degree of trunk
Code first (T51-T65) to identify chemical and intent
Use additional external cause code to identify place (Y92)

T21.40 Corrosion of unspecified degree of trunk, unspecified site

T21.41 Corrosion of unspecified degree of chest wall
Corrosion of unspecified degree of breast

T21.42 Corrosion of unspecified degree of abdominal wall
Corrosion of unspecified degree of flank
Corrosion of unspecified degree of groin

T21.43 Corrosion of unspecified degree of upper back
Corrosion of unspecified degree of interscapular region

T21.44 Corrosion of unspecified degree of lower back

T21.45 Corrosion of unspecified degree of buttock
Corrosion of unspecified degree of anus

T21.46 Corrosion of unspecified degree of male genital region ♂
Corrosion of unspecified degree of penis
Corrosion of unspecified degree of scrotum
Corrosion of unspecified degree of testis

T21.47 Corrosion of unspecified degree of female genital region ♀
Corrosion of unspecified degree of labium (majus) (minus)
Corrosion of unspecified degree of perineum
Corrosion of unspecified degree of vulva
EXCLUDES 2 corrosion of vagina (T28.8)

T21.49 Corrosion of unspecified degree of other site of trunk

T21.5 Corrosion of first degree of trunk
Code first (T51-T65) to identify chemical and intent
Use additional external cause code to identify place (Y92)

T21.50 Corrosion of first degree of trunk, unspecified site

T21.51 Corrosion of first degree of chest wall
Corrosion of first degree of breast

T21.52 Corrosion of first degree of abdominal wall
Corrosion of first degree of flank
Corrosion of first degree of groin

T21.53 Corrosion of first degree of upper back
Corrosion of first degree of interscapular region

T21.54 Corrosion of first degree of lower back

T21.55 Corrosion of first degree of buttock
Corrosion of first degree of anus

T21.56 Corrosion of first degree of male genital region ♂
Corrosion of first degree of penis
Corrosion of first degree of scrotum
Corrosion of first degree of testis

T21.57 Corrosion of first degree of female genital region ♀
Corrosion of first degree of labium (majus) (minus)
Corrosion of first degree of perineum
Corrosion of first degree of vulva
EXCLUDES 2 corrosion of vagina (T28.8)

T21.59 Corrosion of first degree of other site of trunk

T21.6 Corrosion of second degree of trunk
Code first (T51-T65) to identify chemical and intent
Use additional external cause code to identify place (Y92)

T21.60 Corrosion of second degree of trunk, unspecified site

---

7 HAC = Initial encounter only (7th character A, B or C) and not POA.

√x7ᵗʰ **T21.61 Corrosion of second degree of** chest wall
Corrosion of second degree of breast

√x7ᵗʰ **T21.62 Corrosion of second degree of** abdominal wall
Corrosion of second degree of flank
Corrosion of second degree of groin

√x7ᵗʰ **T21.63 Corrosion of second degree of** upper back
Corrosion of second degree of interscapular region

√x7ᵗʰ **T21.64 Corrosion of second degree of** lower back

√x7ᵗʰ **T21.65 Corrosion of second degree of** buttock
Corrosion of second degree of anus

√x7ᵗʰ **T21.66 Corrosion of second degree of** male genital region ♂
Corrosion of second degree of penis
Corrosion of second degree of scrotum
Corrosion of second degree of testis

√x7ᵗʰ **T21.67 Corrosion of second degree of** female genital   ♀
region
Corrosion of second degree of labium (majus) (minus)
Corrosion of second degree of perineum
Corrosion of second degree of vulva
EXCLUDES 2   corrosion of vagina (T28.8)

√x7ᵗʰ **T21.69 Corrosion of second degree of** other site **of trunk**

√5ᵗʰ **T21.7 Corrosion of** third degree **of trunk**
Code first (T51-T65) to identify chemical and intent
Use additional external cause code to identify place (Y92)

7 √x7ᵗʰ **T21.70 Corrosion of third degree of trunk,**   CC
unspecified site
CC Excl: CC with 7th character A: See code: T21.30

7 √x7ᵗʰ **T21.71 Corrosion of third degree of** chest wall   CC
Corrosion of third degree of breast
CC Excl: CC with 7th character A: See code: T21.31

7 √x7ᵗʰ **T21.72 Corrosion of third degree of** abdominal wall   CC
Corrosion of third degree of flank
Corrosion of third degree of groin
CC Excl: CC with 7th character A: See code: T21.32

7 √x7ᵗʰ **T21.73 Corrosion of third degree of** upper back   CC
Corrosion of third degree of interscapular region
CC Excl: CC with 7th character A: See code: T21.33

7 √x7ᵗʰ **T21.74 Corrosion of third degree of** lower back   CC
CC Excl: See code: T21.33

7 √x7ᵗʰ **T21.75 Corrosion of third degree of** buttock   CC
Corrosion of third degree of anus
CC Excl: See code: T21.33

7 √x7ᵗʰ **T21.76 Corrosion of third degree of** male genital   CC ♂
region
Corrosion of third degree of penis
Corrosion of third degree of scrotum
Corrosion of third degree of testis
CC Excl: CC with 7th character A: See code: T21.36

7 √x7ᵗʰ **T21.77 Corrosion of third degree of** female genital   CC ♀
region
Corrosion of third degree of labium (majus) (minus)
Corrosion of third degree of perineum
Corrosion of third degree of vulva
EXCLUDES 2   corrosion of vagina (T28.8)
CC Excl: See code: T21.36

7 √x7ᵗʰ **T21.79 Corrosion of third degree of** other site **of trunk**   CC
CC Excl: CC with 7th character A: See code: T21.30

√4ᵗʰ **T22 Burn and corrosion of shoulder and upper limb, except wrist and hand**
EXCLUDES 2   burn and corrosion of interscapular region (T21.-)
burn and corrosion of wrist and hand (T23.-)

The appropriate 7th character is to be added to each code from category T22.
A   initial encounter
D   subsequent encounter
S   sequela

√5ᵗʰ **T22.0 Burn of** unspecified degree **of shoulder and upper limb, except wrist and hand**
Use additional external cause code to identify the source, place and intent of the burn (X00-X19, X75-X77, X96-X98, Y92)

√x7ᵗʰ **T22.00 Burn of unspecified degree of shoulder and upper limb, except wrist and hand, unspecified site**

√6ᵗʰ **T22.01 Burn of unspecified degree of** forearm

√7ᵗʰ **T22.011 Burn of unspecified degree of** right forearm

√7ᵗʰ **T22.012 Burn of unspecified degree of** left **forearm**

√7ᵗʰ **T22.019 Burn of unspecified degree of** unspecified **forearm**

√6ᵗʰ **T22.02 Burn of unspecified degree of** elbow

√7ᵗʰ **T22.021 Burn of unspecified degree of** right **elbow**

√7ᵗʰ **T22.022 Burn of unspecified degree of** left **elbow**

√7ᵗʰ **T22.029 Burn of unspecified degree of** unspecified **elbow**

√6ᵗʰ **T22.03 Burn of unspecified degree of** upper arm

√7ᵗʰ **T22.031 Burn of unspecified degree of** right **upper arm**

√7ᵗʰ **T22.032 Burn of unspecified degree of** left **upper arm**

√7ᵗʰ **T22.039 Burn of unspecified degree of** unspecified **upper arm**

√6ᵗʰ **T22.04 Burn of unspecified degree of** axilla

√7ᵗʰ **T22.041 Burn of unspecified degree of** right **axilla**

√7ᵗʰ **T22.042 Burn of unspecified degree of** left **axilla**

√7ᵗʰ **T22.049 Burn of unspecified degree of** unspecified **axilla**

√6ᵗʰ **T22.05 Burn of unspecified degree of** shoulder

√7ᵗʰ **T22.051 Burn of unspecified degree of** right **shoulder**

√7ᵗʰ **T22.052 Burn of unspecified degree of** left **shoulder**

√7ᵗʰ **T22.059 Burn of unspecified degree of** unspecified **shoulder**

√6ᵗʰ **T22.06 Burn of unspecified degree of** scapular region

√7ᵗʰ **T22.061 Burn of unspecified degree of** right **scapular region**

√7ᵗʰ **T22.062 Burn of unspecified degree of** left **scapular region**

√7ᵗʰ **T22.069 Burn of unspecified degree of** unspecified **scapular region**

√6ᵗʰ **T22.09 Burn of unspecified degree of** multiple sites **of shoulder and upper limb, except wrist and hand**

√7ᵗʰ **T22.091 Burn of unspecified degree of multiple sites of** right **shoulder and upper limb, except wrist and hand**

√7ᵗʰ **T22.092 Burn of unspecified degree of multiple sites of** left **shoulder and upper limb, except wrist and hand**

√7ᵗʰ **T22.099 Burn of unspecified degree of multiple sites of** unspecified **shoulder and upper limb, except wrist and hand**

√5ᵗʰ **T22.1 Burn of** first degree **of shoulder and upper limb, except wrist and hand**
Use additional external cause code to identify the source, place and intent of the burn (X00-X19, X75-X77, X96-X98, Y92)

√x7ᵗʰ **T22.10 Burn of first degree of shoulder and upper limb, except wrist and hand, unspecified site**

√6ᵗʰ **T22.11 Burn of first degree of** forearm

√7ᵗʰ **T22.111 Burn of first degree of** right **forearm**

√7ᵗʰ **T22.112 Burn of first degree of** left **forearm**

√7ᵗʰ **T22.119 Burn of first degree of** unspecified **forearm**

√6ᵗʰ **T22.12 Burn of first degree of** elbow

√7ᵗʰ **T22.121 Burn of first degree of** right **elbow**

√7ᵗʰ **T22.122 Burn of first degree of** left **elbow**

√7ᵗʰ **T22.129 Burn of first degree of** unspecified **elbow**

√6ᵗʰ **T22.13 Burn of first degree of** upper arm

√7ᵗʰ **T22.131 Burn of first degree of** right **upper arm**

√7ᵗʰ **T22.132 Burn of first degree of** left **upper arm**

√7ᵗʰ **T22.139 Burn of first degree of** unspecified **upper arm**

√6ᵗʰ **T22.14 Burn of first degree of** axilla

√7ᵗʰ **T22.141 Burn of first degree of** right **axilla**

√7ᵗʰ **T22.142 Burn of first degree of** left **axilla**

√7ᵗʰ **T22.149 Burn of first degree of** unspecified **axilla**

√6ᵗʰ **T22.15 Burn of first degree of** shoulder

√7ᵗʰ **T22.151 Burn of first degree of** right **shoulder**

√7ᵗʰ **T22.152 Burn of first degree of** left **shoulder**

---

7   HAC = Initial encounter only (7th character A, B or C) and not POA.

☑ Additional Character Required   √x7ᵗʰ Placeholder Alert   Unacceptable PDx   Manifestation   Hospital Acquired Condition   EXCLUDES 1 Not Coded Here   EXCLUDES 2 Not Included Here

ICD-10-CM 2016   1079

Chapter 19. Injury, Poisoning, and Certain Other Consequences of External Causes

T21.61-T22.152

✓7ᵗʰ **T22.159** Burn of first degree of unspecified shoulder

✓6ᵗʰ **T22.16** Burn of first degree of scapular region

　　✓7ᵗʰ **T22.161** Burn of first degree of right scapular region

　　✓7ᵗʰ **T22.162** Burn of first degree of left scapular region

　　✓7ᵗʰ **T22.169** Burn of first degree of unspecified scapular region

✓6ᵗʰ **T22.19** Burn of first degree of multiple sites of shoulder and upper limb, except wrist and hand

　　✓7ᵗʰ **T22.191** Burn of first degree of multiple sites of right shoulder and upper limb, except wrist and hand

　　✓7ᵗʰ **T22.192** Burn of first degree of multiple sites of left shoulder and upper limb, except wrist and hand

　　✓7ᵗʰ **T22.199** Burn of first degree of multiple sites of unspecified shoulder and upper limb, except wrist and hand

✓5ᵗʰ **T22.2** Burn of second degree of shoulder and upper limb, except wrist and hand

Use additional external cause code to identify the source, place and intent of the burn (X00-X19, X75-X77, X96-X98, Y92)

✓x7ᵗʰ **T22.20** Burn of second degree of shoulder and upper limb, except wrist and hand, unspecified site

✓6ᵗʰ **T22.21** Burn of second degree of forearm

　　✓7ᵗʰ **T22.211** Burn of second degree of right forearm

　　✓7ᵗʰ **T22.212** Burn of second degree of left forearm

　　✓7ᵗʰ **T22.219** Burn of second degree of unspecified forearm

✓6ᵗʰ **T22.22** Burn of second degree of elbow

　　✓7ᵗʰ **T22.221** Burn of second degree of right elbow

　　✓7ᵗʰ **T22.222** Burn of second degree of left elbow

　　✓7ᵗʰ **T22.229** Burn of second degree of unspecified elbow

✓6ᵗʰ **T22.23** Burn of second degree of upper arm

　　✓7ᵗʰ **T22.231** Burn of second degree of right upper arm

　　✓7ᵗʰ **T22.232** Burn of second degree of left upper arm

　　✓7ᵗʰ **T22.239** Burn of second degree of unspecified upper arm

✓6ᵗʰ **T22.24** Burn of second degree of axilla

　　✓7ᵗʰ **T22.241** Burn of second degree of right axilla

　　✓7ᵗʰ **T22.242** Burn of second degree of left axilla

　　✓7ᵗʰ **T22.249** Burn of second degree of unspecified axilla

✓6ᵗʰ **T22.25** Burn of second degree of shoulder

　　✓7ᵗʰ **T22.251** Burn of second degree of right shoulder

　　✓7ᵗʰ **T22.252** Burn of second degree of left shoulder

　　✓7ᵗʰ **T22.259** Burn of second degree of unspecified shoulder

✓6ᵗʰ **T22.26** Burn of second degree of scapular region

　　✓7ᵗʰ **T22.261** Burn of second degree of right scapular region

　　✓7ᵗʰ **T22.262** Burn of second degree of left scapular region

　　✓7ᵗʰ **T22.269** Burn of second degree of unspecified scapular region

✓6ᵗʰ **T22.29** Burn of second degree of multiple sites of shoulder and upper limb, except wrist and hand

　　✓7ᵗʰ **T22.291** Burn of second degree of multiple sites of right shoulder and upper limb, except wrist and hand

　　✓7ᵗʰ **T22.292** Burn of second degree of multiple sites of left shoulder and upper limb, except wrist and hand

　　✓7ᵗʰ **T22.299** Burn of second degree of multiple sites of unspecified shoulder and upper limb, except wrist and hand

✓6ᵗʰ **T22.3** Burn of third degree of shoulder and upper limb, except wrist and hand

Use additional external cause code to identify the source, place and intent of the burn (X00-X19, X75-X77, X96-X98, Y92)

7 ✓x7ᵗʰ **T22.30** Burn of third degree of shoulder and upper limb, except wrist and hand, unspecified site CC
CC Excl: CC with 7th character A: T22.30XA,T22.391-T22.399 with 7th A,T22.70XA,T22.791-T22.799 with 7th A

✓6ᵗʰ **T22.31** Burn of third degree of forearm

　7 ✓7ᵗʰ **T22.311** Burn of third degree of right forearm CC
CC Excl: CC with 7th character A: T22.30XA,T22.311-T22.319 with 7th A,T22.391-T22.399 with 7th A,T22.70XA,T22.711-T22.719 with 7th A,T22.791-T22.799 with 7th A

　7 ✓7ᵗʰ **T22.312** Burn of third degree of left forearm CC
CC Excl: See code: T22.311

　7 ✓7ᵗʰ **T22.319** Burn of third degree of unspecified forearm CC
CC Excl: See code: T22.311

✓6ᵗʰ **T22.32** Burn of third degree of elbow

　7 ✓7ᵗʰ **T22.321** Burn of third degree of right elbow CC
CC Excl: CC with 7th character A: T22.30XA,T22.321-T22.329 with 7th A, T22.391-T22.399 with 7th A,T22.70XA,T22.721-T22.729 with 7th A, T22.791-T22.799 with 7th A

　7 ✓7ᵗʰ **T22.322** Burn of third degree of left elbow CC
CC Excl: See code: T22.321

　7 ✓7ᵗʰ **T22.329** Burn of third degree of unspecified elbow CC
CC Excl: See code: T22.321

✓6ᵗʰ **T22.33** Burn of third degree of upper arm

　7 ✓7ᵗʰ **T22.331** Burn of third degree of right upper arm CC
CC Excl: CC with 7th character A: T22.30XA,T22.331-T22.339 with 7th A,T22.391-T22.399 with 7th A,T22.70XA,T22.731-T22.739 with 7th A, T22.791-T22.799 with 7th A

　7 ✓7ᵗʰ **T22.332** Burn of third degree of left upper arm CC
CC Excl: See code: T22.331

　7 ✓7ᵗʰ **T22.339** Burn of third degree of unspecified upper arm CC
CC Excl: See code: T22.331

✓6ᵗʰ **T22.34** Burn of third degree of axilla

　7 ✓7ᵗʰ **T22.341** Burn of third degree of right axilla CC
CC Excl: CC with 7th character A: T22.30XA,T22.341-T22.349 with 7th A,T22.391-T22.399 with 7th A,T22.70XA,T22.741-T22.749 with 7th A, T22.791-T22.799 with 7th A

　7 ✓7ᵗʰ **T22.342** Burn of third degree of left axilla CC
CC Excl: See code: T22.341

　7 ✓7ᵗʰ **T22.349** Burn of third degree of unspecified axilla CC
CC Excl: See code: T22.341

✓6ᵗʰ **T22.35** Burn of third degree of shoulder

　7 ✓7ᵗʰ **T22.351** Burn of third degree of right shoulder CC
CC Excl: CC with 7th character A: T22.30XA,T22.351-T22.359 with 7th A,T22.391-T22.399 with 7th A,T22.70XA,T22.751-T22.759 with 7th A, T22.791-T22.799 with 7th A

　7 ✓7ᵗʰ **T22.352** Burn of third degree of left shoulder CC
CC Excl: See code: T22.351

　7 ✓7ᵗʰ **T22.359** Burn of third degree of unspecified shoulder CC
CC Excl: See code: T22.351

✓6ᵗʰ **T22.36** Burn of third degree of scapular region

　7 ✓7ᵗʰ **T22.361** Burn of third degree of right scapular region CC
CC Excl: CC with 7th character A: T22.30XA,T22.361-T22.369 with 7th A,T22.391-T22.399 with 7th A,T22.70XA,T22.761-T22.769 with 7th A, T22.791-T22.799 with 7th A

7 　HAC = Initial encounter only (7th character A, B or C) and not POA.

7 ✓7th **T22.362** **Burn of third degree of left scapular region** `CC`
     CC Excl: See code: T22.361

7 ✓7th **T22.369** **Burn of third degree of unspecified scapular region** `CC`
     CC Excl: See code: T22.361

✓6th **T22.39** Burn of third degree of multiple sites of shoulder and upper limb, except wrist and hand

7 ✓7th **T22.391** **Burn of third degree of multiple sites of right shoulder and upper limb, except wrist and hand** `CC`
     CC Excl: CC with 7th character A: T22.30XA,T22.391-T22.399 with 7th A,T22.70XA,T22.791-T22.799 with 7th A

7 ✓7th **T22.392** **Burn of third degree of multiple sites of left shoulder and upper limb, except wrist and hand** `CC`
     CC Excl: See code: T22.391

7 ✓7th **T22.399** **Burn of third degree of multiple sites of unspecified shoulder and upper limb, except wrist and hand** `CC`
     CC Excl: See code: T22.391

✓5th **T22.4** Corrosion of unspecified degree of shoulder and upper limb, except wrist and hand
     Code first (T51-T65) to identify chemical and intent
     Use additional external cause code to identify place (Y92)

✓x7th **T22.40** Corrosion of unspecified degree of shoulder and upper limb, except wrist and hand, unspecified site

✓6th **T22.41** Corrosion of unspecified degree of forearm

     ✓7th **T22.411** Corrosion of unspecified degree of right forearm

     ✓7th **T22.412** Corrosion of unspecified degree of left forearm

     ✓7th **T22.419** Corrosion of unspecified degree of unspecified forearm

✓6th **T22.42** Corrosion of unspecified degree of elbow

     ✓7th **T22.421** Corrosion of unspecified degree of right elbow

     ✓7th **T22.422** Corrosion of unspecified degree of left elbow

     ✓7th **T22.429** Corrosion of unspecified degree of unspecified elbow

✓6th **T22.43** Corrosion of unspecified degree of upper arm

     ✓7th **T22.431** Corrosion of unspecified degree of right upper arm

     ✓7th **T22.432** Corrosion of unspecified degree of left upper arm

     ✓7th **T22.439** Corrosion of unspecified degree of unspecified upper arm

✓6th **T22.44** Corrosion of unspecified degree of axilla

     ✓7th **T22.441** Corrosion of unspecified degree of right axilla

     ✓7th **T22.442** Corrosion of unspecified degree of left axilla

     ✓7th **T22.449** Corrosion of unspecified degree of unspecified axilla

✓6th **T22.45** Corrosion of unspecified degree of shoulder

     ✓7th **T22.451** Corrosion of unspecified degree of right shoulder

     ✓7th **T22.452** Corrosion of unspecified degree of left shoulder

     ✓7th **T22.459** Corrosion of unspecified degree of unspecified shoulder

✓6th **T22.46** Corrosion of unspecified degree of scapular region

     ✓7th **T22.461** Corrosion of unspecified degree of right scapular region

     ✓7th **T22.462** Corrosion of unspecified degree of left scapular region

     ✓7th **T22.469** Corrosion of unspecified degree of unspecified scapular region

✓6th **T22.49** Corrosion of unspecified degree of multiple sites of shoulder and upper limb, except wrist and hand

     ✓7th **T22.491** Corrosion of unspecified degree of multiple sites of right shoulder and upper limb, except wrist and hand

✓7th **T22.492** Corrosion of unspecified degree of multiple sites of left shoulder and upper limb, except wrist and hand

✓7th **T22.499** Corrosion of unspecified degree of multiple sites of unspecified shoulder and upper limb, except wrist and hand

✓5th **T22.5** Corrosion of first degree of shoulder and upper limb, except wrist and hand
     Code first (T51-T65) to identify chemical and intent
     Use additional external cause code to identify place (Y92)

✓x7th **T22.50** Corrosion of first degree of shoulder and upper limb, except wrist and hand unspecified site

✓6th **T22.51** Corrosion of first degree of forearm

     ✓7th **T22.511** Corrosion of first degree of right forearm

     ✓7th **T22.512** Corrosion of first degree of left forearm

     ✓7th **T22.519** Corrosion of first degree of unspecified forearm

✓6th **T22.52** Corrosion of first degree of elbow

     ✓7th **T22.521** Corrosion of first degree of right elbow

     ✓7th **T22.522** Corrosion of first degree of left elbow

     ✓7th **T22.529** Corrosion of first degree of unspecified elbow

✓6th **T22.53** Corrosion of first degree of upper arm

     ✓7th **T22.531** Corrosion of first degree of right upper arm

     ✓7th **T22.532** Corrosion of first degree of left upper arm

     ✓7th **T22.539** Corrosion of first degree of unspecified upper arm

✓6th **T22.54** Corrosion of first degree of axilla

     ✓7th **T22.541** Corrosion of first degree of right axilla

     ✓7th **T22.542** Corrosion of first degree of left axilla

     ✓7th **T22.549** Corrosion of first degree of unspecified axilla

✓6th **T22.55** Corrosion of first degree of shoulder

     ✓7th **T22.551** Corrosion of first degree of right shoulder

     ✓7th **T22.552** Corrosion of first degree of left shoulder

     ✓7th **T22.559** Corrosion of first degree of unspecified shoulder

✓6th **T22.56** Corrosion of first degree of scapular region

     ✓7th **T22.561** Corrosion of first degree of right scapular region

     ✓7th **T22.562** Corrosion of first degree of left scapular region

     ✓7th **T22.569** Corrosion of first degree of unspecified scapular region

✓6th **T22.59** Corrosion of first degree of multiple sites of shoulder and upper limb, except wrist and hand

     ✓7th **T22.591** Corrosion of first degree of multiple sites of right shoulder and upper limb, except wrist and hand

     ✓7th **T22.592** Corrosion of first degree of multiple sites of left shoulder and upper limb, except wrist and hand

     ✓7th **T22.599** Corrosion of first degree of multiple sites of unspecified shoulder and upper limb, except wrist and hand

✓5th **T22.6** Corrosion of second degree of shoulder and upper limb, except wrist and hand
     Code first (T51-T65) to identify chemical and intent
     Use additional external cause code to identify place (Y92)

✓x7th **T22.60** Corrosion of second degree of shoulder and upper limb, except wrist and hand, unspecified site

✓6th **T22.61** Corrosion of second degree of forearm

     ✓7th **T22.611** Corrosion of second degree of right forearm

     ✓7th **T22.612** Corrosion of second degree of left forearm

     ✓7th **T22.619** Corrosion of second degree of unspecified forearm

✓6th **T22.62** Corrosion of second degree of elbow

     ✓7th **T22.621** Corrosion of second degree of right elbow

     ✓7th **T22.622** Corrosion of second degree of left elbow

---

7   HAC = Initial encounter only (7th character A, B or C) and not POA.

✓ Additional Character Required   ✓x7th Placeholder Alert   Unacceptable PDx   Manifestation   Hospital Acquired Condition   **EXCLUDES 1** Not Coded Here   **EXCLUDES 2** Not Included Here

√7ᵗʰ **T22.629** Corrosion of second degree of unspecified elbow

√6ᵗʰ **T22.63** Corrosion of second degree of upper arm

  √7ᵗʰ **T22.631** Corrosion of second degree of right upper arm

  √7ᵗʰ **T22.632** Corrosion of second degree of left upper arm

  √7ᵗʰ **T22.639** Corrosion of second degree of unspecified upper arm

√6ᵗʰ **T22.64** Corrosion of second degree of axilla

  √7ᵗʰ **T22.641** Corrosion of second degree of right axilla

  √7ᵗʰ **T22.642** Corrosion of second degree of left axilla

  √7ᵗʰ **T22.649** Corrosion of second degree of unspecified axilla

√6ᵗʰ **T22.65** Corrosion of second degree of shoulder

  √7ᵗʰ **T22.651** Corrosion of second degree of right shoulder

  √7ᵗʰ **T22.652** Corrosion of second degree of left shoulder

  √7ᵗʰ **T22.659** Corrosion of second degree of unspecified shoulder

√6ᵗʰ **T22.66** Corrosion of second degree of scapular region

  √7ᵗʰ **T22.661** Corrosion of second degree of right scapular region

  √7ᵗʰ **T22.662** Corrosion of second degree of left scapular region

  √7ᵗʰ **T22.669** Corrosion of second degree of unspecified scapular region

√6ᵗʰ **T22.69** Corrosion of second degree of multiple sites of shoulder and upper limb, except wrist and hand

  √7ᵗʰ **T22.691** Corrosion of second degree of multiple sites of right shoulder and upper limb, except wrist and hand

  √7ᵗʰ **T22.692** Corrosion of second degree of multiple sites of left shoulder and upper limb, except wrist and hand

  √7ᵗʰ **T22.699** Corrosion of second degree of multiple sites of unspecified shoulder and upper limb, except wrist and hand

√5ᵗʰ **T22.7** Corrosion of third degree of shoulder and upper limb, except wrist and hand

    Code first (T51-T65) to identify chemical and intent
    Use additional external cause code to identify place (Y92)

7 √x7ᵗʰ **T22.70** **Corrosion of third degree of shoulder and upper limb, except wrist and hand, unspecified site**   CC
    CC Excl: CC with 7th character A: See code: T22.30

√6ᵗʰ **T22.71** Corrosion of third degree of forearm

7 √7ᵗʰ **T22.711** **Corrosion of third degree of right forearm**   CC
    CC Excl: CC with 7th character A: See code: T22.311

7 √7ᵗʰ **T22.712** **Corrosion of third degree of left forearm**   CC
    CC Excl: See code: T22.311

7 √7ᵗʰ **T22.719** **Corrosion of third degree of unspecified forearm**   CC
    CC Excl: See code: T22.311

√6ᵗʰ **T22.72** Corrosion of third degree of elbow

7 √7ᵗʰ **T22.721** **Corrosion of third degree of right elbow**   CC
    CC Excl: CC with 7th character A: See code: T22.321

7 √7ᵗʰ **T22.722** **Corrosion of third degree of left elbow**   CC
    CC Excl: See code: T22.321

7 √7ᵗʰ **T22.729** **Corrosion of third degree of unspecified elbow**   CC
    CC Excl: See code: T22.321

√6ᵗʰ **T22.73** Corrosion of third degree of upper arm

7 √7ᵗʰ **T22.731** **Corrosion of third degree of right upper arm**   CC
    CC Excl: CC with 7th character A: See code: T22.331

7 √7ᵗʰ **T22.732** **Corrosion of third degree of left upper arm**   CC
    CC Excl: See code: T22.331

7 √7ᵗʰ **T22.739** **Corrosion of third degree of unspecified upper arm**   CC
    CC Excl: See code: T22.331

√6ᵗʰ **T22.74** Corrosion of third degree of axilla

7 √7ᵗʰ **T22.741** **Corrosion of third degree of right axilla**   CC
    CC Excl: CC with 7th character A: See code: T22.341

7 √7ᵗʰ **T22.742** **Corrosion of third degree of left axilla**   CC
    CC Excl: See code: T22.341

7 √7ᵗʰ **T22.749** **Corrosion of third degree of unspecified axilla**   CC
    CC Excl: See code: T22.341

√6ᵗʰ **T22.75** Corrosion of third degree of shoulder

7 √7ᵗʰ **T22.751** **Corrosion of third degree of right shoulder**   CC
    CC Excl: CC with 7th character A: See code: T22.351

7 √7ᵗʰ **T22.752** **Corrosion of third degree of left shoulder**   CC
    CC Excl: See code: T22.351

7 √7ᵗʰ **T22.759** **Corrosion of third degree of unspecified shoulder**   CC
    CC Excl: See code: T22.351

√6ᵗʰ **T22.76** Corrosion of third degree of scapular region

7 √7ᵗʰ **T22.761** **Corrosion of third degree of right scapular region**   CC
    CC Excl: CC with 7th character A: See code: T22.361

7 √7ᵗʰ **T22.762** **Corrosion of third degree of left scapular region**   CC
    CC Excl: See code: T22.361

7 √7ᵗʰ **T22.769** **Corrosion of third degree of unspecified scapular region**   CC
    CC Excl: See code: T22.361

√6ᵗʰ **T22.79** Corrosion of third degree of multiple sites of shoulder and upper limb, except wrist and hand

7 √7ᵗʰ **T22.791** **Corrosion of third degree of multiple sites of right shoulder and upper limb, except wrist and hand**   CC
    CC Excl: CC with 7th character A: See code: T22.391

7 √7ᵗʰ **T22.792** **Corrosion of third degree of multiple sites of left shoulder and upper limb, except wrist and hand**   CC
    CC Excl: See code: T22.391

7 √7ᵗʰ **T22.799** **Corrosion of third degree of multiple sites of unspecified shoulder and upper limb, except wrist and hand**   CC
    CC Excl: See code: T22.391

√4ᵗʰ **T23** **Burn and corrosion of wrist and hand**
    AHA: 2015, 1Q, 19

> The appropriate 7th character is to be added to each code from category T23.
> A   initial encounter
> D   subsequent encounter
> S   sequela

√5ᵗʰ **T23.0** Burn of unspecified degree of wrist and hand
    Use additional external cause code to identify the source, place and intent of the burn (X00-X19, X75-X77, X96-X98, Y92)

√6ᵗʰ **T23.00** Burn of unspecified degree of hand, unspecified site

  √7ᵗʰ **T23.001** Burn of unspecified degree of right hand, unspecified site

  √7ᵗʰ **T23.002** Burn of unspecified degree of left hand, unspecified site

  √7ᵗʰ **T23.009** Burn of unspecified degree of unspecified hand, unspecified site

√6ᵗʰ **T23.01** Burn of unspecified degree of thumb (nail)

  √7ᵗʰ **T23.011** Burn of unspecified degree of right thumb (nail)

  √7ᵗʰ **T23.012** Burn of unspecified degree of left thumb (nail)

  √7ᵗʰ **T23.019** Burn of unspecified degree of unspecified thumb (nail)

---

7   HAC = Initial encounter only (7th character A, B or C) and not POA.

Ⓝ Newborn: 0   Ⓟ Pediatric: 0-17   Ⓜ Maternity: 12-55   Ⓐ Adult: 15-124   **MCC** Major CC Condition   **PDxMCC** PDx acts as own MCC   CC CC Condition   **PDxCC** PDx acts as own CC

1082
ICD-10-CM 2016

√6ᵗʰ **T23.02** Burn of unspecified degree of single finger (nail) except thumb

     √7ᵗʰ **T23.021** Burn of unspecified degree of single right finger (nail) except thumb

     √7ᵗʰ **T23.022** Burn of unspecified degree of single left finger (nail) except thumb

     √7ᵗʰ **T23.029** Burn of unspecified degree of unspecified single finger (nail) except thumb

√6ᵗʰ **T23.03** Burn of unspecified degree of multiple fingers (nail), not including thumb

     √7ᵗʰ **T23.031** Burn of unspecified degree of multiple right fingers (nail), not including thumb

     √7ᵗʰ **T23.032** Burn of unspecified degree of multiple left fingers (nail), not including thumb

     √7ᵗʰ **T23.039** Burn of unspecified degree of unspecified multiple fingers (nail), not including thumb

√6ᵗʰ **T23.04** Burn of unspecified degree of multiple fingers (nail), including thumb

     √7ᵗʰ **T23.041** Burn of unspecified degree of multiple right fingers (nail), including thumb

     √7ᵗʰ **T23.042** Burn of unspecified degree of multiple left fingers (nail), including thumb

     √7ᵗʰ **T23.049** Burn of unspecified degree of unspecified multiple fingers (nail), including thumb

√6ᵗʰ **T23.05** Burn of unspecified degree of palm

     √7ᵗʰ **T23.051** Burn of unspecified degree of right palm

     √7ᵗʰ **T23.052** Burn of unspecified degree of left palm

     √7ᵗʰ **T23.059** Burn of unspecified degree of unspecified palm

√6ᵗʰ **T23.06** Burn of unspecified degree of back of hand

     √7ᵗʰ **T23.061** Burn of unspecified degree of back of right hand

     √7ᵗʰ **T23.062** Burn of unspecified degree of back of left hand

     √7ᵗʰ **T23.069** Burn of unspecified degree of back of unspecified hand

√6ᵗʰ **T23.07** Burn of unspecified degree of wrist

     √7ᵗʰ **T23.071** Burn of unspecified degree of right wrist

     √7ᵗʰ **T23.072** Burn of unspecified degree of left wrist

     √7ᵗʰ **T23.079** Burn of unspecified degree of unspecified wrist

√6ᵗʰ **T23.09** Burn of unspecified degree of multiple sites of wrist and hand

     √7ᵗʰ **T23.091** Burn of unspecified degree of multiple sites of right wrist and hand

     √7ᵗʰ **T23.092** Burn of unspecified degree of multiple sites of left wrist and hand

     √7ᵗʰ **T23.099** Burn of unspecified degree of multiple sites of unspecified wrist and hand

√5ᵗʰ **T23.1** Burn of first degree of wrist and hand

Use additional external cause code to identify the source, place and intent of the burn (X00-X19, X75-X77, X96-X98, Y92)

√6ᵗʰ **T23.10** Burn of first degree of hand, unspecified site

     √7ᵗʰ **T23.101** Burn of first degree of right hand, unspecified site

     √7ᵗʰ **T23.102** Burn of first degree of left hand, unspecified site

     √7ᵗʰ **T23.109** Burn of first degree of unspecified hand, unspecified site

√6ᵗʰ **T23.11** Burn of first degree of thumb (nail)

     √7ᵗʰ **T23.111** Burn of first degree of right thumb (nail)

     √7ᵗʰ **T23.112** Burn of first degree of left thumb (nail)

     √7ᵗʰ **T23.119** Burn of first degree of unspecified thumb (nail)

√6ᵗʰ **T23.12** Burn of first degree of single finger (nail) except thumb

     √7ᵗʰ **T23.121** Burn of first degree of single right finger (nail) except thumb

     √7ᵗʰ **T23.122** Burn of first degree of single left finger (nail) except thumb

     √7ᵗʰ **T23.129** Burn of first degree of unspecified single finger (nail) except thumb

√6ᵗʰ **T23.13** Burn of first degree of multiple fingers (nail), not including thumb

     √7ᵗʰ **T23.131** Burn of first degree of multiple right fingers (nail), not including thumb

     √7ᵗʰ **T23.132** Burn of first degree of multiple left fingers (nail), not including thumb

     √7ᵗʰ **T23.139** Burn of first degree of unspecified multiple fingers (nail), not including thumb

√6ᵗʰ **T23.14** Burn of first degree of multiple fingers (nail), including thumb

     √7ᵗʰ **T23.141** Burn of first degree of multiple right fingers (nail), including thumb

     √7ᵗʰ **T23.142** Burn of first degree of multiple left fingers (nail), including thumb

     √7ᵗʰ **T23.149** Burn of first degree of unspecified multiple fingers (nail), including thumb

√6ᵗʰ **T23.15** Burn of first degree of palm

     √7ᵗʰ **T23.151** Burn of first degree of right palm

     √7ᵗʰ **T23.152** Burn of first degree of left palm

     √7ᵗʰ **T23.159** Burn of first degree of unspecified palm

√6ᵗʰ **T23.16** Burn of first degree of back of hand

     √7ᵗʰ **T23.161** Burn of first degree of back of right hand

     √7ᵗʰ **T23.162** Burn of first degree of back of left hand

     √7ᵗʰ **T23.169** Burn of first degree of back of unspecified hand

√6ᵗʰ **T23.17** Burn of first degree of wrist

     √7ᵗʰ **T23.171** Burn of first degree of right wrist

     √7ᵗʰ **T23.172** Burn of first degree of left wrist

     √7ᵗʰ **T23.179** Burn of first degree of unspecified wrist

√6ᵗʰ **T23.19** Burn of first degree of multiple sites of wrist and hand

     √7ᵗʰ **T23.191** Burn of first degree of muiltiple sites of right wrist and hand

     √7ᵗʰ **T23.192** Burn of first degree of multiple sites of left wrist and hand

     √7ᵗʰ **T23.199** Burn of first degree of multiple sites of unspecified wrist and hand

√5ᵗʰ **T23.2** Burn of second degree of wrist and hand

Use additional external cause code to identify the source, place and intent of the burn (X00-X19, X75-X77, X96-X98, Y92)

√6ᵗʰ **T23.20** Burn of second degree of hand, unspecified site

     √7ᵗʰ **T23.201** Burn of second degree of right hand, unspecified site

     √7ᵗʰ **T23.202** Burn of second degree of left hand, unspecified site

     √7ᵗʰ **T23.209** Burn of second degree of unspecified hand, unspecified site

√6ᵗʰ **T23.21** Burn of second degree of thumb (nail)

     √7ᵗʰ **T23.211** Burn of second degree of right thumb (nail)

     √7ᵗʰ **T23.212** Burn of second degree of left thumb (nail)

     √7ᵗʰ **T23.219** Burn of second degree of unspecified thumb (nail)

√6ᵗʰ **T23.22** Burn of second degree of single finger (nail) except thumb

     √7ᵗʰ **T23.221** Burn of second degree of single right finger (nail) except thumb

     √7ᵗʰ **T23.222** Burn of second degree of single left finger (nail) except thumb

     √7ᵗʰ **T23.229** Burn of second degree of unspecified single finger (nail) except thumb

√6ᵗʰ **T23.23** Burn of second degree of multiple fingers (nail), not including thumb

     √7ᵗʰ **T23.231** Burn of second degree of multiple right fingers (nail), not including thumb

     √7ᵗʰ **T23.232** Burn of second degree of multiple left fingers (nail), not including thumb

     √7ᵗʰ **T23.239** Burn of second degree of unspecified multiple fingers (nail), not including thumb

☑ Additional Character Required   ☑x7ᵗʰ Placeholder Alert   Unacceptable PDx   Manifestation   Hospital Acquired Condition   **EXCLUDES 1** Not Coded Here   **EXCLUDES 2** Not Included Here

ICD-10-CM 2016   1083

Chapter 19. Injury, Poisoning, and Certain Other Consequences of External Causes

T23.24–T23.392

✓6ᵗʰ **T23.24** **Burn of second degree of multiple fingers (nail), including thumb**

    ✓7ᵗʰ **T23.241** Burn of second degree of multiple right fingers (nail), including thumb

    ✓7ᵗʰ **T23.242** Burn of second degree of multiple left fingers (nail), including thumb

    ✓7ᵗʰ **T23.249** Burn of second degree of unspecified multiple fingers (nail), including thumb

✓6ᵗʰ **T23.25** **Burn of second degree of palm**

    ✓7ᵗʰ **T23.251** Burn of second degree of right palm

    ✓7ᵗʰ **T23.252** Burn of second degree of left palm

    ✓7ᵗʰ **T23.259** Burn of second degree of unspecified palm

✓6ᵗʰ **T23.26** **Burn of second degree of back of hand**

    ✓7ᵗʰ **T23.261** Burn of second degree of back of right hand

    ✓7ᵗʰ **T23.262** Burn of second degree of back of left hand

    ✓7ᵗʰ **T23.269** Burn of second degree of back of unspecified hand

✓6ᵗʰ **T23.27** **Burn of second degree of wrist**

    ✓7ᵗʰ **T23.271** Burn of second degree of right wrist

    ✓7ᵗʰ **T23.272** Burn of second degree of left wrist

    ✓7ᵗʰ **T23.279** Burn of second degree of unspecified wrist

✓6ᵗʰ **T23.29** **Burn of second degree of multiple sites of wrist and hand**

    ✓7ᵗʰ **T23.291** Burn of second degree of multiple sites of right wrist and hand

    ✓7ᵗʰ **T23.292** Burn of second degree of multiple sites of left wrist and hand

    ✓7ᵗʰ **T23.299** Burn of second degree of multiple sites of unspecified wrist and hand

✓5ᵗʰ **T23.3** **Burn of third degree of wrist and hand**

    Use additional external cause code to identify the source, place and intent of the burn (X00-X19, X75-X77, X96-X98, Y92)

✓6ᵗʰ **T23.30** **Burn of third degree of hand, unspecified site**

    7 ✓7ᵗʰ **T23.301** **Burn of third degree of right hand, unspecified site** CC
      CC Excl: CC with 7th character A: T23.30X-T23.319 with 7th A, T23.391-T23.399 with 7th A, T23.701-T23.719 with 7th A, T23.791-T23.799 with 7th A

    7 ✓7ᵗʰ **T23.302** **Burn of third degree of left hand, unspecified site** CC
      CC Excl: See code: T23.301

    7 ✓7ᵗʰ **T23.309** **Burn of third degree of unspecified hand, unspecified site** CC
      CC Excl: See code: T23.301

✓6ᵗʰ **T23.31** **Burn of third degree of thumb (nail)**

    7 ✓7ᵗʰ **T23.311** **Burn of third degree of right thumb (nail)** CC
      CC Excl: CC with 7th character A: T23.301-T23.319 with 7th A, T23.391-T23.399 with 7th A, T23.701-T23.719 with 7th A, T23.791-T23.799 with 7th A

    7 ✓7ᵗʰ **T23.312** **Burn of third degree of left thumb (nail)** CC
      CC Excl: See code: T23.311

    7 ✓7ᵗʰ **T23.319** **Burn of third degree of unspecified thumb (nail)** CC
      CC Excl: See code: T23.311

✓6ᵗʰ **T23.32** **Burn of third degree of single finger (nail) except thumb**

    7 ✓7ᵗʰ **T23.321** **Burn of third degree of single right finger (nail) except thumb** CC
      CC Excl: CC with 7th character A: T23.301-T23.309 with 7th A, T23.321-T23.329 with 7th, A T23.391-T23.399 with 7th A, T23.701-T23.709 with 7th A, T23.721-T23.729 with 7th A, T23.791-T23.799 with 7th A

    7 ✓7ᵗʰ **T23.322** **Burn of third degree of single left finger (nail) except thumb** CC
      CC Excl: See code: T23.321

    7 ✓7ᵗʰ **T23.329** **Burn of third degree of unspecified single finger (nail) except thumb** CC
      CC Excl: See code: T23.321

✓6ᵗʰ **T23.33** **Burn of third degree of multiple fingers (nail), not including thumb**

    7 ✓7ᵗʰ **T23.331** **Burn of third degree of multiple right fingers (nail), not including thumb** CC
      CC Excl: CC with 7th character A: T23.301-T23.309 with 7th A, T23.331-T23.339 with 7th A, T23.391-T23.399 with 7th A, T23.701-T23.709 with 7th A, T23.731-T23.739 with 7th A, T23.791-T23.799 with 7th A

    7 ✓7ᵗʰ **T23.332** **Burn of third degree of multiple left fingers (nail), not including thumb** CC
      CC Excl: See code: T23.331

    7 ✓7ᵗʰ **T23.339** **Burn of third degree of unspecified multiple fingers (nail), not including thumb** CC
      CC Excl: See code: T23.331

✓6ᵗʰ **T23.34** **Burn of third degree of multiple fingers (nail), including thumb**

    7 ✓7ᵗʰ **T23.341** **Burn of third degree of multiple right fingers (nail), including thumb** CC
      CC Excl: CC with 7th character A: T23.301-T23.309 with 7th A, T23.341-T23.349 with 7th A, T23.391-T23.399 with 7th A, T23.701-T23.709 with 7th A, T23.741-T23.749 with 7th A, T23.791-T23.799 with 7th A

    7 ✓7ᵗʰ **T23.342** **Burn of third degree of multiple left fingers (nail), including thumb** CC
      CC Excl: See code: T23.341

    7 ✓7ᵗʰ **T23.349** **Burn of third degree of unspecified multiple fingers (nail), including thumb** CC
      CC Excl: See code: T23.341

✓6ᵗʰ **T23.35** **Burn of third degree of palm**

    7 ✓7ᵗʰ **T23.351** **Burn of third degree of right palm** CC
      CC Excl: CC with 7th character A: T23.301-T23.309 with 7th A, T23.351-T23.359 with 7th A, T23.391-T23.399 with 7th A, T23.701-T23.709 with 7th A, T23.751-T23.759 with 7th A, T23.791-T23.799 with 7th A

    7 ✓7ᵗʰ **T23.352** **Burn of third degree of left palm** CC
      CC Excl: See code: T23.351

    7 ✓7ᵗʰ **T23.359** **Burn of third degree of unspecified palm** CC
      CC Excl: See code: T23.351

✓6ᵗʰ **T23.36** **Burn of third degree of back of hand**

    7 ✓7ᵗʰ **T23.361** **Burn of third degree of back of right hand** CC
      CC Excl: CC with 7th character A: T23.301-T23.309 with 7th A, T23.361-T23.369 with 7th A, T23.391-T23.399 with 7th A, T23.701-T23.709 with 7th A, T23.761-T23.769 with 7th A, T23.791-T23.799 with 7th A

    7 ✓7ᵗʰ **T23.362** **Burn of third degree of back of left hand** CC
      CC Excl: See code: T23.361

    7 ✓7ᵗʰ **T23.369** **Burn of third degree of back of unspecified hand** CC
      CC Excl: See code: T23.361

✓6ᵗʰ **T23.37** **Burn of third degree of wrist**

    7 ✓7ᵗʰ **T23.371** **Burn of third degree of right wrist** CC
      CC Excl: CC with 7th character A: T23.301-T23.309 with 7th A, T23.371-T23.379 with 7th A, T23.391-T23.399 with 7th A, T23.701-T23.709 with 7th A, T23.771-T23.779 with 7th A, T23.791-T23.799 with 7th A

    7 ✓7ᵗʰ **T23.372** **Burn of third degree of left wrist** CC
      CC Excl: See code: T23.371

    7 ✓7ᵗʰ **T23.379** **Burn of third degree of unspecified wrist** CC
      CC Excl: See code: T23.371

✓6ᵗʰ **T23.39** **Burn of third degree of multiple sites of wrist and hand**

    7 ✓7ᵗʰ **T23.391** **Burn of third degree of multiple sites of right wrist and hand** CC
      CC Excl: See code: T23.301

    7 ✓7ᵗʰ **T23.392** **Burn of third degree of multiple sites of left wrist and hand** CC
      CC Excl: See code: T23.301

---

7   HAC = Initial encounter only (7th character A, B or C) and not POA.

N Newborn: 0   P Pediatric: 0-17   M Maternity: 12-55   A Adult: 15-124   MCC Major CC Condition   PDxMCC PDx acts as own MCC   CC CC Condition   PDxCC PDx acts as own CC

1084   ICD-10-CM 2016

7 ✓7ᵗʰ **T23.399** **Burn of third degree of multiple sites of unspecified wrist and hand**   CC
    CC Excl: See code: T23.301

✓5ᵗʰ **T23.4** **Corrosion of unspecified degree of wrist and hand**
    Code first (T51-T65) to identify chemical and intent
    Use additional external cause code to identify place (Y92)

✓6ᵗʰ **T23.40** **Corrosion of unspecified degree of hand, unspecified site**
    ✓7ᵗʰ **T23.401** **Corrosion of unspecified degree of right hand, unspecified site**
    ✓7ᵗʰ **T23.402** **Corrosion of unspecified degree of left hand, unspecified site**
    ✓7ᵗʰ **T23.409** **Corrosion of unspecified degree of unspecified hand, unspecified site**

✓6ᵗʰ **T23.41** **Corrosion of unspecified degree of thumb (nail)**
    ✓7ᵗʰ **T23.411** **Corrosion of unspecified degree of right thumb (nail)**
    ✓7ᵗʰ **T23.412** **Corrosion of unspecified degree of left thumb (nail)**
    ✓7ᵗʰ **T23.419** **Corrosion of unspecified degree of unspecified thumb (nail)**

✓6ᵗʰ **T23.42** **Corrosion of unspecified degree of single finger (nail) except thumb**
    ✓7ᵗʰ **T23.421** **Corrosion of unspecified degree of single right finger (nail) except thumb**
    ✓7ᵗʰ **T23.422** **Corrosion of unspecified degree of single left finger (nail) except thumb**
    ✓7ᵗʰ **T23.429** **Corrosion of unspecified degree of unspecified single finger (nail) except thumb**

✓6ᵗʰ **T23.43** **Corrosion of unspecified degree of multiple fingers (nail), not including thumb**
    ✓7ᵗʰ **T23.431** **Corrosion of unspecified degree of multiple right fingers (nail), not including thumb**
    ✓7ᵗʰ **T23.432** **Corrosion of unspecified degree of multiple left fingers (nail), not including thumb**
    ✓7ᵗʰ **T23.439** **Corrosion of unspecified degree of unspecified multiple fingers (nail), not including thumb**

✓6ᵗʰ **T23.44** **Corrosion of unspecified degree of multiple fingers (nail), including thumb**
    ✓7ᵗʰ **T23.441** **Corrosion of unspecified degree of multiple right fingers (nail), including thumb**
    ✓7ᵗʰ **T23.442** **Corrosion of unspecified degree of multiple left fingers (nail), including thumb**
    ✓7ᵗʰ **T23.449** **Corrosion of unspecified degree of unspecified multiple fingers (nail), including thumb**

✓6ᵗʰ **T23.45** **Corrosion of unspecified degree of palm**
    ✓7ᵗʰ **T23.451** **Corrosion of unspecified degree of right palm**
    ✓7ᵗʰ **T23.452** **Corrosion of unspecified degree of left palm**
    ✓7ᵗʰ **T23.459** **Corrosion of unspecified degree of unspecified palm**

✓6ᵗʰ **T23.46** **Corrosion of unspecified degree of back of hand**
    ✓7ᵗʰ **T23.461** **Corrosion of unspecified degree of back of right hand**
    ✓7ᵗʰ **T23.462** **Corrosion of unspecified degree of back of left hand**
    ✓7ᵗʰ **T23.469** **Corrosion of unspecified degree of back of unspecified hand**

✓6ᵗʰ **T23.47** **Corrosion of unspecified degree of wrist**
    ✓7ᵗʰ **T23.471** **Corrosion of unspecified degree of right wrist**
    ✓7ᵗʰ **T23.472** **Corrosion of unspecified degree of left wrist**
    ✓7ᵗʰ **T23.479** **Corrosion of unspecified degree of unspecified wrist**

✓6ᵗʰ **T23.49** **Corrosion of unspecified degree of multiple sites of wrist and hand**
    ✓7ᵗʰ **T23.491** **Corrosion of unspecified degree of multiple sites of right wrist and hand**
    ✓7ᵗʰ **T23.492** **Corrosion of unspecified degree of multiple sites of left wrist and hand**
    ✓7ᵗʰ **T23.499** **Corrosion of unspecified degree of multiple sites of unspecified wrist and hand**

✓5ᵗʰ **T23.5** **Corrosion of first degree of wrist and hand**
    Code first (T51-T65) to identify chemical and intent
    Use additional external cause code to identify place (Y92)

✓6ᵗʰ **T23.50** **Corrosion of first degree of hand, unspecified site**
    ✓7ᵗʰ **T23.501** **Corrosion of first degree of right hand, unspecified site**
    ✓7ᵗʰ **T23.502** **Corrosion of first degree of left hand, unspecified site**
    ✓7ᵗʰ **T23.509** **Corrosion of first degree of unspecified hand, unspecified site**

✓6ᵗʰ **T23.51** **Corrosion of first degree of thumb (nail)**
    ✓7ᵗʰ **T23.511** **Corrosion of first degree of right thumb (nail)**
    ✓7ᵗʰ **T23.512** **Corrosion of first degree of left thumb (nail)**
    ✓7ᵗʰ **T23.519** **Corrosion of first degree of unspecified thumb (nail)**

✓6ᵗʰ **T23.52** **Corrosion of first degree of single finger (nail) except thumb**
    ✓7ᵗʰ **T23.521** **Corrosion of first degree of single right finger (nail) except thumb**
    ✓7ᵗʰ **T23.522** **Corrosion of first degree of single left finger (nail) except thumb**
    ✓7ᵗʰ **T23.529** **Corrosion of first degree of unspecified single finger (nail) except thumb**

✓6ᵗʰ **T23.53** **Corrosion of first degree of multiple fingers (nail), not including thumb**
    ✓7ᵗʰ **T23.531** **Corrosion of first degree of multiple right fingers (nail), not including thumb**
    ✓7ᵗʰ **T23.532** **Corrosion of first degree of multiple left fingers (nail), not including thumb**
    ✓7ᵗʰ **T23.539** **Corrosion of first degree of unspecified multiple fingers (nail), not including thumb**

✓6ᵗʰ **T23.54** **Corrosion of first degree of multiple fingers (nail), including thumb**
    ✓7ᵗʰ **T23.541** **Corrosion of first degree of multiple right fingers (nail), including thumb**
    ✓7ᵗʰ **T23.542** **Corrosion of first degree of multiple left fingers (nail), including thumb**
    ✓7ᵗʰ **T23.549** **Corrosion of first degree of unspecified multiple fingers (nail), including thumb**

✓6ᵗʰ **T23.55** **Corrosion of first degree of palm**
    ✓7ᵗʰ **T23.551** **Corrosion of first degree of right palm**
    ✓7ᵗʰ **T23.552** **Corrosion of first degree of left palm**
    ✓7ᵗʰ **T23.559** **Corrosion of first degree of unspecified palm**

✓6ᵗʰ **T23.56** **Corrosion of first degree of back of hand**
    ✓7ᵗʰ **T23.561** **Corrosion of first degree of back of right hand**
    ✓7ᵗʰ **T23.562** **Corrosion of first degree of back of left hand**
    ✓7ᵗʰ **T23.569** **Corrosion of first degree of back of unspecified hand**

✓6ᵗʰ **T23.57** **Corrosion of first degree of wrist**
    ✓7ᵗʰ **T23.571** **Corrosion of first degree of right wrist**
    ✓7ᵗʰ **T23.572** **Corrosion of first degree of left wrist**
    ✓7ᵗʰ **T23.579** **Corrosion of first degree of unspecified wrist**

✓6ᵗʰ **T23.59** **Corrosion of first degree of multiple sites of wrist and hand**
    ✓7ᵗʰ **T23.591** **Corrosion of first degree of multiple sites of right wrist and hand**

---

7   HAC = Initial encounter only (7th character A, B or C) and not POA.

✔ Additional Character Required   ✔7ᵗʰ Placeholder Alert   Unacceptable PDx   Manifestation   Hospital Acquired Condition   **EXCLUDES 1** Not Coded Here   **EXCLUDES 2** Not Included Here

ICD-10-CM 2016   1085

✓7ᵗʰ **T23.592** Corrosion of first degree of multiple sites of **left** wrist and hand

✓7ᵗʰ **T23.599** Corrosion of first degree of multiple sites of **unspecified** wrist and hand

✓5ᵗʰ **T23.6** Corrosion of **second degree** of wrist and hand

Code first (T51-T65) to identify chemical and intent
Use additional external cause code to identify place (Y92)

✓6ᵗʰ **T23.60** Corrosion of second degree of hand, **unspecified site**

✓7ᵗʰ **T23.601** Corrosion of second degree of **right** hand, unspecified site

✓7ᵗʰ **T23.602** Corrosion of second degree of **left** hand, unspecified site

✓7ᵗʰ **T23.609** Corrosion of second degree of **unspecified** hand, unspecified site

✓6ᵗʰ **T23.61** Corrosion of second degree of **thumb (nail)**

✓7ᵗʰ **T23.611** Corrosion of second degree of **right** thumb (nail)

✓7ᵗʰ **T23.612** Corrosion of second degree of **left** thumb (nail)

✓7ᵗʰ **T23.619** Corrosion of second degree of **unspecified** thumb (nail)

✓6ᵗʰ **T23.62** Corrosion of second degree of **single finger** (nail) except thumb

✓7ᵗʰ **T23.621** Corrosion of second degree of single **right** finger (nail) except thumb

✓7ᵗʰ **T23.622** Corrosion of second degree of single **left** finger (nail) except thumb

✓7ᵗʰ **T23.629** Corrosion of second degree of **unspecified** single finger (nail) except thumb

✓6ᵗʰ **T23.63** Corrosion of second degree of **multiple fingers** (nail), not including thumb

✓7ᵗʰ **T23.631** Corrosion of second degree of multiple **right** fingers (nail), not including thumb

✓7ᵗʰ **T23.632** Corrosion of second degree of multiple **left** fingers (nail), not including thumb

✓7ᵗʰ **T23.639** Corrosion of second degree of **unspecified** multiple fingers (nail), not including thumb

✓6ᵗʰ **T23.64** Corrosion of second degree of **multiple fingers** (nail), including thumb

✓7ᵗʰ **T23.641** Corrosion of second degree of multiple **right** fingers (nail), including thumb

✓7ᵗʰ **T23.642** Corrosion of second degree of multiple **left** fingers (nail), including thumb

✓7ᵗʰ **T23.649** Corrosion of second degree of **unspecified** multiple fingers (nail), including thumb

✓6ᵗʰ **T23.65** Corrosion of second degree of **palm**

✓7ᵗʰ **T23.651** Corrosion of second degree of **right** palm

✓7ᵗʰ **T23.652** Corrosion of second degree of **left** palm

✓7ᵗʰ **T23.659** Corrosion of second degree of **unspecified** palm

✓6ᵗʰ **T23.66** Corrosion of second degree of **back of hand**

✓7ᵗʰ **T23.661** Corrosion of second degree back of **right** hand

✓7ᵗʰ **T23.662** Corrosion of second degree back of **left** hand

✓7ᵗʰ **T23.669** Corrosion of second degree back of **unspecified** hand

✓6ᵗʰ **T23.67** Corrosion of second degree of **wrist**

✓7ᵗʰ **T23.671** Corrosion of second degree of **right** wrist

✓7ᵗʰ **T23.672** Corrosion of second degree of **left** wrist

✓7ᵗʰ **T23.679** Corrosion of second degree of **unspecified** wrist

✓6ᵗʰ **T23.69** Corrosion of second degree of **multiple sites** of wrist and hand

✓7ᵗʰ **T23.691** Corrosion of second degree of multiple sites of **right** wrist and hand

✓7ᵗʰ **T23.692** Corrosion of second degree of multiple sites of **left** wrist and hand

✓7ᵗʰ **T23.699** Corrosion of second degree of multiple sites of **unspecified** wrist and hand

✓5ᵗʰ **T23.7** Corrosion of **third degree** of wrist and hand

Code first (T51-T65) to identify chemical and intent
Use additional external cause code to identify place (Y92)

✓6ᵗʰ **T23.70** Corrosion of third degree of hand, **unspecified site**

7 ✓7ᵗʰ **T23.701** Corrosion of third degree of **right** hand, unspecified site   CC
CC Excl: CC with 7th character A: T23.301-T23.319 with 7th A, T23.391-T23.399 with 7th A, T23.701-T23.719 with 7th A, T23.791-T23.799 with 7th A

7 ✓7ᵗʰ **T23.702** Corrosion of third degree of **left** hand, unspecified site   CC
CC Excl: See code: T23.701

7 ✓7ᵗʰ **T23.709** Corrosion of third degree of **unspecified** hand, unspecified site   CC
CC Excl: See code: T23.701

✓6ᵗʰ **T23.71** Corrosion of third degree of **thumb (nail)**

7 ✓7ᵗʰ **T23.711** Corrosion of third degree of **right** thumb (nail)   CC
CC Excl: CC with 7th character A: T23.301-T23.319 with 7th A, T23.391-T23.399 with 7th A, T23.701-T23.719 with 7th A, T23.791-T23.799 with 7th A

7 ✓7ᵗʰ **T23.712** Corrosion of third degree of **left** thumb (nail)   CC
CC Excl: See code: T23.711

7 ✓7ᵗʰ **T23.719** Corrosion of third degree of **unspecified** thumb (nail)   CC
CC Excl: See code: T23.711

✓6ᵗʰ **T23.72** Corrosion of third degree of **single finger** (nail) except thumb

7 ✓7ᵗʰ **T23.721** Corrosion of third degree of single **right** finger (nail) except thumb   CC
CC Excl: CC with 7th character A: T23.301-T23.309 with 7th A, T23.321-T23.329 with 7th A, T23.391-T23.399 with 7th A, T23.701-T23.709 with 7th A, T23.721-T23.729 with 7th A, T23.791-T23.799 with 7th A

7 ✓7ᵗʰ **T23.722** Corrosion of third degree of single **left** finger (nail) except thumb   CC
CC Excl: See code: T23.721

7 ✓7ᵗʰ **T23.729** Corrosion of third degree of **unspecified** single finger (nail) except thumb   CC
CC Excl: See code: T23.721

✓6ᵗʰ **T23.73** Corrosion of third degree of **multiple fingers** (nail), not including thumb

7 ✓7ᵗʰ **T23.731** Corrosion of third degree of multiple **right** fingers (nail), not including thumb   CC
CC Excl: CC with 7th character A: T23.301-T23.309 with 7th A, T23.331-T23.339 with 7th A, T23.391-T23.399 with 7th A, T23.701-T23.709 with 7th A, T23.731-T23.739 with 7th A, T23.791-T23.799 with 7th A

7 ✓7ᵗʰ **T23.732** Corrosion of third degree of multiple **left** fingers (nail), not including thumb   CC
CC Excl: See code: T23.731

7 ✓7ᵗʰ **T23.739** Corrosion of third degree of **unspecified** multiple fingers (nail), not including thumb   CC
CC Excl: See code: T23.731

✓6ᵗʰ **T23.74** Corrosion of third degree of **multiple fingers** (nail), including thumb

7 ✓7ᵗʰ **T23.741** Corrosion of third degree of multiple **right** fingers (nail), including thumb   CC
CC Excl: CC with 7th character A: T23.301-T23.309 with 7th A, T23.341-T23.349 with 7th A, T23.391-T23.399 with 7th A, T23.701-T23.709 with 7th A, T23.741-T23.749 with 7th A, T23.791-T23.799 with 7th A

7 ✓7ᵗʰ **T23.742** Corrosion of third degree of multiple **left** fingers (nail), including thumb   CC
CC Excl: See code: T23.741

---

7   HAC = Initial encounter only (7th character A, B or C) and not POA.

Ⓝ Newborn: 0   Ⓟ Pediatric: 0-17   Ⓜ Maternity: 12-55   Ⓐ Adult: 15-124   **MCC** Major CC Condition   **PDxMCC** PDx acts as own MCC   **CC** CC Condition   **PDxCC** PDx acts as own CC

1086   ICD-10-CM 2016

7 ✓7ᵗʰ **T23.749 Corrosion of third degree of unspecified multiple fingers (nail), including thumb**   CC
CC Excl: See code: T23.741

✓6ᵗʰ **T23.75 Corrosion of third degree of palm**

7 ✓7ᵗʰ **T23.751 Corrosion of third degree of right palm**   CC
CC Excl: CC with 7th character A: T23.301-T23.309 with 7th A, T23.351-T23.359 with 7th A, T23.391-T23.399 with 7th A, T23.701-T23.709 with 7th A, T23.751-T23.759 with 7th A, T23.791-T23.799 with 7th A

7 ✓7ᵗʰ **T23.752 Corrosion of third degree of left palm**   CC
CC Excl: See code: T23.751

7 ✓7ᵗʰ **T23.759 Corrosion of third degree of unspecified palm**   CC
CC Excl: See code: T23.751

✓6ᵗʰ **T23.76 Corrosion of third degree of back of hand**

7 ✓7ᵗʰ **T23.761 Corrosion of third degree of back of right hand**   CC
CC Excl: CC with 7th character A: T23.301-T23.309 with 7th A, T23.361-T23.369 with 7th A, T23.391-T23.399 with 7th A, T23.701-T23.709 with 7th A, T23.761-T23.769 with 7th A, T23.791-T23.799 with 7th A

7 ✓7ᵗʰ **T23.762 Corrosion of third degree of back of left hand**   CC
CC Excl: See code: T23.761

7 ✓7ᵗʰ **T23.769 Corrosion of third degree back of unspecified hand**   CC
CC Excl: See code: T23.761

✓6ᵗʰ **T23.77 Corrosion of third degree of wrist**

7 ✓7ᵗʰ **T23.771 Corrosion of third degree of right wrist**   CC
CC Excl: CC with 7th character A: T23.301-T23.309 with 7th A, T23.371-T23.379 with 7th A, T23.391-T23.399 with 7th A, T23.701-T23.709 with 7th A, T23.771-T23.779 with 7th A, T23.791-T23.799 with 7th A

7 ✓7ᵗʰ **T23.772 Corrosion of third degree of left wrist**   CC
CC Excl: See code: T23.771

7 ✓7ᵗʰ **T23.779 Corrosion of third degree of unspecified wrist**   CC
CC Excl: See code: T23.771

✓6ᵗʰ **T23.79 Corrosion of third degree of multiple sites of wrist and hand**

7 ✓7ᵗʰ **T23.791 Corrosion of third degree of multiple sites of right wrist and hand**   CC
CC Excl: See code: T23.702

7 ✓7ᵗʰ **T23.792 Corrosion of third degree of multiple sites of left wrist and hand**   CC
CC Excl: See code: T23.702

7 ✓7ᵗʰ **T23.799 Corrosion of third degree of multiple sites of unspecified wrist and hand**   CC
CC Excl: See code: T23.702

✓4ᵗʰ **T24 Burn and corrosion of lower limb, except ankle and foot**
EXCLUDES 2   burn and corrosion of ankle and foot (T25.-)
burn and corrosion of hip region (T21.-)

The appropriate 7th character is to be added to each code from category T24.
A   initial encounter
D   subsequent encounter
S   sequela

✓5ᵗʰ **T24.0 Burn of unspecified degree of lower limb, except ankle and foot**
Use additional external cause code to identify the source, place and intent of the burn (X00-X19, X75-X77, X96-X98, Y92)

✓6ᵗʰ **T24.00 Burn of unspecified degree of unspecified site of lower limb, except ankle and foot**

7ᵗʰ **T24.001 Burn of unspecified degree of unspecified site of right lower limb, except ankle and foot**

✓7ᵗʰ **T24.002 Burn of unspecified degree of unspecified site of left lower limb, except ankle and foot**

✓7ᵗʰ **T24.009 Burn of unspecified degree of unspecified site of unspecified lower limb, except ankle and foot**

✓6ᵗʰ **T24.01 Burn of unspecified degree of thigh**

✓7ᵗʰ **T24.011 Burn of unspecified degree of right thigh**

✓7ᵗʰ **T24.012 Burn of unspecified degree of left thigh**

✓7ᵗʰ **T24.019 Burn of unspecified degree of unspecified thigh**

✓6ᵗʰ **T24.02 Burn of unspecified degree of knee**

✓7ᵗʰ **T24.021 Burn of unspecified degree of right knee**

✓7ᵗʰ **T24.022 Burn of unspecified degree of left knee**

✓7ᵗʰ **T24.029 Burn of unspecified degree of unspecified knee**

✓6ᵗʰ **T24.03 Burn of unspecified degree of lower leg**

✓7ᵗʰ **T24.031 Burn of unspecified degree of right lower leg**

✓7ᵗʰ **T24.032 Burn of unspecified degree of left lower leg**

✓7ᵗʰ **T24.039 Burn of unspecified degree of unspecified lower leg**

✓6ᵗʰ **T24.09 Burn of unspecified degree of multiple sites of lower limb, except ankle and foot**

✓7ᵗʰ **T24.091 Burn of unspecified degree of multiple sites of right lower limb, except ankle and foot**

✓7ᵗʰ **T24.092 Burn of unspecified degree of multiple sites of left lower limb, except ankle and foot**

✓7ᵗʰ **T24.099 Burn of unspecified degree of multiple sites of unspecified lower limb, except ankle and foot**

✓5ᵗʰ **T24.1 Burn of first degree of lower limb, except ankle and foot**
Use additional external cause code to identify the source, place and intent of the burn (X00-X19, X75-X77, X96-X98, Y92)

✓6ᵗʰ **T24.10 Burn of first degree of unspecified site of lower limb, except ankle and foot**

✓7ᵗʰ **T24.101 Burn of first degree of unspecified site of right lower limb, except ankle and foot**

✓7ᵗʰ **T24.102 Burn of first degree of unspecified site of left lower limb, except ankle and foot**

✓7ᵗʰ **T24.109 Burn of first degree of unspecified site of unspecified lower limb, except ankle and foot**

✓6ᵗʰ **T24.11 Burn of first degree of thigh**

✓7ᵗʰ **T24.111 Burn of first degree of right thigh**

✓7ᵗʰ **T24.112 Burn of first degree of left thigh**

✓7ᵗʰ **T24.119 Burn of first degree of unspecified thigh**

✓6ᵗʰ **T24.12 Burn of first degree of knee**

✓7ᵗʰ **T24.121 Burn of first degree of right knee**

✓7ᵗʰ **T24.122 Burn of first degree of left knee**

✓7ᵗʰ **T24.129 Burn of first degree of unspecified knee**

✓6ᵗʰ **T24.13 Burn of first degree of lower leg**

✓7ᵗʰ **T24.131 Burn of first degree of right lower leg**

✓7ᵗʰ **T24.132 Burn of first degree of left lower leg**

✓7ᵗʰ **T24.139 Burn of first degree of unspecified lower leg**

✓6ᵗʰ **T24.19 Burn of first degree of multiple sites of lower limb, except ankle and foot**

✓7ᵗʰ **T24.191 Burn of first degree of multiple sites of right lower limb, except ankle and foot**

✓7ᵗʰ **T24.192 Burn of first degree of multiple sites of left lower limb, except ankle and foot**

✓7ᵗʰ **T24.199 Burn of first degree of multiple sites of unspecified lower limb, except ankle and foot**

---

7   HAC = Initial encounter only (7th character A, B or C) and not POA.

√5ᵗʰ **T24.2** Burn of second degree of lower limb, except ankle and foot
Use additional external cause code to identify the source, place and intent of the burn (X00-X19, X75-X77, X96-X98, Y92)

√6ᵗʰ **T24.20** Burn of second degree of unspecified site of lower limb, except ankle and foot

√7ᵗʰ **T24.201** Burn of second degree of unspecified site of right lower limb, except ankle and foot

√7ᵗʰ **T24.202** Burn of second degree of unspecified site of left lower limb, except ankle and foot

√7ᵗʰ **T24.209** Burn of second degree of unspecified site of unspecified lower limb, except ankle and foot

√6ᵗʰ **T24.21** Burn of second degree of thigh

√7ᵗʰ **T24.211** Burn of second degree of right thigh

√7ᵗʰ **T24.212** Burn of second degree of left thigh

√7ᵗʰ **T24.219** Burn of second degree of unspecified thigh

√6ᵗʰ **T24.22** Burn of second degree of knee

√7ᵗʰ **T24.221** Burn of second degree of right knee

√7ᵗʰ **T24.222** Burn of second degree of left knee

√7ᵗʰ **T24.229** Burn of second degree of unspecified knee

√6ᵗʰ **T24.23** Burn of second degree of lower leg

√7ᵗʰ **T24.231** Burn of second degree of right lower leg

√7ᵗʰ **T24.232** Burn of second degree of left lower leg

√7ᵗʰ **T24.239** Burn of second degree of unspecified lower leg

√6ᵗʰ **T24.29** Burn of second degree of multiple sites of lower limb, except ankle and foot

√7ᵗʰ **T24.291** Burn of second degree of multiple sites of right lower limb, except ankle and foot

√7ᵗʰ **T24.292** Burn of second degree of multiple sites of left lower limb, except ankle and foot

√7ᵗʰ **T24.299** Burn of second degree of multiple sites of unspecified lower limb, except ankle and foot

√5ᵗʰ **T24.3** Burn of third degree of lower limb, except ankle and foot
Use additional external cause code to identify the source, place and intent of the burn (X00-X19, X75-X77, X96-X98, Y92)

√6ᵗʰ **T24.30** Burn of third degree of unspecified site of lower limb, except ankle and foot

7 √7ᵗʰ **T24.301** Burn of third degree of unspecified site of right lower limb, except ankle and foot CC
CC Excl: CC with 7th character A: T24.301-T24.309 with 7th A, T24.391-T24.399 with 7th A, T24.701-T24.709 with 7th A, T24.791-T24.799 with 7th A, T25.391-T25.399 with 7th A, T25.791-T25.790 with 7th A

7 √7ᵗʰ **T24.302** Burn of third degree of unspecified site of left lower limb, except ankle and foot CC
CC Excl: See code: T24.301

7 √7ᵗʰ **T24.309** Burn of third degree of unspecified site of unspecified lower limb, except ankle and foot CC
CC Excl: See code: T24.301

√6ᵗʰ **T24.31** Burn of third degree of thigh

7 √7ᵗʰ **T24.311** Burn of third degree of right thigh CC
CC Excl: CC with 7th character A: T24.301-T24.309 with 7th A, T24.311-T24.319 with 7th A, T24.391-T24.399 with 7th A, T24.701-T24.709 with 7th A, T24.711-T24.719 with 7th A, T24.791-T24.799 with 7th A, T25.391-T25.399 with 7th A, T25.791-T25.790 with 7th A

7 √7ᵗʰ **T24.312** Burn of third degree of left thigh CC
CC Excl: See code: T24.311

7 √7ᵗʰ **T24.319** Burn of third degree of unspecified thigh CC
CC Excl: See code: T24.311

√6ᵗʰ **T24.32** Burn of third degree of knee

7 √7ᵗʰ **T24.321** Burn of third degree of right knee CC
CC Excl: CC with 7th character A: T24.301-T24.309 with 7th A, T24.321-T24.329 with 7th A, T24.391-T24.399 with 7th A, T24.701-T24.709 with 7th A, T24.721-T24.729 with 7th A, T24.791-T24.799 with 7th A, T25.391-T25.399 with 7th A, T25.791-T25.790 with 7th A

7 √7ᵗʰ **T24.322** Burn of third degree of left knee CC
CC Excl: See code: T24.321

7 √7ᵗʰ **T24.329** Burn of third degree of unspecified knee CC
CC Excl: See code: T24.321

√6ᵗʰ **T24.33** Burn of third degree of lower leg

7 √7ᵗʰ **T24.331** Burn of third degree of right lower leg CC
CC Excl: CC with 7th character A: T24.301-T24.309 with 7th A, T24.331-T24.339 with 7th A, T24.391-T24.399 with 7th A, T24.701-T24.709 with 7th A, T24.731-T24.739 with 7th A, T24.791-T24.799 with 7th A, T25.391-T25.399 with 7th A, T25.791-T25.790 with 7th A

7 √7ᵗʰ **T24.332** Burn of third degree of left lower leg CC
CC Excl: See code: T24.331

7 √7ᵗʰ **T24.339** Burn of third degree of unspecified lower leg CC
CC Excl: See code: T24.331

√6ᵗʰ **T24.39** Burn of third degree of multiple sites of lower limb, except ankle and foot

7 √7ᵗʰ **T24.391** Burn of third degree of multiple sites of right lower limb, except ankle and foot CC
CC Excl: CC with 7th character A: T24.301-T24.309 with 7th A, T24.391-T24.399 with 7th A, T24.701-T24.709 with 7th A, T24.791-T24.799 with 7th A, T25.391-T25.399 with 7th A, T25.791-T25.799 with 7th A

7 √7ᵗʰ **T24.392** Burn of third degree of multiple sites of left lower limb, except ankle and foot CC
CC Excl: See code: T24.301

7 √7ᵗʰ **T24.399** Burn of third degree of multiple sites of unspecified lower limb, except ankle and foot CC
CC Excl: See code: T24.301

√5ᵗʰ **T24.4** Corrosion of unspecified degree of lower limb, except ankle and foot
Code first (T51-T65) to identify chemical and intent
Use additional external cause code to identify place (Y92)

√6ᵗʰ **T24.40** Corrosion of unspecified degree of unspecified site of lower limb, except ankle and foot

√7ᵗʰ **T24.401** Corrosion of unspecified degree of unspecified site of right lower limb, except ankle and foot

√7ᵗʰ **T24.402** Corrosion of unspecified degree of unspecified site of left lower limb, except ankle and foot

√7ᵗʰ **T24.409** Corrosion of unspecified degree of unspecified site of unspecified lower limb, except ankle and foot

√6ᵗʰ **T24.41** Corrosion of unspecified degree of thigh

√7ᵗʰ **T24.411** Corrosion of unspecified degree of right thigh

√7ᵗʰ **T24.412** Corrosion of unspecified degree of left thigh

√7ᵗʰ **T24.419** Corrosion of unspecified degree of unspecified thigh

√6ᵗʰ **T24.42** Corrosion of unspecified degree of knee

√7ᵗʰ **T24.421** Corrosion of unspecified degree of right knee

√7ᵗʰ **T24.422** Corrosion of unspecified degree of left knee

√7ᵗʰ **T24.429** Corrosion of unspecified degree of unspecified knee

---

7 HAC = Initial encounter only (7th character A, B or C) and not POA.

Ⓝ Newborn: 0 Ⓟ Pediatric: 0-17 Ⓜ Maternity: 12-55 Ⓐ Adult: 15-124 MCC Major CC Condition PDxMCC PDx acts as own MCC CC CC Condition PDxCC PDx acts as own CC

1088 ICD-10-CM 2016

✓6th T24.43 Corrosion of unspecified degree of lower leg

✓7th T24.431 Corrosion of unspecified degree of right lower leg

✓7th T24.432 Corrosion of unspecified degree of left lower leg

✓7th T24.439 Corrosion of unspecified degree of unspecified lower leg

✓6th T24.49 Corrosion of unspecified degree of multiple sites of lower limb, except ankle and foot

✓7th T24.491 Corrosion of unspecified degree of multiple sites of right lower limb, except ankle and foot

✓7th T24.492 Corrosion of unspecified degree of multiple sites of left lower limb, except ankle and foot

✓7th T24.499 Corrosion of unspecified degree of multiple sites of unspecified lower limb, except ankle and foot

✓5th T24.5 Corrosion of first degree of lower limb, except ankle and foot

Code first (T51-T65) to identify chemical and intent

Use additional external cause code to identify place (Y92)

✓6th T24.50 Corrosion of first degree of unspecified site of lower limb, except ankle and foot

✓7th T24.501 Corrosion of first degree of unspecified site of right lower limb, except ankle and foot

✓7th T24.502 Corrosion of first degree of unspecified site of left lower limb, except ankle and foot

✓7th T24.509 Corrosion of first degree of unspecified site of unspecified lower limb, except ankle and foot

✓6th T24.51 Corrosion of first degree of thigh

✓7th T24.511 Corrosion of first degree of right thigh

✓7th T24.512 Corrosion of first degree of left thigh

✓7th T24.519 Corrosion of first degree of unspecified thigh

✓6th T24.52 Corrosion of first degree of knee

✓7th T24.521 Corrosion of first degree of right knee

✓7th T24.522 Corrosion of first degree of left knee

✓7th T24.529 Corrosion of first degree of unspecified knee

✓6th T24.53 Corrosion of first degree of lower leg

✓7th T24.531 Corrosion of first degree of right lower leg

✓7th T24.532 Corrosion of first degree of left lower leg

✓7th T24.539 Corrosion of first degree of unspecified lower leg

✓6th T24.59 Corrosion of first degree of multiple sites of lower limb, except ankle and foot

✓7th T24.591 Corrosion of first degree of multiple sites of right lower limb, except ankle and foot

✓7th T24.592 Corrosion of first degree of multiple sites of left lower limb, except ankle and foot

✓7th T24.599 Corrosion of first degree of multiple sites of unspecified lower limb, except ankle and foot

✓5th T24.6 Corrosion of second degree of lower limb, except ankle and foot

Code first (T51-T65) to identify chemical and intent

Use additional external cause code to identify place (Y92)

✓6th T24.60 Corrosion of second degree of unspecified site of lower limb, except ankle and foot

✓7th T24.601 Corrosion of second degree of unspecified site of right lower limb, except ankle and foot

✓7th T24.602 Corrosion of second degree of unspecified site of left lower limb, except ankle and foot

✓7th T24.609 Corrosion of second degree of unspecified site of unspecified lower limb, except ankle and foot

✓6th T24.61 Corrosion of second degree of thigh

✓7th T24.611 Corrosion of second degree of right thigh

✓7th T24.612 Corrosion of second degree of left thigh

✓7th T24.619 Corrosion of second degree of unspecified thigh

✓6th T24.62 Corrosion of second degree of knee

✓7th T24.621 Corrosion of second degree of right knee

✓7th T24.622 Corrosion of second degree of left knee

✓7th T24.629 Corrosion of second degree of unspecified knee

✓6th T24.63 Corrosion of second degree of lower leg

✓7th T24.631 Corrosion of second degree of right lower leg

✓7th T24.632 Corrosion of second degree of left lower leg

✓7th T24.639 Corrosion of second degree of unspecified lower leg

✓6th T24.69 Corrosion of second degree of multiple sites of lower limb, except ankle and foot

✓7th T24.691 Corrosion of second degree of multiple sites of right lower limb, except ankle and foot

✓7th T24.692 Corrosion of second degree of multiple sites of left lower limb, except ankle and foot

✓7th T24.699 Corrosion of second degree of multiple sites of unspecified lower limb, except ankle and foot

✓5th T24.7 Corrosion of third degree of lower limb, except ankle and foot

Code first (T51-T65) to identify chemical and intent

Use additional external cause code to identify place (Y92)

✓6th T24.70 Corrosion of third degree of unspecified site of lower limb, except ankle and foot

7 **✓7th T24.701** **Corrosion of third degree of unspecified site of right lower limb, except ankle and foot** CC

CC Excl: CC with 7th character A: See code: T24.301

7 **✓7th T24.702** **Corrosion of third degree of unspecified site of left lower limb, except ankle and foot** CC

CC Excl: See code: T24.301

7 **✓7th T24.709** **Corrosion of third degree of unspecified site of unspecified lower limb, except ankle and foot** CC

CC Excl: See code: T24.301

✓6th T24.71 Corrosion of third degree of thigh

7 **✓7th T24.711** **Corrosion of third degree of right thigh** CC

CC Excl: CC with 7th character A: See code: T24.311

7 **✓7th T24.712** **Corrosion of third degree of left thigh** CC

CC Excl: See code: T24.311

7 **✓7th T24.719** **Corrosion of third degree of unspecified thigh** CC

CC Excl: See code: T24.311

✓6th T24.72 Corrosion of third degree of knee

7 **✓7th T24.721** **Corrosion of third degree of right knee** CC

CC Excl: CC with 7th character A: See code: T24.321

7 **✓7th T24.722** **Corrosion of third degree of left knee** CC

CC Excl: See code: T24.321

7 **✓7th T24.729** **Corrosion of third degree of unspecified knee** CC

CC Excl: See code: T24.321

✓6th T24.73 Corrosion of third degree of lower leg

7 **✓7th T24.731** **Corrosion of third degree of right lower leg** CC

CC Excl: CC with 7th character A: See code: T24.331

7 **✓7th T24.732** **Corrosion of third degree of left lower leg** CC

CC Excl: See code: T24.331

7 **✓7th T24.739** **Corrosion of third degree of unspecified lower leg** CC

CC Excl: See code: T24.331

---

7   HAC = Initial encounter only (7th character A, B or C) and not POA.

✓ Additional Character Required   ✓x7th Placeholder Alert   Unacceptable PDx   Manifestation   Hospital Acquired Condition   **EXCLUDES 1** Not Coded Here   **EXCLUDES 2** Not Included Here

Chapter 19. Injury, Poisoning, and Certain Other Consequences of External Causes

T24.79–T25.332

√6ᵗʰ **T24.79** **Corrosion of third degree of** multiple sites **of lower limb, except ankle and foot**

    7 √7ᵗʰ **T24.791** **Corrosion of third degree of multiple sites of** right **lower limb, except ankle and foot** `CC`
       CC Excl: CC with 7th character A: See code: T24.301

    7 √7ᵗʰ **T24.792** **Corrosion of third degree of multiple sites of** left **lower limb, except ankle and foot** `CC`
       CC Excl: See code: T24.301

    7 √7ᵗʰ **T24.799** **Corrosion of third degree of multiple sites of** unspecified **lower limb, except ankle and foot** `CC`
       CC Excl: See code: T24.301

√4ᵗʰ **T25** **Burn and corrosion of ankle and foot**

> The appropriate 7th character is to be added to each code from category T25.
> A   initial encounter
> D   subsequent encounter
> S   sequela

√5ᵗʰ **T25.0** **Burn of unspecified degree of ankle and foot**
    Use additional external cause code to identify the source, place and intent of the burn (X00-X19, X75-X77, X96-X98, Y92)

   √6ᵗʰ **T25.01** **Burn of unspecified degree of** ankle
      √7ᵗʰ **T25.011** **Burn of unspecified degree of** right ankle
      √7ᵗʰ **T25.012** **Burn of unspecified degree of** left ankle
      √7ᵗʰ **T25.019** **Burn of unspecified degree of** unspecified ankle

   √6ᵗʰ **T25.02** **Burn of unspecified degree of** foot
      EXCLUDES 2 *burn of unspecified degree of toe(s) (nail) (T25.03-)*
      √7ᵗʰ **T25.021** **Burn of unspecified degree of** right foot
      √7ᵗʰ **T25.022** **Burn of unspecified degree of** left foot
      √7ᵗʰ **T25.029** **Burn of unspecified degree of** unspecified foot

   √6ᵗʰ **T25.03** **Burn of unspecified degree of** toe(s) (nail)
      √7ᵗʰ **T25.031** **Burn of unspecified degree of** right toe(s) (nail)
      √7ᵗʰ **T25.032** **Burn of unspecified degree of** left toe(s) (nail)
      √7ᵗʰ **T25.039** **Burn of unspecified degree of** unspecified toe(s) (nail)

   √6ᵗʰ **T25.09** **Burn of unspecified degree of** multiple sites **of ankle and foot**
      √7ᵗʰ **T25.091** **Burn of unspecified degree of multiple sites of** right ankle and foot
      √7ᵗʰ **T25.092** **Burn of unspecified degree of multiple sites of** left ankle and foot
      √7ᵗʰ **T25.099** **Burn of unspecified degree of multiple sites of** unspecified ankle and foot

√5ᵗʰ **T25.1** **Burn of first degree of ankle and foot**
    Use additional external cause code to identify the source, place and intent of the burn (X00-X19, X75-X77, X96-X98, Y92)

   √6ᵗʰ **T25.11** **Burn of first degree of** ankle
      √7ᵗʰ **T25.111** **Burn of first degree of** right ankle
      √7ᵗʰ **T25.112** **Burn of first degree of** left ankle
      √7ᵗʰ **T25.119** **Burn of first degree of** unspecified ankle

   √6ᵗʰ **T25.12** **Burn of first degree of** foot
      EXCLUDES 2 *burn of first degree of toe(s) (nail) (T25.13-)*
      √7ᵗʰ **T25.121** **Burn of first degree of** right foot
      √7ᵗʰ **T25.122** **Burn of first degree of** left foot
      √7ᵗʰ **T25.129** **Burn of first degree of** unspecified foot

   √6ᵗʰ **T25.13** **Burn of first degree of** toe(s) (nail)
      √7ᵗʰ **T25.131** **Burn of first degree of** right toe(s) (nail)
      √7ᵗʰ **T25.132** **Burn of first degree of** left toe(s) (nail)
      √7ᵗʰ **T25.139** **Burn of first degree of** unspecified toe(s) (nail)

   √6ᵗʰ **T25.19** **Burn of first degree of** multiple sites **of ankle and foot**
      √7ᵗʰ **T25.191** **Burn of first degree of multiple sites of** right ankle and foot

      √7ᵗʰ **T25.192** **Burn of first degree of multiple sites of** left ankle and foot
      √7ᵗʰ **T25.199** **Burn of first degree of multiple sites of** unspecified ankle and foot

√5ᵗʰ **T25.2** **Burn of second degree of ankle and foot**
    Use additional external cause code to identify the source, place and intent of the burn (X00-X19, X75-X77, X96-X98, Y92)

   √6ᵗʰ **T25.21** **Burn of second degree of** ankle
      √7ᵗʰ **T25.211** **Burn of second degree of** right ankle
      √7ᵗʰ **T25.212** **Burn of second degree of** left ankle
      √7ᵗʰ **T25.219** **Burn of second degree of** unspecified ankle

   √6ᵗʰ **T25.22** **Burn of second degree of** foot
      EXCLUDES 2 *burn of second degree of toe(s) (nail) (T25.23-)*
      √7ᵗʰ **T25.221** **Burn of second degree of** right foot
      √7ᵗʰ **T25.222** **Burn of second degree of** left foot
      √7ᵗʰ **T25.229** **Burn of second degree of** unspecified foot

   √6ᵗʰ **T25.23** **Burn of second degree of** toe(s) (nail)
      √7ᵗʰ **T25.231** **Burn of second degree of** right toe(s) (nail)
      √7ᵗʰ **T25.232** **Burn of second degree of** left toe(s) (nail)
      √7ᵗʰ **T25.239** **Burn of second degree of** unspecified toe(s) (nail)

   √6ᵗʰ **T25.29** **Burn of second degree of** multiple sites **of ankle and foot**
      √7ᵗʰ **T25.291** **Burn of second degree of multiple sites of** right ankle and foot
      √7ᵗʰ **T25.292** **Burn of second degree of multiple sites of** left ankle and foot
      √7ᵗʰ **T25.299** **Burn of second degree of multiple sites of** unspecified ankle and foot

√5ᵗʰ **T25.3** **Burn of** third degree **of ankle and foot**
    Use additional external cause code to identify the source, place and intent of the burn (X00-X19, X75-X77, X96-X98, Y92)

   √6ᵗʰ **T25.31** **Burn of third degree of** ankle
    7 √7ᵗʰ **T25.311** **Burn of third degree of** right ankle `CC`
      CC Excl: CC with 7th character A: T24.301-T24.309 with 7th A, T24.391-T24.399 with 7th A, T24.701-T24.709 with 7th A, T24.791-T24.799 with 7th A, T25.311-T25.319 with 7th A, T25.391-T25.399 with 7th A, T25.711-T25.719 with 7th A, T25.791-T25.790 with 7th A

    7 √7ᵗʰ **T25.312** **Burn of third degree of** left ankle `CC`
      CC Excl: See code: T25.311

    7 √7ᵗʰ **T25.319** **Burn of third degree of** unspecified ankle `CC`
      CC Excl: See code: T25.311

   √6ᵗʰ **T25.32** **Burn of third degree of** foot
      EXCLUDES 2 *burn of third degree of toe(s) (nail) (T25.33-)*
    7 √7ᵗʰ **T25.321** **Burn of third degree of** right foot `CC`
      CC Excl: CC with 7th character A: T24.301-T24.309 with 7th A, T24.391-T24.399 with 7th A, T24.701-T24.709 with 7th A, T24.791-T24.799 with 7th A, T25.321-T25.329 with 7th A, T25.391-T25.399 with 7th A, T25.721-T25.729 with 7th A, T25.791-T25.799 with 7th A

    7 √7ᵗʰ **T25.322** **Burn of third degree of** left foot `CC`
      CC Excl: See code: T25.321

    7 √7ᵗʰ **T25.329** **Burn of third degree of** unspecified foot `CC`
      CC Excl: See code: T25.321

   √6ᵗʰ **T25.33** **Burn of third degree of** toe(s) (nail)
    7 √7ᵗʰ **T25.331** **Burn of third degree of** right toe(s) (nail) `CC`
      CC Excl: CC with 7th character A: T24.301-T24.309 with 7th A, T24.391-T24.399 with 7th A, T24.701-T24.709 with 7th A, T24.791-T24.799 with 7th A, T25.331-T25.339 with 7th A, T25.391-T25.399 with 7th A, T25.731-T25.739 with 7th A, T25.791-T25.799 with 7th A

    7 √7ᵗʰ **T25.332** **Burn of third degree of** left toe(s) (nail) `CC`
      CC Excl: See code: T25.331

---

7   HAC = Initial encounter only (7th character A, B or C) and not POA.

N Newborn: 0   P Pediatric: 0-17   M Maternity: 12-55   A Adult: 15-124   MCC Major CC Condition   PDxMCC PDx acts as own MCC   CC CC Condition   PDxCC PDx acts as own CC

1090   ICD-10-CM 2016

7 ✓7ᵗʰ **T25.339** **Burn of third degree of unspecified toe(s) (nail)** 🄲🄲
CC Excl: See code: T25.331

✓6ᵗʰ **T25.39** Burn of third degree of multiple sites of ankle and foot

7 ✓7ᵗʰ **T25.391** **Burn of third degree of multiple sites of right ankle and foot** 🄲🄲
CC Excl: CC with 7th character A: See code: T25.331

7 ✓7ᵗʰ **T25.392** **Burn of third degree of multiple sites of left ankle and foot** 🄲🄲
CC Excl: See code: T25.331

7 ✓7ᵗʰ **T25.399** **Burn of third degree of multiple sites of unspecified ankle and foot** 🄲🄲
CC Excl: See code: T25.331

✓5ᵗʰ **T25.4** Corrosion of unspecified degree of ankle and foot
Code first (T51-T65) to identify chemical and intent
Use additional external cause code to identify place (Y92)

✓6ᵗʰ **T25.41** Corrosion of unspecified degree of ankle

✓7ᵗʰ **T25.411** Corrosion of unspecified degree of right ankle

✓7ᵗʰ **T25.412** Corrosion of unspecified degree of left ankle

✓7ᵗʰ **T25.419** Corrosion of unspecified degree of unspecified ankle

✓6ᵗʰ **T25.42** Corrosion of unspecified degree of foot
EXCLUDES 2 corrosion of unspecified degree of toe(s) (nail) (T25.43-)

✓7ᵗʰ **T25.421** Corrosion of unspecified degree of right foot

✓7ᵗʰ **T25.422** Corrosion of unspecified degree of left foot

✓7ᵗʰ **T25.429** Corrosion of unspecified degree of unspecified foot

✓6ᵗʰ **T25.43** Corrosion of unspecified degree of toe(s) (nail)

✓7ᵗʰ **T25.431** Corrosion of unspecified degree of right toe(s) (nail)

✓7ᵗʰ **T25.432** Corrosion of unspecified degree of left toe(s) (nail)

✓7ᵗʰ **T25.439** Corrosion of unspecified degree of unspecified toe(s) (nail)

✓6ᵗʰ **T25.49** Corrosion of unspecified degree of multiple sites of ankle and foot

✓7ᵗʰ **T25.491** Corrosion of unspecified degree of multiple sites of right ankle and foot

✓7ᵗʰ **T25.492** Corrosion of unspecified degree of multiple sites of left ankle and foot

✓7ᵗʰ **T25.499** Corrosion of unspecified degree of multiple sites of unspecified ankle and foot

✓5ᵗʰ **T25.5** Corrosion of first degree of ankle and foot
Code first (T51-T65) to identify chemical and intent
Use additional external cause code to identify place (Y92)

✓6ᵗʰ **T25.51** Corrosion of first degree of ankle

✓7ᵗʰ **T25.511** Corrosion of first degree of right ankle

✓7ᵗʰ **T25.512** Corrosion of first degree of left ankle

✓7ᵗʰ **T25.519** Corrosion of first degree of unspecified ankle

✓6ᵗʰ **T25.52** Corrosion of first degree of foot
EXCLUDES 2 corrosion of first degree of toe(s) (nail) (T25.53-)

✓7ᵗʰ **T25.521** Corrosion of first degree of right foot

✓7ᵗʰ **T25.522** Corrosion of first degree of left foot

✓7ᵗʰ **T25.529** Corrosion of first degree of unspecified foot

✓6ᵗʰ **T25.53** Corrosion of first degree of toe(s) (nail)

✓7ᵗʰ **T25.531** Corrosion of first degree of right toe(s) (nail)

✓7ᵗʰ **T25.532** Corrosion of first degree of left toe(s) (nail)

✓7ᵗʰ **T25.539** Corrosion of first degree of unspecified toe(s) (nail)

✓6ᵗʰ **T25.59** Corrosion of first degree of multiple sites of ankle and foot

✓7ᵗʰ **T25.591** Corrosion of first degree of multiple sites of right ankle and foot

✓7ᵗʰ **T25.592** Corrosion of first degree of multiple sites of left ankle and foot

✓7ᵗʰ **T25.599** Corrosion of first degree of multiple sites of unspecified ankle and foot

✓5ᵗʰ **T25.6** Corrosion of second degree of ankle and foot
Code first (T51-T65) to identify chemical and intent
Use additional external cause code to identify place (Y92)

✓6ᵗʰ **T25.61** Corrosion of second degree of ankle

✓7ᵗʰ **T25.611** Corrosion of second degree of right ankle

✓7ᵗʰ **T25.612** Corrosion of second degree of left ankle

✓7ᵗʰ **T25.619** Corrosion of second degree of unspecified ankle

✓6ᵗʰ **T25.62** Corrosion of second degree of foot
EXCLUDES 2 corrosion of second degree of toe(s) (nail) (T25.63-)

✓7ᵗʰ **T25.621** Corrosion of second degree of right foot

✓7ᵗʰ **T25.622** Corrosion of second degree of left foot

✓7ᵗʰ **T25.629** Corrosion of second degree of unspecified foot

✓6ᵗʰ **T25.63** Corrosion of second degree of toe(s) (nail)

✓7ᵗʰ **T25.631** Corrosion of second degree of right toe(s) (nail)

✓7ᵗʰ **T25.632** Corrosion of second degree of left toe(s) (nail)

✓7ᵗʰ **T25.639** Corrosion of second degree of unspecified toe(s) (nail)

✓6ᵗʰ **T25.69** Corrosion of second degree of multiple sites of ankle and foot

✓7ᵗʰ **T25.691** Corrosion of second degree of right ankle and foot

✓7ᵗʰ **T25.692** Corrosion of second degree of left ankle and foot

✓7ᵗʰ **T25.699** Corrosion of second degree of unspecified ankle and foot

✓5ᵗʰ **T25.7** Corrosion of third degree of ankle and foot
Code first (T51-T65) to identify chemical and intent
Use additional external cause code to identify place (Y92)

✓6ᵗʰ **T25.71** Corrosion of third degree of ankle

7 ✓7ᵗʰ **T25.711** **Corrosion of third degree of right ankle** 🄲🄲
CC Excl: CC with 7th character A: T24.301-T24.309 with 7th A, T24.391-T24.399 with 7th A, T24.701-T24.709 with 7th A, T24.791-T24.799 with 7th A, T25.311-T25.319 with 7th A, T25.391-T25.399 with 7th A, T25.711-T25.719 with 7th A, T25.791-T25.799 with 7th A

7 ✓7ᵗʰ **T25.712** **Corrosion of third degree of left ankle** 🄲🄲
CC Excl: See code: T25.711

7 ✓7ᵗʰ **T25.719** **Corrosion of third degree of unspecified ankle** 🄲🄲
CC Excl: See code: T25.711

✓6ᵗʰ **T25.72** Corrosion of third degree of foot
EXCLUDES 2 corrosion of third degree of toe(s) (nail) (T25.73-)

7 ✓7ᵗʰ **T25.721** **Corrosion of third degree of right foot** 🄲🄲
CC Excl: CC with 7th character A: T24.301-T24.309 with 7th A, T24.391-T24.399 with 7th A, T24.701-T24.709 with 7th A, T24.791-T24.799 with 7th A, T25.321-T25.329 with 7th A, T25.391-T25.399 with 7th A, T25.721-T25.729 with 7th A, T25.791-T25.799 with 7th A

7 ✓7ᵗʰ **T25.722** **Corrosion of third degree of left foot** 🄲🄲
CC Excl: See code: T25.721

7 ✓7ᵗʰ **T25.729** **Corrosion of third degree of unspecified foot** 🄲🄲
CC Excl: See code: T25.721

---

7   HAC = Initial encounter only (7th character A, B or C) and not POA.

✓ Additional Character Required   ✓x7ᵗʰ Placeholder Alert   Unacceptable PDx   Manifestation   Hospital Acquired Condition   *EXCLUDES 1* Not Coded Here   *EXCLUDES 2* Not Included Here

✓6th **T25.73** Corrosion of third degree of toe(s) (nail)

    7 ✓7th **T25.731** **Corrosion of third degree of right toe(s) (nail)** CC
         CC Excl: CC with 7th character A: T24.301-T24.309 with 7th A, T24.391-T24.399 with 7th A, T24.701-T24.709 with 7th A, T24.791-T24.799 with 7th A, T25.331-T25.399 with 7th A, T25.731-T25.799 with 7th A

    7 ✓7th **T25.732** **Corrosion of third degree of left toe(s) (nail)** CC
         CC Excl: See code: T25.731

    7 ✓7th **T25.739** **Corrosion of third degree of unspecified toe(s) (nail)** CC
         CC Excl: See code: T25.731

✓6th **T25.79** Corrosion of third degree of multiple sites of ankle and foot

    7 ✓7th **T25.791** **Corrosion of third degree of multiple sites of right ankle and foot** CC
         CC Excl: CC with 7th character A: T24.301-T24.309 with 7th A, T24.391-T24.399 with 7th A, T24.701-T24.709 with 7th A, T24.791-T24.799 with 7th A, T25.391-T25.399 with 7th A, T25.791-T25.799 with 7th A

    7 ✓7th **T25.792** **Corrosion of third degree of multiple sites of left ankle and foot** CC
         CC Excl: See code: T25.791

    7 ✓7th **T25.799** **Corrosion of third degree of multiple sites of unspecified ankle and foot** CC
         CC Excl: See code: T25.791

Burns and corrosions confined to eye and internal organs (T26-T28)

✓4th **T26 Burn and corrosion confined to eye and adnexa**

> The appropriate 7th character is to be added to each code from category T26.
> A   initial encounter
> D   subsequent encounter
> S   sequela

✓5th **T26.0 Burn of eyelid and periocular area**
> Use additional external cause code to identify the source, place and intent of the burn (X00-X19, X75-X77, X96-X98, Y92)

   ✓x7th **T26.00** Burn of unspecified eyelid and periocular area
   ✓x7th **T26.01** Burn of right eyelid and periocular area
   ✓x7th **T26.02** Burn of left eyelid and periocular area

✓5th **T26.1 Burn of cornea and conjunctival sac**
> Use additional external cause code to identify the source, place and intent of the burn (X00-X19, X75-X77, X96-X98, Y92)

   ✓x7th **T26.10** Burn of cornea and conjunctival sac, unspecified eye
   ✓x7th **T26.11** Burn of cornea and conjunctival sac, right eye
   ✓x7th **T26.12** Burn of cornea and conjunctival sac, left eye

✓5th **T26.2 Burn with resulting rupture and destruction of eyeball**
> Use additional external cause code to identify the source, place and intent of the burn (X00-X19, X75-X77, X96-X98, Y92)

   7 ✓x7th **T26.20** **Burn with resulting rupture and destruction of unspecified eyeball** CC
      CC Excl: No Excl

   7 ✓x7th **T26.21** **Burn with resulting rupture and destruction of right eyeball** CC
      CC Excl: No Excl

   7 ✓x7th **T26.22** **Burn with resulting rupture and destruction of left eyeball** CC
      CC Excl: No Excl

✓5th **T26.3 Burns of other specified parts of eye and adnexa**
> Use additional external cause code to identify the source, place and intent of the burn (X00-X19, X75-X77, X96-X98, Y92)

   ✓x7th **T26.30** Burns of other specified parts of unspecified eye and adnexa
   ✓x7th **T26.31** Burns of other specified parts of right eye and adnexa
   ✓x7th **T26.32** Burns of other specified parts of left eye and adnexa

✓5th **T26.4 Burn of eye and adnexa, part unspecified**
> Use additional external cause code to identify the source, place and intent of the burn (X00-X19, X75-X77, X96-X98, Y92)

   ✓x7th **T26.40** Burn of unspecified eye and adnexa, part unspecified
   ✓x7th **T26.41** Burn of right eye and adnexa, part unspecified
   ✓x7th **T26.42** Burn of left eye and adnexa, part unspecified

✓5th **T26.5 Corrosion of eyelid and periocular area**
> Code first (T51-T65) to identify chemical and intent
> Use additional external cause code to identify place (Y92)

   ✓x7th **T26.50** Corrosion of unspecified eyelid and periocular area
   ✓x7th **T26.51** Corrosion of right eyelid and periocular area
   ✓x7th **T26.52** Corrosion of left eyelid and periocular area

✓5th **T26.6 Corrosion of cornea and conjunctival sac**
> Code first (T51-T65) to identify chemical and intent
> Use additional external cause code to identify place (Y92)

   ✓x7th **T26.60** Corrosion of cornea and conjunctival sac, unspecified eye
   ✓x7th **T26.61** Corrosion of cornea and conjunctival sac, right eye
   ✓x7th **T26.62** Corrosion of cornea and conjunctival sac, left eye

✓5th **T26.7 Corrosion with resulting rupture and destruction of eyeball**
> Code first (T51-T65) to identify chemical and intent
> Use additional external cause code to identify place (Y92)

   7 ✓x7th **T26.70** **Corrosion with resulting rupture and destruction of unspecified eyeball** CC
      CC Excl: No Excl

   7 ✓x7th **T26.71** **Corrosion with resulting rupture and destruction of right eyeball** CC
      CC Excl: No Excl

   7 ✓x7th **T26.72** **Corrosion with resulting rupture and destruction of left eyeball** CC
      CC Excl: No Excl

✓5th **T26.8 Corrosions of other specified parts of eye and adnexa**
> Code first (T51-T65) to identify chemical and intent
> Use additional external cause code to identify place (Y92)

   ✓x7th **T26.80** Corrosions of other specified parts of unspecified eye and adnexa
   ✓x7th **T26.81** Corrosions of other specified parts of right eye and adnexa
   ✓x7th **T26.82** Corrosions of other specified parts of left eye and adnexa

✓5th **T26.9 Corrosion of eye and adnexa, part unspecified**
> Code first (T51-T65) to identify chemical and intent
> Use additional external cause code to identify place (Y92)

   ✓x7th **T26.90** Corrosion of unspecified eye and adnexa, part unspecified
   ✓x7th **T26.91** Corrosion of right eye and adnexa, part unspecified
   ✓x7th **T26.92** Corrosion of left eye and adnexa, part unspecified

✓4th **T27 Burn and corrosion of respiratory tract**
> Use additional external cause code to identify the source and intent of the burn (X00-X19, X75-X77, X96-X98)
> Use additional external cause code to identify place (Y92)

> The appropriate 7th character is to be added to each code from category T27.
> A   initial encounter
> D   subsequent encounter
> S   sequela

> **CC Excl:** For CC codes in subcategory T27: CC with 7th character A: T27.0XX-T27.7XX with 7th A, T28.3XX-T28.49X with 7th A, T28.8XX-T28.99X with 7th A

   7 ✓x7th **T27.0** **Burn of larynx and trachea** CC
   7 ✓x7th **T27.1** **Burn involving larynx and trachea with lung** CC
   7 ✓x7th **T27.2** **Burn of other parts of respiratory tract** CC
      Burn of thoracic cavity
   7 ✓x7th **T27.3** **Burn of respiratory tract, part unspecified** CC
      Code first (T51-T65) to identify chemical and intent for codes T27.4-T27.7
   7 ✓x7th **T27.4** **Corrosion of larynx and trachea** CC
   7 ✓x7th **T27.5** **Corrosion involving larynx and trachea with lung** CC
   7 ✓x7th **T27.6** **Corrosion of other parts of respiratory tract** CC
   7 ✓x7th **T27.7** **Corrosion of respiratory tract, part unspecified** CC

---

7   HAC = Initial encounter only (7th character A, B or C) and not POA.

N Newborn: 0   P Pediatric: 0-17   M Maternity: 12-55   A Adult: 15-124   **MCC** Major CC Condition   **PDxMCC** PDx acts as own MCC   **CC** CC Condition   **PDxCC** PDx acts as own CC

✓4ᵗʰ **T28 Burn and corrosion of other internal organs**

Use additional external cause code to identify the source and intent of the burn (X00- X19, X75-X77, X96-X98)

Use additional external cause code to identify place (Y92)

> The appropriate 7th character is to be added to each code from category T28.
> A   initial encounter
> D   subsequent encounter
> S   sequela

✓x7ᵗʰ **T28.0 Burn of mouth and pharynx**

7 ✓x7ᵗʰ **T28.1 Burn of esophagus**   CC

CC Excl: CC with 7th character A: T28.1XXA, T28.3XX-T28.49X with 7th A, T28.6XXA, T28.8XX-T28.99X with 7th A

7 ✓x7ᵗʰ **T28.2 Burn of other parts of alimentary tract**   CC

CC Excl: CC with 7th character A: T28.2XX-T28.49X with 7th A, T28.7XX-T28.99X with 7th A

✓x7ᵗʰ **T28.3 Burn of internal genitourinary organs**

✓5ᵗʰ **T28.4 Burns of other and unspecified internal organs**

✓x7ᵗʰ **T28.40 Burn of unspecified internal organ**

✓6ᵗʰ **T28.41 Burn of ear drum**

✓7ᵗʰ **T28.411 Burn of right ear drum**

✓7ᵗʰ **T28.412 Burn of left ear drum**

✓7ᵗʰ **T28.419 Burn of unspecified ear drum**

✓x7ᵗʰ **T28.49 Burn of other internal organ**

Code first (T51-T65) to identify chemical and intent for T28.5-T28.9-

✓x7ᵗʰ **T28.5 Corrosion of mouth and pharynx**

7 ✓x7ᵗʰ **T28.6 Corrosion of esophagus**   CC

CC Excl: CC with 7th character A: T28.1XXA, T28.3XX-T28.49X with 7th A, T28.6XXA, T28.8XX-T28.99X with 7th A

7 ✓x7ᵗʰ **T28.7 Corrosion of other parts of alimentary tract**   CC

CC Excl: CC with 7th character A: T28.2XX-T28.49X with 7th A, T28.7XX-T28.99X with 7th A

✓x7ᵗʰ **T28.8 Corrosion of internal genitourinary organs**

✓5ᵗʰ **T28.9 Corrosions of other and unspecified internal organs**

✓x7ᵗʰ **T28.90 Corrosions of unspecified internal organs**

✓6ᵗʰ **T28.91 Corrosions of ear drum**

✓7ᵗʰ **T28.911 Corrosions of right ear drum**

✓7ᵗʰ **T28.912 Corrosions of left ear drum**

✓7ᵗʰ **T28.919 Corrosions of unspecified ear drum**

✓x7ᵗʰ **T28.99 Corrosions of other internal organs**

Burns and corrosions of multiple and unspecified body regions (T30-T32)

✓4ᵗʰ **T30 Burn and corrosion, body region unspecified**

T30.0 Burn of unspecified body region, unspecified degree

> NOTE   This code is not for inpatient use. Code to specified site and degree of burns.

Burn NOS   Multiple burns NOS

T30.4 Corrosion of unspecified body region, unspecified degree

> NOTE   This code is not for inpatient use. Code to specified site and degree of corrosion.

Corrosion NOS   Multiple corrosion NOS

✓4ᵗʰ **T31 Burns classified according to extent of body surface involved**

> NOTE   This category is to be used as the primary code only when the site of the burn is unspecified. It should be used as a supplementary code with categories T20-T25 when the site is specified.

CC Excl: For CC codes in category T31: CC or MCC as indicated with 7th A, unless otherwise noted: T31.0-T32.99

T31.0 Burns involving less than 10% of body surface

✓5ᵗʰ **T31.1 Burns involving 10-19% of body surface**

T31.10 Burns involving 10-19% of body surface with 0% to 9% third degree burns   CC

Burns involving 10-19% of body surface NOS

T31.11 Burns involving 10-19% of body surface with 10-19% third degree burns   CC

✓5ᵗʰ **T31.2 Burns involving 20-29% of body surface**

T31.20 Burns involving 20-29% of body surface with 0% to 9% third degree burns   CC

Burns involving 20-29% of body surface NOS

T31.21 Burns involving 20-29% of body surface with 10-19% third degree burns   MCC

T31.22 Burns involving 20-29% of body surface with 20-29% third degree burns   MCC

✓5ᵗʰ **T31.3 Burns involving 30-39% of body surface**

T31.30 Burns involving 30-39% of body surface with 0% to 9% third degree burns   CC

Burns involving 30-39% of body surface NOS

T31.31 Burns involving 30-39% of body surface with 10-19% third degree burns   MCC

T31.32 Burns involving 30-39% of body surface with 20-29% third degree burns   MCC

T31.33 Burns involving 30-39% of body surface 30-39% third degree burns   MCC

✓5ᵗʰ **T31.4 Burns involving 40-49% of body surface**

T31.40 Burns involving 40-49% of body surface with 0% to 9% third degree burns   CC

Burns involving 40-49% of body surface NOS

T31.41 Burns involving 40-49% of body surface with 10-19% third degree burns   MCC

T31.42 Burns involving 40-49% of body surface with 20-29% third degree burns   MCC

T31.43 Burns involving 40-49% of body surface with 30-39% third degree burns   MCC

T31.44 Burns involving 40-49% of body surface with 40-49% third degree burns   MCC

✓5ᵗʰ **T31.5 Burns involving 50-59% of body surface**

T31.50 Burns involving 50-59% of body surface with 0% to 9% third degree burns   CC

Burns involving 50-59% of body surface NOS

T31.51 Burns involving 50-59% of body surface with 10-19% third degree burns   MCC

T31.52 Burns involving 50-59% of body surface with 20-29% third degree burns   MCC

T31.53 Burns involving 50-59% of body surface with 30-39% third degree burns   MCC

T31.54 Burns involving 50-59% of body surface with 40-49% third degree burns   MCC

T31.55 Burns involving 50-59% of body surface with 50-59% third degree burns   MCC

✓5ᵗʰ **T31.6 Burns involving 60-69% of body surface**

T31.60 Burns involving 60-69% of body surface with 0% to 9% third degree burns   CC

Burns involving 60-69% of body surface NOS

T31.61 Burns involving 60-69% of body surface with 10-19% third degree burns   MCC

T31.62 Burns involving 60-69% of body surface with 20-29% third degree burns   MCC

T31.63 Burns involving 60-69% of body surface with 30-39% third degree burns   MCC

T31.64 Burns involving 60-69% of body surface with 40-49% third degree burns   MCC

T31.65 Burns involving 60-69% of body surface with 50-59% third degree burns   MCC

T31.66 Burns involving 60-69% of body surface with 60-69% third degree burns   MCC

✓5ᵗʰ **T31.7 Burns involving 70-79% of body surface**

T31.70 Burns involving 70-79% of body surface with 0% to 9% third degree burns   CC

Burns involving 70-79% of body surface NOS

T31.71 Burns involving 70-79% of body surface with 10-19% third degree burns   MCC

T31.72 Burns involving 70-79% of body surface with 20-29% third degree burns   MCC

T31.73 Burns involving 70-79% of body surface with 30-39% third degree burns   MCC

T31.74 Burns involving 70-79% of body surface with 40-49% third degree burns   MCC

T31.75 Burns involving 70-79% of body surface with 50-59% third degree burns   MCC

T31.76 Burns involving 70-79% of body surface with 60-69% third degree burns   MCC

T31.77 Burns involving 70-79% of body surface with 70-79% third degree burns   MCC

---

7   HAC = Initial encounter only (7th character A, B or C) and not POA.

✓ Additional Character Required   ✓x7ᵗʰ Placeholder Alert   Unacceptable PDx   Manifestation   Hospital Acquired Condition   **EXCLUDES 1** Not Coded Here   *EXCLUDES 2* Not Included Here

ICD-10-CM 2016   1093

✓5ᵗʰ **T31.8** Burns involving 80-89% of body surface

T31.80 **Burns involving 80-89% of body surface with 0% to 9% third degree burns** `CC`
Burns involving 80-89% of body surface NOS

T31.81 **Burns involving 80-89% of body surface with 10-19% third degree burns** `MCC`

T31.82 **Burns involving 80-89% of body surface with 20-29% third degree burns** `MCC`

T31.83 **Burns involving 80-89% of body surface with 30-39% third degree burns** `MCC`

T31.84 **Burns involving 80-89% of body surface with 40-49% third degree burns** `MCC`

T31.85 **Burns involving 80-89% of body surface with 50-59% third degree burns** `MCC`

T31.86 **Burns involving 80-89% of body surface with 60-69% third degree burns** `MCC`

T31.87 **Burns involving 80-89% of body surface with 70-79% third degree burns** `MCC`

T31.88 **Burns involving 80-89% of body surface with 80-89% third degree burns** `MCC`

✓5ᵗʰ **T31.9** Burns involving 90% or more of body surface

T31.90 **Burns involving 90% or more of body surface with 0% to 9% third degree burns** `CC`
Burns involving 90% or more of body surface NOS

T31.91 **Burns involving 90% or more of body surface with 10-19% third degree burns** `MCC`

T31.92 **Burns involving 90% or more of body surface with 20-29% third degree burns** `MCC`

T31.93 **Burns involving 90% or more of body surface with 30-39% third degree burns** `MCC`

T31.94 **Burns involving 90% or more of body surface with 40-49% third degree burns** `MCC`

T31.95 **Burns involving 90% or more of body surface with 50-59% third degree burns** `MCC`

T31.96 **Burns involving 90% or more of body surface with 60-69% third degree burns** `MCC`

T31.97 **Burns involving 90% or more of body surface with 70-79% third degree burns** `MCC`

T31.98 **Burns involving 90% or more of body surface with 80-89% third degree burns** `MCC`

T31.99 **Burns involving 90% or more of body surface with 90% or more third degree burns** `MCC`

✓4ᵗʰ **T32** **Corrosions classified according to extent of body surface involved**
`NOTE` This category is to be used as the primary code only when the site of the corrosion is unspecified. It may be used as a supplementary code with categories T20-T25 when the site is specified.

CC Excl: For CC/MCC codes in category T32: CC or MCC as indicated with 7th A, unless otherwise noted:
See code: T31

T32.0 **Corrosions involving less than 10% of body surface**

✓5ᵗʰ **T32.1** Corrosions involving 10-19% of body surface

T32.10 **Corrosions involving 10-19% of body surface with 0% to 9% third degree corrosion** `CC`
Corrosions involving 10-19% of body surface NOS

T32.11 **Corrosions involving 10-19% of body surface with 10-19% third degree corrosion** `CC`

✓5ᵗʰ **T32.2** Corrosions involving 20-29% of body surface

T32.20 **Corrosions involving 20-29% of body surface with 0% to 9% third degree corrosion** `CC`

T32.21 **Corrosions involving 20-29% of body surface with 10-19% third degree corrosion** `MCC`

T32.22 **Corrosions involving 20-29% of body surface with 20-29% third degree corrosion** `MCC`

✓5ᵗʰ **T32.3** Corrosions involving 30-39% of body surface

T32.30 **Corrosions involving 30-39% of body surface with 0% to 9% third degree corrosion** `CC`

T32.31 **Corrosions involving 30-39% of body surface with 10-19% third degree corrosion** `MCC`

T32.32 **Corrosions involving 30-39% of body surface with 20-29% third degree corrosion** `MCC`

T32.33 **Corrosions involving 30-39% of body surface with 30-39% third degree corrosion** `MCC`

✓5ᵗʰ **T32.4** Corrosions involving 40-49% of body surface

T32.40 **Corrosions involving 40-49% of body surface with 0% to 9% third degree corrosion** `CC`

T32.41 **Corrosions involving 40-49% of body surface with 10-19% third degree corrosion** `MCC`

T32.42 **Corrosions involving 40-49% of body surface with 20-29% third degree corrosion** `MCC`

T32.43 **Corrosions involving 40-49% of body surface with 30-39% third degree corrosion** `MCC`

T32.44 **Corrosions involving 40-49% of body surface with 40-49% third degree corrosion** `MCC`

✓5ᵗʰ **T32.5** Corrosions involving 50-59% of body surface

T32.50 **Corrosions involving 50-59% of body surface with 0% to 9% third degree corrosion** `CC`

T32.51 **Corrosions involving 50-59% of body surface with 10-19% third degree corrosion** `MCC`

T32.52 **Corrosions involving 50-59% of body surface with 20-29% third degree corrosion** `MCC`

T32.53 **Corrosions involving 50-59% of body surface with 30-39% third degree corrosion** `MCC`

T32.54 **Corrosions involving 50-59% of body surface with 40-49% third degree corrosion** `MCC`

T32.55 **Corrosions involving 50-59% of body surface with 50-59% third degree corrosion** `MCC`

✓5ᵗʰ **T32.6** Corrosions involving 60-69% of body surface

T32.60 **Corrosions involving 60-69% of body surface with 0% to 9% third degree corrosion** `CC`

T32.61 **Corrosions involving 60-69% of body surface with 10-19% third degree corrosion** `MCC`

T32.62 **Corrosions involving 60-69% of body surface with 20-29% third degree corrosion** `MCC`

T32.63 **Corrosions involving 60-69% of body surface with 30-39% third degree corrosion** `MCC`

T32.64 **Corrosions involving 60-69% of body surface with 40-49% third degree corrosion** `MCC`

T32.65 **Corrosions involving 60-69% of body surface with 50-59% third degree corrosion** `MCC`

T32.66 **Corrosions involving 60-69% of body surface with 60-69% third degree corrosion** `MCC`

✓5ᵗʰ **T32.7** Corrosions involving 70-79% of body surface

T32.70 **Corrosions involving 70-79% of body surface with 0% to 9% third degree corrosion** `CC`

T32.71 **Corrosions involving 70-79% of body surface with 10-19% third degree corrosion** `MCC`

T32.72 **Corrosions involving 70-79% of body surface with 20-29% third degree corrosion** `MCC`

T32.73 **Corrosions involving 70-79% of body surface with 30-39% third degree corrosion** `MCC`

T32.74 **Corrosions involving 70-79% of body surface with 40-49% third degree corrosion** `MCC`

T32.75 **Corrosions involving 70-79% of body surface with 50-59% third degree corrosion** `MCC`

T32.76 **Corrosions involving 70-79% of body surface with 60-69% third degree corrosion** `MCC`

T32.77 **Corrosions involving 70-79% of body surface with 70-79% third degree corrosion** `MCC`

✓5ᵗʰ **T32.8** Corrosions involving 80-89% of body surface

T32.80 **Corrosions involving 80-89% of body surface with 0% to 9% third degree corrosion** `CC`

T32.81 **Corrosions involving 80-89% of body surface with 10-19% third degree corrosion** `MCC`

T32.82 **Corrosions involving 80-89% of body surface with 20-29% third degree corrosion** `MCC`

T32.83 **Corrosions involving 80-89% of body surface with 30-39% third degree corrosion** `MCC`

T32.84 **Corrosions involving 80-89% of body surface with 40-49% third degree corrosion** `MCC`

T32.85 **Corrosions involving 80-89% of body surface with 50-59% third degree corrosion** `MCC`

T32.86 **Corrosions involving 80-89% of body surface with 60-69% third degree corrosion** `MCC`

T32.87 **Corrosions involving 80-89% of body surface with 70-79% third degree corrosion** `MCC`

T32.88 **Corrosions involving 80-89% of body surface with 80-89% third degree corrosion** `MCC`

Ⓝ Newborn: 0   Ⓟ Pediatric: 0-17   Ⓜ Maternity: 12-55   Ⓐ Adult: 15-124   `MCC` Major CC Condition   `PDxMCC` PDx acts as own MCC   `CC` CC Condition   `PDxCC` PDx acts as own CC

1094   ICD-10-CM 2016

√5ᵗʰ **T32.9 Corrosions involving 90% or more of body surface**

T32.90 **Corrosions involving 90% or more of body surface with 0% to 9% third degree corrosion** `CC`

T32.91 **Corrosions involving 90% or more of body surface with 10-19% third degree corrosion** `MCC`

T32.92 **Corrosions involving 90% or more of body surface with 20-29% third degree corrosion** `MCC`

T32.93 **Corrosions involving 90% or more of body surface with 30-39% third degree corrosion** `MCC`

T32.94 **Corrosions involving 90% or more of body surface with 40-49% third degree corrosion** `MCC`

T32.95 **Corrosions involving 90% or more of body surface with 50-59% third degree corrosion** `MCC`

T32.96 **Corrosions involving 90% or more of body surface with 60-69% third degree corrosion** `MCC`

T32.97 **Corrosions involving 90% or more of body surface with 70-79% third degree corrosion** `MCC`

T32.98 **Corrosions involving 90% or more of body surface with 80-89% third degree corrosion** `MCC`

T32.99 **Corrosions involving 90% or more of body surface with 90% or more third degree corrosion** `MCC`

Frostbite (T33-T34)

EXCLUDES 2   *hypothermia and other effects of reduced temperature (T68, T69-)*

√4ᵗʰ **T33 Superficial frostbite**

INCLUDES   frostbite with partial thickness skin loss

The appropriate 7th character is to be added to each code from category T33.
A   initial encounter
D   subsequent encounter
S   sequela

√5ᵗʰ **T33.0 Superficial frostbite of head**

CC Excl: For CC codes in subcategory T33.0 and T33.1: CC with 7th character A, unless otherwise noted:T33.011-T33.42X with 7th A, T33.60X-T33.72X with 7th A, T33.90X-T34.42X with 7th A, T34.60X-T34.72X with 7th A, T34.90X-T34.99X with 7th A

√6ᵗʰ **T33.01 Superficial frostbite of ear**

7 √7ᵗʰ **T33.011 Superficial frostbite of right ear** `CC`

7 √7ᵗʰ **T33.012 Superficial frostbite of left ear** `CC`

7 √7ᵗʰ **T33.019 Superficial frostbite of unspecified ear** `CC`

7 √x7ᵗʰ **T33.02 Superficial frostbite of nose** `CC`

7 √x7ᵗʰ **T33.09 Superficial frostbite of other part of head** `CC`

7 √x7ᵗʰ **T33.1 Superficial frostbite of neck** `CC`
CC Excl: T33.011-T34.99X with 7th A, T69.021-T69.029 with 7th A

7 √x7ᵗʰ **T33.2 Superficial frostbite of thorax** `CC`
CC Excl: For CC codes in subcategory T33.2: CC with 7th character A, unless otherwise noted: T33.011-T34.99X with 7th A, T69.021-T69.029 with 7th A

7 √x7ᵗʰ **T33.3 Superficial frostbite of abdominal wall, lower back and pelvis** `CC`
CC Excl: See code: T33.2

√5ᵗʰ **T33.4 Superficial frostbite of arm**

EXCLUDES 2   *superficial frostbite of wrist and hand (T33.5-)*

CC Excl: For CC codes in subcategory T33.4: CC with 7th character A, unless otherwise noted: T33.011-T34.99X with 7th A, T69.021-T69.029 with 7th A

7 √x7ᵗʰ **T33.40 Superficial frostbite of unspecified arm** `CC`

7 √x7ᵗʰ **T33.41 Superficial frostbite of right arm** `CC`

7 √x7ᵗʰ **T33.42 Superficial frostbite of left arm** `CC`

√5ᵗʰ **T33.5 Superficial frostbite of wrist, hand, and fingers**

CC Excl: For CC codes in subcategory T33.5: CC with 7th character A, unless otherwise noted: T33.2XX-T33.72X with 7th A, T33.90X-T33.99X with 7th A, T34.2XX-T34.72X with 7th A, T34.90X-T34.99X with 7th A

√6ᵗʰ **T33.51 Superficial frostbite of wrist**

7 √7ᵗʰ **T33.511 Superficial frostbite of right wrist** `CC`

7 √7ᵗʰ **T33.512 Superficial frostbite of left wrist** `CC`

7 √7ᵗʰ **T33.519 Superficial frostbite of unspecified wrist** `CC`

√6ᵗʰ **T33.52 Superficial frostbite of hand**
EXCLUDES 2   *superficial frostbite of fingers (T33.53-)*

7 √7ᵗʰ **T33.521 Superficial frostbite of right hand** `CC`

7 √7ᵗʰ **T33.522 Superficial frostbite of left hand** `CC`

7 √7ᵗʰ **T33.529 Superficial frostbite of unspecified hand** `CC`

√6ᵗʰ **T33.53 Superficial frostbite of finger(s)**

7 √7ᵗʰ **T33.531 Superficial frostbite of right finger(s)** `CC`

7 √7ᵗʰ **T33.532 Superficial frostbite of left finger(s)** `CC`

7 √7ᵗʰ **T33.539 Superficial frostbite of unspecified finger(s)** `CC`

√5ᵗʰ **T33.6 Superficial frostbite of hip and thigh**

CC Excl: For CC codes in subcategory T33.6: CC with 7th character A, unless otherwise noted: T33.011-T34.99X with 7th A, T69.021-T69.029 with 7th A

7 √x7ᵗʰ **T33.60 Superficial frostbite of unspecified hip and thigh** `CC`

7 √x7ᵗʰ **T33.61 Superficial frostbite of right hip and thigh** `CC`

7 √x7ᵗʰ **T33.62 Superficial frostbite of left hip and thigh** `CC`

√5ᵗʰ **T33.7 Superficial frostbite of knee and lower leg**

CC Excl: For CC codes in subcategory T33.7: CC with 7th character A, unless otherwise noted: See code: T33.6

EXCLUDES 2   *superficial frostbite of ankle and foot (T33.8-)*

7 √x7ᵗʰ **T33.70 Superficial frostbite of unspecified knee and lower leg** `CC`

7 √x7ᵗʰ **T33.71 Superficial frostbite of right knee and lower leg** `CC`

7 √x7ᵗʰ **T33.72 Superficial frostbite of left knee and lower leg** `CC`

√5ᵗʰ **T33.8 Superficial frostbite of ankle, foot, and toe(s)**

CC Excl: For CC codes in subcategory T33.8: CC with 7th character A, unless otherwise noted: T33.2XX-T33.42X with 7th A, T33.60X-T33.99X with 7th A, T34.2XX-T34.42X with 7th A, T34.60X-T34.99X with 7th A

√6ᵗʰ **T33.81 Superficial frostbite of ankle**

7 √7ᵗʰ **T33.811 Superficial frostbite of right ankle** `CC`

7 √7ᵗʰ **T33.812 Superficial frostbite of left ankle** `CC`

7 √7ᵗʰ **T33.819 Superficial frostbite of unspecified ankle** `CC`

√6ᵗʰ **T33.82 Superficial frostbite of foot**

7 √7ᵗʰ **T33.821 Superficial frostbite of right foot** `CC`

7 √7ᵗʰ **T33.822 Superficial frostbite of left foot** `CC`

7 √7ᵗʰ **T33.829 Superficial frostbite of unspecified foot** `CC`

√6ᵗʰ **T33.83 Superficial frostbite of toe(s)**

7 √7ᵗʰ **T33.831 Superficial frostbite of right toe(s)** `CC`

7 √7ᵗʰ **T33.832 Superficial frostbite of left toe(s)** `CC`

7 √7ᵗʰ **T33.839 Superficial frostbite of unspecified toe(s)** `CC`

√5ᵗʰ **T33.9 Superficial frostbite of other and unspecified sites**

CC Excl: For CC codes in subcategory T33.9: CC with 7th character A, unless otherwise noted: T33.011-T34.99X with 7th A, T69.021-T69.029 with 7th A

7 √x7ᵗʰ **T33.90 Superficial frostbite of unspecified sites** `CC`
Superficial frostbite NOS

7 √x7ᵗʰ **T33.99 Superficial frostbite of other sites** `CC`
Superficial frostbite of leg NOS
Superficial frostbite of trunk NOS

√4ᵗʰ **T34 Frostbite with tissue necrosis**

The appropriate 7th character is to be added to each code from category T34.
A   initial encounter
D   subsequent encounter
S   sequela

√5ᵗʰ **T34.0 Frostbite with tissue necrosis of head**

CC Excl: For CC codes in subcategory T34.0: CC with 7th character A, unless otherwise noted: T33.011-T33.42 with 7th A, T33.60X-T33.72X with 7th A, T33.90X-T34.42X with 7th A, T34.60X-T34.72X with 7th A, T34.90X-T34.99X with 7th A

---

7   HAC = Initial encounter only (7th character A, B or C) and not POA.

☑ Additional Character Required   √x7ᵗʰ Placeholder Alert   Unacceptable PDx   Manifestation   Hospital Acquired Condition   EXCLUDES 1 Not Coded Here   EXCLUDES 2 Not Included Here

√6ᵗʰ T34.01   **Frostbite with tissue necrosis of ear**

7   √7ᵗʰ **T34.011**   **Frostbite with tissue necrosis of right ear**   CC

7   √7ᵗʰ **T34.012**   **Frostbite with tissue necrosis of left ear**   CC

7   √7ᵗʰ **T34.019**   **Frostbite with tissue necrosis of unspecified ear**   CC

7   √x7ᵗʰ **T34.02**   **Frostbite with tissue necrosis of nose**   CC

7   √x7ᵗʰ **T34.09**   **Frostbite with tissue necrosis of other part of head**   CC

7   √x7ᵗʰ **T34.1**   **Frostbite with tissue necrosis of neck**   CC
CC Excl: CC with 7th character A: T33.011-T33.42X with 7th A, T33.60X-T33.72X with 7th A, T33.90X-T34.42X with 7th A, T34.60X-T34.72X with 7th A, T34.90X-T34.99X with 7th A

7   √x7ᵗʰ **T34.2**   **Frostbite with tissue necrosis of thorax**   CC
CC Excl: CC with 7th character A: T33.011-T34.99X with 7th A, T69.021-T69.029 with 7th A

7   √x7ᵗʰ **T34.3**   **Frostbite with tissue necrosis of abdominal wall, lower back and pelvis**   CC
CC Excl: CC with 7th character A: See code: T34.2

√5ᵗʰ T34.4   **Frostbite with tissue necrosis of arm**
EXCLUDES 2   frostbite with tissue necrosis of wrist and hand (T34.5-)

CC Excl: For CC codes in subcategory T34.4: CC with 7th character A, unless otherwise noted: See code: T34.2

7   √x7ᵗʰ **T34.40**   **Frostbite with tissue necrosis of unspecified arm**   CC

7   √x7ᵗʰ **T34.41**   **Frostbite with tissue necrosis of right arm**   CC

7   √x7ᵗʰ **T34.42**   **Frostbite with tissue necrosis of left arm**   CC

√5ᵗʰ T34.5   **Frostbite with tissue necrosis of wrist, hand, and finger(s)**

CC Excl: For CC codes in subcategory T34.5: CC with 7th character A, unless otherwise noted: T33.2XX-T33.72X with 7th A, T33.90X-T33.99X with 7th A, T34.2XX-T34.72X with 7th A, T34.90X-T34.99X with 7th A

√6ᵗʰ T34.51   **Frostbite with tissue necrosis of wrist**

7   √7ᵗʰ **T34.511**   **Frostbite with tissue necrosis of right wrist**   CC

7   √7ᵗʰ **T34.512**   **Frostbite with tissue necrosis of left wrist**   CC

7   √7ᵗʰ **T34.519**   **Frostbite with tissue necrosis of unspecified wrist**   CC

√6ᵗʰ T34.52   **Frostbite with tissue necrosis of hand**
EXCLUDES 2   frostbite with tissue necrosis of finger(s) (T34.53-)

7   √7ᵗʰ **T34.521**   **Frostbite with tissue necrosis of right hand**   CC

7   √7ᵗʰ **T34.522**   **Frostbite with tissue necrosis of left hand**   CC

7   √7ᵗʰ **T34.529**   **Frostbite with tissue necrosis of unspecified hand**   CC

√6ᵗʰ T34.53   **Frostbite with tissue necrosis of finger(s)**

7   √7ᵗʰ **T34.531**   **Frostbite with tissue necrosis of right finger(s)**   CC

7   √7ᵗʰ **T34.532**   **Frostbite with tissue necrosis of left finger(s)**   CC

7   √7ᵗʰ **T34.539**   **Frostbite with tissue necrosis of unspecified finger(s)**   CC

√5ᵗʰ T34.6   **Frostbite with tissue necrosis of hip and thigh**

CC Excl: For CC codes in subcategory T34.6: CC with 7th character A, unless otherwise noted: T33.011-T34.99X with 7th A, T69.021-T69.029 with 7th A

7   √x7ᵗʰ **T34.60**   **Frostbite with tissue necrosis of unspecified hip and thigh**   CC

7   √x7ᵗʰ **T34.61**   **Frostbite with tissue necrosis of right hip and thigh**   CC

7   √x7ᵗʰ **T34.62**   **Frostbite with tissue necrosis of left hip and thigh**   CC

√5ᵗʰ T34.7   **Frostbite with tissue necrosis of knee and lower leg**
EXCLUDES 2   frostbite with tissue necrosis of ankle and foot (T34.8-)

CC Excl: For CC codes in subcategory T34.7: CC with 7th character A, unless otherwise noted: See code: T34.6

7   √x7ᵗʰ **T34.70**   **Frostbite with tissue necrosis of unspecified knee and lower leg**   CC

7   √x7ᵗʰ **T34.71**   **Frostbite with tissue necrosis of right knee and lower leg**   CC

7   √x7ᵗʰ **T34.72**   **Frostbite with tissue necrosis of left knee and lower leg**   CC

√5ᵗʰ T34.8   **Frostbite with tissue necrosis of ankle, foot, and toe(s)**

CC Excl: For CC codes in subcategory T34.8: CC with 7th character A, unless otherwise noted: T33.2XX-T33.42X with 7th A, T33.60X-T33.99X with 7th A, T34.2XX-T34.42X with 7th A, T34.60X-T34.99X with 7th A

√6ᵗʰ T34.81   **Frostbite with tissue necrosis of ankle**

7   √7ᵗʰ **T34.811**   **Frostbite with tissue necrosis of right ankle**   CC

7   √7ᵗʰ **T34.812**   **Frostbite with tissue necrosis of left ankle**   CC

7   √7ᵗʰ **T34.819**   **Frostbite with tissue necrosis of unspecified ankle**   CC

√6ᵗʰ T34.82   **Frostbite with tissue necrosis of foot**

7   √7ᵗʰ **T34.821**   **Frostbite with tissue necrosis of right foot**   CC

7   √7ᵗʰ **T34.822**   **Frostbite with tissue necrosis of left foot**   CC

7   √7ᵗʰ **T34.829**   **Frostbite with tissue necrosis of unspecified foot**   CC

√6ᵗʰ T34.83   **Frostbite with tissue necrosis of toe(s)**

7   √7ᵗʰ **T34.831**   **Frostbite with tissue necrosis of right toe(s)**   CC

7   √7ᵗʰ **T34.832**   **Frostbite with tissue necrosis of left toe(s)**   CC

7   √7ᵗʰ **T34.839**   **Frostbite with tissue necrosis of unspecified toe(s)**   CC

√5ᵗʰ T34.9   **Frostbite with tissue necrosis of other and unspecified sites**

CC Excl: For CC codes in subcategory T34.9: CC with 7th character A, unless otherwise noted: T33.011-T34.99X with 7th A, T69.021-T69.029 with 7th A

7   √x7ᵗʰ **T34.90**   **Frostbite with tissue necrosis of unspecified sites**   CC
Frostbite with tissue necrosis NOS

7   √x7ᵗʰ **T34.99**   **Frostbite with tissue necrosis of other sites**   CC
Frostbite with tissue necrosis of leg NOS
Frostbite with tissue necrosis of trunk NOS

Poisoning by, adverse effects of and underdosing of drugs, medicaments and biological substances (T36-T50)

INCLUDES   adverse effect of correct substance properly administered
poisoning by overdose of substance
poisoning by wrong substance given or taken in error
underdosing by (inadvertently) (deliberately) taking less substance than prescribed or instructed

Code first, for adverse effects, the nature of the adverse effect, such as:
adverse effect NOS (T88.7)
aspirin gastritis (K29.-)
blood disorders (D56-D76)
contact dermatitis (L23-L25)
dermatitis due to substances taken internally (L27.-)
nephropathy (N14.0-N14.2)

NOTE   The drug giving rise to the adverse effect should be identified by use of codes from categories T36-T50 with fifth or sixth character 5.

Use additional code(s) to specify:
manifestations of poisoning
underdosing or failure in dosage during medical and surgical care (Y63.6, Y63.8-Y63.9)
underdosing of medication regimen (Z91.12-, Z91.13-)

EXCLUDES 1   toxic reaction to local anesthesia in pregnancy (O29.3-)
EXCLUDES 2   abuse and dependence of psychoactive substances (F10-F19)
abuse of non-dependence-producing substances (F55.-)
drug reaction and poisoning affecting newborn (P00-P96)
pathological drug intoxication (inebriation) (F10-F19)

---

7   HAC = Initial encounter only (7th character A, B or C) and not POA.

N Newborn: 0   P Pediatric: 0-17   M Maternity: 12-55   A Adult: 15-124   MCC Major CC Condition   PDxMCC PDx acts as own MCC   CC CC Condition   PDxCC PDx acts as own CC

1096   ICD-10-CM 2016

✓4th **T36** **Poisoning by, adverse effect of and underdosing of systemic antibiotics**

> EXCLUDES1   *antineoplastic antibiotics (T45.1-)*
> *locally applied antibiotic NEC (T49.0)*
> *topically used antibiotic for ear, nose and throat (T49.6)*
> *topically used antibiotic for eye (T49.5)*

> The appropriate 7th character is to be added to each code from category T36.
> A   initial encounter
> D   subsequent encounter
> S   sequela

✓5th **T36.0** **Poisoning by, adverse effect of and underdosing of penicillins**

   ✓6th **T36.0X** **Poisoning by, adverse effect of and underdosing of penicillins**

     ✓7th **T36.0X1** **Poisoning by penicillins, accidental (unintentional)**
       Poisoning by penicillins NOS

     ✓7th **T36.0X2** **Poisoning by penicillins, intentional self-harm**

     ✓7th **T36.0X3** **Poisoning by penicillins, assault**

     ✓7th **T36.0X4** **Poisoning by penicillins, undetermined**

     ✓7th **T36.0X5** **Adverse effect of penicillins**

     ✓7th **T36.0X6** **Underdosing of penicillins**

✓5th **T36.1** **Poisoning by, adverse effect of and underdosing of cephalosporins and other beta-lactam antibiotics**

   ✓6th **T36.1X** **Poisoning by, adverse effect of and underdosing of cephalosporins and other beta-lactam antibiotics**

     ✓7th **T36.1X1** **Poisoning by cephalosporins and other beta-lactam antibiotics, accidental (unintentional)**
       Poisoning by cephalosporins and other beta-lactam antibiotics NOS

     ✓7th **T36.1X2** **Poisoning by cephalosporins and other beta-lactam antibiotics, intentional self-harm**

     ✓7th **T36.1X3** **Poisoning by cephalosporins and other beta-lactam antibiotics, assault**

     ✓7th **T36.1X4** **Poisoning by cephalosporins and other beta-lactam antibiotics, undetermined**

     ✓7th **T36.1X5** **Adverse effect of cephalosporins and other beta-lactam antibiotics**

     ✓7th **T36.1X6** **Underdosing of cephalosporins and other beta-lactam antibiotics**

✓5th **T36.2** **Poisoning by, adverse effect of and underdosing of chloramphenicol group**

   ✓6th **T36.2X** **Poisoning by, adverse effect of and underdosing of chloramphenicol group**

     ✓7th **T36.2X1** **Poisoning by chloramphenicol group, accidental (unintentional)**
       Poisoning by chloramphenicol group NOS

     ✓7th **T36.2X2** **Poisoning by chloramphenicol group, intentional self-harm**

     ✓7th **T36.2X3** **Poisoning by chloramphenicol group, assault**

     ✓7th **T36.2X4** **Poisoning by chloramphenicol group, undetermined**

     ✓7th **T36.2X5** **Adverse effect of chloramphenicol group**

     ✓7th **T36.2X6** **Underdosing of chloramphenicol group**

✓5th **T36.3** **Poisoning by, adverse effect of and underdosing of macrolides**

   ✓6th **T36.3X** **Poisoning by, adverse effect of and underdosing of macrolides**

     ✓7th **T36.3X1** **Poisoning by macrolides, accidental (unintentional)**
       Poisoning by macrolides NOS

     ✓7th **T36.3X2** **Poisoning by macrolides, intentional self-harm**

     ✓7th **T36.3X3** **Poisoning by macrolides, assault**

     ✓7th **T36.3X4** **Poisoning by macrolides, undetermined**

     ✓7th **T36.3X5** **Adverse effect of macrolides**

     ✓7th **T36.3X6** **Underdosing of macrolides**

✓5th **T36.4** **Poisoning by, adverse effect of and underdosing of tetracyclines**

   ✓6th **T36.4X** **Poisoning by, adverse effect of and underdosing of tetracyclines**

     ✓7th **T36.4X1** **Poisoning by tetracyclines, accidental (unintentional)**
       Poisoning by tetracyclines NOS

     ✓7th **T36.4X2** **Poisoning by tetracyclines, intentional self-harm**

     ✓7th **T36.4X3** **Poisoning by tetracyclines, assault**

     ✓7th **T36.4X4** **Poisoning by tetracyclines, undetermined**

     ✓7th **T36.4X5** **Adverse effect of tetracyclines**

     ✓7th **T36.4X6** **Underdosing of tetracyclines**

✓5th **T36.5** **Poisoning by, adverse effect of and underdosing of aminoglycosides**
   Poisoning by, adverse effect of and underdosing of streptomycin

   ✓6th **T36.5X** **Poisoning by, adverse effect of and underdosing of aminoglycosides**

     ✓7th **T36.5X1** **Poisoning by aminoglycosides, accidental (unintentional)**
       Poisoning by aminoglycosides NOS

     ✓7th **T36.5X2** **Poisoning by aminoglycosides, intentional self-harm**

     ✓7th **T36.5X3** **Poisoning by aminoglycosides, assault**

     ✓7th **T36.5X4** **Poisoning by aminoglycosides, undetermined**

     ✓7th **T36.5X5** **Adverse effect of aminoglycosides**

     ✓7th **T36.5X6** **Underdosing of aminoglycosides**

✓5th **T36.6** **Poisoning by, adverse effect of and underdosing of rifampicins**

   ✓6th **T36.6X** **Poisoning by, adverse effect of and underdosing of rifampicins**

     ✓7th **T36.6X1** **Poisoning by rifampicins, accidental (unintentional)**
       Poisoning by rifampicins NOS

     ✓7th **T36.6X2** **Poisoning by rifampicins, intentional self-harm**

     ✓7th **T36.6X3** **Poisoning by rifampicins, assault**

     ✓7th **T36.6X4** **Poisoning by rifampicins, undetermined**

     ✓7th **T36.6X5** **Adverse effect of rifampicins**

     ✓7th **T36.6X6** **Underdosing of rifampicins**

✓5th **T36.7** **Poisoning by, adverse effect of and underdosing of antifungal antibiotics, systemically used**

   ✓6th **T36.7X** **Poisoning by, adverse effect of and underdosing of antifungal antibiotics, systemically used**

     ✓7th **T36.7X1** **Poisoning by antifungal antibiotics, systemically used, accidental (unintentional)**
       Poisoning by antifungal antibiotics, systemically used NOS

     ✓7th **T36.7X2** **Poisoning by antifungal antibiotics, systemically used, intentional self-harm**

     ✓7th **T36.7X3** **Poisoning by antifungal antibiotics, systemically used, assault**

     ✓7th **T36.7X4** **Poisoning by antifungal antibiotics, systemically used, undetermined**

     ✓7th **T36.7X5** **Adverse effect of antifungal antibiotics, systemically used**

     ✓7th **T36.7X6** **Underdosing of antifungal antibiotics, systemically used**

✓5th **T36.8** **Poisoning by, adverse effect of and underdosing of other systemic antibiotics**

   ✓6th **T36.8X** **Poisoning by, adverse effect of and underdosing of other systemic antibiotics**

     ✓7th **T36.8X1** **Poisoning by other systemic antibiotics, accidental (unintentional)**
       Poisoning by other systemic antibiotics NOS

     ✓7th **T36.8X2** **Poisoning by other systemic antibiotics, intentional self-harm**

     ✓7th **T36.8X3** **Poisoning by other systemic antibiotics, assault**

     ✓7th **T36.8X4** **Poisoning by other systemic antibiotics, undetermined**

     ✓7th **T36.8X5** **Adverse effect of other systemic antibiotics**

     ✓7th **T36.8X6** **Underdosing of other systemic antibiotics**

✓ Additional Character Required   ✓x7th Placeholder Alert   Unacceptable PDx   Manifestation   Hospital Acquired Condition   EXCLUDES1 Not Coded Here   EXCLUDES2 Not Included Here

Chapter 19. Injury, Poisoning, and Certain Other Consequences of External Causes

✓5ᵗʰ **T36.9** **Poisoning by, adverse effect of and underdosing of unspecified systemic antibiotic**

     ✓x7ᵗʰ **T36.91** **Poisoning by unspecified systemic antibiotic, accidental (unintentional)**
         Poisoning by systemic antibiotic NOS

     ✓x7ᵗʰ **T36.92** **Poisoning by unspecified systemic antibiotic, intentional self-harm**

     ✓x7ᵗʰ **T36.93** **Poisoning by unspecified systemic antibiotic, assault**

     ✓x7ᵗʰ **T36.94** **Poisoning by unspecified systemic antibiotic, undetermined**

     ✓x7ᵗʰ **T36.95** **Adverse effect of unspecified systemic antibiotic**

     ✓x7ᵗʰ **T36.96** **Underdosing of unspecified systemic antibiotic**

✓4ᵗʰ **T37** **Poisoning by, adverse effect of and underdosing of other systemic anti- infectives and antiparasitics**

     EXCLUDES 1   *anti-infectives topically used for ear, nose and throat (T49.6-)*
         anti-infectives topically used for eye (T49.5-)
         locally applied anti-infectives NEC (T49.0-)

> The appropriate 7th character is to be added to each code from category T37.
> A   initial encounter
> D   subsequent encounter
> S   sequela

✓5ᵗʰ **T37.0** **Poisoning by, adverse effect of and underdosing of sulfonamides**

     ✓6ᵗʰ **T37.0X** **Poisoning by, adverse effect of and underdosing of sulfonamides**

         ✓7ᵗʰ **T37.0X1** **Poisoning by sulfonamides, accidental (unintentional)**
             Poisoning by sulfonamides NOS

         ✓7ᵗʰ **T37.0X2** **Poisoning by sulfonamides, intentional self-harm**

         ✓7ᵗʰ **T37.0X3** **Poisoning by sulfonamides, assault**

         ✓7ᵗʰ **T37.0X4** **Poisoning by sulfonamides, undetermined**

         ✓7ᵗʰ **T37.0X5** **Adverse effect of sulfonamides**

         ✓7ᵗʰ **T37.0X6** **Underdosing of sulfonamides**

✓5ᵗʰ **T37.1** **Poisoning by, adverse effect of and underdosing of antimycobacterial drugs**

     EXCLUDES 1   *rifampicins (T36.6-)*
         streptomycin (T36.5-)

     ✓6ᵗʰ **T37.1X** **Poisoning by, adverse effect of and underdosing of antimycobacterial drugs**

         ✓7ᵗʰ **T37.1X1** **Poisoning by antimycobacterial drugs, accidental (unintentional)**
             Poisoning by antimycobacterial drugs NOS

         ✓7ᵗʰ **T37.1X2** **Poisoning by antimycobacterial drugs, intentional self-harm**

         ✓7ᵗʰ **T37.1X3** **Poisoning by antimycobacterial drugs, assault**

         ✓7ᵗʰ **T37.1X4** **Poisoning by antimycobacterial drugs, undetermined**

         ✓7ᵗʰ **T37.1X5** **Adverse effect of antimycobacterial drugs**

         ✓7ᵗʰ **T37.1X6** **Underdosing of antimycobacterial drugs**

✓5ᵗʰ **T37.2** **Poisoning by, adverse effect of and underdosing of antimalarials and drugs acting on other blood protozoa**

     EXCLUDES 1   *hydroxyquinoline derivatives (T37.8-)*

     ✓6ᵗʰ **T37.2X** **Poisoning by, adverse effect of and underdosing of antimalarials and drugs acting on other blood protozoa**

         ✓7ᵗʰ **T37.2X1** **Poisoning by antimalarials and drugs acting on other blood protozoa, accidental (unintentional)**
             Poisoning by antimalarials and drugs acting on other blood protozoa NOS

         ✓7ᵗʰ **T37.2X2** **Poisoning by antimalarials and drugs acting on other blood protozoa, intentional self-harm**

         ✓7ᵗʰ **T37.2X3** **Poisoning by antimalarials and drugs acting on other blood protozoa, assault**

         ✓7ᵗʰ **T37.2X4** **Poisoning by antimalarials and drugs acting on other blood protozoa, undetermined**

         ✓7ᵗʰ **T37.2X5** **Adverse effect of antimalarials and drugs acting on other blood protozoa**

     ✓7ᵗʰ **T37.2X6** **Underdosing of antimalarials and drugs acting on other blood protozoa**

✓5ᵗʰ **T37.3** **Poisoning by, adverse effect of and underdosing of other antiprotozoal drugs**

     ✓6ᵗʰ **T37.3X** **Poisoning by, adverse effect of and underdosing of other antiprotozoal drugs**

         ✓7ᵗʰ **T37.3X1** **Poisoning by other antiprotozoal drugs, accidental (unintentional)**
             Poisoning by other antiprotozoal drugs NOS

         ✓7ᵗʰ **T37.3X2** **Poisoning by other antiprotozoal drugs, intentional self-harm**

         ✓7ᵗʰ **T37.3X3** **Poisoning by other antiprotozoal drugs, assault**

         ✓7ᵗʰ **T37.3X4** **Poisoning by other antiprotozoal drugs, undetermined**

         ✓7ᵗʰ **T37.3X5** **Adverse effect of other antiprotozoal drugs**

         ✓7ᵗʰ **T37.3X6** **Underdosing of other antiprotozoal drugs**

✓5ᵗʰ **T37.4** **Poisoning by, adverse effect of and underdosing of anthelminthics**

     ✓6ᵗʰ **T37.4X** **Poisoning by, adverse effect of and underdosing of anthelminthics**

         ✓7ᵗʰ **T37.4X1** **Poisoning by anthelminthics, accidental (unintentional)**
             Poisoning by anthelminthics NOS

         ✓7ᵗʰ **T37.4X2** **Poisoning by anthelminthics, intentional self-harm**

         ✓7ᵗʰ **T37.4X3** **Poisoning by anthelminthics, assault**

         ✓7ᵗʰ **T37.4X4** **Poisoning by anthelminthics, undetermined**

         ✓7ᵗʰ **T37.4X5** **Adverse effect of anthelminthics**

         ✓7ᵗʰ **T37.4X6** **Underdosing of anthelminthics**

✓5ᵗʰ **T37.5** **Poisoning by, adverse effect of and underdosing of antiviral drugs**

     EXCLUDES 1   *amantadine (T42.8-)*
         cytarabine (T45.1-)

     ✓6ᵗʰ **T37.5X** **Poisoning by, adverse effect of and underdosing of antiviral drugs**

         ✓7ᵗʰ **T37.5X1** **Poisoning by antiviral drugs, accidental (unintentional)**
             Poisoning by antiviral drugs NOS

         ✓7ᵗʰ **T37.5X2** **Poisoning by antiviral drugs, intentional self-harm**

         ✓7ᵗʰ **T37.5X3** **Poisoning by antiviral drugs, assault**

         ✓7ᵗʰ **T37.5X4** **Poisoning by antiviral drugs, undetermined**

         ✓7ᵗʰ **T37.5X5** **Adverse effect of antiviral drugs**

         ✓7ᵗʰ **T37.5X6** **Underdosing of antiviral drugs**

✓5ᵗʰ **T37.8** **Poisoning by, adverse effect of and underdosing of other specified systemic anti-infectives and antiparasitics**
     Poisoning by, adverse effect of and underdosing of hydroxyquinoline derivatives

     EXCLUDES 1   *antimalarial drugs (T37.2-)*

     ✓6ᵗʰ **T37.8X** **Poisoning by, adverse effect of and underdosing of other specified systemic anti-infectives and antiparasitics**

         ✓7ᵗʰ **T37.8X1** **Poisoning by other specified systemic anti-infectives and antiparasitics, accidental (unintentional)**
             Poisoning by other specified systemic anti-infectives and antiparasitics NOS

         ✓7ᵗʰ **T37.8X2** **Poisoning by other specified systemic anti-infectives and antiparasitics, intentional self-harm**

         ✓7ᵗʰ **T37.8X3** **Poisoning by other specified systemic anti-infectives and antiparasitics, assault**

         ✓7ᵗʰ **T37.8X4** **Poisoning by other specified systemic anti-infectives and antiparasitics, undetermined**

         ✓7ᵗʰ **T37.8X5** **Adverse effect of other specified systemic anti-infectives and antiparasitics**

         ✓7ᵗʰ **T37.8X6** **Underdosing of other specified systemic anti-infectives and antiparasitics**

N Newborn: 0   P Pediatric: 0-17   M Maternity: 12-55   A Adult: 15-124   MCC Major CC Condition   PDxMCC PDx acts as own MCC   CC CC Condition   PDxCC PDx acts as own CC

1098   ICD-10-CM 2016

√5ᵗʰ **T37.9** **Poisoning by, adverse effect of and underdosing of unspecified systemic anti-infective and antiparasitics**

√x7ᵗʰ **T37.91** **Poisoning by unspecified systemic anti-infective and antiparasitics, accidental (unintentional)**
Poisoning by, adverse effect of and underdosing of systemic anti-infective and antiparasitics NOS

√x7ᵗʰ **T37.92** **Poisoning by unspecified systemic anti-infective and antiparasitics, intentional self-harm**

√x7ᵗʰ **T37.93** **Poisoning by unspecified systemic anti-infective and antiparasitics, assault**

√x7ᵗʰ **T37.94** **Poisoning by unspecified systemic anti-infective and antiparasitics, undetermined**

√x7ᵗʰ **T37.95** **Adverse effect of unspecified systemic anti-infective and antiparasitic**

√x7ᵗʰ **T37.96** **Underdosing of unspecified systemic anti-infectives and antiparasitics**

√4ᵗʰ **T38** **Poisoning by, adverse effect of and underdosing of hormones and their synthetic substitutes and antagonists, not elsewhere classified**

> EXCLUDES1   *mineralocorticoids and their antagonists (T50.0-)*
> *oxytocic hormones (T48.0-)*
> *parathyroid hormones and derivatives (T50.9-)*

> The appropriate 7th character is to be added to each code from category T38.
> A   initial encounter
> D   subsequent encounter
> S   sequela

√5ᵗʰ **T38.0** **Poisoning by, adverse effect of and underdosing of glucocorticoids and synthetic analogues**

> EXCLUDES1   *glucocorticoids, topically used (T49.-)*

√6ᵗʰ **T38.0X** **Poisoning by, adverse effect of and underdosing of glucocorticoids and synthetic analogues**

√7ᵗʰ **T38.0X1** **Poisoning by glucocorticoids and synthetic analogues, accidental (unintentional)**
Poisoning by glucocorticoids and synthetic analogues NOS

√7ᵗʰ **T38.0X2** **Poisoning by glucocorticoids and synthetic analogues, intentional self-harm**

√7ᵗʰ **T38.0X3** **Poisoning by glucocorticoids and synthetic analogues, assault**

√7ᵗʰ **T38.0X4** **Poisoning by glucocorticoids and synthetic analogues, undetermined**

√7ᵗʰ **T38.0X5** **Adverse effect of glucocorticoids and synthetic analogues**

√7ᵗʰ **T38.0X6** **Underdosing of glucocorticoids and synthetic analogues**

√5ᵗʰ **T38.1** **Poisoning by, adverse effect of and underdosing of thyroid hormones and substitutes**

√6ᵗʰ **T38.1X** **Poisoning by, adverse effect of and underdosing of thyroid hormones and substitutes**

√7ᵗʰ **T38.1X1** **Poisoning by thyroid hormones and substitutes, accidental (unintentional)**
Poisoning by thyroid hormones and substitutes NOS

√7ᵗʰ **T38.1X2** **Poisoning by thyroid hormones and substitutes, intentional self-harm**

√7ᵗʰ **T38.1X3** **Poisoning by thyroid hormones and substitutes, assault**

√7ᵗʰ **T38.1X4** **Poisoning by thyroid hormones and substitutes, undetermined**

√7ᵗʰ **T38.1X5** **Adverse effect of thyroid hormones and substitutes**

√7ᵗʰ **T38.1X6** **Underdosing of thyroid hormones and substitutes**

√5ᵗʰ **T38.2** **Poisoning by, adverse effect of and underdosing of antithyroid drugs**

√6ᵗʰ **T38.2X** **Poisoning by, adverse effect of and underdosing of antithyroid drugs**

√7ᵗʰ **T38.2X1** **Poisoning by antithyroid drugs, accidental (unintentional)**
Poisoning by antithyroid drugs NOS

√7ᵗʰ **T38.2X2** **Poisoning by antithyroid drugs, intentional self-harm**

√7ᵗʰ **T38.2X3** **Poisoning by antithyroid drugs, assault**

√7ᵗʰ **T38.2X4** **Poisoning by antithyroid drugs, undetermined**

√7ᵗʰ **T38.2X5** **Adverse effect of antithyroid drugs**

√7ᵗʰ **T38.2X6** **Underdosing of antithyroid drugs**

√5ᵗʰ **T38.3** **Poisoning by, adverse effect of and underdosing of insulin and oral hypoglycemic [antidiabetic] drugs**

√6ᵗʰ **T38.3X** **Poisoning by, adverse effect of and underdosing of insulin and oral hypoglycemic [antidiabetic] drugs**

√7ᵗʰ **T38.3X1** **Poisoning by insulin and oral hypoglycemic [antidiabetic] drugs, accidental (unintentional)**
Poisoning by insulin and oral hypoglycemic [antidiabetic] drugs NOS

√7ᵗʰ **T38.3X2** **Poisoning by insulin and oral hypoglycemic [antidiabetic] drugs, intentional self-harm**

√7ᵗʰ **T38.3X3** **Poisoning by insulin and oral hypoglycemic [antidiabetic] drugs, assault**

√7ᵗʰ **T38.3X4** **Poisoning by insulin and oral hypoglycemic [antidiabetic] drugs, undetermined**

√7ᵗʰ **T38.3X5** **Adverse effect of insulin and oral hypoglycemic [antidiabetic] drugs**

√7ᵗʰ **T38.3X6** **Underdosing of insulin and oral hypoglycemic [antidiabetic] drugs**

√5ᵗʰ **T38.4** **Poisoning by, adverse effect of and underdosing of oral contraceptives**
Poisoning by, adverse effect of and underdosing of multiple- and single-ingredient oral contraceptive preparations

√6ᵗʰ **T38.4X** **Poisoning by, adverse effect of and underdosing of oral contraceptives**

√7ᵗʰ **T38.4X1** **Poisoning by oral contraceptives, accidental (unintentional)**
Poisoning by oral contraceptives NOS

√7ᵗʰ **T38.4X2** **Poisoning by oral contraceptives, intentional self-harm**

√7ᵗʰ **T38.4X3** **Poisoning by oral contraceptives, assault**

√7ᵗʰ **T38.4X4** **Poisoning by oral contraceptives, undetermined**

√7ᵗʰ **T38.4X5** **Adverse effect of oral contraceptives**

√7ᵗʰ **T38.4X6** **Underdosing of oral contraceptives**

√5ᵗʰ **T38.5** **Poisoning by, adverse effect of and underdosing of other estrogens and progestogens**
Poisoning by, adverse effect of and underdosing of estrogens and progestogens mixtures and substitutes

√6ᵗʰ **T38.5X** **Poisoning by, adverse effect of and underdosing of other estrogens and progestogens**

√7ᵗʰ **T38.5X1** **Poisoning by other estrogens and progestogens, accidental (unintentional)**
Poisoning by other estrogens and progestogens NOS

√7ᵗʰ **T38.5X2** **Poisoning by other estrogens and progestogens, intentional self-harm**

√7ᵗʰ **T38.5X3** **Poisoning by other estrogens and progestogens, assault**

√7ᵗʰ **T38.5X4** **Poisoning by other estrogens and progestogens, undetermined**

√7ᵗʰ **T38.5X5** **Adverse effect of other estrogens and progestogens**

√7ᵗʰ **T38.5X6** **Underdosing of other estrogens and progestogens**

√5ᵗʰ **T38.6** **Poisoning by, adverse effect of and underdosing of antigonadotrophins, antiestrogens, antiandrogens, not elsewhere classified**
Poisoning by, adverse effect of and underdosing of tamoxifen

√6ᵗʰ **T38.6X** **Poisoning by, adverse effect of and underdosing of antigonadotrophins, antiestrogens, antiandrogens, not elsewhere classified**

√7ᵗʰ **T38.6X1** **Poisoning by antigonadotrophins, antiestrogens, antiandrogens, not elsewhere classified, accidental (unintentional)**
Poisoning by antigonadotrophins, antiestrogens, antiandrogens, not elsewhere classified NOS

☑ Additional Character Required √x7ᵗʰ Placeholder Alert Unacceptable PDx Manifestation Hospital Acquired Condition EXCLUDES1 Not Coded Here EXCLUDES2 Not Included Here

ICD-10-CM 2016   1099

☑7ᵗʰ **T38.6X2** **Poisoning by antigonadotrophins, antiestrogens, antiandrogens, not elsewhere classified, intentional self-harm**

☑7ᵗʰ **T38.6X3** **Poisoning by antigonadotrophins, antiestrogens, antiandrogens, not elsewhere classified, assault**

☑7ᵗʰ **T38.6X4** **Poisoning by antigonadotrophins, antiestrogens, antiandrogens, not elsewhere classified, undetermined**

☑7ᵗʰ **T38.6X5** Adverse effect of antigonadotrophins, antiestrogens, antiandrogens, not elsewhere classified

☑7ᵗʰ **T38.6X6** Underdosing of antigonadotrophins, antiestrogens, antiandrogens, not elsewhere classified

☑5ᵗʰ **T38.7** **Poisoning by, adverse effect of and underdosing of androgens and anabolic congeners**

☑6ᵗʰ **T38.7X** **Poisoning by, adverse effect of and underdosing of androgens and anabolic congeners**

☑7ᵗʰ **T38.7X1** **Poisoning by androgens and anabolic congeners, accidental (unintentional)**
Poisoning by androgens and anabolic congeners NOS

☑7ᵗʰ **T38.7X2** **Poisoning by androgens and anabolic congeners, intentional self-harm**

☑7ᵗʰ **T38.7X3** **Poisoning by androgens and anabolic congeners, assault**

☑7ᵗʰ **T38.7X4** **Poisoning by androgens and anabolic congeners, undetermined**

☑7ᵗʰ **T38.7X5** Adverse effect of androgens and anabolic congeners

☑7ᵗʰ **T38.7X6** Underdosing of androgens and anabolic congeners

☑5ᵗʰ **T38.8** **Poisoning by, adverse effect of and underdosing of other and unspecified hormones and synthetic substitutes**

☑6ᵗʰ **T38.80** **Poisoning by, adverse effect of and underdosing of unspecified hormones and synthetic substitutes**

☑7ᵗʰ **T38.801** **Poisoning by unspecified hormones and synthetic substitutes, accidental (unintentional)**
Poisoning by unspecified hormones and synthetic substitutes NOS

☑7ᵗʰ **T38.802** **Poisoning by unspecified hormones and synthetic substitutes, intentional self-harm**

☑7ᵗʰ **T38.803** **Poisoning by unspecified hormones and synthetic substitutes, assault**

☑7ᵗʰ **T38.804** **Poisoning by unspecified hormones and synthetic substitutes, undetermined**

☑7ᵗʰ **T38.805** Adverse effect of unspecified hormones and synthetic substitutes

☑7ᵗʰ **T38.806** Underdosing of unspecified hormones and synthetic substitutes

☑6ᵗʰ **T38.81** **Poisoning by, adverse effect of and underdosing of anterior pituitary [adenohypophyseal] hormones**

☑7ᵗʰ **T38.811** **Poisoning by anterior pituitary [adenohypophyseal] hormones, accidental (unintentional)**
Poisoning by anterior pituitary [adenohypophyseal] hormones NOS

☑7ᵗʰ **T38.812** **Poisoning by anterior pituitary [adenohypophyseal] hormones, intentional self-harm**

☑7ᵗʰ **T38.813** **Poisoning by anterior pituitary [adenohypophyseal] hormones, assault**

☑7ᵗʰ **T38.814** **Poisoning by anterior pituitary [adenohypophyseal] hormones, undetermined**

☑7ᵗʰ **T38.815** Adverse effect of anterior pituitary [adenohypophyseal] hormones

☑7ᵗʰ **T38.816** Underdosing of anterior pituitary [adenohypophyseal] hormones

☑6ᵗʰ **T38.89** **Poisoning by, adverse effect of and underdosing of other hormones and synthetic substitutes**

☑7ᵗʰ **T38.891** **Poisoning by other hormones and synthetic substitutes, accidental (unintentional)**
Poisoning by other hormones and synthetic substitutes NOS

☑7ᵗʰ **T38.892** **Poisoning by other hormones and synthetic substitutes, intentional self-harm**

☑7ᵗʰ **T38.893** **Poisoning by other hormones and synthetic substitutes, assault**

☑7ᵗʰ **T38.894** **Poisoning by other hormones and synthetic substitutes, undetermined**

☑7ᵗʰ **T38.895** Adverse effect of other hormones and synthetic substitutes

☑7ᵗʰ **T38.896** Underdosing of other hormones and synthetic substitutes

☑5ᵗʰ **T38.9** **Poisoning by, adverse effect of and underdosing of other and unspecified hormone antagonists**

☑6ᵗʰ **T38.90** **Poisoning by, adverse effect of and underdosing of unspecified hormone antagonists**

☑7ᵗʰ **T38.901** **Poisoning by unspecified hormone antagonists, accidental (unintentional)**
Poisoning by unspecified hormone antagonists NOS

☑7ᵗʰ **T38.902** **Poisoning by unspecified hormone antagonists, intentional self-harm**

☑7ᵗʰ **T38.903** **Poisoning by unspecified hormone antagonists, assault**

☑7ᵗʰ **T38.904** **Poisoning by unspecified hormone antagonists, undetermined**

☑7ᵗʰ **T38.905** Adverse effect of unspecified hormone antagonists

☑7ᵗʰ **T38.906** Underdosing of unspecified hormone antagonists

☑6ᵗʰ **T38.99** **Poisoning by, adverse effect of and underdosing of other hormone antagonists**

☑7ᵗʰ **T38.991** **Poisoning by other hormone antagonists, accidental (unintentional)**
Poisoning by other hormone antagonists NOS

☑7ᵗʰ **T38.992** **Poisoning by other hormone antagonists, intentional self-harm**

☑7ᵗʰ **T38.993** **Poisoning by other hormone antagonists, assault**

☑7ᵗʰ **T38.994** **Poisoning by other hormone antagonists, undetermined**

☑7ᵗʰ **T38.995** Adverse effect of other hormone antagonists

☑7ᵗʰ **T38.996** Underdosing of other hormone antagonists

☑4ᵗʰ **T39** **Poisoning by, adverse effect of and underdosing of nonopioid analgesics, antipyretics and antirheumatics**

> The appropriate 7th character is to be added to each code from category T39.
> A   initial encounter
> D   subsequent encounter
> S   sequela

☑5ᵗʰ **T39.0** **Poisoning by, adverse effect of and underdosing of salicylates**

☑6ᵗʰ **T39.01** **Poisoning by, adverse effect of and underdosing of aspirin**
Poisoning by, adverse effect of and underdosing of acetylsalicylic acid

☑7ᵗʰ **T39.011** **Poisoning by aspirin, accidental (unintentional)**

☑7ᵗʰ **T39.012** **Poisoning by aspirin, intentional self-harm**

☑7ᵗʰ **T39.013** **Poisoning by aspirin, assault**

☑7ᵗʰ **T39.014** **Poisoning by aspirin, undetermined**

☑7ᵗʰ **T39.015** Adverse effect of aspirin

☑7ᵗʰ **T39.016** Underdosing of aspirin

☑6ᵗʰ **T39.09** **Poisoning by, adverse effect of and underdosing of other salicylates**

☑7ᵗʰ **T39.091** **Poisoning by salicylates, accidental (unintentional)**
Poisoning by salicylates NOS

Ⓝ Newborn: 0   Ⓟ Pediatric: 0-17   Ⓜ Maternity: 12-55   Ⓐ Adult: 15-124   **MCC** Major CC Condition   **PDxMCC** PDx acts as own MCC   **CC** CC Condition   **PDxCC** PDx acts as own CC

1100   ICD-10-CM 2016

☑7ᵗʰ **T39.Ø92** **Poisoning by salicylates,** intentional self-harm

☑7ᵗʰ **T39.Ø93** **Poisoning by salicylates,** assault

☑7ᵗʰ **T39.Ø94** **Poisoning by salicylates,** undetermined

☑7ᵗʰ **T39.Ø95** Adverse effect **of salicylates**

☑7ᵗʰ **T39.Ø96** Underdosing **of salicylates**

☑5ᵗʰ **T39.1** **Poisoning by, adverse effect of and underdosing of 4-Aminophenol derivatives**

    ☑6ᵗʰ **T39.1X** **Poisoning by, adverse effect of and underdosing of 4-Aminophenol derivatives**

       ☑7ᵗʰ **T39.1X1** **Poisoning by 4-Aminophenol derivatives, accidental (unintentional)**
          Poisoning by 4-Aminophenol derivatives NOS

       ☑7ᵗʰ **T39.1X2** **Poisoning by 4-Aminophenol derivatives, intentional self-harm**

       ☑7ᵗʰ **T39.1X3** **Poisoning by 4-Aminophenol derivatives, assault**

       ☑7ᵗʰ **T39.1X4** **Poisoning by 4-Aminophenol derivatives, undetermined**

       ☑7ᵗʰ **T39.1X5** Adverse effect **of 4-Aminophenol derivatives**

       ☑7ᵗʰ **T39.1X6** Underdosing **of 4-Aminophenol derivatives**

☑5ᵗʰ **T39.2** **Poisoning by, adverse effect of and underdosing of pyrazolone derivatives**

    ☑6ᵗʰ **T39.2X** **Poisoning by, adverse effect of and underdosing of pyrazolone derivatives**

       ☑7ᵗʰ **T39.2X1** **Poisoning by pyrazolone derivatives, accidental (unintentional)**
          Poisoning by pyrazolone derivatives NOS

       ☑7ᵗʰ **T39.2X2** **Poisoning by pyrazolone derivatives, intentional self-harm**

       ☑7ᵗʰ **T39.2X3** **Poisoning by pyrazolone derivatives, assault**

       ☑7ᵗʰ **T39.2X4** **Poisoning by pyrazolone derivatives, undetermined**

       ☑7ᵗʰ **T39.2X5** Adverse effect **of pyrazolone derivatives**

       ☑7ᵗʰ **T39.2X6** Underdosing **of pyrazolone derivatives**

☑5ᵗʰ **T39.3** **Poisoning by, adverse effect of and underdosing of other nonsteroidal anti-inflammatory drugs [NSAID]**

    ☑6ᵗʰ **T39.31** **Poisoning by, adverse effect of and underdosing of propionic acid derivatives**
       Poisoning by, adverse effect of and underdosing of fenoprofen
       Poisoning by, adverse effect of and underdosing of flurbiprofen
       Poisoning by, adverse effect of and underdosing of ibuprofen
       Poisoning by, adverse effect of and underdosing of ketoprofen
       Poisoning by, adverse effect of and underdosing of naproxen
       Poisoning by, adverse effect of and underdosing of oxaprozin

       ☑7ᵗʰ **T39.311** **Poisoning by propionic acid derivatives, accidental (unintentional)**

       ☑7ᵗʰ **T39.312** **Poisoning by propionic acid derivatives, intentional self-harm**

       ☑7ᵗʰ **T39.313** **Poisoning by propionic acid derivatives, assault**

       ☑7ᵗʰ **T39.314** **Poisoning by propionic acid derivatives, undetermined**

       ☑7ᵗʰ **T39.315** Adverse effect **of propionic acid derivatives**

       ☑7ᵗʰ **T39.316** Underdosing **of propionic acid derivatives**

    ☑6ᵗʰ **T39.39** **Poisoning by, adverse effect of and underdosing of other nonsteroidal anti-inflammatory drugs [NSAID]**

       ☑7ᵗʰ **T39.391** **Poisoning by other nonsteroidal anti-inflammatory drugs [NSAID], accidental (unintentional)**
          Poisoning by other nonsteroidal anti-inflammatory drugs NOS

       ☑7ᵗʰ **T39.392** **Poisoning by other nonsteroidal anti-inflammatory drugs [NSAID], intentional self-harm**

☑7ᵗʰ **T39.393** **Poisoning by other nonsteroidal anti-inflammatory drugs [NSAID], assault**

☑7ᵗʰ **T39.394** **Poisoning by other nonsteroidal anti-inflammatory drugs [NSAID], undetermined**

☑7ᵗʰ **T39.395** Adverse effect **of other nonsteroidal anti-inflammatory drugs [NSAID]**

☑7ᵗʰ **T39.396** Underdosing **of other nonsteroidal anti-inflammatory drugs [NSAID]**

☑5ᵗʰ **T39.4** **Poisoning by, adverse effect of and underdosing of antirheumatics, not elsewhere classified**

    EXCLUDES 1   *poisoning by, adverse effect of and underdosing of glucocorticoids (T38.Ø-)*
             poisoning by, adverse effect of and underdosing of salicylates (T39.Ø-)

    ☑6ᵗʰ **T39.4X** **Poisoning by, adverse effect of and underdosing of antirheumatics, not elsewhere classified**

       ☑7ᵗʰ **T39.4X1** **Poisoning by antirheumatics, not elsewhere classified, accidental (unintentional)**
          Poisoning by antirheumatics, not elsewhere classified NOS

       ☑7ᵗʰ **T39.4X2** **Poisoning by antirheumatics, not elsewhere classified, intentional self-harm**

       ☑7ᵗʰ **T39.4X3** **Poisoning by antirheumatics, not elsewhere classified, assault**

       ☑7ᵗʰ **T39.4X4** **Poisoning by antirheumatics, not elsewhere classified, undetermined**

       ☑7ᵗʰ **T39.4X5** Adverse effect **of antirheumatics, not elsewhere classified**

       ☑7ᵗʰ **T39.4X6** Underdosing **of antirheumatics, not elsewhere classified**

☑5ᵗʰ **T39.8** **Poisoning by, adverse effect of and underdosing of other nonopioid analgesics and antipyretics, not elsewhere classified**

    ☑6ᵗʰ **T39.8X** **Poisoning by, adverse effect of and underdosing of other nonopioid analgesics and antipyretics, not elsewhere classified**

       ☑7ᵗʰ **T39.8X1** **Poisoning by other nonopioid analgesics and antipyretics, not elsewhere classified, accidental (unintentional)**
          Poisoning by other nonopioid analgesics and antipyretics, not elsewhere classified NOS

       ☑7ᵗʰ **T39.8X2** **Poisoning by other nonopioid analgesics and antipyretics, not elsewhere classified, intentional self-harm**

       ☑7ᵗʰ **T39.8X3** **Poisoning by other nonopioid analgesics and antipyretics, not elsewhere classified, assault**

       ☑7ᵗʰ **T39.8X4** **Poisoning by other nonopioid analgesics and antipyretics, not elsewhere classified, undetermined**

       ☑7ᵗʰ **T39.8X5** Adverse effect **of other nonopioid analgesics and antipyretics, not elsewhere classified**

       ☑7ᵗʰ **T39.8X6** Underdosing **of other nonopioid analgesics and antipyretics, not elsewhere classified**

☑5ᵗʰ **T39.9** **Poisoning by, adverse effect of and underdosing of unspecified nonopioid analgesic, antipyretic and antirheumatic**

    ☑x7ᵗʰ **T39.91** **Poisoning by unspecified nonopioid analgesic, antipyretic and antirheumatic,** accidental **(unintentional)**
       Poisoning by nonopioid analgesic, antipyretic and antirheumatic NOS

    ☑x7ᵗʰ **T39.92** **Poisoning by unspecified nonopioid analgesic, antipyretic and antirheumatic,** intentional self-harm

    ☑x7ᵗʰ **T39.93** **Poisoning by unspecified nonopioid analgesic, antipyretic and antirheumatic,** assault

    ☑x7ᵗʰ **T39.94** **Poisoning by unspecified nonopioid analgesic, antipyretic and antirheumatic,** undetermined

    ☑x7ᵗʰ **T39.95** Adverse effect **of unspecified nonopioid analgesic, antipyretic and antirheumatic**

    ☑x7ᵗʰ **T39.96** Underdosing **of unspecified nonopioid analgesic, antipyretic and antirheumatic**

☑ Additional Character Required   ☑x7ᵗʰ Placeholder Alert   Unacceptable PDx   Manifestation   Hospital Acquired Condition   *EXCLUDES 1* Not Coded Here   *EXCLUDES 2* Not Included Here

✓4ᵗʰ T40 Poisoning by, adverse effect of and underdosing of narcotics and psychodysleptics [hallucinogens]

> EXCLUDES 2   *drug dependence and related mental and behavioral disorders due to psychoactive substance use (F10-F19-)*

> The appropriate 7th character is to be added to each code from category T40.
> A   initial encounter
> D   subsequent encounter
> S   sequela

✓5ᵗʰ T40.0 Poisoning by, adverse effect of and underdosing of opium
- **✓6ᵗʰ T40.0X Poisoning by, adverse effect of and underdosing of opium**
  - ✓7ᵗʰ **T40.0X1** Poisoning by opium, accidental (unintentional)
    Poisoning by opium NOS
  - ✓7ᵗʰ **T40.0X2** Poisoning by opium, intentional self-harm
  - ✓7ᵗʰ **T40.0X3** Poisoning by opium, assault
  - ✓7ᵗʰ **T40.0X4** Poisoning by opium, undetermined
  - ✓7ᵗʰ **T40.0X5** Adverse effect of opium
  - ✓7ᵗʰ **T40.0X6** Underdosing of opium

✓5ᵗʰ T40.1 Poisoning by and adverse effect of heroin
- **✓6ᵗʰ T40.1X Poisoning by and adverse effect of heroin**
  - ✓7ᵗʰ **T40.1X1** Poisoning by heroin, accidental (unintentional)
    Poisoning by heroin NOS
  - ✓7ᵗʰ **T40.1X2** Poisoning by heroin, intentional self-harm
  - ✓7ᵗʰ **T40.1X3** Poisoning by heroin, assault
  - ✓7ᵗʰ **T40.1X4** Poisoning by heroin, undetermined

✓5ᵗʰ T40.2 Poisoning by, adverse effect of and underdosing of other opioids
- **✓6ᵗʰ T40.2X Poisoning by, adverse effect of and underdosing of other opioids**
  - ✓7ᵗʰ **T40.2X1** Poisoning by other opioids, accidental (unintentional)
    Poisoning by other opioids NOS
  - ✓7ᵗʰ **T40.2X2** Poisoning by other opioids, intentional self-harm
  - ✓7ᵗʰ **T40.2X3** Poisoning by other opioids, assault
  - ✓7ᵗʰ **T40.2X4** Poisoning by other opioids, undetermined
  - ✓7ᵗʰ **T40.2X5** Adverse effect of other opioids
  - ✓7ᵗʰ **T40.2X6** Underdosing of other opioids

✓5ᵗʰ T40.3 Poisoning by, adverse effect of and underdosing of methadone
- **✓6ᵗʰ T40.3X Poisoning by, adverse effect of and underdosing of methadone**
  - ✓7ᵗʰ **T40.3X1** Poisoning by methadone, accidental (unintentional)
    Poisoning by methadone NOS
  - ✓7ᵗʰ **T40.3X2** Poisoning by methadone, intentional self-harm
  - ✓7ᵗʰ **T40.3X3** Poisoning by methadone, assault
  - ✓7ᵗʰ **T40.3X4** Poisoning by methadone, undetermined
  - ✓7ᵗʰ **T40.3X5** Adverse effect of methadone
  - ✓7ᵗʰ **T40.3X6** Underdosing of methadone

✓5ᵗʰ T40.4 Poisoning by, adverse effect of and underdosing of other synthetic narcotics
- **✓6ᵗʰ T40.4X Poisoning by, adverse effect of and underdosing of other synthetic narcotics**
  - ✓7ᵗʰ **T40.4X1** Poisoning by other synthetic narcotics, accidental (unintentional)
    Poisoning by other synthetic narcotics NOS
  - ✓7ᵗʰ **T40.4X2** Poisoning by other synthetic narcotics, intentional self-harm
  - ✓7ᵗʰ **T40.4X3** Poisoning by other synthetic narcotics, assault
  - ✓7ᵗʰ **T40.4X4** Poisoning by other synthetic narcotics, undetermined
  - ✓7ᵗʰ **T40.4X5** Adverse effect of other synthetic narcotics
  - ✓7ᵗʰ **T40.4X6** Underdosing of other synthetic narcotics

✓5ᵗʰ T40.5 Poisoning by, adverse effect of and underdosing of cocaine
- **✓6ᵗʰ T40.5X Poisoning by, adverse effect of and underdosing of cocaine**
  - ✓7ᵗʰ **T40.5X1** Poisoning by cocaine, accidental (unintentional)
    Poisoning by cocaine NOS
  - ✓7ᵗʰ **T40.5X2** Poisoning by cocaine, intentional self-harm
  - ✓7ᵗʰ **T40.5X3** Poisoning by cocaine, assault
  - ✓7ᵗʰ **T40.5X4** Poisoning by cocaine, undetermined
  - ✓7ᵗʰ **T40.5X5** Adverse effect of cocaine
  - ✓7ᵗʰ **T40.5X6** Underdosing of cocaine

✓5ᵗʰ T40.6 Poisoning by, adverse effect of and underdosing of other and unspecified narcotics
- **✓6ᵗʰ T40.60 Poisoning by, adverse effect of and underdosing of unspecified narcotics**
  - ✓7ᵗʰ **T40.601** Poisoning by unspecified narcotics, accidental (unintentional)
    Poisoning by narcotics NOS
  - ✓7ᵗʰ **T40.602** Poisoning by unspecified narcotics, intentional self-harm
  - ✓7ᵗʰ **T40.603** Poisoning by unspecified narcotics, assault
  - ✓7ᵗʰ **T40.604** Poisoning by unspecified narcotics, undetermined
  - ✓7ᵗʰ **T40.605** Adverse effect of unspecified narcotics
  - ✓7ᵗʰ **T40.606** Underdosing of unspecified narcotics
- **✓6ᵗʰ T40.69 Poisoning by, adverse effect of and underdosing of other narcotics**
  - ✓7ᵗʰ **T40.691** Poisoning by other narcotics, accidental (unintentional)
    Poisoning by other narcotics NOS
  - ✓7ᵗʰ **T40.692** Poisoning by other narcotics, intentional self-harm
  - ✓7ᵗʰ **T40.693** Poisoning by other narcotics, assault
  - ✓7ᵗʰ **T40.694** Poisoning by other narcotics, undetermined
  - ✓7ᵗʰ **T40.695** Adverse effect of other narcotics
  - ✓7ᵗʰ **T40.696** Underdosing of other narcotics

✓5ᵗʰ T40.7 Poisoning by, adverse effect of and underdosing of cannabis (derivatives)
- **✓6ᵗʰ T40.7X Poisoning by, adverse effect of and underdosing of cannabis (derivatives)**
  - ✓7ᵗʰ **T40.7X1** Poisoning by cannabis (derivatives), accidental (unintentional)
    Poisoning by cannabis NOS
  - ✓7ᵗʰ **T40.7X2** Poisoning by cannabis (derivatives), intentional self-harm
  - ✓7ᵗʰ **T40.7X3** Poisoning by cannabis (derivatives), assault
  - ✓7ᵗʰ **T40.7X4** Poisoning by cannabis (derivatives), undetermined
  - ✓7ᵗʰ **T40.7X5** Adverse effect of cannabis (derivatives)
  - ✓7ᵗʰ **T40.7X6** Underdosing of cannabis (derivatives)

✓5ᵗʰ T40.8 Poisoning by and adverse effect of lysergide [LSD]
- **✓6ᵗʰ T40.8X Poisoning by and adverse effect of lysergide [LSD]**
  - ✓7ᵗʰ **T40.8X1** Poisoning by lysergide [LSD], accidental (unintentional)
    Poisoning by lysergide [LSD]NOS
  - ✓7ᵗʰ **T40.8X2** Poisoning by lysergide [LSD], intentional self-harm
  - ✓7ᵗʰ **T40.8X3** Poisoning by lysergide [LSD], assault
  - ✓7ᵗʰ **T40.8X4** Poisoning by lysergide [LSD], undetermined

✓5ᵗʰ T40.9 Poisoning by, adverse effect of and underdosing of other and unspecified psychodysleptics [hallucinogens]
- **✓6ᵗʰ T40.90 Poisoning by, adverse effect of and underdosing of unspecified psychodysleptics [hallucinogens]**
  - ✓7ᵗʰ **T40.901** Poisoning by unspecified psychodysleptics [hallucinogens], accidental (unintentional)
  - ✓7ᵗʰ **T40.902** Poisoning by unspecified psychodysleptics [hallucinogens], intentional self-harm
  - ✓7ᵗʰ **T40.903** Poisoning by unspecified psychodysleptics [hallucinogens], assault

Ⓝ Newborn: 0   Ⓟ Pediatric: 0-17   Ⓜ Maternity: 12-55   Ⓐ Adult: 15-124   MCC Major CC Condition   PDxMCC PDx acts as own MCC   CC CC Condition   PDxCC PDx acts as own CC

1102   ICD-10-CM 2016

✓7ᵗʰ **T40.904** **Poisoning by unspecified psychodysleptics [hallucinogens], undetermined**

✓7ᵗʰ **T40.905** Adverse effect of unspecified psychodysleptics [hallucinogens]

✓7ᵗʰ **T40.906** Underdosing of unspecified psychodysleptics

✓6ᵗʰ **T40.99** **Poisoning by, adverse effect of and underdosing of other psychodysleptics [hallucinogens]**

✓7ᵗʰ **T40.991** **Poisoning by other psychodysleptics [hallucinogens], accidental (unintentional)**
Poisoning by other psychodysleptics [hallucinogens] NOS

✓7ᵗʰ **T40.992** **Poisoning by other psychodysleptics [hallucinogens], intentional self-harm**

✓7ᵗʰ **T40.993** **Poisoning by other psychodysleptics [hallucinogens], assault**

✓7ᵗʰ **T40.994** **Poisoning by other psychodysleptics [hallucinogens], undetermined**

✓7ᵗʰ **T40.995** Adverse effect of other psychodysleptics [hallucinogens]

✓7ᵗʰ **T40.996** Underdosing of other psychodysleptics

✓4ᵗʰ **T41** **Poisoning by, adverse effect of and underdosing of anesthetics and therapeutic gases**

EXCLUDES 1 *benzodiazepines (T42.4-)*
cocaine (T40.5-)
complications of anesthesia during labor and delivery (O74.-)
complications of anesthesia during pregnancy (O29.-)
complications of anesthesia during the puerperium (O89.-)
opioids (T40.0-T40.2-)

The appropriate 7th character is to be added to each code from category T41.
A   initial encounter
D   subsequent encounter
S   sequela

✓5ᵗʰ **T41.0** **Poisoning by, adverse effect of and underdosing of inhaled anesthetics**

EXCLUDES 1 *oxygen (T41.5-)*

✓6ᵗʰ **T41.0X** **Poisoning by, adverse effect of and underdosing of inhaled anesthetics**

✓7ᵗʰ **T41.0X1** **Poisoning by inhaled anesthetics, accidental (unintentional)**
Poisoning by inhaled anesthetics NOS

✓7ᵗʰ **T41.0X2** **Poisoning by inhaled anesthetics, intentional self-harm**

✓7ᵗʰ **T41.0X3** **Poisoning by inhaled anesthetics, assault**

✓7ᵗʰ **T41.0X4** **Poisoning by inhaled anesthetics, undetermined**

✓7ᵗʰ **T41.0X5** Adverse effect of inhaled anesthetics

✓7ᵗʰ **T41.0X6** Underdosing of inhaled anesthetics

✓5ᵗʰ **T41.1** **Poisoning by, adverse effect of and underdosing of intravenous anesthetics**
Poisoning by, adverse effect of and underdosing of thiobarbiturates

✓6ᵗʰ **T41.1X** **Poisoning by, adverse effect of and underdosing of intravenous anesthetics**

✓7ᵗʰ **T41.1X1** **Poisoning by intravenous anesthetics, accidental (unintentional)**
Poisoning by intravenous anesthetics NOS

✓7ᵗʰ **T41.1X2** **Poisoning by intravenous anesthetics, intentional self-harm**

✓7ᵗʰ **T41.1X3** **Poisoning by intravenous anesthetics, assault**

✓7ᵗʰ **T41.1X4** **Poisoning by intravenous anesthetics, undetermined**

✓7ᵗʰ **T41.1X5** Adverse effect of intravenous anesthetics

✓7ᵗʰ **T41.1X6** Underdosing of intravenous anesthetics

✓5ᵗʰ **T41.2** **Poisoning by, adverse effect of and underdosing of other and unspecified general anesthetics**

✓6ᵗʰ **T41.20** **Poisoning by, adverse effect of and underdosing of unspecified general anesthetics**

✓7ᵗʰ **T41.201** **Poisoning by unspecified general anesthetics, accidental (unintentional)**
Poisoning by general anesthetics NOS

✓7ᵗʰ **T41.202** **Poisoning by unspecified general anesthetics, intentional self-harm**

✓7ᵗʰ **T41.203** **Poisoning by unspecified general anesthetics, assault**

✓7ᵗʰ **T41.204** **Poisoning by unspecified general anesthetics, undetermined**

✓7ᵗʰ **T41.205** Adverse effect of unspecified general anesthetics

✓7ᵗʰ **T41.206** Underdosing of unspecified general anesthetics

✓6ᵗʰ **T41.29** **Poisoning by, adverse effect of and underdosing of other general anesthetics**

✓7ᵗʰ **T41.291** **Poisoning by other general anesthetics, accidental (unintentional)**
Poisoning by other general anesthetics NOS

✓7ᵗʰ **T41.292** **Poisoning by other general anesthetics, intentional self-harm**

✓7ᵗʰ **T41.293** **Poisoning by other general anesthetics, assault**

✓7ᵗʰ **T41.294** **Poisoning by other general anesthetics, undetermined**

✓7ᵗʰ **T41.295** Adverse effect of other general anesthetics

✓7ᵗʰ **T41.296** Underdosing of other general anesthetics

✓5ᵗʰ **T41.3** **Poisoning by, adverse effect of and underdosing of local anesthetics**
Cocaine (topical)

EXCLUDES 2 *poisoning by cocaine used as a central nervous system stimulant (T40.5X1-T40.5X4)*

✓6ᵗʰ **T41.3X** **Poisoning by, adverse effect of and underdosing of local anesthetics**

✓7ᵗʰ **T41.3X1** **Poisoning by local anesthetics, accidental (unintentional)**
Poisoning by local anesthetics NOS

✓7ᵗʰ **T41.3X2** **Poisoning by local anesthetics, intentional self-harm**

✓7ᵗʰ **T41.3X3** **Poisoning by local anesthetics, assault**

✓7ᵗʰ **T41.3X4** **Poisoning by local anesthetics, undetermined**

✓7ᵗʰ **T41.3X5** Adverse effect of local anesthetics

✓7ᵗʰ **T41.3X6** Underdosing of local anesthetics

✓5ᵗʰ **T41.4** **Poisoning by, adverse effect of and underdosing of unspecified anesthetic**

✓x7ᵗʰ **T41.41** **Poisoning by unspecified anesthetic, accidental (unintentional)**
Poisoning by anesthetic NOS

✓x7ᵗʰ **T41.42** **Poisoning by unspecified anesthetic, intentional self-harm**

✓x7ᵗʰ **T41.43** **Poisoning by unspecified anesthetic, assault**

✓x7ᵗʰ **T41.44** **Poisoning by unspecified anesthetic, undetermined**

✓x7ᵗʰ **T41.45** Adverse effect of unspecified anesthetic

✓x7ᵗʰ **T41.46** Underdosing of unspecified anesthetics

✓5ᵗʰ **T41.5** **Poisoning by, adverse effect of and underdosing of therapeutic gases**

✓6ᵗʰ **T41.5X** **Poisoning by, adverse effect of and underdosing of therapeutic gases**

✓7ᵗʰ **T41.5X1** **Poisoning by therapeutic gases, accidental (unintentional)**
Poisoning by therapeutic gases NOS

✓7ᵗʰ **T41.5X2** **Poisoning by therapeutic gases, intentional self-harm**

✓7ᵗʰ **T41.5X3** **Poisoning by therapeutic gases, assault**

✓7ᵗʰ **T41.5X4** **Poisoning by therapeutic gases, undetermined**

✓7ᵗʰ **T41.5X5** Adverse effect of therapeutic gases

✓7ᵗʰ **T41.5X6** Underdosing of therapeutic gases

✓ Additional Character Required   ✓x7ᵗʰ Placeholder Alert   Unacceptable PDx   Manifestation   Hospital Acquired Condition   *EXCLUDES 1* Not Coded Here   *EXCLUDES 2* Not Included Here

√4ᵗʰ **T42** **Poisoning by, adverse effect of and underdosing of antiepileptic, sedative- hypnotic and antiparkinsonism drugs**

> *EXCLUDES 2*   *drug dependence and related mental and behavioral disorders due to psychoactive substance use (F10- – F19-)*

> The appropriate 7th character is to be added to each code from category T42.
> A   initial encounter
> D   subsequent encounter
> S   sequela

√5ᵗʰ **T42.0** **Poisoning by, adverse effect of and underdosing of hydantoin derivatives**

    √6ᵗʰ **T42.0X** **Poisoning by, adverse effect of and underdosing of hydantoin derivatives**

      √7ᵗʰ **T42.0X1** **Poisoning by hydantoin derivatives, accidental (unintentional)**
         Poisoning by hydantoin derivatives NOS

      √7ᵗʰ **T42.0X2** **Poisoning by hydantoin derivatives, intentional self-harm**

      √7ᵗʰ **T42.0X3** **Poisoning by hydantoin derivatives, assault**

      √7ᵗʰ **T42.0X4** **Poisoning by hydantoin derivatives, undetermined**

      √7ᵗʰ **T42.0X5** **Adverse effect of hydantoin derivatives**

      √7ᵗʰ **T42.0X6** **Underdosing of hydantoin derivatives**

√5ᵗʰ **T42.1** **Poisoning by, adverse effect of and underdosing of iminostilbenes**
     Poisoning by, adverse effect of and underdosing of carbamazepine

    √6ᵗʰ **T42.1X** **Poisoning by, adverse effect of and underdosing of iminostilbenes**

      √7ᵗʰ **T42.1X1** **Poisoning by iminostilbenes, accidental (unintentional)**
         Poisoning by iminostilbenes NOS

      √7ᵗʰ **T42.1X2** **Poisoning by iminostilbenes, intentional self-harm**

      √7ᵗʰ **T42.1X3** **Poisoning by iminostilbenes, assault**

      √7ᵗʰ **T42.1X4** **Poisoning by iminostilbenes, undetermined**

      √7ᵗʰ **T42.1X5** **Adverse effect of iminostilbenes**

      √7ᵗʰ **T42.1X6** **Underdosing of iminostilbenes**

√5ᵗʰ **T42.2** **Poisoning by, adverse effect of and underdosing of succinimides and oxazolidinediones**

    √6ᵗʰ **T42.2X** **Poisoning by, adverse effect of and underdosing of succinimides and oxazolidinediones**

      √7ᵗʰ **T42.2X1** **Poisoning by succinimides and oxazolidinediones, accidental (unintentional)**
         Poisoning by succinimides and oxazolidinediones NOS

      √7ᵗʰ **T42.2X2** **Poisoning by succinimides and oxazolidinediones, intentional self-harm**

      √7ᵗʰ **T42.2X3** **Poisoning by succinimides and oxazolidinediones, assault**

      √7ᵗʰ **T42.2X4** **Poisoning by succinimides and oxazolidinediones, undetermined**

      √7ᵗʰ **T42.2X5** **Adverse effect of succinimides and oxazolidinediones**

      √7ᵗʰ **T42.2X6** **Underdosing of succinimides and oxazolidinediones**

√5ᵗʰ **T42.3** **Poisoning by, adverse effect of and underdosing of barbiturates**

> *EXCLUDES 1*   *poisoning by, adverse effect of and underdosing of thiobarbiturates (T41.1-)*

    √6ᵗʰ **T42.3X** **Poisoning by, adverse effect of and underdosing of barbiturates**

      √7ᵗʰ **T42.3X1** **Poisoning by barbiturates, accidental (unintentional)**
         Poisoning by barbiturates NOS

      √7ᵗʰ **T42.3X2** **Poisoning by barbiturates, intentional self-harm**

      √7ᵗʰ **T42.3X3** **Poisoning by barbiturates, assault**

      √7ᵗʰ **T42.3X4** **Poisoning by barbiturates, undetermined**

      √7ᵗʰ **T42.3X5** **Adverse effect of barbiturates**

      √7ᵗʰ **T42.3X6** **Underdosing of barbiturates**

√5ᵗʰ **T42.4** **Poisoning by, adverse effect of and underdosing of benzodiazepines**

    √6ᵗʰ **T42.4X** **Poisoning by, adverse effect of and underdosing of benzodiazepines**

      √7ᵗʰ **T42.4X1** **Poisoning by benzodiazepines, accidental (unintentional)**
         Poisoning by benzodiazepines NOS

      √7ᵗʰ **T42.4X2** **Poisoning by benzodiazepines, intentional self-harm**

      √7ᵗʰ **T42.4X3** **Poisoning by benzodiazepines, assault**

      √7ᵗʰ **T42.4X4** **Poisoning by benzodiazepines, undetermined**

      √7ᵗʰ **T42.4X5** **Adverse effect of benzodiazepines**

      √7ᵗʰ **T42.4X6** **Underdosing of benzodiazepines**

√5ᵗʰ **T42.5** **Poisoning by, adverse effect of and underdosing of mixed antiepileptics**

    √6ᵗʰ **T42.5X** **Poisoning by, adverse effect of and underdosing of antiepileptics**

      √7ᵗʰ **T42.5X1** **Poisoning by mixed antiepileptics, accidental (unintentional)**
         Poisoning by mixed antiepileptics NOS

      √7ᵗʰ **T42.5X2** **Poisoning by mixed antiepileptics, intentional self-harm**

      √7ᵗʰ **T42.5X3** **Poisoning by mixed antiepileptics, assault**

      √7ᵗʰ **T42.5X4** **Poisoning by mixed antiepileptics, undetermined**

      √7ᵗʰ **T42.5X5** **Adverse effect of mixed antiepileptics**

      √7ᵗʰ **T42.5X6** **Underdosing of mixed antiepileptics**

√5ᵗʰ **T42.6** **Poisoning by, adverse effect of and underdosing of other antiepileptic and sedative-hypnotic drugs**
     Poisoning by, adverse effect of and underdosing of methaqualone
     Poisoning by, adverse effect of and underdosing of valproic acid

> *EXCLUDES 1*   *poisoning by, adverse effect of and underdosing of carbamazepine (T42.1-)*

    √6ᵗʰ **T42.6X** **Poisoning by, adverse effect of and underdosing of other antiepileptic and sedative-hypnotic drugs**

      √7ᵗʰ **T42.6X1** **Poisoning by other antiepileptic and sedative-hypnotic drugs, accidental (unintentional)**
         Poisoning by other antiepileptic and sedative-hypnotic drugs NOS

      √7ᵗʰ **T42.6X2** **Poisoning by other antiepileptic and sedative-hypnotic drugs, intentional self-harm**

      √7ᵗʰ **T42.6X3** **Poisoning by other antiepileptic and sedative-hypnotic drugs, assault**

      √7ᵗʰ **T42.6X4** **Poisoning by other antiepileptic and sedative-hypnotic drugs, undetermined**

      √7ᵗʰ **T42.6X5** **Adverse effect of other antiepileptic and sedative-hypnotic drugs**

      √7ᵗʰ **T42.6X6** **Underdosing of other antiepileptic and sedative-hypnotic drugs**

√5ᵗʰ **T42.7** **Poisoning by, adverse effect of and underdosing of unspecified antiepileptic and sedative-hypnotic drugs**

    √x7ᵗʰ **T42.71** **Poisoning by unspecified antiepileptic and sedative-hypnotic drugs, accidental (unintentional)**
     Poisoning by antiepileptic and sedative-hypnotic drugs NOS

    √x7ᵗʰ **T42.72** **Poisoning by unspecified antiepileptic and sedative-hypnotic drugs, intentional self-harm**

    √x7ᵗʰ **T42.73** **Poisoning by unspecified antiepileptic and sedative-hypnotic drugs, assault**

    √x7ᵗʰ **T42.74** **Poisoning by unspecified antiepileptic and sedative-hypnotic drugs, undetermined**

    √x7ᵗʰ **T42.75** **Adverse effect of unspecified antiepileptic and sedative-hypnotic drugs**

    √x7ᵗʰ **T42.76** **Underdosing of unspecified antiepileptic and sedative-hypnotic drugs**

√5ᵗʰ **T42.8** **Poisoning by, adverse effect of and underdosing of antiparkinsonism drugs and other central muscle-tone depressants**
     Poisoning by, adverse effect of and underdosing of amantadine

    √6ᵗʰ **T42.8X** **Poisoning by, adverse effect of and underdosing of antiparkinsonism drugs and other central muscle-tone depressants**

N Newborn: 0   **P** Pediatric: 0-17   **M** Maternity: 12-55   **A** Adult: 15-124   **MCC** Major CC Condition   **PDxMCC** PDx acts as own MCC   **CC** CC Condition   **PDxCC** PDx acts as own CC

✓7th **T42.8X1** **Poisoning by antiparkinsonism drugs and other central muscle-tone depressants, accidental (unintentional)**
Poisoning by antiparkinsonism drugs and other central muscle-tone depressants NOS

✓7th **T42.8X2** **Poisoning by antiparkinsonism drugs and other central muscle-tone depressants, intentional self-harm**

✓7th **T42.8X3** **Poisoning by antiparkinsonism drugs and other central muscle-tone depressants, assault**

✓7th **T42.8X4** **Poisoning by antiparkinsonism drugs and other central muscle-tone depressants, undetermined**

✓7th **T42.8X5** **Adverse effect of antiparkinsonism drugs and other central muscle-tone depressants**

✓7th **T42.8X6** **Underdosing of antiparkinsonism drugs and other central muscle-tone depressants**

✓4th **T43** **Poisoning by, adverse effect of and underdosing of psychotropic drugs, not elsewhere classified**

EXCLUDES 1   *appetite depressants (T50.5-)*
barbiturates (T42.3-)
benzodiazepines (T42.4-)
methaqualone (T42.6-)
psychodysleptics [hallucinogens] (T40.7-T40.9-)

EXCLUDES 2   *drug dependence and related mental and behavioral disorders due to psychoactive substance use (F10.- – F19.-)*

The appropriate 7th character is to be added to each code from category T43.
A   initial encounter
D   subsequent encounter
S   sequela

✓5th **T43.0** **Poisoning by, adverse effect of and underdosing of tricyclic and tetracyclic antidepressants**

✓6th **T43.01** **Poisoning by, adverse effect of and underdosing of tricyclic antidepressants**

✓7th **T43.011** **Poisoning by tricyclic antidepressants, accidental (unintentional)**
Poisoning by tricyclic antidepressants NOS

✓7th **T43.012** **Poisoning by tricyclic antidepressants, intentional self-harm**

✓7th **T43.013** **Poisoning by tricyclic antidepressants, assault**

✓7th **T43.014** **Poisoning by tricyclic antidepressants, undetermined**

✓7th **T43.015** **Adverse effect of tricyclic antidepressants**

✓7th **T43.016** **Underdosing of tricyclic antidepressants**

✓6th **T43.02** **Poisoning by, adverse effect of and underdosing of tetracyclic antidepressants**

✓7th **T43.021** **Poisoning by tetracyclic antidepressants, accidental (unintentional)**
Poisoning by tetracyclic antidepressants NOS

✓7th **T43.022** **Poisoning by tetracyclic antidepressants, intentional self-harm**

✓7th **T43.023** **Poisoning by tetracyclic antidepressants, assault**

✓7th **T43.024** **Poisoning by tetracyclic antidepressants, undetermined**

✓7th **T43.025** **Adverse effect of tetracyclic antidepressants**

✓7th **T43.026** **Underdosing of tetracyclic antidepressants**

✓5th **T43.1** **Poisoning by, adverse effect of and underdosing of monoamine-oxidase-inhibitor antidepressants**

✓6th **T43.1X** **Poisoning by, adverse effect of and underdosing of monoamine-oxidase-inhibitor antidepressants**

✓7th **T43.1X1** **Poisoning by monoamine-oxidase-inhibitor antidepressants, accidental (unintentional)**
Poisoning by monoamine-oxidase-inhibitor antidepressants NOS

✓7th **T43.1X2** **Poisoning by monoamine-oxidase-inhibitor antidepressants, intentional self-harm**

✓7th **T43.1X3** **Poisoning by monoamine-oxidase-inhibitor antidepressants, assault**

✓7th **T43.1X4** **Poisoning by monoamine-oxidase-inhibitor antidepressants, undetermined**

✓7th **T43.1X5** **Adverse effect of monoamine-oxidase-inhibitor antidepressants**

✓7th **T43.1X6** **Underdosing of monoamine-oxidase-inhibitor antidepressants**

✓5th **T43.2** **Poisoning by, adverse effect of and underdosing of other and unspecified antidepressants**

✓6th **T43.20** **Poisoning by, adverse effect of and underdosing of unspecified antidepressants**

✓7th **T43.201** **Poisoning by unspecified antidepressants, accidental (unintentional)**
Poisoning by antidepressants NOS

✓7th **T43.202** **Poisoning by unspecified antidepressants, intentional self-harm**

✓7th **T43.203** **Poisoning by unspecified antidepressants, assault**

✓7th **T43.204** **Poisoning by unspecified antidepressants, undetermined**

✓7th **T43.205** **Adverse effect of unspecified antidepressants**

✓7th **T43.206** **Underdosing of unspecified antidepressants**

✓6th **T43.21** **Poisoning by, adverse effect of and underdosing of selective serotonin and norepinephrine reuptake inhibitors**
Poisoning by, adverse effect of and underdosing of SSNRI antidepressants

✓7th **T43.211** **Poisoning by selective serotonin and norepinephrine reuptake inhibitors, accidental (unintentional)**

✓7th **T43.212** **Poisoning by selective serotonin and norepinephrine reuptake inhibitors, intentional self-harm**

✓7th **T43.213** **Poisoning by selective serotonin and norepinephrine reuptake inhibitors, assault**

✓7th **T43.214** **Poisoning by selective serotonin and norepinephrine reuptake inhibitors, undetermined**

✓7th **T43.215** **Adverse effect of selective serotonin and norepinephrine reuptake inhibitors**

✓7th **T43.216** **Underdosing of selective serotonin and norepinephrine reuptake inhibitors**

✓6th **T43.22** **Poisoning by, adverse effect of and underdosing of selective serotonin reuptake inhibitors**
Poisoning by, adverse effect of and underdosing of SSRI antidepressants

✓7th **T43.221** **Poisoning by selective serotonin reuptake inhibitors, accidental (unintentional)**

✓7th **T43.222** **Poisoning by selective serotonin reuptake inhibitors, intentional self-harm**

✓7th **T43.223** **Poisoning by selective serotonin reuptake inhibitors, assault**

✓7th **T43.224** **Poisoning by selective serotonin reuptake inhibitors, undetermined**

✓7th **T43.225** **Adverse effect of selective serotonin reuptake inhibitors**

✓7th **T43.226** **Underdosing of selective serotonin reuptake inhibitors**

✓6th **T43.29** **Poisoning by, adverse effect of and underdosing of other antidepressants**

✓7th **T43.291** **Poisoning by other antidepressants, accidental (unintentional)**
Poisoning by other antidepressants NOS

✓7th **T43.292** **Poisoning by other antidepressants, intentional self-harm**

✓7th **T43.293** **Poisoning by other antidepressants, assault**

✓7th **T43.294** **Poisoning by other antidepressants, undetermined**

✓7th **T43.295** **Adverse effect of other antidepressants**

✓7th **T43.296** **Underdosing of other antidepressants**

✓ Additional Character Required   ✓x7th Placeholder Alert   Unacceptable PDx   Manifestation   Hospital Acquired Condition   EXCLUDES 1 Not Coded Here   EXCLUDES 2 Not Included Here

Chapter 19. Injury, Poisoning, and Certain Other Consequences of External Causes

√5ᵗʰ **T43.3 Poisoning by, adverse effect of and underdosing of phenothiazine antipsychotics and neuroleptics**

√6ᵗʰ **T43.3X Poisoning by, adverse effect of and underdosing of phenothiazine antipsychotics and neuroleptics**

√7ᵗʰ **T43.3X1 Poisoning by phenothiazine antipsychotics and neuroleptics, accidental (unintentional)**
Poisoning by phenothiazine antipsychotics and neuroleptics NOS

√7ᵗʰ **T43.3X2 Poisoning by phenothiazine antipsychotics and neuroleptics, intentional self-harm**

√7ᵗʰ **T43.3X3 Poisoning by phenothiazine antipsychotics and neuroleptics, assault**

√7ᵗʰ **T43.3X4 Poisoning by phenothiazine antipsychotics and neuroleptics, undetermined**

√7ᵗʰ **T43.3X5 Adverse effect of phenothiazine antipsychotics and neuroleptics**

√7ᵗʰ **T43.3X6 Underdosing of phenothiazine antipsychotics and neuroleptics**

√5ᵗʰ **T43.4 Poisoning by, adverse effect of and underdosing of butyrophenone and thiothixene neuroleptics**

√6ᵗʰ **T43.4X Poisoning by, adverse effect of and underdosing of butyrophenone and thiothixene neuroleptics**

√7ᵗʰ **T43.4X1 Poisoning by butyrophenone and thiothixene neuroleptics, accidental (unintentional)**
Poisoning by butyrophenone and thiothixene neuroleptics NOS

√7ᵗʰ **T43.4X2 Poisoning by butyrophenone and thiothixene neuroleptics, intentional self-harm**

√7ᵗʰ **T43.4X3 Poisoning by butyrophenone and thiothixene neuroleptics, assault**

√7ᵗʰ **T43.4X4 Poisoning by butyrophenone and thiothixene neuroleptics, undetermined**

√7ᵗʰ **T43.4X5 Adverse effect of butyrophenone and thiothixene neuroleptics**

√7ᵗʰ **T43.4X6 Underdosing of butyrophenone and thiothixene neuroleptics**

√5ᵗʰ **T43.5 Poisoning by, adverse effect of and underdosing of other and unspecified antipsychotics and neuroleptics**

EXCLUDES 1 *poisoning by, adverse effect of and underdosing of rauwolfia (T46.5-)*

√6ᵗʰ **T43.50 Poisoning by, adverse effect of and underdosing of unspecified antipsychotics and neuroleptics**

√7ᵗʰ **T43.501 Poisoning by unspecified antipsychotics and neuroleptics, accidental (unintentional)**
Poisoning by antipsychotics and neuroleptics NOS

√7ᵗʰ **T43.502 Poisoning by unspecified antipsychotics and neuroleptics, intentional self-harm**

√7ᵗʰ **T43.503 Poisoning by unspecified antipsychotics and neuroleptics, assault**

√7ᵗʰ **T43.504 Poisoning by unspecified antipsychotics and neuroleptics, undetermined**

√7ᵗʰ **T43.505 Adverse effect of unspecified antipsychotics and neuroleptics**

√7ᵗʰ **T43.506 Underdosing of unspecified antipsychotics and neuroleptics**

√6ᵗʰ **T43.59 Poisoning by, adverse effect of and underdosing of other antipsychotics and neuroleptics**

√7ᵗʰ **T43.591 Poisoning by other antipsychotics and neuroleptics, accidental (unintentional)**
Poisoning by other antipsychotics and neuroleptics NOS

√7ᵗʰ **T43.592 Poisoning by other antipsychotics and neuroleptics, intentional self-harm**

√7ᵗʰ **T43.593 Poisoning by other antipsychotics and neuroleptics, assault**

√7ᵗʰ **T43.594 Poisoning by other antipsychotics and neuroleptics, undetermined**

√7ᵗʰ **T43.595 Adverse effect of other antipsychotics and neuroleptics**

√7ᵗʰ **T43.596 Underdosing of other antipsychotics and neuroleptics**

√5ᵗʰ **T43.6 Poisoning by, adverse effect of and underdosing of psychostimulants**

EXCLUDES 1 *poisoning by, adverse effect of and underdosing of cocaine (T40.5-)*

√6ᵗʰ **T43.60 Poisoning by, adverse effect of and underdosing of unspecified psychostimulant**

√7ᵗʰ **T43.601 Poisoning by unspecified psychostimulants, accidental (unintentional)**
Poisoning by psychostimulants NOS

√7ᵗʰ **T43.602 Poisoning by unspecified psychostimulants, intentional self-harm**

√7ᵗʰ **T43.603 Poisoning by unspecified psychostimulants, assault**

√7ᵗʰ **T43.604 Poisoning by unspecified psychostimulants, undetermined**

√7ᵗʰ **T43.605 Adverse effect of unspecified psychostimulants**

√7ᵗʰ **T43.606 Underdosing of unspecified psychostimulants**

√6ᵗʰ **T43.61 Poisoning by, adverse effect of and underdosing of caffeine**

√7ᵗʰ **T43.611 Poisoning by caffeine, accidental (unintentional)**
Poisoning by caffeine NOS

√7ᵗʰ **T43.612 Poisoning by caffeine, intentional self-harm**

√7ᵗʰ **T43.613 Poisoning by caffeine, assault**

√7ᵗʰ **T43.614 Poisoning by caffeine, undetermined**

√7ᵗʰ **T43.615 Adverse effect of caffeine**

√7ᵗʰ **T43.616 Underdosing of caffeine**

√6ᵗʰ **T43.62 Poisoning by, adverse effect of and underdosing of amphetamines**
Poisoning by, adverse effect of and underdosing of methamphetamines

√7ᵗʰ **T43.621 Poisoning by amphetamines, accidental (unintentional)**
Poisoning by amphetamines NOS

√7ᵗʰ **T43.622 Poisoning by amphetamines, intentional self-harm**

√7ᵗʰ **T43.623 Poisoning by amphetamines, assault**

√7ᵗʰ **T43.624 Poisoning by amphetamines, undetermined**

√7ᵗʰ **T43.625 Adverse effect of amphetamines**

√7ᵗʰ **T43.626 Underdosing of amphetamines**

√6ᵗʰ **T43.63 Poisoning by, adverse effect of and underdosing of methylphenidate**

√7ᵗʰ **T43.631 Poisoning by methylphenidate, accidental (unintentional)**
Poisoning by methylphenidate NOS

√7ᵗʰ **T43.632 Poisoning by methylphenidate, intentional self-harm**

√7ᵗʰ **T43.633 Poisoning by methylphenidate, assault**

√7ᵗʰ **T43.634 Poisoning by methylphenidate, undetermined**

√7ᵗʰ **T43.635 Adverse effect of methylphenidate**

√7ᵗʰ **T43.636 Underdosing of methylphenidate**

√6ᵗʰ **T43.69 Poisoning by, adverse effect of and underdosing of other psychostimulants**

√7ᵗʰ **T43.691 Poisoning by other psychostimulants, accidental (unintentional)**
Poisoning by other psychostimulants NOS

√7ᵗʰ **T43.692 Poisoning by other psychostimulants, intentional self-harm**

√7ᵗʰ **T43.693 Poisoning by other psychostimulants, assault**

√7ᵗʰ **T43.694 Poisoning by other psychostimulants, undetermined**

√7ᵗʰ **T43.695 Adverse effect of other psychostimulants**

√7ᵗʰ **T43.696 Underdosing of other psychostimulants**

N Newborn: 0   P Pediatric: 0-17   M Maternity: 12-55   A Adult: 15-124   MCC Major CC Condition   PDxMCC PDx acts as own MCC   CC CC Condition   PDxCC PDx acts as own CC

1106

ICD-10-CM 2016

✓5ᵗʰ **T43.8 Poisoning by, adverse effect of and underdosing of other psychotropic drugs**

    ✓6ᵗʰ **T43.8X Poisoning by, adverse effect of and underdosing of other psychotropic drugs**

      ✓7ᵗʰ **T43.8X1 Poisoning by other psychotropic drugs, accidental (unintentional)**
        Poisoning by other psychotropic drugs NOS

      ✓7ᵗʰ **T43.8X2 Poisoning by other psychotropic drugs, intentional self-harm**

      ✓7ᵗʰ **T43.8X3 Poisoning by other psychotropic drugs, assault**

      ✓7ᵗʰ **T43.8X4 Poisoning by other psychotropic drugs, undetermined**

      ✓7ᵗʰ **T43.8X5 Adverse effect of other psychotropic drugs**

      ✓7ᵗʰ **T43.8X6 Underdosing of other psychotropic drugs**

✓5ᵗʰ **T43.9 Poisoning by, adverse effect of and underdosing of unspecified psychotropic drug**

    ✓×7ᵗʰ **T43.91 Poisoning by unspecified psychotropic drug, accidental (unintentional)**
      Poisoning by psychotropic drug NOS

    ✓×7ᵗʰ **T43.92 Poisoning by unspecified psychotropic drug, intentional self-harm**

    ✓×7ᵗʰ **T43.93 Poisoning by unspecified psychotropic drug, assault**

    ✓×7ᵗʰ **T43.94 Poisoning by unspecified psychotropic drug, undetermined**

    ✓×7ᵗʰ **T43.95 Adverse effect of unspecified psychotropic drug**

    ✓×7ᵗʰ **T43.96 Underdosing of unspecified psychotropic drug**

✓4ᵗʰ **T44 Poisoning by, adverse effect of and underdosing of drugs primarily affecting the autonomic nervous system**

> The appropriate 7th character is to be added to each code from category T44.
> A   initial encounter
> D   subsequent encounter
> S   sequela

✓5ᵗʰ **T44.0 Poisoning by, adverse effect of and underdosing of anticholinesterase agents**

    ✓6ᵗʰ **T44.0X Poisoning by, adverse effect of and underdosing of anticholinesterase agents**

      ✓7ᵗʰ **T44.0X1 Poisoning by anticholinesterase agents, accidental (unintentional)**
        Poisoning by anticholinesterase agents NOS

      ✓7ᵗʰ **T44.0X2 Poisoning by anticholinesterase agents, intentional self-harm**

      ✓7ᵗʰ **T44.0X3 Poisoning by anticholinesterase agents, assault**

      ✓7ᵗʰ **T44.0X4 Poisoning by anticholinesterase agents, undetermined**

      ✓7ᵗʰ **T44.0X5 Adverse effect of anticholinesterase agents**

      ✓7ᵗʰ **T44.0X6 Underdosing of anticholinesterase agents**

✓5ᵗʰ **T44.1 Poisoning by, adverse effect of and underdosing of other parasympathomimetics [cholinergics]**

    ✓6ᵗʰ **T44.1X Poisoning by, adverse effect of and underdosing of other parasympathomimetics [cholinergics]**

      ✓7ᵗʰ **T44.1X1 Poisoning by other parasympathomimetics [cholinergics], accidental (unintentional)**
        Poisoning by other parasympathomimetics [cholinergics] NOS

      ✓7ᵗʰ **T44.1X2 Poisoning by other parasympathomimetics [cholinergics], intentional self-harm**

      ✓7ᵗʰ **T44.1X3 Poisoning by other parasympathomimetics [cholinergics], assault**

      ✓7ᵗʰ **T44.1X4 Poisoning by other parasympathomimetics [cholinergics], undetermined**

      ✓7ᵗʰ **T44.1X5 Adverse effect of other parasympathomimetics [cholinergics]**

      ✓7ᵗʰ **T44.1X6 Underdosing of other parasympathomimetics**

✓5ᵗʰ **T44.2 Poisoning by, adverse effect of and underdosing of ganglionic blocking drugs**

    ✓6ᵗʰ **T44.2X Poisoning by, adverse effect of and underdosing of ganglionic blocking drugs**

      ✓7ᵗʰ **T44.2X1 Poisoning by ganglionic blocking drugs, accidental (unintentional)**
        Poisoning by ganglionic blocking drugs NOS

      ✓7ᵗʰ **T44.2X2 Poisoning by ganglionic blocking drugs, intentional self-harm**

      ✓7ᵗʰ **T44.2X3 Poisoning by ganglionic blocking drugs, assault**

      ✓7ᵗʰ **T44.2X4 Poisoning by ganglionic blocking drugs, undetermined**

      ✓7ᵗʰ **T44.2X5 Adverse effect of ganglionic blocking drugs**

      ✓7ᵗʰ **T44.2X6 Underdosing of ganglionic blocking drugs**

T44.3 Poisoning by, adverse effect of and underdosing of other parasympatholytics [anticholinergics and antimuscarinics] and spasmolytics
    Poisoning by, adverse effect of and underdosing of papaverine

    ✓6ᵗʰ **T44.3X Poisoning by, adverse effect of and underdosing of other parasympatholytics [anticholinergics and antimuscarinics] and spasmolytics**

      ✓7ᵗʰ **T44.3X1 Poisoning by other parasympatholytics [anticholinergics and antimuscarinics] and spasmolytics, accidental (unintentional)**
        Poisoning by other parasympatholytics [anticholinergics and antimuscarinics] and spasmolytics NOS

      ✓7ᵗʰ **T44.3X2 Poisoning by other parasympatholytics [anticholinergics and antimuscarinics] and spasmolytics, intentional self-harm**

      ✓7ᵗʰ **T44.3X3 Poisoning by other parasympatholytics [anticholinergics and antimuscarinics] and spasmolytics, assault**

      ✓7ᵗʰ **T44.3X4 Poisoning by other parasympatholytics [anticholinergics and antimuscarinics] and spasmolytics, undetermined**

      ✓7ᵗʰ **T44.3X5 Adverse effect of other parasympatholytics [anticholinergics and antimuscarinics] and spasmolytics**

      ✓7ᵗʰ **T44.3X6 Underdosing of other parasympatholytics [anticholinergics and antimuscarinics] and spasmolytics**

✓5ᵗʰ **T44.4 Poisoning by, adverse effect of and underdosing of predominantly alpha-adrenoreceptor agonists**
    Poisoning by, adverse effect of and underdosing of metaraminol

    ✓6ᵗʰ **T44.4X Poisoning by, adverse effect of and underdosing of predominantly alpha-adrenoreceptor agonists**

      ✓7ᵗʰ **T44.4X1 Poisoning by predominantly alpha-adrenoreceptor agonists, accidental (unintentional)**
        Poisoning by predominantly alpha-adrenoreceptor agonists NOS

      ✓7ᵗʰ **T44.4X2 Poisoning by predominantly alpha-adrenoreceptor agonists, intentional self-harm**

      ✓7ᵗʰ **T44.4X3 Poisoning by predominantly alpha-adrenoreceptor agonists, assault**

      ✓7ᵗʰ **T44.4X4 Poisoning by predominantly alpha-adrenoreceptor agonists, undetermined**

      ✓7ᵗʰ **T44.4X5 Adverse effect of predominantly alpha-adrenoreceptor agonists**

      ✓7ᵗʰ **T44.4X6 Underdosing of predominantly alpha-adrenoreceptor agonists**

✓5ᵗʰ **T44.5 Poisoning by, adverse effect of and underdosing of predominantly beta-adrenoreceptor agonists**
    EXCLUDES 1   *poisoning by, adverse effect of and underdosing of beta-adrenoreceptor agonists used in asthma therapy (T48.6-)*

    ✓6ᵗʰ **T44.5X Poisoning by, adverse effect of and underdosing of predominantly beta-adrenoreceptor agonists**

      ✓7ᵗʰ **T44.5X1 Poisoning by predominantly beta-adrenoreceptor agonists, accidental (unintentional)**
        Poisoning by predominantly beta-adrenoreceptor agonists NOS

✓ Additional Character Required   ✓×7ᵗʰ Placeholder Alert   Unacceptable PDx   Manifestation   Hospital Acquired Condition   **EXCLUDES 1** Not Coded Here   *EXCLUDES 2* Not Included Here

ICD-10-CM 2016   1107

√7ᵗʰ **T44.5X2** **Poisoning by predominantly beta-adrenoreceptor agonists, intentional self-harm**

√7ᵗʰ **T44.5X3** **Poisoning by predominantly beta-adrenoreceptor agonists, assault**

√7ᵗʰ **T44.5X4** **Poisoning by predominantly beta-adrenoreceptor agonists, undetermined**

√7ᵗʰ **T44.5X5** **Adverse effect of predominantly beta-adrenoreceptor agonists**

√7ᵗʰ **T44.5X6** **Underdosing of predominantly beta-adrenoreceptor agonists**

√5ᵗʰ **T44.6** **Poisoning by, adverse effect of and underdosing of alpha-adrenoreceptor antagonists**
> EXCLUDES 1 *poisoning by, adverse effect of and underdosing of ergot alkaloids (T48.0)*

√6ᵗʰ **T44.6X** **Poisoning by, adverse effect of and underdosing of alpha-adrenoreceptor antagonists**

√7ᵗʰ **T44.6X1** **Poisoning by alpha-adrenoreceptor antagonists, accidental (unintentional)**
> Poisoning by alpha-adrenoreceptor antagonists NOS

√7ᵗʰ **T44.6X2** **Poisoning by alpha-adrenoreceptor antagonists, intentional self-harm**

√7ᵗʰ **T44.6X3** **Poisoning by alpha-adrenoreceptor antagonists, assault**

√7ᵗʰ **T44.6X4** **Poisoning by alpha-adrenoreceptor antagonists, undetermined**

√7ᵗʰ **T44.6X5** **Adverse effect of alpha-adrenoreceptor antagonists**

√7ᵗʰ **T44.6X6** **Underdosing of alpha-adrenoreceptor antagonists**

√5ᵗʰ **T44.7** **Poisoning by, adverse effect of and underdosing of beta-adrenoreceptor antagonists**

√6ᵗʰ **T44.7X** **Poisoning by, adverse effect of and underdosing of beta-adrenoreceptor antagonists**

√7ᵗʰ **T44.7X1** **Poisoning by beta-adrenoreceptor antagonists, accidental (unintentional)**
> Poisoning by beta-adrenoreceptor antagonists NOS

√7ᵗʰ **T44.7X2** **Poisoning by beta-adrenoreceptor antagonists, intentional self-harm**

√7ᵗʰ **T44.7X3** **Poisoning by beta-adrenoreceptor antagonists, assault**

√7ᵗʰ **T44.7X4** **Poisoning by beta-adrenoreceptor antagonists, undetermined**

√7ᵗʰ **T44.7X5** **Adverse effect of beta-adrenoreceptor antagonists**

√7ᵗʰ **T44.7X6** **Underdosing of beta-adrenoreceptor antagonists**

√5ᵗʰ **T44.8** **Poisoning by, adverse effect of and underdosing of centrally-acting and adrenergic-neuron- blocking agents**
> EXCLUDES 1 *poisoning by, adverse effect of and underdosing of clonidine (T46.5)*
> *poisoning by, adverse effect of and underdosing of guanethidine (T46.5)*

√6ᵗʰ **T44.8X** **Poisoning by, adverse effect of and underdosing of centrally-acting and adrenergic-neuron-blocking agents**

√7ᵗʰ **T44.8X1** **Poisoning by centrally-acting and adrenergic-neuron-blocking agents, accidental (unintentional)**
> Poisoning by centrally-acting and adrenergic-neuron-blocking agents NOS

√7ᵗʰ **T44.8X2** **Poisoning by centrally-acting and adrenergic-neuron-blocking agents, intentional self-harm**

√7ᵗʰ **T44.8X3** **Poisoning by centrally-acting and adrenergic-neuron-blocking agents, assault**

√7ᵗʰ **T44.8X4** **Poisoning by centrally-acting and adrenergic-neuron-blocking agents, undetermined**

√7ᵗʰ **T44.8X5** **Adverse effect of centrally-acting and adrenergic-neuron-blocking agents**

√7ᵗʰ **T44.8X6** **Underdosing of centrally-acting and adrenergic-neuron-blocking agents**

√5ᵗʰ **T44.9** **Poisoning by, adverse effect of and underdosing of other and unspecified drugs primarily affecting the autonomic nervous system**
> Poisoning by, adverse effect of and underdosing of drug stimulating both alpha and beta-adrenoreceptors

√6ᵗʰ **T44.90** **Poisoning by, adverse effect of and underdosing of unspecified drugs primarily affecting the autonomic nervous system**

√7ᵗʰ **T44.901** **Poisoning by unspecified drugs primarily affecting the autonomic nervous system, accidental (unintentional)**
> Poisoning by unspecified drugs primarily affecting the autonomic nervous system NOS

√7ᵗʰ **T44.902** **Poisoning by unspecified drugs primarily affecting the autonomic nervous system, intentional self-harm**

√7ᵗʰ **T44.903** **Poisoning by unspecified drugs primarily affecting the autonomic nervous system, assault**

√7ᵗʰ **T44.904** **Poisoning by unspecified drugs primarily affecting the autonomic nervous system, undetermined**

√7ᵗʰ **T44.905** **Adverse effect of unspecified drugs primarily affecting the autonomic nervous system**

√7ᵗʰ **T44.906** **Underdosing of unspecified drugs primarily affecting the autonomic nervous system**

√6ᵗʰ **T44.99** **Poisoning by, adverse effect of and underdosing of other drugs primarily affecting the autonomic nervous system**

√7ᵗʰ **T44.991** **Poisoning by other drug primarily affecting the autonomic nervous system, accidental (unintentional)**
> Poisoning by other drugs primarily affecting the autonomic nervous system NOS

√7ᵗʰ **T44.992** **Poisoning by other drug primarily affecting the autonomic nervous system, intentional self-harm**

√7ᵗʰ **T44.993** **Poisoning by other drug primarily affecting the autonomic nervous system, assault**

√7ᵗʰ **T44.994** **Poisoning by other drug primarily affecting the autonomic nervous system, undetermined**

√7ᵗʰ **T44.995** **Adverse effect of other drug primarily affecting the autonomic nervous system**

√7ᵗʰ **T44.996** **Underdosing of other drug primarily affecting the autonomic nervous system**

√4ᵗʰ **T45** **Poisoning by, adverse effect of and underdosing of primarily systemic and hematological agents, not elsewhere classified**

> The appropriate 7th character is to be added to each code from category T45.
> A   initial encounter
> D   subsequent encounter
> S   sequela

√5ᵗʰ **T45.0** **Poisoning by, adverse effect of and underdosing of antiallergic and antiemetic drugs**
> EXCLUDES 1 *poisoning by, adverse effect of and underdosing of phenothiazine-based neuroleptics (T43.3)*

√6ᵗʰ **T45.0X** **Poisoning by, adverse effect of and underdosing of antiallergic and antiemetic drugs**

√7ᵗʰ **T45.0X1** **Poisoning by antiallergic and antiemetic drugs, accidental (unintentional)**
> Poisoning by antiallergic and antiemetic drugs NOS

√7ᵗʰ **T45.0X2** **Poisoning by antiallergic and antiemetic drugs, intentional self-harm**

√7ᵗʰ **T45.0X3** **Poisoning by antiallergic and antiemetic drugs, assault**

√7ᵗʰ **T45.0X4** **Poisoning by antiallergic and antiemetic drugs, undetermined**

√7ᵗʰ **T45.0X5** **Adverse effect of antiallergic and antiemetic drugs**

√7ᵗʰ **T45.0X6** **Underdosing of antiallergic and antiemetic drugs**

√5th **T45.1** **Poisoning by, adverse effect of and underdosing of antineoplastic and immunosuppressive drugs**

> EXCLUDES 1   *poisoning by, adverse effect of and underdosing of tamoxifen (T38.6)*
>
> **AHA:** 2014, 4Q, 22

√6th **T45.1X** **Poisoning by, adverse effect of and underdosing of antineoplastic and immunosuppressive drugs**

√7th **T45.1X1** **Poisoning by antineoplastic and immunosuppressive drugs, accidental (unintentional)**
> Poisoning by antineoplastic and immunosuppressive drugs NOS

√7th **T45.1X2** **Poisoning by antineoplastic and immunosuppressive drugs, intentional self-harm**

√7th **T45.1X3** **Poisoning by antineoplastic and immunosuppressive drugs, assault**

√7th **T45.1X4** **Poisoning by antineoplastic and immunosuppressive drugs, undetermined**

√7th **T45.1X5** **Adverse effect of antineoplastic and immunosuppressive drugs**

√7th **T45.1X6** **Underdosing of antineoplastic and immunosuppressive drugs**

√5th **T45.2** **Poisoning by, adverse effect of and underdosing of vitamins**

> EXCLUDES 2   *poisoning by, adverse effect of and underdosing of iron (T45.4)*
> *poisoning by, adverse effect of and underdosing of nicotinic acid (derivatives) (T46.7)*
> *poisoning by, adverse effect of and underdosing of vitamin K (T45.7)*

√6th **T45.2X** **Poisoning by, adverse effect of and underdosing of vitamins**

√7th **T45.2X1** **Poisoning by vitamins, accidental (unintentional)**
> Poisoning by vitamins NOS

√7th **T45.2X2** **Poisoning by vitamins, intentional self-harm**

√7th **T45.2X3** **Poisoning by vitamins, assault**

√7th **T45.2X4** **Poisoning by vitamins, undetermined**

√7th **T45.2X5** **Adverse effect of vitamins**

√7th **T45.2X6** **Underdosing of vitamins**
> EXCLUDES 1   *vitamin deficiencies (E50-E56)*

√5th **T45.3** **Poisoning by, adverse effect of and underdosing of enzymes**

√6th **T45.3X** **Poisoning by, adverse effect of and underdosing of enzymes**

√7th **T45.3X1** **Poisoning by enzymes, accidental (unintentional)**
> Poisoning by enzymes NOS

√7th **T45.3X2** **Poisoning by enzymes, intentional self-harm**

√7th **T45.3X3** **Poisoning by enzymes, assault**

√7th **T45.3X4** **Poisoning by enzymes, undetermined**

√7th **T45.3X5** **Adverse effect of enzymes**

√7th **T45.3X6** **Underdosing of enzymes**

√5th **T45.4** **Poisoning by, adverse effect of and underdosing of iron and its compounds**

√6th **T45.4X** **Poisoning by, adverse effect of and underdosing of iron and its compounds**

T45.4X1 **Poisoning by iron and its compounds, accidental (unintentional)**
> Poisoning by iron and its compounds NOS

√7th **T45.4X2** **Poisoning by iron and its compounds, intentional self-harm**

√7th **T45.4X3** **Poisoning by iron and its compounds, assault**

√7th **T45.4X4** **Poisoning by iron and its compounds, undetermined**

√7th **T45.4X5** **Adverse effect of iron and its compounds**

√7th **T45.4X6** **Underdosing of iron and its compounds**
> EXCLUDES 1   *iron deficiency (E61.1)*

√5th **T45.5** **Poisoning by, adverse effect of and underdosing of anticoagulants and antithrombotic drugs**

√6th **T45.51** **Poisoning by, adverse effect of and underdosing of anticoagulants**

√7th **T45.511** **Poisoning by anticoagulants, accidental (unintentional)**
> Poisoning by anticoagulants NOS

√7th **T45.512** **Poisoning by anticoagulants, intentional self-harm**

√7th **T45.513** **Poisoning by anticoagulants, assault**

√7th **T45.514** **Poisoning by anticoagulants, undetermined**

√7th **T45.515** **Adverse effect of anticoagulants**
> **AHA:** 2013, 2Q, 34

√7th **T45.516** **Underdosing of anticoagulants**

√6th **T45.52** **Poisoning by, adverse effect of and underdosing of antithrombotic drugs**
> Poisoning by, adverse effect of and underdosing of antiplatelet drugs
>
> EXCLUDES 2   *poisoning by, adverse effect of and underdosing of aspirin (T39.01-)*
> *poisoning by, adverse effect of and underdosing of acetylsalicylic acid (T39.01-)*

√7th **T45.521** **Poisoning by antithrombotic drugs, accidental (unintentional)**
> Poisoning by antithrombotic drug NOS

√7th **T45.522** **Poisoning by antithrombotic drugs, intentional self-harm**

√7th **T45.523** **Poisoning by antithrombotic drugs, assault**

√7th **T45.524** **Poisoning by antithrombotic drugs, undetermined**

√7th **T45.525** **Adverse effect of antithrombotic drugs**

√7th **T45.526** **Underdosing of antithrombotic drugs**

√5th **T45.6** **Poisoning by, adverse effect of and underdosing of fibrinolysis-affecting drugs**

√6th **T45.60** **Poisoning by, adverse effect of and underdosing of unspecified fibrinolysis-affecting drugs**

√7th **T45.601** **Poisoning by unspecified fibrinolysis-affecting drugs, accidental (unintentional)**
> Poisoning by fibrinolysis-affecting drug NOS

√7th **T45.602** **Poisoning by unspecified fibrinolysis-affecting drugs, intentional self-harm**

√7th **T45.603** **Poisoning by unspecified fibrinolysis-affecting drugs, assault**

√7th **T45.604** **Poisoning by unspecified fibrinolysis-affecting drugs, undetermined**

√7th **T45.605** **Adverse effect of unspecified fibrinolysis-affecting drugs**

√7th **T45.606** **Underdosing of unspecified fibrinolysis-affecting drugs**

√6th **T45.61** **Poisoning by, adverse effect of and underdosing of thrombolytic drugs**

√7th **T45.611** **Poisoning by thrombolytic drug, accidental (unintentional)**
> Poisoning by thrombolytic drug NOS

√7th **T45.612** **Poisoning by thrombolytic drug, intentional self-harm**

√7th **T45.613** **Poisoning by thrombolytic drug, assault**

√7th **T45.614** **Poisoning by thrombolytic drug, undetermined**

√7th **T45.615** **Adverse effect of thrombolytic drugs**

√7th **T45.616** **Underdosing of thrombolytic drugs**

√6th **T45.62** **Poisoning by, adverse effect of and underdosing of hemostatic drugs**

√7th **T45.621** **Poisoning by hemostatic drug, accidental (unintentional)**
> Poisoning by hemostatic drug NOS

√7th **T45.622** **Poisoning by hemostatic drug, intentional self-harm**

√7th **T45.623** **Poisoning by hemostatic drug, assault**

√7th **T45.624** **Poisoning by hemostatic drug, undetermined**

√7th **T45.625** **Adverse effect of hemostatic drug**

√7th **T45.626** **Underdosing of hemostatic drugs**

✔ Additional Character Required   ✔x7th Placeholder Alert   Unacceptable PDx   Manifestation   Hospital Acquired Condition   EXCLUDES 1 Not Coded Here   EXCLUDES 2 Not Included Here

ICD-10-CM 2016   1109

✓6ᵗʰ T45.69 Poisoning by, adverse effect of and underdosing of other fibrinolysis-affecting drugs

✓7ᵗʰ **T45.691 Poisoning by other fibrinolysis-affecting drugs, accidental (unintentional)**
Poisoning by other fibrinolysis-affecting drug NOS

✓7ᵗʰ **T45.692 Poisoning by other fibrinolysis-affecting drugs, intentional self-harm**

✓7ᵗʰ **T45.693 Poisoning by other fibrinolysis-affecting drugs, assault**

✓7ᵗʰ **T45.694 Poisoning by other fibrinolysis-affecting drugs, undetermined**

✓7ᵗʰ **T45.695 Adverse effect of other fibrinolysis-affecting drugs**

✓7ᵗʰ **T45.696 Underdosing of other fibrinolysis-affecting drugs**

✓5ᵗʰ T45.7 Poisoning by, adverse effect of and underdosing of anticoagulant antagonists, vitamin K and other coagulants

✓6ᵗʰ T45.7X Poisoning by, adverse effect of and underdosing of anticoagulant antagonists, vitamin K and other coagulants

✓7ᵗʰ **T45.7X1 Poisoning by anticoagulant antagonists, vitamin K and other coagulants, accidental (unintentional)**
Poisoning by anticoagulant antagonists, vitamin K and other coagulants NOS

✓7ᵗʰ **T45.7X2 Poisoning by anticoagulant antagonists, vitamin K and other coagulants, intentional self-harm**

✓7ᵗʰ **T45.7X3 Poisoning by anticoagulant antagonists, vitamin K and other coagulants, assault**

✓7ᵗʰ **T45.7X4 Poisoning by anticoagulant antagonists, vitamin K and other coagulants, undetermined**

✓7ᵗʰ **T45.7X5 Adverse effect of anticoagulant antagonists, vitamin K and other coagulants**

✓7ᵗʰ **T45.7X6 Underdosing of anticoagulant antagonist, vitamin K and other coagulants**
EXCLUDES 1 *vitamin K deficiency (E56.1)*

✓5ᵗʰ T45.8 Poisoning by, adverse effect of and underdosing of other primarily systemic and hematological agents
Poisoning by, adverse effect of and underdosing of liver preparations and other antianemic agents
Poisoning by, adverse effect of and underdosing of natural blood and blood products
Poisoning by, adverse effect of and underdosing of plasma substitute
EXCLUDES 2 *poisoning by, adverse effect of and underdosing of immunoglobulin (T50.Z1)*
poisoning by, adverse effect of and underdosing of iron (T45.4)
transfusion reactions (T80.-)

✓6ᵗʰ T45.8X Poisoning by, adverse effect of and underdosing of other primarily systemic and hematological agents

✓7ᵗʰ **T45.8X1 Poisoning by other primarily systemic and hematological agents, accidental (unintentional)**
Poisoning by other primarily systemic and hematological agents NOS

✓7ᵗʰ **T45.8X2 Poisoning by other primarily systemic and hematological agents, intentional self-harm**

✓7ᵗʰ **T45.8X3 Poisoning by other primarily systemic and hematological agents, assault**

✓7ᵗʰ **T45.8X4 Poisoning by other primarily systemic and hematological agents, undetermined**

✓7ᵗʰ **T45.8X5 Adverse effect of other primarily systemic and hematological agents**

✓7ᵗʰ **T45.8X6 Underdosing of other primarily systemic and hematological agents**

✓5ᵗʰ T45.9 Poisoning by, adverse effect of and underdosing of unspecified primarily systemic and hematological agent

✓x7ᵗʰ **T45.91 Poisoning by unspecified primarily systemic and hematological agent, accidental (unintentional)**
Poisoning by primarily systemic and hematological agent NOS

✓x7ᵗʰ **T45.92 Poisoning by unspecified primarily systemic and hematological agent, intentional self-harm**

✓x7ᵗʰ **T45.93 Poisoning by unspecified primarily systemic and hematological agent, assault**

✓x7ᵗʰ **T45.94 Poisoning by unspecified primarily systemic and hematological agent, undetermined**

✓x7ᵗʰ **T45.95 Adverse effect of unspecified primarily systemic and hematological agent**

✓x7ᵗʰ **T45.96 Underdosing of unspecified primarily systemic and hematological agent**

✓4ᵗʰ T46 Poisoning by, adverse effect of and underdosing of agents primarily affecting the cardiovascular system
EXCLUDES 1 *poisoning by, adverse effect of and underdosing of metaraminol (T44.4)*

The appropriate 7th character is to be added to each code from category T46.
A   initial encounter
D   subsequent encounter
S   sequela

✓5ᵗʰ T46.0 Poisoning by, adverse effect of and underdosing of cardiac-stimulant glycosides and drugs of similar action

✓6ᵗʰ T46.0X Poisoning by, adverse effect of and underdosing of cardiac-stimulant glycosides and drugs of similar action

✓7ᵗʰ **T46.0X1 Poisoning by cardiac-stimulant glycosides and drugs of similar action, accidental (unintentional)**
Poisoning by cardiac-stimulant glycosides and drugs of similar action NOS

✓7ᵗʰ **T46.0X2 Poisoning by cardiac-stimulant glycosides and drugs of similar action, intentional self-harm**

✓7ᵗʰ **T46.0X3 Poisoning by cardiac-stimulant glycosides and drugs of similar action, assault**

✓7ᵗʰ **T46.0X4 Poisoning by cardiac-stimulant glycosides and drugs of similar action, undetermined**

✓7ᵗʰ **T46.0X5 Adverse effect of cardiac-stimulant glycosides and drugs of similar action**

✓7ᵗʰ **T46.0X6 Underdosing of cardiac-stimulant glycosides and drugs of similar action**

T46.1 Poisoning by, adverse effect of and underdosing of calcium-channel blockers

✓6ᵗʰ T46.1X Poisoning by, adverse effect of and underdosing of calcium-channel blockers

✓7ᵗʰ **T46.1X1 Poisoning by calcium-channel blockers, accidental (unintentional)**
Poisoning by calcium-channel blockers NOS

✓7ᵗʰ **T46.1X2 Poisoning by calcium-channel blockers, intentional self-harm**

✓7ᵗʰ **T46.1X3 Poisoning by calcium-channel blockers, assault**

✓7ᵗʰ **T46.1X4 Poisoning by calcium-channel blockers, undetermined**

✓7ᵗʰ **T46.1X5 Adverse effect of calcium-channel blockers**

✓7ᵗʰ **T46.1X6 Underdosing of calcium-channel blockers**

✓5ᵗʰ T46.2 Poisoning by, adverse effect of and underdosing of other antidysrhythmic drugs, not elsewhere classified
EXCLUDES 1 *poisoning by, adverse effect of and underdosing of beta-adrenoreceptor antagonists (T44.7-)*

✓6ᵗʰ T46.2X Poisoning by, adverse effect of and underdosing of other antidysrhythmic drugs

✓7ᵗʰ **T46.2X1 Poisoning by other antidysrhythmic drugs, accidental (unintentional)**
Poisoning by other antidysrhythmic drugs NOS

✓7ᵗʰ **T46.2X2 Poisoning by other antidysrhythmic drugs, intentional self-harm**

✓7ᵗʰ **T46.2X3 Poisoning by other antidysrhythmic drugs, assault**

✓7ᵗʰ **T46.2X4 Poisoning by other antidysrhythmic drugs, undetermined**

✓7ᵗʰ **T46.2X5 Adverse effect of other antidysrhythmic drugs**

✓7ᵗʰ **T46.2X6 Underdosing of other antidysrhythmic drugs**

√5ᵗʰ **T46.3   Poisoning by, adverse effect of and underdosing of coronary vasodilators**

Poisoning by, adverse effect of and underdosing of dipyridamole

> **EXCLUDES 1**   *poisoning by, adverse effect of and underdosing of calcium-channel blockers (T46.1)*

√6ᵗʰ **T46.3X   Poisoning by, adverse effect of and underdosing of coronary vasodilators**

√7ᵗʰ **T46.3X1   Poisoning by coronary vasodilators, accidental (unintentional)**

Poisoning by coronary vasodilators NOS

√7ᵗʰ **T46.3X2   Poisoning by coronary vasodilators, intentional self-harm**

√7ᵗʰ **T46.3X3   Poisoning by coronary vasodilators, assault**

√7ᵗʰ **T46.3X4   Poisoning by coronary vasodilators, undetermined**

√7ᵗʰ **T46.3X5   Adverse effect of coronary vasodilators**

√7ᵗʰ **T46.3X6   Underdosing of coronary vasodilators**

√5ᵗʰ **T46.4   Poisoning by, adverse effect of and underdosing of angiotensin-converting-enzyme inhibitors**

√6ᵗʰ **T46.4X   Poisoning by, adverse effect of and underdosing of angiotensin-converting-enzyme inhibitors**

√7ᵗʰ **T46.4X1   Poisoning by angiotensin-converting-enzyme inhibitors, accidental (unintentional)**

Poisoning by angiotensin-converting-enzyme inhibitors NOS

√7ᵗʰ **T46.4X2   Poisoning by angiotensin-converting-enzyme inhibitors, intentional self-harm**

√7ᵗʰ **T46.4X3   Poisoning by angiotensin-converting-enzyme inhibitors, assault**

√7ᵗʰ **T46.4X4   Poisoning by angiotensin-converting-enzyme inhibitors, undetermined**

√7ᵗʰ **T46.4X5   Adverse effect of angiotensin-converting-enzyme inhibitors**

√7ᵗʰ **T46.4X6   Underdosing of angiotensin-converting-enzyme inhibitors**

√5ᵗʰ **T46.5   Poisoning by, adverse effect of and underdosing of other antihypertensive drugs**

> **EXCLUDES 2**   *poisoning by, adverse effect of and underdosing of beta-adrenoreceptor antagonists (T44.7)*
> *poisoning by, adverse effect of and underdosing of calcium-channel blockers (T46.1)*
> *poisoning by, adverse effect of and underdosing of diuretics (T50.0-T50.2)*

√6ᵗʰ **T46.5X   Poisoning by, adverse effect of and underdosing of other antihypertensive drugs**

√7ᵗʰ **T46.5X1   Poisoning by other antihypertensive drugs, accidental (unintentional)**

Poisoning by other antihypertensive drugs NOS

√7ᵗʰ **T46.5X2   Poisoning by other antihypertensive drugs, intentional self-harm**

√7ᵗʰ **T46.5X3   Poisoning by other antihypertensive drugs, assault**

√7ᵗʰ **T46.5X4   Poisoning by other antihypertensive drugs, undetermined**

√7ᵗʰ **T46.5X5   Adverse effect of other antihypertensive drugs**

√7ᵗʰ **T46.5X6   Underdosing of other antihypertensive drugs**

√5ᵗʰ **T46.6   Poisoning by, adverse effect of and underdosing of antihyperlipidemic and antiarteriosclerotic drugs**

√6ᵗʰ **T46.6X   Poisoning by, adverse effect of and underdosing of antihyperlipidemic and antiarteriosclerotic drugs**

√7ᵗʰ **T46.6X1   Poisoning by antihyperlipidemic and antiarteriosclerotic drugs, accidental (unintentional)**

Poisoning by antihyperlipidemic and antiarteriosclerotic drugs NOS

√7ᵗʰ **T46.6X2   Poisoning by antihyperlipidemic and antiarteriosclerotic drugs, intentional self-harm**

√7ᵗʰ **T46.6X3   Poisoning by antihyperlipidemic and antiarteriosclerotic drugs, assault**

√7ᵗʰ **T46.6X4   Poisoning by antihyperlipidemic and antiarteriosclerotic drugs, undetermined**

√7ᵗʰ **T46.6X5   Adverse effect of antihyperlipidemic and antiarteriosclerotic drugs**

√7ᵗʰ **T46.6X6   Underdosing of antihyperlipidemic and antiarteriosclerotic drugs**

√5ᵗʰ **T46.7   Poisoning by, adverse effect of and underdosing of peripheral vasodilators**

Poisoning by, adverse effect of and underdosing of nicotinic acid (derivatives)

> **EXCLUDES 1**   *poisoning by, adverse effect of and underdosing of papaverine (T44.3)*

√6ᵗʰ **T46.7X   Poisoning by, adverse effect of and underdosing of peripheral vasodilators**

√7ᵗʰ **T46.7X1   Poisoning by peripheral vasodilators, accidental (unintentional)**

Poisoning by peripheral vasodilators NOS

√7ᵗʰ **T46.7X2   Poisoning by peripheral vasodilators, intentional self-harm**

√7ᵗʰ **T46.7X3   Poisoning by peripheral vasodilators, assault**

√7ᵗʰ **T46.7X4   Poisoning by peripheral vasodilators, undetermined**

√7ᵗʰ **T46.7X5   Adverse effect of peripheral vasodilators**

√7ᵗʰ **T46.7X6   Underdosing of peripheral vasodilators**

√5ᵗʰ **T46.8   Poisoning by, adverse effect of and underdosing of antivaricose drugs, including sclerosing agents**

√6ᵗʰ **T46.8X   Poisoning by, adverse effect of and underdosing of antivaricose drugs, including sclerosing agents**

√7ᵗʰ **T46.8X1   Poisoning by antivaricose drugs, including sclerosing agents, accidental (unintentional)**

Poisoning by antivaricose drugs, including sclerosing agents NOS

√7ᵗʰ **T46.8X2   Poisoning by antivaricose drugs, including sclerosing agents, intentional self-harm**

√7ᵗʰ **T46.8X3   Poisoning by antivaricose drugs, including sclerosing agents, assault**

√7ᵗʰ **T46.8X4   Poisoning by antivaricose drugs, including sclerosing agents, undetermined**

√7ᵗʰ **T46.8X5   Adverse effect of antivaricose drugs, including sclerosing agents**

√7ᵗʰ **T46.8X6   Underdosing of antivaricose drugs, including sclerosing agents**

√5ᵗʰ **T46.9   Poisoning by, adverse effect of and underdosing of other and unspecified agents primarily affecting the cardiovascular system**

√6ᵗʰ **T46.90   Poisoning by, adverse effect of and underdosing of unspecified agents primarily affecting the cardiovascular system**

√7ᵗʰ **T46.901   Poisoning by unspecified agents primarily affecting the cardiovascular system, accidental (unintentional)**

√7ᵗʰ **T46.902   Poisoning by unspecified agents primarily affecting the cardiovascular system, intentional self-harm**

√7ᵗʰ **T46.903   Poisoning by unspecified agents primarily affecting the cardiovascular system, assault**

√7ᵗʰ **T46.904   Poisoning by unspecified agents primarily affecting the cardiovascular system, undetermined**

√7ᵗʰ **T46.905   Adverse effect of unspecified agents primarily affecting the cardiovascular system**

√7ᵗʰ **T46.906   Underdosing of unspecified agents primarily affecting the cardiovascular system**

√6ᵗʰ **T46.99   Poisoning by, adverse effect of and underdosing of other agents primarily affecting the cardiovascular system**

√7ᵗʰ **T46.991   Poisoning by other agents primarily affecting the cardiovascular system, accidental (unintentional)**

√7ᵗʰ **T46.992   Poisoning by other agents primarily affecting the cardiovascular system, intentional self-harm**

√7ᵗʰ **T46.993   Poisoning by other agents primarily affecting the cardiovascular system, assault**

☑ Additional Character Required   √x7ᵗʰ Placeholder Alert   Unacceptable PDx   Manifestation   Hospital Acquired Condition   **EXCLUDES 1** Not Coded Here   *EXCLUDES 2* Not Included Here

Chapter 19. Injury, Poisoning, and Certain Other Consequences of External Causes

   ✓7th **T46.994** **Poisoning by other agents primarily affecting the cardiovascular system, undetermined**

   ✓7th **T46.995** Adverse effect of other agents primarily affecting the cardiovascular system

   ✓7th **T46.996** Underdosing of other agents primarily affecting the cardiovascular system

✓4th **T47** **Poisoning by, adverse effect of and underdosing of agents primarily affecting the gastrointestinal system**

> The appropriate 7th character is to be added to each code from category T47.
> A   initial encounter
> D   subsequent encounter
> S   sequela

  ✓5th **T47.0** **Poisoning by, adverse effect of and underdosing of histamine H2-receptor blockers**

    ✓6th **T47.0X** **Poisoning by, adverse effect of and underdosing of histamine H2-receptor blockers**

      ✓7th **T47.0X1** **Poisoning by histamine H2-receptor blockers, accidental (unintentional)**
            Poisoning by histamine H2-receptor blockers NOS

      ✓7th **T47.0X2** **Poisoning by histamine H2-receptor blockers, intentional self-harm**

      ✓7th **T47.0X3** **Poisoning by histamine H2-receptor blockers, assault**

      ✓7th **T47.0X4** **Poisoning by histamine H2-receptor blockers, undetermined**

      ✓7th **T47.0X5** Adverse effect of histamine H2-receptor blockers

      ✓7th **T47.0X6** Underdosing of histamine H2-receptor blockers

  ✓5th **T47.1** **Poisoning by, adverse effect of and underdosing of other antacids and anti-gastric-secretion drugs**

    ✓6th **T47.1X** **Poisoning by, adverse effect of and underdosing of other antacids and anti-gastric-secretion drugs**

      ✓7th **T47.1X1** **Poisoning by other antacids and anti-gastric-secretion drugs, accidental (unintentional)**
            Poisoning by other antacids and anti-gastric-secretion drugs NOS

      ✓7th **T47.1X2** **Poisoning by other antacids and anti-gastric-secretion drugs, intentional self-harm**

      ✓7th **T47.1X3** **Poisoning by other antacids and anti-gastric-secretion drugs, assault**

      ✓7th **T47.1X4** **Poisoning by other antacids and anti-gastric-secretion drugs, undetermined**

      ✓7th **T47.1X5** Adverse effect of other antacids and anti-gastric-secretion drugs

      ✓7th **T47.1X6** Underdosing of other antacids and anti-gastric-secretion drugs

  ✓5th **T47.2** **Poisoning by, adverse effect of and underdosing of stimulant laxatives**

    ✓6th **T47.2X** **Poisoning by, adverse effect of and underdosing of stimulant laxatives**

      ✓7th **T47.2X1** **Poisoning by stimulant laxatives, accidental (unintentional)**
            Poisoning by stimulant laxatives NOS

      ✓7th **T47.2X2** **Poisoning by stimulant laxatives, intentional self-harm**

      ✓7th **T47.2X3** **Poisoning by stimulant laxatives, assault**

      ✓7th **T47.2X4** **Poisoning by stimulant laxatives, undetermined**

      ✓7th **T47.2X5** Adverse effect of stimulant laxatives

      ✓7th **T47.2X6** Underdosing of stimulant laxatives

  ✓5th **T47.3** **Poisoning by, adverse effect of and underdosing of saline and osmotic laxatives**

    ✓6th **T47.3X** **Poisoning by and adverse effect of saline and osmotic laxatives**

      ✓7th **T47.3X1** **Poisoning by saline and osmotic laxatives, accidental (unintentional)**
            Poisoning by saline and osmotic laxatives NOS

      ✓7th **T47.3X2** **Poisoning by saline and osmotic laxatives, intentional self-harm**

      ✓7th **T47.3X3** **Poisoning by saline and osmotic laxatives, assault**

      ✓7th **T47.3X4** **Poisoning by saline and osmotic laxatives, undetermined**

      ✓7th **T47.3X5** Adverse effect of saline and osmotic laxatives

      ✓7th **T47.3X6** Underdosing of saline and osmotic laxatives

  ✓5th **T47.4** **Poisoning by, adverse effect of and underdosing of other laxatives**

    ✓6th **T47.4X** **Poisoning by, adverse effect of and underdosing of other laxatives**

      ✓7th **T47.4X1** **Poisoning by other laxatives, accidental (unintentional)**
            Poisoning by other laxatives NOS

      ✓7th **T47.4X2** **Poisoning by other laxatives, intentional self-harm**

      ✓7th **T47.4X3** **Poisoning by other laxatives, assault**

      ✓7th **T47.4X4** **Poisoning by other laxatives, undetermined**

      ✓7th **T47.4X5** Adverse effect of other laxatives

      ✓7th **T47.4X6** Underdosing of other laxatives

  ✓5th **T47.5** **Poisoning by, adverse effect of and underdosing of digestants**

    ✓6th **T47.5X** **Poisoning by, adverse effect of and underdosing of digestants**

      ✓7th **T47.5X1** **Poisoning by digestants, accidental (unintentional)**
            Poisoning by digestants NOS

      ✓7th **T47.5X2** **Poisoning by digestants, intentional self-harm**

      ✓7th **T47.5X3** **Poisoning by digestants, assault**

      ✓7th **T47.5X4** **Poisoning by digestants, undetermined**

      ✓7th **T47.5X5** Adverse effect of digestants

      ✓7th **T47.5X6** Underdosing of digestants

  ✓5th **T47.6** **Poisoning by, adverse effect of and underdosing of antidiarrheal drugs**

> EXCLUDES 2 poisoning by, adverse effect of and underdosing of systemic antibiotics and other anti-infectives (T36-T37)

    ✓6th **T47.6X** **Poisoning by, adverse effect of and underdosing of antidiarrheal drugs**

      ✓7th **T47.6X1** **Poisoning by antidiarrheal drugs, accidental (unintentional)**
            Poisoning by antidiarrheal drugs NOS

      ✓7th **T47.6X2** **Poisoning by antidiarrheal drugs, intentional self-harm**

      ✓7th **T47.6X3** **Poisoning by antidiarrheal drugs, assault**

      ✓7th **T47.6X4** **Poisoning by antidiarrheal drugs, undetermined**

      ✓7th **T47.6X5** Adverse effect of antidiarrheal drugs

      ✓7th **T47.6X6** Underdosing of antidiarrheal drugs

  ✓5th **T47.7** **Poisoning by, adverse effect of and underdosing of emetics**

    ✓6th **T47.7X** **Poisoning by, adverse effect of and underdosing of emetics**

      ✓7th **T47.7X1** **Poisoning by emetics, accidental (unintentional)**
            Poisoning by emetics NOS

      ✓7th **T47.7X2** **Poisoning by emetics, intentional self-harm**

      ✓7th **T47.7X3** **Poisoning by emetics, assault**

      ✓7th **T47.7X4** **Poisoning by emetics, undetermined**

      ✓7th **T47.7X5** Adverse effect of emetics

      ✓7th **T47.7X6** Underdosing of emetics

  ✓5th **T47.8** **Poisoning by, adverse effect of and underdosing of other agents primarily affecting gastrointestinal system**

    ✓6th **T47.8X** **Poisoning by, adverse effect of and underdosing of other agents primarily affecting gastrointestinal system**

      ✓7th **T47.8X1** **Poisoning by other agents primarily affecting gastrointestinal system, accidental (unintentional)**
            Poisoning by other agents primarily affecting gastrointestinal system NOS

N Newborn: 0   P Pediatric: 0-17   M Maternity: 12-55   A Adult: 15-124   MCC Major CC Condition   PDxMCC PDx acts as own MCC   CC CC Condition   PDxCC PDx acts as own CC

1112   ICD-10-CM 2016

☑7ᵗʰ **T47.8X2** **Poisoning by other agents primarily affecting gastrointestinal system, intentional self-harm**

☑7ᵗʰ **T47.8X3** **Poisoning by other agents primarily affecting gastrointestinal system, assault**

☑7ᵗʰ **T47.8X4** **Poisoning by other agents primarily affecting gastrointestinal system, undetermined**

☑7ᵗʰ **T47.8X5** **Adverse effect of other agents primarily affecting gastrointestinal system**

☑7ᵗʰ **T47.8X6** **Underdosing of other agents primarily affecting gastrointestinal system**

√5ᵗʰ **T47.9** **Poisoning by, adverse effect of and underdosing of unspecified agents primarily affecting the gastrointestinal system**

√x7ᵗʰ **T47.91** **Poisoning by unspecified agents primarily affecting the gastrointestinal system, accidental (unintentional)**
     Poisoning by agents primarily affecting the gastrointestinal system NOS

√x7ᵗʰ **T47.92** **Poisoning by unspecified agents primarily affecting the gastrointestinal system, intentional self-harm**

√x7ᵗʰ **T47.93** **Poisoning by unspecified agents primarily affecting the gastrointestinal system, assault**

√x7ᵗʰ **T47.94** **Poisoning by unspecified agents primarily affecting the gastrointestinal system, undetermined**

√x7ᵗʰ **T47.95** **Adverse effect of unspecified agents primarily affecting the gastrointestinal system**

√x7ᵗʰ **T47.96** **Underdosing of unspecified agents primarily affecting the gastrointestinal system**

√4ᵗʰ **T48** **Poisoning by, adverse effect of and underdosing of agents primarily acting on smooth and skeletal muscles and the respiratory system**

> The appropriate 7th character is to be added to each code from category T48.
> A   initial encounter
> D   subsequent encounter
> S   sequela

√5ᵗʰ **T48.0** **Poisoning by, adverse effect of and underdosing of oxytocic drugs**
     EXCLUDES 1 *poisoning by, adverse effect of and underdosing of estrogens, progestogens and antagonists (T38.4-T38.6)*

√6ᵗʰ **T48.0X** **Poisoning by, adverse effect of and underdosing of oxytocic drugs**

☑7ᵗʰ **T48.0X1** **Poisoning by oxytocic drugs, accidental (unintentional)**
     Poisoning by oxytocic drugs NOS

☑7ᵗʰ **T48.0X2** **Poisoning by oxytocic drugs, intentional self-harm**

☑7ᵗʰ **T48.0X3** **Poisoning by oxytocic drugs, assault**

☑7ᵗʰ **T48.0X4** **Poisoning by oxytocic drugs, undetermined**

☑7ᵗʰ **T48.0X5** **Adverse effect of oxytocic drugs**

☑7ᵗʰ **T48.0X6** **Underdosing of oxytocic drugs**

√5ᵗʰ **T48.1** **Poisoning by, adverse effect of and underdosing of skeletal muscle relaxants [neuromuscular blocking agents]**

√6ᵗʰ **T48.1X** **Poisoning by, adverse effect of and underdosing of skeletal muscle relaxants [neuromuscular blocking agents]**

☑7ᵗʰ **T48.1X1** **Poisoning by skeletal muscle relaxants [neuromuscular blocking agents], accidental (unintentional)**
     Poisoning by skeletal muscle relaxants [neuromuscular blocking agents] NOS

☑7ᵗʰ **T48.1X2** **Poisoning by skeletal muscle relaxants [neuromuscular blocking agents], intentional self-harm**

☑7ᵗʰ **T48.1X3** **Poisoning by skeletal muscle relaxants [neuromuscular blocking agents], assault**

☑7ᵗʰ **T48.1X4** **Poisoning by skeletal muscle relaxants [neuromuscular blocking agents], undetermined**

☑7ᵗʰ **T48.1X5** **Adverse effect of skeletal muscle relaxants [neuromuscular blocking agents]**

☑7ᵗʰ **T48.1X6** **Underdosing of skeletal muscle relaxants [neuromuscular blocking agents]**

√5ᵗʰ **T48.2** **Poisoning by, adverse effect of and underdosing of other and unspecified drugs acting on muscles**

√6ᵗʰ **T48.20** **Poisoning by, adverse effect of and underdosing of unspecified drugs acting on muscles**

☑7ᵗʰ **T48.201** **Poisoning by unspecified drugs acting on muscles, accidental (unintentional)**
     Poisoning by unspecified drugs acting on muscles NOS

☑7ᵗʰ **T48.202** **Poisoning by unspecified drugs acting on muscles, intentional self-harm**

☑7ᵗʰ **T48.203** **Poisoning by unspecified drugs acting on muscles, assault**

☑7ᵗʰ **T48.204** **Poisoning by unspecified drugs acting on muscles, undetermined**

☑7ᵗʰ **T48.205** **Adverse effect of unspecified drugs acting on muscles**

☑7ᵗʰ **T48.206** **Underdosing of unspecified drugs acting on muscles**

√6ᵗʰ **T48.29** **Poisoning by, adverse effect of and underdosing of other drugs acting on muscles**

☑7ᵗʰ **T48.291** **Poisoning by other drugs acting on muscles, accidental (unintentional)**
     Poisoning by other drugs acting on muscles NOS

☑7ᵗʰ **T48.292** **Poisoning by other drugs acting on muscles, intentional self-harm**

☑7ᵗʰ **T48.293** **Poisoning by other drugs acting on muscles, assault**

☑7ᵗʰ **T48.294** **Poisoning by other drugs acting on muscles, undetermined**

☑7ᵗʰ **T48.295** **Adverse effect of other drugs acting on muscles**

☑7ᵗʰ **T48.296** **Underdosing of other drugs acting on muscles**

√5ᵗʰ **T48.3** **Poisoning by, adverse effect of and underdosing of antitussives**

√6ᵗʰ **T48.3X** **Poisoning by, adverse effect of and underdosing of antitussives**

☑7ᵗʰ **T48.3X1** **Poisoning by antitussives, accidental (unintentional)**
     Poisoning by antitussives NOS

☑7ᵗʰ **T48.3X2** **Poisoning by antitussives, intentional self-harm**

☑7ᵗʰ **T48.3X3** **Poisoning by antitussives, assault**

☑7ᵗʰ **T48.3X4** **Poisoning by antitussives, undetermined**

☑7ᵗʰ **T48.3X5** **Adverse effect of antitussives**

☑7ᵗʰ **T48.3X6** **Underdosing of antitussives**

√5ᵗʰ **T48.4** **Poisoning by, adverse effect of and underdosing of expectorants**

√6ᵗʰ **T48.4X** **Poisoning by, adverse effect of and underdosing of expectorants**

☑7ᵗʰ **T48.4X1** **Poisoning by expectorants, accidental (unintentional)**
     Poisoning by expectorants NOS

☑7ᵗʰ **T48.4X2** **Poisoning by expectorants, intentional self-harm**

☑7ᵗʰ **T48.4X3** **Poisoning by expectorants, assault**

☑7ᵗʰ **T48.4X4** **Poisoning by expectorants, undetermined**

☑7ᵗʰ **T48.4X5** **Adverse effect of expectorants**

☑7ᵗʰ **T48.4X6** **Underdosing of expectorants**

√5ᵗʰ **T48.5** **Poisoning by, adverse effect of and underdosing of other anti-common-cold drugs**
     Poisoning by, adverse effect of and underdosing of decongestants
     EXCLUDES 2 *poisoning by, adverse effect of and underdosing of antipyretics, NEC (T39.9-)*
          poisoning by, adverse effect of and underdosing of non-steroidal antiinflammatory drugs (T39.3-)
          poisoning by, adverse effect of and underdosing of salicylates (T39.0-)

√6ᵗʰ **T48.5X** **Poisoning by, adverse effect of and underdosing of other anti-common-cold drugs**

☑ Additional Character Required   √x7ᵗʰ Placeholder Alert   Unacceptable PDx   Manifestation   Hospital Acquired Condition   **EXCLUDES 1** Not Coded Here   **EXCLUDES 2** Not Included Here

ICD-10-CM 2016   1113

Chapter 19. Injury, Poisoning, and Certain Other Consequences of External Causes

√7ᵗʰ **T48.5X1** **Poisoning by other anti-common-cold drugs, accidental (unintentional)**
Poisoning by other anti-common-cold drugs NOS

√7ᵗʰ **T48.5X2** **Poisoning by other anti-common-cold drugs, intentional self-harm**

√7ᵗʰ **T48.5X3** **Poisoning by other anti-common-cold drugs, assault**

√7ᵗʰ **T48.5X4** **Poisoning by other anti-common-cold drugs, undetermined**

√7ᵗʰ **T48.5X5** **Adverse effect of other anti-common-cold drugs**

√7ᵗʰ **T48.5X6** **Underdosing of other anti-common-cold drugs**

√5ᵗʰ **T48.6** **Poisoning by, adverse effect of and underdosing of antiasthmatics, not elsewhere classified**
Poisoning by, adverse effect of and underdosing of beta-adrenoreceptor agonists used in asthma therapy

> EXCLUDES 1   poisoning by, adverse effect of and underdosing of anterior pituitary [adenohypophyseal] hormones (T38.8)
> poisoning by, adverse effect of and underdosing of beta-adrenoreceptor agonists not used in asthma therapy (T44.5)

√6ᵗʰ **T48.6X** **Poisoning by, adverse effect of and underdosing of antiasthmatics**

√7ᵗʰ **T48.6X1** **Poisoning by antiasthmatics, accidental (unintentional)**
Poisoning by antiasthmatics NOS

√7ᵗʰ **T48.6X2** **Poisoning by antiasthmatics, intentional self-harm**

√7ᵗʰ **T48.6X3** **Poisoning by antiasthmatics, assault**

√7ᵗʰ **T48.6X4** **Poisoning by antiasthmatics, undetermined**

√7ᵗʰ **T48.6X5** **Adverse effect of antiasthmatics**

√7ᵗʰ **T48.6X6** **Underdosing of antiasthmatics**

√5ᵗʰ **T48.9** **Poisoning by, adverse effect of and underdosing of other and unspecified agents primarily acting on the respiratory system**

√6ᵗʰ **T48.90** **Poisoning by, adverse effect of and underdosing of unspecified agents primarily acting on the respiratory system**

√7ᵗʰ **T48.901** **Poisoning by unspecified agents primarily acting on the respiratory system, accidental (unintentional)**

√7ᵗʰ **T48.902** **Poisoning by unspecified agents primarily acting on the respiratory system, intentional self-harm**

√7ᵗʰ **T48.903** **Poisoning by unspecified agents primarily acting on the respiratory system, assault**

√7ᵗʰ **T48.904** **Poisoning by unspecified agents primarily acting on the respiratory system, undetermined**

√7ᵗʰ **T48.905** **Adverse effect of unspecified agents primarily acting on the respiratory system**

√7ᵗʰ **T48.906** **Underdosing of unspecified agents primarily acting on the respiratory system**

√6ᵗʰ **T48.99** **Poisoning by, adverse effect of and underdosing of other agents primarily acting on the respiratory system**

√7ᵗʰ **T48.991** **Poisoning by other agents primarily acting on the respiratory system, accidental (unintentional)**

√7ᵗʰ **T48.992** **Poisoning by other agents primarily acting on the respiratory system, intentional self-harm**

√7ᵗʰ **T48.993** **Poisoning by other agents primarily acting on the respiratory system, assault**

√7ᵗʰ **T48.994** **Poisoning by other agents primarily acting on the respiratory system, undetermined**

√7ᵗʰ **T48.995** **Adverse effect of other agents primarily acting on the respiratory system**

√7ᵗʰ **T48.996** **Underdosing of other agents primarily acting on the respiratory system**

√4ᵗʰ **T49** **Poisoning by, adverse effect of and underdosing of topical agents primarily affecting skin and mucous membrane and by ophthalmological, otorhinolaryngological and dental drugs**
Poisoning by, adverse effect of and underdosing of glucocorticoids, topically used

> The appropriate 7th character is to be added to each code from category T49.
> A   initial encounter
> D   subsequent encounter
> S   sequela

√5ᵗʰ **T49.0** **Poisoning by, adverse effect of and underdosing of local antifungal, anti-infective and anti-inflammatory drugs**

√6ᵗʰ **T49.0X** **Poisoning by, adverse effect of and underdosing of local antifungal, anti-infective and anti-inflammatory drugs**

√7ᵗʰ **T49.0X1** **Poisoning by local antifungal, anti-infective and anti-inflammatory drugs, accidental (unintentional)**
Poisoning by local antifungal, anti-infective and anti-inflammatory drugs NOS

√7ᵗʰ **T49.0X2** **Poisoning by local antifungal, anti-infective and anti-inflammatory drugs, intentional self-harm**

√7ᵗʰ **T49.0X3** **Poisoning by local antifungal, anti-infective and anti-inflammatory drugs, assault**

√7ᵗʰ **T49.0X4** **Poisoning by local antifungal, anti-infective and anti-inflammatory drugs, undetermined**

√7ᵗʰ **T49.0X5** **Adverse effect of local antifungal, anti-infective and anti-inflammatory drugs**

√7ᵗʰ **T49.0X6** **Underdosing of local antifungal, anti-infective and anti-inflammatory drugs**

√5ᵗʰ **T49.1** **Poisoning by, adverse effect of and underdosing of antipruritics**

√6ᵗʰ **T49.1X** **Poisoning by, adverse effect of and underdosing of antipruritics**

√7ᵗʰ **T49.1X1** **Poisoning by antipruritics, accidental (unintentional)**
Poisoning by antipruritics NOS

√7ᵗʰ **T49.1X2** **Poisoning by antipruritics, intentional self-harm**

√7ᵗʰ **T49.1X3** **Poisoning by antipruritics, assault**

√7ᵗʰ **T49.1X4** **Poisoning by antipruritics, undetermined**

√7ᵗʰ **T49.1X5** **Adverse effect of antipruritics**

√7ᵗʰ **T49.1X6** **Underdosing of antipruritics**

√5ᵗʰ **T49.2** **Poisoning by, adverse effect of and underdosing of local astringents and local detergents**

√6ᵗʰ **T49.2X** **Poisoning by, adverse effect of and underdosing of local astringents and local detergents**

√7ᵗʰ **T49.2X1** **Poisoning by local astringents and local detergents, accidental (unintentional)**
Poisoning by local astringents and local detergents NOS

√7ᵗʰ **T49.2X2** **Poisoning by local astringents and local detergents, intentional self-harm**

√7ᵗʰ **T49.2X3** **Poisoning by local astringents and local detergents, assault**

√7ᵗʰ **T49.2X4** **Poisoning by local astringents and local detergents, undetermined**

√7ᵗʰ **T49.2X5** **Adverse effect of local astringents and local detergents**

√7ᵗʰ **T49.2X6** **Underdosing of local astringents and local detergents**

√5ᵗʰ **T49.3** **Poisoning by, adverse effect of and underdosing of emollients, demulcents and protectants**

√6ᵗʰ **T49.3X** **Poisoning by, adverse effect of and underdosing of emollients, demulcents and protectants**

√7ᵗʰ **T49.3X1** **Poisoning by emollients, demulcents and protectants, accidental (unintentional)**
Poisoning by emollients, demulcents and protectants NOS

√7ᵗʰ **T49.3X2** **Poisoning by emollients, demulcents and protectants, intentional self-harm**

√7ᵗʰ **T49.3X3** **Poisoning by emollients, demulcents and protectants, assault**

N Newborn: 0   P Pediatric: 0-17   M Maternity: 12-55   A Adult: 15-124   MCC Major CC Condition   PDxMCC PDx acts as own MCC   CC CC Condition   PDxCC PDx acts as own CC

1114   ICD-10-CM 2016

☑7ᵗʰ **T49.3X4** **Poisoning by emollients, demulcents and protectants,** undetermined

☑7ᵗʰ **T49.3X5** Adverse effect **of emollients, demulcents and protectants**

☑7ᵗʰ **T49.3X6** Underdosing **of emollients, demulcents and protectants**

☑5ᵗʰ **T49.4** **Poisoning by, adverse effect of and underdosing of keratolytics, keratoplastics, and other hair treatment drugs and preparations**

     ☑6ᵗʰ **T49.4X** **Poisoning by, adverse effect of and underdosing of** keratolytics, keratoplastics, and other hair treatment drugs and preparations

       ☑7ᵗʰ **T49.4X1** **Poisoning by keratolytics, keratoplastics, and other hair treatment drugs and preparations,** accidental (unintentional)
Poisoning by keratolytics, keratoplastics, and other hair treatment drugs and preparations NOS

       ☑7ᵗʰ **T49.4X2** **Poisoning by keratolytics, keratoplastics, and other hair treatment drugs and preparations,** intentional self-harm

       ☑7ᵗʰ **T49.4X3** **Poisoning by keratolytics, keratoplastics, and other hair treatment drugs and preparations,** assault

       ☑7ᵗʰ **T49.4X4** **Poisoning by keratolytics, keratoplastics, and other hair treatment drugs and preparations,** undetermined

       ☑7ᵗʰ **T49.4X5** Adverse effect **of keratolytics, keratoplastics, and other hair treatment drugs and preparations**

       ☑7ᵗʰ **T49.4X6** Underdosing **of keratolytics, keratoplastics, and other hair treatment drugs and preparations**

☑5ᵗʰ **T49.5** **Poisoning by, adverse effect of and underdosing of ophthalmological drugs and preparations**

     ☑6ᵗʰ **T49.5X** **Poisoning by, adverse effect of and underdosing of** ophthalmological **drugs and preparations**

       ☑7ᵗʰ **T49.5X1** **Poisoning by ophthalmological drugs and preparations,** accidental (unintentional)
Poisoning by ophthalmological drugs and preparations NOS

       ☑7ᵗʰ **T49.5X2** **Poisoning by ophthalmological drugs and preparations,** intentional self-harm

       ☑7ᵗʰ **T49.5X3** **Poisoning by ophthalmological drugs and preparations,** assault

       ☑7ᵗʰ **T49.5X4** **Poisoning by ophthalmological drugs and preparations,** undetermined

       ☑7ᵗʰ **T49.5X5** Adverse effect **of ophthalmological drugs and preparations**

       ☑7ᵗʰ **T49.5X6** Underdosing **of ophthalmological drugs and preparations**

☑5ᵗʰ **T49.6** **Poisoning by, adverse effect of and underdosing of otorhinolaryngological drugs and preparations**

     ☑6ᵗʰ **T49.6X** **Poisoning by, adverse effect of and underdosing of** otorhinolaryngological **drugs and preparations**

       ☑7ᵗʰ **T49.6X1** **Poisoning by otorhinolaryngological drugs and preparations,** accidental (unintentional)
Poisoning by otorhinolaryngological drugs and preparations NOS

       ☑7ᵗʰ **T49.6X2** **Poisoning by otorhinolaryngological drugs and preparations,** intentional self-harm

       ☑7ᵗʰ **T49.6X3** **Poisoning by otorhinolaryngological drugs and preparations,** assault

       ☑7ᵗʰ **T49.6X4** **Poisoning by otorhinolaryngological drugs and preparations,** undetermined

       ☑7ᵗʰ **T49.6X5** Adverse effect **of otorhinolaryngological drugs and preparations**

       ☑7ᵗʰ **T49.6X6** Underdosing **of otorhinolaryngological drugs and preparations**

☑5ᵗʰ **T49.7** **Poisoning by, adverse effect of and underdosing of dental drugs, topically applied**

     ☑6ᵗʰ **T49.7X** **Poisoning by, adverse effect of and underdosing of** dental **drugs, topically applied**

       ☑7ᵗʰ **T49.7X1** **Poisoning by dental drugs, topically applied,** accidental (unintentional)
Poisoning by dental drugs, topically applied NOS

       ☑7ᵗʰ **T49.7X2** **Poisoning by dental drugs, topically applied,** intentional self-harm

       ☑7ᵗʰ **T49.7X3** **Poisoning by dental drugs, topically applied,** assault

       ☑7ᵗʰ **T49.7X4** **Poisoning by dental drugs, topically applied,** undetermined

       ☑7ᵗʰ **T49.7X5** Adverse effect **of dental drugs, topically applied**

       ☑7ᵗʰ **T49.7X6** Underdosing **of dental drugs, topically applied**

☑5ᵗʰ **T49.8** **Poisoning by, adverse effect of and underdosing of other topical agents**
Poisoning by, adverse effect of and underdosing of spermicides

     ☑6ᵗʰ **T49.8X** **Poisoning by, adverse effect of and underdosing of other topical agents**

       ☑7ᵗʰ **T49.8X1** **Poisoning by other topical agents, accidental (unintentional)**
Poisoning by other topical agents NOS

       ☑7ᵗʰ **T49.8X2** **Poisoning by other topical agents, intentional self-harm**

       ☑7ᵗʰ **T49.8X3** **Poisoning by other topical agents, assault**

       ☑7ᵗʰ **T49.8X4** **Poisoning by other topical agents, undetermined**

       ☑7ᵗʰ **T49.8X5** Adverse effect **of other topical agents**

       ☑7ᵗʰ **T49.8X6** Underdosing **of other topical agents**

☑5ᵗʰ **T49.9** **Poisoning by, adverse effect of and underdosing of** unspecified **topical agent**

     ☑ₓ7ᵗʰ **T49.91** **Poisoning by unspecified topical agent, accidental (unintentional)**

     ☑ₓ7ᵗʰ **T49.92** **Poisoning by unspecified topical agent, intentional self-harm**

     ☑ₓ7ᵗʰ **T49.93** **Poisoning by unspecified topical agent, assault**

     ☑ₓ7ᵗʰ **T49.94** **Poisoning by unspecified topical agent, undetermined**

     ☑ₓ7ᵗʰ **T49.95** Adverse effect **of unspecified topical agent**

     ☑ₓ7ᵗʰ **T49.96** Underdosing **of unspecified topical agent**

☑4ᵗʰ **T50** **Poisoning by, adverse effect of and underdosing of diuretics and other and unspecified drugs, medicaments and biological substances**

> The appropriate 7th character is to be added to each code from category T50.
> A   initial encounter
> D   subsequent encounter
> S   sequela

☑5ᵗʰ **T50.0** **Poisoning by, adverse effect of and underdosing of mineralocorticoids and their antagonists**

     ☑6ᵗʰ **T50.0X** **Poisoning by, adverse effect of and underdosing of** mineralocorticoids and their antagonists

       ☑7ᵗʰ **T50.0X1** **Poisoning by mineralocorticoids and their antagonists, accidental (unintentional)**
Poisoning by mineralocorticoids and their antagonists NOS

       ☑7ᵗʰ **T50.0X2** **Poisoning by mineralocorticoids and their antagonists, intentional self-harm**

       ☑7ᵗʰ **T50.0X3** **Poisoning by mineralocorticoids and their antagonists, assault**

       ☑7ᵗʰ **T50.0X4** **Poisoning by mineralocorticoids and their antagonists, undetermined**

       ☑7ᵗʰ **T50.0X5** Adverse effect **of mineralocorticoids and their antagonists**

       ☑7ᵗʰ **T50.0X6** Underdosing **of mineralocorticoids and their antagonists**

√5ᵗʰ **T50.1　Poisoning by, adverse effect of and underdosing of loop [high-ceiling] diuretics**

　　√6ᵗʰ **T50.1X　Poisoning by, adverse effect of and underdosing of loop [high-ceiling] diuretics**

　　　　√7ᵗʰ **T50.1X1　Poisoning by loop [high-ceiling] diuretics, accidental (unintentional)**
　　　　　　　Poisoning by loop [high-ceiling] diuretics NOS

　　　　√7ᵗʰ **T50.1X2　Poisoning by loop [high-ceiling] diuretics, intentional self-harm**

　　　　√7ᵗʰ **T50.1X3　Poisoning by loop [high-ceiling] diuretics, assault**

　　　　√7ᵗʰ **T50.1X4　Poisoning by loop [high-ceiling] diuretics, undetermined**

　　　　√7ᵗʰ **T50.1X5　Adverse effect of loop [high-ceiling] diuretics**

　　　　√7ᵗʰ **T50.1X6　Underdosing of loop [high-ceiling] diuretics**

√5ᵗʰ **T50.2　Poisoning by, adverse effect of and underdosing of carbonic-anhydrase inhibitors, benzothiadiazides and other diuretics**
　　　Poisoning by, adverse effect of and underdosing of acetazolamide

　　√6ᵗʰ **T50.2X　Poisoning by, adverse effect of and underdosing of carbonic-anhydrase inhibitors, benzothiadiazides and other diuretics**

　　　　√7ᵗʰ **T50.2X1　Poisoning by carbonic-anhydrase inhibitors, benzothiadiazides and other diuretics, accidental (unintentional)**
　　　　　　　Poisoning by carbonic-anhydrase inhibitors, benzothiadiazides and other diuretics NOS

　　　　√7ᵗʰ **T50.2X2　Poisoning by carbonic-anhydrase inhibitors, benzothiadiazides and other diuretics, intentional self-harm**

　　　　√7ᵗʰ **T50.2X3　Poisoning by carbonic-anhydrase inhibitors, benzothiadiazides and other diuretics, assault**

　　　　√7ᵗʰ **T50.2X4　Poisoning by carbonic-anhydrase inhibitors, benzothiadiazides and other diuretics, undetermined**

　　　　√7ᵗʰ **T50.2X5　Adverse effect of carbonic-anhydrase inhibitors, benzothiadiazides and other diuretics**

　　　　√7ᵗʰ **T50.2X6　Underdosing of carbonic-anhydrase inhibitors, benzothiadiazides and other diuretics**

√5ᵗʰ **T50.3　Poisoning by, adverse effect of and underdosing of electrolytic, caloric and water-balance agents**
　　　Poisoning by, adverse effect of and underdosing of oral rehydration salts

　　√6ᵗʰ **T50.3X　Poisoning by, adverse effect of and underdosing of electrolytic, caloric and water-balance agents**

　　　　√7ᵗʰ **T50.3X1　Poisoning by electrolytic, caloric and water-balance agents, accidental (unintentional)**
　　　　　　　Poisoning by electrolytic, caloric and water-balance agents NOS

　　　　√7ᵗʰ **T50.3X2　Poisoning by electrolytic, caloric and water-balance agents, intentional self-harm**

　　　　√7ᵗʰ **T50.3X3　Poisoning by electrolytic, caloric and water-balance agents, assault**

　　　　√7ᵗʰ **T50.3X4　Poisoning by electrolytic, caloric and water-balance agents, undetermined**

　　　　√7ᵗʰ **T50.3X5　Adverse effect of electrolytic, caloric and water-balance agents**

　　　　√7ᵗʰ **T50.3X6　Underdosing of electrolytic, caloric and water-balance agents**

√5ᵗʰ **T50.4　Poisoning by, adverse effect of and underdosing of drugs affecting uric acid metabolism**

　　√6ᵗʰ **T50.4X　Poisoning by, adverse effect of and underdosing of drugs affecting uric acid metabolism**

　　　　√7ᵗʰ **T50.4X1　Poisoning by drugs affecting uric acid metabolism, accidental (unintentional)**
　　　　　　　Poisoning by drugs affecting uric acid metabolism NOS

　　　　√7ᵗʰ **T50.4X2　Poisoning by drugs affecting uric acid metabolism, intentional self-harm**

　　　　√7ᵗʰ **T50.4X3　Poisoning by drugs affecting uric acid metabolism, assault**

　　　　√7ᵗʰ **T50.4X4　Poisoning by drugs affecting uric acid metabolism, undetermined**

　　　　√7ᵗʰ **T50.4X5　Adverse effect of drugs affecting uric acid metabolism**

　　　　√7ᵗʰ **T50.4X6　Underdosing of drugs affecting uric acid metabolism**

√5ᵗʰ **T50.5　Poisoning by, adverse effect of and underdosing of appetite depressants**

　　√6ᵗʰ **T50.5X　Poisoning by, adverse effect of and underdosing of appetite depressants**

　　　　√7ᵗʰ **T50.5X1　Poisoning by appetite depressants, accidental (unintentional)**
　　　　　　　Poisoning by appetite depressants NOS

　　　　√7ᵗʰ **T50.5X2　Poisoning by appetite depressants, intentional self-harm**

　　　　√7ᵗʰ **T50.5X3　Poisoning by appetite depressants, assault**

　　　　√7ᵗʰ **T50.5X4　Poisoning by appetite depressants, undetermined**

　　　　√7ᵗʰ **T50.5X5　Adverse effect of appetite depressants**

　　　　√7ᵗʰ **T50.5X6　Underdosing of appetite depressants**

√5ᵗʰ **T50.6　Poisoning by, adverse effect of and underdosing of antidotes and chelating agents**
　　　Poisoning by, adverse effect of and underdosing of alcohol deterrents

　　√6ᵗʰ **T50.6X　Poisoning by, adverse effect of and underdosing of antidotes and chelating agents**

　　　　√7ᵗʰ **T50.6X1　Poisoning by antidotes and chelating agents, accidental (unintentional)**
　　　　　　　Poisoning by antidotes and chelating agents NOS

　　　　√7ᵗʰ **T50.6X2　Poisoning by antidotes and chelating agents, intentional self-harm**

　　　　√7ᵗʰ **T50.6X3　Poisoning by antidotes and chelating agents, assault**

　　　　√7ᵗʰ **T50.6X4　Poisoning by antidotes and chelating agents, undetermined**

　　　　√7ᵗʰ **T50.6X5　Adverse effect of antidotes and chelating agents**

　　　　√7ᵗʰ **T50.6X6　Underdosing of antidotes and chelating agents**

√5ᵗʰ **T50.7　Poisoning by, adverse effect of and underdosing of analeptics and opioid receptor antagonists**

　　√6ᵗʰ **T50.7X　Poisoning by, adverse effect of and underdosing of analeptics and opioid receptor antagonists**

　　　　√7ᵗʰ **T50.7X1　Poisoning by analeptics and opioid receptor antagonists, accidental (unintentional)**
　　　　　　　Poisoning by analeptics and opioid receptor antagonists NOS

　　　　√7ᵗʰ **T50.7X2　Poisoning by analeptics and opioid receptor antagonists, intentional self-harm**

　　　　√7ᵗʰ **T50.7X3　Poisoning by analeptics and opioid receptor antagonists, assault**

　　　　√7ᵗʰ **T50.7X4　Poisoning by analeptics and opioid receptor antagonists, undetermined**

　　　　√7ᵗʰ **T50.7X5　Adverse effect of analeptics and opioid receptor antagonists**

　　　　√7ᵗʰ **T50.7X6　Underdosing of analeptics and opioid receptor antagonists**

√5ᵗʰ **T50.8　Poisoning by, adverse effect of and underdosing of diagnostic agents**

　　√6ᵗʰ **T50.8X　Poisoning by, adverse effect of and underdosing of diagnostic agents**

　　　　√7ᵗʰ **T50.8X1　Poisoning by diagnostic agents, accidental (unintentional)**
　　　　　　　Poisoning by diagnostic agents NOS

　　　　√7ᵗʰ **T50.8X2　Poisoning by diagnostic agents, intentional self-harm**

　　　　√7ᵗʰ **T50.8X3　Poisoning by diagnostic agents, assault**

　　　　√7ᵗʰ **T50.8X4　Poisoning by diagnostic agents, undetermined**

　　　　√7ᵗʰ **T50.8X5　Adverse effect of diagnostic agents**

Ⓝ Newborn: 0　　Ⓟ Pediatric: 0-17　　Ⓜ Maternity: 12-55　　Ⓐ Adult: 15-124　　**MCC** Major CC Condition　　**PDxMCC** PDx acts as own MCC　　**CC** CC Condition　　**PDxCC** PDx acts as own CC

√7ᵗʰ **T50.8X6** Underdosing of diagnostic agents

√5ᵗʰ **T50.A** Poisoning by, adverse effect of and underdosing of bacterial vaccines

√6ᵗʰ **T50.A1** Poisoning by, adverse effect of and underdosing of pertussis vaccine, including combinations with a pertussis component

√7ᵗʰ **T50.A11** Poisoning by pertussis vaccine, including combinations with a pertussis component, accidental (unintentional)

√7ᵗʰ **T50.A12** Poisoning by pertussis vaccine, including combinations with a pertussis component, intentional self-harm

√7ᵗʰ **T50.A13** Poisoning by pertussis vaccine, including combinations with a pertussis component, assault

√7ᵗʰ **T50.A14** Poisoning by pertussis vaccine, including combinations with a pertussis component, undetermined

√7ᵗʰ **T50.A15** Adverse effect of pertussis vaccine, including combinations with a pertussis component

√7ᵗʰ **T50.A16** Underdosing of pertussis vaccine, including combinations with a pertussis component

√6ᵗʰ **T50.A2** Poisoning by, adverse effect of and underdosing of mixed bacterial vaccines without a pertussis component

√7ᵗʰ **T50.A21** Poisoning by mixed bacterial vaccines without a pertussis component, accidental (unintentional)

√7ᵗʰ **T50.A22** Poisoning by mixed bacterial vaccines without a pertussis component, intentional self-harm

√7ᵗʰ **T50.A23** Poisoning by mixed bacterial vaccines without a pertussis component, assault

√7ᵗʰ **T50.A24** Poisoning by mixed bacterial vaccines without a pertussis component, undetermined

√7ᵗʰ **T50.A25** Adverse effect of mixed bacterial vaccines without a pertussis component

√7ᵗʰ **T50.A26** Underdosing of mixed bacterial vaccines without a pertussis component

√6ᵗʰ **T50.A9** Poisoning by, adverse effect of and underdosing of other bacterial vaccines

√7ᵗʰ **T50.A91** Poisoning by other bacterial vaccines, accidental (unintentional)

√7ᵗʰ **T50.A92** Poisoning by other bacterial vaccines, intentional self-harm

√7ᵗʰ **T50.A93** Poisoning by other bacterial vaccines, assault

√7ᵗʰ **T50.A94** Poisoning by other bacterial vaccines, undetermined

√7ᵗʰ **T50.A95** Adverse effect of other bacterial vaccines

√7ᵗʰ **T50.A96** Underdosing of other bacterial vaccines

√5ᵗʰ **T50.B** Poisoning by, adverse effect of and underdosing of viral vaccines

√6ᵗʰ **T50.B1** Poisoning by, adverse effect of and underdosing of smallpox vaccines

√7ᵗʰ **T50.B11** Poisoning by smallpox vaccines, accidental (unintentional)

√7ᵗʰ **T50.B12** Poisoning by smallpox vaccines, intentional self-harm

√7ᵗʰ **T50.B13** Poisoning by smallpox vaccines, assault

√7ᵗʰ **T50.B14** Poisoning by smallpox vaccines, undetermined

√7ᵗʰ **T50.B15** Adverse effect of smallpox vaccines

√7ᵗʰ **T50.B16** Underdosing of smallpox vaccines

√6ᵗʰ **T50.B9** Poisoning by, adverse effect of and underdosing of other viral vaccines

√7ᵗʰ **T50.B91** Poisoning by other viral vaccines, accidental (unintentional)

√7ᵗʰ **T50.B92** Poisoning by other viral vaccines, intentional self-harm

√7ᵗʰ **T50.B93** Poisoning by other viral vaccines, assault

√7ᵗʰ **T50.B94** Poisoning by other viral vaccines, undetermined

√7ᵗʰ **T50.B95** Adverse effect of other viral vaccines

√7ᵗʰ **T50.B96** Underdosing of other viral vaccines

√5ᵗʰ **T50.Z** Poisoning by, adverse effect of and underdosing of other vaccines and biological substances

√6ᵗʰ **T50.Z1** Poisoning by, adverse effect of and underdosing of immunoglobulin

√7ᵗʰ **T50.Z11** Poisoning by immunoglobulin, accidental (unintentional)

√7ᵗʰ **T50.Z12** Poisoning by immunoglobulin, intentional self-harm

√7ᵗʰ **T50.Z13** Poisoning by immunoglobulin, assault

√7ᵗʰ **T50.Z14** Poisoning by immunoglobulin, undetermined

√7ᵗʰ **T50.Z15** Adverse effect of immunoglobulin

√7ᵗʰ **T50.Z16** Underdosing of immunoglobulin

√6ᵗʰ **T50.Z9** Poisoning by, adverse effect of and underdosing of other vaccines and biological substances

√7ᵗʰ **T50.Z91** Poisoning by other vaccines and biological substances, accidental (unintentional)

√7ᵗʰ **T50.Z92** Poisoning by other vaccines and biological substances, intentional self-harm

√7ᵗʰ **T50.Z93** Poisoning by other vaccines and biological substances, assault

√7ᵗʰ **T50.Z94** Poisoning by other vaccines and biological substances, undetermined

√7ᵗʰ **T50.Z95** Adverse effect of other vaccines and biological substances

√7ᵗʰ **T50.Z96** Underdosing of other vaccines and biological substances

√5ᵗʰ **T50.9** Poisoning by, adverse effect of and underdosing of other and unspecified drugs, medicaments and biological substances
AHA: 2015, 1Q, 21

√6ᵗʰ **T50.90** Poisoning by, adverse effect of and underdosing of unspecified drugs, medicaments and biological substances

√7ᵗʰ **T50.901** Poisoning by unspecified drugs, medicaments and biological substances, accidental (unintentional)

√7ᵗʰ **T50.902** Poisoning by unspecified drugs, medicaments and biological substances, intentional self-harm

√7ᵗʰ **T50.903** Poisoning by unspecified drugs, medicaments and biological substances, assault

√7ᵗʰ **T50.904** Poisoning by unspecified drugs, medicaments and biological substances, undetermined

√7ᵗʰ **T50.905** Adverse effect of unspecified drugs, medicaments and biological substances

√7ᵗʰ **T50.906** Underdosing of unspecified drugs, medicaments and biological substances

√6ᵗʰ **T50.99** Poisoning by, adverse effect of and underdosing of other drugs, medicaments and biological substances

√7ᵗʰ **T50.991** Poisoning by other drugs, medicaments and biological substances, accidental (unintentional)

√7ᵗʰ **T50.992** Poisoning by other drugs, medicaments and biological substances, intentional self-harm

√7ᵗʰ **T50.993** Poisoning by other drugs, medicaments and biological substances, assault

√7ᵗʰ **T50.994** Poisoning by other drugs, medicaments and biological substances, undetermined

√7ᵗʰ **T50.995** Adverse effect of other drugs, medicaments and biological substances

√7ᵗʰ **T50.996** Underdosing of other drugs, medicaments and biological substances

Toxic effects of substances chiefly nonmedicinal as to source (T51-T65)

> **NOTE**   When no intent is indicated code to accidental. Undetermined intent is only for use when there is specific documentation in the record that the intent of the toxic effect cannot be determined.

Use additional code(s) for all associated manifestations of toxic effect, such as:
personal history of foreign body fully removed (Z87.821)
respiratory conditions due to external agents (J60-J70)
to identify any retained foreign body, if applicable (Z18.-)

EXCLUDES 1   *contact with and (suspected) exposure to toxic substances (Z77.-)*

✓4ᵗʰ T51   Toxic effect of alcohol

> The appropriate 7th character is to be added to each code from category T51.
> A   initial encounter
> D   subsequent encounter
> S   sequela

✓5ᵗʰ **T51.0**   **Toxic effect of ethanol**
Toxic effect of ethyl alcohol
> **EXCLUDES 2**   *acute alcohol intoxication or 'hangover' effects (F10.129, F10.229, F10.929)*
> *drunkenness (F10.129, F10.229, F10.929)*
> *pathological alcohol intoxication (F10.129, F10.229, F10.929)*

     ✓6ᵗʰ **T51.0X**   **Toxic effect of ethanol**

         ✓7ᵗʰ **T51.0X1**   **Toxic effect of ethanol, accidental (unintentional)**
                 Toxic effect of ethanol NOS

         ✓7ᵗʰ **T51.0X2**   **Toxic effect of ethanol, intentional self-harm**

         ✓7ᵗʰ **T51.0X3**   **Toxic effect of ethanol, assault**

         ✓7ᵗʰ **T51.0X4**   **Toxic effect of ethanol, undetermined**

✓5ᵗʰ **T51.1**   **Toxic effect of methanol**
Toxic effect of methyl alcohol

     ✓6ᵗʰ **T51.1X**   **Toxic effect of methanol**

         ✓7ᵗʰ **T51.1X1**   **Toxic effect of methanol, accidental (unintentional)**
                 Toxic effect of methanol NOS

         ✓7ᵗʰ **T51.1X2**   **Toxic effect of methanol, intentional self-harm**

         ✓7ᵗʰ **T51.1X3**   **Toxic effect of methanol, assault**

         ✓7ᵗʰ **T51.1X4**   **Toxic effect of methanol, undetermined**

✓5ᵗʰ **T51.2**   **Toxic effect of 2-Propanol**
Toxic effect of isopropyl alcohol

     ✓6ᵗʰ **T51.2X**   **Toxic effect of 2-Propanol**

         ✓7ᵗʰ **T51.2X1**   **Toxic effect of 2-Propanol, accidental (unintentional)**
                 Toxic effect of 2-Propanol NOS

         ✓7ᵗʰ **T51.2X2**   **Toxic effect of 2-Propanol, intentional self-harm**

         ✓7ᵗʰ **T51.2X3**   **Toxic effect of 2-Propanol, assault**

         ✓7ᵗʰ **T51.2X4**   **Toxic effect of 2-Propanol, undetermined**

✓5ᵗʰ **T51.3**   **Toxic effect of fusel oil**
Toxic effect of amyl alcohol
Toxic effect of butyl [1-butanol] alcohol
Toxic effect of propyl [1-propanol] alcohol

     ✓6ᵗʰ **T51.3X**   **Toxic effect of fusel oil**

         ✓7ᵗʰ **T51.3X1**   **Toxic effect of fusel oil, accidental (unintentional)**
                 Toxic effect of fusel oil NOS

         ✓7ᵗʰ **T51.3X2**   **Toxic effect of fusel oil, intentional self-harm**

         ✓7ᵗʰ **T51.3X3**   **Toxic effect of fusel oil, assault**

         ✓7ᵗʰ **T51.3X4**   **Toxic effect of fusel oil, undetermined**

✓5ᵗʰ **T51.8**   **Toxic effect of other alcohols**

     ✓6ᵗʰ **T51.8X**   **Toxic effect of other alcohols**

         ✓7ᵗʰ **T51.8X1**   **Toxic effect of other alcohols, accidental (unintentional)**
                 Toxic effect of other alcohols NOS

         ✓7ᵗʰ **T51.8X2**   **Toxic effect of other alcohols, intentional self-harm**

         ✓7ᵗʰ **T51.8X3**   **Toxic effect of other alcohols, assault**

         ✓7ᵗʰ **T51.8X4**   **Toxic effect of other alcohols, undetermined**

✓5ᵗʰ **T51.9**   **Toxic effect of unspecified alcohol**

     ✓x7ᵗʰ **T51.91**   **Toxic effect of unspecified alcohol, accidental (unintentional)**

     ✓x7ᵗʰ **T51.92**   **Toxic effect of unspecified alcohol, intentional self-harm**

     ✓x7ᵗʰ **T51.93**   **Toxic effect of unspecified alcohol, assault**

     ✓x7ᵗʰ **T51.94**   **Toxic effect of unspecified alcohol, undetermined**

✓4ᵗʰ T52   Toxic effect of organic solvents

> **EXCLUDES 1**   *halogen derivatives of aliphatic and aromatic hydrocarbons (T53.-)*

> The appropriate 7th character is to be added to each code from category T52.
> A   initial encounter
> D   subsequent encounter
> S   sequela

✓5ᵗʰ **T52.0**   **Toxic effects of petroleum products**
Toxic effects of ether petroleum
Toxic effects of gasoline [petrol]
Toxic effects of kerosene [paraffin oil]
Toxic effects of naphtha petroleum
Toxic effects of paraffin wax
Toxic effects of spirit petroleum

     ✓6ᵗʰ **T52.0X**   **Toxic effects of petroleum products**

         ✓7ᵗʰ **T52.0X1**   **Toxic effect of petroleum products, accidental (unintentional)**
                 Toxic effects of petroleum products NOS

         ✓7ᵗʰ **T52.0X2**   **Toxic effect of petroleum products, intentional self-harm**

         ✓7ᵗʰ **T52.0X3**   **Toxic effect of petroleum products, assault**

         ✓7ᵗʰ **T52.0X4**   **Toxic effect of petroleum products, undetermined**

✓5ᵗʰ **T52.1**   **Toxic effects of benzene**
> **EXCLUDES 1**   *homologues of benzene (T52.2)*
> *nitroderivatives and aminoderivatives of benzene and its homologues (T65.3)*

     ✓6ᵗʰ **T52.1X**   **Toxic effects of benzene**

         ✓7ᵗʰ **T52.1X1**   **Toxic effect of benzene, accidental (unintentional)**
                 Toxic effects of benzene NOS

         ✓7ᵗʰ **T52.1X2**   **Toxic effect of benzene, intentional self-harm**

         ✓7ᵗʰ **T52.1X3**   **Toxic effect of benzene, assault**

         ✓7ᵗʰ **T52.1X4**   **Toxic effect of benzene, undetermined**

✓5ᵗʰ **T52.2**   **Toxic effects of homologues of benzene**
Toxic effects of toluene [methylbenzene]
Toxic effects of xylene [dimethylbenzene]

     ✓6ᵗʰ **T52.2X**   **Toxic effects of homologues of benzene**

         ✓7ᵗʰ **T52.2X1**   **Toxic effect of homologues of benzene, accidental (unintentional)**
                 Toxic effects of homologues of benzene NOS

         ✓7ᵗʰ **T52.2X2**   **Toxic effect of homologues of benzene, intentional self-harm**

         ✓7ᵗʰ **T52.2X3**   **Toxic effect of homologues of benzene, assault**

         ✓7ᵗʰ **T52.2X4**   **Toxic effect of homologues of benzene, undetermined**

✓5ᵗʰ **T52.3**   **Toxic effects of glycols**

     ✓6ᵗʰ **T52.3X**   **Toxic effects of glycols**

         ✓7ᵗʰ **T52.3X1**   **Toxic effect of glycols, accidental (unintentional)**
                 Toxic effects of glycols NOS

         ✓7ᵗʰ **T52.3X2**   **Toxic effect of glycols, intentional self-harm**

         ✓7ᵗʰ **T52.3X3**   **Toxic effect of glycols, assault**

         ✓7ᵗʰ **T52.3X4**   **Toxic effect of glycols, undetermined**

✓5ᵗʰ **T52.4**   **Toxic effects of ketones**

     ✓6ᵗʰ **T52.4X**   **Toxic effects of ketones**

         ✓7ᵗʰ **T52.4X1**   **Toxic effect of ketones, accidental (unintentional)**
                 Toxic effects of ketones NOS

         ✓7ᵗʰ **T52.4X2**   **Toxic effect of ketones, intentional self-harm**

N Newborn: 0   **P** Pediatric: 0-17   **M** Maternity: 12-55   **A** Adult: 15-124   **MCC** Major CC Condition   **PDxMCC** PDx acts as own MCC   **CC** CC Condition   **PDxCC** PDx acts as own CC

1118   ICD-10-CM 2016

✓7ᵗʰ **T52.4X3** Toxic effect of ketones, assault

✓7ᵗʰ **T52.4X4** Toxic effect of ketones, undetermined

✓5ᵗʰ **T52.8 Toxic effects of other organic solvents**

✓6ᵗʰ **T52.8X Toxic effects of** other organic solvents

✓7ᵗʰ **T52.8X1 Toxic effect of other organic solvents, accidental (unintentional)**
Toxic effects of other organic solvents NOS

✓7ᵗʰ **T52.8X2 Toxic effect of other organic solvents, intentional self-harm**

✓7ᵗʰ **T52.8X3 Toxic effect of other organic solvents, assault**

✓7ᵗʰ **T52.8X4 Toxic effect of other organic solvents, undetermined**

✓5ᵗʰ **T52.9 Toxic effects of** unspecified **organic solvent**

✓x7ᵗʰ **T52.91 Toxic effect of unspecified organic solvent, accidental (unintentional)**

✓x7ᵗʰ **T52.92 Toxic effect of unspecified organic solvent, intentional self-harm**

✓x7ᵗʰ **T52.93 Toxic effect of unspecified organic solvent, assault**

✓x7ᵗʰ **T52.94 Toxic effect of unspecified organic solvent, undetermined**

✓4ᵗʰ **T53 Toxic effect of halogen derivatives of aliphatic and aromatic hydrocarbons**

> The appropriate 7th character is to be added to each code from category T53.
> A   initial encounter
> D   subsequent encounter
> S   sequela

✓5ᵗʰ **T53.0 Toxic effects of carbon tetrachloride**
Toxic effects of tetrachloromethane

✓6ᵗʰ **T53.0X Toxic effects of carbon tetrachloride**

✓7ᵗʰ **T53.0X1 Toxic effect of carbon tetrachloride, accidental (unintentional)**
Toxic effects of carbon tetrachloride NOS

✓7ᵗʰ **T53.0X2 Toxic effect of carbon tetrachloride, intentional self-harm**

✓7ᵗʰ **T53.0X3 Toxic effect of carbon tetrachloride, assault**

✓7ᵗʰ **T53.0X4 Toxic effect of carbon tetrachloride, undetermined**

✓5ᵗʰ **T53.1 Toxic effects of chloroform**
Toxic effects of trichloromethane

✓6ᵗʰ **T53.1X Toxic effects of chloroform**

✓7ᵗʰ **T53.1X1 Toxic effect of chloroform, accidental (unintentional)**
Toxic effects of chloroform NOS

✓7ᵗʰ **T53.1X2 Toxic effect of chloroform, intentional self-harm**

✓7ᵗʰ **T53.1X3 Toxic effect of chloroform, assault**

✓7ᵗʰ **T53.1X4 Toxic effect of chloroform, undetermined**

✓5ᵗʰ **T53.2 Toxic effects of trichloroethylene**
Toxic effects of trichloroethene

✓6ᵗʰ **T53.2X Toxic effects of trichloroethylene**

✓7ᵗʰ **T53.2X1 Toxic effect of trichloroethylene, accidental (unintentional)**
Toxic effects of trichloroethylene NOS

✓7ᵗʰ **T53.2X2 Toxic effect of trichloroethylene, intentional self-harm**

✓7ᵗʰ **T53.2X3 Toxic effect of trichloroethylene, assault**

✓7ᵗʰ **T53.2X4 Toxic effect of trichloroethylene, undetermined**

✓5ᵗʰ **T53.3 Toxic effects of tetrachloroethylene**
Toxic effects of perchloroethylene
Toxic effect of tetrachloroethene

✓6ᵗʰ **T53.3X Toxic effects of tetrachloroethylene**

✓7ᵗʰ **T53.3X1 Toxic effect of tetrachloroethylene, accidental (unintentional)**
Toxic effects of tetrachloroethylene NOS

✓7ᵗʰ **T53.3X2 Toxic effect of tetrachloroethylene, intentional self-harm**

✓7ᵗʰ **T53.3X3 Toxic effect of tetrachloroethylene, assault**

✓7ᵗʰ **T53.3X4 Toxic effect of tetrachloroethylene, undetermined**

✓5ᵗʰ **T53.4 Toxic effects of dichloromethane**
Toxic effects of methylene chloride

✓6ᵗʰ **T53.4X Toxic effects of dichloromethane**

✓7ᵗʰ **T53.4X1 Toxic effect of dichloromethane, accidental (unintentional)**
Toxic effects of dichloromethane NOS

✓7ᵗʰ **T53.4X2 Toxic effect of dichloromethane, intentional self-harm**

✓7ᵗʰ **T53.4X3 Toxic effect of dichloromethane, assault**

✓7ᵗʰ **T53.4X4 Toxic effect of dichloromethane, undetermined**

✓5ᵗʰ **T53.5 Toxic effects of chlorofluorocarbons**

✓6ᵗʰ **T53.5X Toxic effects of chlorofluorocarbons**

✓7ᵗʰ **T53.5X1 Toxic effect of chlorofluorocarbons, accidental (unintentional)**
Toxic effects of chlorofluorocarbons NOS

✓7ᵗʰ **T53.5X2 Toxic effect of chlorofluorocarbons, intentional self-harm**

✓7ᵗʰ **T53.5X3 Toxic effect of chlorofluorocarbons, assault**

✓7ᵗʰ **T53.5X4 Toxic effect of chlorofluorocarbons, undetermined**

✓5ᵗʰ **T53.6 Toxic effects of other halogen derivatives of aliphatic hydrocarbons**

✓6ᵗʰ **T53.6X Toxic effects of other halogen derivatives of aliphatic hydrocarbons**

✓7ᵗʰ **T53.6X1 Toxic effect of other halogen derivatives of aliphatic hydrocarbons, accidental (unintentional)**
Toxic effects of other halogen derivatives of aliphatic hydrocarbons NOS

✓7ᵗʰ **T53.6X2 Toxic effect of other halogen derivatives of aliphatic hydrocarbons, intentional self-harm**

✓7ᵗʰ **T53.6X3 Toxic effect of other halogen derivatives of aliphatic hydrocarbons, assault**

✓7ᵗʰ **T53.6X4 Toxic effect of other halogen derivatives of aliphatic hydrocarbons, undetermined**

✓5ᵗʰ **T53.7 Toxic effects of other halogen derivatives of aromatic hydrocarbons**

✓6ᵗʰ **T53.7X Toxic effects of other halogen derivatives of aromatic hydrocarbons**

✓7ᵗʰ **T53.7X1 Toxic effect of other halogen derivatives of aromatic hydrocarbons, accidental (unintentional)**
Toxic effects of other halogen derivatives of aromatic hydrocarbons NOS

✓7ᵗʰ **T53.7X2 Toxic effect of other halogen derivatives of aromatic hydrocarbons, intentional self-harm**

✓7ᵗʰ **T53.7X3 Toxic effect of other halogen derivatives of aromatic hydrocarbons, assault**

✓7ᵗʰ **T53.7X4 Toxic effect of other halogen derivatives of aromatic hydrocarbons, undetermined**

✓5ᵗʰ **T53.9 Toxic effects of unspecified halogen derivatives of aliphatic and aromatic hydrocarbons**

✓x7ᵗʰ **T53.91 Toxic effect of unspecified halogen derivatives of aliphatic and aromatic hydrocarbons, accidental (unintentional)**

✓x7ᵗʰ **T53.92 Toxic effect of unspecified halogen derivatives of aliphatic and aromatic hydrocarbons, intentional self-harm**

✓x7ᵗʰ **T53.93 Toxic effect of unspecified halogen derivatives of aliphatic and aromatic hydrocarbons, assault**

✓x7ᵗʰ **T53.94 Toxic effect of unspecified halogen derivatives of aliphatic and aromatic hydrocarbons, undetermined**

√4ᵗʰ T54 Toxic effect of corrosive substances

> The appropriate 7th character is to be added to each code from category T54.
> A   initial encounter
> D   subsequent encounter
> S   sequela

√5ᵗʰ **T54.0 Toxic effects of phenol and phenol homologues**

√6ᵗʰ **T54.0X Toxic effects of** phenol and phenol homologues

√7ᵗʰ **T54.0X1 Toxic effect of phenol and phenol homologues, accidental (unintentional)**
Toxic effects of phenol and phenol homologues NOS

√7ᵗʰ **T54.0X2 Toxic effect of phenol and phenol homologues, intentional self-harm**

√7ᵗʰ **T54.0X3 Toxic effect of phenol and phenol homologues, assault**

√7ᵗʰ **T54.0X4 Toxic effect of phenol and phenol homologues, undetermined**

√5ᵗʰ **T54.1 Toxic effects of other corrosive organic compounds**

√6ᵗʰ **T54.1X Toxic effects of** other corrosive organic compounds

√7ᵗʰ **T54.1X1 Toxic effect of other corrosive organic compounds, accidental (unintentional)**
Toxic effects of other corrosive organic compounds NOS

√7ᵗʰ **T54.1X2 Toxic effect of other corrosive organic compounds, intentional self-harm**

√7ᵗʰ **T54.1X3 Toxic effect of other corrosive organic compounds, assault**

√7ᵗʰ **T54.1X4 Toxic effect of other corrosive organic compounds, undetermined**

√5ᵗʰ **T54.2 Toxic effects of corrosive acids and acid-like substances**
Toxic effects of hydrochloric acid
Toxic effects of sulfuric acid

√6ᵗʰ **T54.2X Toxic effects of corrosive** acids and acid-like substances

√7ᵗʰ **T54.2X1 Toxic effect of corrosive acids and acid-like substances, accidental (unintentional)**
Toxic effects of corrosive acids and acid-like substances NOS

√7ᵗʰ **T54.2X2 Toxic effect of corrosive acids and acid-like substances, intentional self-harm**

√7ᵗʰ **T54.2X3 Toxic effect of corrosive acids and acid-like substances, assault**

√7ᵗʰ **T54.2X4 Toxic effect of corrosive acids and acid-like substances, undetermined**

√5ᵗʰ **T54.3 Toxic effects of corrosive alkalis and alkali-like substances**
Toxic effects of potassium hydroxide
Toxic effects of sodium hydroxide

√6ᵗʰ **T54.3X Toxic effects of corrosive** alkalis and alkali-like substances

√7ᵗʰ **T54.3X1 Toxic effect of corrosive alkalis and alkali-like substances, accidental (unintentional)**
Toxic effects of corrosive alkalis and alkali-like substances NOS

√7ᵗʰ **T54.3X2 Toxic effect of corrosive alkalis and alkali-like substances, intentional self-harm**

√7ᵗʰ **T54.3X3 Toxic effect of corrosive alkalis and alkali-like substances, assault**

√7ᵗʰ **T54.3X4 Toxic effect of corrosive alkalis and alkali-like substances, undetermined**

√5ᵗʰ **T54.9 Toxic effects of** unspecified corrosive substance

√x7ᵗʰ **T54.91 Toxic effect of unspecified corrosive substance, accidental (unintentional)**

√x7ᵗʰ **T54.92 Toxic effect of unspecified corrosive substance, intentional self-harm**

√x7ᵗʰ **T54.93 Toxic effect of unspecified corrosive substance, assault**

√x7ᵗʰ **T54.94 Toxic effect of unspecified corrosive substance, undetermined**

√4ᵗʰ T55 Toxic effect of soaps and detergents

> The appropriate 7th character is to be added to each code from category T55.
> A   initial encounter
> D   subsequent encounter
> S   sequela

√5ᵗʰ **T55.0 Toxic effect of soaps**

√6ᵗʰ **T55.0X Toxic effect of** soaps

√7ᵗʰ **T55.0X1 Toxic effect of soaps, accidental (unintentional)**
Toxic effect of soaps NOS

√7ᵗʰ **T55.0X2 Toxic effect of soaps, intentional self-harm**

√7ᵗʰ **T55.0X3 Toxic effect of soaps, assault**

√7ᵗʰ **T55.0X4 Toxic effect of soaps, undetermined**

√5ᵗʰ **T55.1 Toxic effect of detergents**

√6ᵗʰ **T55.1X Toxic effect of** detergents

√7ᵗʰ **T55.1X1 Toxic effect of detergents, accidental (unintentional)**
Toxic effect of detergents NOS

√7ᵗʰ **T55.1X2 Toxic effect of detergents, intentional self-harm**

√7ᵗʰ **T55.1X3 Toxic effect of detergents, assault**

√7ᵗʰ **T55.1X4 Toxic effect of detergents, undetermined**

√4ᵗʰ T56 Toxic effect of metals

> **INCLUDES**   toxic effects of fumes and vapors of metals
> toxic effects of metals from all sources, except medicinal substances
>
> Use additional code to identify any retained metal foreign body, if applicable (Z18.0-, T18.1-)
>
> **EXCLUDES 1**   arsenic and its compounds (T57.0)
> manganese and its compounds (T57.2)

> The appropriate 7th character is to be added to each code from category T56.
> A   initial encounter
> D   subsequent encounter
> S   sequela

√5ᵗʰ **T56.0 Toxic effects of lead and its compounds**

√6ᵗʰ **T56.0X Toxic effects of** lead and its compounds

√7ᵗʰ **T56.0X1 Toxic effect of lead and its compounds, accidental (unintentional)**
Toxic effects of lead and its compounds NOS

√7ᵗʰ **T56.0X2 Toxic effect of lead and its compounds, intentional self-harm**

√7ᵗʰ **T56.0X3 Toxic effect of lead and its compounds, assault**

√7ᵗʰ **T56.0X4 Toxic effect of lead and its compounds, undetermined**

√5ᵗʰ **T56.1 Toxic effects of mercury and its compounds**

√6ᵗʰ **T56.1X Toxic effects of** mercury and its compounds

√7ᵗʰ **T56.1X1 Toxic effect of mercury and its compounds, accidental (unintentional)**
Toxic effects of mercury and its compounds NOS

√7ᵗʰ **T56.1X2 Toxic effect of mercury and its compounds, intentional self-harm**

√7ᵗʰ **T56.1X3 Toxic effect of mercury and its compounds, assault**

√7ᵗʰ **T56.1X4 Toxic effect of mercury and its compounds, undetermined**

√5ᵗʰ **T56.2 Toxic effects of chromium and its compounds**

√6ᵗʰ **T56.2X Toxic effects of** chromium and its compounds

√7ᵗʰ **T56.2X1 Toxic effect of chromium and its compounds, accidental (unintentional)**
Toxic effects of chromium and its compounds NOS

√7ᵗʰ **T56.2X2 Toxic effect of chromium and its compounds, intentional self-harm**

√7ᵗʰ **T56.2X3 Toxic effect of chromium and its compounds, assault**

√7ᵗʰ **T56.2X4 Toxic effect of chromium and its compounds, undetermined**

☑5ᵗʰ **T56.3** Toxic effects of cadmium and its compounds

  ☑6ᵗʰ **T56.3X** Toxic effects of cadmium and its compounds

    ☑7ᵗʰ **T56.3X1** Toxic effect of cadmium and its compounds, accidental (unintentional)
      Toxic effects of cadmium and its compounds NOS

    ☑7ᵗʰ **T56.3X2** Toxic effect of cadmium and its compounds, intentional self-harm

    ☑7ᵗʰ **T56.3X3** Toxic effect of cadmium and its compounds, assault

    ☑7ᵗʰ **T56.3X4** Toxic effect of cadmium and its compounds, undetermined

☑5ᵗʰ **T56.4** Toxic effects of copper and its compounds

  ☑6ᵗʰ **T56.4X** Toxic effects of copper and its compounds

    ☑7ᵗʰ **T56.4X1** Toxic effect of copper and its compounds, accidental (unintentional)
      Toxic effects of copper and its compounds NOS

    ☑7ᵗʰ **T56.4X2** Toxic effect of copper and its compounds, intentional self-harm

    ☑7ᵗʰ **T56.4X3** Toxic effect of copper and its compounds, assault

    ☑7ᵗʰ **T56.4X4** Toxic effect of copper and its compounds, undetermined

☑5ᵗʰ **T56.5** Toxic effects of zinc and its compounds

  ☑6ᵗʰ **T56.5X** Toxic effects of zinc and its compounds

    ☑7ᵗʰ **T56.5X1** Toxic effect of zinc and its compounds, accidental (unintentional)
      Toxic effects of zinc and its compounds NOS

    ☑7ᵗʰ **T56.5X2** Toxic effect of zinc and its compounds, intentional self-harm

    ☑7ᵗʰ **T56.5X3** Toxic effect of zinc and its compounds, assault

    ☑7ᵗʰ **T56.5X4** Toxic effect of zinc and its compounds, undetermined

☑5ᵗʰ **T56.6** Toxic effects of tin and its compounds

  ☑6ᵗʰ **T56.6X** Toxic effects of tin and its compounds

    ☑7ᵗʰ **T56.6X1** Toxic effect of tin and its compounds, accidental (unintentional)
      Toxic effect of tin and its compounds NOS

    ☑7ᵗʰ **T56.6X2** Toxic effect of tin and its compounds, intentional self-harm

    ☑7ᵗʰ **T56.6X3** Toxic effect of tin and its compounds, assault

    ☑7ᵗʰ **T56.6X4** Toxic effect of tin and its compounds, undetermined

☑5ᵗʰ **T56.7** Toxic effects of beryllium and its compounds

  ☑6ᵗʰ **T56.7X** Toxic effects of beryllium and its compounds

    ☑7ᵗʰ **T56.7X1** Toxic effect of beryllium and its compounds, accidental (unintentional)
      Toxic effects of beryllium and its compounds NOS

    ☑7ᵗʰ **T56.7X2** Toxic effect of beryllium and its compounds, intentional self-harm

    ☑7ᵗʰ **T56.7X3** Toxic effect of beryllium and its compounds, assault

    ☑7ᵗʰ **T56.7X4** Toxic effect of beryllium and its compounds, undetermined

☑5ᵗʰ **T56.8** Toxic effects of other metals

  ☑6ᵗʰ **T56.81** Toxic effect of thallium

    ☑7ᵗʰ **T56.811** Toxic effect of thallium, accidental (unintentional)
      Toxic effect of thallium NOS

    ☑7ᵗʰ **T56.812** Toxic effect of thallium, intentional self-harm

    ☑7ᵗʰ **T56.813** Toxic effect of thallium, assault

    ☑7ᵗʰ **T56.814** Toxic effect of thallium, undetermined

  ☑6ᵗʰ **T56.89** Toxic effects of other metals

    ☑7ᵗʰ **T56.891** Toxic effect of other metals, accidental (unintentional)
      Toxic effects of other metals NOS

    ☑7ᵗʰ **T56.892** Toxic effect of other metals, intentional self-harm

    ☑7ᵗʰ **T56.893** Toxic effect of other metals, assault

    ☑7ᵗʰ **T56.894** Toxic effect of other metals, undetermined

☑5ᵗʰ **T56.9** Toxic effects of unspecified metal

  ☑x7ᵗʰ **T56.91** Toxic effect of unspecified metal, accidental (unintentional)

  ☑x7ᵗʰ **T56.92** Toxic effect of unspecified metal, intentional self-harm

  ☑x7ᵗʰ **T56.93** Toxic effect of unspecified metal, assault

  ☑x7ᵗʰ **T56.94** Toxic effect of unspecified metal, undetermined

☑4ᵗʰ **T57** Toxic effect of other inorganic substances

> The appropriate 7th character is to be added to each code from category T57.
> A   initial encounter
> D   subsequent encounter
> S   sequela

☑5ᵗʰ **T57.0** Toxic effect of arsenic and its compounds

  ☑6ᵗʰ **T57.0X** Toxic effect of arsenic and its compounds

    ☑7ᵗʰ **T57.0X1** Toxic effect of arsenic and its compounds, accidental (unintentional)
      Toxic effect of arsenic and its compounds NOS

    ☑7ᵗʰ **T57.0X2** Toxic effect of arsenic and its compounds, intentional self-harm

    ☑7ᵗʰ **T57.0X3** Toxic effect of arsenic and its compounds, assault

    ☑7ᵗʰ **T57.0X4** Toxic effect of arsenic and its compounds, undetermined

☑5ᵗʰ **T57.1** Toxic effect of phosphorus and its compounds
   EXCLUDES 1   *organophosphate insecticides (T60.0)*

  ☑6ᵗʰ **T57.1X** Toxic effect of phosphorus and its compounds

    ☑7ᵗʰ **T57.1X1** Toxic effect of phosphorus and its compounds, accidental (unintentional)
      Toxic effect of phosphorus and its compounds NOS

    ☑7ᵗʰ **T57.1X2** Toxic effect of phosphorus and its compounds, intentional self-harm

    ☑7ᵗʰ **T57.1X3** Toxic effect of phosphorus and its compounds, assault

    ☑7ᵗʰ **T57.1X4** Toxic effect of phosphorus and its compounds, undetermined

☑5ᵗʰ **T57.2** Toxic effect of manganese and its compounds

  ☑6ᵗʰ **T57.2X** Toxic effect of manganese and its compounds

    ☑7ᵗʰ **T57.2X1** Toxic effect of manganese and its compounds, accidental (unintentional)
      Toxic effect of manganese and its compounds NOS

    ☑7ᵗʰ **T57.2X2** Toxic effect of manganese and its compounds, intentional self-harm

    ☑7ᵗʰ **T57.2X3** Toxic effect of manganese and its compounds, assault

    ☑7ᵗʰ **T57.2X4** Toxic effect of manganese and its compounds, undetermined

☑5ᵗʰ **T57.3** Toxic effect of hydrogen cyanide

  ☑6ᵗʰ **T57.3X** Toxic effect of hydrogen cyanide

    ☑7ᵗʰ **T57.3X1** Toxic effect of hydrogen cyanide, accidental (unintentional)
      Toxic effect of hydrogen cyanide NOS

    ☑7ᵗʰ **T57.3X2** Toxic effect of hydrogen cyanide, intentional self-harm

    ☑7ᵗʰ **T57.3X3** Toxic effect of hydrogen cyanide, assault

    ☑7ᵗʰ **T57.3X4** Toxic effect of hydrogen cyanide, undetermined

☑5ᵗʰ **T57.8** Toxic effect of other specified inorganic substances

  ☑6ᵗʰ **T57.8X** Toxic effect of other specified inorganic substances

    ☑7ᵗʰ **T57.8X1** Toxic effect of other specified inorganic substances, accidental (unintentional)
      Toxic effect of other specified inorganic substances NOS

    ☑7ᵗʰ **T57.8X2** Toxic effect of other specified inorganic substances, intentional self-harm

    ☑7ᵗʰ **T57.8X3** Toxic effect of other specified inorganic substances, assault

    ☑7ᵗʰ **T57.8X4** Toxic effect of other specified inorganic substances, undetermined

---

☑ Additional Character Required   ☑x7ᵗʰ Placeholder Alert   Unacceptable PDx   Manifestation   Hospital Acquired Condition   **EXCLUDES 1** Not Coded Here   **EXCLUDES 2** Not Included Here

√5ᵗʰ **T57.9** Toxic effect of unspecified inorganic substance

    √x7ᵗʰ **T57.91** **Toxic effect of unspecified inorganic substance, accidental (unintentional)**

    √x7ᵗʰ **T57.92** **Toxic effect of unspecified inorganic substance, intentional self-harm**

    √x7ᵗʰ **T57.93** **Toxic effect of unspecified inorganic substance, assault**

    √x7ᵗʰ **T57.94** **Toxic effect of unspecified inorganic substance, undetermined**

√4ᵗʰ **T58** **Toxic effect of carbon monoxide**
    INCLUDES asphyxiation from carbon monoxide
        toxic effect of carbon monoxide from all sources

> The appropriate 7th character is to be added to each code from category T58.
> A   initial encounter
> D   subsequent encounter
> S   sequela

√5ᵗʰ **T58.0** **Toxic effect of carbon monoxide from motor vehicle exhaust**
    Toxic effect of exhaust gas from gas engine
    Toxic effect of exhaust gas from motor pump

    √x7ᵗʰ **T58.01** **Toxic effect of carbon monoxide from motor vehicle exhaust, accidental (unintentional)**

    √x7ᵗʰ **T58.02** **Toxic effect of carbon monoxide from motor vehicle exhaust, intentional self-harm**

    √x7ᵗʰ **T58.03** **Toxic effect of carbon monoxide from motor vehicle exhaust, assault**

    √x7ᵗʰ **T58.04** **Toxic effect of carbon monoxide from motor vehicle exhaust, undetermined**

√5ᵗʰ **T58.1** **Toxic effect of carbon monoxide from utility gas**
    Toxic effect of acetylene
    Toxic effect of gas NOS used for lighting, heating, cooking
    Toxic effect of water gas

    √x7ᵗʰ **T58.11** **Toxic effect of carbon monoxide from utility gas, accidental (unintentional)**

    √x7ᵗʰ **T58.12** **Toxic effect of carbon monoxide from utility gas, intentional self-harm**

    √x7ᵗʰ **T58.13** **Toxic effect of carbon monoxide from utility gas, assault**

    √x7ᵗʰ **T58.14** **Toxic effect of carbon monoxide from utility gas, undetermined**

√5ᵗʰ **T58.2** **Toxic effect of carbon monoxide from incomplete combustion of other domestic fuels**
    Toxic effect of carbon monoxide from incomplete combustion of coal, coke, kerosene, wood

    √6ᵗʰ **T58.2X** **Toxic effect of carbon monoxide from incomplete combustion of other domestic fuels**

        √7ᵗʰ **T58.2X1** **Toxic effect of carbon monoxide from incomplete combustion of other domestic fuels, accidental (unintentional)**

        √7ᵗʰ **T58.2X2** **Toxic effect of carbon monoxide from incomplete combustion of other domestic fuels, intentional self-harm**

        √7ᵗʰ **T58.2X3** **Toxic effect of carbon monoxide from incomplete combustion of other domestic fuels, assault**

        √7ᵗʰ **T58.2X4** **Toxic effect of carbon monoxide from incomplete combustion of other domestic fuels, undetermined**

√5ᵗʰ **T58.8** **Toxic effect of carbon monoxide from other source**
    Toxic effect of carbon monoxide from blast furnace gas
    Toxic effect of carbon monoxide from fuels in industrial use
    Toxic effect of carbon monoxide from kiln vapor

    √6ᵗʰ **T58.8X** **Toxic effect of carbon monoxide from other source**

        √7ᵗʰ **T58.8X1** **Toxic effect of carbon monoxide from other source, accidental (unintentional)**

        √7ᵗʰ **T58.8X2** **Toxic effect of carbon monoxide from other source, intentional self-harm**

        √7ᵗʰ **T58.8X3** **Toxic effect of carbon monoxide from other source, assault**

        √7ᵗʰ **T58.8X4** **Toxic effect of carbon monoxide from other source, undetermined**

√5ᵗʰ **T58.9** **Toxic effect of carbon monoxide from unspecified source**

    √x7ᵗʰ **T58.91** **Toxic effect of carbon monoxide from unspecified source, accidental (unintentional)**

    √x7ᵗʰ **T58.92** **Toxic effect of carbon monoxide from unspecified source, intentional self-harm**

    √x7ᵗʰ **T58.93** **Toxic effect of carbon monoxide from unspecified source, assault**

    √x7ᵗʰ **T58.94** **Toxic effect of carbon monoxide from unspecified source, undetermined**

√4ᵗʰ **T59** **Toxic effect of other gases, fumes and vapors**
    INCLUDES aerosol propellants
    EXCLUDES 1 *chlorofluorocarbons (T53.5)*

> The appropriate 7th character is to be added to each code from category T59.
> A   initial encounter
> D   subsequent encounter
> S   sequela

√5ᵗʰ **T59.0** **Toxic effect of nitrogen oxides**

    √6ᵗʰ **T59.0X** **Toxic effect of nitrogen oxides**

        √7ᵗʰ **T59.0X1** **Toxic effect of nitrogen oxides, accidental (unintentional)**
            Toxic effect of nitrogen oxides NOS

        √7ᵗʰ **T59.0X2** **Toxic effect of nitrogen oxides, intentional self-harm**

        √7ᵗʰ **T59.0X3** **Toxic effect of nitrogen oxides, assault**

        √7ᵗʰ **T59.0X4** **Toxic effect of nitrogen oxides, undetermined**

√5ᵗʰ **T59.1** **Toxic effect of sulfur dioxide**

    √6ᵗʰ **T59.1X** **Toxic effect of sulfur dioxide**

        √7ᵗʰ **T59.1X1** **Toxic effect of sulfur dioxide, accidental (unintentional)**
            Toxic effect of sulfur dioxide NOS

        √7ᵗʰ **T59.1X2** **Toxic effect of sulfur dioxide, intentional self-harm**

        √7ᵗʰ **T59.1X3** **Toxic effect of sulfur dioxide, assault**

        √7ᵗʰ **T59.1X4** **Toxic effect of sulfur dioxide, undetermined**

√5ᵗʰ **T59.2** **Toxic effect of formaldehyde**

    √6ᵗʰ **T59.2X** **Toxic effect of formaldehyde**

        √7ᵗʰ **T59.2X1** **Toxic effect of formaldehyde, accidental (unintentional)**
            Toxic effect of formaldehyde NOS

        √7ᵗʰ **T59.2X2** **Toxic effect of formaldehyde, intentional self-harm**

        √7ᵗʰ **T59.2X3** **Toxic effect of formaldehyde, assault**

        √7ᵗʰ **T59.2X4** **Toxic effect of formaldehyde, undetermined**

√5ᵗʰ **T59.3** **Toxic effect of lacrimogenic gas**
    Toxic effect of tear gas

    √6ᵗʰ **T59.3X** **Toxic effect of lacrimogenic gas**

        √7ᵗʰ **T59.3X1** **Toxic effect of lacrimogenic gas, accidental (unintentional)**
            Toxic effect of lacrimogenic gas NOS

        √7ᵗʰ **T59.3X2** **Toxic effect of lacrimogenic gas, intentional self-harm**

        √7ᵗʰ **T59.3X3** **Toxic effect of lacrimogenic gas, assault**

        √7ᵗʰ **T59.3X4** **Toxic effect of lacrimogenic gas, undetermined**

√5ᵗʰ **T59.4** **Toxic effect of chlorine gas**

    √6ᵗʰ **T59.4X** **Toxic effect of chlorine gas**

        √7ᵗʰ **T59.4X1** **Toxic effect of chlorine gas, accidental (unintentional)**
            Toxic effect of chlorine gas NOS

        √7ᵗʰ **T59.4X2** **Toxic effect of chlorine gas, intentional self-harm**

        √7ᵗʰ **T59.4X3** **Toxic effect of chlorine gas, assault**

        √7ᵗʰ **T59.4X4** **Toxic effect of chlorine gas, undetermined**

√5ᵗʰ **T59.5** **Toxic effect of fluorine gas and hydrogen fluoride**

    √6ᵗʰ **T59.5X** **Toxic effect of fluorine gas and hydrogen fluoride**

        √7ᵗʰ **T59.5X1** **Toxic effect of fluorine gas and hydrogen fluoride, accidental (unintentional)**
            Toxic effect of fluorine gas and hydrogen fluoride NOS

        √7ᵗʰ **T59.5X2** **Toxic effect of fluorine gas and hydrogen fluoride, intentional self-harm**

N Newborn: 0   P Pediatric: 0-17   M Maternity: 12-55   A Adult: 15-124   MCC Major CC Condition   PDxMCC PDx acts as own MCC   CC CC Condition   PDxCC PDx acts as own CC

1122   ICD-10-CM 2016

√7ᵗʰ **T59.5X3** Toxic effect of fluorine gas and hydrogen fluoride, **assault**

√7ᵗʰ **T59.5X4** Toxic effect of fluorine gas and hydrogen fluoride, **undetermined**

√5ᵗʰ **T59.6** Toxic effect of hydrogen sulfide

√6ᵗʰ **T59.6X** Toxic effect of hydrogen sulfide

√7ᵗʰ **T59.6X1** Toxic effect of hydrogen sulfide, **accidental (unintentional)**
Toxic effect of hydrogen sulfide NOS

√7ᵗʰ **T59.6X2** Toxic effect of hydrogen sulfide, **intentional self-harm**

√7ᵗʰ **T59.6X3** Toxic effect of hydrogen sulfide, **assault**

√7ᵗʰ **T59.6X4** Toxic effect of hydrogen sulfide, **undetermined**

√5ᵗʰ **T59.7** Toxic effect of carbon dioxide

√6ᵗʰ **T59.7X** Toxic effect of carbon dioxide

√7ᵗʰ **T59.7X1** Toxic effect of carbon dioxide, **accidental (unintentional)**
Toxic effect of carbon dioxide NOS

√7ᵗʰ **T59.7X2** Toxic effect of carbon dioxide, **intentional self-harm**

√7ᵗʰ **T59.7X3** Toxic effect of carbon dioxide, **assault**

√7ᵗʰ **T59.7X4** Toxic effect of carbon dioxide, **undetermined**

√5ᵗʰ **T59.8** Toxic effect of other specified gases, fumes and vapors

√6ᵗʰ **T59.81** Toxic effect of smoke
Smoke inhalation
EXCLUDES 2 toxic effect of cigarette (tobacco) smoke (T65.22-)

√7ᵗʰ **T59.811** Toxic effect of smoke, **accidental (unintentional)**
Toxic effect of smoke NOS
AHA: 2013, 4Q, 121

√7ᵗʰ **T59.812** Toxic effect of smoke, **intentional self-harm**

√7ᵗʰ **T59.813** Toxic effect of smoke, **assault**

√7ᵗʰ **T59.814** Toxic effect of smoke, **undetermined**

√6ᵗʰ **T59.89** Toxic effect of other specified gases, fumes and vapors

√7ᵗʰ **T59.891** Toxic effect of other specified gases, fumes and vapors, **accidental (unintentional)**

√7ᵗʰ **T59.892** Toxic effect of other specified gases, fumes and vapors, **intentional self-harm**

√7ᵗʰ **T59.893** Toxic effect of other specified gases, fumes and vapors, **assault**

√7ᵗʰ **T59.894** Toxic effect of other specified gases, fumes and vapors, **undetermined**

√5ᵗʰ **T59.9** Toxic effect of unspecified gases, fumes and vapors

√x7ᵗʰ **T59.91** Toxic effect of unspecified gases, fumes and vapors, **accidental (unintentional)**

√x7ᵗʰ **T59.92** Toxic effect of unspecified gases, fumes and vapors, **intentional self-harm**

√x7ᵗʰ **T59.93** Toxic effect of unspecified gases, fumes and vapors, **assault**

√x7ᵗʰ **T59.94** Toxic effect of unspecified gases, fumes and vapors, **undetermined**

√4ᵗʰ **T60 Toxic effect of pesticides**
INCLUDES toxic effect of wood preservatives

The appropriate 7th character is to be added to each code from category T60.
A   initial encounter
D   subsequent encounter
S   sequela

√5ᵗʰ **T60.0** Toxic effect of organophosphate and carbamate insecticides

√6ᵗʰ **T60.0X** Toxic effect of organophosphate and carbamate insecticides

√7ᵗʰ **T60.0X1** Toxic effect of organophosphate and carbamate insecticides, **accidental (unintentional)**
Toxic effect of organophosphate and carbamate insecticides NOS

√7ᵗʰ **T60.0X2** Toxic effect of organophosphate and carbamate insecticides, **intentional self-harm**

√7ᵗʰ **T60.0X3** Toxic effect of organophosphate and carbamate insecticides, **assault**

√7ᵗʰ **T60.0X4** Toxic effect of organophosphate and carbamate insecticides, **undetermined**

√5ᵗʰ **T60.1** Toxic effect of halogenated insecticides
EXCLUDES 1 chlorinated hydrocarbon (T53.-)

√6ᵗʰ **T60.1X** Toxic effect of halogenated insecticides

√7ᵗʰ **T60.1X1** Toxic effect of halogenated insecticides, **accidental (unintentional)**
Toxic effect of halogenated insecticides NOS

√7ᵗʰ **T60.1X2** Toxic effect of halogenated insecticides, **intentional self-harm**

√7ᵗʰ **T60.1X3** Toxic effect of halogenated insecticides, **assault**

√7ᵗʰ **T60.1X4** Toxic effect of halogenated insecticides, **undetermined**

√5ᵗʰ **T60.2** Toxic effect of other insecticides

√6ᵗʰ **T60.2X** Toxic effect of other insecticides

√7ᵗʰ **T60.2X1** Toxic effect of other insecticides, **accidental (unintentional)**
Toxic effect of other insecticides NOS

√7ᵗʰ **T60.2X2** Toxic effect of other insecticides, **intentional self-harm**

√7ᵗʰ **T60.2X3** Toxic effect of other insecticides, **assault**

√7ᵗʰ **T60.2X4** Toxic effect of other insecticides, **undetermined**

√5ᵗʰ **T60.3** Toxic effect of herbicides and fungicides

√6ᵗʰ **T60.3X** Toxic effect of herbicides and fungicides

√7ᵗʰ **T60.3X1** Toxic effect of herbicides and fungicides, **accidental (unintentional)**
Toxic effect of herbicides and fungicides NOS

√7ᵗʰ **T60.3X2** Toxic effect of herbicides and fungicides, **intentional self-harm**

√7ᵗʰ **T60.3X3** Toxic effect of herbicides and fungicides, **assault**

√7ᵗʰ **T60.3X4** Toxic effect of herbicides and fungicides, **undetermined**

√5ᵗʰ **T60.4** Toxic effect of rodenticides
EXCLUDES 1 strychnine and its salts (T65.1)
thallium (T56.81-)

√6ᵗʰ **T60.4X** Toxic effect of rodenticides

√7ᵗʰ **T60.4X1** Toxic effect of rodenticides, **accidental (unintentional)**
Toxic effect of rodenticides NOS

√7ᵗʰ **T60.4X2** Toxic effect of rodenticides, **intentional self-harm**

√7ᵗʰ **T60.4X3** Toxic effect of rodenticides, **assault**

√7ᵗʰ **T60.4X4** Toxic effect of rodenticides, **undetermined**

√5ᵗʰ **T60.8** Toxic effect of other pesticides

√6ᵗʰ **T60.8X** Toxic effect of other pesticides

√7ᵗʰ **T60.8X1** Toxic effect of other pesticides, **accidental (unintentional)**
Toxic effect of other pesticides NOS

√7ᵗʰ **T60.8X2** Toxic effect of other pesticides, **intentional self-harm**

√7ᵗʰ **T60.8X3** Toxic effect of other pesticides, **assault**

√7ᵗʰ **T60.8X4** Toxic effect of other pesticides, **undetermined**

√5ᵗʰ **T60.9** Toxic effect of unspecified pesticide

√x7ᵗʰ **T60.91** Toxic effect of unspecified pesticide, **accidental (unintentional)**

√x7ᵗʰ **T60.92** Toxic effect of unspecified pesticide, **intentional self-harm**

√x7ᵗʰ **T60.93** Toxic effect of unspecified pesticide, **assault**

√x7ᵗʰ **T60.94** Toxic effect of unspecified pesticide, **undetermined**

Chapter 19. Injury, Poisoning, and Certain Other Consequences of External Causes

T61–T62.94

√4th **T61 Toxic effect of noxious substances eaten as seafood**

EXCLUDES 1 *allergic reaction to food, such as:*
anaphylactic reaction or shock due to adverse food reaction (T78.0-)
dermatitis (L23.6, L25.4, L27.2)
gastroenteritis (noninfective) (K52.2)
bacterial foodborne intoxications (A05.-)
toxic effect of aflatoxin and other mycotoxins (T64)
toxic effect of cyanides (T65.0-)
toxic effect of harmful algae bloom (T65.82-)
toxic effect of hydrogen cyanide (T57.3-)
toxic effect of mercury (T56.1-)
toxic effect of red tide (T65.82-)

The appropriate 7th character is to be added to each code from category T61.
A   initial encounter
D   subsequent encounter
S   sequela

√5th **T61.0 Ciguatera fish poisoning**

√x7th   **T61.01 Ciguatera fish poisoning, accidental (unintentional)**

√x7th   **T61.02 Ciguatera fish poisoning, intentional self-harm**

√x7th   **T61.03 Ciguatera fish poisoning, assault**

√x7th   **T61.04 Ciguatera fish poisoning, undetermined**

√5th **T61.1 Scombroid fish poisoning**
Histamine-like syndrome

√x7th   **T61.11 Scombroid fish poisoning, accidental (unintentional)**

√x7th   **T61.12 Scombroid fish poisoning, intentional self-harm**

√x7th   **T61.13 Scombroid fish poisoning, assault**

√x7th   **T61.14 Scombroid fish poisoning, undetermined**

√5th **T61.7 Other fish and shellfish poisoning**

√6th   **T61.77 Other fish poisoning**

√7th   **T61.771 Other fish poisoning, accidental (unintentional)**

√7th   **T61.772 Other fish poisoning, intentional self-harm**

√7th   **T61.773 Other fish poisoning, assault**

√7th   **T61.774 Other fish poisoning, undetermined**

√6th   **T61.78 Other shellfish poisoning**

√7th   **T61.781 Other shellfish poisoning, accidental (unintentional)**

√7th   **T61.782 Other shellfish poisoning, intentional self-harm**

√7th   **T61.783 Other shellfish poisoning, assault**

√7th   **T61.784 Other shellfish poisoning, undetermined**

√5th **T61.8 Toxic effect of other seafood**

√6th   **T61.8X Toxic effect of other seafood**

√7th   **T61.8X1 Toxic effect of other seafood, accidental (unintentional)**

√7th   **T61.8X2 Toxic effect of other seafood, intentional self-harm**

√7th   **T61.8X3 Toxic effect of other seafood, assault**

√7th   **T61.8X4 Toxic effect of other seafood, undetermined**

√5th **T61.9 Toxic effect of unspecified seafood**

√x7th   **T61.91 Toxic effect of unspecified seafood, accidental (unintentional)**

√x7th   **T61.92 Toxic effect of unspecified seafood, intentional self-harm**

√x7th   **T61.93 Toxic effect of unspecified seafood, assault**

√x7th   **T61.94 Toxic effect of unspecified seafood, undetermined**

√4th **T62 Toxic effect of other noxious substances eaten as food**

EXCLUDES 1 *allergic reaction to food, such as:*
anaphylactic shock (reaction) due to adverse food reaction (T78.0-)
dermatitis (L23.6, L25.4, L27.2)
gastroenteritis (noninfective) (K52.2)
bacterial food borne intoxications (A05.-)
toxic effect of aflatoxin and other mycotoxins (T64)
toxic effect of cyanides (T65.0-)
toxic effect of hydrogen cyanide (T57.3-)
toxic effect of mercury (T56.1-)

The appropriate 7th character is to be added to each code from category T62.
A   initial encounter
D   subsequent encounter
S   sequela

√5th **T62.0 Toxic effect of ingested mushrooms**

√6th   **T62.0X Toxic effect of ingested mushrooms**

√7th   **T62.0X1 Toxic effect of ingested mushrooms, accidental (unintentional)**
Toxic effect of ingested mushrooms NOS

√7th   **T62.0X2 Toxic effect of ingested mushrooms, intentional self-harm**

√7th   **T62.0X3 Toxic effect of ingested mushrooms, assault**

√7th   **T62.0X4 Toxic effect of ingested mushrooms, undetermined**

√5th **T62.1 Toxic effect of ingested berries**

√6th   **T62.1X Toxic effect of ingested berries**

√7th   **T62.1X1 Toxic effect of ingested berries, accidental (unintentional)**
Toxic effect of ingested berries NOS

√7th   **T62.1X2 Toxic effect of ingested berries, intentional self-harm**

√7th   **T62.1X3 Toxic effect of ingested berries, assault**

√7th   **T62.1X4 Toxic effect of ingested berries, undetermined**

√5th **T62.2 Toxic effect of other ingested (parts of) plant(s)**

√6th   **T62.2X Toxic effect of other ingested (parts of) plant(s)**

√7th   **T62.2X1 Toxic effect of other ingested (parts of) plant(s), accidental (unintentional)**
Toxic effect of other ingested (parts of) plant(s) NOS

√7th   **T62.2X2 Toxic effect of other ingested (parts of) plant(s), intentional self-harm**

√7th   **T62.2X3 Toxic effect of other ingested (parts of) plant(s), assault**

√7th   **T62.2X4 Toxic effect of other ingested (parts of) plant(s), undetermined**

√5th **T62.8 Toxic effect of other specified noxious substances eaten as food**

√6th   **T62.8X Toxic effect of other specified noxious substances eaten as food**

√7th   **T62.8X1 Toxic effect of other specified noxious substances eaten as food, accidental (unintentional)**
Toxic effect of other specified noxious substances eaten as food NOS

√7th   **T62.8X2 Toxic effect of other specified noxious substances eaten as food, intentional self-harm**

√7th   **T62.8X3 Toxic effect of other specified noxious substances eaten as food, assault**

√7th   **T62.8X4 Toxic effect of other specified noxious substances eaten as food, undetermined**

√5th **T62.9 Toxic effect of unspecified noxious substance eaten as food**

√x7th   **T62.91 Toxic effect of unspecified noxious substance eaten as food, accidental (unintentional)**
Toxic effect of unspecified noxious substance eaten as food NOS

√x7th   **T62.92 Toxic effect of unspecified noxious substance eaten as food, intentional self-harm**

√x7th   **T62.93 Toxic effect of unspecified noxious substance eaten as food, assault**

√x7th   **T62.94 Toxic effect of unspecified noxious substance eaten as food, undetermined**

N Newborn: 0   P Pediatric: 0-17   M Maternity: 12-55   A Adult: 15-124   MCC Major CC Condition   PDxMCC PDx acts as own MCC   CC CC Condition   PDxCC PDx acts as own CC

1124   ICD-10-CM 2016

✓4ᵗʰ **T63 Toxic effect of contact with venomous animals and plants**

> INCLUDES   bite or touch of venomous animal
> pricked or stuck by thorn or leaf
> EXCLUDES 2   *ingestion of toxic animal or plant (T61.-, T62.-)*

> The appropriate 7th character is to be added to each code from category T63.
> A   initial encounter
> D   subsequent encounter
> S   sequela

✓5ᵗʰ **T63.0 Toxic effect of** snake venom

   ✓6ᵗʰ **T63.00 Toxic effect of** unspecified **snake venom**

     ✓7ᵗʰ **T63.001 Toxic effect of unspecified snake venom, accidental (unintentional)**
       Toxic effect of unspecified snake venom NOS

     ✓7ᵗʰ **T63.002 Toxic effect of unspecified snake venom, intentional self-harm**

     ✓7ᵗʰ **T63.003 Toxic effect of unspecified snake venom, assault**

     ✓7ᵗʰ **T63.004 Toxic effect of unspecified snake venom, undetermined**

   ✓6ᵗʰ **T63.01 Toxic effect of** rattlesnake **venom**

     ✓7ᵗʰ **T63.011 Toxic effect of rattlesnake venom, accidental (unintentional)**
       Toxic effect of rattlesnake venom NOS

     ✓7ᵗʰ **T63.012 Toxic effect of rattlesnake venom, intentional self-harm**

     ✓7ᵗʰ **T63.013 Toxic effect of rattlesnake venom,** assault

     ✓7ᵗʰ **T63.014 Toxic effect of rattlesnake venom, undetermined**

   ✓6ᵗʰ **T63.02 Toxic effect of** coral snake **venom**

     ✓7ᵗʰ **T63.021 Toxic effect of coral snake venom, accidental (unintentional)**
       Toxic effect of coral snake venom NOS

     ✓7ᵗʰ **T63.022 Toxic effect of coral snake venom, intentional self-harm**

     ✓7ᵗʰ **T63.023 Toxic effect of coral snake venom,** assault

     ✓7ᵗʰ **T63.024 Toxic effect of coral snake venom, undetermined**

   ✓6ᵗʰ **T63.03 Toxic effect of** taipan **venom**

     ✓7ᵗʰ **T63.031 Toxic effect of taipan venom,** accidental **(unintentional)**
       Toxic effect of taipan venom NOS

     ✓7ᵗʰ **T63.032 Toxic effect of taipan venom,** intentional **self-harm**

     ✓7ᵗʰ **T63.033 Toxic effect of taipan venom,** assault

     ✓7ᵗʰ **T63.034 Toxic effect of taipan venom, undetermined**

   ✓6ᵗʰ **T63.04 Toxic effect of** cobra **venom**

     ✓7ᵗʰ **T63.041 Toxic effect of cobra venom,** accidental **(unintentional)**
       Toxic effect of cobra venom NOS

     ✓7ᵗʰ **T63.042 Toxic effect of cobra venom,** intentional **self-harm**

     ✓7ᵗʰ **T63.043 Toxic effect of cobra venom,** assault

     ✓7ᵗʰ **T63.044 Toxic effect of cobra venom, undetermined**

   ✓6ᵗʰ **T63.06 Toxic effect of venom of** other North and South American snake

     ✓7ᵗʰ **T63.061 Toxic effect of venom of other North and South American snake, accidental (unintentional)**
       Toxic effect of venom of other North and South American snake NOS

     ✓7ᵗʰ **T63.062 Toxic effect of venom of other North and South American snake, intentional self-harm**

     ✓7ᵗʰ **T63.063 Toxic effect of venom of other North and South American snake, assault**

     ✓7ᵗʰ **T63.064 Toxic effect of venom of other North and South American snake, undetermined**

   ✓6ᵗʰ **T63.07 Toxic effect of venom of** other Australian snake

     ✓7ᵗʰ **T63.071 Toxic effect of venom of other Australian snake, accidental (unintentional)**
       Toxic effect of venom of other Australian snake NOS

     ✓7ᵗʰ **T63.072 Toxic effect of venom of other Australian snake, intentional self-harm**

     ✓7ᵗʰ **T63.073 Toxic effect of venom of other Australian snake, assault**

     ✓7ᵗʰ **T63.074 Toxic effect of venom of other Australian snake, undetermined**

   ✓6ᵗʰ **T63.08 Toxic effect of venom of** other African and Asian snake

     ✓7ᵗʰ **T63.081 Toxic effect of venom of other African and Asian snake, accidental (unintentional)**
       Toxic effect of venom of other African and Asian snake NOS

     ✓7ᵗʰ **T63.082 Toxic effect of venom of other African and Asian snake, intentional self-harm**

     ✓7ᵗʰ **T63.083 Toxic effect of venom of other African and Asian snake, assault**

     ✓7ᵗʰ **T63.084 Toxic effect of venom of other African and Asian snake, undetermined**

   ✓6ᵗʰ **T63.09 Toxic effect of venom of** other snake

     ✓7ᵗʰ **T63.091 Toxic effect of venom of other snake, accidental (unintentional)**
       Toxic effect of venom of other snake NOS

     ✓7ᵗʰ **T63.092 Toxic effect of venom of other snake, intentional self-harm**

     ✓7ᵗʰ **T63.093 Toxic effect of venom of other snake, assault**

     ✓7ᵗʰ **T63.094 Toxic effect of venom of other snake, undetermined**

✓5ᵗʰ **T63.1 Toxic effect of venom of** other reptiles

   ✓6ᵗʰ **T63.11 Toxic effect of venom of** gila monster

     ✓7ᵗʰ **T63.111 Toxic effect of venom of gila monster, accidental (unintentional)**
       Toxic effect of venom of gila monster NOS

     ✓7ᵗʰ **T63.112 Toxic effect of venom of gila monster, intentional self-harm**

     ✓7ᵗʰ **T63.113 Toxic effect of venom of gila monster, assault**

     ✓7ᵗʰ **T63.114 Toxic effect of venom of gila monster, undetermined**

   ✓6ᵗʰ **T63.12 Toxic effect of venom of** other venomous lizard

     ✓7ᵗʰ **T63.121 Toxic effect of venom of other venomous lizard, accidental (unintentional)**
       Toxic effect of venom of other venomous lizard NOS

     ✓7ᵗʰ **T63.122 Toxic effect of venom of other venomous lizard, intentional self-harm**

     ✓7ᵗʰ **T63.123 Toxic effect of venom of other venomous lizard, assault**

     ✓7ᵗʰ **T63.124 Toxic effect of venom of other venomous lizard, undetermined**

   ✓6ᵗʰ **T63.19 Toxic effect of venom of** other reptiles

     ✓7ᵗʰ **T63.191 Toxic effect of venom of other reptiles, accidental (unintentional)**
       Toxic effect of venom of other reptiles NOS

     ✓7ᵗʰ **T63.192 Toxic effect of venom of other reptiles, intentional self-harm**

     ✓7ᵗʰ **T63.193 Toxic effect of venom of other reptiles, assault**

     ✓7ᵗʰ **T63.194 Toxic effect of venom of other reptiles, undetermined**

✓5ᵗʰ **T63.2 Toxic effect of venom of** scorpion

   ✓6ᵗʰ **T63.2X Toxic effect of venom of scorpion**

     ✓7ᵗʰ **T63.2X1 Toxic effect of venom of scorpion, accidental (unintentional)**
       Toxic effect of venom of scorpion NOS

     ✓7ᵗʰ **T63.2X2 Toxic effect of venom of scorpion, intentional self-harm**

     ✓7ᵗʰ **T63.2X3 Toxic effect of venom of scorpion,** assault

     ✓7ᵗʰ **T63.2X4 Toxic effect of venom of scorpion, undetermined**

Chapter 19. Injury, Poisoning, and Certain Other Consequences of External Causes

T63–T63.2X4

✓5ᵗʰ **T63.3** Toxic effect of venom of spider

  ✓6ᵗʰ **T63.30** Toxic effect of unspecified spider venom

    ✓7ᵗʰ **T63.301** Toxic effect of unspecified spider venom, accidental (unintentional)

    ✓7ᵗʰ **T63.302** Toxic effect of unspecified spider venom, intentional self-harm

    ✓7ᵗʰ **T63.303** Toxic effect of unspecified spider venom, assault

    ✓7ᵗʰ **T63.304** Toxic effect of unspecified spider venom, undetermined

  ✓6ᵗʰ **T63.31** Toxic effect of venom of black widow spider

    ✓7ᵗʰ **T63.311** Toxic effect of venom of black widow spider, accidental (unintentional)

    ✓7ᵗʰ **T63.312** Toxic effect of venom of black widow spider, intentional self-harm

    ✓7ᵗʰ **T63.313** Toxic effect of venom of black widow spider, assault

    ✓7ᵗʰ **T63.314** Toxic effect of venom of black widow spider, undetermined

  ✓6ᵗʰ **T63.32** Toxic effect of venom of tarantula

    ✓7ᵗʰ **T63.321** Toxic effect of venom of tarantula, accidental (unintentional)

    ✓7ᵗʰ **T63.322** Toxic effect of venom of tarantula, intentional self-harm

    ✓7ᵗʰ **T63.323** Toxic effect of venom of tarantula, assault

    ✓7ᵗʰ **T63.324** Toxic effect of venom of tarantula, undetermined

  ✓6ᵗʰ **T63.33** Toxic effect of venom of brown recluse spider

    ✓7ᵗʰ **T63.331** Toxic effect of venom of brown recluse spider, accidental (unintentional)

    ✓7ᵗʰ **T63.332** Toxic effect of venom of brown recluse spider, intentional self-harm

    ✓7ᵗʰ **T63.333** Toxic effect of venom of brown recluse spider, assault

    ✓7ᵗʰ **T63.334** Toxic effect of venom of brown recluse spider, undetermined

  ✓6ᵗʰ **T63.39** Toxic effect of venom of other spider

    ✓7ᵗʰ **T63.391** Toxic effect of venom of other spider, accidental (unintentional)

    ✓7ᵗʰ **T63.392** Toxic effect of venom of other spider, intentional self-harm

    ✓7ᵗʰ **T63.393** Toxic effect of venom of other spider, assault

    ✓7ᵗʰ **T63.394** Toxic effect of venom of other spider, undetermined

✓5ᵗʰ **T63.4** Toxic effect of venom of other arthropods

  ✓6ᵗʰ **T63.41** Toxic effect of venom of centipedes and venomous millipedes

    ✓7ᵗʰ **T63.411** Toxic effect of venom of centipedes and venomous millipedes, accidental (unintentional)

    ✓7ᵗʰ **T63.412** Toxic effect of venom of centipedes and venomous millipedes, intentional self-harm

    ✓7ᵗʰ **T63.413** Toxic effect of venom of centipedes and venomous millipedes, assault

    ✓7ᵗʰ **T63.414** Toxic effect of venom of centipedes and venomous millipedes, undetermined

  ✓6ᵗʰ **T63.42** Toxic effect of venom of ants

    ✓7ᵗʰ **T63.421** Toxic effect of venom of ants, accidental (unintentional)

    ✓7ᵗʰ **T63.422** Toxic effect of venom of ants, intentional self-harm

    ✓7ᵗʰ **T63.423** Toxic effect of venom of ants, assault

    ✓7ᵗʰ **T63.424** Toxic effect of venom of ants, undetermined

  ✓6ᵗʰ **T63.43** Toxic effect of venom of caterpillars

    ✓7ᵗʰ **T63.431** Toxic effect of venom of caterpillars, accidental (unintentional)

    ✓7ᵗʰ **T63.432** Toxic effect of venom of caterpillars, intentional self-harm

    ✓7ᵗʰ **T63.433** Toxic effect of venom of caterpillars, assault

    ✓7ᵗʰ **T63.434** Toxic effect of venom of caterpillars, undetermined

  ✓6ᵗʰ **T63.44** Toxic effect of venom of bees

    ✓7ᵗʰ **T63.441** Toxic effect of venom of bees, accidental (unintentional)

    ✓7ᵗʰ **T63.442** Toxic effect of venom of bees, intentional self-harm

    ✓7ᵗʰ **T63.443** Toxic effect of venom of bees, assault

    ✓7ᵗʰ **T63.444** Toxic effect of venom of bees, undetermined

  ✓6ᵗʰ **T63.45** Toxic effect of venom of hornets

    ✓7ᵗʰ **T63.451** Toxic effect of venom of hornets, accidental (unintentional)

    ✓7ᵗʰ **T63.452** Toxic effect of venom of hornets, intentional self-harm

    ✓7ᵗʰ **T63.453** Toxic effect of venom of hornets, assault

    ✓7ᵗʰ **T63.454** Toxic effect of venom of hornets, undetermined

  ✓6ᵗʰ **T63.46** Toxic effect of venom of wasps
    Toxic effect of yellow jacket

    ✓7ᵗʰ **T63.461** Toxic effect of venom of wasps, accidental (unintentional)

    ✓7ᵗʰ **T63.462** Toxic effect of venom of wasps, intentional self-harm

    ✓7ᵗʰ **T63.463** Toxic effect of venom of wasps, assault

    ✓7ᵗʰ **T63.464** Toxic effect of venom of wasps, undetermined

  ✓6ᵗʰ **T63.48** Toxic effect of venom of other arthropod

    ✓7ᵗʰ **T63.481** Toxic effect of venom of other arthropod, accidental (unintentional)

    ✓7ᵗʰ **T63.482** Toxic effect of venom of other arthropod, intentional self-harm

    ✓7ᵗʰ **T63.483** Toxic effect of venom of other arthropod, assault

    ✓7ᵗʰ **T63.484** Toxic effect of venom of other arthropod, undetermined

✓5ᵗʰ **T63.5** Toxic effect of contact with venomous fish
  EXCLUDES 2 poisoning by ingestion of fish (T61.-)

  ✓6ᵗʰ **T63.51** Toxic effect of contact with stingray

    ✓7ᵗʰ **T63.511** Toxic effect of contact with stingray, accidental (unintentional)

    ✓7ᵗʰ **T63.512** Toxic effect of contact with stingray, intentional self-harm

    ✓7ᵗʰ **T63.513** Toxic effect of contact with stingray, assault

    ✓7ᵗʰ **T63.514** Toxic effect of contact with stingray, undetermined

  ✓6ᵗʰ **T63.59** Toxic effect of contact with other venomous fish

    ✓7ᵗʰ **T63.591** Toxic effect of contact with other venomous fish, accidental (unintentional)

    ✓7ᵗʰ **T63.592** Toxic effect of contact with other venomous fish, intentional self-harm

    ✓7ᵗʰ **T63.593** Toxic effect of contact with other venomous fish, assault

    ✓7ᵗʰ **T63.594** Toxic effect of contact with other venomous fish, undetermined

✓5ᵗʰ **T63.6** Toxic effect of contact with other venomous marine animals
  EXCLUDES 1 sea-snake venom (T63.09)
  EXCLUDES 2 poisoning by ingestion of shellfish (T61.78-)

  ✓6ᵗʰ **T63.61** Toxic effect of contact with Portugese Man-o-war
    Toxic effect of contact with bluebottle

    ✓7ᵗʰ **T63.611** Toxic effect of contact with Portugese Man-o-war, accidental (unintentional)

    ✓7ᵗʰ **T63.612** Toxic effect of contact with Portugese Man-o-war, intentional self-harm

    ✓7ᵗʰ **T63.613** Toxic effect of contact with Portugese Man-o-war, assault

    ✓7ᵗʰ **T63.614** Toxic effect of contact with Portugese Man-o-war, undetermined

  ✓6ᵗʰ **T63.62** Toxic effect of contact with other jellyfish

    ✓7ᵗʰ **T63.621** Toxic effect of contact with other jellyfish, accidental (unintentional)

    ✓7ᵗʰ **T63.622** Toxic effect of contact with other jellyfish, intentional self-harm

N Newborn: 0 **P** Pediatric: 0-17 **M** Maternity: 12-55 **A** Adult: 15-124 **MCC** Major CC Condition **PDxMCC** PDx acts as own MCC **CC** CC Condition **PDxCC** PDx acts as own CC

1126   ICD-10-CM 2016

√7ᵗʰ **T63.623** **Toxic effect of contact with other jellyfish, assault**

√7ᵗʰ **T63.624** **Toxic effect of contact with other jellyfish, undetermined**

√6ᵗʰ **T63.63** **Toxic effect of contact with sea anemone**

√7ᵗʰ **T63.631** **Toxic effect of contact with sea anemone, accidental (unintentional)**

√7ᵗʰ **T63.632** **Toxic effect of contact with sea anemone, intentional self-harm**

√7ᵗʰ **T63.633** **Toxic effect of contact with sea anemone, assault**

√7ᵗʰ **T63.634** **Toxic effect of contact with sea anemone, undetermined**

√6ᵗʰ **T63.69** **Toxic effect of contact with other venomous marine animals**

√7ᵗʰ **T63.691** **Toxic effect of contact with other venomous marine animals, accidental (unintentional)**

√7ᵗʰ **T63.692** **Toxic effect of contact with other venomous marine animals, intentional self-harm**

√7ᵗʰ **T63.693** **Toxic effect of contact with other venomous marine animals, assault**

√7ᵗʰ **T63.694** **Toxic effect of contact with other venomous marine animals, undetermined**

√5ᵗʰ **T63.7** **Toxic effect of contact with venomous plant**

√6ᵗʰ **T63.71** **Toxic effect of contact with venomous marine plant**

√7ᵗʰ **T63.711** **Toxic effect of contact with venomous marine plant, accidental (unintentional)**

√7ᵗʰ **T63.712** **Toxic effect of contact with venomous marine plant, intentional self-harm**

√7ᵗʰ **T63.713** **Toxic effect of contact with venomous marine plant, assault**

√7ᵗʰ **T63.714** **Toxic effect of contact with venomous marine plant, undetermined**

√6ᵗʰ **T63.79** **Toxic effect of contact with other venomous plant**

√7ᵗʰ **T63.791** **Toxic effect of contact with other venomous plant, accidental (unintentional)**

√7ᵗʰ **T63.792** **Toxic effect of contact with other venomous plant, intentional self-harm**

√7ᵗʰ **T63.793** **Toxic effect of contact with other venomous plant, assault**

√7ᵗʰ **T63.794** **Toxic effect of contact with other venomous plant, undetermined**

√5ᵗʰ **T63.8** **Toxic effect of contact with other venomous animals**

√6ᵗʰ **T63.81** **Toxic effect of contact with venomous frog**

EXCLUDES 1   *contact with nonvenomous frog (W62.0)*

√7ᵗʰ **T63.811** **Toxic effect of contact with venomous frog, accidental (unintentional)**

√7ᵗʰ **T63.812** **Toxic effect of contact with venomous frog, intentional self-harm**

√7ᵗʰ **T63.813** **Toxic effect of contact with venomous frog, assault**

√7ᵗʰ **T63.814** **Toxic effect of contact with venomous frog, undetermined**

√6ᵗʰ **T63.82** **Toxic effect of contact with venomous toad**

EXCLUDES 1   *contact with nonvenomous toad (W62.1)*

√7ᵗʰ **T63.821** **Toxic effect of contact with venomous toad, accidental (unintentional)**

√7ᵗʰ **T63.822** **Toxic effect of contact with venomous toad, intentional self-harm**

√7ᵗʰ **T63.823** **Toxic effect of contact with venomous toad, assault**

√7ᵗʰ **T63.824** **Toxic effect of contact with venomous toad, undetermined**

√6ᵗʰ **T63.83** **Toxic effect of contact with other venomous amphibian**

EXCLUDES 1   *contact with nonvenomous amphibian (W62.9)*

√7ᵗʰ **T63.831** **Toxic effect of contact with other venomous amphibian, accidental (unintentional)**

√7ᵗʰ **T63.832** **Toxic effect of contact with other venomous amphibian, intentional self-harm**

√7ᵗʰ **T63.833** **Toxic effect of contact with other venomous amphibian, assault**

√7ᵗʰ **T63.834** **Toxic effect of contact with other venomous amphibian, undetermined**

√6ᵗʰ **T63.89** **Toxic effect of contact with other venomous animals**

√7ᵗʰ **T63.891** **Toxic effect of contact with other venomous animals, accidental (unintentional)**

√7ᵗʰ **T63.892** **Toxic effect of contact with other venomous animals, intentional self-harm**

√7ᵗʰ **T63.893** **Toxic effect of contact with other venomous animals, assault**

√7ᵗʰ **T63.894** **Toxic effect of contact with other venomous animals, undetermined**

√5ᵗʰ **T63.9** **Toxic effect of contact with unspecified venomous animal**

√x7ᵗʰ **T63.91** **Toxic effect of contact with unspecified venomous animal, accidental (unintentional)**

√x7ᵗʰ **T63.92** **Toxic effect of contact with unspecified venomous animal, intentional self-harm**

√x7ᵗʰ **T63.93** **Toxic effect of contact with unspecified venomous animal, assault**

√x7ᵗʰ **T63.94** **Toxic effect of contact with unspecified venomous animal, undetermined**

√4ᵗʰ **T64** **Toxic effect of aflatoxin and other mycotoxin food contaminants**

> The appropriate 7th character is to be added to each code from category T64.
> A   initial encounter
> D   subsequent encounter
> S   sequela

√5ᵗʰ **T64.0** **Toxic effect of aflatoxin**

√x7ᵗʰ **T64.01** **Toxic effect of aflatoxin, accidental (unintentional)**

√x7ᵗʰ **T64.02** **Toxic effect of aflatoxin, intentional self-harm**

√x7ᵗʰ **T64.03** **Toxic effect of aflatoxin, assault**

√x7ᵗʰ **T64.04** **Toxic effect of aflatoxin, undetermined**

√5ᵗʰ **T64.8** **Toxic effect of other mycotoxin food contaminants**

√x7ᵗʰ **T64.81** **Toxic effect of other mycotoxin food contaminants, accidental (unintentional)**

√x7ᵗʰ **T64.82** **Toxic effect of other mycotoxin food contaminants, intentional self-harm**

√x7ᵗʰ **T64.83** **Toxic effect of other mycotoxin food contaminants, assault**

√x7ᵗʰ **T64.84** **Toxic effect of other mycotoxin food contaminants, undetermined**

√4ᵗʰ **T65** **Toxic effect of other and unspecified substances**

> The appropriate 7th character is to be added to each code from category T65.
> A   initial encounter
> D   subsequent encounter
> S   sequela

√5ᵗʰ **T65.0** **Toxic effect of cyanides**

EXCLUDES 1   *hydrogen cyanide (T57.3-)*

√6ᵗʰ **T65.0X** **Toxic effect of cyanides**

√7ᵗʰ **T65.0X1** **Toxic effect of cyanides, accidental (unintentional)**
Toxic effect of cyanides NOS

√7ᵗʰ **T65.0X2** **Toxic effect of cyanides, intentional self-harm**

√7ᵗʰ **T65.0X3** **Toxic effect of cyanides, assault**

√7ᵗʰ **T65.0X4** **Toxic effect of cyanides, undetermined**

√5ᵗʰ **T65.1** **Toxic effect of strychnine and its salts**

√6ᵗʰ **T65.1X** **Toxic effect of strychnine and its salts**

√7ᵗʰ **T65.1X1** **Toxic effect of strychnine and its salts, accidental (unintentional)**
Toxic effect of strychnine and its salts NOS

√7ᵗʰ **T65.1X2** **Toxic effect of strychnine and its salts, intentional self-harm**

√7ᵗʰ **T65.1X3** **Toxic effect of strychnine and its salts, assault**

✔ Additional Character Required   √x7ᵗʰ Placeholder Alert   Unacceptable PDx   Manifestation   Hospital Acquired Condition   EXCLUDES 1 Not Coded Here   EXCLUDES 2 Not Included Here

☑7ᵗʰ **T65.1X4** **Toxic effect of strychnine and its salts,** **undetermined**

☑5ᵗʰ **T65.2** **Toxic effect of tobacco and nicotine**

EXCLUDES 2 *nicotine dependence (F17.-)*

☑6ᵗʰ **T65.21** **Toxic effect of chewing tobacco**

☑7ᵗʰ **T65.211** **Toxic effect of chewing tobacco,** **accidental (unintentional)**
Toxic effect of chewing tobacco NOS

☑7ᵗʰ **T65.212** **Toxic effect of chewing tobacco,** **intentional self-harm**

☑7ᵗʰ **T65.213** **Toxic effect of chewing tobacco, assault**

☑7ᵗʰ **T65.214** **Toxic effect of chewing tobacco,** **undetermined**

☑6ᵗʰ **T65.22** **Toxic effect of tobacco cigarettes**
Toxic effect of tobacco smoke
Use additional code for exposure to second hand tobacco smoke (Z57.31, Z77.22)

☑7ᵗʰ **T65.221** **Toxic effect of tobacco cigarettes,** **accidental (unintentional)**
Toxic effect of tobacco cigarettes NOS

☑7ᵗʰ **T65.222** **Toxic effect of tobacco cigarettes,** **intentional self-harm**

☑7ᵗʰ **T65.223** **Toxic effect of tobacco cigarettes, assault**

☑7ᵗʰ **T65.224** **Toxic effect of tobacco cigarettes,** **undetermined**

☑6ᵗʰ **T65.29** **Toxic effect of other tobacco and nicotine**

☑7ᵗʰ **T65.291** **Toxic effect of other tobacco and nicotine,** **accidental (unintentional)**
Toxic effect of other tobacco and nicotine NOS

☑7ᵗʰ **T65.292** **Toxic effect of other tobacco and nicotine,** **intentional self-harm**

☑7ᵗʰ **T65.293** **Toxic effect of other tobacco and nicotine,** **assault**

☑7ᵗʰ **T65.294** **Toxic effect of other tobacco and nicotine,** **undetermined**

☑5ᵗʰ **T65.3** **Toxic effect of nitroderivatives and aminoderivatives of benzene and its homologues**
Toxic effect of anilin [benzenamine]
Toxic effect of nitrobenzene
Toxic effect of trinitrotoluene

☑6ᵗʰ **T65.3X** **Toxic effect of nitroderivatives and aminoderivatives of benzene and its homologues**

☑7ᵗʰ **T65.3X1** **Toxic effect of nitroderivatives and aminoderivatives of benzene and its homologues, accidental (unintentional)**
Toxic effect of nitroderivatives and aminoderivatives of benzene and its homologues NOS

☑7ᵗʰ **T65.3X2** **Toxic effect of nitroderivatives and aminoderivatives of benzene and its homologues, intentional self-harm**

☑7ᵗʰ **T65.3X3** **Toxic effect of nitroderivatives and aminoderivatives of benzene and its homologues, assault**

☑7ᵗʰ **T65.3X4** **Toxic effect of nitroderivatives and aminoderivatives of benzene and its homologues, undetermined**

☑5ᵗʰ **T65.4** **Toxic effect of carbon disulfide**

☑6ᵗʰ **T65.4X** **Toxic effect of carbon disulfide**

☑7ᵗʰ **T65.4X1** **Toxic effect of carbon disulfide, accidental (unintentional)**
Toxic effect of carbon disulfide NOS

☑7ᵗʰ **T65.4X2** **Toxic effect of carbon disulfide,** **intentional self-harm**

☑7ᵗʰ **T65.4X3** **Toxic effect of carbon disulfide, assault**

☑7ᵗʰ **T65.4X4** **Toxic effect of carbon disulfide,** **undetermined**

☑5ᵗʰ **T65.5** **Toxic effect of nitroglycerin and other nitric acids and esters**
Toxic effect of 1,2,3-Propanetriol trinitrate

☑6ᵗʰ **T65.5X** **Toxic effect of nitroglycerin and other nitric acids and esters**

☑7ᵗʰ **T65.5X1** **Toxic effect of nitroglycerin and other nitric acids and esters, accidental (unintentional)**
Toxic effect of nitroglycerin and other nitric acids and esters NOS

☑7ᵗʰ **T65.5X2** **Toxic effect of nitroglycerin and other nitric acids and esters, intentional self-harm**

☑7ᵗʰ **T65.5X3** **Toxic effect of nitroglycerin and other nitric acids and esters, assault**

☑7ᵗʰ **T65.5X4** **Toxic effect of nitroglycerin and other nitric acids and esters, undetermined**

☑5ᵗʰ **T65.6** **Toxic effect of paints and dyes, not elsewhere classified**

☑6ᵗʰ **T65.6X** **Toxic effect of paints and dyes, not elsewhere classified**

☑7ᵗʰ **T65.6X1** **Toxic effect of paints and dyes, not elsewhere classified, accidental (unintentional)**
Toxic effect of paints and dyes NOS

☑7ᵗʰ **T65.6X2** **Toxic effect of paints and dyes, not elsewhere classified, intentional self-harm**

☑7ᵗʰ **T65.6X3** **Toxic effect of paints and dyes, not elsewhere classified, assault**

☑7ᵗʰ **T65.6X4** **Toxic effect of paints and dyes, not elsewhere classified, undetermined**

☑5ᵗʰ **T65.8** **Toxic effect of other specified substances**

☑6ᵗʰ **T65.81** **Toxic effect of latex**

☑7ᵗʰ **T65.811** **Toxic effect of latex, accidental (unintentional)**
Toxic effect of latex NOS

☑7ᵗʰ **T65.812** **Toxic effect of latex, intentional self-harm**

☑7ᵗʰ **T65.813** **Toxic effect of latex, assault**

☑7ᵗʰ **T65.814** **Toxic effect of latex, undetermined**

☑6ᵗʰ **T65.82** **Toxic effect of harmful algae and algae toxins**
Toxic effect of (harmful) algae bloom NOS
Toxic effect of blue-green algae bloom
Toxic effect of brown tide
Toxic effect of cyanobacteria bloom
Toxic effect of Florida red tide
Toxic effect of pfiesteria piscicida
Toxic effect of red tide

☑7ᵗʰ **T65.821** **Toxic effect of harmful algae and algae toxins, accidental (unintentional)**
Toxic effect of harmful algae and algae toxins NOS

☑7ᵗʰ **T65.822** **Toxic effect of harmful algae and algae toxins, intentional self-harm**

☑7ᵗʰ **T65.823** **Toxic effect of harmful algae and algae toxins, assault**

☑7ᵗʰ **T65.824** **Toxic effect of harmful algae and algae toxins, undetermined**

☑6ᵗʰ **T65.83** **Toxic effect of fiberglass**

☑7ᵗʰ **T65.831** **Toxic effect of fiberglass, accidental (unintentional)**
Toxic effect of fiberglass NOS

☑7ᵗʰ **T65.832** **Toxic effect of fiberglass, intentional self-harm**

☑7ᵗʰ **T65.833** **Toxic effect of fiberglass, assault**

☑7ᵗʰ **T65.834** **Toxic effect of fiberglass, undetermined**

☑6ᵗʰ **T65.89** **Toxic effect of other specified substances**

☑7ᵗʰ **T65.891** **Toxic effect of other specified substances, accidental (unintentional)**
Toxic effect of other specified substances NOS

☑7ᵗʰ **T65.892** **Toxic effect of other specified substances, intentional self-harm**

☑7ᵗʰ **T65.893** **Toxic effect of other specified substances, assault**

☑7ᵗʰ **T65.894** **Toxic effect of other specified substances, undetermined**

☑5ᵗʰ **T65.9** **Toxic effect of unspecified substance**

☑x7ᵗʰ **T65.91** **Toxic effect of unspecified substance, accidental (unintentional)**
Poisoning NOS

☑x7ᵗʰ **T65.92** **Toxic effect of unspecified substance, intentional self-harm**

☑x7ᵗʰ **T65.93** **Toxic effect of unspecified substance, assault**

☑x7ᵗʰ **T65.94** **Toxic effect of unspecified substance, undetermined**

Ⓝ Newborn: 0   Ⓟ Pediatric: 0-17   Ⓜ Maternity: 12-55   Ⓐ Adult: 15-124   MCC Major CC Condition   PDxMCC PDx acts as own MCC   CC CC Condition   PDxCC PDx acts as own CC

1128   ICD-10-CM 2016

Other and unspecified effects of external causes (T66-T78)

✓7ᵗʰ T66 Radiation sickness, unspecified

EXCLUDES 1   specified adverse effects of radiation, such as:
     burns (T20-T31)
     leukemia (C91-C95)
     radiation gastroenteritis and colitis (K52.0)
     radiation pneumonitis (J70.0)
     radiation related disorders of the skin and subcutaneous tissue
       (L55-L59)
     radiation sunburn (L55.-)

The appropriate 7th character is to be added to code T66.
   A   initial encounter
   D   subsequent encounter
   S   sequela

✓4ᵗʰ T67 Effects of heat and light

EXCLUDES 1   erythema [dermatitis] ab igne (L59.0)
     malignant hyperpyrexia due to anesthesia (T88.3)
     radiation-related disorders of the skin and subcutaneous tissue
       (L55-L59)
EXCLUDES 2   burns (T20-T31)
     sunburn (L55.-)
     sweat disorder due to heat (L74-L75)

The appropriate 7th character is to be added to each code from
category T67.
   A   initial encounter
   D   subsequent encounter
   S   sequela

7   ✓7ᵗʰ **T67.0 Heatstroke and sunstroke**   CC
     Heat apoplexy   Siriasis
     Heat pyrexia   Thermoplegia
     Use additional code(s) to identify any associated complications
       of heatstroke, such as:
       coma and stupor (R40.-)
       systemic inflammatory response syndrome (R65.1-)
     CC Excl: CC with 7th character A:T67.[0-9]XXA

✓7ᵗʰ **T67.1 Heat syncope**
     Heat collapse

✓7ᵗʰ **T67.2 Heat cramp**

✓7ᵗʰ **T67.3 Heat exhaustion, anhydrotic**
     Heat prostration due to water depletion
     EXCLUDES 1   heat exhaustion due to salt depletion (T67.4)

✓7ᵗʰ **T67.4 Heat exhaustion due to salt depletion**
     Heat prostration due to salt (and water) depletion

✓7ᵗʰ **T67.5 Heat exhaustion, unspecified**
     Heat prostration NOS

✓7ᵗʰ **T67.6 Heat fatigue, transient**

✓7ᵗʰ **T67.7 Heat edema**

✓7ᵗʰ **T67.8 Other effects of heat and light**

✓7ᵗʰ **T67.9 Effect of heat and light, unspecified**

✓7ᵗʰ T68 Hypothermia

Accidental hypothermia
Hypothermia NOS
Use additional code to identify source of exposure:
   exposure to excessive cold of man-made origin (W93)
   exposure to excessive cold of natural origin (X31)
EXCLUDES 1   hypothermia following anesthesia (T88.51)
     hypothermia not associated with low environmental
       temperature (R68.0)
     hypothermia of newborn (P80.-)
EXCLUDES 2   frostbite (T33-T34)

The appropriate 7th character is to be added to code T68.
   A   initial encounter
   D   subsequent encounter
   S   sequela

✓4ᵗʰ T69 Other effects of reduced temperature

Use additional code to identify source of exposure:
   exposure to excessive cold of man-made origin (W93)
   exposure to excessive cold of natural origin (X31)
EXCLUDES 2   frostbite (T33-T34)

The appropriate 7th character is to be added to each code from
category T69.
   A   initial encounter
   D   subsequent encounter
   S   sequela

✓5ᵗʰ **T69.0 Immersion hand and foot**

     ✓6ᵗʰ **T69.01 Immersion hand**

         ✓7ᵗʰ **T69.011 Immersion hand, right hand**

         ✓7ᵗʰ **T69.012 Immersion hand, left hand**

         ✓7ᵗʰ **T69.019 Immersion hand, unspecified hand**

     ✓6ᵗʰ **T69.02 Immersion foot**
         Trench foot

         **CC Excl: For CC codes in subcategory T69.02: CC
         with 7th character A, unless otherwise noted:**
         T33.2XX-T33.42X with 7th A, T33.60X-T33.72X with
         7th A, T33.90X-T33.99X with 7th A, T34.2XX-
         T34.42X with 7th A, T34.60X-T34.72X with 7th A,
         T34.90X-T34.99X with 7th A, T69.021-T69.029 with
         7th A

    7   ✓7ᵖ **T69.021 Immersion foot, right foot**   CC

    7   ✓7ᵖ **T69.022 Immersion foot, left foot**   CC

    7   ✓7ᵖ **T69.029 Immersion foot, unspecified foot**   CC

✓7ᵗʰ **T69.1 Chilblains**

✓7ᵗʰ **T69.8 Other specified effects of reduced temperature**

✓7ᵗʰ **T69.9 Effect of reduced temperature, unspecified**

✓4ᵗʰ T70 Effects of air pressure and water pressure

The appropriate 7th character is to be added to each code from
category T70.
   A   initial encounter
   D   subsequent encounter
   S   sequela

✓7ᵗʰ **T70.0 Otitic barotrauma**
     Aero-otitis media
     Effects of change in ambient atmospheric pressure or water
       pressure on ears

✓7ᵗʰ **T70.1 Sinus barotrauma**
     Aerosinusitis
     Effects of change in ambient atmospheric pressure on sinuses

✓5ᵗʰ **T70.2 Other and unspecified effects of high altitude**
     EXCLUDES 2   polycythemia due to high altitude (D75.1)

     ✓7ᵗʰ **T70.20 Unspecified effects of high altitude**

     ✓7ᵗʰ **T70.29 Other effects of high altitude**
         Alpine sickness
         Anoxia due to high altitude
         Barotrauma NOS
         Hypobaropathy
         Mountain sickness

7   ✓7ᵗʰ **T70.3 Caisson disease [decompression sickness]**   CC
     Compressed-air disease   Diver's palsy or paralysis
     CC Excl: CC with 7th character A:T70.3XX-T70.9XX with 7th A

✓7ᵗʰ **T70.4 Effects of high-pressure fluids**
     Hydraulic jet injection (industrial)
     Pneumatic jet injection (industrial)
     Traumatic jet injection (industrial)

✓7ᵗʰ **T70.8 Other effects of air pressure and water pressure**

✓7ᵗʰ **T70.9 Effect of air pressure and water pressure, unspecified**

---

7   HAC = Initial encounter only (7th character A, B or C) and not POA.

✓ Additional Character Required   ✓7ᵗʰ Placeholder Alert   Unacceptable PDx   Manifestation   Hospital Acquired Condition   EXCLUDES 1 Not Coded Here   EXCLUDES 2 Not Included Here

✓4th T71   Asphyxiation

Mechanical suffocation   Traumatic suffocation

EXCLUDES 1 *acute respiratory distress (syndrome) (J80)*
anoxia due to high altitude (T70.2)
asphyxia NOS (R09.01)
asphyxia from carbon monoxide (T58.-)
asphyxia from inhalation of food or foreign body (T17.-)
asphyxia from other gases, fumes and vapors (T59.-)
respiratory distress (syndrome) in newborn (P22.-)

The appropriate 7th character is to be added to each code from category T71.
A   initial encounter
D   subsequent encounter
S   sequela

CC Excl: For CC codes in category T71: CC with 7th character A, unless otherwise noted: T71.111-T71.9XX with 7th A

✓5th T71.1   Asphyxiation due to mechanical threat to breathing
Suffocation due to mechanical threat to breathing

✓6th   T71.11   Asphyxiation due to smothering under pillow
7 ✓7th **T71.111   Asphyxiation due to smothering under pillow, accidental**   CC
Asphyxiation due to smothering under pillow NOS

7 ✓7th **T71.112   Asphyxiation due to smothering under pillow, intentional self-harm**   CC

7 ✓7th **T71.113   Asphyxiation due to smothering under pillow, assault**   CC

7 ✓7th **T71.114   Asphyxiation due to smothering under pillow, undetermined**   CC

✓6th   T71.12   Asphyxiation due to plastic bag
7 ✓7th **T71.121   Asphyxiation due to plastic bag, accidental**   CC
Asphyxiation due to plastic bag NOS

7 ✓7th **T71.122   Asphyxiation due to plastic bag, intentional self-harm**   CC

7 ✓7th **T71.123   Asphyxiation due to plastic bag, assault**   CC

7 ✓7th **T71.124   Asphyxiation due to plastic bag, undetermined**   CC

✓6th   T71.13   Asphyxiation due to being trapped in bed linens
7 ✓7th **T71.131   Asphyxiation due to being trapped in bed linens, accidental**   CC
Asphyxiation due to being trapped in bed linens NOS

7 ✓7th **T71.132   Asphyxiation due to being trapped in bed linens, intentional self-harm**   CC

7 ✓7th **T71.133   Asphyxiation due to being trapped in bed linens, assault**   CC

7 ✓7th **T71.134   Asphyxiation due to being trapped in bed linens, undetermined**   CC

✓6th   T71.14   Asphyxiation due to smothering under another person's body (in bed)
7 ✓7th **T71.141   Asphyxiation due to smothering under another person's body (in bed), accidental**   CC
Asphyxiation due to smothering under another person's body (in bed) NOS

7 ✓7th **T71.143   Asphyxiation due to smothering under another person's body (in bed), assault**   CC

7 ✓7th **T71.144   Asphyxiation due to smothering under another person's body (in bed), undetermined**   CC

✓6th   T71.15   Asphyxiation due to smothering in furniture
7 ✓7th **T71.151   Asphyxiation due to smothering in furniture, accidental**   CC
Asphyxiation due to smothering in furniture NOS

7 ✓7th **T71.152   Asphyxiation due to smothering in furniture, intentional self-harm**   CC

7 ✓7th **T71.153   Asphyxiation due to smothering in furniture, assault**   CC

7 ✓7th **T71.154   Asphyxiation due to smothering in furniture, undetermined**   CC

✓6th   T71.16   Asphyxiation due to hanging
Hanging by window shade cord
Use additional code for any associated injuries, such as:
crushing injury of neck (S17.-)
fracture of cervical vertebrae (S12.0-S12.2-)
open wound of neck (S11.-)

7 ✓7th **T71.161   Asphyxiation due to hanging, accidental**   CC
Asphyxiation due to hanging NOS
Hanging NOS

7 ✓7th **T71.162   Asphyxiation due to hanging, intentional self-harm**   CC

7 ✓7th **T71.163   Asphyxiation due to hanging, assault**   CC

7 ✓7th **T71.164   Asphyxiation due to hanging, undetermined**   CC

✓6th   T71.19   Asphyxiation due to mechanical threat to breathing due to other causes
7 ✓7th **T71.191   Asphyxiation due to mechanical threat to breathing due to other causes, accidental**   CC
Asphyxiation due to other causes NOS

7 ✓7th **T71.192   Asphyxiation due to mechanical threat to breathing due to other causes, intentional self-harm**   CC

7 ✓7th **T71.193   Asphyxiation due to mechanical threat to breathing due to other causes, assault**   CC

7 ✓7th **T71.194   Asphyxiation due to mechanical threat to breathing due to other causes, undetermined**   CC

✓5th T71.2   Asphyxiation due to systemic oxygen deficiency due to low oxygen content in ambient air
Suffocation due to systemic oxygen deficiency due to low oxygen content in ambient air

7 ✓x7th **T71.20   Asphyxiation due to systemic oxygen deficiency due to low oxygen content in ambient air due to unspecified cause**   CC

7 ✓x7th **T71.21   Asphyxiation due to cave-in or falling earth**   CC
Use additional code for any associated cataclysm (X34-X38)

✓6th   T71.22   Asphyxiation due to being trapped in a car trunk
✓7th **T71.221   Asphyxiation due to being trapped in a car trunk, accidental**   CC

✓7th **T71.222   Asphyxiation due to being trapped in a car trunk, intentional self-harm**   CC

✓7th **T71.223   Asphyxiation due to being trapped in a car trunk, assault**   CC

✓7th **T71.224   Asphyxiation due to being trapped in a car trunk, undetermined**   CC

✓6th   T71.23   Asphyxiation due to being trapped in a (discarded) refrigerator
✓7th **T71.231   Asphyxiation due to being trapped in a (discarded) refrigerator, accidental**   CC

✓7th **T71.232   Asphyxiation due to being trapped in a (discarded) refrigerator, intentional self-harm**   CC

✓7th **T71.233   Asphyxiation due to being trapped in a (discarded) refrigerator, assault**   CC

✓7th **T71.234   Asphyxiation due to being trapped in a (discarded) refrigerator, undetermined**   CC

7 ✓x7th **T71.29   Asphyxiation due to being trapped in other low oxygen environment**   CC

7 ✓x7th **T71.9   Asphyxiation due to unspecified cause**   CC
Suffocation (by strangulation) due to unspecified cause
Suffocation NOS
Systemic oxygen deficiency due to low oxygen content in ambient air due to unspecified cause
Systemic oxygen deficiency due to mechanical threat to breathing due to unspecified cause
Traumatic asphyxia NOS

---

7 HAC = Initial encounter only (7th character A, B or C) and not POA.

Ⓝ Newborn: 0   Ⓟ Pediatric: 0-17   Ⓜ Maternity: 12-55   Ⓐ Adult: 15-124   **MCC** Major CC Condition   **PDxMCC** PDx acts as own MCC   **CC** CC Condition   **PDxCC** PDx acts as own CC

1130   ICD-10-CM 2016

☑4ᵗʰ **T73** **Effects of other deprivation**

> The appropriate 7th character is to be added to each code from category T73.
> A　initial encounter
> D　subsequent encounter
> S　sequela

√x7ᵗʰ **T73.0** **Starvation**
Deprivation of food

√x7ᵗʰ **T73.1** **Deprivation of water**

√x7ᵗʰ **T73.2** **Exhaustion due to exposure**

√x7ᵗʰ **T73.3** **Exhaustion due to excessive exertion**
Exhaustion due to overexertion

√x7ᵗʰ **T73.8** **Other effects of deprivation**

√x7ᵗʰ **T73.9** **Effect of deprivation, unspecified**

☑4ᵗʰ **T74** **Adult and child abuse, neglect and other maltreatment, confirmed**

> Use additional code, if applicable, to identify any associated current injury
> Use additional external cause code to identify perpetrator, if known (Y07.-)
> *EXCLUDES1* abuse and maltreatment in pregnancy (O9A.3-, O9A.4-, O9A.5-)
> adult and child maltreatment, suspected (T76.-)

> The appropriate 7th character is to be added to each code from category T74.
> A　initial encounter
> D　subsequent encounter
> S　sequela

> **CC Excl: For CC codes in category T74: CC with 7th character A, unless otherwise noted:** T74.01X-T74.92X with 7th A, T76.01X-T76.92X with 7th A

√5ᵗʰ **T74.0** **Neglect or abandonment, confirmed**

√x7ᵗʰ **T74.01** **Adult neglect or abandonment, confirmed** CC A

√x7ᵗʰ **T74.02** **Child neglect or abandonment, confirmed** CC P

√5ᵗʰ **T74.1** **Physical abuse, confirmed**
EXCLUDES2 sexual abuse (T74.2-)

√x7ᵗʰ **T74.11** **Adult physical abuse, confirmed** CC A

√x7ᵗʰ **T74.12** **Child physical abuse, confirmed** CC P
EXCLUDES2 shaken infant syndrome (T74.4)

√5ᵗʰ **T74.2** **Sexual abuse, confirmed**
Rape, confirmed　　　Sexual assault, confirmed

√x7ᵗʰ **T74.21** **Adult sexual abuse, confirmed** CC A

√x7ᵗʰ **T74.22** **Child sexual abuse, confirmed** CC P

√5ᵗʰ **T74.3** **Psychological abuse, confirmed**

√x7ᵗʰ **T74.31** **Adult psychological abuse, confirmed** A

√x7ᵗʰ **T74.32** **Child psychological abuse, confirmed** CC P

√x7ᵗʰ **T74.4** **Shaken infant syndrome** CC P

√5ᵗʰ **T74.9** **Unspecified maltreatment, confirmed**

√x7ᵗʰ **T74.91** **Unspecified adult maltreatment, confirmed** CC A
CC Excl: CC with 7th character A: T74.91X A, T76.91XA

√x7ᵗʰ **T74.92** **Unspecified child maltreatment, confirmed** CC P
CC Excl: CC with 7th character A: T74.01X-T74.92X with 7th A, T76.01X-T76.92X with 7th A

☑4ᵗʰ **T75** **Other and unspecified effects of other external causes**
EXCLUDES1 adverse effects NEC (T78.-)
EXCLUDES2 burns (electric) (T20-T31)

> The appropriate 7th character is to be added to each code from category T75.
> A　initial encounter
> D　subsequent encounter
> S　sequela

√5ᵗʰ **T75.0** **Effects of lightning**
Struck by lightning

√x7ᵗʰ **T75.00** **Unspecified effects of lightning**
Struck by lightning NOS

√x7ᵗʰ **T75.01** **Shock due to being struck by lightning**

√x7ᵗʰ **T75.09** **Other effects of lightning**
Use additional code for other effects of lightning

---

[7] √x7ᵗʰ **T75.1** **Unspecified effects of drowning and nonfatal submersion** CC
Immersion
EXCLUDES1 specified effects of drowning—code to effects
CC Excl: CC with 7th character A: T75.1XXA

√5ᵗʰ **T75.2** **Effects of vibration**

√x7ᵗʰ **T75.20** **Unspecified effects of vibration**

√x7ᵗʰ **T75.21** **Pneumatic hammer syndrome**

√x7ᵗʰ **T75.22** **Traumatic vasospastic syndrome**

√x7ᵗʰ **T75.23** **Vertigo from infrasound**
EXCLUDES1 vertigo NOS (R42)

T75.29 **Other effects of vibration**

√5ᵗʰ **T75.3** **Motion sickness**
Airsickness　　　Travel sickness
Seasickness
Use additional external cause code to identify vehicle or type of motion (Y92.81-, Y93.5-)

√x7ᵗʰ **T75.4** **Electrocution**
Shock from electric current
Shock from electroshock gun (taser)

√5ᵗʰ **T75.8** **Other specified effects of external causes**

√x7ᵗʰ **T75.81** **Effects of abnormal gravitation [G] forces**

√x7ᵗʰ **T75.82** **Effects of weightlessness**

√x7ᵗʰ **T75.89** **Other specified effects of external causes**

☑4ᵗʰ **T76** **Adult and child abuse, neglect and other maltreatment, suspected**

> Use additional code, if applicable, to identify any associated current injury
> *EXCLUDES1* adult and child maltreatment, confirmed (T74.-)
> suspected abuse and maltreatment in pregnancy (O9A.3-, O9A.4-, O9A.5-)
> suspected adult physical and sexual abuse, ruled out (Z04.71)
> suspected adult sexual abused, ruled out (Z04.41)
> suspected child physical abuse, ruled out (Z04.72)
> suspected child sexual abuse, ruled out (Z04.42)

> The appropriate 7th character is to be added to each code from category T76.
> A　initial encounter
> D　subsequent encounter
> S　sequela

> **CC Excl: For CC codes in category T76: CC with 7th character A, unless otherwise noted:** T74.01X-T74.92X with 7th A, T76.01X-T76.92X with 7th A

√5ᵗʰ **T76.0** **Neglect or abandonment, suspected**

√x7ᵗʰ **T76.01** **Adult neglect or abandonment, suspected** CC A

√x7ᵗʰ **T76.02** **Child neglect or abandonment, suspected** CC P

√5ᵗʰ **T76.1** **Physical abuse, suspected**

√x7ᵗʰ **T76.11** **Adult physical abuse, suspected** CC A

√x7ᵗʰ **T76.12** **Child physical abuse, suspected** CC P

√5ᵗʰ **T76.2** **Sexual abuse, suspected**
Rape, suspected　　　Sexual abuse, suspected
EXCLUDES1 alleged abuse, ruled out (Z04.7)

√x7ᵗʰ **T76.21** **Adult sexual abuse, suspected** CC A

√x7ᵗʰ **T76.22** **Child sexual abuse, suspected** CC P

√5ᵗʰ **T76.3** **Psychological abuse, suspected**

√x7ᵗʰ **T76.31** **Adult psychological abuse, suspected** A

√x7ᵗʰ **T76.32** **Child psychological abuse, suspected** CC P

√5ᵗʰ **T76.9** **Unspecified maltreatment, suspected**

√x7ᵗʰ **T76.91** **Unspecified adult maltreatment, suspected** CC A
CC Excl: CC with 7th character A: T74.91XA, T76.91XA

√x7ᵗʰ **T76.92** **Unspecified child maltreatment, suspected** CC P
CC Excl: CC with 7th character A: T74.01-T74.92 with 7th A, T76.01-T76.92 with 7th A

---

[7] HAC = Initial encounter only (7th character A, B or C) and not POA.

☑ Additional Character Required　√x7ᵗʰ Placeholder Alert　Unacceptable PDx　Manifestation　Hospital Acquired Condition　*EXCLUDES1* Not Coded Here　*EXCLUDES2* Not Included Here

Chapter 19. Injury, Poisoning, and Certain Other Consequences of External Causes

T78 Adverse effects, not elsewhere classified
EXCLUDES 2   complications of surgical and medical care NEC (T80-T88)

The appropriate 7th character is to be added to each code from category T78.
A   initial encounter
D   subsequent encounter
S   sequela

CC Excl: For CC codes in category T78: CC with 7th character A, unless otherwise noted: T78.00X-T78.09X with 7th A

✓5ᵗʰ T78.0 Anaphylactic reaction due to food
Anaphylactic reaction due to adverse food reaction
Anaphylactic shock or reaction due to nonpoisonous foods
Anaphylactoid reaction due to food

- ✓x7ᵗʰ **T78.00** Anaphylactic reaction due to **unspecified food** CC
- ✓x7ᵗʰ **T78.01** Anaphylactic reaction due to **peanuts** CC
- ✓x7ᵗʰ **T78.02** Anaphylactic reaction due to **shellfish (crustaceans)** CC
- ✓x7ᵗʰ **T78.03** Anaphylactic reaction due to **other fish** CC
- ✓x7ᵗʰ **T78.04** Anaphylactic reaction due to **fruits and vegetables** CC
- ✓x7ᵗʰ **T78.05** Anaphylactic reaction due to **tree nuts and seeds** CC
  - EXCLUDES 1   anaphylactic reaction due to peanuts (T78.01)
- ✓x7ᵗʰ **T78.06** Anaphylactic reaction due to **food additives** CC
- ✓x7ᵗʰ **T78.07** Anaphylactic reaction due to **milk and dairy products** CC
- ✓x7ᵗʰ **T78.08** Anaphylactic reaction due to **eggs** CC
- ✓x7ᵗʰ **T78.09** Anaphylactic reaction due to **other food products** CC

✓x7ᵗʰ T78.1 Other adverse food reactions, not elsewhere classified
Use additional code to identify the type of reaction
EXCLUDES 1   anaphylactic reaction or shock due to adverse food reaction (T78.0-)
anaphylactic reaction due to food (T78.0-)
bacterial food borne intoxications (A05.-)
EXCLUDES 2   allergic and dietetic gastroenteritis and colitis (K52.2)
allergic rhinitis due to food (J30.5)
dermatitis due to food in contact with skin (L23.6, L24.6, L25.4)
dermatitis due to ingested food (L27.2)

✓x7ᵗʰ T78.2 Anaphylactic shock, unspecified CC
Allergic shock   Anaphylaxis
Anaphylactic reaction
EXCLUDES 1   anaphylactic reaction or shock due to adverse effect of correct medicinal substance properly administered (T88.6)
anaphylactic reaction or shock due to adverse food reaction (T78.0-)
anaphylactic reaction or shock due to serum (T80.5-)

✓x7ᵗʰ T78.3 Angioneurotic edema
Allergic angioedema   Quincke's edema
Giant urticaria
EXCLUDES 1   serum urticaria (T80.6-)
urticaria (L50.-)

✓5ᵗʰ T78.4 Other and unspecified allergy
EXCLUDES 1   specified types of allergic reaction such as:
allergic diarrhea (K52.2)
allergic gastroenteritis and colitis (K52.2)
dermatitis (L23-L25, L27.-)
hay fever (J30.1)

- ✓x7ᵗʰ **T78.40** Allergy, unspecified
  Allergic reaction NOS   Hypersensitivity NOS
- ✓x7ᵗʰ **T78.41** Arthus phenomenon
  Arthus reaction
- ✓x7ᵗʰ **T78.49** Other allergy

✓x7ᵗʰ T78.8 Other adverse effects, not elsewhere classified

Certain early complications of trauma (T79)

✓4ᵗʰ T79 Certain early complications of trauma, not elsewhere classified
EXCLUDES 2   acute respiratory distress syndrome (J80)
complications occurring during or following medical procedures (T80-T88)
complications of surgical and medical care NEC (T80-T88)
newborn respiratory distress syndrome (P22.0)

The appropriate 7th character is to be added to each code from category T79.
A   initial encounter
D   subsequent encounter
S   sequela

✓x7ᵗʰ T79.0 Air embolism (traumatic) MCC
EXCLUDES 1   air embolism complicating abortion or ectopic or molar pregnancy (O00-O07, O08.2)
air embolism complicating pregnancy, childbirth and the puerperium (O88.0)
air embolism following infusion, transfusion, and therapeutic injection (T80.0)
air embolism following procedure NEC (T81.7-)
CC Excl: MCC with 7th A: D78.81-D78.89, E36.8, E89.810-E89.89, H59.011-H59.019, H59.031-H59.099, H59.811-H59.89, H95.811-H95.89, I97.3, L76.81-L76.82, M96.89, N98.1-N98.9, T14.90-T14.91, T79.0XXA, T79.A0X-T80.0XX with 7th A, T81.82XA, T81.89X-T81.9XX with 7th A

✓x7ᵗʰ T79.1 Fat embolism (traumatic) MCC
EXCLUDES 1   fat embolism complicating:
abortion or ectopic or molar pregnancy (O00-O07, O08.2)
pregnancy, childbirth and the puerperium (O88.8)
CC Excl: MCC with 7th A: D78.81-D78.89, E36.8, E89.810-E89.89, H59.011-H59.019, H59.031-H59.099, H59.811-H59.89, H95.811-H95.89, I97.3, L76.81-L76.82, M96.89, N98.1-N98.9, T14.90-T14.91, T79.1XXA, T79.A0X-T79.9XX with 7th A, T81.82XA, T81.89X-T81.9XX with 7th A

✓x7ᵗʰ T79.2 Traumatic secondary and recurrent hemorrhage and seroma CC
CC Excl: CC with 7th character A: D78.81-D78.89, E36.8, E89.810-E89.89, H59.011-H59.019, H59.031-H59.099, H59.811-H59.89, H95.811-H95.89, I97.3, L76.81-L76.82, M96.89, N98.1-N98.9, T14.90-T14.91, T79.2XXA, T79.A0X-T79.9XX with 7th A, T81.82XA, T81.89X-T81.9XX with 7th A

✓x7ᵗʰ T79.4 Traumatic shock MCC
Shock (immediate) (delayed) following injury
EXCLUDES 1   anaphylactic shock due to adverse food reaction (T78.0-)
anaphylactic shock due to correct medicinal substance properly administered (T88.6)
anaphylactic shock due to serum (T80.5-)
anaphylactic shock NOS (T78.2)
anesthetic shock (T88.2)
electric shock (T75.4)
nontraumatic shock NEC (R57.-)
obstetric shock (O75.1)
postprocedural shock (T81.1-)
septic shock (R65.21)
shock complicating abortion or ectopic or molar pregnancy (O00-O07, O08.3)
shock due to lightning (T75.01)
shock NOS (R57.9)
CC Excl: MCC with 7th A: D78.81-D78.89, E36.8, E89.810-E89.89, H59.011-H59.019, H59.031-H59.099, H59.811-H59.89, H95.811-H95.89, I97.3, L76.81-L76.82, M96.89, N98.1-N98.9, T14.90-T14.91, T79.4XXA, T79.A0X-T79.9XX with 7th A, T81.82XA, T81.89X-T81.9XX with 7th A

✓x7ᵗʰ T79.5 Traumatic anuria MCC
Crush syndrome
Renal failure following crushing
CC Excl: MCC with 7th A: D78.01-D78.02, D78.21-D78.89, E36.01-E36.02, E36.8, E89.810-E89.89, G97.51-G97.52, H59.011-H59.019, H59.031-H59.129, H59.311-H59.329, H59.811-H59.89, H95.21-H95.22, H95.41-H95.89, I97.3-I97.42, I97.610-I97.62, J95.61-J95.62, J95.830-J95.831, K91.61-K91.62, K91.840-K91.841, L76.01-L76.02, L76.21-L76.82, M96.810-M96.811, M96.830-M96.89, N98.1-N98.9, N99.61-N99.62, N99.820-N99.821, T14.90-T14.91, T79.5XXA, T79.A0X-T79.9XX with 7th A, T81.10X-T81.19X with 7th A, T81.82XA, T81.89X-T81.9XX with 7th A, T88.2XXA

✓x7ᵗʰ T79.6 Traumatic ischemia of muscle
Traumatic rhabdomyolysis
Volkmann's ischemic contracture
EXCLUDES 2   anterior tibial syndrome (M76.8)
compartment syndrome (traumatic) (T79.A-)
nontraumatic ischemia of muscle (M62.2-)

N Newborn: 0   P Pediatric: 0-17   M Maternity: 12-55   A Adult: 15-124   MCC Major CC Condition   PDxMCC PDx acts as own MCC   CC CC Condition   PDxCC PDx acts as own CC

1132   ICD-10-CM 2016

✓x7ᵗʰ **T79.7 Traumatic subcutaneous emphysema**   CC
    EXCLUDES 1 emphysema NOS (J43)
       emphysema (subcutaneous) resulting from a procedure
       (T81.82)
    CC Excl: CC with 7th character A: D78.81-D78.89, E36.8, E89.810-
    E89.89, H59.011-H59.019, H59.031-H59.099, H59.811-H59.89,
    H95.811-H95.89, I97.3, L76.81-L76.82, M96.89, N98.1-N98.9,
    S21.101-S21.159 with 7th A, S21.301-S21.95X with 7th A, S27.0XX-
    S27.399 with 7th A, S27.50X-S27.809 with 7th A, S27.892-S27.9XX
    with 7th A, S28.1XXA, S29.021A, S29.029A, T14.90-T14.91,
    T79.7XX-T79.9XX with 7th A, T81.82A, T81.89X-T81.9XX with 7th A

✓5ᵗʰ **T79.A Traumatic compartment syndrome**
    EXCLUDES 1 fibromyalgia (M79.7)
       nontraumatic compartment syndrome (M79.A-)
       traumatic ischemic infarction of muscle (T79.6)

✓x7ᵗʰ **T79.A0 Compartment syndrome, unspecified**   CC
    Compartment syndrome NOS
    CC Excl: CC with 7th character A: S31.001A, S31.011A,
    S31.021A, S31.031A, S31.041A, S31.051A, S31.600-
    S31.659 with 7th A, S36.81X-S36.899 with 7th A

✓6ᵗʰ **T79.A1 Traumatic compartment syndrome of upper
    extremity**
    Traumatic compartment syndrome of shoulder, arm,
    forearm, wrist, hand, and fingers

    **CC Excl: For CC codes in category T79.A1: CC
    with 7th character A,unless otherwise noted:**
    M70.80-M70.99, M79.81-M79.9, R29.898

    ✓7ᵗʰ **T79.A11 Traumatic compartment syndrome of**   CC
       right upper extremity

    ✓7ᵗʰ **T79.A12 Traumatic compartment syndrome of**   CC
       left upper extremity

    ✓7ᵗʰ **T79.A19 Traumatic compartment syndrome of**   CC
       unspecified upper extremity

✓6ᵗʰ **T79.A2 Traumatic compartment syndrome of lower
    extremity**
    Traumatic compartment syndrome of hip, buttock,
    thigh, leg, foot, and toes

    **CC Excl: For CC codes in category T79.A2 : CC
    with 7th character A, unless otherwise noted:**
    See code: T79.A1

    ✓7ᵗʰ **T79.A21 Traumatic compartment syndrome of**   CC
       right lower extremity

    ✓7ᵗʰ **T79.A22 Traumatic compartment syndrome of**   CC
       left lower extremity

    ✓7ᵗʰ **T79.A29 Traumatic compartment syndrome of**   CC
       unspecified lower extremity

✓x7ᵗʰ **T79.A3 Traumatic compartment syndrome of abdomen**   CC
    CC Excl: CC with 7th character A: S31.001A, S31.011A,
    S31.021A, S31.031A, S31.041A, S31.051-S31.159 with
    7th A, S31.600-S31.659 with 7th A, S31.831-S31.839
    with 7th A, S36.00X-S37.99X with 7th A, S38.3XX-
    S39.023 with 7th A, T14.90-T14.91, T79.8XX-T79.9XX
    with 7th A

✓x7ᵗʰ **T79.A9 Traumatic compartment syndrome of other sites**   CC
    CC Excl: CC with 7th character A: S31.001A, S31.011A,
    S31.021A, S31.031A, S31.041A, S31.051A, S31.600-
    S31.659 with 7th A, S36.81X-S36.899 with 7th A

✓x7ᵗʰ **T79.8 Other early complications of trauma**

✓x7ᵗʰ **T79.9 Unspecified early complication of trauma**

Complications of surgical and medical care, not elsewhere classified (T80-T88)

Use additional code for adverse effect, if applicable, to identify drug (T36-T50
with fifth or sixth character 5)
Use additional code(s) to identify the specified condition resulting from the
complication
Use additional code to identify devices involved and details of circumstances
(Y62-Y82)
    EXCLUDES 2 any encounters with medical care for postprocedural conditions in
       which no complications are present, such as:
       artificial opening status (Z93.-)
       closure of external stoma (Z43.-)
       fitting and adjustment of external prosthetic device (Z44.-)
       burns and corrosions from local applications and irradiation (T20-T32)
       complications of surgical procedures during pregnancy, childbirth and
       the puerperium (O00-O9A)
       mechanical complication of respirator [ventilator] (J95.850)
       poisoning and toxic effects of drugs and chemicals (T36-T65 with fifth
       or sixth character 1-4 or 6)
       postprocedural fever (R50.82)
       specified complications classified elsewhere, such as:
       cerebrospinal fluid leak from spinal puncture (G97.0)
       colostomy malfunction (K94.0-)
       disorders of fluid and electrolyte imbalance (E86-E87)
       functional disturbances following cardiac surgery (I97.0-I97.1)
       intraoperative and postprocedural complications of specified body
       systems (D78.-, E36.-, E89.-, G97.3-, G97.4, H59.3-, H59.-,
       H95.2-, H95.3, I97.4-, I97.5, J95.6-, J95.7, K91.6-, L76.-,
       M96.-, N99.-)
       ostomy complications (J95.0-, K94-, N99.5-)
       postgastric surgery syndromes (K91.1)
       postlaminectomy syndrome NEC (M96.1)
       postmastectomy lymphedema syndrome (I97.2)
       postsurgical blind-loop syndrome (K91.2)
       ventilator associated pneumonia (J95.851)
    AHA: 2015, 1Q, 15

✓4ᵗʰ **T80 Complications following infusion, transfusion and therapeutic
injection**
    INCLUDES complications following perfusion
    EXCLUDES 2 bone marrow transplant rejection (T86.01)
       febrile nonhemolytic transfusion reaction (R50.84)
       fluid overload due to transfusion (E87.71)
       posttransfusion purpura (D69.51)
       transfusion associated circulatory overload (TACO) (E87.71)
       transfusion (red blood cell) associated hemochromatosis
       (E83.111)
       transfusion related acute lung injury (TRALI) (J95.84)

    The appropriate 7th character is to be added to each code from
    category T80.
    A   initial encounter
    D   subsequent encounter
    S   sequela

7 ✓x7ᵗʰ **T80.0 Air embolism following infusion, transfusion and**   MCC
    therapeutic injection
    CC Excl: MCC with 7th A: T79.0XXA, T80.0XXA

✓x7ᵗʰ **T80.1 Vascular complications following infusion, transfusion**   CC
    and therapeutic injection
    Use additional code to identify the vascular complication
    EXCLUDES 2 extravasation of vesicant agent (T80.81-)
       infiltration of vesicant agent (T80.81-)
       postprocedural vascular complications (T81.7-)
       vascular complications specified as due to prosthetic
       devices, implants and grafts (T82.8-, T83.8,
       T84.8-, T85.8)
    CC Excl: CC with 7th character A: T80.1XXA, T80.810-T80.818
    with 7th A, T80.90XA

✓5ᵗʰ **T80.2 Infections following infusion, transfusion and therapeutic
injection**
    Use additional code to identify the specific infection, such as:
    sepsis (A41.9)
    Use additional code (R65.2-) to identify severe sepsis, if
    applicable
    EXCLUDES 2 infections specified as due to prosthetic devices,
       implants and grafts (T82.6-T82.7, T83.5-T83.6,
       T84.5-T84.7, T85.7)
       postprocedural infections (T81.4)

    **CC Excl: For CC codes in subcategory T80.2: CC with 7th
    character A, unless otherwise noted:** N98.0, T80.211-
    T80.29X with 7th A, T82.7XXA, T88.0XXA

---

7 HAC = Initial encounter only (7th character A, B or C) and not POA.

✓ Additional Character Required   ✓x7ᵗʰ Placeholder Alert   Unacceptable PDx   Manifestation   Hospital Acquired Condition   **EXCLUDES 1** Not Coded Here   EXCLUDES 2 Not Included Here

ICD-10-CM 2016   1133

✓6ᵗʰ **T80.21** **Infection** due to central venous catheter

7 ✓7ᵗʰ **T80.211** **Bloodstream infection** due to central venous catheter [CC]

Catheter-related bloodstream infection (CRBSI) NOS

Central line-associated bloodstream infection (CLABSI)

Bloodstream infection due to Hickman catheter

Bloodstream infection due to peripherally inserted central catheter (PICC)

Bloodstream infection due to portacath (port-a-cath)

Bloodstream infection due to triple lumen catheter

Bloodstream infection due to umbilical venous catheter

7 ✓7ᵗʰ **T80.212** **Local infection** due to central venous catheter [CC]

Exit or insertion site infection

Local infection due to Hickman catheter

Local infection due to peripherally inserted central catheter (PICC)

Local infection due to portacath (port-a-cath)

Local infection due to triple lumen catheter

Local infection due to umbilical venous catheter

Port or reservoir infection

Tunnel infection

7 ✓7ᵗʰ **T80.218** **Other infection** due to central venous catheter [CC]

Other central line-associated infection

Other infection due to Hickman catheter

Other infection due to peripherally inserted central catheter (PICC)

Other infection due to portacath (port-a-cath)

Other infection due to triple lumen catheter

Other infection due to umbilical venous catheter

7 ✓7ᵗʰ **T80.219** **Unspecified** infection due to central venous catheter [CC]

Central line-associated infection NOS

Unspecified infection due to Hickman catheter

Unspecified infection due to peripherally inserted central catheter (PICC)

Unspecified infection due to portacath (port-a-cath)

Unspecified infection due to triple lumen catheter

Unspecified infection due to umbilical venous catheter

✓x7ᵗʰ **T80.22** **Acute infection following transfusion, infusion, or injection of blood and blood products** [CC]

✓x7ᵗʰ **T80.29** **Infection following other infusion, transfusion and therapeutic injection** [CC]

✓5ᵗʰ **T80.3** **ABO incompatibility** reaction due to transfusion of blood or blood products

EXCLUDES 1 *minor blood group antigens reactions (Duffy) (E) (K(ell)) (Kidd) (Lewis) (M) (N) (P) (S) (T80.A)*

CC Excl: CC Excl: For CC/MCC codes in subcategory T80.3: CC with 7th character A, unless otherwise noted: T80.30X-T80.A9X with 7th A, T80.910-T80.92X with 7th A

7 ✓x7ᵗʰ **T80.30** **ABO incompatibility reaction due to transfusion of blood or blood products, unspecified** [CC]

ABO incompatibility blood transfusion NOS

Reaction to ABO incompatibility from transfusion NOS

✓6ᵗʰ **T80.31** **ABO incompatibility** with hemolytic transfusion reaction

7 ✓7ᵗʰ **T80.310** **ABO incompatibility with acute hemolytic transfusion reaction** [CC]

ABO incompatibility with hemolytic transfusion reaction less than 24 hours after transfusion

Acute hemolytic transfusion reaction (AHTR) due to ABO incompatibility

7 ✓7ᵗʰ **T80.311** **ABO incompatibility with delayed hemolytic transfusion reaction** [CC]

ABO incompatibility with hemolytic transfusion reaction 24 hours or more after transfusion

Delayed hemolytic transfusion reaction (DHTR) due to ABO incompatibility

7 ✓7ᵗʰ **T80.319** **ABO incompatibility with hemolytic transfusion reaction, unspecified** [CC]

ABO incompatibility with hemolytic transfusion reaction at unspecified time after transfusion

Hemolytic transfusion reaction (HTR) due to ABO incompatibility NOS

7 ✓x7ᵗʰ **T80.39** **Other ABO incompatibility reaction due to transfusion of blood or blood products** [CC]

Delayed serologic transfusion reaction (DSTR) from ABO incompatibility

Other ABO incompatible blood transfusion

Other reaction to ABO incompatible blood transfusion

✓x7ᵗʰ **T80.4** **Rh incompatibility** reaction due to transfusion of blood or blood products

Reaction due to incompatibility of Rh antigens (C) (c) (D) (E) (e)

CC Excl: For CC/MCC codes in subcategory T80.4: CC with 7th character A, unless otherwise noted: See code: T80.3

✓x7ᵗʰ **T80.40** **Rh incompatibility reaction due to transfusion of blood or blood products, unspecified** [CC]

Reaction due to Rh factor in transfusion NOS

Rh incompatible blood transfusion NOS

✓6ᵗʰ **T80.41** **Rh incompatibility** with hemolytic transfusion reaction

✓7ᵗʰ **T80.410** **Rh incompatibility with acute hemolytic transfusion reaction** [CC]

Acute hemolytic transfusion reaction (AHTR) due to Rh incompatibility

Rh incompatibility with hemolytic transfusion reaction less than 24 hours after transfusion

✓7ᵗʰ **T80.411** **Rh incompatibility with delayed hemolytic transfusion reaction** [CC]

Delayed hemolytic transfusion reaction (DHTR) due to Rh incompatibility

Rh incompatibility with hemolytic transfusion reaction 24 hours or more after transfusion

✓7ᵗʰ **T80.419** **Rh incompatibility with hemolytic transfusion reaction, unspecified** [CC]

Hemolytic transfusion reaction (HTR) due to Rh incompatibility NOS

Rh incompatibility with hemolytic transfusion reaction at unspecified time after transfusion

✓x7ᵗʰ **T80.49** **Other Rh incompatibility reaction due to transfusion of blood or blood products** [CC]

Delayed serologic transfusion reaction (DSTR) from Rh incompatibility

Other reaction to Rh incompatible blood transfusion

CC Excl: CC with 7th character A: T80.30X-T80.419 with 7th A, T80.A9XA, T80.910-T80.92X with 7th A

✓5ᵗʰ **T80.A** **Non-ABO incompatibility** reaction due to transfusion of blood or blood products

Reaction due to incompatibility of minor antigens (Duffy) (Kell) (Kidd) (Lewis) (M) (N) (P) (S)

✓x7ᵗʰ **T80.A0** **Non-ABO incompatibility reaction due to transfusion of blood or blood products, unspecified** [CC]

Non-ABO antigen incompatibility reaction from transfusion NOS

CC Excl: CC with 7th character A, unless otherwise noted: T80.30X-T80.419 with 7th A, T80.A9XA, T80.910-T80.92X with 7th A

✓6ᵗʰ **T80.A1** **Non-ABO incompatibility** with hemolytic transfusion reaction

CC Excl: For CC codes in subcategory T80.A1: CC with 7th character A, unless otherwise noted: See code: T80.A0

7 HAC = Initial encounter only (7th character A, B or C) and not POA.

Ⓝ Newborn: 0   Ⓟ Pediatric: 0-17   Ⓜ Maternity: 12-55   Ⓐ Adult: 15-124   [MCC] Major CC Condition   [PDx MCC] PDx acts as own MCC   [CC] CC Condition   [PDx CC] PDx acts as own CC

1134

ICD-10-CM 2016

√7ᵗʰ **T80.A10** **Non-ABO incompatibility with** acute **hemolytic transfusion reaction**　CC
　　Acute hemolytic transfusion reaction (AHTR) due to non-ABO incompatibility
　　Non-ABO incompatibility with hemolytic transfusion reaction less than 24 hours after transfusion

√7ᵗʰ **T80.A11** **Non-ABO incompatibility with** delayed **hemolytic transfusion reaction**　CC
　　Delayed hemolytic transfusion reaction (DHTR) due to non-ABO incompatibility
　　Non-ABO incompatibility with hemolytic transfusion reaction 24 or more hours after transfusion

√7ᵗʰ **T80.A19** **Non-ABO incompatibility with hemolytic transfusion reaction,** unspecified　CC
　　Hemolytic transfusion reaction (HTR) due to non-ABO incompatibility NOS
　　Non-ABO incompatibility with hemolytic transfusion reaction at unspecified time after transfusion

√x7ᵗʰ **T80.A9** **Other** non-ABO incompatibility reaction due to transfusion of blood or blood products　CC
　　Delayed serologic transfusion reaction (DSTR) from non-ABO incompatibility
　　Other reaction to non-ABO incompatible blood transfusion
　　CC Excl: CC with 7th character A: T80.30X-T80.A9X with 7th A, T80.910-T80.92X with 7th A

√5ᵗʰ **T80.5** **Anaphylactic reaction due to serum**
　　Allergic shock due to serum
　　Anaphylactic shock due to serum
　　Anaphylactoid reaction due to serum
　　Anaphylaxis due to serum
　　EXCLUDES 1　ABO incompatibility reaction due to transfusion of blood or blood products (T80.3-)
　　　allergic reaction or shock NOS (T78.2)
　　　anaphylactic reaction or shock NOS (T78.2)
　　　anaphylactic reaction or shock due to adverse effect of correct medicinal substance properly administered (T88.6)
　　　other serum reaction (T80.6-)

　　CC Excl: For CC/MCC codes in subcategory T80.5: CC with 7th character A, unless otherwise noted: T80.51X-T80.69X with 7th A

√x7ᵗʰ **T80.51** **Anaphylactic reaction due to** administration of blood and blood products　CC

√x7ᵗʰ **T80.52** **Anaphylactic reaction due to** vaccination　CC

√x7ᵗʰ **T80.59** **Anaphylactic reaction due to** other serum　CC

√5ᵗʰ **T80.6** **Other serum reactions**
　　Intoxication by serum　　　Serum sickness
　　Protein sickness　　　　　Serum urticaria
　　Serum rash
　　EXCLUDES 2　serum hepatitis (B16.-)

√x7ᵗʰ **T80.61** **Other serum reaction** due to administration of blood and blood products　CC
　　CC Excl: CC with 7th character A: See code: T80.5

√x7ᵗʰ **T80.62** **Other serum reaction** due to vaccination　CC
　　CC Excl: CC with 7th character A: See code: T80.5

√x7ᵗʰ **T80.69** **Other serum reaction** due to other serum　CC
　　CC Excl: CC with 7th character A: T80.61X-T80.69X with 7th A

√5ᵗʰ **T80.8** **Other complications following infusion, transfusion and therapeutic injection**

√6ᵗʰ **T80.81** **Extravasation of vesicant agent**
　　Infiltration of vesicant agent

√7ᵗʰ **T80.810** **Extravasation of vesicant antineoplastic chemotherapy**　CC
　　Infiltration of vesicant antineoplastic chemotherapy
　　CC Excl: CC with 7th character A: T80.1XXA, T80.810-T80.818 with 7th A, T80.90XA

√7ᵗʰ **T80.818** **Extravasation of other vesicant agent**　CC
　　Infiltration of other vesicant agent
　　CC Excl: CC with 7th character A: See code: T81.810

√x7ᵗʰ **T80.89** **Other complications following infusion, transfusion and therapeutic injection**
　　Delayed serologic transfusion reaction (DSTR), unspecified incompatibility
　　Use additional code to identify graft-versus-host reaction, if applicable, (D89.81-)

√5ᵗʰ **T80.9** **Unspecified complication following infusion, transfusion and therapeutic injection**

√x7ᵗʰ **T80.90** **Unspecified complication** following infusion and therapeutic injection

√6ᵗʰ **T80.91** **Hemolytic transfusion reaction,** unspecified incompatibility
　　EXCLUDES 1　ABO incompatibility with hemolytic transfusion reaction (T80.31-)
　　　Non-ABO incompatibility with hemolytic transfusion reaction (T80.A1-)
　　　Rh incompatibility with hemolytic transfusion reaction (T80.41-)

　　CC Excl: For CC codes in subcategory T80.91: CC with 7th character A, unless otherwise noted: T80.30X-T80.A9X with 7th A, T80.910-T80.92X with 7th A

√7ᵗʰ **T80.910** **Acute hemolytic transfusion reaction, unspecified incompatibility**　CC

√7ᵗʰ **T80.911** **Delayed hemolytic transfusion reaction, unspecified incompatibility**　CC

√7ᵗʰ **T80.919** **Hemolytic transfusion reaction,** unspecified **incompatibility,** unspecified as acute or delayed　CC
　　Hemolytic transfusion reaction NOS

√x7ᵗʰ **T80.92** **Unspecified transfusion reaction**
　　Transfusion reaction NOS

√4ᵗʰ **T81** **Complications of procedures, not elsewhere classified**
　　Use additional code for adverse effect, if applicable, to identify drug (T36-T50 with fifth or sixth character 5)
　　EXCLUDES 2　complications following immunization (T88.0-T88.1)
　　　complications following infusion, transfusion and therapeutic injection (T80.-)
　　　complications of transplanted organs and tissue (T86.-)
　　　specified complications classified elsewhere, such as:
　　　　complication of prosthetic devices, implants and grafts (T82-T85)
　　　　dermatitis due to drugs and medicaments (L23.3, L24.4, L25.1, L27.0-L27.1)
　　　　endosseous dental implant failure (M27.6-)
　　　　floppy iris syndrome (IFIS) (intraoperative) (H21.81)
　　　　intraoperative and postprocedural complications of specific body system (D78.-, E36.-, E89.-, G97.3-, G97.4, H59.3-, H59.-, H95.2-, H95.3, I97.4-, I97.5, J95., K91.-, L76.-, M96.-, N99.-)
　　　　ostomy complications (J95.0-, K94.-, N99.5-)
　　　　plateau iris syndrome (post-iridectomy) (postprocedural) (H21.82)
　　　　poisoning and toxic effects of drugs and chemicals (T36-T65 with fifth or sixth character 1-4 or 6)

　　The appropriate 7th character is to be added to each code from category T81.
　　A　　initial encounter
　　D　　subsequent encounter
　　S　　sequela

√ Additional Character Required　√x7ᵗʰ Placeholder Alert　Unacceptable PDx　Manifestation　Hospital Acquired Condition　*EXCLUDES 1* Not Coded Here　*EXCLUDES 2* Not Included Here

Chapter 19. Injury, Poisoning, and Certain Other Consequences of External Causes

T80.A10–T81

✓5ᵗʰ **T81.1 Postprocedural shock**

Shock during or resulting from a procedure, not elsewhere classified

EXCLUDES 1 anaphylactic shock due to correct substance properly administered (T88.6)
anaphylactic shock due to serum (T80.5-)
anaphylactic shock NOS (T78.2)
anesthetic shock (T88.2)
electric shock (T75.4)
obstetric shock (O75.1)
septic shock (R65.21)
shock following abortion or ectopic or molar pregnancy (O00-O07, O08.3)
traumatic shock (T79.4)

CC Excl: For CC/MCC codes in subcategory T81.1, MCC with 7th A, unless otherwise noted: D78.01-D78.02, D78.21-D78.89, E36.01-E36.02, E36.8, E89.810-E89.89, G97.51-G97.52, H59.011-H59.019, H59.031-H59.129, H59.311-H59.329, H59.811-H59.89, H95.21-H95.22, H95.41-H95.89, I97.3-I97.42, I97.610-I97.62, J95.61-J95.62, J95.830-J95.831, K91.61-K91.62, K91.840-K91.841, L76.01-L76.02, L76.21-L76.82, M96.810-M96.811, M96.830-M96.89, N98.1-N98.9, N99.61-N99.62, N99.820-N99.821, T79.4XXA, T81.10X-T81.19X with 7th A, T81.82XA, T81.89X-T81.9XX with 7th A, T88.2XXA

✓x7ᵗʰ **T81.10 Postprocedural shock unspecified** CC

Collapse NOS during or resulting from a procedure, not elsewhere classified
Postprocedural failure of peripheral circulation
Postprocedural shock NOS

✓x7ᵗʰ **T81.11 Postprocedural cardiogenic shock** MCC

12 ✓x7ᵗʰ **T81.12 Postprocedural septic shock** MCC

Postprocedural endotoxic shock during or resulting from a procedure, not elsewhere classified
Postprocedural gram-negative shock during or resulting from a procedure, not elsewhere classified
Code first underlying infection
Use additional code, to identify any associated acute organ dysfunction, if applicable

✓x7ᵗʰ **T81.19 Other postprocedural shock** MCC

Postprocedural hypovolemic shock

✓5ᵗʰ **T81.3 Disruption of wound, not elsewhere classified**

Disruption of any suture materials or other closure methods

EXCLUDES 1 breakdown (mechanical) of permanent sutures (T85.612)
displacement of permanent sutures (T85.622)
disruption of cesarean delivery wound (O90.0)
disruption of perineal obstetric wound (O90.1)
mechanical complication of permanent sutures NEC (T85.692)

AHA: 2014, 1Q, 23

CC Excl: For CC/MCC codes in subcategory T81.3: CC with 7th character A, unless otherwise noted: D78.81-D78.89, E36.8, E89.810-E89.89, H59.011-H59.019, H59.031-H59.099, H59.811-H59.89, H95.811-H95.89, I97.3, L76.81-L76.82, M96.89, N98.1-N98.9, T81.30X-T81.33X with 7th A, T81.82A, T81.89X-T81.9XX with 7th A

✓x7ᵗʰ **T81.30 Disruption of wound, unspecified** CC

Disruption of wound NOS

✓x7ᵗʰ **T81.31 Disruption of external operation (surgical) wound, not elsewhere classified** CC

Dehiscence of operation wound NOS
Disruption of operation wound NOS
Disruption or dehiscence of closure of cornea
Disruption or dehiscence of closure of mucosa
Disruption or dehiscence of closure of skin and subcutaneous tissue
Full-thickness skin disruption or dehiscence
Superficial disruption or dehiscence of operation wound

EXCLUDES 1 dehiscence of amputation stump (T87.81)

✓x7ᵗʰ **T81.32 Disruption of internal operation (surgical) wound, not elsewhere classified** CC

Deep disruption or dehiscence of operation wound NOS
Disruption or dehiscence of closure of internal organ or other internal tissue
Disruption or dehiscence of closure of muscle or muscle flap
Disruption or dehiscence of closure of ribs or rib cage
Disruption or dehiscence of closure of skull or craniotomy
Disruption or dehiscence of closure of sternum or sternotomy
Disruption or dehiscence of closure of tendon or ligament
Disruption or dehiscence of closure of superficial or muscular fascia

✓x7ᵗʰ **T81.33 Disruption of traumatic injury wound repair** CC

Disruption or dehiscence of closure of traumatic laceration (external) (internal)

4,6,7,8 ✓x7ᵗʰ **T81.4 Infection following a procedure** CC

Intra-abdominal abscess following a procedure
Postprocedural infection, not elsewhere classified
Sepsis following a procedure
Stitch abscess following a procedure
Subphrenic abscess following a procedure
Wound abscess following a procedure
Use additional code to identify infection
Use additional code (R65.2-) to identify severe sepsis, if applicable

EXCLUDES 1 obstetric surgical wound infection (O86.0)
postprocedural fever NOS (R50.82)
postprocedural retroperitoneal abscess (K68.11)

EXCLUDES 2 bleb associated endophthalmitis (H59.4-)
infection due to infusion, transfusion and therapeutic injection (T80.2-)
infection due to prosthetic devices, implants and grafts (T82.6-T82.7, T83.5-T83.6, T84.5-T84.7, T85.7)

AHA: 2014, 1Q, 23
CC Excl: CC with 7th character A: D78.81-D78.89, E36.8, E89.810-E89.89, H59.011-H59.019, H59.031-H59.099, H59.811-H59.89, H95.811-H95.89, I97.3, K68.11, L76.81-L76.82, M96.89, N98.1-N98.9, T81.4XXA, T81.82XA, T81.89X-T81.9XX with 7th A

✓5ᵗʰ **T81.5 Complications of foreign body accidentally left in body following procedure**

AHA: 2014, 4Q, 24

CC Excl: For CC codes in subcategory T81.5: CC with 7th character A, unless otherwise noted: D78.81-D78.89, E36.8, E89.810-E89.89, H59.011-H59.019, H59.031-H59.099, H59.811-H59.89, H95.811-H95.89, I97.3, L76.81-L76.82, M96.89, N98.1-N98.9, T81.500-T81.599 with 7th A, T81.82XA, T81.89X-T81.9XX with 7th A

✓6ᵗʰ **T81.50 Unspecified complication of foreign body accidentally left in body following procedure**

7 ✓7ᵗʰ **T81.500 Unspecified complication of foreign body accidentally left in body following surgical operation** CC

7 ✓7ᵗʰ **T81.501 Unspecified complication of foreign body accidentally left in body following infusion or transfusion** CC

7 ✓7ᵗʰ **T81.502 Unspecified complication of foreign body accidentally left in body following kidney dialysis** CC

7 ✓7ᵗʰ **T81.503 Unspecified complication of foreign body accidentally left in body following injection or immunization** CC

7 ✓7ᵗʰ **T81.504 Unspecified complication of foreign body accidentally left in body following endoscopic examination** CC

7 ✓7ᵗʰ **T81.505 Unspecified complication of foreign body accidentally left in body following heart catheterization** CC

7 ✓7ᵗʰ **T81.506 Unspecified complication of foreign body accidentally left in body following aspiration, puncture or other catheterization** CC

---

4 HAC = as SDx not POA, in combination with PDx E66.01 **AND** one of the following procedure codes: 0D16[0,4,8][7,J,K,Z][9,A,B,L] or 0DV64CZ.

6 HAC = as SDx not POA, in combination with one of the following procedure codes: 0RG[0,1,2,4,6,7,8,A][0,3,4][7,A,J,K,Z][0,1,J]; 0RG[E,F,G,H,J,K][0,3,4][4,7,J,K,Z]Z; 0RG[L,M][0,3,4][4,5,7,J,K,Z]Z; 0RQ[E,F,G,H,J,K,L,M][0,3,4,X]ZZ; 0RU[E,F,G,H,J,K,L,M][0,3,4][7,J,K]Z; 0SG[0,1,3][0,3,4][7,A,J,K,Z][0,1,J]; 0SG[7,8][0,3,4][4,7,J,K,Z]Z.

7 HAC = Initial encounter only (7th character A, B or C) and not POA.

8 HAC = as SDx not POA, in combination with one of the following procedure codes: 02H43[J,K,M]Z; 02H[6,7]3[J,M]Z; 02H[K,L]3JZ; 02HN[0,3,4][J,M]Z; 02PA[0,3,4]MZ; 02PAXMZ; 02WA[0,3,4]MZ; 0JH[6,8][0,3][4,5,6,7,8,9,P]Z; 0JPT[0,3]PZ; 0JWT[0,3]PZ.

12 Unacceptable PDx = initial encounter only (7th character A).

N Newborn: 0 P Pediatric: 0-17 M Maternity: 12-55 A Adult: 15-124 **MCC** Major CC Condition **PDxMCC** PDx acts as own MCC **CC** CC Condition **PDxCC** PDx acts as own CC

1136 ICD-10-CM 2016

7 ✓7ᵗʰ **T81.507** Unspecified complication of foreign body accidentally left in body following removal of catheter or packing ᴄᴄ

7 ✓7ᵗʰ **T81.508** Unspecified complication of foreign body accidentally left in body following other procedure ᴄᴄ

7 ✓7ᵗʰ **T81.509** Unspecified complication of foreign body accidentally left in body following unspecified procedure ᴄᴄ

✓6ᵗʰ **T81.51** Adhesions due to foreign body accidentally left in body following procedure

7 ✓7ᵗʰ **T81.510** Adhesions due to foreign body accidentally left in body following surgical operation ᴄᴄ

7 ✓7ᵗʰ **T81.511** Adhesions due to foreign body accidentally left in body following infusion or transfusion ᴄᴄ

7 ✓7ᵗʰ **T81.512** Adhesions due to foreign body accidentally left in body following kidney dialysis ᴄᴄ

7 ✓7ᵗʰ **T81.513** Adhesions due to foreign body accidentally left in body following injection or immunization ᴄᴄ

7 ✓7ᵗʰ **T81.514** Adhesions due to foreign body accidentally left in body following endoscopic examination ᴄᴄ

7 ✓7ᵗʰ **T81.515** Adhesions due to foreign body accidentally left in body following heart catheterization ᴄᴄ

7 ✓7ᵗʰ **T81.516** Adhesions due to foreign body accidentally left in body following aspiration, puncture or other catheterization ᴄᴄ

7 ✓7ᵗʰ **T81.517** Adhesions due to foreign body accidentally left in body following removal of catheter or packing ᴄᴄ

7 ✓7ᵗʰ **T81.518** Adhesions due to foreign body accidentally left in body following other procedure ᴄᴄ

7 ✓7ᵗʰ **T81.519** Adhesions due to foreign body accidentally left in body following unspecified procedure ᴄᴄ

✓6ᵗʰ **T81.52** Obstruction due to foreign body accidentally left in body following procedure

7 ✓7ᵗʰ **T81.520** Obstruction due to foreign body accidentally left in body following surgical operation ᴄᴄ

7 ✓7ᵗʰ **T81.521** Obstruction due to foreign body accidentally left in body following infusion or transfusion ᴄᴄ

7 ✓7ᵗʰ **T81.522** Obstruction due to foreign body accidentally left in body following kidney dialysis ᴄᴄ

7 ✓7ᵗʰ **T81.523** Obstruction due to foreign body accidentally left in body following injection or immunization ᴄᴄ

7 ✓7ᵗʰ **T81.524** Obstruction due to foreign body accidentally left in body following endoscopic examination ᴄᴄ

7 ✓7ᵗʰ **T81.525** Obstruction due to foreign body accidentally left in body following heart catheterization ᴄᴄ

7 ✓7ᵗʰ **T81.526** Obstruction due to foreign body accidentally left in body following aspiration, puncture or other catheterization ᴄᴄ

7 ✓7ᵗʰ **T81.527** Obstruction due to foreign body accidentally left in body following removal of catheter or packing ᴄᴄ

7 ✓7ᵗʰ **T81.528** Obstruction due to foreign body accidentally left in body following other procedure ᴄᴄ

7 ✓7ᵗʰ **T81.529** Obstruction due to foreign body accidentally left in body following unspecified procedure ᴄᴄ

✓6ᵗʰ **T81.53** Perforation due to foreign body accidentally left in body following procedure

7 ✓7ᵗʰ **T81.530** Perforation due to foreign body accidentally left in body following surgical operation ᴄᴄ

7 ✓7ᵗʰ **T81.531** Perforation due to foreign body accidentally left in body following infusion or transfusion ᴄᴄ

7 ✓7ᵗʰ **T81.532** Perforation due to foreign body accidentally left in body following kidney dialysis ᴄᴄ

7 ✓7ᵗʰ **T81.533** Perforation due to foreign body accidentally left in body following injection or immunization ᴄᴄ

7 ✓7ᵗʰ **T81.534** Perforation due to foreign body accidentally left in body following endoscopic examination ᴄᴄ

7 ✓7ᵗʰ **T81.535** Perforation due to foreign body accidentally left in body following heart catheterization ᴄᴄ

7 ✓7ᵗʰ **T81.536** Perforation due to foreign body accidentally left in body following aspiration, puncture or other catheterization ᴄᴄ

7 ✓7ᵗʰ **T81.537** Perforation due to foreign body accidentally left in body following removal of catheter or packing ᴄᴄ

7 ✓7ᵗʰ **T81.538** Perforation due to foreign body accidentally left in body following other procedure ᴄᴄ

7 ✓7ᵗʰ **T81.539** Perforation due to foreign body accidentally left in body following unspecified procedure ᴄᴄ

✓6ᵗʰ **T81.59** Other complications of foreign body accidentally left in body following procedure

EXCLUDES 2 *obstruction or perforation due to prosthetic devices and implants intentionally left in body (T82.0-T82.5, T83.0-T83.4, T83.7, T84.0-T84.4, T85.0-T85.6)*

7 ✓7ᵗʰ **T81.590** Other complications of foreign body accidentally left in body following surgical operation ᴄᴄ

7 ✓7ᵗʰ **T81.591** Other complications of foreign body accidentally left in body following infusion or transfusion ᴄᴄ

7 ✓7ᵗʰ **T81.592** Other complications of foreign body accidentally left in body following kidney dialysis ᴄᴄ

7 ✓7ᵗʰ **T81.593** Other complications of foreign body accidentally left in body following injection or immunization ᴄᴄ

7 ✓7ᵗʰ **T81.594** Other complications of foreign body accidentally left in body following endoscopic examination ᴄᴄ

7 ✓7ᵗʰ **T81.595** Other complications of foreign body accidentally left in body following heart catheterization ᴄᴄ

7 ✓7ᵗʰ **T81.596** Other complications of foreign body accidentally left in body following aspiration, puncture or other catheterization ᴄᴄ

7 ✓7ᵗʰ **T81.597** Other complications of foreign body accidentally left in body following removal of catheter or packing ᴄᴄ

7 ✓7ᵗʰ **T81.598** Other complications of foreign body accidentally left in body following other procedure ᴄᴄ

7 ✓7ᵗʰ **T81.599** Other complications of foreign body accidentally left in body following unspecified procedure ᴄᴄ

7 HAC = Initial encounter only (7th character A, B or C) and not POA.

✓ Additional Character Required   ✓7ᵗʰ Placeholder Alert   Unacceptable PDx   Manifestation   Hospital Acquired Condition   EXCLUDES 1 Not Coded Here   EXCLUDES 2 Not Included Here

ICD-10-CM 2016   1137

Chapter 19. Injury, Poisoning, and Certain Other Consequences of External Causes

T81.507–T81.599

Chapter 19. Injury, Poisoning, and Certain Other Consequences of External Causes *(side tab)*

T81.6–T82.191 *(side tab)*

√5ᵗʰ **T81.6** **Acute reaction to foreign substance accidentally left during a procedure**

EXCLUDES 2   *complications of foreign body accidentally left in body cavity or operation wound following procedure (T81.5-)*

CC Excl: For CC codes in subcategory T81.6: CC with 7th character A, unless otherwise noted: D78.81-D78.89, E36.8, E89.810-E89.89, H59.011-H59.019, H59.031-H59.099, H59.811-H59.89, H95.811-H95.89, I97.3, L76.81-L76.82, M96.89, N98.1-N98.9, T81.60-T81.69 with 7th A, T81.82XA, T81.89X-T81.9XX with 7th A

7   √x7ᵗʰ   **T81.60**   **Unspecified acute reaction to foreign substance accidentally left during a procedure**   CC

7   √x7ᵗʰ   **T81.61**   **Aseptic peritonitis due to foreign substance accidentally left during a procedure**   CC
     Chemical peritonitis

7   √x7ᵗʰ   **T81.69**   **Other acute reaction to foreign substance accidentally left during a procedure**   CC

√5ᵗʰ **T81.7** **Vascular complications following a procedure, not elsewhere classified**
     Air embolism following procedure NEC
     Phlebitis or thrombophlebitis resulting from a procedure

EXCLUDES 1   *embolism complicating abortion or ectopic or molar pregnancy (O00-O07, O08.2)*
     embolism complicating pregnancy, childbirth and the puerperium (O88.-)
     traumatic embolism (T79.0)

EXCLUDES 2   *embolism due to prosthetic devices, implants and grafts (T82.8-, T83.8, T84.8-, T85.8)*
     embolism following infusion, transfusion and therapeutic injection (T80.0)

√6ᵗʰ **T81.71** **Complication of artery following a procedure, not elsewhere classified**

√7ᵗʰ **T81.710** **Complication of mesenteric artery following a procedure, not elsewhere classified**   CC
     CC Excl: CC with 7th character A: D78.81-D78.89, E36.8, E89.810-E89.89, H59.011-H59.019, H59.031-H59.099, H59.811-H59.89, H95.811-H95.89, I97.3, L76.81-L76.82, M96.89, N98.1-N98.9, T81.710-T81.72X with 7th A, T81.82XA, T81.89X-T81.9XX with 7th A

√7ᵗʰ **T81.711** **Complication of renal artery following a procedure, not elsewhere classified**   CC
     CC Excl: See code: T81.710

√7ᵗʰ **T81.718** **Complication of other artery following a procedure, not elsewhere classified**   CC
     CC Excl: CC with 7th character A: D78.81-D78.89, E36.8, E89.810-E89.89, H59.011-H59.019, H59.031-H59.099, H59.811-H59.89, H95.811-H95.89, I97.3, L76.81-L76.82, M96.89, N98.1-N98.9, T81.718-T81.72X with 7th A, T81.82XA, T81.89X-T81.9XX with 7th A

√7ᵗʰ **T81.719** **Complication of unspecified artery following a procedure, not elsewhere classified**   CC
     CC Excl: See code: T81.718

√x7ᵗʰ **T81.72** **Complication of vein following a procedure, not elsewhere classified**   CC
     CC Excl: See code: T81.718

√5ᵗʰ **T81.8** **Other complications of procedures, not elsewhere classified**

EXCLUDES 2   *hypothermia following anesthesia (T88.51)*
     malignant hyperpyrexia due to anesthesia (T88.3)

13   √x7ᵗʰ   **T81.81**   **Complication of inhalation therapy**

√x7ᵗʰ **T81.82** **Emphysema (subcutaneous) resulting from a procedure**

√x7ᵗʰ **T81.83** **Persistent postprocedural fistula**   CC
     CC Excl: CC with 7th character A: D78.81-D78.89, E36.8, E89.810-E89.89, H59.011-H59.019, H59.031-H59.099, H59.811-H59.89, H95.811-H95.89, I97.3, L76.81-L76.82, M96.89, N98.1-N98.9, T81.82X-T81.9XX with 7th A

√x7ᵗʰ **T81.89** **Other complications of procedures, not elsewhere classified**
     Use additional code to specify complication, such as:
       postprocedural delirium (F05)
     AHA: 2014, 1Q, 23

√x7ᵗʰ **T81.9** **Unspecified complication of procedure**

√4ᵗʰ **T82** **Complications of cardiac and vascular prosthetic devices, implants and grafts**

EXCLUDES 2   *failure and rejection of transplanted organs and tissue (T86.-)*

The appropriate 7th character is to be added to each code from category T82.
A   initial encounter
D   subsequent encounter
S   sequela

√5ᵗʰ **T82.0** **Mechanical complication of heart valve prosthesis**
     Mechanical complication of artificial heart valve

EXCLUDES 1   *mechanical complication of biological heart valve graft (T82.22-)*

CC Excl: For CC codes in subcategory T82.0: CC with 7th character A, unless otherwise noted: D78.81-D78.89, E36.8, E89.810-E89.89, H59.011-H59.019, H59.031-H59.099, H59.811-H59.89, H95.811-H95.89, I97.3, L76.81-L76.82, M96.89, N98.1-N98.9, T81.82XA, T81.89X-T82.09X with 7th A

√x7ᵗʰ **T82.01** **Breakdown (mechanical) of heart valve prosthesis**   CC

√x7ᵗʰ **T82.02** **Displacement of heart valve prosthesis**   CC
     Malposition of heart valve prosthesis

√x7ᵗʰ **T82.03** **Leakage of heart valve prosthesis**   CC

√x7ᵗʰ **T82.09** **Other mechanical complication of heart valve prosthesis**   CC
     Obstruction (mechanical) of heart valve prosthesis
     Perforation of heart valve prosthesis
     Protrusion of heart valve prosthesis

√5ᵗʰ **T82.1** **Mechanical complication of cardiac electronic device**

CC Excl: For CC codes in subcategory T82.1: CC with 7th character A, unless otherwise noted: D78.81-D78.89, E36.8, E89.810-E89.89, H59.011-H59.019, H59.031-H59.099, H59.811-H59.89, H95.811-H95.89, I97.3, L76.81-L76.82, M96.89, N98.1-N98.9, T81.82XA, T81.89X-T81.9XX with 7th A, T82.110-T82.111, T82.120-T82.121, T82.190-T82.191 with 7th A

√6ᵗʰ **T82.11** **Breakdown (mechanical) of cardiac electronic device**

√7ᵗʰ **T82.110** **Breakdown (mechanical) of cardiac electrode**   CC

√7ᵗʰ **T82.111** **Breakdown (mechanical) of cardiac pulse generator (battery)**   CC

√7ᵗʰ **T82.118** **Breakdown (mechanical) of other cardiac electronic device**   CC
     CC Excl: CC with 7th character A: D78.81-D78.89, E36.8, E89.810-E89.89, H59.011-H59.019, H59.031-H59.099, H59.811-H59.89, H95.811-H95.89, I97.3, L76.81-L76.82, M96.89, N98.1-N98.9, T81.82XA, T81.89X-T81.9XX with 7th A, T82.118A, T82.128A, T82.198A, T82.221-T82.228 with 7th A, T82.512A, T82.522A, T82.532A, T82.592A, T82.594A, T82.598A

√7ᵗʰ **T82.119** **Breakdown (mechanical) of unspecified cardiac electronic device**   CC
     CC Excl: No Excl

√6ᵗʰ **T82.12** **Displacement of cardiac electronic device**
     Malposition of cardiac electronic device

√7ᵗʰ **T82.120** **Displacement of cardiac electrode**   CC

√7ᵗʰ **T82.121** **Displacement of cardiac pulse generator (battery)**   CC

√7ᵗʰ **T82.128** **Displacement of other cardiac electronic device**   CC
     CC Excl: See code: T82.118

√7ᵗʰ **T82.129** **Displacement of unspecified cardiac electronic device**   CC
     CC Excl: No Excl

√6ᵗʰ **T82.19** **Other mechanical complication of cardiac electronic device**
     Leakage of cardiac electronic device
     Obstruction of cardiac electronic device
     Perforation of cardiac electronic device
     Protrusion of cardiac electronic device

√7ᵗʰ **T82.190** **Other mechanical complication of cardiac electrode**   CC

√7ᵗʰ **T82.191** **Other mechanical complication of cardiac pulse generator (battery)**   CC

---

7   HAC = Initial encounter only (7th character A, B, or C – specific to category) and not POA.
13   Questionable admission when used as PDx.

N Newborn: 0   P Pediatric: 0-17   M Maternity: 12-55   A Adult: 15-124   **MCC** Major CC Condition   **PDxMCC** PDx acts as own MCC   **CC** CC Condition   **PDxCC** PDx acts as own CC

√7ᵗʰ **T82.198 Other mechanical complication of other cardiac electronic device**
CC Excl: See code: T82.118

√7ᵗʰ **T82.199 Other mechanical complication of unspecified cardiac device**
CC Excl: No Excl

√5ᵗʰ **T82.2 Mechanical complication of coronary artery bypass graft and biological heart valve graft**
EXCLUDES 1 mechanical complication of artificial heart valve prosthesis (T82.0-d)

√6ᵗʰ **T82.21 Mechanical complication of coronary artery bypass graft**

CC Excl: For CC codes in subcategory T82.21: CC with 7th character A, unless otherwise noted: D78.81-D78.89, E36.8, E89.810-E89.89, H59.011-H59.019, H59.031-H59.099, H59.811-H59.89, H95.811-H95.89, I97.3, L76.81-L76.82, M96.89, N98.1-N98.9, T81.82XA, T81.89X-T81.9XX with 7th A, T82.211-T82.218 with 7th A

√7ᵗʰ **T82.211 Breakdown (mechanical) of coronary artery bypass graft**

√7ᵗʰ **T82.212 Displacement of coronary artery bypass graft**
Malposition of coronary artery bypass graft

√7ᵗʰ **T82.213 Leakage of coronary artery bypass graft**

√7ᵗʰ **T82.218 Other mechanical complication of coronary artery bypass graft**
Obstruction, mechanical of coronary artery bypass graft
Perforation of coronary artery bypass graft
Protrusion of coronary artery bypass graft

√6ᵗʰ **T82.22 Mechanical complication of biological heart valve graft**

CC Excl: For CC codes in subcategory T82.22: CC with 7th character A, unless otherwise noted: D78.81-D78.89, E36.8, E89.810-E89.89, H59.011-H59.019, H59.031-H59.099, H59.811-H59.89, H95.811-H95.89, I97.3, L76.81-L76.82, M96.89, N98.1-N98.9, T81.82XA, T81.89X-T81.9XX with 7th A, T82.118A,T82.128A,T82.198A,T82.221-T82.228 with 7th A, T82.512 with 7th A, T82.522 with 7th A, T82.532 with 7th A, T82.592 with 7th A, T82.594 with 7th A, T82.598 with 7th A

√7ᵗʰ **T82.221 Breakdown (mechanical) of biological heart valve graft**

√7ᵗʰ **T82.222 Displacement of biological heart valve graft**
Malposition of biological heart valve graft

√7ᵗʰ **T82.223 Leakage of biological heart valve graft**

√7ᵗʰ **T82.228 Other mechanical complication of biological heart valve graft**
Obstruction of biological heart valve graft
Perforation of biological heart valve graft
Protrusion of biological heart valve graft

√5ᵗʰ **T82.3 Mechanical complication of other vascular grafts**

CC Excl: For CC codes in subcategory T82.3: CC with 7th character A: D78.81-D78.89, E36.8, E89.810-E89.89, H59.011-H59.019, H59.031-H59.099, H59.811-H59.89, H95.811-H95.89, I97.3, L76.81-L76.82, M96.89, N98.1-N98.9, T81.82XA, T81.89X-T81.9XX with 7th A, T82.310-T82.511 with 7th A, T82.513-T82.518 with 7th A, T82.520-T82.521 with 7th A, T82.523-T82.531 with 7th A, T82.533-T82.538 with 7th A, T82.590-T82.591 with 7th A, T82.593A, T82.595A

√6ᵗʰ **T82.31 Breakdown (mechanical) of other vascular grafts**

√7ᵗʰ **T82.310 Breakdown (mechanical) of aortic (bifurcation) graft (replacement)**

√7ᵗʰ **T82.311 Breakdown (mechanical) of carotid arterial graft (bypass)**

√7ᵗʰ **T82.312 Breakdown (mechanical) of femoral arterial graft (bypass)**

√7ᵗʰ **T82.318 Breakdown (mechanical) of other vascular grafts**

√7ᵗʰ **T82.319 Breakdown (mechanical) of unspecified vascular grafts**

√6ᵗʰ **T82.32 Displacement of other vascular grafts**
Malposition of other vascular grafts

√7ᵗʰ **T82.320 Displacement of aortic (bifurcation) graft (replacement)**

√7ᵗʰ **T82.321 Displacement of carotid arterial graft (bypass)**

√7ᵗʰ **T82.322 Displacement of femoral arterial graft (bypass)**

√7ᵗʰ **T82.328 Displacement of other vascular grafts**

√7ᵗʰ **T82.329 Displacement of unspecified vascular grafts**

√6ᵗʰ **T82.33 Leakage of other vascular grafts**

√7ᵗʰ **T82.330 Leakage of aortic (bifurcation) graft (replacement)**

√7ᵗʰ **T82.331 Leakage of carotid arterial graft (bypass)**

√7ᵗʰ **T82.332 Leakage of femoral arterial graft (bypass)**

√7ᵗʰ **T82.338 Leakage of other vascular grafts**

√7ᵗʰ **T82.339 Leakage of unspecified vascular graft**

√6ᵗʰ **T82.39 Other mechanical complication of other vascular grafts**
Obstruction (mechanical) of other vascular grafts
Perforation of other vascular grafts
Protrusion of other vascular grafts

√7ᵗʰ **T82.390 Other mechanical complication of aortic (bifurcation) graft (replacement)**

√7ᵗʰ **T82.391 Other mechanical complication of carotid arterial graft (bypass)**

√7ᵗʰ **T82.392 Other mechanical complication of femoral arterial graft (bypass)**

√7ᵗʰ **T82.398 Other mechanical complication of other vascular grafts**

√7ᵗʰ **T82.399 Other mechanical complication of unspecified vascular grafts**

√5ᵗʰ **T82.4 Mechanical complication of vascular dialysis catheter**
Mechanical complication of hemodialysis catheter
EXCLUDES 1 mechanical complication of intraperitoneal dialysis catheter (T85.62)

CC Excl: For CC codes in subcategory T82.4: CC with 7th character A, unless otherwise noted: See code: T82.3

√x7ᵗʰ **T82.41 Breakdown (mechanical) of vascular dialysis catheter**

√x7ᵗʰ **T82.42 Displacement of vascular dialysis catheter**
Malposition of vascular dialysis catheter

√x7ᵗʰ **T82.43 Leakage of vascular dialysis catheter**

√x7ᵗʰ **T82.49 Other complication of vascular dialysis catheter**
Obstruction (mechanical) of vascular dialysis catheter
Perforation of vascular dialysis catheter
Protrusion of vascular dialysis catheter

√5ᵗʰ **T82.5 Mechanical complication of other cardiac and vascular devices and implants**
EXCLUDES 2 mechanical complication of epidural and subdural infusion catheter (T85.61)

CC Excl: For CC codes in subcategory T82.5: CC with 7th character A, unless otherwise noted: D78.81-D78.89, E36.8, E89.810-E89.89, H59.011-H59.019, H59.031-H59.099, H59.811-H59.89, H95.811-H95.89, I97.3, L76.81-L76.82, M96.89, N98.1-N98.9, T81.82XA, T81.89X-T81.9XX with 7th A, T82.310-T82.511 with 7th A, T82.513-T82.518 with 7th A, T82.520-T82.521 with 7th A, T82.523-T82.531 with 7th A, T82.533-T82.538 with 7th A, T82.590-T82.591 with 7th A, T82.593A, T82.595A

√6ᵗʰ **T82.51 Breakdown (mechanical) of other cardiac and vascular devices and implants**

√7ᵗʰ **T82.510 Breakdown (mechanical) of surgically created arteriovenous fistula**

√7ᵗʰ **T82.511 Breakdown (mechanical) of surgically created arteriovenous shunt**

√7ᵗʰ **T82.512 Breakdown (mechanical) of artificial** CC
heart
CC Excl: CC with 7th character A: D78.81-
D78.89, E36.8, E89.810-E89.89, H59.011-
H59.019, H59.031-H59.099, H59.811-H59.89,
H95.811-H95.89, I97.3, L76.81-L76.82,
M96.89, N98.1-N98.9, T81.82XA, T81.89X-
T81.9XX with 7th A, T82.118A, T82.128A,
T82.198A, T82.221-T82.228 with 7th A,
T82.512A, T82.522A, T82.532A, T82.592A,
T82.594A, T82.598A

√7ᵗʰ **T82.513 Breakdown (mechanical) of balloon** CC
(counterpulsation) device

√7ᵗʰ **T82.514 Breakdown (mechanical) of infusion** CC
catheter

√7ᵗʰ **T82.515 Breakdown (mechanical) of umbrella** CC
device

√7ᵗʰ **T82.518 Breakdown (mechanical) of other** CC
**cardiac and vascular devices and
implants**

√7ᵗʰ **T82.519 Breakdown (mechanical) of** CC
**unspecified cardiac and vascular
devices and implants**
CC Excl: CC with 7th character A: D78.81-
D78.89, E36.8, E89.810-E89.89, H59.011-
H59.019, H59.031-H59.099, H59.811-H59.89,
H95.811-H95.89, I97.3, L76.81-L76.82,
M96.89, N98.1-N98.9, T81.82XA, T81.89X-
T81.9XX with 7th A, T82.519A, T82.539A,
T82.599-T82.9XX with 7th character A,
T85.9XXA

√6ᵗʰ **T82.52 Displacement of other cardiac and vascular devices
and implants**
Malposition of other cardiac and vascular devices and
implants

√7ᵗʰ **T82.520 Displacement of surgically created** CC
arteriovenous fistula

√7ᵗʰ **T82.521 Displacement of surgically created** CC
arteriovenous shunt

√7ᵗʰ **T82.522 Displacement of artificial heart** CC
CC Excl: CC with 7th character A: D78.81-
D78.89, E36.8, E89.810-E89.89, H59.011-
H59.019, H59.031-H59.099, H59.811-H59.89,
H95.811-H95.89, I97.3, L76.81-L76.82,
M96.89, N98.1-N98.9, T81.82XA, T81.89X-
T81.9XX with 7th A, T82.118A, T82.128A,
T82.198A, T82.221-T82.228 with 7th A,
T82.512A, T82.522A, T82.532A, T82.592A,
T82.594A, T82.598A

√7ᵗʰ **T82.523 Displacement of balloon** CC
(counterpulsation) device

√7ᵗʰ **T82.524 Displacement of infusion catheter** CC

√7ᵗʰ **T82.525 Displacement of umbrella device** CC

√7ᵗʰ **T82.528 Displacement of other cardiac and** CC
vascular devices and implants

√7ᵗʰ **T82.529 Displacement of unspecified cardiac** CC
and vascular devices and implants

√6ᵗʰ **T82.53 Leakage of other cardiac and vascular devices and
implants**

√7ᵗʰ **T82.530 Leakage of surgically created** CC
arteriovenous fistula

√7ᵗʰ **T82.531 Leakage of surgically created** CC
arteriovenous shunt

√7ᵗʰ **T82.532 Leakage of artificial heart** CC
CC Excl: CC with 7th character A: D78.81-
D78.89, E36.8, E89.810-E89.89, H59.011-
H59.019, H59.031-H59.099, H59.811-H59.89,
H95.811-H95.89, I97.3, L76.81-L76.82,
M96.89, N98.1-N98.9, T81.82XA, T81.89X-
T81.9XX with 7th A, T82.118A, T82.128A,
T82.198A, T82.221-T82.228 with 7th A,
T82.512A, T82.522A, T82.532A, T82.592A,
T82.594A, T82.598A

√7ᵗʰ **T82.533 Leakage of balloon (counterpulsation)** CC
device

√7ᵗʰ **T82.534 Leakage of infusion catheter** CC

√7ᵗʰ **T82.535 Leakage of umbrella device** CC

√7ᵗʰ **T82.538 Leakage of other cardiac and vascular** CC
devices and implants

√7ᵗʰ **T82.539 Leakage of unspecified cardiac and** CC
vascular devices and implants
CC Excl: CC with 7th character A:D78.81-
D78.89, E36.8, E89.810-E89.89, H59.011-
H59.019, H59.031-H59.099, H59.811-H59.89,
H95.811-H95.89, I97.3, L76.81-L76.82,
M96.89, N98.1-N98.9, T81.82XA, T81.89X-
T81.9XX with 7th A, T82.519A, T82.539A,
T82.599-T82.9XX with 7th A, T85.9XXA

√6ᵗʰ **T82.59 Other mechanical complication of other cardiac and
vascular devices and implants**
Obstruction (mechanical) of other cardiac and vascular
devices and implants
Perforation of other cardiac and vascular devices and
implants
Protrusion of other cardiac and vascular devices and
implants

√7ᵗʰ **T82.590 Other mechanical complication of** CC
surgically created arteriovenous fistula

√7ᵗʰ **T82.591 Other mechanical complication of** CC
surgically created arteriovenous shunt

√7ᵗʰ **T82.592 Other mechanical complication of** CC
artificial heart
CC Excl: CC with 7th character A: D78.81-
D78.89, E36.8, E89.810-E89.89, H59.011-
H59.019, H59.031-H59.099, H59.811-H59.89,
H95.811-H95.89, I97.3, L76.81-L76.82,
M96.89, N98.1-N98.9, T81.82XA, T81.89X-
T81.9XX with 7th A, T82.118A, T82.128A,
T82.198A,T82.221-T82.228 with 7th A,
T82.512A, T82.522A, T82.532A, T82.592A,
T82.594A, T82.598 with 7th A

√7ᵗʰ **T82.593 Other mechanical complication of** CC
balloon (counterpulsation) device

√7ᵗʰ **T82.594 Other mechanical complication of** CC
infusion catheter
CC Excl: CC with 7th character A: D78.81-
D78.89, E36.8, E89.810-E89.89, H59.011-
H59.019, H59.031-H59.099, H59.811-H59.89,
H95.811-H95.89, I97.3, L76.81-L76.82,
M96.89, N98.1-N98.9, T81.82XA, T81.89X-
T81.9XX with 7th A, T82.118A, T82.128A,
T82.198A, T82.310-T82.511 with 7th A,
T82.513-T82.518 with 7th A, T82.520-
T82.521 with 7th A, T82.523-T82.531 with
7th A, T82.533-T82.538 with 7th A, T82.590-
T82.591 with 7th A, T82.593A, T82.595 with
7th A

√7ᵗʰ **T82.595 Other mechanical complication of** CC
umbrella device

√7ᵗʰ **T82.598 Other mechanical complication of** CC
**other cardiac and vascular devices and
implants**
CC Excl: CC with 7th character A: D78.81-
D78.89, E36.8, E89.810-E89.89, H59.011-
H59.019, H59.031-H59.099, H59.811-H59.89,
H95.811-H95.89, I97.3, L76.81-L76.82,
M96.89, N98.1-N98.9, T81.82XA, T81.89X-
T81.9XX with 7th A, T82.118A, T82.128A,
T82.198A,T82.221-T82.228 with 7th A,
T82.512A, T82.522A, T82.532A, T82.592 A,
T82.594A, T82.598A

√7ᵗʰ **T82.599 Other mechanical complication of** CC
**unspecified cardiac and vascular devices
and implants**
CC Excl: CC with 7th character A: D78.81-
D78.89, E36.8, E89.810-E89.89, H59.011-
H59.019, H59.031-H59.099, H59.811-H59.89,
H95.811-H95.89, I97.3, L76.81-L76.82,
M96.89, N98.1-N98.9, T81.82XA, T81.89X-
T81.9XX with 7th A, T82.519A, T82.539A,
T82.599-T82.9XX with 7th A, T85.9XXA

8 √x7ᵗʰ **T82.6 Infection and inflammatory reaction due to cardiac valve** CC
prosthesis
Use additional code to identify infection
CC Excl: CC with 7th character A: D78.81-D78.89, E36.8, E89.810-
E89.89, H59.011-H59.019, H59.031-H59.099, H59.811-H59.89,
H95.811-H95.89, I97.3, L76.81-L76.82, M96.89, N98.1-N98.9,
T81.82XA, T81.89X-T82.09X with 7th A, T82.110-T82.118 with 7th
A, T82.120-T82.128 with 7th A, T82.190-T82.198 with 7th A,
T82.211-T82.9XX with 7th A, T85.310-T85.311 with 7th A, T85.320-
T85.321 with 7th A, T85.390-T85.391 with 7th A, T85.510-T85.9XX
with 7th A, T86.820-T86.829, T86.842-T86.849

---

8 HAC = as SDx not POA, in combination with one of the following procedure codes: 02H43[J,K,M]Z; 02H[6,7]3[J,M]Z; 02H[K,L]3JZ; 02HN[0,3,4][J,M]Z; 02PA[0,3,4]MZ; 02PAXMZ;
02WA[0,3,4]MZ; 0JH[6,8][0,3][4,5,6,7,8,9,P]Z; 0JPT[0,3]PZ; 0JWT[0,3]PZ.

N Newborn: 0   P Pediatric: 0-17   M Maternity: 12-55   A Adult: 15-124   MCC Major CC Condition   PDxMCC PDx acts as own MCC   CC CC Condition   PDxCC PDx acts as own CC

1140

ICD-10-CM 2016

8 ✓x7th **T82.7** Infection and inflammatory reaction due to other cardiac and vascular devices, implants and grafts   CC
    Use additional code to identify infection
    CC Excl: See code: T82.6

✓5th **T82.8** Other specified complications of cardiac and vascular prosthetic devices, implants and grafts

   ✓6th **T82.81** Embolism of cardiac and vascular prosthetic devices, implants and grafts

     ✓7th **T82.817** Embolism of cardiac prosthetic devices, implants and grafts   CC
      CC Excl: CC with 7th character A: D78.81-D78.89, E36.8, E89.810-E89.89, H59.011-H59.019, H59.031-H59.099, H59.811-H59.89, H95.811-H95.89, I97.3, L76.81-L76.82, M96.89, N98.1-N98.9, T81.82XA, T81.89X-T82.09X with 7th A, T82.110-T82.118 with 7th A, T82.120-T82.128 with 7th A, T82.190-T82.198 with 7th A, T82.221-T82.9XX with 7th A, T85.310-T85.311 with 7th A, T85.320-T85.321 with 7th A, T85.390-T85.391 with 7th A, T85.510-T85.9XX with 7th A, T86.820-T86.829, T86.842-T86.849

     ✓7th **T82.818** Embolism of vascular prosthetic devices, implants and grafts   CC
      CC Excl: CC with 7th character A: D78.81-D78.89, E36.8, E89.810-E89.89, H59.011-H59.019, H59.031-H59.099, H59.811-H59.89, H95.811-H95.89, I97.3, L76.81-L76.82, M96.89, N98.1-N98.9, T81.82XA, T81.89X-T82.09X with 7th A, T82.110-T82.118 with 7th A, T82.120-T82.128 with 7th A, T82.190-T82.198 with 7th A, T82.211-T82.9XX with 7th A, T85.310-T85.311 with 7th A, T85.320-T85.321 with 7th A, T85.390-T85.391 with 7th A, T85.510-T85.9XX with 7th A, T86.820-T86.829, T86.842-T86.849

   ✓6th **T82.82** Fibrosis of cardiac and vascular prosthetic devices, implants and grafts

     ✓7th **T82.827** Fibrosis of cardiac prosthetic devices, implants and grafts   CC
      CC Excl: See code: T82.817

     ✓7th **T82.828** Fibrosis of vascular prosthetic devices, implants and grafts   CC
      CC Excl: See code: T82.818

   ✓6th **T82.83** Hemorrhage of cardiac and vascular prosthetic devices, implants and grafts

     ✓7th **T82.837** Hemorrhage of cardiac prosthetic devices, implants and grafts   CC
      CC Excl: See code: T82.817

     ✓7th **T82.838** Hemorrhage of vascular prosthetic devices, implants and grafts   CC
      CC Excl: See code: T82.818

   ✓6th **T82.84** Pain from cardiac and vascular prosthetic devices, implants and grafts

     ✓7th **T82.847** Pain from cardiac prosthetic devices, implants and grafts   CC
      CC Excl: See code: T82.817

     ✓7th **T82.848** Pain from vascular prosthetic devices, implants and grafts   CC
      CC Excl: See code: T82.818

   ✓6th **T82.85** Stenosis of cardiac and vascular prosthetic devices, implants and grafts

     ✓7th **T82.857** Stenosis of cardiac prosthetic devices, implants and grafts   CC
      CC Excl: See code: T82.817

     ✓7th **T82.858** Stenosis of vascular prosthetic devices, implants and grafts   CC
      CC Excl: See code: T82.818

   ✓6th **T82.86** Thrombosis of cardiac and vascular prosthetic devices, implants and grafts

     ✓7th **T82.867** Thrombosis of cardiac prosthetic devices, implants and grafts   CC
      CC Excl: See code: T82.817

     ✓7th **T82.868** Thrombosis of vascular prosthetic devices, implants and grafts   CC
      CC Excl: See code: T82.818

   ✓6th **T82.89** Other specified complication of cardiac and vascular prosthetic devices, implants and grafts

---

     ✓7th **T82.897** Other specified complication of cardiac prosthetic devices, implants and grafts   CC
      CC Excl: See code: T82.817

     ✓7th **T82.898** Other specified complication of vascular prosthetic devices, implants and grafts   CC
      CC Excl: See code: T82.818

✓x7th **T82.9** Unspecified complication of cardiac and vascular prosthetic device, implant and graft   CC
    CC Excl: See code: T82.817

✓4th **T83** Complications of genitourinary prosthetic devices, implants and grafts
   EXCLUDES 2   failure and rejection of transplanted organs and tissue (T86.-)

   The appropriate 7th character is to be added to each code from category T83.
   A   initial encounter
   D   subsequent encounter
   S   sequela

✓5th **T83.0** Mechanical complication of urinary (indwelling) catheter
   EXCLUDES 2   complications of stoma of urinary tract (N99.5-)

   For CC codes in subcategory T83.0: CC with 7th character A, unless otherwise noted: D78.81-D78.89, E36.8, E89.810-E89.89, H59.011-H59.019, H59.031-H59.099, H59.811-H59.89, H95.811-H95.89, I97.3, L76.81-L76.82, M96.89, N98.1-N98.9, N99.510-N99.518, T81.82XA, T81.89X-T81.9XX with 7th A, T83.010A, T83.020A, T83.030A, T83.090A, T83.110-T83.29X with 7th A, T83.410-T83.718 with 7th A, T83.728-T83.9XX with 7th A

   ✓6th **T83.01** Breakdown (mechanical) of urinary (indwelling) catheter

     ✓7th **T83.010** Breakdown (mechanical) of cystostomy catheter   CC

     ✓7th **T83.018** Breakdown (mechanical) of other indwelling urethral catheter

   ✓6th **T83.02** Displacement of urinary (indwelling) catheter
    Malposition of urinary (indwelling) catheter

     ✓7th **T83.020** Displacement of cystostomy catheter   CC

     ✓7th **T83.028** Displacement of other indwelling urethral catheter

   ✓6th **T83.03** Leakage of urinary (indwelling) catheter

     ✓7th **T83.030** Leakage of cystostomy catheter   CC

     ✓7th **T83.038** Leakage of other indwelling urethral catheter

   ✓6th **T83.09** Other mechanical complication of urinary (indwelling) catheter
    Obstruction (mechanical) of urinary (indwelling) catheter
    Perforation of urinary (indwelling) catheter
    Protrusion of urinary (indwelling) catheter

     ✓7th **T83.090** Other mechanical complication of cystostomy catheter   CC

     ✓7th **T83.098** Other mechanical complication of other indwelling urethral catheter

✓5th **T83.1** Mechanical complication of other urinary devices and implants

   CC Excl: For CC codes in subcategory T83.0: CC with 7th character A, unless otherwise noted: See code: T83.0

   ✓6th **T83.11** Breakdown (mechanical) of other urinary devices and implants

     ✓7th **T83.110** Breakdown (mechanical) of urinary electronic stimulator device   CC

     ✓7th **T83.111** Breakdown (mechanical) of urinary sphincter implant   CC

     ✓7th **T83.112** Breakdown (mechanical) of urinary stent   CC

     ✓7th **T83.118** Breakdown (mechanical) of other urinary devices and implants   CC

   ✓6th **T83.12** Displacement of other urinary devices and implants
    Malposition of other urinary devices and implants

     ✓7th **T83.120** Displacement of urinary electronic stimulator device   CC

     ✓7th **T83.121** Displacement of urinary sphincter implant

---

8   HAC = as SDx not POA, in combination with one of the following procedure codes: 02H43[J,K,M]Z; 02H[6,7]3[J,M]Z; 02H[K,L]3JZ; 02HN[0,3,4][J,M]Z; 02PA[0,3,4]MZ; 02PAXMZ; 02WA[0,3,4]MZ; 0JH[6,8][0,3][4,5,6,7,8,9,P]Z; 0JPT[0,3]PZ; 0JWT[0,3]PZ.

✓7ᵗʰ **T83.122** Displacement of urinary stent ▢CC

✓7ᵗʰ **T83.128** Displacement of other urinary devices and implants ▢CC

✓6ᵗʰ **T83.19** Other mechanical complication of other urinary devices and implants
Leakage of other urinary devices and implants
Obstruction (mechanical) of other urinary devices and implants
Perforation of other urinary devices and implants
Protrusion of other urinary devices and implants

✓7ᵗʰ **T83.190** Other mechanical complication of urinary electronic stimulator device ▢CC

✓7ᵗʰ **T83.191** Other mechanical complication of urinary sphincter implant ▢CC

✓7ᵗʰ **T83.192** Other mechanical complication of urinary stent ▢CC

✓7ᵗʰ **T83.198** Other mechanical complication of other urinary devices and implants ▢CC

✓5ᵗʰ **T83.2** Mechanical complication of graft of urinary organ

> **CC Excl:** For CC codes in subcategory T83.0: CC with 7th character A, unless otherwise noted: See code: T83.0

✓x7ᵗʰ **T83.21** Breakdown (mechanical) of graft of urinary organ ▢CC

✓x7ᵗʰ **T83.22** Displacement of graft of urinary organ ▢CC
Malposition of graft of urinary organ

✓x7ᵗʰ **T83.23** Leakage of graft of urinary organ ▢CC

✓x7ᵗʰ **T83.29** Other mechanical complication of graft of urinary organ ▢CC
Obstruction (mechanical) of graft of urinary organ
Perforation of graft of urinary organ
Protrusion of graft of urinary organ

✓5ᵗʰ **T83.3** Mechanical complication of intrauterine contraceptive device

✓x7ᵗʰ **T83.31** Breakdown (mechanical) of intrauterine contraceptive device ♀

✓x7ᵗʰ **T83.32** Displacement of intrauterine contraceptive device ♀
Malposition of intrauterine contraceptive device

✓x7ᵗʰ **T83.39** Other mechanical complication of intrauterine contraceptive device ♀
Leakage of intrauterine contraceptive device
Obstruction (mechanical) of intrauterine contraceptive device
Perforation of intrauterine contraceptive device
Protrusion of intrauterine contraceptive device

✓5ᵗʰ **T83.4** Mechanical complication of other prosthetic devices, implants and grafts of genital tract

> **CC Excl:** For CC codes in subcategory T83.0: CC with 7th character A, unless otherwise noted: See code: T83.0

✓6ᵗʰ **T83.41** Breakdown (mechanical) of other prosthetic devices, implants and grafts of genital tract

✓7ᵗʰ **T83.410** Breakdown (mechanical) of penile (implanted) prosthesis ▢CC ♂

✓7ᵗʰ **T83.418** Breakdown (mechanical) of other prosthetic devices, implants and grafts of genital tract ▢CC

✓6ᵗʰ **T83.42** Displacement of other prosthetic devices, implants and grafts of genital tract
Malposition of other prosthetic devices, implants and grafts of genital tract

✓7ᵗʰ **T83.420** Displacement of penile (implanted) prosthesis ▢CC ♂

✓7ᵗʰ **T83.428** Displacement of other prosthetic devices, implants and grafts of genital tract ▢CC

✓6ᵗʰ **T83.49** Other mechanical complication of other prosthetic devices, implants and grafts of genital tract
Leakage of other prosthetic devices, implants and grafts of genital tract
Obstruction, mechanical of other prosthetic devices, implants and grafts of genital tract
Perforation of other prosthetic devices, implants and grafts of genital tract
Protrusion of other prosthetic devices, implants and grafts of genital tract

✓7ᵗʰ **T83.490** Other mechanical complication of penile (implanted) prosthesis ▢CC ♂

✓7ᵗʰ **T83.498** Other mechanical complication of other prosthetic devices, implants and grafts of genital tract ▢CC

✓5ᵗʰ **T83.5** Infection and inflammatory reaction due to prosthetic device, implant and graft in urinary system
Use additional code to identify infection

7 ✓x7ᵗʰ **T83.51** **Infection and inflammatory reaction due to indwelling urinary catheter** ▢CC
　EXCLUDES 2 complications of stoma of urinary tract (N99.5-)
CC Excl: CC with 7th character A: D78.81-D78.89, E36.8, E89.810-E89.89, H59.011-H59.019, H59.031-H59.099, H59.811-H59.89, H95.811-H95.89, I97.3, L76.81-L76.82, M96.89, N39.0, N98.1-N98.9, N99.510-N99.518, T81.82XA, T81.89X-T81.9XX with 7th A, T83.010A, T83.020A, T83.030A, T83.090A, T83.110-T83.29X with 7th A, T83.410-T83.718 with 7th A, T83.728-T83.9XX with 7th A, T85.310-T85.311 with 7th A, T85.320-T85.321 with 7th A, T85.390-T85.391 with 7th A, T85.510-T85.612 with 7th A, T85.614-T85.622 with 7th A, T85.624-T85.692 with 7th A, T85.694-T85.9XX with 7th A, T86.842-T86.849

✓x7ᵗʰ **T83.59** Infection and inflammatory reaction due to prosthetic device, implant and graft in urinary system ▢CC
CC Excl: CC with 7th character A: D78.81-D78.89, E36.8, E89.810-E89.89, H59.011-H59.019, H59.031-H59.099, H59.811-H59.89, H95.811-H95.89, I97.3, L76.81-L76.82, M96.89, N98.1-N98.9, N99.510-N99.518, T81.82XA, T81.89X-T81.9XX with 7th A, T83.010A, T83.020A, T83.030A, T83.090A, T83.110-T83.29X with 7th A, T83.410-T83.718 with 7th A, T83.728-T83.9XX with 7th A, T85.310-T85.311 with 7th A, T85.320-T85.321 with 7th A, T85.390-T85.391 with 7th A, T85.510-T85.9XX with 7th A, T86.820-T86.829, T86.842-T86.849

✓x7ᵗʰ **T83.6** Infection and inflammatory reaction due to prosthetic device, implant and graft in genital tract ▢CC
Use additional code to identify infection
CC Excl: See code: T83.59

✓5ᵗʰ **T83.7** Complications due to implanted mesh and other prosthetic materials

✓6ᵗʰ **T83.71** Erosion of implanted mesh and other prosthetic materials to surrounding organ or tissue

✓7ᵗʰ **T83.711** Erosion of implanted vaginal mesh and other prosthetic materials to surrounding organ or tissue ♀
Erosion of implanted vaginal mesh and other prosthetic materials into pelvic floor muscles

✓7ᵗʰ **T83.718** Erosion of other implanted mesh and other prosthetic materials to surrounding organ or tissue ▢CC
CC Excl: CC with 7th character A: D78.81-D78.89, E36.8, E89.810-E89.89, H59.011-H59.019, H59.031-H59.099, H59.811-H59.89, H95.811-H95.89, I97.3, L76.81-L76.82, M96.89, N98.1-N98.9, N99.510-N99.518, T81.82XA, T81.89X-T81.9XX with 7th A, T83.010A, T83.020A, T83.030A, T83.090A, T83.110-T83.29X with 7th A, T83.410-T83.718 with 7th A, T83.728-T83.9XX with 7th A

✓6ᵗʰ **T83.72** Exposure of implanted mesh and other prosthetic materials into surrounding organ or tissue

✓7ᵗʰ **T83.721** Exposure of implanted vaginal mesh and other prosthetic materials into vagina ♀
Exposure of implanted vaginal mesh and other prosthetic materials through vaginal wall

✓7ᵗʰ **T83.728** Exposure of other implanted mesh and other prosthetic materials to surrounding organ or tissue ▢CC
CC Excl: See code: T83.718

---

7 HAC = Initial encounter only (7th character A, B or C) and not POA.

☑5ᵗʰ **T83.8** **Other specified complications of** genitourinary prosthetic devices, implants and grafts

> **CC Excl: For CC/MCC codes in subcategory T83.8: CC with 7th character A, unless otherwise noted:** D78.81-D78.89, E36.8, E89.810-E89.89, H59.011-H59.019, H59.031-H59.099, H59.811-H59.89, H95.811-H95.89, I97.3, L76.81-L76.82, M96.89, N98.1-N98.9, N99.510-N99.518, T81.82XA, T81.89X-T81.9XX with 7th A, T83.010A, T83.020A, T83.030 A, T83.090A, T83.110-T83.29X with 7th A, T83.410-T83.718 with 7th A, T83.728-T83.9XX with 7th A, T85.310-T85.311 with 7th A, T85.320-T85.321 with 7th A, T85.390-T85.391 with 7th A, T85.510-T85.9XX with 7th A, T86.820-T86.829, T86.842-T86.849

√x7ᵗʰ **T83.81** **Embolism of** genitourinary prosthetic devices, implants and grafts   CC

√x7ᵗʰ **T83.82** **Fibrosis of** genitourinary prosthetic devices, implants and grafts   CC

√x7ᵗʰ **T83.83** **Hemorrhage of** genitourinary prosthetic devices, implants and grafts   CC

√x7ᵗʰ **T83.84** **Pain from** genitourinary prosthetic devices, implants and grafts   CC

√x7ᵗʰ **T83.85** **Stenosis of** genitourinary prosthetic devices, implants and grafts   CC

√x7ᵗʰ **T83.86** **Thrombosis of** genitourinary prosthetic devices, implants and grafts   CC

√x7ᵗʰ **T83.89** **Other specified complication of** genitourinary prosthetic devices, implants and grafts   CC

√x7ᵗʰ **T83.9** **Unspecified complication of** genitourinary prosthetic device, implant and graft   CC
CC Excl: See code: T83.8

☑4ᵗʰ **T84** **Complications of internal orthopedic prosthetic devices, implants and grafts**
> EXCLUDES 2   failure and rejection of transplanted organs and tissues (T86.-)
> fracture of bone following insertion of orthopedic implant, joint prosthesis or bone plate (M96.6)

> The appropriate 7th character is to be added to each code from category T84.
> A   initial encounter
> D   subsequent encounter
> S   sequela

☑5ᵗʰ **T84.0** **Mechanical complication of** internal joint prosthesis

> **CC Excl: For CC codes in subcategory T84.0: CC with 7th character A, unless otherwise noted:** D78.81-D78.89, E36.8, E89.810-E89.89, H59.011-H59.019, H59.031-H59.099, H59.811-H59.89, H95.811-H95.89, I97.3, L76.81-L76.82, M96.621-M96.69, M96.89, N98.1-N98.9, T81.82XA, T81.89X-T81.9XX with 7th A, T84.010-T84.9XX with 7th A

☑6ᵗʰ **T84.01** **Broken internal joint prosthesis**
Breakage (fracture) of prosthetic joint
Broken prosthetic joint implant
> EXCLUDES 1   periprosthetic joint implant fracture (T84.04)

√7ᵗʰ **T84.010** **Broken internal right hip prosthesis**   CC
√7ᵗʰ **T84.011** **Broken internal left hip prosthesis**   CC
√7ᵗʰ **T84.012** **Broken internal right knee prosthesis**   CC
√7ᵗʰ **T84.013** **Broken internal left knee prosthesis**   CC
√7ᵗʰ **T84.018** **Broken internal joint prosthesis, other site**   CC
> Use additional code to identify the joint (Z96.6-)
√7ᵗʰ **T84.019** **Broken internal joint prosthesis, unspecified site**   CC

☑6ᵗʰ **T84.02** **Dislocation of internal joint prosthesis**
Instability of internal joint prosthesis
Subluxation of internal joint prosthesis
√7ᵗʰ **T84.020** **Dislocation of internal right hip prosthesis**   CC
√7ᵗʰ **T84.021** **Dislocation of internal left hip prosthesis**   CC
√7ᵗʰ **T84.022** **Instability of internal right knee prosthesis**   CC
√7ᵗʰ **T84.023** **Instability of internal left knee prosthesis**   CC
√7ᵗʰ **T84.028** **Dislocation of other internal joint prosthesis**   CC
> Use additional code to identify the joint (Z96.6-)

√7ᵗʰ **T84.029** **Dislocation of unspecified internal joint prosthesis**   CC

☑6ᵗʰ **T84.03** **Mechanical loosening of internal prosthetic joint**
Aseptic loosening of prosthetic joint
√7ᵗʰ **T84.030** **Mechanical loosening of internal right hip prosthetic joint**   CC
√7ᵗʰ **T84.031** **Mechanical loosening of internal left hip prosthetic joint**   CC
√7ᵗʰ **T84.032** **Mechanical loosening of internal right knee prosthetic joint**   CC
√7ᵗʰ **T84.033** **Mechanical loosening of internal left knee prosthetic joint**   CC
√7ᵗʰ **T84.038** **Mechanical loosening of other internal prosthetic joint**   CC
> Use additional code to identify the joint (Z96.6-)
√7ᵗʰ **T84.039** **Mechanical loosening of unspecified internal prosthetic joint**   CC

☑6ᵗʰ **T84.04** **Periprosthetic fracture around internal prosthetic joint**
> EXCLUDES 2   breakage (fracture) of prosthetic joint (T84.01)
√7ᵗʰ **T84.040** **Periprosthetic fracture around internal prosthetic right hip joint**   CC
√7ᵗʰ **T84.041** **Periprosthetic fracture around internal prosthetic left hip joint**   CC
√7ᵗʰ **T84.042** **Periprosthetic fracture around internal prosthetic right knee joint**   CC
√7ᵗʰ **T84.043** **Periprosthetic fracture around internal prosthetic left knee joint**   CC
√7ᵗʰ **T84.048** **Periprosthetic fracture around other internal prosthetic joint**   CC
> Use additional code to identify the joint (Z96.6-)
√7ᵗʰ **T84.049** **Periprosthetic fracture around unspecified internal prosthetic joint**   CC

☑6ᵗʰ **T84.05** **Periprosthetic osteolysis of internal prosthetic joint**
> Use additional code to identify major osseous defect, if applicable (M89.7-)
√7ᵗʰ **T84.050** **Periprosthetic osteolysis of internal prosthetic right hip joint**   CC
√7ᵗʰ **T84.051** **Periprosthetic osteolysis of internal prosthetic left hip joint**   CC
√7ᵗʰ **T84.052** **Periprosthetic osteolysis of internal prosthetic right knee joint**   CC
√7ᵗʰ **T84.053** **Periprosthetic osteolysis of internal prosthetic left knee joint**   CC
√7ᵗʰ **T84.058** **Periprosthetic osteolysis of other internal prosthetic joint**   CC
> Use additional code to identify the joint (Z96.6-)
√7ᵗʰ **T84.059** **Periprosthetic osteolysis of unspecified internal prosthetic joint**   CC

☑6ᵗʰ **T84.06** **Wear of articular bearing surface of internal prosthetic joint**
√7ᵗʰ **T84.060** **Wear of articular bearing surface of internal prosthetic right hip joint**   CC
√7ᵗʰ **T84.061** **Wear of articular bearing surface of internal prosthetic left hip joint**   CC
√7ᵗʰ **T84.062** **Wear of articular bearing surface of internal prosthetic right knee joint**   CC
√7ᵗʰ **T84.063** **Wear of articular bearing surface of internal prosthetic left knee joint**   CC
√7ᵗʰ **T84.068** **Wear of articular bearing surface of other internal prosthetic joint**   CC
> Use additional code to identify the joint (Z96.6-)
√7ᵗʰ **T84.069** **Wear of articular bearing surface of unspecified internal prosthetic joint**   CC

☑6ᵗʰ **T84.09** **Other mechanical complication of internal joint prosthesis**
Prosthetic joint implant failure NOS
√7ᵗʰ **T84.090** **Other mechanical complication of internal right hip prosthesis**   CC
√7ᵗʰ **T84.091** **Other mechanical complication of internal left hip prosthesis**   CC

√7ᵗʰ T84.092 Other mechanical complication of internal **right knee prosthesis** `CC`

√7ᵗʰ T84.093 Other mechanical complication of internal **left knee prosthesis** `CC`

√7ᵗʰ T84.098 Other mechanical complication of **other internal joint prosthesis** `CC`
     Use additional code to identify the joint (Z96.6-)

√7ᵗʰ T84.099 Other mechanical complication of **unspecified internal joint prosthesis** `CC`

√5ᵗʰ T84.1 Mechanical complication of **internal fixation device of bones of limb**

> EXCLUDES 2   *mechanical complication of internal fixation device of bones of feet (T84.2-)*
> *mechanical complication of internal fixation device of bones of fingers (T84.2-)*
> *mechanical complication of internal fixation device of bones of hands (T84.2-)*
> *mechanical complication of internal fixation device of bones of toes (T84.2-)*

> **CC Excl: For CC codes in subcategory T84.1: CC with 7th character A, unless otherwise noted: See code: T84.Ø**

√6ᵗʰ T84.11 Breakdown (mechanical) of internal fixation device of bones of limb

   √7ᵗʰ T84.110 Breakdown (mechanical) of internal fixation device of **right humerus** `CC`

   √7ᵗʰ T84.111 Breakdown (mechanical) of internal fixation device of **left humerus** `CC`

   √7ᵗʰ T84.112 Breakdown (mechanical) of internal fixation device of bone of **right forearm** `CC`

   √7ᵗʰ T84.113 Breakdown (mechanical) of internal fixation device of bone of **left forearm** `CC`

   √7ᵗʰ T84.114 Breakdown (mechanical) of internal fixation device of **right femur** `CC`

   √7ᵗʰ T84.115 Breakdown (mechanical) of internal fixation device of **left femur** `CC`

   √7ᵗʰ T84.116 Breakdown (mechanical) of internal fixation device of bone of **right lower leg** `CC`

   √7ᵗʰ T84.117 Breakdown (mechanical) of internal fixation device of bone of **left lower leg** `CC`

   √7ᵗʰ T84.119 Breakdown (mechanical) of internal fixation device of **unspecified bone of limb** `CC`

√6ᵗʰ T84.12 Displacement of internal fixation device of bones of limb
     Malposition of internal fixation device of bones of limb

   √7ᵗʰ T84.120 Displacement of internal fixation device of **right humerus** `CC`

   √7ᵗʰ T84.121 Displacement of internal fixation device of **left humerus** `CC`

   √7ᵗʰ T84.122 Displacement of internal fixation device of bone of **right forearm** `CC`

   √7ᵗʰ T84.123 Displacement of internal fixation device of bone of **left forearm** `CC`

   √7ᵗʰ T84.124 Displacement of internal fixation device of **right femur** `CC`

   √7ᵗʰ T84.125 Displacement of internal fixation device of **left femur** `CC`

   √7ᵗʰ T84.126 Displacement of internal fixation device of bone of **right lower leg** `CC`

   √7ᵗʰ T84.127 Displacement of internal fixation device of bone of **left lower leg** `CC`

   √7ᵗʰ T84.129 Displacement of internal fixation device of **unspecified bone of limb** `CC`

√6ᵗʰ T84.19 Other mechanical complication of internal fixation device of bones of limb
     Obstruction (mechanical) of internal fixation device of bones of limb
     Perforation of internal fixation device of bones of limb
     Protrusion of internal fixation device of bones of limb

   √7ᵗʰ T84.190 Other mechanical complication of internal fixation device of **right humerus** `CC`

√7ᵗʰ T84.191 Other mechanical complication of internal fixation device of **left humerus** `CC`

√7ᵗʰ T84.192 Other mechanical complication of internal fixation device of bone of **right forearm** `CC`

√7ᵗʰ T84.193 Other mechanical complication of internal fixation device of bone of **left forearm** `CC`

√7ᵗʰ T84.194 Other mechanical complication of internal fixation device of **right femur** `CC`

√7ᵗʰ T84.195 Other mechanical complication of internal fixation device of **left femur** `CC`

√7ᵗʰ T84.196 Other mechanical complication of internal fixation device of bone of **right lower leg** `CC`

√7ᵗʰ T84.197 Other mechanical complication of internal fixation device of bone of **left lower leg** `CC`

√7ᵗʰ T84.199 Other mechanical complication of internal fixation device of **unspecified bone of limb** `CC`

√6ᵗʰ T84.2 Mechanical complication of **internal fixation device of other bones**

> **CC Excl: For CC codes in subcategory T84.2: CC with 7th character A, unless otherwise noted: See code: T84.Ø**

√6ᵗʰ T84.21 Breakdown (mechanical) of internal fixation device of other bones

   √7ᵗʰ T84.210 Breakdown (mechanical) of internal fixation device of bones of **hand and fingers** `CC`

   √7ᵗʰ T84.213 Breakdown (mechanical) of internal fixation device of bones of **foot and toes** `CC`

   √7ᵗʰ T84.216 Breakdown (mechanical) of internal fixation device of **vertebrae** `CC`

   √7ᵗʰ T84.218 Breakdown (mechanical) of internal fixation device of **other bones** `CC`

√6ᵗʰ T84.22 Displacement of internal fixation device of other bones
     Malposition of internal fixation device of other bones

   √7ᵗʰ T84.220 Displacement of internal fixation device of bones of **hand and fingers** `CC`

   √7ᵗʰ T84.223 Displacement of internal fixation device of bones of **foot and toes** `CC`

   √7ᵗʰ T84.226 Displacement of internal fixation device of **vertebrae** `CC`

   √7ᵗʰ T84.228 Displacement of internal fixation device of **other bones** `CC`

√6ᵗʰ T84.29 Other mechanical complication of internal fixation device of other bones
     Obstruction (mechanical) of internal fixation device of other bones
     Perforation of internal fixation device of other bones
     Protrusion of internal fixation device of other bones

   √7ᵗʰ T84.290 Other mechanical complication of internal fixation device of bones of **hand and fingers** `CC`

   √7ᵗʰ T84.293 Other mechanical complication of internal fixation device of bones of **foot and toes** `CC`

   √7ᵗʰ T84.296 Other mechanical complication of internal fixation device of **vertebrae** `CC`

   √7ᵗʰ T84.298 Other mechanical complication of internal fixation device of **other bones** `CC`

√5ᵗʰ T84.3 Mechanical complication of **other bone devices, implants and grafts**

> EXCLUDES 2   *other complications of bone graft (T86.83-)*

> **CC Excl: For CC codes in subcategory T84.3: CC with 7th character A, unless otherwise noted: See code: T84.Ø**

√6ᵗʰ T84.31 Breakdown (mechanical) of other bone devices, implants and grafts

   √7ᵗʰ T84.310 Breakdown (mechanical) of **electronic bone stimulator** `CC`

Ⓝ Newborn: 0   Ⓟ Pediatric: 0-17   Ⓜ Maternity: 12-55   Ⓐ Adult: 15-124   **MCC** Major CC Condition   **PDxMCC** PDx acts as own MCC   **CC** CC Condition   **PDxCC** PDx acts as own CC

1144   ICD-10-CM 2016

✓7ᵗʰ **T84.318** Breakdown (mechanical) of other bone devices, implants and grafts `CC`

✓6ᵗʰ **T84.32** Displacement of other bone devices, implants and grafts
  Malposition of other bone devices, implants and grafts

  ✓7ᵗʰ **T84.320** Displacement of electronic bone stimulator `CC`

  ✓7ᵗʰ **T84.328** Displacement of other bone devices, implants and grafts `CC`
    AHA: 2014, 4Q, 28

✓6ᵗʰ **T84.39** Other mechanical complication of other bone devices, implants and grafts
  Obstruction (mechanical) of other bone devices, implants and grafts
  Perforation of other bone devices, implants and grafts
  Protrusion of other bone devices, implants and grafts

  ✓7ᵗʰ **T84.390** Other mechanical complication of electronic bone stimulator `CC`

  ✓7ᵗʰ **T84.398** Other mechanical complication of other bone devices, implants and grafts `CC`

✓5ᵗʰ **T84.4** Mechanical complication of other internal orthopedic devices, implants and grafts

  CC Excl: For CC codes in subcategory T84.4: CC with 7th character A, unless otherwise noted: See code: T84.0

  ✓6ᵗʰ **T84.41** Breakdown (mechanical) of other internal orthopedic devices, implants and grafts

    ✓7ᵗʰ **T84.410** Breakdown (mechanical) of muscle and tendon graft `CC`

    ✓7ᵗʰ **T84.418** Breakdown (mechanical) of other internal orthopedic devices, implants and grafts `CC`

  ✓6ᵗʰ **T84.42** Displacement of other internal orthopedic devices, implants and grafts
    Malposition of other internal orthopedic devices, implants and grafts

    ✓7ᵗʰ **T84.420** Displacement of muscle and tendon graft `CC`

    ✓7ᵗʰ **T84.428** Displacement of other internal orthopedic devices, implants and grafts `CC`

  ✓6ᵗʰ **T84.49** Other mechanical complication of other internal orthopedic devices, implants and grafts
    Mechanical complication of other internal orthopedic devices, implants and grafts NOS
    Obstruction (mechanical) of other internal orthopedic devices, implants and grafts
    Perforation of other internal orthopedic devices, implants and grafts
    Protrusion of other internal orthopedic devices, implants and grafts

    ✓7ᵗʰ **T84.490** Other mechanical complication of muscle and tendon graft `CC`

    ✓7ᵗʰ **T84.498** Other mechanical complication of other internal orthopedic devices, implants and grafts `CC`

✓5ᵗʰ **T84.5** Infection and inflammatory reaction due to internal joint prosthesis
  Use additional code to identify infection
  AHA: 2015, 1Q, 16

  CC Excl: For CC codes in subcategory T84.5: CC with 7th character A, unless otherwise noted: D78.81-D78.89, E36.8, E89.810-E89.89, H59.011-H59.019, H59.031-H59.099, H59.811-H59.89, H95.811-H95.89, I97.3, L76.81-L76.82, M96.621-M96.69, M96.89, N98.1-N98.9, T81.82XA, T81.89X-T81.9XX with 7th A, T84.010-T84.9XX with 7th A, T85.310-T85.311 with 7th A, T85.320-T85.321, T85.390-T85.391 with 7th A, T85.510-T85.9XX with 7th A, T86.820-T86.829, T86.842-T86.849

  ✓x7ᵗʰ **T84.50** Infection and inflammatory reaction due to unspecified internal joint prosthesis `CC`

  ✓x7ᵗʰ **T84.51** Infection and inflammatory reaction due to internal right hip prosthesis `CC`

  ✓x7ᵗʰ **T84.52** Infection and inflammatory reaction due to internal left hip prosthesis `CC`

  ✓x7ᵗʰ **T84.53** Infection and inflammatory reaction due to internal right knee prosthesis `CC`

  ✓x7ᵗʰ **T84.54** Infection and inflammatory reaction due to internal left knee prosthesis `CC`

  ✓x7ᵗʰ **T84.59** Infection and inflammatory reaction due to other internal joint prosthesis `CC`

✓5ᵗʰ **T84.6** Infection and inflammatory reaction due to internal fixation device
  Use additional code to identify infection

  CC Excl: For CC codes in subcategory T84.6: CC with 7th character A, unless otherwise noted: See code: T84.5

  6 ✓x7ᵗʰ **T84.60** Infection and inflammatory reaction due to internal fixation device of unspecified site `CC`

  ✓6ᵗʰ **T84.61** Infection and inflammatory reaction due to internal fixation device of arm

    6 ✓7ᵗʰ **T84.610** Infection and inflammatory reaction due to internal fixation device of right humerus `CC`

    6 ✓7ᵗʰ **T84.611** Infection and inflammatory reaction due to internal fixation device of left humerus `CC`

    6 ✓7ᵗʰ **T84.612** Infection and inflammatory reaction due to internal fixation device of right radius `CC`

    6 ✓7ᵗʰ **T84.613** Infection and inflammatory reaction due to internal fixation device of left radius `CC`

    6 ✓7ᵗʰ **T84.614** Infection and inflammatory reaction due to internal fixation device of right ulna `CC`

    6 ✓7ᵗʰ **T84.615** Infection and inflammatory reaction due to internal fixation device of left ulna `CC`

    6 ✓7ᵗʰ **T84.619** Infection and inflammatory reaction due to internal fixation device of unspecified bone of arm `CC`

  ✓6ᵗʰ **T84.62** Infection and inflammatory reaction due to internal fixation device of leg

    ✓7ᵗʰ **T84.620** Infection and inflammatory reaction due to internal fixation device of right femur `CC`

    ✓7ᵗʰ **T84.621** Infection and inflammatory reaction due to internal fixation device of left femur `CC`

    ✓7ᵗʰ **T84.622** Infection and inflammatory reaction due to internal fixation device of right tibia `CC`

    ✓7ᵗʰ **T84.623** Infection and inflammatory reaction due to internal fixation device of left tibia `CC`

    ✓7ᵗʰ **T84.624** Infection and inflammatory reaction due to internal fixation device of right fibula `CC`

    ✓7ᵗʰ **T84.625** Infection and inflammatory reaction due to internal fixation device of left fibula `CC`

    ✓7ᵗʰ **T84.629** Infection and inflammatory reaction due to internal fixation device of unspecified bone of leg `CC`

  6 ✓x7ᵗʰ **T84.63** Infection and inflammatory reaction due to internal fixation device of spine `CC`

  6 ✓x7ᵗʰ **T84.69** Infection and inflammatory reaction due to internal fixation device of other site `CC`

6 ✓x7ᵗʰ **T84.7** Infection and inflammatory reaction due to other internal orthopedic prosthetic devices, implants and grafts `CC`
  Use additional code to identify infection
  CC Excl: CC with 7th character A: See code: T84.5

✓5ᵗʰ **T84.8** Other specified complications of internal orthopedic prosthetic devices, implants and grafts

  CC Excl: For CC codes in subcategory T84.8: CC with 7th character A, unless otherwise noted: See code: T84.5

  ✓x7ᵗʰ **T84.81** Embolism due to internal orthopedic prosthetic devices, implants and grafts `CC`

  ✓x7ᵗʰ **T84.82** Fibrosis due to internal orthopedic prosthetic devices, implants and grafts `CC`

---

6 HAC = as SDx not POA, in combination with one of the following procedure codes: 0RG[0,1,2,4,6,7,8,A][0,3,4][7,A,J,K,Z][0,1,J]; 0RG[E,F,G,H,J,K][0,3,4][4,7,J,K,Z]Z; 0RG[L,M][0,3,4][4,5,7,J,K,Z]Z; 0RQ[E,F,G,H,J,K,L,M][0,3,4,X]ZZ; 0RU[E,F,G,H,J,K,L,M][0,3,4][7,J,K]Z; 0SG[0,1,3][0,3,4][7,A,J,K,Z][0,1,J]; 0SG[7,8][0,3,4][4,7,J,K,Z]Z.

✓ Additional Character Required ✓x7ᵗʰ Placeholder Alert   Unacceptable PDx   Manifestation   Hospital Acquired Condition   *EXCLUDES 1* Not Coded Here   *EXCLUDES 2* Not Included Here

√x7ᵗʰ **T84.83** **Hemorrhage due to internal orthopedic prosthetic devices, implants and grafts** CC

√x7ᵗʰ **T84.84** **Pain due to internal orthopedic prosthetic devices, implants and grafts** CC

√x7ᵗʰ **T84.85** **Stenosis due to internal orthopedic prosthetic devices, implants and grafts** CC

√x7ᵗʰ **T84.86** **Thrombosis due to internal orthopedic prosthetic devices, implants and grafts** CC

√x7ᵗʰ **T84.89** **Other specified complication of internal orthopedic prosthetic devices, implants and grafts** CC

√x7ᵗʰ **T84.9** **Unspecified complication of internal orthopedic prosthetic device, implant and graft** CC
    CC Excl: See code: T84.8

√4ᵗʰ **T85** **Complications of other internal prosthetic devices, implants and grafts**
    EXCLUDES 2   *failure and rejection of transplanted organs and tissue (T86.-)*

> The appropriate 7th character is to be added to each code from category T85.
> A   initial encounter
> D   subsequent encounter
> S   sequela

√5ᵗʰ **T85.0** **Mechanical complication of ventricular intracranial (communicating) shunt**

> **CC Excl: For CC codes in subcategory T85.0: CC with 7th character A, unless otherwise noted:** D78.81-D78.89, E36.8, E89.810-E89.89, H59.011-H59.019, H59.031-H59.099, H59.811-H59.89, H95.811-H95.89, I97.3, L76.81-L76.82, M96.89, N98.1-N98.9, T81.82XA, T81.89X-T81.9XX with 7th A, T85.01X-T85.199 with 7th A

√x7ᵗʰ **T85.01** **Breakdown (mechanical) of ventricular intracranial (communicating) shunt** CC

√x7ᵗʰ **T85.02** **Displacement of ventricular intracranial (communicating) shunt** CC
    Malposition of ventricular intracranial (communicating) shunt

√x7ᵗʰ **T85.03** **Leakage of ventricular intracranial (communicating) shunt** CC

√x7ᵗʰ **T85.09** **Other mechanical complication of ventricular intracranial (communicating) shunt** CC
    Obstruction (mechanical) of ventricular intracranial (communicating) shunt
    Perforation of ventricular intracranial (communicating) shunt
    Protrusion of ventricular intracranial (communicating) shunt

√5ᵗʰ **T85.1** **Mechanical complication of implanted electronic stimulator of nervous system**

> **CC Excl: For CC codes in subcategory T85.1: CC with 7th character A, unless otherwise noted:** See code: T85.0

√6ᵗʰ **T85.11** **Breakdown (mechanical) of implanted electronic stimulator of nervous system**

√7ᵗʰ **T85.110** **Breakdown (mechanical) of implanted electronic neurostimulator (electrode) of brain** CC

√7ᵗʰ **T85.111** **Breakdown (mechanical) of implanted electronic neurostimulator (electrode) of peripheral nerve** CC

√7ᵗʰ **T85.112** **Breakdown (mechanical) of implanted electronic neurostimulator (electrode) of spinal cord** CC

√7ᵗʰ **T85.118** **Breakdown (mechanical) of other implanted electronic stimulator of nervous system** CC

√6ᵗʰ **T85.12** **Displacement of implanted electronic stimulator of nervous system**
    Malposition of implanted electronic stimulator of nervous system

√7ᵗʰ **T85.120** **Displacement of implanted electronic neurostimulator (electrode) of brain** CC

√7ᵗʰ **T85.121** **Displacement of implanted electronic neurostimulator (electrode) of peripheral nerve** CC

√7ᵗʰ **T85.122** **Displacement of implanted electronic neurostimulator (electrode) of spinal cord** CC

√7ᵗʰ **T85.128** **Displacement of other implanted electronic stimulator of nervous system** CC

√6ᵗʰ **T85.19** **Other mechanical complication of implanted electronic stimulator of nervous system**
    Leakage of implanted electronic stimulator of nervous system
    Obstruction (mechanical) of implanted electronic stimulator of nervous system
    Perforation of implanted electronic stimulator of nervous system
    Protrusion of implanted electronic stimulator of nervous system

√7ᵗʰ **T85.190** **Other mechanical complication of implanted electronic neurostimulator (electrode) of brain** CC

√7ᵗʰ **T85.191** **Other mechanical complication of implanted electronic neurostimulator (electrode) of peripheral nerve** CC

√7ᵗʰ **T85.192** **Other mechanical complication of implanted electronic neurostimulator (electrode) of spinal cord** CC

√7ᵗʰ **T85.199** **Other mechanical complication of other implanted electronic stimulator of nervous system** CC

√5ᵗʰ **T85.2** **Mechanical complication of intraocular lens**

> **CC Excl: For CC codes in subcategory T85.2: CC with 7th character A, unless otherwise noted:** D78.81-D78.89, E89.810-E89.89, H59.011-H59.019, H59.031-H59.099, H59.811-H59.89, H95.811-H95.89, I97.3, M96.89, N98.1-N98.9, T85.21X-T85.29X with 7th A

√x7ᵗʰ **T85.21** **Breakdown (mechanical) of intraocular lens** CC

√x7ᵗʰ **T85.22** **Displacement of intraocular lens** CC
    Malposition of intraocular lens

√x7ᵗʰ **T85.29** **Other mechanical complication of intraocular lens** CC
    Obstruction (mechanical) of intraocular lens
    Perforation of intraocular lens
    Protrusion of intraocular lens

√5ᵗʰ **T85.3** **Mechanical complication of other ocular prosthetic devices, implants and grafts**
    EXCLUDES 2   *other complications of corneal graft (T86.84-)*

> **CC Excl: For CC codes in subcategory T85.3: CC with 7th character A, unless otherwise noted:** H59.011-H59.019, H59.031-H59.099, H59.811-H59.89, H95.811-H95.89, I97.3, M96.89, N98.1-N98.9, T85.310-T85.311 with 7th A, T85.320-T85.321 with 7th A, T85.390-T85.391 with 7th A, T85.612A, T85.618A, T85.622A, T85.628A, T85.638A, T85.692A, T85.698-T85.9XX with 7th A, T86.842-T86.849

√6ᵗʰ **T85.31** **Breakdown (mechanical) of other ocular prosthetic devices, implants and grafts**

√7ᵗʰ **T85.310** **Breakdown (mechanical) of prosthetic orbit of right eye** CC

√7ᵗʰ **T85.311** **Breakdown (mechanical) of prosthetic orbit of left eye** CC

√7ᵗʰ **T85.318** **Breakdown (mechanical) of other ocular prosthetic devices, implants and grafts**

√6ᵗʰ **T85.32** **Displacement of other ocular prosthetic devices, implants and grafts**
    Malposition of other ocular prosthetic devices, implants and grafts

√7ᵗʰ **T85.320** **Displacement of prosthetic orbit of right eye** CC

√7ᵗʰ **T85.321** **Displacement of prosthetic orbit of left eye** CC

√7ᵗʰ **T85.328** **Displacement of other ocular prosthetic devices, implants and grafts**

√6ᵗʰ **T85.39** **Other mechanical complication of other ocular prosthetic devices, implants and grafts**
    Obstruction (mechanical) of other ocular prosthetic devices, implants and grafts
    Perforation of other ocular prosthetic devices, implants and grafts
    Protrusion of other ocular prosthetic devices, implants and grafts

√7ᵗʰ **T85.390** **Other mechanical complication of prosthetic orbit of right eye** CC

√7ᵗʰ **T85.391** **Other mechanical complication of prosthetic orbit of left eye** CC

Ⓝ Newborn: 0   Ⓟ Pediatric: 0-17   Ⓜ Maternity: 12-55   Ⓐ Adult: 15-124   **MCC** Major CC Condition   **PDxMCC** PDx acts as own MCC   CC Condition   **PDxCC** PDx acts as own CC

1146

ICD-10-CM 2016

√7ᵗʰ **T85.398** **Other mechanical complication of** other **ocular prosthetic devices, implants and grafts**

√5ᵗʰ **T85.4** **Mechanical complication of** breast prosthesis and implant

> **CC Excl: For CC codes in subcategory T85.4: CC with 7th character A, unless otherwise noted:** D78.81-D78.89, E89.810-E89.89, H59.011-H59.019, H59.031-H59.099, H59.811-H59.89, H95.811-H95.89, I97.3, M96.89, N98.1-N98.9, T85.41X-T85.49X with 7th A

√x7ᵗʰ **T85.41** **Breakdown (mechanical) of breast prosthesis and implant** `CC`

√x7ᵗʰ **T85.42** **Displacement of breast prosthesis and implant** `CC`
Malposition of breast prosthesis and implant

√x7ᵗʰ **T85.43** **Leakage of breast prosthesis and implant** `CC`

√x7ᵗʰ **T85.44** **Capsular contracture of breast implant** `CC`

√x7ᵗʰ **T85.49** **Other mechanical complication of breast prosthesis and implant** `CC`
Obstruction (mechanical) of breast prosthesis and implant
Perforation of breast prosthesis and implant
Protrusion of breast prosthesis and implant

√5ᵗʰ **T85.5** **Mechanical complication of** gastrointestinal prosthetic devices, implants and grafts

> **CC Excl: For CC codes in subcategory T85.5: CC with 7th character A, unless otherwise noted:** H95.811-H95.89, I97.3, M96.89, N98.1-N98.9, T85.510-T85.598 with 7th A, T85.612A, T85.618A, T85.622A, T85.628A, T85.638A, T85.692A, T85.698-T85.9XX with 7th A

√6ᵗʰ **T85.51** **Breakdown (mechanical) of gastrointestinal prosthetic devices, implants and grafts**

√7ᵗʰ **T85.510** **Breakdown (mechanical) of bile duct prosthesis** `CC`

√7ᵗʰ **T85.511** **Breakdown (mechanical) of esophageal anti-reflux device** `CC`

√7ᵗʰ **T85.518** **Breakdown (mechanical) of other gastrointestinal prosthetic devices, implants and grafts** `CC`

√6ᵗʰ **T85.52** **Displacement of gastrointestinal prosthetic devices, implants and grafts**
Malposition of gastrointestinal prosthetic devices, implants and grafts

√7ᵗʰ **T85.520** **Displacement of bile duct prosthesis** `CC`

√7ᵗʰ **T85.521** **Displacement of** esophageal anti-reflux device `CC`

√7ᵗʰ **T85.528** **Displacement of other** gastrointestinal prosthetic devices, implants and grafts `CC`

√6ᵗʰ **T85.59** **Other mechanical complication of gastrointestinal prosthetic devices, implants and grafts**
Obstruction, mechanical of gastrointestinal prosthetic devices, implants and grafts
Perforation of gastrointestinal prosthetic devices, implants and grafts
Protrusion of gastrointestinal prosthetic devices, implants and grafts

√7ᵗʰ **T85.590** **Other mechanical complication of bile duct prosthesis** `CC`

√7ᵗʰ **T85.591** **Other mechanical complication of** esophageal anti-reflux device `CC`

√7ᵗʰ **T85.598** **Other mechanical complication of other** gastrointestinal prosthetic devices, implants and grafts `CC`

√5ᵗʰ **T85.6** **Mechanical complication of** other specified internal and external prosthetic devices, implants and grafts

√6ᵗʰ **T85.61** **Breakdown (mechanical) of other specified internal prosthetic devices, implants and grafts**

√7ᵗʰ **T85.610** **Breakdown (mechanical) of epidural and subdural infusion catheter** `CC`
CC Excl: CC with 7th character A: H95.811-H95.89, I97.3, M96.89, N98.1-N98.9, T85.610A, T85.612A, T85.618-T85.620 with 7th A, T85.622A, T85.628-T85.630 with 7th A, T85.638-T85.690 with 7th A, T85.692A, T85.698-T85.9XX with 7th A

√7ᵗʰ **T85.611** **Breakdown (mechanical) of intraperitoneal dialysis catheter** `CC`
EXCLUDES 1 mechanical complication of vascular dialysis catheter (T82.4-)
CC Excl: CC with 7th character A: H95.811-H95.89, I97.3, M96.89, N98.1-N98.9, T85.611-T85.612 with 7th A, T85.614-T85.618 with 7th A, T85.621-T85.622 with 7th A, T85.624-T85.628 with 7th A, T85.631-T85.638 with 7th A, T85.691-T85.692 with 7th A, T85.694-T85.9XX with 7th A

√7ᵗʰ **T85.612** **Breakdown (mechanical) of permanent sutures** `CC`
EXCLUDES 1 mechanical complication of permanent (wire) suture used in bone repair (T84.1-T84.2)
CC Excl: CC with 7th character A: D78.81-D78.89, E89.810-E89.89, H59.011-H59.019, H59.031-H59.099, H59.811-H59.89, H95.811-H95.89, I97.3, M96.89, N98.1-N98.9, T85.310-T85.311 with 7th A, T85.320-T85.321 with 7th A, T85.390-T85.391 with 7th A, T85.510-T85.612 with 7th A, T85.614-T85.622 with 7th A, T85.624-T85.692 with 7th A, T85.694-T85.9XX with 7th A, T86.842-T86.849

√7ᵗʰ **T85.613** **Breakdown (mechanical) of artificial skin graft and decellularized allodermis** `CC`
Failure of artificial skin graft and decellularized allodermis
Non-adherence of artificial skin graft and decellularized allodermis
Poor incorporation of artificial skin graft and decellularized allodermis
Shearing of artificial skin graft and decellularized allodermis
CC Excl: CC with 7th character A: H95.811-H95.89, I97.3, M96.89, N98.1-N98.9, T85.612-T85.613 with 7th A, T85.618A, T85.622-T85.623 with 7th A, T85.628A, T85.638A, T85.692-T85.693 with 7th A, T85.698-T85.9XX with 7th A, T86.820-T86.829

√7ᵗʰ **T85.614** **Breakdown (mechanical) of insulin pump** `CC`
CC Excl: CC with 7th character A: H95.811-H95.89, I97.3, M96.621-M96.69, M96.89, N98.1-N98.9, N99.510-N99.518, T81.82X with 7th A, T81.89X-T82.09X with 7th A, T82.110-T82.118 with 7th A, T82.120-T82.128 with 7th A, T82.190-T82.198 with 7th A, T82.211-T83.010 with 7th A, T83.020A, T83.030A, T83.090A, T83.110-T83.29X with 7th A, T83.410-T83.718 with 7th A, T83.728-T85.29X with 7th A, T85.41X-T85.49X with 7th A, T85.611-T85.612 with 7th A, T85.614-T85.618 with 7th A, T85.621-T85.622 with 7th A, T85.624-T85.628 with 7th A, T85.631-T85.638 with 7th A, T85.691-T85.692 with 7th A, T85.694-T85.9XX with 7th A, T86.820-T86.829

√7ᵗʰ **T85.618** **Breakdown (mechanical) of other specified internal prosthetic devices, implants and grafts** `CC`
CC Excl: CC with 7th character A: D78.81-D78.89, E89.810-E89.89, H59.011-H59.019, H59.031-H59.099, H59.811-H59.89, H95.811-H95.89, I97.3, M96.89, N98.1-N98.9, T85.310-T85.311 with 7th A, T85.320-T85.321 with 7th A, T85.390-T85.391 with 7th A, T85.510-T85.612 with 7th A, T85.614-T85.622 with 7th A, T85.624-T85.692 with 7th A, T85.694-T85.9XX with 7th A, T86.842-T86.849

√6ᵗʰ **T85.62** **Displacement of other specified internal prosthetic devices, implants and grafts**
Malposition of other specified internal prosthetic devices, implants and grafts

√7ᵗʰ **T85.620** **Displacement of epidural and subdural infusion catheter** `CC`
CC Excl: CC with 7th character A: H95.811-H95.89, I97.3, M96.89, N98.1-N98.9, T85.610A, T85.612A, T85.618-T85.620 with 7th A, T85.622A, T85.628-T85.630 with 7th A, T85.638-T85.690 with 7th A, T85.69 A, T85.698-T85.9XX with 7th A

√ Additional Character Required   √x7ᵗʰ Placeholder Alert   Unacceptable PDx   Manifestation   Hospital Acquired Condition   *EXCLUDES 1* Not Coded Here   *EXCLUDES 2* Not Included Here

T85.621 Displacement of intraperitoneal dialysis catheter **CC**
> **EXCLUDES 1** mechanical complication of vascular dialysis catheter (T82.4-)
>
> **CC Excl: CC with 7th character A:** H95.811-H95.89, I97.3, M96.89, N98.1-N98.9, T85.611-T85.612 with 7th A, T85.614-T85.618 with 7th A, T85.621-T85.622 with 7th A, T85.624-T85.628 with 7th A, T85.631-T85.638 with 7th A, T85.691-T85.692 with 7th A, T85.694-T85.9XX with 7th A

T85.622 Displacement of permanent sutures **CC**
> **EXCLUDES 1** mechanical complication of permanent (wire) suture used in bone repair (T84.1-T84.2)
>
> **CC Excl: CC with 7th character A:** D78.81-D78.89, E89.810-E89.89, H59.011-H59.019, H59.031-H59.099, H59.811-H59.89, H95.811-H95.89, I97.3, M96.89, N98.1-N98.9, T85.310-T85.311 with 7th A, T85.320-T85.321 with 7th A, T85.390-T85.391 with 7th A, T85.510-T85.612 with 7th A, T85.614-T85.622 with 7th A, T85.624-T85.692 with 7th A, T85.694-T85.9XX with 7th A, T86.842-T86.849

T85.623 Displacement of artificial skin graft and decellularized allodermis **CC**
> Dislodgement of artificial skin graft and decellularized allodermis
> Displacement of artificial skin graft and decellularized allodermis
>
> **CC Excl: CC with 7th character A:** H95.811-H95.89, I97.3, M96.89, N98.1-N98.9, T85.612-T85.613 with 7th A, T85.618 with 7th A, T85.622-T85.623 with 7th A, T85.628A, T85.638A, T85.692-T85.693 with 7th A, T85.698-T85.9XX with 7th A, T86.820-T86.829

T85.624 Displacement of insulin pump **CC**
> **CC Excl: CC with 7th character A:** H95.811-H95.89, I97.3, M96.621-M96.69, M96.89, N98.1-N98.9, N99.510-N99.518, T81.82X with 7th A, T81.89X-T82.09X with 7th A, T82.110-T82.118 with 7th A, T82.120-T82.128 with 7th A, T82.190-T82.198 with 7th A, T82.211-T83.010 with 7th A, T83.020A, T83.030 with 7th A, T83.090A, T83.110-T83.29X with 7th A, T83.410-T83.718 with 7th A, T83.728-T85.29X with 7th A, T85.41X-T85.49X with 7th A, T85.611-T85.612 with 7th A, T85.614-T85.618 with 7th A, T85.621-T85.622 with 7th A, T85.624-T85.628 with 7th A, T85.631-T85.638 with 7th A, T85.691-T85.692 with 7th A, T85.694-T85.9XX with 7th A, T86.820-T86.829

T85.628 Displacement of other specified internal prosthetic devices, implants and grafts **CC**
> **CC Excl: CC with 7th character A:** D78.81-D78.89, E89.810-E89.89, H59.011-H59.019, H59.031-H59.099, H59.811-H59.89, H95.811-H95.89, I97.3, M96.89, N98.1-N98.9, T85.310-T85.311 with 7th A, T85.320-T85.321 with 7th A, T85.390-T85.391 with 7th A, T85.510-T85.612 with 7th A, T85.614-T85.622 with 7th A, T85.624-T85.692 with 7th A, T85.694-T85.9XX with 7th A, T86.842-T86.849

T85.63 Leakage of other specified internal prosthetic devices, implants and grafts

T85.630 Leakage of epidural and subdural infusion catheter **CC**
> **CC Excl: CC with 7th character A:** See code: T85.620

T85.631 Leakage of intraperitoneal dialysis catheter **CC**
> **EXCLUDES 1** mechanical complication of vascular dialysis catheter (T82.4)
>
> **CC Excl: CC with 7th character A:** See code: T85.621

T85.633 Leakage of insulin pump **CC**
> **CC Excl: CC with 7th character A:** See code: T86.624

T85.638 Leakage of other specified internal prosthetic devices, implants and grafts **CC**
> **CC Excl: CC with 7th character A:** See code: T85.628

T85.69 Other mechanical complication of other specified internal prosthetic devices, implants and grafts
> Obstruction, mechanical of other specified internal prosthetic devices, implants and grafts
> Perforation of other specified internal prosthetic devices, implants and grafts
> Protrusion of other specified internal prosthetic devices, implants and grafts

T85.690 Other mechanical complication of epidural and subdural infusion catheter **CC**
> **CC Excl: CC with 7th character A:** See code: T85.620

T85.691 Other mechanical complication of intraperitoneal dialysis catheter **CC**
> **EXCLUDES 1** mechanical complication of vascular dialysis catheter (T82.4)
>
> **CC Excl: CC with 7th character A:** See code: T85.621

T85.692 Other mechanical complication of permanent sutures **CC**
> **EXCLUDES 1** mechanical complication of permanent (wire) suture used in bone repair (T84.1-T84.2)
>
> **CC Excl: CC with 7th character A:** See code: T85.622

T85.693 Other mechanical complication of artificial skin graft and decellularized allodermis **CC**
> **CC Excl: CC with 7th character A:** See code: T85.623

T85.694 Other mechanical complication of insulin pump **CC**
> **CC Excl: CC with 7th character A:** See code: T85.624

T85.698 Other mechanical complication of other specified internal prosthetic devices, implants and grafts **CC**
> Mechanical complication of nonabsorbable surgical material NOS
>
> **CC Excl: CC with 7th character A:** See code: T85.628

T85.7 Infection and inflammatory reaction due to other internal prosthetic devices, implants and grafts
> Use additional code to identify infection

T85.71 Infection and inflammatory reaction due to peritoneal dialysis catheter **CC**
> **CC Excl: CC with 7th character A:** See code: T85.628

T85.72 Infection and inflammatory reaction due to insulin pump **CC**
> **CC Excl: CC with 7th character A:** D78.81-D78.89, E36.8, E89.810-E89.89, H59.011-H59.019, H59.031-H59.099, H59.811-H59.89, H95.811-H95.89, I97.3, L76.81-L76.82, M96.621-M96.69, M96.89, N98.1-N98.9, N99.510-N99.518, T81.82XA, T81.89X-T82.09X with 7th A, T82.110-T82.118 with 7th A, T82.120-T82.128 with 7th A, T82.190-T82.198 with 7th A, T82.211-T83.010 with 7th A, T83.020A, T83.030A, T83.090A, T83.110-T83.29X with 7th A, T83.410-T83.718 with 7th A, T83.728-T85.9XX with 7th A, T86.820-T86.829, T86.840-T86.849

T85.79 Infection and inflammatory reaction due to other internal prosthetic devices, implants and grafts **CC**
> **CC Excl:** See code: T85.72

T85.8 Other specified complications of internal prosthetic devices, implants and grafts, not elsewhere classified

T85.81 Embolism due to internal prosthetic devices, implants and grafts, not elsewhere classified **CC**
> **CC Excl:** See code: T85.72

T85.82 Fibrosis due to internal prosthetic devices, implants and grafts, not elsewhere classified **CC**
> **CC Excl:** See code: T85.72

T85.83 Hemorrhage due to internal prosthetic devices, implants and grafts, not elsewhere classified **CC**
> **CC Excl:** See code: T85.72

N Newborn: 0   P Pediatric: 0-17   M Maternity: 12-55   A Adult: 15-124   MCC Major CC Condition   PDxMCC PDx acts as own MCC   CC CC Condition   PDxCC PDx acts as own CC

1148	ICD-10-CM 2016

√x7ᵗʰ **T85.84** **Pain** due to internal prosthetic devices, implants and grafts, not elsewhere classified   `CC`
     CC Excl: See code: T85.72

√x7ᵗʰ **T85.85** **Stenosis** due to internal prosthetic devices, implants and grafts, not elsewhere classified   `CC`
     CC Excl: See code: T85.72

√x7ᵗʰ **T85.86** **Thrombosis** due to internal prosthetic devices, implants and grafts, not elsewhere classified   `CC`
     CC Excl: See code: T85.72

√x7ᵗʰ **T85.89** **Other specified complication** of internal prosthetic devices, implants and grafts, not elsewhere classified   `CC`
     CC Excl: See code: T85.72

√x7ᵗʰ **T85.9** **Unspecified complication** of internal prosthetic device, implant and graft
     Complication of internal prosthetic device, implant and graft NOS

√4ᵗʰ **T86** **Complications of transplanted organs and tissue**
     Use additional code to identify other transplant complications, such as:
       graft-versus-host disease (D89.81-)
       malignancy associated with organ transplant (C80.2)
       post-transplant lymphoproliferative disorders (PTLD) (D47.Z1)

√5ᵗʰ **T86.0** **Complications of bone marrow transplant**

> CC Excl: For CC codes in subcategory T86.0: CC with 7th character A, unless otherwise noted: D78.81-D78.89, D89.810-D89.813, E89.810-E89.89, H59.011-H59.019, H59.031-H59.099, H59.811-H59.89, H95.811-H95.89, I97.3, M96.89, N98.1-N98.9, T86.00-T86.09

     T86.00 **Unspecified complication** of bone marrow transplant   `CC`

     T86.01 **Bone marrow transplant rejection**   `CC`

     T86.02 **Bone marrow transplant failure**   `CC`

     T86.03 **Bone marrow transplant infection**   `CC`

     T86.09 **Other complications of bone marrow transplant**   `CC`

√5ᵗʰ **T86.1** **Complications of kidney transplant**

> CC Excl: For CC codes in subcategory T86.1: CC with 7th character A, unless otherwise noted: D78.81-D78.89, E89.810-E89.89, H59.011-H59.019, H59.031-H59.099, H59.811-H59.89, H95.811-H95.89, I97.3, M96.89, N98.1-N98.9, T86.10-T86.19

     T86.10 **Unspecified complication** of kidney transplant   `CC`

     T86.11 **Kidney transplant rejection**   `CC`

     T86.12 **Kidney transplant failure**   `CC`
       AHA: 2013, 1Q, 24

     T86.13 **Kidney transplant infection**   `CC`
       Use additional code to specify infection

     T86.19 **Other complication of kidney transplant**   `CC`

√5ᵗʰ **T86.2** **Complications of heart transplant**
     EXCLUDES 1 complication of:
       artificial heart device (T82.5)
       heart-lung transplant (T86.3)

> CC Excl: For CC codes in subcategory T86.2: CC with 7th character A, unless otherwise noted: D78.81-D78.89, E89.810-E89.89, H59.011-H59.019, H59.031-H59.099, H59.811-H59.89, H95.811-H95.89, I97.3, M96.89, N98.1-N98.9, T86.20-T86.39

     T86.20 **Unspecified complication** of heart transplant   `CC`

     T86.21 **Heart transplant rejection**   `CC`

     T86.22 **Heart transplant failure**   `CC`

     T86.23 **Heart transplant infection**   `CC`
       Use additional code to specify infection

√6ᵗʰ   **T86.29** **Other complications of heart transplant**

     T86.290 **Cardiac allograft vasculopathy**   `CC`
       EXCLUDES 1 atherosclerosis of coronary arteries (I25.75-, I25.76-, I25.81-)

     T86.298 **Other complications of heart transplant**

√5ᵗʰ **T86.3** **Complications of heart-lung transplant**

> CC Excl: For CC codes in subcategory T86.3: CC with 7th character A, unless otherwise noted: See code: T86.2

     T86.30 **Unspecified complication** of heart-lung transplant   `PDx CC` `CC`

     T86.31 **Heart-lung transplant rejection**   `PDx CC` `CC`

     T86.32 **Heart-lung transplant failure**   `PDx CC` `CC`

     T86.33 **Heart-lung transplant infection**   `PDx CC`
       Use additional code to specify infection

     T86.39 **Other complications of heart-lung transplant**   `PDx CC`

√5ᵗʰ **T86.4** **Complications of liver transplant**

     T86.40 **Unspecified complication** of liver transplant   `CC`

> CC Excl: For CC codes in subcategory T86.4: CC with 7th character A, unless otherwise noted: D78.81-D78.89, E89.810-E89.89, H59.011-H59.019, H59.031-H59.099, H59.811-H59.89, H95.811-H95.89, I97.3, M96.89, N98.1-N98.9, T86.40-T86.49

     T86.41 **Liver transplant rejection**   `CC`

     T86.42 **Liver transplant failure**   `CC`

     T86.43 **Liver transplant infection**
       Use additional code to identify infection, such as: cytomegalovirus (CMV) infection (B25.-)

     T86.49 **Other complications of liver transplant**   `CC`

T86.5 **Complications of stem cell transplant**   `CC`
     Complications from stem cells from peripheral blood
     Complications from stem cells from umbilical cord

> CC Excl: For CC codes in subcategory T86.5: CC with 7th character A, unless otherwise noted: D78.81-D78.89, E89.810-E89.89, H59.011-H59.019, H59.031-H59.099, H59.811-H59.89, H95.811-H95.89, I97.3, M96.89, N98.1-N98.9, T86.5, T86.830-T86.839

√5ᵗʰ **T86.8** **Complications of other transplanted organs and tissues**

√6ᵗʰ   **T86.81** **Complications of lung transplant**
     EXCLUDES 1 complication of heart-lung transplant (T86.3-)

> CC Excl: For CC codes in subcategory T86.81: CC with 7th character A, unless otherwise noted: D78.81-D78.89, E89.810-E89.89, H59.011-H59.019, H59.031-H59.099, H59.811-H59.89, H95.811-H95.89, I97.3, M96.89, N98.1-N98.9, T86.810-T86.819

     T86.810 **Lung transplant rejection**   `CC`

     T86.811 **Lung transplant failure**   `CC`

     T86.812 **Lung transplant infection**   `CC`
       Use additional code to specify infection

     T86.818 **Other complications of lung transplant**   `CC`

     T86.819 **Unspecified complication of lung transplant**   `CC`

√6ᵗʰ   **T86.82** **Complications of skin graft (allograft) (autograft)**
     EXCLUDES 2 complication of artificial skin graft (T85.693)

> CC Excl: For CC codes in subcategory T86.82: CC with 7th character A, unless otherwise noted: D78.81-D78.89, E89.810-E89.89, H59.011-H59.019, H59.031-H59.099, H59.811-H59.89, H95.811-H95.89, I97.3, M96.89, N98.1-N98.9, T85.613A, T85.623A, T85.693A, T86.820-T86.829

     T86.820 **Skin graft (allograft) rejection**   `CC`

     T86.821 **Skin graft (allograft) (autograft) failure**   `CC`

     T86.822 **Skin graft (allograft) (autograft) infection**   `CC`
       Use additional code to specify infection

     T86.828 **Other complications of skin graft (allograft) (autograft)**   `CC`

     T86.829 **Unspecified complication of skin graft (allograft) (autograft)**   `CC`

√6ᵗʰ   **T86.83** **Complications of bone graft**
     EXCLUDES 2 mechanical complications of bone graft (T84.3-)

> CC Excl: For CC codes in subcategory T86.83: CC with 7th character A, unless otherwise noted: H95.811-H95.89, I97.3, M96.89, N98.1-N98.9, T86.5, T86.830-T86.839

     T86.830 **Bone graft rejection**   `CC`

     T86.831 **Bone graft failure**   `CC`

     T86.832 **Bone graft infection**   `CC`
       Use additional code to specify infection

     T86.838 **Other complications of bone graft**   `CC`

     T86.839 **Unspecified complication of bone graft**   `CC`

✓6ᵗʰ T86.84 Complications of corneal transplant
     EXCLUDES 2 mechanical complications of corneal graft (T85.3-)

T86.840 Corneal transplant rejection CC
CC Excl: CC with 7th character A: H59.011-H59.019, H59.031-H59.099, H59.811-H59.89, H95.811-H95.89, I97.3, M96.89, N98.1-N98.9, T85.318A, T85.328A, T85.398A, T86.840-T86.841

T86.841 Corneal transplant failure CC
CC Excl: See code: T86.840

T86.842 Corneal transplant infection CC
Use additional code to specify infection
CC Excl: CC with 7th character A: H59.011-H59.019, H59.031-H59.099, H59.811-H59.89, H95.811-H95.89, I97.3, M96.621-M96.69, M96.89, N98.1-N98.9, N99.510-N99.518, T81.82XA, T81.89X-T82.09X with 7th A, T82.110-T82.118 with 7th A, T82.120-T82.128 with 7th A, T82.190-T82.198 with 7th A, T82.211-T83.010 with 7th A, T83.020A, T83.030A, T83.090A, T83.110-T83.29X with 7th A, T83.410-T83.718 with 7th A, T83.728-T85.49X with 7th A, T85.612A, T85.618A, T85.622A, T85.628A, T85.638A, T85.692A, T85.698-T85.9XX with 7th A, T86.820-T86.829, T86.840-T86.849

T86.848 Other complications of corneal transplant CC
CC Excl: See code: T86.842

T86.849 Unspecified complication of corneal transplant CC
CC Excl: See code: T86.842

✓6ᵗʰ T86.85 Complication of intestine transplant

T86.850 Intestine transplant rejection CC
CC Excl: CC with 7th character A: D47.Z1, D78.81-D78.89, E89.810-E89.89, H59.011-H59.019, H59.031-H59.099, H59.811-H59.89, H95.811-H95.89, I97.3, M96.89, N98.1-N98.9, T86.850-T86.859, T86.90-T86.99

T86.851 Intestine transplant failure CC
CC Excl: See code: T86.850

T86.852 Intestine transplant infection CC
Use additional code to specify infection
CC Excl: See code: T86.850

T86.858 Other complications of intestine transplant CC
CC Excl: See code: T86.850

T86.859 Unspecified complication of intestine transplant CC
CC Excl: See code: T86.850

✓6ᵗʰ T86.89 Complications of other transplanted tissue
Transplant failure or rejection of pancreas

T86.890 Other transplanted tissue rejection CC
CC Excl: CC with 7th character A: D78.81-D78.89, E89.810-E89.89, H59.011-H59.019, H59.031-H59.099, H59.811-H59.89, H95.811-H95.89, I97.3, M96.89, N98.1-N98.9, T86.890-T86.899

T86.891 Other transplanted tissue failure CC
CC Excl: See code: T86.890

T86.892 Other transplanted tissue infection CC
Use additional code to specify infection
CC Excl: See code: T86.890

T86.898 Other complications of other transplanted tissue CC
CC Excl: See code: T86.890

T86.899 Unspecified complication of other transplanted tissue CC
CC Excl: See code: T86.890

✓5ᵗʰ T86.9 Complication of unspecified transplanted organ and tissue

T86.90 Unspecified complication of unspecified transplanted organ and tissue CC
CC Excl: CC with 7th character A: D47.Z1, D78.81-D78.89, E89.810-E89.89, H59.011-H59.019, H59.031-H59.099, H59.811-H59.89, H95.811-H95.89, I97.3, M96.89, N98.1-N98.9, T86.850-T86.859, T86.90-T86.99

T86.91 Unspecified transplanted organ and tissue rejection CC
CC Excl: See code: T86.90

T86.92 Unspecified transplanted organ and tissue failure CC
CC Excl: See code: T86.90

T86.93 Unspecified transplanted organ and tissue infection CC
Use additional code to specify infection
CC Excl: See code: T86.90

T86.99 Other complications of unspecified transplanted organ and tissue CC
CC Excl: See code: T86.90

✓4ᵗʰ T87 Complications peculiar to reattachment and amputation

✓5ᵗʰ T87.0 Complications of reattached (part of) upper extremity

✓6ᵗʰ T87.0X Complications of reattached (part of) upper extremity

CC Excl: For CC codes in subcategory T87.0X: CC with 7th character A, unless otherwise noted: D78.81-D78.89, E36.8, E89.810-E89.89, H59.011-H59.019, H59.031-H59.099, H59.811-H59.89, H95.811-H95.89, I97.3, L76.81-L76.82, M96.89, N98.1-N98.9, T81.82XA, T81.89X-T81.9XX with 7th A, T87.0X1-T87.0X9

T87.0X1 Complications of reattached (part of) right upper extremity CC

T87.0X2 Complications of reattached (part of) left upper extremity CC

T87.0X9 Complications of reattached (part of) unspecified upper extremity CC

✓5ᵗʰ T87.1 Complications of reattached (part of) lower extremity

✓6ᵗʰ T87.1X Complications of reattached (part of) lower extremity

CC Excl: For CC codes in subcategory T87.1X: CC with 7th character A, unless otherwise noted: D78.81-D78.89, E36.8, E89.810-E89.89, H59.011-H59.019, H59.031-H59.099, H59.811-H59.89, H95.811-H95.89, I97.3, L76.81-L76.82, M96.89, N98.1-N98.9, T81.82XA, T81.89X-T81.9XX with 7th A, T87.1X1-T87.1X9

T87.1X1 Complications of reattached (part of) right lower extremity CC

T87.1X2 Complications of reattached (part of) left lower extremity CC

T87.1X9 Complications of reattached (part of) unspecified lower extremity CC

T87.2 Complications of other reattached body part CC
CC Excl: CC with 7th character A: D78.81-D78.89, E36.8, E89.810-E89.89, H59.011-H59.019, H59.031-H59.099, H59.811-H59.89, H95.811-H95.89, I97.3, L76.81-L76.82, M96.89, N98.1-N98.9, T81.82XA, T81.89X-T81.9XX with 7th A, T87.2

✓5ᵗʰ T87.3 Neuroma of amputation stump

T87.30 Neuroma of amputation stump, unspecified extremity

T87.31 Neuroma of amputation stump, right upper extremity

T87.32 Neuroma of amputation stump, left upper extremity

T87.33 Neuroma of amputation stump, right lower extremity

T87.34 Neuroma of amputation stump, left lower extremity

✓5ᵗʰ T87.4 Infection of amputation stump

CC Excl: For CC codes in subcategory T87.4: CC with 7th character A, unless otherwise noted: D78.81-D78.89, E36.8, E89.810-E89.89, H59.011-H59.019, H59.031-H59.099, H59.811-H59.89, H95.811-H95.89, I97.3, L76.81-L76.82, M96.89, N98.1-N98.9, T81.82XA, T81.89X-T81.9XX with 7th A, T87.40-T87.9

T87.40 Infection of amputation stump, unspecified extremity CC

T87.41 Infection of amputation stump, right upper extremity CC

T87.42 Infection of amputation stump, left upper extremity CC

T87.43 Infection of amputation stump, right lower extremity CC

T87.44 Infection of amputation stump, left lower extremity CC

N Newborn: 0   P Pediatric: 0-17   M Maternity: 12-55   A Adult: 15-124   **MCC** Major CC Condition   **PDxMCC** PDx acts as own MCC   **CC** CC Condition   **PDxCC** PDx acts as own CC

1150

ICD-10-CM 2016

√5ᵗʰ **T87.5** **Necrosis** of amputation stump

     T87.50 **Necrosis** of amputation stump, **unspecified extremity**

     T87.51 **Necrosis** of amputation stump, **right upper extremity**

     T87.52 **Necrosis** of amputation stump, **left upper extremity**

     T87.53 **Necrosis** of amputation stump, **right lower extremity**

     T87.54 **Necrosis** of amputation stump, **left lower extremity**

√5ᵗʰ **T87.8** **Other** complications of amputation stump

     T87.81 **Dehiscence** of amputation stump

     T87.89 **Other** complications of amputation stump
         Amputation stump contracture
         Amputation stump contracture of next proximal joint
         Amputation stump flexion
         Amputation stump edema
         Amputation stump hematoma
         EXCLUDES 2   *phantom limb syndrome (G54.6-G54.7)*

T87.9 **Unspecified** complications of amputation stump

√4ᵗʰ **T88** **Other** complications of surgical and medical care, not elsewhere classified
     EXCLUDES 2   *complication following infusion, transfusion and therapeutic injection (T80.-)*
         complication following procedure NEC (T81.-)
         complications of anesthesia in labor and delivery (O74.-)
         complications of anesthesia in pregnancy (O29.-)
         complications of anesthesia in puerperium (O89.-)
         complications of devices, implants and grafts (T82-T85)
         complications of obstetric surgery and procedure (O75.4)
         dermatitis due to drugs and medicaments (L23.3, L24.4, L25.1, L27.0-L27.1)
         poisoning and toxic effects of drugs and chemicals (T36-T65 with fifth or sixth character 1-4 or 6)
         specified complications classified elsewhere

> The appropriate 7th character is to be added to each code from category T88.
> A   initial encounter
> D   subsequent encounter
> S   sequela

√x7ᵗʰ **T88.0** **Infection following immunization**   CC
     Sepsis following immunization
     CC Excl: CC with 7th character A: N98.0, T80.211-T80.29X with 7th A, T82.7XXA, T88.0XXA

√x7ᵗʰ **T88.1** **Other complications following immunization, not elsewhere classified**   CC
     Generalized vaccinia
     Rash following immunization
     EXCLUDES 1   *vaccinia not from vaccine (B08.011)*
     EXCLUDES 2   *anaphylactic shock due to serum (T80.5-)*
         other serum reactions (T80.6-)
         postimmunization arthropathy (M02.2)
         postimmunization encephalitis (G04.02)
         postimmunization fever (R50.83)
     CC Excl: CC with 7th character A: T88.1X

√x7ᵗʰ **T88.2** **Shock due to anesthesia**   CC
     Use additional code for adverse effect, if applicable, to identify drug (T41.- with fifth or sixth character 5)
     EXCLUDES 1   *complications of anesthesia (in):*
         labor and delivery (O74.-)
         postprocedural shock NOS (T81.1-)
         pregnancy (O29.-)
         puerperium (O89.-)
     CC Excl: CC with 7th character A: D78.01-D78.02, D78.21-D78.89, E36.01-E36.02, E36.8, E89.810-E89.89, G97.51-G97.52, H59.011-H59.019, H59.031-H59.129, H59.311-H59.329, H59.811-H59.89, H95.21-H95.22, H95.41-H95.89, I97.3-I97.42, I97.610-I97.62, J95.61-J95.62, J95.830-J95.831, K91.61-K91.62, K91.840-K91.841, L76.01-L76.02, L76.21-L76.82, M96.810-M96.811, M96.830-M96.89, N98.1-N98.9, N99.61-N99.62, N99.820-N99.821, T79.4XXA, T81.10X-T81.19X with 7th A, T81.82XA, T81.89X-T81.9XX with 7th A, T88.2XXA

√x7ᵗʰ **T88.3** **Malignant hyperthermia due to anesthesia**   CC
     Use additional code for adverse effect, if applicable, to identify drug (T41.- with fifth or sixth character 5)
     CC Excl: CC with 7th character A: D78.01-D78.02, D78.21-D78.89, E36.01-E36.02, E36.8, E89.810-E89.89, G97.51-G97.52, H59.011-H59.019, H59.031-H59.129, H59.311-H59.329, H59.811-H59.89, H95.21-H95.22, H95.41-H95.89, I97.3-I97.42, I97.610-I97.62, J95.61-J95.62, J95.830-J95.831, K91.61-K91.62, K91.840-K91.841, L76.01-L76.02, L76.21-L76.82, M96.810-M96.811, M96.830-M96.89, N98.1-N98.9, N99.61-N99.62, N99.820-N99.821, T79.4XXA, T81.10X-T81.19X with 7th A, T81.82XA, T81.89X-T81.9XX with 7th A, T88.2XX-T88.3XX with 7th A

13 √x7ᵗʰ **T88.4** **Failed or difficult intubation**

√5ᵗʰ **T88.5** **Other complications of anesthesia**
     Use additional code for adverse effect, if applicable, to identify drug (T41.- with fifth or sixth character 5)

     √x7ᵗʰ **T88.51** **Hypothermia following anesthesia**

     √x7ᵗʰ **T88.52** **Failed moderate sedation during procedure**
         Failed conscious sedation during procedure
         EXCLUDES 2   *personal history of failed moderate sedation (Z92.83)*

     √x7ᵗʰ **T88.59** **Other complications of anesthesia**

√x7ᵗʰ **T88.6** **Anaphylactic reaction due to adverse effect of correct drug or medicament properly administered**   CC
     Anaphylactic shock due to adverse effect of correct drug or medicament properly administered
     Anaphylactoid reaction NOS
     Use additional code for adverse effect, if applicable, to identify drug (T41.- with fifth or sixth character 5)
     EXCLUDES 1   *anaphylactic reaction due to serum (T80.5-)*
         anaphylactic shock or reaction due to adverse food reaction (T78.0-)
     CC Excl: CC with 7th character A: T78.00X-T78.09X with 7th A

13 √x7ᵗʰ **T88.7** **Unspecified adverse effect of drug or medicament**
     Drug hypersensitivity NOS
     Drug reaction NOS
     Use additional code for adverse effect, if applicable, to identify drug (T41.- with fifth or sixth character 5)
     EXCLUDES 1   *specified adverse effects of drugs and medicaments (A00-R94 and T80-T88.6, T88.8)*

13 √x7ᵗʰ **T88.8** **Other specified complications of surgical and medical care, not elsewhere classified**
     Use additional code to identify the complication

13 √x7ᵗʰ **T88.9** **Complication of surgical and medical care, unspecified**

✔ Additional Character Required   √x7ᵗʰ Placeholder Alert   Unacceptable PDx   Manifestation   Hospital Acquired Condition   EXCLUDES 1 Not Coded Here   EXCLUDES 2 Not Included Here

Chapter 20. External Causes of Morbidity (VØØ–Y99)

Chapter Specific Guidelines with Coding Examples

The chapter specific guidelines from the ICD-10-CM Official Guidelines for Coding and Reporting have been provided below. Along with these guidelines are coding examples, contained in the shaded boxes, that have been developed to help illustrate the coding and/or sequencing guidance found in these guidelines.

The external causes of morbidity codes should never be sequenced as the first-listed or principal diagnosis.

External cause codes are intended to provide data for injury research and evaluation of injury prevention strategies. These codes capture how the injury or health condition happened (cause), the intent (unintentional or accidental; or intentional, such as suicide or assault), the place where the event occurred, the activity of the patient at the time of the event, and the person's status (e.g., civilian, military).

There is no national requirement for mandatory ICD-10-CM external cause code reporting. Unless a provider is subject to a state-based external cause code reporting mandate or these codes are required by a particular payer, reporting of ICD-10-CM codes in Chapter 20, External Causes of Morbidity, is not required. In the absence of a mandatory reporting requirement, providers are encouraged to voluntarily report external cause codes, as they provide valuable data for injury research and evaluation of injury prevention strategies.

a. General external cause coding guidelines

1) **Used with any code in the range of A00.0–T88.9, Z00–Z99**

   An external cause code may be used with any code in the range of A00.0–T88.9, Z00–Z99, classification that is a health condition due to an external cause. Though they are most applicable to injuries, they are also valid for use with such things as infections or diseases due to an external source, and other health conditions, such as a heart attack that occurs during strenuous physical activity.

   > Actinic reticuloid due to tanning bed use
   >
   > **L57.1**   **Actinic reticuloid**
   >
   > **W89.1XXA**   **Exposure to tanning bed, initial encounter**
   >
   > *Explanation:* An external cause code may be used with any code in the range of A00.0–T88.9, Z00–Z99, classifications that describe health conditions due to an external cause. Code W89.1 Exposure to tanning bed requires a seventh character of A to report this initial encounter, with a placeholder X for the fifth and sixth characters.

2) **External cause code used for length of treatment**

   Assign the external cause code, with the appropriate 7th character (initial encounter, subsequent encounter or sequela) for each encounter for which the injury or condition is being treated.

   Most categories in chapter 20 have a 7th character requirement for each applicable code. Most categories in this chapter have three 7th character values: A, initial encounter, D, subsequent encounter and S, sequela. While the patient may be seen by a new or different provider over the course of treatment for an injury or condition, assignment of the 7th character for external cause should match the 7th character of the code assigned for the associated injury or condition for the encounter.

3) **Use the full range of external cause codes**

   Use the full range of external cause codes to completely describe the cause, the intent, the place of occurrence, and if applicable, the activity of the patient at the time of the event, and the patient's status, for all injuries, and other health conditions due to an external cause.

4) **Assign as many external cause codes as necessary**

   Assign as many external cause codes as necessary to fully explain each cause. If only one external code can be recorded, assign the code most related to the principal diagnosis.

5) **The selection of the appropriate external cause code**

   The selection of the appropriate external cause code is guided by the Alphabetic Index of External Causes and by Inclusion and Exclusion notes in the Tabular List.

6) **External cause code can never be a principal diagnosis**

   An external cause code can never be a principal (first-listed) diagnosis.

7) **Combination external cause codes**

   Certain of the external cause codes are combination codes that identify sequential events that result in an injury, such as a fall which results in striking against an object. The injury may be due to either event or both. The combination external cause code used should correspond to the sequence of events regardless of which caused the most serious injury.

   > Toddler tripped and fell while walking and struck his head on an end table, sustaining a scalp contusion
   >
   > **S00.03XA**   **Contusion of scalp, initial encounter**
   >
   > **W01.190A**   **Fall on same level from slipping, tripping and stumbling with subsequent striking against furniture, initial encounter**
   >
   > *Explanation:* Combination external cause codes identify sequential events that result in an injury, such as a fall resulting in striking against an object. The injury may be due to either or both events.

8) **No external cause code needed in certain circumstances**

   No external cause code from Chapter 20 is needed if the external cause and intent are included in a code from another chapter (e.g. T36.0X1-Poisoning by penicillins, accidental (unintentional)).

b. Place of occurrence guideline

Codes from category Y92, Place of occurrence of the external cause, are secondary codes for use after other external cause codes to identify the location of the patient at the time of injury or other condition.

Generally, a place of occurrence code is assigned only once, at the initial encounter for treatment. However, in the rare instance that a new injury occurs during hospitalization, an additional place of occurrence code may be assigned. No 7th characters are used for Y92.

Do not use place of occurrence code Y92.9 if the place is not stated or is not applicable.

> A farmer was working in his barn and sustained a foot contusion when the horse stepped on his left foot
>
> **S90.32XA**   **Contusion of left foot, initial encounter**
>
> **W55.19XA**   **Other contact with horse, initial encounter**
>
> **Y92.71**   **Barn as the place of occurrence of the external cause**
>
> *Explanation:* A place-of-occurrence code from category Y92 is assigned at the initial encounter to identify the location of the patient at the time the injury occurred.

c. Activity code

Assign a code from category Y93, Activity code, to describe the activity of the patient at the time the injury or other health condition occurred.

An activity code is used only once, at the initial encounter for treatment. Only one code from Y93 should be recorded on a medical record.

The activity codes are not applicable to poisonings, adverse effects, misadventures or sequela.

Do not assign Y93.9, Unspecified activity, if the activity is not stated.

A code from category Y93 is appropriate for use with external cause and intent codes if identifying the activity provides additional information about the event.

> Ranch hand who was grooming a horse sustained a foot contusion when the horse stepped on his left foot
>
> **S90.32XA**   **Contusion of left foot, initial encounter**
>
> **W55.19XA**   **Other contact with horse, initial encounter**
>
> **Y93.K3**   **Activity, grooming and shearing an animal**
>
> *Explanation:* One activity code from category Y93 is assigned at the initial encounter only to describe the activity of the patient at the time the injury occurred.

d. Place of occurrence, activity, and status codes used with other external cause code

When applicable, place of occurrence, activity, and external cause status codes are sequenced after the main external cause code(s). Regardless of the number of external cause codes assigned, there should be only one place of occurrence code, one activity code, and one external cause status code assigned to an encounter.

e. If the reporting format limits the number of external cause codes

If the reporting format limits the number of external cause codes that can be used in reporting clinical data, report the code for the cause/intent most related to the principal diagnosis. If the format permits, capture of additional external cause codes, the cause/intent, including medical misadventures, of the additional events should be reported rather than the codes for place, activity, or external status.

f. Multiple external cause coding guidelines

More than one external cause code is required to fully describe the external cause of an illness or injury. The assignment of external cause codes should be sequenced in the following priority:

If two or more events cause separate injuries, an external cause code should be assigned for each cause. The first-listed external cause code will be selected in the following order:

External codes for child and adult abuse take priority over all other external cause codes.

See Section I.C.19., Child and Adult abuse guidelines.

External cause codes for terrorism events take priority over all other external cause codes except child and adult abuse.

External cause codes for cataclysmic events take priority over all other external cause codes except child and adult abuse and terrorism.

External cause codes for transport accidents take priority over all other external cause codes except cataclysmic events, child and adult abuse and terrorism.

Activity and external cause status codes are assigned following all causal (intent) external cause codes.

The first-listed external cause code should correspond to the cause of the most serious diagnosis due to an assault, accident, or self-harm, following the order of hierarchy listed above.

30-year-old man accidentally discharged his hunting rifle, sustaining an open gunshot wound to the right thigh, which caused him to fall down the stairs, resulting in closed displaced comminuted fracture of his left radial shaft

S71.101A	**Unspecified open wound, right thigh, initial encounter**
W33.02XA	**Accidental discharge of hunting rifle, initial encounter**
S52.352A	**Displaced comminuted fracture of shaft of radius, left arm, initial encounter for closed fracture**
W10.9XXA	**Fall (on) (from) unspecified stairs and steps, initial encounter**

Explanation: If two or more events cause separate injuries, an external cause code should be assigned for each cause.

---

g. Child and adult abuse guideline

Adult and child abuse, neglect and maltreatment are classified as assault. Any of the assault codes may be used to indicate the external cause of any injury resulting from the confirmed abuse.

For confirmed cases of abuse, neglect and maltreatment, when the perpetrator is known, a code from Y07, Perpetrator of maltreatment and neglect, should accompany any other assault codes.

See Section I.C.19. Adult and child abuse, neglect and other maltreatment

h. Unknown or Undetermined Intent Guideline

If the intent (accident, self-harm, assault) of the cause of an injury or other condition is unknown or unspecified, code the intent as accidental intent. All transport accident categories assume accidental intent.

1) Use of undetermined intent

External cause codes for events of undetermined intent are only for use if the documentation in the record specifies that the intent cannot be determined.

i. Sequelae (late effects) of external cause guidelines

1) Sequelae external cause codes

Sequela are reported using the external cause code with the 7th character "S" for sequela. These codes should be used with any report of a late effect or sequela resulting from a previous injury.

See Section I.B.10 Sequela (Late Effects)

2) Sequela external cause code with a related current injury

A sequela external cause code should never be used with a related current nature of injury code.

3) Use of sequela external cause codes for subsequent visits

Use a late effect external cause code for subsequent visits when a late effect of the initial injury is being treated. Do not use a late effect external cause code for subsequent visits for follow-up care (e.g., to assess healing, to receive rehabilitative therapy) of the injury when no late effect of the injury has been documented.

j. Terrorism guidelines

1) Cause of injury identified by the Federal Government (FBI) as terrorism

When the cause of an injury is identified by the Federal Government (FBI) as terrorism, the first-listed external cause code should be a code from category Y38, Terrorism. The definition of terrorism employed by the FBI is found at the inclusion note at the beginning of category Y38. Use additional code for place of occurrence (Y92.-). More than one Y38 code may be assigned if the injury is the result of more than one mechanism of terrorism.

2) Cause of an injury is suspected to be the result of terrorism

When the cause of an injury is suspected to be the result of terrorism a code from category Y38 should not be assigned. Suspected cases should be classified as assault.

3) Code Y38.9, Terrorism, secondary effects

Assign code Y38.9, Terrorism, secondary effects, for conditions occurring subsequent to the terrorist event. This code should not be assigned for conditions that are due to the initial terrorist act.

It is acceptable to assign code Y38.9 with another code from Y38 if there is an injury due to the initial terrorist event and an injury that is a subsequent result of the terrorist event.

k. External cause status

A code from category Y99, External cause status, should be assigned whenever any other external cause code is assigned for an encounter, including an Activity code, except for the events noted below. Assign a code from category Y99, External cause status, to indicate the work status of the person at the time the event occurred. The status code indicates whether the event occurred during military activity, whether a non-military person was at work, whether an individual including a student or volunteer was involved in a non-work activity at the time of the causal event.

A code from Y99, External cause status, should be assigned, when applicable, with other external cause codes, such as transport accidents and falls. The external cause status codes are not applicable to poisonings, adverse effects, misadventures or late effects.

Do not assign a code from category Y99 if no other external cause codes (cause, activity) are applicable for the encounter.

An external cause status code is used only once, at the initial encounter for treatment. Only one code from Y99 should be recorded on a medical record.

Do not assign code Y99.9, Unspecified external cause status, if the status is not stated.

Chapter 20. External Causes of Morbidity (V00-Y99)

NOTE This chapter permits the classification of environmental events and circumstances as the cause of injury, and other adverse effects. Where a code from this section is applicable, it is intended that it shall be used secondary to a code from another chapter of the Classification indicating the nature of the condition. Most often, the condition will be classifiable to Chapter 19, Injury, poisoning and certain other consequences of external causes (S00-T88). Other conditions that may be stated to be due to external causes are classified in Chapters I to XVIII. For these conditions, codes from Chapter 20 should be used to provide additional information as to the cause of the condition.

This chapter contains the following blocks:

V00-X58	Accidents
V00-V99	Transport accidents
V00-V09	Pedestrian injured in transport accident
V10-V19	Pedal cycle rider injured in transport accident
V20-V29	Motorcycle rider injured in transport accident
V30-V39	Occupant of three-wheeled motor vehicle injured in transport accident
V40-V49	Car occupant injured in transport accident
V50-V59	Occupant of pick-up truck or van injured in transport accident
V60-V69	Occupant of heavy transport vehicle injured in transport accident
V70-V79	Bus occupant injured in transport accident
V80-V89	Other land transport accidents
V90-V94	Water transport accidents
V95-V97	Air and space transport accidents
V98-V99	Other and unspecified transport accidents
W00-X58	Other external causes of accidental injury
W00-W19	Slipping, tripping, stumbling and falls
W20-W49	Exposure to inanimate mechanical forces
W50-W64	Exposure to animate mechanical forces
W65-W74	Accidental non-transport drowning and submersion
W85-W99	Exposure to electric current, radiation and extreme ambient air temperature and pressure
X00-X08	Exposure to smoke, fire and flames
X10-X19	Contact with heat and hot substances
X30-X39	Exposure to forces of nature
X52-X58	Accidental exposure to other specified factors
X71-X83	Intentional self-harm
X92-Y08	Assault
Y21-Y33	Event of undetermined intent
Y35-Y38	Legal intervention, operations of war, military operations, and terrorism
Y62-Y84	Complications of medical and surgical care
Y62-Y69	Misadventures to patients during surgical and medical care
Y70-Y82	Medical devices associated with adverse incidents in diagnostic and therapeutic use
Y83-Y84	Surgical and other medical procedures as the cause of abnormal reaction of the patient, or of later complication, without mention of misadventure at the time of the procedure
Y90-Y99	Supplementary factors related to causes of morbidity classified elsewhere

Accidents (V00-X58)

Transport accidents (V00-V99)

NOTE This section is structured in 12 groups. Those relating to land transport accidents (V01-V89) reflect the victim's mode of transport and are subdivided to identify the victim's 'counterpart' or the type of event. The vehicle of which the injured person is an occupant is identified in the first two characters since it is seen as the most important factor to identify for prevention purposes. A transport accident is one in which the vehicle involved must be moving or running or in use for transport purposes at the time of the accident.

Use additional code to identify:
airbag injury (W22.1)
type of street or road (Y92.4-)
use of cellular telephone and other electronic equipment at the time of the transport accident (Y93.C-)

EXCLUDES 1 *agricultural vehicles in stationary use or maintenance (W31.-)*
assault by crashing of motor vehicle (Y03.-)
automobile or motor cycle in stationary use or maintenance—code to type of accident
crashing of motor vehicle, undetermined intent (Y32)
intentional self-harm by crashing of motor vehicle (X82)

EXCLUDES 2 *transport accidents due to cataclysm (X34-X38)*

NOTE Definitions of transport vehicles:

(a) A transport accident is any accident involving a device designed primarily for, or used at the time primarily for, conveying persons or good from one place to another.

(b) A public highway [trafficway] or street is the entire width between property lines (or other boundary lines) of land open to the public as a matter of right or custom for purposes of moving persons or property from one place to another. A roadway is that part of the public highway designed, improved and customarily used for vehicular traffic.

(c) A traffic accident is any vehicle accident occurring on the public highway [i.e. originating on, terminating on, or involving a vehicle partially on the highway]. A vehicle accident is assumed to have occurred on the public highway unless another place is specified, except in the case of accidents involving only off-road motor vehicles, which are classified as nontraffic accidents unless the contrary is stated.

(d) A nontraffic accident is any vehicle accident that occurs entirely in any place other than a public highway.

(e) A pedestrian is any person involved in an accident who was not at the time of the accident riding in or on a motor vehicle, railway train, streetcar or animal-drawn or other vehicle, or on a pedal cycle or animal. This includes, a person changing a tire or working on a parked car. It also includes the use of a pedestrian conveyance such as a baby carriage, ice-skates, roller skates, a skateboard, nonmotorized or motorized wheelchair, motorized mobility scooter, or nonmotorized scooter.

(f) A driver is an occupant of a transport vehicle who is operating or intending to operate it.

(g) A passenger is any occupant of a transport vehicle other than the driver, except a person traveling on the outside of the vehicle.

(h) A person on the outside of a vehicle is any person being transported by a vehicle but not occupying the space normally reserved for the driver or passengers, or the space intended for the transport of property. This includes the body, bumper, fender, roof, running board or step of a vehicle.

(i) A pedal cycle is any land transport vehicle operated solely by nonmotorized pedals including a bicycle or tricycle.

(j) A pedal cyclist is any person riding a pedal cycle or in a sidecar or trailer attached to a pedal cycle.

(k) A motorcycle is a two-wheeled motor vehicle with one or two riding saddles and sometimes with a third wheel for the support of a sidecar. The sidecar is considered part of the motorcycle.

(l) A motorcycle rider is any person riding a motorcycle or in a sidecar or trailer attached to the motorcycle.

(m) A three-wheeled motor vehicle is a motorized tricycle designed primarily for on-road use. This includes a motor-driven tricycle, a motorized rickshaw, or a three-wheeled motor car.

(n) A car [automobile] is a four-wheeled motor vehicle designed primarily for carrying up to 7 persons. A trailer being towed by the car is considered part of the car.

(o) A pick-up truck or van is a four or six-wheeled motor vehicle designed for carrying passengers as well as property or cargo weighing less than the local limit for classification as a heavy goods vehicle, and not requiring a special driver's license. This includes a minivan and a sport-utility vehicle (SUV).

(p) A heavy transport vehicle is a motor vehicle designed primarily for carrying property, meeting local criteria for classification as a heavy goods vehicle in terms of weight and requiring a special driver's license.

(q) A bus (coach) is a motor vehicle designed or adapted primarily for carrying more than 10 passengers, and requiring a special driver's license.

(r) A railway train or railway vehicle is any device, with or without freight or passenger cars couple to it, designed for traffic on a railway track. This includes subterranean (subways) or elevated trains.

(s) A streetcar, is a device designed and used primarily for transporting passengers within a municipality, running on rails, usually subject to normal traffic control signals, and operated principally on a right-of-way that forms part of the roadway. This includes a tram or trolley that runs on rails. A trailer being towed by a streetcar is considered part of the streetcar.

(t) A special vehicle mainly used on industrial premises is a motor vehicle designed primarily for use within the buildings and premises of industrial or commercial establishments. This includes battery-powered trucks, forklifts, coal-cars in a coal mine, logging cars and trucks used in mines or quarries.

(u) A special vehicle mainly used in agriculture is a motor vehicle designed specifically for use in farming and agriculture (horticulture), to work the land, tend and harvest crops and transport materials on the farm. This includes harvesters, farm machinery and tractor and trailers.

(v) A special construction vehicle is a motor vehicle designed specifically for use on construction and demolition sites. This includes bulldozers, diggers, earth levellers, dump trucks. backhoes, front-end loaders, pavers, and mechanical shovels.

N Newborn: 0 | P Pediatric: 0-17 | M Maternity: 12-55 | A Adult: 15-124 | MCC Major CC Condition | PDxMCC PDx acts as own MCC | CC CC Condition | PDxCC PDx acts as own CC

1154

ICD-10-CM 2016

(w) A special all-terrain vehicle is a motor vehicle of special design to enable it to negotiate over rough or soft terrain, snow or sand. This includes snow mobiles, All-terrain vehicles (ATV), and dune buggies. It does not include passenger vehicle designated as Sport Utility Vehicles. (SUV)

(x) A watercraft is any device designed for transporting passengers or goods on water. This includes motor or sailboats, ships, and hovercraft.

(y) An aircraft is any device for transporting passengers or goods in the air. This includes hot-air balloons, gliders, helicopters and airplanes.

(z) A military vehicle is any motorized vehicle operating on a public roadway owned by the military and being operated by a member of the military

Pedestrian injured in transport accident (V00-V09)

INCLUDES   person changing tire on transport vehicle
             person examining engine of vehicle broken down in (on side of) road
EXCLUDES 1   fall due to non-transport collision with other person (W03)
             pedestrian on foot falling (slipping) on ice and snow (W00.-)
             struck or bumped by another person (W51)

√4ᵗʰ **V00 Pedestrian conveyance accident**

Use additional place of occurrence and activity external cause codes, if known (Y92-, Y93-)

EXCLUDES 1   collision with another person without fall (W51)
             fall due to person on foot colliding with another person on foot (W03)
             fall from non-moving wheelchair, nonmotorized scooter and motorized mobility scooter without collision (W05.-)
             pedestrian (conveyance) collision with other land transport vehicle (V01-V09)
             pedestrian on foot falling (slipping) on ice and snow (W00.-)

> The appropriate 7th character is to be added to each code from category V00.
> A   initial encounter
> D   subsequent encounter
> S   sequela

√5ᵗʰ **V00.0 Pedestrian on foot injured in collision with pedestrian conveyance**

√x7ᵗʰ **V00.01 Pedestrian on foot injured in collision with roller-skater**

√x7ᵗʰ **V00.02 Pedestrian on foot injured in collision with skateboarder**

√x7ᵗʰ **V00.09 Pedestrian on foot injured in collision with other pedestrian conveyance**

√5ᵗʰ **V00.1 Rolling-type pedestrian conveyance accident**

EXCLUDES 1   accident with babystroller (V00.82-)
             accident with motorized mobility scooter (V00.83-)
             accident with wheelchair (powered) (V00.81-)

√6ᵗʰ **V00.11 In-line roller-skate accident**

√7ᵗʰ **V00.111 Fall from in-line roller-skates**

√7ᵗʰ **V00.112 In-line roller-skater colliding with stationary object**

√7ᵗʰ **V00.118 Other in-line roller-skate accident**
EXCLUDES 1   roller-skater collision with other land transport vehicle (V01-V09 with 5th character 1)

√6ᵗʰ **V00.12 Non-in-line roller-skate accident**

√7ᵗʰ **V00.121 Fall from non-in-line roller-skates**

√7ᵗʰ **V00.122 Non-in-line roller-skater colliding with stationary object**

√7ᵗʰ **V00.128 Other non-in-line roller-skating accident**
EXCLUDES 1   roller-skater collision with other land transport vehicle (V01-V09 with 5th character 1)

√6ᵗʰ **V00.13 Skateboard accident**

√7ᵗʰ **V00.131 Fall from skateboard**

√7ᵗʰ **V00.132 Skateboarder colliding with stationary object**

√7ᵗʰ **V00.138 Other skateboard accident**
EXCLUDES 1   skateboarder collision with other land transport vehicle (V01-V09 with 5th character 2)

√6ᵗʰ **V00.14 Scooter (nonmotorized) accident**
EXCLUDES 1   motorscooter accident (V20-V29)

√7ᵗʰ **V00.141 Fall from scooter (nonmotorized)**

√7ᵗʰ **V00.142 Scooter (nonmotorized) colliding with stationary object**

√7ᵗʰ **V00.148 Other scooter (nonmotorized) accident**
EXCLUDES 1   scooter (nonmotorized) collision with other land transport vehicle (V01-V09 with fifth character 9)

√6ᵗʰ **V00.15 Heelies accident**
Rolling shoe
Wheeled shoe
Wheelies accident

√7ᵗʰ **V00.151 Fall from heelies**

√7ᵗʰ **V00.152 Heelies colliding with stationary object**

√7ᵗʰ **V00.158 Other heelies accident**

√6ᵗʰ **V00.18 Accident on other rolling-type pedestrian conveyance**

√7ᵗʰ **V00.181 Fall from other rolling-type pedestrian conveyance**

√7ᵗʰ **V00.182 Pedestrian on other rolling-type pedestrian conveyance colliding with stationary object**

√7ᵗʰ **V00.188 Other accident on other rolling-type pedestrian conveyance**

√5ᵗʰ **V00.2 Gliding-type pedestrian conveyance accident**

√6ᵗʰ **V00.21 Ice-skates accident**

√7ᵗʰ **V00.211 Fall from ice-skates**

√7ᵗʰ **V00.212 Ice-skater colliding with stationary object**

√7ᵗʰ **V00.218 Other ice-skates accident**
EXCLUDES 1   ice-skater collision with other land transport vehicle (V01-V09 with 5th digit 9)

√6ᵗʰ **V00.22 Sled accident**

√7ᵗʰ **V00.221 Fall from sled**

√7ᵗʰ **V00.222 Sledder colliding with stationary object**

√7ᵗʰ **V00.228 Other sled accident**
EXCLUDES 1   sled collision with other land transport vehicle (V01-V09 with 5th digit 9)

√6ᵗʰ **V00.28 Other gliding-type pedestrian conveyance accident**

√7ᵗʰ **V00.281 Fall from other gliding-type pedestrian conveyance**

√7ᵗʰ **V00.282 Pedestrian on other gliding-type pedestrian conveyance colliding with stationary object**

√7ᵗʰ **V00.288 Other accident on other gliding-type pedestrian conveyance**
EXCLUDES 1   gliding-type pedestrian conveyance collision with other land transport vehicle (V01-V09 with 5th digit 9)

√5ᵗʰ **V00.3 Flat-bottomed pedestrian conveyance accident**

√6ᵗʰ **V00.31 Snowboard accident**

√7ᵗʰ **V00.311 Fall from snowboard**

√7ᵗʰ **V00.312 Snowboarder colliding with stationary object**

√7ᵗʰ **V00.318 Other snowboard accident**
EXCLUDES 1   snowboarder collision with other land transport vehicle (V01-V09 with 5th digit 9)

√6ᵗʰ **V00.32 Snow-ski accident**

√7ᵗʰ **V00.321 Fall from snow-skis**

√7ᵗʰ **V00.322 Snow-skier colliding with stationary object**

√7ᵗʰ **V00.328 Other snow-ski accident**
EXCLUDES 1   snow-skier collision with other land transport vehicle (V01-V09 with 5th digit 9)

√6ᵗʰ **V00.38 Other flat-bottomed pedestrian conveyance accident**

√7ᵗʰ **V00.381 Fall from other flat-bottomed pedestrian conveyance**

√7ᵗʰ **V00.382 Pedestrian on other flat-bottomed pedestrian conveyance colliding with stationary object**

√7ᵗʰ **V00.388 Other accident on other flat-bottomed pedestrian conveyance**

✔ Additional Character Required   √x7ᵗʰ Placeholder Alert   Unacceptable PDx   Manifestation   Hospital Acquired Condition   EXCLUDES 1 Not Coded Here   EXCLUDES 2 Not Included Here

Chapter 20. External Causes of Morbidity

✓5ᵗʰ **V00.8** **Accident on other pedestrian conveyance**

✓6ᵗʰ   **V00.81** **Accident with wheelchair (powered)**

✓7ᵗʰ   **V00.811** **Fall from moving wheelchair (powered)**
        EXCLUDES 1 *fall from non-moving wheelchair (W05.0)*

✓7ᵗʰ   **V00.812** **Wheelchair (powered) colliding with stationary object**

✓7ᵗʰ   **V00.818** **Other accident with wheelchair (powered)**

✓6ᵗʰ   **V00.82** **Accident with babystroller**

✓7ᵗʰ   **V00.821** **Fall from babystroller**

✓7ᵗʰ   **V00.822** **Babystroller colliding with stationary object**

✓7ᵗʰ   **V00.828** **Other accident with babystroller**

✓6ᵗʰ   **V00.83** **Accident with motorized mobility scooter**

     V00.831 **Fall from motorized mobility scooter**
        EXCLUDES 1 *fall from non-moving motorized mobility scooter (W05.2)*

     V00.832 **Motorized mobility scooter colliding with stationary object**

     V00.838 **Other accident with motorized mobility scooter**

✓6ᵗʰ   **V00.89** **Accident on other pedestrian conveyance**

✓7ᵗʰ   **V00.891** **Fall from other pedestrian conveyance**

✓7ᵗʰ   **V00.892** **Pedestrian on other pedestrian conveyance colliding with stationary object**

✓7ᵗʰ   **V00.898** **Other accident on other pedestrian conveyance**
        EXCLUDES 1 *other pedestrian (conveyance) collision with other land transport vehicle (V01-V09 with 5th digit 9)*

✓4ᵗʰ **V01** **Pedestrian injured in collision with pedal cycle**

> The appropriate 7th character is to be added to each code from category V01.
> A   initial encounter
> D   subsequent encounter
> S   sequela

✓5ᵗʰ   **V01.0** **Pedestrian injured in collision with pedal cycle in nontraffic accident**

✓x7ᵗʰ   **V01.00** **Pedestrian on foot injured in collision with pedal cycle in nontraffic accident**
        Pedestrian NOS injured in collision with pedal cycle in nontraffic accident

✓x7ᵗʰ   **V01.01** **Pedestrian on roller-skates injured in collision with pedal cycle in nontraffic accident**

✓x7ᵗʰ   **V01.02** **Pedestrian on skateboard injured in collision with pedal cycle in nontraffic accident**

✓x7ᵗʰ   **V01.09** **Pedestrian with other conveyance injured in collision with pedal cycle in nontraffic accident**
        Pedestrian with babystroller injured in collision with pedal cycle in nontraffic accident
        Pedestrian on ice-skates injured in collision with pedal cycle in nontraffic accident
        Pedestrian on nonmotorized scooter injured in collision with pedal cycle in nontraffic accident
        Pedestrian on sled injured in collision with pedal cycle in nontraffic accident
        Pedestrian on snowboard injured in collision with pedal cycle in nontraffic accident
        Pedestrian on snow-skis injured in collision with pedal cycle in nontraffic accident
        Pedestrian in wheelchair (powered) injured in collision with pedal cycle in nontraffic accident
        Pedestrian in motorized mobility scooter injured in collision with pedal cycle in nontraffic accident

✓5ᵗʰ   **V01.1** **Pedestrian injured in collision with pedal cycle in traffic accident**

✓x7ᵗʰ   **V01.10** **Pedestrian on foot injured in collision with pedal cycle in traffic accident**
        Pedestrian NOS injured in collision with pedal cycle in traffic accident

✓x7ᵗʰ   **V01.11** **Pedestrian on roller-skates injured in collision with pedal cycle in traffic accident**

✓x7ᵗʰ   **V01.12** **Pedestrian on skateboard injured in collision with pedal cycle in traffic accident**

✓x7ᵗʰ   **V01.19** **Pedestrian with other conveyance injured in collision with pedal cycle in traffic accident**
        Pedestrian with babystroller injured in collision with pedal cycle in traffic accident
        Pedestrian on ice-skates injured in collision with pedal cycle in traffic accident
        Pedestrian on nonmotorized scooter injured in collision with pedal cycle in traffic accident
        Pedestrian on sled injured in collision with pedal cycle in traffic accident
        Pedestrian on snowboard injured in collision with pedal cycle in traffic accident
        Pedestrian on snow-skis injured in collision with pedal cycle in traffic accident
        Pedestrian in wheelchair (powered) injured in collision with pedal cycle in traffic accident
        Pedestrian in motorized mobility scooter injured in collision with pedal cycle in traffic accident

✓5ᵗʰ   **V01.9** **Pedestrian injured in collision with pedal cycle, unspecified whether traffic or nontraffic accident**

✓x7ᵗʰ   **V01.90** **Pedestrian on foot injured in collision with pedal cycle, unspecified whether traffic or nontraffic accident**
        Pedestrian NOS injured in collision with pedal cycle, unspecified whether traffic or nontraffic accident

✓x7ᵗʰ   **V01.91** **Pedestrian on roller-skates injured in collision with pedal cycle, unspecified whether traffic or nontraffic accident**

✓x7ᵗʰ   **V01.92** **Pedestrian on skateboard injured in collision with pedal cycle, unspecified whether traffic or nontraffic accident**

✓x7ᵗʰ   **V01.99** **Pedestrian with other conveyance injured in collision with pedal cycle, unspecified whether traffic or nontraffic accident**
        Pedestrian with babystroller injured in collision with pedal cycle, unspecified whether traffic or nontraffic accident
        Pedestrian on ice-skates injured in collision with pedal cycle unspecified, whether traffic or nontraffic accident
        Pedestrian on nonmotorized scooter injured in collision with pedal cycle, unspecified whether traffic or nontraffic accident
        Pedestrian on sled injured in collision with pedal cycle unspecified, whether traffic or nontraffic accident
        Pedestrian on snowboard injured in collision with pedal cycle, unspecified whether traffic or nontraffic accident
        Pedestrian on snow-skis injured in collision with pedal cycle, unspecified whether traffic or nontraffic accident
        Pedestrian in wheelchair (powered) injured in collision with pedal cycle, unspecified whether traffic or nontraffic accident
        Pedestrian in motorized mobility scooter injured in collision with pedal cycle, unspecified whether traffic or nontraffic accident

✓4ᵗʰ **V02** **Pedestrian injured in collision with two- or three-wheeled motor vehicle**

> The appropriate 7th character is to be added to each code from category V02.
> A   initial encounter
> D   subsequent encounter
> S   sequela

✓5ᵗʰ   **V02.0** **Pedestrian injured in collision with two- or three-wheeled motor vehicle in nontraffic accident**

✓x7ᵗʰ   **V02.00** **Pedestrian on foot injured in collision with two- or three-wheeled motor vehicle in nontraffic accident**
        Pedestrian NOS injured in collision with two- or three-wheeled motor vehicle in nontraffic accident

✓x7ᵗʰ   **V02.01** **Pedestrian on roller-skates injured in collision with two- or three-wheeled motor vehicle in nontraffic accident**

✓x7ᵗʰ   **V02.02** **Pedestrian on skateboard injured in collision with two- or three-wheeled motor vehicle in nontraffic accident**

Ⓝ Newborn: 0   Ⓟ Pediatric: 0-17   Ⓜ Maternity: 12-55   Ⓐ Adult: 15-124   **MCC** Major CC Condition   **PDxMCC** PDx acts as own MCC   **CC** CC Condition   **PDxCC** PDx acts as own CC

1156   ICD-10-CM 2016

√x7th **V02.09** **Pedestrian with other conveyance injured in collision with two- or three-wheeled motor vehicle in nontraffic accident**
Pedestrian with babystroller injured in collision with two- or three-wheeled motor vehicle in nontraffic accident
Pedestrian on ice-skates injured in collision with two- or three-wheeled motor vehicle in nontraffic accident
Pedestrian on nonmotorized scooter injured in collision with two- or three-wheeled motor vehicle in nontraffic accident
Pedestrian on sled injured in collision with two- or three-wheeled motor vehicle in nontraffic accident
Pedestrian on snowboard injured in collision with two- or three-wheeled motor vehicle in nontraffic accident
Pedestrian on snow-skis injured in collision with two- or three-wheeled motor vehicle in nontraffic accident
Pedestrian in wheelchair (powered) injured in collision with two- or three-wheeled motor vehicle in nontraffic accident
Pedestrian in motorized mobility scooter injured in collision with two- or three-wheeled motor vehicle in nontraffic accident

√5th **V02.1** **Pedestrian injured in collision with two- or three-wheeled motor vehicle in traffic accident**

√x7th **V02.10** **Pedestrian on foot injured in collision with two- or three-wheeled motor vehicle in traffic accident**
Pedestrian NOS injured in collision with two- or three-wheeled motor vehicle in traffic accident

√x7th **V02.11** **Pedestrian on roller-skates injured in collision with two- or three-wheeled motor vehicle in traffic accident**

√x7th **V02.12** **Pedestrian on skateboard injured in collision with two- or three-wheeled motor vehicle in traffic accident**

√x7th **V02.19** **Pedestrian with other conveyance injured in collision with two- or three-wheeled motor vehicle in traffic accident**
Pedestrian with babystroller injured in collision with two- or three-wheeled motor vehicle in traffic accident
Pedestrian on ice-skates injured in collision with two- or three-wheeled motor vehicle in traffic accident
Pedestrian on nonmotorized scooter injured in collision with two- or three-wheeled motor vehicle in traffic accident
Pedestrian on sled injured in collision with two- or three-wheeled motor vehicle in traffic accident
Pedestrian on snowboard injured in collision with two- or three-wheeled motor vehicle in traffic accident
Pedestrian on snow-skis injured in collision with two- or three-wheeled motor vehicle in traffic accident
Pedestrian in wheelchair (powered) injured in collision with two- or three-wheeled motor vehicle in traffic accident
Pedestrian in motorized mobility scooter injured in collision with two- or three-wheeled motor vehicle in traffic accident

√5th **V02.9** **Pedestrian injured in collision with two- or three-wheeled motor vehicle, unspecified whether traffic or nontraffic accident**

√x7th **V02.90** **Pedestrian on foot injured in collision with two- or three-wheeled motor vehicle, unspecified whether traffic or nontraffic accident**
Pedestrian NOS injured in collision with two- or three-wheeled motor vehicle, unspecified whether traffic or nontraffic accident

√x7th **V02.91** **Pedestrian on roller-skates injured in collision with two- or three-wheeled motor vehicle, unspecified whether traffic or nontraffic accident**

√x7th **V02.92** **Pedestrian on skateboard injured in collision with two- or three-wheeled motor vehicle, unspecified whether traffic or nontraffic accident**

√x7th **V02.99** **Pedestrian with other conveyance injured in collision with two- or three-wheeled motor vehicle, unspecified whether traffic or nontraffic accident**
Pedestrian with babystroller injured in collision with two- or three-wheeled motor vehicle, unspecified whether traffic or nontraffic accident
Pedestrian on ice-skates injured in collision with two- or three-wheeled motor vehicle, unspecified whether traffic or nontraffic accident
Pedestrian on nonmotorized scooter injured in collision with two- or three-wheeled motor vehicle, unspecified whether traffic or nontraffic accident
Pedestrian on sled injured in collision with two- or three-wheeled motor vehicle, unspecified whether traffic or nontraffic accident
Pedestrian on snowboard injured in collision with two- or three-wheeled motor vehicle, unspecified whether traffic or nontraffic accident
Pedestrian on snow-skis injured in collision with two- or three-wheeled motor vehicle, unspecified whether traffic or nontraffic accident
Pedestrian in wheelchair (powered) injured in collision with two- or three-wheeled motor vehicle, unspecified whether traffic or nontraffic accident
Pedestrian in motorized mobility scooter injured in collision with two- or three-wheeled motor vehicle, unspecified whether traffic or nontraffic accident

√4th **V03** **Pedestrian injured in collision with car, pick-up truck or van**

The appropriate 7th character is to be added to each code from category V03.
A   initial encounter
D   subsequent encounter
S   sequela

√5th **V03.0** **Pedestrian injured in collision with car, pick-up truck or van in nontraffic accident**

√x7th **V03.00** **Pedestrian on foot injured in collision with car, pick-up truck or van in nontraffic accident**
Pedestrian NOS injured in collision with car, pick-up truck or van in nontraffic accident

√x7th **V03.01** **Pedestrian on roller-skates injured in collision with car, pick-up truck or van in nontraffic accident**

√x7th **V03.02** **Pedestrian on skateboard injured in collision with car, pick-up truck or van in nontraffic accident**

√x7th **V03.09** **Pedestrian with other conveyance injured in collision with car, pick-up truck or van in nontraffic accident**
Pedestrian with babystroller injured in collision with car, pick-up truck or van in nontraffic accident
Pedestrian on ice-skates injured in collision with car, pick-up truck or van in nontraffic accident
Pedestrian on nonmotorized scooter injured in collision with car, pick-up truck or van in nontraffic accident
Pedestrian on sled injured in collision with car, pick-up truck or van in nontraffic accident
Pedestrian on snowboard injured in collision with car, pick-up truck or van in nontraffic accident
Pedestrian on snow-skis injured in collision with car, pick-up truck or van in nontraffic accident
Pedestrian in wheelchair (powered) injured in collision with car, pick-up truck or van in nontraffic accident
Pedestrian in motorized mobility scooter injured in collision with car, pick-up truck or van in nontraffic accident

√5th **V03.1** **Pedestrian injured in collision with car, pick-up truck or van in traffic accident**

√x7th **V03.10** **Pedestrian on foot injured in collision with car, pick-up truck or van in traffic accident**
Pedestrian NOS injured in collision with car, pick-up truck or van in traffic accident

√x7th **V03.11** **Pedestrian on roller-skates injured in collision with car, pick-up truck or van in traffic accident**

√x7th **V03.12** **Pedestrian on skateboard injured in collision with car, pick-up truck or van in traffic accident**

√x7ᵗʰ **V03.19** **Pedestrian** with other conveyance **injured in collision with car, pick-up truck or van in traffic accident**
  Pedestrian with babystroller injured in collision with car, pick-up truck or van in traffic accident
  Pedestrian on ice-skates injured in collision with car, pick-up truck or van in traffic accident
  Pedestrian on nonmotorized scooter injured in collision with car, pick-up truck or van in traffic accident
  Pedestrian on sled injured in collision with car, pick-up truck or van in traffic accident
  Pedestrian on snowboard injured in collision with car, pick-up truck or van in traffic accident
  Pedestrian on snow-skis injured in collision with car, pick-up truck or van in traffic accident
  Pedestrian in wheelchair (powered) injured in collision with car, pick-up truck or van in traffic accident
  Pedestrian in motorized mobility scooter injured in collision with car, pick-up truck or van in traffic accident

√5ᵗʰ **V03.9** **Pedestrian injured in collision with car, pick-up truck or van,** unspecified whether traffic or nontraffic accident

√7ᵗʰ **V03.90** **Pedestrian** on foot **injured in collision with car, pick-up truck or van, unspecified whether traffic or nontraffic accident**
  Pedestrian NOS injured in collision with car, pick-up truck or van, unspecified whether traffic or nontraffic accident

√x7ᵗʰ **V03.91** **Pedestrian** on roller-skates **injured in collision with car, pick-up truck or van, unspecified whether traffic or nontraffic accident**

√x7ᵗʰ **V03.92** **Pedestrian** on skateboard **injured in collision with car, pick-up truck or van, unspecified whether traffic or nontraffic accident**

√x7ᵗʰ **V03.99** **Pedestrian** with other conveyance **injured in collision with car, pick-up truck or van, unspecified whether traffic or nontraffic accident**
  Pedestrian with babystroller injured in collision with car, pick-up truck or van, unspecified whether traffic or nontraffic accident
  Pedestrian on ice-skates injured in collision with car, pick-up truck or van, unspecified whether traffic or nontraffic accident
  Pedestrian on nonmotorized scooter injured in collision with car, pick-up truck or van, unspecified whether traffic or nontraffic accident
  Pedestrian on sled injured in collision with car, pick-up truck or van in nontraffic accident
  Pedestrian on snowboard injured in collision with car, pick-up truck or van, unspecified whether traffic or nontraffic accident
  Pedestrian on snow-skis injured in collision with car, pick-up truck or van, unspecified whether traffic or nontraffic accident
  Pedestrian in wheelchair (powered) injured in collision with car, pick-up truck or van, unspecified whether traffic or nontraffic accident
  Pedestrian in motorized mobility scooter injured in collision with car, pick-up truck or van, unspecified whether traffic or nontraffic accident

√4ᵗʰ **V04** **Pedestrian injured in collision with heavy transport vehicle or bus**
  EXCLUDES 1 *pedestrian injured in collision with military vehicle (V09.01, V09.21)*

  The appropriate 7th character is to be added to each code from category V04.
  A   initial encounter
  D   subsequent encounter
  S   sequela

√5ᵗʰ **V04.0** **Pedestrian injured in collision with heavy transport vehicle or bus** in nontraffic accident

√x7ᵗʰ **V04.00** **Pedestrian** on foot **injured in collision with heavy transport vehicle or bus in nontraffic accident**
  Pedestrian NOS injured in collision with heavy transport vehicle or bus in nontraffic accident

√x7ᵗʰ **V04.01** **Pedestrian** on roller-skates **injured in collision with heavy transport vehicle or bus in nontraffic accident**

√x7ᵗʰ **V04.02** **Pedestrian** on skateboard **injured in collision with heavy transport vehicle or bus in nontraffic accident**

√x7ᵗʰ **V04.09** **Pedestrian** with other conveyance **injured in collision with heavy transport vehicle or bus in nontraffic accident**
  Pedestrian with babystroller injured in collision with heavy transport vehicle or bus in nontraffic accident
  Pedestrian on ice-skates injured in collision with heavy transport vehicle or bus in nontraffic accident
  Pedestrian on nonmotorized scooter injured in collision with heavy transport vehicle or bus in nontraffic accident
  Pedestrian on sled injured in collision with heavy transport vehicle or bus in nontraffic accident
  Pedestrian on snowboard injured in collision with heavy transport vehicle or bus in nontraffic accident
  Pedestrian on snow-skis injured in collision with heavy transport vehicle or bus in nontraffic accident
  Pedestrian in wheelchair (powered) injured in collision with heavy transport vehicle or bus in nontraffic accident
  Pedestrian in motorized mobility scooter injured in collision with heavy transport vehicle or bus in nontraffic accident

√5ᵗʰ **V04.1** **Pedestrian injured in collision with heavy transport vehicle or bus** in traffic accident

√x7ᵗʰ **V04.10** **Pedestrian** on foot **injured in collision with heavy transport vehicle or bus in traffic accident**
  Pedestrian NOS injured in collision with heavy transport vehicle or bus in traffic accident

√x7ᵗʰ **V04.11** **Pedestrian** on roller-skates **injured in collision with heavy transport vehicle or bus in traffic accident**

√x7ᵗʰ **V04.12** **Pedestrian** on skateboard **injured in collision with heavy transport vehicle or bus in traffic accident**

√x7ᵗʰ **V04.19** **Pedestrian** with other conveyance **injured in collision with heavy transport vehicle or bus in traffic accident**
  Pedestrian with babystroller injured in collision with heavy transport vehicle or bus in traffic accident
  Pedestrian on ice-skates injured in collision with heavy transport vehicle or bus in traffic accident
  Pedestrian on nonmotorized scooter injured in collision with heavy transport vehicle or bus in traffic accident
  Pedestrian on sled injured in collision with heavy transport vehicle or bus in traffic accident
  Pedestrian on snowboard injured in collision with heavy transport vehicle or bus in traffic accident
  Pedestrian on snow-skis injured in collision with heavy transport vehicle or bus in traffic accident
  Pedestrian in wheelchair (powered) injured in collision with heavy transport vehicle or bus in traffic accident
  Pedestrian in motorized mobility scooter injured in collision with heavy transport vehicle or bus in traffic accident

√5ᵗʰ **V04.9** **Pedestrian injured in collision with heavy transport vehicle or bus,** unspecified whether traffic or nontraffic accident

√x7ᵗʰ **V04.90** **Pedestrian** on foot **injured in collision with heavy transport vehicle or bus, unspecified whether traffic or nontraffic accident**
  Pedestrian NOS injured in collision with heavy transport vehicle or bus, unspecified whether traffic or nontraffic accident

√x7ᵗʰ **V04.91** **Pedestrian** on roller-skates **injured in collision with heavy transport vehicle or bus, unspecified whether traffic or nontraffic accident**

√x7ᵗʰ **V04.92** **Pedestrian** on skateboard **injured in collision with heavy transport vehicle or bus, unspecified whether traffic or nontraffic accident**

Ⓝ Newborn: 0   Ⓟ Pediatric: 0-17   Ⓜ Maternity: 12-55   Ⓐ Adult: 15-124   MCC Major CC Condition   PDxMCC PDx acts as own MCC   CC CC Condition   PDxCC PDx acts as own CC

1158   ICD-10-CM 2016

√x7ᵗʰ V04.99 Pedestrian with other conveyance injured in collision with heavy transport vehicle or bus, unspecified whether traffic or nontraffic accident
> Pedestrian with babystroller injured in collision with heavy transport vehicle or bus, unspecified whether traffic or nontraffic accident
> Pedestrian on ice-skates injured in collision with heavy transport vehicle or bus, unspecified whether traffic or nontraffic accident
> Pedestrian on nonmotorized scooter injured in collision with heavy transport vehicle or bus, unspecified whether traffic or nontraffic accident
> Pedestrian on sled injured in collision with heavy transport vehicle or bus, unspecified whether traffic or nontraffic accident
> Pedestrian on snowboard injured in collision with heavy transport vehicle or bus, unspecified whether traffic or nontraffic accident
> Pedestrian on snow-skis injured in collision with heavy transport vehicle or bus, unspecified whether traffic or nontraffic accident
> Pedestrian in wheelchair (powered) injured in collision with heavy transport vehicle or bus, unspecified whether traffic or nontraffic accident
> Pedestrian in motorized mobility scooter injured in collision with heavy transport vehicle or bus, unspecified whether traffic or nontraffic accident

√4ᵗʰ V05 Pedestrian injured in collision with railway train or railway vehicle

> The appropriate 7th character is to be added to each code from category V05.
> A   initial encounter
> D   subsequent encounter
> S   sequela

√5ᵗʰ V05.0 Pedestrian injured in collision with railway train or railway vehicle in nontraffic accident

√x7ᵗʰ V05.00 Pedestrian on foot injured in collision with railway train or railway vehicle in nontraffic accident
> Pedestrian NOS injured in collision with railway train or railway vehicle in nontraffic accident

√x7ᵗʰ V05.01 Pedestrian on roller-skates injured in collision with railway train or railway vehicle in nontraffic accident

√x7ᵗʰ V05.02 Pedestrian on skateboard injured in collision with railway train or railway vehicle in nontraffic accident

√x7ᵗʰ V05.09 Pedestrian with other conveyance injured in collision with railway train or railway vehicle in nontraffic accident
> Pedestrian with babystroller injured in collision with railway train or railway vehicle in nontraffic accident
> Pedestrian on ice-skates injured in collision with railway train or railway vehicle in nontraffic accident
> Pedestrian on nonmotorized scooter injured in collision with railway train or railway vehicle in nontraffic accident
> Pedestrian on sled injured in collision with railway train or railway vehicle in nontraffic accident
> Pedestrian on snowboard injured in collision with railway train or railway vehicle in nontraffic accident
> Pedestrian on snow-skis injured in collision with railway train or railway vehicle in nontraffic accident
> Pedestrian in wheelchair (powered) injured in collision with railway train or railway vehicle in nontraffic accident
> Pedestrian in motorized mobility scooter injured in collision with railway train or railway vehicle in nontraffic accident

√5ᵗʰ V05.1 Pedestrian injured in collision with railway train or railway vehicle in traffic accident

√x7ᵗʰ V05.10 Pedestrian on foot injured in collision with railway train or railway vehicle in traffic accident
> Pedestrian NOS injured in collision with railway train or railway vehicle in traffic accident

√x7ᵗʰ V05.11 Pedestrian on roller-skates injured in collision with railway train or railway vehicle in traffic accident

√x7ᵗʰ V05.12 Pedestrian on skateboard injured in collision with railway train or railway vehicle in traffic accident

√x7ᵗʰ V05.19 Pedestrian with other conveyance injured in collision with railway train or railway vehicle in traffic accident
> Pedestrian with babystroller injured in collision with railway train or railway vehicle in traffic accident
> Pedestrian on ice-skates injured in collision with railway train or railway vehicle in traffic accident
> Pedestrian on nonmotorized scooter injured in collision with railway train or railway vehicle in traffic accident
> Pedestrian on sled injured in collision with railway train or railway vehicle in traffic accident
> Pedestrian on snowboard injured in collision with railway train or railway vehicle in traffic accident
> Pedestrian on snow-skis injured in collision with railway train or railway vehicle in traffic accident
> Pedestrian in wheelchair (powered) injured in collision with railway train or railway vehicle in traffic accident
> Pedestrian in motorized mobility scooter injured in collision with railway train or railway vehicle in traffic accident

√5ᵗʰ V05.9 Pedestrian injured in collision with railway train or railway vehicle, unspecified whether traffic or nontraffic accident

√x7ᵗʰ V05.90 Pedestrian on foot injured in collision with railway train or railway vehicle, unspecified whether traffic or nontraffic accident
> Pedestrian NOS injured in collision with railway train or railway vehicle, unspecified whether traffic or nontraffic accident

√x7ᵗʰ V05.91 Pedestrian on roller-skates injured in collision with railway train or railway vehicle, unspecified whether traffic or nontraffic accident

√x7ᵗʰ V05.92 Pedestrian on skateboard injured in collision with railway train or railway vehicle, unspecified whether traffic or nontraffic accident

√x7ᵗʰ V05.99 Pedestrian with other conveyance injured in collision with railway train or railway vehicle, unspecified whether traffic or nontraffic accident
> Pedestrian with babystroller injured in collision with railway train or railway vehicle, unspecified whether traffic or nontraffic
> Pedestrian on ice-skates injured in collision with railway train or railway vehicle, unspecified whether traffic or nontraffic
> Pedestrian on nonmotorized scooter injured in collision with railway train or railway vehicle, unspecified whether traffic or nontraffic
> Pedestrian on sled injured in collision with railway train or railway vehicle, unspecified whether traffic or nontraffic
> Pedestrian on snowboard injured in collision with railway train or railway vehicle, unspecified whether traffic or nontraffic
> Pedestrian on snow-skis injured in collision with railway train or railway vehicle, unspecified whether traffic or nontraffic
> Pedestrian in wheelchair (powered) injured in collision with railway train or railway vehicle, unspecified whether traffic or nontraffic
> Pedestrian in motorized mobility scooter injured in collision with railway train or railway vehicle, unspecified whether traffic or nontraffic

√4ᵗʰ V06 Pedestrian injured in collision with other nonmotor vehicle
> **INCLUDES** collision with animal-drawn vehicle, animal being ridden, nonpowered streetcar
> **EXCLUDES 1** pedestrian injured in collision with pedestrian conveyance (V00.0-)

> The appropriate 7th character is to be added to each code from category V06.
> A   initial encounter
> D   subsequent encounter
> S   sequela

√5ᵗʰ V06.0 Pedestrian injured in collision with other nonmotor vehicle in nontraffic accident

√x7ᵗʰ V06.00 Pedestrian on foot injured in collision with other nonmotor vehicle in nontraffic accident
> Pedestrian NOS injured in collision with other nonmotor vehicle in nontraffic accident

√x7ᵗʰ V06.01 Pedestrian on roller-skates injured in collision with other nonmotor vehicle in nontraffic accident

✔ Additional Character Required   √x7ᵗʰ Placeholder Alert   Unacceptable PDx   Manifestation   Hospital Acquired Condition   **EXCLUDES 1** Not Coded Here   **EXCLUDES 2** Not Included Here

ICD-10-CM 2016   1159

√x7ᵗʰ **V06.02** **Pedestrian on skateboard injured in collision with other nonmotor vehicle in nontraffic accident**

√x7ᵗʰ **V06.09** **Pedestrian with other conveyance injured in collision with other nonmotor vehicle in nontraffic accident**
Pedestrian with babystroller injured in collision with other nonmotor vehicle in nontraffic accident
Pedestrian on ice-skates injured in collision with other nonmotor vehicle in nontraffic accident
Pedestrian on nonmotorized scooter injured in collision with other nonmotor vehicle in nontraffic accident
Pedestrian on sled injured in collision with other nonmotor vehicle in nontraffic accident
Pedestrian on snowboard injured in collision with other nonmotor vehicle in nontraffic accident
Pedestrian on snow-skis injured in collision with other nonmotor vehicle in nontraffic accident
Pedestrian in wheelchair (powered) injured in collision with other nonmotor vehicle in nontraffic accident
Pedestrian in motorized mobility scooter injured in collision with other nonmotor vehicle in nontraffic accident

√5ᵗʰ **V06.1** **Pedestrian injured in collision with other nonmotor vehicle in traffic accident**

√x7ᵗʰ **V06.10** **Pedestrian on foot injured in collision with other nonmotor vehicle in traffic accident**
Pedestrian NOS injured in collision with other nonmotor vehicle in traffic accident

√x7ᵗʰ **V06.11** **Pedestrian on roller-skates injured in collision with other nonmotor vehicle in traffic accident**

√x7ᵗʰ **V06.12** **Pedestrian on skateboard injured in collision with other nonmotor vehicle in traffic accident**

√x7ᵗʰ **V06.19** **Pedestrian with other conveyance injured in collision with other nonmotor vehicle in traffic accident**
Pedestrian with babystroller injured in collision with other nonmotor vehicle in nontraffic accident
Pedestrian on ice-skates injured in collision with other nonmotor vehicle in traffic accident
Pedestrian on nonmotorized scooter injured in collision with other nonmotor vehicle in traffic accident
Pedestrian on sled injured in collision with other nonmotor vehicle in traffic accident
Pedestrian on snowboard injured in collision with other nonmotor vehicle in traffic accident
Pedestrian on snow-skis injured in collision with other nonmotor vehicle in traffic accident
Pedestrian in wheelchair (powered) injured in collision with other nonmotor vehicle in traffic accident
Pedestrian in motorized mobility scooter injured in collision with other nonmotor vehicle in traffic accident

√5ᵗʰ **V06.9** **Pedestrian injured in collision with other nonmotor vehicle, unspecified whether traffic or nontraffic accident**

√x7ᵗʰ **V06.90** **Pedestrian on foot injured in collision with other nonmotor vehicle, unspecified whether traffic or nontraffic accident**
Pedestrian NOS injured in collision with other nonmotor vehicle, unspecified whether traffic or nontraffic accident

√x7ᵗʰ **V06.91** **Pedestrian on roller-skates injured in collision with other nonmotor vehicle, unspecified whether traffic or nontraffic accident**

√x7ᵗʰ **V06.92** **Pedestrian on skateboard injured in collision with other nonmotor vehicle, unspecified whether traffic or nontraffic accident**

√x7ᵗʰ **V06.99** **Pedestrian with other conveyance injured in collision with other nonmotor vehicle, unspecified whether traffic or nontraffic accident**
Pedestrian with babystroller injured in collision with other nonmotor vehicle, unspecified whether traffic or nontraffic accident
Pedestrian on ice-skates injured in collision with other nonmotor vehicle, unspecified whether traffic or nontraffic accident
Pedestrian on nonmotorized scooter injured in collision with other nonmotor vehicle, unspecified whether traffic or nontraffic accident
Pedestrian on sled injured in collision with other nonmotor vehicle, unspecified whether traffic or nontraffic accident
Pedestrian on snowboard injured in collision with other nonmotor vehicle, unspecified whether traffic or nontraffic accident
Pedestrian on snow-skis injured in collision with other nonmotor vehicle, unspecified whether traffic or nontraffic accident
Pedestrian in wheelchair (powered) injured in collision with other nonmotor vehicle, unspecified whether traffic or nontraffic accident
Pedestrian in motorized mobility scooter injured in collision with other nonmotor vehicle, unspecified whether traffic or nontraffic accident

√4ᵗʰ **V09** **Pedestrian injured in other and unspecified transport accidents**

The appropriate 7th character is to be added to each code from category V09.
A   initial encounter
D   subsequent encounter
S   sequela

√5ᵗʰ **V09.0** **Pedestrian injured in nontraffic accident involving other and unspecified motor vehicles**

√x7ᵗʰ **V09.00** **Pedestrian injured in nontraffic accident involving unspecified motor vehicles**

√x7ᵗʰ **V09.01** **Pedestrian injured in nontraffic accident involving military vehicle**

√x7ᵗʰ **V09.09** **Pedestrian injured in nontraffic accident involving other motor vehicles**
Pedestrian injured in nontraffic accident by special vehicle

√x7ᵗʰ **V09.1** **Pedestrian injured in unspecified nontraffic accident**

√5ᵗʰ **V09.2** **Pedestrian injured in traffic accident involving other and unspecified motor vehicles**

√x7ᵗʰ **V09.20** **Pedestrian injured in traffic accident involving unspecified motor vehicles**

√x7ᵗʰ **V09.21** **Pedestrian injured in traffic accident involving military vehicle**

√x7ᵗʰ **V09.29** **Pedestrian injured in traffic accident involving other motor vehicles**

√x7ᵗʰ **V09.3** **Pedestrian injured in unspecified traffic accident**

√x7ᵗʰ **V09.9** **Pedestrian injured in unspecified transport accident**

Pedal cycle rider injured in transport accident (V10–V19)
INCLUDES   any non-motorized vehicle, excluding an animal-drawn vehicle, or a sidecar or trailer attached to the pedal cycle
EXCLUDES 2   *rupture of pedal cycle tire (W37.0)*

√4ᵗʰ **V10** **Pedal cycle rider injured in collision with pedestrian or animal**
EXCLUDES 1   *pedal cycle rider collision with animal-drawn vehicle or animal being ridden (V16.-)*

The appropriate 7th character is to be added to each code from category V10.
A   initial encounter
D   subsequent encounter
S   sequela

√x7ᵗʰ **V10.0** **Pedal cycle driver injured in collision with pedestrian or animal in nontraffic accident**

√x7ᵗʰ **V10.1** **Pedal cycle passenger injured in collision with pedestrian or animal in nontraffic accident**

√x7ᵗʰ **V10.2** **Unspecified pedal cyclist injured in collision with pedestrian or animal in nontraffic accident**

√x7ᵗʰ **V10.3** **Person boarding or alighting a pedal cycle injured in collision with pedestrian or animal**

√x7ᵗʰ **V10.4** **Pedal cycle driver injured in collision with pedestrian or animal in traffic accident**

N Newborn: 0   P Pediatric: 0-17   M Maternity: 12-55   A Adult: 15-124   **MCC** Major CC Condition   **PDxMCC** PDx acts as own MCC   **CC** CC Condition   **PDxCC** PDx acts as own CC

√x7ᵗʰ **V10.5** Pedal cycle passenger injured in collision with pedestrian or animal in traffic accident

√x7ᵗʰ **V10.9** Unspecified pedal cyclist injured in collision with pedestrian or animal in traffic accident

√4ᵗʰ **V11 Pedal cycle rider injured in collision with other pedal cycle**

The appropriate 7th character is to be added to each code from category V11.
A   initial encounter
D   subsequent encounter
S   sequela

√x7ᵗʰ **V11.0** Pedal cycle driver injured in collision with other pedal cycle in nontraffic accident

√x7ᵗʰ **V11.1** Pedal cycle passenger injured in collision with other pedal cycle in nontraffic accident

√x7ᵗʰ **V11.2** Unspecified pedal cyclist injured in collision with other pedal cycle in nontraffic accident

√x7ᵗʰ **V11.3** Person boarding or alighting a pedal cycle injured in collision with other pedal cycle

√x7ᵗʰ **V11.4** Pedal cycle driver injured in collision with other pedal cycle in traffic accident

√x7ᵗʰ **V11.5** Pedal cycle passenger injured in collision with other pedal cycle in traffic accident

√x7ᵗʰ **V11.9** Unspecified pedal cyclist injured in collision with other pedal cycle in traffic accident

√4ᵗʰ **V12 Pedal cycle rider injured in collision with two- or three-wheeled motor vehicle**

The appropriate 7th character is to be added to each code from category V12.
A   initial encounter
D   subsequent encounter
S   sequela

√x7ᵗʰ **V12.0** Pedal cycle driver injured in collision with two- or three-wheeled motor vehicle in nontraffic accident

√x7ᵗʰ **V12.1** Pedal cycle passenger injured in collision with two- or three-wheeled motor vehicle in nontraffic accident

√x7ᵗʰ **V12.2** Unspecified pedal cyclist injured in collision with two- or three-wheeled motor vehicle in nontraffic accident

√x7ᵗʰ **V12.3** Person boarding or alighting a pedal cycle injured in collision with two- or three-wheeled motor vehicle

√x7ᵗʰ **V12.4** Pedal cycle driver injured in collision with two- or three-wheeled motor vehicle in traffic accident

√x7ᵗʰ **V12.5** Pedal cycle passenger injured in collision with two- or three-wheeled motor vehicle in traffic accident

√x7ᵗʰ **V12.9** Unspecified pedal cyclist injured in collision with two- or three-wheeled motor vehicle in traffic accident

√4ᵗʰ **V13 Pedal cycle rider injured in collision with car, pick-up truck or van**

The appropriate 7th character is to be added to each code from category V13.
A   initial encounter
D   subsequent encounter
S   sequela

√x7ᵗʰ **V13.0** Pedal cycle driver injured in collision with car, pick-up truck or van in nontraffic accident

√x7ᵗʰ **V13.1** Pedal cycle passenger injured in collision with car, pick-up truck or van in nontraffic accident

√x7ᵗʰ **V13.2** Unspecified pedal cyclist injured in collision with car, pick-up truck or van in nontraffic accident

√x7ᵗʰ **V13.3** Person boarding or alighting a pedal cycle injured in collision with car, pick-up truck or van

√x7ᵗʰ **V13.4** Pedal cycle driver injured in collision with car, pick-up truck or van in traffic accident

√x7ᵗʰ **V13.5** Pedal cycle passenger injured in collision with car, pick-up truck or van in traffic accident

√x7ᵗʰ **V13.9** Unspecified pedal cyclist injured in collision with car, pick-up truck or van in traffic accident

√4ᵗʰ **V14 Pedal cycle rider injured in collision with heavy transport vehicle or bus**

EXCLUDES1   pedal cycle rider injured in collision with military vehicle (V19.81)

The appropriate 7th character is to be added to each code from category V14.
A   initial encounter
D   subsequent encounter
S   sequela

√x7ᵗʰ **V14.0** Pedal cycle driver injured in collision with heavy transport vehicle or bus in nontraffic accident

√x7ᵗʰ **V14.1** Pedal cycle passenger injured in collision with heavy transport vehicle or bus in nontraffic accident

√x7ᵗʰ **V14.2** Unspecified pedal cyclist injured in collision with heavy transport vehicle or bus in nontraffic accident

√x7ᵗʰ **V14.3** Person boarding or alighting a pedal cycle injured in collision with heavy transport vehicle or bus

√x7ᵗʰ **V14.4** Pedal cycle driver injured in collision with heavy transport vehicle or bus in traffic accident

√x7ᵗʰ **V14.5** Pedal cycle passenger injured in collision with heavy transport vehicle or bus in traffic accident

√x7ᵗʰ **V14.9** Unspecified pedal cyclist injured in collision with heavy transport vehicle or bus in traffic accident

√4ᵗʰ **V15 Pedal cycle rider injured in collision with railway train or railway vehicle**

The appropriate 7th character is to be added to each code from category V15.
A   initial encounter
D   subsequent encounter
S   sequela

√x7ᵗʰ **V15.0** Pedal cycle driver injured in collision with railway train or railway vehicle in nontraffic accident

√x7ᵗʰ **V15.1** Pedal cycle passenger injured in collision with railway train or railway vehicle in nontraffic accident

√x7ᵗʰ **V15.2** Unspecified pedal cyclist injured in collision with railway train or railway vehicle in nontraffic accident

√x7ᵗʰ **V15.3** Person boarding or alighting a pedal cycle injured in collision with railway train or railway vehicle

√x7ᵗʰ **V15.4** Pedal cycle driver injured in collision with railway train or railway vehicle in traffic accident

√x7ᵗʰ **V15.5** Pedal cycle passenger injured in collision with railway train or railway vehicle in traffic accident

√x7ᵗʰ **V15.9** Unspecified pedal cyclist injured in collision with railway train or railway vehicle in traffic accident

√4ᵗʰ **V16 Pedal cycle rider injured in collision with other nonmotor vehicle**

INCLUDES   collision with animal-drawn vehicle, animal being ridden, streetcar

The appropriate 7th character is to be added to each code from category V16.
A   initial encounter
D   subsequent encounter
S   sequela

√x7ᵗʰ **V16.0** Pedal cycle driver injured in collision with other nonmotor vehicle in nontraffic accident

√x7ᵗʰ **V16.1** Pedal cycle passenger injured in collision with other nonmotor vehicle in nontraffic accident

√x7ᵗʰ **V16.2** Unspecified pedal cyclist injured in collision with other nonmotor vehicle in nontraffic accident

√x7ᵗʰ **V16.3** Person boarding or alighting a pedal cycle injured in collision with other nonmotor vehicle in nontraffic accident

√x7ᵗʰ **V16.4** Pedal cycle driver injured in collision with other nonmotor vehicle in traffic accident

√x7ᵗʰ **V16.5** Pedal cycle passenger injured in collision with other nonmotor vehicle in traffic accident

√x7ᵗʰ **V16.9** Unspecified pedal cyclist injured in collision with other nonmotor vehicle in traffic accident

✓4ᵗʰ V17 Pedal cycle rider injured in collision with fixed or stationary object

> The appropriate 7th character is to be added to each code from category V17.
> A   initial encounter
> D   subsequent encounter
> S   sequela

✓x7ᵗʰ **V17.0 Pedal cycle driver injured in collision with fixed or stationary object in nontraffic accident**

✓x7ᵗʰ **V17.1 Pedal cycle passenger injured in collision with fixed or stationary object in nontraffic accident**

✓x7ᵗʰ **V17.2 Unspecified pedal cyclist injured in collision with fixed or stationary object in nontraffic accident**

✓x7ᵗʰ **V17.3 Person boarding or alighting a pedal cycle injured in collision with fixed or stationary object**

✓x7ᵗʰ **V17.4 Pedal cycle driver injured in collision with fixed or stationary object in traffic accident**

✓x7ᵗʰ **V17.5 Pedal cycle passenger injured in collision with fixed or stationary object in traffic accident**

✓x7ᵗʰ **V17.9 Unspecified pedal cyclist injured in collision with fixed or stationary object in traffic accident**

✓4ᵗʰ V18 Pedal cycle rider injured in noncollision transport accident

> INCLUDES fall or thrown from pedal cycle (without antecedent collision)
> overturning pedal cycle NOS
> overturning pedal cycle without collision

> The appropriate 7th character is to be added to each code from category V18.
> A   initial encounter
> D   subsequent encounter
> S   sequela

✓x7ᵗʰ **V18.0 Pedal cycle driver injured in noncollision transport accident in nontraffic accident**

✓x7ᵗʰ **V18.1 Pedal cycle passenger injured in noncollision transport accident in nontraffic accident**

✓x7ᵗʰ **V18.2 Unspecified pedal cyclist injured in noncollision transport accident in nontraffic accident**

✓x7ᵗʰ **V18.3 Person boarding or alighting a pedal cycle injured in noncollision transport accident**

✓x7ᵗʰ **V18.4 Pedal cycle driver injured in noncollision transport accident in traffic accident**

✓x7ᵗʰ **V18.5 Pedal cycle passenger injured in noncollision transport accident in traffic accident**

✓x7ᵗʰ **V18.9 Unspecified pedal cyclist injured in noncollision transport accident in traffic accident**

✓4ᵗʰ V19 Pedal cycle rider injured in other and unspecified transport accidents

> The appropriate 7th character is to be added to each code from category V19.
> A   initial encounter
> D   subsequent encounter
> S   sequela

✓5ᵗʰ **V19.0 Pedal cycle driver injured in collision with other and unspecified motor vehicles in nontraffic accident**

✓x7ᵗʰ **V19.00 Pedal cycle driver injured in collision with unspecified motor vehicles in nontraffic accident**

✓x7ᵗʰ **V19.09 Pedal cycle driver injured in collision with other motor vehicles in nontraffic accident**

✓5ᵗʰ **V19.1 Pedal cycle passenger injured in collision with other and unspecified motor vehicles in nontraffic accident**

✓x7ᵗʰ **V19.10 Pedal cycle passenger injured in collision with unspecified motor vehicles in nontraffic accident**

✓x7ᵗʰ **V19.19 Pedal cycle passenger injured in collision with other motor vehicles in nontraffic accident**

✓5ᵗʰ **V19.2 Unspecified pedal cyclist injured in collision with other and unspecified motor vehicles in nontraffic accident**

✓x7ᵗʰ **V19.20 Unspecified pedal cyclist injured in collision with unspecified motor vehicles in nontraffic accident**
> Pedal cycle collision NOS, nontraffic

✓x7ᵗʰ **V19.29 Unspecified pedal cyclist injured in collision with other motor vehicles in nontraffic accident**

✓x7ᵗʰ **V19.3 Pedal cyclist (driver) (passenger) injured in unspecified nontraffic accident**
> Pedal cycle accident NOS, nontraffic
> Pedal cyclist injured in nontraffic accident NOS

✓5ᵗʰ **V19.4 Pedal cycle driver injured in collision with other and unspecified motor vehicles in traffic accident**

✓x7ᵗʰ **V19.40 Pedal cycle driver injured in collision with unspecified motor vehicles in traffic accident**

✓x7ᵗʰ **V19.49 Pedal cycle driver injured in collision with other motor vehicles in traffic accident**

✓5ᵗʰ **V19.5 Pedal cycle passenger injured in collision with other and unspecified motor vehicles in traffic accident**

✓x7ᵗʰ **V19.50 Pedal cycle passenger injured in collision with unspecified motor vehicles in traffic accident**

✓x7ᵗʰ **V19.59 Pedal cycle passenger injured in collision with other motor vehicles in traffic accident**

✓5ᵗʰ **V19.6 Unspecified pedal cyclist injured in collision with other and unspecified motor vehicles in traffic accident**

✓x7ᵗʰ **V19.60 Unspecified pedal cyclist injured in collision with unspecified motor vehicles in traffic accident**
> Pedal cycle collision NOS (traffic)

✓x7ᵗʰ **V19.69 Unspecified pedal cyclist injured in collision with other motor vehicles in traffic accident**

✓5ᵗʰ **V19.8 Pedal cyclist (driver) (passenger) injured in other specified transport accidents**

✓x7ᵗʰ **V19.81 Pedal cyclist (driver) (passenger) injured in transport accident with military vehicle**

✓x7ᵗʰ **V19.88 Pedal cyclist (driver) (passenger) injured in other specified transport accidents**

✓x7ᵗʰ **V19.9 Pedal cyclist (driver) (passenger) injured in unspecified traffic accident**
> Pedal cycle accident NOS

Motorcycle rider injured in transport accident (V20-V29)

INCLUDES moped
motorcycle with sidecar
motorized bicycle
motor scooter
EXCLUDES 1 three-wheeled motor vehicle (V30-V39)

✓4ᵗʰ V20 Motorcycle rider injured in collision with pedestrian or animal

> EXCLUDES 1 motorcycle rider collision with animal-drawn vehicle or animal being ridden (V26.-)

> The appropriate 7th character is to be added to each code from category V20.
> A   initial encounter
> D   subsequent encounter
> S   sequela

✓x7ᵗʰ **V20.0 Motorcycle driver injured in collision with pedestrian or animal in nontraffic accident**

✓x7ᵗʰ **V20.1 Motorcycle passenger injured in collision with pedestrian or animal in nontraffic accident**

✓x7ᵗʰ **V20.2 Unspecified motorcycle rider injured in collision with pedestrian or animal in nontraffic accident**

✓x7ᵗʰ **V20.3 Person boarding or alighting a motorcycle injured in collision with pedestrian or animal**

✓x7ᵗʰ **V20.4 Motorcycle driver injured in collision with pedestrian or animal in traffic accident**

✓x7ᵗʰ **V20.5 Motorcycle passenger injured in collision with pedestrian or animal in traffic accident**

✓x7ᵗʰ **V20.9 Unspecified motorcycle rider injured in collision with pedestrian or animal in traffic accident**

✓4ᵗʰ V21 Motorcycle rider injured in collision with pedal cycle

> The appropriate 7th character is to be added to each code from category V21.
> A   initial encounter
> D   subsequent encounter
> S   sequela

✓x7ᵗʰ **V21.0 Motorcycle driver injured in collision with pedal cycle in nontraffic accident**

✓x7ᵗʰ **V21.1 Motorcycle passenger injured in collision with pedal cycle in nontraffic accident**

✓x7ᵗʰ **V21.2 Unspecified motorcycle rider injured in collision with pedal cycle in nontraffic accident**

N Newborn: 0   P Pediatric: 0-17   M Maternity: 12-55   A Adult: 15-124   MCC Major CC Condition   PDxMCC PDx acts as own MCC   CC CC Condition   PDxCC PDx acts as own CC

1162

ICD-10-CM 2016

✓x7ᵗʰ **V21.3** Person boarding or alighting a motorcycle injured in collision with pedal cycle

✓x7ᵗʰ **V21.4** Motorcycle driver injured in collision with pedal cycle in traffic accident

✓x7ᵗʰ **V21.5** Motorcycle passenger injured in collision with pedal cycle in traffic accident

✓x7ᵗʰ **V21.9** Unspecified motorcycle rider injured in collision with pedal cycle in traffic accident

✓4ᵗʰ **V22** **Motorcycle rider injured in collision with two- or three-wheeled motor vehicle**

> The appropriate 7th character is to be added to each code from category V22.
> A   initial encounter
> D   subsequent encounter
> S   sequela

✓x7ᵗʰ **V22.0** Motorcycle driver injured in collision with two- or three-wheeled motor vehicle in nontraffic accident

✓x7ᵗʰ **V22.1** Motorcycle passenger injured in collision with two- or three-wheeled motor vehicle in nontraffic accident

✓x7ᵗʰ **V22.2** Unspecified motorcycle rider injured in collision with two- or three-wheeled motor vehicle in nontraffic accident

✓x7ᵗʰ **V22.3** Person boarding or alighting a motorcycle injured in collision with two- or three-wheeled motor vehicle

✓x7ᵗʰ **V22.4** Motorcycle driver injured in collision with two- or three-wheeled motor vehicle in traffic accident

✓x7ᵗʰ **V22.5** Motorcycle passenger injured in collision with two- or three-wheeled motor vehicle in traffic accident

✓x7ᵗʰ **V22.9** Unspecified motorcycle rider injured in collision with two- or three-wheeled motor vehicle in traffic accident

✓4ᵗʰ **V23** **Motorcycle rider injured in collision with car, pick-up truck or van**

> The appropriate 7th character is to be added to each code from category V23.
> A   initial encounter
> D   subsequent encounter
> S   sequela

✓x7ᵗʰ **V23.0** Motorcycle driver injured in collision with car, pick-up truck or van in nontraffic accident

✓x7ᵗʰ **V23.1** Motorcycle passenger injured in collision with car, pick-up truck or van in nontraffic accident

✓x7ᵗʰ **V23.2** Unspecified motorcycle rider injured in collision with car, pick-up truck or van in nontraffic accident

✓x7ᵗʰ **V23.3** Person boarding or alighting a motorcycle injured in collision with car, pick-up truck or van

✓x7ᵗʰ **V23.4** Motorcycle driver injured in collision with car, pick-up truck or van in traffic accident

✓x7ᵗʰ **V23.5** Motorcycle passenger injured in collision with car, pick-up truck or van in traffic accident

✓x7ᵗʰ **V23.9** Unspecified motorcycle rider injured in collision with car, pick-up truck or van in traffic accident

✓4ᵗʰ **V24** **Motorcycle rider injured in collision with heavy transport vehicle or bus**

> **EXCLUDES 1**   motorcycle rider injured in collision with military vehicle (V29.81)

> The appropriate 7th character is to be added to each code from category V24.
> A   initial encounter
> D   subsequent encounter
> S   sequela

✓x7ᵗʰ **V24.0** Motorcycle driver injured in collision with heavy transport vehicle or bus in nontraffic accident

✓x7ᵗʰ **V24.1** Motorcycle passenger injured in collision with heavy transport vehicle or bus in nontraffic accident

✓x7ᵗʰ **V24.2** Unspecified motorcycle rider injured in collision with heavy transport vehicle or bus in nontraffic accident

✓x7ᵗʰ **V24.3** Person boarding or alighting a motorcycle injured in collision with heavy transport vehicle or bus

✓x7ᵗʰ **V24.4** Motorcycle driver injured in collision with heavy transport vehicle or bus in traffic accident

✓x7ᵗʰ **V24.5** Motorcycle passenger injured in collision with heavy transport vehicle or bus in traffic accident

✓x7ᵗʰ **V24.9** Unspecified motorcycle rider injured in collision with heavy transport vehicle or bus in traffic accident

✓4ᵗʰ **V25** **Motorcycle rider injured in collision with railway train or railway vehicle**

> The appropriate 7th character is to be added to each code from category V25.
> A   initial encounter
> D   subsequent encounter
> S   sequela

✓x7ᵗʰ **V25.0** Motorcycle driver injured in collision with railway train or railway vehicle in nontraffic accident

✓x7ᵗʰ **V25.1** Motorcycle passenger injured in collision with railway train or railway vehicle in nontraffic accident

✓x7ᵗʰ **V25.2** Unspecified motorcycle rider injured in collision with railway train or railway vehicle in nontraffic accident

✓x7ᵗʰ **V25.3** Person boarding or alighting a motorcycle injured in collision with railway train or railway vehicle

✓x7ᵗʰ **V25.4** Motorcycle driver injured in collision with railway train or railway vehicle in traffic accident

✓x7ᵗʰ **V25.5** Motorcycle passenger injured in collision with railway train or railway vehicle in traffic accident

✓x7ᵗʰ **V25.9** Unspecified motorcycle rider injured in collision with railway train or railway vehicle in traffic accident

✓4ᵗʰ **V26** **Motorcycle rider injured in collision with other nonmotor vehicle**

> **INCLUDES**   collision with animal-drawn vehicle, animal being ridden, streetcar

> The appropriate 7th character is to be added to each code from category V26.
> A   initial encounter
> D   subsequent encounter
> S   sequela

✓x7ᵗʰ **V26.0** Motorcycle driver injured in collision with other nonmotor vehicle in nontraffic accident

✓x7ᵗʰ **V26.1** Motorcycle passenger injured in collision with other nonmotor vehicle in nontraffic accident

✓x7ᵗʰ **V26.2** Unspecified motorcycle rider injured in collision with other nonmotor vehicle in nontraffic accident

✓x7ᵗʰ **V26.3** Person boarding or alighting a motorcycle injured in collision with other nonmotor vehicle

✓x7ᵗʰ **V26.4** Motorcycle driver injured in collision with other nonmotor vehicle in traffic accident

✓x7ᵗʰ **V26.5** Motorcycle passenger injured in collision with other nonmotor vehicle in traffic accident

✓x7ᵗʰ **V26.9** Unspecified motorcycle rider injured in collision with other nonmotor vehicle in traffic accident

✓4ᵗʰ **V27** **Motorcycle rider injured in collision with fixed or stationary object**

> The appropriate 7th character is to be added to each code from category V27.
> A   initial encounter
> D   subsequent encounter
> S   sequela

✓x7ᵗʰ **V27.0** Motorcycle driver injured in collision with fixed or stationary object in nontraffic accident

✓x7ᵗʰ **V27.1** Motorcycle passenger injured in collision with fixed or stationary object in nontraffic accident

✓x7ᵗʰ **V27.2** Unspecified motorcycle rider injured in collision with fixed or stationary object in nontraffic accident

✓x7ᵗʰ **V27.3** Person boarding or alighting a motorcycle injured in collision with fixed or stationary object

✓x7ᵗʰ **V27.4** Motorcycle driver injured in collision with fixed or stationary object in traffic accident

✓x7ᵗʰ **V27.5** Motorcycle passenger injured in collision with fixed or stationary object in traffic accident

✓x7ᵗʰ **V27.9** Unspecified motorcycle rider injured in collision with fixed or stationary object in traffic accident

---

✓ Additional Character Required   ✓x7ᵗʰ Placeholder Alert   Unacceptable PDx   Manifestation   Hospital Acquired Condition   **EXCLUDES 1** Not Coded Here   **EXCLUDES 2** Not Included Here

Chapter 20. External Causes of Morbidity *(side margin)*

V28–V31.9 *(side margin)*

✓4ᵗʰ **V28 Motorcycle rider injured in noncollision transport accident**
   INCLUDES fall or thrown from motorcycle (without antecedent collision)
            overturning motorcycle NOS
            overturning motorcycle without collision

The appropriate 7th character is to be added to each code from category V28.
A   initial encounter
D   subsequent encounter
S   sequela

✓x7ᵗʰ **V28.0 Motorcycle driver injured in noncollision transport accident in nontraffic accident**

✓x7ᵗʰ **V28.1 Motorcycle passenger injured in noncollision transport accident in nontraffic accident**

✓x7ᵗʰ **V28.2 Unspecified motorcycle rider injured in noncollision transport accident in nontraffic accident**

✓x7ᵗʰ **V28.3 Person boarding or alighting a motorcycle injured in noncollision transport accident**

✓x7ᵗʰ **V28.4 Motorcycle driver injured in noncollision transport accident in traffic accident**

✓x7ᵗʰ **V28.5 Motorcycle passenger injured in noncollision transport accident in traffic accident**

✓x7ᵗʰ **V28.9 Unspecified motorcycle rider injured in noncollision transport accident in traffic accident**

✓4ᵗʰ **V29 Motorcycle rider injured in other and unspecified transport accidents**

The appropriate 7th character is to be added to each code from category V29.
A   initial encounter
D   subsequent encounter
S   sequela

✓5ᵗʰ **V29.0 Motorcycle driver injured in collision with other and unspecified motor vehicles in nontraffic accident**

  ✓x7ᵗʰ **V29.00 Motorcycle driver injured in collision with unspecified motor vehicles in nontraffic accident**

  ✓x7ᵗʰ **V29.09 Motorcycle driver injured in collision with other motor vehicles in nontraffic accident**

✓5ᵗʰ **V29.1 Motorcycle passenger injured in collision with other and unspecified motor vehicles in nontraffic accident**

  ✓x7ᵗʰ **V29.10 Motorcycle passenger injured in collision with unspecified motor vehicles in nontraffic accident**

  ✓x7ᵗʰ **V29.19 Motorcycle passenger injured in collision with other motor vehicles in nontraffic accident**

✓5ᵗʰ **V29.2 Unspecified motorcycle rider injured in collision with other and unspecified motor vehicles in nontraffic accident**

  ✓x7ᵗʰ **V29.20 Unspecified motorcycle rider injured in collision with unspecified motor vehicles in nontraffic accident**
      Motorcycle collision NOS, nontraffic

  ✓x7ᵗʰ **V29.29 Unspecified motorcycle rider injured in collision with other motor vehicles in nontraffic accident**

✓x7ᵗʰ **V29.3 Motorcycle rider (driver) (passenger) injured in unspecified nontraffic accident**
    Motorcycle accident NOS, nontraffic
    Motorcycle rider injured in nontraffic accident NOS

✓5ᵗʰ **V29.4 Motorcycle driver injured in collision with other and unspecified motor vehicles in traffic accident**

  ✓x7ᵗʰ **V29.40 Motorcycle driver injured in collision with unspecified motor vehicles in traffic accident**

  ✓x7ᵗʰ **V29.49 Motorcycle driver injured in collision with other motor vehicles in traffic accident**

✓5ᵗʰ **V29.5 Motorcycle passenger injured in collision with other and unspecified motor vehicles in traffic accident**

  ✓x7ᵗʰ **V29.50 Motorcycle passenger injured in collision with unspecified motor vehicles in traffic accident**

  ✓x7ᵗʰ **V29.59 Motorcycle passenger injured in collision with other motor vehicles in traffic accident**

✓5ᵗʰ **V29.6 Unspecified motorcycle rider injured in collision with other and unspecified motor vehicles in traffic accident**

  ✓x7ᵗʰ **V29.60 Unspecified motorcycle rider injured in collision with unspecified motor vehicles in traffic accident**
      Motorcycle collision NOS (traffic)

  ✓x7ᵗʰ **V29.69 Unspecified motorcycle rider injured in collision with other motor vehicles in traffic accident**

✓5ᵗʰ **V29.8 Motorcycle rider (driver) (passenger) injured in other specified transport accidents**

  ✓x7ᵗʰ **V29.81 Motorcycle rider (driver) (passenger) injured in transport accident with military vehicle**

  ✓x7ᵗʰ **V29.88 Motorcycle rider (driver) (passenger) injured in other specified transport accidents**

✓x7ᵗʰ **V29.9 Motorcycle rider (driver) (passenger) injured in unspecified traffic accident**
    Motorcycle accident NOS

Occupant of three-wheeled motor vehicle injured in transport accident (V30-V39)

  INCLUDES motorized tricycle
           motorized rickshaw
           three-wheeled motor car
  EXCLUDES 1 all-terrain vehicles (V86.-)
           motorcycle with sidecar (V20-V29)
           vehicle designed primarily for off-road use (V86.-)

✓4ᵗʰ **V30 Occupant of three-wheeled motor vehicle injured in collision with pedestrian or animal**
  EXCLUDES 1 three-wheeled motor vehicle collision with animal-drawn vehicle or animal being ridden (V36.-)

The appropriate 7th character is to be added to each code from category V30.
A   initial encounter
D   subsequent encounter
S   sequela

✓x7ᵗʰ **V30.0 Driver of three-wheeled motor vehicle injured in collision with pedestrian or animal in nontraffic accident**

✓x7ᵗʰ **V30.1 Passenger in three-wheeled motor vehicle injured in collision with pedestrian or animal in nontraffic accident**

✓x7ᵗʰ **V30.2 Person on outside of three-wheeled motor vehicle injured in collision with pedestrian or animal in nontraffic accident**

✓x7ᵗʰ **V30.3 Unspecified occupant of three-wheeled motor vehicle injured in collision with pedestrian or animal in nontraffic accident**

✓x7ᵗʰ **V30.4 Person boarding or alighting a three-wheeled motor vehicle injured in collision with pedestrian or animal**

✓x7ᵗʰ **V30.5 Driver of three-wheeled motor vehicle injured in collision with pedestrian or animal in traffic accident**

✓x7ᵗʰ **V30.6 Passenger in three-wheeled motor vehicle injured in collision with pedestrian or animal in traffic accident**

✓x7ᵗʰ **V30.7 Person on outside of three-wheeled motor vehicle injured in collision with pedestrian or animal in traffic accident**

✓x7ᵗʰ **V30.9 Unspecified occupant of three-wheeled motor vehicle injured in collision with pedestrian or animal in traffic accident**

✓4ᵗʰ **V31 Occupant of three-wheeled motor vehicle injured in collision with pedal cycle**

The appropriate 7th character is to be added to each code from category V31.
A   initial encounter
D   subsequent encounter
S   sequela

✓x7ᵗʰ **V31.0 Driver of three-wheeled motor vehicle injured in collision with pedal cycle in nontraffic accident**

✓x7ᵗʰ **V31.1 Passenger in three-wheeled motor vehicle injured in collision with pedal cycle in nontraffic accident**

✓x7ᵗʰ **V31.2 Person on outside of three-wheeled motor vehicle injured in collision with pedal cycle in nontraffic accident**

✓x7ᵗʰ **V31.3 Unspecified occupant of three-wheeled motor vehicle injured in collision with pedal cycle in nontraffic accident**

✓x7ᵗʰ **V31.4 Person boarding or alighting a three-wheeled motor vehicle injured in collision with pedal cycle**

✓x7ᵗʰ **V31.5 Driver of three-wheeled motor vehicle injured in collision with pedal cycle in traffic accident**

✓x7ᵗʰ **V31.6 Passenger in three-wheeled motor vehicle injured in collision with pedal cycle in traffic accident**

✓x7ᵗʰ **V31.7 Person on outside of three-wheeled motor vehicle injured in collision with pedal cycle in traffic accident**

✓x7ᵗʰ **V31.9 Unspecified occupant of three-wheeled motor vehicle injured in collision with pedal cycle in traffic accident**

N Newborn: 0 P Pediatric: 0-17 M Maternity: 12-55 A Adult: 15-124 MCC Major CC Condition PDxMCC PDx acts as own MCC CC CC Condition PDxCC PDx acts as own CC

1164   ICD-10-CM 2016

✅4ᵗʰ **V32 Occupant of three-wheeled motor vehicle injured in collision with two- or three-wheeled motor vehicle**

> The appropriate 7th character is to be added to each code from category V32.
> A   initial encounter
> D   subsequent encounter
> S   sequela

√x7ᵗʰ **V32.0 Driver** of three-wheeled motor vehicle injured in collision with two- or three-wheeled motor vehicle in nontraffic accident

√x7ᵗʰ **V32.1 Passenger** in three-wheeled motor vehicle injured in collision with two- or three-wheeled motor vehicle in nontraffic accident

√x7ᵗʰ **V32.2 Person on outside** of three-wheeled motor vehicle injured in collision with two- or three-wheeled motor vehicle in nontraffic accident

√x7ᵗʰ **V32.3 Unspecified** occupant of three-wheeled motor vehicle injured in collision with two- or three-wheeled motor vehicle in nontraffic accident

√x7ᵗʰ **V32.4 Person boarding or alighting** a three-wheeled motor vehicle injured in collision with two- or three-wheeled motor vehicle

√x7ᵗʰ **V32.5 Driver** of three-wheeled motor vehicle injured in collision with two- or three-wheeled motor vehicle in traffic accident

√x7ᵗʰ **V32.6 Passenger** in three-wheeled motor vehicle injured in collision with two- or three-wheeled motor vehicle in traffic accident

√x7ᵗʰ **V32.7 Person on outside** of three-wheeled motor vehicle injured in collision with two- or three-wheeled motor vehicle in traffic accident

√x7ᵗʰ **V32.9 Unspecified** occupant of three-wheeled motor vehicle injured in collision with two- or three-wheeled motor vehicle in traffic accident

✅4ᵗʰ **V33 Occupant of three-wheeled motor vehicle injured in collision with car, pick-up truck or van**

> The appropriate 7th character is to be added to each code from category V33.
> A   initial encounter
> D   subsequent encounter
> S   sequela

√x7ᵗʰ **V33.0 Driver** of three-wheeled motor vehicle injured in collision with car, pick-up truck or van in nontraffic accident

√x7ᵗʰ **V33.1 Passenger** in three-wheeled motor vehicle injured in collision with car, pick-up truck or van in nontraffic accident

√x7ᵗʰ **V33.2 Person on outside** of three-wheeled motor vehicle injured in collision with car, pick-up truck or van in nontraffic accident

√x7ᵗʰ **V33.3 Unspecified** occupant of three-wheeled motor vehicle injured in collision with car, pick-up truck or van in nontraffic accident

√x7ᵗʰ **V33.4 Person boarding or alighting** a three-wheeled motor vehicle injured in collision with car, pick-up truck or van

√x7ᵗʰ **V33.5 Driver** of three-wheeled motor vehicle injured in collision with car, pick-up truck or van in traffic accident

√x7ᵗʰ **V33.6 Passenger** in three-wheeled motor vehicle injured in collision with car, pick-up truck or van in traffic accident

√x7ᵗʰ **V33.7 Person on outside** of three-wheeled motor vehicle injured in collision with car, pick-up truck or van in traffic accident

√x7ᵗʰ **V33.9 Unspecified** occupant of three-wheeled motor vehicle injured in collision with car, pick-up truck or van in traffic accident

✅4ᵗʰ **V34 Occupant of three-wheeled motor vehicle injured in collision with heavy transport vehicle or bus**

> **EXCLUDES 1**   occupant of three-wheeled motor vehicle injured in collision with military vehicle (V39.81)

> The appropriate 7th character is to be added to each code from category V34.
> A   initial encounter
> D   subsequent encounter
> S   sequela

√x7ᵗʰ **V34.0 Driver** of three-wheeled motor vehicle injured in collision with heavy transport vehicle or bus in nontraffic accident

√x7ᵗʰ **V34.1 Passenger** in three-wheeled motor vehicle injured in collision with heavy transport vehicle or bus in nontraffic accident

√x7ᵗʰ **V34.2 Person on outside** of three-wheeled motor vehicle injured in collision with heavy transport vehicle or bus in nontraffic accident

√x7ᵗʰ **V34.3 Unspecified** occupant of three-wheeled motor vehicle injured in collision with heavy transport vehicle or bus in nontraffic accident

√x7ᵗʰ **V34.4 Person boarding or alighting** a three-wheeled motor vehicle injured in collision with heavy transport vehicle or bus

√x7ᵗʰ **V34.5 Driver** of three-wheeled motor vehicle injured in collision with heavy transport vehicle or bus in traffic accident

√x7ᵗʰ **V34.6 Passenger** in three-wheeled motor vehicle injured in collision with heavy transport vehicle or bus in traffic accident

√x7ᵗʰ **V34.7 Person on outside** of three-wheeled motor vehicle injured in collision with heavy transport vehicle or bus in traffic accident

√x7ᵗʰ **V34.9 Unspecified** occupant of three-wheeled motor vehicle injured in collision with heavy transport vehicle or bus in traffic accident

✅4ᵗʰ **V35 Occupant of three-wheeled motor vehicle injured in collision with railway train or railway vehicle**

> The appropriate 7th character is to be added to each code from category V35.
> A   initial encounter
> D   subsequent encounter
> S   sequela

√x7ᵗʰ **V35.0 Driver** of three-wheeled motor vehicle injured in collision with railway train or railway vehicle in nontraffic accident

√x7ᵗʰ **V35.1 Passenger** in three-wheeled motor vehicle injured in collision with railway train or railway vehicle in nontraffic accident

√x7ᵗʰ **V35.2 Person on outside** of three-wheeled motor vehicle injured in collision with railway train or railway vehicle in nontraffic accident

√x7ᵗʰ **V35.3 Unspecified** occupant of three-wheeled motor vehicle injured in collision with railway train or railway vehicle in nontraffic accident

√x7ᵗʰ **V35.4 Person boarding or alighting** a three-wheeled motor vehicle injured in collision with railway train or railway vehicle

√x7ᵗʰ **V35.5 Driver** of three-wheeled motor vehicle injured in collision with railway train or railway vehicle in traffic accident

√x7ᵗʰ **V35.6 Passenger** in three-wheeled motor vehicle injured in collision with railway train or railway vehicle in traffic accident

√x7ᵗʰ **V35.7 Person on outside** of three-wheeled motor vehicle injured in collision with railway train or railway vehicle in traffic accident

√x7ᵗʰ **V35.9 Unspecified** occupant of three-wheeled motor vehicle injured in collision with railway train or railway vehicle in traffic accident

✅4ᵗʰ **V36 Occupant of three-wheeled motor vehicle injured in collision with other nonmotor vehicle**

> **INCLUDES**   collision with animal-drawn vehicle, animal being ridden, streetcar

> The appropriate 7th character is to be added to each code from category V36.
> A   initial encounter
> D   subsequent encounter
> S   sequela

√x7ᵗʰ **V36.0 Driver** of three-wheeled motor vehicle injured in collision with other nonmotor vehicle in nontraffic accident

√x7ᵗʰ **V36.1 Passenger** in three-wheeled motor vehicle injured in collision with other nonmotor vehicle in nontraffic accident

√x7ᵗʰ **V36.2 Person on outside** of three-wheeled motor vehicle injured in collision with other nonmotor vehicle in nontraffic accident

√x7ᵗʰ **V36.3 Unspecified** occupant of three-wheeled motor vehicle injured in collision with other nonmotor vehicle in nontraffic accident

√x7ᵗʰ **V36.4 Person boarding or alighting** a three-wheeled motor vehicle injured in collision with other nonmotor vehicle

√x7ᵗʰ **V36.5 Driver** of three-wheeled motor vehicle injured in collision with other nonmotor vehicle in traffic accident

√x7ᵗʰ **V36.6 Passenger** in three-wheeled motor vehicle injured in collision with other nonmotor vehicle in traffic accident

√x7ᵗʰ **V36.7 Person on outside** of three-wheeled motor vehicle injured in collision with other nonmotor vehicle in traffic accident

√x7ᵗʰ **V36.9 Unspecified** occupant of three-wheeled motor vehicle injured in collision with other nonmotor vehicle in traffic accident

✅ Additional Character Required   √x7ᵗʰ Placeholder Alert   Unacceptable PDx   Manifestation   Hospital Acquired Condition   **EXCLUDES 1** Not Coded Here   **EXCLUDES 2** Not Included Here

ICD-10-CM 2016   1165

Chapter 20. External Causes of Morbidity

V37–V39.9

√4ᵗʰ **V37** **Occupant of three-wheeled motor vehicle injured in collision with fixed or stationary object**

> The appropriate 7th character is to be added to each code from category V37.
> A   initial encounter
> D   subsequent encounter
> S   sequela

√x7ᵗʰ **V37.0** **Driver** of three-wheeled motor vehicle injured in collision with fixed or stationary object in nontraffic accident

√x7ᵗʰ **V37.1** **Passenger** in three-wheeled motor vehicle injured in collision with fixed or stationary object in nontraffic accident

√x7ᵗʰ **V37.2** **Person on outside** of three-wheeled motor vehicle injured in collision with fixed or stationary object in nontraffic accident

√x7ᵗʰ **V37.3** **Unspecified** occupant of three-wheeled motor vehicle injured in collision with fixed or stationary object in nontraffic accident

√x7ᵗʰ **V37.4** **Person boarding or alighting** a three-wheeled motor vehicle injured in collision with fixed or stationary object

√x7ᵗʰ **V37.5** **Driver** of three-wheeled motor vehicle injured in collision with fixed or stationary object in traffic accident

√x7ᵗʰ **V37.6** **Passenger** in three-wheeled motor vehicle injured in collision with fixed or stationary object in traffic accident

√x7ᵗʰ **V37.7** **Person on outside** of three-wheeled motor vehicle injured in collision with fixed or stationary object in traffic accident

√x7ᵗʰ **V37.9** **Unspecified** occupant of three-wheeled motor vehicle injured in collision with fixed or stationary object in traffic accident

√4ᵗʰ **V38** **Occupant of three-wheeled motor vehicle injured in noncollision transport accident**

> INCLUDES   fall or thrown from three-wheeled motor vehicle
> overturning of three-wheeled motor vehicle NOS
> overturning of three-wheeled motor vehicle without collision

> The appropriate 7th character is to be added to each code from category V38.
> A   initial encounter
> D   subsequent encounter
> S   sequela

√x7ᵗʰ **V38.0** **Driver** of three-wheeled motor vehicle injured in noncollision transport accident in nontraffic accident

√x7ᵗʰ **V38.1** **Passenger** in three-wheeled motor vehicle injured in noncollision transport accident in nontraffic accident

√x7ᵗʰ **V38.2** **Person on outside** of three-wheeled motor vehicle injured in noncollision transport accident in nontraffic accident

√x7ᵗʰ **V38.3** **Unspecified** occupant of three-wheeled motor vehicle injured in noncollision transport accident in nontraffic accident

√x7ᵗʰ **V38.4** **Person boarding or alighting** a three-wheeled motor vehicle injured in noncollision transport accident

√x7ᵗʰ **V38.5** **Driver** of three-wheeled motor vehicle injured in noncollision transport accident in traffic accident

√x7ᵗʰ **V38.6** **Passenger** in three-wheeled motor vehicle injured in noncollision transport accident in traffic accident

√x7ᵗʰ **V38.7** **Person on outside** of three-wheeled motor vehicle injured in noncollision transport accident in traffic accident

√x7ᵗʰ **V38.9** **Unspecified** occupant of three-wheeled motor vehicle injured in noncollision transport accident in traffic accident

√4ᵗʰ **V39** **Occupant of three-wheeled motor vehicle injured in other and unspecified transport accidents**

> The appropriate 7th character is to be added to each code from category V39.
> A   initial encounter
> D   subsequent encounter
> S   sequela

√5ᵗʰ **V39.0** **Driver** of three-wheeled motor vehicle injured in collision with other and unspecified motor vehicles in nontraffic accident

     √x7ᵗʰ **V39.00** **Driver** of three-wheeled motor vehicle injured in collision with unspecified motor vehicles in nontraffic accident

     √x7ᵗʰ **V39.09** **Driver** of three-wheeled motor vehicle injured in collision with other motor vehicles in nontraffic accident

√5ᵗʰ **V39.1** **Passenger** in three-wheeled motor vehicle injured in collision with other and unspecified motor vehicles in nontraffic accident

     √x7ᵗʰ **V39.10** **Passenger** in three-wheeled motor vehicle injured in collision with unspecified motor vehicles in nontraffic accident

     √x7ᵗʰ **V39.19** **Passenger** in three-wheeled motor vehicle injured in collision with other motor vehicles in nontraffic accident

√5ᵗʰ **V39.2** **Unspecified** occupant of three-wheeled motor vehicle injured in collision with other and unspecified motor vehicles in nontraffic accident

     √x7ᵗʰ **V39.20** **Unspecified** occupant of three-wheeled motor vehicle injured in collision with unspecified motor vehicles in nontraffic accident
> Collision NOS involving three-wheeled motor vehicle, nontraffic

     √x7ᵗʰ **V39.29** **Unspecified** occupant of three-wheeled motor vehicle injured in collision with other motor vehicles in nontraffic accident

√x7ᵗʰ **V39.3** **Occupant (driver) (passenger)** of three-wheeled motor vehicle injured in unspecified nontraffic accident
> Accident NOS involving three-wheeled motor vehicle, nontraffic
> Occupant of three-wheeled motor vehicle injured in nontraffic accident NOS

√5ᵗʰ **V39.4** **Driver** of three-wheeled motor vehicle injured in collision with other and unspecified motor vehicles in traffic accident

     √x7ᵗʰ **V39.40** **Driver** of three-wheeled motor vehicle injured in collision with unspecified motor vehicles in traffic accident

     √x7ᵗʰ **V39.49** **Driver** of three-wheeled motor vehicle injured in collision with other motor vehicles in traffic accident

√5ᵗʰ **V39.5** **Passenger** in three-wheeled motor vehicle injured in collision with other and unspecified motor vehicles in traffic accident

     √x7ᵗʰ **V39.50** **Passenger** in three-wheeled motor vehicle injured in collision with unspecified motor vehicles in traffic accident

     √x7ᵗʰ **V39.59** **Passenger** in three-wheeled motor vehicle injured in collision with other motor vehicles in traffic accident

√5ᵗʰ **V39.6** **Unspecified** occupant of three-wheeled motor vehicle injured in collision with other and unspecified motor vehicles in traffic accident

     √x7ᵗʰ **V39.60** **Unspecified** occupant of three-wheeled motor vehicle injured in collision with unspecified motor vehicles in traffic accident
> Collision NOS involving three-wheeled motor vehicle (traffic)

     √x7ᵗʰ **V39.69** **Unspecified** occupant of three-wheeled motor vehicle injured in collision with other motor vehicles in traffic accident

√5ᵗʰ **V39.8** **Occupant (driver) (passenger)** of three-wheeled motor vehicle injured in other specified transport accidents

     √x7ᵗʰ **V39.81** **Occupant (driver) (passenger)** of three-wheeled motor vehicle injured in transport accident with military vehicle

     √x7ᵗʰ **V39.89** **Occupant (driver) (passenger)** of three-wheeled motor vehicle injured in other specified transport accidents

√x7ᵗʰ **V39.9** **Occupant (driver) (passenger)** of three-wheeled motor vehicle injured in unspecified traffic accident
> Accident NOS involving three-wheeled motor vehicle

N Newborn: 0   P Pediatric: 0-17   M Maternity: 12-55   A Adult: 15-124   MCC Major CC Condition   PDxMCC PDx acts as own MCC   CC CC Condition   PDxCC PDx acts as own CC

1166   ICD-10-CM 2016

Car occupant injured in transport accident (V40-V49)

INCLUDES　a four-wheeled motor vehicle designed primarily for carrying passengers
automobile (pulling a trailer or camper)

EXCLUDES 1　bus (V50-V59)
minibus (V50-V59)
minivan (V50-V59)
motorcoach (V70-V79)
pick-up truck (V50-V59)
sport utility vehicle (SUV) (V50-V59)

✓4th **V40　Car occupant injured in collision with pedestrian or animal**

　　EXCLUDES 1　car collision with animal-drawn vehicle or animal being ridden (V46.-)

The appropriate 7th character is to be added to each code from category V40.
A　initial encounter
D　subsequent encounter
S　sequela

✓x7th **V40.0　Car driver** injured in collision with pedestrian or animal in nontraffic accident

✓x7th **V40.1　Car passenger** injured in collision with pedestrian or animal in nontraffic accident

✓x7th **V40.2　Person on outside** of car injured in collision with pedestrian or animal in nontraffic accident

✓x7th **V40.3　Unspecified** car occupant injured in collision with pedestrian or animal in nontraffic accident

✓x7th **V40.4　Person boarding or alighting** a car injured in collision with pedestrian or animal

✓x7th **V40.5　Car driver** injured in collision with pedestrian or animal in traffic accident

✓x7th **V40.6　Car passenger** injured in collision with pedestrian or animal in traffic accident

✓x7th **V40.7　Person on outside** of car injured in collision with pedestrian or animal in traffic accident

✓x7th **V40.9　Unspecified** car occupant injured in collision with pedestrian or animal in traffic accident

✓4th **V41　Car occupant injured in collision with pedal cycle**

The appropriate 7th character is to be added to each code from category V41.
A　initial encounter
D　subsequent encounter
S　sequela

✓x7th **V41.0　Car driver** injured in collision with pedal cycle in nontraffic accident

✓x7th **V41.1　Car passenger** injured in collision with pedal cycle in nontraffic accident

✓x7th **V41.2　Person on outside** of car injured in collision with pedal cycle in nontraffic accident

✓x7th **V41.3　Unspecified** car occupant injured in collision with pedal cycle in nontraffic accident

✓x7th **V41.4　Person boarding or alighting** a car injured in collision with pedal cycle

✓x7th **V41.5　Car driver** injured in collision with pedal cycle in traffic accident

✓x7th **V41.6　Car passenger** injured in collision with pedal cycle in traffic accident

✓x7th **V41.7　Person on outside** of car injured in collision with pedal cycle in traffic accident

✓x7th **V41.9　Unspecified** car occupant injured in collision with pedal cycle in traffic accident

✓4th **V42　Car occupant injured in collision with two- or three-wheeled motor vehicle**

The appropriate 7th character is to be added to each code from category V42.
A　initial encounter
D　subsequent encounter
S　sequela

✓x7th **V42.0　Car driver** injured in collision with two- or three-wheeled motor vehicle in nontraffic accident

✓x7th **V42.1　Car passenger** injured in collision with two- or three-wheeled motor vehicle in nontraffic accident

✓x7th **V42.2　Person on outside** of car injured in collision with two- or three-wheeled motor vehicle in nontraffic accident

✓x7th **V42.3　Unspecified** car occupant injured in collision with two- or three-wheeled motor vehicle in nontraffic accident

✓x7th **V42.4　Person boarding or alighting** a car injured in collision with two- or three-wheeled motor vehicle

✓x7th **V42.5　Car driver** injured in collision with two- or three-wheeled motor vehicle in traffic accident

✓x7th **V42.6　Car passenger** injured in collision with two- or three-wheeled motor vehicle in traffic accident

✓x7th **V42.7　Person on outside** of car injured in collision with two- or three-wheeled motor vehicle in traffic accident

✓x7th **V42.9　Unspecified** car occupant injured in collision with two- or three-wheeled motor vehicle in traffic accident

✓4th **V43　Car occupant injured in collision with car, pick-up truck or van**

The appropriate 7th character is to be added to each code from category V43.
A　initial encounter
D　subsequent encounter
S　sequela

✓5th **V43.0　Car driver** injured in collision with car, pick-up truck or van in nontraffic accident

　✓x7th **V43.01　Car driver** injured in collision with sport utility vehicle in nontraffic accident

　✓x7th **V43.02　Car driver** injured in collision with other type car in nontraffic accident

　✓x7th **V43.03　Car driver** injured in collision with pick-up truck in nontraffic accident

　✓x7th **V43.04　Car driver** injured in collision with van in nontraffic accident

✓5th **V43.1　Car passenger** injured in collision with car, pick-up truck or van in nontraffic accident

　✓x7th **V43.11　Car passenger** injured in collision with sport utility vehicle in nontraffic accident

　✓x7th **V43.12　Car passenger** injured in collision with other type car in nontraffic accident

　✓x7th **V43.13　Car passenger** injured in collision with pick-up in nontraffic accident

　✓x7th **V43.14　Car passenger** injured in collision with van in nontraffic accident

✓5th **V43.2　Person on outside** of car injured in collision with car, pick-up truck or van in nontraffic accident

　✓x7th **V43.21　Person on outside** of car injured in collision with sport utility vehicle in nontraffic accident

　✓x7th **V43.22　Person on outside** of car injured in collision with other type car in nontraffic accident

　✓x7th **V43.23　Person on outside** of car injured in collision with pick-up truck in nontraffic accident

　✓x7th **V43.24　Person on outside** of car injured in collision with van in nontraffic accident

✓5th **V43.3　Unspecified** car occupant injured in collision with car, pick-up truck or van in nontraffic accident

　✓x7th **V43.31　Unspecified** car occupant injured in collision with sport utility vehicle in nontraffic accident

　✓x7th **V43.32　Unspecified** car occupant injured in collision with other type car in nontraffic accident

　✓x7th **V43.33　Unspecified** car occupant injured in collision with pick-up truck in nontraffic accident

　✓x7th **V43.34　Unspecified** car occupant injured in collision with van in nontraffic accident

✓5th **V43.4　Person boarding or alighting** a car injured in collision with car, pick-up truck or van

　✓x7th **V43.41　Person boarding or alighting** a car injured in collision with sport utility vehicle

　✓x7th **V43.42　Person boarding or alighting** a car injured in collision with other type car

　✓x7th **V43.43　Person boarding or alighting** a car injured in collision with pick-up truck

　✓x7th **V43.44　Person boarding or alighting** a car injured in collision with van

✓5th **V43.5　Car driver** injured in collision with car, pick-up truck or van in traffic accident

　✓x7th **V43.51　Car driver** injured in collision with sport utility vehicle in traffic accident

---

✓ Additional Character Required　　✓x7th Placeholder Alert　　Unacceptable PDx　　Manifestation　　Hospital Acquired Condition　　EXCLUDES 1 Not Coded Here　　EXCLUDES 2 Not Included Here

√x7ᵗʰ **V43.52** Car driver injured in collision with other type car in traffic accident

√x7ᵗʰ **V43.53** Car driver injured in collision with pick-up truck in traffic accident

√x7ᵗʰ **V43.54** Car driver injured in collision with van in traffic accident

√5ᵗʰ **V43.6** Car passenger injured in collision with car, pick-up truck or van in traffic accident

√x7ᵗʰ **V43.61** Car passenger injured in collision with sport utility vehicle in traffic accident

√x7ᵗʰ **V43.62** Car passenger injured in collision with other type car in traffic accident

√x7ᵗʰ **V43.63** Car passenger injured in collision with pick-up truck in traffic accident

√x7ᵗʰ **V43.64** Car passenger injured in collision with van in traffic accident

√5ᵗʰ **V43.7** Person on outside of car injured in collision with car, pick-up truck or van in traffic accident

√x7ᵗʰ **V43.71** Person on outside of car injured in collision with sport utility vehicle in traffic accident

√x7ᵗʰ **V43.72** Person on outside of car injured in collision with other type car in traffic accident

√x7ᵗʰ **V43.73** Person on outside of car injured in collision with pick-up truck in traffic accident

√x7ᵗʰ **V43.74** Person on outside of car injured in collision with van in traffic accident

√5ᵗʰ **V43.9** Unspecified car occupant injured in collision with car, pick-up truck or van in traffic accident

√x7ᵗʰ **V43.91** Unspecified car occupant injured in collision with sport utility vehicle in traffic accident

√x7ᵗʰ **V43.92** Unspecified car occupant injured in collision with other type car in traffic accident

√x7ᵗʰ **V43.93** Unspecified car occupant injured in collision with pick-up truck in traffic accident

√x7ᵗʰ **V43.94** Unspecified car occupant injured in collision with van in traffic accident

√4ᵗʰ **V44** Car occupant injured in collision with heavy transport vehicle or bus

EXCLUDES 1 *car occupant injured in collision with military vehicle (V49.81)*

The appropriate 7th character is to be added to each code from category V44.
A   initial encounter
D   subsequent encounter
S   sequela

√x7ᵗʰ **V44.0** Car driver injured in collision with heavy transport vehicle or bus in nontraffic accident

√x7ᵗʰ **V44.1** Car passenger injured in collision with heavy transport vehicle or bus in nontraffic accident

√x7ᵗʰ **V44.2** Person on outside of car injured in collision with heavy transport vehicle or bus in nontraffic accident

√x7ᵗʰ **V44.3** Unspecified car occupant injured in collision with heavy transport vehicle or bus in nontraffic accident

√x7ᵗʰ **V44.4** Person boarding or alighting a car injured in collision with heavy transport vehicle or bus

√x7ᵗʰ **V44.5** Car driver injured in collision with heavy transport vehicle or bus in traffic accident

√x7ᵗʰ **V44.6** Car passenger injured in collision with heavy transport vehicle or bus in traffic accident

√x7ᵗʰ **V44.7** Person on outside of car injured in collision with heavy transport vehicle or bus in traffic accident

√x7ᵗʰ **V44.9** Unspecified car occupant injured in collision with heavy transport vehicle or bus in traffic accident

√4ᵗʰ **V45** Car occupant injured in collision with railway train or railway vehicle

The appropriate 7th character is to be added to each code from category V45.
A   initial encounter
D   subsequent encounter
S   sequela

√x7ᵗʰ **V45.0** Car driver injured in collision with railway train or railway vehicle in nontraffic accident

√x7ᵗʰ **V45.1** Car passenger injured in collision with railway train or railway vehicle in nontraffic accident

√x7ᵗʰ **V45.2** Person on outside of car injured in collision with railway train or railway vehicle in nontraffic accident

√x7ᵗʰ **V45.3** Unspecified car occupant injured in collision with railway train or railway vehicle in nontraffic accident

√x7ᵗʰ **V45.4** Person boarding or alighting a car injured in collision with railway train or railway vehicle

√x7ᵗʰ **V45.5** Car driver injured in collision with railway train or railway vehicle in traffic accident

√x7ᵗʰ **V45.6** Car passenger injured in collision with railway train or railway vehicle in traffic accident

√x7ᵗʰ **V45.7** Person on outside of car injured in collision with railway train or railway vehicle in traffic accident

√x7ᵗʰ **V45.9** Unspecified car occupant injured in collision with railway train or railway vehicle in traffic accident

√4ᵗʰ **V46** Car occupant injured in collision with other nonmotor vehicle

INCLUDES collision with animal-drawn vehicle, animal being ridden, streetcar

The appropriate 7th character is to be added to each code from category V46.
A   initial encounter
D   subsequent encounter
S   sequela

√x7ᵗʰ **V46.0** Car driver injured in collision with other nonmotor vehicle in nontraffic accident

√x7ᵗʰ **V46.1** Car passenger injured in collision with other nonmotor vehicle in nontraffic accident

√x7ᵗʰ **V46.2** Person on outside of car injured in collision with other nonmotor vehicle in nontraffic accident

√x7ᵗʰ **V46.3** Unspecified car occupant injured in collision with other nonmotor vehicle in nontraffic accident

√x7ᵗʰ **V46.4** Person boarding or alighting a car injured in collision with other nonmotor vehicle

√x7ᵗʰ **V46.5** Car driver injured in collision with other nonmotor vehicle in traffic accident

√x7ᵗʰ **V46.6** Car passenger injured in collision with other nonmotor vehicle in traffic accident

√x7ᵗʰ **V46.7** Person on outside of car injured in collision with other nonmotor vehicle in traffic accident

√x7ᵗʰ **V46.9** Unspecified car occupant injured in collision with other nonmotor vehicle in traffic accident

√4ᵗʰ **V47** Car occupant injured in collision with fixed or stationary object

The appropriate 7th character is to be added to each code from category V47.
A   initial encounter
D   subsequent encounter
S   sequela

√5ᵗʰ **V47.0** Car driver injured in collision with fixed or stationary object in nontraffic accident

√x7ᵗʰ **V47.01** Driver of sport utility vehicle injured in collision with fixed or stationary object in nontraffic accident

√x7ᵗʰ **V47.02** Driver of other type car injured in collision with fixed or stationary object in nontraffic accident

√5ᵗʰ **V47.1** Car passenger injured in collision with fixed or stationary object in nontraffic accident

√x7ᵗʰ **V47.11** Passenger of sport utility vehicle injured in collision with fixed or stationary object in nontraffic accident

√x7ᵗʰ **V47.12** Passenger of other type car injured in collision with fixed or stationary object in nontraffic accident

√x7ᵗʰ **V47.2** Person on outside of car injured in collision with fixed or stationary object in nontraffic accident

√5ᵗʰ **V47.3** Unspecified car occupant injured in collision with fixed or stationary object in nontraffic accident

√x7ᵗʰ **V47.31** Unspecified occupant of sport utility vehicle injured in collision with fixed or stationary object in nontraffic accident

√x7ᵗʰ **V47.32** Unspecified occupant of other type car injured in collision with fixed or stationary object in nontraffic accident

√x7ᵗʰ **V47.4** Person boarding or alighting a car injured in collision with fixed or stationary object

Ⓝ Newborn: 0   Ⓟ Pediatric: 0-17   Ⓜ Maternity: 12-55   Ⓐ Adult: 15-124   **MCC** Major CC Condition   **PDxMCC** PDx acts as own MCC   **CC** CC Condition   **PDxCC** PDx acts as own CC

1168

ICD-10-CM 2016

✓5ᵗʰ **V47.5** Car driver injured in collision with fixed or stationary object in traffic accident

     ✓x7ᵗʰ **V47.51** Driver of sport utility vehicle injured in collision with fixed or stationary object in traffic accident

     ✓x7ᵗʰ **V47.52** Driver of other type car injured in collision with fixed or stationary object in traffic accident

✓5ᵗʰ **V47.6** Car passenger injured in collision with fixed or stationary object in traffic accident

     ✓x7ᵗʰ **V47.61** Passenger of sport utility vehicle injured in collision with fixed or stationary object in traffic accident

     ✓x7ᵗʰ **V47.62** Passenger of other type car injured in collision with fixed or stationary object in traffic accident

✓x7ᵗʰ **V47.7** Person on outside of car injured in collision with fixed or stationary object in traffic accident

✓5ᵗʰ **V47.9** Unspecified car occupant injured in collision with fixed or stationary object in traffic accident

     ✓x7ᵗʰ **V47.91** Unspecified occupant of sport utility vehicle injured in collision with fixed or stationary object in traffic accident

     ✓x7ᵗʰ **V47.92** Unspecified occupant of other type car injured in collision with fixed or stationary object in traffic accident

✓4ᵗʰ **V48** Car occupant injured in noncollision transport accident

     INCLUDES   overturning car NOS
                  overturning car without collision

> The appropriate 7th character is to be added to each code from category V48.
> A   initial encounter
> D   subsequent encounter
> S   sequela

✓x7ᵗʰ **V48.0** Car driver injured in noncollision transport accident in nontraffic accident

✓x7ᵗʰ **V48.1** Car passenger injured in noncollision transport accident in nontraffic accident

✓x7ᵗʰ **V48.2** Person on outside of car injured in noncollision transport accident in nontraffic accident

✓x7ᵗʰ **V48.3** Unspecified car occupant injured in noncollision transport accident in nontraffic accident

✓x7ᵗʰ **V48.4** Person boarding or alighting a car injured in noncollision transport accident

✓x7ᵗʰ **V48.5** Car driver injured in noncollision transport accident in traffic accident

✓x7ᵗʰ **V48.6** Car passenger injured in noncollision transport accident in traffic accident

✓x7ᵗʰ **V48.7** Person on outside of car injured in noncollision transport accident in traffic accident

✓x7ᵗʰ **V48.9** Unspecified car occupant injured in noncollision transport accident in traffic accident

✓4ᵗʰ **V49** Car occupant injured in other and unspecified transport accidents

> The appropriate 7th character is to be added to each code from category V49.
> A   initial encounter
> D   subsequent encounter
> S   sequela

✓5ᵗʰ **V49.0** Driver injured in collision with other and unspecified motor vehicles in nontraffic accident

     ✓x7ᵗʰ **V49.00** Driver injured in collision with unspecified motor vehicles in nontraffic accident

     ✓x7ᵗʰ **V49.09** Driver injured in collision with other motor vehicles in nontraffic accident

✓5ᵗʰ **V49.1** Passenger injured in collision with other and unspecified motor vehicles in nontraffic accident

     ✓x7ᵗʰ **V49.10** Passenger injured in collision with unspecified motor vehicles in nontraffic accident

     ✓x7ᵗʰ **V49.19** Passenger injured in collision with other motor vehicles in nontraffic accident

✓5ᵗʰ **V49.2** Unspecified car occupant injured in collision with other and unspecified motor vehicles in nontraffic accident

     ✓x7ᵗʰ **V49.20** Unspecified car occupant injured in collision with unspecified motor vehicles in nontraffic accident
             Car collision NOS, nontraffic

     ✓x7ᵗʰ **V49.29** Unspecified car occupant injured in collision with other motor vehicles in nontraffic accident

✓x7ᵗʰ **V49.3** Car occupant (driver) (passenger) injured in unspecified nontraffic accident
     Car accident NOS, nontraffic
     Car occupant injured in nontraffic accident NOS

✓5ᵗʰ **V49.4** Driver injured in collision with other and unspecified motor vehicles in traffic accident

     ✓x7ᵗʰ **V49.40** Driver injured in collision with unspecified motor vehicles in traffic accident

     ✓x7ᵗʰ **V49.49** Driver injured in collision with other motor vehicles in traffic accident

✓5ᵗʰ **V49.5** Passenger injured in collision with other and unspecified motor vehicles in traffic accident

     ✓x7ᵗʰ **V49.50** Passenger injured in collision with unspecified motor vehicles in traffic accident

     ✓x7ᵗʰ **V49.59** Passenger injured in collision with other motor vehicles in traffic accident

✓5ᵗʰ **V49.6** Unspecified car occupant injured in collision with other and unspecified motor vehicles in traffic accident

     ✓x7ᵗʰ **V49.60** Unspecified car occupant injured in collision with unspecified motor vehicles in traffic accident
             Car collision NOS (traffic)

     ✓x7ᵗʰ **V49.69** Unspecified car occupant injured in collision with other motor vehicles in traffic accident

✓5ᵗʰ **V49.8** Car occupant (driver) (passenger) injured in other specified transport accidents

     ✓x7ᵗʰ **V49.81** Car occupant (driver) (passenger) injured in transport accident with military vehicle

     ✓x7ᵗʰ **V49.88** Car occupant (driver) (passenger) injured in other specified transport accidents

✓x7ᵗʰ **V49.9** Car occupant (driver) (passenger) injured in unspecified traffic accident
     Car accident NOS

Occupant of pick-up truck or van injured in transport accident (V50-V59)

     INCLUDES   a four or six wheel motor vehicle designed primarily for carrying passengers and property but weighing less than the local limit for classification as a heavy goods vehicle
                minibus
                minivan
                sport utility vehicle (SUV)
                truck
                van
     EXCLUDES 1   *heavy transport vehicle (V60-V69)*

✓4ᵗʰ **V50** Occupant of pick-up truck or van injured in collision with pedestrian or animal
     EXCLUDES 1   *pick-up truck or van collision with animal-drawn vehicle or animal being ridden (V56.-)*

> The appropriate 7th character is to be added to each code from category V50.
> A   initial encounter
> D   subsequent encounter
> S   sequela

✓x7ᵗʰ **V50.0** Driver of pick-up truck or van injured in collision with pedestrian or animal in nontraffic accident

✓x7ᵗʰ **V50.1** Passenger in pick-up truck or van injured in collision with pedestrian or animal in nontraffic accident

✓x7ᵗʰ **V50.2** Person on outside of pick-up truck or van injured in collision with pedestrian or animal in nontraffic accident

✓x7ᵗʰ **V50.3** Unspecified occupant of pick-up truck or van injured in collision with pedestrian or animal in nontraffic accident

✓x7ᵗʰ **V50.4** Person boarding or alighting a pick-up truck or van injured in collision with pedestrian or animal

✓x7ᵗʰ **V50.5** Driver of pick-up truck or van injured in collision with pedestrian or animal in traffic accident

✓x7ᵗʰ **V50.6** Passenger in pick-up truck or van injured in collision with pedestrian or animal in traffic accident

✓x7ᵗʰ **V50.7** Person on outside of pick-up truck or van injured in collision with pedestrian or animal in traffic accident

✓x7ᵗʰ **V50.9** Unspecified occupant of pick-up truck or van injured in collision with pedestrian or animal in traffic accident

---

✓ Additional Character Required   ✓x7ᵗʰ Placeholder Alert   Unacceptable PDx   Manifestation   Hospital Acquired Condition   **EXCLUDES 1** Not Coded Here   **EXCLUDES 2** Not Included Here

✓4ᵗʰ **V51 Occupant of pick-up truck or van injured in collision with pedal cycle**

> The appropriate 7th character is to be added to each code from category V51.
> A   initial encounter
> D   subsequent encounter
> S   sequela

✓x7ᵗʰ **V51.0 Driver** of pick-up truck or van injured in collision with pedal cycle in nontraffic accident

✓x7ᵗʰ **V51.1 Passenger** in pick-up truck or van injured in collision with pedal cycle in nontraffic accident

✓x7ᵗʰ **V51.2 Person on outside** of pick-up truck or van injured in collision with pedal cycle in nontraffic accident

✓x7ᵗʰ **V51.3 Unspecified** occupant of pick-up truck or van injured in collision with pedal cycle in nontraffic accident

✓x7ᵗʰ **V51.4 Person boarding or alighting** a pick-up truck or van injured in collision with pedal cycle

✓x7ᵗʰ **V51.5 Driver** of pick-up truck or van injured in collision with pedal cycle in traffic accident

✓x7ᵗʰ **V51.6 Passenger** in pick-up truck or van injured in collision with pedal cycle in traffic accident

✓x7ᵗʰ **V51.7 Person on outside** of pick-up truck or van injured in collision with pedal cycle in traffic accident

✓x7ᵗʰ **V51.9 Unspecified** occupant of pick-up truck or van injured in collision with pedal cycle in traffic accident

✓4ᵗʰ **V52 Occupant of pick-up truck or van injured in collision with two- or three-wheeled motor vehicle**

> The appropriate 7th character is to be added to each code from category V52.
> A   initial encounter
> D   subsequent encounter
> S   sequela

✓x7ᵗʰ **V52.0 Driver** of pick-up truck or van injured in collision with two- or three-wheeled motor vehicle in nontraffic accident

✓x7ᵗʰ **V52.1 Passenger** in pick-up truck or van injured in collision with two- or three-wheeled motor vehicle in nontraffic accident

✓x7ᵗʰ **V52.2 Person on outside** of pick-up truck or van injured in collision with two- or three-wheeled motor vehicle in nontraffic accident

✓x7ᵗʰ **V52.3 Unspecified** occupant of pick-up truck or van injured in collision with two- or three-wheeled motor vehicle in nontraffic accident

✓x7ᵗʰ **V52.4 Person boarding or alighting** a pick-up truck or van injured in collision with two- or three-wheeled motor vehicle

✓x7ᵗʰ **V52.5 Driver** of pick-up truck or van injured in collision with two- or three-wheeled motor vehicle in traffic accident

✓x7ᵗʰ **V52.6 Passenger** in pick-up truck or van injured in collision with two- or three-wheeled motor vehicle in traffic accident

✓x7ᵗʰ **V52.7 Person on outside** of pick-up truck or van injured in collision with two- or three-wheeled motor vehicle in traffic accident

✓x7ᵗʰ **V52.9 Unspecified** occupant of pick-up truck or van injured in collision with two- or three-wheeled motor vehicle in traffic accident

✓4ᵗʰ **V53 Occupant of pick-up truck or van injured in collision with car, pick-up truck or van**

> The appropriate 7th character is to be added to each code from category V53.
> A   initial encounter
> D   subsequent encounter
> S   sequela

✓x7ᵗʰ **V53.0 Driver** of pick-up truck or van injured in collision with car, pick-up truck or van in nontraffic accident

✓x7ᵗʰ **V53.1 Passenger** in pick-up truck or van injured in collision with car, pick-up truck or van in nontraffic accident

✓x7ᵗʰ **V53.2 Person on outside** of pick-up truck or van injured in collision with car, pick-up truck or van in nontraffic accident

✓x7ᵗʰ **V53.3 Unspecified** occupant of pick-up truck or van injured in collision with car, pick-up truck or van in nontraffic accident

✓x7ᵗʰ **V53.4 Person boarding or alighting** a pick-up truck or van injured in collision with car, pick-up truck or van

✓x7ᵗʰ **V53.5 Driver** of pick-up truck or van injured in collision with car, pick-up truck or van in traffic accident

✓x7ᵗʰ **V53.6 Passenger** in pick-up truck or van injured in collision with car, pick-up truck or van in traffic accident

✓x7ᵗʰ **V53.7 Person on outside** of pick-up truck or van injured in collision with car, pick-up truck or van in traffic accident

✓x7ᵗʰ **V53.9 Unspecified** occupant of pick-up truck or van injured in collision with car, pick-up truck or van in traffic accident

✓4ᵗʰ **V54 Occupant of pick-up truck or van injured in collision with heavy transport vehicle or bus**

> **EXCLUDES 1**   occupant of pick-up truck or van injured in collision with military vehicle (V59.81)

> The appropriate 7th character is to be added to each code from category V54.
> A   initial encounter
> D   subsequent encounter
> S   sequela

✓x7ᵗʰ **V54.0 Driver** of pick-up truck or van injured in collision with heavy transport vehicle or bus in nontraffic accident

✓x7ᵗʰ **V54.1 Passenger** in pick-up truck or van injured in collision with heavy transport vehicle or bus in nontraffic accident

✓x7ᵗʰ **V54.2 Person on outside** of pick-up truck or van injured in collision with heavy transport vehicle or bus in nontraffic accident

✓x7ᵗʰ **V54.3 Unspecified** occupant of pick-up truck or van injured in collision with heavy transport vehicle or bus in nontraffic accident

✓x7ᵗʰ **V54.4 Person boarding or alighting** a pick-up truck or van injured in collision with heavy transport vehicle or bus

✓x7ᵗʰ **V54.5 Driver** of pick-up truck or van injured in collision with heavy transport vehicle or bus in traffic accident

✓x7ᵗʰ **V54.6 Passenger** in pick-up truck or van injured in collision with heavy transport vehicle or bus in traffic accident

✓x7ᵗʰ **V54.7 Person on outside** of pick-up truck or van injured in collision with heavy transport vehicle or bus in traffic accident

✓x7ᵗʰ **V54.9 Unspecified** occupant of pick-up truck or van injured in collision with heavy transport vehicle or bus in traffic accident

✓4ᵗʰ **V55 Occupant of pick-up truck or van injured in collision with railway train or railway vehicle**

> The appropriate 7th character is to be added to each code from category V55.
> A   initial encounter
> D   subsequent encounter
> S   sequela

✓x7ᵗʰ **V55.0 Driver** of pick-up truck or van injured in collision with railway train or railway vehicle in nontraffic accident

✓x7ᵗʰ **V55.1 Passenger** in pick-up truck or van injured in collision with railway train or railway vehicle in nontraffic accident

✓x7ᵗʰ **V55.2 Person on outside** of pick-up truck or van injured in collision with railway train or railway vehicle in nontraffic accident

✓x7ᵗʰ **V55.3 Unspecified** occupant of pick-up truck or van injured in collision with railway train or railway vehicle in nontraffic accident

✓x7ᵗʰ **V55.4 Person boarding or alighting** a pick-up truck or van injured in collision with railway train or railway vehicle

✓x7ᵗʰ **V55.5 Driver** of pick-up truck or van injured in collision with railway train or railway vehicle in traffic accident

✓x7ᵗʰ **V55.6 Passenger** in pick-up truck or van injured in collision with railway train or railway vehicle in traffic accident

✓x7ᵗʰ **V55.7 Person on outside** of pick-up truck or van injured in collision with railway train or railway vehicle in traffic accident

✓x7ᵗʰ **V55.9 Unspecified** occupant of pick-up truck or van injured in collision with railway train or railway vehicle in traffic accident

✓4ᵗʰ **V56 Occupant of pick-up truck or van injured in collision with other nonmotor vehicle**

> **INCLUDES**   collision with animal-drawn vehicle, animal being ridden, streetcar

> The appropriate 7th character is to be added to each code from category V56.
> A   initial encounter
> D   subsequent encounter
> S   sequela

✓x7ᵗʰ **V56.0 Driver** of pick-up truck or van injured in collision with other nonmotor vehicle in nontraffic accident

✓x7ᵗʰ **V56.1 Passenger** in pick-up truck or van injured in collision with other nonmotor vehicle in nontraffic accident

√x7ᵗʰ **V56.2** Person on outside of pick-up truck or van injured in collision with other nonmotor vehicle in nontraffic accident

√x7ᵗʰ **V56.3** Unspecified occupant of pick-up truck or van injured in collision with other nonmotor vehicle in nontraffic accident

√x7ᵗʰ **V56.4** Person boarding or alighting a pick-up truck or van injured in collision with other nonmotor vehicle

√x7ᵗʰ **V56.5** Driver of pick-up truck or van injured in collision with other nonmotor vehicle in traffic accident

√x7ᵗʰ **V56.6** Passenger in pick-up truck or van injured in collision with other nonmotor vehicle in traffic accident

√x7ᵗʰ **V56.7** Person on outside of pick-up truck or van injured in collision with other nonmotor vehicle in traffic accident

√x7ᵗʰ **V56.9** Unspecified occupant of pick-up truck or van injured in collision with other nonmotor vehicle in traffic accident

√4ᵗʰ **V57 Occupant of pick-up truck or van injured in collision with fixed or stationary object**

> The appropriate 7th character is to be added to each code from category V57.
> A   initial encounter
> D   subsequent encounter
> S   sequela

√x7ᵗʰ **V57.0** Driver of pick-up truck or van injured in collision with fixed or stationary object in nontraffic accident

√x7ᵗʰ **V57.1** Passenger in pick-up truck or van injured in collision with fixed or stationary object in nontraffic accident

√x7ᵗʰ **V57.2** Person on outside of pick-up truck or van injured in collision with fixed or stationary object in nontraffic accident

√x7ᵗʰ **V57.3** Unspecified occupant of pick-up truck or van injured in collision with fixed or stationary object in nontraffic accident

√x7ᵗʰ **V57.4** Person boarding or alighting a pick-up truck or van injured in collision with fixed or stationary object

√x7ᵗʰ **V57.5** Driver of pick-up truck or van injured in collision with fixed or stationary object in traffic accident

√x7ᵗʰ **V57.6** Passenger in pick-up truck or van injured in collision with fixed or stationary object in traffic accident

√x7ᵗʰ **V57.7** Person on outside of pick-up truck or van injured in collision with fixed or stationary object in traffic accident

√x7ᵗʰ **V57.9** Unspecified occupant of pick-up truck or van injured in collision with fixed or stationary object in traffic accident

√4ᵗʰ **V58 Occupant of pick-up truck or van injured in noncollision transport accident**

> INCLUDES   overturning pick-up truck or van NOS
>   overturning pick-up truck or van without collision

> The appropriate 7th character is to be added to each code from category V58.
> A   initial encounter
> D   subsequent encounter
> S   sequela

√x7ᵗʰ **V58.0** Driver of pick-up truck or van injured in noncollision transport accident in nontraffic accident

√x7ᵗʰ **V58.1** Passenger in pick-up truck or van injured in noncollision transport accident in nontraffic accident

√x7ᵗʰ **V58.2** Person on outside of pick-up truck or van injured in noncollision transport accident in nontraffic accident

√x7ᵗʰ **V58.3** Unspecified occupant of pick-up truck or van injured in noncollision transport accident in nontraffic accident

√x7ᵗʰ **V58.4** Person boarding or alighting a pick-up truck or van injured in noncollision transport accident

√x7ᵗʰ **V58.5** Driver of pick-up truck or van injured in noncollision transport accident in traffic accident

√x7ᵗʰ **V58.6** Passenger in pick-up truck or van injured in noncollision transport accident in traffic accident

√x7ᵗʰ **V58.7** Person on outside of pick-up truck or van injured in noncollision transport accident in traffic accident

√x7ᵗʰ **V58.9** Unspecified occupant of pick-up truck or van injured in noncollision transport accident in traffic accident

√4ᵗʰ **V59 Occupant of pick-up truck or van injured in other and unspecified transport accidents**

> The appropriate 7th character is to be added to each code from category V59.
> A   initial encounter
> D   subsequent encounter
> S   sequela

√5ᵗʰ **V59.0** Driver of pick-up truck or van injured in collision with other and unspecified motor vehicles in nontraffic accident

√x7ᵗʰ **V59.00** Driver of pick-up truck or van injured in collision with unspecified motor vehicles in nontraffic accident

√x7ᵗʰ **V59.09** Driver of pick-up truck or van injured in collision with other motor vehicles in nontraffic accident

√5ᵗʰ **V59.1** Passenger in pick-up truck or van injured in collision with other and unspecified motor vehicles in nontraffic accident

√x7ᵗʰ **V59.10** Passenger in pick-up truck or van injured in collision with unspecified motor vehicles in nontraffic accident

√x7ᵗʰ **V59.19** Passenger in pick-up truck or van injured in collision with other motor vehicles in nontraffic accident

√5ᵗʰ **V59.2** Unspecified occupant of pick-up truck or van injured in collision with other and unspecified motor vehicles in nontraffic accident

√x7ᵗʰ **V59.20** Unspecified occupant of pick-up truck or van injured in collision with unspecified motor vehicles in nontraffic accident
     Collision NOS involving pick-up truck or van, nontraffic

√x7ᵗʰ **V59.29** Unspecified occupant of pick-up truck or van injured in collision with other motor vehicles in nontraffic accident

√x7ᵗʰ **V59.3** Occupant (driver) (passenger) of pick-up truck or van injured in unspecified nontraffic accident
     Accident NOS involving pick-up truck or van, nontraffic
     Occupant of pick-up truck or van injured in nontraffic accident NOS

√5ᵗʰ **V59.4** Driver of pick-up truck or van injured in collision with other and unspecified motor vehicles in traffic accident

√x7ᵗʰ **V59.40** Driver of pick-up truck or van injured in collision with unspecified motor vehicles in traffic accident

√x7ᵗʰ **V59.49** Driver of pick-up truck or van injured in collision with other motor vehicles in traffic accident

√5ᵗʰ **V59.5** Passenger in pick-up truck or van injured in collision with other and unspecified motor vehicles in traffic accident

√x7ᵗʰ **V59.50** Passenger in pick-up truck or van injured in collision with unspecified motor vehicles in traffic accident

√x7ᵗʰ **V59.59** Passenger in pick-up truck or van injured in collision with other motor vehicles in traffic accident

√5ᵗʰ **V59.6** Unspecified occupant of pick-up truck or van injured in collision with other and unspecified motor vehicles in traffic accident

√x7ᵗʰ **V59.60** Unspecified occupant of pick-up truck or van injured in collision with unspecified motor vehicles in traffic accident
     Collision NOS involving pick-up truck or van (traffic)

√x7ᵗʰ **V59.69** Unspecified occupant of pick-up truck or van injured in collision with other motor vehicles in traffic accident

√5ᵗʰ **V59.8** Occupant (driver) (passenger) of pick-up truck or van injured in other specified transport accidents

√x7ᵗʰ **V59.81** Occupant (driver) (passenger) of pick-up truck or van injured in transport accident with military vehicle

√x7ᵗʰ **V59.88** Occupant (driver) (passenger) of pick-up truck or van injured in other specified transport accidents

√x7ᵗʰ **V59.9** Occupant (driver) (passenger) of pick-up truck or van injured in unspecified traffic accident
     Accident NOS involving pick-up truck or van

✔ Additional Character Required   √x7ᵗʰ Placeholder Alert   Unacceptable PDx   Manifestation   Hospital Acquired Condition   EXCLUDES 1 Not Coded Here   EXCLUDES 2 Not Included Here

ICD-10-CM 2016   1171

Chapter 20. External Causes of Morbidity

Occupant of heavy transport vehicle injured in transport accident (V60-V69)

INCLUDES   18 wheeler
           armored car
           panel truck

EXCLUDES 1   *bus*
           motorcoach

✓4ᵗʰ **V60 Occupant of heavy transport vehicle injured in collision with pedestrian or animal**

     EXCLUDES 1   *heavy transport vehicle collision with animal-drawn vehicle or animal being ridden (V66.-)*

     The appropriate 7th character is to be added to each code from category V60.
     A   initial encounter
     D   subsequent encounter
     S   sequela

✓x7ᵗʰ **V60.0 Driver** of heavy transport vehicle injured in collision with **pedestrian or animal** in nontraffic accident

✓x7ᵗʰ **V60.1 Passenger** in heavy transport vehicle injured in collision with **pedestrian or animal** in nontraffic accident

✓x7ᵗʰ **V60.2 Person on outside** of heavy transport vehicle injured in collision with pedestrian or animal in nontraffic accident

✓x7ᵗʰ **V60.3 Unspecified** occupant of heavy transport vehicle injured in collision with pedestrian or animal in nontraffic accident

✓x7ᵗʰ **V60.4 Person boarding or alighting** a heavy transport vehicle injured in collision with pedestrian or animal

✓x7ᵗʰ **V60.5 Driver** of heavy transport vehicle injured in collision with **pedestrian or animal** in traffic accident

✓x7ᵗʰ **V60.6 Passenger** in heavy transport vehicle injured in collision with **pedestrian or animal** in traffic accident

✓x7ᵗʰ **V60.7 Person on outside** of heavy transport vehicle injured in collision with pedestrian or animal in traffic accident

✓x7ᵗʰ **V60.9 Unspecified** occupant of heavy transport vehicle injured in collision with pedestrian or animal in traffic accident

✓4ᵗʰ **V61 Occupant of heavy transport vehicle injured in collision with pedal cycle**

     The appropriate 7th character is to be added to each code from category V61.
     A   initial encounter
     D   subsequent encounter
     S   sequela

✓x7ᵗʰ **V61.0 Driver** of heavy transport vehicle injured in collision with **pedal cycle** in nontraffic accident

✓x7ᵗʰ **V61.1 Passenger** in heavy transport vehicle injured in collision with **pedal cycle** in nontraffic accident

✓x7ᵗʰ **V61.2 Person on outside** of heavy transport vehicle injured in collision with **pedal cycle** in nontraffic accident

✓x7ᵗʰ **V61.3 Unspecified** occupant of heavy transport vehicle injured in collision with **pedal cycle** in nontraffic accident

✓x7ᵗʰ **V61.4 Person boarding or alighting** a heavy transport vehicle injured in collision with pedal cycle while boarding or alighting

✓x7ᵗʰ **V61.5 Driver** of heavy transport vehicle injured in collision with **pedal cycle** in traffic accident

✓x7ᵗʰ **V61.6 Passenger** in heavy transport vehicle injured in collision with **pedal cycle** in traffic accident

✓x7ᵗʰ **V61.7 Person on outside** of heavy transport vehicle injured in collision with **pedal cycle** in traffic accident

✓x7ᵗʰ **V61.9 Unspecified** occupant of heavy transport vehicle injured in collision with pedal cycle in traffic accident

✓4ᵗʰ **V62 Occupant of heavy transport vehicle injured in collision with two- or three-wheeled motor vehicle**

     The appropriate 7th character is to be added to each code from category V62.
     A   initial encounter
     D   subsequent encounter
     S   sequela

✓x7ᵗʰ **V62.0 Driver** of heavy transport vehicle injured in collision with **two- or three-wheeled motor vehicle** in nontraffic accident

✓x7ᵗʰ **V62.1 Passenger** in heavy transport vehicle injured in collision with **two- or three-wheeled motor vehicle** in nontraffic accident

✓x7ᵗʰ **V62.2 Person on outside** of heavy transport vehicle injured in collision with two- or three-wheeled motor vehicle in nontraffic accident

✓x7ᵗʰ **V62.3 Unspecified** occupant of heavy transport vehicle injured in collision with two- or three-wheeled motor vehicle in nontraffic accident

✓x7ᵗʰ **V62.4 Person boarding or alighting** a heavy transport vehicle injured in collision with two- or three-wheeled motor vehicle

✓x7ᵗʰ **V62.5 Driver** of heavy transport vehicle injured in collision with **two- or three-wheeled motor vehicle** in traffic accident

✓x7ᵗʰ **V62.6 Passenger** in heavy transport vehicle injured in collision with **two- or three-wheeled motor vehicle** in traffic accident

✓x7ᵗʰ **V62.7 Person on outside** of heavy transport vehicle injured in collision with two- or three-wheeled motor vehicle in traffic accident

✓x7ᵗʰ **V62.9 Unspecified** occupant of heavy transport vehicle injured in collision with two- or three-wheeled motor vehicle in traffic accident

✓4ᵗʰ **V63 Occupant of heavy transport vehicle injured in collision with car, pick-up truck or van**

     The appropriate 7th character is to be added to each code from category V63.
     A   initial encounter
     D   subsequent encounter
     S   sequela

✓x7ᵗʰ **V63.0 Driver** of heavy transport vehicle injured in collision with **car, pick-up truck or van** in nontraffic accident

✓x7ᵗʰ **V63.1 Passenger** in heavy transport vehicle injured in collision with **car, pick-up truck or van** in nontraffic accident

✓x7ᵗʰ **V63.2 Person on outside** of heavy transport vehicle injured in collision with car, pick-up truck or van in nontraffic accident

✓x7ᵗʰ **V63.3 Unspecified** occupant of heavy transport vehicle injured in collision with car, pick-up truck or van in nontraffic accident

✓x7ᵗʰ **V63.4 Person boarding or alighting** a heavy transport vehicle injured in collision with car, pick-up truck or van

✓x7ᵗʰ **V63.5 Driver** of heavy transport vehicle injured in collision with **car, pick-up truck or van** in traffic accident

✓x7ᵗʰ **V63.6 Passenger** in heavy transport vehicle injured in collision with **car, pick-up truck or van** in traffic accident

✓x7ᵗʰ **V63.7 Person on outside** of heavy transport vehicle injured in collision with car, pick-up truck or van in traffic accident

✓x7ᵗʰ **V63.9 Unspecified** occupant of heavy transport vehicle injured in collision with car, pick-up truck or van in traffic accident

✓4ᵗʰ **V64 Occupant of heavy transport vehicle injured in collision with heavy transport vehicle or bus**

     EXCLUDES 1   *occupant of heavy transport vehicle injured in collision with military vehicle (V69.81)*

     The appropriate 7th character is to be added to each code from category V64.
     A   initial encounter
     D   subsequent encounter
     S   sequela

✓x7ᵗʰ **V64.0 Driver** of heavy transport vehicle injured in collision with **heavy transport vehicle or bus** in nontraffic accident

✓x7ᵗʰ **V64.1 Passenger** in heavy transport vehicle injured in collision with **heavy transport vehicle or bus** in nontraffic accident

✓x7ᵗʰ **V64.2 Person on outside** of heavy transport vehicle injured in collision with heavy transport vehicle or bus in nontraffic accident

✓x7ᵗʰ **V64.3 Unspecified** occupant of heavy transport vehicle injured in collision with heavy transport vehicle or bus in nontraffic accident

✓x7ᵗʰ **V64.4 Person boarding or alighting** a heavy transport vehicle injured in collision with heavy transport vehicle or bus while boarding or alighting

✓x7ᵗʰ **V64.5 Driver** of heavy transport vehicle injured in collision with **heavy transport vehicle or bus** in traffic accident

✓x7ᵗʰ **V64.6 Passenger** in heavy transport vehicle injured in collision with **heavy transport vehicle or bus** in traffic accident

✓x7ᵗʰ **V64.7 Person on outside** of heavy transport vehicle injured in collision with heavy transport vehicle or bus in traffic accident

✓x7ᵗʰ **V64.9 Unspecified** occupant of heavy transport vehicle injured in collision with heavy transport vehicle or bus in traffic accident

N Newborn: 0   P Pediatric: 0-17   M Maternity: 12-55   A Adult: 15-124   MCC Major CC Condition   PDxMCC PDx acts as own MCC   CC CC Condition   PDxCC PDx acts as own CC

1172

ICD-10-CM 2016

☑4ᵗʰ **V65** **Occupant of heavy transport vehicle injured in collision with railway train or railway vehicle**

> The appropriate 7th character is to be added to each code from category V65.
> A   initial encounter
> D   subsequent encounter
> S   sequela

√x7ᵗʰ **V65.0** Driver of heavy transport vehicle injured in collision with railway train or railway vehicle in nontraffic accident

√x7ᵗʰ **V65.1** Passenger in heavy transport vehicle injured in collision with railway train or railway vehicle in nontraffic accident

√x7ᵗʰ **V65.2** Person on outside of heavy transport vehicle injured in collision with railway train or railway vehicle in nontraffic accident

√x7ᵗʰ **V65.3** Unspecified occupant of heavy transport vehicle injured in collision with railway train or railway vehicle in nontraffic accident

√x7ᵗʰ **V65.4** Person boarding or alighting a heavy transport vehicle injured in collision with railway train or railway vehicle

√x7ᵗʰ **V65.5** Driver of heavy transport vehicle injured in collision with railway train or railway vehicle in traffic accident

√x7ᵗʰ **V65.6** Passenger in heavy transport vehicle injured in collision with railway train or railway vehicle in traffic accident

√x7ᵗʰ **V65.7** Person on outside of heavy transport vehicle injured in collision with railway train or railway vehicle in traffic accident

√x7ᵗʰ **V65.9** Unspecified occupant of heavy transport vehicle injured in collision with railway train or railway vehicle in traffic accident

☑4ᵗʰ **V66** **Occupant of heavy transport vehicle injured in collision with other nonmotor vehicle**

> INCLUDES   collision with animal-drawn vehicle, animal being ridden, streetcar

> The appropriate 7th character is to be added to each code from category V66.
> A   initial encounter
> D   subsequent encounter
> S   sequela

√x7ᵗʰ **V66.0** Driver of heavy transport vehicle injured in collision with other nonmotor vehicle in nontraffic accident

√x7ᵗʰ **V66.1** Passenger in heavy transport vehicle injured in collision with other nonmotor vehicle in nontraffic accident

√x7ᵗʰ **V66.2** Person on outside of heavy transport vehicle injured in collision with other nonmotor vehicle in nontraffic accident

√x7ᵗʰ **V66.3** Unspecified occupant of heavy transport vehicle injured in collision with other nonmotor vehicle in nontraffic accident

√x7ᵗʰ **V66.4** Person boarding or alighting a heavy transport vehicle injured in collision with other nonmotor vehicle

√x7ᵗʰ **V66.5** Driver of heavy transport vehicle injured in collision with other nonmotor vehicle in traffic accident

√x7ᵗʰ **V66.6** Passenger in heavy transport vehicle injured in collision with other nonmotor vehicle in traffic accident

√x7ᵗʰ **V66.7** Person on outside of heavy transport vehicle injured in collision with other nonmotor vehicle in traffic accident

√x7ᵗʰ **V66.9** Unspecified occupant of heavy transport vehicle injured in collision with other nonmotor vehicle in traffic accident

☑4ᵗʰ **V67** **Occupant of heavy transport vehicle injured in collision with fixed or stationary object**

> The appropriate 7th character is to be added to each code from category V67.
> A   initial encounter
> D   subsequent encounter
> S   sequela

√x7ᵗʰ **V67.0** Driver of heavy transport vehicle injured in collision with fixed or stationary object in nontraffic accident

√x7ᵗʰ **V67.1** Passenger in heavy transport vehicle injured in collision with fixed or stationary object in nontraffic accident

√x7ᵗʰ **V67.2** Person on outside of heavy transport vehicle injured in collision with fixed or stationary object in nontraffic accident

√x7ᵗʰ **V67.3** Unspecified occupant of heavy transport vehicle injured in collision with fixed or stationary object in nontraffic accident

√x7ᵗʰ **V67.4** Person boarding or alighting a heavy transport vehicle injured in collision with fixed or stationary object

√x7ᵗʰ **V67.5** Driver of heavy transport vehicle injured in collision with fixed or stationary object in traffic accident

√x7ᵗʰ **V67.6** Passenger in heavy transport vehicle injured in collision with fixed or stationary object in traffic accident

√x7ᵗʰ **V67.7** Person on outside of heavy transport vehicle injured in collision with fixed or stationary object in traffic accident

√x7ᵗʰ **V67.9** Unspecified occupant of heavy transport vehicle injured in collision with fixed or stationary object in traffic accident

☑4ᵗʰ **V68** **Occupant of heavy transport vehicle injured in noncollision transport accident**

> INCLUDES   overturning heavy transport vehicle NOS
> overturning heavy transport vehicle without collision

> The appropriate 7th character is to be added to each code from category V68.
> A   initial encounter
> D   subsequent encounter
> S   sequela

√x7ᵗʰ **V68.0** Driver of heavy transport vehicle injured in noncollision transport accident in nontraffic accident

√x7ᵗʰ **V68.1** Passenger in heavy transport vehicle injured in noncollision transport accident in nontraffic accident

√x7ᵗʰ **V68.2** Person on outside of heavy transport vehicle injured in noncollision transport accident in nontraffic accident

√x7ᵗʰ **V68.3** Unspecified occupant of heavy transport vehicle injured in noncollision transport accident in nontraffic accident

√x7ᵗʰ **V68.4** Person boarding or alighting a heavy transport vehicle injured in noncollision transport accident

√x7ᵗʰ **V68.5** Driver of heavy transport vehicle injured in noncollision transport accident in traffic accident

√x7ᵗʰ **V68.6** Passenger in heavy transport vehicle injured in noncollision transport accident in traffic accident

√x7ᵗʰ **V68.7** Person on outside of heavy transport vehicle injured in noncollision transport accident in traffic accident

√x7ᵗʰ **V68.9** Unspecified occupant of heavy transport vehicle injured in noncollision transport accident in traffic accident

☑4ᵗʰ **V69** **Occupant of heavy transport vehicle injured in other and unspecified transport accidents**

> The appropriate 7th character is to be added to each code from category V69.
> A   initial encounter
> D   subsequent encounter
> S   sequela

√6ᵗʰ **V69.0** Driver of heavy transport vehicle injured in collision with other and unspecified motor vehicles in nontraffic accident

    √x7ᵗʰ **V69.00** Driver of heavy transport vehicle injured in collision with unspecified motor vehicles in nontraffic accident

    √x7ᵗʰ **V69.09** Driver of heavy transport vehicle injured in collision with other motor vehicles in nontraffic accident

√5ᵗʰ **V69.1** Passenger in heavy transport vehicle injured in collision with other and unspecified motor vehicles in nontraffic accident

    √x7ᵗʰ **V69.10** Passenger in heavy transport vehicle injured in collision with unspecified motor vehicles in nontraffic accident

    √x7ᵗʰ **V69.19** Passenger in heavy transport vehicle injured in collision with other motor vehicles in nontraffic accident

√5ᵗʰ **V69.2** Unspecified occupant of heavy transport vehicle injured in collision with other and unspecified motor vehicles in nontraffic accident

    √x7ᵗʰ **V69.20** Unspecified occupant of heavy transport vehicle injured in collision with unspecified motor vehicles in nontraffic accident
      Collision NOS involving heavy transport vehicle, nontraffic

    √x7ᵗʰ **V69.29** Unspecified occupant of heavy transport vehicle injured in collision with other motor vehicles in nontraffic accident

√x7ᵗʰ **V69.3** Occupant (driver) (passenger) of heavy transport vehicle injured in unspecified nontraffic accident
    Accident NOS involving heavy transport vehicle, nontraffic
    Occupant of heavy transport vehicle injured in nontraffic accident NOS

✓ Additional Character Required   √x7ᵗʰ Placeholder Alert   Unacceptable PDx   Manifestation   Hospital Acquired Condition   EXCLUDES 1 Not Coded Here   EXCLUDES 2 Not Included Here

ICD-10-CM 2016   1173

Chapter 20. External Causes of Morbidity

√5ᵗʰ **V69.4** **Driver of heavy transport vehicle injured in collision with other and unspecified motor vehicles** in traffic accident

√x7ᵗʰ **V69.40** **Driver of heavy transport vehicle injured in collision with unspecified motor vehicles** in traffic accident

√x7ᵗʰ **V69.49** **Driver of heavy transport vehicle injured in collision with other motor vehicles** in traffic accident

√5ᵗʰ **V69.5** **Passenger in heavy transport vehicle injured in collision with other and unspecified motor vehicles** in traffic accident

√x7ᵗʰ **V69.50** **Passenger in heavy transport vehicle injured in collision** with unspecified motor vehicles **in traffic accident**

√x7ᵗʰ **V69.59** **Passenger in heavy transport vehicle injured in collision** with other motor vehicles **in traffic accident**

√5ᵗʰ **V69.6** **Unspecified occupant of heavy transport vehicle injured in collision with other and unspecified motor vehicles** in traffic accident

√x7ᵗʰ **V69.60** **Unspecified occupant of heavy transport vehicle injured in collision** with unspecified motor vehicles **in traffic accident**
Collision NOS involving heavy transport vehicle (traffic)

√x7ᵗʰ **V69.69** **Unspecified occupant of heavy transport vehicle injured in collision** with other motor vehicles **in traffic accident**

√5ᵗʰ **V69.8** **Occupant (driver) (passenger) of heavy transport vehicle injured in other specified transport accidents**

√x7ᵗʰ **V69.81** **Occupant (driver) (passenger) of heavy transport vehicle injured in transport accidents** with military vehicle

√x7ᵗʰ **V69.88** **Occupant (driver) (passenger) of heavy transport vehicle injured** in other specified transport accidents

√x7ᵗʰ **V69.9** **Occupant (driver) (passenger) of heavy transport vehicle injured in** unspecified traffic accident
Accident NOS involving heavy transport vehicle

Bus occupant injured in transport accident (V70-V79)

INCLUDES   motorcoach
EXCLUDES 1   *minibus (V50-V59)*

√4ᵗʰ **V70** **Bus occupant injured in collision with pedestrian or animal**

EXCLUDES 1   *bus collision with animal-drawn vehicle or animal being ridden (V76.-)*

The appropriate 7th character is to be added to each code from category V70.
A   initial encounter
D   subsequent encounter
S   sequela

√x7ᵗʰ **V70.0** **Driver of bus injured in collision with pedestrian or animal** in nontraffic accident

√x7ᵗʰ **V70.1** **Passenger on bus injured in collision with pedestrian or animal** in nontraffic accident

√x7ᵗʰ **V70.2** **Person on outside of bus injured in collision with pedestrian or animal** in nontraffic accident

√x7ᵗʰ **V70.3** **Unspecified occupant of bus injured in collision with pedestrian or animal** in nontraffic accident

√x7ᵗʰ **V70.4** **Person boarding or alighting from bus injured in collision with pedestrian or animal**

√x7ᵗʰ **V70.5** **Driver of bus injured in collision with pedestrian or animal** in traffic accident

√x7ᵗʰ **V70.6** **Passenger on bus injured in collision with pedestrian or animal** in traffic accident

√x7ᵗʰ **V70.7** **Person on outside of bus injured in collision with pedestrian or animal** in traffic accident

√x7ᵗʰ **V70.9** **Unspecified occupant of bus injured in collision with pedestrian or animal** in traffic accident

√4ᵗʰ **V71** **Bus occupant injured in collision with pedal cycle**

The appropriate 7th character is to be added to each code from category V71.
A   initial encounter
D   subsequent encounter
S   sequela

√x7ᵗʰ **V71.0** **Driver of bus injured in collision with pedal cycle** in nontraffic accident

√x7ᵗʰ **V71.1** **Passenger on bus injured in collision with pedal cycle** in nontraffic accident

√x7ᵗʰ **V71.2** **Person on outside of bus injured in collision with pedal cycle** in nontraffic accident

√x7ᵗʰ **V71.3** **Unspecified occupant of bus injured in collision with pedal cycle** in nontraffic accident

√x7ᵗʰ **V71.4** **Person boarding or alighting from bus injured in collision with pedal cycle**

√x7ᵗʰ **V71.5** **Driver of bus injured in collision with pedal cycle** in traffic accident

√x7ᵗʰ **V71.6** **Passenger on bus injured in collision with pedal cycle** in traffic accident

√x7ᵗʰ **V71.7** **Person on outside of bus injured in collision with pedal cycle** in traffic accident

√x7ᵗʰ **V71.9** **Unspecified occupant of bus injured in collision with pedal cycle** in traffic accident

√4ᵗʰ **V72** **Bus occupant injured in collision with two- or three-wheeled motor vehicle**

The appropriate 7th character is to be added to each code from category V72.
A   initial encounter
D   subsequent encounter
S   sequela

√x7ᵗʰ **V72.0** **Driver of bus injured in collision with two- or three-wheeled motor vehicle** in nontraffic accident

√x7ᵗʰ **V72.1** **Passenger on bus injured in collision with two- or three-wheeled motor vehicle** in nontraffic accident

√x7ᵗʰ **V72.2** **Person on outside of bus injured in collision with two- or three-wheeled motor vehicle** in nontraffic accident

√x7ᵗʰ **V72.3** **Unspecified occupant of bus injured in collision with two- or three-wheeled motor vehicle** in nontraffic accident

√x7ᵗʰ **V72.4** **Person boarding or alighting from bus injured in collision with two- or three-wheeled motor vehicle**

√x7ᵗʰ **V72.5** **Driver of bus injured in collision with two- or three-wheeled motor vehicle** in traffic accident

√x7ᵗʰ **V72.6** **Passenger on bus injured in collision with two- or three-wheeled motor vehicle** in traffic accident

√x7ᵗʰ **V72.7** **Person on outside of bus injured in collision with two- or three-wheeled motor vehicle** in traffic accident

√x7ᵗʰ **V72.9** **Unspecified occupant of bus injured in collision with two- or three-wheeled motor vehicle** in traffic accident

√4ᵗʰ **V73** **Bus occupant injured in collision with car, pick-up truck or van**

The appropriate 7th character is to be added to each code from category V73.
A   initial encounter
D   subsequent encounter
S   sequela

√x7ᵗʰ **V73.0** **Driver of bus injured in collision with car, pick-up truck or van** in nontraffic accident

√x7ᵗʰ **V73.1** **Passenger on bus injured in collision with car, pick-up truck or van** in nontraffic accident

√x7ᵗʰ **V73.2** **Person on outside of bus injured in collision with car, pick-up truck or van** in nontraffic accident

√x7ᵗʰ **V73.3** **Unspecified occupant of bus injured in collision with car, pick-up truck or van** in nontraffic accident

√x7ᵗʰ **V73.4** **Person boarding or alighting from bus injured in collision with car, pick-up truck or van**

√x7ᵗʰ **V73.5** **Driver of bus injured in collision with car, pick-up truck or van** in traffic accident

√x7ᵗʰ **V73.6** **Passenger on bus injured in collision with car, pick-up truck or van** in traffic accident

√x7ᵗʰ **V73.7** **Person on outside of bus injured in collision with car, pick-up truck or van** in traffic accident

√x7ᵗʰ **V73.9** **Unspecified occupant of bus injured in collision with car, pick-up truck or van** in traffic accident

√4ᵗʰ **V74** **Bus occupant injured in collision with heavy transport vehicle or bus**

EXCLUDES 1   *bus occupant injured in collision with military vehicle (V79.81)*

The appropriate 7th character is to be added to each code from category V74.
A   initial encounter
D   subsequent encounter
S   sequela

√x7ᵗʰ **V74.0** **Driver of bus injured in collision with heavy transport vehicle or bus** in nontraffic accident

N Newborn: 0   P Pediatric: 0-17   M Maternity: 12-55   A Adult: 15-124   MCC Major CC Condition   PDxMCC PDx acts as own MCC   CC CC Condition   PDxCC PDx acts as own CC

1174   ICD-10-CM 2016

√x7ᵗʰ **V74.1** Passenger on bus injured in collision with heavy transport vehicle or bus in nontraffic accident

√x7ᵗʰ **V74.2** Person on outside of bus injured in collision with heavy transport vehicle or bus in nontraffic accident

√x7ᵗʰ **V74.3** Unspecified occupant of bus injured in collision with heavy transport vehicle or bus in nontraffic accident

√x7ᵗʰ **V74.4** Person boarding or alighting from bus injured in collision with heavy transport vehicle or bus

√x7ᵗʰ **V74.5** Driver of bus injured in collision with heavy transport vehicle or bus in traffic accident

√x7ᵗʰ **V74.6** Passenger on bus injured in collision with heavy transport vehicle or bus in traffic accident

√x7ᵗʰ **V74.7** Person on outside of bus injured in collision with heavy transport vehicle or bus in traffic accident

√x7ᵗʰ **V74.9** Unspecified occupant of bus injured in collision with heavy transport vehicle or bus in traffic accident

√4ᵗʰ **V75** **Bus occupant injured in collision with railway train or railway vehicle**

> The appropriate 7th character is to be added to each code from category V75.
> A   initial encounter
> D   subsequent encounter
> S   sequela

√x7ᵗʰ **V75.0** Driver of bus injured in collision with railway train or railway vehicle in nontraffic accident

√x7ᵗʰ **V75.1** Passenger on bus injured in collision with railway train or railway vehicle in nontraffic accident

√x7ᵗʰ **V75.2** Person on outside of bus injured in collision with railway train or railway vehicle in nontraffic accident

√x7ᵗʰ **V75.3** Unspecified occupant of bus injured in collision with railway train or railway vehicle in nontraffic accident

√x7ᵗʰ **V75.4** Person boarding or alighting from bus injured in collision with railway train or railway vehicle

√x7ᵗʰ **V75.5** Driver of bus injured in collision with railway train or railway vehicle in traffic accident

√x7ᵗʰ **V75.6** Passenger on bus injured in collision with railway train or railway vehicle in traffic accident

√x7ᵗʰ **V75.7** Person on outside of bus injured in collision with railway train or railway vehicle in traffic accident

√x7ᵗʰ **V75.9** Unspecified occupant of bus injured in collision with railway train or railway vehicle in traffic accident

√4ᵗʰ **V76** **Bus occupant injured in collision with other nonmotor vehicle**
> INCLUDES   collision with animal-drawn vehicle, animal being ridden, streetcar

> The appropriate 7th character is to be added to each code from category V76.
> A   initial encounter
> D   subsequent encounter
> S   sequela

√x7ᵗʰ **V76.0** Driver of bus injured in collision with other nonmotor vehicle in nontraffic accident

√x7ᵗʰ **V76.1** Passenger on bus injured in collision with other nonmotor vehicle in nontraffic accident

√x7ᵗʰ **V76.2** Person on outside of bus injured in collision with other nonmotor vehicle in nontraffic accident

√x7ᵗʰ **V76.3** Unspecified occupant of bus injured in collision with other nonmotor vehicle in nontraffic accident

√x7ᵗʰ **V76.4** Person boarding or alighting from bus injured in collision with other nonmotor vehicle

√x7ᵗʰ **V76.5** Driver of bus injured in collision with other nonmotor vehicle in traffic accident

√x7ᵗʰ **V76.6** Passenger on bus injured in collision with other nonmotor vehicle in traffic accident

√x7ᵗʰ **V76.7** Person on outside of bus injured in collision with other nonmotor vehicle in traffic accident

√x7ᵗʰ **V76.9** Unspecified occupant of bus injured in collision with other nonmotor vehicle in traffic accident

√4ᵗʰ **V77** **Bus occupant injured in collision with fixed or stationary object**

> The appropriate 7th character is to be added to each code from category V77.
> A   initial encounter
> D   subsequent encounter
> S   sequela

√x7ᵗʰ **V77.0** Driver of bus injured in collision with fixed or stationary object in nontraffic accident

√x7ᵗʰ **V77.1** Passenger on bus injured in collision with fixed or stationary object in nontraffic accident

√x7ᵗʰ **V77.2** Person on outside of bus injured in collision with fixed or stationary object in nontraffic accident

√x7ᵗʰ **V77.3** Unspecified occupant of bus injured in collision with fixed or stationary object in nontraffic accident

√x7ᵗʰ **V77.4** Person boarding or alighting from bus injured in collision with fixed or stationary object

√x7ᵗʰ **V77.5** Driver of bus injured in collision with fixed or stationary object in traffic accident

√x7ᵗʰ **V77.6** Passenger on bus injured in collision with fixed or stationary object in traffic accident

√x7ᵗʰ **V77.7** Person on outside of bus injured in collision with fixed or stationary object in traffic accident

√x7ᵗʰ **V77.9** Unspecified occupant of bus injured in collision with fixed or stationary object in traffic accident

√4ᵗʰ **V78** **Bus occupant injured in noncollision transport accident**
> INCLUDES   overturning bus NOS
> overturning bus without collision

> The appropriate 7th character is to be added to each code from category V78.
> A   initial encounter
> D   subsequent encounter
> S   sequela

√x7ᵗʰ **V78.0** Driver of bus injured in noncollision transport accident in nontraffic accident

√x7ᵗʰ **V78.1** Passenger on bus injured in noncollision transport accident in nontraffic accident

√x7ᵗʰ **V78.2** Person on outside of bus injured in noncollision transport accident in nontraffic accident

√x7ᵗʰ **V78.3** Unspecified occupant of bus injured in noncollision transport accident in nontraffic accident

√x7ᵗʰ **V78.4** Person boarding or alighting from bus injured in noncollision transport accident

√x7ᵗʰ **V78.5** Driver of bus injured in noncollision transport accident in traffic accident

√x7ᵗʰ **V78.6** Passenger on bus injured in noncollision transport accident in traffic accident

√x7ᵗʰ **V78.7** Person on outside of bus injured in noncollision transport accident in traffic accident

√x7ᵗʰ **V78.9** Unspecified occupant of bus injured in noncollision transport accident in traffic accident

√4ᵗʰ **V79** **Bus occupant injured in other and unspecified transport accidents**

> The appropriate 7th character is to be added to each code from category V79.
> A   initial encounter
> D   subsequent encounter
> S   sequela

√5ᵗʰ **V79.0** Driver of bus injured in collision with other and unspecified motor vehicles in nontraffic accident

   √x7ᵗʰ **V79.00** Driver of bus injured in collision with unspecified motor vehicles in nontraffic accident

   √x7ᵗʰ **V79.09** Driver of bus injured in collision with other motor vehicles in nontraffic accident

√5ᵗʰ **V79.1** Passenger on bus injured in collision with other and unspecified motor vehicles in nontraffic accident

   √x7ᵗʰ **V79.10** Passenger on bus injured in collision with unspecified motor vehicles in nontraffic accident

   √x7ᵗʰ **V79.19** Passenger on bus injured in collision with other motor vehicles in nontraffic accident

☑ Additional Character Required   √x7ᵗʰ Placeholder Alert   Unacceptable PDx   Manifestation   Hospital Acquired Condition   EXCLUDES 1 Not Coded Here   EXCLUDES 2 Not Included Here

ICD-10-CM 2016   1175

✓5ᵗʰ **V79.2** Unspecified **bus** occupant injured in collision with other and unspecified motor vehicles in nontraffic accident

     ✓x7ᵗʰ **V79.20** Unspecified bus occupant injured in collision with unspecified motor vehicles in nontraffic accident
       Bus collision NOS, nontraffic

     ✓x7ᵗʰ **V79.29** Unspecified bus occupant injured in collision with other motor vehicles in nontraffic accident

✓x7ᵗʰ **V79.3** Bus occupant (driver) (passenger) injured in unspecified nontraffic accident
     Bus accident NOS, nontraffic
     Bus occupant injured in nontraffic accident NOS

✓5ᵗʰ **V79.4** Driver of bus injured in collision with other and unspecified motor vehicles in traffic accident

     ✓x7ᵗʰ **V79.40** Driver of bus injured in collision with unspecified motor vehicles in traffic accident

     ✓x7ᵗʰ **V79.49** Driver of bus injured in collision with other motor vehicles in traffic accident

✓5ᵗʰ **V79.5** Passenger on bus injured in collision with other and unspecified motor vehicles in traffic accident

     ✓x7ᵗʰ **V79.50** Passenger on bus injured in collision with unspecified motor vehicles in traffic accident

     ✓x7ᵗʰ **V79.59** Passenger on bus injured in collision with other motor vehicles in traffic accident

✓5ᵗʰ **V79.6** Unspecified **bus** occupant injured in collision with other and unspecified motor vehicles in traffic accident

     ✓x7ᵗʰ **V79.60** Unspecified bus occupant injured in collision with unspecified motor vehicles in traffic accident
       Bus collision NOS (traffic)

     ✓x7ᵗʰ **V79.69** Unspecified bus occupant injured in collision with other motor vehicles in traffic accident

✓5ᵗʰ **V79.8** Bus occupant (driver) (passenger) injured in other specified transport accidents

     ✓x7ᵗʰ **V79.81** Bus occupant (driver) (passenger) injured in transport accidents with military vehicle

     ✓x7ᵗʰ **V79.88** Bus occupant (driver) (passenger) injured in other specified transport accidents

✓x7ᵗʰ **V79.9** Bus occupant (driver) (passenger) injured in unspecified traffic accident
     Bus accident NOS

Other land transport accidents (V80-V89)

✓4ᵗʰ **V80** Animal-rider or occupant of animal-drawn vehicle injured in transport accident

> The appropriate 7th character is to be added to each code from category V80.
> A   initial encounter
> D   subsequent encounter
> S   sequela

✓5ᵗʰ **V80.0** Animal-rider or occupant of animal drawn vehicle injured by fall from or being thrown from animal or animal-drawn vehicle in noncollision accident

     ✓6ᵗʰ **V80.01** Animal-rider injured by fall from or being thrown from animal in noncollision accident

       ✓7ᵗʰ **V80.010** Animal-rider injured by fall from or being thrown from horse in noncollision accident

       ✓7ᵗʰ **V80.018** Animal-rider injured by fall from or being thrown from other animal in noncollision accident

     ✓x7ᵗʰ **V80.02** Occupant of animal-drawn vehicle injured by fall from or being thrown from animal-drawn vehicle in noncollision accident
       Overturning animal-drawn vehicle NOS
       Overturning animal-drawn vehicle without collision

✓5ᵗʰ **V80.1** Animal-rider or occupant of animal-drawn vehicle injured in collision with pedestrian or animal

     EXCLUDES 1 *animal-rider or animal-drawn vehicle collision with animal-drawn vehicle or animal being ridden (V80.7)*

     ✓x7ᵗʰ **V80.11** Animal-rider injured in collision with pedestrian or animal

     ✓x7ᵗʰ **V80.12** Occupant of animal-drawn vehicle injured in collision with pedestrian or animal

✓5ᵗʰ **V80.2** Animal-rider or occupant of animal-drawn vehicle injured in collision with pedal cycle

     ✓x7ᵗʰ **V80.21** Animal-rider injured in collision with pedal cycle

     ✓x7ᵗʰ **V80.22** Occupant of animal-drawn vehicle injured in collision with pedal cycle

✓5ᵗʰ **V80.3** Animal-rider or occupant of animal-drawn vehicle injured in collision with two- or three-wheeled motor vehicle

     ✓x7ᵗʰ **V80.31** Animal-rider injured in collision with two- or three-wheeled motor vehicle

     ✓x7ᵗʰ **V80.32** Occupant of animal-drawn vehicle injured in collision with two- or three-wheeled motor vehicle

✓5ᵗʰ **V80.4** Animal-rider or occupant of animal-drawn vehicle injured in collision with car, pick-up truck, van, heavy transport vehicle or bus

     EXCLUDES 1 *animal-rider injured in collision with military vehicle (V80.910)*
       occupant of animal-drawn vehicle injured in collision with military vehicle (V80.920)

     ✓x7ᵗʰ **V80.41** Animal-rider injured in collision with car, pick-up truck, van, heavy transport vehicle or bus

     ✓x7ᵗʰ **V80.42** Occupant of animal-drawn vehicle injured in collision with car, pick-up truck, van, heavy transport vehicle or bus

✓5ᵗʰ **V80.5** Animal-rider or occupant of animal-drawn vehicle injured in collision with other specified motor vehicle

     ✓x7ᵗʰ **V80.51** Animal-rider injured in collision with other specified motor vehicle

     ✓x7ᵗʰ **V80.52** Occupant of animal-drawn vehicle injured in collision with other specified motor vehicle

✓5ᵗʰ **V80.6** Animal-rider or occupant of animal-drawn vehicle injured in collision with railway train or railway vehicle

     ✓x7ᵗʰ **V80.61** Animal-rider injured in collision with railway train or railway vehicle

     ✓x7ᵗʰ **V80.62** Occupant of animal-drawn vehicle injured in collision with railway train or railway vehicle

✓5ᵗʰ **V80.7** Animal-rider or occupant of animal-drawn vehicle injured in collision with other nonmotor vehicles

     ✓6ᵗʰ **V80.71** Animal-rider or occupant of animal-drawn vehicle injured in collision with animal being ridden

       ✓7ᵗʰ **V80.710** Animal-rider injured in collision with other animal being ridden

       ✓7ᵗʰ **V80.711** Occupant of animal-drawn vehicle injured in collision with animal being ridden

     ✓6ᵗʰ **V80.72** Animal-rider or occupant of animal-drawn vehicle injured in collision with other animal-drawn vehicle

       ✓7ᵗʰ **V80.720** Animal-rider injured in collision with animal-drawn vehicle

       ✓7ᵗʰ **V80.721** Occupant of animal-drawn vehicle injured in collision with other animal-drawn vehicle

     ✓6ᵗʰ **V80.73** Animal-rider or occupant of animal-drawn vehicle injured in collision with streetcar

       ✓7ᵗʰ **V80.730** Animal-rider injured in collision with streetcar

       ✓7ᵗʰ **V80.731** Occupant of animal-drawn vehicle injured in collision with streetcar

     ✓6ᵗʰ **V80.79** Animal-rider or occupant of animal-drawn vehicle injured in collision with other nonmotor vehicles

       ✓7ᵗʰ **V80.790** Animal-rider injured in collision with other nonmotor vehicles

       ✓7ᵗʰ **V80.791** Occupant of animal-drawn vehicle injured in collision with other nonmotor vehicles

✓5ᵗʰ **V80.8** Animal-rider or occupant of animal-drawn vehicle injured in collision with fixed or stationary object

     ✓x7ᵗʰ **V80.81** Animal-rider injured in collision with fixed or stationary object

     ✓x7ᵗʰ **V80.82** Occupant of animal-drawn vehicle injured in collision with fixed or stationary object

✓5ᵗʰ **V80.9** Animal-rider or occupant of animal-drawn vehicle injured in other and unspecified transport accidents

     ✓6ᵗʰ **V80.91** Animal-rider injured in other and unspecified transport accidents

       ✓7ᵗʰ **V80.910** Animal-rider injured in transport accident with military vehicle

☑7ᵗʰ **V80.918** **Animal-rider injured** in other transport accident

☑7ᵗʰ **V80.919** **Animal-rider injured** in unspecified transport accident
Animal rider accident NOS

☑6ᵗʰ **V80.92** Occupant of animal-drawn vehicle injured in other and unspecified transport accidents

☑7ᵗʰ **V80.920** **Occupant of animal-drawn vehicle injured** in transport accident with military vehicle

☑7ᵗʰ **V80.928** **Occupant of animal-drawn vehicle injured** in other transport accident

☑7ᵗʰ **V80.929** **Occupant of animal-drawn vehicle injured** in unspecified transport accident
Animal-drawn vehicle accident NOS

☑4ᵗʰ **V81** Occupant of railway train or railway vehicle injured in transport accident

INCLUDES derailment of railway train or railway vehicle
person on outside of train

EXCLUDES 1 streetcar (V82.-)

The appropriate 7th character is to be added to each code from category V81.
A   initial encounter
D   subsequent encounter
S   sequela

☑x7ᵗʰ **V81.0** **Occupant of railway train or railway vehicle injured in collision with motor vehicle** in nontraffic accident
EXCLUDES 1 occupant of railway train or railway vehicle injured due to collision with military vehicle (V81.83)

☑x7ᵗʰ **V81.1** **Occupant of railway train or railway vehicle injured in collision with motor vehicle** in traffic accident
EXCLUDES 1 occupant of railway train or railway vehicle injured due to collision with military vehicle (V81.83)

☑x7ᵗʰ **V81.2** **Occupant of railway train or railway vehicle injured in collision with or** hit by rolling stock

☑x7ᵗʰ **V81.3** **Occupant of railway train or railway vehicle injured in collision with** other object
Railway collision NOS

☑x7ᵗʰ **V81.4** **Person injured** while boarding or alighting **from railway train or railway vehicle**

☑x7ᵗʰ **V81.5** **Occupant of railway train or railway vehicle injured** by fall in railway train **or railway vehicle**

☑x7ᵗʰ **V81.6** **Occupant of railway train or railway vehicle injured** by fall from railway train **or railway vehicle**

☑x7ᵗʰ **V81.7** **Occupant of railway train or railway vehicle injured in derailment without antecedent collision**

☑5ᵗʰ **V81.8** **Occupant of railway train or railway vehicle injured in** other specified railway accidents

☑x7ᵗʰ **V81.81** **Occupant of railway train or railway vehicle injured due to** explosion or fire on train

☑x7ᵗʰ **V81.82** **Occupant of railway train or railway vehicle injured due to** object falling onto **train**
Occupant of railway train or railway vehicle injured due to falling earth onto train
Occupant of railway train or railway vehicle injured due to falling rocks onto train
Occupant of railway train or railway vehicle injured due to falling snow onto train
Occupant of railway train or railway vehicle injured due to falling trees onto train

☑x7ᵗʰ **V81.83** **Occupant of railway train or railway vehicle injured due to** collision with military vehicle

☑x7ᵗʰ **V81.89** **Occupant of railway train or railway vehicle injured due to** other specified railway accident

☑x7ᵗʰ **V81.9** **Occupant of railway train or railway vehicle injured in unspecified railway accident**
Railway accident NOS

☑4ᵗʰ **V82** Occupant of powered streetcar injured in transport accident

INCLUDES interurban electric car
person on outside of streetcar
tram (car)
trolley (car)

EXCLUDES 1 bus (V70-V79)
motorcoach (V70-V79)
nonpowered streetcar (V76.-)
train (V81.-)

The appropriate 7th character is to be added to each code from category V82.
A   initial encounter
D   subsequent encounter
S   sequela

☑x7ᵗʰ **V82.0** **Occupant of streetcar injured in collision with motor vehicle** in nontraffic accident

☑x7ᵗʰ **V82.1** **Occupant of streetcar injured in collision with motor vehicle** in traffic accident

☑x7ᵗʰ **V82.2** **Occupant of streetcar injured in collision with or** hit by rolling stock

☑x7ᵗʰ **V82.3** **Occupant of streetcar injured in collision with** other object
EXCLUDES 1 collision with animal-drawn vehicle or animal being ridden (V82.8)

☑x7ᵗʰ **V82.4** **Person injured** while boarding or alighting **from streetcar**

☑x7ᵗʰ **V82.5** **Occupant of streetcar injured by** fall in streetcar
EXCLUDES 1 fall in streetcar:
while boarding or alighting (V82.4)
with antecedent collision (V82.0-V82.3)

☑x7ᵗʰ **V82.6** **Occupant of streetcar injured by** fall from streetcar
EXCLUDES 1 fall from streetcar:
while boarding or alighting (V82.4)
with antecedent collision (V82.0-V82.3)

☑x7ᵗʰ **V82.7** **Occupant of streetcar injured in** derailment without antecedent collision
EXCLUDES 1 occupant of streetcar injured in derailment with antecedent collision (V82.0-V82.3)

☑x7ᵗʰ **V82.8** **Occupant of streetcar injured in** other specified transport accidents
Streetcar collision with military vehicle
Streetcar collision with train or nonmotor vehicles

☑x7ᵗʰ **V82.9** **Occupant of streetcar injured in** unspecified traffic accident
Streetcar accident NOS

☑4ᵗʰ **V83** Occupant of special vehicle mainly used on industrial premises injured in transport accident

INCLUDES battery-powered airport passenger vehicle
battery-powered truck (baggage) (mail)
coal-car in mine
forklift (truck)
logging car
self-propelled industrial truck
station baggage truck (powered)
tram, truck, or tub (powered) in mine or quarry

EXCLUDES 1 special construction vehicles (V85.-)
special industrial vehicle in stationary use or maintenance (W31.-)

The appropriate 7th character is to be added to each code from category V83.
A   initial encounter
D   subsequent encounter
S   sequela

☑x7ᵗʰ **V83.0** **Driver** of special industrial vehicle injured **in traffic accident**

☑x7ᵗʰ **V83.1** **Passenger** of special industrial vehicle injured **in traffic accident**

☑x7ᵗʰ **V83.2** **Person on outside** of special industrial vehicle injured **in traffic accident**

☑x7ᵗʰ **V83.3** **Unspecified occupant** of special industrial vehicle injured **in traffic accident**

☑x7ᵗʰ **V83.4** **Person injured while** boarding or alighting **from special industrial vehicle**

☑x7ᵗʰ **V83.5** **Driver** of special industrial vehicle injured **in nontraffic accident**

☑x7ᵗʰ **V83.6** **Passenger** of special industrial vehicle injured **in nontraffic accident**

☑x7ᵗʰ **V83.7** **Person on outside** of special industrial vehicle injured **in nontraffic accident**

☑ Additional Character Required   ☑x7ᵗʰ Placeholder Alert   Unacceptable PDx   Manifestation   Hospital Acquired Condition   **EXCLUDES 1** Not Coded Here   **EXCLUDES 2** Not Included Here

ICD-10-CM 2016   1177

√x7ᵗʰ **V83.9** **Unspecified occupant** of special industrial vehicle injured in nontraffic accident
Special-industrial-vehicle accident NOS

√4ᵗʰ **V84** **Occupant of special vehicle mainly used in agriculture injured in transport accident**
INCLUDES   self-propelled farm machinery
tractor (and trailer)
EXCLUDES1   animal-powered farm machinery accident (W30.8-)
contact with combine harvester (W30.0)
special agricultural vehicle in stationary use or maintenance (W30.-)

> The appropriate 7th character is to be added to each code from category V84.
> A   initial encounter
> D   subsequent encounter
> S   sequela

√x7ᵗʰ **V84.0** **Driver** of special agricultural vehicle injured in traffic accident

√x7ᵗʰ **V84.1** **Passenger** of special agricultural vehicle injured in traffic accident

√x7ᵗʰ **V84.2** **Person on outside** of special agricultural vehicle injured in traffic accident

√x7ᵗʰ **V84.3** **Unspecified** occupant of special agricultural vehicle injured in traffic accident

√x7ᵗʰ **V84.4** **Person injured while** boarding or alighting from special agricultural vehicle

√x7ᵗʰ **V84.5** **Driver** of special agricultural vehicle injured in nontraffic accident

√x7ᵗʰ **V84.6** **Passenger** of special agricultural vehicle injured in nontraffic accident

√x7ᵗʰ **V84.7** **Person on outside** of special agricultural vehicle injured in nontraffic accident

√x7ᵗʰ **V84.9** **Unspecified** occupant of special agricultural vehicle injured in nontraffic accident
Special-agricultural vehicle accident NOS

√4ᵗʰ **V85** **Occupant of special construction vehicle injured in transport accident**
INCLUDES   bulldozer
digger
dump truck
earth-leveller
mechanical shovel
road-roller
EXCLUDES1   special industrial vehicle (V83.-)
special construction vehicle in stationary use or maintenance (W31.-)

> The appropriate 7th character is to be added to each code from category V85.
> A   initial encounter
> D   subsequent encounter
> S   sequela

√x7ᵗʰ **V85.0** **Driver** of special construction vehicle injured in traffic accident

√x7ᵗʰ **V85.1** **Passenger** of special construction vehicle injured in traffic accident

√x7ᵗʰ **V85.2** **Person on outside** of special construction vehicle injured in traffic accident

√x7ᵗʰ **V85.3** **Unspecified** occupant of special construction vehicle injured in traffic accident

√x7ᵗʰ **V85.4** **Person injured while** boarding or alighting from special construction vehicle

√x7ᵗʰ **V85.5** **Driver** of special construction vehicle injured in nontraffic accident

√x7ᵗʰ **V85.6** **Passenger** of special construction vehicle injured in nontraffic accident

√x7ᵗʰ **V85.7** **Person on outside** of special construction vehicle injured in nontraffic accident

√x7ᵗʰ **V85.9** **Unspecified** occupant of special construction vehicle injured in nontraffic accident
Special-construction-vehicle accident NOS

√4ᵗʰ **V86** **Occupant of special all-terrain or other off-road motor vehicle, injured in transport accident**
EXCLUDES1   special all-terrain vehicle in stationary use or maintenance (W31.-)
sport-utility vehicle (V50-V59)
three-wheeled motor vehicle designed for on-road use (V30-V39)

> The appropriate 7th character is to be added to each code from category V86.
> A   initial encounter
> D   subsequent encounter
> S   sequela

√5ᵗʰ **V86.0** **Driver** of special all-terrain or other off-road motor vehicle injured in traffic accident

√x7ᵗʰ **V86.01** **Driver** of ambulance or fire engine injured in traffic accident

√x7ᵗʰ **V86.02** **Driver** of snowmobile injured in traffic accident

√x7ᵗʰ **V86.03** **Driver** of dune buggy injured in traffic accident

√x7ᵗʰ **V86.04** **Driver** of military vehicle injured in traffic accident

√x7ᵗʰ **V86.09** **Driver** of other special all-terrain or other off-road motor vehicle injured in traffic accident
Driver of dirt bike injured in traffic accident
Driver of go cart injured in traffic accident
Driver of golf cart injured in traffic accident

√5ᵗʰ **V86.1** **Passenger** of special all-terrain or other off-road motor vehicle injured in traffic accident

√x7ᵗʰ **V86.11** **Passenger** of ambulance or fire engine injured in traffic accident

√x7ᵗʰ **V86.12** **Passenger** of snowmobile injured in traffic accident

√x7ᵗʰ **V86.13** **Passenger** of dune buggy injured in traffic accident

√x7ᵗʰ **V86.14** **Passenger** of military vehicle injured in traffic accident

√x7ᵗʰ **V86.19** **Passenger** of other special all-terrain or other off-road motor vehicle injured in traffic accident
Passenger of dirt bike injured in traffic accident
Passenger of go cart injured in traffic accident
Passenger of golf cart injured in traffic accident

√5ᵗʰ **V86.2** **Person on outside** of special all-terrain or other off-road motor vehicle injured in traffic accident

√x7ᵗʰ **V86.21** **Person on outside** of ambulance or fire engine injured in traffic accident

√x7ᵗʰ **V86.22** **Person on outside** of snowmobile injured in traffic accident

√x7ᵗʰ **V86.23** **Person on outside** of dune buggy injured in traffic accident

√x7ᵗʰ **V86.24** **Person on outside** of military vehicle injured in traffic accident

√x7ᵗʰ **V86.29** **Person on outside** of other special all-terrain or other off-road motor vehicle injured in traffic accident
Person on outside of dirt bike injured in traffic accident
Person on outside of go cart injured in traffic accident
Person on outside of golf cart injured in traffic accident

√5ᵗʰ **V86.3** **Unspecified** occupant of special all-terrain or other off-road motor vehicle injured in traffic accident

√x7ᵗʰ **V86.31** **Unspecified** occupant of ambulance or fire engine injured in traffic accident

√x7ᵗʰ **V86.32** **Unspecified** occupant of snowmobile injured in traffic accident

√x7ᵗʰ **V86.33** **Unspecified** occupant of dune buggy injured in traffic accident

√x7ᵗʰ **V86.34** **Unspecified** occupant of military vehicle injured in traffic accident

√x7ᵗʰ **V86.39** **Unspecified** occupant of other special all-terrain or other off-road motor vehicle injured in traffic accident
Unspecified occupant of dirt bike injured in traffic accident
Unspecified occupant of go cart injured in traffic accident
Unspecified occupant of golf cart injured in traffic accident

√5ᵗʰ **V86.4** **Person injured while** boarding or alighting from special all-terrain or other off-road motor vehicle

√x7ᵗʰ **V86.41** **Person injured while boarding or alighting from** ambulance or fire engine

✓x7ᵗʰ **V86.42** **Person injured while boarding or alighting from** snowmobile

✓x7ᵗʰ **V86.43** **Person injured while boarding or alighting from** dune buggy

✓x7ᵗʰ **V86.44** **Person injured while boarding or alighting from** military vehicle

✓x7ᵗʰ **V86.49** **Person injured while boarding or alighting from** other **special all-terrain or other off-road motor vehicle**
Person injured while boarding or alighting from dirt bike
Person injured while boarding or alighting from go cart
Person injured while boarding or alighting from golf cart

✓5ᵗʰ **V86.5** Driver **of special all-terrain or other off-road motor vehicle** injured in nontraffic accident

✓x7ᵗʰ **V86.51** **Driver of** ambulance **or** fire engine **injured in** nontraffic accident

✓x7ᵗʰ **V86.52** **Driver of** snowmobile **injured in nontraffic accident**

✓x7ᵗʰ **V86.53** **Driver of** dune buggy **injured in nontraffic accident**

✓x7ᵗʰ **V86.54** **Driver of** military vehicle **injured in nontraffic accident**

✓x7ᵗʰ **V86.59** **Driver of** other **special all-terrain or other off-road motor vehicle injured in nontraffic accident**
Driver of dirt bike injured in nontraffic accident
Driver of go cart injured in nontraffic accident
Driver of golf cart injured in nontraffic accident

✓5ᵗʰ **V86.6** Passenger **of special all-terrain or other off-road motor vehicle** injured in nontraffic accident

✓x7ᵗʰ **V86.61** **Passenger of** ambulance **or** fire engine **injured in** nontraffic accident

✓x7ᵗʰ **V86.62** **Passenger of** snowmobile **injured in nontraffic** accident

✓x7ᵗʰ **V86.63** **Passenger of** dune buggy **injured in nontraffic** accident

✓x7ᵗʰ **V86.64** **Passenger of** military vehicle **injured in nontraffic** accident

✓x7ᵗʰ **V86.69** **Passenger of** other **special all-terrain or other off-road motor vehicle injured in nontraffic accident**
Passenger of dirt bike injured in nontraffic accident
Passenger of go cart injured in nontraffic accident
Passenger of golf cart injured in nontraffic accident

✓5ᵗʰ **V86.7** Person on outside **of special all-terrain or other off-road motor vehicle** injured in nontraffic accident

✓x7ᵗʰ **V86.71** **Person on outside of** ambulance **or** fire engine **injured in nontraffic accident**

✓x7ᵗʰ **V86.72** **Person on outside of** snowmobile **injured in** nontraffic accident

✓x7ᵗʰ **V86.73** **Person on outside of** dune buggy **injured in** nontraffic accident

✓x7ᵗʰ **V86.74** **Person on outside of** military **vehicle injured in** nontraffic accident

✓x7ᵗʰ **V86.79** **Person on outside of** other **special all-terrain or other off-road motor vehicles injured in nontraffic** accident
Person on outside of dirt bike injured in nontraffic accident
Person on outside of go cart injured in nontraffic accident
Person on outside of golf cart injured in nontraffic accident

✓5ᵗʰ **V86.9** Unspecified occupant **of special all-terrain or other off-road motor vehicle** injured in nontraffic accident

✓x7ᵗʰ **V86.91** **Unspecified occupant of** ambulance **or** fire engine **injured in nontraffic accident**

✓x7ᵗʰ **V86.92** **Unspecified occupant of** snowmobile **injured in** nontraffic accident

✓x7ᵗʰ **V86.93** **Unspecified occupant of** dune buggy **injured in** nontraffic accident

✓x7ᵗʰ **V86.94** **Unspecified occupant of** military vehicle **injured in** nontraffic accident

✓x7ᵗʰ **V86.99** **Unspecified occupant of** other **special all-terrain or other off-road motor vehicle injured in nontraffic accident**
All-terrain motor-vehicle accident NOS
Off-road motor-vehicle accident NOS
Other motor-vehicle accident NOS
Unspecified occupant of dirt bike injured in nontraffic accident
Unspecified occupant of go cart injured in nontraffic accident
Unspecified occupant of golf cart injured in nontraffic accident

✓4ᵗʰ **V87** **Traffic accident of specified type but victim's mode of transport unknown**

EXCLUDES 1 *collision involving:*
pedal cycle (V10-V19)
pedestrian (V01-V09)

The appropriate 7th character is to be added to each code from category V87.
A   initial encounter
D   subsequent encounter
S   sequela

✓x7ᵗʰ **V87.0** **Person injured in collision between** car and two- or three-wheeled powered vehicle **(traffic)**

✓x7ᵗʰ **V87.1** **Person injured in collision between** other motor vehicle and two- or three-wheeled motor vehicle **(traffic)**

✓x7ᵗʰ **V87.2** **Person injured in collision between** car and pick-up truck or van **(traffic)**

✓x7ᵗʰ **V87.3** **Person injured in collision between** car and bus **(traffic)**

✓x7ᵗʰ **V87.4** **Person injured in collision between** car and heavy transport vehicle **(traffic)**

✓x7ᵗʰ **V87.5** **Person injured in collision between** heavy transport vehicle and bus **(traffic)**

✓x7ᵗʰ **V87.6** **Person injured in collision between** railway train or railway vehicle and car **(traffic)**

✓x7ᵗʰ **V87.7** **Person injured in collision between** other specified motor vehicles **(traffic)**

✓x7ᵗʰ **V87.8** **Person injured in** other specified noncollision transport accidents **involving** motor vehicle **(traffic)**

✓x7ᵗʰ **V87.9** **Person injured in** other specified (collision)(noncollision) transport accidents **involving** nonmotor vehicle **(traffic)**

✓4ᵗʰ **V88** **Nontraffic accident of specified type but victim's mode of transport unknown**

EXCLUDES 1 *collision involving:*
pedal cycle (V10-V19)
pedestrian (V01-V09)

The appropriate 7th character is to be added to each code from category V88.
A   initial encounter
D   subsequent encounter
S   sequela

✓x7ᵗʰ **V88.0** **Person injured in collision between** car and two- or three-wheeled motor vehicle, nontraffic

✓x7ᵗʰ **V88.1** **Person injured in collision between** other motor vehicle and two- or three-wheeled motor vehicle, nontraffic

✓x7ᵗʰ **V88.2** **Person injured in collision between** car and pick-up truck or van, nontraffic

✓x7ᵗʰ **V88.3** **Person injured in collision between** car and bus, nontraffic

✓x7ᵗʰ **V88.4** **Person injured in collision between** car and heavy transport vehicle, nontraffic

✓x7ᵗʰ **V88.5** **Person injured in collision between** heavy transport vehicle and bus, nontraffic

✓x7ᵗʰ **V88.6** **Person injured in collision between** railway train or railway vehicle and car, nontraffic

✓x7ᵗʰ **V88.7** **Person injured in collision between** other specified motor vehicle, nontraffic

✓x7ᵗʰ **V88.8** **Person injured in** other specified noncollision transport accidents **involving** motor vehicle, nontraffic

✓x7ᵗʰ **V88.9** **Person injured in** other specified (collision)(noncollision) transport accidents **involving** nonmotor vehicle, nontraffic

✓ Additional Character Required   ✓x7ᵗʰ Placeholder Alert   Unacceptable PDx   Manifestation   Hospital Acquired Condition   **EXCLUDES 1** Not Coded Here   **EXCLUDES 2** Not Included Here

ICD-10-CM 2016   1179

✓4ᵗʰ **V89 Motor- or nonmotor-vehicle accident, type of vehicle unspecified**

> The appropriate 7th character is to be added to each code from category V89.
> A   initial encounter
> D   subsequent encounter
> S   sequela

✓x7ᵗʰ **V89.0 Person injured in unspecified motor-vehicle accident, nontraffic**
Motor-vehicle accident NOS, nontraffic

✓x7ᵗʰ **V89.1 Person injured in unspecified nonmotor-vehicle accident, nontraffic**
Nonmotor-vehicle accident NOS (nontraffic)

✓x7ᵗʰ **V89.2 Person injured in unspecified motor-vehicle accident, traffic**
Motor-vehicle accident [MVA] NOS
Road (traffic) accident [RTA] NOS

✓x7ᵗʰ **V89.3 Person injured in unspecified nonmotor-vehicle accident, traffic**
Nonmotor-vehicle traffic accident NOS

✓x7ᵗʰ **V89.9 Person injured in unspecified vehicle accident**
Collision NOS

Water transport accidents (V90-V94)

✓4ᵗʰ **V90 Drowning and submersion due to accident to watercraft**
> **EXCLUDES 1**   civilian water transport accident involving military watercraft (V94.81-)
> fall into water not from watercraft (W16.-)
> military watercraft accident in military or war operations (Y36.0-, Y37.0-)
> water-transport-related drowning or submersion without accident to watercraft (V92.-)

> The appropriate 7th character is to be added to each code from category V90.
> A   initial encounter
> D   subsequent encounter
> S   sequela

✓5ᵗʰ **V90.0 Drowning and submersion due to watercraft overturning**

✓x7ᵗʰ **V90.00 Drowning and submersion due to merchant ship overturning**

✓x7ᵗʰ **V90.01 Drowning and submersion due to passenger ship overturning**
Drowning and submersion due to Ferry-boat overturning
Drowning and submersion due to Liner overturning

✓x7ᵗʰ **V90.02 Drowning and submersion due to fishing boat overturning**

✓x7ᵗʰ **V90.03 Drowning and submersion due to other powered watercraft overturning**
Drowning and submersion due to Hovercraft (on open water) overturning
Drowning and submersion due to Jet ski overturning

✓x7ᵗʰ **V90.04 Drowning and submersion due to sailboat overturning**

✓x7ᵗʰ **V90.05 Drowning and submersion due to canoe or kayak overturning**

✓x7ᵗʰ **V90.06 Drowning and submersion due to (nonpowered) inflatable craft overturning**

✓x7ᵗʰ **V90.08 Drowning and submersion due to other unpowered watercraft overturning**
Drowning and submersion due to windsurfer overturning

✓x7ᵗʰ **V90.09 Drowning and submersion due to unspecified watercraft overturning**
Drowning and submersion due to boat NOS overturning
Drowning and submersion due to ship NOS overturning
Drowning and submersion due to watercraft NOS overturning

✓5ᵗʰ **V90.1 Drowning and submersion due to watercraft sinking**

✓x7ᵗʰ **V90.10 Drowning and submersion due to merchant ship sinking**

✓x7ᵗʰ **V90.11 Drowning and submersion due to passenger ship sinking**
Drowning and submersion due to Ferry-boat sinking
Drowning and submersion due to Liner sinking

✓x7ᵗʰ **V90.12 Drowning and submersion due to fishing boat sinking**

✓x7ᵗʰ **V90.13 Drowning and submersion due to other powered watercraft sinking**
Drowning and submersion due to Hovercraft (on open water) sinking
Drowning and submersion due to Jet ski sinking

✓x7ᵗʰ **V90.14 Drowning and submersion due to sailboat sinking**

✓x7ᵗʰ **V90.15 Drowning and submersion due to canoe or kayak sinking**

✓x7ᵗʰ **V90.16 Drowning and submersion due to (nonpowered) inflatable craft sinking**

✓x7ᵗʰ **V90.18 Drowning and submersion due to other unpowered watercraft sinking**

✓x7ᵗʰ **V90.19 Drowning and submersion due to unspecified watercraft sinking**
Drowning and submersion due to boat NOS sinking
Drowning and submersion due to ship NOS sinking
Drowning and submersion due to watercraft NOS sinking

✓5ᵗʰ **V90.2 Drowning and submersion due to falling or jumping from burning watercraft**

✓x7ᵗʰ **V90.20 Drowning and submersion due to falling or jumping from burning merchant ship**

✓x7ᵗʰ **V90.21 Drowning and submersion due to falling or jumping from burning passenger ship**
Drowning and submersion due to falling or jumping from burning Ferry-boat
Drowning and submersion due to falling or jumping from burning Liner

✓x7ᵗʰ **V90.22 Drowning and submersion due to falling or jumping from burning fishing boat**

✓x7ᵗʰ **V90.23 Drowning and submersion due to falling or jumping from other burning powered watercraft**
Drowning and submersion due to falling and jumping from burning Hovercraft (on open water)
Drowning and submersion due to falling and jumping from burning Jet ski

✓x7ᵗʰ **V90.24 Drowning and submersion due to falling or jumping from burning sailboat**

✓x7ᵗʰ **V90.25 Drowning and submersion due to falling or jumping from burning canoe or kayak**

✓x7ᵗʰ **V90.26 Drowning and submersion due to falling or jumping from burning (nonpowered) inflatable craft**

✓x7ᵗʰ **V90.27 Drowning and submersion due to falling or jumping from burning water-skis**

✓x7ᵗʰ **V90.28 Drowning and submersion due to falling or jumping from other burning unpowered watercraft**
Drowning and submersion due to falling and jumping from burning surf-board
Drowning and submersion due to falling and jumping from burning windsurfer

✓x7ᵗʰ **V90.29 Drowning and submersion due to falling or jumping from unspecified burning watercraft**
Drowning and submersion due to falling or jumping from burning boat NOS
Drowning and submersion due to falling or jumping from burning ship NOS
Drowning and submersion due to falling or jumping from burning watercraft NOS

✓5ᵗʰ **V90.3 Drowning and submersion due to falling or jumping from crushed watercraft**

✓x7ᵗʰ **V90.30 Drowning and submersion due to falling or jumping from crushed merchant ship**

✓x7ᵗʰ **V90.31 Drowning and submersion due to falling or jumping from crushed passenger ship**
Drowning and submersion due to falling and jumping from crushed Ferry boat
Drowning and submersion due to falling and jumping from crushed Liner

✓x7ᵗʰ **V90.32 Drowning and submersion due to falling or jumping from crushed fishing boat**

✓x7ᵗʰ **V90.33 Drowning and submersion due to falling or jumping from other crushed powered watercraft**
Drowning and submersion due to falling and jumping from crushed Hovercraft
Drowning and submersion due to falling and jumping from crushed Jet ski

✓x7ᵗʰ **V90.34 Drowning and submersion due to falling or jumping from crushed sailboat**

Ⓝ Newborn: 0   Ⓟ Pediatric: 0-17   Ⓜ Maternity: 12-55   Ⓐ Adult: 15-124   MCC Major CC Condition   PDxMCC PDx acts as own MCC   CC CC Condition   PDxCC PDx acts as own CC

1180   ICD-10-CM 2016

✓x7ᵗʰ **V90.35** **Drowning and submersion due to falling or jumping from crushed canoe or kayak**

✓x7ᵗʰ **V90.36** **Drowning and submersion due to falling or jumping from crushed (nonpowered) inflatable craft**

✓x7ᵗʰ **V90.37** **Drowning and submersion due to falling or jumping from crushed water-skis**

✓x7ᵗʰ **V90.38** **Drowning and submersion due to falling or jumping from other crushed unpowered watercraft**
Drowning and submersion due to falling and jumping from crushed surf-board
Drowning and submersion due to falling and jumping from crushed windsurfer

✓x7ᵗʰ **V90.39** **Drowning and submersion due to falling or jumping from crushed unspecified watercraft**
Drowning and submersion due to falling and jumping from crushed boat NOS
Drowning and submersion due to falling and jumping from crushed ship NOS
Drowning and submersion due to falling and jumping from crushed watercraft NOS

✓5ᵗʰ **V90.8** **Drowning and submersion due to other accident to watercraft**

✓x7ᵗʰ **V90.80** **Drowning and submersion due to other accident to merchant ship**

✓x7ᵗʰ **V90.81** **Drowning and submersion due to other accident to passenger ship**
Drowning and submersion due to other accident to Ferry-boat
Drowning and submersion due to other accident to Liner

✓x7ᵗʰ **V90.82** **Drowning and submersion due to other accident to fishing boat**

✓x7ᵗʰ **V90.83** **Drowning and submersion due to other accident to other powered watercraft**
Drowning and submersion due to other accident to Hovercraft (on open water)
Drowning and submersion due to other accident to Jet ski

✓x7ᵗʰ **V90.84** **Drowning and submersion due to other accident to sailboat**

✓x7ᵗʰ **V90.85** **Drowning and submersion due to other accident to canoe or kayak**

✓x7ᵗʰ **V90.86** **Drowning and submersion due to other accident to (nonpowered) inflatable craft**

✓x7ᵗʰ **V90.87** **Drowning and submersion due to other accident to water-skis**

✓x7ᵗʰ **V90.88** **Drowning and submersion due to other accident to other unpowered watercraft**
Drowning and submersion due to other accident to surf-board
Drowning and submersion due to other accident to windsurfer

✓x7ᵗʰ **V90.89** **Drowning and submersion due to other accident to unspecified watercraft**
Drowning and submersion due to other accident to boat NOS
Drowning and submersion due to other accident to ship NOS
Drowning and submersion due to other accident to watercraft NOS

✓4ᵗʰ **V91** **Other injury due to accident to watercraft**
     INCLUDES   any injury except drowning and submersion as a result of an accident to watercraft
     EXCLUDES 1   *civilian water transport accident involving military watercraft (V94.81-)*
military watercraft accident in military or war operations (Y36, Y37.-)
     EXCLUDES 2   *drowning and submersion due to accident to watercraft (V90.-)*

The appropriate 7th character is to be added to each code from category V91.
A   initial encounter
D   subsequent encounter
S   sequela

✓5ᵗʰ **V91.0** **Burn due to watercraft on fire**
     EXCLUDES 1   *burn from localized fire or explosion on board ship without accident to watercraft (V93.-)*

✓x7ᵗʰ **V91.00** **Burn due to merchant ship on fire**

✓x7ᵗʰ **V91.01** **Burn due to passenger ship on fire**
Burn due to Ferry-boat on fire
Burn due to Liner on fire

✓x7ᵗʰ **V91.02** **Burn due to fishing boat on fire**

✓x7ᵗʰ **V91.03** **Burn due to other powered watercraft on fire**
Burn due to Hovercraft (on open water) on fire
Burn due to Jet ski on fire

✓x7ᵗʰ **V91.04** **Burn due to sailboat on fire**

✓x7ᵗʰ **V91.05** **Burn due to canoe or kayak on fire**

✓x7ᵗʰ **V91.06** **Burn due to (nonpowered) inflatable craft on fire**

✓x7ᵗʰ **V91.07** **Burn due to water-skis on fire**

✓x7ᵗʰ **V91.08** **Burn due to other unpowered watercraft on fire**

✓x7ᵗʰ **V91.09** **Burn due to unspecified watercraft on fire**
Burn due to boat NOS on fire
Burn due to ship NOS on fire
Burn due to watercraft NOS on fire

✓5ᵗʰ **V91.1** **Crushed between watercraft and other watercraft or other object due to collision**
Crushed by lifeboat after abandoning ship in a collision
     NOTE   Select the specified type of watercraft that the victim was on at the time of the collision

✓x7ᵗʰ **V91.10** **Crushed between merchant ship and other watercraft or other object due to collision**

✓x7ᵗʰ **V91.11** **Crushed between passenger ship and other watercraft or other object due to collision**
Crushed between Ferry-boat and other watercraft or other object due to collision
Crushed between Liner and other watercraft or other object due to collision

✓x7ᵗʰ **V91.12** **Crushed between fishing boat and other watercraft or other object due to collision**

✓x7ᵗʰ **V91.13** **Crushed between other powered watercraft and other watercraft or other object due to collision**
Crushed between Hovercraft (on open water) and other watercraft or other object due to collision
Crushed between Jet ski and other watercraft or other object due to collision

✓x7ᵗʰ **V91.14** **Crushed between sailboat and other watercraft or other object due to collision**

✓x7ᵗʰ **V91.15** **Crushed between canoe or kayak and other watercraft or other object due to collision**

✓x7ᵗʰ **V91.16** **Crushed between (nonpowered) inflatable craft and other watercraft or other object due to collision**

✓x7ᵗʰ **V91.18** **Crushed between other unpowered watercraft and other watercraft or other object due to collision**
Crushed between surfboard and other watercraft or other object due to collision
Crushed between windsurfer and other watercraft or other object due to collision

✓x7ᵗʰ **V91.19** **Crushed between unspecified watercraft and other watercraft or other object due to collision**
Crushed between boat NOS and other watercraft or other object due to collision
Crushed between ship NOS and other watercraft or other object due to collision
Crushed between watercraft NOS and other watercraft or other object due to collision

✓5ᵗʰ **V91.2** **Fall due to collision between watercraft and other watercraft or other object**
Fall while remaining on watercraft after collision
     NOTE   Select the specified type of watercraft that the victim was on at the time of the collision.
     EXCLUDES 1   *crushed between watercraft and other watercraft and other object due to collision (V91.1-)*
drowning and submersion due to falling from crushed watercraft (V90.3-)

✓x7ᵗʰ **V91.20** **Fall due to collision between merchant ship and other watercraft or other object**

✓x7ᵗʰ **V91.21** **Fall due to collision between passenger ship and other watercraft or other object**
Fall due to collision between Ferry-boat and other watercraft or other object
Fall due to collision between Liner and other watercraft or other object

✓x7ᵗʰ **V91.22** **Fall due to collision between fishing boat and other watercraft or other object**

✓ Additional Character Required   ✓x7ᵗʰ Placeholder Alert   Unacceptable PDx   Manifestation   Hospital Acquired Condition   EXCLUDES 1 Not Coded Here   EXCLUDES 2 Not Included Here

√x7ᵗʰ **V91.23** **Fall due to collision between** other powered watercraft **and other watercraft or other object**
Fall due to collision between Hovercraft (on open water) and other watercraft or other object
Fall due to collision between Jet ski and other watercraft or other object

√x7ᵗʰ **V91.24** **Fall due to collision between** sailboat **and other watercraft or other object**

√x7ᵗʰ **V91.25** **Fall due to collision between** canoe or kayak **and other watercraft or other object**

√x7ᵗʰ **V91.26** **Fall due to collision between** (nonpowered) inflatable craft **and other watercraft or other object**

√x7ᵗʰ **V91.29** **Fall due to collision between** unspecified **watercraft and other watercraft or other object**
Fall due to collision between boat NOS and other watercraft or other object
Fall due to collision between ship NOS and other watercraft or other object
Fall due to collision between watercraft NOS and other watercraft or other object

√5ᵗʰ **V91.3** **Hit or struck by falling object due to accident to watercraft**
Hit or struck by falling object (part of damaged watercraft or other object) after falling or jumping from damaged watercraft
EXCLUDES 2 *drowning or submersion due to fall or jumping from damaged watercraft (V90.2-, V90.3-)*

√x7ᵗʰ **V91.30** **Hit or struck by falling object due to accident to** merchant ship

√x7ᵗʰ **V91.31** **Hit or struck by falling object due to accident to** passenger ship
Hit or struck by falling object due to accident to Ferry-boat
Hit or struck by falling object due to accident to Liner

√x7ᵗʰ **V91.32** **Hit or struck by falling object due to accident to** fishing boat

√x7ᵗʰ **V91.33** **Hit or struck by falling object due to accident to** other powered **watercraft**
Hit or struck by falling object due to accident to Hovercraft (on open water)
Hit or struck by falling object due to accident to Jet ski

√x7ᵗʰ **V91.34** **Hit or struck by falling object due to accident to** sailboat

√x7ᵗʰ **V91.35** **Hit or struck by falling object due to accident to** canoe or kayak

√x7ᵗʰ **V91.36** **Hit or struck by falling object due to accident to** (nonpowered) inflatable craft

√x7ᵗʰ **V91.37** **Hit or struck by falling object due to accident to** water-skis
Hit by water-skis after jumping off of waterskis

√x7ᵗʰ **V91.38** **Hit or struck by falling object due to accident to** other unpowered **watercraft**
Hit or struck by surf-board after falling off damaged surf-board
Hit or struck by object after falling off damaged windsurfer

√x7ᵗʰ **V91.39** **Hit or struck by falling object due to accident to** unspecified **watercraft**
Hit or struck by falling object due to accident to boat NOS
Hit or struck by falling object due to accident to ship NOS
Hit or struck by falling object due to accident to watercraft NOS

√5ᵗʰ **V91.8** **Other injury due to other accident to watercraft**

√x7ᵗʰ **V91.80** **Other injury due to other accident to** merchant ship

√x7ᵗʰ **V91.81** **Other injury due to other accident to** passenger ship
Other injury due to other accident to Ferry-boat
Other injury due to other accident to Liner

√x7ᵗʰ **V91.82** **Other injury due to other accident to** fishing boat

√x7ᵗʰ **V91.83** **Other injury due to other accident to** other powered **watercraft**
Other injury due to other accident to Hovercraft (on open water)
Other injury due to other accident to Jet ski

√x7ᵗʰ **V91.84** **Other injury due to other accident to** sailboat

√x7ᵗʰ **V91.85** **Other injury due to other accident to** canoe or kayak

√x7ᵗʰ **V91.86** **Other injury due to other accident to** (nonpowered) inflatable craft

√x7ᵗʰ **V91.87** **Other injury due to other accident to** water-skis

√x7ᵗʰ **V91.88** **Other injury due to other accident to** other unpowered **watercraft**
Other injury due to other accident to surf-board
Other injury due to other accident to windsurfer

√x7ᵗʰ **V91.89** **Other injury due to other accident to** unspecified **watercraft**
Other injury due to other accident to boat NOS
Other injury due to other accident to ship NOS
Other injury due to other accident to watercraft NOS

√4ᵗʰ **V92** **Drowning and submersion due to accident on board watercraft, without accident to watercraft**
EXCLUDES 1 *civilian water transport accident involving military watercraft (V94.81-)*
drowning or submersion due to accident to watercraft (V90-V91)
drowning or submersion of diver who voluntarily jumps from boat not involved in an accident (W16.711, W16.721)
fall into water without watercraft (W16.-)
military watercraft accident in military or war operations (Y36, Y37)

> The appropriate 7th character is to be added to each code from category V92.
> A   initial encounter
> D   subsequent encounter
> S   sequela

√5ᵗʰ **V92.0** **Drowning and submersion due to** fall off **watercraft**
Drowning and submersion due to fall from gangplank of watercraft
Drowning and submersion due to fall overboard watercraft
EXCLUDES 2 *hitting head on object or bottom of body of water due to fall from watercraft (V94.0-)*

√x7ᵗʰ **V92.00** **Drowning and submersion due to fall off** merchant ship

√x7ᵗʰ **V92.01** **Drowning and submersion due to fall off** passenger ship
Drowning and submersion due to fall off Ferry-boat
Drowning and submersion due to fall off Liner

√x7ᵗʰ **V92.02** **Drowning and submersion due to fall off** fishing boat

√x7ᵗʰ **V92.03** **Drowning and submersion due to fall off** other powered **watercraft**
Drowning and submersion due to fall off Hovercraft (on open water)
Drowning and submersion due to fall off Jet ski

√x7ᵗʰ **V92.04** **Drowning and submersion due to fall off** sailboat

√x7ᵗʰ **V92.05** **Drowning and submersion due to fall off** canoe or kayak

√x7ᵗʰ **V92.06** **Drowning and submersion due to fall off** (nonpowered) inflatable craft

√x7ᵗʰ **V92.07** **Drowning and submersion due to fall off** water-skis
EXCLUDES 1 *drowning and submersion due to falling off burning water-skis (V90.27)*
drowning and submersion due to falling off crushed water-skis (V90.37)
hit by boat while water-skiing NOS (V94.X)

√x7ᵗʰ **V92.08** **Drowning and submersion due to fall off** other unpowered **watercraft**
Drowning and submersion due to fall off surf-board
Drowning and submersion due to fall off windsurfer
EXCLUDES 1 *drowning and submersion due to fall off burning unpowered watercraft (V90.28)*
drowning and submersion due to fall off crushed unpowered watercraft (V90.38)
drowning and submersion due to fall off damaged unpowered watercraft (V90.88)
drowning and submersion due to rider of nonpowered watercraft being hit by other watercraft (V94.-)
other injury due to rider of nonpowered watercraft being hit by other watercraft (V94.-)

√x7ᵗʰ **V92.09** **Drowning and submersion due to fall off** unspecified **watercraft**
Drowning and submersion due to fall off boat NOS
Drowning and submersion due to fall off ship
Drowning and submersion due to fall off watercraft NOS

√5ᵗʰ **V92.1** **Drowning and submersion due to being** thrown overboard **by motion of watercraft**
EXCLUDES 1   *drowning and submersion due to fall off surf-board (V92.08)*
drowning and submersion due to fall off water-skis (V92.07)
drowning and submersion due to fall off windsurfer (V92.08)

√x7ᵗʰ **V92.10** **Drowning and submersion due to being thrown overboard by motion of** merchant ship

√x7ᵗʰ **V92.11** **Drowning and submersion due to being thrown overboard by motion of** passenger ship
Drowning and submersion due to being thrown overboard by motion of Ferry-boat
Drowning and submersion due to being thrown overboard by motion of Liner

√x7ᵗʰ **V92.12** **Drowning and submersion due to being thrown overboard by motion of** fishing boat

√x7ᵗʰ **V92.13** **Drowning and submersion due to being thrown overboard by motion of** other powered **watercraft**
Drowning and submersion due to being thrown overboard by motion of Hovercraft

√x7ᵗʰ **V92.14** **Drowning and submersion due to being thrown overboard by motion of** sailboat

√x7ᵗʰ **V92.15** **Drowning and submersion due to being thrown overboard by motion of** canoe or kayak

√x7ᵗʰ **V92.16** **Drowning and submersion due to being thrown overboard by motion of (nonpowered)** inflatable craft

√x7ᵗʰ **V92.19** **Drowning and submersion due to being thrown overboard by motion of** unspecified **watercraft**
Drowning and submersion due to being thrown overboard by motion of boat NOS
Drowning and submersion due to being thrown overboard by motion of ship NOS
Drowning and submersion due to being thrown overboard by motion of watercraft NOS

√5ᵗʰ **V92.2** **Drowning and submersion due to being** washed overboard **from watercraft**
Code first any associated cataclysm (X37.0-)

√x7ᵗʰ **V92.20** **Drowning and submersion due to being washed overboard from** merchant ship

√x7ᵗʰ **V92.21** **Drowning and submersion due to being washed overboard from** passenger ship
Drowning and submersion due to being washed overboard from Ferry-boat
Drowning and submersion due to being washed overboard from Liner

√x7ᵗʰ **V92.22** **Drowning and submersion due to being washed overboard from** fishing boat

√x7ᵗʰ **V92.23** **Drowning and submersion due to being washed overboard from** other powered **watercraft**
Drowning and submersion due to being washed overboard from Hovercraft (on open water)
Drowning and submersion due to being washed overboard from Jet ski

√x7ᵗʰ **V92.24** **Drowning and submersion due to being washed overboard from** sailboat

√x7ᵗʰ **V92.25** **Drowning and submersion due to being washed overboard from** canoe or kayak

√x7ᵗʰ **V92.26** **Drowning and submersion due to being washed overboard from (nonpowered)** inflatable craft

√x7ᵗʰ **V92.27** **Drowning and submersion due to being washed overboard from** water-skis
EXCLUDES 1   *drowning and submersion due to fall off water-skis (V92.07)*

√x7ᵗʰ **V92.28** **Drowning and submersion due to being washed overboard from** other unpowered **watercraft**
Drowning and submersion due to being washed overboard from surf-board
Drowning and submersion due to being washed overboard from windsurfer

√x7ᵗʰ **V92.29** **Drowning and submersion due to being washed overboard from** unspecified **watercraft**
Drowning and submersion due to being washed overboard from boat NOS
Drowning and submersion due to being washed overboard from ship NOS
Drowning and submersion due to being washed overboard from watercraft NOS

√4ᵗʰ **V93** **Other injury due to accident on board watercraft, without accident to watercraft**
EXCLUDES 1   *civilian water transport accident involving military watercraft (V94.81-)*
other injury due to accident to watercraft (V91.-)
military watercraft accident in military or war operations (Y36, Y37.-)
EXCLUDES 2   *drowning and submersion due to accident on board watercraft, without accident to watercraft (V92.-)*

The appropriate 7th character is to be added to each code from category V93.
A   initial encounter
D   subsequent encounter
S   sequela

√5ᵗʰ **V93.0** **Burn due to localized fire on board watercraft**
EXCLUDES 1   *burn due to watercraft on fire (V91.0-)*

√x7ᵗʰ **V93.00** **Burn due to localized fire on board** merchant vessel

√x7ᵗʰ **V93.01** **Burn due to localized fire on board** passenger vessel
Burn due to localized fire on board Ferry-boat
Burn due to localized fire on board Liner

√x7ᵗʰ **V93.02** **Burn due to localized fire on board** fishing boat

√x7ᵗʰ **V93.03** **Burn due to localized fire on board** other powered **watercraft**
Burn due to localized fire on board Hovercraft
Burn due to localized fire on board Jet ski

√x7ᵗʰ **V93.04** **Burn due to localized fire on board** sailboat

√x7ᵗʰ **V93.09** **Burn due to localized fire on board** unspecified **watercraft**
Burn due to localized fire on board boat NOS
Burn due to localized fire on board ship NOS
Burn due to localized fire on board watercraft NOS

√5ᵗʰ **V93.1** **Other burn on board watercraft**
Burn due to source other than fire on board watercraft
EXCLUDES 1   *burn due to watercraft on fire (V91.0-)*

√x7ᵗʰ **V93.10** **Other burn on board** merchant vessel

√x7ᵗʰ **V93.11** **Other burn on board** passenger vessel
Other burn on board Ferry-boat
Other burn on board Liner

√x7ᵗʰ **V93.12** **Other burn on board** fishing boat

√x7ᵗʰ **V93.13** **Other burn on board** other powered **watercraft**
Other burn on board Hovercraft
Other burn on board Jet ski

√x7ᵗʰ **V93.14** **Other burn on board** sailboat

√x7ᵗʰ **V93.19** **Other burn on board** unspecified **watercraft**
Other burn on board boat NOS
Other burn on board ship NOS
Other burn on board watercraft NOS

√5ᵗʰ **V93.2** **Heat exposure on board watercraft**
EXCLUDES 1   *exposure to man-made heat not aboard watercraft (W92)*
exposure to natural heat while on board watercraft (X30)
exposure to sunlight while on board watercraft (X32)
EXCLUDES 2   *burn due to fire on board watercraft (V93.0-)*

√x7ᵗʰ **V93.20** **Heat exposure on board** merchant ship

√x7ᵗʰ **V93.21** **Heat exposure on board** passenger ship
Heat exposure on board Ferry-boat
Heat exposure on board Liner

√x7ᵗʰ **V93.22** **Heat exposure on board** fishing boat

√x7ᵗʰ **V93.23** **Heat exposure on board** other powered **watercraft**
Heat exposure on board hovercraft

√x7ᵗʰ **V93.24** **Heat exposure on board** sailboat

√x7ᵗʰ **V93.29** **Heat exposure on board** unspecified **watercraft**
Heat exposure on board boat NOS
Heat exposure on board ship NOS
Heat exposure on board watercraft NOS

Chapter 20. External Causes of Morbidity

V92.09–V93.29

✓5ᵗʰ **V93.3 Fall on board watercraft**
>EXCLUDES 1 *fall due to collision of watercraft (V91.2-)*

✓x7ᵗʰ **V93.30 Fall on board merchant ship**

✓x7ᵗʰ **V93.31 Fall on board passenger ship**
Fall on board Ferry-boat
Fall on board Liner

✓x7ᵗʰ **V93.32 Fall on board fishing boat**

✓x7ᵗʰ **V93.33 Fall on board other powered watercraft**
Fall on board Hovercraft (on open water)
Fall on board Jet ski

✓x7ᵗʰ **V93.34 Fall on board sailboat**

✓x7ᵗʰ **V93.35 Fall on board canoe or kayak**

✓x7ᵗʰ **V93.36 Fall on board (nonpowered) inflatable craft**

✓x7ᵗʰ **V93.38 Fall on board other unpowered watercraft**

✓x7ᵗʰ **V93.39 Fall on board unspecified watercraft**
Fall on board boat NOS
Fall on board ship NOS
Fall on board watercraft NOS

✓5ᵗʰ **V93.4 Struck by falling object on board watercraft**
Hit by falling object on board watercraft
>EXCLUDES 1 *struck by falling object due to accident to watercraft (V91.3)*

✓x7ᵗʰ **V93.40 Struck by falling object on merchant ship**

✓x7ᵗʰ **V93.41 Struck by falling object on passenger ship**
Struck by falling object on Ferry-boat
Struck by falling object on Liner

✓x7ᵗʰ **V93.42 Struck by falling object on fishing boat**

✓x7ᵗʰ **V93.43 Struck by falling object on other powered watercraft**
Struck by falling object on Hovercraft

✓x7ᵗʰ **V93.44 Struck by falling object on sailboat**

✓x7ᵗʰ **V93.48 Struck by falling object on other unpowered watercraft**

✓x7ᵗʰ **V93.49 Struck by falling object on unspecified watercraft**

✓5ᵗʰ **V93.5 Explosion on board watercraft**
Boiler explosion on steamship
>EXCLUDES 2 *fire on board watercraft (V93.0-)*

✓x7ᵗʰ **V93.50 Explosion on board merchant ship**

✓x7ᵗʰ **V93.51 Explosion on board passenger ship**
Explosion on board Ferry-boat
Explosion on board Liner

✓x7ᵗʰ **V93.52 Explosion on board fishing boat**

✓x7ᵗʰ **V93.53 Explosion on board other powered watercraft**
Explosion on board Hovercraft
Explosion on board Jet ski

✓x7ᵗʰ **V93.54 Explosion on board sailboat**

✓x7ᵗʰ **V93.59 Explosion on board unspecified watercraft**
Explosion on board boat NOS
Explosion on board ship NOS
Explosion on board watercraft NOS

✓5ᵗʰ **V93.6 Machinery accident on board watercraft**
>EXCLUDES 1 *machinery explosion on board watercraft (V93.4-)*
>*machinery fire on board watercraft (V93.0-)*

✓x7ᵗʰ **V93.60 Machinery accident on board merchant ship**

✓x7ᵗʰ **V93.61 Machinery accident on board passenger ship**
Machinery accident on board Ferry-boat
Machinery accident on board Liner

✓x7ᵗʰ **V93.62 Machinery accident on board fishing boat**

✓x7ᵗʰ **V93.63 Machinery accident on board other powered watercraft**
Machinery accident on board Hovercraft

✓x7ᵗʰ **V93.64 Machinery accident on board sailboat**

✓x7ᵗʰ **V93.69 Machinery accident on board unspecified watercraft**
Machinery accident on board boat NOS
Machinery accident on board ship NOS
Machinery accident on board watercraft NOS

✓5ᵗʰ **V93.8 Other injury due to other accident on board watercraft**
Accidental poisoning by gases or fumes on watercraft

✓x7ᵗʰ **V93.80 Other injury due to other accident on board merchant ship**

✓x7ᵗʰ **V93.81 Other injury due to other accident on board passenger ship**
Other injury due to other accident on board Ferry-boat
Other injury due to other accident on board Liner

✓x7ᵗʰ **V93.82 Other injury due to other accident on board fishing boat**

✓x7ᵗʰ **V93.83 Other injury due to other accident on board other powered watercraft**
Other injury due to other accident on board Hovercraft
Other injury due to other accident on board Jet ski

✓x7ᵗʰ **V93.84 Other injury due to other accident on board sailboat**

✓x7ᵗʰ **V93.85 Other injury due to other accident on board canoe or kayak**

✓x7ᵗʰ **V93.86 Other injury due to other accident on board (nonpowered) inflatable craft**

✓x7ᵗʰ **V93.87 Other injury due to other accident on board water-skis**
Hit or struck by object while waterskiing

✓x7ᵗʰ **V93.88 Other injury due to other accident on board other unpowered watercraft**
Hit or struck by object while surfing
Hit or struck by object while on board windsurfer

✓x7ᵗʰ **V93.89 Other injury due to other accident on board unspecified watercraft**
Other injury due to other accident on board boat NOS
Other injury due to other accident on board ship NOS
Other injury due to other accident on board watercraft NOS

✓4ᵗʰ **V94 Other and unspecified water transport accidents**
>EXCLUDES 1 *military watercraft accidents in military or war operations (Y36, Y37)*

> The appropriate 7th character is to be added to each code from category V94.
> A   initial encounter
> D   subsequent encounter
> S   sequela

✓x7ᵗʰ **V94.0 Hitting object or bottom of body of water due to fall from watercraft**
>EXCLUDES 2 *drowning and submersion due to fall from watercraft (V92.0-)*

✓5ᵗʰ **V94.1 Bather struck by watercraft**
Swimmer hit by watercraft

✓x7ᵗʰ **V94.11 Bather struck by powered watercraft**

✓x7ᵗʰ **V94.12 Bather struck by nonpowered watercraft**

✓5ᵗʰ **V94.2 Rider of nonpowered watercraft struck by other watercraft**

✓x7ᵗʰ **V94.21 Rider of nonpowered watercraft struck by other nonpowered watercraft**
Canoer hit by other nonpowered watercraft
Surfer hit by other nonpowered watercraft
Windsurfer hit by other nonpowered watercraft

✓x7ᵗʰ **V94.22 Rider of nonpowered watercraft struck by powered watercraft**
Canoer hit by motorboat
Surfer hit by motorboat
Windsurfer hit by motorboat

✓5ᵗʰ **V94.3 Injury to rider of (inflatable) watercraft being pulled behind other watercraft**

✓x7ᵗʰ **V94.31 Injury to rider of (inflatable) recreational watercraft being pulled behind other watercraft**
Injury to rider of inner-tube pulled behind motor boat

✓x7ᵗʰ **V94.32 Injury to rider of non-recreational watercraft being pulled behind other watercraft**
Injury to occupant of dingy being pulled behind boat or ship
Injury to occupant of life-raft being pulled behind boat or ship

✓x7ᵗʰ **V94.4 Injury to barefoot water-skier**
Injury to person being pulled behind boat or ship

✓5ᵗʰ **V94.8 Other water transport accident**

✓6ᵗʰ **V94.81 Water transport accident involving military watercraft**

✓7ᵗʰ **V94.810 Civilian watercraft involved in water transport accident with military watercraft**
Passenger on civilian watercraft injured due to accident with military watercraft

✓7ᵗʰ **V94.811 Civilian in water injured by military watercraft**

✓7ᵗʰ **V94.818 Other water transport accident involving military watercraft**

Ⓝ Newborn: 0   Ⓟ Pediatric: 0-17   Ⓜ Maternity: 12-55   Ⓐ Adult: 15-124   MCC Major CC Condition   PDxMCC PDx acts as own MCC   CC CC Condition   PDxCC PDx acts as own CC

1184
ICD-10-CM 2016

√x7ᵗʰ **V94.89** **Other water transport accident**

√x7ᵗʰ **V94.9** **Unspecified water transport accident**
Water transport accident NOS

Air and space transport accidents (V95-V97)

EXCLUDES 1 *military aircraft accidents in military or war operations (Y36, Y37)*

√4ᵗʰ **V95** **Accident to powered aircraft causing injury to occupant**

The appropriate 7th character is to be added to each code from category V95.
A   initial encounter
D   subsequent encounter
S   sequela

√5ᵗʰ **V95.0** **Helicopter accident injuring occupant**

√x7ᵗʰ **V95.00** **Unspecified helicopter accident injuring occupant**

√x7ᵗʰ **V95.01** **Helicopter crash injuring occupant**

√x7ᵗʰ **V95.02** **Forced landing of helicopter injuring occupant**

√x7ᵗʰ **V95.03** **Helicopter collision injuring occupant**
Helicopter collision with any object, fixed, movable or moving

√x7ᵗʰ **V95.04** **Helicopter fire injuring occupant**

√x7ᵗʰ **V95.05** **Helicopter explosion injuring occupant**

√x7ᵗʰ **V95.09** **Other helicopter accident injuring occupant**

√5ᵗʰ **V95.1** **Ultralight, microlight or powered-glider accident injuring occupant**

√x7ᵗʰ **V95.10** **Unspecified ultralight, microlight or powered-glider accident injuring occupant**

√x7ᵗʰ **V95.11** **Ultralight, microlight or powered-glider crash injuring occupant**

√x7ᵗʰ **V95.12** **Forced landing of ultralight, microlight or powered-glider injuring occupant**

√x7ᵗʰ **V95.13** **Ultralight, microlight or powered-glider collision injuring occupant**
Ultralight, microlight or powered-glider collision with any object, fixed, movable or moving

√x7ᵗʰ **V95.14** **Ultralight, microlight or powered-glider fire injuring occupant**

√x7ᵗʰ **V95.15** **Ultralight, microlight or powered-glider explosion injuring occupant**

√x7ᵗʰ **V95.19** **Other ultralight, microlight or powered-glider accident injuring occupant**

√5ᵗʰ **V95.2** **Other private fixed-wing aircraft accident injuring occupant**

√x7ᵗʰ **V95.20** **Unspecified accident to other private fixed-wing aircraft, injuring occupant**

√x7ᵗʰ **V95.21** **Other private fixed-wing aircraft crash injuring occupant**

√x7ᵗʰ **V95.22** **Forced landing of other private fixed-wing aircraft injuring occupant**

√x7ᵗʰ **V95.23** **Other private fixed-wing aircraft collision injuring occupant**
Other private fixed-wing aircraft collision with any object, fixed, movable or moving

√x7ᵗʰ **V95.24** **Other private fixed-wing aircraft fire injuring occupant**

√x7ᵗʰ **V95.25** **Other private fixed-wing aircraft explosion injuring occupant**

√x7ᵗʰ **V95.29** **Other accident to other private fixed-wing aircraft injuring occupant**

√5ᵗʰ **V95.3** **Commercial fixed-wing aircraft accident injuring occupant**

√x7ᵗʰ **V95.30** **Unspecified accident to commercial fixed-wing aircraft injuring occupant**

√x7ᵗʰ **V95.31** **Commercial fixed-wing aircraft crash injuring occupant**

√x7ᵗʰ **V95.32** **Forced landing of commercial fixed-wing aircraft injuring occupant**

√x7ᵗʰ **V95.33** **Commercial fixed-wing aircraft collision injuring occupant**
Commercial fixed-wing aircraft collision with any object, fixed, movable or moving

√x7ᵗʰ **V95.34** **Commercial fixed-wing aircraft fire injuring occupant**

√x7ᵗʰ **V95.35** **Commercial fixed-wing aircraft explosion injuring occupant**

√x7ᵗʰ **V95.39** **Other accident to commercial fixed-wing aircraft injuring occupant**

√5ᵗʰ **V95.4** **Spacecraft accident injuring occupant**

√x7ᵗʰ **V95.40** **Unspecified spacecraft accident injuring occupant**

√x7ᵗʰ **V95.41** **Spacecraft crash injuring occupant**

√x7ᵗʰ **V95.42** **Forced landing of spacecraft injuring occupant**

√x7ᵗʰ **V95.43** **Spacecraft collision injuring occupant**
Spacecraft collision with any object, fixed, moveable or moving

√x7ᵗʰ **V95.44** **Spacecraft fire injuring occupant**

√x7ᵗʰ **V95.45** **Spacecraft explosion injuring occupant**

√x7ᵗʰ **V95.49** **Other spacecraft accident injuring occupant**

√x7ᵗʰ **V95.8** **Other powered aircraft accidents injuring occupant**

√x7ᵗʰ **V95.9** **Unspecified aircraft accident injuring occupant**
Aircraft accident NOS
Air transport accident NOS

√4ᵗʰ **V96** **Accident to nonpowered aircraft causing injury to occupant**

The appropriate 7th character is to be added to each code from category V96.
A   initial encounter
D   subsequent encounter
S   sequela

√5ᵗʰ **V96.0** **Balloon accident injuring occupant**

√x7ᵗʰ **V96.00** **Unspecified balloon accident injuring occupant**

√x7ᵗʰ **V96.01** **Balloon crash injuring occupant**

√x7ᵗʰ **V96.02** **Forced landing of balloon injuring occupant**

√x7ᵗʰ **V96.03** **Balloon collision injuring occupant**
Balloon collision with any object, fixed, moveable or moving

√x7ᵗʰ **V96.04** **Balloon fire injuring occupant**

√x7ᵗʰ **V96.05** **Balloon explosion injuring occupant**

√x7ᵗʰ **V96.09** **Other balloon accident injuring occupant**

√5ᵗʰ **V96.1** **Hang-glider accident injuring occupant**

√x7ᵗʰ **V96.10** **Unspecified hang-glider accident injuring occupant**

√x7ᵗʰ **V96.11** **Hang-glider crash injuring occupant**

√x7ᵗʰ **V96.12** **Forced landing of hang-glider injuring occupant**

√x7ᵗʰ **V96.13** **Hang-glider collision injuring occupant**
Hang-glider collision with any object, fixed, moveable or moving

√x7ᵗʰ **V96.14** **Hang-glider fire injuring occupant**

√x7ᵗʰ **V96.15** **Hang-glider explosion injuring occupant**

√x7ᵗʰ **V96.19** **Other hang-glider accident injuring occupant**

√5ᵗʰ **V96.2** **Glider (nonpowered) accident injuring occupant**

√x7ᵗʰ **V96.20** **Unspecified glider (nonpowered) accident injuring occupant**

√x7ᵗʰ **V96.21** **Glider (nonpowered) crash injuring occupant**

√x7ᵗʰ **V96.22** **Forced landing of glider (nonpowered) injuring occupant**

√x7ᵗʰ **V96.23** **Glider (nonpowered) collision injuring occupant**
Glider (nonpowered) collision with any object, fixed, moveable or moving

√x7ᵗʰ **V96.24** **Glider (nonpowered) fire injuring occupant**

√x7ᵗʰ **V96.25** **Glider (nonpowered) explosion injuring occupant**

√x7ᵗʰ **V96.29** **Other glider (nonpowered) accident injuring occupant**

√x7ᵗʰ **V96.8** **Other nonpowered-aircraft accidents injuring occupant**
Kite carrying a person accident injuring occupant

√x7ᵗʰ **V96.9** **Unspecified nonpowered-aircraft accident injuring occupant**
Nonpowered-aircraft accident NOS

√4ᵗʰ **V97** **Other specified air transport accidents**

The appropriate 7th character is to be added to each code from category V97.
A   initial encounter
D   subsequent encounter
S   sequela

√x7ᵗʰ **V97.0** **Occupant of aircraft injured in other specified air transport accidents**
Fall in, on or from aircraft in air transport accident
EXCLUDES 1 *accident while boarding or alighting aircraft (V97.1)*

√x7ᵗʰ **V97.1** **Person injured while boarding or alighting from aircraft**

☑ Additional Character Required   √x7ᵗʰ Placeholder Alert   Unacceptable PDx   Manifestation   Hospital Acquired Condition   *EXCLUDES 1* Not Coded Here   *EXCLUDES 2* Not Included Here

Chapter 20. External Causes of Morbidity *(left margin)*

✓5ᵗʰ **V97.2 Parachutist accident**

   ✓x7ᵗʰ **V97.21 Parachutist entangled in object**
        Parachutist landing in tree

   ✓x7ᵗʰ **V97.22 Parachutist injured on landing**

   ✓x7ᵗʰ **V97.29 Other parachutist accident**

✓5ᵗʰ **V97.3 Person on ground injured in air transport accident**

   ✓x7ᵗʰ **V97.31 Hit by object falling from aircraft**
        Hit by crashing aircraft
        Injured by aircraft hitting house
        Injured by aircraft hitting car

   ✓x7ᵗʰ **V97.32 Injured by rotating propeller**

   ✓x7ᵗʰ **V97.33 Sucked into jet engine**

   ✓x7ᵗʰ **V97.39 Other injury to person on ground due to air transport accident**

✓5ᵗʰ **V97.8 Other air transport accidents, not elsewhere classified**
    EXCLUDES 1 *aircraft accident NOS (V95.9)*
        exposure to changes in air pressure during ascent or descent (W94.-)

   ✓6ᵗʰ **V97.81 Air transport accident involving military aircraft**

      ✓7ᵗʰ **V97.810 Civilian aircraft involved in air transport accident with military aircraft**
          Passenger in civilian aircraft injured due to accident with military aircraft

      ✓7ᵗʰ **V97.811 Civilian injured by military aircraft**

      ✓7ᵗʰ **V97.818 Other air transport accident involving military aircraft**

   ✓x7ᵗʰ **V97.89 Other air transport accidents, not elsewhere classified**
        Injury from machinery on aircraft

Other and unspecified transport accidents (V98-V99)

EXCLUDES 1 *vehicle accident, type of vehicle unspecified (V89.-)*

✓4ᵗʰ **V98 Other specified transport accidents**

> The appropriate 7th character is to be added to each code from category V98.
> A   initial encounter
> D   subsequent encounter
> S   sequela

✓x7ᵗʰ **V98.0 Accident to, on or involving cable-car, not on rails**
    Caught or dragged by cable-car, not on rails
    Fall or jump from cable-car, not on rails
    Object thrown from or in cable-car, not on rails

✓x7ᵗʰ **V98.1 Accident to, on or involving land-yacht**

✓x7ᵗʰ **V98.2 Accident to, on or involving ice yacht**

✓x7ᵗʰ **V98.3 Accident to, on or involving ski lift**
    Accident to, on or involving ski chair-lift
    Accident to, on or involving ski-lift with gondola

✓x7ᵗʰ **V98.8 Other specified transport accidents**

✓x7ᵗʰ **V99 Unspecified transport accident**

> The appropriate 7th character is to be added to code V99.
> A   initial encounter
> D   subsequent encounter
> S   sequela

OTHER EXTERNAL CAUSES OF ACCIDENTAL INJURY (W00-X58)

Slipping, tripping, stumbling and falls (W00-W19)

EXCLUDES 1 *assault involving a fall (Y01-Y02)*
    fall from animal (V80.-)
    fall (in) (from) machinery (in operation) (W28-W31)
    fall (in) (from) transport vehicle (V01-V99)
    intentional self-harm involving a fall (X80-X81)
EXCLUDES 2 *at risk for fall (history of fall) Z91.81*
    fall (in) (from) burning building (X00.-)
    fall into fire (X00-X04, X08-X09)

✓4ᵗʰ **W00 Fall due to ice and snow**
    INCLUDES pedestrian on foot falling (slipping) on ice and snow
    EXCLUDES 1 *fall on (from) ice and snow involving pedestrian conveyance (V00.-)*
        fall from stairs and steps not due to ice and snow (W10.-)

> The appropriate 7th character is to be added to each code from category W00.
> A   initial encounter
> D   subsequent encounter
> S   sequela

✓x7ᵗʰ **W00.0 Fall on same level due to ice and snow**

✓x7ᵗʰ **W00.1 Fall from stairs and steps due to ice and snow**

✓x7ᵗʰ **W00.2 Other fall from one level to another due to ice and snow**

✓x7ᵗʰ **W00.9 Unspecified fall due to ice and snow**

✓4ᵗʰ **W01 Fall on same level from slipping, tripping and stumbling**
    INCLUDES fall on moving sidewalk
    EXCLUDES 1 *fall due to bumping (striking) against object (W18.0-)*
        fall in shower or bathtub (W18.2-)
        fall on same level NOS (W18.30)
        fall on same level from slipping, tripping and stumbling due to ice or snow (W00.0)
        fall off or from toilet (W18.1-)
        slipping, tripping and stumbling NOS (W18.40)
        slipping, tripping and stumbling without falling (W18.4-)

> The appropriate 7th character is to be added to each code from category W01.
> A   initial encounter
> D   subsequent encounter
> S   sequela

✓x7ᵗʰ **W01.0 Fall on same level from slipping, tripping and stumbling without subsequent striking against object**
    Falling over animal

✓5ᵗʰ **W01.1 Fall on same level from slipping, tripping and stumbling with subsequent striking against object**

   ✓x7ᵗʰ **W01.10 Fall on same level from slipping, tripping and stumbling with subsequent striking against unspecified object**

   ✓6ᵗʰ **W01.11 Fall on same level from slipping, tripping and stumbling with subsequent striking against sharp object**

      ✓7ᵗʰ **W01.110 Fall on same level from slipping, tripping and stumbling with subsequent striking against sharp glass**

      ✓7ᵗʰ **W01.111 Fall on same level from slipping, tripping and stumbling with subsequent striking against power tool or machine**

      ✓7ᵗʰ **W01.118 Fall on same level from slipping, tripping and stumbling with subsequent striking against other sharp object**

      ✓7ᵗʰ **W01.119 Fall on same level from slipping, tripping and stumbling with subsequent striking against unspecified sharp object**

   ✓6ᵗʰ **W01.19 Fall on same level from slipping, tripping and stumbling with subsequent striking against other object**

      ✓7ᵗʰ **W01.190 Fall on same level from slipping, tripping and stumbling with subsequent striking against furniture**

      ✓7ᵗʰ **W01.198 Fall on same level from slipping, tripping and stumbling with subsequent striking against other object**

✓x7ᵗʰ **W03 Other fall on same level due to collision with another person**
    Fall due to non-transport collision with other person
    EXCLUDES 1 *collision with another person without fall (W51)*
        crushed or pushed by a crowd or human stampede (W52)
        fall involving pedestrian conveyance (V00-V09)
        fall due to ice or snow (W00)
        fall on same level NOS (W18.30)
    AHA: 2012, 4Q, 108

> The appropriate 7th character is to be added to code W03.
> A   initial encounter
> D   subsequent encounter
> S   sequela

N Newborn: 0   P Pediatric: 0-17   M Maternity: 12-55   A Adult: 15-124   MCC Major CC Condition   PDxMCC PDx acts as own MCC   CC CC Condition   PDxCC PDx acts as own CC

1186   ICD-10-CM 2016

✓x7th **W04 Fall while being carried or supported by other persons**
Accidentally dropped while being carried

> The appropriate 7th character is to be added to code W04.
> A   initial encounter
> D   subsequent encounter
> S   sequela

✓4th **W05 Fall from non-moving wheelchair, nonmotorized scooter and motorized mobility scooter**
> *EXCLUDES 1*   *fall from moving motorized mobility scooter (V00.831)*
> *fall from moving wheelchair (powered) (V00.811)*
> *fall from nonmotorized scooter (V00.141)*

> The appropriate 7th character is to be added to each code from category W05.
> A   initial encounter
> D   subsequent encounter
> S   sequela

✓x7th **W05.0 Fall from non-moving wheelchair**

✓x7th **W05.1 Fall from non-moving nonmotorized scooter**

✓x7th **W05.2 Fall from non-moving motorized mobility scooter**

✓x7th **W06 Fall from bed**

> The appropriate 7th character is to be added to code W06.
> A   initial encounter
> D   subsequent encounter
> S   sequela

✓x7th **W07 Fall from chair**

> The appropriate 7th character is to be added to code W07.
> A   initial encounter
> D   subsequent encounter
> S   sequela

✓x7th **W08 Fall from other furniture**

> The appropriate 7th character is to be added to code W08.
> A   initial encounter
> D   subsequent encounter
> S   sequela

✓4th **W09 Fall on and from playground equipment**
> *EXCLUDES 1*   *fall involving recreational machinery (W31)*

> The appropriate 7th character is to be added to each code from category W09.
> A   initial encounter
> D   subsequent encounter
> S   sequela

✓x7th **W09.0 Fall on or from playground slide**

✓x7th **W09.1 Fall from playground swing**

✓x7th **W09.2 Fall on or from jungle gym**

✓x7th **W09.8 Fall on or from other playground equipment**

✓4th **W10 Fall on and from stairs and steps**
> *EXCLUDES 1*   *Fall from stairs and steps due to ice and snow (W00.1)*

> The appropriate 7th character is to be added to each code from category W10.
> A   initial encounter
> D   subsequent encounter
> S   sequela

✓x7th **W10.0 Fall (on)(from) escalator**

✓x7th **W10.1 Fall (on)(from) sidewalk curb**

✓x7th **W10.2 Fall (on)(from) incline**
Fall (on) (from) ramp

✓x7th **W10.8 Fall (on) (from) other stairs and steps**

✓x7th **W10.9 Fall (on) (from) unspecified stairs and steps**

✓x7th **W11 Fall on and from ladder**

> The appropriate 7th character is to be added code W11.
> A   initial encounter
> D   subsequent encounter
> S   sequela

✓x7th **W12 Fall on and from scaffolding**

> The appropriate 7th character is to be added code W12.
> A   initial encounter
> D   subsequent encounter
> S   sequela

✓4th **W13 Fall from, out of or through building or structure**

> The appropriate 7th character is to be added to each code from category W13.
> A   initial encounter
> D   subsequent encounter
> S   sequela

✓x7th **W13.0 Fall from, out of or through balcony**
Fall from, out of or through railing

✓x7th **W13.1 Fall from, out of or through bridge**

✓x7th **W13.2 Fall from, out of or through roof**

✓x7th **W13.3 Fall through floor**

✓x7th **W13.4 Fall from, out of or through window**
> *EXCLUDES 2*   *fall with subsequent striking against sharp glass (W01.110)*

✓x7th **W13.8 Fall from, out of or through other building or structure**
Fall from, out of or through viaduct
Fall from, out of or through wall
Fall from, out of or through flag-pole

✓x7th **W13.9 Fall from, out of or through building, not otherwise specified**
> *EXCLUDES 1*   *collapse of a building or structure (W20.-)*
> *fall or jump from burning building or structure (X00.-)*

✓x7th **W14 Fall from tree**

> The appropriate 7th character is to be added to code W14.
> A   initial encounter
> D   subsequent encounter
> S   sequela

✓x7th **W15 Fall from cliff**

> The appropriate 7th character is to be added to code W15.
> A   initial encounter
> D   subsequent encounter
> S   sequela

✓4th **W16 Fall, jump or diving into water**
> *EXCLUDES 1*   *accidental non-watercraft drowning and submersion not involving fall (W65-W74)*
> *effects of air pressure from diving (W94.-)*
> *fall into water from watercraft (V90-V94)*
> *hitting an object or against bottom when falling from watercraft (V94.0)*
> *EXCLUDES 2*   *striking or hitting diving board (W21.4)*

> The appropriate 7th character is to be added to each code from category W16.
> A   initial encounter
> D   subsequent encounter
> S   sequela

✓5th **W16.0 Fall into swimming pool**
Fall into swimming pool NOS
> *EXCLUDES 1*   *fall into empty swimming pool (W17.3)*

✓6th **W16.01 Fall into swimming pool striking water surface**

✓7th **W16.011 Fall into swimming pool striking water surface causing drowning and submersion**
> *EXCLUDES 1*   *drowning and submersion while in swimming pool without fall (W67)*

✓7th **W16.012 Fall into swimming pool striking water surface causing other injury**

✓6th **W16.02 Fall into swimming pool striking bottom**

✓7th **W16.021 Fall into swimming pool striking bottom causing drowning and submersion**
> *EXCLUDES 1*   *drowning and submersion while in swimming pool without fall (W67)*

✓7th **W16.022 Fall into swimming pool striking bottom causing other injury**

✓ Additional Character Required   ✓x7th Placeholder Alert   Unacceptable PDx   Manifestation   Hospital Acquired Condition   *EXCLUDES 1* Not Coded Here   *EXCLUDES 2* Not Included Here

ICD-10-CM 2016   1187

✓6th **W16.03 Fall into swimming pool** striking wall

    ✓7th **W16.031 Fall into swimming pool striking wall causing** drowning **and submersion**
        EXCLUDES 1 *drowning and submersion while in swimming pool without fall (W67)*

    ✓7th **W16.032 Fall into swimming pool striking wall causing** other injury

✓5th **W16.1 Fall into natural body of water**
    Fall into lake   Fall into river
    Fall into open sea   Fall into stream

  ✓6th **W16.11 Fall into natural body of water** striking water surface

    ✓7th **W16.111 Fall into natural body of water striking water surface causing** drowning **and submersion**
        EXCLUDES 1 *drowning and submersion while in natural body of water without fall (W69)*

    ✓7th **W16.112 Fall into natural body of water striking water surface causing** other injury

  ✓6th **W16.12 Fall into natural body of water** striking bottom

    ✓7th **W16.121 Fall into natural body of water striking bottom causing** drowning and submersion
        EXCLUDES 1 *drowning and submersion while in natural body of water without fall (W69)*

    ✓7th **W16.122 Fall into natural body of water striking bottom causing** other injury

  ✓6th **W16.13 Fall into natural body of water** striking side

    ✓7th **W16.131 Fall into natural body of water striking side causing** drowning **and submersion**
        EXCLUDES 1 *drowning and submersion while in natural body of water without fall (W69)*

    ✓7th **W16.132 Fall into natural body of water striking side causing** other injury

✓5th **W16.2 Fall in (into) filled bathtub or bucket of water**

  ✓6th **W16.21 Fall in (into)** filled bathtub
    EXCLUDES 1 *fall into empty bathtub (W18.2)*

    ✓7th **W16.211 Fall in (into) filled bathtub causing** drowning **and submersion**
        EXCLUDES 1 *drowning and submersion while in filled bathtub without fall (W65)*

    ✓7th **W16.212 Fall in (into) filled bathtub causing** other injury

  ✓6th **W16.22 Fall in (into)** bucket of water

    ✓7th **W16.221 Fall in (into) bucket of water causing** drowning **and submersion**

    ✓7th **W16.222 Fall in (into) bucket of water causing** other injury

✓5th **W16.3 Fall into other water**
    Fall into fountain   Fall into reservoir

  ✓6th **W16.31 Fall into other water** striking water surface

    ✓7th **W16.311 Fall into other water striking water surface causing** drowning **and submersion**
        EXCLUDES 1 *drowning and submersion while in other water without fall (W73)*

    ✓7th **W16.312 Fall into other water striking water surface causing** other injury

  ✓6th **W16.32 Fall into other water** striking bottom

    ✓7th **W16.321 Fall into other water striking bottom causing** drowning **and submersion**
        EXCLUDES 1 *drowning and submersion while in other water without fall (W73)*

    ✓7th **W16.322 Fall into other water striking bottom causing** other injury

  ✓6th **W16.33 Fall into other water** striking wall

    ✓7th **W16.331 Fall into other water striking wall causing** drowning **and submersion**
        EXCLUDES 1 *drowning and submersion while in other water without fall (W73)*

    ✓7th **W16.332 Fall into other water striking wall causing** other injury

✓5th **W16.4 Fall into unspecified water**

  ✓x7th **W16.41 Fall into unspecified water causing** drowning **and submersion**

  ✓x7th **W16.42 Fall into unspecified water causing** other injury

✓5th **W16.5 Jumping or diving into swimming pool**

  ✓6th **W16.51 Jumping or diving into swimming pool** striking water surface

    ✓7th **W16.511 Jumping or diving into swimming pool striking water surface causing** drowning **and submersion**
        EXCLUDES 1 *drowning and submersion while in swimming pool without jumping or diving (W67)*

    ✓7th **W16.512 Jumping or diving into swimming pool striking water surface causing** other injury

  ✓6th **W16.52 Jumping or diving into swimming pool** striking bottom

    ✓7th **W16.521 Jumping or diving into swimming pool striking bottom causing** drowning **and submersion**
        EXCLUDES 1 *drowning and submersion while in swimming pool without jumping or diving (W67)*

    ✓7th **W16.522 Jumping or diving into swimming pool striking bottom causing** other injury

  ✓6th **W16.53 Jumping or diving into swimming pool** striking wall

    ✓7th **W16.531 Jumping or diving into swimming pool striking wall causing** drowning **and submersion**
        EXCLUDES 1 *drowning and submersion while in swimming pool without jumping or diving (W67)*

    ✓7th **W16.532 Jumping or diving into swimming pool striking wall causing** other injury

✓5th **W16.6 Jumping or diving into** natural body of water
    Jumping or diving into lake
    Jumping or diving into open sea
    Jumping or diving into river
    Jumping or diving into stream

  ✓6th **W16.61 Jumping or diving into natural body of water** striking water surface

    ✓7th **W16.611 Jumping or diving into natural body of water striking water surface causing** drowning **and submersion**
        EXCLUDES 1 *drowning and submersion while in natural body of water without jumping or diving (W69)*

    ✓7th **W16.612 Jumping or diving into natural body of water striking water surface causing** other injury

  ✓6th **W16.62 Jumping or diving into natural body of water** striking bottom

    ✓7th **W16.621 Jumping or diving into natural body of water striking bottom causing** drowning **and submersion**
        EXCLUDES 1 *drowning and submersion while in natural body of water without jumping or diving (W69)*

    ✓7th **W16.622 Jumping or diving into natural body of water striking bottom causing** other injury

✓5th **W16.7 Jumping or diving** from boat
    EXCLUDES 1 *Fall from boat into water—see watercraft accident (V90-V94)*

  ✓6th **W16.71 Jumping or diving from boat** striking water surface

    ✓7th **W16.711 Jumping or diving from boat striking water surface causing** drowning **and submersion**

    ✓7th **W16.712 Jumping or diving from boat striking water surface causing** other injury

  ✓6th **W16.72 Jumping or diving from boat** striking bottom

    ✓7th **W16.721 Jumping or diving from boat striking bottom causing** drowning **and submersion**

    ✓7th **W16.722 Jumping or diving from boat striking bottom causing** other injury

✓5th **W16.8 Jumping or diving into other water**
Jumping or diving into fountain
Jumping or diving into reservoir

    ✓6th **W16.81 Jumping or diving into other water striking water surface**

        ✓7th **W16.811 Jumping or diving into other water striking water surface causing drowning and submersion**
EXCLUDES 1 *drowning and submersion while in other water without jumping or diving (W73)*

        ✓7th **W16.812 Jumping or diving into other water striking water surface causing other injury**

    ✓6th **W16.82 Jumping or diving into other water striking bottom**

        ✓7th **W16.821 Jumping or diving into other water striking bottom causing drowning and submersion**
EXCLUDES 1 *drowning and submersion while in other water without jumping or diving (W73)*

        ✓7th **W16.822 Jumping or diving into other water striking bottom causing other injury**

    ✓6th **W16.83 Jumping or diving into other water striking wall**

        ✓7th **W16.831 Jumping or diving into other water striking wall causing drowning and submersion**
EXCLUDES 1 *drowning and submersion while in other water without jumping or diving (W73)*

        ✓7th **W16.832 Jumping or diving into other water striking wall causing other injury**

✓5th **W16.9 Jumping or diving into unspecified water**

    ✓x7th **W16.91 Jumping or diving into unspecified water causing drowning and submersion**

    ✓x7th **W16.92 Jumping or diving into unspecified water causing other injury**

✓4th **W17 Other fall from one level to another**

> The appropriate 7th character is to be added to each code from category W17.
> A   initial encounter
> D   subsequent encounter
> S   sequela

    ✓x7th **W17.0 Fall into well**

    ✓x7th **W17.1 Fall into storm drain or manhole**

    ✓x7th **W17.2 Fall into hole**
Fall into pit

    ✓x7th **W17.3 Fall into empty swimming pool**
EXCLUDES 1 *fall into filled swimming pool (W16.0-)*

    ✓x7th **W17.4 Fall from dock**

    ✓5th **W17.8 Other fall from one level to another**

        ✓x7th **W17.81 Fall down embankment (hill)**

        ✓x7th **W17.82 Fall from (out of) grocery cart**
Fall due to grocery cart tipping over

        ✓x7th **W17.89 Other fall from one level to another**
Fall from cherry picker
Fall from lifting device
Fall from mobile elevated work platform [MEWP]
Fall from sky lift

✓4th **W18 Other slipping, tripping and stumbling and falls**

> The appropriate 7th character is to be added to each code from category W18.
> A   initial encounter
> D   subsequent encounter
> S   sequela

    ✓5th **W18.0 Fall due to bumping against object**
Striking against object with subsequent fall
EXCLUDES 1 *fall on same level due to slipping, tripping, or stumbling with subsequent striking against object (W01.1-)*

        ✓x7th **W18.00 Striking against unspecified object with subsequent fall**

        ✓x7th **W18.01 Striking against sports equipment with subsequent fall**

        ✓x7th **W18.02 Striking against glass with subsequent fall**

        ✓x7th **W18.09 Striking against other object with subsequent fall**

✓5th **W18.1 Fall from or off toilet**

    ✓x7th **W18.11 Fall from or off toilet without subsequent striking against object**
Fall from (off) toilet NOS

    ✓x7th **W18.12 Fall from or off toilet with subsequent striking against object**

✓x7th **W18.2 Fall in (into) shower or empty bathtub**
EXCLUDES 1 *fall in full bathtub causing drowning or submersion (W16.21-)*

✓5th **W18.3 Other and unspecified fall on same level**

    ✓x7th **W18.30 Fall on same level, unspecified**

    ✓x7th **W18.31 Fall on same level due to stepping on an object**
Fall on same level due to stepping on an animal
EXCLUDES 1 *slipping, tripping and stumbling without fall due to stepping on animal (W18.41)*

    ✓x7th **W18.39 Other fall on same level**

✓5th **W18.4 Slipping, tripping and stumbling without falling**
EXCLUDES 1 *collision with another person without fall (W51)*

    ✓x7th **W18.40 Slipping, tripping and stumbling without falling, unspecified**

    ✓x7th **W18.41 Slipping, tripping and stumbling without falling due to stepping on object**
Slipping, tripping and stumbling without falling due to stepping on animal
EXCLUDES 1 *slipping, tripping and stumbling with fall due to stepping on animal (W18.31)*

    ✓x7th **W18.42 Slipping, tripping and stumbling without falling due to stepping into hole or opening**

    ✓x7th **W18.43 Slipping, tripping and stumbling without falling due to stepping from one level to another**

    ✓x7th **W18.49 Other slipping, tripping and stumbling without falling**

✓x7th **W19 Unspecified fall**
Accidental fall NOS
AHA: 2012, 4Q, 95

> The appropriate 7th character is to be added to code W19.
> A   initial encounter
> D   subsequent encounter
> S   sequela

Exposure to inanimate mechanical forces (W20-W49)

EXCLUDES 1 *assault (X92-Y08)*
contact or collision with animals or persons (W50-W64)
exposure to inanimate mechanical forces involving military or war operations (Y36-, Y37-)
intentional self-harm (X71-X83)

✓4th **W20 Struck by thrown, projected or falling object**
Code first any associated:
cataclysm (X34-X39)
lightning strike (T75.00)
EXCLUDES 1 *falling object in machinery accident (W24, W28-W31)*
falling object in transport accident (V01-V99)
object set in motion by explosion (W35-W40)
object set in motion by firearm (W32-W34)
struck by thrown sports equipment (W21.-)

> The appropriate 7th character is to be added to each code from category W20.
> A   initial encounter
> D   subsequent encounter
> S   sequela

    ✓x7th **W20.0 Struck by falling object in cave-in**
EXCLUDES 2 *asphyxiation due to cave-in (T71.21)*

    ✓x7th **W20.1 Struck by object due to collapse of building**
EXCLUDES 1 *struck by object due to collapse of burning building (X00.2, X02.2)*

    ✓x7th **W20.8 Other cause of strike by thrown, projected or falling object**
EXCLUDES 1 *struck by thrown sports equipment (W21.-)*

✓ Additional Character Required   ✓x7th Placeholder Alert   Unacceptable PDx   Manifestation   Hospital Acquired Condition   **EXCLUDES 1** Not Coded Here   **EXCLUDES 2** Not Included Here

Chapter 20. External Causes of Morbidity

W21–W27.0

✓4ᵗʰ **W21 Striking against or struck by sports equipment**
     EXCLUDES 1   *assault with sports equipment (Y08.0-)*
              striking against or struck by sports equipment with subsequent
              fall (W18.01)

     The appropriate 7th character is to be added to each code from
     category W21.
     A   initial encounter
     D   subsequent encounter
     S   sequela

     ✓5ᵗʰ **W21.0 Struck by hit or thrown ball**
         ✓x7ᵗʰ **W21.00 Struck by hit or thrown ball, unspecified type**
         ✓x7ᵗʰ **W21.01 Struck by football**
         ✓x7ᵗʰ **W21.02 Struck by soccer ball**
         ✓x7ᵗʰ **W21.03 Struck by baseball**
         ✓x7ᵗʰ **W21.04 Struck by golf ball**
         ✓x7ᵗʰ **W21.05 Struck by basketball**
         ✓x7ᵗʰ **W21.06 Struck by volleyball**
         ✓x7ᵗʰ **W21.07 Struck by softball**
         ✓x7ᵗʰ **W21.09 Struck by other hit or thrown ball**

     ✓5ᵗʰ **W21.1 Struck by bat, racquet or club**
         ✓x7ᵗʰ **W21.11 Struck by baseball bat**
         ✓x7ᵗʰ **W21.12 Struck by tennis racquet**
         ✓x7ᵗʰ **W21.13 Struck by golf club**
         ✓x7ᵗʰ **W21.19 Struck by other bat, racquet or club**

     ✓5ᵗʰ **W21.2 Struck by hockey stick or puck**
         ✓6ᵗʰ **W21.21 Struck by hockey stick**
             ✓7ᵗʰ **W21.210 Struck by ice hockey stick**
             ✓7ᵗʰ **W21.211 Struck by field hockey stick**
         ✓6ᵗʰ **W21.22 Struck by hockey puck**
             ✓7ᵗʰ **W21.220 Struck by ice hockey puck**
             ✓7ᵗʰ **W21.221 Struck by field hockey puck**

     ✓5ᵗʰ **W21.3 Struck by sports foot wear**
         ✓x7ᵗʰ **W21.31 Struck by shoe cleats**
             Stepped on by shoe cleats
         ✓x7ᵗʰ **W21.32 Struck by skate blades**
             Skated over by skate blades
         ✓x7ᵗʰ **W21.39 Struck by other sports foot wear**

     ✓x7ᵗʰ **W21.4 Striking against diving board**
             Use additional code for subsequent falling into water, if
             applicable (W16.-)

     ✓5ᵗʰ **W21.8 Striking against or struck by other sports equipment**
         ✓x7ᵗʰ **W21.81 Striking against or struck by football helmet**
         ✓x7ᵗʰ **W21.89 Striking against or struck by other sports equipment**
     ✓x7ᵗʰ **W21.9 Striking against or struck by unspecified sports equipment**

✓4ᵗʰ **W22 Striking against or struck by other objects**
     EXCLUDES 1   *striking against or struck by object with subsequent fall*
              (W18.09)

     The appropriate 7th character is to be added to each code from
     category W22.
     A   initial encounter
     D   subsequent encounter
     S   sequela

     ✓5ᵗʰ **W22.0 Striking against stationary object**
         EXCLUDES 1   *striking against stationary sports equipment (W21.8)*
         ✓x7ᵗʰ **W22.01 Walked into wall**
         ✓x7ᵗʰ **W22.02 Walked into lamppost**
         ✓x7ᵗʰ **W22.03 Walked into furniture**
         ✓6ᵗʰ **W22.04 Striking against wall of swimming pool**
             ✓7ᵗʰ **W22.041 Striking against wall of swimming pool**
                    causing drowning and submersion
                    EXCLUDES 1   *drowning and submersion while*
                               swimming without striking
                               against wall (W67)
             ✓7ᵗʰ **W22.042 Striking against wall of swimming pool**
                    causing other injury
         ✓x7ᵗʰ **W22.09 Striking against other stationary object**
     ✓5ᵗʰ **W22.1 Striking against or struck by automobile airbag**
         ✓x7ᵗʰ **W22.10 Striking against or struck by unspecified automobile**
                 airbag

         ✓x7ᵗʰ **W22.11 Striking against or struck by driver side automobile**
                 airbag
         ✓x7ᵗʰ **W22.12 Striking against or struck by front passenger side**
                 automobile airbag
         ✓x7ᵗʰ **W22.19 Striking against or struck by other automobile**
                 airbag
     ✓x7ᵗʰ **W22.8 Striking against or struck by other objects**
             Striking against or struck by object NOS
         EXCLUDES 1   *struck by thrown, projected or falling object (W20.-)*

✓4ᵗʰ **W23 Caught, crushed, jammed or pinched in or between objects**
     EXCLUDES 1   *injury caused by cutting or piercing instruments (W25-W27)*
              injury caused by firearms malfunction (W32.1, W33.1-, W34.1-)
              injury caused by lifting and transmission devices (W24.-)
              injury caused by machinery (W28-W31)
              injury caused by nonpowered hand tools (W27.-)
              injury caused by transport vehicle being used as a means of
                 transportation (V01-V99)
              injury caused by struck by thrown, projected or falling object
                 (W20.-)

     The appropriate 7th character is to be added to each code from
     category W23.
     A   initial encounter
     D   subsequent encounter
     S   sequela

     ✓x7ᵗʰ **W23.0 Caught, crushed, jammed, or pinched between moving**
                    objects
     ✓x7ᵗʰ **W23.1 Caught, crushed, jammed, or pinched between stationary**
                    objects

✓4ᵗʰ **W24 Contact with lifting and transmission devices, not elsewhere**
classified
     EXCLUDES 1   *transport accidents (V01-V99)*

     The appropriate 7th character is to be added to each code from
     category W24.
     A   initial encounter
     D   subsequent encounter
     S   sequela

     ✓x7ᵗʰ **W24.0 Contact with lifting devices, not elsewhere classified**
             Contact with chain hoist
             Contact with drive belt
             Contact with pulley (block)
     ✓x7ᵗʰ **W24.1 Contact with transmission devices, not elsewhere classified**
             Contact with transmission belt or cable

✓x7ᵗʰ **W25 Contact with sharp glass**
     Code first any associated:
         injury due to flying glass from explosion or firearm discharge (W32-
         W40)
         transport accident (V00-V99)
     EXCLUDES 1   *fall on same level due to slipping, tripping and stumbling with*
              subsequent striking against sharp glass (W01.10)
              striking against sharp glass with subsequent fall (W18.02)

     The appropriate 7th character is to be added to code W25.
     A   initial encounter
     D   subsequent encounter
     S   sequela

✓4ᵗʰ **W26 Contact with knife, sword or dagger**

     The appropriate 7th character is to be added to each code from
     category W26.
     A   initial encounter
     D   subsequent encounter
     S   sequela

     ✓x7ᵗʰ **W26.0 Contact with knife**
         EXCLUDES 1   *contact with electric knife (W29.1)*
     ✓x7ᵗʰ **W26.1 Contact with sword or dagger**

✓4ᵗʰ **W27 Contact with nonpowered hand tool**

     The appropriate 7th character is to be added to each code from
     category W27.
     A   initial encounter
     D   subsequent encounter
     S   sequela

     ✓x7ᵗʰ **W27.0 Contact with workbench tool**
             Contact with auger   Contact with handsaw
             Contact with axe   Contact with screwdriver
             Contact with chisel

Ⓝ Newborn: 0   Ⓟ Pediatric: 0-17   Ⓜ Maternity: 12-55   Ⓐ Adult: 15-124   **MCC** Major CC Condition   **PDxMCC** PDx acts as own MCC   **CC** CC Condition   **PDxCC** PDx acts as own CC

1190   ICD-10-CM 2016

√x7ᵗʰ **W27.1 Contact with garden tool**
    Contact with hoe
    Contact with nonpowered lawn mower
    Contact with pitchfork
    Contact with rake

√x7ᵗʰ **W27.2 Contact with scissors**

√x7ᵗʰ **W27.3 Contact with needle (sewing)**
    EXCLUDES1   *contact with hypodermic needle (W46.-)*

√x7ᵗʰ **W27.4 Contact with kitchen utensil**
    Contact with fork
    Contact with ice-pick
    Contact with can-opener NOS

√x7ᵗʰ **W27.5 Contact with paper-cutter**

√x7ᵗʰ **W27.8 Contact with other nonpowered hand tool**
    Contact with nonpowered sewing machine
    Contact with shovel

√x7ᵗʰ **W28 Contact with powered lawn mower**
    Powered lawn mower (commercial) (residential)
    EXCLUDES1   *contact with nonpowered lawn mower (W27.1)*
    EXCLUDES2   *exposure to electric current (W86.-)*

    The appropriate 7th character is to be added to code W28.
    A   initial encounter
    D   subsequent encounter
    S   sequela

√4ᵗʰ **W29 Contact with other powered hand tools and household machinery**
    EXCLUDES1   *contact with commercial machinery (W31.82)*
    contact with hot household appliance (X15)
    contact with nonpowered hand tool (W27.-)
    exposure to electric current (W86)

    The appropriate 7th character is to be added to each code from category W29.
    A   initial encounter
    D   subsequent encounter
    S   sequela

√x7ᵗʰ **W29.0 Contact with powered kitchen appliance**
    Contact with blender   Contact with garbage disposal
    Contact with can-opener   Contact with mixer

√x7ᵗʰ **W29.1 Contact with electric knife**

√x7ᵗʰ **W29.2 Contact with other powered household machinery**
    Contact with electric fan
    Contact with powered dryer (clothes) (powered) (spin)
    Contact with washing-machine
    Contact with sewing machine

√x7ᵗʰ **W29.3 Contact with powered garden and outdoor hand tools and machinery**
    Contact with chainsaw
    Contact with edger
    Contact with garden cultivator (tiller)
    Contact with hedge trimmer
    Contact with other powered garden tool
    EXCLUDES1   *contact with powered lawn mower (W28)*

√x7ᵗʰ **W29.4 Contact with nail gun**

√x7ᵗʰ **W29.8 Contact with other powered powered hand tools and household machinery**
    Contact with do-it-yourself tool NOS

√4ᵗʰ **W30 Contact with agricultural machinery**
    INCLUDES   animal-powered farm machine
    EXCLUDES1   *agricultural transport vehicle accident (V01-V99)*
    explosion of grain store (W40.8)
    exposure to electric current (W86.-)

    The appropriate 7th character is to be added to each code from category W30.
    A   initial encounter
    D   subsequent encounter
    S   sequela

√x7ᵗʰ **W30.0 Contact with combine harvester**
    Contact with reaper   Contact with thresher

√x7ᵗʰ **W30.1 Contact with power take-off devices (PTO)**

√x7ᵗʰ **W30.2 Contact with hay derrick**

√x7ᵗʰ **W30.3 Contact with grain storage elevator**
    EXCLUDES1   *explosion of grain store (W40.8)*

√5ᵗʰ **W30.8 Contact with other specified agricultural machinery**

√x7ᵗʰ **W30.81 Contact with agricultural transport vehicle in stationary use**
    Contact with agricultural transport vehicle under repair, not on public roadway
    EXCLUDES1   *agricultural transport vehicle accident (V01-V99)*

√x7ᵗʰ **W30.89 Contact with other specified agricultural machinery**

√x7ᵗʰ **W30.9 Contact with unspecified agricultural machinery**
    Contact with farm machinery NOS

√4ᵗʰ **W31 Contact with other and unspecified machinery**
    EXCLUDES1   *contact with agricultural machinery (W30.-)*
    contact with machinery in transport under own power or being towed by a vehicle (V01-V99)
    exposure to electric current (W86)

    The appropriate 7th character is to be added to each code from category W31.
    A   initial encounter
    D   subsequent encounter
    S   sequela

√x7ᵗʰ **W31.0 Contact with mining and earth-drilling machinery**
    Contact with bore or drill (land) (seabed)
    Contact with shaft hoist
    Contact with shaft lift
    Contact with undercutter

√x7ᵗʰ **W31.1 Contact with metalworking machines**
    Contact with abrasive wheel
    Contact with forging machine
    Contact with lathe
    Contact with mechanical shears
    Contact with metal drilling machine
    Contact with milling machine
    Contact with power press
    Contact with rolling-mill
    Contact with metal sawing machine

√x7ᵗʰ **W31.2 Contact with powered woodworking and forming machines**
    Contact with band saw   Contact with overhead plane
    Contact with bench saw   Contact with powered saw
    Contact with circular saw   Contact with radial saw
    Contact with molding machine   Contact with sander
    EXCLUDES1   *nonpowered woodworking tools (W27.0)*

√x7ᵗʰ **W31.3 Contact with prime movers**
    Contact with gas turbine
    Contact with internal combustion engine
    Contact with steam engine
    Contact with water driven turbine

√5ᵗʰ **W31.8 Contact with other specified machinery**

√x7ᵗʰ **W31.81 Contact with recreational machinery**
    Contact with roller coaster

√x7ᵗʰ **W31.82 Contact with other commercial machinery**
    Contact with commercial electric fan
    Contact with commercial kitchen appliances
    Contact with commercial powered dryer (clothes) (powered) (spin)
    Contact with commercial washing-machine
    Contact with commercial sewing machine
    EXCLUDES1   *contact with household machinery (W29.-)*
    contact with powered lawn mower (W28)

√x7ᵗʰ **W31.83 Contact with special construction vehicle in stationary use**
    Contact with special construction vehicle under repair, not on public roadway
    EXCLUDES1   *special construction vehicle accident (V01-V99)*

√x7ᵗʰ **W31.89 Contact with other specified machinery**

√x7ᵗʰ **W31.9 Contact with unspecified machinery**
    Contact with machinery NOS

✔ Additional Character Required   √x7ᵗʰ Placeholder Alert   Unacceptable PDx   Manifestation   Hospital Acquired Condition   EXCLUDES1 Not Coded Here   EXCLUDES2 Not Included Here

✓4ᵗʰ **W32 Accidental handgun discharge and malfunction**

INCLUDES accidental discharge and malfunction of gun for single hand use
accidental discharge and malfunction of pistol
accidental discharge and malfunction of revolver
handgun discharge and malfunction NOS

EXCLUDES 1 *accidental airgun discharge and malfunction (W34.010, W34.110)*
accidental BB gun discharge and malfunction (W34.010, W34.110)
accidental pellet gun discharge and malfunction (W34.010, W34.110)
accidental shotgun discharge and malfunction (W33.01, W33.11)
assault by handgun discharge (X93)
handgun discharge involving legal intervention (Y35.0-)
handgun discharge involving military or war operations (Y36.4-)
intentional self-harm by handgun discharge (X72)
Very pistol discharge and malfunction (W34.09, W34.19)

The appropriate 7th character is to be added to each code from category W32.
A   initial encounter
D   subsequent encounter
S   sequela

✓x7ᵗʰ **W32.0 Accidental handgun discharge**

✓x7ᵗʰ **W32.1 Accidental handgun malfunction**
Injury due to explosion of handgun (parts)
Injury due to malfunction of mechanism or component of handgun
Injury due to recoil of handgun
Powder burn from handgun

✓4ᵗʰ **W33 Accidental rifle, shotgun and larger firearm discharge and malfunction**

INCLUDES rifle, shotgun and larger firearm discharge and malfunction NOS

EXCLUDES 1 *accidental airgun discharge and malfunction (W34.010, W34.110)*
accidental BB gun discharge and malfunction (W34.010, W34.110)
accidental handgun discharge and malfunction (W32.-)
accidental pellet gun discharge and malfunction (W34.010, W34.110)
assault by rifle, shotgun and larger firearm discharge (X94)
firearm discharge involving legal intervention (Y35.0-)
firearm discharge involving military or war operations (Y36.4-)
intentional self-harm by rifle, shotgun and larger firearm discharge (X73)

The appropriate 7th character is to be added to each code from category W33.
A   initial encounter
D   subsequent encounter
S   sequela

✓5ᵗʰ **W33.0 Accidental rifle, shotgun and larger firearm discharge**

✓x7ᵗʰ **W33.00 Accidental discharge of unspecified larger firearm**
Discharge of unspecified larger firearm NOS

✓x7ᵗʰ **W33.01 Accidental discharge of shotgun**
Discharge of shotgun NOS

✓x7ᵗʰ **W33.02 Accidental discharge of hunting rifle**
Discharge of hunting rifle NOS

✓x7ᵗʰ **W33.03 Accidental discharge of machine gun**
Discharge of machine gun NOS

✓x7ᵗʰ **W33.09 Accidental discharge of other larger firearm**
Discharge of other larger firearm NOS

✓5ᵗʰ **W33.1 Accidental rifle, shotgun and larger firearm malfunction**
Injury due to explosion of rifle, shotgun and larger firearm (parts)
Injury due to malfunction of mechanism or component of rifle, shotgun and larger firearm
Injury due to piercing, cutting, crushing or pinching due to (by) slide trigger mechanism, scope or other gun part
Injury due to recoil of rifle, shotgun and larger firearm
Powder burn from rifle, shotgun and larger firearm

✓x7ᵗʰ **W33.10 Accidental malfunction of unspecified larger firearm**
Malfunction of unspecified larger firearm NOS

✓x7ᵗʰ **W33.11 Accidental malfunction of shotgun**
Malfunction of shotgun NOS

✓x7ᵗʰ **W33.12 Accidental malfunction of hunting rifle**
Malfunction of hunting rifle NOS

✓x7ᵗʰ **W33.13 Accidental malfunction of machine gun**
Malfunction of machine gun NOS

✓x7ᵗʰ **W33.19 Accidental malfunction of other larger firearm**
Malfunction of other larger firearm NOS

✓4ᵗʰ **W34 Accidental discharge and malfunction from other and unspecified firearms and guns**

The appropriate 7th character is to be added to each code from category W34.
A   initial encounter
D   subsequent encounter
S   sequela

✓5ᵗʰ **W34.0 Accidental discharge from other and unspecified firearms and guns**

✓x7ᵗʰ **W34.00 Accidental discharge from unspecified firearms or gun**
Discharge from firearm NOS
Gunshot wound NOS
Shot NOS

✓6ᵗʰ **W34.01 Accidental discharge of gas, air or spring-operated guns**

✓7ᵗʰ **W34.010 Accidental discharge of airgun**
Accidental discharge of BB gun
Accidental discharge of pellet gun

✓7ᵗʰ **W34.011 Accidental discharge of paintball gun**
Accidental injury due to paintball discharge

✓7ᵗʰ **W34.018 Accidental discharge of other gas, air or spring-operated gun**

✓x7ᵗʰ **W34.09 Accidental discharge from other specified firearms**
Accidental discharge from Very pistol [flare]

✓5ᵗʰ **W34.1 Accidental malfunction from other and unspecified firearms and guns**

✓x7ᵗʰ **W34.10 Accidental malfunction from unspecified firearms or gun**
Firearm malfunction NOS

✓6ᵗʰ **W34.11 Accidental malfunction of gas, air or spring-operated guns**

✓7ᵗʰ **W34.110 Accidental malfunction of airgun**
Accidental malfunction of BB gun
Accidental malfunction of pellet gun

✓7ᵗʰ **W34.111 Accidental malfunction of paintball gun**
Accidental injury due to paintball gun malfunction

✓7ᵗʰ **W34.118 Accidental malfunction of other gas, air or spring-operated gun**

✓x7ᵗʰ **W34.19 Accidental malfunction from other specified firearms**
Accidental malfunction from Very pistol [flare]

✓x7ᵗʰ **W35 Explosion and rupture of boiler**
EXCLUDES 1 *explosion and rupture of boiler on watercraft (V93.4)*

The appropriate 7th character is to be added to code W35.
A   initial encounter
D   subsequent encounter
S   sequela

✓4ᵗʰ **W36 Explosion and rupture of gas cylinder**

The appropriate 7th character is to be added to each code from category W36.
A   initial encounter
D   subsequent encounter
S   sequela

✓x7ᵗʰ **W36.1 Explosion and rupture of aerosol can**

✓x7ᵗʰ **W36.2 Explosion and rupture of air tank**

✓x7ᵗʰ **W36.3 Explosion and rupture of pressurized-gas tank**

✓x7ᵗʰ **W36.8 Explosion and rupture of other gas cylinder**

✓x7ᵗʰ **W36.9 Explosion and rupture of unspecified gas cylinder**

✓4ᵗʰ **W37 Explosion and rupture of pressurized tire, pipe or hose**

The appropriate 7th character is to be added to each code from category W37.
A   initial encounter
D   subsequent encounter
S   sequela

✓x7ᵗʰ **W37.0 Explosion of bicycle tire**

✓x7ᵗʰ **W37.8 Explosion and rupture of other pressurized tire, pipe or hose**

N Newborn: 0   P Pediatric: 0-17   M Maternity: 12-55   A Adult: 15-124   MCC Major CC Condition   PDxMCC PDx acts as own MCC   CC CC Condition   PDxCC PDx acts as own CC

1192   ICD-10-CM 2016

✓x7ᵗʰ **W38 Explosion and rupture of other specified pressurized devices**

> The appropriate 7th character is to be added to code W38.
> A   initial encounter
> D   subsequent encounter
> S   sequela

✓x7ᵗʰ **W39 Discharge of firework**

> The appropriate 7th character is to be added to code W39.
> A   initial encounter
> D   subsequent encounter
> S   sequela

✓4ᵗʰ **W40 Explosion of other materials**

> **EXCLUDES 1**   assault by explosive material (X96)
>   explosion involving legal intervention (Y35.1-)
>   explosion involving military or war operations (Y36.0-, Y36.2-)
>   intentional self-harm by explosive material (X75)

> The appropriate 7th character is to be added to each code from category W40.
> A   initial encounter
> D   subsequent encounter
> S   sequela

✓x7ᵗʰ **W40.0 Explosion of blasting material**
> Explosion of blasting cap
> Explosion of detonator
> Explosion of dynamite
> Explosion of explosive (any) used in blasting operations

✓x7ᵗʰ **W40.1 Explosion of explosive gases**
> Explosion of acetylene   Explosion of fire damp
> Explosion of butane   Explosion of gasoline fumes
> Explosion of coal gas   Explosion of methane
> Explosion in mine NOS   Explosion of propane
> Explosion of explosive gas

✓x7ᵗʰ **W40.8 Explosion of other specified explosive materials**
> Explosion in dump NOS   Explosion in grain store
> Explosion in factory NOS   Explosion in munitions
> **EXCLUDES 1**   explosion involving legal intervention (Y35.1-)
>   explosion involving military or war operations (Y36.0-, Y36.2-)

✓x7ᵗʰ **W40.9 Explosion of unspecified explosive materials**
> Explosion NOS

✓4ᵗʰ **W42 Exposure to noise**

> The appropriate 7th character is to be added to each code from category W42.
> A   initial encounter
> D   subsequent encounter
> S   sequela

✓x7ᵗʰ **W42.0 Exposure to supersonic waves**

✓x7ᵗʰ **W42.9 Exposure to other noise**
> Exposure to sound waves NOS

✓4ᵗʰ **W45 Foreign body or object entering through skin**

> **EXCLUDES 2**   contact with hand tools (nonpowered) (powered) (W27-W29)
>   contact with knife, sword or dagger (W26.-)
>   contact with sharp glass (W25.-)
>   struck by objects (W20-W22)

> The appropriate 7th character is to be added to each code from category W45.
> A   initial encounter
> D   subsequent encounter
> S   sequela

✓x7ᵗʰ **W45.0 Nail entering through skin**

✓x7ᵗʰ **W45.1 Paper entering through skin**
> Paper cut

✓x7ᵗʰ **W45.2 Lid of can entering through skin**

✓x7ᵗʰ **W45.8 Other foreign body or object entering through skin**
> Splinter in skin NOS

✓4ᵗʰ **W46 Contact with hypodermic needle**

> The appropriate 7th character is to be added to each code from category W46.
> A   initial encounter
> D   subsequent encounter
> S   sequela

✓x7ᵗʰ **W46.0 Contact with hypodermic needle**
> Hypodermic needle stick NOS

✓x7ᵗʰ **W46.1 Contact with contaminated hypodermic needle**

✓4ᵗʰ **W49 Exposure to other inanimate mechanical forces**
> **INCLUDES**   exposure to abnormal gravitational [G] forces
>   exposure to inanimate mechanical forces NEC
> **EXCLUDES 1**   exposure to inanimate mechanical forces involving military or war operations (Y36.-, Y37.-)

> The appropriate 7th character is to be added to each code from category W49.
> A   initial encounter
> D   subsequent encounter
> S   sequela

✓5ᵗʰ **W49.0 Item causing external constriction**

    ✓x7ᵗʰ **W49.01 Hair causing external constriction**

    ✓x7ᵗʰ **W49.02 String or thread causing external constriction**

    ✓x7ᵗʰ **W49.03 Rubber band causing external constriction**

    ✓x7ᵗʰ **W49.04 Ring or other jewelry causing external constriction**

    ✓x7ᵗʰ **W49.09 Other specified item causing external constriction**

✓x7ᵗʰ **W49.9 Exposure to other inanimate mechanical forces**

Exposure to animate mechanical forces (W50-W64)
> **EXCLUDES 1**   Toxic effect of contact with venomous animals and plants (T63.-)

✓4ᵗʰ **W50 Accidental hit, strike, kick, twist, bite or scratch by another person**
> Hit, strike, kick, twist, bite, or scratch by another person NOS
> **EXCLUDES 1**   assault by bodily force (Y04)
>   struck by objects (W20-W22)

> The appropriate 7th character is to be added to each code from category W50.
> A   initial encounter
> D   subsequent encounter
> S   sequela

✓x7ᵗʰ **W50.0 Accidental hit or strike by another person**
> Hit or strike by another person NOS

✓x7ᵗʰ **W50.1 Accidental kick by another person**
> Kick by another person NOS

✓x7ᵗʰ **W50.2 Accidental twist by another person**
> Twist by another person NOS

✓x7ᵗʰ **W50.3 Accidental bite by another person**
> Human bite   Bite by another person NOS

✓x7ᵗʰ **W50.4 Accidental scratch by another person**
> Scratch by another person NOS

✓x7ᵗʰ **W51 Accidental striking against or bumped into by another person**
> **EXCLUDES 1**   assault by striking against or bumping into by another person (Y04.2)
>   fall due to collision with another person (W03)

> The appropriate 7th character is to be added to code W51.
> A   initial encounter
> D   subsequent encounter
> S   sequela

✓x7ᵗʰ **W52 Crushed, pushed or stepped on by crowd or human stampede**
> Crushed, pushed or stepped on by crowd or human stampede with or without fall

> The appropriate 7th character is to be added to code W52.
> A   initial encounter
> D   subsequent encounter
> S   sequela

✓4ᵗʰ **W53 Contact with rodent**
> **INCLUDES**   Contact with saliva, feces or urine of rodent

> The appropriate 7th character is to be added to each code from category W53.
> A   initial encounter
> D   subsequent encounter
> S   sequela

✓5ᵗʰ **W53.0 Contact with mouse**

    ✓x7ᵗʰ **W53.01 Bitten by mouse**

    ✓x7ᵗʰ **W53.09 Other contact with mouse**

✓5ᵗʰ **W53.1 Contact with rat**

    ✓x7ᵗʰ **W53.11 Bitten by rat**

    ✓x7ᵗʰ **W53.19 Other contact with rat**

✓5ᵗʰ **W53.2 Contact with squirrel**

    ✓x7ᵗʰ **W53.21 Bitten by squirrel**

    ✓x7ᵗʰ **W53.29 Other contact with squirrel**

✓ Additional Character Required   ✓x7ᵗʰ Placeholder Alert   Unacceptable PDx   Manifestation   Hospital Acquired Condition   **EXCLUDES 1** Not Coded Here   **EXCLUDES 2** Not Included Here

✓5ᵗʰ W53.8 Contact with other rodent

　　✓x7ᵗʰ **W53.81 Bitten by** other rodent

　　✓x7ᵗʰ **W53.89 Other** contact with other rodent

✓4ᵗʰ W54 Contact with dog

　　INCLUDES　Contact with saliva, feces or urine of dog

　　The appropriate 7th character is to be added to each code from category W54.
　　A　initial encounter
　　D　subsequent encounter
　　S　sequela

✓x7ᵗʰ **W54.0 Bitten by dog**

✓x7ᵗʰ **W54.1 Struck by dog**
　　　　Knocked over by dog

✓x7ᵗʰ **W54.8 Other** contact with dog

✓4ᵗʰ W55 Contact with other mammals

　　INCLUDES　Contact with saliva, feces or urine of mammal
　　EXCLUDES 1　animal being ridden—see transport accidents
　　　　　　　bitten or struck by dog (W54)
　　　　　　　bitten or struck by rodent (W53.-)
　　　　　　　contact with marine mammals (W56.-)

　　The appropriate 7th character is to be added to each code from category W55.
　　A　initial encounter
　　D　subsequent encounter
　　S　sequela

✓5ᵗʰ **W55.0 Contact with** cat

　　✓x7ᵗʰ **W55.01 Bitten by cat**

　　✓x7ᵗʰ **W55.03 Scratched by cat**

　　✓x7ᵗʰ **W55.09 Other** contact with cat

✓5ᵗʰ **W55.1 Contact with** horse

　　✓x7ᵗʰ **W55.11 Bitten by horse**

　　✓x7ᵗʰ **W55.12 Struck by horse**

　　✓x7ᵗʰ **W55.19 Other** contact with horse

✓5ᵗʰ **W55.2 Contact with** cow
　　　　Contact with bull

　　✓x7ᵗʰ **W55.21 Bitten by cow**

　　✓x7ᵗʰ **W55.22 Struck by cow**
　　　　　　Gored by bull

　　✓x7ᵗʰ **W55.29 Other** contact with cow

✓5ᵗʰ **W55.3 Contact with other** hoof stock
　　　　Contact with goats　　　　Contact with sheep

　　✓x7ᵗʰ **W55.31 Bitten by other hoof stock**

　　✓x7ᵗʰ **W55.32 Struck by other hoof stock**
　　　　　　Gored by goat　　　　Gored by ram

　　✓x7ᵗʰ **W55.39 Other** contact with other hoof stock

✓5ᵗʰ **W55.4 Contact with** pig

　　✓x7ᵗʰ **W55.41 Bitten by pig**

　　✓x7ᵗʰ **W55.42 Struck by pig**

　　✓x7ᵗʰ **W55.49 Other** contact with pig

✓5ᵗʰ **W55.5 Contact with** raccoon

　　✓x7ᵗʰ **W55.51 Bitten by raccoon**

　　✓x7ᵗʰ **W55.52 Struck by raccoon**

　　✓x7ᵗʰ **W55.59 Other** contact with raccoon

✓5ᵗʰ **W55.8 Contact with other** mammals

　　✓x7ᵗʰ **W55.81 Bitten by other mammals**

　　✓x7ᵗʰ **W55.82 Struck by other mammals**

　　✓x7ᵗʰ **W55.89 Other** contact with other mammals

✓4ᵗʰ W56 Contact with nonvenomous marine animal

　　EXCLUDES 1　contact with venomous marine animal (T63.-)

　　The appropriate 7th character is to be added to each code from category W56.
　　A　initial encounter
　　D　subsequent encounter
　　S　sequela

✓5ᵗʰ **W56.0 Contact with** dolphin

　　✓x7ᵗʰ **W56.01 Bitten by dolphin**

　　✓x7ᵗʰ **W56.02 Struck by dolphin**

　　✓x7ᵗʰ **W56.09 Other** contact with dolphin

✓5ᵗʰ **W56.1 Contact with** sea lion

　　✓x7ᵗʰ **W56.11 Bitten by sea lion**

　　✓x7ᵗʰ **W56.12 Struck by sea lion**

　　✓x7ᵗʰ **W56.19 Other** contact with sea lion

✓5ᵗʰ **W56.2 Contact with** orca
　　　　Contact with killer whale

　　✓x7ᵗʰ **W56.21 Bitten by orca**

　　✓x7ᵗʰ **W56.22 Struck by orca**

　　✓x7ᵗʰ **W56.29 Other** contact with orca

✓5ᵗʰ **W56.3 Contact with other** marine mammals

　　✓x7ᵗʰ **W56.31 Bitten by other marine mammals**

　　✓x7ᵗʰ **W56.32 Struck by other marine mammals**

　　✓x7ᵗʰ **W56.39 Other** contact with other marine mammals

✓5ᵗʰ **W56.4 Contact with** shark

　　✓x7ᵗʰ **W56.41 Bitten by shark**

　　✓x7ᵗʰ **W56.42 Struck by shark**

　　✓x7ᵗʰ **W56.49 Other** contact with shark

✓5ᵗʰ **W56.5 Contact with other** fish

　　✓x7ᵗʰ **W56.51 Bitten by other fish**

　　✓x7ᵗʰ **W56.52 Struck by other fish**

　　✓x7ᵗʰ **W56.59 Other** contact with other fish

✓5ᵗʰ **W56.8 Contact with other** nonvenomous marine animals

　　✓x7ᵗʰ **W56.81 Bitten by other nonvenomous marine animals**

　　✓x7ᵗʰ **W56.82 Struck by other nonvenomous marine animals**

　　✓x7ᵗʰ **W56.89 Other** contact with other nonvenomous marine animals

✓x7ᵗʰ W57 Bitten or stung by nonvenomous insect and other nonvenomous arthropods

　　EXCLUDES 1　contact with venomous insects and arthropods (T63.2-, T63.3-, T63.4-)

　　The appropriate 7th character is to be added to code W57.
　　A　initial encounter
　　D　subsequent encounter
　　S　sequela

✓4ᵗʰ W58 Contact with crocodile or alligator

　　The appropriate 7th character is to be added to each code from category W58.
　　A　initial encounter
　　D　subsequent encounter
　　S　sequela

✓5ᵗʰ **W58.0 Contact with** alligator

　　✓x7ᵗʰ **W58.01 Bitten by alligator**

　　✓x7ᵗʰ **W58.02 Struck by alligator**

　　✓x7ᵗʰ **W58.03 Crushed by alligator**

　　✓x7ᵗʰ **W58.09 Other** contact with alligator

✓5ᵗʰ **W58.1 Contact with** crocodile

　　✓x7ᵗʰ **W58.11 Bitten by crocodile**

　　✓x7ᵗʰ **W58.12 Struck by crocodile**

　　✓x7ᵗʰ **W58.13 Crushed by crocodile**

　　✓x7ᵗʰ **W58.19 Other** contact with crocodile

✓4ᵗʰ W59 Contact with other nonvenomous reptiles

　　EXCLUDES 1　contact with venomous reptile (T63.0-, T63.1-)

　　The appropriate 7th character is to be added to each code from category W59.
　　A　initial encounter
　　D　subsequent encounter
　　S　sequela

✓5ᵗʰ **W59.0 Contact with** nonvenomous lizards

　　✓x7ᵗʰ **W59.01 Bitten by nonvenomous lizards**

　　✓x7ᵗʰ **W59.02 Struck by nonvenomous lizards**

　　✓x7ᵗʰ **W59.09 Other** contact with nonvenomous lizards
　　　　　　Exposure to nonvenomous lizards

✓5ᵗʰ **W59.1 Contact with** nonvenomous snakes

　　✓x7ᵗʰ **W59.11 Bitten by nonvenomous snake**

　　✓x7ᵗʰ **W59.12 Struck by nonvenomous snake**

　　✓x7ᵗʰ **W59.13 Crushed by nonvenomous snake**

　　✓x7ᵗʰ **W59.19 Other** contact with nonvenomous snake

Ⓝ Newborn: 0　Ⓟ Pediatric: 0-17　Ⓜ Maternity: 12-55　Ⓐ Adult: 15-124　MCC Major CC Condition　PDxMCC PDx acts as own MCC　CC CC Condition　PDxCC PDx acts as own CC

1194
ICD-10-CM 2016

✓5ᵗʰ **W59.2 Contact with turtles**
> EXCLUDES1   contact with tortoises (W59.8-)

✓x7ᵗʰ **W59.21 Bitten by turtle**

✓x7ᵗʰ **W59.22 Struck by turtle**

✓x7ᵗʰ **W59.29 Other contact with turtle**
> Exposure to turtles

✓5ᵗʰ **W59.8 Contact with other nonvenomous reptiles**

✓x7ᵗʰ **W59.81 Bitten by other nonvenomous reptiles**

✓x7ᵗʰ **W59.82 Struck by other nonvenomous reptiles**

✓x7ᵗʰ **W59.83 Crushed by other nonvenomous reptiles**

✓x7ᵗʰ **W59.89 Other contact with other nonvenomous reptiles**

✓x7ᵗʰ **W60 Contact with nonvenomous plant thorns and spines and sharp leaves**
> EXCLUDES1   contact with venomous plants (T63.7-)

> The appropriate 7th character is to be added to code W60.
> A   initial encounter
> D   subsequent encounter
> S   sequela

✓4ᵗʰ **W61 Contact with birds (domestic) (wild)**
> INCLUDES   contact with excreta of birds

> The appropriate 7th character is to be added to each code from category W61.
> A   initial encounter
> D   subsequent encounter
> S   sequela

✓5ᵗʰ **W61.0 Contact with parrot**

✓x7ᵗʰ **W61.01 Bitten by parrot**

✓x7ᵗʰ **W61.02 Struck by parrot**

✓x7ᵗʰ **W61.09 Other contact with parrot**
> Exposure to parrots

✓5ᵗʰ **W61.1 Contact with macaw**

✓x7ᵗʰ **W61.11 Bitten by macaw**

✓x7ᵗʰ **W61.12 Struck by macaw**

✓x7ᵗʰ **W61.19 Other contact with macaw**
> Exposure to macaws

✓5ᵗʰ **W61.2 Contact with other psittacines**

✓x7ᵗʰ **W61.21 Bitten by other psittacines**

✓x7ᵗʰ **W61.22 Struck by other psittacines**

✓x7ᵗʰ **W61.29 Other contact with other psittacines**
> Exposure to other psittacines

✓5ᵗʰ **W61.3 Contact with chicken**

✓x7ᵗʰ **W61.32 Struck by chicken**

✓x7ᵗʰ **W61.33 Pecked by chicken**

✓x7ᵗʰ **W61.39 Other contact with chicken**
> Exposure to chickens

✓5ᵗʰ **W61.4 Contact with turkey**

✓x7ᵗʰ **W61.42 Struck by turkey**

✓x7ᵗʰ **W61.43 Pecked by turkey**

✓x7ᵗʰ **W61.49 Other contact with turkey**

✓5ᵗʰ **W61.5 Contact with goose**

✓x7ᵗʰ **W61.51 Bitten by goose**

✓x7ᵗʰ **W61.52 Struck by goose**

✓x7ᵗʰ **W61.59 Other contact with goose**

✓5ᵗʰ **W61.6 Contact with duck**

✓x7ᵗʰ **W61.61 Bitten by duck**

✓x7ᵗʰ **W61.62 Struck by duck**

✓x7ᵗʰ **W61.69 Other contact with duck**

✓5ᵗʰ **W61.9 Contact with other birds**

✓x7ᵗʰ **W61.91 Bitten by other birds**

✓x7ᵗʰ **W61.92 Struck by other birds**

✓x7ᵗʰ **W61.99 Other contact with other birds**
> Contact with bird NOS

✓4ᵗʰ **W62 Contact with nonvenomous amphibians**
> EXCLUDES1   contact with venomous amphibians (T63.81-R63.83)

> The appropriate 7th character is to be added to each code from category W62.
> A   initial encounter
> D   subsequent encounter
> S   sequela

✓x7ᵗʰ **W62.0 Contact with nonvenomous frogs**

✓x7ᵗʰ **W62.1 Contact with nonvenomous toads**

✓x7ᵗʰ **W62.9 Contact with other nonvenomous amphibians**

✓x7ᵗʰ **W64 Exposure to other animate mechanical forces**
> INCLUDES   exposure to nonvenomous animal NOS
> EXCLUDES1   contact with venomous animal (T63.-)

> The appropriate 7th character is to be added to code W64.
> A   initial encounter
> D   subsequent encounter
> S   sequela

Accidental non-transport drowning and submersion (W65-W74)
> EXCLUDES1   accidental drowning and submersion due to fall into water (W16.-)
> accidental drowning and submersion due to water transport accident (V90.-, V92.-)
> EXCLUDES2   accidental drowning and submersion due to cataclysm (X34-X39)

✓x7ᵗʰ **W65 Accidental drowning and submersion while in bath-tub**
> EXCLUDES1   accidental drowning and submersion due to fall in (into) bathtub (W16.211)

> The appropriate 7th character is to be added to code W65.
> A   initial encounter
> D   subsequent encounter
> S   sequela

✓x7ᵗʰ **W67 Accidental drowning and submersion while in swimming-pool**
> EXCLUDES1   accidental drowning and submersion due to fall into swimming pool (W16.011, W16.021, W16.031)
> accidental drowning and submersion due to striking into wall of swimming pool (W22.041)

> The appropriate 7th character is to be added to code W67.
> A   initial encounter
> D   subsequent encounter
> S   sequela

✓x7ᵗʰ **W69 Accidental drowning and submersion while in natural water**
> Accidental drowning and submersion while in lake
> Accidental drowning and submersion while in open sea
> Accidental drowning and submersion while in river
> Accidental drowning and submersion while in stream
> EXCLUDES1   accidental drowning and submersion due to fall into natural body of water (W16.111, W16.121, W16.131)

> The appropriate 7th character is to be added to code W69.
> A   initial encounter
> D   subsequent encounter
> S   sequela

✓x7ᵗʰ **W73 Other specified cause of accidental non-transport drowning and submersion**
> Accidental drowning and submersion while in quenching tank
> Accidental drowning and submersion while in reservoir
> EXCLUDES1   accidental drowning and submersion due to fall into other water (W16.311, W16.321, W16.331)

> The appropriate 7th character is to be added to code W73.
> A   initial encounter
> D   subsequent encounter
> S   sequela

✓x7ᵗʰ **W74 Unspecified cause of accidental drowning and submersion**
> Drowning NOS

> The appropriate 7th character is to be added to code W74.
> A   initial encounter
> D   subsequent encounter
> S   sequela

✓ Additional Character Required   ✓x7ᵗʰ Placeholder Alert   Unacceptable PDx   Manifestation   Hospital Acquired Condition   EXCLUDES1 Not Coded Here   EXCLUDES2 Not Included Here

ICD-10-CM 2016   1195

Chapter 20. External Causes of Morbidity

W85–W99

Exposure to electric current, radiation and extreme ambient air temperature and pressure (W85-W99)

EXCLUDES 1   exposure to:
  failure in dosage of radiation or temperature during surgical and
    medical care (Y63.2-Y63.5)
  lightning (T75.Ø-)
  natural cold (X31)
  natural heat (X3Ø)
  natural radiation NOS (X39)
  radiological procedure and radiotherapy (Y84.2)
  sunlight (X32)

✓x7ᵗʰ W85 Exposure to electric transmission lines
Broken power line

The appropriate 7th character is to be added to code W85.
A   initial encounter
D   subsequent encounter
S   sequela

✓4ᵗʰ W86 Exposure to other specified electric current

The appropriate 7th character is to be added to each code from
category W86.
A   initial encounter
D   subsequent encounter
S   sequela

✓7ᵗʰ **W86.Ø** Exposure to domestic wiring and appliances

✓7ᵗʰ **W86.1** Exposure to industrial wiring, appliances and electrical machinery
  Exposure to conductors
  Exposure to control apparatus
  Exposure to electrical equipment and machinery
  Exposure to transformers

✓7ᵗʰ **W86.8** Exposure to other electric current
  Exposure to wiring and appliances in or on farm (not farmhouse)
  Exposure to wiring and appliances outdoors
  Exposure to wiring and appliances in or on public building
  Exposure to wiring and appliances in or on residential
    institutions
  Exposure to wiring and appliances in or on schools

✓4ᵗʰ W88 Exposure to ionizing radiation
EXCLUDES 1   exposure to sunlight (X32)

The appropriate 7th character is to be added to each code from
category W88.
A   initial encounter
D   subsequent encounter
S   sequela

✓7ᵗʰ **W88.Ø** Exposure to X-rays

✓7ᵗʰ **W88.1** Exposure to radioactive isotopes

✓7ᵗʰ **W88.8** Exposure to other ionizing radiation

✓4ᵗʰ W89 Exposure to man-made visible and ultraviolet light
INCLUDES   exposure to welding light (arc)
EXCLUDES 2   exposure to sunlight (X32)

The appropriate 7th character is to be added to each code from
category W89.
A   initial encounter
D   subsequent encounter
S   sequela

✓7ᵗʰ **W89.Ø** Exposure to welding light (arc)

✓7ᵗʰ **W89.1** Exposure to tanning bed

✓7ᵗʰ **W89.8** Exposure to other man-made visible and ultraviolet light

✓7ᵗʰ **W89.9** Exposure to unspecified man-made visible and ultraviolet light

✓4ᵗʰ W9Ø Exposure to other nonionizing radiation
EXCLUDES 1   exposure to sunlight (X32)

The appropriate 7th character is to be added to each code from
category W9Ø.
A   initial encounter
D   subsequent encounter
S   sequela

✓7ᵗʰ **W9Ø.Ø** Exposure to radiofrequency

✓7ᵗʰ **W9Ø.1** Exposure to infrared radiation

✓7ᵗʰ **W9Ø.2** Exposure to laser radiation

✓7ᵗʰ **W9Ø.8** Exposure to other nonionizing radiation

✓x7ᵗʰ W92 Exposure to excessive heat of man-made origin

The appropriate 7th character is to be added to code W92.
A   initial encounter
D   subsequent encounter
S   sequela

✓4ᵗʰ W93 Exposure to excessive cold of man-made origin

The appropriate 7th character is to be added to each code from
category W93.
A   initial encounter
D   subsequent encounter
S   sequela

✓5ᵗʰ **W93.Ø** Contact with or inhalation of dry ice

    ✓x7ᵗʰ **W93.Ø1** Contact with dry ice

    ✓x7ᵗʰ **W93.Ø2** Inhalation of dry ice

✓5ᵗʰ **W93.1** Contact with or inhalation of liquid air

    ✓x7ᵗʰ **W93.11** Contact with liquid air
  Contact with liquid hydrogen
  Contact with liquid nitrogen

    ✓x7ᵗʰ **W93.12** Inhalation of liquid air
  Inhalation of liquid hydrogen
  Inhalation of liquid nitrogen

✓x7ᵗʰ **W93.2** Prolonged exposure in deep freeze unit or refrigerator

✓x7ᵗʰ **W93.8** Exposure to other excessive cold of man-made origin

✓4ᵗʰ W94 Exposure to high and low air pressure and changes in air pressure

The appropriate 7th character is to be added to each code from
category W94.
A   initial encounter
D   subsequent encounter
S   sequela

✓x7ᵗʰ **W94.Ø** Exposure to prolonged high air pressure

✓5ᵗʰ **W94.1** Exposure to prolonged low air pressure

    ✓x7ᵗʰ **W94.11** Exposure to residence or prolonged visit at high altitude

    ✓x7ᵗʰ **W94.12** Exposure to other prolonged low air pressure

✓5ᵗʰ **W94.2** Exposure to rapid changes in air pressure during ascent

    ✓x7ᵗʰ **W94.21** Exposure to reduction in atmospheric pressure while surfacing from deep-water diving

    ✓x7ᵗʰ **W94.22** Exposure to reduction in atmospheric pressure while surfacing from underground

    ✓x7ᵗʰ **W94.23** Exposure to sudden change in air pressure in aircraft during ascent

    ✓x7ᵗʰ **W94.29** Exposure to other rapid changes in air pressure during ascent

✓5ᵗʰ **W94.3** Exposure to rapid changes in air pressure during descent

    ✓x7ᵗʰ **W94.31** Exposure to sudden change in air pressure in aircraft during descent

    ✓x7ᵗʰ **W94.32** Exposure to high air pressure from rapid descent in water

    ✓x7ᵗʰ **W94.39** Exposure to other rapid changes in air pressure during descent

✓x7ᵗʰ W99 Exposure to other man-made environmental factors

The appropriate 7th character is to be added to code W99.
A   initial encounter
D   subsequent encounter
S   sequela

Ⓝ Newborn: 0   Ⓟ Pediatric: 0-17   Ⓜ Maternity: 12-55   Ⓐ Adult: 15-124   **MCC** Major CC Condition   **PDxMCC** PDx acts as own MCC   **CC** CC Condition   **PDxCC** PDx acts as own CC

1196   ICD-10-CM 2016

Exposure to smoke, fire and flames (X00-X08)

EXCLUDES 1   arson (X97)
EXCLUDES 2   explosions (W35-W40)
           lightning (T75.0-)
           transport accident (V01-V99)

✓4th X00   Exposure to uncontrolled fire in building or structure

INCLUDES   conflagration in building or structure

Code first any associated cataclysm

EXCLUDES 2   exposure to ignition or melting of nightwear (X05)
           exposure to ignition or melting of other clothing and apparel
           (X06.-)
           exposure to other specified smoke, fire and flames (X08.-)

The appropriate 7th character is to be added to each code from
category X00.
A   initial encounter
D   subsequent encounter
S   sequela

- ✓x7th **X00.0**   Exposure to flames in uncontrolled fire in building or structure
- ✓x7th **X00.1**   Exposure to smoke in uncontrolled fire in building or structure
- ✓x7th **X00.2**   Injury due to collapse of burning building or structure in uncontrolled fire
  - **EXCLUDES 1**   injury due to collapse of building not on fire (W20.1)
- ✓x7th **X00.3**   Fall from burning building or structure in uncontrolled fire
- ✓x7th **X00.4**   Hit by object from burning building or structure in uncontrolled fire
- ✓x7th **X00.5**   Jump from burning building or structure in uncontrolled fire
- ✓x7th **X00.8**   Other exposure to uncontrolled fire in building or structure

✓4th X01   Exposure to uncontrolled fire, not in building or structure

INCLUDES   exposure to forest fire

The appropriate 7th character is to be added to each code from
category X01.
A   initial encounter
D   subsequent encounter
S   sequela

- ✓x7th **X01.0**   Exposure to flames in uncontrolled fire, not in building or structure
- ✓x7th **X01.1**   Exposure to smoke in uncontrolled fire, not in building or structure
- ✓x7th **X01.3**   Fall due to uncontrolled fire, not in building or structure
- ✓x7th **X01.4**   Hit by object due to uncontrolled fire, not in building or structure
- ✓x7th **X01.8**   Other exposure to uncontrolled fire, not in building or structure

✓4th X02   Exposure to controlled fire in building or structure

INCLUDES   exposure to fire in fireplace
           exposure to fire in stove

The appropriate 7th character is to be added to each code from
category X02.
A   initial encounter
D   subsequent encounter
S   sequela

- ✓x7th **X02.0**   Exposure to flames in controlled fire in building or structure
- ✓x7th **X02.1**   Exposure to smoke in controlled fire in building or structure
- ✓x7th **X02.2**   Injury due to collapse of burning building or structure in controlled fire
  - **EXCLUDES 1**   injury due to collapse of building not on fire (W20.1)
- ✓x7th **X02.3**   Fall from burning building or structure in controlled fire
- ✓x7th **X02.4**   Hit by object from burning building or structure in controlled fire
- ✓x7th **X02.5**   Jump from burning building or structure in controlled fire
- ✓x7th **X02.8**   Other exposure to controlled fire in building or structure

✓4th X03   Exposure to controlled fire, not in building or structure

INCLUDES   exposure to bon fire
           exposure to camp-fire
           exposure to trash fire

The appropriate 7th character is to be added to each code from
category X03.
A   initial encounter
D   subsequent encounter
S   sequela

- ✓x7th **X03.0**   Exposure to flames in controlled fire, not in building or structure
- ✓x7th **X03.1**   Exposure to smoke in controlled fire, not in building or structure
- ✓x7th **X03.3**   Fall due to controlled fire, not in building or structure
- ✓x7th **X03.4**   Hit by object due to controlled fire, not in building or structure
- ✓x7th **X03.8**   Other exposure to controlled fire, not in building or structure

✓x7th X04   Exposure to ignition of highly flammable material

Exposure to ignition of gasoline
Exposure to ignition of kerosene
Exposure to ignition of petrol

EXCLUDES 2   exposure to ignition or melting of nightwear (X05)
           exposure to ignition or melting of other clothing and apparel
           (X06)

The appropriate 7th character is to be added to code X04.
A   initial encounter
D   subsequent encounter
S   sequela

✓x7th X05   Exposure to ignition or melting of nightwear

EXCLUDES 2   exposure to uncontrolled fire in building or structure (X00.-)
           exposure to uncontrolled fire, not in building or structure (X01.-)
           exposure to controlled fire in building or structure (X02.-)
           exposure to controlled fire, not in building or structure (X03.-)
           exposure to ignition of highly flammable materials (X04.-)

The appropriate 7th character is to be added to code X05.
A   initial encounter
D   subsequent encounter
S   sequela

✓4th X06   Exposure to ignition or melting of other clothing and apparel

EXCLUDES 2   exposure to uncontrolled fire in building or structure (X00.-)
           exposure to uncontrolled fire, not in building or structure (X01.-)
           exposure to controlled fire in building or structure (X02.-)
           exposure to controlled fire, not in building or structure (X03.-)
           exposure to ignition of highly flammable materials (X04.-)

The appropriate 7th character is to be added to each code from
category X06.
A   initial encounter
D   subsequent encounter
S   sequela

- ✓x7th **X06.0**   Exposure to ignition of plastic jewelry
- ✓x7th **X06.1**   Exposure to melting of plastic jewelry
- ✓x7th **X06.2**   Exposure to ignition of other clothing and apparel
- ✓x7th **X06.3**   Exposure to melting of other clothing and apparel

✓4th X08   Exposure to other specified smoke, fire and flames

The appropriate 7th character is to be added to each code from
category X08.
A   initial encounter
D   subsequent encounter
S   sequela

- ✓5th **X08.0**   Exposure to bed fire
  Exposure to mattress fire
  - ✓x7th **X08.00**   Exposure to bed fire due to unspecified burning material
  - ✓x7th **X08.01**   Exposure to bed fire due to burning cigarette
  - ✓x7th **X08.09**   Exposure to bed fire due to other burning material
- ✓5th **X08.1**   Exposure to sofa fire
  - ✓x7th **X08.10**   Exposure to sofa fire due to unspecified burning material
  - ✓x7th **X08.11**   Exposure to sofa fire due to burning cigarette
  - ✓x7th **X08.19**   Exposure to sofa fire due to other burning material
- ✓5th **X08.2**   Exposure to other furniture fire
  - ✓x7th **X08.20**   Exposure to other furniture fire due to unspecified burning material

---

✓ Additional Character Required   ✓x7th Placeholder Alert   Unacceptable PDx   Manifestation   Hospital Acquired Condition   **EXCLUDES 1** Not Coded Here   **EXCLUDES 2** Not Included Here

√x7ᵗʰ **X08.21**   **Exposure to other furniture fire due to** burning **cigarette**

√x7ᵗʰ **X08.29**   **Exposure to other furniture fire due to** other **burning material**

√x7ᵗʰ **X08.8**   **Exposure to** other **specified smoke, fire and flames**

Contact with heat and hot substances (X10-X19)

EXCLUDES 1   *exposure to excessive natural heat (X30)*
                exposure to fire and flames (X00-X09)

√4ᵗʰ **X10**   **Contact with hot drinks, food, fats and cooking oils**

> The appropriate 7th character is to be added to each code from category X10.
> A   initial encounter
> D   subsequent encounter
> S   sequela

√x7ᵗʰ **X10.0**   **Contact with hot drinks**

√x7ᵗʰ **X10.1**   **Contact with hot food**

√x7ᵗʰ **X10.2**   **Contact with fats and cooking oils**

√4ᵗʰ **X11**   **Contact with hot tap-water**

   INCLUDES   contact with boiling tap-water
                contact with boiling water NOS
   EXCLUDES 1   *contact with water heated on stove (X12)*

> The appropriate 7th character is to be added to each code from category X11.
> A   initial encounter
> D   subsequent encounter
> S   sequela

√x7ᵗʰ **X11.0**   **Contact with hot water in bath or tub**
     EXCLUDES 1   *contact with running hot water in bath or tub (X11.1)*

√x7ᵗʰ **X11.1**   **Contact with running hot water**
     Contact with hot water running out of hose
     Contact with hot water running out of tap

√x7ᵗʰ **X11.8**   **Contact with other hot tap-water**
     Contact with hot water in bucket
     Contact with hot tap-water NOS

√x7ᵗʰ **X12**   **Contact with other hot fluids**
     Contact with water heated on stove
     EXCLUDES 1   *hot (liquid) metals (X18)*

> The appropriate 7th character is to be added to code X12.
> A   initial encounter
> D   subsequent encounter
> S   sequela

√4ᵗʰ **X13**   **Contact with steam and other hot vapors**

> The appropriate 7th character is to be added to each code from category X13.
> A   initial encounter
> D   subsequent encounter
> S   sequela

√x7ᵗʰ **X13.0**   **Inhalation of steam and other hot vapors**

√x7ᵗʰ **X13.1**   **Other contact with steam and other hot vapors**

√4ᵗʰ **X14**   **Contact with hot air and other hot gases**

> The appropriate 7th character is to be added to each code from category X14.
> A   initial encounter
> D   subsequent encounter
> S   sequela

√x7ᵗʰ **X14.0**   **Inhalation of hot air and gases**

√x7ᵗʰ **X14.1**   **Other contact with hot air and other hot gases**

√4ᵗʰ **X15**   **Contact with hot household appliances**

   EXCLUDES 1   *contact with heating appliances (X16)*
                contact with powered household appliances (W29.-)
                exposure to controlled fire in building or structure due to household appliance (X02.8)
                exposure to household appliances electrical current (W86.0)

> The appropriate 7th character is to be added to each code from category X15.
> A   initial encounter
> D   subsequent encounter
> S   sequela

√x7ᵗʰ **X15.0**   **Contact with hot stove (kitchen)**

√x7ᵗʰ **X15.1**   **Contact with hot toaster**

√x7ᵗʰ **X15.2**   **Contact with** hotplate

√x7ᵗʰ **X15.3**   **Contact with hot** saucepan or skillet

√x7ᵗʰ **X15.8**   **Contact with** other **hot household appliances**
     Contact with cooker   Contact with light bulbs
     Contact with kettle

√x7ᵗʰ **X16**   **Contact with hot heating appliances, radiators and pipes**

   EXCLUDES 1   *contact with powered appliances (W29.-)*
                exposure to controlled fire in building or structure due to appliance (X02.8)
                exposure to industrial appliances electrical current (W86.1)

> The appropriate 7th character is to be added to code X16.
> A   initial encounter
> D   subsequent encounter
> S   sequela

√x7ᵗʰ **X17**   **Contact with hot engines, machinery and tools**

   EXCLUDES 1   *contact with hot heating appliances, radiators and pipes (X16)*
                contact with hot household appliances (X15)

> The appropriate 7th character is to be added to code X17.
> A   initial encounter
> D   subsequent encounter
> S   sequela

√x7ᵗʰ **X18**   **Contact with other hot metals**
     Contact with liquid metal

> The appropriate 7th character is to be added to code X18.
> A   initial encounter
> D   subsequent encounter
> S   sequela

√x7ᵗʰ **X19**   **Contact with other heat and hot substances**

   EXCLUDES 1   *objects that are not normally hot, e.g., an object made hot by a house fire (X00-X09)*

> The appropriate 7th character is to be added to code X19.
> A   initial encounter
> D   subsequent encounter
> S   sequela

Exposure to forces of nature (X30-X39)

√x7ᵗʰ **X30**   **Exposure to excessive** natural heat
     Exposure to excessive heat as the cause of sunstroke
     Exposure to heat NOS
   EXCLUDES 1   *excessive heat of man-made origin (W92)*
                exposure to man-made radiation (W89)
                exposure to sunlight (X32)
                exposure to tanning bed (W89)

> The appropriate 7th character is to be added to code X30.
> A   initial encounter
> D   subsequent encounter
> S   sequela

√x7ᵗʰ **X31**   **Exposure to excessive** natural cold
     Excessive cold as the cause of chilblains NOS
     Excessive cold as the cause of immersion foot or hand
     Exposure to cold NOS
     Exposure to weather conditions
   EXCLUDES 1   *cold of man-made origin (W93.-)*
                contact with or inhalation of dry ice (W93.-)
                contact with or inhalation of liquefied gas (W93.-)

> The appropriate 7th character is to be added to code X31.
> A   initial encounter
> D   subsequent encounter
> S   sequela

√x7ᵗʰ **X32**   **Exposure to sunlight**

   EXCLUDES 1   *radiation-related disorders of the skin and subcutaneous tissue (L55-L59)*
                man-made radiation (tanning bed) (W89)

> The appropriate 7th character is to be added to code X32.
> A   initial encounter
> D   subsequent encounter
> S   sequela

√x7ᵗʰ **X34**   **Earthquake**

   EXCLUDES 2   *tidal wave (tsunami) due to earthquake (X37.41)*

> The appropriate 7th character is to be added to code X34.
> A   initial encounter
> D   subsequent encounter
> S   sequela

N Newborn: 0   P Pediatric: 0-17   M Maternity: 12-55   A Adult: 15-124   MCC Major CC Condition   PDxMCC PDx acts as own MCC   CC CC Condition   PDxCC PDx acts as own CC

1198   ICD-10-CM 2016

☑x7th **X35 Volcanic eruption**
EXCLUDES 2 *tidal wave (tsunami) due to volcanic eruption (X37.41)*

> The appropriate 7th character is to be added to code X35.
> A   initial encounter
> D   subsequent encounter
> S   sequela

☑4th **X36 Avalanche, landslide and other earth movements**
INCLUDES   victim of mudslide of cataclysmic nature
EXCLUDES 1 *earthquake (X34)*
EXCLUDES 2 *transport accident involving collision with avalanche or landslide not in motion (V01-V99)*

> The appropriate 7th character is to be added to each code from category X36.
> A   initial encounter
> D   subsequent encounter
> S   sequela

☑x7th **X36.0 Collapse of dam or man-made structure causing earth movement**

☑x7th **X36.1 Avalanche, landslide, or mudslide**

☑4th **X37 Cataclysmic storm**

> The appropriate 7th character is to be added to each code from category X37.
> A   initial encounter
> D   subsequent encounter
> S   sequela

☑x7th **X37.0 Hurricane**
> Storm surge   Typhoon

☑x7th **X37.1 Tornado**
> Cyclone   Twister

☑x7th **X37.2 Blizzard (snow)(ice)**

☑x7th **X37.3 Dust storm**

☑5th **X37.4 Tidalwave**

> ☑x7th **X37.41 Tidal wave due to earthquake or volcanic eruption**
> Tidal wave NOS   Tsunami

> ☑x7th **X37.42 Tidal wave due to storm**

> ☑x7th **X37.43 Tidal wave due to landslide**

☑x7th **X37.8 Other cataclysmic storms**
> Cloudburst   Torrential rain
> EXCLUDES 2 *flood (X38)*

☑x7th **X37.9 Unspecified cataclysmic storm**
> Storm NOS
> EXCLUDES 1 *collapse of dam or man-made structure causing earth movement (X39.0)*

☑x7th **X38 Flood**
> Flood arising from remote storm
> Flood of cataclysmic nature arising from melting snow
> Flood resulting directly from storm
> EXCLUDES 1 *collapse of dam or man-made structure causing earth movement (X39.0)*
> *tidal wave NOS (X37.41)*
> *tidal wave caused by storm (X37.2)*

> The appropriate 7th character is to be added to code X38.
> A   initial encounter
> D   subsequent encounter
> S   sequela

☑4th **X39 Exposure to other forces of nature**

> The appropriate 7th character is to be added to each code from category X39.
> A   initial encounter
> D   subsequent encounter
> S   sequela

☑5th **X39.0 Exposure to natural radiation**
> EXCLUDES 1 *contact with and (suspected) exposure to radon and other naturally occuring radiation (Z77.122)*
> *exposure to man-made radiation (W88-W90)*
> *exposure to sunlight (X32)*

> ☑x7th **X39.01 Exposure to radon**

> ☑x7th **X39.08 Exposure to other natural radiation**

☑x7th **X39.8 Other exposure to forces of nature**

Accidental exposure to other specified factors (X52, X58)

☑x7th **X52 Prolonged stay in weightless environment**
> Weightlessness in spacecraft (simulator)

> The appropriate 7th character is to be added to code X52.
> A   initial encounter
> D   subsequent encounter
> S   sequela

☑x7th **X58 Exposure to other specified factors**
> Accident NOS   Exposure NOS

> The appropriate 7th character is to be added to code X58.
> A   initial encounter
> D   subsequent encounter
> S   sequela

Intentional self-harm (X71-X83)
Purposely self-inflicted injury
Suicide (attempted)

☑4th **X71 Intentional self-harm by drowning and submersion**

> The appropriate 7th character is to be added to each code from category X71.
> A   initial encounter
> D   subsequent encounter
> S   sequela

☑x7th **X71.0 Intentional self-harm by drowning and submersion while in bathtub**

☑x7th **X71.1 Intentional self-harm by drowning and submersion while in swimming pool**

☑x7th **X71.2 Intentional self-harm by drowning and submersion after jump into swimming pool**

☑x7th **X71.3 Intentional self-harm by drowning and submersion in natural water**

☑x7th **X71.8 Other intentional self-harm by drowning and submersion**

☑x7th **X71.9 Intentional self-harm by drowning and submersion, unspecified**

☑x7th **X72 Intentional self-harm by handgun discharge**
> Intentional self-harm by gun for single hand use
> Intentional self-harm by pistol
> Intentional self-harm by revolver
> EXCLUDES 1 *Very pistol (X74.8)*

> The appropriate 7th character is to be added to code X72.
> A   initial encounter
> D   subsequent encounter
> S   sequela

☑4th **X73 Intentional self-harm by rifle, shotgun and larger firearm discharge**
> EXCLUDES 1 *airgun (X74.01)*

> The appropriate 7th character is to be added to each code from category X73.
> A   initial encounter
> D   subsequent encounter
> S   sequela

☑x7th **X73.0 Intentional self-harm by shotgun discharge**

☑x7th **X73.1 Intentional self-harm by hunting rifle discharge**

☑x7th **X73.2 Intentional self-harm by machine gun discharge**

☑x7th **X73.8 Intentional self-harm by other larger firearm discharge**

☑x7th **X73.9 Intentional self-harm by unspecified larger firearm discharge**

☑4th **X74 Intentional self-harm by other and unspecified firearm and gun discharge**

> The appropriate 7th character is to be added to each code from category X74.
> A   initial encounter
> D   subsequent encounter
> S   sequela

☑5th **X74.0 Intentional self-harm by gas, air or spring-operated guns**

> ☑x7th **X74.01 Intentional self-harm by airgun**
> Intentional self-harm by BB gun discharge
> Intentional self-harm by pellet gun discharge

> ☑x7th **X74.02 Intentional self-harm by paintball gun**

> ☑x7th **X74.09 Intentional self-harm by other gas, air or spring-operated gun**

☑ Additional Character Required   ☑x7th Placeholder Alert   Unacceptable PDx   Manifestation   Hospital Acquired Condition   EXCLUDES 1 Not Coded Here   EXCLUDES 2 Not Included Here

ICD-10-CM 2016

X35–X74.09

1199

Chapter 20. External Causes of Morbidity

√x7th **X74.8** **Intentional self-harm by** other firearm discharge
Intentional self-harm by Very pistol [flare] discharge

√x7th **X74.9** **Intentional self-harm by** unspecified firearm discharge

√x7th **X75** **Intentional self-harm by explosive material**

> The appropriate 7th character is to be added to code X75.
> A   initial encounter
> D   subsequent encounter
> S   sequela

√x7th **X76** **Intentional self-harm by smoke, fire and flames**

> The appropriate 7th character is to be added to code X76.
> A   initial encounter
> D   subsequent encounter
> S   sequela

√4th **X77** **Intentional self-harm by steam, hot vapors and hot objects**

> The appropriate 7th character is to be added to each code from
> category X77.
> A   initial encounter
> D   subsequent encounter
> S   sequela

√x7th **X77.0** **Intentional self-harm by** steam or hot vapors

√x7th **X77.1** **Intentional self-harm by** hot tap water

√x7th **X77.2** **Intentional self-harm by** other hot fluids

√x7th **X77.3** **Intentional self-harm by** hot household appliances

√x7th **X77.8** **Intentional self-harm by** other hot objects

√x7th **X77.9** **Intentional self-harm by** unspecified hot objects

√4th **X78** **Intentional self-harm by sharp object**

> The appropriate 7th character is to be added to each code from
> category X78.
> A   initial encounter
> D   subsequent encounter
> S   sequela

√x7th **X78.0** **Intentional self-harm by** sharp glass

√x7th **X78.1** **Intentional self-harm by** knife

√x7th **X78.2** **Intentional self-harm by** sword or dagger

√x7th **X78.8** **Intentional self-harm by** other sharp object

√x7th **X78.9** **Intentional self-harm by** unspecified sharp object

√x7th **X79** **Intentional self-harm by blunt object**

> The appropriate 7th character is to be added to code X79.
> A   initial encounter
> D   subsequent encounter
> S   sequela

√x7th **X80** **Intentional self-harm by jumping from a high place**
Intentional fall from one level to another

> The appropriate 7th character is to be added to code X80.
> A   initial encounter
> D   subsequent encounter
> S   sequela

√4th **X81** **Intentional self-harm by jumping or lying in front of moving object**

> The appropriate 7th character is to be added to each code from
> category X81.
> A   initial encounter
> D   subsequent encounter
> S   sequela

√x7th **X81.0** **Intentional self-harm by jumping or lying in front of** motor vehicle

√x7th **X81.1** **Intentional self-harm by jumping or lying in front of** (subway) train

√x7th **X81.8** **Intentional self-harm by jumping or lying in front of** other moving object

√4th **X82** **Intentional self-harm by crashing of motor vehicle**

> The appropriate 7th character is to be added to each code from
> category X82.
> A   initial encounter
> D   subsequent encounter
> S   sequela

√x7th **X82.0** **Intentional collision of motor vehicle with** other motor vehicle

√x7th **X82.1** **Intentional collision of motor vehicle with** train

√x7th **X82.2** **Intentional collision of motor vehicle with** tree

√x7th **X82.8** **Other intentional self-harm by crashing of motor vehicle**

√4th **X83** **Intentional self-harm by other specified means**

> **EXCLUDES 1**   intentional self-harm by poisoning or contact with toxic
> substance—see Table of Drugs and Chemicals

> The appropriate 7th character is to be added to each code from
> category X83.
> A   initial encounter
> D   subsequent encounter
> S   sequela

√x7th **X83.0** **Intentional self-harm by** crashing of aircraft

√x7th **X83.1** **Intentional self-harm by** electrocution

√x7th **X83.2** **Intentional self-harm by** exposure to extremes of cold

√x7th **X83.8** **Intentional self-harm by** other specified means

Assault (X92-Y08)

INCLUDES   homicide
injuries inflicted by another person with intent to injure or kill, by
any means

EXCLUDES 1   injuries due to legal intervention (Y35.-)
injuries due to operations of war (Y36.-)
injuries due to terrorism (Y38.-)

√4th **X92** **Assault by drowning and submersion**

> The appropriate 7th character is to be added to each code from
> category X92.
> A   initial encounter
> D   subsequent encounter
> S   sequela

√x7th **X92.0** **Assault by drowning and submersion while in** bathtub

√x7th **X92.1** **Assault by drowning and submersion while in** swimming pool

√x7th **X92.2** **Assault by drowning and submersion** after push into swimming pool

√x7th **X92.3** **Assault by drowning and submersion** in natural water

√x7th **X92.8** **Other assault by drowning and submersion**

√x7th **X92.9** **Assault by drowning and submersion,** unspecified

√x7th **X93** **Assault by** handgun discharge
Assault by discharge of gun for single hand use
Assault by discharge of pistol
Assault by discharge of revolver
EXCLUDES 1   Very pistol (X95.8)

> The appropriate 7th character is to be added to code X93.
> A   initial encounter
> D   subsequent encounter
> S   sequela

√4th **X94** **Assault by** rifle, shotgun and larger firearm discharge
EXCLUDES 1   airgun (X95.01)

> The appropriate 7th character is to be added to each code from
> category X94.
> A   initial encounter
> D   subsequent encounter
> S   sequela

√x7th **X94.0** **Assault by** shotgun

√x7th **X94.1** **Assault by** hunting rifle

√x7th **X94.2** **Assault by** machine gun

√x7th **X94.8** **Assault by** other larger firearm discharge

√x7th **X94.9** **Assault by** unspecified larger firearm discharge

√4th **X95** **Assault by other and unspecified firearm and gun discharge**

> The appropriate 7th character is to be added to each code from
> category X95.
> A   initial encounter
> D   subsequent encounter
> S   sequela

√5th **X95.0** **Assault by** gas, air or spring-operated guns

> √x7th **X95.01** **Assault by** airgun discharge
> Assault by BB gun discharge
> Assault by pellet gun discharge

> √x7th **X95.02** **Assault by** paintball gun discharge

> √x7th **X95.09** **Assault by** other gas, air or spring-operated gun

√x7th **X95.8** **Assault by** other firearm discharge
Assault by Very pistol [flare] discharge

N Newborn: 0   **P** Pediatric: 0-17   **M** Maternity: 12-55   **A** Adult: 15-124   **MCC** Major CC Condition   **PDx MCC** PDx acts as own MCC   **CC** CC Condition   **PDx CC** PDx acts as own CC

1200

ICD-10-CM 2016

√x7th **X95.9**   **Assault by unspecified firearm discharge**

√4th **X96**   **Assault by explosive material**
> EXCLUDES1   *incendiary device (X97)*
> *terrorism involving explosive material (Y38.2-)*

> The appropriate 7th character is to be added to each code from category X96.
> A   initial encounter
> D   subsequent encounter
> S   sequela

√x7th **X96.0**   **Assault by antipersonnel bomb**
> EXCLUDES1   *antipersonnel bomb use in military or war (Y36.2-)*

√x7th **X96.1**   **Assault by gasoline bomb**

√x7th **X96.2**   **Assault by letter bomb**

√x7th **X96.3**   **Assault by fertilizer bomb**

√x7th **X96.4**   **Assault by pipe bomb**

√x7th **X96.8**   **Assault by other specified explosive**

√x7th **X96.9**   **Assault by unspecified explosive**

√x7th **X97**   **Assault by smoke, fire and flames**
> Assault by arson   Assault by incendiary device
> Assault by cigarettes

> The appropriate 7th character is to be added to code X97.
> A   initial encounter
> D   subsequent encounter
> S   sequela

√4th **X98**   **Assault by steam, hot vapors and hot objects**

> The appropriate 7th character is to be added to each code from category X98.
> A   initial encounter
> D   subsequent encounter
> S   sequela

√x7th **X98.0**   **Assault by steam or hot vapors**

√x7th **X98.1**   **Assault by hot tap water**

√x7th **X98.2**   **Assault by hot fluids**

√x7th **X98.3**   **Assault by hot household appliances**

√x7th **X98.8**   **Assault by other hot objects**

√x7th **X98.9**   **Assault by unspecified hot objects**

√4th **X99**   **Assault by sharp object**
> EXCLUDES1   *assault by strike by sports equipment (Y08.0-)*

> The appropriate 7th character is to be added to each code from category X99.
> A   initial encounter
> D   subsequent encounter
> S   sequela

√x7th **X99.0**   **Assault by sharp glass**

√x7th **X99.1**   **Assault by knife**

√x7th **X99.2**   **Assault by sword or dagger**

√x7th **X99.8**   **Assault by other sharp object**

√x7th **X99.9**   **Assault by unspecified sharp object**
> Assault by stabbing NOS

√x7th **Y00**   **Assault by blunt object**
> EXCLUDES1   *assault by strike by sports equipment (Y08.0-)*

> The appropriate 7th character is to be added to code Y00.
> A   initial encounter
> D   subsequent encounter
> S   sequela

√x7th **Y01**   **Assault by pushing from high place**

> The appropriate 7th character is to be added to code Y01.
> A   initial encounter
> D   subsequent encounter
> S   sequela

√4th **Y02**   **Assault by pushing or placing victim in front of moving object**

> The appropriate 7th character is to be added to each code from category Y02.
> A   initial encounter
> D   subsequent encounter
> S   sequela

√x7th **Y02.0**   **Assault by pushing or placing victim in front of motor vehicle**

√x7th **Y02.1**   **Assault by pushing or placing victim in front of (subway) train**

√x7th **Y02.8**   **Assault by pushing or placing victim in front of other moving object**

√4th **Y03**   **Assault by crashing of motor vehicle**

> The appropriate 7th character is to be added to each code from category Y03.
> A   initial encounter
> D   subsequent encounter
> S   sequela

√x7th **Y03.0**   **Assault by being hit or run over by motor vehicle**

√x7th **Y03.8**   **Other assault by crashing of motor vehicle**

√4th **Y04**   **Assault by bodily force**
> EXCLUDES1   *assault by:*
> *submersion (X92.-)*
> *use of weapon (X93-X95, X99, Y00)*

> The appropriate 7th character is to be added to each code from category Y04.
> A   initial encounter
> D   subsequent encounter
> S   sequela

√x7th **Y04.0**   **Assault by unarmed brawl or fight**

√x7th **Y04.1**   **Assault by human bite**

√x7th **Y04.2**   **Assault by strike against or bumped into by another person**

√x7th **Y04.8**   **Assault by other bodily force**
> Assault by bodily force NOS

√4th **Y07**   **Perpetrator of assault, maltreatment and neglect**
> NOTE   Codes from this category are for use only in cases of confirmed abuse (T74.-)
> Selection of the correct perpetrator code is based on the relationship between the perpetrator and the victim
> INCLUDES   perpetrator of abandonment
> perpetrator of emotional neglect
> perpetrator of mental cruelty
> perpetrator of physical abuse
> perpetrator of physical neglect
> perpetrator of sexual abuse
> perpetrator of torture

√5th **Y07.0**   **Spouse or partner, perpetrator of maltreatment and neglect**
> NOTE   Spouse or partner, perpetrator of maltreatment and neglect against spouse or partner

    Y07.01   **Husband, perpetrator of maltreatment and neglect**

    Y07.02   **Wife, perpetrator of maltreatment and neglect**

    Y07.03   **Male partner, perpetrator of maltreatment and neglect**

    Y07.04   **Female partner, perpetrator of maltreatment and neglect**

√5th **Y07.1**   **Parent (adoptive) (biological), perpetrator of maltreatment and neglect**

    Y07.11   **Biological father, perpetrator of maltreatment and neglect**

    Y07.12   **Biological mother, perpetrator of maltreatment and neglect**

    Y07.13   **Adoptive father, perpetrator of maltreatment and neglect**

    Y07.14   **Adoptive mother, perpetrator of maltreatment and neglect**

√5th **Y07.4**   **Other family member, perpetrator of maltreatment and neglect**

   √6th **Y07.41**   **Sibling, perpetrator of maltreatment and neglect**
> EXCLUDES1   *stepsibling, perpetrator of maltreatment and neglect (Y07.435, Y07.436)*

     Y07.410   **Brother, perpetrator of maltreatment and neglect**

     Y07.411   **Sister, perpetrator of maltreatment and neglect**

   √6th **Y07.42**   **Foster parent, perpetrator of maltreatment and neglect**

     Y07.420   **Foster father, perpetrator of maltreatment and neglect**

     Y07.421   **Foster mother, perpetrator of maltreatment and neglect**

   √6th **Y07.43**   **Stepparent or stepsibling, perpetrator of maltreatment and neglect**

     Y07.430   **Stepfather, perpetrator of maltreatment and neglect**

√ Additional Character Required   √x7th Placeholder Alert   Unacceptable PDx   Manifestation   Hospital Acquired Condition   EXCLUDES1 Not Coded Here   EXCLUDES2 Not Included Here

Chapter 20. External Causes of Morbidity

Y07.432   **Male friend of parent (co-residing in household), perpetrator of maltreatment and neglect**

Y07.433   **Stepmother, perpetrator of maltreatment and neglect**

Y07.434   **Female friend of parent (co-residing in household), perpetrator of maltreatment and neglect**

Y07.435   **Stepbrother, perpetrator or maltreatment and neglect**

Y07.436   **Stepsister, perpetrator of maltreatment and neglect**

✓6ᵗʰ **Y07.49**   **Other family member, perpetrator of maltreatment and neglect**

Y07.490   **Male cousin, perpetrator of maltreatment and neglect**

Y07.491   **Female cousin, perpetrator of maltreatment and neglect**

Y07.499   **Other family member, perpetrator of maltreatment and neglect**

✓5ᵗʰ **Y07.5**   **Non-family member, perpetrator of maltreatment and neglect**

Y07.50   **Unspecified non-family member, perpetrator of maltreatment and neglect**

✓6ᵗʰ **Y07.51**   **Daycare provider, perpetrator of maltreatment and neglect**

Y07.510   **At-home childcare provider, perpetrator of maltreatment and neglect**

Y07.511   **Daycare center childcare provider, perpetrator of maltreatment and neglect**

Y07.512   **At-home adultcare provider, perpetrator of maltreatment and neglect**

Y07.513   **Adultcare center provider, perpetrator of maltreatment and neglect**

Y07.519   **Unspecified daycare provider, perpetrator of maltreatment and neglect**

✓6ᵗʰ **Y07.52**   **Healthcare provider, perpetrator of maltreatment and neglect**

Y07.521   **Mental health provider, perpetrator of maltreatment and neglect**

Y07.528   **Other therapist or healthcare provider, perpetrator of maltreatment and neglect**
     Nurse, perpetrator of maltreatment and neglect
     Occupational therapist, perpetrator of maltreatment and neglect
     Physical therapist, perpetrator of maltreatment and neglect
     Speech therapist, perpetrator of maltreatment and neglect

Y07.529   **Unspecified healthcare provider, perpetrator of maltreatment and neglect**

Y07.53   **Teacher or instructor, perpetrator of maltreatment and neglect**
     Coach, perpetrator of maltreatment and neglect

Y07.59   **Other non-family member, perpetrator of maltreatment and neglect**

Y07.9   **Unspecified perpetrator of maltreatment and neglect**

✓4ᵗʰ **Y08**   **Assault by other specified means**

> The appropriate 7th character is to be added to each code from category Y08.
> A   initial encounter
> D   subsequent encounter
> S   sequela

✓5ᵗʰ **Y08.0**   **Assault by strike by sport equipment**

✓x7ᵗʰ **Y08.01**   **Assault by strike by hockey stick**

✓x7ᵗʰ **Y08.02**   **Assault by strike by baseball bat**

✓x7ᵗʰ **Y08.09**   **Assault by strike by other specified type of sport equipment**

✓5ᵗʰ **Y08.8**   **Assault by other specified means**

✓x7ᵗʰ **Y08.81**   **Assault by crashing of aircraft**

✓x7ᵗʰ **Y08.89**   **Assault by other specified means**

Y09   **Assault by unspecified means**
Assassination (attempted) NOS   Manslaughter (attempted) NOS
Homicide (attempted) NOS   Murder (attempted) NOS

Event of undetermined intent (Y21-Y33)

Undetermined intent is only for use when there is specific documentation in the record that the intent of the injury cannot be determined. If no such documentation is present, code to accidental (unintentional)

✓4ᵗʰ **Y21**   **Drowning and submersion, undetermined intent**

> The appropriate 7th character is to be added to each code from category Y21.
> A   initial encounter
> D   subsequent encounter
> S   sequela

✓x7ᵗʰ **Y21.0**   **Drowning and submersion while in bathtub, undetermined intent**

✓x7ᵗʰ **Y21.1**   **Drowning and submersion after fall into bathtub, undetermined intent**

✓x7ᵗʰ **Y21.2**   **Drowning and submersion while in swimming pool, undetermined intent**

✓x7ᵗʰ **Y21.3**   **Drowning and submersion after fall into swimming pool, undetermined intent**

✓x7ᵗʰ **Y21.4**   **Drowning and submersion in natural water, undetermined intent**

✓x7ᵗʰ **Y21.8**   **Other drowning and submersion, undetermined intent**

✓x7ᵗʰ **Y21.9**   **Unspecified drowning and submersion, undetermined intent**

✓x7ᵗʰ **Y22**   **Handgun discharge, undetermined intent**
Discharge of gun for single hand use, undetermined intent
Discharge of pistol, undetermined intent
Discharge of revolver, undetermined intent
> EXCLUDES 2   *Very pistol (Y24.8)*

> The appropriate 7th character is to be added to code Y22.
> A   initial encounter
> D   subsequent encounter
> S   sequela

✓4ᵗʰ **Y23**   **Rifle, shotgun and larger firearm discharge, undetermined intent**
> EXCLUDES 2   *airgun (Y24.0)*

> The appropriate 7th character is to be added to each code from category Y23.
> A   initial encounter
> D   subsequent encounter
> S   sequela

✓x7ᵗʰ **Y23.0**   **Shotgun discharge, undetermined intent**

✓x7ᵗʰ **Y23.1**   **Hunting rifle discharge, undetermined intent**

✓x7ᵗʰ **Y23.2**   **Military firearm discharge, undetermined intent**

✓x7ᵗʰ **Y23.3**   **Machine gun discharge, undetermined intent**

✓x7ᵗʰ **Y23.8**   **Other larger firearm discharge, undetermined intent**

✓x7ᵗʰ **Y23.9**   **Unspecified larger firearm discharge, undetermined intent**

✓4ᵗʰ **Y24**   **Other and unspecified firearm discharge, undetermined intent**

> The appropriate 7th character is to be added to each code from category Y24.
> A   initial encounter
> D   subsequent encounter
> S   sequela

✓x7ᵗʰ **Y24.0**   **Airgun discharge, undetermined intent**
     BB gun discharge, undetermined intent
     Pellet gun discharge, undetermined intent

✓x7ᵗʰ **Y24.8**   **Other firearm discharge, undetermined intent**
     Paintball gun discharge, undetermined intent
     Very pistol [flare] discharge, undetermined intent

✓x7ᵗʰ **Y24.9**   **Unspecified firearm discharge, undetermined intent**

Ⓝ Newborn: 0   Ⓟ Pediatric: 0-17   Ⓜ Maternity: 12-55   Ⓐ Adult: 15-124   **MCC** Major CC Condition   **PDxMCC** PDx acts as own MCC   **CC** CC Condition   **PDxCC** PDx acts as own CC

1202

ICD–10-CM 2016

✓x7ᵗʰ Y25 Contact with explosive material, undetermined intent

> The appropriate 7th character is to be added to code Y25.
> A   initial encounter
> D   subsequent encounter
> S   sequela

✓x7ᵗʰ Y26 Exposure to smoke, fire and flames, undetermined intent

> The appropriate 7th character is to be added to code Y26.
> A   initial encounter
> D   subsequent encounter
> S   sequela

✓4ᵗʰ Y27 Contact with steam, hot vapors and hot objects, undetermined intent

> The appropriate 7th character is to be added to each code from category Y27.
> A   initial encounter
> D   subsequent encounter
> S   sequela

✓x7ᵗʰ   **Y27.0 Contact with steam and hot vapors, undetermined intent**
✓x7ᵗʰ   **Y27.1 Contact with hot tap water, undetermined intent**
✓x7ᵗʰ   **Y27.2 Contact with hot fluids, undetermined intent**
✓x7ᵗʰ   **Y27.3 Contact with hot household appliance, undetermined intent**
✓x7ᵗʰ   **Y27.8 Contact with other hot objects, undetermined intent**
✓x7ᵗʰ   **Y27.9 Contact with unspecified hot objects, undetermined intent**

✓4ᵗʰ Y28 Contact with sharp object, undetermined intent

> The appropriate 7th character is to be added to each code from category Y28.
> A   initial encounter
> D   subsequent encounter
> S   sequela

✓x7ᵗʰ   **Y28.0 Contact with sharp glass, undetermined intent**
✓x7ᵗʰ   **Y28.1 Contact with knife, undetermined intent**
✓x7ᵗʰ   **Y28.2 Contact with sword or dagger, undetermined intent**
✓x7ᵗʰ   **Y28.8 Contact with other sharp object, undetermined intent**
✓x7ᵗʰ   **Y28.9 Contact with unspecified sharp object, undetermined intent**

✓x7ᵗʰ Y29 Contact with blunt object, undetermined intent

> The appropriate 7th character is to be added to code Y29.
> A   initial encounter
> D   subsequent encounter
> S   sequela

✓x7ᵗʰ Y30 Falling, jumping or pushed from a high place, undetermined intent
> Victim falling from one level to another, undetermined intent

> The appropriate 7th character is to be added to code Y30.
> A   initial encounter
> D   subsequent encounter
> S   sequela

✓x7ᵗʰ Y31 Falling, lying or running before or into moving object, undetermined intent

> The appropriate 7th character is to be added to code Y31.
> A   initial encounter
> D   subsequent encounter
> S   sequela

✓x7ᵗʰ Y32 Crashing of motor vehicle, undetermined intent

> The appropriate 7th character is to be added to code Y32.
> A   initial encounter
> D   subsequent encounter
> S   sequela

✓x7ᵗʰ Y33 Other specified events, undetermined intent

> The appropriate 7th character is to be added to code Y33.
> A   initial encounter
> D   subsequent encounter
> S   sequela

Legal intervention, operations of war, military operations, and terrorism (Y35-Y38)

✓4ᵗʰ Y35 Legal intervention
> INCLUDES   any injury sustained as a result of an encounter with any law enforcement official, serving in any capacity at the time of the encounter, whether on-duty or off-duty. Includes: injury to law enforcement official, suspect and bystander

> The appropriate 7th character is to be added to each code from category Y35.
> A   initial encounter
> D   subsequent encounter
> S   sequela

✓5ᵗʰ   **Y35.0 Legal intervention involving firearm discharge**

    ✓6ᵗʰ   **Y35.00 Legal intervention involving unspecified firearm discharge**
       Legal intervention involving gunshot wound
       Legal intervention involving shot NOS

       ✓7ᵗʰ   **Y35.001 Legal intervention involving unspecified firearm discharge, law enforcement official injured**

       ✓7ᵗʰ   **Y35.002 Legal intervention involving unspecified firearm discharge, bystander injured**

       ✓7ᵗʰ   **Y35.003 Legal intervention involving unspecified firearm discharge, suspect injured**

    ✓6ᵗʰ   **Y35.01 Legal intervention involving injury by machine gun**

       ✓7ᵗʰ   **Y35.011 Legal intervention involving injury by machine gun, law enforcement official injured**

       ✓7ᵗʰ   **Y35.012 Legal intervention involving injury by machine gun, bystander injured**

       ✓7ᵗʰ   **Y35.013 Legal intervention involving injury by machine gun, suspect injured**

    ✓6ᵗʰ   **Y35.02 Legal intervention involving injury by handgun**

       ✓7ᵗʰ   **Y35.021 Legal intervention involving injury by handgun, law enforcement official injured**

       ✓7ᵗʰ   **Y35.022 Legal intervention involving injury by handgun, bystander injured**

       ✓7ᵗʰ   **Y35.023 Legal intervention involving injury by handgun, suspect injured**

    ✓6ᵗʰ   **Y35.03 Legal intervention involving injury by rifle pellet**

       ✓7ᵗʰ   **Y35.031 Legal intervention involving injury by rifle pellet, law enforcement official injured**

       ✓7ᵗʰ   **Y35.032 Legal intervention involving injury by rifle pellet, bystander injured**

       ✓7ᵗʰ   **Y35.033 Legal intervention involving injury by rifle pellet, suspect injured**

    ✓6ᵗʰ   **Y35.04 Legal intervention involving injury by rubber bullet**

       ✓7ᵗʰ   **Y35.041 Legal intervention involving injury by rubber bullet, law enforcement official injured**

       ✓7ᵗʰ   **Y35.042 Legal intervention involving injury by rubber bullet, bystander injured**

       ✓7ᵗʰ   **Y35.043 Legal intervention involving injury by rubber bullet, suspect injured**

    ✓6ᵗʰ   **Y35.09 Legal intervention involving other firearm discharge**

       ✓7ᵗʰ   **Y35.091 Legal intervention involving other firearm discharge, law enforcement official injured**

       ✓7ᵗʰ   **Y35.092 Legal intervention involving other firearm discharge, bystander injured**

       ✓7ᵗʰ   **Y35.093 Legal intervention involving other firearm discharge, suspect injured**

✓5ᵗʰ   **Y35.1 Legal intervention involving explosives**

    ✓6ᵗʰ   **Y35.10 Legal intervention involving unspecified explosives**

       ✓7ᵗʰ   **Y35.101 Legal intervention involving unspecified explosives, law enforcement official injured**

       ✓7ᵗʰ   **Y35.102 Legal intervention involving unspecified explosives, bystander injured**

       ✓7ᵗʰ   **Y35.103 Legal intervention involving unspecified explosives, suspect injured**

✓ Additional Character Required   ✓x7ᵗʰ Placeholder Alert   Unacceptable PDx   Manifestation   Hospital Acquired Condition   **EXCLUDES 1** Not Coded Here   **EXCLUDES 2** Not Included Here

ICD-10-CM 2016   1203

✓6ᵗʰ **Y35.11** **Legal intervention involving injury by dynamite**
  ✓7ᵗʰ **Y35.111** **Legal intervention involving injury by dynamite, law enforcement official injured**
  ✓7ᵗʰ **Y35.112** **Legal intervention involving injury by dynamite, bystander injured**
  ✓7ᵗʰ **Y35.113** **Legal intervention involving injury by dynamite, suspect injured**

✓6ᵗʰ **Y35.12** **Legal intervention involving injury by explosive shell**
  ✓7ᵗʰ **Y35.121** **Legal intervention involving injury by explosive shell, law enforcement official injured**
  ✓7ᵗʰ **Y35.122** **Legal intervention involving injury by explosive shell, bystander injured**
  ✓7ᵗʰ **Y35.123** **Legal intervention involving injury by explosive shell, suspect injured**

✓6ᵗʰ **Y35.19** **Legal intervention involving other explosives**
  Legal intervention involving injury by grenade
  Legal intervention involving injury by mortar bomb
  ✓7ᵗʰ **Y35.191** **Legal intervention involving other explosives, law enforcement official injured**
  ✓7ᵗʰ **Y35.192** **Legal intervention involving other explosives, bystander injured**
  ✓7ᵗʰ **Y35.193** **Legal intervention involving other explosives, suspect injured**

✓5ᵗʰ **Y35.2** **Legal intervention involving gas**
  Legal intervention involving asphyxiation by gas
  Legal intervention involving poisoning by gas

  ✓6ᵗʰ **Y35.20** **Legal intervention involving unspecified gas**
    ✓7ᵗʰ **Y35.201** **Legal intervention involving unspecified gas, law enforcement official injured**
    ✓7ᵗʰ **Y35.202** **Legal intervention involving unspecified gas, bystander injured**
    ✓7ᵗʰ **Y35.203** **Legal intervention involving unspecified gas, suspect injured**

  ✓6ᵗʰ **Y35.21** **Legal intervention involving injury by tear gas**
    ✓7ᵗʰ **Y35.211** **Legal intervention involving injury by tear gas, law enforcement official injured**
    ✓7ᵗʰ **Y35.212** **Legal intervention involving injury by tear gas, bystander injured**
    ✓7ᵗʰ **Y35.213** **Legal intervention involving injury by tear gas, suspect injured**

  ✓6ᵗʰ **Y35.29** **Legal intervention involving other gas**
    ✓7ᵗʰ **Y35.291** **Legal intervention involving other gas, law enforcement official injured**
    ✓7ᵗʰ **Y35.292** **Legal intervention involving other gas, bystander injured**
    ✓7ᵗʰ **Y35.293** **Legal intervention involving other gas, suspect injured**

✓5ᵗʰ **Y35.3** **Legal intervention involving blunt objects**
  Legal intervention involving being hit or struck by blunt object

  ✓6ᵗʰ **Y35.30** **Legal intervention involving unspecified blunt objects**
    ✓7ᵗʰ **Y35.301** **Legal intervention involving unspecified blunt objects, law enforcement official injured**
    ✓7ᵗʰ **Y35.302** **Legal intervention involving unspecified blunt objects, bystander injured**
    ✓7ᵗʰ **Y35.303** **Legal intervention involving unspecified blunt objects, suspect injured**

  ✓6ᵗʰ **Y35.31** **Legal intervention involving baton**
    ✓7ᵗʰ **Y35.311** **Legal intervention involving baton, law enforcement official injured**
    ✓7ᵗʰ **Y35.312** **Legal intervention involving baton, bystander injured**
    ✓7ᵗʰ **Y35.313** **Legal intervention involving baton, suspect injured**

  ✓6ᵗʰ **Y35.39** **Legal intervention involving other blunt objects**
    ✓7ᵗʰ **Y35.391** **Legal intervention involving other blunt objects, law enforcement official injured**
    ✓7ᵗʰ **Y35.392** **Legal intervention involving other blunt objects, bystander injured**

  ✓7ᵗʰ **Y35.393** **Legal intervention involving other blunt objects, suspect injured**

✓5ᵗʰ **Y35.4** **Legal intervention involving sharp objects**
  Legal intervention involving being cut by sharp objects
  Legal intervention involving being stabbed by sharp objects

  ✓6ᵗʰ **Y35.40** **Legal intervention involving unspecified sharp objects**
    ✓7ᵗʰ **Y35.401** **Legal intervention involving unspecified sharp objects, law enforcement official injured**
    ✓7ᵗʰ **Y35.402** **Legal intervention involving unspecified sharp objects, bystander injured**
    ✓7ᵗʰ **Y35.403** **Legal intervention involving unspecified sharp objects, suspect injured**

  ✓6ᵗʰ **Y35.41** **Legal intervention involving bayonet**
    ✓7ᵗʰ **Y35.411** **Legal intervention involving bayonet, law enforcement official injured**
    ✓7ᵗʰ **Y35.412** **Legal intervention involving bayonet, bystander injured**
    ✓7ᵗʰ **Y35.413** **Legal intervention involving bayonet, suspect injured**

  ✓6ᵗʰ **Y35.49** **Legal intervention involving other sharp objects**
    ✓7ᵗʰ **Y35.491** **Legal intervention involving other sharp objects, law enforcement official injured**
    ✓7ᵗʰ **Y35.492** **Legal intervention involving other sharp objects, bystander injured**
    ✓7ᵗʰ **Y35.493** **Legal intervention involving other sharp objects, suspect injured**

✓5ᵗʰ **Y35.8** **Legal intervention involving other specified means**

  ✓6ᵗʰ **Y35.81** **Legal intervention involving manhandling**
    ✓7ᵗʰ **Y35.811** **Legal intervention involving manhandling, law enforcement official injured**
    ✓7ᵗʰ **Y35.812** **Legal intervention involving manhandling, bystander injured**
    ✓7ᵗʰ **Y35.813** **Legal intervention involving manhandling, suspect injured**

  ✓6ᵗʰ **Y35.89** **Legal intervention involving other specified means**
    ✓7ᵗʰ **Y35.891** **Legal intervention involving other specified means, law enforcement official injured**
    ✓7ᵗʰ **Y35.892** **Legal intervention involving other specified means, bystander injured**
    ✓7ᵗʰ **Y35.893** **Legal intervention involving other specified means, suspect injured**

✓5ᵗʰ **Y35.9** **Legal intervention, means unspecified**
  ✓x7ᵗʰ **Y35.91** **Legal intervention, means unspecified, law enforcement official injured**
  ✓x7ᵗʰ **Y35.92** **Legal intervention, means unspecified, bystander injured**
  ✓x7ᵗʰ **Y35.93** **Legal intervention, means unspecified, suspect injured**

✓4ᵗʰ **Y36** **Operations of war**
  INCLUDES injuries to military personnel and civilians caused by war, civil insurrection, and peacekeeping missions
  EXCLUDES 1 *injury to military personnel occurring during peacetime military operations (Y37.-)*
  military vehicles involved in transport accidents with non-military vehicle during peacetime (V09.01, V09.21, V19.81, V29.81, V39.81, V49.81, V59.81, V69.81, V79.81)
  AHA: 2014, 3Q, 4

  The appropriate 7th character is to be added to each code from category Y36.
  A   initial encounter
  D   subsequent encounter
  S   sequela

✓5ᵗʰ **Y36.0** **War operations involving explosion of marine weapons**

  ✓6ᵗʰ **Y36.00** **War operations involving explosion of unspecified marine weapon**
    War operations involving underwater blast NOS
    ✓7ᵗʰ **Y36.000** **War operations involving explosion of unspecified marine weapon, military personnel**
    ✓7ᵗʰ **Y36.001** **War operations involving explosion of unspecified marine weapon, civilian**

☑6ᵗʰ Y36.01   **War operations involving explosion of depth-charge**
- ☑7ᵗʰ Y36.010   **War operations involving explosion of depth-charge, military personnel**
- ☑7ᵗʰ Y36.011   **War operations involving explosion of depth-charge, civilian**

☑6ᵗʰ Y36.02   **War operations involving explosion of marine mine**
War operations involving explosion of marine mine, at sea or in harbor
- ☑7ᵗʰ Y36.020   **War operations involving explosion of marine mine, military personnel**
- ☑7ᵗʰ Y36.021   **War operations involving explosion of marine mine, civilian**

☑6ᵗʰ Y36.03   **War operations involving explosion of sea-based artillery shell**
- ☑7ᵗʰ Y36.030   **War operations involving explosion of sea-based artillery shell, military personnel**
- ☑7ᵗʰ Y36.031   **War operations involving explosion of sea-based artillery shell, civilian**

☑6ᵗʰ Y36.04   **War operations involving explosion of torpedo**
- ☑7ᵗʰ Y36.040   **War operations involving explosion of torpedo, military personnel**
- ☑7ᵗʰ Y36.041   **War operations involving explosion of torpedo, civilian**

☑6ᵗʰ Y36.05   **War operations involving accidental detonation of onboard marine weapons**
- ☑7ᵗʰ Y36.050   **War operations involving accidental detonation of onboard marine weapons, military personnel**
- ☑7ᵗʰ Y36.051   **War operations involving accidental detonation of onboard marine weapons, civilian**

☑6ᵗʰ Y36.09   **War operations involving explosion of other marine weapons**
- ☑7ᵗʰ Y36.090   **War operations involving explosion of other marine weapons, military personnel**
- ☑7ᵗʰ Y36.091   **War operations involving explosion of other marine weapons, civilian**

☑5ᵗʰ Y36.1   **War operations involving destruction of aircraft**

☑6ᵗʰ Y36.10   **War operations involving unspecified destruction of aircraft**
- ☑7ᵗʰ Y36.100   **War operations involving unspecified destruction of aircraft, military personnel**
- ☑7ᵗʰ Y36.101   **War operations involving unspecified destruction of aircraft, civilian**

☑6ᵗʰ Y36.11   **War operations involving destruction of aircraft due to enemy fire or explosives**
War operations involving destruction of aircraft due to air to air missile
War operations involving destruction of aircraft due to explosive placed on aircraft
War operations involving destruction of aircraft due to rocket propelled grenade [RPG]
War operations involving destruction of aircraft due to small arms fire
War operations involving destruction of aircraft due to surface to air missile
- ☑7ᵗʰ Y36.110   **War operations involving destruction of aircraft due to enemy fire or explosives, military personnel**
- ☑7ᵗʰ Y36.111   **War operations involving destruction of aircraft due to enemy fire or explosives, civilian**

☑6ᵗʰ Y36.12   **War operations involving destruction of aircraft due to collision with other aircraft**
- ☑7ᵗʰ Y36.120   **War operations involving destruction of aircraft due to collision with other aircraft, military personnel**
- ☑7ᵗʰ Y36.121   **War operations involving destruction of aircraft due to collision with other aircraft, civilian**

☑6ᵗʰ Y36.13   **War operations involving destruction of aircraft due to onboard fire**
- ☑7ᵗʰ Y36.130   **War operations involving destruction of aircraft due to onboard fire, military personnel**
- ☑7ᵗʰ Y36.131   **War operations involving destruction of aircraft due to onboard fire, civilian**

☑6ᵗʰ Y36.14   **War operations involving destruction of aircraft due to accidental detonation of onboard munitions and explosives**
- ☑7ᵗʰ Y36.140   **War operations involving destruction of aircraft due to accidental detonation of onboard munitions and explosives, military personnel**
- ☑7ᵗʰ Y36.141   **War operations involving destruction of aircraft due to accidental detonation of onboard munitions and explosives, civilian**

☑6ᵗʰ Y36.19   **War operations involving other destruction of aircraft**
- ☑7ᵗʰ Y36.190   **War operations involving other destruction of aircraft, military personnel**
- ☑7ᵗʰ Y36.191   **War operations involving other destruction of aircraft, civilian**

☑5ᵗʰ Y36.2   **War operations involving other explosions and fragments**
> EXCLUDES 1   *war operations involving explosion of aircraft (Y36.1-)*
> *war operations involving explosion of marine weapons (Y36.0-)*
> *war operations involving explosion of nuclear weapons (Y36.5-)*
> *war operations involving explosion occurring after cessation of hostilities (Y36.8-)*

☑6ᵗʰ Y36.20   **War operations involving unspecified explosion and fragments**
War operations involving air blast NOS
War operations involving blast NOS
War operations involving blast fragments NOS
War operations involving blast wave NOS
War operations involving blast wind NOS
War operations involving explosion NOS
War operations involving explosion of bomb NOS
- ☑7ᵗʰ Y36.200   **War operations involving unspecified explosion and fragments, military personnel**
- ☑7ᵗʰ Y36.201   **War operations involving unspecified explosion and fragments, civilian**

☑6ᵗʰ Y36.21   **War operations involving explosion of aerial bomb**
- ☑7ᵗʰ Y36.210   **War operations involving explosion of aerial bomb, military personnel**
- ☑7ᵗʰ Y36.211   **War operations involving explosion of aerial bomb, civilian**

☑6ᵗʰ Y36.22   **War operations involving explosion of guided missile**
- ☑7ᵗʰ Y36.220   **War operations involving explosion of guided missile, military personnel**
- ☑7ᵗʰ Y36.221   **War operations involving explosion of guided missile, civilian**

☑6ᵗʰ Y36.23   **War operations involving explosion of improvised explosive device [IED]**
War operations involving explosion of person-borne improvised explosive device [IED]
War operations involving explosion of vehicle-borne improvised explosive device [IED]
War operations involving explosion of roadside improvised explosive device [IED]
- ☑7ᵗʰ Y36.230   **War operations involving explosion of improvised explosive device [IED], military personnel**
- ☑7ᵗʰ Y36.231   **War operations involving explosion of improvised explosive device [IED], civilian**

☑6ᵗʰ Y36.24   **War operations involving explosion due to accidental detonation and discharge of own munitions or munitions launch device**
- ☑7ᵗʰ Y36.240   **War operations involving explosion due to accidental detonation and discharge of own munitions or munitions launch device, military personnel**
- ☑7ᵗʰ Y36.241   **War operations involving explosion due to accidental detonation and discharge of own munitions or munitions launch device, civilian**

☑ Additional Character Required   ☑x7ᵗʰ Placeholder Alert   Unacceptable PDx   ■ Manifestation   Hospital Acquired Condition   **EXCLUDES 1** Not Coded Here   **EXCLUDES 2** Not Included Here

ICD-10-CM 2016   1205

✓6th **Y36.25 War operations involving fragments from munitions**

    ✓7th **Y36.250 War operations involving fragments from munitions, military personnel**

    ✓7th **Y36.251 War operations involving fragments from munitions, civilian**

✓6th **Y36.26 War operations involving fragments of improvised explosive device [IED]**

    War operations involving fragments of person-borne improvised explosive device [IED]
    War operations involving fragments of vehicle-borne improvised explosive device [IED]
    War operations involving fragments of roadside improvised explosive device [IED]

    ✓7th **Y36.260 War operations involving fragments of improvised explosive device [IED], military personnel**

    ✓7th **Y36.261 War operations involving fragments of improvised explosive device [IED], civilian**

✓6th **Y36.27 War operations involving fragments from weapons**

    ✓7th **Y36.270 War operations involving fragments from weapons, military personnel**

    ✓7th **Y36.271 War operations involving fragments from weapons, civilian**

✓6th **Y36.29 War operations involving other explosions and fragments**

    War operations involving explosion of grenade
    War operations involving explosions of land mine
    War operations involving shrapnel NOS

    ✓7th **Y36.290 War operations involving other explosions and fragments, military personnel**

    ✓7th **Y36.291 War operations involving other explosions and fragments, civilian**

✓5th **Y36.3 War operations involving fires, conflagrations and hot substances**

    War operations involving smoke, fumes, and heat from fires, conflagrations and hot substances

    EXCLUDES 1   *war operations involving fires and conflagrations aboard military aircraft (Y36.1-)*
          war operations involving fires and conflagrations aboard military watercraft (Y36.0-)
          war operations involving fires and conflagrations caused indirectly by conventional weapons (Y36.2-)
          war operations involving fires and thermal effects of nuclear weapons (Y36.53-)

    ✓6th **Y36.30 War operations involving unspecified fire, conflagration and hot substance**

      ✓7th **Y36.300 War operations involving unspecified fire, conflagration and hot substance, military personnel**

      ✓7th **Y36.301 War operations involving unspecified fire, conflagration and hot substance, civilian**

    ✓6th **Y36.31 War operations involving gasoline bomb**

      War operations involving incendiary bomb
      War operations involving petrol bomb

      ✓7th **Y36.310 War operations involving gasoline bomb, military personnel**

      ✓7th **Y36.311 War operations involving gasoline bomb, civilian**

    ✓6th **Y36.32 War operations involving incendiary bullet**

      ✓7th **Y36.320 War operations involving incendiary bullet, military personnel**

      ✓7th **Y36.321 War operations involving incendiary bullet, civilian**

    ✓6th **Y36.33 War operations involving flamethrower**

      ✓7th **Y36.330 War operations involving flamethrower, military personnel**

      ✓7th **Y36.331 War operations involving flamethrower, civilian**

    ✓6th **Y36.39 War operations involving other fires, conflagrations and hot substances**

      ✓7th **Y36.390 War operations involving other fires, conflagrations and hot substances, military personnel**

      ✓7th **Y36.391 War operations involving other fires, conflagrations and hot substances, civilian**

✓5th **Y36.4 War operations involving firearm discharge and other forms of conventional warfare**

    ✓6th **Y36.41 War operations involving rubber bullets**

      ✓7th **Y36.410 War operations involving rubber bullets, military personnel**

      ✓7th **Y36.411 War operations involving rubber bullets, civilian**

    ✓6th **Y36.42 War operations involving firearms pellets**

      ✓7th **Y36.420 War operations involving firearms pellets, military personnel**

      ✓7th **Y36.421 War operations involving firearms pellets, civilian**

    ✓6th **Y36.43 War operations involving other firearms discharge**

      War operations involving bullets NOS

      EXCLUDES 1   *war operations involving munitions fragments (Y36.25-)*
          war operations involving incendiary bullets (Y36.32-)

      ✓7th **Y36.430 War operations involving other firearms discharge, military personnel**

      ✓7th **Y36.431 War operations involving other firearms discharge, civilian**

    ✓6th **Y36.44 War operations involving unarmed hand to hand combat**

      EXCLUDES 1   *war operations involving combat using blunt or piercing object (Y36.45-)*
          war operations involving intentional restriction of air and airway (Y36.46-)
          war operations involving unintentional restriction of air and airway (Y36.47-)

      ✓7th **Y36.440 War operations involving unarmed hand to hand combat, military personnel**

      ✓7th **Y36.441 War operations involving unarmed hand to hand combat, civilian**

    ✓6th **Y36.45 War operations involving combat using blunt or piercing object**

      ✓7th **Y36.450 War operations involving combat using blunt or piercing object, military personnel**

      ✓7th **Y36.451 War operations involving combat using blunt or piercing object, civilian**

    ✓6th **Y36.46 War operations involving intentional restriction of air and airway**

      ✓7th **Y36.460 War operations involving intentional restriction of air and airway, military personnel**

      ✓7th **Y36.461 War operations involving intentional restriction of air and airway, civilian**

    ✓6th **Y36.47 War operations involving unintentional restriction of air and airway**

      ✓7th **Y36.470 War operations involving unintentional restriction of air and airway, military personnel**

      ✓7th **Y36.471 War operations involving unintentional restriction of air and airway, civilian**

    ✓6th **Y36.49 War operations involving other forms of conventional warfare**

      ✓7th **Y36.490 War operations involving other forms of conventional warfare, military personnel**

      ✓7th **Y36.491 War operations involving other forms of conventional warfare, civilian**

✓5th **Y36.5 War operations involving nuclear weapons**

    War operations involving dirty bomb NOS

    ✓6th **Y36.50 War operations involving unspecified effect of nuclear weapon**

      ✓7th **Y36.500 War operations involving unspecified effect of nuclear weapon, military personnel**

      ✓7th **Y36.501 War operations involving unspecified effect of nuclear weapon, civilian**

    ✓6th **Y36.51 War operations involving direct blast effect of nuclear weapon**

      War operations involving blast pressure of nuclear weapon

      ✓7th **Y36.510 War operations involving direct blast effect of nuclear weapon, military personnel**

N Newborn: 0   P Pediatric: 0-17   M Maternity: 12-55   A Adult: 15-124   MCC Major CC Condition   PDxMCC PDx acts as own MCC   CC CC Condition   PDxCC PDx acts as own CC

1206   ICD-10-CM 2016

✓7ᵗʰ Y36.511 **War operations involving direct blast effect of nuclear weapon, civilian**

✓6ᵗʰ Y36.52 **War operations involving** indirect blast **effect of nuclear weapon**
War operations involving being thrown by blast of nuclear weapon
War operations involving being struck or crushed by blast debris of nuclear weapon

✓7ᵗʰ Y36.520 **War operations involving indirect blast effect of nuclear weapon, military personnel**

✓7ᵗʰ Y36.521 **War operations involving indirect blast effect of nuclear weapon, civilian**

✓6ᵗʰ Y36.53 **War operations involving** thermal radiation **effect of nuclear weapon**
War operations involving direct heat from nuclear weapon
War operation involving fireball effects from nuclear weapon

✓7ᵗʰ Y36.530 **War operations involving thermal radiation effect of nuclear weapon, military personnel**

✓7ᵗʰ Y36.531 **War operations involving thermal radiation effect of nuclear weapon, civilian**

✓6ᵗʰ Y36.54 **War operation involving** nuclear radiation **effects of nuclear weapon**
War operation involving acute radiation exposure from nuclear weapon
War operation involving exposure to immediate ionizing radiation from nuclear weapon
War operation involving fallout exposure from nuclear weapon
War operation involving secondary effects of nuclear weapons

✓7ᵗʰ Y36.540 **War operation involving nuclear radiation effects of nuclear weapon, military personnel**

✓7ᵗʰ Y36.541 **War operation involving nuclear radiation effects of nuclear weapon, civilian**

✓6ᵗʰ Y36.59 **War operation involving** other **effects of nuclear weapons**

✓7ᵗʰ Y36.590 **War operation involving other effects of nuclear weapons, military personnel**

✓7ᵗʰ Y36.591 **War operation involving other effects of nuclear weapons, civilian**

✓5ᵗʰ Y36.6 **War operations involving biological weapons**

✓6ᵗʰ Y36.6X **War operations involving** biological weapons

✓7ᵗʰ Y36.6X0 **War operations involving biological weapons, military personnel**

✓7ᵗʰ Y36.6X1 **War operations involving biological weapons, civilian**

✓5ᵗʰ Y36.7 **War operations involving chemical weapons and other forms of unconventional warfare**
EXCLUDES 1 *war operations involving incendiary devices (Y36.3-, Y36.5-)*

✓6ᵗʰ Y36.7X **War operations involving** chemical weapons **and other forms of** unconventional warfare

✓7ᵗʰ Y36.7X0 **War operations involving chemical weapons and other forms of unconventional warfare, military personnel**

✓7ᵗʰ Y36.7X1 **War operations involving chemical weapons and other forms of unconventional warfare, civilian**

✓5ᵗʰ Y36.8 **War operations occurring** after cessation of hostilities
War operations classifiable to categories Y36.0-Y36.8 but occurring after cessation of hostilities

✓6ᵗʰ Y36.81 **Explosion of** mine **placed during war operations but exploding after cessation of hostilities**

✓7ᵗʰ Y36.810 **Explosion of mine placed during war operations but exploding after cessation of hostilities, military personnel**

✓7ᵗʰ Y36.811 **Explosion of mine placed during war operations but exploding after cessation of hostilities, civilian**

✓6ᵗʰ Y36.82 **Explosion of** bomb **placed during war operations but exploding after cessation of hostilities**

✓7ᵗʰ Y36.820 **Explosion of bomb placed during war operations but exploding after cessation of hostilities, military personnel**

✓7ᵗʰ Y36.821 **Explosion of bomb placed during war operations but exploding after cessation of hostilities, civilian**

✓6ᵗʰ Y36.88 **Other** war operations occurring after cessation of hostilities

✓7ᵗʰ Y36.880 **Other war operations occurring after cessation of hostilities, military personnel**

✓7ᵗʰ Y36.881 **Other war operations occurring after cessation of hostilities, civilian**

✓6ᵗʰ Y36.89 Unspecified **war operations occurring after cessation of hostilities**

✓7ᵗʰ Y36.890 **Unspecified war operations occurring after cessation of hostilities, military personnel**

✓7ᵗʰ Y36.891 **Unspecified war operations occurring after cessation of hostilities, civilian**

✓5ᵗʰ Y36.9 **Other and unspecified war operations**

✓x7ᵗʰ Y36.90 **War operations, unspecified**

✓x7ᵗʰ Y36.91 **War operations** involving unspecified weapon of mass destruction [WMD]

✓x7ᵗʰ Y36.92 **War operations** involving friendly fire

✓4ᵗʰ **Y37 Military operations**
INCLUDES injuries to military personnel and civilians occurring during peacetime on military property and during routine military exercises and operations
EXCLUDES 1 *military aircraft involved in aircraft accident with civilian aircraft (V97.81-)*
military vehicles involved in transport accident with civilian vehicle (V09.01, V09.21, V19.81, V29.81, V39.81, V49.81, V59.81, V69.81, V79.81)
military watercraft involved in water transport accident with civilian watercraft (V94.81-)
war operations (Y36.-)

The appropriate 7th character is to be added to each code from category Y37.
A initial encounter
D subsequent encounter
S sequela

✓5ᵗʰ Y37.0 **Military operations involving** explosion of marine weapons

✓6ᵗʰ Y37.00 **Military operations involving explosion of** unspecified marine weapon
Military operations involving underwater blast NOS

✓7ᵗʰ Y37.000 **Military operations involving explosion of unspecified marine weapon, military personnel**

✓7ᵗʰ Y37.001 **Military operations involving explosion of unspecified marine weapon, civilian**

✓6ᵗʰ Y37.01 **Military operations involving explosion of** depth-charge

✓7ᵗʰ Y37.010 **Military operations involving explosion of depth-charge, military personnel**

✓7ᵗʰ Y37.011 **Military operations involving explosion of depth-charge, civilian**

✓6ᵗʰ Y37.02 **Military operations involving explosion of** marine mine
Military operations involving explosion of marine mine, at sea or in harbor

✓7ᵗʰ Y37.020 **Military operations involving explosion of marine mine, military personnel**

✓7ᵗʰ Y37.021 **Military operations involving explosion of marine mine, civilian**

✓6ᵗʰ Y37.03 **Military operations involving explosion of** sea-based artillery shell

✓7ᵗʰ Y37.030 **Military operations involving explosion of sea-based artillery shell, military personnel**

✓7ᵗʰ Y37.031 **Military operations involving explosion of sea-based artillery shell, civilian**

✓6ᵗʰ Y37.04 **Military operations involving explosion of** torpedo

✓7ᵗʰ Y37.040 **Military operations involving explosion of torpedo, military personnel**

Chapter 20. External Causes of Morbidity

✓7ᵗʰ **Y37.041** **Military operations involving explosion of torpedo, civilian**

✓6ᵗʰ **Y37.05** **Military operations involving accidental detonation of onboard marine weapons**

    ✓7ᵗʰ **Y37.050** **Military operations involving accidental detonation of onboard marine weapons, military personnel**

    ✓7ᵗʰ **Y37.051** **Military operations involving accidental detonation of onboard marine weapons, civilian**

✓6ᵗʰ **Y37.09** **Military operations involving explosion of other marine weapons**

    ✓7ᵗʰ **Y37.090** **Military operations involving explosion of other marine weapons, military personnel**

    ✓7ᵗʰ **Y37.091** **Military operations involving explosion of other marine weapons, civilian**

✓5ᵗʰ **Y37.1** **Military operations involving destruction of aircraft**

✓6ᵗʰ **Y37.10** **Military operations involving unspecified destruction of aircraft**

    ✓7ᵗʰ **Y37.100** **Military operations involving unspecified destruction of aircraft, military personnel**

    ✓7ᵗʰ **Y37.101** **Military operations involving unspecified destruction of aircraft, civilian**

✓6ᵗʰ **Y37.11** **Military operations involving destruction of aircraft due to enemy fire or explosives**

    Military operations involving destruction of aircraft due to air to air missile

    Military operations involving destruction of aircraft due to explosive placed on aircraft

    Military operations involving destruction of aircraft due to rocket propelled grenade [RPG]

    Military operations involving destruction of aircraft due to small arms fire

    Military operations involving destruction of aircraft due to surface to air missile

    ✓7ᵗʰ **Y37.110** **Military operations involving destruction of aircraft due to enemy fire or explosives, military personnel**

    ✓7ᵗʰ **Y37.111** **Military operations involving destruction of aircraft due to enemy fire or explosives, civilian**

✓6ᵗʰ **Y37.12** **Military operations involving destruction of aircraft due to collision with other aircraft**

    ✓7ᵗʰ **Y37.120** **Military operations involving destruction of aircraft due to collision with other aircraft, military personnel**

    ✓7ᵗʰ **Y37.121** **Military operations involving destruction of aircraft due to collision with other aircraft, civilian**

✓6ᵗʰ **Y37.13** **Military operations involving destruction of aircraft due to onboard fire**

    ✓7ᵗʰ **Y37.130** **Military operations involving destruction of aircraft due to onboard fire, military personnel**

    ✓7ᵗʰ **Y37.131** **Military operations involving destruction of aircraft due to onboard fire, civilian**

✓6ᵗʰ **Y37.14** **Military operations involving destruction of aircraft due to accidental detonation of onboard munitions and explosives**

    ✓7ᵗʰ **Y37.140** **Military operations involving destruction of aircraft due to accidental detonation of onboard munitions and explosives, military personnel**

    ✓7ᵗʰ **Y37.141** **Military operations involving destruction of aircraft due to accidental detonation of onboard munitions and explosives, civilian**

✓6ᵗʰ **Y37.19** **Military operations involving other destruction of aircraft**

    ✓7ᵗʰ **Y37.190** **Military operations involving other destruction of aircraft, military personnel**

    ✓7ᵗʰ **Y37.191** **Military operations involving other destruction of aircraft, civilian**

✓5ᵗʰ **Y37.2** **Military operations involving other explosions and fragments**

EXCLUDES 1 *military operations involving explosion of aircraft (Y37.1-)*

military operations involving explosion of marine weapons (Y37.0-)

military operations involving explosion of nuclear weapons (Y37.5-)

✓6ᵗʰ **Y37.20** **Military operations involving unspecified explosion and fragments**

    Military operations involving air blast NOS

    Military operations involving blast NOS

    Military operations involving blast fragments NOS

    Military operations involving blast wave NOS

    Military operations involving blast wind NOS

    Military operations involving explosion NOS

    Military operations involving explosion of bomb NOS

    ✓7ᵗʰ **Y37.200** **Military operations involving unspecified explosion and fragments, military personnel**

    ✓7ᵗʰ **Y37.201** **Military operations involving unspecified explosion and fragments, civilian**

✓6ᵗʰ **Y37.21** **Military operations involving explosion of aerial bomb**

    ✓7ᵗʰ **Y37.210** **Military operations involving explosion of aerial bomb, military personnel**

    ✓7ᵗʰ **Y37.211** **Military operations involving explosion of aerial bomb, civilian**

✓6ᵗʰ **Y37.22** **Military operations involving explosion of guided missile**

    ✓7ᵗʰ **Y37.220** **Military operations involving explosion of guided missile, military personnel**

    ✓7ᵗʰ **Y37.221** **Military operations involving explosion of guided missile, civilian**

✓6ᵗʰ **Y37.23** **Military operations involving explosion of improvised explosive device [IED]**

    Military operations involving explosion of person-borne improvised explosive device [IED]

    Military operations involving explosion of vehicle-borne improvised explosive device [IED]

    Military operations involving explosion of roadside improvised explosive device [IED]

    ✓7ᵗʰ **Y37.230** **Military operations involving explosion of improvised explosive device [IED], military personnel**

    ✓7ᵗʰ **Y37.231** **Military operations involving explosion of improvised explosive device [IED], civilian**

✓6ᵗʰ **Y37.24** **Military operations involving explosion due to accidental detonation and discharge of own munitions or munitions launch device**

    ✓7ᵗʰ **Y37.240** **Military operations involving explosion due to accidental detonation and discharge of own munitions or munitions launch device, military personnel**

    ✓7ᵗʰ **Y37.241** **Military operations involving explosion due to accidental detonation and discharge of own munitions or munitions launch device, civilian**

✓6ᵗʰ **Y37.25** **Military operations involving fragments from munitions**

    ✓7ᵗʰ **Y37.250** **Military operations involving fragments from munitions, military personnel**

    ✓7ᵗʰ **Y37.251** **Military operations involving fragments from munitions, civilian**

✓6ᵗʰ **Y37.26** **Military operations involving fragments of improvised explosive device [IED]**

    Military operations involving fragments of person-borne improvised explosive device [IED]

    Military operations involving fragments of vehicle-borne improvised explosive device [IED]

    Military operations involving fragments of roadside improvised explosive device [IED]

    ✓7ᵗʰ **Y37.260** **Military operations involving fragments of improvised explosive device [IED], military personnel**

    ✓7ᵗʰ **Y37.261** **Military operations involving fragments of improvised explosive device [IED], civilian**

N Newborn: 0   P Pediatric: 0-17   M Maternity: 12-55   A Adult: 15-124   MCC Major CC Condition   PDxMCC PDx acts as own MCC   CC CC Condition   PDxCC PDx acts as own CC

1208   ICD-10-CM 2016

√6ᵗʰ **Y37.27 Military operations involving fragments from weapons**

√7ᵗʰ **Y37.270 Military operations involving fragments from weapons, military personnel**

√7ᵗʰ **Y37.271 Military operations involving fragments from weapons, civilian**

√6ᵗʰ **Y37.29 Military operations involving other explosions and fragments**
Military operations involving explosion of grenade
Military operations involving explosions of land mine
Military operations involving shrapnel NOS

√7ᵗʰ **Y37.290 Military operations involving other explosions and fragments, military personnel**

√7ᵗʰ **Y37.291 Military operations involving other explosions and fragments, civilian**

√5ᵗʰ **Y37.3 Military operations involving fires, conflagrations and hot substances**
Military operations involving smoke, fumes, and heat from fires, conflagrations and hot substances

EXCLUDES 1   *military operations involving fires and conflagrations aboard military aircraft (Y37.1-)*
military operations involving fires and conflagrations aboard military watercraft (Y37.0-)
military operations involving fires and conflagrations caused indirectly by conventional weapons (Y37.2-)
military operations involving fires and thermal effects of nuclear weapons (Y36.53-)

√6ᵗʰ **Y37.30 Military operations involving unspecified fire, conflagration and hot substance**

√7ᵗʰ **Y37.300 Military operations involving unspecified fire, conflagration and hot substance, military personnel**

√7ᵗʰ **Y37.301 Military operations involving unspecified fire, conflagration and hot substance, civilian**

√6ᵗʰ **Y37.31 Military operations involving gasoline bomb**
Military operations involving incendiary bomb
Military operations involving petrol bomb

√7ᵗʰ **Y37.310 Military operations involving gasoline bomb, military personnel**

√7ᵗʰ **Y37.311 Military operations involving gasoline bomb, civilian**

√6ᵗʰ **Y37.32 Military operations involving incendiary bullet**

√7ᵗʰ **Y37.320 Military operations involving incendiary bullet, military personnel**

√7ᵗʰ **Y37.321 Military operations involving incendiary bullet, civilian**

√6ᵗʰ **Y37.33 Military operations involving flamethrower**

√7ᵗʰ **Y37.330 Military operations involving flamethrower, military personnel**

√7ᵗʰ **Y37.331 Military operations involving flamethrower, civilian**

√6ᵗʰ **Y37.39 Military operations involving other fires, conflagrations and hot substances**

√7ᵗʰ **Y37.390 Military operations involving other fires, conflagrations and hot substances, military personnel**

√7ᵗʰ **Y37.391 Military operations involving other fires, conflagrations and hot substances, civilian**

√5ᵗʰ **Y37.4 Military operations involving firearm discharge and other forms of conventional warfare**

√6ᵗʰ **Y37.41 Military operations involving rubber bullets**

√7ᵗʰ **Y37.410 Military operations involving rubber bullets, military personnel**

√7ᵗʰ **Y37.411 Military operations involving rubber bullets, civilian**

√6ᵗʰ **Y37.42 Military operations involving firearms pellets**

√7ᵗʰ **Y37.420 Military operations involving firearms pellets, military personnel**

√7ᵗʰ **Y37.421 Military operations involving firearms pellets, civilian**

√6ᵗʰ **Y37.43 Military operations involving other firearms discharge**
Military operations involving bullets NOS

EXCLUDES 1   *military operations involving munitions fragments (Y37.25-)*
military operations involving incendiary bullets (Y37.32-)

√7ᵗʰ **Y37.430 Military operations involving other firearms discharge, military personnel**

√7ᵗʰ **Y37.431 Military operations involving other firearms discharge, civilian**

√6ᵗʰ **Y37.44 Military operations involving unarmed hand to hand combat**

EXCLUDES 1   *military operations involving combat using blunt or piercing object (Y37.45-)*
military operations involving intentional restriction of air and airway (Y37.46-)
military operations involving unintentional restriction of air and airway (Y37.47-)

√7ᵗʰ **Y37.440 Military operations involving unarmed hand to hand combat, military personnel**

√7ᵗʰ **Y37.441 Military operations involving unarmed hand to hand combat, civilian**

√6ᵗʰ **Y37.45 Military operations involving combat using blunt or piercing object**

√7ᵗʰ **Y37.450 Military operations involving combat using blunt or piercing object, military personnel**

√7ᵗʰ **Y37.451 Military operations involving combat using blunt or piercing object, civilian**

√6ᵗʰ **Y37.46 Military operations involving intentional restriction of air and airway**

√7ᵗʰ **Y37.460 Military operations involving intentional restriction of air and airway, military personnel**

√7ᵗʰ **Y37.461 Military operations involving intentional restriction of air and airway, civilian**

√6ᵗʰ **Y37.47 Military operations involving unintentional restriction of air and airway**

√7ᵗʰ **Y37.470 Military operations involving unintentional restriction of air and airway, military personnel**

√7ᵗʰ **Y37.471 Military operations involving unintentional restriction of air and airway, civilian**

√6ᵗʰ **Y37.49 Military operations involving other forms of conventional warfare**

√7ᵗʰ **Y37.490 Military operations involving other forms of conventional warfare, military personnel**

√7ᵗʰ **Y37.491 Military operations involving other forms of conventional warfare, civilian**

√5ᵗʰ **Y37.5 Military operations involving nuclear weapons**
Military operation involving dirty bomb NOS

√6ᵗʰ **Y37.50 Military operations involving unspecified effect of nuclear weapon**

√7ᵗʰ **Y37.500 Military operations involving unspecified effect of nuclear weapon, military personnel**

√7ᵗʰ **Y37.501 Military operations involving unspecified effect of nuclear weapon, civilian**

√6ᵗʰ **Y37.51 Military operations involving direct blast effect of nuclear weapon**
Military operations involving blast pressure of nuclear weapon

√7ᵗʰ **Y37.510 Military operations involving direct blast effect of nuclear weapon, military personnel**

√7ᵗʰ **Y37.511 Military operations involving direct blast effect of nuclear weapon, civilian**

Chapter 20. External Causes of Morbidity

Y37.52–Y38.3X2

√6ᵗʰ **Y37.52 Military operations involving indirect blast effect of nuclear weapon**
Military operations involving being thrown by blast of nuclear weapon
Military operations involving being struck or crushed by blast debris of nuclear weapon

√7ᵗʰ **Y37.520 Military operations involving indirect blast effect of nuclear weapon, military personnel**

√7ᵗʰ **Y37.521 Military operations involving indirect blast effect of nuclear weapon, civilian**

√6ᵗʰ **Y37.53 Military operations involving thermal radiation effect of nuclear weapon**
Military operations involving direct heat from nuclear weapon
Military operation involving fireball effects from nuclear weapon

√7ᵗʰ **Y37.530 Military operations involving thermal radiation effect of nuclear weapon, military personnel**

√7ᵗʰ **Y37.531 Military operations involving thermal radiation effect of nuclear weapon, civilian**

√6ᵗʰ **Y37.54 Military operation involving nuclear radiation effects of nuclear weapon**
Military operation involving acute radiation exposure from nuclear weapon
Military operation involving exposure to immediate ionizing radiation from nuclear weapon
Military operation involving fallout exposure from nuclear weapon
Military operation involving secondary effects of nuclear weapons

√7ᵗʰ **Y37.540 Military operation involving nuclear radiation effects of nuclear weapon, military personnel**

√7ᵗʰ **Y37.541 Military operation involving nuclear radiation effects of nuclear weapon, civilian**

√6ᵗʰ **Y37.59 Military operation involving other effects of nuclear weapons**

√7ᵗʰ **Y37.590 Military operation involving other effects of nuclear weapons, military personnel**

√7ᵗʰ **Y37.591 Military operation involving other effects of nuclear weapons, civilian**

√5ᵗʰ **Y37.6 Military operations involving biological weapons**

√6ᵗʰ **Y37.6X Military operations involving biological weapons**

√7ᵗʰ **Y37.6X0 Military operations involving biological weapons, military personnel**

√7ᵗʰ **Y37.6X1 Military operations involving biological weapons, civilian**

√5ᵗʰ **Y37.7 Military operations involving chemical weapons and other forms of unconventional warfare**
EXCLUDES 1 military operations involving incendiary devices (Y36.3-, Y36.5-)

√6ᵗʰ **Y37.7X Military operations involving chemical weapons and other forms of unconventional warfare**

√7ᵗʰ **Y37.7X0 Military operations involving chemical weapons and other forms of unconventional warfare, military personnel**

√7ᵗʰ **Y37.7X1 Military operations involving chemical weapons and other forms of unconventional warfare, civilian**

√5ᵗʰ **Y37.9 Other and unspecified military operations**

√x7ᵗʰ **Y37.90 Military operations, unspecified**

√x7ᵗʰ **Y37.91 Military operations involving unspecified weapon of mass destruction [WMD]**

√x7ᵗʰ **Y37.92 Military operations involving friendly fire**

√4ᵗʰ **Y38 Terrorism**
NOTE These codes are for use to identify injuries resulting from the unlawful use of force or violence against persons or property to intimidate or coerce a Government, the civilian population, or any segment thereof, in furtherance of political or social objective.
Use additional code for place of occurrence (Y92.-)

The appropriate 7th character is to be added to each code from category Y38.
A initial encounter
D subsequent encounter
S sequela

√5ᵗʰ **Y38.0 Terrorism involving explosion of marine weapons**
Terrorism involving depth-charge
Terrorism involving marine mine
Terrorism involving mine NOS, at sea or in harbor
Terrorism involving sea-based artillery shell
Terrorism involving torpedo
Terrorism involving underwater blast

√6ᵗʰ **Y38.0X Terrorism involving explosion of marine weapons**

√7ᵗʰ **Y38.0X1 Terrorism involving explosion of marine weapons, public safety official injured**

√7ᵗʰ **Y38.0X2 Terrorism involving explosion of marine weapons, civilian injured**

√7ᵗʰ **Y38.0X3 Terrorism involving explosion of marine weapons, terrorist injured**

√5ᵗʰ **Y38.1 Terrorism involving destruction of aircraft**
Terrorism involving aircraft burned
Terrorism involving aircraft exploded
Terrorism involving aircraft being shot down
Terrorism involving aircraft used as a weapon

√6ᵗʰ **Y38.1X Terrorism involving destruction of aircraft**

√7ᵗʰ **Y38.1X1 Terrorism involving destruction of aircraft, public safety official injured**

√7ᵗʰ **Y38.1X2 Terrorism involving destruction of aircraft, civilian injured**

√7ᵗʰ **Y38.1X3 Terrorism involving destruction of aircraft, terrorist injured**

√5ᵗʰ **Y38.2 Terrorism involving other explosions and fragments**
Terrorism involving antipersonnel (fragments) bomb
Terrorism involving blast NOS
Terrorism involving explosion NOS
Terrorism involving explosion of breech block
Terrorism involving explosion of cannon block
Terrorism involving explosion (fragments) of artillery shell
Terrorism involving explosion (fragments) of bomb
Terrorism involving explosion (fragments) of grenade
Terrorism involving explosion (fragments) of guided missile
Terrorism involving explosion (fragments) of land mine
Terrorism involving explosion of mortar bomb
Terrorism involving explosion of munitions
Terrorism involving explosion (fragments) of rocket
Terrorism involving explosion (fragments) of shell
Terrorism involving shrapnel
Terrorism involving mine NOS, on land
EXCLUDES 1 terrorism involving explosion of nuclear weapon (Y38.5)
terrorism involving suicide bomber (Y38.81)

√6ᵗʰ **Y38.2X Terrorism involving other explosions and fragments**

√7ᵗʰ **Y38.2X1 Terrorism involving other explosions and fragments, public safety official injured**

√7ᵗʰ **Y38.2X2 Terrorism involving other explosions and fragments, civilian injured**

√7ᵗʰ **Y38.2X3 Terrorism involving other explosions and fragments, terrorist injured**

√5ᵗʰ **Y38.3 Terrorism involving fires, conflagration and hot substances**
Terrorism involving conflagration NOS
Terrorism involving fire NOS
Terrorism involving petrol bomb
EXCLUDES 1 terrorism involving fire or heat of nuclear weapon (Y38.5)

√6ᵗʰ **Y38.3X Terrorism involving fires, conflagration and hot substances**

√7ᵗʰ **Y38.3X1 Terrorism involving fires, conflagration and hot substances, public safety official injured**

√7ᵗʰ **Y38.3X2 Terrorism involving fires, conflagration and hot substances, civilian injured**

N Newborn: 0   P Pediatric: 0-17   M Maternity: 12-55   A Adult: 15-124   MCC Major CC Condition   PDxMCC PDx acts as own MCC   CC CC Condition   PDxCC PDx acts as own CC

1210   ICD-10-CM 2016

✓7th **Y38.3X3** **Terrorism involving fires, conflagration and hot substances,** terrorist **injured**

✓5th **Y38.4** **Terrorism involving firearms**
　　　Terrorism involving carbine bullet
　　　Terrorism involving machine gun bullet
　　　Terrorism involving pellets (shotgun)
　　　Terrorism involving pistol bullet
　　　Terrorism involving rifle bullet
　　　Terrorism involving rubber (rifle) bullet

　　✓6th **Y38.4X** **Terrorism involving** firearms
　　　　✓7th **Y38.4X1** **Terrorism involving firearms,** public safety official **injured**
　　　　✓7th **Y38.4X2** **Terrorism involving firearms,** civilian **injured**
　　　　✓7th **Y38.4X3** **Terrorism involving firearms,** terrorist **injured**

✓5th **Y38.5** **Terrorism involving nuclear weapons**
　　　Terrorism involving blast effects of nuclear weapon
　　　Terrorism involving exposure to ionizing radiation from nuclear weapon
　　　Terrorism involving fireball effect of nuclear weapon
　　　Terrorism involving heat from nuclear weapon

　　✓6th **Y38.5X** **Terrorism involving** nuclear weapons
　　　　✓7th **Y38.5X1** **Terrorism involving nuclear weapons,** public safety official **injured**
　　　　✓7th **Y38.5X2** **Terrorism involving nuclear weapons,** civilian **injured**
　　　　✓7th **Y38.5X3** **Terrorism involving nuclear weapons,** terrorist **injured**

✓5th **Y38.6** **Terrorism involving biological weapons**
　　　Terrorism involving anthrax　　Terrorism involving smallpox
　　　Terrorism involving cholera

　　✓6th **Y38.6X** **Terrorism involving** biological weapons
　　　　✓7th **Y38.6X1** **Terrorism involving biological weapons,** public safety official **injured**
　　　　✓7th **Y38.6X2** **Terrorism involving biological weapons,** civilian **injured**
　　　　✓7th **Y38.6X3** **Terrorism involving biological weapons,** terrorist **injured**

✓5th **Y38.7** **Terrorism involving chemical weapons**
　　　Terrorism involving gases, fumes, chemicals
　　　Terrorism involving hydrogen cyanide
　　　Terrorism involving phosgene
　　　Terrorism involving sarin

　　✓6th **Y38.7X** **Terrorism involving** chemical weapons
　　　　✓7th **Y38.7X1** **Terrorism involving chemical weapons,** public safety official **injured**
　　　　✓7th **Y38.7X2** **Terrorism involving chemical weapons,** civilian **injured**
　　　　✓7th **Y38.7X3** **Terrorism involving chemical weapons,** terrorist **injured**

✓5th **Y38.8** **Terrorism involving other and unspecified means**
　　　Y38.80 **Terrorism involving unspecified means**
　　　　　Terrorism NOS
　　✓6th **Y38.81** **Terrorism involving** suicide bomber
　　　　✓7th **Y38.811** **Terrorism involving suicide bomber,** public safety official **injured**
　　　　✓7th **Y38.812** **Terrorism involving suicide bomber,** civilian **injured**
　　✓6th **Y38.89** **Terrorism involving** other **means**
　　　　Terrorism involving drowning and submersion
　　　　Terrorism involving lasers
　　　　Terrorism involving piercing or stabbing instruments
　　　　✓7th **Y38.891** **Terrorism involving other means,** public safety official **injured**
　　　　✓7th **Y38.892** **Terrorism involving other means,** civilian **injured**
　　　　✓7th **Y38.893** **Terrorism involving other means,** terrorist **injured**

✓5th **Y38.9** **Terrorism, secondary effects**
　　　NOTE This code is for use to identify injuries occurring subsequent to a terrorist attack, not those that are due to the initial terrorist attack.

　　✓6th **Y38.9X** **Terrorism,** secondary effects

✓7th **Y38.9X1** **Terrorism, secondary effects,** public safety official **injured**
✓7th **Y38.9X2** **Terrorism, secondary effects,** civilian **injured**

Complications of medical and surgical care (Y62-Y84)

INCLUDES complications of medical devices
surgical and medical procedures as the cause of abnormal reaction of the patient, or of later complication, without mention of misadventure at the time of the procedure

Misadventures to patients during surgical and medical care (Y62-Y69)

EXCLUDES 2 *breakdown or malfunctioning of medical device (during procedure) (after implantation) (ongoing use) (Y70-Y82)*
surgical and medical procedures as the cause of abnormal reaction of the patient, without mention of misadventure at the time of the procedure (Y83-Y84)

✓4th **Y62** **Failure of** sterile precautions **during surgical and medical care**
　　Y62.0 **Failure of sterile precautions during** surgical operation
　　Y62.1 **Failure of sterile precautions during** infusion or transfusion
　　Y62.2 **Failure of sterile precautions during** kidney dialysis and other perfusion
　　Y62.3 **Failure of sterile precautions during** injection or immunization
　　Y62.4 **Failure of sterile precautions during** endoscopic examination
　　Y62.5 **Failure of sterile precautions during** heart catheterization
　　Y62.6 **Failure of sterile precautions during** aspiration, puncture and other catheterization
　　Y62.8 **Failure of sterile precautions during** other surgical and medical care
　　Y62.9 **Failure of sterile precautions during** unspecified surgical and medical care

✓4th **Y63** **Failure in** dosage **during surgical and medical care**
　　EXCLUDES 2 *accidental overdose of drug or wrong drug given in error (T36-T50)*
　　Y63.0 **Excessive amount of blood or other fluid given during transfusion or infusion**
　　Y63.1 **Incorrect dilution of fluid used during infusion**
　　Y63.2 **Overdose of radiation given during therapy**
　　Y63.3 **Inadvertent exposure of patient to radiation during medical care**
　　Y63.4 **Failure in dosage in electroshock or insulin-shock therapy**
　　Y63.5 **Inappropriate temperature in local application and packing**
　　Y63.6 **Underdosing and nonadministration of necessary drug, medicament or biological substance**
　　Y63.8 **Failure in dosage during other surgical and medical care**
　　Y63.9 **Failure in dosage during unspecified surgical and medical care**

✓4th **Y64** **Contaminated** medical or biological **substances**
　　Y64.0 **Contaminated medical or biological substance,** transfused or infused
　　Y64.1 **Contaminated medical or biological substance,** injected or used for immunization
　　Y64.8 **Contaminated medical or biological substance administered** by other means
　　Y64.9 **Contaminated medical or biological substance administered** by unspecified means
　　　　Administered contaminated medical or biological substance NOS

✓4th **Y65** **Other misadventures during surgical and medical care**
　　Y65.0 **Mismatched blood in transfusion**
　　Y65.1 **Wrong fluid used in infusion**
　　Y65.2 **Failure in suture or ligature during surgical operation**
　　Y65.3 **Endotracheal tube wrongly placed during anesthetic procedure**
　　Y65.4 **Failure to introduce or to remove other tube or instrument**
　　✓5th **Y65.5** **Performance of** wrong procedure (operation)
　　　　11**Y65.51** **Performance of wrong procedure (operation) on correct patient**
　　　　　　Wrong device implanted into correct surgical site
　　　　　　EXCLUDES 1 *performance of correct procedure (operation) on wrong side or body part (Y65.53)*

---

11 Wrong procedure performed edit applies.

✓ Additional Character Required　✓7th Placeholder Alert　Unacceptable PDx　　Manifestation　　Hospital Acquired Condition　　**EXCLUDES 1** Not Coded Here　**EXCLUDES 2** Not Included Here

ICD-10-CM 2016　　1211

11 Y65.52 Performance of procedure (operation) on patient not scheduled for surgery
Performance of procedure (operation) intended for another patient
Performance of procedure (operation) on wrong patient

11 Y65.53 Performance of correct procedure (operation) on wrong side or body part
Performance of correct procedure (operation) on wrong side
Performance of correct procedure (operation) on wrong site

Y65.8 Other specified misadventures **during surgical and medical care**

Y66 Nonadministration of surgical and medical care
Premature cessation of surgical and medical care
EXCLUDES 1 *DNR status (Z66)*
palliative care (Z51.5)

Y69 Unspecified misadventure during surgical and medical care

Medical devices associated with adverse incidents in diagnostic and therapeutic use (Y70-Y82)

INCLUDES breakdown or malfunction of medical devices (during use) (after implantation) (ongoing use)

EXCLUDES 1 *misadventure to patients during surgical and medical care, classifiable to (Y62-Y69)*
later complications following use of medical devices without breakdown or malfunctioning of device (Y83-Y84)

✓4ᵗʰ Y70 Anesthesiology devices associated with adverse incidents

Y70.0 Diagnostic and monitoring anesthesiology devices associated with adverse incidents

Y70.1 Therapeutic (nonsurgical) and rehabilitative anesthesiology devices associated with adverse incidents

Y70.2 Prosthetic and other implants, materials and accessory anesthesiology devices associated with adverse incidents

Y70.3 Surgical instruments, materials and anesthesiology devices (including sutures) associated with adverse incidents

Y70.8 Miscellaneous anesthesiology devices associated with adverse incidents, not elsewhere classified

✓4ᵗʰ Y71 Cardiovascular devices associated with adverse incidents

Y71.0 Diagnostic and monitoring cardiovascular devices associated with adverse incidents

Y71.1 Therapeutic (nonsurgical) and rehabilitative cardiovascular devices associated with adverse incidents

Y71.2 Prosthetic and other implants, materials and accessory cardiovascular devices associated with adverse incidents

Y71.3 Surgical instruments, materials and cardiovascular devices (including sutures) associated with adverse incidents

Y71.8 Miscellaneous cardiovascular devices associated with adverse incidents, not elsewhere classified

✓4ᵗʰ Y72 Otorhinolaryngological devices associated with adverse incidents

Y72.0 Diagnostic and monitoring otorhinolaryngological devices associated with adverse incidents

Y72.1 Therapeutic (nonsurgical) and rehabilitative otorhinolaryngological devices associated with adverse incidents

Y72.2 Prosthetic and other implants, materials and accessory otorhinolaryngological devices associated with adverse incidents

Y72.3 Surgical instruments, materials and otorhinolaryngological devices (including sutures) associated with adverse incidents

Y72.8 Miscellaneous otorhinolaryngological devices associated with adverse incidents, not elsewhere classified

✓4ᵗʰ Y73 Gastroenterology and urology devices associated with adverse incidents

Y73.0 Diagnostic and monitoring gastroenterology and urology devices associated with adverse incidents

Y73.1 Therapeutic (nonsurgical) and rehabilitative gastroenterology and urology devices associated with adverse incidents

Y73.2 Prosthetic and other implants, materials and accessory gastroenterology and urology devices associated with adverse incidents

Y73.3 Surgical instruments, materials and gastroenterology and urology devices (including sutures) associated with adverse incidents

Y73.8 Miscellaneous gastroenterology and urology devices associated with adverse incidents, not elsewhere classified

✓4ᵗʰ Y74 General hospital and personal-use devices associated with adverse incidents

Y74.0 Diagnostic and monitoring general hospital and personal-use devices associated with adverse incidents

Y74.1 Therapeutic (nonsurgical) and rehabilitative general hospital and personal-use devices associated with adverse incidents

Y74.2 Prosthetic and other implants, materials and accessory general hospital and personal-use devices associated with adverse incidents

Y74.3 Surgical instruments, materials and general hospital and personal-use devices (including sutures) associated with adverse incidents

Y74.8 Miscellaneous general hospital and personal-use devices associated with adverse incidents, not elsewhere classified

✓4ᵗʰ Y75 Neurological devices associated with adverse incidents

Y75.0 Diagnostic and monitoring neurological devices associated with adverse incidents

Y75.1 Therapeutic (nonsurgical) and rehabilitative neurological devices associated with adverse incidents

Y75.2 Prosthetic and other implants, materials and neurological devices associated with adverse incidents

Y75.3 Surgical instruments, materials and neurological devices (including sutures) associated with adverse incidents

Y75.8 Miscellaneous neurological devices associated with adverse incidents, not elsewhere classified

✓4ᵗʰ Y76 Obstetric and gynecological devices associated with adverse incidents

Y76.0 Diagnostic and monitoring obstetric and gynecological devices associated with adverse incidents ♀

Y76.1 Therapeutic (nonsurgical) and rehabilitative obstetric and gynecological devices associated with adverse incidents ♀

Y76.2 Prosthetic and other implants, materials and accessory obstetric and gynecological devices associated with adverse incidents ♀

Y76.3 Surgical instruments, materials and obstetric and gynecological devices (including sutures) associated with adverse incidents ♀

Y76.8 Miscellaneous obstetric and gynecological devices associated with adverse incidents, not elsewhere classified ♀

✓4ᵗʰ Y77 Ophthalmic devices associated with adverse incidents

Y77.0 Diagnostic and monitoring ophthalmic devices associated with adverse incidents

Y77.1 Therapeutic (nonsurgical) and rehabilitative ophthalmic devices associated with adverse incidents

Y77.2 Prosthetic and other implants, materials and accessory ophthalmic devices associated with adverse incidents

Y77.3 Surgical instruments, materials and ophthalmic devices (including sutures) associated with adverse incidents

Y77.8 Miscellaneous ophthalmic devices associated with adverse incidents, not elsewhere classified

✓4ᵗʰ Y78 Radiological devices associated with adverse incidents

Y78.0 Diagnostic and monitoring radiological devices associated with adverse incidents

Y78.1 Therapeutic (nonsurgical) and rehabilitative radiological devices associated with adverse incidents

Y78.2 Prosthetic and other implants, materials and accessory radiological devices associated with adverse incidents

Y78.3 Surgical instruments, materials and radiological devices (including sutures) associated with adverse incidents

Y78.8 Miscellaneous radiological devices associated with adverse incidents, not elsewhere classified

✓4ᵗʰ Y79 Orthopedic devices associated with adverse incidents

Y79.0 Diagnostic and monitoring orthopedic devices associated with adverse incidents

Y79.1 Therapeutic (nonsurgical) and rehabilitative orthopedic devices associated with adverse incidents

Y79.2 Prosthetic and other implants, materials and accessory orthopedic devices associated with adverse incidents

---

11 Wrong procedure performed edit applies.

Y79.3   Surgical instruments, materials and orthopedic devices (including sutures) associated with adverse incidents

Y79.8   Miscellaneous orthopedic devices associated with adverse incidents, not elsewhere classified

✅4ᵗʰ **Y80   Physical medicine devices associated with adverse incidents**

Y80.0   Diagnostic and monitoring physical medicine devices associated with adverse incidents

Y80.1   Therapeutic (nonsurgical) and rehabilitative physical medicine devices associated with adverse incidents

Y80.2   Prosthetic and other implants, materials and accessory physical medicine devices associated with adverse incidents

Y80.3   Surgical instruments, materials and physical medicine devices (including sutures) associated with adverse incidents

Y80.8   Miscellaneous physical medicine devices associated with adverse incidents, not elsewhere classified

✅4ᵗʰ **Y81   General- and plastic-surgery devices associated with adverse incidents**

Y81.0   Diagnostic and monitoring general- and plastic-surgery devices associated with adverse incidents

Y81.1   Therapeutic (nonsurgical) and rehabilitative general- and plastic-surgery devices associated with adverse incidents

Y81.2   Prosthetic and other implants, materials and accessory general- and plastic-surgery devices associated with adverse incidents

Y81.3   Surgical instruments, materials and general- and plastic-surgery devices (including sutures) associated with adverse incidents

Y81.8   Miscellaneous general- and plastic-surgery devices associated with adverse incidents, not elsewhere classified

✅4ᵗʰ **Y82   Other and unspecified medical devices associated with adverse incidents**

Y82.8   Other medical devices associated with adverse incidents

Y82.9   Unspecified medical devices associated with adverse incidents

Surgical and other medical procedures as the cause of abnormal reaction of the patient, or of later complication, without mention of misadventure at the time of the procedure (Y83-Y84)

EXCLUDES 1   misadventures to patients during surgical and medical care, classifiable to (Y62-Y69)

✅4ᵗʰ **Y83   Surgical operation and other surgical procedures as the cause of abnormal reaction of the patient, or of later complication, without mention of misadventure at the time of the procedure**

Y83.0   Surgical operation with transplant of whole organ as the cause of abnormal reaction of the patient, or of later complication, without mention of misadventure at the time of the procedure

Y83.1   Surgical operation with implant of artificial internal device as the cause of abnormal reaction of the patient, or of later complication, without mention of misadventure at the time of the procedure

Y83.2   Surgical operation with anastomosis, bypass or graft as the cause of abnormal reaction of the patient, or of later complication, without mention of misadventure at the time of the procedure

Y83.3   Surgical operation with formation of external stoma as the cause of abnormal reaction of the patient, or of later complication, without mention of misadventure at the time of the procedure

Y83.4   Other reconstructive surgery as the cause of abnormal reaction of the patient, or of later complication, without mention of misadventure at the time of the procedure

Y83.5   Amputation of limb(s) as the cause of abnormal reaction of the patient, or of later complication, without mention of misadventure at the time of the procedure

Y83.6   Removal of other organ (partial) (total) as the cause of abnormal reaction of the patient, or of later complication, without mention of misadventure at the time of the procedure

Y83.8   Other surgical procedures as the cause of abnormal reaction of the patient, or of later complication, without mention of misadventure at the time of the procedure

Y83.9   Surgical procedure, unspecified as the cause of abnormal reaction of the patient, or of later complication, without mention of misadventure at the time of the procedure

✅4ᵗʰ **Y84   Other medical procedures as the cause of abnormal reaction of the patient, or of later complication, without mention of misadventure at the time of the procedure**

Y84.0   Cardiac catheterization as the cause of abnormal reaction of the patient, or of later complication, without mention of misadventure at the time of the procedure

Y84.1   Kidney dialysis as the cause of abnormal reaction of the patient, or of later complication, without mention of misadventure at the time of the procedure

Y84.2   Radiological procedure and radiotherapy as the cause of abnormal reaction of the patient, or of later complication, without mention of misadventure at the time of the procedure

Y84.3   Shock therapy as the cause of abnormal reaction of the patient, or of later complication, without mention of misadventure at the time of the procedure

Y84.4   Aspiration of fluid as the cause of abnormal reaction of the patient, or of later complication, without mention of misadventure at the time of the procedure

Y84.5   Insertion of gastric or duodenal sound as the cause of abnormal reaction of the patient, or of later complication, without mention of misadventure at the time of the procedure

Y84.6   Urinary catheterization as the cause of abnormal reaction of the patient, or of later complication, without mention of misadventure at the time of the procedure

Y84.7   Blood-sampling as the cause of abnormal reaction of the patient, or of later complication, without mention of misadventure at the time of the procedure

Y84.8   Other medical procedures as the cause of abnormal reaction of the patient, or of later complication, without mention of misadventure at the time of the procedure
    AHA: 2014, 4Q, 24

Y84.9   Medical procedure, unspecified as the cause of abnormal reaction of the patient, or of later complication, without mention of misadventure at the time of the procedure

Supplementary factors related to causes of morbidity classified elsewhere (Y90-Y99)

NOTE   These categories may be used to provide supplementary information concerning causes of morbidity. They are not to be used for single-condition coding.

✅4ᵗʰ **Y90   Evidence of alcohol involvement determined by blood alcohol level**

Code first any associated alcohol related disorders (F10)

Y90.0   Blood alcohol level of less than 20 mg/100 ml

Y90.1   Blood alcohol level of 20-39 mg/100 ml

Y90.2   Blood alcohol level of 40-59 mg/100 ml

Y90.3   Blood alcohol level of 60-79 mg/100 ml

Y90.4   Blood alcohol level of 80-99 mg/100 ml

Y90.5   Blood alcohol level of 100-119 mg/100 ml

Y90.6   Blood alcohol level of 120-199 mg/100 ml

Y90.7   Blood alcohol level of 200-239 mg/100 ml

Y90.8   Blood alcohol level of 240 mg/100 ml or more

Y90.9   Presence of alcohol in blood, level not specified

✅4ᵗʰ **Y92   Place of occurrence of the external cause**

The following category is for use, when relevant, to identify the place of occurrence of the external cause. Use in conjunction with an activity code.

Place of occurrence should be recorded only at the initial encounter for treatment

✅5ᵗʰ   Y92.0   Non-institutional (private) residence as the place of occurrence of the external cause

    EXCLUDES 1   abandoned or derelict house (Y92.89)
      home under construction but not yet occupied (Y92.6-)
      institutional place of residence (Y92.1-)

    ✅6ᵗʰ   Y92.00   Unspecified non-institutional (private) residence as the place of occurrence of the external cause

       Y92.000   Kitchen of unspecified non-institutional (private) residence as the place of occurrence of the external cause

       Y92.001   Dining room of unspecified non-institutional (private) residence as the place of occurrence of the external cause

✅ Additional Character Required   ✅×7ᵗʰ Placeholder Alert   Unacceptable PDx   Manifestation   Hospital Acquired Condition   EXCLUDES 1 Not Coded Here   EXCLUDES 2 Not Included Here

ICD-10-CM 2016   1213

Y92.002 **Bathroom** of unspecified non-institutional (private) residence single-family (private) house as the place of occurrence of the external cause

Y92.003 **Bedroom** of unspecified non-institutional (private) residence as the place of occurrence of the external cause

Y92.007 **Garden or yard** of unspecified non-institutional (private) residence as the place of occurrence of the external cause

Y92.008 **Other** place in unspecified non-institutional (private) residence as the place of occurrence of the external cause

Y92.009 **Unspecified** place in unspecified non-institutional (private) residence as the place of occurrence of the external cause
　　　Home (NOS) as the place of occurrence of the external cause

√6ᵗʰ **Y92.01** **Single-family** non-institutional (private) house as the place of occurrence of the external cause
　　　Farmhouse as the place of occurrence of the external cause
　　　　EXCLUDES 1　barn (Y92.71)
　　　　　chicken coop or hen house (Y92.72)
　　　　　farm field (Y92.73)
　　　　　orchard (Y92.74)
　　　　　single family mobile home or trailer (Y92.02-)
　　　　　slaughter house (Y92.86)

Y92.010 **Kitchen** of single-family (private) house as the place of occurrence of the external cause

Y92.011 **Dining room** of single-family (private) house as the place of occurrence of the external cause

Y92.012 **Bathroom** of single-family (private) house as the place of occurrence of the external cause

Y92.013 **Bedroom** of single-family (private) house as the place of occurrence of the external cause

Y92.014 **Private driveway** to single-family (private) house as the place of occurrence of the external cause

Y92.015 **Private garage** of single-family (private) house as the place of occurrence of the external cause

Y92.016 **Swimming-pool** in single-family (private) house or garden as the place of occurrence of the external cause

Y92.017 **Garden or yard** in single-family (private) house as the place of occurrence of the external cause

Y92.018 **Other** place in single-family (private) house as the place of occurrence of the external cause

Y92.019 **Unspecified** place in single-family (private) house as the place of occurrence of the external cause

√6ᵗʰ **Y92.02** **Mobile home** as the place of occurrence of the external cause

Y92.020 **Kitchen** in mobile home as the place of occurrence of the external cause

Y92.021 **Dining room** in mobile home as the place of occurrence of the external cause

Y92.022 **Bathroom** in mobile home as the place of occurrence of the external cause

Y92.023 **Bedroom** in mobile home as the place of occurrence of the external cause

Y92.024 **Driveway** of mobile home as the place of occurrence of the external cause

Y92.025 **Garage** of mobile home as the place of occurrence of the external cause

Y92.026 **Swimming-pool** of mobile home as the place of occurrence of the external cause

Y92.027 **Garden or yard** of mobile home as the place of occurrence of the external cause

Y92.028 **Other** place in mobile home as the place of occurrence of the external cause

Y92.029 **Unspecified** place in mobile home as the place of occurrence of the external cause

√6ᵗʰ **Y92.03** **Apartment** as the place of occurrence of the external cause
　　　Condominium as the place of occurrence of the external cause
　　　Co-op apartment as the place of occurrence of the external cause

Y92.030 **Kitchen** in apartment as the place of occurrence of the external cause

Y92.031 **Bathroom** in apartment as the place of occurrence of the external cause

Y92.032 **Bedroom** in apartment as the place of occurrence of the external cause

Y92.038 **Other** place in apartment as the place of occurrence of the external cause

Y92.039 **Unspecified** place in apartment as the place of occurrence of the external cause

√6ᵗʰ **Y92.04** **Boarding-house** as the place of occurrence of the external cause

Y92.040 **Kitchen** in boarding-house as the place of occurrence of the external cause

Y92.041 **Bathroom** in boarding-house as the place of occurrence of the external cause

Y92.042 **Bedroom** in boarding-house as the place of occurrence of the external cause

Y92.043 **Driveway** of boarding-house as the place of occurrence of the external cause

Y92.044 **Garage** of boarding-house as the place of occurrence of the external cause

Y92.045 **Swimming-pool** of boarding-house as the place of occurrence of the external cause

Y92.046 **Garden or yard** of boarding-house as the place of occurrence of the external cause

Y92.048 **Other** place in boarding-house as the place of occurrence of the external cause

Y92.049 **Unspecified** place in boarding-house as the place of occurrence of the external cause

√6ᵗʰ **Y92.09** **Other** non-institutional residence as the place of occurrence of the external cause

Y92.090 **Kitchen** in other non-institutional residence as the place of occurrence of the external cause

Y92.091 **Bathroom** in other non-institutional residence as the place of occurrence of the external cause

Y92.092 **Bedroom** in other non-institutional residence as the place of occurrence of the external cause

Y92.093 **Driveway** of other non-institutional residence as the place of occurrence of the external cause

Y92.094 **Garage** of other non-institutional residence as the place of occurrence of the external cause

Y92.095 **Swimming-pool** of other non-institutional residence as the place of occurrence of the external cause

Y92.096 **Garden** or yard of other non-institutional residence as the place of occurrence of the external cause

Y92.098 **Other** place in other non-institutional residence as the place of occurrence of the external cause

Y92.099 **Unspecified** place in other non-institutional residence as the place of occurrence of the external cause

√5ᵗʰ **Y92.1** **Institutional** (nonprivate) residence as the place of occurrence of the external cause

Y92.10 **Unspecified** residential institution as the place of occurrence of the external cause

√6ᵗʰ **Y92.11** **Children's home and orphanage** as the place of occurrence of the external cause

Y92.110 **Kitchen** in children's home and orphanage as the place of occurrence of the external cause

Y92.111 **Bathroom** in children's home and orphanage as the place of occurrence of the external cause

Ⓝ Newborn: 0　Ⓟ Pediatric: 0-17　Ⓜ Maternity: 12-55　Ⓐ Adult: 15-124　MCC Major CC Condition　PDx MCC PDx acts as own MCC　CC CC Condition　PDx CC PDx acts as own CC

Y92.002–Y92.111

1214　　　　ICD-10-CM 2016

Y92.112   **Bedroom** in children's home and orphanage as the place of occurrence of the external cause

Y92.113   **Driveway** of children's home and orphanage as the place of occurrence of the external cause

Y92.114   **Garage** of children's home and orphanage as the place of occurrence of the external cause

Y92.115   **Swimming-pool** of children's home and orphanage as the place of occurrence of the external cause

Y92.116   **Garden or yard** of children's home and orphanage as the place of occurrence of the external cause

Y92.118   **Other** place in children's home and orphanage as the place of occurrence of the external cause

Y92.119   **Unspecified** place in children's home and orphanage as the place of occurrence of the external cause

✓6ᵗʰ   **Y92.12**   **Nursing home** as the place of occurrence of the external cause

     Home for the sick as the place of occurrence of the external cause
     Hospice as the place of occurrence of the external cause

Y92.120   **Kitchen** in nursing home as the place of occurrence of the external cause

Y92.121   **Bathroom** in nursing home as the place of occurrence of the external cause

Y92.122   **Bedroom** in nursing home as the place of occurrence of the external cause

Y92.123   **Driveway** of nursing home as the place of occurrence of the external cause

Y92.124   **Garage** of nursing home as the place of occurrence of the external cause

Y92.125   **Swimming-pool** of nursing home as the place of occurrence of the external cause

Y92.126   **Garden or yard** of nursing home as the place of occurrence of the external cause

Y92.128   **Other** place in nursing home as the place of occurrence of the external cause

Y92.129   **Unspecified** place in nursing home as the place of occurrence of the external cause

✓6ᵗʰ   **Y92.13**   **Military base** as the place of occurrence of the external cause

     EXCLUDES 1   *military training grounds (Y92.83)*

Y92.130   **Kitchen** on military base as the place of occurrence of the external cause

Y92.131   **Mess hall** on military base as the place of occurrence of the external cause

Y92.133   **Barracks** on military base as the place of occurrence of the external cause

Y92.135   **Garage** on military base as the place of occurrence of the external cause

Y92.136   **Swimming-pool** on military base as the place of occurrence of the external cause

Y92.137   **Garden or yard** on military base as the place of occurrence of the external cause

Y92.138   **Other** place on military base as the place of occurrence of the external cause

Y92.139   **Unspecified** place military base as the place of occurrence of the external cause

✓6ᵗʰ   **Y92.14**   **Prison** as the place of occurrence of the external cause

Y92.140   **Kitchen** in prison as the place of occurrence of the external cause

Y92.141   **Dining room** in prison as the place of occurrence of the external cause

Y92.142   **Bathroom** in prison as the place of occurrence of the external cause

Y92.143   **Cell** of prison as the place of occurrence of the external cause

Y92.146   **Swimming-pool** of prison as the place of occurrence of the external cause

Y92.147   **Courtyard** of prison as the place of occurrence of the external cause

Y92.148   **Other** place in prison as the place of occurrence of the external cause

Y92.149   **Unspecified** place in prison as the place of occurrence of the external cause

✓6ᵗʰ   **Y92.15**   **Reform school** as the place of occurrence of the external cause

Y92.150   **Kitchen** in reform school as the place of occurrence of the external cause

Y92.151   **Dining room** in reform school as the place of occurrence of the external cause

Y92.152   **Bathroom** in reform school as the place of occurrence of the external cause

Y92.153   **Bedroom** in reform school as the place of occurrence of the external cause

Y92.154   **Driveway** of reform school as the place of occurrence of the external cause

Y92.155   **Garage** of reform school as the place of occurrence of the external cause

Y92.156   **Swimming-pool** of reform school as the place of occurrence of the external cause

Y92.157   **Garden or yard** of reform school as the place of occurrence of the external cause

Y92.158   **Other** place in reform school as the place of occurrence of the external cause

Y92.159   **Unspecified** place in reform school as the place of occurrence of the external cause

✓6ᵗʰ   **Y92.16**   **School dormitory** as the place of occurrence of the external cause

     EXCLUDES 1   *reform school as the place of occurrence of the external cause (Y92.15-)*
         school buildings and grounds as the place of occurrence of the external cause (Y92.2-)
         school sports and athletic areas as the place of occurrence of the external cause (Y92.3-)

Y92.160   **Kitchen** in school dormitory as the place of occurrence of the external cause

Y92.161   **Dining room** in school dormitory as the place of occurrence of the external cause

Y92.162   **Bathroom** in school dormitory as the place of occurrence of the external cause

Y92.163   **Bedroom** in school dormitory as the place of occurrence of the external cause

Y92.168   **Other** place in school dormitory as the place of occurrence of the external cause

Y92.169   **Unspecified** place in school dormitory as the place of occurrence of the external cause

✓6ᵗʰ   **Y92.19**   **Other specified residential institution** as the place of occurrence of the external cause

Y92.190   **Kitchen** in other specified residential institution as the place of occurrence of the external cause

Y92.191   **Dining** room in other specified residential institution as the place of occurrence of the external cause

Y92.192   **Bathroom** in other specified residential institution as the place of occurrence of the external cause

Y92.193   **Bedroom** in other specified residential institution as the place of occurrence of the external cause

Y92.194   **Driveway** of other specified residential institution as the place of occurrence of the external cause

Y92.195   **Garage** of other specified residential institution as the place of occurrence of the external cause

Y92.196   **Pool** of other specified residential institution as the place of occurrence of the external cause

Y92.197   **Garden or yard** of other specified residential institution as the place of occurrence of the external cause

Y92.198   **Other** place in other specified residential institution as the place of occurrence of the external cause

Y92.199   **Unspecified** place in other specified residential institution as the place of occurrence of the external cause

---

✓ Additional Character Required   ✓x7ᵗʰ Placeholder Alert   Unacceptable PDx   Manifestation   Hospital Acquired Condition   **EXCLUDES 1** Not Coded Here   **EXCLUDES 2** Not Included Here

√5th **Y92.2 School, other institution and public administrative area as the place of occurrence of the external cause**

Building and adjacent grounds used by the general public or by a particular group of the public

EXCLUDES 1 *building under construction as the place of occurrence of the external cause (Y92.6)*

residential institution as the place of occurrence of the external cause (Y92.1)

school dormitory as the place of occurrence of the external cause (Y92.16-)

sports and athletics area of schools as the place of occurrence of the external cause (Y92.3-)

√6th **Y92.21 School (private) (public) (state) as the place of occurrence of the external cause**

Y92.210 Daycare center as the place of occurrence of the external cause

Y92.211 Elementary school as the place of occurrence of the external cause

Kindergarten as the place of occurrence of the external cause

Y92.212 Middle school as the place of occurrence of the external cause

Y92.213 High school as the place of occurrence of the external cause

AHA: 2012, 4Q, 108

Y92.214 College as the place of occurrence of the external cause

University as the place of occurrence of the external cause

Y92.215 Trade school as the place of occurrence of the external cause

Y92.218 Other school as the place of occurrence of the external cause

Y92.219 Unspecified school as the place of occurrence of the external cause

Y92.22 Religious institution as the place of occurrence of the external cause

Church as the place of occurrence of the external cause

Mosque as the place of occurrence of the external cause

Synagogue as the place of occurrence of the external cause

√6th **Y92.23 Hospital as the place of occurrence of the external cause**

EXCLUDES 1 *ambulatory (outpatient) health services establishments (Y92.53-)*

home for the sick as the place of occurrence of the external cause (Y92.12-)

hospice as the place of occurrence of the external cause (Y92.12-)

nursing home as the place of occurrence of the external cause (Y92.12-)

Y92.230 Patient room in hospital as the place of occurrence of the external cause

Y92.231 Patient bathroom in hospital as the place of occurrence of the external cause

Y92.232 Corridor of hospital as the place of occurrence of the external cause

Y92.233 Cafeteria of hospital as the place of occurrence of the external cause

Y92.234 Operating room of hospital as the place of occurrence of the external cause

Y92.238 Other place in hospital as the place of occurrence of the external cause

Y92.239 Unspecified place in hospital as the place of occurrence of the external cause

√6th **Y92.24 Public administrative building as the place of occurrence of the external cause**

Y92.240 Courthouse as the place of occurrence of the external cause

Y92.241 Library as the place of occurrence of the external cause

Y92.242 Post office as the place of occurrence of the external cause

Y92.243 City hall as the place of occurrence of the external cause

Y92.248 Other public administrative building as the place of occurrence of the external cause

√6th **Y92.25 Cultural building as the place of occurrence of the external cause**

Y92.250 Art Gallery as the place of occurrence of the external cause

Y92.251 Museum as the place of occurrence of the external cause

Y92.252 Music hall as the place of occurrence of the external cause

Y92.253 Opera house as the place of occurrence of the external cause

Y92.254 Theater (live) as the place of occurrence of the external cause

Y92.258 Other cultural public building as the place of occurrence of the external cause

Y92.26 Movie house or cinema as the place of occurrence of the external cause

Y92.29 Other specified public building as the place of occurrence of the external cause

Assembly hall as the place of occurrence of the external cause

Clubhouse as the place of occurrence of the external cause

√5th **Y92.3 Sports and athletics area as the place of occurrence of the external cause**

√6th **Y92.31 Athletic court as the place of occurrence of the external cause**

EXCLUDES 1 *tennis court in private home or garden (Y92.09)*

Y92.310 Basketball court as the place of occurrence of the external cause

Y92.311 Squash court as the place of occurrence of the external cause

Y92.312 Tennis court as the place of occurrence of the external cause

Y92.318 Other athletic court as the place of occurrence of the external cause

√6th **Y92.32 Athletic field as the place of occurrence of the external cause**

Y92.320 Baseball field as the place of occurrence of the external cause

Y92.321 Football field as the place of occurrence of the external cause

Y92.322 Soccer field as the place of occurrence of the external cause

Y92.328 Other athletic field as the place of occurrence of the external cause

Cricket field as the place of occurrence of the external cause

Hockey field as the place of occurrence of the external cause

√6th **Y92.33 Skating rink as the place of occurrence of the external cause**

Y92.330 Ice skating rink (indoor) (outdoor) as the place of occurrence of the external cause

Y92.331 Roller skating rink as the place of occurrence of the external cause

Y92.34 Swimming pool (public) as the place of occurrence of the external cause

EXCLUDES 1 *swimming pool in private home or garden (Y92.016)*

Y92.39 Other specified sports and athletic area as the place of occurrence of the external cause

Golf-course as the place of occurrence of the external cause

Gymnasium as the place of occurrence of the external cause

Riding-school as the place of occurrence of the external cause

Stadium as the place of occurrence of the external cause

N Newborn: 0   P Pediatric: 0-17   M Maternity: 12-55   A Adult: 15-124   MCC Major CC Condition   PDxMCC PDx acts as own MCC   CC CC Condition   PDxCC PDx acts as own CC

1216   ICD-10-CM 2016

✓5th **Y92.4 Street, highway and other paved roadways as the place of occurrence of the external cause**
> EXCLUDES 1 *private driveway of residence (Y92.014, Y92.024, Y92.043, Y92.093, Y92.113, Y92.123, Y92.154, Y92.194)*

✓6th **Y92.41 Street and highway as the place of occurrence of the external cause**

Y92.410 Unspecified street and highway as the place of occurrence of the external cause
> Road NOS as the place of occurrence of the external cause

Y92.411 Interstate highway as the place of occurrence of the external cause
> Freeway as the place of occurrence of the external cause
> Motorway as the place of occurrence of the external cause

Y92.412 Parkway as the place of occurrence of the external cause

Y92.413 State road as the place of occurrence of the external cause

Y92.414 Local residential or business street as the place of occurrence of the external cause

Y92.415 Exit ramp or entrance ramp of street or highway as the place of occurrence of the external cause

✓6th **Y92.48 Other paved roadways as the place of occurrence of the external cause**

Y92.480 Sidewalk as the place of occurrence of the external cause

Y92.481 Parking lot as the place of occurrence of the external cause

Y92.482 Bike path as the place of occurrence of the external cause

Y92.488 Other paved roadways as the place of occurrence of the external cause

✓5th **Y92.5 Trade and service area as the place of occurrence of the external cause**
> EXCLUDES 1 *garage in private home (Y92.015)*
> *schools and other public administration buildings (Y92.2-)*

✓6th **Y92.51 Private commercial establishments as the place of occurrence of the external cause**

Y92.510 Bank as the place of occurrence of the external cause

Y92.511 Restaurant or café as the place of occurrence of the external cause

Y92.512 Supermarket, store or market as the place of occurrence of the external cause

Y92.513 Shop (commercial) as the place of occurrence of the external cause

✓6th **Y92.52 Service areas as the place of occurrence of the external cause**

Y92.520 Airport as the place of occurrence of the external cause

Y92.521 Bus station as the place of occurrence of the external cause

Y92.522 Railway station as the place of occurrence of the external cause

Y92.523 Highway rest stop as the place of occurrence of the external cause

Y92.524 Gas station as the place of occurrence of the external cause
> Petroleum station as the place of occurrence of the external cause
> Service station as the place of occurrence of the external cause

✓6th **Y92.53 Ambulatory health services establishments as the place of occurrence of the external cause**

Y92.530 Ambulatory surgery center as the place of occurrence of the external cause
> Outpatient surgery center, including that connected with a hospital as the place of occurrence of the external cause
> Same day surgery center, including that connected with a hospital as the place of occurrence of the external cause

Y92.531 Health care provider office as the place of occurrence of the external cause
> Physician office as the place of occurrence of the external cause

Y92.532 Urgent care center as the place of occurrence of the external cause

Y92.538 Other ambulatory health services establishments as the place of occurrence of the external cause

Y92.59 Other trade areas as the place of occurrence of the external cause
> Office building as the place of occurrence of the external cause
> Casino as the place of occurrence of the external cause
> Garage (commercial) as the place of occurrence of the external cause
> Hotel as the place of occurrence of the external cause
> Radio or television station as the place of occurrence of the external cause
> Shopping mall as the place of occurrence of the external cause
> Warehouse as the place of occurrence of the external cause

✓5th **Y92.6 Industrial and construction area as the place of occurrence of the external cause**

Y92.61 Building [any] under construction as the place of occurrence of the external cause

Y92.62 Dock or shipyard as the place of occurrence of the external cause
> Dockyard as the place of occurrence of the external cause
> Dry dock as the place of occurrence of the external cause
> Shipyard as the place of occurrence of the external cause

Y92.63 Factory as the place of occurrence of the external cause
> Factory building as the place of occurrence of the external cause
> Factory premises as the place of occurrence of the external cause
> Industrial yard as the place of occurrence of the external cause

Y92.64 Mine or pit as the place of occurrence of the external cause
> Mine as the place of occurrence of the external cause

Y92.65 Oil rig as the place of occurrence of the external cause
> Pit (coal) (gravel) (sand) as the place of occurrence of the external cause

Y92.69 Other specified industrial and construction area as the place of occurrence of the external cause
> Gasworks as the place of occurrence of the external cause
> Power-station (coal) (nuclear) (oil) as the place of occurrence of the external cause
> Tunnel under construction as the place of occurrence of the external cause
> Workshop as the place of occurrence of the external cause

✓5th **Y92.7 Farm as the place of occurrence of the external cause**
> Ranch as the place of occurrence of the external cause
> EXCLUDES 1 *farmhouse and home premises of farm (Y92.01-)*

Y92.71 Barn as the place of occurrence of the external cause

Y92.72 Chicken coop as the place of occurrence of the external cause
> Hen house as the place of occurrence of the external cause

Y92.73 Farm field as the place of occurrence of the external cause

Y92.74 Orchard as the place of occurrence of the external cause

Y92.79 Other farm location as the place of occurrence of the external cause

✓5th **Y92.8 Other places as the place of occurrence of the external cause**

✓6th **Y92.81 Transport vehicle as the place of occurrence of the external cause**
> EXCLUDES 1 *transport accidents (V00-V99)*

Y92.810 Car as the place of occurrence of the external cause

✔ Additional Character Required   ✔x7th Placeholder Alert   Unacceptable PDx   Manifestation   Hospital Acquired Condition   EXCLUDES 1 Not Coded Here   EXCLUDES 2 Not Included Here

Chapter 20. External Causes of Morbidity

Y92.811   **Bus** as the place of occurrence of the external cause

Y92.812   **Truck** as the place of occurrence of the external cause

Y92.813   **Airplane** as the place of occurrence of the external cause

Y92.814   **Boat** as the place of occurrence of the external cause

Y92.815   **Train** as the place of occurrence of the external cause

Y92.816   **Subway car** as the place of occurrence of the external cause

Y92.818   **Other transport vehicle** as the place of occurrence of the external cause

✓6ᵗʰ **Y92.82**   **Wilderness area**

Y92.820   **Desert** as the place of occurrence of the external cause

Y92.821   **Forest** as the place of occurrence of the external cause

Y92.828   **Other wilderness area** as the place of occurrence of the external cause
Swamp as the place of occurrence of the external cause
Mountain as the place of occurrence of the external cause
Marsh as the place of occurrence of the external cause
Prairie as the place of occurrence of the external cause

✓6ᵗʰ **Y92.83**   **Recreation area** as the place of occurrence of the external cause

Y92.830   **Public park** as the place of occurrence of the external cause

Y92.831   **Amusement park** as the place of occurrence of the external cause

Y92.832   **Beach** as the place of occurrence of the external cause
Seashore as the place of occurrence of the external cause

Y92.833   **Campsite** as the place of occurrence of the external cause

Y92.834   **Zoological garden (Zoo)** as the place of occurrence of the external cause

Y92.838   **Other recreation area** as the place of occurrence of the external cause

Y92.84   **Military training ground** as the place of occurrence of the external cause

Y92.85   **Railroad track** as the place of occurrence of the external cause

Y92.86   **Slaughter house** as the place of occurrence of the external cause

Y92.89   **Other specified places** as the place of occurrence of the external cause
Derelict house as the place of occurrence of the external cause

Y92.9   **Unspecified place or not applicable**

✓4ᵗʰ **Y93**   **Activity codes**

> **NOTE**   Category Y93 is provided for use to indicate the activity of the person seeking healthcare for an injury or health condition, such as a heart attack while shoveling snow, which resulted from, or was contributed to, by the activity. These codes are appropriate for use for both acute injuries, such as those from chapter 19, and conditions that are due to the long-term, cumulative effects of an activity, such as those from chapter 13. They are also appropriate for use with external cause codes for cause and intent if identifying the activity provides additional information on the event. These codes should be used in conjunction with codes for external cause status (Y99) and place of occurrence (Y92).

This section contains the following broad activity categories:

Y93.Ø   Activities involving walking and running
Y93.1   Activities involving water and water craft
Y93.2   Activities involving ice and snow
Y93.3   Activities involving climbing, rappelling, and jumping off
Y93.4   Activities involving dancing and other rhythmic movement
Y93.5   Activities involving other sports and athletics played individually
Y93.6   Activities involving other sports and athletics played as a team or group
Y93.7   Activities involving other specified sports and athletics
Y93.A   Activities involving other cardiorespiratory exercise
Y93.B   Activities involving other muscle strengthening exercises
Y93.C   Activities involving computer technology and electronic devices
Y93.D   Activities involving arts and handcrafts
Y93.E   Activities involving personal hygiene and interior property and clothing maintenance
Y93.F   Activities involving caregiving
Y93.G   Activities involving food preparation, cooking and grilling
Y93.H   Activities involving exterior property and land maintenance, building and construction
Y93.I   Activities involving roller coasters and other types of external motion
Y93.J   Activities involving playing musical instrument
Y93.K   Activities involving animal care
Y93.8   Activities, other specified
Y93.9   Activity, unspecified

✓5ᵗʰ **Y93.Ø**   **Activities involving walking and running**
> **EXCLUDES 1**   *activity, walking an animal (Y93.K1)*
> *activity, walking or running on a treadmill (Y93.A1)*

Y93.Ø1   **Activity, walking, marching and hiking**
Activity, walking, marching and hiking on level or elevated terrain
> **EXCLUDES 1**   *activity, mountain climbing (Y93.31)*

Y93.Ø2   **Activity, running**

✓5ᵗʰ **Y93.1**   **Activities involving water and water craft**
> **EXCLUDES 1**   *activities involving ice (Y93.2-)*

Y93.11   **Activity, swimming**

Y93.12   **Activity, springboard and platform diving**

Y93.13   **Activity, water polo**

Y93.14   **Activity, water aerobics and water exercise**

Y93.15   **Activity, underwater diving and snorkeling**
Activity, SCUBA diving

Y93.16   **Activity, rowing, canoeing, kayaking, rafting and tubing**
Activity, canoeing, kayaking, rafting and tubing in calm and turbulent water

Y93.17   **Activity, water skiing and wake boarding**

Y93.18   **Activity, surfing, windsurfing and boogie boarding**
Activity, water sliding

Y93.19   **Activity, other involving water and watercraft**
Activity involving water NOS
Activity, parasailing
Activity, water survival training and testing

✓5ᵗʰ **Y93.2**   **Activities involving ice and snow**
> **EXCLUDES 1**   *activity, shoveling ice and snow (Y93.H1)*

Y93.21   **Activity, ice skating**
Activity, figure skating (singles) (pairs)
Activity, ice dancing
> **EXCLUDES 1**   *activity, ice hockey (Y93.22)*

Y93.22   **Activity, ice hockey**

Y93.23   **Activity, snow (alpine) (downhill) skiing, snow boarding, sledding, tobogganing and snow tubing**
> **EXCLUDES 1**   *activity, cross country skiing (Y93.24)*

Y93.24   **Activity, cross country skiing**
Activity, nordic skiing

Ⓝ Newborn: 0   Ⓟ Pediatric: 0-17   Ⓜ Maternity: 12-55   Ⓐ Adult: 15-124   **MCC** Major CC Condition   **PDxMCC** PDx acts as own MCC   **CC** CC Condition   **PDxCC** PDx acts as own CC

1218   ICD-10-CM 2016

Y93.29   **Activity, other involving** ice and snow
Activity involving ice and snow NOS

✓5ᵗʰ **Y93.3**   **Activities involving climbing, rappelling and jumping off**
    EXCLUDES 1   *activity, hiking on level or elevated terrain (Y93.01)*
                activity, jumping rope (Y93.56)
                activity, trampoline jumping (Y93.44)

Y93.31   **Activity, mountain climbing, rock climbing and wall climbing**

Y93.32   **Activity, rappelling**

Y93.33   **Activity, BASE jumping**
Activity, Building, Antenna, Span, Earth jumping

Y93.34   **Activity, bungee jumping**

Y93.35   **Activity, hang gliding**

Y93.39   **Activity, other involving climbing, rappelling and jumping off**

✓5ᵗʰ **Y93.4**   **Activities involving dancing and other rhythmic movement**
    EXCLUDES 1   *activity, martial arts (Y93.75)*

Y93.41   **Activity, dancing**
AHA: 2012, 4Q, 108

Y93.42   **Activity, yoga**

Y93.43   **Activity, gymnastics**
Activity, rhythmic gymnastics
    EXCLUDES 1   *activity, trampolining (Y93.44)*

Y93.44   **Activity, trampolining**

Y93.45   **Activity, cheerleading**

Y93.49   **Activity, other involving dancing and other rhythmic movements**

✓5ᵗʰ **Y93.5**   **Activities involving other sports and athletics played individually**
    EXCLUDES 1   *activity, dancing (Y93.41)*
                activity, gymnastic (Y93.43)
                activity, trampolining (Y93.44)
                activity, yoga (Y93.42)

Y93.51   **Activity, roller skating (inline) and skateboarding**

Y93.52   **Activity, horseback riding**

Y93.53   **Activity, golf**

Y93.54   **Activity, bowling**

Y93.55   **Activity, bike riding**

Y93.56   **Activity, jumping rope**

Y93.57   **Activity, non-running track and field events**
    EXCLUDES 1   *activity, running (any form) (Y93.02)*

Y93.59   **Activity, other involving other sports and athletics played individually**
    EXCLUDES 1   *activities involving climbing, rappelling, and jumping (Y93.3-)*
                activities involving ice and snow (Y93.2-)
                activities involving walking and running (Y93.0-)
                activities involving water and watercraft (Y93.1-)

✓5ᵗʰ **Y93.6**   **Activities involving other sports and athletics played as a team or group**
    EXCLUDES 1   *activity, ice hockey (Y93.22)*
                activity, water polo (Y93.13)

Y93.61   **Activity, American tackle football**
Activity, football NOS

Y93.62   **Activity, American flag or touch football**

Y93.63   **Activity, rugby**

Y93.64   **Activity, baseball**
Activity, softball

Y93.65   **Activity, lacrosse and field hockey**

Y93.66   **Activity, soccer**

Y93.67   **Activity, basketball**

Y93.68   **Activity, volleyball (beach) (court)**

Y93.6A   **Activity, physical games generally associated with school recess, summer camp and children**   P
Activity, capture the flag   Activity, four square
Activity, dodge ball   Activity, kickball

Y93.69   **Activity, other involving other sports and athletics played as a team or group**
Activity, cricket

✓5ᵗʰ **Y93.7**   **Activities involving other specified sports and athletics**

Y93.71   **Activity, boxing**

Y93.72   **Activity, wrestling**

Y93.73   **Activity, racquet and hand sports**
Activity, handball   Activity, squash
Activity, racquetball   Activity, tennis

Y93.74   **Activity, frisbee**
Activity, ultimate frisbee

Y93.75   **Activity, martial arts**
Activity, combatives

Y93.79   **Activity, other specified sports and athletics**
    EXCLUDES 1   *sports and athletics activities specified in categories Y93.0-Y93.6*

✓5ᵗʰ **Y93.A**   **Activities involving other cardiorespiratory exercise**
Activities involving physical training

Y93.A1   **Activity, exercise machines primarily for cardiorespiratory conditioning**
Activity, elliptical and stepper machines
Activity, stationary bike
Activity, treadmill

Y93.A2   **Activity, calisthenics**
Activity, jumping jacks
Activity, warm up and cool down

Y93.A3   **Activity, aerobic and step exercise**

Y93.A4   **Activity, circuit training**

Y93.A5   **Activity, obstacle course**
Activity, challenge course
Activity, confidence course

Y93.A6   **Activity, grass drills**
Activity, guerilla drills

Y93.A9   **Activity, other involving cardiorespiratory exercise**
    EXCLUDES 1   *activities involving cardiorespiratory exercise specified in categories Y93.0-Y93.7*

✓5ᵗʰ **Y93.B**   **Activities involving other muscle strengthening exercises**

Y93.B1   **Activity, exercise machines primarily for muscle strengthening**

Y93.B2   **Activity, push-ups, pull-ups, sit-ups**

Y93.B3   **Activity, free weights**
Activity, barbells   Activity, dumbbells

Y93.B4   **Activity, pilates**

Y93.B9   **Activity, other involving muscle strengthening exercises**
    EXCLUDES 1   *activities involving muscle strengthening specified in categories Y93.0-Y93.A*

✓5ᵗʰ **Y93.C**   **Activities involving computer technology and electronic devices**
    EXCLUDES 1   *activity, electronic musical keyboard or instruments (Y93.J-)*

Y93.C1   **Activity, computer keyboarding**
Activity, electronic game playing using keyboard or other stationary device

Y93.C2   **Activity, hand held interactive electronic device**
Activity, cellular telephone and communication device
Activity, electronic game playing using interactive device
    EXCLUDES 1   *activity, electronic game playing using keyboard or other stationary device (Y93.C1)*

Y93.C9   **Activity, other involving computer technology and electronic devices**

✓5ᵗʰ **Y93.D**   **Activities involving arts and handcrafts**
    EXCLUDES 1   *activities involving playing musical instrument (Y93.J-)*

Y93.D1   **Activity, knitting and crocheting**

Y93.D2   **Activity, sewing**

Y93.D3   **Activity, furniture building and finishing**
Activity, furniture repair

Y93.D9   **Activity, other involving arts and handcrafts**

✓5ᵗʰ **Y93.E**   **Activities involving personal hygiene and interior property and clothing maintenance**
    EXCLUDES 1   *activities involving cooking and grilling (Y93.G-)*
                activities involving exterior property and land maintenance, building and construction (Y93.H-)
                activities involving caregiving (Y93.F-)
                activity, dishwashing (Y93.G1)
                activity, food preparation (Y93.G1)
                activity, gardening (Y93.H2)

Y93.E1   **Activity, personal bathing and showering**

Y93.E2   **Activity, laundry**

Y93.E3   **Activity, vacuuming**

Y93.E4   **Activity, ironing**

Chapter 20. External Causes of Morbidity

Y93.E5   **Activity,** floor mopping and cleaning

Y93.E6   **Activity,** residential relocation
> Activity, packing up and unpacking involved in moving to a new residence

Y93.E8   **Activity,** other personal hygiene

Y93.E9   **Activity,** other interior property and clothing maintenance

☑5ᵗʰ **Y93.F**   **Activities involving** caregiving
> Activity involving the provider of caregiving

Y93.F1   **Activity, caregiving,** bathing

Y93.F2   **Activity, caregiving,** lifting

Y93.F9   **Activity,** other caregiving

☑5ᵗʰ **Y93.G**   **Activities involving food preparation, cooking and grilling**

Y93.G1   **Activity, food** preparation and clean up
> Activity, dishwashing

Y93.G2   **Activity,** grilling and smoking food

Y93.G3   **Activity,** cooking and baking
> Activity, use of stove, oven and microwave oven

Y93.G9   **Activity,** other involving cooking and grilling

☑5ᵗʰ **Y93.H**   **Activities involving exterior property and land maintenance, building and construction**

Y93.H1   **Activity,** digging, shoveling and raking
> Activity, dirt digging
> Activity, raking leaves
> Activity, snow shoveling

Y93.H2   **Activity,** gardening and landscaping
> Activity, pruning, trimming shrubs, weeding

Y93.H3   **Activity,** building and construction

Y93.H9   **Activity,** other involving exterior property and land maintenance, building and construction

☑5ᵗʰ **Y93.I**   **Activities involving roller coasters and other types of external motion**

Y93.I1   **Activity,** rollercoaster riding

Y93.I9   **Activity,** other involving external motion

☑5ᵗʰ **Y93.J**   **Activities involving playing musical instrument**
> Activity involving playing electric musical instrument

Y93.J1   **Activity,** piano playing
> Activity, musical keyboard (electronic) playing

Y93.J2   **Activity,** drum and other percussion instrument playing

Y93.J3   **Activity,** string instrument playing

Y93.J4   **Activity,** winds and brass instrument playing

☑5ᵗʰ **Y93.K**   **Activities involving** animal care
> **EXCLUDES 1**   activity, horseback riding (Y93.52)

Y93.K1   **Activity,** walking an animal

Y93.K2   **Activity,** milking an animal

Y93.K3   **Activity,** grooming and shearing an animal

Y93.K9   **Activity,** other involving animal care

☑5ᵗʰ **Y93.8**   **Activities, other specified**

Y93.81   **Activity,** refereeing a sports activity

Y93.82   **Activity,** spectator at an event

Y93.83   **Activity,** rough housing and horseplay

Y93.84   **Activity,** sleeping

Y93.89   **Activity,** other specified

Y93.9   **Activity,** unspecified

Y95   **Nosocomial condition**
> **AHA:** 2013, 4Q, 119

☑4ᵗʰ **Y99**   **External cause status**
> **NOTE**   A single code from category Y99 should be used in conjunction with the external cause code(s) assigned to a record to indicate the status of the person at the time the event occurred.

Y99.0   **Civilian activity done for income or pay**
> Civilian activity done for financial or other compensation
> **EXCLUDES 1**   military activity (Y99.1)
>   volunteer activity (Y99.2)

Y99.1   **Military activity**
> **EXCLUDES 1**   activity of off duty military personnel (Y99.8)

Y99.2   **Volunteer activity**
> **EXCLUDES 1**   activity of child or other family member assisting in compensated work of other family member (Y99.8)

Y99.8   **Other external cause status**
> Activity NEC
> Activity of child or other family member assisting in compensated work of other family member
> Hobby not done for income
> Leisure activity
> Off-duty activity of military personnel
> Recreation or sport not for income or while a student
> Student activity
> **EXCLUDES 1**   civilian activity done for income or compensation (Y99.0)
>   military activity (Y99.1)
> **AHA:** 2012, 4Q, 108

Y99.9   **Unspecified external cause status**

Ⓝ Newborn: 0   ℙ Pediatric: 0-17   Ⓜ Maternity: 12-55   Ⓐ Adult: 15-124   **MCC** Major CC Condition   **PDxMCC** PDx acts as own MCC   **CC** CC Condition   **PDxCC** PDx acts as own CC

1220   ICD-10-CM 2016

Chapter 21. Factors Influencing Health Status and Contact with Health Services (Z00–Z99)

Chapter Specific Guidelines with Coding Examples

The chapter specific guidelines from the ICD-10-CM Official Guidelines for Coding and Reporting have been provided below. Along with these guidelines are coding examples, contained in the shaded boxes, that have been developed to help illustrate the coding and/or sequencing guidance found in these guidelines.

Note: The chapter specific guidelines provide additional information about the use of Z codes for specified encounters.

a. Use of Z codes in any healthcare setting

Z codes are for use in any healthcare setting. Z codes may be used as either a first-listed (principal diagnosis code in the inpatient setting) or secondary code, depending on the circumstances of the encounter. Certain Z codes may only be used as first-listed or principal diagnosis.

Patient with middle lobe lung cancer admitted for initiation of chemotherapy

Z51.11   **Encounter for antineoplastic chemotherapy**

C34.2   **Malignant neoplasm of middle lobe, bronchus or lung**

Explanation: A Z code can be used as first-listed in this situation based on guidelines in this chapter as well as chapter 2, "Neoplasms."

Patient has chronic lymphocytic leukemia for which the patient had previous chemotherapy and is now in remission

C91.11   **Chronic lymphocytic leukemia of B-cell type in remission**

Z92.21   **Personal history of antineoplastic chemotherapy**

*Explanation:*The personal history Z code is used to describe a secondary (supplementary) diagnosis to identify that this patient has had chemotherapy in the past.

---

b. Z Codes indicate a reason for an encounter

Z codes are not procedure codes. A corresponding procedure code must accompany a Z code to describe any procedure performed.

c. Categories of Z codes

1) Contact/exposure

Category Z20 indicates contact with, and suspected exposure to, communicable diseases. These codes are for patients who do not show any sign or symptom of a disease but are suspected to have been exposed to it by close personal contact with an infected individual or are in an area where a disease is epidemic.

Category Z77, Other contact with and (suspected) exposures hazardous to health, indicates contact with and suspected exposures hazardous to health.

Contact/exposure codes may be used as a first-listed code to explain an encounter for testing, or, more commonly, as a secondary code to identify a potential risk.

2) Inoculations and vaccinations

Code Z23 is for encounters for inoculations and vaccinations. It indicates that a patient is being seen to receive a prophylactic inoculation against a disease. Procedure codes are required to identify the actual administration of the injection and the type(s) of immunizations given. Code Z23 may be used as a secondary code if the inoculation is given as a routine part of preventive health care, such as a well-baby visit.

3) Status

Status codes indicate that a patient is either a carrier of a disease or has the sequelae or residual of a past disease or condition. This includes such things as the presence of prosthetic or mechanical devices resulting from past treatment. A status code is informative, because the status may affect the course of treatment and its outcome. A status code is distinct from a history code. The history code indicates that the patient no longer has the condition.

A status code should not be used with a diagnosis code from one of the body system chapters, if the diagnosis code includes the information provided by the status code. For example, code Z94.1, Heart transplant status, should not be used with a code from subcategory T86.2, Complications of heart transplant. The status code does not provide

additional information. The complication code indicates that the patient is a heart transplant patient.

For encounters for weaning from a mechanical ventilator, assign a code from subcategory J96.1, Chronic respiratory failure, followed by code Z99.11, Dependence on respirator [ventilator] status.

The status Z codes/categories are:

Z14   Genetic carrier

      Genetic carrier status indicates that a person carries a gene, associated with a particular disease, which may be passed to offspring who may develop that disease. The person does not have the disease and is not at risk of developing the disease.

Z15   Genetic susceptibility to disease

      Genetic susceptibility indicates that a person has a gene that increases the risk of that person developing the disease.

      Codes from category Z15 should not be used as principal or first-listed codes. If the patient has the condition to which he/she is susceptible, and that condition is the reason for the encounter, the code for the current condition should be sequenced first. If the patient is being seen for follow-up after completed treatment for this condition, and the condition no longer exists, a follow-up code should be sequenced first, followed by the appropriate personal history and genetic susceptibility codes. If the purpose of the encounter is genetic counseling associated with procreative management, code Z31.5, Encounter for genetic counseling, should be assigned as the first-listed code, followed by a code from category Z15. Additional codes should be assigned for any applicable family or personal history.

Z16   Resistance to antimicrobial drugs

      This code indicates that a patient has a condition that is resistant to antimicrobial drug treatment. Sequence the infection code first.

Z17   Estrogen receptor status

Z18   Retained foreign body fragments

Z21   Asymptomatic HIV infection status

      This code indicates that a patient has tested positive for HIV but has manifested no signs or symptoms of the disease.

Z22   Carrier of infectious disease

      Carrier status indicates that a person harbors the specific organisms of a disease without manifest symptoms and is capable of transmitting the infection.

Z28.3   Underimmunization status

Z33.1   Pregnant state, incidental

      This code is a secondary code only for use when the pregnancy is in no way complicating the reason for visit. Otherwise, a code from the obstetric chapter is required.

Z66   Do not resuscitate

      This code may be used when it is documented by the provider that a patient is on do not resuscitate status at any time during the stay.

Z67   Blood type

Z68   Body mass index (BMI)

Z74.01   Bed confinement status

Z76.82   Awaiting organ transplant status

Z78   Other specified health status

      Code Z78.1, Physical restraint status, may be used when it is documented by the provider that a patient has been put in restraints during the current encounter. Please note that this code should not be reported when it is documented by the provider that a patient is temporarily restrained during a procedure.

Z79   Long-term (current) drug therapy

      Codes from this category indicate a patient's continuous use of a prescribed drug (including such things as aspirin therapy) for the long-term treatment of a condition or for prophylactic use. It is not for use for patients who have addictions to drugs. This subcategory is not for use of medications for detoxification or maintenance programs to prevent withdrawal symptoms in patients with drug dependence (e.g., methadone maintenance for opiate dependence). Assign the appropriate code for the drug dependence instead.

Assign a code from Z79 if the patient is receiving a medication for an extended period as a prophylactic measure (such as for the prevention of deep vein thrombosis) or as treatment of a chronic condition (such as arthritis) or a disease requiring a lengthy course of treatment (such as cancer). Do not assign a code from category Z79 for medication being administered for a brief period of time to treat an acute illness or injury (such as a course of antibiotics to treat acute bronchitis).

Z88	Allergy status to drugs, medicaments and biological substances
	Except: Z88.9, Allergy status to unspecified drugs, medicaments and biological substances status
Z89	Acquired absence of limb
Z90	Acquired absence of organs, not elsewhere classified
Z91.0-	Allergy status, other than to drugs and biological substances
Z92.82	Status post administration of tPA (rtPA) in a different facility within the last 24 hours prior to admission to a current facility

Assign code Z92.82, Status post administration of tPA (rtPA) in a different facility within the last 24 hours prior to admission to current facility, as a secondary diagnosis when a patient is received by transfer into a facility and documentation indicates they were administered tissue plasminogen activator (tPA) within the last 24 hours prior to admission to the current facility.

This guideline applies even if the patient is still receiving the tPA at the time they are received into the current facility.

The appropriate code for the condition for which the tPA was administered (such as cerebrovascular disease or myocardial infarction) should be assigned first.

Code Z92.82 is only applicable to the receiving facility record and not to the transferring facility record.

Z93	Artificial opening status
Z94	Transplanted organ and tissue status
Z95	Presence of cardiac and vascular implants and grafts
Z96	Presence of other functional implants
Z97	Presence of other devices
Z98	Other postprocedural states

Assign code Z98.85, Transplanted organ removal status, to indicate that a transplanted organ has been previously removed. This code should not be assigned for the encounter in which the transplanted organ is removed. The complication necessitating removal of the transplant organ should be assigned for that encounter.

See section I.C19. for information on the coding of organ transplant complications.

Z99	Dependence on enabling machines and devices, not elsewhere classified

Note: Categories Z89-Z90 and Z93-Z99 are for use only if there are no complications or malfunctions of the organ or tissue replaced, the amputation site or the equipment on which the patient is dependent.

4) History (of)

There are two types of history Z codes, personal and family. Personal history codes explain a patient's past medical condition that no longer exists and is not receiving any treatment, but that has the potential for recurrence, and therefore may require continued monitoring.

Family history codes are for use when a patient has a family member(s) who has had a particular disease that causes the patient to be at higher risk of also contracting the disease.

Personal history codes may be used in conjunction with follow-up codes and family history codes may be used in conjunction with screening codes to explain the need for a test or procedure. History codes are also acceptable on any medical record regardless of the reason for visit. A history of an illness, even if no longer present, is important information that may alter the type of treatment ordered.

The history Z code categories are:

Z80	Family history of primary malignant neoplasm
Z81	Family history of mental and behavioral disorders
Z82	Family history of certain disabilities and chronic diseases (leading to disablement)
Z83	Family history of other specific disorders
Z84	Family history of other conditions
Z85	Personal history of malignant neoplasm

Z86	Personal history of certain other diseases
Z87	Personal history of other diseases and conditions
Z91.4-	Personal history of psychological trauma, not elsewhere classified
Z91.5	Personal history of self-harm
Z91.8-	Other specified personal risk factors, not elsewhere classified
	Except: Z91.83, Wandering in diseases classified elsewhere
Z92	Personal history of medical treatment
	Except: Z92.0, Personal history of contraception
	Except: Z92.82, Status post administration of tPA (rtPA) in a different facility within the last 24 hours prior to admission to a current facility

5) Screening

Screening is the testing for disease or disease precursors in seemingly well individuals so that early detection and treatment can be provided for those who test positive for the disease (e.g., screening mammogram).

The testing of a person to rule out or confirm a suspected diagnosis because the patient has some sign or symptom is a diagnostic examination, not a screening. In these cases, the sign or symptom is used to explain the reason for the test.

A screening code may be a first-listed code if the reason for the visit is specifically the screening exam. It may also be used as an additional code if the screening is done during an office visit for other health problems. A screening code is not necessary if the screening is inherent to a routine examination, such as a pap smear done during a routine pelvic examination.

Should a condition be discovered during the screening then the code for the condition may be assigned as an additional diagnosis.

> Prostate screening of healthy 50-year-old male patient; PSA noted to be elevated but normal digital rectal exam
>
> **Z12.5**   **Encounter for screening for malignant neoplasm of prostate**
>
> **R97.2**   **Elevated prostate specific antigen [PSA]**
>
> *Explanation:* The patient had no signs or symptoms of any prostate-related illness prior to coming in for the screening. The screening code is appropriately used as the first-listed code to signify that this was for routine screening. The elevated PSA is reported as a secondary diagnosis to reflect that an abnormal lab value was found as a result of the screening procedure(s).

The Z code indicates that a screening exam is planned. A procedure code is required to confirm that the screening was performed.

The screening Z codes/categories:

Z11	Encounter for screening for infectious and parasitic diseases
Z12	Encounter for screening for malignant neoplasms
Z13	Encounter for screening for other diseases and disorders
	Except: Z13.9, Encounter for screening, unspecified
Z36	Encounter for antenatal screening for mother

6) Observation

There are two observation Z code categories. They are for use in very limited circumstances when a person is being observed for a suspected condition that is ruled out. The observation codes are not for use if an injury or illness or any signs or symptoms related to the suspected condition are present. In such cases the diagnosis/symptom code is used with the corresponding external cause code.

The observation codes are to be used as principal diagnosis only. Additional codes may be used in addition to the observation code but only if they are unrelated to the suspected condition being observed.

Codes from subcategory Z03.7, Encounter for suspected maternal and fetal conditions ruled out, may either be used as a first-listed or as an additional code assignment depending on the case. They are for use in very limited circumstances on a maternal record when an encounter is for a suspected maternal or fetal condition that is ruled out during that encounter (for example, a maternal or fetal condition may be suspected due to an abnormal test result). These codes should not be used when the condition is confirmed. In those cases, the confirmed condition should be coded. In addition, these codes are not for use if an illness or any signs or symptoms related to the suspected condition or problem are present. In such cases the diagnosis/symptom code is used.

Additional codes may be used in addition to the code from subcategory Z03.7, but only if they are unrelated to the suspected condition being evaluated.

Codes from subcategory Z03.7 may not be used for encounters for antenatal screening of mother. *See Section I.C.21. Screening.*

For encounters for suspected fetal condition that are inconclusive following testing and evaluation, assign the appropriate code from category O35, O36, O40 or O41.

The observation Z code categories:

Z03   Encounter for medical observation for suspected diseases and conditions ruled out

Z04   Encounter for examination and observation for other reasons

       Except: Z04.9, Encounter for examination and observation for unspecified reason

7) Aftercare

Aftercare visit codes cover situations when the initial treatment of a disease has been performed and the patient requires continued care during the healing or recovery phase, or for the long-term consequences of the disease. The aftercare Z code should not be used if treatment is directed at a current, acute disease. The diagnosis code is to be used in these cases. Exceptions to this rule are codes Z51.0, Encounter for antineoplastic radiation therapy, and codes from subcategory Z51.1, Encounter for antineoplastic chemotherapy and immunotherapy. These codes are to be first-listed, followed by the diagnosis code when a patient's encounter is solely to receive radiation therapy, chemotherapy, or immunotherapy for the treatment of a neoplasm. If the reason for the encounter is more than one type of antineoplastic therapy, code Z51.0 and a code from subcategory Z51.1 may be assigned together, in which case one of these codes would be reported as a secondary diagnosis.

The aftercare Z codes should also not be used for aftercare for injuries. For aftercare of an injury, assign the acute injury code with the appropriate 7th character (for subsequent encounter).

The aftercare codes are generally first-listed to explain the specific reason for the encounter. An aftercare code may be used as an additional code when some type of aftercare is provided in addition to the reason for admission and no diagnosis code is applicable. An example of this would be the closure of a colostomy during an encounter for treatment of another condition.

Aftercare codes should be used in conjunction with other aftercare codes or diagnosis codes to provide better detail on the specifics of an aftercare encounter visit, unless otherwise directed by the classification. Should a patient receive multiple types of antineoplastic therapy during the same encounter, code Z51.0, Encounter for antineoplastic radiation therapy, and codes from subcategory Z51.1, Encounter for antineoplastic chemotherapy and immunotherapy, may be used together on a record. The sequencing of multiple aftercare codes depends on the circumstances of the encounter.

Certain aftercare Z code categories need a secondary diagnosis code to describe the resolving condition or sequelae. For others, the condition is included in the code title.

Additional Z code aftercare category terms include fitting and adjustment, and attention to artificial openings.

Status Z codes may be used with aftercare Z codes to indicate the nature of the aftercare. For example code Z95.1, Presence of aortocoronary bypass graft, may be used with code Z48.812, Encounter for surgical aftercare following surgery on the circulatory system, to indicate the surgery for which the aftercare is being performed. A status code should not be used when the aftercare code indicates the type of status, such as using Z43.0, Encounter for attention to tracheostomy, with Z93.0, Tracheostomy status.

The aftercare Z category/codes:

Z42   Encounter for plastic and reconstructive surgery following medical procedure or healed injury

Z43   Encounter for attention to artificial openings

Z44   Encounter for fitting and adjustment of external prosthetic device

Z45   Encounter for adjustment and management of implanted device

Z46   Encounter for fitting and adjustment of other devices

Z47   Orthopedic aftercare

Z48   Encounter for other postprocedural aftercare

Z49   Encounter for care involving renal dialysis

Z51   Encounter for other aftercare

8) Follow-up

The follow-up codes are used to explain continuing surveillance following completed treatment of a disease, condition, or injury. They imply that the condition has been fully treated and no longer exists. They should not be confused with aftercare codes, or injury codes with a 7th character for subsequent encounter, that explain ongoing care of a healing condition

or its sequelae. Follow-up codes may be used in conjunction with history codes to provide the full picture of the healed condition and its treatment. The follow-up code is sequenced first, followed by the history code.

A follow-up code may be used to explain multiple visits. Should a condition be found to have recurred on the follow-up visit, then the diagnosis code for the condition should be assigned in place of the follow-up code.

The follow-up Z code categories:

Z08   Encounter for follow-up examination after completed treatment for malignant neoplasm

Z09   Encounter for follow-up examination after completed treatment for conditions other than malignant neoplasm

Z39   Encounter for maternal postpartum care and examination

Follow-up for patient several months after completing a regime of IV antibiotics for recurrent pneumonia; lungs are clear and pneumonia is resolved

Z09   **Encounter for follow-up examination after completed treatment for conditions other than malignant neoplasm**

Z87.01   **Personal history of pneumonia (recurrent)**

Explanation: Code Z09 identifies the follow-up visit as being unrelated to a malignant neoplasm, and code Z87 describes the condition that has now resolved.

Follow-up for patient several months after completing a regime of IV antibiotics for recurrent pneumonia; pneumonia has recurred, and a new antibiotic regimen has been prescribed

J18.9   **Pneumonia, unspecified organism**

Explanation: Since the follow-up exam for pneumonia determined that the pneumonia was not resolved or recurred, code Z09 Encounter for follow-up examination after completed treatment for conditions other than malignant neoplasm, no longer applies. Instead the first-listed code describes the pneumonia.

---

9) Donor

Codes in category Z52, Donors of organs and tissues, are used for living individuals who are donating blood or other body tissue. These codes are only for individuals donating for others, not for self-donations. They are not used to identify cadaveric donations.

10) Counseling

Counseling Z codes are used when a patient or family member receives assistance in the aftermath of an illness or injury, or when support is required in coping with family or social problems. They are not used in conjunction with a diagnosis code when the counseling component of care is considered integral to standard treatment.

The counseling Z codes/categories:

Z30.0-   Encounter for general counseling and advice on contraception

Z31.5   Encounter for genetic counseling

Z31.6-   Encounter for general counseling and advice on procreation

Z32.2   Encounter for childbirth instruction

Z32.3   Encounter for childcare instruction

Z69   Encounter for mental health services for victim and perpetrator of abuse

Z70   Counseling related to sexual attitude, behavior and orientation

Z71   Persons encountering health services for other counseling and medical advice, not elsewhere classified

Z76.81   Expectant mother prebirth pediatrician visit

11) Encounters for obstetrical and reproductive services

See Section I.C.15. Pregnancy, Childbirth, and the Puerperium, for further instruction on the use of these codes.

Z codes for pregnancy are for use in those circumstances when none of the problems or complications included in the codes from the Obstetrics chapter exist (a routine prenatal visit or postpartum care). Codes in category Z34, Encounter for supervision of normal pregnancy, are always first-listed and are not to be used with any other code from the OB chapter.

Codes in category Z3A, Weeks of gestation, may be assigned to provide additional information about the pregnancy. The date of the admission should be used to determine weeks of gestation for inpatient admissions that encompass more than one gestational week.

The outcome of delivery, category Z37, should be included on all maternal delivery records. It is always a secondary code. Codes in category Z37 should not be used on the newborn record.

Z codes for family planning (contraceptive) or procreative management and counseling should be included on an obstetric record either during the pregnancy or the postpartum stage, if applicable.

Z codes/categories for obstetrical and reproductive services:

Z30	Encounter for contraceptive management
Z31	Encounter for procreative management
Z32.2	Encounter for childbirth instruction
Z32.3	Encounter for childcare instruction
Z33	Pregnant state
Z34	Encounter for supervision of normal pregnancy
Z36	Encounter for antenatal screening of mother
Z3A	Weeks of gestation
Z37	Outcome of delivery
Z39	Encounter for maternal postpartum care and examination
Z76.81	Expectant mother prebirth pediatrician visit

12) Newborns and infants

See Section I.C.16. Newborn (Perinatal) Guidelines, for further instruction on the use of these codes.

Newborn Z codes/categories:

Z76.1	Encounter for health supervision and care of foundling
Z00.1-	Encounter for routine child health examination
Z38	Liveborn infants according to place of birth and type of delivery

13) Routine and administrative examinations

The Z codes allow for the description of encounters for routine examinations, such as, a general check-up, or, examinations for administrative purposes, such as, a pre-employment physical. The codes are not to be used if the examination is for diagnosis of a suspected condition or for treatment purposes. In such cases the diagnosis code is used. During a routine exam, should a diagnosis or condition be discovered, it should be coded as an additional code. Pre-existing and chronic conditions and history codes may also be included as additional codes as long as the examination is for administrative purposes and not focused on any particular condition.

Some of the codes for routine health examinations distinguish between "with" and "without" abnormal findings. Code assignment depends on the information that is known at the time the encounter is being coded. For example, if no abnormal findings were found during the examination, but the encounter is being coded before test results are back, it is acceptable to assign the code for "without abnormal findings." When assigning a code for "with abnormal findings," additional code(s) should be assigned to identify the specific abnormal finding(s).

> 12-month-old boy admitted for well-child visit; pediatrician notices some eczema on the child's scalp and back of the knees
>
> **Z00.121   Encounter for routine child health examination with abnormal findings**
>
> **L30.9   Dermatitis, unspecified**
>
> *Explanation:* The Z code identifying that this is a routine well-child visit is reported first. Because an abnormal finding (eczema) was documented, a code for this condition may also be appended.

Pre-operative examination and pre-procedural laboratory examination Z codes are for use only in those situations when a patient is being cleared for a procedure or surgery and no treatment is given.

The Z codes/categories for routine and administrative examinations:

Z00	Encounter for general examination without complaint, suspected or reported diagnosis
Z01	Encounter for other special examination without complaint, suspected or reported diagnosis
Z02	Encounter for administrative examination Except: Z02.9, Encounter for administrative examinations, unspecified
Z32.0-	Encounter for pregnancy test

14) Miscellaneous Z codes

The miscellaneous Z codes capture a number of other health care encounters that do not fall into one of the other categories. Certain of these codes identify the reason for the encounter; others are for use as additional codes that provide useful information on circumstances that may affect a patient's care and treatment.

Prophylactic Organ Removal

For encounters specifically for prophylactic removal of an organ (such as prophylactic removal of breasts due to a genetic susceptibility to cancer or a family history of cancer), the principal or first-listed code should be a code from category Z40, Encounter for prophylactic surgery, followed by the appropriate codes to identify the associated risk factor (such as genetic susceptibility or family history).

If the patient has a malignancy of one site and is having prophylactic removal at another site to prevent either a new primary malignancy or metastatic disease, a code for the malignancy should also be assigned in addition to a code from subcategory Z40.0, Encounter for prophylactic surgery for risk factors related to malignant neoplasms. A Z40.0 code should not be assigned if the patient is having organ removal for treatment of a malignancy, such as the removal of the testes for the treatment of prostate cancer.

Miscellaneous Z codes/categories:

Z28	Immunization not carried out Except: Z28.3, Underimmunization status
Z40	Encounter for prophylactic surgery
Z41	Encounter for procedures for purposes other than remedying health state Except: Z41.9, Encounter for procedure for purposes other than remedying health state, unspecified
Z53	Persons encountering health services for specific procedures and treatment, not carried out
Z55	Problems related to education and literacy
Z56	Problems related to employment and unemployment
Z57	Occupational exposure to risk factors
Z58	Problems related to physical environment
Z59	Problems related to housing and economic circumstances
Z60	Problems related to social environment
Z62	Problems related to upbringing
Z63	Other problems related to primary support group, including family circumstances
Z64	Problems related to certain psychosocial circumstances
Z65	Problems related to other psychosocial circumstances
Z72	Problems related to lifestyle
Z73	Problems related to life management difficulty
Z74	Problems related to care provider dependency Except: Z74.01, Bed confinement status
Z75	Problems related to medical facilities and other health care
Z76.0	Encounter for issue of repeat prescription
Z76.3	Healthy person accompanying sick person
Z76.4	Other boarder to healthcare facility
Z76.5	Malingerer [conscious simulation]
Z91.1-	Patient's noncompliance with medical treatment and regimen
Z91.83	Wandering in diseases classified elsewhere
Z91.89	Other specified personal risk factors, not elsewhere classified

15) Nonspecific Z codes

Certain Z codes are so non-specific, or potentially redundant with other codes in the classification, that there can be little justification for their use in the inpatient setting. Their use in the outpatient setting should be limited to those instances when there is no further documentation to permit more precise coding. Otherwise, any sign or symptom or any other reason for visit that is captured in another code should be used.

Nonspecific Z codes/categories:

Z02.9	Encounter for administrative examinations, unspecified
Z04.9	Encounter for examination and observation for unspecified reason
Z13.9	Encounter for screening, unspecified
Z41.9	Encounter for procedure for purposes other than remedying health state, unspecified
Z52.9	Donor of unspecified organ or tissue
Z86.59	Personal history of other mental and behavioral disorders
Z88.9	Allergy status to unspecified drugs, medicaments and biological substances status
Z92.0	Personal history of contraception

16)Z codes that may only be principal/first-listed diagnosis

The following Z codes/categories may only be reported as the principal/first-listed diagnosis, except when there are multiple encounters on the same day and the medical records for the encounters are combined:

Z00   Encounter for general examination without complaint, suspected or reported diagnosis
          Except: Z00.6

Z01   Encounter for other special examination without complaint, suspected or reported diagnosis

Z02   Encounter for administrative examination

Z03   Encounter for medical observation for suspected diseases and conditions ruled out

Z04   Encounter for examination and observation for other reasons

Z33.2   Encounter for elective termination of pregnancy

Z31.81   Encounter for male factor infertility in female patient

Z31.82   Encounter for Rh incompatibility status

Z31.83   Encounter for assisted reproductive fertility procedure cycle

Z31.84   Encounter for fertility preservation procedure

Z34   Encounter for supervision of normal pregnancy

Z39   Encounter for maternal postpartum care and examination

Z38   Liveborn infants according to place of birth and type of delivery

Z42   Encounter for plastic and reconstructive surgery following medical procedure or healed injury

Z51.0   Encounter for antineoplastic radiation therapy

Z51.1-   Encounter for antineoplastic chemotherapy and immunotherapy

Z52   Donors of organs and tissues
          Except: Z52.9, Donor of unspecified organ or tissue

Z76.1   Encounter for health supervision and care of foundling

Z76.2   Encounter for health supervision and care of other healthy infant and child

Z99.12   Encounter for respirator [ventilator] dependence during power failure

Female patient seen at 32 weeks' gestation to check the progress of her first pregnancy

Z34.03   **Encounter for supervision of normal first pregnancy, third trimester**

Z3A.32   **32 weeks gestation of pregnancy**

Explanation: Category Z34 is appropriate as a first-listed diagnosis. Category Z3A helps to clarify at which point in the pregnancy the patient was provided supervision.

Chapter 21. Factors Influencing Health Status and Contact With Health Services (Z00-Z99)

NOTE   Z codes represent reasons for encounters. A corresponding procedure code must accompany a Z code if a procedure is performed. Categories Z00-Z99 are provided for occasions when circumstances other than a disease, injury or external cause classifiable to categories A00-Y89 are recorded as "diagnoses" or "problems". This can arise in two main ways:

(a) When a person who may or may not be sick encounters the health services for some specific purpose, such as to receive limited care or service for a current condition, to donate an organ or tissue, to receive prophylactic vaccination (immunization), or to discuss a problem which is in itself not a disease or injury.

(b) When some circumstance or problem is present which influences the person's health status but is not in itself a current illness or injury.

This chapter contains the following blocks:

Z00-Z13	Persons encountering health services for examinations
Z14-Z15	Genetic carrier and genetic susceptibility to disease
Z16	Resistance to antimicrobial drugs
Z17	Estrogen receptor status
Z18	Retained foreign body fragments
Z20-Z28	Persons with potential health hazards related to communicable diseases
Z30-Z39	Persons encountering health services in circumstances related to reproduction
Z40-Z53	Encounters for other specific health care
Z55-Z65	Persons with potential health hazards related to socioeconomic and psychosocial circumstances
Z66	Do not resuscitate status
Z67	Blood type
Z68	Body mass index (BMI)
Z69-Z76	Persons encountering health services in other circumstances
Z77-Z99	Persons with potential health hazards related to family and personal history and certain conditions influencing health status

Persons encountering health services for examinations (Z00-Z13)

NOTE   Nonspecific abnormal findings disclosed at the time of these examinations are classified to categories R70-R94.

EXCLUDES 1   *examinations related to pregnancy and reproduction (Z30-Z36, Z39-)*

✓4ᵗʰ **Z00**   **Encounter for general examination without complaint, suspected or reported diagnosis**

     EXCLUDES 1   *encounter for examination for administrative purposes (Z02.-)*
     EXCLUDES 2   *encounter for pre-procedural examinations (Z01.81-)*
          special screening examinations (Z11-Z13)

✓5ᵗʰ **Z00.0**   **Encounter for general adult medical examination**

Encounter for adult periodic examination (annual) (physical) and any associated laboratory and radiologic examinations

     EXCLUDES 1   *encounter for examination of sign or symptom—code to sign or symptom*
          general health check-up of infant or child (Z00.12-)

     Z00.00   **Encounter for general adult medical examination without abnormal findings**   A

Encounter for adult health check-up NOS

     Z00.01   **Encounter for general adult medical examination with abnormal findings**   A

Use additional code to identify abnormal findings

✓5ᵗʰ **Z00.1**   **Encounter for newborn, infant and child health examinations**

     ✓6ᵗʰ **Z00.11**   **Newborn health examination**

Health check for child under 29 days old
Use additional code to identify any abnormal findings

          EXCLUDES 1   *health check for child over 28 days old (Z00.12-)*

         Z00.110   **Health examination for newborn under 8 days old**   N

Health check for newborn under 8 days old

         Z00.111   **Health examination for newborn 8 to 28 days old**   N

Health check for newborn 8 to 28 days old
Newborn weight check

     ✓6ᵗʰ **Z00.12**   **Encounter for routine child health examination**

Encounter for development testing of infant or child
Health check (routine) for child over 28 days old

          EXCLUDES 1   *health check for child under 29 days old (Z00.11-)*
               health supervision of foundling or other healthy infant or child (Z76.1-Z76.2)
               newborn health examination (Z00.11-)

         Z00.121   **Encounter for routine child health examination with abnormal findings**   P

Use additional code to identify abnormal findings

         Z00.129   **Encounter for routine child health examination without abnormal findings**   P

Encounter for routine child health examination NOS

     Z00.2   **Encounter for examination for period of rapid growth in childhood**   P

     Z00.3   **Encounter for examination for adolescent development state**   P

Encounter for puberty development state

     Z00.5   **Encounter for examination of potential donor of organ and tissue**

     Z00.6   **Encounter for examination for normal comparison and control in clinical research program**

Examination of participant or control in clinical research program

✓5ᵗʰ **Z00.7**   **Encounter for examination for period of delayed growth in childhood**

     Z00.70   **Encounter for examination for period of delayed growth in childhood without abnormal findings**   P

     Z00.71   **Encounter for examination for period of delayed growth in childhood with abnormal findings**   P

Use additional code to identify abnormal findings

     Z00.8   **Encounter for other general examination**

Encounter for health examination in population surveys

✓4ᵗʰ **Z01**   **Encounter for other special examination without complaint, suspected or reported diagnosis**

     INCLUDES   routine examination of specific system
     NOTE   Codes from category Z01 represent the reason for the encounter. A separate procedure code is required to identify any examinations or procedures performed.
     EXCLUDES 1   *encounter for examination for administrative purposes (Z02.-)*
          encounter for examination for suspected conditions, proven not to exist (Z03.-)
          encounter for laboratory and radiologic examinations as a component of general medical examination (Z00.0-)
          encounter for laboratory, radiologic and imaging examinations for sign(s) and symptom(s)—code to the sign(s) or symptom(s)
     EXCLUDES 2   *screening examinations (Z11-Z13)*

✓5ᵗʰ **Z01.0**   **Encounter for examination of eyes and vision**

     EXCLUDES 1   *examination for driving license (Z02.4)*

     Z01.00   **Encounter for examination of eyes and vision without abnormal findings**

Encounter for examination of eyes and vision NOS

     Z01.01   **Encounter for examination of eyes and vision with abnormal findings**

Use additional code to identify abnormal findings

✓5ᵗʰ **Z01.1**   **Encounter for examination of ears and hearing**

     Z01.10   **Encounter for examination of ears and hearing without abnormal findings**

Encounter for examination of ears and hearing NOS

     ✓6ᵗʰ **Z01.11**   **Encounter for examination of ears and hearing with abnormal findings**

         Z01.110   **Encounter for hearing examination following failed hearing screening**

         Z01.118   **Encounter for examination of ears and hearing with other abnormal findings**

Use additional code to identify abnormal findings

     Z01.12   **Encounter for hearing conservation and treatment**

✓5ᵗʰ **Z01.2**   **Encounter for dental examination and cleaning**

     Z01.20   **Encounter for dental examination and cleaning without abnormal findings**

Encounter for dental examination and cleaning NOS

     Z01.21   **Encounter for dental examination and cleaning with abnormal findings**

Use additional code to identify abnormal findings

N Newborn: 0   P Pediatric: 0-17   M Maternity: 12-55   A Adult: 15-124   **MCC** Major CC Condition   **PDxMCC** PDx acts as own MCC   **CC** CC Condition   **PDxCC** PDx acts as own CC

Chapter 21. Factors Influencing Health Status and Contact with Health Services

✓5ᵗʰ **Z01.3 Encounter for examination of** blood pressure

  Z01.30 Encounter for examination of blood pressure without abnormal findings
       Encounter for examination of blood pressure NOS

  Z01.31 Encounter for examination of blood pressure with abnormal findings
       Use additional code to identify abnormal findings

✓5ᵗʰ **Z01.4 Encounter for** gynecological **examination**
   EXCLUDES 2   pregnancy examination or test (Z32.0-)
           routine examination for contraceptive maintenance (Z30.4-)

  ✓6ᵗʰ **Z01.41 Encounter for** routine **gynecological examination**
       Encounter for general gynecological examination with or without cervical smear
       Encounter for gynecological examination (general) (routine) NOS
       Encounter for pelvic examination (annual) (periodic)
       Use additional code:
         for screening for human papillomavirus, if applicable, (Z11.51)
         for screening vaginal pap smear, if applicable (Z12.72)
         to identify acquired absence of uterus, if applicable (Z90.71-)
     EXCLUDES 1   gynecologic examination status-post hysterectomy for malignant condition (Z08)
            screening cervical pap smear not a part of a routine gynecological examination (Z12.4)

    Z01.411 Encounter for gynecological examination (general) (routine) with abnormal findings ♀

    Z01.419 Encounter for gynecological examination (general) (routine) without abnormal findings ♀
        Use additional code to identify abnormal findings

  Z01.42 Encounter for cervical smear to confirm findings **of recent normal smear following initial abnormal smear** ♀

✓5ᵗʰ **Z01.8 Encounter for** other **specified** special **examinations**

  ✓6ᵗʰ **Z01.81 Encounter for** preprocedural **examinations**
       Encounter for preoperative examinations
       Encounter for radiological and imaging examinations as part of preprocedural examination

    Z01.810 Encounter for preprocedural cardiovascular examination

    Z01.811 Encounter for preprocedural respiratory **examination**

    Z01.812 Encounter for preprocedural laboratory **examination**
        Blood and urine tests prior to treatment or procedure

    Z01.818 Encounter for other **preprocedural examination**
        Encounter for preprocedural examination NOS
        Encounter for examinations prior to antineoplastic chemotherapy

  Z01.82 Encounter for allergy testing
     EXCLUDES 1   encounter for antibody response examination (Z01.84)

  Z01.83 Encounter for blood typing
       Encounter for Rh typing

  Z01.84 Encounter for antibody response examination
       Encounter for immunity status testing
     EXCLUDES 1   encounter for allergy testing (Z01.82)

  Z01.89 Encounter for other **specified special examinations**

✓4ᵗʰ **Z02 Encounter for** administrative **examination**

  Z02.0 Encounter for examination for admission to educational institution
       Encounter for examination for admission to preschool (education)
       Encounter for examination for re-admission to school following illness or medical treatment

  Z02.1 Encounter for pre-employment **examination**

  Z02.2 Encounter for examination for admission to residential institution
     EXCLUDES 1   examination for admission to prison (Z02.89)

  Z02.3 Encounter for examination for recruitment to armed forces

  Z02.4 Encounter for examination for driving license

  Z02.5 Encounter for examination for participation in sport
     EXCLUDES 1   blood-alcohol and blood-drug test (Z02.83)

  Z02.6 Encounter for examination for insurance purposes

✓5ᵗʰ **Z02.7 Encounter for** issue of medical certificate
     EXCLUDES 1   encounter for general medical examination (Z00-Z01, Z02.0-Z02.6, Z02.8-Z02.9)

  Z02.71 Encounter for disability determination
       Encounter for issue of medical certificate of incapacity
       Encounter for issue of medical certificate of invalidity

  Z02.79 Encounter for issue of other **medical certificate**

✓5ᵗʰ **Z02.8 Encounter for** other **administrative examinations**

  Z02.81 Encounter for paternity testing

  Z02.82 Encounter for adoption services

  Z02.83 Encounter for blood-alcohol and blood-drug test
       Use additional code for findings of alcohol or drugs in blood (R78.-)

  Z02.89 Encounter for other **administrative examinations**
       Encounter for examination for admission to prison
       Encounter for examination for admission to summer camp
       Encounter for immigration examination
       Encounter for naturalization examination
       Encounter for premarital examination
     EXCLUDES 1   health supervision of foundling or other healthy infant or child (Z76.1-Z76.2)

  Z02.9 Encounter for administrative examinations, unspecified

✓4ᵗʰ **Z03 Encounter for** medical observation **for suspected diseases and conditions ruled out**
   NOTE   This category is to be used when a person without a diagnosis is suspected of having an abnormal condition, without signs or symptoms, which requires study, but after examination and observation, is ruled out. This category is also for use for administrative and legal observation status.
   EXCLUDES 1   contact with and (suspected) exposures hazardous to health (Z77.-)
           newborn observation for suspected condition, ruled out (P00-P04)
           person with feared complaint in whom no diagnosis is made (Z71.1)
           signs or symptoms under study—code to signs or symptoms

  Z03.6 Encounter for observation for suspected toxic effect from ingested substance **ruled out**
       Encounter for observation for suspected adverse effect from drug
       Encounter for observation for suspected poisoning

✓5ᵗʰ **Z03.7 Encounter for suspected** maternal and fetal conditions **ruled out**
       Encounter for suspected maternal and fetal conditions not found
     EXCLUDES 1   known or suspected fetal anomalies affecting management of mother, not ruled out (O26-, O35-, O36-, O40-, O41-)

  Z03.71 Encounter for suspected problem with amniotic cavity and membrane ruled out Ⓜ ♀
       Encounter for suspected oligohydramnios ruled out
       Encounter for suspected polyhydramnios ruled out

  Z03.72 Encounter for suspected placental problem **ruled out** Ⓜ ♀

  Z03.73 Encounter for suspected fetal anomaly **ruled out** Ⓜ ♀

  Z03.74 Encounter for suspected problem with fetal growth **ruled out** Ⓜ ♀

  Z03.75 Encounter for suspected cervical shortening **ruled out** Ⓜ ♀

  Z03.79 Encounter for other **suspected maternal and fetal conditions ruled out** Ⓜ ♀

✓5ᵗʰ **Z03.8 Encounter for** observation **for other suspected diseases and conditions ruled out**

  ✓6ᵗʰ **Z03.81 Encounter for observation for suspected** exposure to biological agents **ruled out**

    Z03.810 Encounter for observation for suspected exposure to anthrax **ruled out**

    Z03.818 Encounter for observation for suspected exposure to other **biological agents ruled out**

  Z03.89 Encounter for observation for other **suspected diseases and conditions ruled out**

☑ Additional Character Required   ✓x7ᵗʰ Placeholder Alert   Unacceptable PDx   Manifestation   Hospital Acquired Condition   *EXCLUDES 1* Not Coded Here   *EXCLUDES 2* Not Included Here

Z01.3–Z03.89

✓4ᵗʰ Z04 Encounter for examination and observation for other reasons

INCLUDES encounter for examination for medicolegal reasons

NOTE This category is to be used when a person without a diagnosis is suspected of having an abnormal condition, without signs or symptoms, which requires study, but after examination and observation, is ruled-out. This category is also for use for administrative and legal observation status.

Z04.1 Encounter for examination and observation following transport accident

EXCLUDES 1 encounter for examination and observation following work accident (Z04.2)

Z04.2 Encounter for examination and observation following work accident

Z04.3 Encounter for examination and observation following other accident

✓5ᵗʰ Z04.4 Encounter for examination and observation following alleged rape

Encounter for examination and observation of victim following alleged rape

Encounter for examination and observation of victim following alleged sexual abuse

Z04.41 Encounter for examination and observation following alleged adult rape Ⓐ

Suspected adult rape, ruled out

Suspected adult sexual abuse, ruled out

Z04.42 Encounter for examination and observation following alleged child rape Ⓟ

Suspected child rape, ruled out

Suspected child sexual abuse, ruled out

Z04.6 Encounter for general psychiatric examination, requested by authority

✓5ᵗʰ Z04.7 Encounter for examination and observation following alleged physical abuse

Z04.71 Encounter for examination and observation following alleged adult physical abuse Ⓐ

Suspected adult physical abuse, ruled out

EXCLUDES 1 confirmed case of adult physical abuse (T74.-)

encounter for examination and observation following alleged adult sexual abuse (Z04.41)

suspected case of adult physical abuse, not ruled out (T76.-)

Z04.72 Encounter for examination and observation following alleged child physical abuse Ⓟ

Suspected child physical abuse, ruled out

EXCLUDES 1 confirmed case of child physical abuse (T74.-)

encounter for examination and observation following alleged child sexual abuse (Z04.42)

suspected case of child physical abuse, not ruled out (T76.-)

Z04.8 Encounter for examination and observation for other specified reasons

Encounter for examination and observation for request for expert evidence

Z04.9 Encounter for examination and observation for unspecified reason

Encounter for observation NOS

Z08 Encounter for follow-up examination after completed treatment for malignant neoplasm

Medical surveillance following completed treatment

Use additional code to identify any acquired absence of organs (Z90.-)

Use additional code to identify the personal history of malignant neoplasm (Z85.-)

EXCLUDES 1 aftercare following medical care (Z43-Z49, Z51)

Z09 Encounter for follow-up examination after completed treatment for conditions other than malignant neoplasm

Medical surveillance following completed treatment

Use additional code to identify any applicable history of disease code (Z86-, Z87-)

EXCLUDES 1 aftercare following medical care (Z43-Z49, Z51)

surveillance of contraception (Z30.4-)

surveillance of prosthetic and other medical devices (Z44-Z46)

AHA: 2015, 1Q, 8

✓4ᵗʰ Z11 Encounter for screening for infectious and parasitic diseases

NOTE Screening is the testing for disease or disease precursors in asymptomatic individuals so that early detection and treatment can be provided for those who test positive for the disease.

EXCLUDES 1 encounter for diagnostic examination—code to sign or symptom

Z11.0 Encounter for screening for intestinal infectious diseases

Z11.1 Encounter for screening for respiratory tuberculosis

Z11.2 Encounter for screening for other bacterial diseases

Z11.3 Encounter for screening for infections with a predominantly sexual mode of transmission

EXCLUDES 2 encounter for screening for human immunodeficiency virus [HIV] (Z11.4)

encounter for screening for human papillomavirus (Z11.51)

Z11.4 Encounter for screening for human immunodeficiency virus [HIV]

✓5ᵗʰ Z11.5 Encounter for screening for other viral diseases

EXCLUDES 2 encounter for screening for viral intestinal disease (Z11.0)

Z11.51 Encounter for screening for human papillomavirus (HPV)

Z11.59 Encounter for screening for other viral diseases

Z11.6 Encounter for screening for other protozoal diseases and helminthiases

EXCLUDES 2 encounter for screening for protozoal intestinal disease (Z11.0)

Z11.8 Encounter for screening for other infectious and parasitic diseases

Encounter for screening for chlamydia

Encounter for screening for rickettsial

Encounter for screening for spirochetal

Encounter for screening for mycoses

Z11.9 Encounter for screening for infectious and parasitic diseases, unspecified

✓4ᵗʰ Z12 Encounter for screening for malignant neoplasms

NOTE Screening is the testing for disease or disease precursors in asymptomatic individuals so that early detection and treatment can be provided for those who test positive for the disease.

Use additional code to identify any family history of malignant neoplasm (Z80.-)

EXCLUDES 1 encounter for diagnostic examination—code to sign or symptom

Z12.0 Encounter for screening for malignant neoplasm of stomach

✓5ᵗʰ Z12.1 Encounter for screening for malignant neoplasm of intestinal tract

Z12.10 Encounter for screening for malignant neoplasm of intestinal tract, unspecified

Z12.11 Encounter for screening for malignant neoplasm of colon

Encounter for screening colonoscopy NOS

Z12.12 Encounter for screening for malignant neoplasm of rectum

Z12.13 Encounter for screening for malignant neoplasm of small intestine

Z12.2 Encounter for screening for malignant neoplasm of respiratory organs

✓5ᵗʰ Z12.3 Encounter for screening for malignant neoplasm of breast

Z12.31 Encounter for screening mammogram for malignant neoplasm of breast

EXCLUDES 1 inconclusive mammogram (R92.2)

AHA: 2015, 1Q, 24

Z12.39 Encounter for other screening for malignant neoplasm of breast

Z12.4 Encounter for screening for malignant neoplasm of cervix ♀

Encounter for screening pap smear for malignant neoplasm of cervix

EXCLUDES 1 encounter for screening for human papillomavirus (Z11.51)

when screening is part of general gynecological examination (Z01.4-)

Z12.5 Encounter for screening for malignant neoplasm of prostate ♂

Z12.6 Encounter for screening for malignant neoplasm of bladder

Ⓝ Newborn: 0   Ⓟ Pediatric: 0-17   Ⓜ Maternity: 12-55   Ⓐ Adult: 15-124   MCC Major CC Condition   PDxMCC PDx acts as own MCC   CC CC Condition   PDxCC PDx acts as own CC

1228

ICD-10-CM 2016

Z04–Z12.6

✓5th Z12.7 Encounter for screening for malignant neoplasm of other **genitourinary organs**

    Z12.71 Encounter for screening for malignant neoplasm of testis   ♂

    Z12.72 Encounter for screening for malignant neoplasm of vagina   ♀
        Vaginal pap smear status-post hysterectomy for non-malignant condition
        Use additional code to identify acquired absence of uterus (Z90.71-)
        EXCLUDES 1 *vaginal pap smear status-post hysterectomy for malignant conditions (Z08)*

    Z12.73 Encounter for screening for malignant neoplasm of ovary   ♀

    Z12.79 Encounter for screening for malignant neoplasm of other **genitourinary organs**

✓5th Z12.8 Encounter for screening for malignant neoplasm of other **sites**

    Z12.81 Encounter for screening for malignant neoplasm of oral cavity

    Z12.82 Encounter for screening for malignant neoplasm of nervous system

    Z12.83 Encounter for screening for malignant neoplasm of skin

    Z12.89 Encounter for screening for malignant neoplasm of other **sites**

Z12.9 Encounter for screening for malignant neoplasm, site unspecified

✓4th Z13 Encounter for screening for other **diseases and disorders**
    NOTE   Screening is the testing for disease or disease precursors in asymptomatic individuals so that early detection and treatment can be provided for those who test positive for the disease.
    EXCLUDES 1 *encounter for diagnostic examination—code to sign or symptom*

Z13.0 Encounter for screening for diseases of the blood and blood-forming organs **and certain disorders involving the** immune mechanism

Z13.1 Encounter for screening for diabetes mellitus

✓5th Z13.2 Encounter for screening for nutritional, metabolic and other endocrine disorders

    Z13.21 Encounter for screening for nutritional **disorder**

    ✓6th Z13.22 Encounter for screening for metabolic **disorder**

        Z13.220 Encounter for screening for lipoid **disorders**
            Encounter for screening for cholesterol level
            Encounter for screening for hypercholesterolemia
            Encounter for screening for hyperlipidemia

        Z13.228 Encounter for screening for other metabolic disorders

    Z13.29 Encounter for screening for other **suspected endocrine disorder**
        EXCLUDES 1 *encounter for screening for diabetes mellitus (Z13.1)*

Z13.4 Encounter for screening for certain developmental **disorders in** childhood   P
    Encounter for screening for developmental handicaps in early childhood
    EXCLUDES 1 *routine development testing of infant or child (Z00.1-)*

Z13.5 Encounter for screening for eye and ear **disorders**
    EXCLUDES 2 *encounter for general hearing examination (Z01.1-)*
                encounter for general vision examination (Z01.0-)

Z13.6 Encounter for screening for cardiovascular **disorders**

✓5th Z13.7 Encounter for screening for genetic and chromosomal **anomalies**
    EXCLUDES 1 *genetic testing for procreative management (Z31.4-)*

    Z13.71 Encounter for nonprocreative screening for genetic disease carrier status

    Z13.79 Encounter for other **screening for genetic and chromosomal anomalies**

✓5th Z13.8 Encounter for screening for other **specified diseases and disorders**
    EXCLUDES 2 *screening for malignant neoplasms (Z12.-)*

    ✓6th Z13.81 Encounter for screening for digestive system **disorders**

        Z13.810 Encounter for screening for upper gastrointestinal **disorder**

        Z13.811 Encounter for screening for lower gastrointestinal **disorder**
            EXCLUDES 1 *encounter for screening for intestinal infectious disease (Z11.0)*

        Z13.818 Encounter for screening for other **digestive system disorders**

    ✓6th Z13.82 Encounter for screening for musculoskeletal **disorder**

        Z13.820 Encounter for screening for osteoporosis

        Z13.828 Encounter for screening for other **musculoskeletal disorder**

    Z13.83 Encounter for screening for respiratory **disorder NEC**
        EXCLUDES 1 *encounter for screening for respiratory tuberculosis (Z11.1)*

    Z13.84 Encounter for screening for dental **disorders**

    ✓6th Z13.85 Encounter for screening for nervous system **disorders**

        Z13.850 Encounter for screening for traumatic brain injury

        Z13.858 Encounter for screening for other **nervous system disorders**

    Z13.88 Encounter for screening for disorder due to exposure to contaminants
        EXCLUDES 1 *those exposed to contaminants without suspected disorders (Z57-Z77-)*

    Z13.89 Encounter for screening for other **disorder**
        Encounter for screening for genitourinary disorders

Z13.9 Encounter for screening, unspecified

Genetic carrier and genetic susceptibility to disease (Z14-Z15)

✓4th Z14 Genetic carrier

  ✓5th Z14.0 Hemophilia A carrier

    Z14.01 Asymptomatic hemophilia A carrier

    Z14.02 Symptomatic hemophilia A carrier

  Z14.1 Cystic fibrosis carrier

  Z14.8 Genetic carrier of other **disease**

✓4th Z15 Genetic susceptibility to disease
    Confirmed abnormal gene
    Use additional code, if applicable, for any associated family history of the disease (Z80-Z84)
    EXCLUDES 1 *chromosomal anomalies (Q90-Q99)*

  ✓5th Z15.0 Genetic susceptibility to malignant neoplasm
    Code first, if applicable, any current malignant neoplasm (C00-C75, C81-C96)
    Use additional code, if applicable, for any personal history of malignant neoplasm (Z85.-)

    Z15.01 Genetic susceptibility to malignant neoplasm of breast

    Z15.02 Genetic susceptibility to malignant neoplasm of ovary   ♀

    Z15.03 Genetic susceptibility to malignant neoplasm of prostate   ♂

    Z15.04 Genetic susceptibility to malignant neoplasm of endometrium   ♀

    Z15.09 Genetic susceptibility to other malignant neoplasm

  ✓5th Z15.8 Genetic susceptibility to other disease

    Z15.81 Genetic susceptibility to multiple endocrine neoplasia [MEN]
        EXCLUDES 1 *multiple endocrine neoplasia [MEN] syndromes (E31.2-)*

    Z15.89 Genetic susceptibility to other **disease**

✓ Additional Character Required   ✓x7th Placeholder Alert   Unacceptable PDx   Manifestation   Hospital Acquired Condition   EXCLUDES 1 Not Coded Here   EXCLUDES 2 Not Included Here

ICD-10-CM 2016   1229

Resistance to antimicrobial drugs (Z16)

✓4ᵗʰ Z16 Resistance to antimicrobial drugs
> **NOTE** The codes in this category are provided for use as additional codes to identify the resistance and non-responsiveness of a condition to antimicrobial drugs.
>
> Code first the infection
> **EXCLUDES 1** *Methicillin resistant Staphylococcus aureus infection (A49.02)*
> *Methicillin resistant Staphylococcus aureus infection in diseases classified elsewhere (B95.62)*
> *Methicillin resistant Staphylococcus aureus pneumonia (J15.212)*
> *Sepsis due to Methicillin resistant Staphylococcus aureus (A41.02)*

✓5ᵗʰ Z16.1 Resistance to beta lactam antibiotics
- **Z16.10 Resistance to unspecified beta lactam antibiotics**
- **Z16.11 Resistance to penicillins**
  - Resistance to amoxicillin
  - Resistance to ampicillin
- **Z16.12 Extended spectrum beta lactamase (ESBL) resistance**
- **Z16.19 Resistance to other specified beta lactam antibiotics**
  - Resistance to cephalosporins

✓5ᵗʰ Z16.2 Resistance to other antibiotics
- **Z16.20 Resistance to unspecified antibiotic**
  - Resistance to antibiotics NOS
- **Z16.21 Resistance to vancomycin**
- **Z16.22 Resistance to vancomycin related antibiotics**
- **Z16.23 Resistance to quinolones and fluoroquinolones**
- **Z16.24 Resistance to multiple antibiotics**
- **Z16.29 Resistance to other single specified antibiotic**
  - Resistance to aminoglycosides
  - Resistance to macrolides
  - Resistance to sulfonamides
  - Resistance to tetracyclines

✓5ᵗʰ Z16.3 Resistance to other antimicrobial drugs
> **EXCLUDES 1** *resistance to antibiotics (Z16.1-, Z16.2-)*
- **Z16.30 Resistance to unspecified antimicrobial drugs**
  - Drug resistance NOS
- **Z16.31 Resistance to antiparasitic drug(s)**
  - Resistance to quinine and related compounds
- **Z16.32 Resistance to antifungal drug(s)**
- **Z16.33 Resistance to antiviral drug(s)**
- **✓6ᵗʰ Z16.34 Resistance to antimycobacterial drug(s)**
  - Resistance to tuberculostatics
  - **Z16.341 Resistance to single antimycobacterial drug**
    - Resistance to antimycobacterial drug NOS
  - **Z16.342 Resistance to multiple antimycobacterial drugs**
- **Z16.35 Resistance to multiple antimicrobial drugs**
  > **EXCLUDES 1** *Resistance to multiple antibiotics only (Z16.24)*
- **Z16.39 Resistance to other specified antimicrobial drug**

Estrogen receptor status (Z17)

✓4ᵗʰ Z17 Estrogen receptor status
> Code first malignant neoplasm of breast (C50.-)
- **Z17.0 Estrogen receptor positive status [ER+]**
- **Z17.1 Estrogen receptor negative status [ER-]**

Retained foreign body fragment (Z18)

✓4ᵗʰ Z18 Retained foreign body fragments
- Embedded fragment (status)
- Embedded splinter (status)
- Retained foreign body status
> **EXCLUDES 1** *artificial joint prosthesis status (Z96.6-)*
> *foreign body accidentally left during a procedure (T81.5-)*
> *foreign body entering through orifice (T15-T19)*
> *in situ cardiac device (Z95.-)*
> *organ or tissue replaced by means other than transplant (Z96.-, Z97.-)*
> *organ or tissue replaced by transplant (Z94.-)*
> *personal history of retained foreign body fully removed (Z87.821)*
> *superficial foreign body (non-embedded splinter)—code to superficial foreign body, by site*

✓5ᵗʰ Z18.0 Retained radioactive fragments
- **Z18.01 Retained depleted uranium fragments**
- **Z18.09 Other retained radioactive fragments**
  - Other retained depleted isotope fragments
  - Retained nontherapeutic radioactive fragments

✓5ᵗʰ Z18.1 Retained metal fragments
> **EXCLUDES 1** *retained radioactive metal fragments (Z18.01-Z18.09)*
- **Z18.10 Retained metal fragments, unspecified**
  - Retained metal fragment NOS
- **Z18.11 Retained magnetic metal fragments**
- **Z18.12 Retained nonmagnetic metal fragments**

Z18.2 Retained plastic fragments
- Acrylics fragments
- Diethylhexylphthalates fragments
- Isocyanate fragments

✓5ᵗʰ Z18.3 Retained organic fragments
- **Z18.31 Retained animal quills or spines**
- **Z18.32 Retained tooth**
- **Z18.33 Retained wood fragments**
- **Z18.39 Other retained organic fragments**

✓5ᵗʰ Z18.8 Other specified retained foreign body
- **Z18.81 Retained glass fragments**
- **Z18.83 Retained stone or crystalline fragments**
  - Retained concrete or cement fragments
- **Z18.89 Other specified retained foreign body fragments**

Z18.9 Retained foreign body fragments, unspecified material

Persons with potential health hazards related to communicable diseases (Z20-Z28)

✓4ᵗʰ Z20 Contact with and (suspected) exposure to communicable diseases
> **EXCLUDES 1** *carrier of infectious disease (Z22.-)*
> *diagnosed current infectious or parasitic disease—see Alphabetic Index*
> **EXCLUDES 2** *personal history of infectious and parasitic diseases (Z86.1-)*

✓5ᵗʰ Z20.0 Contact with and (suspected) exposure to intestinal infectious diseases
- **Z20.01 Contact with and (suspected) exposure to intestinal infectious diseases due to Escherichia coli (E. coli)**
- **Z20.09 Contact with and (suspected) exposure to other intestinal infectious diseases**

Z20.1 Contact with and (suspected) exposure to tuberculosis

Z20.2 Contact with and (suspected) exposure to infections with a predominantly sexual mode of transmission

Z20.3 Contact with and (suspected) exposure to rabies

Z20.4 Contact with and (suspected) exposure to rubella

Z20.5 Contact with and (suspected) exposure to viral hepatitis

Z20.6 Contact with and (suspected) exposure to human immunodeficiency virus [HIV]
> **EXCLUDES 1** *asymptomatic human immunodeficiency virus [HIV] HIV infection status (Z21)*

Z20.7 Contact with and (suspected) exposure to pediculosis, acariasis and other infestations

✓5ᵗʰ Z20.8 Contact with and (suspected) exposure to other communicable diseases
- **✓6ᵗʰ Z20.81 Contact with and (suspected) exposure to other bacterial communicable diseases**
  - **Z20.810 Contact with and (suspected) exposure to anthrax**
  - **Z20.811 Contact with and (suspected) exposure to meningococcus**
  - **Z20.818 Contact with and (suspected) exposure to other bacterial communicable diseases**
- **✓6ᵗʰ Z20.82 Contact with and (suspected) exposure to other viral communicable diseases**
  - **Z20.820 Contact with and (suspected) exposure to varicella**
  - **Z20.828 Contact with and (suspected) exposure to other viral communicable diseases**
- **Z20.89 Contact with and (suspected) exposure to other communicable diseases**

Z20.9 Contact with and (suspected) exposure to unspecified communicable disease

N Newborn: 0 P Pediatric: 0-17 M Maternity: 12-55 A Adult: 15-124 MCC Major CC Condition PDxMCC PDx acts as own MCC CC CC Condition PDxCC PDx acts as own CC

1230
ICD-10-CM 2016

13Z21 Asymptomatic human immunodeficiency virus [HIV] infection status
HIV positive NOS
Code first human immunodeficiency virus [HIV] disease complicating pregnancy, childbirth and the puerperium, if applicable (O98.7-)
EXCLUDES 1   acquired immunodeficiency syndrome (B20)
contact with human immunodeficiency virus [HIV] (Z20.6)
exposure to human immunodeficiency virus [HIV] (Z20.6)
human immunodeficiency virus [HIV] disease (B20)
inconclusive laboratory evidence of human immunodeficiency virus [HIV] (R75)

✓4th **Z22 Carrier of infectious disease**
Colonization status
Suspected carrier

Z22.0 Carrier of typhoid

Z22.1 Carrier of other intestinal infectious diseases

Z22.2 Carrier of diphtheria

✓5th **Z22.3 Carrier of other specified bacterial diseases**

     Z22.31 Carrier of bacterial disease due to meningococci

     ✓6th **Z22.32 Carrier of bacterial disease due to staphylococci**

       Z22.321 Carrier or suspected carrier of Methicillin susceptible Staphylococcus aureus
MSSA colonization

       Z22.322 Carrier or suspected carrier of Methicillin resistant Staphylococcus aureus
MRSA colonization

     ✓6th **Z22.33 Carrier of bacterial disease due to streptococci**

       Z22.330 Carrier of Group B streptococcus

       Z22.338 Carrier of other streptococcus

     Z22.39 Carrier of other specified bacterial diseases

Z22.4 Carrier of infections with a predominantly sexual mode of transmission

✓5th **Z22.5 Carrier of viral hepatitis**

     Z22.50 Carrier of unspecified viral hepatitis

     Z22.51 Carrier of viral hepatitis B
Hepatitis B surface antigen [HBsAg] carrier

     Z22.52 Carrier of viral hepatitis C

     Z22.59 Carrier of other viral hepatitis

Z22.6 Carrier of human T-lymphotropic virus type-1 [HTLV-1] infection

Z22.8 Carrier of other infectious diseases

Z22.9 Carrier of infectious disease, unspecified

Z23 Encounter for immunization
Code first any routine childhood examination
NOTE   Procedure codes are required to identify the types of immunizations given

✓4th **Z28 Immunization not carried out and underimmunization status**
Vaccination not carried out

✓5th **Z28.0 Immunization not carried out because of contraindication**

     Z28.01 Immunization not carried out because of acute illness of patient

     Z28.02 Immunization not carried out because of chronic illness or condition of patient

     Z28.03 Immunization not carried out because of immune compromised state of patient

     Z28.04 Immunization not carried out because of patient allergy to vaccine or component

     Z28.09 Immunization not carried out because of other contraindication

Z28.1 Immunization not carried out because of patient decision for reasons of belief or group pressure
Immunization not carried out because of religious belief

✓5th **Z28.2 Immunization not carried out because of patient decision for other and unspecified reason**

     Z28.20 Immunization not carried out because of patient decision for unspecified reason

     Z28.21 Immunization not carried out because of patient refusal

     Z28.29 Immunization not carried out because of patient decision for other reason

Z28.3 Underimmunization status
Delinquent immunization status
Lapsed immunization schedule status

✓5th **Z28.8 Immunization not carried out for other reason**

     Z28.81 Immunization not carried out due to patient having had the disease

     Z28.82 Immunization not carried out because of caregiver refusal
Immunization not carried out because of guardian refusal
Immunization not carried out because of parent refusal
EXCLUDES 1   immunization not carried out because of caregiver refusal because of religious belief (Z28.1)

     Z28.89 Immunization not carried out for other reason

Z28.9 Immunization not carried out for unspecified reason

Persons encountering health services in circumstances related to reproduction (Z30-Z39)

✓4th **Z30 Encounter for contraceptive management**

✓5th **Z30.0 Encounter for general counseling and advice on contraception**

     ✓6th **Z30.01 Encounter for initial prescription of contraceptives**
EXCLUDES 1   encounter for surveillance of contraceptives (Z30.4-)

       Z30.011 Encounter for initial prescription of contraceptive pills ♀

       Z30.012 Encounter for prescription of emergency contraception ♀
Encounter for postcoital contraception

       Z30.013 Encounter for initial prescription of injectable contraceptive ♀

       Z30.014 Encounter for initial prescription of intrauterine contraceptive device ♀
EXCLUDES 1   encounter for insertion of intrauterine contraceptive device (Z30.430, Z30.432)

       Z30.018 Encounter for initial prescription of other contraceptives ♀

       Z30.019 Encounter for initial prescription of contraceptives, unspecified ♀

     Z30.02 Counseling and instruction in natural family planning to avoid pregnancy

     Z30.09 Encounter for other general counseling and advice on contraception
Encounter for family planning advice NOS

Z30.2 Encounter for sterilization

✓5th **Z30.4 Encounter for surveillance of contraceptives**

     Z30.40 Encounter for surveillance of contraceptives, unspecified

     Z30.41 Encounter for surveillance of contraceptive pills ♀
Encounter for repeat prescription for contraceptive pill

     Z30.42 Encounter for surveillance of injectable contraceptive ♀

     ✓6th **Z30.43 Encounter for surveillance of intrauterine contraceptive device**

       Z30.430 Encounter for insertion of intrauterine contraceptive device ♀

       Z30.431 Encounter for routine checking of intrauterine contraceptive device ♀

       Z30.432 Encounter for removal of intrauterine contraceptive device ♀

       Z30.433 Encounter for removal and reinsertion of intrauterine contraceptive device ♀
Encounter for replacement of intrauterine contraceptive device

     Z30.49 Encounter for surveillance of other contraceptives ♀

Z30.8 Encounter for other contraceptive management
Encounter for postvasectomy sperm count
Encounter for routine examination for contraceptive maintenance
EXCLUDES 1   sperm count following sterilization reversal (Z31.42)
sperm count for fertility testing (Z31.41)

Z30.9 Encounter for contraceptive management, unspecified

---

13   Questionable admission when used as PDx.

✅ Additional Character Required   ✓x7th Placeholder Alert   Unacceptable PDx   Manifestation   Hospital Acquired Condition   EXCLUDES 1 Not Coded Here   EXCLUDES 2 Not Included Here

✓4ᵗʰ **Z31 Encounter for procreative management**
     EXCLUDES 1   *complications associated with artificial fertilization (N98.-)*
        female infertility (N97.-)
        male infertility (N46.-)

   Z31.0 Encounter for reversal of previous sterilization

✓5ᵗʰ **Z31.4 Encounter for procreative investigation and testing**
     EXCLUDES 1   *postvasectomy sperm count (Z30.8)*

     Z31.41 Encounter for fertility testing
       Encounter for fallopian tube patency testing
       Encounter for sperm count for fertility testing

     Z31.42 Aftercare following sterilization reversal
       Sperm count following sterilization reversal

✓6ᵗʰ   **Z31.43 Encounter for genetic testing of female for procreative management**
       Use additional code for recurrent pregnancy loss, if applicable (N96, O26.2-)
       EXCLUDES 1   *nonprocreative genetic testing (Z13.7-)*

       Z31.430 Encounter of female for testing for genetic disease carrier status for procreative management ♀

       Z31.438 Encounter for other genetic testing of female for procreative management ♀

✓6ᵗʰ   **Z31.44 Encounter for genetic testing of male for procreative management**
       EXCLUDES 1   *nonprocreative genetic testing (Z13.7-)*

       Z31.440 Encounter of male for testing for genetic disease carrier status for procreative management ♂

       Z31.441 Encounter for testing of male partner of patient with recurrent pregnancy loss Ⓐ♂

       Z31.448 Encounter for other genetic testing of male for procreative management Ⓐ♂

     Z31.49 Encounter for other procreative investigation and testing

   Z31.5 Encounter for genetic counseling

✓5ᵗʰ **Z31.6 Encounter for general counseling and advice on procreation**

     Z31.61 Procreative counseling and advice using natural family planning

     Z31.62 Encounter for fertility preservation counseling
       Encounter for fertility preservation counseling prior to cancer therapy
       Encounter for fertility preservation counseling prior to surgical removal of gonads

     Z31.69 Encounter for other general counseling and advice on procreation

✓5ᵗʰ **Z31.8 Encounter for other procreative management**

     Z31.81 Encounter for male factor infertility in female patient ♀

     Z31.82 Encounter for Rh incompatibility status ♀
       AHA: 2014, 4Q, 17

     Z31.83 Encounter for assisted reproductive fertility procedure cycle ♀
       Patient undergoing in vitro fertilization cycle
       Use additional code to identify the type of infertility
       EXCLUDES 1   *pre-cycle diagnosis and testing—code to reason for encounter*

     Z31.84 Encounter for fertility preservation procedure
       Encounter for fertility preservation procedure prior to cancer therapy
       Encounter for fertility preservation procedure prior to surgical removal of gonads

     Z31.89 Encounter for other procreative management

   Z31.9 Encounter for procreative management, unspecified

✓4ᵗʰ **Z32 Encounter for pregnancy test and childbirth and childcare instruction**

✓5ᵗʰ **Z32.0 Encounter for pregnancy test**

     Z32.00 Encounter for pregnancy test, result unknown ♀
       Encounter for pregnancy test NOS

     Z32.01 Encounter for pregnancy test, result positive Ⓜ♀

     Z32.02 Encounter for pregnancy test, result negative ♀

   Z32.2 Encounter for childbirth instruction

   Z32.3 Encounter for childcare instruction
     Encounter for prenatal or postpartum childcare instruction

---

✓4ᵗʰ **Z33 Pregnant state**

   Z33.1 Pregnant state, incidental Ⓜ♀
     Pregnant state NOS
     EXCLUDES 1   *complications of pregnancy (O00-O9A)*

   Z33.2 Encounter for elective termination of pregnancy Ⓜ♀
     EXCLUDES 1   *early fetal death with retention of dead fetus (O02.1)*
       late fetal death (O36.4)
       spontaneous abortion (O03)

✓4ᵗʰ **Z34 Encounter for supervision of normal pregnancy**
     EXCLUDES 1   *any complication of pregnancy (O00-O9A)*
       encounter for pregnancy test (Z32.0-)
       encounter for supervision of high risk pregnancy (O09.-)
   AHA: 2014, 4Q, 17

✓5ᵗʰ **Z34.0 Encounter for supervision of normal first pregnancy**

     Z34.00 Encounter for supervision of normal first pregnancy, unspecified trimester Ⓜ♀

     Z34.01 Encounter for supervision of normal first pregnancy, first trimester Ⓜ♀

     Z34.02 Encounter for supervision of normal first pregnancy, second trimester Ⓜ♀

     Z34.03 Encounter for supervision of normal first pregnancy, third trimester Ⓜ♀

✓5ᵗʰ **Z34.8 Encounter for supervision of other normal pregnancy**

     Z34.80 Encounter for supervision of other normal pregnancy, unspecified trimester Ⓜ♀

     Z34.81 Encounter for supervision of other normal pregnancy, first trimester Ⓜ♀

     Z34.82 Encounter for supervision of other normal pregnancy, second trimester Ⓜ♀

     Z34.83 Encounter for supervision of other normal pregnancy, third trimester Ⓜ♀

✓5ᵗʰ **Z34.9 Encounter for supervision of normal pregnancy, unspecified**

     Z34.90 Encounter for supervision of normal pregnancy, unspecified, unspecified trimester Ⓜ♀

     Z34.91 Encounter for supervision of normal pregnancy, unspecified, first trimester Ⓜ♀

     Z34.92 Encounter for supervision of normal pregnancy, unspecified, second trimester Ⓜ♀

     Z34.93 Encounter for supervision of normal pregnancy, unspecified, third trimester Ⓜ♀

   Z36 Encounter for antenatal screening of mother Ⓜ♀
     EXCLUDES 1   *abnormal findings on antenatal screening of mother (O28.-)*
       diagnostic examination—code to sign or symptom
       encounter for suspected maternal and fetal conditions ruled out (Z03.7-)
       suspected fetal condition affecting management of pregnancy—code to condition in Chapter 15
     EXCLUDES 2   *genetic counseling and testing (Z31.43-, Z31.5)*
       routine prenatal care (Z34)

✓4ᵗʰ **Z3A Weeks of gestation**
     NOTE   Codes from category Z3A are for use, only on the maternal record, to indicate the weeks of gestation of the pregnancy.
     Code first complications of pregnancy, childbirth and the puerperium (O00-O9A)
     AHA: 2014, 3Q, 17; 2014, 2Q, 9; 2013, 2Q, 33

✓5ᵗʰ **Z3A.0 Weeks of gestation of pregnancy, unspecified or less than 10 weeks**

     Z3A.00 Weeks of gestation of pregnancy not specified Ⓜ♀

     Z3A.01 Less than 8 weeks gestation of pregnancy Ⓜ♀

     Z3A.08 8 weeks gestation of pregnancy Ⓜ♀

     Z3A.09 9 weeks gestation of pregnancy Ⓜ♀

✓5ᵗʰ **Z3A.1 Weeks of gestation of pregnancy, weeks 10-19**

     Z3A.10 10 weeks gestation of pregnancy Ⓜ♀

     Z3A.11 11 weeks gestation of pregnancy Ⓜ♀

     Z3A.12 12 weeks gestation of pregnancy Ⓜ♀

     Z3A.13 13 weeks gestation of pregnancy Ⓜ♀

     Z3A.14 14 weeks gestation of pregnancy Ⓜ♀

     Z3A.15 15 weeks gestation of pregnancy Ⓜ♀

     Z3A.16 16 weeks gestation of pregnancy Ⓜ♀

     Z3A.17 17 weeks gestation of pregnancy Ⓜ♀

     Z3A.18 18 weeks gestation of pregnancy Ⓜ♀

     Z3A.19 19 weeks gestation of pregnancy Ⓜ♀

✓5ᵗʰ **Z3A.2 Weeks of gestation of pregnancy, weeks 20-29**

     Z3A.20 20 weeks gestation of pregnancy Ⓜ♀

     Z3A.21 21 weeks gestation of pregnancy Ⓜ♀

Ⓝ Newborn: 0   Ⓟ Pediatric: 0-17   Ⓜ Maternity: 12-55   Ⓐ Adult: 15-124   **MCC** Major CC Condition   **PDxMCC** PDx acts as own MCC   **CC** CC Condition   **PDxCC** PDx acts as own CC

1232

ICD-10-CM 2016

Z31–Z3A.21

Z3A.22	22 weeks gestation of pregnancy	M ♀
Z3A.23	23 weeks gestation of pregnancy	M ♀
Z3A.24	24 weeks gestation of pregnancy	M ♀
Z3A.25	25 weeks gestation of pregnancy	M ♀
Z3A.26	26 weeks gestation of pregnancy	M ♀
Z3A.27	27 weeks gestation of pregnancy	M ♀
Z3A.28	28 weeks gestation of pregnancy	M ♀
Z3A.29	29 weeks gestation of pregnancy	M ♀

✓5ᵗʰ **Z3A.3 Weeks of gestation of pregnancy, weeks 30-39**

Z3A.30	30 weeks gestation of pregnancy	M ♀
Z3A.31	31 weeks gestation of pregnancy	M ♀
Z3A.32	32 weeks gestation of pregnancy	M ♀
Z3A.33	33 weeks gestation of pregnancy	M ♀
Z3A.34	34 weeks gestation of pregnancy	M ♀
Z3A.35	35 weeks gestation of pregnancy	M ♀
Z3A.36	36 weeks gestation of pregnancy	M ♀
Z3A.37	37 weeks gestation of pregnancy	M ♀
Z3A.38	38 weeks gestation of pregnancy	M ♀
Z3A.39	39 weeks gestation of pregnancy	M ♀

✓5ᵗʰ **Z3A.4 Weeks of gestation of pregnancy, weeks 40 or greater**
AHA: 2014, 4Q, 23

Z3A.40	40 weeks gestation of pregnancy	M ♀
Z3A.41	41 weeks gestation of pregnancy	M ♀
Z3A.42	42 weeks gestation of pregnancy	M ♀
Z3A.49	Greater than 42 weeks gestation of pregnancy	M ♀

✓4ᵗʰ **Z37 Outcome of delivery**
> NOTE   This category is intended for use as an additional code to identify the outcome of delivery on the mother's record. It is not for use on the newborn record.
> EXCLUDES 1   *stillbirth (P95)*

Z37.0 Single live birth   M ♀
AHA: 2014, 2Q, 9

Z37.1	Single stillbirth	M ♀
Z37.2	Twins, both liveborn	M ♀
Z37.3	Twins, one liveborn and one stillborn	M ♀
Z37.4	Twins, both stillborn	M ♀

✓5ᵗʰ **Z37.5 Other multiple births, all liveborn**

Z37.50	Multiple births, unspecified, all liveborn	M ♀
Z37.51	Triplets, all liveborn	M ♀
Z37.52	Quadruplets, all liveborn	M ♀
Z37.53	Quintuplets, all liveborn	M ♀
Z37.54	Sextuplets, all liveborn	M ♀
Z37.59	Other multiple births, all liveborn	M ♀

✓5ᵗʰ **Z37.6 Other multiple births, some liveborn**

Z37.60	Multiple births, unspecified, some liveborn	M ♀
Z37.61	Triplets, some liveborn	M ♀
Z37.62	Quadruplets, some liveborn	M ♀
Z37.63	Quintuplets, some liveborn	M ♀
Z37.64	Sextuplets, some liveborn	M ♀
Z37.69	Other multiple births, some liveborn	M ♀

Z37.7	Other multiple births, all stillborn	M ♀
Z37.9	Outcome of delivery, unspecified	M ♀
	Multiple birth NOS	
	Single birth NOS	

✓4ᵗʰ **Z38 Liveborn infants according to place of birth and type of delivery**
> NOTE   This category is for use as the principal code on the initial record of a newborn baby. It is to be used for the initial birth record only. It is not to be used on the mother's record.

✓5ᵗʰ **Z38.0 Single liveborn infant, born in hospital**
Single liveborn infant, born in birthing center or other health care facility

Z38.00	Single liveborn infant, delivered vaginally	N
Z38.01	Single liveborn infant, delivered by cesarean	N
Z38.1	Single liveborn infant, born outside hospital	N
Z38.2	Single liveborn infant, unspecified as to place of birth	N
	Single liveborn infant NOS	

✓5ᵗʰ **Z38.3 Twin liveborn infant, born in hospital**

Z38.30	Twin liveborn infant, delivered vaginally	N
Z38.31	Twin liveborn infant, delivered by cesarean	N
Z38.4	Twin liveborn infant, born outside hospital	N
Z38.5	Twin liveborn infant, unspecified as to place of birth	N

✓5ᵗʰ **Z38.6 Other multiple liveborn infant, born in hospital**

Z38.61	Triplet liveborn infant, delivered vaginally	N
Z38.62	Triplet liveborn infant, delivered by cesarean	N
Z38.63	Quadruplet liveborn infant, delivered vaginally	N
Z38.64	Quadruplet liveborn infant, delivered by cesarean	N
Z38.65	Quintuplet liveborn infant, delivered vaginally	N
Z38.66	Quintuplet liveborn infant, delivered by cesarean	N
Z38.68	Other multiple liveborn infant, delivered vaginally	N
Z38.69	Other multiple liveborn infant, delivered by cesarean	N
Z38.7	Other multiple liveborn infant, born outside hospital	N
Z38.8	Other multiple liveborn infant, unspecified as to place of birth	N

✓4ᵗʰ **Z39 Encounter for maternal postpartum care and examination**

Z39.0 Encounter for care and examination of mother immediately after delivery   M ♀
Care and observation in uncomplicated cases when the delivery occurs outside a healthcare facility
> EXCLUDES 1   *care for postpartum complication—see Alphabetic index*

Z39.1 Encounter for care and examination of lactating mother   M ♀
Encounter for supervision of lactation
> EXCLUDES 1   *disorders of lactation (O92.-)*

Z39.2 Encounter for routine postpartum follow-up   M ♀

Encounters for other specific health care (Z40-Z53)

> NOTE   Categories Z40-Z53 are intended for use to indicate a reason for care. They may be used for patients who have already been treated for a disease or injury, but who are receiving aftercare or prophylactic care, or care to consolidate the treatment, or to deal with a residual state.
> EXCLUDES 2   *follow-up examination for medical surveillance after treatment (Z08-Z09)*

✓4ᵗʰ **Z40 Encounter for prophylactic surgery**
> EXCLUDES 1   *organ donations (Z52.-)*
> *therapeutic organ removal—code to condition*

✓5ᵗʰ **Z40.0 Encounter for prophylactic surgery for risk factors related to malignant neoplasms**
Admission for prophylactic organ removal
Use additional code to identify risk factor

Z40.00	Encounter for prophylactic removal of unspecified organ	
Z40.01	Encounter for prophylactic removal of breast	
Z40.02	Encounter for prophylactic removal of ovary	♀
Z40.09	Encounter for prophylactic removal of other organ	
Z40.8	Encounter for other prophylactic surgery	
Z40.9	Encounter for prophylactic surgery, unspecified	

✓4ᵗʰ **Z41 Encounter for procedures for purposes other than remedying health state**

Z41.1 Encounter for cosmetic surgery
Encounter for cosmetic breast implant
Encounter for cosmetic procedure
> EXCLUDES 1   *encounter for plastic and reconstructive surgery following medical procedure or healed injury (Z42.-)*
> *encounter for post-mastectomy breast implantation (Z42.1)*

Z41.2	Encounter for routine and ritual male circumcision	♂
Z41.3	Encounter for ear piercing	
Z41.8	Encounter for other procedures for purposes other than remedying health state	
Z41.9	Encounter for procedure for purposes other than remedying health state, unspecified	

✓4ᵗʰ **Z42 Encounter for plastic and reconstructive surgery following medical procedure or healed injury**
> EXCLUDES 1   *encounter for cosmetic plastic surgery (Z41.1)*
> *encounter for plastic surgery for treatment of current injury—code to relevant injury*

Z42.1 Encounter for breast reconstruction following mastectomy   A
> EXCLUDES 1   *deformity and disproportion of reconstructed breast (N65.1-)*

✓ Additional Character Required   ✓x7ᵗʰ Placeholder Alert   Unacceptable PDx   Manifestation   Hospital Acquired Condition   EXCLUDES 1 Not Coded Here   EXCLUDES 2 Not Included Here

Z42.8 Encounter for *other plastic and reconstructive surgery following medical procedure or healed injury*

√4ᵗʰ **Z43 Encounter for attention to artificial openings**

> INCLUDES closure of artificial openings
> passage of sounds or bougies through artificial openings
> reforming artificial openings
> removal of catheter from artificial openings
> toilet or cleansing of artificial openings
>
> EXCLUDES 1 *artificial opening status only, without need for care (Z93.-)*
> *complications of external stoma (J95.0-, K94.-, N99.5-)*
> EXCLUDES 2 *fitting and adjustment of prosthetic and other devices (Z44-Z46)*

Z43.0 Encounter for attention to *tracheostomy*

Z43.1 Encounter for attention to *gastrostomy*   CC
> **CC Excl:** Z43.1

Z43.2 Encounter for attention to *ileostomy*

Z43.3 Encounter for attention to *colostomy*

Z43.4 Encounter for attention to other artificial *openings of digestive tract*

Z43.5 Encounter for attention to *cystostomy*

Z43.6 Encounter for attention to other artificial *openings of urinary tract*
> Encounter for attention to nephrostomy
> Encounter for attention to ureterostomy
> Encounter for attention to urethrostomy

Z43.7 Encounter for attention to artificial *vagina*

Z43.8 Encounter for attention to *other* artificial openings

Z43.9 Encounter for attention to *unspecified* artificial opening

√4ᵗʰ **Z44 Encounter for fitting and adjustment of external prosthetic device**

> INCLUDES removal or replacement of external prosthetic device
> EXCLUDES 1 *malfunction or other complications of device—see Alphabetical Index*
> *presence of prosthetic device (Z97.-)*

√5ᵗʰ **Z44.0** Encounter for fitting and adjustment of *artificial arm*

√6ᵗʰ **Z44.00** Encounter for fitting and adjustment of *unspecified* artificial arm

Z44.001 Encounter for fitting and adjustment of unspecified *right* artificial arm

Z44.002 Encounter for fitting and adjustment of unspecified *left* artificial arm

Z44.009 Encounter for fitting and adjustment of unspecified artificial arm, *unspecified* arm

√6ᵗʰ **Z44.01** Encounter for fitting and adjustment of *complete* artificial arm

Z44.011 Encounter for fitting and adjustment of complete *right* artificial arm

Z44.012 Encounter for fitting and adjustment of complete *left* artificial arm

Z44.019 Encounter for fitting and adjustment of complete artificial arm, *unspecified* arm

√6ᵗʰ **Z44.02** Encounter for fitting and adjustment of *partial* artificial arm

Z44.021 Encounter for fitting and adjustment of partial artificial *right* arm

Z44.022 Encounter for fitting and adjustment of partial artificial *left* arm

Z44.029 Encounter for fitting and adjustment of partial artificial arm, *unspecified* arm

√5ᵗʰ **Z44.1** Encounter for fitting and adjustment of *artificial leg*

√6ᵗʰ **Z44.10** Encounter for fitting and adjustment of *unspecified* artificial leg

Z44.101 Encounter for fitting and adjustment of unspecified *right* artificial leg

Z44.102 Encounter for fitting and adjustment of unspecified *left* artificial leg

Z44.109 Encounter for fitting and adjustment of unspecified artificial leg, *unspecified* leg

√6ᵗʰ **Z44.11** Encounter for fitting and adjustment of *complete* artificial leg

Z44.111 Encounter for fitting and adjustment of complete *right* artificial leg

Z44.112 Encounter for fitting and adjustment of complete *left* artificial leg

Z44.119 Encounter for fitting and adjustment of complete artificial leg, *unspecified* leg

√6ᵗʰ **Z44.12** Encounter for fitting and adjustment of *partial* artificial leg

Z44.121 Encounter for fitting and adjustment of partial artificial *right* leg

Z44.122 Encounter for fitting and adjustment of partial artificial *left* leg

Z44.129 Encounter for fitting and adjustment of partial artificial leg, *unspecified* leg

√5ᵗʰ **Z44.2** Encounter for fitting and adjustment of *artificial eye*
> EXCLUDES 1 *mechanical complication of ocular prosthesis (T85.3)*

Z44.20 Encounter for fitting and adjustment of artificial eye, *unspecified*

Z44.21 Encounter for fitting and adjustment of artificial *right* eye

Z44.22 Encounter for fitting and adjustment of artificial *left* eye

√5ᵗʰ **Z44.3** Encounter for fitting and adjustment of *external breast prosthesis*
> EXCLUDES 1 *complications of breast implant (T85.4-)*
> *encounter for adjustment or removal of breast implant (Z45.81-)*
> *encounter for initial breast implant insertion for cosmetic breast augmentation (Z41.1)*
> *encounter for breast reconstruction following mastectomy (Z42.1)*

Z44.30 Encounter for fitting and adjustment of external breast prosthesis, *unspecified* breast   ♀

Z44.31 Encounter for fitting and adjustment of external *right* breast prosthesis   ♀

Z44.32 Encounter for fitting and adjustment of external *left* breast prosthesis   ♀

Z44.8 Encounter for fitting and adjustment of *other* external prosthetic devices

Z44.9 Encounter for fitting and adjustment of *unspecified* external prosthetic device

√4ᵗʰ **Z45 Encounter for adjustment and management of implanted device**

> INCLUDES removal or replacement of implanted device
> EXCLUDES 1 *malfunction or other complications of device—see Alphabetical Index*
> *presence of prosthetic and other devices (Z95-Z97)*
> EXCLUDES 2 *encounter for fitting and adjustment of non-implanted device (Z46.-)*

√5ᵗʰ **Z45.0** Encounter for adjustment and management of *cardiac device*

√6ᵗʰ **Z45.01** Encounter for adjustment and management of cardiac *pacemaker*
> EXCLUDES 1 *encounter for adjustment and management of automatic implantable cardiac defibrillator with synchronous cardiac pacemaker (Z45.02)*

¹³**Z45.010** Encounter for checking and testing of cardiac pacemaker *pulse generator [battery]*
> Encounter for replacing cardiac pacemaker pulse generator [battery]

¹³**Z45.018** Encounter for adjustment and management of *other* part of cardiac pacemaker

¹³**Z45.02** Encounter for adjustment and management of automatic implantable cardiac defibrillator
> Encounter for adjustment and management of automatic implantable cardiac defibrillator with synchronous cardiac pacemaker

¹³**Z45.09** Encounter for adjustment and management of other cardiac device

Z45.1 Encounter for adjustment and management of *infusion pump*

Z45.2 Encounter for adjustment and management of *vascular access device*
> Encounter for adjustment and management of vascular catheters
> EXCLUDES 1 *encounter for adjustment and management of renal dialysis catheter (Z49.01)*

√5ᵗʰ **Z45.3** Encounter for adjustment and management of implanted devices *of the special senses*

Z45.31 Encounter for adjustment and management of implanted *visual* substitution device

---

¹³ Questionable admission when used as PDx.

N Newborn: 0   P Pediatric: 0-17   M Maternity: 12-55   A Adult: 15-124   MCC Major CC Condition   PDxMCC PDx acts as own MCC   CC CC Condition   PDxCC PDx acts as own CC

1234   ICD-10-CM 2016

✓6ᵗʰ Z45.32 Encounter for adjustment and management of implanted hearing device
> EXCLUDES 1 *Encounter for fitting and adjustment of hearing aide (Z46.1)*

Z45.320 Encounter for adjustment and management of bone conduction device

Z45.321 Encounter for adjustment and management of cochlear device

Z45.328 Encounter for adjustment and management of other implanted hearing device

✓5ᵗʰ Z45.4 Encounter for adjustment and management of implanted nervous system device

Z45.41 Encounter for adjustment and management of cerebrospinal fluid drainage device
> Encounter for adjustment and management of cerebral ventricular (communicating) shunt

Z45.42 Encounter for adjustment and management of neuropacemaker (brain) (peripheral nerve) (spinal cord)

Z45.49 Encounter for adjustment and management of other implanted nervous system device
> AHA: 2014, 3Q, 19

✓5ᵗʰ Z45.8 Encounter for adjustment and management of other implanted devices

✓6ᵗʰ Z45.81 Encounter for adjustment or removal of breast implant
> Encounter for elective implant exchange (different material) (different size)
> Encounter removal of tissue expander without synchronous insertion of permanent implant
> EXCLUDES 1 *complications of breast implant (T85.4-)*
> *encounter for initial breast implant insertion for cosmetic breast augmentation (Z41.1)*
> *encounter for breast reconstruction following mastectomy (Z42.1)*

Z45.811 Encounter for adjustment or removal of right breast implant ♀

Z45.812 Encounter for adjustment or removal of left breast implant ♀

Z45.819 Encounter for adjustment or removal of unspecified breast implant ♀

Z45.82 Encounter for adjustment or removal of myringotomy device (stent) (tube)

Z45.89 Encounter for adjustment and management of other implanted devices
> AHA: 2014, 4Q, 26-28

Z45.9 Encounter for adjustment and management of unspecified implanted device

✓4ᵗʰ Z46 Encounter for fitting and adjustment of other devices
> INCLUDES removal or replacement of other device
> EXCLUDES 1 *malfunction or other complications of device—see Alphabetical Index*
> EXCLUDES 2 *encounter for fitting and management of implanted devices (Z45.-)*
> *issue of repeat prescription only (Z76.0)*
> *presence of prosthetic and other devices (Z95-Z97)*

Z46.0 Encounter for fitting and adjustment of spectacles and contact lenses

Z46.1 Encounter for fitting and adjustment of hearing aid
> EXCLUDES 1 *encounter for adjustment and management of implanted hearing device (Z45.32-)*

Z46.2 Encounter for fitting and adjustment of other devices related to nervous system and special senses
> EXCLUDES 2 *encounter for adjustment and management of implanted nervous system device (Z45.4-)*
> *encounter for adjustment and management of implanted visual substitution device (Z45.31)*

Z46.3 Encounter for fitting and adjustment of dental prosthetic device
> Encounter for fitting and adjustment of dentures

Z46.4 Encounter for fitting and adjustment of orthodontic device

✓5ᵗʰ Z46.5 Encounter for fitting and adjustment of other gastrointestinal appliance and device
> EXCLUDES 1 *encounter for attention to artificial openings of digestive tract (Z43.1-Z43.4)*

Z46.51 Encounter for fitting and adjustment of gastric lap band

Z46.59 Encounter for fitting and adjustment of other gastrointestinal appliance and device

Z46.6 Encounter for fitting and adjustment of urinary device
> EXCLUDES 2 *attention to artificial openings of urinary tract (Z43.5, Z43.6)*

✓6ᵗʰ Z46.8 Encounter for fitting and adjustment of other specified devices

Z46.81 Encounter for fitting and adjustment of insulin pump
> Encounter for insulin pump instruction and training
> Encounter for insulin pump titration

Z46.82 Encounter for fitting and adjustment of non-vascular catheter

Z46.89 Encounter for fitting and adjustment of other specified devices
> Encounter for fitting and adjustment of wheelchair
> AHA: 2014, 4Q, 26-28

Z46.9 Encounter for fitting and adjustment of unspecified device

✓4ᵗʰ Z47 Orthopedic aftercare
> EXCLUDES 1 *aftercare for healing fracture—code to fracture with 7th character D*

Z47.1 Aftercare following joint replacement surgery
> Use additional code to identify the joint (Z96.6-)

Z47.2 Encounter for removal of internal fixation device
> EXCLUDES 1 *encounter for adjustment of internal fixation device for fracture treatment—code to fracture with appropriate 7th character*
> *encounter for removal of external fixation device—code to fracture with 7th character D*
> *infection or inflammatory reaction to internal fixation device (T84.6-)*
> *mechanical complication of internal fixation device (T84.1-)*

✓5ᵗʰ Z47.3 Aftercare following explantation of joint prosthesis
> Aftercare following explantation of joint prosthesis, staged procedure
> Encounter for joint prosthesis insertion following prior explantation of joint prosthesis
> AHA: 2015, 1Q, 16

Z47.31 Aftercare following explantation of shoulder joint prosthesis
> EXCLUDES 1 *acquired absence of shoulder joint following prior explantation of shoulder joint prosthesis (Z89.23-)*
> *shoulder joint prosthesis explantation status (Z89.23-)*

Z47.32 Aftercare following explantation of hip joint prosthesis
> EXCLUDES 1 *acquired absence of hip joint following prior explantation of hip joint prosthesis (Z89.62-)*
> *hip joint prosthesis explantation status (Z89.62-)*

Z47.33 Aftercare following explantation of knee joint prosthesis
> EXCLUDES 1 *acquired absence of knee joint following prior explantation of knee prosthesis (Z89.52-)*
> *knee joint prosthesis explantation status (Z89.52-)*

✓5ᵗʰ Z47.8 Encounter for other orthopedic aftercare

Z47.81 Encounter for orthopedic aftercare following surgical amputation
> Use additional code to identify the limb amputated (Z89.-)

Z47.82 Encounter for orthopedic aftercare following scoliosis surgery

Z47.89 Encounter for other orthopedic aftercare
> AHA: 2015, 1Q, 8

☑ Additional Character Required   ✓x7ᵗʰ Placeholder Alert   Unacceptable PDx   Manifestation   Hospital Acquired Condition   EXCLUDES 1 Not Coded Here   EXCLUDES 2 Not Included Here

ICD-10-CM 2016   1235

✓4ᵗʰ Z48 Encounter for other postprocedural aftercare

> **EXCLUDES 1** encounter for follow-up examination after completed treatment (Z08-Z09)
>
> **EXCLUDES 2** encounter for attention to artificial openings (Z43.-)
> encounter for fitting and adjustment of prosthetic and other devices (Z44-Z46)
>
> **AHA:** 2015, 1Q, 6-7

✓5ᵗʰ Z48.0 Encounter for attention to dressings, sutures and drains

> **EXCLUDES 1** encounter for planned postprocedural wound closure (Z48.1)

Z48.00 Encounter for change or removal of nonsurgical wound dressing
Encounter for change or removal of wound dressing NOS

Z48.01 Encounter for change or removal of surgical wound dressing

Z48.02 Encounter for removal of sutures
Encounter for removal of staples

Z48.03 Encounter for change or removal of drains

Z48.1 Encounter for planned postprocedural wound closure

> **EXCLUDES 1** encounter for attention to dressings and sutures (Z48.0-)

✓5ᵗʰ Z48.2 Encounter for aftercare following organ transplant

Z48.21 Encounter for aftercare following heart transplant `PDxCC` `CC`
CC Excl: D47.Z1,T86.20-T86.23,T86.290,T86.298,T86.30-T86.39,T86.850-T86.859,T86.90-T86.99,Z94.1,Z94.3, Z94.89- Z94.9

Z48.22 Encounter for aftercare following kidney transplant `PDxCC` `CC`
CC Excl: D47.Z1,T86.10-T86.13, T86.19, T86.850-T86.859,T86.90-T86.99,Z94.0,Z94.89-Z94.9

Z48.23 Encounter for aftercare following liver transplant `PDxCC` `CC`
CC Excl: D47.Z1,T86.40-T86.43,T86.49,T86.850-T86.859,T86.90-T86.99, Z94.4,Z94.89-Z94.9

Z48.24 Encounter for aftercare following lung transplant `PDxCC` `CC`
CC Excl: D47.Z1, T86.810-T86.819,T86.49,T86.850-T86.859,T86.90-T86.99,Z94.2,Z94.89-Z94.9

✓6ᵗʰ Z48.28 Encounter for aftercare following multiple organ transplant

Z48.280 Encounter for aftercare following heart-lung transplant `PDxCC` `CC`
CC Excl: See Code: Z48.21

Z48.288 Encounter for aftercare following multiple organ transplant

✓6ᵗʰ Z48.29 Encounter for aftercare following other organ transplant

Z48.290 Encounter for aftercare following bone marrow transplant `PDxCC` `CC`
CC Excl: D47.Z1, T86.810-T86.813,T86.00-T86.09,T86.850-T86.859,T86.90-T86.99,Z94.9

Z48.298 Encounter for aftercare following other organ transplant

Z48.3 Aftercare following surgery for neoplasm
Use additional code to identify the neoplasm

✓5ᵗʰ Z48.8 Encounter for other specified postprocedural aftercare

✓6ᵗʰ Z48.81 Encounter for surgical aftercare following surgery on specified body systems

> **NOTE** These codes identify the body system requiring aftercare. They are for use in conjunction with other aftercare codes to fully explain the aftercare encounter. The condition treated should also be coded if still present.
>
> **EXCLUDES 1** aftercare for injury—code the injury with 7th character D
> aftercare following surgery for neoplasm (Z48.3)
>
> **EXCLUDES 2** aftercare following organ transplant (Z48.2-)
> orthopedic aftercare (Z47.-)

Z48.810 Encounter for surgical aftercare following surgery on the sense organs

Z48.811 Encounter for surgical aftercare following surgery on the nervous system

> **EXCLUDES 2** encounter for surgical aftercare following surgery on the sense organs (Z48.810)

Z48.812 Encounter for surgical aftercare following surgery on the circulatory system
AHA: 2012, 4Q, 96

Z48.813 Encounter for surgical aftercare following surgery on the respiratory system

Z48.814 Encounter for surgical aftercare following surgery on the teeth or oral cavity

Z48.815 Encounter for surgical aftercare following surgery on the digestive system

Z48.816 Encounter for surgical aftercare following surgery on the genitourinary system

> **EXCLUDES 1** encounter for aftercare following sterilization reversal (Z31.42)

Z48.817 Encounter for surgical aftercare following surgery on the skin and subcutaneous tissue

Z48.89 Encounter for other specified surgical aftercare

✓4ᵗʰ Z49 Encounter for care involving renal dialysis

> Code also associated end stage renal disease (N18.6)

✓5ᵗʰ Z49.0 Preparatory care for renal dialysis
Encounter for dialysis instruction and training

Z49.01 Encounter for fitting and adjustment of extracorporeal dialysis catheter
Removal or replacement of renal dialysis catheter
Toilet or cleansing of renal dialysis catheter

Z49.02 Encounter for fitting and adjustment of peritoneal dialysis catheter

✓5ᵗʰ Z49.3 Encounter for adequacy testing for dialysis

Z49.31 Encounter for adequacy testing for hemodialysis

Z49.32 Encounter for adequacy testing for peritoneal dialysis
Encounter for peritoneal equilibration test

✓4ᵗʰ Z51 Encounter for other aftercare

> Code also condition requiring care
>
> **EXCLUDES 1** follow-up examination after treatment (Z08-Z09)

Z51.0 Encounter for antineoplastic radiation therapy

✓5ᵗʰ Z51.1 Encounter for antineoplastic chemotherapy and immunotherapy

> **EXCLUDES 2** encounter for chemotherapy and immunotherapy for nonneoplastic condition—code to condition

Z51.11 Encounter for antineoplastic chemotherapy

Z51.12 Encounter for antineoplastic immunotherapy

Z51.5 Encounter for palliative care

✓5ᵗʰ Z51.8 Encounter for other specified aftercare

> **EXCLUDES 1** holiday relief care (Z75.5)

Z51.81 Encounter for therapeutic drug level monitoring
Code also any long-term (current) drug therapy (Z79.-)

> **EXCLUDES 1** encounter for blood-drug test for administrative or medicolegal reasons (Z02.83)

14 Z51.89 Encounter for other specified aftercare
AHA: 2012, 4Q, 95-97

✓4ᵗʰ Z52 Donors of organs and tissues

> **INCLUDES** autologous and other living donors
>
> **EXCLUDES 1** cadaveric donor—omit code
> examination of potential donor (Z00.5)
>
> **AHA:** 2012, 4Q, 99

✓5ᵗʰ Z52.0 Blood donor

✓6ᵗʰ Z52.00 Unspecified blood donor
Z52.000 Unspecified donor, whole blood
Z52.001 Unspecified donor, stem cells
Z52.008 Unspecified donor, other blood

✓6ᵗʰ Z52.01 Autologous blood donor
Z52.010 Autologous donor, whole blood
Z52.011 Autologous donor, stem cells
Z52.018 Autologous donor, other blood

✓6ᵗʰ Z52.09 Other blood donor
Volunteer donor
Z52.090 Other blood donor, whole blood
Z52.091 Other blood donor, stem cells
Z52.098 Other blood donor, other blood

✓5ᵗʰ Z52.1 Skin donor
Z52.10 Skin donor, unspecified

---

14 Unacceptable PDx unless a secondary diagnosis is present.

N Newborn: 0   **P** Pediatric: 0-17   **M** Maternity: 12-55   **A** Adult: 15-124   **MCC** Major CC Condition   **PDxMCC** PDx acts as own MCC   **CC** CC Condition   **PDxCC** PDx acts as own CC

Z52.11   **Skin donor,** autologous

Z52.19   **Skin donor,** other

✓5ᵗʰ   **Z52.2**   **Bone donor**

     Z52.20   **Bone donor,** unspecified

     Z52.21   **Bone donor,** autologous

     Z52.29   **Bone donor,** other

Z52.3   **Bone marrow donor**

Z52.4   **Kidney donor**

Z52.5   **Cornea donor**

Z52.6   **Liver donor**

✓5ᵗʰ   **Z52.8**   **Donor of** other specified organs or tissues

     ✓6ᵗʰ   **Z52.81**   **Egg (Oocyte) donor**

         Z52.810   **Egg (Oocyte) donor** under age 35, anonymous **recipient** ♀

             Egg donor under age 35 NOS

         Z52.811   **Egg (Oocyte) donor** under age 35, designated **recipient** ♀

         Z52.812   **Egg (Oocyte) donor** age 35 and over, anonymous **recipient** ♀

             Egg donor age 35 and over NOS

         Z52.813   **Egg (Oocyte) donor** age 35 and over, designated **recipient** ♀

         Z52.819   **Egg (Oocyte) donor,** unspecified ♀

     Z52.89   **Donor of** other specified organs or tissues

Z52.9   **Donor of** unspecified organ or tissue

     Donor NOS

✓4ᵗʰ   **Z53**   **Persons encountering health services for specific procedures and treatment, not carried out**

     ✓5ᵗʰ   **Z53.0**   **Procedure and treatment not carried out because of** contraindication

         Z53.01   **Procedure and treatment not carried out due to** patient smoking

         Z53.09   **Procedure and treatment not carried out because of** other contraindication

     Z53.1   **Procedure and treatment not carried out because of patient's decision for** reasons of belief and group pressure

     ✓5ᵗʰ   **Z53.2**   **Procedure and treatment not carried out because of patient's decision for** other and unspecified reasons

         Z53.20   **Procedure and treatment not carried out because of patient's decision for** unspecified reasons

         Z53.21   **Procedure and treatment not carried out due to** patient leaving prior to being seen by health care provider

         Z53.29   **Procedure and treatment not carried out because of patient's decision for** other reasons

     Z53.8   **Procedure and treatment not carried out for** other reasons

     Z53.9   **Procedure and treatment not carried out,** unspecified reason

Persons with potential health hazards related to socioeconomic and psychosocial circumstances (Z55-Z65)

✓4ᵗʰ   **Z55**   **Problems related to education and literacy**

     EXCLUDES 1   *disorders of psychological development (F80-F89)*

     Z55.0   **Illiteracy and low-level literacy**

     Z55.1   **Schooling unavailable and unattainable**

     Z55.2   **Failed school examinations**

     Z55.3   **Underachievement in school**

     Z55.4   **Educational maladjustment and discord with teachers and classmates**

     Z55.8   **Other problems related to education and literacy**

         Problems related to inadequate teaching

     Z55.9   **Problems related to education and literacy, unspecified**

         Academic problems NOS

✓4ᵗʰ   **Z56**   **Problems related to employment and unemployment**

     EXCLUDES 2   *occupational exposure to risk factors (Z57.-)*

             problems related to housing and economic circumstances (Z59.-)

     Z56.0   **Unemployment, unspecified**

     Z56.1   **Change of job**

     Z56.2   **Threat of job loss**

     Z56.3   **Stressful work schedule**

     Z56.4   **Discord with boss and workmates**

     Z56.5   **Uncongenial work environment**

         Difficult conditions at work

Z56.6   **Other physical and mental strain related to work**

✓5ᵗʰ   **Z56.8**   **Other problems related to employment**

     Z56.81   **Sexual harassment on the job**

     Z56.82   **Military deployment status**

         Individual (civilian or military) currently deployed in theater or in support of military war, peacekeeping and humanitarian operations

     Z56.89   **Other problems related to employment**

Z56.9   **Unspecified problems related to employment**

     Occupational problems NOS

✓4ᵗʰ   **Z57**   **Occupational exposure to risk factors**

     Z57.0   **Occupational exposure to** noise

     Z57.1   **Occupational exposure to** radiation

     Z57.2   **Occupational exposure to** dust

     ✓5ᵗʰ   **Z57.3**   **Occupational exposure to** other air contaminants

         Z57.31   **Occupational exposure to environmental** tobacco smoke

             EXCLUDES 2   *exposure to environmental tobacco smoke (Z77.22)*

         Z57.39   **Occupational exposure to other** air contaminants

     Z57.4   **Occupational exposure to** toxic agents in agriculture

         Occupational exposure to solids, liquids, gases or vapors in agriculture

     Z57.5   **Occupational exposure to** toxic agents in other industries

         Occupational exposure to solids, liquids, gases or vapors in other industries

     Z57.6   **Occupational exposure to** extreme temperature

     Z57.7   **Occupational exposure to** vibration

     Z57.8   **Occupational exposure to** other risk factors

     Z57.9   **Occupational exposure to** unspecified risk factor

✓4ᵗʰ   **Z59**   **Problems related to housing and economic circumstances**

     EXCLUDES 2   *problems related to upbringing (Z62.-)*

     Z59.0   **Homelessness**

     Z59.1   **Inadequate housing**

         Lack of heating

         Restriction of space

         Technical defects in home preventing adequate care

         Unsatisfactory surroundings

         EXCLUDES 1   *problems related to the natural and physical environment (Z77.1-)*

     Z59.2   **Discord with neighbors, lodgers and landlord**

     Z59.3   **Problems related to living in residential institution**

         Boarding-school resident

         EXCLUDES 1   *institutional upbringing (Z62.2)*

     Z59.4   **Lack of adequate food and safe drinking water**

         Inadequate drinking water supply

         EXCLUDES 1   *effects of hunger (T73.0)*

             inappropriate diet or eating habits (Z72.4)

             malnutrition (E40-E46)

     Z59.5   **Extreme poverty**

     Z59.6   **Low income**

     Z59.7   **Insufficient social insurance and welfare support**

     Z59.8   **Other problems related to housing and economic circumstances**

         Foreclosure on loan   Problems with creditors

         Isolated dwelling

     Z59.9   **Problem related to housing and economic circumstances, unspecified**

✓4ᵗʰ   **Z60**   **Problems related to social environment**

     Z60.0   **Problems of adjustment to life-cycle transitions**

         Empty nest syndrome   Problem with adjustment

         Phase of life problem   to retirement [pension]

     Z60.2   **Problems related to living alone**

     Z60.3   **Acculturation difficulty**

         Problem with migration

         Problem with social transplantation

     Z60.4   **Social exclusion and rejection**

         Exclusion and rejection on the basis of personal characteristics, such as unusual physical appearance, illness or behavior.

         EXCLUDES 1   *target of adverse discrimination such as for racial or religious reasons (Z60.5)*

     Z60.5   **Target of (perceived) adverse discrimination and persecution**

         EXCLUDES 1   *social exclusion and rejection (Z60.4)*

     Z60.8   **Other problems related to social environment**

     Z60.9   **Problem related to social environment, unspecified**

✓ Additional Character Required   ✓x7ᵗʰ Placeholder Alert   Unacceptable PDx   Manifestation   Hospital Acquired Condition   EXCLUDES 1 Not Coded Here   EXCLUDES 2 Not Included Here

☑4ᵗʰ **Z62** **Problems related to upbringing**
Current and past negative life events in childhood
Current and past problems of a child related to upbringing
EXCLUDES 2   *maltreatment syndrome (T74.-)*
     problems related to housing and economic circumstances (Z59.-)

Z62.0 **Inadequate parental supervision and control**

Z62.1 **Parental overprotection**

☑5ᵗʰ **Z62.2** **Upbringing away from parents**
     EXCLUDES 1   *problems with boarding school (Z59.3)*

   Z62.21 **Child in welfare custody**   P
       Child in care of non-parental family member
       Child in foster care
       EXCLUDES 2   *problem for parent due to child in welfare custody (Z63.5)*

   Z62.22 **Institutional upbringing**
       Child living in orphanage or group home

   Z62.29 **Other upbringing away from parents**

Z62.3 **Hostility towards and scapegoating of child**   P

Z62.6 **Inappropriate (excessive) parental pressure**

☑5ᵗʰ **Z62.8** **Other specified problems related to upbringing**

   ☑6ᵗʰ **Z62.81** **Personal history of abuse in childhood**

     Z62.810 **Personal history of physical and sexual abuse in childhood**
         EXCLUDES 1   *current child physical abuse (T74.12, T76.12)*
             current child sexual abuse (T74.22, T76.22)

     Z62.811 **Personal history of psychological abuse in childhood**
         EXCLUDES 1   *current child psychological abuse (T74.32, T76.32)*

     Z62.812 **Personal history of neglect in childhood**
         EXCLUDES 1   *current child neglect (T74.02, T76.02)*

     Z62.819 **Personal history of unspecified abuse in childhood**
         EXCLUDES 1   *current child abuse NOS (T74.92, T76.92)*

   ☑6ᵗʰ **Z62.82** **Parent-child conflict**
     Z62.820 **Parent-biological child conflict**
       Parent-child problem NOS
     Z62.821 **Parent-adopted child conflict**
     Z62.822 **Parent-foster child conflict**

   ☑6ᵗʰ **Z62.89** **Other specified problems related to upbringing**
     Z62.890 **Parent-child estrangement NEC**
     Z62.891 **Sibling rivalry**
     Z62.898 **Other specified problems related to upbringing**

Z62.9 **Problem related to upbringing, unspecified**

☑4ᵗʰ **Z63** **Other problems related to primary support group, including family circumstances**
     EXCLUDES 2   *maltreatment syndrome (T74-, T76)*
         parent-child problems (Z62.-)
         problems related to negative life events in childhood (Z62.-)
         problems related to upbringing (Z62.-)

Z63.0 **Problems in relationship with spouse or partner**
     EXCLUDES 1   *counseling for spousal or partner abuse problems (Z69.1)*
         counseling related to sexual attitude, behavior, and orientation (Z70.-)

Z63.1 **Problems in relationship with in-laws**

☑5ᵗʰ **Z63.3** **Absence of family member**
     EXCLUDES 1   *absence of family member due to disappearance and death (Z63.4)*
         absence of family member due to separation and divorce (Z63.5)

   Z63.31 **Absence of family member due to military deployment**
       Individual or family affected by other family member being on military deployment
       EXCLUDES 1   *family disruption due to return of family member from military deployment (Z63.71)*

   Z63.32 **Other absence of family member**

Z63.4 **Disappearance and death of family member**
     Assumed death of family member
     Bereavement
     AHA: 2014, 1Q, 25

Z63.5 **Disruption of family by separation and divorce**
     Marital estrangement

Z63.6 **Dependent relative needing care at home**

☑5ᵗʰ **Z63.7** **Other stressful life events affecting family and household**

   Z63.71 **Stress on family due to return of family member from military deployment**
       Individual or family affected by family member having returned from military deployment (current or past conflict)

   Z63.72 **Alcoholism and drug addiction in family**

   Z63.79 **Other stressful life events affecting family and household**
       Anxiety (normal) about sick person in family
       Health problems within family
       Ill or disturbed family member
       Isolated family

Z63.8 **Other specified problems related to primary support group**
     Family discord NOS
     Family estrangement NOS
     High expressed emotional level within family
     Inadequate family support NOS
     Inadequate or distorted communication within family

Z63.9 **Problem related to primary support group, unspecified**
     Relationship disorder NOS

☑4ᵗʰ **Z64** **Problems related to certain psychosocial circumstances**

Z64.0 **Problems related to unwanted pregnancy**   M ♀

Z64.1 **Problems related to multiparity**   ♀

Z64.4 **Discord with counselors**
     Discord with probation officer
     Discord with social worker

☑4ᵗʰ **Z65** **Problems related to other psychosocial circumstances**

Z65.0 **Conviction in civil and criminal proceedings without imprisonment**

Z65.1 **Imprisonment and other incarceration**

Z65.2 **Problems related to release from prison**

Z65.3 **Problems related to other legal circumstances**
     Arrest
     Child custody or support proceedings
     Litigation
     Prosecution

Z65.4 **Victim of crime and terrorism**
     Victim of torture

Z65.5 **Exposure to disaster, war and other hostilities**
     EXCLUDES 1   *target of perceived discrimination or persecution (Z60.5)*

Z65.8 **Other specified problems related to psychosocial circumstances**

Z65.9 **Problem related to unspecified psychosocial circumstances**

Do not resuscitate status (Z66)

Z66 **Do not resuscitate**
     DNR status

Blood type (Z67)

☑4ᵗʰ **Z67** **Blood type**

☑5ᵗʰ **Z67.1** **Type A blood**
   Z67.10 **Type A blood, Rh positive**
   Z67.11 **Type A blood, Rh negative**

☑5ᵗʰ **Z67.2** **Type B blood**
   Z67.20 **Type B blood, Rh positive**
   Z67.21 **Type B blood, Rh negative**

☑5ᵗʰ **Z67.3** **Type AB blood**
   Z67.30 **Type AB blood, Rh positive**
   Z67.31 **Type AB blood, Rh negative**

☑5ᵗʰ **Z67.4** **Type O blood**
   Z67.40 **Type O blood, Rh positive**
   Z67.41 **Type O blood, Rh negative**

☑5ᵗʰ **Z67.9** **Unspecified blood type**
   Z67.90 **Unspecified blood type, Rh positive**
   Z67.91 **Unspecified blood type, Rh negative**

N Newborn: 0   P Pediatric: 0-17   M Maternity: 12-55   A Adult: 15-124   **MCC** Major CC Condition   **PDxMCC** PDx acts as own MCC   **CC** CC Condition   **PDxCC** PDx acts as own CC

1238

ICD-10-CM 2016

Body mass index [BMI] (Z68)

✓4ᵗʰ Z68 Body mass index [BMI]
Kilograms per meters squared
> **NOTE** BMI adult codes are for use for persons 21 years of age or older.
> BMI pediatric codes are for use for persons 2-20 years of age. These percentiles are based on the growth charts published by the Centers for Disease Control and Prevention (CDC)

Z68.1 Body mass index [BMI] 19 or less, adult   CC A
> **CC Excl:** E66.01-E66.1,E66.8-E66.9, Z68.1,Z68.20-Z68.39, Z68.1-Z68.54

✓5ᵗʰ Z68.2 Body mass index [BMI] 20-29, adult

Z68.20	Body mass index [BMI] 20.0-20.9, adult	A
Z68.21	Body mass index [BMI] 21.0-21.9, adult	A
Z68.22	Body mass index [BMI] 22.0-22.9, adult	A
Z68.23	Body mass index [BMI] 23.0-23.9, adult	A
Z68.24	Body mass index [BMI] 24.0-24.9, adult	A
Z68.25	Body mass index [BMI] 25.0-25.9, adult	A
Z68.26	Body mass index [BMI] 26.0-26.9, adult	A
Z68.27	Body mass index [BMI] 27.0-27.9, adult	A
Z68.28	Body mass index [BMI] 28.0-28.9, adult	A
Z68.29	Body mass index [BMI] 29.0-29.9, adult	A

✓5ᵗʰ Z68.3 Body mass index [BMI] 30-39, adult

Z68.30	Body mass index [BMI] 30.0-30.9, adult	A
Z68.31	Body mass index [BMI] 31.0-31.9, adult	A
Z68.32	Body mass index [BMI] 32.0-32.9, adult	A
Z68.33	Body mass index [BMI] 33.0-33.9, adult	A
Z68.34	Body mass index [BMI] 34.0-34.9, adult	A
Z68.35	Body mass index [BMI] 35.0-35.9, adult	A
Z68.36	Body mass index [BMI] 36.0-36.9, adult	A
Z68.37	Body mass index [BMI] 37.0-37.9, adult	A
Z68.38	Body mass index [BMI] 38.0-38.9, adult	A
Z68.39	Body mass index [BMI] 39.0-39.9, adult	A

✓5ᵗʰ Z68.4 Body mass index [BMI] 40 or greater, adult
> **CC Excl:** For CC codes in subcategory Z68.4: CC with 7th character A, unless otherwise noted: E65-E66.1, E66.8-E66.9, Z68.1-Z68.54

Z68.41	Body mass index [BMI] 40.0-44.9, adult	CC A
Z68.42	Body mass index [BMI] 45.0-49.9, adult	CC A
Z68.43	Body mass index [BMI] 50-59.9, adult	CC A
Z68.44	Body mass index [BMI] 60.0-69.9, adult	CC A
Z68.45	Body mass index [BMI] 70 or greater, adult	CC A

✓5ᵗʰ Z68.5 Body mass index [BMI] pediatric

Z68.51	Body mass index [BMI] pediatric, less than 5th percentile for age	P
Z68.52	Body mass index [BMI] pediatric, 5th percentile to less than 85th percentile for age	P
Z68.53	Body mass index [BMI] pediatric, 85th percentile to less than 95th percentile for age	P
Z68.54	Body mass index [BMI] pediatric, greater than or equal to 95th percentile for age	P

Persons encountering health services in other circumstances (Z69-Z76)

✓4ᵗʰ Z69 Encounter for mental health services for victim and perpetrator of abuse
Counseling for victims and perpetrators of abuse

✓5ᵗʰ Z69.0 Encounter for mental health services for child abuse problems

✓6ᵗʰ Z69.01 Encounter for mental health services for parental child abuse

Z69.010 Encounter for mental health services for victim of parental child abuse   P

Z69.011 Encounter for mental health services for perpetrator of parental child abuse   P
> **EXCLUDES 1** encounter for mental health services for non-parental child abuse (Z69.02-)

✓6ᵗʰ Z69.02 Encounter for mental health services for non-parental child abuse

Z69.020 Encounter for mental health services for victim of non-parental child abuse   P

Z69.021 Encounter for mental health services for perpetrator of non-parental child abuse

✓5ᵗʰ Z69.1 Encounter for mental health services for spousal or partner abuse problems

Z69.11 Encounter for mental health services for victim of spousal or partner abuse

Z69.12 Encounter for mental health services for perpetrator of spousal or partner abuse

✓5ᵗʰ Z69.8 Encounter for mental health services for victim or perpetrator of other abuse

Z69.81 Encounter for mental health services for victim of other abuse
Encounter for rape victim counseling

Z69.82 Encounter for mental health services for perpetrator of other abuse

✓4ᵗʰ Z70 Counseling related to sexual attitude, behavior and orientation
Encounter for mental health services for sexual attitude, behavior and orientation
> **EXCLUDES 2** contraceptive or procreative counseling (Z30-Z31)

Z70.0 Counseling related to sexual attitude

Z70.1 Counseling related to patient's sexual behavior and orientation
Patient concerned regarding impotence
Patient concerned regarding non-responsiveness
Patient concerned regarding promiscuity
Patient concerned regarding sexual orientation

Z70.2 Counseling related to sexual behavior and orientation of third party
Advice sought regarding sexual behavior and orientation of child
Advice sought regarding sexual behavior and orientation of partner
Advice sought regarding sexual behavior and orientation of spouse

Z70.3 Counseling related to combined concerns regarding sexual attitude, behavior and orientation

Z70.8 Other sex counseling
Encounter for sex education

Z70.9 Sex counseling, unspecified

✓4ᵗʰ Z71 Persons encountering health services for other counseling and medical advice, not elsewhere classified
> **EXCLUDES 2** contraceptive or procreation counseling (Z30-Z31)
> sex counseling (Z70.-)

Z71.0 Person encountering health services to consult on behalf of another person
Person encountering health services to seek advice or treatment for non-attending third party
> **EXCLUDES 2** anxiety (normal) about sick person in family (Z63.7)
> expectant (adoptive) parent(s) pre-birth pediatrician visit (Z76.81)

Z71.1 Person with feared health complaint in whom no diagnosis is made
Person encountering health services with feared condition which was not demonstrated
Person encountering health services in which problem was normal state
"Worried well"
> **EXCLUDES 1** medical observation for suspected diseases and conditions proven not to exist (Z03.-)

Z71.2 Person consulting for explanation of examination or test findings

Z71.3 Dietary counseling and surveillance
Use additional code for any associated underlying medical condition
Use additional code to identify body mass index (BMI), if known (Z68.-)

✓5ᵗʰ Z71.4 Alcohol abuse counseling and surveillance
Use additional code for alcohol abuse or dependence (F10.-)

Z71.41 Alcohol abuse counseling and surveillance of alcoholic

Z71.42 Counseling for family member of alcoholic
Counseling for significant other, partner, or friend of alcoholic

✓5ᵗʰ Z71.5 Drug abuse counseling and surveillance
Use additional code for drug abuse or dependence (F11-F16, F18-F19)

Z71.51 Drug abuse counseling and surveillance of drug abuser

✓ Additional Character Required   ✓x7ᵗʰ Placeholder Alert   Unacceptable PDx   Manifestation   Hospital Acquired Condition   **EXCLUDES 1** Not Coded Here   **EXCLUDES 2** Not Included Here

Chapter 21. Factors Influencing Health Status and Contact with Health Services

Z71.52   **Counseling for** family member of drug abuser
Counseling for significant other, partner, or friend of drug abuser

Z71.6   **Tobacco abuse counseling**
Use additional code for nicotine dependence (F17.-)

Z71.7   **Human immunodeficiency virus [HIV] counseling**

✓5ᵗʰ **Z71.8**   **Other specified counseling**
EXCLUDES 2   *counseling for contraception (Z30.0-)*
counseling for genetics (Z31.5)
counseling for procreative management (Z31.6-)

Z71.81   **Spiritual or religious counseling**

Z71.89   **Other specified counseling**

Z71.9   **Counseling, unspecified**
Encounter for medical advice NOS

✓4ᵗʰ **Z72**   **Problems related to lifestyle**
EXCLUDES 2   *problems related to life-management difficulty (Z73.-)*
problems related to socioeconomic and psychosocial circumstances (Z55-Z65)

Z72.0   **Tobacco use**
Tobacco use NOS
EXCLUDES 1   *history of tobacco dependence (Z87.891)*
nicotine dependence (F17.2-)
tobacco dependence (F17.2-)
tobacco use during pregnancy (O99.33-)

Z72.3   **Lack of physical exercise**

Z72.4   **Inappropriate diet and eating habits**
EXCLUDES 1   *behavioral eating disorders of infancy or childhood (F98.2- F98.3)*
eating disorders (F50.-)
lack of adequate food (Z59.4)
malnutrition and other nutritional deficiencies (E40-E64)

✓5ᵗʰ **Z72.5**   **High risk sexual behavior**
Promiscuity
EXCLUDES 1   *paraphilias (F65)*

Z72.51   **High risk heterosexual behavior**

Z72.52   **High risk homosexual behavior**

Z72.53   **High risk bisexual behavior**

Z72.6   **Gambling and betting**
EXCLUDES 1   *compulsive or pathological gambling (F63.0)*

Z72.8   **Other problems related to lifestyle**

✓6ᵗʰ **Z72.81**   **Antisocial behavior**
EXCLUDES 1   *conduct disorders (F91.-)*

Z72.810   **Child and adolescent antisocial behavior**   P
Antisocial behavior (child) (adolescent) without manifest psychiatric disorder
Delinquency NOS
Group delinquency
Offenses in the context of gang membership
Stealing in company with others
Truancy from school

Z72.811   **Adult antisocial behavior**   A
Adult antisocial behavior without manifest psychiatric disorder

✓6ᵗʰ **Z72.82**   **Problems related to sleep**

Z72.820   **Sleep deprivation**
Lack of adequate sleep
EXCLUDES 1   *insomnia (G47.0-)*

Z72.821   **Inadequate sleep hygiene**
Bad sleep habits
Irregular sleep habits
Unhealthy sleep wake schedule
EXCLUDES 1   *insomnia (F51.0-, G47.0-)*

Z72.89   **Other problems related to lifestyle**
Self-damaging behavior

Z72.9   **Problem related to lifestyle, unspecified**

✓4ᵗʰ **Z73**   **Problems related to life management difficulty**
EXCLUDES 2   *problems related to socioeconomic and psychosocial circumstances (Z55-Z65)*

Z73.0   **Burn-out**

Z73.1   **Type A behavior pattern**

Z73.2   **Lack of relaxation and leisure**

Z73.3   **Stress, not elsewhere classified**
Physical and mental strain NOS
EXCLUDES 1   *stress related to employment or unemployment (Z56.-)*

Z73.4   **Inadequate social skills, not elsewhere classified**

Z73.5   **Social role conflict, not elsewhere classified**

Z73.6   **Limitation of activities due to disability**
EXCLUDES 1   *care-provider dependency (Z74.-)*

✓5ᵗʰ **Z73.8**   **Other problems related to life management difficulty**

✓6ᵗʰ **Z73.81**   **Behavioral insomnia of childhood**

Z73.810   **Behavioral insomnia of childhood, sleep-onset association type**   P

Z73.811   **Behavioral insomnia of childhood, limit setting type**   P

Z73.812   **Behavioral insomnia of childhood, combined type**   P

Z73.819   **Behavioral insomnia of childhood, unspecified type**   P

Z73.82   **Dual sensory impairment**

Z73.89   **Other problems related to life management difficulty**

Z73.9   **Problem related to life management difficulty, unspecified**

✓4ᵗʰ **Z74**   **Problems related to care provider dependency**
EXCLUDES 2   *dependence on enabling machines or devices NEC (Z99.-)*

✓5ᵗʰ **Z74.0**   **Reduced mobility**

Z74.01   **Bed confinement status**
Bedridden

Z74.09   **Other reduced mobility**
Chair ridden
Reduced mobility NOS
EXCLUDES 2   *wheelchair dependence (Z99.3)*

Z74.1   **Need for assistance with personal care**

Z74.2   **Need for assistance at home and no other household member able to render care**

Z74.3   **Need for continuous supervision**

Z74.8   **Other problems related to care provider dependency**

Z74.9   **Problem related to care provider dependency, unspecified**

✓4ᵗʰ **Z75**   **Problems related to medical facilities and other health care**

Z75.0   **Medical services not available in home**
EXCLUDES 1   *no other household member able to render care (Z74.2)*

Z75.1   **Person awaiting admission to adequate facility elsewhere**

Z75.2   **Other waiting period for investigation and treatment**

Z75.3   **Unavailability and inaccessibility of health-care facilities**
EXCLUDES 1   *bed unavailable (Z75.1)*

Z75.4   **Unavailability and inaccessibility of other helping agencies**

Z75.5   **Holiday relief care**

Z75.8   **Other problems related to medical facilities and other health care**

Z75.9   **Unspecified problem related to medical facilities and other health care**

✓4ᵗʰ **Z76**   **Persons encountering health services in other circumstances**

Z76.0   **Encounter for issue of repeat prescription**
Encounter for issue of repeat prescription for appliance
Encounter for issue of repeat prescription for medicaments
Encounter for issue of repeat prescription for spectacles
EXCLUDES 2   *issue of medical certificate (Z02.7)*
repeat prescription for contraceptive (Z30.4-)

Z76.1   **Encounter for health supervision and care of foundling**

Z76.2   **Encounter for health supervision and care of other healthy infant and child**   P
Encounter for medical or nursing care or supervision of healthy infant under circumstances such as adverse socioeconomic conditions at home
Encounter for medical or nursing care or supervision of healthy infant under circumstances such as awaiting foster or adoptive placement
Encounter for medical or nursing care or supervision of healthy infant under circumstances such as maternal illness
Encounter for medical or nursing care or supervision of healthy infant under circumstances such as number of children at home preventing or interfering with normal care

Z76.3   **Healthy person accompanying sick person**

Z76.4   **Other boarder to healthcare facility**
EXCLUDES 1   *homelessness (Z59.0)*

Z76.5   **Malingerer [conscious simulation]**
Person feigning illness (with obvious motivation)
EXCLUDES 1   *factitious disorder (F68.1-)*
peregrinating patient (F68.1-)

N Newborn: 0   P Pediatric: 0-17   M Maternity: 12-55   A Adult: 15-124   MCC Major CC Condition   PDx MCC PDx acts as own MCC   CC CC Condition   PDx CC PDx acts as own CC

✓5ᵗʰ **Z76.8** **Persons encountering health services in other specified circumstances**

Z76.81 **Expectant parent(s) prebirth pediatrician visit**
Pre-adoption pediatrician visit for adoptive parent(s)

Z76.82 **Awaiting organ transplant status**
Patient waiting for organ availability

Z76.89 **Persons encountering health services in other specified circumstances**
Persons encountering health services NOS
AHA: 2014, 2Q, 10

Persons with potential health hazards related to family and personal history and certain conditions influencing health status (Z77-Z99)

Code also any follow-up examination (Z08-Z09)

✓4ᵗʰ **Z77** **Other contact with and (suspected) exposures hazardous to health**

INCLUDES   contact with and (suspected) exposures to potential hazards to health

EXCLUDES 2   *contact with and (suspected) exposure to communicable diseases (Z20.-)*
exposure to (parental) (environmental) tobacco smoke in the perinatal period (P96.81)
newborn (suspected to be) affected by noxious substances transmitted via placenta or breast milk (P04.-)
occupational exposure to risk factors (Z57.-)
retained foreign body (Z18.-)
retained foreign body fully removed (Z87.821)
toxic effects of substances chiefly nonmedicinal as to source (T51-T65)

✓5ᵗʰ **Z77.0** **Contact with and (suspected) exposure to** hazardous, chiefly nonmedicinal, chemicals

✓6ᵗʰ **Z77.01** **Contact with and (suspected) exposure to hazardous metals**

Z77.010 **Contact with and (suspected) exposure to arsenic**

Z77.011 **Contact with and (suspected) exposure to lead**

Z77.012 **Contact with and (suspected) exposure to uranium**
EXCLUDES 1   *retained depleted uranium fragments (Z18.01)*

Z77.018 **Contact with and (suspected) exposure to** other **hazardous metals**
Contact with and (suspected) exposure to chromium compounds
Contact with and (suspected) exposure to nickel dust

✓6ᵗʰ **Z77.02** **Contact with and (suspected) exposure to hazardous aromatic compounds**

Z77.020 **Contact with and (suspected) exposure to aromatic amines**

Z77.021 **Contact with and (suspected) exposure to benzene**

Z77.028 **Contact with and (suspected) exposure to** other **hazardous aromatic compounds**
Aromatic dyes NOS
Polycyclic aromatic hydrocarbons

✓6ᵗʰ **Z77.09** **Contact with and (suspected) exposure to other hazardous, chiefly** nonmedicinal, chemicals

Z77.090 **Contact with and (suspected) exposure to asbestos**

Z77.098 **Contact with and (suspected) exposure to** other **hazardous, chiefly nonmedicinal, chemicals**
Dyes NOS

✓5ᵗʰ **Z77.1** **Contact with and (suspected) exposure to environmental pollution and** hazards in the physical environment

✓6ᵗʰ **Z77.11** **Contact with and (suspected) exposure to environmental pollution**

Z77.110 **Contact with and (suspected) exposure to** air **pollution**

Z77.111 **Contact with and (suspected) exposure to** water **pollution**

Z77.112 **Contact with and (suspected) exposure to** soil **pollution**

Z77.118 **Contact with and (suspected) exposure to** other **environmental pollution**

✓6ᵗʰ **Z77.12** **Contact with and (suspected) exposure to hazards in the physical environment**

Z77.120 **Contact with and (suspected) exposure to** mold (toxic)

Z77.121 **Contact with and (suspected) exposure to** harmful algae and algae toxins
Contact with and (suspected) exposure to (harmful) algae bloom NOS
Contact with and (suspected) exposure to blue-green algae bloom
Contact with and (suspected) exposure to brown tide
Contact with and (suspected) exposure to cyanobacteria bloom
Contact with and (suspected) exposure to Florida red tide
Contact with and (suspected) exposure to pfiesteria piscicida
Contact with and (suspected) exposure to red tide

Z77.122 **Contact with and (suspected) exposure to** noise

Z77.123 **Contact with and (suspected) exposure to** radon and other naturally occuring radiation
EXCLUDES 2   *radiation exposure as the cause of a confirmed condition (W88-W90, X39.0-)*
radiation sickness NOS (T66)

Z77.128 **Contact with and (suspected) exposure to** other hazards in the physical environment

✓5ᵗʰ **Z77.2** **Contact with and (suspected) exposure to** other **hazardous substances**

Z77.21 **Contact with and (suspected) exposure to potentially hazardous** body fluids

Z77.22 **Contact with and (suspected) exposure to** environmental tobacco smoke (acute) (chronic)
Exposure to second hand tobacco smoke (acute) (chronic)
Passive smoking (acute) (chronic)
EXCLUDES 1   *nicotine dependence (F17.-)*
tobacco use (Z72.0)
EXCLUDES 2   *occupational exposure to environmental tobacco smoke (Z57.31)*

Z77.29 **Contact with and (suspected) exposure to** other **hazardous substances**

Z77.9 Other contact with and (suspected) exposures hazardous to health

✓4ᵗʰ **Z78** **Other specified health status**

EXCLUDES 2   *asymptomatic human immunodeficiency virus [HIV] infection status (Z21)*
postprocedural status (Z93- Z99)
sex reassignment status (Z87.890)

Z78.0 **Asymptomatic menopausal state**   A ♀
Menopausal state NOS
Postmenopausal status NOS
EXCLUDES 2   *symptomatic menopausal state (N95.1)*

Z78.1 **Physical restraint status**
EXCLUDES 1   *physical restraint due to a procedure - omit code*

Z78.9 **Other specified health status**

✓4ᵗʰ **Z79** **Long term (current) drug therapy**
INCLUDES   long term (current) drug use for prophylactic purposes
Code also any therapeutic drug level monitoring (Z51.81)
EXCLUDES 2   *drug abuse and dependence (F11-F19)*
drug use complicating pregnancy, childbirth, and the puerperium (O99.32-)

✓5ᵗʰ **Z79.0** **Long term (current) use of anticoagulants and antithrombotics/antiplatelets**
EXCLUDES 2   *long term (current) use of aspirin (Z79.82)*

Z79.01 **Long term (current) use of** anticoagulants

Z79.02 **Long term (current) use of antithrombotics/antiplatelets**

Z79.1 **Long term (current) use of** non-steroidal anti-inflammatories (NSAID)
EXCLUDES 2   *long term (current) use of aspirin (Z79.82)*

Z79.2 **Long term (current) use of** antibiotics

Z79.3 **Long term (current) use of** hormonal contraceptives
Long term (current) use of birth control pill or patch

Z79.4 **Long term (current) use of** insulin

✓ Additional Character Required   ✓x7ᵗʰ Placeholder Alert   Unacceptable PDx   Manifestation   Hospital Acquired Condition   EXCLUDES 1 Not Coded Here   EXCLUDES 2 Not Included Here

ICD-10-CM 2016   1241

✓5ᵗʰ Z79.5   Long term (current) use of steroids

     Z79.51   Long term (current) use of inhaled steroids

     Z79.52   Long term (current) use of systemic steroids

✓5ᵗʰ Z79.8   Other long term (current) drug therapy

     ✓6ᵗʰ Z79.81   Long term (current) use of agents affecting estrogen receptors and estrogen levels

         Code first, if applicable:

         malignant neoplasm of breast (C50.-)

         malignant neoplasm of prostate (C61)

         Use additional code, if applicable, to identify:

         estrogen receptor positive status (Z17.0)

         family history of breast cancer (Z80.3)

         genetic susceptibility to malignant neoplasm (cancer) (Z15.0-)

         personal history of breast cancer (Z85.3)

         personal history of prostate cancer (Z85.46)

         postmenopausal status (Z78.0)

         EXCLUDES 1   hormone replacement therapy (postmenopausal) (Z79.890)

         Z79.810   Long term (current) use of selective estrogen receptor modulators (SERMs)

             Long term (current) use of raloxifene (Evista)

             Long term (current) use of tamoxifen (Nolvadex)

             Long term (current) use of toremifene (Fareston)

         Z79.811   Long term (current) use of aromatase inhibitors

             Long term (current) use of anastrozole (Arimidex)

             Long term (current) use of exemestane (Aromasin)

             Long term (current) use of letrozole (Femara)

         Z79.818   Long term (current) use of other **agents affecting estrogen receptors and estrogen levels**

             Long term (current) use of estrogen receptor downregulators

             Long term (current) use of fulvestrant (Faslodex)

             Long term (current) use of gonadotropin-releasing hormone (GnRH) agonist

             Long term (current) use of goserelin acetate (Zoladex)

             Long term (current) use of leuprolide acetate (leuprorelin) (Lupron)

             Long term (current) use of megestrol acetate (Megace)

     Z79.82   Long term (current) use of aspirin

     Z79.83   Long term (current) use of bisphosphonates

     ✓6ᵗʰ Z79.89   Other long term (current) drug therapy

         Z79.890   Hormone replacement therapy (postmenopausal) ♀

         Z79.891   Long term (current) use of opiate analgesic

             Long term (current) use of methadone for pain management

             EXCLUDES 1   methodone use NOS (F11.2-)

                              use of methadone for treatment of heroin addiction (F11.2-)

         Z79.899   Other long term (current) drug therapy

✓4ᵗʰ Z80   Family history of primary malignant neoplasm

     Z80.0   Family history of malignant neoplasm of digestive organs

         Conditions classifiable to C15-C26

     Z80.1   Family history of malignant neoplasm of trachea, bronchus and lung

         Conditions classifiable to C33-C34

     Z80.2   Family history of malignant neoplasm of other respiratory and intrathoracic organs

         Conditions classifiable to C30-C32, C37-C39

     Z80.3   Family history of malignant neoplasm of breast

         Conditions classifiable to C50-

     ✓5ᵗʰ Z80.4   Family history of malignant neoplasm of genital organs

         Conditions classifiable to C51-C63

         Z80.41   Family history of malignant neoplasm of ovary

         Z80.42   Family history of malignant neoplasm of prostate

         Z80.43   Family history of malignant neoplasm of testis

         Z80.49   Family history of malignant neoplasm of other genital organs

     ✓5ᵗʰ Z80.5   Family history of malignant neoplasm of urinary tract

         Conditions classifiable to C64-C68

         Z80.51   Family history of malignant neoplasm of kidney

         Z80.52   Family history of malignant neoplasm of bladder

         Z80.59   Family history of malignant neoplasm of other urinary tract organ

     Z80.6   Family history of leukemia

         Conditions classifiable to C91-C95

     Z80.7   Family history of other **malignant neoplasms of** lymphoid, hematopoietic and related tissues

         Conditions classifiable to C81-C90, C96-

     Z80.8   Family history of malignant neoplasm of other organs or systems

         Conditions classifiable to C00-C14, C40-C49, C69-C79

     Z80.9   Family history of malignant neoplasm, unspecified

         Conditions classifiable to C80.1

✓4ᵗʰ Z81   Family history of mental and behavioral disorders

     Z81.0   Family history of intellectual disabilities

         Conditions classifiable to F70-F79

     Z81.1   Family history of alcohol abuse and dependence

         Conditions classifiable to F10-

     Z81.2   Family history of tobacco abuse and dependence

         Conditions classifiable to F17-

     Z81.3   Family history of other psychoactive substance abuse and dependence

         Conditions classifiable to F11-F16, F18-F19

     Z81.4   Family history of other substance abuse and dependence

         Conditions classifiable to F55

     Z81.8   Family history of other mental and behavioral disorders

         Conditions classifiable elsewhere in F01-F99

✓4ᵗʰ Z82   Family history of certain disabilities and chronic diseases (leading to disablement)

     Z82.0   Family history of epilepsy **and other diseases of the nervous system**

         Conditions classifiable to G00-G99

     Z82.1   Family history of blindness and visual loss

         Conditions classifiable to H54-

     Z82.2   Family history of deafness and hearing loss

         Conditions classifiable to H90-H91

     Z82.3   Family history of stroke

         Conditions classifiable to I60-I64

     ✓5ᵗʰ Z82.4   Family history of ischemic heart disease and other diseases of the circulatory system

         Conditions classifiable to I00-I52, I65-I99

         Z82.41   Family history of sudden cardiac death

         Z82.49   Family history of ischemic heart disease **and other diseases of the circulatory system**

     Z82.5   Family history of asthma **and other chronic lower respiratory diseases**

         Conditions classifiable to J40-J47

         EXCLUDES 2   family history of other diseases of the respiratory system (Z83.6)

     ✓5ᵗʰ Z82.6   Family history of arthritis and other diseases of the musculoskeletal system and connective tissue

         Conditions classifiable to M00-M99

         Z82.61   Family history of arthritis

         Z82.62   Family history of osteoporosis

         Z82.69   Family history of other **diseases of the musculoskeletal system and connective tissue**

     ✓5ᵗʰ Z82.7   Family history of congenital malformations, deformations and chromosomal abnormalities

         Conditions classifiable to Q00-Q99

         Z82.71   Family history of polycystic kidney

         Z82.79   Family history of other **congenital malformations, deformations and chromosomal abnormalities**

     Z82.8   Family history of other disabilities and chronic diseases leading to disablement, **not elsewhere classified**

✓4ᵗʰ Z83   Family history of other specific disorders

     EXCLUDES 2   contact with and (suspected) exposure to communicable disease in the family (Z20.-)

     Z83.0   Family history of human immunodeficiency virus [HIV] disease

         Conditions classifiable to B20

Ⓝ Newborn: 0   Ⓟ Pediatric: 0-17   Ⓜ Maternity: 12-55   Ⓐ Adult: 15-124   **MCC** Major CC Condition   **PDxMCC** PDx acts as own MCC   **CC** CC Condition   **PDxCC** PDx acts as own CC

1242

ICD-10-CM 2016

Z83.1 Family history of other infectious and parasitic diseases
Conditions classifiable to A00-B19, B25-B94, B99

Z83.2 Family history of diseases of the blood and blood-forming organs **and certain disorders involving the immune mechanism**
Conditions classifiable to D50-D89

Z83.3 Family history of diabetes mellitus
Conditions classifiable to E08-E13

✓5th **Z83.4 Family history of other endocrine, nutritional and metabolic diseases**
Conditions classifiable to E00-E07, E15-E88

    Z83.41 Family history of multiple endocrine neoplasia [MEN] syndrome

    Z83.49 Family history of other endocrine, nutritional and metabolic diseases

✓5th **Z83.5 Family history of eye and ear disorders**

    ✓6th **Z83.51 Family history of** eye disorders
    Conditions classifiable to H00-H53, H55-H59
    EXCLUDES 2 family history of blindness and visual loss (Z82.1)

        Z83.511 Family history of glaucoma

        Z83.518 Family history of other specified eye disorder

    Z83.52 Family history of ear disorders
    Conditions classifiable to H60-H83, H92-H95
    EXCLUDES 2 family history of deafness and hearing loss (Z82.2)

Z83.6 Family history of other diseases of the respiratory system
Conditions classifiable to J00-J39, J60-J99
EXCLUDES 2 family history of asthma and other chronic lower respiratory diseases (Z82.5)

✓5th **Z83.7 Family history of diseases of the digestive system**
Conditions classifiable to K00-K93

    Z83.71 Family history of colonic polyps
    EXCLUDES 1 family history of malignant neoplasm of digestive organs (Z80.0)

    Z83.79 Family history of other diseases of the digestive system

✓4th **Z84 Family history of other conditions**

Z84.0 Family history of diseases of the skin and subcutaneous tissue
Conditions classifiable to L00-L99

Z84.1 Family history of disorders of kidney and ureter
Conditions classifiable to N00-N29

Z84.2 Family history of other diseases of the genitourinary system
Conditions classifiable to N30-N99

Z84.3 Family history of consanguinity

✓5th **Z84.8 Family history of other specified conditions**

    Z84.81 Family history of carrier of genetic disease

    Z84.89 Family history of other specified conditions

✓4th **Z85 Personal history of malignant neoplasm**
Code first any follow-up examination after treatment of malignant neoplasm (Z08)
Use additional code to identify:
  alcohol use and dependence (F10.-)
  exposure to environmental tobacco smoke (Z77.22)
  history of tobacco use (Z87.891)
  occupational exposure to environmental tobacco smoke (Z57.31)
  tobacco dependence (F17.-)
  tobacco use (Z72.0)
EXCLUDES 2 personal history of benign neoplasm (Z86.01-)
  personal history of carcinoma-in-situ (Z86.00-)

✓5th **Z85.0 Personal history of malignant neoplasm of** digestive organs

    Z85.00 Personal history of malignant neoplasm of unspecified digestive organ

    Z85.01 Personal history of malignant neoplasm of esophagus
    Conditions classifiable to C15

    ✓6th **Z85.02 Personal history of malignant neoplasm of** stomach

        Z85.020 Personal history of malignant carcinoid tumor of stomach
        Conditions classifiable to C7A.092

        Z85.028 Personal history of other malignant neoplasm of stomach
        Conditions classifiable to C16

✓6th **Z85.03 Personal history of malignant neoplasm of** large intestine

    Z85.030 Personal history of malignant carcinoid tumor of large intestine
    Conditions classifiable to C7A.022-C7A.025, C7A.029

    Z85.038 Personal history of other malignant neoplasm of large intestine
    Conditions classifiable to C18

✓6th **Z85.04 Personal history of malignant neoplasm of** rectum, rectosigmoid junction, and anus

    Z85.040 Personal history of malignant carcinoid tumor of rectum
    Conditions classifiable to C7A.026

    Z85.048 Personal history of other malignant neoplasm of rectum, rectosigmoid junction, and anus
    Conditions classifiable to C19-C21

Z85.05 Personal history of malignant neoplasm of liver
Conditions classifiable to C22

✓6th **Z85.06 Personal history of malignant neoplasm of** small intestine

    Z85.060 Personal history of malignant carcinoid tumor of small intestine
    Conditions classifiable to C7A.01-

    Z85.068 Personal history of other malignant neoplasm of small intestine
    Conditions classifiable to C17

Z85.07 Personal history of malignant neoplasm of pancreas
Conditions classifiable to C25

Z85.09 Personal history of malignant neoplasm of other digestive organs

✓5th **Z85.1 Personal history of malignant neoplasm of** trachea, bronchus and lung

    ✓6th **Z85.11 Personal history of malignant neoplasm of** bronchus and lung

        Z85.110 Personal history of malignant carcinoid tumor of bronchus and lung
        Conditions classifiable to C7A.090

        Z85.118 Personal history of other malignant neoplasm of bronchus and lung
        Conditions classifiable to C34

    Z85.12 Personal history of malignant neoplasm of trachea
    Conditions classifiable to C33

✓5th **Z85.2 Personal history of malignant neoplasm of other** respiratory and intrathoracic organs

    Z85.20 Personal history of malignant neoplasm of unspecified respiratory organ

    Z85.21 Personal history of malignant neoplasm of larynx
    Conditions classifiable to C32

    Z85.22 Personal history of malignant neoplasm of nasal cavities, middle ear, and accessory sinuses
    Conditions classifiable to C30-C31

    ✓6th **Z85.23 Personal history of malignant neoplasm of** thymus

        Z85.230 Personal history of malignant carcinoid tumor of thymus
        Conditions classifiable to C7A.091

        Z85.238 Personal history of other malignant neoplasm of thymus
        Conditions classifiable to C37

    Z85.29 Personal history of malignant neoplasm of other respiratory and intrathoracic organs

Z85.3 Personal history of malignant neoplasm of breast
Conditions classifiable to C50.-

✓5th **Z85.4 Personal history of malignant neoplasm of** genital organs
Conditions classifiable to C51-C63

    Z85.40 Personal history of malignant neoplasm of unspecified female genital organ ♀

    Z85.41 Personal history of malignant neoplasm of cervix uteri ♀

    Z85.42 Personal history of malignant neoplasm of other parts of uterus ♀

    Z85.43 Personal history of malignant neoplasm of ovary ♀

    Z85.44 Personal history of malignant neoplasm of other female genital organs ♀

    Z85.45 Personal history of malignant neoplasm of unspecified male genital organ ♂

☑ Additional Character Required   ✓7th Placeholder Alert   Unacceptable PDx   Manifestation   Hospital Acquired Condition   *EXCLUDES 1* Not Coded Here   *EXCLUDES 2* Not Included Here

Z85.46 **Personal history of malignant neoplasm of prostate** ♂

Z85.47 **Personal history of malignant neoplasm of** testis ♂

Z85.48 **Personal history of malignant neoplasm of epididymis** ♂

Z85.49 **Personal history of malignant neoplasm of** other male genital organs ♂

✓5ᵗʰ **Z85.5** **Personal history of malignant neoplasm of** urinary tract
Conditions classifiable to C64-C68

Z85.50 **Personal history of malignant neoplasm of** unspecified urinary tract organ

Z85.51 **Personal history of malignant neoplasm of** bladder

✓6ᵗʰ **Z85.52** **Personal history of malignant neoplasm of** kidney
EXCLUDES 1 *personal history of malignant neoplasm of renal pelvis (Z85.53)*

Z85.520 **Personal history of malignant** carcinoid tumor of kidney
Conditions classifiable to C7A.093

Z85.528 **Personal history of** other malignant neoplasm of kidney
Conditions classifiable to C64

Z85.53 **Personal history of malignant neoplasm of** renal pelvis

Z85.54 **Personal history of malignant neoplasm of** ureter

Z85.59 **Personal history of malignant neoplasm of** other urinary tract organ

Z85.6 **Personal history of** leukemia
Conditions classifiable to C91-C95
EXCLUDES 1 *leukemia in remission C91.0-C95.9 with 5th character 1*

✓5ᵗʰ **Z85.7** **Personal history of other malignant neoplasms of lymphoid, hematopoietic and related tissues**

Z85.71 **Personal history of** Hodgkin lymphoma
Conditions classifiable to C81

Z85.72 **Personal history of** non-Hodgkin lymphomas
Conditions classifiable to C82-C85

Z85.79 **Personal history of** other malignant neoplasms of lymphoid, hematopoietic and related tissues
Conditions classifiable to C88-C90, C96
EXCLUDES 1 *multiple myeloma in remission (C90.01)*
plasma cell leukemia in remission (C90.11)
plasmacytoma in remission (C90.21)

✓5ᵗʰ **Z85.8** **Personal history of malignant neoplasms of other organs and systems**
Conditions classifiable to C00-C14, C40-C49, C69-C79, C7A.098

✓6ᵗʰ **Z85.81** **Personal history of malignant neoplasm of** lip, oral cavity, and pharynx

Z85.810 **Personal history of malignant neoplasm of** tongue

Z85.818 **Personal history of malignant neoplasm of** other sites of lip, oral cavity, and pharynx

Z85.819 **Personal history of malignant neoplasm of** unspecified site of lip, oral cavity, and pharynx

✓6ᵗʰ **Z85.82** **Personal history of malignant neoplasm of** skin

Z85.820 **Personal history of malignant** melanoma of skin
Conditions classifiable to C43

Z85.821 **Personal history of** Merkel cell carcinoma
Conditions classifiable to C4A

Z85.828 **Personal history of** other malignant neoplasm of skin
Conditions classifiable to C44

✓6ᵗʰ **Z85.83** **Personal history of malignant neoplasm of** bone and soft tissue

Z85.830 **Personal history of malignant neoplasm of** bone

Z85.831 **Personal history of malignant neoplasm of** soft tissue
EXCLUDES 2 *personal history of malignant neoplasm of skin (Z85.82-)*

✓6ᵗʰ **Z85.84** **Personal history of malignant neoplasm of** eye and nervous tissue

Z85.840 **Personal history of malignant neoplasm of** eye

Z85.841 **Personal history of malignant neoplasm of** brain

Z85.848 **Personal history of malignant neoplasm of** other parts of nervous tissue

✓6ᵗʰ **Z85.85** **Personal history of malignant neoplasm of** endocrine glands

Z85.850 **Personal history of malignant neoplasm of** thyroid

Z85.858 **Personal history of malignant neoplasm of** other endocrine glands

Z85.89 **Personal history of malignant neoplasm of** other organs and systems

Z85.9 **Personal history of malignant neoplasm,** unspecified
Conditions classifiable to C7A.00, C80.1

✓4ᵗʰ **Z86** **Personal history of certain other diseases**
Code first any follow-up examination after treatment (Z09)

✓5ᵗʰ **Z86.0** **Personal history of in-situ and benign neoplasms and neoplasms of uncertain behavior**
EXCLUDES 2 *personal history of malignant neoplasms (Z85.-)*

✓6ᵗʰ **Z86.00** **Personal history of** in-situ neoplasm

Z86.000 **Personal history of in-situ neoplasm of** breast

Z86.001 **Personal history of in-situ neoplasm of** cervix uteri ♀

Z86.008 **Personal history of in-situ neoplasm of** other site

✓6ᵗʰ **Z86.01** **Personal history of** benign neoplasm

Z86.010 **Personal history of** colonic polyps

Z86.011 **Personal history of benign neoplasm of** the brain

Z86.012 **Personal history of benign** carcinoid tumor

Z86.018 **Personal history of** other benign neoplasm

Z86.03 **Personal history of** neoplasm of uncertain behavior

✓5ᵗʰ **Z86.1** **Personal history of** infectious and parasitic diseases
Conditions classifiable to A00-B89, B99
EXCLUDES 1 *personal history of infectious diseases specific to a body system*
sequelae of infectious and parasitic diseases (B90-B94)

Z86.11 **Personal history of** tuberculosis

Z86.12 **Personal history of** poliomyelitis

Z86.13 **Personal history of** malaria

Z86.14 **Personal history of** Methicillin resistant Staphylococcus aureus infection
Personal history of MRSA infection

Z86.19 **Personal history of** other infectious and parasitic diseases

Z86.2 **Personal history of diseases of the** blood and blood-forming organs and certain disorders involving the immune mechanism
Conditions classifiable to D50-D89

✓5ᵗʰ **Z86.3** **Personal history of** endocrine, nutritional and metabolic diseases
Conditions classifiable to E00-E88

Z86.31 **Personal history of** diabetic foot ulcer
EXCLUDES 2 *current diabetic foot ulcer (E08.621, E09.621, E10.621, E11.621, E13.621)*

Z86.32 **Personal history of** gestational diabetes ♀
Personal history of conditions classifiable to O24.4-
EXCLUDES 1 *gestational diabetes mellitus in current pregnancy (O24.4-)*

Z86.39 **Personal history of** other endocrine, nutritional and metabolic disease

✓5ᵗʰ **Z86.5** **Personal history of** mental and behavioral disorders
Conditions classifiable to F40-F59

Z86.51 **Personal history of** combat and operational stress reaction Ⓐ

Z86.59 **Personal history of** other mental and behavioral disorders

✓5ᵗʰ **Z86.6** **Personal history of diseases of the** nervous system and sense organs
Conditions classifiable to G00-G99, H00-H95
EXCLUDES 2 *personal history of anaphylactic shock (Z87.892)*

Z86.61 **Personal history of** infections of the central nervous system
Personal history of encephalitis
Personal history of meningitis

Z86.69 **Personal history of** other diseases of the nervous system and sense organs

---

Ⓝ Newborn: 0   Ⓟ Pediatric: 0-17   Ⓜ Maternity: 12-55   Ⓐ Adult: 15-124   **MCC** Major CC Condition   **PDx MCC** PDx acts as own MCC   **CC** CC Condition   **PDx CC** PDx acts as own CC

1244

ICD-10-CM 2016

✓5ᵗʰ Z86.7 Personal history of diseases of the circulatory system
Conditions classifiable to I00-I99
EXCLUDES 2   old myocardial infarction (I25.2)
     personal history of anaphylactic shock (Z87.892)
     postmyocardial infarction syndrome (I24.1)

✓6ᵗʰ Z86.71 Personal history of venous thrombosis and embolism

Z86.711 Personal history of pulmonary embolism

Z86.718 Personal history of other venous thrombosis and embolism

Z86.72 Personal history of thrombophlebitis

Z86.73 Personal history of transient ischemic attack (TIA), and cerebral infarction without residual deficits
Personal history of prolonged reversible ischemic neurological deficit (PRIND)
Personal history of stroke NOS without residual deficits
EXCLUDES 1   personal history of traumatic brain injury (Z87.820)
     sequelae of cerebrovascular disease (I69.-)
AHA: 2012, 4Q, 92

Z86.74 Personal history of sudden cardiac arrest
Personal history of sudden cardiac death successfully resuscitated

Z86.79 Personal history of other diseases of the circulatory system

✓4ᵗʰ Z87 Personal history of other diseases and conditions
Code first any follow-up examination after treatment (Z09)

✓5ᵗʰ Z87.0 Personal history of diseases of the respiratory system
Conditions classifiable to J00-J99

Z87.01 Personal history of pneumonia (recurrent)

Z87.09 Personal history of other diseases of the respiratory system

✓5ᵗʰ Z87.1 Personal history of diseases of the digestive system
Conditions classifiable to K00-K93

Z87.11 Personal history of peptic ulcer disease

Z87.19 Personal history of other diseases of the digestive system

Z87.2 Personal history of diseases of the skin and subcutaneous tissue
Conditions classifiable to L00-L99
EXCLUDES 2   personal history of diabetic foot ulcer (Z86.31)

✓5ᵗʰ Z87.3 Personal history of diseases of the musculoskeletal system and connective tissue
Conditions classifiable to M00-M99
EXCLUDES 2   personal history of (healed) traumatic fracture (Z87.81)

✓6ᵗʰ Z87.31 Personal history of (healed) nontraumatic fracture

Z87.310 Personal history of (healed) osteoporosis fracture
Personal history of (healed) fragility fracture
Personal history of (healed) collapsed vertebra due to osteoporosis

Z87.311 Personal history of (healed) other pathological fracture
Personal history of (healed) collapsed vertebra NOS
EXCLUDES 2   personal history of osteoporosis fracture (Z87.310)

Z87.312 Personal history of (healed) stress fracture
Personal history of (healed) fatigue fracture

Z87.39 Personal history of other diseases of the musculoskeletal system and connective tissue

✓5ᵗʰ Z87.4 Personal history of diseases of genitourinary system
Conditions classifiable to N00-N99

✓6ᵗʰ Z87.41 Personal history of dysplasia of the female genital tract
EXCLUDES 1   personal history of malignant neoplasm of female genital tract (Z85.40-Z85.44)

Z87.410 Personal history of cervical dysplasia ♀

Z87.411 Personal history of vaginal dysplasia ♀

Z87.412 Personal history of vulvar dysplasia ♀

Z87.42 Personal history of other diseases of the female genital tract ♀

✓6ᵗʰ Z87.43 Personal history of diseases of the male genital organs

Z87.430 Personal history of prostatic dysplasia ♂
EXCLUDES 1   personal history of malignant neoplasm of prostate (Z85.46)

Z87.438 Personal history of other diseases of male genital organs ♂

✓6ᵗʰ Z87.44 Personal history of diseases of the urinary system
EXCLUDES 1   personal history of malignant neoplasm of cervix uteri (Z85.41)

Z87.440 Personal history of urinary (tract) infections

Z87.441 Personal history of nephrotic syndrome

Z87.442 Personal history of urinary calculi
Personal history of kidney stones

Z87.448 Personal history of other diseases of urinary system

✓5ᵗʰ Z87.5 Personal history of complications of pregnancy, childbirth and the puerperium
Conditions classifiable to O00-O9A
EXCLUDES 2   recurrent pregnancy loss (N96)

Z87.51 Personal history of pre-term labor ♀
EXCLUDES 1   current pregnancy with history of pre-term labor (O09.21-)

Z87.59 Personal history of other complications of pregnancy, childbirth and the puerperium ♀
Personal history of trophoblastic disease

✓5ᵗʰ Z87.7 Personal history of (corrected) congenital malformations
Conditions classifiable to Q00-Q89 that have been repaired or corrected
EXCLUDES 1   congenital malformations that have been partially corrected or repaired but which still require medical treatment—code to condition
EXCLUDES 2   other postprocedural states (Z98.-)
     personal history of medical treatment (Z92.-)
     presence of cardiac and vascular implants and grafts (Z95.-)
     presence of other devices (Z97.-)
     presence of other functional implants (Z96.-)
     transplanted organ and tissue status (Z94.-)

✓6ᵗʰ Z87.71 Personal history of (corrected) congenital malformations of genitourinary system

Z87.710 Personal history of (corrected) hypospadias ♂

Z87.718 Personal history of other specified (corrected) congenital malformations of genitourinary system

✓6ᵗʰ Z87.72 Personal history of (corrected) congenital malformations of nervous system and sense organs

Z87.720 Personal history of (corrected) congenital malformations of eye

Z87.721 Personal history of (corrected) congenital malformations of ear

Z87.728 Personal history of other specified (corrected) congenital malformations of nervous system and sense organs

✓6ᵗʰ Z87.73 Personal history of (corrected) congenital malformations of digestive system

Z87.730 Personal history of (corrected) cleft lip and palate

Z87.738 Personal history of other specified (corrected) congenital malformations of digestive system

Z87.74 Personal history of (corrected) congenital malformations of heart and circulatory system

Z87.75 Personal history of (corrected) congenital malformations of respiratory system

Z87.76 Personal history of (corrected) congenital malformations of integument, limbs and musculoskeletal system

✓6ᵗʰ Z87.79 Personal history of other (corrected) congenital malformations

Z87.790 Personal history of (corrected) congenital malformations of face and neck

Z87.798 Personal history of other (corrected) congenital malformations

---

☑ Additional Character Required   ✓x7ᵗʰ Placeholder Alert   Unacceptable PDx   Manifestation   Hospital Acquired Condition   *EXCLUDES 1* Not Coded Here   *EXCLUDES 2* Not Included Here

✓5ᵗʰ Z87.8 Personal history of other specified conditions
    EXCLUDES 2   *personal history of self harm (Z91.5)*

    Z87.81 Personal history of (healed) traumatic fracture
      EXCLUDES 2   *personal history of (healed) nontraumatic fracture (Z87.31-)*

    ✓6ᵗʰ Z87.82 Personal history of other (healed) physical injury and trauma
      Conditions classifiable to S00-T88, except traumatic fractures

      Z87.820 Personal history of traumatic brain injury
        EXCLUDES 1   *personal history of transient ischemic attack (TIA), and cerebral infarction without residual deficits (Z86.73)*

      Z87.821 Personal history of retained foreign body fully removed

      Z87.828 Personal history of other (healed) physical injury and trauma

    ✓6ᵗʰ Z87.89 Personal history of other specified conditions
      Z87.890 Personal history of sex reassignment
      Z87.891 Personal history of nicotine dependence
        EXCLUDES 1   *current nicotine dependence (F17.2-)*

      Z87.892 Personal history of anaphylaxis
        Code also allergy status such as:
        allergy status to drugs, medicaments and biological substances (Z88.-)
        allergy status, other than to drugs and biological substances (Z91.0-)

      Z87.898 Personal history of other specified conditions
        AHA: 2013, 1Q, 21

✓4ᵗʰ Z88 Allergy status to drugs, medicaments and biological substances
    EXCLUDES 2   *allergy status, other than to drugs and biological substances (Z91.0-)*

    Z88.0 Allergy status to penicillin
    Z88.1 Allergy status to other antibiotic agents status
    Z88.2 Allergy status to sulfonamides status
    Z88.3 Allergy status to other anti-infective agents status
    Z88.4 Allergy status to anesthetic agent status
    Z88.5 Allergy status to narcotic agent status
    Z88.6 Allergy status to analgesic agent status
    Z88.7 Allergy status to serum and vaccine status
    Z88.8 Allergy status to other drugs, medicaments and biological substances status
    Z88.9 Allergy status to unspecified drugs, medicaments and biological substances status

✓4ᵗʰ Z89 Acquired absence of limb
    INCLUDES   amputation status
        postprocedural loss of limb
        post-traumatic loss of limb
    EXCLUDES 1   *acquired deformities of limbs (M20-M21)*
        congenital absence of limbs (Q71-Q73)

    ✓5ᵗʰ Z89.0 Acquired absence of thumb and other finger(s)
      ✓6ᵗʰ Z89.01 Acquired absence of thumb
        Z89.011 Acquired absence of right thumb
        Z89.012 Acquired absence of left thumb
        Z89.019 Acquired absence of unspecified thumb

      ✓6ᵗʰ Z89.02 Acquired absence of other finger(s)
        EXCLUDES 2   *acquired absence of thumb (Z89.01-)*
        Z89.021 Acquired absence of right finger(s)
        Z89.022 Acquired absence of left finger(s)
        Z89.029 Acquired absence of unspecified finger(s)

    ✓5ᵗʰ Z89.1 Acquired absence of hand and wrist
      ✓6ᵗʰ Z89.11 Acquired absence of hand
        Z89.111 Acquired absence of right hand
        Z89.112 Acquired absence of left hand
        Z89.119 Acquired absence of unspecified hand

      ✓6ᵗʰ Z89.12 Acquired absence of wrist
        Disarticulation at wrist
        Z89.121 Acquired absence of right wrist
        Z89.122 Acquired absence of left wrist
        Z89.129 Acquired absence of unspecified wrist

✓5ᵗʰ Z89.2 Acquired absence of upper limb above wrist
    ✓6ᵗʰ Z89.20 Acquired absence of upper limb, unspecified level
      Z89.201 Acquired absence of right upper limb, unspecified level
      Z89.202 Acquired absence of left upper limb, unspecified level
      Z89.209 Acquired absence of unspecified upper limb, unspecified level
        Acquired absence of arm NOS

    ✓6ᵗʰ Z89.21 Acquired absence of upper limb below elbow
      Z89.211 Acquired absence of right upper limb below elbow
      Z89.212 Acquired absence of left upper limb below elbow
      Z89.219 Acquired absence of unspecified upper limb below elbow

    ✓6ᵗʰ Z89.22 Acquired absence of upper limb above elbow
      Disarticulation at elbow
      Z89.221 Acquired absence of right upper limb above elbow
      Z89.222 Acquired absence of left upper limb above elbow
      Z89.229 Acquired absence of unspecified upper limb above elbow

    ✓6ᵗʰ Z89.23 Acquired absence of shoulder
      Acquired absence of shoulder joint following explantation of shoulder joint prosthesis, with or without presence of antibiotic-impregnated cement spacer
      Z89.231 Acquired absence of right shoulder
      Z89.232 Acquired absence of left shoulder
      Z89.239 Acquired absence of unspecified shoulder

✓5ᵗʰ Z89.4 Acquired absence of toe(s), foot, and ankle
    ✓6ᵗʰ Z89.41 Acquired absence of great toe
      Z89.411 Acquired absence of right great toe
      Z89.412 Acquired absence of left great toe
      Z89.419 Acquired absence of unspecified great toe

    ✓6ᵗʰ Z89.42 Acquired absence of other toe(s)
      EXCLUDES 2   *acquired absence of great toe (Z89.41-)*
      Z89.421 Acquired absence of other right toe(s)
      Z89.422 Acquired absence of other left toe(s)
      Z89.429 Acquired absence of other toe(s), unspecified side

    ✓6ᵗʰ Z89.43 Acquired absence of foot
      Z89.431 Acquired absence of right foot
      Z89.432 Acquired absence of left foot
      Z89.439 Acquired absence of unspecified foot

    ✓6ᵗʰ Z89.44 Acquired absence of ankle
      Disarticulation of ankle
      Z89.441 Acquired absence of right ankle
      Z89.442 Acquired absence of left ankle
      Z89.449 Acquired absence of unspecified ankle

✓5ᵗʰ Z89.5 Acquired absence of leg below knee
    ✓6ᵗʰ Z89.51 Acquired absence of leg below knee
      Z89.511 Acquired absence of right leg below knee
      Z89.512 Acquired absence of left leg below knee
      Z89.519 Acquired absence of unspecified leg below knee

    ✓6ᵗʰ Z89.52 Acquired absence of knee
      Acquired absence of knee joint following explantation of knee joint prosthesis, with or without presence of antibiotic-impregnated cement spacer
      Z89.521 Acquired absence of right knee
      Z89.522 Acquired absence of left knee
      Z89.529 Acquired absence of unspecified knee

✓5ᵗʰ Z89.6 Acquired absence of leg above knee
    ✓6ᵗʰ Z89.61 Acquired absence of leg above knee
      Acquired absence of leg NOS
      Disarticulation at knee
      Z89.611 Acquired absence of right leg above knee
      Z89.612 Acquired absence of left leg above knee
      Z89.619 Acquired absence of unspecified leg above knee

ℕ Newborn: 0   ℙ Pediatric: 0-17   ℳ Maternity: 12-55   𝔸 Adult: 15-124   MCC Major CC Condition   PDxMCC PDx acts as own MCC   CC CC Condition   PDxCC PDx acts as own CC

1246   ICD-10-CM 2016

✓6ᵗʰ **Z89.62 Acquired absence of hip**
 Acquired absence of hip joint following explantation of hip joint prosthesis, with or without presence of antibiotic-impregnated cement spacer
 Disarticulation at hip
  Z89.621 Acquired absence of right hip joint
  Z89.622 Acquired absence of left hip joint
  Z89.629 Acquired absence of unspecified hip joint
 Z89.9 Acquired absence of limb, unspecified

✓4ᵗʰ **Z90 Acquired absence of organs, not elsewhere classified**
 INCLUDES   postprocedural or post-traumatic loss of body part NEC
 EXCLUDES 1 congenital absence—see Alphabetical Index
 EXCLUDES 2 postprocedural absence of endocrine glands (E89.-)

 ✓5ᵗʰ **Z90.0 Acquired absence of part of head and neck**
  Z90.01 Acquired absence of eye
  Z90.02 Acquired absence of larynx
  Z90.09 Acquired absence of other part of head and neck
   Acquired absence of nose
   EXCLUDES 2 teeth (K08.1)

 ✓5ᵗʰ **Z90.1 Acquired absence of breast and nipple**
  Z90.10 Acquired absence of unspecified breast and nipple
  Z90.11 Acquired absence of right breast and nipple
  Z90.12 Acquired absence of left breast and nipple
  Z90.13 Acquired absence of bilateral breasts and nipples
 Z90.2 Acquired absence of lung [part of]
 Z90.3 Acquired absence of stomach [part of]
 ✓5ᵗʰ **Z90.4 Acquired absence of other specified parts of digestive tract**
  ✓6ᵗʰ **Z90.41 Acquired absence of pancreas**
   Use additional code to identify any associated:
    insulin use (Z79.4)
    diabetes mellitus, postpancreatectomy (E13.-)
   Z90.410 Acquired total absence of pancreas
    Acquired absence of pancreas NOS
   Z90.411 Acquired partial absence of pancreas
  Z90.49 Acquired absence of other specified parts of digestive tract
 Z90.5 Acquired absence of kidney
 Z90.6 Acquired absence of other parts of urinary tract
  Acquired absence of bladder
 ✓5ᵗʰ **Z90.7 Acquired absence of genital organ(s)**
  EXCLUDES 1 personal history of sex reassignment (Z87.890)
  EXCLUDES 2 female genital mutilation status (N90.81-)

  ✓6ᵗʰ **Z90.71 Acquired absence of cervix and uterus**
   Z90.710 Acquired absence of both cervix and uterus ♀
    Acquired absence of uterus NOS
    Status post total hysterectomy
   Z90.711 Acquired absence of uterus with remaining cervical stump ♀
    Status post partial hysterectomy with remaining cervical stump
   Z90.712 Acquired absence of cervix with remaining uterus ♀
  ✓6ᵗʰ **Z90.72 Acquired absence of ovaries**
   Z90.721 Acquired absence of ovaries, unilateral ♀
   Z90.722 Acquired absence of ovaries, bilateral ♀
  Z90.79 Acquired absence of other genital organ(s)
 ✓5ᵗʰ **Z90.8 Acquired absence of other organs**
  Z90.81 Acquired absence of spleen
  Z90.89 Acquired absence of other organs

✓4ᵗʰ **Z91 Personal risk factors, not elsewhere classified**
 EXCLUDES 2 contact with and (suspected) exposures hazardous to health (Z77.-)
   exposure to pollution and other problems related to physical environment (Z77.1-)
   personal history of physical injury and trauma (Z87.81, Z87.82-)
   occupational exposure to risk factors (Z57.-)

 ✓5ᵗʰ **Z91.0 Allergy status, other than to drugs and biological substances**
  EXCLUDES 2 allergy status to drugs, medicaments, and biological substances (Z88.-)

  ✓6ᵗʰ **Z91.01 Food allergy status**
   EXCLUDES 2 food additives allergy status (Z91.02)
   Z91.010 Allergy to peanuts
   Z91.011 Allergy to milk products
    EXCLUDES 1 lactose intolerance (E73.-)

   Z91.012 Allergy to eggs
   Z91.013 Allergy to seafood
    Allergy to shellfish
    Allergy to octopus or squid ink
   Z91.018 Allergy to other foods
    Allergy to nuts other than peanuts
  Z91.02 Food additives allergy status
 ✓6ᵗʰ **Z91.03 Insect allergy status**
  Z91.030 Bee allergy status
  Z91.038 Other insect allergy status
 ✓6ᵗʰ **Z91.04 Nonmedicinal substance allergy status**
  Z91.040 Latex allergy status
   Latex sensitivity status
  Z91.041 Radiographic dye allergy status
   Allergy status to contrast media used for diagnostic X-ray procedure
  Z91.048 Other nonmedicinal substance allergy status
 Z91.09 Other allergy status, other than to drugs and biological substances

 ✓5ᵗʰ **Z91.1 Patient's noncompliance with medical treatment and regimen**
  Z91.11 Patient's noncompliance with dietary regimen
  ✓6ᵗʰ **Z91.12 Patient's intentional underdosing of medication regimen**
   Code first underdosing of medication (T36-T50) with fifth or sixth character 6
   EXCLUDES 1 adverse effect of prescribed drug taken as directed—code to adverse effect
     poisoning (overdose)—code to poisoning
   Z91.120 Patient's intentional underdosing of medication regimen due to financial hardship
   Z91.128 Patient's intentional underdosing of medication regimen for other reason
  ✓6ᵗʰ **Z91.13 Patient's unintentional underdosing of medication regimen**
   Code first underdosing of medication (T36-T50) with fifth or sixth character 6
   EXCLUDES 1 adverse effect of prescribed drug taken as directed—code to adverse effect
     poisoning (overdose)—code to poisoning
   Z91.130 Patient's unintentional underdosing of medication regimen due to age-related debility
   Z91.138 Patient's unintentional underdosing of medication regimen for other reason
  Z91.14 Patient's other noncompliance with medication regimen
   Patient's underdosing of medication NOS
  Z91.15 Patient's noncompliance with renal dialysis
  Z91.19 Patient's noncompliance with other medical treatment and regimen
 ✓5ᵗʰ **Z91.4 Personal history of psychological trauma, not elsewhere classified**
  ✓6ᵗʰ **Z91.41 Personal history of adult abuse**
   EXCLUDES 2 personal history of abuse in childhood (Z62.81-)
   Z91.410 Personal history of adult physical and sexual abuse 🅐
    EXCLUDES 1 current adult physical abuse (T74.11, T76.11)
      current adult sexual abuse (T74.21, T76.11)
   Z91.411 Personal history of adult psychological abuse 🅐
   Z91.412 Personal history of adult neglect 🅐
    EXCLUDES 1 current adult neglect (T74.01, T76.01)
   Z91.419 Personal history of unspecified adult abuse 🅐
  Z91.49 Other personal history of psychological trauma, not elsewhere classified
 Z91.5 Personal history of self-harm
  Personal history of parasuicide
  Personal history of self-poisoning
  Personal history of suicide attempt

✓5ᵗʰ Z91.8   Other specified personal risk factors, not elsewhere classified

    Z91.81   History of falling
         At risk for falling

    Z91.82   Personal history of military deployment   A
         Individual (civilian or military) with past history of military war, peacekeeping and humanitarian deployment (current or past conflict)
         Returned from military deployment

    Z91.83   *Wandering in diseases classified elsewhere*
         Code first underlying disorder such as:
           Alzheimer's disease (G30.-)
           autism or pervasive developmental disorder (F84.-)
           intellectual disabilities (F70-F79)
           unspecified dementia with behavioral disturbance (F03.9-)

    Z91.89   Other specified personal risk factors, not elsewhere classified

✓4ᵗʰ Z92   Personal history of medical treatment
    EXCLUDES 2   postprocedural states (Z98.-)

    Z92.0   Personal history of contraception
         EXCLUDES 1   counseling or management of current contraceptive practices (Z30.-)
            long term (current) use of contraception (Z79.3)
            presence of (intrauterine) contraceptive device (Z97.5)

    ✓5ᵗʰ Z92.2   Personal history of drug therapy
         EXCLUDES 2   long term (current) drug therapy (Z79.-)

        Z92.21   Personal history of antineoplastic chemotherapy

        Z92.22   Personal history of monoclonal drug therapy

        Z92.23   Personal history of estrogen therapy

        ✓6ᵗʰ Z92.24   Personal history of steroid therapy

            Z92.240   Personal history of inhaled steroid therapy

            Z92.241   Personal history of systemic steroid therapy
                 Personal history of steroid therapy NOS

        Z92.25   Personal history of immunosupression therapy
            EXCLUDES 2   personal history of steroid therapy (Z92.24)

        Z92.29   Personal history of other drug therapy

    Z92.3   Personal history of irradiation
         Personal history of exposure to therapeutic radiation
         EXCLUDES 1   exposure to radiation in the physical environment (Z77.12)
            occupational exposure to radiation (Z57.1)

    ✓5ᵗʰ Z92.8   Personal history of other medical treatment

        Z92.81   Personal history of extracorporeal membrane oxygenation (ECMO)

        Z92.82   Status post administration of tPA (rtPA) in a different facility within the last 24 hours prior to admission to current facility
            Code first condition requiring tPA administration, such as:
              acute cerebral infarction (I63.-)
              acute myocardial infarction (I21-, I22-)
            AHA: 2013, 4Q, 124

        Z92.83   Personal history of failed moderate sedation
            Personal history of failed conscious sedation
            EXCLUDES 2   failed moderate sedation during procedure (T88.52)

        Z92.89   Personal history of other medical treatment

✓4ᵗʰ Z93   Artificial opening status
    EXCLUDES 1   artificial openings requiring attention or management (Z43.-)
            complications of external stoma (J95.0-, K94.-, N99.5-)

    Z93.0   Tracheostomy status
         AHA: 2013, 4Q, 129

    Z93.1   Gastrostomy status

    Z93.2   Ileostomy status

    Z93.3   Colostomy status

    Z93.4   Other artificial openings of gastrointestinal tract status

    ✓5ᵗʰ Z93.5   Cystostomy status

        Z93.50   Unspecified cystostomy status

        Z93.51   Cutaneous-vesicostomy status

        Z93.52   Appendico-vesicostomy status

        Z93.59   Other cystostomy status

    Z93.6   Other artificial openings of urinary tract status
         Nephrostomy status
         Ureterostomy status
         Urethrostomy status

    Z93.8   Other artificial opening status

    Z93.9   Artificial opening status, unspecified

✓4ᵗʰ Z94   Transplanted organ and tissue status
    INCLUDES   organ or tissue replaced by heterogenous or homogenous transplant
    EXCLUDES 1   complications of transplanted organ or tissue—see Alphabetical Index
    EXCLUDES 2   presence of vascular grafts (Z95.-)

    Z94.0   Kidney transplant status   CC
         CC Excl: D47.Z1,T86.10-T86.13, T86.19, T86.850-T86.859,T86.90-T86.99,Z94.0,Z94.89-Z94.9

    Z94.1   Heart transplant status   CC
         EXCLUDES 1   artificial heart status (Z95.812)
            heart-valve replacement status (Z95.2-Z95.4)
         CC Excl: D47.Z1, T86.20-T86.39, T86.850-T86.859, T86.90-T86.99, Z94.1, Z94.3, Z94.89-Z94.9

    Z94.2   Lung transplant status   CC
         CC Excl: D47.Z1, T86.810-T86.819,T86.850-T86.859,T86.90-T86.99,Z94.2,Z94.89-Z94.9

    Z94.3   Heart and lungs transplant status   PDxCC CC
         CC Excl: See Code: Z94.1

    Z94.4   Liver transplant status   CC
         CC Excl: D47.Z1,T86.40-T86.43,T86.49,T86.850-T86.859,T86.90-T86.99, Z94.4,Z94.89-Z94.9

    Z94.5   Skin transplant status
         Autogenous skin transplant status

    Z94.6   Bone transplant status

    Z94.7   Corneal transplant status

    ✓5ᵗʰ Z94.8   Other transplanted organ and tissue status

        Z94.81   Bone marrow transplant status   CC
            CC Excl: D47.Z1, T86.810-T86.813,T86.00-T86.09,T86.850-T86.859,T86.90-T86.99,Z94.9

        Z94.82   Intestine transplant status   CC
            CC Excl: D47.Z1, T86.830-T86.839, T86.90-T86.99, Z94.82, Z94.89-Z94.9

        Z94.83   Pancreas transplant status   CC
            CC Excl: D47.Z1,T86.850-T86.99,Z94.83,Z94.9

        Z94.84   Stem cells transplant status   CC
            CC Excl: D47.Z1,T86.850-T86.859,T86.90-T86.99,Z94.83,Z94.9

        Z94.89   Other transplanted organ and tissue status

    Z94.9   Transplanted organ and tissue status, unspecified

✓4ᵗʰ Z95   Presence of cardiac and vascular implants and grafts
    EXCLUDES 1   complications of cardiac and vascular devices, implants and grafts (T82.-)

    Z95.0   Presence of cardiac pacemaker
         EXCLUDES 1   adjustment or management of cardiac device (Z45.0)
            presence of automatic (implantable) cardiac defibrillator with synchronous cardiac pacemaker (Z95.810)

    Z95.1   Presence of aortocoronary bypass graft

    Z95.2   Presence of prosthetic heart valve
         Presence of heart valve NOS

    Z95.3   Presence of xenogenic heart valve

    Z95.4   Presence of other heart-valve replacement

    Z95.5   Presence of coronary angioplasty implant and graft
         EXCLUDES 1   coronary angioplasty status without implant and graft (Z98.61)

    ✓5ᵗʰ Z95.8   Presence of other cardiac and vascular implants and grafts

        ✓6ᵗʰ Z95.81   Presence of other cardiac implants and grafts

            Z95.810   Presence of automatic (implantable) cardiac defibrillator
                 Presence of automatic (implantable) cardiac defibrillator with synchronous cardiac pacemaker

            Z95.811   Presence of heart assist device   CC
                 CC Excl: D47.Z1, I46.2-I46.9, I49.01, R09.2, R57.0-R57.8, T86.20-T86.39, T86.850-T86.859, T86.90-T86.99, Z94.1, Z94.3, Z95.811-Z95.812

            Z95.812   Presence of fully implantable artificial heart   CC
                 CC Excl: See code: Z95.811

            Z95.818   Presence of other cardiac implants and grafts

---

N Newborn: 0   P Pediatric: 0-17   M Maternity: 12-55   A Adult: 15-124   **MCC** Major CC Condition   **PDxMCC** PDx acts as own MCC   **CC** CC Condition   **PDxCC** PDx acts as own CC

1248   ICD-10-CM 2016

✓6ᵗʰ **Z95.82 Presence of other vascular implants and grafts**

Z95.820 Peripheral vascular angioplasty status with implants and grafts
> EXCLUDES 1   *peripheral vascular angioplasty without implant and graft (Z98.62)*

Z95.828 Presence of other vascular implants and grafts
> Presence of intravascular prosthesis NEC

Z95.9 Presence of cardiac and vascular implant and graft, unspecified

✓4ᵗʰ **Z96 Presence of other functional implants**
> EXCLUDES 2   *complications of internal prosthetic devices, implants and grafts (T82-T85)*
> *fitting and adjustment of prosthetic and other devices (Z44-Z46)*

Z96.0 Presence of urogenital implants

Z96.1 Presence of intraocular lens
> Presence of pseudophakia

✓5ᵗʰ **Z96.2 Presence of otological and audiological implants**

Z96.20 Presence of otological and audiological implant, unspecified

Z96.21 Cochlear implant status

Z96.22 Myringotomy tube(s) status

Z96.29 Presence of other otological and audiological implants
> Presence of bone-conduction hearing device
> Presence of eustachian tube stent
> Stapes replacement

Z96.3 Presence of artificial larynx

✓5ᵗʰ **Z96.4 Presence of endocrine implants**

Z96.41 Presence of insulin pump (external) (internal)

Z96.49 Presence of other endocrine implants

Z96.5 Presence of tooth-root and mandibular implants

✓5ᵗʰ **Z96.6 Presence of orthopedic joint implants**

Z96.60 Presence of unspecified orthopedic joint implant

✓6ᵗʰ **Z96.61 Presence of artificial shoulder joint**

Z96.611 Presence of right artificial shoulder joint

Z96.612 Presence of left artificial shoulder joint

Z96.619 Presence of unspecified artificial shoulder joint

✓6ᵗʰ **Z96.62 Presence of artificial elbow joint**

Z96.621 Presence of right artificial elbow joint

Z96.622 Presence of left artificial elbow joint

Z96.629 Presence of unspecified artificial elbow joint

✓6ᵗʰ **Z96.63 Presence of artificial wrist joint**

Z96.631 Presence of right artificial wrist joint

Z96.632 Presence of left artificial wrist joint

Z96.639 Presence of unspecified artificial wrist joint

✓6ᵗʰ **Z96.64 Presence of artificial hip joint**
> Hip-joint replacement (partial) (total)

Z96.641 Presence of right artificial hip joint

Z96.642 Presence of left artificial hip joint

Z96.643 Presence of artificial hip joint, bilateral

Z96.649 Presence of unspecified artificial hip joint

✓6ᵗʰ **Z96.65 Presence of artificial knee joint**

Z96.651 Presence of right artificial knee joint

Z96.652 Presence of left artificial knee joint

Z96.653 Presence of artificial knee joint, bilateral

Z96.659 Presence of unspecified artificial knee joint

✓6ᵗʰ **Z96.66 Presence of artificial ankle joint**

Z96.661 Presence of right artificial ankle joint

Z96.662 Presence of left artificial ankle joint

Z96.669 Presence of unspecified artificial ankle joint

✓6ᵗʰ **Z96.69 Presence of other orthopedic joint implants**

Z96.691 Finger-joint replacement of right hand

Z96.692 Finger-joint replacement of left hand

Z96.693 Finger-joint replacement, bilateral

Z96.698 Presence of other orthopedic joint implants

Z96.7 Presence of other bone and tendon implants
> Presence of skull plate

✓5ᵗʰ **Z96.8 Presence of other specified functional implants**

Z96.81 Presence of artificial skin

Z96.89 Presence of other specified functional implants

Z96.9 Presence of functional implant, unspecified

✓4ᵗʰ **Z97 Presence of other devices**
> EXCLUDES 1   *complications of internal prosthetic devices, implants and grafts (T82-T85)*
> *fitting and adjustment of prosthetic and other devices (Z44-Z46)*
> EXCLUDES 2   *presence of cerebrospinal fluid drainage device (Z98.2)*

Z97.0 Presence of artificial eye

✓5ᵗʰ **Z97.1 Presence of artificial limb (complete) (partial)**

Z97.10 Presence of artificial limb (complete) (partial), unspecified

Z97.11 Presence of artificial right arm (complete) (partial)

Z97.12 Presence of artificial left arm (complete) (partial)

Z97.13 Presence of artificial right leg (complete) (partial)

Z97.14 Presence of artificial left leg (complete) (partial)

Z97.15 Presence of artificial arms, bilateral (complete) (partial)

Z97.16 Presence of artificial legs, bilateral (complete) (partial)

Z97.2 Presence of dental prosthetic device (complete) (partial)
> Presence of dentures (complete) (partial)

Z97.3 Presence of spectacles and contact lenses

Z97.4 Presence of external hearing-aid

Z97.5 Presence of (intrauterine) contraceptive device ♀
> EXCLUDES 1   *checking, reinsertion or removal of contraceptive device (Z30.43)*

Z97.8 Presence of other specified devices

✓4ᵗʰ **Z98 Other postprocedural states**
> EXCLUDES 2   *aftercare (Z43-Z49, Z51)*
> *follow-up medical care (Z08- Z09)*
> *postprocedural complication—see Alphabetical Index*

Z98.0 Intestinal bypass and anastomosis status
> EXCLUDES 2   *bariatric surgery status (Z98.84)*
> *gastric bypass status (Z98.84)*
> *obesity surgery status (Z98.84)*

Z98.1 Arthrodesis status

Z98.2 Presence of cerebrospinal fluid drainage device
> Presence of CSF shunt

Z98.3 Post therapeutic collapse of lung status
> Code first underlying disease

✓5ᵗʰ **Z98.4 Cataract extraction status**
> Use additional code to identify intraocular lens implant status (Z96.1)
> EXCLUDES 1   *aphakia (H27.0)*

Z98.41 Cataract extraction status, right eye

Z98.42 Cataract extraction status, left eye

Z98.49 Cataract extraction status, unspecified eye

✓5ᵗʰ **Z98.5 Sterilization status**
> EXCLUDES 1   *female infertility (N97.-)*
> *male infertility (N46.-)*

Z98.51 Tubal ligation status ♀

Z98.52 Vasectomy status Ⓐ♂

✓5ᵗʰ **Z98.6 Angioplasty status**

Z98.61 Coronary angioplasty status
> EXCLUDES 1   *coronary angioplasty status with implant and graft (Z95.5)*

Z98.62 Peripheral vascular angioplasty status
> EXCLUDES 1   *peripheral vascular angioplasty status with implant and graft (Z95.820)*

✓5ᵗʰ **Z98.8 Other specified postprocedural states**

✓6ᵗʰ **Z98.81 Dental procedure status**

Z98.810 Dental sealant status

Z98.811 Dental restoration status
> Dental crown status
> Dental fillings status

Z98.818 Other dental procedure status

Z98.82 Breast implant status
> EXCLUDES 1   *breast implant removal status (Z98.86)*

✓ Additional Character Required   ✓x7ᵗʰ Placeholder Alert   Unacceptable PDx   Manifestation   Hospital Acquired Condition   EXCLUDES 1 Not Coded Here   EXCLUDES 2 Not Included Here

Z98.83   **Filtering (vitreous) bleb after glaucoma surgery status**
     EXCLUDES 1   *inflammation (infection) of postprocedural bleb (H59.4-)*

Z98.84   **Bariatric surgery status**
     Gastric banding status
     Gastric bypass status for obesity
     Obesity surgery status
     EXCLUDES 1   *bariatric surgery status complicating pregnancy, childbirth, or the puerperium (O99.84)*
     EXCLUDES 2   *intestinal bypass and anastomosis status (Z98.0)*

Z98.85   **Transplanted organ removal status**
     Transplanted organ previously removed due to complication, failure, rejection or infection
     EXCLUDES 1   *encounter for removal of transplanted organ—code to complication of transplanted organ (T86.-)*

Z98.86   **Personal history of breast implant removal**

✓6ᵗʰ **Z98.87**   **Personal history of in utero procedure**
     Z98.870   **Personal history of in utero procedure during pregnancy** ♀
         EXCLUDES 2   *complications from in utero procedure for current pregnancy (O35.7)*
             supervision of current pregnancy with history of in utero procedure during previous pregnancy (O09.82-)
     Z98.871   **Personal history of in utero procedure while a fetus**

Z98.89   **Other specified postprocedural states**
     Personal history of surgery, not elsewhere classified

✓4ᵗʰ **Z99**   **Dependence on enabling machines and devices, not elsewhere classified**
     EXCLUDES 1   *cardiac pacemaker status (Z95.0)*

Z99.0   **Dependence on aspirator**

✓5ᵗʰ **Z99.1**   **Dependence on respirator**
     Dependence on ventilator

     CC Excl: For CC codes in subcategory Z99.1: CC with 7th character A, unless otherwise noted: J95.850, Z99.0-Z99.12, Z99.81- Z99.89

     Z99.11   **Dependence on respirator [ventilator] status**   CC
         AHA: 2015, 1Q, 21
     Z99.12   **Encounter for respirator [ventilator] dependence during power failure**   CC
         EXCLUDES 1   *mechanical complication of respirator [ventilator] (J95.850)*

Z99.2   **Dependence on renal dialysis**
     Hemodialysis status
     Peritoneal dialysis status
     Presence of arteriovenous shunt for dialysis
     Renal dialysis status NOS
     EXCLUDES 1   *encounter for fitting and adjustment of dialysis catheter (Z49.0-)*
             noncompliance with renal dialysis (Z91.15)
     AHA: 2013, 4Q, 125

Z99.3   **Dependence on wheelchair**
     Wheelchair confinement status
     Code first cause of dependence, such as:
         muscular dystrophy (G71.0)
         obesity (E66.-)

✓5ᵗʰ **Z99.8**   **Dependence on other enabling machines and devices**
     Z99.81   **Dependence on supplemental oxygen**
         Dependence on long-term oxygen
         AHA: 2013, 4Q, 129
     Z99.89   **Dependence on other enabling machines and devices**
         Dependence on machine or device NOS

NOTES

NOTES

NOTES

NOTES

Appendixes

Appendix A: 10 Steps to Correct Coding

Follow the 10 steps below to correctly code encounters for health care services.

Step 1: Identify the reason for the visit or encounter (i.e., a sign, symptom, diagnosis and/or condition).

The medical record documentation should accurately reflect the patient's condition, using terminology that includes specific diagnoses and symptoms or clearly states the reasons for the encounter.

Choosing the main term that best describes the reason chiefly responsible for the service provided is the most important step in coding. If symptoms are present and documented but a definitive diagnosis has not yet been determined, code the symptoms. **For outpatient cases, do not code conditions that are referred to as "rule out," "suspected," "probable," or "questionable."** Diagnoses often are not established at the time of the initial encounter/visit and may require two or more visits to be established. Code only what is documented in the available records and only to the highest degree of certainty known at the time of the patient's visit, unless it is an inpatient medical record, in which case uncertain diagnoses may be reported if documented at the time of discharge.

Step 2: After selecting the reason for the encounter, always consult the alphabetic index before verifying code selection in the tabular section.

The most critical rule is to begin code selection in the *alphabetic index*. Never turn first to the tabular list. The index provides cross-references, essential and nonessential modifiers, and inclusion terms not found in the tabular list. To prevent coding errors, always use both the alphabetic index (to identify a code) and the tabular list (to verify a code), as the index does not include the important instructional notes found in the tabular list. An added benefit of using the tabular list, which groups like things together, is that while looking at one code in the list, a coder might see a more specific one that would have been missed had the coder relied solely on the alphabetic index. Additionally, many of the codes require a fourth, fifth, sixth, or seventh, character to be valid, and many of these characters can be found only in the tabular list.

Step 3: Locate the main term entry.

The alphabetic index is a listing of conditions, which may be expressed as nouns or eponyms, with critical use of adjectives. Some conditions known by several names have multiple main entries. Reasons for encounters may be located under general terms such as admission, encounter, and examination. Other general terms such as history of, status post, or presence (of) are used to locate factors influencing health.

Step 4: Read cross-references listed with the main term or the subterm.

Cross-references such as *"see"* and *"see also"* are identified by italicized type and should always be checked to ensure that all alternative terms are researched.

Step 5: Review entries for modifiers.

Nonessential modifiers are the terms in parentheses following the main term entry. These parenthetical terms are supplementary words or explanatory information that may or may not appear in the diagnostic statement and do not affect code selection. The subterms listed under the main term are essential modifiers that do affect coding assignment. Each line of indent represents a more specific code entry. The nonessential modifiers apply to the subterms following a main term except when they are mutually exclusive, in which case the subterm takes precedence. For example, if "acute" is listed as a nonessential modifier but there is a subentry for "chronic," then the nonessential modifier of "acute" does not apply.

Step 6: Interpret abbreviations, cross-references, default codes, additional characters, and brackets.

The abbreviation NEC (not elsewhere classified) that follows some main terms or subterms indicates that there is no specific code for the condition even though the medical documentation may be very specific. The code next to the main term is called the default code. It represents the condition most commonly associated with the main term or the unspecified code for the main term. Additional characters may be required to construct the code; the tabular list must be referenced to determine what those specific characters should be. The alphabetic index uses brackets [] to enclose manifestation codes that can be used only as secondary codes to the underlying condition code immediately preceding it. Both codes must be reported in this multiple-coding situation.

Step 7: Choose a potential code and locate it in the tabular list.

The coder must follow any Includes, Excludes 1 and Excludes 2 notes, and other instructional notes, such as "Code first" and "Use additional code," listed in the tabular list for the chapter, category, subcategory, and subclassification level of code selection that direct the coder to use a different or additional code. Any codes in the tabular range, A00.0- through T88.9-, may be used to identify the diagnostic reason for the encounter. The tabular list encompasses many codes describing disease and injury classifications (e.g., infectious and parasitic diseases, neoplasms, symptoms, nervous and circulatory system etc.).

Codes that describe symptoms and signs, as opposed to definitive diagnoses, should be used for reporting purposes when an established diagnosis has not been made (confirmed) by the physician. Chapter 18 of the ICD-10-CM code book, "Symptoms, Signs, and Abnormal Clinical and Laboratory Findings" (codes R00.--R99), contains many, but not all, codes for symptoms.

ICD-10-CM classifies encounters with health care providers for circumstances other than a disease or injury using codes in chapter 21, "Factors Influencing Health Status and Contact with Health Services" (codes Z00–Z99.8). Circumstances other than a disease or injury often are recorded as chiefly responsible for the encounter.

Step 8: Determine whether the code is at the highest level of specificity.

A code is invalid if it has not been coded to the full number of characters (greatest level of specificity) required. Codes in ICD-10-CM can contain from three up to seven alphanumeric characters. A three-character code is to be used only if the category is not further subdivided into four-, five-, or six-character codes. Placeholder character X is used both to allow for future expansion and as a placeholder for empty characters in a code that requires a seventh character but has no fourth, fifth, or sixth character. Certain categories require seventh characters that apply to all codes in that category. Always check the category level for applicable seventh characters for that category.

Step 9: Assign the code.

Having reviewed all relevant information concerning the possible code choices, assign the code that most completely describes the condition.

Repeat steps one through nine for all additional documented conditions that meet the following criteria:

- Conditions that currently exist at the time of the visit
- Conditions that require or affect patient care, treatment, or management

Step 10: Sequence codes correctly.

Sequencing is the order in which the codes are listed on the claim. List first the ICD-10-CM code for the diagnosis, condition, problem, or other reason for the encounter/visit, which is shown in the medical record to be chiefly responsible for the services provided. List additional codes that describe any coexisting conditions. Follow the official coding guidelines (see section II, "Selection of Principal Diagnosis"; section III, "Reporting Additional Diagnoses"; and section IV, "Diagnostic Coding and Reporting Guidelines for Outpatient Services") on proper sequencing of codes.

Coding Examples

Diagnosis: Anorexia

Step 1: The reason for the encounter was the condition, anorexia.

Step 2: Consult the alphabetic index.

Step 3: Locate the main term "Anorexia."

Step 4: There are no cross-references to check.

Step 5: Note that there are two possible subterms (essential modifiers), "hysterical" and "nervosa," neither of which is documented in this instance and therefore cannot be used in code selection. The code listed next to the main term is called the default code selection.

Step 6: There are no abbreviations, cross-references, additional character icons, or brackets.

Step 7: Turn to code R63.0 in the tabular list and read the instructional notes. In this case the Excludes 1 note indicates that anorexia nervosa and loss of appetite determined to be of nonorganic origin should be coded to a code from chapter 5. The diagnostic statement does not indicate nonorganic origin.

Step 8: There is no further division of the category past the fourth character subcategory. Therefore, the subcategory code level is the highest level of specificity.

Step 9: The default code, R63.0 Anorexia, is the correct code selection

Step 10: Since anorexia is listed as the chief reason for the health care encounter, the first-listed, or principal, diagnosis is R63.0. Note that this is a chapter 18 symptom code but can be assigned since the provider did not establish a more definitive diagnosis.

Diagnosis: Acute bronchitis

Step 1: The reason for the encounter was the condition, acute bronchitis.

Step 2: Consult the alphabetic index.

Step 3: Locate the main term "Bronchitis."

Step 4: There are cross-references to interpret.

Step 5: Review entries for modifiers. Since "acute" is not listed as a nonessential modifier, read past the "with" modifier until you find the subterm "acute or subacute" with a nonessential modifier of "with bronchospasm or obstruction," code J20.9.

Step 6: There are no abbreviations, cross-references, additional character icons, or brackets.

Step 7: Since there are no more appropriate subterms, turn to code J20.9 in the tabular list. The Includes note under category J20 does refer to other alternative terms for acute bronchitis. Note that the inclusion term list is not exhaustive but is only a representative selection of diagnoses that are included in the subcategory. The Excludes 1 note refers bronchitis and tracheobronchitis NOS to category J40. There are several Excludes 2 notes that, if applicable, can be coded in addition to this code.

Step 8: Note that the subcategories included in J20 represent acute bronchitis due to various infectious organisms that would be selected if identified in the documentation. In this case, the organism was not identified and there is no further division of the category past the fourth character subcategory. Therefore, the subcategory code level is the highest level of specificity.

Step 9: Assign code J20.9 Acute bronchitis, unspecified.

Step 10: Repeat steps 1-9 for any additional code assignments.

Diagnosis: Infectious diarrhea

Step 1: The reason for the encounter was the condition, infectious diarrhea.

Step 2: Consult the alphabetic index.

Step 3: Locate the main term "Diarrhea" in the alphabetic index.

Step 4: There are no cross-references to check.

Step 5: Review entries for modifiers. Note that the nonessential modifiers (in parentheses) after the main term do not include the term "infectious," which means that the coder should search the subterms for the term "infectious." The subterm "infectious" refers to code A09.

Step 6: There are no abbreviations, cross-references, additional character icons, or brackets.

Step 7: Locate code A09 in the tabular list, and read all instructional notes under the main category and subcategories. The Includes notes does not list the term "infectious diarrhea" under code A09; however, as instructed by the alphabetic index, you should code the condition to A09. The ICD-10-CM code book implies that infectious diarrhea is the same as infectious gastroenteritis, enteritis, and colitis.

Step 8: There is no further division of the category past the third-character category level. Therefore, the category code level is the highest level of specificity. The final code assignment would be A09.

Step 9: Assign code A09 Infectious gastroenteritis and colitis, unspecified.

Step 10: Since infectious diarrhea is listed as the chief reason for the health care encounter, the first-listed, or principal, diagnosis is A09.

Diagnosis: Decubitus ulcer of right elbow with skin loss and necrosis of subcutaneous tissue

Step 1: The reason for the encounter was the condition, decubitus ulcer.

Step 2: Consult the alphabetic index.

Step 3: Locate the main term "Ulcer" in the alphabetic index.

Step 4: There are no cross-references to check.

Step 5: This entry does not have any important nonessential modifiers; however, there are other terms such as ulcerated, ulcerating, etc., that are included as main terms. Locate the subterm "decubitus" and note that there is an italicized cross-reference to "see Ulcer, pressure, by site." Go to the subterm "pressure" and locate "elbow," which refers to code L89.0-.

Step 6: Note that the code L89.0 is followed by a dash and an additional character icon, which indicate that more characters are required. From here, the tabular list can be consulted at code L89.0-.

Step 7: Locate code L89.0 in the tabular list, and check the category level L89 for any instructional, Includes, and Excludes 1 and 2 notes. Note that "decubitus" is an Includes note under L89 Pressure ulcer. Excludes 2 notes indicate that if this were documented as a diabetic pressure ulcer, it would be necessary to use a code from chapter 4.

Step 8: Read through the subcategory codes under L89.0 and note that the fifth character describes laterality. Locate the right elbow at subcategory L89.01. See that an additional sixth character is now needed to complete the code. The sixth character specifies the stage of the ulcer, which can be determined either by the specific documentation of the stage (e.g., stage 1, stage 2) or in this case, a description that matches one of the Includes notes that follow each stage code. For example, the description in this case of "skin loss and necrosis of the subcutaneous tissue" matches the Includes notes under L89.013 Pressure ulcer of right elbow, stage 3.

Step 9: Assign code L89.013 Pressure ulcer of right elbow, stage 3

Step 10: Since the decubitus ulcer is listed as the chief reason for the health care encounter, the first-listed, or principal, diagnosis is L89.013. However, according to the Code first instructional note at the L89 category level, gangrene would be sequenced before the pressure ulcer if it were documented.

Diagnosis: First visit for bimalleolar fracture of the right ankle due to trauma

Step 1: The reason for the encounter was the condition, bimalleolar fracture of the right ankle.

Step 2: Consult the alphabetic index.

Step 3: Locate the main term "Fracture" in the alphabetic index.

Step 4: Note that the first main term for Fracture is pathological with cross-reference to "see also Fracture, traumatic." Locate the main term "Fracture, traumatic."

Step 5: Review entries for nonessential modifiers. Locate the subterms "ankle," "bimalleolar." Note that "displaced" is a nonessential modifier following "bimalleolar," indicating that S82.84- is the default code unless the fracture is specified as nondisplaced.

Step 6: Note that code S82.84- is followed by a dash and an additional character icon, both of which indicate that more characters are required. From here, the tabular list can be consulted at code S82.84.

Step 7: Locate code S82.84 Bimalleolar fracture of lower leg, in the tabular list and check the category level S82 for any instructional, Includes, and Excludes 1 and 2 notes. See the instructional notes indicating that fractures not specified as displaced or nondisplaced default to displaced, and fractures not designated as open or closed default to closed. See also the list of appropriate seventh characters to be added to all codes from category S82.

Step 8: Read through the subcategory codes under S82.84, and note that the sixth character specifies displaced or nondisplaced and laterality. Locate the displaced bimalleolar fracture of the right lower leg at code S82.841. See that an additional seventh character is still needed to complete the code. The seventh character specifies the type of encounter and whether the fracture is open or closed. Use character A listed in the box at the category level to describe initial encounter, closed fracture.

Step 9: Assign code S82.841A Displaced bimalleolar fracture of right lower leg, initial encounter for closed fracture.

Step 10: Since this is an injury code, code additionally any external cause, place of occurrence, and activity codes, with the injury (fracture) sequenced first.

Appendix B: Valid 3-character ICD-10-CM Codes

A09	Infectious gastroenteritis and colitis, unspecified
A33	Tetanus neonatorum
A34	Obstetrical tetanus
A35	Other tetanus
A46	Erysipelas
A55	Chlamydial lymphogranuloma (venereum)
A57	Chancroid
A58	Granuloma inguinale
A64	Unspecified sexually transmitted disease
A65	Nonvenereal syphilis
A70	Chlamydia psittaci infections
A78	Q fever
A86	Unspecified viral encephalitis
A89	Unspecified viral infection of central nervous system
A90	Dengue fever [classical dengue]
A91	Dengue hemorrhagic fever
A94	Unspecified arthropod-borne viral fever
A99	Unspecified viral hemorrhagic fever
B03	Smallpox
B04	Monkeypox
B09	Unspecified viral infection characterized by skin and mucous membrane lesions
B20	Human immunodeficiency virus [HIV] disease
B49	Unspecified mycosis
B54	Unspecified malaria
B59	Pneumocystosis
B64	Unspecified protozoal disease
B72	Dracunculiasis
B75	Trichinellosis
B79	Trichuriasis
B80	Enterobiasis
B86	Scabies
B89	Unspecified parasitic disease
B91	Sequelae of poliomyelitis
B92	Sequelae of leprosy
C01	Malignant neoplasm of base of tongue
C07	Malignant neoplasm of parotid gland
C12	Malignant neoplasm of pyriform sinus
C19	Malignant neoplasm of rectosigmoid junction
C20	Malignant neoplasm of rectum
C23	Malignant neoplasm of gallbladder
C33	Malignant neoplasm of trachea
C37	Malignant neoplasm of thymus
C52	Malignant neoplasm of vagina
C55	Malignant neoplasm of uterus, part unspecified
C58	Malignant neoplasm of placenta
C61	Malignant neoplasm of prostate
C73	Malignant neoplasm of thyroid gland
D34	Benign neoplasm of thyroid gland
D45	Polycythemia vera
D62	Acute posthemorrhagic anemia
D65	Disseminated intravascular coagulation [defibrination A syndrome]
D66	Hereditary factor VIII deficiency
D67	Hereditary factor IX deficiency
D71	Functional disorders of polymorphonuclear neutrophils
D77	Other disorders of blood and blood-forming organs in diseases classified elsewhere
E02	Subclinical iodine-deficiency hypothyroidism
E15	Nondiabetic hypoglycemic coma
E35	Disorders of endocrine glands in diseases classified elsewhere
E40	Kwashiorkor
E41	Nutritional marasmus
E42	Marasmic kwashiorkor

E43	Unspecified severe protein-calorie malnutrition
E45	Retarded development following protein-calorie malnutrition
E46	Unspecified protein-calorie malnutrition
E52	Niacin deficiency [pellagra]
E54	Ascorbic acid deficiency
E58	Dietary calcium deficiency
E59	Dietary selenium deficiency
E60	Dietary zinc deficiency
E65	Localized adiposity
E68	Sequelae of hyperalimentation
F04	Amnestic disorder due to known physiological condition
F05	Delirium due to known physiological condition
F09	Unspecified mental disorder due to known physiological condition
F21	Schizotypal disorder
F22	Delusional disorders
F23	Brief psychotic disorder
F24	Shared psychotic disorder
F28	Other psychotic disorder not due to a substance or known physiological condition
F29	Unspecified psychosis not due to a substance or known physiological condition
F39	Unspecified mood [affective] disorder
F42	Obsessive-compulsive disorder
F53	Puerperal psychosis
F54	Psychological and behavioral factors associated with disorders or diseases classified elsewhere
F59	Unspecified behavioral syndromes associated with physiological disturbances and physical factors
F66	Other sexual disorders
F69	Unspecified disorder of adult personality and behavior
F70	Mild intellectual disabilities
F71	Moderate intellectual disabilities
F72	Severe intellectual disabilities
F73	Profound intellectual disabilities
F78	Other intellectual disabilities
F79	Unspecified intellectual disabilities
F82	Specific developmental disorder of motor function
F88	Other disorders of psychological development
F89	Unspecified disorder of psychological development
F99	Mental disorder, not otherwise specified
G01	Meningitis in bacterial diseases classified elsewhere
G02	Meningitis in other infectious and parasitic diseases classified elsewhere
G07	Intracranial and intraspinal abscess and granuloma in diseases classified elsewhere
G08	Intracranial and intraspinal phlebitis and thrombophlebitis
G09	Sequelae of inflammatory diseases of central nervous system
G10	Huntington's disease
G14	Postpolio syndrome
G20	Parkinson's disease
G26	Extrapyramidal and movement disorders in diseases classified elsewhere
G35	Multiple sclerosis
G53	Cranial nerve disorders in diseases classified elsewhere
G55	Nerve root and plexus compressions in diseases classified elsewhere
G59	Mononeuropathy in diseases classified elsewhere
G63	Polyneuropathy in diseases classified elsewhere
G64	Other disorders of peripheral nervous system
G92	Toxic encephalopathy
G94	Other disorders of brain in diseases classified elsewhere
H22	Disorders of iris and ciliary body in diseases classified elsewhere
H28	Cataract in diseases classified elsewhere
H32	Chorioretinal disorders in diseases classified elsewhere
H36	Retinal disorders in diseases classified elsewhere

H42	Glaucoma in diseases classified elsewhere
I00	Rheumatic fever without heart involvement
I10	Essential (primary) hypertension
I32	Pericarditis in diseases classified elsewhere
I38	Endocarditis, valve unspecified
I39	Endocarditis and heart valve disorders in diseases classified elsewhere
I41	Myocarditis in diseases classified elsewhere
I43	Cardiomyopathy in diseases classified elsewhere
I52	Other heart disorders in diseases classified elsewhere
I76	Septic arterial embolism
I81	Portal vein thrombosis
I96	Gangrene, not elsewhere classified
J00	Acute nasopharyngitis (common cold)
J13	Pneumonia due to Streptococcus pneumoniae
J14	Pneumonia due to Hemophilus influenzae
J17	Pneumonia in diseases classified elsewhere
J22	Unspecified acute lower respiratory infection
J36	Peritonsillar abscess
J40	Bronchitis, not specified as acute or chronic
J42	Unspecified chronic bronchitis
J60	Coalworker's pneumoconiosis
J61	Pneumoconiosis due to asbestos and other mineral fibers
J64	Unspecified pneumoconiosis
J65	Pneumoconiosis associated with tuberculosis
J80	Acute respiratory distress syndrome
J82	Pulmonary eosinophilia, not elsewhere classified
J90	Pleural effusion, not elsewhere classified
J99	Respiratory disorders in diseases classified elsewhere
K23	Disorders of esophagus in diseases classified elsewhere
K30	Functional dyspepsia
K36	Other appendicitis
K37	Unspecified appendicitis
K67	Disorders of peritoneum in infectious diseases classified elsewhere
K77	Liver disorders in diseases classified elsewhere
K87	Disorders of gallbladder, biliary tract and pancreas in diseases classified elsewhere
L00	Staphylococcal scalded skin syndrome
L14	Bullous disorders in diseases classified elsewhere
L22	Diaper dermatitis
L26	Exfoliative dermatitis
L42	Pityriasis rosea
L45	Papulosquamous disorders in diseases classified elsewhere
L52	Erythema nodosum
L54	Erythema in diseases classified elsewhere
L62	Nail disorders in diseases classified elsewhere
L80	Vitiligo
L83	Acanthosis nigricans
L84	Corns and callosities
L86	Keratoderma in diseases classified elsewhere
L88	Pyoderma gangrenosum
L99	Other disorders of skin and subcutaneous tissue in diseases classified elsewhere
N08	Glomerular disorders in diseases classified elsewhere
N10	Acute tubulo-interstitial nephritis
N12	Tubulo-interstitial nephritis, not specified as acute or chronic
N16	Renal tubulo-interstitial disorders in diseases classified elsewhere
N19	Unspecified kidney failure
N22	Calculus of urinary tract in diseases classified elsewhere
N23	Unspecified renal colic
N29	Other disorders of kidney and ureter in diseases classified elsewhere
N33	Bladder disorders in diseases classified elsewhere
N37	Urethral disorders in diseases classified elsewhere
N51	Disorders of male genital organs in diseases classified elsewhere
N61	Inflammatory disorders of breast
N62	Hypertrophy of breast
N63	Unspecified lump in breast

N72	Inflammatory disease of cervix uteri
N74	Female pelvic inflammatory disorders in diseases classified elsewhere
N86	Erosion and ectropion of cervix uteri
N96	Recurrent pregnancy loss
O68	Labor and delivery complicated by abnormality of fetal acid-base balance
O76	Abnormality in fetal heart rate and rhythm complicating labor and delivery
O80	Encounter for full-term uncomplicated delivery
O82	Encounter for cesarean delivery without indication
O85	Puerperal sepsis
O94	Sequelae of complication of pregnancy, childbirth, and the puerperium
P09	Abnormal findings on neonatal screening
P53	Hemorrhagic disease of newborn
P60	Disseminated intravascular coagulation of newborn
P84	Other problems with newborn
P90	Convulsions of newborn
P95	Stillbirth
Q02	Microcephaly
R05	Cough
R12	Heartburn
R17	Unspecified jaundice
R21	Rash and other nonspecific skin eruption
R32	Unspecified urinary incontinence
R34	Anuria and oliguria
R37	Sexual dysfunction, unspecified
R42	Dizziness and giddiness
R51	Headache
R52	Pain, unspecified
R54	Age-related physical debility
R55	Syncope and collapse
R58	Hemorrhage, not elsewhere classified
R61	Generalized hyperhidrosis
R64	Cachexia
R69	Illness, unspecified
R75	Inconclusive laboratory evidence of human immunodeficiency virus [HIV]
R81	Glycosuria
R99	Ill-defined and unknown cause of mortality
T07	Unspecified multiple injuries
Y09	Assault by unspecified means
Y66	Nonadministration of surgical and medical care
Y69	Unspecified misadventure during surgical and medical care
Y95	Nosocomial condition
Z08	Encounter for follow-up examination after completed treatment for malignant neoplasm
Z09	Encounter for follow-up examination after completed treatment for conditions other than malignant neoplasm
Z21	Asymptomatic human immunodeficiency virus [HIV] infection status
Z23	Encounter for immunization
Z36	Encounter for antenatal screening of mother
Z66	Do not resuscitate

Appendix C: Pharmacology List 2016

This section enables the coder to quickly review drugs, drug actions, and indications that are often associated with overlooked or undocumented diagnoses. The coder should review the patient's medication record and know what condition the physician is treating with the prescribed medication based on documentation in the medical record. When documentation is lacking, the coder can reference this section to locate the drug, determine the drug action, confirm drug indications, and when necessary query the physician.

Drug	Drug Action	Indications
Accupril [quinapril]	ACE inhibitor; antihypertensive	Congestive heart failure; essential hypertension
Acetaminophen and codeine [acetaminophen/codeine phosphate]	Analgesic	Pain, moderate to severe
Actemra [tocilizumab]	Antirheumatic	Rheumatoid arthritis
Actonel [risedronate]	Electrolytic and renal agent; bone resorption inhibitor	Decrease bone loss in multiple myeloma patients; Paget's disease; hyperparathyroidism; osteoporosis
Adalat CC [nifedipine]	Calcium channel blocker	Vasospastic angina; chronic stable angina; essential hypertension
Aldactone [spironolactone]	Cardiovascular agent; antihypertensive agent; diuretic; electrolytic and renal agent	Treatment of severe heart failure; ascites associated with cirrhosis; hypokalemia
Allegra [fexofenadine/ hydrochloride pseudoephedrine]	Antihistamine	Seasonal allergic rhinitis
Allopurinol [allopurinol]	Antigout	Gouty arthritis, renal calculus, hyperuricemia, hyperuricemia secondary to leukemia, hyperuricemia secondary to lymphoma
Alphagan P [brimonidine]	Antiglaucoma agent (ophthalmic) antihypertensive, ocular	Open angle glaucoma or another condition in which pressure in the eye is too high (ocular hypertension)
Alprazolam [alprazolam]	Antianxiety; sedative/hypnotic	
Altace [ramipril]	ACE inhibitor; antihypertensive	Congestive heart failure, essential hypertension
Amaryl [glimepiride]	Blood glucose regulator	Diabetes mellitus
Ambien [zolpidem]	Sedative/hypnotic	Insomnia
Abilify [aripiprazole]	Antipsychotic	Depression, bipolar disorder, schizophrenia, autism symptoms
Amikacin [amikacin sulfate]	Aminoglycoside antibiotic	Active in treatment of gram-negative bacterial infections such as *Pseudomonas, Escherichia coli (E. coli), Proteus, Klebsiella-Enterobacter-Serratia*
Aminophylline [aminophylline]	Bronchodilator, pulmonary vasodilator, smooth muscle relaxant	Relief and/or prevention of symptoms from asthma and reversible bronchospasms in bronchitis and emphysema
Amitriptyline hydrochloride [amitriptyline hydrochloride]	Anorexiant/CNS stimulant; antidepressant	Depression
Amoxicillin, Amoxil [amoxicillin]	Penicillin	Effective for infections with a broad spectrum of bactericidal activity against many gram-positive and gram-negative micro-organisms; otitis media, gonorrhea, skin, respiratory, gastrointestinal, and genitourinary infections
Amrix [cyclobenzaprine hydrochloride]	Muscle relaxant	Adjunct to rest and physical therapy for muscle spasms
Ancef [cefazoline sodium]	Semisynthetic cephalosporin antibiotic	Respiratory tract infections due to *Streptococcus pneumoniae, Klebsiella species, Haemophilus influenzae (H. influenzae), Staphylococcus aureus*, and group A betahemolytic streptococci; urinary tract infections due to *E. coli, Proteus mirabilis, Klebsiella* species and some strains of Enterobacter and enterococci; skin and skin structure infections, biliary tract infections, bone and joint infections, genital infections, septicemia, and endocarditis
Antabuse [disulfiram]	Alcohol treatment	Alcoholism
Anzemet [dolasetron mesylate]	Antiemetic/ antinauseant	Management of nausea/vomiting following surgery or from effects of chemotherapy or cancer
Aranesp [darbepoetin alfa]	Erythropoiesis-stimulating agent (ESA)	Treat lower than normal blood cells (anemia) from disorders such as CKD and neoplasms
Aricept [donepezil hydrochloride]	Acetylcholine sterase inhibitor	Symptoms of mild to moderate Alzheimer's disease; can improve thinking ability in some patients
Arthrotec [diclofenac/misoprostol]	Analgesic	Treatment of patients with arthritis who may develop stomach ulcers from taking nonsteroidal anti-inflammatory drugs (NSAIDs) alone; used to help relieve some symptoms of arthritis, such as inflammation, swelling, stiffness, and joint pain
Atenolol [atenolol]	Antianginal; antihypertensive; beta blocker	Chronic stable angina pectoris; essential hypertension; reduces cardiovascular mortality in those with definite or suspected acute myocardial infarction
Ativan [lorazepam]	Antianxiety; sedative/hypnotic	Anxiety disorder associated with depressive symptoms; controls tension, agitation, irritability, and insomnia
Atrovent [ipratropium bromide]	Antiasthmatic/bronchodilator	Chronic bronchitis, emphysema; bronchial asthma
Augmentin [amoxicillin/clavulanate]	Antibacterial	Middle ear, lower respiratory, sinus, skin and skin structures, and urinary tract infections
Avapro [irbesartan]	Antihypertensive	Hypertension
Axid [nizatidine]	Histamine H2-receptor antagonist	Acid/peptic disorder; gastroesophageal reflux; duodenal, gastric, and peptic ulcers

Drug	Drug Action	Indications
Bactrim [sulfamethoxazole trimethoprim]	Antibacterial	Treatment of urinary tract infections, acute otitis media, acute exacerbation of chronic bronchitis, shigellosis, and pneumocystis carinii
Bactroban [mupirocin]	Dermatologic; topical anti-infective	Topical treatment of impetigo
Beconase AQ [beclomethasone dipropionate monohydrate]	Corticosteroids; antiasthmatic	Bronchial asthma, prevention of nasal polyps, perennial allergies, seasonal allergies and vasomotor rhinitis
Betoptic [betaxolol hydrochloride]	Cardioselective beta-adrenergic receptor blocking agent	Lowers intraocular pressure; also used for treatment of ocular hypertension and chronic open-angle glaucoma
Biaxin [clarithromycin]	Macrolide	Acid/peptic disorder or ulcer, acute exacerbation chronic bronchitis, human immunodeficiency virus, lower and upper respiratory tract infection, sinus infection, prophylaxis mycobacterium avium complex, pharyngitis, pneumonia, tonsillitis
Buspirone [buspirone hydrochloride]	Antianxiety	Generalized anxiety disorder
Butorphanol Tartrate [butorphanol tartrate]	Narcotic analgesic	Moderate to severe postsurgical pain
Calan [verapamil hydrochloride]	Antianginal; antiarrhythmic, antiarthritic, antihypertensive, calcium channel blocker	Angina pectoris at rest and chronic stable, arrhythmia, atrial fibrillation, atrial flutter, paroxysmal supraventricular tachycardia, ventricular arrhythmia, essential hypertension
Cardizem CD, Tiazac [diltiazem hydrochloride]	Antianginal, antiarrhythmic, antihypertensive, channel blocker, coronary vasodilator	Chronic stable angina, atrial fibrillation, atrial flutter, essential hypertension, paroxysmal supraventricular tachycardia
Cardura [doxazosin mesylate]	Antihypertensive	Benign prostatic hyperplasia, essential hypertension
Catapres, Clonidine [clonidine]	Antihypertensive	Hypertension
Ceftin [cefuroxime axetil]	Antibiotic: second generation cephalosporins	Acute exacerbation and chronic bronchitis, middle ear infection, sexually transmitted gonorrhea infection, upper respiratory tract infection, urinary tract infection, pharyngitis, tonsillitis
Cefprozil [cefprozil]	Antibiotic: second generation cephalosporins	Acute exacerbation and chronic bronchitis, lower respiratory tract infection, upper respiratory tract infection, pharyngitis, tonsillitis
Celebrex [celecoxib]	Antirheumatic, nonsteroidal anti-inflammatory	Relief of some symptoms caused by arthritis, such as inflammation, swelling, stiffness, and joint pain
Celexa [citalopram hydrobromide]	Antidepressant	Depression
Chantix [varenicline]	Smoking cessation aid	Nicotine addiction, smoking
Cipro [ciprofloxacin]	Anti-infective; quinolone	Cystitis, infectious diarrhea, gonorrhea, bone and joint infection, gastrointestinal tract infection, lower and upper respiratory tract infection, sinus infection, urinary tract infection, nosocomial pneumonia, chronic prostatitis
Claritin [loratadine/ pseudoephedrine sulfate]	Antihistamine	Seasonal allergic rhinitis, chronic idiopathic urticaria
Clonazepam, Klonopin [clonazepam]	Anticonvulsant	Absence, akinetic and myoclonic epilepsy, Lennox-Gastaut syndrome
Cogentin [benztropine mesylate]	Antiparkinsonism	Parkinson's disease
Colace [docusate sodium]	Gastrointestinal agent; laxative, stool softener	Constipation
Combivent [ipratropium bromide/albuterol sulfate]	Antiasthmatic/bronchodilator	Chronic bronchitis, emphysema; bronchial asthma
Compro [prochlorperazine] suppository form only	Antiemetic, antipsychotic	Nausea, vomiting, and manic phase of bipolar syndrome or schizophrenia
Cortisporin [hydrocortisone acetate/neomycin sulfate]	Topical anti-infective, topical steroid	Dermatosis
Coumadin [warfarin sodium]	Thrombolytic agent/anticoagulant	Prophylaxis and treatment of venous thrombosis, treatment of atrial fibrillation with embolization (pulmonary embolism), arrhythmias, myocardial infarction, and stroke prevention
Cozaar [losartan]	Antihypertensive	Essential hypertension
Crestor [rosuvastatin calcium]	HMG-CoA reductase inhibitor (statin)	Hypercholesterolemia, hyperlipidemia, hyperproteinemia
Crixivan [indinavir sulfate]	HIV inhibitor	HIV, asymptomatic HIV
Cytomel [liothyronine sodium]	Thyroid hormone	Treatment of hypothyroidism or prevention of euthyroid goiters
Daypro [oxaprozin]	Nonsteroidal anti-inflammatory drug (NSAID)	Osteoarthritis and rheumatoid arthritis
Depakote [divalproex]	Anticonvulsant	Bipolar affective disorder; complex absence, complex partial and mixed pattern epilepsy; migraine headache
Desogen [desogestrel/ethinyl estradiol]	Contraceptive; estrogen/progestin	Contraception
Detrol [tolterodine tartrate]	Muscarinic receptor antagonist	Overactive bladders in patients with urinary frequency, urgency, or urge incontinence
Diflucan [fluconazole]	Antifungal agent	Oropharyngeal and esophageal candidiasis and cryptococcal meningitis in AIDS patients
Digoxin [digoxin]	Cardiotonic glycoside	Heart failure, atrial flutter, atrial fibrillation, and supraventricular tachycardia
Dilantin [phenytoin sodium]	Anticonvulsant	Control of grand mal and psychomotor seizures

Drug	Drug Action	Indications
Diovan [valsartan]	Ace inhibitor	Essential hypertension
Effexor XR [venlafaxine]	Antidepressant	Depression
Epinephrine [epinephrine]	Bronchodilator, cardiotonic	Most commonly used to relieve respiratory distress due to bronchospasm and to restore cardiac rhythm in cardiac arrest
Epivir, Epivir-HBV [lamivudine]	HIV and HBV inhibitor	HIV, hepatitis B (HBV), asymptomatic HIV
ERY-TAB [erythromycin]	Acne product; macrolide; ocular anti-infective; topical anti-infective	Acne vulgaris, intestinal amebiasis, infectious conjunctivitis, diphtheria, endocarditis, prevention, erythrasma treatment of infections: endocervical, gynecologic, lower and upper respiratory tract, ophthalmic, rectal; skin and skin structures, and urethral; Legionnaires' disease, pelvic inflammatory disease, pertussis, pneumonia, rheumatic fever, prophylaxis, syphilis
Estrace [estradiol]	Estrogen therapy	Vaginal cream used to treat vaginal and vulvar atrophy
Estraderm, Climara [estradiol]	Estrogen therapy	Osteoporosis prevention and to treat menopausal symptoms, vaginal and vulvar atrophy, hypoestrogenism, ovarian failure
Evista [raloxifene hydrochloride]	Estrogen receptor modulator, selective osteoporosis prophylactic	Prevention of thinning of the bones (osteoporosis) only in postmenopausal women
Flavoxate hydrochloride [flavoxate hydrochloride]	Urinary tract spasmolytic	Relief of dysuria, urgency, nocturia, suprapubic pain, frequency, and incontinence associated with cystitis, prostatitis, urethritis, and urethrocystitis/urethrotrigonitis
Flomax [tamsulosin hydrochloride]	Benign prostatic hypertrophy therapy agent	Signs and symptoms of benign enlargement of the prostate (benign prostatic hyperplasia or BPH)
Flonase [fluticasone propionate]	Corticosteroid-inhalation/nasal; topical steroid	Corticosteroid-responsive dermatosis; perennial allergic and seasonal allergic rhinitis
Flovent HFA [fluticasone propionate]	Corticosteroid-inhalation/nasal; topical steroid	Corticosteroid-responsive dermatosis, perennial allergic and seasonal allergic rhinitis
Fosamax [alendronate sodium]	Calcium metabolism	Osteoporosis; Paget's disease
Fosinopril sodium [fosinopril sodium]	ACE inhibitor; antihypertensive	Essential hypertension
Glucophage [metformin hydrochloride]	Blood glucose regulator	Diabetes mellitus antihyperglycemic drug used in the management of non-insulin-dependent diabetes mellitus (NIDDM)
Glucotrol [glipizide]	Oral blood-glucose-lowering agent	Adjunct to diet for the control of hyperglycemia in patients with noninsulin dependent diabetes mellitus (NIDDM, type II)
Glyburide (micronized) [glyburide]	Blood glucose regulator	Diabetes mellitus
Heparin sodium [heparin sodium]	Anticoagulant	Prophylaxis and treatment of venous thrombosis, pulmonary embolism; prevention of cerebral thrombosis, and treatment of consumptive coagulopathies
Hydrochlorothiazide [hydrochlorothiazide]	Diuretic, antihypertensive	Management of hypertension and in adjunctive therapy for edema associated with congestive heart failure, hepatic cirrhosis, corticosteroid, and estrogen therapy
Hydrocodone bitartrate and acetaminophen [acetaminophen/hydrocodone bitartrate]	Analgesic, general; analgesic-narcotic; antitussive/expectorant	Pain, moderate to severe
Hyzaar [hydrochlorothiazide/losartan/potassium]	Antihypertensive	Hypertension
Imitrex [sumatriptan succinate]	Antimigraine	Migraine headache
Inderal [propranolol hydrochloride]	Beta-adrenergic blocking agent	Management of hypertension, long-term management of angina pectoris due to coronary atherosclerosis, cardiac arrhythmias
Isordil [isosorbide dinitrate]	Smooth muscle relaxant	Acute anginal attacks
Isuprel [isoproterenol hydrochloride]	Adrenergic agent	Bronchodilator for asthma, chronic pulmonary emphysema, bronchitis, and other conditions accompanied by bronchospasm; can be used in cardiogenic shock cases
K-Tab, Klor-Con [potassium chloride]	Replaces potassium and maintains potassium level	Hypokalemia
Keflex [cephalexin]	Antibacterial	Bone, middle ear, skin and skin structures, upper respiratory tract and urinary tract infections; acute prostatitis
Klonopin [clonazepam]	Anticonvulsant, anxiolytic - benzodiazepine	Epilepsy, seizures, panic disorder
Lamisil [terbinafine hydrochloride]	Antifungal	*Tinea cruris* (jock itch), *T. pedis* (athlete's foot), *T. corporis* (ringworm)
Lanoxin [digoxin]	Cardiotonic glycoside	Congestive heart failure
Lasix [furosemide]	Antihypertensive; diuretic	Management of edema associated with congestive heart failure, renal disease, including nephrotic syndrome and hypertension
Lescol [fluvastatin]	HMG-CoA reductase inhibitor (statin)	Hypercholesterolemia; hyperlipidemia; hyperlipoproteinemia
Levaquin [levofloxacin]	Fluoroquinolone antibacterial	Acute exacerbation chronic bronchitis; cellulitis; furuncle; impetigo; infections of the lower and upper respiratory tract, sinus, skin and skin structures, and urinary tract; pneumonia, community-acquired; pyoderma
Levoxyl [levothyroxine sodium]	Synthetic thyroid hormone	Euthyroid goiter; hypothyroidism

Drug	Drug Action	Indications
Lexapro [escitalopram oxalate]	Antidepressant—selective serotonin reuptake inhibitor (SSRI)	Depression, anxiety
Librium [chlordiazepoxide hydrochloride]	Antianxiety agent	Acute withdrawal symptoms, especially from alcohol, or for other anxiety-producing conditions
Lidocaine [lidocaine hydrochloride]	Antiarrhythmic	Management of ventricular arrhythmias or during cardiac manipulation, such as cardiac surgery
Lipitor [atorvastatin calcium]	HMG-CoA reductase inhibitor (statin)	Hypercholesterolemia, hyperlipidemia, hyperproteinemia
Lithium [lithium carbonate]	Antimanic	Control of manic episodes in bipolar disorders
Lomotil [diphenoxylate hydrochloride with atropine]	Antidiarrheal	Treatment of symptoms of chronic and functional diarrhea
Lopid [gemfibrozil]	Lipid regulating agent	Hypercholesterolemia, hyperlipidemia, hyperlipoproteinemia, hypertriglyceridemia
Lopressor [metoprolol tartrate]	Antihypertensive, betablocker antianginal; antihypertensive; betablocker	Essential hypertension therapy, angina pectoris, and myocardial infarction
Lorazepam [lorazepam]	Antianxiety; sedative/hypnotic	Anxiety disorder associated with depressive symptoms; controls tension, agitation, irritability, and insomnia
Lotensin [benazepril]	ACE inhibitor; antihypertensive	Essential hypertension
Lotrel [amlodipine/benazepril]	Antihypertensive	Hypertension
Lotrisone [clotrimazole/ betamethasone]	Antifungal-corticosteroid	Relief of redness, swelling, itching, and other discomfort of fungus infections
Lovastatin [lovastatin]	HMG-CoA reductase inhibitor (statin)	Hypercholesterolemia; hyperlipidemia, hyperlipoproteinemia
Macrodantin [nitrofurantoin]	Antibacterial	Urinary tract infection; prophylaxis
Meclinzine hydrochloride [meclizine hydrochloride]	Antihistamine	Management of nausea and vomiting, and dizziness associated with motion sickness
Medrol [methylprednisolone]	Glucocorticoid; anti-inflammatory	Acute/chronic adrenal insufficiency, congenital adrenal hyperplasia, adrenal insufficiency secondary to pituitary insufficiency; nonendocrine disorders include arthritis, rheumatic carditis, bronchial asthma, cerebral edema, and allergic, collagen, intestinal tract, liver, ocular, renal, and skin diseases
Methergine [methylergonovine maleate]	Oxytocic agent	Routine management of postpartum hemorrhage after delivery of placenta
Miacalcin [calcitonin salmon]	Calcitonin; a peptide hormone	Hypercalcemia, osteoporosis, postmenopausal symptoms, Paget's disease
Monoket [isosorbide mononitrate]	Antianginal; coronary vasodilator, nitrate	Angina pectoris
Motrin [ibuprofen]	Analgesic, general; analgesic, non-narcotic; antiarthritic; antigout; antipyretic; NSAID	Osteoarthritis and rheumatoid arthritis, dysmenorrhea, fever; pain, mild to moderate
Multaq [dronedarone]	Cardiac rhythm regulator	Treatment of patients with recent episodes of atrial fibrillation or atrial flutter
Nabumetone [nabumetone]	Non-steroidal anti-inflammatory drug (NSAID)	Osteoarthritis and rheumatoid arthritis
Naprosyn [naproxen]	Anti-inflammatory analgesic, general; analgesic, non-narcotic; antiarthritic; antigout; NSAID	Rheumatoid, gouty arthritis and osteoarthritis; ankylosing spondylitis; bursitis; dysmenorrhea; pain, mild to moderate; tendonitis
Nefazodone hydrochloride [nefazodone hydrochloride]	Antidepressant	Depression
Nembutal sodium [pentobarbital sodium]	Sedative; hypnotic	Adjunct medication in diagnostic procedures or for emergency use with convulsive disorders
Neurontin [gabapentin]	Anticonvulsant	Epilepsy, partial
Nexium [esomeprazole magnesium]	Proton pump inhibitor	Gastroesophageal reflux disease (GERD), erosive esophagitis
Nitropress [sodium nitroprusside]	Vasodilator	Potent, rapid action in reducing blood pressure in hypertensive crisis or for controlling bleeding during anesthesia by producing controlled hypotension
Nitrostat [nitroglycerin]	Muscle relaxant antianginal; antihypertensive; coronary vasodilator	Prophylaxis and treatment of angina pectoris; heart failure associated with myocardial infarction; hypertension, perioperative; surgery, adjunct
Norpace [disopyramide]	Antiarrhythmic	Coronary artery disease, for prevention, recurrence and control of unifocal, multifocal, and paired PVCs
Norvasc [amlodipine besylate]	Calcium channel blocker	Hypertension, chronic stable angina, and vasospastic angina
Onglyza [saxagliptin]	Blood glucose regulator	Adjunct to diet and exercise for the control of hyperglycemia in patients with noninsulin-dependent diabetes mellitus (NIDDM, type II)
Orphenadrine citrate [orphenadrine citrate]	Muscle relaxant	Acute spasms, tension, and post-trauma cases
Ortho-Novum [norethindrone/ethinyl estradiol]	Contraceptive; estrogen/progestin	Contraception
Oxazepam [oxazepam]	Antianxiety	Anxiety, tension, and alcohol withdrawal
Pavabid [papaverine hydrochloride]	Vasodilator	Relief of cerebral and peripheral ischemia
Paxil [paroxetine]	Antidepressant	Anxiety with panic disorder and depression; obsessive-compulsive disorder

Drug	Drug Action	Indications
Penicillin-VK [penicillin V potassium]	Natural penicillin	Chorea, prevention; endocarditis, prevention, secondary to tooth extraction; erysipelas; infections of the skin and skin structures, upper respiratory tract; rheumatic fever, prophylaxis; scarlet fever; Vincent's gingivitis; Vincent's pharyngitis
Pepcid [famotidine]	Histamine H2-receptor inhibitor	Acid/peptic disorder; adenoma, secretory; gastroesophageal reflux; duodenal and gastric ulcer; Zollinger-Ellison syndrome
Percocet, Roxicet [oxycodone and acetaminophen]	Analgesic, general; analgesic-narcotic	Pain, moderate to severe
Persantine [dipyridamole]	Platelet inhibitor	Therapy for chronic angina pectoris, preventing clots post heart valve surgery
Phenobarbital [phenobarbital sodium]	Barbiturate	Grand mal epilepsy
Pitocin [oxytocin]	Synthetic oxytocin	Induction or stimulation of labor at term
Plasmanate [plasma, plasma protein fraction]	Blood volume expander	Hypovolemic shock, burn patients, and hemorrhages when whole blood is unavailable
Plavix [clopidogrel bisulfate]	Antithrombotic platelet aggregation inhibitor	Lessening of the chance of heart attack or stroke
Plendil [felodipine]	Antihypertensive; calcium channel blocker	Essential hypertension
Pravachol [pravastatin]	HMG-CoA reductase inhibitor (statin)	Hypercholesterolemia, hyperlipidemia, hyperlipoproteinemia
Prednisone [prednisone]	Adrenocorticoid, corticosteroid	Used for its immunosuppressant effects and for relief of inflammations; used in arthritis, polymyositis and other systemic diseases
Pregnyl [chorionic gonadotropin]	Gonadotropic hormone	Prepubertal cryptorchidism, hypogonadism, corpus luteum insufficiency and infertility
Premarin [conjugated estrogens]	Antineoplastic; estrogen	Vasomotor symptoms associated with menopause; atrophic vaginitis; kraurosis vulvae, female hypogonadism; primary ovarian failure
Prempro [conjugated estrogens/medroxyproges- terone]	Estrogen/progestin	Menopause, osteoporosis, atrophic vaginitis
Prevacid [lansoprazole]	Proton pump inhibitor (PPI)	Acid/peptic disorder, erosive esophagitis, duodenal ulcer, Zollinger-Ellison syndrome
Prinivil [lisinopril]	Synthetic peptide derivative, long-acting angiotensin converting enzyme inhibitor	Congestive heart failure, essential hypertension
Prilosec [omeprazole]	Proton pump inhibitor	Acid/peptic disorder; endocrine adenoma; erosive esophagitis; systemic mastocytosis; gastroesophageal reflux; duodenal, peptic and gastric ulcer; Zollinger-Ellison syndrome
Procardia [nifedipine]	Antianginal agent; calcium channel blocker	Management of vasospastic angina and chronic stable angina, essential hypertension
Promethazine hydrochloride [promethazine hydrochloride]	Anesthesia, adjunct to; antiemetic; antihistamine; antitussive/expectorant; sedative/hypnotic; vertigo/motion sickness/vomiting	Anesthesia; adjunct; angioedema; conjunctivitis; dermographism; hypersensitivity, motion sickness; pain; perennial, seasonal, and allergic rhinitis; sedation, obstetrical; urticaria
Protonix [pantoprazole]	Proton pump inhibitor (PPI)	Short-term treatment and maintenance therapy of erosive esophagitis associated with gastroesophageal reflux disease (GERD)
Proventil-HFA [albuterol sulfate]	Antiasthmatic/bronchodilator	Asthma
Provera/Depo-Provera [medroxyprogesterone acetate]	Antineoplastic; contraceptive; progestin	Amenorrhea; carcinoma, endometrium, adjunct; carcinoma, renal; contraception; hemorrhage
Prozac [fluoxetine hydrochloride]	Serotonin reuptake inhibitor	Bulimia nervosa; depression; obsessive-compulsive disorder
Qnasl [beclomethasone dipropionate]	Corticosteroid	Perennial allergies, seasonal allergies, and vasomotor rhinitis
Quinidine gluconate [quinidine gluconate]	Antiarrhythmic	Management of cardiac arrhythmias
Qvar [beclomethasone dipropionate]	Corticosteroids; antiasthmatic	Prevention and control of symptoms related to asthma
Restoril [temazepam]	Sedative/hypnotic	Insomnia
Retrovir [zidovudine]	Antiretroviral agent	Indicated in symptomatic HIV infection
Risperdal [risperidone]	Antipsychotic/antimanic	Schizophrenia; bipolar I disorder
Ritalin [methylphenidate hydrochloride]	Central nervous system (CNS) stimulant	Treatment of depression and hyperkinetic activity in children
Sabril [vigabatrin]	Anticonvulsant	Refractory complex partial seizures
Septra [sulfamethoxazole trimethoprim]	Antibacterial	Treatment of urinary tract infections, acute otitis media, acute exacerbations of chronic bronchitis, and shigellosis
Serevent [salmeterol xinafoate]	Bronchodilator	Asthma
Sinemet [carbidopa, levodopa]	Antiparkinsonian	Parkinson's disease
Singulair [montelukast]	Antiasthmatic, leukotriene receptor antagonist	Treatment of mild to moderate asthma to decrease the symptoms of asthma and the number of acute asthma attacks
Soltamox [tamoxifen citrate]	Antineoplastic; hormonal/biological response modifier	Breast cancer
Solu-Medrol [methylprednisolone sodium succinate]	Adrenocorticosteroid	Anti-inflammatory and antiallergenic for shock and ulcerative colitis

Appendix C: Pharmacology List 2016

Drug	Drug Action	Indications
Synthroid, Levothroid [levothyroxine sodium]	Thyroid hormone	Treatment of hypothyroidism
Tagamet [cimetidine]	Acid reducer	Treatment of active duodenal ulcer, short-term treatment of active, benign gastric ulcer, and treatment of pathological hypersecretory conditions
Tegretol [carbamazepine]	Anticonvulsant; analgesic	Epilepsy, especially with complex symptomatology; specific analgesic for trigeminal neuralgia
Tenormin [atenolol]	Antianginal; antihypertensive; beta blocker	Treatment of hypertension; lowering blood pressure lowers the risk of fatal and nonfatal cardiovascular events, primarily strokes and myocardial infarctions
Terazosin hydrochloride [terazosin hydrochloride]	Alphablocker; antihypertensive; diuretic	Benign prostatic hypertrophy; essential hypertension
Tobradex [tobramycin and dexamethasone]	Aminoglycoside ocular anti-infective; anti-inflammatory	Infectious conjunctivitis; dermatosis, corticosteroid-responsive with secondary infection; foreign body in eye; corneal inflammation; uveitis
Toprol-XL [metoprolol succinate]	Antianginal antihypertensive beta blocker	Angina pectoris, essential hypertension
Trazodone hydrochloride [trazodone hydrochloride]	Antidepressant	Depression
Triamterene and hydrochlorothiazide [triamterene/ hydrochlorothiazide]	Antihypertensive, diuretic	Edema; essential hypertension
Trimethoprim [trimethoprim]	Antibacterial	Acute exacerbation chronic bronchitis; travelers' diarrhea; infections of the middle, lower respiratory tract, and urinary tract; pneumonia, pneumocystis; shigellosis
Trivora-28 [ethinyl estradiol/ levonorgestrel]	Contraceptive, estrogen/progestin	Contraception
Ultram [tramadol]	Analgesic, non-narcotic	Pain, moderate to moderately severe
Uniphyl [theophylline]	Bronchodilator, pulmonary vasodilator, smooth muscle relaxant	Treatment of bronchial obstruction in asthma and chronic obstructive pulmonary disease
Valium [diazepam]	Antianxiety, muscle relaxant, anticonvulsant	Anxiety, tension, withdrawal from alcohol, muscle spasms and anticonvulsant therapy; epilepsy, generalized tonic-clonic; status epilepticus; stiff-man syndrome; tetanus
Vasotec [enalaprilat]	ACE inhibitor, antihypertensive	Congestive heart failure; essential hypertension
Ventolin HFA [albuterol, albuterol sulfate]	Antiasthmatic/bronchodilator	Asthma
Verapamil HCL, Calan [verapamil hydrochloride]	Antianginal, antiarrhythmic, antiarthritic, antihypertensive, calcium channel blocker	Angina pectoris, chronic stable angina, atrial fibrillation, atrial flutter, paroxysmal supraventricular tachycardia, ventricular arrhythmia, essential hypertension
Viagra [sildenafil citrate]	Phosphodiesterase-5 (PDE5) inhibitor	Erectile dysfunction
Victoza [liraglutide recombinant]	Glucagon-like peptide-1 (GLP-1) receptor agonist	Adjunct to diet and exercise for the control of hyperglycemia in patients with noninsulin-dependent diabetes mellitus (NIDDM, type II)
Vistaril [hydroxyzine pamoate]	Antianxiety agent, antiemetic	Treatment of nausea and vomiting, for reducing narcotic requirement in surgery and as tranquilizer for tension, anxiety, or agitation states
Wellbutrin SR, Welbutrin XL [bupropion hydrochloride]	Antidepressant; CNS	Depression; smoking cessation
Xalatan [latanoprost]	Prostaglandin F2α analogue	Glaucoma, open-angle; ocular hypertension
Xanax, Xanax XR [alprazolam]	Antianxiety; sedative/hypnotic	Anxiety disorders with panic disorder and depression
Xigris [drotrecogin alfa]	Biologic response modifier	Severe sepsis
Zantac [ranitidine hydrochloride]	Histamine H2-receptors inhibitor	Acid/peptic disorder, erosive esophagitis, gastrointestinal hypersecretion, mastocytosis, gastroesophageal reflux, peptic ulcer, Zollinger-Ellison syndrome
Zestoretic [lisinopril and hydrochlorothiazide]	ACE inhibitor; antihypertensive	Congestive heart failure; essential hypertension
Zestril [lisinopril]	ACE inhibitor; antihypertensive	Congestive heart failure; essential hypertension
Ziac [bisoprolol fumarate/ hydrochlorothiazide]	Antihypertensive	Essential hypertension
Zithromax [azithromycin]	Macrolide	Infections of the cervix, lower respiratory tract, skin and skin structures, urethra, nongonococcal; mycobacterium avium complex; pharyngitis, streptococcal pneumonia; tonsillitis
Zocor [simvastatin]	HMG-CoA reductase inhibitor (statin)	Hypercholesterolemia, hyperlipidemia, hyperlipoproteinemia, hypertriglyceridemia
Zoloft [sertraline hydrochloride]	Antidepressant	Anxiety with panic disorder and depression; obsessive-compulsive disorder
Zovirax [acyclovir]	Antiviral	Genital herpes and herpes zoster infections
Zyloprim [allopurinol]	Antigout	Gouty arthritis, renal calculus, hyperuricemia, hyperuricemia secondary to leukemia, hyperuricemia secondary to lymphoma
Zyprexa [olanzapine]	Antipsychotic/antimanic	Psychotic disorders; schizophrenia
Zyrtec [cetirizine hydrochloride]	Antihistamine	Perennial allergic and seasonal allergic rhinitis; chronic urticaria

Appendix D: Z Codes for Long-Term Drug Use with Associated Drugs

Z79.01 **Long term (current) use of anticoagulants**
Arixtra
Coumadin
Eliquis
Heparin
Jantoven
Lovenox
Pradaxa
Warfarin
Xarelto

Z79.02 **Long term (current) use of antithrombotics/antiplatelets**
Aggrenox
Aggrastat
Clopidogrel
Clopidogrel bisulfate
Effient
Persantine
Plavix
Pletal
Pradaxa
Ticlid

Z79.1 **Long term (current) use of non-steroidal anti-inflammatories (NSAID)**
Advil
Aleve
Anaprox
Celebrex
Clinoril
Daypro
Feldene
Ibuprofen
Indocin
Lodine
Motrin
Nalfon
Naprosyn
Orudis
Ponstel
Relafen
Tolectin
Toradol
Voltaren

Z79.2 **Long term (current) use of antibiotics**
Amikin
Amoxicillin
Amoxil
Ampicillin
Ancef

Augmentin
Azactam
Azithromycin
Bactrim
Cefaclor
Ceftriaxone
Cephalexin
Cephalosporin
Cipro
Ciprofloxacin
Clarithromycin
Cleocin
Clindamycin
Co-trimoxazole
Daptomycin
Dificid
Doxycycline
Ertapenem
ERYC
Erythromycin
Factive
Flagyl
Flucloxacillin
Gentamicin
Isoniazid
Invanz
Keflex
Levaquin
Macrobid
Merrem
Metronidazole
Minocin
Nitrofurantoin
Omnipen
Ornidazole
Penicillin G
Penicillin V
Polycillin
Primaxin
Rifampicin
Rocephin
Septra
Streptomycin
Tazicef
Tazocin
Tetracycline HCl
Timentin
Trimethoprim
Tobramycin
Unipen
Vancocin
Vancomycin
Vibramycin

Zinacef
Zithromax
Zosyn
Zyvox

Z79.3 **Long term (current) use of hormonal contraceptives**
Oral
　Combined oral contraceptive
　Progestin-only pills
Patch
　Ortho Evra
　Injectable
　DMPA—depo medroxyprogesterone acetate
Vaginal Ring
　NuvaRing
Implantable rods
　Implanon

Z79.4 **Long term (current) use of insulin**
Apidra
Humalog
Humulin
Lantus
Levemir
Novolin
NovoLog
Velosulin

Z79.51 **Long term (current) use of inhaled steroids**
Advair
Aerospan
Alvesco
Asmanex Twisthaler
Dulera
Flovent
Pulmicort
Qvar
Symbicort

Z79.52 **Long term (current) use of systemic steroids**
Cortef
Cortisone acetate
Depo-Medrol
Dexamethasone
Hydrocortisone
Kenalog
Medrol
Methylprednisolone
Prednisolone
Prednisone
Solu-Medrol

Z79.810 Long term (current) use of selective estrogen receptor modulators (SERMs)
Evista
Fareston
Nolvadex
Osphena
Raloxifene
Soltamox
Tamoxifen
Toremifene

Z79.811 Long term (current) use of aromatase inhibitors
Anastrozole
Arimidex
Aromasin
Exemestane
Femara
Letrozole

Z79.818 Long term (current) use of other agents affecting estrogen receptors and estrogen levels
Eligard
Faslodex
Fulvestrant
Lupron
Megace
Supprelin La
Synarel
Trelstar
Vantas
Viadur
Zoladex

Z79.82 Long term (current) use of aspirin
Bayer
Ecotrin
Bufferin

Z79.83 Long term (current) use of bisphosphonates
Actonel
Aredia

Atelvia
Binosto
Boniva
Didronel
Fosamax
Reclast
Zometa

Z79.890 Hormone replacement therapy (postmenopausal)
Activella
Alora
Angeliq
Climara
Enjuvia
Estrace
Estratest
EstroGel
Femring
Femtrace
Menostar
Premarin
Provera
Vivelle

Z79.891 Long term (current) use of opiate analgesic
Astramorph
Avinza
Buprenex
Buprenorphine
Codeine
Demerol
Dilaudid
Duragesic
Duramorph
Fentanyl
Fentora
Fioricet with codeine
Hydrocodone
Hydromorphone
Kadian
Lorcet

Lortab
Methadone HCL
Methadose
Morphine
MS Contin
Norco
Oxycodone
OxyContin
Percocet
Roxicodone
Sublimaze
Tylenol with codeine
Ultram

Z79.899 Other long term (current) drug therapy]
Actimmune
Antineoplastic/chemotherapy
Astagraf XL
Avonex
Cellcept
Cyclosporin
Envarsus XR
Gengraf
Imuran
Interferon
Monoclonal antibodies
Neoral
Orthoclone OKT3
Peginterferon
Prograf
Protopic
Rapamune
Rebif
Sandimmune
Simulect
Sirolimus
Sylatron
Tacrolimus
Torisel
Zenapax

Appendix E: Major Complication and Comorbidity (MCC) Code List

A02.1	A52.14	B58.81	G03.0	I40.9	I63.232	J09.X1	K25.2	K66.1
A02.21	A54.81	B59	G03.8	I41	I63.239	J10.00	K25.4	K67
A02.22	A54.86	B77.81	G03.9	I46.2	I63.29	J10.01	K25.5	K68.12
A06.4	A80.0	D57.00	G04.00	I46.8	I63.30	J10.08	K25.6	K68.19
A06.5	A80.1	D57.01	G04.01	I46.9	I63.311	J11.00	K26.0	K68.9
A06.6	A80.2	D57.02	G04.02	I49.01	I63.312	J11.08	K26.1	K70.41
A17.0	A80.30	D57.211	G04.2	I49.02	I63.319	J12.0	K26.2	K71.11
A17.1	A80.39	D57.212	G04.30	I50.21	I63.321	J12.1	K26.4	K72.00
A17.81	A83.0	D57.219	G04.31	I50.23	I63.322	J12.2	K26.5	K72.01
A17.82	A83.1	D57.411	G04.32	I50.31	I63.329	J12.3	K26.6	K72.11
A17.83	A83.2	D57.412	G04.39	I50.33	I63.331	J12.81	K27.0	K72.91
A17.89	A83.3	D57.419	G04.81	I50.41	I63.332	J12.89	K27.1	K75.0
A18.31	A83.4	D57.811	G04.89	I50.43	I63.339	J12.9	K27.2	K75.1
A19.0	A83.5	D57.812	G04.90	I51.1	I63.341	J13	K27.4	K76.2
A19.1	A83.6	D57.819	G04.91	I51.2	I63.342	J14	K27.5	K76.3
A19.2	A83.8	D59.3	G05.3	I60.00	I63.349	J15.0	K27.6	K76.7
A19.8	A83.9	D60.0	G05.4	I60.01	I63.39	J15.1	K28.0	K80.67
A19.9	A84.0	D60.1	G06.0	I60.02	I63.40	J15.20	K28.1	K82.2
A20.0	A84.1	D60.8	G06.1	I60.10	I63.411	J15.211	K28.2	K83.1
A20.1	A84.8	D60.9	G06.2	I60.11	I63.412	J15.212	K28.4	K83.2
A20.2	A84.9	D61.1	G07	I60.12	I63.419	J15.29	K28.5	K85.0
A20.3	A85.2	D61.2	G08	I60.20	I63.421	J15.3	K28.6	K85.1
A20.7	A92.30	D61.3	G21.0	I60.21	I63.422	J15.4	K29.01	K85.2
A20.8	A92.31	D61.810	G37.4	I60.22	I63.429	J15.5	K29.21	K85.3
A20.9	A92.32	D61.811	G40.301	I60.30	I63.431	J15.6	K29.31	K85.8
A22.1	A92.39	D61.89	G40.311	I60.31	I63.432	J15.7	K29.41	K85.9
A22.7	B00.3	D65	G40.319	I60.32	I63.439	J15.8	K29.51	L89.003
A26.7	B00.4	D66	G70.01	I60.4	I63.441	J15.9	K29.61	L89.004
A27.81	B00.7	D67	G80.0	I60.50	I63.442	J16.0	K29.71	L89.013
A32.7	B00.82	E03.5	G82.50	I60.51	I63.449	J16.8	K29.81	L89.014
A33	B01.11	E05.01	G82.51	I60.52	I63.49	J17	K29.91	L89.023
A35	B01.12	E05.11	G82.52	I60.6	I63.50	J18.0	K31.811	L89.024
A37.01	B01.2	E05.21	G82.53	I60.7	I63.511	J18.1	K31.82	L89.103
A37.11	B02.1	E05.31	G83.5	I60.8	I63.512	J18.8	K35.2	L89.104
A37.81	B02.24	E05.41	G92	I60.9	I63.519	J18.9	K35.3	L89.113
A37.91	B05.0	E05.81	G93.40	I61.0	I63.521	J68.1	K40.10	L89.114
A39.0	B05.2	E05.91	G93.41	I61.1	I63.522	J69.0	K40.11	L89.123
A39.1	B06.01	E08.00	G93.49	I61.2	I63.529	J69.1	K40.40	L89.124
A39.2	B10.01	E08.01	G93.5	I61.3	I63.531	J69.8	K40.41	L89.133
A39.3	B10.09	E08.10	G93.6	I61.4	I63.532	J81.0	K41.10	L89.134
A39.4	B15.0	E08.11	G93.7	I61.5	I63.539	J84.81	K41.11	L89.143
A39.50	B16.0	E08.641	G93.82	I61.6	I63.541	J84.83	K41.40	L89.144
A39.51	B16.2	E09.00	G95.11	I61.8	I63.542	J84.841	K41.41	L89.153
A39.52	B17.11	E09.01	G95.19	I61.9	I63.549	J84.842	K42.1	L89.154
A39.53	B19.0	E09.10	I21.01	I62.00	I63.59	J84.843	K43.1	L89.203
A39.81	B19.11	E09.11	I21.02	I62.01	I63.6	J84.848	K43.4	L89.204
A40.0	B19.21	E09.641	I21.09	I62.02	I63.8	J85.0	K43.7	L89.213
A40.1	B20	E10.10	I21.11	I62.03	I63.9	J85.1	K44.1	L89.214
A40.3	B25.0	E10.11	I21.19	I62.1	I67.0	J85.2	K45.1	L89.223
A40.8	B25.2	E10.641	I21.21	I63.00	I67.83	J85.3	K46.1	L89.224
A40.9	B26.1	E11.00	I21.29	I63.011	I71.00	J86.0	K55.0	L89.303
A41.01	B26.2	E11.01	I21.3	I63.012	I71.01	J86.9	K55.21	L89.304
A41.02	B37.1	E11.641	I21.4	I63.019	I71.02	J93.0	K56.2	L89.313
A41.1	B37.5	E13.00	I22.0	I63.02	I71.03	J95.1	K57.01	L89.314
A41.2	B37.6	E13.01	I22.1	I63.031	I71.1	J95.2	K57.11	L89.323
A41.3	B37.7	E13.10	I22.2	I63.032	I71.3	J95.3	K57.13	L89.324
A41.4	B38.4	E13.11	I22.8	I63.039	I71.5	J95.821	K57.21	L89.43
A41.50	B39.0	E13.641	I22.9	I63.09	I71.8	J95.822	K57.31	L89.44
A41.51	B39.1	E40	I23.4	I63.10	I74.01	J96.00	K57.33	L89.503
A41.52	B39.2	E41	I23.5	I63.111	I77.71	J96.01	K57.41	L89.504
A41.53	B44.0	E42	I25.42	I63.112	I77.72	J96.02	K57.51	L89.513
A41.59	B45.1	E43	I26.01	I63.119	I77.73	J96.20	K57.53	L89.514
A41.81	B46.0	E84.0	I26.02	I63.12	I77.74	J96.21	K57.81	L89.523
A41.89	B46.1	E84.11	I26.09	I63.131	I77.79	J96.22	K57.91	L89.524
A41.9	B46.2	E88.3	I26.90	I63.132	I81	J96.90	K57.93	L89.603
A42.7	B46.3	G00.0	I26.92	I63.139	I82.0	J96.91	K63.1	L89.604
A48.0	B46.4	G00.1	I26.99	I63.19	I82.220	J96.92	K63.81	L89.613
A48.1	B46.5	G00.2	I33.0	I63.20	I82.221	J98.5	K65.0	L89.614
A48.3	B46.8	G00.3	I33.9	I63.211	I85.01	K22.11	K65.1	L89.623
A50.41	B46.9	G00.8	I40.0	I63.212	I85.11	K22.3	K65.2	L89.624
A50.42	B50.9	G00.9	I40.1	I63.219	J04.11	K22.6	K65.3	L89.813
A51.41	B58.2	G01	I40.8	I63.22	J04.31	K25.0	K65.8	L89.814
A52.13	B58.3	G02		I63.231	J05.11	K25.1	K65.9	L89.893

L89.894	O41.1023	O46.011	O88.812	P54.1	Q79.59	S06.313A	S06.5X2A	S12.250B
L89.93	O41.1024	O46.012	O88.813	P54.2	Q89.4	S06.314A	S06.5X3A	S12.251B
L89.94	O41.1025	O46.013	O88.82	P54.3	Q93.81	S06.315A	S06.5X4A	S12.290B
M31.1	O41.1029	O46.021	O88.83	P56.0	R09.2	S06.316A	S06.5X5A	S12.291B
M72.6	O41.1030	O46.022	O90.3	P56.90	R40.20	S06.317A	S06.5X6A	S12.300B
N00.0	O41.1031	O46.023	O90.4	P56.99	R40.2110	S06.318A	S06.5X7A	S12.301B
N00.1	O41.1032	O46.091	O99.42	P57.0	R40.2111	S06.319A	S06.5X8A	S12.330B
N00.2	O41.1033	O46.092	P10.0	P57.8	R40.2112	S06.320A	S06.5X9A	S12.331B
N00.3	O41.1034	O46.093	P10.1	P57.9	R40.2113	S06.321A	S06.6X0A	S12.34XB
N00.4	O41.1035	O60.02	P10.3	P59.1	R40.2114	S06.322A	S06.6X1A	S12.350B
N00.5	O41.1039	O60.03	P10.4	P59.20	R40.2120	S06.323A	S06.6X2A	S12.351B
N00.6	O41.1210	O60.12X0	P10.8	P59.29	R40.2121	S06.324A	S06.6X3A	S12.390B
N00.7	O41.1211	O60.12X1	P10.9	P60	R40.2122	S06.325A	S06.6X4A	S12.391B
N00.8	O41.1212	O60.12X2	P11.0	P61.0	R40.2123	S06.326A	S06.6X5A	S12.400B
N00.9	O41.1213	O60.12X3	P11.2	P61.5	R40.2124	S06.327A	S06.6X6A	S12.401B
N01.0	O41.1214	O60.12X4	P11.9	P74.0	R40.2210	S06.328A	S06.6X7A	S12.430B
N01.1	O41.1215	O60.12X5	P22.0	P77.1	R40.2211	S06.329A	S06.6X8A	S12.431B
N01.2	O41.1219	O60.12X9	P23.0	P77.2	R40.2212	S06.330A	S06.6X9A	S12.44XB
N01.3	O41.1220	O60.13X0	P23.1	P77.3	R40.2213	S06.331A	S06.816A	S12.450B
N01.4	O41.1221	O60.13X1	P23.2	P77.9	R40.2214	S06.332A	S06.817A	S12.451B
N01.5	O41.1222	O60.13X2	P23.3	P78.0	R40.2220	S06.333A	S06.818A	S12.490B
N01.6	O41.1223	O60.13X3	P23.4	P83.2	R40.2221	S06.334A	S06.826A	S12.491B
N01.7	O41.1224	O60.13X4	P23.5	P90	R40.2222	S06.335A	S06.827A	S12.500B
N01.8	O41.1225	O60.13X5	P23.6	P91.0	R40.2223	S06.336A	S06.828A	S12.501B
N01.9	O41.1229	O60.13X9	P23.8	P91.1	R40.2224	S06.337A	S06.896A	S12.530B
N15.1	O41.1230	O60.14X0	P23.9	P91.2	R40.2310	S06.338A	S06.897A	S12.531B
N17.0	O41.1231	O60.14X1	P24.01	P91.3	R40.2311	S06.339A	S06.898A	S12.54XB
N17.1	O41.1232	O60.14X2	P24.11	P91.4	R40.2312	S06.340A	S06.9X6A	S12.550B
N17.2	O41.1233	O60.14X3	P24.21	P91.5	R40.2313	S06.341A	S06.9X7A	S12.551B
N18.6	O41.1234	O60.14X4	P24.31	P91.63	R40.2314	S06.342A	S06.9X8A	S12.590B
N73.3	O41.1235	O60.14X5	P24.81	P92.01	R40.2320	S06.343A	S11.011A	S12.591B
O03.2	O41.1239	O60.14X9	P25.0	Q00.0	R40.2321	S06.344A	S11.012A	S12.600B
O03.31	O41.1410	O60.22X0	P25.1	Q00.1	R40.2322	S06.345A	S11.013A	S12.601B
O03.32	O41.1411	O60.22X1	P25.2	Q00.2	R40.2323	S06.346A	S11.014A	S12.630B
O03.81	O41.1412	O60.22X2	P25.3	Q04.0	R40.2324	S06.347A	S11.015A	S12.631B
O03.82	O41.1413	O60.22X3	P25.8	Q04.1	R40.2340	S06.348A	S11.019A	S12.64XB
O04.7	O41.1414	O60.22X4	P26.0	Q04.2	R40.2341	S06.349A	S11.021A	S12.650B
O04.81	O41.1415	O60.22X5	P26.1	Q04.3	R40.2342	S06.350A	S11.022A	S12.651B
O04.82	O41.1419	O60.22X9	P26.8	Q20.0	R40.2343	S06.351A	S11.023A	S12.690B
O07.2	O41.1420	O60.23X0	P26.9	Q20.1	R40.2344	S06.352A	S11.024A	S12.691B
O07.31	O41.1421	O60.23X1	P27.0	Q20.2	R53.2	S06.353A	S11.025A	S12.8XXA
O07.32	O41.1422	O60.23X2	P27.1	Q20.3	R57.0	S06.354A	S11.029A	S14.0XXA
O08.2	O41.1423	O60.23X3	P27.8	Q20.4	R57.1	S06.355A	S11.031A	S14.101A
O08.3	O41.1424	O60.23X4	P27.9	Q21.3	R57.8	S06.356A	S11.032A	S14.102A
O08.4	O41.1425	O60.23X5	P28.5	Q22.0	R65.11	S06.357A	S11.033A	S14.103A
O10.42	O41.1429	O60.23X9	P28.81	Q22.4	R65.20	S06.358A	S11.034A	S14.104A
O11.1	O41.1430	O67.0	P29.3	Q22.5	R65.21	S06.359A	S11.035A	S14.105A
O11.2	O41.1431	O71.02	P29.81	Q22.6	S02.0XXB	S06.360A	S11.039A	S14.106A
O11.3	O41.1432	O71.03	P35.1	Q22.8	S02.10XB	S06.361A	S12.000B	S14.107A
O14.12	O41.1433	O71.1	P35.2	Q22.9	S02.110B	S06.362A	S12.001B	S14.108A
O14.13	O41.1434	O75.1	P35.3	Q23.4	S02.111B	S06.363A	S12.01XB	S14.111A
O14.22	O41.1435	O75.3	P35.8	Q24.2	S02.112B	S06.364A	S12.02XB	S14.112A
O14.23	O41.1439	O85	P35.9	Q24.4	S02.113B	S06.365A	S12.030B	S14.113A
O15.02	O44.11	O86.81	P36.0	Q24.6	S02.118B	S06.366A	S12.031B	S14.114A
O15.03	O44.12	O86.89	P36.10	Q25.5	S02.119B	S06.367A	S12.040B	S14.115A
O15.1	O44.13	O87.1	P36.19	Q25.6	S02.19XB	S06.368A	S12.041B	S14.116A
O15.2	O45.001	O88.011	P36.2	Q25.71	S02.91XB	S06.369A	S12.090B	S14.117A
O22.31	O45.002	O88.012	P36.30	Q25.72	S06.0X6A	S06.370A	S12.091B	S14.118A
O22.32	O45.003	O88.013	P36.39	Q25.79	S06.1X0A	S06.376A	S12.100B	S14.121A
O22.33	O45.011	O88.02	P36.4	Q28.2	S06.1X1A	S06.377A	S12.101B	S14.122A
O24.02	O45.012	O88.03	P36.5	Q28.3	S06.1X2A	S06.378A	S12.110B	S14.123A
O24.12	O45.013	O88.111	P36.8	Q33.2	S06.1X3A	S06.380A	S12.111B	S14.124A
O24.32	O45.021	O88.112	P36.9	Q33.3	S06.1X4A	S06.386A	S12.112B	S14.125A
O24.82	O45.022	O88.113	P37.0	Q33.6	S06.1X5A	S06.387A	S12.120B	S14.126A
O34.31	O45.023	O88.12	P37.1	Q39.0	S06.1X6A	S06.388A	S12.121B	S14.127A
O34.32	O45.091	O88.13	P37.2	Q39.1	S06.1X7A	S06.4X0A	S12.130B	S14.128A
O34.33	O45.092	O88.211	P37.3	Q39.2	S06.1X8A	S06.4X1A	S12.131B	S14.131A
O41.1010	O45.093	O88.212	P37.4	Q39.3	S06.1X9A	S06.4X2A	S12.14XB	S14.132A
O41.1011	O45.8X1	O88.213	P37.8	Q39.4	S06.2X0A	S06.4X3A	S12.150B	S14.133A
O41.1012	O45.8X2	O88.22	P37.9	Q44.2	S06.2X7A	S06.4X4A	S12.151B	S14.134A
O41.1013	O45.8X3	O88.23	P52.21	Q44.3	S06.2X8A	S06.4X5A	S12.190B	S14.135A
O41.1014	O45.91	O88.311	P52.22	Q79.0	S06.306A	S06.4X6A	S12.191B	S14.136A
O41.1015	O45.92	O88.312	P52.4	Q79.1	S06.307A	S06.4X7A	S12.200B	S14.137A
O41.1019	O45.93	O88.313	P52.5	Q79.2	S06.308A	S06.4X8A	S12.201B	S14.138A
O41.1020	O46.001	O88.32	P52.6	Q79.3	S06.311A	S06.4X9A	S12.230B	S14.141A
O41.1021	O46.002	O88.33	P52.8	Q79.4	S06.312A	S06.5X0A	S12.231B	S14.142A
O41.1022	O46.003	O88.811	P52.9	Q79.51	S06.312A	S06.5X1A	S12.24XB	S14.143A

Appendix E: Major Complication and Comorbidity (MCC) Code List

S14.144A	S22.058B	S25.312A	S31.631A	S32.316B	S32.464B	S34.123A	S37.091A	S42.399B
S14.145A	S22.059B	S25.319A	S31.632A	S32.391B	S32.465A	S34.124A	S37.092A	S42.401B
S14.146A	S22.060B	S25.321A	S31.633A	S32.392B	S32.465B	S34.125A	S37.099A	S42.402B
S14.147A	S22.061B	S25.322A	S31.634A	S32.399B	S32.466A	S34.129A	S42.201B	S42.409B
S14.148A	S22.062B	S25.329A	S31.635A	S32.401A	S32.466B	S34.131A	S42.202B	S42.411B
S14.151A	S22.068B	S25.391A	S31.639A	S32.401B	S32.471A	S34.132A	S42.209B	S42.412B
S14.152A	S22.069B	S25.392A	S31.640A	S32.402A	S32.471B	S34.139A	S42.211B	S42.413B
S14.153A	S22.070B	S25.399A	S31.641A	S32.402B	S32.472A	S34.3XXA	S42.212B	S42.414B
S14.154A	S22.071B	S25.401A	S31.642A	S32.409A	S32.472B	S35.00XA	S42.213B	S42.415B
S14.155A	S22.072B	S25.402A	S31.643A	S32.409B	S32.473A	S35.01XA	S42.214B	S42.416B
S14.156A	S22.078B	S25.409A	S31.644A	S32.411A	S32.473B	S35.02XA	S42.215B	S42.421B
S14.157A	S22.079B	S25.411A	S31.645A	S32.411B	S32.474A	S35.09XA	S42.216B	S42.422B
S14.158A	S22.080B	S25.412A	S31.649A	S32.412A	S32.474B	S35.10XA	S42.221B	S42.423B
S21.301A	S22.081B	S25.419A	S31.650A	S32.412B	S32.475A	S35.11XA	S42.222B	S42.424B
S21.302A	S22.082B	S25.421A	S31.651A	S32.413A	S32.475B	S35.12XA	S42.223B	S42.425B
S21.309A	S22.088B	S25.422A	S31.652A	S32.413B	S32.476A	S35.19XA	S42.224B	S42.426B
S21.311A	S22.089B	S25.429A	S31.653A	S32.414A	S32.476B	S35.211A	S42.225B	S42.431B
S21.312A	S22.20XB	S25.491A	S31.654A	S32.414B	S32.481A	S35.212A	S42.226B	S42.432B
S21.319A	S22.21XB	S25.492A	S31.655A	S32.415A	S32.481B	S35.218A	S42.231B	S42.433B
S21.321A	S22.22XB	S25.499A	S31.659A	S32.415B	S32.482A	S35.219A	S42.232B	S42.434B
S21.322A	S22.23XB	S26.020A	S32.000B	S32.416A	S32.482B	S35.221A	S42.239B	S42.435B
S21.329A	S22.24XB	S26.021A	S32.001B	S32.416B	S32.483A	S35.222A	S42.241B	S42.436B
S21.331A	S22.31XB	S26.022A	S32.002B	S32.421A	S32.483B	S35.228A	S42.242B	S42.441B
S21.332A	S22.32XB	S26.12XA	S32.008B	S32.421B	S32.484A	S35.229A	S42.249B	S42.442B
S21.339A	S22.39XB	S26.92XA	S32.009B	S32.422A	S32.484B	S35.231A	S42.251B	S42.443B
S21.341A	S22.41XB	S27.1XXA	S32.010B	S32.422B	S32.485A	S35.232A	S42.252B	S42.444B
S21.342A	S22.42XB	S27.2XXA	S32.011B	S32.423A	S32.485B	S35.238A	S42.253B	S42.445B
S21.349A	S22.43XB	S27.331A	S32.012B	S32.423B	S32.486A	S35.239A	S42.254B	S42.446B
S21.351A	S22.49XB	S27.332A	S32.018B	S32.424A	S32.486B	S35.291A	S42.255B	S42.447B
S21.352A	S22.5XXA	S27.339A	S32.019B	S32.424B	S32.491A	S35.292A	S42.256B	S42.448B
S21.359A	S22.5XXB	S27.401A	S32.020B	S32.425A	S32.491B	S35.298A	S42.261B	S42.449B
S21.401A	S22.9XXB	S27.402A	S32.021B	S32.425B	S32.492A	S35.299A	S42.262B	S42.451B
S21.402A	S24.0XXA	S27.409A	S32.022B	S32.426A	S32.492B	S35.311A	S42.263B	S42.452B
S21.409A	S24.101A	S27.411A	S32.028B	S32.426B	S32.499A	S35.318A	S42.264B	S42.453B
S21.411A	S24.102A	S27.412A	S32.029B	S32.431A	S32.499B	S35.319A	S42.265B	S42.454B
S21.412A	S24.103A	S27.419A	S32.030B	S32.431B	S32.501B	S35.321A	S42.266B	S42.455B
S21.419A	S24.104A	S27.421A	S32.031B	S32.432A	S32.502B	S35.328A	S42.291B	S42.456B
S21.421A	S24.111A	S27.422A	S32.032B	S32.432B	S32.509B	S35.329A	S42.292B	S42.461B
S21.422A	S24.112A	S27.429A	S32.038B	S32.433A	S32.511B	S35.331A	S42.293B	S42.462B
S21.429A	S24.113A	S27.431A	S32.039B	S32.433B	S32.512B	S35.338A	S42.294B	S42.463B
S21.431A	S24.114A	S27.432A	S32.040B	S32.434A	S32.519B	S35.339A	S42.295B	S42.464B
S21.432A	S24.131A	S27.439A	S32.041B	S32.434B	S32.591B	S35.341A	S42.296B	S42.465B
S21.439A	S24.132A	S27.491A	S32.042B	S32.435A	S32.592B	S35.348A	S42.301B	S42.466B
S21.441A	S24.133A	S27.492A	S32.048B	S32.435B	S32.599B	S35.349A	S42.302B	S42.471B
S21.442A	S24.134A	S27.499A	S32.049B	S32.436A	S32.601B	S35.401A	S42.309B	S42.472B
S21.449A	S24.141A	S27.812A	S32.050B	S32.436B	S32.602B	S35.402A	S42.321B	S42.473B
S21.451A	S24.142A	S27.813A	S32.051B	S32.441A	S32.609B	S35.403A	S42.322B	S42.474B
S21.452A	S24.143A	S27.818A	S32.052B	S32.441B	S32.611B	S35.404A	S42.323B	S42.475B
S21.459A	S24.144A	S27.819A	S32.058B	S32.442A	S32.612B	S35.405A	S42.324B	S42.476B
S22.000B	S24.151A	S31.001A	S32.059B	S32.442B	S32.613B	S35.406A	S42.325B	S42.491B
S22.001B	S24.152A	S31.011A	S32.10XB	S32.443A	S32.614B	S35.411A	S42.326B	S42.492B
S22.002B	S24.153A	S31.021A	S32.110B	S32.443B	S32.615B	S35.412A	S42.331B	S42.493B
S22.008B	S24.154A	S31.031A	S32.111B	S32.444A	S32.616B	S35.413A	S42.332B	S42.494B
S22.009B	S25.00XA	S31.041A	S32.112B	S32.444B	S32.691B	S35.414A	S42.333B	S42.495B
S22.010B	S25.01XA	S31.051A	S32.119B	S32.445A	S32.692B	S35.415A	S42.334B	S42.496B
S22.011B	S25.02XA	S31.600A	S32.120B	S32.445B	S32.699B	S35.416A	S42.335B	S42.90XB
S22.012B	S25.09XA	S31.601A	S32.121B	S32.446A	S32.810B	S35.491A	S42.336B	S42.91XB
S22.018B	S25.101A	S31.602A	S32.122B	S32.446B	S32.811B	S35.492A	S42.341B	S42.92XB
S22.019B	S25.102A	S31.603A	S32.129B	S32.451A	S32.82XB	S35.493A	S42.342B	S45.001A
S22.020B	S25.109A	S31.604A	S32.130B	S32.451B	S32.89XB	S35.494A	S42.343B	S45.002A
S22.021B	S25.111A	S31.605A	S32.131B	S32.452A	S32.9XXB	S35.495A	S42.344B	S45.009A
S22.022B	S25.112A	S31.609A	S32.132B	S32.452B	S34.01XA	S35.496A	S42.345B	S45.011A
S22.028B	S25.119A	S31.610A	S32.139B	S32.453A	S34.02XA	S35.50XA	S42.346B	S45.012A
S22.029B	S25.121A	S31.611A	S32.14XB	S32.453B	S34.101A	S35.511A	S42.351B	S45.019A
S22.030B	S25.122A	S31.612A	S32.15XB	S32.454A	S34.102A	S35.512A	S42.352B	S45.091A
S22.031B	S25.129A	S31.613A	S32.16XB	S32.454B	S34.103A	S35.513A	S42.353B	S45.092A
S22.032B	S25.191A	S31.614A	S32.17XB	S32.455A	S34.104A	S35.514A	S42.354B	S45.099A
S22.038B	S25.192A	S31.615A	S32.19XB	S32.455B	S34.105A	S35.515A	S42.355B	S52.001B
S22.039B	S25.199A	S31.619A	S32.2XXB	S32.456A	S34.109A	S35.516A	S42.356B	S52.001C
S22.040B	S25.20XA	S31.620A	S32.301B	S32.456B	S34.111A	S35.59XA	S42.361B	S52.002B
S22.041B	S25.21XA	S31.621A	S32.302B	S32.461A	S34.112A	S36.031A	S42.362B	S52.002C
S22.042B	S25.22XA	S31.622A	S32.309B	S32.461B	S34.113A	S36.032A	S42.363B	S52.009B
S22.048B	S25.29XA	S31.623A	S32.311B	S32.462A	S34.114A	S36.115A	S42.364B	S52.009C
S22.049B	S25.301A	S31.624A	S32.312B	S32.462B	S34.115A	S36.116A	S42.365B	S52.021B
S22.050B	S25.302A	S31.625A	S32.313B	S32.463A	S34.119A	S37.061A	S42.366B	S52.021C
S22.051B	S25.309A	S31.629A	S32.314B	S32.463B	S34.121A	S37.062A	S42.391B	S52.022B
S22.052B	S25.311A	S31.630A	S32.315B	S32.464A	S34.122A	S37.069A	S42.392B	S52.022C

Appendix E: Major Complication and Comorbidity (MCC) Code List

S52.023B	S52.202C	S52.292B	S52.381C	S52.614B	S72.042C	S72.121B	S72.309A	S72.361C
S52.023C	S52.209B	S52.292C	S52.382B	S52.614C	S72.043A	S72.121C	S72.309B	S72.362A
S52.024B	S52.209C	S52.299B	S52.382C	S52.615B	S72.043B	S72.122A	S72.309C	S72.362B
S52.024C	S52.221B	S52.299C	S52.389B	S52.615C	S72.043C	S72.122B	S72.321A	S72.362C
S52.025B	S52.221C	S52.301B	S52.389C	S52.616B	S72.044A	S72.122C	S72.321B	S72.363A
S52.025C	S52.222B	S52.301C	S52.391B	S52.616C	S72.044B	S72.123A	S72.321C	S72.363B
S52.026B	S52.222C	S52.302B	S52.391C	S52.691B	S72.044C	S72.123B	S72.322A	S72.363C
S52.026C	S52.223B	S52.302C	S52.392B	S52.691C	S72.045A	S72.123C	S72.322B	S72.364A
S52.031B	S52.223C	S52.309B	S52.392C	S52.692B	S72.045B	S72.124A	S72.322C	S72.364B
S52.031C	S52.224B	S52.309C	S52.399B	S52.692C	S72.045C	S72.124B	S72.323A	S72.364C
S52.032B	S52.224C	S52.321B	S52.399C	S52.699B	S72.046A	S72.124C	S72.323B	S72.365A
S52.032C	S52.225B	S52.321C	S52.501B	S52.699C	S72.046B	S72.125A	S72.323C	S72.365B
S52.033B	S52.225C	S52.322B	S52.501C	S52.90XB	S72.046C	S72.125B	S72.324A	S72.365C
S52.033C	S52.226B	S52.322C	S52.502B	S52.90XC	S72.051A	S72.125C	S72.324B	S72.366A
S52.034B	S52.226C	S52.323B	S52.502C	S52.91XB	S72.051B	S72.126A	S72.324C	S72.366B
S52.034C	S52.231B	S52.323C	S52.509B	S52.91XC	S72.051C	S72.126B	S72.325A	S72.366C
S52.035B	S52.231C	S52.324B	S52.509C	S52.92XB	S72.052A	S72.126C	S72.325B	S72.391A
S52.035C	S52.232B	S52.324C	S52.511B	S52.92XC	S72.052B	S72.131A	S72.325C	S72.391B
S52.036B	S52.232C	S52.325B	S52.511C	S72.001A	S72.052C	S72.131B	S72.326A	S72.391C
S52.036C	S52.233B	S52.325C	S52.512B	S72.001B	S72.059A	S72.131C	S72.326B	S72.392A
S52.041B	S52.233C	S52.326B	S52.512C	S72.001C	S72.059B	S72.132A	S72.326C	S72.392B
S52.041C	S52.234B	S52.326C	S52.513B	S72.002A	S72.059C	S72.132B	S72.331A	S72.392C
S52.042B	S52.234C	S52.331B	S52.513C	S72.002B	S72.061A	S72.132C	S72.331B	S72.399A
S52.042C	S52.235B	S52.331C	S52.514B	S72.002C	S72.061B	S72.133A	S72.331C	S72.399B
S52.043B	S52.235C	S52.332B	S52.514C	S72.009A	S72.061C	S72.133B	S72.332A	S72.399C
S52.043C	S52.236B	S52.332C	S52.515B	S72.009B	S72.062A	S72.133C	S72.332B	S72.401B
S52.044B	S52.236C	S52.333B	S52.515C	S72.009C	S72.062B	S72.134A	S72.332C	S72.401C
S52.044C	S52.241B	S52.333C	S52.516B	S72.011A	S72.062C	S72.134B	S72.333A	S72.402B
S52.045B	S52.241C	S52.334B	S52.516C	S72.011B	S72.063A	S72.134C	S72.333B	S72.402C
S52.045C	S52.242B	S52.334C	S52.531B	S72.011C	S72.063B	S72.135A	S72.333C	S72.409B
S52.046B	S52.242C	S52.335B	S52.531C	S72.012A	S72.063C	S72.135B	S72.334A	S72.409C
S52.046C	S52.243B	S52.335C	S52.532B	S72.012B	S72.064A	S72.135C	S72.334B	S72.411B
S52.091B	S52.243C	S52.336B	S52.532C	S72.012C	S72.064B	S72.136A	S72.334C	S72.411C
S52.091C	S52.244B	S52.336C	S52.539B	S72.019A	S72.064C	S72.136B	S72.335A	S72.412B
S52.092B	S52.244C	S52.341B	S52.539C	S72.019B	S72.065A	S72.136C	S72.335B	S72.412C
S52.092C	S52.245B	S52.341C	S52.541B	S72.019C	S72.065B	S72.141A	S72.335C	S72.413B
S52.099B	S52.245C	S52.342B	S52.541C	S72.021A	S72.065C	S72.141B	S72.336A	S72.413C
S52.099C	S52.246B	S52.342C	S52.542B	S72.021B	S72.066A	S72.141C	S72.336B	S72.414B
S52.101B	S52.246C	S52.343B	S52.542C	S72.021C	S72.066B	S72.142A	S72.336C	S72.414C
S52.101C	S52.251B	S52.343C	S52.549B	S72.022A	S72.066C	S72.142B	S72.341A	S72.415B
S52.102B	S52.251C	S52.344B	S52.549C	S72.022B	S72.091A	S72.142C	S72.341B	S72.415C
S52.102C	S52.252B	S52.344C	S52.551B	S72.022C	S72.091B	S72.143A	S72.341C	S72.416B
S52.109B	S52.252C	S52.345B	S52.551C	S72.023A	S72.091C	S72.143B	S72.342A	S72.416C
S52.109C	S52.253B	S52.345C	S52.552B	S72.023B	S72.092A	S72.143C	S72.342B	S72.421B
S52.121B	S52.253C	S52.346B	S52.552C	S72.023C	S72.092B	S72.144A	S72.342C	S72.421C
S52.121C	S52.254B	S52.346C	S52.559B	S72.024A	S72.092C	S72.144B	S72.343A	S72.422B
S52.122B	S52.254C	S52.351B	S52.559C	S72.024B	S72.099A	S72.144C	S72.343B	S72.422C
S52.122C	S52.255B	S52.351C	S52.561B	S72.024C	S72.099B	S72.145A	S72.343C	S72.423B
S52.123B	S52.255C	S52.352B	S52.561C	S72.025A	S72.099C	S72.145B	S72.344A	S72.423C
S52.123C	S52.256B	S52.352C	S52.562B	S72.025B	S72.101A	S72.145C	S72.344B	S72.424B
S52.124B	S52.256C	S52.353B	S52.562C	S72.025C	S72.101B	S72.146A	S72.344C	S72.424C
S52.124C	S52.261B	S52.353C	S52.569B	S72.026A	S72.101C	S72.146B	S72.345A	S72.425B
S52.125B	S52.261C	S52.354B	S52.569C	S72.026B	S72.102A	S72.146C	S72.345B	S72.425C
S52.125C	S52.262B	S52.354C	S52.571B	S72.026C	S72.102B	S72.21XA	S72.345C	S72.426B
S52.126B	S52.262C	S52.355B	S52.571C	S72.031A	S72.102C	S72.21XB	S72.346A	S72.426C
S52.126C	S52.263B	S52.355C	S52.572B	S72.031B	S72.109A	S72.21XC	S72.346B	S72.431B
S52.131B	S52.263C	S52.356B	S52.572C	S72.031C	S72.109B	S72.22XA	S72.346C	S72.431C
S52.131C	S52.264B	S52.356C	S52.579B	S72.032A	S72.109C	S72.22XB	S72.351A	S72.432B
S52.132B	S52.264C	S52.361B	S52.579C	S72.032B	S72.111A	S72.22XC	S72.351B	S72.432C
S52.132C	S52.265B	S52.361C	S52.591B	S72.032C	S72.111B	S72.23XA	S72.351C	S72.433B
S52.133B	S52.265C	S52.362B	S52.591C	S72.033A	S72.111C	S72.23XB	S72.352A	S72.433C
S52.133C	S52.266B	S52.362C	S52.592B	S72.033B	S72.112A	S72.23XC	S72.352B	S72.434B
S52.134B	S52.266C	S52.363B	S52.592C	S72.033C	S72.112B	S72.24XA	S72.352C	S72.434C
S52.134C	S52.271B	S52.363C	S52.599B	S72.034A	S72.112C	S72.24XB	S72.353A	S72.435B
S52.135B	S52.271C	S52.364B	S52.599C	S72.034B	S72.113A	S72.24XC	S72.353B	S72.435C
S52.135C	S52.272B	S52.364C	S52.601B	S72.034C	S72.113B	S72.25XA	S72.353C	S72.436B
S52.136B	S52.272C	S52.365B	S52.601C	S72.035A	S72.113C	S72.25XB	S72.354A	S72.436C
S52.136C	S52.279B	S52.365C	S52.602B	S72.035B	S72.114A	S72.25XC	S72.354B	S72.441B
S52.181B	S52.279C	S52.366B	S52.602C	S72.035C	S72.114B	S72.26XA	S72.354C	S72.441C
S52.181C	S52.281B	S52.366C	S52.609B	S72.036A	S72.114C	S72.26XB	S72.355A	S72.442B
S52.182B	S52.281C	S52.371B	S52.609C	S72.036B	S72.115A	S72.26XC	S72.355B	S72.442C
S52.182C	S52.282B	S52.371C	S52.611B	S72.036C	S72.115B	S72.301A	S72.355C	S72.443B
S52.189B	S52.282C	S52.372B	S52.611C	S72.041A	S72.115C	S72.301B	S72.356A	S72.443C
S52.189C	S52.283B	S52.372C	S52.612B	S72.041B	S72.116A	S72.301C	S72.356B	S72.444B
S52.201B	S52.283C	S52.379B	S52.612C	S72.041C	S72.116B	S72.302A	S72.356C	S72.444C
S52.201C	S52.291B	S52.379C	S52.613B	S72.042A	S72.116C	S72.302B	S72.361A	S72.445B
S52.202B	S52.291C	S52.381B	S52.613C	S72.042B	S72.121A	S72.302C	S72.361B	S72.445C

S72.446B	S75.001A	S82.116C	S82.191C	S82.252C	S82.433C	S82.831C	T31.62	T32.72
S72.446C	S75.002A	S82.121B	S82.192B	S82.253B	S82.434B	S82.832B	T31.63	T32.73
S72.451B	S75.009A	S82.121C	S82.192C	S82.253C	S82.434C	S82.832C	T31.64	T32.74
S72.451C	S75.011A	S82.122B	S82.199B	S82.254C	S82.435B	S82.839B	T31.65	T32.75
S72.452B	S75.012A	S82.122C	S82.199C	S82.254C	S82.435C	S82.839C	T31.66	T32.76
S72.452C	S75.019A	S82.123B	S82.201B	S82.255B	S82.436B	S82.861B	T31.71	T32.77
S72.453B	S75.021A	S82.123C	S82.201C	S82.255C	S82.436C	S82.861C	T31.72	T32.81
S72.453C	S75.022A	S82.124B	S82.202B	S82.256B	S82.441B	S82.862B	T31.73	T32.82
S72.454B	S75.029A	S82.124C	S82.202C	S82.256C	S82.441C	S82.862C	T31.74	T32.83
S72.454C	S75.091A	S82.125B	S82.209B	S82.261B	S82.442B	S82.863B	T31.75	T32.84
S72.455B	S75.092A	S82.125C	S82.209C	S82.261C	S82.442C	S82.863C	T31.76	T32.85
S72.455C	S75.099A	S82.126B	S82.221B	S82.262B	S82.443B	S82.864B	T31.77	T32.86
S72.456B	S75.101A	S82.126C	S82.221C	S82.262C	S82.443C	S82.864C	T31.81	T32.87
S72.456C	S75.102A	S82.131B	S82.222B	S82.263B	S82.444B	S82.865B	T31.82	T32.88
S72.461B	S75.109A	S82.131C	S82.222C	S82.263C	S82.444C	S82.865C	T31.83	T32.91
S72.461C	S75.111A	S82.132B	S82.223B	S82.264B	S82.445B	S82.866B	T31.84	T32.92
S72.462B	S75.112A	S82.132C	S82.223C	S82.264C	S82.445C	S82.866C	T31.85	T32.93
S72.462C	S75.119A	S82.133B	S82.224B	S82.265B	S82.446B	S85.001A	T31.86	T32.94
S72.463B	S75.121A	S82.133C	S82.224C	S82.265C	S82.446C	S85.002A	T31.87	T32.95
S72.463C	S75.122A	S82.134B	S82.225B	S82.266B	S82.451B	S85.009A	T31.88	T32.96
S72.464B	S75.129A	S82.134C	S82.225C	S82.266C	S82.451C	S85.011A	T31.91	T32.97
S72.464C	S75.191A	S82.135B	S82.226B	S82.291B	S82.452B	S85.012A	T31.92	T32.98
S72.465B	S75.192A	S82.135C	S82.226C	S82.291C	S82.452C	S85.019A	T31.93	T32.99
S72.465C	S75.199A	S82.136B	S82.231B	S82.292B	S82.453B	S85.091A	T31.94	T79.0XXA
S72.466B	S79.001A	S82.136C	S82.231C	S82.292C	S82.453C	S85.092A	T31.95	T79.1XXA
S72.466C	S79.002A	S82.141B	S82.232B	S82.299B	S82.454B	S85.099A	T31.96	T79.4XXA
S72.491B	S79.009A	S82.141C	S82.232C	S82.299C	S82.454C	S85.501A	T31.97	T79.5XXA
S72.491C	S79.011A	S82.142B	S82.233B	S82.401B	S82.455B	S85.502A	T31.98	T80.0XXA
S72.492B	S79.012A	S82.142C	S82.233C	S82.401C	S82.455C	S85.509A	T31.99	T81.11XA
S72.492C	S79.019A	S82.143B	S82.234B	S82.402B	S82.456B	S85.511A	T32.21	T81.12XA
S72.499B	S79.091A	S82.143C	S82.234C	S82.402C	S82.456C	S85.512A	T32.22	T81.19XA
S72.499C	S79.092A	S82.144B	S82.235B	S82.409B	S82.461B	S85.519A	T32.31	
S72.8X1A	S79.099A	S82.144C	S82.235C	S82.409C	S82.461C	S85.591A	T32.32	
S72.8X1B	S82.101B	S82.145B	S82.236B	S82.421B	S82.462B	S85.592A	T32.33	
S72.8X1C	S82.101C	S82.145C	S82.236C	S82.421C	S82.462C	S85.599A	T32.41	
S72.8X2A	S82.102B	S82.146B	S82.241B	S82.422B	S82.463B	T31.21	T32.42	
S72.8X2B	S82.102C	S82.146C	S82.241C	S82.422C	S82.463C	T31.22	T32.43	
S72.8X2C	S82.109B	S82.151B	S82.242B	S82.423B	S82.464B	T31.31	T32.44	
S72.8X9A	S82.109C	S82.151C	S82.242C	S82.423C	S82.464C	T31.32	T32.51	
S72.8X9B	S82.111B	S82.152B	S82.243B	S82.424B	S82.465B	T31.33	T32.52	
S72.8X9C	S82.111C	S82.152C	S82.243C	S82.424C	S82.465C	T31.41	T32.53	
S72.90XA	S82.112B	S82.153B	S82.244B	S82.425B	S82.466B	T31.42	T32.54	
S72.90XB	S82.112C	S82.153C	S82.244C	S82.425C	S82.466C	T31.43	T32.55	
S72.90XC	S82.113B	S82.154B	S82.245B	S82.426B	S82.491B	T31.44	T32.61	
S72.91XA	S82.113C	S82.154C	S82.245C	S82.426C	S82.491C	T31.51	T32.62	
S72.91XB	S82.114B	S82.155B	S82.246B	S82.431B	S82.492B	T31.52	T32.63	
S72.91XC	S82.114C	S82.155C	S82.246C	S82.431C	S82.492C	T31.53	T32.64	
S72.92XA	S82.115B	S82.156B	S82.251B	S82.432B	S82.499B	T31.54	T32.65	
S72.92XB	S82.115C	S82.156C	S82.251C	S82.432C	S82.499C	T31.55	T32.66	
S72.92XC	S82.116B	S82.191B	S82.252B	S82.433B	S82.831B	T31.61	T32.71	

Appendix F: Complication and Comorbidity (CC) Code List

A00.0	A18.11	A32.89	A51.32	A75.2	B00.53	B37.84	B57.5	B77.9
A00.1	A18.12	A32.9	A51.39	A75.3	B00.59	B37.89	B58.00	B78.0
A00.9	A18.13	A34	A51.42	A75.9	B00.81	B38.0	B58.01	B78.7
A01.00	A18.14	A36.0	A51.43	A77.0	B00.89	B38.1	B58.09	B78.9
A01.01	A18.15	A36.1	A51.44	A77.1	B01.0	B38.2	B58.1	B79
A01.02	A18.16	A36.2	A51.45	A77.2	B01.81	B38.3	B58.82	B80
A01.03	A18.17	A36.3	A51.46	A77.3	B01.89	B38.7	B58.83	B81.0
A01.04	A18.18	A36.81	A51.49	A77.40	B01.9	B38.81	B58.89	B81.1
A01.05	A18.2	A36.82	A52.00	A77.41	B02.0	B38.89	B58.9	B81.2
A01.09	A18.32	A36.83	A52.01	A77.49	B02.21	B38.9	B60.0	B81.3
A01.1	A18.39	A36.84	A52.02	A77.8	B02.22	B39.3	B60.10	B81.4
A01.2	A18.4	A36.85	A52.03	A77.9	B02.23	B40.0	B60.19	B81.8
A01.3	A18.50	A36.86	A52.04	A78	B02.29	B40.1	B60.2	B82.0
A01.4	A18.51	A36.89	A52.05	A79.0	B02.30	B40.2	B65.0	B97.21
A02.0	A18.52	A36.9	A52.06	A79.1	B02.31	B40.3	B65.1	B97.33
A02.23	A18.53	A37.00	A52.09	A79.81	B02.32	B40.7	B65.2	B97.34
A02.24	A18.54	A37.10	A52.10	A79.89	B02.33	B40.81	B65.3	B97.35
A02.25	A18.59	A37.80	A52.11	A79.9	B02.34	B40.89	B65.8	C15.3
A02.29	A18.6	A37.90	A52.12	A81.00	B02.39	B40.9	B65.9	C15.4
A02.8	A18.7	A38.0	A52.15	A81.01	B02.7	B41.7	B66.0	C15.5
A02.9	A18.81	A38.1	A52.16	A81.09	B02.8	B41.8	B66.1	C15.8
A03.0	A18.82	A38.8	A52.17	A81.1	B03	B41.9	B66.2	C15.9
A04.0	A18.83	A38.9	A52.19	A81.2	B04	B44.1	B66.3	C16.0
A04.1	A18.84	A39.82	A52.2	A81.81	B05.1	B44.2	B66.4	C16.1
A04.2	A18.85	A39.83	A52.3	A81.82	B05.4	B44.7	B66.5	C16.2
A04.3	A18.89	A39.84	A52.71	A81.83	B05.81	B44.81	B66.8	C16.3
A04.4	A21.0	A39.89	A52.72	A81.89	B05.89	B44.89	B67.0	C16.4
A04.5	A21.1	A39.9	A52.73	A81.9	B06.00	B44.9	B67.1	C16.5
A04.6	A21.2	A42.0	A52.74	A82.0	B06.02	B45.0	B67.2	C16.6
A04.7	A21.3	A42.1	A52.75	A82.1	B06.09	B45.2	B67.31	C16.8
A04.8	A21.7	A42.2	A52.76	A82.9	B06.81	B45.3	B67.32	C16.9
A04.9	A21.8	A42.81	A52.77	A85.0	B06.82	B45.7	B67.39	C17.0
A05.0	A21.9	A42.82	A52.78	A85.1	B06.89	B45.8	B67.4	C17.1
A05.1	A22.0	A42.89	A52.79	A85.8	B08.3	B45.9	B67.5	C17.2
A05.2	A22.2	A42.9	A54.00	A86	B08.71	B47.0	B67.61	C17.3
A05.3	A22.8	A43.0	A54.01	A87.0	B15.9	B47.1	B67.69	C17.8
A05.4	A22.9	A43.1	A54.02	A87.1	B16.1	B47.9	B67.7	C17.9
A05.5	A23.8	A43.8	A54.03	A87.2	B16.9	B48.2	B67.8	C18.0
A05.8	A23.9	A43.9	A54.09	A87.8	B17.0	B48.3	B67.90	C18.1
A06.0	A24.0	A44.0	A54.1	A87.9	B17.10	B48.4	B67.99	C18.2
A06.1	A24.1	A44.1	A54.21	A88.0	B17.2	B48.8	B68.0	C18.3
A06.2	A24.2	A44.8	A54.22	A88.8	B17.8	B49	B68.1	C18.4
A06.3	A24.3	A44.9	A54.23	A89	B17.9	B50.0	B68.9	C18.5
A06.81	A24.9	A48.51	A54.24	A90	B18.0	B50.8	B69.0	C18.6
A06.82	A25.0	A48.52	A54.29	A91	B18.1	B51.0	B69.1	C18.7
A06.89	A25.1	A50.01	A54.30	A92.0	B18.8	B51.8	B69.81	C18.8
A07.1	A25.9	A50.02	A54.31	A92.1	B18.9	B51.9	B69.89	C18.9
A07.2	A27.0	A50.03	A54.32	A92.2	B19.10	B52.0	B69.9	C19
A07.3	A27.89	A50.04	A54.33	A92.4	B19.9	B52.8	B70.0	C20
A07.4	A27.9	A50.05	A54.39	A92.8	B25.1	B52.9	B70.1	C21.0
A07.8	A28.0	A50.06	A54.40	A92.9	B25.8	B53.0	B71.0	C21.1
A07.9	A28.1	A50.07	A54.41	A93.0	B25.9	B53.1	B71.1	C21.2
A08.0	A28.2	A50.08	A54.42	A93.1	B26.0	B53.8	B71.8	C21.8
A08.11	A28.8	A50.09	A54.43	A93.2	B26.3	B54	B72	C22.0
A08.19	A28.9	A50.2	A54.49	A93.8	B26.81	B55.0	B73.00	C22.1
A08.2	A30.0	A50.30	A54.82	A94	B26.82	B55.1	B73.01	C22.2
A08.31	A30.1	A50.31	A54.83	A95.0	B26.83	B55.2	B73.02	C22.3
A08.32	A30.2	A50.32	A54.84	A95.1	B26.84	B55.9	B73.09	C22.4
A08.39	A30.3	A50.39	A54.85	A95.9	B26.85	B56.0	B73.1	C22.7
A09	A30.4	A50.40	A54.89	A96.0	B26.89	B56.1	B74.0	C22.8
A15.0	A30.5	A50.43	A54.9	A96.1	B33.1	B56.9	B74.1	C22.9
A15.4	A30.8	A50.44	A68.0	A96.8	B33.20	B57.0	B74.2	C23
A15.5	A30.9	A50.45	A68.1	A96.9	B33.21	B57.1	B74.3	C24.0
A15.6	A31.0	A50.49	A68.9	A98.0	B33.22	B57.2	B74.4	C24.1
A15.7	A31.1	A50.51	A69.1	A98.1	B33.23	B57.30	B74.8	C24.8
A15.8	A31.2	A50.52	A69.20	A98.2	B34.3	B57.31	B74.9	C24.9
A15.9	A31.8	A50.53	A69.21	A98.5	B37.0	B57.32	B75	C25.0
A17.9	A31.9	A50.54	A69.22	A98.8	B37.41	B57.39	B76.0	C25.1
A18.01	A32.0	A50.55	A69.23	A99	B37.49	B57.40	B76.1	C25.2
A18.02	A32.11	A50.56	A69.29	B00.2	B37.81	B57.41	B76.8	C25.3
A18.03	A32.12	A50.57	A70	B00.50	B37.82	B57.42	B76.9	C25.4
A18.09	A32.81	A50.59	A75.0	B00.51	B37.83	B57.49	B77.0	C25.7
A18.10	A32.82	A51.31	A75.1	B00.52			B77.89	C25.8

C25.9	C48.2	C77.2	C81.04	C82.11	C82.98	C84.05	C85.12	C91.60
C33	C48.8	C77.3	C81.05	C82.12	C82.99	C84.06	C85.13	C91.61
C34.00	C49.0	C77.4	C81.06	C82.13	C83.00	C84.07	C85.14	C91.62
C34.01	C49.10	C77.5	C81.07	C82.14	C83.01	C84.08	C85.15	C91.90
C34.02	C49.11	C77.8	C81.08	C82.15	C83.02	C84.09	C85.16	C91.91
C34.10	C49.12	C77.9	C81.09	C82.16	C83.03	C84.10	C85.17	C91.92
C34.11	C49.20	C78.00	C81.10	C82.17	C83.04	C84.11	C85.18	C91.A0
C34.12	C49.21	C78.01	C81.11	C82.18	C83.05	C84.12	C85.19	C91.A1
C34.2	C49.22	C78.02	C81.12	C82.19	C83.06	C84.13	C85.20	C91.A2
C34.30	C49.3	C78.1	C81.13	C82.20	C83.07	C84.14	C85.21	C91.Z0
C34.31	C49.4	C78.2	C81.14	C82.21	C83.08	C84.15	C85.22	C91.Z1
C34.32	C49.5	C78.30	C81.15	C82.22	C83.09	C84.16	C85.23	C91.Z2
C34.80	C49.6	C78.39	C81.16	C82.23	C83.10	C84.17	C85.24	C92.00
C34.81	C49.8	C78.4	C81.17	C82.24	C83.11	C84.18	C85.25	C92.01
C34.82	C49.9	C78.5	C81.18	C82.25	C83.12	C84.19	C85.26	C92.02
C34.90	C56.1	C78.6	C81.19	C82.26	C83.13	C84.40	C85.27	C92.10
C34.91	C56.2	C78.7	C81.20	C82.27	C83.14	C84.41	C85.28	C92.11
C34.92	C56.9	C78.80	C81.21	C82.28	C83.15	C84.42	C85.29	C92.12
C37	C64.1	C78.89	C81.22	C82.29	C83.16	C84.43	C85.80	C92.20
C38.0	C64.2	C79.00	C81.23	C82.30	C83.17	C84.44	C85.81	C92.21
C38.1	C64.9	C79.01	C81.24	C82.31	C83.18	C84.45	C85.82	C92.22
C38.2	C65.1	C79.02	C81.25	C82.32	C83.19	C84.46	C85.83	C92.30
C38.3	C65.2	C79.10	C81.26	C82.33	C83.30	C84.47	C85.84	C92.31
C38.4	C65.9	C79.11	C81.27	C82.34	C83.31	C84.48	C85.85	C92.32
C38.8	C66.1	C79.19	C81.28	C82.35	C83.32	C84.49	C85.86	C92.40
C40.00	C66.2	C79.2	C81.29	C82.36	C83.33	C84.60	C85.87	C92.41
C40.01	C66.9	C79.31	C81.30	C82.37	C83.34	C84.61	C85.88	C92.42
C40.02	C68.0	C79.32	C81.31	C82.38	C83.35	C84.62	C85.89	C92.50
C40.10	C68.1	C79.40	C81.32	C82.39	C83.36	C84.63	C85.90	C92.51
C40.11	C68.8	C79.49	C81.33	C82.40	C83.37	C84.64	C85.91	C92.52
C40.12	C68.9	C79.51	C81.34	C82.41	C83.38	C84.65	C85.92	C92.60
C40.20	C70.0	C79.52	C81.35	C82.42	C83.39	C84.66	C85.93	C92.61
C40.21	C70.1	C79.60	C81.36	C82.43	C83.50	C84.67	C85.94	C92.62
C40.22	C70.9	C79.61	C81.37	C82.44	C83.51	C84.68	C85.95	C92.90
C40.30	C71.0	C79.62	C81.38	C82.45	C83.52	C84.69	C85.96	C92.91
C40.31	C71.1	C79.70	C81.39	C82.46	C83.53	C84.70	C85.97	C92.92
C40.32	C71.2	C79.71	C81.40	C82.47	C83.54	C84.71	C85.98	C92.A0
C40.80	C71.3	C79.72	C81.41	C82.48	C83.55	C84.72	C85.99	C92.A1
C40.81	C71.4	C79.81	C81.42	C82.49	C83.56	C84.73	C86.0	C92.A2
C40.82	C71.5	C79.82	C81.43	C82.50	C83.57	C84.74	C86.1	C92.Z0
C40.90	C71.6	C79.89	C81.44	C82.51	C83.58	C84.75	C86.2	C92.Z1
C40.91	C71.7	C79.9	C81.45	C82.52	C83.59	C84.76	C86.3	C92.Z2
C40.92	C71.8	C7A.00	C81.46	C82.53	C83.70	C84.77	C86.4	C93.00
C41.0	C71.9	C7A.010	C81.47	C82.54	C83.71	C84.78	C86.5	C93.01
C41.1	C72.0	C7A.011	C81.48	C82.55	C83.72	C84.79	C86.6	C93.02
C41.2	C72.1	C7A.012	C81.49	C82.56	C83.73	C84.90	C88.2	C93.10
C41.3	C72.20	C7A.019	C81.70	C82.57	C83.74	C84.91	C88.3	C93.11
C41.4	C72.21	C7A.020	C81.71	C82.58	C83.75	C84.92	C88.4	C93.12
C41.9	C72.22	C7A.021	C81.72	C82.59	C83.76	C84.93	C88.8	C93.30
C45.0	C72.30	C7A.022	C81.73	C82.60	C83.77	C84.94	C88.9	C93.31
C45.1	C72.31	C7A.023	C81.74	C82.61	C83.78	C84.95	C90.00	C93.32
C45.2	C72.32	C7A.024	C81.75	C82.62	C83.79	C84.96	C90.01	C93.90
C46.0	C72.40	C7A.025	C81.76	C82.63	C83.80	C84.97	C90.02	C93.91
C46.1	C72.41	C7A.026	C81.77	C82.64	C83.81	C84.98	C90.10	C93.92
C46.2	C72.42	C7A.029	C81.78	C82.65	C83.82	C84.99	C90.11	C93.Z0
C46.3	C72.50	C7A.090	C81.79	C82.66	C83.83	C84.A0	C90.12	C93.Z1
C46.4	C72.59	C7A.091	C81.90	C82.67	C83.84	C84.A1	C90.20	C93.Z2
C46.50	C72.9	C7A.092	C81.91	C82.68	C83.85	C84.A2	C90.21	C94.00
C46.51	C74.00	C7A.093	C81.92	C82.69	C83.86	C84.A3	C90.22	C94.01
C46.52	C74.01	C7A.094	C81.93	C82.80	C83.87	C84.A4	C90.30	C94.02
C46.7	C74.02	C7A.095	C81.94	C82.81	C83.88	C84.A5	C90.31	C94.20
C46.9	C74.10	C7A.096	C81.95	C82.82	C83.89	C84.A6	C90.32	C94.21
C47.0	C74.11	C7A.098	C81.96	C82.83	C83.90	C84.A7	C91.00	C94.22
C47.10	C74.12	C7A.1	C81.97	C82.84	C83.91	C84.A8	C91.01	C94.30
C47.11	C74.90	C7A.8	C81.98	C82.85	C83.92	C84.A9	C91.02	C94.31
C47.12	C74.91	C7B.01	C81.99	C82.86	C83.93	C84.Z0	C91.10	C94.32
C47.20	C74.92	C7B.02	C82.00	C82.87	C83.94	C84.Z1	C91.11	C94.40
C47.21	C75.0	C7B.03	C82.01	C82.88	C83.95	C84.Z2	C91.12	C94.41
C47.22	C75.1	C7B.04	C82.02	C82.89	C83.96	C84.Z3	C91.30	C94.42
C47.3	C75.2	C7B.09	C82.03	C82.90	C83.97	C84.Z4	C91.31	C94.6
C47.4	C75.3	C7B.8	C82.04	C82.91	C83.98	C84.Z5	C91.32	C94.80
C47.5	C75.4	C80.0	C82.05	C82.92	C83.99	C84.Z6	C91.40	C94.81
C47.6	C75.5	C80.2	C82.06	C82.93	C84.00	C84.Z7	C91.41	C94.82
C47.8	C75.8	C81.00	C82.07	C82.94	C84.01	C84.Z8	C91.42	C95.00
C47.9	C75.9	C81.01	C82.08	C82.95	C84.02	C84.Z9	C91.50	C95.01
C48.0	C77.0	C81.02	C82.09	C82.96	C84.03	C85.10	C91.51	C95.02
C48.1	C77.1	C81.03	C82.10	C82.97	C84.04	C85.11	C91.52	C95.10

Appendix F: Complication and Comorbidity (CC) Code List

C95.11	D80.9	E70.318	E74.09	F10.188	F14.151	F19.232	G03.1	G40.823
C95.12	D81.0	E70.319	E74.20	F10.19	F14.20	F19.239	G03.2	G40.824
C95.90	D81.1	E70.320	E74.21	F10.221	F14.221	F19.250	G04.1	G40.89
C95.91	D81.2	E70.321	E74.29	F10.230	F14.222	F19.251	G10	G40.911
C95.92	D81.3	E70.328	E74.4	F10.231	F14.229	F19.259	G11.0	G40.919
C96.0	D81.4	E70.329	E74.8	F10.232	F14.23	F19.26	G11.1	G40.A11
C96.2	D81.5	E70.330	E75.00	F10.239	F14.250	F19.27	G11.2	G40.A19
C96.4	D81.6	E70.331	E75.01	F10.24	F14.251	F19.280	G11.3	G40.B01
C96.5	D81.7	E70.338	E75.02	F10.251	F14.259	F19.281	G11.4	G40.B09
C96.6	D81.89	E70.339	E75.09	F10.259	F14.280	F19.282	G11.8	G40.B11
C96.9	D81.9	E70.39	E75.10	F10.27	F14.281	F19.288	G11.9	G40.B19
C96.A	D82.0	E70.40	E75.11	F10.280	F14.282	F19.921	G12.0	G43.601
C96.Z	D82.1	E70.41	E75.19	F10.281	F14.288	F19.930	G12.1	G43.609
D46.22	D83.0	E70.49	E75.23	F10.288	F14.921	F19.931	G12.20	G43.611
D46.C	D83.1	E70.5	E75.25	F10.29	F14.950	F19.932	G12.21	G43.619
D47.0	D83.2	E70.8	E75.29	F10.921	F14.951	F19.939	G12.22	G45.0
D47.1	D83.8	E70.9	E75.4	F10.94	F15.121	F19.950	G12.29	G45.1
D47.9	D83.9	E71.0	E76.01	F10.951	F15.150	F19.951	G12.8	G45.2
D47.Z1	D84.8	E71.110	E76.02	F10.959	F15.151	F19.97	G12.9	G45.3
D47.Z9	D84.9	E71.111	E76.03	F10.980	F15.20	F20.0	G21.11	G45.8
D58.8	D89.810	E71.118	E76.1	F10.981	F15.221	F20.1	G21.19	G45.9
D58.9	D89.811	E71.120	E76.210	F10.988	F15.222	F20.2	G21.2	G46.0
D59.0	D89.812	E71.121	E76.211	F10.99	F15.23	F20.5	G21.3	G46.1
D59.1	D89.813	E71.128	E76.219	F11.121	F15.250	F20.81	G21.8	G46.2
D59.2	E06.0	E71.19	E76.22	F11.150	F15.251	F20.89	G21.9	G60.1
D59.4	E08.52	E71.2	E76.29	F11.151	F15.259	F23	G23.0	G61.0
D59.9	E09.52	E71.310	E76.3	F11.20	F15.280	F30.10	G23.1	G61.81
D61.01	E10.52	E71.311	E76.8	F11.221	F15.281	F30.11	G23.2	G62.81
D61.09	E11.52	E71.312	E76.9	F11.222	F15.282	F30.12	G23.8	G70.80
D61.818	E13.52	E71.313	E78.71	F11.23	F15.288	F30.13	G23.9	G70.81
D61.82	E15	E71.314	E78.72	F11.250	F15.921	F30.2	G24.02	G71.0
D61.9	E22.1	E71.318	E79.1	F11.251	F15.93	F30.9	G24.09	G71.2
D62	E22.2	E71.32	E79.2	F11.259	F15.950	F31.0	G24.2	G72.0
D68.0	E22.8	E71.39	E79.8	F11.281	F15.951	F31.10	G24.8	G72.1
D68.1	E22.9	E71.50	E79.9	F11.282	F16.121	F31.11	G25.82	G72.2
D68.2	E23.0	E71.510	E80.0	F11.288	F16.150	F31.12	G25.9	G72.81
D68.311	E23.2	E71.511	E80.1	F11.921	F16.151	F31.13	G31.81	G73.1
D68.312	E24.0	E71.518	E80.20	F11.93	F16.20	F31.2	G31.82	G73.3
D68.318	E24.2	E71.520	E80.21	F11.950	F16.221	F31.30	G32.0	G80.1
D68.32	E24.3	E71.521	E80.29	F11.951	F16.250	F31.31	G32.81	G80.2
D68.4	E24.4	E71.522	E80.3	F12.121	F16.251	F31.32	G36.0	G80.3
D68.51	E24.8	E71.528	E84.19	F12.150	F16.259	F31.4	G36.1	G81.00
D68.52	E24.9	E71.529	E84.8	F12.151	F16.280	F31.5	G36.8	G81.01
D68.59	E27.0	E71.53	E84.9	F12.221	F16.283	F31.60	G36.9	G81.02
D68.61	E27.1	E71.540	E85.0	F12.250	F16.288	F31.61	G37.0	G81.03
D68.62	E27.2	E71.541	E85.1	F12.251	F16.921	F31.62	G37.1	G81.04
D68.69	E27.3	E71.542	E85.2	F12.921	F16.950	F31.63	G37.2	G81.10
D68.8	E27.40	E71.548	E85.3	F12.950	F16.951	F31.64	G37.3	G81.11
D68.9	E27.49	E72.00	E85.4	F12.951	F17.203	F31.81	G37.5	G81.12
D69.0	E27.5	E72.01	E85.8	F13.121	F17.213	F31.89	G37.8	G81.13
D69.3	E32.1	E72.02	E85.9	F13.150	F17.223	F32.0	G37.9	G81.14
D69.41	E34.0	E72.03	E87.0	F13.151	F17.293	F32.1	G40.001	G81.90
D69.42	E36.01	E72.04	E87.1	F13.20	F18.121	F32.2	G40.009	G81.91
D74.0	E36.02	E72.09	E87.2	F13.221	F18.150	F32.3	G40.011	G81.92
D74.8	E36.11	E72.10	E87.3	F13.230	F18.151	F33.0	G40.019	G81.93
D74.9	E36.12	E72.11	E87.4	F13.231	F18.17	F33.1	G40.101	G81.94
D75.81	E44.0	E72.12	E88.40	F13.232	F18.20	F33.2	G40.109	G82.20
D76.1	E44.1	E72.19	E88.41	F13.239	F18.221	F33.3	G40.111	G82.21
D76.2	E45	E72.20	E88.42	F13.250	F18.250	F33.40	G40.119	G82.22
D76.3	E46	E72.21	E88.49	F13.251	F18.251	F33.8	G40.201	G83.0
D78.01	E51.11	E72.22	E89.1	F13.259	F18.259	F33.9	G40.209	G83.4
D78.02	E51.12	E72.23	E89.6	F13.26	F18.27	F34.8	G40.211	G90.3
D78.11	E51.2	E72.29	E89.810	F13.27	F18.280	F34.9	G40.219	G90.50
D78.12	E51.8	E72.3	E89.811	F13.280	F18.288	F50.00	G40.411	G90.511
D78.21	E51.9	E72.4	E89.89	F13.281	F18.921	F50.01	G40.419	G90.512
D78.22	E53.0	E72.50	F01.51	F13.282	F18.950	F50.02	G40.501	G90.513
D78.81	E55.0	E72.51	F02.81	F13.288	F18.951	F50.2	G40.509	G90.519
D78.89	E64.0	E72.52	F03.91	F13.921	F18.97	F68.10	G40.801	G90.521
D80.0	E66.2	E72.53	F05	F13.930	F19.121	F68.12	G40.802	G90.522
D80.1	E70.0	E72.59	F06.0	F13.931	F19.150	F72	G40.803	G90.523
D80.2	E70.1	E72.8	F06.2	F13.932	F19.151	F73	G40.804	G90.529
D80.3	E70.20	E72.9	F10.121	F13.939	F19.17	F84.0	G40.811	G90.59
D80.4	E70.21	E74.00	F10.14	F13.950	F19.20	F84.2	G40.812	G91.0
D80.5	E70.29	E74.01	F10.151	F13.951	F19.221	F84.3	G40.813	G91.1
D80.6	E70.30	E74.02	F10.159	F13.97	F19.222	F84.5	G40.814	G91.2
D80.7	E70.310	E74.03	F10.180	F14.121	F19.230	F84.8	G40.821	G91.3
D80.8	E70.311	E74.04	F10.181	F14.150	F19.231	F84.9	G40.822	G91.8

G91.9	H30.90	H44.022	H59.119	I23.8	I50.1	I70.438	I75.012	I82.503
G93.1	H30.91	H44.023	H59.121	I24.0	I50.20	I70.439	I75.013	I82.509
G95.0	H30.92	H44.029	H59.122	I24.1	I50.22	I70.441	I75.019	I82.511
G95.20	H30.93	H44.111	H59.123	I24.8	I50.30	I70.442	I75.021	I82.512
G95.29	H31.321	H44.112	H59.129	I24.9	I50.32	I70.443	I75.022	I82.513
G95.81	H31.322	H44.113	H59.211	I25.110	I50.40	I70.444	I75.023	I82.519
G95.89	H31.323	H44.119	H59.212	I25.3	I50.42	I70.448	I75.029	I82.521
G95.9	H31.329	H44.121	H59.213	I25.700	I51.0	I70.449	I75.81	I82.522
G96.0	H31.401	H44.122	H59.219	I25.710	I51.81	I70.461	I75.89	I82.523
G96.11	H31.402	H44.123	H59.221	I25.711	I62.9	I70.462	I76	I82.529
G97.0	H31.403	H44.129	H59.222	I25.718	I67.3	I70.463	I77.2	I82.531
G97.2	H31.409	H44.131	H59.223	I25.719	I67.4	I70.468	I77.4	I82.532
G97.31	H31.411	H44.132	H59.229	I25.720	I67.5	I70.469	I77.5	I82.533
G97.32	H31.412	H44.133	H59.311	I25.721	I67.6	I70.531	I80.10	I82.539
G97.41	H31.413	H44.139	H59.312	I25.728	I67.7	I70.532	I80.11	I82.541
G97.48	H31.419	H44.19	H59.313	I25.729	I67.81	I70.533	I80.12	I82.542
G97.49	H31.421	H46.00	H59.319	I25.730	I67.82	I70.534	I80.13	I82.543
G97.51	H31.422	H46.01	H59.321	I25.731	I67.841	I70.538	I80.201	I82.549
G97.52	H31.423	H46.02	H59.322	I25.738	I67.848	I70.539	I80.202	I82.591
G97.81	H31.429	H46.03	H59.323	I25.739	I67.89	I70.541	I80.203	I82.592
G97.82	H33.121	H46.10	H59.329	I25.750	I68.2	I70.542	I80.209	I82.593
G99.0	H33.122	H46.11	H59.811	I25.751	I69.051	I70.543	I80.211	I82.599
G99.2	H33.123	H46.12	H59.812	I25.758	I69.052	I70.544	I80.212	I82.5Y1
H05.011	H33.129	H46.13	H59.813	I25.759	I69.053	I70.548	I80.213	I82.5Y2
H05.012	H33.20	H46.8	H59.819	I25.760	I69.054	I70.549	I80.219	I82.5Y3
H05.013	H33.21	H46.9	H59.88	I25.761	I69.059	I70.561	I80.221	I82.5Y9
H05.019	H33.22	H47.10	H59.89	I25.768	I69.151	I70.562	I80.222	I82.5Z1
H05.021	H33.23	H47.11	H60.20	I25.769	I69.152	I70.563	I80.223	I82.5Z2
H05.022	H33.40	H47.41	H60.21	I25.790	I69.153	I70.568	I80.229	I82.5Z3
H05.023	H33.41	H47.42	H60.22	I25.791	I69.154	I70.569	I80.231	I82.5Z9
H05.029	H33.42	H47.43	H60.23	I25.798	I69.159	I70.631	I80.232	I82.601
H05.031	H33.43	H47.49	H70.001	I25.799	I69.251	I70.632	I80.233	I82.602
H05.032	H33.8	H47.511	H70.002	I25.810	I69.252	I70.633	I80.239	I82.603
H05.033	H34.00	H47.512	H70.003	I25.811	I69.253	I70.634	I80.291	I82.609
H05.039	H34.01	H47.519	H70.009	I25.812	I69.254	I70.638	I80.292	I82.611
H20.00	H34.02	H47.521	H70.011	I27.0	I69.259	I70.639	I80.293	I82.612
H20.011	H34.03	H47.522	H70.012	I27.1	I69.351	I70.641	I80.299	I82.613
H20.012	H34.10	H47.529	H70.013	I27.82	I69.352	I70.642	I82.1	I82.619
H20.013	H34.11	H47.531	H70.019	I28.0	I69.353	I70.643	I82.210	I82.621
H20.019	H34.12	H47.532	H70.091	I28.1	I69.354	I70.644	I82.211	I82.622
H20.021	H34.13	H47.539	H70.092	I30.0	I69.359	I70.648	I82.290	I82.623
H20.022	H34.211	H47.621	H70.093	I30.1	I69.851	I70.649	I82.291	I82.629
H20.023	H34.212	H47.622	H70.099	I30.8	I69.852	I70.661	I82.3	I82.701
H20.029	H34.213	H47.629	H95.21	I30.9	I69.853	I70.662	I82.401	I82.702
H20.031	H34.219	H47.631	H95.22	I31.0	I69.854	I70.663	I82.402	I82.703
H20.032	H34.231	H47.632	H95.31	I31.1	I69.859	I70.668	I82.403	I82.709
H20.033	H34.232	H47.639	H95.32	I31.2	I69.951	I70.669	I82.409	I82.711
H20.039	H34.233	H47.641	H95.41	I31.3	I69.952	I70.731	I82.411	I82.712
H20.9	H34.239	H47.642	H95.42	I31.4	I69.953	I70.732	I82.412	I82.713
H21.331	H34.811	H47.649	H95.811	I31.8	I69.954	I70.733	I82.413	I82.719
H21.332	H34.812	H49.811	H95.812	I31.9	I69.959	I70.734	I82.419	I82.721
H21.333	H34.813	H49.812	H95.813	I32	I70.261	I70.738	I82.421	I82.722
H21.339	H34.819	H49.813	H95.819	I38	I70.262	I70.739	I82.422	I82.723
H30.101	H34.9	H49.819	H95.88	I39	I70.263	I70.741	I82.423	I82.729
H30.102	H35.70	H53.121	H95.89	I42.0	I70.268	I70.742	I82.429	I82.811
H30.103	H35.721	H53.122	I01.0	I42.1	I70.269	I70.743	I82.431	I82.812
H30.109	H35.722	H53.123	I01.1	I42.2	I70.331	I70.744	I82.432	I82.813
H30.111	H35.723	H53.129	I01.2	I42.3	I70.332	I70.748	I82.433	I82.819
H30.112	H35.729	H53.131	I01.8	I42.4	I70.333	I70.749	I82.439	I82.890
H30.113	H35.731	H53.132	I01.9	I42.5	I70.334	I70.761	I82.441	I82.891
H30.119	H35.732	H53.133	I02.0	I42.6	I70.338	I70.762	I82.442	I82.90
H30.121	H35.739	H53.139	I02.9	I42.7	I70.339	I70.763	I82.443	I82.91
H30.122	H35.82	H59.011	I09.0	I42.8	I70.341	I70.768	I82.449	I82.A11
H30.123	H40.211	H59.012	I09.2	I42.9	I70.342	I70.769	I82.491	I82.A12
H30.129	H40.212	H59.013	I09.81	I43	I70.343	I70.92	I82.492	I82.A13
H30.131	H40.213	H59.019	I12.0	I44.2	I70.344	I73.01	I82.493	I82.A19
H30.132	H40.219	H59.031	I13.0	I45.2	I70.348	I74.09	I82.499	I82.A21
H30.133	H44.001	H59.032	I13.11	I45.3	I70.349	I74.10	I82.4Y1	I82.A22
H30.139	H44.002	H59.033	I13.2	I45.89	I70.361	I74.11	I82.4Y2	I82.A23
H30.141	H44.003	H59.039	I20.0	I47.0	I70.362	I74.19	I82.4Y3	I82.A29
H30.142	H44.009	H59.091	I20.1	I47.1	I70.363	I74.2	I82.4Y9	I82.B11
H30.143	H44.011	H59.092	I23.0	I47.2	I70.368	I74.3	I82.4Z1	I82.B12
H30.149	H44.012	H59.093	I23.1	I48.1	I70.369	I74.4	I82.4Z2	I82.B13
H30.891	H44.013	H59.099	I23.2	I48.3	I70.431	I74.5	I82.4Z3	I82.B19
H30.892	H44.019	H59.111	I23.3	I48.4	I70.432	I74.8	I82.4Z9	I82.B21
I30.893	H44.021	H59.112	I23.6	I48.92	I70.433	I74.9	I82.501	I82.B22
H30.899	H44.021	H59.113	I23.7	I49.2	I70.434	I75.011	I82.502	I82.B23

Appendix F: Complication and Comorbidity (CC) Code List

I82.B29	I97.89	J96.10	K51.219	K80.12	K94.23	L05.02	L97.319	M00.111
I82.C11	J05.10	J96.11	K51.30	K80.13	K94.30	L08.1	L97.321	M00.112
I82.C12	J18.2	J96.12	K51.311	K80.18	K94.31	L10.0	L97.322	M00.119
I82.C13	J21.0	J98.11	K51.312	K80.19	K94.32	L10.1	L97.323	M00.121
I82.C19	J21.1	J98.19	K51.313	K80.21	K94.33	L10.2	L97.324	M00.122
I82.C21	J21.8	K04.0	K51.314	K80.30	K94.39	L10.3	L97.329	M00.129
I82.C22	J21.9	K04.4	K51.318	K80.31	K95.01	L10.4	L97.401	M00.131
I82.C23	J36	K11.3	K51.319	K80.32	K95.09	L10.5	L97.402	M00.132
I82.C29	J39.0	K11.4	K51.40	K80.33	K95.81	L10.81	L97.403	M00.139
I83.201	J39.1	K12.2	K51.411	K80.34	K95.89	L10.89	L97.404	M00.141
I83.202	J44.0	K22.10	K51.412	K80.35	L02.01	L10.9	L97.409	M00.142
I83.203	J44.1	K25.3	K51.413	K80.36	L02.211	L12.0	L97.411	M00.149
I83.204	J45.21	K26.3	K51.414	K80.37	L02.212	L12.30	L97.412	M00.151
I83.205	J45.22	K27.3	K51.418	K80.40	L02.213	L12.31	L97.413	M00.152
I83.208	J45.31	K28.3	K51.419	K80.41	L02.214	L12.35	L97.414	M00.159
I83.209	J45.32	K31.0	K51.50	K80.42	L02.215	L12.8	L97.419	M00.161
I83.211	J45.41	K31.1	K51.511	K80.43	L02.216	L12.9	L97.421	M00.162
I83.212	J45.42	K31.5	K51.512	K80.44	L02.219	L49.3	L97.422	M00.169
I83.213	J45.51	K31.6	K51.513	K80.45	L02.31	L49.4	L97.423	M00.171
I83.214	J45.52	K35.80	K51.514	K80.46	L02.411	L49.5	L97.424	M00.172
I83.215	J45.901	K35.89	K51.518	K80.47	L02.412	L49.6	L97.429	M00.179
I83.218	J45.902	K40.00	K51.519	K80.51	L02.413	L49.7	L97.801	M00.18
I83.219	J47.0	K40.01	K51.80	K80.60	L02.414	L49.8	L97.802	M00.19
I83.221	J47.1	K40.30	K51.811	K80.61	L02.415	L49.9	L97.803	M00.20
I83.222	J67.7	K40.31	K51.812	K80.62	L02.416	L51.1	L97.804	M00.211
I83.223	J67.8	K41.00	K51.813	K80.63	L02.419	L51.2	L97.809	M00.212
I83.224	J67.9	K41.01	K51.814	K80.64	L02.511	L51.3	L97.811	M00.219
I83.225	J68.0	K41.30	K51.818	K80.65	L02.512	L53.0	L97.812	M00.221
I83.228	J70.0	K41.31	K51.819	K80.66	L02.519	L53.1	L97.813	M00.222
I83.229	J70.1	K42.0	K51.90	K80.71	L02.611	L53.2	L97.814	M00.229
I85.00	J80	K43.0	K51.911	K80.81	L02.612	L53.3	L97.819	M00.231
I85.10	J81.1	K43.3	K51.912	K81.0	L02.619	L76.01	L97.821	M00.232
I87.011	J82	K43.6	K51.913	K81.2	L02.811	L76.02	L97.822	M00.239
I87.012	J84.01	K44.0	K51.914	K82.0	L02.818	L76.11	L97.823	M00.241
I87.013	J84.02	K45.0	K51.918	K82.1	L02.91	L76.12	L97.824	M00.242
I87.019	J84.03	K46.0	K51.919	K82.3	L03.111	L76.21	L97.829	M00.249
I87.031	J84.09	K50.00	K52.0	K83.0	L03.112	L76.22	L97.901	M00.251
I87.032	J84.114	K50.011	K52.1	K83.3	L03.113	L88	L97.902	M00.252
I87.033	J84.116	K50.012	K55.1	K86.0	L03.114	L97.101	L97.903	M00.259
I87.039	J84.117	K50.013	K55.8	K86.1	L03.115	L97.102	L97.904	M00.261
I87.1	J84.2	K50.014	K55.9	K86.2	L03.116	L97.103	L97.909	M00.262
I87.311	J84.82	K50.018	K56.0	K86.3	L03.119	L97.104	L97.911	M00.269
I87.312	J84.9	K50.019	K56.1	K90.1	L03.121	L97.109	L97.912	M00.271
I87.313	J90	K50.10	K56.3	K90.2	L03.122	L97.111	L97.913	M00.272
I87.319	J91.0	K50.111	K56.49	K90.3	L03.123	L97.112	L97.914	M00.279
I87.331	J91.8	K50.112	K56.5	K90.4	L03.124	L97.113	L97.919	M00.28
I87.332	J93.11	K50.113	K56.60	K90.81	L03.125	L97.114	L97.921	M00.29
I87.333	J93.12	K50.114	K56.69	K90.89	L03.126	L97.119	L97.922	M00.80
I87.339	J93.81	K50.118	K56.7	K90.9	L03.129	L97.121	L97.923	M00.811
I96	J93.82	K50.119	K57.00	K91.2	L03.211	L97.122	L97.924	M00.812
I97.110	J93.83	K50.80	K57.12	K91.3	L03.212	L97.123	L97.929	M00.819
I97.111	J93.9	K50.811	K57.20	K91.61	L03.221	L97.124	L98.3	M00.821
I97.120	J94.0	K50.812	K57.32	K91.62	L03.222	L97.129	M00.00	M00.822
I97.121	J94.2	K50.813	K57.40	K91.71	L03.311	L97.201	M00.011	M00.829
I97.130	J94.8	K50.814	K57.52	K91.72	L03.312	L97.202	M00.012	M00.831
I97.131	J95.00	K50.818	K57.80	K91.81	L03.313	L97.203	M00.019	M00.832
I97.190	J95.01	K50.819	K57.92	K91.82	L03.314	L97.204	M00.021	M00.839
I97.191	J95.02	K50.90	K59.2	K91.83	L03.315	L97.209	M00.022	M00.841
I97.410	J95.03	K50.911	K59.3	K91.840	L03.316	L97.211	M00.029	M00.842
I97.411	J95.04	K50.912	K61.0	K91.841	L03.317	L97.212	M00.031	M00.849
I97.418	J95.09	K50.913	K61.1	K91.850	L03.319	L97.213	M00.032	M00.851
I97.42	J95.4	K50.914	K61.2	K91.858	L03.321	L97.214	M00.039	M00.852
I97.51	J95.5	K50.918	K61.3	K91.86	L03.322	L97.219	M00.041	M00.859
I97.52	J95.61	K50.919	K61.4	K91.89	L03.323	L97.221	M00.042	M00.861
I97.610	J95.62	K51.00	K62.5	K92.0	L03.324	L97.222	M00.049	M00.862
I97.611	J95.71	K51.011	K62.6	K92.1	L03.325	L97.223	M00.051	M00.869
I97.618	J95.72	K51.012	K63.0	K92.2	L03.326	L97.224	M00.052	M00.871
I97.62	J95.811	K51.013	K63.2	K92.81	L03.327	L97.229	M00.059	M00.872
I97.710	J95.812	K51.014	K63.3	K94.01	L03.329	L97.301	M00.061	M00.879
I97.711	J95.830	K51.018	K65.4	K94.02	L03.811	L97.302	M00.062	M00.88
I97.790	J95.831	K51.019	K68.11	K94.03	L03.818	L97.303	M00.069	M00.89
I97.791	J95.84	K51.20	K76.6	K94.09	L03.891	L97.304	M00.071	M00.9
I97.810	J95.850	K51.211	K77	K94.11	L03.898	L97.309	M00.072	M01.X0
I97.811	J95.851	K51.212	K80.00	K94.12	L03.90	L97.311	M00.079	M01.X11
I97.820	J95.859	K51.213	K80.01	K94.13	L03.91	L97.312	M00.08	M01.X12
I97.821	J95.88	K51.214	K80.10	K94.19	L05.01	L97.313	M00.09	M01.X19
I97.88	J95.89	K51.218	K80.11	K94.22		L97.314	M00.10	M01.X21

MØ1.X22	MØ2.841	M32.12	M48.57XA	M8Ø.Ø29P	M8Ø.839K	M84.35ØK	M84.441K	M84.5ØXA
MØ1.X29	MØ2.842	M33.ØØ	M48.58XA	M8Ø.Ø31A	M8Ø.839P	M84.35ØP	M84.441P	M84.5ØXK
MØ1.X31	MØ2.849	M33.Ø1	M5Ø.ØØ	M8Ø.Ø31K	M8Ø.841A	M84.351K	M84.442A	M84.5ØXP
MØ1.X32	MØ2.851	M33.Ø2	M5Ø.Ø1	M8Ø.Ø31P	M8Ø.841K	M84.351P	M84.442K	M84.511A
MØ1.X39	MØ2.852	M33.Ø9	M5Ø.Ø2	M8Ø.Ø32A	M8Ø.841P	M84.352K	M84.442P	M84.511K
MØ1.X41	MØ2.859	M33.1Ø	M5Ø.Ø3	M8Ø.Ø32K	M8Ø.842A	M84.352P	M84.443A	M84.511P
MØ1.X42	MØ2.861	M33.11	M51.Ø4	M8Ø.Ø32P	M8Ø.842K	M84.353K	M84.443K	M84.512A
MØ1.X49	MØ2.862	M33.12	M51.Ø5	M8Ø.Ø39A	M8Ø.842P	M84.353P	M84.443P	M84.512K
MØ1.X51	MØ2.869	M33.19	M51.Ø6	M8Ø.Ø39K	M8Ø.849A	M84.359K	M84.444A	M84.512P
MØ1.X52	MØ2.871	M33.2Ø	M6Ø.ØØØ	M8Ø.Ø39P	M8Ø.849K	M84.359P	M84.444K	M84.519A
MØ1.X59	MØ2.872	M33.21	M6Ø.ØØ1	M8Ø.Ø41A	M8Ø.849P	M84.361K	M84.444P	M84.519K
MØ1.X61	MØ2.879	M33.22	M6Ø.ØØ2	M8Ø.Ø41K	M8Ø.851A	M84.361P	M84.445A	M84.519P
MØ1.X62	MØ2.88	M33.29	M6Ø.ØØ3	M8Ø.Ø41P	M8Ø.851K	M84.362K	M84.445K	M84.521A
MØ1.X69	MØ2.89	M33.9Ø	M6Ø.ØØ4	M8Ø.Ø42A	M8Ø.851P	M84.362P	M84.445P	M84.521K
MØ1.X71	MØ5.4Ø	M33.91	M6Ø.ØØ5	M8Ø.Ø42K	M8Ø.852A	M84.363K	M84.446A	M84.521P
MØ1.X72	MØ5.411	M33.92	M6Ø.ØØ9	M8Ø.Ø42P	M8Ø.852K	M84.363P	M84.446K	M84.522A
MØ1.X79	MØ5.412	M33.99	M6Ø.Ø11	M8Ø.Ø49A	M8Ø.852P	M84.364K	M84.446P	M84.522K
MØ1.X8	MØ5.419	M34.81	M6Ø.Ø12	M8Ø.Ø49K	M8Ø.859A	M84.364P	M84.451A	M84.522P
MØ1.X9	MØ5.421	M34.82	M6Ø.Ø19	M8Ø.Ø49P	M8Ø.859K	M84.369K	M84.451K	M84.529A
MØ2.1Ø	MØ5.422	M35.Ø3	M6Ø.Ø21	M8Ø.Ø51A	M8Ø.859P	M84.369P	M84.451P	M84.529K
MØ2.111	MØ5.429	M35.1	M6Ø.Ø22	M8Ø.Ø51K	M8Ø.861A	M84.371K	M84.452A	M84.529P
MØ2.112	MØ5.431	M35.2	M6Ø.Ø29	M8Ø.Ø51P	M8Ø.861K	M84.371P	M84.452K	M84.531A
MØ2.119	MØ5.432	M35.5	M6Ø.Ø31	M8Ø.Ø52A	M8Ø.861P	M84.372K	M84.452P	M84.531K
MØ2.121	MØ5.439	M35.8	M6Ø.Ø32	M8Ø.Ø52K	M8Ø.862A	M84.372P	M84.453A	M84.531P
MØ2.122	MØ5.441	M36.Ø	M6Ø.Ø39	M8Ø.Ø52P	M8Ø.862K	M84.373K	M84.453K	M84.532A
MØ2.129	MØ5.442	M46.2Ø	M6Ø.Ø41	M8Ø.Ø59A	M8Ø.862P	M84.373P	M84.453P	M84.532K
MØ2.131	MØ5.449	M46.21	M6Ø.Ø42	M8Ø.Ø59K	M8Ø.869A	M84.374K	M84.454A	M84.532P
MØ2.132	MØ5.451	M46.22	M6Ø.Ø43	M8Ø.Ø59P	M8Ø.869K	M84.374P	M84.454K	M84.533A
MØ2.139	MØ5.452	M46.23	M6Ø.Ø44	M8Ø.Ø61A	M8Ø.869P	M84.375K	M84.454P	M84.533K
MØ2.141	MØ5.459	M46.24	M6Ø.Ø45	M8Ø.Ø61K	M8Ø.871A	M84.375P	M84.459A	M84.533P
MØ2.142	MØ5.461	M46.25	M6Ø.Ø46	M8Ø.Ø61P	M8Ø.871K	M84.376K	M84.459K	M84.534A
MØ2.149	MØ5.462	M46.26	M6Ø.Ø51	M8Ø.Ø62A	M8Ø.871P	M84.376P	M84.459P	M84.534K
MØ2.151	MØ5.469	M46.27	M6Ø.Ø52	M8Ø.Ø62K	M8Ø.872A	M84.377K	M84.461A	M84.539A
MØ2.152	MØ5.471	M46.28	M6Ø.Ø59	M8Ø.Ø62P	M8Ø.872K	M84.377P	M84.461K	M84.539K
MØ2.159	MØ5.472	M46.3Ø	M6Ø.Ø61	M8Ø.Ø69A	M8Ø.872P	M84.378K	M84.461P	M84.539P
MØ2.161	MØ5.479	M46.31	M6Ø.Ø62	M8Ø.Ø69K	M8Ø.879A	M84.378P	M84.462A	M84.541A
MØ2.162	MØ5.49	M46.32	M6Ø.Ø69	M8Ø.Ø69P	M8Ø.879K	M84.379K	M84.462K	M84.541K
MØ2.169	M25.ØØ	M46.33	M6Ø.Ø7Ø	M8Ø.Ø71A	M8Ø.879P	M84.379P	M84.462P	M84.541P
MØ2.171	M25.Ø11	M46.34	M6Ø.Ø71	M8Ø.Ø71K	M8Ø.88XA	M84.38XK	M84.463A	M84.542A
MØ2.172	M25.Ø12	M46.35	M6Ø.Ø72	M8Ø.Ø71P	M8Ø.88XK	M84.38XP	M84.463K	M84.542K
MØ2.179	M25.Ø19	M46.36	M6Ø.Ø73	M8Ø.Ø72A	M8Ø.88XP	M84.4ØXA	M84.463P	M84.542P
MØ2.18	M25.Ø21	M46.37	M6Ø.Ø74	M8Ø.Ø72K	M84.3ØXK	M84.4ØXK	M84.464A	M84.549A
MØ2.19	M25.Ø22	M46.38	M6Ø.Ø75	M8Ø.Ø72P	M84.3ØXP	M84.4ØXP	M84.464K	M84.549K
MØ2.3Ø	M25.Ø29	M46.39	M6Ø.Ø76	M8Ø.Ø79A	M84.311K	M84.411A	M84.464P	M84.549P
MØ2.311	M25.Ø31	M47.Ø11	M6Ø.Ø77	M8Ø.Ø79K	M84.311P	M84.411K	M84.469A	M84.55ØA
MØ2.312	M25.Ø32	M47.Ø12	M6Ø.Ø78	M8Ø.Ø79P	M84.312K	M84.411P	M84.469K	M84.55ØK
MØ2.319	M25.Ø39	M47.Ø13	M6Ø.Ø8	M8Ø.Ø8XA	M84.312P	M84.412A	M84.469P	M84.55ØP
MØ2.321	M25.Ø41	M47.Ø14	M6Ø.Ø9	M8Ø.Ø8XK	M84.319K	M84.412K	M84.471A	M84.551A
MØ2.322	M25.Ø42	M47.Ø15	M62.82	M8Ø.Ø8XP	M84.319P	M84.412P	M84.471K	M84.551K
MØ2.329	M25.Ø49	M47.Ø16	M79.A11	M8Ø.8ØXA	M84.321K	M84.419A	M84.471P	M84.551P
MØ2.331	M25.Ø51	M47.Ø19	M79.A12	M8Ø.8ØXK	M84.321P	M84.419K	M84.472A	M84.552A
MØ2.332	M25.Ø52	M47.Ø21	M79.A19	M8Ø.8ØXP	M84.322K	M84.419P	M84.472K	M84.552K
MØ2.339	M25.Ø59	M47.Ø22	M79.A21	M8Ø.811A	M84.322P	M84.421A	M84.472P	M84.553A
MØ2.341	M25.Ø61	M47.Ø29	M79.A22	M8Ø.811K	M84.329K	M84.421K	M84.473A	M84.553K
MØ2.342	M25.Ø62	M47.1Ø	M79.A29	M8Ø.811P	M84.329P	M84.421P	M84.473K	M84.553P
MØ2.349	M25.Ø69	M47.11	M79.A3	M8Ø.812A	M84.331K	M84.422A	M84.473P	M84.559A
MØ2.351	M25.Ø71	M47.12	M79.A9	M8Ø.812K	M84.331P	M84.422K	M84.474A	M84.559K
MØ2.352	M25.Ø72	M47.13	M8Ø.ØØXA	M8Ø.812P	M84.332K	M84.422P	M84.474K	M84.559P
MØ2.359	M25.Ø73	M47.14	M8Ø.ØØXK	M8Ø.819A	M84.332P	M84.429A	M84.474P	M84.561A
MØ2.361	M25.Ø74	M47.15	M8Ø.ØØXP	M8Ø.819K	M84.333K	M84.429K	M84.475A	M84.561K
MØ2.362	M25.Ø75	M47.16	M8Ø.Ø11A	M8Ø.819P	M84.333P	M84.429P	M84.475K	M84.561P
MØ2.369	M25.Ø76	M48.3Ø	M8Ø.Ø11K	M8Ø.821A	M84.334K	M84.431A	M84.475P	M84.562A
MØ2.371	M25.Ø8	M48.31	M8Ø.Ø11P	M8Ø.821K	M84.334P	M84.431K	M84.476A	M84.562K
MØ2.372	M3Ø.Ø	M48.32	M8Ø.Ø12A	M8Ø.821P	M84.339K	M84.431P	M84.476K	M84.562P
MØ2.379	M3Ø.1	M48.33	M8Ø.Ø12K	M8Ø.822A	M84.339P	M84.432A	M84.476P	M84.563A
MØ2.38	M3Ø.2	M48.34	M8Ø.Ø12P	M8Ø.822K	M84.341K	M84.432K	M84.477A	M84.563K
MØ2.39	M3Ø.3	M48.35	M8Ø.Ø19A	M8Ø.822P	M84.341P	M84.432P	M84.477K	M84.563P
MØ2.8Ø	M3Ø.8	M48.36	M8Ø.Ø19K	M8Ø.829A	M84.342K	M84.433A	M84.477P	M84.564A
MØ2.811	M31.Ø	M48.37	M8Ø.Ø19P	M8Ø.829K	M84.342P	M84.433K	M84.478A	M84.564K
MØ2.812	M31.2	M48.38	M8Ø.Ø21A	M8Ø.829P	M84.343K	M84.433P	M84.478K	M84.564P
MØ2.819	M31.3Ø	M48.5ØXA	M8Ø.Ø21K	M8Ø.831A	M84.343P	M84.434A	M84.478P	M84.569A
MØ2.821	M31.31	M48.51XA	M8Ø.Ø21P	M8Ø.831K	M84.344K	M84.434K	M84.479A	M84.569K
MØ2.822	M31.4	M48.52XA	M8Ø.Ø22A	M8Ø.831P	M84.344P	M84.434P	M84.479K	M84.569P
MØ2.829	M31.7	M48.53XA	M8Ø.Ø22K	M8Ø.832A	M84.345K	M84.439A	M84.479P	M84.571A
MØ2.831	M31.8	M48.54XA	M8Ø.Ø22P	M8Ø.832K	M84.345P	M84.439K	M84.48XA	M84.571K
MØ2.832	M31.9	M48.55XA	M8Ø.Ø29A	M8Ø.832P	M84.346K	M84.441	M84.48XK	
MØ2.839	M32.11	M48.56XA	M8Ø.Ø29K	M8Ø.839A	M84.346P	M84.441A	M84.48XP	

Appendix F: Complication and Comorbidity (CC) Code List

M84.571P	M84.659K	M86.159	M86.472	M87.038	M87.221	M87.377	M96.631	N18.4
M84.572A	M84.659P	M86.161	M86.479	M87.039	M87.222	M87.378	M96.632	N18.5
M84.572K	M84.661A	M86.162	M86.48	M87.041	M87.229	M87.379	M96.639	N20.1
M84.572P	M84.661K	M86.169	M86.49	M87.042	M87.231	M87.38	M96.65	N20.2
M84.573A	M84.661P	M86.171	M86.50	M87.043	M87.232	M87.39	M96.661	N25.1
M84.573K	M84.662A	M86.172	M86.511	M87.044	M87.233	M87.80	M96.662	N25.81
M84.573P	M84.662K	M86.179	M86.512	M87.045	M87.234	M87.811	M96.669	N28.0
M84.574A	M84.662P	M86.18	M86.519	M87.046	M87.235	M87.812	M96.671	N28.84
M84.574K	M84.663A	M86.19	M86.521	M87.050	M87.236	M87.819	M96.672	N28.85
M84.574P	M84.663K	M86.20	M86.522	M87.051	M87.237	M87.821	M96.679	N28.86
M84.575A	M84.663P	M86.211	M86.529	M87.052	M87.238	M87.822	M96.69	N30.00
M84.575K	M84.664A	M86.212	M86.531	M87.059	M87.239	M87.829	M96.810	N30.01
M84.575P	M84.664K	M86.219	M86.532	M87.061	M87.241	M87.831	M96.811	N30.40
M84.576A	M84.664P	M86.221	M86.539	M87.062	M87.242	M87.832	M96.820	N30.41
M84.576K	M84.669A	M86.222	M86.541	M87.063	M87.243	M87.833	M96.821	N32.1
M84.576P	M84.669K	M86.229	M86.542	M87.064	M87.244	M87.834	M96.830	N32.2
M84.58XA	M84.669P	M86.231	M86.549	M87.065	M87.245	M87.835	M96.831	N34.0
M84.58XK	M84.671A	M86.232	M86.551	M87.066	M87.246	M87.836	M96.89	N36.0
M84.58XP	M84.671K	M86.239	M86.552	M87.071	M87.250	M87.837	M99.10	N39.0
M84.60XA	M84.671P	M86.241	M86.559	M87.072	M87.251	M87.838	M99.11	N41.0
M84.60XK	M84.672A	M86.242	M86.561	M87.073	M87.252	M87.839	M99.18	N41.2
M84.60XP	M84.672K	M86.249	M86.562	M87.074	M87.256	M87.841	N02.0	N43.1
M84.611A	M84.672P	M86.251	M86.569	M87.075	M87.261	M87.842	N02.1	N44.00
M84.611K	M84.673A	M86.252	M86.571	M87.076	M87.262	M87.843	N02.2	N44.01
M84.611P	M84.673K	M86.259	M86.572	M87.077	M87.263	M87.844	N02.3	N44.02
M84.612A	M84.673P	M86.261	M86.579	M87.078	M87.264	M87.845	N02.4	N44.03
M84.612K	M84.674A	M86.262	M86.58	M87.079	M87.265	M87.849	N02.5	N44.04
M84.612P	M84.674K	M86.269	M86.59	M87.08	M87.266	M87.850	N02.6	N45.4
M84.619A	M84.674P	M86.271	M86.60	M87.09	M87.271	M87.851	N02.7	N48.30
M84.619K	M84.675A	M86.272	M86.611	M87.10	M87.272	M87.852	N02.8	N48.31
M84.619P	M84.675K	M86.279	M86.612	M87.111	M87.273	M87.859	N02.9	N48.32
M84.621A	M84.675P	M86.28	M86.619	M87.112	M87.274	M87.861	N03.0	N48.33
M84.621K	M84.676A	M86.29	M86.621	M87.119	M87.275	M87.862	N03.1	N48.39
M84.621P	M84.676K	M86.30	M86.622	M87.121	M87.276	M87.863	N03.2	N70.01
M84.622A	M84.676P	M86.311	M86.629	M87.122	M87.277	M87.864	N03.3	N70.02
M84.622K	M84.68XA	M86.312	M86.631	M87.129	M87.278	M87.865	N03.4	N70.03
M84.622P	M84.68XK	M86.319	M86.632	M87.131	M87.279	M87.869	N03.5	N71.0
M84.629A	M84.68XP	M86.321	M86.639	M87.132	M87.28	M87.871	N03.6	N73.0
M84.629K	M86.00	M86.322	M86.641	M87.133	M87.29	M87.872	N03.7	N73.4
M84.629P	M86.011	M86.329	M86.642	M87.134	M87.30	M87.873	N03.8	N75.1
M84.631A	M86.012	M86.331	M86.649	M87.135	M87.311	M87.874	N03.9	N76.4
M84.631K	M86.019	M86.332	M86.651	M87.136	M87.312	M87.875	N04.0	N76.81
M84.631P	M86.021	M86.339	M86.652	M87.137	M87.319	M87.876	N04.1	N82.0
M84.632A	M86.022	M86.341	M86.659	M87.138	M87.321	M87.877	N04.2	N82.1
M84.632K	M86.029	M86.342	M86.661	M87.139	M87.322	M87.878	N04.3	N82.2
M84.632P	M86.031	M86.349	M86.662	M87.141	M87.329	M87.879	N04.4	N82.3
M84.633A	M86.032	M86.351	M86.669	M87.142	M87.331	M87.88	N04.5	N82.4
M84.633K	M86.039	M86.352	M86.671	M87.143	M87.332	M87.89	N04.6	N82.5
M84.633P	M86.041	M86.359	M86.672	M87.144	M87.333	M87.9	N04.7	N82.8
M84.634A	M86.042	M86.361	M86.679	M87.145	M87.334	M90.50	N04.8	N82.9
M84.634K	M86.049	M86.362	M86.68	M87.146	M87.335	M90.511	N04.9	N83.51
M84.634P	M86.051	M86.369	M86.69	M87.150	M87.336	M90.512	N05.2	N83.52
M84.639A	M86.052	M86.371	M86.8X0	M87.151	M87.337	M90.519	N05.3	N83.53
M84.639K	M86.059	M86.372	M86.8X1	M87.152	M87.338	M90.521	N05.4	N98.0
M84.639P	M86.061	M86.379	M86.8X2	M87.159	M87.339	M90.522	N05.5	N98.1
M84.641A	M86.062	M86.38	M86.8X3	M87.161	M87.341	M90.529	N06.2	N98.2
M84.641K	M86.069	M86.39	M86.8X4	M87.162	M87.342	M90.531	N06.3	N98.3
M84.641P	M86.071	M86.40	M86.8X5	M87.163	M87.343	M90.532	N06.4	N98.8
M84.642A	M86.072	M86.411	M86.8X6	M87.164	M87.344	M90.539	N06.5	N98.9
M84.642K	M86.079	M86.412	M86.8X7	M87.165	M87.345	M90.541	N07.2	N99.510
M84.642P	M86.08	M86.419	M86.8X8	M87.166	M87.346	M90.542	N07.3	N99.511
M84.649A	M86.09	M86.421	M86.8X9	M87.171	M87.350	M90.549	N07.4	N99.512
M84.649K	M86.10	M86.422	M86.9	M87.172	M87.351	M90.551	N07.5	N99.518
M84.649P	M86.111	M86.429	M87.00	M87.173	M87.352	M90.552	N10	N99.61
M84.650A	M86.112	M86.431	M87.011	M87.174	M87.353	M90.559	N11.1	N99.62
M84.650K	M86.119	M86.432	M87.012	M87.175	M87.361	M90.561	N11.8	N99.71
M84.650P	M86.121	M86.439	M87.019	M87.176	M87.362	M90.562	N11.9	N99.72
M84.651A	M86.122	M86.441	M87.021	M87.177	M87.363	M90.569	N12	N99.820
M84.651K	M86.129	M86.442	M87.022	M87.178	M87.364	M90.571	N13.1	N99.821
M84.651P	M86.131	M86.449	M87.029	M87.179	M87.365	M90.572	N13.2	O00.0
M84.652A	M86.132	M86.451	M87.031	M87.180	M87.366	M90.579	N13.30	O00.1
M84.652K	M86.139	M86.452	M87.032	M87.188	M87.371	M90.58	N13.39	O00.2
M84.652P	M86.141	M86.459	M87.033	M87.19	M87.372	M90.59	N13.4	O00.8
M84.653A	M86.142	M86.461	M87.034	M87.20	M87.373	M96.0	N13.6	O00.9
M84.653K	M86.149	M86.462	M87.035	M87.211	M87.374	M96.621	N13.8	O03.0
M84.653P	M86.151	M86.469	M87.036	M87.212	M87.375	M96.622	N17.8	O03.30
M84.659A	M86.152	M86.471	M87.037	M87.219	M87.376	M96.629	N17.9	O03.33

O03.34	O22.40	O30.103	O36.0910	O71.5	O99.321	Q04.8	Q43.7	Q87.5
O03.35	O22.41	O30.111	O36.0911	O71.6	O99.322	Q05.0	Q43.8	Q87.81
O03.36	O22.42	O30.112	O36.0912	O71.7	O99.323	Q05.1	Q43.9	Q87.89
O03.37	O22.43	O30.113	O36.0913	O72.0	O99.324	Q05.2	Q44.0	Q89.01
O03.38	O22.50	O30.121	O36.0914	O72.1	O99.325	Q05.3	Q44.1	Q89.09
O03.39	O22.51	O30.122	O36.0915	O72.2	O99.354	Q05.4	Q44.4	Q89.3
O03.5	O22.52	O30.123	O36.0919	O75.2	O99.355	Q07.02	Q44.5	Q89.7
O03.7	O22.53	O30.191	O36.0920	O86.11	O99.411	Q07.03	Q44.6	Q89.8
O03.80	O22.8X1	O30.192	O36.0921	O86.12	O99.412	Q20.5	Q44.7	Q91.0
O03.83	O22.8X2	O30.193	O36.0922	O86.13	O99.413	Q21.0	Q45.0	Q91.1
O03.84	O22.8X3	O30.201	O36.0923	O86.19	O99.43	Q21.1	Q45.1	Q91.2
O03.85	O22.8X9	O30.202	O36.0924	O86.20	O99.830	Q21.2	Q45.2	Q91.3
O03.86	O22.90	O30.203	O36.0925	O86.21	O99.834	Q22.1	Q45.3	Q91.4
O03.87	O23.01	O30.211	O36.0929	O86.22	O99.835	Q22.2	Q60.0	Q91.5
O03.88	O23.02	O30.212	O36.0930	O86.29	P10.2	Q22.3	Q60.1	Q91.6
O03.89	O23.03	O30.213	O36.0931	O86.4	P12.2	Q23.0	Q60.2	Q91.7
O04.5	O23.11	O30.221	O36.0932	O87.0	P28.0	Q23.1	Q60.3	Q93.3
O04.80	O23.12	O30.222	O36.0933	O87.2	P28.10	Q23.2	Q60.4	Q93.4
O04.83	O23.13	O30.223	O36.0934	O87.3	P28.11	Q23.3	Q60.5	Q93.5
O04.84	O23.21	O30.291	O36.0935	O87.8	P28.19	Q24.0	Q60.6	Q93.7
O04.85	O23.22	O30.292	O36.0939	O88.319	P28.2	Q24.1	Q61.00	Q93.88
O04.86	O23.23	O30.293	O36.4XX0	O98.011	P28.3	Q24.3	Q61.01	Q93.89
O04.87	O23.31	O30.801	O36.4XX1	O98.012	P28.4	Q24.5	Q61.02	Q93.9
O04.88	O23.32	O30.802	O36.4XX2	O98.013	P35.0	Q25.0	Q61.11	R04.2
O04.89	O23.33	O30.803	O36.4XX3	O98.02	P38.1	Q25.1	Q61.19	R04.81
O07.0	O23.41	O30.811	O36.4XX4	O98.03	P38.9	Q25.2	Q61.2	R04.89
O07.1	O23.42	O30.812	O36.4XX5	O98.111	P39.0	Q25.3	Q61.3	R04.9
O07.30	O23.43	O30.813	O36.4XX9	O98.112	P39.2	Q25.4	Q61.4	R06.3
O07.33	O23.511	O30.821	O41.01X0	O98.113	P39.3	Q25.8	Q61.5	R09.01
O07.34	O23.512	O30.822	O41.01X1	O98.12	P39.4	Q25.9	Q61.8	R17
O07.35	O23.513	O30.823	O41.01X2	O98.13	P39.8	Q26.0	Q61.9	R18.0
O07.36	O23.521	O30.891	O41.01X3	O98.211	P39.9	Q26.1	Q62.0	R18.8
O07.37	O23.522	O30.892	O41.01X4	O98.212	P52.0	Q26.2	Q62.10	R29.0
O07.38	O23.523	O30.893	O41.01X5	O98.213	P52.1	Q26.3	Q62.11	R29.1
O07.39	O23.591	O31.8X10	O41.01X9	O98.22	P52.3	Q26.4	Q62.12	R29.5
O08.0	O23.592	O31.8X11	O41.02X0	O98.23	P53	Q26.8	Q62.2	R39.0
O08.1	O23.593	O31.8X12	O41.02X1	O98.311	P54.4	Q26.9	Q62.31	R40.3
O08.5	O23.91	O31.8X13	O41.02X2	O98.312	P61.2	Q27.30	Q62.32	R41.4
O08.6	O23.92	O31.8X14	O41.02X3	O98.313	P61.3	Q27.4	Q62.39	R44.0
O08.7	O23.93	O31.8X15	O41.02X4	O98.32	P61.4	Q28.0	Q64.10	R44.2
O08.81	O24.011	O31.8X19	O41.02X5	O98.33	P61.6	Q28.1	Q64.11	R44.3
O08.82	O24.012	O31.8X20	O41.02X9	O98.411	P70.2	Q28.8	Q64.12	R45.851
O08.83	O24.013	O31.8X21	O41.03X0	O98.412	P70.8	Q28.9	Q64.19	R47.01
O08.89	O24.019	O31.8X22	O41.03X1	O98.413	P71.0	Q31.1	Q64.2	R56.00
O08.9	O24.03	O31.8X23	O41.03X2	O98.42	P71.1	Q31.2	Q64.31	R56.01
O10.011	O24.111	O31.8X24	O41.03X3	O98.43	P71.2	Q31.3	Q64.32	R56.1
O10.012	O24.112	O31.8X25	O41.03X4	O98.511	P71.3	Q31.5	Q64.33	R57.9
O10.013	O24.113	O31.8X29	O41.03X5	O98.512	P71.4	Q31.8	Q64.39	R64
O10.02	O24.119	O31.8X30	O41.03X9	O98.513	P71.8	Q31.9	Q67.5	R65.10
O10.411	O24.13	O31.8X31	O44.01	O98.52	P71.9	Q32.0	Q67.8	R71.0
O10.412	O24.311	O31.8X32	O44.02	O98.53	P72.0	Q32.1	Q68.1	R78.81
O10.413	O24.312	O31.8X33	O44.03	O98.611	P72.1	Q32.2	Q74.3	R82.0
O10.43	O24.313	O31.8X34	O47.02	O98.612	P72.2	Q32.3	Q76.3	R82.1
O10.911	O24.319	O31.8X35	O47.03	O98.613	P72.8	Q32.4	Q76.425	S01.101A
O10.912	O24.33	O31.8X39	O47.1	O98.62	P74.5	Q33.0	Q76.426	S01.102A
O10.913	O24.811	O33.0	O60.10X0	O98.63	P74.6	Q33.4	Q76.427	S01.109A
O10.92	O24.812	O36.0110	O60.10X1	O98.711	P74.8	Q39.5	Q76.428	S02.0XXA
O12.11	O24.813	O36.0111	O60.10X2	O98.712	P76.1	Q39.6	Q76.429	S02.0XXK
O12.12	O24.819	O36.0112	O60.10X3	O98.713	P83.0	Q39.8	Q76.6	S02.10XA
O12.13	O24.83	O36.0113	O60.10X4	O98.72	P83.30	Q39.9	Q76.7	S02.10XK
O12.21	O24.911	O36.0114	O60.10X5	O98.73	P83.39	Q41.0	Q76.8	S02.110A
O12.22	O24.912	O36.0115	O60.10X9	O98.811	P91.60	Q41.1	Q76.9	S02.110K
O12.23	O24.913	O36.0119	O60.20X0	O98.812	P91.61	Q41.2	Q77.2	S02.111A
O14.02	O24.919	O36.0120	O60.20X1	O98.813	P91.62	Q41.8	Q78.0	S02.111K
O14.03	O24.93	O36.0121	O60.20X2	O98.82	P93.0	Q41.9	Q78.2	S02.112A
O14.92	O26.611	O36.0122	O60.20X3	O98.83	P93.8	Q42.0	Q79.6	S02.112K
O14.93	O26.612	O36.0123	O60.20X4	O98.911	P94.0	Q42.1	Q85.1	S02.113A
O16.1	O26.613	O36.0124	O60.20X5	O98.912	P96.1	Q42.2	Q85.8	S02.113K
O16.2	O26.62	O36.0125	O60.20X9	O98.913	P96.2	Q42.3	Q85.9	S02.118A
O16.3	O26.831	O36.0129	O63.9	O98.92	Q01.0	Q42.8	Q87.1	S02.118K
O20.0	O26.832	O36.0130	O68	O98.93	Q01.1	Q42.9	Q87.2	S02.119A
O20.9	O26.833	O36.0131	O70.2	O99.111	Q01.2	Q43.1	Q87.3	S02.119K
O22.20	O26.872	O36.0132	O70.3	O99.112	Q01.8	Q43.2	Q87.40	S02.19XA
O22.21	O26.873	O36.0133	O70.4	O99.113	Q01.9	Q43.3	Q87.410	S02.19XK
O22.22	O26.879	O36.0134	O71.2	O99.119	Q04.4	Q43.4	Q87.418	S02.2XXB
O22.23	O30.101	O36.0135	O71.3	O99.12	Q04.5	Q43.5	Q87.42	S02.2XXK
O22.30	O30.102	O36.0139	O71.4	O99.13	Q04.6	Q43.6	Q87.43	S02.3XXA

Appendix F: Complication and Comorbidity (CC) Code List

S02.3XXB	S04.22XA	S06.813A	S12.110K	S12.500A	S15.122A	S22.019K	S22.23XA	S27.893A
S02.3XXK	S04.30XA	S06.814A	S12.111A	S12.500K	S15.129A	S22.020A	S22.23XK	S27.898A
S02.400A	S04.31XA	S06.815A	S12.111K	S12.501A	S15.191A	S22.020K	S22.24XA	S27.899A
S02.400B	S04.32XA	S06.819A	S12.112A	S12.501K	S15.192A	S22.021A	S22.24XK	S27.9XXA
S02.400K	S04.40XA	S06.821A	S12.112K	S12.530A	S15.199A	S22.021K	S22.31XA	S28.1XXA
S02.401A	S04.41XA	S06.822A	S12.120A	S12.530K	S15.201A	S22.022A	S22.31XK	S29.021A
S02.401B	S04.42XA	S06.823A	S12.120K	S12.531A	S15.202A	S22.022K	S22.32XA	S29.029A
S02.401K	S04.50XA	S06.824A	S12.121A	S12.531K	S15.209A	S22.028A	S22.32XK	S32.000A
S02.402A	S04.51XA	S06.825A	S12.121K	S12.54XA	S15.211A	S22.028K	S22.39XA	S32.000K
S02.402B	S04.52XA	S06.829A	S12.130A	S12.54XK	S15.212A	S22.029A	S22.39XK	S32.001A
S02.402K	S04.60XA	S06.891A	S12.130K	S12.550A	S15.219A	S22.029K	S22.41XA	S32.001K
S02.411A	S04.61XA	S06.892A	S12.131A	S12.550K	S15.221A	S22.030A	S22.41XK	S32.002A
S02.411B	S04.62XA	S06.893A	S12.131K	S12.551A	S15.222A	S22.030K	S22.42XA	S32.002K
S02.411K	S04.70XA	S06.894A	S12.14XA	S12.551K	S15.229A	S22.031A	S22.42XK	S32.008A
S02.412A	S04.71XA	S06.895A	S12.14XK	S12.590A	S15.291A	S22.031K	S22.43XA	S32.008K
S02.412B	S04.72XA	S06.899A	S12.150A	S12.590K	S15.292A	S22.032A	S22.43XK	S32.009A
S02.412K	S04.811A	S06.9X1A	S12.150K	S12.591A	S15.299A	S22.032K	S22.49XA	S32.009K
S02.413A	S04.812A	S06.9X2A	S12.151A	S12.591K	S15.301A	S22.038A	S22.49XK	S32.010A
S02.413B	S04.819A	S06.9X3A	S12.151K	S12.600A	S15.302A	S22.038K	S22.5XXA	S32.010K
S02.413K	S04.891A	S06.9X4A	S12.190A	S12.600K	S15.309A	S22.039A	S22.9XXA	S32.011A
S02.42XA	S04.892A	S06.9X5A	S12.190K	S12.601A	S15.311A	S22.039K	S22.9XXK	S32.011K
S02.42XB	S04.899A	S06.9X9A	S12.191A	S12.601K	S15.312A	S22.040A	S25.501A	S32.012A
S02.42XK	S04.9XXA	S07.0XXA	S12.191K	S12.630A	S15.319A	S22.040K	S25.502A	S32.012K
S02.5XXK	S05.20XA	S07.1XXA	S12.200A	S12.630K	S15.321A	S22.041A	S25.509A	S32.018A
S02.600A	S05.21XA	S07.8XXA	S12.200K	S12.631A	S15.322A	S22.041K	S25.511A	S32.018K
S02.600B	S05.22XA	S07.9XXA	S12.201A	S12.631K	S15.329A	S22.042A	S25.512A	S32.019A
S02.600K	S05.30XA	S09.0XXA	S12.201K	S12.64XA	S15.391A	S22.042K	S25.519A	S32.019K
S02.609A	S05.31XA	S09.20XA	S12.230A	S12.64XK	S15.392A	S22.048A	S25.591A	S32.020A
S02.609B	S05.32XA	S09.21XA	S12.230K	S12.650A	S15.399A	S22.048K	S25.592A	S32.020K
S02.609K	S05.40XA	S09.22XA	S12.231A	S12.650K	S15.8XXA	S22.049A	S25.599A	S32.021A
S02.61XA	S05.41XA	S09.301A	S12.231K	S12.651A	S15.9XXA	S22.049K	S25.801A	S32.021K
S02.61XB	S05.42XA	S09.302A	S12.24XA	S12.651K	S17.0XXA	S22.050A	S25.802A	S32.022A
S02.61XK	S05.50XA	S09.309A	S12.24XK	S12.690A	S17.8XXA	S22.050K	S25.809A	S32.022K
S02.62XA	S05.51XA	S09.311A	S12.250A	S12.690K	S17.9XXA	S22.051A	S25.811A	S32.028A
S02.62XB	S05.52XA	S09.312A	S12.250K	S12.691A	S21.101A	S22.051K	S25.812A	S32.028K
S02.62XK	S05.70XA	S09.313A	S12.251A	S12.691K	S21.102A	S22.052A	S25.819A	S32.029A
S02.63XA	S05.71XA	S09.319A	S12.251K	S12.9XXA	S21.109A	S22.052K	S25.891A	S32.029K
S02.63XB	S05.72XA	S09.391A	S12.290A	S13.0XXA	S21.111A	S22.058A	S25.892A	S32.030A
S02.63XK	S05.8X1A	S09.392A	S12.290K	S13.101A	S21.112A	S22.058K	S25.899A	S32.030K
S02.64XA	S05.8X2A	S09.399A	S12.291A	S13.110A	S21.119A	S22.059A	S25.90XA	S32.031A
S02.64XB	S05.8X9A	S11.10XA	S12.291K	S13.111A	S21.121A	S22.059K	S25.91XA	S32.031K
S02.64XK	S05.91XA	S11.11XA	S12.300A	S13.120A	S21.122A	S22.060A	S25.99XA	S32.032A
S02.65XA	S05.92XA	S11.12XA	S12.300K	S13.121A	S21.129A	S22.060K	S26.00XA	S32.032K
S02.65XB	S06.0X1A	S11.13XA	S12.301A	S13.130A	S21.131A	S22.061A	S26.01XA	S32.038A
S02.65XK	S06.0X2A	S11.14XA	S12.301K	S13.131A	S21.132A	S22.061K	S26.09XA	S32.038K
S02.66XA	S06.0X3A	S11.15XA	S12.330A	S13.140A	S21.139A	S22.062A	S26.10XA	S32.039A
S02.66XB	S06.0X4A	S11.20XA	S12.330K	S13.141A	S21.141A	S22.062K	S26.11XA	S32.039K
S02.66XK	S06.0X5A	S11.21XA	S12.331A	S13.150A	S21.142A	S22.068A	S26.19XA	S32.040A
S02.67XA	S06.0X7A	S11.22XA	S12.331K	S13.151A	S21.149A	S22.068K	S26.90XA	S32.040K
S02.67XB	S06.0X8A	S11.23XA	S12.34XA	S13.160A	S21.151A	S22.069A	S26.91XA	S32.041A
S02.67XK	S06.0X9A	S11.24XA	S12.34XK	S13.161A	S21.152A	S22.069K	S26.99XA	S32.041K
S02.69XA	S06.2X1A	S11.25XA	S12.350A	S13.170A	S21.159A	S22.070A	S27.0XXA	S32.042A
S02.69XB	S06.2X2A	S12.000A	S12.350K	S13.171A	S21.90XA	S22.070K	S27.301A	S32.042K
S02.69XK	S06.2X3A	S12.000K	S12.351A	S13.180A	S21.91XA	S22.071A	S27.302A	S32.048A
S02.8XXA	S06.2X4A	S12.001A	S12.351K	S13.181A	S21.92XA	S22.071K	S27.309A	S32.048K
S02.8XXB	S06.2X5A	S12.001K	S12.390A	S13.20XA	S21.93XA	S22.072A	S27.311A	S32.049A
S02.8XXK	S06.2X9A	S12.01XA	S12.390K	S13.29XA	S21.94XA	S22.072K	S27.312A	S32.049K
S02.91XA	S06.301A	S12.01XK	S12.391A	S15.001A	S21.95XA	S22.078A	S27.319A	S32.050A
S02.91XK	S06.302A	S12.02XA	S12.391K	S15.002A	S22.000A	S22.078K	S27.321A	S32.050K
S02.92XA	S06.303A	S12.02XK	S12.400A	S15.009A	S22.000K	S22.079A	S27.322A	S32.051A
S02.92XB	S06.304A	S12.030A	S12.400K	S15.011A	S22.001A	S22.079K	S27.329A	S32.051K
S02.92XK	S06.305A	S12.030K	S12.401A	S15.012A	S22.001K	S22.080A	S27.391A	S32.052A
S04.011A	S06.309A	S12.031A	S12.401K	S15.019A	S22.002A	S22.080K	S27.392A	S32.052K
S04.012A	S06.371A	S12.031K	S12.430A	S15.021A	S22.002K	S22.081A	S27.399A	S32.058A
S04.019A	S06.372A	S12.040A	S12.430K	S15.022A	S22.008A	S22.081K	S27.50XA	S32.058K
S04.02XA	S06.373A	S12.040K	S12.431A	S15.029A	S22.008K	S22.082A	S27.51XA	S32.059A
S04.031A	S06.374A	S12.041A	S12.431K	S15.091A	S22.009A	S22.082K	S27.52XA	S32.059K
S04.032A	S06.375A	S12.041K	S12.44XA	S15.092A	S22.009K	S22.088A	S27.53XA	S32.10XA
S04.039A	S06.379A	S12.090A	S12.44XK	S15.099A	S22.010A	S22.088K	S27.59XA	S32.10XK
S04.041A	S06.381A	S12.090K	S12.450A	S15.101A	S22.010K	S22.089A	S27.60XA	S32.110A
S04.042A	S06.382A	S12.091A	S12.450K	S15.102A	S22.011A	S22.089K	S27.63XA	S32.110K
S04.049A	S06.383A	S12.091K	S12.451A	S15.109A	S22.011K	S22.20XA	S27.69XA	S32.111A
S04.10XA	S06.384A	S12.100A	S12.451K	S15.111A	S22.012A	S22.20XK	S27.802A	S32.111K
S04.11XA	S06.385A	S12.100K	S12.490A	S15.112A	S22.012K	S22.21XA	S27.803A	S32.112A
S04.12XA	S06.389A	S12.101A	S12.490K	S15.119A	S22.018A	S22.21XK	S27.808A	S32.112K
S04.20XA	S06.811A	S12.101K	S12.491A	S15.121A	S22.018K	S22.22XA	S27.809A	S32.119A
S04.21XA	S06.812A	S12.110A	S12.491K		S22.019A	S22.22XK	S27.892A	S32.119K

S32.120A	S32.445K	S32.89XA	S36.490A	S37.60XA	S42.033K	S42.142B	S42.223P	S42.292K
S32.120K	S32.446K	S32.89XK	S36.498A	S37.62XA	S42.033P	S42.142K	S42.224A	S42.292P
S32.121A	S32.451K	S32.9XXA	S36.499A	S37.63XA	S42.034B	S42.142P	S42.224K	S42.293A
S32.121K	S32.452K	S32.9XXK	S36.500A	S37.69XA	S42.034K	S42.143B	S42.224P	S42.293P
S32.122A	S32.453K	S35.531A	S36.501A	S37.812A	S42.034P	S42.143K	S42.225A	S42.294A
S32.122K	S32.454K	S35.532A	S36.502A	S37.813A	S42.035B	S42.143P	S42.225K	S42.294K
S32.129A	S32.455K	S35.533A	S36.503A	S37.818A	S42.035K	S42.144B	S42.225P	S42.294P
S32.129K	S32.456K	S35.534A	S36.508A	S37.819A	S42.035P	S42.144K	S42.226A	S42.295A
S32.130A	S32.461K	S35.535A	S36.509A	S37.892A	S42.036B	S42.144P	S42.226K	S42.295K
S32.130K	S32.462K	S35.536A	S36.510A	S37.893A	S42.036K	S42.145B	S42.226P	S42.296A
S32.131A	S32.463K	S35.8X1A	S36.511A	S37.898A	S42.036P	S42.145K	S42.231A	S42.296K
S32.131K	S32.464K	S35.8X8A	S36.512A	S37.899A	S42.101B	S42.145P	S42.231K	S42.296P
S32.132A	S32.465K	S35.8X9A	S36.513A	S37.90XA	S42.101K	S42.146B	S42.231P	S42.301A
S32.132K	S32.466K	S35.90XA	S36.518A	S37.92XA	S42.101P	S42.146K	S42.232A	S42.301K
S32.139A	S32.471K	S35.91XA	S36.519A	S37.93XA	S42.102B	S42.146P	S42.232K	S42.301P
S32.139K	S32.472K	S35.99XA	S36.520A	S37.99XA	S42.102K	S42.151B	S42.232P	S42.302A
S32.14XA	S32.473K	S36.00XA	S36.521A	S42.001A	S42.102P	S42.151K	S42.239A	S42.302K
S32.14XK	S32.474K	S36.020A	S36.522A	S42.001K	S42.109B	S42.151P	S42.239K	S42.302P
S32.15XA	S32.475K	S36.021A	S36.523A	S42.001P	S42.109K	S42.152B	S42.239P	S42.309A
S32.15XK	S32.476K	S36.029A	S36.528A	S42.002B	S42.109P	S42.152K	S42.241A	S42.309K
S32.16XA	S32.481K	S36.030A	S36.529A	S42.002K	S42.111B	S42.152P	S42.241K	S42.309P
S32.16XK	S32.482K	S36.039A	S36.530A	S42.002P	S42.111K	S42.153B	S42.241P	S42.311A
S32.17XA	S32.483K	S36.09XA	S36.531A	S42.009B	S42.111P	S42.153K	S42.242A	S42.311K
S32.17XK	S32.484K	S36.112A	S36.532A	S42.009K	S42.112B	S42.153P	S42.242P	S42.311P
S32.19XA	S32.485K	S36.113A	S36.533A	S42.009P	S42.112K	S42.154B	S42.249A	S42.312A
S32.19XK	S32.486K	S36.114A	S36.538A	S42.011B	S42.112P	S42.154K	S42.249K	S42.312K
S32.2XXA	S32.491K	S36.118A	S36.539A	S42.011K	S42.113B	S42.154P	S42.249P	S42.312P
S32.2XXK	S32.492K	S36.119A	S36.590A	S42.011P	S42.113K	S42.155B	S42.251A	S42.319A
S32.301A	S32.499K	S36.122A	S36.591A	S42.012B	S42.113P	S42.155K	S42.251K	S42.319K
S32.301K	S32.501A	S36.123A	S36.592A	S42.012K	S42.114B	S42.155P	S42.251P	S42.319P
S32.302A	S32.501K	S36.128A	S36.593A	S42.012P	S42.114K	S42.156B	S42.252A	S42.321A
S32.302K	S32.502A	S36.129A	S36.598A	S42.013B	S42.114P	S42.156K	S42.252K	S42.321K
S32.309A	S32.502K	S36.13XA	S36.599A	S42.013K	S42.115B	S42.156P	S42.252P	S42.321P
S32.309K	S32.509A	S36.200A	S36.60XA	S42.013P	S42.115K	S42.191B	S42.253A	S42.322A
S32.311A	S32.509K	S36.201A	S36.61XA	S42.014B	S42.115P	S42.191K	S42.253K	S42.322K
S32.311K	S32.511A	S36.202A	S36.62XA	S42.014K	S42.116B	S42.191P	S42.253P	S42.322P
S32.312A	S32.511K	S36.209A	S36.63XA	S42.014P	S42.116K	S42.192B	S42.254A	S42.323A
S32.312K	S32.512A	S36.220A	S36.69XA	S42.015B	S42.116P	S42.192K	S42.254K	S42.323K
S32.313A	S32.512K	S36.221A	S36.81XA	S42.015P	S42.121B	S42.192P	S42.254P	S42.323P
S32.313K	S32.519A	S36.222A	S36.892A	S42.016B	S42.121K	S42.199B	S42.255A	S42.324A
S32.314A	S32.519K	S36.229A	S36.893A	S42.016K	S42.121P	S42.199K	S42.255K	S42.324K
S32.314K	S32.591A	S36.230A	S36.898A	S42.016P	S42.122B	S42.199P	S42.255P	S42.324P
S32.315A	S32.591K	S36.231A	S36.899A	S42.017B	S42.122K	S42.201A	S42.256A	S42.325A
S32.315K	S32.592A	S36.232A	S36.90XA	S42.017K	S42.122P	S42.201K	S42.256K	S42.325K
S32.316A	S32.592K	S36.239A	S36.92XA	S42.017P	S42.123B	S42.201P	S42.256P	S42.325P
S32.316K	S32.599A	S36.240A	S36.93XA	S42.018B	S42.123K	S42.202A	S42.261A	S42.326A
S32.391A	S32.599K	S36.241A	S36.99XA	S42.018K	S42.123P	S42.202K	S42.261K	S42.326K
S32.391K	S32.601A	S36.242A	S37.001A	S42.018P	S42.124B	S42.202P	S42.261P	S42.326P
S32.392A	S32.601K	S36.249A	S37.002A	S42.019B	S42.124K	S42.209A	S42.262A	S42.331A
S32.392K	S32.602A	S36.250A	S37.009A	S42.019K	S42.124P	S42.209K	S42.262K	S42.331K
S32.399A	S32.602K	S36.251A	S37.011A	S42.019P	S42.125B	S42.209P	S42.262P	S42.332A
S32.399K	S32.609A	S36.252A	S37.012A	S42.021B	S42.125K	S42.211A	S42.263A	S42.332K
S32.401K	S32.609K	S36.259A	S37.019A	S42.021K	S42.125P	S42.211K	S42.263K	S42.332P
S32.402K	S32.611A	S36.260A	S37.021A	S42.021P	S42.126B	S42.211P	S42.263P	S42.333A
S32.409K	S32.611K	S36.261A	S37.022A	S42.022B	S42.126K	S42.212A	S42.264A	S42.333K
S32.411K	S32.612A	S36.262A	S37.029A	S42.022K	S42.126P	S42.212K	S42.264K	S42.333P
S32.412K	S32.612K	S36.269A	S37.031A	S42.022P	S42.131B	S42.212P	S42.264P	S42.334A
S32.413K	S32.613A	S36.290A	S37.032A	S42.023B	S42.131K	S42.213A	S42.265A	S42.334K
S32.414K	S32.613K	S36.291A	S37.039A	S42.023K	S42.131P	S42.213K	S42.265K	S42.334P
S32.415K	S32.614A	S36.292A	S37.041A	S42.023P	S42.132B	S42.213P	S42.265P	S42.335A
S32.416K	S32.614K	S36.299A	S37.042A	S42.024B	S42.132K	S42.214A	S42.266A	S42.335K
S32.421K	S32.615A	S36.30XA	S37.049A	S42.024K	S42.132P	S42.214K	S42.266K	S42.335P
S32.422K	S32.615K	S36.32XA	S37.051A	S42.024P	S42.133B	S42.214P	S42.266P	S42.336A
S32.423K	S32.616A	S36.33XA	S37.052A	S42.025B	S42.133K	S42.215A	S42.271A	S42.336K
S32.424K	S32.616K	S36.39XA	S37.059A	S42.025K	S42.133P	S42.215K	S42.271K	S42.336P
S32.425K	S32.691A	S36.400A	S37.10XA	S42.025P	S42.134B	S42.215P	S42.271P	S42.341A
S32.426K	S32.691K	S36.408A	S37.12XA	S42.026B	S42.134K	S42.216A	S42.272A	S42.341K
S32.431K	S32.692A	S36.409A	S37.13XA	S42.026K	S42.134P	S42.216K	S42.272K	S42.341P
S32.432K	S32.692K	S36.410A	S37.19XA	S42.026P	S42.135B	S42.216P	S42.272P	S42.342A
S32.433K	S32.699A	S36.418A	S37.20XA	S42.031B	S42.135K	S42.221A	S42.279A	S42.342K
S32.434K	S32.699K	S36.419A	S37.22XA	S42.031K	S42.135P	S42.221K	S42.279K	S42.342P
S32.435K	S32.810A	S36.420A	S37.23XA	S42.031P	S42.136B	S42.221P	S42.279P	S42.343A
S32.436K	S32.810K	S36.428A	S37.29XA	S42.032B	S42.136K	S42.222A	S42.291A	S42.343K
S32.441K	S32.811A	S36.429A	S37.30XA	S42.032K	S42.136P	S42.222K	S42.291K	S42.342A
S32.442K	S32.811K	S36.430A	S37.32XA	S42.032P	S42.141B	S42.222P	S42.291P	S42.343A
S32.443K	S32.82XA	S36.438A	S37.33XA	S42.032P	S42.141K	S42.223A	S42.292A	S42.343K
S32.444K	S32.82XK	S36.439A	S37.39XA	S42.033B	S42.141P	S42.223K	S42.292A	S42.343P

Appendix F: Complication and Comorbidity (CC) Code List

S42.344A	S42.415P	S42.454K	S42.92XA	S46.329A	S49.099K	S52.012A	S52.036R	S52.112K
S42.344K	S42.416A	S42.454P	S42.92XK	S46.821A	S49.099P	S52.012K	S52.041K	S52.112P
S42.344P	S42.416K	S42.455A	S42.92XP	S46.822A	S49.101A	S52.012P	S52.041M	S52.119A
S42.345A	S42.416P	S42.455K	S43.201A	S46.829A	S49.101K	S52.019A	S52.041N	S52.119K
S42.345K	S42.421A	S42.455P	S43.202A	S46.921A	S49.101P	S52.019K	S52.041P	S52.119P
S42.345P	S42.421K	S42.456A	S43.203A	S46.922A	S49.102A	S52.019P	S52.041Q	S52.121K
S42.346A	S42.421P	S42.456K	S43.204A	S46.929A	S49.102K	S52.021K	S52.041R	S52.121M
S42.346K	S42.422A	S42.456P	S43.205A	S48.011A	S49.102P	S52.021M	S52.042K	S52.121N
S42.346P	S42.422K	S42.461A	S43.206A	S48.012A	S49.109A	S52.021N	S52.042M	S52.121P
S42.351A	S42.422P	S42.461K	S43.211A	S48.019A	S49.109K	S52.021P	S52.042N	S52.121Q
S42.351K	S42.423A	S42.461P	S43.212A	S48.021A	S49.109P	S52.021Q	S52.042P	S52.121R
S42.351P	S42.423K	S42.462A	S43.213A	S48.022A	S49.111A	S52.021R	S52.042Q	S52.122K
S42.352A	S42.423P	S42.462K	S43.214A	S48.029A	S49.111K	S52.022K	S52.042R	S52.122M
S42.352K	S42.424A	S42.462P	S43.215A	S48.111A	S49.111P	S52.022M	S52.043K	S52.122N
S42.352P	S42.424K	S42.463A	S43.216A	S48.112A	S49.112A	S52.022N	S52.043M	S52.122P
S42.353A	S42.424P	S42.463K	S43.221A	S48.119A	S49.112K	S52.022P	S52.043N	S52.122Q
S42.353K	S42.425A	S42.463P	S43.222A	S48.121A	S49.112P	S52.022Q	S52.043P	S52.122R
S42.353P	S42.425K	S42.464A	S43.223A	S48.122A	S49.119A	S52.022R	S52.043Q	S52.123K
S42.354A	S42.425P	S42.464K	S43.224A	S48.129A	S49.119K	S52.023K	S52.043R	S52.123M
S42.354K	S42.426A	S42.464P	S43.225A	S48.911A	S49.119P	S52.023M	S52.044K	S52.123N
S42.354P	S42.426K	S42.465A	S43.226A	S48.912A	S49.121A	S52.023N	S52.044M	S52.123P
S42.355A	S42.426P	S42.465K	S45.101A	S48.919A	S49.121K	S52.023P	S52.044N	S52.123Q
S42.355K	S42.431A	S42.465P	S45.102A	S48.921A	S49.121P	S52.023Q	S52.044P	S52.123R
S42.355P	S42.431K	S42.466A	S45.109A	S48.922A	S49.122A	S52.023R	S52.044Q	S52.124K
S42.356A	S42.431P	S42.466K	S45.111A	S48.929A	S49.122K	S52.024K	S52.044R	S52.124M
S42.356K	S42.432A	S42.466P	S45.112A	S49.001A	S49.122P	S52.024M	S52.045K	S52.124N
S42.356P	S42.432K	S42.471A	S45.119A	S49.001K	S49.129A	S52.024N	S52.045M	S52.124P
S42.361A	S42.432P	S42.471K	S45.191A	S49.001P	S49.129K	S52.024P	S52.045N	S52.124Q
S42.361K	S42.433A	S42.471P	S45.192A	S49.002A	S49.129P	S52.024Q	S52.045P	S52.124R
S42.361P	S42.433K	S42.472A	S45.199A	S49.002K	S49.131A	S52.024R	S52.045Q	S52.125K
S42.362A	S42.433P	S42.472K	S45.201A	S49.002P	S49.131K	S52.025K	S52.045R	S52.125M
S42.362K	S42.434A	S42.472P	S45.202A	S49.009A	S49.131P	S52.025M	S52.046K	S52.125N
S42.362P	S42.434K	S42.473A	S45.209A	S49.009K	S49.132A	S52.025N	S52.046M	S52.125P
S42.363A	S42.434P	S42.473K	S45.211A	S49.009P	S49.132K	S52.025P	S52.046N	S52.125Q
S42.363K	S42.435A	S42.473P	S45.212A	S49.011A	S49.132P	S52.025Q	S52.046P	S52.125R
S42.363P	S42.435K	S42.474A	S45.219A	S49.011K	S49.139A	S52.025R	S52.046Q	S52.126K
S42.364A	S42.435P	S42.474K	S45.291A	S49.011P	S49.139K	S52.026K	S52.046R	S52.126M
S42.364K	S42.436A	S42.474P	S45.292A	S49.012A	S49.139P	S52.026M	S52.091K	S52.126N
S42.364P	S42.436K	S42.475A	S45.299A	S49.012K	S49.141A	S52.026N	S52.091M	S52.126P
S42.365A	S42.436P	S42.475K	S45.301A	S49.012P	S49.141K	S52.026P	S52.091N	S52.126Q
S42.365K	S42.441A	S42.475P	S45.302A	S49.019A	S49.141P	S52.026Q	S52.091P	S52.126R
S42.365P	S42.441K	S42.476A	S45.309A	S49.019K	S49.142A	S52.026R	S52.091Q	S52.131K
S42.366A	S42.441P	S42.476K	S45.311A	S49.019P	S49.142K	S52.031K	S52.091R	S52.131M
S42.366K	S42.442A	S42.476P	S45.312A	S49.021A	S49.142P	S52.031M	S52.092K	S52.131N
S42.366P	S42.442K	S42.481A	S45.319A	S49.021K	S49.149A	S52.031N	S52.092M	S52.131P
S42.391A	S42.442P	S42.481K	S45.391A	S49.021P	S49.149K	S52.031P	S52.092N	S52.131Q
S42.391K	S42.443A	S42.481P	S45.392A	S49.022A	S49.149P	S52.031Q	S52.092P	S52.131R
S42.391P	S42.443K	S42.482A	S45.399A	S49.022K	S49.191A	S52.031R	S52.092Q	S52.132K
S42.392A	S42.443P	S42.482K	S45.801A	S49.022P	S49.191K	S52.032K	S52.092R	S52.132M
S42.392K	S42.444A	S42.482P	S45.802A	S49.029A	S49.191P	S52.032M	S52.099K	S52.132N
S42.392P	S42.444K	S42.489A	S45.809A	S49.029K	S49.192A	S52.032N	S52.099M	S52.132P
S42.399A	S42.444P	S42.489K	S45.811A	S49.029P	S49.192K	S52.032P	S52.099N	S52.132Q
S42.399K	S42.445A	S42.489P	S45.812A	S49.031A	S49.192P	S52.032Q	S52.099P	S52.132R
S42.399P	S42.445K	S42.491A	S45.819A	S49.031K	S49.199A	S52.032R	S52.099Q	S52.133K
S42.401A	S42.445P	S42.491K	S45.891A	S49.031P	S49.199K	S52.033K	S52.099R	S52.133M
S42.401K	S42.446A	S42.491P	S45.892A	S49.032A	S49.199P	S52.033M	S52.101K	S52.133N
S42.401P	S42.446K	S42.492A	S45.899A	S49.032K	S52.001K	S52.033N	S52.101M	S52.133P
S42.402A	S42.446P	S42.492K	S45.901A	S49.032P	S52.001M	S52.033P	S52.101N	S52.133Q
S42.402K	S42.447A	S42.492P	S45.902A	S49.039A	S52.001N	S52.033Q	S52.101P	S52.133R
S42.402P	S42.447K	S42.493A	S45.909A	S49.039K	S52.001P	S52.033R	S52.101Q	S52.134K
S42.409A	S42.447P	S42.493K	S45.911A	S49.039P	S52.001Q	S52.034K	S52.101R	S52.134M
S42.409K	S42.448A	S42.493P	S45.912A	S49.041A	S52.001R	S52.034M	S52.102K	S52.134N
S42.409P	S42.448K	S42.494A	S45.919A	S49.041K	S52.002K	S52.034N	S52.102M	S52.134P
S42.411A	S42.448P	S42.494K	S45.991A	S49.041P	S52.002M	S52.034P	S52.102N	S52.134Q
S42.411K	S42.449A	S42.494P	S45.992A	S49.042A	S52.002N	S52.034Q	S52.102P	S52.134R
S42.411P	S42.449K	S42.495A	S45.999A	S49.042K	S52.002P	S52.034R	S52.102Q	S52.135K
S42.412A	S42.449P	S42.495K	S46.021A	S49.042P	S52.002Q	S52.035K	S52.102R	S52.135M
S42.412K	S42.451A	S42.495P	S46.022A	S49.049A	S52.002R	S52.035M	S52.109K	S52.135N
S42.412P	S42.451K	S42.496A	S46.029A	S49.049K	S52.009K	S52.035N	S52.109M	S52.135P
S42.413A	S42.451P	S42.496K	S46.121A	S49.049P	S52.009M	S52.035P	S52.109N	S52.135Q
S42.413K	S42.452A	S42.496P	S46.122A	S49.091A	S52.009N	S52.035Q	S52.109P	S52.135R
S42.413P	S42.452K	S42.90XA	S46.129A	S49.091K	S52.009P	S52.035R	S52.109Q	S52.136K
S42.414A	S42.452P	S42.90XK	S46.221A	S49.091P	S52.009Q	S52.036K	S52.109R	S52.136M
S42.414K	S42.453A	S42.90XP	S46.222A	S49.092A	S52.009R	S52.036M	S52.111A	S52.136N
S42.414P	S42.453K	S42.91XA	S46.229A	S49.092K	S52.011A	S52.036N	S52.111K	S52.136P
S42.415A	S42.453P	S42.91XK	S46.321A	S49.092P	S52.011K	S52.036P	S52.111P	S52.136Q
S42.415K	S42.454A	S42.91XP	S46.322A	S49.099A	S52.011P	S52.036Q	S52.112A	S52.136R

Appendix F: Complication and Comorbidity (CC) Code List

S52.181K	S52.225K	S52.244K	S52.263K	S52.292P	S52.326M	S52.345M	S52.364M	S52.399M
S52.181M	S52.225M	S52.244M	S52.263N	S52.292Q	S52.326N	S52.345N	S52.364N	S52.399N
S52.181N	S52.225N	S52.244P	S52.263P	S52.299A	S52.326P	S52.345P	S52.364P	S52.399P
S52.181P	S52.225P	S52.244Q	S52.263Q	S52.299K	S52.326Q	S52.345Q	S52.364Q	S52.399Q
S52.181Q	S52.225Q	S52.244R	S52.263R	S52.299M	S52.326R	S52.345R	S52.364R	S52.399R
S52.181R	S52.225R	S52.245A	S52.264A	S52.299N	S52.331A	S52.346A	S52.365A	S52.501A
S52.182K	S52.226A	S52.245K	S52.264K	S52.299P	S52.331K	S52.346K	S52.365K	S52.501K
S52.182M	S52.226K	S52.245M	S52.264M	S52.299Q	S52.331M	S52.346M	S52.365M	S52.501M
S52.182N	S52.226M	S52.245P	S52.264N	S52.301A	S52.331N	S52.346N	S52.365N	S52.501N
S52.182P	S52.226N	S52.245Q	S52.264P	S52.301K	S52.331P	S52.346P	S52.365P	S52.501P
S52.182Q	S52.226P	S52.245R	S52.264Q	S52.301M	S52.331Q	S52.346Q	S52.365Q	S52.501Q
S52.182R	S52.226Q	S52.246A	S52.264R	S52.301N	S52.331R	S52.346R	S52.365R	S52.501R
S52.189K	S52.226R	S52.246K	S52.265A	S52.301P	S52.332A	S52.351A	S52.366A	S52.502A
S52.189M	S52.231A	S52.246M	S52.265K	S52.301Q	S52.332K	S52.351K	S52.366K	S52.502K
S52.189N	S52.231K	S52.246P	S52.265M	S52.302A	S52.332M	S52.351M	S52.366M	S52.502M
S52.189P	S52.231M	S52.246Q	S52.265N	S52.302K	S52.332N	S52.351N	S52.366N	S52.502N
S52.189Q	S52.231N	S52.246R	S52.265P	S52.302M	S52.332P	S52.351P	S52.366P	S52.502P
S52.189R	S52.231P	S52.251A	S52.265Q	S52.302N	S52.332Q	S52.351Q	S52.366Q	S52.502Q
S52.201A	S52.231Q	S52.251K	S52.265R	S52.302P	S52.332R	S52.351R	S52.366R	S52.502R
S52.201K	S52.231R	S52.251M	S52.266A	S52.302Q	S52.333A	S52.352A	S52.371A	S52.509A
S52.201M	S52.232A	S52.251N	S52.266K	S52.309A	S52.333K	S52.352K	S52.371K	S52.509K
S52.201N	S52.232K	S52.251P	S52.266M	S52.309K	S52.333M	S52.352M	S52.371M	S52.509M
S52.201P	S52.232M	S52.251Q	S52.266N	S52.309M	S52.333N	S52.352N	S52.371N	S52.509N
S52.201Q	S52.232N	S52.251R	S52.266P	S52.309N	S52.333P	S52.352P	S52.371P	S52.509P
S52.201R	S52.232P	S52.252A	S52.266Q	S52.309P	S52.333Q	S52.352Q	S52.371Q	S52.509Q
S52.202A	S52.232Q	S52.252K	S52.266R	S52.309Q	S52.333R	S52.352R	S52.371R	S52.509R
S52.202K	S52.232R	S52.252M	S52.271K	S52.309R	S52.334A	S52.353A	S52.372A	S52.511A
S52.202M	S52.233A	S52.252N	S52.271M	S52.311A	S52.334K	S52.353K	S52.372K	S52.511K
S52.202N	S52.233K	S52.252P	S52.271N	S52.311K	S52.334M	S52.353M	S52.372M	S52.511M
S52.202P	S52.233M	S52.252Q	S52.271P	S52.311P	S52.334N	S52.353N	S52.372P	S52.511N
S52.202Q	S52.233N	S52.252R	S52.271Q	S52.312A	S52.334P	S52.353P	S52.372Q	S52.511P
S52.202R	S52.233P	S52.253A	S52.271R	S52.312K	S52.334Q	S52.353Q	S52.372R	S52.511Q
S52.209A	S52.233Q	S52.253K	S52.272K	S52.312P	S52.334R	S52.353R	S52.379A	S52.511R
S52.209K	S52.233R	S52.253M	S52.272M	S52.319A	S52.335A	S52.354A	S52.379K	S52.512A
S52.209M	S52.234A	S52.253N	S52.272N	S52.319K	S52.335K	S52.354K	S52.379M	S52.512K
S52.209N	S52.234K	S52.253P	S52.272Q	S52.319P	S52.335M	S52.354M	S52.379N	S52.512M
S52.209P	S52.234M	S52.253Q	S52.272R	S52.321A	S52.335N	S52.354N	S52.379P	S52.512N
S52.209Q	S52.234N	S52.253R	S52.279K	S52.321K	S52.335P	S52.354P	S52.379Q	S52.512Q
S52.209R	S52.234P	S52.254A	S52.279M	S52.321M	S52.335Q	S52.354Q	S52.379R	S52.512R
S52.211A	S52.234Q	S52.254K	S52.279N	S52.321N	S52.335R	S52.354R	S52.381A	S52.513A
S52.211K	S52.234R	S52.254M	S52.279P	S52.321P	S52.336A	S52.355A	S52.381K	S52.513K
S52.211P	S52.235A	S52.254N	S52.279Q	S52.321Q	S52.336K	S52.355K	S52.381M	S52.513M
S52.212A	S52.235K	S52.254P	S52.279R	S52.321R	S52.336M	S52.355M	S52.381N	S52.513N
S52.212K	S52.235M	S52.254Q	S52.281A	S52.322A	S52.336N	S52.355N	S52.381P	S52.513P
S52.212P	S52.235N	S52.254R	S52.281K	S52.322K	S52.336P	S52.355P	S52.381Q	S52.513Q
S52.219A	S52.235P	S52.255A	S52.281M	S52.322M	S52.336Q	S52.355Q	S52.381R	S52.513R
S52.219K	S52.235Q	S52.255K	S52.281N	S52.322N	S52.336R	S52.355R	S52.382A	S52.514A
S52.219P	S52.235R	S52.255M	S52.281P	S52.322P	S52.341A	S52.356A	S52.382K	S52.514K
S52.221A	S52.236A	S52.255N	S52.281Q	S52.322Q	S52.341K	S52.356K	S52.382M	S52.514M
S52.221K	S52.236K	S52.255P	S52.281R	S52.322R	S52.341M	S52.356M	S52.382N	S52.514N
S52.221M	S52.236M	S52.255Q	S52.282A	S52.323A	S52.341N	S52.356N	S52.382P	S52.514Q
S52.221N	S52.236N	S52.255R	S52.282K	S52.323K	S52.341P	S52.356P	S52.382Q	S52.514R
S52.221P	S52.236P	S52.256A	S52.282M	S52.323M	S52.341Q	S52.356Q	S52.382R	S52.515A
S52.221Q	S52.236Q	S52.256K	S52.282N	S52.323N	S52.341R	S52.356R	S52.389A	S52.515K
S52.221R	S52.236R	S52.256M	S52.282P	S52.323P	S52.342A	S52.361A	S52.389K	S52.515M
S52.222A	S52.241A	S52.256N	S52.282Q	S52.323Q	S52.342K	S52.361K	S52.389M	S52.515N
S52.222K	S52.241K	S52.256P	S52.282R	S52.323R	S52.342M	S52.361M	S52.389N	S52.515Q
S52.222M	S52.241M	S52.256Q	S52.283A	S52.324A	S52.342N	S52.361N	S52.389P	S52.515R
S52.222N	S52.241N	S52.256R	S52.283K	S52.324K	S52.342P	S52.361P	S52.389Q	S52.516A
S52.222P	S52.241P	S52.261A	S52.283M	S52.324M	S52.342Q	S52.361Q	S52.389R	S52.516K
S52.222Q	S52.241Q	S52.261K	S52.283N	S52.324N	S52.342R	S52.361R	S52.391A	S52.516M
S52.222R	S52.241R	S52.261M	S52.283P	S52.324P	S52.343A	S52.362A	S52.391K	S52.516N
S52.223A	S52.242A	S52.261N	S52.283Q	S52.324Q	S52.343K	S52.362K	S52.391M	S52.516Q
S52.223K	S52.242K	S52.261P	S52.283R	S52.324R	S52.343M	S52.362M	S52.391N	S52.516R
S52.223M	S52.242M	S52.261Q	S52.291A	S52.325A	S52.343N	S52.362N	S52.391P	S52.521A
S52.223N	S52.242N	S52.261R	S52.291K	S52.325K	S52.343P	S52.362P	S52.391Q	S52.521K
S52.223P	S52.242P	S52.262A	S52.291M	S52.325M	S52.343Q	S52.362Q	S52.391R	S52.521P
S52.223Q	S52.242Q	S52.262K	S52.291N	S52.325N	S52.343R	S52.362R	S52.392A	S52.522A
S52.223R	S52.242R	S52.262M	S52.291P	S52.325P	S52.344A	S52.363A	S52.392K	S52.522K
S52.224A	S52.243A	S52.262N	S52.291Q	S52.325Q	S52.344K	S52.363K	S52.392M	S52.522P
S52.224K	S52.243K	S52.262P	S52.291R	S52.325R	S52.344M	S52.363M	S52.392N	S52.529A
S52.224M	S52.243M	S52.262Q	S52.292A	S52.326A	S52.344N	S52.363N	S52.392P	S52.529K
S52.224N	S52.243N	S52.262R	S52.292K	S52.326K	S52.344P	S52.363P	S52.392Q	S52.529P
S52.224P	S52.243P	S52.263A	S52.292M		S52.344Q	S52.363Q	S52.392R	
S52.224Q	S52.243Q		S52.292N		S52.344R	S52.363R	S52.399A	
S52.224-R	S52.243R				S52.345A	S52.364A	S52.399K	
S52.225A	S52.244A				S52.345K	S52.364K		

S52.531A	S52.569A	S52.612A	S52.91XQ	S56.426A	S59.091K	S59.239A	S62.034P	S62.143K
S52.531K	S52.569K	S52.612K	S52.91XR	S56.427A	S59.091P	S59.239K	S62.035B	S62.143P
S52.531M	S52.569M	S52.612M	S52.92XA	S56.428A	S59.092A	S59.239P	S62.035P	S62.144B
S52.531N	S52.569N	S52.612N	S52.92XK	S56.429A	S59.092K	S59.241A	S62.036B	S62.144K
S52.531P	S52.569P	S52.612P	S52.92XM	S56.521A	S59.092P	S59.241K	S62.036K	S62.144P
S52.531Q	S52.569Q	S52.612Q	S52.92XN	S56.522A	S59.099A	S59.241P	S62.036P	S62.145B
S52.531R	S52.569R	S52.612R	S52.92XP	S56.529A	S59.099K	S59.242A	S62.101B	S62.145K
S52.532A	S52.571A	S52.613A	S52.92XQ	S56.821A	S59.099P	S59.242K	S62.101K	S62.145P
S52.532K	S52.571K	S52.613K	S52.92XR	S56.822A	S59.101K	S59.242P	S62.101P	S62.146B
S52.532M	S52.571M	S52.613M	S55.001A	S56.829A	S59.101P	S59.249A	S62.102B	S62.146K
S52.532N	S52.571N	S52.613N	S55.002A	S56.921A	S59.102K	S59.249K	S62.102K	S62.146P
S52.532P	S52.571P	S52.613P	S55.009A	S56.922A	S59.102P	S59.249P	S62.102P	S62.151B
S52.532Q	S52.571Q	S52.613Q	S55.011A	S56.929A	S59.109K	S59.291A	S62.109B	S62.151K
S52.532R	S52.571R	S52.613R	S55.012A	S58.011A	S59.109P	S59.291K	S62.109K	S62.151P
S52.539A	S52.572A	S52.614A	S55.019A	S58.012A	S59.111K	S59.291P	S62.109P	S62.152B
S52.539K	S52.572K	S52.614K	S55.091A	S58.019A	S59.111P	S59.292A	S62.111B	S62.152K
S52.539M	S52.572M	S52.614M	S55.092A	S58.021A	S59.112K	S59.292K	S62.111K	S62.152P
S52.539N	S52.572N	S52.614N	S55.099A	S58.022A	S59.112P	S59.292P	S62.111P	S62.153B
S52.539P	S52.572P	S52.614P	S55.101A	S58.029A	S59.119K	S59.299A	S62.112B	S62.153K
S52.539Q	S52.572Q	S52.614Q	S55.102A	S58.111A	S59.119P	S59.299K	S62.112K	S62.153P
S52.539R	S52.572R	S52.614R	S55.109A	S58.112A	S59.121K	S59.299P	S62.112P	S62.154B
S52.541A	S52.579A	S52.615A	S55.111A	S58.119A	S59.121P	S62.001B	S62.113B	S62.154K
S52.541K	S52.579K	S52.615K	S55.112A	S58.121A	S59.122K	S62.001K	S62.113K	S62.154P
S52.541M	S52.579M	S52.615M	S55.119A	S58.122A	S59.122P	S62.001P	S62.113P	S62.155B
S52.541N	S52.579N	S52.615N	S55.191A	S58.129A	S59.129K	S62.002B	S62.114B	S62.155K
S52.541P	S52.579P	S52.615P	S55.192A	S58.911A	S59.129P	S62.002K	S62.114K	S62.155P
S52.541Q	S52.579Q	S52.615Q	S55.199A	S58.912A	S59.131K	S62.002P	S62.114P	S62.156B
S52.541R	S52.579R	S52.615R	S55.201A	S58.919A	S59.131P	S62.009B	S62.115B	S62.156K
S52.542A	S52.591A	S52.616A	S55.202A	S58.921A	S59.132K	S62.009K	S62.115K	S62.156P
S52.542K	S52.591K	S52.616K	S55.209A	S58.922A	S59.132P	S62.009P	S62.115P	S62.161B
S52.542M	S52.591M	S52.616M	S55.211A	S58.929A	S59.139K	S62.011B	S62.116B	S62.161K
S52.542N	S52.591N	S52.616N	S55.212A	S59.001A	S59.139P	S62.011K	S62.116K	S62.161P
S52.542P	S52.591P	S52.616P	S55.219A	S59.001K	S59.141K	S62.011P	S62.116P	S62.162B
S52.542Q	S52.591Q	S52.616Q	S55.291A	S59.001P	S59.141P	S62.012B	S62.121B	S62.162K
S52.542R	S52.591R	S52.616R	S55.292A	S59.002A	S59.142K	S62.012K	S62.121K	S62.162P
S52.549A	S52.592A	S52.621A	S55.299A	S59.002K	S59.142P	S62.012P	S62.121P	S62.163B
S52.549K	S52.592K	S52.621K	S55.801A	S59.002P	S59.149K	S62.013B	S62.122K	S62.163K
S52.549M	S52.592M	S52.621P	S55.802A	S59.009A	S59.149P	S62.013K	S62.122P	S62.163P
S52.549N	S52.592N	S52.622A	S55.809A	S59.009K	S59.191K	S62.013P	S62.123B	S62.164B
S52.549P	S52.592P	S52.622K	S55.811A	S59.009P	S59.191P	S62.014B	S62.123K	S62.164K
S52.549Q	S52.592Q	S52.622P	S55.812A	S59.011A	S59.192K	S62.014K	S62.123P	S62.164P
S52.549R	S52.592R	S52.629A	S55.819A	S59.011K	S59.192P	S62.014P	S62.124B	S62.165B
S52.551A	S52.599A	S52.629K	S55.891A	S59.011P	S59.199K	S62.015B	S62.124K	S62.165K
S52.551K	S52.599K	S52.629P	S55.892A	S59.012A	S59.199P	S62.015K	S62.124P	S62.165P
S52.551M	S52.599M	S52.691A	S55.899A	S59.012K	S59.201A	S62.015P	S62.125B	S62.166B
S52.551N	S52.599N	S52.691K	S55.901A	S59.012P	S59.201K	S62.016B	S62.125K	S62.166K
S52.551P	S52.599P	S52.691M	S55.902A	S59.019A	S59.201P	S62.016K	S62.125P	S62.166P
S52.551Q	S52.599Q	S52.691N	S55.909A	S59.019K	S59.202A	S62.016P	S62.126B	S62.171B
S52.551R	S52.599R	S52.691P	S55.911A	S59.019P	S59.202K	S62.021B	S62.126K	S62.171K
S52.552A	S52.601A	S52.691Q	S55.912A	S59.021A	S59.202P	S62.021K	S62.126P	S62.171P
S52.552K	S52.601K	S52.691R	S55.919A	S59.021K	S59.209A	S62.021P	S62.131B	S62.172B
S52.552M	S52.601M	S52.692A	S55.991A	S59.021P	S59.209K	S62.022B	S62.131K	S62.172K
S52.552N	S52.601N	S52.692K	S55.992A	S59.022A	S59.209P	S62.022K	S62.131P	S62.172P
S52.552P	S52.601P	S52.692M	S55.999A	S59.022K	S59.211A	S62.022P	S62.132B	S62.173B
S52.552Q	S52.601Q	S52.692N	S56.021A	S59.022P	S59.211K	S62.023B	S62.132K	S62.173K
S52.552R	S52.601R	S52.692P	S56.022A	S59.029A	S59.211P	S62.023K	S62.132P	S62.173P
S52.559A	S52.602A	S52.692Q	S56.029A	S59.029K	S59.212A	S62.023P	S62.133B	S62.174B
S52.559K	S52.602K	S52.692R	S56.121A	S59.029P	S59.212K	S62.024B	S62.133K	S62.174K
S52.559M	S52.602M	S52.699A	S56.122A	S59.031A	S59.212P	S62.024K	S62.133P	S62.174P
S52.559N	S52.602N	S52.699K	S56.123A	S59.031K	S59.219A	S62.024P	S62.134B	S62.175B
S52.559P	S52.602P	S52.699M	S56.124A	S59.031P	S59.219K	S62.025B	S62.134K	S62.175K
S52.559Q	S52.602Q	S52.699N	S56.125A	S59.032A	S59.219P	S62.025K	S62.134P	S62.175P
S52.559R	S52.602R	S52.699P	S56.126A	S59.032K	S59.221A	S62.025P	S62.135B	S62.176B
S52.561A	S52.609A	S52.699Q	S56.127A	S59.032P	S59.221K	S62.026B	S62.135K	S62.176K
S52.561K	S52.609K	S52.699R	S56.128A	S59.039A	S59.221P	S62.026K	S62.135P	S62.176P
S52.561M	S52.609M	S52.90XA	S56.129A	S59.039K	S59.222A	S62.026P	S62.136B	S62.181B
S52.561N	S52.609N	S52.90XK	S56.221A	S59.039P	S59.222K	S62.031B	S62.136K	S62.181K
S52.561P	S52.609P	S52.90XM	S56.222A	S59.041A	S59.222P	S62.031K	S62.136P	S62.181P
S52.561Q	S52.609Q	S52.90XN	S56.229A	S59.041K	S59.229A	S62.031P	S62.141B	S62.182B
S52.561R	S52.609R	S52.90XP	S56.321A	S59.041P	S59.229K	S62.032B	S62.141K	S62.182K
S52.562A	S52.611A	S52.90XQ	S56.322A	S59.042A	S59.229P	S62.032K	S62.141P	S62.182P
S52.562K	S52.611K	S52.90XR	S56.329A	S59.042K	S59.231A	S62.032P	S62.142B	S62.183B
S52.562M	S52.611M	S52.91XA	S56.421A	S59.042P	S59.231K	S62.033B	S62.142K	S62.183K
S52.562N	S52.611N	S52.91XK	S56.422A	S59.049A	S59.231P	S62.033K	S62.142P	S62.183P
S52.562P	S52.611P	S52.91XM	S56.423A	S59.049K	S59.232A	S62.033P	S62.143B	S62.184B
S52.562Q	S52.611Q	S52.91XN	S56.424A	S59.049P	S59.232K	S62.034B	S62.143K	ICD-10-CM 2016
S52.562R	S52.611R	S52.91XP	S56.425A	S59.091A	S59.232P	S62.034K	S62.143B	S62.184P

S62.185B	S62.246P	S62.316K	S62.342B	S62.367P	S62.525K	S62.624B	S62.649P	S65.092A
S62.185K	S62.251B	S62.316P	S62.342K	S62.368B	S62.525P	S62.624K	S62.650B	S65.099A
S62.185P	S62.251K	S62.317B	S62.342P	S62.368K	S62.526B	S62.624P	S62.650K	S65.101A
S62.186B	S62.251P	S62.317K	S62.343B	S62.368P	S62.526K	S62.625B	S62.650P	S65.102A
S62.186K	S62.252B	S62.317P	S62.343K	S62.369B	S62.526P	S62.625K	S62.651B	S65.109A
S62.186P	S62.252K	S62.318B	S62.343P	S62.369K	S62.600B	S62.625P	S62.651K	S65.111A
S62.201B	S62.252P	S62.318K	S62.344B	S62.369P	S62.600K	S62.626B	S62.651P	S65.112A
S62.201K	S62.253B	S62.318P	S62.344K	S62.390B	S62.600P	S62.626K	S62.652B	S65.119A
S62.201P	S62.253K	S62.319B	S62.344P	S62.390K	S62.601B	S62.626P	S62.652K	S65.191A
S62.202B	S62.253P	S62.319K	S62.345B	S62.390P	S62.601K	S62.627B	S62.652P	S65.192A
S62.202K	S62.254B	S62.319P	S62.345K	S62.391B	S62.601P	S62.627K	S62.653B	S65.199A
S62.202P	S62.254K	S62.320B	S62.345P	S62.391K	S62.602B	S62.627P	S62.653K	S65.201A
S62.209B	S62.254P	S62.320K	S62.346B	S62.391P	S62.602K	S62.628B	S62.653P	S65.202A
S62.209K	S62.255B	S62.320P	S62.346K	S62.392B	S62.602P	S62.628K	S62.654B	S65.209A
S62.209P	S62.255K	S62.321B	S62.346P	S62.392K	S62.603B	S62.628P	S62.654K	S65.211A
S62.211B	S62.255P	S62.321K	S62.347B	S62.392P	S62.603K	S62.629B	S62.654P	S65.212A
S62.211K	S62.256B	S62.321P	S62.347K	S62.393B	S62.603P	S62.629K	S62.655B	S65.219A
S62.211P	S62.256K	S62.322B	S62.347P	S62.393K	S62.604B	S62.629P	S62.655K	S65.291A
S62.212B	S62.256P	S62.322K	S62.348B	S62.393P	S62.604K	S62.630B	S62.655P	S65.292A
S62.212K	S62.291B	S62.322P	S62.348K	S62.394B	S62.604P	S62.630K	S62.656B	S65.299A
S62.212P	S62.291K	S62.323B	S62.348P	S62.394K	S62.605B	S62.630P	S62.656K	S65.301A
S62.213B	S62.291P	S62.323K	S62.349B	S62.394P	S62.605K	S62.631B	S62.656P	S65.302A
S62.213K	S62.292B	S62.323P	S62.349K	S62.395B	S62.605P	S62.631K	S62.657B	S65.309A
S62.213P	S62.292K	S62.324B	S62.349P	S62.395K	S62.606B	S62.631P	S62.657K	S65.311A
S62.221B	S62.292P	S62.324K	S62.350B	S62.395P	S62.606K	S62.632B	S62.657P	S65.312A
S62.221K	S62.299B	S62.324P	S62.350K	S62.396B	S62.606P	S62.632K	S62.658B	S65.319A
S62.221P	S62.299K	S62.325B	S62.350P	S62.396K	S62.607B	S62.632P	S62.658K	S65.391A
S62.222B	S62.299P	S62.325K	S62.351B	S62.396P	S62.607K	S62.633B	S62.658P	S65.392A
S62.222K	S62.300B	S62.325P	S62.351K	S62.397B	S62.607P	S62.633K	S62.659B	S65.399A
S62.222P	S62.300K	S62.326B	S62.351P	S62.397K	S62.608B	S62.633P	S62.659K	S65.401A
S62.223B	S62.300P	S62.326K	S62.352B	S62.397P	S62.608K	S62.634B	S62.659P	S65.402A
S62.223K	S62.301B	S62.326P	S62.352K	S62.398B	S62.608P	S62.634K	S62.660B	S65.409A
S62.223P	S62.301K	S62.327B	S62.352P	S62.398K	S62.609B	S62.634P	S62.660K	S65.411A
S62.224B	S62.301P	S62.327K	S62.353B	S62.398P	S62.609K	S62.635B	S62.660P	S65.412A
S62.224K	S62.302B	S62.327P	S62.353K	S62.399B	S62.609P	S62.635K	S62.661B	S65.419A
S62.224P	S62.302K	S62.328B	S62.353P	S62.399K	S62.610B	S62.635P	S62.661K	S65.491A
S62.225B	S62.302P	S62.328K	S62.354B	S62.399P	S62.610K	S62.636B	S62.661P	S65.492A
S62.225K	S62.303B	S62.328P	S62.354K	S62.501B	S62.610P	S62.636K	S62.662B	S65.499A
S62.225P	S62.303K	S62.329B	S62.354P	S62.501K	S62.611B	S62.636P	S62.662K	S65.500A
S62.226B	S62.303P	S62.329K	S62.355B	S62.501P	S62.611K	S62.637B	S62.662P	S65.501A
S62.226K	S62.304B	S62.329P	S62.355K	S62.502B	S62.611P	S62.637K	S62.663B	S65.502A
S62.226P	S62.304K	S62.330B	S62.355P	S62.502K	S62.612B	S62.637P	S62.663K	S65.503A
S62.231B	S62.304P	S62.330K	S62.356B	S62.502P	S62.612K	S62.638B	S62.663P	S65.504A
S62.231K	S62.305B	S62.330P	S62.356K	S62.509B	S62.612P	S62.638K	S62.664B	S65.505A
S62.231P	S62.305K	S62.331B	S62.356P	S62.509K	S62.613B	S62.638P	S62.664K	S65.506A
S62.232B	S62.305P	S62.331K	S62.357B	S62.509P	S62.613K	S62.639B	S62.664P	S65.507A
S62.232K	S62.306B	S62.331P	S62.357K	S62.511B	S62.613P	S62.639K	S62.665B	S65.508A
S62.232P	S62.306K	S62.332B	S62.357P	S62.511K	S62.614B	S62.639P	S62.665K	S65.509A
S62.233B	S62.306P	S62.332K	S62.358B	S62.511P	S62.614K	S62.640B	S62.665P	S65.510A
S62.233K	S62.307B	S62.332P	S62.358K	S62.512B	S62.614P	S62.640K	S62.666B	S65.511A
S62.233P	S62.307K	S62.333B	S62.358P	S62.512K	S62.615B	S62.640P	S62.666K	S65.512A
S62.234B	S62.307P	S62.333K	S62.359B	S62.512P	S62.615K	S62.641B	S62.666P	S65.513A
S62.234K	S62.308B	S62.333P	S62.359K	S62.513B	S62.615P	S62.641K	S62.667B	S65.514A
S62.234P	S62.308K	S62.334B	S62.359P	S62.513K	S62.616B	S62.641P	S62.667K	S65.515A
S62.235B	S62.308P	S62.334K	S62.360B	S62.513P	S62.616K	S62.642B	S62.667P	S65.516A
S62.235K	S62.309B	S62.334P	S62.360K	S62.514B	S62.616P	S62.642K	S62.668B	S65.517A
S62.235P	S62.309K	S62.335B	S62.360P	S62.514K	S62.617B	S62.642P	S62.668K	S65.518A
S62.236B	S62.309P	S62.335K	S62.361B	S62.514P	S62.617K	S62.643B	S62.668P	S65.519A
S62.236K	S62.310B	S62.335P	S62.361K	S62.515B	S62.617P	S62.643K	S62.669B	S65.590A
S62.236P	S62.310K	S62.336B	S62.361P	S62.515K	S62.618B	S62.643P	S62.669K	S65.591A
S62.241B	S62.310P	S62.336K	S62.362B	S62.515P	S62.618K	S62.644B	S62.669P	S65.592A
S62.241K	S62.311B	S62.336P	S62.362K	S62.516B	S62.618P	S62.644K	S62.90XB	S65.593A
S62.241P	S62.311K	S62.337B	S62.362P	S62.516K	S62.619B	S62.644P	S62.90XK	S65.594A
S62.242B	S62.311P	S62.337K	S62.363B	S62.516P	S62.619K	S62.645B	S62.90XP	S65.595A
S62.242K	S62.312B	S62.337P	S62.363K	S62.521B	S62.619P	S62.645K	S62.91XB	S65.596A
S62.242P	S62.312K	S62.338B	S62.363P	S62.521K	S62.620B	S62.645P	S62.91XK	S65.597A
S62.243B	S62.312P	S62.338K	S62.364B	S62.521P	S62.620K	S62.646B	S62.91XP	S65.598A
S62.243K	S62.313B	S62.338P	S62.364K	S62.522B	S62.620P	S62.646K	S62.92XB	S65.599A
S62.243P	S62.313K	S62.339B	S62.364P	S62.522K	S62.621B	S62.646P	S62.92XK	S65.801A
S62.244B	S62.313P	S62.339K	S62.365B	S62.522P	S62.621K	S62.647B	S62.92XP	S65.802A
S62.244K	S62.314B	S62.339P	S62.365K	S62.523B	S62.621P	S62.647K	S65.001A	S65.809A
S62.244P	S62.314K	S62.340B	S62.365P	S62.523K	S62.622B	S62.647P	S65.002A	S65.811A
S62.245B	S62.314P	S62.340K	S62.366B	S62.523P	S62.622K	S62.648B	S65.009A	S65.812A
S62.245K	S62.315B	S62.340P	S62.366K	S62.524B	S62.622P	S62.648K	S65.011A	S65.819A
S62.245P	S62.315K	S62.341B	S62.366P	S62.524K	S62.623B	S62.648P	S65.012A	S65.891A
S62.246B	S62.315P	S62.341K	S62.367B	S62.524P	S62.623K	S62.649B	S65.019A	S65.892A
S62.246K	S62.316B	S62.341P	S62.367K	S62.525B	S62.623P	S62.649K	S65.091A	S65.899A

Appendix F: Complication and Comorbidity (CC) Code List

S65.901A	S72.002R	S72.033Q	S72.061P	S72.112N	S72.133M	S72.24XK	S72.331R	S72.352Q
S65.902A	S72.009K	S72.033R	S72.061Q	S72.112P	S72.133N	S72.24XM	S72.332K	S72.352R
S65.909A	S72.009M	S72.034K	S72.061R	S72.112Q	S72.133P	S72.24XN	S72.332M	S72.353K
S65.911A	S72.009N	S72.034M	S72.062K	S72.112R	S72.133Q	S72.24XP	S72.332N	S72.353M
S65.912A	S72.009P	S72.034N	S72.062M	S72.113K	S72.133R	S72.24XQ	S72.332P	S72.353N
S65.919A	S72.009Q	S72.034P	S72.062N	S72.113M	S72.134K	S72.24XR	S72.332Q	S72.353P
S65.991A	S72.009R	S72.034Q	S72.062P	S72.113N	S72.134M	S72.25XK	S72.332R	S72.353Q
S65.992A	S72.011K	S72.034R	S72.062Q	S72.113P	S72.134N	S72.25XM	S72.333K	S72.353R
S65.999A	S72.011M	S72.035K	S72.062R	S72.113Q	S72.134P	S72.25XN	S72.333M	S72.354K
S66.021A	S72.011N	S72.035M	S72.063K	S72.113R	S72.134Q	S72.25XP	S72.333N	S72.354M
S66.022A	S72.011P	S72.035N	S72.063M	S72.114K	S72.134R	S72.25XQ	S72.333P	S72.354N
S66.029A	S72.011Q	S72.035P	S72.063N	S72.114M	S72.135K	S72.25XR	S72.333Q	S72.354P
S66.120A	S72.011R	S72.035Q	S72.063P	S72.114N	S72.135M	S72.26XK	S72.333R	S72.354Q
S66.121A	S72.012K	S72.035R	S72.063Q	S72.114P	S72.135N	S72.26XM	S72.334K	S72.354R
S66.122A	S72.012M	S72.036K	S72.063R	S72.114Q	S72.135P	S72.26XN	S72.334M	S72.355K
S66.123A	S72.012N	S72.036M	S72.064K	S72.114R	S72.135Q	S72.26XP	S72.334N	S72.355M
S66.124A	S72.012P	S72.036N	S72.064M	S72.115K	S72.135R	S72.26XQ	S72.334P	S72.355N
S66.125A	S72.012Q	S72.036P	S72.064N	S72.115M	S72.136K	S72.26XR	S72.334Q	S72.355P
S66.126A	S72.012R	S72.036Q	S72.064P	S72.115N	S72.136M	S72.301K	S72.334R	S72.355Q
S66.127A	S72.019K	S72.036R	S72.064Q	S72.115P	S72.136N	S72.301M	S72.335K	S72.355R
S66.128A	S72.019M	S72.041K	S72.064R	S72.115Q	S72.136P	S72.301N	S72.335M	S72.356K
S66.129A	S72.019N	S72.041M	S72.065K	S72.115R	S72.136Q	S72.301P	S72.335N	S72.356M
S66.221A	S72.019P	S72.041N	S72.065M	S72.116K	S72.136R	S72.301Q	S72.335P	S72.356N
S66.222A	S72.019Q	S72.041P	S72.065N	S72.116M	S72.141K	S72.301R	S72.335Q	S72.356P
S66.229A	S72.019R	S72.041Q	S72.065P	S72.116N	S72.141M	S72.302K	S72.335R	S72.356Q
S66.320A	S72.021K	S72.041R	S72.065Q	S72.116P	S72.141N	S72.302M	S72.336K	S72.356R
S66.321A	S72.021M	S72.042K	S72.065R	S72.116Q	S72.141P	S72.302N	S72.336M	S72.361K
S66.322A	S72.021N	S72.042M	S72.066K	S72.116R	S72.141Q	S72.302P	S72.336N	S72.361M
S66.323A	S72.021P	S72.042N	S72.066M	S72.121K	S72.141R	S72.302Q	S72.336P	S72.361N
S66.324A	S72.021Q	S72.042P	S72.066N	S72.121M	S72.142K	S72.302R	S72.336Q	S72.361P
S66.325A	S72.021R	S72.042Q	S72.066P	S72.121N	S72.142M	S72.309K	S72.336R	S72.361Q
S66.326A	S72.022K	S72.042R	S72.066Q	S72.121P	S72.142N	S72.309M	S72.341K	S72.361R
S66.327A	S72.022M	S72.043K	S72.066R	S72.121Q	S72.142P	S72.309N	S72.341M	S72.362K
S66.328A	S72.022N	S72.043M	S72.091K	S72.121R	S72.142Q	S72.309P	S72.341N	S72.362M
S66.329A	S72.022P	S72.043N	S72.091M	S72.122K	S72.142R	S72.309Q	S72.341P	S72.362N
S66.421A	S72.022Q	S72.043P	S72.091N	S72.122M	S72.143K	S72.309R	S72.341Q	S72.362P
S66.422A	S72.022R	S72.043Q	S72.091P	S72.122N	S72.143M	S72.321K	S72.341R	S72.362Q
S66.429A	S72.023K	S72.043R	S72.091Q	S72.122P	S72.143N	S72.321M	S72.342K	S72.362R
S66.520A	S72.023M	S72.044K	S72.091R	S72.122Q	S72.143P	S72.321N	S72.342M	S72.363K
S66.521A	S72.023N	S72.044M	S72.092K	S72.122R	S72.143Q	S72.321P	S72.342N	S72.363M
S66.522A	S72.023P	S72.044N	S72.092M	S72.123K	S72.143R	S72.321Q	S72.342P	S72.363N
S66.523A	S72.023Q	S72.044P	S72.092N	S72.123M	S72.144K	S72.321R	S72.342Q	S72.363P
S66.524A	S72.023R	S72.044Q	S72.092P	S72.123N	S72.144M	S72.322K	S72.342R	S72.363Q
S66.525A	S72.024K	S72.044R	S72.092Q	S72.123P	S72.144N	S72.322M	S72.343K	S72.363R
S66.526A	S72.024M	S72.045K	S72.092R	S72.123Q	S72.144P	S72.322N	S72.343M	S72.364K
S66.527A	S72.024N	S72.045M	S72.099K	S72.123R	S72.144Q	S72.322P	S72.343N	S72.364M
S66.528A	S72.024P	S72.045N	S72.099M	S72.124K	S72.144R	S72.322Q	S72.343P	S72.364N
S66.529A	S72.024Q	S72.045P	S72.099N	S72.124M	S72.145K	S72.322R	S72.343Q	S72.364P
S66.821A	S72.024R	S72.045Q	S72.099P	S72.124N	S72.145M	S72.323K	S72.343R	S72.364Q
S66.822A	S72.025K	S72.045R	S72.099Q	S72.124P	S72.145N	S72.323M	S72.344K	S72.364R
S66.829A	S72.025M	S72.046K	S72.099R	S72.124Q	S72.145P	S72.323N	S72.344M	S72.365K
S66.921A	S72.025N	S72.046M	S72.101K	S72.124R	S72.145Q	S72.323P	S72.344N	S72.365M
S66.922A	S72.025P	S72.046N	S72.101M	S72.125K	S72.145R	S72.323Q	S72.344P	S72.365N
S66.929A	S72.025Q	S72.046P	S72.101N	S72.125M	S72.146K	S72.323R	S72.344Q	S72.365P
S68.411A	S72.025R	S72.046Q	S72.101P	S72.125N	S72.146M	S72.324K	S72.344R	S72.365Q
S68.412A	S72.026K	S72.046R	S72.101Q	S72.125P	S72.146N	S72.324M	S72.345K	S72.365R
S68.419A	S72.026M	S72.051K	S72.101R	S72.125Q	S72.146P	S72.324N	S72.345M	S72.366K
S68.421A	S72.026N	S72.051M	S72.102K	S72.125R	S72.146Q	S72.324P	S72.345N	S72.366M
S68.422A	S72.026P	S72.051N	S72.102M	S72.126K	S72.146R	S72.324Q	S72.345P	S72.366N
S68.429A	S72.026Q	S72.051P	S72.102N	S72.126M	S72.21XK	S72.324R	S72.345Q	S72.366P
S68.711A	S72.026R	S72.051Q	S72.102P	S72.126N	S72.21XM	S72.325K	S72.345R	S72.366Q
S68.712A	S72.031K	S72.051R	S72.102Q	S72.126P	S72.21XN	S72.325M	S72.346K	S72.366R
S68.719A	S72.031M	S72.052K	S72.102R	S72.126Q	S72.21XP	S72.325N	S72.346M	S72.391K
S68.721A	S72.031N	S72.052M	S72.109K	S72.126R	S72.21XQ	S72.325P	S72.346N	S72.391M
S68.722A	S72.031P	S72.052N	S72.109M	S72.131K	S72.21XR	S72.325Q	S72.346P	S72.391N
S68.729A	S72.031Q	S72.052P	S72.109N	S72.131M	S72.22XK	S72.325R	S72.346Q	S72.391P
S72.001K	S72.031R	S72.052Q	S72.109P	S72.131N	S72.22XM	S72.326K	S72.346R	S72.391Q
S72.001M	S72.032K	S72.052R	S72.109Q	S72.131P	S72.22XN	S72.326M	S72.351K	S72.391R
S72.001N	S72.032M	S72.059K	S72.109R	S72.131Q	S72.22XP	S72.326N	S72.351M	S72.392K
S72.001P	S72.032N	S72.059M	S72.111K	S72.131R	S72.22XQ	S72.326P	S72.351N	S72.392M
S72.001Q	S72.032P	S72.059N	S72.111M	S72.132K	S72.22XR	S72.326Q	S72.351P	S72.392N
S72.001R	S72.032Q	S72.059P	S72.111N	S72.132M	S72.23XK	S72.326R	S72.351Q	S72.392P
S72.002K	S72.032R	S72.059Q	S72.111P	S72.132N	S72.23XM	S72.331K	S72.351R	S72.392Q
S72.002M	S72.033K	S72.059R	S72.111Q	S72.132P	S72.23XN	S72.331M	S72.352K	S72.392R
S72.002N	S72.033M	S72.061K	S72.111R	S72.132Q	S72.23XP	S72.331N	S72.352M	S72.399K
S72.002P	S72.033N	S72.061M	S72.112K	S72.132R	S72.23XQ	S72.331P	S72.352N	S72.399M
S72.002Q	S72.033P	S72.061N	S72.112M	S72.133K	S72.23XR	S72.331Q	S72.352P	S72.399N

S72.399P	S72.422P	S72.441P	S72.456P	S72.8X1N	S75.802A	S79.101A	S82.009N	S82.023B
S72.399Q	S72.422Q	S72.441Q	S72.456Q	S72.8X1P	S75.809A	S79.101K	S82.009P	S82.023C
S72.399R	S72.422R	S72.441R	S72.456R	S72.8X1Q	S75.811A	S79.101P	S82.009Q	S82.023K
S72.401A	S72.423A	S72.442A	S72.461A	S72.8X1R	S75.812A	S79.102A	S82.009R	S82.023M
S72.401K	S72.423K	S72.442K	S72.461K	S72.8X2K	S75.819A	S79.102K	S82.011A	S82.023N
S72.401M	S72.423M	S72.442M	S72.461M	S72.8X2M	S75.891A	S79.102P	S82.011B	S82.023P
S72.401N	S72.423N	S72.442N	S72.461N	S72.8X2N	S75.892A	S79.109A	S82.011C	S82.023Q
S72.401P	S72.423P	S72.442P	S72.461P	S72.8X2P	S75.899A	S79.109K	S82.011K	S82.023R
S72.401Q	S72.423Q	S72.442Q	S72.461Q	S72.8X2Q	S75.901A	S79.109P	S82.011M	S82.024A
S72.401R	S72.423R	S72.442R	S72.461R	S72.8X2R	S75.902A	S79.111A	S82.011N	S82.024B
S72.402A	S72.424A	S72.443A	S72.462A	S72.8X9K	S75.909A	S79.111K	S82.011P	S82.024C
S72.402K	S72.424K	S72.443K	S72.462K	S72.8X9N	S75.911A	S79.111P	S82.011Q	S82.024K
S72.402M	S72.424M	S72.443M	S72.462M	S72.8X9P	S75.912A	S79.112A	S82.011R	S82.024M
S72.402N	S72.424N	S72.443N	S72.462N	S72.8X9Q	S75.919A	S79.112K	S82.012A	S82.024N
S72.402P	S72.424P	S72.443P	S72.462P	S72.8X9R	S75.991A	S79.112P	S82.012B	S82.024P
S72.402Q	S72.424Q	S72.443Q	S72.462Q	S72.90XK	S75.992A	S79.119A	S82.012C	S82.024Q
S72.402R	S72.424R	S72.443R	S72.462R	S72.90XM	S75.999A	S79.119K	S82.012K	S82.024R
S72.409A	S72.425A	S72.444A	S72.463A	S72.90XN	S76.021A	S79.119P	S82.012M	S82.025A
S72.409K	S72.425K	S72.444K	S72.463K	S72.90XP	S76.022A	S79.121A	S82.012N	S82.025B
S72.409M	S72.425M	S72.444M	S72.463M	S72.90XQ	S76.029A	S79.121K	S82.012P	S82.025C
S72.409N	S72.425N	S72.444N	S72.463N	S72.90XR	S76.121A	S79.121P	S82.012Q	S82.025K
S72.409P	S72.425P	S72.444P	S72.463P	S72.91XK	S76.122A	S79.122A	S82.012R	S82.025M
S72.409Q	S72.425Q	S72.444Q	S72.463Q	S72.91XM	S76.129A	S79.122K	S82.013A	S82.025N
S72.409R	S72.425R	S72.444R	S72.463R	S72.91XN	S76.221A	S79.122P	S82.013B	S82.025P
S72.411A	S72.426A	S72.445A	S72.464A	S72.91XP	S76.222A	S79.129A	S82.013C	S82.025Q
S72.411K	S72.426K	S72.445K	S72.464K	S72.91XQ	S76.229A	S79.129K	S82.013K	S82.025R
S72.411M	S72.426M	S72.445M	S72.464M	S72.91XR	S76.321A	S79.129P	S82.013M	S82.026A
S72.411N	S72.426N	S72.445N	S72.464N	S72.92XK	S76.322A	S79.131A	S82.013N	S82.026B
S72.411P	S72.426P	S72.445P	S72.464P	S72.92XM	S76.329A	S79.131K	S82.013P	S82.026C
S72.411Q	S72.426Q	S72.445Q	S72.464Q	S72.92XN	S76.821A	S79.131P	S82.013Q	S82.026K
S72.411R	S72.426R	S72.445R	S72.464R	S72.92XP	S76.822A	S79.132A	S82.013R	S82.026M
S72.412A	S72.431A	S72.446A	S72.465A	S72.92XQ	S76.829A	S79.132K	S82.014A	S82.026N
S72.412K	S72.431K	S72.446K	S72.465K	S72.92XR	S76.921A	S79.132P	S82.014B	S82.026P
S72.412M	S72.431M	S72.446M	S72.465M	S73.001A	S76.922A	S79.139A	S82.014C	S82.026Q
S72.412N	S72.431N	S72.446N	S72.465N	S73.002A	S76.929A	S79.139K	S82.014K	S82.026R
S72.412P	S72.431P	S72.446P	S72.465P	S73.003A	S77.00XA	S79.139P	S82.014M	S82.031A
S72.412Q	S72.431Q	S72.446Q	S72.465Q	S73.004A	S77.01XA	S79.141A	S82.014N	S82.031B
S72.412R	S72.431R	S72.446R	S72.465R	S73.005A	S77.02XA	S79.141K	S82.014P	S82.031C
S72.413A	S72.432A	S72.451A	S72.466A	S73.006A	S77.10XA	S79.141P	S82.014Q	S82.031K
S72.413K	S72.432K	S72.451K	S72.466K	S73.011A	S77.11XA	S79.142A	S82.014R	S82.031M
S72.413M	S72.432M	S72.451M	S72.466M	S73.012A	S77.12XA	S79.142K	S82.015A	S82.031N
S72.413N	S72.432N	S72.451N	S72.466N	S73.013A	S78.011A	S79.142P	S82.015B	S82.031P
S72.413P	S72.432P	S72.451P	S72.466P	S73.014A	S78.012A	S79.149A	S82.015C	S82.031Q
S72.413Q	S72.432Q	S72.451Q	S72.466Q	S73.015A	S78.019A	S79.149K	S82.015K	S82.031R
S72.413R	S72.432R	S72.451R	S72.466R	S73.016A	S78.021A	S79.149P	S82.015M	S82.032A
S72.414A	S72.433A	S72.452A	S72.471A	S73.021A	S78.022A	S79.191A	S82.015N	S82.032B
S72.414K	S72.433K	S72.452K	S72.471K	S73.022A	S78.029A	S79.191K	S82.015P	S82.032C
S72.414M	S72.433M	S72.452M	S72.471P	S73.023A	S78.111A	S79.191P	S82.015Q	S82.032K
S72.414N	S72.433N	S72.452N	S72.472A	S73.024A	S78.112A	S79.192A	S82.015R	S82.032M
S72.414P	S72.433P	S72.452P	S72.472K	S73.025A	S78.119A	S79.192K	S82.016A	S82.032N
S72.414Q	S72.433Q	S72.452Q	S72.472P	S73.026A	S78.121A	S79.192P	S82.016B	S82.032P
S72.414R	S72.433R	S72.452R	S72.479A	S73.031A	S78.122A	S79.199A	S82.016C	S82.032Q
S72.415A	S72.434A	S72.453A	S72.479K	S73.032A	S78.129A	S79.199K	S82.016K	S82.032R
S72.415K	S72.434K	S72.453K	S72.479P	S73.033A	S78.911A	S79.199P	S82.016M	S82.033A
S72.415M	S72.434M	S72.453M	S72.491A	S73.034A	S78.912A	S82.001A	S82.016N	S82.033B
S72.415N	S72.434N	S72.453N	S72.491K	S73.035A	S78.919A	S82.001B	S82.016P	S82.033C
S72.415P	S72.434P	S72.453P	S72.491M	S73.036A	S78.921A	S82.001C	S82.016Q	S82.033K
S72.415Q	S72.434Q	S72.453Q	S72.491N	S73.041A	S78.922A	S82.001K	S82.016R	S82.033M
S72.415R	S72.434R	S72.453R	S72.491P	S73.042A	S78.929A	S82.001M	S82.021A	S82.033N
S72.416A	S72.435A	S72.454A	S72.491Q	S73.043A	S79.001K	S82.001N	S82.021B	S82.033P
S72.416K	S72.435K	S72.454K	S72.491R	S73.044A	S79.001P	S82.001P	S82.021C	S82.033Q
S72.416M	S72.435M	S72.454M	S72.492A	S73.045A	S79.002K	S82.001Q	S82.021K	S82.033R
S72.416N	S72.435N	S72.454N	S72.492K	S73.046A	S79.002P	S82.001R	S82.021M	S82.034A
S72.416P	S72.435P	S72.454P	S72.492M	S75.201A	S79.009K	S82.002A	S82.021N	S82.034B
S72.416Q	S72.435Q	S72.454Q	S72.492N	S75.202A	S79.009P	S82.002B	S82.021P	S82.034C
S72.416R	S72.435R	S72.454R	S72.492P	S75.209A	S79.011K	S82.002C	S82.021Q	S82.034K
S72.421A	S72.436A	S72.455A	S72.492Q	S75.211A	S79.011P	S82.002K	S82.021R	S82.034M
S72.421K	S72.436K	S72.455K	S72.492R	S75.212A	S79.012K	S82.002M	S82.022A	S82.034N
S72.421M	S72.436M	S72.455M	S72.499A	S75.219A	S79.012P	S82.002N	S82.022B	S82.034P
S72.421N	S72.436N	S72.455N	S72.499K	S75.221A	S79.019K	S82.002P	S82.022C	S82.034Q
S72.421P	S72.436P	S72.455P	S72.499M	S75.222A	S79.019P	S82.002Q	S82.022K	S82.034R
S72.421Q	S72.436Q	S72.455Q	S72.499N	S75.229A	S79.091K	S82.002R	S82.022M	S82.035A
S72.421R	S72.436R	S72.455R	S72.499P	S75.291A	S79.091P	S82.009A	S82.022N	S82.035B
S72.422A	S72.441A	S72.456A	S72.499Q	S75.292A	S79.092K	S82.009B	S82.022P	S82.035C
S72.422K	S72.441K	S72.456K	S72.499R	S75.299A	S79.092P	S82.009C	S82.022Q	S82.035K
S72.422M	S72.441M	S72.456M	S72.8X1K	S75.801A	S79.099K	S82.009K	S82.022R	S82.035M
S72.422N	S72.441N	S72.456N	S72.8X1M	S75.802A	S79.099P	S82.009M	S82.023A	S82.035N

Appendix F: Complication and Comorbidity (CC) Code List

S82.035P	S82.092C	S82.116Q	S82.135Q	S82.154Q	S82.222N	S82.241N	S82.256N	S82.302K
S82.035Q	S82.092K	S82.116R	S82.135R	S82.154R	S82.222P	S82.241P	S82.256P	S82.302M
S82.035R	S82.092M	S82.121A	S82.136A	S82.155A	S82.222Q	S82.241Q	S82.256Q	S82.302N
S82.036A	S82.092N	S82.121K	S82.136K	S82.155K	S82.222R	S82.241R	S82.256R	S82.302P
S82.036B	S82.092P	S82.121M	S82.136M	S82.155M	S82.223A	S82.242A	S82.261A	S82.302Q
S82.036C	S82.092Q	S82.121N	S82.136N	S82.155N	S82.223K	S82.242K	S82.261K	S82.302R
S82.036K	S82.092R	S82.121P	S82.136P	S82.155P	S82.223M	S82.242M	S82.261M	S82.309B
S82.036M	S82.099A	S82.121Q	S82.136Q	S82.155Q	S82.223N	S82.242N	S82.261N	S82.309C
S82.036N	S82.099B	S82.121R	S82.136R	S82.155R	S82.223P	S82.242P	S82.261P	S82.309K
S82.036P	S82.099C	S82.122A	S82.141A	S82.156A	S82.223Q	S82.242Q	S82.261Q	S82.309M
S82.036Q	S82.099K	S82.122K	S82.141K	S82.156K	S82.223R	S82.242R	S82.261R	S82.309N
S82.036R	S82.099M	S82.122M	S82.141M	S82.156M	S82.224A	S82.243A	S82.262A	S82.309P
S82.041A	S82.099N	S82.122N	S82.141N	S82.156N	S82.224K	S82.243K	S82.262K	S82.309Q
S82.041B	S82.099P	S82.122P	S82.141P	S82.156P	S82.224M	S82.243M	S82.262M	S82.309R
S82.041C	S82.099Q	S82.122Q	S82.141Q	S82.156Q	S82.224N	S82.243N	S82.262N	S82.311A
S82.041K	S82.099R	S82.122R	S82.141R	S82.156R	S82.224P	S82.243P	S82.262P	S82.311K
S82.041M	S82.101A	S82.123A	S82.142A	S82.161A	S82.224Q	S82.243Q	S82.262Q	S82.311P
S82.041N	S82.101K	S82.123K	S82.142K	S82.161K	S82.224R	S82.243R	S82.262R	S82.312A
S82.041P	S82.101M	S82.123M	S82.142M	S82.161P	S82.225A	S82.244A	S82.263A	S82.312K
S82.041Q	S82.101N	S82.123N	S82.142N	S82.162A	S82.225K	S82.244K	S82.263K	S82.312P
S82.041R	S82.101P	S82.123P	S82.142P	S82.162K	S82.225M	S82.244M	S82.263M	S82.319A
S82.042A	S82.101Q	S82.123Q	S82.142Q	S82.162P	S82.225N	S82.244N	S82.263N	S82.319K
S82.042B	S82.101R	S82.123R	S82.142R	S82.169A	S82.225P	S82.244P	S82.263P	S82.319P
S82.042C	S82.102A	S82.124A	S82.143A	S82.169K	S82.225Q	S82.244Q	S82.263Q	S82.391B
S82.042K	S82.102K	S82.124K	S82.143K	S82.169P	S82.225R	S82.244R	S82.263R	S82.391C
S82.042M	S82.102M	S82.124M	S82.143M	S82.191A	S82.226A	S82.245A	S82.264A	S82.391K
S82.042N	S82.102N	S82.124N	S82.143N	S82.191K	S82.226K	S82.245K	S82.264K	S82.391M
S82.042P	S82.102P	S82.124P	S82.143P	S82.191M	S82.226M	S82.245M	S82.264M	S82.391N
S82.042Q	S82.102Q	S82.124Q	S82.143Q	S82.191N	S82.226N	S82.245N	S82.264N	S82.391P
S82.042R	S82.102R	S82.124R	S82.143R	S82.191P	S82.226P	S82.245P	S82.264P	S82.391Q
S82.043A	S82.109A	S82.125A	S82.144A	S82.191Q	S82.226Q	S82.245Q	S82.264Q	S82.391R
S82.043B	S82.109K	S82.125K	S82.144K	S82.191R	S82.226R	S82.245R	S82.264R	S82.392B
S82.043C	S82.109M	S82.125M	S82.144M	S82.192A	S82.231A	S82.246A	S82.265A	S82.392C
S82.043K	S82.109N	S82.125N	S82.144N	S82.192K	S82.231K	S82.246K	S82.265K	S82.392K
S82.043M	S82.109P	S82.125P	S82.144P	S82.192M	S82.231M	S82.246M	S82.265M	S82.392M
S82.043N	S82.109Q	S82.125Q	S82.144Q	S82.192N	S82.231N	S82.246N	S82.265N	S82.392N
S82.043P	S82.109R	S82.125R	S82.144R	S82.192P	S82.231P	S82.246P	S82.265P	S82.392P
S82.043Q	S82.111A	S82.126A	S82.145A	S82.192Q	S82.231Q	S82.246Q	S82.265Q	S82.392Q
S82.043R	S82.111K	S82.126K	S82.145K	S82.192R	S82.231R	S82.246R	S82.265R	S82.392R
S82.044A	S82.111M	S82.126M	S82.145M	S82.199A	S82.232A	S82.251A	S82.266A	S82.399B
S82.044B	S82.111N	S82.126N	S82.145N	S82.199K	S82.232K	S82.251K	S82.266K	S82.399C
S82.044C	S82.111P	S82.126P	S82.145P	S82.199M	S82.232M	S82.251M	S82.266M	S82.399K
S82.044K	S82.111Q	S82.126Q	S82.145Q	S82.199N	S82.232N	S82.251N	S82.266N	S82.399M
S82.044M	S82.111R	S82.126R	S82.145R	S82.199P	S82.232P	S82.251P	S82.266P	S82.399N
S82.044N	S82.112A	S82.131A	S82.146A	S82.199Q	S82.232Q	S82.251Q	S82.266Q	S82.399P
S82.044P	S82.112K	S82.131K	S82.146K	S82.199R	S82.232R	S82.251R	S82.266R	S82.399Q
S82.044Q	S82.112M	S82.131M	S82.146M	S82.201A	S82.233A	S82.252A	S82.291A	S82.399R
S82.044R	S82.112N	S82.131N	S82.146N	S82.201K	S82.233K	S82.252K	S82.291K	S82.401K
S82.045A	S82.112P	S82.131P	S82.146P	S82.201M	S82.233M	S82.252M	S82.291M	S82.401M
S82.045B	S82.112Q	S82.131Q	S82.146Q	S82.201N	S82.233N	S82.252N	S82.291N	S82.401N
S82.045C	S82.112R	S82.131R	S82.146R	S82.201P	S82.233P	S82.252P	S82.291P	S82.401P
S82.045K	S82.113A	S82.132A	S82.151A	S82.201Q	S82.233Q	S82.252Q	S82.291Q	S82.401Q
S82.045M	S82.113K	S82.132K	S82.151K	S82.201R	S82.233R	S82.252R	S82.291R	S82.401R
S82.045N	S82.113M	S82.132M	S82.151M	S82.202A	S82.234A	S82.253A	S82.292A	S82.402K
S82.045P	S82.113N	S82.132N	S82.151N	S82.202K	S82.234K	S82.253K	S82.292K	S82.402M
S82.045Q	S82.113P	S82.132P	S82.151P	S82.202M	S82.234M	S82.253M	S82.292M	S82.402N
S82.045R	S82.113Q	S82.132Q	S82.151Q	S82.202N	S82.234N	S82.253N	S82.292N	S82.402P
S82.046A	S82.113R	S82.132R	S82.151R	S82.202P	S82.234P	S82.253P	S82.292P	S82.402Q
S82.046B	S82.114A	S82.133A	S82.152A	S82.202Q	S82.234Q	S82.253Q	S82.292Q	S82.402R
S82.046C	S82.114K	S82.133K	S82.152K	S82.202R	S82.234R	S82.253R	S82.292R	S82.409K
S82.046K	S82.114M	S82.133M	S82.152M	S82.209A	S82.235A	S82.254A	S82.299A	S82.409M
S82.046M	S82.114N	S82.133N	S82.152N	S82.209K	S82.235K	S82.254K	S82.299K	S82.409N
S82.046N	S82.114P	S82.133P	S82.152P	S82.209M	S82.235M	S82.254M	S82.299M	S82.409P
S82.046P	S82.114Q	S82.133Q	S82.152Q	S82.209N	S82.235N	S82.254N	S82.299N	S82.409Q
S82.046Q	S82.114R	S82.133R	S82.152R	S82.209P	S82.235P	S82.254P	S82.299P	S82.409R
S82.046R	S82.115A	S82.134A	S82.153A	S82.209Q	S82.235Q	S82.254Q	S82.299Q	S82.421K
S82.091A	S82.115K	S82.134K	S82.153K	S82.209R	S82.235R	S82.254R	S82.299R	S82.421M
S82.091B	S82.115M	S82.134M	S82.153M	S82.221A	S82.236A	S82.255A	S82.301B	S82.421N
S82.091C	S82.115N	S82.134N	S82.153N	S82.221K	S82.236K	S82.255K	S82.301C	S82.421P
S82.091K	S82.115P	S82.134P	S82.153P	S82.221M	S82.236M	S82.255M	S82.301K	S82.421Q
S82.091M	S82.115Q	S82.134Q	S82.153Q	S82.221N	S82.236N	S82.255N	S82.301M	S82.421R
S82.091N	S82.115R	S82.134R	S82.153R	S82.221P	S82.236P	S82.255P	S82.301N	S82.422K
S82.091P	S82.116A	S82.135A	S82.154A	S82.221Q	S82.236Q	S82.255Q	S82.301P	S82.422M
S82.091Q	S82.116K	S82.135K	S82.154K	S82.221R	S82.236R	S82.255R	S82.301Q	S82.422N
S82.091R	S82.116M	S82.135M	S82.154M	S82.222A	S82.241A	S82.256A	S82.301R	S82.422P
S82.092A	S82.116N	S82.135N	S82.154N	S82.222K	S82.241K	S82.256K	S82.302B	S82.422Q
S82.092B	S82.116P	S82.135P	S82.154P	S82.222M	S82.241M	S82.256M	S82.302C	S82.422R

S82.423K	S82.443R	S82.464Q	S82.56XP	S82.839N	S82.854C	S82.873K	S82.92XR	S86.122A
S82.423M	S82.444K	S82.464R	S82.56XQ	S82.839P	S82.854K	S82.873M	S85.101A	S86.129A
S82.423N	S82.444M	S82.465K	S82.56XR	S82.839Q	S82.854M	S82.873N	S85.102A	S86.221A
S82.423P	S82.444N	S82.465M	S82.61XB	S82.839R	S82.854N	S82.873P	S85.109A	S86.222A
S82.423Q	S82.444P	S82.465N	S82.61XC	S82.841B	S82.854P	S82.873Q	S85.111A	S86.229A
S82.423R	S82.444Q	S82.465P	S82.61XK	S82.841C	S82.854Q	S82.873R	S85.112A	S86.321A
S82.424K	S82.444R	S82.465Q	S82.61XM	S82.841K	S82.854R	S82.874B	S85.119A	S86.322A
S82.424M	S82.445K	S82.465R	S82.61XN	S82.841M	S82.855B	S82.874C	S85.121A	S86.329A
S82.424N	S82.445M	S82.466K	S82.61XP	S82.841N	S82.855C	S82.874K	S85.122A	S86.821A
S82.424P	S82.445N	S82.466M	S82.61XQ	S82.841P	S82.855K	S82.874M	S85.129A	S86.822A
S82.424Q	S82.445P	S82.466N	S82.61XR	S82.841Q	S82.855M	S82.874N	S85.131A	S86.829A
S82.424R	S82.445Q	S82.466P	S82.62XB	S82.841R	S82.855N	S82.874P	S85.132A	S86.921A
S82.425K	S82.445R	S82.466Q	S82.62XC	S82.842B	S82.855P	S82.874Q	S85.139A	S86.922A
S82.425M	S82.446K	S82.466R	S82.62XK	S82.842C	S82.855Q	S82.874R	S85.141A	S86.929A
S82.425N	S82.446M	S82.491K	S82.62XM	S82.842K	S82.855R	S82.875B	S85.142A	S88.011A
S82.425P	S82.446N	S82.491M	S82.62XN	S82.842M	S82.856B	S82.875C	S85.149A	S88.012A
S82.425Q	S82.446P	S82.491N	S82.62XP	S82.842N	S82.856C	S82.875K	S85.151A	S88.019A
S82.425R	S82.446Q	S82.491P	S82.62XQ	S82.842P	S82.856K	S82.875M	S85.152A	S88.021A
S82.426K	S82.446R	S82.491Q	S82.62XR	S82.842Q	S82.856M	S82.875N	S85.159A	S88.022A
S82.426M	S82.451K	S82.491R	S82.63XB	S82.842R	S82.856N	S82.875P	S85.161A	S88.029A
S82.426N	S82.451M	S82.492K	S82.63XC	S82.843B	S82.856P	S82.875Q	S85.162A	S88.111A
S82.426P	S82.451N	S82.492M	S82.63XK	S82.843C	S82.856Q	S82.875R	S85.169A	S88.112A
S82.426Q	S82.451P	S82.492N	S82.63XM	S82.843K	S82.856R	S82.876B	S85.171A	S88.119A
S82.426R	S82.451Q	S82.492P	S82.63XN	S82.843M	S82.861K	S82.876C	S85.172A	S88.121A
S82.431K	S82.451R	S82.492Q	S82.63XP	S82.843N	S82.861M	S82.876K	S85.179A	S88.122A
S82.431M	S82.452K	S82.492R	S82.63XQ	S82.843P	S82.861N	S82.876M	S85.181A	S88.129A
S82.431N	S82.452M	S82.499K	S82.63XR	S82.843Q	S82.861P	S82.876N	S85.182A	S88.911A
S82.431P	S82.452N	S82.499M	S82.64XB	S82.843R	S82.861Q	S82.876P	S85.189A	S88.912A
S82.431Q	S82.452P	S82.499N	S82.64XC	S82.844B	S82.861R	S82.876Q	S85.201A	S88.919A
S82.431R	S82.452Q	S82.499P	S82.64XK	S82.844C	S82.862K	S82.876R	S85.202A	S88.921A
S82.432K	S82.452R	S82.499Q	S82.64XM	S82.844K	S82.862M	S82.891B	S85.209A	S88.922A
S82.432M	S82.453K	S82.499R	S82.64XN	S82.844M	S82.862N	S82.891C	S85.211A	S88.929A
S82.432N	S82.453M	S82.51XB	S82.64XP	S82.844N	S82.862P	S82.891K	S85.212A	S89.001A
S82.432P	S82.453N	S82.51XC	S82.64XQ	S82.844P	S82.862Q	S82.891M	S85.219A	S89.001K
S82.432Q	S82.453P	S82.51XK	S82.64XR	S82.844Q	S82.862R	S82.891N	S85.291A	S89.001P
S82.432R	S82.453Q	S82.51XM	S82.65XB	S82.844R	S82.863K	S82.891P	S85.292A	S89.002A
S82.433K	S82.453R	S82.51XN	S82.65XC	S82.845B	S82.863M	S82.891Q	S85.299A	S89.002K
S82.433M	S82.454K	S82.51XP	S82.65XK	S82.845C	S82.863N	S82.891R	S85.301A	S89.002P
S82.433N	S82.454M	S82.51XQ	S82.65XM	S82.845K	S82.863P	S82.892B	S85.302A	S89.009A
S82.433P	S82.454N	S82.51XR	S82.65XN	S82.845M	S82.863Q	S82.892C	S85.309A	S89.009K
S82.433Q	S82.454P	S82.52XB	S82.65XP	S82.845N	S82.863R	S82.892K	S85.311A	S89.009P
S82.433R	S82.454Q	S82.52XC	S82.65XQ	S82.845P	S82.864K	S82.892M	S85.312A	S89.011A
S82.434K	S82.454R	S82.52XK	S82.65XR	S82.845Q	S82.864M	S82.892N	S85.319A	S89.011K
S82.434M	S82.455K	S82.52XM	S82.66XB	S82.845R	S82.864N	S82.892P	S85.391A	S89.011P
S82.434N	S82.455M	S82.52XN	S82.66XC	S82.846B	S82.864P	S82.892Q	S85.392A	S89.012A
S82.434P	S82.455N	S82.52XP	S82.66XK	S82.846C	S82.864Q	S82.892R	S85.399A	S89.012K
S82.434Q	S82.455P	S82.52XQ	S82.66XM	S82.846K	S82.864R	S82.899B	S85.401A	S89.012P
S82.434R	S82.455Q	S82.52XR	S82.66XN	S82.846M	S82.865K	S82.899C	S85.402A	S89.019A
S82.435K	S82.455R	S82.53XB	S82.66XP	S82.846N	S82.865M	S82.899K	S85.409A	S89.019K
S82.435M	S82.456K	S82.53XC	S82.66XQ	S82.846P	S82.865N	S82.899M	S85.411A	S89.019P
S82.435N	S82.456M	S82.53XK	S82.66XR	S82.846Q	S82.865P	S82.899N	S85.412A	S89.021A
S82.435P	S82.456N	S82.53XM	S82.811K	S82.846R	S82.865Q	S82.899P	S85.419A	S89.021K
S82.435Q	S82.456P	S82.53XN	S82.811P	S82.851B	S82.865R	S82.899Q	S85.491A	S89.021P
S82.435R	S82.456Q	S82.53XP	S82.812K	S82.851C	S82.866K	S82.899R	S85.492A	S89.022A
S82.436K	S82.456R	S82.53XQ	S82.812P	S82.851K	S82.866M	S82.90XB	S85.499A	S89.022K
S82.436M	S82.461K	S82.53XR	S82.819K	S82.851M	S82.866N	S82.90XC	S85.801A	S89.022P
S82.436N	S82.461M	S82.54XB	S82.819P	S82.851N	S82.866P	S82.90XK	S85.802A	S89.029A
S82.436P	S82.461N	S82.54XC	S82.821K	S82.851P	S82.866Q	S82.90XM	S85.809A	S89.029K
S82.436Q	S82.461P	S82.54XK	S82.821P	S82.851Q	S82.866R	S82.90XN	S85.811A	S89.029P
S82.436R	S82.461Q	S82.54XM	S82.822K	S82.851R	S82.871B	S82.90XP	S85.812A	S89.031A
S82.441K	S82.461R	S82.54XN	S82.822P	S82.852B	S82.871C	S82.90XQ	S85.819A	S89.031K
S82.441M	S82.462K	S82.54XP	S82.829K	S82.852C	S82.871K	S82.90XR	S85.891A	S89.031P
S82.441N	S82.462M	S82.54XQ	S82.829P	S82.852K	S82.871M	S82.91XB	S85.892A	S89.032A
S82.441P	S82.462N	S82.54XR	S82.831K	S82.852M	S82.871N	S82.91XC	S85.899A	S89.032K
S82.441Q	S82.462P	S82.55XB	S82.831M	S82.852N	S82.871P	S82.91XK	S85.901A	S89.032P
S82.441R	S82.462Q	S82.55XC	S82.831N	S82.852P	S82.871Q	S82.91XM	S85.902A	S89.039A
S82.442K	S82.462R	S82.55XK	S82.831P	S82.852Q	S82.871R	S82.91XN	S85.909A	S89.039K
S82.442M	S82.463K	S82.55XM	S82.831Q	S82.852R	S82.872B	S82.91XP	S85.911A	S89.039P
S82.442N	S82.463M	S82.55XN	S82.831R	S82.853B	S82.872C	S82.91XQ	S85.912A	S89.041A
S82.442P	S82.463N	S82.55XP	S82.832K	S82.853C	S82.872K	S82.91XR	S85.919A	S89.041K
S82.442Q	S82.463P	S82.55XQ	S82.832M	S82.853K	S82.872M	S82.92XB	S85.991A	S89.041P
S82.442R	S82.463Q	S82.55XR	S82.832N	S82.853M	S82.872N	S82.92XC	S85.992A	S89.042A
S82.443K	S82.463R	S82.56XB	S82.832P	S82.853N	S82.872P	S82.92XK	S85.999A	S89.042K
S82.443M	S82.464K	S82.56XC	S82.832Q	S82.853P	S82.872Q	S82.92XM	S86.021A	S89.042P
S82.443N	S82.464M	S82.56XK	S82.832R	S82.853Q	S82.872R	S82.92XN	S86.022A	S89.049A
S82.443P	S82.464N	S82.56XM	S82.839K	S82.853R	S82.873B	S82.92XP	S86.029A	S89.049K
S82.443Q	S82.464P	S82.56XN	S82.839M	S82.854B	S82.873C	S82.92XQ	S86.121A	S89.049P

S89.091A	S89.312K	S92.036K	S92.115B	S92.156P	S92.242K	S92.331B	S92.416P	S92.902K
S89.091K	S89.312P	S92.036P	S92.115K	S92.191B	S92.242P	S92.331K	S92.421K	S92.902P
S89.091P	S89.319K	S92.041B	S92.115P	S92.191K	S92.243B	S92.331P	S92.421P	S92.909B
S89.092A	S89.319P	S92.041K	S92.116B	S92.191P	S92.243P	S92.332K	S92.422K	S92.909P
S89.092K	S89.321K	S92.041P	S92.116K	S92.192B	S92.244B	S92.332P	S92.422P	S92.911K
S89.092P	S89.321P	S92.042B	S92.116P	S92.192K	S92.244K	S92.333B	S92.423K	S92.911P
S89.099A	S89.322K	S92.042K	S92.121B	S92.192P	S92.244P	S92.333K	S92.423P	S92.912K
S89.099K	S89.322P	S92.042P	S92.121K	S92.199B	S92.245B	S92.333P	S92.424K	S92.912P
S89.099P	S89.329K	S92.043B	S92.121P	S92.199K	S92.245K	S92.334K	S92.424P	S92.919K
S89.101K	S89.329P	S92.043K	S92.122B	S92.199P	S92.245P	S92.334K	S92.425K	S92.919P
S89.101P	S89.391K	S92.043P	S92.122K	S92.201B	S92.246B	S92.334P	S92.425P	S95.001A
S89.102K	S89.391P	S92.044B	S92.122P	S92.201K	S92.246K	S92.335B	S92.426K	S95.002A
S89.102P	S89.392K	S92.044K	S92.123B	S92.201P	S92.246P	S92.335K	S92.426P	S95.009A
S89.109K	S89.392P	S92.044P	S92.123K	S92.202B	S92.251B	S92.335P	S92.491K	S95.011A
S89.109P	S89.399K	S92.045B	S92.123P	S92.202K	S92.251K	S92.336B	S92.491P	S95.012A
S89.111K	S89.399P	S92.045K	S92.124B	S92.202P	S92.251P	S92.336K	S92.492K	S95.019A
S89.111P	S92.001K	S92.045P	S92.124K	S92.209B	S92.252B	S92.336P	S92.492P	S95.091A
S89.112K	S92.001P	S92.046B	S92.124P	S92.209K	S92.252K	S92.341B	S92.499K	S95.092A
S89.112P	S92.002B	S92.046K	S92.125B	S92.209P	S92.252P	S92.341K	S92.499P	S95.099A
S89.119K	S92.002K	S92.046P	S92.125K	S92.211B	S92.253B	S92.341P	S92.501K	S95.101A
S89.119P	S92.002P	S92.051B	S92.125P	S92.211K	S92.253K	S92.342B	S92.501P	S95.102A
S89.121K	S92.009B	S92.051K	S92.126B	S92.211P	S92.253P	S92.342K	S92.502K	S95.109A
S89.121P	S92.009K	S92.051P	S92.126K	S92.212B	S92.254B	S92.342P	S92.502P	S95.111A
S89.122K	S92.009P	S92.052B	S92.126P	S92.212K	S92.254K	S92.343B	S92.503K	S95.112A
S89.122P	S92.011B	S92.052K	S92.131B	S92.212P	S92.254P	S92.343K	S92.503P	S95.119A
S89.129K	S92.011K	S92.052P	S92.131K	S92.213B	S92.255B	S92.343P	S92.504K	S95.191A
S89.129P	S92.011P	S92.053B	S92.131P	S92.213K	S92.255K	S92.344B	S92.504P	S95.192A
S89.131K	S92.012B	S92.053K	S92.132B	S92.213P	S92.255P	S92.344K	S92.505K	S95.199A
S89.131P	S92.012K	S92.053P	S92.132K	S92.214B	S92.256B	S92.344P	S92.505P	S95.201A
S89.132K	S92.012P	S92.054B	S92.132P	S92.214K	S92.256K	S92.345B	S92.506K	S95.202A
S89.132P	S92.013B	S92.054K	S92.133B	S92.214P	S92.256P	S92.345K	S92.506P	S95.209A
S89.139K	S92.013K	S92.054P	S92.133P	S92.215B	S92.301B	S92.345P	S92.511K	S95.211A
S89.139P	S92.013P	S92.055B	S92.134B	S92.215K	S92.301K	S92.346B	S92.511P	S95.212A
S89.141K	S92.014B	S92.055K	S92.134K	S92.215P	S92.301P	S92.346K	S92.512K	S95.219A
S89.141P	S92.014K	S92.055P	S92.134P	S92.216B	S92.302B	S92.346P	S92.512P	S95.291A
S89.142K	S92.014P	S92.056B	S92.135B	S92.216K	S92.302K	S92.351B	S92.513K	S95.292A
S89.142P	S92.015B	S92.056K	S92.135K	S92.216P	S92.302P	S92.351K	S92.513P	S95.299A
S89.149K	S92.015K	S92.056P	S92.135P	S92.221B	S92.309B	S92.351P	S92.514K	S95.801A
S89.149P	S92.015P	S92.061B	S92.136B	S92.221K	S92.309K	S92.352B	S92.514P	S95.802A
S89.191K	S92.016B	S92.061K	S92.136K	S92.221P	S92.309P	S92.352K	S92.515K	S95.809A
S89.191P	S92.016K	S92.061P	S92.136P	S92.222B	S92.311B	S92.352P	S92.515P	S95.811A
S89.192K	S92.016P	S92.062B	S92.141B	S92.222K	S92.311K	S92.353B	S92.516K	S95.812A
S89.192P	S92.021B	S92.062K	S92.141K	S92.222P	S92.311P	S92.353K	S92.516P	S95.819A
S89.199K	S92.021K	S92.062P	S92.141P	S92.223B	S92.312B	S92.353P	S92.521K	S95.891A
S89.199P	S92.021P	S92.063B	S92.142B	S92.223K	S92.312K	S92.354B	S92.521P	S95.892A
S89.201K	S92.022B	S92.063K	S92.142K	S92.223P	S92.312P	S92.354K	S92.522K	S95.899A
S89.201P	S92.022K	S92.063P	S92.142P	S92.224B	S92.313B	S92.354P	S92.522P	S95.901A
S89.202K	S92.022P	S92.064B	S92.143B	S92.224K	S92.313K	S92.355B	S92.523K	S95.902A
S89.202P	S92.023B	S92.064K	S92.143K	S92.224P	S92.313P	S92.355K	S92.523P	S95.909A
S89.209K	S92.023K	S92.064P	S92.143P	S92.225B	S92.314B	S92.355P	S92.524K	S95.911A
S89.209P	S92.023P	S92.065B	S92.144B	S92.225K	S92.314K	S92.356B	S92.524P	S95.912A
S89.211K	S92.024B	S92.065K	S92.144K	S92.225P	S92.314P	S92.356K	S92.525K	S95.919A
S89.211P	S92.024K	S92.065P	S92.144P	S92.226B	S92.315B	S92.356P	S92.525P	S95.991A
S89.212K	S92.024P	S92.066B	S92.145B	S92.226K	S92.315K	S92.401K	S92.526K	S95.992A
S89.212P	S92.025B	S92.066K	S92.145K	S92.226P	S92.315P	S92.401P	S92.526P	S95.999A
S89.219K	S92.025K	S92.066P	S92.145P	S92.231B	S92.316B	S92.402K	S92.531K	S96.021A
S89.219P	S92.025P	S92.101B	S92.146B	S92.231K	S92.316K	S92.402P	S92.531P	S96.022A
S89.221K	S92.026B	S92.101K	S92.146K	S92.231P	S92.316P	S92.403K	S92.532K	S96.029A
S89.221P	S92.026K	S92.101P	S92.146P	S92.232B	S92.321B	S92.403P	S92.532P	S96.121A
S89.222K	S92.026P	S92.102B	S92.151B	S92.232K	S92.321K	S92.404K	S92.533K	S96.122A
S89.222P	S92.031B	S92.102K	S92.151K	S92.232P	S92.321P	S92.404P	S92.533P	S96.129A
S89.229K	S92.031K	S92.102P	S92.151P	S92.233B	S92.322B	S92.405K	S92.534K	S96.221A
S89.229P	S92.031P	S92.109B	S92.152B	S92.233K	S92.322K	S92.405P	S92.534P	S96.222A
S89.291K	S92.032B	S92.109K	S92.152K	S92.234B	S92.322P	S92.406K	S92.535K	S96.229A
S89.291P	S92.032K	S92.109P	S92.152P	S92.234K	S92.323B	S92.406P	S92.535P	S96.821A
S89.292K	S92.032P	S92.111B	S92.153B	S92.234P	S92.323K	S92.411K	S92.536K	S96.822A
S89.292P	S92.033B	S92.111K	S92.153K	S92.235B	S92.323P	S92.411P	S92.536P	S96.829A
S89.299K	S92.033K	S92.111P	S92.153P	S92.235K	S92.324B	S92.412K	S92.591K	S96.921A
S89.299P	S92.033P	S92.112B	S92.154B	S92.235P	S92.324K	S92.412P	S92.591P	S96.922A
S89.301K	S92.034B	S92.112K	S92.154K	S92.236B	S92.324P	S92.413K	S92.592K	S96.929A
S89.301P	S92.034K	S92.112P	S92.154P	S92.236K	S92.325B	S92.413P	S92.592P	S98.011A
S89.302K	S92.034P	S92.113B	S92.155B	S92.236P	S92.325K	S92.414K	S92.599K	S98.012A
S89.302P	S92.035B	S92.113K	S92.155K	S92.241B	S92.325P	S92.414P	S92.599P	S98.019A
S89.309K	S92.035K	S92.113P	S92.155P	S92.241K	S92.326B	S92.414P	S92.901B	S98.021A
S89.309P	S92.035P	S92.114B	S92.156B	S92.241P	S92.326K	S92.415K	S92.901K	S98.022A
S89.311K	S92.035P	S92.114K	S92.156B	S92.241P	S92.326K	S92.415P	S92.901P	S98.022A
S89.311P	S92.036B	S92.114P	S92.156K	S92.242B	S92.326P	S92.416K	S92.902B	S98.029A

S98.311A	T22.311A	T23.722A	T26.70XA	T34.1XXA	T74.02XA	T81.32XA	T82.199A	T82.867A
S98.312A	T22.312A	T23.729A	T26.71XA	T34.2XXA	T74.11XA	T81.33XA	T82.211A	T82.868A
S98.319A	T22.319A	T23.731A	T26.72XA	T34.3XXA	T74.12XA	T81.4XXA	T82.212A	T82.897A
S98.321A	T22.321A	T23.732A	T27.0XXA	T34.40XA	T74.21XA	T81.500A	T82.213A	T82.898A
S98.322A	T22.322A	T23.739A	T27.1XXA	T34.41XA	T74.22XA	T81.501A	T82.218A	T82.9XXA
S98.329A	T22.329A	T23.741A	T27.2XXA	T34.42XA	T74.31XA	T81.502A	T82.221A	T83.010A
S98.911A	T22.331A	T23.742A	T27.3XXA	T34.511A	T74.32XA	T81.503A	T82.222A	T83.020A
S98.912A	T22.332A	T23.749A	T27.4XXA	T34.512A	T74.4XXA	T81.504A	T82.223A	T83.030A
S98.919A	T22.339A	T23.751A	T27.5XXA	T34.519A	T74.91XA	T81.505A	T82.228A	T83.090A
S98.921A	T22.341A	T23.752A	T27.6XXA	T34.521A	T74.92XA	T81.506A	T82.310A	T83.110A
S98.922A	T22.342A	T23.759A	T27.7XXA	T34.522A	T75.1XXA	T81.507A	T82.311A	T83.111A
S98.929A	T22.349A	T23.761A	T28.1XXA	T34.529A	T76.01XA	T81.508A	T82.312A	T83.112A
T17.400A	T22.351A	T23.762A	T28.2XXA	T34.531A	T76.02XA	T81.509A	T82.318A	T83.118A
T17.408A	T22.352A	T23.769A	T28.6XXA	T34.532A	T76.11XA	T81.510A	T82.319A	T83.120A
T17.410A	T22.359A	T23.771A	T28.7XXA	T34.539A	T76.12XA	T81.511A	T82.320A	T83.121A
T17.418A	T22.361A	T23.772A	T31.10	T34.60XA	T76.21XA	T81.512A	T82.321A	T83.122A
T17.420A	T22.362A	T23.779A	T31.11	T34.61XA	T76.22XA	T81.513A	T82.322A	T83.128A
T17.428A	T22.369A	T23.791A	T31.20	T34.62XA	T76.91XA	T81.514A	T82.328A	T83.190A
T17.490A	T22.391A	T23.792A	T31.30	T34.70XA	T76.92XA	T81.515A	T82.329A	T83.191A
T17.498A	T22.392A	T23.799A	T31.40	T34.71XA	T78.00XA	T81.516A	T82.330A	T83.192A
T17.500A	T22.399A	T24.301A	T31.50	T34.72XA	T78.01XA	T81.517A	T82.331A	T83.198A
T17.508A	T22.70XA	T24.302A	T31.60	T34.811A	T78.02XA	T81.518A	T82.332A	T83.21XA
T17.510A	T22.711A	T24.309A	T31.70	T34.812A	T78.03XA	T81.519A	T82.338A	T83.22XA
T17.518A	T22.712A	T24.311A	T31.80	T34.819A	T78.04XA	T81.520A	T82.339A	T83.23XA
T17.520A	T22.719A	T24.312A	T31.90	T34.821A	T78.05XA	T81.521A	T82.390A	T83.29XA
T17.528A	T22.721A	T24.319A	T32.10	T34.822A	T78.06XA	T81.522A	T82.391A	T83.410A
T17.590A	T22.722A	T24.321A	T32.11	T34.829A	T78.07XA	T81.523A	T82.392A	T83.418A
T17.598A	T22.729A	T24.322A	T32.20	T34.831A	T78.08XA	T81.524A	T82.398A	T83.420A
T17.800A	T22.731A	T24.329A	T32.30	T34.832A	T78.09XA	T81.525A	T82.399A	T83.428A
T17.808A	T22.732A	T24.331A	T32.40	T34.839A	T78.2XXA	T81.526A	T82.41XA	T83.490A
T17.810A	T22.739A	T24.332A	T32.50	T34.90XA	T79.2XXA	T81.527A	T82.42XA	T83.498A
T17.818A	T22.741A	T24.339A	T32.60	T34.99XA	T79.7XXA	T81.528A	T82.43XA	T83.51XA
T17.820A	T22.742A	T24.391A	T32.70	T67.0XXA	T79.A0XA	T81.529A	T82.49XA	T83.59XA
T17.828A	T22.749A	T24.392A	T32.80	T69.021A	T79.A11A	T81.530A	T82.510A	T83.6XXA
T17.890A	T22.751A	T24.399A	T32.90	T69.022A	T79.A12A	T81.531A	T82.511A	T83.718A
T17.898A	T22.752A	T24.701A	T33.011A	T69.029A	T79.A19A	T81.532A	T82.512A	T83.728A
T20.30XA	T22.759A	T24.702A	T33.012A	T70.3XXA	T79.A21A	T81.533A	T82.513A	T83.81XA
T20.311A	T22.761A	T24.709A	T33.019A	T71.111A	T79.A22A	T81.534A	T82.514A	T83.82XA
T20.312A	T22.762A	T24.711A	T33.02XA	T71.112A	T79.A29A	T81.535A	T82.515A	T83.83XA
T20.319A	T22.769A	T24.712A	T33.09XA	T71.113A	T79.A3XA	T81.536A	T82.518A	T83.84XA
T20.32XA	T22.791A	T24.719A	T33.1XXA	T71.114A	T79.A9XA	T81.537A	T82.519A	T83.85XA
T20.33XA	T22.792A	T24.721A	T33.2XXA	T71.121A	T80.1XXA	T81.538A	T82.520A	T83.86XA
T20.34XA	T22.799A	T24.722A	T33.3XXA	T71.122A	T80.211A	T81.539A	T82.521A	T83.89XA
T20.35XA	T23.301A	T24.729A	T33.40XA	T71.123A	T80.212A	T81.590A	T82.522A	T83.9XXA
T20.36XA	T23.302A	T24.731A	T33.41XA	T71.124A	T80.218A	T81.591A	T82.523A	T84.010A
T20.37XA	T23.309A	T24.732A	T33.42XA	T71.131A	T80.219A	T81.592A	T82.524A	T84.011A
T20.39XA	T23.311A	T24.739A	T33.511A	T71.132A	T80.22XA	T81.593A	T82.525A	T84.012A
T20.70XA	T23.312A	T24.791A	T33.512A	T71.133A	T80.29XA	T81.594A	T82.528A	T84.013A
T20.711A	T23.319A	T24.792A	T33.519A	T71.134A	T80.30XA	T81.595A	T82.529A	T84.018A
T20.712A	T23.321A	T24.799A	T33.521A	T71.141A	T80.310A	T81.596A	T82.530A	T84.019A
T20.719A	T23.322A	T25.311A	T33.522A	T71.143A	T80.311A	T81.597A	T82.531A	T84.020A
T20.72XA	T23.329A	T25.312A	T33.529A	T71.144A	T80.319A	T81.598A	T82.532A	T84.021A
T20.73XA	T23.331A	T25.319A	T33.531A	T71.151A	T80.39XA	T81.599A	T82.533A	T84.022A
T20.74XA	T23.332A	T25.321A	T33.532A	T71.152A	T80.40XA	T81.60XA	T82.534A	T84.023A
T20.75XA	T23.339A	T25.322A	T33.539A	T71.153A	T80.410A	T81.61XA	T82.535A	T84.028A
T20.76XA	T23.341A	T25.329A	T33.60XA	T71.154A	T80.411A	T81.69XA	T82.538A	T84.029A
T20.77XA	T23.342A	T25.331A	T33.61XA	T71.161A	T80.419A	T81.710A	T82.539A	T84.030A
T20.79XA	T23.349A	T25.332A	T33.62XA	T71.162A	T80.49XA	T81.711A	T82.590A	T84.031A
T21.30XA	T23.351A	T25.339A	T33.70XA	T71.163A	T80.51XA	T81.718A	T82.591A	T84.032A
T21.31XA	T23.352A	T25.391A	T33.71XA	T71.164A	T80.52XA	T81.719A	T82.592A	T84.033A
T21.32XA	T23.359A	T25.392A	T33.72XA	T71.191A	T80.59XA	T81.72XA	T82.593A	T84.038A
T21.33XA	T23.361A	T25.399A	T33.811A	T71.192A	T80.61XA	T81.83XA	T82.594A	T84.039A
T21.34XA	T23.362A	T25.711A	T33.812A	T71.193A	T80.62XA	T82.01XA	T82.595A	T84.040A
T21.35XA	T23.369A	T25.712A	T33.819A	T71.194A	T80.69XA	T82.02XA	T82.598A	T84.041A
T21.36XA	T23.371A	T25.719A	T33.821A	T71.20XA	T80.810A	T82.03XA	T82.599A	T84.042A
T21.37XA	T23.372A	T25.721A	T33.822A	T71.21XA	T80.818A	T82.09XA	T82.6XXA	T84.043A
T21.39XA	T23.379A	T25.722A	T33.829A	T71.221A	T80.910A	T82.110A	T82.7XXA	T84.048A
T21.70XA	T23.391A	T25.729A	T33.831A	T71.222A	T80.911A	T82.111A	T82.817A	T84.049A
T21.71XA	T23.392A	T25.731A	T33.832A	T71.223A	T80.919A	T82.118A	T82.818A	T84.050A
T21.72XA	T23.399A	T25.732A	T33.839A	T71.224A	T80.A0XA	T82.119A	T82.827A	T84.051A
T21.73XA	T23.701A	T25.739A	T33.90XA	T71.231A	T80.A10A	T82.120A	T82.828A	T84.052A
T21.74XA	T23.702A	T25.791A	T33.99XA	T71.232A	T80.A11A	T82.121A	T82.837A	T84.053A
T21.75XA	T23.709A	T25.792A	T34.011A	T71.233A	T80.A19A	T82.128A	T82.838A	T84.058A
T21.76XA	T23.711A	T25.799A	T34.012A	T71.234A	T80.A9XA	T82.129A	T82.847A	T84.059A
T21.77XA	T23.712A	T26.20XA	T34.019A	T71.29XA	T81.10XA	T82.190A	T82.848A	T84.060A
T21.79XA	T23.719A	T26.21XA	T34.02XA	T71.9XXA	T81.30XA	T82.191A	T82.857A	T84.061A
T22.30XA	T23.721A	T26.22XA	T34.09XA	T74.01XA	T81.31XA	T82.198A	T82.858A	T84.062A

T84.063A	T84.195A	T84.54XA	T85.110A	T85.590A	T85.85XA	T86.812	T86.99	Z94.1
T84.068A	T84.196A	T84.59XA	T85.111A	T85.591A	T85.86XA	T86.818	T87.0X1	Z94.2
T84.069A	T84.197A	T84.60XA	T85.112A	T85.598A	T85.89XA	T86.819	T87.0X2	Z94.3
T84.090A	T84.199A	T84.610A	T85.118A	T85.610A	T86.00	T86.820	T87.0X9	Z94.4
T84.091A	T84.210A	T84.611A	T85.120A	T85.611A	T86.01	T86.821	T87.1X1	Z94.81
T84.092A	T84.213A	T84.612A	T85.121A	T85.612A	T86.02	T86.822	T87.1X2	Z94.82
T84.093A	T84.216A	T84.613A	T85.122A	T85.613A	T86.03	T86.828	T87.1X9	Z94.83
T84.098A	T84.218A	T84.614A	T85.128A	T85.614A	T86.09	T86.829	T87.2	Z94.84
T84.099A	T84.220A	T84.615A	T85.190A	T85.618A	T86.10	T86.830	T87.40	Z95.811
T84.110A	T84.223A	T84.619A	T85.191A	T85.620A	T86.11	T86.831	T87.41	Z95.812
T84.111A	T84.226A	T84.620A	T85.192A	T85.621A	T86.12	T86.832	T87.42	Z99.11
T84.112A	T84.228A	T84.621A	T85.199A	T85.622A	T86.13	T86.838	T87.43	Z99.12
T84.113A	T84.290A	T84.622A	T85.21XA	T85.623A	T86.19	T86.839	T87.44	
T84.114A	T84.293A	T84.623A	T85.22XA	T85.624A	T86.20	T86.840	T88.0XXA	
T84.115A	T84.296A	T84.624A	T85.29XA	T85.628A	T86.21	T86.841	T88.1XXA	
T84.116A	T84.298A	T84.625A	T85.310A	T85.630A	T86.22	T86.842	T88.2XXA	
T84.117A	T84.310A	T84.629A	T85.311A	T85.631A	T86.23	T86.848	T88.3XXA	
T84.119A	T84.318A	T84.63XA	T85.320A	T85.633A	T86.290	T86.849	T88.6XXA	
T84.120A	T84.320A	T84.69XA	T85.321A	T85.638A	T86.298	T86.850	Z43.1	
T84.121A	T84.328A	T84.7XXA	T85.390A	T85.690A	T86.30	T86.851	Z48.21	
T84.122A	T84.390A	T84.81XA	T85.391A	T85.691A	T86.31	T86.852	Z48.22	
T84.123A	T84.398A	T84.82XA	T85.41XA	T85.692A	T86.32	T86.858	Z48.23	
T84.124A	T84.410A	T84.83XA	T85.42XA	T85.693A	T86.33	T86.859	Z48.24	
T84.125A	T84.418A	T84.84XA	T85.43XA	T85.694A	T86.39	T86.890	Z48.280	
T84.126A	T84.420A	T84.85XA	T85.44XA	T85.698A	T86.40	T86.891	Z48.290	
T84.127A	T84.428A	T84.86XA	T85.49XA	T85.71XA	T86.41	T86.892	Z68.1	
T84.129A	T84.490A	T84.89XA	T85.510A	T85.72XA	T86.42	T86.898	Z68.41	
T84.190A	T84.498A	T84.9XXA	T85.511A	T85.79XA	T86.43	T86.899	Z68.42	
T84.191A	T84.50XA	T85.01XA	T85.518A	T85.81XA	T86.49	T86.90	Z68.43	
T84.192A	T84.51XA	T85.02XA	T85.520A	T85.82XA	T86.5	T86.91	Z68.44	
T84.193A	T84.52XA	T85.03XA	T85.521A	T85.83XA	T86.810	T86.92	Z68.45	
T84.194A	T84.53XA	T85.09XA	T85.528A	T85.84XA	T86.811	T86.93	Z94.0	

Appendix G: Lists of Principal Diagnoses That Are Their Own CC and Their Own MCC

Principal Diagnoses That Are Their Own CC

B25.1	I70.368	I70.562	I70.749	K51.513	M02.331	M05.459	M90.559
B52.0	I70.369	I70.563	I70.761	K51.514	M02.332	M05.461	M90.561
D57.211	I70.431	I70.568	I70.762	K51.812	M02.339	M05.462	M90.562
D57.411	I70.432	I70.569	I70.763	K51.813	M02.341	M05.469	M90.569
E08.52	I70.433	I70.631	I70.768	K51.814	M02.342	M05.471	M90.571
E09.52	I70.434	I70.632	I70.769	K51.912	M02.349	M05.472	M90.572
E10.52	I70.438	I70.633	I73.01	K51.913	M02.351	M05.479	M90.579
E11.52	I70.439	I70.634	K50.012	K51.914	M02.352	M05.49	M90.58
E13.52	I70.441	I70.638	K50.013	K57.00	M02.359	M32.11	M90.59
I25.110	I70.442	I70.639	K50.014	K57.01	M02.361	M32.12	N11.1
I25.700	I70.443	I70.641	K50.112	K57.20	M02.362	M33.02	N13.1
I25.710	I70.444	I70.642	K50.113	K57.21	M02.369	M33.12	N13.2
I25.720	I70.448	I70.643	K50.114	K57.40	M02.371	M33.22	O12.21
I25.730	I70.449	I70.644	K50.812	K57.41	M02.372	M33.92	O12.22
I25.750	I70.461	I70.648	K50.813	K57.52	M02.379	M34.81	O12.23
I25.760	I70.462	I70.649	K50.814	K57.80	M02.38	M34.82	T86.30
I25.790	I70.463	I70.661	K50.912	K57.81	M02.39	M35.03	T86.31
I70.331	I70.468	I70.662	K50.913	K80.30	M05.40	M90.50	T86.32
I70.332	I70.469	I70.663	K50.914	K80.31	M05.411	M90.511	T86.33
I70.333	I70.531	I70.668	K51.012	K80.32	M05.412	M90.512	T86.39
I70.334	I70.532	I70.669	K51.013	K80.33	M05.419	M90.519	Z48.21
I70.338	I70.533	I70.731	K51.014	K80.34	M05.421	M90.521	Z48.22
I70.339	I70.534	I70.732	K51.212	K80.35	M05.422	M90.522	Z48.23
I70.341	I70.538	I70.733	K51.213	K80.36	M05.429	M90.529	Z48.24
I70.342	I70.539	I70.734	K51.214	K80.37	M05.431	M90.531	Z48.280
I70.343	I70.541	I70.738	K51.312	M02.30	M05.432	M90.532	Z48.290
I70.344	I70.542	I70.739	K51.313	M02.311	M05.439	M90.539	Z94.3
I70.348	I70.543	I70.741	K51.314	M02.312	M05.441	M90.541	
I70.349	I70.544	I70.742	K51.412	M02.319	M05.442	M90.542	
I70.361	I70.548	I70.743	K51.413	M02.321	M05.449	M90.549	
I70.362	I70.549	I70.744	K51.414	M02.322	M05.451	M90.551	
I70.363	I70.561	I70.748	K51.512	M02.329	M05.452	M90.552	

Principal Diagnoses That Are Their Own MCC

A22.7	B44.0	L89.004	L89.133	L89.224	L89.513	L89.814	S06.1X5A
A26.7	B45.1	L89.013	L89.134	L89.303	L89.514	L89.893	S06.1X6A
A32.7	B77.81	L89.014	L89.143	L89.304	L89.523	L89.894	S06.1X7A
A37.01	I26.01	L89.023	L89.144	L89.313	L89.524	L89.93	S06.1X8A
A37.11	I26.02	L89.024	L89.153	L89.314	L89.603	L89.94	S06.1X9A
A37.81	I26.09	L89.103	L89.154	L89.323	L89.604	R65.21	
A37.91	K70.41	L89.104	L89.203	L89.324	L89.613	S06.1X0A	
A54.86	K71.11	L89.113	L89.204	L89.43	L89.614	S06.1X1A	
B25.0	K72.01	L89.114	L89.213	L89.44	L89.623	S06.1X2A	
B25.2	K72.11	L89.123	L89.214	L89.503	L89.624	S06.1X3A	
B37.7	L89.003	L89.124	L89.223	L89.504	L89.813	S06.1X4A	

Appendix H: Present on Admission (POA) Tutorial

Present-on-admission (POA) indicators are required on all diagnoses and external cause-of-injury codes for all inpatient acute care hospital discharges, according to the requirement outlined in the Deficit Reduction Act of 2005, section 5001(c). The only exception is for a select group of codes that have been designated as exempt from the POA regulations. Certain facilities are also exempt from this reporting requirement and include the following:

- Critical access hospitals
- Long-term care hospitals
- Cancer hospitals
- Inpatient psychiatric hospitals
- Inpatient rehabilitation facilities
- Veterans Administration/Department of Defense Hospitals
- Children's inpatient facilities

The POA indicator guidelines are not intended to replace the official *ICD-10-CM Official Guidelines for Coding and Reporting*. Nor will the POA guidelines supersede the Uniform Hospital Discharge Data Set (UHDDS) definition of principal diagnosis, defined as the condition established after study to be chiefly responsible for occasioning the admission of the patient to the hospital. The definition of "additional diagnoses" also remains the same. Coders must report all conditions that coexist at the time of admission, develop subsequently, or that affect the treatment received and/or the length of stay. This significantly affects assignment of the POA indicators. Because the POA indicator should accurately reflect the patient's conditions upon admission, review of POA guidelines as well as the *ICD-10-CM Official Guidelines for Coding and Reporting* is required.

The following is a summary of the POA guidelines:

- A POA condition is defined not only as one that is clearly present at the time of admission, but also one that was clearly present but not diagnosed until after the time of admission.

- Present on admission is defined as present at the time the order for an inpatient admission is made, whether or not the patient's episode of care originated in the emergency department, ambulatory surgery area, or other outpatient area. Conditions that develop during an outpatient encounter are considered present on admission.

- A POA indicator is assigned to the principal diagnosis, secondary diagnoses, and the external cause-of-injury codes.

- The POA guidelines are not intended to replace any of the other *ICD-10-CM Official Guidelines for Coding and Reporting*.

- The intent of the POA guidelines is not to determine whether or not a condition should be coded, but rather how to apply the POA indicator.

The following reporting options, with definitions, should be used to indicate whether a condition was POA:

Y   Yes: Present at the time of inpatient admission

N   No: Not present at the time of inpatient admission

U   Unknown: Documentation is insufficient to determine if condition is present on admission

W   Clinically undetermined: Provider is unable to clinically determine whether condition was or was not present on admission

Unreported/not used—(exempt from POA reporting)—Most ICD-10-CM codes require the assignment of a POA indicator. However, there are some diagnoses that are considered exempt from the POA reporting. For these exempt conditions the POA field should be left blank.

Timeframe for POA identification and documentation

There is no timeframe during the encounter in which a condition must be diagnosed to be considered present on admission. In many cases, it is not clinically possible for the provider to determine a definitive diagnosis until well into the admission, after labs, imaging, and other tests have been performed and results examined. In these cases the condition is still considered to be present on admission, indicated with Y.

Examples

- A patient was admitted for diagnostic work-up for cachexia. The final diagnosis was malignant neoplasm of lung with metastasis.

  Assign Y in the POA field for the malignant neoplasm, which was clearly present on admission, although it was not diagnosed until after the admission occurred.

- A patient with severe cough and difficulty breathing was diagnosed during his hospitalization to have lung cancer.

  Assign Y in the POA field for the lung cancer. Even though the cancer was not diagnosed until after admission, it is a chronic condition that was clearly present before the patient's admission.

- A urine culture was obtained on admission. The provider documented urinary tract infection when the culture results became available a few days later.

  Assign Y to the urinary tract infection since the diagnosis is based on test results from a specimen obtained on admission. It may not be possible for a provider to make a definitive diagnosis for a period of time after admission. There is no required timeframe as to when a provider must identify or document a condition for it to be considered present on admission.

Condition is on the "Exempt from Reporting" list

Several codes are exempt from POA reporting. An abbreviated list of exempt codes can be found following appendix I, "Present on Admission Reporting Guidelines," at the beginning of the code book, while a detailed list of codes can be found as an official download at http://www.cms.gov/Medicare/Coding/ICD10/Downloads/2015-POA-Exempt-List.zip. The POA field is left blank for codes excluded from POA reporting.

Note: Codes from chapter 19, "Injury, Poisoning and Certain Other Consequences of External Causes," and chapter 20, "External Causes of Morbidity" included in the exempt from reporting list are *only* those codes with a seventh character representing a subsequent encounter or sequela. These same codes but with a seventh character representing an "initial" encounter are *not* excluded.

Examples

- A patient was admitted for inpatient surgery on a burn contracture from scar tissue from a burn five years ago.

  Assign Y for the principal condition of the scar; however, the secondary code for the specifics of the burn injury with a seventh character for sequela is left blank since it is excluded from POA reporting.

- A patient was admitted to inpatient for a PEG tube insertion because of residual dysphagia due to a recent CVA.

  No POA indicator is assigned for the dysphagia following a CVA. Codes under I69.- are defined as sequela of cerebrovascular disease and are exempt from POA reporting.

- A patient was admitted to inpatient for corrective surgery for a malunion of a closed femur fracture.

  No POA indicator is assigned for the malunion of a closed fracture because the seventh character for malunion of fractures is considered a subsequent encounter and is exempt from POA reporting.

- A patient was admitted for breast reconstruction following mastectomy.

  The POA indicator field is left blank as this Z code is exempt from POA reporting.

- A patient was admitted for changing the battery in his AICD as it is at the end of its useful life.

  The POA indicator field is left blank as this Z code is exempt from POA reporting.

POA Explicitly documented

If the provider explicitly documents a condition as being present on admission or not present on admission, assign the appropriate Y or N POA indicator based on that documentation. If there is conflicting documentation by different providers, query the attending physician.

Examples

- Even though sepsis is not diagnosed in the ED, the discharge summary states that the patient presented with sepsis at the time of admission.

  The provider explicitly stated that the sepsis was present on admission and therefore the Y POA indicator should be used.

- The patient was admitted with chills and cough and two days later diagnosed with pneumonia. The discharge summary documents that the pneumonia was not present on admission.

  Although the patient showed some symptoms of pneumonia on admission, the provider may have clinical evidence (e.g., chest x-rays, cultures) that indicates that pneumonia did not develop until after admission. Since this was explicitly stated in the discharge summary, the appropriate POA indicator is N.

- A consult note states that a patient came in with renal failure while the discharge summary states that the renal failure was not present on admission.

  When in doubt and there is conflicting documentation, query the attending physician.

Conditions diagnosed prior to inpatient admission

Conditions that were diagnosed prior to admission—for example, chronic conditions such as hypertension, diabetes, and asthma—are assigned the POA indicator of Y. A tip to help establish that a condition was POA is to check the patient's medication history for drugs that are routinely prescribed for these types of chronic conditions.

Examples

- The history and physical states that the patient has a history of hypertension and seizure disorder, and it is noted that the patient is currently on Atenolol and Dilantin.

  The hypertension and seizure disorder existed prior to admission; therefore, the appropriate POA indicator is Y. Verification that the patient is on long-term use of Atenolol and Dilantin can help solidify that these conditions are currently being treated.

- A 56-year-old male was admitted as an inpatient for multi-trauma wounds. Because the patient was unconscious on admission, his medical history was unknown. A progress note two days into the stay noted that the patient was on Metformin for history of type 2 diabetes.

  The timeframe of the diagnosis is irrelevant to POA. Even though it was not discovered until two days into the encounter that the patient had a history of DM2, the DM2 was still present prior to this admission and would be identified as such with the Y POA indicator.

- A patient was admitted to an inpatient facility from the ED. The admitting provider indicated that the patient had a current history of lung cancer and chronic kidney disease.

  Both of these conditions are indicated with Y, present on admission.

- During the course of an eight-day inpatient stay with surgery, a patient was diagnosed postoperatively with hypertension and discharged on Metoprolol.

  The hypertension was not diagnosed prior to admission and would be reported with an N POA indicator.

Conditions diagnosed during the admission but clearly present before admission

The POA indictor Y is assigned for conditions that clearly presented with applicable signs and symptoms but may have not been definitively diagnosed until later on, or even at the end of the encounter. Even if the presenting diagnosis was documented on admission as suspected, possible, or rule out, or written as a differential diagnosis and later confirmed, it is still considered present on admission.

Examples

- A patient was admitted with jaundice, fatigue, and mental confusion. Differential diagnosis on admission lists possible liver failure. The definitive diagnosis of liver failure is not made until two days after admission.

  Assign Y to the liver failure since the symptoms were present on admission and the differential diagnosis listed "possible" liver failure on admission even though the final diagnosis was two days later.

- An aid worker recently returned from Afghanistan presents to the ED with hematemesis, chest pain, and fever. Patient is put into inpatient isolation with suspected TB documented on the H & P. TB is confirmed the next day.

  The POA indicator Y is assigned because, even though the TB was only "suspected" on admission, it was confirmed the next day.

Condition develops during outpatient encounter prior to inpatient admission

Assign Y for any condition that develops during an outpatient encounter such as same-day surgery, observation, or extended recovery prior to a written order for inpatient admission. This also pertains to conditions that develop in facilities such as transitional care units, skilled nursing homes, long-term care, hospice, or rehabilitation facilities with the patient transferring to inpatient hospital admission.

Examples

- A patient underwent outpatient surgery. During the recovery period, the patient developed atrial fibrillation and was subsequently admitted to the hospital as an inpatient.

  Assign Y on the POA field for the atrial fibrillation since it developed prior to a written order for inpatient admission.

- A patient was treated in observation and while in observation fell out of bed and broke a hip. The patient was subsequently admitted as an inpatient to treat the hip fracture.

  Assign Y on the POA field for the hip fracture since it developed prior to a written order for inpatient admission.

- An elderly patient underwent outpatient surgery with plans to go home after the surgery. In recovery, the patient developed shortness of breath, chest pain, and fever. A sputum sample was taken, and the surgeon decided to admit the patient to inpatient. The next day the patient was diagnosed with staphylococcal pneumonia based on sputum results and admitting chest x-ray.

  Assign Y to the staphylococcal pneumonia even though it was not diagnosed until the day following the admission. Even though the patient had undergone outpatient surgery, the sputum sample, signs, and symptoms were evident prior to the inpatient admission.

Documentation does not indicate whether condition was present on admission

If the documentation in the medical record is unclear as to the presence of a condition on admission, assign a U for unknown. This should be used sparingly and, if possible, the physician should be queried for further clarification.

Example

- A wheelchair-bound patient was admitted in respiratory failure from a long-term care facility to an inpatient hospital with severe aspiration pneumonia. A progress note three days into the admission listed a pressure ulcer stage 2 on the lower back.

  Assign U for the stage 2 pressure ulcer if unknown whether it was present on admission. Since the patient was wheelchair-bound and critically ill on admission, it is possible that the ulcer was present and not immediately addressed. The admitting physician can be queried to clarify, or a U is assigned if that is not possible.

Documentation states it cannot be determined whether the condition was or was not present on admission

A W is assigned when the documentation states that it cannot be clinically determined whether the condition was POA or not.

Examples

- An elderly patient was admitted with multi-trauma injuries from a motor vehicle accident. Two days into the admission, a urinary tract infection was diagnosed. No labs or urine cultures had been taken on admission as focus was stabilization from traumatic wounds. Documentation from the provider in a progress note stated that it was not clinically possible to determine whether the UTI was present on admission.

  Assign W for the UTI as it was specifically stated that it was not clinically possible to determine whether it was present on admission.

- A patient was admitted with high fever and pneumonia. The patient rapidly deteriorated and became septic. The discharge diagnosis listed sepsis and pneumonia. The documentation was unclear as to whether the sepsis was present on admission or developed shortly after admission.

  Query the physician as to whether the sepsis was present on admission, developed shortly after admission, or it cannot be clinically determined as to whether it was or was not present on admission.

Chronic condition with acute exacerbation during the admission

If a single code identifies only the chronic condition and not the acute exacerbation, assign Y. For instance, when there is no code for the acute exacerbation of a chronic condition as in acute exacerbation of chronic leukemia, the Y is assigned for the chronic leukemia.

For a single combination code that identifies both the chronic and acute exacerbation, see the combination code instructions.

Example

- Documentation on admission stated that the patient had chronic myelomonocytic leukemia. A progress note three days into the stay stated that the patient had, since admission, developed an acute exacerbation of his myelomonocytic leukemia.

  There is no code for an acute exacerbation of chronic myelomonocytic leukemia; therefore, assign Y since the chronic leukemia (either not specified as in remission, or in relapse) is represented by a single code and was present on admission.

Acute and Chronic conditions

Assign Y to acute conditions present on admission and N to acute conditions not present at the time of admission.

Assign Y to conditions specified as chronic, even though they may not be diagnosed until after admission.

See the POA guidelines for combination codes for a single code that identifies both the acute and chronic condition.

Examples

- A patient was admitted to the hospital for coronary artery bypass surgery. Postoperatively he developed a pulmonary embolism.

  Assign N in the POA field for the pulmonary embolism. This is an acute condition that was not present on admission.

- A patient admitted with sepsis due to pneumonia and acute respiratory failure developed acute renal failure on day three.

  Assign Y for the sepsis, pneumonia, and acute respiratory failure, which were all acute conditions, present on admission. Assign N for the acute renal failure; even though it is an acute condition, it was not present until after the patient was admitted.

- A patient admitted with hypoglycemia, weakness, confusion, and slurred speech was diagnosed the next day with type 2 diabetes.

  Assign Y to the type 2 diabetes since it is a chronic condition that was present on admission, even though it was not diagnosed until the next day.

Combination Codes

If any part of a combination code is not present on admission, assign N. If all parts of a combination code are present on admission, assign Y.

Examples

- Obstructive chronic bronchitis was diagnosed on admission, with exacerbation occurring later in the encounter.

  The POA indicator N would be assigned to COPD with exacerbation if the exacerbation did not happen until after the admission.

- A patient with chronic diastolic heart failure decompensated after admission.

  Assign N to the code for acute on chronic diastolic (congestive) heart failure. Although the heart failure was present on admission, the acute decompensation of the failure was not.

- A patient with viral hepatitis B progressed to hepatic coma after admission.

  Assign N for the viral hepatitis B with hepatic coma because a condition described by part of the code description did not develop until after admission.

- A patient with known systolic congestive heart failure was admitted to the hospital with decompensated systolic heart failure.

  Assign Y in the POA field for the acute on chronic systolic (congestive) heart failure as both the chronic and acute parts of the condition were present on admission.

If symptoms related to two conditions were present at the time of admission and the final diagnosis includes suspected, comparative, or contrasting diagnoses, the POA indicators for both conditions are Y.

Example

- A patient presented with chills, and the discharge summary indicates the chills were due to either pneumonia or urinary tract infection.

  Assign Y for both pneumonia and urinary tract infection. A patient may present with chills but may improve clinically and be discharged or transferred before a definitive determination of the final diagnosis can be made.

Assign Y for infection codes that include the organism if the infection was present on admission even though the culture results are not available until after admission.

Example

- A patient was septic on admission with blood, sputum, and urine cultures taken. Two days later, *E. coli* was determined to be the causal organism.

  Assign Y even though the test results were not confirmed until after admission.

Conditions documented as possible, probable, suspected, or rule out at the time of discharge or conditions documented as impending or threatened at the time of discharge

If the final diagnosis contains language identifying a condition as possible, probable, suspected, or rule out, or as an impending or threatened diagnosis but the diagnosis is based on signs and symptoms that were present on admission, the POA indicator is Y. If those signs and symptoms were not present on admission, the appropriate POA indicator is N.

Examples

- A patient underwent inpatient surgery, after which the patient developed fever and was treated aggressively. The physician's final diagnosis documented "possible postoperative infection following surgery."

  Assign N on the POA field for the postoperative infection since final diagnoses that contain the terms "possible," "probable," "suspected," or "rule out" and that are based on symptoms or clinical findings that were not present on admission should be reported as N.

- A patient with prior cardiac intervention history was admitted with chest pain. After two days, the chest pain diminished with no underlying cause found. The discharge summary stated, "Suspected costochondritis or coronary artery spasm. Pain resolved. Follow up at regular cardiology office visit."

  Since the chest pain was present on admission, both suspected conditions of costochondritis and coronary artery spasm are represented by the POA indicator of Y.

- A patient was admitted with a known history of coronary atherosclerosis, status post myocardial infarction five years ago, and was then admitted for treatment of impending myocardial infarction. The patient was transferred to a larger facility with a cath lab. The final diagnosis was documented as "impending myocardial infarction."

  Assign Y to the impending myocardial infarction because the condition is present on admission.

Same diagnosis code for two or more conditions

When two or more separate conditions are classified to the same diagnosis code in the same encounter, assign Y if all conditions represented by the single code were present on admission and N if any of the conditions were not present on admission.

Examples

- A patient was admitted with diabetes type 2 with ketoacidosis.

  Assign Y since both the diabetes and ketoacidosis were present on admission.

- A patient involved in a car accident was admitted with hemorrhage to the abdomen secondary to the trauma; shortly after being admitted the patient also developed a seroma as a result of the trauma.

  The secondary traumatic hemorrhage was present on admission, and the traumatic seroma did not develop until after admission. Both of these conditions are classified to one code, but because both conditions were not present when the patient was admitted, a POA of N should be assigned.

Obstetrical conditions

The POA assignment for obstetrical conditions is not affected by whether the patient delivers during the encounter but rather by whether the pregnancy complication was or was not present at the time of admission. If two or more conditions are classified to a single code, all conditions represented by that single code must be present on admission to correctly assign a Y. If all conditions are not present at the time of admission, the appropriate POA indicator is N. Several obstetrics codes are listed in the POA exclusion list; for obstetrics codes that are not on the exclusion list, all applicable POA guidelines apply.

Examples

- A female patient was admitted to the hospital and underwent a normal delivery.

  Leave the "present on admission" (POA) field blank. Code O80 Normal delivery, is on the "exempt from reporting" list.

- A patient was admitted in late pregnancy due to excessive vomiting and dehydration. During admission, the patient went into premature labor.

  Assign Y for the excessive vomiting and the dehydration. Assign N for the premature labor.

- A patient was admitted in active labor. During the stay, a breast abscess was noted when the mother attempted to breastfeed. The provider was unable to clinically determine whether the abscess was present on admission.

  Assign W for the breast abscess since the provider was unable to clinically determine whether the abscess was present on admission.

- A patient was admitted in active labor. After 12 hours of labor, it was noted that the infant was in fetal distress, and a cesarean section was performed.

  Assign N for the fetal distress even if it is used for the principal diagnosis, since it did not develop until later in the admission. In obstetrics cases, the principal diagnosis may have a POA indicator of N.

Perinatal and congenital conditions

Newborns are not considered admitted until after birth; therefore all conditions that develop in utero, occur during delivery, or are present at birth are represented by the POA indicator Y. Any conditions that develop after birth and admission are represented by N.

The congenital conditions and anomalies listed in chapter 16 are considered present on admission and are represented by the POA indicator Y.

All the congenital malformations, deformations, and chromosomal abnormalities represented by the codes in chapter 17, categories Q00–Q99, are exempt from POA reporting.

Examples

- A single liveborn infant was delivered in the hospital via cesarean section. The physician documented fetal bradycardia during labor as the final diagnosis in the newborn record.

  Assign Y because the bradycardia developed prior to the newborn admission (birth).

- A newborn developed diarrhea, which was believed to be due to the hospital baby formula.

  Assign N because the diarrhea developed after admission.

- A newborn was diagnosed with cephalhematoma due to birth injury.

  Assign Y because the injury occurred during delivery.

- A newborn was diagnosed with congenital pneumonia.

  Assign Y for the congenital pneumonia. Congenital conditions from chapter 16 are always considered present on admission and require the POA indicator.

- A newborn was diagnosed with congenital hydrocephalus.

  There should be no POA indicator assigned. This condition is coded in chapter 17 and is excluded from POA reporting.

- A 10-year-old boy was admitted for complications of spina bifida with hydrocephalus.

  No POA indicator is assigned. This condition is coded in chapter 17 and is excluded from POA reporting.

External cause and injury codes

If an injury or poisoning occurred prior to or at the time of admission and the seventh character indicates an initial encounter or active treatment, the code for the injury/poisoning is reported with POA indicator Y. Injury and poisoning codes S00–T88 with the seventh character indicating subsequent or sequela are exempt from POA indicators since, in order to be a subsequent or sequela encounter, the condition must have occurred before the admission. Many of the external causes of morbidity codes from chapters V, W, and X are also exempt from POA reporting when the seventh character of S or D, representing subsequent or sequela encounters, are used.

Coders should be extremely careful in assigning the appropriate POA indicator if a patient suffers an injury while an inpatient. For example, if a patient falls from the hospital bed and fractures a hip, the codes representing that injury (along with the appropriate initial-encounter seventh character) should be assigned N for the corresponding POA indicator.

Examples

- A 12-year-old was admitted for treatment of fractured arm from falling out of a tree house.

  The injury itself and the cause of the injury are both assigned a Y POA indicator. **Note:** *The injury code and external cause code POA indicators should always match.*

- A patient admitted for pneumonia sustained a laceration of the right arm after falling and hitting his arm against a cart in the hospital room, requiring stitches.

  Assign N for the laceration for the right arm because it was not present on admission.

- A patient was admitted for manipulation of a knee contracture due to a scar from a burn injury 10 years ago.

  Assign Y for the code for the scar, but leave blank the POA indicator for the burn injury with the seventh character of S for sequela. Sequela and subsequent-encounter codes in chapter 19 are exempt from POA reporting.

Appendix I: Hospital Acquired Conditions

Hospital-acquired conditions (HACs) are conditions considered reasonably preventable through the application of evidence-based guidelines. These conditions, in and of themselves, are either a complication or comorbidity (CC) or major complication or comorbidity (MCC) that as a secondary diagnosis will move the MS-DRG assignment from a lower-paying MS-DRG to a higher-paying MS-DRG. However, if these conditions are not present on admission (meaning they developed during the hospital admission), the CC or MCC designation is nullified and the case will not group to the higher-paying MS-DRG based solely upon the reporting of the HAC code. As many of these HACs are conditional, the following lists the specific HAC conditions and any associated stipulations. The resources used to compile this list are the ICD-10-CM/PCS MS-DRG v32 Definitions Manual and the *Federal Register*, volume 80, no. 83, April 30, 2015 ("Hospital Inpatient Prospective Payment Systems for Acute Care Hospitals and the Long Term Care Hospital Prospective Payment System Policy Changes and FY2016 Rates; Proposed Rule").

HAC 01: Foreign Object Retained After Surgery

Secondary diagnosis not POA:

T81.500A
T81.501A
T81.502A
T81.503A
T81.504A
T81.505A
T81.506A
T81.507A
T81.508A
T81.509A
T81.510A
T81.511A
T81.512A
T81.513A
T81.514A
T81.515A
T81.516A
T81.517A
T81.518A
T81.519A
T81.520A
T81.521A
T81.522A
T81.523A
T81.524A
T81.525A
T81.526A
T81.527A
T81.528A
T81.529A
T81.530A
T81.531A
T81.532A
T81.533A
T81.534A
T81.535A
T81.536A
T81.537A
T81.538A
T81.539A
T81.590A
T81.591A
T81.592A
T81.593A
T81.594A
T81.595A
T81.596A
T81.597A
T81.598A
T81.599A
T81.60XA
T81.61XA
T81.69XA

HAC 02: Air Embolism

Secondary diagnosis not POA:

T80.0XXA

HAC 03: Blood Incompatibility

Secondary diagnosis not POA:

T80.30XA
T80.310A
T80.311A
T80.319A
T80.39XA

HAC 04: Stage III and IV Pressure Ulcers

Secondary diagnosis not POA:

L89.003
L89.004
L89.013
L89.014
L89.023
L89.024
L89.103
L89.104
L89.113
L89.114
L89.123
L89.124
L89.133
L89.134
L89.143
L89.144
L89.153
L89.154
L89.203
L89.204
L89.213
L89.214
L89.223
L89.224
L89.303
L89.304
L89.313
L89.314
L89.323
L89.324
L89.43
L89.44
L89.503
L89.504
L89.513
L89.514
L89.523
L89.524
L89.603
L89.604
L89.613
L89.614
L89.623
L89.624
L89.813
L89.814
L89.893
L89.894
L89.93
L89.94

HAC 05: Falls and Trauma

Secondary diagnosis not POA:

M99.10
M99.11
M99.18
S02.0XXA
S02.0XXB
S02.10XA
S02.10XB
S02.110A
S02.110B
S02.111A
S02.111B
S02.112A
S02.112B
S02.113A
S02.113B
S02.118A
S02.118B
S02.119A
S02.119B
S02.19XA
S02.19XB
S02.2XXB
S02.3XXA
S02.3XXB
S02.400A
S02.400B
S02.401A
S02.401B
S02.402A
S02.402B
S02.411A
S02.411B
S02.412A
S02.412B
S02.413A
S02.413B
S02.42XA
S02.42XB
S02.600A
S02.600B
S02.609A
S02.609B
S02.61XA
S02.61XB
S02.62XA
S02.62XB
S02.63XA
S02.63XB
S02.64XA
S02.64XB
S02.65XA
S02.65XB
S02.66XA
S02.66XB
S02.67XA
S02.67XB
S02.69XA
S02.69XB
S02.8XXA
S02.8XXB
S02.91XA
S02.91XB
S02.92XA
S02.92XB
S06.0X1A
S06.0X2A
S06.0X3A
S06.0X4A
S06.0X5A
S06.0X6A
S06.0X7A
S06.0X8A
S06.0X9A
S06.1X1A
S06.1X2A
S06.1X3A
S06.1X4A
S06.1X5A
S06.1X6A
S06.1X7A
S06.1X8A
S06.1X9A
S06.2X1A
S06.2X2A
S06.2X3A
S06.2X4A
S06.2X5A
S06.2X6A
S06.2X7A
S06.2X8A
S06.2X9A
S06.301A
S06.302A
S06.303A
S06.304A
S06.305A
S06.306A
S06.307A
S06.308A
S06.309A
S06.310A
S06.311A
S06.312A
S06.313A
S06.314A
S06.315A
S06.316A
S06.317A
S06.318A
S06.319A
S06.320A
S06.321A
S06.322A
S06.323A
S06.324A
S06.325A
S06.326A
S06.327A
S06.328A
S06.329A
S06.330A
S06.331A
S06.332A
S06.333A
S06.334A
S06.335A
S06.336A
S06.337A
S06.338A
S06.339A
S06.340A
S06.341A
S06.342A
S06.343A
S06.344A
S06.345A
S06.346A
S06.347A
S06.348A
S06.349A
S06.350A
S06.351A
S06.352A
S06.353A
S06.354A
S06.355A
S06.356A
S06.357A
S06.358A
S06.359A
S06.360A
S06.361A
S06.362A
S06.363A
S06.364A
S06.365A
S06.366A
S06.367A
S06.368A
S06.369A
S06.370A
S06.371A
S06.372A
S06.373A
S06.374A
S06.375A
S06.376A
S06.377A
S06.378A
S06.379A
S06.380A
S06.381A
S06.382A
S06.383A
S06.384A
S06.385A
S06.386A
S06.387A
S06.388A
S06.389A
S06.4X0A
S06.4X1A
S06.4X2A
S06.4X3A
S06.4X4A
S06.4X5A
S06.4X6A
S06.4X7A
S06.4X8A
S06.4X9A
S06.5X0A
S06.5X1A
S06.5X2A
S06.5X3A
S06.5X4A
S06.5X5A
S06.5X6A
S06.5X7A
S06.5X8A
S06.5X9A
S06.6X0A
S06.6X1A
S06.6X2A
S06.6X3A
S06.6X4A
S06.6X5A
S06.6X6A
S06.6X7A
S06.6X8A
S06.6X9A
S06.811A
S06.812A
S06.813A
S06.814A
S06.815A
S06.816A
S06.817A
S06.818A
S06.819A
S06.821A
S06.822A
S06.823A
S06.824A
S06.825A
S06.826A
S06.827A
S06.828A
S06.829A
S06.891A
S06.892A
S06.893A
S06.894A
S06.895A
S06.896A
S06.897A
S06.898A
S06.899A
S06.9X1A
S06.9X2A
S06.9X3A
S06.9X4A

HAC 05: Falls and Trauma (continued)

S06.9X5A	S12.300A	S13.110A	S22.020A	S22.23XB	S32.039B
S06.9X6A	S12.300B	S13.111A	S22.020B	S22.24XA	S32.040A
S06.9X7A	S12.301A	S13.120A	S22.021A	S22.24XB	S32.040B
S06.9X8A	S12.301B	S13.121A	S22.021B	S22.31XA	S32.041A
S06.9X9A	S12.330A	S13.130A	S22.022A	S22.31XB	S32.041B
S07.0XXA	S12.330B	S13.131A	S22.022B	S22.32XA	S32.042A
S07.1XXA	S12.331A	S13.140A	S22.028A	S22.32XB	S32.042B
S07.8XXA	S12.331B	S13.141A	S22.028B	S22.39XA	S32.048A
S07.9XXA	S12.34XA	S13.150A	S22.029A	S22.39XB	S32.048B
S12.000A	S12.34XB	S13.151A	S22.029B	S22.41XA	S32.049A
S12.000B	S12.350A	S13.160A	S22.030A	S22.41XB	S32.049B
S12.001A	S12.350B	S13.161A	S22.030B	S22.42XA	S32.050A
S12.001B	S12.351A	S13.170A	S22.031A	S22.42XB	S32.050B
S12.01XA	S12.351B	S13.171A	S22.031B	S22.43XA	S32.051A
S12.01XB	S12.390A	S13.180A	S22.032A	S22.43XB	S32.051B
S12.02XA	S12.390B	S13.181A	S22.032B	S22.49XA	S32.052A
S12.02XB	S12.391A	S13.20XA	S22.038A	S22.49XB	S32.052B
S12.030A	S12.391B	S13.29XA	S22.038B	S22.5XXA	S32.058A
S12.030B	S12.400A	S14.101A	S22.039A	S22.5XXB	S32.058B
S12.031A	S12.400B	S14.102A	S22.039B	S22.9XXA	S32.059A
S12.031B	S12.401A	S14.103A	S22.040A	S22.9XXB	S32.059B
S12.040A	S12.401B	S14.104A	S22.040B	S24.101A	S32.10XA
S12.040B	S12.430A	S14.105A	S22.041A	S24.102A	S32.10XB
S12.041A	S12.430B	S14.106A	S22.041B	S24.103A	S32.110A
S12.041B	S12.431A	S14.107A	S22.042A	S24.104A	S32.110B
S12.090A	S12.431B	S14.109A	S22.042B	S24.109A	S32.111A
S12.090B	S12.44XA	S14.111A	S22.048A	S24.111A	S32.111B
S12.091A	S12.44XB	S14.112A	S22.048B	S24.112A	S32.112A
S12.091B	S12.450A	S14.113A	S22.049A	S24.113A	S32.112B
S12.100A	S12.450B	S14.114A	S22.049B	S24.114A	S32.119A
S12.100B	S12.451A	S14.115A	S22.050A	S24.131A	S32.119B
S12.101A	S12.451B	S14.116A	S22.050B	S24.132A	S32.120A
S12.101B	S12.490A	S14.117A	S22.051A	S24.133A	S32.120B
S12.110A	S12.490B	S14.121A	S22.051B	S24.134A	S32.121A
S12.110B	S12.491A	S14.122A	S22.052A	S24.151A	S32.121B
S12.111A	S12.491B	S14.123A	S22.052B	S24.152A	S32.122A
S12.111B	S12.500A	S14.124A	S22.058A	S24.153A	S32.122B
S12.112A	S12.500B	S14.125A	S22.058B	S24.154A	S32.129A
S12.112B	S12.501A	S14.126A	S22.059A	S32.000A	S32.129B
S12.120A	S12.501B	S14.127A	S22.059B	S32.000B	S32.130A
S12.120B	S12.530A	S14.131A	S22.060A	S32.001A	S32.130B
S12.121A	S12.530B	S14.132A	S22.060B	S32.001B	S32.131A
S12.121B	S12.531A	S14.133A	S22.061A	S32.002A	S32.131B
S12.130A	S12.531B	S14.134A	S22.061B	S32.002B	S32.132A
S12.130B	S12.54XA	S14.135A	S22.062A	S32.008A	S32.132B
S12.131A	S12.54XB	S14.136A	S22.062B	S32.008B	S32.139A
S12.131B	S12.550A	S14.137A	S22.068A	S32.009A	S32.139B
S12.14XA	S12.550B	S14.151A	S22.068B	S32.009B	S32.14XA
S12.14XB	S12.551A	S14.152A	S22.069A	S32.010A	S32.14XB
S12.150A	S12.551B	S14.153A	S22.069B	S32.010B	S32.15XA
S12.150B	S12.590A	S14.154A	S22.070A	S32.011A	S32.15XB
S12.151A	S12.590B	S14.155A	S22.070B	S32.011B	S32.16XA
S12.151B	S12.591A	S14.156A	S22.071A	S32.012A	S32.16XB
S12.190A	S12.591B	S14.157A	S22.071B	S32.012B	S32.17XA
S12.190B	S12.600A	S17.0XXA	S22.072A	S32.018A	S32.17XB
S12.191A	S12.600B	S17.8XXA	S22.072B	S32.018B	S32.19XA
S12.191B	S12.601A	S17.9XXA	S22.078A	S32.019A	S32.19XB
S12.200A	S12.601B	S22.000A	S22.078B	S32.019B	S32.2XXA
S12.200B	S12.630A	S22.000B	S22.079A	S32.020A	S32.2XXB
S12.201A	S12.630B	S22.001A	S22.079B	S32.020B	S32.301A
S12.201B	S12.631A	S22.001B	S22.080A	S32.021A	S32.301B
S12.230A	S12.631B	S22.002A	S22.080B	S32.021B	S32.302A
S12.230B	S12.64XA	S22.002B	S22.081A	S32.022A	S32.302B
S12.231A	S12.64XB	S22.008A	S22.081B	S32.022B	S32.309A
S12.231B	S12.650A	S22.008B	S22.082A	S32.028A	S32.309B
S12.24XA	S12.650B	S22.009A	S22.082B	S32.028B	S32.311A
S12.24XB	S12.651A	S22.009B	S22.088A	S32.029A	S32.311B
S12.250A	S12.651B	S22.010A	S22.088B	S32.029B	S32.312A
S12.250B	S12.690A	S22.010B	S22.089A	S32.030A	S32.312B
S12.251A	S12.690B	S22.011A	S22.089B	S32.030B	S32.313A
S12.251B	S12.691A	S22.011B	S22.20XA	S32.031A	S32.313B
S12.290A	S12.691B	S22.012A	S22.20XB	S32.031B	S32.314A
S12.290B	S12.8XXA	S22.012B	S22.21XA	S32.032A	S32.314B
S12.291A	S12.9XXA	S22.018A	S22.21XB	S32.032B	S32.315A
S12.291B	S13.0XXA	S22.018B	S22.22XA	S32.038A	S32.315B
	S13.100A	S22.019A	S22.22XB	S32.038B	S32.316A
	S13.101A	S22.019B	S22.23XA	S32.039A	S32.316B

HAC 05: Falls and Trauma (continued)

S32.391A	S32.462B	S32.692A	S42.133B	S42.263A	S42.355B
S32.391B	S32.463A	S32.692B	S42.134B	S42.263B	S42.356A
S32.392A	S32.463B	S32.699A	S42.135B	S42.264A	S42.356B
S32.392B	S32.464A	S32.699B	S42.136B	S42.264B	S42.361A
S32.399A	S32.464B	S32.810A	S42.141B	S42.265A	S42.361B
S32.399B	S32.465A	S32.810B	S42.142B	S42.265B	S42.362A
S32.401A	S32.465B	S32.811A	S42.143B	S42.266A	S42.362B
S32.401B	S32.466A	S32.811B	S42.144B	S42.266B	S42.363A
S32.402A	S32.466B	S32.82XA	S42.145B	S42.271A	S42.363B
S32.402B	S32.471A	S32.82XB	S42.146B	S42.272A	S42.364A
S32.409A	S32.471B	S32.89XA	S42.151B	S42.279A	S42.364B
S32.409B	S32.472A	S32.89XB	S42.152B	S42.291A	S42.365A
S32.411A	S32.472B	S32.9XXA	S42.153B	S42.291B	S42.365B
S32.411B	S32.473A	S32.9XXB	S42.154B	S42.292A	S42.366A
S32.412A	S32.473B	S34.101A	S42.155B	S42.292B	S42.366B
S32.412B	S32.474A	S34.102A	S42.156B	S42.293A	S42.391A
S32.413A	S32.474B	S34.103A	S42.191B	S42.293B	S42.391B
S32.413B	S32.475A	S34.104A	S42.192B	S42.294A	S42.392A
S32.414A	S32.475B	S34.105A	S42.199B	S42.294B	S42.392B
S32.414B	S32.476A	S34.109A	S42.201A	S42.295A	S42.399A
S32.415A	S32.476B	S34.111A	S42.201B	S42.295B	S42.399B
S32.415B	S32.481A	S34.112A	S42.202A	S42.296A	S42.401A
S32.416A	S32.481B	S34.113A	S42.202B	S42.296B	S42.401B
S32.416B	S32.482A	S34.114A	S42.209A	S42.301A	S42.402A
S32.421A	S32.482B	S34.115A	S42.209B	S42.301B	S42.402B
S32.421B	S32.483A	S34.119A	S42.211A	S42.302A	S42.409A
S32.422A	S32.483B	S34.121A	S42.211B	S42.302B	S42.409B
S32.422B	S32.484A	S34.122A	S42.212A	S42.309A	S42.411A
S32.423A	S32.484B	S34.123A	S42.212B	S42.309B	S42.411B
S32.423B	S32.485A	S34.124A	S42.213A	S42.311A	S42.412A
S32.424A	S32.485B	S34.125A	S42.213B	S42.312A	S42.412B
S32.424B	S32.486A	S34.129A	S42.214A	S42.319A	S42.413A
S32.425A	S32.486B	S34.131A	S42.214B	S42.321A	S42.413B
S32.425B	S32.491A	S34.132A	S42.215A	S42.321B	S42.414A
S32.426A	S32.491B	S34.139A	S42.215B	S42.322A	S42.414B
S32.426B	S32.492A	S34.3XXA	S42.216A	S42.322B	S42.415A
S32.431A	S32.492B	S42.001B	S42.216B	S42.323A	S42.415B
S32.431B	S32.499A	S42.002B	S42.221A	S42.323B	S42.416A
S32.432A	S32.499B	S42.009B	S42.221B	S42.324A	S42.416B
S32.432B	S32.501A	S42.011B	S42.222A	S42.324B	S42.421A
S32.433A	S32.501B	S42.012B	S42.222B	S42.325A	S42.421B
S32.433B	S32.502A	S42.013B	S42.223A	S42.325B	S42.422A
S32.434A	S32.502B	S42.014B	S42.223B	S42.326A	S42.422B
S32.434B	S32.509A	S42.015B	S42.224A	S42.326B	S42.423A
S32.435A	S32.509B	S42.016B	S42.224B	S42.331A	S42.423B
S32.435B	S32.511A	S42.017B	S42.225A	S42.331B	S42.424A
S32.436A	S32.511B	S42.018B	S42.225B	S42.332A	S42.424B
S32.436B	S32.512A	S42.019B	S42.226A	S42.332B	S42.425A
S32.441A	S32.512B	S42.021B	S42.226B	S42.333A	S42.425B
S32.441B	S32.519A	S42.022B	S42.231A	S42.333B	S42.426A
S32.442A	S32.519B	S42.023B	S42.231B	S42.334A	S42.426B
S32.442B	S32.591A	S42.024B	S42.232A	S42.334B	S42.431A
S32.443A	S32.591B	S42.025B	S42.232B	S42.335A	S42.431B
S32.443B	S32.592A	S42.026B	S42.239A	S42.335B	S42.432A
S32.444A	S32.592B	S42.031B	S42.239B	S42.336A	S42.432B
S32.444B	S32.599A	S42.032B	S42.241A	S42.336B	S42.433A
S32.445A	S32.599B	S42.033B	S42.241B	S42.341A	S42.433B
S32.445B	S32.601A	S42.034B	S42.242A	S42.341B	S42.434A
S32.446A	S32.601B	S42.035B	S42.242B	S42.342A	S42.434B
S32.446B	S32.602A	S42.036B	S42.249A	S42.342B	S42.435A
S32.451A	S32.602B	S42.101B	S42.249B	S42.343A	S42.435B
S32.451B	S32.609A	S42.102B	S42.251A	S42.343B	S42.436A
S32.452A	S32.609B	S42.109B	S42.251B	S42.344A	S42.436B
S32.452B	S32.611A	S42.111B	S42.252A	S42.344B	S42.441A
S32.453A	S32.611B	S42.112B	S42.252B	S42.345A	S42.441B
S32.453B	S32.612A	S42.113B	S42.253A	S42.345B	S42.442A
S32.454A	S32.612B	S42.114B	S42.253B	S42.346A	S42.442B
S32.454B	S32.613A	S42.115B	S42.254A	S42.346B	S42.443A
S32.455A	S32.613B	S42.116B	S42.254B	S42.351A	S42.443B
S32.455B	S32.614A	S42.121B	S42.255A	S42.351B	S42.444A
S32.456A	S32.614B	S42.122B	S42.255B	S42.352A	S42.444B
S32.456B	S32.615A	S42.123B	S42.256A	S42.352B	S42.445A
S32.461A	S32.615B	S42.124B	S42.256B	S42.353A	S42.445B
S32.461B	S32.616A	S42.125B	S42.261A	S42.353B	S42.446A
S32.462A	S32.616B	S42.126B	S42.261B	S42.354A	S42.446B
	S32.691A	S42.131B	S42.262A	S42.354B	S42.447A
	S32.691B	S42.132B	S42.262B	S42.355A	S42.447B

HAC 05: Falls and Trauma (continued)

S42.448A	S43.223A	S52.043B	S52.225A	S52.266C	S52.342B
S42.448B	S43.224A	S52.043C	S52.225B	S52.271B	S52.342C
S42.449A	S43.225A	S52.044B	S52.225C	S52.271C	S52.343A
S42.449B	S43.226A	S52.044C	S52.226A	S52.272B	S52.343B
S42.451A	S49.001A	S52.045B	S52.226B	S52.272C	S52.343C
S42.451B	S49.002A	S52.045C	S52.226C	S52.279B	S52.344A
S42.452A	S49.009A	S52.046B	S52.231A	S52.279C	S52.344B
S42.452B	S49.011A	S52.046C	S52.231B	S52.281A	S52.344C
S42.453A	S49.012A	S52.091B	S52.231C	S52.281B	S52.345A
S42.453B	S49.019A	S52.091C	S52.232A	S52.281C	S52.345B
S42.454A	S49.021A	S52.092B	S52.232B	S52.282A	S52.345C
S42.454B	S49.022A	S52.092C	S52.232C	S52.282B	S52.346A
S42.455A	S49.029A	S52.099B	S52.233A	S52.282C	S52.346B
S42.455B	S49.031A	S52.099C	S52.233B	S52.283A	S52.346C
S42.456A	S49.032A	S52.101B	S52.233C	S52.283B	S52.351A
S42.456B	S49.039A	S52.101C	S52.234A	S52.283C	S52.351B
S42.461A	S49.041A	S52.102B	S52.234B	S52.291A	S52.351C
S42.461B	S49.042A	S52.102C	S52.234C	S52.291B	S52.352A
S42.462A	S49.049A	S52.109B	S52.235A	S52.291C	S52.352B
S42.462B	S49.091A	S52.109C	S52.235B	S52.292A	S52.352C
S42.463A	S49.092A	S52.111A	S52.235C	S52.292B	S52.353A
S42.463B	S49.099A	S52.112A	S52.236A	S52.292C	S52.353B
S42.464A	S49.101A	S52.119A	S52.236B	S52.299A	S52.353C
S42.464B	S49.102A	S52.121B	S52.236C	S52.299B	S52.354A
S42.465A	S49.109A	S52.121C	S52.241A	S52.299C	S52.354B
S42.465B	S49.111A	S52.122B	S52.241B	S52.301A	S52.354C
S42.466A	S49.112A	S52.122C	S52.241C	S52.301B	S52.355A
S42.466B	S49.119A	S52.123B	S52.242A	S52.301C	S52.355B
S42.471A	S49.121A	S52.123C	S52.242B	S52.302A	S52.355C
S42.471B	S49.122A	S52.124B	S52.242C	S52.302B	S52.356A
S42.472A	S49.129A	S52.124C	S52.243A	S52.302C	S52.356B
S42.472B	S49.131A	S52.125B	S52.243B	S52.309A	S52.356C
S42.473A	S49.132A	S52.125C	S52.243C	S52.309B	S52.361A
S42.473B	S49.139A	S52.126B	S52.244A	S52.309C	S52.361B
S42.474A	S49.141A	S52.126C	S52.244B	S52.311A	S52.361C
S42.474B	S49.142A	S52.131B	S52.244C	S52.312A	S52.362A
S42.475A	S49.149A	S52.131C	S52.245A	S52.319A	S52.362B
S42.475B	S49.191A	S52.132B	S52.245B	S52.321A	S52.362C
S42.476A	S49.192A	S52.132C	S52.245C	S52.321B	S52.363A
S42.476B	S49.199A	S52.133B	S52.246A	S52.321C	S52.363B
S42.481A	S52.001B	S52.133C	S52.246B	S52.322A	S52.363C
S42.482A	S52.001C	S52.134B	S52.246C	S52.322B	S52.364A
S42.489A	S52.002B	S52.134C	S52.251A	S52.322C	S52.364B
S42.491A	S52.002C	S52.135B	S52.251B	S52.323A	S52.364C
S42.491B	S52.009B	S52.135C	S52.251C	S52.323B	S52.365A
S42.492A	S52.009C	S52.136B	S52.252A	S52.323C	S52.365B
S42.492B	S52.011A	S52.136C	S52.252B	S52.324A	S52.365C
S42.493A	S52.012A	S52.181B	S52.252C	S52.324B	S52.366A
S42.493B	S52.019A	S52.181C	S52.253A	S52.324C	S52.366B
S42.494A	S52.021B	S52.182B	S52.253B	S52.325A	S52.366C
S42.494B	S52.021C	S52.182C	S52.253C	S52.325B	S52.371A
S42.495A	S52.022B	S52.189B	S52.254A	S52.325C	S52.371B
S42.495B	S52.022C	S52.189C	S52.254B	S52.326A	S52.371C
S42.496A	S52.023B	S52.201A	S52.254C	S52.326B	S52.372A
S42.496B	S52.023C	S52.201B	S52.255A	S52.326C	S52.372B
S42.90XA	S52.024B	S52.201C	S52.255B	S52.331A	S52.372C
S42.90XB	S52.024C	S52.202A	S52.255C	S52.331B	S52.379A
S42.91XA	S52.025B	S52.202B	S52.256A	S52.331C	S52.379B
S42.91XB	S52.025C	S52.202C	S52.256B	S52.332A	S52.379C
S42.92XA	S52.026B	S52.209A	S52.256C	S52.332B	S52.381A
S42.92XB	S52.026C	S52.209B	S52.261A	S52.332C	S52.381B
S43.201A	S52.031B	S52.209C	S52.261B	S52.333A	S52.381C
S43.202A	S52.031C	S52.211A	S52.261C	S52.333B	S52.382A
S43.203A	S52.032B	S52.212A	S52.262A	S52.333C	S52.382B
S43.204A	S52.032C	S52.219A	S52.262B	S52.334A	S52.382C
S43.205A	S52.033B	S52.221A	S52.262C	S52.334B	S52.389A
S43.206A	S52.033C	S52.221B	S52.263A	S52.334C	S52.389B
S43.211A	S52.034B	S52.221C	S52.263B	S52.335A	S52.389C
S43.212A	S52.034C	S52.222A	S52.263C	S52.335B	S52.391A
S43.213A	S52.035B	S52.222B	S52.264A	S52.335C	S52.391B
S43.214A	S52.035C	S52.222C	S52.264B	S52.336A	S52.391C
S43.215A	S52.036B	S52.223A	S52.264C	S52.336B	S52.392A
S43.216A	S52.036C	S52.223B	S52.265A	S52.336C	S52.392B
S43.221A	S52.041B	S52.223C	S52.265B	S52.341A	S52.392C
S43.222A	S52.041C	S52.224A	S52.265C	S52.341B	S52.399A
	S52.042B	S52.224B	S52.266A	S52.341C	S52.399B
	S52.042C	S52.224C	S52.266B	S52.342A	S52.399C

HAC 05: Falls and Trauma (continued)

S52.501A	S52.591A	S59.209A	S62.172B	S62.333B	S62.615B
S52.501B	S52.591B	S59.211A	S62.173B	S62.334B	S62.616B
S52.501C	S52.591C	S59.212A	S62.174B	S62.335B	S62.617B
S52.502A	S52.592A	S59.219A	S62.175B	S62.336B	S62.618B
S52.502B	S52.592B	S59.221A	S62.176B	S62.337B	S62.619B
S52.502C	S52.592C	S59.222A	S62.181B	S62.338B	S62.620B
S52.509A	S52.599A	S59.229A	S62.182B	S62.339B	S62.621B
S52.509B	S52.599B	S59.231A	S62.183B	S62.340B	S62.622B
S52.509C	S52.599C	S59.232A	S62.184B	S62.341B	S62.623B
S52.511A	S52.601A	S59.239A	S62.185B	S62.342B	S62.624B
S52.511B	S52.601B	S59.241A	S62.186B	S62.343B	S62.625B
S52.511C	S52.601C	S59.242A	S62.201B	S62.344B	S62.626B
S52.512A	S52.602A	S59.249A	S62.202B	S62.345B	S62.627B
S52.512B	S52.602B	S59.291A	S62.209B	S62.346B	S62.628B
S52.512C	S52.602C	S59.292A	S62.211B	S62.347B	S62.629B
S52.513A	S52.609A	S59.299A	S62.212B	S62.348B	S62.630B
S52.513B	S52.609B	S62.001B	S62.213B	S62.349B	S62.631B
S52.513C	S52.609C	S62.002B	S62.221B	S62.350B	S62.632B
S52.514A	S52.611A	S62.009B	S62.222B	S62.351B	S62.633B
S52.514B	S52.611B	S62.011B	S62.223B	S62.352B	S62.634B
S52.514C	S52.611C	S62.012B	S62.224B	S62.353B	S62.635B
S52.515A	S52.612A	S62.013B	S62.225B	S62.354B	S62.636B
S52.515B	S52.612B	S62.014B	S62.226B	S62.355B	S62.637B
S52.515C	S52.612C	S62.015B	S62.231B	S62.356B	S62.638B
S52.516A	S52.613A	S62.016B	S62.232B	S62.357B	S62.639B
S52.516B	S52.613B	S62.021B	S62.233B	S62.358B	S62.640B
S52.516C	S52.613C	S62.022B	S62.234B	S62.359B	S62.641B
S52.521A	S52.614A	S62.023B	S62.235B	S62.360B	S62.642B
S52.522A	S52.614B	S62.024B	S62.236B	S62.361B	S62.643B
S52.529A	S52.614C	S62.025B	S62.241B	S62.362B	S62.644B
S52.531A	S52.615A	S62.026B	S62.242B	S62.363B	S62.645B
S52.531B	S52.615B	S62.031B	S62.243B	S62.364B	S62.646B
S52.531C	S52.615C	S62.032B	S62.244B	S62.365B	S62.647B
S52.532A	S52.616A	S62.033B	S62.245B	S62.366B	S62.648B
S52.532B	S52.616B	S62.034B	S62.246B	S62.367B	S62.649B
S52.532C	S52.616C	S62.035B	S62.251B	S62.368B	S62.650B
S52.539A	S52.621A	S62.036B	S62.252B	S62.369B	S62.651B
S52.539B	S52.622A	S62.101B	S62.253B	S62.390B	S62.652B
S52.539C	S52.629A	S62.102B	S62.254B	S62.391B	S62.653B
S52.541A	S52.691A	S62.109B	S62.255B	S62.392B	S62.654B
S52.541B	S52.691B	S62.111B	S62.256B	S62.393B	S62.655B
S52.541C	S52.691C	S62.112B	S62.291B	S62.394B	S62.656B
S52.542A	S52.692A	S62.113B	S62.292B	S62.395B	S62.657B
S52.542B	S52.692B	S62.114B	S62.299B	S62.396B	S62.658B
S52.542C	S52.692C	S62.115B	S62.300B	S62.397B	S62.659B
S52.549A	S52.699A	S62.116B	S62.301B	S62.398B	S62.660B
S52.549B	S52.699B	S62.121B	S62.302B	S62.399B	S62.661B
S52.549C	S52.699C	S62.122B	S62.303B	S62.501B	S62.662B
S52.551A	S52.90XA	S62.123B	S62.304B	S62.502B	S62.663B
S52.551B	S52.90XB	S62.124B	S62.305B	S62.509B	S62.664B
S52.551C	S52.90XC	S62.125B	S62.306B	S62.511B	S62.665B
S52.552A	S52.91XA	S62.126B	S62.307B	S62.512B	S62.666B
S52.552B	S52.91XB	S62.131B	S62.308B	S62.513B	S62.667B
S52.552C	S52.91XC	S62.132B	S62.309B	S62.514B	S62.668B
S52.559A	S52.92XA	S62.133B	S62.310B	S62.515B	S62.669B
S52.559B	S52.92XB	S62.134B	S62.311B	S62.516B	S62.90XB
S52.559C	S52.92XC	S62.135B	S62.312B	S62.521B	S62.91XB
S52.561A	S59.001A	S62.136B	S62.313B	S62.522B	S62.92XB
S52.561B	S59.002A	S62.141B	S62.314B	S62.523B	S72.001A
S52.561C	S59.009A	S62.142B	S62.315B	S62.524B	S72.001B
S52.562A	S59.011A	S62.143B	S62.316B	S62.525B	S72.001C
S52.562B	S59.012A	S62.144B	S62.317B	S62.526B	S72.002A
S52.562C	S59.019A	S62.145B	S62.318B	S62.600B	S72.002B
S52.569A	S59.021A	S62.146B	S62.319B	S62.601B	S72.002C
S52.569B	S59.022A	S62.151B	S62.320B	S62.602B	S72.009A
S52.569C	S59.029A	S62.152B	S62.321B	S62.603B	S72.009B
S52.571A	S59.031A	S62.153B	S62.322B	S62.604B	S72.009C
S52.571B	S59.032A	S62.154B	S62.323B	S62.605B	S72.011A
S52.571C	S59.039A	S62.155B	S62.324B	S62.606B	S72.011B
S52.572A	S59.041A	S62.156B	S62.325B	S62.607B	S72.011C
S52.572B	S59.042A	S62.161B	S62.326B	S62.608B	S72.012A
S52.572C	S59.049A	S62.162B	S62.327B	S62.609B	S72.012B
S52.579A	S59.091A	S62.163B	S62.328B	S62.610B	S72.012C
S52.579B	S59.092A	S62.164B	S62.329B	S62.611B	S72.019A
S52.579C	S59.099A	S62.165B	S62.330B	S62.612B	S72.019B
	S59.201A	S62.166B	S62.331B	S62.613B	S72.019C
	S59.202A	S62.171B	S62.332B	S62.614B	S72.021A

HAC 05: Falls and Trauma (continued)

S72.021B	S72.065B	S72.141A	S72.335C	S72.411B	S72.453A
S72.021C	S72.065C	S72.141B	S72.336A	S72.411C	S72.453B
S72.022A	S72.066A	S72.141C	S72.336B	S72.412A	S72.453C
S72.022B	S72.066B	S72.142A	S72.336C	S72.412B	S72.454A
S72.022C	S72.066C	S72.142B	S72.341A	S72.412C	S72.454B
S72.023A	S72.091A	S72.142C	S72.341B	S72.413A	S72.454C
S72.023B	S72.091B	S72.143A	S72.341C	S72.413B	S72.455A
S72.023C	S72.091C	S72.143B	S72.342A	S72.413C	S72.455B
S72.024A	S72.092A	S72.143C	S72.342B	S72.414A	S72.455C
S72.024B	S72.092B	S72.144A	S72.342C	S72.414B	S72.456A
S72.024C	S72.092C	S72.144B	S72.343A	S72.414C	S72.456B
S72.025A	S72.099A	S72.144C	S72.343B	S72.415A	S72.456C
S72.025B	S72.099B	S72.145A	S72.343C	S72.415B	S72.461A
S72.025C	S72.099C	S72.145B	S72.344A	S72.415C	S72.461B
S72.026A	S72.101A	S72.145C	S72.344B	S72.416A	S72.461C
S72.026B	S72.101B	S72.146A	S72.344C	S72.416B	S72.462A
S72.026C	S72.101C	S72.146B	S72.345A	S72.416C	S72.462B
S72.031A	S72.102A	S72.146C	S72.345B	S72.421A	S72.462C
S72.031B	S72.102B	S72.21XA	S72.345C	S72.421B	S72.463A
S72.031C	S72.102C	S72.21XB	S72.346A	S72.421C	S72.463B
S72.032A	S72.109A	S72.21XC	S72.346B	S72.422A	S72.463C
S72.032B	S72.109B	S72.22XA	S72.346C	S72.422B	S72.464A
S72.032C	S72.109C	S72.22XB	S72.351A	S72.422C	S72.464B
S72.033A	S72.111A	S72.22XC	S72.351B	S72.423A	S72.464C
S72.033B	S72.111B	S72.23XA	S72.351C	S72.423B	S72.465A
S72.033C	S72.111C	S72.23XB	S72.352A	S72.423C	S72.465B
S72.034A	S72.112A	S72.23XC	S72.352B	S72.424A	S72.465C
S72.034B	S72.112B	S72.24XA	S72.352C	S72.424B	S72.466A
S72.034C	S72.112C	S72.24XB	S72.353A	S72.424C	S72.466B
S72.035A	S72.113A	S72.24XC	S72.353B	S72.425A	S72.466C
S72.035B	S72.113B	S72.25XA	S72.353C	S72.425B	S72.471A
S72.035C	S72.113C	S72.25XB	S72.354A	S72.425C	S72.472A
S72.036A	S72.114A	S72.25XC	S72.354B	S72.426A	S72.479A
S72.036B	S72.114B	S72.26XA	S72.354C	S72.426B	S72.491A
S72.036C	S72.114C	S72.26XB	S72.355A	S72.426C	S72.491B
S72.041A	S72.115A	S72.26XC	S72.355B	S72.431A	S72.491C
S72.041B	S72.115B	S72.301A	S72.355C	S72.431B	S72.492A
S72.041C	S72.115C	S72.301B	S72.356A	S72.431C	S72.492B
S72.042A	S72.116A	S72.301C	S72.356B	S72.432A	S72.492C
S72.042B	S72.116B	S72.302A	S72.356C	S72.432B	S72.499A
S72.042C	S72.116C	S72.302B	S72.361A	S72.432C	S72.499B
S72.043A	S72.121A	S72.302C	S72.361B	S72.433A	S72.499C
S72.043B	S72.121B	S72.309A	S72.361C	S72.433B	S72.8X1A
S72.043C	S72.121C	S72.309B	S72.362A	S72.433C	S72.8X1B
S72.044A	S72.122A	S72.309C	S72.362B	S72.434A	S72.8X1C
S72.044B	S72.122B	S72.321A	S72.362C	S72.434B	S72.8X2A
S72.044C	S72.122C	S72.321B	S72.363A	S72.434C	S72.8X2B
S72.045A	S72.123A	S72.321C	S72.363B	S72.435A	S72.8X2C
S72.045B	S72.123B	S72.322A	S72.363C	S72.435B	S72.8X9A
S72.045C	S72.123C	S72.322B	S72.364A	S72.435C	S72.8X9B
S72.046A	S72.124A	S72.322C	S72.364B	S72.436A	S72.8X9C
S72.046B	S72.124B	S72.323A	S72.364C	S72.436B	S72.90XA
S72.046C	S72.124C	S72.323B	S72.365A	S72.436C	S72.90XB
S72.051A	S72.125A	S72.323C	S72.365B	S72.441A	S72.90XC
S72.051B	S72.125B	S72.324A	S72.365C	S72.441B	S72.91XA
S72.051C	S72.125C	S72.324B	S72.366A	S72.441C	S72.91XB
S72.052A	S72.126A	S72.324C	S72.366B	S72.442A	S72.91XC
S72.052B	S72.126B	S72.325A	S72.366C	S72.442B	S72.92XA
S72.052C	S72.126C	S72.325B	S72.391A	S72.442C	S72.92XB
S72.059A	S72.131A	S72.325C	S72.391B	S72.443A	S72.92XC
S72.059B	S72.131B	S72.326A	S72.391C	S72.443B	S73.001A
S72.059C	S72.131C	S72.326B	S72.392A	S72.443C	S73.002A
S72.061A	S72.132A	S72.326C	S72.392B	S72.444A	S73.003A
S72.061B	S72.132B	S72.331A	S72.392C	S72.444B	S73.004A
S72.061C	S72.132C	S72.331B	S72.399A	S72.444C	S73.005A
S72.062A	S72.133A	S72.331C	S72.399B	S72.445A	S73.006A
S72.062B	S72.133B	S72.332A	S72.399C	S72.445B	S73.011A
S72.062C	S72.133C	S72.332B	S72.401A	S72.445C	S73.012A
S72.063A	S72.134A	S72.332C	S72.401B	S72.446A	S73.013A
S72.063B	S72.134B	S72.333A	S72.401C	S72.446B	S73.014A
S72.063C	S72.134C	S72.333B	S72.402A	S72.446C	S73.015A
S72.064A	S72.135A	S72.333C	S72.402B	S72.451A	S73.016A
S72.064B	S72.135B	S72.334A	S72.402C	S72.451B	S73.021A
S72.064C	S72.135C	S72.334B	S72.409A	S72.451C	S73.022A
S72.065A	S72.136A	S72.334C	S72.409B	S72.452A	S73.023A
	S72.136B	S72.335A	S72.409C	S72.452B	S73.024A
	S72.136C	S72.335B	S72.411A	S72.452C	S73.025A

HAC 05: Falls and Trauma (continued)

S73.026A	S82.021C	S82.113B	S82.155A	S82.245C	S82.424C
S73.031A	S82.022A	S82.113C	S82.155B	S82.246A	S82.425B
S73.032A	S82.022B	S82.114A	S82.155C	S82.246B	S82.425C
S73.033A	S82.022C	S82.114B	S82.156A	S82.246C	S82.426B
S73.034A	S82.023A	S82.114C	S82.156B	S82.251A	S82.426C
S73.035A	S82.023B	S82.115A	S82.156C	S82.251B	S82.431B
S73.036A	S82.023C	S82.115B	S82.161A	S82.251C	S82.431C
S73.041A	S82.024A	S82.115C	S82.162A	S82.252A	S82.432B
S73.042A	S82.024B	S82.116A	S82.169A	S82.252B	S82.432C
S73.043A	S82.024C	S82.116B	S82.191A	S82.252C	S82.433B
S73.044A	S82.025A	S82.116C	S82.191B	S82.253A	S82.433C
S73.045A	S82.025B	S82.121A	S82.191C	S82.253B	S82.434B
S73.046A	S82.025C	S82.121B	S82.192A	S82.253C	S82.434C
S77.00XA	S82.026A	S82.121C	S82.192B	S82.254A	S82.435B
S77.01XA	S82.026B	S82.122A	S82.192C	S82.254B	S82.435C
S77.02XA	S82.026C	S82.122B	S82.199A	S82.254C	S82.436B
S77.10XA	S82.031A	S82.122C	S82.199B	S82.255A	S82.436C
S77.11XA	S82.031B	S82.123A	S82.199C	S82.255B	S82.441B
S77.12XA	S82.031C	S82.123B	S82.201A	S82.255C	S82.441C
S79.001A	S82.032A	S82.123C	S82.201B	S82.256A	S82.442B
S79.002A	S82.032B	S82.124A	S82.201C	S82.256B	S82.442C
S79.009A	S82.032C	S82.124B	S82.202A	S82.256C	S82.443B
S79.011A	S82.033A	S82.124C	S82.202B	S82.261A	S82.443C
S79.012A	S82.033B	S82.125A	S82.202C	S82.261B	S82.444B
S79.019A	S82.033C	S82.125B	S82.209A	S82.261C	S82.444C
S79.091A	S82.034A	S82.125C	S82.209B	S82.262A	S82.445B
S79.092A	S82.034B	S82.126A	S82.209C	S82.262B	S82.445C
S79.099A	S82.034C	S82.126B	S82.221A	S82.262C	S82.446B
S79.101A	S82.035A	S82.126C	S82.221B	S82.263A	S82.446C
S79.102A	S82.035B	S82.131A	S82.221C	S82.263B	S82.451B
S79.109A	S82.035C	S82.131B	S82.222A	S82.263C	S82.451C
S79.111A	S82.036A	S82.131C	S82.222B	S82.264A	S82.452B
S79.112A	S82.036B	S82.132A	S82.222C	S82.264B	S82.452C
S79.119A	S82.036C	S82.132B	S82.223A	S82.264C	S82.453B
S79.121A	S82.041A	S82.132C	S82.223B	S82.265A	S82.453C
S79.122A	S82.041B	S82.133A	S82.223C	S82.265B	S82.454B
S79.129A	S82.041C	S82.133B	S82.224A	S82.265C	S82.454C
S79.131A	S82.042A	S82.133C	S82.224B	S82.266A	S82.455B
S79.132A	S82.042B	S82.134A	S82.224C	S82.266B	S82.455C
S79.139A	S82.042C	S82.134B	S82.225A	S82.266C	S82.456B
S79.141A	S82.043A	S82.134C	S82.225B	S82.291A	S82.456C
S79.142A	S82.043B	S82.135A	S82.225C	S82.291B	S82.461B
S79.149A	S82.043C	S82.135B	S82.226A	S82.291C	S82.461C
S79.191A	S82.044A	S82.135C	S82.226B	S82.292A	S82.462B
S79.192A	S82.044B	S82.136A	S82.226C	S82.292B	S82.462C
S79.199A	S82.044C	S82.136B	S82.231A	S82.292C	S82.463B
S82.001A	S82.045A	S82.136C	S82.231B	S82.299A	S82.463C
S82.001B	S82.045B	S82.141A	S82.231C	S82.299B	S82.464B
S82.001C	S82.045C	S82.141B	S82.232A	S82.299C	S82.464C
S82.002A	S82.046A	S82.141C	S82.232B	S82.301B	S82.465B
S82.002B	S82.046B	S82.142A	S82.232C	S82.301C	S82.465C
S82.002C	S82.046C	S82.142B	S82.233A	S82.302B	S82.466B
S82.009A	S82.091A	S82.142C	S82.233B	S82.302C	S82.466C
S82.009B	S82.091B	S82.143A	S82.233C	S82.309B	S82.491B
S82.009C	S82.091C	S82.143B	S82.234A	S82.309C	S82.491C
S82.011A	S82.092A	S82.143C	S82.234B	S82.311A	S82.492B
S82.011B	S82.092B	S82.144A	S82.234C	S82.312A	S82.492C
S82.011C	S82.092C	S82.144B	S82.235A	S82.319A	S82.499B
S82.012A	S82.099A	S82.144C	S82.235B	S82.391B	S82.499C
S82.012B	S82.099B	S82.145A	S82.235C	S82.391C	S82.51XB
S82.012C	S82.099C	S82.145B	S82.236A	S82.392B	S82.51XC
S82.013A	S82.101A	S82.145C	S82.236B	S82.392C	S82.52XB
S82.013B	S82.101B	S82.146A	S82.236C	S82.399B	S82.52XC
S82.013C	S82.101C	S82.146B	S82.241A	S82.399C	S82.53XB
S82.014A	S82.102A	S82.146C	S82.241B	S82.401B	S82.53XC
S82.014B	S82.102B	S82.151A	S82.241C	S82.401C	S82.54XB
S82.014C	S82.102C	S82.151B	S82.242A	S82.402B	S82.54XC
S82.015A	S82.109A	S82.151C	S82.242B	S82.402C	S82.55XB
S82.015B	S82.109B	S82.152A	S82.242C	S82.409B	S82.55XC
S82.015C	S82.109C	S82.152B	S82.243A	S82.409C	S82.56XB
S82.016A	S82.111A	S82.152C	S82.243B	S82.421B	S82.56XC
S82.016B	S82.111B	S82.153A	S82.243C	S82.421C	S82.61XB
S82.016C	S82.111C	S82.153B	S82.244A	S82.422B	S82.61XC
S82.021A	S82.112A	S82.153C	S82.244B	S82.422C	S82.62XB
S82.021B	S82.112B	S82.154A	S82.244C	S82.423B	S82.62XC
	S82.112C	S82.154B	S82.245A	S82.423C	S82.63XB
	S82.113A	S82.154C	S82.245B	S82.424B	S82.63XC

HAC 05: Falls and Trauma (continued)

S82.64XB	S89.011A	S92.143B	S92.355B	T22.741A	T24.339A
S82.64XC	S89.012A	S92.144B	S92.356B	T22.742A	T24.391A
S82.65XB	S89.019A	S92.145B	S92.901B	T22.749A	T24.392A
S82.65XC	S89.021A	S92.146B	S92.902B	T22.751A	T24.399A
S82.66XB	S89.022A	S92.151B	S92.909B	T22.752A	T24.701A
S82.66XC	S89.029A	S92.152B	T20.30XA	T22.759A	T24.702A
S82.831B	S89.031A	S92.153B	T20.311A	T22.761A	T24.709A
S82.831C	S89.032A	S92.154B	T20.312A	T22.762A	T24.711A
S82.832B	S89.039A	S92.155B	T20.319A	T22.769A	T24.712A
S82.832C	S89.041A	S92.156B	T20.32XA	T22.791A	T24.719A
S82.839B	S89.042A	S92.191B	T20.33XA	T22.792A	T24.721A
S82.839C	S89.049A	S92.192B	T20.34XA	T22.799A	T24.722A
S82.841B	S89.091A	S92.199B	T20.35XA	T23.301A	T24.729A
S82.841C	S89.092A	S92.201B	T20.36XA	T23.302A	T24.731A
S82.842B	S89.099A	S92.202B	T20.37XA	T23.309A	T24.732A
S82.842C	S92.001B	S92.209B	T20.39XA	T23.311A	T24.739A
S82.843B	S92.002B	S92.211B	T20.70XA	T23.312A	T24.791A
S82.843C	S92.009B	S92.212B	T20.711A	T23.319A	T24.792A
S82.844B	S92.011B	S92.213B	T20.712A	T23.321A	T24.799A
S82.844C	S92.012B	S92.214B	T20.719A	T23.322A	T25.311A
S82.845B	S92.013B	S92.215B	T20.72XA	T23.329A	T25.312A
S82.845C	S92.014B	S92.216B	T20.73XA	T23.331A	T25.319A
S82.846B	S92.015B	S92.221B	T20.74XA	T23.332A	T25.321A
S82.846C	S92.016B	S92.222B	T20.75XA	T23.339A	T25.322A
S82.851B	S92.021B	S92.223B	T20.76XA	T23.341A	T25.329A
S82.851C	S92.022B	S92.224B	T20.77XA	T23.342A	T25.331A
S82.852B	S92.023B	S92.225B	T20.79XA	T23.349A	T25.332A
S82.852C	S92.024B	S92.226B	T21.30XA	T23.351A	T25.339A
S82.853B	S92.025B	S92.231B	T21.31XA	T23.352A	T25.391A
S82.853C	S92.026B	S92.232B	T21.32XA	T23.359A	T25.392A
S82.854B	S92.031B	S92.233B	T21.33XA	T23.361A	T25.399A
S82.854C	S92.032B	S92.234B	T21.34XA	T23.362A	T25.711A
S82.855B	S92.033B	S92.235B	T21.35XA	T23.369A	T25.712A
S82.855C	S92.034B	S92.236B	T21.36XA	T23.371A	T25.719A
S82.856B	S92.035B	S92.241B	T21.37XA	T23.372A	T25.721A
S82.856C	S92.036B	S92.242B	T21.39XA	T23.379A	T25.722A
S82.861B	S92.041B	S92.243B	T21.70XA	T23.391A	T25.729A
S82.861C	S92.042B	S92.244B	T21.71XA	T23.392A	T25.731A
S82.862B	S92.043B	S92.245B	T21.72XA	T23.399A	T25.732A
S82.862C	S92.044B	S92.246B	T21.73XA	T23.701A	T25.739A
S82.863B	S92.045B	S92.251B	T21.74XA	T23.702A	T25.791A
S82.863C	S92.046B	S92.252B	T21.75XA	T23.709A	T25.792A
S82.864B	S92.051B	S92.253B	T21.76XA	T23.711A	T25.799A
S82.864C	S92.052B	S92.254B	T21.77XA	T23.712A	T26.20XA
S82.865B	S92.053B	S92.255B	T21.79XA	T23.719A	T26.21XA
S82.865C	S92.054B	S92.256B	T22.30XA	T23.721A	T26.22XA
S82.866B	S92.055B	S92.301B	T22.311A	T23.722A	T26.70XA
S82.866C	S92.056B	S92.302B	T22.312A	T23.729A	T26.71XA
S82.871B	S92.061B	S92.309B	T22.319A	T23.731A	T26.72XA
S82.871C	S92.062B	S92.311B	T22.321A	T23.732A	T27.0XXA
S82.872B	S92.063B	S92.312B	T22.322A	T23.739A	T27.1XXA
S82.872C	S92.064B	S92.313B	T22.329A	T23.741A	T27.2XXA
S82.873B	S92.065B	S92.314B	T22.331A	T23.742A	T27.3XXA
S82.873C	S92.066B	S92.315B	T22.332A	T23.749A	T27.4XXA
S82.874B	S92.101B	S92.316B	T22.339A	T23.751A	T27.5XXA
S82.874C	S92.102B	S92.321B	T22.341A	T23.752A	T27.6XXA
S82.875B	S92.109B	S92.322B	T22.342A	T23.759A	T27.7XXA
S82.875C	S92.111B	S92.323B	T22.349A	T23.761A	T28.1XXA
S82.876B	S92.112B	S92.324B	T22.351A	T23.762A	T28.2XXA
S82.876C	S92.113B	S92.325B	T22.352A	T23.769A	T28.6XXA
S82.891B	S92.114B	S92.326B	T22.359A	T23.771A	T28.7XXA
S82.891C	S92.115B	S92.331B	T22.361A	T23.772A	T31.10
S82.892B	S92.116B	S92.332B	T22.362A	T23.779A	T31.11
S82.892C	S92.121B	S92.333B	T22.369A	T23.791A	T31.20
S82.899B	S92.122B	S92.334B	T22.391A	T23.792A	T31.21
S82.899C	S92.123B	S92.335B	T22.392A	T23.799A	T31.22
S82.90XB	S92.124B	S92.336B	T22.399A	T24.301A	T31.30
S82.90XC	S92.125B	S92.341B	T22.70XA	T24.302A	T31.31
S82.91XB	S92.126B	S92.342B	T22.711A	T24.309A	T31.32
S82.91XC	S92.131B	S92.343B	T22.712A	T24.311A	T31.33
S82.92XB	S92.132B	S92.344B	T22.719A	T24.312A	T31.40
S82.92XC	S92.133B	S92.345B	T22.721A	T24.319A	T31.41
S89.001A	S92.134B	S92.346B	T22.722A	T24.321A	T31.42
S89.002A	S92.135B	S92.351B	T22.729A	T24.322A	T31.43
S89.009A	S92.136B	S92.352B	T22.731A	T24.329A	T31.44
	S92.141B	S92.353B	T22.732A	T24.331A	T31.50
	S92.142B	S92.354B	T22.739A	T24.332A	T31.51

HAC 05: Falls and Trauma (continued)

T31.52	T32.10	T32.85	T33.811A	T34.821A	T71.20XA
T31.53	T32.11	T32.86	T33.812A	T34.822A	T71.21XA
T31.54	T32.20	T32.87	T33.819A	T34.829A	T71.29XA
T31.55	T32.21	T32.88	T33.821A	T34.831A	T71.9XXA
T31.60	T32.22	T32.90	T33.822A	T34.832A	T75.1XXA
T31.61	T32.30	T32.91	T33.829A	T34.839A	
T31.62	T32.31	T32.92	T33.831A	T34.90XA	**HAC 06: Catheter Associated Urinary Tract Infection (UTI)**
T31.63	T32.32	T32.93	T33.832A	T34.99XA	
T31.64	T32.33	T32.94	T33.839A	T67.0XXA	Secondary diagnosis not POA:
T31.65	T32.40	T32.95	T33.90XA	T69.021A	T83.51XA
T31.66	T32.41	T32.96	T33.99XA	T69.022A	
T31.70	T32.42	T32.97	T34.011A	T69.029A	**With or Without**
T31.71	T32.43	T32.98	T34.012A	T70.3XXA	Secondary diagnosis (also not POA) of:
T31.72	T32.44	T32.99	T34.019A	T71.111A	B37.41
T31.73	T32.50	T33.011A	T34.02XA	T71.112A	B37.49
T31.74	T32.51	T33.012A	T34.09XA	T71.113A	N10
T31.75	T32.52	T33.019A	T34.1XXA	T71.114A	N11.9
T31.76	T32.53	T33.02XA	T34.2XXA	T71.121A	N12
T31.77	T32.54	T33.09XA	T34.3XXA	T71.122A	N13.6
T31.80	T32.55	T33.1XXA	T34.40XA	T71.123A	N15.1
T31.81	T32.60	T33.2XXA	T34.41XA	T71.124A	N28.84
T31.82	T32.61	T33.3XXA	T34.42XA	T71.131A	N28.85
T31.83	T32.62	T33.40XA	T34.511A	T71.132A	N28.86
T31.84	T32.63	T33.41XA	T34.512A	T71.133A	N30.00
T31.85	T32.64	T33.42XA	T34.519A	T71.134A	N30.01
T31.86	T32.65	T33.511A	T34.521A	T71.141A	N34.0
T31.87	T32.66	T33.512A	T34.522A	T71.143A	N39.0
T31.88	T32.70	T33.519A	T34.529A	T71.144A	
T31.90	T32.71	T33.521A	T34.531A	T71.151A	**HAC 07: Vascular Catheter Associated Infection**
T31.91	T32.72	T33.522A	T34.532A	T71.152A	
T31.92	T32.73	T33.529A	T34.539A	T71.153A	Secondary diagnosis not POA:
T31.93	T32.74	T33.531A	T34.60XA	T71.154A	T80.211A
T31.94	T32.75	T33.532A	T34.61XA	T71.161A	T80.212A
T31.95	T32.76	T33.539A	T34.62XA	T71.162A	T80.218A
T31.96	T32.77	T33.60XA	T34.70XA	T71.163A	T80.219A
T31.97	T32.80	T33.61XA	T34.71XA	T71.164A	
T31.98	T32.81	T33.62XA	T34.72XA	T71.191A	
T31.99	T32.82	T33.70XA	T34.811A	T71.192A	
	T32.83	T33.71XA	T34.812A	T71.193A	
	T32.84	T33.72XA	T34.819A	T71.194A	

Appendix I: Hospital Acquired Conditions

HAC 08: Surgical Site Infection of Mediastinitis Following Coronary Bypass Graft (CABG) Procedures

Secondary diagnosis not POA:
J98.5

AND

Any of the following procedures:

0210093 Bypass Coronary Artery, One Site from Coronary Artery with Autologous Venous Tissue, Open Approach

0210098 Bypass Coronary Artery, One Site from Right Internal Mammary with Autologous Venous Tissue, Open Approach

0210099 Bypass Coronary Artery, One Site from Left Internal Mammary with Autologous Venous Tissue, Open Approach

021009C Bypass Coronary Artery, One Site from Thoracic Artery with Autologous Venous Tissue, Open Approach

021009F Bypass Coronary Artery, One Site from Abdominal Artery with Autologous Venous Tissue, Open Approach

021009W Bypass Coronary Artery, One Site from Aorta with Autologous Venous Tissue, Open Approach

02100A3 Bypass Coronary Artery, One Site from Coronary Artery with Autologous Arterial Tissue, Open Approach

02100A8 Bypass Coronary Artery, One Site from Right Internal Mammary with Autologous Arterial Tissue, Open Approach

02100A9 Bypass Coronary Artery, One Site from Left Internal Mammary with Autologous Arterial Tissue, Open Approach

02100AC Bypass Coronary Artery, One Site from Thoracic Artery with Autologous Arterial Tissue, Open Approach

02100AF Bypass Coronary Artery, One Site from Abdominal Artery with Autologous Arterial Tissue, Open Approach

02100AW Bypass Coronary Artery, One Site from Aorta with Autologous Arterial Tissue, Open Approach

02100J3 Bypass Coronary Artery, One Site from Coronary Artery with Synthetic Substitute, Open Approach

02100J8 Bypass Coronary Artery, One Site from Right Internal Mammary with Synthetic Substitute, Open Approach

02100J9 Bypass Coronary Artery, One Site from Left Internal Mammary with Synthetic Substitute, Open Approach

02100JC Bypass Coronary Artery, One Site from Thoracic Artery with Synthetic Substitute, Open Approach

02100JF Bypass Coronary Artery, One Site from Abdominal Artery with Synthetic Substitute, Open Approach

02100JW Bypass Coronary Artery, One Site from Aorta with Synthetic Substitute, Open Approach

02100K3 Bypass Coronary Artery, One Site from Coronary Artery with Nonautologous Tissue Substitute, Open Approach

02100K8 Bypass Coronary Artery, One Site from Right Internal Mammary with Nonautologous Tissue Substitute, Open Approach

02100K9 Bypass Coronary Artery, One Site from Left Internal Mammary with Nonautologous Tissue Substitute, Open Approach

02100KC Bypass Coronary Artery, One Site from Thoracic Artery with Nonautologous Tissue Substitute, Open Approach

02100KF Bypass Coronary Artery, One Site from Abdominal Artery with Nonautologous Tissue Substitute, Open Approach

02100KW Bypass Coronary Artery, One Site from Aorta with Nonautologous Tissue Substitute, Open Approach

02100Z3 Bypass Coronary Artery, One Site from Coronary Artery, Open Approach

02100Z8 Bypass Coronary Artery, One Site from Right Internal Mammary, Open Approach

02100Z9 Bypass Coronary Artery, One Site from Left Internal Mammary, Open Approach

02100ZC Bypass Coronary Artery, One Site from Thoracic Artery, Open Approach

02100ZF Bypass Coronary Artery, One Site from Abdominal Artery, Open Approach

0210493 Bypass Coronary Artery, One Site from Coronary Artery with Autologous Venous Tissue, Percutaneous Endoscopic Approach

0210498 Bypass Coronary Artery, One Site from Right Internal Mammary with Autologous Venous Tissue, Percutaneous Endoscopic Approach

0210499 Bypass Coronary Artery, One Site from Left Internal Mammary with Autologous Venous Tissue, Percutaneous Endoscopic Approach

021049C Bypass Coronary Artery, One Site from Thoracic Artery with Autologous Venous Tissue, Percutaneous Endoscopic Approach

021049F Bypass Coronary Artery, One Site from Abdominal Artery with Autologous Venous Tissue, Percutaneous Endoscopic Approach

021049W Bypass Coronary Artery, One Site from Aorta with Autologous Venous Tissue, Percutaneous Endoscopic Approach

02104A3 Bypass Coronary Artery, One Site from Coronary Artery with Autologous Arterial Tissue, Percutaneous Endoscopic Approach

02104A8 Bypass Coronary Artery, One Site from Right Internal Mammary with Autologous Arterial Tissue, Percutaneous Endoscopic Approach

02104A9 Bypass Coronary Artery, One Site from Left Internal Mammary with Autologous Arterial Tissue, Percutaneous Endoscopic Approach

02104AC Bypass Coronary Artery, One Site from Thoracic Artery with Autologous Arterial Tissue, Percutaneous Endoscopic Approach

02104AF Bypass Coronary Artery, One Site from Abdominal Artery with Autologous Arterial Tissue, Percutaneous Endoscopic Approach

02104AW Bypass Coronary Artery, One Site from Aorta with Autologous Arterial Tissue, Percutaneous Endoscopic Approach

02104J3 Bypass Coronary Artery, One Site from Coronary Artery with Synthetic Substitute, Percutaneous Endoscopic Approach

02104J8 Bypass Coronary Artery, One Site from Right Internal Mammary with Synthetic Substitute, Percutaneous Endoscopic Approach

02104J9 Bypass Coronary Artery, One Site from Left Internal Mammary with Synthetic Substitute, Percutaneous Endoscopic Approach

02104JC Bypass Coronary Artery, One Site from Thoracic Artery with Synthetic Substitute, Percutaneous Endoscopic Approach

02104JF Bypass Coronary Artery, One Site from Abdominal Artery with Synthetic Substitute, Percutaneous Endoscopic Approach

02104JW Bypass Coronary Artery, One Site from Aorta with Synthetic Substitute, Percutaneous Endoscopic Approach

02104K3 Bypass Coronary Artery, One Site from Coronary Artery with Nonautologous Tissue Substitute, Percutaneous Endoscopic Approach

02104K8 Bypass Coronary Artery, One Site from Right Internal Mammary with Nonautologous Tissue Substitute, Percutaneous Endoscopic Approach

02104K9 Bypass Coronary Artery, One Site from Left Internal Mammary with Nonautologous Tissue Substitute, Percutaneous Endoscopic Approach

02104KC Bypass Coronary Artery, One Site from Thoracic Artery with Nonautologous Tissue Substitute, Percutaneous Endoscopic Approach

02104KF Bypass Coronary Artery, One Site from Abdominal Artery with Nonautologous Tissue Substitute, Percutaneous Endoscopic Approach

02104KW Bypass Coronary Artery, One Site from Aorta with Nonautologous Tissue Substitute, Percutaneous Endoscopic Approach

02104Z3 Bypass Coronary Artery, One Site from Coronary Artery, Percutaneous Endoscopic Approach

02104Z8 Bypass Coronary Artery, One Site from Right Internal Mammary, Percutaneous Endoscopic Approach

02104Z9 Bypass Coronary Artery, One Site from Left Internal Mammary, Percutaneous Endoscopic Approach

02104ZC Bypass Coronary Artery, One Site from Thoracic Artery, Percutaneous Endoscopic Approach

02104ZF Bypass Coronary Artery, One Site from Abdominal Artery, Percutaneous Endoscopic Approach

0211093 Bypass Coronary Artery, Two Sites from Coronary Artery with Autologous Venous Tissue, Open Approach

0211098 Bypass Coronary Artery, Two Sites from Right Internal Mammary with Autologous Venous Tissue, Open Approach

0211099 Bypass Coronary Artery, Two Sites from Left Internal Mammary with Autologous Venous Tissue, Open Approach

021109C Bypass Coronary Artery, Two Sites from Thoracic Artery with Autologous Venous Tissue, Open Approach

021109F Bypass Coronary Artery, Two Sites from Abdominal Artery with Autologous Venous Tissue, Open Approach

021109W Bypass Coronary Artery, Two Sites from Aorta with Autologous Venous Tissue, Open Approach

02110A3 Bypass Coronary Artery, Two Sites from Coronary Artery with Autologous Arterial Tissue, Open Approach

02110A8 Bypass Coronary Artery, Two Sites from Right Internal Mammary with Autologous Arterial Tissue, Open Approach

HAC 08: Surgical Site Infection of Mediastinitis Following Coronary Bypass Graft (CABG) Procedures (continued)

Ø2110A9   Bypass Coronary Artery, Two Sites from Left Internal Mammary with Autologous Arterial Tissue, Open Approach

Ø2110AC   Bypass Coronary Artery, Two Sites from Thoracic Artery with Autologous Arterial Tissue, Open Approach

Ø2110AF   Bypass Coronary Artery, Two Sites from Abdominal Artery with Autologous Arterial Tissue, Open Approach

Ø2110AW   Bypass Coronary Artery, Two Sites from Aorta with Autologous Arterial Tissue, Open Approach

Ø2110J3   Bypass Coronary Artery, Two Sites from Coronary Artery with Synthetic Substitute, Open Approach

Ø2110J8   Bypass Coronary Artery, Two Sites from Right Internal Mammary with Synthetic Substitute, Open Approach

Ø2110J9   Bypass Coronary Artery, Two Sites from Left Internal Mammary with Synthetic Substitute, Open Approach

Ø2110JC   Bypass Coronary Artery, Two Sites from Thoracic Artery with Synthetic Substitute, Open Approach

Ø2110JF   Bypass Coronary Artery, Two Sites from Abdominal Artery with Synthetic Substitute, Open Approach

Ø2110JW   Bypass Coronary Artery, Two Sites from Aorta with Synthetic Substitute, Open Approach

Ø2110K3   Bypass Coronary Artery, Two Sites from Coronary Artery with Nonautologous Tissue Substitute, Open Approach

Ø2110K8   Bypass Coronary Artery, Two Sites from Right Internal Mammary with Nonautologous Tissue Substitute, Open Approach

Ø2110K9   Bypass Coronary Artery, Two Sites from Left Internal Mammary with Nonautologous Tissue Substitute, Open Approach

Ø2110KC   Bypass Coronary Artery, Two Sites from Thoracic Artery with Nonautologous Tissue Substitute, Open Approach

Ø2110KF   Bypass Coronary Artery, Two Sites from Abdominal Artery with Nonautologous Tissue Substitute, Open Approach

Ø2110KW   Bypass Coronary Artery, Two Sites from Aorta with Nonautologous Tissue Substitute, Open Approach

Ø2110Z3   Bypass Coronary Artery, Two Sites from Coronary Artery, Open Approach

Ø2110Z8   Bypass Coronary Artery, Two Sites from Right Internal Mammary, Open Approach

Ø2110Z9   Bypass Coronary Artery, Two Sites from Left Internal Mammary, Open Approach

Ø2110ZC   Bypass Coronary Artery, Two Sites from Thoracic Artery, Open Approach

Ø2110ZF   Bypass Coronary Artery, Two Sites from Abdominal Artery, Open Approach

Ø211493   Bypass Coronary Artery, Two Sites from Coronary Artery with Autologous Venous Tissue, Percutaneous Endoscopic Approach

Ø211498   Bypass Coronary Artery, Two Sites from Right Internal Mammary with Autologous Venous Tissue, Percutaneous Endoscopic Approach

Ø211499   Bypass Coronary Artery, Two Sites from Left Internal Mammary with Autologous Venous Tissue, Percutaneous Endoscopic Approach

Ø21149C   Bypass Coronary Artery, Two Sites from Thoracic Artery with Autologous Venous Tissue, Percutaneous Endoscopic Approach

Ø21149F   Bypass Coronary Artery, Two Sites from Abdominal Artery with Autologous Venous Tissue, Percutaneous Endoscopic Approach

Ø21149W   Bypass Coronary Artery, Two Sites from Aorta with Autologous Venous Tissue, Percutaneous Endoscopic Approach

Ø2114A3   Bypass Coronary Artery, Two Sites from Coronary Artery with Autologous Arterial Tissue, Percutaneous Endoscopic Approach

Ø2114A8   Bypass Coronary Artery, Two Sites from Right Internal Mammary with Autologous Arterial Tissue, Percutaneous Endoscopic Approach

Ø2114A9   Bypass Coronary Artery, Two Sites from Left Internal Mammary with Autologous Arterial Tissue, Percutaneous Endoscopic Approach

Ø2114AC   Bypass Coronary Artery, Two Sites from Thoracic Artery with Autologous Arterial Tissue, Percutaneous Endoscopic Approach

Ø2114AF   Bypass Coronary Artery, Two Sites from Abdominal Artery with Autologous Arterial Tissue, Percutaneous Endoscopic Approach

Ø2114AW   Bypass Coronary Artery, Two Sites from Aorta with Autologous Arterial Tissue, Percutaneous Endoscopic Approach

Ø2114J3   Bypass Coronary Artery, Two Sites from Coronary Artery with Synthetic Substitute, Percutaneous Endoscopic Approach

Ø2114J8   Bypass Coronary Artery, Two Sites from Right Internal Mammary with Synthetic Substitute, Percutaneous Endoscopic Approach

Ø2114J9   Bypass Coronary Artery, Two Sites from Left Internal Mammary with Synthetic Substitute, Percutaneous Endoscopic Approach

Ø2114JC   Bypass Coronary Artery, Two Sites from Thoracic Artery with Synthetic Substitute, Percutaneous Endoscopic Approach

Ø2114JF   Bypass Coronary Artery, Two Sites from Abdominal Artery with Synthetic Substitute, Percutaneous Endoscopic Approach

Ø2114JW   Bypass Coronary Artery, Two Sites from Aorta with Synthetic Substitute, Percutaneous Endoscopic Approach

Ø2114K3   Bypass Coronary Artery, Two Sites from Coronary Artery with Nonautologous Tissue Substitute, Percutaneous Endoscopic Approach

Ø2114K8   Bypass Coronary Artery, Two Sites from Right Internal Mammary with Nonautologous Tissue Substitute, Percutaneous Endoscopic Approach

Ø2114K9   Bypass Coronary Artery, Two Sites from Left Internal Mammary with Nonautologous Tissue Substitute, Percutaneous Endoscopic Approach

Ø2114KC   Bypass Coronary Artery, Two Sites from Thoracic Artery with Nonautologous Tissue Substitute, Percutaneous Endoscopic Approach

Ø2114KF   Bypass Coronary Artery, Two Sites from Abdominal Artery with Nonautologous Tissue Substitute, Percutaneous Endoscopic Approach

Ø2114KW   Bypass Coronary Artery, Two Sites from Aorta with Nonautologous Tissue Substitute, Percutaneous Endoscopic Approach

Ø2114Z3   Bypass Coronary Artery, Two Sites from Coronary Artery, Percutaneous Endoscopic Approach

Ø2114Z8   Bypass Coronary Artery, Two Sites from Right Internal Mammary, Percutaneous Endoscopic Approach

Ø2114Z9   Bypass Coronary Artery, Two Sites from Left Internal Mammary, Percutaneous Endoscopic Approach

Ø2114ZC   Bypass Coronary Artery, Two Sites from Thoracic Artery, Percutaneous Endoscopic Approach

Ø2114ZF   Bypass Coronary Artery, Two Sites from Abdominal Artery, Percutaneous Endoscopic Approach

Ø212093   Bypass Coronary Artery, Three Sites from Coronary Artery with Autologous Venous Tissue, Open Approach

Ø212098   Bypass Coronary Artery, Three Sites from Right Internal Mammary with Autologous Venous Tissue, Open Approach

Ø212099   Bypass Coronary Artery, Three Sites from Left Internal Mammary with Autologous Venous Tissue, Open Approach

Ø21209C   Bypass Coronary Artery, Three Sites from Thoracic Artery with Autologous Venous Tissue, Open Approach

Ø21209F   Bypass Coronary Artery, Three Sites from Abdominal Artery with Autologous Venous Tissue, Open Approach

Ø21209W   Bypass Coronary Artery, Three Sites from Aorta with Autologous Venous Tissue, Open Approach

Ø2120A3   Bypass Coronary Artery, Three Sites from Coronary Artery with Autologous Arterial Tissue, Open Approach

Ø2120A8   Bypass Coronary Artery, Three Sites from Right Internal Mammary with Autologous Arterial Tissue, Open Approach

Ø2120A9   Bypass Coronary Artery, Three Sites from Left Internal Mammary with Autologous Arterial Tissue, Open Approach

Ø2120AC   Bypass Coronary Artery, Three Sites from Thoracic Artery with Autologous Arterial Tissue, Open Approach

Ø2120AF   Bypass Coronary Artery, Three Sites from Abdominal Artery with Autologous Arterial Tissue, Open Approach

Ø2120AW   Bypass Coronary Artery, Three Sites from Aorta with Autologous Arterial Tissue, Open Approach

Ø2120J3   Bypass Coronary Artery, Three Sites from Coronary Artery with Synthetic Substitute, Open Approach

Ø2120J8   Bypass Coronary Artery, Three Sites from Right Internal Mammary with Synthetic Substitute, Open Approach

Ø2120J9   Bypass Coronary Artery, Three Sites from Left Internal Mammary with Synthetic Substitute, Open Approach

Ø2120JC   Bypass Coronary Artery, Three Sites from Thoracic Artery with Synthetic Substitute, Open Approach

Ø2120JF   Bypass Coronary Artery, Three Sites from Abdominal Artery with Synthetic Substitute, Open Approach

Ø2120JW   Bypass Coronary Artery, Three Sites from Aorta with Synthetic Substitute, Open Approach

HAC 08: Surgical Site Infection of Mediastinitis Following Coronary Bypass Graft (CABG) Procedures (continued)

Ø2120K3 Bypass Coronary Artery, Three Sites from Coronary Artery with Nonautologous Tissue Substitute, Open Approach

Ø2120K8 Bypass Coronary Artery, Three Sites from Right Internal Mammary with Nonautologous Tissue Substitute, Open Approach

Ø2120K9 Bypass Coronary Artery, Three Sites from Left Internal Mammary with Nonautologous Tissue Substitute, Open Approach

Ø2120KC Bypass Coronary Artery, Three Sites from Thoracic Artery with Nonautologous Tissue Substitute, Open Approach

Ø2120KF Bypass Coronary Artery, Three Sites from Abdominal Artery with Nonautologous Tissue Substitute, Open Approach

Ø2120KW Bypass Coronary Artery, Three Sites from Aorta with Nonautologous Tissue Substitute, Open Approach

Ø2120Z3 Bypass Coronary Artery, Three Sites from Coronary Artery, Open Approach

Ø2120Z8 Bypass Coronary Artery, Three Sites from Right Internal Mammary, Open Approach

Ø2120Z9 Bypass Coronary Artery, Three Sites from Left Internal Mammary, Open Approach

Ø2120ZC Bypass Coronary Artery, Three Sites from Thoracic Artery, Open Approach

Ø2120ZF Bypass Coronary Artery, Three Sites from Abdominal Artery, Open Approach

Ø212493 Bypass Coronary Artery, Three Sites from Coronary Artery with Autologous Venous Tissue, Percutaneous Endoscopic Approach

Ø212498 Bypass Coronary Artery, Three Sites from Right Internal Mammary with Autologous Venous Tissue, Percutaneous Endoscopic Approach

Ø212499 Bypass Coronary Artery, Three Sites from Left Internal Mammary with Autologous Venous Tissue, Percutaneous Endoscopic Approach

Ø21249C Bypass Coronary Artery, Three Sites from Thoracic Artery with Autologous Venous Tissue, Percutaneous Endoscopic Approach

Ø21249F Bypass Coronary Artery, Three Sites from Abdominal Artery with Autologous Venous Tissue, Percutaneous Endoscopic Approach

Ø21249W Bypass Coronary Artery, Three Sites from Aorta with Autologous Venous Tissue, Percutaneous Endoscopic Approach

Ø2124A3 Bypass Coronary Artery, Three Sites from Coronary Artery with Autologous Arterial Tissue, Percutaneous Endoscopic Approach

Ø2124A8 Bypass Coronary Artery, Three Sites from Right Internal Mammary with Autologous Arterial Tissue, Percutaneous Endoscopic Approach

Ø2124A9 Bypass Coronary Artery, Three Sites from Left Internal Mammary with Autologous Arterial Tissue, Percutaneous Endoscopic Approach

Ø2124AC Bypass Coronary Artery, Three Sites from Thoracic Artery with Autologous Arterial Tissue, Percutaneous Endoscopic Approach

Ø2124AF Bypass Coronary Artery, Three Sites from Abdominal Artery with Autologous Arterial Tissue, Percutaneous Endoscopic Approach

Ø2124AW Bypass Coronary Artery, Three Sites from Aorta with Autologous Arterial Tissue, Percutaneous Endoscopic Approach

Ø2124J3 Bypass Coronary Artery, Three Sites from Coronary Artery with Synthetic Substitute, Percutaneous Endoscopic Approach

Ø2124J8 Bypass Coronary Artery, Three Sites from Right Internal Mammary with Synthetic Substitute, Percutaneous Endoscopic Approach

Ø2124J9 Bypass Coronary Artery, Three Sites from Left Internal Mammary with Synthetic Substitute, Percutaneous Endoscopic Approach

Ø2124JC Bypass Coronary Artery, Three Sites from Thoracic Artery with Synthetic Substitute, Percutaneous Endoscopic Approach

Ø2124JF Bypass Coronary Artery, Three Sites from Abdominal Artery with Synthetic Substitute, Percutaneous Endoscopic Approach

Ø2124JW Bypass Coronary Artery, Three Sites from Aorta with Synthetic Substitute, Percutaneous Endoscopic Approach

Ø2124K3 Bypass Coronary Artery, Three Sites from Coronary Artery with Nonautologous Tissue Substitute, Percutaneous Endoscopic Approach

Ø2124K8 Bypass Coronary Artery, Three Sites from Right Internal Mammary with Nonautologous Tissue Substitute, Percutaneous Endoscopic Approach

Ø2124K9 Bypass Coronary Artery, Three Sites from Left Internal Mammary with Nonautologous Tissue Substitute, Percutaneous Endoscopic Approach

Ø2124KC Bypass Coronary Artery, Three Sites from Thoracic Artery with Nonautologous Tissue Substitute, Percutaneous Endoscopic Approach

Ø2124KF Bypass Coronary Artery, Three Sites from Abdominal Artery with Nonautologous Tissue Substitute, Percutaneous Endoscopic Approach

Ø2124KW Bypass Coronary Artery, Three Sites from Aorta with Nonautologous Tissue Substitute, Percutaneous Endoscopic Approach

Ø2124Z3 Bypass Coronary Artery, Three Sites from Coronary Artery, Percutaneous Endoscopic Approach

Ø2124Z8 Bypass Coronary Artery, Three Sites from Right Internal Mammary, Percutaneous Endoscopic Approach

Ø2124Z9 Bypass Coronary Artery, Three Sites from Left Internal Mammary, Percutaneous Endoscopic Approach

Ø2124ZC Bypass Coronary Artery, Three Sites from Thoracic Artery, Percutaneous Endoscopic Approach

Ø2124ZF Bypass Coronary Artery, Three Sites from Abdominal Artery, Percutaneous Endoscopic Approach

Ø213093 Bypass Coronary Artery, Four or More Sites from Coronary Artery with Autologous Venous Tissue, Open Approach

Ø213098 Bypass Coronary Artery, Four or More Sites from Right Internal Mammary with Autologous Venous Tissue, Open Approach

Ø213099 Bypass Coronary Artery, Four or More Sites from Left Internal Mammary with Autologous Venous Tissue, Open Approach

Ø21309C Bypass Coronary Artery, Four or More Sites from Thoracic Artery with Autologous Venous Tissue, Open Approach

Ø21309F Bypass Coronary Artery, Four or More Sites from Abdominal Artery with Autologous Venous Tissue, Open Approach

Ø21309W Bypass Coronary Artery, Four or More Sites from Aorta with Autologous Venous Tissue, Open Approach

Ø2130A3 Bypass Coronary Artery, Four or More Sites from Coronary Artery with Autologous Arterial Tissue, Open Approach

Ø2130A8 Bypass Coronary Artery, Four or More Sites from Right Internal Mammary with Autologous Arterial Tissue, Open Approach

Ø2130A9 Bypass Coronary Artery, Four or More Sites from Left Internal Mammary with Autologous Arterial Tissue, Open Approach

Ø2130AC Bypass Coronary Artery, Four or More Sites from Thoracic Artery with Autologous Arterial Tissue, Open Approach

Ø2130AF Bypass Coronary Artery, Four or More Sites from Abdominal Artery with Autologous Arterial Tissue, Open Approach

Ø2130AW Bypass Coronary Artery, Four or More Sites from Aorta with Autologous Arterial Tissue, Open Approach

Ø2130J3 Bypass Coronary Artery, Four or More Sites from Coronary Artery with Synthetic Substitute, Open Approach

Ø2130J8 Bypass Coronary Artery, Four or More Sites from Right Internal Mammary with Synthetic Substitute, Open Approach

Ø2130J9 Bypass Coronary Artery, Four or More Sites from Left Internal Mammary with Synthetic Substitute, Open Approach

Ø2130JC Bypass Coronary Artery, Four or More Sites from Thoracic Artery with Synthetic Substitute, Open Approach

Ø2130JF Bypass Coronary Artery, Four or More Sites from Abdominal Artery with Synthetic Substitute, Open Approach

Ø2130JW Bypass Coronary Artery, Four or More Sites from Aorta with Synthetic Substitute, Open Approach

Ø2130K3 Bypass Coronary Artery, Four or More Sites from Coronary Artery with Nonautologous Tissue Substitute, Open Approach

Ø2130K8 Bypass Coronary Artery, Four or More Sites from Right Internal Mammary with Nonautologous Tissue Substitute, Open Approach

Ø2130K9 Bypass Coronary Artery, Four or More Sites from Left Internal Mammary with Nonautologous Tissue Substitute, Open Approach

Ø2130KC Bypass Coronary Artery, Four or More Sites from Thoracic Artery with Nonautologous Tissue Substitute, Open Approach

Ø2130KF Bypass Coronary Artery, Four or More Sites from Abdominal Artery with Nonautologous Tissue Substitute, Open Approach

Ø2130KW Bypass Coronary Artery, Four or More Sites from Aorta with Nonautologous Tissue Substitute, Open Approach

HAC 08: Surgical Site Infection of Mediastinitis Following Coronary Bypass Graft (CABG) Procedures (continued)

Ø213ØZ3   Bypass Coronary Artery, Four or More Sites from Coronary Artery, Open Approach

Ø213ØZ8   Bypass Coronary Artery, Four or More Sites from Right Internal Mammary, Open Approach

Ø213ØZ9   Bypass Coronary Artery, Four or More Sites from Left Internal Mammary, Open Approach

Ø213ØZC   Bypass Coronary Artery, Four or More Sites from Thoracic Artery, Open Approach

Ø213ØZF   Bypass Coronary Artery, Four or More Sites from Abdominal Artery, Open Approach

Ø213493   Bypass Coronary Artery, Four or More Sites from Coronary Artery with Autologous Venous Tissue, Percutaneous Endoscopic Approach

Ø213498   Bypass Coronary Artery, Four or More Sites from Right Internal Mammary with Autologous Venous Tissue, Percutaneous Endoscopic Approach

Ø213499   Bypass Coronary Artery, Four or More Sites from Left Internal Mammary with Autologous Venous Tissue, Percutaneous Endoscopic Approach

Ø21349C   Bypass Coronary Artery, Four or More Sites from Thoracic Artery with Autologous Venous Tissue, Percutaneous Endoscopic Approach

Ø21349F   Bypass Coronary Artery, Four or More Sites from Abdominal Artery with Autologous Venous Tissue, Percutaneous Endoscopic Approach

Ø21349W   Bypass Coronary Artery, Four or More Sites from Aorta with Autologous Venous Tissue, Percutaneous Endoscopic Approach

Ø2134A3   Bypass Coronary Artery, Four or More Sites from Coronary Artery with Autologous Arterial Tissue, Percutaneous Endoscopic Approach

Ø2134A8   Bypass Coronary Artery, Four or More Sites from Right Internal Mammary with Autologous Arterial Tissue, Percutaneous Endoscopic Approach

Ø2134A9   Bypass Coronary Artery, Four or More Sites from Left Internal Mammary with Autologous Arterial Tissue, Percutaneous Endoscopic Approach

Ø2134AC   Bypass Coronary Artery, Four or More Sites from Thoracic Artery with Autologous Arterial Tissue, Percutaneous Endoscopic Approach

Ø2134AF   Bypass Coronary Artery, Four or More Sites from Abdominal Artery with Autologous Arterial Tissue, Percutaneous Endoscopic Approach

Ø2134AW   Bypass Coronary Artery, Four or More Sites from Aorta with Autologous Arterial Tissue, Percutaneous Endoscopic Approach

Ø2134J3   Bypass Coronary Artery, Four or More Sites from Coronary Artery with Synthetic Substitute, Percutaneous Endoscopic Approach

Ø2134J8   Bypass Coronary Artery, Four or More Sites from Right Internal Mammary with Synthetic Substitute, Percutaneous Endoscopic Approach

Ø2134J9   Bypass Coronary Artery, Four or More Sites from Left Internal Mammary with Synthetic Substitute, Percutaneous Endoscopic Approach

Ø2134JC   Bypass Coronary Artery, Four or More Sites from Thoracic Artery with Synthetic Substitute, Percutaneous Endoscopic Approach

Ø2134JF   Bypass Coronary Artery, Four or More Sites from Abdominal Artery with Synthetic Substitute, Percutaneous Endoscopic Approach

Ø2134JW   Bypass Coronary Artery, Four or More Sites from Aorta with Synthetic Substitute, Percutaneous Endoscopic Approach

Ø2134K3   Bypass Coronary Artery, Four or More Sites from Coronary Artery with Nonautologous Tissue Substitute, Percutaneous Endoscopic Approach

Ø2134K8   Bypass Coronary Artery, Four or More Sites from Right Internal Mammary with Nonautologous Tissue Substitute, Percutaneous Endoscopic Approach

Ø2134K9   Bypass Coronary Artery, Four or More Sites from Left Internal Mammary with Nonautologous Tissue Substitute, Percutaneous Endoscopic Approach

Ø2134KC   Bypass Coronary Artery, Four or More Sites from Thoracic Artery with Nonautologous Tissue Substitute, Percutaneous Endoscopic Approach

Ø2134KF   Bypass Coronary Artery, Four or More Sites from Abdominal Artery with Nonautologous Tissue Substitute, Percutaneous Endoscopic Approach

Ø2134KW   Bypass Coronary Artery, Four or More Sites from Aorta with Nonautologous Tissue Substitute, Percutaneous Endoscopic Approach

Ø2134Z3   Bypass Coronary Artery, Four or More Sites from Coronary Artery, Percutaneous Endoscopic Approach

Ø2134Z8   Bypass Coronary Artery, Four or More Sites from Right Internal Mammary, Percutaneous Endoscopic Approach

Ø2134Z9   Bypass Coronary Artery, Four or More Sites from Left Internal Mammary, Percutaneous Endoscopic Approach

Ø2134ZC   Bypass Coronary Artery, Four or More Sites from Thoracic Artery, Percutaneous Endoscopic Approach

Ø2134ZF   Bypass Coronary Artery, Four or More Sites from Abdominal Artery, Percutaneous Endoscopic Approach

HAC 09: Manifestations of Poor Glycemic Control

Secondary diagnosis not POA:

E08.00
E08.01
E08.10
E09.00
E09.01
E09.10
E10.10
E11.00
E11.01
E13.00
E13.01
E13.10
E15

HAC 10: Deep Vein Thrombosis (DVT) or Pulmonary Embolism (PE) with Total Knee or Hip Replacement

Secondary diagnosis not POA:

I26.02
I26.09

I26.92
I26.99
I82.401
I82.402
I82.403
I82.409
I82.411
I82.412
I82.413
I82.419
I82.421
I82.422
I82.423
I82.429
I82.431
I82.432
I82.433
I82.439
I82.441
I82.442
I82.443
I82.449
I82.491
I82.492
I82.493
I82.499
I82.4Y1
I82.4Y2
I82.4Y3
I82.4Y9
I82.4Z1
I82.4Z2
I82.4Z3
I82.4Z9

AND

Any of the following procedures:

ØSR9Ø19   Replacement of Right Hip Joint with Metal Synthetic Substitute, Cemented, Open Approach

ØSR9Ø1A   Replacement of Right Hip Joint with Metal Synthetic Substitute, Uncemented, Open Approach

ØSR9Ø1Z   Replacement of Right Hip Joint with Metal Synthetic Substitute, Open Approach

ØSR9Ø29   Replacement of Right Hip Joint with Metal on Polyethylene Synthetic Substitute, Cemented, Open Approach

ØSR9Ø2A   Replacement of Right Hip Joint with Metal on Polyethylene Synthetic Substitute, Uncemented, Open Approach

ØSR9Ø2Z   Replacement of Right Hip Joint with Metal on Polyethylene Synthetic Substitute, Open Approach

ØSR9Ø39   Replacement of Right Hip Joint with Ceramic Synthetic Substitute, Cemented, Open Approach

ØSR9Ø3A   Replacement of Right Hip Joint with Ceramic Synthetic Substitute, Uncemented, Open Approach

ØSR9Ø3Z   Replacement of Right Hip Joint with Ceramic Synthetic Substitute, Open Approach

ØSR9Ø49   Replacement of Right Hip Joint with Ceramic on Polyethylene Synthetic Substitute, Cemented, Open Approach

ØSR9Ø4A   Replacement of Right Hip Joint with Ceramic on Polyethylene Synthetic Substitute, Uncemented, Open Approach

ØSR9Ø4Z   Replacement of Right Hip Joint with Ceramic on Polyethylene Synthetic Substitute, Open Approach

ØSR9Ø7Z   Replacement of Right Hip Joint with Autologous Tissue Substitute, Open Approach

HAC 10: Deep Vein Thrombosis (DVT) or Pulmonary Embolism (PE) with Total Knee or Hip Replacement (continued)

ØSR90J9 Replacement of Right Hip Joint with Synthetic Substitute, Cemented, Open Approach

ØSR90JA Replacement of Right Hip Joint with Synthetic Substitute, Uncemented, Open Approach

ØSR90JZ Replacement of Right Hip Joint with Synthetic Substitute, Open Approach

ØSR90KZ Replacement of Right Hip Joint with Nonautologous Tissue Substitute, Open Approach

ØSRAØØ9 Replacement of Right Hip Joint, Acetabular Surface with Polyethylene Synthetic Substitute, Cemented, Open Approach

ØSRAØØA Replacement of Right Hip Joint, Acetabular Surface with Polyethylene Synthetic Substitute, Uncemented, Open Approach

ØSRAØØZ Replacement of Right Hip Joint, Acetabular Surface with Polyethylene Synthetic Substitute, Open Approach

ØSRAØ19 Replacement of Right Hip Joint, Acetabular Surface with Metal Synthetic Substitute, Cemented, Open Approach

ØSRAØ1A Replacement of Right Hip Joint, Acetabular Surface with Metal Synthetic Substitute, Uncemented, Open Approach

ØSRAØ1Z Replacement of Right Hip Joint, Acetabular Surface with Metal Synthetic Substitute, Open Approach

ØSRAØ39 Replacement of Right Hip Joint, Acetabular Surface with Ceramic Synthetic Substitute, Cemented, Open Approach

ØSRAØ3A Replacement of Right Hip Joint, Acetabular Surface with Ceramic Synthetic Substitute, Uncemented, Open Approach

ØSRAØ3Z Replacement of Right Hip Joint, Acetabular Surface with Ceramic Synthetic Substitute, Open Approach

ØSRAØ7Z Replacement of Right Hip Joint, Acetabular Surface with Autologous Tissue Substitute, Open Approach

ØSRAØJ9 Replacement of Right Hip Joint, Acetabular Surface with Synthetic Substitute, Cemented, Open Approach

ØSRAØJA Replacement of Right Hip Joint, Acetabular Surface with Synthetic Substitute, Uncemented, Open Approach

ØSRAØJZ Replacement of Right Hip Joint, Acetabular Surface with Synthetic Substitute, Open Approach

ØSRAØKZ Replacement of Right Hip Joint, Acetabular Surface with Nonautologous Tissue Substitute, Open Approach

ØSRBØ19 Replacement of Left Hip Joint with Metal Synthetic Substitute, Cemented, Open Approach

ØSRBØ1A Replacement of Left Hip Joint with Metal Synthetic Substitute, Uncemented, Open Approach

ØSRBØ1Z Replacement of Left Hip Joint with Metal Synthetic Substitute, Open Approach

ØSRBØ29 Replacement of Left Hip Joint with Metal on Polyethylene Synthetic Substitute, Cemented, Open Approach

ØSRBØ2A Replacement of Left Hip Joint with Metal on Polyethylene Synthetic Substitute, Uncemented, Open Approach

ØSRBØ2Z Replacement of Left Hip Joint with Metal on Polyethylene Synthetic Substitute, Open Approach

ØSRBØ39 Replacement of Left Hip Joint with Ceramic Synthetic Substitute, Cemented, Open Approach

ØSRBØ3A Replacement of Left Hip Joint with Ceramic Synthetic Substitute, Uncemented, Open Approach

ØSRBØ3Z Replacement of Left Hip Joint with Ceramic Synthetic Substitute, Open Approach

ØSRBØ49 Replacement of Left Hip Joint with Ceramic on Polyethylene Synthetic Substitute, Cemented, Open Approach

ØSRBØ4A Replacement of Left Hip Joint with Ceramic on Polyethylene Synthetic Substitute, Uncemented, Open Approach

ØSRBØ4Z Replacement of Left Hip Joint with Ceramic on Polyethylene Synthetic Substitute, Open Approach

ØSRBØ7Z Replacement of Left Hip Joint with Autologous Tissue Substitute, Open Approach

ØSRBØJ9 Replacement of Left Hip Joint with Synthetic Substitute, Cemented, Open Approach

ØSRBØJA Replacement of Left Hip Joint with Synthetic Substitute, Uncemented, Open Approach

ØSRBØJZ Replacement of Left Hip Joint with Synthetic Substitute, Open Approach

ØSRBØKZ Replacement of Left Hip Joint with Nonautologous Tissue Substitute, Open Approach

ØSRCØ7Z Replacement of Right Knee Joint with Autologous Tissue Substitute, Open Approach

ØSRCØJ9 Replacement of Right Knee Joint with Synthetic Substitute, Cemented, Open Approach

ØSRCØJA Replacement of Right Knee Joint with Synthetic Substitute, Uncemented, Open Approach

ØSRCØJZ Replacement of Right Knee Joint with Synthetic Substitute, Open Approach

ØSRCØKZ Replacement of Right Knee Joint with Nonautologous Tissue Substitute, Open Approach

ØSRDØ7Z Replacement of Left Knee Joint with Autologous Tissue Substitute, Open Approach

ØSRDØJ9 Replacement of Left Knee Joint with Synthetic Substitute, Cemented, Open Approach

ØSRDØJA Replacement of Left Knee Joint with Synthetic Substitute, Uncemented, Open Approach

ØSRDØJZ Replacement of Left Knee Joint with Synthetic Substitute, Open Approach

ØSRDØKZ Replacement of Left Knee Joint with Nonautologous Tissue Substitute, Open Approach

ØSREØØ9 Replacement of Left Hip Joint, Acetabular Surface with Polyethylene Synthetic Substitute, Cemented, Open Approach

ØSREØØA Replacement of Left Hip Joint, Acetabular Surface with Polyethylene Synthetic Substitute, Uncemented, Open Approach

ØSREØØZ Replacement of Left Hip Joint, Acetabular Surface with Polyethylene Synthetic Substitute, Open Approach

ØSREØ19 Replacement of Left Hip Joint, Acetabular Surface with Metal Synthetic Substitute, Cemented, Open Approach

ØSREØ1A Replacement of Left Hip Joint, Acetabular Surface with Metal Synthetic Substitute, Uncemented, Open Approach

ØSREØ1Z Replacement of Left Hip Joint, Acetabular Surface with Metal Synthetic Substitute, Open Approach

ØSREØ39 Replacement of Left Hip Joint, Acetabular Surface with Ceramic Synthetic Substitute, Cemented, Open Approach

ØSREØ3A Replacement of Left Hip Joint, Acetabular Surface with Ceramic Synthetic Substitute, Uncemented, Open Approach

ØSREØ3Z Replacement of Left Hip Joint, Acetabular Surface with Ceramic Synthetic Substitute, Open Approach

ØSREØ7Z Replacement of Left Hip Joint, Acetabular Surface with Autologous Tissue Substitute, Open Approach

ØSREØJ9 Replacement of Left Hip Joint, Acetabular Surface with Synthetic Substitute, Cemented, Open Approach

ØSREØJA Replacement of Left Hip Joint, Acetabular Surface with Synthetic Substitute, Uncemented, Open Approach

ØSREØJZ Replacement of Left Hip Joint, Acetabular Surface with Synthetic Substitute, Open Approach

ØSREØKZ Replacement of Left Hip Joint, Acetabular Surface with Nonautologous Tissue Substitute, Open Approach

ØSRRØ19 Replacement of Right Hip Joint, Femoral Surface with Metal Synthetic Substitute, Cemented, Open Approach

ØSRRØ1A Replacement of Right Hip Joint, Femoral Surface with Metal Synthetic Substitute, Uncemented, Open Approach

ØSRRØ1Z Replacement of Right Hip Joint, Femoral Surface with Metal Synthetic Substitute, Open Approach

ØSRRØ39 Replacement of Right Hip Joint, Femoral Surface with Ceramic Synthetic Substitute, Cemented, Open Approach

ØSRRØ3A Replacement of Right Hip Joint, Femoral Surface with Ceramic Synthetic Substitute, Uncemented, Open Approach

ØSRRØ3Z Replacement of Right Hip Joint, Femoral Surface with Ceramic Synthetic Substitute, Open Approach

ØSRRØ7Z Replacement of Right Hip Joint, Femoral Surface with Autologous Tissue Substitute, Open Approach

ØSRRØJ9 Replacement of Right Hip Joint, Femoral Surface with Synthetic Substitute, Cemented, Open Approach

ØSRRØJA Replacement of Right Hip Joint, Femoral Surface with Synthetic Substitute, Uncemented, Open Approach

ØSRRØJZ Replacement of Right Hip Joint, Femoral Surface with Synthetic Substitute, Open Approach

ØSRRØKZ Replacement of Right Hip Joint, Femoral Surface with Nonautologous Tissue Substitute, Open Approach

ØSRSØ19 Replacement of Left Hip Joint, Femoral Surface with Metal Synthetic Substitute, Cemented, Open Approach

ØSRSØ1A Replacement of Left Hip Joint, Femoral Surface with Metal Synthetic Substitute, Uncemented, Open Approach

ØSRSØ1Z Replacement of Left Hip Joint, Femoral Surface with Metal Synthetic Substitute, Open Approach

ØSRSØ39 Replacement of Left Hip Joint, Femoral Surface with Ceramic Synthetic Substitute, Cemented, Open Approach

ØSRSØ3A Replacement of Left Hip Joint, Femoral Surface with Ceramic Synthetic Substitute, Uncemented, Open Approach

HAC 10: Deep Vein Thrombosis (DVT) or Pulmonary Embolism (PE) with Total Knee or Hip Replacement (continued)

ØSRSØ3Z   Replacement of Left Hip Joint, Femoral Surface with Ceramic Synthetic Substitute, Open Approach

ØSRSØ7Z   Replacement of Left Hip Joint, Femoral Surface with Autologous Tissue Substitute, Open Approach

ØSRSØJ9   Replacement of Left Hip Joint, Femoral Surface with Synthetic Substitute, Cemented, Open Approach

ØSRSØJA   Replacement of Left Hip Joint, Femoral Surface with Synthetic Substitute, Uncemented, Open Approach

ØSRSØJZ   Replacement of Left Hip Joint, Femoral Surface with Synthetic Substitute, Open Approach

ØSRSØKZ   Replacement of Left Hip Joint, Femoral Surface with Nonautologous Tissue Substitute, Open Approach

ØSRTØ7Z   Replacement of Right Knee Joint, Femoral Surface with Autologous Tissue Substitute, Open Approach

ØSRTØJ9   Replacement of Right Knee Joint, Femoral Surface with Synthetic Substitute, Cemented, Open Approach

ØSRTØJA   Replacement of Right Knee Joint, Femoral Surface with Synthetic Substitute, Uncemented, Open Approach

ØSRTØJZ   Replacement of Right Knee Joint, Femoral Surface with Synthetic Substitute, Open Approach

ØSRTØKZ   Replacement of Right Knee Joint, Femoral Surface with Nonautologous Tissue Substitute, Open Approach

ØSRUØ7Z   Replacement of Left Knee Joint, Femoral Surface with Autologous Tissue Substitute, Open Approach

ØSRUØJ9   Replacement of Left Knee Joint, Femoral Surface with Synthetic Substitute, Cemented, Open Approach

ØSRUØJA   Replacement of Left Knee Joint, Femoral Surface with Synthetic Substitute, Uncemented, Open Approach

ØSRUØJZ   Replacement of Left Knee Joint, Femoral Surface with Synthetic Substitute, Open Approach

ØSRUØKZ   Replacement of Left Knee Joint, Femoral Surface with Nonautologous Tissue Substitute, Open Approach

ØSRVØ7Z   Replacement of Right Knee Joint, Tibial Surface with Autologous Tissue Substitute, Open Approach

ØSRVØJ9   Replacement of Right Knee Joint, Tibial Surface with Synthetic Substitute, Cemented, Open Approach

ØSRVØJA   Replacement of Right Knee Joint, Tibial Surface with Synthetic Substitute, Uncemented, Open Approach

ØSRVØJZ   Replacement of Right Knee Joint, Tibial Surface with Synthetic Substitute, Open Approach

ØSRVØKZ   Replacement of Right Knee Joint, Tibial Surface with Nonautologous Tissue Substitute, Open Approach

ØSRWØ7Z   Replacement of Left Knee Joint, Tibial Surface with Autologous Tissue Substitute, Open Approach

ØSRWØJ9   Replacement of Left Knee Joint, Tibial Surface with Synthetic Substitute, Cemented, Open Approach

ØSRWØJA   Replacement of Left Knee Joint, Tibial Surface with Synthetic Substitute, Uncemented, Open Approach

ØSRWØJZ   Replacement of Left Knee Joint, Tibial Surface with Synthetic Substitute, Open Approach

ØSRWØKZ   Replacement of Left Knee Joint, Tibial Surface with Nonautologous Tissue Substitute, Open Approach

ØSU9ØBZ   Supplement Right Hip Joint with Resurfacing Device, Open Approach

ØSUAØBZ   Supplement Right Hip Joint, Acetabular Surface with Resurfacing Device, Open Approach

ØSUBØBZ   Supplement Left Hip Joint with Resurfacing Device, Open Approach

ØSUEØBZ   Supplement Left Hip Joint, Acetabular Surface with Resurfacing Device, Open Approach

ØSURØBZ   Supplement Right Hip Joint, Femoral Surface with Resurfacing Device, Open Approach

ØSUSØBZ   Supplement Left Hip Joint, Femoral Surface with Resurfacing Device, Open Approach

HAC 11: Surgical Site Infection Following Bariatric Surgery

Principal diagnosis of:
E66.Ø1

AND

Secondary diagnosis not POA:
K68.11
K95.Ø1
K95.81
T81.4XXA

AND

Any of the following procedures:

ØD16Ø79   Bypass Stomach to Duodenum with Autologous Tissue Substitute, Open Approach

ØD16Ø7A   Bypass Stomach to Jejunum with Autologous Tissue Substitute, Open Approach

ØD16Ø7B   Bypass Stomach to Ileum with Autologous Tissue Substitute, Open Approach

ØD16Ø7L   Bypass Stomach to Transverse Colon with Autologous Tissue Substitute, Open Approach

ØD16ØJ9   Bypass Stomach to Duodenum with Synthetic Substitute, Open Approach

ØD16ØJA   Bypass Stomach to Jejunum with Synthetic Substitute, Open Approach

ØD16ØJB   Bypass Stomach to Ileum with Synthetic Substitute, Open Approach

ØD16ØJL   Bypass Stomach to Transverse Colon with Synthetic Substitute, Open Approach

ØD16ØK9   Bypass Stomach to Duodenum with Nonautologous Tissue Substitute, Open Approach

ØD16ØKA   Bypass Stomach to Jejunum with Nonautologous Tissue Substitute, Open Approach

ØD16ØKB   Bypass Stomach to Ileum with Nonautologous Tissue Substitute, Open Approach

ØD16ØKL   Bypass Stomach to Transverse Colon with Nonautologous Tissue Substitute, Open Approach

ØD16ØZ9   Bypass Stomach to Duodenum, Open Approach

ØD16ØZA   Bypass Stomach to Jejunum, Open Approach

ØD16ØZB   Bypass Stomach to Ileum, Open Approach

ØD16ØZL   Bypass Stomach to Transverse Colon, Open Approach

ØD16479   Bypass Stomach to Duodenum with Autologous Tissue Substitute, Percutaneous Endoscopic Approach

ØD1647A   Bypass Stomach to Jejunum with Autologous Tissue Substitute, Percutaneous Endoscopic Approach

ØD1647B   Bypass Stomach to Ileum with Autologous Tissue Substitute, Percutaneous Endoscopic Approach

ØD1647L   Bypass Stomach to Transverse Colon with Autologous Tissue Substitute, Percutaneous Endoscopic Approach

ØD164J9   Bypass Stomach to Duodenum with Synthetic Substitute, Percutaneous Endoscopic Approach

ØD164JA   Bypass Stomach to Jejunum with Synthetic Substitute, Percutaneous Endoscopic Approach

ØD164JB   Bypass Stomach to Ileum with Synthetic Substitute, Percutaneous Endoscopic Approach

ØD164JL   Bypass Stomach to Transverse Colon with Synthetic Substitute, Percutaneous Endoscopic Approach

ØD164K9   Bypass Stomach to Duodenum with Nonautologous Tissue Substitute, Percutaneous Endoscopic Approach

ØD164KA   Bypass Stomach to Jejunum with Nonautologous Tissue Substitute, Percutaneous Endoscopic Approach

ØD164KB   Bypass Stomach to Ileum with Nonautologous Tissue Substitute, Percutaneous Endoscopic Approach

ØD164KL   Bypass Stomach to Transverse Colon with Nonautologous Tissue Substitute, Percutaneous Endoscopic Approach

ØD164Z9   Bypass Stomach to Duodenum, Percutaneous Endoscopic Approach

ØD164ZA   Bypass Stomach to Jejunum, Percutaneous Endoscopic Approach

ØD164ZB   Bypass Stomach to Ileum, Percutaneous Endoscopic Approach

ØD164ZL   Bypass Stomach to Transverse Colon, Percutaneous Endoscopic Approach

ØD16879   Bypass Stomach to Duodenum with Autologous Tissue Substitute, Via Natural or Artificial Opening Endoscopic

ØD1687A   Bypass Stomach to Jejunum with Autologous Tissue Substitute, Via Natural or Artificial Opening Endoscopic

ØD1687B   Bypass Stomach to Ileum with Autologous Tissue Substitute, Via Natural or Artificial Opening Endoscopic

ØD1687L   Bypass Stomach to Transverse Colon with Autologous Tissue Substitute, Via Natural or Artificial Opening Endoscopic

ØD168J9   Bypass Stomach to Duodenum with Synthetic Substitute, Via Natural or Artificial Opening Endoscopic

ØD168JA   Bypass Stomach to Jejunum with Synthetic Substitute, Via Natural or Artificial Opening Endoscopic

ØD168JB   Bypass Stomach to Ileum with Synthetic Substitute, Via Natural or Artificial Opening Endoscopic

ØD168JL   Bypass Stomach to Transverse Colon with Synthetic Substitute, Via Natural or Artificial Opening Endoscopic

ØD168K9   Bypass Stomach to Duodenum with Nonautologous Tissue Substitute, Via Natural or Artificial Opening Endoscopic

ØD168KA   Bypass Stomach to Jejunum with Nonautologous Tissue Substitute, Via Natural or Artificial Opening Endoscopic

ØD168KB   Bypass Stomach to Ileum with Nonautologous Tissue Substitute, Via Natural or Artificial Opening Endoscopic

Appendix I: Hospital Acquired Conditions

HAC 11: Surgical Site Infection Following Bariatric Surgery (continued)

ØD168KL Bypass Stomach to Transverse Colon with Nonautologous Tissue Substitute, Via Natural or Artificial Opening Endoscopic

ØD168Z9 Bypass Stomach to Duodenum, Via Natural or Artificial Opening Endoscopic

ØD168ZA Bypass Stomach to Jejunum, Via Natural or Artificial Opening Endoscopic

ØD168ZB Bypass Stomach to Ileum, Via Natural or Artificial Opening Endoscopic

ØD168ZL Bypass Stomach to Transverse Colon, Via Natural or Artificial Opening Endoscopic

ØDV64CZ Restriction of Stomach with Extraluminal Device, Percutaneous Endoscopic Approach

HAC 12: Surgical Site Infection Following Certain Orthopedic Procedures of the Spine, Shoulder, and Elbow

Secondary diagnosis not POA:

K68.11
T81.4XXA
T84.60XA
T84.610A
T84.611A
T84.612A
T84.613A
T84.614A
T84.615A
T84.619A
T84.63XA
T84.69XA
T84.7XXA

AND

Any of the following procedures:

ØRG0070 Fusion of Occipital-cervical Joint with Autologous Tissue Substitute, Anterior Approach, Anterior Column, Open Approach

ØRG0071 Fusion of Occipital-cervical Joint with Autologous Tissue Substitute, Posterior Approach, Posterior Column, Open Approach

ØRG007J Fusion of Occipital-cervical Joint with Autologous Tissue Substitute, Posterior Approach, Anterior Column, Open Approach

ØRG00A0 Fusion of Occipital-cervical Joint with Interbody Fusion Device, Anterior Approach, Anterior Column, Open Approach

ØRG00A1 Fusion of Occipital-cervical Joint with Interbody Fusion Device, Posterior Approach, Posterior Column, Open Approach

ØRG00AJ Fusion of Occipital-cervical Joint with Interbody Fusion Device, Posterior Approach, Anterior Column, Open Approach

ØRG00J0 Fusion of Occipital-cervical Joint with Synthetic Substitute, Anterior Approach, Anterior Column, Open Approach

ØRG00J1 Fusion of Occipital-cervical Joint with Synthetic Substitute, Posterior Approach, Posterior Column, Open Approach

ØRG00JJ Fusion of Occipital-cervical Joint with Synthetic Substitute, Posterior Approach, Anterior Column, Open Approach

ØRG00K0 Fusion of Occipital-cervical Joint with Nonautologous Tissue Substitute, Anterior Approach, Anterior Column, Open Approach

ØRG00K1 Fusion of Occipital-cervical Joint with Nonautologous Tissue Substitute, Posterior Approach, Posterior Column, Open Approach

ØRG00KJ Fusion of Occipital-cervical Joint with Nonautologous Tissue Substitute, Posterior Approach, Anterior Column, Open Approach

ØRG00Z0 Fusion of Occipital-cervical Joint, Anterior Approach, Anterior Column, Open Approach

ØRG00Z1 Fusion of Occipital-cervical Joint, Posterior Approach, Posterior Column, Open Approach

ØRG00ZJ Fusion of Occipital-cervical Joint, Posterior Approach, Anterior Column, Open Approach

ØRG0370 Fusion of Occipital-cervical Joint with Autologous Tissue Substitute, Anterior Approach, Anterior Column, Percutaneous Approach

ØRG0371 Fusion of Occipital-cervical Joint with Autologous Tissue Substitute, Posterior Approach, Posterior Column, Percutaneous Approach

ØRG037J Fusion of Occipital-cervical Joint with Autologous Tissue Substitute, Posterior Approach, Anterior Column, Percutaneous Approach

ØRG03A0 Fusion of Occipital-cervical Joint with Interbody Fusion Device, Anterior Approach, Anterior Column, Percutaneous Approach

ØRG03A1 Fusion of Occipital-cervical Joint with Interbody Fusion Device, Posterior Approach, Posterior Column, Percutaneous Approach

ØRG03AJ Fusion of Occipital-cervical Joint with Interbody Fusion Device, Posterior Approach, Anterior Column, Percutaneous Approach

ØRG03J0 Fusion of Occipital-cervical Joint with Synthetic Substitute, Anterior Approach, Anterior Column, Percutaneous Approach

ØRG03J1 Fusion of Occipital-cervical Joint with Synthetic Substitute, Posterior Approach, Posterior Column, Percutaneous Approach

ØRG03JJ Fusion of Occipital-cervical Joint with Synthetic Substitute, Posterior Approach, Anterior Column, Percutaneous Approach

ØRG03K0 Fusion of Occipital-cervical Joint with Nonautologous Tissue Substitute, Anterior Approach, Anterior Column, Percutaneous Approach

ØRG03K1 Fusion of Occipital-cervical Joint with Nonautologous Tissue Substitute, Posterior Approach, Posterior Column, Percutaneous Approach

ØRG03KJ Fusion of Occipital-cervical Joint with Nonautologous Tissue Substitute, Posterior Approach, Anterior Column, Percutaneous Approach

ØRG03Z0 Fusion of Occipital-cervical Joint, Anterior Approach, Anterior Column, Percutaneous Approach

ØRG03Z1 Fusion of Occipital-cervical Joint, Posterior Approach, Posterior Column, Percutaneous Approach

ØRG03ZJ Fusion of Occipital-cervical Joint, Posterior Approach, Anterior Column, Percutaneous Approach

ØRG0470 Fusion of Occipital-cervical Joint with Autologous Tissue Substitute, Anterior Approach, Anterior Column, Percutaneous Endoscopic Approach

ØRG0471 Fusion of Occipital-cervical Joint with Autologous Tissue Substitute, Posterior Approach, Posterior Column, Percutaneous Endoscopic Approach

ØRG047J Fusion of Occipital-cervical Joint with Autologous Tissue Substitute, Posterior Approach, Anterior Column, Percutaneous Endoscopic Approach

ØRG04A0 Fusion of Occipital-cervical Joint with Interbody Fusion Device, Anterior Approach, Anterior Column, Percutaneous Endoscopic Approach

ØRG04A1 Fusion of Occipital-cervical Joint with Interbody Fusion Device, Posterior Approach, Posterior Column, Percutaneous Endoscopic Approach

ØRG04AJ Fusion of Occipital-cervical Joint with Interbody Fusion Device, Posterior Approach, Anterior Column, Percutaneous Endoscopic Approach

ØRG04J0 Fusion of Occipital-cervical Joint with Synthetic Substitute, Anterior Approach, Anterior Column, Percutaneous Endoscopic Approach

ØRG04J1 Fusion of Occipital-cervical Joint with Synthetic Substitute, Posterior Approach, Posterior Column, Percutaneous Endoscopic Approach

ØRG04JJ Fusion of Occipital-cervical Joint with Synthetic Substitute, Posterior Approach, Anterior Column, Percutaneous Endoscopic Approach

ØRG04K0 Fusion of Occipital-cervical Joint with Nonautologous Tissue Substitute, Anterior Approach, Anterior Column, Percutaneous Endoscopic Approach

ØRG04K1 Fusion of Occipital-cervical Joint with Nonautologous Tissue Substitute, Posterior Approach, Posterior Column, Percutaneous Endoscopic Approach

ØRG04KJ Fusion of Occipital-cervical Joint with Nonautologous Tissue Substitute, Posterior Approach, Anterior Column, Percutaneous Endoscopic Approach

ØRG04Z0 Fusion of Occipital-cervical Joint, Anterior Approach, Anterior Column, Percutaneous Endoscopic Approach

ØRG04Z1 Fusion of Occipital-cervical Joint, Posterior Approach, Posterior Column, Percutaneous Endoscopic Approach

ØRG04ZJ Fusion of Occipital-cervical Joint, Posterior Approach, Anterior Column, Percutaneous Endoscopic Approach

ØRG1070 Fusion of Cervical Vertebral Joint with Autologous Tissue Substitute, Anterior Approach, Anterior Column, Open Approach

ØRG1071 Fusion of Cervical Vertebral Joint with Autologous Tissue Substitute, Posterior Approach, Posterior Column, Open Approach

ØRG107J Fusion of Cervical Vertebral Joint with Autologous Tissue Substitute, Posterior Approach, Anterior Column, Open Approach

ØRG10A0 Fusion of Cervical Vertebral Joint with Interbody Fusion Device, Anterior Approach, Anterior Column, Open Approach

ØRG10A1 Fusion of Cervical Vertebral Joint with Interbody Fusion Device, Posterior Approach, Posterior Column, Open Approach

ØRG10AJ Fusion of Cervical Vertebral Joint with Interbody Fusion Device, Posterior Approach, Anterior Column, Open Approach

HAC 12: Surgical Site Infection Following Certain Orthopedic Procedures of the Spine, Shoulder, and Elbow (continued)

ØRG1ØJØ Fusion of Cervical Vertebral Joint with Synthetic Substitute, Anterior Approach, Anterior Column, Open Approach

ØRG1ØJ1 Fusion of Cervical Vertebral Joint with Synthetic Substitute, Posterior Approach, Posterior Column, Open Approach

ØRG1ØJJ Fusion of Cervical Vertebral Joint with Synthetic Substitute, Posterior Approach, Anterior Column, Open Approach

ØRG1ØKØ Fusion of Cervical Vertebral Joint with Nonautologous Tissue Substitute, Anterior Approach, Anterior Column, Open Approach

ØRG1ØK1 Fusion of Cervical Vertebral Joint with Nonautologous Tissue Substitute, Posterior Approach, Posterior Column, Open Approach

ØRG1ØKJ Fusion of Cervical Vertebral Joint with Nonautologous Tissue Substitute, Posterior Approach, Anterior Column, Open Approach

ØRG1ØZØ Fusion of Cervical Vertebral Joint, Anterior Approach, Anterior Column, Open Approach

ØRG1ØZ1 Fusion of Cervical Vertebral Joint, Posterior Approach, Posterior Column, Open Approach

ØRG1ØZJ Fusion of Cervical Vertebral Joint, Posterior Approach, Anterior Column, Open Approach

ØRG137Ø Fusion of Cervical Vertebral Joint with Autologous Tissue Substitute, Anterior Approach, Anterior Column, Percutaneous Approach

ØRG1371 Fusion of Cervical Vertebral Joint with Autologous Tissue Substitute, Posterior Approach, Posterior Column, Percutaneous Approach

ØRG137J Fusion of Cervical Vertebral Joint with Autologous Tissue Substitute, Posterior Approach, Anterior Column, Percutaneous Approach

ØRG13AØ Fusion of Cervical Vertebral Joint with Interbody Fusion Device, Anterior Approach, Anterior Column, Percutaneous Approach

ØRG13A1 Fusion of Cervical Vertebral Joint with Interbody Fusion Device, Posterior Approach, Posterior Column, Percutaneous Approach

ØRG13AJ Fusion of Cervical Vertebral Joint with Interbody Fusion Device, Posterior Approach, Anterior Column, Percutaneous Approach

ØRG13JØ Fusion of Cervical Vertebral Joint with Synthetic Substitute, Anterior Approach, Anterior Column, Percutaneous Approach

ØRG13J1 Fusion of Cervical Vertebral Joint with Synthetic Substitute, Posterior Approach, Posterior Column, Percutaneous Approach

ØRG13JJ Fusion of Cervical Vertebral Joint with Synthetic Substitute, Posterior Approach, Anterior Column, Percutaneous Approach

ØRG13KØ Fusion of Cervical Vertebral Joint with Nonautologous Tissue Substitute, Anterior Approach, Anterior Column, Percutaneous Approach

ØRG13K1 Fusion of Cervical Vertebral Joint with Nonautologous Tissue Substitute, Posterior Approach, Posterior Column, Percutaneous Approach

ØRG13KJ Fusion of Cervical Vertebral Joint with Nonautologous Tissue Substitute, Posterior Approach, Anterior Column, Percutaneous Approach

ØRG13ZØ Fusion of Cervical Vertebral Joint, Anterior Approach, Anterior Column, Percutaneous Approach

ØRG13Z1 Fusion of Cervical Vertebral Joint, Posterior Approach, Posterior Column, Percutaneous Approach

ØRG13ZJ Fusion of Cervical Vertebral Joint, Posterior Approach, Anterior Column, Percutaneous Approach

ØRG147Ø Fusion of Cervical Vertebral Joint with Autologous Tissue Substitute, Anterior Approach, Anterior Column, Percutaneous Endoscopic Approach

ØRG1471 Fusion of Cervical Vertebral Joint with Autologous Tissue Substitute, Posterior Approach, Posterior Column, Percutaneous Endoscopic Approach

ØRG147J Fusion of Cervical Vertebral Joint with Autologous Tissue Substitute, Posterior Approach, Anterior Column, Percutaneous Endoscopic Approach

ØRG14AØ Fusion of Cervical Vertebral Joint with Interbody Fusion Device, Anterior Approach, Anterior Column, Percutaneous Endoscopic Approach

ØRG14A1 Fusion of Cervical Vertebral Joint with Interbody Fusion Device, Posterior Approach, Posterior Column, Percutaneous Endoscopic Approach

ØRG14AJ Fusion of Cervical Vertebral Joint with Interbody Fusion Device, Posterior Approach, Anterior Column, Percutaneous Endoscopic Approach

ØRG14JØ Fusion of Cervical Vertebral Joint with Synthetic Substitute, Anterior Approach, Anterior Column, Percutaneous Endoscopic Approach

ØRG14J1 Fusion of Cervical Vertebral Joint with Synthetic Substitute, Posterior Approach, Posterior Column, Percutaneous Endoscopic Approach

ØRG14JJ Fusion of Cervical Vertebral Joint with Synthetic Substitute, Posterior Approach, Anterior Column, Percutaneous Endoscopic Approach

ØRG14KØ Fusion of Cervical Vertebral Joint with Nonautologous Tissue Substitute, Anterior Approach, Anterior Column, Percutaneous Endoscopic Approach

ØRG14K1 Fusion of Cervical Vertebral Joint with Nonautologous Tissue Substitute, Posterior Approach, Posterior Column, Percutaneous Endoscopic Approach

ØRG14KJ Fusion of Cervical Vertebral Joint with Nonautologous Tissue Substitute, Posterior Approach, Anterior Column, Percutaneous Endoscopic Approach

ØRG14ZØ Fusion of Cervical Vertebral Joint, Anterior Approach, Anterior Column, Percutaneous Endoscopic Approach

ØRG14Z1 Fusion of Cervical Vertebral Joint, Posterior Approach, Posterior Column, Percutaneous Endoscopic Approach

ØRG14ZJ Fusion of Cervical Vertebral Joint, Posterior Approach, Anterior Column, Percutaneous Endoscopic Approach

ØRG2Ø7Ø Fusion of 2 or more Cervical Vertebral Joints with Autologous Tissue Substitute, Anterior Approach, Anterior Column, Open Approach

ØRG2Ø71 Fusion of 2 or more Cervical Vertebral Joints with Autologous Tissue Substitute, Posterior Approach, Posterior Column, Open Approach

ØRG2Ø7J Fusion of 2 or more Cervical Vertebral Joints with Autologous Tissue Substitute, Posterior Approach, Anterior Column, Open Approach

ØRG2ØAØ Fusion of 2 or more Cervical Vertebral Joints with Interbody Fusion Device, Anterior Approach, Anterior Column, Open Approach

ØRG2ØA1 Fusion of 2 or more Cervical Vertebral Joints with Interbody Fusion Device, Posterior Approach, Posterior Column, Open Approach

ØRG2ØAJ Fusion of 2 or more Cervical Vertebral Joints with Interbody Fusion Device, Posterior Approach, Anterior Column, Open Approach

ØRG2ØJØ Fusion of 2 or more Cervical Vertebral Joints with Synthetic Substitute, Anterior Approach, Anterior Column, Open Approach

ØRG2ØJ1 Fusion of 2 or more Cervical Vertebral Joints with Synthetic Substitute, Posterior Approach, Posterior Column, Open Approach

ØRG2ØJJ Fusion of 2 or more Cervical Vertebral Joints with Synthetic Substitute, Posterior Approach, Anterior Column, Open Approach

ØRG2ØKØ Fusion of 2 or more Cervical Vertebral Joints with Nonautologous Tissue Substitute, Anterior Approach, Anterior Column, Open Approach

ØRG2ØK1 Fusion of 2 or more Cervical Vertebral Joints with Nonautologous Tissue Substitute, Posterior Approach, Posterior Column, Open Approach

ØRG2ØKJ Fusion of 2 or more Cervical Vertebral Joints with Nonautologous Tissue Substitute, Posterior Approach, Anterior Column, Open Approach

ØRG2ØZØ Fusion of 2 or more Cervical Vertebral Joints, Anterior Approach, Anterior Column, Open Approach

ØRG2ØZ1 Fusion of 2 or more Cervical Vertebral Joints, Posterior Approach, Posterior Column, Open Approach

ØRG2ØZJ Fusion of 2 or more Cervical Vertebral Joints, Posterior Approach, Anterior Column, Open Approach

ØRG237Ø Fusion of 2 or more Cervical Vertebral Joints with Autologous Tissue Substitute, Anterior Approach, Anterior Column, Percutaneous Approach

ØRG2371 Fusion of 2 or more Cervical Vertebral Joints with Autologous Tissue Substitute, Posterior Approach, Posterior Column, Percutaneous Approach

ØRG237J Fusion of 2 or more Cervical Vertebral Joints with Autologous Tissue Substitute, Posterior Approach, Anterior Column, Percutaneous Approach

ØRG23AØ Fusion of 2 or more Cervical Vertebral Joints with Interbody Fusion Device, Anterior Approach, Anterior Column, Percutaneous Approach

ØRG23A1 Fusion of 2 or more Cervical Vertebral Joints with Interbody Fusion Device, Posterior Approach, Posterior Column, Percutaneous Approach

ØRG23AJ Fusion of 2 or more Cervical Vertebral Joints with Interbody Fusion Device, Posterior Approach, Anterior Column, Percutaneous Approach

HAC 12: Surgical Site Infection Following Certain Orthopedic Procedures of the Spine, Shoulder, and Elbow (continued)

ØRG23JØ Fusion of 2 or more Cervical Vertebral Joints with Synthetic Substitute, Anterior Approach, Anterior Column, Percutaneous Approach

ØRG23J1 Fusion of 2 or more Cervical Vertebral Joints with Synthetic Substitute, Posterior Approach, Posterior Column, Percutaneous Approach

ØRG23JJ Fusion of 2 or more Cervical Vertebral Joints with Synthetic Substitute, Posterior Approach, Anterior Column, Percutaneous Approach

ØRG23KØ Fusion of 2 or more Cervical Vertebral Joints with Nonautologous Tissue Substitute, Anterior Approach, Anterior Column, Percutaneous Approach

ØRG23K1 Fusion of 2 or more Cervical Vertebral Joints with Nonautologous Tissue Substitute, Posterior Approach, Posterior Column, Percutaneous Approach

ØRG23KJ Fusion of 2 or more Cervical Vertebral Joints with Nonautologous Tissue Substitute, Posterior Approach, Anterior Column, Percutaneous Approach

ØRG23ZØ Fusion of 2 or more Cervical Vertebral Joints, Anterior Approach, Anterior Column, Percutaneous Approach

ØRG23Z1 Fusion of 2 or more Cervical Vertebral Joints, Posterior Approach, Posterior Column, Percutaneous Approach

ØRG23ZJ Fusion of 2 or more Cervical Vertebral Joints, Posterior Approach, Anterior Column, Percutaneous Approach

ØRG247Ø Fusion of 2 or more Cervical Vertebral Joints with Autologous Tissue Substitute, Anterior Approach, Anterior Column, Percutaneous Endoscopic Approach

ØRG2471 Fusion of 2 or more Cervical Vertebral Joints with Autologous Tissue Substitute, Posterior Approach, Posterior Column, Percutaneous Endoscopic Approach

ØRG247J Fusion of 2 or more Cervical Vertebral Joints with Autologous Tissue Substitute, Posterior Approach, Anterior Column, Percutaneous Endoscopic Approach

ØRG24AØ Fusion of 2 or more Cervical Vertebral Joints with Interbody Fusion Device, Anterior Approach, Anterior Column, Percutaneous Endoscopic Approach

ØRG24A1 Fusion of 2 or more Cervical Vertebral Joints with Interbody Fusion Device, Posterior Approach, Posterior Column, Percutaneous Endoscopic Approach

ØRG24AJ Fusion of 2 or more Cervical Vertebral Joints with Interbody Fusion Device, Posterior Approach, Anterior Column, Percutaneous Endoscopic Approach

ØRG24JØ Fusion of 2 or more Cervical Vertebral Joints with Synthetic Substitute, Anterior Approach, Anterior Column, Percutaneous Endoscopic Approach

ØRG24J1 Fusion of 2 or more Cervical Vertebral Joints with Synthetic Substitute, Posterior Approach, Posterior Column, Percutaneous Endoscopic Approach

ØRG24JJ Fusion of 2 or more Cervical Vertebral Joints with Synthetic Substitute, Posterior Approach, Anterior Column, Percutaneous Endoscopic Approach

ØRG24KØ Fusion of 2 or more Cervical Vertebral Joints with Nonautologous Tissue Substitute, Anterior Approach, Anterior Column, Percutaneous Endoscopic Approach

ØRG24K1 Fusion of 2 or more Cervical Vertebral Joints with Nonautologous Tissue Substitute, Posterior Approach, Posterior Column, Percutaneous Endoscopic Approach

ØRG24KJ Fusion of 2 or more Cervical Vertebral Joints with Nonautologous Tissue Substitute, Posterior Approach, Anterior Column, Percutaneous Endoscopic Approach

ØRG24ZØ Fusion of 2 or more Cervical Vertebral Joints, Anterior Approach, Anterior Column, Percutaneous Endoscopic Approach

ØRG24Z1 Fusion of 2 or more Cervical Vertebral Joints, Posterior Approach, Posterior Column, Percutaneous Endoscopic Approach

ØRG24ZJ Fusion of 2 or more Cervical Vertebral Joints, Posterior Approach, Anterior Column, Percutaneous Endoscopic Approach

ØRG407Ø Fusion of Cervicothoracic Vertebral Joint with Autologous Tissue Substitute, Anterior Approach, Anterior Column, Open Approach

ØRG4071 Fusion of Cervicothoracic Vertebral Joint with Autologous Tissue Substitute, Posterior Approach, Posterior Column, Open Approach

ØRG407J Fusion of Cervicothoracic Vertebral Joint with Autologous Tissue Substitute, Posterior Approach, Anterior Column, Open Approach

ØRG40AØ Fusion of Cervicothoracic Vertebral Joint with Interbody Fusion Device, Anterior Approach, Anterior Column, Open Approach

ØRG40A1 Fusion of Cervicothoracic Vertebral Joint with Interbody Fusion Device, Posterior Approach, Posterior Column, Open Approach

ØRG40AJ Fusion of Cervicothoracic Vertebral Joint with Interbody Fusion Device, Posterior Approach, Anterior Column, Open Approach

ØRG40JØ Fusion of Cervicothoracic Vertebral Joint with Synthetic Substitute, Anterior Approach, Anterior Column, Open Approach

ØRG40J1 Fusion of Cervicothoracic Vertebral Joint with Synthetic Substitute, Posterior Approach, Posterior Column, Open Approach

ØRG40JJ Fusion of Cervicothoracic Vertebral Joint with Synthetic Substitute, Posterior Approach, Anterior Column, Open Approach

ØRG40KØ Fusion of Cervicothoracic Vertebral Joint with Nonautologous Tissue Substitute, Anterior Approach, Anterior Column, Open Approach

ØRG40K1 Fusion of Cervicothoracic Vertebral Joint with Nonautologous Tissue Substitute, Posterior Approach, Posterior Column, Open Approach

ØRG40KJ Fusion of Cervicothoracic Vertebral Joint with Nonautologous Tissue Substitute, Posterior Approach, Anterior Column, Open Approach

ØRG40ZØ Fusion of Cervicothoracic Vertebral Joint, Anterior Approach, Anterior Column, Open Approach

ØRG40Z1 Fusion of Cervicothoracic Vertebral Joint, Posterior Approach, Posterior Column, Open Approach

ØRG40ZJ Fusion of Cervicothoracic Vertebral Joint, Posterior Approach, Anterior Column, Open Approach

ØRG437Ø Fusion of Cervicothoracic Vertebral Joint with Autologous Tissue Substitute, Anterior Approach, Anterior Column, Percutaneous Approach

ØRG4371 Fusion of Cervicothoracic Vertebral Joint with Autologous Tissue Substitute, Posterior Approach, Posterior Column, Percutaneous Approach

ØRG437J Fusion of Cervicothoracic Vertebral Joint with Autologous Tissue Substitute, Posterior Approach, Anterior Column, Percutaneous Approach

ØRG43AØ Fusion of Cervicothoracic Vertebral Joint with Interbody Fusion Device, Anterior Approach, Anterior Column, Percutaneous Approach

ØRG43A1 Fusion of Cervicothoracic Vertebral Joint with Interbody Fusion Device, Posterior Approach, Posterior Column, Percutaneous Approach

ØRG43AJ Fusion of Cervicothoracic Vertebral Joint with Interbody Fusion Device, Posterior Approach, Anterior Column, Percutaneous Approach

ØRG43JØ Fusion of Cervicothoracic Vertebral Joint with Synthetic Substitute, Anterior Approach, Anterior Column, Percutaneous Approach

ØRG43J1 Fusion of Cervicothoracic Vertebral Joint with Synthetic Substitute, Posterior Approach, Posterior Column, Percutaneous Approach

ØRG43JJ Fusion of Cervicothoracic Vertebral Joint with Synthetic Substitute, Posterior Approach, Anterior Column, Percutaneous Approach

ØRG43KØ Fusion of Cervicothoracic Vertebral Joint with Nonautologous Tissue Substitute, Anterior Approach, Anterior Column, Percutaneous Approach

ØRG43K1 Fusion of Cervicothoracic Vertebral Joint with Nonautologous Tissue Substitute, Posterior Approach, Posterior Column, Percutaneous Approach

ØRG43KJ Fusion of Cervicothoracic Vertebral Joint with Nonautologous Tissue Substitute, Posterior Approach, Anterior Column, Percutaneous Approach

ØRG43ZØ Fusion of Cervicothoracic Vertebral Joint, Anterior Approach, Anterior Column, Percutaneous Approach

ØRG43Z1 Fusion of Cervicothoracic Vertebral Joint, Posterior Approach, Posterior Column, Percutaneous Approach

ØRG43ZJ Fusion of Cervicothoracic Vertebral Joint, Posterior Approach, Anterior Column, Percutaneous Approach

ØRG447Ø Fusion of Cervicothoracic Vertebral Joint with Autologous Tissue Substitute, Anterior Approach, Anterior Column, Percutaneous Endoscopic Approach

ØRG4471 Fusion of Cervicothoracic Vertebral Joint with Autologous Tissue Substitute, Posterior Approach, Posterior Column, Percutaneous Endoscopic Approach

ØRG447J Fusion of Cervicothoracic Vertebral Joint with Autologous Tissue Substitute, Posterior Approach, Anterior Column, Percutaneous Endoscopic Approach

ØRG44AØ Fusion of Cervicothoracic Vertebral Joint with Interbody Fusion Device, Anterior Approach, Anterior Column, Percutaneous Endoscopic Approach

HAC 12: Surgical Site Infection Following Certain Orthopedic Procedures of the Spine, Shoulder, and Elbow (continued)

ØRG44A1   Fusion of Cervicothoracic Vertebral Joint with Interbody Fusion Device, Posterior Approach, Posterior Column, Percutaneous Endoscopic Approach

ØRG44AJ   Fusion of Cervicothoracic Vertebral Joint with Interbody Fusion Device, Posterior Approach, Anterior Column, Percutaneous Endoscopic Approach

ØRG44JØ   Fusion of Cervicothoracic Vertebral Joint with Synthetic Substitute, Anterior Approach, Anterior Column, Percutaneous Endoscopic Approach

ØRG44J1   Fusion of Cervicothoracic Vertebral Joint with Synthetic Substitute, Posterior Approach, Posterior Column, Percutaneous Endoscopic Approach

ØRG44JJ   Fusion of Cervicothoracic Vertebral Joint with Synthetic Substitute, Posterior Approach, Anterior Column, Percutaneous Endoscopic Approach

ØRG44KØ   Fusion of Cervicothoracic Vertebral Joint with Nonautologous Tissue Substitute, Anterior Approach, Anterior Column, Percutaneous Endoscopic Approach

ØRG44K1   Fusion of Cervicothoracic Vertebral Joint with Nonautologous Tissue Substitute, Posterior Approach, Posterior Column, Percutaneous Endoscopic Approach

ØRG44KJ   Fusion of Cervicothoracic Vertebral Joint with Nonautologous Tissue Substitute, Posterior Approach, Anterior Column, Percutaneous Endoscopic Approach

ØRG44ZØ   Fusion of Cervicothoracic Vertebral Joint, Anterior Approach, Anterior Column, Percutaneous Endoscopic Approach

ØRG44Z1   Fusion of Cervicothoracic Vertebral Joint, Posterior Approach, Posterior Column, Percutaneous Endoscopic Approach

ØRG44ZJ   Fusion of Cervicothoracic Vertebral Joint, Posterior Approach, Anterior Column, Percutaneous Endoscopic Approach

ØRG6Ø7Ø   Fusion of Thoracic Vertebral Joint with Autologous Tissue Substitute, Anterior Approach, Anterior Column, Open Approach

ØRG6Ø71   Fusion of Thoracic Vertebral Joint with Autologous Tissue Substitute, Posterior Approach, Posterior Column, Open Approach

ØRG6Ø7J   Fusion of Thoracic Vertebral Joint with Autologous Tissue Substitute, Posterior Approach, Anterior Column, Open Approach

ØRG6ØAØ   Fusion of Thoracic Vertebral Joint with Interbody Fusion Device, Anterior Approach, Anterior Column, Open Approach

ØRG6ØA1   Fusion of Thoracic Vertebral Joint with Interbody Fusion Device, Posterior Approach, Posterior Column, Open Approach

ØRG6ØAJ   Fusion of Thoracic Vertebral Joint with Interbody Fusion Device, Posterior Approach, Anterior Column, Open Approach

ØRG6ØJØ   Fusion of Thoracic Vertebral Joint with Synthetic Substitute, Anterior Approach, Anterior Column, Open Approach

ØRG6ØJ1   Fusion of Thoracic Vertebral Joint with Synthetic Substitute, Posterior Approach, Posterior Column, Open Approach

ØRG6ØJJ   Fusion of Thoracic Vertebral Joint with Synthetic Substitute, Posterior Approach, Anterior Column, Open Approach

ØRG6ØKØ   Fusion of Thoracic Vertebral Joint with Nonautologous Tissue Substitute, Anterior Approach, Anterior Column, Open Approach

ØRG6ØK1   Fusion of Thoracic Vertebral Joint with Nonautologous Tissue Substitute, Posterior Approach, Posterior Column, Open Approach

ØRG6ØKJ   Fusion of Thoracic Vertebral Joint with Nonautologous Tissue Substitute, Posterior Approach, Anterior Column, Open Approach

ØRG6ØZØ   Fusion of Thoracic Vertebral Joint, Anterior Approach, Anterior Column, Open Approach

ØRG6ØZ1   Fusion of Thoracic Vertebral Joint, Posterior Approach, Posterior Column, Open Approach

ØRG6ØZJ   Fusion of Thoracic Vertebral Joint, Posterior Approach, Anterior Column, Open Approach

ØRG637Ø   Fusion of Thoracic Vertebral Joint with Autologous Tissue Substitute, Anterior Approach, Anterior Column, Percutaneous Approach

ØRG6371   Fusion of Thoracic Vertebral Joint with Autologous Tissue Substitute, Posterior Approach, Posterior Column, Percutaneous Approach

ØRG637J   Fusion of Thoracic Vertebral Joint with Autologous Tissue Substitute, Posterior Approach, Anterior Column, Percutaneous Approach

ØRG63AØ   Fusion of Thoracic Vertebral Joint with Interbody Fusion Device, Anterior Approach, Anterior Column, Percutaneous Approach

ØRG63A1   Fusion of Thoracic Vertebral Joint with Interbody Fusion Device, Posterior Approach, Posterior Column, Percutaneous Approach

ØRG63AJ   Fusion of Thoracic Vertebral Joint with Interbody Fusion Device, Posterior Approach, Anterior Column, Percutaneous Approach

ØRG63JØ   Fusion of Thoracic Vertebral Joint with Synthetic Substitute, Anterior Approach, Anterior Column, Percutaneous Approach

ØRG63J1   Fusion of Thoracic Vertebral Joint with Synthetic Substitute, Posterior Approach, Posterior Column, Percutaneous Approach

ØRG63JJ   Fusion of Thoracic Vertebral Joint with Synthetic Substitute, Posterior Approach, Anterior Column, Percutaneous Approach

ØRG63KØ   Fusion of Thoracic Vertebral Joint with Nonautologous Tissue Substitute, Anterior Approach, Anterior Column, Percutaneous Approach

ØRG63K1   Fusion of Thoracic Vertebral Joint with Nonautologous Tissue Substitute, Posterior Approach, Posterior Column, Percutaneous Approach

ØRG63KJ   Fusion of Thoracic Vertebral Joint with Nonautologous Tissue Substitute, Posterior Approach, Anterior Column, Percutaneous Approach

ØRG63ZØ   Fusion of Thoracic Vertebral Joint, Anterior Approach, Anterior Column, Percutaneous Approach

ØRG63Z1   Fusion of Thoracic Vertebral Joint, Posterior Approach, Posterior Column, Percutaneous Approach

ØRG63ZJ   Fusion of Thoracic Vertebral Joint, Posterior Approach, Anterior Column, Percutaneous Approach

ØRG647Ø   Fusion of Thoracic Vertebral Joint with Autologous Tissue Substitute, Anterior Approach, Anterior Column, Percutaneous Endoscopic Approach

ØRG6471   Fusion of Thoracic Vertebral Joint with Autologous Tissue Substitute, Posterior Approach, Posterior Column, Percutaneous Endoscopic Approach

ØRG647J   Fusion of Thoracic Vertebral Joint with Autologous Tissue Substitute, Posterior Approach, Anterior Column, Percutaneous Endoscopic Approach

ØRG64AØ   Fusion of Thoracic Vertebral Joint with Interbody Fusion Device, Anterior Approach, Anterior Column, Percutaneous Endoscopic Approach

ØRG64A1   Fusion of Thoracic Vertebral Joint with Interbody Fusion Device, Posterior Approach, Posterior Column, Percutaneous Endoscopic Approach

ØRG64AJ   Fusion of Thoracic Vertebral Joint with Interbody Fusion Device, Posterior Approach, Anterior Column, Percutaneous Endoscopic Approach

ØRG64JØ   Fusion of Thoracic Vertebral Joint with Synthetic Substitute, Anterior Approach, Anterior Column, Percutaneous Endoscopic Approach

ØRG64J1   Fusion of Thoracic Vertebral Joint with Synthetic Substitute, Posterior Approach, Posterior Column, Percutaneous Endoscopic Approach

ØRG64JJ   Fusion of Thoracic Vertebral Joint with Synthetic Substitute, Posterior Approach, Anterior Column, Percutaneous Endoscopic Approach

ØRG64KØ   Fusion of Thoracic Vertebral Joint with Nonautologous Tissue Substitute, Anterior Approach, Anterior Column, Percutaneous Endoscopic Approach

ØRG64K1   Fusion of Thoracic Vertebral Joint with Nonautologous Tissue Substitute, Posterior Approach, Posterior Column, Percutaneous Endoscopic Approach

ØRG64KJ   Fusion of Thoracic Vertebral Joint with Nonautologous Tissue Substitute, Posterior Approach, Anterior Column, Percutaneous Endoscopic Approach

ØRG64ZØ   Fusion of Thoracic Vertebral Joint, Anterior Approach, Anterior Column, Percutaneous Endoscopic Approach

ØRG64Z1   Fusion of Thoracic Vertebral Joint, Posterior Approach, Posterior Column, Percutaneous Endoscopic Approach

ØRG64ZJ   Fusion of Thoracic Vertebral Joint, Posterior Approach, Anterior Column, Percutaneous Endoscopic Approach

ØRG7Ø7Ø   Fusion of 2 to 7 Thoracic Vertebral Joints with Autologous Tissue Substitute, Anterior Approach, Anterior Column, Open Approach

ØRG7Ø71   Fusion of 2 to 7 Thoracic Vertebral Joints with Autologous Tissue Substitute, Posterior Approach, Posterior Column, Open Approach

ØRG7Ø7J   Fusion of 2 to 7 Thoracic Vertebral Joints with Autologous Tissue Substitute, Posterior Approach, Anterior Column, Open Approach

ØRG7ØAØ   Fusion of 2 to 7 Thoracic Vertebral Joints with Interbody Fusion Device, Anterior Approach, Anterior Column, Open Approach

HAC 12: Surgical Site Infection Following Certain Orthopedic Procedures of the Spine, Shoulder, and Elbow (continued)

ØRG70A1 Fusion of 2 to 7 Thoracic Vertebral Joints with Interbody Fusion Device, Posterior Approach, Posterior Column, Open Approach

ØRG70AJ Fusion of 2 to 7 Thoracic Vertebral Joints with Interbody Fusion Device, Posterior Approach, Anterior Column, Open Approach

ØRG70J0 Fusion of 2 to 7 Thoracic Vertebral Joints with Synthetic Substitute, Anterior Approach, Anterior Column, Open Approach

ØRG70J1 Fusion of 2 to 7 Thoracic Vertebral Joints with Synthetic Substitute, Posterior Approach, Posterior Column, Open Approach

ØRG70JJ Fusion of 2 to 7 Thoracic Vertebral Joints with Synthetic Substitute, Posterior Approach, Anterior Column, Open Approach

ØRG70K0 Fusion of 2 to 7 Thoracic Vertebral Joints with Nonautologous Tissue Substitute, Anterior Approach, Anterior Column, Open Approach

ØRG70K1 Fusion of 2 to 7 Thoracic Vertebral Joints with Nonautologous Tissue Substitute, Posterior Approach, Posterior Column, Open Approach

ØRG70KJ Fusion of 2 to 7 Thoracic Vertebral Joints with Nonautologous Tissue Substitute, Posterior Approach, Anterior Column, Open Approach

ØRG70Z0 Fusion of 2 to 7 Thoracic Vertebral Joints, Anterior Approach, Anterior Column, Open Approach

ØRG70Z1 Fusion of 2 to 7 Thoracic Vertebral Joints, Posterior Approach, Posterior Column, Open Approach

ØRG70ZJ Fusion of 2 to 7 Thoracic Vertebral Joints, Posterior Approach, Anterior Column, Open Approach

ØRG7370 Fusion of 2 to 7 Thoracic Vertebral Joints with Autologous Tissue Substitute, Anterior Approach, Anterior Column, Percutaneous Approach

ØRG7371 Fusion of 2 to 7 Thoracic Vertebral Joints with Autologous Tissue Substitute, Posterior Approach, Posterior Column, Percutaneous Approach

ØRG737J Fusion of 2 to 7 Thoracic Vertebral Joints with Autologous Tissue Substitute, Posterior Approach, Anterior Column, Percutaneous Approach

ØRG73A0 Fusion of 2 to 7 Thoracic Vertebral Joints with Interbody Fusion Device, Anterior Approach, Anterior Column, Percutaneous Approach

ØRG73A1 Fusion of 2 to 7 Thoracic Vertebral Joints with Interbody Fusion Device, Posterior Approach, Posterior Column, Percutaneous Approach

ØRG73AJ Fusion of 2 to 7 Thoracic Vertebral Joints with Interbody Fusion Device, Posterior Approach, Anterior Column, Percutaneous Approach

ØRG73J0 Fusion of 2 to 7 Thoracic Vertebral Joints with Synthetic Substitute, Anterior Approach, Anterior Column, Percutaneous Approach

ØRG73J1 Fusion of 2 to 7 Thoracic Vertebral Joints with Synthetic Substitute, Posterior Approach, Posterior Column, Percutaneous Approach

ØRG73JJ Fusion of 2 to 7 Thoracic Vertebral Joints with Synthetic Substitute, Posterior Approach, Anterior Column, Percutaneous Approach

ØRG73K0 Fusion of 2 to 7 Thoracic Vertebral Joints with Nonautologous Tissue Substitute, Anterior Approach, Anterior Column, Percutaneous Approach

ØRG73K1 Fusion of 2 to 7 Thoracic Vertebral Joints with Nonautologous Tissue Substitute, Posterior Approach, Posterior Column, Percutaneous Approach

ØRG73KJ Fusion of 2 to 7 Thoracic Vertebral Joints with Nonautologous Tissue Substitute, Posterior Approach, Anterior Column, Percutaneous Approach

ØRG73Z0 Fusion of 2 to 7 Thoracic Vertebral Joints, Anterior Approach, Anterior Column, Percutaneous Approach

ØRG73Z1 Fusion of 2 to 7 Thoracic Vertebral Joints, Posterior Approach, Posterior Column, Percutaneous Approach

ØRG73ZJ Fusion of 2 to 7 Thoracic Vertebral Joints, Posterior Approach, Anterior Column, Percutaneous Approach

ØRG7470 Fusion of 2 to 7 Thoracic Vertebral Joints with Autologous Tissue Substitute, Anterior Approach, Anterior Column, Percutaneous Endoscopic Approach

ØRG7471 Fusion of 2 to 7 Thoracic Vertebral Joints with Autologous Tissue Substitute, Posterior Approach, Posterior Column, Percutaneous Endoscopic Approach

ØRG747J Fusion of 2 to 7 Thoracic Vertebral Joints with Autologous Tissue Substitute, Posterior Approach, Anterior Column, Percutaneous Endoscopic Approach

ØRG74A0 Fusion of 2 to 7 Thoracic Vertebral Joints with Interbody Fusion Device, Anterior Approach, Anterior Column, Percutaneous Endoscopic Approach

ØRG74A1 Fusion of 2 to 7 Thoracic Vertebral Joints with Interbody Fusion Device, Posterior Approach, Posterior Column, Percutaneous Endoscopic Approach

ØRG74AJ Fusion of 2 to 7 Thoracic Vertebral Joints with Interbody Fusion Device, Posterior Approach, Anterior Column, Percutaneous Endoscopic Approach

ØRG74J0 Fusion of 2 to 7 Thoracic Vertebral Joints with Synthetic Substitute, Anterior Approach, Anterior Column, Percutaneous Endoscopic Approach

ØRG74J1 Fusion of 2 to 7 Thoracic Vertebral Joints with Synthetic Substitute, Posterior Approach, Posterior Column, Percutaneous Endoscopic Approach

ØRG74JJ Fusion of 2 to 7 Thoracic Vertebral Joints with Synthetic Substitute, Posterior Approach, Anterior Column, Percutaneous Endoscopic Approach

ØRG74K0 Fusion of 2 to 7 Thoracic Vertebral Joints with Nonautologous Tissue Substitute, Anterior Approach, Anterior Column, Percutaneous Endoscopic Approach

ØRG74K1 Fusion of 2 to 7 Thoracic Vertebral Joints with Nonautologous Tissue Substitute, Posterior Approach, Posterior Column, Percutaneous Endoscopic Approach

ØRG74KJ Fusion of 2 to 7 Thoracic Vertebral Joints with Nonautologous Tissue Substitute, Posterior Approach, Anterior Column, Percutaneous Endoscopic Approach

ØRG74Z0 Fusion of 2 to 7 Thoracic Vertebral Joints, Anterior Approach, Anterior Column, Percutaneous Endoscopic Approach

ØRG74Z1 Fusion of 2 to 7 Thoracic Vertebral Joints, Posterior Approach, Posterior Column, Percutaneous Endoscopic Approach

ØRG74ZJ Fusion of 2 to 7 Thoracic Vertebral Joints, Posterior Approach, Anterior Column, Percutaneous Endoscopic Approach

ØRG8070 Fusion of 8 or More Thoracic Vertebral Joints with Autologous Tissue Substitute, Anterior Approach, Anterior Column, Open Approach

ØRG8071 Fusion of 8 or More Thoracic Vertebral Joints with Autologous Tissue Substitute, Posterior Approach, Posterior Column, Open Approach

ØRG807J Fusion of 8 or More Thoracic Vertebral Joints with Autologous Tissue Substitute, Posterior Approach, Anterior Column, Open Approach

ØRG80A0 Fusion of 8 or More Thoracic Vertebral Joints with Interbody Fusion Device, Anterior Approach, Anterior Column, Open Approach

ØRG80A1 Fusion of 8 or More Thoracic Vertebral Joints with Interbody Fusion Device, Posterior Approach, Posterior Column, Open Approach

ØRG80AJ Fusion of 8 or More Thoracic Vertebral Joints with Interbody Fusion Device, Posterior Approach, Anterior Column, Open Approach

ØRG80J0 Fusion of 8 or More Thoracic Vertebral Joints with Synthetic Substitute, Anterior Approach, Anterior Column, Open Approach

ØRG80J1 Fusion of 8 or More Thoracic Vertebral Joints with Synthetic Substitute, Posterior Approach, Posterior Column, Open Approach

ØRG80JJ Fusion of 8 or More Thoracic Vertebral Joints with Synthetic Substitute, Posterior Approach, Anterior Column, Open Approach

ØRG80K0 Fusion of 8 or More Thoracic Vertebral Joints with Nonautologous Tissue Substitute, Anterior Approach, Anterior Column, Open Approach

ØRG80K1 Fusion of 8 or More Thoracic Vertebral Joints with Nonautologous Tissue Substitute, Posterior Approach, Posterior Column, Open Approach

ØRG80KJ Fusion of 8 or More Thoracic Vertebral Joints with Nonautologous Tissue Substitute, Posterior Approach, Anterior Column, Open Approach

ØRG80Z0 Fusion of 8 or More Thoracic Vertebral Joints, Anterior Approach, Anterior Column, Open Approach

ØRG80Z1 Fusion of 8 or More Thoracic Vertebral Joints, Posterior Approach, Posterior Column, Open Approach

ØRG80ZJ Fusion of 8 or More Thoracic Vertebral Joints, Posterior Approach, Anterior Column, Open Approach

ØRG8370 Fusion of 8 or More Thoracic Vertebral Joints with Autologous Tissue Substitute, Anterior Approach, Anterior Column, Percutaneous Approach

ØRG8371 Fusion of 8 or More Thoracic Vertebral Joints with Autologous Tissue Substitute, Posterior Approach, Posterior Column, Percutaneous Approach

ØRG837J Fusion of 8 or More Thoracic Vertebral Joints with Autologous Tissue Substitute, Posterior Approach, Anterior Column, Percutaneous Approach

HAC 12: Surgical Site Infection Following Certain Orthopedic Procedures of the Spine, Shoulder, and Elbow (continued)

ØRG83AØ Fusion of 8 or More Thoracic Vertebral Joints with Interbody Fusion Device, Anterior Approach, Anterior Column, Percutaneous Approach

ØRG83A1 Fusion of 8 or More Thoracic Vertebral Joints with Interbody Fusion Device, Posterior Approach, Posterior Column, Percutaneous Approach

ØRG83AJ Fusion of 8 or More Thoracic Vertebral Joints with Interbody Fusion Device, Posterior Approach, Anterior Column, Percutaneous Approach

ØRG83JØ Fusion of 8 or More Thoracic Vertebral Joints with Synthetic Substitute, Anterior Approach, Anterior Column, Percutaneous Approach

ØRG83J1 Fusion of 8 or More Thoracic Vertebral Joints with Synthetic Substitute, Posterior Approach, Posterior Column, Percutaneous Approach

ØRG83JJ Fusion of 8 or More Thoracic Vertebral Joints with Synthetic Substitute, Posterior Approach, Anterior Column, Percutaneous Approach

ØRG83KØ Fusion of 8 or More Thoracic Vertebral Joints with Nonautologous Tissue Substitute, Anterior Approach, Anterior Column, Percutaneous Approach

ØRG83K1 Fusion of 8 or More Thoracic Vertebral Joints with Nonautologous Tissue Substitute, Posterior Approach, Posterior Column, Percutaneous Approach

ØRG83KJ Fusion of 8 or More Thoracic Vertebral Joints with Nonautologous Tissue Substitute, Posterior Approach, Anterior Column, Percutaneous Approach

ØRG83ZØ Fusion of 8 or More Thoracic Vertebral Joints, Anterior Approach, Anterior Column, Percutaneous Approach

ØRG83Z1 Fusion of 8 or More Thoracic Vertebral Joints, Posterior Approach, Posterior Column, Percutaneous Approach

ØRG83ZJ Fusion of 8 or More Thoracic Vertebral Joints, Posterior Approach, Anterior Column, Percutaneous Approach

ØRG847Ø Fusion of 8 or More Thoracic Vertebral Joints with Autologous Tissue Substitute, Anterior Approach, Anterior Column, Percutaneous Endoscopic Approach

ØRG8471 Fusion of 8 or More Thoracic Vertebral Joints with Autologous Tissue Substitute, Posterior Approach, Posterior Column, Percutaneous Endoscopic Approach

ØRG847J Fusion of 8 or More Thoracic Vertebral Joints with Autologous Tissue Substitute, Posterior Approach, Anterior Column, Percutaneous Endoscopic Approach

ØRG84AØ Fusion of 8 or More Thoracic Vertebral Joints with Interbody Fusion Device, Anterior Approach, Anterior Column, Percutaneous Endoscopic Approach

ØRG84A1 Fusion of 8 or More Thoracic Vertebral Joints with Interbody Fusion Device, Posterior Approach, Posterior Column, Percutaneous Endoscopic Approach

ØRG84AJ Fusion of 8 or More Thoracic Vertebral Joints with Interbody Fusion Device, Posterior Approach, Anterior Column, Percutaneous Endoscopic Approach

ØRG84JØ Fusion of 8 or More Thoracic Vertebral Joints with Synthetic Substitute, Anterior Approach, Anterior Column, Percutaneous Endoscopic Approach

ØRG84J1 Fusion of 8 or More Thoracic Vertebral Joints with Synthetic Substitute, Posterior Approach, Posterior Column, Percutaneous Endoscopic Approach

ØRG84JJ Fusion of 8 or More Thoracic Vertebral Joints with Synthetic Substitute, Posterior Approach, Anterior Column, Percutaneous Endoscopic Approach

ØRG84KØ Fusion of 8 or More Thoracic Vertebral Joints with Nonautologous Tissue Substitute, Anterior Approach, Anterior Column, Percutaneous Endoscopic Approach

ØRG84K1 Fusion of 8 or More Thoracic Vertebral Joints with Nonautologous Tissue Substitute, Posterior Approach, Posterior Column, Percutaneous Endoscopic Approach

ØRG84KJ Fusion of 8 or More Thoracic Vertebral Joints with Nonautologous Tissue Substitute, Posterior Approach, Anterior Column, Percutaneous Endoscopic Approach

ØRG84ZØ Fusion of 8 or More Thoracic Vertebral Joints, Anterior Approach, Anterior Column, Percutaneous Endoscopic Approach

ØRG84Z1 Fusion of 8 or More Thoracic Vertebral Joints, Posterior Approach, Posterior Column, Percutaneous Endoscopic Approach

ØRG84ZJ Fusion of 8 or More Thoracic Vertebral Joints, Posterior Approach, Anterior Column, Percutaneous Endoscopic Approach

ØRGAØ7Ø Fusion of Thoracolumbar Vertebral Joint with Autologous Tissue Substitute, Anterior Approach, Anterior Column, Open Approach

ØRGAØ71 Fusion of Thoracolumbar Vertebral Joint with Autologous Tissue Substitute, Posterior Approach, Posterior Column, Open Approach

ØRGAØ7J Fusion of Thoracolumbar Vertebral Joint with Autologous Tissue Substitute, Posterior Approach, Anterior Column, Open Approach

ØRGAØAØ Fusion of Thoracolumbar Vertebral Joint with Interbody Fusion Device, Anterior Approach, Anterior Column, Open Approach

ØRGAØA1 Fusion of Thoracolumbar Vertebral Joint with Interbody Fusion Device, Posterior Approach, Posterior Column, Open Approach

ØRGAØAJ Fusion of Thoracolumbar Vertebral Joint with Interbody Fusion Device, Posterior Approach, Anterior Column, Open Approach

ØRGAØJØ Fusion of Thoracolumbar Vertebral Joint with Synthetic Substitute, Anterior Approach, Anterior Column, Open Approach

ØRGAØJ1 Fusion of Thoracolumbar Vertebral Joint with Synthetic Substitute, Posterior Approach, Posterior Column, Open Approach

ØRGAØJJ Fusion of Thoracolumbar Vertebral Joint with Synthetic Substitute, Posterior Approach, Anterior Column, Open Approach

ØRGAØKØ Fusion of Thoracolumbar Vertebral Joint with Nonautologous Tissue Substitute, Anterior Approach, Anterior Column, Open Approach

ØRGAØK1 Fusion of Thoracolumbar Vertebral Joint with Nonautologous Tissue Substitute, Posterior Approach, Posterior Column, Open Approach

ØRGAØKJ Fusion of Thoracolumbar Vertebral Joint with Nonautologous Tissue Substitute, Posterior Approach, Anterior Column, Open Approach

ØRGAØZØ Fusion of Thoracolumbar Vertebral Joint, Anterior Approach, Anterior Column, Open Approach

ØRGAØZ1 Fusion of Thoracolumbar Vertebral Joint, Posterior Approach, Posterior Column, Open Approach

ØRGAØZJ Fusion of Thoracolumbar Vertebral Joint, Posterior Approach, Anterior Column, Open Approach

ØRGA37Ø Fusion of Thoracolumbar Vertebral Joint with Autologous Tissue Substitute, Anterior Approach, Anterior Column, Percutaneous Approach

ØRGA371 Fusion of Thoracolumbar Vertebral Joint with Autologous Tissue Substitute, Posterior Approach, Posterior Column, Percutaneous Approach

ØRGA37J Fusion of Thoracolumbar Vertebral Joint with Autologous Tissue Substitute, Posterior Approach, Anterior Column, Percutaneous Approach

ØRGA3AØ Fusion of Thoracolumbar Vertebral Joint with Interbody Fusion Device, Anterior Approach, Anterior Column, Percutaneous Approach

ØRGA3A1 Fusion of Thoracolumbar Vertebral Joint with Interbody Fusion Device, Posterior Approach, Posterior Column, Percutaneous Approach

ØRGA3AJ Fusion of Thoracolumbar Vertebral Joint with Interbody Fusion Device, Posterior Approach, Anterior Column, Percutaneous Approach

ØRGA3JØ Fusion of Thoracolumbar Vertebral Joint with Synthetic Substitute, Anterior Approach, Anterior Column, Percutaneous Approach

ØRGA3J1 Fusion of Thoracolumbar Vertebral Joint with Synthetic Substitute, Posterior Approach, Posterior Column, Percutaneous Approach

ØRGA3JJ Fusion of Thoracolumbar Vertebral Joint with Synthetic Substitute, Posterior Approach, Anterior Column, Percutaneous Approach

ØRGA3KØ Fusion of Thoracolumbar Vertebral Joint with Nonautologous Tissue Substitute, Anterior Approach, Anterior Column, Percutaneous Approach

ØRGA3K1 Fusion of Thoracolumbar Vertebral Joint with Nonautologous Tissue Substitute, Posterior Approach, Posterior Column, Percutaneous Approach

ØRGA3KJ Fusion of Thoracolumbar Vertebral Joint with Nonautologous Tissue Substitute, Posterior Approach, Anterior Column, Percutaneous Approach

ØRGA3ZØ Fusion of Thoracolumbar Vertebral Joint, Anterior Approach, Anterior Column, Percutaneous Approach

ØRGA3Z1 Fusion of Thoracolumbar Vertebral Joint, Posterior Approach, Posterior Column, Percutaneous Approach

ØRGA3ZJ Fusion of Thoracolumbar Vertebral Joint, Posterior Approach, Anterior Column, Percutaneous Approach

HAC 12: Surgical Site Infection Following Certain Orthopedic Procedures of the Spine, Shoulder, and Elbow (continued)

ØRGA47Ø Fusion of Thoracolumbar Vertebral Joint with Autologous Tissue Substitute, Anterior Approach, Anterior Column, Percutaneous Endoscopic Approach

ØRGA471 Fusion of Thoracolumbar Vertebral Joint with Autologous Tissue Substitute, Posterior Approach, Posterior Column, Percutaneous Endoscopic Approach

ØRGA47J Fusion of Thoracolumbar Vertebral Joint with Autologous Tissue Substitute, Posterior Approach, Anterior Column, Percutaneous Endoscopic Approach

ØRGA4AØ Fusion of Thoracolumbar Vertebral Joint with Interbody Fusion Device, Anterior Approach, Anterior Column, Percutaneous Endoscopic Approach

ØRGA4A1 Fusion of Thoracolumbar Vertebral Joint with Interbody Fusion Device, Posterior Approach, Posterior Column, Percutaneous Endoscopic Approach

ØRGA4AJ Fusion of Thoracolumbar Vertebral Joint with Interbody Fusion Device, Posterior Approach, Anterior Column, Percutaneous Endoscopic Approach

ØRGA4JØ Fusion of Thoracolumbar Vertebral Joint with Synthetic Substitute, Anterior Approach, Anterior Column, Percutaneous Endoscopic Approach

ØRGA4J1 Fusion of Thoracolumbar Vertebral Joint with Synthetic Substitute, Posterior Approach, Posterior Column, Percutaneous Endoscopic Approach

ØRGA4JJ Fusion of Thoracolumbar Vertebral Joint with Synthetic Substitute, Posterior Approach, Anterior Column, Percutaneous Endoscopic Approach

ØRGA4KØ Fusion of Thoracolumbar Vertebral Joint with Nonautologous Tissue Substitute, Anterior Approach, Anterior Column, Percutaneous Endoscopic Approach

ØRGA4K1 Fusion of Thoracolumbar Vertebral Joint with Nonautologous Tissue Substitute, Posterior Approach, Posterior Column, Percutaneous Endoscopic Approach

ØRGA4KJ Fusion of Thoracolumbar Vertebral Joint with Nonautologous Tissue Substitute, Posterior Approach, Anterior Column, Percutaneous Endoscopic Approach

ØRGA4ZØ Fusion of Thoracolumbar Vertebral Joint, Anterior Approach, Anterior Column, Percutaneous Endoscopic Approach

ØRGA4Z1 Fusion of Thoracolumbar Vertebral Joint, Posterior Approach, Posterior Column, Percutaneous Endoscopic Approach

ØRGA4ZJ Fusion of Thoracolumbar Vertebral Joint, Posterior Approach, Anterior Column, Percutaneous Endoscopic Approach

ØRGE04Z Fusion of Right Sternoclavicular Joint with Internal Fixation Device, Open Approach

ØRGE07Z Fusion of Right Sternoclavicular Joint with Autologous Tissue Substitute, Open Approach

ØRGE0JZ Fusion of Right Sternoclavicular Joint with Synthetic Substitute, Open Approach

ØRGE0KZ Fusion of Right Sternoclavicular Joint with Nonautologous Tissue Substitute, Open Approach

ØRGE0ZZ Fusion of Right Sternoclavicular Joint, Open Approach

ØRGE34Z Fusion of Right Sternoclavicular Joint with Internal Fixation Condition, Percutaneous Approach

ØRGE37Z Fusion of Right Sternoclavicular Joint with Autologous Tissue Substitute, Percutaneous Approach

ØRGE3JZ Fusion of Right Sternoclavicular Joint with Synthetic Substitute, Percutaneous Approach

ØRGE3KZ Fusion of Right Sternoclavicular Joint with Nonautologous Tissue Substitute, Percutaneous Approach

ØRGE3ZZ Fusion of Right Sternoclavicular Joint, Percutaneous Approach

ØRGE44Z Fusion of Right Sternoclavicular Joint with Internal Fixation Device, Percutaneous Endoscopic Approach

ØRGE47Z Fusion of Right Sternoclavicular Joint with Autologous Tissue Substitute, Percutaneous Endoscopic Approach

ØRGE4JZ Fusion of Right Sternoclavicular Joint with Synthetic Substitute, Percutaneous Endoscopic Approach

ØRGE4KZ Fusion of Right Sternoclavicular Joint with Nonautologous Tissue Substitute, Percutaneous Endoscopic Approach

ØRGE4ZZ Fusion of Right Sternoclavicular Joint, Percutaneous Endoscopic Approach

ØRGF04Z Fusion of Left Sternoclavicular Joint with Internal Fixation Device, Open Approach

ØRGF07Z Fusion of Left Sternoclavicular Joint with Autologous Tissue Substitute, Open Approach

ØRGF0JZ Fusion of Left Sternoclavicular Joint with Synthetic Substitute, Open Approach

ØRGF0KZ Fusion of Left Sternoclavicular Joint with Nonautologous Tissue Substitute, Open Approach

ØRGF0ZZ Fusion of Left Sternoclavicular Joint, Open Approach

ØRGF34Z Fusion of Left Sternoclavicular Joint with Internal Fixation Device, Percutaneous Approach

ØRGF37Z Fusion of Left Sternoclavicular Joint with Autologous Tissue Substitute, Percutaneous Approach

ØRGF3JZ Fusion of Left Sternoclavicular Joint with Synthetic Substitute, Percutaneous Approach

ØRGF3KZ Fusion of Left Sternoclavicular Joint with Nonautologous Tissue Substitute, Percutaneous Approach

ØRGF3ZZ Fusion of Left Sternoclavicular Joint, Percutaneous Approach

ØRGF44Z Fusion of Left Sternoclavicular Joint with Internal Fixation Device, Percutaneous Endoscopic Approach

ØRGF47Z Fusion of Left Sternoclavicular Joint with Autologous Tissue Substitute, Percutaneous Endoscopic Approach

ØRGF4JZ Fusion of Left Sternoclavicular Joint with Synthetic Substitute, Percutaneous Endoscopic Approach

ØRGF4KZ Fusion of Left Sternoclavicular Joint with Nonautologous Tissue Substitute, Percutaneous Endoscopic Approach

ØRGF4ZZ Fusion of Left Sternoclavicular Joint, Percutaneous Endoscopic Approach

ØRGG04Z Fusion of Right Acromioclavicular Joint with Internal Fixation Device, Open Approach

ØRGG07Z Fusion of Right Acromioclavicular Joint with Autologous Tissue Substitute, Open Approach

ØRGG0JZ Fusion of Right Acromioclavicular Joint with Synthetic Substitute, Open Approach

ØRGG0KZ Fusion of Right Acromioclavicular Joint with Nonautologous Tissue Substitute, Open Approach

ØRGG0ZZ Fusion of Right Acromioclavicular Joint, Open Approach

ØRGG34Z Fusion of Right Acromioclavicular Joint with Internal Fixation Device, Percutaneous Approach

ØRGG37Z Fusion of Right Acromioclavicular Joint with Autologous Tissue Substitute, Percutaneous Approach

ØRGG3JZ Fusion of Right Acromioclavicular Joint with Synthetic Substitute, Percutaneous Approach

ØRGG3KZ Fusion of Right Acromioclavicular Joint with Nonautologous Tissue Substitute, Percutaneous Approach

ØRGG3ZZ Fusion of Right Acromioclavicular Joint, Percutaneous Approach

ØRGG44Z Fusion of Right Acromioclavicular Joint with Internal Fixation Device, Percutaneous Endoscopic Approach

ØRGG47Z Fusion of Right Acromioclavicular Joint with Autologous Tissue Substitute, Percutaneous Endoscopic Approach

ØRGG4JZ Fusion of Right Acromioclavicular Joint with Synthetic Substitute, Percutaneous Endoscopic Approach

ØRGG4KZ Fusion of Right Acromioclavicular Joint with Nonautologous Tissue Substitute, Percutaneous Endoscopic Approach

ØRGG4ZZ Fusion of Right Acromioclavicular Joint, Percutaneous Endoscopic Approach

ØRGH04Z Fusion of Left Acromioclavicular Joint with Internal Fixation Device, Open Approach

ØRGH07Z Fusion of Left Acromioclavicular Joint with Autologous Tissue Substitute, Open Approach

ØRGH0JZ Fusion of Left Acromioclavicular Joint with Synthetic Substitute, Open Approach

ØRGH0KZ Fusion of Left Acromioclavicular Joint with Nonautologous Tissue Substitute, Open Approach

ØRGH0ZZ Fusion of Left Acromioclavicular Joint, Open Approach

ØRGH34Z Fusion of Left Acromioclavicular Joint with Internal Fixation Device, Percutaneous Approach

ØRGH37Z Fusion of Left Acromioclavicular Joint with Autologous Tissue Substitute, Percutaneous Approach

ØRGH3JZ Fusion of Left Acromioclavicular Joint with Synthetic Substitute, Percutaneous Approach

ØRGH3KZ Fusion of Left Acromioclavicular Joint with Nonautologous Tissue Substitute, Percutaneous Approach

ØRGH3ZZ Fusion of Left Acromioclavicular Joint, Percutaneous Approach

ØRGH44Z Fusion of Left Acromioclavicular Joint with Internal Fixation Device, Percutaneous Endoscopic Approach

ØRGH47Z Fusion of Left Acromioclavicular Joint with Autologous Tissue Substitute, Percutaneous Endoscopic Approach

ØRGH4JZ Fusion of Left Acromioclavicular Joint with Synthetic Substitute, Percutaneous Endoscopic Approach

ØRGH4KZ Fusion of Left Acromioclavicular Joint with Nonautologous Tissue Substitute, Percutaneous Endoscopic Approach

ØRGH4ZZ Fusion of Left Acromioclavicular Joint, Percutaneous Endoscopic Approach

ØRGJ04Z Fusion of Right Shoulder Joint with Internal Fixation Device, Open Approach

ØRGJ07Z Fusion of Right Shoulder Joint with Autologous Tissue Substitute, Open Approach

HAC 12: Surgical Site Infection Following Certain Orthopedic Procedures of the Spine, Shoulder, and Elbow (continued)

ØRGJØJZ — Fusion of Right Shoulder Joint with Synthetic Substitute, Open Approach

ØRGJØKZ — Fusion of Right Shoulder Joint with Nonautologous Tissue Substitute, Open Approach

ØRGJØZZ — Fusion of Right Shoulder Joint, Open Approach

ØRGJ34Z — Fusion of Right Shoulder Joint with Internal Fixation Device, Percutaneous Approach

ØRGJ37Z — Fusion of Right Shoulder Joint with Autologous Tissue Substitute, Percutaneous Approach

ØRGJ3JZ — Fusion of Right Shoulder Joint with Synthetic Substitute, Percutaneous Approach

ØRGJ3KZ — Fusion of Right Shoulder Joint with Nonautologous Tissue Substitute, Percutaneous Approach

ØRGJ3ZZ — Fusion of Right Shoulder Joint, Percutaneous Approach

ØRGJ44Z — Fusion of Right Shoulder Joint with Internal Fixation Device, Percutaneous Endoscopic Approach

ØRGJ47Z — Fusion of Right Shoulder Joint with Autologous Tissue Substitute, Percutaneous Endoscopic Approach

ØRGJ4JZ — Fusion of Right Shoulder Joint with Synthetic Substitute, Percutaneous Endoscopic Approach

ØRGJ4KZ — Fusion of Right Shoulder Joint with Nonautologous Tissue Substitute, Percutaneous Endoscopic Approach

ØRGJ4ZZ — Fusion of Right Shoulder Joint, Percutaneous Endoscopic Approach

ØRGKØ4Z — Fusion of Left Shoulder Joint with Internal Fixation Device, Open Approach

ØRGKØ7Z — Fusion of Left Shoulder Joint with Autologous Tissue Substitute, Open Approach

ØRGKØJZ — Fusion of Left Shoulder Joint with Synthetic Substitute, Open Approach

ØRGKØKZ — Fusion of Left Shoulder Joint with Nonautologous Tissue Substitute, Open Approach

ØRGKØZZ — Fusion of Left Shoulder Joint, Open Approach

ØRGK34Z — Fusion of Left Shoulder Joint with Internal Fixation Device, Percutaneous Approach

ØRGK37Z — Fusion of Left Shoulder Joint with Autologous Tissue Substitute, Percutaneous Approach

ØRGK3JZ — Fusion of Left Shoulder Joint with Synthetic Substitute, Percutaneous Approach

ØRGK3KZ — Fusion of Left Shoulder Joint with Nonautologous Tissue Substitute, Percutaneous Approach

ØRGK3ZZ — Fusion of Left Shoulder Joint, Percutaneous Approach

ØRGK44Z — Fusion of Left Shoulder Joint with Internal Fixation Device, Percutaneous Endoscopic Approach

ØRGK47Z — Fusion of Left Shoulder Joint with Autologous Tissue Substitute, Percutaneous Endoscopic Approach

ØRGK4JZ — Fusion of Left Shoulder Joint with Synthetic Substitute, Percutaneous Endoscopic Approach

ØRGK4KZ — Fusion of Left Shoulder Joint with Nonautologous Tissue Substitute, Percutaneous Endoscopic Approach

ØRGK4ZZ — Fusion of Left Shoulder Joint, Percutaneous Endoscopic Approach

ØRGLØ4Z — Fusion of Right Elbow Joint with Internal Fixation Device, Open Approach

ØRGLØ5Z — Fusion of Right Elbow Joint with External Fixation Device, Open Approach

ØRGLØ7Z — Fusion of Right Elbow Joint with Autologous Tissue Substitute, Open Approach

ØRGLØJZ — Fusion of Right Elbow Joint with Synthetic Substitute, Open Approach

ØRGLØKZ — Fusion of Right Elbow Joint with Nonautologous Tissue Substitute, Open Approach

ØRGLØZZ — Fusion of Right Elbow Joint, Open Approach

ØRGL34Z — Fusion of Right Elbow Joint with Internal Fixation Device, Percutaneous Approach

ØRGL35Z — Fusion of Right Elbow Joint with External Fixation Device, Percutaneous Approach

ØRGL37Z — Fusion of Right Elbow Joint with Autologous Tissue Substitute, Percutaneous Approach

ØRGL3JZ — Fusion of Right Elbow Joint with Synthetic Substitute, Percutaneous Approach

ØRGL3KZ — Fusion of Right Elbow Joint with Nonautologous Tissue Substitute, Percutaneous Approach

ØRGL3ZZ — Fusion of Right Elbow Joint, Percutaneous Approach

ØRGL44Z — Fusion of Right Elbow Joint with Internal Fixation Device, Percutaneous Endoscopic Approach

ØRGL45Z — Fusion of Right Elbow Joint with External Fixation Device, Percutaneous Endoscopic Approach

ØRGL47Z — Fusion of Right Elbow Joint with Autologous Tissue Substitute, Percutaneous Endoscopic Approach

ØRGL4JZ — Fusion of Right Elbow Joint with Synthetic Substitute, Percutaneous Endoscopic Approach

ØRGL4KZ — Fusion of Right Elbow Joint with Nonautologous Tissue Substitute, Percutaneous Endoscopic Approach

ØRGL4ZZ — Fusion of Right Elbow Joint, Percutaneous Endoscopic Approach

ØRGMØ4Z — Fusion of Left Elbow Joint with Internal Fixation Device, Open Approach

ØRGMØ5Z — Fusion of Left Elbow Joint with External Fixation Device, Open Approach

ØRGMØ7Z — Fusion of Left Elbow Joint with Autologous Tissue Substitute, Open Approach

ØRGMØJZ — Fusion of Left Elbow Joint with Synthetic Substitute, Open Approach

ØRGMØKZ — Fusion of Left Elbow Joint with Nonautologous Tissue Substitute, Open Approach

ØRGMØZZ — Fusion of Left Elbow Joint, Open Approach

ØRGM34Z — Fusion of Left Elbow Joint with Internal Fixation Device, Percutaneous Approach

ØRGM35Z — Fusion of Left Elbow Joint with External Fixation Device, Percutaneous Approach

ØRGM37Z — Fusion of Left Elbow Joint with Autologous Tissue Substitute, Percutaneous Approach

ØRGM3JZ — Fusion of Left Elbow Joint with Synthetic Substitute, Percutaneous Approach

ØRGM3KZ — Fusion of Left Elbow Joint with Nonautologous Tissue Substitute, Percutaneous Approach

ØRGM3ZZ — Fusion of Left Elbow Joint, Percutaneous Approach

ØRGM44Z — Fusion of Left Elbow Joint with Internal Fixation Device, Percutaneous Endoscopic Approach

ØRGM45Z — Fusion of Left Elbow Joint with External Fixation Device, Percutaneous Endoscopic Approach

ØRGM47Z — Fusion of Left Elbow Joint with Autologous Tissue Substitute, Percutaneous Endoscopic Approach

ØRGM4JZ — Fusion of Left Elbow Joint with Synthetic Substitute, Percutaneous Endoscopic Approach

ØRGM4KZ — Fusion of Left Elbow Joint with Nonautologous Tissue Substitute, Percutaneous Endoscopic Approach

ØRGM4ZZ — Fusion of Left Elbow Joint, Percutaneous Endoscopic Approach

ØRQEØZZ — Repair Right Sternoclavicular Joint, Open Approach

ØRQE3ZZ — Repair Right Sternoclavicular Joint, Percutaneous Approach

ØRQE4ZZ — Repair Right Sternoclavicular Joint, Percutaneous Endoscopic Approach

ØRQEXZZ — Repair Right Sternoclavicular Joint, External Approach

ØRQFØZZ — Repair Left Sternoclavicular Joint, Open Approach

ØRQF3ZZ — Repair Left Sternoclavicular Joint, Percutaneous Approach

ØRQF4ZZ — Repair Left Sternoclavicular Joint, Percutaneous Endoscopic Approach

ØRQFXZZ — Repair Left Sternoclavicular Joint, External Approach

ØRQGØZZ — Repair Right Acromioclavicular Joint, Open Approach

ØRQG3ZZ — Repair Right Acromioclavicular Joint, Percutaneous Approach

ØRQG4ZZ — Repair Right Acromioclavicular Joint, Percutaneous Endoscopic Approach

ØRQGXZZ — Repair Right Acromioclavicular Joint, External Approach

ØRQHØZZ — Repair Left Acromioclavicular Joint, Open Approach

ØRQH3ZZ — Repair Left Acromioclavicular Joint, Percutaneous Approach

ØRQH4ZZ — Repair Left Acromioclavicular Joint, Percutaneous Endoscopic Approach

ØRQHXZZ — Repair Left Acromioclavicular Joint, External Approach

ØRQJØZZ — Repair Right Shoulder Joint, Open Approach

ØRQJ3ZZ — Repair Right Shoulder Joint, Percutaneous Approach

ØRQJ4ZZ — Repair Right Shoulder Joint, Percutaneous Endoscopic Approach

ØRQJXZZ — Repair Right Shoulder Joint, External Approach

ØRQKØZZ — Repair Left Shoulder Joint, Open Approach

ØRQK3ZZ — Repair Left Shoulder Joint, Percutaneous Approach

ØRQK4ZZ — Repair Left Shoulder Joint, Percutaneous Endoscopic Approach

ØRQKXZZ — Repair Left Shoulder Joint, External Approach

ØRQLØZZ — Repair Right Elbow Joint, Open Approach

ØRQL3ZZ — Repair Right Elbow Joint, Percutaneous Approach

ØRQL4ZZ — Repair Right Elbow Joint, Percutaneous Endoscopic Approach

ØRQLXZZ — Repair Right Elbow Joint, External Approach

ØRQMØZZ — Repair Left Elbow Joint, Open Approach

ØRQM3ZZ — Repair Left Elbow Joint, Percutaneous Approach

ØRQM4ZZ — Repair Left Elbow Joint, Percutaneous Endoscopic Approach

HAC 12: Surgical Site Infection Following Certain Orthopedic Procedures of the Spine, Shoulder, and Elbow (continued)

ØRQMXZZ Repair Left Elbow Joint, External Approach

ØRUEØ7Z Supplement Right Sternoclavicular Joint with Autologous Tissue Substitute, Open Approach

ØRUEØJZ Supplement Right Sternoclavicular Joint with Synthetic Substitute, Open Approach

ØRUEØKZ Supplement Right Sternoclavicular Joint with Nonautologous Tissue Substitute, Open Approach

ØRUE37Z Supplement Right Sternoclavicular Joint with Autologous Tissue Substitute, Percutaneous Approach

ØRUE3JZ Supplement Right Sternoclavicular Joint with Synthetic Substitute, Percutaneous Approach

ØRUE3KZ Supplement Right Sternoclavicular Joint with Nonautologous Tissue Substitute, Percutaneous Approach

ØRUE47Z Supplement Right Sternoclavicular Joint with Autologous Tissue Substitute, Percutaneous Endoscopic Approach

ØRUE4JZ Supplement Right Sternoclavicular Joint with Synthetic Substitute, Percutaneous Endoscopic Approach

ØRUE4KZ Supplement Right Sternoclavicular Joint with Nonautologous Tissue Substitute, Percutaneous Endoscopic Approach

ØRUFØ7Z Supplement Left Sternoclavicular Joint with Autologous Tissue Substitute, Open Approach

ØRUFØJZ Supplement Left Sternoclavicular Joint with Synthetic Substitute, Open Approach

ØRUFØKZ Supplement Left Sternoclavicular Joint with Nonautologous Tissue Substitute, Open Approach

ØRUF37Z Supplement Left Sternoclavicular Joint with Autologous Tissue Substitute, Percutaneous Approach

ØRUF3JZ Supplement Left Sternoclavicular Joint with Synthetic Substitute, Percutaneous Approach

ØRUF3KZ Supplement Left Sternoclavicular Joint with Nonautologous Tissue Substitute, Percutaneous Approach

ØRUF47Z Supplement Left Sternoclavicular Joint with Autologous Tissue Substitute, Percutaneous Endoscopic Approach

ØRUF4JZ Supplement Left Sternoclavicular Joint with Synthetic Substitute, Percutaneous Endoscopic Approach

ØRUF4KZ Supplement Left Sternoclavicular Joint with Nonautologous Tissue Substitute, Percutaneous Endoscopic Approach

ØRUGØ7Z Supplement Right Acromioclavicular Joint with Autologous Tissue Substitute, Open Approach

ØRUGØJZ Supplement Right Acromioclavicular Joint with Synthetic Substitute, Open Approach

ØRUGØKZ Supplement Right Acromioclavicular Joint with Nonautologous Tissue Substitute, Open Approach

ØRUG37Z Supplement Right Acromioclavicular Joint with Autologous Tissue Substitute, Percutaneous Approach

ØRUG3JZ Supplement Right Acromioclavicular Joint with Synthetic Substitute, Percutaneous Approach

ØRUG3KZ Supplement Right Acromioclavicular Joint with Nonautologous Tissue Substitute, Percutaneous Approach

ØRUG47Z Supplement Right Acromioclavicular Joint with Autologous Tissue Substitute, Percutaneous Endoscopic Approach

ØRUG4JZ Supplement Right Acromioclavicular Joint with Synthetic Substitute, Percutaneous Endoscopic Approach

ØRUG4KZ Supplement Right Acromioclavicular Joint with Nonautologous Tissue Substitute, Percutaneous Endoscopic Approach

ØRUHØ7Z Supplement Left Acromioclavicular Joint with Autologous Tissue Substitute, Open Approach

ØRUHØJZ Supplement Left Acromioclavicular Joint with Synthetic Substitute, Open Approach

ØRUHØKZ Supplement Left Acromioclavicular Joint with Nonautologous Tissue Substitute, Open Approach

ØRUH37Z Supplement Left Acromioclavicular Joint with Autologous Tissue Substitute, Percutaneous Approach

ØRUH3JZ Supplement Left Acromioclavicular Joint with Synthetic Substitute, Percutaneous Approach

ØRUH3KZ Supplement Left Acromioclavicular Joint with Nonautologous Tissue Substitute, Percutaneous Approach

ØRUH47Z Supplement Left Acromioclavicular Joint with Autologous Tissue Substitute, Percutaneous Endoscopic Approach

ØRUH4JZ Supplement Left Acromioclavicular Joint with Synthetic Substitute, Percutaneous Endoscopic Approach

ØRUH4KZ Supplement Left Acromioclavicular Joint with Nonautologous Tissue Substitute, Percutaneous Endoscopic Approach

ØRUJØ7Z Supplement Right Shoulder Joint with Autologous Tissue Substitute, Open Approach

ØRUJØJZ Supplement Right Shoulder Joint with Synthetic Substitute, Open Approach

ØRUJØKZ Supplement Right Shoulder Joint with Nonautologous Tissue Substitute, Open Approach

ØRUJ37Z Supplement Right Shoulder Joint with Autologous Tissue Substitute, Percutaneous Approach

ØRUJ3JZ Supplement Right Shoulder Joint with Synthetic Substitute, Percutaneous Approach

ØRUJ3KZ Supplement Right Shoulder Joint with Nonautologous Tissue Substitute, Percutaneous Approach

ØRUJ47Z Supplement Right Shoulder Joint with Autologous Tissue Substitute, Percutaneous Endoscopic Approach

ØRUJ4JZ Supplement Right Shoulder Joint with Synthetic Substitute, Percutaneous Endoscopic Approach

ØRUJ4KZ Supplement Right Shoulder Joint with Nonautologous Tissue Substitute, Percutaneous Endoscopic Approach

ØRUKØ7Z Supplement Left Shoulder Joint with Autologous Tissue Substitute, Open Approach

ØRUKØJZ Supplement Left Shoulder Joint with Synthetic Substitute, Open Approach

ØRUKØKZ Supplement Left Shoulder Joint with Nonautologous Tissue Substitute, Open Approach

ØRUK37Z Supplement Left Shoulder Joint with Autologous Tissue Substitute, Percutaneous Approach

ØRUK3JZ Supplement Left Shoulder Joint with Synthetic Substitute, Percutaneous Approach

ØRUK3KZ Supplement Left Shoulder Joint with Nonautologous Tissue Substitute, Percutaneous Approach

ØRUK47Z Supplement Left Shoulder Joint with Autologous Tissue Substitute, Percutaneous Endoscopic Approach

ØRUK4JZ Supplement Left Shoulder Joint with Synthetic Substitute, Percutaneous Endoscopic Approach

ØRUK4KZ Supplement Left Shoulder Joint with Nonautologous Tissue Substitute, Percutaneous Endoscopic Approach

ØRULØ7Z Supplement Right Elbow Joint with Autologous Tissue Substitute, Open Approach

ØRULØJZ Supplement Right Elbow Joint with Synthetic Substitute, Open Approach

ØRULØKZ Supplement Right Elbow Joint with Nonautologous Tissue Substitute, Open Approach

ØRUL37Z Supplement Right Elbow Joint with Autologous Tissue Substitute, Percutaneous Approach

ØRUL3JZ Supplement Right Elbow Joint with Synthetic Substitute, Percutaneous Approach

ØRUL3KZ Supplement Right Elbow Joint with Nonautologous Tissue Substitute, Percutaneous Approach

ØRUL47Z Supplement Right Elbow Joint with Autologous Tissue Substitute, Percutaneous Endoscopic Approach

ØRUL4JZ Supplement Right Elbow Joint with Synthetic Substitute, Percutaneous Endoscopic Approach

ØRUL4KZ Supplement Right Elbow Joint with Nonautologous Tissue Substitute, Percutaneous Endoscopic Approach

ØRUMØ7Z Supplement Left Elbow Joint with Autologous Tissue Substitute, Open Approach

ØRUMØJZ Supplement Left Elbow Joint with Synthetic Substitute, Open Approach

ØRUMØKZ Supplement Left Elbow Joint with Nonautologous Tissue Substitute, Open Approach

ØRUM37Z Supplement Left Elbow Joint with Autologous Tissue Substitute, Percutaneous Approach

ØRUM3JZ Supplement Left Elbow Joint with Synthetic Substitute, Percutaneous Approach

ØRUM3KZ Supplement Left Elbow Joint with Nonautologous Tissue Substitute, Percutaneous Approach

ØRUM47Z Supplement Left Elbow Joint with Autologous Tissue Substitute, Percutaneous Endoscopic Approach

ØRUM4JZ Supplement Left Elbow Joint with Synthetic Substitute, Percutaneous Endoscopic Approach

ØRUM4KZ Supplement Left Elbow Joint with Nonautologous Tissue Substitute, Percutaneous Endoscopic Approach

ØSGØØ7Ø Fusion of Lumbar Vertebral Joint with Autologous Tissue Substitute, Anterior Approach, Anterior Column, Open Approach

ØSGØØ71 Fusion of Lumbar Vertebral Joint with Autologous Tissue Substitute, Posterior Approach, Posterior Column, Open Approach

ØSGØØ7J Fusion of Lumbar Vertebral Joint with Autologous Tissue Substitute, Posterior Approach, Anterior Column, Open Approach

HAC 12: Surgical Site Infection Following Certain Orthopedic Procedures of the Spine, Shoulder, and Elbow (continued)

ØSG00AØ Fusion of Lumbar Vertebral Joint with Interbody Fusion Device, Anterior Approach, Anterior Column, Open Approach

ØSG00A1 Fusion of Lumbar Vertebral Joint with Interbody Fusion Device, Posterior Approach, Posterior Column, Open Approach

ØSG00AJ Fusion of Lumbar Vertebral Joint with Interbody Fusion Device, Posterior Approach, Anterior Column, Open Approach

ØSG00JØ Fusion of Lumbar Vertebral Joint with Synthetic Substitute, Anterior Approach, Anterior Column, Open Approach

ØSG00J1 Fusion of Lumbar Vertebral Joint with Synthetic Substitute, Posterior Approach, Posterior Column, Open Approach

ØSG00JJ Fusion of Lumbar Vertebral Joint with Synthetic Substitute, Posterior Approach, Anterior Column, Open Approach

ØSG00KØ Fusion of Lumbar Vertebral Joint with Nonautologous Tissue Substitute, Anterior Approach, Anterior Column, Open Approach

ØSG00K1 Fusion of Lumbar Vertebral Joint with Nonautologous Tissue Substitute, Posterior Approach, Posterior Column, Open Approach

ØSG00KJ Fusion of Lumbar Vertebral Joint with Nonautologous Tissue Substitute, Posterior Approach, Anterior Column, Open Approach

ØSG00ZØ Fusion of Lumbar Vertebral Joint, Anterior Approach, Anterior Column, Open Approach

ØSG00Z1 Fusion of Lumbar Vertebral Joint, Posterior Approach, Posterior Column, Open Approach

ØSG00ZJ Fusion of Lumbar Vertebral Joint, Posterior Approach, Anterior Column, Open Approach

ØSG037Ø Fusion of Lumbar Vertebral Joint with Autologous Tissue Substitute, Anterior Approach, Anterior Column, Percutaneous Approach

ØSG0371 Fusion of Lumbar Vertebral Joint with Autologous Tissue Substitute, Posterior Approach, Posterior Column, Percutaneous Approach

ØSG037J Fusion of Lumbar Vertebral Joint with Autologous Tissue Substitute, Posterior Approach, Anterior Column, Percutaneous Approach

ØSG03AØ Fusion of Lumbar Vertebral Joint with Interbody Fusion Device, Anterior Approach, Anterior Column, Percutaneous Approach

ØSG03A1 Fusion of Lumbar Vertebral Joint with Interbody Fusion Device, Posterior Approach, Posterior Column, Percutaneous Approach

ØSG03AJ Fusion of Lumbar Vertebral Joint with Interbody Fusion Device, Posterior Approach, Anterior Column, Percutaneous Approach

ØSG03JØ Fusion of Lumbar Vertebral Joint with Synthetic Substitute, Anterior Approach, Anterior Column, Percutaneous Approach

ØSG03J1 Fusion of Lumbar Vertebral Joint with Synthetic Substitute, Posterior Approach, Posterior Column, Percutaneous Approach

ØSG03JJ Fusion of Lumbar Vertebral Joint with Synthetic Substitute, Posterior Approach, Anterior Column, Percutaneous Approach

ØSG03KØ Fusion of Lumbar Vertebral Joint with Nonautologous Tissue Substitute, Anterior Approach, Anterior Column, Percutaneous Approach

ØSG03K1 Fusion of Lumbar Vertebral Joint with Nonautologous Tissue Substitute, Posterior Approach, Posterior Column, Percutaneous Approach

ØSG03KJ Fusion of Lumbar Vertebral Joint with Nonautologous Tissue Substitute, Posterior Approach, Anterior Column, Percutaneous Approach

ØSG03ZØ Fusion of Lumbar Vertebral Joint, Anterior Approach, Anterior Column, Percutaneous Approach

ØSG03Z1 Fusion of Lumbar Vertebral Joint, Posterior Approach, Posterior Column, Percutaneous Approach

ØSG03ZJ Fusion of Lumbar Vertebral Joint, Posterior Approach, Anterior Column, Percutaneous Approach

ØSG0470 Fusion of Lumbar Vertebral Joint with Autologous Tissue Substitute, Anterior Approach, Anterior Column, Percutaneous Endoscopic Approach

ØSG0471 Fusion of Lumbar Vertebral Joint with Autologous Tissue Substitute, Posterior Approach, Posterior Column, Percutaneous Endoscopic Approach

ØSG047J Fusion of Lumbar Vertebral Joint with Autologous Tissue Substitute, Posterior Approach, Anterior Column, Percutaneous Endoscopic Approach

ØSG04AØ Fusion of Lumbar Vertebral Joint with Interbody Fusion Device, Anterior Approach, Anterior Column, Percutaneous Endoscopic Approach

ØSG04A1 Fusion of Lumbar Vertebral Joint with Interbody Fusion Device, Posterior Approach, Posterior Column, Percutaneous Endoscopic Approach

ØSG04AJ Fusion of Lumbar Vertebral Joint with Interbody Fusion Device, Posterior Approach, Anterior Column, Percutaneous Endoscopic Approach

ØSG04JØ Fusion of Lumbar Vertebral Joint with Synthetic Substitute, Anterior Approach, Anterior Column, Percutaneous Endoscopic Approach

ØSG04J1 Fusion of Lumbar Vertebral Joint with Synthetic Substitute, Posterior Approach, Posterior Column, Percutaneous Endoscopic Approach

ØSG04JJ Fusion of Lumbar Vertebral Joint with Synthetic Substitute, Posterior Approach, Anterior Column, Percutaneous Endoscopic Approach

ØSG04KØ Fusion of Lumbar Vertebral Joint with Nonautologous Tissue Substitute, Anterior Approach, Anterior Column, Percutaneous Endoscopic Approach

ØSG04K1 Fusion of Lumbar Vertebral Joint with Nonautologous Tissue Substitute, Posterior Approach, Posterior Column, Percutaneous Endoscopic Approach

ØSG04KJ Fusion of Lumbar Vertebral Joint with Nonautologous Tissue Substitute, Posterior Approach, Anterior Column, Percutaneous Endoscopic Approach

ØSG04ZØ Fusion of Lumbar Vertebral Joint, Anterior Approach, Anterior Column, Percutaneous Endoscopic Approach

ØSG04Z1 Fusion of Lumbar Vertebral Joint, Posterior Approach, Posterior Column, Percutaneous Endoscopic Approach

ØSG04ZJ Fusion of Lumbar Vertebral Joint, Posterior Approach, Anterior Column, Percutaneous Endoscopic Approach

ØSG1070 Fusion of 2 or More Lumbar Vertebral Joints with Autologous Tissue Substitute, Anterior Approach, Anterior Column, Open Approach

ØSG1071 Fusion of 2 or More Lumbar Vertebral Joints with Autologous Tissue Substitute, Posterior Approach, Posterior Column, Open Approach

ØSG107J Fusion of 2 or More Lumbar Vertebral Joints with Autologous Tissue Substitute, Posterior Approach, Anterior Column, Open Approach

ØSG10AØ Fusion of 2 or More Lumbar Vertebral Joints with Interbody Fusion Device, Anterior Approach, Anterior Column, Open Approach

ØSG10A1 Fusion of 2 or More Lumbar Vertebral Joints with Interbody Fusion Device, Posterior Approach, Posterior Column, Open Approach

ØSG10AJ Fusion of 2 or More Lumbar Vertebral Joints with Interbody Fusion Device, Posterior Approach, Anterior Column, Open Approach

ØSG10JØ Fusion of 2 or More Lumbar Vertebral Joints with Synthetic Substitute, Anterior Approach, Anterior Column, Open Approach

ØSG10J1 Fusion of 2 or More Lumbar Vertebral Joints with Synthetic Substitute, Posterior Approach, Posterior Column, Open Approach

ØSG10JJ Fusion of 2 or More Lumbar Vertebral Joints with Synthetic Substitute, Posterior Approach, Anterior Column, Open Approach

ØSG10KØ Fusion of 2 or More Lumbar Vertebral Joints with Nonautologous Tissue Substitute, Anterior Approach, Anterior Column, Open Approach

ØSG10K1 Fusion of 2 or More Lumbar Vertebral Joints with Nonautologous Tissue Substitute, Posterior Approach, Posterior Column, Open Approach

ØSG10KJ Fusion of 2 or More Lumbar Vertebral Joints with Nonautologous Tissue Substitute, Posterior Approach, Anterior Column, Open Approach

ØSG10ZØ Fusion of 2 or More Lumbar Vertebral Joints, Anterior Approach, Anterior Column, Open Approach

ØSG10Z1 Fusion of 2 or More Lumbar Vertebral Joints, Posterior Approach, Posterior Column, Open Approach

ØSG10ZJ Fusion of 2 or More Lumbar Vertebral Joints, Posterior Approach, Anterior Column, Open Approach

ØSG1370 Fusion of 2 or More Lumbar Vertebral Joints with Autologous Tissue Substitute, Anterior Approach, Anterior Column, Percutaneous Approach

ØSG1371 Fusion of 2 or More Lumbar Vertebral Joints with Autologous Tissue Substitute, Posterior Approach, Posterior Column, Percutaneous Approach

ØSG137J Fusion of 2 or More Lumbar Vertebral Joints with Autologous Tissue Substitute, Posterior Approach, Anterior Column, Percutaneous Approach

Appendix I: Hospital Acquired Conditions

HAC 12: Surgical Site Infection Following Certain Orthopedic Procedures of the Spine, Shoulder, and Elbow (continued)

ØSG13AØ Fusion of 2 or More Lumbar Vertebral Joints with Interbody Fusion Device, Anterior Approach, Anterior Column, Percutaneous Approach

ØSG13A1 Fusion of 2 or More Lumbar Vertebral Joints with Interbody Fusion Device, Posterior Approach, Posterior Column, Percutaneous Approach

ØSG13AJ Fusion of 2 or More Lumbar Vertebral Joints with Interbody Fusion Device, Posterior Approach, Anterior Column, Percutaneous Approach

ØSG13JØ Fusion of 2 or More Lumbar Vertebral Joints with Synthetic Substitute, Anterior Approach, Anterior Column, Percutaneous Approach

ØSG13J1 Fusion of 2 or More Lumbar Vertebral Joints with Synthetic Substitute, Posterior Approach, Posterior Column, Percutaneous Approach

ØSG13JJ Fusion of 2 or More Lumbar Vertebral Joints with Synthetic Substitute, Posterior Approach, Anterior Column, Percutaneous Approach

ØSG13KØ Fusion of 2 or More Lumbar Vertebral Joints with Nonautologous Tissue Substitute, Anterior Approach, Anterior Column, Percutaneous Approach

ØSG13K1 Fusion of 2 or More Lumbar Vertebral Joints with Nonautologous Tissue Substitute, Posterior Approach, Posterior Column, Percutaneous Approach

ØSG13KJ Fusion of 2 or More Lumbar Vertebral Joints with Nonautologous Tissue Substitute, Posterior Approach, Anterior Column, Percutaneous Approach

ØSG13ZØ Fusion of 2 or More Lumbar Vertebral Joints, Anterior Approach, Anterior Column, Percutaneous Approach

ØSG13Z1 Fusion of 2 or More Lumbar Vertebral Joints, Posterior Approach, Posterior Column, Percutaneous Approach

ØSG13ZJ Fusion of 2 or More Lumbar Vertebral Joints, Posterior Approach, Anterior Column, Percutaneous Approach

ØSG147Ø Fusion of 2 or More Lumbar Vertebral Joints with Autologous Tissue Substitute, Anterior Approach, Anterior Column, Percutaneous Endoscopic Approach

ØSG1471 Fusion of 2 or More Lumbar Vertebral Joints with Autologous Tissue Substitute, Posterior Approach, Posterior Column, Percutaneous Endoscopic Approach

ØSG147J Fusion of 2 or More Lumbar Vertebral Joints with Autologous Tissue Substitute, Posterior Approach, Anterior Column, Percutaneous Endoscopic Approach

ØSG14AØ Fusion of 2 or More Lumbar Vertebral Joints with Interbody Fusion Device, Anterior Approach, Anterior Column, Percutaneous Endoscopic Approach

ØSG14A1 Fusion of 2 or More Lumbar Vertebral Joints with Interbody Fusion Device, Posterior Approach, Posterior Column, Percutaneous Endoscopic Approach

ØSG14AJ Fusion of 2 or More Lumbar Vertebral Joints with Interbody Fusion Device, Posterior Approach, Anterior Column, Percutaneous Endoscopic Approach

ØSG14JØ Fusion of 2 or More Lumbar Vertebral Joints with Synthetic Substitute, Anterior Approach, Anterior Column, Percutaneous Endoscopic Approach

ØSG14J1 Fusion of 2 or More Lumbar Vertebral Joints with Synthetic Substitute, Posterior Approach, Posterior Column, Percutaneous Endoscopic Approach

ØSG14JJ Fusion of 2 or More Lumbar Vertebral Joints with Synthetic Substitute, Posterior Approach, Anterior Column, Percutaneous Endoscopic Approach

ØSG14KØ Fusion of 2 or More Lumbar Vertebral Joints with Nonautologous Tissue Substitute, Anterior Approach, Anterior Column, Percutaneous Endoscopic Approach

ØSG14K1 Fusion of 2 or More Lumbar Vertebral Joints with Nonautologous Tissue Substitute, Posterior Approach, Posterior Column, Percutaneous Endoscopic Approach

ØSG14KJ Fusion of 2 or More Lumbar Vertebral Joints with Nonautologous Tissue Substitute, Posterior Approach, Anterior Column, Percutaneous Endoscopic Approach

ØSG14ZØ Fusion of 2 or More Lumbar Vertebral Joints, Anterior Approach, Anterior Column, Percutaneous Endoscopic Approach

ØSG14Z1 Fusion of 2 or More Lumbar Vertebral Joints, Posterior Approach, Posterior Column, Percutaneous Endoscopic Approach

ØSG14ZJ Fusion of 2 or More Lumbar Vertebral Joints, Posterior Approach, Anterior Column, Percutaneous Endoscopic Approach

ØSG3Ø7Ø Fusion of Lumbosacral Joint with Autologous Tissue Substitute, Anterior Approach, Anterior Column, Open Approach

ØSG3Ø71 Fusion of Lumbosacral Joint with Autologous Tissue Substitute, Posterior Approach, Posterior Column, Open Approach

ØSG3Ø7J Fusion of Lumbosacral Joint with Autologous Tissue Substitute, Posterior Approach, Anterior Column, Open Approach

ØSG3ØAØ Fusion of Lumbosacral Joint with Interbody Fusion Device, Anterior Approach, Anterior Column, Open Approach

ØSG3ØA1 Fusion of Lumbosacral Joint with Interbody Fusion Device, Posterior Approach, Posterior Column, Open Approach

ØSG3ØAJ Fusion of Lumbosacral Joint with Interbody Fusion Device, Posterior Approach, Anterior Column, Open Approach

ØSG3ØJØ Fusion of Lumbosacral Joint with Synthetic Substitute, Anterior Approach, Anterior Column, Open Approach

ØSG3ØJ1 Fusion of Lumbosacral Joint with Synthetic Substitute, Posterior Approach, Posterior Column, Open Approach

ØSG3ØJJ Fusion of Lumbosacral Joint with Synthetic Substitute, Posterior Approach, Anterior Column, Open Approach

ØSG3ØKØ Fusion of Lumbosacral Joint with Nonautologous Tissue Substitute, Anterior Approach, Anterior Column, Open Approach

ØSG3ØK1 Fusion of Lumbosacral Joint with Nonautologous Tissue Substitute, Posterior Approach, Posterior Column, Open Approach

ØSG3ØKJ Fusion of Lumbosacral Joint with Nonautologous Tissue Substitute, Posterior Approach, Anterior Column, Open Approach

ØSG3ØZØ Fusion of Lumbosacral Joint, Anterior Approach, Anterior Column, Open Approach

ØSG3ØZ1 Fusion of Lumbosacral Joint, Posterior Approach, Posterior Column, Open Approach

ØSG3ØZJ Fusion of Lumbosacral Joint, Posterior Approach, Anterior Column, Open Approach

ØSG337Ø Fusion of Lumbosacral Joint with Autologous Tissue Substitute, Anterior Approach, Anterior Column, Percutaneous Approach

ØSG3371 Fusion of Lumbosacral Joint with Autologous Tissue Substitute, Posterior Approach, Posterior Column, Percutaneous Approach

ØSG337J Fusion of Lumbosacral Joint with Autologous Tissue Substitute, Posterior Approach, Anterior Column, Percutaneous Approach

ØSG33AØ Fusion of Lumbosacral Joint with Interbody Fusion Device, Anterior Approach, Anterior Column, Percutaneous Approach

ØSG33A1 Fusion of Lumbosacral Joint with Interbody Fusion Device, Posterior Approach, Posterior Column, Percutaneous Approach

ØSG33AJ Fusion of Lumbosacral Joint with Interbody Fusion Device, Posterior Approach, Anterior Column, Percutaneous Approach

ØSG33JØ Fusion of Lumbosacral Joint with Synthetic Substitute, Anterior Approach, Anterior Column, Percutaneous Approach

ØSG33J1 Fusion of Lumbosacral Joint with Synthetic Substitute, Posterior Approach, Posterior Column, Percutaneous Approach

ØSG33JJ Fusion of Lumbosacral Joint with Synthetic Substitute, Posterior Approach, Anterior Column, Percutaneous Approach

ØSG33KØ Fusion of Lumbosacral Joint with Nonautologous Tissue Substitute, Anterior Approach, Anterior Column, Percutaneous Approach

ØSG33K1 Fusion of Lumbosacral Joint with Nonautologous Tissue Substitute, Posterior Approach, Posterior Column, Percutaneous Approach

ØSG33KJ Fusion of Lumbosacral Joint with Nonautologous Tissue Substitute, Posterior Approach, Anterior Column, Percutaneous Approach

ØSG33ZØ Fusion of Lumbosacral Joint, Anterior Approach, Anterior Column, Percutaneous Approach

ØSG33Z1 Fusion of Lumbosacral Joint, Posterior Approach, Posterior Column, Percutaneous Approach

ØSG33ZJ Fusion of Lumbosacral Joint, Posterior Approach, Anterior Column, Percutaneous Approach

ØSG347Ø Fusion of Lumbosacral Joint with Autologous Tissue Substitute, Anterior Approach, Anterior Column, Percutaneous Endoscopic Approach

HAC 12: Surgical Site Infection Following Certain Orthopedic Procedures of the Spine, Shoulder, and Elbow (continued)

ØSG3471 Fusion of Lumbosacral Joint with Autologous Tissue Substitute, Posterior Approach, Posterior Column, Percutaneous Endoscopic Approach

ØSG347J Fusion of Lumbosacral Joint with Autologous Tissue Substitute, Posterior Approach, Anterior Column, Percutaneous Endoscopic Approach

ØSG34AØ Fusion of Lumbosacral Joint with Interbody Fusion Device, Anterior Approach, Anterior Column, Percutaneous Endoscopic Approach

ØSG34A1 Fusion of Lumbosacral Joint with Interbody Fusion Device, Posterior Approach, Posterior Column, Percutaneous Endoscopic Approach

ØSG34AJ Fusion of Lumbosacral Joint with Interbody Fusion Device, Posterior Approach, Anterior Column, Percutaneous Endoscopic Approach

ØSG34JØ Fusion of Lumbosacral Joint with Synthetic Substitute, Anterior Approach, Anterior Column, Percutaneous Endoscopic Approach

ØSG34J1 Fusion of Lumbosacral Joint with Synthetic Substitute, Posterior Approach, Posterior Column, Percutaneous Endoscopic Approach

ØSG34JJ Fusion of Lumbosacral Joint with Synthetic Substitute, Posterior Approach, Anterior Column, Percutaneous Endoscopic Approach

ØSG34KØ Fusion of Lumbosacral Joint with Nonautologous Tissue Substitute, Anterior Approach, Anterior Column, Percutaneous Endoscopic Approach

ØSG34K1 Fusion of Lumbosacral Joint with Nonautologous Tissue Substitute, Posterior Approach, Posterior Column, Percutaneous Endoscopic Approach

ØSG34KJ Fusion of Lumbosacral Joint with Nonautologous Tissue Substitute, Posterior Approach, Anterior Column, Percutaneous Endoscopic Approach

ØSG34ZØ Fusion of Lumbosacral Joint, Anterior Approach, Anterior Column, Percutaneous Endoscopic Approach

ØSG34Z1 Fusion of Lumbosacral Joint, Posterior Approach, Posterior Column, Percutaneous Endoscopic Approach

ØSG34ZJ Fusion of Lumbosacral Joint, Posterior Approach, Anterior Column, Percutaneous Endoscopic Approach

ØSG7Ø4Z Fusion of Right Sacroiliac Joint with Internal Fixation Device, Open Approach

ØSG7Ø7Z Fusion of Right Sacroiliac Joint with Autologous Tissue Substitute, Open Approach

ØSG7ØJZ Fusion of Right Sacroiliac Joint with Synthetic Substitute, Open Approach

ØSG7ØKZ Fusion of Right Sacroiliac Joint with Nonautologous Tissue Substitute, Open Approach

ØSG7ØZZ Fusion of Right Sacroiliac Joint, Open Approach

ØSG734Z Fusion of Right Sacroiliac Joint with Internal Fixation Device, Percutaneous Approach

ØSG737Z Fusion of Right Sacroiliac Joint with Autologous Tissue Substitute, Percutaneous Approach

ØSG73JZ Fusion of Right Sacroiliac Joint with Synthetic Substitute, Percutaneous Approach

ØSG73KZ Fusion of Right Sacroiliac Joint with Nonautologous Tissue Substitute, Percutaneous Approach

ØSG73ZZ Fusion of Right Sacroiliac Joint, Percutaneous Approach

ØSG744Z Fusion of Right Sacroiliac Joint with Internal Fixation Device, Percutaneous Endoscopic Approach

ØSG747Z Fusion of Right Sacroiliac Joint with Autologous Tissue Substitute, Percutaneous Endoscopic Approach

ØSG74JZ Fusion of Right Sacroiliac Joint with Synthetic Substitute, Percutaneous Endoscopic Approach

ØSG74KZ Fusion of Right Sacroiliac Joint with Nonautologous Tissue Substitute, Percutaneous Endoscopic Approach

ØSG74ZZ Fusion of Right Sacroiliac Joint, Percutaneous Endoscopic Approach

ØSG8Ø4Z Fusion of Left Sacroiliac Joint with Internal Fixation Device, Open Approach

ØSG8Ø7Z Fusion of Left Sacroiliac Joint with Autologous Tissue Substitute, Open Approach

ØSG8ØJZ Fusion of Left Sacroiliac Joint with Synthetic Substitute, Open Approach

ØSG8ØKZ Fusion of Left Sacroiliac Joint with Nonautologous Tissue Substitute, Open Approach

ØSG8ØZZ Fusion of Left Sacroiliac Joint, Open Approach

ØSG834Z Fusion of Left Sacroiliac Joint with Internal Fixation Device, Percutaneous Approach

ØSG837Z Fusion of Left Sacroiliac Joint with Autologous Tissue Substitute, Percutaneous Approach

ØSG83JZ Fusion of Left Sacroiliac Joint with Synthetic Substitute, Percutaneous Approach

ØSG83KZ Fusion of Left Sacroiliac Joint with Nonautologous Tissue Substitute, Percutaneous Approach

ØSG83ZZ Fusion of Left Sacroiliac Joint, Percutaneous Approach

ØSG844Z Fusion of Left Sacroiliac Joint with Internal Fixation Device, Percutaneous Endoscopic Approach

ØSG847Z Fusion of Left Sacroiliac Joint with Autologous Tissue Substitute, Percutaneous Endoscopic Approach

ØSG84JZ Fusion of Left Sacroiliac Joint with Synthetic Substitute, Percutaneous Endoscopic Approach

ØSG84KZ Fusion of Left Sacroiliac Joint with Nonautologous Tissue Substitute, Percutaneous Endoscopic Approach

ØSG84ZZ Fusion of Left Sacroiliac Joint, Percutaneous Endoscopic Approach

HAC 13: Surgical Site Infection (SSI) Following Cardiac Implantable Electronic Device (CIED) Procedures

Secondary diagnosis not POA:

K68.11
T81.4XXA
T82.6XXA
T82.7XXA

AND

Any of the following procedures:

02H43JZ Insertion of Pacemaker Lead into Coronary Vein, Percutaneous Approach

02H43KZ Insertion of Defibrillator Lead into Coronary Vein, Percutaneous Approach

02H43MZ Insertion of Cardiac Lead into Coronary Vein, Percutaneous Approach

02H63JZ Insertion of Pacemaker Lead into Right Atrium, Percutaneous Approach

02H63MZ Insertion of Cardiac Lead into Right Atrium, Percutaneous Approach

02H73JZ Insertion of Pacemaker Lead into Left Atrium, Percutaneous Approach

02H73MZ Insertion of Cardiac Lead into Left Atrium, Percutaneous Approach

02HK3JZ Insertion of Pacemaker Lead into Right Ventricle, Percutaneous Approach

02HL3JZ Insertion of Pacemaker Lead into Left Ventricle, Percutaneous Approach

02HNØJZ Insertion of Pacemaker Lead into Pericardium, Open Approach

02HNØMZ Insertion of Cardiac Lead into Pericardium, Open Approach

02HN3JZ Insertion of Pacemaker Lead into Pericardium, Percutaneous Approach

02HN3MZ Insertion of Cardiac Lead into Pericardium, Percutaneous Approach

02HN4JZ Insertion of Pacemaker Lead into Pericardium, Percutaneous Endoscopic Approach

02HN4MZ Insertion of Cardiac Lead into Pericardium, Percutaneous Endoscopic Approach

02PAØMZ Removal of Cardiac Lead from Heart, Open Approach

02PA3MZ Removal of Cardiac Lead from Heart, Percutaneous Approach

02PA4MZ Removal of Cardiac Lead from Heart, Percutaneous Endoscopic Approach

02PAXMZ Removal of Cardiac Lead from Heart, External Approach

02WAØMZ Revision of Cardiac Lead in Heart, Open Approach

02WA3MZ Revision of Cardiac Lead in Heart, Percutaneous Approach

02WA4MZ Revision of Cardiac Lead in Heart, Percutaneous Endoscopic Approach

ØJH6Ø4Z Insertion of Pacemaker, Single Chamber into Chest Subcutaneous Tissue and Fascia, Open Approach

ØJH6Ø5Z Insertion of Pacemaker, Single Chamber Rate Responsive into Chest Subcutaneous Tissue and Fascia, Open Approach

ØJH6Ø6Z Insertion of Pacemaker, Dual Chamber into Chest Subcutaneous Tissue and Fascia, Open Approach

ØJH6Ø7Z Insertion of Cardiac Resynchronization Pacemaker Pulse Generator into Chest Subcutaneous Tissue and Fascia, Open Approach

ØJH6Ø8Z Insertion of Defibrillator Generator into Chest Subcutaneous Tissue and Fascia, Open Approach

ØJH6Ø9Z Insertion of Cardiac Resynchronization Defibrillator Pulse Generator into Chest Subcutaneous Tissue and Fascia, Open Approach

ØJH6ØPZ Insertion of Cardiac Rhythm Related Device into Chest Subcutaneous Tissue and Fascia, Open Approach

ØJH634Z Insertion of Pacemaker, Single Chamber into Chest Subcutaneous Tissue and Fascia, Percutaneous Approach

ØJH635Z Insertion of Pacemaker, Single Chamber Rate Responsive into Chest Subcutaneous Tissue and Fascia, Percutaneous Approach

ØJH636Z Insertion of Pacemaker, Dual Chamber into Chest Subcutaneous Tissue and Fascia, Percutaneous Approach

HAC 13: Surgical Site Infection (SSI) Following Cardiac Implantable Electronic Device (CIED) Procedures (continued)

ØJH637Z　Insertion of Cardiac Resynchronization Pacemaker Pulse Generator into Chest Subcutaneous Tissue and Fascia, Percutaneous Approach

ØJH638Z　Insertion of Defibrillator Generator into Chest Subcutaneous Tissue and Fascia, Percutaneous Approach

ØJH639Z　Insertion of Cardiac Resynchronization Defibrillator Pulse Generator into Chest Subcutaneous Tissue and Fascia, Percutaneous Approach

ØJH63PZ　Insertion of Cardiac Rhythm Related Device into Chest Subcutaneous Tissue and Fascia, Percutaneous Approach

ØJH8Ø4Z　Insertion of Pacemaker, Single Chamber into Abdomen Subcutaneous Tissue and Fascia, Open Approach

ØJH8Ø5Z　Insertion of Pacemaker, Single Chamber Rate Responsive into Abdomen Subcutaneous Tissue and Fascia, Open Approach

ØJH8Ø6Z　Insertion of Pacemaker, Dual Chamber into Abdomen Subcutaneous Tissue and Fascia, Open Approach

ØJH8Ø7Z　Insertion of Cardiac Resynchronization Pacemaker Pulse Generator into Abdomen Subcutaneous Tissue and Fascia, Open Approach

ØJH8Ø8Z　Insertion of Defibrillator Generator into Abdomen Subcutaneous Tissue and Fascia, Open Approach

ØJH8Ø9Z　Insertion of Cardiac Resynchronization Defibrillator Pulse Generator into Abdomen Subcutaneous Tissue and Fascia, Open Approach

ØJH8ØPZ　Insertion of Cardiac Rhythm Related Device into Abdomen Subcutaneous Tissue and Fascia, Open Approach

ØJH834Z　Insertion of Pacemaker, Single Chamber into Abdomen Subcutaneous Tissue and Fascia, Percutaneous Approach

ØJH835Z　Insertion of Pacemaker, Single Chamber Rate Responsive into Abdomen Subcutaneous Tissue and Fascia, Percutaneous Approach

ØJH836Z　Insertion of Pacemaker, Dual Chamber into Abdomen Subcutaneous Tissue and Fascia, Percutaneous Approach

ØJH837Z　Insertion of Cardiac Resynchronization Pacemaker Pulse Generator into Abdomen Subcutaneous Tissue and Fascia, Percutaneous Approach

ØJH838Z　Insertion of Defibrillator Generator into Abdomen Subcutaneous Tissue and Fascia, Percutaneous Approach

ØJH839Z　Insertion of Cardiac Resynchronization Defibrillator Pulse Generator into Abdomen Subcutaneous Tissue and Fascia, Percutaneous Approach

ØJH83PZ　Insertion of Cardiac Rhythm Related Device into Abdomen Subcutaneous Tissue and Fascia, Percutaneous Approach

ØJPTØPZ　Removal of Cardiac Rhythm Related Device from Trunk Subcutaneous Tissue and Fascia, Open Approach

ØJPT3PZ　Removal of Cardiac Rhythm Related Device from Trunk Subcutaneous Tissue and Fascia, Percutaneous Approach

ØJWTØPZ　Revision of Cardiac Rhythm Related Device in Trunk Subcutaneous Tissue and Fascia, Open Approach

ØJWT3PZ　Revision of Cardiac Rhythm Related Device in Trunk Subcutaneous Tissue and Fascia, Percutaneous Approach

HAC 14: Iatrogenic Pneumothorax with Venous Catheterization

Secondary diagnosis not POA:
J95.811

AND

Any of the following procedures:

Ø5HM33Z　Insertion of Infusion Device into Right Internal Jugular Vein, Percutaneous Approach

Ø5HN33Z　Insertion of Infusion Device into Left Internal Jugular Vein, Percutaneous Approach

Ø5HP33Z　Insertion of Infusion Device into Right External Jugular Vein, Percutaneous Approach

Ø5HQ33Z　Insertion of Infusion Device into Left External Jugular Vein, Percutaneous Approach

ØJH63XZ　Insertion of Vascular Access Device into Chest Subcutaneous Tissue and Fascia, Percutaneous Approach

Peripheral Nervous System

Brain

Cranial Nerves

Eye

Sclera
Cornea
Iris
Pupil
Anterior chamber
Posterior chamber
Ciliary body
Conjunctiva

Choroid (uvea)
Vitreous body
Lens
Hyaloid canal
Lamina cribosa
Optic nerve
Optic disk
Fovea
Retina

Globe (Eyeball)

Posterior Pole of Globe

Macula
Fovea
Optic disk

Ciliary body
Conjunctival veins
Canal of Schlemm
Trabecular mesh
Anterior chamber
Iris
Lens

Flow of Aqueous Humor

Lacrimal System

Superior and inferior lobes of lacrimal gland
Medial angle
Lacrimal canaliculi
Nasolacrimal sac
Lacrimal ducts
Lacrimal caruncle
Superior, inferior lacrimal puncta
Left eye

Ear and Mastoid

Helix
Antihelix
Concha
Mastoid process
External auditory meatus
Tragus
Antitragus

Middle Ear

Osseus labyrinth
Auditory ossicles: Stapes
Incus
Malleus
External auditory canal
Cochlea (round window)
Semicircular canals
Utricle and saccule
CN VIII
Cochlea in bone
Eustachian tube
Pharynx

Exposed view of middle and inner ear

Arteries

Veins

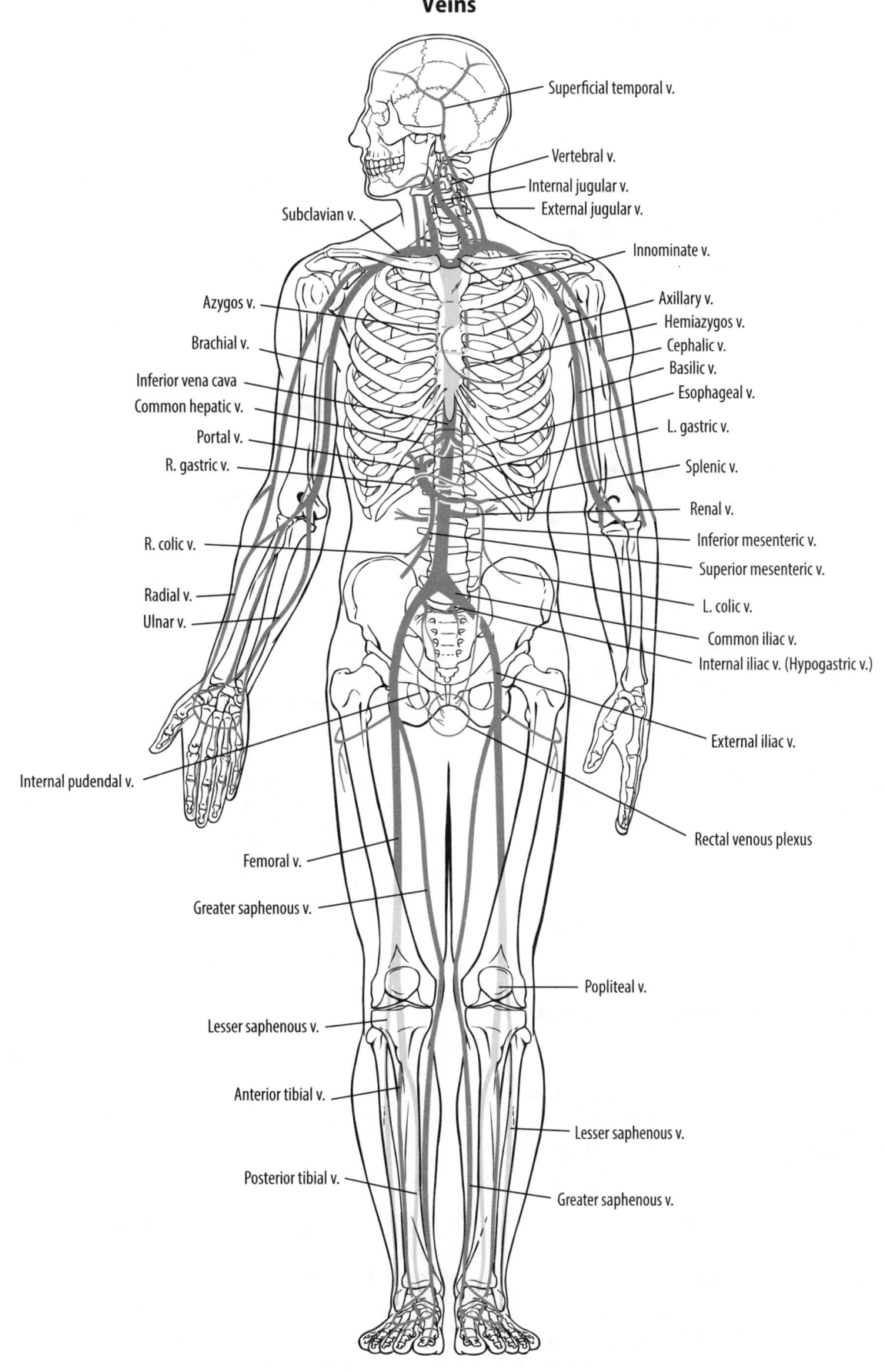

Anatomy of Heart

Arteries of Heart

Cerebrovascular Arteries

Veins of Head and Neck

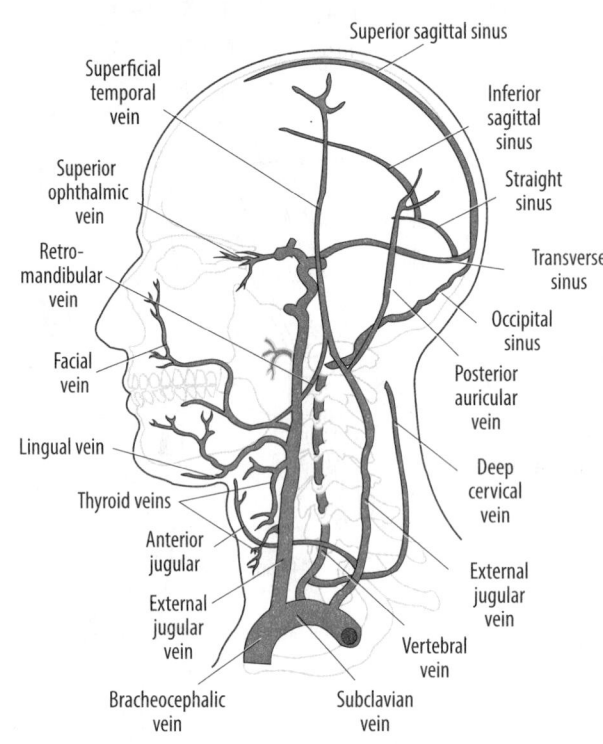

Lymphatic System of Head and Neck

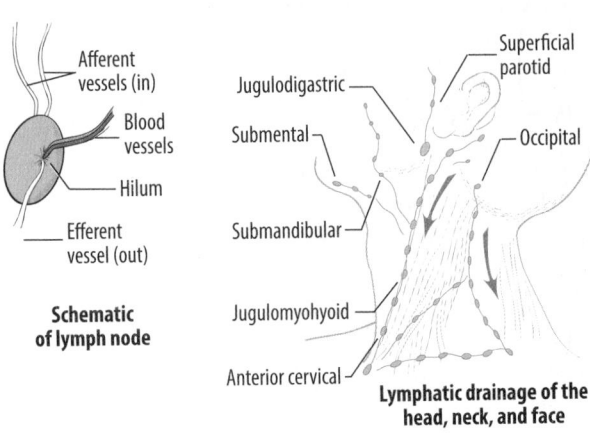

Schematic of lymph node

Lymphatic drainage of the head, neck, and face

Lymph Nodes

Respiratory System

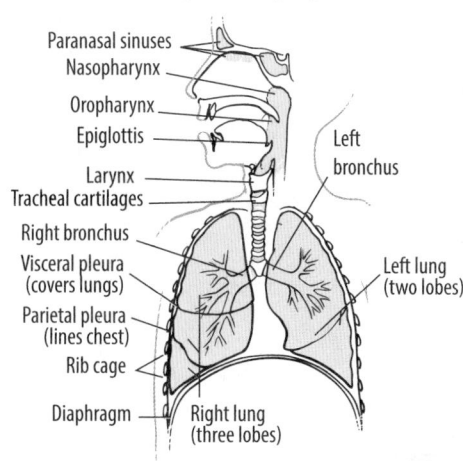

Paranasal sinuses
Nasopharynx
Oropharynx
Epiglottis
Larynx
Tracheal cartilages
Right bronchus
Visceral pleura (covers lungs)
Parietal pleura (lines chest)
Rib cage
Diaphragm
Left bronchus
Left lung (two lobes)
Right lung (three lobes)

Paranasal Sinuses

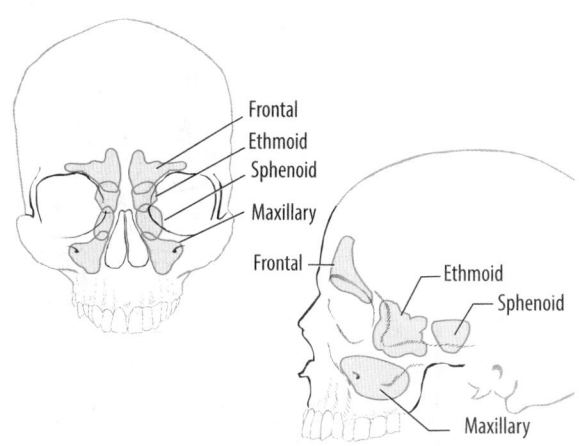

Frontal
Ethmoid
Sphenoid
Maxillary
Frontal
Ethmoid
Sphenoid
Maxillary

Oral Cavity

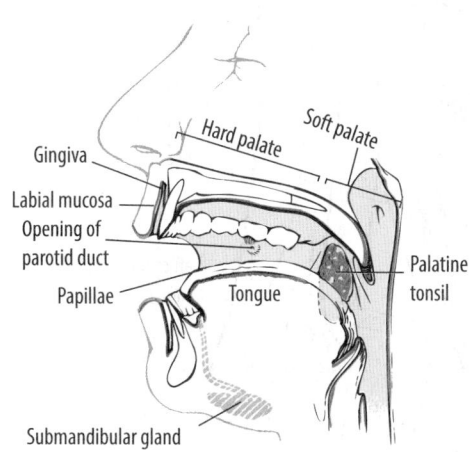

Gingiva
Labial mucosa
Opening of parotid duct
Papillae
Submandibular gland
Hard palate
Soft palate
Tongue
Palatine tonsil

Pancreas

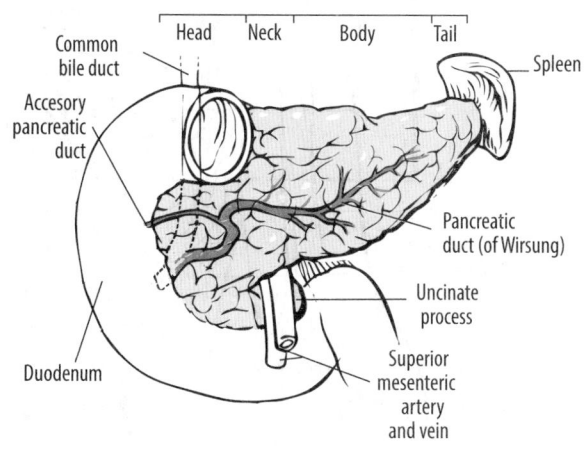

Head   Neck   Body   Tail
Common bile duct
Accesory pancreatic duct
Duodenum
Spleen
Pancreatic duct (of Wirsung)
Uncinate process
Superior mesenteric artery and vein

Gallbladder and Bile Ducts

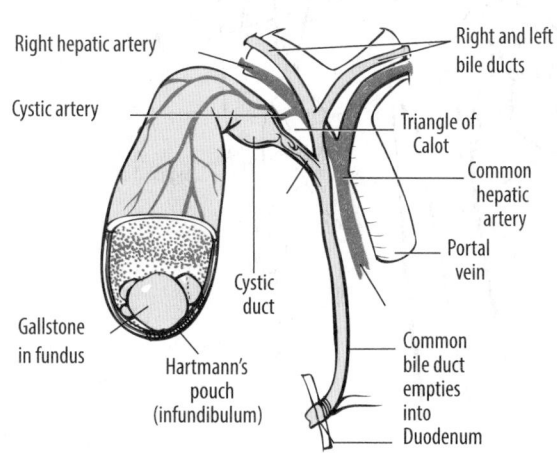

Right hepatic artery
Cystic artery
Gallstone in fundus
Hartmann's pouch (infundibulum)
Cystic duct
Right and left bile ducts
Triangle of Calot
Common hepatic artery
Portal vein
Common bile duct empties into Duodenum

Liver

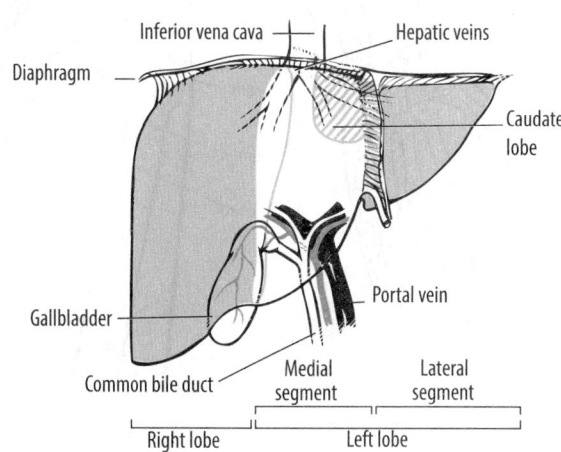

Inferior vena cava
Diaphragm
Gallbladder
Common bile duct
Hepatic veins
Caudate lobe
Portal vein
Medial segment
Lateral segment
Right lobe
Left lobe

Gastrointestinal System

Endocrine System

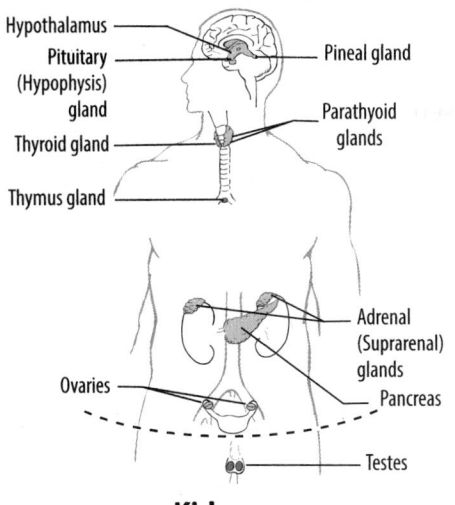

Dorsal View of Parathyroid Gland

Kidney

Urinary System

Male Pelvic Organs

Female Genitourinary System

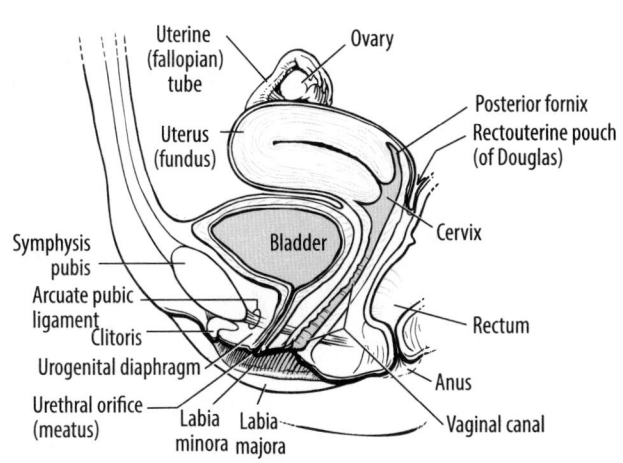

Joints

Shoulder (Anterior View)

Shoulder (Posterior View)

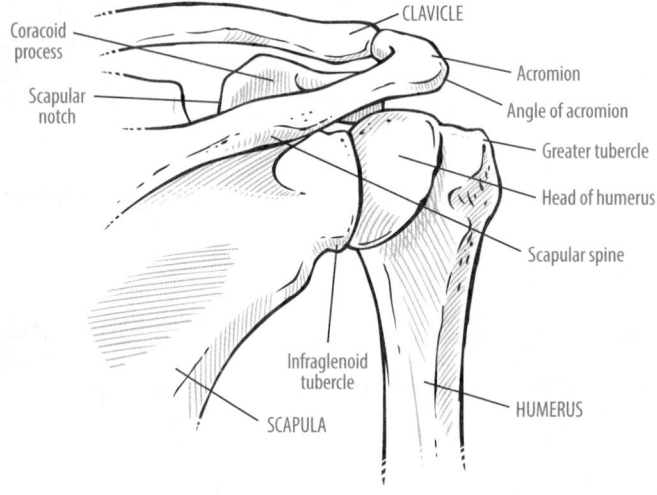

Joints
Elbow (Anterior View)

Elbow (Posterior View)

Hand

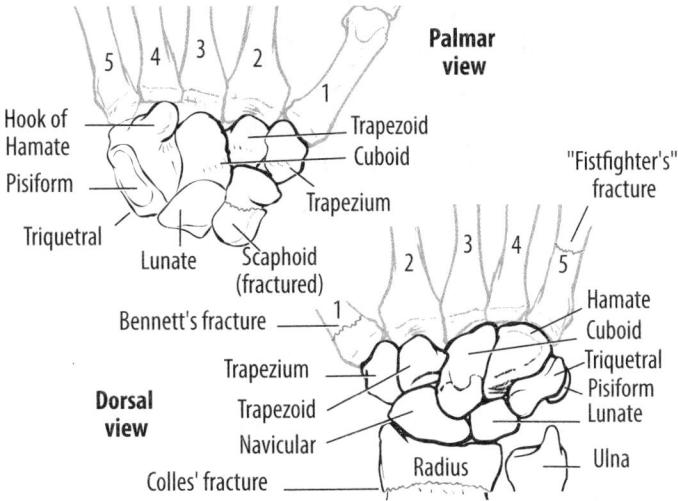

Joints

Hip (Anterior View)

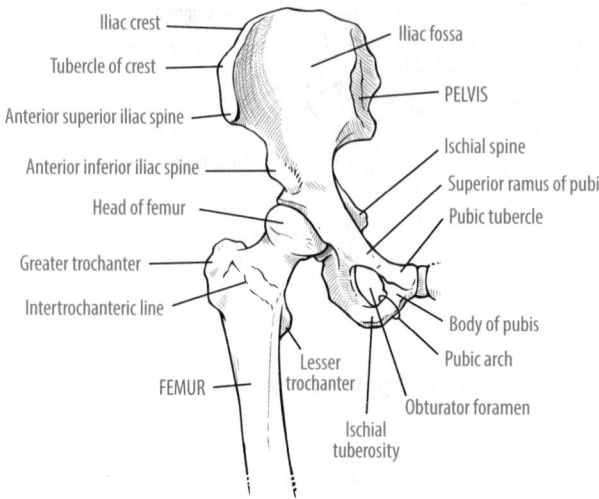

Iliac crest
Tubercle of crest
Anterior superior iliac spine
Anterior inferior iliac spine
Head of femur
Greater trochanter
Intertrochanteric line
FEMUR
Lesser trochanter
Ischial tuberosity
Iliac fossa
PELVIS
Ischial spine
Superior ramus of pubis
Pubic tubercle
Body of pubis
Pubic arch
Obturator foramen

Hip (Posterior View)

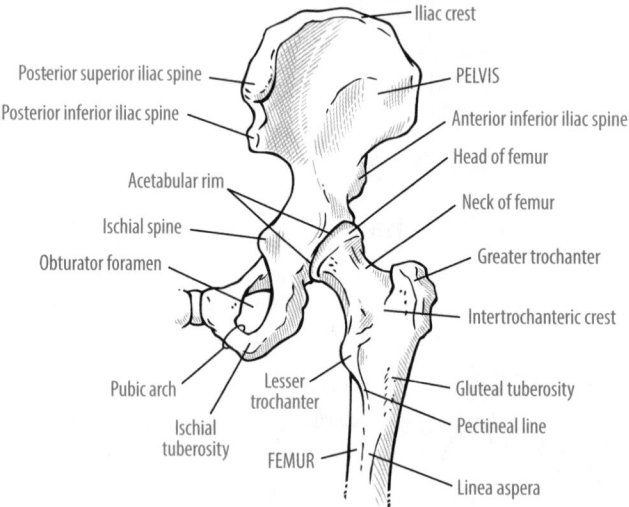

Posterior superior iliac spine
Posterior inferior iliac spine
Acetabular rim
Ischial spine
Obturator foramen
Pubic arch
Ischial tuberosity
Lesser trochanter
FEMUR
Iliac crest
PELVIS
Anterior inferior iliac spine
Head of femur
Neck of femur
Greater trochanter
Intertrochanteric crest
Gluteal tuberosity
Pectineal line
Linea aspera

Joints

Knee (Anterior View)

Knee (Posterior View)

Right Foot

Bones/Joints

Muscles

Step 4:
Professional Resources

"Nothing is particularly hard if you divide it into small jobs."

— Henry Ford

As you reach higher and more specialized levels of coding, we want to applaud you for taking this step in your career. You won't be disappointed. Specialized coders are like rare gems—*they are harder to find and greatly valued* in the profession.

— Carol J. Buck, MS, CPC, CCS-P

— Jackie L. Grass, CPC

Track your progress!

See the checklist in the back of this book to learn more about your steps toward coding success!

BB-04

PROFESSIONAL
EDITION

2016
ICD-10-CM
FOR HOSPITALS

INCLUDES
NETTER'S
ANATOMY
ART

Carol J. Buck
MS, CPC, CCS-P

Former Program Director
Medical Secretary Programs
Northwest Technical College
East Grand Forks, Minnesota

ELSEVIER

ELSEVIER
SAUNDERS

3251 Riverport Lane
St. Louis, Missouri 63043

2016 ICD-10-CM HOSPITAL EDITION

ISBN: 978-0-323-27975-8
eISBN: 978-0-323-29183-5

Notice

Knowledge and best practice in this field are constantly changing. As new research and experience broaden our understanding, changes in research methods, professional practices, or medical treatment may become necessary.

Practitioners and researchers must always rely on their own experience and knowledge in evaluating and using any information, methods, compounds, or experiments described herein. In using such information or methods they should be mindful of their own safety and the safety of others, including parties for whom they have a professional responsibility.

With respect to any drug or pharmaceutical products identified, readers are advised to check the most current information provided (i) on procedures featured or (ii) by the manufacturer of each product to be administered, to verify the recommended dose or formula, the method and duration of administration, and contraindications. It is the responsibility of practitioners, relying on their own experience and knowledge of their patients, to make diagnoses, to determine dosages and the best treatment for each individual patient, and to take all appropriate safety precautions.

To the fullest extent of the law, neither the Publisher nor the authors, contributors, or editors, assume any liability for any injury and/or damage to persons or property as a matter of products liability, negligence or otherwise, or from any use or operation of any methods, products, instructions, or ideas contained in the material herein.

Library of Congress Cataloging-in-Publication Data

Buck, Carol J., author.
  2016 ICD-10-CM for hospitals / Carol J. Buck. -- Professional edition.
     p. ; cm.
  Includes index.
  ISBN 978-0-323-27975-8 (spiral bound) -- ISBN 978-0-323-29185-3 (eISBN)
  I. Title.
  [DNLM: 1. International statistical classification of diseases and related health problems. 10th revision. Clinical modification. 2. Disease--classification. 3. Forms and Records Control--methods. 4. International Classification of Diseases. 5. Medical Records. WB 15]
  RB115
  616.001'2--dc23
                                                                          2014011896

Director, Private Sector Education & Professional/References: Jeanne R. Olson
Content Development Manager: Luke Held
Publishing Services Manager: Jeffrey Patterson
Project Manager: Lisa A. P. Bushy
Senior Designer: Julia Dummitt

Printed in Canada

 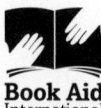 Working together to grow libraries in developing countries

ELSEVIER   Book Aid International

www.elsevier.com • www.bookaid.org

Last digit is the print number: 9   8   7   6   5   4   3   2   1